NEOPLASTIC HEMATOPATHOLOGY

Second Edition

NEOPLASTIC HEMATOPATHOLOGY

Second Edition

EDITED BY

Daniel M. Knowles, M.D.
David D. Thompson Professor and Chair
Department of Pathology
Weill Medical College of Cornell University
Pathologist-in-Chief
New York–Presbyterian Hospital
New York, New York

LIPPINCOTT WILLIAMS & WILKINS
A **Wolters Kluwer** Company
Philadelphia • Baltimore • New York • London
Buenos Aires • Hong Kong • Sydney • Tokyo

Acquisitions Editor: Ruth W. Weinberg
Developmental Editor: Joyce A. Murphy
Production Editor: Kim Yi
Manufacturing Manager: Colin Warnock
Cover Designer: QT Design
Compositor: Maryland Composition, Inc.
Printer: Courier Westford

530 Walnut Street
Philadelphia, PA 19106 USA
LWW.com

Printed in the USA

Library of Congress Cataloging-in-Publication Data

Neoplastic hematopathology / edited by Daniel M. Knowles.—2nd ed.
p. ; cm.
Includes bibliographical references and index.
ISBN 0-683-30246-9 (alk. paper)
1. Lymphoproliferative disorders—Cytopathology. 2. Hematopoietic system—Cancer—Cytopathology. I. Knowles, Daniel M.
[DNLM: 1. Hematopoietic System—pathology. 2. Bone Marrow Diseases—pathology. 3. Leukemia—pathology. 4. Lymphoproliferative Disorders—pathology. 5. Neoplasms—pathology. WH 140 N438 2000]
RC646.2 .N46 2000
616.99'442—dc21

00-041238

---

10 9 8 7 6 5 4 3 2 1

To my parents,
to Marian, my wife and best friend,
and to Tyler, our son and inspiration

Contents

Contributing Authors

Ruth Achten, M.D. *Fellow of the FWO Flanders, Department of Morphology and Medical Imaging and Department of Pathology, University Hospitals K.U. Leuven. Minderbroedersstraat 12, B-3000 Leuven, Belgium*

Ioannis Anagnostopoulos, M.D. *Institute of Pathology, Klinikum Benjamin Franklin, Free University of Berlin, Hindenburgdamm 30, D-12200 Berlin, Germany*

John Anastasi, M.D. *Associate Professor of Pathology, Department of Pathology, University of Chicago, 5841 South Maryland Avenue, MC0008, Chicago, Illinois 60637*

James O. Armitage, M.D. *Dean, College of Medicine, University of Nebraska Medical Center, 983332 Nebraska Medical Center, Omaha, Nebraska 68198*

Peter M. Banks, M.D. *Clinical Professor of Pathology, Department of Pathology, University of North Carolina at Chapel Hill, 816 Brinkhous-Bullit Building, Chapel Hill, North Carolina 27599-7525; and Director, Department of Hematopathology, Carolinas Medical Center, 1000 Blythe Boulevard, Charlotte, North Carolina 28203*

Frederick G. Behm, M.D. *Associate Member and Vice-Chair, Department of Pathology, St. Jude Children's Research Hospital, 332 North Lauderdale, Memphis, Tennessee 38105*

Jonathan Ben-Ezra, M.D. *Professor of Pathology and Director of Hematopathology, Medical College of Virginia, Campus of Virginia Commonwealth University, 403 North 13th Street, Richmond, Virginia 23298-0250*

Kishor Bhatia, Ph.D. *Grants Review Branch, Division of Extramural Affairs, National Cancer Institute, 6116 Executive Boulevard, Bethesda, Maryland 20852*

Mitchell A. Bitter, M.D. *Clinical Professor, Department of Pathology, University of Colorado Health Sciences Center, 4200 East 9th Avenue, Denver, Colorado 80262; and Hematopathologist, Department of Pathology, Presbyterian/St. Luke's Medical Center, 1719 East 19th Avenue, Denver, Colorado 80218*

Michael J. Borowitz, M.D., Ph.D. *Professor, Department of Pathology and Director, Hematologic Pathology, Johns Hopkins Medical Institutions, 600 North Wolfe Street, Baltimore, Maryland 21287-6417*

Richard D. Brunning, M.D. *Professor Emeritus, Department of Laboratory Medicine and Pathology, University of Minnesota, 420 Delaware Street, SE, Box 609-Mayo, Minneapolis, Minnesota 55455*

Jerome S. Burke, M.D. *Clinical Professor, Department of Pathology, Stanford University Medical Center, 300 Pasteur Drive, Stanford, California 94305; and Director, Department of Anatomic Pathology, Alta Bates Medical Center, 2450 Ashby Avenue, Berkeley, California 94705*

Elias Campo, M.D. *Associate Professor, Department of Cell Biology and Pathology, Medical School, University of Barcelona, Casanovas, 146, 08036, Barcelona, Spain; and Chief, Hematopathology Section, Laboratory of Pathology, Hospital Clinic, Villarroel, 170, 08036, Barcelona, Spain*

Paolo Casali, M.D. *Professor of Pathology, Microbiology and Immunology, Department of Pathology, Weill Medical College of Cornell University, 1300 York Avenue, New York, New York 10021*

Daniel Catovsky, M.D. *Professor and Head, Academic Department of Haematology and Cytogenetics, Institute of Cancer Research, Royal Marsden Hospital, 203 Fulham Road, London SW3 6JJ, United Kingdom*

Ethel Cesarman M.D., Ph.D. *Associate Professor of Pathology, Department of Pathology, Weill Medical College of Cornell University, 1300 York Avenue, New York, New York 10021*

Amy Chadburn, M.D. *Associate Professor of Pathology, Department of Pathology, Weill Medical College of Cornell University, 1300 York Avenue, New York, New York 10021*

Jeffrey Cossman, M.D. *Oscar Benwood Hunter Professor of Pathology, Georgetown University Medical Center, NW 103 Medical-Dental Building, 3900 Reservoir Road, NW, Washington, DC 20007*

Riccardo Dalla-Favera, M.D. *Joanne and Percy Uris Professor of Pathology and Genetics Development, Department of Pathology, and Director, Institute of Cancer Genetics, Columbia University, 1150 St. Nicholas Avenue, New York, New York 10032*

Friederike Dallenbach, M.D. *Institute of Pathology, Klinikum Benjamin Franklin, Free University of Berlin, Hindenburgdamm 30, D-12200 Berlin, Germany*

Chris De Wolf-Peeters, M.D. *Professor of Pathology and Head of Department, Department of Morphology and Medical Imaging, K.U. Leuven; and Deputy Director, Department of Pathology, University Hospitals K.U. Leuven, Minderbroedersstraat 12, B-3000 Leuven, Belgium*

Joseph A. DiGiuseppe, M.D., Ph.D. *Assistant Professor, Department of Laboratory Medicine, University of Connecticut School of Medicine, 263 Farmington Avenue, Farmington, Connecticut 06030; and Director, Special Hematology Laboratory, Department of Pathology and Laboratory Medicine, Hartford Hospital, 80 Seymour Street, Hartford, Connecticut 06102-5037*

James R. Downing, M.D., Ph.D. *Professor, Department of Pathology, College of Medicine, The University of Tennessee, Memphis, 899 Madison Avenue, Memphis, Tennessee 38163; and Chairman, Department of Pathology, D4047, St. Jude Children's Research Hospital, 332 North Lauderdale, Memphis, Tennessee 38105*

Milton R. Drachenberg, M.D., Ph.D. *Fellow in Hematopathology, Los Angeles County/University of Southern California Medical Center, Los Angeles, California 90033*

Falko Fend, M.D. *Associate Professor, Institute of Pathology, Technical University Munich, Ismaningerstr. 22, D-81675 Munich, Germany*

Judith A. Ferry, M.D. *Associate Professor, Department of Pathology, Harvard Medical School, 25 Shattuck Street, Boston, Massachusetts 02215; and Associate Pathologist, Massachusetts General Hospital, 55 Fruit Street, Boston, Massachusetts 02114*

Douglas B. Flieder, M.D. *Assistant Professor, Department of Pathology, Weill Medical College of Cornell University, 1300 York Avenue, New York, New York 10021*

M. Kathryn Foucar, M.D. *Professor, Department of Pathology, University of New Mexico Health Sciences Center-BMSB 335, 915 Camino de Salud, NE, Albuquerque, New Mexico 87131-5301; and Medical Director, Tri Core Reference Labs, 4700 Lincoln NE, Albuquerque, New Mexico 87109*

Glauco Frizzera, M.D. *Professor, Department of Pathology, Weill Medical College of Cornell University; and Chief of Hematopathology, New York-Presbyterian Hospital, 525 East 68th Street, New York, New York 10021*

Thomas M. Grogan, M.D. *Professor of Pathology, Department of Pathology, Arizona Health Sciences Center, Room 5212, 1501 North Campbell Avenue, Tucson, Arizona 85274*

Nancy Lee Harris, M.D. *Professor of Pathology, Department of Pathology, Harvard Medical School, 25 Shattuck Street, Boston, Massachusetts 02215; and Director of Pathology Training Programs, Department of Pathology, Massachusetts General Hospital, 55 Fruit Street, Warren Building Room 219, Boston, Massachusetts 02114*

Antonio M. Hernandez, M.D. *Clinical Assistant Professor, Los Angeles County/University of Southern California Medical Center, Los Angeles, California 90033*

Hans P. Horny, M.D. *Professor of Pathology, Institute of Pathology, University of Tübingen, Liebermeister Str. 8, 72076 Tübingen, Germany*

Peter G. Isaacson, M.D. *Professor and Head, Department of Histopathology, Royal Free and University College Medical School, Rockefeller Building, University Street, London WC1E 6JJ, United Kingdom*

Elaine S. Jaffe, M.D. *Chief, Hematopathology Section, Laboratory of Pathology, Division of Clinical Sciences, National Cancer Institute, 10 Center Drive M5C-1500, Bethesda, Maryland 20892*

Marshall E. Kadin, M.D. *Associate Professor, Department of Pathology, Harvard Medical School; and Director of Hematopathology, Department of Pathology, Beth Israel Deaconess Medical Center, 330 Brookline Avenue, Boston, Massachusetts 02215*

Daniel M. Knowles, M.D. *David D. Thompson Professor and Chairman, Department of Pathology, Weill Medical College of Cornell University, 1300 York Avenue; and Pathologist-in-Chief, New York–Presbyterian Hospital, New York, New York 10021*

Steven H. Kroft, M.D. *Assistant Professor, Department of Pathology, University of Texas Southwestern Medical School; and Medical Director, Hematology Laboratory, Parkland Memorial Hospital, 5323 Harry Hines Boulevard, Dallas, Texas 75390-9073*

Michelle M. Le Beau, Ph.D. *Professor, Department of Medicine, Section of Hematology/Oncology, University of Chicago, 5841 South Maryland Avenue, Box MC2115, Chicago, Illinois 60637*

Catherine P. Leith, M.B., B. Chir. *Associate Professor, Department of Pathology, University of New Mexico, 915 Camino de Salud NE, Albuquerque, New Mexico 87131; and Staff Pathologist, Department of Pathology, University Hospital, 2211 Lomas Boulevard NE, Albuquerque, New Mexico 87106*

Chin-Yang Li, M.D. *Professor, Laboratory Medicine and Pathology, Mayo Medical School; and Consultant, Department of Laboratory Medicine and Pathology, Mayo Clinic, 200 First Street, S.W., Rochester, Minnesota 55905*

Ian T. Magrath, M.B., F.R.C.P., F.R.C. Path. *Professor of Pediatrics, Department of Pediatrics, University of the Uniformed Services in the Health Sciences, Bethesda, Maryland; and President, International Network for Cancer Treatment and Research, Rue Engeland 642, R-1180 Brussels, Belgium*

Estella Matutes, M.D. *Senior Lecturer, Academic Haematology and Cytogenetics, Institute of Cancer Research; and Consultant, Haematology, Department of Academic Haematology, Royal Marsden Hospital, Fulham Road, London SW3 6JJ, United Kingdom*

Robert W. McKenna, M.D. *Executive Chair, Department of Pathology, University of Texas Southwestern Medical Center, 5323 Harry Hines Boulevard; and Department Chairman, Department of Pathology, Parkland Health and Hospital Systems, 5201 Harry Hines Boulevard, Dallas, Texas 75235*

Malcolm A.S. Moore, M.D., Ph.D. *Member, Department of Cell Biology, Sloan-Kettering Institute; and Attending, Division of Medical Oncology, Memorial Sloan-Kettering Cancer Center, 1275 York Avenue, New York, New York 10021*

Angela Murray, M.S. *Immunopathology Laboratory Manager, Department of Pathology, New York–Presbyterian Hospital, 525 East 68th Street, New York, New York 10021*

Bharat N. Nathwani, M.D. *Professor of Pathology, Chief of Hematopathology, Department of Hematopathology, University of Southern California School of Medicine, 2011 Zonal Avenue, HMR 209, Los Angeles, California 90033; and Chief of Hematopathology, Department of Pathology, Los Angeles County University of Southern California Health Care Network General Hospital, Room 2422, Los Angeles, California 90033*

Richard S. Neiman, M.D. *Professor of Laboratory Medicine and Medicine, Indiana University School of Medicine; and Director of Hematopathology, Department of Pathology and Laboratory Medicine/ Hematopathology, Riley Hospital for Children, Room 0969, 702 Barnhill Drive, Indianapolis, Indiana 46202-5200*

Attilio Orazi, M.D., M.R.C. Path. *Professor, Department of Pathology, College of Physicians and Surgeons of Columbia University; and Director, Division of Hematopathology, Department of Pathology, Columbia-Presbyterian Medical Center, 630 West 168th Street, New York, New York 10032*

Langxing Pan, M.D., Ph.D. *Assistant Professor, Department of Pathology, Weill Medical College of Cornell University, 1300 York Avenue, New York, New York 10021*

Reza M. Parwaresch, M.D., Dr. H.C. *Professor of Pathology, Director, Institute of Hematopathology and Lymphnode Registry Kiel, Christian-Albrechts Universität zu Kiel, Michaelis Str. 11, 24105 Kiel, Germany*

LoAnn C. Peterson, M.D. *Professor of Pathology, Northwestern University Medical School; and Director of Hematopathology, Northwestern Memorial Hospital, 251 East Huron Street, Chicago, Illinois 60611*

Geraldine S. Pinkus, M.D. *Professor of Pathology, Department of Pathology, Harvard Medical School, Boston, Massachusetts; and Director, Hematopathology Division, Department of Pathology, Brigham and Women's Hospital, 75 Francis Street, Boston, Massachusetts 02115*

William C. Pitts, M.D. *Director of Anatomic Pathology, Community Medical Centers, Fresno and R Streets, Fresno, California 93701*

Mark Raffeld, M.D. *Chief of Specialized Diagnostic Unit, Laboratory of Pathology, National Cancer Institute, 9000 Rockville Pike, Bethesda, Maryland 20892*

Jonathan W. Said, M.D. *Professor and Chief, Division of Anatomic Pathology, University of California Los Angeles School of Medicine, 10833 Le Conte Avenue, Los Angeles, California 90095*

Elaine J. Schattner, M.D. *Assistant Professor, Division of Hematology and Medical Oncology, Department of Medicine, Cornell University; and Immunology Program, Weill Graduate School of Medical Sciences of Cornell University, 1300 York Avenue, New York, New York 10021*

Verena Schemmel, M.D. *Department of Paediatric Medicine, Hochschule Hannover, Care-Nueberg-Straße 1, 30625, Hannover, Germany*

Bertram Schnitzer, M.D. *Professor, Department of Pathology, University of Michigan, 1301 Catherine, Ann Arbor, Michigan 48109-0602; and Director, Department of Hematopathology, University of Michigan Health Systems, 1500 East Medical Center Drive, Ann Arbor, Michigan 48109*

Robert A. Soslow, M.D. *Associate Attending Pathologist, Department of Pathology, Memorial Sloan-Kettering Cancer Center, 1275 York Avenue, New York, New York 10021*

Catherine M. Spier, M.D. *Associate Professor, Department of Pathology, University of Arizona, and Director, Hematopathology and Immunology, Department of Pathology, University Medical Center, 1501 North Campbell Avenue, Tucson, Arizona 85724*

Louis Staudt *Senior Investigator, National Cancer Institute, National Institutes of Health, Bethesda, Maryland*

Harald Stein *Professor and Chairman of Pathology, Institut fur Pathologie, Klinikum Benjamin Franklin, Free University of Berlin, Hindenburgdamm 30, D-12200, Berlin, Germany*

Wayne Tam *Hematopathology Fellow, Department of Pathology, Weill Medical College of Cornell University, 1300 York Avenue; and Research Fellow, Institute of Cancer Genetics, Columbia University, New York, New York 10021*

Anna Tierens *Consultant Hematopathologist, Department of Pathology, The Norwegian Radiumhospital and Institution for Cancer Research, Montebello, 0310 Oslo, Norway*

James W. Vardiman, M.D. *Professor, Department of Pathology, University of Chicago, 5841 South Maryland Avenue, MC 0008, Chicago, Illinois 60637*

Roger A. Warnke, M.D. *Professor and Pathologist, Department of Pathology, Stanford University, 300 Pasteur Drive, Stanford, California 94305-5324*

Shaw Watanabe, M.D., D.M.S. *Professor, Department of Applied Bioscience, Tokyo University of Agriculture, 1-1-1, Sakuragaoka, Tokyo 156-8502, Japan*

Dennis D. Weisenburger, M.D. *Professor, Department of Pathology and Microbiology, University of Nebraska Medical Center; and Chief of Hematopathology Section, Department of Pathology and Microbiology, Nebraska Health System Hospitals, 983135 Nebraska Medical Center, Omaha, Nebraska 68198-3135*

Lawrence M. Weiss, M.D. *Chairman, Division of Pathology, City of Hope National Medical Center, 1500 East Duarte Road, Duarte, California 91010*

Cheryl L. Willman, M.D. *Director, University of New Mexico Cancer Center; and Professor, Department of Pathology, University of New Mexico, 2325 Camino de Salud NE, Albuquerque, New Mexico 87131*

Gary S. Wood, M.D. *Professor, Department of Dermatology, Pathology, and Oncology, Case Western Reserve University, 10900 Euclid Avenue, Cleveland, Ohio 44106; and Chief, Department of Dermatology, Louis Stokes VA Medical Center, 10701 East Boulevard, Cleveland, Ohio 44106*

Lung T. Yam, M.D. *Professor, Department of Medicine, University of Louisville, School of Medicine, HSC, Louisville, Kentucky 40292; and Chief, Department of Hematology, VA Medical Center, 800 Zorn Avenue, Louisville, Kentucky 40206*

Samuel A. Yousem, M.D. *Professor of Pathology, Department of Pathology, University of Pittsburgh Medical Center, 200 Lothrop Street, Pittsburgh, Pennsylvania 15213*

Preface to the First Edition

Pathologists have traditionally experienced difficulty in diagnosing hematologic neoplasms. One factor that accounts for these difficulties is that malignant lymphoma and leukemia cells often exhibit cytomorphologic features that mimic those of normal differentiating hematolymphoid cells. A second and perhaps more significant factor for many years was the lack of knowledge and understanding of the hematopoietic and immune systems. This prevented pathologists from comprehending the origin and nature of hematologic neoplasms and their relation to the normal cellular components of the hematopoietic and immune systems. The unprecedented explosion of new scientific information concerning the hematopoietic and immune systems that has taken place during the past 20 years, however, has generated the scientific bases for the reliable and reproducible diagnosis and classification of most hematologic neoplasms.

Modern hematopathology began in the early 1970s soon after immunologists discovered that lymphocytes are divisible into two distinct subpopulations. B cells and T cells, that vary according to their differentiation process, anatomic localization, and functional properties and are distinguishable according to their differential expression of various surface membrane and cytoplasmic antigens and receptors. Pathologists soon discovered that many neoplastic lymphoid cells also express B- and T-cell-associated markers, presumptive evidence of their B or T cell origin. They also discovered that benign, reactive lymphoid proliferations are polyclonal (i.e., contain mixtures of B and T cells), whereas many non-Hodgkin's lymphomas and lymphoid leukemias are monoclonal B cell proliferations (i.e., contain a predominance of B cells that express only one immunoglobulin light chain class, either κ or λ). These discoveries led to the use of cell marker analysis (the routine classification of lymphoid neoplasms as B- or T-cell derived) as an adjunct to morphologic interpretation in the diagnosis of lymphoid neoplasia, encouraged the correlation of morphologic features with immunologic cell markers, and fostered the development of new terminology and classification schemes.

The second phase of modern hematopathology, the monoclonal antibody era, began in the early 1980s when an array of highly specific monoclonal antibodies that detect B cell, T cell, monocyte/macrophage and myeloid lineage, differentiation, and subset-associated antigens became commercially available. During the same time, several comparatively inexpensive fluorescent-activated cell sorters that permit rapid, accurate, and objective analysis and sorting of cell populations also became available. In addition, several very sensitive immunohistochemical staining techniques, particularly the avidin-biotin-complex immunoperoxidase and alkaline phosphatase/antialkaline phosphatase methods, were developed and the reagents were made available in kit form for use in routine pathology laboratories. The combined commercial availability of sensitive and specific monoclonal antibodies and immunohistochemical reagents and affordable fluorescent-activated cell sorters resulted in the establishment of specialized hematopathology laboratories that routinely perform immunophenotypic analysis. The result has been an enormous collective experience with immunophenotypic analysis in the diagnosis and classification of hematologic neoplasms. This experience has allowed us to document the immunophenotypic profiles exhibited by nearly all the major clinicopathologic categories of hematologic neoplasia and to establish guidelines for their immunodiagnosis, resulting in a substantial improvement in diagnostic accuracy and greatly facilitating our understanding of the relation between malignant hematolymphoid cells and normal cells of the hematopoietic and immune systems.

The third and current phase of modern hematopathology, the molecular biology era, began in the mid 1980s. The development of the Southern blot hybridization technique, the cloning of the immunoglobulin and T cell receptor genes, and the preparation and dissemination of the DNA probes that detect clonal rearrangements of these genes have provided pathologists with a sensitive, accurate, and objective method for determining the lineage and clonality of lymphoid neoplasms. This approach has allowed for the determination of the lineage of neoplasms that exhibit immature, ambiguous, and anomalous immunophenotypes; the determination of the monoclonal nature of lymphoid proliferations of an uncertain nature; and the detection of clonal B and T cell populations that are undetectable by morphologic examination and/or by immunophenotypic analysis. The availability of many additional DNA probes and the development of DNA amplification techniques such as the polymerase chain reaction now allow us to detect routinely oncogenes, chromosomal translocations, and viral sequences as well, thereby facilitating the investigation of the pathogenesis of hematologic neoplasia.

Unfortunately, this sudden and rapid growth has generated a constantly changing and often confusing and conflicting literature. The rapid turnover of knowledge in hematopathology and the increasing reliance on new scientific techniques by hematopathologists have left many experienced pathologists (unfamiliar with the changing concepts and who are unable to perform these modern diagnostic techniques) uncomfortable in rendering definitive diagnostic opinions concerning hematolymphoid proliferations. Pathologists in training have often been discouraged from studying hematopathology for the same reasons. Furthermore, no single source of information that encompasses the morphologic, immunologic, and molecular aspects of hematolymphoid neoplasia has been available to pathologists (to guide them in daily practice) or to pathologists in training (to assist them in acquiring the basic tenets of knowledge of modern hematopathology) until now.

This book represents the first definitive textbook of modern hematopathology. It is aimed at providing a thorough overview of the morphologic, immunologic, and molecular genetic characteristics of the benign and malignant proliferations derived from the hematopoietic and immune systems. The volume begins with a review of our current understanding of the structural and functional characteristics of the hematopoietic and immune systems, followed by chapters that describe the currently available immunologic markers and their application in the flow cytometric and immunohistochemical analysis of hematologic neoplasms, the structure and function of the antigen receptor genes and oncogenes and their application in the diagnosis and classification of hematologic neoplasms, and an overview of the role of cytogenetics. Practical guidelines for the organization and operation of a hematopathology laboratory and for the technical evaluation of lymph node biopsies also are provided. The role of fine needle biopsy and imprint cytology in the diagnosis and classification of hematologic neoplasms is discussed next. These background chapters are followed by twenty-one chapters that describe in detail the benign, reactive lymphoid proliferations that stimulate malignant lymphoma, Hodgkin's disease, each major clinicopathologic category of non-Hodgkin's lymphoma, and the extranodal lymphoid hyperplasias and malignant lymphomas. This is followed by practical guidelines for the handling and cytochemical and immunohistochemical analysis of bone marrow specimens. The final chapters deal with bone marrow involvement by malignant lymphoma, the acute and chronic lymphoid and myeloid leukemias, the myeloproliferative disorders, histiocytic and dendritic cell proliferations, mast cell disease, and the splenic manifestations of hematolymphoid neoplasia.

This volume is a multiauthored text by necessity. The vast amount of information currently available that concerns the clinical and biologic aspects of the numerous and diverse categories of hematopoietic neoplasia precludes any one individual from successfully preparing a definitive, accurate, and up-to-date reference work on neoplastic hematopathology. For that reason, a sincere effort was made to select for the preparation of each chapter experts who have been closely associated with the growth and development of and who have made significant contributions to that particular aspect of hematopathology. The result is that the list of contributors to this textbook represents a veritable Who's Who in hematopathology. These are the very same investigators who have been largely responsible for the many exciting and important developments that have taken place in hematopathology during the past 20 years. Each expert has responded with excitement and enthusiasm for this project. I am grateful to them for their support of and participation in the preparation of *Neoplastic Hematopathology.*

Daniel M. Knowles, M.D.

Preface

Since publication of the first edition in 1992, our knowledge in all facets of hematopathology (i.e., morphology, immunology, and molecular biology) has continued to grow unabated.

In 1992, a lack of consensus on lymphoma classification existed, the Working Formulation was the standard in the United States and the Kiel Classification was the standard in most European countries. However, as our conceptual understanding of newly as well as previously recognized lymphoma entities grew, it became increasingly obvious that both classifications had inherent deficiencies. For example, the Working Formulation categories were broadly defined to accommodate the classification of all lymphomas but did not permit the recognition and distinction of specific disease entities [i.e., mantle cell lymphoma, the low-grade extranodal B-cell lymphomas arising in mucosa-associated lymphoid tissue (MALT), and peripheral T-cell lymphomas]. In addition to other shortcomings, the Kiel Classification neglected to include extranodal lymphomas and failed to distinguish MALT lymphomas.

A group of 19 expert hematopathologists from the United States, Europe, and Asia, designating themselves the International Lymphoma Study Group (ILSG), began to meet informally in 1991 to exchange ideas and information concerning the lymphomas. In 1993, the ILSG undertook the task to reach consensus on a list of ''real'' lymphoma entities based upon a combination of clinical, morphologic, immunophenotypic, and molecular genetic characteristics. This consensus list was published in 1994 and designated the Revised European–American Lymphoma (REAL) Classification since it represented a revision of the current European and American lymphoma classifications. Shortly thereafter, the reproducibility and clinical utility of the REAL classification was validated in a multi-observer study of 1,300 cases of non-Hodgkin's lymphoma gathered from several institutions around the world.

Since 1995, members of the American and European Hematopathology Societies have been collaborating on a new World Health Organization (WHO) Classification of hematologic malignancies. The WHO Classification employs an updated version of the REAL Classification for the lymphomas and expands the tenets of the REAL Classification to codify the myeloid and histiocytic neoplasms. The WHO Classification will replace all existing classifications and thus represents the first classification of hematologic malignancies in which true international consensus has been achieved.

By the time the first edition of this book was published, four international white cell differentiation antigen workshops had taken place and leukocyte antigens CD1 through CDw78 had been defined. Since then, two more workshops have been convened, leading to the further clarification of the structural and functional properties of these antigens and the expanded recognition of distinct leukocyte antigens through CD166. Thus, in the eight year interval between the publication of the first and second editions of this book, the number of distinct monoclonal antibody-defined leukocyte antigens has doubled.

In 1992, immunophenotypic characterization of lymphoproliferative disorders involving solid tissues was most often performed by immunohistochemical staining of frozen tissue sections. Most monoclonal antibodies commercially available at that time were not immunoreactive in paraffin tissue sections; only a few antigens, principally CD3, CD15, CD20, CD30, CD43, and CD45, were detectable in paraffin tissue sections. However, during the past several years, a concerted effort by many investigators to prepare paraffin-reactive monoclonal antibodies has resulted in an explosion of new antibody reagents capable of detecting most of the additional leukocyte antigens that are critical to immunophenotypic analysis, including for example, CD1a, CD4, CD5, CD8, CD10, and CD79α, in paraffin tissue sections. In addition, several investigators have developed heat-based antigen retrieval techniques capable of ''unmasking'' heretofore undetectable antigens in paraffin tissue sections. These techniques have further expanded the spectrum of paraffin-reactive monoclonal antibodies as well as enhanced the sensitivity and reproducibility of antigen detection in paraffin tissue sections. Finally, efficient, reliable automated immunohistochemical staining instruments have been introduced and widely accepted. As a consequence, at the present time, unlike in 1992, immunophenotypic characterization of the majority of lymphoproliferative disorders involving solid tissues are performed by the immunohistochemical staining of paraffin tissue sections, and, in many instances, by using automated instrumentation. These advances obviated the special requirements and technical difficulties associated with frozen tissue section immunohistochemistry, which has resulted in a marked expansion of the routine immunophenotypic analysis of hematologic malignancies.

By 1992, molecular characterization of the hematologic malignancies had become an established facet of hematopathology. However, the laborious, time-consuming, and relatively insensitive Southern blot technique restricted such studies to a few specialized laboratories. The introduction of simpler, more rapid, and far more sensitive polymerase chain reaction-based assays has resulted in a marked expansion of studies aimed at deciphering the molecular pathology of the hematologic malignancies. In addition, numerous significant discoveries in basic molecular biology have occurred since 1992. One example is the discovery of the *BCL-6* gene, a transcriptional repressor belonging to the POZ/Zinc finger family of transcriptional factors, which appears to play an important role in germinal center formation. Rearrangements of the *BCL-6* gene preferentially occur in diffuse large B-cell lymphomas where they may be associated with extranodal disease and a better prognosis. Another example is the discovery of the Kaposi's sarcoma-associated herpes virus, also referred to as human herpesvirus-8, which is a novel gamma 2-herpesvirus present in virtually all Kaposi's sarcoma lesions. This virus also has been found to be highly associated with an uncommonly occurring subset of unusual non-Hodgkin's lymphomas referred to as *primary effusion lymphomas,* which appear to originate in the body cavities as an effusion in the absence of an identifiable tumor mass. The combination of these and other scientific discoveries and the ever-widening use of molecular biological techniques in the study of hematologic malignancies has contributed significantly to our understanding of the role of molecular genetic lesions in the pathogenesis and the clinical and biological behavior of hematologic malignancies.

Our enhanced knowledge and understanding of the morphologic, immunologic, and molecular genetic characteristics of the hematologic malignancies and the lesions that simulate them necessitated that this book be updated. That is precisely what we have done. This second edition represents a thorough revision and marked expansion of the first edition to reflect our increased knowledge and current concepts of hematopathology. Each chapter appearing in the first edition has been revised; indeed, nearly all of them have been entirely rewritten. The result is that this book represents the definitive textbook of modern hematopathology.

This book is aimed at providing a thorough overview of the morphologic, immunologic, and molecular genetic characteristics of the benign and malignant proliferations derived from the cellular elements that comprise the hematopoietic and immune systems. The book begins with a review of our current understanding of the structural and functional characteristics of the hematopoietic and immune systems, followed by chapters that describe the currently available immunologic markers and their application in the flow cytometric and immunohistochemical analysis of hematologic neoplasms, the normal histology and immunoarchitecture of the lymphoid organs, the structure and function of the antigen receptor genes and oncogenes and their application in the diagnosis and classification of hematologic neoplasms, and an overview of the role of cytogenetics. Practical guidelines for the organization and operation of a hematopathology laboratory and for the technical evaluation of lymph node biopsies also are provided. The role of fine needle biopsy and imprint cytology in the diagnosis and classification of hematologic neoplasms is discussed next. These background chapters are followed by 23 chapters that describe in detail the benign, reactive lymphoid proliferations that simulate malignant lymphoma, the atypical lymphoproliferative disorders, Hodgkin's disease, the current classification of the non-Hodgkin's lymphomas and Hodgkin's disease and the clinical significance of these classifications, each major clinicopathologic category of non-Hodgkin's lymphoma, and the extranodal lymphoid hyperplasias and malignant lymphomas. This is followed by practical guides for the handling and cytochemical and immunohistochemical analysis of bone marrow specimens. The final chapters deal with bone marrow involvement by malignant lymphoma, acute and chronic lymphoid and myeloid leukemias, myeloproliferative disorders, histiocytic and dendritic cell proliferations, mast cell disease, and the splenic manifestations of hematolymphoid neoplasia.

This book is a multiauthored text by necessity. The vast amount of information concerning the clinical, pathologic, and biologic aspects of the numerous and diverse categories of hematopoietic neoplasia currently available precludes any one individual from successfully preparing a definitive, accurate, and up-to-date reference work on neoplastic hematopathology. For that reason, a sincere effort was made to select for the preparation of each chapter experts who have been closely associated with the growth and development, and who have made significant contributions to that particular aspect of hematopathology. The result is that the list of contributors represents a veritable Who's Who in hematopathology. These are the very same investigators who have been largely responsible for many of the exciting and important developments that have taken place in hematopathology during the past 25 years. Each expert responded with excitement and enthusiasm for this project. I am grateful to each of them for their support and participation in the preparation of the second edition of *Neoplastic Hematopathology*.

Daniel M. Knowles, M.D.

Acknowledgments

The opportunity to thank publicly those persons who have contributed substantially to one's professional development and career comes infrequently; therefore, I would like to take this opportunity to do precisely that. I express my sincere appreciation to Dr. Henry Rappaport for his stimulating lectures in hematopathology, which I attended as a medical student at the University of Chicago and which sparked my initial interest in hematopathology; to Dr. Henry Rappaport's surgical pathology faculty and house staff at the University of Chicago for inspiring me as a senior medical student to become a surgical pathologist; to Dr. Ralph Williams for introducing me to research during a medical student elective in his laboratory at the University of New Mexico, for assisting me in the preparation of my first abstract and paper, and for guiding me toward academic medicine; to Dr. Donald West King for accepting me into the pathology training program at the Columbia University College of Physicians & Surgeons and for providing an extraordinarily flexible training program that was a wonderful, nurturing environment that allowed me to grow personally and professionally; to Drs. Raffaele Lattes, Nathan Lane, Marianne Wolff, and Karl Perzin for training me in surgical pathology and for establishing a superior standard of diagnostic excellence to which I shall always aspire; to the late Dr. Henry Kunkel, the finest scientific intellect I have ever known, and to his staff at the Rockefeller University for guiding my training in laboratory research; to Dr. Vittorio Defendi, Chairman of Pathology at New York University and Dr. Michael Shelanski, Chairman of Pathology at the Columbia University College of Physicians & Surgeons, for their friendship and uncompromising support while I was a member of their departments; to the other members of the International Lymphoma Study Group for making the annual scientific meetings intellectually stimulating and personally rewarding; to Dr. Robert Michaels and Dr. Antonio M. Gotto, former and present Dean of the Weill Medical College of Cornell University, respectively, and to Dr. David B. Skinner and Dr. Herbert Pardes, former and present President and Chief Executive Officer of New York Presbyterian Hospital, respectively, for their generous support of me and the Department of Pathology; to all the Basic Science and Clinical Departmental Chairs at the Weill Medical College for their warm collegiality; and to my faculty for making our department better clinically and academically.

In addition, I thank the numerous physicians with whom I have worked and collaborated during the past 20 years, but especially Drs. Riccardo Dalla-Favera, James Halper, Giorgio Inghirami, Pier Giuseppe-Pelicci, and Chang Yi Wang. I also thank all of the fellows, residents, graduate students, technicians, and secretaries who have worked for me during the past 20 years and have helped my Hematopathology Laboratory grow and prosper. In this regard I give special thanks to two of my former fellows: Dr. Ethel Cesarman, now a successful independent research scientist and colleague, whose intelligence and creativity have inspired my laboratory for many years, and Dr. Amy Chadburn, now a successful hematopathologist and colleague who oversees the daily operation of the Hematopathology Laboratory and who has taken on many other responsibilities for me while I worked on this project; to Angela Murray, my laboratory manager whose intelligence, enthusiasm, devotion, and hard work have been responsible for many of the successes of my laboratory during the past 15 years; to Gina Imperato, my Departmental Administrator, whose extraordinary abilities, dedication, and support have contributed so much to my success as Chairman of Pathology at the Weill Medical College of Cornell University; and to Susan Roman, my administrative assistant, whose presence makes each workday easier and more pleasant. I also thank Timothy Satterfield of Williams and Wilkins for convincing me to prepare the first edition of this textbook 10 years ago and the staff at Lippincott Williams & Wilkins for being so helpful during the preparation of both editions of this textbook.

I thank each contributor to this textbook for their time and effort in the preparation of their chapters and for being so tolerant of my editorial changes and constant nagging to complete their sections on schedule. This textbook owes its title, *Neoplastic Hematopathology,* to the highly acclaimed "Tutorial on Neoplastic

Hematopathology,'' developed by Dr. Henry Rappaport, which has been successfully conducted annually for 30 consecutive years under the direction initially of Dr. Henry Rappaport, later Dr. Richard Brunning, and now me. I pay my respects to all of the individuals who have taught in the Tutorial and thereby have contributed to my education and to that of thousands of others in hematopathology. And lastly, but most importantly, I express my deepest and most sincere gratitude to Marian, my wife, who graciously supported me while I labored on most evenings and weekends for the past two years on this project. I could not have completed this textbook without her support and understanding.

Neoplastic Hematopathology

Second Edition

CHAPTER 1

The Hematopoietic System and Hematopoiesis

Malcolm A. S. Moore

Blood cell formation, or hematopoiesis, is a complex process encompassing the continuous generation of a spectrum of highly specialized, differentiated cell types whose life span can be measured in hours or years. What is particularly remarkable is the continual generation of these multiple lineages from a population of rare, pluripotent, self-renewing stem cells under steady-state conditions and under conditions of increased demand for one or a number of lineages. In adult humans for example, the bone marrow produces approximately 10^{10} erythrocytes and 4×10^8 leukocytes every hour. Historically, descriptive histologic and anatomic techniques revealed much of the organization of the morphologically recognizable components of the system, but these methods failed to reveal the complexities of the progenitor and stem cell compartments and the dynamics of hematopoiesis. Cell kinetic analysis using radioisotope labeling techniques provided insight into cellular dynamics, and the development of functional assays using *in vitro* and *in vivo* clonogenic systems provided insight into the more primitive compartments. Phenotypic analysis, particularly using CD antigens as differentiation markers, has been a powerful tool for analysis of lineage and differentiation stage.

The last decade has seen a remarkable revolution in understanding hematopoiesis at the molecular level. We are close to defining hematopoiesis as the consequence of a pattern of expression of more than 50 gene products, variously defined as hematopoietic growth factors, cytokines, and chemokines, that are produced within hematopoietic tissues and orchestrate the complex process of multilineage proliferation and differentiation. Dysregulation of this complex pattern of autocrine, paracrine, and endocrine regulation provides a molecular basis for immunohematopathology.

The hematopoietic system can be divided into three main compartments. The first, most primitive, and self-sustaining compartment consists of pluripotential stem cells. The second compartment consists of progenitor cells with various degrees of lineage restriction and little or no self-renewal capacity. The third compartment consists of morphologically identifiable, lineage-restricted, maturing cells, which can be further subdivided into mitotically active populations and postmitotic mature granulocytes, red blood cells, and platelets. The maintenance of the balance between stem cell self-renewal and commitment to terminally differentiate along one or more hematopoietic lineages underlies the hematopoietic homeostasis necessary for the continuous production of the different types of hematopoietic cells required under normal conditions and for the transient, increased production in situations of stress.

HEMATOPOIETIC STEM CELLS

Nearly 40 years ago, it was shown that mouse hematopoietic tissues contained a class of cells (colony-forming units–spleen [CFU-S]) capable of giving rise to macroscopic colonies containing more than 10^6 cells in the spleens of lethally irradiated, syngeneic recipients (1). The colonies originated from pluripotent cells; they generated granulocyte, megakaryocyte, and erythroid elements, and some colonies contained CFU-S capable of secondary spleen colony formation. Direct measurement of the localization of intravenously injected CFU-S indicated a seeding efficiency at 3 to 24 hours of 8% to 10% in marrow and spleen (2). After correcting for this seeding factor, the number of CFU-S is 100 to $250/10^5$ marrow cells. CFU-S are heterogeneous and the later-appearing, day-12 CFU-SI originate from more primitive cells than CFU-SII, which form colonies at 7 to 10 days (3). The frequency of CFU-SII and the ability to separate the bulk of these from long-term repopulating cells indicates that they represent a compartment of pluripotent preprogenitors of importance to short-term hematopoietic regeneration after myelosuppressive insult or transplantation (4).

Measurement of the stem cell population requires assays that are selective for pluripotent, preferably lymphomyeloid potent, cells with extensive self-renewal potential. Reconsti-

M. A. S. Moore: Memorial Sloan-Kettering Cancer Center, New York, New York 10021 tution of lethally irradiated mice with limiting dilutions of a stem cell source provides an assay for cells capable of repopulating the lymphoid and myeloid compartments for at least 6 to 12 months. Such an assay requires that the donor cells are marked to allow their progeny to be distinguished from any surviving endogenous stem cells (5). In practice, the assay population is mixed with cells capable of supporting short-term hematopoiesis and a competitive repopulation assay established. In this way, subtle differences in stem cell self-renewal potential, such as that caused by age, can be detected.

In attempts to establish *in vivo* assays for human stem cells, two xenograft systems have been used. The immunoincompetent nonobese diabetic/severe combined immunodeficient (NOD/SCID) mice, when injected with adult or, more efficiently, neonatal or fetal hematopoietic cells or CD34$^+$ selected populations, show substantial numbers (5% to 20%) of human CD45$^+$ cells of myeloid morphology (CD14, CD15, CD33), including CD34$^+$ subsets and B lymphocytes (CD19$^+$) in marrow and, to a much lesser extent, in the spleen and circulation (6). The extent of engraftment is usually evaluated at 5 weeks, but evidence of stable engraftment for much longer and the ability to repassage into a second group of mice support the view that this system assays a human stem cell. In limiting dilution assays, the SCID repopulating cell (SRC) has been estimated at 1 : 20,000 nucleated marrow cells. Injection of human stem cell sources into immunoincompetent, first-trimester, fetal lambs has shown that stable, multilineage, human engraftment is obtained and persists into postnatal life with, ultimately, adult sheep that are stable human hematopoietic chimeras (7). The major expansion of hematopoiesis that can result from injection of relatively few candidate stem cells and the stable long-term chimerism obtained makes this the gold standard for human stem cell assays, although one that is not generally available. A search continues for a phenotypic characterization of human stem cells that would permit their quantitation by flow cytofluorometry or their separation from contaminating tumor cells or T cells for autologous or allogeneic transplantation. Most hematopoietic stem cells (HSCs) and progenitors of all lineages express CD34, and there has been extensive clinical transplantation of purified CD34$^+$ populations in autologous and allogeneic situations. A rare population of stem cells lacks detectable CD34 and, in the mouse, is capable of long-term repopulation (8); the human equivalent was detected in the NOD/SCID (9) and fetal lamb (10) assays. Engraftment kinetics in the lamb model have suggested that the CD34$^-$ stem cells may be superior to the CD34$^+$ stem cells in long-term expansion potential. It is possible that CD34 antigen is modulated on the surface of stem cells, possibly not expressed by deeply quiescent cells, and is upregulated as cells enter the proliferative pool.

HSCs develop from hemangioblasts that have endothelial and hematopoietic potential, and these more primitive cells express CD34 (and the vascular endothelial growth factor receptor [VEGFR]-FLK-1) (11). An intriguing report, which stated that purified neural stem cells could reconstitute hematopoiesis in lethally irradiated mice (12), has raised critical issues about the plasticity of the differentiated state of stem cells. Despite unsubstantiated claims, there is no good evidence that a common stem cell exists with the capacity to generate hematopoiesis and hematopoietic stromal elements. A separate mesenchymal stem cell, capable of generating bone, cartilage, and marrow stroma, does exist within the bone marrow, and it is discussed in the context of the hematopoietic microenvironment.

A search for cells phenotypically and perhaps functionally equivalent to the embryonic hemangioblasts in adult humans has not proved fruitful but has led to the identification of a bone marrow–derived, circulating, endothelial progenitor that could form endothelial linings to artificial arterial grafts in dogs (13). This cell in humans is CD34$^+$ and KDR$^+$ (human VEGFR$^+$) and, unlike young differentiated endothelium, expresses a stem cell antigen found on HSCs (AC133) (14). The human endothelial progenitor cell comprises 1% to 2% of the granulocyte colony-stimulating factor (G-CSF) mobilized peripheral blood CD34$^+$ population and 1% to 2% of umbilical cord CD34$^+$ cells and may play a role in neovascularization and repair of damaged endothelium throughout the body. This cell population has been shown to differentiate only into endothelium.

HSCs are characterized by low or absent expression of antigens that mark later differentiation stages (Table 1.1). The phenotype CD34$^+$, CD38$^-$, and CD45RA^{low} and CD71^{low} characterizes less than 1% of the total CD34$^+$ population and contains more than 75% of HSC. Human leukocyte antigen-DR (HLA-DR) is absent or expressed at low levels on adult HSCs but is present on fetal and neonatal HSCs (15). THY-1 antigen is present on mouse and human HSCs and on a proportion of committed progenitors (16). The multidrug resistance-1 gene *(MDR1)* is strongly expressed on HSCs, and expression of the P-glycoprotein confers on these cells the ability to exclude the mitochondrial binding dye rhodamine 123 (17). The rhodamine^{low} HSC phenotype can also be attributed to HSCs in quiescence (G_0), with reduced or absent mitochondria. An epitope on a 5 transmembrane-spanning receptor protein recognized by monoclonal antibody AC133 has been shown to characterize human HSCs, including cells with immunodeficient NOD/SCID and fetal lamb engrafting potential (18). Like CD34, it is also expressed on myeloid progenitors, but unlike CD34, it is not expressed on erythroid progenitors.

In Vitro Hematopoietic Stem Cell Assays

In vitro HSC assays are based on clonal or limiting dilution expansion of cells in the presence of cytokine combinations, marrow stromal support, or both (Table 1.1). The high proliferative potential–colony forming unit (HPP-CFU) assay detects cells that are quiescent in normal marrow, resistant to 5-fluorouracil (5-FU) or 4-hydroperoxycyclophosphamide (4-HC), and form colonies in semisolid culture sys-

TABLE 1.1. *Phenotype and functional assays for hematopoietic stem cells and progenitors*

Stem cells	Frequency/10^5	Progenitors	Percentage[a]
Phenotype[a]			
CD34, CD38-ve, Thy-1, Kit	10–30	CD34, CD38	1–3
Flt3, CD45RA^{low}, CD71^{low}, CD33^{low}	10–30	CD34, CD33, CD54	0.3–1
HLA-DR$^{-/low}$, MDR1^{hi}, Rh^{dull}	10–30	CD19, CD7, CD24	
AC133, Lin-ve	3–10	CD34, CD9, CD18, CD31, CD44, CD29	0.5–2
CD34-ve, Lin-ve	1–2	HLA-DR, MDR^{low}, Rh^{bright}	1–3
Assay			
CRU	1–5	CFU-GM	0.2
SRC	2–5	BFU-E	0.1
HPP-CFU-1	0.2–1	CFU-Meg	0.025
CFUblast	10–40	CFU-GEMM	0.01
LTHC-IC	2–5	CFU-SI day 12	0.01
Delta assay	2–5	CFU-SII day 8	0.02
CAFC wk 5	2–5	CAFC wk 2	0.15
Stromal BL-CFC	1–3	HPP-CFU-2, -3	0.02
LTC-IC	2–5		

CRU, competitive repopulating unit (mouse); SRC, NOD/SCID repopulating cell; HPP-CFU, high proliferative potential CFU, types 1, 2, or 3 (mouse); LTHC-IC, long-term hematopoietic culture-initiating cell (stroma-free assay); LTC-IC, long-term culture-initiating cell assay (5wk on stroma); CAFC, cobblestone area–forming cells (at 2 or 5 wk on stroma); CFU-S, spleen colony–forming units scored at 8 or 12 days (mouse); BFU-E, burst-forming units–erythroid; CFU, colony-forming units; GM, granulocyte-macrophage; Meg, megakaryocyte, GEMM, granulocyte, erythroid, macrophage, and megakaryocyte.

[a] Phenotype of human marrow only. Frequency and percentage are for normal human marrow or for mouse marrow if there is no human equivalent.

tems larger than 0.5 mm in diameter containing more than 10^5 cells (19,20). This compartment is heterogeneous, embracing primitive, self-renewing, pluripotent cells (HPP-CFU-1) with a stringent requirement for multiple synergistic cytokines for stimulation, through HPP-CFU-2, with less restricted cytokine requirements, and HPP-CFU-3, stimulated by interleukin-3 (IL-3) alone, with limited or absent self-renewal potential. Most cells sorted using stem cell phenotypic characteristics are capable of forming colonies of blast cells *in vitro*, and many of these become HPP colonies if cultured for 2 to 4 weeks.

In the murine system, two distinct populations of CFU blasts (CFU-B1) exist—one stimulated by Kit ligand, with or without potentiation by other growth factors, and a second set stimulated by Flk ligand, with potentiation through gp130 signaling by IL-11, IL-6, or leukemia-inhibitory factor (LIF) (19,20–22). The frequency of CFU-B1 (up to 40 per 10^5 in rodent marrow) is considerably in excess of documented stem cells measured by long-term competitive repopulation (competitive repopulating units [CRU]), and most do not generate secondary CFU-B1, but in contrast to lineage-committed, progenitor-derived colonies, blast colonies are composed predominantly of committed progenitors of multiple lineages. CFU-B1 represent a transit population of preprogenitor cells that are more differentiated than stem cells and probably closely related to CFU-SII but a major amplification compartment of importance to short-term hematopoietic recovery, such as after bone marrow transplantation.

Multiple limiting dilution passage, or recloning assays (i.e., Delta assays) involve expansion of 5-FU– or 4-HC–resistant cells or selected CD34$^+$ populations with multiple cytokine stimulation. Cumulative expansion of progenitors and total cells provide an index of proliferative potential of the input population, and when carried out at limiting dilutions, they can be used to quantitate long-term hematopoietic culture-initiating cells (LTHC-IC) (19,23–25). The *in vitro* assays that most reflect *in vivo*, long-term repopulating capacity are those in which hematopoietic cells are cocultured for 5 to 8 weeks on bone marrow stroma. This assay developed from the system of stromal-supported long-term bone marrow culture, first described in the mouse by Dexter (26). On adaptation to human use, it was shown that bone marrow cells lacking HLA-DR expression sustained long-term hematopoiesis on human marrow stroma and generated secondary colony-forming units–granulocyte macrophage (CFU-GM) and burst-forming units–erythroid (BFU-E) for at least 5 weeks. In contrast, HLA-DR$^+$ populations containing all the committed progenitors, including BFU-E and CFU-GM, did not sustain long-term hematopoiesis (27). By establishing a linear relationship between secondary CFU-GM produced after 5 weeks and an input population of long-term culture-initiating cells (LTC-IC) and by demonstrating the close phenotypic and functional relationship between these and *in vivo* CRU, this assay has become the most accepted *in vitro* surrogate stem cell assay (28). The LTC-IC assay may be modified to allow subsets of murine LTC-IC to express myeloid and lymphoid differentiation potential (29). Limiting dilution analysis shows that such lymphomyelopotent LTC-IC are present in normal murine marrow at a frequency of 1 per 10^5 cells, which is on the order of the frequency of CRUs.

Closely related to LTC-IC are cells forming foci of dark-phase cells growing beneath the stromal layer. These cobblestone area–forming cells are considered to be committed progenitors when scored at 2 to 3 weeks but are measured as HSC. LTC-IC frequencies in marrow are in the range of 0.5% of the total $CD34^+$ population and between 0.25% to 1% in mobilized peripheral blood or umbilical cord blood.

Regulation of Stem Cell Self-Renewal and Differentiation

The relative contribution of cell-intrinsic stochastic mechanisms or cell-extrinsic deterministic or instructive mechanism to hematopoietic differentiation is still under debate. With the discovery of the extensive family of diffusible regulators of hematopoiesis, much attention has been directed at their mechanism of action–specifically whether they play an instructive role or are simply permissive or selective, permitting the survival or proliferation of independently committed cells. Ogawa and colleagues (30) demonstrated by single-cell recloning studies that stochastic events accounted for the random assortment of blood cell lineages obtained by recloning pluripotent progenitors. At the level of committed progenitor (e.g., CFU-E), the presence of erythropoietin is absolutely required for terminal erythroid differentiation, and in its absence, the erythropoietin receptor (EPOR)–expressing cell undergoes apoptosis. Erythropoietin plays a permissive role, allowing an erythroid-committed, receptor-expressing cell to fulfill its preprogrammed differentiation fate. Most growth factors are not essential for lineage determination, as shown in cytokine-knockout mice. Mice lacking erythropoietin, G-CSF, or granulocyte macrophage colony-stimulating factor (GM-CSF) still generate near-normal numbers of specific progenitors that respond normally to these factors.

Analysis of the fate of individual sorted stem cells from human fetal liver revealed extensive functional heterogeneity when they were cultured in the presence of a combination of cytokines (e.g., FK-2/FLT-3 ligand, KIT ligand, IL-3, IL-6, G-CSF) (31). Cells with the highest overall proliferative potential could be recognized by their slow growth kinetics. Most subclones derived from slow-growing $CD34^+CD38^-$ cells were fast-growing clones with low proliferative potential. However, a minority of subclones showed growth kinetics similar to the parental clones, and this heterogeneity was preserved through four to six generations. This continuous generation of functional heterogeneity among the clonal progeny of HSCs supports the view that stem cell fate is controlled intrinsically. The mechanism involved in the heritable functional heterogeneity within stem cell clonal progeny most probably involves asymmetric cell division resulting in one daughter cell more committed to terminal differentiation and the other daughter being similar to the mother cell. The potential for asymmetric division is supported by direct observation of slow-growing $CD34^+CD38^-$ HSCs. Such cells exhibit a distinct polarity; they are small and motile, having a ''comma'' shape with most of the cellular volume preceding a cytoplasmic tail of one- to two-cell diameters. In an analysis of cytokine-stimulated cultures of single $CD34^+CD38^-$ cells from fetal liver, cord blood, and adult marrow, about 40% of initial cell divisions were asymmetric, with one of the daughter cells becoming quiescent while the other proliferated exponentially (32).

The highly conserved mechanism implicated in asymmetric cell division of neural progenitors in *Drosophila* and mammals involves the expression of one of the members of the Notch family of transmembrane receptors and signaling through interaction with one of its ligands, such as Delta or Serrate/Jagged (33). Cleavage orientation and asymmetric inheritance of Notch-1 in daughter cells has been reported in mammalian neurogenesis (34). A further mechanism involving blocking of Notch signal transduction by asymmetric distribution of a Notch-binding protein, Numb, confers distinct fate to daughter cells (35). The expression of Notch-1 and -2 on $CD34^+$ cells and the expression of the Notch ligands Jagged and Delta-like by hematopoietic stroma supports a role for this signaling system in primitive hematopoiesis and is supported by experimental evidence of altered probabilities of generation of primitive progenitors such as CFU-Mix after activation of Notch (36). The relatively modest changes observed in the various experimental systems may reflect the experimental difficulties in optimally engaging this signaling system or to the existence of powerful systems to limit or counteract Notch signaling with its potential to completely block differentiation if unrestrained. Very small changes in the probability that a stem cell will self renew or differentiate have major long-term consequences for the stability of the stem cell pool, at the one extreme leading to its exhaustion with hematopoietic failure and at the other to overabundance of stem cells at the expense of differentiation, with potential leukemogenicity.

Molecular studies of receptor signaling also support the role of stochastic determinism. Although most hematopoietic growth factors have specific private ligand binding domains, many receptors share common or public signaling domains and have similar or overlapping downstream signaling pathways, making it difficult to see how a unique deterministic signal could be delivered. In studies in which hybrid receptors are generated by combining the ligand-binding domain, such as of MPL, and the cytoplasmic domain of, for example, the G-CSF receptor (G-CSFR) under the control of the MPL regulatory element, thrombopoietin is able to support survival and proliferation of cells expressing the receptor without changing commitment bias, arguing against a deterministic role for growth factors in lineage commitment (37).

The importance of receptor expression to the differentiation process has led to various studies of patterns of receptor expression on pluripotent cells. Radiolabeled ligand binding studies using highly purified progenitors and stem cells have shown that there is considerable heterogeneity in terms of the percent of the population expressing receptors and the number of receptors per cells (38). Numbers of receptors were frequently very low (<100/cell) or undetectable, even though biologic responses to the ligand could be demonstrated (e.g., macrophage colony stimulating factor [M-CSF], GM-CSF). Similar results have been obtained by reverse transcriptase–polymerase chain reaction (RT-PCR) analysis of single multipotent progenitor cells. Detailed molecular analysis of multipotential stem cells has shown that lineage-specific genes (e.g., globin, myeloperoxidase, IGH, CD3d) are in a primed state, characterized by open chromatin and some low-level sporadic expression (39). Many different lineage-affiliated components can be expressed in the same cell. This low-level multigene activity can be built on or amplified by random forces that influence transcription or by means of positive or negative reinforcement through extracellular signalling through stochastically expressed receptor molecules.

Homeobox genes *(HOX)* have been implicated in controlling stem cell fate, with overexpression of certain members increasing the probability of self-renewal. Homeobox genes are a family of transcription factors that were originally described as developmental regulators responsible for the correct sequence of segmentation production. The expression of *HOX* genes usually coincides with the development of the mesodermal germ layer from which the hematopoietic system is derived. The positional arrangement of the *HOX* genes on human chromosome 7p14-7p15 *(HOXA)*, Cr 17 q21-17q22 *(HOXB)*, Cr 12 q12-q13 *(HOXC)*, and Cr 2 q31-q37 *(HOXD)* correlates with their expression in body parts. In hematopoiesis, the *HOX* genes at the 3′ end are generally expressed in the stem cell compartment, and those at the 5′ end are expressed predominantly in committed progenitors (40). Those of the *HOXA* cluster are expressed primarily in myelomonocytic cells, those of *HOXB* in myelomonocytic and erythropoietic cells, and those of *HOXC* in lymphopoietic cells. Overexpression of *HOXB8* in marrow cells leads to increased IL-3 production and increased self-renewal of stem cells; overexpression of *HOXB4* results in a 50-fold enhancement of primitive stem cell numbers in primary and secondary mouse transplantation models, and *HOXA10* overexpression leads to increased progenitor cells and a dramatic increase in megakaryocytes and primitive blast cells and can result in a disorder resembling chronic myelocytic leukemia (40).

Hematopoietic Stem Cell Migration

A critical property of the stem cell is its ability to migrate from site to site, as exemplified by stem cell migration streams among yolk sac, aorta-gonad-mesonephros, fetal liver, thymus, spleen, and marrow during the course of fetal development. Of equal importance in the adult is the ability of stem cells to be released from the marrow into the circulation and to migrate to other intramedullary and extramedullary sites. The normal frequency of $CD34^+$ cells in the circulation is 40 per 10^5 white blood cells. This frequency rises to more than 1,000 per 10^5 after G-CSF treatment and more than 300 per 10^5 after GM-CSF treatment (41). The most primitive stem cell fraction usually comprises less than 1% of the total $CD34^+$ population, and a higher proportion of these primitive cells are found in $CD34^+$ cells mobilized by GM-CSF and particularly by the combination of G-CSF and KIT ligand (i.e., stem cell factor) (25).

Certain mechanisms by which circulating stem cells exit the blood and reenter the marrow (i.e., possess a marrow-homing capacity) are critical to successful bone marrow transplantation. The process involves chemokines for navigation and adhesive interactions to guide the cells to their appropriate niches within the marrow microenvironment. In addition to adhesive interactions, stem cells, like differentiated leukocytes, are required to undergo deformation, extension of cytoplasmic projections, and generation of contractile forces as they move (e.g., in transit through marrow sinusoidal endothelium). Studies have revealed remarkable pseudopod morphologies expressed by purified human $CD34^+$ cells (42). The migration characteristics of fluorescein-labeled $CD34^+$ cells were observed using time-lapse fluorescent microscopy. The cells were observed to extend long, thin pseudopods of two morphologies. Tenupodia are very thin and form in linear segments. They adhere to the substrate, can bifurcate multiple times, and can connect cells more than 300 μm apart. Magnupodia are much thicker and have been observed to extend more than 330 μm away from cells. Magnupods are flexible structures that exhibit rapid dynamic motion. Both forms of pseudopod can adhere to surfaces coated with fibronectin, collagen IV, and laminin. The deployment of these podia during *in vitro* cell migration, suggests that they perform sensory and mechanical functions.

$CD34^+$ homing to bone marrow sinusoidal endothelium may be mediated through selectins, such as L-selectin and E-selectin, followed by firm adhesion mediated by vascular cell adhesion molecule-1 (VCAM-1)/very late antigen-4 (VLA-4) and intracellular adhesion molecule-1 (ICAM-1)/lymphocyte function associated-1 (LFA-1) ligand pairs followed by interaction with junctional adhesion molecules such as platelet-endothelial cytoadhesion molecule (PECAM). The concept that integrins are important for stem or progenitor cell trafficking is supported by the finding that circulatory progenitors express lower levels of the β_1 integrin VLA-4 and the β_2 integrin LFA-1 but have comparable levels of PECAM compared with progenitors in the bone marrow (43,44). VCAM-1 is the dominant bone marrow endothelial addressin in hematopoietic homing of $VLA\text{-}4^+$ $CD34^+$ cells, and treating cells with anti-VLA-4 reduces homing to marrow by 30% to 50%, and antibody to VLA-4 (integrin $\alpha_4\beta_1$) mobilizes progenitors (45). The log number of cells transplanted that expressed CD44, L-selectin, VLA-5, but not VLA-4, LFA-1, ICAM-1, LFA-3, or THY-1 correlated with time required to reach a platelet count of 20,000/mL (46). The higher proportion of $CD34^+$ $L\text{-}selectin^+$ or

$CD44^+$ cells in leukapheresis product than in bone marrow may be one explanation for more rapid reconstitution with the former. Hematopoietic growth factors IL-3, KIT ligand (47), and thrombopoietin (48) rapidly (30 minutes) upregulate VLA-4 and VLA-5 on primitive (predominantly $CD34^+$ $CD38^-$ but not $CD38^+$ cells) human hematopoietic cells promoting their adhesion to VLA-4 and fibronectin. PECAM ligands heparin and chondroitin sulfate enhance VLA-4 adhesive activity of $CD34^+$ cells. The KIT receptor has also been implicated in adhesion of hematopoietic cells to stromal cells (44), and KIT expression is reduced on mobilized cells (49). Anti-VLA-4 or anti-VCAM-1 with cytokines G-CSF, KIT ligand, and FLT-3 ligand enhances mobilization (45). WWv and Sl/Sld mice with mutations in *Kit* and its ligand, respectively, have impaired responses to anti-VLA-4. Signaling through Kit is required for this mobilization, and it does not result from simple de-adhesion. This is a novel example of integrin-cytokine cosignaling.

Although it is attractive to ascribe some unique form of adhesion mechanism to selectively trap stem cells only within the hematopoietic vasculature, it is equally plausible that physical trapping of cells within the marrow is relatively nonspecific, but that the microenvironment provides selective growth or survival advantages for HSCs or provides specific chemotactic signals promoting egress of HSCs from the circulation. Homing of circulating stem cells to the marrow involves activation of the CXCR4 chemokine receptor, expressed on up to 60% of circulating $CD34^+$ cells and more than 80% of the most primitive $CD34^+CD38^-$ subpopulations, by the bone marrow–derived chemokine stromal cell–derived factor-1 (SDF-1) (50). Subsequent chemotaxis results in rapid transendothelial migration of cells, detected in the *in vitro* cobblestone area-forming cells (CAFC) and LTC-IC assays and by the NOD/SCID *in vivo* repopulation assay, and blocking of chemotaxis or *in vivo* stem cell engraftment can be achieved by use of antibodies to CXCR4 (51,52).

Hematopoietic Stem Cell Proliferation, Telomerase, and Proliferative Senescence

Proliferation of normal somatic cells is associated with progressive shortening of the telomeric ends of the chromosomes that at birth comprise of 10,000 to 12,000 base pairs (bp) of tandem repeats of TAAGGG. In human leukocytes, some 50 bp of telomeric DNA are lost per year of normal life (53), with a particularly rapid loss in the first year of life. *In vitro*, similar telomere shortening is seen, with 50 to 80 bp lost per population doubling in cultures of $CD34^+$ cells (54), and telomeric loss of 400 to 1,500 bp is associated with allogeneic or autologous stem cell transplantation (55). When cells achieve a critical degree of telomere shortening, they enter proliferative senescence and fail to divide further or undergo apoptosis. This has been called the *Hayflick limit*, named after the investigator who first drew an association between the restricted *in vitro* life span on nontransformed fibroblasts, age and population doubling potential (56).

Cells can escape from senescence and "crisis" by undergoing mutational events leading to the upregulation of the ribonucleoprotein telomerase, which can elongate telomeric ends. Acting in concert with oncogenes or mutated tumor suppressor genes, telomerase expression is associated with the malignant phenotype and is found in 85% to 90% of all human cancers (57). It is also expressed normally at high levels in testes and ovaries, where it is required to maintain the telomeric integrity of the germline. It is induced in T and B lymphocytes on antigen or mitogen stimulation and is constitutively expressed in the thymus and germinal centers. Within the hematopoietic system, telomerase is expressed in proliferating $CD34^+$ cells of progenitor ($CD38^+$) and stem cell–enriched ($CD38^-$) subsets, and it is rapidly induced within 24 to 48 hours of exposure of noncycling $CD34^+$ cells to cytokines (54). Paradoxically, progressive telomere shortening is observed in proliferating $CD34^+$ cells that are expressing telomerase, suggesting that levels of enzymatic activity are insufficient to totally protect the cells from telomere erosion or that some other mechanisms, possibly involving telomere binding proteins, may inhibit enzyme action.

Despite the tremendous proliferation occurring throughout life within the hematopoietic system, proliferative senescence is unlikely to contribute to any observed hematopoietic pathology within a normal life span. However, excessive hematopoietic proliferation associated with repeated cycles of myelosuppressive chemotherapy and stem cell damage or with stem cell transplantation may lead to accelerated telomere shortening (55,58). This may predispose to cytogenetic instability and aneuploidy, which characterizes myelodysplastic syndrome and secondary leukemia seen at greatly increased frequency as a complication of therapy of patients with malignant lymphoma, multiple myeloma, and aplastic anemia. Studies have shown that introduction of the catalytic component of human telomerase into normal human fibroblasts leads to high levels of telomerase expression and "immortalization" of the cells that continuously grow for hundreds of population doublings beyond their normal point of senescence, with retention of normal phenotype and with no evidence of transformation (59).

HEMATOPOIETIC PROGENITOR CELLS

In the mid-1960s, *in vitro* colony assays in semisolid medium were developed that initially allowed detection of colonies of granulocytes and macrophages in the presence of crude sources of "colony-stimulating activity," subsequently identified as GM-, G-, and M-CSF (60,61). Extensive characterization of these CFU-GM revealed that they were committed granulocyte-macrophage progenitors and more differentiated than CFU-S. Subsequently, with different sources of stimuli, clonal assays for early (BFU-E) and late (CFU-E) erythroid progenitors were developed; the former required a combination of erythropoietin and GM-CSF or IL-3, and the latter required only erythropoietin (Fig. 1.1).

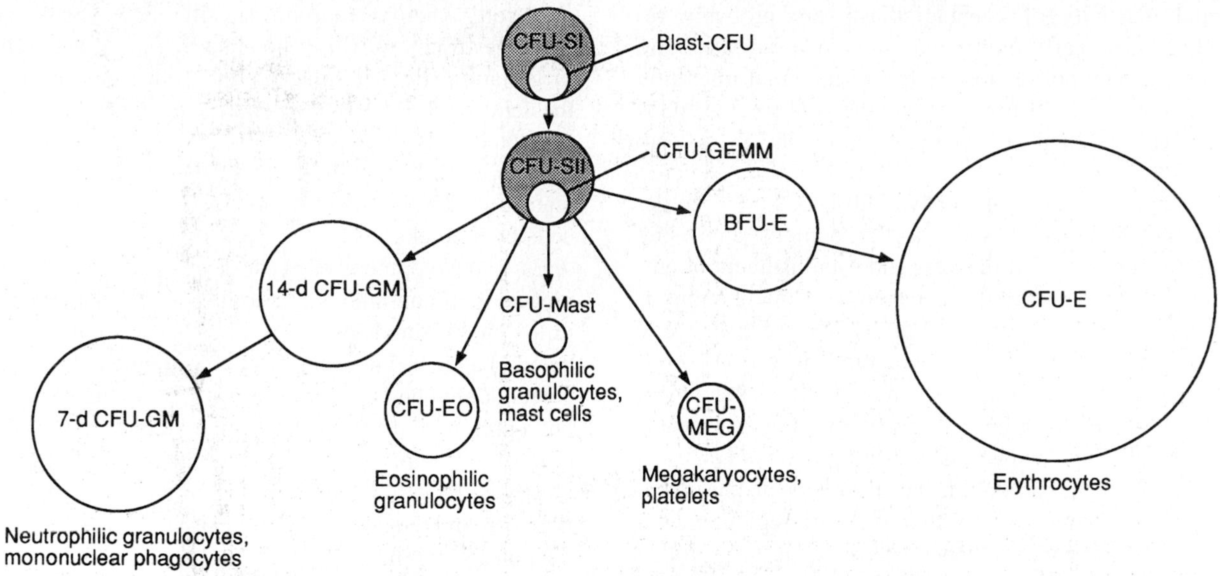

FIG. 1.1 Types of colony-forming units (CFU) and their origins. The area of the circles is approximately proportional to the frequency of the various types of CFUs in normal bone marrow. *In vitro* assays for blast-CFU and CFU-GEMM (erythroid, granulocyte, macrophage and megakaryocytic lineages) probably identify a proportion of CFU-SI (spleen CFU at about 12 days) and CFU-SII (spleen CFU at about 10 days, adjusted for seeding efficiency), respectively. The totipotent immunohematopoietic stem cells, able to reconstitute lethally irradiated animals, are probably more primitive than CFU-SI. BFU-E, burst-forming units–erythroid; CFU-E, colony-forming units–erythrocyte; CFU-EO, colony-forming units—eosinophil; CFU-GM, colony-forming units–granulocyte-macrophage; CFU-MEG, colony-forming units–megakaryocyte.

Colonies of endoreduplicating megakaryocytes were also shown to develop from diploid megakaryocyte progenitors (CFU-Meg) in the presence of GM-CSF or IL-3 with IL-6, IL-11, LIF, or with thrombopoietin alone. In all cases, the progenitors appeared to be restricted to one or, at most, two lineages and had no self-renewal capacity. A rarer pluripotent cell capable of forming mixed colonies containing erythroid, granulocyte, macrophage, and megakaryocytic lineages was called the CFU-GEMM or CFU-Mix, but the inability to detect secondary CFU-GEMM after recloning of primary mixed colonies indicated that this pluripotent progenitor lacked self-renewal potential. The relative proportion of progenitors and stem cell detected in the various assays is shown schematically in Figure 1.1.

DEVELOPMENT AND STRUCTURE OF THE HEMATOPOIETIC SYSTEM

Embryonic Hematopoiesis

Blood formation during vertebrate embryogenesis involves a sequence of events beginning with mesodermal induction by agents such as fibroblast growth factor or activin, followed by mesodermal patterning induced by bone morphogenic protein-4 (BMP-4) and cell specification by hematopoietic-specific transcription factors (e.g., GATA-1, GATA-2, stem cell leukemia [SCL]). GATA-1 regulates most if not all erythroid-specific genes and is absolutely required for terminal erythroid differentiation, and GATA-2 is required for maintenance or proliferation of hematopoietic progenitors. The first site of hematopoiesis is extraembryonic and occurs in the visceral yolk sac, where mesodermal cells aggregate into clusters to form blood islands that consist of an inner core of blood cells and an external layer of endothelial cells. Yolk sac hematopoiesis begins at 3 weeks' gestation in humans and 7.5 days' gestation in mice and consists predominantly of large nucleated primitive erythrocytes expressing embryonic hemoglobin and primitive macrophages (62,63). Hematopoietic progenitors (CFU-GM) appear within the yolk sac as soon as hematopoiesis is established (62) and shortly thereafter. By 8.5 days' gestation in the mouse, they appear within the embryo proper in the paraaortic splanchnopleure (64). Cells with *in vivo* CFU-S–forming potential and long-term repopulating capacity develop at 9.5 to 10.5 days in the aorto-gonadal-mesonephros (AGM) region, before their appearance in the developing liver, where they are first detected by 10.5 to 11 days or at the 23-somite stage (65). Specific regions of the dorsal aorta within the AGM region of mouse (9 to 10 days) and human (4 to 6 weeks) embryos and in the umbilical and omphalomesenteric arteries consist of structures in which a core of hemocytoblasts is circumscribed by endothelial cells (64,65). These structures, like the yolk sac blood islands, are probably sites where $CD34^+$, KIT^+, and $FLK\text{-}1^+$ ($VEGFR^+$) hemangioblasts differentiate into angioblastic endothelial progenitors and hemoblastic pluripotential HSCs. Cells with the developmental plasticity of hemangioblasts are probably restricted to these early embryonic and yolk sac sites, and thereafter, hematopoiesis results from sequential migration of streams of stem cells moving from the yolk sac and AGM to fetal liver and then to developing bone marrow, spleen, and thymus.

This dynamic interchange of lympho-HSCs between developing hematopoietic tissues was first demonstrated using sex chromosomes as cell markers and establishment of embryonic vascular anastomoses between developing embryos of the opposite sex, occurring naturally in certain dizygotic twins, or artificially established by parabiosis (66). As originally formulated, this model of hematopoietic development was called the *yolk sac migration hypothesis,* because it envisioned the yolk sac blood islands as a unique site of hemangioblast development (66). With the discovery of the prehepatic onset of hematopoiesis in the AGM region, it was proposed that the yolk sac was a transient site of primitive generation erythropoiesis and that definitive generation stem cells arose *de novo* in the AGM and subsequently migrated to the fetal liver (65). The main evidence for the importance of the AGM was that it was shown to contain *in vivo* repopulating cells capable of multilineage hematopoietic regeneration when transplanted into adult irradiated mice, as measured by CFU-S assay and long-term repopulation. Such cells appeared at the same time as they appeared in the yolk sac in the mouse, although in greater numbers, and they expanded between day 9 and day 11 to a greater degree (65). However, multilineage stem cells with the capacity for long-term repopulation of adult mice are present in the early yolk sac but require "conditioning" by residence in the liver (e.g., by direct injection into the liver of busulfan-treated newborn mice) before they are capable of repopulating the adult bone marrow and generating definitive hematopoiesis (67). That early stem cells that colonize the fetal liver lack the homing mechanisms necessary for localizing in the adult marrow or use a different homing mechanism is not surprising. The SDF-1–CXCR4 chemotaxis mechanism used by adult or neonatal stem cells for homing to the marrow can be knocked out in CXCR4 or SDF-1 $-/-$ mice that die perinatally because of failure of onset of hematopoiesis in the marrow but have extensive hepatic hematopoiesis, suggesting that stem cell trafficking to liver from a site such as yolk sac involves a different homing mechanism (68,69).

Hepatic Hematopoiesis

Four- to 5-week embryos (5- to 6-mm crown-rump length [CRL]) have approximately 2×10^6 cells in the yolk sac, of which 2,000 to 4,000 are BFU-E, CFU-E, and CFU-GM. By 6- to 9-mm CRL, most progenitors disappear from the yolk sac and begin to appear in the liver rudiment by 5 weeks. The first blood cells to appear in the liver are macrophages, followed by erythroid elements. The first morphologically identifiable thrombocytes are present in the fetal circulation at 8 to 9 weeks' gestation, and levels similar to those of adult blood are reached around the 18th week of gestation, whereas morphologically recognizable neutrophils are absent in liver or bone marrow until the 16th week of gestation. Between the 5th and 10th week of gestation, the fetal liver increases in size, with the total number of nucleated cells increasing from 2×10^6 to 1×10^8. The number of BFU-E, CFU-E, and CFU-GM increases up to a plateau of approximately 500 colonies/3×10^5 nucleated cells by 7 weeks.

Early development of erythrocytes occurs in hepatocyte niches, with continuous maturation within the sinusoids or in the blood islands of erythroid cells surrounding a central macrophage. In later stages of development, erythroblasts are randomly interspersed within the liver parenchyma, without a preferential localization among the sinusoids. Production of granulocytes and monocyte-macrophages occurs mostly in the vascular areas of the portal triads, where erythropoiesis and megakaryocytopoiesis are less evident. B lymphopoiesis originates within the mammalian fetal liver, which functions as a primary B-lymphoid organ supporting stem cell to B lymphocyte differentiation. In birds, the fetal liver is not a site of hematopoiesis, and B-lymphocyte development first develops in a specialized primary lymphoid organ, the bursa of Fabricius, that is colonized by immigrant stem cells (66). The spleen, which is a hematopoietic organ in nonhuman mammals, is not a significant site of hematopoiesis in the human fetus.

Definitive Hematopoiesis: Bone Marrow

Before hematopoiesis begins within the fetal bone (<15 weeks' gestation), a process of calcification of the cartilage prototypes of the bones occurs. As calcification proceeds, the central cells in the bone rudiments die, creating spaces that represent the initial marrow cavity. This space is invaded by a periosteal bud, formed by capillaries, osteogenic cells, and mesenchymal cells that contribute to the marrow vasculature, endosteal bone, and mesenchymal fixed tissue elements of the marrow stroma. The prehematopoietic stroma in the medullary spaces of the bone consists of loose connective tissue attached to bone trabeculae with large sinusoids, reticular cells, and morphologically undifferentiated mononuclear cells, including immigrant $CD34^+$ stem cells trafficking from the fetal liver. Early hematopoietic islands composed of a mixtures of differentiating and immature cells start to appear, and by 22 weeks of gestation, marrow hematopoiesis is very active (70).

The bone marrow is characterized by a double vasculature, with the nutrient artery entering the medullary cavity through the nutrient foramen and running parallel to the long axis in the central part of the cavity. The second blood source derives from branches of the periosteal arteries that join with the tributaries of the nutrient artery to form a subendosteal plexus of the capillaries. These capillaries are continuous with the sinusoids that converge to the central sinus and then to the emissary veins that exit the medullary cavity. The sinusoidal endothelial cells play a critical role in egress of leukocytes, platelets. and red cells from the marrow and in the trafficking of stem cells between the marrow and the circulating pool. Like the stromal mesenchymal cells, they are also a source of a variety of cytokines and chemokines that influence every facet of hematopoietic development and function. In the intersinusoidal spaces are alkaline-positive reticular cells that have extensive cytoplasmic extensions that establish intimate contact with processes of other reticular cells and with hematopoietic cells. Reticular cells also support the sinusoidal endothelium, covering a high proportion of the endothelial abluminal surface and, together with the endothelium, forming a blood-marrow barrier that regulates cell migration and possibly diffusion of chemokines and cytokines.

Other components of the marrow stroma include typical fibroblasts that are probably preadipocytes, endosteal cells, and adipocytes. The latter lipid-engorged cells are the main component of the yellow nonhematopoietic marrow. An inverse relationship exists between the number of marrow adipocytes and marrow hematopoietic activity. During periods of hematopoietic stress, marrow adipose cells undergo lipolysis and decrease in number. During periods of decreased hematopoiesis, there is an increase in marrow adipocyte number and lipid content.

Phenotypic characterization of stromal elements of the marrow has been undertaken on primary marrow material (71,72) and on stroma developing in long-term bone marrow culture (73). It has been hypothesized that distinct stromal cells form niches within the marrow microenvironment that selectively regulate stem cell function. This microenvironment is a complex, three-dimensional structure composed of many cell types and abundant extracellular matrix. Many data on the role of the microenvironment have been derived by analysis of the adherent layers of long-term bone marrow cultures, and investigators have established panels of immortalized marrow or fetal liver stromal lines of murine or human origin (74,75). Most such lines share the ability to produce an array of cytokines but differ markedly in their ability to support long-term maintenance of stem cells with *in vivo* repopulating potential, with the latter property retained only by a small minority of lines.

A minor subset of $CD34^+$ cells coexpress epitopes recognized by an anti-stromal antibody STRO-1, and they function as stromal precursors (72). They are also the same population of CFU-F, comprising 1 per 5,000 to 10,000 marrow mononuclear cells that form fibroblast colonies (76). Approximately 40% of CFU-F colonies were further induced to form osteogenic tissue when transplanted *in vivo*, and approximately 15% produced a bone marrow organ containing a full spectrum of stromal types, including bone cells. CFU-F form colonies "spontaneously" in serum-containing cultures, but under serum-free conditions, they are absolutely dependent on an exogenous source of growth factor, particularly a combination of platelet-derived growth factor (PDGF) and epidermal growth factor (EGF). The cytokines interferon-2α (IFN-1α) and IL-4 were found to be potent inhibitors of CFU-F colony formation stimulated by EGF or PDGF.

On direct marrow cytospin, 0.6% of cells express VECAM-1 and low-affinity nerve growth factor receptors (NGFRs) (77). These adventitial reticular cells form spindle cells in culture and in the marrow comprise a network of dendritic $NGFR^+$ cells throughout the marrow and concentrated at the trabecular and vascular margins. These cells are star shaped, with long and convoluted dendritic projections, and branch with each other to form a complex system of lacunae on which hematopoietic cells are arranged, whereas others have an elongated, spindle-like morphology. $NGFR^+$ cells are also positive for alkaline phosphatase, reticulin, collagen type II, and vimentin and appear in fetal marrow before hematopoietic activity begins, originating from the vessel adventitia, and then radiate into the bone marrow cavity (76).

α-Smooth muscle actin (α-SMA)–positive cells comprise a significant proportion of polygonal stromal cells developing in marrow culture, but in marrow biopsies, α-SMA^+ cells are confined to areas of vascular smooth muscle. Human fibrotic marrow stroma contains α-SMA^+ cells that closely resemble myofibroblasts in other fibrotic tissue.

The existence of multipotent mesenchymal stem cells in marrow has been confirmed by the isolation of cells with the potential to differentiate in culture into osteoblasts, chondrocytes, adipocytes, and myoblasts (78). Intriguing data suggest that these cells can contribute to stromal populations in various sites, including marrow and spleen, when intravenously injected into irradiated mice (78). Cytokines whose receptors share the gp130 protein can modulate stromal cell commitment to adipocyte and osteoblast differentiation pathways. IL-6, IL-11, LIF, and oncostatin M (OSM) inhibit hydrocortisone-induced adipocyte differentiation in a dose-dependent manner, and LIF and OSM modulate the steady-state mRNA level of a unique osteoblastic gene marker, osteocalcin (79). Various cytokines, of which IL-1 and tumor necrosis factor (TNF) have been most extensively evaluated, induce production of a spectrum of hematopoietic growth factors by stromal cells (discussed later in more detail in the section on hematopoietic growth factors). In particular, induction of G-CSF, GM-CSF, IL-6, IL-7, IL-11, LIF, and M-CSF by IL-1 or TNF treatment of stroma leads to enhanced proliferation and differentiation of hematopoietic progenitors in coculture. Because the differentiated progeny include macrophages that can secrete IL-1 and TNF, cytokine feedback further modulates the microenvironmental milieu.

Cell adhesion molecules (CAMs) play a major role in mediating interactions between primitive hematopoietic progenitors and various components of the bone marrow stroma. CAMs can be classified into five main groups, including integrin, selectin, immunoglobulin, cadherin, and mucin-like molecular families. Among the mucin-like molecules expressed within the hematopoietic system are the L-selectin ligands CD34, GlyCAM-1, PSGL-1 (CD162), and MAd-

CAM-1 and integrin $\alpha_4\beta_7$. Other members include CD43 (sialophorin), CD45RA, CD68, and tactile (CD96) (80). At least four of these are expressed at high levels on primitive hematopoietic precursors (i.e., CD34, CD43, CD45RA, and CD162). A novel transmembrane isoform of the mucin-like glycoprotein, MGC-24 (CD164), is expressed by progenitor cells and marrow stromal cells, and functional studies have demonstrated its role in adhesion of progenitors to bone marrow stromal cells *in vitro* and suggest that CD164 represents a potent signaling molecule with the capacity to suppress hematopoietic cell proliferation (80).

The VLA-4/VCAM-1, the VLA-5/fibronectin, and the LFA-1/ICAM pathways have also been implicated in adhesive interactions with cultured bone marrow stroma. Anti-VLA-4 (anti-α_4 integrin, anti-CD49d) but not anti-β_2 integrin (anti-CD18) treatment selectively mobilized a wide range of immature hematopoietic progenitors into the bloodstream (up to 200-fold) (45). Both target ligands for VLA-4 (i.e., VCAM-1 and CS-1 region alternatively spliced non–type III connecting segment of human plasma fibrinogen) are constitutively expressed by marrow stroma, and levels of membrane-bound VCAM-1 are upregulated after exposure of stromal cells to IL-1, TNF or IL-4, and antibodies to VLA-4 block myelopoiesis and lymphopoiesis in long-term marrow stromal cultures (81).

Hematopoietic stromal cells produce and are intimately associated with a variety of proteins, proteoglycans, and glycosaminoglycans that comprise the marrow extracellular matrix. Elements of the extracellular matrix include collage, fibronectin, laminin, heparin sulfate, chondroitin sulfate, hemonectin, and hyaluronic acid. The extracellular matrix may influence hematopoiesis in various ways. Matrix elements bind cytokines and chemokines and in doing so may block their activity or enhance activity by stabilization and concentration at sites of hematopoietic cell binding. "Compartmentalized" growth factors may serve to define microenvironmental niches and may act in concert with membrane-bound growth factors to provide a very local form of growth control. Matrix elements can function as ligands for hematopoietic adhesion molecules (81).

ERYTHROPOIESIS

During the course of fetal development, erythropoiesis takes place sequentially in the yolk sac, paraaortic region, liver, and bone marrow. This involves migration of stem cells between these anatomic sites and a shift from primitive megaloblastic erythropoiesis, with embryonic type hemoglobins and nucleated erythrocytes, to definitive monoblastic erythropoiesis, with fetal or adult type hemoglobin.

Erythropoiesis in the yolk sac begins between the 14th and 19th day of gestation and is characterized by expression of hemoglobins Gower-1 ($\zeta_2\epsilon_2$), Portland ($\zeta_2\gamma_2$), and Gower ($\alpha_2\epsilon_2$). At 4 weeks, GATA-1 expression and CD34$^+$ cells appear in the paraaortic region in contact with the endothelium. At 5 weeks of gestation, the number of early erythroid precursors (BFU-E) rapidly decline in the yolk sac, whereas a consistent number of the more mature CFU-E remain. At the same time, BFU-E appear in the circulation, and their numbers increase rapidly in the liver and rapidly increase through the 7th or 8th week of gestation. Primitive megaloblasts increase rapidly in the liver until the 6th to 7th week of gestation and then decline. Definitive erythroblasts continue to increase from the 6th week, until definitive erythropoiesis clearly dominates primitive megaloblastic erythropoiesis (82). Starting at 5 to 6 weeks, stem cells proliferating in the liver gradually develop their differentiation program, and their erythroid progeny undergo parallel switches of morphology (megaloblast to monoblast) and globin synthesis ($\zeta \rightarrow \alpha$ and $\epsilon \rightarrow \gamma$).

The liver remains the major source of erythropoiesis from month 3 through 6, and some hepatic erythropoiesis is still observed at birth. Except for the initial phase of megaloblastic erythropoiesis, the erythroblasts in the liver show normoblastic characteristics, accumulate fetal hemoglobin ($\alpha_2\beta_2$), and give rise to nonnucleated erythrocytes. Erythropoiesis in the bone marrow initiates in the fifth month of gestation and becomes predominant in the last 3 months of gestation.

The sum of the erythropoietic cells and mature erythrocytes is called the *erythron*. As with other lineages, the erythron is composed of morphologically unrecognizable precursor cells and maturing cells. The total volume of the erythron is approximately 100 mL (4×10^{12} cells) and releases 25 mL (2×10^{11} cells) of erythrocytes daily to maintain a circulating pool of approximately 2 to 5×10^{12} erythrocytes, with a half-life of 90 days (83).

The stochastic generation of early erythroid progenitors (BFU-E) from pluripotent progenitors and stem cells occurs in the presence of the early-acting cytokine KIT ligand, together with additional factors such as IL-3 and GM-CSF, and it is erythropoietin independent. The differentiation of BFU-E to CFU-E is erythropoietin dependent, but in the adult, it requires the synergy of erythropoietin with IL-3, GM-CSF, IL-9, or KIT ligand. In fetal life, BFU-E can develop with erythropoietin alone, indicating an independence from a source of synergistic activity or an increased sensitivity allowing response to low levels of factors produced by accessory cells or present in the serum component of the culture medium. The final erythroid maturation from the CFU-E, which is closely related to the proerythroblast, occurs in the presence of erythropoietin alone. The erythroid "burst" that develops in 14 days in semisolid culture from a BFU-E exhibits a characteristic pattern of 3 to 20 multiple, separate erythroid colonies, each composed of 64 to 128 maturing erythroid cells. Each of these subcolonies represents a CFU-E that undergoes five to six divisions over 5 to 7 days before terminal maturation. In the absence of erythropoietin, CFU-E undergo rapid apoptosis *in vivo* or *in vitro*; in the absence of KIT ligand or IL-3/GM-CSF, BFU-E also undergo apoptosis and cannot be maintained by erythropoietin alone. Regulation of erythropoiesis is based on its production by renal cortical cells under the control of an oxygen sensor mechanism (84). Extrarenal sources of erythropoietin include the liver, which can contribute less than 10% of total erythropoietin requirements, requiring treatment with recombinant erythropoietin, as in anephric patients on renal dialysis.

The proerythroblasts or pronormoblasts become recognizable when the primitive erythroid cells initiate ribosome assembly and hemoglobin synthesis. The pronormoblast is a round or slightly oval cell with a diameter of 12 to 20 μm, a large nucleus with fine chromatin and one or more nuclei, scarce cytoplasm that stains deep blue, and often a visible Golgi apparatus. Proerythroblasts undergo a series of three or four divisions while cytoplasmic maturation progresses. With a generation time of 12 hours, the proerythroblasts give rise to two daughter cells, basophilic erythroblasts, which are smaller than proerythroblasts and range in size from 10 to 18 μm. These cells have a lower nuclear to cytoplasmic ratio, a strongly basophilic cytoplasm, and a rather coarse chromatin pattern with condensed masses near the nuclear membrane. The transit time of the basophilic erythroblasts is 20 hours, almost twice that of the proerythroblasts, and there are therefore approximately four times more basophilic erythroblasts than proerythroblasts in the bone marrow. Basophilic erythroblasts mature, accumulate more RNA and hemoglobin, and divide to form polychromatic erythroblasts. These are much smaller cells (diameter of 10 to 15 μm) with lower nuclear to cytoplasmic ratio, coarse chromatin pattern, and cytoplasm that exhibits polychromatophilic staining because of the accumulation of RNA and hemoglobin. This is the last stage able to undergo mitosis; however, hemoglobin acts as a regulator of cell division, and an increase in the mean cellular hemoglobin concentration (MCHC) may prevent mitosis, whereas a decrease in MCHC may induce an additional mitosis with formation of microcytic and hypochromic erythrocytes.

The polychromatophilic erythroblast divides after a transit time of 30 hours, forming two orthochromatic (or late polychromatophilic) erythroblasts. These nondividing cells have a diameter of 10 to 12 μm, a small nucleus with heavy condensed chromatin, and acidophilic cytoplasm, similar to that of mature erythrocytes, because of the accumulation of hemoglobin. The maturation time from orthochromatic erythroblast to erythrocyte is approximately 48 hours. The inactive nuclear chromatin is condensed and moved to one side of the cell. Actin filaments, which during erythroid differentiation move from a cytoplasmic localization to become associated with spectrin and other proteins of the membrane skeleton, form a contractile ring at the base of the eccentrically located nucleus, determining a membrane constriction that results in enucleation (85). The condensed pyknotic nucleus is extruded through the erythroblast membrane together with part of the membrane and a thin layer of cytoplasm containing 5% to 10% of the synthesized hemoglobin. The extruded nucleus is then engulfed and digested by neighboring macrophages. After extrusion of the nucleus, the cells are called reticulocytes. The remaining mitochondria and ribosomes that cluster together and are stained by basophilic dyes, giving these cells the morphologic appearance responsible for their name.

Reticulocytes reside in the marrow for 2 days and then are released into the bloodstream. The release of the reticulocytes from the marrow coincides with decrease or loss of membrane adhesion molecules, including receptors for fibronectin (86). Reticulocytes continue hemoglobin synthesis for several days after being released. The total hemoglobin produced in this period represents 10% to 30% of the total content of the erythrocytes. When mitochondria and ribosomes dissociate and disappear, the reticulocyte transforms into mature erythrocytes. Imperfect reticulocytes are detained and lysed in the bone marrow. Those that escape this selection undergo a second selection in the spleen, where they are lysed or, in some cases, repaired by removal of remaining nuclei or nuclear fragments.

Several changes occur in the expression of surface molecules during the maturation of erythroid cells. Class I human leukocyte antigen (HLA) molecules are expressed on progenitor cells and are lost only during late differentiation, whereas class II HLA molecules are expressed only on progenitor cells. Blood group antigens A, B, H, Rh (D), and I are present on erythroblasts and mature erythrocytes. Glycophorin A, a major 55-kd transmembrane glycoprotein of erythrocytes, appears in erythroblasts at the time of initiation of hemoglobin synthesis and is absent from proerythroblasts. Major changes in the membrane components during erythropoietic cell differentiation result from the formation of the erythroid membrane skeleton, of which the heterodimeric protein spectrin, cross-linked by actin, is the principal component (85). CD34 and CD38 antigens are present on erythroid progenitor cells and are lost during differentiation. The transferrin receptor (CD71 antigen) is expressed from the progenitor cell to the reticulocyte stage, until hemoglobin synthesis ceases. The receptor for erythropoietin is present on BFU-E and CFU-E, and its expression decreases on more mature erythroid cells.

GRANULOCYTE-MACROPHAGE PRODUCTION

Granulocytes and mononuclear phagocytes (i.e., monocyte-macrophages) originate from a common progenitor, the CFU-GM, comprising 0.1% to 0.2% of the nucleated bone marrow cell population. Stochastic mechanisms result in the generation of progeny restricted to eosinophils or neutrophil pathways or to a pathway through a $CD14^+$ intermediate to monocytes, macrophages, myeloid dendritic cells, or osteoclasts. GM-CSF and IL-3 can support differentiation into all lineages, whereas G-CSF promotes exclusively neutrophil differentiation, M-CSF promotes monocyte-macrophage differentiation, and IL-5 promotes eosinophil differentiation. Dendritic cell differentiation is promoted by a combination of GM-CSF and TNF-α or IL-4.

Neutrophil Granulocytes

Neutrophils first appear in fetal life at the beginning of the second trimester, although their progenitors (CFU-GM) are detectable at the very earliest stages of hematopoietic development (4 weeks). In the adult, mature neutrophils have a half-life of 6 hours, and on the order of 10^{11} are generated each day. To sustain this remarkable steady-state production, a flux of precursors into the myeloblast pool of approximately 0.4×10^7 cells/kg/hour is required (87). The myeloblast has a diameter of 15 to 18 μm and a large, slightly oblong nucleus with fine granular chromatin and two or more pale nucleoli, eccentrically surrounded by narrow rims of deep blue cytoplasm with conventional staining. A clear perinuclear zone is lacking, and small granules are usually present. These myeloblasts divide on average every 16 hours, and the appearance of primary granules indicates maturation to the promyelocyte stage. Promyelocytes are up to 20 μm in diameter and have copious amounts of cytoplasm that stains blue and shows a marked Golgi apparatus. The nucleus is eccentrically located, with somewhat granular chromatin and fading nucleoli, and the cytoplasm contains 0.8-μm-diameter primary granules loaded with lysosomal enzymes, including myeloperoxidase, acid phosphatase, elastase, cathepsins, arylsulfatase, and lysozyme.

With promyelocyte maturation, the primary granules increase to several dozen, ultimately overlying the nucleus. A promyelocyte division occurs on average at 20 hours (87). After cessation of primary granule synthesis, transition to neutrophilic myelocytes occurs. Myelocytes are the last myeloid precursors capable of cell division, and they divide twice, with a cycle of 54 hours each division. Amplification within this myeloid lineage with increased mature neutrophil output can be produced by increasing G-CSF stimulation, shortening of the transit time and increasing cell doublings within the myelocyte compartments. Myelocytes undergo maturation with acquisition of specific secondary granules of 0.5 μm diameter, resulting in the characteristic pale pink cytoplasmic staining of these cells. The nucleus is pushed to one side and partly flattened, with coarse and clumped nuclear chromatin. The specific secondary granules lack peroxidase and are rich in lysozyme, collagenase, plasminogen activator, aminopeptidase, vitamin B_{12}–binding protein, and lactoferrin. Alkaline phosphatase is expressed in a smaller subpopulation of specific granules.

A minimum of 3 hours is required for myelocytes to mature to metamyelocytes of 14 to 16 μm diameter, and they are characterized by an indented, kidney-shaped nucleus with clumped chromatin, eccentrically embedded in finely granular, pink cytoplasm with abundant secondary granules. Metamyelocytes mature in about 30 hours to band or stab forms of 13 μm diameter with a horseshoe-shaped nucleus and clumps of chromatin and, in some cases, the beginning of nuclear segmentation. Band cells mature to polymorphonuclear neutrophils (PMNs) in approximately 50 hours. The PMN nucleus is segmented into two to five lobes, and the fine predominantly secondary granules stain the cytoplasm faint pink. Various CD antigens can be used to characterize the different stages of differentiation from the earliest progenitor through to the mature neutrophil (Fig. 1.2).

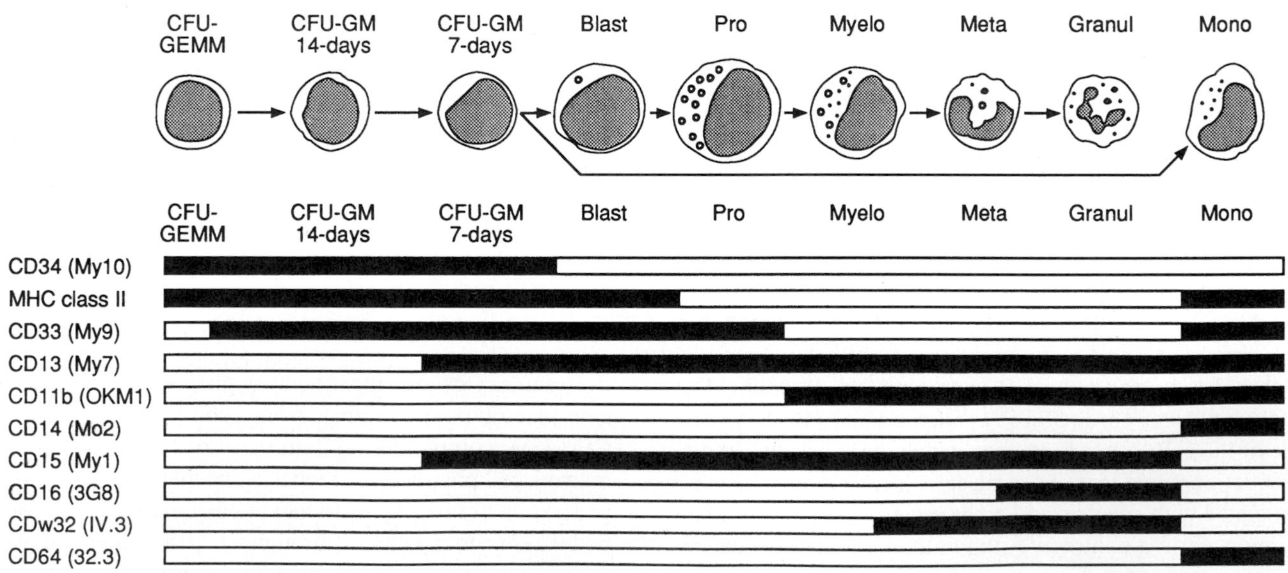

FIG. 1.2 Expression of differentiation markers during neutrophil or monocyte differentiation. The various surface antigens are indicated by the cluster of differentiation (CD) number, followed in parentheses by a representative antibody recognizing the antigen. The black bars indicate the stage of differentiation at which the antigens are expressed. CFU-GEMM, colony-forming units–erythrocyte, granulocyte, macrophage, and megakaryocyte; CFU-GM, colony-forming units–granulocyte-macrophage; Blast, myeloblast; Pro, promyelocyte; Myelo, myelocyte; Meta, metamyelocyte; Granul, granulocyte; Mono, monocyte.

Mature neutrophils may reside in the marrow for 2 to 3 days before being released, and this large pool, called the neutrophil reserve, is immediately available for mobilization in response to inflammatory signals and is responsible for the early neutrophilia in infections. The rapid emargination of neutrophils seen in inflammation is facilitated by dilation of postcapillary venules and increased vascular permeability. Mobilization of the marrow neutrophil reserve is rapidly followed by increased marrow granulopoiesis. This may be caused by removal of a negative feedback mediated by mature cells or removal from marrow of a large ''sink'' of mature neutrophils capable of receptor binding and internalizing G-CSF, freeing G-CSF for progenitor stimulation. Under conditions of increased neutrophil demand, the emergence time of neutrophils from the bone marrow can be reduced from 6 days to 48 hours.

The mature neutrophil life span in the circulation is influenced by cytokines, such as GM-CSF, which prolongs neutrophil survival and acts as a neutrophil migration inhibitory factor, suppressing neutrophil egress from the circulation. The expression of the chemokine receptors CXCR1 and CXCR2 on neutrophils is responsible for their chemotactic migration to sites of inflammation and infection in response to chemokines such as IL-8, granulopcyte chemoattractant protein-2 (GCP-2), and growth-related oncogene (GRO). The functional activation of neutrophils by cytokines and chemokines is discussed further in later sections.

Eosinophilic Granulocytes

Production of eosinophils from pluripotent CFU-GM or oligopotent CFU-GM involves the concatenate action of IL-3 or GM-CSF and IL-5 (88). Although IL-3 or GM-CSF can generate eosinophil and eosinophil-mixed colonies, IL-5 is the prime regulator of eosinopoiesis. Eosinophils cannot be distinguished from other granulocyte precursors before the promyelocyte stage at which point they can be distinguished by their abundant large peroxidase-positive specific granules. Mature eosinophils are characterized by a nucleus with two or three nuclear lobes. The granules are in the shape of biconcave disks that are 1.0 μm across and 0.6 μm thick, containing a lamellated crystalloid core encapsulated by a less dense matrix. The core contains phospholipids, melanin, and basic proteins rich in arginine and lysine that bind to acidic macromolecules, including heparin, and produce a strong eosin stain. The matrix contains peroxidase, arylsulfatase, and other hydrolytic enzymes. The mature eosinophil expresses different types of complement receptors: Fcγ receptors (CD16 and CD32) and Fcϵ receptors. Eosinophils, like neutrophils, have phagocytic and cytotoxic activity and have NADPH-dependent oxidase and respiratory burst capabilities.

Eosinophils remain in the circulation for only a short time, and one half migrate to the tissues in their first circulation. The chemokine receptor CCR3, expressed on eosinophils, and the chemokine eotaxin mediate eosinophil chemotaxis and eosinophil localization at sites of eotaxin production, such as asthmatic lungs or allergic infiltrates.

Basophilic Granulocytes and Mast Cells

Basophils are rare myeloid cells, representing only 0.1% of nucleated blood cells and 0.3% of marrow cells. They originate from progenitors different from the CFU-GM and can be found among the progeny of CFU-GEMM, and a bipotential eosinophil-basophil CFU has been reported (89). IL-3 and KIT ligand induce the formation of basophil colonies. Mature adult basophils are characterized by numerous large metachromatic, purple-black–stained granules. The specific basophil granules are first formed at the myelocyte stage, continue to be produced during maturation, and persist in mature cells. The granules have a diameter of 0.4 to 0.8 μm, have a round or oblong shape, and are surrounded by a membrane. They contain heparin, histamine, lipids, and proteoglycans, but they are devoid of hydrolytic enzymes, and the presence of peroxidase is controversial. Basophils do not express many of the antigens characteristic of neutrophils and monocytes, but they express the Fcγ receptor CD32 and the high-affinity Fcϵ receptor.

Tissue mast cells share a number of features in common with basophils and are derived from a bone marrow precursor, generally not through a basophil intermediate stage. Mast cell development, including sustained proliferation of relatively mature mast cells, depends on KIT ligand, also known as mast cell growth factor. Profound defects in the development of mast cells, including tissue mast cells, are seen in mice with mutations involving KIT ligand or its receptor KIT. Additional factors capable of stimulating mast cell proliferation and differentiation include IL-3 and IL-4, and these cytokines synergize with KIT ligand.

Monocytes and Macrophages

Bone marrow monocyte precursors, circulating monocytes, fixed tissue macrophages (e.g., Kupffer cells of the liver), and osteoclasts form the *mononuclear phagocyte system,* a term that replaced the earlier *reticuloendothelial system.* These cells ultimately arise from marrow bipotential CFU-GM progenitors on stimulation by GM-CSF, IL-3, or M-CSF. Monoblasts are the first recognizable cell type in the differentiation of monocytes and macrophages, although the most immature forms are difficult to distinguish from myeloblasts. These cells are medium-size blasts (16 μm diameter), with deep blue cytoplasm on Wright-Giemsa staining and a large, eccentric, and indented nucleus with one or two large nucleoli. Maturation of promonoblast/CFU-GM to monocytes requires at least three successive divisions, with a transit time of approximately 54 hours. The progeny of monoblasts are promonocytes, large (16 to 18 μm diameter), with blue cytoplasm, a few neutral red-staining structures near the nuclear indentation, an irregular cell margin, peroxidase-positive granules, and limited phagocytic and locomotive function.

Promonocytes undergo two divisions before maturing to monocytes. Because there is no significant reserve of monocytes in the bone marrow, these cells are rare and difficult to identify without histochemical staining (i.e., peroxidase, fluoride-sensitive nonspecific esterase) or monoclonal antibody staining ($CD14^+$). Monocytes are the largest blood cell (15 to 18 μm diameter), with abundant, gray-blue cytoplasm containing many granules and vacuoles and a bulky nucleus with a variably indented, reniform, or lobular shape. Monocyte functions include active migration and chemotaxis, phagocytosis, NADPH-dependent oxidase and respiratory burst capability, bactericidal activity, and cytotoxicity, including antibody-dependent cell-mediated cytotoxicity (ADCC). On activation by GM-CSF and M-CSF or by TNF and interferon-γ (IFN-γ), with or without endotoxin stimulation, these functional activities are activated, and a spectrum of chemokines and cytokines are secreted that mediate host defense and participate in the inflammatory process (see section on cytokines and chemokines).

Young monocytes enter the circulation when incompletely differentiated, persist in the peripheral blood with a half-life of 3 days, and then migrate into tissues where they mature into tissue macrophages, with some capacity for proliferation under the control of M-CSF. Marker studies in allogeneic marrow transplant patients indicate that tissue macrophages are replaced within 3 months. Monocytes can also differentiate into dendritic cells (DCs).

Dendritic Cells and Langerhans Cells

DCs are irregularly shaped and have numerous cell membrane processes, including spiny dendrites, bulbous pseudopods, and lamellipodia or veils. The mature DCs lack phagocytic capacity and are nonadherent. They express high levels of class II MHC molecules and CD40, CD83, and CD1a but lack the monocyte-macrophage marker CD14 (90,91). These cells are professional antigen presenters, stimulating primary T-cell responses and the autologous mixed lymphocyte reaction, which probably is related to the primary response to exogenous antigen. DCs have a heterogeneous lineage and can arise from lymphoid or myeloid precursors. $CD34^+$ precursors in normal marrow generate dendritic colonies when stimulated with GM-CSF and TNF. Large numbers of functionally mature DCs can also be generated over 12 to 14 days in suspension cultures of $CD34^+$ cells with these same cytokines, and absolute recovery is enhanced by addition of KIT or FLT-3 ligands (probably by expanding production of CFU-GM progenitors) (92). Development of DCs in this system occurs through an intermediate $CD14^+$, HLA-DR^+, and FMS (i.e., M-CSF receptor)–positive cell that lacks myeloperoxidase and nonspecific esterase. These cells possess substantial phagocytic capacity and are bipotential, generating typical adherent $CD14^+$ phagocytic macrophages in the presence of M-CSF and of $CD14^-$, FMS^-, $CD1a^+$, $CD83^+$, HLA-DR^+ DCs in the presence of GM-CSF and TNF (93).

Blood monocytes also differentiate into DCs without proliferation, and in the presence of GM-CSF, this pathway is reversible, but exposure to proinflammatory cytokines such as TNF induces an apparently irreversible maturation to DCs with downmodulation of FMS (90,91). GM-CSF TNF, and IL-4 are widely used to induce DC development from blood monocytes. $CD40^-$–CD40 ligand interactions play a central role in antigen presentation and T-cell–dependent effector function, and CD40 ligation alone promotes differentiation of monocytes into functional DCs in the absence of GM-CSF or IL-4 (94). Physiologic conditions inducing monocyte differentiation to DCs include a combination of phagocytosis and transendothelial migration. In one *in vitro* model, monocytes first cross a layer of endothelial cells and lodge in an underlying collagen matrix, mimicking entry of monocytes into tissues from the circulation (95). A proportion of these cells then "reverse transmigrate" and become DCs, mimicking migration of DCs out of tissues into the lymphatics. The cells that remain in the collagen "tissue" become macrophages. The phagocytosis process provides a strong stimulus for DC maturation, and the endothelium may be a source of GM-CSF and proinflammatory cytokines.

The Langerhans cells (LC) of the skin provide a clear model of the life history of DCs. These cells develop from myeloid precursors, probably $CD34^+$ cells expressing homing cutaneous lymphocyte-associated antigen, that move through the circulation and enter the epidermis. LCs express high levels of MHC class II molecules but differ from mature DCs in expressing Fc receptors, expressing CD1a, and in possessing Birbeck granules and the associated LAG antigen (96,97). At this stage, the cells are poor T-cell activators but are capable of phagocytosis, receptor-mediated endocytosis, and antigen processing. After a variable period of sentry duty in the skin, they leave, bearing samples of antigen from the local environment, moving through the afferent lymph as "veiled" cells, and entering the draining lymph node to become mature DCs. They have lost phagocytic capacity at this stage but have acquired the capacity to present antigen and stimulate T cells. This change is associated with a drop in FcγIIR, CD1a, and Birbeck granules and increase in class II MHC, B7-2, and CD40 expression.

A thymic origin for DCs has been established in which early thymic precursors in the presence of TNF and IL-1, together with IL-3, IL-7, KIT ligand, FLT-3 ligand, and CD40 ligand (but not GM-CSF), generate functional DCs coexpressing DC markers and several markers normally associated with lymphoid cells, including CD8α, CD2, and CD25 (97). The evidence for a lymphoid-related population of DCs in humans is less compelling, and human DCs, even in the thymus, do not express CD8α, although they do express CD4. Murine pro-B lymphocytes expressing CD19 can also be induced by IL-1, IL-7, IL-3, TNF, FLT-3 ligand, and KIT ligand to develop into DCs with T-cell stimulatory properties and with DC markers CD11c, DEC205, CD80, CD86, and high-density MHC class II molecules (98).

Osteoclasts

Morphogenesis and remodeling of bone involves the synthesis of bone matrix by osteoblasts and coordinated resorption of bone by osteoclasts. Osteoblasts arise from mesenchymal stem cells and osteoclasts differentiate from hematopoietic monocyte-macrophage precursors. $CD14^+$ adherent human monocytes differentiate into tartrate-resistant acid phosphatase (TRAP)–positive, osteoclast-like multinucleate giant cells in the presence of GM-CSF and IL-4 (99). Increased osteoclast activity is seen in many osteopenic disorders, including postmenopausal osteoporosis, and increased osteoclastic activity leads to increased bone resorption and crippling bone damage. Mice with mutations of M-CSF (CSF-1) have osteopetrosis and exhibit arrest of osteoclastogenesis at the preosteoclast stage. Several factors influence osteoclastogenesis at different stages, including M-CSF, IL-1, TGF-β, TGF-α, TNF-α, IL-6 IL-11, calcitonin, vitamin D_3, and parathyroid hormone.

A new TNF family molecule, osteprotegerin (OPGL), also known as osteoclast differentiation factor, can activate mature osteoclasts and mediate osteoclastogenesis in the presence of M-CSF (100,101). OPGL is produced by osteoblasts, stromal cells, and activated T cells, and it signals through a TNF-receptor family member, RANK, which is expressed on DCs, T cells, and hematopoietic precursors. OPGL is an osteoclast differentiation factor and a regulator of interaction of T cells and DCs. Mice with a disrupted *opgl* gene show severe osteopetrosis and a defect in tooth eruption, and they completely lack osteoclasts as a result of an inability of osteoblasts to support osteoclastogenesis (101). Although DCs appear normal the deficient mice exhibit defects in early differentiation of T and B lymphocytes. OPGL appears necessary for the progression of $CD25^+CD44^-$ precursors to $CD25^-CD44^-$ thymocytes at the stage of pre-T-cell receptor (pTCR) expression. It appears also to be necessary for the maturation of pro-B cells to pre-B cells. The mice also lack all lymph nodes but have normal splenic structure and Peyer's patches. OPGL is a regulator of lymph node organogenesis and lymphocyte development and is essential for osteoclast differentiation *in vivo*.

MEGAKARYOCYTOPOIESIS

Regulation of human megakaryocytopoiesis and platelet production is a complex process that consists of two distinct stages or compartments: a dividing compartment and a compartment of nondividing cells that increase their size by polyploidization or nuclear endoreduplication and ultimately fragment into platelets. Morphologically, three stages of maturation are distinguished. Stage I (i.e., megakaryoblast) is a 15- to 20-μm cell with an oval, indented nucleus and basophilic cytoplasm because of abundant ribosomes. Stage II (i.e., promegakaryocyte) is a 20- to 80-μm cell, is less basophilic, and has developing granules. Stage III (i.e., megakaryocyte), has a diameter of 20 to 150 μm and a more acidophilic cytoplasm. Almost all cells at stage I have a 4N DNA content, whereas most cells in stage III are 32N or even 64N.

The time from diploid precursor to complete polyploidization is at least 5 days. Megakaryocytes develop from $CD34^+$ pluripotent stem cells through a primitive megakaryocyte progenitor (burst forming unit–megakaryocyte [BFU-MK]) and a more differentiated megakaryocyte progenitor (colony forming unit–megakaryocyte [CFU-MK]) that also express CD34 antigen. The expression of platelet proteins, especially glycoprotein IIb/IIIa (CD41a), occurs at an early stage of the megakaryocyte lineage and precedes polyploidization (102,103). Factor VIII antigen, factor V, and β-thromboglobulin are present from the megakaryoblast stage. Megakaryocytes and platelets also express the Fcγ receptor CD32 and the thrombopoietin receptor MPL. Immunofluorescence and ultrastructural studies reveal a population of immature blastic megakaryocytes expressing GPIIIa subdivided into $CD34^+$, in which α granules are rare, and $CD34^-$, in which α granules are more developed and demarcation membranes are exhibited. Proliferation and polyploidization capacity is higher in the $CD34^+$ GPIIIa subset, and 10% of these cells can give rise to megakaryocyte colonies containing a maximum of 16 cells (102). GPIb is expressed on sixfold fewer cells than GPIIIa but can be detected on a few $CD34^+$ cells. Overall, less than 2% of marrow $CD34^+$ cells express GP and CD34 expression is related to the capacity of megakaryocyte precursors to accomplish DNA synthesis (cell division or endomitosis).

The process of megakaryocytopoiesis and platelet production is regulated by numerous cytokines, of which thrombopoietin is the most significant. The extent to which the mechanisms of proliferation or of endoreduplication are independently regulated or are interdependent is still debated. Thrombopoietin regulates megakaryocyte proliferation, maturation, and endoreduplication, and it induces platelet production *in vitro* (104,105). Whether platelet production *in vivo* is mediated by thrombopoietin alone or in combination with other factors is unknown. It has been shown that NF-E2 (a hematopoietic specific transcription factor of erythroid cells and megakaryocytes) knockout mice, despite physiologic levels of thrombopoietin and increased numbers of megakaryocytes, have a profound reduction in platelet count, implying that the final stages of platelet formation and release may be regulated by as yet undefined cellular signaling pathways (106). Bone marrow stromal cells have been shown to inhibit platelet release, suggesting that megakaryocytes may have to exit the marrow microenvironment to release platelets (107).

Megakaryocytopoiesis occurs in the adult predominantly in the extravascular compartment of the bone marrow, with mature megakaryocytes appearing in proximity to bone marrow sinusoidal endothelial cells. Adherence of megakaryocytes to marrow stromal cell extracellular matrix induces extension of pseudopodia and final fragmentation into platelet-like particles (108). Megakaryocytes express certain adhesion molecules that enable them to interact with resting and activated endothelium. Electron microscopic analysis of marrow biopsies shows that megakaryocytes residing on the subluminal surface of the endothelial cells are capable of transmigrating through the endothelial junctions (109,110). Several studies suggest that megakaryocytes generated in the marrow also have the capacity to egress as whole cells and travel to the lungs, where they fragment into platelets (111).

The spleen and liver may also play a role in extramedullary platelet production. The extent to which extramedullary platelet production contributes to overall thrombocytosis is controversial. In rodent studies, even during periods of intense stimulation of thrombopoiesis, megakaryocytes, including naked nuclei or large cytoplasmic fragments, were rare in liver and lung tissue while greatly increased in marrow and spleen, and they increased in the former tissues after splenectomy or marrow ablation by strontium 90 treatment (112).

There is an active search for factors regulating transmigration of megakaryocytes or their pseudopods and platelet release into the marrow sinusoids. One mechanism involves expression of the G-protein–coupled chemokine receptor CXCR4 on mature polyploid megakaryocytes (113). The ligand for CXCR4, SDF-1, mediates transendothelial chemotaxis of mature megakaryocytes and activation of endothelium by IL-1, increasing SDF-1–induced megakaryocyte migration threefold (113) (Fig. 1.3). Neutralizing antibodies to the endothelial-specific adhesion molecule, E-selectin, blocked transendothelial migration of megakaryocytes, suggesting that cellular interactions of megakaryocytes with marrow endothelium is critical for migration. At the end of platelet release, senescent megakaryocytes may consist of a large nucleus enveloped by a thin layer of cytoplasm, and this state has been referred to as denuded megakaryocyte (DMK). Usually, marrow biopsies from normal individuals contain only very small numbers of DMKs; however, they are a common feature in various pathologic conditions influencing the megakaryocyte lineage, such as human immunodeficiency virus type 1 (HIV-1) disease or chronic myeloproliferative disorders (114). Macrophages are frequently located in the vicinity of degenerating megakaryocytes and extend processes that partially or completely engulf the dying cells (115).

Apoptosis may represent a physiologic event for end-stage megakaryocytes, and a peculiarity of apoptosis in these cells seems to be that it mainly involves the cell nucleus and a short rim of cytoplasm surrounding the nucleus (114). Identification of apoptotic megakaryocytes in normal marrow biopsies is difficult because of the speed of the apoptotic process and the presence in the marrow of resident marrow

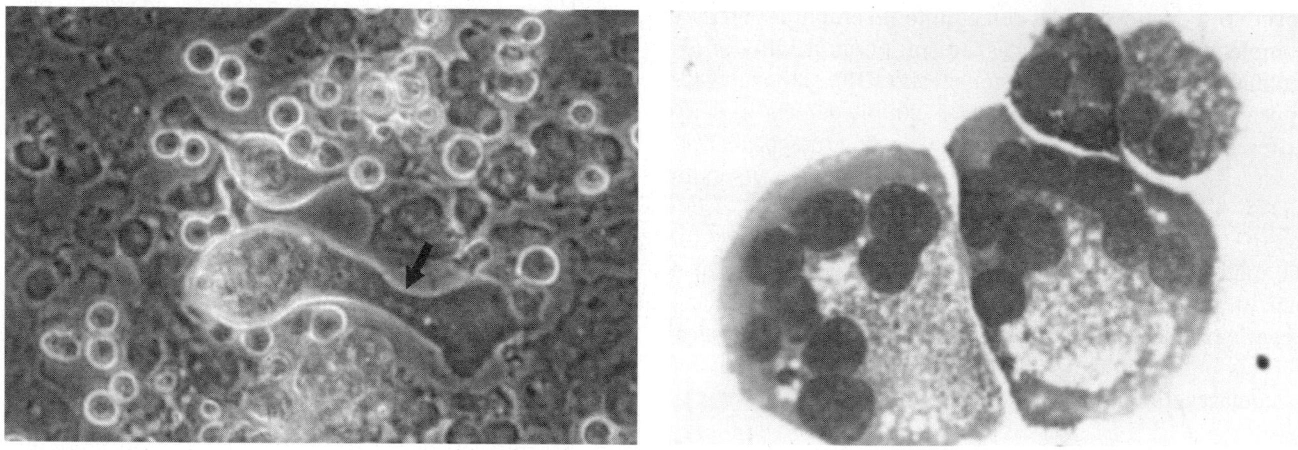

A B

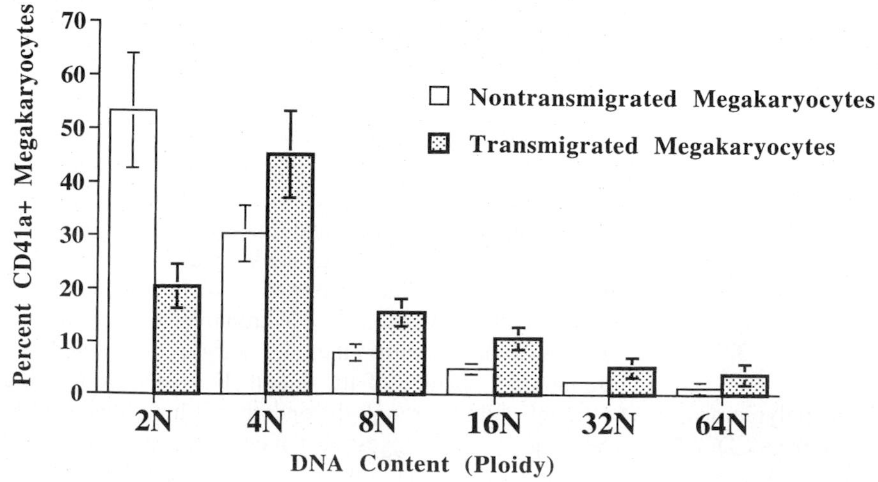

C

FIG. 1.3 Ploidy analysis of migrated megakaryocytes. **A:** Attachment of megakaryocytes to bone marrow endothelial cells (BMEC), results in profound morphologic changes, including a unilateral pseudopod formation *(arrow)*. **B:** Light microscopy of Wright-Giemsa–stained, transmigrated megakaryocytes in response to SDF-1 (200 ng/mL) demonstrated a predominance of polyploid megakaryocytes. **C:** Ploidy analysis of migrated megakaryocytes in response to SDF-1 demonstrated a predominance of polyploid megakaryocytes (n = 4, $p <$ 0.05 for 4, 18, 16, and 32 N). (Adapted from Hamada T, Mohle R, Hesselgesser J. Transendothelial migration of megakaryocytes in response to stromal cell–derived factor 1 (SDF-1) enhances platelet formation. *J Exp Med* 1998; 188:539–548., with permiossion.)

macrophages that clear apoptotic bodies very rapidly. *In vitro* studies showed that thrombopoietin, but not IL-3 or erythropoietin, showed some protection of megakaryocytes from apoptosis at early culture times but had no significant effect at later times (114). This suggests that the terminal phase of the megakaryocyte life span is characterized by the onset of apoptosis, which can be modulated only to a certain extent by thrombopoietin. Normal bone marrow contains 6 $\times 10^6$ megakaryocytes/kg body weight, and each megakaryocyte releases a thousand platelets (116). The role of thrombopoietin in regulation of platelet production is reviewed in the section on cytokines in this chapter.

CYTOKINES AFFECTING HEMATOPOIESIS

A complex family of cytokines with pleiotropic and frequently overlapping activity orchestrates the process of steady-state lymphohematopoiesis and acute responses involving specific cell lineages (Fig. 1.4). For historical reasons, hematopoietic growth factors have been named after

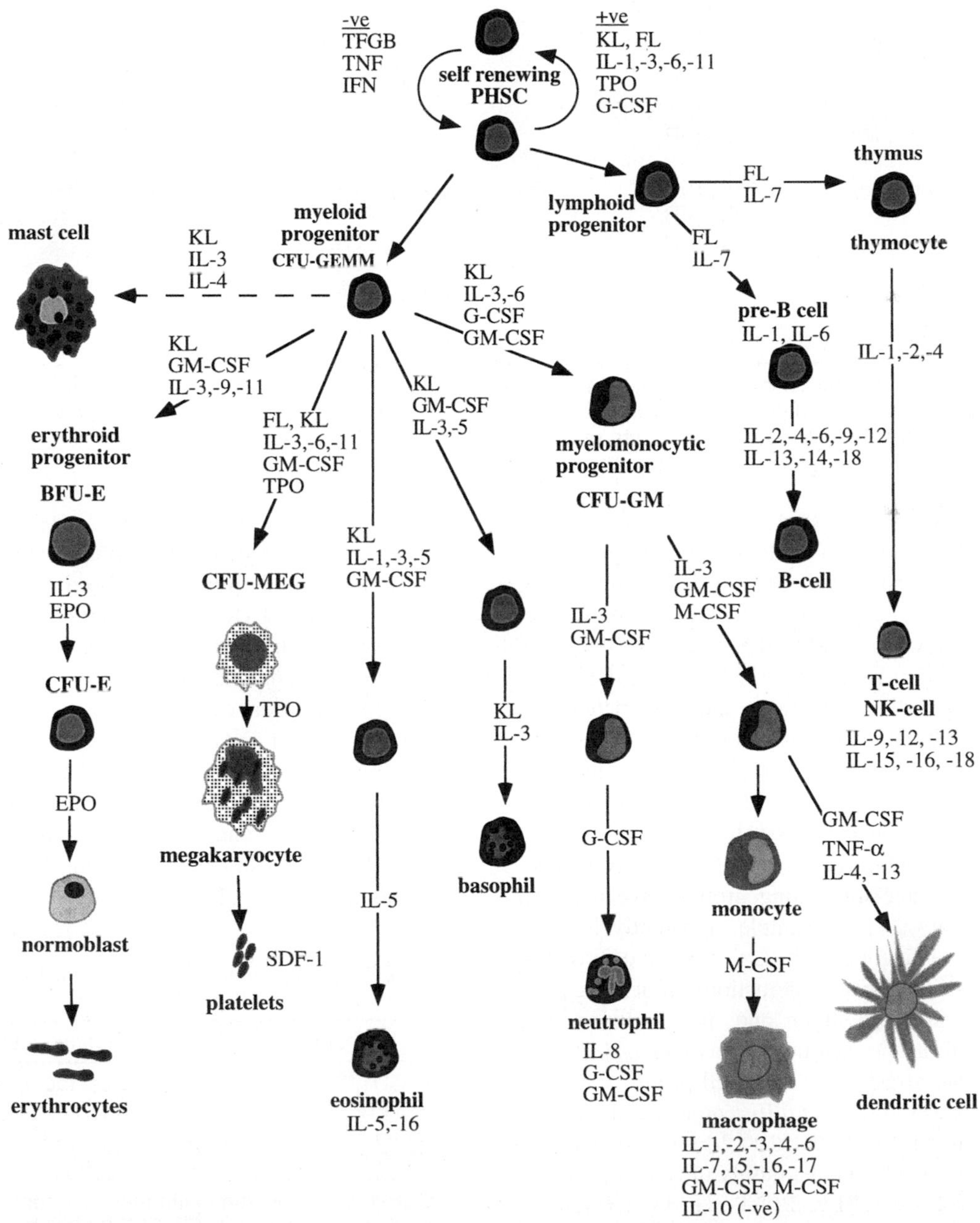

FIG. 1.4 Hematopoiesis and activity of cytokines within the lymphohematopoietic system. Factors are shown where they have primary or synergistic roles at specific stages of differentiation, influencing proliferation and differentiation. At some points, such as for the macrophage, cytokines are shown that affect the function of the mature cell.

TABLE 1.2. *Cytokines, source, receptors, and signal transducers*

Cytokine	Source	Receptor	Common receptor	JAK	STAT
G-CSF	M, F, E	G-CSFR		1, 2	5
GM-CSF	T, M, F, E	GM-CSFRα	β-common	1, 2	5
M-CSF	M, F, E FMS				
Epo	K, L	EpoR		2	5
Tpo	L, E	MPL		2	?
IL-1α, -β	M, E, F, B, T	IL-1R			
IL-2	T	IL-2Rα	IL-2Rγ, IL-2Rβ	1, 3	5
IL-3	T, NK	IL-3Rα	β-common	1, 2	5
IL-4	T	IL-4Rα	IL-2Rγ, IL-13Rα	1, 3	6
IL-5	T	IL-5Rα	β-common	1, 2	5
IL-6	M, E, F, B	IL-6R	gp130	1, 2, TYK-2	1, 3
IL-7	F	IL-7Rα	IL-2Rγ	1, 3	?
IL-8	M, E	CXCR1, 2			
IL-9	T	IL-9Rα	IL-2Rγ	1, 3	?
IL-10	T, B, M	IL-10R		?	?
IL-11	F, E	IL-11Rα	gp130	2	1, 3
IL-12	M, Ma, DC	IL-12p40, IL-12Rβ		2, TYK-2	4
IL-13	T, NK, Ma	IL-13Rα	IL-4Rα, IL-13Rγ	?	6
IL-14	B	?	?	?	?
IL-15	M, K, L	IL-15Rα	IL-2Rγ, IL-2Rβ	1, 3	?
IL-16	T	IL-16R			
IL-17	T	IL-17R			
IL-18	M, K, L, DC	IL-18R			
LIF	M, T, F, E, L	?	gp130, LIFR-1, -2, TYK-2	1, 3	
KL	F, E	KIT			
FL	F, E	FLK-2/FLT-3			

E, endothelium; F, fibroblast/mesenchymal cells; M, monocyte/macrophage; T, T lymphocyte; B, B lymphocyte; K, kidney; L, liver; NK, natural killer; DC, dendritic cell; Ma, mast cell; IL, interleukin; CSF, colony-stimulating factor; G, granulocyte; GM, granulocyte-macrophage; Epo, erythopoietin; LIF, leukemia inhibitory factor; KL, KIT ligand; FL, FMS ligand; Tpo, thrombopoeitin.

the lineage they regulate (e.g., erythropoietin, thrombopoietin) or after an assay that permitted their detection (e.g., G-CSF, M-CSF). The nomenclature for interleukins was derived to indicate a cytokine produced by and acting on leukocytes. Of the 18 identified interleukins, many can be produced by nonleukocytic populations and have actions on cells outside the hematopoietic system and on leukocytes and their progenitors. Still other cytokines are identified by their receptors (e.g., KIT ligand, FLK-2/FLT-3 ligands). Early attempts to functionally classify hematopoietic growth factors into early-acting or late-acting groups or as lineage-specific or multilineage-stimulating groups have not held up to detailed analysis. For example, apparently lineage-specific, late-acting factors, such as G-CSF and thrombopoietin, have potent synergistic interactions influencing pluripotential stem cell proliferation and differentiation, and early-acting, multilineage factors, such as KIT and FLK-2/FLT-3 ligands, can affect early stem cell proliferation and differentiation, as well as highly differentiated cells such as mast cells (KIT ligand) or DCs (FLK-2/FLT-3 ligand).

The cytokines signal through a family of type III tyrosine kinase receptors (i.e., KIT, FLK-2/FLT-3, FMS, αβ platelet-derived growth factor R [PDGFR]), or through a large family of structurally related hematopoietin receptors (Tables 1.2, 1.3). The conserved extracellular motifs of these receptors are derived from the fibronectin type III module. Different family members contain one to three chains. All such receptors are associated with one or more members of a family of Janus kinases (JAKs). These kinases couple ligand binding to tyrosine phosphorylation, both of known signaling proteins and of a unique family of transcription factors called the signal transducers and activators of transcription (STATs) (Table 1.2) (117).

The receptors for IL-3, IL-5, and GM-CSF each consist of a ligand-binding α chain associated with a common β chain whose membrane proximal domain associates with JAK-2, leading to signal transduction (118). The receptors for a number of cytokines, including IL-6, IL-11, ciliary

TABLE 1.3. *Tyrosine kinase class III receptors and their ligands*

Receptor	Ligand
KIT (CD117)	Steel factor, KIT ligand, SCF
FLT-3/FLK-2	FL, FLT-3 ligand
CSF-1R FMS (CD115)	M-CSF, CSF-1
PDGFR (α, β)	PDGF

CSF-1R, colonly-stimulating factor-1 receptor; CSF-1, colony-stimulating factor-1; FL, FLT-3 ligand; FLK, fetal liver kinase; FLT, FMS-like tyrosine kinase; FLT-3, FMS-like tyrosine kinase-3; FMS, older designation for CSF-1R; M-CSF, macrophage colony-stimulating factor; PDGFR, platelet-derived growth factor receptor, SCF, stem cell factor.

neurotrophic factor (CNTF), oncostatin m (OSM), ciliary neutrophic factor-1 (CT-1), and leukemia inhibitory factor (LIF), all use ligand-specific binding chains that associate with gp130 or a related signaling protein that associates with and activates JAK-1 and JAK-2 (119). A third category is receptors (i.e., erythropoietin, thrombopoietin, G-CSF, growth hormone, and prolactin) consisting of single chains that associate with JAK-2 through a receptor membrane–proximal domain. The IL-2 receptor family (i.e., IL-2, IL-4, IL-7, IL-9, and IL-15) and the interferon receptor family (i.e., IFN-α/β, IFN-γ, and IL-10) represent an association pattern in which two chains are required for signaling. The IL-2 receptor contains α, β, and γ_c chains; the cytoplasmic domains of the latter two are required for signal transduction. The receptors for IL-4, IL-7, IL-9, and IL-15 each contain a ligand-specific α chain and a γ_c chain. JAK-1 associates with the IL-2 receptor β chain, and JAK-3 associates with the γ_c chain and ligand-induced receptor aggregation brings JAK-1 and JAK-3 together. The IL-4Rα is shared between receptors for IL-4 and IL-13. In all cases, the primary function of the ligand is to mediate receptor aggregation and resulting homotypic or heterotypic aggregation of JAKs. The sharing of receptor subunits among different cytokine receptors accounts in part for the redundancy that is characteristic of the cytokine family (120).

The signaling cascade that ultimately results in the appropriate cellular response to the initial stimulus is under strict regulatory control. A growing family of cytokine-inducible SRC homology-2 (SH2) domain proteins (CISs), also called suppressors of cytokine signaling (SOCS), have been identified (121,122). These molecules are negative regulators of JAK-STAT signaling. CIS-1 is induced by EPOR, IL-3R, or IL-2R signaling through STAT-5 and binds to the receptors, thereby inhibiting further activation of STAT-5 (123). SOCS-1 is an inhibitor of IL-6 signaling induced through gp130 and STAT-3 and inhibiting JAK tyrosine kinase activity (124). CIS-3 is strongly induced by IFN-γ, probably through STAT-1 and inhibits signaling through binding to JAKs (121).

GRANULOCYTE COLONY-STIMULATING FACTOR

The purification and molecular cloning of G-CSF was performed between 1984 and 1986 (125,126), and clinical development commenced in 1986 with approval for clinical use in cancer patients treated with chemotherapy (127). Human G-CSF is a glycoprotein of 19,600 daltons and structurally has four antiparallel α helices arranged to form a helical bundle. G-CSF is encoded by a single gene on chromosome 17q21-22. The factor is produced constitutively at all levels by many tissues, particularly by monocytes and macrophages, endothelial cells, and fibroblasts (Table 1.2), and high serum levels are induced by a variety of inflammatory stimuli, including bacterial lipopolysaccharides (LPSs) (128). The G-CSF receptor is encoded by a single gene on chromosome 1p35-p34.3. Receptors are expressed on mature neutrophils (500 to 3,000 per cell), are found at the myeloblast-promyelocyte stage, and are present on pluripotent stem cells (38). The binding of G-CSF to its receptor decreases the number of available surface receptors because the receptor complex is rapidly internalized and degraded. G-CSF gene (−/−) mice have overtly normal postnatal development, but have a 70% to 90% reduction in neutrophils, a reduction in CFU-GM, and a reduced capacity to mobilize neutrophils on challenge with infectious agents (129).

In vitro, G-CSF stimulates selectively neutrophil granulocyte colony formation, but in synergy with other factors such as KIT ligand, it enhances proliferation of pluripotent progenitors, including stem cells. Evidence supports a mostly stochastic model of hematopoiesis, in which cytokines provide important growth and survival signals but do not direct terminal differentiation (Fig 1.4). Ecotropic expression of the G-CSFR into normal hematopoietic progenitors results in G-CSF–dependent differentiation of these cells into mature granulocytes, macrophages, megakaryocytes, and erythroid cells (130).

In vivo administration of G-CSF causes an increase in neutrophil granulocyte production, with a dose-dependent reduction in their maturation time in the marrow and with an expansion of the promyelocyte and myelocyte compartment (131). Unlike GM-CSF, there is no effect on leukocyte half-life or margination. G-CSF is a potent activator of PMNs, mobilizing secretory vesicles (i.e., leukocyte alkaline phosphatase and CD11b) and inducing the release of specific granules (i.e., lactoferrin, CD11b, and CD66b) and azurophil granules (i.e., elastase and α_1-antitrypsin complexes) (128). G-CSF enhances PMN superoxide release, which enhances respiratory burst metabolism. G-CSF has also been shown *in vitro* to downregulate allogeneic immune responses of peripheral blood mononuclear cells by inhibiting TNF-α production at a posttranscriptional level.

Administration of G-CSF causes a significant increase in circulating CD34$^+$ cells, including primitive subsets (CD34$^+$THY-1$^+$,CD38$^-$) with levels of circulating CD34$^+$ progenitors of up to 35 time normal usually achieved by day 5 (132,133). Extensive clinical application of G-CSF mobilized peripheral blood stem cells in autologous and allogeneic transplantation has resulted because of the ease with which large numbers of CD34$^+$ cells can be obtained by apheresis and the more rapid platelet and neutrophil recovery observed relative to results with conventional marrow transplantation. Recombinant human G-CSF (Filgrastim) was initially used as an adjunct to chemotherapy for ameliorating neutropenia, one of the major side effects of cancer chemotherapy (134). Its use led to reduced infections and hospital admissions. It has been approved for treatment of myelosuppression after bone marrow transplantation, severe chronic neutropenia (idiopathic and congenital), acute leukemia, aplastic anemia, and myelodysplastic syndrome. It has also proved effective for reversing the neutropenia associated with acquired immunodeficiency syndrome (AIDS) (134).

MACROPHAGE COLONY-STIMULATING FACTOR

More than 30 years ago, a colony-stimulating factor was identified in serum, urine, and a fibroblast cell line–conditioned medium that had a restricted ability to stimulate the development of colonies containing only macrophages (135,136). One unit of M-CSF was defined as the amount of factor required to stimulate a single murine macrophage colony in the linear part of the dose-response curve, representing 0.44 fmol of murine M-CSF. This sensitive bioassay facilitated the purification of the factor that in the mouse was a protein of 70 kd composed of two 35-kd polypeptide chains with disulfide bonds (137). The M-CSF gene is located on chromosome 1p13-p21 (138). As a result of alternative splicing of exon 6, three spliced variants of biologically active M-CSF are produced, a short or α form, with a leader sequence of 32 amino acids followed by 256 amino acids; a long or β form of 554 amino acids; and a γ form of 438 amino acids (139,140). The COOH terminus anchors some forms of M-CSF in an active cell-associated form, with the native secreted form of M-CSFα being generated by cotranslational *N*-linked glycosylation and proteolytic cleavage at or near amino acid 158.

The 18 cysteines in the 49-kd homodimeric species form three intermolecular and three intramolecular disulfide bonds, rendering the protein resistant to proteolytic cleavage. The dimer consists of two bundles of four α helices laid end to end, with an interchain disulfide bond (141). M-CSF is present in normal plasma at levels of 100 to 200 units/mL, and most tissues produce M-CSF transcripts of several sizes. This ubiquitous expression may reflect production by cells common to many organs (e.g., macrophages, endothelial cells, fibroblasts, mesothelial cells) (142). Fluctuations in levels of circulating M-CSF reflect a balance between production and excretion, with M-CSF receptors on Kupffer cells in the liver and splenic macrophages responsible for significant clearance by specific binding of M-CSF, with subsequent endocytosis and intracellular destruction (143). Adherence and bacterial LPS are potent inducing stimuli for monocyte and macrophage M-CSF production, with further enhancement by cyclooxygenase inhibitors and inhibition by prostaglandin E, which participates in a negative feedback loop (142,144).

The M-CSF receptor is encoded by the *FMS* oncogene and consists of an extracellular ligand-binding domain joined through a single membrane-spanning helix to a cytoplasmic protein kinase domain (145). On ligand binding, the receptor undergoes noncovalent dimerization, autophosphorylation, and signaling followed by covalent dimerization through disulfide bonds leading to further modification, tyrosine dephosphorylation, and internalization. Signaling involves tyrosine phosphorylation of TYK-2, a protein kinase of the JAK family, and the STAT-1, STAT-3, and STAT-5 transcription factors (144) (Table 1.2). High-affinity (K_d = 10^{-13} M) M-CSF binding sites are expressed at levels of $10 \times 10^4 - 10 \times 10^5$ per cell on mature monocytes, macrophages, and osteoclasts. During maturation, the number of receptors increases, but the proliferative response to M-CSF declines.

There is strong evidence that M-CSF is involved in survival, proliferation, and differentiation on at least some monocyte-macrophage populations; there is also evidence that the factor functions as a macrophage activator as part of an inflammatory host defense response. Acute events after M-CSF interaction with monocytes include increased cell spreading, membrane ruffling and receptor turnover, and induction of a variety of cytokines (e.g., IL-1, G-CSF, TNF, IL-6). The latter response may only be observed with adherent cells. M-CSF activation enhances macrophage phagocytosis, bacteriocidal, and amebicidal capacity and upregulates FcRγ and ADCC (142). At the progenitor level, highly purified populations are stimulated by M-CSF alone and by GM-CSF and IL-3, with a frequency indicating that many progenitors have receptors for all three growth factors (Fig 1.4). Cultures of marrow cells initiated with M-CSF followed by delayed addition of GM-CSF formed colonies of granulocytes and macrophage indistinguishable from those initiated with GM-CSF (146). This indicates that M-CSF sustains a progenitor population with the potential to form granulocytes, although it is responsible only for macrophage-lineage terminal differentiation. In the murine system, multipotent high proliferative potential cells, including stem cells respond to M-CSF but only in synergistic interaction with IL-1, IL-6, IL-3, or KIT ligand (20,147).

Insight into the physiologic importance of M-CSF has come from studies of the osteoporotic (op/op) mouse characterized by an autosomal recessive inactivating mutation of the M-CSF gene, resulting in absence of M-CSF (148). The mice are toothless, and the marrow cavities are occluded by bone overgrowth caused by an osteoclast deficit. Although a specific osteoclast CSF supports proliferation of osteoclast progenitors and formation of colonies of tartrate-resistant acid phosphatase–positive osteoclasts, M-CSF may play a role in later development of osteoclasts by stimulating their motility, spreading, and survival. Quantitative defects in macrophage populations also characterize op/op mice with marrow macrophages at 1% of control and without splenic marginal zone macrophages. Clinical trials of recombinant human CSF revealed that treatment leads to expansion of circulating mononuclear phagocytes, enhanced macrophage ADCC and phagocytosis, reduced platelet levels, and a reduction in serum cholesterol (149). The cholesterol-lowering effect may be attributed to enhanced macrophage activities of neutral and acidic cholesteryl ester hydrolases, enhancing net hydrolysis of acidic cholesterol ester (150).

GRANULOCYTE-MACROPHAGE COLONY-STIMULATING FACTOR

GM-CSF shares with several other hematopoietic growth factors a pair of α helices stabilized by disulfide bonds between cysteine residues. The mature molecule of amino acids has a molecular mass of 23 kd and glycosylation at two *N*-linked glycosylation sites (151). The GM-CSF gene is located on chromosome 5q23-31 in proximity to the IL-3 gene. The long arm of chromosome 5 contains a clustering of hematopoietic regulatory genes that includes GM-CSF, IL-3, IL-4, IL-5, M-CSF, and the receptors for PDGF and M-CSF (i.e., FMS) (152). Deletion of the long arm of chromosome 5 from 5q11-21 to 5q22-34 is associated with primary and familial myelodysplastic syndrome and therapy-related leukemia, but it is more likely that the candidate for pathogenesis if 5q- is the interferon regulatory factor-1 gene mapping to 5q31.1 (153). GM-CSF is an inducible product of a variety of cell types. It is produced by antigen-, lectin-, or IL-2–stimulated T lymphocytes; antigen-, LPS-, or IL-1–stimulated B lymphocytes; macrophages activated by LPS, phagocytosis, or adherence; and IL-1– or TNF-stimulated fibroblasts and endothelieal cells (Table 1.2) (154). In these various inducible cells, the accumulation of GM-CSF mRNA results from an increased transcription rate and post-transcriptional stabilization of the mRNA.

The GM-CSF receptor α chain is encoded by a gene within the pseudoautonomous region, an area of homology between the ends of the human sex chromosomes that undergoes obligatory exchange between the X and Y chromosomes during meiosis, thereby behaving ''pseudo-autosomally'' (155). The common β subunit of GM-CSF is shared with IL-3 and IL-5 receptors and is encoded by a gene located on chromosome 22q12-13. The receptor is expressed at levels of 50 to 500 receptors per cell on myeloid progenitors, neutrophils, monocytes, eosinophils, and DCs but not lymphoid or erythroid cell populations (154). The signal transduction pathway involves physical association of β_c with JAK-2, with subsequent activation of STAT-1, STAT-2, and STAT-5. A second pathway involves activation of RAS and MAP kinases, with consequent activation of FOS and JUN (117).

The biologic effects of GM-CSF initially were related to its ability to stimulate proliferation and differentiation of myeloid-committed progenitors (CFU-GM). GM-CSF can promote proliferation and differentiation of eosinophils, basophils, megakaryocytes, and erythroid and DCs in synergy with other factors (e.g., with erythropoietin for erythropoiesis, with TNF or IL-4 for dendritic differentiation). With KIT ligand or FLT-3 ligand, it stimulates multipotent progenitors and stem cells, including HPP-CFU (20). GM-CSF promotes survival of myeloid cells, including mature neutrophils, by suppressing apoptosis. The pleiotropic functions of GM-CSF extend to enhancement of innate and specific immune responses, which can be initiated alone or in synergy with other cytokines such as TNF. It enhances antibody-dependent cell killing and phagocytosis by neutrophils and macrophages, and it acts as a neutrophil migration and adhesion inhibitory factor. GM-CSF also enhances FcγRII receptor and class II MHC expression on monocytes and neutrophils and stimulates monocyte-macrophage cytokine, leukotriene, and prostaglandin release (154).

Mice in which the GM-CSF gene is knocked out exhibit normal steady-state hematopoiesis, suggesting functional redundancy of the myeloid regulatory factors or lack of a role for the factor in normal hematopoiesis (129). A universal abnormality in these mice is pulmonary pathology with similarities to human alveolar proteinosis and that involves accumulation of pulmonary surfactant protein and associated opportunistic infection. Mice lacking GM-CSF and G-CSF have a greater degree of neutropenia at birth and higher mortality than those lacking G-CSF only, but in adults, neutrophil levels were comparable (129). More surprising is the normality of hematopoiesis in β_c/IL-3 double-mutant mice that lack entire GM-CSF, IL-3, and IL-5 function (156). The mice showed normal hematopoietic parameters except for reduced numbers of eosinophils and lack of an eosinophil response to *Listeria monocytogenes.* Hematopoietic recovery after administration of the myelosuppressive drug 5-FU was unimpaired, indicating that these three cytokines were dispensable for hematopoiesis in emergency and steady states.

Excess levels of GM-CSF achieved by intravenous or subcutaneous injections of glycosylated or nonglycosylated recombinant human GM-CSF in primates and humans results in leukocytosis involving elevation of neutrophils, eosinophils, monocytes, and to a lesser extent, lymphocytes. The therapeutic applications of GM-CSF were initially restricted to amelioration of chemotherapy-induced myelotoxicity, allowing dose intensification (154,157). It has also proved effective for radioprotection. Sustained administration of GM-CSF alone or in combination with cyclophosphamide induces mobilization of $CD34^+$ cells, including stem and progenitor populations, into the circulation (24). The apheresis product can then be used for autologous or allogeneic transplantation (154,157). The capacity of GM-CSF to enhance the ability of neutrophils and monocytes to phagocytose and destroy bacteria *in vitro* and its ability *in vivo* to protect mice against lethal infections of *Salmonella aureus* and *Pseudomonas aeruginosa* suggests a clinical use of the cytokine in treating bacterial and fungal infections. It has proved effective in the adjuvant treatment of opportunistic fungal infections in AIDS patients. GM-CSF also is a potent stimulator of sustained specific antitumor immunity and is used in various cancer vaccine strategies (157). A cholesterol-lowering effect of GM-CSF has been reported and may be mediated by enhancement of macrophage functions in lipid metabolism and an increase in very-light-density lipoprotein receptor expression (157,158).

ERYTHROPOIETIN

Erythropoietin is a late-acting, lineage-specific hematopoietic growth factor that supports proliferation and maturation of progenitor cells committed to erythropoiesis. The existence of erythropoietin was demonstrated in 1953 by

Erslev (159), who showed that administration of serum from anemic rabbits increased erythropoiesis in normal rabbits. In 1977, human urinary erythropoietin was purified (160), and in 1985, the gene encoding erythropoietin was cloned, and recombinant erythropoietin became available (161,162). The gene encoding erythropoietin is found in the human chromosomal region 7q11-q22. Human erythropoietin is a glycoprotein (M_r of 24,000 to 39,000) with a polypeptide backbone 166 amino acids. There are four cysteine residues involved in interchain disulfide bonds. Carbohydrate modification of erythropoietin accounts for approximately 30% of the weight of the hormone, and *N*-linked carbohydrate side chains are essential for full activity *in vivo* because of rapid clearance of the desialated hormone from the circulation.

Erythropoietin is produced mainly in the kidney, with less than 10% produced by the liver. Erythropoietin mRNA is expressed in renal interstitial cells near the proximal tubules in the cortex, and levels can rise up to 100-fold in response to hypoxia or anemia, partly because of an increased transcription rate of the erythropoietin gene (163,164). The gene for the erythropoietin receptor has been cloned and assigned to human chromosome 19p (164). The receptor (M_r of 66,000) belongs to the hematopoietin receptor superfamily (165). The receptors are expressed at levels of 100 to 2,000 per cell and are expressed at the BFU-E stage, increasing in number with maturation to CFU-E and disappearing from more mature cells (166). The cellular action of erythropoietin begins at the BFU-E stage, and together with KIT ligand, IL-3, and GM-CSF, it promotes erythroid differentiation (Fig. 1.4). The erythropoietin receptor can physically associate with the common β chain of the IL-3 and GM-CSF receptor, providing a molecular explanation of the synergistic effect of erythropoietin and IL-3/GM-CSF (167). Erythropoietin alone at low concentrations prevents apoptosis of CFU-E, and at higher concentrations, it is mitogenic, stimulating the formation of colonies of 64 to 128 orthochromatic erythroblasts within 7 days.

In vivo treatment with erythropoietin induces polycythemia in the normal individual. Recombinant erythropoietin has been approved for treatment of anemia associated with renal failure and in anephric patients. It has also reduced blood transfusion requirements in cancer patients receiving myelosuppressive chemotherapy and counteracted the anemia frequently seen in AIDS patients treated with zidovudine (AZT) (164).

THROMBOPOIETIN

Before the discovery of thrombopoietin, four cytokines—IL-3, IL-6, IL-11, and LIF—were thought to function as thrombopoietins because of their effects on megakaryocyte development. IL-6 with IL-3 stimulates megakaryocyte colony (CFU-MK) development and supports development of mature megakaryocytes *in vitro* (Fig. 1.4). *In vivo* studies with IL-6 showed only modest platelet elevations; however, it may play a role in reactive thrombocytosis in inflammatory or neoplastic conditions (168). IL-6, IL-11, and LIF share a common signal transduction pathway, gp130 (119,169) (Table 1.2). Preclinical studies of IL-11 showed significant elevation of platelet counts after marrow transplantation. Randomized trials of IL-11 in adult cancer patients with severe thrombocytopenia caused by chemotherapy demonstrated a significant reduction in the number of platelet transfusions (170).

The existence of a lineage-specific factor regulating platelet production was doubted until the discovery of the orphan cytokine receptor MPL (171). The expression of MPL was found to be restricted to progenitor cells, megakaryocytes, and platelets, and MPL antisense oligonucleotides selectively inhibited megakaryopoiesis (172). Several groups used MPL as a purification tool to isolate and clone its ligand (173–175), and others purified the ligand using standard chromatography techniques (176,177).

Human thrombopoietin is composed of an amino-terminal domain of 153 amino acids, showing 50% similarity to erythropoietin and a unique 181–amino acid C-terminal domain that is highly glycosylated (173–175). A recombinant, truncated form of thrombopoietin, consisting of only the erythropoietin-like domain, was fully functional *in vitro* and has been evaluated *in vivo* in primates and in clinical trials in a pegelated form as megakaryocyte growth and development factor (MGDF) (178,179). In cancer patients, up to a 10-fold increase in platelets was observed with doses of 1.0 μg/kg/day for 12 days, with no alteration in platelet-activation status. In a primate model of marrow-suppressive chemotherapy, MGDF and G-CSF combinations eliminated the thrombocytopenia and neutropenia (179). Clinical trials of MGDF were terminated because some patients developed thrombocytopenia from autoantibodies to endogenous thrombopoietin. Breaking of self-tolerance and development of cross-reacting antibodies to endogenous thrombopoietin was also seen in animal studies after human thrombopoietin administration (180,181). There is no evidence that cross-reacting antibodies would develop if species-appropriate, full-length glycosylated thrombopoietin were administered. Chronic overexpression of thrombopoietin in rodent models by retroviral (182) or adenoviral (183) gene transfer produced increases in platelet counts of 10- to 20-fold but ultimately led to development of myelofibrosis and osteosclerosis. The twofold to five fold elevation of TGF-β_1 and PDGF in the serum of thrombopoietin-overexpressing mice (182) and the absence of fibrosis in chronically thrombocytopenic mice bearing the NOD and SCID mutations (183) provide clues to the pathophysiology of human myelofibrosis.

Mice deficient in genes for Mpl or thrombopoietin exhibit a dramatic 85% to 90% drop in platelet count and megakaryocytes in marrow and spleen (184). Megakaryocyte progenitors are decreased but so are erythroid and myeloid progenitors, indicating that thrombopoietin acts on a very early pluripotent stem or progenitor cell. Evidence for an action of thrombopoietin on stem cells has been obtained in studies showing expression of Mpl on murine or human populations, highly enriched for stem cells (185,186). There is also evidence that thrombopoietin directly promotes survival and suppresses apoptosis of human primitive $CD34^+CD38^-$ bone marrow cells (187). In combination with the FLK-2/FLT-3 ligand, thrombopoietin produces prolonged (24 weeks) and extensive (2×10^5-fold) expansion of cord blood cells with stem cell properties (i.e., LTC-IC) (188). Thrombopoietin acts directly on hematopoietic progenitors to induce megakaryocytic differentiation but also acts synergistically (e.g., KIT ligand, FLT-3 ligand) and addictively (e.g., IL-6, IL-3) with early- and late-acting hematopoietic growth factors to stimulate megakaryocyte production (189,190).

Thrombopoietin is expressed in various tissues and is abundant in the liver, kidney, muscle, brain, and intestine and moderately expressed in marrow, spleen, and lung. However, acute thrombocytopenia does not affect thrombopoietin gene expression or transcription in the major thrombopoietin-producing tissues or in the tissues sustaining megakaryocytopoiesis (189,190). Thrombopoietin levels appear to be regulated by platelet mass (189), being expressed constitutively and sequestered by platelets through high affinity (K_d ~ 100 to 400 pM) binding to Mpl. Platelets from Mpl-knockout mice do not bind thrombopoietin, and their clearance of thrombopoietin is fivefold slower than in wild-type mice (191). Megakaryocyte mass may also play a role in regulating circulating thrombopoietin levels, because idiopathic thrombocytopenia purpura patients and mice deficient in NF-E2 transcription factor are highly thrombocytopenic but have elevated numbers of megakaryocytes in the marrow and normal thrombopoietin levels (192,193).

INTERLEUKINS

Interleukin-1

IL-1 is a proinflammatory cytokine that exists as an α and a β form (194). These separate gene products have similar biologic activities. IL-1α is synthesized at a 31-kd precursor (pro-IL-1α), which is fully active but remains within the cytoplasm until released by cell death. The 17-kd form results from cleavage by extracellular proteases or by membrane-associated cysteine proteases called calpains. Pro-IL-1α can be myristoylated and transported to the cell surface, particularly on B lymphocytes and monocytes, where it can function as an active "membrane" form. IL-1β mRNA is rapidly induced in cells such as monocytes by a variety of stimulants, including adherence, but there is a dissociation between transcription and translation, with most of the mRNA degrading with no significant translation into pro-IL-1β (194). Addition of endotoxin or IL-1 itself results in augmented translation.

After synthesis, pro-IL-1β remains cytosolic, is only marginally active and has no membrane form. Release of mature IL-1β involves specific processing involving aspartic acid-alanine peptide cleavage by the IL-1β–converting enzyme (ICE). Two IL-1 receptors (IL-1RI and IL-1RII) and a receptor accessory protein IL-1RAcP have been identified (195). All three molecules are members of the immunoglobulin superfamily, each comprising three IgG-like domains and sharing significant homology. IL-1RI is a 80-kd glycoprotein encoded by a gene on chromosome 2. It is expressed at levels of 50 to 200 receptors per cell on lymphocytes, endothelial cells, fibroblasts, smooth muscle cells, keratinocytes, and HSCs. Complexing of the receptor with IL-1RAcP increases the IL-1 binding affinity, with signal transduction occurring in cells with less than 10 receptors. IL-1RI is the primary signal transducing receptor, and the IL-1RII, with only a short 29–amino acid cytosolic domain, appears to act as a "decoy" molecule, tightly binding IL-1β and preventing its binding to IL-1RI. The extracellular domains of both receptors are found as "soluble" molecules in the circulation of normal individuals and in inflammatory fluids.

The competition between IL-1 binding to signaling and nonsignaling receptors and the ratios of the latter molecules determine the extent and duration of the IL-1–dependent proinflammatory response. The IL-1R signal transduction system is efficient because fewer than 10 ligand-occupied receptors are required per cell to elicit a strong response. A major component of the signaling pathway involves activation of the transcription factor NF-κB, which is of central importance to inflammatory and immune responses, and signaling studies have focused on activation of a kinase, which results in phosphorylation of the inhibitory I-κB molecule that precedes its proteolytic degradation with release of active NF-κB (195).

IL-1 is produced by virtually all nucleated cell types and has a broad spectrum of activities, including induction of acute-phase responses, fever, mediation of catabolic response in inflammation, breakdown of cartilage, proliferation of fibroblasts, and nonspecific resistance to infection (Table 1.2). In studies of hematopoiesis, IL-1 was shown to have an activity identical to hematopoietin-1 (196), that synergizes with M-CSF or IL-3 to stimulate murine HPP-CFU (147). Pluripotent progenitors, including stem cell populations can be expanded *in vitro* by IL-1 and IL-3 or KIT ligand (197,198) and such *ex vivo* treated populations produced faster engraftment with fewer cells on transplantation (198). IL-1 had a direct effect on human $CD34^+$ cells (199), and in synergy with factors such as KIT ligand, IL-3, IL-6, and erythropoietin, it has been used to expand $CD34^+$ cells that were subsequently used for autologous transplantation (200). The synergistic activity may be accounted for in part by the ability of IL-1 to upregulate receptors for M-CSF, GM-CSF, IL-3, and SCF (201).

A second major effect of IL-1 on hematopoiesis is indirect, resulting from its ability to rapidly induce cytokine production (e.g., G-CSF, GM-CSF, M-CSF, IL-6, IL-11) by bone marrow stromal cells, endothelial cells, or macrophages (201). In animal models, IL-1 is radioprotective (202), and it protects stem cells from damage after cyclophosphamide treatment (203). The mechanisms involved include induction in early hematopoietic cells of manganese superoxide dismutase that scavenges free oxygen radicals (204) and aldehyde dehydrogenase that inactivates the active form of cyclophosphamide (203). *In vivo*, IL-1 was shown to accelerate neutrophil and platelet recovery after high-dose 5-FU treatment and to synergize with G-CSF in further accelerating neutrophil recovery (147). Clinical studies have demonstrated a protective effect from radiation damage when used with radiolabeled monoclonal antibody therapy for cancer (201). It has also been shown to stimulate neutrophil recovery and platelet elevation in cancer patients receiving high-dose chemotherapy. However, its toxicity profile, associated with release of acute-phase reactants, precludes the use of dosages sufficient to have a meaningful clinical effect on hematopoietic recovery (204a).

The biologic effects of IL-1 on T cells include induction of a variety of lymphokines, including IL-2 production, increased high-affinity IL-2R expression, and enhancement of IL-2 induction of lymphokine-activated killer (LAK) cell activity (205). Its action on B cells includes costimulation of proliferation and induction of maturation of pre-B cells.

Interleukin-2

IL-2 is the prototype of a class of cytokines that affects lymphoid proliferation and function and shares the common γ_c chain of the IL-2 receptor for signaling (e.g., IL-4, IL-7, IL-9, IL-13, IL-15). The factor was first identified as a 15-kd glycoprotein human T-cell growth factor (206) and was subsequently shown to be central to the regulation of the immune response. It is produced by activated helper T cells of the T_H1 type and by large granular lymphocytes. It is a 133–amino acid polypeptide that undergoes posttranslational modification through glycosylation and is encoded by a gene on chromosome 4q26-28 (207,208). Its production is transcriptionally regulated by T-cell receptor ligation, intracellular Ca^{2+} elevation induced by immunomodulators, or CD28 activation by B7-2 ligand expressed on activated lymphoid cells or DCs (209).

Signaling occurs through a high affinity heteromeric receptor consisting of a p55 IL-2Rα chain, a p75 IL-2β chain, and a p64 common IL-2γ_c (209,210) (Table 1.2). The IL-2β chain is expressed constitutively on monocytes and natural killer (NK) cells and functions as a low-affinity receptor. In addition to stimulating long-term proliferation of antigen-stimulated T cells and LAK cells, IL-2 induces rapid activation of NK and LAK cells with cytolytic activity induced within hours of IL-2 exposure and persisting for several days. ADCC activity through binding of antibodies to FcRγ-III is also enhanced (211). It is also a T-cell chemotactic factor, particularly for LAK cells expressing IL-2Rα/γ. Activated B cells also respond to IL-2 with enhanced proliferation, and it is a late-acting factor for B cells making IgM. Macrophages constitutively express the IL-2β/γ chains and respond to IL-2 by production of TGF-β and TNF-α and with augmented cytotoxicity against tumor cells.

Interleukin-3

In the early 1980s, a murine factor was purified from conditioned medium and shown to stimulate multiple different murine hematopoietic lineages. The factor was initially called multi-CSF but subsequently renamed IL-3 (212). The human IL-3, which is species restricted in its activity, is a glycoprotein of 25 to 30 kd, with a core protein of 14.6 kd consisting of 152 amino acids with a 19–amino acid signal peptide (213). The gene encoding IL-3 is located on the long arm of chromosome 5 (5q23-32), only 9 kilobases from the gene for GM-CSF. IL-3 mRNA is not detectable in unstimulated T cells but is produced by activated T cells, NK cells, and mast cells after a transient increase in gene transcription and mRNA stabilization. It is probably a local acting factor because it does not normally circulate at detectable levels in the blood. Measurable amounts of IL-3 are produced in a subgroup of patients suffering from extensive graft-versus-host disease. The receptor for IL-3 consists of two subunits, a 70-kd ligand-binding subunit (IL-3Rα), and a 120-kd signal transducing chain (β_c) that is shared by GM-CSF and IL-3 (214,215) (Table 1.2).

IL-3 stimulates colony formation by a spectrum of progenitors, including CFU-GEMM, CFU-GM, and neutrophil-, eosinophil-, and basophil-restricted progenitors, and acts in synergy with other factors, such as CFU-Meg and BFU-E (215,216). The common IL-3/GM-CSF receptor β_c chain functionally and physically associates with the EPOR, suggesting that these receptors exist as a large supercomplex and offering a molecular explanation of the synergistic effects of IL-3 and GM-CSF with erythropoietin during erythropoiesis (167). In assays of more primitive blast cell colonies and HPP-CFU, IL-3 stimulates in synergy with factors such as IL-1, IL-6, IL-11, G-CSF, KIT ligand, and FLT-3 ligand (20). In addition to growth stimulation and shortening of doubling time of early hematopoietic cells, it also has an anti-apoptotic action on progenitor populations at concentrations lower than necessary to initiate proliferation. IL-3 alters the function of mature phagocytes, acting as a survival factor for monocytes and inducing macrophage secretion of TNF-α, IL-1β, and IL-6 (217).

There are conflicting reports on the effects of brief cytokine exposure on marrow repopulating ability. Tavassoli (218) reported that 2- to 3-hour preincubation of mouse bone marrow with IL-3 enhanced repopulating ability, possibly because of upregulation of homing receptors. In contrast, van der Loo and Ploemacher (219) found that a similar preincubation with IL-3 or with IL-3, IL-12, and KIT ligand led to sustained decrease in marrow and spleen seeding of early and late CAFC and a reduction in day-12 CFU-S seeding from 11.4% to 7.3%, together with a decrease in long-term repopulation.

IL-3 addition can lead to a reduction in the long-term repopulating ability of cultured marrow (220–222). Its addition to combinations of FLT-3 ligand and thrombopoietin inhibited the long-term generation of LTC-IC in cord blood cultures (188). This negative regulation by IL-3 acts at the level of the stem cell self-renewal versus differentiation decision and appears to be mediated by the common receptor signaling subunit β_c and the additional IL-3 signaling protein βIL-3, which is specific to IL-3 and is found in mice but not humans (222). In apparent contradiction to the inhibitory effects of IL-3 on stem cells *in vitro*, *in vivo* treatment of NOD/SCID mice engrafted with human $CD34^+$ cells with hIL-3 resulted in substantial expansion of the most primitive stem cell population (223). In preclinical studies in primates, IL-3 administration after intensive myelosuppressive chemotherapy dramatically enhanced myeloid recovery and reduced the duration of neutropenia (224). Numerous clinical trials have shown the beneficial effect of IL-3 after cytotoxic therapy, in the posttransplant period after bone marrow transplantation, and in a variety of neutropenic settings (215).

Interleukin-4

IL-4 was first identified as a cytokine capable of costimulating murine B-cell proliferation (225). It is produced by activated T_H2 cells, NK cells, and basophil or mast cells. The secreted protein of 129 amino acids is a 15- to 19-kd glycoprotein comprising a four-α-helices bundle resembling GM-CSF, M-CSF, and growth hormone (226). The IL-4 gene is on chromosome 5q23q-31, near the genes for IL-3, IL-5, IL-9, IL-13, and GM-CSF. IL-4 binds with high affinity to a specific 140-kd glycoprotein receptor that has the conserved WSXWS box of the class 1 cytokine receptor superfamily. This receptor forms a heterodimer with the IL-2 common receptor component (IL-2Rγ_c) with a twofold to threefold increased IL-4 binding affinity (227) (Table 1.2). Relatively low numbers of receptors (100 to 1,000 per cell) are found on nearly every cell type, including lymphoid, myeloid, macrophage, fibroblast, epithelial, and endothelial cells. A distinct low-affinity receptor has been reported at the cell surface and as a soluble form and is apparently unrelated to the p140 (228). Signal transduction involves activation of JAK-1, JAK-3, and STATs.

The effects on B cells include costimulation of proliferation and upregulation of surface immunoglobulin, CD40, CD23, and low-affinity IgE-binding Fc receptors, with augmented antigen presentation toward T cells (229). IL-4 induces B-cell production of IL-6 and TNF and induces isotype switching with enhanced IgE and IgG4 production.

The differentiation of $CD4^+$ helper T cells into T_H1 or T_H2 subsets is driven by various cytokines. IL-4 directs T_H2 maturation and the cytokine repertoire of these cells includes IL-4, IL-5, IL-6, IL-10, and IL-13, all cytokines involved in humoral immunity and allergic response. The lymphokine has an autocrine effect on T_H2 cell proliferation and induces CD23 on activated T cells. The effect on macrophages includes enhanced antigen presentation because of upregulation of MHC class II molecules and a powerful antiinflammatory action by means of a blocking action on proinflammatory cytokine (e.g., IL-1, IL-6, IL-8, TNF-α), chemokine (e.g., IP-10), and collagenase production (230). In synergy with GM-CSF, IL-4 induces monocyte differentiation to DCs (91) (Fig. 1.4).

Numerous synergistic effects of IL-4 on hematopoiesis have been reported, although generally of a modest nature. With IL-3 and KIT ligand, it stimulates multipotent progenitors and acts as a cofactor with G-CSF in stimulating neutrophil progenitors, possibly by upregulating the G-CSFR (231). It is a mast cell growth factor but directly inhibits IL-3–stimulated macrophage colony formation (232). Its potential clinical role is in cancer immunotherapy and in diseases where its immunomodulatory and antiinflammatory properties would be of benefit.

Interleukin-5

IL-5 is a homodimeric glycoprotein of 40 to 45 kd that is encoded by a gene in the cytokine gene cluster on chromosome 5q31. It has a pleiotropic effect on the immune system and inflammation, and its most obvious activities are on eosinophil development and function, although it has additional effects on murine B cells (233). It is secreted by activated T_H2 lymphocytes, and it is produced by LPS-, IL-1–, or IL-2–activated microvascular endothelium (234).

IL-5 induces terminal eosinophil differentiation from eosinophil committed progenitors and, in synergy with IL-3, from more primitive tripotent or pluripotent precursors (88) (Fig. 1.4). IL-5 prolongs eosinophil survival by delaying apoptotic death, increases eosinophil adhesion to endothelial cells, induces eosinophil chemotaxis, and enhances eosinophil effector function. The expression of IL-5 by eosinophils at the sites of allergic inflammation may provide an important autocrine pathway for maintaining the effector function and viability of recruited eosinophils in, for example, the asthmatic lung. IL-5 and IL-5R −/− mice unexpectedly have normal basal levels of eosinophils, but they have impairment in the ability to mount an eosinopoietic response to and kill a parasitic worm infection that is normally controlled by eosinophils (233). IL-5 was initially identified by its ability to support the growth and differentiation of murine B cells, and in mice (but not humans), it is involved in the development of primitive B cells and production of natural antibody and of secretory IgA antibody in mucosal lymphoid cells (235).

The IL-5 receptor (IL-5R) consists of an α and β chain. The former specifically binds IL-5 with low affinity, and the latter does not bind ligand by itself but does form a high-affinity receptor in combination with the α chain. The β chain is the common β chain that binds with IL-3Rα and GM-CSFRα, is required for signaling, and provides a molecular basis for the functional redundancy of these cytokines. JAK-2 and JAK-1 are constitutively associated with the IL-5Rα and β_c subunit, respectively, and are activated on IL-5 stimulation (235) (Table 1.2).

Interleukin-6

IL-6 is a pleiotropic cytokine that acts on a variety of cells, playing a role in the immune response, inflammation, and hematopoiesis and acting on the endocrine and nervous system (Table 1.2). It induces the differentiation of B cells to antibody-producing plasma cells. Transgenic mice overexpressing IL-6 show massive plasmacytosis, hypergammaglobulinemia, increased acute-phase proteins, and increased megakaryocytes and eventually develop plasmacytomas (236). IL-6–deficient mice show reduced IgG responses and a striking reduction in mucosal IgA-producing cells. Such mice have a defective ability to generate cytotoxic T cells against certain viruses, and the inflammatory acute-phase response after tissue damage or infection is severely compromised. IL-6 is a necessary component of the fever response to IL-1 and LPS. IL-6 belongs to a cytokine subfamily that exhibits functional redundancy, structural similarity, and sharing of a receptor subunit. The members of this family include IL-6, LIF, CNTF, OSM, IL-11, and CT-1, and their functional redundancy is largely explained by their sharing of the receptor subunit, gp130 (Table 1.2) (119).

The IL-6 receptor complex consists of an 80-kd IL-6–binding molecule (IL-6Rα), a member of the type I cytokine receptor superfamily, and a signal transducer, gp130. The cytoplasmic domain of IL-6Rα is not necessary for signal transduction, and the soluble form of the extracellular domain can form a complex with IL-6 that associates with gp130 to initiate signaling. The complete structure of the IL-6R is a hexamer composed of two molecules each of IL-6, IL6-R, and gp130. JAK-1, JAK-2, and TYK-2 associate constitutively with gp130 and are tyrosine phosphorylated in response to cytokine signaling. IL-6 can activate STAT-3, STAT-1, and STAT-5. In addition to JAK-STAT signal-transduction, gp130 activates the RAS-MAP kinase pathway through SRC homology phosphotyrosine phosphatase-2 (SHP-2) (119,236).

Interleukin-7

IL-7 is a 25-kd glycoprotein that was originally defined as a pre-B-cell growth factor implicated in pro-B-cell proliferation, but it was subsequently shown to participate in proliferation and differentiation of T cells (Fig. 1.4). It is produced by stromal cells within the marrow, fetal liver, and thymus and signals through an IL-7Rα–specific receptor chain that heterodimerizes with the IL-2Rγ_c chain (Table 1.2). IL-7 has been shown to form a heterodimer with a cofactor of 30 kd, also produced by stromal cells, and this complex selectively stimulates proliferation and presumptive differentiation of pre-pro-B cells in long-term culture, priming the cells to respond to monomeric IL-7 (237).

The cytokine stimulates proliferation of immature $CD4^-$ and $CD8^-$ thymocyte subsets and early B cells. It upregulates IL-2 and IL-2R on mature T cells participating in their activation and proliferation. It is a cofactor for V(D)J rearrangements of the T-cell receptor β gene and sustains recombination-activating gene-1 product (RAG-1) and RAG-2 expression in the embryonic thymus, where it is abundantly expressed (238).

IL-7 receptors are expressed on monocyte-macrophages, and IL-7 has been shown to enhance their tumoricidal activity and induce production of IL-1, IL-6, TNF, and IL-8. $CD56^+$ NK cells can be generated from $CD34^+$ cells in the presence of IL-7. Effects on myelopoiesis have been reported to include synergistic enhancement of colony formation in combination with IL-3, GM-CSF, and M-CSF in mice and with G-CSF and KIT ligand in humans (239). *In vivo* administration of IL-7 causes a threefold to fivefold increase in lymphocytes in spleen and lymph nodes, with elevation of B cell, T cell, NK cell, and macrophage populations, and the $CD8^+$ cells increase disproportionally to $CD4^+$ cells (240). *In vivo* administration of IL-7 also results in mobilization of stem cells, with long-term repopulating potential from the marrow into the circulation (241). A potential clinical application of IL-7 follows from this stem cell mobilizing action and from its ability to accelerate lymphoid repopulation in cyclophosphamide-treated mice. In IL-7–knockout mice, there is a massive reduction in the cellularity of the thymus, spleen, and lymph nodes, with a 20-fold reduction in CD4 and CD8 thymocytes and a block in the B-cell lineage between the pro-B and pre-B stage.

Interleukin-8

A monocyte-derived neutrophil chemotactic factor (MDNCF) was first isolated from LPS-stimulated human monocyte culture supernatants and was subsequently renamed IL-8 in view of its multiple functions (242). Perhaps unfortunately named, IL-8 is in fact a member of the CXC family of chemokines, a large family of proteins of 92 to 125 amino acids with leader sequences of 20 to 25 amino acids. Chemokines such as IL-8 signal through seven transmembrane domain receptors that use heterotrimeric GTP-binding proteins as signal transducers (see the section on chemokines). The biologic activities of IL-8 include neutrophil chemotaxis and neutrophil activation as measured by release of lysosomal enzymes, induction of respiratory bursts, reactive oxygen generation, and increased expression of adhesion molecules (243). IL-8 also induces chemotaxis of $CD4^+$ and $CD8^+$ T lymphocytes. IL-8 may also have effects on certain nonleukocytic cell populations, including endothelial cells, fibroblasts, and melanocytes. A pathogenic role for IL-8 in acute respiratory distress syndrome has been proposed, leading to neutrophil infiltration into the lungs (244).

Interleukin-9

IL-9 is a T-cell–derived lymphokine, initially designated P40 after its identification in the mouse as a growth factor for certain T_H cell clones. It is a 32- to 39-kd protein produced by activated $CD4^+$ T cells of the T_H2 subtype and by naive $CD4^+$ T cells. Increased IL-9 production is linked to T-cell receptor–mediated signals, and IL-1 can act as a co-stimulator. The IL-9 gene is located on chromosome 5q31-32 in the hematopoietic regulatory gene cluster (245). The high-affinity receptor is a heterodimer composed of the IL-9Rα chain that binds to the IL-2Rγ_c chain. Receptor activation leads to stimulation of proliferation of $CD4^+$ and $CD8^+$ T cells, including cytotoxic T lymphocytes, on their activation by IL-2, antigen, or lectin. IL-9 potentiates the proliferation of thymocytes in the presence of IL-2 and of mast cells in the presence of IL-3. It potentiates IL-4–induced IgE synthesis by B cells. Effects on *in vitro* erythropoiesis have been reported, with enhancement of erythroid burst formation by purified adult progenitors in synergy with erythropoietin and synergizing to stimulate CFU-mix and CFU-GM in addition to BFU-E with fetal liver progenitors (246).

Interleukin-10

IL-10 was discovered after a search for a product of T_H2 cells that could inhibit proliferation, effector function (e.g., cytokine secretion), and possibly development of T_H1 cells in a manner analogous to inhibition of T_H2 proliferation by the T_H1 cytokine IFN-γ. A T_H2-derived cytokine was identified by its ability to inhibit T_H1 production of cytokines that included IFN-γ (247,248). Based on its primary structure, IL-10 is a member of the four-α-helix bundle of cytokines and has an open reading frame of 178 amino acids, including a hydrophobic leader sequence (247,248). Human IL-10 is a nonglycosylated 18-kd polypeptide expressed as a noncovalent homodimer. There is a strong homology in the mature coding sequence of IL-10 and the BCRF-1 open reading frame of the Epstein-Barr virus (EBV) genome that has been designated viral IL-10 (247,248). IL-10 is not strictly a $CD4^+$ T-cell product, because it is also expressed by $CD8^+$ T cells, activated B cells, malignant B cells, monocytes, macrophages, and keratinocytes. Its production is influenced by cytokine feedback mechanisms; for example, IL-4 and IFN-γ inhibits its production by activated monocytes and macrophages. Its action is as an inhibitor of cytokine production at the mRNA and protein level, suppressing production of IFN-γ, GM-CSF, TNF-α, and TFN-β by activated T cells. IL-10 also inhibits macrophage accessory cell-dependent synthesis of IFN-γ and TNF-α. IL-10 is a potent suppressor of activated macrophage production of important activating or chemotactic cytokines (i.e., IL-1α, IL-β, IL-6, IL-8, TNF-α, GM-CSF, and G-CSF), and it directly inhibits neutrophil and macrophage phagocytic and bactericidal activity (248).

The cytokine has been implicated as a major mediator of sepsis-induced impairment of antibacterial host defense and the evolution of bacterial pneumonia (249). In this regard, IL-10 plays contrasting roles in the septic response. It is a vital downmodulator of the often lethal overabundance of proinflammatory cytokines, and administration of IL-10 confers significant protection. When bacterial pneumonia ensues, elevated production of endogenous IL-10 may suppress proactive innate immunity by its action on macrophages and neutrophils (249). Elevated levels of prostaglandin E_2, produced by activated monocytes and macrophages, is a primary inducer of IL-10 production by these same cells, while also inhibiting their production of proinflammatory cytokines, including IL-12 and IFN-γ.

Interleukin-11

IL-11 was identified during a search for marrow stroma–derived factors capable of supporting hematopoiesis. Expression cloning of IL-11 was undertaken using a cDNA library generated from a primate marrow stromal cell line (250). IL-11 precursor protein consists of 199 amino acids, including a 21–amino acid leader sequence with a molecular mass of 19,154 daltons. It belongs to the four-helix bundle family of cytokines and is encoded by a gene mapping to chromosome 19q13.3-19q13.4 (251). The cytokine is expressed *in vivo* in a wide range of normal tissues, including fibroblasts, mesenchymal cells, endothelium, keratinocytes, muscle cells, osteoblasts, and neural tissue. Expression in these cells is modulated by several proinflammatory cytokines (e.g., IL-1α, IL-1β, TGF-β) and agonists.

IL-11 signals through the common gp130 receptor, shared with IL-6, LIF, and CNTF. The IL-11 receptor α chain has the conserved 5–amino acid motif (WSXWS) of the hematopoietin receptor superfamily, and the extracellular domain shares sequence similarity with the α chains of the IL-6 and CNTF receptors. Low-affinity binding of IL-11 to IL-11Rα occurs but is not sufficient for signal transduction, and the generation of high-affinity receptors requires coexpression of IL-11Rα and gp130 (Table 1.2). Activation of this receptor complex is followed by activation of JAK-2 and then STAT or the RAS-MAP kinase pathway (251).

IL-11 has pleiotropic effects on hematopoietic cells,, osteogenic cells, intestinal epithelium, and neural tissue. It is also a potent stimulator of acute-phase reactants, an inhibitor of adipogenesis, and an inducer of a febrile response. It is a potent synergistic factor acting with a variety of cytokines (e.g., IL-3, IL-4, IL-7, IL-12, IL-13, KIT ligand, FLT-3 ligand, GM-CSF) to stimulate proliferation of primitive stem cells and progenitors. IL-11 can act directly on erythroid progenitors (BFU-E), independent of the presence of other hematopoietic growth factors, except erythropoietin (252). In animals, it increased the cycling rate and absolute numbers of myeloid progenitors in marrow and spleen but had no effect on peripheral leukocyte counts. *In vitro*, it acts synergistically with IL-3 and thrombopoietin or KIT ligand to stimulate production, differentiation, and maturation of megakaryocytes, and *in vivo*, it resulted in marked stimulation of megakaryopoiesis with modest platelet elevation (251,253).

A number of multicenter, randomized, placebo-controlled

trials of IL-11 have been undertaken in cancer patients and have shown a significant reduction in platelet transfusion requirements after high-dose chemotherapy, resulting in U.S. Food and Drug Administration approval of the cytokine for treatment of chemotherapy-associated thrombocytopenia (251,254). There are suggestions that IL-11 may act as a paracrine or autocrine growth factor for cells of the hematopoietic microenvironment. It enhances the *in vitro* development of adherent marrow stroma from normal or aplastic anemia patients (255) and may be linked to the evolution of myelofibrosis because it appears to modulate megakaryocyte-dependent marrow fibroblast proliferation (256). IL-11 may be involved in normal growth control of gastrointestinal epithelial cells, reversibly inhibiting their proliferation (257). IL-11 may also be an important osteoblast-derived paracrine regulator of bone metabolism influencing osteoblasts and osteoclasts (258).

Interleukin-12

IL-12 was first identified as a factor secreted by EBV-transformed lymphoblastoid B cells that induced IFN-γ production and enhancement of cell-mediated toxicity of T and NK cells and had a comitogenic effect on resting T cells (259). The purified factor was a unique heterodimer of 70 kd formed by two covalently linked glycosylated chains of 40 kd (p40) and 35 kd (p35). The p35 cDNA sequence encodes a 219–amino acid polypeptide with some homology to IL-6 and G-CSF. P40, a 328–amino acid polypeptide with a 22–amino acid hydrophobic signal sequence, is apparently related to the hematopoietin receptor superfamily and is characterized by an alanine-modified WSXWS motif (260). The gene for p40 maps to 5q31-q33, close to genes encoding several cytokines and receptors, and the completely unrelated gene for p35 is encoded on 3q12.3-3q13.2 (261). The IL-12 receptor consists of a 666–amino acid type 1 transmembrane protein with a 516–amino acid extracellular domain (262). It is a member of the hematopoietin receptor superfamily and is homologous to gp130 and to LIF-Rβ and G-CSFR (Table 1.2). The receptor is expressed at a level of 1,000 to 9,000 receptors per activated T cell or NK cell.

IL-12 is a major proinflammatory cytokine produced by cells involved in early innate resistance to infection including monocytes, macrophages, neutrophils, mast cells, and keratinocytes and by professional antigen-presenting cells (e.g., DCs, cutaneous LCs) (261). IL-12 enhances cell-mediated responses while suppressing antibody responses by preferentially stimulating T_H1 cell populations and inhibiting induction of T_H2 cell populations. The differentiation of $CD4^+$ helper T cells into T_H1 or T_H2 subsets is driven by varying cytokine production. IL-12 preferentially directs the development of naive T cells to T_H1 cells involved in cell-mediated immune response, which on activation secrete IL-2, IFN-γ, TNF-α, TNF-β, and GM-CSF. IL-12 is particularly effective in inducing INF-γ production by T and NK cells, as well as TNF-α, GM-CSF, M-CSF, IL-3, IL-8, and IL-2. IL-12 has little effect on resting T and NK cells but directly induces proliferation of preactivated cells. IL-12 directly enhances NK cytotoxicity, in part by increasing transcription of granzyme A and B and the lytic protein perforin. In addition to its effects on lymphoid populations, IL-12 has been shown to act synergistically with, among others, IL-3 and KIT ligand to enhance survival and proliferation of stem cells, pluripotent progenitors (including myeloid–B lymphoid precursors), and lineage-committed progenitors (263,264).

Interleukin-13

IL-13 is a 13-kd protein produced by activated T_H0/T_H2 cells, mast cells, and NK cells (265,266). It is 30% identical to IL-4 at the amino acid level and shares with that cytokine a critical role in modulating B lymphocytes and monocytes. In humans, the gene for IL-13 is located on chromosome 5, together with genes for IL-3, IL-4, and GM-CSF (267).

IL-13 signals through a receptor complex consisting of a unique IL-13Rα, which associates with IL-4Rα and a common γ chain to form a high-affinity receptor (Table 1.2) (268). In NK and T cells, IL-13 is a potent regulator of STAT-6 and JAK-3 (269). IL-13 enhances the expression of MHC class II molecules and CD33 on monocytes and B cells and, like IL-4, induces an Ig class switch to IgE in B cells and elicits B-cell proliferation. Like IL-4, it has antiinflammatory activities, suppressing the IL-1α–initiated secretion of IL-1β, IL-8, and IL-1 receptor antagonist by human peripheral blood mononuclear cells (270). It also induces the formation of arachidonic acid products that inhibit the proinflammatory actions of the leukotriene B_4. Unlike IL-4, it increases IL-2–induced IFN-γ production and cytolytic activity and the proliferation of primary human T and NK cells. A synergistic effect of IL-13 with KIT ligand, G-CSF, or GM-CSF has been observed on the proliferation of primitive murine Lin-ve, Sca-1^+ hematopoietic progenitor cells, with IL-13 promoting exclusively macrophage differentiation (271). The pathophysiologic features of allergic asthma are thought to result from the activity of T_H2 cytokines, particularly IL-4 and IL-5, with eosinophils as primary effector cells. Studies using blocking antibody to IL-13Rα in a mouse asthma model have shown that IL-13 is necessary and sufficient for expression of allergic asthma (272).

Interleukin-14

A high-molecular-weight B-cell growth factor produced by malignant non-Hodgkin's lymphoma cells has been called IL-14 (273). Expression of receptors for the cytokine on malignant B cells suggested that autocrine or paracrine production of IL-14 may play a role in the rapid proliferation of aggressive lymphoma. It induces B-cell proliferation, inhibits immunoglobulin secretion, and selectively expands certain B cells (205).

Interleukin-15

IL-15 is a 14- to 18-kd cytokine with biologic activities similar to those of IL-2 (274). It triggers and regulates innate immune responses after bacterial and viral infections. It is produced by LPS-activated monocytes and by a variety of tissues, including heart, liver, lung, and kidney but not activated T cells. It signals through a heterotrimeric receptor composed of the β and γ chains of the IL-2R and its own high-affinity binding α chain, structurally related to the α chain of the IL-2R (Table 1.2) (275).

The factor acts as a T-cell growth factor and a T-cell chemoattractant. In synergy with IL-12, it induces IFN-γ production by purified CD4$^+$T cells. It costimulates with IL-12 the proliferation of NK cells, is an NK survival factor, and induces production of proinflammatory cytokines (e.g., IFN-γ, GM-CSF, TNF-α) by these cells. It induces the proliferation and immunoglobulin synthesis of tonsillar B cells stimulated with CD40 ligand. It also a potent autocrine regulator of macrophage proinflammatory cytokine production and promotes monocyte production of IL-12 and IL-17 (276,277). In chronic inflammatory disorders, IL-15 may play a role in a self-perpetuating cycle, with IL-15–stimulated CD4$^+$ T cells activating monocytes to release IL-12, which synergizes with IL-15 to induce an IL-12 response and IFN-γ production (277). Reports that IL-15 induces mRNA for perforin and granzymes in lymphocytes, activates human peripheral blood lymphocytes for perforin-mediated lysis of tumor cells, induces the generation of cytotoxic T lymphocytes, and promotes maturation of cytotoxic NK cells have led to the suggestion that this cytokine plays an important role in antitumor immunity (278).

Interleukin-16

IL-16 is a multifunctional cytokine that induces its effects after interaction with CD4. It is a chemoattractant for CD4$^+$ T cells, monocytes, and eosinophils, and it upregulates the IL-2R (279). IL-16 is synthesized as an approximately 80-kd precursor molecule, pro-IL-16, which lacks a signal peptide but is processed by cleavage at residue 515, resulting in secretion of a 121–amino acid C-terminal peptide that autoaggregates to form bioactive multimers. It has no homology with other cytokines, but like IL-1, it is proteolytically cleaved on cell activation by ICE. Widespread expression of pro-IL-16 in lymphoid tissue and circulating lymphocytes has been identified by immunohistochemistry. By flow cytometric analysis, more than 70% of CD4$^+$ and CD8$^+$ T cells constitutively express pro-IL-16 protein, and it is proteolytically processed by cell activation. CD8$^+$ T cells constitutively express a significant pool of mature IL-16 peptide, but CD4$^+$ T cells constitutively express little or no mature IL-16 peptide, requiring cell activation to secrete mature IL-16 (280).

Interleukin-17

IL-17 is a novel cytokine, apparently secreted only by activated CD4 T cells, that activates mesenchymal cells, leading to their production of a proinflammatory spectrum of factors. IL-17 was cloned from a T-cell CD4 library and shown to possess a unique 155–amino acid sequence with a 19–amino acid signal peptide (281). The protein core of 15 kd, on glycosylation and dimerization through cysteine bonds, generates active molecules of 30 and 38 kd.

The lymphokine induces stromal fibroblast production of IL-1β, G-CSF, IFN-γ, IL-6, IL-8, prostaglandin E, and LIF and induces macrophage production of TNF-α, IL-β, IL-6, IL-10, and IL-12 (281,282). TNF-α and IFN-γ had an additive effect on IL-1 induction of IL-6, and the combination of IL-17 and TNF-α promotes GM-CSF release by synovial fibroblasts. Keratinocytes express IL-17R and IL-17, both directly and in synergy with IFN-γ or TNF-α (or both); IL-17 stimulates synthesis and release of IL-8 and augments ICAM-1 expression by these cells (283). By virtue of its ability to induce certain hematopoietic growth factors, IL-17 sustains the maturation of CD34$^+$ progenitors to neutrophils when cultured with fibroblasts (284). In mice, delivery of high levels of IL-17 by adenovector resulted in a 10-fold rise in neutrophils with marked splenic myelopoiesis, partially explained by acute induction of elevated levels of G-CSF (285).

Interleukin-18

IL-18 was first identified as an IFN-γ–inducing agent in endotoxic shock, and the cloned gene product induces IFN-γ production by T cells (286). IL-18 mRNA predicts for a protein precursor of 192 amino acids with an unusual leader sequence of 35 amino acids and an active protein of 18.3 kd. IL-18–producing tissues include kidney, liver, skeletal muscle, lung, bone, and skin, and specific cell types include osteoblasts, keratinocytes, monocyte-macrophages, and DCs (Table 1.2) (287). IL-18 lacks a conventional signal sequence, and an aspartate-specific protease has been implicated in its processing. One such protease, ICE, has been shown to liberate active IL-18. In ICE-deficient mice, which are deficient in IL-1β production, their failure to produce IFN-γ on LPS stimulation can be attributed to failure to process pro-IL-18 to its active form (288). The receptor for IL-18 was shown to be identical to a receptor isolated earlier on the basis of homology to the IL-1R (289). The IL-18R signals through the IL-1 receptor–associated kinase (IRAK) pathway to induce nuclear translocation of p65/p50 NF-κB complex.

Exposure to IL-18 enhances host defense and aids resistance to bacterial, fungal, and parasitic pathogens. Antigenically stimulated T_H1 T cells exposed to IL-18 secrete IL-2 and GM-CSF in addition to IFN-γ, and they proliferate at a greater rate than nontreated cells. IL-18 alone stimulates low-level IFN-γ production by NK cells but induces a remarkable increase when combined with IL-2 or IL-12. Purified B cells also produce IFN-γ in response to anti-CD40 antibody, IL-12, and IL-18. IL-18 inhibits osteoclast formation through T-cell ($CD4^+$ or $CD8^+$) production of GM-CSF (287). IL-18 production by mature osteoblasts may be one mechanism to limit osteoclast formation acting through T-cell GM-CSF induction.

HEMATOPOIETIC REGULATORS SIGNALING THROUGH CLASS III RECEPTOR TYROSINE KINASES

Receptor tyrosine kinases comprise several classes and can be divided into at least four groups according to their amino acid sequences. Of greatest importance to hematopoietic regulation are the class III receptor tyrosine kinases that share structural characteristics such as five heavily glycosylated immunoglobulin-like domains in their extracellular domain and an interrupted kinase domain in their catalytic intracellular region. This class (Table 1.3) includes the protooncogene *KIT*, corresponding to the ''*white spotting locus*'' in the mouse; *FMS*, encoding the CSF-1 or M-CSF receptor; and the α and β forms of the PGDF receptor. Another member of this family is the murine gene for fetal liver kinase-2 *(Flk2)* (290) and its human equivalent, designated FMS-like tyrosine kinase-3 *(FLT3)* (291). The encoded Flk-2 and FLT-3 are nearly identical in amino acid sequence, differing only in two amino acids in the extracellular domain and 31 amino acids near the C-terminus in the cytoplasmic domain.

KIT LIGAND

Mutations at the *Steel* and *White spotting* loci in mice cause macrocytic anemia, infertility, and depigmentation. The complementary relationship between the *S1* and *W* mutations implied that their gene products function in one biochemical pathway. This was confirmed by the demonstration that the *S1* and *W* loci encode a ligand-receptor pair—the Kit receptor tyrosine kinase, the gene product of the protooncogene *Kit* (292,293) and its ligand (i.e., Kit ligand, SCF, steel factor) (294,295). Mice bearing the *S1* mutation have normal stem cells but a defective hematopoietic environment because of absent or truncated ligand production, whereas *W* mutants have intrinsic stem cell defects because of Kit receptor mutations. W anemic mice can be ''cured'' by intravenous injection of S1 marrow, whereas correction of S1 anemia requires grafting of intact hematopoietic microenvironment, such as a neonatal spleen from a W mouse.

Two alternatively spliced KIT ligand RNA transcripts encode two cell-associated KIT ligand proteins, KL-1 and KL-2, of 248 and 220 amino acids, respectively, and differing in their sequences N-terminal of the transmembrane segment (296). Both transcripts are expressed in a tissue-specific fashion. The presence of a major proteolytic cleavage site on KL-1 provides a mechanism for production of a biologically active, soluble form of KIT ligand, whereas KL-2 provides a differentially more stable, cell-associated form of KIT ligand. Analysis of the phenotype of W anemic mice with receptor defects and S1 mice with total deletion of Kit ligand or with expression of a truncated, soluble ligand with no transmembrane forms (S1 Dicke) or mice engineered to express only the KL-2 splice variant has provided insight into the crucial role of this signaling system in hematopoiesis. Normal, *in vitro*, long-term hematopoiesis can be sustained by coculture of S1/S1 HSCs on W marrow stroma but not in the reverse combination (297).

A hallmark of mice carrying *W* and *S1* mutations is a profound effect on mast cell development, with mice lacking virtually all mast cells. The erythroid defect is manifest as a reduced mean hematocrit percentage and increased mean erythrocyte volume, with diminished response to hypoxia and blood loss. Marrow cellularity and erythroid, myeloid, and megakaryocyte progenitors are all decreased, and mutant mice display an increased sensitivity to total body irradiation.

KIT receptors are expressed on the most primitive populations of hematopoietic cells, including stem cells and committed progenitors, and tissue mast cells exhibit high levels of KIT (296). Soluble KIT ligand is a potent mast cell growth factor on its own and a potent synergistic factor when combined with a variety of cytokines (e.g., Il-3, GM-CSF, G-CSF, erythropoietin, thrombopoietin) in stimulating early and late progenitor populations of myeloid, erythroid, and megakaryocyte lineage. Soluble KIT ligand also promotes survival of primitive hematopoietic cells, preventing their apoptosis on growth-factor deprivation or gamma irradiation (298). KIT ligand also has important effects on cell–extracellular matrix and cell-cell interactions. Interaction of KIT with cells expressing membrane forms of KIT ligand mediate adhesion (e.g., of mast cells to fibroblasts). KIT ligand also induces adhesion of marrow cells to a fibronectin matrix by an inside-out mechanism, requiring KIT kinase activity. This is mediated by $\alpha_5\beta_1$ integrins, and the concentration of KIT ligand needed to induce adhesion is about 20 times lower than that required for proliferation (299,300).

Potential clinical uses of KIT ligand have been limited by adverse events involving dermal mast cell activation with pruritic wheal formation and 10% to 20% of patients developing allergic-like reactions characterized by urticaria and, in some cases, laryngeal edema. Lower doses of KIT ligand (SCF) have been used in conjunction with G-CSF for mobilization of $CD34^+$ cells, resulting in significant improvement in the quantity of CD34 cells harvested and in their quality as measured by *ex vivo* expansion potential and stem cell content (25,301).

FLK-2/FLT-3 LIGAND

The FLK-2/FLT-3 receptor is activated by a cognate molecule called the FLT-3 ligand. The human and murine ligands have been cloned and shown to encode a type I transmembrane protein and a soluble protein (291,302,303). Genetic mapping localizes the FLT-3 ligand gene to human chromosome 19q13.3 (304,305). Alternative splicing of a putative sixth exon can lead to the generation of a soluble form of the ligand by insertion of a stop codon into the reading frame (305). Other FLT-3 ligand isoforms that contain an extra exon encode proteins that are soluble or a long version of the transmembrane protein. cDNA has been isolated that arises from a failure to splice out an intron, resulting in a protein in which the entire C-terminus of the protein is replaced, leading to a biologically active cell-bound protein resistant to proteolytic cleavage and unable to generate a soluble form of the ligand (305).

FLK-2/FLT-3 ligand promotes the survival and stimulates proliferation, differentiation, and mobilization of early murine and human precursors, differing from KIT ligand in that it does not potentiate erythropoiesis nor stimulate mast cells (305). Unlike KIT ligand, it does potentiate the growth of pro-B cells (304). It primarily acts as a synergistic factor, maximally stimulating colony formation or *in vitro* $CD34^+$ cell proliferation when combined with IL-3, IL-6, KIT ligand, GM-CSF, or thrombopoietin (306). Of all the cytokines, FLT-3 ligand appears to be the most effective synergistic factor in promoting stem cell self-renewal, resulting in expansion of stem cell numbers *in vitro*, as measured by LTC-IC assay, with cord blood cells (188) and adult bone marrow (307) when combined with thrombopoietin. FLK-2/FLT-3 ligand enhances the rate of growth of IL-3–dependent colonies by shortening the duration of the G_1 phase of each cell cycle, an effect abrogated by addition of TGF-β (308). FLK-2/FLT-3 ligand is an important cofactor for the growth of primitive B-cell progenitors, synergizing with IL-6, IL-11, or G-CSF to support formation of multilineage colonies from mouse marrow, of which about 30% are lymphohematopoietic and give B-cell colonies when replaced into secondary cultures with IL-7 and KIT ligand (309). FLK-2/FLT-3 ligand also synergizes with IL-7 in promoting expansion and differentiation of human fetal marrow pro-B cells *in vitro* (310).

In vivo treatment of mice and primates with FLT-3 ligand demonstrated that it is a potent mobilizer of hematopoietic progenitors and, when combined with G-CSF, gives much higher mobilization levels than does either cytokine alone. Dramatic numeric increases in DCs of T lymphocyte and myeloid derivation are seen after FLT-3 ligand treatment in spleen, marrow, peripheral blood, peritoneal cavity, thymus, lymph nodes, liver, and lung (311,312). Up to 15% to 20% of splenocytes are DCs, in contrast to 0.5% in controls, and a high percentage (10% to 15%) of $CD8^+$ cells express DC markers. Combinations of FLT-3 ligand and IL-12 significantly increase the numbers of functionally active DC recovered from marrow and spleen (313), and these cytokine combinations had a synergistic antitumor effect.

CHEMOKINES

Chemokines comprise a family of more than 50 small, secretory or membrane bound proteins of 6 to 14 kd (Table 1.4). They are characterized by four conserved cysteines forming two essential disulfide bonds. The α or CXC and the β or CC subgroups are distinguished according to the position of the first two cysteines, which are adjacent (CC) or separated by one amino acid (CXC) (314,315). Genes for each subfamily are clustered on separate chromosomes; α-chemokine genes are on chromosome 4q12-21, and β-chemokine genes are on chromosome 17q11-23. Two additional factors, lymphotactin and fractalkine/neurotactin, are included in the chemokine family; the former has two instead of four conserved cysteines, and the latter has three amino acids between the first two cysteines (CX_3C) (314,315).

The receptors for chemokines are heptahelical and are coupled to GTP-binding proteins. Five receptors for CXC chemokines and nine receptors for CC chemokines have been characterized (Table 1.5). The versatility and redundancy of the chemokine signaling system is demonstrated by the recognition that most receptors recognize more than one chemokine, and several chemokines bind to more than one receptor (Table 1.5).

The chemokines were initially thought of as proinflammatory agents because they are inducible by inflammatory stimuli and attract leukocytes that mediate inflammation, but is clear that they are involved in the normal function of the immunohematopoietic system and the migration of immature blood cells, naive lymphocytes, and DCs. Additional interest in the chemokines followed the discovery in 1996 that some of their receptors function as binding sites for AIDS viruses (316).

The prototypic CXC chemokine is IL-8 (reviewed earlier). It is an ELR chemokine that shares a common three amino acid motif close to the N terminus, between it and the first cysteine. Other members include the growth related oncogene (GRO) family of neutrophil-specific chemoattractants, also secreted by activated mononuclear cells, and epithelium-derived neutrophil-activating peptide-78 (ENA-78) and GCP-2. The earliest member of the non-ELR CXC family to be purified was platelet factor-4 (PF-4). It is a very weak neutrophil chemotactic agent, but it attracts fibroblasts, and like the IFN-γ-inducible chemokine IP-10, it inhibits endothelial cell proliferation and is antiangiogenic (314,315). Monokine induced by interferon-γ (MIG) is another IFN-γ–inducible chemokine isolated from macrophages and, like IP-10, has chemoattractant activity for tumor-infiltrating lymphocytes.

The CXC chemokine SDF-1, which signals through CXCR4, was isolated from bone marrow stromal cells and was shown to be an early B-cell growth-stimulating factor (317). It is a major regulator of leukocyte (e.g., lymphocyte, monocyte) migration and promotes chemotaxis of primitive hematopoietic progenitors and stem cells (see section on stem cells) and of megakaryocytes and platelets (see section on megakaryopoiesis). Mice with knocked-out SDF-1 or CXCR5 have similar phenotypes involving *in utero* or perinatal mortality associated with failure of bone marrow development, reduced B lymphopoiesis, and severe defects in ventricular septal development (68,69). There are also defects

TABLE 1.4. *Chemokine superfamily*

CXC-chemokines	
IL-8	Interleukin-8
GRO-α	Growth-related oncogene-α
GRO-β	Growth-related oncogene-β (MIP-2α)
GRO-γ	Growth-related oncogene-γ (MIP-2β)
NAP-2	Neutrophil activating peptide
ENA-78	Epithelial-derived neutrophil attractant-78
GCP-2	Granulocyte chemoattractant protein-2
PF-4	Platelet factor-4
IP-10	Interferon-γ–inducible protein-10
SDF-1α	Stromal cell–derived factor-1α (PBSF)
SDF-1β	Stromal cell–derived factor-1β
BLC	B-lymphocyte chemoattractant (BCA-1)
MIG	Monokine induced by interferon-γ
CC-chemokines	
MCP-1	Monocyte chemoattractant protein-1 (MCAF)
MCP-2	Monocyte chemoattractant protein-2
MCP-3	Monocyte chemoattractant protein-3
MCP-4	Monocyte chemoattractant protein-4
Eotaxin	Eosinophil chemotactic factor
MPIF-1	Myeloid progenitor inhibitory factor-1 (MIP-3, CKβ-8)
MPIF-2	Myeloid progenitor inhibitory factor-2 (eotaxin-2)
RANTES	Regulated on activation of normal T-cell expressed and secreted
MIP-1α	Macrophage inflammatory protein-1α
MIP-1β	Macrophage inflammatory protein-1β
MIP-3α	Macrophage inflammatory protein-3α (LARC)
MIP-3β	Macrophage inflammatory protein-3β (ELC, CKβ-11, SCYA-19)
MCIF	Macrophage colony inhibitory factor (HCC-1, NCC-2, CKβ-1, SCYA-14)
TARC	Thymus and activation-regulated chemokine
MDC	Macrophage-derived chemokine
PARC	Pulmonary and activation-regulated chemokine (DCCK-1/MIP-4α, SCYA-18
SLC	Secondary lymphoid tissue chemokine (6–ckine, exodus-2)
LKN-1	Leukotactin (MIP-5)
I-309	Small inducible cytokine subfamily A-1 (SCYA-1)

LARC, liver and activation-regulated chemokine; CK, creatine kinase.

TABLE 1.5. *Chemokine receptors: ligand specificity and cellular localization*

Receptor	Ligand	Receptor expression
CXCR1	IL-8, GCP-2	Neu, M, T, NK
CXCR2	IL-8, GRO-α, GRO-β, GRO-γ, GCP-2, NAP-2, ENA-78, LIX	Neu, M, act./mem.T, naive B, act.B, NK,
CXCR3	IP-10, MIG, SLC,	act./mem.T, T_H1, M
CXCR4	SDF-1	Ty, act./mem.T, T_H1, T_H2, naive B, act.B, PreB, M, Plt, Meg, SC, PC, DC
CXCR5	BLC	naive B,
CCR1	MIP-1α, RANTES, MCP-3, LKN-1, MPIF-1, MCIF	M, T_H2, T_H1, act./mem.
CCR2	MCP-1, -2, -3, -4, -5,	M, act./mem.T, T_H1, T_H2, naive B, act. B, Bas
CCR3	RANTES, LKN-1, MCP-2, -3, -4, Eotaxin, MPIF-2, RANTES	act./mem.T, DC, T_H2, Eos, PC, SC, Bas,
CCR4	TARC, MDC,	T_H2, act./mem.T, Bas, Plt
CCR5	RANTES, MIP-1α, MIP-1β	Ty, T_H1, T_H2, act./mem.T, M, B, DC
CCR6	MIP-3α	act./mem.T, B
CCR7	MIP-3β, SLC, MCP-1	Ty, act./mem.T, T_H1, T_H2 B, naive B, act B, PreB,
CCR8	I-309, TARC, MIP-1β	T act./mem.,Ty, T_H2,
XCR1	Lymphotactin	T
CX_3C	Fractalkine	act./mem.T

Ty, thymocyte; T, T lymphocyte; act., activated; mem., memory; B, B lymphocyte; PreB, B-cell progenitors; M, monocyte/macrophage; DC, dendritic cells; Eos, eosinophil; Neu, neutrophil; Bas, basophil, Plt, Platelets; Meg, megakaryocytes; SC, stem cells; PC, progenitor cells; for cytokines, see Table 1.4.

in cerebellar architecture, indicating a chemotactic role for SDF-1 in neuronal migration. Defective vascularization of the gastrointestinal tract indicates a role for CXCR4 receptor in organ-specific vascular development. The SDF-1/CXCR4 system points to an potentially important role of chemokines in morphogenesis where cells that form tissues may initially be kept in close contact by chemoattractants.

The prototypic CC chemokine MCAF/MCP-1 was identified as a monocyte chemotactic and activating factor. It induces intracellular calcium influx, respiratory burst, release of lysosomal enzymes, and expression of adhesion molecules such as β_2 integrins; enhances tumoricidal activity; and induces production of tissue factor and proinflammatory cytokines such as IL-6 and IL-1 (318). MCP-1 induces chemotaxis of basophils and induces their release of histamine and leukotriene. It is also chemotactic for $CD4^+$ and $CD8^+$ T lymphocytes and, *in vitro*, for NK cells. Three chemokines, MCP-2, -3 and -4, are closely related to MCP-1 and display similar activity against monocytes, T lymphocytes, and NK cells, although there are differences in potency. MCP-2, -3, and -4, but not MCP-1, exhibit potent eosinophil chemotactic and activating effects on eosinophils, whereas only MCP-3 is chemotactic for DCs.

Macrophage inflammatory protein-1 (MIP-1) was initially purified as an 8-kd protein doublet produced by endotoxin-stimulated macrophages that induced neutrophil accumulation at sites of injection. The protein preparation was later shown to be composed of two highly related proteins: MIP-1β and MIP-1α. MIP-1 is induced during T-cell activation and induces activated T-cell adhesion to endothelium, facilitating their egress from the circulation. MIP-1α is chemotactic for activated $CD8^+$ T cells, and MIP-1β is chemotactic for activated $CD4^+$ T cells, and both are chemotactic for activated naive and memory T cells (319). Both MIP-1 forms activate NK function in $CD56^+$ cells (320). Macrophages produce and respond to both forms of MIP-1, and the response involves induction of secretion of TNF, IL-1, and IL-6; the MIP-1 complex induces macrophage chemotaxis. A marrow macrophage-derived inhibitor, CFU-S proliferation inhibitory factor, was shown to be identical to MIP-1α (321). MIP-1α inhibits proliferation of primitive pluripotent cells with extensive proliferative potential (e.g., CFU-S, CFU-GEMM) but is not active on true stem cells with long-term *in vivo* reconstituting ability (319).

The regulated on activation, normally T-cell expressed and secreted (RANTES) molecule is produced by mitogen- or antigen-activated T cells and is nearly as potent a monocyte chemoattractant as MCP-1 but is much less effective in stimulating exocytosis. It promotes transendothelial chemotaxis of CD4 and CD8 cells, and it attracts and activates NK cells. It is an important chemoattractant for eosinophils and induces histamine release by basophils (320).

Leukotactin-1 (i.e., MIP-5) and two murine chemokines (i.e., macrophage inflammatory protein-related proteins-1 and -2) are classified as C6 β-chemokines because they contain six rather than four conserved cysteines (322). Leukotactin is a potent chemoattractant for neutrophils, monocytes, and lymphocytes, inducing calcium flux in CCR1- and CCR3-expressing cells. It also suppresses colony formation by human granulocyte-macrophage, erythroid, and multipotent progenitor cells stimulated by combinations of growth factors. In methylcellulose hematopoietic progenitor clonogenic assays, a number of chemokines have been identified as suppressive (i.e., MIP-1α, GRO-β, PF4, IL-8, MCP-1, IP-10, and CCF18), and mixtures are synergistic in their suppression (321).

Fractalkine is the prototype member of a fourth class of chemokines bearing a CX3C fingerprint (323). The molecule exists as a membrane-anchored or as a shed 95-kd glycoprotein; the latter has potent chemotactic activity for T cells and monocytes, and the former, induced on activated endothelium, promotes leukocyte adhesion.

RANTES, MIP-1α, and MIP-1β were the first chemokines shown to chemoattract lymphocytes (314,315). The monocyte chemoattractants MCP-1 through MCP-4 are also potent attractants of T lymphocytes, NK cells, and DCs. Modulation of receptors CCR1, CCR2, and CCR5 on lymphocytes determines their response to chemokines. IL-2 upregulates these receptors, but antigen stimulation downmodulates them. T lymphocytes may migrate in response to chemokines after IL-2 stimulation but not during antigen-induced activation. After viral infection or in delayed-type hypersensitivity reactions, production of IP-10 and MIG is induced by IFN-γ, which inhibits the production of most other chemokines; these CXC chemokines then chemoattract CXCR3-expressing IL-2–activated T lymphocytes. The T_H1 and T_H2 populations of $CD4^+$ helper T cells differentially express different chemokine receptors (Table 1.5), with CCR5 expressed preferentially by T_H1 cells, whereas CCR3 and CCR4 characterize T_H2 cells. The complex interplay of chemokines in the development and trafficking of lymphocytes is shown in Figure 1.5.

The interaction of DCs with B and T cells and their trafficking from sites where they process antigens (e.g., skin LCs) to sites where they present antigen to lymphocytes in lymph nodes and spleen is regulated by chemokines. The CC chemokines MCP-3, MIP-1α, RANTES, and MIP-3β and the CXC chemokine SDF-1 elicit chemotactic migration and increased intracellular Ca^{2+} in DCs, with responsiveness to the different chemokines depending on maturation stage (314,315). Several M- and T-tropic strains of HIV can enter DCs through CCR5 and CXCR4 (or a non-CXCR4 SDF-1 receptor), respectively, and entry can be blocked by a CCR5 ligand RANTES and the CXCR4 ligand SDF-1 (316,324). CCR3, the eotaxin receptor, is expressed on DCs and may be used as an entry coreceptor for dual-tropic HIV strains (325). Mature, but not immature (HLA-DR^{lo}, $CD83^-$), DCs express CCR7 and respond to MIP-3β. Immature, but not mature, DCs, respond to MCP-3, MIP-1α, and RANTES (326). These latter chemokines can mediate migration of immature DCs located in peripheral sites, whereas MIP-3β can direct migration of antigen-carrying DCs from

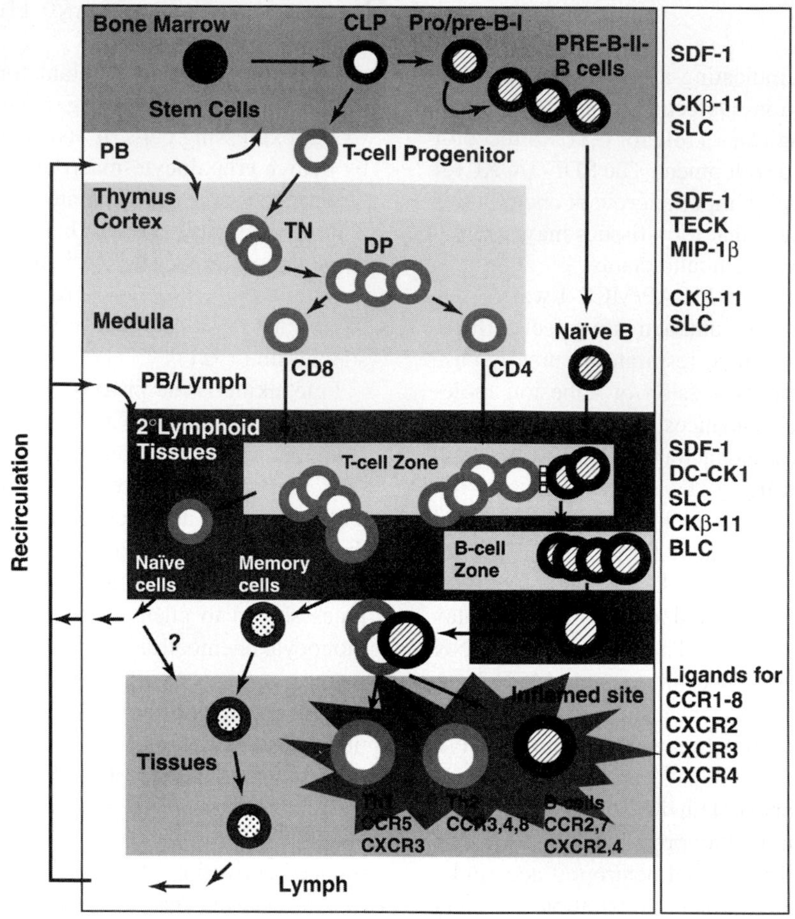

FIG. 1.5 Chemokines and the development and trafficking of lymphocytes. Lymphocytes at different developmental stages have different sensitivities to chemokines. Developing lymphocytes differentially express chemokine receptors to modulate their chemotactic sensitivity to certain chemokines, which enables them to find and be localized at certain microenvironments or niches in primary, secondary, or tertiary lymphoid tissues. Early common lymphoid progenitors (CLP) for T cells and B cells originate from bone marrow. Trafficking of bone marrow hematopoietic progenitor cells is likely to be regulated by stromal cell–derived factor 1 (SDF-1) and perhaps other unidentified chemokines. Thymic T-cell progenitors undergo several differentiation stages to become SP thymocytes. At the Dp thymocyte stage, thymocytes undergo selection processes that allow only functional thymocytes with no reactivity to self-antigens to proceed into the SP stages. Chemokines such as SDF-1, macrophage inflammatory protein-1β (MIP-1β, TECK, and CKβ-11 differentially attract thymocyte subsets, a possible trafficking signal for thymocyte migration in thymus. Mature SP T cells migrate and recirculate to secondary lymphoid tissues until they meet specific antigens for activation. T cells are localized in T-cell zones in lymph nodes, spleen, or Peyer's patches. Chemokines such as SDF-1, SLC (secondary lymphoid tissue chemokine), CKβ-11, and DC-CK1 can be involved in the migration of naive T cells to T-cell zones. These chemokines are expressed in secondary lymphoid tissues or, more specifically, in T-cell zones. B cells with specific surface antigen receptors are generated in bone marrow. They also undergo antigen-dependent selection at an immature (IgD^+IgM^-) stage. Mature (naive) IgD^+IgM^+ B cells migrate to peripheral lymphoid tissues. SDF-1, CKβ-11, SLC, and BLC (B-lymphocyte chemoattractant) are possible chemoattractants for the migration of naive B cells to secondary lymphoid tissues. Naive B cells catch, internalize, and process antigens in the secondary lymphoid tissues and present them to T cells in the T-cell zones. With the help of T cells (cytokines and cognate interaction), B cells proliferate and differentiate. Activated B cells form germinal centers and go through affinity maturation and somatic mutation in the germinal centers in B-cell areas (i.e., follicles) of the secondary lymphoid tissues. The efficacious B-cell chemoattractant, BLC, is expressed in the follicles of the secondary lymphoid tissues. BLC and its receptor CXCR5 are essential to form and maintain the germinal centers. Activation at germinal centers of the secondary lymphoid tissues also modulates chemotactic responsiveness, but not receptor expression (CXCR4), of B cells to SDF-1. Most chemokine receptors (CCR1 to CCR8, CXCR2, CXCR3, and CXCR4) appear to be involved in the migration of effector or memory lymphocytes. CCR7 or CXCR4 ligands (SLC, CKβ-11, and SDF-1) are also chemotactively active for activated lymphocytes. Antibody-producing B cells (i.e., plasma cells) are found in the secondary lymphoid tissues (i.e., red pulp of spleen and the medulla and deep cortex of lymph nodes) and in the bone marrow, a major site of antibody production. SDF-1, produced from bone marrow stromal cells, can attract plasma cells to the bone marrow. (Adapted from Kim CH, Broxmeyer HE. Chemokines: signal lamps for trafficking of T and B cells for development and effector function. *J Leukoc Biol* 1999;65:6–15, with permission.)

peripheral inflammatory sites, where DCs are stimulated to upregulate CCR7, to lymphoid organs. A CC chemokine DC-CK-1/PARK is specifically expressed at high levels by DCs present in germinal centers and T-cell areas of secondary lymphoid organs (327). It specifically attracts naive T cells to the DC and plays an important role in the induction of an immune response.

The involvement of chemokines in allergy follows from the observation that eotaxin, RANTES, and MCP-3 activate eosinophil and basophil leukocytes. Eotaxin in particular is expressed in the lungs of animals with asthma and in human tissues where eosinophils accumulate (328). Lymphocytes expressing the eotaxin receptor CCR3 are also found with eosinophils in allergic infiltrates.

SUMMARY AND CONCLUSIONS

The complexity of hematopoiesis presents a challenge to those dedicated to understanding the normal steady-state equilibrium between the stem cell compartment and the mature cells in the circulation. It is even more of a challenge to understand pathologic perturbations. For more than 100 years, the main tools remained the stained cells and the microscope. Modern hematology then encompassed immunologic profiling using the CD antigens and *in vitro* culture techniques that revealed the potentialities of the rare, morphologically identifiable stem and progenitor cells.

A considerable portion of this review has been taken up with a description of the cytokine and chemokine families that are involved in the proliferation, differentiation, and function of blood cells. An understanding of these factors at the cellular and molecular level is critical to an understanding of hematopoiesis. The profound alteration in patterns of hematopoiesis produced by resetting the level of a single hematopoietic growth factor is amply illustrated in the cases of erythropoietin, thrombopoietin, or G-CSF, and more subtle alterations are seen with perturbations of virtually every one of these regulatory molecules. From the knowledge of normal patterns of production and response of these regulatory macromolecules, it is increasingly possible to define perturbations in these patterns at the molecular level that are the cause or consequence of hematopathology. In particular, neoplastic transformation leads to perturbation in production of these regulators and in response of the transformed cells to normal cytokine or chemokine signaling. With a more complete understanding of normal control of hematopoietic growth and differentiation, a better understanding of the leukemic phenotype should be possible. This should allow the development of strategies to restore a more regulated pattern of behavior on cells that have escaped from normal growth control.

REFERENCES

1. Till JE, McCulloch EA. A direct measurement of the radiation sensitivity of normal mouse bone marrow cells. *Radiat Res* 1961;14: 213–222.
2. Hendrikx PJ, Martens ACM, Hagenbeek A, et al. Homing of fluorescently labeled murine hematopoietic stem cells. *Exp Hematol* 1996; 24:129–140.
3. Magli MC, Iscove NN, Odartchenko N. The transient nature of early hematopoietic spleen colonies. *Nature* 1982;295:527–529.
4. Moore MAS. Stem cell proliferation: Ex vivo and in vivo observations. *Stem Cells* 1997;15(Suppl 1):239–251.
5. Harrison DE, Stone M, Astle CM. Effects of transplantation on the primitive immunohematopoietic stem cell. *J Exp Med* 1990;172: 431–437.
6. Bhatia M, Wang JCY, Kapp U, et al. Purification of primitive human hematopoietic cells capable of repopulating immune-deficient mice. *Proc Natl Acad Sci USA* 1997;94:5320–5325.
7. Shimizu Y, Ogawa M, Kobayashi M, et al. Engraftment of cultured human hematopoietic cells in sheep. *Blood* 1998;91:3688–3692.
8. Osawa M, Hanada K, Hamada H, et al. Long-term lymphohematopoietic reconstitution by a single CD34$^+$ low/negative hematopoietic stem cell. *Science* 1996;273:242–245.
9. Bhatia M, Bonnet D, Murdoch B, et al. A newly discovered class of human hematopoietic cells with SCID-repopulating activity. *Nat Med* 1998;Sept 4(9):1038–1044.
10. Zanjani ED, Almeida-Porada G, Livingston AG, et al. Human bone marrow CD34$^-$ cells engraft in vivo and undergo multilineage expression that includes giving rise to CD34$^+$ cells. *Exp Hematol* 1998;26: 353–360.
11. Kennedy M, Firpo M, Choi K, et al. A common precursor for primitive erythropoiesis and definitive haematopoiesis. *Nature* 1997;386: 488–493.
12. Bjornson CRR, Rietze RL, Reynolds BA, et al. Turning brain into blood: a hematopoietic fate adopted by adult neural stem cells in vivo. *Science* 1999;283:534–537.
13. Shi Q, Rafii S, Wu MH-D, et al. Evidence for circulating bone marrow-derived endothelial cells. *Blood* 1998;92:362–367.
14. Peichev M, Naiyer AJ, Hicklin D, et al. Expression of VEGFR-2 and AC133 by circulating human CD34$^+$ cells identifies a population of functional endothelial precursors. *Blood.* 2000;95(3):952–958.
15. Pettengell R, Moore MAS. Hematopoietic stem cells: proliferation, purification, and clinical applications. In: Quesenberry PJ, Stein GS, Forget BG, Weissman SM, eds. *Stem cell biology and gene therapy.* New York: Wiley-Liss, 1998:133–159.
16. Lansdorp PM. Self-renewal of stem cells. *Biol Blood Marrow Transplant* 1997;3:171–178.
17. Chaudhary PM, Robinson IB. Expression and activity of p-glycoprotein, a multidrug efflux pump in human hematopoietic stem cells. *Cell* 1991;66:85–94.
18. Yin AH, Miraglia S, Zanjani ED, et al. AC133, a novel marker for human hematopoietic stem and progenitor cells. *Blood* 1997;90: 5002–5012.
19. Moore MAS. Clinical implications of positive and negative hematopoietic stem cell regulators [Review Stratton Lecture]. *Blood* 1991; 78:1–19.
20. Muench MO, Schneider JG, Moore MAS. Interactions among colony stimulating factors, IL-1β, IL-6 and Kit-ligand (KL) in the regulation of primitive murine hematopoietic cells. *Exp Hematol* 1992;20: 339–349.
21. Ogawa M. Differentiation and proliferation of hematopoietic stem cells. *Blood* 1993;81:2844–2853.
22. Metcalf D. Pre-Progenitor cells: a proposed new category of hematopoietic precursor cells. *Leukemia* 1997;12:1–3.
23. Srour EF, Bregni M, Traycoff CM, et al. Long-term hematopoietic culture-initiating cells are more abundant in mobilized peripheral blood grafts than in bone marrow but have a more limited ex vivo expansion potential. *Blood* 1996;22:68–81.
24. Moore MAS, Hoskins I. Ex vivo expansion of cord blood derived stem cells and progenitors. *Blood Cells* 1994;20:468–481.
25. Shapiro F, Yao T-J, Moskowitz C, et al. Effects of prior therapy on the in vitro proliferative potential of stem cell factor plus Filgrastim-mobilized CD34-positive progenitor cells. *Clin Cancer Res* 1997;3: 1571–1578.
26. Dexter TM, Allen TD, Lajth A. Conditions controlling the proliferation of hematopoietic stem cells in vitro. *J Cell Physiol* 1977;91: 335–344.
27. Moore MAS, Broxmeyer HE, Sheridan APC, et al. Continuous human

bone marrow culture: Ia antigen characterization of probable human pluripotential stem cells. *Blood* 1980;55:682–690.
28. Sutherland HJ, Lansdorp PM, Henkelman DH, et al. Functional characterization of individual human hematopoietic stem cells cultured at limiting dilution on supportive marrow stromal layers. *Proc Natl Acad Sci USA* 1990;87:3584–3588.
29. Lemieux ME, Rebel VI, Lansdorp P, et al. Characterization and purification of a primitive hematopoietic cell type in adult mouse marrow capable of lymphomyeloid differentiation in long-term marrow "switch" cultures. *Blood* 1995;86:1339–1347.
30. Ogawa M, Porter PN, Nakahata T. Renewal and commitment of hematopoietic stem cells (an interpretative review). *Blood* 1983;61: 823–829.
31. Brummendorf TH, Dragowska W, Zijlmans J, et al. Asymmetric cell divisions sustain long-term hematopoiesis from single-sorted human fetal liver cells. *J Exp Med* 1998;188:1117–1127.
32. Huang S, Francis K, Law P, et al. Kinetics and symmetry of initial cell division of human $CD34^+/CD38^-$ cells from different ontogenic age. *Biol Blood Marrow Transplant* 1998;4:107(abst).
33. Lin H, Schagat T. Neuroblasts: a model for the asymmetric division of stem cells. *Trends Genet* 1997;13:33–39.
34. Chenn A, McConnell SK. Cleavage, orientation, and the asymmetric inheritance of Notch-1 immunoreactivity in mammalian neurogenesis. *Cell* 1995;82:631–641.
35. Rhym M, Jan L, Jan YN. Asymmetric distribution of numb protein during division of the sensory organ precursor confers distinct fates to daughter cells. *Cell* 1994;76:477–491.
36. Moore MAS, Han W, Ye Q. Notch signaling during hematopoiesis. In: Zon L, ed. Hematopoiesis: a developmental approach. New York: Oxford University Press, 1999.
37. Enver T, Heyworth CM, Dexter TM. Do stem cells play dice? *Blood* 1998;92:348–351.
38. McKinstry WJ, Chung-Leung L, Rasko JEJ, et al. Cytokine receptor expression on hematopoietic stem and progenitor cells. *Blood* 1997; 89:65–71.
39. Hu M, Krause D, Greaves M, et al. Multilineage gene expression precedes commitment in the hematopoietic system. *Genes Dev* 1997; 11:774–780.
40. Rich IN. Homeobox genes and hematopoiesis: an emerging picture for genomic therapy. *J Hematother* 1998;7:515–520.
41. Ho AD, Young D, Maruyama M, et al. Pluripotent and lineage-committed $CD34^+$ subsets in leukapheresis products mobilized by G-CSF, GM-CSF, vs. a combination of both. *Exp Hematol* 1996;24: 1460–1468.
42. Francis K, Ramakrishna R, Holloway W, et al. Two new pseudopod morphologies displayed by the human hematopoietic KG1a progenitor cell line and by primary human $CD34^+$ cells. *Blood* 1998;92: 3616–3623.
43. Mohle RS, Murea M, Kirsch M, et al. Differential expression of L-selectin, VAL-4, and LAF-1 on $CD34^+$ progenitor cells from bone marrow and peripheral blood during G-CSF enhanced recovery. *Exp Hematol* 1995;23:1535–1542.
44. Kodama H, Nose M, Niida S, et al. Involvement of the c-kit receptor in the adhesion of hematopoietic cells to stromal cells. *Exp Hematol* 1994;22:979–984.
45. Papayannopoulou T, Craddock C. Homing and trafficking of hematopoietic progenitor cells. *Acta Haematol* 1997;97:97–104.
46. Watanaba T, Dave B, Heimann DG, et al. Cell adhesion molecule expression on $CD34^+$ cells in grafts and time to myeloid and platelet recovery after autologous stem cell transplantation. *Exp Hematol* 1998;26:10–18.
47. Kovach NL, Tin N, Yednock T, et al. Stem cell factor modulates avidity of alpha 4 beta 1 and alpha 5 beta 1 integrins expressed on hematopoietic cell lines. *Blood* 1995;85:159–167.
48. Cui L, Ramsfjell V, Borge OJ, et al. Thrombopoietin promotes adhesion of primitive human hematopoietic cells to fibronectin and vascular cell adhesion molecule-1: role of activation of very late antigen (VLA)-4 and VLA-5. *J Immunol* 1997;159:1961–1969.
49. To LB, Haylock DN, Dowse T, et al. A comparative study of the phenotype and proliferative capacity of peripheral blood (PB) $CD34^+$ cells mobilized by four different protocols and those of steady state PB and bone marrow $CD34^+$ cells. *Blood* 1994;84:2930–2939.
50. Mohle R, Bautz F, Rafii S, et al. The chemokine receptor CXCR-4 is expressed on $CD34^+$ hematopoietic progenitors and leukemic cells and mediates transendothelial migration induced by stromal cell-derived factor-1. *Blood* 1998;91:4523–4530.
51. Jo D-Y, Rafii S, Hamada T, et al. Chemotaxis of primitive hematopoietic cells in response to stromal cell-derived factor-1. *J Clin Invest.* 2000;105(1):101–111.
52. Peled A, Petit I, Kollet O, et al. Dependence of human stem cell engraftment and repopulation of NOD/SCID mice on CXCR4. *Science* 1999;283:845–848.
53. Vazir H, Dragowska W, Allsop RC, et al. Evidence for a mitotic clock in human hematopoietic stem cells: loss of telomeric DNA with age. *Proc Natl Acad Sci USA* 1994;91:9857–9860.
54. Engelhardt M, Kumar R, Albanell J, et al. Telomerase regulation, cell cycle, and telomere stability in primitive hematopoietic cells. *Blood* 1997;90:182–193.
55. Notaro R, Cimmino A, Tabarini D, et al. In vivo telomere dynamics of human hematopoietic ste cells. *Proc Natl Acad Sci USA* 1997;94: 13782–13785.
56. Hayflick L, Moorhead P. The limited in vitro lifetime of human diploid cell strains. *Exp Cell Res* 1961;25:585–621.
57. Holt SE, Shay JW, Wright WE. Refining the telomere-telomerase hypothesis of aging and cancer. *Nat Biotech* 1996;14:836–839.
58. Engelhardt M, Ozkaynak MF, Drullinsky P, et al. Telomerase activity and telomere length in pediatric patients with malignancies undergoing chemotherapy. *Leukemia* 1998;12:13–24.
59. Bodnar AG, Ouellette M, Frolkis M, et al. Extension of lifespan by introduction of telomerase into normal human cells. *Science* 1998; 279:349–352.
60. Bradley TR, Metcalf D. The growth of mouse bone marrow cells in vitro. *Aust J Exp Biol Med* 1966;44:287–299.
61. Pluznik DH, Sach L. The cloning of normal "mast" cells in tissue culture. *J Cell Physiol* 1965;66:319–324.
62. Moore MAS, Metcalf D. Ontogeny of the haemopoietic system: Yolk sac origin of in vivo and in vitro colony forming cell in the developing mouse embryo. *Br J Haematol* 1970;18:279–296.
63. Labastie M-C, Cortes F, Romeo P-H, et al. Molecular identify of hematopoietic precursor cells emerging in the human embryo. *Blood* 1998;92:3624–3635.
64. Ogawa M, Kizumoto M, Nishikawa S, et al. Expression of α4-Integrin defines the earliest precursor of hematopoietic cell lineage diverged from endothelial cells. *Blood* 1999;93:1168–1177.
65. Medvinsky A, Dzzierzak E. Definitive hematopoiesis is autonomously initiated by the AGM region. *Cell* 1996;86:897–906.
66. Moore MAS, Owen JJT. Stem cell migration in developing myeloid and lymphoid systems. *Lancet* 1967;2:658–659.
67. Yoder MC, Hiatt K, Dutt P, et al. Characterization of definitive lymphohematopoietic stem cells in the day 9 murine yolk sac. *Immunity* 1997;7:335–344.
68. Nagasawa T, Hirota S, Tachibana K, et al. Defects of B-cell lymphopoiesis and bone-marrow myelopoiesis in mice lacking the CXC chemokine PBSF/SDF-1. *Nature* 1996;382:635–638.
69. Zou Y-R, Kottmann AH, Kuroda M, et al. Function of the chemokine receptor CXCR4 in haematopoiesis and in cerebellar development. *Nature* 1998;393:595–599.
70. Chervenick PA, Zucker-Franklin D, Moore MAS. In vitro and in vivo hematopoiesis. In: Zucker-Franklin D, Greaves MF, Grossi CE, et al. *Atlas of blood cells.* Milan: Edi-Ermes, 1988:1–27.
71. Wilkins BS, Jones DB. Immunophenotypic characterization of stromal cells in aspirated human bone marrow samples. *Exp Hematol* 1998;26:1061–1067.
72. Simmons PJ, Torok-Storb B. CD34 Expression by stromal precursors in normal human adult bone marrow. *Blood* 1991;78:2848–2853.
73. Moore MAS, Sheridan APC, Allen TD, et al. Prolonged hematopoiesis in a primate bone marrow culture system: characteristics of stem cell production and the hematopoietic microenvironment. *Blood* 1979;54: 775–793.
74. Wineman J, Moork K, Lemischka I, et al. Functional hetergeneity of the hematopoietic microenvironment: rare stromal elements maintain long-term repopulating stem cells. *Blood* 1996;87:4082–4090.
75. Roecklein BA, Torok-Storb B. Functionally distinct human marrow stromal cell lines immortalized by transduction with the human papillomavirus E6/E7 genes. *Blood* 1995;85:997–1005.
76. Castro-Malaspina H, Gay RE, Resnick G, et al. Characterization of

human bone marrow fibroblast colony-forming cells (CFU-F) and their progeny. *Blood* 1980;56:289–301.
77. Cattoretti G, Schiro R, Orazi A, et al. Bone marrow stroma in humans: anti-nerve growth factor receptor antibodies selectively stain reticular cells in vivo and in vitro. *Blood* 1993;81:1726–1738.
78. Prockop DJ. Marrow stromal cells as stem cells for non-hematopoietic tissues. *Science* 1997;276:71–74.
79. Gimble JM, Wanker F, Wang CS, et al. Regulation of bone marrow stromal cell differentiation by cytokines whose receptors share the gp130 protein. *J Cell Biochem* 1994;54:122–133.
80. Zannettino ACW, Buhring H-J, Niutta S, et al. The sialomucin CD164 (MGC-24v) is an adhesive glycoprotein expressed by human hematopoietic progenitors and bone marrow stromal cells that serves as a potent negative regulator of hematopoiesis. *Blood* 1998;92: 2613–2678.
81. Heinrich MC, Bagby GC. The role of hematopoietic stromal cells in the regulation of hematopoiesis. In: Cacciola E, Deisseroth AB, Giustolisi R, eds. *Hematopoietic growth factors: oncogenesis and cytokines in clinical hematology.* Basel: Kruger, 1994:22–48.
82. Migliaccio G, Migliaccio AR, Petti S, et al. Human embryonic hemopoiesis: kinetics of progenitors and precursors underlying the yolk sac–liver transition. *J Clin Invest* 1986;78:51–60.
83. Jandl JH. *Blood.* Boston: Little, Brown, 1987.
84. Koury St, Koury MJ, Bondurant MC, et al. Quantitation of erythropoietin-producing cells in kidneys of mice by in situ hybridization: correlation with hematocrit, renal erythropoietin mRNA, and serum erythropoietin concentration. *Blood* 1989;74:645–651.
85. Lazarides E, Woods C. Biogenesis of the red blood cell mem brane–skeleton and the control of erythroid morphogenesis. *Annu Rev Biol* 1989;5:427–452.
86. Tsai S, Emerson SG, Sieff CA, et al. Differential binding of erythroid and myeloid progenitors to fibroblasts and fibronectin. *Blood* 1987; 69:1587–1594.
87. Cronkite EP. Analytical review of structure and regulation of hemopoiesis. *Blood Cells* 1988;14:313–328.
88. Warren DJ, Moore MAS. Synergism among interleukin 1, interleukin 3, and interleukin 5 in the production of eosinophils from primitive hemopoietic stem cells. *J Immunol* 1988;140:94–99.
89. Denburg JA. Heterogeneity of human peripheral blood eosinophil-type colonies: evidence for a common basophil-eosinophil progenitor. *Blood* 1985;66:312–318.
90. Hart DNJ. Dendritic cells: unique leukocyte population which control the primary immune response. *Blood* 1997;90:3245–3287.
91. Banchereau J, Steinman RM. Dendritic cells and the control of immunity. *Nature* 1998;392:245–252.
92. Young JW, Szabolcs P, Moore MAS. Identification of dendritic cell colony-forming units among normal human $CD34^+$ bone marrow progenitors that are expanded by c-kit-ligand and yield pure dendritic cell colonies in the presence of granulocyte/macrophage colony-stimulating factor and tumor necrosis factor a. *J Exp Med* 1995;182: 1111–1120.
93. Szabolcs P, Avigan D, Gezelter S, et al. Dendritic cells and macrophages can mature independently from a human bone marrow-derived, post-colony-forming unit intermediate. *Blood* 1996;87:4520–4530.
94. Brossard P, Grunebach F, Stuhler G, et al. Generation of functional human dendritic cells from adherent peripheral blood monocytes by CD40 ligation in the absence of granulocyte-macrophage colony-stimulating factor. *Blood* 1998;92:4238–4247.
95. Randolph GJ, Beaulieu S, Lebecque S, et al. Differentiation of monocytes into dendritic cells in a model of transendothelial trafficking. *Science* 1998;282:480–483.
96. Strobl H, Riedl E, Bell-Fernandez C, et al. Epidermal Langerhans cell development and differentiation. *Immunology* 1997;198:588–605.
97. Shortman K, Caix C. Dendritic cell development: multiple pathways to nature's adjuvants. *Stem Cells* 1997;15:409–419.
98. Bjorck P, Kincade PW. Cutting edge: $CD19^+$ pro-B cells can give rise to dendritic cells in vitro. *J Immunol* 1998;161:5795–5999.
99. Akagawa KS, Takasuka N, Nozaki Y, et al. Generation of $CD1^+RelB^+$ dendritic cells and tartrate-resistant acid phosphatase-positive osteoclast-like multinucleate giant cells from human monocytes. *Blood* 1996;88:4029–4039.
100. Lacey DL, Timms E, Tan HL, et al. Osteoprotegerin ligand is a cytokine that regulates osteoclast differentiation and activation. *Cell* 1998; 93:165–176.
101. Kong Y-Y, Yoshida H, Sarosi I, et al. OPGL is a key regulator of osteoclastogenesis, lymphocyte development, and lymph node organogenesis. *Nature* 1999;397:315–323.
102. Debili N, Issaad C, Masse J-M, et al. Expression of CD34 and platelet glycoproteins during human megakaryocytic differentiation. *Blood* 1992;80:3022–3035.
103. Zucker-Franklin D, Yang J-S, Grusky G. Characterization of glycoprotein IIb/IIIa positive cells in human umbilical cord blood: their potential usefulness as megakaryocyte progenitors. *Blood* 1992;79: 347–355.
104. Zucker-Franklin D, Kaushansky K. Effect of thrombopoietin on the development of megakaryocytes and platelets: an ultrastructural analysis. *Blood* 1996;88:1632–1638.
105. De Sauvage FJ, Carver-Moore K, Luoh S-M, et al. Physiological regulation of early and late stages of megakaryocytopoiesis by thrombopoietin. *J Exp Med* 1996;183:651–656.
106. Shivdasani RA, Fielder P, Keller GA, et al. Regulation of the serum concentration of thrombopoietin in thrombocytopenic NF-E2 knockout mice. *Blood* 1997;90:1821–1827.
107. Nagahisa H, Nagata Y, Ohnuki T, et al. Bone marrow stromal cells produce thrombopoietin and simulate megakaryocyte growth and maturation but suppress proplatelet formation. *Blood* 1996;87: 1309–1316.
108. Levine RF, Eldor A, Hyam E, et al. Megakaryocyte interaction with subendothelial extracellular matrix is associated with adhesion, platelet-like shape change and thromboxane A2 production. *Blood* 1985; 66:570–576.
109. Avraham HS, Cowley SY, Chi SJ, et al. Characterization of adhesive interactions between human endothelial cells and megakaryocytes. *J Clin Invest* 1993;91:2378–2384.
110. Hagiwara T, Nagasawa T, Nagahisa H, et al. Expression of adhesion molecules on cytoplasmic processes of human megakaryocytes. *Exp Hematol* 1996;24:690–695.
111. Levine RF, Eldor A, Shoff PK, et al. Circulating megakaryocytes: delivery of large numbers of intact, mature megakaryocytes to the lungs. *Eur J Haematol* 1993;51:233–246.
112. Davis RE, Stenberg PE, Levin J, et al. Localization of megakaryocytes in normal mice and following administration of platelet antiserum, 5-fluorouracil, or radiostrontium: evidence for the site of platelet production. *Exp Hematol* 1997;25:638–648.
113. Hamada T, Mohle R, Hesselgesser J. Transendothelial migration of megakaryocytes in response to stromal cell–derived factor 1 (SDF-1) enhances platelet formation. *J Exp Med* 1998;188:539–548.
114. Zauli G, Vitale M, Falcieri E, et al. In vitro senescence and apoptotic cell death of human megakaryocytes. *Blood* 1997;90:2234–2243.
115. Radley JM, Holder CJ. Fate of senescent megakaryocytes in the bone marrow. *Br J Haemataol* 1983;53:277–287.
116. Harker LA, Finch CA. Thrombokinetics in man. *J Clin Invest* 1969; 48:963–974.
117. Ihle NJ. Cytokine receptor signalling. *Nature* 1995;377:591–594.
118. Bagley CJ, Woodcock JM, Stomaski FC, et al. The structural and functional basis of cytokine receptor activation: lessons from the common β subunit of the granulocyte-macrophage colony-stimulating factor, interleukin-3 (IL-3), and IL-5 receptors. *Blood* 1997;89: 1471–1482.
119. Hirano T, Nakajima K, Hibi M. Signaling mechanisms through gp 130: a model of the cytokine system. *Cytokine Growth Factor Rev* 1997;8:241–252.
120. Metcalf D. Hematopoietic regulators: redundancy or sublety? *Blood* 1993;82:3515–3523.
121. Yoshimura A. The CIS family: negative regulators of JAK-STAT signaling. *Cytokine Growth Factor Rev* 1998;9:197–204.
122. Nicholson SE, Hilton DJ. The SOCS proteins: a new family of negative regulators of signal transduction. *J Leukoc Biol* 1998;63:665–668.
123. Yoshimura A, Ohkubo T, Kiguchi T, et al. A novel cytokine-inducible gene CIS encodes an SH2-containing protein that binds to tyrosine-phosphoryated interleukin 3 and erythropoietin receptors. *EMBO J* 1995;14:2816–2826.
124. Starr R, Willson TA, Viney EM, et al. A family of cytokine-inducible inhibitors of signalling. *Nature* 1997;387:917–920.
125. Welte K, Platzer E, Lu L, et al. Purification and biochemical characterization of human pluripotent hematopoietic colony-stimulating factor. *Proc Natl Acad Sci USA* 1985;82:152–1530.
126. Souza LM, Boone TC, Gabrilove JL, et al. Recombinant human granulocyte colony-stimulating factor: effects on normal and leukemic myeloid cells. *Science* 1986;232:61–65.

127. Gabrilove JL, Jakubowski A, Scher H, et al. Effect of granulocyte colony-stimulating factor on neutropenia and associated morbidity due to chemotherapy for transitional-cell carcinoma of the urothelium. *N Engl J Med* 1988;318:1414–1422.
128. Moore MAS. Hematopoietic growth factors. In: Kelley WN, ed. *Textbook of internal medicine,* 3rd ed. Philadelphia: Lippincott-Raven, 1997:1522–1525.
129. Metcalf D. The granulocyte-macrophage regulators: reappraisal by gene inactivation. *Exp Hematol* 1995;23:569–572.
130. Jacob J, Huag JS, Raptis S, et al. Specific signals generated by the cytoplasmic domain of the granulocyte colony-stimulating factor (G-CSF) receptor are not required for G-CSF–dependent granulocyte differentiation. *Blood* 1998;92:353–361.
131. Roberts AW, Nicola NA. Granulocyte colony-stimulating factor. In: Garland JM, Quesenberry PJ, Hilton DJ, eds. *Colony stimulating factors:* molecular and cellular biology, 2nd ed. New York: Marcel Dekker, 1997:203–225.
132. Anderlini P, Przepiorka D, Champlin R, et al. Biological and clinical effects of granulocyte-colony-stimulating factor in normal individuals. *Blood* 1996;88:2819–2825.
133. Welte K, Gabrilove J, Bronchud MH, et al. Filgrastim (r-metHuG-CSF): the first 10 years. *Blood* 1996;88:1907–1929.
134. Johnston EM, Crawford J. Hematopoietic growth factors in the reduction of chemotherapeutic toxicity. *Semin Oncol* 1998;25:552–561.
135. Robinson W, Metcalf D, Bradley TR. Stimulation by normal and leukemic mouse sera of colony formation in vitro by mouse bone marrow cells. *J Cell Physiol* 1967;69:83–92.
136. Stanley ER, Metcalf D. Partial purification and some properties of the factor in normal and leukaemic human urine stimulating mouse bone marrow colony growth in vitro. *Aust J Exp Biol Med Sci* 1969; 47:467–483.
137. Stanley ER, Heard PM. Factors regulating macrophage production and growth: purification and some properties of the colony-stimulating factor from medium conditioned by mouse L cells. *J Biol Chem* 1977;252:4305–4312.
138. Morris SW, Valentine MB, Shapiro DN, et al. Reassignment of the human CSF-1 gene to chromosome 1p13-p21. *Blood* 1991;78: 2013–2020.
139. Kawasaki ES, Ladner MB, Wang AM, et al. Molecular cloning of a complementary DNA encoding human macrophage-specific colony-stimulating factor (CSF-1). *Science* 1985;230:291–296.
140. Wong GG, Temple PA, Leary AC, et al. Human CSF-1: molecular cloning and expression of 4 kb cDNA encoding the human urinary protein. *Science* 1987;235:1504–1508.
141. Glocker MO, Arbogast B, Schreurs J, et al. Assignment of the inter- and intramolecular disulfide linkages in recombinant human macrophage colony-stimulating factor using fast atom bombardment mass spectrometry. *Biochemistry* 1993;32:482–488.
142. Moore MAS. Macrophage colony-stimulating factor. In: Garland JM, Quesenberry PJ, Hilton DJ, eds. *Colony stimulating factors: molecular and cellular biology,* 2nd ed. New York: Marcel Dekker, 1997: 255–289.
143. Bartocci A, Mastrogiannis DS, Migliorati G, et al. Macrophages specifically regulate the concentration of their own growth factor in the circulation. *Proc Natl Acad Sci USA* 1987;84:6179–6183.
144. Hamilton JA. Coordinate and noncoordinate colony-stimulating factor formation by human monocytes. *J Leukoc Biol* 1994;55:355–361.
145. Sherr CJ. Colony-stimulating factor-1 receptor. *Blood* 1990;75:1–12.
146. Rothstein G, Rhondeau SM, Peters CA, et al. Stimulation of neutrophil production in CSF-1 responsive clones. *Blood* 1988;72:898–902.
147. Moore MAS, Warren DJ. Synergy of interleukin 1 and granulocyte colony-stimulating factor: *in vivo* stimulation of stem-cell recovery and hematopoietic regeneration following 5-fluorouracil treatment of mice. *Proc Natl Acad Sci USA* 1987;84:7134–7138.
148. Wiktor-Jedrzejczak W, Bartocci A, et al. Total absence of colony-stimulating factor 1 in the macrophage-deficient osteopetrotic (op/op) mouse. *Proc Natl Acad Sci USA* 1990;87:4828–4832.
149. Sanda MG, Yang JC, Topalian SL, et al. Intravenous administration of recombinant human macrophage colony-stimulating factor to patients with metastatic cancer: a phase I study. *J Clin Oncol* 1992;10: 1643–1649.
150. Inaba T, Shimano H, Gotoda T, et al. Macrophage colony-stimulating factor regulates both activities of neutral and acidic cholesteryl ester hydrolases in human monocyte-derived macrophages. *J Clin Invest* 1993;92:750–757.
151. Wong GG, Witek J, Temple PA, et al. Human GM-CSF: molecular cloning of the complementary DNA and purification of the natural and recombinant proteins. *Science* 1985;228:810–815.
152. Van Leeuwen BH, Martinson ME, Webb GC, et al. Molecular organization of the cytokine gene cluster, involving the human IL-3, IL-4, IL-5, and GM-CSF genes, on human chromosome 5. *Blood* 1989;73: 1142–1148.
153. Willman CL, Sever CE, Pallavicini MG, et al. Deletion of IRF-1 mapping to chromosome 5q31.1, in human leukemia and preleukemic myelodysplasia. *Science* 1993;259:968–971.
154. Rasko JEJ. Granulocyte-macrophage colony-stimulating factor and its receptor. In: Garland JM, Quesenberry PJ, Hilton DJ, eds. *Colony stimulating factors: molecular and cellular biology,* 2nd ed. New York: Marcel Dekker, 1997:163–202.
155. Gough NM, Gearing DP, Nicola NA, et al. Localization of the human GM-CSF receptor gene to the X-Y pseudoautosomal region. *Nature* 1990;345:734–736.
156. Nishinakamura R, Miyajima A, Mee PJ, et al. Hematopoiesis in mice lacking the entire granulocyte-macrophage colony-stimulating factor/interleukin-3/interleukin-5 functions. *Blood* 1996;88:2458–2464.
157. Armitage JO. Emerging applications of recombinant human granulocyte-macrophage colony-stimulating factor. *Blood* 1998;92: 4491–4508.
158. Ishibashi T, Yokoyama K, Shindo J, et al. Potent cholesterol-lowering effect by human granulocyte-macrophage colony-stimulating factor in rabbits: possible implication of enhancement of macrophage functions and an increase in mRNA for VLDL receptor. *Arterioscler Thromb* 1994;14:1534–1541.
159. Erslev A. Humoral regulation of red cell production. *Blood* 1953;8: 349–357.
160. Miyake T, Kung CK, Goldwasser E. Purification of human erythropoietin. *J Biol Chem* 1977;252:5558–5564.
161. Jacobs K, Shoemaker C, Rudersdorf R, et al. Isolation and characterization of genomic and cDNA clones of human erythropoietin. *Nature* 1985;313:806–810.
162. Lin FK, Suggs S, Lin CH, et al. Cloning and expression of the human erythropoietin gene. *Proc Natl Acad Sci USA* 1985;82:7580–7584.
163. Koury ST, Koury MJ, Bondurant MC, et al. Quantitation of erythropoietin-producing cells in kidneys of mice by in situ hybridization: correlation with hematocrit, renal erythropoietin mRNA, and serum erythropoietin concentration. *Blood* 1989;74:645–651.
164. Watowich SS. Erythropoietin. In: Garland JM, Quesenberry PJ, Hilton DJ, eds. *Colony stimulating factors: molecular and cellular biology,* 2nd ed. New York: Marcel Dekker, 1997:291–313.
165. Watowich SS, Hilton DJ, Lodish HF. Activation and inhibition of erythropoietin receptor function: role of receptor dimerization. *Mol Cell Biol* 1994;14:3535–3549.
166. Sawada K, Krantz SB, Dai CH, et al. Purification of human blood burst-forming units—erythroid and demonstration of the evolution of erythropoietin receptors. *J Cell Physiol* 1990;142:219–230.
167. Jubinsky PT, Krijanovski OI, Nathan DG, et al. The β chain of the interleukin-3 receptor functionally associates with the erythropoietin receptor. *Blood* 1997;90:1867–1873.
168. Kaushansky K, Broudy VC, Lin N, et al. Thrombopoietin, the Mpl ligand, is essential for full megakaryocyte development. *Proc Natl Acad Sci USA* 1995;92:3234–3238.
169. Yin T, Taga T, Tsang M-S, et al. Involvement of IL-6 signal transducer gp130 in IL-11–mediated signal transduction. *J Immunol* 1993;151: 2555–2561.
170. Tepler I, Elias L, Smith JW, et al. A randomized placebo-controlled trial of recombinant human interleukin-11 in cancer patients with severe thrombocytopenia due to chemotherapy. *Blood* 1996;87: 3607–3614.
171. Vigon I, Momon JP, Cocault L, et al. Molecular cloning and characterization of mpl, the human homolog of the v-*mpl* oncogene: Identification of a member of the hematopoietic growth factor receptor superfamily. *Proc Natl Acad Sci USA* 1992;89:5640–5644.
172. Methia M, Louache F, Vainchenker W, et al. Oligodeoxynucleotides antisense to the proto-oncogene c-*mpl* specifically inhibit in vitro megakaryocytopoiesis. *Blood* 1993;82:1395–1401.
173. De Sauvage FJ, Haas PE, Spencer SD, et al. Stimulation of megakary-

ocytopoiesis and thrombopoiesis by the c-Mpl ligand. *Nature* 1994;369:533–538.
174. Lok S, Kaushansky K, Holly RD, et al. Cloning and expression of murine thrombopoietin cDNA and stimulation of platelet production in vivo. *Nature* 1994;369:565–568.
175. Bartley TD, Bogenberger J, Hunt P, et al. Identification and cloning of a megakaryocyte growth and development factor that is a ligand for the cytokine receptor Mpl. *Cell* 1994;77:1117–1124.
176. Sohma Y, Akahori H, Seki N, et al. Molecular cloning and chromosomal localization of the human thrombopoietin gene. *FEBS Lett* 1994;353:57–61.
177. Kuter DJ, Beeler DL, Rosenberg RD. The purification of megapoietin: a physiological regulator of megakaryocyte growth and platelet production. *Proc Natl Acad Sci USA* 1994;91:11104–11108.
178. O'Malley CJ, Rasko JEJ, Basser RL, et al. Administration of pegylated recombinant human megakaryocyte growth and development factor to humans stimulates the production of functional platelets that show no evidence of in vivo activation. *Blood* 1996;88:3288–3298.
179. Harker LA, Marzec UM, Kelly AB, et al. Prevention of thrombocytopenia and neutropenia in a nonhuman primate model of marrow suppressive chemotherapy by combining pegylated recombinant human megakaryocyte growth and development factor and recombinant human granulocyte colony-stimulating factor. *Blood* 1997;89:155–165.
180. Dale DC, Nichol JL, Rich DA, et al. Chronic thrombocytopenia is induced in dogs by development of cross-reacting antibodies to the MpL ligand. *Blood* 1997;90:3456–3461.
181. Narumi K, Suzuki M, Song W, et al. Intermittent, repetitive corticosteroid-induced upregulation of platelet levels after adenovirus-mediated transfer to the liver of a chimeric glucocorticoid-responsive promoter controlling the thrombopoietin cDNA. *Blood* 1998;92:822–833.
182. Yan X-Q, Lacey D, Hill D, et al. A model of myelofibrosis and osteosclerosis in mice induced by overexpressing thrombopoietin (mpl ligand): reversal of disease by bone marrow transplantation. *Blood* 1996;88:402–409.
183. Frey BM, Rafii S, Teterson M, et al. Adenovector-mediated expression of human thrombopoietin cDNA in immune-compromised mice: insights into the pathophysiology of osteomyelofibrosis. *J Immunol* 1998;160:691–699.
184. Bunting S, Widmer R, Lipari T, et al. Normal platelets and megakaryocytes are produced in vivo in the absence of thrombopoietin. *Blood* 1997;90:3423–3429.
185. Solar GP, Kerr WG, Zeigler FC, et al. Role of c-mpl in early hematopoiesis. *Blood* 1998;92:4–10.
186. Kaushansky K. Thrombopoietin and the hematopoietic stem cell. *Blood* 1998;92:1–3.
187. Borge OJ, Ramsfjell V, Cui L, et al. Ability of early acting cytokines to directly promote survival and suppress apoptosis of human primitive $CD34^+CD38^-$ bone marrow cells with multilineage potential at the single cell level: key role of thrombopoietin. *Blood* 1997;90:2282–2292.
188. Piacibello W, Sanavio F, Garetto, L, et al. Extensive amplification and self-renewal of human primitive hematopoietic stem cells from cord blood. *Blood* 1997;89:2644–2653.
189. Stoffel R, Wiestner A, Skoda RC. Thrombopoietin in thrombocytopenic mice: evidence against regulation at the mRNA level and for a direct regulatory role of platelets. *Blood* 1996;87:567–573.
190. Eaton DL, de Sauvage FJ. Thrombopoietin: the primary regulator of megakaryocytopoiesis and thrombopoiesis. *Exp Hematol* 1997;25:1–7.
191. Fielder PJ, Gurney AL, Stefanich E, et al. Regulation of thrombopoietin levels by c-mpl–mediated binding to platelets. *Blood* 1996;87:2154–2161.
192. Emmons RVB, Reid DM, Cohen RL, et al. Human thrombopoietin levels are high when thrombocytopenia is due to megakaryocyte deficiency and low when due to platelet destruction. *Blood* 1996;87:4068–4071.
193. Shivdasani RA, Rosenblatt MF, Zucker-Franklin D, et al. Transcription factor NF-E2 is required for platelet formation independent of the action of thrombopoietin/MGDF in megakaryocyte development. *Cell* 1995;81:695–704.
194. Dinarello CA. Interleukin 1. *Cytokine Growth Factor Rev* 1997;8:253–265.
195. Auron PE. The Interleukin 1 receptor: ligand interactions and signal transduction. *Cytokine Growth Factor Rev* 1998;9:221–237.
196. Stanley ER, Bartocci A, Patinkin D, et al. Regulation of very primitive multipotent hematopoietic cells by hemopoietin-1. *Cell* 1986;45:667–674.
197. Iscove NN, Shaw AR, Keller G. Net increase of pluripotent hematopoietic precursors in suspension culture in response to IL-1 and IL-3. *J Immunol* 1989;142:2332–2337.
198. Muench MO, Firpo MT, Moore MAS. Bone marrow transplantation with interleukin-1 plus kit-ligand ex vivo expanded bone marrow accelerates hematopoietic reconstitution in mice without the loss of stem cell lineage and proliferative potential. *Blood* 1993;81:3463–3473.
199. Kobayashi M, Imamura M, Gotohda Y, et al. Synergistic effect of interleukin-1β and interleukin-3 on the expansion of human hematopoietic progenitor cells iin liquid culture. *Blood* 1991;78:1947–1953.
200. Brugger W, Heimfeld S, Bemeson RJ, et al. Reconstitution of hematopoiesis after high-dose chemotherapy by autologous progenitor cells generated ex vivo. *N Engl J Med* 1995;333:283–287.
201. Zucali JR, DuBois CM, Oppenheim JJ. Hematopoietic effects of Interleukin-1. In: Garland JM, Quesenberry PJ, Hilton DJ, eds. *Colony stimulating factors: molecular and cellular biology,* 2nd ed. New York: Marcel Dekker, 1997:347–368.
202. Neta R, Douches S, Oppenheim JJ. IL-1 is a radioprotector. *J Immunol* 1986;136:2483–2485.
203. Moreb J, Zucali JR, Zhang Y, et al. Role of aldehyde dehydrogenase in the protection of hematopoietic progenitor cells from 4-hydroperoxycyclophosphamide by interleukin-1β and tumor necrosis factor. *Cancer Res* 1992;52:1770–1774.
204. Eastgate J, Moreb J, Nick HS, et al. A role for manganese superoxide dismutase in radioprotection of hematopoietic stem cells by IL-1. *Blood* 1993;81:639–646.
204a. Crown J, Jakubowski A, Kemeny N, et al. A phase 1 trial of recombinant human interleukin-1β alone and in combination with myelosuppressive doses of 5-fluorouracil in patients with gastrointestinal cancer. *Blood* 1991;78:1420–1427.
205. Tushinski RJ, Mule JJ. Biology of cytokines: the interleukins. In: De Vita VT Jr, Hellman S, Rosenberg SA, eds. *Biologic therapy of cancer,* 2nd ed. Philadelphia: JB Lippincott, 1995:87–94.
206. Morgan DA, Ruscetti FW, Gallo R. Selective in vitro growth of T lymphocytes from normal human bone marrow. *Science* 1976;193:1007–1008.
207. Welte K, Wang CY, Mertelsmann R, et al. Purification of human interleukin-2 to apparent homogeneity and its molecular heterogeneity. *J Exp Med* 1982;156:454–464.
208. Taniguchi T, Matsui H, Fujita T, et al. Structure and expression of a cloned cDNA for human interleukin-2. *Nature* 1983;302:305–310.
209. Lin J-X, Leonard WJ. Signaling from the IL-2 receptor to the nucleus. *Cytokine Growth Factor Rev* 1997;8:313–332.
210. Waldmann TA. The multi-subunit interleukin-2 receptor. *Annu Rev Biochem* 1989;58:875–911.
211. Lotz MT. Biological therapy with Interleukin-1: preclinical studies. In: DeVita VT Jr, Hellman S, Rosenberg SA, eds. *Biologic therapy of cancer,* 2nd ed. Philadelphia: JB Lippincott, 1995:207–233.
212. Ihle JN, Keller J, Oroszlan S, et al. Biological properties of homogeneous interleukin-3. I. Demonstration of WEHI-3 growth factor activity, mast cell growth factor activity, P-cell stimulating factor activity, colony-stimulating factor activity, and histamine-producing factor activity. *J Immunol* 1983;131:282–287.
213. Yang YC, Ciarletta AB, Temple PA, et al. Human IL-3 (multi-CSF): identification by expression cloning of a novel hematopoietic growth factor related to murine IL-3. *Cell* 1986;47:3–10.
214. Sato N, Miyajima A. A multimeric cytokine receptor: common versus specific functions. *Curr Opin Cell Biol* 1994;6:174–179.
215. Yang Y-C. Human Interleukin-3: an overview. In: Garland JM, Quesenberry PJ, Hilton DJ, eds. *Colony stimulating factors: molecular and cellular biology,* 2nd ed. New York: Marcel Dekker, 1997:227–254.
216. Moore MAS. Interleukin 3: an overview. In: Schrader J, ed: Lymphokines, vol 15. New York: Academic Press, 1988:219–280.
217. Thomassen MJ, Antal JM, Connors MJ, et al. Immunomodulatory effects of recombinant interleukin-3 treatment on human alveolar macrophages and monocytes. *J Immunother* 1993;14:43–50.
218. Tavassoli M, Konno M, Shiota Y, et al. Enhancement of the grafting efficiency of transplanted marrow cells by preincubation with interleu-

kin-3 and granulocyte-macrophage colony-stimulating factor. *Blood* 1991;77:1599–1606.
219. Van der Loo NCM, Ploemacher RE. Marrow- and spleen-seeding efficiencies of all murine hematopoietic stem cell subsets are decreased by preincubation with hematopoietic growth factors. *Blood* 1995;85:2598–2606.
220. Peters SO, Kittler ELW, Ramshaw HS, et al. Ex vivo expansion of murine marrow cells with interleukin-3 (IL-3), IL-6, IL-11, and stem cell factor leads to impaired engraftment in irradiated hosts. *Blood* 1996;87:30–37.
221. Ogawa M, Yonemura Y, Ku H. In vitro expansion of hematopoietic stem cells. *Stem Cells* 1997;15(Suppl 1):7–11.
222. Matsunaga T, Hirayama F, Yonemura Y, Murray R, Ogawa M. Negative regulation by interleukin-3 (IL-3) of mouse early B-cell progenitors and stem cells in culture: transduction of negative signals by βc and βIL-3 proteins of IL-3 receptor and absence of negative regulation by granulocyte-macrophage colony-stimulating factor. *Blood* 1998; 92:901–907.
223. Cashman JD, Eaves CJ. Human growth factor-enhanced regeneration of transplantable human hematopoietic stem cells in nonobese diabetic/severe combined immunodeficient mice. *Blood* 1999;93: 481–487.
224. Gillio AP, Gasparetto C, Laver J, et al. Effects of Interleukin-3 on hematopoietic recovery after 5-fluorouracil or cyclophosphamide treatment of cynomolgus primates. *J Clin Invest* 1990;85:1560–1565.
225. Howard M, Farrar J, Hilfiker M, et al. Identification of a T-cell derived B cell growth factor distinct from interleukin-2. *J Exp Med* 1982;155: 914–921.
226. Yokota T, Otsuka T, Mosmann T, et al. Isolation and characterization of a human interleukin cDNA clone, homologous to mouse B-cell stimulatory factor 1, that expressed B-cell-stimulatory activities. *Proc Natl Acad Sci USA* 1986;83:5894–5898.
227. Keegan AD, Nelms K, Wang LM, et al. Interleukin-4 receptor: signaling mechanisms. *Immunol Today* 1994;15:423–432.
228. Fanslow WC, Spriggs MK, Rauch CT, et al. Identification of a distinct low-affinity receptor for human interleukin-4 on pre-B cells. *Blood* 1993;81:2998–3005.
229. O'Garra A, Spits H. The immunobiology of interleukin-4. *Res Immunol* 1993;144:567–643.
230. Saeland S, Banchereau J. The role of interleukin-4 in normal and malignant human hematopoiesis. In: Garland JM, Quesenberry PJ, Hilton DJ, eds. *Colony stimulating factors: molecular and cellular biology,* 2nd ed. New York: Marcel Dekker, 1997:315–346.
231. Rennick D, Yang G, Muller-Sieburg C, et al. Interleukin-4 (B-cell stimulatory factor 1) can enhance or antagonize the factor-dependent growth of hematopoietic progenitor cells. *Proc Natl Acad Sci USA* 1987;84:6889–6893.
232. Jansen JH, Wientjens G-JHM, Fibbe WE, et al. Inhibition of human macrophage colony formation by interleukin-4. *J Exp Med* 1989;170: 577–582.
233. Sanderson CJ. Interleukin-5. In: Garland JM, Quesenberry PJ, Hilton DJ, eds. *Colony stimulating factors: molecular and cellular biology,* 2nd ed. New York: Marcel Dekker, 1997:405–420.
234. Mohle R, Salemi P, Moore MAS, et al. Expression of interleukin-5 by human bone marrow microvascular endothelial cells: implications for the regulation of eosinophilopoiesis in vivo. *Br J Haematol* 1997; 99:732–738.
235. Takatsu K. Interleukin 5 and B cell differentiation. *Cytokine Growth Factor Rev* 1998;9:25–35.
236. Hirano T. Interleukin 6 and its receptor: ten years later. *Intern Rev Immunol* 1998;16:249–284.
237. Lai L, Chen F, McKenna S, et al. Identification of an IL-7–associated pre-pro-B cell growth-stimulating factor (PPBSF). II. PPBSF is a covalently linked heterodimer of IL-7 and a M_r 30,000 cofactor. *J Immunol* 1998;160:2280–2286.
238. Muegge K, Vila MP, Durum SK. Interleukin-7: a cofactor for V(D)J rearrangement of the T cell receptor β gene. *Science* 1993;261:93–95.
239. Jacobsen FW, Rusten LS, Jacobsen SE. Direct synergistic effects of interleukin-7 on in vitro myelopoiesis of human CD34$^+$ bone marrow progenitors. *Blood* 1994;84:775–779.
240. Komschlies KL, Grzegorzewski KJ, Wiltrout RH. Diverse immunological and hematological effects of interleukin-7: implications for clinical application. *J Leukoc Biol* 1995;58:623–633.
241. Grzegorzewski KJ, Komschlies KL, Jacobsen SEW, et al. Mobilization of long-term reconstituting hematopoietic stem cells in mice by recombinant human interleukin 7. *J Exp Med* 1995;181:369–374.
242. Yoshimura T, Matsushima K, Tanaka S, et al. Purification of a human monocyte-derived neutrophil chemotactic factor that has peptide sequence similarity to other host defence cytokines. *Proc Natl Acad Sci USA* 1987;84:9233–9237.
243. Mukaida N, Harada A, Matsushima K. Interleukin-8 (IL-8) and monocyte chemotactic and activating factor (MCAF/MCP-1), chemokines essentially involved in inflammatory and immune reactions. *Cytokine Growth Factor Rev* 1998;9:9–23.
244. Donnelly SC, Striter RM, Kunkel SL, et al. Interleukin-8 and development of adult respiratory distress syndrome in at-risk patient groups. *Lancet* 1993;341:643–647.
245. Kelleher K, Bean K, Clark SC, et al. Human interleukin-9 genomic sequence, chromosomal location, and sequences essential for its expression in human T-cell leukemia virus (HTLV)-1–transformed human T cells. *Blood* 1991;77:1436–1441.
246. Holbrook ST, Ohls RK, Schibler KR, et al. Effect of interleukin-9 on clonogenic maturation and cell-cycle status of fetal and adult hematopoietic progenitors. *Blood* 1991;77:2129–2134.
247. Fiorentino DF, Bond MW, Mosmann TR. Two types of mouse helper T cell. IV. Th2 clones secrete a factor that inhibits cytokine production by Th1 clones. *J Exp Med* 1989;170:2081–2095.
248. Moore KW, O'Garra A, Malefyt R de W, et al. Interleukin-10. *Annu Rev Immunol* 1993;11:165–190.
249. Steinhauser ML, Hogaboam CM, Kunkel SL, et al. IL-10 is a major mediator of sepsis-induced impairment in lung antibacterial host defense. *J Immunol* 1999;162:392–399.
250. Paul SR, Bennett F, Calvetti JA, et al. Molecular cloning of a cDNA encoding interleukin 11, a stromal cell-derived lymphopoietic and hematopoietic cytokine. *Proc Natl Acad Sci USA* 1990;87: 7512–7516.
251. Du X, Williams DA. Interleukin-11: review of molecular, cell biology, and clinical use. *Blood* 1997;89:3897–3908.
252. Rodriguez M-H, Arnaud S, Blanchet JP. IL-11 directly stimulates murine and human erythroid burst formation in semisolid cultures. *Exp Hematol* 1995;23:545–550.
253. Bruno E, Briddell RA, Cooper RJ, et al. Effects of recombinant interleukin-11 on human megakaryocyte progenitor cells. *Exp Hematol* 1991;19:378–381.
254. Tepler I, Elias L, Smith W II, et al. A randomized placebo-controlled trial of recombinant human interleukin-11 in cancer patients with severe thrombocytopenia due to chemotherapy. *Blood* 1996;87: 3607–3614.
255. Keller DC, Du XX, Srour ER, et al. Interleukin-11 inhibits adipogenesis and stimulates myelopoiesis in long-term marrow cultures. *Blood* 1993;82:1428–1435.
256. Wickenhauser C, Hillienhof A, Jungheim K, et al. Detection and quantification of transforming growth factor beta (TGF-b) and platelet-derived growth factor (DGF) release by normal human megakaryocytes. *Leukemia* 1995;9:310–315.
257. Peterson RL, Trepicchio WL, Bossa MM, et al. G1 growth arrest and reduced proliferation of intestinal epithelial cells induced by rhIL-11 may mediate protection against mucositis. *Blood* 1995;86(Suppl 1): 311a*(abst).*
258. Romas E, Udagawa N, Zhou H, et al. The role of gp130-mediated signals in osteoclast development: regulation of interleukin-11 production by osteoblasts and distribution of its receptor in bone marrow cultures. *J Exp Med* 1996;183:2581–2591.
259. Kobayashi M, Fitz L, Ryan M, et al. Identification and purification of natural killer cell stimulatory factor (NKSF), a cytokine with multiple biological effects on human lymphocytes. *J Exp Med* 1989;170: 827–846.
260. Wolf SF, Temple PA, Kobayashi M, et al. Cloning of cDNA for natural killer cell stimulatory factor, a heterodimeric cytokine with multiple biological effects on T and natural killer cells. *J Immunol* 1991;146:3074–3081.
261. Trinchieri G. Interleukin-12: a proinflammatory cytokine with immunoregulatory functions that bridge innate resistance and antigen-specific adaptive immunity. *Annu Rev Immunol* 1995;13:251–276.
262. Chua AO, Chizzonite R, Desai BB, et al. Expression cloning of a human IL-12 receptor component: a new member of the cytokine receptor superfamily with strong homology to GP130. *J Immunol* 1994;153:128–136.

263. Jacobsen SEW, Veiby OP, Smeland EB. Cytotoxic lymphocyte maturation factor (interleukin 12) is a synergistic growth factor for hematopoietic stem cells. *J Exp Med* 1993;178:413–418.
264. Hirayama F, Katayama N, Neben S, et al. Synergistic interaction between interleukin-12 and Steel factor in support of proliferation of murine lymphohematopoietic progenitors in culture. *Blood* 1994;83: 92–98.
265. Minty A, Chalon P, Derocq J-M, et al. Interleukin-13 is a new human lymphokine regulating inflammatory and immune responses. *Nature* 1993;362:248–250.
266. Hoshino T, Winkler-Pickett RT, Mason AT, et al. IL-13 production by NK cells: IL-13-producing NK and T cells are present in vivo in the absence of IFN-γ. *J Immunol* 1999;162:51–59.
267. McKenzie ANJ, Li X, Largaespada DA, et al. Structural comparison and chromosomal localization of the human and mouse IL-13 genes. *J Immunol* 1993;150:5436–5444.
268. Hilton DJ, Zhang J-G, Metcalf D, et al. Cloning and characterization of a binding subunit of the interleukin-13 receptor that is also a component of the interleukin-4 receptor. *Proc Natl Acad Sci USA* 1996;93: 497–501.
269. Yu C-R, Kirken RA, Malabarba MG, et al. Differential regulation of the Janus kinase-STAT pathway and biological function of IL-13 in primary human NK and T cells: a comparative study with IL-4. *J Immunol* 1998;161:218–227.
270. Deleuran B, Iversen L, Deleuran M, et al. Interleukin 13 suppresses cytokine production and stimulates production of 15-HETE in PBMC. *Cytokine* 1995;7:319–324.
271. Jacobsen SEW, Okkenhaug C, Veiby OP, et al. Interleukin 13: novel role in direct regulation of proliferation and differentiation of primitive hematopoietic progenitor cells. *J Exp Med* 1994;180:75–82.
272. Wills-Karp M, Luyimbazi J, Xu X, et al. Interleukin-13: central mediator of allergic asthma. *Science* 1998;282:2258–2261.
273. Ford R, Tamayo A, Martin B, et al. Identification of B-cell growth factors (interleukin-14; high molecular weight-B-cell growth factors) in effusion fluids from patients with aggressive B-cell lymphomas. *Blood* 1995;86:283–293.
274. Grabstein KH, Eisenman J, Shanebeck K, et al. Cloning of a novel T cell growth factor that interacts with the β chain of the IL-2 receptor. *Science* 1994;264:965–968.
275. Giri JG, Anderson DM, Kumaki S, et al. IL-15, a novel T cell growth factor that shares activities and receptor components with IL-2. *J Leukoc Biol* 1995;57:763–766.
276. Alleva DG, Kaser SB, Monroy MA, et al. IL-15 functions as a potent autocrine regulator of macrophage proinflammatory cytokine production: evidence for differential receptor subunit utilization associated with stimulation or inhibition. *J Immunol* 1997;159:2941–2951.
277. Avice M-N, Demeure CE, Delespesse G, et al. IL-15 promotes IL-12 production by human monocytes via T cell–dependent contact and may contribute to IL-12–mediated IFN-γ secretion by $CD4^+$ T cells in the absence of TCR ligation. *J Immunol* 1998;161:3408–3415.
278. Chapoval AI, Fuller JA, Kremlev SG, Kamdar SJ, et al. Combination chemotherapy and IL-15 administration induce permanent tumor regression in a mouse lung tumor model: NK and T cell-mediated effects antagonized by B cells. *J Immunol* 1998;161:6977–6984.
279. Center DM, Kornfeld H, Cruikshank WW. Interleukin 16 and its function as a CD4 ligand. *Immunol Today* 1996;17:476–481.
280. Chupp GL, Wright EA, Wu D, et al. Tissue and T cell distribution of precursor and mature IL-16. *J Immunol* 1998;161:3114–3119.
281. Yao Z, Painter SL, Fanslow WC, et al. Human IL-17: a novel cytokine derived from T cells. *J Immunol* 1995;155:5483–5486.
282. Chabaud M, Fossiez F, Taupin J-L, et al. Enhancing effect of IL-17 on IL-1–induced IL-6 and leukemia inhibitory factor production by rheumatoid arthritis synoviocytes and its regulation by Th2 cytokines. *J Immunol* 1998;161:409–414.
283. Albanesi C, Cavani A, Girolomoni G. IL-17 is produced by nickel-specific T lymphocytes and regulates ICAM-1 expression and chemokine production in human ketarinocytes: synergistic or antagonistic effects with IFN-γ and TNF-α. *J Immunol* 1999;162:494–502.
284. Fossiez F, Djossou O, Chomarat P, et al. T-cell interleukin-17 induces stromal cells to produce proinflammatory and hematopoietic cytokines. *J Exp Med* 1996;183:2593–2603.
285. Schwarzenberger P, La Russa V, Miller A, et al. IL-17 stimulates granolopoiesis in mice: Use of an alternate, novel gene therapy-derived method for in vivo evaluation of cytokines. *J Immunol* 1998; 161:6383–6389.
286. Okamura H, Tsutsi H, Komatsu T, et al. Cloning of a new cytokine that induces IFN-gamma production by T cells. *Nature* 1995;378: 88–91.
287. Gillespie MT, Horwood NJ. Interleukin-18: perspectives on the newest interleukin. *Cytokine Growth Factor Rev* 1998;9:109–116.
288. Gu Y, Kuida K, Tsutsui H, et al. Activation of interferon-gamma inducing factor mediated by interleukin-1β converting enzyme. *Science* 1997;275:206–209.
289. Torigoe K, Ushio S, Okura T, et al. Purification and characterization of the human interleukin-18 receptor. *J Biol Chem* 1997;272: 25737–25742.
290. Matthews W, Jordan CT, Gavin M, et al. A receptor tyrosine kinase cDNA isolated from a population of enriched primitive hematopoietic cells and exhibiting close genetic linkage to c-kit. *Proc Natl Acad Sci USA* 1991;88:9026–9030.
291. Lyman SD, James L, Vanden BT, et al. Molecular cloning of a ligand for the flt3/flk2 tyrosine kinase receptor. A proliferative factor for primitive hematopoietic cells. *Cell* 1993;75:1157–1167.
292. Chabot B, Stephenson DA, Chapman VM, et al. The proto-oncogene c-kit encoding a transmembrane tyrosine kinase receptor maps to the mouse W locus. *Nature* 1986;335:88–89.
293. Nocka K, Majumder S, Chabot B, et al. Expression of c-kit gene products in known cellular targets of W mutations in normal and W mutant mice—evidence for impaired c-kit kinase in mutant mice. *Genes Dev* 1989;3:816–826.
294. Nocka K, Huang E, Beier DR, et al. The hematopoietic growth factor KL is encoded by the SL locus and is the ligand of the c-kit receptor, the gene product of the W locus. *Cell* 1990;63:225–333.
295. Zsebo KM, Wypych J, McNiece IK, et al. Identification, purification, and biological characterization of hematopoietic stem cell factor from buffalo rat liver conditioned medium. *Cell* 1990;63:195–201.
296. Besmer P. Kit-ligand-stem cell factor. In: Garland JM, Quesenberry PJ, Hilton DJ, eds. *Colony stimulating factors: molecular and cellular biology,* 2nd ed. New York: Marcel Dekker, 1997:369–404.
297. Dexter TM, Moore MAS. *In vitro* duplication and ''cure'' of haemopoietic defects in genetically anaemic mice. *Nature* 1977;269: 412–414.
298. Keller JR, Ortiz M, Ruscetti FW. Steel factor (c-kit ligand) promotes the survivial of hematopoietic stem/progenitor cells in the absence of cell division. *Blood* 1995;86:1757–1764.
299. Levesque JP, Leavesley DI, Niutta S, et al. Cytokines increase human hematopoietic cells adhesiveness by activation of very late antigen (VLA)-4 and VLA-5 integrins. *J Exp Med* 1995;181:1805–1815.
300. Broudy VC. Stem cell factor and hematopoiesis. *Blood* 1997;90: 1345–1364.
301. Weaver A, Ryder D, Crowther D, et al. Increased numbers of long-term culture-initiating cells in the apheresis product of patients randomized to receive increasing doses of stem cell factor administered in combination with chemotherapy and a standard dose of granulocyte colony-stimulating factor. *Blood* 1996;88:3323–3328.
302. Lyman SD, James L, Zappone J, et al. Characterization of the protein encoded by flt3 (flk2) receptor-like tyrosine kinase gene. *Oncogene* 1993;8:815–822.
303. Hannum C, Culpepper J, Campbell D, et al. Ligand for Flt3/flk2 receptor regulates growth of hematopoietic stem cells and is encoded by variant RNAs. *Nature* 1994;68:643–648.
304. Shurin MR, Esche C, Lotze MT. FLT3: receptor and ligand. Biology and potential clinical application. *Cytokines Growth Factor Rev* 1998; 9:37–48.
305. Lyman SD, James L, Escobar S, et al. Identification of soluble and membrane-bound isoforms of the murine flt3 ligand generated by alternative splicing of mRNAs. *Oncogene* 1995;10:149–157.
306. Shapiro F, Pytowski B, Rafii S, et al. The effects of Flk-2/flt3 ligand as compared with c-kit ligand on short-term and long-term proliferation of $CD34^+$ hematopoietic progenitors elicited from human fetal liver, umbilical cord blood, bone marrow, and mobilized peripheral blood. *J Hematother* 1996;5:655–662.
307. Petzer AL, Zandstra PW, Piret JM, et al. Differential cytokine effects on primitive ($CD34^+/CD38^-$) human hematopoietic cells: novel responses to Flt3-ligand and thrombopoietin. *J Exp Med* 1996;183: 2551–2258.
308. Ohishi K, Katayama N, Itoh R, et al. Accelerated cell-cycling of hema-

topoietic progenitors by the flt3 ligand that is modulated by transforming growth factor-β. *Blood* 1996;87:1718–1727.
309. Hirayama F, Lyman SD, Clark SC, et al. The flt3 ligand supports proliferation of lymphohematopoietic progenitors and early B-lymphoid progenitors. *Blood* 1995;85:1762–1768.
310. Namikawa R, Muench MO, de Vries JE, et al. The FLK2/FLT3 ligand synergizes with interleukin-7 in promoting stromal-cell–independent expansion and differentiation of human fetal pro-B cells in vitro. *Blood* 1996;87:1881–1890.
311. Brasel K, McKenna HJ, Morrissey PJ, et al. Hematologic effects of flt3 ligand in vivo in mice. *Blood* 1996;88:2004–2012.
312. Maraskovsky E, Brasel K, Teepe M, et al. Dramatic increase in the numbers of functionally mature dendritic cells in Flt3 ligand-treated mice: multiple dendritic cell subpopulations identified. *J Exp Med* 1996;184:1953–1962.
313. Shurin MR, Esche C, Lotze MT. FLT3: receptor and ligand. Biology and potential clinical application. *Cytokine Growth Factor Rev* 1998; 9:37–48.
314. Rollins BJ. Chemokines. *Blood* 1997;90:909–928.
315. Kim CH, Broxmeyer HE. Chemokines: signal lamps for trafficking of T and B cells for development and effector function. *J Leukoc Biol* 1999;65:6–15.
316. Dragic T, Litwin V, Allaway GP, et al. HIV-1 entry into $CD4^+$ cells is mediated by the chemokine receptor CC-FKR-5. *Nature* 1996;381: 667–673.
317. Nagasawa T, Kikutani H, Kishimoto T. Molecular cloning and structure of a pre-B-cell growth-stimulating factor. *Proc Natl Acad Sci USA* 1994;91:2305–2309.
318. Matsushima K, Larsen CG, DuBois GC, et al. Purification and characterization of a novel monocyte chemotactic and activating factor produced by a human monocytic cell line. *J Exp Med* 1989;167: 1883–1893.
319. Plumb MA, Wright E. Macrophage inflammatory protein-1α. In: Garland JM, Quesenberry PJ, Hilton DJ, eds. *Colony stimulating factors: molecular and cellular biology,* 2nd ed. New York: Marcel Dekker, 1997:421–444.
320. Rollins BJ. Chemokines. *Blood* 1997;90:909–928.
321. Graham GJ, Wright EG, Hewick R, et al. Identification and characterization of an inhibitor of hematopoietic stem cell proliferation. *Nature* 1990;344:442–444.
322. Youn B-S, Zhang SM, Lee EK, et al. Molecular cloning of leukotactin-1: a novel human β-chemokine, a chemoattractant for neutrophils, monocytes, and lymphocytes, and a potent agonist at CC chemokine receptors 1 and 3. *J Immunol* 1997;159:5201–5205.
323. Bazan JF, Bacon KB, Hardiman G, et al. A new class of membrane-bound chemokine with a CX_3C motif. *Nature* 1997;385:640–644.
324. Oberlin E, Amara A, Bachelerie F, et al. The CXC chemokine SDF-1 is the ligand for LESTR/fusin and prevents infection by T cell line-adapted HIV-1. *Nature* 1996;382:833–835.
325. Rubbert A, Combadiere C, Ostrowski M, et al. Dendritic cells express multiple chemokine receptors used as coreceptors for HIV entry. *J Immunol* 1998;160:3933–3941.
326. Adema GJ, Hargers F, Verstraten R, et al. A dendritic-cell–derived C-C chemokine that preferentially attracts naive T cells. *Nature* 1997; 387:713–717.
327. Yanagihara S, Komura E, Nagafune J, et al. EBI1/CCR7 is a new member of dendritic cell chemokine receptor that is up-regulated upon maturation. *J Immunol* 1998;161:3096–3102.
328. Baggiolini M. Chemokines and leukocyte traffic. *Nature* 1998;392: 565–568.

CHAPTER 2

The Immune System: Structure and Function

Elaine J. Schattner and Paolo Casali

GENERAL PRINCIPLES

The immune system encompasses a complex network of cell types, ligand-receptor pairs, and interrelated signaling pathways that have evolved to facilitate specific and effective responses to invading pathogens. Humans are exposed constantly to viruses, bacteria, fungi, and parasites that, if unchecked, can cause morbidity and mortality. The skin represents an effective barrier to most microbial agents. Nevertheless, some infectious pathogens can enter through the skin, airway, gut, genitourinary tract, eye, or other sites. In most circumstances, bacteria are destroyed before they penetrate the epithelial layer by local microbicidal factors such as fatty acids in the skin, acid pH in the stomach, and lysozyme in tears. At the epithelial surface of the skin, normal bacterial flora protect the host from invasive pathogens by competing with them for space and nutrients and in some cases by generating specific antibacterial factors, such as colicins produced by *Escherichia coli.* Similar mechanisms of protection occur through bacterial colonization of the small intestine, upper respiratory tract, and genitourinary area.

After microorganisms break through these barriers to infection, macrophages, natural killer (NK) cells, and other components of the innate response provide a broad but imperfect immediate defense. Complete eradication of an infectious agent, in general, depends on the induction of an appropriate adaptive immune response, which entails high-affinity interactions between specific receptors and many diverse antigens, selection and preferential growth of clones that recognize particular structures, and immunologic memory. On antigen encounter, immune effector cells proliferate and differentiate, resulting in the generation and secretion of cytokines, antibodies, and other protective factors. The development of adaptive immunity is tightly regulated, such that the host destroys foreign cells and organisms but not itself. Elaborate mechanisms have evolved to facilitate distinction of self from foreign antigens and for functional deletion of autoreactive lymphocytes.

Besides restrictions on the molecular and cellular targets of immunity, there are limitations on the duration and magnitude of the responses that are achieved largely through control of cell cycle and induction of apoptosis. Most immune effector cells are programmed to undergo cell death after specific activation events, such that they are deleted after the relevant antigen has been eradicated. Failure to control the immune response can result in pathogenic inflammatory states, autoimmunity, and lymphoproliferative disease.

History of Immunology

Historical references to acquired, specific immunity can be found in *The History of the Peloponnesian War*, in which Thucydides observed that individuals who survived the Athenian plague were relatively unaffected by a second exposure and were able to nurse the sick and dying in a recurrent epidemic (1,2). Starting in the first half of the second millennium AD, Chinese, Turkish, Persians, and others practiced various methods of smallpox inoculation in children (3). However, the basic concepts of contagion and infection were not generally accepted in the Occidental world. The contention of Girolamo Fracastoro of Padua, in 1546, that infection is spread by contagious seminaria, tiny and imperceptible germ or seedlike particles, was revolutionary (2,4,5).

Some consider Edward Jenner to be the founder of modern immunology. Jenner reported in 1798 that inoculation of humans with vaccinia (cowpox) afforded protection against smallpox (3,6). In his practice as a physician in Gloucestershire, England, Jenner observed that material from pustules

E. J. Schattner: Division of Hematology and Medical Oncology, Department of Medicine, Cornell University, and Immunology Program, Weill Graduate School of Medical Sciences of Cornell University, New York, New York 10021

P. Casali: Division of Molecular Immunology, Department of Pathology and Department of Microbiology and Immunology, Weill Medical College, and Immunology Program, Weill Graduate School of Medical Sciences of Cornell University, New York, New York 10021 of horses' hoofs was transmitted to the nipples of cows by farm workers. He observed that milkmaids who developed lesions on their hands and wrists after handling such cows were thereafter immune to smallpox infection. The term *vaccination* is derived from Jenner's deduction that inoculation with vaccinia conferred later protection to the organism that causes smallpox, and it is still used to describe methods of inducing immunity by inoculation. Although some cultural practices throughout the world reflected a pragmatic understanding of infection and immunity, there was little formal appreciation for specific immune mechanisms until after Robert Koch's identification of microorganisms as the cause of infectious disease. Koch's important observation that anthrax could be transmitted from a culture system to animals, reported in 1876 (7), was followed shortly by Louis Pasteur's demonstration that vaccination could protect animals from infections such as cholera and anthrax (3,8).

These advances in the last part of the 19th century spurred investigations regarding specific mechanisms of microbial immunity in animals and in humans. Based on their work at the Pasteur Institute, Emile Roux and Elexandre Yersin reported the purification of a soluble toxin from the supernatants of microbial cultures of diphtheria (2,3). At the Koch Institute, Emile von Behring and Shibasaburo Kitasato soon discovered that vaccination of animals with diphtheria or tetanus toxins led to production of a humoral substance that inhibited the toxin's effect (9,10). The term *antibody* refers to this factor, which is produced after immunization and has a neutralizing effect on the potency of microbial antigens.

Shortly after this central finding, Paul Ehrlich postulated that antibodies function as cellular receptors for specific antigens, such as foodstuff, to which they bind directly (2,11). Ehrlich speculated that antibody engagement by antigen for which it is specific would result in antibody shedding from the cell surface and production of more antibody by that cell, thereby offering the foundation for the concept of clonal activation and selection. During the early 20th century, a variety of hypotheses were proposed to explain the extreme diversity and specificity of antibody formation in mammals (2). Linus Pauling and others proposed *instructive theories,* according to which the structure and specificity of an antibody was shaped by its physical interaction with a particular antigen. Niels Jerne posed the first *selection model* for antibody affinity and maturation (12). His work was followed by that of Burnet, Talmage, and Lederberg, who postulated that when an antigen binds to an antibody at the cell surface the cell becomes activated, proliferates, and differentiates into an antibody-secreting plasma cell. These investigators' original observations and ideas, expounded in the late 1950s, provide the basis for our modern theory of clonal selection and expansion in B cells (13,14).

TABLE 2.1. *Cells of the immune system*

Cell type	Primary function
Lymphocytes	
B lymphocyte	Antibody production, antigen presentation
T lymphocyte	Regulation of the cellular and humoral responses, cytotoxicity
Natural killer cell	Cytotoxicity
Phagocytic and antigen presenting cells	
Monocyte	Circulating macrophage precursor, phagocytosis
Macrophage	Phagocytosis, cytokine secretion
Dendritic cell	Antigen presentation, generation of antigen-specific, cytotoxic T-cell reponse
Follicular dendritic cell[a]	Nonhematopoetic (stromal) germinal center cell, antigen capture
Myeloid cells	
Neutrophil	Phagocytosis, early response to bacteria, fungi
Eosinophil	Immunity to parasites
Basophil	Unknown
Mast cell	Vascular permeability, mucosal immunity

[a] Follicular dendritic cells do not internalize and process antigen for major histocompatibility complex–restricted display.

Cellular Components of the Immune System

The mammalian defense mechanisms against infectious agents include three major categories of immune effector cells: lymphocytes, antigen-presenting cells (APCs), and myeloid cells (Table 2.1). All the cellular components of the immune system are derived from hematopoietic progenitor cells in the bone marrow (Fig. 2.1). Each cell type has evolved such that it is highly specialized for function in specific immune responses. For example, neutrophils play a central role in the early response to pathogens by binding bacterial cell wall components such as lipopolysaccharide (LPS). They phagocytose bacteria that have been opsonized by the alternative complement pathway, in the absence of antigen-specific antibodies, and destroy microorganisms through the production of toxic oxygen metabolites and proteases. Professional APCs, such as monocytes, macrophages, and dendritic cells (DCs), are characterized by the capacity to internalize foreign particles, digest them, and display antigen fragments in the context of major histocompatibility complex (MHC) proteins to initiate a coordinated immune response against the processed peptides.

T and B lymphocytes constitute the main effector cells of adaptive immunity. Progenitor lymphocytes are distinguished by expression of the recombination-activating genes *RAG1* and *RAG2*, which mediate rearrangement of genes encoding the B-cell receptor (BCR) and the T-cell receptor (TCR) for antigen present at the surface of the mature elements. Mature lymphocytes express unique surface receptors for antigen, generated as products of rearranged segments. Although the developmental origin of NK cells is not certain,

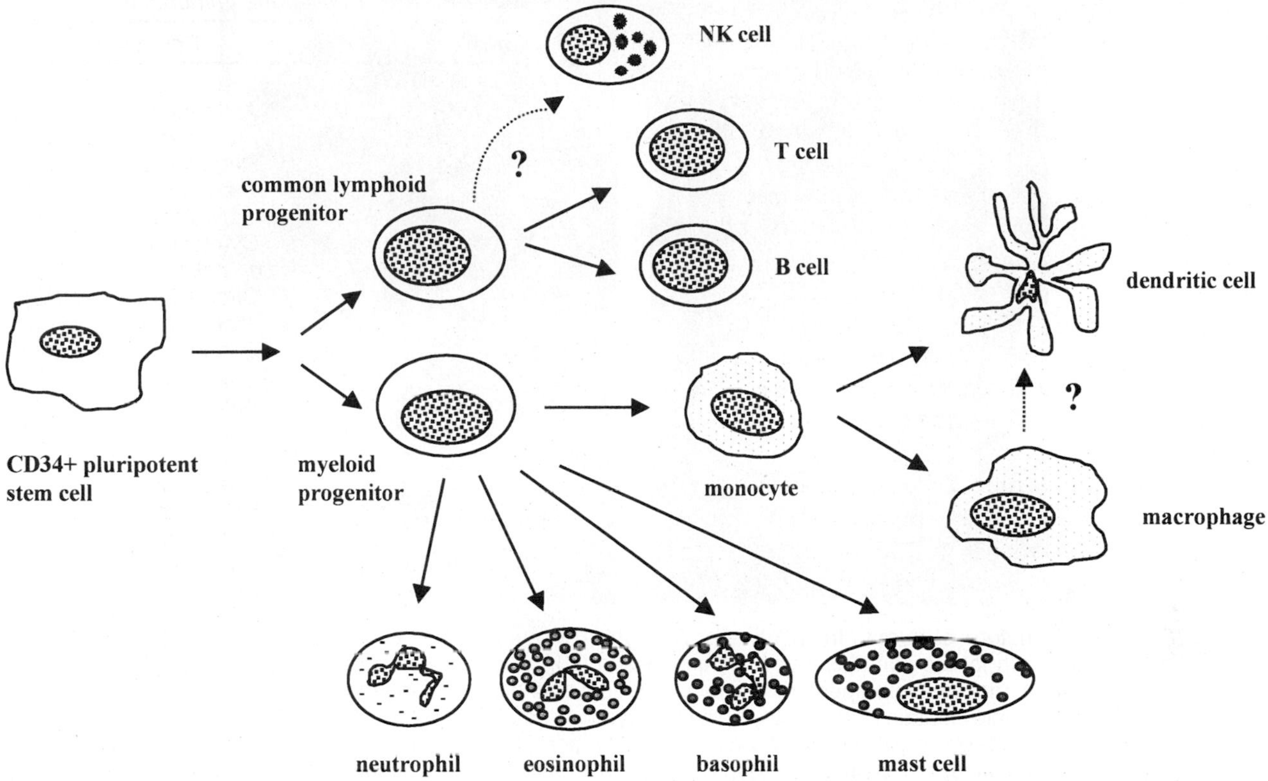

FIG. 2.1. Origin of immune effector cells from hematopoietic progenitors. Pluripotent $CD34^{+}$ stem cells in the bone marrow are the source of immune effector cells. Lymphoid cells, which arise from putative lymphoid progenitors, include natural killer (NK), T, and B cells; myeloid cells include the granulocytes (i.e., neutrophils, eosinophils, basophils, and mast cells), monocytes, and macrophages. Dendritic cells include several cell types of distinct cellular origins. Some dendritic cells are derived from circulating monocytic cells.

these cells are usually categorized with T lymphocytes because they share certain morphologic features, cell-surface antigens, and cytotoxic capacity.

Primary and Secondary Lymphoid Organs

The primary, or central, lymphoid organs are those in which lymphoid precursors are generated. The lymphoid progenitor cells, derived from pluripotent hematopoietic cells, are produced in blood islands of the yolk sac in early fetal development, later in the fetal liver and spleen, and finally in the bone marrow of the perinatal and adult human. Naive lymphocytes circulate through the bloodstream and are delivered to the lymph nodes through specialized venules. An extensive network of lymphatic vessels drain lymph fluid from the extracellular tissues, such that antigen and APCs from those spaces are delivered and trapped in the lymph nodes. The secondary, or peripheral, lymphoid organs, are the major sites of adaptive immunity and include the lymph nodes, spleen, and mucosa-associated lymphoid tissue (MALT).

Bone Marrow

The bone marrow is a soft tissue compartment containing stromal cells, adipocytes, hematopoietic precursors, and differentiated blood cells, including lymphocytes, myeloid cells, and monocytes. Pluripotent stem cells undergo lineage commitment and differentiation in a process that is determined by direct interaction with cellular and matrix components of the bone marrow microenvironment and by soluble factors (15,16). Like all immune cells, B and T lymphocytes are generated in the bone marrow, but only the B lymphocytes undergo maturation in that environment. Within the bone marrow compartment, B-lineage commitment and differentiation require the presence of bone marrow stromal cells that support B-cell development through expression of specific cell adhesion molecules and B-cell growth factors such as the stem cell factor (SCF) and KIT ligand. Cytokines such as interleukin (IL)-7 and stromal cell–derived factor-1 (SDF-1) are present at high levels in the bone marrow microenvironment and regulate early B-cell development (17–20) (see Chapter 1).

Thymus

In humans, the thymus is mature at birth and functions primarily during the first 15 years of life. The thymic medulla is derived from endodermal cells of the third pharyngeal pouch and the cortex from ectodermal cells of the third brachial cleft. At approximately the seventh week of gesta-

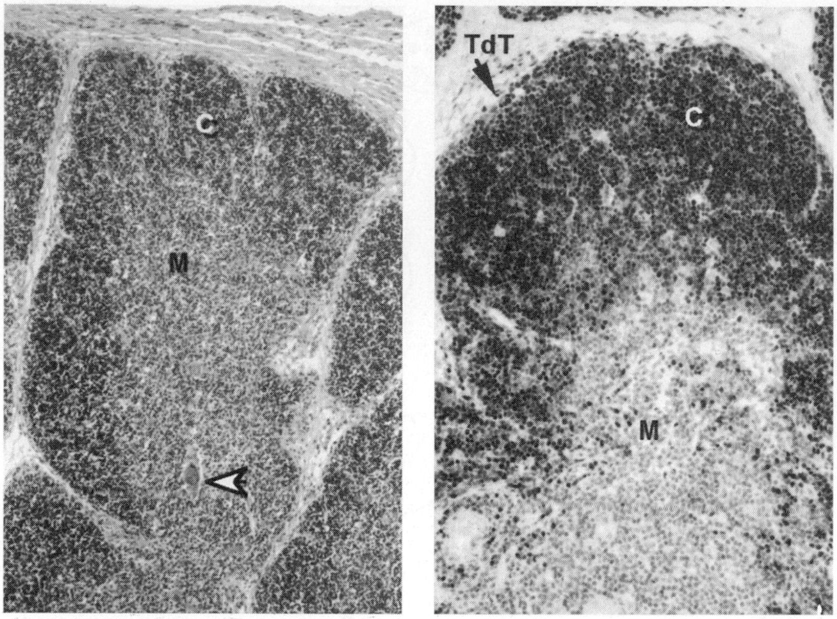

FIG. 2.2. Structure of human thymic tissue. **A:** Light micrograph of a section from a human thymus shows that each lobule contains thymic cortical tissue (C), which appears dark because of numerous proliferating thymocytes interspersed with thymic cortical epithelial cells and macrophages. The medulla (M) of each lobule contains mature thymocytes, thymic medullary epithelial cells, macrophages, and dendritic cells. The arrow points to a Hassall's corpuscle (hematoxylin and eosin stain, original magnification: 100× magnification). **B:** Immunohistochemical stain for terminal deoxynucleotidyl transferase (TdT) demonstrates specific expression in the cortex, where T-cell receptor gene rearrangements occur in developing thymocytes (immunoperoxidase stain, original magnification: 200× magnification). (Courtesy of Amy Chadburn, M.D., Weill Medical College of Cornell University.)

tion, prothymocytes from the yolk sac and liver migrate to the thymus. Later, cells migrate from the bone marrow. Thymic precursors infiltrate the thymus and interact there with MHC-expressing cortical epithelial cells, macrophages, medullary DCs, and Langerhans cells which, in the presence of cytokines and other factors, guide the process of T-cell development and selection (Fig. 2.2). Ultimately, only approximately 2% of prothymocytes survive the thymic ''education'' process and are released into the circulation, from which they enter the secondary lymphoid organs and participate in adaptive immunity (21–24) (see Chapter 6).

Spleen

The spleen is a center for several basic immune functions, including clearance of infectious pathogens, elimination of aged and abnormal blood cells, and constitution of humoral immunity. The spleen comprises red pulp tissue, which is primarily a site of erythrocyte destruction, and white pulp, which is composed of specialized lymphoid centers dispersed throughout the red pulp (Fig. 2.3). The white pulp structures are discrete regions that surround the central arterioles. Within the white pulp there are T-cell–enriched periarteriolar lymphoid sheaths (PALS), B-cell–rich germinal centers (GCs), and marginal zones that circumferentially envelop each GC and associated mantle zone.

In contrast to lymph node GCs, to which antigen is delivered through the lymphatic system, antigen enters the splenic white pulp regions directly through the bloodstream. The spleen is necessary for the early adaptive response to circulating pathogens such as occurs in bacterial sepsis. Besides the lymphoid elements found predominantly in the white pulp, the spleen contains numerous macrophages in the sinusoids. These macrophages clear from the bloodstream microorganisms that have been primed for phagocytosis by antibody and complement deposition at their surface (25–27) (see Chapters 6 and 53).

Lymph Nodes

The lymphoid follicles occur in the outer lymph node cortex and in some cases contain GCs (Fig. 2.4). These highly organized structures are crucial in controlling the adaptive immune response, which occurs through interactions among T cells, B cells, DCs, and follicular dendritic cells (FDCs). B cells of the mantle zone, surrounding the GC, express immunoglobulin M (IgM) and IgD, and they are thought to be mainly naive. In the course of an immune response to antigen, these IgM^+, IgD^+ B cells migrate into the GC, where they proliferate and mature in a process that is determined by their affinity for antigen and by the presence of helper T cells that recognize the same antigen. There is a

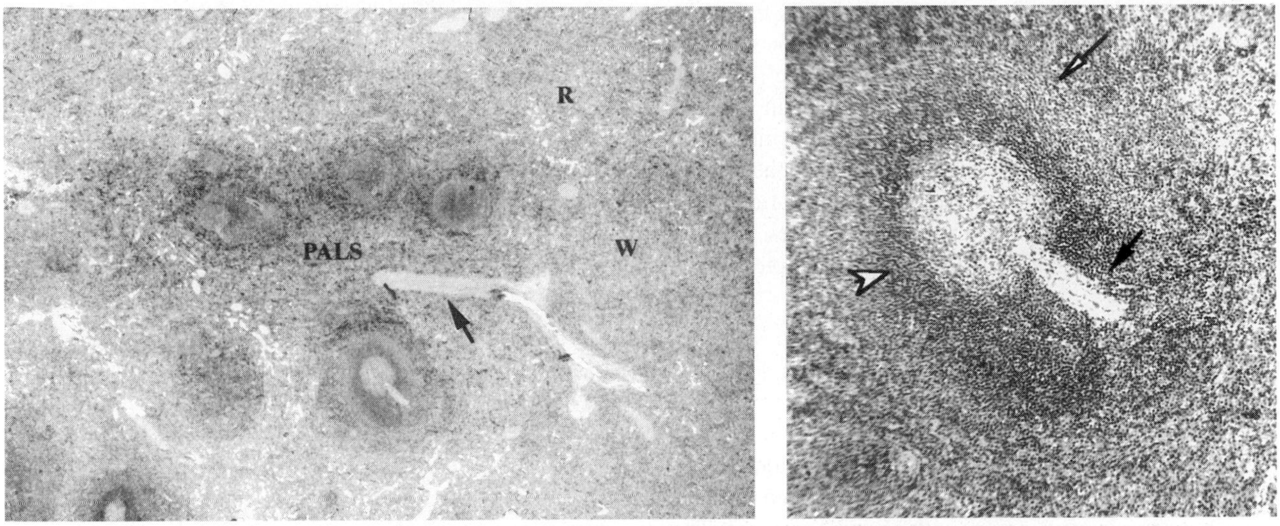

FIG. 2.3. Human splenic architecture. **A:** Light micrograph of a human splenic section demonstrates white pulp (W) with central arteriole *(arrow)*, periarteriolar lymphoid sheaths (PALS), numerous follicles, and red pulp (R) with sinusoids (hematoxylin and eosin stain, original magnification: 54× magnification). **B:** High-power view of a splenic germinal center (GC) includes the arteriole (A), mantle zone *(arrowhead)*, and the surrounding marginal zone *(arrow)* (hematoxylin and eosin stain, original magnification: 200× magnification). (Courtesy of Amy Chadburn, M.D., Weill Medical College of Cornell University.)

high rate of cellular proliferation and apoptosis in the dark zone, where B centroblasts undergo immunoglobulin gene hypermutation. The centrocytes, occupying the light or apical zone of the GC, have survived the affinity maturation process. The most differentiated B cell, the plasma cell, exits the lymph node through efferent lymphatics and returns to the circulation through the thoracic duct (28–30) (see Chapter 6).

Musoca-Associated Lymphoid Tissue

Specialized lymphoid compartments underlie the mucosal surfaces such as the lumen of the gut, the bronchial epithelium, and occur also in glandular tissues such as the breast, prostate, parotid, and lacrimal glands. The best-characterized of these tissues are Peyer's patches, which are lymphoid follicles present throughout the small intestine just beneath

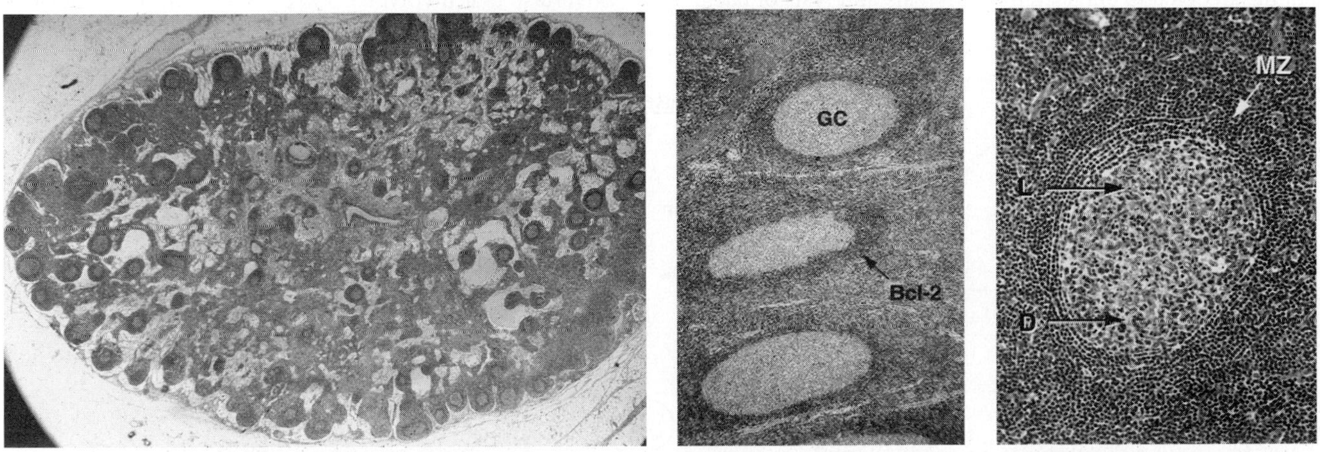

FIG. 2.4. Lymph node structure and compartments. **A:** Low-power light micrograph of a benign human lymph node with numerous reactive follicles (GCs) in the cortex (hematoxylin and eosin stain, original magnification: 20× magnification). **B:** Immunohistochemistry for BCL-2 reveals high levels of expression in the mantle zone (immunoperoxidase stain, original magnification: 130× magnification). **C:** High-power view of a single GC, with dark and light zones and a surrounding mantle zone (hematoxylin and eosin stain, original magnification: 260× magnification). (Courtesy of Amy Chadburn, M.D., Weill Medical College of Cornell University.)

the epithelial surface. A subset of epithelial cells lining the small intestine, called M cells, are specialized for vectorial transport of bacteria and other antigens from the intestinal lumen to the lymphoid tissue beneath. Within Peyer's patches, most lymphocytes are memory B cells of intermediate size that resemble marginal zone B cells of the spleen. Like the GC, the MALT follicle contains T-cell–rich zones and a conserved overall structure that facilitates antigen-dependent B-cell differentiation (31,32) (see Chapters 6, 33, and 35).

INNATE IMMUNITY AND THE EARLY RESPONSE TO INFECTIOUS AGENTS

Elements of the innate immune response provide the initial, early resistance to pathogens and do not depend on high-affinity interactions of receptors with specific antigens. The innate response is immediate and broad but nonspecific, and it does not generate immunologic memory. Our understanding of innate immunity stems partly from the pioneering work of Elie Metchnikoff, a Russian zoologist who determined that microbial organisms could be engulfed and destroyed by phagocytic cells such as macrophages (2,33,34). Metchnikoff appreciated the power of a response in which unprimed cells are immediately available to combat a wide range of common pathogens. After a microorganism breaks through physical barriers to invasion, such as the epithelial surface, components of the innate immune system, like a guarding infantry, are ready to attack (Fig. 2.5). The innate response functions promptly to reduce the load of invading pathogens and facilitates the development of an effective, adaptive response later (35,36).

The most phylogenetically primitive innate system of defense is the complement system, a broad network of proteins that has evolved to enhance phagocytosis and lysis of bacteria and viruses. Cellular elements of the innate response include phagocytic cells, such as monocytes, macrophages, and neutrophils, and ''nonrestricted'' cytotoxic cells such as NK cells. Other lymphocytes with specific receptors for antigen, such as T cells and B-1 B cells, also play a role in the early response to pathogens.

Complement Activation: Alternative, Lectin, and Classic Pathways

The term *complement* refers to a multi-enzymatic cascade of heat-labile plasma proteins that augments, or complements, antibody-mediated opsonization of bacteria (37). These proteins, together with their specific inhibitors, represent a conserved effector system that targets circulating microorganisms for destruction. In humans, there are three pathways by which complement can be activated at the pathogen surface: the classic, lectin, and alternative pathways (38–40). Each cascade involves distinct initiating events, but all converge at a central point, the production of a protease called C3 convertase, which activates the central C3 component and leads to the generation of opsonization-enhancing intermediates, production of inflammatory mediators, and formation of the terminal membrane attack complex (MAC).

The alternative and lectin pathways of complement activation provide the most immediate lines of defense because their activity does not require the presence or generation of antibody (39,41). The lectin pathway is initiated directly by mannose residues in microbial pathogens, which bind mannan-binding lectin (MBL) and trigger a complement cascade in an antibody-independent manner (38,42). The alternative pathway is activated readily by components of the surfaces of bacteria and viruses and leads to the generation of a C3-convertase that involves C3 itself (Fig. 2.6). Once activated

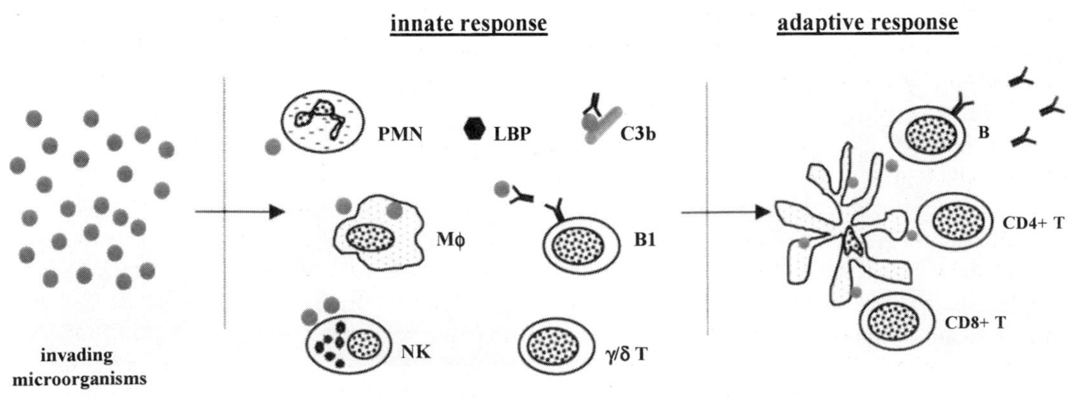

FIG. 2.5. The innate response provides the first line of protection against common pathogens. The immediate response to invading microorganisms includes cellular elements, such as polymorphonuclear leukocytes (PMNs), macrophages, natural killer (NK) cells, B-1 cells, and $\gamma\delta$ T cells, and soluble elements, such as complement component 3b, lipopolysaccharide (LPS)-binding protein (LBP), and natural antibodies that directly recognize and bind carbohydrate and lipid structures. In the later, adaptive response, antigen-presenting cells (APCs) process and present microbial glycoprotein components, favoring expansion of T and B lymphocytes that bind antigen with high affinity.

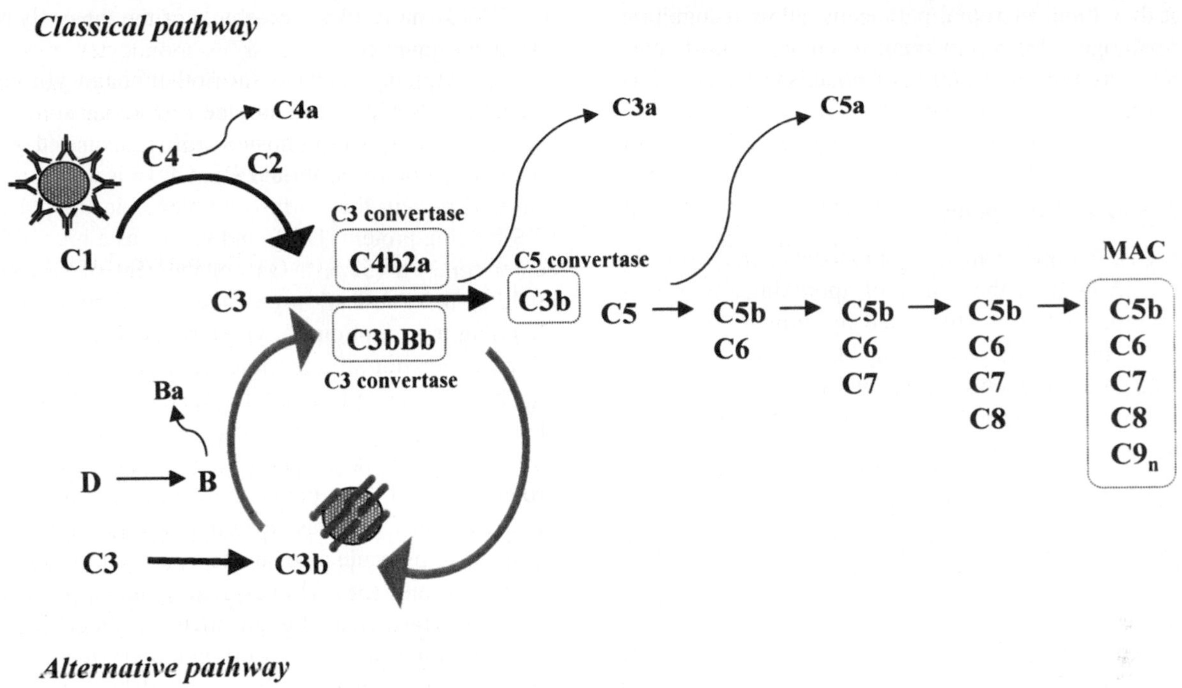

FIG. 2.6. Classic complement activation and membrane attack complex (MAC) formation. The classic complement pathway is activated directly by antigen-antibody complexes and is initiated by proteases of the C1 complex. C1s is a serine protease that cleaves the complement components C4 and C2. These initial steps generate the C4bC2a C3 convertase. Alternatively, C3 undergoes autolytic cleavage, and the active fragment, together with component D, cleaves component B to generate the C3bBb convertase. The C3 amplification loop of the alternative pathway yields rapid escalation in the rate of complement deposition after initiation of either pathway. After C3b is generated and binds to the microbial cell surface, it gives rise to C4b2a3b, or C5 convertase. C5b activates and sequentially binds the other MAC components C6, C7, C8, and multiple C9 molecules to form the terminal MAC. The C3a, C4a, and C5a peptides are potent anaphylatoxins, which accelerate local inflammation by causing increased vascular permeability and mast cell activation.

by a C3 convertase generated through one of the three pathways of complement activation, C3, an abundant plasma protein, undergoes continuous autolysis. The larger cleavage product, C3b, binds covalently to bacterial membrane structures, resulting in their priming and opsonization for engulfment by phagocytes expressing the C3b receptor, called complement receptor-1 (CR1). CR1 is expressed in a variety of cell types, including erythrocytes, neutrophils, B cells, macrophages, and other APCs (43). In host cells, a complex system of complement regulatory proteins inactivate C3b, such that neither opsonization nor MAC formation occur (44). These include decay-accelerating factor (DAF, CD55), and components H and I. Thus, autolysis of C3 in the plasma facilitates complement fixation at the surface of invasive microorganisms in the absence of specific antibody. At the same time, autologous cells are protected from spontaneous complement activation by host inhibitory factors and control elements.

The classic complement pathway is triggered directly by antigen-antibody complexes and is initiated by proteases of the C1 complex. In the first step, recruitment of the first complement component C1q by IgG or IgM bound to a pathogen results in C1r activation and C1s cleavage at the pathogen surface. C1s is a serine protease that cleaves the complement components C4 and C2. These initial reactions generate the C4b2a C3 convertase and cause release of the biologically active C4a peptide, which, like the related C3a and C5a peptides, is a potent anaphylatoxin and inflammatory mediator. These anaphylatoxins induce local inflammation mediated by increased vascular permeability and mast cell activation. In the plasma, C4b is readily inactivated by hydrolysis, and if it is dissociated from the pathogen surface, it cannot function in subsequent steps of complement activation.

Regardless of the activating pathway, once generated, the C3 convertases cleave C3 to generate C3b and active C3a peptide. C3b binds directly to the microbial cell surface, giving rise to a C4b2a3b complex, or C5 convertase. This cleaves C5 to yield C5a peptide and C5b. C5b activates and sequentially binds the other MAC components C6, C7, and C8. The C567 complex incorporates C8, which leads to polymerization of multiple C9 molecules and generation of the terminal MAC, a perforin-like, ringed structure that by inserting into the lipid bilayer forms pores in the plasma membrane and facilitates cell lysis (45,46). Thus, the complement components are activated in a rapid and controlled fashion such that they bind microbial pathogens, allow recognition of those pathogens by complement receptors on host cells, and directly promote destruction of organisms by pore formation and microbial cell lysis.

Monocytes and Macrophages

Monocytes mature from myelomonocytic precursors in the bone marrow over the course of approximately 6 days through a process that is stimulated by growth factors including IL-3 and granulocyte colony-stimulating factor (G-CSF). After leaving the bone marrow, monocytes circulate for 1 to 3 days in the bloodstream. These cells, which ultimately become macrophages or DCs, are highly adapted for innate immune functions such as phagocytosis. Monocytes express the LPS receptor (CD14) at high levels, as well as Fc receptors for IgG (FcγRI and FcγRIIa; CD64 and CD32, respectively) and for IgA (FcαRI, CD89). Compared with more differentiated APCs, such as macrophages and DCs and consistent with their limited capacity in antigen display, circulating monocytes express only low levels of MHC class II (MHC-II) molecules and CD86. Although monocytes are heterogeneous in size, morphology, and expression of cell-surface antigens, in the bloodstream these cells cannot be distinguished by their final destination.

In the tissues, differentiated monocytes include Kuppfer cells in the liver, interstitial and alveolar macrophages in the lung, reactive microglial cells in the brain, and multinucleated giant cells of granuloma (47,48) (see Chapter 1). Tissue macrophages are differentiated monocytes that have penetrated the extravascular space by diapedesis across the endothelial cell wall. At sites of infection, macrophages bind and engulf extracellular pathogens. Macrophage activation is largely dependent on their interaction with type 1 helper T cells (T_H1 cells), which stimulate macrophages by secretion of interferon-γ (IFN-γ) and other factors. Peptides derived from the digested microbes are displayed in the context of MHC-II molecules, thereby driving the early steps of adaptive immunity. Activated macrophages generate nitric oxide, which has potent activity against diverse microbial pathogens and against cytokines, proteases, and toxic oxygen radicals (49,50). Mice deficient in inducible nitric oxide synthase are vulnerable to infection by intracellular pathogens such as mycobacteria and *Listeria* (51).

Macrophages reside in tissues that can be damaged by the inflammatory mediators they produce. Without engulfment of target organisms by macrophages, damage would ensue from release of toxic enzymes and metabolites into the tissue. Although macrophages are effective in eradicating pathogens contained within intracellular vesicles, they are not useful in destroying some organisms such as parasites too large to be ingested by a single cell. Activated macrophages express augmented levels of CD40 and CD80, two molecules critical for costimulation of T cells. Peptides derived from the digested microbes are displayed in the context of MHC-II molecules, thereby driving the early steps of adaptive immunity.

Monocytes, macrophages, and other phagocytic cells such as neutrophils express membrane-bound and soluble CD14, a glycosyl phosphatidylinositol (GPI)–anchored scavenger receptor that binds bacterial LPS. CD14 is a conserved lipid transport protein that forms complexes in the plasma with LPS-binding protein (LBP) and serves as a high-affinity receptor for LPS (52,53). On engagement of surface CD14 by LPS, there follows a cascade of inflammatory events, including transcription of cytokines, such as IL-1 and IFN-γ, and expression of adhesion molecules (Fig. 2.7). CD14, which lacks a cytoplasmic tail, transduces signals to the nucleus through the signaling capacity of a nearby receptor that is the mammalian homologue of the *Drosophila* Toll protein (54–57). Like many conserved structures in the immune system, CD14 has several distinct functions. For example, this molecule also serves as a receptor for apoptotic cell membranes (58). However, in contrast to the LPS response, CD14-mediated engulfment of apoptotic cell fragments does not instigate an inflammatory reaction. Macrophages clear cellular and infectious debris at sites of cell death and infection through their capacity to bind and engulf apoptotic cell fragments in the absence of inflammation (see Chapter 6).

Myeloid Cells

Granulocytes and monocytes are derived from a common myeloid progenitor cell in the bone marrow. Myeloid cells are distinguished by the occurrence of dense cytoplasmic granules in the cytoplasm. The term *polymorphonuclear leukocytes* refers to the heavily indented nuclei that characterize mature myeloid forms. There are four major classes of granulocytes: neutrophils, eosinophils, basophils, and mast cells (see Chapter 1).

Neutrophils

Neutrophils are the most common myeloid cells and are among the principal effectors of the innate response to bacteria and fungi (Fig. 2.8A). Neutrophils can directly bind and engulf many bacteria, which are cleared in the absence of humoral immunity (59–61). However, some bacterial envelopes have evolved to escape recognition by leukocyte receptors for microbial products, such as CD14, and are engulfed only after opsonization by complement or antibody. Regardless of the stimulus and method by which phagocytosis occurs, after bacteria enter the neutrophilic granules, they are subject to a low pH environment and a variety of potent antimicrobial factors. These include toxic proteases, such as cathepsins, lysozyme, elastase, and defensins, as well as toxic oxygen metabolites (62,63).

Circulating neutrophils bear highly specialized receptors at the surface to facilitate chemotaxis and locomotion to sites of inflammation. The initial interaction of circulating

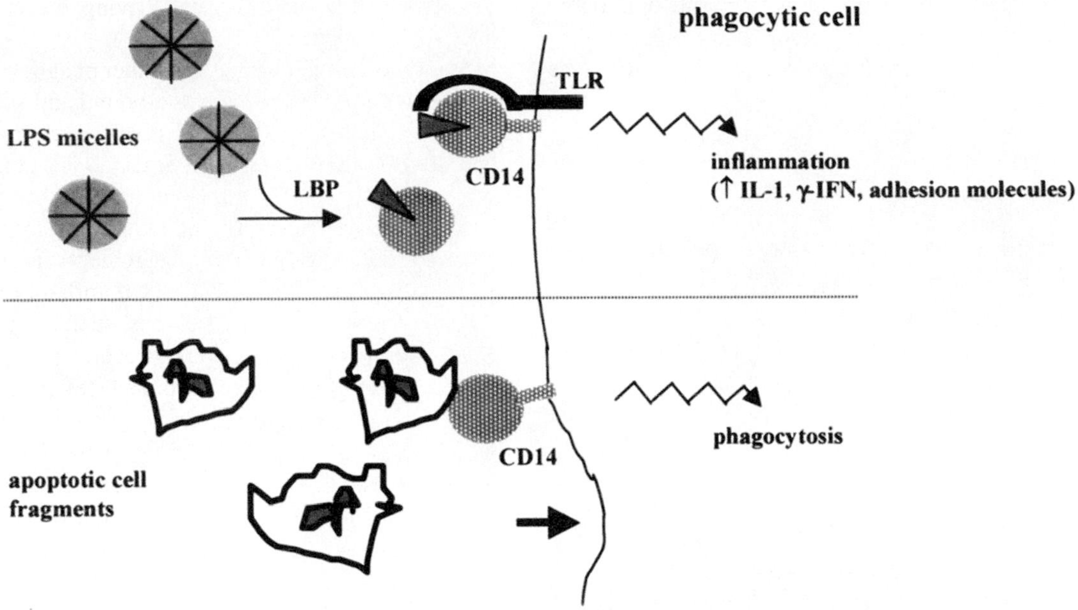

FIG. 2.7. CD14 is a multifunctional receptor that binds lipopolysaccharide (LPS) and membranes of apoptotic cells. CD14 is a high-affinity LPS receptor expressed in macrophages, polymorphonuclear leukocytes (PMNs), and monocytes. This glycosyl phosphatidylinositol (GPI)–anchored lipid transport protein associates with the toll-like receptor (TLR), which on LPS binding instigates a potent inflammatory response. Transcriptional activation results in rapid generation of interleukin-1 (IL-1), tumor necrosis factor-α (TNF-α), and interferon-α (IFN-α). CD14 has affinity for apoptotic cell membranes. However, on binding of apoptotic cell fragments to CD14, the material is internalized and destroyed in the absence of inflammation.

neutrophils with vascular endothelial cells constitutes the rolling phase of leukocyte trafficking, and is mediated by adhesion molecules called *selectins* (CD62). Selectins are cell-surface glycoproteins that contain lectin elements and adhere to specific carbohydrate moieties. The leukocyte selectins, called L-selectins (CD62L), bind structures such as sialyl Lewis^X in endothelial cell-surface glycoproteins, such that the phagocytic cells are slowed as they traverse small blood vessels. At sites of inflammation, bacterial LPS and host-derived inflammatory mediators such as leukotriene B_4, the complement component C5a, and tumor necrosis factor-α (TNF-α), upregulate endothelial cell expression of E- and P-selectins (CD62E and CD62P). These molecules recognize specific carbohydrate residues in leukocyte glycoproteins and facilitate brief adhesion of the leukocytes to the endothelium of inflamed tissue (64–66).

The second, or tethering, phase of leukocyte migration is mediated by integrins and intercellular adhesion molecules (ICAMs). There are three leukocyte integrins, all of which are expressed in phagocytic cells and each of which contains a common β chain (β_2, CD18) and a distinct α chain (67,68). The three β_2 integrins are the lymphocyte function-associated antigen-1 (LFA-1, CD11a/CD18), MAC-1 (CR3, CD11b/CD18), and CD11c/CD18. The ICAMs are widely expressed imunoglobulin-related molecules that mediate intercellular adhesion and leukocyte activation and that serve as counterreceptors for LFA-1 and MAC-1 at the endothelial cell surface. When inflammation occurs, IL-8 and other factors augment neutrophil expression of LFA-1 and MAC-1, such that the leukocytes firmly adhere to the vascular endothelial cell surface where ICAM is expressed. This interaction also facilitates diapedesis of the neutrophils from the blood vessel lumen into the tissue compartment (69).

Throughout this process, locomotion, contraction, and pseudopod extension in the neutrophils are carried out by a network of cytoskeletal proteins, including actin filaments, myosin, and gelsolin. Neutrophil transmigration into the extravascular space depends on homotypic adhesion of platelet-endothelial cell adhesion molecule (PECAM, CD31), expressed by the leukocytes and endothelial cells. In the final phase of leukocyte transmigration, penetration of the neutrophils into the affected tissue requires proteases to digest the basement membrane, and also chemotactic factors (64,70).

Activation of the neutrophil is induced on binding of LPS to its receptor, crosslinking of Fc receptors (FcRs), or other stimuli at the cell surface. A *respiratory burst* occurs in which toxic oxygen metabolites such as hydrogen peroxide (H_2O_2) and superoxide (O_2^-) are generated. The enzyme responsible for superoxide generation is the membrane-associated electron transport complex NADPH oxidase, which catalyzes the transfer of electrons from NADPH to O_2. After hydrogen peroxide is generated from superoxides and water by superoxide dismutase, the myeloperoxidase enzyme produces hypochlorous acid (HOCl), a potent oxidant that can

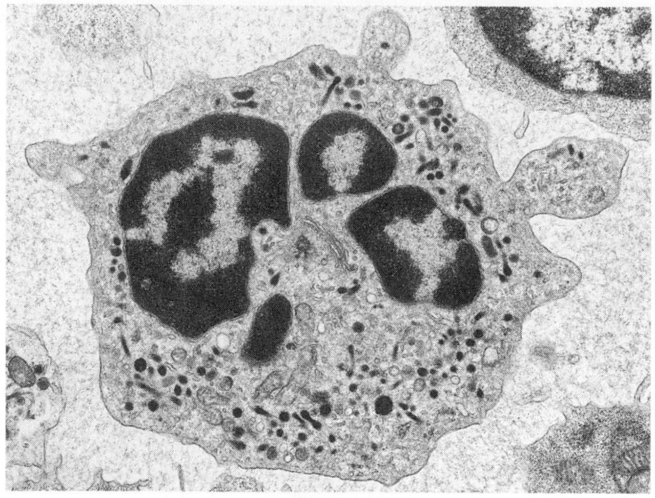

A

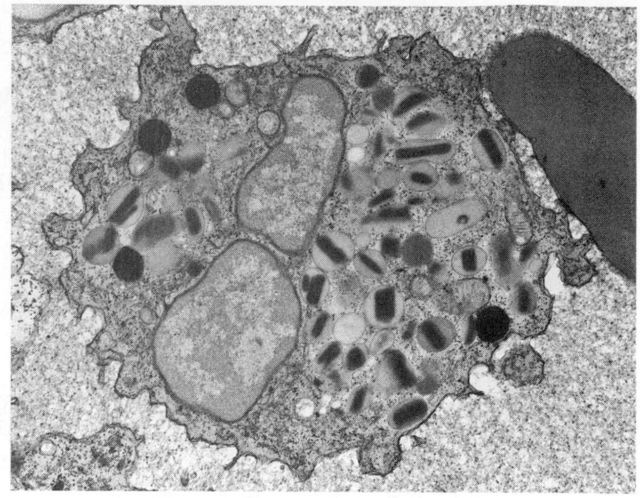

B

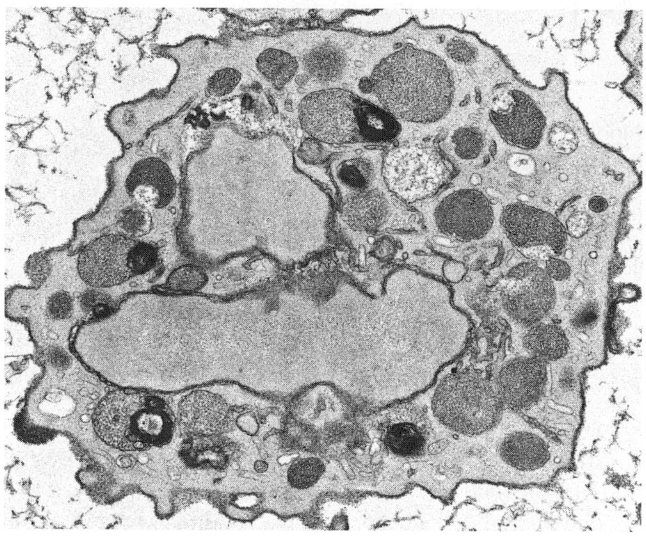

C

FIG. 2.8. Electron micrographs of human myeloid cells. **A:** Neutrophil (original magnification: 14,000× magnification). **B:** Electron micrograph of a human peripheral blood eosinophil showing bilobed nucleus; irregular, blunt surface processes; granules; and mitochondria. Dark cytoplasmic particles are monoparticulate glycogen. Four large, round, osmiophilic lipoic bodies are present. Specific granules are elongated, membrane-bound structures with dense crystal and lightly dense matrix. Primary granules do not have central crystals. **C:** Electron micrograph of a peripheral blood basophil with a polylobed nucleus; irregular, broad-surface processes; and secretory granules filled with particles. Concentric, dense membranous arrays subcompartmentalize some granules. (Courtesy of Ann M. Dvorak, M.D., Harvard Medical School. Reprinted from references 60, 75, and 82 with permission.)

destroy amino acids, amines, thiols, thioesters, nucleotides, and other molecular components. Hypochlorous acid is the neutrophil component responsible for the greenish color and characteristic odor that occur where large numbers of neutrophils are present, such as in microbial abscesses and in solid tumors of neutrophils, called chloromas (59,61,62,71).

Eosinophils

Eosinophils play a central role in immunity to parasitic organisms (72,73). These cells have bilobed nuclei and are characterized by granules containing arginine-rich, basic proteins that bind the acidic eosin stain with high affinity, which results in a red appearance (Fig. 2.8B). Eosinophils resemble neutrophils in several developmental and functional respects and are nearly indistinguishable from neutrophils up to the point of specific granule generation. In the mature form, they share common mechanisms of locomotion, phagocytosis, and microbial killing. Eosinophil growth and maturation in the bone marrow are promoted by granulocyte macrophage colony stimulating factor (GM-CSF), IL-3, and IL-5 (74). Among the specific eosinophilic granule contents are eosinophil peroxidase, collagenase, cationic protein, eosinophil-derived neurotoxin, leukotrienes, and platelet-activating factor (75,76).

Eosinophils can exert damaging effects in the tissues because of their capacity to extrude toxic granule contents; extravasation of circulating eosinophils is regulated by factors such as the chemokine eotaxin (77). Eosinophils produce and secrete IL-5, overexpression of which occurs in diseases characterized by eosinophilia (74,78). Eosinophils in the circulation do not usually bind significant amounts of IgE. Like basophils and mast cells, eosinophils express the low-affinity IgE receptor CD23 (79) and the high-affinity IgE receptor FcϵRI, but they express the high-affinity receptor only on activation (80). Some infectious particles, such as parasitic worms, are too large for single cells to ingest. Eosinophils recognize IgE bound to the surface of such parasites, which results in eosinophil adhesion to the parasites, crosslinking of FϵRI, and discharge of eosinophil granule contents. These damaging materials are administered by eosinophil adhesion and granule extrusion to the parasites in the extracellular space.

Mast Cells and Basophils

Mast cells are critical mediators of local and system hypersensitivity reactions such as anaphylaxis. These cells modulate vascular permeability through the contents of their distinctive granules (Fig. 2.8C). These large cells are not common in the circulation, but are relatively abundant in the connective tissues lining blood vessels, particularly in the dermis, and in the submucosal tissues lining the gastrointestinal and respiratory tracts (81,82). Mast cell granules contain histamine, heparin, leukotrienes, proteases, and cytokines, including TNF-α (83–85). On activation of the mast cell, degranulation occurs, resulting in local vasodilation. There is an immediate increase in passage of circulating inflammatory cells, such as neutrophils and macrophages, into the tissue. Lymphatic flow to and from the area is also augmented, enhancing delivery of antigen from the tissue to the regional lymph node. Histamines and leukotrienes released by the mast cells affect smooth muscle in the gut and bronchi, causing contractions that foster the mechanical elimination of invading pathogens from these mucosal sites.

Mast cells constitutively express FcϵRI receptors (79,86,87). These bind monomeric IgE with high affinity, such that a significant proportion of IgE in many individuals is effectively adsorbed by these cells and by basophils. IgE crosslinking by antigen, however, is necessary for mast cell activation and degranulation to occur. In atopic individuals, mast cells are present in the tissues with IgE bound to FcϵRI, and on ingestion of the appropriate antigen, anaphylaxis can occur in a matter of seconds. Similarly, inhalation of specific allergens results in mast cell degranulation along the respiratory mucosa. The *wheel and flare reaction*, characteristic of an ectopic response to subcutaneous injection, is mediated by mast cells within the dermis (81).

Basophils represent less than 1% of the normal circulating myeloid cells (88). They contain large cytoplasmic granules of heparin and other sulfated or carboxylated acidic proteins that appear blue after exposure to Wright-Giemsa stain. Basophils are closely related to mast cells and are sometimes considered as their circulating counterpart. Although the distinct function of basophils is largely unknown, these cells appear to play a role in the innate response to some infectious agents (85). Like mast cells, basophils express FcϵRI receptors, which bind monomeric IgE. In most individuals, a significant proportion of IgE is bound to the basophils and mast cells (79,86).

Natural Killer Cells and Receptors

Natural Killer (NK) cells account for approximately 10% of the circulating lymphocytes in adults, but are common in the cord blood and at the fetomaternal interface in pregnancy (89). These cells are morphologically similar to lymphocytes and have cytotoxic capacity due to granules that contain perforins and granzymes (90,91). NK cells are thought to have a central role in fetal and graft tolerance and in immune recognition of certain tumors. These cells express a diverse repertoire of inhibitory and activation receptors that, through their specific interactions with nonclassic MHC-I–related molecules, function to identify and discern among targets for autologous cytotoxic killing (89,92,93).

There are two broad categories of NK cell receptors: the C-type lectin-like receptors, and immunoglobulin domain-containing receptors (Fig. 2.9). In general, each NK cell expresses multiple receptors of each kind. The C-type lectin receptors consist of disulfide-linked, type 2 integral membrane proteins that occur as heterodimers at the cell surface. In humans, the best studied of these receptors are heterodim-

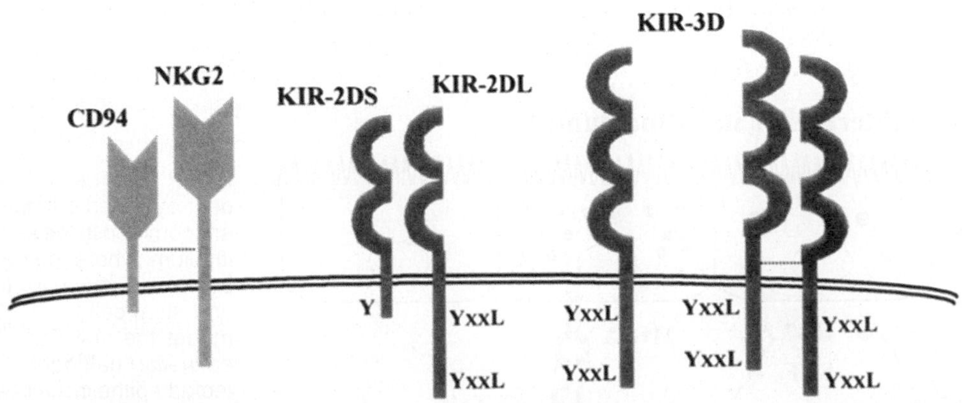

FIG. 2.9. Natural killer (NK) cell receptors. The C-type lectin NK receptors include the invariant CD94, which lacks a cytoplasmic tail and occurs as a heterodimer with NKG2. The human killer inhibitory receptors (KIRs) contain two (KIR2D) or three (KIR3D) immunoglobulin (Ig) domains. These molecules contain cytoplasmic immunoreceptor tyrosine-based inhibitory motif (ITIM) signaling elements.

ers of CD94 with associated NKG-2 proteins. CD94 occurs as an invariant chain and lacks a cytoplasmic tail. It is expressed together with an NKG-2 protein, through which signals are transduced. The NKG-2 proteins have diverse structures, suitable for recognition of distinct human leukocyte antigen (HLA) molecules. One variant of this receptor called NKG2D, binds MICA, an MHC-I type of molecule expressed by stressed and malignant epithelial cells. Engagement of NKG2D by MICA results in NK cell activation and cytotoxicity (94).

The human killer inhibitory receptors (KIRs) are immunoglobulin-related molecules that, despite their distinct structure from that of the C-type lectin receptors, bear similar patterns of cell recognition, HLA class I ligand binding, and cytosolic signaling mechanisms (89,93). The human KIR family includes various *KIR2D-* and *KIR3D*-encoded receptors, which contain two or three immunoglobulin domains in the extracellular portion of the molecule, respectively. There appear to be at least twelve KIR-encoding genes in humans, which occur at chromosome 19q13.4. Within any individual, there are expressed KIR molecules with highly diverse extracellular, transmembrane, and cytoplasmic amino acid sequences that arise from allelic polymorphisms and alternative mRNA splicing (93). Killer inhibitory receptors recognize MHC-I molecules and in general, KIR engagement by MHC-I inhibits NK-mediated cytotoxicity against autologous cells. However, in some malignancies, viral infections, or other circumstances, reduction in MHC-I expression allows for NK-mediated cytotoxicity because of the loss of KIR-mediated inhibitory signals.

The KIRS signal through conserved elements in the cytosolic segments called immunoreceptor tyrosine activation motifs (ITAMs) and immunoreceptor tyrosine inhibitory motifs (ITIMs). Immunoreceptor tyrosine activation motifs are conserved recognition sequences for SRC homology-2 (SH2)–type tyrosine kinases that contain two linked tyrosine-containing sequences, such as $YXX(L/I)X_{6\text{-}8}YXX(L/I)$ (i.e., amino acid sequences with Y [tyrosine], L [leucine], I [isoleucine], and X [any amino acid) (95–97). The ITIMs resemble ITAM signaling domains but are distinguished by the occurrence of a hydrophobic residue preceding the motif at the -2 position and by the capacity to transmit negative signals (98–100). These critical sequences are essential for regulation of NK cell activation and cytotoxicity. Immunoreceptor tyrosine activation motif and ITIM elements also occur in the cytosolic domains of other multichain immune receptor recognition (MIRR) proteins, such as the BCR, TCR, and FcRs (see Chapters 1, 3, and 6).

$\gamma\delta$ T Cells

The $\gamma\delta$ T cells represent only a small proportion of the peripheral blood lymphocytes in humans and mice, but they are highly prevalent in the peripheral tissues such as skin, intestinal tract, and mammary ducts, where they play a central role in the early response to infectious pathogens (101). Their growth is supported by IL-7 and SCF, which can be secreted by epithelial cells (102,103). In mice and in humans, the $\gamma\delta$ TCR repertoire is quite restricted, such that oligoclonal populations are evident in the skin and gut. The $\gamma\delta$ TCRs are skewed for binding of common pathogenic microbes and may be selected by environmental factors and infections in the host (104). The $\gamma\delta$ T cells are activated by cells expressing MICA (MHC-I chain-related gene A) and MICB (MHC-I chain-related gene B) gene products, and through these interactions can destroy infected or transformed epithelial cells in a manner independent of classic MHC (Fig. 2.10) (105–107). Like the other components of the innate system, $\gamma\delta$ T cells are present at sites of early infection and can mediate cytotoxicity in the absence of antigen-specific priming (see Chapters 3 and 6).

Natural Antibodies

Natural antibodies represent a primitive humoral response to common microbial elements such as bacterial polysaccharides and LPS. These "T-independent" antigens can stimulate naive B lymphocytes directly, in the absence of T cell-

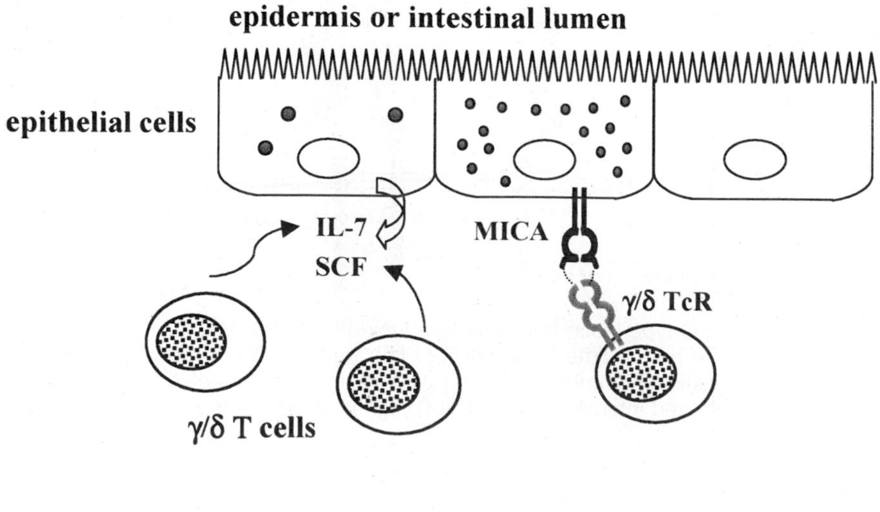

FIG. 2.10. The $\gamma\delta$ T cells recognize and destroy inflamed epithelial cells. They are common in the skin and intestinal epithelium, where their growth is promoted by factors such as interleukin-7 (IL-7) and stem cell factor (SCF). These cells mount the first line of defense against epithelial pathogens. Stressed or infected epithelial cells express MICA and MICB, major histocompatibility complex (MHC) class I–related gene products that are recognized by $\gamma\delta$ T cells. These interactions promote an early, cytotoxic response independent of MHC-restricted antigen presentation.

derived costimulatory signals, to proliferate and secrete immunoglobulin. Most natural antibodies are polyreactive and bind antigen with relatively low affinity compared with the tightly regulated, highly specific immunoglobulin generated through the adaptive response. However, because most natural antibodies are IgM and therefore pentameric, the overall avidity with which they bind antigen is relatively high. In general, natural antibodies are produced by B-1 cells, a distinct subset of B cells that appear early in ontogeny and phylogeny.

Natural antibodies provide an effective barrier to common bacteria (108). Because of their relatively broad reactivity, they can bind many antigens of the self (i.e., autoantigens); these provide the templates for pathogenic antibodies in certain autoimmune diseases such as systemic lupus erythematosus, rheumatoid arthritis, and Sjögren's syndrome (109–111).

Fc Receptors

The FcRs mediate immunoglobulin recognition by immune effector cells such as phagocytes, thereby facilitating the ancillary role of these cells in humoral immunity. These molecules constitute a family of single-chain, low-affinity receptors for the Fc region of specific immunoglobulin subtypes (112,113). The FcγRI, FcγRIIa, FcγRIIc, and FcγRIIIa isoforms are expressed by monocytes, macrophages, neutrophils, and other phagocytic cells (Table 2.2). These FcRs are MIRR-type transmembrane proteins, with ITAMs in the cytoplasmic tail that transduce activation signals on FcR engagement. In a subset of FcRs (FcγRI, FcγRIII, and FcϵRI), intracellular signals are transmitted by a nearby γ chain, which resembles the ζ chain associated with the TCR (113). Particles coated with immunoglobulin, such as microbial pathogens or, in some situations, blood cells, bind cells expressing FcRs to induce phagocytosis and cytotoxicity.

Some FcRs have highly specialized functions. For example, the polymeric IgA and IgM receptor (pIgR) binds and transports polymeric IgA or IgM across epithelial cells (114). Another receptor, FcRn, is expressed primarily in the fetus and newborn. This molecule transports IgG from the maternal circulation across the placenta to the fetus and later from ingested breast milk in the intestinal lumen across the intestinal mucosa to the newborn (115). The inhibitory receptor for IgG, FcγRIIb, is expressed primarily in B cells, where it plays an important role in downregulation of the humoral response. This receptor has a cytoplasmic ITIM, which transmits negative signals, such that B-cell proliferation and antibody production are reduced on crosslinking of FcγRIIb by IgG. Tyrosine phosphorylation of the FcγRIIb ITIM impedes positive signaling through the BCR, in part by interference with the RAS pathway and by consumption of lipid mediators of Ca^{2+} mobilization in B cells (100,116,117) (see Chapter 3).

Links Between Innate and Adaptive Immunity

Many links exist between the humoral and cellular mediators of the innate immune response and the later, antigen-specific adaptive responses. For example, macrophages readily ingest bacteria and other microorganisms. At the same time, macrophages initiate the adaptive response by processing antigen for recognition by antigen-specific T cells and by secretion of inflammatory cytokines. Likewise, the complement system functions in innate and adaptive immunity. It can be activated directly by bacteria and viruses through the alternative and lectin pathways, but it is activated also through the classic pathway on binding of specific antibodies to antigen. Moreover, complement improves the ef-

TABLE 2.2. *Human Fc receptors*

FcR subtype	Molecular group	Ligand	Function	Sites of constitutive expression
FcαRI	CD89	IgA	Phagocytosis, cytotoxicity	Neutrophils, macrophages, eosinophils
FcγRI	CD64	IgG (high affinity)	Phagocytosis	Phagocytic cells (macrophages, neutrophils, eosinophils), dendritic cells
FcγRIIa	CD32	IgG	Phagocytosis, granule release in eosinophils	Phagocytic cells, platelets
FcγRIIb		IgG	Inhibitory receptor	B cells
FcγRIIc		IgG	Phagocytosis, granule release in eosinophils	Phagocytic cells, platelets, Langerhans cells
FcγRIIIa	CD16	IgG	Cytotoxicity	Natural killer cells, phagocytic cells, Langerhans cells
FcγRIIIb		IgG	Granule release	Neutrophils
FcϵRI		IgE (high affinity)	Granule release	Mast cells, basophils
FcϵRII	CD23	IgE (low affinity)	Inhibitory receptor	B cells, activated monocytes
Fcμ, FcαR (pIgR)		IgA, polymeric IgM	Transcytosis across epithelial cells	Glandular epithelium
FcRn		IgG	Maternal-fetal transfer of IgG	Fetus, newborn gut

fectiveness of antigen-specific humoral immunity by enhancing opsonization of microbes and by engaging phagocytes that express complement receptors. One complement receptor, CD21 (C3d receptor, complement receptor-2) is expressed in B cells, where it functions as an integral part of the coreceptor for antigen. On binding the C3 split product C3d at the pathogen surface, CD21 links that antigen with the BCR coreceptor complex and thereby augments the antigen's capacity to signal through the BCR (118). Mast cells and basophils, which primarily function in the innate response, express CD154 (CD40 ligand) on activation and, in the presence of IL-4, thereby stimulate B-cell differentiation and production of IgE (119). Through these diverse molecular and cellular interactions, the elements of innate immunity generate an initial barrier to infection and contribute to the generation of adaptive immunity and immunologic memory (35).

B LYMPHOCYTES AND THE GENERATION OF IMMUNOGLOBULIN DIVERSITY

B lymphocytes can be defined as cells that produce immunoglobulin molecules, which bind, neutralize, and eradicate microbial pathogens and toxic substances. The term *B* was originally coined as a designation for the bursa of Fabricius, the avian organ in which immunoglobulin-producing cells arise. Conveniently, the nomenclature is appropriate also for the bone marrow, where immunoglobulin-producing cells are generated in mammals. Immunoglobulin is expressed at the surface of mature B cells, where it serves as the receptor (BCR) for antigen. On activation, the B cell secretes an antibody with identical specificity for antigen. In humans, the immune system has evolved such that an individual can generate at least 10^{10} distinct B-cell clones and therefore immunoglobulin molecules with distinct specificity. The intricate process by which B cells mature and differentiate to provide such a diverse and potent repertoire of B-cell clones is strictly regulated at each step.

Immunoglobulin Gene Structure and Functional Diversity

Diversity among the lymphocyte antigen receptors is generated at several levels (120–123). First, variation in the genomic, or inherited, BCR (immunoglobulin) and TCR genes provides the structural substrate for distinct antigen-binding domains. Second, recombination events during lymphocyte differentiation result in a still greater range of receptor structures. In mature B cells, somatic hypermutation and receptor editing afford another layer of diversity. All seven antigen receptor gene complexes, which are the immunoglobulin heavy (H) and light (κ and λ) chains and the TCR α, β, γ, and δ chains, share some common organizational features (Fig. 2.11). The inherited (germline) genes are retained in all nonhematopoietic cells, with multiple homologous but nonidentical copies of each gene segment type, called V for variable segment, D for diversity segment, J for joining segment, and C for constant segment. For example, the *IGH* locus on human chromosome 14 contains 51 functional V segments, 27 D segments, six J segments, and nine C regions (which encode each of the nine heavy chain isotypes: μ, δ, γ_1, γ_2, γ_3, γ_4, α_1, α_2, and ϵ) (124,125). The recombinase complex mediates the process of DNA recombination in developing B cells, such that the segments are connected in an orderly manner to generate a functional immunoglobulin VDJ-H, followed by Vκ-Jκ or Vλ-Jλ gene segments. The pairing of two identical and unique H chains with two identical Vκ-Jκ or Vλ-Jλ chains yields a unique antigen-binding structure (121,123) (see Chapter 7).

Isotype switching refers to the process by which B cells convert from the expression of the antigen binding site in the context of a given immunoglobulin isotype, such as IgM, to another isotype, such as IgG, IgA, or IgE. This process affords functional immunoglobulin diversity because of the generation of structurally distinct immunoglobulin molecules with preserved (identical) antigen-binding domains (126). In the immunoglobulin molecule, the two identical heavy chains each have a molecular mass of approximately 50 kd and are linked by a disulfide bond (Fig. 2.12). The identical light chains each have a molecular mass of approximately 25 kd and are each linked to a heavy chain by a disulfide bond (127,128). Each molecule includes a repeated structural motif, or immunoglobulin domain, which consists of approximately 110 amino acids. This sequence motif is highly conserved and occurs in many other proteins important in regulating cell contact and adhesion (Table 2.3).

Within an antibody molecule, there are four immunoglob-

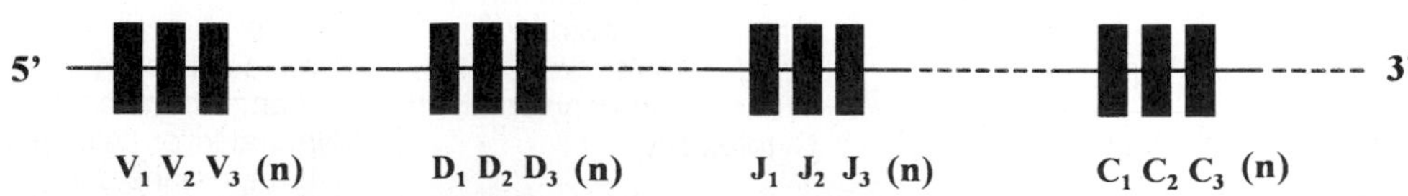

FIG. 2.11. Schematic representation of the antigen receptor genes. All seven antigen receptor genes (*IGH*; those for the κ and λ chains; and those for the T-cell receptor [TCR] α, β, γ, and δ chains) share a basic structural motif. The inherited (germline) genes are retained in all nonhematopoietic cells, with multiple, homologous but nonidentical copies of each segment type, called V for the variable segment, D for the diversity segment, J for the joining segment, and C for the constant segment. The recombinase complex mediates the process of DNA recombination, such that the segments are connected in an orderly manner to generate a functional immunoglobulin (Ig) or TCR chain.

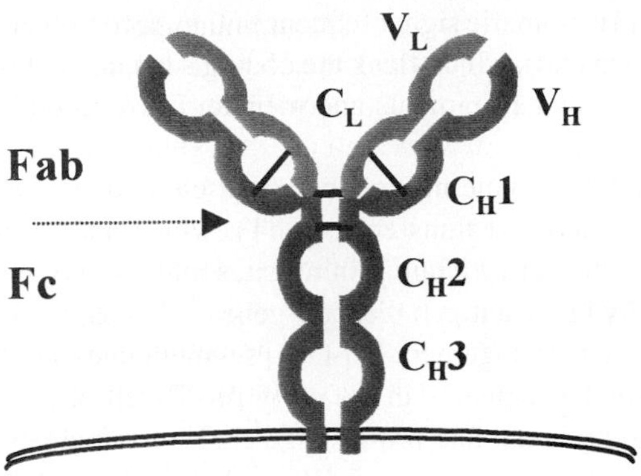

FIG. 2.12. Prototypic immunoglobulin (Ig) molecule. Each Ig monomer consists of two heavy (H) and two light (L, κ or λ) chains, which together form the V (variable, antigen-binding) and C (constant) regions. The H chains each include four conserved Ig domains of approximately 110 amino acids, called V_H, C_H1, C_H2, and C_H3. The L chains each include two Ig domains, called V_L and C_L. The heavy chains are linked by disulfide bonds, and each light chain associates with one heavy chain. Together, the V_H and C_H segments are the most diverse in amino acid sequence and confer most of the specificity for antigen binding. The section between the second and third C_H domains is the hinge region, which confers flexibility in Ig binding and is sensitive to proteolytic cleavage. Papain exposure generates two large Ig fragments, the antigen-binding Fab, and the constant, crystallizable fragment Fc.

TABLE 2.3. *Immunoglobulin superfamily proteins*

Receptor type	Specific function
Immune recognition	
Ig	B-cell antigen receptor
TCR	T-cell antigen receptor
β_2-microglobulin	MHC-I–associated invariant chain
MHC-I (α_3 domain)	Antigen presentation
MHC-II	Antigen presentation
CD80	B7-1; expressed in APCs; binds CD28 and CTLA-4
CD86	B7-2; expressed in APCs; binds CD28 and CTLA-4
CD28	Low-affinity receptor for CD80, CD86
CTLA-4	High-affinity receptor for CD80, CD86
CD4	Co-engagement of MHC-II
CD8	Co-engagement of MHC-I
FcRs	Bind Fc portions of Ig
KIRs	NK receptors bind MHC-I ligands
Adhesion	
CD2	LFA-2
CD31	PECAM
CD54	ICAM-1
CD102	ICAM-2
CD50	ICAM-3
CD56	NCAM
CD106	VCAM-1
Other functions	
CD19	Amplifies signals through BCR
CD22	Regulates signals through BCR

APC, antigen-presenting cell; BCR, B-cell receptor; CD, clusters of differentiation; CTLA-4, cytotoxic T-lymphocyte–associated molecule-4; ICAM-1, intercellular cell adhesion molecule-1; Ig, immunoglobulin; KIR, killer inhibitory receptor; LFA-2, leukocyte function antigen-2; MHC, major histocompatibility complex; NCAM, neural cell adhesion molecule; NK, natural killer; PECAM, platelet–endothelial cell adhesion molecule; TCR, T-cell receptor; VCAM, vascular cell adhesion molecule.

ulin domains in each heavy chain and two in each light chain, linked in such a way as to form a flexible hinge region. This section of the molecule is susceptible to papain cleavage, which generates two fragment antigen binding (Fab) regions and one fragment crystallizable (Fc) region. The Fab portions comprise the variable segments of each chain and all immunoglobulin components with specificity for antigen. The Fc fragment of each antibody includes nonvariable segments and heavy chain determinants that are essential for effector function and binding to FcRs (113,128).

Immature B cells express IgM at the surface and are the earliest B cells to leave the bone marrow. In the circulation, these B cells acquire surface IgD in addition to IgM due to alternative splicing of transcripts within individual cells, thereby completing the transition to mature B cells. In the mature naive B cells, IgM is secreted as part of the initial response to antigen if appropriate T-cell–derived signals are provided. The secreted form of IgM occurs as a 970-kd pentamer, previously called macroglobulin (129,130). The pentameric IgM includes a 15-kd peptide, or J chain, which links the individual IgM components. Further differentiation signals, provided largely by helper T (T_H) cells, result in isotype switching and production of IgG, IgA, or IgE. These isotypes are not generated contemporaneously within individual cells but serve distinct effector functions adapted for specific immune compartments and inflammatory responses.

IgG is the most common immunoglobulin form. Unlike IgM, it is monomeric in the membrane-bound and secreted forms. IgG is associated with long-term immunity, conferred by memory B cells, and is critical in the eradication of antigens in the extravascular space, as IgM cannot pass the endothelial cell barrier. Antigen bound by IgG is eliminated by phagocytic cells such as neutrophils and macrophages, which express FcRs that bind the Fc portions of IgG1 and IgG3. Both IgG and IgM can activate the complement cascade.

IgA is produced in B cells of the MALT tissues such as the gut, lacrimal glands, parotid glands, and breast ducts. It functions primarily in mucosal immunity. The secreted form of IgA is dimeric and, like IgM, includes a J chain (131). Some bacterial species, such as *Neisseria gonorrhoeae* and *Neisseria meningitidis,* produce ectoenzymes that cleave IgA, enhancing their capacity to infect and survive in mucosal epithelia (132).

Of the human immunoglobulin isotypes, IgE has the shortest half-life and is present at the lowest concentration in serum. It occurs only as a monomer and provides immunity to parasitic organisms. IgE binds to high-affinity IgE FcRs (FcϵRI) in eosinophils, mast cells, and basophils, thereby triggering activation and release of granules in those cells (79). Activated B cells express a low-affinity receptor for IgE, FcϵII (CD23), which functions through a negative feedback loop to inhibit IgE production in B cells (133).

B-Cell Ontogeny

Pro-B cells are the earliest committed B-cell elements and are derived from lymphoid progenitor cells in the bone marrow (Fig. 2.13). These cells have limited capacity for self-renewal and can be identified by the presence of certain cell-surface structures such as the BCR accessory chains CD79a and CD79b (Igα and Igβ). In the developing B cell, immunoglobulin gene rearrangements are mediated by a V(D)J recombinase complex, which includes the recombination activation gene products RAG-1 and RAG-2, DNA-dependent protein kinase (DNA-PK), a DNA ligase, and KU-70 and KU-80 (134). RAG-1 and RAG-2 are expressed at high levels in the early pro-B-cell stage, during which *IGH* gene rearrangements occur, and again at the pre-B-cell stage, during which immunoglobulin light-chain gene rearrangements are ongoing. These enzymes recognize conserved heptameric and nanomeric signal sequences (i.e., recombination signal sequences), which flank the coding sequences of individual V, D, and J segments and mediate DNA recombination (Fig. 2.14).

Another enzyme in the recombinase complex is terminal deoxynucleotidyl transferase (TdT), which adds N-nucleotides at the heavy chain joining sites and thereby increases diversity in the antigen receptor genes (135). Human B cells acquire a rearrangement V_H-D-J_H segment due to joining of the D and J segments in the early pro-B-cell phase and V-DJ joining in the late pro-B stage (121). In a human B cell, D-J joining can occur separately on both chromosomes, and either of two rearranged DJ segments is theoretically available for juxtaposition with a V gene in late pro-B cells.

Pre-B cells express the product of an intact, fully rearranged *IGH* gene, called μ. This molecule is stabilized at the cell surface in association with two small proteins, VpreB and λ5, which through noncovalent linkage form a surrogate light chain (136). The pre-B-cell receptor (pre-BCR), which is essential for B-cell development and maturation, consists of two μ chains and two surrogate light chains and, in some mammalian species, the BCR-associated signaling molecules CD79a and CD79b (137). The pre-BCR is expressed

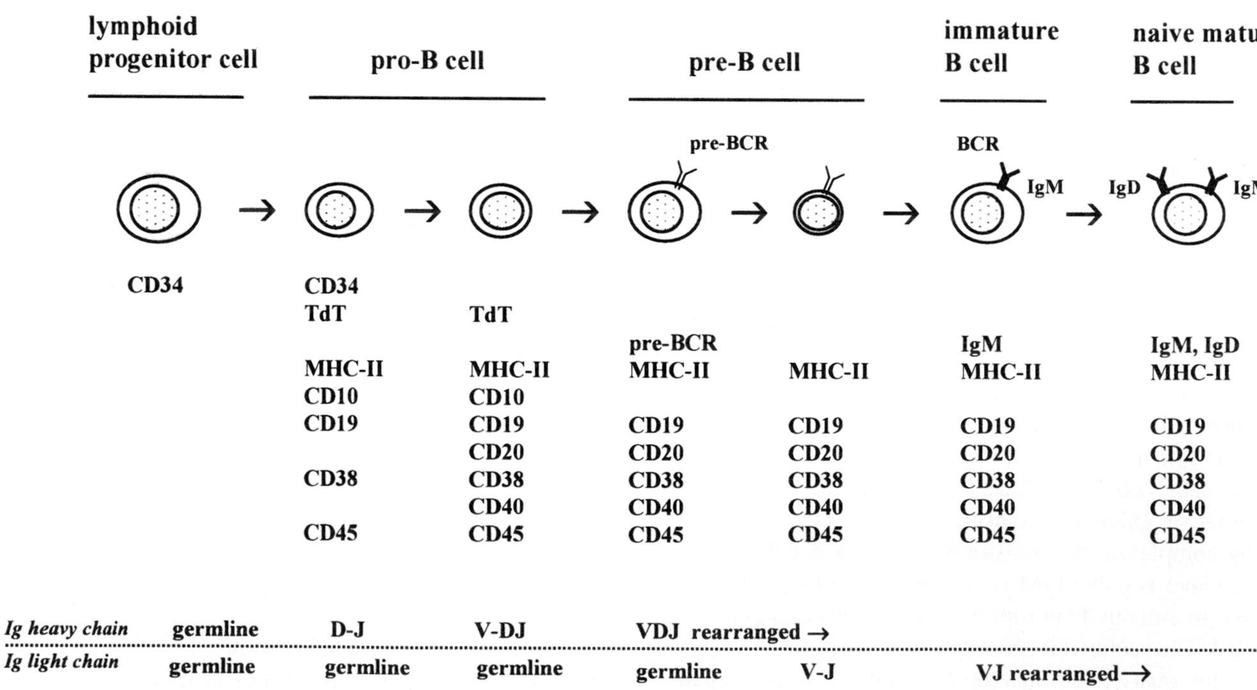

FIG. 2.13. Antigen-independent B-cell ontogeny. Progenitor B cells in the bone marrow undergo stochastic rearrangements of immunoglobulin (Ig) gene segments. The earliest recombination events occur in the pro-B cell stage. On production of an intact IGH, the cells express the pre-B-cell receptor (pre-BCR), which includes Ig heavy and surrogate light chains. Large pre-B cells proliferate in the bone marrow, generating numerous progeny with identical heavy chains. These daughter cells are subject to recombination at the κ and λ loci, which usually results in production of a light chain and, in combination with IGH, a complete and unique Ig molecule. The earliest mature B cells express IgM. Naive B cells express IgD and IgM due to alternative splicing of the Ig transcript such that it includes the δ or μ constant segment.

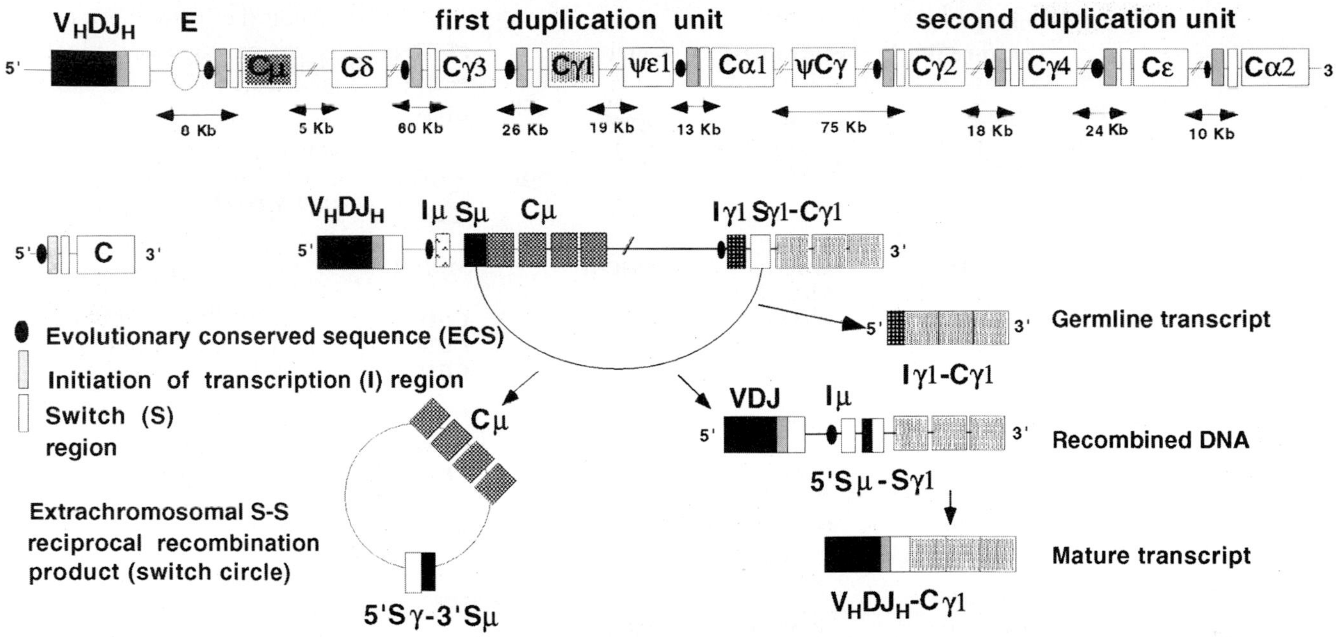

FIG. 2.14. Organization of the human immunoglobulin heavy (Ig H) chain locus on chromosome 14 and mechanisms of Ig H chain gene switch recombination. The human H chain locus is organized in two main clusters of genes, possibly resulting from the duplication of a primordial single locus. Each cluster consists of several H chain gene complexes, each of them comprising 4 or 5 exons (C_H1, Hinge, C_H2, C_H3, C_H4). The first cluster begins with $C\mu$ and ends with ϕC_γ; the second cluster begins with $C_\gamma 2$ and ends with $C_\alpha 2$. Each Ig class or isotype exon complex is preceded upstream by a switch region (S), an I region, and an ECS. Switch recombination causes the recombined V(D)J gene segment, which is initially expressed with the C_μ gene, to be subsequently expressed with one of seven downstream C_H genes ($C_\gamma 1$ is shown). Isotype switching, with the exception of switching to IgD, is effected by a deletional DNA recombination event called switch recombination, which occurs between tandemly repeated S regions. As depicted for C_μ to $C_\gamma 1$ switching, the switch recombination event forms a composite switch region that includes an upstream segment from the S_μ and a downstream segment from the S_γ region of the targeted H chain. The resulting intervening sequence is looped out as a switch or S circle. S circles are reciprocal recombination products; they encompass 5′ to 3′ the residual 5′ sequence of the S region of the downstream Ig H chain gene that was the target of recombination. Germline transcription precedes switch recombination to the same isotype. All germline I_H-C_H transcripts have the same structure, initiating 5′ to the tandem repeats of the S region (I region), proceeding through the C_H gene, and terminating at the normal poly(A) site for secreted or membrane-bound Ig H-chain mRNA.

transiently, and its emergence coincides with cessation of RAG-1 and RAG-2 synthesis, ensuring that each cell at this stage generates only a single *IGH* gene product (136). In the murine system, pre-β-cell division is usually sustained through five or six generations, such that a single pre-B cell with an intact μ chain generates 2^5 to 2^6 progeny.

Gene rearrangement at the immunoglobulin κ and λ loci occur at the next stage, that of the small pre-B cell, in which RAG-1 and RAG-2 are expressed again. $V_\kappa J_\kappa$ gene rearrangements precede those of $V_\lambda J_\lambda$ genes, which occur only if $V_\kappa J_\kappa$ rearrangements fail to yield an open reading frame sequence. If none of the κ rearrangements on the first chromosome tried is productive, the κ locus of the homologous chromosome undergoes the same process. Approximately 33% of pre-B cells fail to generate a productive V-J rearrangement at the κ locus, in which case the recombination complex is activated at the λ locus on chromosome 22. Because of redundancy at the light-chain loci and the capacity for trying multiple rearrangements at each locus on each chromosome, only a small fraction of human pre-B cells do not form a functional immunoglobulin κ or λ chain. Most pre-B cells generate an intact immunoglobulin molecule and become immature B cells, expressing a surface IgM BCR.

Immature B cells express IgM at the surface and thereby are able to interact directly with antigen for which they are specific. Whereas gene rearrangements leading to productive or nonproductive immunoglobulin H and L chains in pro-B and pre-B cells are stochastic and do not depend on affinity of the immunoglobulin gene product for antigen, once B cells acquire IgM at the surface, their fate is determined largely by the presence or absence of antigen to which they bind. From this stage on, B-cell growth and differentiation are antigen dependent. For example, crosslinking of IgM in immature B cells results in apoptosis (138). In healthy

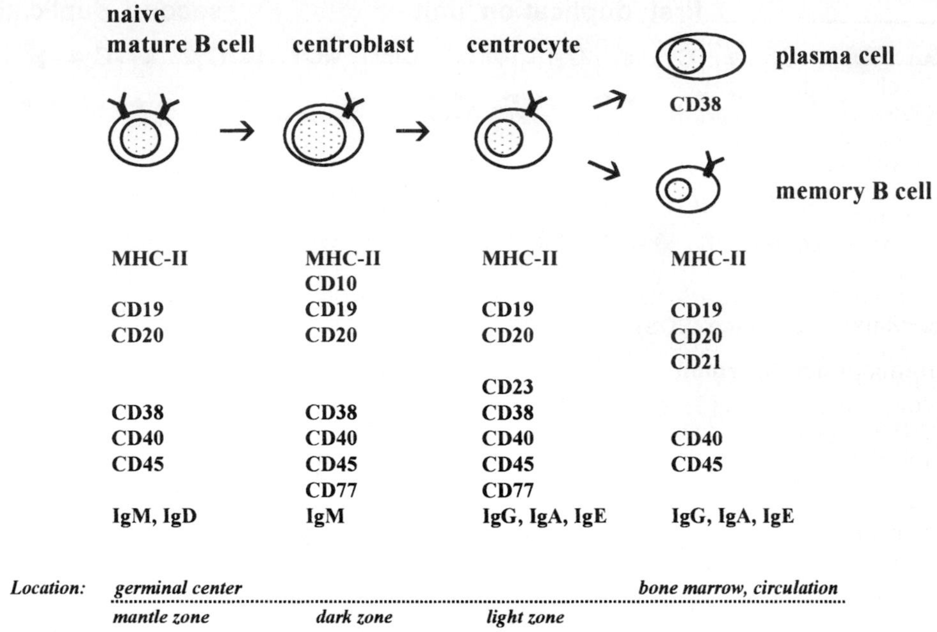

FIG. 2.15. Antigen-dependent B cell ontogeny. Naive mature B cells express immunoglobulins IgM and IgD. On recognition of antigen in the context of T-cell–derived signals, these cells enter the primary follicles and initiate germinal center (GC) formation. Undifferentiated GC B cells, called centroblasts, proliferate in the dark zone, where they undergo somatic mutation and Ig gene recombination. There is a high rate of apoptosis among GC centroblasts. The B cells that bind antigen and receive cognate T-cell "help" survive the affinity maturation process and differentiate into centrocytes, which fill the light zone. Differentiated centrocytes can exit the lymph node as plasma cells or as memory B cells.

individuals, immature B cells with affinity for autologous structures, such as those that bind multivalent repetitive ligands, are deleted in the bone marrow and do not enter the circulation.

In the peripheral circulation, most immature, IgM$^+$ B cells become mature, IgM$^+$IgD$^+$ B cells that can enter the spleen, lymph nodes, and MALT tissues (Fig. 2.15). In the spleen and the lymph nodes, naive B cells are located primarily in the mantle zone. These cells proliferate and enter the GC in response to stimuli such as antigen binding, IL-4, and costimulatory signals from T cells. The centroblasts, or early GC B cells, are found primarily in the dark zone (27). These cells are subject to somatic hypermutation and recombination events at the immunoglobulin gene loci (139–141). Based on their responsiveness to antigen bound to FDCs and presented by APCs, and receipt of costimulatory signals, some centroblasts differentiate as they traverse the GC, from which they exit as long-term memory B cells or as plasma cells. The factors that determine whether a B-cell differentiates into a memory cell, which expresses surface immunoglobulin (sIg), or undergoes terminal differentiation into a plasma cell, are poorly understood (26) (see Chapters 3, 6, and 7).

B-Cell Activation

B-cell activation is a tightly regulated process that integrates signals from the BCR, costimulatory interactions with T lymphocytes, and soluble factors such as cytokines. The principal mediators of B-cell activation are the BCR (sIg) and its associated signaling apparatus, which includes CD79a and CD79b; the B-cell coreceptor components CD19, CD21, and CD81; and other nearby surface proteins such as CD22 and CD45 (Table 2.4). In itself, sIg is incompetent in signal transduction because the nonsecretory, transmembrane form penetrates the B-cell cytoplasm by only a few amino acids. The cytosol contains protein tyrosine kinases (PTKs), phosphatases, adaptor proteins, and other signaling elements that integrate and control the response to BCR engagement. The two structures most closely linked to sIg are CD79a and CD79b, which each contain an ITAM sequence in the cytoplasmic domain (193,194,222). ITAMS contain essential phosphorylation sites that are recognized by SH2-related tyrosine kinases. In the B-cell resting state, there is a dynamic equilibrium among partially activated ITAMs, phosphatases, and cytosolic PTKs (194,223).

The BCR shares several basic features with other MIRRs, which include the TCR, most FcRs, and a subset of NK receptors (193,194). The structures of these complex, immunoglobulin domain–containing molecules facilitate separation and compartmentalization of ligand binding and signal transduction. On crosslinking of the antigen receptor, there can occur highly divergent outcomes, such as apoptosis in naive, immature B cells and proliferation in GC B cells (96,154,192). Several PTKs are associated with the BCR, including SRC family kinases, BTK, and the ZAP-70 (zeta

TABLE 2.4. *Common B-cell surface antigens*

Molecule	Features	References
Ig	B-cell receptor to antigen	122, 128
MHC-I	Mediates antigen-specific $CD8^+$ T-cell responses	142, 143
MHC-II	Mediates antigen-specific $CD4^+$ T-cell responses;	142, 144
CD5	In B-1 cells; modulates BCR reponse	145–147
CD10	Common acute lymphoblastic leukemia antigen; zinc metalloproteinase expressed in pro-B cells, GC centroblasts	148–150
CD19	Coexpressed with BCR; phosphorylated on BCR engagement; amplifies BCR-mediated signals	151–154
CD20	Phosphoprotein with four transmembrane domains, probable Ca^{2+} channel	155–158
CD21	CR2 (complement component C3d receptor, Epstein-Barr virus receptor); coexpressed with BCR; ligand for CD23	118, 159–162
CD22	Ig superfamily member activates SHP-1, which inhibits BCR-mediated signaling	154, 163–165
CD23	Low-affinity IgE receptor; induced by CD40 ligation in B cells; binds CD21	162, 166–168
CD27	TNFR-type protein; ligand is CD70; expressed in memory B cells	169, 170
CD30	TNFR-type activation antigen binds CD153; inhibits CD40-mediated signals	171, 172
CD38	NAD glycohydrolase	173–175
CD39	Ecto-ADPase; B-cell function is unknown	176, 177
CD40	TNFR type molecule expressed in all B cells; binds CD154; transduces B-cell survival, proliferation, and differentiation signals	178, 179
CD45	Leukocyte common antigen; phosphatase	98, 180
CD54	Intracellular cell adhesion molecule-1	181, 182
CD70	TNF-type ligand expressed in activated lymphocytes; ligand for CD27; putative role in T-cell–dependent B-cell differentiation	183–185
CD71	Transferrin receptor	186–188
CD72	C-type lectin, ligand for CD5	189
CD77	Glycosphingolipid expressed in GC B cells, "Burkitt's lymphoma antigen"	190, 191
CD79a, b	Igα, β; Ig accessory molecules; cytoplasmic domains contain ITAM regions for transmitting BCR-induced signals	192–194
CD80	B7-1; Ig superfamily member; binds to CD28 and CTLA-4 in T cells	195–199
CD81	Target of antiproliferative antibody-1; four transmembrane domain protein associates with BCR; receptor for hepatitis C	200–202
CD86	B7-2; Ig superfamily member; binds to CD28 and CTLA-4 in T cells	198, 199, 203, 204
CD95	FAS; APO-1; TNFR family member expressed in activated lymphocytes; initiates apoptotic signals	205–209
CD120a	TNFRI; p55; transduces death signals through death domain	210–212
CD120b	TNFRII; p75	210, 213
CD124	IL-4 receptor	214, 215
CD125	IL-5 receptor	216
CD126	IL-6 receptor α subunit	217
CD130	Common subunit of IL-6, IL-11, oncostatin M, and leukemia inhibitory factory receptors	218, 219
CD138	Syndecan-1; heparan sulphate proteoglycan	220, 221

BCR, B-cell receptor; CD, clusters of differentiation; CTLA-4, cytotoxic T-lymphocyte–associated molecule-4; GC, germinal center; Ig, immunoglobulin; IL, interleukin; ITAM, immunoreceptor tyrosine-based activation motif; SHP, SRC homology-2 (SH2) domain–containing tyrosine phosphatase; TNFR, tumor necrosis factor receptor.

chain–associated protein)–like kinase SYK) (96,193,224, 225). One of the first events on antigen receptor cross-linking is phosphorylation of the CD79a and CD79b ITAMs by SRC-type PTKs such as LYN, BLK, and FYN (193). On phosphorylation of these ITAM residues, downstream signaling events are initiated along several pathways. SYC is activated and recruited to the complex, followed by translocation of phospholipase Cγ2 (PLCγ2) to the cell membrane, cleavage of phosphatidylinositol 4,5-bisphosphate (PIP_2) to yield diacylglycerol (DAG) and 1,4,5-triphosphate (IP_3), with subsequent Ca^{2+} flux and increase of intracellular Ca^{2+} concentration. Simultaneously, there occur DAG-mediated activation of protein kinase C (PKC) and RAS-mediated initiation of the mitogen-activated protein (MAP) kinase cascade (96). Ultimately, these rapid metabolic changes in the B-cell cytosol lead to activation of nuclear transcriptional factors such as nuclear factor-κB (NF-κB), and DNA synthesis.

Several phosphatases are associated with the BCR complex, which regulates kinase activation in response to sIg engagement (98,226). These include the widely expressed CD45 (leukocyte common antigen) tyrosine phosphatase, a large glycosylated membrane receptor that occurs in various isoforms of M_r 180 to 220 kd (180,227). These isoforms are generated by alternative splicing and by glycosylation of specific residues in the formed protein, which can be altered by the occurrence and affinity of antigen binding to the cell. CD45 removes inhibitory phosphates from SH2-type kinases, facilitating ITAM phosphorylation on sIg crosslinking by antigen. Additional phosphatases that play an important role in B-cell activation include the SRC homology inositol polyphosphate 5′-phosphatase (SHIP) and the phosphotyrosine phosphatases (SHP-1 and SHP-2) (228). In general, these phosphatases generate negative signals through their interactions with ITIM elements of inhibitory receptors such as FcγRIIb.

CD19, CD21 (receptor for the C3d or complement receptor-2), and CD81 (target of antiproliferative antibody-1 [TAPA-1]) colocalize with immunoglobulin and form the B-cell coreceptor complex (Fig. 2.16). CD19 is an immunoglobulin superfamily transmembrane protein expressed in B cells from the early pre-B-cell stage through that just before the plasma cell (154). When phosphorylated, CD19 associates with phosphatidyl inositol 3 (PI3) kinase and amplifies signals initiated on BCR engagement. CD19 augments sIg-mediated signals to such an extent that DNA synthesis induced on BCR crosslinking is increased by approximately 100-fold relative to that which occurs in the absence of CD19 (152,153). CD19 signaling is modulated by SHIP, which dephosphorylates CD19 and thereby dampens the B-cell response to BCR engagement. Surface immunoglobulin crosslinking also results in tyrosine phosphorylation of CD22, which activates the tyrosine phosphatase SHP-1, an inhibitor of BCR signaling (165,229). CD21 is the receptor for complement component C3d and serves as a receptor for Epstein-Barr virus (EBV). CD81 (TAPA-1) was identified as a receptor for the hepatitis C viral envelope protein E2 (200,201).

Although the precise function of CD20 in B-cell survival and differentiation is not established, this molecule is the focus of numerous studies primarily because its engagement by antibody can trigger B-cell apoptosis (230). It is the target antigen for several monoclonal antibodies that have been used to induce death of malignant B cells *in vitro*, in murine models, and in humans (231). CD20 is a nonglycosylated protein of 33 to 37 kd that contains four transmembrane-spanning domains and appears to function as a calcium channel (158). Expression of CD20 is highly B cell specific, and it can be detected at high levels at the surface of B cells from the pre-B-cell stage almost to the point of terminal differentiation. Crosslinking of CD20 results in activation of cytoplasmic kinases, phosphorylation of phospholipase C-γ (PLC-γ), and mobilization of intracellular Ca^{2+} stores (232). Based on evidence that Ca^{2+} chelation can inhibit apoptosis in B cells exposed to monoclonal antibody to CD20, some investigators have suggested that CD20-mediated cell death occurs as a function of Ca^{2+}-dependent apoptotic pathways (230).

B-1 Cells

B-1 cells are a distinct subset of B cells committed to the production of natural antibodies. These are mainly polyreactive IgM with moderate to high affinity for bacterial antigens, including repetitive carbohydrate structures. These cells appear early in phylogeny and ontogeny, and they are distinguished from conventional B-2 cells by expression of surface CD5 (145,233). B-1 cells are abundant in the neonate; in the umbilical cord, more than 90% of B cells are $CD5^+$. In adult humans, B-1 cells are found in relatively high proportion in the spleen and in the peritoneal and

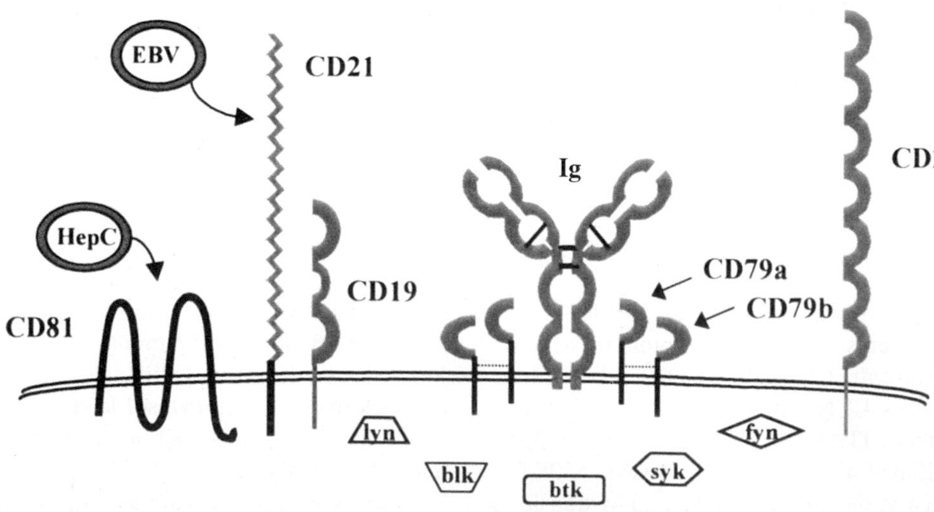

FIG. 2.16. B-cell receptor (BCR) complex. The BCR consists of surface immunoglobulin (sIg), which lacks a cytosolic signaling domain, and the closely associated Igα and Igβ chains (CD79a and CD79b), which contain cytosolic immunoreceptor tyrosine-based activation motifs (ITAMs) that are necessary for BCR-mediated signal transduction and through which these molecules interact with cytosolic protein tyrosine kinases (PTKs). The co-receptor complex also includes CD19, CD21, and CD81. CD21 is a receptor for Epstein-Barr virus, and CD81 is a receptor for hepatitis C virus.

pleural cavities (111). B-1 cells are thought to give rise to the neoplastic elements in chronic lymphocytic leukemia (CLL) (234,235).

B-1 cells are distinguished from other B cells by expression of CD5, a cysteine-rich, 67-kd, transmembrane protein of the macrophage "scavenger receptor" family (147,236). Molecules with demonstrated affinity include CD72 (189 237), the lymphocyte-activation molecule gp35-37 (CD5L) (238), and the framework region of the *IGH*-encoded V segment (239). In T cells, CD5 acts as a negative regulator of TCR-induced signal transduction (240), and in murine B-1 cells, CD5 inhibits nuclear translocation of NF-κB on BCR engagement (146). In T and B cells, the cytoplasmic domain of CD5 associates with the β subunit of the serine/threonine kinase casein kinase-2 (CK-2), an important regulator of inhibitor of kappa B (I-κB) phosphorylation (147,241). CD5 appears to modulate the response to antigen receptor engagement and, in autoreactive B lymphocytes, may limit cellular activation and proliferation in the context of antigen binding.

T LYMPHOCYTES AND THE MAJOR HISTOCOMPATIBILITY COMPLEX: RESTRICTION AND FUNCTION

T cells represent 50% to 70% of the circulating lymphocytes in humans. Like B cells, T lymphocytes bear highly diversified surface antigen receptors that bind antigen specifically. The TCR structure is closely related to that of immunoglobulin, with diverse antigen-binding regions, the sequences of which are generated through an orderly process of V, D, and J gene rearrangements (242,243). In contrast to immunoglobulin, the TCR is neither secreted nor shed from the cell surface, and the TCR does not bind soluble proteins or other antigens in the circulation. T cells instead identify and bind peptide antigens displayed at the host cell surface by specialized and highly polymorphic glycoproteins of the MHC system (142,244).

There are two major T-cell subsets that are distinguished by expression of the TCR complex type I ($\gamma\delta$) or type 2 ($\alpha\beta$). Most T cells in the peripheral blood, lymph nodes, and spleen are $\alpha\beta$ (type 2) T cells. These T cells are CD4$^+$ (helper) or CD8$^+$ (suppressor) T cells. In general, CD4$^+$ T cells recognize peptides at the APC surface in the context of MHC class II (MHC-II) molecules, and CD8$^+$ T cells recognize peptides in the context of MHC class I (MHC-I) molecules (Fig. 2.17).

CD4$^+$ T cells comprise two major subtypes, T_H1 and T_H2 T cells. In general, T_H1 cells promote and mediate cellular immunity through the generation and secretion of cytokines such as IL-2 and IFN-γ, which activate macrophages and other T cells. T_H2 cells induce humoral immunity through expression of costimulatory molecules and by secretion of cytokines such as IL-4 that promote proliferation and differentiation of B cells (245,246).

Major Histocompatibility Complex

The MHC (i.e., HLA in humans) genes encompass a large region of DNA on human chromosome 6 (247). There are two broad categories of MHC antigens, called MHC class I (MHC-I) and MHC class II (MHC-II) (142). Whereas MHC-I antigens are expressed in all nucleated cells and platelets, under most circumstances, MHC-II antigens are expressed only in APCs such as macrophages, DCs, and B cells. The MHC-I molecules each comprise two noncovalently linked proteins: a 44-kd heavy, or α, chain, encoded at the MHC locus, and a 12-kd invariant chain, termed β_2-microglobulin, encoded on chromosome 15 (248). At each MHC-I locus,

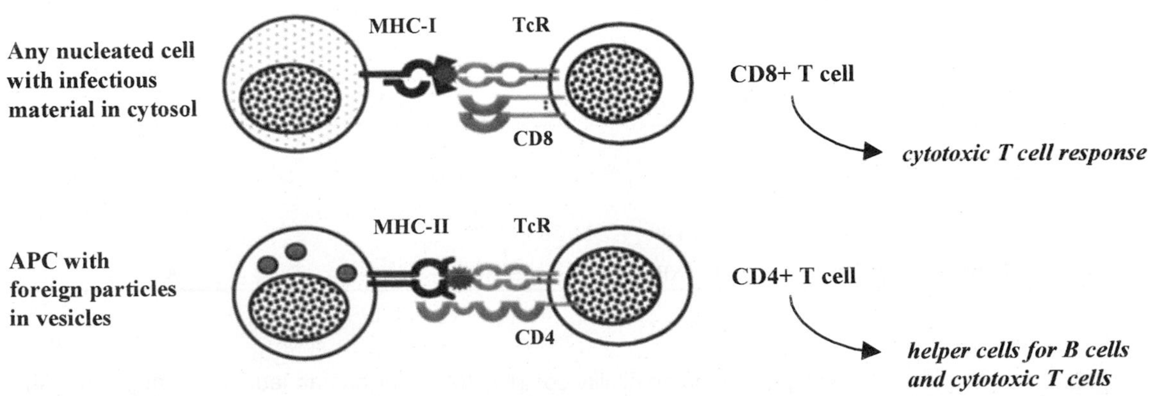

FIG. 2.17. Recognition of antigen by CD4$^+$ and CD8$^+$ T cells in the context of the major histocompatibility complex (MHC). CD4$^+$ T cells identify peptides displayed by MHC class II molecules. These peptides are degraded components of extracellular microbes that have been engulfed by macropinocytosis or internalized after receptor binding, or of intravesicular, intracellular pathogens. In general, CD4$^+$ T-cell activation results in augmentation of the humoral response. In contrast, CD8$^+$ T cells recognize peptides presented at the cell surface in the context of MHC class I molecules, which are usually derived from intracellular cytosolic pathogens. Activation of antigen-specific CD8$^+$ T cells results in cytotoxicity directed at infected cells.

there are three distinct α-chain subloci, called HLA-A, HLA-B, and HLA-C, each with highly polymorphic alleles. Together the three subloci determine the MHC-I haplotype for that chromosome (249). MHC-II molecules contain two noncovalently bound chains of 33 and 29 kd, designated α and β, which are each anchored to the cell surface by a membrane-spanning domain. At the MHC-II locus, the MHC-II α- and β-chain genes occur in clusters, called HLA-DR, -DP, -DQ, and others (250). In many haplotypes, the HLA-DR cluster contains an additional, or alternate, β-chain allele, such that the chromosome includes genes for four distinct and complete MHC-II molecules. Because MHC molecules are polyallelic and expressed in a codominant fashion, a human with nonoverlapping haplotypes on each chromosome can express six distinct MHC-I molecules and as many as eight MHC-II molecules.

The MHC locus on human chromosome 6 contains nearly 200 genes (Fig. 2.18). Besides those encoding MHC-I and MHC-II, there are genes for several immunoregulatory proteins such as transporters associated with antigen-processing (TAP) protein-1 and -2 and the proteosome components LMP-2 and LMP-7. The MHC-I locus also encodes some proteins important in cellular stress responses, such as the heat shock protein (HSP). In the MHC-II region, there are genes encoding HLA-DM and HLA-DO chains (DN-α and DO-β). These MHC-II–like molecules are not expressed at the cell surface, but they instead facilitate MHC-II peptide interaction and loading within the endosomal MHC-II compartment (MIIC) vesicles (251–253). The MHC-III region genes include those for TNF-α and TNF-β complement components C2, factor B, and C4; and MICA and MICB. The loci for some genes linked to specific human diseases but of unknown immune function occur at the MHC locus. These include the genes encoding 21-hydroxylase and those that serve as markers for hereditary hemachromatosis (254,255).

Antigen Processing and Presentation

CD8$^+$ T cells recognize peptides presented at the cell surface by MHC-I molecules, whereas CD4$^+$ T cells identify peptides in the context of MHC-II molecules. This difference reflects distinct mechanisms that have evolved to direct the immune response to infectious pathogens in specific cellular compartments (142). In general, MHC-I molecules transport and display peptides from viruses or other cytosolic pathogens, and infected cells are targeted for recognition by cytotoxic CD8$^+$ T cells. Our understanding of how microbial antigens are processed and then displayed as short peptides for immune recognition by T cells was facilitated by solving the structure of MHC-I by x-ray crystallography (248,256,257). The MHC-I heavy chain includes three extracellular domains, called α1, α2, and α3, and a transmembrane domain. The α1 and α2 regions form a cleftlike structure in which peptides are transported and presented (Fig. 2.19). The α3 region contains an immunoglobulin domain. The MHC-I invariable chain, β_2-microglobulin, is noncovalently attached to the heavy chain in the extracellular portion and contains an immunoglobulin domain. In the antigen-binding cleft of each MHC-I lies a peptide of 8 to 10 amino acids, fixed by hydrophobic anchor residues. Between the anchor sites in the MHC-I groove, the peptide fragment and polymorphic cleft sequence generate a unique quarternary structure for T-cell recognition and discrimination. MHC proteins have evolved such that a cell encoding only six distinct MHC-I molecules can display peptides derived from innumerable pathogens (248).

The process of MHC-I–associated antigen display depends on controlled generation of peptides in the cytosol and their subsequent loading onto MHC-I molecules (Fig. 2.20). In mammalian cells, cytosolic proteins are marked for degradation by ubiquitin and reduced to small peptides by large, multi-protease complexes called *proteosomes* (258).

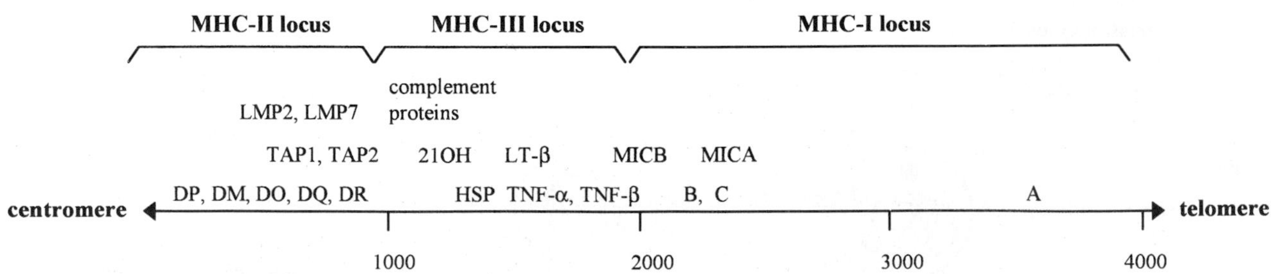

FIG. 2.18. Map of human major histocompatibility complex (MHC, or human leukocyte antigen [HLA]) locus on chromosome 6. This simplified map of the MHC locus represents the three main loci and selected genes. The MHC-II locus includes MHC-II genes such as DP, DM, DO, DQ, and DR, as well as genes for the proteosome components, the latent membrane protein (LMP)-2 and LMP-7, and transporters associated with antigen-processing (TAP) proteins, TAP-1 and TAP-2. The MHC class III region includes genes for complement components such as C2, C4, and factor B, as well as 21-hydroxylase (21OH), heat shock protein-70 (HSP-70), tumor necrosis factor-α (TNF-α), lymphotoxin-β (LT-β), and TNF-β (i.e., LT-α). Class I genes include the B, C, and A clusters, as shown, in addition to MICA and MICB, MHC class I–related gene products. (Adapted from Campbell RD, Trowsdale J. Map of the human MHC. *Immunol Today* 1993;14:349–352.)

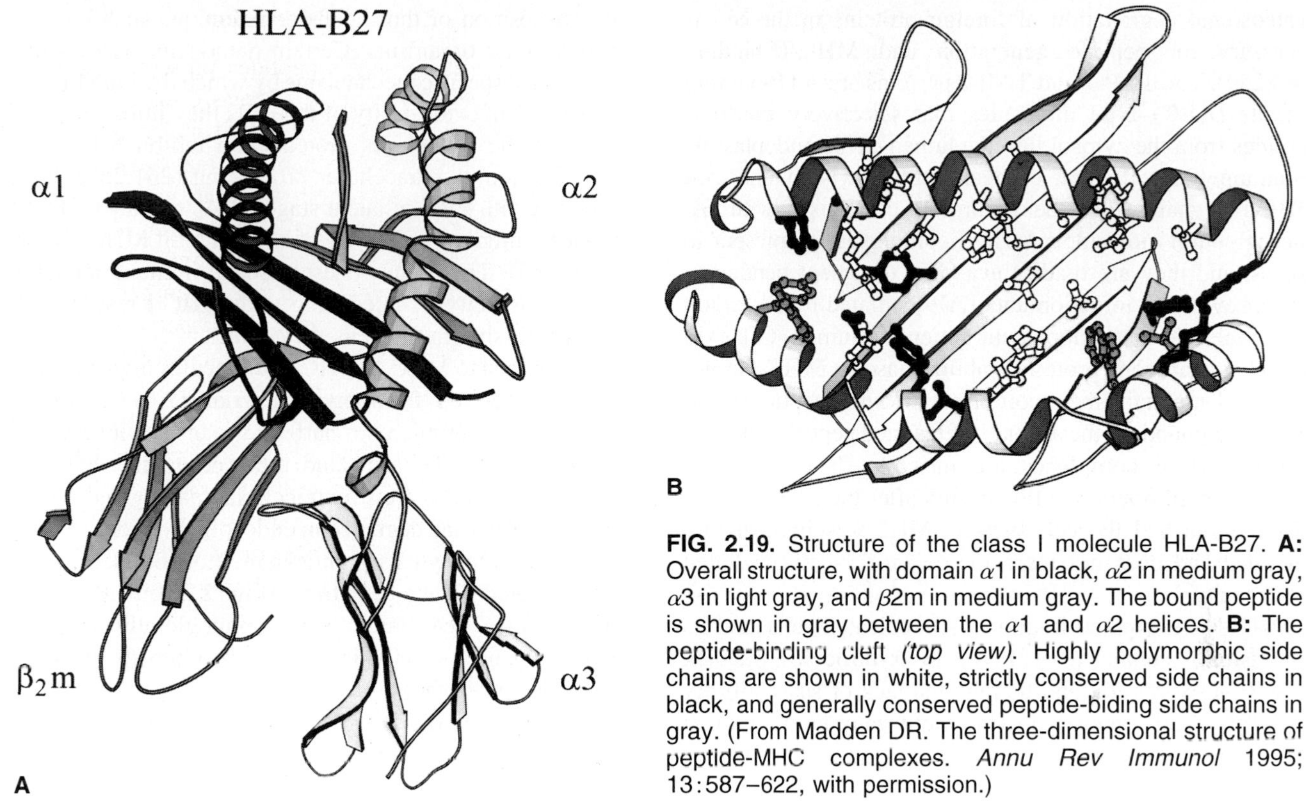

FIG. 2.19. Structure of the class I molecule HLA-B27. **A:** Overall structure, with domain α1 in black, α2 in medium gray, α3 in light gray, and β2m in medium gray. The bound peptide is shown in gray between the α1 and α2 helices. **B:** The peptide-binding cleft *(top view)*. Highly polymorphic side chains are shown in white, strictly conserved side chains in black, and generally conserved peptide-biding side chains in gray. (From Madden DR. The three-dimensional structure of peptide-MHC complexes. *Annu Rev Immunol* 1995; 13:587–622, with permission.)

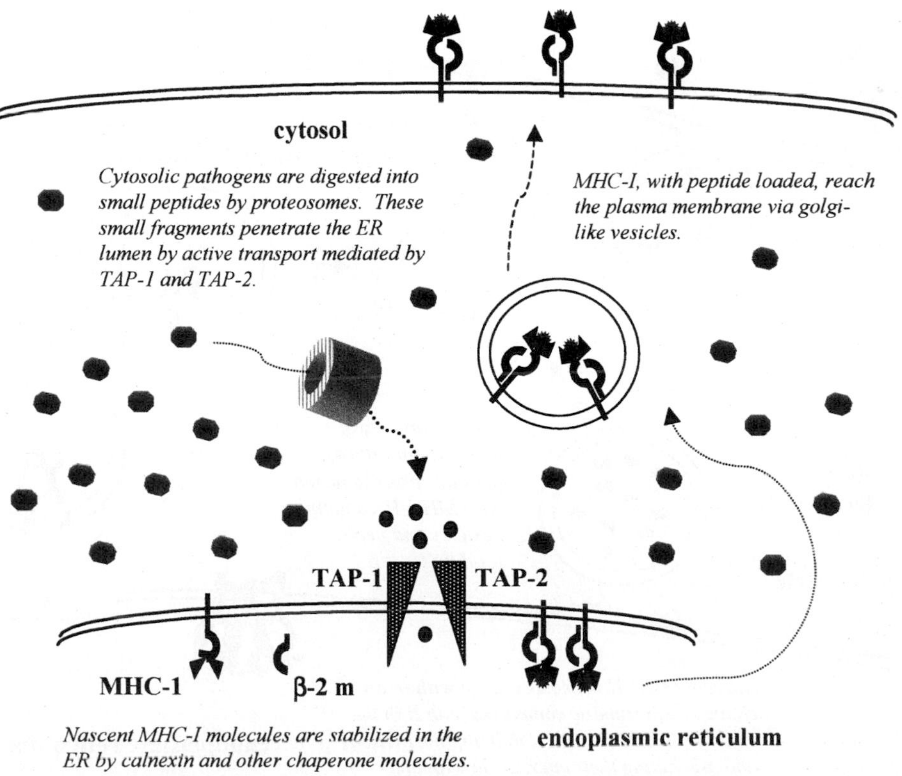

cytosol
Cytosolic pathogens are digested into small peptides by proteosomes. These small fragments penetrate the ER lumen by active transport mediated by TAP-1 and TAP-2.
MHC-I, with peptide loaded, reach the plasma membrane via golgi-like vesicles.
TAP-1
TAP-2
MHC-1
β-2 m
Nascent MHC-I molecules are stabilized in the ER by calnexin and other chaperone molecules.
endoplasmic reticulum

FIG. 2.20. Major histocompatibility (MHC) class I peptide loading occurs after proteosomal degradation of cytosolic antigens. Nascent MHC-I and β_2-microglobulin (β-2m) are stabilized by tapasin and other proteins in the endoplasmic reticulum. After digestion of cytosolic material by proteosomes, peptides are inserted into the endoplasmic reticulum by means of transporters associated with antigen-processing (TAP) proteins, TAP-1 and TAP-2. After peptide insertion and binding, MHC-I folds in such a way as to be released from chaperone molecules. The MHC-1 complexes with peptides travel to the cell surface through Golgi-like vesicles.

Proteosomal degradation of foreign proteins in the cell is necessary for peptide generation and MHC-I binding (143,259). The TAP-1 and TAP-2 proteins are ATP-binding cassette (ABC)–type molecules that selectively transport peptides from the cytosol into the lumen of the endoplasmic reticulum (260). In that compartment, newly synthesized MHC-I α chains form heterodimeric complexes with β_2-microglobulin molecules. MHC-I complexes are present in excess, and they are readily available to accept peptide in case of cytosolic infection and TAP-mediated translocation of peptide into the endoplasmic reticulum lumen. Calnexin and other chaperone proteins stabilize nascent MHC-I molecules and maintain their conformation until peptide is inserted and bound. In the absence of inserted peptide, unchaperoned MHC-I complexes are unstable. If cleavage or dissociation of bound peptide occurs after the MHC-I complex has reached the cell surface, MHC-I is immediately degraded and does not mark the cell for T-cell–mediated cytotoxicity.

MHC-I is expressed in almost all nucleated cells, and its expression is enhanced by IFN-γ. In erythrocytes, the lack of MHC-I expression and thereby the lack of susceptibility to $CD8^+$ T-cell–mediated cytotoxicity may be a factor in the disposition of those cells to infections such as malaria and *Babesia* organisms. Certain pathogenic viruses in humans have specific mechanisms by which they inhibit MHC-I–dependent cytotoxicity of the cells they infect. For example, specific adenovirus proteins can inhibit MHC-1 gene transcription or intracellular processing (261,262). In cells infected with EBV in latent stage, G-A_2 repeats in the EBV nuclear antigen-1 (EBNA-1) protein inhibit MHC-1 expression (263). Thus some viruses escape immune recognition and cytotoxicity by interfering with MHC-I restricted antigen processing in the cells they infect.

In contrast to MHC-I, MHC-II molecules bind and present peptides derived from mycobacteria, *Listeria monocytogenes,* and other microbes harbored in intracellular vesicles. MHC-II molecules affix and transport to the cell-surface peptide fragments from extracellular pathogens that have been engulfed and degraded in endosomal vesicles, as occurs after macropinocytosis of antigen or, more often, after receptor-mediated uptake of antigen (Fig. 2.21). In B cells, this may involve FcR binding to immunoglobulin complexed with antigen, or specific interaction between sIg and antigen at the B-cell surface.

In general, MHC-II molecules bind and present peptides

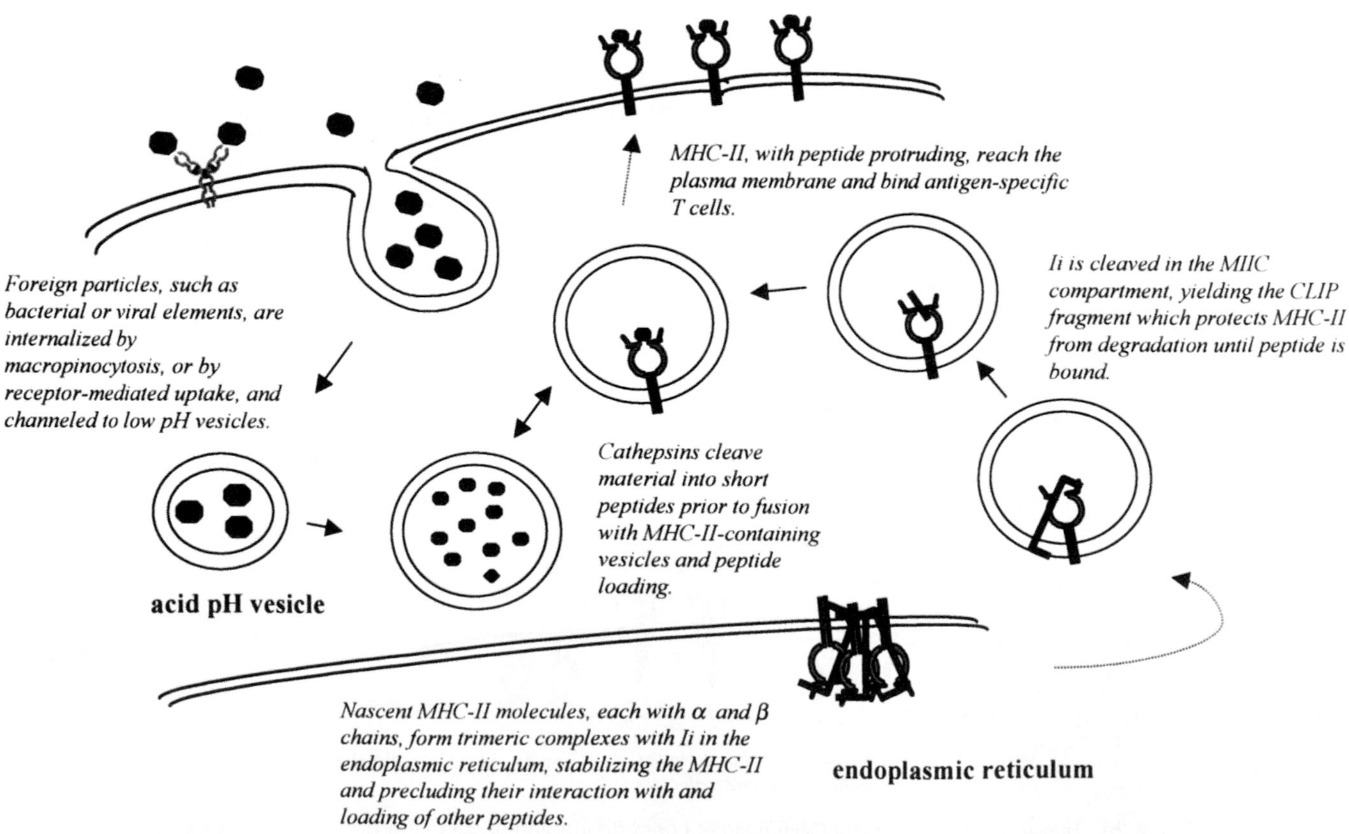

FIG. 2.21. Major histocompatibility (MHC) class II peptide loading occurs in specialized vesicles after cleavage of the invariant chain (Ii). MHC-II is generated and bound to Ii in the endoplasmic reticulum lumen and exits to MHC-II compartment (MIIC) vesicles. These fuse with acid pH vesicles in which foreign material has been digested. In the MIIC compartment, Ii is clipped, and peptides are loaded before transport of the MHC-II complexes to the cell surface.

of at least 13 amino acids in such a manner that the peptides protrude from the cleft. In the endoplasmic reticulum, newly synthesized MHC-II α and β chains form heterodimeric complexes that bind calnexin and the MHC-II–associated invariant chain (Ii). The physical relationship between MHC-II and Ii precludes interaction of partially synthesized host proteins with the MHC-II peptide-binding groove (264,265). The Ii chain also targets MHC-II proteins to low-pH endosomal vesicles, called MIIC (MHC-II compartment), where Ii is cleaved. One of the cleavage products, class II–associated invariant chain peptide (CLIP), remains bound to MHC-II in such a manner that peptides can bind only after their interaction with another MHC-encoded molecule in the vesicle, HLA-DM. Within MIIC vesicles, foreign antigens are destroyed by acid proteases such as cathepsins B, D, and L. Peptide loading onto MHC-II in the MIIC compartment is strictly regulated by MHC-related accessory molecules including HLA-DM and DO (264,266). After CLIP is generated, MHC-II molecules that do not bind peptide are rapidly degraded in the endosomal compartment.

T-Cell Receptor

The TCR consists of two transmembrane glycoprotein chains linked by a disulfide bond. Each TCR chain contains two immunoglobulin domains, which form constant and variable regions, a positively charged intramembrane segment, and a small cytoplasmic tail. Like those for immunoglobulin, the genes encoding the TCR undergo an orderly recombinatorial process during T-cell development, such that each cell expresses a unique TCR of the $\alpha\beta$ or $\gamma\delta$ type. The δ-chain locus is embedded within the TCR α-chain gene locus. There are at least four δV regions, which are dispersed among the V regions for the α chain, and three D, three J, and a single C region, all of which occur in the intron between the V and J segments of the α chain (267). Antigen recognition by the TCR occurs primarily at the third complementarity-determining region (CDR3), where there is tremendous structural diversity (242,243,268) (see Chapter 7).

Much like BCR, TCR-induced T-cell activation involves several coreceptor molecules, associated cytoplasmic kinases, and phosphatases (269–272) (Table 2.5). The CD3 complex includes the γ, δ, ϵ, and ζ chains (Fig. 2.22). Although transcription of the CD3 genes is controlled separately from that of the TCR chains, CD3 is coexpressed with the TCR and colocalizes with the TCR at the cell surface. The CD3 γ, δ, and ϵ chains each contain a single ITAM motif that is critical for signal transduction on ligand binding to the TCR. The ζ chains each contain three ITAM regions, and the phosphorylation state of the six ζ ITAMs in any TCR complex can reflect subtle differences in ligand quantity and binding affinity (301). TCR signaling is initiated through

TABLE 2.5. *T-cell surface antigens*

Molecule	Features	References
TcR	T-cell receptor for antigen	242, 243
MHC-I	Mediates antigen-specific $CD8^+$ T-cell responses	143, 273
CD2	LFA-2; T-cell adhesion and activation	274, 275
CD3	TCR-associated molecule; necessary for TCR expression and signaling	269, 276
CD4	TCR co-receptor; binds MHC-II; receptor for HIV	276
CD5	Scavenger receptor type protein; negative regulator of TCR-mediated signal transduction	240
CD7	Ig superfamily receptor regulates cell adhesion; cytoplasmic domain associates with PI_3 kinase	277
CD8	TCR co-receptor; binds MHC-I	276
CD10	Neprolysin; zinc metalloproteinase; unknown role in T cells	278
CD11a	α_1 integrin associates with CD18 to form LFA-1	279
CD25	TAC; IL-2 receptor β chain	280, 281
CD28	Abundant, low-affinity costimulatory ligand for CD80 and CD86	198, 282, 283
CD30	TNFR family member mediates intrathymic T-cell deletion; expressed in activated mature T cells; binds CD153	284, 285
CD44	Hermes antigen; mediates cell adhesion	286, 287
CD45	Leukocyte common antigen; phophatase	98, 180
CD95	FAS, APO-1; TNFR-type molecule expressed in activated lymphocytes; mediates death signals	207, 208
CD120a	TNFRI, p55; mediates death signals	210–212, 288
CD120b	TNFRII, p75; lacks death domain	210, 213
CD124	IL-4 receptor	289
CD127	IL-7 receptor	290
CD134	OX40; TNFR family member	291, 292
CD152	CTLA-4; high-affinity ligand for CD80 and CD86; inhibits T-cell activation	293–295
CD153	CD30 ligand	284
CD154	CD40 ligand; gp39; TBAM	296–300

CTLA-4, cytotoxic T-lymphocyte–associated molecule-4; HIV, human immunodeficiency virus; IL, interleukin; LFA, leukocyte function antigen; MHC, major histocompatibility complex; TBAM, T- and B-cell–activating molecule; TCR, T-cell receptor; TNFR, tumor necrosis factor receptor.

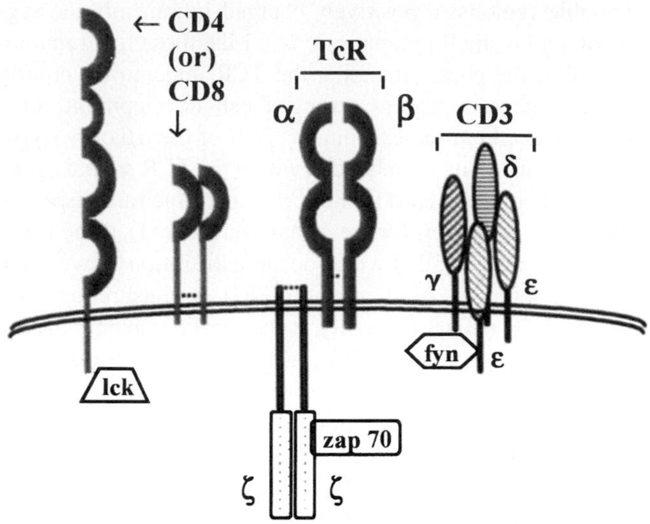

FIG. 2.22. T-cell receptor (TCR) complex. The type II TCR consists of two transmembrane chains, α and β, that penetrate the cytoplasm with only a few amino acids. The ζ chains are intimately associated, and transduce signals through nearby protein tyrosine kinases (PTKs) and cytosolic phosphatases such as ζ-associated protein-70 (ZAP-70). The TCR complex also includes CD3, which comprises four transmembrane proteins (two ϵ, one γ, and one δ) with cytosolic immunoreceptor tyrosine-based activation motifs (ITAMs).

activation of two SRC-related PTKs: LCK, which associates with the cytoplasmic domains of CD4 and CD8, and FYN, which associates with the ζ and ϵ chains (269,272). On TCR engagement by MHC with appropriate peptide, CD4 binds to MHC-II, or CD8 binds to MHC-I, resulting in activation of LCK, phosphorylation of TCR ITAMs, and recruitment of ZAP-70. Transphosphorylation of ZAP-70 by SRC-type PTKs leads to phosphorylation of downstream cytosolic substrates, triggering of PLC-γ and signal transduction by RAS-dependent cytosolic kinase cascades (271,272).

T-Cell Ontogeny

Progenitor cells arriving in the thymus from the bone marrow mature through their interaction with the thymic stroma and soluble factors such as IL-2 and IL-7 (23,290,302). The earliest thymocytes express CD34 and CD7 and are pluripotent, in that they retain the capacity to be induced *in vitro* to differentiate into cells of several types besides T cells, such as DCs or NK cells (303–305). T-cell development in the thymus is characterized by distinct and sequential patterns of surface antigen expression and by the progressive and orderly rearrangements of the genes encoding the TCR (22,24,306,307). The earliest definitive T cells are characterized by expression of CD2 and CD44 (Fig. 2.23). These cells evolve in the subcapsular region of the thymic cortex and are sometimes referred to as triple-negative cells, because they do not yet express CD3, CD4, or CD8. Alternatively, these early prothymocytes are considered early double-negative T cells, because of the lack of CD4 and CD8. At this stage, the TCR β chain retains the germline configuration. These prothymocytes can give rise to $\alpha\beta$ or $\gamma\delta$ T cells or to intrathymic DCs.

In the next phase, prothymocytes express the IL-2 receptor β chain (CD25, TAC), CD44 expression is reduced, and rearrangements occur in the gene encoding the TCR β chain.

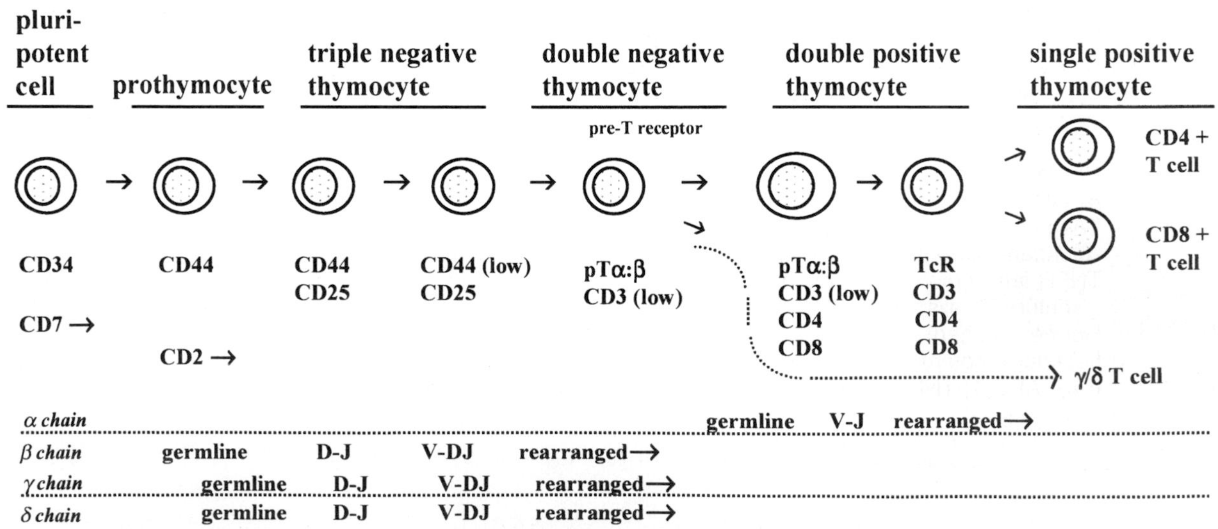

FIG. 2.23. T-cell ontogeny. Pluripotent cells arriving in the thymus differentiate into CD2$^+$ cells, after which they undergo an orderly sequence of T-cell receptor (TCR) gene rearrangements, first involving the β chain gene, followed by the γ and δ segments and, if the $\gamma\delta$ gene product is unsuccessful, the α chain segment. Each stage of T-cell maturation is characterized by a particular pattern of antigens at the surface. Triple-negative thymocytes lack CD3; double-negative thymocytes lack CD4 and CD8; and double-positive thymocytes express CD4 and CD8. Mature $\alpha\beta$ (type 2) thymocytes express CD4 or CD8.

Rearrangements of the γ and δ genes occur simultaneously with α-chain gene rearrangement, all of which take place before rearrangements of the α chain. Thus, mature T cells either of type ($\alpha\beta$ or $\gamma\delta$) demonstrate nongermline patterns of γ and δ TCR genes. Although relatively little is known about differentiation along the type I pathway, most T cells that generate a functional $\gamma\delta$ TCR become type I cells (308). After the β chain is generated, it binds to a surrogate α chain, called pre-T-cell α (pTα), to generate a pre-TCR that forms a complex with CD3 at the prothymocyte surface (309,310). At this stage of double-negative prothymocytes, cells are distinguished by surface expression of the pre-TCR. Cell-surface expression of the pre-TCR is necessary for thymocyte maturation, in part because of the regulatory capacity of associated signaling molecules such as the SRC family PTK Lck (311,312). In double-negative prothymocytes, there is a burst of cell proliferation. At this point, signaling through the pre-TCR and associated PTKs inhibits RAG-1 and RAG-2 expression, which impedes additional gene rearrangements in the β chain, resulting in the generation of numerous progeny with identical TCR β chains.

Also important at this stage is the interaction of the thymocytes with CD81 (TAPA-1), a 26-kd transmembrane protein expressed at the surface of human thymocytes. Crosslinking of CD81 results in augmented expression of thymocyte adhesion molecules such as LFA-1 (313,314). After proliferating, type II cells express the coreceptors CD4 and CD8, and are referred to as double-positive thymocytes. In cells that have not produced a suitable $\gamma\delta$ TCR, reactivation of the *RAG1* and *RAG2* genes results in recombination at the α-chain locus (315) and, in most cells, generation of an intact $\alpha\beta$ TCR.

Thymic education occurs in the double-positive stage of thymocyte differentiation, during which cells are selected for their capacity to bind MHC and for their lack of autoreactivity (316). Positive selection of thymocytes requires their interaction with thymic cortical epithelial cells expressing MHC complexed with autologous peptides derived from histones, ribosomal proteins, and other cellular components (317). Through this process, most thymocytes are rejected for export to the periphery based on their failure to recognize autologous MHC and are induced to undergo apoptosis in the thymic medulla. Double-positive thymocytes that interact successfully with MHC-I develop into CD8$^+$ T cells, and those that bind appropriately to MHC-II develop into CD4$^+$ T cells (318). In a parallel process, referred to as *negative selection,* thymocytes that bind peptides derived from autologous structures with high affinity are eliminated (319). Of the double-positive T cells in the thymus, only a small fraction survive the selection process to be released into the circulation as mature CD4$^+$ or CD8$^+$ T cells. The rapid production and deletion of thymocytes is evident on histologic examination of the thymic medulla, which reveals a tremendous amount of apoptosis and tingible body macrophages (see Chapters 3 and 6).

T-Cell Activation and Function

TCR engagement by peptide in the context of MHC is necessary but not sufficient to trigger a full and appropriate T-cell response to antigen (320). Rather, T-cell activation, proliferation, and differentiation require additional, costimulatory signals, which are mediated largely through CD28. CD28 binds CD80 (B7-1), which is expressed by activated APCs including B cells, DCs, and monocytes, or CD86 (B7-2), which is expressed in those cells and in resting monocytes. When engaged by CD80 or CD86, CD28 signaling initiates T-cell transcriptional activation and proliferation (198,282,283). If engaged, another receptor for CD80 and CD86, called CTLA-4 (CD28 homologue cytotoxic T lymphocyte antigen-4, CD152), dampens T-cell proliferation (293,295). CTLA-4 is expressed minimally in resting T cells, but its expression is augmented upon TCR and CD28-mediated T-cell activation. Once CTLA-4 is present at the T-cell surface, which occurs approximately 2 days after initial stimulation, it binds CD80 and CD86 with higher affinity than does CD28 and transmits growth-inhibitory signals. Through the discordant expression of CD28 and CTLA-4 and their differential affinity for the same ligands, signaling through these two competitive receptors allows for nearly opposite T-cell responses to the APC. Whereas in the initial response to antigen, costimulatory signals from CD80 and CD86 induce T-cell activation and expansion, later in the course of the same immune response, these signals inhibit T-cell growth (293).

T cells in which antigen receptor crosslinking occurs but to which costimulatory signals are not delivered from the APC are rendered anergic (321). The requirement for combined TCR and CD28 engagement in the T cell minimizes the occurrence of T-cell response to self-antigen and, possibly, autoimmunity. Occasionally, T cells with specificity for autologous peptides escape negative selection in the thymus. If such autoreactive T cells were to encounter antigen to which they bind in the peripheral tissue, the requirement for costimulation would prevent T-cell activation in the context of TCR engagement alone (Fig. 2.24). The term *tolerance* often refers to the acquired unresponsiveness, or anergy, of lymphocytes recognizing a particular antigen or antigens. T-cell anergy, induced by TCR engagement in the absence of costimulatory signals from APCs, affords protection from tissue damage in case of T-cell affinity for autologous structures.

Activated T cells express and secrete a variety of cytokines, called *interleukins* (Table 2.6). There are several broad categories of cytokines, which include interleukins, interferons, hematopoietins, and chemokines (334). In general, these are small proteins that act locally within the immunologic "synapse," such as between a T cell and an APC, and which mediate their effects by binding to high-affinity receptors in target cells (334,379). Distinct patterns of T-cell cytokine production exist and are determined by the nature of the inducing stimulus, such as an infectious agent,

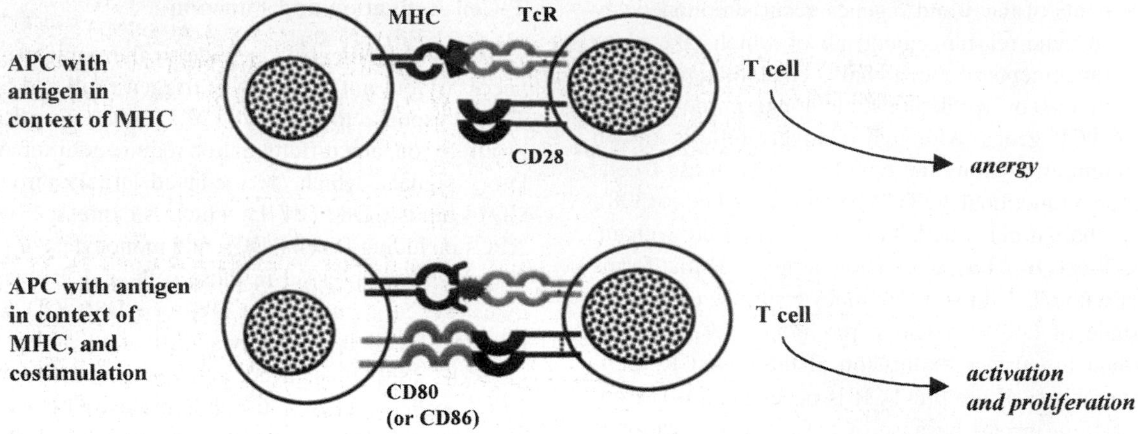

FIG. 2.24. T-cell anergy occurs in the absence of costimulation. Engagement of the T-cell receptor (TCR) by antigen is insufficient to induce T-cell proliferation, activation, and cytokine secretion. The T cell requires costimulatory signals through CD28 and B7-1 (CD80 or CD86) to generate a response.

TABLE 2.6. *Cytokines*

Molecule	Cell source	Major functions	References
Interleukins			
IL-1	Macrophages, most nucleated cells	Diffuse proinflammatory and catabolic effects, activation of endothelial cells, phagocytic cells, lymphocytes	322, 323
IL-2	$CD4^+$, some $CD8^+$	T-cell growth factor; induces T-cell proliferation and affects NK and B-cell growth	324–327
IL-3	Most T cells, thymic epithelial cells; myeloid cells	Hematopoeisis	328–332
IL-4	$CD4^+$ (T_H2), NK, basophils	B-cell growth factor; induces B-cell differentiation, IgE generation, B- and T-cell survival	215, 333, 334
IL-5	$CD4^+$ (T_H2), basophils	Eosinophil growth, also B-cell differentiation, IgA transcription	335–338
IL-6	T cells, macrophages	B-cell differentiation and Ig production, T-cell activation, and acute-phase response (with IL-1)	219, 339–341
IL-7	Bone marrow stromal cells, fetal liver, thymic epithelial cells	Growth factor for pre-B cells, T lymphocytes	17, 342, 343
IL-8	Macrophages	Neutrophil activation and chemotaxis; activation of T cells, endothelial cells, fibroblasts	344–346
IL-9	$CD4^+$ T cells	Mast cell activation, T-cell proliferation (with IL-2)	347
IL-10	T cells, macrophages, B cells	Suppression of macrophage function and cytokine secretion, T_H1 inhibition	348–350
IL-11	Stromal fibroblasts	Hematopoeisis, acute phase response (fever)	351–353
IL-12	DCs, B cells, macrophages	Stimulation of T_H1 response, NK cell activation	354–357
IL-13	T cells, mast cells, NK cells	B-cell survival and differentiation, inhibits macrophage activity	358–363
IL-14	B cells	B-cell activation and proliferation	364, 365
Il-15	T cells	T-cell growth factor; diffuse proinflammatory effects, innate immunity, intestinal epithelial cell growth	327, 366
IL-16	$CD8^+$ T cells	Lymphocyte chemoattractant factor, binds CD4	367, 368
IL-17	Activated $CD4^+$ T cells	Mesenchymal inflammation	369, 370
IL-18	Kidney, liver, muscle, other	Induces IFN-γ production by T cells	371, 372
Other T-cell–derived cytokines			
GM-CSF	Most T cells	Promotes granulocyte, macrophage, DC growth	373, 374
IFN-γ	$CD4^+$ T (T_H1), some $CD8^+$ T	Macrophage activation	375, 376
TGF-β	$CD4^+$T	Inhibits B-cell growth, stimulates fibroblast growth	377, 378

DCs, dendritic cells; GM-CSF, granulocyte-macrophage colony-stimulating factor; IFN, interferon; IL, interleukin; NK, natural killer; TGF, transforming growth factor; T_H, helper T cell subset.

and are affected also by host factors, such as medication and inherited disposition.

The patterns of cytokine production by T cells determine the cellular responses to specific pathogens (246,380). In the normal host, intracellular pathogens such as *Leishmania major* stimulate T_H1 cells, which promote macrophage activation and growth through the generation and secretion of cytokines, including IL-2, TNF-α, and IFN-γ (245). In contrast, extracellular bacteria such as pneumococci, *Clostridium*, and tetanus-causing organisms elicit T_H2 cell responses, which foster humoral immunity through production of IL-4, IL-5, IL-10, IL-13, and TGF-β (Fig. 2.25). The T_H1/T_H2 balance varies with different infectious conditions and for the same infectious agent with different stages of disease. For example, in patients with human immunodeficiency virus (HIV) disease, there occurs a gross diminution in the number of $CD4^+$ T cells and qualitative changes in the function of those cells. In late stages of certain diseases, including acquired immunodeficiency syndrome (AIDS), there occur abnormal patterns of cytokine production by the $CD4^+$ T cells, characterized by relatively high amounts of IL-4, IL-5, and IL-10 (381). This T_H2-type cytokine pattern may contribute to polyclonal B-cell expansion, excessive immunoglobulin production, and eosinophilia that is often seen in patients with AIDS (381,382).

The interleukin and cytokine receptors are multimeric transmembrane structures that in some cases include common protein chains and signaling motifs. One of the best studied of these molecules, the high-affinity IL-2 receptor, consists of α, β, and γ chains (280,281). The β and γ chains are expressed constitutively in most T cells and constitute a low-affinity receptor for IL-2. On T-cell activation, the α chain is induced, generating an intact high-affinity IL-2 receptor. Activated T cells secrete and bind IL-2, which results in cell cycle progression and clonal expansion. The IL-2 receptor γ chain serves also as a component of the receptors for IL-4, IL-7, IL-9, and IL-15. Humans deficient in this common γ chain suffer from X-linked severe combined

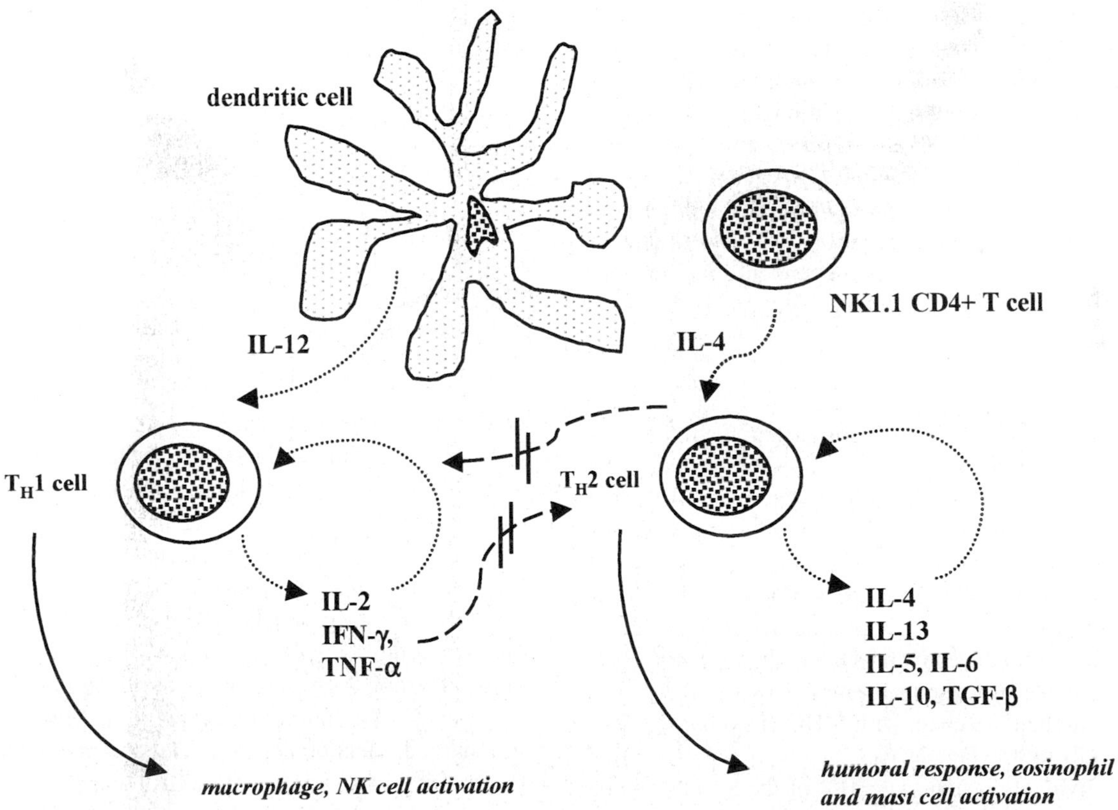

FIG. 2.25. Type 1 and type 2 helper T cells (T_H1 and T_H2) have distinct roles in cellular immunity. Mature $CD4^+$ T cells can be categorized in terms of the cytokine profile, based on their propensity to augment cellular or humoral responses. Dendritic cells secreting interleukin (IL)-12 induce a T_H1 response, characterized by T-cell production of IL-2, interferon-γ (IFN-γ), and tumor necrosis factor-α (TNF-α). These factors promote macrophage and natural killer (NK) cell activation and are essential for clearance of intracellular organisms such as the protozoan *Leishmania major.* The T_H2 response, induced by NK1.1 $CD4^+$ T cells, results in T-cell generation and secretion of IL-4, IL-5, IL-6, IL-10, and transforming growth factor-β (TGF-β). These cytokines promote B-cell differentiation, immunoglobulin production, and activation of eosinophils and mast cells. IFN-γ, produced by T_H1 cells, inhibits T_H2-cell development. IL-4, IL-10, and other T_H2-derived factors can suppress macrophage activation and T_H1 cell growth.

immunodeficiency (SCID), which is characterized by the absence of the cytokine response pathways necessary for T- and B-cell development. The sharing of cytokine receptor components occurs among receptors for other cytokines. For example, there is a common β chain in the IL-3, IL-5, and GM-CSF receptors and in certain chemokine receptors such as that for IL-8.

The intracellular signals instigated from cytokines binding to their receptors are mediated largely by the JAK (Janus kinase) family of kinases. The JAKs are constitutively associated with the cytoplasmic domains of specific membrane receptors and become activated on ligand binding. These enzymes have a key role in transmitting the lymphocyte response to interferons, interleukins, and other ligands for which the receptors lack intrinsic kinase activity (383,384). On receptor activation by ligand, a series of phosphorylation events occurs that results in JAK-mediated activation of STAT (signal transducer and activator of transcription). The relationships among the four known mammalian JAKs and the seven STATs are somewhat promiscuous, such that one STAT can be activated by multiple JAKs (384). The STATs each contain a single tyrosine phosphorylation site, an SH2 domain, a DNA binding domain, and protein-protein interaction domains, and on activation, they enter the cell nucleus. Although tyrosine phosphorylation is thought to be the most critical event for STAT activation, serine phosphorylation can also affect STAT activation and DNA binding capacity (385,386). Ultimately, phosphorylated STATs bind to their response elements on DNA, resulting in transcription of STAT target genes and a cytokine-dependent inflammatory response.

T-Cell Superantigens

Recognition of TCR by the appropriate antigen is the basis for the induction of an adaptive response and provides the specificity of this process. However, certain antigens are capable of binding multiple antigen receptors and are referred to as superantigens. T-cell superantigens are microbial products that avidly bind the products of one or more TCR Vβ gene families (387–389). These bind MHC-II molecules at a site distinct from the conventional antigen-binding cleft, and so are capable of forming bridges between T cells expressing a particular Vβ chain with MHC-II expressing cells such as B cells (390) (Fig. 2.26).

In any individual, as many as 30% of the T cells can be activated by any one superantigen, and the effects can be profound. Direct activation of T cells through the TCR Vβ chain, independent of the α chain and CDR, results in rapid, inappropriate cytokine release by many T cells. These cytokines include IFN-γ, which activates macrophages to produce TNF-α, the main mediator of toxic shock syndrome. Production and release of IFN-γ is a perilous but not singular outcome of T-cell stimulation by superantigens. Depending on the nature of the superantigens and the differentiation state of the T cell, the affected T cell may proliferate and

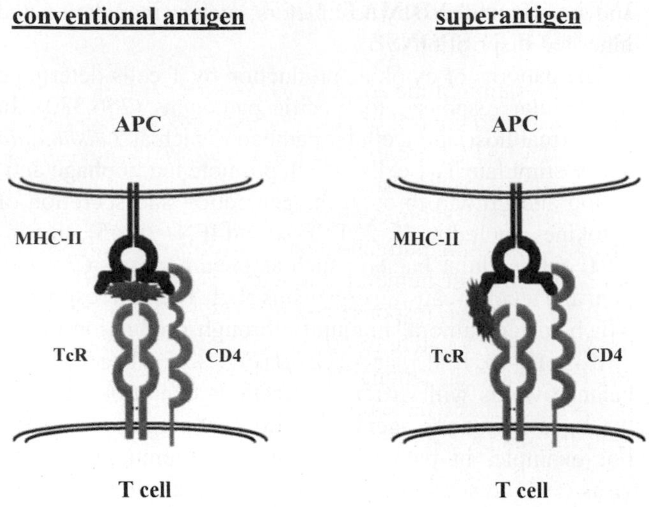

FIG. 2.26. T-cell superantigens bind the T-cell receptor (TCR) β chain directly. Conventional antigens are bound and displayed in the MHC peptide-binding groove, where they interact specifically with the TCR complementarity-determining region (CDR). In contrast, superantigens bind the TCR β chain directly, outside of the CDR, resulting in a bridge between the antigen-presenting cell (APC) and any T cell expressing a β chain for which the superantigen has affinity.

differentiate or undergo apoptosis. Two of the more common T-cell superantigens are *Staphylococcus aureus* enterotoxins (391,392), which cause food poisoning, and toxic shock syndrome toxin-1, which is responsible for toxic shock syndrome.

B-cell superantigens also exist. They are microbial products that directly bind conserved framework regions within immunoglobulin V segments, such as the HIV protein gp120 (393) and *Staphylococcus aureus* protein A (394).

Viral T-cell superantigens have been studied most extensively in the murine system. The genes encoding endogenous superantigens of the mouse mammary tumor virus (MMTV) are vertically transmitted in infected strains of mice due to integration of viral genes into the murine chromosome (395). The MMTV gene products were originally called minor lymphocyte stimulating (Mls) antigens, because these proteins induced strong T-cell responses in mixed lymphocyte reactions (396–398). In mice that express the Mls antigens, there is a marked effect on negative selection in the thymus. Double-positive thymocytes with TCRs that recognize MMTV antigens are deleted, and the mice are thereby tolerized to these superantigens (399,400). In infected mice, viral particles are produced in the mammary glands and transmitted in breast milk. After infecting B cells in the progeny, viral replication would not be feasible except for the encoded superantigen, which triggers B-cell division by stimulating T cells to express CD154 and IL-4. Through these complex interactions involving host cells and viral gene products, MMTV-encoded superantigens promote host tolerance to viral proteins and foster viral replication in the infected cells.

INDUCTION AND MATURATION OF THE IMMUNE RESPONSE

Orchestration of the adaptive response to antigen requires integration and control of numerous antigen-responsive elements. The APCs are essential in the initial phases of the adaptive response, because these are the cells that process antigens for T-cell recognition in the context of MHC, thereby promoting antigen-specific cytotoxic responses and T-cell–dependent humoral immunity. The induction of an effective adaptive response requires transport of antigen to the GC, Peyer's patch, or other secondary lymphoid organ, where interactions among DCs, T lymphocytes, and B lymphocytes facilitate development of highly specific and long-term immunity.

Dendritic Cells and Initiation of the Adaptive Response

DCs comprise a heterogeneous group of highly specialized APCs of distinct developmental origins (305,356,401). These cells are distinguished by their stellate shape, which is suited to antigen capture, peptide presentation, and interaction with other immune effector cells (Fig. 2.27). Dendritic cells include cells of myeloid origin, such as Langerhans cells of the skin, and cells of lymphoid origin, such as thymic DCs. Factors that promote DC maturation from bone marrow–derived monocytes include GM-CSF, IL-4, and TNF-α (401,402). When monocytes exit the circulation and enter the tissues by diapedesis, factors in the subendothelial cell matrix such as chemokines, adhesion molecules, and glycoproteins affect DC differentiation (403). The process of phagocytosis, triggered in monocytes and immature DCs by FcR engagement, also promotes DC maturation. In general, monocytes and immature DCs take up antigen in tissues and then migrate to lymph nodes, where they differentiate into mature DCs and participate in the adaptive response.

Albeit low in number, DCs can be found in almost all nonlymphoid tissues with the exception of the central nervous system, testis, and eye. At the surface, DCs express many, diverse structures including MHC-I and MHC-II molecules, adhesion molecules, receptors for antigen uptake, cytokine and chemokine receptors, and TNF receptor (TNFR)–type molecules (402). DCs express high levels of CD1 antigens, which are highly conserved, MHC-related molecules that recognize lipid and glycolipid structures such as mycolic acid (404,405). There are at least five CD1 proteins, called CD1a, -b, -c, -d, and -e, which in humans are encoded by distinct genes on chromosome 1q. The CD1 proteins have limited homology to MHC-1, and like MHC-1, they are expressed at the surface in noncovalent association with β_2-microglobulin. CD1d is essential in immunity to GPI-linked antigens, such as those in the membranes of *Plasmodium falciparum, Trypanosoma brucei,* and *Leishmania mexicana* (406). CD1-mediated binding of nonprotein antigens is essential in stimulation of $CD4^+$ T cells and NK cells that recognize these structures (407). Because CD1 can be expressed independently of MHC-I and MHC-II, the CD1

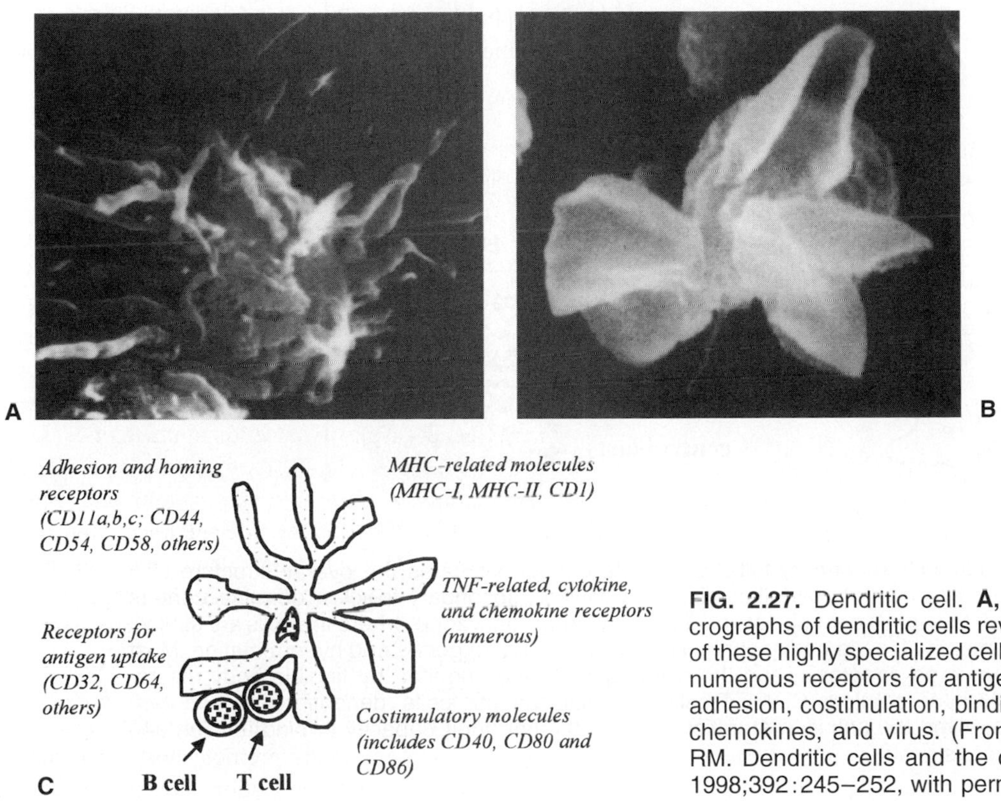

FIG. 2.27. Dendritic cell. **A, B:** Scanning electron micrographs of dendritic cells reveal the stellate morphology of these highly specialized cells. **C:** Dendritic cells express numerous receptors for antigen uptake and presentation, adhesion, costimulation, binding of TNF-related proteins, chemokines, and virus. (From Banchereau J, Steinman RM. Dendritic cells and the control of immunity. *Nature* 1998;392:245–252, with permission.)

system plays a particular role in MHC-independent antigen presentation and T-cell stimulation. One specialized cell type, the $CD4^+$, NK1.1 T cell, helps to initiate the T_H2 type response on recognition and binding of glycolipid structures in the context of CD1d (405,406).

In the tissues, DCs capture antigen, display peptides, and mediate the effector responses of helper and cytotoxic T cells. An example of DC-mediated T-cell function is the delayed-type hypersensitivity (DTH) reaction, as occurs after injection of tuberculin antigens into the skin of an individual who has previously been exposed to *Mycobacterium tuberculosis.* In the initial response, macrophages and DCs bind and engulf microbial antigens, which results in cytokine secretion and recruitment of T cells to the site of infection. The subsequent infiltration of mature T_H cells at the site, and the specific stimulation of those T cells with affinity for specific antigens presented by MHC-expressing DCs, results in delayed-type hypersensitivity. As much as DCs have a role in the generation of DTH and T_H functions, there is substantial evidence that these powerful APCs are key regulators of the antigen-specific cytotoxic T-cell responses, as is sometimes induced against microbial or tumor antigens. The ''license to kill'' model suggests that, on presentation of antigen by DC, antigen-specific $CD4^+$ T cells induce DC maturation and efficacy by engagement of CD40 at the APC surface (408–410). Consequent expression of costimulatory and adhesion molecules by the DC allows and facilitates generation of $CD8^+$ effector T cells specific for that antigen (411–414). Thus, DCs represent an important regulatory link between helper T and killer cells, by requiring T_H-mediated costimulatory signals for induction of the cytotoxic response (see Chapters 1, 3, and 6).

The Germinal Center Reaction: Induction of Immunoglobulin Class Switching, Somatic Hypermutation, and Generation of Memory

GCs are the principal sites of affinity maturation and adaptive immune expansion (28,29). Before entry into the GC, naive B cells from the bone marrow circulate in the peripheral blood and permeate the T-cell–rich zones of secondary lymphoid organs such as the splenic PALS and GC mantle zone. On encounter with antigen, which is often presented by DCs, these IgM^+IgD^+ B cells are induced to proliferate and initiate the GC reaction. Studies in antigen-primed mice indicate that within 3 days of antigen exposure, small clusters of IgM-expressing centroblasts emerge in the central section of primary follicles. This primary humoral response to antigen occurs rapidly and results in the loss of B-cell surface IgD and the production and secretion of IgM with relatively low affinity for the inducing pathogen. Approximately 1 week after inoculation, tingible body macrophages are evident in the GC. These macrophages function to clear cells that have undergone apoptosis, and generate a starry-sky appearance evident on histologic examination (28). At this point, activated T cells, DCs, and differentiated, immunoglobulin-secreting B cells, called centrocytes, constitute the light zone of the GC (Fig. 2.28). As the concentration of antigen decreases, antibody-producing cells revert to a resting phenotype. The cells are prepared for restimulation at any subsequent exposure to antigen.

After primary immunization, most GC B cells express IgM, whereas after secondary and any subsequent immunization, they mainly express IgG (415) or, in the case of MALT lymphoid centers (Peyer's patches), IgA (416). The adaptive humoral response is generated through the interac-

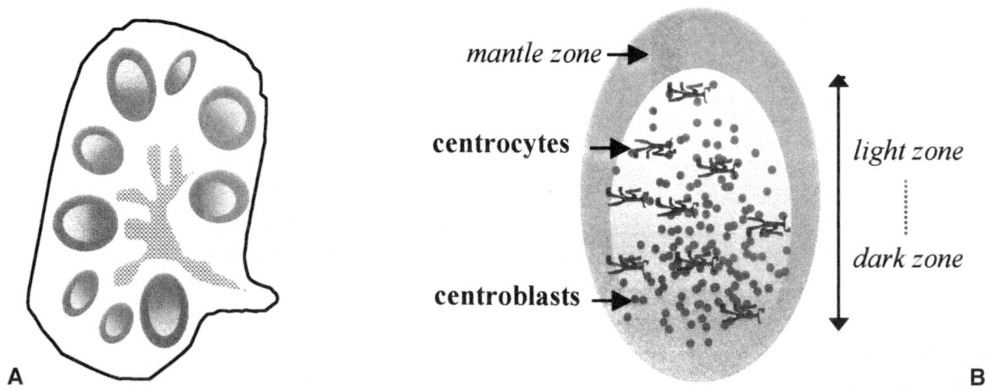

FIG. 2.28. Lymph node with secondary follicles. **A:** The cartoon indicates the overall structure of a reactive lymph node with a central, medullary sinus and multiple secondary follicles, germinal centers (GCs). **B:** Undifferentiated, IgM^+ centroblasts proliferate in the GC dark zone, where the cells are subject to somatic rearrangements of the Ig heavy-chain (H) and light-chain (L) genes and hypermutation. Most of the centroblasts undergo apoptosis, and the cell fragments are engulfed by tingible body macrophages. The GC light zone contains $CD4^+$ T cells, follicular dendritic cells, dendritic cells, and centrocytes that have survived the affinity maturation process through their capacity to bind antigen and receipt of costimulatory signals.

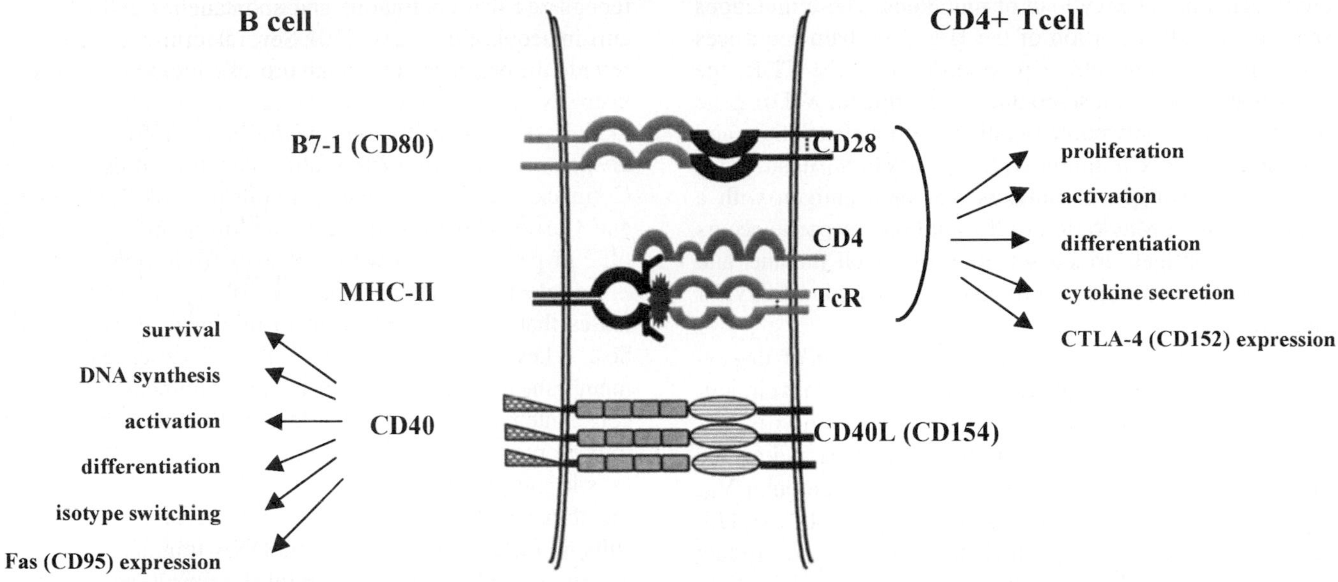

FIG. 2.29. Cognate interaction between $CD4^+$ T cells and B cells. $CD4^+$ T cells recognize antigen presented by major histocompatibility complex class II (MHC-II) molecules, resulting in cognate interaction and delivery of costimulatory signals. T cells constitutively express CD28, a receptor for CD80 and CD86 (B7-1 and B7-2), which occur at the antigen-presenting cell (APC) surface. Ligation of CD28 by CD80 or CD86 results in T cell-activation, proliferation, and differentiation. Concomitant T-cell receptor (TCR) and CD28 engagement in the T cell result in expression of cytotoxic T-lymphocyte–associated molecule-4 (CTLA-4) (not shown), a high-affinity receptor for CD80 and CD86 that transduces inhibitory signals and thereby downmodulates T-cell activation. On the B-cell side, ligation of CD40 by activated, antigen-specific T cells expressing CD154 (CD40L) initially promotes survival, proliferation, and differentiation. At the same time, CD40 ligation results in expression of CD95 (FAS), which primes the B cell for activation-induced cell death on elimination of antigen.

tion of antigen-specific B lymphocytes with $CD4^+$ T lymphocytes responding to the same antigen in the GC. Naive IgM^+ B cells enter the GC where they undergo rapid cycles of division and also apoptosis. In the GC, B-cell survival, proliferation, and differentiation require engagement by two distinct ligands, which are antigen and CD154 (CD40L). CD154 is a TNF-related molecule that is expressed transiently by $CD4^+$ T cells after engagement of the TCR (297,300,417). It provides potent and essential costimulatory signals to B cells that express CD40, a member of the TNFR family of cell-surface proteins (418,419). CD40 ligation in B cells occurs as a function of cognate interaction, during which antigen-specific $CD4^+$ T cells recognize and bind antigen in the context of MHC-II (Fig. 2.29). This interaction results in B-cell survival, transcriptional activation, differentiation, and isotype switching (179,420,421). In humans, CD154 deficiency causes the hyper-IgM syndrome, characterized by high levels of IgM and severely reduced levels of IgG and IgA. Patients with this disease suffer from lack of B-cell differentiation and lack of IgG, IgA and IgE because of the inability of affected T cells to induce isotype switching in B cells (299,422,423).

Immunoglobulin class switching is the process whereby a B cell substitutes the constant portion of the expressed BCR and immunoglobulin without changing the specificity of the variable, antigen-specific portion of the receptor. A few days into a primary response, antigen-specific B cells switch the primary IgM isotype to a secondary isotype: IgG, IgA, or IgE. Changing the constant portion of the molecule endows the antibody with a novel biologic activity. For instance, the polymeric structure of the primary receptor, IgM, allows for effective clearance of invading microorganisms in the circulating blood during the early stages of infections but hampers IgM from egressing into the extravascular space. In later stages of infection, antibody distribution outside of the vasculature is necessary for eradication of invading pathogens, and this is a functional feature of antibodies of the IgG class. Neither IgG or IgM, however, are effectively secreted through epithelial surfaces, such as those of the intestine and the respiratory tree. This requires the constant portion of IgA. Thus, immunoglobulin class switching is an important component, together with somatic hypermutation, of the maturation of the antibody response to antigen and the adaptation of the antibody response to the nature of the invading microorganism.

In normal humans, GC B cells that bind antigen and receive costimulatory signals from T cells are induced to proliferate and differentiate into plasma or memory cells. *Somatic hypermutation* is the process whereby the expressed H chain V(D)J and light chain $V_\kappa J_\kappa$ or $V_\lambda J_\lambda$ gene segments are targeted by a heavy load of mutations. These mutations spare the constant portion of the H and L chain sequences and appear to concentrate preferentially in the CDR, the areas that come in close contact with antigen. V(D)J gene mutations are mostly point mutations, although deletions and insertions also occur and provide the structural substrate for selection by antigen of mutants that bind antigen with a higher strength. Maturation of the antibody response occurs because of antigen-driven selection of B-cell mutants and consequent generation of antibodies with a high affinity for antigen (139,424).

Centroblasts undergo somatic hypermutation of the expressed immunoglobulin V(D)J genes and in certain circumstances undergo receptor editing. Receptor editing is mediated by the reactivation of the RAG enzymes and results in the replacement of the GC B-cell immunoglobulin V_H, V_κ, or V_λ segment with a new V segment (140,141,425, 426). In general, cells in which the new V gene product binds antigen with higher affinity survive and proliferate in the GC environment, as long as T-cell help is still present, whereas those that do not bind antigen undergo cell death. This process of affinity maturation results in the rapid evolution and domination of the B-cell clones that bind antigen with high affinity.

REGULATION OF THE IMMUNE RESPONSE

The physiologic response to an infectious agent requires complex molecular signaling pathways that induce activation, proliferation, and differentiation of specific immune cellular components. At the same time, host survival depends on coordination and limitation of the inflammatory response. Apoptosis, or programmed cell death, is a highly conserved process by which aged cells, surplus immune effector cells, and infected cells are eliminated. The genes that control the apoptosis machinery are highly conserved from *Caenorhabditis elegans* to humans. In this section, we review the fundamental aspects of apoptosis in mammalian cells and consider several families of proteins that regulate apoptosis, such as TNF-type ligands and their receptors, B-cell lymphoma-2 (BCL-2)–related proteins, and caspases. These molecules are considered in the context of the adaptive immune response to antigen.

Apoptosis

The essential role of cell death in development was first recognized by embryologists, who appreciated that massive deletion of cells in developing limbs is controlled by genetic, hormonal, and other factors (427,428). Pathologists described the formation and engulfment of *Councilman's bodies* in dying tissues, such as in hepatocytes after exposure to noxious agents (429). In the 1960s, cancer researchers studying the kinetics of tumor growth and cell proliferation recognized that continuous and spontaneous cell death occurs in neoplastic tissues (430). Several terms were coined to refer to the organized cell death process, including *shrinkage necrosis* (431), *popcorn-type cytolysis* (432), *zeiosis* (433,434), and *extrusion subdivision* (435). The term *apoptosis* (*άπόπτωσισ*) is attributed to Professor James Cormack, a classic scholar and colleague of Kerr, Wyllie, and Currie (436,437). It refers to "dropping" or "falling off" of petals from flowers or leaves from trees.

Apoptosis is an active process involving endogenous proteases that regulate cell death to minimize damage to the host. A key feature of apoptosis is the maintenance of plasma membrane integrity, which ensures containment of the dying cell contents before phagocytic engulfment or breakdown into apoptotic bodies. Cytoskeletal changes result in characteristic morphologic features, including cell shrinkage and membrane blebbing (Fig. 2.30). Endonuclease activation results in nuclear condensation and DNA fragmentation. This process provides a mechanism for the physiologic elimination of cells that are produced in excess, improperly developed, or genetically damaged. Apoptosis can be contrasted with cell death by necrosis, a passive process resulting from acute cellular injury characterized by rapid cell swelling and lysis.

Apoptosis in immunity is essential at several levels. First, it is necessary for achieving tolerance to self antigens through elimination of autoreactive T lymphocytes in the thymus and of autoreactive B cells in the bone marrow or GC. In mature peripheral T and B lymphocytes, activation-induced cell death (AICD) is critical in downmodulating the immune response, such that the proliferation and expansion of cells responding to a particular antigen is limited. In the context of infection, apoptosis allows for the controlled destruction of infected cells by NK and cytotoxic T cells.

Perforins and Granzymes

Cytotoxic T lymphocytes and NK cells can induce apoptosis in nearby cells by releasing cytotoxic granules into the target cell or by ligand-receptor dependent mechanisms (91,438). There are two major categories of cytotoxic granules in T and NK cells, called perforins and granzymes, both of which exert their effects in a Ca^{2+}-dependent manner. Perforins are proteins that polymerize such that they form cylindrical structures with lipophilic outer and hydrophobic inner sections (Fig. 2.31). These insert into the lipid bilayer such that they form pores in the target cell membrane and are similar in structure to the MAC in the terminal step of complement-mediated cell lysis. Perforin-mediated cytotoxicity is important in suppressing infection by noncytopathic viruses such as lymphocytic choriomeningitis virus (in mice) and in protection against certain intracellular bacteria such as *Listeria monocytogenes* in humans. However, perforins are not necessary for cytolysis of cells infected with cytopathic viruses such as vaccinia and vesicular stomatitis virus (90).

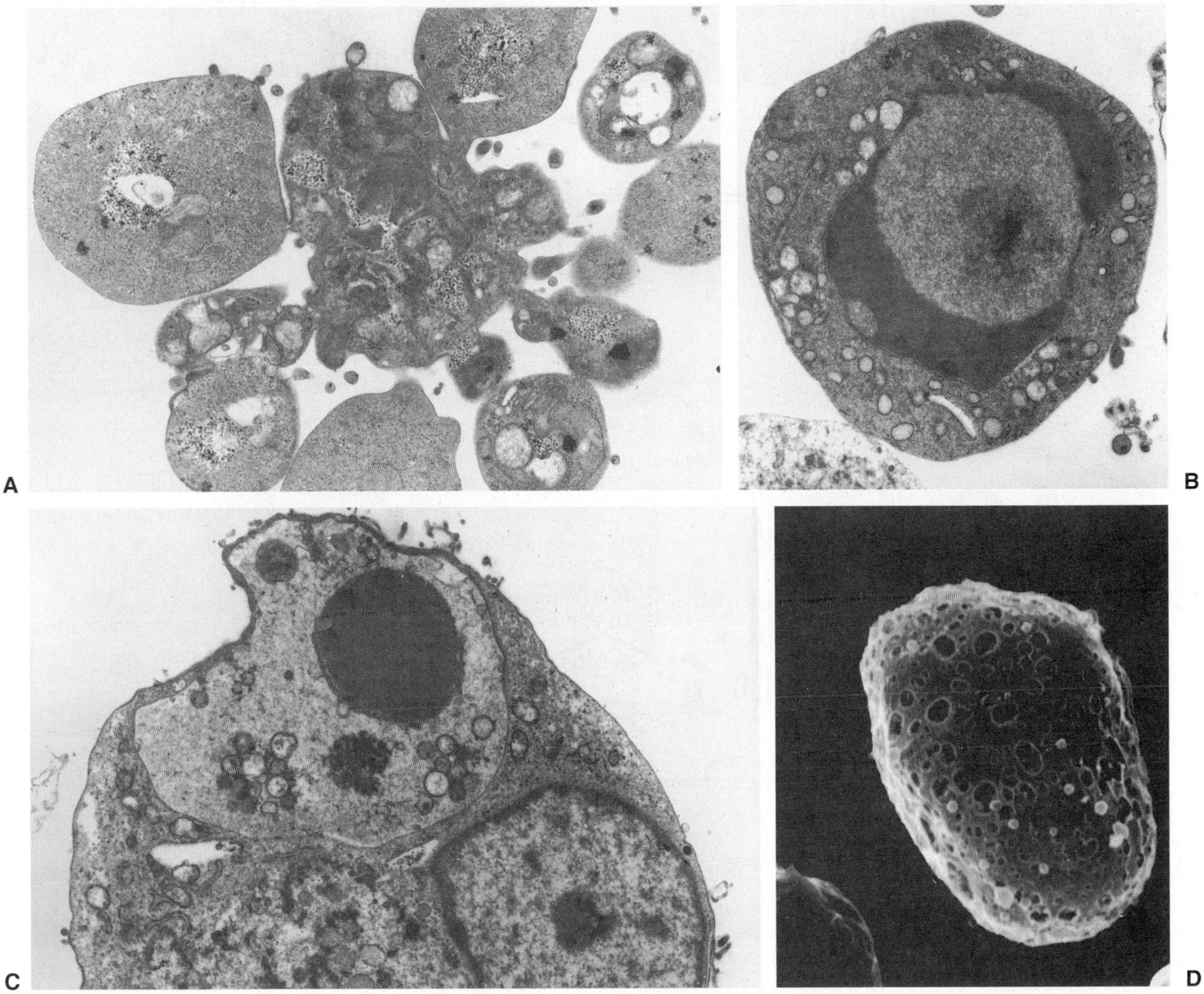

FIG. 2.30. Apoptotic cells. **A:** Murine lymphocyte explodes into multiple membrane-bound apoptotic bodies after treatment with glucocorticoid. **B:** Characteristic nuclear changes in an apoptotic thymocyte. **C:** Phagocytosis by one rat sarcoma cell (nucleus at bottom right) of another cell (nucleus at top) after myc expression in low serum conditions. **D:** Scanning micrograph of late apoptosis in a thymocyte. (Courtesy of Andrew H. Wyllie, Department of Pathology, Cambridge University, Cambridge, England.)

Related to the perforins are granzymes, a family of serine proteases that can bind and activate caspases (91,439,440). Like perforins, granzymes are stored in granules of cytotoxic effector cells. It appears that perforins have only modest killing potential in themselves, whereas these proteins are effective and necessary for killing by cells that also express granzyme A (441). Some investigators have suggested that perforins act primarily by inducing pore formation in target cell membranes, after which granzymes enter the target cell and activate caspases. Alternatively, granzymes can enter target cells by endocytosis in a perforin-independent manner that depends on the presence of specific receptors at the target cell surface (442). Inside the cell, granzymes cause apoptosis by caspase activation. For example, granzyme B binds to and cleaves one of the terminal caspases, caspase-3.

Caspases

Caspases (cysteinyl aspartate specific enzymes) are IL-1β–converting enzyme (ICE)–like cytoplasmic proteases that mediate the process of apoptosis. These cysteine proteases are homologous to the *C. elegans* gene product Ced-3, which is essential to the death process in nematodes. Caspases occur in the cytosol as proenzymes of 30 to 50 kd and are sequentially cleaved at specific aspartic acid residues to generate mature enzymes. There are at least 13 mammalian caspases identified, which can be categorized according to

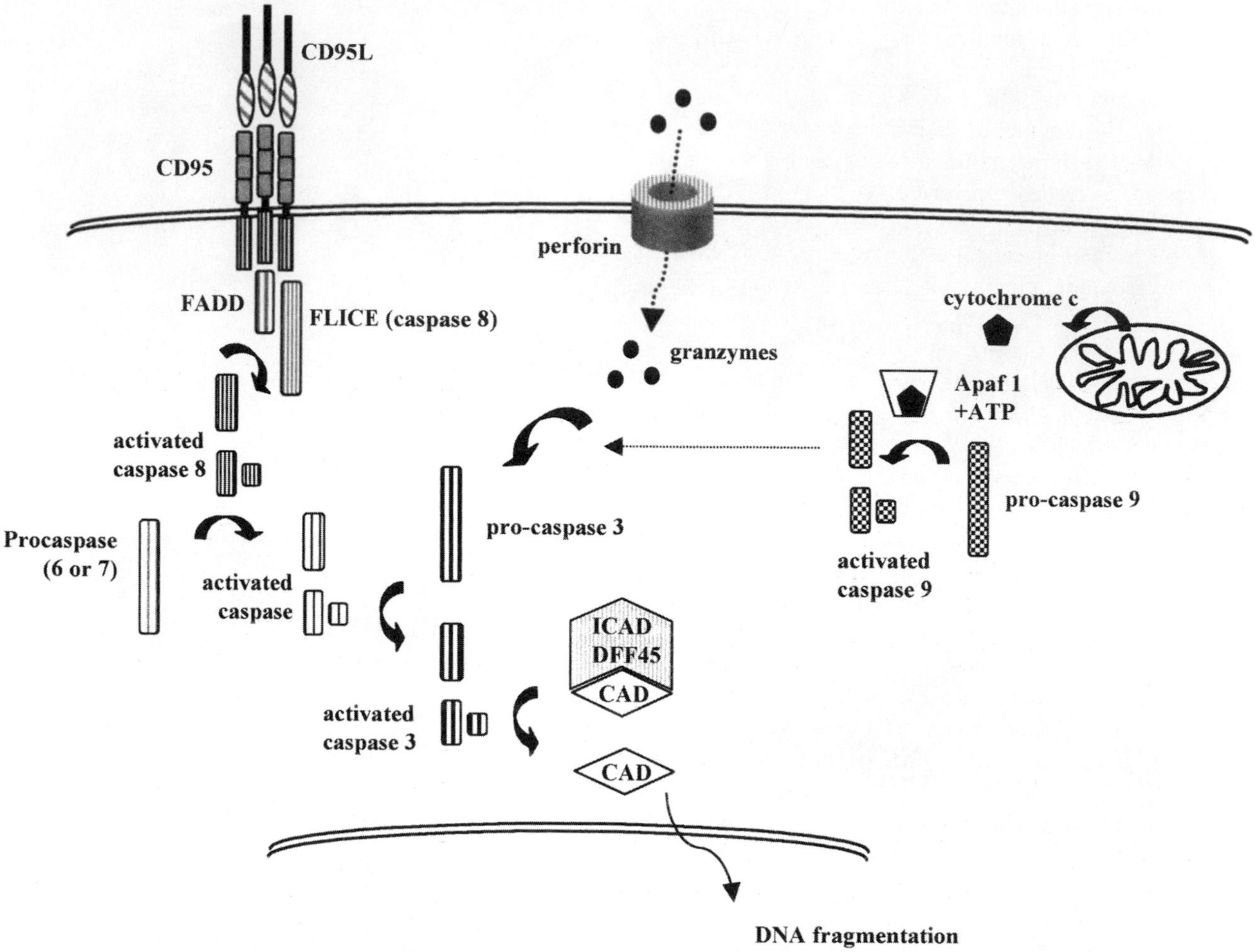

FIG. 2.31. Mechanisms of apoptosis in mammalian cells induced by receptor-ligand interactions at the cell surface, by cytotoxic granules, and by intracellular stress or metabolic derangements. One example of receptor-mediated apoptosis is that induced on trimerization of CD95 (FAS) by CD95L (FASL). FAS ligation results in recruitment of FADD to the receptor complex and activation of FLICE (caspase-8). These events at the cell surface trigger a cascade of downstream proteolytic cleavage events and activation of effector caspases. Most caspases occur in the cytosol as proenzymes that are cleaved to yield three fragments, two of which remain associated and constitute the activated caspase form. Ultimately, the inhibitor of caspase-activated DNAse (ICAD, in murine systems, or DNA fragmentation factor-45 [DFF-45] in humans is cleaved by caspase-3, releasing CAD, which enters the nucleus and cleaves DNA. Granzymes, contained in the granules of cytotoxic cells, induce apoptosis in target cells after entry through endocytosis or perforin-generated pores. Intracellular stress or metabolic changes, such as occur during growth factor withdrawal or radiation exposure, result in the release of cytochrome *c* from the mitochondria. Cytochrome *c* can effect caspase cleavage through its interaction with APAF-1. The release of cytochrome *c* and subsequent activation of APAF-1 are regulated by members of the BCL-2 family of proteins (not shown).

function and by their relative placement in the apoptosis signaling cascade. Overall, the ICE-like caspases (including caspase-1, -4, and -5) are distinguished from the death-effector caspases by their proinflammatory effects. The primary substrate of caspase-1 is the proenzyme pro-IL-1β (443–445).

Caspases that mediate apoptosis, the death-inducing caspases, are classified by their particular recognition sequences for proteolytic cleavage and by their relative location in the signaling cascade as ''initiator'' or ''effector'' caspases. For example, caspase-8 (FLICE) is an initiator caspase that interacts with CD95 (FAS)–associated adaptor proteins near the plasma membrane. In the absence of inhibitors to caspase-8, triggering of CD95 by its ligand results in trimerization of the receptor, recruitment of adaptor proteins, and cleavage of caspase-8. Caspase-8 activation initiates a chain of proteolytic events in the cytosol involving downstream caspases such as caspase-6 and -7 and the ''executioner'' caspase-3.

Based on observations that FAS-mediated apoptosis can occur in the presence of inhibitors to protein and RNA synthesis (207) and can be induced in enucleated cells (446), it is evident that all of the signaling components necessary for inducing apoptosis are present in the cytoplasm of healthy, growing cells. The intracellular caspase enzyme machinery can be likened to a loaded gun, ready to implement cell death on receptor engagement.

In 1998, a team of investigators led by Shigekazu Nagata reported the isolation, cloning, and characterization of the ultimate target of caspase activation, a caspase-activated DNase (CAD) (447). Caspase-activated DNAse is synthesized in mammalian cells together with its inhibitor (ICAD in the murine system, or DFF45, DNA fragmentation factor 45, in humans), which is a substrate for caspase-3 (448,449). In healthy cells, CAD exists in the cytoplasm bound to its inhibitor, ICAD. On activation of caspase-3, ICAD is cleaved, which results in release and nuclear translocation of CAD. In the nucleus, CAD rapidly cleaves chromosomal DNA. Signals initiated by specific death receptors at the cell surface are implemented through a series of proteolytic events that activate proenzymes in the cytoplasm and release activity of a potent endonuclease. The physiologic substrates for caspases are diverse and include over 40 proteins. These include nuclear lamina, gelsolin, fodrin, poly-ADP ribose polymerase (PARP), and BCL-2 (445). Of interest are several viral gene products that have specific caspase-inhibitory functions. These include the cowpox viral protein CrmA, a serpin-type protein that specifically inhibits the initiator caspase-8 (450). Downstream caspase-3, -6, and -7 are inhibited by the baculovirus protein p35 (451,452). Endogenous caspase inhibitors also occur, and are called inhibitors of apoptosis (IAPs).

BCL-2 Protein Family

The BCL-2 protein was originally identified by its overexpression in follicular lymphomas because of a translocation involving the *BCL2* locus on chromosome 18q21 and the immunoglobulin heavy-chain region at 14q32 (453). This outer mitochondrial membrane protein and related family members are potent regulators of apoptosis in normal and malignant cells. There are at least 14 mammalian BCL-2 family members, all of which bear homology to the Ced-9 gene product of *C. elegans* (454). These proteins have complex structures with multiple and independent functional domains ''like a Swiss army knife'' (455). A remarkable finding regarding BCL-2 family members was the determination of the three-dimensional structure of BCL-XL (redesignated as BCL-2L1 for BCL2-like-1 protein), which is highly similar to that of diphtheria toxin (456). BCL-2, BCL-XL, and BAX (BCL2-associated X protein) are thought to function, at least in part, through their capacity to form ion channels in the bipolar lipid membrane (457). Alternatively, some serve primarily as adaptor, or docking proteins, which act primarily by binding to and regulating the activity of other BCL-2 family members.

Human BCl-2 is a 26-kd structure with four BCL-2 homology (BH) domains (Fig. 2.32). It is normally expressed at high levels in T cells of the thymic cortex, in B cells of the GC mantle zone, and in memory B cells (458). Although the precise mechanism by which BCL-XL inhibits apoptosis is uncertain, it appears that at least one important feature of this molecule is its capacity to preclude release of cytochrome c from the mitochondrion, an important step in activation of caspase-9 (459). BCL-XL and BCL-XS are two distinct protein products generated by the long and short

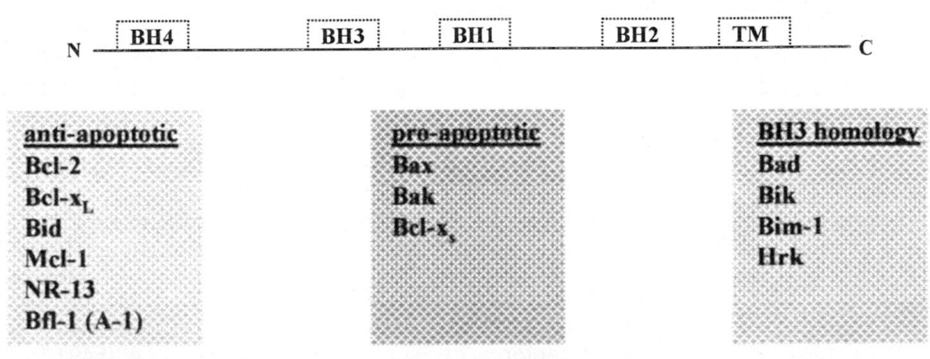

FIG. 2.32. B-cell lymphoma-2 (BCL-2)–related proteins. BCL-2 protein family members contain one to four BCL-2 homology (BH) domains and a transmembrane domain. The proteins are thought to form ion channels in bipolar membranes such as that of the mitochondrion. Expression of BCL-2, BCL-XL (redesignated as BCL-2L1 for BCL2-like-1), BID (BH3-interacting domain [death agonist]), MCL-1 (myeloid cell leukemia sequence-1), NR-13, or A-1 generally results in inhibition of apoptosis, whereas expression of BAX (BCL-2–associated X protein), BAK (BCL-2–antagonist/killer), or BCL-XS (redesignated BCL-2L1 for BCL2-like-1) can promote cell death. The precise functions of BAD (BCL-2–antagonist of cell death), BIK (BCL-2–interacting killer [apoptosis inducing]), BIM-1 (redesignated as BCL-2L11 [apoptosis facilitator)], and HRK (harakin, a BCL-2–interacting protein), which contain only BH3 homology segments, are not established.

forms of the differentially spliced BCL-X transcript, respectively (460). Whereas BCL-XL inhibits apoptosis in many cell systems, BCL-XS promotes cell death. One example of BCL-XL function occurs in developing thymocytes, where BCL-XL expression promotes survival during the double-positive stage, before selection by antigen binding (460,461). Similarly, BCL-XL expression in immature bone marrow B cells raises the threshold for apoptosis on crosslinking of the BCR (462). Under some circumstances, this permits survival of B cells with low and intermediate affinity for self antigens, which then may be subject to receptor editing. In GC B cells CD40 ligation results in induction of BCL-XL, thereby favoring survival of B cells receiving costimulatory signals from $CD4^+$ T cells in the context of BCR engagement (463).

Tumor Necrosis Family Receptors and Ligands

The TNF-related molecules and their receptors are critical mediators of lymphocyte proliferation, differentiation, and apoptosis (171,211). The ligands are a diverse molecular group; there is less homology among the ligands than the receptors (Fig. 2.33). The regulation of expression of TNF-type ligands is strict. These molecules are expressed only transiently at the surface of activated cells, from which they are cleaved by metalloproteinases (464–466). Most TNF family members can be detected in membrane-bound form at the cell surface and also in soluble form in the plasma. For some TNF-related molecules such as FAS ligand (FASL), circulating soluble ligand can act as a competitive inhibitor of the more potent, cell-bound ligand (467). The TNFRs are type II transmembrane proteins that lack intrinsic enzymatic activity and instead transmit messages through their interaction with cytoplasmic adaptor, or docking, proteins such as the TNFR-associated factors (TRAFs). A subset of the TNFRs contain death domains, through which they recruit to the cell surface and interact with adaptor proteins necessary for caspase recruitment and activation. Most TNFRs, including CD120a (TNFR-1) and CD120b (TNFR-2), CD30, CD40, and CD95 (FAS), require trimerization at the plasma membrane for signals to be transduced in the cytoplasm. Although it is beyond the scope of this chapter to describe the structure and function of all the known TNF receptors and ligands, we discuss several of the key molecular pairs because of the importance of these molecules in the physiology and regulation of the immune response.

TNF-α was originally characterized by its capacity to induce cell death in tumor cells (468,469). This potent inflammatory mediator is expressed and secreted by a variety of cell types, including helper and cytotoxic T cells, some B cells, and macrophages. In patients with septic shock, high levels of circulating TNF-α induce fever, endothelial cell damage, and vital organ destruction. The two receptors for TNF-α are called TNFR-1 and TNFR-2. The cytotoxic functions of TNF-α are mediated primarily by TNFR-1, which in its cytoplasm has a death domain sequence through which it binds death effector proteins (470). Alternatively, cross-

FIG. 2.33. Tumor necrosis factor (TNF)–related ligands and receptors. The TNF-type ligands are a relatively diverse group of proteins that regulate proliferation, differentiation, and apoptosis of lymphocytes and other TNF receptor (TNFR)–expressing cells. There is little structural homology among the TNF-type ligands, whereas the receptors share common structural motifs, including extracellular cysteine-rich domains, where binding occurs; transmembrane domains; and cytosolic death domains or TNFR-associated factor (TRAF) binding domains. Most TNF-related molecules occur at the cell surface and in soluble forms. Two exceptions are lymphotoxin-α (LT-α, also called TNF-β), which occurs only in soluble form, and nerve growth factor (NGF), which binds the TNFR-like NGFR (p75) but does not exhibit homology to other TNF-related molecules. LT-β is generated as a heterotrimer, with two soluble LT-α components linked to a single, cell-bound LT-β chain. A subset of TNFR family members contain cytosolic death domain sequences through which, on trimerization, they recruit and activate death effector molecules. Other TNFR family members do not transmit death signals, but they recruit and interact with cytoplasmic signaling elements such as TRAFs and phosphatases. Decoy receptors for FASL (DCR-3) and TRAIL (DCR-1, DCR-2) bind ligand but do not transmit signals because of an absent or truncated cytosolic domain. A few TNFR-type molecules occur in soluble form; these include DCR-3, osteoprotegerin, and poxvirus gene products, which bind and neutralize TNF ligands (479,487).

Ligand	Receptor	Reference
TNF-α	TNFRI, TNFRII	211,470,488
LT-α	TNFRI, TNFRII	288,489
LT-β	LT-β receptor	490,491
CD70	CD27	170
CD153	CD30	284,285
CD154	CD40	178,179,410,492
CD95L	CD95,DcR3	211,288,479,492,493
OX40L	OX40	494
CD137L	CD137	494
(NGF)	NGFR	495
APO-3L	DR3	211
APO-2L	DR4, DR5, DcR1, DcR2	211
OPGL	OPG, RANK	496,497
	poxvirus protein	498

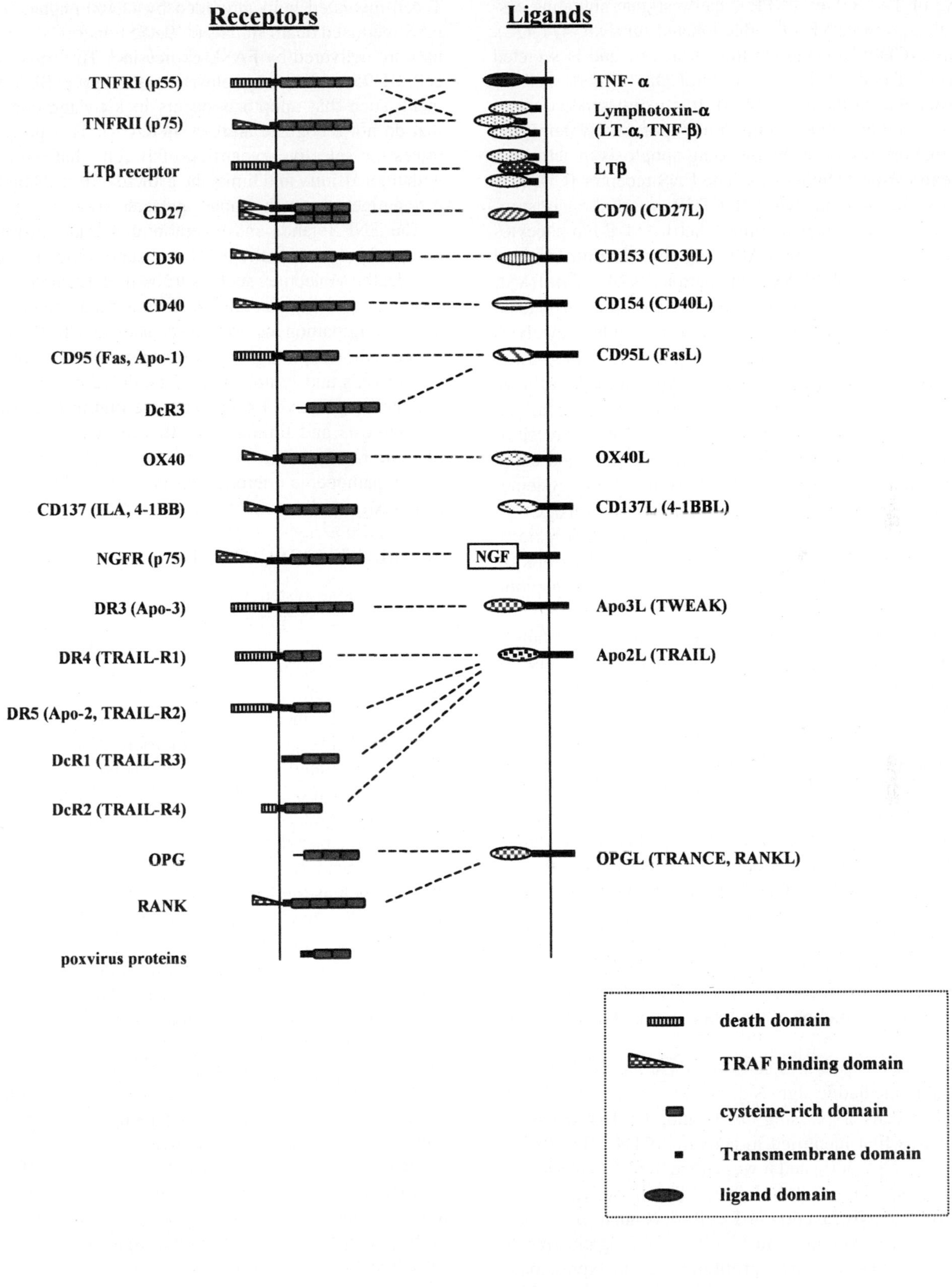
Receptors
Ligands
TNFRI (p55)
TNFRII (p75)
LTβ receptor
CD27
CD30
CD40
CD95 (Fas, Apo-1)
DcR3
OX40
CD137 (ILA, 4-1BB)
NGFR (p75)
DR3 (Apo-3)
DR4 (TRAIL-R1)
DR5 (Apo-2, TRAIL-R2)
DcR1 (TRAIL-R3)
DcR2 (TRAIL-R4)
OPG
RANK
poxvirus proteins
TNF- α
Lymphotoxin-α
(LT-α, TNF-β)
LTβ
CD70 (CD27L)
CD153 (CD30L)
CD154 (CD40L)
CD95L (FasL)
OX40L
CD137L (4-1BBL)
NGF
Apo3L (TWEAK)
Apo2L (TRAIL)
OPGL (TRANCE, RANKL)
death domain
TRAF binding domain
cysteine-rich domain
Transmembrane domain
ligand domain

linking of TNFR-1 or TNFR-2 can instigate signaling cascades that promote NF-κB induction and survival (471,472).

FASL (CD95L) occurs at the surface of and is secreted by $CD4^+$ T cells of the T_H1 subset, $CD8^+$ T cells, cells of the testis, and of the retina (473). It is expressed at sites of immune privilege, where it minimizes potentially damaging inflammatory responses by inducing apoptosis in activated, FAS-expressing lymphocytes. The FAS receptor (CD95) is expressed in T lymphocytes after TCR crosslinking or stimuli such as environmental stress. Activated T lymphocytes expressing both FAS and FASL can commit fratricide and even suicide by FAS-FASL interactions (474–476). FASL is expressed in some human tumor cells such as melanoma and metastatic colon cancer, where it may induce cytolysis of tumor-infiltrating cytotoxic T lymphocytes (477,478). A related mechanism by which some malignant cells achieve immune evasion is by gene amplification, expression, and secretion of a soluble, FASL-binding "decoy" receptor (DCR-3), such as occurs in some primary lung and colon cancer tumors. The DCR-3 molecule contains four cysteine-rich domains that resemble the extracellular portion of CD95 but lacks the transmembrane and intracellular DD regions. Tumor cells can escape FASL-induced cytolysis by secreting a protein that binds FASL but does not transduce apoptotic signals (479).

CD30 (Ki-1 antigen) was one of the first TNFR family members described, as it was identified in Hodgkin's disease specimens using a monoclonal antibody derived from mice injected with Reed-Sternberg cell-line cells (480). Subsequently, it was determined that CD30 is expressed in activated T and B cells and in the malignant cells of Hodgkin's disease, anaplastic large cell lymphoma, and some other B- and T-cell malignancies (171,481). CD30 has a large extracellular domain compared with that of other TNFR family members, and it lacks a cytoplasmic death domain. The ligand for CD30, CD153 (CD30L) is expressed in the thymic medulla, where it appears to be necessary for negative selection in double-positive thymocytes (285,482). The function of CD30 in activated, peripheral T cells is not established. In human B cells, CD30 ligation impedes CD40-mediated signals such as induction of the transcriptional regulator NF-κB (172).

CD40 is expressed in B cells and most APCs, where it is essential in mediating signals derived from activated T cells and other cells expressing its ligand, CD154 (CD40L). CD154 was first identified in activated $CD4^+$ T cells and T-cell lines (297,300), and it was called TRAP (TNF-related activation protein) or T-BAM (T-cell/B-cell–activating molecule) based on its function in T-cell–dependent B-cell activation and differentiation. In B cells, CD40 ligation results in transcriptional activation, proliferation, and expression of activation antigens, including CD80 and CD86 (B7) (483), CD23 (168), and FAS (209,484) (Fig. 2.29). On engagement by $CD4^+$ T cells expressing CD154 in cognate interaction, activated GC centroblasts are induced to proliferate and differentiate. At the same time, B cells are primed by $CD4^+$ T cell-mediated help, provided by CD40 engagement, for FAS-mediated death signals (209,485). In the GC, these signals are delivered by FASL-expressing, T_H1 cells. In the B cell, CD95-mediated apoptosis is inhibited by BCR engagement, such that apoptosis occurs in activated centroblasts that do not recognize antigen (484,486). This process promotes the selective expansion of B cells that bind antigen with high affinity and limits the growth of B cells that recognize antigen that is no longer present.

The TNF ligands and receptors constitute an important group of proteins that regulate cell survival, differentiation, and death. Molecules such as TNF-α, generated in macrophages and other cells, function in the initial, innate response to invading pathogens. Molecules such as CD30 and CD40 regulate the adaptive response by providing regulatory signals in DCs and lymphocytes. The death receptor proteins and their respective ligands are essential in the instigation of apoptosis and limitation of the adaptive response. The growing family of decoy receptors, generated by host cells and by pathogenic microbes, provides an additional level of complexity to these molecular systems.

SUMMARY AND CONCLUSIONS

The immune system includes a wide range of cellular and molecular signaling elements that function to protect individuals from damaging foreign particles. In healthy persons, the immune system provides immediate and long-term responses to infection by bacteria, viruses, fungi, and parasites. Innate immune mechanisms afford early recognition, neutralization, and engulfment of microorganisms. Adaptive responses, generated largely by T and B lymphocytes through their interaction with APCs, confer highly specific and long-term immunity.

During the past three decades, developments in immunology have elucidated the biology of specific hematologic neoplasms, such as the leukemias and lymphomas and of solid tumors such as renal cell carcinoma and melanoma. Vaccine strategies, which are being tried for diverse tumors such as multiple myeloma and melanoma, depend on antigen presentation and the coordinated response induced by DCs and T lymphocytes. Passive immunotherapies, based on the infusion of monoclonal antibodies to particular antigens or delivery of cytokines, are engineered based on information regarding cell-surface antigens and their particular functions. Adaptive immunotherapies, by which autologous DCs, T lymphocytes, or other cells are cultivated and manipulated *ex vivo* to generate an expanded, tumor-reactive effector cell population, are based on principles of antigen recognition, tolerance, and cell-mediated cytotoxicity. Our understanding of the pathophysiology of specific neoplasms and our capacity to treat them effectively rests in our expanding knowledge of normal host defenses.

REFERENCES

1. Thucydides. *The history of the Peloponnesian war*. Livingstone R, trans. New York: Oxford University Press, 1960.

2. Silverstein AM. *A history of immunology*. San Diego: Academic Press, 1989.
3. Parish HJ. *A history of immunization*. Edinburgh: E & S Livingstone, 1965.
4. De Contagione FG. Contagiosis morbis et eorum curatione (1546). Wright WC, trans [originally published in New York: GP Putnam's Sons, 1930]. In: Brock TD, ed. *Milestones in microbiology*. Washington, DC: American Society for Microbiology, 1975.
5. Bulloch W. *The history of bacteriology*. London: Oxford University Press, 1938.
6. Jenner E. An inquiry into the causes and effects of the variolae vaccinae, a disease discovered in some of the western counties of England, particularly Gloucestershire, and known by the name of the Cow Pox (1798) [abridged from facsimile edition published in Milan: R Van Lier, 1923]. In: Brock TD, ed. *Milestones in microbiology*. Washington, DC: American Society for Microbiology, 1975.
7. Koch R. Untersuchungen über Bakterien V. Die Aetiologie der Milzbrand-Krankheit, begründet auf die Entwicklungsgeschichte des Bacillus Anthracis (1877). Brock TD, trans. from *Beitr Biol Pflanzen* 1877;2:277–310. In: Brock TD, ed. *Milestones in microbiology*. Washington, DC: American Society for Microbiology, 1975.
8. Pasteur L. Sur les virus-vaccins du choléra des poules et du charbon (1881). Brock TD, trans, from Comptes rendus des travaux du Congrès international des directeurs des stations agronomiques, session de Versailles, June 1881:151–162. In: Brock TD, ed. *Milestones in microbiology*. Washington, DC: American Society for Microbiology, 1975.
9. von Behring E, Kitasato S. Ueber das Zustandekommen der Diptherie-Immunität und der Tetanus-Immunität bei Thieren (1890). Brock TD, trans, from *Deutsche Med Wochenschr* 1890;16:1113–1114. In: Brock TD, ed. *Milestones in microbiology*. Washington, DC: American Society for Microbiology, 1975.
10. Fox H. Baron Shibasaburo Kitasato. *Ann Med Hist Series* 1934;2: 491–499.
11. Ehrlich P. *Collected studies on immunity*. New York: John Wiley & Sons, 1906.
12. Jerne NK. The natural selection theory of antibody formation; ten years later. In: Cairns J, Stent GS, Watson JD, eds. *Phage and the origins of molecular biology*. Cold Spring Harbor, NY: Cold Spring Harbor Laboratory of Quantitative Biology, 1966.
13. Burnet FM. *The clonal selection theory of acquired immunity*. Cambridge: The University Press, 1959.
14. Silverstein AM. A history of theories of antibody formation. *Cell Immunol* 1985;91:263–283.
15. Watowich SS, Wu H, Socolovsky M, et al. Cytokine receptor signal transduction and the control of hematopoietic cell development. *Annu Rev Cell Dev Biol* 1996;12:91–128.
16. Rafii S, Mohle R, Shapiro F, et al. Regulation of hematopoiesis by microvascular endothelium. *Leuk Lymphoma* 1997;27:375–386.
17. Rosenberg N, Kincade PW. B-lineage differentiation in normal and transformed cells and the microenvironment that supports it. *Curr Opin Immunol* 1994;6:203–211.
18. Nagasawa T, Hirota S, Tachibana K, et al. Defects of B-cell lymphopoiesis and bone-marrow myelopoiesis in mice lacking the CXC chemokine PBSF/SDF-1. *Nature* 1996;382:635–638.
19. Namikawa R, Muench MO, de Vries JE, Roncarolo MG. The FLK2/FLT3 ligand synergizes with interleukin-7 in promoting stromal-cell–independent expansion and differentiation of human fetal pro-B cells in vitro. *Blood* 1996;87:1881–1890.
20. Le Bien TW. B-cell lymphopoiesis in mouse and man. *Curr Opin Immunol* 1998;10:188–195.
21. Shortman K, Egerton M, Spangrude GJ, et al. The generation and fate of thymocytes. *Semin Immunol* 1990;2:3–12.
22. Haynes BF, Heinly CS. Early human T cell development: analysis of the human thymus at the time of initial entry of hematopoietic stem cells into the fetal thymic microenvironment. *J Exp Med* 1995;181: 1445–1458.
23. Anderson G, Moore NC, Owen JJ, et al. Cellular interactions in thymocyte development. *Annu Rev Immunol* 1996;14:73–99.
24. Res P, Spits H. Developmental stages in the human thymus. *Semin Immunol* 1999;11:39–46.
25. Kelsoe G, Zheng B. Sites of B-cell activation in vivo. *Curr Opin Immunol* 1993;5:418–422.
26. Liu Y-J, Banchereau J. The paths and molecular controls of peripheral B-cell development. *Immunologist* 1996;4:55–66.
27. MacLennan IC, Gulbranson-Judge A, Toellner KM, et al. The changing preference of T and B cells for partners as T-dependent antibody responses develop. *Immunol Rev* 1997;156:53–66.
28. Kroese FG, Timens W, Nieuwenhuis P. Germinal center reaction and B lymphocytes: morphology and function. *Curr Top Pathol* 1990;84: 103–148.
29. MacLennan IC. Germinal centers. *Annu Rev Immunol* 1994;12: 117–139.
30. Liu YJ, Grouard G, de Bouteiller O, et al. Follicular dendritic cells and germinal centers. *Int Rev Cytol* 1996;166:139–179.
31. Kerneis S, Bogdanova A, Kraehenbuhl JP, et al. Conversion by Peyer's patch lymphocytes of human enterocytes into M cells that transport bacteria. *Science* 1997;277:949–952.
32. Spencer J, Finn T, Pulford KA, et al. The human gut contains a novel population of B lymphocytes which resemble marginal zone cells. *Clin Exp Immunol* 1985;62:607–612.
33. Metchnikoff E. Lectures on the comparative pathology of inflammation [delivered at the Pasteur Institute in 1891]. Starling FA and Starling EH, trans. New York: Dover, 1968.
34. Metchnicoff O. *Life of Elie Metchnicoff.* Boston: Houghton Mifflin, 1921.
35. Fearon DT, Locksley RM. The instructive role of innate immunity in the acquired immune response. *Science* 1996;272:50–53.
36. Carroll MC, Prodeus AP. Linkages of innate and adaptive immunity. *Curr Opin Immunol* 1998;10:36–40.
37. Ehrlich P. Zur theorie der lysenwirkung. *Berl Klin Wochenschr* 1899; 36:6–9.
38. Holmskov U, Malhotra R, Sim RB, et al. Collectins: collagenous C-type lectins of the innate immune defense system. *Immunol Today* 1994;15:67–74.
39. Carroll MC. The role of complement and complement receptors in induction and regulation of immunity. *Annu Rev Immunol* 1998;16: 545–568.
40. Lambris JD, Reid KB, Volanakis JE. The evolution, structure, biology and pathophysiology of complement. *Immunol Today* 1999;20: 207–211.
41. Morgan BP. Physiology and pathophysiology of complement: progress and trends. *Crit Rev Clin Lab Sci* 1995;32:265–298.
42. Thiel S, Vorup-Jensen T, Stover CM, et al. A second serine protease associated with mannan-binding lectin that activates complement. *Nature* 1997;386:506–510.
43. Fearon DT. Identification of the membrane glycoprotein that is the C3b receptor of the human erythrocyte, polymorphonuclear leukocyte, B lymphocyte, and monocyte. *J Exp Med* 1980;152:20–30.
44. Medof ME, Iida K, Mold C, et al. Unique role of the complement receptor CR1 in the degradation of C3b associated with immune complexes. *J Exp Med* 1982;156:1739–1754.
45. Young JD, Cohn ZA, Podack ER. The ninth component of complement and the pore-forming protein (perforin 1) from cytotoxic T cells: structural, immunological, and functional similarities. *Science* 1986; 233:184–190.
46. Liu CC, Persechini PM, Young JD. Perforin and lymphocyte-mediated cytolysis. *Immunol Rev* 1995;146:145–175.
47. Johnston RB Jr. Current concepts: immunology. Monocytes and macrophages. *N Engl J Med* 1988;318:747–752.
48. Ziegler-Heitbrock HW. Heterogeneity of human blood monocytes: the $CD14^+$ $CD16^+$ subpopulation. *Immunol Today* 1996;17:424–428.
49. Paulnock DM. Macrophage activation by T cells. *Curr Opin Immunol* 1992;4:344–349.
50. MacMicking J, Xie QW, Nathan C. Nitric oxide and macrophage function. *Annu Rev Immunol* 1997;15:323–350.
51. MacMicking JD, Nathan C, Hom G, et al. Altered responses to bacterial infection and endotoxic shock in mice lacking inducible nitric oxide synthase. *Cell* 1995;81:641–650.
52. Wright SD. CD14 and innate recognition of bacteria. *J Immunol* 1995; 155:6–8.
53. Su GL, Simmons RL, Wang SC. Lipopolysaccharide binding protein participation in cellular activation by LPS. *Crit Rev Immunol* 1995; 15:201–214.
54. Medzhitov R, Preston-Hurlburt P, Janeway CA Jr. A human homo-

logue of the *Drosophila* toll protein signals activation of adaptive immunity. *Nature* 1997;388:394–397.
55. Yang RB, Mark MR, Gray A, et al. Toll-like receptor-2 mediates lipopolysaccharide-induced cellular signalling. *Nature* 1998;395: 284–288.
56. Kirschning CJ, Wesche H, Merrill Ayres T, et al. Human toll-like receptor 2 confers responsiveness to bacterial lipopolysaccharide. *J Exp Med* 1998;188:2091–2097.
57. Modlin RL, Brightbill HD. The Toll of innate immunity on microbial pathogens. *N Engl J Med* 1999;340:1834–1835.
58. Devitt A, Moffatt OD, Raykundalia C, et al. Human CD14 mediates recognition and phagocytosis of apoptotic cells. *Nature* 1998;392: 505–509.
59. Marcinkiewicz J. Neutrophil chloramines: missing links between innate and acquired immunity. *Immunol Today* 1997;18:577–580.
60. Dvorak AM. Human peripheral blood neutrophil. *Blood* 1995;85: 3333.
61. Hampton MB, Kettle AJ, Winterbourn CC. Inside the neutrophil phagosome: oxidants, myeloperoxidase, and bacterial killing. *Blood* 1998;92:3007–3017.
62. Borregaard N. Current concepts about neutrophil granule physiology. *Curr Opin Hematol* 1996;3:11–18.
63. Matzner Y. Neutrophil pathophysiology. *Semin Hematol* 1997;34: 265–266.
64. Springer TA. Traffic signals for lymphocyte recirculation and leukocyte emigration: the multistep paradigm. *Cell* 1994;76:301–314.
65. McEver RP, Moore KL, Cummings RD. Leukocyte trafficking mediated by selectin-carbohydrate interactions. *J Biol Chem* 1995;270: 11025–11028.
66. Edwards SW, Watson F. The cell biology of phagocytes. *Immunol Today* 1995;16:508–510.
67. Gahmberg CG. Leukocyte adhesion: CD11/CD18 integrins and intercellular adhesion molecules. *Curr Opin Cell Biol* 1997;9:643–650.
68. Stewart M, Thiel M, Hogg N. Leukocyte integrins. *Curr Opin Cell Biol* 1995;7:690–696.
69. Brown E. Neutrophil adhesion and the therapy of inflammation. *Semin Hematol* 1997;34:319–326.
70. Newman PJ. The biology of PECAM-1. *J Clin Invest* 1997;99:3–8.
71. Tsunawaki S, Mizunari H, Namiki H, et al. NADPH-binding component of the respiratory burst oxidase system: studies using neutrophil membranes from patients with chronic granulomatous disease lacking the beta-subunit of cytochrome b_{558}. *J Exp Med* 1994;179:291–297.
72. Walsh GM. Human eosinophils: their accumulation, activation and fate. *Br J Haematol* 1997;97:701–709.
73. Weller PF. Human eosinophils. *J Allergy Clin Immunol* 1997;100: 283–287.
74. Rothenberg ME. Eosinophilia. *N Engl J Med* 1998;338:1592–1600.
75. Dvorak AM, Ackerman SJ, Weller PF. Subcellular morphology and biochemistry of eosinophils. In: Harris JR, ed. *Megakaryocytes, platelets, macrophages and eosinophils,* 2. London: Plenum Publishing, 1991.
76. Weller PF. Eosinophils: structure and functions. *Curr Opin Immunol* 1994;6:85–90.
77. Ponath PD, Qin S, Post TW, et al. Molecular cloning and characterization of a human eotaxin receptor expressed selectively on eosinophils. *J Exp Med* 1996;183:2437–2448.
78. Dubucquoi S, Desreumaux P, Janin A, et al. Interleukin 5 synthesis by eosinophils: association with granules and immunoglobulin-dependent secretion. *J Exp Med* 1994;179:703–708.
79. Sutton BJ, Gould HJ. The human IgE network. *Nature* 1993;366: 421–428.
80. Garman SC, Kinet JP, Jardetzky TS. Crystal structure of the human high-affinity IgE receptor. *Cell* 1998;95:951–961.
81. Marshall JS, Bienenstock J. The role of mast cells in inflammatory reactions of the airways, skin and intestine. *Curr Opin Immunol* 1994; 6:853–859.
82. Dvorak AM. The fine structure of human basophils and mast cells. In: Holgate ST, ed. *Mast cells, mediators and disease.* Dordrecht, The Netherlands: Kluwer Academic Publishers, 1988.
83. Schwartz LB. Mast cells: function and contents. *Curr Opin Immunol* 1994;6:91–97.
84. Church MK, Levi-Schaffer F. The human mast cell. *J Allergy Clin Immunol* 1997;99:155–160.
85. Abraham SN, Arock M. Mast cells and basophils in innate immunity. *Semin Immunol* 1998;10:373–381.
86. Conrad DH, Squire CM, Bartlett WC, et al. Fc epsilon receptors. *Curr Opin Immunol* 1991;3:859–864.
87. Torigoe C, Inman JK, Metzger H. An unusual mechanism for ligand antagonism. *Science* 1998;281:568–572.
88. Dvorak AM. Cell biology of the basophil. *Int Rev Cytol* 1998;180: 87–236.
89. Yokoyama WM. Natural killer cell receptors. *Curr Opin Immunol* 1998;10:298–305.
90. Kagi D, Ledermann B, Burki K, et al. Molecular mechanisms of lymphocyte-mediated cytotoxicity and their role in immunological protection and pathogenesis in vivo. *Annu Rev Immunol* 1996;14:207–232.
91. Moretta A. Molecular mechanisms in cell-mediated cytotoxicity. *Cell* 1997;90:13–18.
92. Valiante NM, Uhrberg M, Shilling HG, et al. Functionally and structurally distinct NK cell receptor repertoires in the peripheral blood of two human donors. *Immunity* 1997;7:739–751.
93. Lanier LL. NK cell receptors. *Annu Rev Immunol* 1998;16:359–393.
94. Bauer S, Groh V, Wu J, et al. Activation of NK cells and T cells by NKG2D, a receptor for stress-inducible MICA. *Science* 1999;285: 727–729.
95. Reth M. Antigen receptor tail clue. *Nature* 1989;338:383–384.
96. De Franco AL. The complexity of signaling pathways activated by the BCR. *Curr Opin Immunol* 1997;9:296–308.
97. Rudd CE. Adaptors and molecular scaffolds in immune cell signaling. *Cell* 1999;96:5–8.
98. Neel BG. Role of phosphatases in lymphocyte activation. *Curr Opin Immunol* 1997;9:405–420.
99. Unkeless JC, Jin J. Inhibitory receptors, ITIM sequences and phosphatases. *Curr Opin Immunol* 1997;9:338–343.
100. Coggeshall KM. Inhibitory signaling by B cell Fc gamma RIIb. *Curr Opin Immunol* 1998;10:306–312.
101. Boismenu R, Havran WL. An innate view of gamma delta T cells. *Curr Opin Immunol* 1997;9:57–63.
102. Laky K, Lefrancois L, von Freeden-Jeffry U, et al. The role of IL-7 in thymic and extrathymic development of TCR gamma delta cells. *J Immunol* 1998;161:707–713.
103. Madrigal-Estebas L, McManus R, Byrne B, et al. Human small intestinal epithelial cells secrete interleukin-7 and differentially express two different interleukin-7 mRNA transcripts: implications for extrathymic T-cell differentiation. *Hum Immunol* 1997;58:83–90.
104. Chowers Y, Holtmeier W, Harwood J, et al. The V delta 1 T cell receptor repertoire in human small intestine and colon. *J Exp Med* 1994;180:183–190.
105. Bahram S, Bresnahan M, Geraghty DE, Spies T. A second lineage of mammalian major histocompatibility complex class I genes. *Proc Natl Acad Sci U S A* 1994;91:6259–6263.
106. Bukowski JF, Morita CT, Brenner MB. Recognition and destruction of virus-infected cells by human gamma delta CTL. *J Immunol* 1994; 153:5133–5140.
107. Groh V, Steinle A, Bauer S, et al. Recognition of stress-induced MHC molecules by intestinal epithelial gamma delta T cells. *Science* 1998; 279:1737–1740.
108. Boes M, Prodeus AP, Schmidt T, et al. A critical role of natural immunoglobulin M in immediate defense against systemic bacterial infection. *J Exp Med* 1998;188:2381–2386.
109. Hayakawa K, Asano M, Shinton SA, et al. Positive selection of natural autoreactive B cells. *Science* 1999;285:113–116.
110. Casali P, Notkins AL. $CD5^+$ B lymphocytes, polyreactive antibodies and the human B-cell repertoire. *Immunol Today* 1989;10:364–368.
111. Kasaian MT, Casali P. Autoimmunity-prone B-1 (CD5 B) cells, natural antibodies and self recognition. *Autoimmunity* 1993;15:315–329.
112. Hulett MD, Hogarth PM. Molecular basis of Fc receptor function. *Adv Immunol* 1994;57:1–127.
113. Daeron M. Fc receptor biology. *Annu Rev Immunol* 1997;15:203–234.
114. Mostov KE. Transepithelial transport of immunoglobulins. *Annu Rev Immunol* 1994;12:63–84.
115. Simister NE, Mostov KE. An Fc receptor structurally related to MHC class I antigens. *Nature* 1989;337:184–187.

116. Hunziker W, Koch T, Whitney JA, et al. Fc receptor phosphorylation during receptor-mediated control of B-cell activation. *Nature* 1990; 345:628–632.
117. Ravetch JV. Fc receptors. *Curr Opin Immunol* 1997;9:121–125.
118. Fearon DT, Carter RH. The CD19/CR2/TAPA-1 complex of B lymphocytes: linking natural to acquired immunity. *Annu Rev Immunol* 1995;13:127–149.
119. Gauchat JF, Henchoz S, Mazzei G, et al. Induction of human IgE synthesis in B cells by mast cells and basophils. *Nature* 1993;365: 340–343.
120. Tonegawa S. Somatic generation of antibody diversity. *Nature* 1983; 302:575–581.
121. Alt FW, Blackwell TK, Yancopoulos GD. Development of the primary antibody repertoire. *Science* 1987;238:1079–1087.
122. Casali P, Silberstein LESE. Immunoglobulin gene expression in development and disease. *Ann NY Acad Sci* 1995;764.
123. Grawunder U, West RB, Lieber MR. Antigen receptor gene rearrangement. *Curr Opin Immunol* 1998;10:172–180.
124. Cook GP, Tomlinson IM. The human immunoglobulin VH repertoire. *Immunol Today* 1995;16:237–242.
125. Matsuda F, Honjo T. Organization of the human immunoglobulin heavy-chain locus. *Adv Immunol* 1996;62:1–29.
126. Stavnezer J. Immunoglobulin class switching. *Curr Opin Immunol* 1996;8:199–205.
127. Edelman GM. Antibody structure and molecular immunology. *Science* 1973;180:830–840.
128. Eisen HN. *General Immunology*. Philadelphia: JB Lippincott, 1990.
129. Kehry M, Ewald S, Douglas R, et al. The immunoglobulin mu chains of membrane-bound and secreted IgM molecules differ in their C-terminal segments. *Cell* 1980;21:393–406.
130. Davis AC, Shulman MJ. IgM—molecular requirements for its assembly and function. *Immunol Today* 1989;10:118–122, 127–118.
131. Brandtzaeg P, Prydz H. Direct evidence for an integrated function of J chain and secretory component in epithelial transport of immunoglobulins. *Nature* 1984;311:71–73.
132. Plaut AG, Gilbert JV, Artenstein MS, et al. *Neisseria gonorrhoeae* and *Neisseria meningitidis:* extracellular enzyme cleaves human immunoglobulin A. *Science* 1975;190:1103–1105.
133. Flores-Romo L, Shields J, Humbert Y, et al. Inhibition of an in vivo antigen-specific IgE response by antibodies to CD23. *Science* 1993; 261:1038–1041.
134. Ramsden DA, van Gent DC, Gellert M. Specificity in V(D)J recombination: new lessons from biochemistry and genetics. *Curr Opin Immunol* 1997;9:114–120.
135. Komori T, Okada A, Stewart V, et al. Lack of N regions in antigen receptor variable region genes of TdT-deficient lymphocytes. *Science* 1993;261:1171–1175.
136. Ghia P, ten Boekel E, Rolink AG, et al. B-cell development: a comparison between mouse and man. *Immunol Today* 1998;19:480–485.
137. Torres RM, Flaswinkel H, Reth M, et al. Aberrant B cell development and immune response in mice with a compromised BCR complex. *Science* 1996;272:1804–1808.
138. Norvell A, Mandik L, Monroe JG. Engagement of the antigen-receptor on immature murine B lymphocytes results in death by apoptosis. *J Immunol* 1995;154:4404–4413.
139. Jacob J, Kelsoe G, Rajewsky K, et al. Intraclonal generation of antibody mutants in germinal centres. *Nature* 1991;354:389–392.
140. Hikida M, Mori M, Takai T, et al. Reexpression of RAG-1 and RAG-2 genes in activated mature mouse B cells. *Science* 1996;274: 2092–2094.
141. Papavasiliou F, Casellas R, Suh H, et al. V(D)J recombination in mature B cells: a mechanism for altering antibody responses. *Science* 1997;278:298–301.
142. Germain RN. MHC-dependent antigen processing and peptide presentation: providing ligands for T lymphocyte activation. *Cell* 1994;76: 287–299.
143. Pamer E, Cresswell P. Mechanisms of MHC class I—restricted antigen processing. *Annu Rev Immunol* 1998;16:323–358.
144. Kovats S, Drover S, Marshall WH, et al. Coordinate defects in human histocompatibility leukocyte antigen class II expression and antigen presentation in bare lymphocyte syndrome. *J Exp Med* 1994;179: 2017–2022.
145. Kantor A. A new nomenclature for B cells. *Immunol Today* 1991;12: 388.
146. Bikah G, Carey J, Ciallella JR, et al. CD5-mediated negative regulation of antigen receptor-induced growth signals in B-1 B cells. *Science* 1996;274:1906–1909.
147. Raman C, Kuo A, Deshane J, et al. Regulation of casein kinase 2 by direct interaction with cell surface receptor CD5. *J Biol Chem* 1998; 273:19183–19189.
148. Shipp MA, Stefano GB, D'Adamio L, et al. Downregulation of enkephalin-mediated inflammatory responses by CD10/neutral endopeptidase 24.11. *Nature* 1990;347:394–396.
149. Ganju RK, Shpektor RG, Brenner DG, Shipp MA. CD10/neutral endopeptidase 24.11 is phosphorylated by casein kinase II and coassociates with other phosphoproteins including the lyn src-related kinase. *Blood* 1996;88:4159–4165.
150. Le Bien TW, McCormack RT. The common acute lymphoblastic leukemia antigen (CD10)—emancipation from a functional enigma. *Blood* 1989;73:625–635.
151. Stamenkovic I, Seed B. CD19, the earliest differentiation antigen of the B cell lineage, bears three extracellular immunoglobulin-like domains and an Epstein-Barr virus-related cytoplasmic tail. *J Exp Med* 1988;168:1205–1210.
152. Carter RH, Fearon DT. CD19: lowering the threshold for antigen receptor stimulation of B lymphocytes. *Science* 1992;256:105–107.
153. O'Rourke LM, Tooze R, Turner M, et al. CD19 as a membrane-anchored adaptor protein of B lymphocytes: costimulation of lipid and protein kinases by recruitment of Vav. *Immunity* 1998;8:635–645.
154. O'Rourke L, Tooze R, Fearon DT. Co-receptors of B lymphocytes. *Curr Opin Immunol* 1997;9:324–329.
155. Nadler LM, Stashenko P, Hardy R, et al. A monoclonal antibody defining a lymphoma-associated antigen in man. *J Immunol* 1980; 125:570–577.
156. Einfeld DA, Brown JP, Valentine MA, et al. Molecular cloning of the human B cell CD20 receptor predicts a hydrophobic protein with multiple transmembrane domains. *EMBO J* 1988;7:711–717.
157. Tedder TF, Streuli M, Schlossman SF, et al. Isolation and structure of a cDNA encoding the B1 (CD20) cell-surface antigen of human B lymphocytes. *Proc Natl Acad Sci USA* 1988;85:208–212.
158. Tedder TF, Engel P. CD20: a regulator of cell-cycle progression of B lymphocytes. *Immunol Today* 1994;15:450–454.
159. Weis JJ, Tedder TF, Fearon DT. Identification of a 145,000 Mr membrane protein as the C3d receptor (CR2) of human B lymphocytes. *Proc Natl Acad Sci USA* 1984;81:881–885.
160. Fremeaux-Bacchi V, Bernard I, Maillet F, et al. Human lymphocytes shed a soluble form of CD21 (the C3dg/Epstein-Barr virus receptor, CR2) that binds iC3b and CD23. *Eur J Immunol* 1996;26:1497–1503.
161. Makar KW, Pham CT, Dehoff MH, et al. An intronic silencer regulates B lymphocyte cell- and stage-specific expression of the human complement receptor type 2 (CR2, CD21) gene. *J Immunol* 1998;160: 1268–1278.
162. Aubry JP, Pochon S, Graber P, et al. CD21 is a ligand for CD23 and regulates IgE production. *Nature* 1992;358:505–507.
163. Stamenkovic I, Sgroi D, Aruffo A, et al. The B lymphocyte adhesion molecule CD22 interacts with leukocyte common antigen CD45RO on T cells and alpha-2,6-sialyltransferase, CD75, on B cells. *Cell* 1991;66:1133–1144.
164. Doody GM, Dempsey PW, Fearon DT. Activation of B lymphocytes: integrating signals from CD19, CD22 and Fc gamma RIIb1. *Curr Opin Immunol* 1996;8:378–382.
165. Tedder TF, Tuscano J, Sato S, et al. CD22, a B lymphocyte-specific adhesion molecule that regulates antigen receptor signaling. *Annu Rev Immunol* 1997;15:481–504.
166. Gordon J. B-cell signalling via the C-type lectins CD23 and CD72. *Immunol Today* 1994;15:411–417.
167. Punnonen J, Aversa G, Cocks BG, et al. Interleukin 13 induces interleukin 4–independent IgG4 and IgE synthesis and CD23 expression by human B cells. *Proc Natl Acad Sci USA* 1993;90:3730–3734.
168. Saeland S, Duvert V, Moreau I, et al. Human B cell precursors proliferate and express CD23 after CD40 ligation. *J Exp Med* 1993;178: 113–120.
169. Klein U, Goossens T, Fischer M, et al. Somatic hypermutation in

normal and transformed human B cells. *Immunol Rev* 1998;162: 261–280.
170. Lens SM, Tesselaar K, van Oers MH, et al. Control of lymphocyte function through CD27-CD70 interactions. *Semin Immunol* 1998;10: 491–499.
171. Gruss HJ, Dower SK. Tumor necrosis factor ligand superfamily: involvement in the pathology of malignant lymphomas. *Blood* 1995; 85:3378–3404.
172. Cerutti A, Schaffer A, Shah S, et al. CD30 is a CD40-inducible molecule that negatively regulates CD40-mediated immunoglobulin class switching in non-antigen-selected human B cells. *Immunity* 1998;9: 247–256.
173. Kumagai M, Coustan-Smith E, Murray DJ, et al. Ligation of CD38 suppresses human B lymphopoiesis. *J Exp Med* 1995;181:1101–1110.
174. Liu YJ, Arpin C, de Bouteiller O, et al. Sequential triggering of apoptosis, somatic mutation and isotype switch during germinal center development. *Semin Immunol* 1996;8:169–177.
175. Lund FE, Cockayne DA, Randall TD, et al. CD38: a new paradigm in lymphocyte activation and signal transduction. *Immunol Rev* 1998; 161:79–93.
176. Maliszewski CR, Delespesse GJ, Schoenborn MA, et al. The CD39 lymphoid cell activation antigen. Molecular cloning and structural characterization. *J Immunol* 1994;153:3574–3583.
177. Kaczmarek E, Koziak K, Sevigny J, et al. Identification and characterization of CD39/vascular ATP diphosphohydrolase. *J Biol Chem* 1996;271:33116–33122.
178. Uckun FM, Gajl-Peczalska K, Myers DE, et al. Temporal association of CD40 antigen expression with discrete stages of human B-cell ontogeny and the efficacy of anti-CD40 immunotoxins against clonogenic B-lineage acute lymphoblastic leukemia as well as B-lineage non-Hodgkin's lymphoma cells. *Blood* 1990;76:2449–2456.
179. van Kooten C, Banchereau J. Functions of CD40 on B cells, dendritic cells and other cells. *Curr Opin Immunol* 1997;9:330–337.
180. Trowbridge IS, Thomas ML. CD45: an emerging role as a protein tyrosine phosphatase required for lymphocyte activation and development. *Annu Rev Immunol* 1994;12:85–116.
181. Diamond MS, Staunton DE, de Fougerolles AR, et al. ICAM-1 (CD54): a counter-receptor for Mac-1 (CD11b/CD18). *J Cell Biol* 1990;111:3129–3139.
182. Springer TA. Adhesion receptors of the immune system. *Nature* 1990; 346:425–434.
183. Goodwin RG, Alderson MR, Smith CA, et al. Molecular and biological characterization of a ligand for CD27 defines a new family of cytokines with homology to tumor necrosis factor. *Cell* 1993;73: 447–456.
184. Lens SM, Keehnen RM, van Oers MH, et al. Identification of a novel subpopulation of germinal center B cells characterized by expression of IgD and CD70. *Eur J Immunol* 1996;26:1007–1011.
185. Jacquot S, Kobata T, Iwata S, et al. CD154/CD40 and CD70/CD27 interactions have different and sequential functions in T cell-dependent B cell responses: enhancement of plasma cell differentiation by CD27 signaling. *J Immunol* 1997;159:2652–2657.
186. McClelland A, Kuhn LC, Ruddle FH. The human transferrin receptor gene: genomic organization, and the complete primary structure of the receptor deduced from a cDNA sequence. *Cell* 1984;39:267–274.
187. Kuhn LC, McClelland A, Ruddle FH. Gene transfer, expression, and molecular cloning of the human transferrin receptor gene. *Cell* 1984; 37:95–103.
188. Collawn JF, Stangel M, Kuhn LA, et al. Transferrin receptor internalization sequence YXRF implicates a tight turn as the structural recognition motif for endocytosis. *Cell* 1990;63:1061–1072.
189. Van de Velde H, von Hoegen I, Luo W, et al. The B-cell surface protein CD72/Lyb-2 is the ligand for CD5. *Nature* 1991;351:662–665.
190. Wiels J, Fellous M, Tursz T. Monoclonal antibody against a Burkitt lymphoma-associated antigen. *Proc Natl Acad Sci USA* 1981;78: 6485–6488.
191. Mangeney M, Richard Y, Coulaud D, et al. CD77: an antigen of germinal center B cells entering apoptosis. *Eur J Immunol* 1991;21: 1131–1140.
192. Pleiman CM, D'Ambrosio D, Cambier JC. The B-cell antigen receptor complex: structure and signal transduction. *Immunol Today* 1994;15: 393–399.
193. Kurosaki T. Molecular mechanisms in B cell antigen receptor signaling. *Curr Opin Immunol* 1997;9:309–318.
194. Tamir I, Cambier JC. Antigen receptor signaling: integration of protein tyrosine kinase functions. *Oncogene* 1998;17:1353–1364.
195. Yokochi T, Holly RD, Clark EA. B lymphoblast antigen (BB-1) expressed on Epstein-Barr virus–activated B cell blasts, B lymphoblastoid cell lines, and Burkitt's lymphomas. *J Immunol* 1982;128: 823–827.
196. Freedman AS, Freeman G, Horowitz JC, et al. B7, a B-cell–restricted antigen that identifies preactivated B cells. *J Immunol* 1987;139: 3260–3267.
197. Linsley PS, Clark EA, Ledbetter JA. T-cell antigen CD28 mediates adhesion with B cells by interacting with activation antigen B7/BB-1. *Proc Natl Acad Sci USA* 1990;87:5031–5035.
198. Lenschow DJ, Walunas TL, Bluestone JA. CD28/B7 system of T cell costimulation. *Annu Rev Immunol* 1996;14:233–258.
199. Reiser H, Stadecker MJ. Costimulatory B7 molecules in the pathogenesis of infectious and autoimmune diseases. *N Engl J Med* 1996;335: 1369–1377.
200. Levy S, Todd SC, Maecker HT. CD81 (TAPA-1): a molecule involved in signal transduction and cell adhesion in the immune system. *Annu Rev Immunol* 1998;16:89–109.
201. Pileri P, Uematsu Y, Campagnoli S, et al. Binding of hepatitis C virus to CD81. *Science* 1998;282:938–941.
202. Horvath G, Serru V, Clay D, et al. CD19 is linked to the integrin-associated tetraspans CD9, CD81, and CD82. *J Biol Chem* 1998;273: 30537–30543.
203. Freeman GJ, Gribben JG, Boussiotis VA, et al. Cloning of B7-2: a CTLA-4 counter-receptor that costimulates human T cell proliferation. *Science* 1993;262:909–911.
204. Azuma M, Ito D, Yagita H, et al. B70 antigen is a second ligand for CTLA-4 and CD28. *Nature* 1993;366:76–79.
205. Trauth BC, Klas C, Peters AM, et al. Monoclonal antibody-mediated tumor regression by induction of apoptosis. *Science* 1989;245: 301–305.
206. Yonehara S, Ishii A, Yonehara M. A cell-killing monoclonal antibody (anti-Fas) to a cell surface antigen co-downregulated with the receptor of tumor necrosis factor. *J Exp Med* 1989;169:1747–1756.
207. Itoh N, Yonehara S, Ishii A, et al. The polypeptide encoded by the cDNA for human cell surface antigen Fas can mediate apoptosis. *Cell* 1991;66:233–243.
208. Oehm A, Behrmann I, Falk W, et al. Purification and molecular cloning of the APO-1 cell surface antigen, a member of the tumor necrosis factor/nerve growth factor receptor superfamily. Sequence identity with the Fas antigen. *J Biol Chem* 1992;267:10709–10715.
209. Schattner EJ, Elkon KB, Yoo DH, et al. CD40 ligation induces Apo-1/Fas expression on human B lymphocytes and facilitates apoptosis through the Apo-1/Fas pathway. *J Exp Med* 1995;182:1557–1565.
210. Baker SJ, Reddy EP. Modulation of life and death by the TNF receptor superfamily. *Oncogene* 1998;17:3261–3270.
211. Ashkenazi A, Dixit VM. Death receptors: signaling and modulation. *Science* 1998;281:1305–1308.
212. Jiang Y, Woronicz JD, Liu W, Goeddel DV. Prevention of constitutive TNF receptor 1 signaling by silencer of death domains. *Science* 1999; 283:543–546.
213. Beltinger CP, White PS, Maris JM, et al. Physical mapping and genomic structure of the human TNFR2 gene. *Genomics* 1996;35:94–100.
214. Keegan AD, Nelms K, Wang LM, et al. Interleukin 4 receptor: signaling mechanisms. *Immunol Today* 1994;15:423–432.
215. Nelms K, Huang H, Ryan J, et al. Interleukin-4 receptor signalling mechanisms and their biological significance. *Adv Exp Med Biol* 1998; 452:37–43.
216. Devos R, Plaetinck G, Cornelis S, et al. Interleukin-5 and its receptor: a drug target for eosinophilia associated with chronic allergic disease. *J Leukoc Biol* 1995;57:813–819.
217. Yamasaki K, Taga T, Hirata Y, et al. Cloning and expression of the human interleukin-6 (BSF-2/IFN beta 2) receptor. *Science* 1988;241: 825–828.
218. Hibi M, Murakami M, Saito M, et al. Molecular cloning and expression of an IL-6 signal transducer, gp130. *Cell* 1990;63:1149–1157.
219. Taga T, Kishimoto T. Gp130 and the interleukin-6 family of cytokines. *Annu Rev Immunol* 1997;15:797–819.

220. Turner CA Jr, Mack DH, Davis MM. Blimp-1, a novel zinc finger-containing protein that can drive the maturation of B lymphocytes into immunoglobulin-secreting cells. *Cell* 1994;77:297–306.
221. Carey DJ. Syndecans: multifunctional cell-surface co-receptors. *Biochem J* 1997;327:1–16.
222. Cambier JC, Campbell KS. Membrane immunoglobulin and its accomplices: new lessons from an old receptor. *FASEB J* 1992;6: 3207–3217.
223. Siminovitch KA, Neel BG. Regulation of B cell signal transduction by SH2-containing protein-tyrosine phosphatases. *Semin Immunol* 1998; 10:329–347.
224. Corey SJ, Anderson SM. Src-related protein tyrosine kinases in hematopoiesis. *Blood* 1999;93:1–14.
225. Schwartzberg PL. The many faces of Src: multiple functions of a prototypical tyrosine kinase. *Oncogene* 1998;17:1463–1468.
226. Bolen JB, Brugge JS. Leukocyte protein tyrosine kinases: potential targets for drug discovery. *Annu Rev Immunol* 1997;15:371–404.
227. Fischer EH, Charbonneau H, Tonks NK. Protein tyrosine phosphatases: a diverse family of intracellular and transmembrane enzymes. *Science* 1991;253:401–406.
228. Ono M, Okada H, Bolland S, et al. Deletion of SHIP or SHP-1 reveals two distinct pathways for inhibitory signaling. *Cell* 1997;90:293–301.
229. Doody GM, Justement LB, Delibrias CC, et al. A role in B cell activation for CD22 and the protein tyrosine phosphatase SHP. *Science* 1995;269:242–244.
230. Shan D, Ledbetter JA, Press OW. Apoptosis of malignant human B cells by ligation of CD20 with monoclonal antibodies. *Blood* 1998; 91:1644–1652.
231. McLaughlin P, Grillo-Lopez AJ, Link BK, et al. Rituximab chimeric anti-CD20 monoclonal antibody therapy for relapsed indolent lymphoma: half of patients respond to a four-dose treatment program. *J Clin Oncol* 1998;16:2825–2833.
232. Deans JP, Schieven GL, Shu GL, et al. Association of tyrosine and serine kinases with the B cell surface antigen CD20. Induction via CD20 of tyrosine phosphorylation and activation of phospholipase C-gamma 1 and PLC phospholipase C-gamma 2. *J Immunol* 1993;151: 4494–4504.
233. Hardy RR, Li YS, Hayakawa K. Distinctive developmental origins and specificities of the $CD5^+$ B-cell subset. *Semin Immunol* 1996;8: 37–44.
234. Caligaris-Cappio F. B-chronic lymphocytic leukemia: a malignancy of anti-self B cells. *Blood* 1996;87:2615–2620.
235. Kipps TJ, Carson DA. Autoantibodies in chronic lymphocytic leukemia and related systemic autoimmune diseases. *Blood* 1993;81: 2475–2487.
236. Resnick D, Pearson A, Krieger M. The SRCR superfamily: a family reminiscent of the Ig superfamily. *Trends Biochem Sci* 1994;19:5–8.
237. Luo W, Van de Velde H, von Hoegen I, et al. Ly-1 (CD5), a membrane glycoprotein of mouse T lymphocytes and a subset of B cells, is a natural ligand of the B cell surface protein Lyb-2 (CD72). *J Immunol* 1992;148:1630–1634.
238. Biancone L, Bowen MA, Lim A, et al. Identification of a novel inducible cell-surface ligand of CD5 on activated lymphocytes. *J Exp Med* 1996;184:811–819.
239. Pospisil R, Fitts MG, Mage RG. CD5 is a potential selecting ligand for B cell surface immunoglobulin framework region sequences. *J Exp Med* 1996;184:1279–1284.
240. Tarakhovsky A, Kanner SB, Hombach J, et al. A role for CD5 in TCR-mediated signal transduction and thymocyte selection. *Science* 1995;269:535–537.
241. Barroga CF, Stevenson JK, Schwarz EM, et al. Constitutive phosphorylation of I kappa B alpha by casein kinase II. *Proc Natl Acad Sci USA* 1995;92:7637–7641.
242. Davis MM, Bjorkman PJ. T-cell antigen receptor genes and T-cell recognition. *Nature* 1988;334:395–402.
243. Bentley GA, Mariuzza RA. The structure of the T cell antigen receptor. *Annu Rev Immunol* 1996;14:563–590.
244. Bevan MJ, Hogquist KA, Jameson SC. Selecting the T cell receptor repertoire. *Science* 1994;264:796–797.
245. Abbas AK, Murphy KM, Sher A. Functional diversity of helper T lymphocytes. *Nature* 1996;383:787–793.
246. Del Prete G. The concept of type-1 and type-2 helper T cells and their cytokines in humans. *Int Rev Immunol* 1998;16:427–455.
247. Campbell RD, Trowsdale J. Map of the human MHC. *Immunol Today* 1993;14:349–352.
248. Madden DR. The three-dimensional structure of peptide-MHC complexes. *Annu Rev Immunol* 1995;13:587–622.
249. Parham P, Adams EJ, Arnett KL. The origins of HLA-A,B,C polymorphism. *Immunol Rev* 1995;143:141–180.
250. Newell WR, Trowsdale J, Beck S. MHCDB: database of the human MHC (release 2). *Immunogenetics* 1996;45:6–8.
251. Sanderson F, Kleijmeer MJ, Kelly A, et al. Accumulation of HLA-DM, a regulator of antigen presentation, in MHC class II compartments. *Science* 1994;266:1566–1569.
252. Denzin LK, Sant'Angelo DB, Hammond C, et al. Negative regulation by HLA-DO of MHC class II-restricted antigen processing. *Science* 1997;278:106–109.
253. Kropshofer H, Vogt AB, Thery C, et al. A role for HLA-DO as a cochaperone of HLA-DM in peptide loading of MHC class II molecules. *EMBO J* 1998;17:2971–2981.
254. Thomson G. HLA disease associations: models for the study of complex human genetic disorders. *Crit Rev Clin Lab Sci* 1995;32: 183–219.
255. Lebron JA, Bennett MJ, Vaughn DE, et al. Crystal structure of the hemochromatosis protein HFE and characterization of its interaction with transferrin receptor. *Cell* 1998;93:111–123.
256. Bjorkman PJ, Saper MA, Samraoui B, et al. Structure of the human class I histocompatibility antigen, HLA-A2. *Nature* 1987;329: 506–512.
257. Madden DR, Gorga JC, Strominger JL, et al. The three-dimensional structure of HLA-B27 at 2.1 A resolution suggests a general mechanism for tight peptide binding to MHC. *Cell* 1992;70:1035–1048.
258. Weissman AM. Regulating protein degradation by ubiquitination. *Immunol Today* 1997;18:189–198.
259. Gaczynska M, Rock KL, Goldberg AL. Gamma-interferon and expression of MHC genes regulate peptide hydrolysis by proteasomes. *Nature* 1993;365:264–267.
260. Kelly A, Powis SH, Kerr LA, et al. Assembly and function of the two ABC transporter proteins encoded in the human major histocompatibility complex. *Nature* 1992;355:641–644.
261. Routes JM, Metz BA, Cook JL. Endogenous expression of E1A in human cells enhances the effect of adenovirus E3 on class I major histocompatibility complex antigen expression. *J Virol* 1993;67: 3176–3181.
262. Andersson M, Paabo S, Nilsson T, et al. Impaired intracellular transport of class I MHC antigens as a possible means for adenoviruses to evade immune surveillance. *Cell* 1985;43:215–222.
263. Levitskaya J, Coram M, Levitsky V, et al. Inhibition of antigen processing by the internal repeat region of the Epstein-Barr virus nuclear antigen-1. *Nature* 1995;375:685–688.
264. Cresswell P. Assembly, transport, and function of MHC class II molecules. *Annu Rev Immunol* 1994;12:259–293.
265. Bakke O, Dobberstein B. MHC class II-associated invariant chain contains a sorting signal for endosomal compartments. *Cell* 1990;63: 707–716.
266. Nakagawa T, Roth W, Wong P, et al. Cathepsin L: critical role in Ii degradation and CD4 T cell selection in the thymus. *Science* 1998; 280:450–453.
267. Krangel MS, Hernandez-Munain C, Lauzurica P, et al. Developmental regulation of V(D)J recombination at the TCR alpha/delta locus. *Immunol Rev* 1998;165:131–147.
268. Garcia KC, Teyton L, Wilson IA. Structural basis of T cell recognition. *Annu Rev Immunol* 1999;17:369–397.
269. Weiss A, Littman DR. Signal transduction by lymphocyte antigen receptors. *Cell* 1994;76:263–274.
270. Chan AC, Desai DM, Weiss A. The role of protein tyrosine kinases and protein tyrosine phosphatases in T cell antigen receptor signal transduction. *Annu Rev Immunol* 1994;12:555–592.
271. Chu DH, Morita CT, Weiss A. The Syk family of protein tyrosine kinases in T-cell activation and development. *Immunol Rev* 1998;165: 167–180.
272. Clements JL, Koretzky GA. Recent developments in lymphocyte acti-

vation: linking kinases to downstream signaling events. *J Clin Invest* 1999;103:925–929.
273. Bjorkman PJ, Saper MA, Samraoui B, et al. The foreign antigen binding site and T cell recognition regions of class I histocompatibility antigens. *Nature* 1987;329:512–518.
274. Boussiotis VA, Freeman GJ, Griffin JD, et al. CD2 is involved in maintenance and reversal of human alloantigen-specific clonal anergy. *J Exp Med* 1994;180:1665–1673.
275. Wyss DF, Choi JS, Li J, et al. Conformation and function of the N-linked glycan in the adhesion domain of human CD2. *Science* 1995; 269:1273–1278.
276. Janeway CA Jr. The T cell receptor as a multicomponent signalling machine: CD4/CD8 coreceptors and CD45 in T cell activation. *Annu Rev Immunol* 1992;10:645–674.
277. Chan AS, Mobley JL, Fields GB, et al CD7-mediated regulation of integrin adhesiveness on human T cells involves tyrosine phosphorylation-dependent activation of phosphatidylinositol 3-kinase. *J Immunol* 1997;159:934–942.
278. Shipp MA, Look AT. Hematopoietic differentiation antigens that are membrane-associated enzymes: cutting is the key! *Blood* 1993;82: 1052–1070.
279. Dustin ML, Springer TA. T-cell receptor cross-linking transiently stimulates adhesiveness through LFA-1. *Nature* 1989;341:619–624.
280. Minami Y, Kono T, Miyazaki T, et al. The IL-2 receptor complex: its structure, function, and target genes. *Annu Rev Immunol* 1993;11: 245–268.
281. Theze J, Alzari PM, Bertoglio J. Interleukin 2 and its receptors: recent advances and new immunological functions. *Immunol Today* 1996; 17:481–486.
282. June CH, Bluestone JA, Nadler LM, et al. The B7 and CD28 receptor families. *Immunol Today* 1994;15:321–331.
283. Bluestone JA. New perspectives of CD28-B7–mediated T cell costimulation. *Immunity* 1995;2:555–559.
284. Smith CA, Gruss HJ, Davis T, et al. CD30 antigen, a marker for Hodgkin's lymphoma, is a receptor whose ligand defines an emerging family of cytokines with homology to TNF. *Cell* 1993;73:1349–1360.
285. Romagnani P, Annunziato F, Manetti R, et al. High CD30 ligand expression by epithelial cells and Hassal's corpuscles in the medulla of human thymus. *Blood* 1998;91:3323–3332.
286. Taher TE, Smit L, Griffioen AW, et al. Signaling through CD44 is mediated by tyrosine kinases. Association with p56lck in T lymphocytes. *J Biol Chem* 1996;271:2863–2867.
287. Ilangumaran S, Briol A, Hoessli DC. CD44 selectively associates with active Src family protein tyrosine kinases Lck and Fyn in glycosphingolipid-rich plasma membrane domains of human peripheral blood lymphocytes. *Blood* 1998;91:3901–3908.
288. Zheng L, Fisher G, Miller RE, et al. Induction of apoptosis in mature T cells by tumour necrosis factor. *Nature* 1995;377:348–351.
289. Lischke A, Moriggl R, Brandlein S, et al. The interleukin-4 receptor activates STAT5 by a mechanism that relies upon common gamma-chain. *J Biol Chem* 1998;273:31222–31229.
290. Akashi K, Kondo M, Weissman IL. Role of interleukin-7 in T-cell development from hematopoietic stem cells. *Immunol Rev* 1998;165: 13–28.
291. Latza U, Durkop H, Schnittger S, et al. The human OX40 homolog: cDNA structure, expression and chromosomal assignment of the ACT35 antigen. *Eur J Immunol* 1994;24:677–683.
292. Imura A, Hori T, Imada K, et al. The human OX40/gp34 system directly mediates adhesion of activated T cells to vascular endothelial cells. *J Exp Med* 1996;183:2185–2195.
293. Waterhouse P, Penninger JM, Timms E, et al. Lymphoproliferative disorders with early lethality in mice deficient in Ctla-4. *Science* 1995; 270:985–988.
294. Lee KM, Chuang E, Griffin M, et al. Molecular basis of T cell inactivation by CTLA-4. *Science* 1998;282:2263–2266.
295. Saito T. Negative regulation of T cell activation. *Curr Opin Immunol* 1998;10:313–321.
296. Noelle RJ, Roy M, Shepherd DM, et al. A 39-kDa protein on activated helper T cells binds CD40 and transduces the signal for cognate activation of B cells. *Proc Natl Acad Sci USA* 1992;89:6550–6554.
297. Graf D, Korthauer U, Mages HW, et al. Cloning of TRAP, a ligand for CD40 on human T cells. *Eur J Immunol* 1992;22:3191–3194.
298. Hollenbaugh D, Grosmaire LS, Kullas CD, et al. The human T cell antigen gp39, a member of the TNF gene family, is a ligand for the CD40 receptor: expression of a soluble form of gp39 with B cell co-stimulatory activity. *EMBO J* 1992;11:4313–4321.
299. Aruffo A, Farrington M, Hollenbaugh D, et al. The CD40 ligand, gp39, is defective in activated T cells from patients with X-linked hyper-IgM syndrome. *Cell* 1993;72:291–300.
300. Lederman S, Yellin MJ, Krichevsky A, et al. Identification of a novel surface protein on activated $CD4^+$ T cells that induces contact-dependent B cell differentiation (help). *J Exp Med* 1992;175:1091–1101.
301. Kersh EN, Shaw AS, Allen PM. Fidelity of T cell activation through multistep T cell receptor zeta phosphorylation. *Science* 1998;281: 572–575.
302. van Ewijk W. T-cell differentiation is influenced by thymic microenvironments. *Annu Rev Immunol* 1991;9:591–615.
303. Sanchez MJ, Muench MO, Roncarolo MG, et al. Identification of a common T/natural killer cell progenitor in human fetal thymus. *J Exp Med* 1994;180:569–576.
304. Spits H, Blom B, Jaleco AC, et al. Early stages in the development of human T, natural killer and thymic dendritic cells. *Immunol Rev* 1998;165:75–86.
305. Res PCM, Couwenberg F, Vyth-Dreese FA, Spits H. Expression of pTa mRNA in a committed dendritic cell precursor in the human thymus. *Blood* 1999;94:2647–2657.
306. von Boehmer H. The developmental biology of T lymphocytes. *Annu Rev Immunol* 1988;6:309–326.
307. Petrie HT, Hugo P, Scollay R, et al. Lineage relationships and developmental kinetics of immature thymocytes: CD3, CD4, and CD8 acquisition in vivo and in vitro. *J Exp Med* 1990;172:1583–1588.
308. Killeen N, Irving BA, Pippig S, et al. Signaling checkpoints during the development of T lymphocytes. *Curr Opin Immunol* 1998;10: 360–367.
309. Zuniga-Pflucker JC, Lenardo MJ. Regulation of thymocyte development from immature progenitors. *Curr Opin Immunol* 1996;8: 215–224.
310. von Boehmer H, Fehling HJ. Structure and function of the pre-T cell receptor. *Annu Rev Immunol* 1997;15:433–452.
311. von Boehmer H, Aifantis I, Azogui O, et al. Crucial function of the pre-T-cell receptor (TCR) in TCR beta selection, TCR beta allelic exclusion and alpha beta versus gamma delta lineage commitment. *Immunol Rev* 1998;165:111–119.
312. Schmedt C, Saijo K, Niidome T, et al. Csk controls antigen receptor-mediated development and selection of T-lineage cells. *Nature* 1998; 394:901–904.
313. Boismenu R, Rhein M, Fischer WH, et al. A role for CD81 in early T cell development. *Science* 1996;271:198–200.
314. Todd SC, Lipps SG, Crisa L, et al. CD81 expressed on human thymocytes mediates integrin activation and interleukin 2–dependent proliferation. *J Exp Med* 1996;184:2055–2060.
315. Yoshikai Y, Clark SP, Taylor S, et al. Organization and sequences of the variable, joining and constant region genes of the human T-cell receptor alpha-chain. *Nature* 1985;316:837–840.
316. Sebzda E, Mariathasan S, Ohteki T, et al. Selection of the T cell repertoire. *Annu Rev Immunol* 1999;17:829–874.
317. von Boehmer H. Positive selection of lymphocytes. *Cell* 1994;76: 219–228.
318. Zuniga-Pflucker JC, Jones LA, Chin LT, et al. CD4 and CD8 act as co-receptors during thymic selection of the T cell repertoire. *Semin Immunol* 1991;3:167–175.
319. Nossal GJ. Negative selection of lymphocytes. *Cell* 1994;76:229–239.
320. McAdam AJ, Schweitzer AN, Sharpe AH. The role of B7 co-stimulation in activation and differentiation of $CD4^+$ and $CD8^+$ T cells. *Immunol Rev* 1998;165:231–247.
321. Powell JD, Ragheb JA, Kitagawa-Sakakida S, et al. Molecular regulation of interleukin-2 expression by CD28 co-stimulation and anergy. *Immunol Rev* 1998;165:287–300.
322. Dinarello CA. Biologic basis for interleukin-1 in disease. *Blood* 1996; 87:2095–2147.
323. Dinarello CA. Interleukin-1, interleukin-1 receptors and interleukin-1 receptor antagonist. *Int Rev Immunol* 1998;16:457–499.
324. Morgan DA, Ruscetti FW, Gallo R. Selective in vitro growth of T

lymphocytes from normal human bone marrows. *Science* 1976;193:1007–1008.
325. Smith KA. Interleukin-2: inception, impact, and implications. *Science* 1988;240:1169–1176.
326. Caligiuri MA, Zmuidzinas A, Manley TJ, et al. Functional consequences of interleukin 2 receptor expression on resting human lymphocytes: identification of a novel natural killer cell subset with high affinity receptors. *J Exp Med* 1990;171:1509–1526.
327. Di Santo JP. Cytokines: shared receptors, distinct functions. *Curr Biol* 1997;7:R424–426.
328. Yang YC, Ciarletta AB, Temple PA, et al. Human IL-3 (multi-CSF): identification by expression cloning of a novel hematopoietic growth factor related to murine IL-3. *Cell* 1986;47:3–10.
329. Donahue RE, Seehra J, Metzger M, et al. Human IL-3 and GM-CSF act synergistically in stimulating hematopoiesis in primates. *Science* 1988;241:1820–1823.
330. Kitamura T, Sato N, Arai K, et al. Expression cloning of the human IL-3 receptor cDNA reveals a shared beta subunit for the human IL-3 and GM-CSF receptors. *Cell* 1991;66:1165–1174.
331. Kurimoto Y, de Weck AL, Dahinden CA. Interleukin 3–dependent mediator release in basophils triggered by C5a. *J Exp Med* 1989;170:467–479.
332. Kita H, Ohnishi T, Okubo Y, et al. Granulocyte/macrophage colony-stimulating factor and interleukin 3 release from human peripheral blood eosinophils and neutrophils. *J Exp Med* 1991;174:745–748.
333. Solari R, Quint D, Obray H, et al. Purification and characterization of recombinant human interleukin 4: biological activities, receptor binding and the generation of monoclonal antibodies. *Biochem J* 1989;262:897–908.
334. Paul WE, Seder RA. Lymphocyte responses and cytokines. *Cell* 1994;76:241–251.
335. Milburn MV, Hassell AM, Lambert MH, et al. A novel dimer configuration revealed by the crystal structure at 2.4 A resolution of human interleukin-5. *Nature* 1993;363:172–176.
336. Leung DY, Martin RJ, Szefler SJ, et al. Dysregulation of interleukin 4, interleukin 5, and interferon gamma gene expression in steroid-resistant asthma. *J Exp Med* 1995;181:33–40.
337. Takatsu K. Interleukin 5 and B cell differentiation. *Cytokine Growth Factor Rev* 1998;9:25–35.
338. Denburg JA. Bone marrow in atopy and asthma: hematopoietic mechanisms in allergic inflammation. *Immunol Today* 1999;20:111–113.
339. Titus RG, Sherry B, Cerami A. The involvement of TNF, IL-1 and IL-6 in the immune response to protozoan parasites. *Immunol Today* 1991;12:A13–16.
340. Kishimoto T, Akira S, Taga T. Interleukin-6 and its receptor: a paradigm for cytokines. *Science* 1992;258:593–597.
341. Hirano T. Interleukin 6 and its receptor: ten years later. *Int Rev Immunol* 1998;16:249–284.
342. Muegge K, Vila MP, Durum SK. Interleukin-7: a cofactor for V(D)J rearrangement of the T cell receptor beta gene. *Science* 1993;261:93–95.
343. Komschlies KL, Grzegorzewski KJ, Wiltrout RH. Diverse immunological and hematological effects of interleukin 7: implications for clinical application. *J Leukoc Biol* 1995;58:623–633.
344. Koch AE, Polverini PJ, Kunkel SL, et al. Interleukin-8 as a macrophage-derived mediator of angiogenesis. *Science* 1992;258:1798–1801.
345. Horuk R. The interleukin-8–receptor family: from chemokines to malaria. *Immunol Today* 1994;15:169–174.
346. Mukaida N, Harada A, Matsushima K. Interleukin-8 (IL-8) and monocyte chemotactic and activating factor (MCAF/MCP-1), chemokines essentially involved in inflammatory and immune reactions. *Cytokine Growth Factor Rev* 1998;9:9–23.
347. Demoulin JB, Renauld JC. Interleukin 9 and its receptor: an overview of structure and function. *Int Rev Immunol* 1998;16:345–364.
348. Moore KW, O'Garra A, de Waal Malefyt R, et al. Interleukin-10. *Annu Rev Immunol* 1993;11:165–190.
349. Roth I, Corry DB, Locksley RM, et al. Human placental cytotrophoblasts produce the immunosuppressive cytokine interleukin 10. *J Exp Med* 1996;184:539–548.
350. Brandtzaeg P, Osnes L, Ovstebo R, et al. Net inflammatory capacity of human septic shock plasma evaluated by a monocyte-based target cell assay: identification of interleukin-10 as a major functional deactivator of human monocytes. *J Exp Med* 1996;184:51–60.
351. Yang YC. Interleukin 11: an overview. *Stem Cells* (Dayt) 1993;11:474–486.
352. Zhang XG, Gu JJ, Lu ZY, et al. Ciliary neurotropic factor, interleukin 11, leukemia inhibitory factor, and oncostatin M are growth factors for human myeloma cell lines using the interleukin 6 signal transducer gp130. *J Exp Med* 1994;179:1337–1342.
353. Du X, Williams DA. Interleukin-11: review of molecular, cell biology, and clinical use. *Blood* 1997;89:3897–3908.
354. Altare F, Durandy A, Lammas D, et al. Impairment of mycobacterial immunity in human interleukin-12 receptor deficiency. *Science* 1998;280:1432–1435.
355. Gately MK, Renzetti LM, Magram J, et al. The interleukin-12/interleukin-12–receptor system: role in normal and pathologic immune responses. *Annu Rev Immunol* 1998;16:495–521.
356. Rissoan MC, Soumelis V, Kadowaki N, et al. Reciprocal control of T helper cell and dendritic cell differentiation. *Science* 1999;283:1183–1186.
357. Trinchieri G, Scott P. Interleukin-12: basic principles and clinical applications. *Curr Top Microbiol Immunol* 1999;238:57–78.
358. Burd PR, Thompson WC, Max EE, et al. Activated mast cells produce interleukin 13. *J Exp Med* 1995;181:1373–1380.
359. Grunig G, Warnock M, Wakil AE, et al. Requirement for IL-13 independently of IL-4 in experimental asthma. *Science* 1998;282:2261–2263.
360. Wills Karp M, Luyimbazi J, Xu X, et al. Interleukin-13: central mediator of allergic asthma. *Science* 1998;282:2258–2261.
361. Ogata H, Ford D, Kouttab N, et al. Regulation of interleukin-13 receptor constituents on mature human B lymphocytes. *J Biol Chem* 1998;273:9864–9871.
362. Chomarat P, Banchereau J. Interleukin-4 and interleukin-13: their similarities and discrepancies. *Int Rev Immunol* 1998;17:1–52.
363. Chiaramonte MG, Schopf LR, Neben TY, et al. IL-13 is a key regulatory cytokine for Th2 cell-mediated pulmonary granuloma formation and IgE responses induced by Schistosoma mansoni eggs. *J Immunol* 1999;162:920–930.
364. Uckun FM, Fauci AS, Chandan-Langlie M, et al. Detection and characterization of human high molecular weight B cell growth factor receptors on leukemic B cells in chronic lymphocytic leukemia. *J Clin Invest* 1989;84:1595–1608.
365. Ambrus JL Jr, Pippin J, Joseph A, et al. Identification of a cDNA for a human high molecular-weight B-cell growth factor. *Proc Natl Acad Sci USA* 1996;93:8154.
366. Carson WE, Giri JG, Lindemann MJ, et al. Interleukin (IL) 15 is a novel cytokine that activates human natural killer cells via components of the IL-2 receptor. *J Exp Med* 1994;180:1395–1403.
367. Center DM, Kornfeld H, Cruikshank WW. Interleukin 16 and its function as a CD4 ligand. *Immunol Today* 1996;17:476–481.
368. Cruikshank WW, Kornfeld H, Center DM. Signaling and functional properties of interleukin-16. *Int Rev Immunol* 1998;16:523–540.
369. Fossiez F, Djossou O, Chomarat P, et al. T cell interleukin-17 induces stromal cells to produce proinflammatory and hematopoietic cytokines. *J Exp Med* 1996;183:2593–2603.
370. Fossiez F, Banchereau J, Murray R, et al. Interleukin-17. *Int Rev Immunol* 1998;16:541–551.
371. Dinarello CA. IL-18: a T_H1-inducing, proinflammatory cytokine and new member of the IL-1 family. *J Allergy Clin Immunol* 1999;103:11–24.
372. Fehniger TA, Shah MH, Turner MJ, et al. Differential cytokine and chemokine gene expression by human NK cells following activation with IL-18 or IL-15 in combination with IL-12: implications for the innate immune response. *J Immunol* 1999;162:4511–4520.
373. Wong GG, Witek JS, Temple PA, et al. Human GM-CSF: molecular cloning of the complementary DNA and purification of the natural and recombinant proteins. *Science* 1985;228:810–815.
374. van Leeuwen BH, Martinson ME, Webb GC, et al. Molecular organization of the cytokine gene cluster, involving the human IL-3, IL-4, IL-5, and GM-CSF genes, on human chromosome 5. *Blood* 1989;73:1142–1148.
375. Strober W, Kelsall B, Fuss I, et al. Reciprocal IFN-gamma and TGF-

beta responses regulate the occurrence of mucosal inflammation. *Immunol Today* 1997;18:61–64.

376. Boehm U, Klamp T, Groot M, et al. Cellular responses to interferon-gamma. *Annu Rev Immunol* 1997;15:749–795.
377. Horwitz DA, Gray JD, Ohtsuka K, et al. The immunoregulatory effects of NK cells: the role of TGF-beta and implications for autoimmunity. *Immunol Today* 1997;18:538–542.
378. Letterio JJ, Roberts AB. Regulation of immune responses by TGF-beta. *Annu Rev Immunol* 1998;16:137–161.
379. Grakoui A, Bromley SK, Sumen C, et al. The immunological synapse: a molecular machine controlling T cell activation. *Science* 1999;285:221–227.
380. Romagnani S. The Thl/Th2 paradigm. *Immunol Today* 1997;18:263–266.
381. Clerici M, Shearer GM. The Thl-Th2 hypothesis of HIV infection: new insights. *Immunol Today* 1994;15:575–581.
382. Monroe JG, Silberstein LE. HIV-mediated B-lymphocyte activation and lymphomagenesis. *J Clin Immunol* 1995;15:61–68.
383. Ivashkiv LB. Cytokines and STATs: how can signals achieve specificity? *Immunity* 1995;3:1–4.
384. Darnell JE Jr. STATs and gene regulation. *Science* 1997;277:1630–1635.
385. Zhang X, Blenis J, Li HC, et al. Requirement of serine phosphorylation for formation of STAT-promoter complexes. *Science* 1995;267:1990–1994.
386. Wen Z, Zhong Z, Darnell JE Jr. Maximal activation of transcription by Statl and Stat3 requires both tyrosine and serine phosphorylation. *Cell* 1995;82:241–250.
387. Dellabona P, Peccoud J, Kappler J, et al. Superantigens interact with MHC class II molecules outside of the antigen groove. *Cell* 1990;62:1115–1121.
388. Herman A, Kappler JW, Marrack P, et al. Superantigens: mechanism of T-cell stimulation and role in immune responses. *Annu Rev Immunol* 1991;9:745–772.
389. Webb SR, Gascoigne NR. T-cell activation by superantigens. *Curr Opin Immunol* 1994;6:467–475.
390. Tumang JR, Posnett DN, Cole BC, et al. Helper T cell-dependent human B cell differentiation mediated by a mycoplasmal superantigen bridge. *J Exp Med* 1990;171:2153–2158.
391. Choi YW, Herman A, DiGiusto D, et al. Residues of the variable region of the T-cell-receptor beta-chain that interact with *S. aureus* toxin superantigens. *Nature* 1990;346:471–473.
392. Marrack P, Blackman M, Kushnir E, et al. The toxicity of staphylococcal enterotoxin B in mice is mediated by T cells. *J Exp Med* 1990;171:455–464.
393. Berberian L, Goodglick L, Kipps TJ, et al. Immunoglobulin VH3 gene products: natural ligands for HIV gp120. *Science* 1993;261:1588–1591.
394. Hillson JL, Karr NS, Oppliger IR, et al. The structural basis of germline-encoded VH3 immunoglobulin binding to staphylococcal protein A. *J Exp Med* 1993;178:331–336.
395. Marrack P, Kushnir E, Kappler J. A maternally inherited superantigen encoded by a mammary tumour virus. *Nature* 1991;349:524–526.
396. Pullen AM, Wade T, Marrack P, et al. Identification of the region of T cell receptor beta chain that interacts with the self-superantigen MIs-1a. *Cell* 1990;61:1365–1374.
397. Frankel WN, Rudy C, Coffin JM, et al. Linkage of Mls genes to endogenous mammary tumour viruses of inbred mice. *Nature* 1991;349:526–528.
398. Luther SA, Acha-Orbea H. Immune response to mouse mammary tumour virus. *Curr Opin Immunol* 1996;8:498–502.
399. Dyson PJ, Knight AM, Fairchild S, et al. Genes encoding ligands for deletion of V beta 11 T cells cosegregate with mammary tumour virus genomes. *Nature* 1991;349:531–532.
400. Woodland DL, Happ MP, Gollob KJ, et al. An endogenous retrovirus mediating deletion of alpha beta T cells? *Nature* 1991;349:529–530.
401. Cella M, Sallusto F, Lanzavecchia A. Origin, maturation and antigen presenting function of dendritic cells. *Curr Opin Immunol* 1997;9:10–16.
402. Banchereau J, Steinman RM. Dendritic cells and the control of immunity. *Nature* 1998;392:245–252.
403. Randolph GJ, Beaulieu S, Lebecque S, et al. Differentiation of monocytes into dendritic cells in a model of transendothelial trafficking. *Science* 1998;282:480–483.
404. Porcelli SA, Segelke BW, Sugita M, et al. The CD1 family of lipid antigen-presenting molecules. *Immunol Today* 1998;19:362–368.
405. Porcelli SA, Modlin RL. The CD1 system: antigen-presenting molecules for T cell recognition of lipids and glycolipids. *Annu Rev Immunol* 1999;17:297–329.
406. Schofield L, McConville MJ, Hansen D, et al. CD1d-restricted immunoglobulin G formation to GPI-anchored antigens mediated by NKT cells. *Science* 1999;283:225–229.
407. Grant EP, Degano M, Rosat JP, et al. Molecular recognition of lipid antigens by T cell receptors. *J Exp Med* 1999;189:195–205.
408. Ridge JP, Di Rosa F, Matzinger P. A conditioned dendritic cell can be a temporal bridge between a $CD4^+$ T-helper and a T-killer cell. *Nature* 1998;393:474–478.
409. Bennett SR, Carbone FR, Karamalis F, et al. Help for cytotoxic-T-cell responses is mediated by CD40 signalling. *Nature* 1998;393:478–480.
410. Schoenberger SP, Toes RE, van der Voort EI, et al. T-cell help for cytotoxic T lymphocytes is mediated by CD40-CD40L interactions. *Nature* 1998;393:480–483.
411. Bender A, Sapp M, Feldman M, et al. Dendritic cells as immunogens for human CTL responses. *Adv Exp Med Biol* 1997;417:383–387.
412. Nestle FO, Alijagic S, Gilliet M, et al. Vaccination of melanoma patients with peptide- or tumor lysate-pulsed dendritic cells. *Nat Med* 1998;4:328–332.
413. Pardoll DM. Cancer vaccines. *Nat Med* 1998;4:525–531.
414. Sotomayor EM, Borrello I, Tubb E, et al. Conversion of tumor-specific $CD4^+$ T-cell tolerance to T-cell priming through in vivo ligation of CD40. *Nat Med* 1999;5:780–787.
415. Kraal G, Weissman IL, Butcher EC. Germinal centre B cells: antigen specificity and changes in heavy chain class expression. *Nature* 1982;298:377–379.
416. Butcher EC, Rouse RV, Coffman RL, et al. Surface phenotype of Peyer's patch germinal center cells: implications for the role of germinal centers in B cell differentiation. *J Immunol* 1982;129:2698–2707.
417. Spriggs MK, Armitage RJ, Strockbine L, et al. Recombinant human CD40 ligand stimulates B cell proliferation and immunoglobulin E secretion. *J Exp Med* 1992;176:1543–1550.
418. Ledbetter JA, Shu G, Gallagher M, et al. Augmentation of normal and malignant B cell proliferation by monoclonal antibody to the B cell-specific antigen BP50 (CDW40). *J Immunol* 1987;138:788–794.
419. Stamenkovic I, Clark EA, Seed B. A B-lymphocyte activation molecule related to the nerve growth factor receptor and induced by cytokines in carcinomas. *EMBO J* 1989;8:1403–1410.
420. Liu YJ, Joshua DE, Williams GT, et al. Mechanism of antigen-driven selection in germinal centres. *Nature* 1989;342:929–931.
421. Lalmanach-Girard AC, Chiles TC, Parker DC, et al. T cell-dependent induction of NF-kappa B in B cells. *J Exp Med* 1993;177:1215–1219.
422. Di Santo JP, Bonnefoy JY, Gauchat JF, et al. CD40 ligand mutations in X-linked immunodeficiency with hyper-IgM. *Nature* 1993;361:541–543.
423. Allen RC, Armitage RJ, Conley ME, et al. CD40 ligand gene defects responsible for X-linked hyper-IgM syndrome. *Science* 1993;259:990–993.
424. Berek C, Berger A, Apel M. Maturation of the immune response in germinal centers. *Cell* 1991;67:1121–1129.
425. Han S, Zheng B, Schatz DG, et al. Neoteny in lymphocytes: Ragl and Rag2 expression in germinal center B cells. *Science* 1996;274:2094–2097.
426. Han S, Dillon SR, Zheng B, et al. V(D)J recombinase activity in a subset of germinal center B lymphocytes. *Science* 1997;278:301–305.
427. Glücksmann A. Cell death in normal vertebrate ontogeny. *Biol Rev Camb Philos Soc* 1951;26:59–86.
428. Saunders JW Jr. Death in embryonic systems. *Science* 1966;154:604–612.
429. Klion FM, Schaffner F. The ultrastructure of acidophilic ''councilman-like'' bodies in the liver. *Am J Pathol* 1966;48:755–767.
430. Iversen OH. Kinetics of cellular proliferation and cell loss in human carcinomas: a discussion of methods available for in vivo studies. *Eur J Cancer* 1967;3:389–394.

431. Kerr JF. Shrinkage necrosis: a distinct mode of cellular death. *J Pathol* 1971;105:13–20.
432. Pratt NE, Sodicoff M. Ultrastructural injury following x-irradiation of rat parotid gland acinar cells. *Arch Oral Biol* 1972;17:1177–1186.
433. Costero I, Pomerat CM. Cultivation of neurons from the adult human cerebral and cerebellar cortices. *Am J Anat* 1951;89:405–467.
434. Sanderson CJ. The mechanism of T cell mediated cytotoxicity. II. Morphological studies of cell death by time-lapse microcinematography. *Proc R Soc Lond B Biol Sci* 1976;192:241–255.
435. Mullinger AM, Johnson RT. Perturbation of mammalian cell division. III. The topography and kinetics of extrusion subdivision. *J Cell Sci* 1976;22:243–285.
436. Kerr JF, Wyllie AH, Currie AR. Apoptosis: a basic biological phenomenon with wide-ranging implications in tissue kinetics. *Br J Cancer* 1972;26:239–257.
437. Wyllie AH, Kerr JF, Currie AR. Cell death: the significance of apoptosis. *Int Rev Cytol* 1980;68:251–306.
438. Shresta S, Pham CT, Thomas DA, et al. How do cytotoxic lymphocytes kill their targets? *Curr Opin Immunol* 1998;10:581–587.
439. Smyth MJ, Trapani JA. Granzymes: exogenous proteinases that induce target cell apoptosis. *Immunol Today* 1995;16:202–206.
440. Talanian RV, Yang X, Turbov J, et al. Granule-mediated killing: pathways for granzyme B-initiated apoptosis. *J Exp Med* 1997;186: 1323–1331.
441. Shiver JW, Su L, Henkart PA. Cytotoxicity with target DNA breakdown by rat basophilic leukemia cells expressing both cytolysin and granzyme A. *Cell* 1992;71;315–322.
442. Froelich CJ, Orth K, Turbov J, et al. New paradigm for lymphocyte granule-mediated cytotoxicity. Target cells bind and internalize granzyme B, but an endosomolytic agent is necessary for cytosolic delivery and subsequent apoptosis. *J Biol Chem* 1996;271:29073–29079.
443. Nagata S. Apoptosis by death factor. *Cell* 1997;88:355–365.
444. Salvesen GS, Dixit VM. Caspases: intracellular signaling by proteolysis. *Cell* 1997;91:443–446.
445. Thornberry NA, Lazebnik Y. Caspases: enemies within. *Science* 1998; 281:1312–1316.
446. Schulze-Osthoff K, Walczak H, Droge W, et al. Cell nucleus and DNA fragmentation are not required for apoptosis. *J Cell Biol* 1994; 127:15–20.
447. Enari M, Sakahira H, Yokoyama H, et al. A caspase-activated DNase that degrades DNA during apoptosis, and its inhibitor ICAD. *Nature* 1998;391:43–50.
448. Sakahira H, Enari M, Nagata S. Cleavage of CAD inhibitor in CAD activation and DNA degradation during apoptosis. *Nature* 1998;391: 96–99.
449. Liu X, Zou H, Slaughter C, et al. DFF, a heterodimeric protein that functions downstream of caspase-3 to trigger DNA fragmentation during apoptosis. *Cell* 1997;89:175–184.
450. Tewari M, Quan LT, O'Rourke K, et al. Yama/CPP32 beta, a mammalian homolog of CED-3, is a CrmA-inhibitable protease that cleaves the death substrate poly(ADP-ribose) polymerase. *Cell* 1995;81: 801–809.
451. Bump NJ, Hackett M, Hugunin M, et al. Inhibition of ICE family proteases by baculovirus antiapoptotic protein p35. *Science* 1995;269: 1885–1888.
452. Beidler DR, Tewari M, Friesen PD, et al. The baculovirus p35 protein inhibits Fas- and tumor necrosis factor-induced apoptosis. *J Biol Chem* 1995;270:16526–16528.
453. Bakhshi A, Jensen JP, Goldman P, et al. Cloning the chromosomal breakpoint of t(14;18) human lymphomas: clustering around JH on chromosome 14 and near a transcriptional unit on 18. *Cell* 1985;41: 899–906.
454. Adams JM, Cory S. The Bcl-2 protein family: arbiters of cell survival. *Science* 1998;281:1322–1326.
455. Reed JC. Double identity for proteins of the Bcl-2 family. *Nature* 1997;387:773–776.
456. Muchmore SW, Sattler M, Liang H, et al. X-ray and NMR structure of human Bcl-xL, an inhibitor of programmed cell death. *Nature* 1996; 381:335–341.
457. Minn AJ, Velez P, Schendel SL, et al. Bcl-x(L) forms an ion channel in synthetic lipid membranes. *Nature* 1997;385:353–357.
458. Korsmeyer SJ. Bcl-2 initiates a new category of oncogenes: regulators of cell death. *Blood* 1992;80:879–886.
459. Yang J, Liu X, Bhalla K, et al. Prevention of apoptosis by Bcl-2: release of cytochrome c from mitochondria blocked. *Science* 1997; 275:1129–1132.
460. Boise LH, Gonzalez-Garcia M, Postema CE, et al. Bcl-x, a bcl-2–related gene that functions as a dominant regulator of apoptotic cell death. *Cell* 1993;74:597–608.
461. Ma A, Pena JC, Chang B, et al. Bclx regulates the survival of double-positive thymocytes. *Proc Natl Acad Sci USA* 1995;92:4763–4767.
462. Fang W, Weintraub BC, Dunlap B, et al. Self-reactive B lymphocytes overexpressing Bcl-xL escape negative selection and are tolerized by clonal anergy and receptor editing. *Immunity* 1998;9:35–45.
463. Wang Z, Karras JG, Howard RG, et al. Induction of bcl-x by CD40 engagement rescues sIg-induced apoptosis in murine B cells. *J Immunol* 1995;155:3722–3725.
464. Black RA, Rauch CT, Kozlosky CJ, et al. A metalloproteinase disintegrin that releases tumour necrosis factor-alpha from cells. *Nature* 1997;385:729–733.
465. Moss ML, Jin SL, Milla ME, et al. Cloning of a disintegrin metalloproteinase that processes precursor tumour-necrosis factor-alpha. *Nature* 1997;385:733–736.
466. Yamamoto S, Higuchi Y, Yoshiyama K, et al. ADAM family proteins in the immune system. *Immunol Today* 1999;20:278–284.
467. Masat T, Tanaka I, Masashi A, et al. Downregulation of Fas ligand by shedding. *Nat Med* 1998;4:31–36.
468. Beutler B, Greenwald D, Hulmes JD, et al. Identity of tumour necrosis factor and the macrophage-secreted factor cachectin. *Nature* 1985; 316:552–554.
469. Beutler B, Cerami A. The biology of cachectin/TNF—a primary mediator of the host response. *Annu Rev Immunol* 1989;7:625–655.
470. Wallach D, Varfolomeev EE, Malinin NL, et al. Tumor Necrosis Factor Receptor and Fas signaling mechanisms. *Annu Rev Immunol* 1999;17:331–367.
471. Liu ZG, Hsu H, Goeddel DV, et al. Dissection of TNF receptor 1 effector functions: JNK activation is not linked to apoptosis while NF-kappaB activation prevents cell death. *Cell* 1996;87:565–576.
472. Kelliher MA, Grimm S, Ishida Y, et al. The death domain kinase RIP mediates the TNF-induced NF-kappaB signal. *Immunity* 1998;8: 297–303.
473. Griffith TS, Brunner T, Fletcher SM, et al. Fas ligand-induced apoptosis as a mechanism of immune privilege. *Science* 1995;270: 1189–1192.
474. Dhein J, Walczak H, Baumler C, et al. Autocrine T-cell suicide mediated by APO-1/(Fas/CD95). *Nature* 1995;373:438–441.
475. Brunner T, Mogil RJ, LaFace D, et al. Cell-autonomous Fas (CD95)/ Fas-ligand interaction mediates activation-induced apoptosis in T-cell hybridomas. *Nature* 1995;373:441–444.
476. Ju ST, Panka DJ, Cui H, et al. Fas (CD95)/FasL interactions required for programmed cell death after T-cell activation. *Nature* 1995;373: 444–448.
477. Hahne M, Rimoldi D, Schroter M, et al. Melanoma cell expression of Fas (Apo-1/CD95) ligand: implications for tumor immune escape. *Science* 1996;274:1363–1366.
478. O'Connell J, O'Sullivan GC, Collins JK, et al. The Fas counterattack: Fas-mediated T cell killing by colon cancer cells expressing Fas ligand. *J Exp Med* 1996;184:1075–1082.
479. Pitti RM, Marsters SA, Lawrence DA, et al. Genomic amplification of a decoy receptor for Fas ligand in lung and colon cancer. *Nature* 1998;396:699–703.
480. Schwab U, Stein H, Gerdes J, et al. Production of a monoclonal antibody specific for Hodgkin and Sternberg-Reed cells of Hodgkin's disease and a subset of normal lymphoid cells. *Nature* 1982;299: 65–67.
481. Froese P, Lemke H, Gerdes J, et al. Biochemical characterization and biosynthesis of the Ki-1 antigen in Hodgkin-derived and virus-transformed human B and T lymphoid cell lines. *J Immunol* 1987; 139:2081–2087.
482. Amakawa R, Hakem A, Kundig TM, et al. Impaired negative selection of T cells in Hodgkin's disease antigen CD30-deficient mice. *Cell* 1996;84:551–562.
483. Ranheim EA, Kipps TJ. Activated T cells induce expression of B7/ BB1 on normal or leukemic B cells through a CD40-dependent signal. *J Exp Med* 1993;177:925–935.

484. Rothstein TL, Wang JK, Panka DJ, et al. Protection against Fas-dependent Th1–mediated apoptosis by antigen receptor engagement in B cells. *Nature* 1995;374:163–165.
485. Schattner EJ, Mascarenhas J, Bishop J, et al. $CD4^+$ T-cell induction of Fas-mediated apoptosis in Burkitt's lymphoma B cells. *Blood* 1996; 88:1375–1382.
486. Schneider TJ, Fischer GM, Donohoe TJ, et al. A novel gene coding for a Fas apoptosis inhibitory molecule (FAIM) isolated from inducibly Fas-resistant B lymphocytes. *J Exp Med* 1999;189:949–956.
487. Smith CA, Farrah T, Goodwin RG. The TNF receptor superfamily of cellular and viral proteins: activation, costimulation, and death. *Cell* 1994;76:959–962.
488. Jones EY, Stuart DI, Walker NP. Structure of tumour necrosis factor. *Nature* 1989;338:225–228.
489. Ware CF, Van Arsdale TL, Crowe PD, et al. The ligands and receptors of the lymphotoxin system. *Curr Top Microbiol Immunol* 1995;198: 175–218.
490. Browning JL, Ngam-ek A, Lawton P, et al. Lymphotoxin beta, a novel member of the TNF family that forms a heteromeric complex with lymphotoxin on the cell surface. *Cell* 1993;72:847–856.
491. Crowe PD, Van Arsdale TL, Walter BN, et al. A lymphotoxin-beta-specific receptor. *Science* 1994;264:707–710.
492. Rathmell JC, Townsend SE, Xu JC, et al. Expansion or elimination of B cells in vivo: dual roles for CD40- and Fas (CD95)-ligands modulated by the B cell antigen receptor. *Cell* 1996;87:319–329.
493. Green DR, Ware CF. Fas-ligand: privilege and peril. *Proc Natl Acad Sci USA* 1997;94:5986–5990.
494. Arch RH, Thompson CB. 4-1BB and Ox40 are members of a tumor necrosis factor (TNF)-nerve growth factor receptor subfamily that bind TNF receptor-associated factors and activate nuclear factor kappaB. *Mol Cell Biol* 1998;18:558–565.
495. Casaccia-Bonnefil P, Carter BD, Dobrowsky RT, et al. Death of oligodendrocytes mediated by the interaction of nerve growth factor with its receptor p75. *Nature* 1996;383:716–719.
496. Kong YY, Yoshida H, Sarosi I, et al. OPGL is a key regulator of osteoclastogenesis, lymphocyte development and lymph-node organogenesis. *Nature* 1999;397:315–323.
497. Green EA, Flavell RA. TRANCE-RANK, a new signal pathway involved in lymphocyte development and T cell activation. *J Exp Med* 1999;189:1017–1020.
498. Bertin J, Armstrong RC, Ottilie S, et al. Death effector domain-containing herpesvirus and poxvirus proteins inhibit both Fas- and TNFR1-induced apoptosis. *Proc Natl Acad Sci USA* 1997;94: 1172–1176.

CHAPTER 3

Immunophenotypic Markers Useful in the Diagnosis and Classification of Hematopoietic Neoplasms

Daniel M. Knowles

It was known for many years that leukemias and lymphomas represent a large, clinically and morphologically diverse spectrum of malignant neoplasms (1). However, virtually no understanding of the biologic basis for this heterogeneity and very little accurate insight into the histogeneses or pathogeneses of these diseases existed prior to the 1970s. At that time, advances in cellular immunology led to the discovery that normal lymphoid cells are divisible according to their expression of various cell surface antigens and receptors into distinct subsets populating discrete microenvironments and subserving different functions (2) (see Chapters 2 and 6). These discoveries prompted some investigators to analyze leukemias and lymphomas for these same cell surface antigens and receptors and perform the first immunophenotypic analyses of malignant hematopoietic cells (3–5).

The widespread application of cellular immunologic techniques to the analysis of leukemias and lymphomas at that time was hampered by several factors. These included the lack of standardized, commercially available reagents of high quality; difficulties in adapting technically-demanding, labor-intensive, and time-consuming cellular immunologic assays to diagnostic pathology laboratories; the expense of equipping a cellular immunology laboratory; and the difficulty and expense of recruiting appropriately skilled technical personnel. For these reasons, these procedures largely remained the province of a few specialized research laboratories.

This situation changed dramatically in the 1980s because of the development, characterization, and commercial distribution of monoclonal antibodies (MAbs) capable of detecting a wide spectrum of lymphohematopoietic lineage–, differentiation-, and subset-associated antigens (6–9). This coincided with the development of reasonably priced, operator-friendly fluorescent activated cell sorters and highly sensitive frozen tissue section immunohistochemical staining assays such as avidin-biotin complex immunoperoxidase (10,11) and alkaline phosphatase–antialkaline phosphatase (12). MAb reagents obviated the numerous problems, such as sensitivity, specificity, and availability, associated with heteroantisera. Modern fluorescent activated cell sorters represent sophisticated instrumentation capable of accurate and objective identification and quantitation of lymphoid cell populations (see Chapter 5). The immunohistochemical techniques are relatively easy to perform and readily adapted to most pathology laboratories. Indeed, even automated instrumentation capable of performing immunohistochemical assays is now available and widely utilized (see Chapter 4).

These developments prompted numerous investigators to characterize hematopoietic neoplasms with the continuously expanding panels of commercially available MAbs using cytofluorometric or immunohistochemical techniques (6–9,13,14). Literally thousands of commercially and privately generated MAb reagents have been characterized in a succession of international workshops leading to the worldwide adoption of a standard nomenclature (15–20). These multitudinous studies have resulted in a voluminous literature concerning the distribution of reactivity of several hundred different MAbs with benign and malignant hematopoietic cells. The end result has been twofold: First, immunophenotypic analysis has been universally accepted as a useful and often necessary adjunct to the morphologic diagnosis of leukemias and lymphomas and has become established widely in research, commercial, and hospital laboratories. Second, immunophenotypic analysis has resulted in novel insights into the histogenesis and pathogenesis of the hema-

D. M. Knowles: Department of Pathology, Weill Medical College of Cornell University, New York, New York 10021 topoietic neoplasms that were not possible based on morphologic examination alone. In this chapter, we discuss the different methodologic approaches to immunophenotypic analysis, the characteristics and distribution of reactivity of the principal conventional cell markers and MAb reagents used in cell suspension and frozen and paraffin tissue section immunophenotyping, the immunophenotypic characteristics of normal developing hematopoietic cells, and criteria useful in immunodiagnosis. The immunophenotypic profiles of each of the major categories of hematopoietic neoplasia are discussed by the authors of other chapters.

METHODOLOGIC APPROACHES

General Comments

Considerable confusion often surrounds the planning, performance, and interpretation of the results of immunophenotypic analysis of a hematologic specimen. In part, this confusion emanates from an incomplete understanding of the nature and special characteristics of each one of the vast array of antigens and receptors expressed by hematopoietic cells, and a lack of awareness of the advantages, disadvantages, and limitations of the various methodologic approaches used to detect these lymphohematopoietic cell markers. Not all lymphohematopoietic cell markers are detectable using the same methodologic approach. Although many of them are detectable by using multiple approaches, others are optimally demonstrated by only one method (6).

For example, the vast majority of lymphohematopoietic cell markers are surface membrane molecules that are masked or even destroyed by the harsh fixatives routinely employed in pathology laboratories. They are detectable only if methodologic systems that preserve cell membrane integrity, such as viable cell suspensions and frozen tissue sections, and not formalin-fixed, paraffin-embedded tissue sections, are used (6). On the other hand, certain lymphohematopoietic cell markers are expressed in the cytoplasm (cytoplasmic immunoglobulin) (21) or in the nucleus (terminal deoxynucleotidyl transferase [TdT]) (22) and not on the cell membrane. In these instances, the cells or tissue must be fixed under carefully controlled conditions that permit optimal penetration of the antibody reagent and reliable detection of the antigen. Some antigens such as B-cell lineage–restricted antigen CD20 possess both a surface membrane component, detectable in cell suspensions or frozen tissue sections with MAb B1 (23,24), and a cytoplasmic component, detectable in routinely fixed and paraffin-embedded tissue sections with MAb L26 (25).

The various methodologic approaches to the immunophenotypic analysis of hematopoietic neoplasms can be subdivided into three broad categories. These are cytofluorometric analysis of cell suspensions or immunohistochemical analysis of cytocentrifuge slides prepared from cell suspensions, immunohistochemical analysis of frozen tissue sections, and immunohistochemical analysis of routinely fixed and paraffin-embedded tissue sections. Each one of these three distinct approaches possesses certain advantages and disadvantages as well as special features that render it ideally suited to detect particular lymphohematopoietic cell markers or to be used in specific immunodiagnostic situations.

Cell Suspensions

The sterile isolation of mononuclear cells and the preparation of a viable cell suspension is the classic approach employed by cellular immunologists to analyze hematopoietic cells. This approach is employed necessarily in the immunophenotypic analysis of peripheral blood and bodily fluid (i.e., ascites, pleural effusion, and cerebrospinal fluid) samples. This approach can be used for solid lymphoid tissues and for aspirated bone marrow as well. In these instances, the lymphoid tissue can be disrupted mechanically with a scalpel and forceps, and the small tissue fragments, or bony spicules in the case of bone marrow, are crushed with the flat rubber bottom of the plunger from a sterile plastic syringe. This technique produces a single-cell suspension, which can be centrifuged, if necessary, over a ficoll-hypaque density gradient to obtain a purified population of viable mononuclear cells devoid of erythrocytes, granulocytes, dead cells, and cellular debris (see Chapter 11). These viable, metabolically active cells can then be analyzed for their expression of multiple cell markers by direct and indirect immunofluorescent cytofluorometric analysis, and the percentages of cells expressing each marker can be determined readily (see Chapter 5). Alternatively, the cells may be placed onto glass microscope slides by cytocentrifugation and analyzed for surface membrane or cytoplasmic antigens using various immunohistochemical techniques (see Chapters 4, 11 and 38).

The major advantage of the cell-suspension approach is that it offers the greatest flexibility with regard to cell marker analysis. Once isolated, the cells can be manipulated so as to allow detection of surface membrane, cytoplasmic, or intranuclear antigens or more than one antigen simultaneously. This approach also permits accurate quantitation of the percentage of cells expressing each marker. Two- and three-color cytofluorometric analysis can be employed to demonstrate multiple antigen expression by the same cell population. Distinct and separate cell populations present within the same sample can be preferentially gated and analyzed. This approach supplies the investigator with cells for immunogenotypic analyses, proliferation and ploidy analyses, and functional and any other studies requiring the *in vitro* culture of sterile, viable mononuclear cells. The cell-suspension approach allows the investigator to identify and quantitate the largest number and range of lymphohematopoietic cell markers and also offers the greatest latitude of choice of additional immunologic and molecular diagnostic assays.

Some of the principal disadvantages of this approach are the requirement of freshly obtained tissue samples and the expense of establishing a flow cytometry facility. Most pathologists consider the greatest disadvantage to be the loss of the ability to view the topographic distribution of the immunostained lymphohematopoietic cell populations in tissue sections. For this reason, some pathologists believe that immunohistochemical staining of tissue sections is the only correct approach to the immunophenotypic analysis of solid hematologic specimens. They are wrong. If cell suspensions are properly obtained from solid tissue specimens and correctly analyzed, and the results are correlated with the histopathologic sections, immunophenotypic analysis of cell suspensions results in a correct immunodiagnosis in the vast majority of patients; erroneous results can be avoided easily (see Chapter 5).

Frozen Tissue Sections

Historically, the immunohistochemical analysis of frozen tissue sections, usually by avidin-biotin immunoperoxidase or alkaline phophatase–antialkaline phosphatase, has been the most commonly employed methodologic approach in the immunophenotypic analysis of solid hematologic specimens. The vast majority of cell surface membrane antigens and receptors are preserved intact if tissue is rapidly and properly frozen and therefore are demonstrable with a variety of immunohistochemical techniques (6) (see Chapter 4).

The principal advantage of this approach is that it allows the pathologist to view the topographic distribution and the *in situ* organization of the immunostained lymphohematopoietic cell populations in tissue sections that can be correlated with the permanent histologic sections. This approach is also ideal for analyzing small tissue specimens (i.e., cutaneous punch, needle core, and stereotactic biopsy specimens and sclerotic or partially necrotic tissue specimens) in which a representative and quantitatively sufficient cell suspension cannot be prepared. The other principal advantage of this approach is the low cost of establishing, equipping, and operating the laboratory facility. This approach allows the investigator to semiquantitate the immunostained cell populations. Two-color immunohistochemical staining can be performed in order to view the topographic relationship between two distinct cell populations or, for example, to simultaneously detect distinct surface membrane and cytoplasmic antigens expressed by the same cell.

One of the principal disadvantages of this approach is the often poor cytomorphologic detail of the immunostained cells. Another disadvantage is the relative inability to manipulate the tissue optimally to detect the range of lymphohematopoietic markers detectable in cell suspension. For example, immunoglobulin and other antigens, such as CD3 and CD22, detected in frozen tissue sections may represent surface or cytoplasmic expression. It may not be possible to be certain if one, the other, or both are expressed in a specific patient. Also, some of the cell markers detectable in paraffin tissue sections or properly fixed cell suspensions, such as S-100 protein and cytoplasmic immunoglobin (cIg), are not easily detected in frozen tissue sections (see Chapter 4).

Paraffin Tissue Sections

The third methodologic approach is the immunohistochemical staining of routinely fixed and paraffin-embedded tissue sections. The harsh fixtures and embedding procedures routinely employed in tissue processing usually result in the masking or even destruction of most lymphohematopoietic cell surface membrane antigens and receptors but preserve cytoplasmic antigens. Surface membrane immunoglobulin (sIg) and the vast majority of lymphohematopoietic cell surface antigens detectable by MAbs in cell suspensions and frozen tissue sections are not detectable in paraffin tissue sections using standard immunohistochemical procedures (6). Because the monoclonal nature of the majority of B-cell lymphomas is established on the basis of exclusive surface expression of κ or λ light chains, the majority of B-cell lymphomas lack cIg, and sIg is masked or destroyed by fixation; the immunohistochemical analysis of paraffin tissue sections is not generally useful in establishing the monoclonality of a B-cell proliferation. However, cIg is detectable in plasma cells in paraffin tissue sections (26). Immunohistochemical analysis of paraffin tissue sections is useful in determining the clonal nature of plasma cell proliferations containing cIg.

Until relatively recently, immunophenotypic analysis of paraffin tissue sections was not often helpful and infrequently employed in the immunodiagnosis of lymphohematopoietic neoplasms. The description of two MAbs reactive with leukocytes in routinely fixed, paraffin-embedded tissue sections in the early 1980s (27), however, opened the door to the development and characterization of antibodies reactive with lymphohematopoietic cells in routinely processed tissue sections. During the past 10 years, many MAbs that detect fixation and paraffin-resistant B-cell, T-cell, monocyte-macrophage, and other lymphohematopoietic antigens in formalin-fixed, paraffin-embedded tissue sections have been prepared and characterized (19,20). In addition, the recent development of antigen-retrieval techniques (28) has enhanced further the ability to detect lymphohematopoietic antigens in paraffin tissue sections. The availability of these reagents and techniques has resulted in a dramatic increase in the use of this methodologic approach for immunophenotypic analysis in diagnostic pathology. This approach has proven extremely helpful in a variety of immunodiagnostic situations, such as distinguishing between epithelial malignancies and non-Hodgkin's lymphoma (NHL), between NHL and Hodgkin's disease, and between B- and T-cell NHLs. Paraffin tissue section immunohistochemistry also has been very helpful, for example, in delineating the immunophenotypic profile of the Reed-Sternberg cell of Hodgkin's disease (see Chapters 17 and 18). There is no doubt that the development of paraffin-reactive MAbs and antigen-retrieval techniques that further enhance their use has increased greatly the ability of pathologists to recognize and accurately diagnose hematopoietic neoplasms.

The principal advantage of this approach is the ability to

use routinely processed pathologic specimens. This obviates the need to make special arrangements to handle tissue specimens under sterile, fresh, and unfixed conditions, avoiding the disruption of the normal flow of specimens from clinical physician to pathologist. Also, some tissue specimens arrive in the pathology laboratory already in fixative, and fresh tissue is simply not available. Immunophenotypic analysis can be performed in these instances nonetheless. This also means that immunophenotypic analysis can be performed on virtually every pathologic specimen, rendering archival material, even after storage for many years, amenable to retrospective immunophenotypic analysis. The performance of immunophenotypic analysis in paraffin tissue sections permits the reservation of fresh tissue for studies that absolutely require it, such as many molecular genetic analyses. Additional advantages include the excellent cytomorphology of the immunostained slides, their permanency, and the ease and low cost of establishing and maintaining this type of laboratory facility. For all these reasons, this methodologic approach is ideally suited for small pathology laboratories and community hospitals in which flow cytometry facilities may not be cost-effective to establish and operate.

Despite the development of antigen-retrieval techniques and the availability of a greatly increased number of MAbs applicable to paraffin tissue sections, however, not every lymphohematopoietic antigen is detectable in paraffin tissue sections. This remains the principal disadvantage of this approach. The other principal disadvantage is that even these fixation- and paraffin-resistant antigens are differentially susceptible to various fixatives and the duration of fixation. Not all of these MAbs work equally well in every routinely processed pathologic specimen. The antigen retrieval prestaining conditions must be modified for each antibody, and each antibody should be titered according to the particular fixative employed (formalin, B5, Bouin's, and so forth) (see Chapter 4).

Optimal Approach

There is no one (correct) way to approach the immunophenotypic analysis of all hematologic specimens. The ideal methodologic approach is one tailored to meet the needs and situation of the particular laboratory, the individual pathologic specimen, and the specific diagnostic problem. A hematopathology laboratory serving a large medical institution should arrange to receive all hematologic specimens fresh and unfixed and should possess the ability to use all of the methodologic approaches described here. This permits the hematopathologist to serve the patient and the patient's physician in the best manner possible: as a consultant. The hematopathologist then has the opportunity to select the methodologic approach (cell suspension, frozen tissue sections, or paraffin tissue sections) that is optimal for the particular hematologic specimen and the specific diagnostic problem.

The pathologist at the small community hospital who lacks the facilities to perform immunophenotypic studies should cryopreserve a representative portion of every pathologic specimen in which cell marker studies may be helpful. Following review of the histopathologic sections, an informed decision to either discard the tissue or submit it on dry ice to a reference laboratory for immunophenotypic, and possibly immunogenotypic, analysis can be made. If the pathologist does not have the resources to freeze tissue and transport frozen tissue, fresh unfixed tissue generally can be transported safely in tissue culture media by same-day or overnight courier services. The practicing hematologist or oncologist similarly can arrange to transport freshly drawn peripheral blood and bone marrow aspiration samples. Finally, paraffin tissue sections and blocks can be transported easily by overnight mail to a reference laboratory capable of performing such studies. Therefore, every clinical physician and pathologist should be able at least to arrange for the performance of immunophenotypic analyses, if they cannot perform the studies themselves.

CONVENTIONAL IMMUNOPHENOTYPIC MARKERS

Background

During the late 1960s and early 1970s, cellular immunologists discovered that human peripheral blood lymphocytes, despite similar cytomorphologic appearances, are actually divisable into two major populations. These were designated *B cells* and *T cells* based on their organs of derivation, the bone marrow and the thymus, respectively. Cellular immunologists discovered that B and T cells undergo distinctive differentiation processes, possess characteristic and distinctive anatomic localizations within the central and peripheral lymphoid organs and tissues, and subserve different functions. B cells differentiate into antibody-producing plasma cells and thereby serve as effector cells for the humoral arm of the immune system. T cells serve as effector cells in cell-mediated immunity and also perform immunoregulatory functions, including help and suppression of B-cell differentiation into antibody-producing plasma cells (see Chapter 2).

Immunologists also discovered that sIg is expressed exclusively by B cells and that sheep erythrocytes (E) bind spontaneously to human T cells, a phenomenon referred to as *E rosette formation*. The sIg and E rosette formation became the classic cell surface markers useful in detecting and distinguishing between human B and T cells reliably. Studies concerning the binding of antigen–antibody complexes and antibody-coated sheep erythrocytes to human peripheral blood mononuclear cells led to the discovery of complement and Fc receptors. The preparation of heteroantisera by immunization with benign and malignant lymphoid cells led to the discovery of terminal deoxynucleotidyl transferase (TdT), the common acute lymphoblastic leukemia antigen (CALLA), and a panel of primitive but sometimes useful antisera for detecting T and B cell subpopulations. Studies with human alloantisera led to the discovery of the major histocompatibility complex (MHC) class II (HLA-DR) antigens (2–6). These immunophenotypic markers, developed and characterized prior to the MAb era, have been referred to as *conventional* cell markers. Their application led to the initial insights into the histogenesis of many lymphoid neoplasms. Many of the assays originally used to detect these markers are no longer employed routinely; these markers often are detected with MAbs, but most of them remain valuable as immunophenotypic markers in the diagnosis and classification of hematopoietic neoplasms.

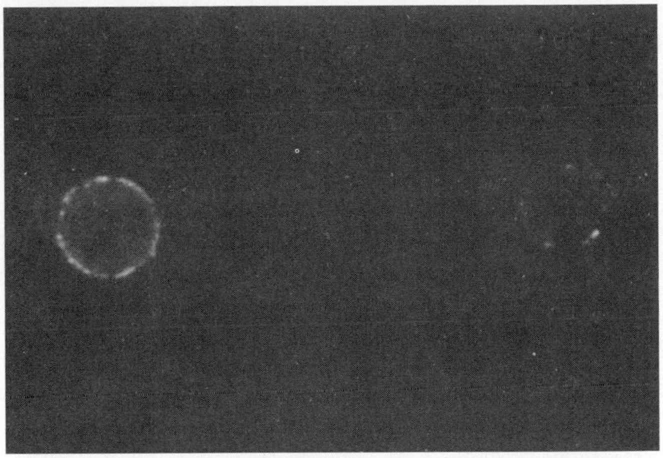

FIG. 3.1. Normal peripheral blood lymphocytes stained with an $F(ab')_2$ fragment preparation of rhodamine-conjugated rabbit antihuman immunoglobulin. The immunofluorescent detection of intrinsic surface membrane immunoglobulin (sIg) permits the identification of two B cells in this field. These B cells exhibit the typical speckled pattern of immunofluorescent staining for sIg. The variable density of sIg, reflected by the variable staining intensity, is a feature of normal polyclonal B cells (original magnification: 600× magnification). (From Knowles DM. Non-Hodgkin's lymphomas: I. Immunologic and enzymatic markers useful in their evaluation. In: Fenoglio CM, Wolff M, eds. *Progress in surgical pathology*, vol 2. New York: Masson Publishing, 1980:71–105, with permission.)

Surface Immunoglobulin

Intrinsic sIg is expressed uniquely by B cells and serves as the antigen-recognition molecule for B cells. Therefore, it remains the classic and specific marker of this lymphocyte population. Each of the immunoglobulin heavy chain classes can be expressed on the B cell membrane, and an individual B cell can express more than one heavy chain class. The majority of mature peripheral B cells expresses surface IgM, with or without IgD (29,30). Less than 10% of mature, peripheral sIg-positive (sIg^+) B cells express IgG or IgA if suitable precautions are taken to avoid cytophilic uptake of immunoglobulin from the serum (29–32).

The first heavy chain class of Ig to appear on the B-cell membrane during B-cell ontogeny is IgM. The large majority of immature B cells expresses only IgM and in high density. As development proceeds, the average amount of sIgM decreases, and an increasing amount of IgD appears on the B-cell membrane (33). The IgM and IgD molecules that coexist in the cell membrane cap independently but share the same idiotype and have the same light chain (34–36). If a given B cell interacts with its specific antigen, B-cell activation and differentiation occurs. During these events, B cells bearing sIgM, sIgD, and sIgG appear. These cells then lose IgD and later IgM as the result of a productive isotype gene rearrangement switch. Some of these B cells progress in their differentiation process and become antibody-producing cells, that is, plasma cells. During this process, different subpopulations of memory B cells expressing sIgM or sIgG may be derived (37).

Approximately two thirds of mature, peripheral sIg^+ B cells express κ light chains, and the remaining one third expresses λ light chains. Individual B cells express κ or λ light chains but not both (29). The clonality of a given B-cell population may be inferred from the uniformity of light chain class expression. A vast predominance of κ or λ light chain–bearing B cells indicates monoclonality; a mixture of κ and λ chain–bearing B cells suggests polyclonality. B-cell monoclonality usually implies a neoplastic B-cell proliferation; polyclonality generally implies a reactive, nonneoplastic proliferation.

The sIg density of normal mature peripheral B cells is heterogeneous, as is readily apparent from the immunofluorescent examination of polyclonal B cells (Fig. 3.1). More sensitive approaches, such as cytofluorometric analysis, demonstrate that there is a continuous distribution of immunoglobulin on B-cell membranes (4). Monoclonal B-cell populations often show a more restricted range of sIg density.

Surface immunoglobulin may be detected on viable cells in suspension by cytofluorometric analysis following direct immunofluorescent staining with fluorochrome-conjugated heterologous antisera raised against whole or Fab fragments of human immunoglobulin molecules (polyvalent antisera). Class-specific antisera monospecific for μ, δ, γ, α, κ, and λ determinants (monovalent antisera) may be used to determine the precise isotype of sIg^+ B cells and to infer their monoclonal or polyclonal nature. Alternatively, indirect immunofluorescent staining using monoclonal anti-human immunoglobulin antibodies may be employed (see Chapter 5). The sIg also may be detected in cytocentrifuge slides prepared from cells in suspension (Fig. 3.2) and in frozen tissue sections (Fig. 3.3) employing various immunohistochemical techniques (see Chapter 4).

A discussion of the technical details concerning the demonstration of sIg expression by B cells is beyond the scope of this chapter; moreover, this topic has been reviewed extensively elsewhere (38–41). A few relevant points should be mentioned briefly. Some of these remarks are also applicable to the demonstration of other cell markers.

Accurate quantitation of the percentage of sIg^+ B cells

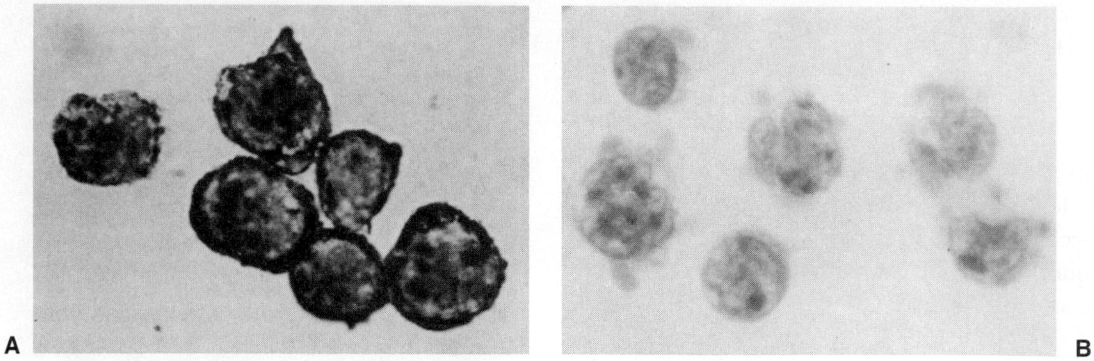

FIG. 3.2. Daudi lymphoblastoid cell line cells stained with an $F(ab')_2$ preparation of peroxidase-conjugated rabbit antihuman immunoglobulin antisera monospecific for μ (**A**) and α determinants (**B**). **A:** The deposition of abundant dark brown pigment on the cell surface indicates the presence of surface IgM. **B:** The absence of brown pigment from the cell surface indicates the absence of surface IgA. Nuclear detail is discernable because of a nuclear fast red counterstain (original magnification: 600× magnification). (From Knowles DM, Winchester RJ, Kunkel HG. A comparison of peroxidase fluorochrome-conjugated antisera for the demonstration of surface and intracellular antigens. *Clin Immunol Immunopathol* 1977;7:410–425, with permission.)

in cell suspension by immunofluorescence or in frozen tissue sections by immunohistochemical staining may be hampered by several technical problems. First, immunoglobulin present in the serum may be absorbed passively nonspecifically by Fc receptors present on cells, often non-B cells, which do not actually synthesize their own sIg. This sIg is referred to as *cytophilic antibody*; it does not represent intrinsic membrane sIg, that is, immunoglobulin actually synthesized by the cell carrying it. These cells may include, for example, monocytes or macrophages, granulocytes, large granular lymphocytes (LGLs) or natural killer (NK) cells, and activated T cells (32,38,39). In the case of cells in suspension, overnight incubation of isolated mononuclear cells in tissue culture medium with 5% to 10% fetal calf serum usually

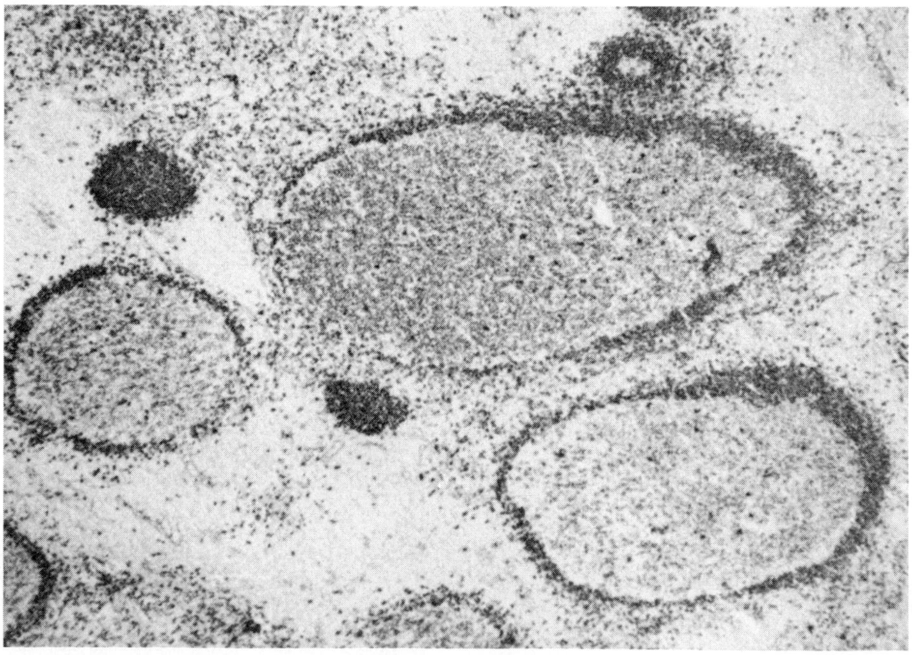

FIG. 3.3. Indirect immunoperoxidase staining of a frozen tissue section of tonsil with an $F(ab')_2$ fragment preparation of sheep antihuman immunoglobulin antisera monospecific for δ determinants. The surface immunoglobulin (sIg)–positive B cells expressing IgD are predominantly localized in the primary and secondary follicles, with smaller numbers scattered in the interfollicular areas. The crescent-shaped mantle zone of each follicle expresses high-density sIgD in comparison with the germinal centers, which express sIgD in lower density or not all (immunoperoxidase stain, original magnification: 40× magnification).

allows shedding of passively absorbed cytophilic Ig. Alternatively, sIg may be removed by trypsin or pronase treatment and the cells cultured *in vitro* overnight. Intrinsic sIg is resynthesized by the cell; passively absorbed cytophilic immunoglobulin is not resynthesized (38,39). Frozen tissue sections should be washed in phosphate-buffered saline and preincubated with nonimmune serum of the animal in which the anti-human immunoglobulin antibody was prepared prior to immunostaining. These procedures help to ensure that the immunoglobulin detected is actually intrinsic membrane sIg synthesized by the cell carrying it and not cytophilic immunoglobulin passively absorbed from the serum.

Second, fluorochrome-conjugated antibodies used to identify sIg^+ B cells may bind nonspecifically to Fc receptors in the total absence of sIg. Two mechanisms may account for this reaction: IgG antibody may aggregate spontaneously (these aggregates have a high Fc receptor affinity), or soluble immune complexes generated after addition of the labeled antibody may bind to Fc receptors and thereby simulate an sIg^+ B cell. Some commercial antisera contain large amounts of soluble immune complexes. It is precisely these mechanisms that led to the incorrect reports in the older literature that up to 35% of peripheral blood lymphocytes are B cells and that they primarily express sIgG or sIgA. These difficulties are best circumvented by using $F(ab')_2$ antibody fragments prepared by pepsin digestion (32). Pepsin digests the Fc portion of antibody molecules, producing bivalent $F(ab')_2$ antibody fragments. These $F(ab')_2$ antibody fragments do not bind to Fc receptors and thereby avoid nonspecific staining (4) (see Chapter 11 and Appendix 10). Cell marker laboratories should employ $F(ab')_2$ reagents and appropriate incubation procedures routinely to allow shedding of cytophilic antibody, so as to obviate the difficulties discussed here.

Approximately 80% of all NHLs occurring in the Western hemisphere are of B cell origin, and the majority expresses monotypic sIg (42–44). Therefore, lymphoid proliferations are examined routinely for the presence and clonal nature of sIg expression. Demonstration of the monoclonal or polyclonal nature of sIg expression by a B-cell proliferation is the operational basis for classic immunophenotypic analysis (6). Traditionally, it has been inferred routinely that monoclonal B-cell proliferations are neoplastic and polyclonal B-cell proliferations are nonneoplastic (45–47). The sIg isotypes expressed by B-cell NHLs and lymphoid leukemias parallel those of normal B cells. The most common heavy chain class is IgM, with or without IgD. IgG and IgA heavy chain classes are expressed much less frequently (48,49). Certain sIg isotypes, however, are associated preferentially with certain categories of lymphoid malignancy. For example, a higher proportion of hairy cell leukemias than of other lymphoid leukemias and NHLs express sIgG (50). About two thirds of B-cell NHLs and lymphoid leukemias express κ light chains, and the remaining one third express λ light chains (42–49).

Cytoplasmic (Intracellular) Immunoglobulin

Cytoplasmic (intracellular) immunoglobulin is present within B cells at two points during ontogeny: during the immature, pre-B cell stage and again during the secretory (plasma cell) stage. Pre-B cells contain cytoplasmic μ heavy chains but lack cytoplasmic light chains and sIg (51). Small numbers of these cells populate the fetal liver and normal bone marrow but not normal adult lymphoid tissues (51). The majority of mature circulating and lymphoid tissue sIg^+ B cells lack cIg (29). All B cells, however, possess the capacity to differentiate into immunoglobulin-producing (secretory) plasma cells following interaction with their specific antigen. If this occurs, $sIgMD^+$ B cells undergo an immunoglobulin heavy chain switch, begin to lose sIg, and acquire cIg. During this process, plasma cells expressing different immunoglobulin heavy chain classes on the membrane and in the cytoplasm may be encountered (52). Terminally differentiated IgG-secreting plasma cells, however, lack sIg. The cIg contained within plasma cells is complete and consists of both heavy and light chains (29).

Unlike sIg, which is detectable in viable cells in suspension or in minimally fixed frozen tissue sections, the detection of cIg requires permeabilization of the cell membrane by fixative to allow penetration of the anti-Ig reagents. Therefore, in the case of viable cell suspensions, cIg usually is detected by immunofluorescent (21) or immunoperoxidase (40) staining of alcohol-fixed cytocentrifuge smears prepared from the cell suspension (Fig. 3.4). Alternatively,

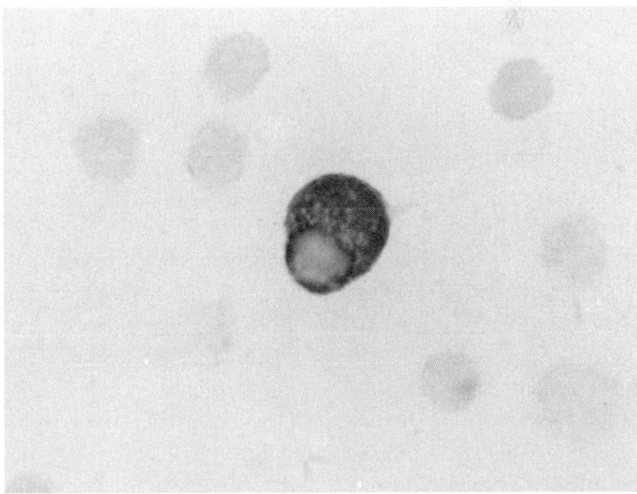

FIG. 3.4. The mononuclear cells were isolated from a benign, reactive lymph node and placed into cell suspension, and alcohol-fixed cytospin smears were prepared by cytocentrifugation. These smears then were stained with peroxidase-conjugated rabbit antihuman immunoglobulin antisera monospecific for γ heavy chains. A single plasma cell displays abundant cytoplasmic brown reaction product, indicating the presence of intracellular IgG. The remaining cells lack the brown reaction product, indicating absence of intracellular IgG (immunoperoxidase stain, original magnification: 600× magnification).

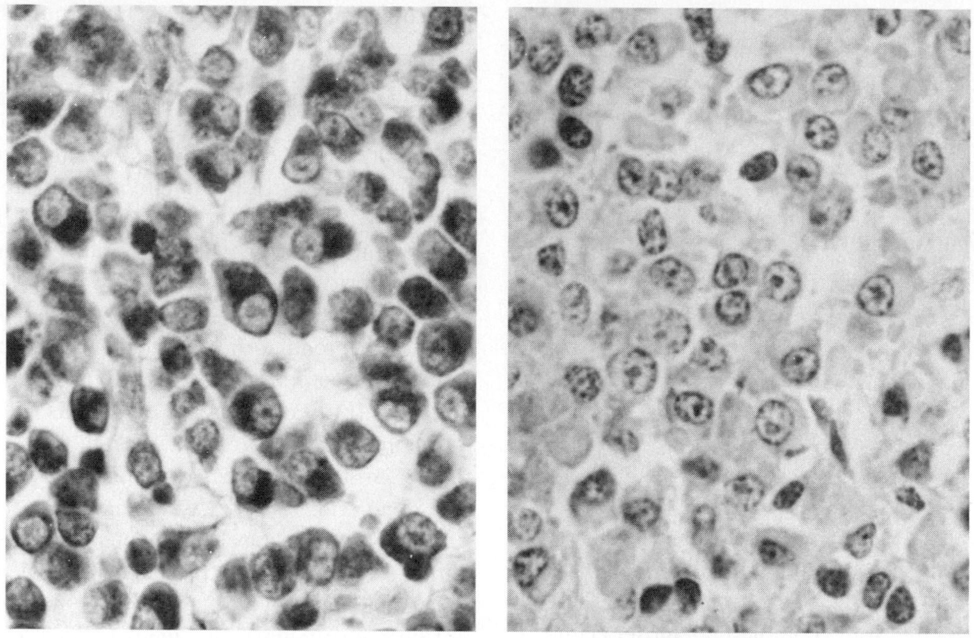

A B

FIG. 3.5. Bouin's solution–fixed, paraffin-embedded tissue sections prepared from an orbital plasmacytoma immunostained with peroxidase-conjugated antisera monospecific for λ (**A**) and κ (**B**) light chain determinants. **A:** The deposition of abundant intracellular brown reaction product indicates the presence of cytoplasmic λ light chains in nearly all of the plasma cells. **B:** The absence of brown reaction product indicates the absence of cytoplasmic κ light chains from these plasma cells. These immunostaining results are indicative of a clonal plasma cell proliferation. This orbital plasmacytoma represented the clinical presentation of a disseminated IgD λ multiple myeloma, (immunoperoxidase stain, original magnification: 600× magnification). (From Knowles DM, Halper JP, Trokel S, et al. Immunofluorescent and immunoperoxidase characteristics of IgD λ myeloma involving the orbit. *Am J Ophthalmol* 1978; 85:485–494, with permission.)

cIg is demonstrable by immunohistochemical staining of routinely fixed and paraffin-embedded tissue sections (26,40,53) (Fig. 3.5). The cIg also is sometimes detectable in frozen tissue sections (54). The cIg is not always demonstrable in frozen tissue sections that have been minimally fixed with a gentle fixative. The cIg-containing plasma cells sometimes may be misinterpreted as cIg-negative (cIg^-) if frozen sections are immunostained but correctly identified as cIg^+ if appropriately fixed cell suspension cytocentrifuge smears or paraffin tissue sections are immunostained.

Because the majority of B-cell NHLs lack easily detectable cIg, there is usually little reason to examine most NHLs for cIg, unless suggested by their clinical, pathologic, or other immunologic features. The demonstration of cytoplasmic μ heavy chains without light chains in malignant lymphoblasts assists in defining precursor B-cell lymphoblastic lymphoma or leukemia (51). Also, demonstrating clonal cIg heavy or light chains is useful in the immunodiagnosis of plasma cell dyscrasias, including Waldenström's macroglobulinemia and multiple myeloma (26,40,53,54) (see Chapter 42).

Sheep Erythrocyte Rosette

Washed, unsensitized sheep erythrocytes bind spontaneously to viable, metabolically active human T cells *in vitro*, a phenomenon referred to as *E rosette formation* (55–58). Virtually all normal thymocytes and mature peripheral blood and lymphoid tissue T cells form spontaneous E rosettes (58,59). Rosette formation between sheep erythrocytes and human peripheral T cells is a temperature-dependent reaction. The E rosettes formed between sheep erythrocytes and mature, peripheral T cells persist or increase following incubation at 4°C but disassociate at 37°C (heat-labile E rosettes) (55). The temperature dependence of this reaction does not apply to thymocytes; the majority of thymocytes form E rosettes that do not disassociate at 37°C (heat-stable E rosettes) (56,60). T-cell neoplasms derived from mature, peripheral T cells—that is, cutaneous and peripheral T-cell lymphomas—form heat-labile E rosettes (61); those derived from thymocytes—that is, precursor T-cell lymphoblastic lymphoma or leukemia—form heat-stable E rosettes (60) (Fig. 3.6).

At one time, E rosette formation was the best T-cell marker available, and it was employed widely in clinical and investigative situations (4). Interlaboratory methodologic differences and numerous variables (e.g., individual sheep variation, age of the sheep erythrocytes, use of various pretreatments), however, influence the results of the E rosette assay (58,62,63), sometimes leading to conflicting results. Also, the E rosette assay cannot be performed reproducibly

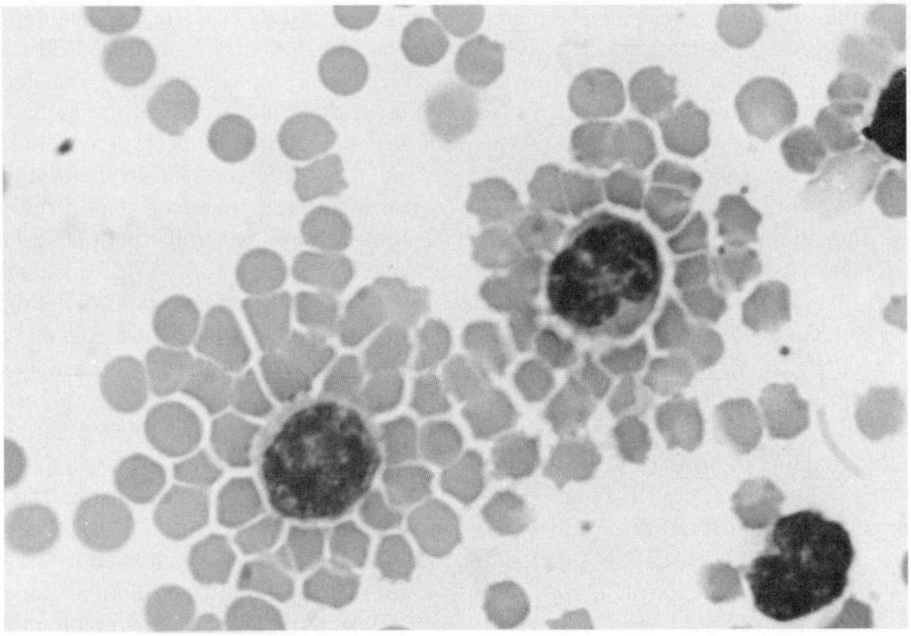

FIG. 3.6. The mononuclear cells were isolated from a lymph node diffusely replaced by a peripheral T-cell lymphoma and incubated with washed, unsensitized sheep erythrocytes to evaluate rosette formation. The rosetted cells then were placed onto glass microscope slides by cytocentrifugation and counterstained with a Wright-Giemsa stain (original magnification: 950× magnification). Two cytomorphologically malignant cells bind numerous sheep erythrocytes, thereby exhibiting evidence of rosette formation.

in frozen tissue sections (4,64,65). Several MAbs that detect the E rosette receptor have been prepared (66–69); they have been clustered as CD2 (15). These MAbs now are employed routinely to detect the E rosette receptor in frozen tissue sections as well as in cell suspensions and obviate the difficulties associated with the reproducible performance and interpretation of the E rosette assay (see CD2 below).

Fc Receptors

Receptors for the Fc portion of immunoglobulin molecules have been referred to simply as *Fc receptors*. Initially it was suggested that predominantly peripheral blood sIg^+ B cells and monocytes bear receptors for the Fc portion of IgG (70). It soon became apparent that a large proportion of peripheral blood T cells possesses Fc receptors for IgM ($T\mu$ cells), and a smaller proportion possesses Fc receptors for IgG ($T\gamma$ cells) (71,72). B cells lacking sIg and large granular lymphocytes or NK cells also were found to bear Fc receptors (2,73–75). We now know that Fc receptors constitute a large family of related but distinct antigens expressed by multiple lymphohematopoietic cell populations (see Chapter 2).

The different assays initially employed to detect Fc receptors often preferentially detected different Fc receptor–bearing cell populations (65,76–78). For example, B-cell Fc receptors were identified with fluorosceine-labeled, heat-aggregated human IgG (79,80) or radiolabeled soluble antigen–antibody complexes (70). Monocyte-macrophage Fc receptors were identified in cell suspensions and frozen tissue sections with a rosetting assay using sheep erythrocytes coated with IgG antibody (65,81). Numerous MAbs that specifically detect these various Fc receptors, however, have been developed during the past decade. These MAbs have replaced the various *in vitro* assays for detecting Fc receptor–positive cells and have resulted in an increased understanding of the biologic functions of the various Fc receptors (see Chapter 2). These MAb reagents are discussed subsequently in this chapter.

Complement Receptors

Lymphocytes bearing receptors for the third component of complement (C3) initially were identified with the EAC rosette assay, that is, sheep erythrocytes (E) coated with IgM antibody (A) and complement (C) (82). The EAC rosette assay may be performed in cell suspension (82) and in frozen tissue sections (83). Hence, cells bearing complement receptors (CRs) sometimes were referred to as *EAC rosette–positive* cells and CRs as *EAC receptors*. The CR-positive cells initially were identified as B cells (82), but monocytes, macrophages, and granulocytes also were found to express CRs (84,85), although normal human B cells have receptors for both C3b and C3d (86) but monocytes, macrophages, and granulocytes only have receptors for C3b (84,85). Because most EAC reagents are prepared from whole serums that contain a mixture of C3b and C3d, however, they adhere to B lymphocytes, monocytes or macrophages, and granulocytes. For this reason, and also because of numerous methodologic variables (87), like the E rosette assay, the EAC rosette assay no longer is employed routinely in immunophenotypic analysis.

We now recognize three different types of cellular receptors for the major cleavage fragments of C3. These are as CR types 1 (CR1), 2 (CR2), and 3 (CR3). These receptors have distinct structures and binding sites in the C3 molecule. The C3b receptor (CR1) is a polymorphic 220-kd surface membrane glycoprotein (88,89) that has primary specificity for C3b but also may bind iC3b (90) and C4b (91). CR1 is expressed by B cells, monocytes or macrophages, granulocytes, erythrocytes, a subset of T cells (92), and follicular dendritic cells (93,94). CR1 is recognized by several MAbs that have been clustered as CD35 (95). The C3d receptor (CR2) is a 140-kd single chain glycoprotein (96,97) that serves as the receptor for the Epstein-Barr virus (EBV) on B cells (98), as well as for C3d (96,97). CR2 is expressed by mature B cells (99–101) and follicular dendritic cells (93,94). CR2 is recognized by many MAbs clustered as CD21 (102), including B2 (103), HB5 (99), and OKB7 (104,105). The iC3b receptor (CR3) consists of two polypeptide chains, a 155-kd α chain and a 95-kd β chain (106,107). The β chain is shared with two other leukocyte surface antigens that have a unique α chain, lymphocyte function associated antigen-1 (LFA-1) and p150,95 (108). Several MAbs, including OKM1 (109) and Mo1 (110), recognize the α chain; these MAbs have been clustered as CD11b (111). CR3 is expressed by monocytes and macrophages, granulocytes (109,110,112), follicular dendritic cells (93,94), and large granular lymphocytes and NK cells (113). These CRs are identified routinely using MAbs.

Terminal Deoxynucleotidyl Transferase

Terminal deoxynucleotidyl transferase, encoded by a 35-kilobase (kb) gene on chromosome 10q23-25 (114), is a unique intranuclear DNA polymerase that catalyzes the random addition of deoxynucleotidyl residues on the 3′-hydroxyl termini of single-stranded DNA and of oligodeoxynucleotidyl primers in the absence of a template (22,115–117). B and T cells recognize antigens by specialized antigen-recognition receptors on their surfaces, immunoglobulin and T-cell receptors (TCRs), respectively (118,119) (see Chapters 2 and 7). TdT expends its DNA polymerase function during immunoglobulin and TCR gene rearrangement as a nonessential, tissue-specific component of VDJ recombinase (120). Diversity in the immunoglobulin and TCR repertoires is generated in developing B and T cells by the combinatorial association of different sets of gene segments encoding variable regions of receptor chains (118,119). Additional diversity is created at the junction of recombining gene segments by mechanisms that involve the deletion of a variable number of nucleotides followed by the template-dependent and template-independent inclusion of non–germline-encoded nucleotides called *N regions* (121). It is believed that TdT is responsible for the template-independent addition of N regions (120–125).

Terminal deoxynucleotidyl transferase is expressed by precursor B and T cells at the earliest recognizable stages of lymphoid cell ontogeny (126). Under normal conditions, TdT^+ cells are confined to the thymus and bone marrow, in which these precursor cells reside; TdT^+ cells are not normally observed in the peripheral blood or in peripheral lymphoid tissue (116,127–129). The presence of TdT^+ cells in such circumstances is considered diagnostic of precursor lymphoblastic lymphoma or leukemia (129). TdT is not expressed by myeloid, erythroid, or megakaryocytic precursors or by epithelial, mesenchymal, or germ cells (129).

Terminal deoxynucleotidyl transferase–positive cells represent about 2% to 7% of bone marrow cells in neonates and children up to 5 years of age and 1% to 2% of normal adult bone marrow cells (130,131). The age-adjusted decline of TdT^+ cells is likely related to the loss of bone marrow precursor cells (132). In normal bone marrow, the sparse TdT^+ cells are dispersed randomly in the interstitium (133). Under certain physiologic conditions, such as regenerating bone marrow and following bone marrow transplantation, TdT^+ cells may account for up to 20% of the bone marrow cellularity (130,131). Although a variety of cell populations make up the thymus, thymocytes (precursor and other immature T cells) constitute the majority of the cells (134–136). Thymocytes are divisable into immunophenotypically distinct subsets, representing different developmental stages of T-cell ontogeny, that preferentially reside in the cortex (immature) or medulla (mature) (134–136). Essentially all cortical thymocytes express TdT, and all medullary thymocytes except for a small subset lack TdT (135–137) (Fig. 3.7).

Although the functional role of TdT in lymphocyte onto-

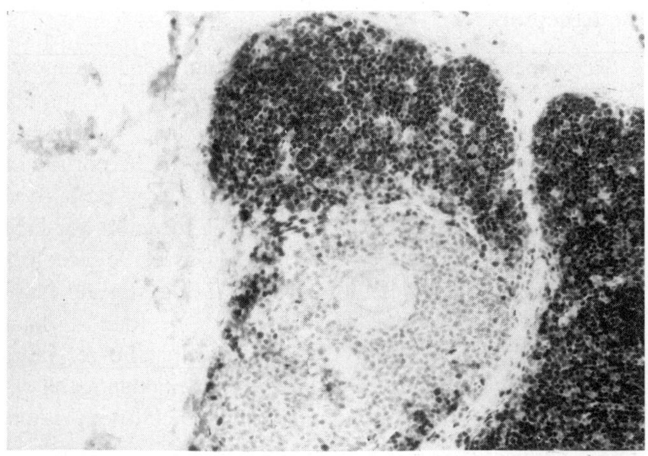

FIG. 3.7. Formalin-fixed, paraffin-embedded tissue section of human thymus immunostained with an anti–terminal deoxynucleotidyl transferase (TdT) antibody. All of the cortical thymocytes express strong intranuclear TdT positivity; only small numbers of thymocytes residing in the medullary thymus express TdT (immunoperoxidase stain, original magnification: 100× magnification).

geny has been debated for many years, its usefulness as a marker of immature hematopoietic cells was recognized early and has been exploited widely in the diagnosis and characterization of NHLs and acute leukemias (116). Virtually all malignant lymphoblasts comprising essentially all cases of precursor B- and T-cell lymphoblastic lymphoma or leukemia and cases of chronic myelogenous leukemia in lymphoid blast crisis express TdT (115,116,127,128, 138–144). None of the malignant lymphoid cells comprising essentially any cases of nonlymphoblastic NHL express TdT (130,140,143,145). Initially it was believed that the majority of acute myeloid leukemias (AMLs) similarly lack TdT (116,138,146,147), but the interpretation and significance of TdT expression by acute leukemias has become increasingly confusing because of the growing recognition of mixed-lineage leukemias (148). Approximately 20% of patients with AML apparently have TdT^+ malignant cells (149–157). In these patients, however, the proportion of TdT^+ blasts coexpressing myeloid-associated antigens is variable and often represents only a small subset of the malignant cell population. In most series, TdT^+ AML is diagnosed if as few as 5% to 10% TdT^+ malignant cells are identified (157). The clinical and prognostic significance of TdT expression in AML has been controversial (157). The use of TdT determination in the diagnostic evaluation and characterization of acute leukemias should be performed in the context of a thorough immunophenotypic analysis, including relevant enzymatic markers (129).

Immunophenotypic analysis represents a useful tool for monitoring minimal residual disease following chemotherapy and for detecting the reemergence of malignant blasts during clinically apparent complete remission of acute leukemia (158–162). In the case of precursor B- and T-cell lymphoblastic lymphoma or leukemia, clinically silent, diffuse infiltration of lymphoblasts can occur in ''privileged'' sites such as the testes and central nervous system as well as the bone marrow and peripheral blood (129). The immunophenotypic detection of such cells is useful in predicting leukemia relapse and guiding early corrective therapy (163). The immunocytochemical demonstration of TdT^+ cells in cerebrospinal fluid samples is diagnostic of precursor lymphoblastic lymphoma or leukemia, because TdT^+ cells are not found there under normal conditions (164). The immunohistochemical demonstration of TdT^+ cells in the testis is similarly diagnostic (165), as is the cytofluorometric or immunocytochemical demonstration of TdT^+ cells in the peripheral blood (129). This is not entirely true in the case of the bone marrow, because normal and regenerating bone marrow contains small numbers of benign TdT^+ cells (130,131). Certain antigen combinations not usually expressed by normal bone marrow cells, however, often can be considered immunodiagnostic of malignancy (129). These include, for example, the coexpression of TdT with cytoplasmic CD3 (cCD3), and/or CD5 and/or CD1 or with CD13 and/or CD33 and/or CDw65 and/or CD56 (158–162,166).

Functional biochemical assays have been used widely to detect TdT activity in leukolysates of bone marrow or tissue extracts (127,139). Biochemical assays simple enough to be performed in clinical laboratories using commerically avail able reagents have been described (167). For the purpose of routine immunophenotypic analysis, however, these biochemical assays have been replaced progressively by immunocytochemical and immunohistochemical assays, which offer the advantages of technical simplicity, applicability to smears and tissue sections, and the ability to evaluate cell morphology (129) (Fig. 3.8).

The immunofluorescent detection of TdT is very sensitive and for many years was the preferred method for analyzing peripheral blood and bone marrow aspiration smears and cytocentrifuge preparations (4,116,117,168). Immunofluorescence also lends itself to dual-marker analysis of TdT and surface membrane antigens (149,169,170). The development of methods to fix cells in suspension so as to permeabilize the cell membrane and the nuclear envelope to permit the penetration of antibodies allowed the demonstration of TdT by cytofluorometric analysis (171–175). TdT determination can be incorporated into routine quantitative and multiparametric cytofluorometric analysis of cells in suspension (see Chapter 5). Immunoperoxidase and immunoalkaline phosphatase techniques (176–178) have come to be preferred by pathologists, however, because they permit enhanced cytomorphologic evaluation and provide a permanent record. Dual-marker evaluation by immunoenzymatic techniques is also possible (179,180). Both immunofluorescent and immunoenzymatic techniques have been adapted successfully to frozen tissue sections (133,134,181). The immunohistochemical detection of TdT in formalin-fixed, paraffin-embedded tissue sections has been accomplished using a modified peroxidase–antiperoxidase technique in conjunction with a 0.1% DNAase digestion, overnight incubation with anti-TdT, and repeated bridge peroxidase–antiperoxidase applications (182,183). The recent introduction of antigen-retrieval techniques (28) has vastly simplified the immunohistochemical determination of TdT by obviating the need for DNAase digestions and prolonged incubations and has increased greatly the sensitivity of detection as well (184,185) (Fig. 3.9). These tissue section approaches permit evaluation of the topographic distribution of TdT^+ cells in a given sample and enhance our understanding of tissue microenvironments. Obviously, these tissue section approaches are particularly useful in those frequent diagnostic situations in which only tissue, and often only fixed tissue, is available. The choice of fixatives, the preferred commercially available anti-TdT heteroantisera or MAbs, and conditions surrounding the optimal determination of TdT have been reviewed in detail by Chilosi and Pizzolo (129).

Common Acute Lymphoblastic Leukemia Antigen

The common acute lymphoblastic leukemia antigen originally was recognized with a heteroantiserum raised in rabbits by immunizing with the malignant lymphoblasts obtained

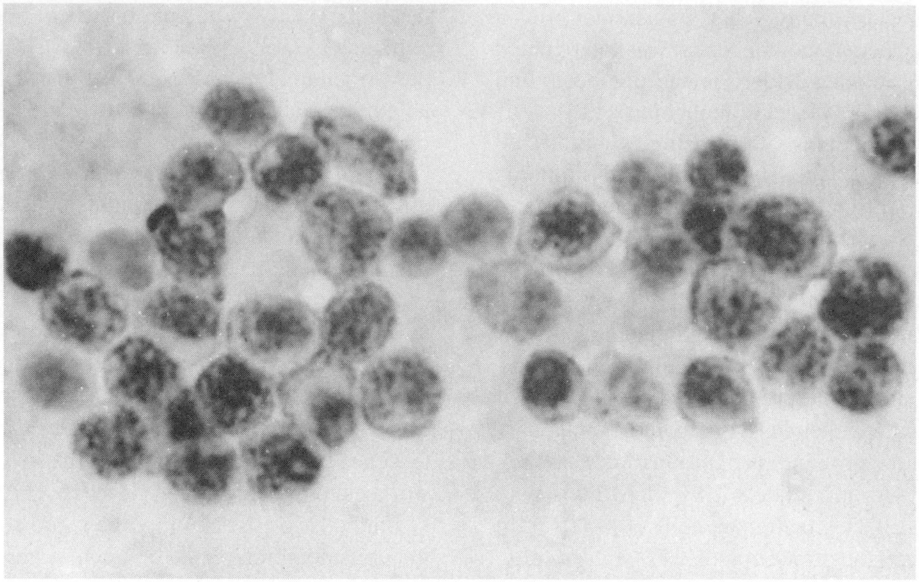

FIG. 3.8. The malignant lymphoblasts isolated from the peripheral blood of a young boy presenting with precursor T-cell acute lymphoblastic leukemia were placed onto glass microscope slides by cytocentrifugation and then immunostained for terminal deoxynucleotidyl transferase. The malignant lymphoblasts show abundant intranuclear staining consistent with terminal deoxynucleotidyl transferase positivity (immunoperoxidase stain, original magnification: 1,000× magnification).

from a case of ''non-B, non-T cell'' acute lymphoblastic leukemia (186). Expression of this antigen was demonstrated on small numbers of TdT and HLA-DR antigen–positive cells in the bone marrow and fetal liver that were believed to be lymphohematopoietic precursor cells (187–189). Myeloid and erythroid progenitor cells and mature peripheral B and T cells were found to lack CALLA expression (187–189). Consequently, it was believed initially that CALLA expression was limited to non-B, non-T cell acute lymphoblastic leukemias and the normal lymphohematopoietic precursors from which these acute leukemias are derived (186–190). Shortly thereafter, however, several MAbs that recognize CALLA were prepared (191–193); they were clustered as CD10 at the First International Leukocyte Differentiation Workshop (15). The availability of these MAbs led to numerous additional studies that resulted in the realization that CALLA (CD10) is not a leukemia-specific antigen, nor is it B- or T-cell lineage–restricted. A review of the current status of CD10 is presented elsewhere in this chapter.

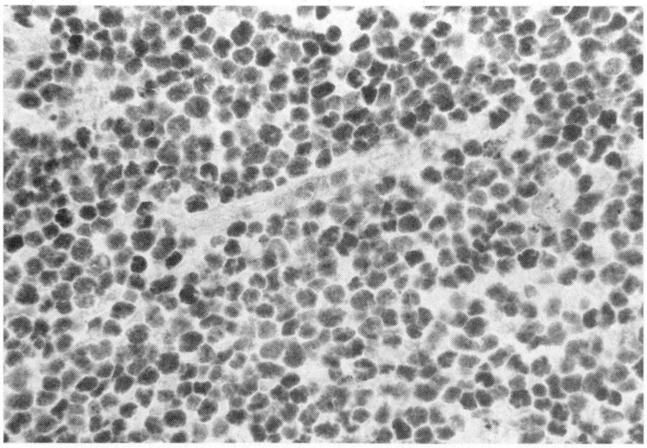

FIG. 3.9. Formalin-fixed, paraffin-embedded tissue section of a precusor T-cell lymphoblastic lymphoma/leukemia immunostained with an anti–terminal deoxynucleotidyl transferase antibody. The malignant lymphoblasts express strong intranuclear terminal deoxynucleotidyl transferase positivity (immunoperoxidase stain, original magnification: 400× magnification).

HLA-DR (Immune-Associated) Antigens

The ability to distinguish self from nonself is a fundamental protective mechanism characteristic of virtually all multicellular organisms. The highly polymorphic cell surface structures involved in this recognition system initially were identified in mice, in which they became known as the *major histocompatibility complex* (MHC). Later, the human equivalent of the MHC, known as the human leukocyte antigen (HLA) system, was identified and mapped to chromosome 6. Three classes of MHC or HLA molecules, designated I, II, and III, have been identified. Three separate class I loci, termed *HLA-A*, *HLA-B*, and *HLA-C*, have been demonstrated; they encode classic transplantation antigens. Class I molecules comprise a glycosylated 45-kd polypeptide chain noncovalently associated with a nonpolymorphic 12-kd polypeptide, β_2-microglobulin. Class II genes, encoded in the *HLAD* region, are organized into three gene families called *DR*, *DQ*, and *DP*. They are identical to the murine immune response genes known to control murine responses to different antigens. Class II molecules are genetically polymorphic heterodimeric glycoproteins comprising noncovalently linked α and β chains 33 to 34 kd and 26 to 29 kd in molecular weight, respectively, depending on the locus. Class I gene products are recognized primarily by cytotoxic T cells. Class II gene products, often called *immune-associated antigens*, are involved primarily in the activation of helper T cells. The class III genes encode several components of the complement system (194) (see Chapter 2).

Human HLA-DR (immune-associated) antigens were detected and studied initially using alloantisera (74,195,196), then using heteroantisera (75,196), and finally with MAbs (197,198). Originally, HLA-DR antigens were believed to be present exclusively on B cells (195), but they quickly were discovered on antigen-presenting cells, that is, monocytes/macrophages (74,196,199) and Langerhans' cells (200,201). We now know that HLA-DR antigens actually are distributed widely on hematopoietic cells and even are expressed on some nonhematopoietic cells (199), especially in certain pathologic conditions (194). HLA-DR antigens are expressed at the earliest stages of lymphohematopoietic cell development (202–204). They are expressed throughout B-cell ontogeny until the plasma cell (secretory) stage, at which they are lost (205). They are also present on hematopoietic progenitor cells (CFU-GEMM) and granulocyte-macrophage, erythroid, and megakaryocytic precursors (203,206–211). HLA-DR antigen expression is differentiation-linked in these lineages, the pattern being expression on the progenitor cell and the first cytologically distinct stage of lineage-specific maturation followed by disappearance on the more mature stages. HLA-DR antigens are expressed on myeloblasts but are lost during maturation to the promyelocyte stage (203). Similarly, they are expressed on proerythroblasts and megakaryocytes but are absent from erythrocytes beyond the basophilic normoblast stage and platelets (203,206,207,209,210). HLA-DR antigens are present throughout monocyte/macrophage differentiation and are expressed variably by peripheral blood monocytes and tissue macrophages (212). They are expressed on all dendritic cell populations (213), including Langerhans' cells (200,201), interdigitating dendritic cells (213), and follicular dendritic cells (dendritic reticulum cells) (93). HLA-DR antigens also are expressed at the earliest stages of T-cell ontogeny (204) but quickly are lost, and the vast majority of thymocytes and mature peripheral circulating and lymphoid tissue T cells are HLA-DR$^-$ (75,196,202,214). *In vitro* and *in vivo* activated T cells, however, express HLA-DR antigens (215–217).

HLA-DR antigen expression on malignant hematopoietic cells mirrors HLA-DR expression on benign hematopoietic cells. HLA-DR antigens are expressed on the vast majority of B-cell neoplasms. Greater than 90% of TdT$^+$ precursor B-cell lymphoblastic lymphomas/leukemias and mature (TdT$^-$) sIg$^+$ as well as sIg$^-$ B-cell NHLs and lymphoid leukemias express HLA-DR antigens (6–8,218) (Fig. 3.10). This includes those neoplasms lacking B cell–restricted antigens and whose B-cell derivation can be demonstrated only by immunoglobulin gene rearrangement analysis (219,220). Virtually the only mature (TdT$^-$) B-cell neoplasms lacking HLA-DR expression are those undergoing plasma cell differentiation. HLA-DR antigens are expressed variably by

A

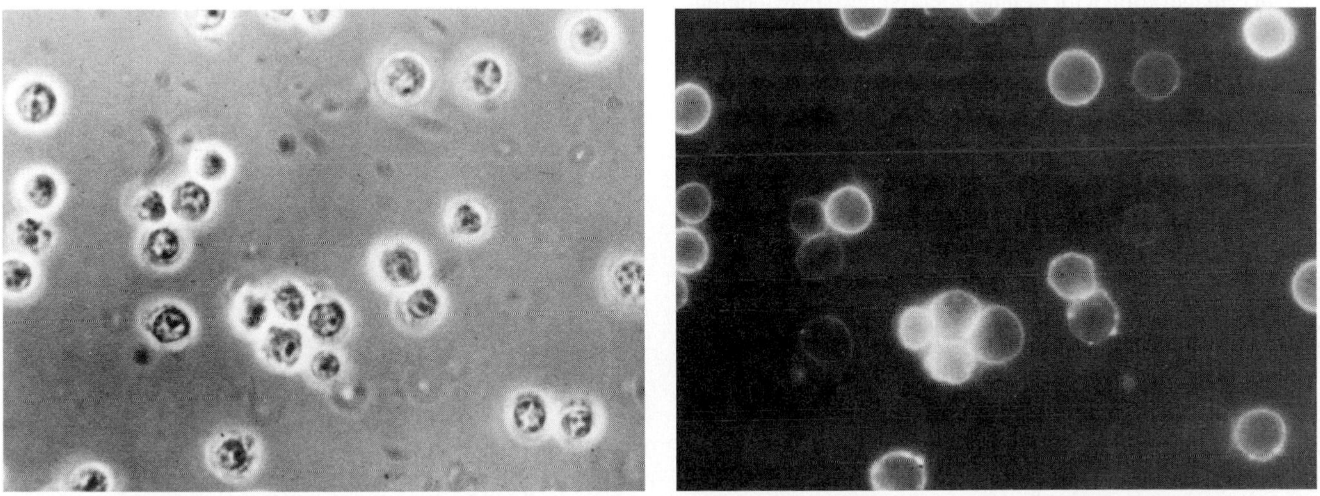

B

FIG. 3.10. The mononuclear cells isolated from the peripheral blood of a patient with B-cell chronic lymphocytic leukemia were stained in cell suspension by direct immunofluorescence with rhodamine-conjugated antihuman HLA-DR (Ia) heteroantisera. **A:** The cells viewed by phase microscopy. **B:** The same field viewed by fluorescent microscopy. The B cells display a bright, ring-like pattern of fluorescent staining, indicating the presence of HLA-DR (Ia) antigens. The occasional negative cells represent residual benign T cells (original magnification: 500× magnification). (From Knowles DM. Non-Hodgkin's lymphomas: I. Immunologic and enzymatic markers useful in their evaluation. In: Fenoglio CM, Wolff M, eds. *Progress in surgical pathology,* vol 2. New York: Masson Publishing, 1980:71–105, with permission.)

the less mature plasma cells of Waldenström's macroglobulinemia and lymphoplasmacytoid lymphoma (205,214) and are absent from the terminally differentiated plasma cells of multiple myeloma (205). Only rare TdT$^+$ precursor T-cell lymphoblastic lymphomas/leukemias express HLA-DR antigens (221,222). HLA-DR antigens, however, are expressed variably by all categories of postthymic T-cell neoplasia (13,14). For example, approximately 75% or more of cutaneous T-cell lymphomas (223–226), 60% to 70% of peripheral T-cell lymphomas (227–229), and 30% of adult T-cell lymphomas/leukemias (230,231) express HLA-DR antigens. HLA-DR antigens are expressed by approximately 90% of French–American–British (FAB) M1 and M2 AMLs (232–234), greater than 95% of FAB M4 and M5 AMLs (232–234), and in cases of acute myelofibrosis (235), but only rarely by FAB M3 acute myeloid (promyelocytic) leukemias (232–234). HLA-DR antigens are expressed in approximately 90% of patients with chronic myelogenous leukemia in myeloid and lymphoid blast crisis (232,236,237) but are not expressed in chronic myelogenous leukemia (203). HLA-DR antigens also have been described in a variety of nonhematopoietic neoplasms, most commonly malignant melanomas (238–240).

MONOCLONAL ANTIBODY–DEFINED IMMUNOPHENOTYPIC MARKERS

Background and Nomenclature

Around 1980, Kung, Goldstein, and colleagues (242) employed the hybridoma technology developed by Kohler and Milstein (241) to prepare the OKT MAbs. These investigators, in collaboration with Reinherz and Schlossman, demonstrated that the OKT MAbs recognize antigens expressed by T cells at specific points during normal T-cell ontogeny and by functionally distinct T-cell subsets (137,242–244). Their findings led to the proposal of the first hypothetical schema of normal human T-cell differentiation (243,244). According to this scheme, maturing T cells serially acquire and lose various MAb-defined cell surface antigens as they differentiate from prothymocytes into mature, peripheral immunocompetent T cells (243,244). Immunophenotypic studies with these MAb reagents led to considerable advances in our understanding of the histogenesis of T-cell neoplasms and their relationship to normal T-cell ontogeny.

Subsequently, numerous investigators prepared and distributed large numbers of MAbs detecting identical, closely related, or novel T-cell antigens as well as other lymphohematopoietic antigens. These MAbs sometimes were poorly characterized prior to their release. Moreover, investigators and commercial distributors employed their own personal, diverse, and randomly selected terminology to designate their MAbs. Consequently, users of these reagents often were presented with multiple distinct MAbs, designated by seemingly nonsensical abbreviations of inapparent significance, which often detected identical or closely related antigens. For example, multiple MAbs (A50, T1, T101, Leu1, and UCHT2) detect the same gp67 antigen expressed by benign and malignant T cells and B-cell chronic lymphocytic leukemia cells (15). This complex and confusing terminology served as a formidable barrier for physicians entering the field and attempting to understand the immunodiagnostic literature, and it impeded the widespread implementation of these reagents in the diagnosis and classification of hematopoietic neoplasms.

In order to alleviate problems in nomenclature, the World Health Organization, in conjunction with the International Union of Immunological Societies, the Institut National de la Sante et de la Recherche Medicale, and the Medical Research Council, sponsored the First International Workshop on Human Leukocyte Differentiation Antigens in 1982 (15). Data were collected on the reactivities of numerous MAbs with specific target cells, and statistical methods were employed to define groups of antibodies with similar reactivity. Each distinct MAb group was designated a cluster of differentiation (CD). For example, MAbs A50, T1, T101, Leu1, and UCHT2 were clustered together as CD5 (15). Since then, five more International Leukocyte Differentiation Antigen Workshops have been conducted (16–20). These meetings have provided a forum for objectively defining the reactivity of the vast array of privately and commercially generated MAbs and for designating them with a standardized, internationally accepted nomenclature.

Monoclonal Antibodies Useful in Immunophenotypic Analysis

Literally thousands of MAbs generated by numerous commercial and private laboratories have been evaluated during the first six International Leukocyte Differentiation Antigen Workshops (15–20). Many of these MAbs detect identical antigens or different epitopes of the same antigen, and only a finite number of distinct MAb CD clusters have been defined thus far (Table 3.1). A detailed description of the structure, function, and expression of selected MAb CD clusters useful in cell suspension, frozen tissue section, or paraffin tissue section immunophenotypic analysis is presented subsequently.

Panhematopoietic Cell Antigens

CD45

The CD45 MAb cluster, commonly referred to as *leukocyte common antigen* (LCA), was defined at the third workshop by numerous antibodies (245). LCA represents a family of proteins that are equivalent to murine Ly-5 (246). The LCA proteins belong to a broader family of protein tyrosine phosphatases that includes a minimum of 16 other members, including at least seven other transmembrane proteins (247). CD45 is expressed on the surface membrane of virtually all lymphohematopoietic cells and their progenitors, except

TABLE 3.1. *Leukocyte differentiation antigens*

CD designation	Representative assigned monoclonal antibodies	kd	Comments	Principal reactivity
CD1a	T6, Leu-6, NA1/34, O10	gp49	Non-peptide antigen-presenting molecule; lymphocyte activation signal?	Cortical Thy, LC, IDC
CD1b	WM-25, 4A76	gp43	Non-peptide antigen-presenting molecule; lymphocyte activation signal?	Cortical Thy, LC, IDC
CD1c	L161, M241, PHM3	gp45	Non-peptide antigen-presenting molecule; lymphocyte activation signal?	Cortical Thy, LC, IDC, B subset
CD2	T11, 9.6, OKT11, Leu5	gp50	E-rosette receptor; LFA-2 receptor for CD58, CD48, CD59, and CD15; adhesion and signal transducing molecule	Thy, T, NK
CD2R	T11.3, VIT13	gp50	E-rosette receptor; LFA-2 receptor for CD58, CD48, CD59, and CD15; adhesion and signal transducing molecule	Act T
CD3	T3, Leu4, UCHT1, CD3	gp/p25, 21, 20, 16	Assembly and expression of TCR complex	Precursor T, Thy (cytoplasmic, surface), T (surface)
CD4	OKT4, Leu3a, T4, NCL-CD4	gp55	Binds to MHC class II; HIV receptor	T subset, M
CD5	Leu1, T101, T1, UCHT2	gp67	Costimulatory molecule	Thy, T, B subset
CD6	T12, VIT12	gp100/130	Adhesion molecule	T subset, B subset
CD7	3A1, Leu9, 4A, WT1	gp40	Possible coactivation/adhesion modulating molecule	Precursor T, T subset, T, NK
CD8	T8, Leu2a, UCHT4, NCL-CD8	gp68	Binds to MHC class I	T subset, NK
CD9	BA-2, ALB-6	p24	Adhesion? Activation?	Plt, Precursor B, Act T
CD10	J5, BA-3, VILA1	gp100	Zinc metalloprotease; neutral endopeptidase 24.11	Precursor B, B subset, G
CD11a	2F12, CRIS3	gp180/(95)	LFA-1α; leukocyte adhesion	Leukocytes, broad
CD11b	Mo1, OKM1	gp170/(95)	CR3; iC3b receptor; adherence; chemotaxis	G, M, NK
CD11c	LeuM5, L29, B-lyb	gp150/(95)	Adherence; chemotaxis	G, M, NK
CDw12	M67	p90–120	Function unknown	G, M, NK
CD13	My7, MCS-2	gp150	Zinc metalloprotease; aminopeptidase N	G, M
CD14	Mo2, My4, LeuM3	gp55	GPI-linked; receptor for lipopolysaccharide	M, (G), LC
CD15	My-1, LeuM1, IG10	X-hapten	Lacto-N-Fucopentaose III; Lewis antigen; Cell adhesion?	G, (M), Reed-Sternberg cells
CD15s	2F3, SNH-3	Sialyl Le^x	Cell adhesion; ligand for E-, P-, and L-selectin (CD62E, P and L)	G, M, NK, Act T, Act B
CD16	3G8, B73.1, NCL-CD16	gp50–65	Low affinity receptor for IgG; FcγRIIIa: Transmembrane; FcγRIIIb: GPI-linked; regulation of NK cytotoxicity and cytokine production	NK, Act M, Macrophages, G
CDw17	GO35, Huly-M13	Carbohydrate	Lactosylceramide; phagocytosis?	G, M, Plt, B subset
CD18	M232, MHM23	(180)/95	β chain of CD11a,b,c; leukocyte adhesion	Leukocytes, broad
CD19	B4, Leu12	gp95	Signal transduction molecule	Precursor B, B
CD20	B1, Leu16, L26	p33	Regulates cell cycle progession	Precursor B subset, B
CD21	B2, OKB7, HB-5	gp140	CR2; C3d/EBV receptor	B subset, FDC, T subset
CD22	HD39, To15, S-HCL1	gp140	Adhesion molecule: signaling molecule	Precursor B, B

(continued)

TABLE 3.1. *Continued.*

CD designation	Representative assigned monoclonal antibodies	kd	Comments	Principal reactivity
CD23	Blast-2, Leu20, MHM6	gp45	Low-affinity receptor for IgE (FcϵRII)	Act B, Act M, Eo, FDC subset
CD24	BA-1, VIB-E3, OKB2	gp35–45	Homologous to mouse heat stable antigen; GPI-linked on G	Precursor B, B, G
CD25	Tac, 7G7/B6	gp55	IL-2R α chain	Act T, Act B, Act M
CD26	BA5, TS145	gp110	Dipeptidyl peptidase IV	Act T, Act B, Act NK
CD27	VIT14, OKT18A	gp55	Receptor for CD70; costimulatory molecule	Thy subset, T, NK, B subset
CD28	9.3, KOLT2	gp44	Receptor for CD80/CD86; Costimulatory molecule	T subset, PC
CD29	K20, 4B4	gp130	Integrin β1; adhesion receptor	Leukocytes, broad
CD30	Ki-1, Ber-H2	gp120	Cell activation; Intracellular signaling	Act T, Act B, Reed-Sternberg cells
CD31	SG134, TM3	gp135	PECAM-1; adhesion receptor; transendothelial migration	Plt, M, G, B, (T)
CD32	2E1, IV.3	gp32	Low affinity IgG receptor (FcγRII)	M, G, B, Eo, Bas, Plt
CD33	My9, LeuM9, L4F3	gp67	Sialic acid-dependent cell adhesion molecule	Precursor myeloid, M
CD34	My10, BI-3C5, QBEND10	gp105–120	Cell adhesion	Hematopoietic progenitor cells, Endothelium
CD35	To5, CB04, J3D3	gp160–280	CR1; C3b/C4b receptor (immune adherence); regulates complement activation	G, M, E, B, FDC, T subset
CD36	5F1, OKM5	gp88	Plt GPIV (GPIIIb); cell adhesion	Plt, M, (B)
CD37	HD28, HH1	gp52-40	Signal transduction	B, (T), (M), (G)
CD38	OKT10, T16, Leu17	p45	ADP-ribosyl cyclase; regulator of cell activation and proliferation	Lymphoid progenitor cells, NK, Act T, PC
CD39	AC2, OKT28, G28-10	gp70–100	Possible ectoapyrase	B subset, Act T, NK, M, LC, DC
CD40	G28-5, S2C6	gp48	Costimulatory molecule, survival receptor	B, FDC, IDC, (M)
CD41	CLB-Thromb/7, PMB6.4	gp140	Integrin α11β; GPIIb; mediates platelet adhesion	Plt
CD42a–d	FMC25, PHN89, G1–27, V3	gp22/160/22/82	GPX, Ibα/Ibβ, V complex; receptor for von Willebrand factor; mediates platelet adhesion to subendothelial matrices	Plt
CD43	Leu22, MT1, DF-T1	gp115–135	Leukosialin (Sialophorin); antiadhesion (barrier) molecule	Thy, T, G, M, NK, Act B, PC
CD44	F10-44-2, GRHL 1	gp85	Pgp-1; hermes; lymphocyte homing receptor; costimulatory molecule	Leukocytes, broad
CD45	T29/33, 2811	gp180/190/205/220	Leukocyte common antigen (LCA); Regulator of leukocyte activation	Leukocytes, broad
CD45RA	4KB5, MB1, MT2	gp205/220	Restricted LCA; regulator of leukocyte activation	Naive/resting T, B, M, NK
CD45RB	PD7/26	gp190/205/220	Restricted LCA; regulator of leukocyte activation	T subset, B, G, M
CD45RO	UCHL-1, OPD4, A6	gp180	Restricted LCA; regulator of leukocyte activation	Cortical Thy, Act/memory T, M, G
CD46	HulyM5, J4B	gp66/56	Membrane cofactor protein	Leukocytes, broad
CD47	BRIC126	gp47–52	Adhesion receptor	Leukocytes, broad
CD48	WM68, J4–57	gp41	GPI-linked; adhesion molecule	Leukocytes
CD49a–f	GoH3, B5G10, CLB-thromb/4	gp25/135–gp200	Integrin-α1–α6; VLA-1α to VLA6α; adhesion receptors	Wide range
CD50	BU68	gp110–140	ICAM-3; ligand for LFA-1; costimulatory molecule	Leukocytes, broad
CD51	13C2, 23C6	gp150	α chain of vitronectin receptor; (β chain is CD61); adhesion molecule	Plt
CD52	097, YTH66.9	gp8–9	CAMPATH-1; Function unknown	B, T, NK, M
CD53	H129, H136	gp32–42	Signal transduction	B, T, M, NK, G
CD54	OKT27, MY13, RR1/1	gp90	ICAM-1; LFA-1 ligand; adhesion receptor	B, T, M, G, Endothelium

TABLE 3.1. *Continued.*

CD designation	Representative assigned monoclonal antibodies	kd	Comments	Principal reactivity
CD55	H4	gp72	Decay acceleration factor; GPI-linked	All hematopoietic cells
CD56	KH1, Leu19, N901, 123C3	gp135–220	N-CAM; Homotypic and heterotypic adhesion	NK, Act T
CD57	HNK1	gp110	Function unknown	NK subset, T subset, Neuroectodermal cells
CD58	G26, TS2/9	gp55–70	GPI-linked; LFA3; ligand for CD2; costimulatory molecule	Leukocytes, broad
CD59	MEM-43, YTH53.1	gp20	GPI-linked; protectin; inhibition of terminal complement pathway	Most cells
CDw60	MT32	Carbohydrate	Function unknown	Plt, T subset
CD61	CLB-thromb/1, Y2/51	gp110	GPIIIa; $\beta 3$ chain of vitronectin receptor (α chain is CD51)	Plt
CD62E	H4/18,H18/7	gp115	E-selectin; ELAM-1; mediates leukocyte rolling	Endothelium
CD62L	Leu8, Dreg 56	gp74	L-selectin; receptor for lymphocyte homing: receptor for lymphocyte rolling	B, T, M, G, NK
CD62P	CLB-Thromb/6	gp140	P-selectin; PADGEM; platelet adhesion; phagocyte binding; binds to CD162	Act Plt
CD63	CLB-gran/12	gp55	Function unknown	Act Plt, M, G
CD64	32.3	gp72	High affinity Fc receptor for IgG (FcγRI); endocytosis; phagocytosis; antibody dependent cell-mediated cytotoxicity	M, (G)
CD65	VIM8, HE10	Carbohydrate	Type II chain fucoganglioside; function unknown	G, M
CD65s	V1M2	Carbohydrate	Sialylated CD65; potential E- or P-selectin ligand	G, M
CD66a–f	CLB-gran/10, G0F5, B13.9, B6.2	gp35/54–72 90/95–100/ 140–180/ 180	Carcinoembryonic antigen family; homophilic and heterophilic adhesion; E-selectin binding	G, Epithelial cells G
CD68	Ki-M6, Ki-M7, Y2/131, KP1, PGM1	gp110	A macrosialin; function unknown	M, G
CD69	Leu23, MLR3, L78	p32/28	Activation inducer molecule; leukocyte activation	Act leukocytes
CD70	Ki-24, BU69	p29	Ligand for CD27; costimulation of B and T cells	Act B, Act T
CD71	OKT9, T9, VIP-1	gp95	Transferrin receptor; iron uptake	Precursor E, All proliferating cells
CD72	S-HCL2, BU-40	gp39–43	Ligand for CD5	Precursor B, B
CD73	1E9.28.1, 7G2.2.11	p69	Ecto-5′ nucleotidase; GPI-linked	B subset, T subset
CD74	LN2, BU43, BU45	p33/35/41	MHC class II-associated invariant chain	B, M, Act T, LC, DC
CDw75	LN1, OKB4, HH2	Unknown	Possible ligand for CD22	B subset, E, (T subset)
CDw76	HD66, CRIS-4	Unknown	Function unknown	B, T subset
CD77	38.13, KH1, 5B5	Carbohydrate	Transducer of an apoptopic signal	B subset
CDw78	Leu21, BA612G2	Unknown	Function unknown	Precursor B, B, Act B, M
CD79a	HM47, HM57, JCB117	gp40–45	Ig-a; component of B cell receptor; signal transduction	Precursor B, B, Act B
CD79b	SN8, B29/123, CH3-1	gp37	Ig-b; component of B cell receptor; signal transduction	Precursor B, B, Act B
CD80	B7, BB1	gp60	Ligand for CD28 and CD152; costimulatory molecule	B subset, Act T

(continued)

TABLE 3.1. *Continued.*

CD designation	Representative assigned monoclonal antibodies	kd	Comments	Principal reactivity
CD81	1D6, 5A6	p26	Signal transduction	Leukocytes, broad
CD82	4F9, C33, IA4	gp45–90	Costimulation	Leukocytes, broad
CD83	HB15a, HB15b	gp45	Function unknown	Act B, LC, IDC, DC
CD84	2G7, 152-1D5	gp64–82	Function unknown	B, Act B, M, T subset, Plt
CD85	VMP55, H47	gp110	Possible role in T-cell activation	B, Act B, PC, M, T subset, NK subset
CD86	BU63, FUN-1	gp80	B7-2/B70; ligand for CD28 and CD152; costimulatory molecule	IDC, LC, DC, M, B subset, Act B
CD87	V1M5, IID7	gp55	Urokinase plasminogen activator receptor; facilitates pericellular proteolysis by invading inflammatory and neoplastic cells; GPI-linked	T subset, M subset, NK subset, G subset, Endothelium
CD88	4C8	gp43	Complement C5a receptor	G, Eo, M
CD89	My43, A3, A77	gp65	IgA Fc receptor (Fc2R); Induces phagocytosis, degranulation, respiratory burst	Precursor myeloid, G, M
CD90	5E10, V45	gp18	Thy-1; may contribute to hematopoietic stem cell and neuronal cell differentiation	High endothelium, hematopoietic stem cells
CD91	A2MRb-1, A2MRa-1	gp600	α_2-macroglobulin receptor; Endocystosis-mediating	M, Multiple noncell types
CDw92	V1M15, V1M15b	gp70	Function unknown	M, G, (B), (T)
CDw93	V1MD2, X2	gp110–120	Function unknown	M, G, Endothelium
CD94	HP-3D9, NKH3	p30	Assembled with other C-type lectins; forms inhibitory or activating receptors for HLA class I	NK, T subset
CD95	APO-1, CH11, 7C11	p43	Receptor molecule for Fas ligand, which mediates apoptosis-inducing signals	Act B, Act T, Thy subset
CD96	G8.5	gp160	Adhesion of activated T and NK cells during the late phase of immune response	Act NK, Act T, (NK), (T)
CD97	V1M3, BL-Ac/F2	gp75–85	Adhesion molecule; CD55 ligand	M, N, Act B, Act T, (B), (T)
CD98	MEM-108, BU53, 4F2	gp80/p45	Regulates T-cell proliferation	Thy, Act T, (leukocytes)
CD99	0662, L129	gp32	M1C2 gene product; Modulates T-cell adhesion; Induces apoptosis of $CD4^+CD8^+$ thymocytes	Thy, T, Act T, NK, G, E, many nonhematopoietic cells and tumors
CD99R	D44, FMC-29	gp32	Modulates T cell adhesion; Induces apoptosis of $CD4^+CD8^+$ thymocytes	Cortical Thy, Act T, NK, G, E, (T), (many non-hematopoietic cells and tumors)
CD100	A8, BB18	gp150	Physically associated with CD45 and a serine kinase; costimulatory molecule for T cells	Act T, T, B subset, (M), (N), (NK)
CD101	BB27, BA27, BC27	gp130	Costimulatory molecule	M, G, DC, Act T
CD102	6D5, B-R7	gp55–65	ICAM-2; Ligand for LFA-1; costimulatory molecule	Endothelium, (M), (T), (B)
CD103	HML-1, B-1y7	gp25/150	Integrin-α E subunit; receptor for E-cadherin	Intraepithelial lymphocytes in MALT, Lamina propria T cells
CD104	AA3, ASC-3	gp205–220	Integrin β4; receptor for laminins; hemidesmosome formation; cell migration toward basement membrane	Epithelium, Schwann cells
CD105	1G2, 44G4, E-9	gp180	Endoglin; transforming growth factor-β coreceptor	Epithelium, Act M, Macrophages, Precursor B subset

TABLE 3.1. *Continued.*

CD designation	Representative assigned monoclonal antibodies	kd	Comments	Principal reactivity
CD106	2G7, Hu8/4	gp110	VCAM-1; mediates cell–cell adhesion and signaling with α4 integrin bearing cells	Act Endothelium, FDC, IDC
CD107a	H5G11, BB6	gp110–120	Lysosome-associated membrane protein-1; function unknown; cell adhesion?	Degranulated Plt
CD107b	H4B4	gp110–120	Lysosome-associated membrane protein-2; function unknown; cell adhesion?	Degranulated Plt
CDw108	MEM-121, H8, N-L156	gp80	JMH human blood antigen; Function unknown; GPI-linked	E, (B), (T)
CD109	8A3, 7D1	gp170	Function unknown	Act Plt, Act T, Endothelium
CD114	129,LMM741	gp130	Granulocyte-colony stimulating factor receptor	Myeloid progenitor cells, G, M
CD115	7-7A3-14	gp150	Macrophage-colony stimulating factor receptor	Progenitor M, M, Osteoclasts
CD116	2B7-17-A, S-50, SC06	gp80	Granulocyte-macrophage colony stimulating factor (GM-CSF) receptor α subunit; low affinity GM-CSF binding	G and M progenitors, G, M, Meg subset, Eo
CD117	17F11, 4B5.B8	gp145	c-KIT; stem cell factor receptor	Hematopoietic stem and progenitor cells, Mast cells
CDw119	G1R 208, G1R-301	gp80–95	Human interferon γ receptor α chain; ligand trafficking through the cell	Most cells except E
CD120a	htr9	p55	Tumor necrosis factor receptor type I	Most cells
CD120b	utr1	p75	Tumor necrosis factor receptor type II	Most cells
CD121a	M1, 6B5	gp80	Interleukin-I receptor type I; signaling receptor	Most cells
CDw121b	M2	gp65	Interleukin-1 receptor type II; negative regulator of IL-1	Most cells
CD122	Mik-β1, Tu27	gp70–75	Common subunit for 1L-2R and 1L-15R; signal transduction	T, B, NK, M, Act T
CD123	7G3, S-12, 9F5	gp70	1L-3R α subunit; low affinity 1L-3 binding	Myeloid progenitors, G, Eo, M, Mast cells, B subset, Endothelial cell subset
CD124	hIL-4R-M57	gp140	1L-4 and 1L-13 receptor	Act B, Act T, B, T, M, (NK), (G)
CDw125	KM1257, KM1266	gp160	1L-5 receptor α chain	Eo, Bas, Act B
CD126	MT18, PM1, M11	gp80	Low affinity receptor for 1L-6	T, M, Act B
CD127	h1L-7R-M20		1L-7 receptor	Precursor B, T, (B)
CDw128	9H1, 10H2	gp67–70	IL-8R types I,II; CXCR 1/2; Neutrophil chemotaxis and activation; T-cell chemotaxis; histamine and leukotriene release from basophils	G, M, (NK), (T subset)
CD130	AM64, B-K5, B-T6, B-58, GPX7	gp130–140	Common subunit for 1L-6, 1L-11, oncostatin M, leukemia inhibitory factor, ciliary neurotrophic factor and cardiotrophin 1 receptor	Most cells
CDw131	3D7, S-16	gp140	Common β subunit of 1L-3, 1L-5, and GM-CSF receptors	Myeloid progenitors, G, Eo, M, B subset, Mast cells
CD132	3B5, 3G11, AG184	gp164	Common γ subunit of 1L-2, 1L-4, 1L-7, 1L-9 and 1L-15 receptors	B, T, G, M, NK, Act T
CD134	L106	gp50	Receptor for OX40 ligand; Costimulatory molecule; adhesion molecule	Medullary thy, T, Act T
CD135	M22, 4G8, BV10	gp155	Growth factor receptor for early hematopoietic progenitors; receptor tyrosine kinase; Costimulatory molecule; Survival receptor	Myelomonocytic progenitors, Precursor B

(continued)

TABLE 3.1. *Continued.*

CD designation	Representative assigned monoclonal antibodies	kd	Comments	Principal reactivity
CDw136	1D1, 1D2	gp180	Macrophage-stimulating protein receptor; chemotactic migration; cytokine induction; phagocytosis; cell differentiation; morphological change	M, Epithelium, Developing bones
CDw137	4B4, M121	gp39	Receptor for 4-1BB ligand; costimulatory molecule	Act T, T
CD138	B-B4, 1D4, F59-2E9, MI15	gp85–92	Snydecan-1; extracellular matrix receptor	PC, B subset, Epithelium
CD139	CAT13.4G9, BU30	gp209–228	Function unknown	Precursor B, B, Act B, FDC, (M), (G), (Eo), E
CD140a	16A1, PR292	gp170–190	Platelet derived growth factor α receptor	Mesenchymal cells
CD140b	28D4, PR7212	gp170–190	Platelet derived growth factor β receptor	M, G, Mesenchymal cells
CD141	1A4, KA-4	gp75	Thrombomodulin; cofactor in the thrombin-mediated activation of protein C	Endothelium, M, G, Meg, Plt, Keratinocytes
CD142	MTFH-1, V-D8, TF10-1D10	gp45	Tissue factor; initiator of the blood clotting cascade; cell surface receptor for factor VII	Endothelium, M, Keratinocytes, Epithelium
CD143	9B9, 3A5	gp170	Angiotensin-converting enzyme; peptidyl dipeptidase	Selected endothelium Epithelium, Neuronal cells
CD144	BV6, BV9, hec1	gp135	VE-cadherin; control of endothelial permeability, growth, and migration	Endothelium
CD145	7E9, P7A5	gp25/90/110	Function unknown	Endothelium
CD146	Muc18, MN3, MuBA 18.2	gp118	Function unknown; adhesion? Cell–cell contact?	Endothelium, Act T
CD147	I32,HB4,HIM6	gp50–60	Neurothelin/basigin; potential adhesion molecule	Leukocytes (Broad) E, Plt, Epithelium, Endothelium
CD148	143-41, A3, MEM133, MEM120	gp200–260 gp120–130	Protein phosphatase Function unknown	M, G, DC, Act T, (B), (T), (NK),(Plt), B, T, M, NK, (G), (Eo), (Plt)
CDw150	A12, 1PO-3	gp75–95	Signaling lymphocyte activation molecule (SLAM); costimulatory molecule	Thy, DC, T subset, B subset, Act B
CD151	14A2, H1, 11B1.G4	gp28–32	Integrin-associated protein; transmembrane signaling; homotypic adhesion	Meg, Plt, Endothelium, Epithelium
CD152	11D4, 7F8	gp33	Cytotoxic T lymphocyte-associated molecule-4 (CTLA-4); receptor for CD80/CD86; negative regulator of T cell activation	Act T, Act B
CD153	M80, M81, M82	gp40	Ligand for CD30; costimulatory for T cells	B, Act T, Act M, G
CD154	TRAP-1, 5C8, M79	gp33	Ligand for CD40; essential germinal center formation and antibody class switching; costimulatory molecule	Act T
CD155	D171, PV404	gp80–90	Poliovirus receptor	M, Neurons
CD156	1-11-G, 3-2-c	gp60	Metalloprotease	M, G
CD157	Mo5, Bec7, RF3	gp42–45	ADP-ribosyl cyclase; GPI-linked	M, G, Bone marrow stromal cells, Endothelium
CD158a	EB6, HP-3E4	gp50/58	Receptor for HLA-C alleles (CW2,3,4,5 and 6)	NK, T subset
CD158b	CH-L, GL183	gp50/58	Receptor for HLA-C alleles (CW1,3,7 and 8)	NK, T subset
CD161	DX12, HP-3G10	gp80	Regulation of NK cell cytolytic activity; regulation of thymocyte precursor proliferation	NK, Thy subset, T subset
CD162	PL1, PL2	gp110	P-selectin glycoprotein ligand-1; Receptor for leukocyte rolling	G, M, T, B subset

TABLE 3.1. *Continued.*

CD designation	Representative assigned monoclonal antibodies	kd	Comments	Principal reactivity
CD163	GHi/61, D11, Ber-Mac3, Ki-M8	gp110	Function unknown	M, Macrophage
CD164	105.A5, 103B.2/9E10	gp80	Adhesion of hematopoietic progenitor cell to cultured bone marrow stroma	M, Bone marrow stromal cells, Epithelium
CD165	ADL, SN2	gp37	Adhesion of thymocytes to thymic epithelial cells	Plt, (Leukocytes, broad), Thy, Thymic epithelium
CD166	3A6, J4–81, HAL8.2	gp100	Activated leukocyte cell adhesion molecule (ALCAM); ligand for CD6	Endothelium, Act T, Act M, Thymic epithelium, Neurons

This list reports the clusters of differentiation as defined at the Sixth International Workshop on Human Leukocyte Differentiation Antigens (20). The CD designation defines the antibody clusters.

Thy, thymocytes; LC, Langerhans cell; IDC, Interdigitating dendritic cell; FDC, Follicular dendritic cell; Act, activated; B, B cells; T, T cells; G, neutrophils; M, monocytes; Eo, eosinophils; Bas, basophils; NK, natural killer cells; Plt, platelets; PC, plasma cells; E, erythrocytes; CR, complement receptor, FcR, receptor for the Fc portion of Ig; GPI, glycosyl phosphatidylinositol; MHC, major histocompatibility complex; LCA, leukocyte common antigen; LFA, leukocyte function antigen; IL-2R; interleukin-2 receptor; TCR, T-cell receptor; NCAM, neuronal cell adhesion molecule, ICAM, intercellular cell adhesion molecule.

megakaryocytes and erythroid cells, and thus represents a panhematopoietic cell marker. CD45 is not expressed by any nonlymphohematopoietic cells (248). In addition, many anti-CD45 MAbs are immunoreactive in routinely fixed, paraffin-embedded tissue sections. For these reasons, anti-CD45 MAbs have become among the most widely utilized immunodiagnostic reagents in pathology (249).

All the LCA proteins are encoded by a single gene located on 1q31-32 (250). The gene is composed of 33 exons that code for the cDNA sequence and 3′ and 5′ nontranslated regions (251). The protein consists of a large globular cytoplasmic domain of 707 amino acids coded by exons 17 through 32, a transmembrane region of 22 amino acids coded by exon 16, and a rod-like external domain of 391, 438, 486, 504 or 552 amino acids, depending on the pattern of exon splicing, coded by exons 3 through 15 (251,252). The cytoplasmic domain is highly conserved among mammalian species. It consists of two homologous subdomains, coded by exons 17 through 24 and 25 through 32, that are separated by a short spacer region (247,252,253). Both subdomains possess significant homology with placental tyrosine phosphatase (254), and CD45 proteins possess intrinsic tyrosine phosphatase activity (255). The external domain is less conserved. It consists of an O-linked region and two cysteine-rich subdomains, all of which are heavily glycosylated (249,252).

The heterogeneity of the LCA protein family is a result of the differential usage of three exons, termed *A*, *B*, and *C*, within the LCA gene. These exons code for amino acid sequences of different lengths, which are located in the O-linked region within the external domain of LCA (256). They generate eight different mRNAs (257,258) and at least five distinct LCA proteins (256) (Table 3.2). The expression of these individual CD45 proteins is controlled in a cell type–specific fashion that has been conserved throughout mammalian evolution (259–263).

The LCA protein family has been implicated in a variety of immunologic processes and is of critical importance to

TABLE 3.2. *Protein isoforms of CD45 proteins and antibody reactivities*

Known Isoforms of CD45 Proteins			Immunoprecipitation band, kd	Antibody reactivity				Cell expression
				CD45	CD45RA	CD45RB	CD45RO	
A	B	C	220	+	+	+	–	Pre-B and B cells
A	B	—	205	+	+	+	–	Naive T cells
—	B	C	205	+	–	+	–	T cells
—	B	—	190	+	–	+	–	Macrophages; T cells; plasma cell subset; marginal zone B cells
—	—	—	180	+	–	–	+	Macrophages; granulocytes; thymocytes; memory T cells; transformed B cells; preplasma cells

From Weiss LM, Arber DA, Chang KL. CD45: A review. *Appl Immunohistochem* 1993;1:166–181, with permission.

the function of both T and B lymphocytes (249). CD45 molecules appear to be involved in promoting cell-to-cell interactions and intracellular signaling (248,249). For example, antigen-induced T-cell proliferation appears to require CD45 (264). CD45 is required for both T-cell antigen receptor and CD2-mediated activation of T-cell protein tyrosine kinase (265). CD45-deficient T-cell clones have impaired responses to TCR stimuli (266). CD45 is linked physically to both CD2 and the TCR on the surface of memory T cells (267,268). It is believed that LFA-1 is associated with the exon A–encoded region, and that CD4 and CD8 are associated with the exon C–encoded region of CD45. CD2 may be associated with a receptor formed when exons A, B, and C are absent (269). Although the precise interactions have not been delineated, the external domain is believed to function as a receptor for one or more as yet undetermined ligands (249). The structural differences among the external domains of the different CD45 proteins probably determine the specific target stimuli for the different cell types expressing CD45 (249). CD45 proteins also may be important in B-cell function. Experimental data suggest that the CD45 expressed on B cells occurs as a component of a protein complex associated with the B-cell antigen receptor, and that CD45 may regulate signal transduction by modulating the phophorylation state of the antigen receptor subunits (249). Finally, CD45 proteins are potent inhibitors of NK cell cytolysis (270), which may be mediated through carbohydrate structures on the external domain of CD45 (271). These and other functional activities of the CD45 molecules are reviewed in more detail elsewhere (248,249).

Numerous MAbs that detect members of the LCA family have been described (249) (Table 3.3). Those antibodies that recognize epitopes common to all members of the LCA family are clustered as CD45 (272). These MAbs immunoprecipitate four chains with molecular weights of 220 kd (ABC isoform), 205 kd (two distinct AB and BC isoforms), 190 kd (B isoform), and 180 kd (O isoform) (245). Those antibodies that only recognize a subset of the LCA isoforms are clustered as CD45R (restricted) (245,272,273) (Fig. 3.11). The CD45R antibodies are subclustered further by employing the suffixes *A*, *B*, and *O* to indicate those MAbs that recognize LCA proteins containing the exon A sequence (CD45RA), containing the exon B sequence (CD45RB), and lacking the A, B, and C exon sequences (CD45RO) (273). MAbs that specifically recognize proteins containing the C exon sequence have not been identified (249). Therefore, anti-CD45RA antibodies immunoprecipitate 220- and 205-kd proteins; anti-CD45RB antibodies immunoprecipitate 220-, 205-, and 190-kd proteins; and anti-CD45RO antibodies only immunoprecipitate the 180-kd protein (245,274,275) (Table 3.2). In addition to the numerous antibodies that can be assigned to the CD45 cluster or to the CD45R subclusters, numerous other MAbs, such as MT3 (276), whose CD45 epitopes have not been well characterized, also exist (249). In addition, there are MAbs that specifically recognize the carbohydrate structures that are added to the LCA proteins posttranslationally (277).

CD45 proteins are major components of the lymphoid cell surface membrane, accounting for much of the membrane carbohydrate and about 10% of the lymphoid cell surface (253). Ultrastructural studies have localized MAb PD7-2B11 immune reactivity predominantly to the surface membrane and occasionally to the paranuclear regions of lymphoid cells (278). Consequently, the pattern of CD45 immune reactivity at the light microscopic level usually is strong linear membrane staining (27,278,279). Granular membranous, diffuse cytoplasmic, and focal paranuclear (Golgi region) positivity, however, also have been noted (278,279).

CD45 expression appears to occur very early in B-cell ontogeny, apparently prior to immunoglobulin gene rearrangement, and continues throughout B-cell differentiation until about the preplasma cell stage (249). Most immature and mature B cells strongly express the 220-kd isoform and are recognized by anti-CD45, anti-CD45RA, and anti-CD45RB but not by anti-CD45RO MAbs (280,281). These include primary follicle and mantle zone B cells (280,281). Germinal center B cells exhibit similar, albeit often weaker and more variable, reactivity with most anti-CD45, anti-CD45RA, and anti-CD45RB MAbs, especially those whose immunoreactivity is very sensitive to neuraminidase (280,281). Marginal zone B cells express the 190-kd isoform in addition to the 220-kd isoform (280,281). Transformed B cells and preplasma cells tend to lose the 220-kd isoform and begin to produce the 180-kd isoform and may be reactive with anti-CD45RO MAbs (281,282). Plasma cells may lose the 180-kd isoform but produce the 190-kd isoform and be

TABLE 3.3. *Classification of anti-CD45 monoclonal antibodies characterized using cell lines expressing individual CD45 determinants in various studies*

CD45	GAP8.3, anti-HLe, BMAC1, BMAC2, BMAC3, F10-89-4, 13.4, EO1, CMRF.12, 71.4, VIT200, 71.5, G1–14, G25-1, 9.4, TT52, 1–33, S-80, F101–139, 6RT42, 4B2, YTH24.5(830), YTH54.12, T29/33, MEM28, ?2B11[a]
CD45RA	Anti-2H4, 3AC5, F8-11-13, E7, CMRF.11, 73.5.17, G1–15, 10G3, 111-1C5(829), Leu18, 2A10, 5A9, MMT-1, 5E7, 4F4, HB-11, MB1
CD45RB	PD7, MT3[b]
CD45RO	UCHL1, A6, OPD4

[a] 2B11 only reacts against AB transfectant.
[b] MT3 only reacts against B and AB transfectants.
From Weiss LM, Arber DA, Chang KL. CD45: A review. *Appl Immunohistochem* 1993;1:166–181, with permission.

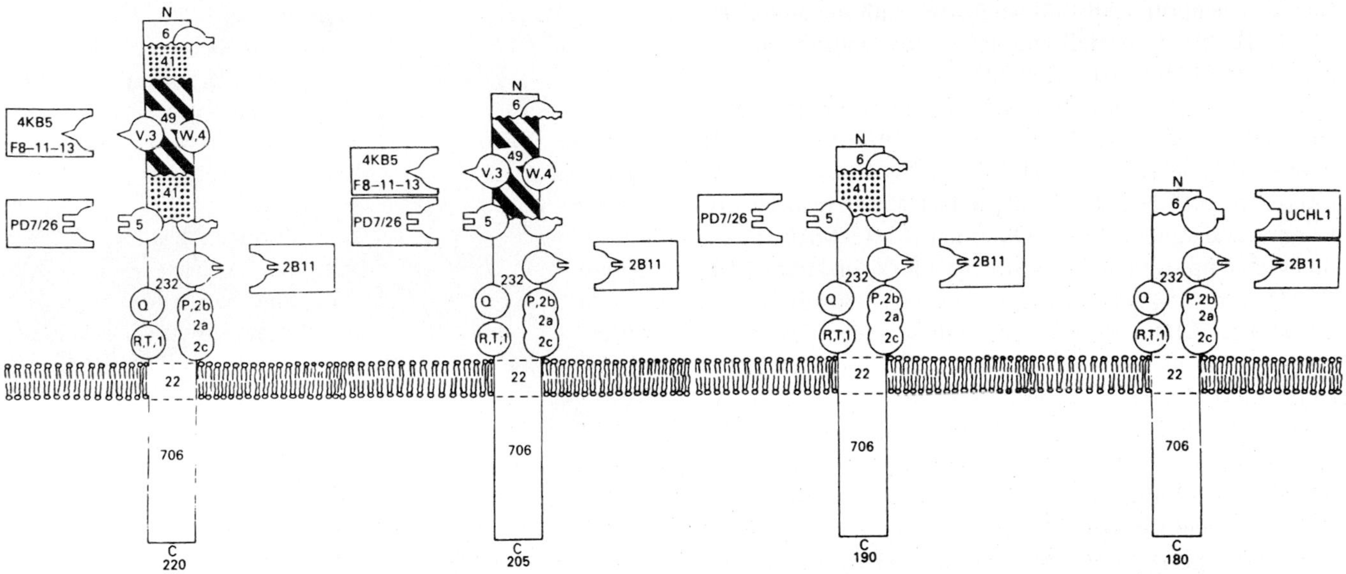

FIG. 3.11. Schematic representation of the four major molecular species of the leukocyte common antigen. The antibodies binding to the antigen are indicated. The shaded portions bearing antibody binding sites for 4KB5 and F8-11-13 are spliced out in the lower molecular weight forms; the binding sites of other anti–leukocyte common antigen antibodies such as 2B11 are conserved in all forms. Molecular weights in kilodaltons are indicated beneath each molecule. (From Norton AJ, Isaacson PG. Lymphoma phenotyping in formalin-fixed and paraffin wax-embedded tissues: I. Range of antibodies and staining patterns. *Histopathology* 1989;14:437–446, with permission.)

recognizable with MAb MT3 (CD45RB) but not with anti-CD45RA or anti-CD45RO MAbs (283). Finally, a subset of plasma cells may lack CD45 proteins entirely (249).

T cells exhibit a more complicated pattern of CD45 protein expression than do B cells. The pattern of CD45 protein expression reflects changes during T-cell activation and functional differences among T-cell subsets (284–287). The most immature thymocytes express only the 180-kd isoform and are recognized only by anti-CD45 and anti-CD45RO MAbs (288). As T-cell differentiation procedes, the 190-kd isoform and the 205-kd (exon BC) isoform are expressed by both the CD4$^+$ and the CD8$^+$ T-cell subsets (286,289) and also are recognizable by anti-CD45RB MAbs, such as MT3 (249). Mature T cells generally express at least one additional CD45 protein, depending on their functional states (287). Naive T cells express the 205-kd (exon AB) isoform and therefore are CD45RA$^+$CD45RO$^-$. In contrast, memory T cells express the 180-kd isoform and therefore are CD45RA$^-$CD45RO$^+$ (287). CD45RA$^+$ T cells rapidly become CDR45RO$^+$ and slowly lose their CD45RA expression on mitogen and antigen stimulation (290). Approximately equivalent numbers of CD45RO$^+$ and CD45RA$^+$ T cells reside in the paracortical regions of lymph nodes (280,288). CD45RO$^+$ T cells comprise almost exclusively the T-cell population of germinal centers and the lamina propria of the gastrointestinal tract (288). A small population of CD45RA$^+$CD45RO$^+$ T cells, probably representing recently activated cells, are particularly prevalent in the intestinal submucosa (288). The CD45RO$^+$ T cells responsible for immunologic memory tend to be larger and to have a faster dividing time and a shorter lifespan than CD45RA$^+$ T cells (249,287,291). They tend to express low levels of molecules associated with T-cell activation and higher levels of lymphocyte adhesion molecules than CD45RA$^+$ T cells (249,287). CD45RA$^+$ T cells tend to produce a wide range of cytokines (249,287). The immunophenotypic features and functional and other properties of these cells are discussed in more detail elsewhere (249,287).

Myeloid and erythroid stem cells and primitive erythroid burst-forming units (E-BFUs) express the 180-kd isoform and are recognized by anti-CD45 and anti-CD45RO MAbs. More mature erythroid cells lack CD45 proteins (292). Granulocyte-macrophage colony-forming units (GM-CFUs) lack CD45RO; mature myeloid cells and monocytes/macrophages generally express CD45RO (292). Monocytes/macrophages and myeloid cells, however, possess a much smaller amount of surface membrane CD45 (mCD45) proteins than lymphoid cells (249). Consequently, CD45 expression by these cell populations often appears to be weak or absent in routine immunodiagnosis (249). Specific monocyte/macrophage subpopulations such as sinus histiocytes, epithelioid histiocytes, and multinucleated giant cells may express CD45RA and CD45RB (278,293,294). Plasmacytoid monocytes weakly express CD45RA and lack CD45RO (295). Mast cells express CD45 (249). CD1$^+$ dendritic cells, including Langerhans cells, express CD45 but express CD45RA, CD45RB, and CD45RO at very low or undetectable levels (27,249,296). Interdigitating dendritic cells and follicular dendritic cells are unreactive with the anti-CD45 MAb PD7-2B11 cocktail but are reactive with the alleged anti-CD45 MAb L3B12 (293,297).

We and most other investigators routinely employ a PD7 and 2B11 MAb cocktail (27,278,279), MAb 4KB5 (298–300), and MAb UCHL1 (274,299,301,302) or A6 (303) to detect CD45, CD45RA, and CD45RO, respectively, in immunodiagnosis (249). Other anti-CD45 MAbs sometimes are employed in diagnostic pathology, including MB1 (CD45RA) (304,305), MT2 (CD45RA) (304,305), and OPD4 (CD45RO) (306,307). All of these antibodies are immunoreactive in frozen tissue sections and also in formalin- and B5-fixed, paraffin-embedded tissue sections (249), although the intensity of immunoreactivity generally is slightly less in fixed tissues (27,249).

Monoclonal antibody 2B11 has been categorized as an anti-CD45 antibody because it recognizes all four (220-, 205-, 190-, and 180-kd) CD45 isoforms and has an appropriately wide pattern of immune reactivity (27,273,308). MAb 2B11 reacts only focally, however, with germinal center and mantle zone B cells (27) and does not react with the CD45 epitope on CD1a$^+$ epidermal and tonsillar epithelial dendritic cells (296). MAb PD7 reacts with the 220-, 205-, and 190-kd isoforms (CD45RB) but not with the 180-kd isoform detected by anti-CD45RO antibodies (27,273,308). MAbs 2B11 and PD7 are commercially available as a CD45-CD45RB MAb cocktail, which is the immunodiagnostic reagent that is employed most commonly to demonstrate CD45 (LCA) expression by benign and malignant lymphohematopoietic cells (249).

This anti-CD45 MAb cocktail displays variable immunoreactivity with lymphohematopoietic cell populations. It is variably reactive with cortical thymocytes but strongly reactive with medullary thymocytes (27,278,309). It is diffusely reactive with the T- and B-cell zones of lymph nodes, tonsils, and spleen. Germinal center B cells, however, exhibit stronger expression than mantle zone B cells, and interfollicular immunoblasts exhibit weaker expression than the surrounding small lymphocytes (27,278,309). It is only weakly or not at all reactive with plasma cells (27,278). It is not reactive with the sinusoidal cells of the spleen (278,309). It reacts variably with cells of macrophage and dendritic cell derivation (27,278). Usually, it does not react with interdigitating dendritic cells, germinal center tingible body macrophages, or follicular dendritic cells but reacts variably with epithelioid histiocytes, Langhans-type giant cells, and sinus histiocytes (278). This MAb cocktail also is reactive with mast cells but is essentially unreactive with megakaryocytes, erthyroid cells, and myeloid cells, except in some myeloproliferative disorders, in which myeloblasts and promyelocytes may be positive (27,278).

Anti-CD45 MAbs are extremely useful in evaluating lymphoid malignancy, because they are immunoreactive with the vast majority of B- and T-cell NHLs and lymphoid leukemias but not with epithelial and mesenchymal neoplasms (27,249,278,310–312) (Figs. 3.12, 3.13). This allows immediate separation of these clinicopathologically distinct categories of human neoplasia and instantly resolves many difficult diagnostic dilemmas. This anti-CD45 MAb cocktail reacts with approximately 97% of B-cell and 89% of T-cell NHLs (95% overall) in paraffin tissue sections (278,279,309, 313–317). Among B-cell lymphomas, only occasional cases of precursor B cell lymphoblastic lymphoma/leukemia and immunoblastic lymphoma do not express CD45

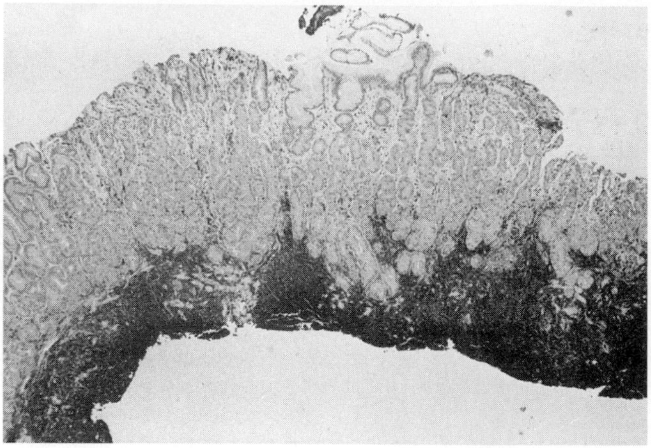

FIG. 3.12. Formalin-fixed, paraffin-embedded tissue section of a portion of gastric mucosa containing a B-cell non-Hodgkin's lymphoma that has been immunostained for CD45. The monoclonal anti-CD45 antibody is immunoreactive with the lymphoma cells infiltrating the gastric mucosa; the gastric mucosa is CD45-negative. This permits easy visualization of the lymphomatous B-cell population in this tissue specimen (immunoperoxidase stain, original magnification: 40× magnification).

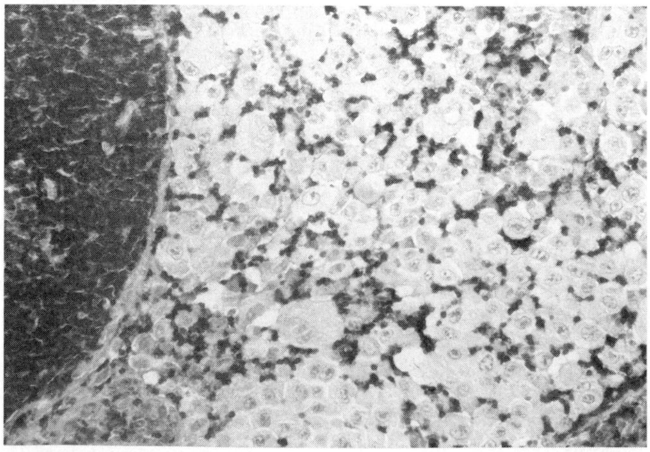

FIG. 3.13. Formalin-fixed, paraffin-embedded tissue section of a lymph node involved by malignant melanoma, which has been immunostained for CD45. The malignant melanoma cells, which are primarily present in the interfollicular areas, are CD45-negative. The residual germinal center and other benign lymphoid cells express CD45 (immunoperoxidase stain, original magnification: 400× magnification).

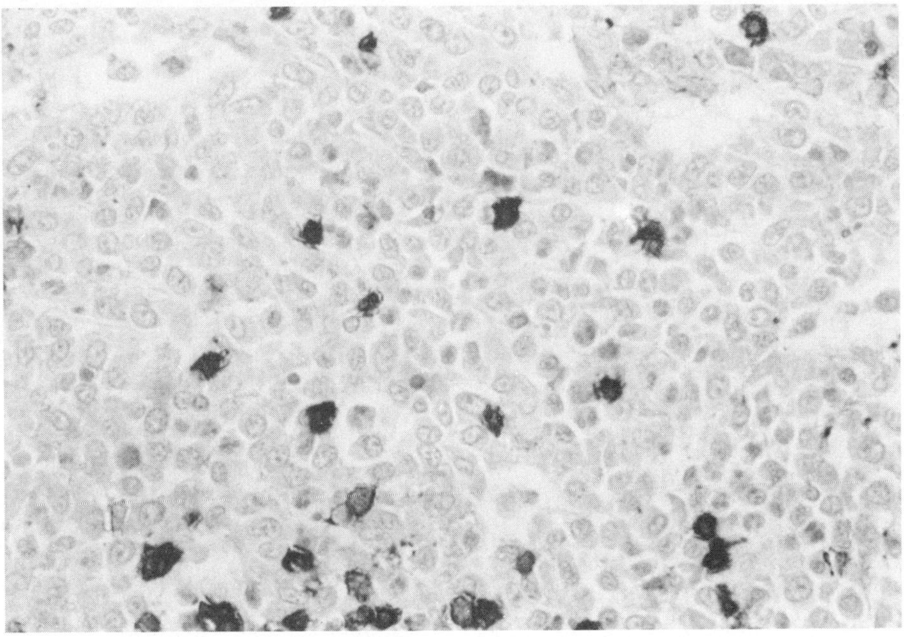

FIG. 3.14. Bouin's solution–fixed, paraffin-embedded tissue section of a bone marrow biopsy specimen diffusely infiltrated by multiple myeloma that has been immunostained with a monoclonal anti-CD45 antibody. CD45 (leukocyte common antigen) is expressed in high density on scattered residual normal hematopoietic cells, but the myeloma plasma cells are conspicuously negative (immunoperoxidase stain, original magnification: 400× magnification).

(315,318–321). Essentially all patients with chronic lymphocytic leukemia and hairy cell leukemia express CD45 (278,320,322–325). Only variable proportions of the circulating malignant B cells in Waldenstrom's macroglobulinemia, however, express CD45 (282). In addition, most malignant plasma cells in the majority of plasmacytomas and multiple myelomas lack CD45 (27,278,326) (Fig. 3.14). An equivalent percentage, approximately 92%, of cutaneous T-cell lymphomas and peripheral T-cell lymphomas, but only about 84% of precursor T-cell lymphoblastic lymphomas and leukemias, express CD45 (278,279,309,313–317,319, 320). Only about 50% to 60% of $CD30^+$ anaplastic large cell lymphomas express CD45 (278,315,318,327–331) (Fig 3.15). The lack of CD45 expression by some B- and T-cell NHLs and plasma cell neoplasms probably reflects the normal physiologic changes in CD45 expression that occur during B- and T-cell differentiation and activation (248).

This anti-CD45 MAb cocktail is reactive with the Reed-Sternberg cells and variants in only about 5% or less of cases of nodular sclerosis, mixed cellularity, and lymphocyte depletion Hodgkin's disease in paraffin tissue sections (278,279,314,315,319,328,330,332–335). The rate of immunoreactivity has been reported to be much higher in frozen tissue sections and in plastic-embedded tissue sections, however (336,337). The latter findings raise the possibility that CD45 is present, but in a quantity below the detectable threshold, in paraffin tissue sections (249). In contrast with classic Hodgkin's disease, this anti-CD45 MAb cocktail is reactive with the Reed-Sternberg cells and variants in about two thirds or more of cases of nodular lymphocytic and histiocytic (L&H) lymphocyte predominance Hodgkin's disease in paraffin tissue sections (278,279,315,319,332–335, 338).

Anti-CD45 MAbs are immunoreactive with the majority of AMLs, although the proportion of $CD45^+$ patients detected by cytofluorometric analysis is greater than that detected by immunohistochemical staining of paraffin tissue sections (278,320,339–344). The 2B11-PD7 MAb cocktail also has been found to be reactive in patients with mast cell disease (278). In general, however, the various anti-CD45 MAbs display variable reactivity with neoplasms of histiocytic and dendritic cell derivation (345–350).

The 2B11-PD7 MAb cocktail is usually reactive in routinely processed paraffin tissue sections that have been preserved in a wide array of fixatives, including 10% neutral buffered formalin, formol saline, B5, Bouin's, and Zenker's (278,279,309,323,351,352). Nonetheless, immunoreactivity patterns differ based on the type and length of time of fixation. Formalin may be the best fixative for tissues fixed up to 24 hours (352,353), and it is thoroughly adequate for immunohistochemical staining even after 90 hours of fixation. Some investigators believe that B5 is superior to all other fixatives, because more cells react more intensely with this MAb cocktail in B5-fixed tissue (278). Other investigators believe that B5-fixed tissue has high background staining (279). Trypsinization often increases background staining and does not appear to increase reactivity consistently (278,351). The new antigen-retrieval techniques, however,

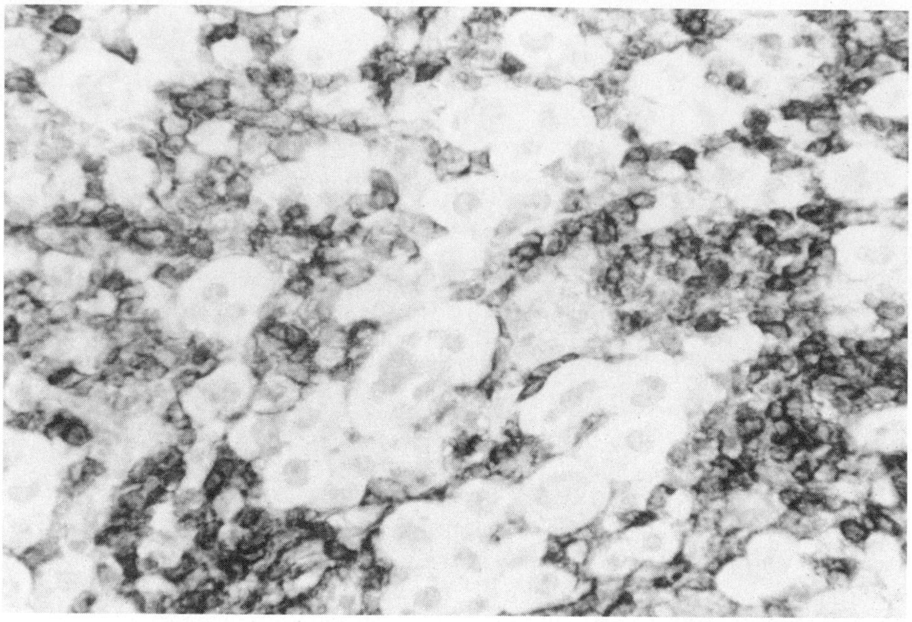

FIG. 3.15. Paraffin tissue section of a lymph node diffusely infiltrated by a CD30 positive anaplastic large cell lymphoma. The malignant lymphoma cells are CD45-negative. Numerous residual small benign lymphocytes are CD45-positive and serve as an internal positive control (immunoperoxidase stain, original magnification: 400× magnification).

yield excellent staining results and circumvent many of these issues and problems (see Chapter 4).

Although it has not been completely characterized (272), MAb 4KB5 has been clustered as an anti-CD45RA antibody because it recognizes the 220-, 205- (AB exon), and 190-kd isoforms. It is preferentially reactive with B cells (298–300,354,355) and is used frequently as a B-cell marker (249). MAb 4KB5 is immunoreactive with the B-cell zones of benign lymph nodes, tonsils, and spleen, with the mantle zone B cells showing far stronger positivity than germinal center B cells (298,323,325,356). MAb 4KB5 also is immunoreactive with interfollicular B immunoblasts in lymph nodes and tonsils (323) and with marginal zone lymphocytes in the spleen but not with plasma cells (356). In addition, MAb 4KB5 reacts with some monocytes, macrophages, and granulocytes, but membrane positivity by bone marrow elements is observed uncommonly (325).

Monoclonal antibody 4KB5 is immunoreactive with approximately 75% of all B-cell NHLs. This includes more than 90% of small lymphocytic lymphomas and chronic lymphocytic leukemias (including those with plasmacytoid features), mantle cell lymphomas, and marginal zone lymphomas, more than 80% of follicle center lymphomas, and the great majority of precursor B-cell lymphoblastic lymphomas/leukemias. It is also reactive in all cases of hairy cell leukemia. MAb 4KB5 reacts, however, with only approximately 70% of immunoblastic and Burkitt's lymphomas and less than 20% of plasmacytomas (315,317,320, 322,323,325,354,356,357). MAb 4KB5 reacts with only about 6% of T-cell NHLs overall, most of which are peripheral T-cell lymphomas and almost none of which are cutaneous T-cell lymphomas or precursor T-cell lymphoblastic lymphomas or leukemias (315,317,320,322,325,354).

Monoclonal antibody 4KB5 reacts with the Reed-Sternberg cells and variants in about 50% of patients with nodular L&H Hodgkin's disease but only very rarely with those in classic Hodgkin's disease (315,319,325,330,358). It reacts with approximately 20% of cases of AML classified as FAB M1 through M5 (325,340–342) but does not react with FAB M6 acute myeloid (erythroblastic) leukemia or chronic myelogenous leukemia (320,322,325,340).

This antibody appears to react optimally in tissues that have been fixed in either B5 or formalin. Again, however, the time spent in fixative is a crucial factor in obtaining optimal staining results (322,325,353). Adequate MAb 4KB5 staining also is obtained with Bouin's solution–fixed tissue but not with tissue fixed in Zenker's solution (322). Trypsinization decreases the staining intensity of MAb 4KB5 (322,353).

Monoclonal antibodies UCHL1 (302) and A6 (303) are two anti-CD45RO MAbs that appear to identify close epitopes on the same molecule (296,303). MAb OPD4 also recognizes the 180-kd CD45RO isoform (306) but exhibits a slightly different pattern of immune reactivity than MAbs UCHL1 and A6 (307,359).

Monoclonal antibody UCHL1 reacts with approximately 90% of cortical thymocytes, 50% of medullary thymocytes (301,360), approximately 50% to 70% of $CD2^+$ and $CD3^+$ peripheral blood and lymphoid tissue T cells (274,352), and approximately 75% of CD4 and 33% of CD8 T cells (352) but rarely, if ever, with B cells (299,352,360), as seen on cytofluorometric analysis. MAb OPD4 reacts with approxi-

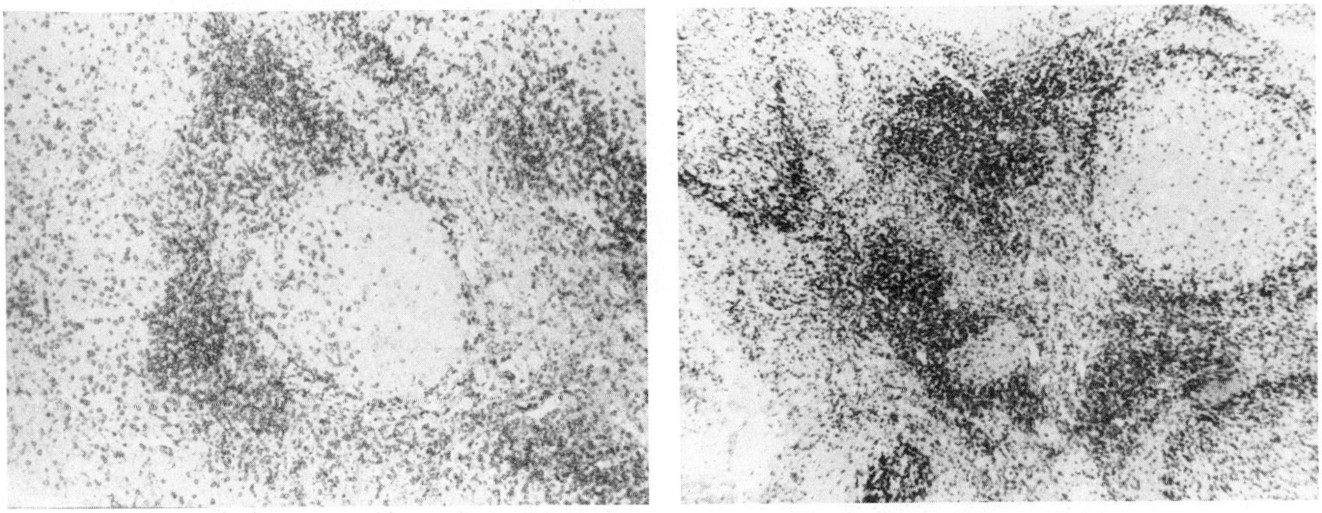

A B

FIG. 3.16. Formalin-fixed, paraffin-embedded tissue sections of a benign lymph node immunostained with monoclonal antibodies (MAbs) UCHL-1 (**A**) and A6 (**B**), which detect CD45RO. The patterns of immunoreactivity of these two antibodies in paraffin tissue sections are comparable to that of anti-pan-T cell antibodies in frozen tissue sections. MAb A6, however, generally exhibits stronger immunoreactivity than does MAb UCHL-1 (immunoperoxidase stain, original magnification: 100× magnification).

mately 30% of peripheral blood CD3 T cells, including 50% of CD4 T cells and 15% of CD8 T cells, and less than 2% of B cells by cytofluorometric analysis (306).

Monoclonal antibodies UCHL1, A6, and OPD4 characteristically show crisp ring-like membrane staining of hematopoietic cells in both frozen and paraffin tissue sections (301,306,325,361). Ultrastructural immunohistochemical studies have localized MAb UCHL1 immunoreactivity to the surface membrane (305). In addition, rare large lymphoid cells and monocytes and macrophages exhibit faint cytoplasmic positivity (301). Cytoplasmic as well as surface positivity can be seen in myeloid cells, the stronger cytoplasmic positivity being present in the more mature myeloid cells (342).

Monoclonal antibody UCHL1 has a pattern of immunoreactivity in both frozen and paraffin tissue sections of benign hematolymphoid tissues that is comparable to that of anti-pan T cell antibodies in frozen tissue sections (301). It reacts with lymph node and tonsil paracortical lymphocytes, splenic periarteriolar lymphoid sheath lymphocytes, and scattered lymphoid cells within the germinal centers of these tissues (299,301,325,360) (Fig. 3.16). MAb OPD4 appears to detect fewer T cells and displays a pattern of immune reactivity comparable to that of anti-CD4 MAbs in frozen tissue sections (306) (Fig. 3.17). Monoclonal antibody UCHL1 reacts with small lymphocytes in the bone marrow (341), and MAb OPD4 reacts with some of these cells as well (306). A proportion of monocytes and macrophages, primarily those located in the sinusoids, also react with MAb UCHL1, but with less intensity than with benign lymphocytes (301,313,323,325). MAb OPD4 exhibits a lower level of immune reactivity with monocytes and macrophages than does MAb UCHL1 or A6 (359). It is unreactive with tingible body macrophages and interdigitating dendritic cells (306). In general, MAb UCHL1 does not react with erythroid precursors, megakaryocytes, or myeloblasts, but it occasionally reacts weakly with promyelocytes, and as myeloid cells mature, they exhibit cytoplasmic positivity (301,342). The most strongly positive myeloid cells are neutrophils, which appear to exhibit both membrane and cytoplasmic positivity, but this is usually weaker than that of benign T cells

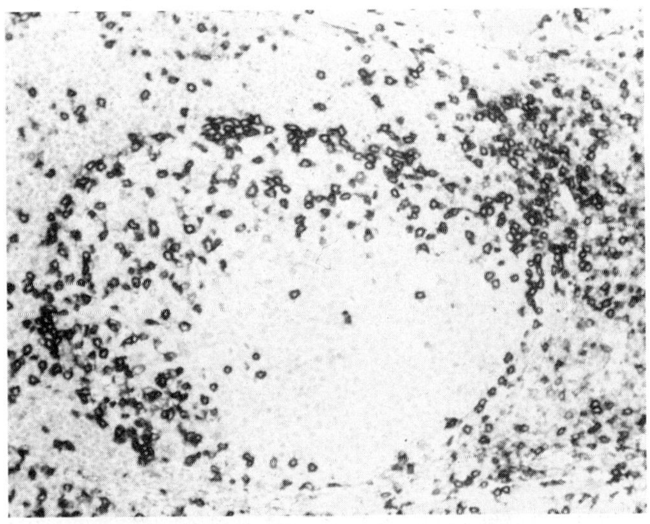

FIG. 3.17. Formalin-fixed, paraffin-embedded tissue section of a benign lymph node immunostained with monoclonal antibody OPD4, which detects CD45RO. Monoclonal antibody OPD4 appears to detect fewer T cells than other anti-CD45RO antibodies in paraffin-embedded tissue sections and displays immune reactivity comparable to that of anti-CD4 monoclonal antibodies in frozen tissue sections (immunoperoxidase stain, original magnification: 200× magnification).

(301,313,342). MAb OPD4 is not reactive with normal bone marrow elements, that is, erythroid precursors, myeloid cells, and megakaryocytes (306). The only nonhematopoietic cell type reported to show membrane reactivity with MAb UCHL1 is the placental Hofbauer cell (301). MAb OPD4 is unreactive with nonhematopoietic tissues (306).

Monoclonal antibody UCHL1 reacts with approximately 77% of all T-cell NHLs in paraffin tissue sections. This includes more than 80% of all cutaneous T-cell lymphomas, including mycosis fungoides, about 80% of peripheral T-cell lymphomas (303,313,316,317,319,320,325,339,354,360,361) (Fig. 3.18), and about 50% of T-cell anaplastic large cell lymphomas (315,329,330,361,362). Consistent with the lack of expression of the CD45RO isoform by immature thymocytes, MAb UCHL1 is reactive with only a little more than 50% of precursor T-cell lymphoblastic lymphomas and leukemias (301,313,315-317,319,320,323,339,354,360). In contrast, MAb UCHL1 exhibits strong membrane reactivity with less than 5% of B-cell NHLs, predominantly diffuse large B-cell lymphomas, in paraffin tissue sections (303,313,315,317,319,320,323,325,339,354,360,361) (Fig. 3.19). MAbs UCHL1 and A6 are not reactive with B-cell chronic lymphocytic leukemia, hairy cell leukemia, or plasmacytoma/multiple myeloma (301,303,320,322,325,354,361).

The distribution of immune reactivity of MAb A6 with T- and B-cell NHLs is similar to that of MAb UCHL1, although MAB A6 may react with a slightly higher proportion of T-cell tumors (303). MAb OPD4 reacts with slightly more than 50% of T-cell and with less than 5% of B-cell NHLs (306,307,352) (Fig 3.20). Although the distribution of MAb OPD4 reactivity is similar to that of CD4 in benign lymphoid tissues, MAb OPD4 does not react preferentially with $CD4^+$ T-cell lymphomas (307). MAb OPD4 reacts with approximately equivalent proportions of $CD4^+$ (58%) and $CD4^-$ (64%) postthymic T-cell lymphomas (307). It reacts with only about 20% of precursor T-cell lymphoblastic lymphomas/leukemias (306,307).

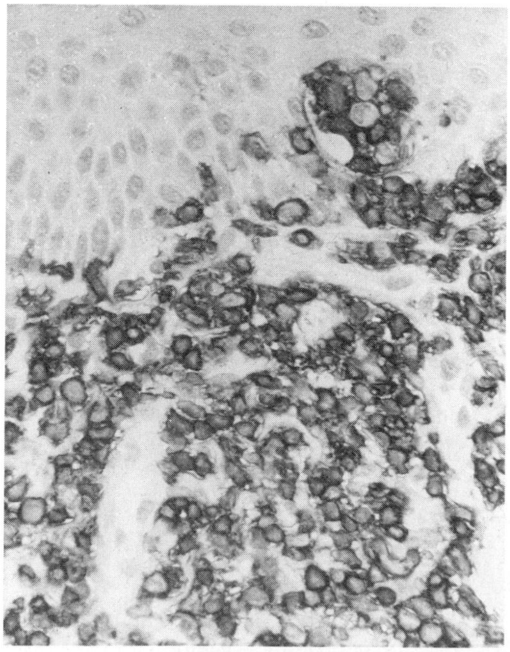

FIG. 3.18. Formalin-fixed, paraffin-embedded tissue section of skin involved by mycosis fungoides that has been immunostained with monoclonal antibody UCHL-1. The majority of the malignant mycosis fungoides T cells strongly express CD45RO (immunoperoxidase stain, original magnification: 400× magnification).

Monoclonal antibodies UCHL1, A6, and OPD4 react only rarely, if at all, with the Reed-Sternberg cells and variants of Hodgkin's disease in paraffin tissue sections (301,305,306,315,319,325,360,361). UCHL1-reactive Reed-Sternberg cells, however, were identified plastic-embedded tissue sections from more than 70% of patients with Hodgkin's disease in one study (337), suggesting that this antibody may exhibit immunoreactivity with Reed-Sternberg cells in these preparations.

Monoclonal antibody UCHL1 is immunoreactive with about 25% of FAB M1 through M5 AMLs but not with FAB M6 or M7 AMLs (301,320,325,339–341). This antibody is also immunoreactive with the more differentiated myeloid cells in some patients with chronic myelogenous leukemia (325,339,342). Membrane and/or cytoplasmic positivity may be present in these patients (341,342). MAb OPD4 has been unreactive with the few acute and chronic myeloid leukemias studied (306). Anti-CD45RO MAbs have exhibited variable immunoreactivity with the few histiocytic and dendritic cell tumors studied (322,339,349,360).

Monoclonal antibody UCHL1 reacts with tissues preserved in a variety of fixatives, including neutral buffered formalin, formol saline, Bouin's solution, B5, and Zenker's solution (319,322,325,341,354). MAb UCHL1, however, appears to react with more cells more intensely in more patients in tissues processed after fixation in either B5 or formalin (307,322,325,353,361). Many immunohistochemists believe that the immunoreactivity is more crisp and intense in B5- than in formalin-fixed tissue. Others believe that the background staining in B5-fixed tissues is unacceptable (325). The amount of time spent in fixative influences UCHL1 reactivity. This MAb reacts best with tissues fixed in B5 for between 3 and 21 hours. Immunohistochemical results are suboptimal if tissue is fixed in B5 for more than 60 hours (352). MAb UCHL1 works well, however, in tissues that have been fixed for up to 90 hours in formalin (352). Enzymatic treatment of tissue appears to increase the intensity of UCHL1 immunoreactivity, but it also increases the background staining (322,353). MAb OPD4 appears to work relatively well in tissues that have been fixed in either buffered formalin or B5 (306,307,352). Its reactivity is decreased in tissues fixed in nonbuffered formalin, ethanol, or Bouin's solution (307,352). Again, however, antigen-retrieval techniques circumvent many of these issues.

There is no evidence to suggest that any benign, normal nonlymphohematopoietic cell populations express members

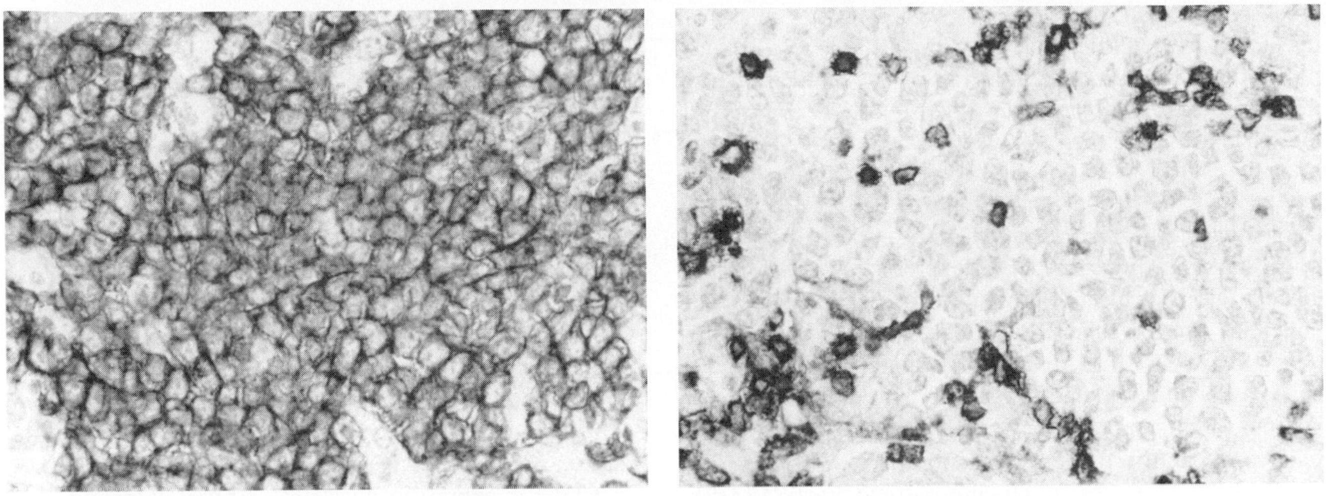

FIG. 3.19. Formalin-fixed, paraffin-embedded tissue sections of a B-cell non-Hodgkin's lymphoma immunostained with monoclonal antibodies L26 (**A**) and UCHL-1 (**B**). **A:** Monoclonal antibody L26 reacts strongly with the large neoplastic B cells but does not react with residual small lymphocytes (predominately T cells) or vascular endothelium. **B:** Monoclonal antibody UCHL-1 reacts strongly with benign residual T cells but not with the large malignant lymphoma cells (immunoperoxidase stain, original magnification: 400× magnification).

of the LCA protein family (249). Extensive studies generally have demonstrated a complete lack of expression of CD45 proteins by nonhematopoietic neoplasms, including carcinomas, sarcomas, malignant melanomas, germ cell tumors, and neuroepithelial neoplasms (27,278,279,312,320). Rare exceptions have been reported (363–365), the significance of which is unclear. For all intents and purposes, CD45 expression by a neoplastic cell population almost definitely rules out a nonhematopoietic neoplasm.

B-Cell Lineage–Associated Antigens

CD10

CALLA initially was identified and its distribution of expression documented with a heteroantiserum (186–190). Five MAbs recognizing CALLA, including J5 (191) and BA-3 (192), were clustered as CD10 at the first workshop (15). Multiple additional MAbs, many of which are commercially available (366), were included in the CD10 cluster

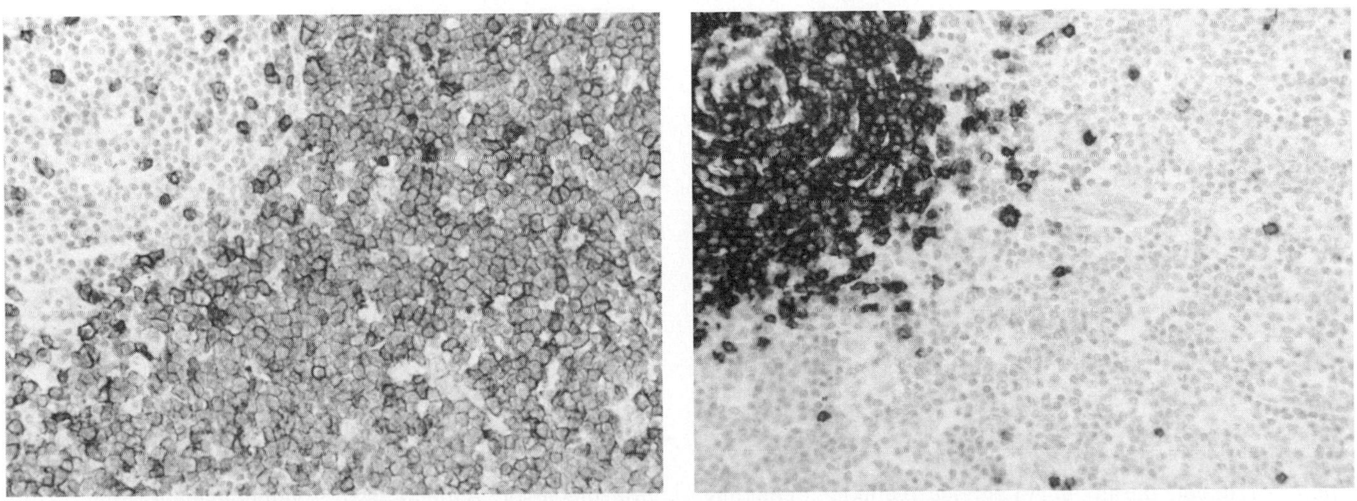

FIG. 3.20. Formalin-fixed, paraffin-embedded tissue sections of a peripheral T-cell lymphoma immunostained with monoclonal antibodies OPD4 (**A**) and L26 (**B**). **A:** Monoclonal antibody OPD4 reacts strongly with the interfollicular neoplastic T cells but reacts with only small numbers of scattered lymphocytes, presumably benign CD4 T cells, within the residual benign germinal center. **B:** Monoclonal antibody L26 strongly reacts with the B cells present within a residual benign germinal center but does not react with the neoplastic T cells (immunoperoxidase stain, original magnification: 250× magnification).

in subsequent workshops (367,368). These MAbs appear to detect the same or closely related epitopes (367,368). Prior to the identification of CALLA, a cell surface zinc-dependent metalloprotease now known as *neutral endopeptidase* EC 3.4. 24.11 was described as a neutral mettaloendopeptidase in kidney and as an enkephalinase in brain. It is now known that this enzyme is identical to CD10 (369–371), and the designation *CD10–neutral endopeptidase* sometimes is used for this reason. Although CD10 is expressed by many different cell types, it is most helpful in the categorization of acute leukemias and the subclassification of NHLs. Most of the available anti-CD10 MAbs are applicable in cytofluorometric analysis or in frozen tissue section immunohistochemistry; some of the antibodies have been reported to be immunoreactive in paraffin tissue sections (366).

The CD10 gene, present on chromosome 3q21-27 (372), is composed of 24 exons spanning more than 80 kb (373). Several different CD10 cDNAs have been found that result from alternative splicing of unique 5′ untranslated region sequences into a common exon. The different tissue specificities of the enzyme as well as the developmentally regulated expression of CD10 may be related to this alternative splicing (373–375). Biochemical analyses also suggest that tissue-specific differences exist in the resultant glycoprotein. The molecular mass of CD10 varies from 90 kd in fibroblasts and renal tubules, to 100 kd in lymphoid progenitor cells, to 110 kd in neutrophils (376,377).

CD10 is a monomeric 749–amino acid type II integral membrane peptide (378). It contains a hydrophobic 24–amino acid transmembrane region, which also functions as a signal peptide, and a 25–amino acid residue cytoplasmic amino-terminal domain. The extracellular region contains a pentapeptide sequence that is characteristically associated with zinc binding and catalytic activity in cell surface and zinc-dependent metalloproteases. Tissue-specific differences in the molecular mass of CD10 may be related to differences in the glycosylation patterns of six potential N-linked glycosylation sites on the extracellular region (378). The extracellular region also contains 12 cysteine residues that form disulfide bonds that are essential for enzymatic activity (369,378,379). CD10 is phosphorylated by casein kinase II, a serine and threonine kinase that increases in activity following peptide signaling (366). CD10 also has been shown to coassociate with other tyrosine phosphoproteins, including LYN-SRC-related kinase (380).

Cell surface CD10 is a zinc metalloprotease enzyme that acts to reduce the cellular response to peptide hormones by regulating local peptide concentrations (381,382). The surface CD10 molecule hydrolyzes peptide bonds on the amino side of the hydrophobic amino acid Val, Phe, Ile, or Tyr, thereby reducing the amount of peptide available for binding to the hormone receptor and, in turn, reducing signal transduction (366). CD10 hydrolyzes a variety of substances, including, for example, bombesin-like peptides, endothelins, enkephalin, angiotensin, and inflammatory peptides (366). Because of its wide biologic activity, CD10 has many biologic effects, but the function of CD10 is not well defined in lymphocytes (366). It has been suggested that CD10 plays a role in the regulation of B-cell development (383). This may occur through direct inactivation of a peptide that stimulates B-cell growth and differentiation or activation of another substance that then inactivates such development (383).

A variety of substances affect the amount of surface CD10 and, consequently, its enzymatic activity. Glucocorticoids, tumor necrosis factor (TNF), and granulocyte-macrophage colony stimulating factor (GM-CSF), among others, increase surface CD10 activity (379,384). Anti-CD10 antibodies, phorbol esters, certain growth factors, and transfection of cells with the EBV latent membrane protein gene result in decreased cell surface expression of CD10 (385–388).

CD10 is expressed by a wide variety of nonneoplastic hematopoietic, epithelial, and mesenchymal stromal cells (366,376,377,389). Among hematopoietic cells, CD10 is expressed by mature granulocytes but not by immature myeloid cells (377,390,391), suggesting that its expression is maturation-related. In contrast with the myeloid cell lineage, CD10 usually is not expressed by mature peripheral blood lymphocytes but is expressed by a subpopulation of immature lymphoid cells that can be identified in normal bone marrow (392,393) and thymus (394) and in fetal liver and spleen (395).

The $CD10^+$ lymphoid cells in the bone marrow are believed to represent hematogones, for example, progenitor cells (396). The bone marrow $CD19^+CD10^+$ B cells appear to be a separate population, distinct from the more mature $CD20^+CD21^+CD22^+$ B-cell population (397,398). They may resemble small lymphocytes or larger FAB L1 lymphoblasts morphologically (366). Although some of these cells apparently do not express B- or T-cell lineage–associated antigens, others have the $TdT^+CD34^+CD19^+CD10^+$ immunophenotype characteristic of precursor B cells (366). Although some investigators have suggested that CD10 expression by bone marrow lymphoid cells is limited to B-cell precursors (398), it has been reported that a significant proportion of bone marrow T-cell precursors express CD10 as well (399). The percentage of $CD10^+$ cells in the bone marrow generally decreases with age, from 13% to 40% in the fetus (395,398,399), to 2% to 27% in children (189,393), to less than 1% to 7% in younger adults (189,385,392,393,400,401), to 1% in elderly adults (399). In the fetus, almost all bone marrow B cells express CD10 (395,402). The number of $CD10^+$ B cells, which usually are also TdT^+, may increase in regenerating bone marrow and following bone marrow transplantation (399,403–405). If this occurs in patients who have histories of precursor lymphoblastic lymphoma/leukemia, distinguishing these nonneoplastic cells from residual or recurrent malignant lymphoblasts can be problemmatic. These cells, however, morphologically resemble small lymphocytes or hematogones and often can be distinguished from a patient's malignant lymphoblasts by further immunophenotypic characterization (366). They do not exhibit evidence of monoclonality (405). Finally, the majority of fetal liver and spleen B cells are CD10$^+$ (395,406). CD10$^+$ precursor lymphoid cells are not increased in adult liver or spleen or in nonneoplastic lymph nodes or tonsils at any age (189,395,406).

Some normal T cells in the thymus, many of which also express CD34, express CD10. This expression is strongest in those immature thymocytes that are CD3$^-$ or CD3^{low} and CD4$^-$CD8$^-$, moderate in those that are CD4$^+$CD8$^+$ or CD4$^-$CD8$^+$, and weakest or absent in those that are CD4$^+$CD8$^-$ (407).

Although most nonneoplastic CD10$^+$ B cells are progenitor cells, nonneoplastic mature sIg$^+$ B cells residing in peripheral lymphoid tissue germinal centers also may express CD10 (408,409) (Fig. 3.21). It has been suggested that such expression is a marker of early B-cell activation. B cells can acquire CD10 at an early stage and lose CD10 at a later stage of B-cell activation (410). The lymph node germinal center is the site for B-cell activation and proliferation (see Chapter 2).

Although the early studies suggested that CALLA (CD10) is only expressed by so-called common-type acute lymphoblastic leukemia, it is known now that CD10 is expressed by other acute leukemias as well as by many NHLs (366). Approximately 90% of patients with precursor B-cell lymphoblastic lymphoma/leukemia and chronic myelogenous leukemia in lymphoid blast crisis and about 25% of those with sIg$^+$ FAB L3 acute lymphoblastic (Burkitt's) leukemia and precursor T-cell lymphoblastic lymphoma/leukemia express CD10 (7,144,191,411–416). Only a small proportion, less than 3%, of AMLs express CD10 (343,417–420).

Many investigators have suggested that CD10 expression in precursor B- and T-cell lymphoblastic lymphoma/leukemia has prognostic significance (366). Decreased survival

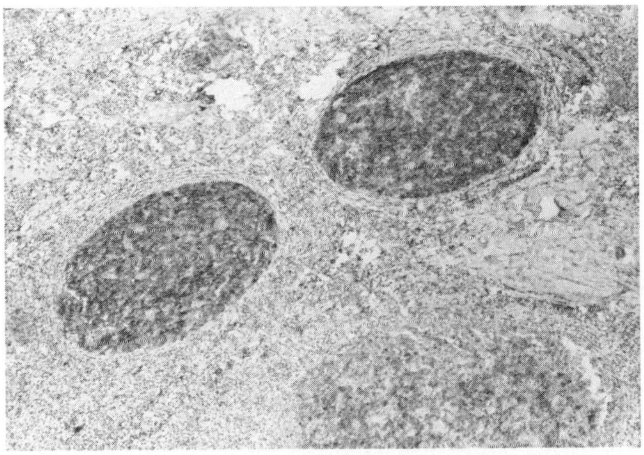

FIG. 3.21. Frozen tissue section of a benign lymph node immunostained with a monoclonal anti-CD10 antibody. The germinal centers are highlighted because of the preferential immune reactivity of this antibody with the germinal center B-cell population (immunoperoxidase stain, original magnification: 100× magnification).

has been associated with a lack of CD10 expression in precursor B-cell lymphoblastic lymphoma/leukemia occurring in infants (421) and children (422,423). Also, the degree of CD10 antigen density on precursor B-cell lymphoblasts may have prognostic significance (424). Apparently, white women, the group with the best prognosis, have the highest CD10 antigen density; black men, a group with poor prognosis, have the lowest CD10 antigen density on precursor B-cell lymphoblasts (424). High CD10 density also has been shown to correlate with hyperdiploidy, a good prognostic indicator; low and undetectable CD10 expression have been associated with the translocations t(1;19) and t(4;11), respectively (425), both poor prognostic indicators, in precursor B-cell lymphoblastic lymphoma/leukemia. A better prognosis also has been associated with CD10 expression in precursor T-cell lymphoblastic lymphoma/leukemia. A greater proportion of children and adults who have CD10$^+$ precursor T-cell lymphoblasts achieve complete remission and disease-free survival (411,426–428).

A large number of studies has investigated CD10 expression by B-cell NHLs, chronic lymphoid leukemias, and plasma cell neoplasms (366). These studies have found that CD10 is expressed by approximately 90% of precursor B-cell lymphoblastic lymphomas (comparable to precursor B-cell acute lymphoblastic leukemia), by 90% of Burkitt's lymphomas (a significantly higher proportion than in the closely related FAB L3 acute lymphoblastic [Burkitt's] leukemias), by about 60% of follicle center lymphomas, and infrequently or not at all by other categories of B-cell neoplasia. About 30% of diffuse large B-cell lymphomas and 20% of large B-cell immunoblastic lymphomas have been reported to express CD10, but many of these cases probably represent transformed follicle center lymphomas. More than 20% of patients categorized as having diffuse small cleaved cell lymphoma have been reported to be CD10$^+$, although many of these patients probably have mantle cell lymphomas, about 15% of which express CD10. Almost 30% of patients with splenic B-cell lymphoma with circulating villous lymphocytes are CD10$^+$. Approximately 20% of hairy cell leukemias have been said to express CD10, but this percentage may be artificially inflated because it is based largely on one study (429). Expression of CD10 is very uncommon or absent among patients with small lymphocytic lymphoma/chronic lymphocytic leukemia, lymphoplasmacytoid lymphoma, prolymphocytic leukemia, CD11c$^+$ chronic lymphoproliferative disorder, marginal zone lymphoma, or splenic marginal zone lymphoma (366). CD10$^+$ tumor cells are present in approximately one third of patients with plasmacytoma/multiple myeloma. These CD10$^+$ myelomas have been reported to be more clinically aggressive and to be associated with a poorer chance of survival (430–432) (see Chapter 42).

With the exception of precursor T-cell lymphoblastic lymphoma, CD10 expression among T-cell neoplasms is very uncommon (366). CD10 is not expressed by T-cell chronic lymphocytic leukemia, T-cell prolymphocytic leukemia, adult T-cell lymphoma/leukemia, cutaneous T-cell lymphoma, peripheral and angiocentric T-cell lymphoma, anaplastic large cell lymphoma, or lymphoproliferative disorders of LGL/NK cell derivation (366). In addition, the Reed-Sternberg cells of Hodgkin's disease are CD10$^-$ (332,366).

Because CD10 is expressed widely among benign nonhematopoietic cells (366), it should not be too surprising that CD10 is expressed by a variety of nonhematopoietic neoplasms of epithelial and mesenchymal cell origin (366). These include pulmonary carcinomas (433–436), thymic carcinomas (437), cutaneous and ocular malignant melanomas (385,438,439), and mesotheliomas (436), among others (366).

Anti-CD10 MAbs exhibit a wide range of immune reactivity. Consequently, caution must be exercised if these MAbs are employed in immunophenotypic analysis. If utilized in the proper context and in conjunction with other immunophenotypic markers, they are helpful in the diagnosis and classification of hematologic neoplasms. This is especially true in the case of precursor T- and B-cell lymphoblastic lymphoma/leukemia, in which CD10 expression also carries prognostic significance; among the low-grade B-cell NHLs; and in the case of Burkitt's lymphoma.

CD19

The CD19 molecule is a 95-kd glycosylated type I integral membrane protein whose expression is limited to B cells and follicular dendritic cells (440,441). CD19 originally was identified by MAb B4 (442) and later by MAb Leu12 (443). The CD19 cluster was established at the second workshop (102). These and the additional antibodies added to the CD19 cluster at subsequent workshops appear to detect the same or identical epitopes (102,444,445). These antibodies are employed most commonly to detect CD19$^+$ B cells in suspension by cytofluorometric analysis or in frozen tissue sections by immunohistochemistry. These antibodies are not reactive in routinely fixed and paraffin-embedded tissue sections.

The human CD19 gene has been mapped to 16p11 (446). It consists of 15 exons with a very similar overall structure and the 5′ and 3′ flanking regions share sequence homologies (447). CD19 is a member of the immunoglobulin gene superfamily. Its roughly 280–amino acid extracellular region contains two C2-type immunoglobulin-like domains separated by a smaller potentially disulfide-linked domain (448). The extensive, highly charged cytoplasmic domain of 242–amino acid residues is well conserved across species, suggesting that it is important for CD19 function (449).

CD19 noncovalently associates with CD21 and also associates with other cell surface proteins, such as CD81 and Leu13, to form a multimolecular signal transduction complex independent of the antigen receptor that is unique to B cells (450,451). Because CD21 is expressed much later during B-cell maturation than CD19 and CD81, the composition of this complex may vary during B-cell development so that signalling by this complex is regulated developmentally. MAb binding to CD19 likely initiates multiple intracellular signal transduction cascades, either through CD19 directly or through other members of the CD19 complex (440). Engagement of CD19 likely plays an important role in antigen-specific responses by mature B cells and is also likely to be central to other signal-transduction systems (440). CD19 may function as a central signaling element that is linked to multiple cell surface receptors (440). A physical and functional association between CD19 and sIg has been postulated (452). No biochemical indication of a direct physical association between the CD19-CD21 complex and the sIg receptor complex exists (440). The signaling capability of CD19 is not dependent on sIg expression, because CD19 is functionally active in B-cell precursors lacking antigen receptors (453–455). Additional studies are necessary to determine the role of the CD19-CD21 complex in B-cell function *in vivo*. The CD19-CD21 complex appears to play an important role in the activation and growth regulation of B cells (440).

The development of CD19-deficient and human CD19 transgenic mice that overexpress CD19 have provided additional insight into the role of CD19 in B-cell development and activation (456–458). B cells from CD19-deficient mice are hyporesponsive to transmembrane signals, leading to significant defects during the later stages of B-cell maturation, clonal expansion, and differentiation (457). Germinal center formation is reduced significantly in CD19-deficient mice (457). B cells from human CD19 trangenic mice are hyperresponsive to a variety of transmembrane signals (456,457,459). CD19 overexpression leads to severe impairment of B-cell development, characterized by a decreased number of mature B cells in the bone marrow and periphery, suggesting that CD19 plays an important role in negative selection during B-cell development in the bone marrow (456). The development of CD5$^+$ B cells is diminished severely in CD19-deficient mice but augmented markedly, along with autoantibody production, in human CD19 transgenic mice (460). These findings have led to the hypothesis that CD19 serves as a general response regulator that defines B-cell signaling thresholds critical for early clonal selection, the maintenance and expansion of the peripheral B-cell pool, the generation of B-1 lymphocytes, and the development of autoantibodies (445).

CD19 appears to be the earliest B-cell lineage–restricted antigen demonstrable in fetal tissues (442). CD19 precedes all other B cell–restricted antigens in early B-cell ontogeny. It is expressed by progenitor B cells in the bone marrow, presumably around the time of immunoglobulin heavy chain gene rearrangement, after HLA-DR expression. CD19 expression persists throughout all stages of B-cell maturation but is lost on terminal differentiation to plasma cells (100,442,461). CD19 is expressed by greater than 95% of peripheral blood, lymphoid tissue, and splenic B cells but is not expressed by immature, mature, or activated T cells, monocytes or macrophages, or granulocytes (442,443).

CD19 is an excellent B-cell lineage–restricted pan-B cell

marker for enumerating or isolating normal B cells and also for evaluating lymphoid malignancies. CD19 is expressed by approximately 90% of all precursor B-cell lymphoblastic lymphomas/leukemias and patients with chronic myelogenous leukemia in lymphoid blast crisis. It also is expressed by more than 95% of mature (TdT$^-$) sIg$^+$ and sIg$^-$ B-cell NHLs and nonlymphoblastic lymphoid leukemias, including hairy cell leukemia. CD19 is expressed variably by Waldenström's macroglobulinemia but usually is absent from multiple myeloma. Conversely, CD19 is not expressed by precursor T-cell lymphoblastic lymphomas/leukemias or by postthymic (peripheral) T-cell lymphomas and leukemias (7,8,218,442,443,461,462). Lymphoid antigens, including CD19, occasionally are expressed in patients with FAB M0, M1, and M2 AML and in chronic myelogenous leukemia in myeloid blast crisis (462). CD19 expression in AML may be associated with the translocation t(9;22), a poor prognostic indicator, or t(8;21), a favorable prognostic indicator (418,463). CD19 is not expressed by Langerhans cell histiocytosis or true histiocytic and dendritic cell neoplasms (462).

CD20

The CD20 molecule is a membrane-embedded, nonglycosylated, phosphorylated 35- to 37-kd protein that initially was recognized by MAb B1 in 1980 (23). The CD20 cluster was established at the second workshop with MAbs B1, B19 (IF5), and 2H7 (102). Numerous additional MAbs have been clustered as CD20 since then (356,367,464,465). Unlike B1 and some of these other MAbs, MAb L26, first described by Ishii and colleagues in 1984 (466), recognizes the intracellular cytoplasmic tail of CD20 (467) and has no surface membrane reactivity (466,468). It is used exclusively in the detection of CD20 in routinely fixed, paraffin-embedded tissue sections (25,469), in which its reactivity parallels that of MAb B1 in frozen tissue sections (25). It was assigned to the CD20 cluster as cCD20 at the fifth workshop (464). Several other anti-CD20 MAbs that react in paraffin and frozen tissue sections and also can be used to label cells in suspension are available commercially (470). B1 (or Leu16) and L26 remain the antibodies most widely used to detect CD20 in cell suspensions and frozen tissue sections and in paraffin tissue sections, respectively.

The human CD20 gene is a single-copy gene located on chromosome 11q12-q13, near the site of the t(11;14) (q13; q32) translocation (471). The CD20 gene is 16 kbp long and comprises eight exons, six of which encode the protein (472). A sequence element, known as the *BAT box*, located in the most proximal region of the promoter between bases −214 and −201, is important in the high constitutive expression of CD20 in mature B cells and the induction of CD20 in pre-B cells (473). The BAT box also may be important in B cell–specific expression of CD21 (473).

The entire CD20 open reading frame has been cloned and sequenced (474–476). The predicted amino acid sequence contains 297 residues and has a molecular mass of 33,097 d. Only 44 of these amino acid residues are extracellular; both the carboxyl terminus and the amino terminus lie within the cytoplasm. The protein contains three extensive hydrophobic regions that traverse the membrane (474–476). The CD20 molecule structure, with its proposed multiple membrane spanning regions, resembles an ion channel (472). Multiple forms of CD20 result from different patterns of phosphorylation of the CD20 protein (472,477–479). The form with a 33 kd molecular weight represents 75% to 80% of the cell surface CD20. Two additional forms, with molecular weights of 34.5 and 36 kd, account for the remaining 20% to 25% of mCD20 (480). The CD20 protein has no major sequence homology to other known proteins (470).

Although the precise physiologic role of the CD20 molecule remains unknown, studies have shown that it is involved in the regulation of B-cell activation, proliferation, and differentiation (470). Some anti-CD20 MAbs trigger resting B cells to enter the cell cycle or induce IgM production (481); others inhibit B-cell activation (479). Anti-CD20 MAbs B1 and B19 interact with close but distinct epitopes (480,482). MAb B19 directly stimulates small, resting B cells to proliferate (477), initiating the transition from the G_0 to the G_1 phase of the cell cycle (482) and increasing the level of mRNA expression for the *MYC* gene (483). Also, similar to anti-immunoglobulin, MAb B19 can induce increased expression of MHC class II antigens (477,478,482). In contrast, MAb B1 inhibits B-cell proliferation to various activation signals and prevents entry of the cells into the S and $G_2 + M$ phases of the cell cycle (484). Both MAbs B1 and B19 are protein inhibitors of B-cell differentiation to immunoglobulin-secreting cells (484). In addition, the CD20 molecule downregulates both constitutive and interleukin-4 (IL-4)–induced CD23 expression on EBV-transformed B cells, primarily because of an increase in cleavage of the CD23 molecule at the B-cell surface (485). It has been hypothesized that the CD20 molecule is an integral component of a calcium channel or regulates a calcium channel (486). This is supported by studies suggesting that the CD20 protein structure is similar to that of other calcium channel–forming structures (487). It appears that CD20 directly regulates transmembrane calcium conductance in B cells; it has been suggested that multimeric complexes of CD20 may form calcium conductive ion channels in the plasma membrane of B cells (485). Other structural and functional aspects of CD20 have been reviewed in detail by Chang, Arber, and Weiss (470).

CD20 appears on the B-cell surface between immunoglobulin light chain gene rearrangement and the expression of intact sIg. CD20 apparently is expressed after CD19 and CD10 expression but before cytoplasmic μ chain expression. CD20 continues to be expressed throughout B-cell differentiation and is lost only prior to terminal differentiation of B cells into plasma cells (218,511,488–490). CD20 is expressed by both resting and activated B cells, although its expression is fourfold greater on activated than on resting B cells (491,492). CD20 antigen density is greater than that

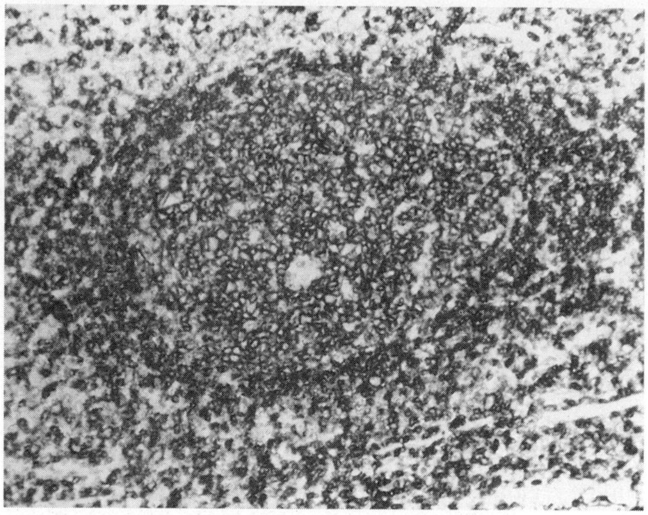

FIG. 3.22. Formalin-fixed, paraffin-embedded tissue section of a benign lymph node immunostained with monoclonal anti-CD20 antibody L26. CD20 is expressed strongly by virtually all germinal center and mantle zone B cells as well as by scattered interfollicular B cells (immunoperoxidase stain, original magnification: 200× magnification).

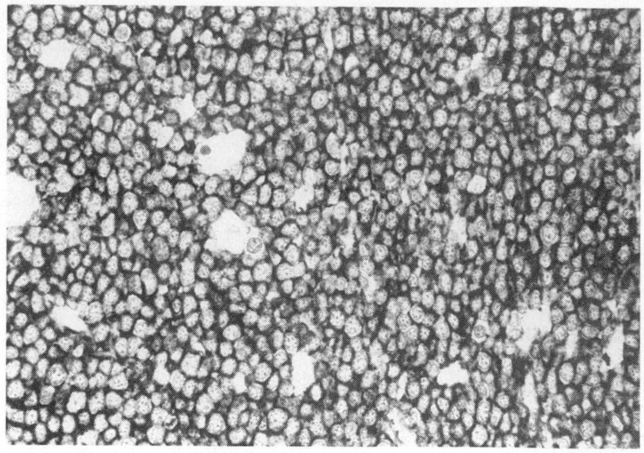

FIG. 3.23. Formalin-fixed, paraffin-embedded tissue section of mantle cell lymphoma immunostained with monoclonal anti-CD20 antibody L26. Virtually all of the neoplastic B cells strongly express CD20 (immunoperoxidase stain, original magnification: 250× magnification).

of CD19 on peripheral blood B cells, making it the preferred choice for B-cell enumeration by flow cytometry (470). CD20 is expressed strongly by virtually all germinal center and mantle zone B cells in mature, peripheral lymphoid tissues (25,322,469,493) (Fig. 3.22). CD20 antigen density is greater on the germinal center than on the mantle zone B cells (493). CD20 also is expressed by scattered interfollicular B cells with the morphology of immunoblasts (25,466,468,469) but not by plasma cells (466,469), and it is expressed by thymic medullary B cells (494). It has been reported that CD20 expression is increased on B cells from HIV-infected individuals, and that this increase tends to be greater in individuals who have more advanced disease (495). This increased expression may reflect polyclonal B-cell activation and hypergammaglobulinemia (496).

Hutlin and colleagues (497) reported that a minor human T-cell subset expresses low levels of CD20 or a cross-reacting antigen. They found the $CD20^{dim}$ T cells to be immunophenotypically heterogeneous and, compared with $CD20^{-}$ T cells, more likely to be $\gamma\delta^{+}$ and $CD8^{+}CD45RO^{+}$ and less likely to be $CD38^{+}$ or $CD4^{+}$ (497). The $CD20^{dim}$ T cells were distinct from $CD5^{dim}$ B cells (497). A small subset of peripheral blood $CD20^{+}$ T cells also has been identified by another group (498). Except for B cells and, possibly, weak expression by a minor T-cell subset, CD20 is not expressed by other hematolymphoid cells including benign, normal precursor T cells, immature and mature myeloid and erythroid cells, megakaryocytes, monocytes/macrophages, Langerhans cells, dendritic cells, and mesenchymal cells (23,25,102,353,466,469,499).

CD20 expression, whether determined by cytofluorometric analysis of cell suspensions or by immunohistochemical analysis of frozen or paraffin tissue sections, is a sensitive and highly specific marker of B cell lineage neoplasms. Virtually all the malignant B cells in greater than 95% of patients with small lymphocytic lymphoma/chronic lymphocytic leukemia, mantle cell lymphoma, marginal zone lymphoma, follicle center cell lymphoma, large cell lymphoma, Burkitt's lymphoma, prolymphocytic leukemia, and hairy cell leukemia express CD20. This is true irrespective of the location of disease and the presence or absence of sIg expression by the neoplastic B cells (Figs. 3.23–3.25). CD20 expression by the malignant B-cell population comprising patients with plasmacytoid small lymphocytic lymphoma, Waldenström's macroglobulinemia, and immunoblastic lymphoma is slightly more variable and is related to the

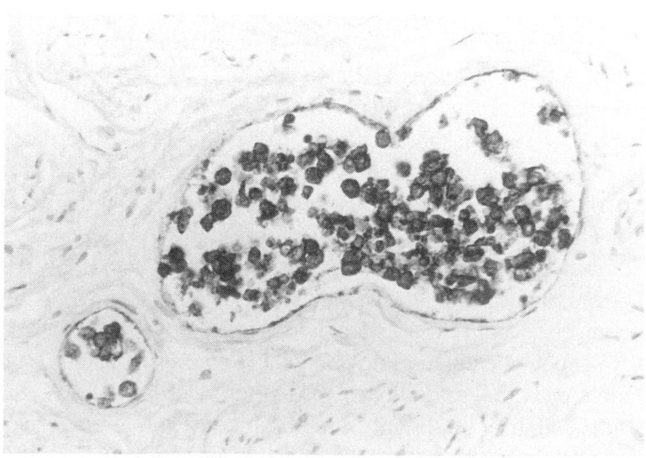

FIG. 3.24. Formalin-fixed, paraffin-embedded tissue section of B-cell intravascular lymphomatosis immunostained with monoclonal anti-CD20 antibody L26. The malignant B cells present within the vascular lumens strongly express CD20 and are readily identifiable (immunoperoxidase stain, original magnification: 250× magnification).

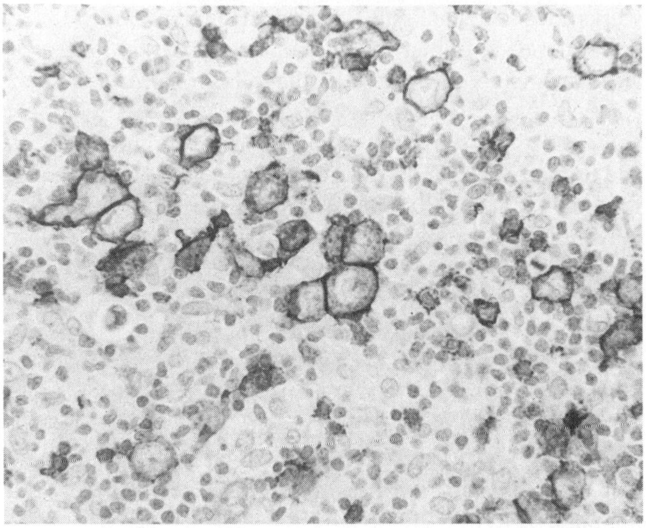

FIG. 3.25. Formalin-fixed, paraffin-embedded tissue section of a T cell–rich B-cell lymphoma (pseudoperipheral T-cell lymphoma) immunostained with monoclonal anti-CD20 antibody L26. The large neoplastic B cells strongly express CD20 and are easily recognizable among the numerous CD20-negative residual benign T cells (immunoperoxidase stain, original magnification: 400× magnification).

degree of plasma cell differentiation (7,8,23–25,218,318, 320,462,469,500–502). Originally, CD20 was thought to be consistently absent from malignant plasma cells, mirroring its lack of expression by benign plasma cells (25,322,466, 469,501). More recent studies, however, have suggested that a variable proportion of myeloma plasma cells in 6 to 20% of patients express CD20 (503–506). CD20 expression does not appear to correlate with plasma cell morphology (503). Some investigators have suggested that patients with CD20$^+$ multiple myeloma have a more aggressive clinical course, however (506). The malignant lymphoblasts in only about 50% of precursor B-cell lymphoblastic lymphomas/leukemias express CD20 (7,25,218,320,328,340,461,469,501). This is because CD20 follows HLA-DR, TdT, CD19, and CD10 expression in B-cell ontogeny (218,461,488,489), and therefore only those B-lineage lymphoblasts that have attained that level of B-cell maturation express CD20 (218,461). The malignant blasts in about 50% of patients with chronic myelogenous leukemias in lymphoid blast crisis express CD20 (24,236), for the same reasons.

In more than 90% of patients with nodular L&H (lymphocyte predominance) Hodgkin's disease, the majority of the L&H cells express CD20 (315,332,469,507–515) (Fig. 3.26). Among the nodular sclerosis, mixed cellularity, and lymphocyte depletion subtypes of Hodgkin's disease, a variable but often small proportion of the Reed-Sternberg cells and variants in about 25% of patients express CD20 (315,332,469,507-510,513,514,516–519). In paraffin tissue sections immunostained with MAb L26, the L&H cells and Reed-Sternberg cells and variants exhibit strong, distinct membrane positivity, accompanied by strong paranuclear globular positivity (332,508,516,517). Occasionally, weak cytoplasmic positivity also is observed (508). CD20 expression appears to be strongest in patients with lymphocyte predominance Hodgkin's disease (508). In addition to the

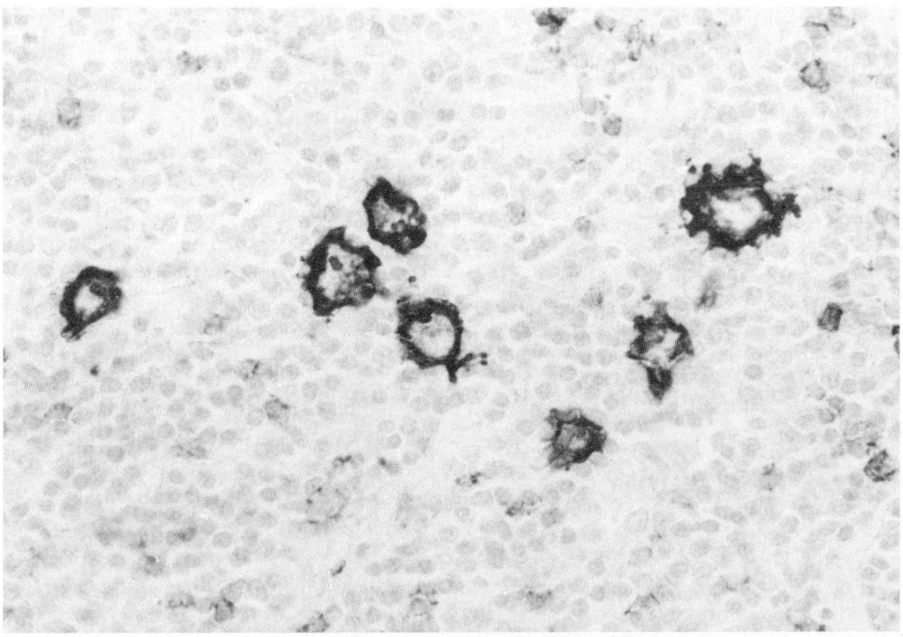

FIG. 3.26. Formalin-fixed, paraffin-embedded tissue section of lymphocyte predominance Hodgkin's disease immunostained with monoclonal anti-CD20 antibody L26. The Reed-Sternberg cells and Reed-Sternberg cell variants exhibit strong and distinct membrane staining with monoclonal antibody L26 (immunoperoxidase stain, original magnification: 400× magnification).

malignant cells, approximately 50% of the background small lymphocytes of nodular lymphocyte predominance Hodgkin's disease express CD20 (508). Careful attention to CD20 expression may be useful in distinguishing among Hodgkin's disease, anaplastic large cell lymphoma, and T cell–rich B-cell lymphoma (470,520) (see Fig. 3.25).

A subset of $CD20^{dim}$-positive normal T cells has been described (497,498) and rare $CD20^+$ T cell neoplasms have been reported. The latter includes a $CD20^+$ EBV-containing peripheral T-cell lymphoma (498) and rare cases of $CD20^+$ precursor T-cell lymphoblastic lymphoma/leukemia (521). Despite these reports, CD20 expression remains a highly specific marker of B-cell lineage neoplasms. Among six large immunohistochemical surveys, not a single one of 168 T-cell lymphomas expressed CD20, based on their uniform nonreactivity with MAbs B1 or L26 (24,315,320,502,522, 523) (Fig. 3.27). Among 854 patients with childhood and adult AML collected from 70 separate studies, only 3% contained any $CD20^+$ malignant cells (524). Traweek (343) identified $CD20^+$ malignant cells in only one of 204 AMLs; Hanson and associates (525) found $CD20^+$ malignant cells in 2 of 52 acute biphenotypic leukemias. Traweek and colleagues (344) reported less than 10% $CD20^+$ malignant cells in 1 of 28 granulocytic sarcomas, and none were found among 30 granulocytic sarcomas in another study (526). Patients with true histiocytic lymphoma, Langerhans cell histiocytosis (320,322,527), and nonhematopoietic neoplasms (25,501) similarly lack CD20. Chilosi and coworkers (528) have reported CD20 expression by the neoplastic epithelial cells in a subset of human thymomas.

Monoclonal antibody L26 is immunoreactive in tissue processed in a variety of fixatives, including buffered formalin, B5, formol saline, and acid formalin (25,322,353,501). Although some investigators have reported that MAb L26 works adequately in tissue fixed with Bouin's solution (322), our experience is that L26 immunoreactivity is lost, or is at best variable, in tissues that have been fixed in Bouin's solution. Also, it has been noted that MAb L26 does not work well in tissues processed in Zenker's solution (322), and furthermore that decalcification may alter L26 immunoreactivity (25). CD20 expression is believed to be stronger in B5-fixed than in formalin-fixed tissues (501,508), because MAb L26 reacted with 97% of B5-fixed, compared with 89% of formalin-fixed, B-cell lymphomas in one study (501). Many immunohistochemists believe that optimal immunoreactivity with MAb L26 occurs in tissue processed after B5 fixation (25,353,501,508). In addition, although some investigators claim that trypsinization increases L26 immunoreactivity, most immunohistochemists have found that pretreatment with trypsin decreases or abolishes L26 immunoreactivity (322,353,469).

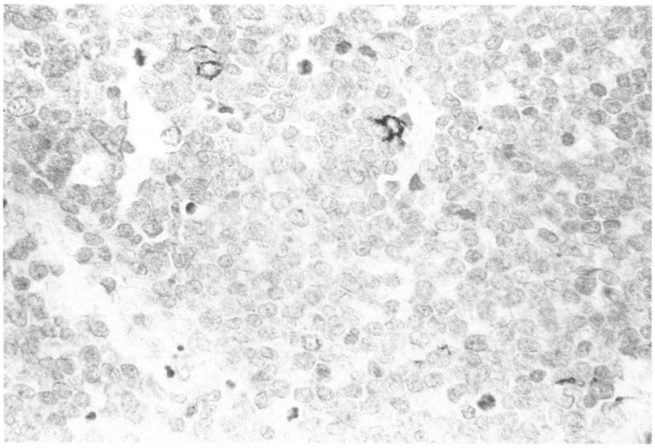

FIG. 3.27. Formalin-fixed, paraffin-embedded tissue section of a precursor T-cell lymphoblastic lymphoma immunostained with monoclonal anti-CD20 antibody L26. Only rare residual benign B cells express CD20. The malignant T lymphoblasts are CD20-negative (immunoperoxidase stain, original magnification: 400× magnification).

CD21

The CD21 cluster was established at the second workshop (102). The prototype antibody was MAb B2 (103). Numerous additional MAbs, including for example HB5 (99), OKB1, and OKB7 (104,105), have been added to this cluster since then (356,367,529,530). These and other anti-CD21 MAbs identify at least six distinct CD21 epitopes (531,532). CD21 belongs to a family of complement regulatory proteins that includes CD35 (CR1), C4-binding protein, factor H, and CD55 (decay-accelerating factor) (533,534). The CD21 molecule serves as the receptor on B cells for the iC3b, C3d,g and C3d fragments of the third component of complement (96,97) and hence also is known as CR2. CD21 also serves as the receptor for EBV on human B cells (98).

Cell surface CD21 is a 140-kd glycoprotein encoded by a gene located at 1q32 that is tightly linked to genes for CD35, CD55, and C4-binding protein (533). It has been suggested that CD21 and CD35 are the result of duplication of the same ancestral gene sequence (535). The CD21 gene consists of an extracellular domain, a 28–amino acid transmembrane domain and a 34–amino acid C-terminal cytoplasmic tail (530). The extracellular domain is comprised of 15 or 16 compactly folded units of 60 to 70 amino acid residues each, called *short consensus repeats*, that are organized into at least five groups and account for at least six distinct epitopes (536). The cytoplasmic domain contains potential protein kinase C and tyrosine kinase phosphorylation sites (533). Several allelic forms of CR2 are known (533).

CD21 noncovalently associates with CD19 and also associates with other cell surface proteins such as CD81 and Leu13 to form a multimolecular signal transduction complex that is unique to B cells (450,451) (CD19). The CD19-CD21 complex appears to play an important role in the activation and growth regulation of B cells (440). Because the short cytoplasmic domain of CD21 is believed to be incapable of transducing signals across the plasma membrane, the association of CD21 with CD19 and CD81 provides a molecular explanation for the signaling capacity of this receptor (440). CD21 may serve as an iC3b and C3d,g ligand-binding unit for the CD19-CD21 complex (440). This complex does not require CD21 for signal transduction, however (537). The several distinct CD21 epitopes, when binding their specific ligands, result in differential transmembrane signalling (530). CD21 ligands specifically binding to the C3d,g-EBV binding site of CD21 strongly enhance B-cell activation through a selective FOS-dependent signaling pathway (538). The role of CD21 as a C3d,g receptor suggests a link between complement activation and B cell function (440). In addition, CD21 has been shown to bind CD23, a low-affinity receptor for human IgE (FcεRII). Interaction between CD21 and CD23 is believed to play a role in B- and T-cell interaction and in the control of IgE production (539–541). No functional differences have been detected among the different allelic forms of CR2 (533,542).

CD21 is expressed by mature B cells, follicular dendritic cells, subsets of normal thymocytes and T cells, and certain epithelial cells (529,533). CD21 appears later than CD19 and CD20 in B-cell ontogeny; CD21 is not expressed by precursor and immature B cells in the fetal liver and bone marrow (99). Mature B cells first express CD21 in the third trimester of fetal life (534). CD21 is lost from B cells during the early stages of activation and is absent from activated B cells that still express CD19 and CD20 (100,102). CD21 is not expressed by plasma cells (99,100). CD21 has a narrower window of expression by B cells than do CD19 and CD20. CD21 is expressed by most, but not all, peripheral blood and lymphoid tissue B cells, but CD21 expression by lymphoid tissue B cells is generally stronger (101). In lymphoid tissues, CD21 expression is absent or weak on germinal center B cells, moderate on mantle zone B cells, and strong on marginal zone B cells (530,543,544). CD21 expression is minimal or absent on bone marrow B cells (102). Follicular dendritic cells strongly express C3d receptors (CD21) (101,499,545,546) that are identical to those expressed on B cells (545) (Fig. 3.28). Low-density CD21 expression by some thymocytes and mature T cells has been described (547,548), the biologic significance of which is unclear (529). CD21 is not expressed by monocytes or macrophages, NK cells, granulocytes, or other nonlymphoid hematopoietic cells (530). CD21 is expressed, however, by some epithelial cells (549,550); it is likely that it mediates EBV adsorption to these cells (551).

CD21 is expressed by most B-cell chronic lymphocytic leukemias, follicle center cell lymphomas, and mantle cell lymphomas but by only approximately 50% or less of large B-cell lymphomas (99,101–103,462). CD21 is expressed by endemic (African) but not sporadic (Western) Burkitt's lymphomas (102). CD21 is not expressed by hairy cell leukemias, lymphoplasmacytoid lymphomas, Waldenström's macroglobulinemia, or multiple myeloma or by most precursor B-cell lymphoblastic lymphomas/leukemias (99,101–103,218,462). CD21 expression by some T-cell neoplasms, including occasional precursor T cell lymphoblastic lymphomas/leukemias, has been described (102,552,553). AMLs do not express CD21 (102).

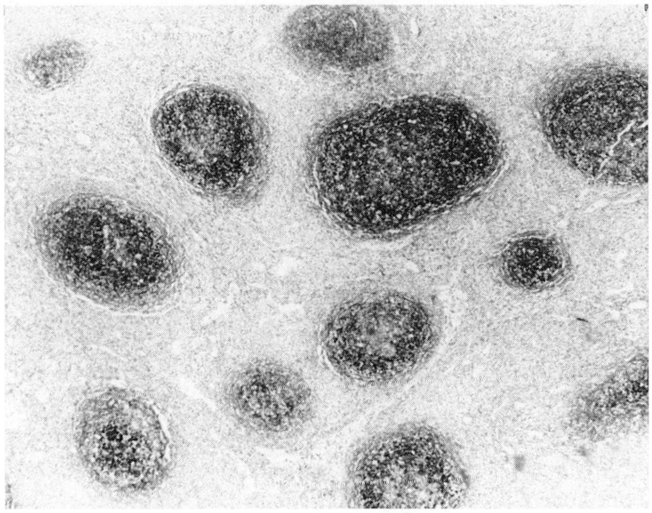

FIG. 3.28. Frozen tissue section of a benign lymph node immunostained with monoclonal anti-CD21 antibody B2. The germinal centers are highlighted because of the strong immune reactivity of MAb B2 with follicular dendritic cells (immunoperoxidase stain, original magnification: 40× magnification).

CD22

The CD22 cluster was defined at the second workshop (102) by MAbs HD39 (B3) (554), S-HCL1 (Leu14) (555), and To15 (556), among others. Additional antibodies have been added to the CD22 cluster in subsequent workshops (557). CD22 is a B-cell lineage–restricted glycosylated type I integral membrane protein whose gene has been mapped to chromosome 19q13, a region to which adhesion receptors with sequence homology to CD22 also have been mapped (558). The human CD22 gene consists of 15 exons with similar overall structure (558). It is a member of the immunoglobulin gene superfamily. It consists of an extracellular region composed of an amino-terminal V-type immunoglobulin-like domain followed by six C-type immunoglobulin-like domains (559) and a cytoplasmic tail (560). The two amino-terminal immunoglobulin-like domains exhibit significant amino acid sequence homologies with CD33, myelin-associated glycoprotein, and the neural adhesion molecule N-CAM (560). The cytoplasmic tail contains a region with homology to a motif found in the cytoplasmic domains of several signal-transduction molecules termed the *antigen receptor recognition homology 1 motif* (561). Two molecular species of CD22 exist, a complete 140-kd form and a minor 130-kd isoform that lacks the fourth immunoglobulin-like domain (562). Different anti-CD22 MAbs recognize distinct epitopes, most of which correspond to specific immunoglobulin-like domains (563).

It is likely that the CD22 molecule functions as an adhesion receptor and as a signaling molecule that probably plays a significant role in B-cell activation (560). CD22 has been shown to mediate adhesion to B and T lymphocytes, neutrophils, monocytes, and red blood cells (559,562,564). The engagement of CD22 with MAb that blocks the binding of CD22 to its ligands results in rapid CD22 tyrosine phosphorylation and an increased association of LYN and SRC kinases as well as phosphatidylinositol 3-kinase with the cytoplasmic portion of CD22 (565). An association between protein tyrosine phosphatase 1C and the cytoplasmic domain of CD22 also has been demonstrated (566,567). The precise functional role of CD22 *in vivo* and its natural ligands remains unclear (560).

CD22 is expressed in the cytoplasm at the earliest stages of pre-B cell differentiation; approximately 80% of TdT^+ bone marrow precursor B cells express cCD22 (568,569). cCD22 and CD19 appear at about the same time during B-cell ontogeny, and prior to CD20. CD22 is not exported to the cell surface until the mature, resting B-cell stage (554,569). Surface CD22 expression accompanies or follows surface IgM and precedes or accompanies surface IgD expression (568,570). Although approximately 95% of peripheral blood B cells contain cCD22, only about 75% express surface CD22 (102,555,568,569). Following mitogen activation *in vitro*, CD22 expression transiently increases but then rapidly decreases and is lost during the terminal stages of B-cell differentiation prior to the plasma cell stage (102,554,569). In lymph nodes, tonsils, and other benign lymphoid tissues, mantle zone (resting mature) B cells strongly express CD22; germinal center (activated or differentiating) B cells express considerably lower levels of CD22 (101,102) (Fig. 3.29). CD22 is not expressed by T cells, monocytes/macrophages (with the exception of occasional weak staining of epithelioid histiocytes), follicular dendritic cells, granulocytes, or nonlymphoid tissues (101,102,571).

The pattern of CD22 expression among B-cell neoplasms is heterogeneous and does not appear to be differentiation- or activation-related. Virtually 100% of hairy cell leukemias and B-prolymphocytic leukemias, 70% of follicle center cell and large B-cell lymphomas, and more than 50% of precursor B-cell lymphoblastic lymphomas/leukemias express surface or cCD22 (102,462,555,569,571,572). The intensity of immunoreactivity is greatest on hairy cell and prolymphocytic leukemias (462,555,571). Different investigators have reported that from 25% to 90% of B-cell chronic lymphocytic leukemias express CD22 (101,571). Waldenström's macroglobulinemia and lymphoplasmacytoid lymphomas generally express CD22, but multiple myeloma is consistently $CD22^-$ (571). Precursor and postthymic T-cell NHLs and lymphoid leukemias consistently lack CD22 (102,571,572). CD22 is a valuable marker for distinguishing B- and T-cell neoplasms. Anti-CD22 MAbs react with a small proportion of AMLs, but in these instances the antibodies appear to be detecting a high molecular weight cytoplasmic protein that cross-reacts with CD22 (571,572).

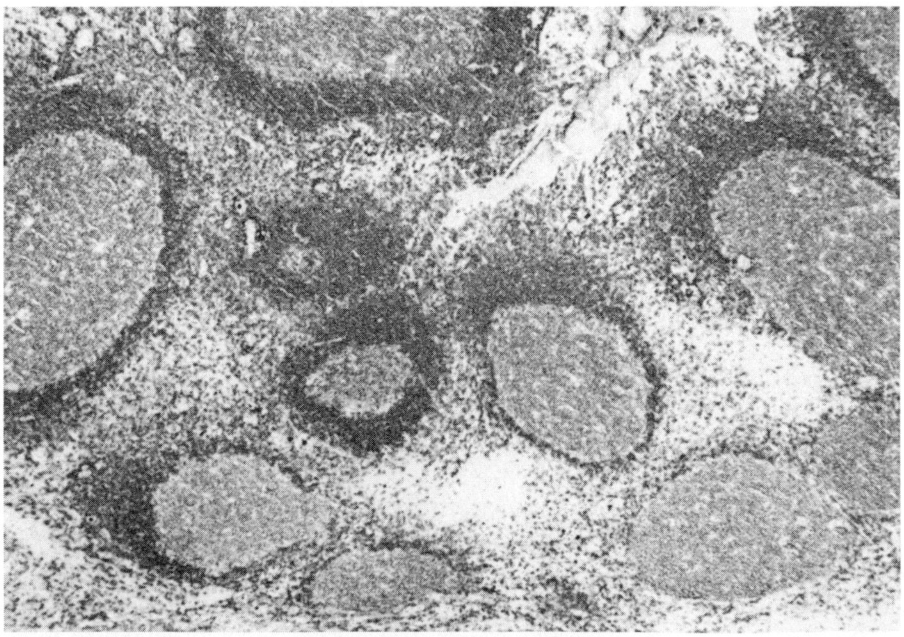

FIG. 3.29. Frozen tissue section of tonsil immunostained for B-cell lineage–associated antigen CD22. The primary and secondary follicles (B-cell zones) express CD22, as do occasional small numbers of interfollicular B cells. The mantle zone (resting mature) B cells express CD22 in higher density than the majority of germinal center (activated or differentiating) B cells (immunoperoxidase stain, original magnification: 40× magnification).

CD23

The CD23 cluster was established at the second workshop (102) by MAbs BLAST-2 (573) and MHM6 (574). Since then, many additional anti-CD23 MAbs have been prepared and characterized (575,576). CD23 has been identified independently as a cell surface marker specifically expressed on EBV-transformed B cells (577) or as a B-cell activation antigen (BLAST-2) (573) and as the low-affinity receptor for IgE (FcϵRII) on human lymphoblastoid cells (578,579).

Cell surface CD23 is a 45-kd glycoprotein (101) encoded by a gene mapped to 19p13 (580). CD23 is a type II integral membrane glycoprotein comprised of a 23–amino acid amino-terminal intracytoplasmic tail, a 20–amino acid transmembrane domain, and a 277 amino acid carboxyl-terminal extracellular region (581). CD23 is associated spatially with MHC class II antigens (582). CD23 does not belong to the immunoglobulin gene superfamily (581). Two human CD23 isoforms (A and B), differing by six amino acids in their intracytoplasmic domains, are generated after alternate splicing of exon 2 of the same CD23 gene (581). mCD23 has a half-life of only 1 or 2 hours. Processing at the cell surface releases soluble fragments of CD23 of varying molecular weight (16 kd, 25 kd, 33 kd) (583). The soluble fragments of CD23 isoforms A and B are identical (584).

Since its discovery as the low-affinity receptor for IgE (FcϵRII) on B cells (578,579), it has been suggested that CD23 plays an important role in the regulation of IgE production. Soluble CD23 enhances IgE synthesis (585), and anti-CD23 MAb profoundly suppresses IgE synthesis (586) *in vitro*. Also, polyclonal anti-CD23 antibodies inhibit an *in vivo* antigen-specific IgE response (587). The other established function of cell surface CD23 is to facilitate antigen presentation by B cells to T cells by efficient trapping of IgE immune complexes (582,588). CD23 type A isoform likely is involved in antigen presentation (576). The precise function of CD23 type B isoform on activated B cells is unclear (576). It is involved in the IgE-dependent biologic activities of inflammatory cells (576), however, including the release of TNF-α and IL-1, and the generation of superoxides (539). In contrast with cell surface CD23, the biologic activities of soluble CD23 are largely IgE-dependent (581). Soluble CD23 is a proinflammatory molecule in that it triggers monocytes to release TNF-α, IL-1, IL-6, and GM-CSF and causes an increase in oxidative products (589,590). Soluble CD23 also potently costimulates IL-2- or IL-12-induced interferon-γ by T cells (589). CD23 probably plays a role in inflammatory diseases (581).

The CD23 antigen differs from other B-cell lineage–restricted antigens in that it is expressed weakly or not at all on resting, mature peripheral blood and lymphoid tissue B cells (102,573,591) but appears on B cells within 24 hours following their activation with various stimuli, both *in vitro* and *in vivo* (102,573). In lymphoid tissue, CD23 expression is absent or variably present on only a small fraction of mantle zone (resting mature) B cells, is absent from splenic marginal zone B cells, but is present on a variable proportion of germinal center (activated) B cells (101,102,444,592). The CD23 type A isoform is restricted to resting B cells; the CD23 type B isoform is expressed on activated B cells (584). CD23 expression on B cells is dramatically and rapidly upregulated after EBV, phorbol ester, and IL-4 activation (573,593,594). CD23 only is expressed and its expression induced, however, on mature sIgMD$^+$ B cells and not on B cells that have already lost surface IgD, undergone isotype switch, and express surface IgG, IgA, or IgE (591). CD23 type B isoform only also is expressed by monocytes, eosinophils, Langerhan's cells, follicular dendritic cells in the light zone (Fig. 3.30), and subpopulations of T cells, platelets, and thymic epithelium (582,595–597). CD23 is not expressed by precursor B cells, plasma cells, or myeloid cells (573,582,597). CD23 similarly is not expressed by normal nonlymphoid tissue (592).

The CD23 gene appears to be abnormally expressed and regulated in B-cell chronic lymphocytic leukemia (581). CD23 is expressed strongly by the neoplastic B cells in the majority of these patients (101,573,592), and they often have elevated levels of soluble CD23 (581). It even has been suggested that soluble CD23 serum levels are useful in identifying those patients who are at risk of developing disease progression at an early stage and is a significant prognostic marker for survival (598). CD23 also frequently is expressed by follicle center cell lymphomas (101,102,462,573,592). In contrast, CD23 usually is not expressed by mantle cell lymphomas or by nodal or extranodal marginal zone lymphomas (462,599,600) (Fig. 3.30). Consequently, it is often useful to consider CD23 expression in the differential diagnosis of small B-cell neoplasms. CD23 typically is not expressed by the vast majority of patients with hairy cell

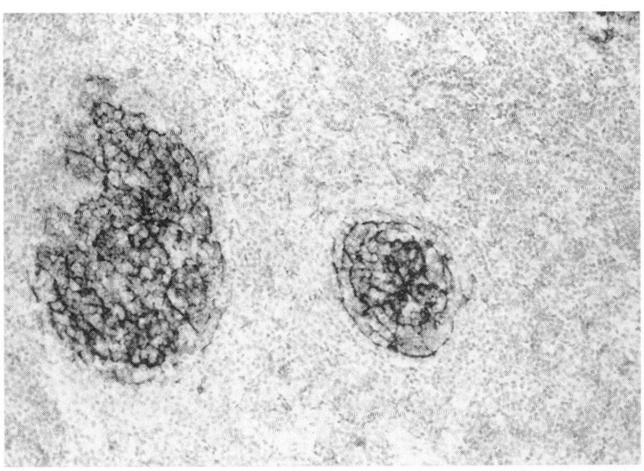

FIG. 3.30. Frozen tissue section of a benign lymph node immunostained with monoclonal anti-CD23 antibody BLAST-2. The follicular dendritic cell population in the light zone of the germinal center expresses CD23 (immunoperoxidase stain, original magnification: 100× magnification).

leukemia, plasmacytoma/multiple myeloma, precursor B- and T-cell lymphoblastic lymphoma/leukemia, postthymic T-cell neoplasia, or acute and chronic myeloid leukemia (102,462,573,592,600).

CD24

The CD24 cluster was established at the first workshop (15) by the prototype MAb BA-1 (601). Many other antibodies, including OKB2 (104,105), have been added to this cluster since (602). The CD24 gene has been mapped to 6p21 (603). CD24 is a glycosyl phosphatidylinositol-anchored (604) single-chain sialoglycoprotein with a molecular mass of 35 to 45 kd (605). CD24 consists of a short, mature peptide core of 31 to 35 amino acids of about 4 kd, which directs the extensive N- and O-linked glycosylation (606). About 90% of the molecular mass of CD24 consists of carbohydrate structures (606). Anti-CD24 MAbs recognize at least four distinct peptide and oligosaccharide epitopes (607,608).

The cellular function of human CD24 is uncertain (609). Human CD24 is structurally homologous to the murine heat stable antigen (606), however, and these molecules share similar patterns of cellular expression during B-cell ontogeny in the bone marrow (609). Therefore, CD24 may play a functional role similar to that of heat stable antigen in early B-cell development and intercellular adhesion (609). These molecules also may have similar functional roles in the activation of mature B cells (609).

CD24 is a pan-B cell antigen. It is expressed virtually throughout B-cell differentiation, beginning with $CD34^+$ progenitor B cells in the bone marrow and continuing through mature $sIgMD^+$ B cells until the onset of plasma cell differentiation; CD24 is not expressed by plasma cells (101,601,610–612). In lymphoid tissues, CD24 is expressed by primary follicular and mantle zone B cells but is absent or only expressed weakly by germinal center B cells (356). CD24 is not expressed by T cells, monocytes, or red blood cells but is expressed by mature granulocytes (101,601,604) and therefore is not B cell lineage–restricted. CD24 also is expressed by kidney and other epithelia and cells of neural crest origin (408,613,614).

CD24 is expressed by the vast majority of precursor B cell lymphoblastic lymphomas/leukemias and by chronic myelogenous leukemia in lymphoid blast crisis and also by virtually all mature (TdT^-) sIg^+ and sIg^- B-cell NHLs and lymphoid leukemias except for nodal and extranodal marginal zone lymphomas. CD24 similarly is not expressed by plasmacytoma/multiple myeloma (101,462,601,615). CD24 is not expressed by precursor T-cell lymphoblastic lymphomas/leukemias or by postthymic T-cell neoplasms (101,601). It is expressed by $CD13^+CD33^+$ small myeloblasts in the bone marrow of patients who have chronic myelogenous leukemia and chronic myelogenous leukemia in myeloid blast crisis (616) and also by tumors of neuroectodermal origin (613). As in the case of other MAbs that recognize pan-B cell antigens, anti-CD24 MAbs such as BA-1 have been used to purge the bone marrow of acute lymphoblastic leukemia cells in autologous bone marrow transplantation (615).

CD79

Antibodies against mb-1/Ig-α and B29/Ig-β were clustered as $CD79_\alpha$ and $CD79_\beta$, respectively, at the fifth workshop (617). $CD79_\alpha$ and $CD79_\beta$ form disulfide-linked heterodimers that noncovalently associate with sIg to constitute the B-cell antigen receptor complex on the surface of mature B cells (618–620). All sIg isotypes can be expressed together with $CD79_\alpha$ and $CD79_\beta$ (620). This multimeric complex functions in antigen recognition and internalization and in signal transduction (621). Its expression is restricted to the B-cell lineage (618–620,622). The anti-$CD79_\alpha$ MAbs include HM47 (622) and HM57 (622), and the anti-$CD79_\beta$ MAbs include SN8 (623) and B29-123 (617). JCB117 (624) was clustered as $CD79_\alpha$ and CH3-1 and CH3-2 (625) were clustered as $CD79_\beta$ at the sixth workshop (621). MAbs HM47, HM57, and B29-123 were subclustered as $CD79_\alpha$cy and $CD79_\beta$cy, respectively, because they detect intracytoplasmic epitopes (617). Three of these four anti-$CD79_\beta$ MAbs, but none of the three anti-$CD79_\alpha$ MAbs, react with viable B cells, suggesting limited accessibility of their epitopes if the $CD79_\alpha$ chain is assembled with $CD79_\beta$ and IgM as the multimeric B-cell antigen receptor complex (621). Among these antibodies, MAb HM57 has proven to be the most suitable for the detection of cCD79 by cytofluorometric analysis following cell fixation and permeabilization (626). MAb JCB117 recognizes sodium dodecyl sulfate–denatured $CD79_\alpha$ in western blot analysis (624). The $CD79_\alpha$ epitope recognized by MAb JCB117 similarly is either inaccessible or absent on viable B cells (624); it is not useful in cytofluorometric analysis (624). MAb JCB117 is immunoreactive, however, with B cells in formalin-fixed, paraffin-embedded tissue sections (624) and is of considerable utility in diagnostic pathology.

$CD79_\alpha$ is encoded by the *MB1* gene located on 19q13.2 (627). $CD79_\alpha$ is a membrane glycoprotein comprised of a leader peptide of 32 amino acids and extracellular, transmembrane, and intracytoplasmic domains of 111, 22, and 61 amino acids, respectively, with a predicted relative molecular mass of 22 kd (628). $CD79_\beta$ is encoded by the B29 gene located on 17q23 (629,630). $CD79_\beta$ is a membrane glycoprotein comprised of a 30–amino acid leader peptide and extracellular, transmembrane and intracytoplasmic domains of 129, 22, and 48 amino acids, respectively, with a predicted relative molecular mass of 26 kd (629). The extracellular portion of $CD79_\alpha$ constitutes a C2-type immunoglobulin-like domain, and that of $CD79_\beta$ constitutes a V-type immunoglobulin-like domain. The molecular sizes of immunoprecipitated $CD79_\alpha$ and $CD79_\beta$ molecules are heterogeneous because of differential glycosylation (621). The difference in molecular size depends on the maturational stages of B cells and the isotypes of immunoglobulins constituting the B-cell receptor (621).

$CD79_\alpha$ and $CD79_\beta$ form disulfide-linked heterodimers that associate with sIg noncovalently to constitute multimeric B-cell antigen receptor complexes (621). These $CD79_\alpha$-$CD79_\beta$ heterodimers are essential and sufficient for surface expression of the B-cell antigen receptor and for signal transmission into the cytoplasm following antigen binding to sIg (621). Consensus sequences in the cytoplasmic tails of $CD79_\alpha$ and $CD79_\beta$ bind with several protein tyrosine kinases, including LYN, FYN, BTH, and SYK (621). Phosphorylation signals through these kinases switch on downstream signal-transduction pathways, which result in B-cell activation, differentiation, and sometimes apoptosis (621). Although the functional role of each kinase is not fully understood, the signals caused by these kinases are critical to B-cell maturation (631,632). $CD79_\alpha$ and $CD79_\beta$ appear to play distinctive roles in B-cell activation and maturation (633–636).

Among normal hematopoietic cells, CD79 expression is restricted to the B cell lineage (618–620,622). CD79 expression begins at the progenitor B cell stage and continues througout B-cell differentiation, ceasing around the onset of plasma cell differentiation (621,622,624,625). In human lymphoid tissues, $CD79_\alpha$ is expressed more strongly by mantle zone B cells than by germinal center B cells, suggesting that CD79 expression is downregulated by the activation of mature B cells (621) (Fig. 3.31). $CD79_\alpha$ also is expressed by splenic marginal zone B cells and by at least some plasma cells (622). Analogous to T-cell–lineage restricted antigen CD3, CD79 is expressed initially in the cytoplasm, and prior to μ heavy chain expression (622). More than 80% of the normal TdT^+, μ-negative progenitor B cells in the bone marrow contain $CD79_\beta$ (625). Approximately 25% of the $cCD79_\beta{}^+$ cells in the bone marrow are μ-negative; all μ-positive pre-B and B cells express $CD79_\beta$ (621). Surface expression of CD79 appears to correlate with that of μ chain or immunoglobulin (621). Almost all $CD79_\beta{}^+$ cells in the bone marrow express surface μ heavy chain; $CD79_\beta{}^-$ cells express μ heavy chain. Surface expression of CD79 does not occur until μ heavy chain and light chains are synthesized in the late pre-B cell stage (621). Essentially all mature circulating B cells express CD79 (618–620,622). $CD79_\beta$ continues to be expressed following isotype switching and then is downregulated at the terminally differentiated plasma cell stage (625,637). The cell surface expression of $CD79_\alpha$ has not been studied directly because of the unavailability of anti-$CD79_\alpha$ MAbs that are reactive with viable B cells. Also, the anti-$CD79_\alpha$ MAbs react with cytoplasmic determinants and cannot distinguish between surface and $cCD79_\alpha$. The surface expression of $CD79_\alpha$, however, should be similar to that of $CD79_\beta$, because these molecules generally are expressed as heterodimers on the cell surface (621).

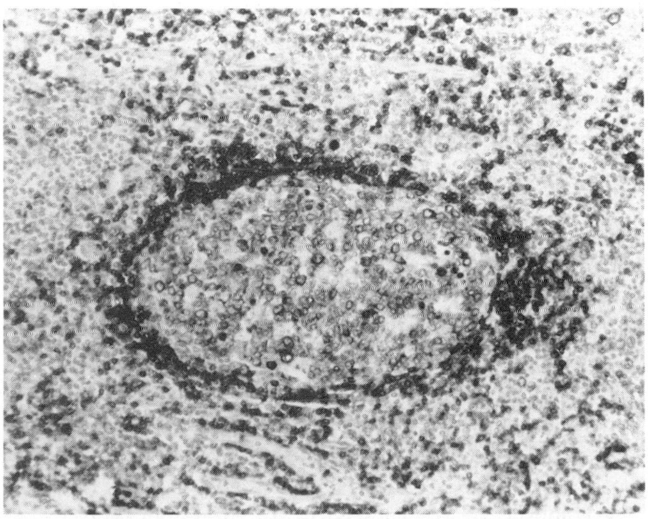

FIG. 3.31. Formalin-fixed, paraffin-embedded tissue section of a benign lymph node immunostained with monoclonal anti-CD79α antibody JCB117. CD79α is expressed more strongly by mantle zone B cells than by germinal center B cells, thus accentuating the mantle zone surrounding the germinal center in this lymphoid follicle (immunoperoxidase stain, original magnification: 200× magnification).

Nearly all patients with precursor B cell lymphoblastic lymphoma/leukemia or chronic myelogenous leukemia in lymphoid blast crisis express $CD79_\alpha$ (622,624,638). More than 95% of all mature (TdT^-) sIg^+ as well as sIg^- NHLs and lymphoid leukemias also express $CD79_\alpha$ (622,624,639). Anti-$CD79_\alpha$ MAb JCB117 is immunoreactive with about 50% of plasmacytomas/multiple myelomas (624). Initially, several investigators reported that all precursor T-cell lymphoblastic lymphomas/leukemias and mature (TdT^-) postthymic NHLs and lymphoid leukemias lack $CD79_\alpha$ (622,624,638,639). All leukemias of myeloid cell derivation, except for those displaying clonal immunoglobulin heavy chain gene rearrangements and lymphoid cell antigens and therefore considered biphenotypic, also were reported to lack $CD79_\alpha$ (624,638). More recent studies suggest that anti-$CD79_\alpha$ MAb JCB117 reacts with many precursor T-cell lymphoblastic lymphomas/leukemias (Gatter K, personal communication, 1998). In addition, anti-$CD79_\alpha$ MAb HM57 is immunoreactive with a small but significant proportion of AMLs, nearly all of which represent cases of FAB M3 AML (acute promyelocytic leukemia) exhibiting the translocation t(15;17) (640). The majority of the L&H cells in most patients wth nodular L&H lymphocyte predominance Hodgkin's disease and a variable but generally small proportion of the Reed-Sternberg cells and variants in about 20% of patients with classic Hodgkin's disease express $CD79_\alpha$ (641). In summary, $CD79_\alpha$ serves as an excellent B-cell marker for malignant B-cell populations at all but the terminal stages of B-cell differentiation and is often helpful in distinguishing B and T-cell neoplasms. CD79 expression, however, is not restricted entirely to neoplasms of B-cell lineage derivation.

CD138

This molecule was defined by plasma cell–specific MAbs B-B2, B-B4 (642), and MI15 (643), which were described at the fifth workshop (642,643), and clustered as CD138 at the sixth workshop (644). CD138 was given the name *syndecan-1*, coming from the Greek *syndein* meaning to bind together, because it appears to bind together components of the cellular microenvironment with the cytoskeleton (644). Syndecan-1 is a member of the family of transmembrane heparan sulfate proteoglycans (645). Because it has been recognized only recently, CD138, including its cellular expression, has been best studied in the mouse (646–648) and remains incompletely studied in the human.

Syndecan-1 is a member of the family of transmembrane heparan sulfate proteoglycans (645). The syndecan-1 core protein is a 30-kd single-chain molecule comprised of extracellular, transmembrane, and intracellular domains of 234, 25, and 34 amino acids, respectively (645). The protein bears heparan sulfates and sometimes chondroitin sulfates (644). Five putative glycosoaminoglycan attachment sites are located in the ectodomain, and a putative protease cleavage site is present at its carboxyl terminus (644). The different molecular weights achieved with different anti-CD138 MAbs in immunoprecipitation and western blotting studies most likely reflect the variable glycosoaminoglycan pattern on syndecan-1 (644). All four anti-CD138 MAbs react with the extracellular domain but appear to recognize two close but distinct epitopes (645).

CD138 is an extracellular matrix receptor that permits epithelial organization (649). CD138 may be involved in the organization of cells into tissues and organs (644). A variety of components, such as collagen, fibronectin, thrombin, antithrombin III, and basic fibroblast growth factor, bind to CD138 through heparan sulfates (644). The binding is influenced by the size and composition of the heparan sulfates, which is dependent on the cells producing them (650). CD138 may be responsible for the nonthrombogenic property of the vascular endothelial cell surface (644). A role for CD138 in B-cell stage-specific adhesion in murine B cells has been suggested (651). Mature human plasma cells probably adhere to bone marrow stromal matrix through CD138, because CD138 is involved in their adhesion to type I collagen (652).

Although many antibodies are plasma cell reactive, only the anti-CD138 MAbs appear to be plasma cell–specific (644). Among human hematopoietic cells, only cIg-containing plasma cells express CD138. CD34$^+$ progenitor cells, mature peripheral blood, bone marrow, and tonsil B and T cells, monocytes, granulocytes, platelets, and red blood cells do not express CD138 (643,644,653).

Monoclonal anti-CD138 antibodies are immunoreactive in 60% (643) to 100% (653) of patients in multiple myeloma. CD138 expression is variable among myeloma plasma cells, however; 70% to 100% of the cells within an individual malignant plasma cell population express CD138 (644). The apparent absence of CD138 expression by malignant plasma cells may be because of variation in expression (643), may be related to the differentiation stage of the malignant plasma cells (652), or may result from the sensitivity of CD138 to proteolytic cleavage (642). Anti-CD138 MAbs B-B2 and B-B4 also are immunoreactive with most B-cell chronic lymphocytic leukemias (642) and with the primary effusion lymphomas containing Kaposi's sarcoma–associated herpesvirus (654) (see Chapter 28). CD138 MAbs are not immunoreactive with precursor B-cell lymphoblastic lymphomas/leukemias, Burkitt's lymphoma cell lines, or EBV-infected lymphoblastoid cell lines (643). The further and more definitive elucidation of the immunoreactivity of these MAbs with hematologic malignancies requires additional studies.

Among nonhematopoietic tissues, CD138 is expressed by fibroblasts, endothelial cells, simple and stratified epithelia, and stratified keratinocytes (646–648). Its expression by human keratinocytes is induced by differentiation and suppressed by malignant transformation (655). A correlation between loss of CD138 expression and poor clinical outcome in squamous cell carcinoma of the head and neck has been described (656).

T-Cell Lineage–Associated Antigens

CD1

CD1 was the first human leukocyte differentiation antigen to be defined by MAbs (657) and was recognized as the first cluster of differentiation at the first workshop (15). Initially, CD1 was believed to be limited in expression to immature (cortical) thymocytes (137,657) and thought to represent the human homologue of the murine thymus leukemia antigen (658). Subsequent immunoprecipitation studies demonstrated the existence of three distinct CD1 molecules designated *CD1a*, *CD1b*, and *CD1c* (659–661) and, more recently, a fourth molecule designated *CD1d* (662). MAbs T6 (137), neutrophil antigen 1 (NA1)-34 (657), and Leu6 (663) detect CD1a, MAb 4A76 (664) detects CD1b, and MAb M241 (665) detects CD1c. Many other anti-CD1a, anti-CD1b, and anti-CD1c MAbs have been characterized during subsequent workshops (666,667). All of these MAbs are immunoreactive with viable cells in suspension, in cytocentrifuge preparations, and in frozen tissue sections, but not in paraffin tissue sections. Anti-CD1a MAb O10 (668) detects a fixation-resistant epitope of CD1a and is immunoreactive in paraffin tissue sections prepared from tissue specimens that have been fixed routinely in formalin, Bouin's or Zenker's solution, or B5 (669,670). The immunoreactivity of MAb O10 in routinely fixed, paraffin-embedded tissue sections is comparable to that of other anti-CD1a MAbs in frozen tissue sections (669,670). This antibody should find wide applicability in diagnostic pathology, especially in the immunodiagnosis of Langerhans'cell histiocytosis.

Each CD1 molecule consists of a glycosylated type I transmembrane polypeptide α chain of 49 kd (CD1a), 45 kd (CD1b), or 43 kd (CD1c) that is noncovalently associated with 12-kd β_2-microglobulin and bears a distinct set of epitopes (659–661,671–673). On the basis of sequence homology, CD1 molecules can be classified into two groups: Group 1 includes CD1a, CD1b, and CD1c molecules, and group 2 includes CD1d molecules and their homologues in other species (674). The human CD1 locus contains five genes (*CD1A*, *CD1B*, *CD1C*, *CD1D*, and *CD1E*) covering approximately 190 kb within q22-23 in chromosome 1 (675). The *CD1* genes consist of multiple exons with functional domains of the polypeptide encoded by separate exons (5′-untranslated leader, α_1, α_2, α_3, transmembrane and cytoplasmic 3′-untranslated) (667). The α_1, α_2 ,and α_3 domains encode nonpolymorphic extracellular domains of approximately 90 amino acid residues in length (676). In addition to the different CD1 genes, this antigen possesses considerable complexity, which arises through alternative splicing (667). The alternative splicing pattern is tissue-specific and gives rise to membrane-attached and soluble forms (667).

The CD1 molecules represent a family of MHC class I–like glycoproteins belonging to the immunoglobulin gene superfamily (676,677). Unlike MHC class I molecules, however, they are not polymorphic (678) and they possess a highly restricted tissue distribution. The *CD1* genes are not MHC-linked, because they have been mapped to chromosome 1 (675). In contrast with the MHC-encoded products, CD1 molecules have been shown to restrict T-cell responses to nonpeptide lipid and glycolipid antigens (679). It has been shown that anti-CD1 MAbs can modulate the response of thymocytes by certain bacterial superantigens (680). CD1 molecules could be involved in the delivery of signals for lymphocyte activation. The expression of CD1 molecules on thymocytes has been related to a role in thymic T-cell development (675). It also has been suggested that CD1 may act as a restriction element for T$\gamma\delta$ cells (681).

CD1 has a restricted distribution. Within the T-cell lineage, CD1 is not expressed at the very early stages of T-cell ontogeny (204). CD1a, CD1b, and CD1c are expressed by approximately 70% of all thymocytes. This includes the majority of CD4$^+$CD8$^+$ (double-positive) thymocytes but not the CD4$^+$CD8$^-$ or CD4$^-$CD8$^+$ (single-positive) thymocytes. CD1 molecules are expressed by the majority of cortical thymocytes and are absent from most medullary thymocytes (137,657,682) (Fig. 3.32). *CD1D* gene products also are expressed at low levels in the thymus (667). Similarly, CD1 is not expressed by resting mature peripheral blood and lymphoid tissue T cells (137,657,682). CD1 has been detected, however, in the cytoplasm of activated T cells (683). CD1 expression by benign T cells is mirrored by malignant T cells. Precursor T-cell lymphoblastic lymphomas/leukemias expressing immature (cortical) thymocyte phenotypes, but not those expressing prothymocyte or medullary thymocyte phenotypes, are CD1$^+$ (7,13,14,137,144,222, 462,684). All postthymic (TdT$^-$) T-cell neoplasms, including cutaneous and peripheral T-cell lymphoma, the Sézary syndrome, T-cell chronic lymphocytic and prolymphocytic leukemia, adult T-cell lymphoma/leukemia, anaplastic large cell lymphoma, and LGL/NK cell leukemia consistently lack CD1 expression (6-8,13,14,462,600).

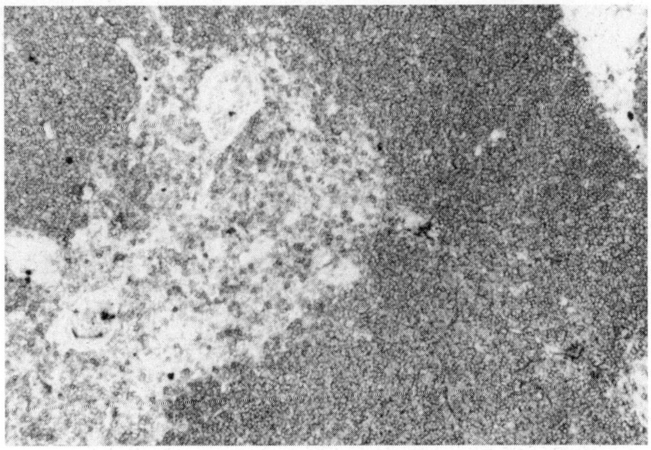

FIG. 3.32. Frozen tissue section of thymus immunostained for CD1a. Essentially all of the cortical thymocytes but only a proportion of the more mature medullary thymocytes express CD1a (immunoperoxidase stain, original magnification: 100× magnification).

Epidermal Langerhans cells express CD1a (669,685,686); dermal and mucosal dendritic cells express CD1a and variably express CD1c (682,687); afferent lymph veiled cells express CD1b (688); and interdigitating dendritic cells express CD1a, CD1b, and CD1c (669,682) (Fig. 3.33). The proliferating cellular component of eosinophilic granuloma, Letterer-Siwe disease, and the Hand-Schüller-Christian syn-

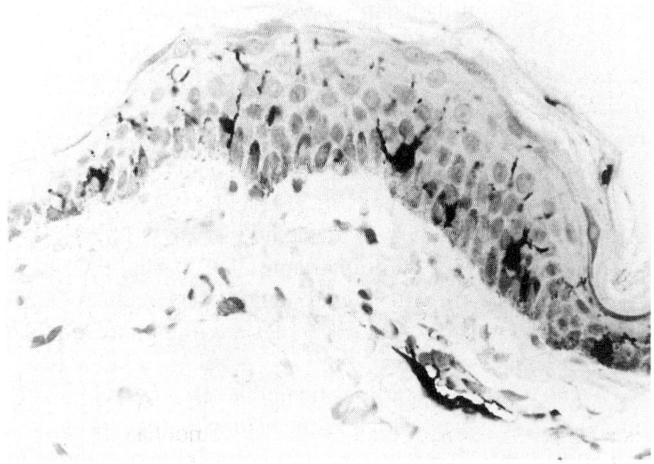

FIG. 3.33. Formalin-fixed, paraffin-embedded tissue section of normal human skin immunostained with a monoclonal anti-CD1a antibody. Epidermal Langerhans cells and dermal dendritic cells are highlighted by their strong expression of CD1a in the absence of the expression of this antigen by other cutaneous cell populations (immunoperoxidase stain, original magnification: 400× magnification).

drome, now collectively referred to as *Langerhans cell histiocytosis* (*histiocytosis X*) is derived from these dendritic cell populations (689) and similarly expresses CD1 (669,670,682,689,690) (see Chapter 51). Benign monocytes/macrophages and follicular dendritic cells and their neoplastic counterparts lack CD1 (297,691–693) (see Chapter 51). CD1a, CD1b and CD1c expression, however, can be induced on monocytes by GM-CSF alone or by GM-CSF plus IL-4 (667), and CD1 molecules have been detected on AMLs (694).

CD1c is expressed by more than 90% of cord blood B cells that express IgM but not IgG. CD1c also is expressed by approximately 50% of spleen B cells, by a smaller proportion of tonsil B cells, and by a small number of circulating B cells in older children and adults who achieve full immunologic competence (695–697). The CD5 B-cell subset is distributed evenly between $CD1c^+$ and $CD1c^-$ B cells (696). Following *in vitro* activation, CD1c is upregulated on $CD1c^+$ B cells and is induced *de novo* on a portion of the $CD1c^-$ B cells (696). In normal lymph nodes and spleen, the $CD1c^+$ B cell subset is localized preferentially to the mantle zone of lymphoid follicles; germinal center B cells are $CD1c^-$ (682). CD1c also is expressed by malignant B-cell populations but not simply those derived from mantle zone B cells. Approximately one third of mature (TdT^-) B-cell NHLs and chronic lymphocytic leukemias are $CD1c^+$ (696,697). Resting mature and activated normal B cells and malignant B cells appear to be consistently $CD1a^-CD1b^-$ (695,696). CD1c antigen expression may prove useful in studying B-cell ontogeny and in identifying and dissecting normal and neoplastic B-cell populations.

CD2

Human T cells were originally distinguished from human B cells based on their ability to spontaneously bind sheep erythrocytes and thereby form E rosettes (55–57). This phenomenon is mediated by the CD2 molecule, initially termed the *sheep red blood cell receptor*, which is expressed by the majority of immature and mature T cells and is believed to play a crucial role in the adhesion and activation processes of T cells (698–700). The CD2 MAb cluster was established at the first workshop (15) to include MAbs T11 (68) and 9.6 (66). Numerous additional anti-CD2 MAbs since have been prepared, characterized, and clustered as CD2 (701–704). None of these antibodies are immunoreactive in paraffin tissue sections.

CD2 is a 50-kd type I transmembrane glycoprotein of 351 amino acid residues, which is encoded by a gene located on 1p13 (705). CD2 consists of two domains and belongs to the immunoglobulin gene superfamily (706). Domain 1 is a V-type immunoglobulina-like domain that mediates its adhesion functions through CD58, CD48, and CD59 binding. Domain 2 is a C2-type immunoglobulin-like domain that contains an activation-related epitope of CD2 designated *CD2R* (706), which facilitates T-cell activation (700).

Three distinct epitope groups, $T11_1$, $T11_2$, and $T11_3$, have been defined on the human CD2 molecule based on their distribution on resting and activated T cells and their ability to bind sheep erythrocytes and thereby form E rosettes (698,707). $T11_1$ and $T11_2$ are expressed on both resting and activated T cells (707,708); $T11_3$ expression is restricted to activated T cells (698,707). The $T11_3$ epitope now is designated CD2R (restricted) (702) for this reason. The $T11_1$ epitope is responsible for sheep erythrocyte binding. Consequently, the E rosette phenomenon is inhibited by MAbs such as T11 that are directed against the $T11_1$ epitope (66–68), but not by MAbs directed against the $T11_2$ and $T11_3$ epitopes (707). Individual anti-CD2 MAbs are unable to induce T-cell activation, but several combinations of anti-CD2 MAbs that detect two distinct CD2 epitopes, $T11_1$, $T11_2$ or $T11_3$, are mitogenic (698,707,709). As many as seven functionally distinct CD2 epitopic regions may be identified on this basis (710).

The *in vitro* activation of human T cells can occur through either of two pathways. The antigen-dependent pathway involves the triggering of the TCR-CD3 complex (711–713). The CD2 molecule appears to be involved in the physiologic T-cell activation pathway that occurs after antigen-specific T-cell activation of the TCR-CD3 complex (709), however, because it has been shown to positively regulate TCR-CD3-mediated activation signals (714). The alternative pathway involves triggering of the CD2 molecule (66,68,707). Activation through CD2, however, appears to require a functional TCR-CD3 complex at the cell surface, and especially a functional TCR ζ chain (715). This suggests that the receptors have similar pathways, and T-cell stimulation through both CD2 and TCR-CD3 is mediated through an IL-2-dependent pathway (707).

The functional responses of T cells to pertubations of various combinations of CD2 epitopes are complex. They probably reflect the complexity of signaling induced by combinations of multiple natural ligands of CD2 (716). LFA-3 (CD58), also a member of the immunoglobulin gene superfamily, is the primary ligand for CD2 (717,718). CD59, a complement regulatory protein, CD48, and CD15 also act as ligands for CD2 (719–721). It is possible that additional ligands exist, especially for the CD2R region. MAbs directed against LFA-3 block CD2-dependent adhesion of T cells to other cells (717,722). Furthermore, LFA-3 (CD58) binds to CD2 and with a nonmitogenic anti-CD2 MAb activates T cells (723).

CD2 is one of the earliest T-cell lineage–restricted antigens to appear during T-cell ontogeny; rare $CD2^+$ cells can be found in the bone marrow (204). Although we know that CD2 appears after CD7 but before CD1, its temporal relationship with CD3 is less clear. At one time, CD2 was believed to be expressed prior to CD3 (698), but the evidence now suggests that CD3 is present in the cytoplasm prior to CD2. The functional role of CD2 in thymic ontogeny remains unsettled (708). CD2-LFA-3 interaction is known to mediate thymocyte–thymic epithelium adhesion (724), a reaction that may be important in prothymocyte homing. CD2 is expressed by about 95% of cortical and medullary thymocytes and nearly all mature peripheral blood and lymphoid tissue T cells (66–68,698) and by approximately 80% to 90% of NK cells (725), but not by B cells or any other lymphohematopoietic or nonhematopoietic cell populations (66–68,698). A small subset of mature $CD3^+CD2^-$ T cells has been identified in the peripheral blood, however (708). Nonetheless, CD2 can be considered one of the four pan-T cell antigens, the others being CD3, CD5, and CD7, and is very useful in identifying and isolating virtually all normal T cells.

CD2 is also very useful in the immunophenotypic analysis of lymphoid malignancies. CD2 is expressed by the vast majority of precursor T-cell lymphoblastic lymphomas/leukemias and mature (TdT^-) postthymic NHLs and lymphoid leukemias, including cutaneous and peripheral T-cell lymphoma, adult T-cell lymphoma/leukemia, Sézary syndrome, T-cell chronic lymphocytic and prolymphocytic leukemia, and LGL and NK cell leukemia (6–8,13,14,227,462). As in the case of pan-T cell antigens CD3, CD5, and CD7, however, CD2 may be deleted aberrantly in some malignant T-cell populations (14,726), most commonly among the postthymic peripheral T-cell lymphomas (14,227,726,727). In contrast, CD2 is not expressed by virtually any precursor B-cell lymphoblastic lymphomas/leukemias or mature (TdT^-) sIg^+ or sIg^- B-cell NHLs and lymphoid leukemias (6–8,14,462). One exception is the rare patients with biphenotypic acute lymphoblastic leukemia who coexpress CD2 and CD19 but lack CD3, sIg, and cytoplasmic μ heavy chain (728). Their leukemic cells may represent the malignant counterparts of rare, transiently occurring, normal biphenotypic $CD2^+CD19^+$ precursor lymphoid cells (728). Rare sIg^+ B cell NHLs and lymphoid leukemias form E rosettes based on the anti-sheep red blood cell antibody activity of their sIg and not through the CD2 molecule (214).

In addition, CD2 is expressed by a small proportion of AMLs (729), but this expression is not entirely random. CD2 expression is associated specifically with FAB M3 AML (730) and its microgranular variant (FAB M3v) (731). CD2 expression by an $HLA\text{-}DR^-$ AML is highly associated with M3 morphology and the translocation t(11;17) (343,463,732). CD2 expression also occurs in the M4EO subtype of FAB M4 AML (733,734), which is associated with chromosome 16 abnormalities and a better prognosis (735,736). CD2 has been reported variably to be present or absent on the Reed-Sternberg cells and variants of Hodgkin's disease over the years and has remained controversial (462). Most investigators believe that the malignant cells of Hodgkin's disease are $CD2^-$ (see Chapter 18). CD2 is not expressed by true histiocytic and dendritic cell neoplasms, including Langerhans cell histiocytosis (462) (see Chapter 51).

CD3

The CD3 cluster initially was defined at the first workshop (15) by MAbs T3 (737) and UCHT1 (738), among others. Since then, many additional MAbs, including OKT3 (242) and Leu4 (739), have been added to the CD3 cluster (740). CD3 expression is restricted to the T-cell lineage, in which it is present virtually throughout T-cell differentiation. Monoclonal anti-CD3 antibodies are utilized widely in the identification, enumeration, and isolation of benign, normal T cells and in the immunophenotypic analysis of lymphohematopoietic malignancies (6–8,14,462,726). Anti-CD3 MAbs are useful for detecting CD3, and consequently T cells, in viable cell suspensions by flow cytometry, in cytocentrifuge smears by immunocytochemistry, and in frozen tissue sections by immunohistochemistry, but not in formalin-fixed, paraffin-embedded tissue sections. Polyclonal CD3, an anti-CD3 heteroantiserum prepared by immunization with amino acids 156 through 168 of the CD3ϵ chain (741), displays immunoreactivity in paraffin tissue sections rivaling that of anti-CD3 MAbs in frozen tissue sections (741–743). The heteroantiserum polyclonal CD3 is used extensively in diagnostic pathology because of its applicability to paraffin tissue sections prepared from routinely fixed and processed tissue specimens (502,743). An MAb that detects the extracellular domain of the ϵ subunit of CD3 and is immunoreactive in routinely fixed and paraffin-embedded tissue sections has been described (744). Its sensitivity and reliability under these conditions have not yet been investigated thoroughly.

The CD3 complex is composed of six polypeptides with usually four distinct glycoprotein chains: γ (25 kd), δ (21 kd), ϵ (20 kd), and ζ (16 kd). Three different dimers ($\gamma\epsilon$, $\delta\epsilon$, and $\zeta\zeta$) constitute the CD3 complex (119). The designation *CD3* generally has been employed to include only the CD3 γ, δ, and ϵ chains but sometimes is used to include the ζ chain as well (740). CD3γ, CD3δ, and CD3ϵ are composed of 160–, 160–, and 185–amino acid residues: 89 to 104 residues for the extracellular domain, 26 or 27 residues for the transmembrane domain, and 44 to 55 residues for the intracellular domain. These chains contain a single immunoglobulin-like domain in their extracellular regions and belong to the immunoglobulin gene superfamily (740). The three genes encoding the CD3 γ, δ, and ϵ chains are located in close proximity on 11q23 (745,746), and their sequences are highly homologous (740). Most likely they have been produced by gene duplication (740).

The CD3 ζ chain is completely different from the CD3 γ, δ, and ϵ chains (747). The CD3 ζ chain is a 16-kd glycoprotein with a much shorter (nine amino acid residue) extracellular region and a longer (112 amino acid residue) cytoplasmic domain than CD3 γ, δ, and ϵ and has no N-linked sugars (740). It is expressed either as a disulfide-linked homodimer or as a heterodimer with the η chain (748). The η chain is an alternatively spliced product from the same gene as CD3ζ. The ζ chain is related to the γ chain of the IgE Fc receptor and also can associate with Fcγ receptor III (CD16) (749). The gene encoding the CD3 ζ and η chains has been mapped to 1q22-25 (750), a different gene than those encoding the CD3 γ, δ, and ϵ chains (745,746).

The TCR complex is formed by the noncovalent association of the CD3 complex with the TCR$\alpha\beta$ or, alternatively, the TCR$\gamma\delta$ heterodimer (119). All TCR chains contain one or two positively charged amino acids within the transmembrane region; each CD3 γ, δ, or ϵ chain contains negatively charged amino acids within its transmembrane region (740). The intereaction between the positively charged amino acids in TCR chains and the negatively charged amino acids in CD3 chains is critical for the stable expression of the functional TCR-CD3 complex (740).

The CD3 complex is critical in regulating the cell surface expression of the TCR complex (740). The CD3 complex is assembled in the endoplasmic reticulum after synthesis of the individual chains. Only the completely assembled octameric complex TCR$\alpha\beta$-CD3$\alpha\beta$-CD3$\delta\epsilon$-CD3$\zeta\zeta$ can be transferred to the cell surface. The incomplete complex TCR$\alpha\beta$-CD3$\gamma\epsilon$-CD3$\delta\epsilon$, in the absence of association with the CD3 ζ chain, is targeted for lysosomal degradation. The CD3 ζ chain determines the rate of assembly and also signals the switch from lysosomal degradation to transportation to the plasma membrane (751).

Monoclonal anti-CD3 antibodies can stimulate all mature, peripheral T cells to proliferate, release lymphokines, and display nonspecific cytotoxicity (752–756), mimicking T-cell stimulation by antigens and mitogens. These properties require the presence of accessory cells that interact with the Fc portion of the MAb and provide a critical signal to the T cell (757–760). The mitogenic properties of anti-CD3 MAbs have led to our understanding that the CD3 complex is responsible for mediating signal transduction to the intracellular environment of T cells on antigen recognition by the TCR (761). The CD3 γ, δ, and ϵ chains and the CD3 ζ chain function as distinct signaling molecules (762). Each CD3 chain contains an immunoreceptor tyrosine-based activation motif (ITAM), also called a *Reth motif*, within its cytoplasmic domain (763). The CD3 γ, δ, and ϵ chains contain one ITAM each; the CD3 ζ chain contains three ITAMs (763). Signaling functions of the CD3 chains are mediated through these ITAMs in the cytoplasmic region (740). The different ITAMs of the TCR-CD3 complex can interact with different cytosolic effectors, thereby generating diversity of signaling by the TCR complex (764).

The CD3 complex is also important for the internalization of the TCR-CD3 complex on T-cell activation. If T cells are activated, the entire TCR-CD3 complex is internalized rapidly, and T cells thus become functionally unresponsive (740). Furthermore, the CD3 complex plays an important role in thymocyte differentiation by constituting a previously unknown pre-TCR complex and a clonotype-independent CD3 complex on immature thymocytes (740).

Investigators initially believed that CD3 was expressed by only a small proportion of normal thymocytes (137,243) and was expressed uncommonly by precursor T-cell lymphoblastic lymphomas/leukemias (137,765,766). These findings were based, however, on analyses of isolated thymocytes and malignant lymphoblasts in suspension using

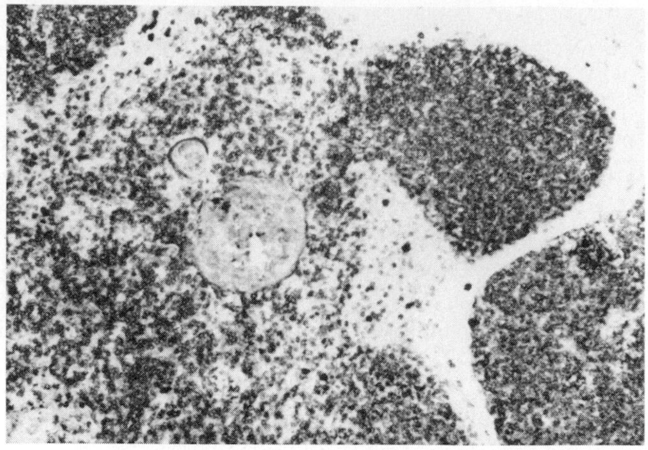

FIG. 3.34. Frozen tissue section of human thymus immunostained for CD3. Essentially all of the thymocytes are CD3-positive. This uniform expression of CD3 is because of the combination of cytoplasmic CD3 expression by the majority of cortical thymocytes and surface membrane CD3 expression by the majority of medullary thymocytes (immunoperoxidase stain, original magnification: 100× magnification).

immunofluorescent and cytofluorometric techniques that detect surface membrane antigens and not cytoplasmic antigens. Immunohistochemical studies on frozen tissue sections demonstrated that CD3 is present in the cytoplasm prior to its expression on the cell surface membrane of thymocytes (767) and that more than 95% of thymocytes express mCD3 or cCD3 (768,769) (Fig. 3.34). CD3 was similarly shown to be frequently expressed in the cytoplasm of malignant T-cell lymphoblasts (144,767,768). Other studies have demonstrated that CD3δ and CD3ϵ proteins are detectable in the cytoplasm of virtually all mCD3$^-$ acute lymphoblastic leukemias (769), including those that have not yet rearranged their TCRB gene (770). Therefore, CD3 gene transcription is one of the earliest events to occur in T-cell ontogeny, beginning during the prothymocyte stage prior to entrance into the thymus (770). Putative cCD3$^+$mCD3$^-$ thymocytes that express CD45 and CD7 and lack expression of TdT, HLA-DR, TCR$\alpha\beta$, and TCR$\gamma\beta$ have been identified in the fetal yolk sac and liver in the 7th gestational week prior to the formation of the thymus gland (771,772). After the 10th week of gestation mCD3$^+$ cells emerge in the fetal liver (771,772). After 10.5 weeks of gestation, approximately 95% of fetal thymocytes are cCD3$^+$, but a smaller proportion are mCD3$^+$ (771). As common thymocytes differentiate into mature medullary thymocytes and subsequently into mature peripheral T cells, cCD3 is lost (768,769). mCD3 is expressed by virtually all mature peripheral blood and lymphoid tissue T cells but not by B cells, monocytes/macrophages, myeloid cells, or any other hematopoietic or nonhematopoietic cell populations (242–244,742,743,768,769) (Fig 3.35). The only exception among hematopoietic cells is NK cells, which may express cCD3 but do not express mCD3 (773). The only exception among nonhematopoietic

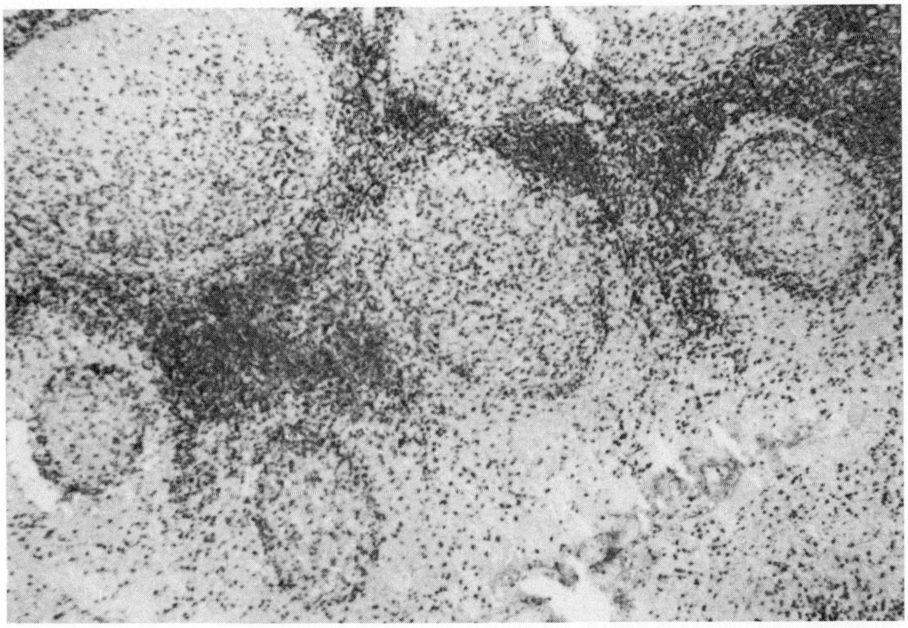

A

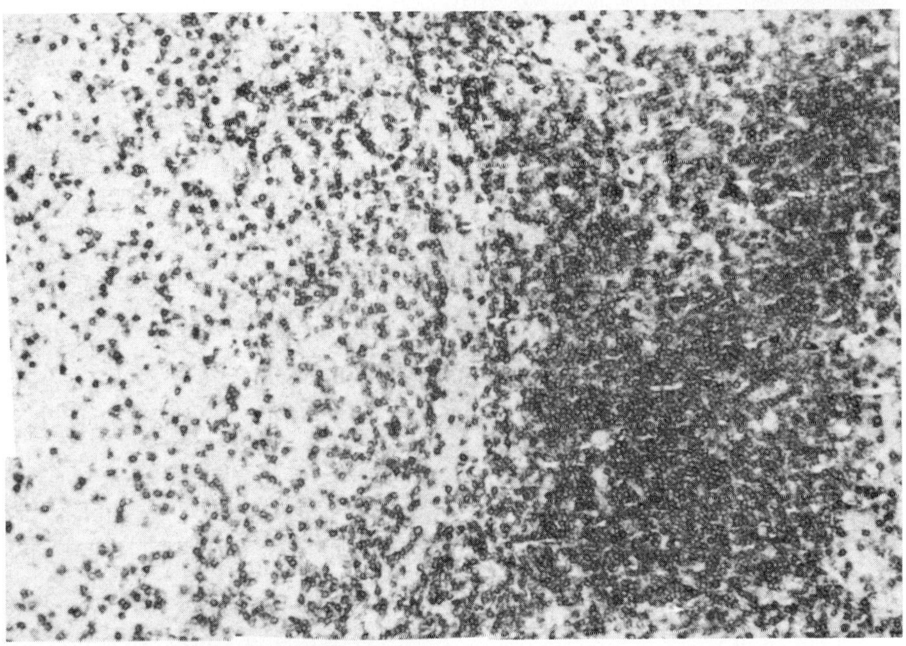

B

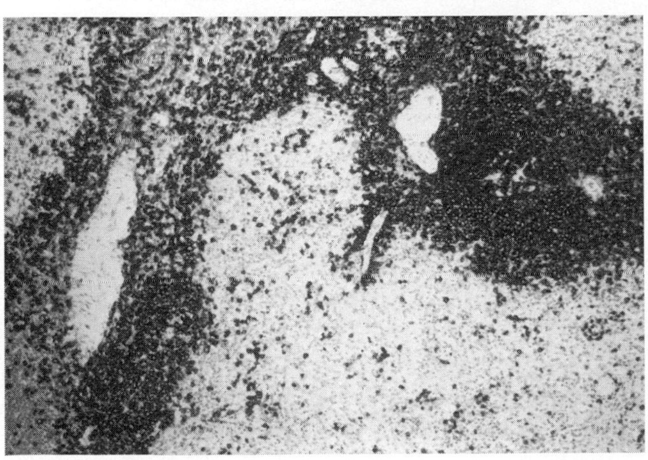

C

FIG. 3.35. Frozen tissue sections of tonsil (**A,B**) and spleen (**C**) immunostained for CD3 (immunoperoxidase stain). **A:** CD3-positive T cells principally occupy the interfollicular (T-cell) region (original magnification: 40× magnification). **B:** Higher magnification shows that, in addition to making up the large majority of the interfollicular cells, CD3-positive T cells are also present in small numbers throughout the germinal center (original magnification: 100× magnification). **C:** CD3-positive T cells principally occupy the periarteriolar lymphoid sheath (T-cell) region within the spleen (original magnification: 40× magnification).

cells appears to be cerebellar Purkinje cells, which react with MAbs Leu4 and UCHT1 but not with MAb OKT3 (774). CD3 is a pan-T cell restricted antigen.

The majority of anti-CD3 MAbs, including Leu4 and UCHT-1, recognize epitopes mapping to the CD3 ϵ subunit (769,775). Although MAbs Leu4 and UCHT-1 detect cCD3 in cytocentrifuge preparations, however, MAb T3 detects surface mCD3 but not cCD3 in these preparations, and many other anti-CD3 MAbs are not reactive at all in cytocentrifuge preparations (769). Selection of the appropriate MAb reagent can be crucial to the accurate demonstration of cCD3. In addition, the paraffin-immunoreactive heteroantiserum polyclonal CD3 similarly detects the CD3 ϵ subunit (741). Polyclonal CD3 is immunoreactive in tissues that have been fixed in formalin, Bouin's solution, and B5, as well as in those that have been decalcified (307,340,741–743) (Fig. 3.36). Proteolytic treatment of the paraffin tissue sec-tionswith enzymes such as pepsin and trypsin or the use of other antigen-retrieval techniques, however, is generally necessary to detect CD3 properly in fixed tissues (502,742,743).

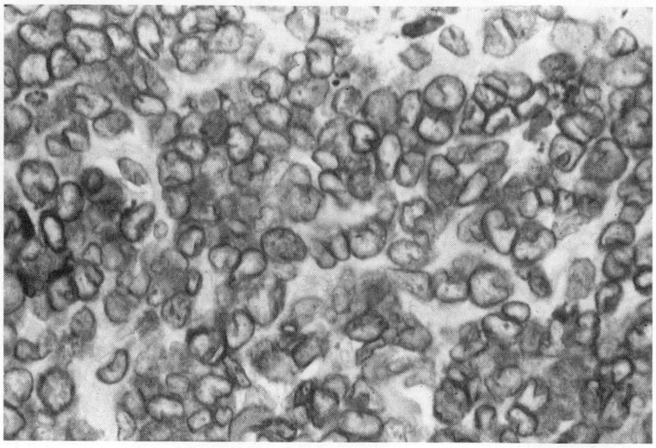

FIG. 3.37. Formalin-fixed, paraffin-embedded tissue section of a precursor T-cell lymphoblastic lymphoma/leukemia immunostained with polyclonal antibody CD3. Essentially all of the malignant T lymphoblasts strongly express CD3 (immunoperoxidase stain, original magnification: 630× magnification).

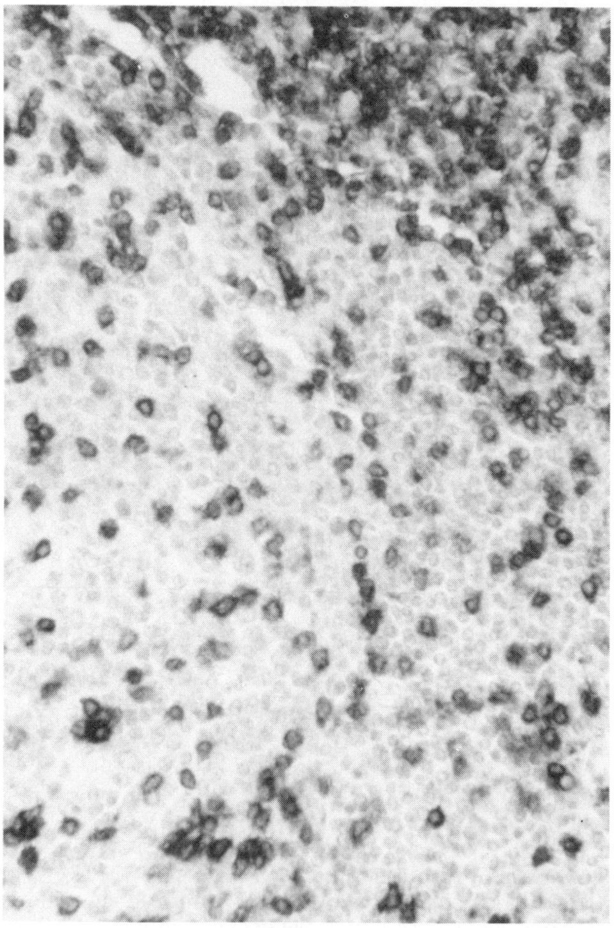

FIG. 3.36. Formalin-fixed, paraffin-embedded tissue section of tonsil immunostained with polyclonal CD3. The pattern of reactivity of polyclonal CD3 in paraffin tissue sections parallels that of anti-CD3 monoclonal antibodies in frozen tissue sections. Note the reactivity of polyclonal CD3 with the majority of interfollicular T cells and small numbers of T cells at the border between the germinal center and the mantle zone and also within the germinal center (immunoperoxidase stain, original magnification: 250× magnification).

Because CD3 is restricted to the T-cell lineage and is expressed virtually throughout T-cell differentiation, it represents the most specific as well as the most sensitive T-cell lineage marker available for the immunophenotypic analysis of lymphohematopoietic malignancies (462). The evaluation of CD3 expression is particularly useful in distinguishing precursor T-cell lymphoblastic lymphomas/leukemias, which consistently express cCD3, from precursor B-cell lymphoblastic lymphomas/leukemias, AMLs, granulocytic sarcomas, and chronic myelogenous leukemia in myeloid or lymphoid blast crisis, which uniformly lack cCD3 (6–8,14,322,340,462,743,768–770) (Fig. 3.37). Precursor T-cell lymphoblastic/leukemias exhibiting late cortical and medullary thymocyte phenotypes express mCD3 in addition to, or instead of, cCD3 (462). The majority of T-cell malignancies belonging to all the clinicopathologic categories of mature (postthymic) T-cell neoplasia—cutaneous and peripheral T-cell lymphoma, Sézary syndrome, adult T-cell lymphoma/leukemia, T-cell chronic lymphocytic and prolymphocytic leukemia, and anaplastic large cell lymphoma—express mCD3 but not cCD3 (6–8,14,227,462,726, 727,741–743). As in the case of the other pan-T cell antigens (CD2,CD5,and CD7), however, CD3 may be deleted aberrantly in some malignant T-cell populations (14,726). Aberrant deletion of CD3 occurs most frequently among the peripheral T-cell lymphomas and the anaplastic large cell lymphomas (14,726,727). Cases of LGL NK cell leukemia are divisable into two broad categories, those in which a T-cell phenotype is expressed and those in which an NK cell phenotype is expressed (776). In the former cases CD3 usually is expressed and clonal TCRβ gene rearrangements exhibited; in the latter cases CD3 usually is not expressed and the TCRβ germline configuration is exhibited (777,778).

Polyclonal CD3 is generally immunoreactive in paraffin tissue sections of those T-cell malignancies with which anti-CD3 MAbs are immunoreactive in cell suspensions, cytocentrifuge preparations, and frozen tissue sections (502,741–743). In addition, polyclonal CD3 is sometimes immunoreactive in paraffin tissue sections of T-cell neoplasms with which anti-CD3 MAbs are not immunoreactive in frozen tissue sections (742,743). The latter cases primarily are precursor T-cell lymphoblastic lymphomas/leukemias in which the malignant lymphoblasts express cCD3 but not mCD3 (340,741,742).

CD3 essentially is never expressed by precursor B-cell lymphoblastic lymphomas/leukemias or by mature (TdT$^-$) B-cell NHLs and lymphoid leukemias, regardless of clinicopathologic category (6–8,14,307,340,462,502,741–743) (Fig. 3.38). The only exception appears to be exceedingly rare patients with biphenotypic lymphoma (779), the nature and origin of which are unclear. The expression of T cell–associated antigens, including CD3, by the Reed-Sternberg cells and variants of classic Hodgkin's disease, has been controversial. Most investigators believe that these malignant cells do not express CD3 (see Chapter 18). Similarly, CD3 is not expressed by histiocytic and dendritic cell neoplasms or by nonhematopoietic tumors (see Chapters 30 and 52). CD3 expression by a hematologic neoplasm almost certainly indicates a T cell–lineage derivation.

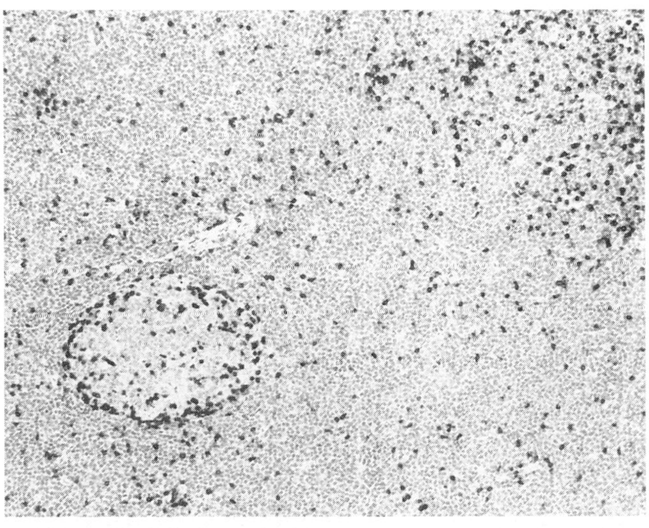

FIG. 3.38. Formalin-fixed, paraffin-embedded tissue section of a lymph node involved by mantle cell lymphoma that has been immunostained with polyclonal antibody CD3. The neoplastic B-cell population is CD3-negative. The only CD3-positive cells are scattered residual benign T cells, some of which surround a residual benign germinal center. This pattern of immune reactivity helps to accentuate the mantle zone pattern of distribution of this lymphoma (immunoperoxidase stain, original magnification: 200× magnification).

CD4 and CD8

Shortly after the discovery that lymphocytes are divisible into B cells and T cells, it became clear that T cells are heterogeneous and that discrete subsets of T cells subserve distinct functions such as help, suppression, and cytotoxicity (780). Helper T cells were identified initially based on their expression of Fc receptors for IgM (Tμ cells) (71) and their nonreactivity with the anti-TH_2 heteroantiserum (781). Suppressor or cytotoxic T cells initially were identified based on their expression of Fc receptors for IgG (Tγcells) (71,72) and their reactivity with the anti-TH_2 heteroantiserum (781). Later, helper or inducer and suppressor or cytotoxic T cells were recognized by their expression of the CD4 and CD8 molecules, respectively (739,782). The CD4 cluster was defined by MAbs T4 (783) and Leu3a (784), among others, at the first workshop (15). The CD8 cluster was defined by MAbs Leu2a (784), T8 (785), and others at the first workshop (15) as well. Many anti-CD4 and anti-CD8 MAbs have been added to the CD4 and CD8 clusters since then (666,701,786–789). Although they are immunoreactive with viable cells in suspension, in cytocentrifuge preparations, and in frozen tissue sections, none of these anti-CD4 and anti-CD8 MAbs are immunoreactive in paraffin tissue sections. MAb OPD4, which originally was thought to recognize CD4 in paraffin tissue sections (306), actually detects CD45RO (359). Anti-CD4 and anti-CD8 MAbs (NCL-CD4 and NCL-CD8, respectively) that are immunoreactive in routinely fixed and paraffin-embedded tissue sections following antigen retrieval, however, recently have been described and characterized preliminarily (790). These antibodies should prove to be very useful reagents in diagnostic pathology.

The CD4 and CD8 molecules are nonpolymorphic, integral surface membrane glycoproteins belonging to the immunoglobulin gene superfamily that are preferentially expressed by mutually exclusive, functionally distinct T-cell populations (791). The CD4 molecule is a 55-kd glycoprotein consisting of a 370 amino acid residue extracellular region comprising two C2-type and two V-type immunoglobulin-like domains, a 25-residue transmembrane domain, and a 38-residue cytoplasmic domain (791–793). The *CD4* gene has been mapped to the short arm of chromosome 12 (794).

The CD8 cell surface molecule is a 68-kd type I transmembrane glycoprotein composed of a 32- to 34-kd α chain and a 30- to 32-kd β chain, which are disulfide-linked to form $\alpha\beta$ heterodimers (795). CD8 also may be expressed as $\alpha\alpha$ homodimers (795). The CD8 molecule is expressed primarily as an $\alpha\beta$ heterodimer by the majority of thymocytes and by MHC class I restricted mature T cells. Variable proportions (donor-related) of TCR$\gamma\delta$ T cells and CD8$^+$CD16$^+$ peripheral blood NK cells express CD8$\alpha\alpha$ homodimers (796). CD8β cell surface expression is strictly dependent on CD8α expression (797). CD8α can, but CD8β cannot, form homodimers.

Both the CD8 α and β chains consist of extracellular, transmembrane, and intracellular domains (795,798). The mature CD8α protein possesses a 214 amino acid residue extracellular region that contains a V-type immunoglobulin-like domain, followed by a 25-residue transmembrane domain, and a 28-residue cytoplasmic tail (795). The mature CD8β protein consists of a 143 amino acid residue extracellular domain that contains a similar V-type immunoglobulin-like domain, an immunoglobulin J region–like short sequence, and one N-linked glycosylation site, followed by a 27-residue transmembrane domain and a 19-residue cytoplasmic tail (797,799,800).

The *CD8A* gene is located on chromosome 2, near the κ locus (801). The *CD8B* gene has six exons spanning approximately 7 kb (802). There are two recently duplicated genes for CD8β, *CD8B1* and *CD8B2*, which differ only by nine nucleotides in their coding regions (803). The *CD8B1* gene lies approximately 25 kb upstream from the *CD8A* gene in the same transcriptional orientation on chromosome 2 (803). Although both *CD8B* genes appear functional, all forms of CD8 mRNA are derived by alternative splicing from *CD8B1* transcripts (803).

A soluble form of CD8α which lacks the transmembrane domain is produced by an alternative splicing mechanism (804). Soluble CD8 is detectable in the supernatants of $CD8^+$ T cell leukemia cell lines and in the sera of patients who have $CD8^+$ T cell leukemia (805). An increase in soluble CD8α has been reported in the sera of patients with AIDS (806).

$CD4^+$ T cells almost invariably recognize foreign antigens as peptides presented by MHC class II molecules (807,808). CD4 appears to bind to the nonpolymorphic regions of MHC class II molecules (808–811), leading to the formation of a ternary complex with the TCR. During the antigen-recognition process by the TCR-CD3 complex, MHC class II molecules are engaged in simultaneous interaction with TCR and CD4, leading to the coclustering of CD4 and TCR and to T-cell activation (788). Conversely, if preceded by ligation of CD4 with anti-CD4 MAbs or other ligands, signaling through TCR-CD3 results in T-cell unresponsiveness because of the induction of activation-dependent cell death by apoptosis (812). In the absence of antigen recognition and TCR-mediated signaling, the interaction of CD4 with MHC class II molecules generates a signal inhibiting T cell–B cell adhesion (813).

$CD8^+$ T cells recognize foreign antigens as peptides presented by MHC class I molecules (807,808,811). By interacting with the nonpolymorphic domain of the same MHC class I molecules that interact with the TCR, CD8 can mediate a function as a coreceptor in TCR-ligand binding and T-cell activation (814).

The CD4 molecule also serves as the primary cellular receptor for HIV (815,816) by interacting with the gp120 subunit of the viral envelope glycoprotein. Actual entry of HIV particles into target cells requires other more recently identified non-CD4 cellular receptors, however (817). One of these HIV coreceptors, CXCR4, binds the $CD4^-$ gp120 complex (818). Other ligands that have been identified are IL-16 (819) and gp17 (820). IL-16 is a chemoattractant factor for $CD4^+$ cells and serves to decrease immune responses and HIV replication (819); the function of gp17 is unknown (788). Mounting evidence suggests that the role played by CD4 during the life cycle of HIV in T cells is not limited strictly to its ability to bind the virus, however; CD4 probably plays other roles that are important to the productive infection process as well (788).

The cytoplasmic tails of CD4 and CD8 associate with $p56^{lck}$, an SRC-like T lymphocyte–specific protein tyrosine kinase (821–823) that is related structurally to receptor kinases such as the receptor for epidermal growth factor and platelet-derived growth factor (824). This association would appear to permit CD4 and CD8 to tranduce intracellular signals if triggered by ligand binding (825,826). The CD4 and CD8 molecules may act as the ligand-binding component of the complex; $p56^{lck}$ may generate signals linked to the activation or downregulation of T-cell growth. This association may constitute the underlying molecular basis for CD4 and CD8 function, either independently or in conjunction with the TCR-CD3 complex (825).

In summary, the multiple facets of CD4 and CD8 function are dependent on molecular interactions with MHC class II and I antigens, the TCR-CD3 complex, the intracellular T cell–specific protein tyrosine kinase $p56^{lck}$ and, in the case of CD4, the HIV envelope glycoprotein gp120 (788). It has been shown that distinct patterns of intracellular protein phosphorylation may be related to functionally distinct CD4 epitopes (827) and that CD3 dimer formation may account for distinct CD4-mediated functions (828,829). CD8 also plays an important role in the positive selection of T cells in the thymus (830,831).

The CD4 and CD8 antigens appear during the common thymocyte stage in T-cell ontogeny (137,243,244,770,832). CD4 and CD8 are expressed by approximately 80% to 90% and 70% to 80% of normal thymocytes, respectively (137,243,244,739) (Fig. 3.39). Thereafter, CD4 and CD8 are retained by those maturing thymocytes destined to become helper or inducer and suppressor or cytotoxic T cells, respectively (137,243,244,770,832). CD4 is expressed by about 55% to 65% of mature peripheral T cells, specifically the helper or inducer T-cell subset. CD8 is expressed by about 25% to 35% of mature peripheral T cells, specifically the suppressor or cytotoxic T-cell subset (243,244,739,782). This phenotype–function association, however, is not universal. Subpopulations of suppressor or cytotoxic T cells can be identified among $CD4^+$ T cells (833,834) (see Chapter 2). CD4 also is expressed on the surface and in the cytoplasm of monocytes and macrophages (297) and by Langerhans cells and other dendritic cells (213,297). CD8 also is expressed in low density by approximately 30% of NK cells (725). CD4 and CD8 are not expressed by B cells (6–8,137,242–244,739,782).

$CD4^+CD8^+$ T cells are phenotypically and functionally heterogeneous. For example, $CD4^+$ T cells can be subdivided into functionally distinct and largely reciprocal subsets

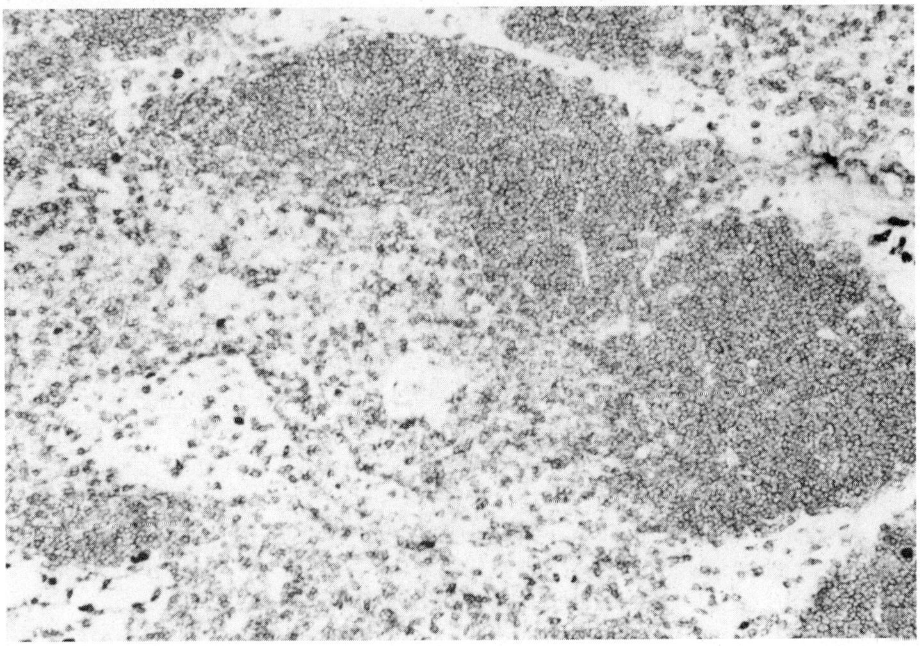

FIG. 3.39. Frozen tissue section of thymus immunostained for CD8 by immunoperoxidase. Nearly all of the cortical (immature) thymocytes express CD8. However, only a small number of medullary (mature) thymocytes, specifically those destined to become suppressor or cytotoxic T cells, express CD8 (immunoperoxidase stain, original magnification: 100× magnification).

based on their differential expression of CD45RA, CD45RO, and the CD29-VLA β chain (248,274,835–837). The $CD4^+CD45RO^+CD45RA^-CD29^{high}$ memory (helper–inducer) subset responds maximally to recall antigen and provides marked helper function for B-cell IgG synthesis (274,837). In contrast, the $CD4^+CD45RO^-CD45RA^+CD29^{low}$ naive (suppressor–inducer) subset responds poorly to recall antigen and does not provide helper function but can induce CD8 T cells to suppress IgG synthesis (274,835–837). Many cell surface molecules, such as CD2, CD26, LFA-1, LFA-3, ICAM-1, and CD44, have been reported to be preferentially expressed on $CD4^+CD45RO^+CD45RA^-CD29^{high}$ memory T cells and reported to play key roles in the function of the helper population (838,839). The definition and characterization of additional molecules associated with $CD4^+CD8^+$ T cells, such as CD27, CD28, and CD60 among others, is necessary to facilitate our further understanding of the complex biology of human T cells under both physiologic and pathologic conditions (see Chapter 2).

Several different epitopes of the CD4 antigen have been identified (840,841). Epitope mapping has demonstrated that most anti-CD4 MAbs, including Leu3a (784), are directed against CDR-like loops in CD4 domain 1 (788). MAb OKT4 is directed against CD4 domain 3, however (788). This has considerable relevance for the immunophenotypic identification of $CD4^+$ T cells in at least two situations. First, the CD4 epitope detected by MAb OKT4 is absent from CD4 T cells in about 4% of the African-American population because of genetic polymorphism (842). The CD4 T cells in these individuals are detectable with MAb Leu3a (843; Knowles, unpublished observations). Second, CD4 T cells are detectable in cell suspension by flow cytometry but not in frozen tissue sections by immunohistochemistry using MAb OKT4 (844). CD4 T cells, however, are detectable in frozen tissue sections using a cocktail composed of two anti-CD4 MAbs such as OKT4b and OKT4d (Knowles, unpublished observations) or Leu3a and Leu3b (726), which detect independent, non–cross-blocking epitopes on the CD4 molecule (739).

The determination of CD4 and CD8 expression is a critically important component of the immunophenotypic analysis of benign and malignant lymphohematopoietic cell populations. First, anti-CD4 and anti-CD8 MAbs are employed routinely and extensively to identify and quantitate the benign, normal, mature peripheral blood and lymphoid tissue T-cell subsets, that is, $CD4^+CD8^-$ and $CD4^-CD8^+$, that are associated commonly with helper or inducer and suppressor or cytotoxic functions, respectively (see Chapters 2 and 6). The demonstration of these T-cell subsets in peripheral blood by flow cytometry, in cytocentrifuge smears by immunocytochemistry, and in frozen tissue sections by immunohistochemistry has permitted numerous investigators to characterize the distribution of these functionally distinct T-cell subsets in a wide spectrum of human diseases. Determination of the absolute number of $CD4^+$ T cells in the peripheral blood of HIV-infected individuals is the basis for the classification of HIV-related illness and AIDS (845,846) (see Chapter 28).

Second, determination of CD4 and CD8 expression is extremely useful in the immunodiagnosis and classification of lymphohematopoietic malignancies (6–8,13,14,462,726). Analogous to their simultaneous expression by the majority of normal thymocytes, CD4 and CD8 are coexpressed by the majority of precursor T-cell lymphoblastic lymphomas/leukemias. Most of the remaining patients, representative of the medullary thymocyte stage, express CD4 or CD8 but not both. Rare patients representative of the earliest stages of T-cell ontogeny lack both CD4 and CD8 (13,14,144,222,462). The majority of cases belonging to nearly all clinicopathologic categories of mature, postthymic (TdT^-) T-cell NHL and lymphoid leukemia, including cutaneous and peripheral T-cell lymphoma, adult T-cell lymphoma/leukemia, and chronic lymphocytic and prolymphocytic leukemia, is derived from the helper or inducer T-cell subset and is $CD4^+CD8^-$ (6–8,13,14,231,462,600,726,847,848) (Fig. 3.40). This is especially true in the case of mycosis fungoides and the Sézary syndrome, in which only rare patients express the $CD4^-CD8^+$ phenotype (6-8,13,14,462,600,726,847, 848). Among the other clinicopathologic categories, a larger proportion of patients is $CD4^-CD8^+$ (227,462,726,727). A notable exception is LGL/NK cell leukemia, in which the vast majority of patients lacks CD4 and most express CD8 (776–778). Analogous with their benign, nonneoplastic counterparts, malignant T-cell populations generally exhibit subset restriction; that is, they express either CD4 or CD8 but not both. As in the case of other T cell–associated antigens, however, CD4 or CD8 may be expressed aberrantly or deleted from neoplastic T cells (14,726). Occasional postthymic T-cell NHLs and lymphoid leukemias express the $CD4^+CD8^+$ phenotype, and rare patients express the $CD4^-CD8^-$ phenotype (13,14,227,726,727). Therefore, anti-CD4 and anti-CD8 MAbs are important in the evaluation of two immunodiagnostic criteria of T-cell neoplasia, subset restriction and anomalous antigen expression.

In contrast, CD4 and CD8 essentially are never expressed by patients with precursor B-cell lymphoblastic lymphoma/leukemia, chronic myelogenous leukemia in lymphoid blast crisis, or mature (TdT^-) B-cell NHLs and lymphoid leukemias, regardless of clinicopathologic category (6–8,461,462). CD4 and CD8 are similarly absent from the Reed-Sternberg cells and variants of Hodgkin's disease (see Chapter 18). Nonetheless, CD4 expression is not necessarily indicative of the T cell–lineage derivation of a hematologic neoplasm. Some AMLs, especially FAB M0 and M1 AML, as well as those exhibiting monocytic derivation (FAB M4 and M5 AML), may express CD4 (730). Also, neoplasms of monocyte-macrophage derivation, that is, true histiocytic neoplasms, similarly often express CD4 (462) (see Chapter 51).

CD5

The CD5 molecule was one of the first MAb-defined lymphocyte surface membrane molecules to be recognized (849,850). The CD5 cluster was established at the first workshop (15). Some of the best known and most widely utilized anti-CD5 MAbs are Leu1 (851), OKT1 (849), and T101 (852), but numerous additional anti-CD5 MAbs are commercially available (853). These MAbs are capable of detecting CD5 in viable cell suspensions by flow cytometry, in cytocentrifuge smears by immunocytochemistry, and in frozen tissue sections by immunohistochemistry, but not in paraffin tissue sections (853). Recently, two MAbs, NCL-CD5 and NCL-CD5-4C7, claimed to be capable of detecting CD5 in routinely fixed, paraffin-embedded tissue sections after antigen retrieval have become available. The initial studies sug-

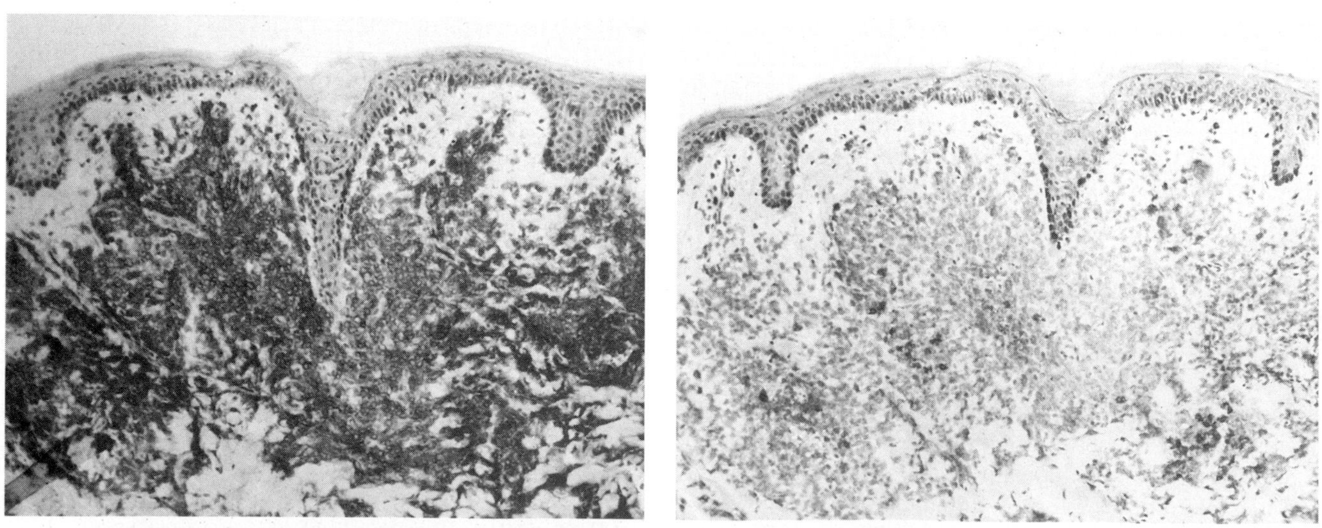

FIG. 3.40. Frozen tissue section of skin involved by mycosis fungoides, which has been immunostained with a monoclonal anti-CD4 antibody (**A**) and a monoclonal anti-CD8 antibody (**B**). Virtually all of the neoplastic T cells infiltrating the dermis express CD4 but lack CD8. Only small numbers of residual benign CD8 T cells are identified (immunoperoxidase stain, original magnification: 100× magnification).

gest that detection of CD5 under these conditions by the MAb NCL-CD5 is suboptimal, however (854). On the other hand, MAb NCL-CD5-4C7 appears to provide better results under these conditions (855) and may prove to be a useful reagent in diagnostic pathology.

The CD5 molecule is a 67-kd glycoprotein with structural features characteristic of receptor molecules. It consists of a signal peptide, a 347–amino acid extracellular segment, a transmembrane region, and a 93–amino acid intracellular segment suitable for signal transduction (856). The extracellular region consists of three scavenger receptor cysteine-rich domains, the first two of which are separated by a highly conserved proline and threonine-rich connecting peptide (856). Most anti-CD5 MAbs are directed against conformational or linear epitopes involving the first extracellular domain (857). Human CD5 is equivalent to the murine Ly-1 antigen; both are believed to be distantly related members of the immunoglobulin gene superfamily (858). The gene encoding CD5 has been mapped to 11q13 (858).

Initially, anti-CD5 MAbs were considered anti–T cell reagents based on their reactivity with virtually all immature (thymic) and mature (postthymic) peripheral T cells (849,851). Further studies, however, demonstrated that the vast majority of B-cell chronic lymphocytic leukemias also express CD5 (850,852,859,860) and that a small but significant population of CD5 B cells normally circulates in the peripheral blood and resides in fetal and adult peripheral lymphoid tissue (861–863). It is believed that the CD5 gene's product is expressed in an identical manner in both B and T cells (864). CD5 is not expressed by monocytes/macrophages, Langerhans cells, or interdigitating dendritic cells, although MAbs Leu1 and UCHT2 have been reported to immunoreact with a subset of circulating dendritic cells (865).

CD5 is expressed by virtually all immature (thymic) and mature (postthymic) peripheral T cells at all stages of T-cell differentiation (137,243,849–851). CD5 expression is acquired intrathymically by $CD34^+$ precursor T cells (866), which differentiate into $CD3^+CD4^+CD8^+$ T cells but not into NK cells (867). CD5 expression is weak on these precursor T cells and increases progressively during T-cell maturation (868). A small subpopulation of $CD3^+CD5^-$ T cells exists that increases following bone marrow and renal transplantation (869–871). These $CD3^+CD5^-$ T cells are thought to be cytotoxic; about one third of them express TCR$\gamma\delta$ (869,872). The TCR$\gamma\delta$ is preferentially expressed on $CD5^{dim}$ or $CD5^-$ T cells (872). $CD5^{bright+}$ mature T cells express the IL-2 receptor; $CD5^{dim+}$, less mature T cells do not express the IL-2 receptor (873).

Although its precise functional role is unclear, CD5 has been shown to physically associate with the antigen-specific receptor complex present on both T and B cells (874,875) and is believed to modulate signaling through that complex. CD5 sustains and enhances TCR-CD3-mediated proliferative responses in peripheral T cells (876), although it acts as a negative regulator of TCR-CD3 signaling in thymocytes (877). The interaction of CD5 with the TCR-CD3 complex apparently represents an alternative signaling pathway within the TCR complex (878). In addition, CD5 may generate T-cell activation signals independent of the TCR-CD3 complex (879–881). The combination of immobilized anti-CD5 MAbs with phorbol 12-myristate 13-acetate results in T-cell proliferation by an IL-2-dependent mechanism, suggesting a role for CD5 as an independent signal-transducing molecule (880,882,883). CD5 also has been shown to regulate the responsiveness of T cells to IL-1 (884). The recent reports of putative ligands for CD5, CD72 on resting B cells (885), and gp35-37 on activated B cells (886) support a role for CD5 in modulating antibody-mediated immune responses that are dependent on T cell–B cell interaction (857).

The omentum is believed to be the site of origin of $CD5^+$ B cells (887). These cells first appear in the fetus in the peritoneal and pleural cavities as early as gestational week 15, at which time they are absent from the bone marrow (888). Later, they become prominent in the fetal spleen, in which 60% or more B cells may express CD5 (889–891). The number of fetal peripheral blood CD5 B cells also increases with gestational age until it stabilizes at 36 weeks (892). At birth, nearly 70% of cord blood B cells and approximately 50% of newborn peripheral blood B cells express CD5 (893,894). The percentage of peripheral blood $CD5^+$ B cells drops to almost adult levels within the first year of life (895).

CD5 expression by B cells is usually weak, or dim, compared with its strong, or bright, expression by mature T cells (853). This has made precise identification of these cells difficult and sometimes controversial, resulting in reports of variable percentages of $CD5^+$ B cells in different anatomic locations (853). $CD5^+$ B cells generally, however, make up 15% to 25% of peripheral blood, 8% to 26% of splenic, 10% of tonsillar, and as many as 50% of intrathymic B cells (862,896–899).

The significance of the nonneoplastic $CD5^+$ B-cell population has been controversial. Some investigators believe that CD5 expression by B cells is a sign of activation (900,901). Other investigators believe that $CD5^+$ B cells represent a distinct B-cell lineage that predominates in the fetus and expands in specific disease states (902–905). Several differences between $CD5^+$ and $CD5^-$ B cells have been demonstrated; these are reviewed elsewhere (853) (see Chapter 2). Briefly, $CD5^+$ B cells are committed to the production of antibodies, principally IgM but also IgG and IgA, which represent the expression of a restricted number of immunoglobulin heavy and light chain genes (906,907), and which bind to a large number of self and non-self antigens (902,908). These low-affinity polyreactive antibodies, often called *autoantibodies*, may be better termed *natural antibodies* (853). Approximately 50% of the autoantibody-associated cross-reactive idiotype-bearing B cells express CD5 (909). It has been suggested that the natural antibodies generated by $CD5^+$ B cells represent the first line of defense against invading pathogens in the fetus and neonate (902,910).

Differences in CD5 antigen expression and CD5 mRNA production among B cells have led to a proposed nomenclature for the distinct B-cell populations (911). It is proposed that B-1 cells include the $CD5^+$ B-cell population, designated *B-1a* cells, and those $CD5^-$ B cells that are associated with polyreactive antibody production, designated *B-1b* cells (911). The latter cells contain CD5 mRNA (912). The conventional B cells that lack CD5 and do not produce polyreactive antibodies or CD5 mRNA are designated *B-2* cells (911). Two models of $CD5^+$ B-cell development have been hypothesized. The ''lineage model'' proposes that precursor B cells are committed to the B-1a, B-1b, or B-2 lineage prior to immunoglobulin variable region gene rearrangement. The ''differentiation pathway model'' proposes that CD5 expression occurs secondary to expression and engagement of the B-cell surface receptor for antigen (913–915).

Alterations, especially expansion, of the $CD5^+$ B-cell population (B-1a cells) have been reported in many nonneoplastic disease states, including a wide range of autoimmune disorders. These patients generally have an increased percentage and often an increased absolute number of $CD5^+$ B cells. The disease-associated abnormalities in CD5 expression have been reviewed by Arber and Weiss (853).

The evaluation of CD5 expression is extremely useful in the immunophenotypic analysis of lymphohematopoietic malignancies. Among acute leukemias, CD5 expression represents a fairly specific and sensitive marker of the T-cell lineage (853). CD5 is expressed by approximately 90% of precursor T-cell lymphoblastic lymphomas/leukemias but not by precursor B-cell lymphoblastic/lymphomas/leukemias or by chronic myelogenous leukemia in lymphoid blast crisis (6–8,13,14,144,222,462,853). Also, CD5 is expressed by less than 5% of AMLs (including chronic myelogenous leukemia in myeloid blast crisis), primarily those expressing other lymphoid antigens (524,916,917). The frequency of aberrant CD5 expression in AML is less than that of other lymphoid antigens (420). In addition, aberrant CD5 expression in AML does not appear to have any prognostic significance (417,917).

CD5 also is expressed by all categories of postthymic (TdT^-) T-cell neoplasia (6–8,13,14,227,726,727,853,918). As in the case of pan-T cell antigens CD2, CD3, and CD7, however, CD5 may be deleted aberrantly in T-cell malignancies (14,726), and this varies according to the clinicopathologic category (853). CD5 is expressed by virtually 100% of T-cell prolymphocytic leukemias, more than 90% of adult T-cell lymphoma/leukemias, about 85% of cutaneous T-cell lymphomas, but less than 70% of peripheral T-cell lymphomas (853), and by less than 50% of LGL/NK cell leukemias, reflecting the true NK cell origin of some of these latter proliferations (853). Consequently, CD5 is expressed by only about 75% of post-thymic T cell neoplasms overall (853).

In addition, CD5 is expressed commonly by certain clinicopathologic categories of small B-cell NHL and lymphoid leukemia; it is uncommonly, rarely, or not at all expressed by all other categories of B-cell neoplasia. CD5 is expressed by approximately 90% of chronic lymphocytic leukemias, 70% of small lymphocytic lymphomas, 90% of mantle cell lymphomas with circulating lymphoma cells, and 80% of mantle cell lymphomas with lymph node–only disease (853), thus making CD5 one of the defining criteria for these categories of B-cell neoplasia (462,600) (Fig. 3.41). The majority of patients with chronic lymphocytic leukemia with increased numbers of prolymphocytes (chronic lymphocytic leukemia/prolymphocytic leukemia) also express CD5; only about 20% of those with prolymphocytic leukemia express CD5 (853). Also, only about 30% of patients with plasmacytoid small lymphocytic lymphomas express CD5 (853). CD5 may be retained or lost during large cell transformation of chronic lymphocytic leukemia or small lymphocytic lymphoma (Richter's syndrome) (919). It generally is believed that the minor lymphoid tissue $CD5^+$ B-cell population represents the benign counterpart of these malignant $CD5^+$ B-cell populations (853) (see Chapters 21, 22 and 40). Similarly, most neoplastic $CD5^+$ B-cell populations characteristically express CD5 in low density (853).

CD5 is expressed by only about 20% of patients with splenic lymphoma with villous lymphocytes and by no or fewer than 5% of patients with hairy cell leukemia, follicle center cell lymphoma, nodal or extranodal marginal zone lymphoma, large cell lymphoma, Burkitt's lymphoma, or precursor B-cell lymphoblastic lymphoma/leukemia (853). Unlike small lymphocytic lymphoma and mantle cell lymphoma, circulating lymphoma cells associated with the other categories of B-cell NHL do not characteristically express CD5 (853). The lack of CD5 expression generally is considered one of the defining criteria for nodal and extranodal marginal zone lymphoma (462,600,853) (see Chapters 23 and 33). Consequently, determination of the presence or absence of CD5 is an important aspect of the immunophenotypic evaluation of small B-cell neoplasms (462,600,853, 920).

Except for a few notable exceptions, other hematopoietic and nonhematopoietic neoplasms lack CD5. It generally is believed that the Reed-Sternberg cells and variants of Hodgkin's disease lack CD5 (853) (see Chapter 18). Also, CD5 is not expressed by patients with plasmacytoma/multiple myeloma (921,922), Langerhans cell histiocytosis (527), or true histiocytic and dendritic cell neoplasms (see Chapter 51). CD5 has been reported to be expressed by thymic carcinomas but not by other epithelial malignancies (923).

In conclusion, although CD5 is widely considered to be a pan-T cell antigen, as initially described, it also defines a small but highly significant B-cell subset and may be expressed on some other hematopoietic cells as well. Determination of the expression or absence of CD5, in conjunction with other B and T cell–associated antigens, is extremely valuable in the immunodiagnosis and classification of T-cell neoplasms and the small B-cell neoplasms.

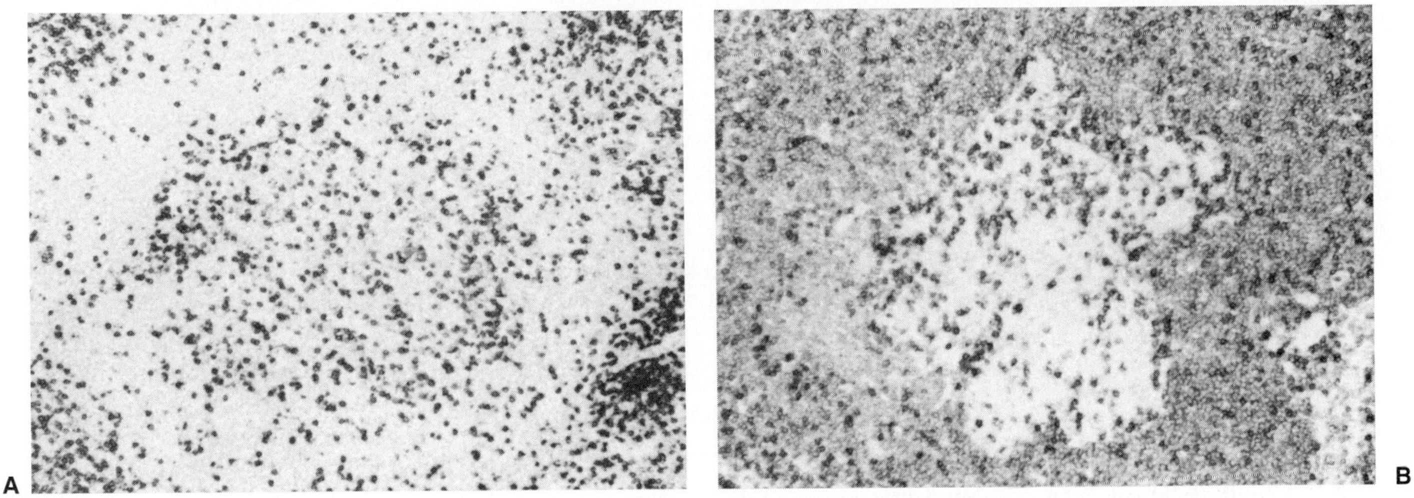

FIG. 3.41. Frozen tissue sections of a mantle cell lymphoma growing in a mantle zone pattern immunostained for CD3 (**A**) and CD5 (**B**). **A:** CD3 positive T cells are evenly distributed throughout the germinal center, are present in small numbers in the mantle zone, and are present in considerably larger numbers in the interfollicular (T-cell) region. **B:** Two distinct CD5-positive cell populations can be identified. Strongly positive CD5 cells are distributed evenly throughout the germinal center and are present in small numbers in the mantle zone and in considerably larger numbers in the interfollicular (T-cell) zone. This strongly positive CD5 cell population is identical in distribution to the CD3-positive T-cell population and represents residual benign T cells. A weakly positive CD5 cell population completely occupies the mantle zone. These cells are CD3-negative and therefore do not represent T cells. Additional immunostains demonstrated that these mantle zone lymphocytes express B-cell lineage–associated antigen CD22 and exclusively express κ light chains. This is a CD5-positive B cell mantle cell lymphoma growing in a mantle zone distribution (immunoperoxidase stain, original magnification: 100× magnification).

CD7

CD7 is a membrane-bound 40-kd glycoprotein that was defined at the first workshop (15) by MAbs 3A1 (924) and 4A (925). Nine additional MAbs, including WT1 (926) and 4H9 (Leu9) (927), were included in the CD7 cluster in the second workshop (928), and multiple additional MAbs were included in subsequent workshops (666,929). Many of these MAbs are commercially available. These anti-CD7 MAbs are applicable in cytofluorometric analysis and in frozen tissue section immunohistochemistry; none are capable of detecting CD7 in formalin-fixed, paraffin-embedded tissue sections (930).

The CD7 gene, located on 17q25 (931), is a member of the immunoglobulin gene superfamily and shares sequence homology with Igκ and TCRγ genes (932). The human CD7 gene is comprised of four exons and three introns that span 3280 bp. Each of the four exons corresponds to the functional domains of the CD7 glycoprotein (933,934). CD7 consists of a single V-type immunoglobulin-like domain at the amino terminus followed by a membrane-proximal ''stalk'' region, a hydrophobic membrane-spanning region, and a 39 amino acid residue cytoplasmic domain (932).

The exact function of CD7 is not known (930). It had been reported that the CD7 molecule functioned as the Fc receptor for IgM (Fcμ) on the surface of T cells (935). It was later shown, however, that the Fcμ receptor on NK cells is a specific immunoglobulin-binding structure, distinct from CD7 or CD16 (936). Other early studies suggested that CD7 is involved in T-cell activation, because its expression is upregulated on phytohemagglutinin- and concanavalin A–stimulated T cells (924,925,937,938). CD7 upregulation is an early event in T-cell activation (939), and although certain studies suggest that CD7 is involved directly in this process, its precise role is unclear (930). The intracellular mechanism of CD7 signal transduction similarly is unknown (930). CD7 is phosphorylated in resting T cells (940). After activation, CD7 becomes hyperphosphorylated; this is linked to progression of the cell to proliferation (941). CD7 expression is downregulated on T cells after treatment with phorbol esters (942). Also, most anti-CD7 MAbs induce modulation of CD7, and soluble MAbs partially inhibit the allogeneic mixed lymphocyte reaction (943).

CD7 is the first T-cell lineage–associated antigen to appear during T-cell ontogeny (937). Haynes and colleagues (772,937,944) demonstrated that $CD45^{+}CD7^{+}TCR\gamma\delta^{-}$ $CD2^{-}CD3^{-}CD4^{-}CD8^{-}$ (triple-negative) precursor T cells appear in 7-week-old fetal tissues prior to colonization of the epithelial thymic rudiment by hematopoietic cells. These $CD7^{+}$ triple-negative cells are pleuripotential stem cells capable of giving rise to $\alpha\beta$- and $\gamma\delta$-expressing T cells as well as erythroid, megakaryocytic, and myeloid cells (937,945). The thymus is colonized by bone marrow and liver precursor cells termed *prothymocytes* that express TdT, HLA-DR, and CD34 (204,221,937). The prothymocytes continue to express TdT and HLA-DR, begin to lose CD34, and acquire cell surface CD7. As these T cells mature under the influence of the thymic epithelium, they gain and lose various other T-cell lineage– and subset-associated antigens in serial fashion and also undergo TCR gene rearrangement (930) (see below). CD7 is retained, however, throughout intrathymic differentiation and is expressed on essentially all thymocytes, including the large prothymocytes residing in the subcapsular cortex (772,924,937,946,947). The function of the CD7 molecule with respect to T-cell ontogeny is unclear. The fact that CD7 is the first T-cell lineage–associated antigen to appear in T-cell differentiation, that it persists throughout T-cell differentiation, and that it is absent from the precursor T cells of children who have severe combined immunodeficiency disease (948) suggests that the CD7 molecule may play an important role in T-cell ontogeny (930).

As medullary thymocytes peripheralize to become mature T cells, they lose TdT and cCD3 but retain CD7. Approximately 85% of peripheral T cells, including all those that are $CD8^+$ and about 90% of those that are $CD4^+$, express CD7, as determined by cytofluorometric analysis (924,946,947). Frozen tissue section immunohistochemistry of benign, reactive lymphoid tissues has produced comparable findings (726). The only other $CD7^+$ cell population is NK cells, approximately 80% of which bear cell surface CD7 (725). B cells and normal epithelial and mesenchymal cells do not express CD7 (930).

CD7 is a very useful and important immunophenotypic marker in the evaluation of hematologic malignancy. The demonstration of CD7 expression is extremely useful in distinguishing between precursor T- and B-cell lymphoblastic lymphomas/leukemias. CD7 is expressed strongly by more than 95% of TdT^+ precursor T-cell lymphoblastic lymphomas/leukemias (13,14,144,222,684,926,927,949), including those displaying the least mature immunophenotypes and those lacking clonal TCR gene rearrangements (221,950,951). In contrast, CD7 expression is consistently absent from precursor B-cell lymphoblastic lymphomas and leukemias (13,14,926,927). CD7 expression by an acute leukemia, however, does not necessarily imply a T cell–lineage derivation. Depending on the series, from 5 to 20% of *de novo* AMLs, as well as a small proportion of patients with chronic myelogenous leukemia in myeloid blast crisis, express CD7 (343,524,952–962). The preponderance of these cases appear to belong to the FAB M0 and M1 categories (730,953), but cases belonging to the FAB M4 and M5 categories (963,964) and cases expressing TdT (965) have been described. Determination of CD7 expression by AMLs is important because $CD7^+$ and $CD7^-$ AMLs display numerous statistically significant clinical differences (930). Included among these are a higher incidence of central nervous system relapse, a poorer response to conventional antileukemia chemotherapy, and a less favorable outcome for $CD7^+$ than $CD7^-$ AMLs (953,961,966). A $CD7^+$ stem cell leukemia, once again displaying distinctive clinical characteristics and a poor response to conventional antileukemia therapy, also has been described (967–969). Whether the latter cases represent a distinct clinicopathologic entity or merely variants of $CD7^+$ acute lymphoblastic or myeloid leukemia remains to be determined (930).

CD7 also is expressed by virtually all clinicopathologic categories of postthymic (TdT^-) T-cell lymphoma and leukemia (7,8,13,14,227,462,726,727) with the exception of adult T-cell lymphoma/leukemia, in which CD7 is conspicuously absent (231). One or more of the four pan-T cell antigens (CD2, CD3, CD5, and CD7) may be deleted aberrantly in malignant postthymic T-cell populations, and among these CD7 is the most frequently deleted (14,726). Picker and colleagues (726) discovered aberrant deletion of CD7 in 56% of patients with postthymic T-cell lymphoma overall. In particular, CD7 expression is generally absent in about two thirds of patients with patch- or plaque-stage mycosis fungoides (726) and in most with tumor-stage mycosis fungoides (726) and the Sézary syndrome (223,847,848). Many clinically aggressive NK cell lymphomas/leukemias but only approximately 50% of clinically indolent LGL/NK cell leukemias express CD7 (930).

The absence of one or more of these pan-T cell antigens is an extremely useful criterion in the immunodiagnosis of T-cell neoplasia (14,726). Caution should be exercised, however, in relying on the absence of CD7 expression as an immunodiagnostic marker of T-cell neoplasia in the absence of other criteria. This is because a significant proportion of benign T cells (generally less than 50%) in selected benign cutaneous lymphoid proliferations lack CD7 (970). This could represent a benign expansion of the normally occurring $CD7^-CD4^+$ T-cell subset. Also, the peripheral blood T cells and intrasynovial lymphocytes of patients who have rheumatoid arthritis exhibit markedly diminished CD7 expression (971).

In contrast, CD7 is not expressed by virtually any mature (TdT^-) sIg^+ or sIg^- B-cell NHLs or lymphoid leukemias (7,8,462,926,927). The Reed-Sternberg cells and variants of Hodgkin's disease similarly lack CD7, as do Langerhans cell histiocytosis, true histiocytic and dendritic cell neoplasms, carcinomas, melanomas, and sarcomas (930) (see Chapters 18, 30, and 51).

T Cell Receptor $\alpha\beta$, $\gamma\delta$

The TCR represents the antigen recognition molecule on T cells (972), analogous to immunoglobulin on B cells (118) (see Chapter 7). The TCR molecules are expressed in association with an invariant transmembrane signaling component, the CD3 complex (119). Two forms of the TCR exist. Each is a heterodimeric structure consisting of two disulfide bond–linked glycosylated polypeptide chains (118). TCR$\alpha\beta$ consists of a 49-kd α chain and a 43-kd β chain (711,973). TCR$\gamma\delta$ consists of a 55-kd γ chain and a 40-kd δ chain (974,975). More than 90% of thymocytes and mature peripheral T cells but less than 5% of postnatal thymus and adult peripheral blood and lymphoid tissue T cells utilize the

TCR$\alpha\beta$ heterodimer (975–979) (see Chapter 2). TCR$\alpha\beta$- and TCR$\gamma\delta$-bearing T cells represent mutually exclusive cell populations (980).

Several MAbs recognizing framework determinants of TCR β chains have been described, including WT31 (976), βF_1 (978), and βF_2 (981). MAb WT31 reacts with surface TCR$\alpha\beta$ on viable T cells; MAbs βF_1 and βF_2 do not (981). For this reason, MAb WT31 provides optimal results if employed in the flow cytometric analysis of viable cells in suspension, and MAbs βF_1 and βF_2 provide optimal results (βF_1 generally better than βF_2) if used in the immunohistochemical staining of frozen tissue sections (981; Knowles, unpublished observations). These anti-TCR$\alpha\beta$ MAbs react with more than 90% of cortical and medullary thymocytes and mature, peripheral T cells circulating in the peripheral blood and residing in adult lymphoid tissue (976,978,981, 982). The pattern of distribution of reactivity is comparable to that of anti-CD3 MAbs (981,982). The vast majority of T cells in benign reactive proliferations coexpress TCR$\alpha\beta$ and CD3 (982).

T-cell receptor $\alpha\beta$ is expressed inconsistently by malignant T-cell populations. MAb βF_1 reacts with only about 60% of precursor T-cell lymphoblastic lymphomas/leukemias (981–983), making TCR$\alpha\beta$ less commonly expressed than pan-T cell antigens CD7, CD3, CD5, and CD2 by these tumors (982). MAb βF_1 reacts with only about two thirds of postthymic T-cell neoplasms and often shows discordance with CD3 expression (981–983). Only about 20% of sinonasal postthymic T-cell neoplasms react with MAb βF_1 (983). These neoplasms have been classified preliminarily among the peripheral T cell lymphomas, but they frequently lack CD3 and other pan-T cell antigens and express NK cell–associated antigens (982,983). Aberrant immunophenotypic expression of TCR$\alpha\beta$ by neoplastic T cells may be related to abnormal or asynchronous gene expression, analogous to that of other pan-T cell antigens (982). Anti-TCR$\alpha\beta$ MAbs display no or only weak nonspecific immunoreactivity with B-cell NHLs and nonhematopoietic malignancies (981,982).

Monoclonal antibodies recognizing TCR$\gamma\delta$ framework determinants also have been described recently (984,985). Flow cytometric and immunohistochemical studies employing these MAbs have demonstrated that

- T-cell receptor $\gamma\delta$ thymocytes reside predominantly in the thymic medulla and in the corticomedullary junction.
- Variable, but generally small, numbers of TCR$\gamma\delta$ T cells circulate in the peripheral blood and reside in the interfollicular and paracortical (T-cell) zones of all adult lymphoid tissues.
- All peripheral blood TCR$\gamma\delta$ cells express CD3, CD2, CD5, and CD7 antigens.
- Approximately 40% of TCR$\gamma\delta$ cells express CD8, but at lower density than TCR$\alpha\beta$ T cells.
- Only 1% to 4% of peripheral blood TCR$\gamma\delta$ cells express CD4.
- T-cell receptor $\gamma\delta$ T cells are in G_0 or G_1 phase and lack proliferation/activation-associated antigens.
- T-cell receptor $\gamma\delta$ cells variably express multiple cell surface antigens associated with various cell lineages (979, 980,986).

These findings suggest that TCR$\gamma\delta$ cells are a heterogeneous population of mature, resting CD3 T cells that may subserve multiple functions, including a primary role in suppressor or cytotoxic phenomena (979).

Approximately 10% to 20% of CD3$^+$TCR$\alpha\beta^-$ precursor T-cell lymphoblastic lymphomas and two thirds of CD3$^+$TCR$\alpha\beta^-$ precursor T-cell acute lymphoblastic leukemias express TCR$\gamma\delta$ (987,988). These TCR$\gamma\delta^+$ tumors are often CD4$^-$CD8$^-$ (987), the phenotype most commonly associated with normal TCR$\gamma\delta$ T cells (979). Postthymic T-cell NHLs and lymphoid leukemias, even those that are CD3$^+$TCR$\alpha\beta^-$, infrequently express TCR$\gamma\delta$ (987). The vast majority of TCR$\alpha\beta$ negative T-cell neoplasms also is TCR$\gamma\delta^-$.

Large Granular Lymphocyte– or Natural Killer Cell–Associated Antigens

CD16

The CD16 antigen, a 50- to 70-kd glycoprotein, is the low-affinity receptor for aggregated (complexed) IgG (FcγRIII) (989). Two distinct forms of the CD16 antigen exist, FcγR-IIIa and FcγRIIIb. They are encoded by two linked, highly homologous genes, *FCGRIIIA* and *FCGRIIIB*, located on 1q23 (990), whose expression is cell specific. The genetic heterogeneity of FcγRIII generates alternative membrane-anchored proteins with distinct signaling capacities if cross-linked by immune complexes (991). The CD16 molecule FcγRIIIa is an integral membrane protein that is expressed on NK cells, activated monocytes, and tissue macrophages. The CD16 molecule FcγRIIIb is a glycosyl phosphatidylinositol–linked glycoprotein that is expressed only on the surface of neutrophils (990,992,993). The neutrophils of individuals who have paroxysmal nocturnal hemoglobinuria may lack CD16 (994). Polymorphism of the *FCGRIIIB* gene results in two codominant allelic variants, NA1 and NA2), with different glycosylation patterns based on amino acid substitutions (995). These antigens exhibit phenotypic frequencies in caucasians of 46% and 88%, respectively (996). FcγRIIIa exhibits cell-specific size heterogeneity; monocyte FcγRIIIa is more glycosylated than NK cell FcγRIIIa (997). FcγRIIIb NA1 and NA2 also can be distinguished by size and by NA1- and NA2-specific MAbs (996).

The CD16 cluster was established at the second workshop (998). Numerous MAbs have been generated against CD16, including B73.1 (Leu11c) (999,1000), VEP13 (1001), PEN1 (1002), MG38 (1003), ID3 (1003), and others (95,998,1003–1005). Many investigators have documented the differential cellular specificity and functional characteristics of anti-CD16 MAbs (992,996,999,1003,1006–1008). The differential reactivities of these MAbs reflect their specificity for different FcγRIII epitopes and the variable FcγRIII glycosylation patterns as well as their immunoglobulin classes and binding affinities (1006). For example, MAb PEN1 is strongly reactive with FcγRIIIa and therefore with NK cells, activated monocytes and tissue macrophages, and NA2-positive neutrophils (1002). MAb ID3 is FcγRIIIb-specific and therefore is reactive with neutrophils but not with the other CD16$^+$ cell populations (1009). MAb MG38 is specific for the NA1 allelic variant of FcγRIIIb and thus only reacts with NA1-positive neutrophils (1010). The MAb reagent selected for the identification and quantitation of CD16$^+$ cell populations in immunophenotypic analysis is important. Generally speaking, MAb 3G8 exhibits maximum reactivity and is among the anti-CD16 MAbs most commonly employed in cytofluorometric analysis and frozen tissue section immunohistochemistry. Anti-CD16 MAb NCL-CD16 is useful in paraffin tissue sections following the application of antigen-retrieval procedures.

The CD16 molecule represents the functional receptor structure on NK cells responsible for mediating antibody-dependent cell-mediated cytotoxicity (ADCC) (1011). FcγRIII-mediated NK cell activation leads to induction of cytolytic activity, a rise in intracellular calcium, tyrosine phosphorylation of many regulatory proteins, and the secretion of cytokines such as TNF-α and IFN-γ (1012–1014). The tyrosine kinase p72^{syk} is phosphorylated and activated after stimulation of NK cells with anti-CD16 MAbs (1015). CD16-mediated activation of NK cells is p21^{ras} dependent (1016). Also, with respect to CD16-mediated signal transduction in NK cells, p56^{lck} is associated with CD16 (1017). Treatment with some anti-CD16 MAbs can induce apoptosis of IL-2-activated NK cells (1018). Despite the presence of CD16, neutrophils cannot mediate ADCC function (1011,1012). Therefore, it has been suggested that, on granulocytes, CD16 may act as an adhesion structure to bind immune complexes for subsequent cellular activation by other types of FcR (1012).

Those anti-CD16 MAbs that recognize FcγRIIIa, for example MAbs 3G8 and PEN1, react with approximately 15% to 20% of peripheral blood lymphocytes (999,1006,1008); with a much smaller proportion (<5%) of those in tonsil, spleen, and bone marrow; and with almost none in lymph node and thymus (999). These CD16$^+$ peripheral blood lymphocytes belong to the phenotypically and functionally distinct NK cell population (999,1006). The NK cell population is divisable into two distinct subpopulations based on the expression of CD16 and CD56. Approximately 90% of peripheral blood NK cells express abundant CD16 and low levels of CD56 (1019). These CD16^{bright}CD56^{dim} NK cells display LGL morphology; lack B and T cell–associated antigens, with the exception of CD2 on 80% to 90% of the cells and low-density CD8 on 20% to 50% of the cells (999,1000,1006,1019); proliferate poorly in response to exogenous cytokines; and contain virtually all NK and K cell functional activity (999,1007,1019). The remaining 10% of peripheral blood NK cells are CD16$^{dim/negative}$CD56^{bright}. These cells may or may not exhibit LGL morphology, do proliferate in response to exogenous cytokines, and do not mediate strong cytolytic activity (1019,1020). The majority of leukocytes present in the placental bed during trophoblast infiltration of the uterine decidua are CD3$^-$ NK cells (1021). In contrast with the peripheral blood, the majority of the decidual NK cells is CD16$^{dim/negative}$CD56^{bright}, and only a small proportion is CD16^{bright} (1021–1023). Whether these decidual CD16$^{dim/negative}$CD56^{bright} NK cells represent precursors of the apparently more mature CD16^{bright}CD56^{dim} peripheral blood NK cells or a distinct NK cell subset with special functional properties is unclear. These CD56^{bright} NK cells may participate in the maternal response to fetal implantation, however (1024).

These same anti-CD16 MAbs react with a variable proportion, approximately 35% to 75%, of cultured monocytes (1008), but not with resting unstimulated monocytes (1006,1007). A minor subset of peripheral blood and lymphoid tissue CD16$^+$CD14$^+$ "small monocytes," however, has been described (1025). These cells exhibit monocyte morphology, express monocyte and not NK cell antigens, exhibit light-scattering properties intermediate between typical monocytes and lymphocytes, and possess distinct functional properties (1025). The number of CD16$^+$ monocytes can be elevated substantially in patients with HIV infection, sepsis, and metastatic cancer (1019).

These anti-CD16 MAbs display heterogeneous reactivity with tissue macrophages and can be subdivided into two broad groups based on this reactivity. Some of these antibodies, including 3G8, ID3, and MG38, have a limited distribution of immune reactivity. They react weakly or not at all with renal, pulmonary, and placental macrophages and with Kupffer cells and only react with a subpopulation of thymic macrophages (1026). In contrast, other anti-CD16 antibodies, including PEN1 and GRM1, display wider patterns of immune reactivity. These antibodies react strongly with renal, pulmonary, placental, and thymic macrophages and with Kupffer cells. They are also immunoreactive with Langerhans cells, interfollicular macrophages in the tonsil and red pulp macrophages in the spleen (1026).

In addition, those anti-CD16 MAbs that recognize FcγRIIIb-NA1 and FcγRIIIb-NA2 react with more than 95% of neutrophils (990,992) and a subset of eosinophils (1019) but not with basophils (1027). Finally, CD16 is expressed by a small subset of T cells that expresses either $\alpha\beta$ or $\gamma\delta$ TCRs and is capable of ADCC function (1028).

CD16 expression among malignant hematopoietic cell populations largely mirrors its expression among benign hematopoietic cells. Consequently, CD16 is expressed primarily by LGL/NK cell lymphoproliferative disorders. These are broadly divided into those of T-cell NK cell origin, based on the presence or absence of CD3 expression and clonal TCR gene rearrangements (776,778,1029). The patients with T-cell LGL leukemia express CD3 and clonal TCR gene rearrangements, usually are TCR$\alpha\beta^+$CD4$^-$CD8$^+$CD56$^-$ CD5 7$^+$, and variably express CD16 (778). The variability of CD16 expression among these patients may be a result simply of the differential reactivity of anti-CD16 MAbs; all $CD3^+$ T cell LGL leukemias may actually express CD16 (778). The patients with LGL/NK leukemia lack CD3 and clonal TCR gene rearrangements, express CD16, and usually are $TCR\alpha\beta^- CD4^- CD8^- CD56^+ CD57^-$ (778). CD16 also is expressed occasionally by the clinically and biologically distinctive group of $CD56^+$ nasal and related extranodal angiocentric T- or NK cell lymphomas (1030–1033) (see Chapters 29, 43). A small number of precursor T-cell lymphoblastic lymphomas/leukemias express NK cell–associated antigens CD16, CD56, or CD57 as well (1034–1038). These neoplasms exhibit typical lymphoblastic morphology and immunophenotypic profiles, including TdT expression, but may be clinically and biologically distinctive (see Chapter 26). Finally, CD16 is expressed variably by malignant neoplasms of monocyte/macrophage and Langerhans cell origin (462) (see Chapter 51). CD16 is not expressed by B-cell lymphomas or leukemias, plasma cell neoplasms, or AMLs (462).

CD56

The CD56 antigen is a membrane glycoprotein with a molecular mass of 175 to 220 kd under nonreducing conditions (1039,1040) that originally was identified in the chicken brain and designated the *neuronal cell adhesion molecule* (NCAM) (1041). Lanier and coworkers (1042) demonstrated that the molecule detected by MAb NKH-1 (1040) is identical to the 140-kd isoform of human NCAM. Subsequently, the CD56 cluster was established at the fourth workshop (1043), based on its recognition by MAbs NKH-1 (1040), Leu19 (1039), and N901 (1044), among others. CD56 (NCAM) is a member of the immunoglobulin superfamily (1045–1047). It mediates neuronal homophilic adhesion and plays a role in neuronal cell differentiation during embryogenesis (1048). The function of CD56 on human NK cells and T cells remains unclear (1049). CD56 expression is not essential for NK cell function; CD56 is absent from rodent NK cells and NK and T-cell development and function appear normal in mice with disrupted NCAM genes (1050).

CD56 is encoded by a single gene located on 11q23-24 that generates a wide variety of glycoprotein isoforms by alternative splicing (1046). More than 24 distinct mRNAs of CD56 (NCAM) may be expressed (1051). The three major isoforms of CD56 differ mainly in overall size and in the type of membrane attachment. Two transmembrane-anchored glycoproteins of 140 kd and 180 kd, respectively, and a 120-kd glycosyl phosphatidylinositol–anchored glycoprotein result from the use of different exons for the carboxyl terminus of the molecule (1046,1052–1054). Further heterogeneity is created by alternative splicing of small exons that encode segments of the extracellular domain, including a muscle-specific domain (1051,1055,1056). NK cells and T cells only express the 140-kd transmembrane isoform. The extracellular domain of the 140-kd isoform contains 689 amino acid residues composed of five C2-type immunoglobulin-like domains and two fibronectin type III segments. The cytoplasmic domain consists of 119 amino acid residues (1045–1047). CD56 is modified posttranslationally by the addition of O-linked and N-linked oligosaccharides as well as α-2-8-linked polysialic acid and by sulfation (1057). All of these modifications play critical roles in the regulation of NCAM-mediated cell adhesion and are essential for the correct differentiation of various tissues (1045).

Anti-CD56 MAbs, along with anti-CD16 MAbs, are the most useful antibodies currently available for the identification and isolation of human NK cells (1049). The anti-CD56 MAbs are applicable in cytofluorometric analysis and with immunohistochemistry using frozen but not paraffin tissue sections. MAb 123C3 detects CD56, however, on routine formalin-fixed, paraffin-embedded tissue sections after suitable antigen-retrieval procedures, comparable to those of MAb NKH-1 in frozen tissue sections (1058).

The presence and intensity of CD56 and CD16 expression permits division of the NK cell population into two distinct subsets. Anti-CD56 MAbs react with virtually all peripheral blood, mucosal, and uterine decidual NK cells and are pan-NK cell markers (1019,1020,1024,1059). Approximately 90% of peripheral blood NK cells express low levels of CD56 and abundant CD16. These $CD16^{bright}CD56^{dim}$ NK cells exhibit LGL morphology, proliferate poorly in response to exogenous cytokines, and mediate non-MHC-restricted cytotoxicity (1019,1020,1039,1040). The remaining 10% of peripheral blood $CD16^{dim/negative}CD56^{bright}$ NK cells may or may not exhibit LGL morphology, do proliferate in response to exogenous cytokines, and do not mediate strong cytolytic activity (1019,1020). The physiologic role of $CD56^{bright}$ NK cells *in vivo* and their developmental relationship with the $CD56^{dim}$ NK cell population has not been elucidated. CD56 is upregulated, however, on $CD56^{dim}$ NK cells following *in vitro* and *in vivo* activation (1060,1061).

CD56 also is expressed by a small subset (5%) of peripheral blood $CD3^+$ T cells (1039,1062). Most of these $CD3^+CD56^+$ T cells express TCR $\alpha\beta$, pan-T cell antigens CD2 and CD5, and subset antigen CD8 and not CD4 and lack CD16 (1019,1039,1062). These $CD3^+CD56^+CD16^-$ T cells constitute a unique subset of cytotoxic T cells possessing LGL morphology that exhibit spontaneous non-MHC-restricted cytotoxicity (1039). CD56 also is expressed on many cytotoxic and noncytotoxic IL-2-dependent T-cell lines and clones expressing either CD4 or CD8 that are maintained in long-term culture (1063). CD56 is not expressed on thymocytes, B cells, plasma cells, monocytes, or granulocytes (505,1039,1040,1044,1064,1065).

CD56 is present in all three germ layers during early development (1066) and is expressed by several embryonic tissues (1066), including smooth (1067) and striated muscle (1068). In the adult, however, CD56, is restricted mainly to neural cells (1045). CD56 (NCAM) is expressed variably, but generally weakly, in human brain, including in the cerebrum, cerebellum, spinal cord, and other regions; the expression seen depends on the anti-CD56 MAb employed (1069).

CD56 is expressed by only about 2% of all NHLs overall and, with rare exception, only those of NK or T-cell origin (1030,1031). LGL/NK cell lymphoproliferative disorders are divided broadly into those of T-cell and those of NK cell origin (778). Patients with LGL/NK leukemia lack CD3 and TCR$\alpha\beta$ and usually are $CD4^-CD8^-CD16^+CD57^-$ (778). Those with T-cell LGL leukemia express CD3 and TCR$\alpha\beta$ and usually are $CD4^-CD8^+CD16^+CD56^-CD57^+$ (778). A clinically aggressive $CD56^+$ variant of T-cell LGL leukemia also has been described (1070). In addition, CD56 characteristically is expressed by a clinically and biologically distinctive group of nasal and related extranodal angiocentric T- and NK cell lymphomas that sometimes express CD16 and generally lack CD57 (1030–1033,1071). CD56 also often is expressed by hepatosplenic $\gamma\delta$ T-cell lymphoma (1071,1072) and by S-100 protein–positive T-cell lymphoma (1071). A small number of peripheral T-cell lymphomas, which have been referred to as *NK-like T-cell lymphomas*, also express CD56 (1073). Although not expressed by benign polyclonal plasma cells, CD56 is expressed by monoclonal plasma cells in about 75% of patients with multiple myeloma (505,1064). Patients who have $CD56^-$ myeloma appear generally to have aggressive disease (1064) (see Chapter 42). Measurement of serum CD56 (NCAM) levels has been proposed as a useful prognostic marker in patients who have multiple myeloma (1074). CD56, CD16, or CD57 expression also has been reported in some precursor T-cell lymphoblastic lymphomas/leukemias (1034–1038), which may be clinically and biologically distinctive (see Chapter 26). Finally, CD56 frequently is expressed by the uncommonly occurring and incompletely understood microvillous large B-cell lymphomas (1075) (see Chapter 25).

In addition, CD56 is expressed by some AMLs (462), in particular by some FAB M5 AMLs (418), and by a recently described clinicopathologic entity referred to as *myeloid/NK cell acute leukemia* (1076). The $CD56^+$ malignant blasts making up the latter form of acute leukemia resemble FAB M3v AML morphologically and FAB M3 AML immunophenotypically but lack the translocation t(15;17) and rearrangements of the retinoic acid receptor-α locus (1076).

Among malignant nonhematopoietic neoplasms, CD56 is expressed strongly by neuroectodermally derived tumors, including neuroblastomas, medulloblastomas, astrocytomas, (1069,1077), malignant Schwannomas (1068), and small cell lung carcinomas (1077–1079), as well as by Wilm's tumors (1080), rhabdomyosarcomas (1068), and a small proportion of carcinomas arising in various organs (1081).

CD57

The CD57 cluster was established at the fourth workshop (1082). The CD57 antigen originally was recognized by MAb HNK-1 (Leu7) (1083) and believed to be selectively expressed by human NK and K cells (1083,1084). It soon was realized that CD57 is expressed widely, including by some T-cell subpopulations (1085), by some neural and neuroendocrine cells, and by various neoplasms (1086), and is not an NK cell–specific marker. MAb HNK-1 (Leu7) and many other anti-CD57 MAbs are immunoreactive in routine formalin-fixed, paraffin-embedded tissue sections (1086). For this reason, CD57 has become employed widely in the immunodiagnostic evaluation of benign and malignant hematopoietic and nonhematopoietic cell populations (1086).

The CD57 antigen is a 110-kd glycoprotein (1083,1087,1088) encoded by a gene that appears to be located on chromosome 11 (1089). Little else, however, other than its expression, is known about CD57. The molecular structure, ligands, associated molecules, biochemical activity, and cellular function of CD57 and its relevance to human disease are unknown (1082).

Monoclonal antibody HNK-1 (Leu7) reacts with approximately 10% to 25% of peripheral blood lymphoid cells, including a subset of the $CD16^+$ NK cell population (1083–1085,1090), and a distinct T-ell subpopulation that expresses T cell—associated antigens CD2, CD3, and CD5 (1085,1091,1092). CD57 is not expressed by peripheral blood B cells, monocytes, granulocytes, erythrocytes, or platelets (1083,1091).

The absolute number and percentage of peripheral blood $CD57^+$ lymphoid cells vary with age. CD57 is virtually undetectable on fetal and cord blood lymphoid cells, although $CD16^+$ and $CD56^+$ NK cells are present (1093,1094). In the newborn, less than 1% to approximately 4% of peripheral blood lymphoid cells express CD57 (1095,1096). The percentage of $CD57^+$ lymphoid cells increases throughout life, averaging about 5% in children younger than 15 years of age (1095), rising to 10% to 20% in adults (1097), and increasing to 20% to 40% in individuals older than 80 years of age (1098). In adults, 50% to 60% of $CD57^+$ peripheral blood lymphoid cells are NK cells, and the remaining 40% to 50% are T cells (1098).

Four peripheral blood mononuclear cell subpopulations can be defined on the basis of CD16 and CD57 expression (1091). The $CD16^+CD57^+$ subset contains substantial NK activity; the $CD16^-CD57^-$ subset contains no NK activity. The $CD16^-CD57^+$ subpopulation, which includes a predominance of $CD3^+CD8^+$ T cells that frequently express CD11b (1099), exhibits weak NK activity. The $CD16^+CD57^+$ subset displays variable NK activity (1091). In addition, the variable expression of CD57 by $CD56^+$ and $CD56^-$ NK cells suggests that other NK cell subpopulations exist as well (1100). CD57 is expressed by about 50% to 60% of $CD56^{dim}$ NK cells and is downregulated on these cells after activation. CD57 is not expressed by $CD56^{bright}$ NK cells (1019,1020).

Those $CD3^+$ T cells that express CD57 are almost entirely $CD8^+$ T cells, although a small percentage does express CD4 (1091). $CD57^+$ T cells probably represent a stage of T-cell differentiation that occurs late in the immune response rather than a separate T-cell lineage (1086). This is supported by the fact that IL-2 and IL-4 can induce CD57 expression on $CD57^-$ T cells of both the CD4 and CD8 types (1083). $CD57^+CD3^+CD8^+$ T cells differ phenotypically and functionally from the more common $CD57^-CD3^+CD8^+$ antigen-specific cytotoxic T cells (1086). $CD57^+$ T cells have less dense CD3 expression than do $CD57^-$ T cells (1101). $CD57^+CD3^+CD8^+$ T cells express CD45RA but not CD45RO (1102), consistent with naive T cells, but differ from other naive T cells in that they fail to lose CD45RA if stimulated by alloantigens (1102). They also differ from other T cells in their increased ability to acquire HLA-DR and in their lack of antigen-specific cytotoxic activity against allogeneic target cells (1102). They also exhibit lower proliferative responses to phytohemagglutinin or mitogenic anti-CD3 antibodies than $CD57^-$ T cells (1103). In healthy individuals, $CD57^+CD3^+CD8^+$ T cells actually suppress the generation of cytotoxic T cells to autologous EBV-transformed B-lymphoblastoid cell lines (1104). $CD57^+CD3^+CD8^+$ T cells preferentially mediate lectin-dependent cytotoxicity and anti-CD3-induced cytotoxicity compared with $CD57^-$ T cells (1101). Anti CD2 antibodies block the cytolytic functions of these cells and can induce their apoptosis (1105).

Elevations of peripheral blood $CD57^+$ mononuclear cells, predominantly $CD3^+CD8^+$ T cells, have been identified in a variety of disease states (1086), including HIV infection (1106), rheumatoid arthritis (1107,1108), and Crohn's disease (1109), as well as in healthy cytomegalovirus carriers (1100) and after bone marrow and solid organ transplantation (1110–1112). At least some of the peripheral blood elevations in $CD57^+$ cells occurring in rheumatoid arthritis patients represent clonal proliferations of LGLs (1113). The relationship between the number and type of $CD57^+$ mononuclear cells and various diseases has been reviewed by Arber and Weiss (1086).

$CD57^+$ lymphoid cells are rare in the thymus (1114,1115) and bone marrow (1085). In lymph nodes and tonsil, $CD57^+$ lymphoid cells are located primarily in the germinal center (1114–1117). Unlike the peripheral blood $CD57^+$ lymphoid cells, these lymphoid tissue germinal center $CD57^+$ cells are $CD3^+$ T cells that express CD4 and not CD8 (1118,1119). They do not exhibit, however, the usual helper activity of CD4 T cells (1119). $CD3^+CD4^+CD57^-$ T cells generally lie outside the germinal center (1114–1117). Similarly, in the spleen, $CD57^+$ lymphoid cells are located primarily within the germinal center of the white pulp (1114,1115) or form a rim around the central white pulp (1114).

Anti-CD57 MAbs also react with normal cellular elements, that is, oligodendroglia and Schwann cells, and the myelin sheaths of the peripheral and central nervous system (1120), apparently based on the recognition of myelin-associated glycoprotein (1088,1121,1122). Anti-CD57 MAbs recognize part of the myeloid-associated protein that has a similar molecular mass (110 kd) to CD57 (1088,1123). Some neural cell adhesion molecules contain a carbohydrate epitope that is recognized by anti-CD57 MAbs (1124,1125). Anti-CD57 MAbs react with other neural adhesion molecules as well (1121,1126–1129). These are usually glycosphinogolipids that contain sulfated glucuronic acid (1130). Apparently, the sulfate group is essential for CD57 antibody binding to these antigens (1131). Among humans, this sulfated antigen is present in fetal brain and in adult peripheral nervous tissue but not in the postnatal central nervous system (1131,1132).

Anti-CD57 MAbs are also immunoreactive with prostatic epithelium, renal loops of Henle and proximal tubular cells, adrenal medullary cells, pancreatic islet cells, gastric chief cells, chromaffin cells of the intestine, epithelial cells of the outer cortex of the thymus, and select cells of the fetal bronchus (1133–1136).

The most common $CD57^+$ lymphoproliferative disorder, by far, is LGL/NK cell leukemia. Approximately 70% of these patients overall express CD57 (1086). These disorders are divided broadly into those of T-cell and NK cell origin based on the presence or absence of CD3 expression and clonal TCR gene rearrangements (776,778,1029). The T-cell LGL leukemias are usually $CD57^+CD8^+$. The LGL/NK leukemias are $CD3^-CD16^+$ and may be subtyped by the presence or absence of CD57 (778,1029). CD57 expression among these disorders may be clinically relevant, because it has been suggested that $CD57^-$ LGL/NK cell leukemias are associated with an increased mortality rate (1137) (see Chapter 43). Less than 10% of the $CD56^+$ nasal and related extranodal angiocentric T/NK cell lymphomas express CD57 (1030,1138) (see Chapter 29). CD57, CD16, or CD56 expression has been described in occasional precursor T-cell lymphoblastic lymphomas/leukemias (1034–1038), which may be clinically and biologically distinctive (see Chapter 26). CD57 is not expressed by B-cell lymphomas or leukemias, plasma cell neoplasms, AMLs, or Langerhans cell histiocytosis (1086).

Although most hematopoietic tumors do not express CD57, some are associated with an increased number of nonneoplastic $CD57^+$ lymphoid cells (1086). For example, the number of $CD57^+$ lymphoid cells is increased in patients with nodular L&H (lymphocyte predominance) Hodgkin's disease. Here, they are $CD4^+$ (1139) and surround the $CD20^+$ L&H cells (1140). Their presence around the L&H cells may be useful in the differential diagnosis of nodular L&H Hodgkin's disease from nodular sclerosis Hodgkin's disease, T cell–rich B-cell lymphoma and follicular lymphoma, in which this phenomenon is not observed (1140).

CD57 is expressed by a wide range of neoplasms of epithelial, neural, neuroendocrine, and mesenchymal origin (1086). This includes more than 95% of prostatic adenocarcinomas, papillary thyroid carcinomas, pheochromocytomas, and thymomas; about 90% of oligodendrogliomas; about 75% or more of carcinoid tumors, paragangliomas, granular cell tumors, dysgerminomas, glioblastomas, neuroblastomas, and esthesioneuroblastomas; about 50% or more of small cell lung carcinomas, benign and malignant schwannomas, neurofibromas, astrocytomas, follicular and medullary thyroid carcinomas, and mesotheliomas; and a variable but smaller proportion of thymic carcinomas, adenocarcinomas, ganglioneuroblastomas, medulloblastomas, meningiomas, and sarcomas of diverse histogenesis (1086). The proportion of CD57^{+} cells and the intensity of expression vary considerably among these neoplasms (1086). Anti-CD57 MAbs must be used in conjunction with other antibodies, such as those to S-100 protein, cytokeratin, neuron-specific enolase, chromogranin, and synaptophysin, in the immunodiagnostic evaluation of these and related neoplasms.

Monocyte-Macrophage and Myeloid-Associated Antigens

CD11b

CD11b, also known as Mac-1 and CR3 (CR3), belongs to the leukocyte integrin receptor family of cellular adhesion molecules, which plays a critical role in the cellular adhesion reactions of leukocytes (108). Mac-1 was one of the first integrin molecules to be recognized; it was identified initially in the mouse (1141) and later in the human (109,110,1142). The CD11 cluster, which was preliminarily established at the first workshop (15), included MAb Mo1 (110). The CD11b cluster was distinguished from CD18 and established as a separate cluster at the third workshop (245) when it was discovered that MAb Mo1 is specific for CR3, the receptor for the complement component, iC3b. This cluster also includes MAbs OKM1 (109) and MY8 (112), among others (111).

The integrin receptors are heterodimeric molecules comprised of noncovalently associated α and β subunits (1143,1144). Different subfamilies of integrins displaying distinctive cell and organ distributions have been identified. Leukocytes express the $\beta 2$ subfamily of integrins, which consists of four molecules that have identical 95-kd β chains (CD18), but have structurally and antigenically distinct α chains. These are LFA-1 or CD11a-CD18, Mac-1 or CR3 (CD11b-CD18), p150,95 (CD11c-CD18), and the recently described $\alpha d\beta 2$ (presumably CD11d-CD18) (1145,1146). These molecules play critical roles in cell adhesion in the immune system and in the inflammatory response (1147). Expression of the CD11b subunit on the leukocyte cell surface requires the presence of an intact $\beta 2$ (CD18) subunit (1148). Individuals who have mutated CD18 genes, a condition known as *leukocyte adhesion deficiency-1* (1148,1149), produce abnormal or very small amounts of the 95-kd β chain and do not express any of the $\beta 2$ integrins (1148). These individuals exhibit profound abnormalities in leukocyte adhesion-dependent function, resulting in defective inflammatory responses to bacterial infections (1150). They develop recurrent life-threatening bacterial infections and often die at early ages (1148,1149). Anti-CD11b MAbs are directed against the 155-kd α chain and immunoprecipitate both the α and β subunits (1151). Multiple epitopes have been identified (107), and the existence of two functional domains has been proposed: one involved in iC3b binding and the other in promoting certain granulocyte adhesion-dependent functions (1151).

Like the other $\beta 2$ integrin α subunits, the human CD11b gene is located on chromosome 16, band p11-p13 (1152). CD11b is a type I transmembrane protein consisting of 1,137 amino acid residues comprised of an extracellular domain of 1,092 amino acids, a transmembrane domain of 26 amino acids, and a cytoplasmic domain of 19 amino acids (1153). The amino-terminal extracellular domain contains seven short homologous repeating sequences of about 60 residues each (I–VII), of which the last three (V–VII) contain "EF hand"-like divalent cation-binding domains. Inserted between domains II and III is the 187-residue "I" or inserted domain, which contains an additional metal-binding site (1154) and ligand iC3b, fibrinogen, and ICAM-1 binding sites. Many anti-CD11b MAbs, including Mo1, react with epitopes on the I domain (1155).

CD11b (Mac-1) is a multifunctional receptor that binds to a multiplicity of soluble and cellular ligands, including ICAM-1, fibrinogen, iC3b, and coagulation factor X (1156). CD11b mediates the adherence of neutrophils and monocytes to endothelium, and subsequently neutrophil extravasation to sites of inflammation (1156). It also mediates neutrophil homotypic aggregation, chemotaxis, and phagocytosis of iC3b-coated particles (1157–1159). Mac-1 engages in cis interactions with receptors such as FcγRII and FcγRIII, which are believed to lead to signaling events in myeloid cells (1160).

CD11b is expressed by more than 90% of peripheral blood monocytes, granulocytes (110,112), and NK cells (725), as well as by tissue macrophages, including sinus histiocytes; germinal center tingible body macrophages; epithelioid histiocytes in lymph nodes, tonsil, and spleen; alveolar macrophages; Kupffer cells (1161); and follicular dendritic cells (546). CD11b also is expressed by about 30% of bone marrow cells (112). It is expressed on all bone marrow myeloid cells beginning with the promyelocyte stage; myeloid precursor cells (GM-CFUs) lack CD11b (112). Monocyte and granulocyte CD11b expression is upregulated by inflammatory stimuli such as IL-1, GM-CSF, and interferon-γ (1156). CD11b is not expressed by mature, resting B or T cells, erythrocytes, or platelets (112). CD11b similarly is not expressed by interdigitating dendritic cells, Langerhans' cells, splenic macrophages, or endothelial cells (1161). A minor CD8^{+} T-cell subset has been reported to express CD11b (1162), but these cells may be NK cells, because they exhibit LGL morphology and express CD57 (1163).

CD11b is expressed by approximately 30% to 40% of all pediatric and adult AMLs (418,420,730,916). This includes virtually no FAB M6 (erythroblastic) or M7 (megakaryoblastic) AMLs, a small proportion of FAB M3 AMLs, approximately 25% to 70% of FAB M0, M1, and M2 (nonmonocytic) AMLs, and more than 75% of FAB M4 and M5 (monocytic) AMLs (112,730,1164–1166). CD11b also is expressed by approximately 75% of patients with chronic myelogenous leukemias (112) and 60% of those with chronic myelogenous leukemia in myeloid blast crisis (CML-MBC) but is absent in cases of chronic myelogenous leukemia in lymphoid blast crisis (CML-LBC) (112,236,1167). The reported variability in immunoreactivity appears to be related largely to the MAb reagent used—OKM1, Mo1, or MY8 (1166,1168). Anti-CD11b MAbs may be useful in confirming the cytomorphologic diagnosis of AML. More importantly, perhaps, CD11b expression in adult AML is an independent prognostic indicator and is significantly predictive of a shorter duration of survival (420). CD11b also is expressed by a small number of acute biphenotypic leukemias (525) and is expressed variably by $CD3^+$ T-cell LGL leukemias, $CD3^-$ LGL/NK leukemias (462,600,788,1169), $CD56^+$ nasal and related extranodal angiocentric T-cell NK cell lymphomas (1030), and $CD56^+$ NK-like peripheral T-cell lymphomas (1073) (see Chapters 29 and 43). The true frequency of CD11b expression among these disorders is unknown because immunophenotypic analysis of these disorders often has not included examination of CD11b (1031,1032,1071,1073,1169). CD11b is not expressed by other postthymic T-cell lymphomas and leukemias (462,600). Similarly, CD11b is not expressed by B-cell lymphomas and leukemias, with the exception of hairy cell leukemia (462,600) (see Chapter 41). Finally, CD11b is expressed variably by neoplasms of histiocytic derivation (see Chapter 51).

CD11c

The CD11 cluster was established preliminarily at the first workshop (15). CD11c, also known as p150,95 and CR4, was identified biochemically as a protein containing a 150-kd subunit that is noncovalently associated with the 95-kd β subunit common to LFA-1 and Mac-1 (108). Later, the antigen recognized by MAb S-HCL3 (Leu M5) on hairy cell leukemia (555) was found to be identical to p150,95 (1170,1171). The CD11c cluster subsequently was established at the third workshop (245).

CD11c complexes with the β subunit of the integrin family, CD18, to form the cell surface heterodimer CD11c-CD18 (p150,95) (108,1170–1172). CD11c-CD18 is one of four members of the leukocyte integrin family, the other three being LFA-1 (CD11a-CD18), Mac-1 or CR3 (CD11b-CD18), and the recently described $\alpha d\beta 2$ (presumably CD11d-CD18) (1145,1146,1170,1171). MAbs that specifically recognize the p150,95 heterodimer are actually specific for its 150-kd α subunit, CD11c.

Like the other $\beta 2$ integrin α subunits, the human CD11c gene is located on chromosome 16, band p11-p13 (1152). This gene spans about 30 kb and consists of 31 exons grouped in five clusters (1152). The structure of CD11c is similar to that of the other $\beta 2$ integrin α subunits. CD11c is a type I transmembrane glycoprotein of 1,163 amino acid residues comprised of a short signal sequence, a large extracellular domain of 1,088 residues, a transmembrane region, and a short cytoplasmic tail of 35 residues. The amino-terminal extracellular domain contains an I domain of 187 residues and three tandem putative divalent cation-binding EF hand–like repeats. Each of the three putative divalent cation-binding sites is encoded by a separate exon; the I domain is distributed over four exons (1173).

Similar to CR3 (CD11b-CD18), p150,95 specifically recognizes the iC3b fragment in a cation-dependent manner (1174–1176). Therefore, one of the primary functions of monocyte-macrophage and granulocyte CD11c molecules is to clear opsonized particles and immune complexes (1176). In addition, like CD11b-CD18, leukocyte integrin CD11c-CD18 is an adhesion molecule. It mediates monocyte-granulocyte adhesion to endothelium during inflammatory responses (1177), fibrinogen binding (1178), neutrophil adhesion to serum-coated surfaces, and chemotaxis and adhesion of peripheral blood monocytes (1179–1181). Its activities reflect those of Mac-1, with which it acts synergistically (1160). CD11c-CD18 (p150,95) also has been implicated in B-cell activation, cytotoxic T lymphocyte–mediated killing, and the respiratory burst in granulocytes (1182–1184).

CD11c is expressed strongly by peripheral blood monocytes (1185,1186). After extravasation *in vivo*, p150,95 is upregulated during the differentiation of peripheral blood monocytes into tissue macrophages (1187,1188). Therefore, CD11c also is expressed strongly by tissue macrophages, including sinus histiocytes and germinal center tingible body macrophages of lymph node, tonsil, and spleen; thymic macrophages; alveolar macrophages; splenic macrophages (1185,1186); and microglia (1189) (Fig. 3.42). Granulocytes also express CD11c, although less strongly than monocytes/macrophages (1185,1186). In addition to cell surface expression, p150,95 is present in a large intracellular pool in monocytes and granulocytes, which can be mobilized rapidly to the cell surface on induction by inflammatory mediators (1171,1188,1190).

In addition to its constitutive expression by monocytes/macrophages, and granulocytes, approximately 50% of benign $CD4^-CD8^+$ T cells express p150,95 following *in vitro* activation (1191). Similarly, p150,95 expression is upregulated on B cells after activation with phorbol esters (1183). p150,95 expression also has been observed on variable proportions of epithelioid histiocytes (1161), NK cells (1019,1170,1171,1187,1188), interdigitating dendritic cells (1161), and Kupffer cells (1161). CD11c is not expressed by follicular dendritic cells, cutaneous Langerhans cells, or endothelial cells (1161).

CD11c (p150,95) is expressed in virtually all patients with hairy cell leukemia (555,1192), as well as the variant form of hairy cell leukemia (1193) (see Chapter 41). Initially it was believed that p150,95 was not expressed by any other NHLs or lymphoid leukemias (555) and hence was a highly specific immunodiagnostic marker for hairy cell leukemia (555,1192). We now know that p150,95 also is expressed by occasional chronic lymphoid leukemias that exhibit features intermediate between CLL and hairy cell leukemia (1194) and are reported as a distinct disease category (1195), as well as on CLL cells following stimulation with phorbol

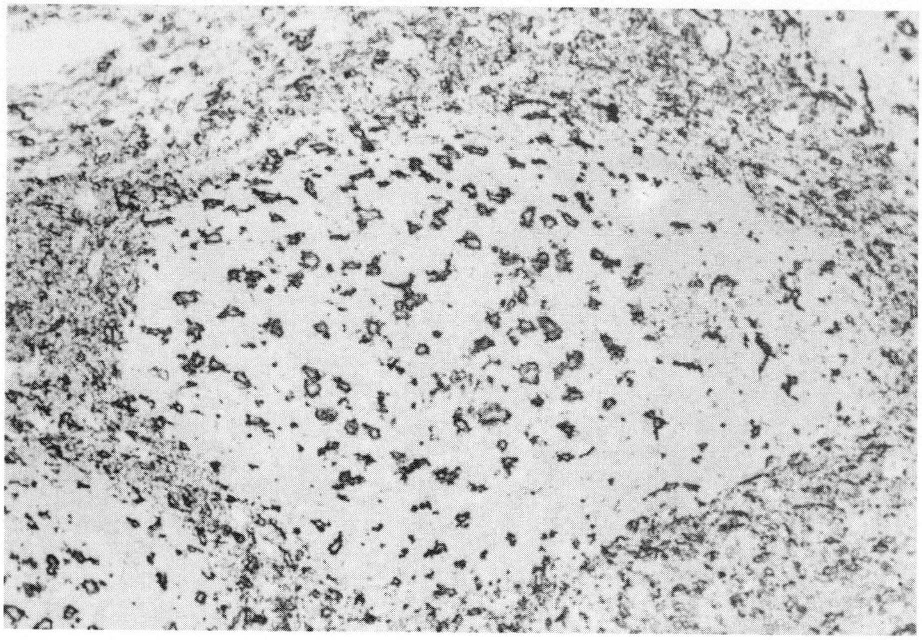

FIG. 3.42. Frozen tissue section of tonsil immunostained for CD11c with monoclonal antibody LeuM5. CD11c is expressed in high density by germinal center tingible body macrophages and also by macrophages within the interfollicular tissue (immunoperoxidase stain, original magnification: 100× magnification).

ester (1196). CD11c also is expressed in almost 50% of patients with splenic lymphoma with villous lymphocytes (1197), as well as a high proportion of patients with marginal zone B-cell lymhomas (see Chapters 23 and 33). In addition, it appears that the majority of CD4$^-$CD8$^+$ postthymic T-cell neoplasms, including the NK-like T-cell lymphomas described by Macon and colleagues (1073); occasional CD4$^+$CD8$^-$ postthymic T-cell neoplasms (1191,1198); and some NHLs of uncertain lineage express p150,95 (1199). CD11c is not expressed, however, by precursor B- and T-cell lymphoblastic lymphomas/leukemias. CD11c also is expressed by about 30% of AMLs overall (730). This includes virtually no FAB M6 (erythroblastic), M7 (megakaryoblastic), or M3 AMLs; 30% of FAB M0 and M1 AMLs; 50% of FAB M2 AMLs; and 60% or more of FAB M4 and M5 (monocytic) AMLs (730,964,1200), a distribution similar to that of CD11b (730,1200). The majority of cells in chronic myelogenous leukemia also expresses CD11c. CD11c is expressed variably among neoplasms of histiocytic derivation (see Chapter 51). CD11c remains a useful immunodiagnostic marker for hairy cell leukemia and hairy cell leukemia variant, but its utility extends to other disease categories as well, in which it is used in conjunction with other judiciously selected immunodiagnostic reagents.

CD13

The CD13 molecule originally was recognized using MAb MY7 (112) and established as a cluster at the first workshop (15). Many other anti-CD13 MAbs, including MCS-2 (1201) and LeuM7, have been described (95,1202,1203). CD13 subsequently was discovered to be identical to aminopeptidase N (APN) (1204), a prominent membrane-bound zinc-binding metalloprotease on the brush border of the small intestine and renal proximal tubules (1204,1205). APN plays a role in the metabolism of biologically active peptides by various cell populations, including granulocytes, macrophages, small intestinal and renal tubular epithelium, and the synaptic membranes of cells from the central nervous system (379).

The gene encoding CD13 has been mapped to 15q25-26, which coincides with the region assigned to the *FES* protooncogene, another gene specifically expressed by myeloid cells (1206). The CD13 cell surface molecule is a 150-kd type II integral membrane protein comprised of 967 amino acids and having 11 potential sites for asparagine-linked oligosaccharide addition (1204,1205). It is composed of a large extracellular carboxyl-terminal domain, a short intracellular amino-terminal segment, and a hydrophobic signal sequence that is retained and functions as the transmembrane domain (1204,1205). The extracellular domain includes a polypeptide consensus sequence that is essential for zinc coordination and the catalytic activity of metalloproteases (1207,1208). At least three different subpopulations of CD13-APN molecules possessing glycosylation differences have been described (1209,1210). These variations in O-linked glycosylation produce epitopes that account for the different binding patterns of different anti-CD13 MAbs. An intracellular 130-kd precursor CD13 molecule, differing from the mature 150-kd molecule only in the composition of its carbohydrate chains, also exists (1211).

Aminopeptidase N catalyzes the removal of single amino acids from the amino-terminal end of small peptides and probably plays a role in their final digestion (1212). For example, CD13-APN participates in trimming peptides bound to MHC class II molecules (1213). CD13-APN on the surface of neutrophils, in cooperation with the coexpressed enzyme CD10–neutral endopeptidase, participates in the cleavage and inactivation of the chemotactic peptide f-Met-Leu-Phe (1214,1215). CD13-APN on the surface of monocytes cleaves and inactivates the biologically active peptide tuftsin (1216,1217). In the intestine, CD13-APN probably plays a role in the final stages of digestion of small peptides (1212). CD13-APN also has been shown to function as a receptor for coronaviruses (1218), RNA viruses that are responsible for about 20% of common upper respiratory tract infections.

Within the hematopoietic system, CD13 is expressed by about 40% of GM-CFUs, and by all cells of these lineages as they mature (1219). CD13 is expressed by the majority of peripheral blood granulocytes, 25% of monocytes, and 6% of normal bone marrow cells (112), including all stages of myeloid differentiation from the myeloblast through the granulocyte (1219). CD13 is not expressed by erythroid precursors (E-CFUs, E-BFUs) or by mature erythrocytes (112,1219). CD13 similarly is not expressed by progenitor, mature, or activated B and T cells (112,1219). The lineage-restricted pattern of CD13 expression within the hematopoietic system suggests that this molecule may play an important physiologic role in myeloid differentiation (1203).

Among hematopoietic malignancies, CD13 is a pan-myeloid marker. CD13 is expressed by approximately 65% to 95% of pediatric and adult FAB M0 through M6 AMLs, and a smaller proportion of FAB M7 AMLs (about 90% of AMLs overall), depending on the anti-CD13 MAb employed (112,232,343,417,420,462,730,916,1166,1168, 1220–1222). CD13 often is expressed by immature (FAB M0 and M1) AMLs lacking CD33 expression or cytochemical evidence of myeloid differentiation (232,233,1222). The detection of CD13 by immunocytochemistry is more sensitive than by flow cytometry, because CD13 is expressed initially in the cytoplasm (1220). CD13 also is expressed by about 90% of patients with chronic myelogenous leukemia, CML-MBC (112,232,1168,1220), and acute myelofibrosis (235). CD13 generally is expressed by 80% or more of the blasts present within an individual AML (1168), except in patients with FAB M6 AML, in whom CD13 expression is more variable (1221). In contrast, CD13 is not usually expressed in patients with CML-LBC (112,232,1168). CD13 is expressed by about 10% of precursor B-cell lymphoblastic lymphomas/leukemias (232,343,1168,1223) and rare precursor T-cell lymphoblastic lymphomas/leukemias (426,525,1168). Nevertheless, if used in conjunction with other MAb reagents and cytochemistry, anti-CD13 MAbs are very useful in identifying acute leukemias belonging to all categories of AML and distinguising them from acute lymphoblastic leukemia (ALL). In addition, mature B- and T-cell lymphomas and leukemias are uniformly CD13$^-$ (232,1168). CD13 expression by leukemic blasts has been correlated with lower complete remission and survival rates among patients who have AML (1224,1225) and a worse prognosis among adults who have ALL (1168,1223). Other investigators have failed to confirm these findings (420,426).

Outside of the hematopoietic system, CD13 is expressed by renal proximal tubular and intestinal brush border epithelium, bone marrow stromal cells, epithelial cells lining the bile duct canaliculi, fibroblasts, osteoclasts, endothelial cells, and the perineurium of peripheral nerve trunks (95,1226,1227). Among nonhematopoietic malignancies, CD13 expression has been identified in renal cell, hepatocellular, and cholangiocarcinoma cell lines (1228,1229) and in a variety of benign and malignant mesenchymal tumors (1226).

CD14

The CD14 cluster was established at the second workshop (111). The CD14 molecule is a 53- to 55-kd glycoprotein recognized by MAbs MY4 (112), Mo2 (110) and LeuM3 (1230), among many others (95,1231–1233). These MAbs appear to detect four or more epitopes of the CD14 molecule (1234,1235). CD14 is composed of 365 amino acids and is anchored to the cell membrane by glycosyl phosphatidylinositol (1236,1237); it belongs to the family of glycosyl phosphatidylinositol (PI)–linked proteins (1238). CD14 is expressed strongly on the surface of monocytes and macrophages and weakly on the surface of neutrophils (110,112,1239,1240). The monocytes from patients with paroxysmal nocturnal hemaglobulinuria, a hereditary disorder characterized by the absence of PI-linked proteins (1241), lack CD14 (1236,1237). In addition, soluble forms of CD14 that lack the glycosyl phosphatidylinositol anchor are detectable in the serum and also in the urine of nephrotic patients (1236,1239,1241,1242). Soluble CD14 is generated by two distinct mechanisms that result in molecules of different molecular weight. A 48-kd soluble form of CD14 is shed from the cell surface as a result of proteolytic cleavage (1236,1243–1245). A second soluble form of CD14 of higher molecular weight is released from cells prior to the addition of the glycosyl phosphatidylinositol anchor (1246,1247).

The gene encoding CD14 maps to 5q23-31, a region known to contain a cluster of genes encoding several growth factors and growth factor receptors such as GM-CSF, platelet-derived growth factor, and IL-3 (1248). The CD14 gene is included in the "critical region" that frequently is deleted in certain myeloid leukemias (1249). The inference is that CD14 also may represent some form of myeloid growth factor or receptor and play a role in leukemiagenesis.

The membrane form of CD14 serves as a high-affinity cell surface receptor for lipopolysaccharide complexes and for serum lipopolysaccharide-binding protein (1250,1251). In this CD14-dependent pathway of lipopolysaccharide-induced activation, monocytes/macrophages and neutrophils release cytokines such as TNF-α in response to very low concentrations of lipopolysaccharide (1245,1251). This activation pathway appears to be a major pathway mediating the initial events occurring in gram-negative endotoxin shock (1252). In addition, soluble CD14 functions as a ligand for lipopolysaccharide and is required for the LPS-induced activation of cells lacking mCD14, such as endothelial cells (1253,1254). If endothelial cells are activated with lipopolysaccharide-CD14, they release cytokines such as IL-6 and IL-8 and upregulate the expression of adhesion molecules ICAM-1 and VCAM-1 (1253,1254). Functional characterization of the CD14 molecule *in vitro* suggests the existence of at least two functional epitopes of CD14, distinct from the lipopolysaccharide binding site, that may be tissue-specific (1235,1255).

CD14 is expressed in high density by more than 90% of peripheral blood monocytes (110,112,1230,1256), by 5% to 10% of normal bone marrow cells (primarily monocytes) (112), and by virtually all tissue phagocytic macrophages in all anatomic sites (1230,1256) and is expressed weakly by about 30% of granulocytes (1230). CD14 is absent from GM-CFUs; it appears at the promonocyte stage of maturation (112). CD14 is not expressed by immature, mature resting, or activated T cells, erythrocytes, or platelets (112,1230). Initially, CD14 was believed to be absent from B cells as well (112,1230). CD14 is detectable, however, in very low density on a variable proportion (donor-related) of peripheral blood B cells (1257) and on lymphoid tissue mantle zone B cells (1258) by MAb MY4, but not by MAb LeuM3 (1257,1258).

CD14 is expressed by approximately 15% to 20% of pediatric and adult AMLs overall, rendering this antigen considerably less useful than CD13 and CD33 to confirm a morphologic diagnosis of AML (343,420,916). Anti-CD14 MAbs are useful in subclassifying AMLs, because of their preferential immunoreactivity with those AMLs exhibiting monocytic differentiation; CD14 is expressed by approximately 50% to 90% of FAB M4 and M5 (monocytic) AMLs (112,233,343,730,1166,1168). In contrast, CD14 is not usually expressed by FAB M0 AMLs (1222), is expressed only weakly in some FAB M6 AMLs (1221), and is expressed by only about 25% or less of FAB M1, M2 and M3 AMLs (112,233,343,730,1166,1168). In addition, CD14 is expressed only occasionally in paients with CML-MBC (236) and acute myelofibrosis (235). The apparent variable expression of CD14 within each FAB category appears to be dependent on the MAb reagent utilized (233,964,1166,1168) and reflects the epitotic heterogeneity of CD14 (1234,1235). CD14 antigen expression may have prognostic value. The expression of CD14 by malignant myeloblasts (as detected by MAb MY4) has been associated with an increased incidence of extramedullary and central nervous system involvement (1224) and a lower complete remission rate in AML (420,1224). CD14 is expressed only rarely by precursor B-cell lymphoblastic lymphoma/leukemia (525).

CD14 is also detectable in approximately 90% of B-cell chronic lymphocytic leukemias (1257,1259) and 80% of follicular and 40% of diffuse B-cell NHLs with MAb MY4, but not with MAbs LeuM3 or Mo2 (1258). Anti-CD14 MAb MY4 is also immunoreactive with rare T-cell NHLs (1258). This is further evidence that MAbs MY4 and LeuM3 detect distinct CD14 epitopes. The immunoreactivity of MAb MY4 and other antimyeloid cell MAbs with B-cell chronic lymphocytic leukemias has been shown to be highly associated with their ability to produce IL-1 (1259).

CD33

Monoclonal antibodies MY9 (232), L4F3, and LiB2 (1260) were characterized at the second workshop (111) and clustered as CD33 at the third workshop (95). Additional MAbs have been added to the CD33 cluster since then (1261–1263). These anti-CD33 MAbs appear to recognize identical or spatially related epitopes (1264). CD33 is a member of the immunoglobulin gene superfamily, which is expressed exclusively by cells of the myeloid lineage (1263). CD33 shares homology with myelin-associated glycoprotein, CD22, and sialoadhesin and also has functional characteristics of the sialoadhesin family, which are sialic acid–dependent cytoadhesion molecules (1263). The precise biologic role for the CD33 molecule is unknown.

The gene encoding CD33 has been localized to 19q13.1-13.3 (1265). CD33 is a 67-kd glycoprotein composed of 364 amino acids (1265). It is comprised of a signal peptide (amino acid residues 1–17), an extracellular domain of 241 amino acid residues that includes an IgV domain (residues 18–121) and an IgC2 type domain (residues 156–219), a transmembrane spanning domain (residues 260–282), and a cytoplasmic tail (residues 283–364). There are five consensus sites for the addition of asparagine-linked oligosaccharide chains (1266).

CD33 is expressed by committed hematopoietic progenitors, including multipotent stem cells (GEMM-CFU), early erythroid progenitors (E-BFU), all bone marrow and peripheral blood granulocyte and macrophage progenitors (GM-CFUs), and mast cells (232,1260,1264,1267,1268). In contrast, the earliest hematopoietic stem cells capable of self-renewal that lack evidence of differentiation along a specific hematopoietic lineage lack CD33 (1269). CD33 also is expressed by approximately 30% of all normal bone marrow cells, including myeloblasts, promyelocytes, and myelocytes, and by all peripheral blood monocytes and tissue macrophages (232,1264). CD33 antigen density decreases from the myeloblast to the myelocyte stage and is absent or only minimally expressed by terminally differentiated granulocytes (232,1260,1267). The lack of reactivity of anti-CD33 MAbs with granulocytes and mature bone marrow myeloid cells distinguishes them from all other antimyeloid cell MAbs (232). CD33 is expressed throughout monocyte differentiation (232). CD33 is not expressed by granulocytes, erythrocytes, platelets, thymocytes, or immature, resting mature, or activated B and T cells (232,1260,1264,1267). CD33 is not expressed on nonhematopoietic cells (1270,1271). It has been suggested that CD33 is the only truly myeloid lineage–restricted antigen (232,1261,1265), because the majority of the other published antimyeloid cell MAbs react with nonmyeloid cells including activated lymphocytes (232,1265). CD33 is, however, variably expressed by epidermal Langerhans cells (1272), although these cells express other myeloid- and monocyte-associated antigens and even may be derived from GM-CFUs (1273).

In the case of hematopoietic malignancies, CD33, like CD13, is a panmyeloid antigen. CD33 is expressed by approximately 65% to nearly 100% of pediatric and adult FAB M0 through M7 AMLs (about 90% of AMLs overall) (232,343,417,462,730,916,1166–1168,1221,1222). CD33 may be expressed by immature (FAB M0 and M1) AMLs lacking CD13 or cytochemical evidence of myeloid differentiation (232,233). CD33 also is expressed in more than 90% of patients with CML-MBC (232,1167) and acute myelofibrosis (235). In general, CD33 is expressed by all of the cells in an individual blast cell population (1168), except in patients with FAB M6 AML, in whom it often is expressed by a variable proportion of the blasts (1221). CD33 also is expressed in TdT$^+$ AMLs (1167), in about 10% of precursor B-cell lymphoblastic lymphomas/leukemias (343,1223), and in rare precursor T-cell lymphoblastic lymphomas/leukemias (343,426,525). If employed in conjunction with other immunophenotypic markers, however, anti-CD33 MAbs are very useful in identifying acute leukemias belonging to all categories of AML and distinguishing them from ALL. Also, mature B- and T-cell lymphomas and leukemias are consistently CD33$^-$ (232). Anti-CD33 MAbs have been employed therapeutically as well. They have been used to purge residual leukemic myeloblasts prior to autologous bone marrow transplantation for patients with AML in remission (1274,1275). They also have been coupled to iodine-131 in immunotherapeutic trials (1276).

CD68

Six MAbs, Ki-M6, Ki-M7, Y1-82A, EBM-11, Y2-131, and KP1 (1277–1281) were assigned to the CD68 cluster at the fourth workshop (1282); MAb PG-M1 (1283) was added to the CD68 cluster at the fifth workshop (1284). These antibodies bind to lentil lectin–Sepharose and precipitate identical 110-kd antigens (1285). Although all these MAbs apparently recognize the same molecular weight antigen, inhibition studies indicate that they detect distinct epitopes (1282,1285,1286). All anti-CD68 MAbs display immunoreactivity in frozen tissue sections, and several of them display variable immunoreactivity in formalin-, Bouin's solution–, or B5-fixed tissues following proteolytic digestion (1287). MAbs KP1 and PG-M1 recognize formalin-resistant CD68 epitopes most easily and most consistently and this immune reactivity is enhanced after proteolysis (1287). Consequently, MAbs KP1 and PG-M1 are the most commonly employed anti-CD68 antibodies in diagnostic pathology (1287).

CD68 is a heavily glycosylated lysosomal transmembrane protein that belongs to a family of lysosomal glycoprotein–plasma membrane shuttling proteins that play a role in endocytosis or lysosomal trafficking (1288). cDNA clones have been identified for the 110-kd molecule and also for a smaller 70-kd molecule. The longer clone encodes a 351–amino acid peptide and the shorter clone encodes a 295–amino acid peptide. The difference represents an internal deletion that probably represents an artifact of the cloning process (1285). Multiple isoforms of the CD68 molecule probably do not exist (1285). Human CD68 exhibits a strong similarity with murine macrosialin (1289). The chromosomal location of the gene encoding CD68 remains unknown.

The 110-kd CD68 antigen is expressed primarily intracellularly, principally within the acidic granules of monocytes and macrophages, and also is found extracellularly in human serum (1282,1285,1286,1290). Immunoelectronmicroscopic studies have localized CD68 to the outer membranes of lysosomes and phagosomes of macrophages and a subset of the primary granules of neutrophils (1277,1278,1291). Some anti-CD68 MAbs, however, exhibit some immune reactivity with the interior of lysosomes and phagosomes (1277,1278). CD68 also can be detected in small amounts on the surface membranes of some normal human cells, including monocytes, macrophages, neutrophils, basophils, and NK cells (1280–1282,1290). The function of CD68 is unknown. The experimental evidence suggests that CD68 plays a role in the generation of oxygen radicals during the respiratory burst in phagocytosing cells (1287).

In contrast with the relatively uniform immunoreactivity of MAbs belonging to many leukocyte antigen clusters, anti-CD68 MAbs exhibit variable immunoreactivity with the same cell populations (1287), presumably because they detect distinct epitopes (1282,1283,1285,1286). All anti-CD68 MAbs react strongly with peripheral blood monocytes but show variable immune reactivity with other cells (1287). For example, MAb KP1 also reacts with neutrophils, basophils, and large lymphocytes and represents the least specific anti-CD68 MAb for evaluating cells in the peripheral blood (1290). In contrast, MAb PG-M1 appears to be completely specific for monocytes; it does not react with other peripheral blood cells (1283). The large lymphocytes that react with some anti-CD68 antibodies appear to represent LGLs, because these cells possess granules that contain serine esterases (1287). Also, MAb KP1 reacts, but MAb PG-M1 does not, with myeloid precursors in the bone marrow (1281,1283). All anti-CD68 MAbs react with a subset of megakaryocytes, but none react with erythroid precursors (692,1279,1280,1281,1283,1292).

Although the proportion of CD68 immunoreactive tissue macrophages seen varies slightly according to the antibody employed, all anti-CD68 MAbs react with all tissue macrophages in all anatomic sites. This includes tingible body

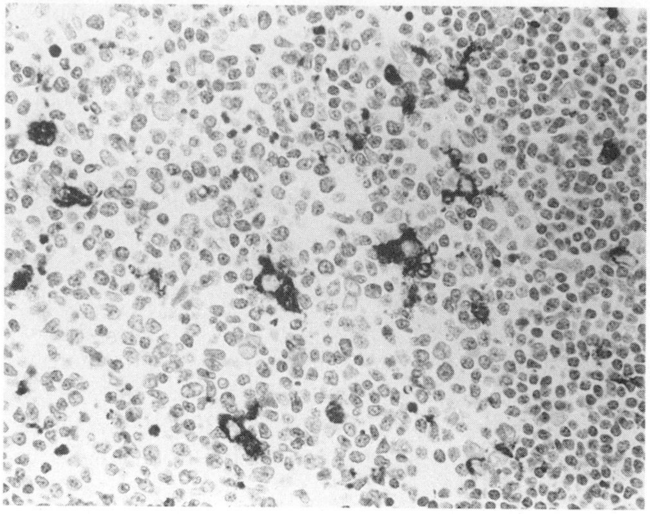

FIG. 3.43. Formalin-fixed, paraffin-embedded tissue section of a benign lymph node immunostained with monoclonal anti-CD68 antibody PGM1. The tingible body macrophages present within the germinal center strongly express CD68; the follicular dendritic cell, B-cell, T-cell, and other cell populations lack CD68 (immunoperoxidase stain, original magnification: 400× magnification).

macrophages, sinus histiocytes, and interfollicular macrophages in lymph nodes, tonsil, and spleen; macrophages in the red pulp of the spleen, the skin, gastrointestinal tract, thymus, and lung; and Kupffer cells (692,1277–1281,1283, 1290,1292–1295) (Fig. 3.43). Anti-CD68 MAbs are also immunoreactive with the epithelioid histiocytes and multinucleated giant cells in granulomas, plasmacytoid monocytes, the foamy histiocytes of Gaucher's disease, sea-blue histiocytes, pseudo-Gaucher cells, the benign multinucleated giant cells in giant cell tumor of bone, resting microglia, mast cells, and osteoclasts (1277,1279–1281,1283,1292-1294, 1296–1298). These antibodies are not generally immunoreactive with cutaneous Langerhans cells, follicular dendritic cells, interdigitating dendritic cells, indeterminate dendritic cells, or B and T cells (692,1277,1278,1281–1283,1292, 1299). An exception is occasional interdigitating dendritic cells in dermatopathic lymphadenitis, which may display dot-like reactivity with MAb KP1 in paraffin tissue sections (692,1279,1281). Some granulocytes display faint immunoreactivity with MAb KP1 (1281). Recently it also has been shown that CD68 is expressed by some peripheral blood B cells (1300).

Among normal nonhematopoietic tissues, MAb PG-M1 appears to be the most specific, and MAb KP1 the least specific, anti-CD68 antibody for detecting monocytes and macrophages (1287). All anti-CD68 MAbs, with the exception of PG-M1, react with hepatocytes and renal tubules (1290). Also in contrast with MAb PG-M1, MAb KP1 variably reacts with renal glomeruli, pancreatic acini and islets, epidermis, sweat glands, and endothelial cells (1290). MAb PG-M1 has been reported to react with synovial cells (1283).

Because anti-CD68 MAbs detect distinct epitopes, it is not surprising that they display a variable distribution of immune reactivity with malignant cell populations. MAb KP1 reacts with nearly all AMLs and with most granulocytic sarcomas, the neoplastic cells displaying bright granular cytoplasmic positivity (340,344,1301), suggesting that CD68 is a useful immunodiagnostic marker for AML. In contrast, MAb PG-M1 is strongly immunoreactive with FAB M4 and M5 AML but is unreactive with FAB M1, M2, or M3 AML (1283), suggesting that MAb PG-M1 is specific for those types of AML exhibiting monocytic differentiation. Both KP1 and PG-M1 are immunoreactive with the proliferating mast cells in patients with of mast cell disease (1279,1296,1301), with true histiocytic lymphoma (1302–1304), and with variable proportions of the proliferating Langerhans cells in Langerhans cell histiocytosis (527,1279,1305).

Most anti-CD68 MAbs, including PG-M1, show no evidence of immunoreactivity with B- or T-cell NHLs or Hodgkin's disease (1280,1283,1293,1294). A notable exception is MAb KP1, which reacts with the majority of hairy cell leukemias (1281,1301) and approximately 20% of B-cell NHLs of diverse histopathologic subtypes, most commonly small lymphocytic lymphoma/chronic lymphocytic leukemia and mantle cell lymphoma (1301,1306). In these patients, the immunoreactive pattern usually consists of localized, cytoplasmic dot-like or finely granular positivity (1287), patterns distinctly different from that observed in myeloid and histiocytic malignancies (1287). CD68 is weakly expressed by about 50% of precursor B-cell acute lymphoblastic leukemias (1300). MAb KP1 is unreactive with T-cell NHLs or Hodgkin's disease (330,1301,1306).

Monoclonal anti-CD68 antibodies also exhibit immune reactivity with a variety of nonhematopoietic tumors, consistent with their lysosomal content (1287). MAb KP1 reacts strongly with virtually all granular cell tumors (1283,1307), with the Schwann cells of benign neural tumors (1294,1308), and with a variable proportion of atypical fibroxanthomas (1309), malignant fibrous histiocytomas (1294,1310,1311), renal cell adenocarcinomas, malignant melanomas, meningiomas, and glioblastomas, among a few others (1283, 1294,1312,1313). Caution should be exercised in interpreting the immunoreactivity of anti-CD68 MAbs (1287). Because these antibodies are organelle- rather than cell lineage–specific, their immune reactivity with a given neoplasm does not necessarily imply a histiocytic derivation (1308).

Progenitor Cell–Associated Antigens

CD34

The CD34 antigen originally was defined by MAb My10 (1314) and BI-3C5 (1315), which were clustered as CD34 at the third workshop (95). Many additional anti-CD34 MAbs have been characterized since then; a minimum of 16 different MAbs were shown to belong to the CD34 cluster at the fifth workshop (1316). Anti-CD34 MAbs define an antigen that is expressed selectively on hematopoietic progenitor cells (1314,1315), vascular endothelium, and some tissue fibroblasts (1317,1318). Anti-CD34 MAbs are divisible into three groups according to the susceptibility of their epitopes to enzymatic cleavage with neuraminadase, glycoprotease, and chymopapain (1319). Anti-CD34 MAbs are applicable in cytofluorometric analysis and in frozen tissue section immunohistochemistry (1320). In addition, some of them, including My10 and QBEND10, are immunoreactive with CD34 in routinely prepared, formalin-fixed, paraffin-embedded tissue sections (1320). The complex pattern of reactivity of anti-CD34 Mabs is dependent on the variation of glycosylated epitopes (1319). The expression of the glycosylation-dependent epitopes is regulated by the glycosyltransferase activity of the cell, which may change during maturation of the progenitor cells.

The gene for CD34 is located on 1q32, a region that contains genes encoding several adhesion matrix, hematopoietic signaling, and regulatory molecules (1321). The human CD34 molecule is a heavily glycosylated type I transmembrane cell surface glycoprotein of approximately 110 kd (1322). The protein backbone of the CD34 molecule is estimated at 40 kd (1323). There are two forms of the CD34 molecule, which are generated by alternative splicing (1324,1325). A large part of the molecular weight of CD34 consists of extracellular sugar groups that are attached covalently to the protein core. The glycosylation of this core appears to be determined by the protein sequence (1320). The extracellular portion of CD34 contains high percentages of serine and threonine residues, which serve as anchorage sites for the numerous O-linked sugars present on this molecule. Also, nine potential sites for N-linked glycosylation are present on the extracellular part of CD34. Both CD34 forms contain complete and identical extracellular and transmembrane domains. The full-length form of CD34 has an intracellular domain that contains several consensus sites for protein kinase C phosphorylation as well as phosphorylation by other kinases. The truncated form of CD34 lacks most of the intracellular domain, including many of the potential phosphorylation sites (1322,1323).

The function of the CD34 molecule is unknown. It may play a role in cell adhesion (1322). The highly glycosylated nature of CD34 could allow it to serve as a ligand for lectins (1320); the mouse homologue of human CD34 has been shown to be a ligand for L-selectin (1326). $CD34^+$ hematopoietic precursor cells might bind to lectin-expressing stromal cells in the bone marrow in this manner (1320). The finding that CD34 expression is inversely correlated with the expression of cell surface molecules ELAM-1 and ICAM-1 suggests a modulatory role in cell adhesion for CD34 as well (1327). The presence of several phosphorylation sites on the cytoplasmic portion of CD34 suggests still another function for this molecule (1327). CD34 can be phosphorylated in response to protein kinase C activators (1328,1329), suggesting a role for CD34 in signal transduction (1320).

Anti-CD34 MAbs label hematopoietic progenitor cells more specifically than any other MAbs currently available. CD34 is expressed by approximately 1 to 2% of normal bone marrow mononuclear cells (1314,1330,1331). This percentage is similar whether detected by cytofluorometric analysis or immunohistochemistry (1331). The percentage does not appear to increase in hyperplastic or regenerating bone marrow (1331,1332). The cells are larger than lymphocytes, are granular, and resemble blasts morphologically. They include lymphoblasts, myeloblasts, monoblasts, erythroblasts, and megakaryoblasts. These $CD34^+$ cells uniformly express HLA-DR but lack antigens associated with mature B cells, T cells, NK cells, monocytes, and granulocytes (1330). CD34 is expressed by all assayed unipotent and multipotent progenitor cells, including C-CFU, E-BFU, E-CFUs, GM-CFU, GEMM-CFU, BFU-MK, and MK-CFU (1314,1333–1337). $CD34^+$ bone marrow cells account for more than 90% of all immature hematopoietic cells detected by *in vitro* colony forming assays (1314). Purified $CD34^+$ bone marrow cells have been shown to reconstitute hematopoiesis in lethally irradiated baboons (1338,1339) and in patients with solid tumors following marrow ablative therapy (1340). CD34 is lost progressively from hematopoietic progenitor cells in parallel with advancing maturational stage (1335). CD34 also is expressed by all TdT^+ bone marrow cells and thus encompasses the entire TdT^+ HLA-$DR^+CD19^+CD10^+$ precursor B-cell population in pediatric and adult bone marrow (570,1314,1341). Precursors of stromal cells capable of creating a microenvironment supportive of hematopoiesis also are included in the $CD34^+$ bone marrow population (1342,1343).

CD34 is not expressed by normal peripheral blood B or T cells, monocytes, granulocytes, erythrocytes, or platelets or by *in vitro* activated peripheral blood mononuclear cells (1314,1315). $CD34^+$ cells generally are undetectable in peripheral blood samples of normal individuals by flow cytometry (1344). $CD34^+$ cells can be detected in the peripheral blood after chemotherapy or treatment with cytokines (1344–1346).

Within postfetal lymphoid tissues, CD34 antigen–positive hematopoietic progenitor cells can be identified in greatest numbers in the spleen, where they reside at the interface of mature T cells in the marginal zone and mature B cells in the mantle zone. They also can be identified in small groups in the hepatic portal triads and rarely in Peyer's patches (1347). $CD34^+$ cells are not identifiable in lymph node, kidney, or skin (1347). A subset of immature thymocytes that express CD34 has been identified by cytofluorometric analysis (1348).

The specificity of CD34 expression for the early stages of normal hematopoiesis is reflected in its expression by leukemic cells. CD34 is expressed by the malignant blasts in approximately 40% of pediatric and adult AMLs overall, including TdT^+ AML (1167,1314,1315,1349). Although CD34 is expressed by nearly all FAB M0 and M1 AMLs (730,1222) and the majority of M6 (erythroblastic) (1221) and M7 (megakaryoblastic) AMLs (235,1167,1350), it is expressed variably by decreasing proportions of more mature categories of AML, usually being absent from FAB M5 AML (462,730). CD34 also is expressed by patients with CML-MBC (1315) and by approximately one third of those with granulocytic sarcomas (344). The expression of CD34 in myelodysplastic syndromes appears to be predictive of transformation and poor survival (1351). CD34 also is expressed by about 75% of precursor B-cell acute lymphoblastic leukemias, including CML-LBC (1167,1315,1352–1354), and less than 5% of precursor T-cell acute lymphoblastic leukemia (1354).

$CD34^+$ AMLs tend to be morphologically and immunophenotypically less mature than $CD34^-$ ones. Among AMLs, those expressing CD34 are significantly more likely to exhibit FAB M1 or M2 or even unclassifiable morphology and to lack CD15 or CD33. $CD34^+$ AMLs are more likely to arise following chemotherapy and often exhibit loss or partial deletion of chromosome 7 (1349), a karyotypic feature frequently associated with therapy-induced or secondary leukemias (1355,1356). The presenting clinical characteristics of patients with $CD34^+$ or $CD34^-$ precursor B-cell acute lymphoblastic leukemia are similar, except that $CD34^+$ patients are more likely to have white blood cell counts less than 50×10^9 and $CD34^-$ patients exhibit an increased incidence of central nervous system involvement at diagnosis (1352). The leukemic blasts from patients with $CD34^+$ precursor B-cell acute lymphoblastic leukemia are significantly more likely to coexpress CD9, CD13, and CD22, to lack cytoplasmic μ and CD20, and to be hyperdiploid (1352). Some of these immunologic and genetic markers are known to confer a good prognosis. Nonetheless, CD34 expression appears to be an independent favorable prognostic factor for early event-free survival in precursor B-cell acute lymphoblastic leukemia (1352). CD34 expression is associated with a poor prognosis in AML (1357–1359) and a favorable prognosis in acute lymphoblastic leukemia. CD34 is not expressed by postthymic (TdT^-) T-cell neoplasms, nonlymphoblastic B-cell NHLs, B-cell lymphoid leukemias, chronic myelogenous leukemia, or the Reed-Sternberg cells of Hodgkin's disease (1167,1314,1315,1320, 1332).

CD34 also is expressed variably by normal vascular endothelium (1317,1360) but apparently not by normal lymphatic endothelium (1317,1361,1362). It is not surprising that CD34 is expressed by a wide spectrum of benign and malignant vascular neoplasms, including hemangiomas, Kaposi's sarcoma, and angiosarcomas, among others (1360–1365). For reasons that are unclear, CD34 also is expressed by a diverse group of additional neoplasms, including for example hemangiopericytomas, nerve sheath tumors, epithelioid sarcomas, smooth muscle tumors and gastrointestinal stromal tumors (1320). CD34 is not expressed generally by carcinomas, malignant melanomas, or most sarcomas (1320). Anti-CD34 MAbs often are very helpful in the differential diagnosis of numerous neoplasms encountered in routine surgical pathology (1320).

Nonlineage Antigens

CD15

The numerous MAbs that belong to this cluster include MMA (LeuM1) (1366), My1 (1367), IG10 (1368), and VIM-D5 (1369), among many others (1370). These antibodies were generated by immunization and screening with a variety of human and mouse hematopoietic and carcinoma cell lines (1366–1369,1371). It gradually became recognized that this heterogeneous collection of MAbs possess similar patterns of immune reactivity, and they were clustered as CD15 at the second workshop (111).

These antibodies recognize a specific sugar sequence occurring in the glycolipid lacto-N-fucopentaose III ceramide, in several higher glycolipids and in glycoproteins (1372):

$$\begin{array}{l} \text{Gal } \beta1\rightarrow4\text{G1}_c\text{NA}_c\ \beta1\rightarrow3\text{Gal } \beta1\rightarrow\text{R} \\ \qquad\quad 3 \\ \qquad\quad \uparrow \\ \qquad\ \text{Fuc}_{\alpha}1 \end{array}$$

This sugar sequence, which also is referred to as *X hapten* (1373) *Le*^{x} (1374,1375), or *stage-specific embryonic antigen* (1371), is highly immunogenic in mice (1372), which accounts for the large number of MAbs in this cluster. Immunoprecipitation studies using various anti-CD15 antibodies have demonstrated five distinct bands with molecular weights between 105 and 200 kd (1376). The vast majority of anti-CD15 Mabs belong to the IgM isotype (1370) and do not react with the sialylated form of CD15, which now is designated *CD15s* (1377). The fact that these MAbs are applicable in routinely prepared, formalin-fixed, paraffin-embedded tissue sections has resulted in their widespread use in diagnostic surgical pathology.

Because CD15 is a carbohydrate antigen, it is not a direct gene product. Instead it represents a common haptenic determinant present on different molecular species in a single cell and is a result of specific modifications of previously existing antigens (1260). The antigens detected by anti-CD15 MAbs show great similarity to blood group antigens (1370). The glycolipid lacto-N-fucopentaose III, which has the sugar sequence detected by anti-CD15 MAbs, possesses a structure similar to the Lewis a blood group antigens (1378). The glycolipid lacto-N-fucopentaose III is not present in human myeloid cells or in all CD15-expressing leukemic cell lines (1372). Also, it is absent or present in only small amounts in benign, human epithelium (1374,1378). Lacto-N-fucopentaose III is present in many benign human epithelial cells (1374), and a substance containing the recognized sugar sequence (X hapten) is present on granulocytes and some AML cells (1372,1373). The function of CD15 has been studied extensively but has not been delineated.

Immunofluorescent and cytofluorometric analyses have

demonstrated that CD15 is expressed by the majority of day 7 bone marrow GM-CFUs and myeloblasts, 90% or more of myeloid cells past the myeloblast stage, and virtually all peripheral blood granulocytes, including eosinophils and basophils (1260,1366,1367), with antigenic expression increasing with myeloid maturation (1367,1379). CD15 is expressed in variable density by more than 90% of peripheral blood monocytes (1366) but is expressed by only small numbers of tissue macrophages (1380) and is absent from dendritic cells (1256). CD15 is not expressed by erythroid progenitors (E-BFU, E-CFU) (1260), mature erythrocytes (1260,1366,1367), or platelets (1366,1367). CD15 is similarly absent from immature and mature, resting peripheral blood and lymphoid tissue B and T cells (1260,1366,1367, 1379) and NK cells (1366).

Immunohistochemical staining with LeuM1 and the other major anti-CD15 MAbs results in nearly identical patterns of immune reactivity in frozen and paraffin tissue sections (1380,1381). CD15$^+$ cells may exhibit cytoplasmic or membrane staining, which can be intensified by neuraminidase treatment in some instances (333,336,1380,1382). Myeloid cells show intense cCD15 positivity that often overshadows membrane positivity in tissue sections (1383).

Only rare mononuclear cells in tonsil and lymph node tissue sections express CD15, the majority of which appear to be histiocytes exhibiting faint juxtanuclear or Golgi region positivity (333,336,1366,1380,1384,1385). Small lymphocytes in the interfollicular areas as well as tingible body macrophages, follicular dendritic cells, interdigitating dendritic cells, sinus histiocytes, and epithelioid histiocytes, however, have been reported occasionally to express CD15 (334,336,1385,1386). In some patients, it is necessary to pretreat paraffin tissue sections with neuraminidase in order to detect CD15 expression by any cells other than granulocytes, however (336,1380). In the thymus, only the epithelial cells of Hassall's corpuscles express CD15 (1383,1385). In the spleen, only granulocytes and rare scattered mononuclear cells within the red pulp express CD15 (1380,1385). In the bone marrow, granulocytes at all stages of maturation exhibit both cytoplasmic and membranous CD15 positivity, with the more mature cells exhibiting the strongest positivity (1383,1385). Erythroid precursors, megakaryocytes, lymphocytes, and plasma cells lack CD15 (1380,1383). CD15 is expressed by a wide range of epithelial cells, including those of the gastrointestinal tract, liver, pancreas, kidney, bladder, breast, and salivary glands (1376,1380,1383,1384, 1387–1390).

The demonstration of CD15 expression by normal human cells does differ slightly with different anti-CD15 MAbs (1370). For example, although all of the antibodies react with mature granulocytes (1366–1369,1372) their reactivity with less mature granulocytes varies (1370). They exhibit the greatest variability in reactivity with normal peripheral blood monocytes, however (1370). MAb LeuM1 exhibits strong immune reactivity (1366); MAbs My1, VIM-D5, and IG10 exhibit weak or no immune reactivity (1367–1389), with normal peripheral blood monocytes.

If investigated by cytofluorometric analysis, approximately 50% to 70% of FAB M1, M2, and M3 and 75% to 90% of FAB M4 and M5 AMLs are found to express CD15, depending on the MAb reagent employed (730,1166,1168, 1225,1368,1391,1392). CD15 also is expressed in virtually all patients with chronic myelogenous leukemia (1366–1368,1383) and in approximately one third of those with chronic myelogenous leukemia in myeloid blast crisis (237). CD15 usually is expressed by 80% or more of the leukemic blasts in a given AML (1168). A much higher percentage of AMLs are found to be CD15$^+$ by cytofluorometric analysis than by paraffin tissue section immunohistochemistry (1370), although 50% or more of granulocytic sarcomas are found to be CD15$^+$ in paraffin tissue sections (339,1393). Neuraminidase pretreatment increases the immunoreactivity of anti-CD15 antibodies with AMLs in paraffin tissue sections (1394,1395). The prognostic significance, if any, of CD15 expression by AMLs has been controversial and remains unclear (1370).

In contrast, CD15 is expressed by less than 5% of patients with precursor B- or T-cell lymphoblastic lymphoma/leukemia (237,414,1367,1396–1398) and rarely or not at all in those with chronic myelogenous leukemia in lymphoid blast crisis (237). At least some of these cases may represent examples of acute mixed lineage leukemia (237). The prognostic significance of CD15 expression among these patients remains unclear (1370), although CD15 expression occurs most commonly in CD10$^-$ precursor B-cell acute lymphoblastic leukemias, which generally have a poor prognosis (1398).

Monoclonal anti-CD15 antibodies are employed most commonly in the immunodiagnosis of Hodgkin's disease in paraffin tissue sections (1370). Essentially all anti-CD15 MAbs are immunoreactive with the Reed-Sternberg cells and variants of Hodgkin's disease under these conditions (1370). CD15$^+$ Reed-Sternberg cells and variants may exhibit membranous, diffuse cytoplasmic, granular cytoplasmic, blush-like paranuclear or bright globular juxtanuclear cytoplasmic staining (332–335,507,1380,1385, 1399). The most frequent staining pattern is juxtanuclear (Golgi region) positivity, with or without membrane positivity (332,335,1380,1399) (Fig. 3.44). The diffuse cytoplasmic positivity observed in patients with lymphocyte predominance Hodgkin's disease (334,1400) has been interpreted as false positivity by some investigators (1401). Immunoultrastructural studies have shown that anti-CD15 MAbs react with the plasma membranes, rough endoplasmic reticulum, and lysosomal granules of Reed-Sternberg cells, the latter appearing to be continuous with the perinuclear membrane vesicles and possibly the Golgi apparatus, thereby accounting for the juxtanuclear staining (1402).

A review of the early literature by Hall and D'Ardenne (1403) revealed that about 80% of 571 cases of Hodgkin's disease examined for CD15 expression contained CD15$^+$

A 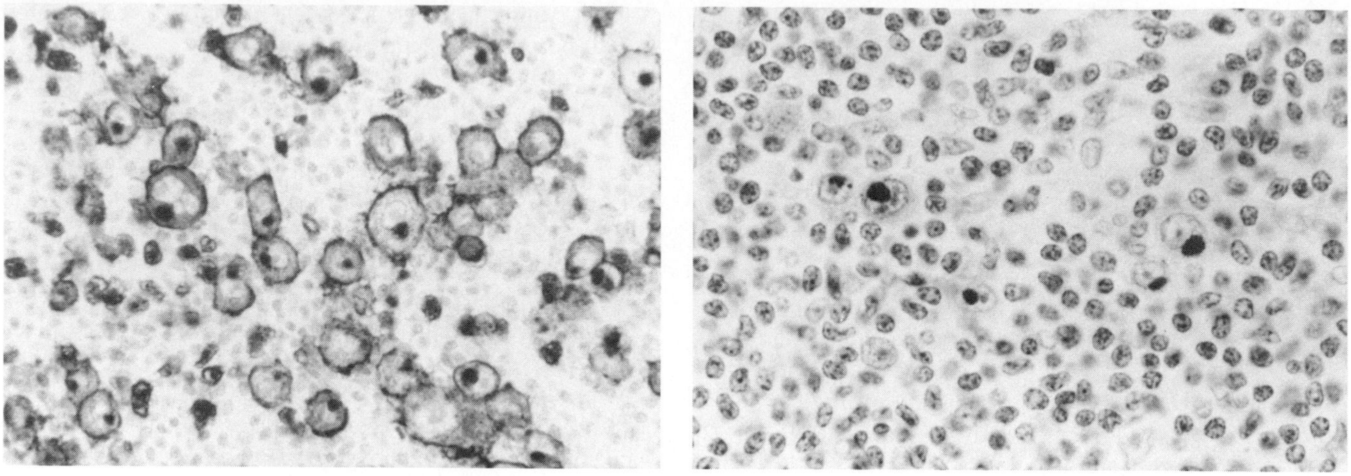 B

FIG. 3.44. Formalin-fixed (**A**) and B5-fixed (**B**) paraffin-embedded tissue sections of Hodgkin's disease immunostained for CD15 with MAb LeuM1 (immunoperoxidase stain). **A:** The numerous Reed-Sternberg cells and Reed-Sternberg cell variants exhibit membranous, cytoplasmic, or bright globular juxtanuclear staining (original magnification: 630× magnification). **B:** The Reed-Sternberg cells and Reed-Sternberg cell variants exhibit prominent globular juxtanuclear cytoplasmic staining without membranous or diffuse cytoplasmic staining original magnification: 400× magnification).

Reed-Sternberg cells and variants. More recent studies have found similar results (314,334,335,337,509,516,518, 1404–1407). CD15 expression in Hodgkin's disease varies, however, according to the histopathologic category. The Reed-Sternberg cells and variants in almost 90% of patients with nodular sclerosis, mixed cellularity and lymphocyte depletion Hodgkin's disease express CD15. In contrast, the Reed-Sternberg cells and variants in only about one third of patients with lymphocyte predominance Hodgkin's disease express CD15 (314,315,319,332–337,507,509,516,518, 1380,1381,1385,1386,1389,1399,1401,1403–1411). The nodular L&H subtype of lymphocyte predominance Hodgkin's disease is least likely to contain CD15$^+$ cells (315,1385,1401,1409,1411). It has been suggested that the sialylated form of CD15 is present in the L&H cells of lymphocyte predominance Hodgkin's disease, limiting its detection (1382). Enzymatic treatment, especially with neuraminidase, increases the number of L&H cells detectable in the latter cases (315,336,1382). The use of such enzymatic treatments may account for the larger number of CD15$^+$ cases of lymphocyte predominance Hodgkin's disease reported in some series (338,1399,1400,1410).

CD15 expression in Hodgkin's disease also varies among separate lesions occurring in an individual patient and among Reed-Sternberg cells and variants within an individual lesion. Chu and colleagues reported marked variability of CD15 expression in Hodgkin's disease lesions in simultaneous and consecutive lymph node biopsy specimens obtained from the same patient (513). Also, a variable proportion (a few, some, many, or all) of the Reed-Sternberg cells and variants in an individual Hodgkin's disease lesion express CD15 (1370). Immunohistochemical staining for CD15 often identifies more malignant Hodgkin's cells than are evident from the examination of routine histologic sections (333) (Fig. 3.45).

The incidence of CD15 expression among NHLs varies considerably among reports in the literature (1370). It appears that CD15 is expressed by approximately 20% of T-cell and about 5% of B-cell NHLs (313,314,319,320,333, 334,338,339,1380,1381,1384,1385,1389,1396,1407,1412–1416), the majority of which display large cell, primarily immunoblastic, morphology or have undergone morphologic transformation from a low-grade to a high-grade neoplasm, for example advanced (tumor) stage mycosis fungoides (319,320,334,338,1386,1389,1412,1414,1415,1417). Very few or no patients with small lymphocytic lymphoma or chronic lymphocytic leukemia, other low-grade B-cell NHLs, hairy cell leukemia, or T-cell chronic lymphocytic leukemia express CD15 (320,338,1201,1380,1384,1385, 1416). The incidence of CD15 expression in anaplastic large cell lymphoma has ranged from 0 to 20% in various series (315,327,329,330,333,1418,1419). In some of these cases, however, CD15 positivity occurs only as small granules within the cytoplasm (327) of only a small proportion of the malignant cells (330,333). Conceivably, also, some of these cases may represent Hodgkin's disease rather than anaplastic large cell lymphoma; it is sometimes difficult to distinguish between these entities (1370).

Among the malignant cells making up T-cell NHLs, it is those with the morphologic features of Reed-Sternberg cells that most commonly express CD15 (320,334,1389,1396, 1412). Neoplastic mononuclear cells without Reed-Sternberg–like features also may be CD15$^+$, however (1385,1396,1412,1414,1415). The pattern of CD15 expres-

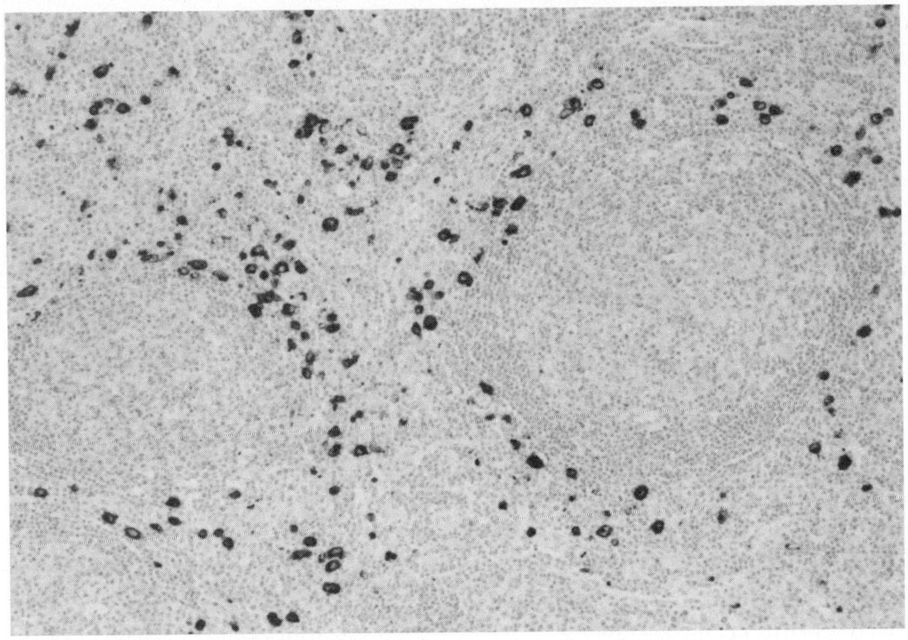

FIG. 3.45. Formalin-fixed, paraffin-embedded tissue section of interfollicular Hodgkin's disease immunostained for CD15 with monoclonal antibody LeuM1. The numerous Reed-Sternberg cells and Reed-Sternberg cell variants present in the interfollicular areas and surrounding two residual benign germinal centers are identified readily and highlighted by immunostaining. More of these calls are identified by immunostaining than are readily apparent from examining routine histologic sections (immunoperoxidase stain, original magnification: 100× magnification).

sion cannot be used to reliably distinguish between NHL and Hodgkin's disease, because the lymphoma cells may exhibit membranous and perinuclear (Golgi) staining, similar to that seen in the Reed-Sternberg cells of Hodgkin's disease (334,1389,1396,1410,1412). In some patients they show only weak membranous, focal punctate, or weak diffuse cytoplasmic positivity (313,327,1396,1412,1414, 1417). In some patients with mycosis fungoides, the small neoplastic cerebriform cells exhibit focal punctate cCD15 positivity (1381,1412). Occasional patients with anaplastic multiple myeloma express CD15 (1389); those with true histiocytic lymphoma uncommonly express CD15 (338,339,1385,1399).

Because a wide spectrum of benign epithelial cells express CD15, it should not be surprising that a wide array of carcinomas express CD15 (1370). Sheibani and coworkers (1389) reported that 56% of all carcinomas studied, including adenocarcinomas, squamous cell carcinomas, and small and large cell undifferentiated carcinomas of diverse origin, expressed CD15. These tumors usually display focal areas of diffuse, strong cytoplasmic positivity (1370,1389). These findings have been confirmed and expanded by many other investigators (1383,1390,1416,1420,1421). They must be kept in mind to avoid misinterpreting a focus of metastatic carcinoma in a lymph node as Hodgkin's disease (1370). In addition, CD15 is expressed by thymomas, carcinoid tumors, and a minority of sarcomas and meningiomas, but not by malignant melanomas or germ cell tumors (1389).

CD30

The CD30 molecule initially was recognized on the Reed-Sternberg cells of Hodgkin's disease by MAb Ki-1 (1409), which was prepared by immunizing with the alleged Hodgkin's disease cell line L428 (1422). The immunoreactivity of MAb Ki-1 is generally weak, however, and is restricted to the cell membrane in frozen tissue sections; this antibody is not immunoreactive in paraffin tissue sections because its epitope is denatured by fixation (1423). Several additional MAbs, including Ber-H2 (1423), were included in the CD30 cluster in the fourth workshop (1424). MAb Ber-H2 recognizes a fixation-resistant CD30 epitope and exhibits stronger and broader immunoreactivity than does MAb Ki-1 (1423). Consequently, Ber-H2 has become the anti-CD30 MAb of choice in diagnostic pathology to demonstrate CD30 expression.

Monoclonal antibody Ber-H2 is immunoreactive in tissues processed in a variety of fixatives, including formalin, Bouin's solution, and B5, although some observers have suggested that Ber-H2 immunoreactivity is diminished in B5-fixed tissues (320,334,353,357,1423,1425). Immunohistochemical staining with MAb Ber-H2 usually results in circumferential membranous and paranuclear (Golgi region) dot-like positivity (327,331,334,1423,1426). Weak, diffuse cytoplasmic Ber-H2 immunoreactivity is considered irrelevant diagnostically (1423).

The human gene for CD30 has been localized to 1p36

(1427). Deletions, translocations, inversions and duplications affecting this band have been reported frequently in Hodgkin's disease (1428) and in some NHLs as well (1429). Band 1p36 also is the location of the *TNF2* gene (1430). In addition, this is a preferential site for viral integration; *EBV1* is located on 1p35 (1431).

The cDNAs that code for the precursor CD30 apoprotein have been cloned (1432). The cDNA sequence reveals a type I transmembrane protein with a 595–amino acid open reading frame with a molecular mass of 64 kd (1432). Structural analysis of the polypeptide predicts an 18-residue leader peptide, an extracellular domain of 365 residues, a single transmembrane domain of 24 residues, and a cytoplasmic domain of 188 residues. The extracellular domain can be divided into six internal cysteine-rich motifs of about 40 amino acids each (1432). This domain bears significant homology with that of members of the TNF receptor–nerve growth factor receptor superfamily, establishing CD30 as a member of this family (1432). Other members of this family include low-affinity nerve growth factor receptor, TNF receptors 1 and 2, CD27, CD40, and Fas-APO-1 antigen, among others (1433).

The anti-CD30 MAb Ki-1 recognizes two independently synthesized molecules, a membrane-associated glycoprotein and an intracellular protein (1434). Investigators regard the membrane-associated glycoprotein as the true CD30 antigen (1424,1434,1435). The intracellular molecule is a 57-kd protein kinase (1436) that is phosphorylated at serine residues but is not glycosylated (1434). The membrane-associated molecule has a molecular mass of 105 to 120 kd and also is phophorylated at serine residues. It contains a glycosidically O- and N-bound carbohydrate portion, which includes about 15 kd of sialic acid in the terminal positions (1423,1434,1437). The 105- to 120-kd membrane-bound glycoprotein is produced by glycosylation of an 84 kd nonphosphorylated precursor during its passage through the Golgi complex (1434,1437).

The 105- to 120-kd membrane bound molecule is catabolized to a membrane-associated intermediate form that is further processed to an 85- to 90-kd soluble molecule (1424). Soluble CD30 is detectable in CD30 cell line supernatants, in the serum of patients with CD30$^+$ malignancies or infectious mononucleosis (1438–1440), and in patients who have hepatitis B infection (1441), but not in the sera of healthy normal blood donors. The mechanism of soluble CD30 secretion and its function are unknown. CD30 shedding occurs as an active process of viable CD30$^+$ cells and does not represent merely release from dead and dying cells (1442). In patients who have CD30$^+$ malignancies, there is a correlation between the tumor cell mass and the serum level of soluble CD30. The level of soluble CD30 drops immediately after initiation of therapy, and disease relapse often is accompanied by an increasing serum level of soluble CD30 (1442).

The human CD30 ligand (CD30L) has been identified and its gene cloned and localized to 9q33 (1443). CD30L was clustered as CD153 at the sixth workshop (1444). Significant homology exists between the extracellular domain of CD30L (CD153) and a family of cytokines having homology with TNF, including TNF-α, TNF-β, CD27L, and CD40L (1443). Recombinant CD30L exhibits pleiotropic cytokine activities (1443). These include inducing proliferation of activated T cells in the presence of an anti-CD3 costimulus and enhancing proliferation of the alleged Hodgkin's disease cell line HDLM-2 (1443). CD30L mRNA expression is inducible on T cells and macrophages, and it has been suggested that autocrine and paracrine mechanisms may be operational (1443). These findings further establish CD30 as a cytokine receptor belonging to the TNF receptor–nerve growth factor receptor superfamily.

The precise physiologic role of CD30 and the nature of its interaction with CD30L are unclear. However, CD30 signaling appears to involve binding of TNF receptor–associated factors to the cytoplasmic domain (1445). Signaling through CD30 may induce activation or apoptosis (1446,1447). CD30-CD30L interactions are believed to be involved with negative selection of both $\alpha\beta$ and $\gamma\delta$ T cells in the thymus (1447).

CD30 expression is associated with activation; CD30 is not expressed by resting peripheral blood B or T cells or monocytes (1423). The expression of CD30 is induced on B cells following stimulation with *Staphylococcus aureus* Cowan-1 and on T cells following stimulation with phytohemagglutinin or with autologous and allogeneic stimulator cells (1423,1424,1448). CD30 also is expressed on EBV-transformed B cells and human T-cell lymphotropic virus type 1 transfected T-cell lines (1423,1449). CD30 expression by activated T cells is preceded by the expression of CD38, CD71, CD25, epithelial membrane antigen, HLA-DR, and CD15 and followed by expression of CD11c (1450). Monocytes stimulated with interferon-γ or lipopolysaccharide remain CD30$^-$ (1423).

Occasional large CD30$^+$ B and T cells are scattered around lymphoid follicles, and some large CD30$^+$ B cells are present at the margin of germinal centers in normal and reactive lymph nodes and tonsils and in extranodal lymphoid tissue (334,1409,1422,1423,1449). Most of these CD30$^+$ lymphoid cells appear to be proliferating, because they also express Ki-67 (1451). The number of CD30$^+$ lymphoid cells may increase significantly in some reactive conditions, such as in infectious mononucleosis and toxoplasmic lymphadenitis (1449,1452). Tissue macrophages generally lack CD30, but they may express CD30 in granulomatous lesions and in certain other disorders (1453,1454). The activated tissue macrophages encountered in virus-associated hemophagocytic syndrome and hemophagocytic lymphohistiocytosis are CD30$^-$, however (1455). Occasional medullary thymocytes may express CD30 (1423,1424). Rare CD30$^+$ large cells may be observed in the white pulp of fetal spleen (1444). Germinal center T cells, mantle zone B cells, cortical thymocytes, thymic epithelium, cutaneous Langerhans cells, interdigitating dendritic cells, and developing hematolymphoid cells in fetal liver and bone marrow do not express

CD30 (1409,1422–1424,1449,1456). The diffuse cCD30 immunoreactivity observed in plasma cells (1423) is believed to represent an artifact (1426). MAb Ber-H2 is essentially unreactive with normal nonhematopoietic tissues except for pancreatic acini, cerebral cortical neurons, and cerebellar Purkinje cells (1423,1424).

Variable proportions of Reed-Sternberg cells and variants present in about 90% of patients with nodular sclerosis, mixed cellularity, and lymphocyte depletion Hodgkin's disease are found to express CD30 if MAb Ber-H2 is used in paraffin tissue sections (Fig. 3.46). The proportion of $CD30^+$ patients is comparable among these different categories. The $CD30^+$ Hodgkin's cells are readily identifiable in about 90% of patients and infrequent and difficult to find in the remaining 10% of cases (315,330,334,518,1406,1423, 1457,1458). These $CD30^+$ Hodgkin's cells usually display strong membrane, bright globular or dot-like paranuclear (Golgi region), and weak cytoplasmic immunoreactivity (334,1423) (Fig. 3.46). In contrast, the Hodgkin's cells present in less than 25% of patients with lymphocyte predominance Hodgkin's disease are found to express CD30 if MAb Ber-H2 is employed in paraffin tissue sections (315,330,334, 518,1406,1423,1457,1458). Moreover, these $CD30^+$ Hodgkin's cells generally display weak immunoreactivity that is limited to the cell membrane (334).

In 1985, the examination of large panels of diverse hematologic neoplasms for their immunoreactivity with anti-CD30 Mabs led to the identification of a distinct clinicopathologic entity designated *anaplastic large cell lymphoma* (1449). Previously, this entity had been classified variously as malignant histiocytosis, anaplastic carcinoma, amelanotic melanoma, and so forth.

CD30 is expressed characteristically by all the neoplastic cells making up most anaplastic large cell lymphomas (315,327,329,330,362,510,1419,1449,1459). In nearly all instances, the $CD30^+$ neoplastic cells display strong membrane and bright globular paranuclear positivity, similar to that observed in the Reed-Sternberg cells of non–lymphocyte predominance Hodgkin's disease (327,329,331,1419) (Fig. 3.47). This has led to the widespread use of the terms *Ki-1* and *CD30* lymphoma as synonomous with anaplastic large cell lymphoma (329,330,510,1419,1449,1459). Occasional cases of $CD30^-$ anaplastic large cell lymphoma have been reported, however (327), and among NHLs, CD30 expression is not limited to anaplastic large cell lymphoma. Approximately 15% to 20% of B-cell and 30% of T-cell NHLs other than anaplastic large cell lymphoma are immunoreactive with anti-CD30 MAb Ber-H2 in paraffin tissue sections (320,323,518,1423,1449,1458). Among B-cell NHLs, CD30 is expressed most frequently by immunoblastic lymphomas, but all major categories, with the exception of precursor lymphoblastic lymphoma/leukemia, may express CD30 (320,323,518,1423,1449,1458). CD30 frequently is expressed by the Kaposi's sarcoma–associated herpesvirus containing primary effusion lymphomas, which display morphologic features bridging immunoblastic and anaplastic large cell lymphoma (1460) (see Chapter 28). In many of these patients, the malignant cells display only focal paranuclear dot-like or weak diffuse cytoplasmic positivity, but they may display the same immunoreactive staining

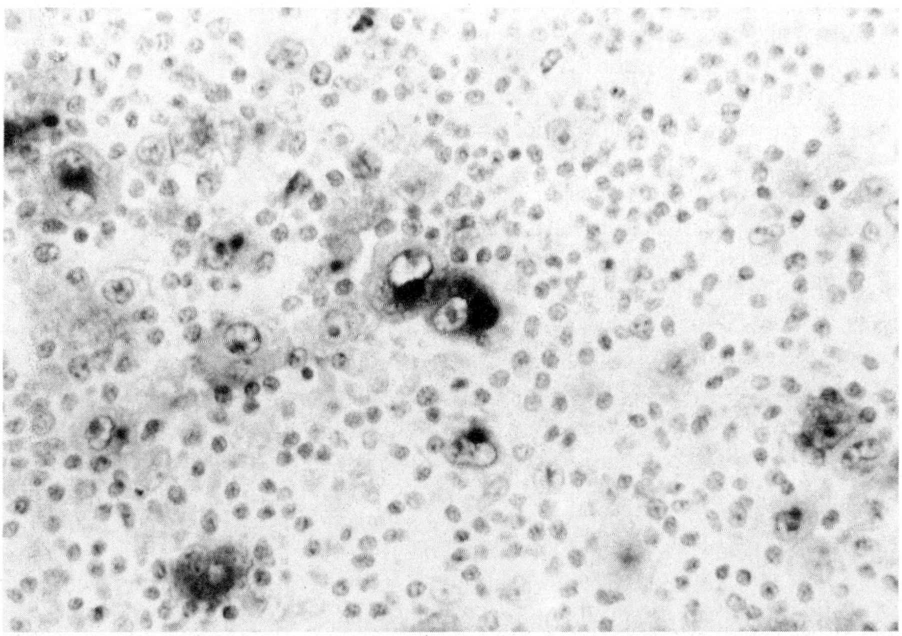

FIG. 3.46. Formalin-fixed, paraffin-embedded tissue section of Hodgkin's disease immunostained for CD30 using monoclonal antibody BerH2 by alkaline phosphatase–anti-alkaline phosphatase (original magnification: 400× magnification). The Reed-Sternberg cells and Reed-Sternberg cell variants show prominent juxtanuclear Golgi region and diffuse cytoplasmic staining with monoclonal antibody BerH2.

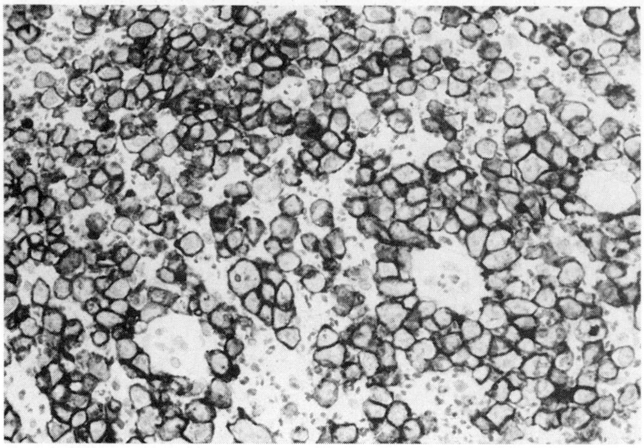

FIG. 3.47. Formalin-fixed, paraffin-embedded tissue section of an anaplastic large cell lymphoma immunostained with monoclonal anti-CD30 antibody BerH2. Virtually all of the tumor cells express CD30 (immunoperoxidase stain, original magnification: 200× magnification).

pattern as that seen in Hodgkin's disease and anaplastic large cell lymphoma (323,1423,1458–1462). With the exception of precursor lymphoblastic lymphoma/leukemia, CD30 similarly is expressed by all major categories of T-cell NHL, including cutaneous T-cell lymphoma, peripheral T-cell lymphoma, and adult T-cell lymphoma/leukemia (320,357,518,1423,1458). In these cases, however, CD30 expression usually is limited to a subset of the malignant cells. Also, a variable proportion of the large, atypical Reed-Sternberg–like cells of lymphomatoid papulosis express CD30 (357,1449,1463). Occasional multiple myelomas or plasmacytomas express CD30 (323,1423,1464). CD30 is not expressed in hairy cell leukemia (320,323,1423) or Langerhans cell histiocytosis (527,1423). Whether CD30 is expressed in histiocytic and dendritic cell neoplasms is not entirely clear, because of the difficulties encountered in defining these neoplasms as well as their rarity (1426).

Nonhematolymphoid neoplasms generally do not express CD30 (1426). The most notable exception is embryonal carcinoma and the embryonal elements in mixed germ cell tumors, which are consistently immunoreactive with MAb Ber-H2 in paraffin tissue sections (1465). Occasional pancreatic, salivary gland, and other carcinomas and malignant melanomas express weak, diffuse cCD30 positivity (1423), but this probably represents nonspecific staining (1426).

CD43

Three MAbs, namely MT-1, Leu22 (L60), and DF-T1, found to be immunoreactive with T cells in formalin-fixed, paraffin-embedded tissue sections, were discovered to recognize the same molecular target, sialophorin (also known as *leukosialin, leukocyte sialoglycoprotein, large sialoglycoprotein,* and *gpL115*) (1466,1467). These antibodies were clustered as CD43 at the third workshop (245). Numerous additional MAbs have been included in the CD43 cluster since then (1468–1470). Paraffin-reactive MAbs MT-1, Leu 22 (L60) and DF-T1 remain the most commonly employed anti-CD43 antibodies in routine diagnostic pathology (1471). $CD43^+$ cells display strong, crisp membrane immune reactivity with these anti-CD43 MAbs in routinely prepared, formalin-fixed, paraffin-embedded tissue sections (304,319,323,358,1472).

The discovery that the CD43 molecule is deficient in amount on the T cells of patients who have the congenital T-cell immunodeficiency disorder Wiskott-Aldrich syndrome (1473) prompted extensive investigation of the CD43 molecule (1471). Also discovered was that a higher molecular weight isoform of CD43 is present on the T cells of a subgroup of these patients (1474). The human sialophorin gene has been localized to chromosome 16, excluding a CD43 defect as the primary genetic defect in the Wiskott-Aldrich syndrome, however (1475,1476). The CD43 defects on the T cells of patients with Wiskott-Aldrich syndrome have been interpreted variously as resulting from ineffective or pseudoactivation of their T cells or a defect in glycosylating enzymes (1474).

CD43 is an integral membrane mucin, that is, a heavily O-glycosylated and sialylated type I transmembrane glycoprotein (60% carbohydrate) (1475,1476). It has been described as the leukocyte equivalent of the O-glycosylated sialoglycoprotein glycophorin A, which is specific for the erythroid lineage (1477), and is similar to the glycoprotein Ib molecule on platelets (1473,1478). The mature polypeptide chain of CD43 consists of 381 amino acid residues. The extracellular domain of 239 residues carries one N-glycan chain and about 70 to 85 O-linked oligosaccharides (1475,1476). The highly conserved cytoplasmic domain is phosphorylated constitutively on serine residues, and the level of phosphorylation increases at cell activation (1479).

Two CD43 isoforms on white blood cells have been characterized: a 115-kd CD43 on resting T cells and monocytes in which the O-glycans are predominantly tetrasaccharides, and a 135-kd CD43 on neutrophils, platelets (low levels), and some activated T cells in which the O-glycans are predominantly branched hexasaccharides (1474,1480,1481). The reported molecular weight of the same isoform differs depending on the laboratory conditions (1469), but these isoforms possess the same number of sialylated O-linked carbohydrate units, the same number of N-linked units, and identical polypeptide cores (1481,1482). CD43 is lost rapidly from the lymphocyte and neutrophil surface by proteolytic shedding after activation with various stimuli (1483). A soluble form of CD43, called *galactoglycoprotein*, is present in plasma (1484).

CD43 appears to be involved in intercellular adhesion. It remains unclear, however, whether its role is primarily proadhesive and costimulatory (1485,1486) or antiadhesive, that is, serving as a "barrier molecule" mediating repulsion between leukocytes and other cells (1487–1489). CD43 is downregulated as part of diverse cell activation events

(1490), consistent with its hypothesized function as a barrier molecule. Cross-linking of CD43 by specific MAbs may induce activation in T cells (1485,1486,1491) or monocytes (1492) and induces apoptosis in hematopoietic progenitor cells (1479,1493).

Anti-CD43 MAbs exhibit slight variations in their immunoreactivity with benign and malignant hematolymphoid cells, apparently because of differential binding to different epitopes of the CD43 molecule (1471). A minimum of four distinct CD43 epitopes have been identified (1494). Most anti-CD43 MAbs react with carbohydrate-dependent epitopes, and the heterogeneity of immune reactivity also reflects the existence of CD43 glycosylation variants on different cell types. Some anti-CD43 MAbs detect carbohydrate-independent epitopes (1494), but despite the variability in their immune reactivity with various hematopoietic cell populations, all anti-CD43 MAbs react with the vast majority of thymocytes and mature T cells (1471).

CD43 often is thought of as a T-cell lineage–associated antigen. Anti-CD43 MAbs MT1 and Leu22 react with more than 95% of thymocytes and 95% and 85% of $CD3^+$ mature peripheral blood and tonsil T cells, respectively (CD43 being absent from a subset of tonsil $CD8^+$ T cells) (352,1467). CD43 is expressed, however, by essentially all white blood cells, except resting mature B cells. This includes activated B cells, plasma cells, NK cells, granulocytes, and monocytes/macrophages (1468,1495). Approximately 95% of $CD34^+$ cord blood cells, including partially committed myeloid, erythroid, and lymphoid progenitors, as well as stem cells, express CD43 (1469). Erythroblasts, megakaryocytes (1496), and bone marrow $CD34^+$ cells (1497) express CD43 as well. It even has been reported that about 5% to 8% of nonneoplastic, resting, mature peripheral B cells express CD43, as shown by cytofluorometric analysis (1498).

Most of our information concerning CD43 expression has come from immunohistochemical studies performed on routinely prepared, formalin-fixed, paraffin-embedded lymphoid tissue sections employing MAbs MT1, Leu22, and DF-T1 (1471). Using this approach it has been possible to study certain nonneoplastic cell populations with considerably more ease (1471). In these studies, anti-CD43 MAbs have been found to react with essentially all cortical thymocytes but with only approximately half of medullary thymocytes (304,358,1384,1467). They react with the vast majority of lymph node and tonsil paracortical and interfollicular lymphocytes and splenic periarteriolar lymphoid sheath lymphocytes, and with only occasional germinal center and mantle zone small lymphocytes, that is, the T cells. They are unreactive with the majority of germinal center and mantle zone lymphocytes, that is, the B cells, but are reactive with plasma cells and rare lymphoplasmacytoid cells (304,323,358,726, 1384,1467,1468,1472) (Figs. 3.48, 3.49). CD43 expression among monocytes/macrophages is variable. Germinal center tingible body macrophages occasionally express CD43, albeit weakly and sometimes cytoplasmic (1384). Interdigitating dendritic cells, epithelioid histiocytes, and multinucleated giant cells usually are $CD43^+$. Follicular dendritic cells

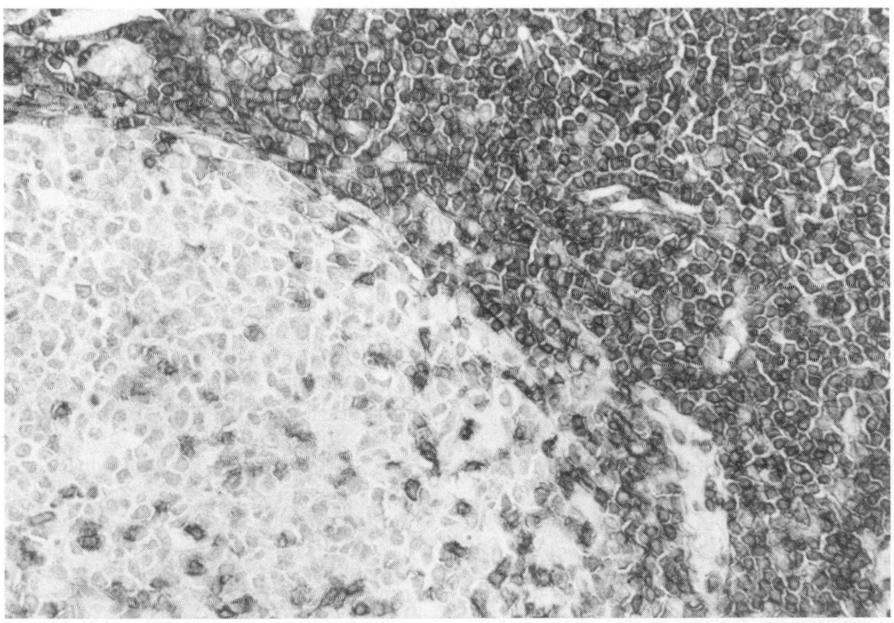

FIG. 3.48. Formalin-fixed, paraffin-embedded tissue section of lymph node stained for CD43 with monoclonal antibody Leu22. This antibody has a distribution of reactivity in routinely processed paraffin tissue sections comparable to that of anti-CD3 monoclonal antibodies in frozen tissue sections (immunoperoxidase stain, original magnification: 250× magnification). (From Wieczorek R, Buck D, Bindl J, et al. Monoclonal antibody Leu22 (L60) permits the demonstration of some neoplastic T cells in routinely fixed and paraffin-embedded tissue sections. *Hum Pathol* 1988;19:1434–1443, with permission.)

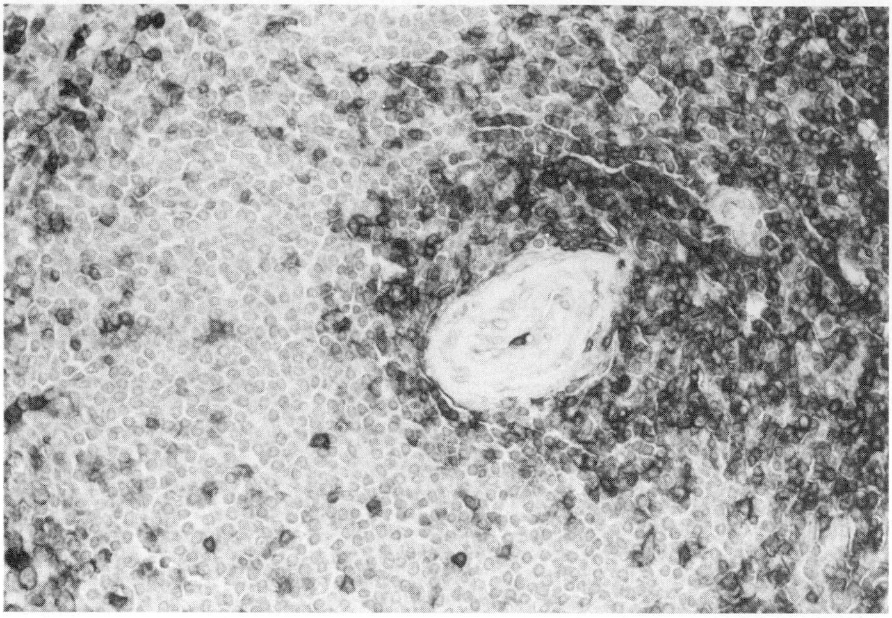

FIG. 3.49. Formalin-fixed, paraffin-embedded tissue section of spleen immunostained for CD43 with monoclonal antibody Leu22. This antibody reacts with the periarteriolar lymphoid sheath lymphocytes comparable to the reactivity of anti-CD3 monoclonal antibodies in frozen tissue sections of spleen (immunoperoxidase stain, original magnification: 250× magnification). (From Wieczorek R, Buck D, Bindl J, et al. Monoclonal antibody Leu22 (L60) permits the demonstration of some neoplastic T cells in routinely fixed and paraffin-embedded tissue sections. *Hum Pathol* 1988;19:1434–1443, with permission.)

consistently lack CD43, and sinusoidal histiocytes usually lack CD43 as well (726,1468,1472).

Comparable immunohistochemical studies of paraffin tissue sections of bone marrow demonstrate that myeloid cells at all stages of maturation, including granulocytes, as well as erythroid precursors and megakaryocytes express CD43; mature red blood cells lack CD43 (304,358,1384,1467). Other cells of the hematolymphoid system, including cutaneous Langerhans cells, Kupffer cells, and plasmacytoid T cells (thought to be of myeloid or monocytic derivation) also express CD43 (313,1499). CD43 is not expressed by normal epithelial cells, endothelial cells, fibroblasts, or muscle or nerve tissue (358,1384,1468).

Monoclonal anti-CD43 antibodies are employed infrequently in cytofluorometric analysis. The experience in the literature concerning CD43 expression in hematologic neoplasia is based largely on immunohistochemical studies performed in routinely prepared, formalin-fixed, paraffin-embedded tissue sections (1471). CD43 is expressed by most precursor T-cell, and approximately 75% of precursor B-cell, lymphoblastic lymphomas/leukemias (304,313,320, 328,340,354,358, 1384,1467). Hence, CD43 expression is not useful in the lineage assignment of malignant lymphoblasts. Furthermore, more than 95% of patients with FAB M1 through M5 AML and 90% or more of granulocytic sarcomas express CD43; FAB M6 (acute erythroblastic) leukemias lack CD43 (339–341,344,1393,1467,1472,1500). The determination of CD43 antigen expression is of limited usefulness in determining the lineage of an acute leukemia. Caution must be utilized in interpreting the "CD43-only" immunophenotype expressed by a suspected NHL, because this could represent a T-cell, B-cell, or myeloid neoplasm (1501).

Approximately 85% of patients with mycosis fungoides, nonepidermatropic cutaneous T-cell lymphoma, or peripheral T-cell lymphoma (307,313,315,317,319,320,352,354, 357,358,361,1384,1472), and 75% of those with anaplastic large cell lymphoma (315,329,330,518,522) express CD43 (Figs. 3.50–3.52). CD43 also is expressed, however, by almost 30% of all nonlymphoblastic B-cell NHLs. This includes about two thirds of patiens with small lymphocytic lymphoma/chronic lymphocytic leukemia and mantle cell lymphoma, most with Burkitt's lymphoma, 10% to 20% with large cell and immunoblastic lymphomas, and about 10% with follicle center cell lymphomas (304,317,319,320,323, 354,357,358,1467,1472,1502) (Fig. 3.53). Hairy cell leukemia does not express CD43 (323,1467,1468,1472). $CD43^+$ B cell NHLs usually express CD20 and other B-cell lineage–associated antigens (1471). Immunohistochemical detection of CD43 expression by nonneoplastic B cells is extremely uncommon (1471). Consequently, the immunohistochemical demonstration of CD20 and CD43 coexpression can be extremely useful in distinguishing a B-cell NHL from a nonneoplastic lymphoid proliferation (1502,1503).

Among other hematopoietic neoplasms, CD43 is ex-

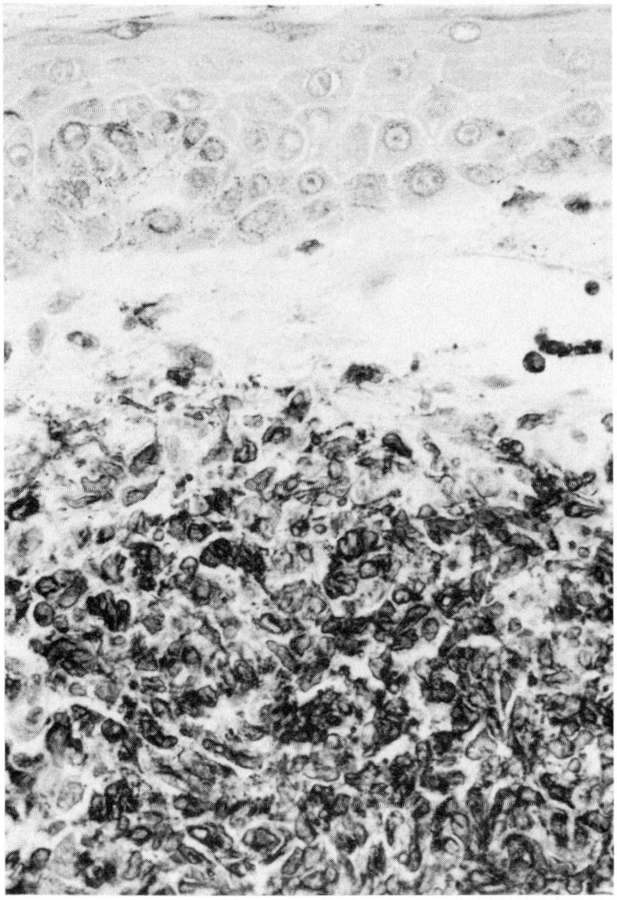

FIG. 3.50. Bouin's solution–fixed, paraffin-embedded tissue section of a $CD3^+CD4^+CD8^-$ cutaneous T-cell lymphoma originally processed in 1980 and subsequently immunostained by monclonal antibody Leu22 in 1988 by immunoperoxidase. Despite 8 years of storage of the tissue in paraffin, the section shows strong reactivity of Leu22 with essentially all of the cerebriform neoplastic T cells (immunoperoxidase stain, original magnification: 400× magnification). (From Wieczorek R, Buck D, Bindl J, et al. Monoclonal antibody Leu22 (L60) permits the demonstration of some neoplastic T cells in routinely fixed and paraffin-embedded tissue sections. *Hum Pathol* 1988;19:1434–1443, with permission.)

pressed by Reed-Sternberg cells and variants in a vanishingly small number of patients with nodular sclerosis, mixed cellularity, or lymphocyte depletion Hodgkin's disease. In patients with lymphocyte predominance Hodgkin's disease, these cells consistently lack CD43 (315,319,334,358,361, 1384,1472). CD43 also is expressed in about 50% of plasmacytomas and multiple myelomas (304,323,361,726,1468, 1472). Patients with Langerhans cell histiocytosis (304) and mast cell disease express CD43, as do some with true histiocytic lymphoma (320,358,1384,1467). Rare nonhematopoietic tumors, such as breast carcinoma and malignant melanoma, have been reported to be $CD43^+$ (1472). In these cases, however, the tumor cells display diffuse cytoplasmic positivity, in contrast with the surface membrane positivity observed in hematologic neoplasms (1472).

CD71

Monoclonal antibody OKT9 initially was believed to detect an immature thymocyte-associated antigen, because it was discovered to react with about 10% of thymocytes (137). Later it was found to react with large B-cell lymphomas exhibiting plasmacytoid differentiation (1504). Its specificity for immature T cells was questioned, and the notion that MAb OKT9 reactivity is related to cellular activation was advanced (1504). Goding and Burns (1505) and Sutherland and colleagues (1506) subsequently demonstrated that MAb OKT9 actually detects the transferrin receptor on actively proliferating (dividing) cells. The transferrin receptor binds transferrin and hence mediates iron uptake (1507). In addition to OKT9, other MAbs that detect the transferrin receptor were discovered, and these were clustered as CD71 at the fourth workshop (1508). Numerous MAbs have been added to the CD71 cluster since then (1509,1510).

The transferrin receptor (CD71) is a 95-kd type II membrane glycoprotein that occurs as a 190-kd disulfide-linked homodimer on the cell surface (671). CD71 consists of a short amino-terminal cytoplasmic domain of 61 amino acid residues that mediates internalization and recycling (1511), a transmembrane region of 28 amino acid residues, and a large intracellular domain of 671 residues that binds transferrin (1511). CD71 is encoded by a gene mapped to 3q26.2 (1510).

The molecular mechanism by which transferrin receptor expression is regulated by the level of available iron within the cell has been investigated extensively. These studies have led to the elucidation of a novel posttranscriptional process mediated by five "iron-regulatory elements" in the 3′ untranslated region of transferrin receptor mRNA (1512). CD71 is of interest from other perspectives as well. In particular, the transferrin receptor (CD71) is a member of the class of transport receptors that participate in receptor-mediated endocytosis (1511). Because transferrin receptors are endocytosed rapidly and expressed selectively on brain capillary endothelial cells but not in other capillary endothelial cells, anti-CD71 MAbs have been investigated as potential agents for transporting drugs or growth factors across the blood-brain barrier for therapeutic purposes (1513,1514). Anti-CD71 MAbs also have been used to inhibit proliferation and to target cytotoxic molecules to proliferating cells (1515). CD71 can be released into the circulation as a proteolytic fragment of the extracellular domain. Serum levels of soluble CD71 may be of diagnostic value in a variety of hematological diseases (1516,1517). CD71 is of more clinical and biologic interest than merely as a lymphocyte activation antigen (1509).

The transferrin receptor is essential for iron transport into proliferating cells (1507). Because growing cells require iron, receptors for the iron-binding protein transferrin always are expressed on proliferating cells (1507). CD71 antigen expression by both benign and malignant cells is associated strongly with proliferation, although this expression is not

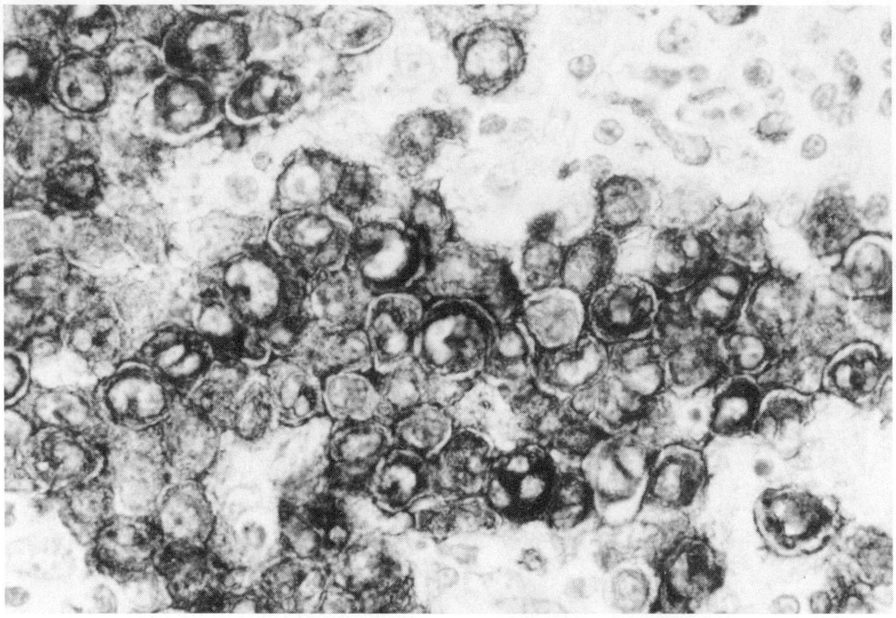

FIG. 3.51. Bouin's solution–fixed, paraffin-embedded tissue section of cutaneous T-cell lymphoma of non-mycosis fungoides type originally processed in 1978 and subsequently immunostained in 1988 with monoclonal antibody Leu22 by immunoperoxidase. Leu22 displays strong membrane, cytoplasmic, or focal paranuclear Golgi region staining in the majority of the large neoplastic T cells (immunoperoxidase stain, original magnification: 630× magnification). (From Wieczorek R, Buck D, Bindl J, et al. Monoclonal antibody Leu22 (L60) permits the demonstration of some neoplastic T cells in routinely fixed and paraffin-embedded tissue sections. *Hum Pathol* 1988;19:1434–1443, with permission.)

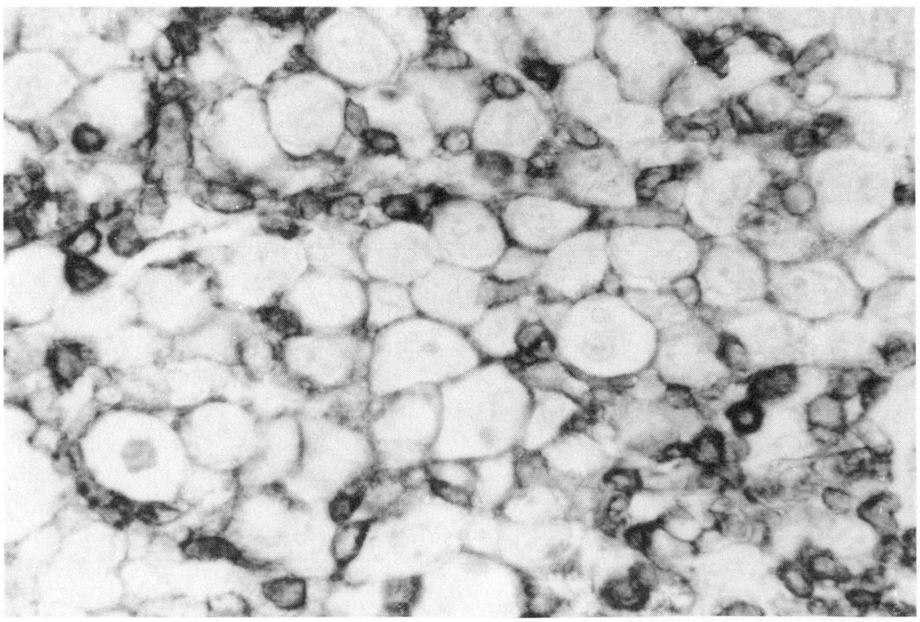

FIG. 3.52. B5-fixed, paraffin-embedded tissue section of a CD30-positive anaplastic large cell lymphoma immunostained with monoclonal antibody Leu22. The antibody displays distinct linear membrane staining of virtually all of the large anaplastic tumor cells. It shows much stronger membrane staining of the numerous residual small benign T cells (immunoperoxidase stain, original magnification: 400× magnification).

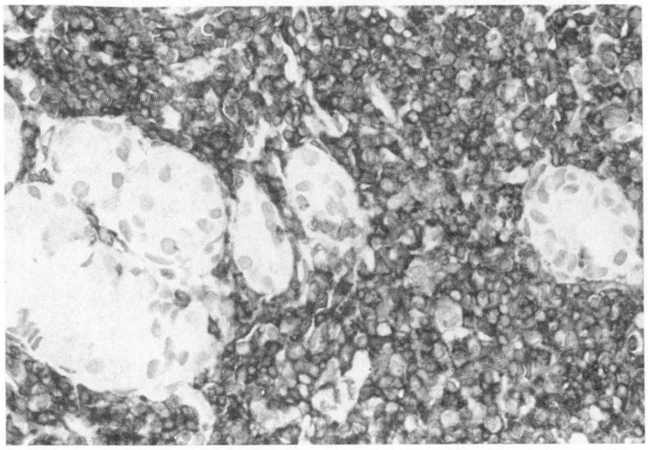

FIG. 3.53. Formalin-fixed, paraffin-embedded tissue section of a gastric lymphoma of mucosa-associated lymphoid tissue, which has been immunostained with monoclonal anti-CD43 antibody Leu22. Approximately 30% of all nonlymphoblastic B-cell non-Hodgkin's lymphomas express CD43. The coexpression of CD20 and CD43 is a useful immunophenotypic criterion of B-cell malignancy in immunodiagnosis (immunoperoxidase stain, original magnification: 400× magnification).

cell cycle–dependent (1506). CD71 is a prototypic activation antigen associated with increased proliferative activity in most tissues (1509). CD71 is expressed by actively proliferating cells belonging to all hematopoietic lineages, some nonhematopoietic lineages, mitogen and allogeneic-activated B and T cells, capillary endothelium in brain, and some fetal tissues (liver and thymus). CD71 is not expressed by mature, resting peripheral blood and lymphoid tissue B and T cells, monocytes, granulocytes and erythrocytes (671,1506,1508,1518–1520). CD71, however, also is expressed on cells such as erythroblasts that require large amounts of iron for metabolic purposes other than growth (1509).

Among lymphoid neoplasms, CD71 is expressed by the malignant lymphoblasts of precursor T-cell lymphoblastic lymphomas/leukemias exhibiting prothymocyte and thymocyte phenotypes (7,13,14,144,765) and is expressed variably by postthymic T-cell neoplasms, especially peripheral T cell-lymphomas (13,14), and by B-cell large cell immunoblastic lymphomas (1504,1521). Indolent, low-grade NHLs and lymphoid leukemias with a low proliferative index generally contain no or only a small number of $CD71^+$ neoplastic cells (1521,1522).

Platelet-Associated Antigens

CD9

The CD9 cluster was defined at the first workshop by MAbs BA-2 (1523) and DU-ALL-1 (1524), among others (15). Many additional MAbs have been added to the CD9 cluster in subsequent workshops (102,1525–1528). CD9 is a member of the transmembrane 4 superfamily of proteins, which also is known as *tetraspans* (1529). Tetraspans are expressed by many cell types and show a different subcellular distribution; the function of the tetraspans is not yet known (1529). CD9 is a 24-kd single chain membrane protein (p24) (1523) that is encoded by 12p13 (1530). Anti-CD9 MAbs have a variety of functions; the most important and best understood is the induction of platelet activation through the interaction of the bound anti-CD9 MAb with the Fc receptor FcγRII (1527,1528).

Although initially considered anti-B cell antibodies, anti-CD9 MAbs have been categorized among the antiplatelet antibodies since the third workshop (1525). CD9 is expressed by platelets and also is found in the α granules of platelets. CD9 is not expressed by the majority of mature peripheral blood and lymphoid tissue B or T cells or by other normal circulating lymphohematopoietic cells (7,1523,1528, 1530). CD9 is expressed, however, by mitogen-stimulated T cells (1531) and mast cells (1268). CD9 also is expressed by lymphoid progenitor cells in the bone marrow, specifically by 3% to 5% of bone marrow mononuclear cells that are TdT^+, sIg^-, and $CD2^-$, and is coexpressed by about 50% of the TdT^+ bone marrow mononuclear cell population (1523,1532). CD9 is not expressed by normal pleuripotential (GEMM-CFU) or committed (GM-CFU, E-BFU, E-CFU) hematopoietic progenitor cells (1532). Anti-CD9 MAbs have a wide range of immune reactivity with normal human cells and tissues, including endothelial cells, cardiac and vascular smooth muscle cells, various epithelia, glomeruli and renal tubules, and brain and peripheral nerves (1526).

CD9 expression by malignant cells is not strictly lineage-, differentiation-, or activation-related. CD9 is expressed by 75% or more of precursor B-cell lymphoblastic lymphomas/leukemias, approximately 50% of B-cell chronic lymphocytic leukemias, and some B-cell prolymphocytic leukemias, multiple myelomas, T-cell neoplasias, and AMLs, especially FAB M7 (megakaryoblastic) AML (7,1523,1524,1527, 1533–1536). CD9 also is expressed variably by neuroblastomas and by some epithelial neoplasms (1523,1532,1536). Anti-CD9 MAbs have been employed therapeutically to purge $CD9^+$ acute lymphoblastic leukemia cells from the bone marrow for autologous transplantation (101). In addition, the peripheral blood CD9 concentration has been used as an indicator of HIV production (1537). Anti-CD9 MAbs no longer are used routinely in immunophenotypic analysis, except for the obvious necessity to use them in cytofluorometric analysis to identify patients with acute lymphoblastic leukemia who are candidates for anti-CD9 MAb purging.

Proliferation-Associated Antigens

Pathologists always have had considerable interest in determining the proliferation rate of human neoplasms. It has been thought that this information is important in grading neoplasms, predicting their clinical behavior and prognosis, and sometimes distinguishing benign and malignant proliferations. Various methods directed at different parts of the cell cycle have been developed for this purpose. Historically, pathologists have enumerated the number of mitotic figures per high power field visualized through a light microscope. More recently, DNA synthesis (S phase) has been assayed by measuring labeled DNA precursor incorporation, such as tritiated thymidine, or a nucleotide analogue, such as bromodeoxyuridine; DNA content has been quantitated by flow cytometry; and proliferation rates have been assayed by the silver staining of proteins associated with nucleolar organizer regions (1538). Each of these approaches has obvious disadvantages, as well as advantages, rendering each of them a less than perfect indication of the true proliferation fraction of a tumor. This led to a search for proliferation-associated antigens that can be assayed immunohistochemically.

Gerdes and colleagues generated MAb Ki-67 (1539), which detects a huge nuclear nonhistone protein doublet of 345 and 395 kd (1540), encoded by a gene localized to 10q25-qter (1541), and which is expressed at the end of G_1, S, G_2, and M phases of the cell cycle; it is not expressed in G_0 (1542). MAb Ki-67 detects a human nuclear cell proliferation-associated antigen. Ki-67 antigen synthesis and expression start at the beginning of S phase and rise through S phase and G_2 to reach maximal expression in mitosis (1543). After mitosis, during G_1, either the Ki-67 antigen is rapidly degraded or the epitope is modified or lost (1543); the detectable half-life is 1 hour or less (1544). Ki-67 antigen synthesis starts again at the beginning of S phase (1543). Cells expressing Ki-67 in G_1 represent the first daughter cells returning to G_1 after mitosis (1543). During interphase, the Ki-67 antigen is localized predominantly to the nucleolar cortex and in the dense fibrillar components (1545). It has been suggested that the Ki-67 antigen is associated with the so-called nuclear matrix–intermediate filament scaffold (1545). With progression from S into G_2, the Ki-67 antigen is associated tightly with chromatin, and at mitosis, all Ki-67 immunoreactivity is colocalized with chromatids (1546). Although Ki-67 expression appears to be an absolute requirement for proliferation (1547), the precise function of Ki-67 remains unclear. It has been proposed that Ki-67 represents a major structural protein with DNA binding properties that plays a primary role in maintaining higher-order structure for DNA during the process of mitosis (1548).

Monoclonal antibody Ki-67 is immunoreactive with permeablized cells in suspension (1549), in cytocentifuge slide preparations, and in frozen tissue sections (1539), providing a simple and reliable means of rapidly evaluating the growth fraction, that is, the number of cells in cell cycle in benign, normal, and neoplastic cell populations. MAb Ki-67 is not immunoreactive, however, in routinely prepared, formalin-fixed, paraffin-embedded tissue sections, even after the application of antigen retrieval procedures (1539,1549,1550).

Additional MAbs, designated *MIB-1*, *MIB-2*, and *MIB-3* (1551), and rabbit (1552) and sheep (1553) polyclonal anti-Ki-67 antibodies have been raised against peptides from recombinant fragments of the gene for Ki-67. All of these monoclonal and polyclonal antibodies react with the mature Ki-67 protein and exhibit an immunoreactive pattern identical with that of MAb Ki-67 in frozen tissue sections (1551–1553). All of these antibodies can be regarded as true Ki-67 equivalents. Furthermore, the rabbit and sheep anti-Ki-67 heteroantisera and MAbs MIB-1 and MIB-3 are immunoreactive with the nuclei of the proliferative cell compartment of benign and neoplastic tissues in routinely prepared, formalin-fixed, paraffin-embedded tissue sections following antigen retrieval by microwave irradiation (1551–1553). The nuclear staining pattern observed in paraffin tissue sections with these antibodies parallels that of MAb Ki-67 in frozen tissue sections and coincides with data on normal cell proliferation obtained by measuring the nuclear incorporation of radioactively labelled DNA precursors (1539). The immune reactivity of these antibodies with paraffin-resistant epitopes in microwave-irradiated paraffin tissue sections is not inhibited or altered by decalcification or depigmentation techniques (1550). The rabbit and sheep anti-Ki-67 heteroantisera are particularly useful for facilitating parallel evaluation of the growth fraction of a tumor and expression of a particular membrane antigen by dual immunostaining in combination with MAbs (1552,1553).

Monoclonal and polyclonal anti-Ki-67 antibodies detect the proliferative compartment of benign normal human tissues. They react with cortical thymocytes but with only occasional medullary thymocytes (Fig.3.54), and not with Hassal's corpuscles (1539,1550). In peripheral lymphoid tissues, they react with many germinal center lymphoid cells and scattered paracortical immunoblasts and with only very small numbers of other lymphoid cells (1539,1550). They also react with the basal cells of squamous epithelium, with the mucosal neck and deep crypt cells of gastrointestinal epithelium, and with many undifferentiated spermatogonia (1539,1550,1552,1553). MAb Ki-67 exhibits cross-reactivity with the cytoplasm of squamous epithelium in frozen tissue sections (1540,1551–1553). The sheep and rabbit anti-Ki-67 heteroantisera and MAb MIB-1 do not exhibit this nonspecific cytoplasmic staining (1539,1552,1553). Anti-Ki-67 antibodies are not immunoreactive with cells known to be in a resting or quiesent state, that is, mature resting B and T cells, monocytes and macrophages, fibroblasts, muscle cells, hepatocytes, gastric parietal cells, intestinal Paneth cells, renal epithelium and brain cells, and so forth (1539,1550). Although in comparison with the assessment of cell proliferation measured by tritiated thymidine uptake, for a variety of reasons, Ki-67-MIB-1 positivity may either underestimate or overestimate the growth fraction (1543,1546,1554). The applicability and clinical relevance of Ki-67-MIB-1 expression for assessing cell proliferation has been demonstrated in numerous studies (1555).

Other antibodies have been generated that detect proliferation-associated antigens. MAb JC1 recognizes a nuclear protein associated with cell proliferation that is distinct from Ki-67 (1556). MAbs PC10 (1557) and 19F4 (1558) recognize proliferating cell nuclear antigen, a 36-kd nuclear protein

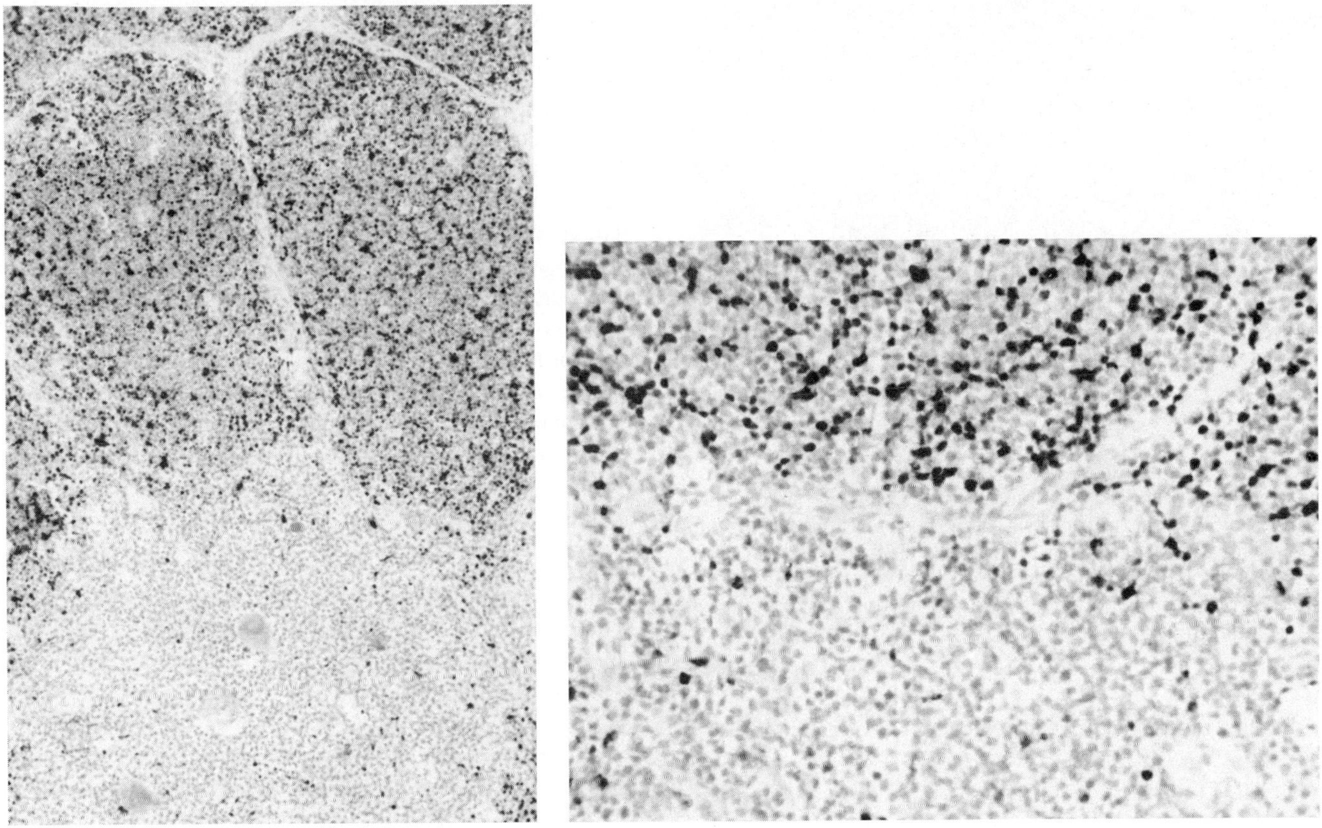

A B

FIG. 3.54. Frozen tissue section of thymus immunostained with monoclonal antibody Ki-67 (immunoperoxidase stain). This antibody recognizes a proliferation-associated antigen expressed by cycling cells but not by resting cells and thereby provides a simple means of evaluating the growth fraction of normal and neoplastic human cell populations. **A:** Numerous Ki-67-positive cells are present in the cortical thymus, which contains numerous proliferating thymocytes. In contrast, only small numbers of Ki-67-positive cells are identified in the medullary thymus, which consists predominantly of resting, mature thymocytes (original magnification: 100× magnification). **B:** Higher magnification shows the marked difference between the number of Ki-67-positive cells in the cortical thymus (*above*) and medullary thymus (*below*) (original magnification: 250× magnification).

associated with DNA polymerase δ (1559,1560), which is present throughout the cell cycle in proliferating cells. These antibodies are similarly immunoreactive in conventionally processed tissues following microwave irradiation (1556–1558). In comparative immunohistochemical studies, however, MAb MIB-1 and polyclonal Ki-67 appear to be superior to these other antibodies with respect to their specific immune reactivity with the proliferative compartment in normal tissues, as defined immunohistochemically by MAb Ki-67 in frozen tissue sections, or by tritiated thymidine uptake, specificity of nuclear versus cytoplasmic staining, and cleanliness of background (1538,1561,1562). MAb MIB-1 and polyclonal Ki-67 appear to be the best antibody reagents available for measuring proliferation fraction in conventionally processed tissues in diagnostic immunopathology (1538,1561). MAb MIB-1 has been shown to be immunoreactive in paraffin tissue sections obtained from paraffin blocks stored for as long as 60 years (1550). The immunohistochemical demonstration of Ki-67-MIB-1 positivity in paraffin tissue sections has become the most popular approach among pathologists for measuring the growth fraction of benign and malignant cell populations in both newly accessioned and archival pathologic specimens.

Multiple studies have been performed utilizing the immune reactivity of MAbs Ki-67 and MIB-1 to determine the growth fraction of malignant tumors (1563–1572), including malignant lymphomas (1573–1576), and correlating the findings with histologic grade, clinical behavior, and prognosis (Fig. 3.55). Among malignant lymphomas, the proportion of Ki-67$^+$MIB-1$^+$ cells generally parallels the malignant grade of the histopathologic category of NHL (1573–1576). There is a highly significant correlation between the proportions of Ki-67$^+$ cells and the subclassification of NHLs into low- and high-grade categories (1573–1575). For example, only approximately 1% to 15% (median 8%) of small lymphocytic lymphoma or chronic lymphocytic leukemia cells are Ki-67$^+$; 60% to 95% (median 63%) of Burkitt's lymphoma cells are Ki-67$^+$ (1573). The wide range of Ki-67 proliferation indices in each clinicopathologic category indicates that the growth fractions of

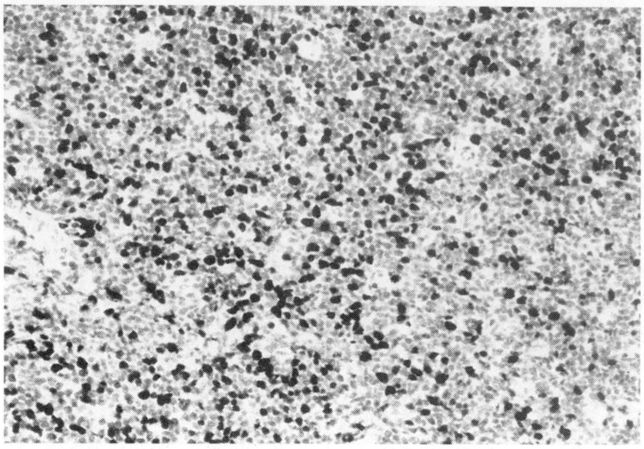

FIG. 3.55. Frozen tissue section of a lymph node involved by mantle cell lymphoma immunostained with monoclonal antibody Ki-67. Scattered neoplastic cells exhibit immunoreactivity with Ki-67 indicating those cells that are cycling. This determination is useful in indicating the proliferating cell population or growth fraction of a malignant tumor (immunoperoxidase stain, original magnification: 200× magnification).

individual tumors within each category are quite heterogeneous, however (1573–1576). On this basis, it has been suggested that the determination of the growth fraction in NHLs may have prognostic value. In one study of patients who had low-grade NHLs, those whose NHLs had relatively high Ki-67 proliferation indices had a worse survival rate than those whose NHL had a low Ki-67 proliferation index (1575). In a study of patients with diffuse large cell lymphoma, Ki-67 expression was found to be an independent predictor of duration of survival (1576). Those patients whose diffuse large cell lymphomas contained less than 60% Ki-67$^+$ malignant cells had a median duration of survival of 39 months; those whose comparable lymphomas contained more than 60% Ki-67$^+$ cells had a statistically significantly lower median duration of survival of only 8 months (1576). Some potential drawbacks to the use of Ki-67 expression to assess the growth fraction of a tumor are the marked intratumor heterogeneity of Ki-67 expression and the variations in proliferation indices over the life span of a tumor, among others.

IMMUNOPHENOTYPIC CHARACTERISTICS OF NORMAL HEMATOPOIETIC CELLS

Background

Extensive immunophenotypic studies of normal and neoplastic B and T cells using large panels of MAbs in conjunction with cytofluorometric and immunohistochemical techniques have led to the creation of schema of normal B- and T-cell differentiation (6,7,14,218,461). In these schema, discrete developmental stages are defined according to reactivity with a panel of MAbs that detect differentiation and subset-associated antigens. The central thesis in these immunophenotyping studies is that lymphoid neoplasms represent clonal proliferations of neoplastic cells frozen or blocked at a particular stage in B- or T-cell ontogeny. This thesis may not be entirely correct; also, differentiation is a continuous and not a discrete process, so these schema are overly simplified. Neoplastic cell immunophenotypes that do not reflect these differentiation schema have been encountered. Whether this is because the models of normal B- and T-cell differentiation are incorrect, because the normal counterparts of some malignant lymphoid cells are identified uncommonly, or because they aberrantly express B- and T-cell differentiation antigens has not yet been determined. These schema are helpful, however, in understanding the immunophenotypes of malignant lymphoid cell populations and their relationship to normal T- and B-cell differentiation.

B Cells

By definition, a B lymphocyte is capable of producing immunoglobulin. Mammalian B cells are generated in the bone marrow and undergo differentiation (B-cell ontogeny) by direct interaction with cellular components and soluble factors within the bone marrow microenvironment (1577). B-cell ontogeny can be divided into several discrete stages according to the expression of B cell–restricted and associated cytoplasmic and surface membrane antigens. These stages can be referred to as *progenitor B cell*, *pre-pre-B cell*, *pre-B cell*, *immature B cell*, and *resting mature B cell*. Further differentiation into activated or differentiating B cells and secretory B cells (plasma cells) is antigen-dependent and occurs in the peripheral lymphoid tissues (Fig. 3.56) (see Chapter 2). The B-cell markers employed to define these stages can be subgrouped broadly according to the stages they detect. Antigens that span B-cell ontogeny—CD19, CD20, and CD22—are referred to as *pan-B cell* antigens. Antigens that are not expressed on resting mature B cells but are expressed following activation, such as CD23, are referred to as *activation* antigens.

According to current concepts of B-cell differentiation (6–8,129,218,397,461,569,618,1335) (Fig. 3.56), the earliest identifiable B cells, that is, progenitor B cells, retain the immunoglobulin genes in the germline configuration and express intranuclear TdT, HLA-DR, CD34, and cCD79. Progenitor B cells acquire B-cell lineage–associated antigens CD19 and CD22 and undergo immunoglobulin heavy chain gene rearrangement to become pre-pre-B cells. They then acquire CD10, followed by B cell–associated antigen CD20. They begin to lose CD34 and continue to acquire CD20 and to express mCD79 and cytoplasmic μ heavy chains without light chains as they enter the pre-B cell stage. Pre-B cells lose TdT, CD34, cytoplasmic μ heavy chains, and CD10; retain CD19, CD22, CD20, and CD79; undergo immunoglobulin light chain gene rearrangement; and acquire CD21 and sIgM to become immature B cells. CD5 is expressed by a subset of immature B cells. As normal development proceeds, the average amount of sIgM decreases, an increasing amount of sIgD appears, and the cells become resting

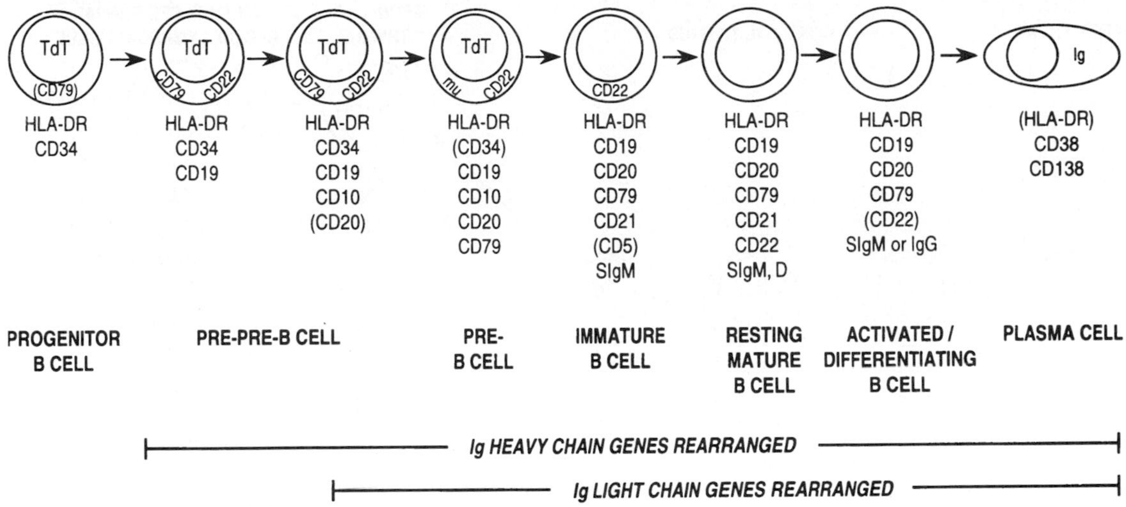

FIG. 3.56. Schematic representation of B-cell ontogeny. The parentheses indicate that only a subpopulation of these cells expresses this marker.

mature (naive) B cells. The resting mature (naive) B cell is a small lymphocyte that expresses HLA-DR, CD19, CD22, CD79, CD21, and sIgMD; is in the G_0 stage of the cell cycle; and has not yet undergone the events associated with activation. The naive B cell is the first B cell to exit the bone marrow and circulate in the peripheral blood, from which it can enter the lymph nodes, spleen, and mucosa-associated lymphoid tissues. In lymph nodes naive B cells are located primarily in the mantle zone.

After binding with antigen or mitogens, resting mature B cells are activated and enter the germinal center in which they proliferate to enter the activated–differentiating stage. Activation is accompanied by a distinct sequence of cell surface antigenic changes (100). B cells expressing sIgM, sIgD, and sIgG appear. These cells lose sIgD and later sIgM as well as CD21. They simultaneously acquire certain antigens associated with B-cell activation as well as growth factor receptors and other important regulatory molecules, including, for example, CD23, CD25 (IL-2 receptor), and CD71 (transferrin receptor). Proliferating B cells subsequently interact with additional lymphokines that halt cell division and induce the cells to differentiate into Ig-producing (secretory) B cells. This differentiative stage is accompanied by the gradual but progressive loss of sIg, HLA-DR, CD19, CD22, CD20, CD79 and the activation-associated antigens, as well as the acquisition of new antigens, including CD38 and CD138, which are expressed on plasma cells. The molecular events and other immunophenotypic changes that occur during antigen-independent and antigen-dependent B-cell differentiation are discussed in Chapters 2, 6, and 7.

T Cells

T-cell ontogeny, that is, the differentiation of lymphoid precursor cells in the bone marrow into mature, peripheral immunocompetent T cells, can be divided operationally into several discrete stages according to the expression of T-cell lineage–restricted and associated cytoplasmic and surface membrane antigens. These stages can be referred to as *prothymocyte, immature thymocyte, common thymocyte, mature thymocyte, and mature peripheral T cell* (6,7,13,14,137,243) (Fig. 3.57). Antigens that span T-cell ontogeny—CD2, CD3, CD5, and CD7—are referred to as *pan-T cell* antigens. Antigens that are preferentially expressed on the helper or inducer and suppressor or cytotoxic T cell subsets, CD4 and CD8, respectively, are referred to as *subset-restricted* antigens.

As discussed in Chapter 2 and summarized previously here, two distinct types of TCR exist: the "classic" TCR composed of an α and β chain (711,973) and the "alternative" or "second" TCR composed of a γ and δ chain (974,975). The majority (at least 90%) of thymocytes and mature human peripheral blood and lymphoid tissue T cells express TCR$\alpha\beta$ (977); only a small minority (less than 5%) express TCR$\gamma\delta$ (979). Although notable exceptions exist (987,988), the majority of human T-cell neoplasms are clonal proliferations of TCR$\alpha\beta$ and not TCR$\gamma\delta$ T cells (981–983,987). For the purposes of this discussion, a hypothetical scheme encompassing only the correlative immunophenotypic changes and TCR gene rearrangements occurring in the classic linear TCR$\alpha\beta$ T-cell differentiation pathway is presented. Hypothetical schema of T-cell ontogeny that include $\alpha\beta$ and $\gamma\delta$ cell differentiation pathways have been presented and discussed elsewhere (937,1578) (see Chapter 2).

According to current concepts of lymphoid cell differentiation (7,8,14,137,243,244,770, 771,937,1579) (Fig. 3.57), the majority of bone marrow pleuripotential lymphoid precursor cells express intranuclear TdT, HLA-DR, and CD34 antigens and retain the immunoglobulin and TCR genes in the germline configuration. Prothymocytes are the earliest identifiable T-cell precursors to appear in the bone marrow.

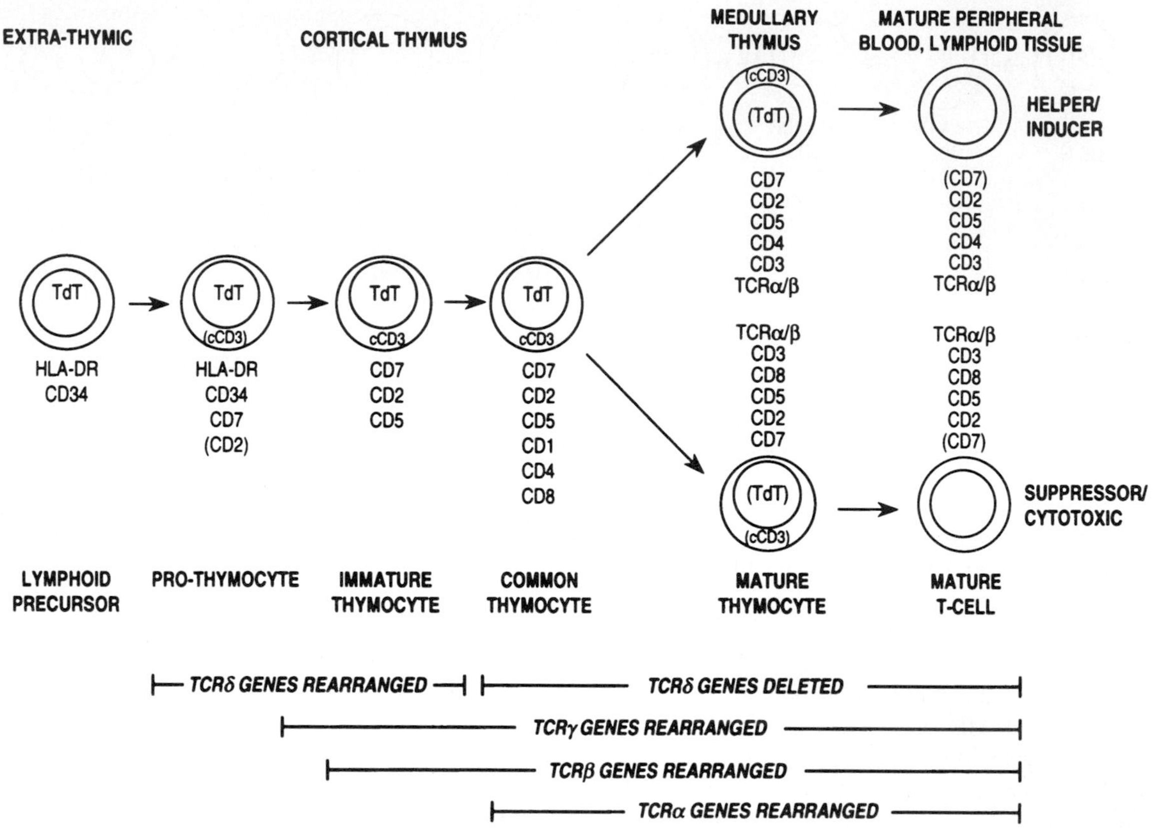

FIG. 3.57. Schematic representation of T-cell ontogeny. The parentheses indicate that only a subpopulation of these cells expresses this marker.

In addition to TdT, HLA-DR, and CD34, prothymocytes express CD7, generally believed to be the first T-cell lineage–restricted antigen to appear during T-cell ontogeny (204,221,937). $CD7^+CD3^-CD4^-CD8^-$ precursor T cells, referred to as *triple negative*, can be identified in 7-week fetal tissues prior to the development of the thymus (937). These prothymocytes, however, also appear to variably express cCD3 and CD2. CD3 gene transcription apparently begins during the prothymocyte stage, prior to entrance into the thymus, and cCD3ϵ appears after CD7 but before CD2 (770,771). These $CD7^+cCD3^+$ and $CD7^+cCD3^-$ prothymocytes then migrate to and colonize the epithelial thymic rudiment, which may be mediated by antigen molecules such as CD44, which also are expressed by these prothymocytes (1580,1581). These T-cell precursors undergo all further maturation under the influence of the thymic epithelium (1582,1583). T-cell development in the thymus is characterized by distinct and sequential patterns of surface antigen expression and loss, accompanied by the progressive and orderly rearrangements of the genes encoding the TCR (1582,1583). The prothymocytes lose HLA-DR and CD34, continue to acquire cCD3 and CD2 as well as CD5, and undergo rearrangement of the TCRδ gene, immediately followed by rearrangement of the TCRγ and TCRβ genes, to become the immature thymocyte population. Immature thymocytes retain cCD3, CD7, CD2, and CD5 and acquire CD1, CD4, and CD8 to become common thymocytes, which make up approximately 70% of all thymocytes. Thymocytes that coexpress CD4 and CD8 are referred to as *double-positive*. The prothymocyte, immature thymocyte, and common thymocyte populations reside in the cortex. Common thymocytes lose CD1, undergo TCRδ gene deletion followed by TCRα gene rearrangement, acquire the completely assembled TCR-CD3 surface membrane complex, and differentiate along one of two pathways, either retaining CD4 and losing CD8 or retaining CD8 and losing CD4, to become mature (medullary) thymocytes. These cells variably express cCD3 and TdT. The mature thymocytes subsequently peripheralize, losing cCD3 and TdT entirely, and become the mature $CD4^+$-$CD8^-$ (helper-inducer) and $CD4^-CD8^+$(suppressor-cytotoxic) T-cell subsets, respectively. In addition to the T-cell differentiation–associated antigens discussed here and illustrated in Figure 3.57, thymocytes variably express a wide range of other molecules, including CD38, CD71 (the transferrin receptor) and various integrins and other receptors (1584) (see Chapters 2 and 6). Antigen expression on T cells after activation is discussed in Chapters 2 and 6.

Accessory Cells

Monocytes/Macrophages

Macrophages and their ability to phagocytize foreign particles have been recognized for more than 100 years (1585).

The heterogeneity of the cell populations that previously have been lumped together as macrophages or "histiocytes" and their diverse functional properties, which include antigen presentation to B and T cells and the synthesis of immunoregulatory substances, have been recognized widely only during the past 20 years (212). Because of the recent evidence that these cell populations play an integrated, multifaceted role in humoral and cellular immunity considerably beyond simple phagocytosis, the former designation *mononuclear phagocyte system* (1586,1587) appears to be a misnomer. This prompted Foucar and Foucar to propose the alternative designation *mononuclear phagocyte and immunoregulatory effector (M-PIRE) system* (212) to convey more accurately the diverse yet integrated functional role these cells play in the immune system. In their proposal, the M-PIRE system includes monocytes, macrophages, the multiple dendritic cell populations including Langerhans cells and follicular dendritic cells (dendritic reticulum cells), and their bone marrow precursors. There is some evidence to suggest that all these cells share a common cell of origin (692,1273) and that transitions between them may occur (1588) (see Chapter 1). This concept remains controversial, however, and many investigators consider monocytes and macrophages, dendritic cells, and follicular dendritic cells to represent three distinct cell lineages. These cell populations exhibit distinctive morphology and possess unique immunophenotypic and functional properties; they are discussed separately here.

Mononuclear phagocytes (monocytes and macrophages) and polymorphonuclear phagocytes (neutrophilic granulocytes) originate from a common committed bone marrow precursor cell, the GM-CFU (see Chapter 1). The first recognizable cell in the monocyte-macrophage lineage is the monoblast from which promonocytes and later mature monocytes derive. Young monocytes remain in the bone marrow for only a brief time, enter the circulation incompletely differentiated, persist in the peripheral blood with a half-life of 3 days, and then migrate by diapedesis across endothelial cell walls into tissues, in which they become ubiquitously distributed and mature into tissue macrophages (1589). Following migration from the intravascular space into solid tissues, monocytes generally do not return to the circulation. Some monocytes specifically localize in the liver to become Kupffer cells and some in the lungs to become alveolar macrophages; others become germinal center tingible body macrophages, lymph node sinus histiocytes, epithelioid histiocytes, T-zone macrophages, microglial cells, Bilroth cord cells, and osteoclasts (1590). Some investigators have suggested that immunophenotypically distinct monocyte subsets preferentially migrate to specific tissues to become particular cell types, because a variety of patterns of antigenic expression have been identified on peripheral blood monocyte populations (1591–1593).

Monocytes/macrophages represent the third cell population, in addition to B cells and T cells, involved in humoral and cellular immunity. They play a crucial role in the immune system as antigen-presenting cells, interacting with other leukocytes in a bidirectional fashion. Their other principal functions include host defense against invading tumor cells and foreign organisms, particularly the ingestion and killing of obligate intracellular microorganisms; ingestion and removal of senescent cells; secretion of products that affect hematopoiesis, lymphocyte and macrophage function, coagulation and other diverse immune activities; and modulation of tumor growth and tissue remodeling (212) (see Chapter 2).

The earliest stages in the monocyte lineage have not been well characterized. We know that these cells undergo cytochemical and immunophenotypic alterations as they differentiate from monoblasts to mature monocytes. Bone marrow monoblasts and promonocytes contain the enzymes acid phosphatase, nonspecific esterase, and lysozyme within their cytoplasm and express CD45 (LCA), MHC class I (HLA-A, HLA-B, HLA-C) and class II (HLA-DR) antigens, CD11b, CD13, CD14, CD15, and CD33 (112,212,232,1219,1366, 1587,1590). Mature circulating monocytes, in addition, contain α_1-antitrypsin and α_1-anti-chymotrypsin and express CD4, CD11c, CD21, CD25, and the Fcγ receptors CD32 and CD64, as well as CD68, although heterogeneity within this immunophenotypic profile has been described (112,212,663,1230,1280,1290,1587,1593–1596). Phagocytic tissue macrophages express cytochemical and immunophenotypic profiles very similar to those of mature circulating monocytes, although these cell populations exhibit considerably more immunophenotypic heterogeneity than peripheral blood monocytes, especially with respect to expression of CD11b, CD13, and CD33 (212,249,297,663, 691,693,1161,1185,1590,1592–1597). In addition, they express CD16 (1026) but generally do not express CD15 (1380). This immunophenotypic heterogeneity may reflect distinct monocyte and macrophage subpopulations, functional status, or alterations induced by the antigenic environment or the immune system (212). The vast majority of the antigens expressed by monocytes and macrophages are not unique to this lineage; most of them also are expressed by granulocytes or B- and T-cell immune response accessory cells, that is, dendritic cells. This may reflect the common origin of myelomonocytic cells and the related functional properties of monocytes and macrophages and dendritic cells. One exception appears to be the CD68 epitope detected by MAb PG-M1, which appears to be specific for monocytes and macrophages and is not expressed by any other cell populations, including myeloid cells and granulocytes (1283) (Fig. 3.43). MAb PG-M1 and other anti-CD68 MAbs are not generally reactive with cutaneous Langerhans cells, indeterminate dendritic cells, interdigitating dendritic cells, or follicular dendritic cells (1283,1290). Monocytes and macrophages do not express S-100 protein or CD1 (297,691–693).

Langerhans Cells and Dendritic Cells

Langerhans (1598) initially identified what came to be known as *Langerhans cells* in the suprabasal epidermis by their distinctive dendritic morphology upon impregnating human skin with gold salts in 1868. Almost 100 years later, in 1961, Langerhans cells were identified by the presence of a characteristic cytoplasmic organelle, the Birbeck granule, with the electron microscope (1599). It is now known that Langerhans cells represent only one subset of a large family of morphologically distinctive potent antigen-presenting cells referred to as *dendritic cells*.

Dendritic cells comprise a complex system composed of several distinct cell populations occupying discrete portions of lymphoid and nonlymphoid organs that is interconnected by defined pathways of movement. In each site, the dendritic cells share morphologic, immunophenotypic, and functional characteristics, the most notable being the ability to capture antigens in an immunogenic form *in situ* and initiate T cell–mediated immunity (213,1600–1602) (see Chapter 2). The dendritic cell system consists of cutaneous and mucosal Langerhans and indeterminate cells, interstitial dendritic cells, afferent lymph veiled cells, peripheral blood dendritic cells, lymphoid dendritic cells, and interdigitating dendritic cells (213). Follicular dendritic cells (dendritic reticulum cells) appear to be distinct from these dendritic cell populations (1601); they are discussed subsequently here. Dendritic cells are present in lymphoid tissue, including lymph node, tonsil, thymus, and spleen, and nonlymphoid tissue, including skin, heart, lung, liver, and the gastrointestinal tract; they also circulate in the peripheral blood and afferent lymph (213). The precise origin of dendritic cells and the ontogenic relationships among the various dendritic cell subpopulations, monocytes and macrophages, and follicular dendritic cells are not yet completely understood. Dendritic cells appear to represent one or more distinct mononuclear cell lineages derived from bone marrow pleuripotent stem cells (213,1603,1604) (see Chapter 1).

Dendritic cells share many properties with monocytes and macrophages. At each anatomic site, however, dendritic cells exhibit distinctive unifying cytomorphologic, ultrastructural, histochemical, immunophenotypic, and functional properties that serve to distinguish them from monocytes/macrophages (213,1600–1602). For example, dendritic cells are nonadherent and non- or minimally phagocytic and possess low levels of Fc receptors but high levels of MHC class II antigens. In contrast, monocytes/macrophages are adherent and phagocytic and possess abundant Fc receptors but variable levels of MHC class II antigens (213). Dendritic cells lack lysozyme, α_1-antitrypsin, and α_1-antichymotrypsin; contain low or undetectable levels of nonspecific esterase and acid phosphatase; but strongly express S-100 protein, cytochemical properties that are opposite those of monocytes/macrophages (297,1600–1602,1605,1606).

Epidermal Langerhans cells represent the best-characterized dendritic cell population. Ultrastructurally, Langerhans cells have clear cytoplasm devoid of tonofilaments, desmosomes, and melanosomes; a lobulated and frequently convoluted nucleus containing very delicate chromatin; numerous cytoplasmic extensions; and the distinctive cytoplasmic organelle referred to as the *Birbeck granule* (1607). Langerhans cells represent an important component of the cutaneous immune system. *In vitro* studies have demonstrated their ability to present antigens to T cells, stimulate allogeneic and syngeneic mixed leukocyte reactions, and secrete lymphokines (213). These cells also are required for the generation of cutaneous delayed hypersensitivity (213). Among all dendritic cell populations, only Langerhans cells appear to be able to process and present whole antigens (1608). Langerhans cells can leave the epidermis, move into the dermis, and subsequently travel through afferent lymphatics to draining lymphoid organs (688,1609). Cells with Birbeck granules have been found in lymph and in normal lymph nodes (1610,1611) and in increased numbers in dermatopathic lymphadenopathy (1611,1612). In culture, Langerhans cells enlarge, express more MHC class II and adhesion molecules, and lose Fc receptors and Birbeck granules (1613,1614), resembling peripheral blood and lymphoid dendritic cells (1613,1615). Most investigators believe that the Birbeck granule is not a constant morphologic marker of Langerhans cells but rather a morphologic expression of the epidermal microenvironment or a specific functional state of Langerhans cells (1272,1616,1617). The cells residing in the epidermis, dermis, and mucosa that resemble Langerhans cells morphologically, cytochemically, and phenotypically but lack Birbeck granules have been referred to as *indeterminate cells* (1618–1621). They have been postulated to represent Langerhans cell precursors (1617,1622) and are considered to belong to the Langerhans cell lineage (1604). Mucosal indeterminate cells may serve in a functional capacity analogous to epidermal Langerhans cells (1623).

Veiled cells having distinctive dendritic morphology and other structural and functional dendritic cell properties have been identified in the afferent, but not in the efferent, lymph (688,1624). Veiled cells may represent migrating dendritic cells, in particular Langerhans cells in transit from the skin into lymph nodes in which they become interdigitating dendritic cells. It is well known that Langerhans cells and interdigitating dendritic cells often are dramatically increased in number in the lymph node paracortex in dermatopathic lymphadenopathy (1625,1626). Dendritic cells also circulate in the peripheral blood, in which they make up less than 0.1% of peripheral blood leukocytes (1627). Peripheral blood dendritic cells may be *en route* from the bone marrow to lymphoid and nonlymphoid tissues and are another possible source for veiled cells (213,1627).

Interdigitating dendritic cells are present within lymph nodes, tonsil, spleen, and other lymphoid tissue. They resemble Langerhans cells morphologically, except for the frequent absence of Birbeck granules, and immunophenotypically, except for the lower frequency of CD1 expression (1626,1628,1629). They are characteristically located in T-cell domains, that is, the paracortex and interfollicular areas of lymph nodes and tonsils, and the periarteriolar lymphoid sheath of the spleen (1630). They are typically surrounded by helper T cells (297,844). Interdigitating dendritic cells are present in the thymic medulla as well (1631,1632), in which they also may express CD1 (1633).

$CD1^+$ dendritic cells, including Langerhans cells, express the panhematopoietic cell antigen CD45, consistent with a bone marrow derivation (27,296); interdigitating dendritic cells and follicular dendritic cells do not express CD45 (297). Dendritic cells lack the lineage markers characteristic of B cells (CD19, CD20), T cells (CD2, CD3, CD5), and LGLs and NK cells (CD16, CD56, CD57) (297,1627). No panhuman dendritic cell lineage-restricted antigen has been identified. Dendritic cells display, however, an immunophenotypic profile that is unique among leukocytes and is consistent with their functional properties: antigen presentation (abundant MHC class I and II molecules), active clustering with T cells (high levels of several adhesins), and weak phagocytosis (low levels of Fc and CRs) (Fig. 3.58).

Dendritic cells express abundant MHC class II molecules, including HLA-DR, HLA-DP, and HLA-DQ (200,201,297, 1627) and the class II associated invariant chain, CD74 (1627,1634), consistent with their strong antigen-presenting cell function. They also express abundant polymorphic class I products (297,1627,1635). CD1, which is not encoded in the MHC but is class I–like and may act as a restriction element for $\gamma\delta$ T cells (681), is abundant on dendritic cells in the skin and mucosa (CD1a) (297,685,686,1636) (Fig. 3.33) and in afferent lymph (CD1b) (688).

Integrin and adhesion molecules contribute to cell binding and homing, both of which are important features of dendritic cell function. Consequently, dendritic cells can have high levels of CD11c (1627,1637). Peripheral blood, but not cutaneous, dendritic cells express CD11a (LFA-1) (1614,1627). Dendritic cells also can have high levels of other adhesins, including CD29 (β_1 integrin), CD54 (ICAM-1), and CD58 (LFA-3) (213,1613,1627). Moreover, they synthesize high levels of IL-2 (1638).

Dendritic cells are not actively phagocytic. Consistent with this, there is little or no expression of Fcγ receptors (CD16,CD32,CD64) or C3 receptors (CD11b,CD21,CD35) (213). An exception is freshly isolated epidermal Langerhans cells, which express FcγRII (CD32) (1602,1615); on culturing, these cells lose CD32 (1614,1639). This finding is in keeping with the fact that only freshly isolated Langerhans cells actively process and present native proteins (213). Low-affinity FcϵRII (CD23) are upregulated on epidermal Langerhans cells with IL-4 and interferon-γ (1640), consistent with data implicating Langerhans cells in the transport of contact allergens (213).

Many of these antigens are expressed homogeneously on dendritic cells populating different sites. There are exceptions, however. Some of these differences may occur as dendritic cells mature and migrate or may reflect local environmental factors (213). For example, Langerhans cells and interdigitating dendritic cells strongly express S-100 protein (Fig. 3.59) and weakly and variably express CD4 (297,663,1605,1606,1626), like other dendritic cells. Epidermal and mucosal Langerhans cells and indeterminate cells, however, appear to be the only dendritic cells that consistently express CD1 (685,1619,1620,1623,1636). A significantly larger proportion of epidermal and mucosal Langerhans cells and indeterminate cells express CD1 than express HLA-DR. Consequently, CD1 is a better marker of these cell populations (1617,1623,1636). The $CD1^+$ interdigitating dendritic cells located in the lymph node paracor-

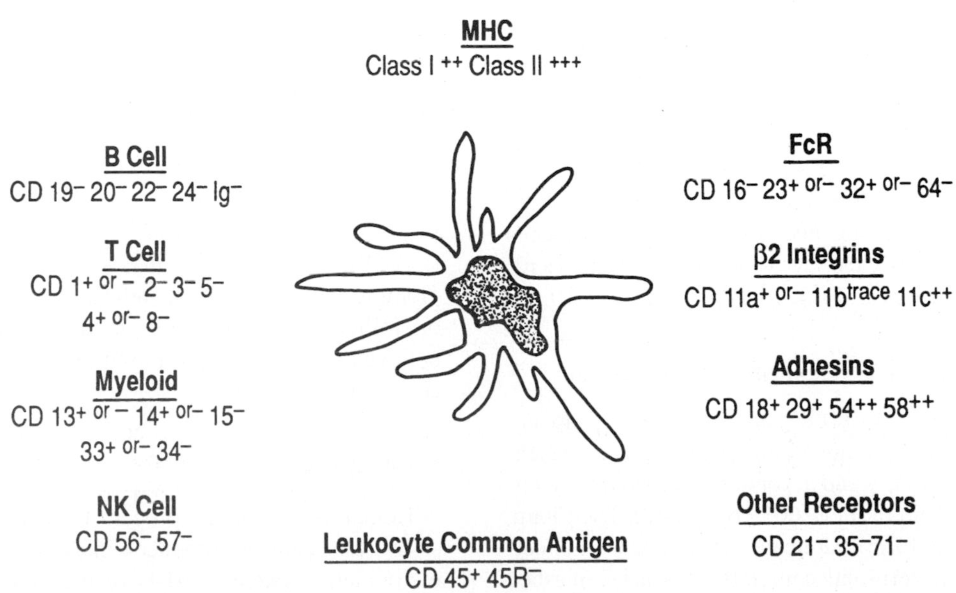

FIG. 3.58. The immunophenotypic characteristics of dendritic cells. (Adapted from Steinman RM. The dendritic cell system and its role in immunogenicity. *Annu Rev Immunol* 1991;9:271–296, with permission.)

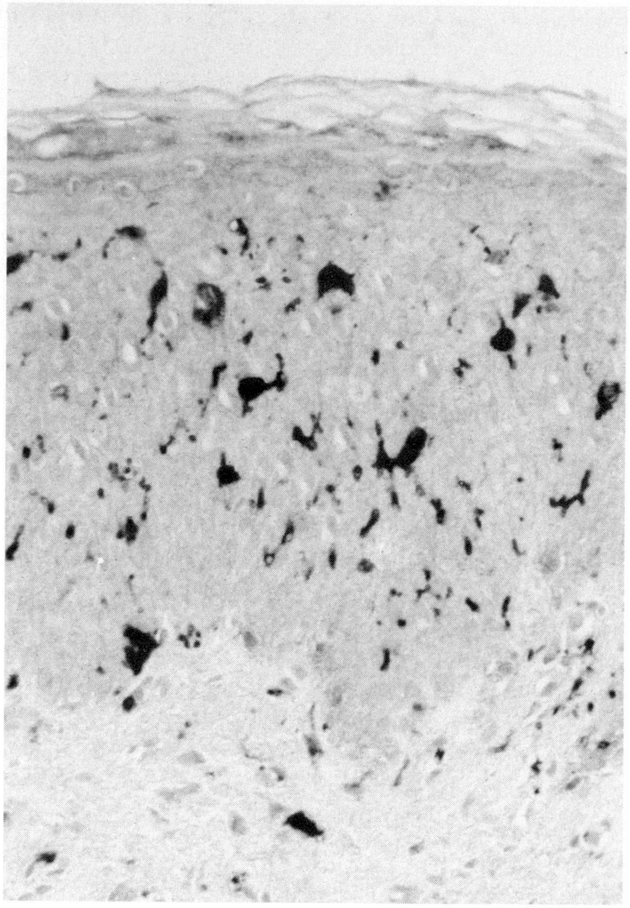

FIG. 3.59. Formalin-fixed, paraffin-embedded tissue section of skin immunostained for S-100 protein. The numerous epidermal Langerhans cells and their processes can be identified because of their strong expression of S-100 (immunoperoxidase stain, original magnification: 250× magnification).

tex probably represent $CD1^+$ Langerhans cells or indeterminate cells that have migrated from the skin and epithelia (297). In addition, Langerhans cells and interdigitating dendritic cells weakly and variably express CD14 (297,1272), and Langerhans cells variably express CD33 (1272). Langerhans cells contain formalin-resistant sulphydryl-dependent adenosinetriphosphatase (1607). Dendritic cells lack reactivity with anti-CD68 MAb PG-M1, which specifically detects monocytes and macrophages (1283,1290).

Follicular Dendritic Cells (Dendritic Reticulum Cells)

Follicular dendritic cells (1601) are specialized, nonphagocytic accessory cells that are found only in B cell–dependent areas, that is, primary and secondary lymphoid follicles, of peripheral lymphoid tissue (1601,1641,1642). Their long, branching processes form a delicate three-dimensional network within which germinal center B cells are enmeshed (1641,1642). Follicular dendritic cells can be identified by their light microscopic and ultrastructural morphology (clear indented nucleus, peripheral condensed nuclear chromatin, small distinct nucleolus, and desmosome-linked cytoplasmic extensions), and restricted occurrence in germinal centers (1641,1642). Follicular dendritic cells bind antigen-antibody complexes through receptors for the C3b fragment of complement (1642), and possibly also through Fc receptors (93). They are believed to play an important role in the retention of antigen in lymphoid follicles, the presentation of antigen to germinal center B cells, and the generation of memory B cells (1642). They also appear capable of trapping lymphoid cells (1641). On isolation they often form multicell clusters associated with entrapped B cells (93,1643). They also may be involved in B-cell homing, because neoplastic B cells of follicle center origin accumulate within a meshwork of follicular dendritic cells, even if the neoplasm is present in nonlymphoid tissue, whereas neoplastic B cells not of follicle center origin do not (1644). Neoplastic follicles, however, contain significantly fewer follicular dendritic cells than do benign hyperplastic follicles (1645).

Analysis of isolated follicular dendritic cells and follicular dendritic cells in touch imprints and tissue sections has demonstrated that they express cytochemical and immunophenotypic characteristics of monocytes/macrophages, namely, acid phosphatase, nonspecific esterase, α_1-antitrypsin, α_1-antichymotrypsin, CD45, MHC class I and II molecules (93,297,1592,1643,1646), and all three categories of complement (C3) receptor, CR1 (CD35), CR2 (CD21) (see Fig. 3.28), and CR3 (CD11b), as well as the Fcγ receptor CD32 (93,94,533,546,1642,1647). The presence of CR1, CR2, and CR3 on follicular dendritic cells is a surface characteristic not found in any other cell type that optimally allows follicular dendritic cells to bind antigen–antibody complexes bearing any type of C3 fragment (94). Follicular dendritic cells also express CD14 in low density and variably express CD4 faintly (93,297). A subset of follicular dendritic cells in the light zone of the germinal center also expresses CD23 (see Fig. 3.30), which is the low-affinity receptor for IgE (579) and also one of the ligands for CD21, allowing them to bind complexes containing CD21 with higher affinity, as well as to intereact with IgE (582,596). Follicular dendritic cells do not appear to constitutively express CD45 or mature lineage-restricted pan-B and pan-T cell antigens (93,94,1643), and they uniformly lack expression of S-100 protein and CD1 (297,691–693,1643). Finally, surface membrane immunoglobulin of the IgM, IgG, and IgA isotypes is demonstrable on follicular dendritic cells in tissue sections, but this is believed to be cytophilic immunoglobulin bound by Fc receptors (93,1643,1646).

Myeloid Cells

Hematopoiesis is the process by which blood cells such as myeloid cells are produced in the bone marrow. The hematopoietic system consists of pleuripotent hematopoietic stem cells, progenitor cells that are committed to differentiate along one or more pathways, and nonproliferating mature cells that subserve specialized functions. Mature myeloid cells are derived from a population of pleuripotential hematopoietic stem cells having the capacity for both self-renewal and differentiation. The progeny of these stem cells include several committed precursor cells that give rise separately to granulocytes and monocytes/macrophages, erythroid cells, and megakaryocytes under the influence of regulatory substances. Neutrophilic granulocytes and monocytes/macrophages originate from a common committed precursor cell, the GM-CFU. The precursor cells generated from GM-CFU are committed randomly to becoming G- or M-CFUs that can be induced to proliferate and differentiate into granulocytes or monocytes/macrophages by lineage-specific factors. On maturation in the bone marrow, the mature blood cells enter the peripheral circulation and, in some instances, home to other tissues (see Chapter 1).

Numerous studies have shown that developing myeloid cells express differentiation-associated antigens, that is, antigens whose expression changes during the process of maturation. These myeloid-associated antigens can be used to identify as well as to isolate developing myeloid cells at different points in their maturation (see Chapter 1). The expression of myeloid-associated antigens during normal bone marrow myelopoiesis is portrayed schematically in Figure 3.60. Briefly, the earliest progenitor cells, the GEMM-CFUs, express MHC class II (HLA-DR) antigens, the hematopoietic precursor cell antigen CD34, and acquire panmyeloid antigen CD33 early in their maturation to 14-day GM-CFUs. In addition to these antigens, 7-day GM-CFUs acquire panmyeloid antigens CD13 and CD15. These cells serially lose CD34 as they mature into myeloblasts, HLA-DR antigens as they mature into promyelocytes, and CD33 as they mature into myelocytes; they retain CD13 and CD15 and acquire CD11b. Metamyelocytes and granulocytes retain CD13, CD15, and CD11b and also acquire CD16 (see Chapter 1).

Large Granular Lymphocytes/Natural Killer Cells

Natural killer cells originally were defined functionally on the basis of their unique ability to lyse autologous and allogeneic tumor cells (1648), virus-infected cells (1649), and certain normal target cells in the absence of previous sensitization or activation (1650). The origin of NK cells is controversial, but they probably represent a third lineage of lymphoid cells (1651). Several lines of evidence suggest that NK cells originate from lymphoid progenitor cells (1652,1653). They differentiate in the bone marrow and, unlike T cells, do not require the presence of the thymus for their maturation (1650). NK cells leave the bone marrow at a very early stage of maturation. Hence, mature NK cells are almost absent from the bone marrow (999). Most NK cells are found in the peripheral blood and spleen, in which they comprise approximately 15% and 3% of lymphocytes, respectively (999). Fewer NK cells are found in tonsil and bone marrow, and almost none are found in lymph nodes, thymus, or other lymphoid organs (999) (see Chapter 2).

Natural killer cells have the morphology of LGLs. These are medium to large lymphocytes with a low nuclear to cytoplasmic ratio. They possess abundant cytoplasm containing azurophilic granules and an indented or kidney-shaped nucleus (1650). The azurophilic granules contain substances that are believed to play roles in their cytotoxic activity (1654,1655). In humans, LGLs account for most NK activity. Not all LGLs, however, possess NK activity. In particular, large agranular lymphocytes (LAL), which lack cytoplasmic azurophilic granules but are otherwise morpho-

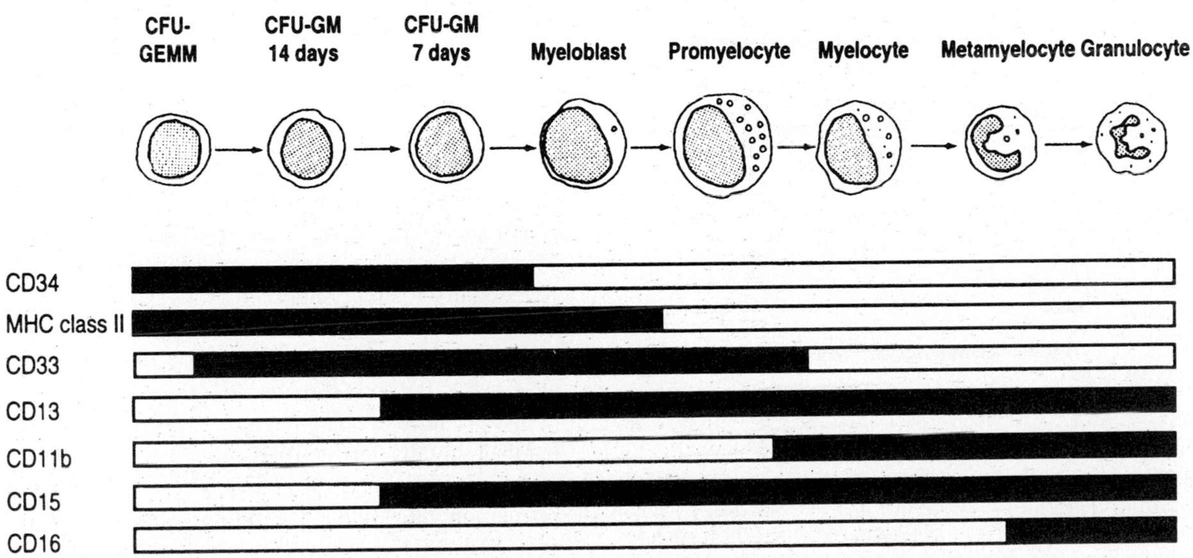

FIG. 3.60. Schematic representation of immunophenotypic expression of myeloid-associated antigens during normal myelopoiesis. The *black bar* indicates expression and the *white bar* indicates lack of expression of the particular antigen.

logically and immunophenotypically identical to LGLs, are present in the spleen and to a lesser extent in other lymphoid organs. These large agranular lymphocytes may represent the immature form of LGLs (1650).

The *in vivo* functions of NK cells are incompletely understood. NK cells play a role in the defense against malignant cells and virus-infected cells and also may serve important regulatory functions in hematopoiesis (1650) (see Chapter 1). NK cells, which do not require prior antigen sensitization, lyse their target cells in the absence of MHC restriction (1650). The receptors recognized by NK cells in this process are unknown (1650). NK cells also efficiently lyse IgG-sensitized target cells through ADCC. Here, the recognition element on NK cells is CD16, the low-affinity Fc receptor for IgG (1006). Although resting mature NK cells are functionally cytotoxic, their activity is increased by certain cytokines, including IL-2 and interferons (1649,1656). NK cells are also powerful producers of lymphokines (1657) (see Chapter 1).

NK cells represent a morphologically and functionally homogeneous but immunophenotypically heterogeneous cell population (Fig. 3.61). They express a variety of surface and cytoplasmic molecules, the majority of which they share with monocytes and macrophages, granulocytes (CD11b, CD16), and T cells (CD2, CD7, CD8) (999,1650). Essentially all peripheral blood mononuclear cells with the morphologic appearance of LGLs and accounting for all NK and

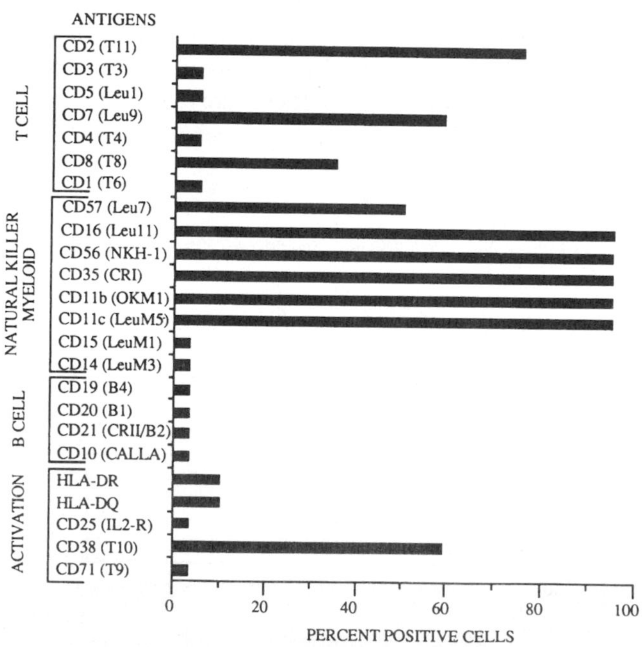

FIG. 3.61. Immunophenotypic profile of freshly isolated human natural killer cells. (Adapted from Lanier LL, Phillips JH. A map of the cell surface antigens expressed on resting and activated human natural killer cells. In: Reinherz EI, Haynes BF, Nadler LM, et al., eds. *Leucocyte typing II: human, myeloid and hematopoietic cells.* New York: Springer-Verlag, 1986: 157–170.)

killer functional activity express CD16 (999,1006), the IgG Fc receptor III (1000,1006) that mediates ADCC (1006). Virtually this entire $CD16^+$ NK cell population also expresses low levels of CD56 (NCAM) (1039,1040) and the vast majority express CD11b (113,999,1006,1658), the iC3b receptor (CR3) (107). Approximately 20% to 70% of NK cells (variably donor-related) express CD57 (1006). A variable proportion of NK cells express T cell–associated antigens as follows: CD2 (80–90%) (999,1000,1006), CD7 (50–60%) (113), low-density CD8 (20–50%) (999,1000,1006); and CD38 (113). CD11b, CD16, and CD56 also are expressed on minor T-cell subpopulations (1028,1039,1162), supporting the hypothesis that NK cells are more closely related to T cells than to myeloid cells. NK cells, however, lack other T-cell antigens such as CD3, CD4, and CD5 (999,1006,1091). They also lack all B cell–associated antigens (999,1000,1006,1091). Whether or not a proportion of NK cells express MHC class II (HLA-DR) antigens has been controversial (1006).

IMMUNOPHENOTYPIC CRITERIA USEFUL IN THE IMMUNODIAGNOSIS OF LYMPHOID NEOPLASIA

Background

Normal mature lymphoid tissue occurring in lymph nodes and in extranodal sites such as Waldeyer's ring and the gastrointestinal tract is composed of a mixture of T cells, B cells, macrophages, and small numbers of other minor cell populations. Benign, reactive lymphoid proliferations occurring in nodal and extranodal sites recapitulate the immunoarchitecture of normal mature lymphoid tissues (5,6,47, 1659). T cells nearly always make up between 50% and 75% of the total lymphocyte population within these proliferations. One exception is marked follicular (B-cell) hyperplasia, in which less than half the lymphocytes may be T cells. Another exception is benign, reactive pleural effusions in which T cells often are 80% or more of the total lymphocyte population (5,47,1659). In all these instances, greater than 95% of the T lymphocytes express pan-T cell associated antigens CD2, CD3, and CD5 (68,243,244,726,850) and approximately 80% to 90% express CD7 (726,924,946,947). The T-cell population consists of two mutually exclusive and functionally distinct subpopulations, $CD4^+CD8^-$ (helper-inducer) and $CD4^-CD8^+$ (suppressor-cytotoxic) T cells (243,244). Less than 5% of mature peripheral $CD3^+$ T cells are $CD4^-CD8^-$ (1660), and less than 2% are $CD4^+CD8^+$ (844). The ratio of CD4 to CD8 T cells may be quite variable but usually falls between 1.0 and 5.0 (1659). B cells usually make up between 20% and 50% of the total lymphocyte population, the notable exceptions being the ones mentioned previously (5,47). Virtually all the B cells express pan-B cell associated antigens CD19 and CD20 (23,442,443), among others, and a variable proportion coexpress sIg (29,38,214). Each individual B cell may express more than one heavy chain, most commonly IgM and IgD, but expresses only one light chain, κ or λ (29). Approximately two thirds of mature peripheral sIg^+ B cells express κ light chains, and the remaining one third express λ light chains (29). Normally, the ratio of κ to γ light chain–positive B cells is approximately 2:1 (5,29,214), although this ratio may vary somewhat (47). B cells residing in the germinal centers often lack sIg (726) and, therefore, cell suspensions and frozen tissue sections of lymphoid proliferations exhibiting marked follicular hyperplasia frequently contain sizable numbers of sIg^- B cells. Monocytes and macrophages and the various other minor cell populations usually do not enter into routine immunophenotypic analysis unless they are overrepresented in the specimen (5,47,214). Several immunophenotypic criteria especially applicable to cell suspensions and frozen tissue sections exist that are useful in the immunodiagnosis of lymphoid neoplasia. These criteria generally exploit the distinctive features of the immunophenotypic profiles of lymphoid neoplasms that are not observed among those of normal lymphoid tissue and benign, reactive lymphoid proliferations.

B-Cell Neoplasms

The B-cell population present in benign, reactive lymphoid proliferations occurring in lymph nodes and extranodal tissues represents the progeny of multiple B-cell clones; κ- and λ-expressing B cells are present in approximately a 2:1 ratio, comparable to normal lymphoid tissue and peripheral blood. In contrast, neoplastic B cells making up the NHLs and lymphoid leukemias represent the clonal progeny of a single neoplastic cell. Because individual B cells express κ or λ light chains, but never both (29), neoplastic B-cell populations that express sIg exclusively express κ or λ light chains (5,6,42–44,47). For this reason, the clonality of a particular B-cell population may be inferred from the uniformity of its immunoglobulin light chain class expression (isotypic exclusion). A mixture of κ- and λ-positive B cells indicates polyclonality; a vast predominance of κ or λ light chain–positive B cells indicates monoclonality (Fig. 3.62). Approximately 80% of NHLs and lymphoid leukemias occurring in the Western Hemisphere are of B-cell origin; about two thirds of them express monotypic sIg (42–44,726). The immunophenotypic demonstration of a monoclonal B-cell population generally has been considered to indicate a B-cell neoplasm, whereas that of a polyclonal B-cell proliferation generally has been considered to indicate a benign, reactive, nonneoplastic proliferation (45–47). These suppositions provide the operational basis for the immunophenotypic marker analysis of lymphoproliferative disorders (6).

Definitive immunophenotypic criteria for the definition of B-cell monoclonality, however, have been difficult to establish and suggested guidelines have not been uniformly accepted. Many years ago, Taylor considered "a κ/λ light chain ratio ≥3:1 or a λ/κ light chain ratio ≥2:1" as indicative of B-cell monoclonality (1661). We and others, however, have encountered many examples of benign, reactive nodal and extranodal lymphoid proliferations that represent clear exceptions to these criteria. At least some of the cases reported by Levy and coworkers (1662) and by Palutke and colleagues (1663) as morphologically benign lymphoid hyperplasias expressing monoclonal sIg represent such examples. Levy and colleagues (1662) and we also have noticed that lymph nodes exhibiting florid follicular hyperplasia and the other histopathologic features associated with toxoplasmic lymphadenitis are among those benign lymph nodes most frequently found to have κ:λ light chain ratios above or below normal. Most commonly, these ratios fall in the ranges from 0.3 through 1.0 and 3.0 through 7.0. These criteria are clearly too restrictive, and κ:λ ratios in these ranges should not be used to diagnose B-cell neoplasia in the absence of morphologic evidence. Strict adherence to these criteria would result in the misinterpretation of a small proportion of benign lymphoid proliferations as malignant lymphoma. Obviously, the true monoclonal, oligoclonal, or polyclonal nature of these proliferations can be determined easily using immunoglobulin gene rearrangement analysis (1664–1666) (see Chapter 7).

For these reasons, most investigators have adopted a more liberal definition of polyclonality and taken a more cautious approach in defining immunophenotypic criteria of B-cell monoclonality. It has been recommended that immunoglobulin light chain restriction be defined by the presence of a vast predominance (at least 10:1) of B cells expressing one light chain class, either κ or λ (726). Precise numbers can be generated by cytofluorometric analysis. In frozen tissue sections, sheets of B cells exhibiting light chain isotypic restriction should be identified in order to satisfy these criteria. Those cases in which there is a clear admixture of κ and λ light chain–positive B cells in frozen tissue sections with only a slight predominance of one light chain over the other should not be considered monoclonal B-cell proliferations (Fig. 3.62). These criteria appear to have been accepted by other investigators and generally fit our experience as well. A histopathologically benign and reactive appearing lymphoid proliferation should not be considered malignant simply because of a slight predominance of B cells expressing one light chain class. The results of immunophenotypic analysis should be interpreted in conjunction with the clinical and morphologic findings. Failure to do so may result in erroneous conclusions, with grave consequences for the patient. Marked discrepancies between histopathology and the results of immunophenotypic analysis probably should be resolved by immunogenotypic analysis or, if necessary, by a repeat biopsy.

In addition to immunoglobulin light chain restriction, the absence of immunoglobulin light chain expression is also a useful criterion of B-cell neoplasia. Among 297 B-cell NHLs and lymphoid leukemias in one study (726), one third lacked sIg expression. This included as many as 30% to 40% of the lymphomas displaying diffuse large cell and follicular

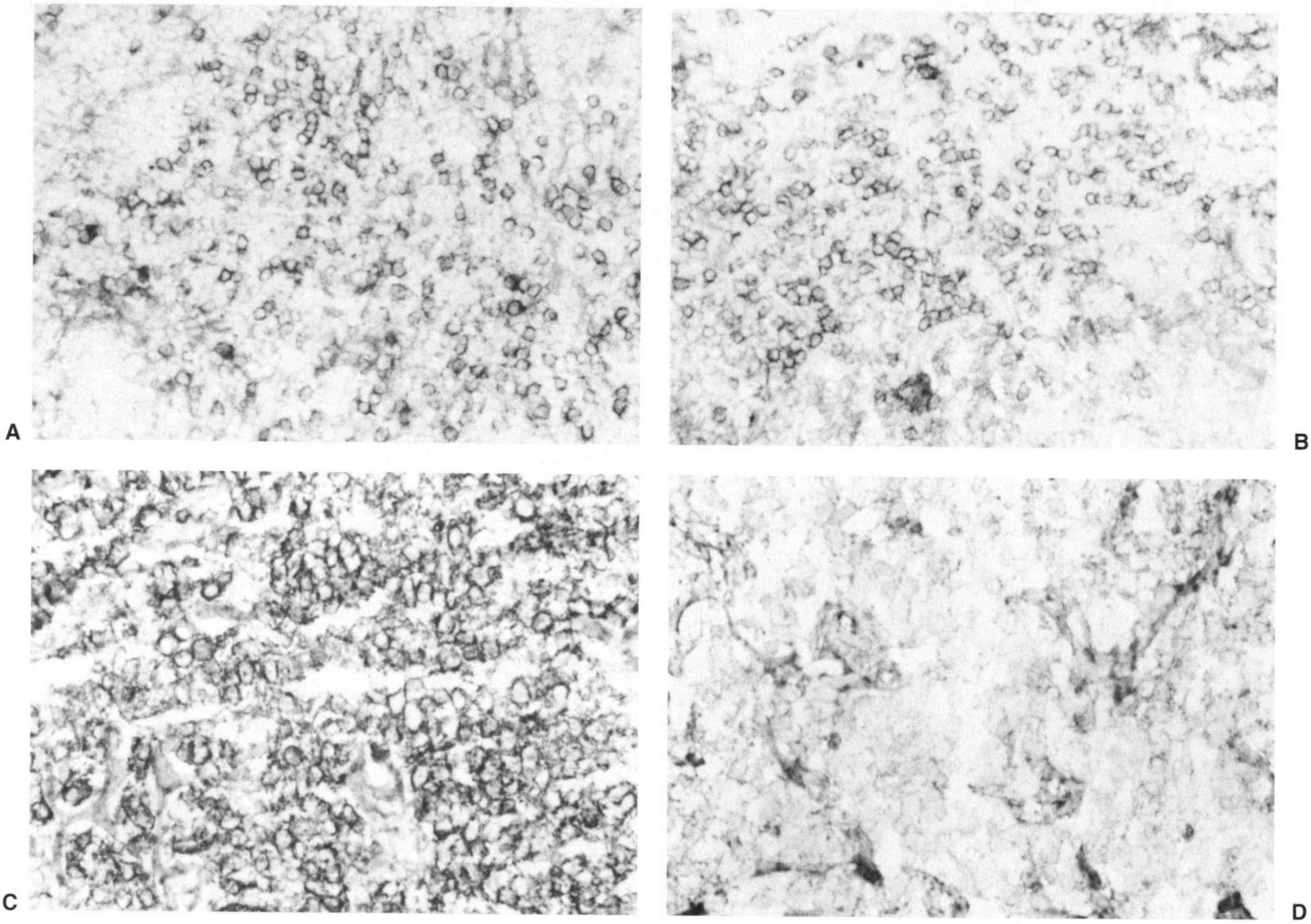

FIG. 3.62. Frozen tissue sections of an orbital lymphoid hyperplasia (**A,B**) and an orbital malignant lymphoma (**C,D**) immunostained for κ (**A,C**) and λ (**B,D**) light chains by immunoperoxidase. **A,B:** Approximately equivalent proportions of the cells present in this benign reactive lymphoid proliferation express κ light chains and λ light chains, consistent with a polyclonal B-cell proliferation (original magnification: 250× magnification). **C,D:** Virtually all of the cells present within this orbital malignant lymphoma express κ light chains (**C**) and virtually none express λ light chains (**D**), consistent with a monoclonal B-cell proliferation (original magnification: 400× magnification).

and diffuse mixed small and large cell histologies. A diffuse B-cell proliferation devoid of immunoglobulin light chain expression most likely is a malignant lymphoma (726). Immunoglobulin light chain expression, however, normally is weak or absent on germinal center B cells (726). For this reason, the immunoglobulin light chain–negative B-cell phenotype is not abnormal or unusual in this situation, and caution should be exercised in applying this criterion to follicular B-cell proliferations.

Expression of the CD5 antigen by a B-cell proliferation is another immunodiagnostic criterion useful in defining B cell neoplasia. Normally CD5 is expressed by virtually all mature peripheral T cells (849–851) but only a minor B-cell subset (902,908). For all intents and purposes, CD5 B cells are not readily identifiable in normal lymphoid tissue or benign reactive lymphoid proliferations if routinely examined by single-color flow cytometry or immunohistochemical analysis of frozen tissue sections. More than 90% of B-cell small lymphocytic lymphomas/chronic lymphocytic leukemias and mantle cell lymphomas, however, and about 5% of follicle center cell and large B-cell lymphomas express the CD5 antigen (726,853,918,919). The demonstration of a distinct CD5 B-cell proliferation in nodal and extranodal tissues is virtually diagnostic of malignant lymphoma (Fig. 3.41).

Although these represent the major immunophenotypic criteria for B-cell neoplasia, the anomalous expression of other antigens has been recommended as also satisfying immunodiagnostic criteria for B-cell neoplasia (726). These include reactivity of a B-cell population with MAb Leu22 (CD43) in frozen or paraffin tissue sections (Fig. 3.53); the loss of expression of pan-B cell antigen CD19, CD20, or

CD22 by a B-cell population; and the lack of LFA-1 expression (726). These additional immunophenotypic criteria for B-cell malignancy are discussed in detail elsewhere (726).

T-Cell Neoplasms

At least five immunophenotypic criteria exist that are helpful in the immunodiagnosis of T-cell neoplasia. In increasing order of utility, these are marked T-cell predominance, T-cell subset antigen restriction, anomalous T-cell subset antigen expression, a precursor T-cell immunophenotype, and anomalous deletion of one or more pan-T cell antigens (14,726).

A lymphoid proliferation composed of 80% or more T cells, especially one containing a marked predominance of $CD4^+CD8^-$ or $CD4^-CD8^+$ T cells, raises the possibility of a T-cell neoplasm. Neither T-cell predominance nor T-cell subset antigen restriction, however, are in themselves sufficient to warrant a definitive diagnosis of T-cell neoplasia. Many benign cutaneous lymphoid infiltrates consist of a preponderance of T cells and, in many instances, the $CD4^+CD8^-$ T-cell subset predominates, sometimes to a marked degree. In addition, marked quantitative alterations in the numbers of benign CD4 and CD8 T cells occur in the peripheral blood and lymphoid tissues for a variety of reasons. For example, it is not unusual for peripheral blood and even lymphoid tissue CD4:CD8 T-cell ratios of 0.4 or less to occur in the advanced stages of AIDS (see Chapter 28). Hodgkin's disease lesions often contain an increased proportion of T cells, sometimes 80% or more, and an elevated CD4:CD8 T-cell subset ratio, often in excess of 5:1 (1659,1667). Alternatively, a decreased CD4:CD8 T-cell subset ratio sometimes is observed in the lesional tissue in Hodgkin's disease (1659,1667). T-cell predominance and T-cell subset antigen restriction are two immunodiagnostic criteria that should be used with considerable caution. In practice, they are only truly useful in those instances in which the infiltrating cell population satisfies morphologic criteria of malignancy. Morphologically malignant infiltrates that express T-cell lineage–associated antigens and exhibit T-cell subset antigen restriction may be considered T-cell neoplasms.

Anomalous T-cell subset antigen expression is a more useful criterion in the immunodiagnosis of T-cell neoplasia. Essentially all mature peripheral blood and lymphoid tissue T cells express either the CD4 or the CD8 antigen, but not both; $CD4^+CD8^-$ and $CD4^-CD8^+$ T cells represent mutually exclusive and functionally distinct T-cell subsets (243,244,844,1660). The presence of a $CD4^+CD8^+$ (double-positive) or a $CD4^-CD8^-$ (double-negative) T-cell proliferation is distinctly abnormal and extremely suspicious for a malignant T-cell proliferation. Certain immunophenotypic pitfalls can result in the identification of what appears to be a $CD4^-CD8^-$ T-cell proliferation but really is not. First, the CD4 epitope detected by MAb OKT4 is absent from CD4 T cells in about 4% of the African-American population because of genetic polymorphism (842). The CD4 T cells in these individuals are detectable with MAb Leu3a (843). Second, CD4 T cells are stained weakly in frozen tissue sections using MAb OKT4 (844) but are readily detectable using cocktails composed of two anti-CD4 MAbs such as Leu3a and Leu3b (726) or OKT4b and OKT4d (Knowles, unpublished observations), which detect independent, non-cross-blocking epitopes on the CD4 molecule (739). Third, a benign, reactive expansion of the $CD4^-CD8^-$ T-cell subset sometimes is observed in the peripheral blood of individuals with AIDS (1668). In our experience, however, the expression of the double-positive or double-negative immunophenotype is indicative of a T-cell lymphoproliferative disorder if these three situations have been ruled out.

Precursor T cells, that is those expressing TdT or CD1, are found in the thymus and only rarely, if ever, are identified in the peripheral blood or peripheral lymphoid tissue of normal healthy adults (127–129). The majority of the T cells making up the thymus exhibit a spectrum of immature immunophenotypes consistent with various stages of intrathymic T-cell differentiation (137,243,244). The presence of benign T cells expressing a precursor T-cell immunophenotype (TdT^+CD1^+) outside of the thymus is so abnormal as to be essentially diagnostic of precursor T-cell neoplasia. In these situations, however, those cells expressing the immature markers TdT or CD1 should be evaluated for the expression of T-cell lineage and other markers before making a definitive diagnosis of T-cell neoplasia.

In general, the single most useful criterion in the immunodiagnosis of T-cell neoplasia is the conspicuous absence of one or more of the pan-T cell antigens (CD2, CD3, CD5, CD7) by 50% or more of the cells making up a T-cell proliferation (14,726,727) (Fig. 3.63). In addition, Picker and colleagues (982) suggested that the expression of TCR$\alpha\beta$ chain framework antigens detectable with MAbs WT31 (976) and β (978) is also useful in this regard. As many as one third of peripheral T-cell lymphomas, but not benign T-cell proliferations, display discordant expression of CD3 and TCR α and β chain antigens (982). Approximately two thirds of patients with patch- or plaque-stage mycosis fungoides exhibit deletion of pan-T cell antigen CD7 (726). Approximately 75% of peripheral T-cell lymphomas and nearly all patients with advanced (tumor) stage mycosis fungoides exhibit deletion of one or more pan-T cell antigens (726). CD7 is deleted most commonly, followed by CD5, CD2, and CD3 (726). Pan-T cell antigen loss is a useful and practical immunodiagnostic criterion of T-cell neoplasia. Even this criterion should be employed with caution. In our experience, some morphologically benign cutaneous lymphoid infiltrates contain a marked reduction in $CD7^+$ T cells. These cells may represent a benign expansion of the normally occurring $CD7^-CD4^+$ T-cell subset (947). Also, one or more of these pan-T cell antigens may be deleted in lymphomatoid papulosis (1669,1670), a cutaneous T-cell lymphoproliferative

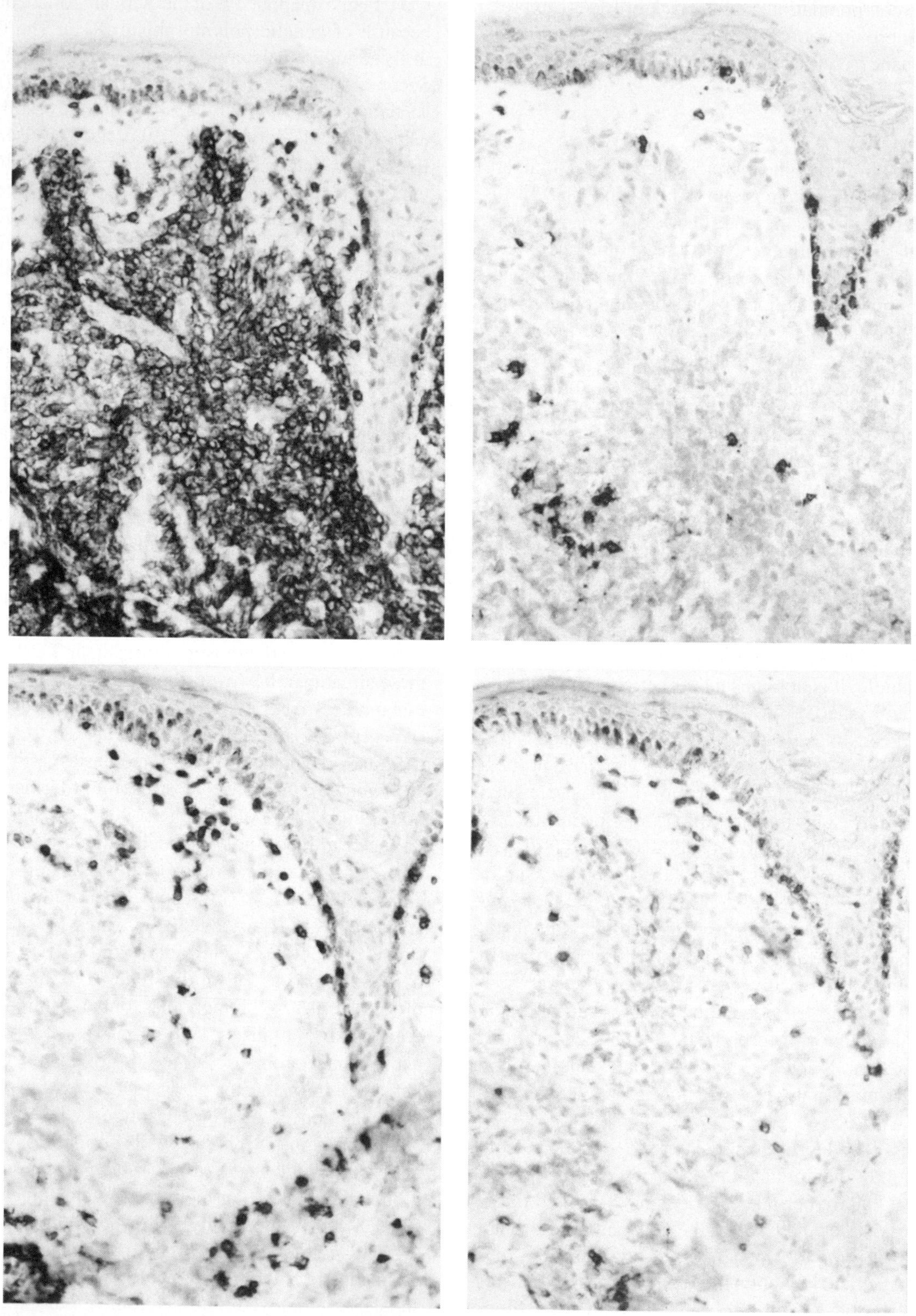

A B C D

FIG. 3.63. Frozen tissue sections of a cutaneous T-cell lymphoma of non-mycosis fungoides type immunostained for CD4 (**A**), CD8 (**B**), CD3 (**C**), and CD5 (**D**) antigens by immunoperoxidase. Greater than 90% of the cells are CD4-positive and less than 5% are CD8-positive, indicating that the vast majority of the cells belong to the $CD4^+CD8^-$ subset. Less than 10% of the cells, presumably residual benign T cells, express pan-T cell antigens CD3 or CD5. Therefore, most of the $CD4^+CD8^-$ cells lack two pan-T cell antigens that are expressed by essentially all normal T cells. The combination of marked subset antigen restriction and pan-T cell antigen deletion is strong evidence in support of a diagnosis of T-cell lymphoma (immunoperoxidase stain, original magnification: 100× magnification).

disorder with a benign indolent course in the majority of patients (1671,1672).

Although these immunophenotypic criteria are useful in the immunodiagnosis of T-cell neoplasia, no immunophenotypic marker of T-cell clonality, comparable to immunoglobulin light chain isotypic exclusion to infer B-cell clonality (6,44–47), exists. It is not always possible to distinguish between certain clinicopathologic entities that share overlapping morphologic and immunophenotypic characteristics such as peripheral T-cell lymphoma and mixed cellularity Hodgkin's disease or to determine if an abnormal peripheral blood or lymphoid tissue CD4:CD8 ratio represents a clonal neoplastic expansion of one T-cell subset or merely a quantitative alteration in the normal T-cell subpopulations. The presence of residual benign T and B cells within a T-cell neoplasm may obscure the immunophenotypic identification of neoplastic T cells and the application of these immunodiagnostic criteria. In these instances, it is often necessary to perform immunophenotypic analysis in paraffin tissue sections and correlate the findings with those of cell suspension or frozen tissue section immunophenotypic analysis or, alternatively, to employ immunogenotypic approaches (see Chapter 9).

New immunophenotypic criteria useful in the immunodiagnosis of T-cell neoplasia most likely will emerge in the future. For example, studies suggest that the TCR β chain uses a limited number of variable-region segments that rarely if ever are altered by somatic mutations (1673). The product of these variable-region segments can be identified with MAbs (1674). Each MAb that detects a particular variable-region segment or family reacts with a small proportion, approximately 5%, of normal peripheral T cells. Eventually, it should be possible to produce a panel of variable region–specific MAbs that identify most or possibly all T-cell specificities (1674). Each individual MAb in such a panel would react with only a subset of T cells in benign polyclonal T-cell proliferations but would react with a large proportion of the T cells making up an individual T-cell neoplasm.

Hodgkin's Disease

The lesional tissue of Hodgkin's disease usually consists predominantly of host response cells (T cells, B cells, plasma cells, histiocytes, neutrophils, eosinophils) and generally contains only small numbers of Reed-Sternberg cells and Reed-Sternberg cell variants, i.e., the malignant cell of Hodgkin's disease (1675–1677). The majority of patients with nodular sclerosis and mixed cellularity Hodgkin's disease has a proponderance of T cells that can comprise 80% or more of the total lymphocyte population (1659,1678,1679). Patients with lymphocyte predominance Hodgkin's disease usually contain smaller numbers of T cells and larger numbers of B cells (508,1680). In each instance, however, the T cells express all of the pan-T cell associated antigens, and both CD4 and CD8 T-cell subsets are represented, although the CD4:CD8 ratio often is increased beyond 4.0 (1659). Both κ and λ light chain–positive B cells usually are present in the normal ratio. The immunophenotypic profile of the Reed-Sternberg cell and its variants has been well documented and includes expression of MHC class II antigens, CD15, CD25, and CD30, as well as B-cell lineage–associated antigens in some instances (334–337,1380,1385,1423) (Figs. 3.44–3.46). In general, however, Reed-Sternberg cells and variants are present only in very small numbers, if at all, in cell suspensions prepared from tissue involved by Hodgkin's disease. The immunophenotypic identification of these cells in frozen tissue sections often is complicated by the inability to unequivocally identify them morphologically; also, they may be obscured by the more abundant cellular elements that surround them in immunostained frozen tissue sections. In cell suspensions and in frozen tissue sections, the immunophenotypic characteristics of tissue involved by Hodgkin's disease often overlap those of benign, reactive lymphoid proliferations (1659). For these reasons, the immunodiagnosis of Hodgkin's disease and its differentiation from the benign lymphoproliferative disorders and various B- and T-cell NHLs that simulate Hodgkin's disease usually is best performed by immunophenotypic analysis of paraffin tissue sections (see Chapters 17, 18).

SUMMARY AND CONCLUSIONS

Immunophenotypic analysis emerged as an ancillary technique in the diagnosis and classification of malignant lymphomas and lymphoid leukemias in the early 1970s. At that time, such analyses consisted of the detection of sIg or cIg to identify B cells and the demonstration of sheep E rosette formation to identify T cells. Subsequently, other phenotypic markers, such as HLA-DR antigen, Fc receptors, CRs, CALLA, and TdT, were described and utilized. The application of these markers to the study of hematopoietic neoplasms led to the demonstration that the majority of NHLs and lymphoid leukemias are of B- or T-cell origin, that so-called histiocytic lymphomas are also usually of B- or T-cell and only rarely of true histiocytic origin, and that T-cell neoplasms are broadly divisable into thymic and postthymic categories. These phenotypic markers also found a role in the diagnosis, classification, and prognosis of hematopoietic neoplasms.

The modern era of immunophenotypic analysis began in the early 1980s with the commercial availability of MAbs, highly specific and sensitive reagents capable of detecting B-cell, T-cell, monocyte/macrophage, and myeloid lineage–associated as well as subset and differentiation-associated antigens. The only drawback to the use of these reagents generally has been the requirement that they be applied to freshly isolated viable cells in suspension or frozen tissue. During the past several years, however, antigen-retrieval immunohistochemical techniques and a wide spectrum of MAbs that detect antigens in routinely processed, fixed, and paraffin-embedded tissue have been developed. The availability of these reagents and techniques worldwide has led to a large collective experience in the immunophenotypic analysis of normal and malignant hematopoietic cells by flow cytometry and by the immunohistochemical staining of frozen and paraffin tissue sections. The result is that normal hematopoietic cells and the neoplasms derived from these cells have become well characterized immunophenotypically, and the constellation of immunophenotypic features that characterize them has been delineated. In many instances, these immunophenotypic profiles are sufficiently characteristic of a particular category of hematopoietic neoplasia to be helpful in diagnosis and classification. This has had important clinical implications. Many of these MAbs also define surface membrane and cytoplasmic molecules that serve important biologic functions; immunophenotypic analysis also has played a role in improving our understanding of normal lymphocyte biology and physiology. The principal characteristics of the major MAb-defined antigens and their distribution of reactivity on benign and malignant hematopoietic cells are summarized in this chapter.

ACKNOWLEDGMENTS

The author gives thanks and sincere appreciation to Drs. Amy Chadburn and Elizabeth Hyjek for supplying many of the photomicrographs; Awilda Melendez-Cruz, Carol Taymor, and Susan Roman for assistance in preparing the manuscript; and to Al Lamme, FBPA, and Scientific Photographic Services, Edgewater, New Jersey, for preparing the photomicrographs and figures.

REFERENCES

1. Rappaport H. Tumors of the hematopoietic system. In: *Atlas of tumor pathology*, section 3, fascicle 8. Washington: US Armed Forces Institute of Pathology, 1966.
2. Chess L, Schlossman SF. Human lymphocyte subpopulations. *Adv Immunol* 1977;25:213–241.
3. Mann RB, Jaffe ES, Berard CW. Malignant lymphoma: a conceptual understanding of morphologic diversity. *Am J Pathol* 1979;94: 105–192.
4. Knowles DM. Non-Hodgkin's lymphomas: I. Immunologic and enzymatic markers useful in their evaluation. In: Fenoglio CM, Wolff M, eds. *Progress in surgical pathology,* vol 2. New York: Masson Publishing, 1980;71–105.
5. Knowles DM. Non-Hodgkin's lymphomas: II. Current immunologic concepts. In: Fenoglio CM, Wolff M, eds. *Progress in surgical pathology,* vol 2. New York: Masson Publishing, 1980;107–143.
6. Knowles DM. Lymphoid cell markers: their distribution and usefulness in the immunophenotypic analyses of lymphoid neoplasms. *Am J Surg Pathol* 1985;9[Suppl]:85–108.
7. Foon KA, Todd RF. Immunologic classification of leukemia and lymphoma. *Blood* 1986;68:1–31.
8. Freedman AS, Nadler LM. Cell surface markers in hematologic malignancies. *Semin Oncol* 1987;14:193–212.
9. Griffin JD. The use of monoclonal antibodies in the characterization of myeloid leukemias. *Hematol Pathol* 1987;1:81–91.
10. Hsu SM, Raine L, Fanger H. Use of avidin-biotin-peroxidase complex (ABC) in immunoperoxidase techniques: a comparison between ABC and unlabeled antibody (PAP) procedures. *J Histochem Cytochem* 1981;29:577–580.
11. Hsu SM, Raine L, Fanger N. The use of anti-avidin antibody and avidin-biotin-peroxidase complex in immunoperoxidase techniques. *Am J Clin Pathol* 1981;75:816–821.
12. Cordell JL, Falini B, Erber WN, et al. Immunoenzymatic labeling of monoclonal antibodies using immune complexes of alkaline phosphatase and monoclonal anti-alkaline phosphatase (APAAP) complexes. *J Histochem Cytochem* 1984;32:219–229.
13. Knowles DM. The human T-cell leukemias: clinical, cytomorphologic, immunophenotypic, and genotypic characteristics. *Hum Pathol* 1986;17:14–33.
14. Knowles DM. Immunophenotypic and antigen receptor gene rearrangement analysis in T cell neoplasia. *Am J Pathol* 1989;134: 761–785.
15. Bernard A, Boumsell L, Hill C. Joint report of the First International Workshop on Human Leucocyte Differentiation Antigens by the investigators of the participating laboratories. In: Bernard A, Boumsell L, Dausset J, et al, eds. *Leukocyte typing: human leucocyte differentiation antigens selected by monoclonal antibodies.* New York: Springer-Verlag, 1984.
16. Reinherz EL, Haynes BF, Nadler LM, et al, eds. *Leukocyte typing II*, vols I–III, New York: Springer-Verlag, 1986.
17. McMichael AJ, Beverley PCL, Cobbold S, et al, eds. *Leukocyte typing III: white cell differentiation antigens.* Oxford: Oxford University Press, 1987.
18. Knapp W, Dorken B, Gilks WR, et al, eds. *Leukocyte typing IV: white cell differentiation antigens.* New York: Oxford University Press, 1989.
19. Schlossman SF, Boumsell L, Gilks WR, et al, eds. *Leukocyte typing V: white cell differentiation antigens.* New York: Oxford University Press, 1995.
20. Kishimoto T, Kikutani H, von dem Borne AEGK, et al, eds. *Leukocyte typing VI: white cell differentiation antigens.* New York: Garland Publishing, 1998.
21. Hijmans W, Schmit HRE, Klein F. An immunofluorescence procedure for the detection of intracellular immunoglobulins. *Clin Exp Immunol* 1969;4:457–472.
22. Bollum FJ. Terminal deoxynucleotidyl transferase. In: Boyer PD, ed. *The enzymes*, vol 10. New York: Academic Press, 1974:145–171.
23. Stashenko P, Nadler LM, Hardy R, et al. Characterization of a human B lymphocyte specific antigen. *J Immunol* 1980;125:1678–1685.
24. Nadler L, Ritz J, Hardy R, et al. A unique cell surface antigen identifying lymphoid malignancies of B cell origin. *J Clin Invest* 1981; 67:134–140.
25. Cartun RW, Coles FB, Pastuszak WT. Utilization of monoclonal antibody L26 in the identification and confirmation of B-cell lymphomas: a sensitive and specific marker applicable to formalin- and B5-fixed, paraffin-embedded tissues. *Am J Pathol* 1987;129: 415–421.
26. Taylor CR, Mason DY. The immunohistological detection of intracellular immunoglobulin in formalin-paraffin sections from multiple myeloma and related conditions using the immunoperoxidase technique. *Clin Exp Immunol* 1974;18:417–429.
27. Warnke RA, Gatter KC, Falini B, et al. Diagnosis of human lymphoma with monoclonal antileukocyte antibodies. *N Engl J Med* 1983;309:1275–1281.
28. Gown AM, de Wever N, Battifora H. Microwave-based antigenic unmasking: a revolutionary new technique for routine immunohistochemistry. *Appl Immunohistochem* 1993;1:256–266.
29. Pernis B. Lymphocyte membrane immunoglobulins: an overview. In: Littman GW, Good RA, eds. *Immunoglobulins.* New York: Plenum Press, 1978:359–372.
30. Abney ER, Cooper MD, Kearney JF, et al. Sequential expression of immunoglobulin on developing mouse B lymphocytes: a systematic survey that suggests a model for the generation of immunoglobulin isotype diversity. *J Immunol* 1978;120:2041–2049.
31. Fu SM, Winchester RJ, Kunkel HG. Occurrence of IgM, IgD and free light chains on human lymphocytes. *J Exp Med* 1974;139:451–456.
32. Winchester RJ, Fu SM, Hoffman TJ, et al. IgG on lymphocyte surfaces: technical problems and the significance of a third cell population. *J Immunol* 1975;114:1210–1212.
33. Gathings WE, Kubagawa H, Cooper M. A distinctive pattern of B cell immaturity in perinatal humans. *Immunol Rev* 1981;57:107–126.
34. Rowe DS, Hug K, Forni L, et al. Immunoglobulin D as a lymphocyte receptor. *J Exp Med* 1973;138:965–972.
35. Fu SM, Winchester RJ, Feizi T, et al. Idiotypic specificity of surface

immunoglobulin and the maturation of leukemic bone marrow derived lymphocytes. *Proc Natl Acad Sci USA* 1974;71:4487–4490.
36. Fu SM, Winchester RJ, Kunkel HG. Similar idiotype specificity for the membrane IgD and IgM of human B lymphocytes. *J Immunol* 1975;114:250–252.
37. Black SJ, Van der Loo W, et al. Expression of IgD by murine lymphocytes: loss of surface IgD indicates maturation of memory B cells. *J Exp Med* 1978;147:984–996.
38. Winchester RJ: Technique of surface immunofluorescence applied to the analysis of the lymphocyte. In: Bloom BR, David JR, eds. *In vitro methods in cell-mediated and tumor immunity.* New York: Academic Press, 1976:171–186.
39. Winchester RJ, Ross GD. Methods for enumerating lymphocyte populations. In: Rose NR, Fredman J, eds. *Manual of clinical immunology.* Washington: American Society for Microbiology, 1980: 213–228.
40. Knowles DM, Winchester RJ, Kunkel HG. A comparison of peroxidase and fluorochrome conjugated antisera for the demonstration of surface and intracellular antigens. *Clin Immunol Immunopathol* 1977;7:410–425.
41. Preud'homme JL, Gugliemi P, Labaume S. Lymphocyte markers in human leukemias and lymphomas: methodologic remarks. *Semin Hematol* 1984;21:296–301.
42. Lukes RJ, Taylor CR, Parker JW, et al. A morphologic and immunologic surface marker study of 299 cases of non-Hodgkin's lymphomas and related leukemias. *Am J Pathol* 1978;90:461–486.
43. Lukes RJ, Parker JW, Taylor CR, et al. Immunologic approach to non Hodgkin's lymphomas and related leukemias: analysis of the results of multiparameter studies of 425 cases. *Semin Hematol* 1978; 15:322–335.
44. Tubbs RR, Fishleder A, Weiss RA, et al. Immunohistologic cellular phenotypes of lymphoproliferative disorders: comprehensive evaluation of 564 cases including 257 non-Hodgkin's lymphomas classified by the International Working Formulation. *Am J Pathol* 1983;113: 207–221.
45. Levy R, Warnke R, Dorfman RF, et al. The monoclonality of human B cell lymphomas. *J Exp Med* 1977;145:1014–1028.
46. Brubaker DB, Whiteside TL. Differentiation between benign and malignant human lymph nodes by means of immunologic markers. *Cancer* 1979;43:1165–1176.
47. Knowles DM, Halper JP, Jakobiec FA. The immunologic characterization of 40 extranodal lymphoid infiltrates: usefulness in distinguishing between benign pseudolymphoma and malignant lymphoma. *Cancer* 1982;49: 2321–2335.
48. Preud'homme JL, Seligmann M. Surface bound immunoglobulin as a cell marker in human lymphoproliferative diseases. *Blood* 1972; 40:777–794.
49. Landaas TO, Godal T, Marton PF, et al. Cell-associated immunoglobulin in human non-Hodgkin lymphomas. *Acta Pathol Microbiol Scand Sect A* 1981;89:91–101.
50. Kluin-Nelemans HC, Krouwels MM, Jansen JH, et al. Hairy cell leukemia preferentially expresses the IgG3 subclass. *Blood* 1990; 75:972–975.
51. Vogler LB, Crist WM, Bockman DE, et al. Pre-B-cell leukemia: a new phenotype of childhood lymphoblastic leukemia. *N Engl J Med* 1978;298:972–978.
52. Pernis B, Forni L, Amante L. Immunoglobulins as cell receptors. *Ann NY Acad Sci* 1971;190:420–429.
53. Pinkus GS, Said JW. Specific identification of intracellular immunoglobulin in paraffin sections of multiple myeloma and macroglobulinemia using an immunoperoxidase technique. *Am J Pathol* 1977; 87:47–58.
54. Wood GS, Warnke RA. The immunologic phenotype of bone marrow biopsies and aspirates: frozen section techniques. *Blood* 1982; 59:913–922.
55. Lay WH, Mendes NF, Bianco C, et al. Binding of sheep red blood cells to a large population of human lymphocytes. *Nature* 1971;230: 531–532.
56. Jondal M, Holm G, Wigzell H. Surface markers on human T and B lymphocytes: I. A large population of lymphocytes forming nonimmune rosettes with sheep red blood cells. *J Exp Med* 1972;136: 207–215.
57. Wybran J, Carr MC, Fudenberg HH. The human rosette forming cell as a marker of a population of thymus-derived cells. *J Clin Invest* 1972;51:2537–2543.
58. Hoffman T, Kunkel HG. The E rosette test. In: Bloom BR, David JR, eds. *In vitro methods in cell-mediated and tumor immunity.* New York: Academic Press, 1976;71–82.
59. Bloom BR, Cohn ZA, David J, et al. Evaluation of in vitro methods for characterization of lymphocytes and macrophages. In: Bloom BR, David JR, eds. *In vitro methods in cell-mediated and tumor immunity.* New York: Academic Press, 1976;3–25.
60. Borella L, Sen L. E receptors on blasts from untreated acute lymphocytic leukemia (ALL): comparison of temperature dependence of E rosettes formed by normal and leukemic lymphoid cells. *J Immunol* 1975;114:187–190.
61. Siegal FP, Filippa DA, Koziner B. Surface markers in leukemias and lymphomas. *Am J Pathol* 1978;90:451–460.
62. Kaplan ME, Woodson M, Clark C. Detection of human T lymphocytes by rosette formation with AET-treated sheep red cells. In: Bloom BR, David JR, eds. *In vitro methods in cell-mediated and tumor immunity.* New York: Academic Press, 1976;83–88.
63. Mahowald ML, Handweiger BS, Capertone IM, et al. A comparative study of procedures for sheep erythrocyte-human T lymphocyte rosette formation. *J Immunol Methods* 1977;15:239–245.
64. Edelson RL, Smith RW, Frank MM, et al. Identification of subpopulations of mononuclear cells in cutaneous infiltrates: I. Differentiation between B cells, T cells and histiocytes. *J Invest Dermatol* 1973;61:82–89.
65. Frank MM, Jaffe ES, Green I. Detection of specific mononuclear cell receptors in tissue sections. In: Bloom BR, David JR, eds. *In vitro methods in cell-mediated and tumor immunity.* New York: Academic Press, 1976;203–215.
66. Kamoun MP, Martin PJ, Hansen JA, et al. Identification of a human T-lymphocyte surface protein associated with the E-rosette receptor. *J Exp Med* 1981;153:207–212.
67. Howard FD, Ledbetter JA, Wong J, et al. A human T lymphocyte differentiation marker defined by monoclonal antibodies that block E-rosette formation. *J Immunol* 1981;126:2117–2122.
68. Verbi W, Greaves M, Schneider C, et al. Monoclonal antibodies OKT11 and OKT11A have pan-T reactivity and block sheep erythrocyte "receptors." *Eur J Immunol* 1981;12:81–86.
69. Bernard A, Gelin C, Raynal B, et al. Phenomenon of human T-cells rosetting with sheep erythrocytes analyzed with monoclonal antibodies. *J Exp Med* 1982;155:1317–1333.
70. Basten A, Miller J, Sprent J, et al. A receptor for antibody on B lymphocytes: I. Method of detection and functional significance. *J Exp Med* 1972;135:610–626.
71. Moretta L, Ferrarini M, Mingeri MC, et al. Subpopulations of human T cells identified by receptors for immunoglobulin and mitogen responsiveness. *J Immunol* 1976;117:2171–2174.
72. Moretta L, Webb SR, Grossi CE, et al. Functional analysis of two human T-cell subpopulations: help and suppression of B-cell responses by T cells bearing receptors for IgM or IgG. *J Exp Med* 1977;146:184–200.
73. Perlmann P, Perlmann H, Muller-Eberhard HJ. Cytolytic lymphocytic cells with complement receptor in human blood: induction of cytolysis by IgG antibody but not by target cell bound C3. *J Exp Med* 1975;141:287–296.
74. Winchester RJ, Fu SM, Wernet P, et al. Recognition by pregnancy serums of non-HL-A alloantigens selectively expressed on B lymphocytes. *J Exp Med* 1975;141:924–929.
75. Chess L, Evans R, Humphryes RE, et al. Inhibition of antibody dependent cellular cytoxicity and immunoglobulin synthesis by an antiserum prepared against a human B-cell Ia-like molecule. *J Exp Med* 1976;144:113–122.
76. Arbeit RD, Henkart PA, Dickler HB. Lymphocyte binding of heat-aggregated and antigen complexed immunoglobulin. In: Bloom BR, David JR, eds. *In vitro methods in cell-mediated and tumor immunity.* New York: Academic Press, 1976:143–154.
77. Froland SS, Wisloff F. A rosette technique for identification of human lymphocytes with Fc receptors. In: Bloom BR, David JR, eds. *In vitro methods in cell-mediated and tumor immunity.* New York: Academic Press, 1976;137–142.
78. Winchester RJ, Hoffman T, Ferrarini M, et al. Comparison of various tests for Fc receptors on different human lymphocyte subpopulations. *Clin Exp Immunol* 1979;37:126–133.

79. Dickler HB, Kunkel HG: Interaction of aggregated gammaglobulin with B lymphocytes. *J Exp Med* 1972;136:191–196.
80. Dickler HB. Studies of the human lymphocyte receptor for heat-aggregated or antigen complexed immunoglobulin. *J Exp Med* 1974; 140:508–522.
81. Huber H, Douglas SD, Fudenberg HH. The IgG receptor: an immunological marker for the characterization of mononuclear cells. *Immunology* 1969;17:7–21.
82. Bianco C, Patrick R, Nussenzweig V. A population of lymphocytes bearing a membrane receptor for antigen-antibody-complement complexes: I. Separation and characterization. *J Exp Med* 1970;132: 702–720.
83. Dukor P, Bianco C, Nussenzweig V. Tissue localization of lymphocytes bearing a membrane receptor for antigen-antibody-complement complexes. *Proc Natl Acad Sci USA* 1970;67:991–997.
84. Eden A, Miller GW, Nussenzweig V. Human lymphocytes bear membrane receptors for C3b and C3d. *J Clin Invest* 1973;52: 3239–3242.
85. Reynolds HY, Atkinson, JP, Newball HH, et al. Receptors for immunoglobulin and complement on human alveolar macrophages. *J Immunol* 1975;114:1813–1819.
86. Ross GD, Polley MJ, Rabellino EM, et al. Two different complement receptors on human lymphocytes: one specific for C3b and one specific for C3b inactivator cleaved C3b. *J Exp Med* 1973;138:798–811.
87. Ross GD, Polley MJ. Detection of complement receptor lymphocytes (CRL). In: Bloom BR, David JR, eds. *In vitro methods in cell-mediated and tumor immunity.* New York: Academic Press, 1976; 123–136.
88. Dykman TR, Cole JL, Iida K, et al. Polymorphism of human erythrocyte C3b/C4b receptor. *Proc Natl Acad Sci USA* 1983;80: 1698–1702.
89. Dykman TR, Hatch JA, Atkinson JP. Polymorphism of the human C3b/C4b receptor: identification of a third allele and analysis of receptor phenotypes in families and patients with systemic lupus erythematosus. *J Exp Med* 1984;159:691–703.
90. Medof ME, Iida K, Mold C, et al Unique role of the complement receptor CR1 in the degradation of C3b associated with immune complexes. *J Exp Med* 1982;156:1739–1754.
91. Cooper NR. Immune adherence by the fourth component of complement. *Science* 1969;165:396–398.
92. Fearon DT, Wong WW. Complement ligand-receptor interactions that mediate biological responses. *Ann Rev Immunol* 1983;1: 243–271.
93. Heinen E, Lilet-Leclercq C, Mason DY, et al. Isolation of follicular dendritic cells from human tonsils and adenoids: II. Immunocytochemical characterization. *Eur J Immunol* 1984;14:267–273.
94. Reynes M, Aubert JP, Cohen JHM, et al. Human follicular dendritic cells express CR1, CR2, and CR3 complement receptor antigens. *J Immunol* 1985;135:2687–2694.
95. Hogg N, Horton MA. Myeloid antigens: new and previously defined clusters. In: McMichael AJ, Beverley PCL, Cobbold S, et al, eds. *Leucocyte typing III: white cell differentiation antigens.* Oxford: Oxford University Press, 1987;576–621.
96. Iida K, Nadler LM, Nussenzweig V. Identification of the membrane receptor for the complement C3d by means of a monoclonal antibody. *J Exp Med* 1983;158:1021–1033.
97. Weis JJ, Tedder TF, Fearon DT. Identification of a 145,000 Mr membrane protein as the C3d receptor (CR2) of human B lymphocytes. *Proc Natl Acad Sci USA* 1984;81:881–885.
98. Fingeroth JD, Weis JJ, Tedder TF, et al. Epstein-Barr virus receptor of human B lymphocytes is the C3d receptor CR2. *Proc Natl Acad Sci USA* 1984;81:4510–4514.
99. Tedder TF, Clement LT, Cooper MD. Expression of C3d receptors during human B cell differentiation: immunofluorescence analysis with the HB-5 monoclonal antibody. *J Immunol* 1984;133:678–683.
100. Boyd AW, Anderson KC, Freedman AS, et al. Studies of in vitro activation and differentiation of human B lymphocytes: I. Phenotypic and functional characterization of the B cell population responding to anti-Ig antibody. *J Immunol* 1985;134:1516–1523.
101. Zola H. The surface antigens of human B lymphocytes. *Immunol Today* 1987;8:308–315.
102. Nadler LM. B cell/leukemia panel workshop: summary and comments. In: Reinherz EL, Haynes BF, Nadler LM, et al, eds. *Leucocyte typing II*, vol 2. New York: Springer Verlag, 1986:3–43.
103. Nadler LM, Stashenko P, Hardy R, et al. Characterization of a human B cell-specific antigen (B2) distinct from B1. *J Immunol* 1981;126: 1941–1947.
104. Mittler RS, Talle MA, Carpenter K, et al. Generation and characterization of monoclonal antibodies reactive with human B lymphocytes. *J Immunol* 1983;131:1754–1761.
105. Knowles DM, Tolidjian B, Marboe CC, et al. Distribution of antigens defined by OKB monoclonal antibodies on benign and malignant lymphoid cells and on nonlymphoid tissues. *Blood* 1984;63: 886–896.
106. Arnaout MA, Todd RF, Dana N, et al. Inhibition of phagocytosis of complement C3- or immunoglobulin G-coated particles and of C3bi binding by monoclonal antibodies to a monocyte-granulocyte membrane glycoprotein (Mo1). *J Clin Invest* 1983;72:171–179.
107. Wright SD, Weitz JI, Huang AJ, et al. Complement receptor type three (CD11b/CD18) of human polymorphonuclear leukocytes recognizes fibrinogen. *Proc Natl Acad Sci USA* 1988;85: 7734–7738.
108. Sanchez-Madrid F, Nagy JA, Robbins E, et al. A human leukocyte differentiation antigen family with distinct α-subunits and a common β-subunit: the lymphocyte function-associated antigen (LFA-1), the C3bi complement receptor (OKM1/Mac-1), and the p150,95 molecule. *J Exp Med* 1983;158:1785–1803.
109. Breard J, Reinherz EL, Kung PC, et al. A monoclonal antibody reactive with human peripheral blood monocytes. *J Immunol* 1980; 124:1943–1948.
110. Todd RF, Nadler LM, Schlossman SF. Antigens on human monocytes identified by monoclonal antibodies. *J Immunol* 1981;126: 1435–1442.
111. Bernstein ID, Self S. Joint report of the myeloid section of the Second International Workshop on Human Leukocyte Differentiation Antigens. In: Reinherz EL, Haynes BF, Nadler LM, et al, eds. *Leukocyte typing II: human myeloid and hematopoietic cells*, vol 3. New York: Springer Verlag, 1986:1–25.
112. Griffin JD, Ritz J, Nadler LM, et al. Expression of myeloid differentiation antigens on normal and malignant myeloid cells. *J Clin Invest* 1981;68:932–941.
113. Ortaldo JR, Sharrow SO, Timonen T, et al. Determination of surface antigens in highly purified human NK cells by flow cytometry with monoclonal antibodies. *J Immunol* 1981;127:2401–2409.
114. Peterson RC, Cheung LC, Mattaliano RJ, et al. Molecular cloning of human terminal deoxynucleotidyl transferase. *Proc Natl Acad Sci USA* 1984;81:4363–4367.
115. McCaffrey R, Smoler DF, Baltimore D. Terminal deoxynucleotidyl transferase in a case of childhood acute lymphoblastic leukemia. *Proc Natl Acad Sci USA* 1973; 70:523–525.
116. Bollum FJ. Terminal deoxynucleotidyl transferase as a hematopoietic cell marker. *Blood* 1979;54:1203–1215.
117. Bollum FJ. Terminal transferase: past to present. In: Bertazzoni U, Bollum FJ, eds. *Terminal transferase in immunobiology and leukemia.* New York: Plenum Press, 1982;1–11.
118. Waldmann TA. The arrangement of immunoglobulin and T cell receptor genes in human lymphoproliferative disorders. *Adv Immunol* 1987;40:247–321.
119. Clavers H, Alarcon B, Wileman T, et al. The T cell receptor/CD3 complex: a dynamic protein ensemble. *Annu Rev Immunol* 1988;6: 629–662.
120. Alt FW, Oltz EM, Young F, et al. VDJ recombination. *Immunol Today* 1992;13:306–314.
121. Alt FW, Baltimore D. Joining of immunoglobulin heavy chain gene segments: implications from a chromosome with evidence of three D-JH fusions. *Proc Natl Acad Sci USA* 1982;79:4118–4122.
122. Baltimore D. Is terminal deoxynucleotidyl transferase a somatic mutagen in lymphocytes? *Nature* 1974;248:409–411.
123. Desiderio SV, Yancopoulos GD, Paskind M, et al. Insertion of N regions into heavy-chain genes is correlated with expression of terminal deoxytransferase in B cells. *Nature* 1984;311:752–755.
124. Landau NR, Schatz DG, Rosa M, et al. Increased frequency of N-region insertion in a murine pre-B cell line infected with a terminal deoxynucleotidyl transferase retroviral expression vector. *Mol Cell Biol* 1987;7:3237–3243.
125. Bonati A, Zanelli P, Ferrari S, et al. TCR β-chain gene rearrangement and expression during human thymic ontogenesis. *Blood* 1992;79: 1472–1483.
126. Silverstone AE, Cantor H, Goldstein G, et al. Terminal deoxynucleo-

tidyl transferase is found in prothymocytes. *J Exp Med* 1976;144: 543–548.
127. McCaffrey R, Harrison TA, Parkman P, et al. Terminal deoxynucleotidyl transferase activity in human leukemic cells and in normal thymocytes. *N Engl J Med* 1975;292:775–780.
128. McCaffrey RP. Case records of the Massachusetts General Hospital: weekly clinicopathological exercises. *N Engl J Med* 1978;299: 296–303.
129. Chilosi M, Pizzolo G. Review of terminal deoxynucleotidyl transferase: biological aspects, methods of detection, and selected diagnostic applications. *Appl Immunohistochem* 1995;3:209–221.
130. Bearman RM, Winberg CD, Maslow WC, et al. Terminal deoxynucleotidyl transferase activity in neoplastic and non-neoplastic hematopoietic cells. *Am J Clin Pathol* 1981;75:794–802.
131. Muehleck SD, McKenna RW, Gale PF, et al. Terminal deoxynucleotidyl transferase (TdT)-positive cells in bone marrow in the absence of hematologic malignancy. *Am J Clin Pathol* 1983;79:277–284.
132. Pahwa RN, Modak MJ, McMorrow T, et al. Terminal deoxynucleotidyl transferase (TdT) enzyme in thymus and bone marrow: I. Age-associated decline of TdT in humans and mice. *Cell Immunol* 1981; 58:39–48.
133. Chilosi M, Pizzolo G, Fiore-Donati L, et al. Routine immunofluorescent and histochemical analysis of bone marrow involvement by lymphoma/leukemia: the use of cryostat sections. *Br J Cancer* 1983; 48:763–775.
134. Janossy G, Thomas JA, Bollum FJ, et al. The human thymic microenvironment: an immunohistologic study. *J Immunol* 1980;125: 202–212.
135. Janossy G, Bofill M, Trejdosiewicz LK, et al. Cellular differentiation of lymphoid subpopulations and their microenvironments in the human thymus. In: Muller-Hermelink HK, ed. *The human thymus: histopathology and pathology*. Berlin: Springer-Verlag, 1986; 89–125.
136. Boyd RL, Tucek CL, Godfrey DI, et al. The thymic microenvironment. *Immunol Today* 1993;14:445–459.
137. Reinherz EL, Kung PC, Goldstein G, et al. Discrete stages of human intrathymic differentiation: analysis of normal thymocytes and leukemic lymphoblasts of T-cell lineage. *Proc Natl Acad Sci USA* 1980; 77:1588–1592.
138. Kung PC, Long JC, McCaffrey RP, et al. Terminal deoxynucleotidyl transferase in the diagnosis of leukemia and malignant lymphoma. *Am J Med* 1978;64:788–794.
139. Mertelsmann R, Mertelsmann I, Koziner B, et al. Improved biochemical assay for terminal deoxynucleotidyl transferase in human blood cells: results in 89 adult patients with lymphoid leukemias and malignant lymphomas in leukemic phase. *Leukemia* 1978;2:57–69.
140. Jaffe ES, Berard CW. Lymphoblastic lymphoma: a term rekindled with new precision. *Ann Intern Med* 1978;89:415–417.
141. Sarin PS, Anderson PN, Gallo RC. Terminal deoxynucleotidyl transferase activities in human blood leukocytes and lymphoblast cell lines: high levels in lymphoblast cell lines and in blast cells of some patients with chronic myelogenous leukemia in acute phase. *Blood* 1976;47:11–20.
142. Marks SM, Baltimore D, McCaffrey R. Terminal transferase as a predictor of initial responsiveness to vincristine and prednisone in blastic crisis chronic myelogenous leukemia. *N Engl J Med* 1978; 298:812–814.
143. Murphy S, Jaffe ES. Terminal transferase activity and lymphoblastic neoplasms. *N Engl J Med* 1984;311:1373–1374.
144. Weiss L, Bindl JM, Picozzi VJ, et al. Lymphoblastic lymphoma: an immunophenotype study of 26 cases with comparison to T cell acute lymphoblastic leukemia. *Blood* 1986;67:474–478.
145. Braziel RM, Keneklis T, Donlon JA, et al. Terminal deoxynucleotidyl transferase in non-Hodgkin's lymphoma. *Am J Clin Pathol* 1983; 80:655–659.
146. Cuttner J, Seremetis S, Najfeld V, et al. TdT-positive acute leukemia with monocytoid characteristics: clinical, cytochemical, cytogenetic, and immunologic findings. *Blood* 1984;64:237–243.
147. Stark AN, MacKarill ID, Limbert HJ, et al. TdT expression in acute myeloid leukemia. *Blut* 1988;56:33–38.
148. Stass S, Mirro J. Unexpected heterogeneity in acute leukemia: mixed lineages and lineage switch. *Hum Pathol* 1985;16:864–866.
149. Janossy G, Hoffbrand AV, Greaves MF, et al. Terminal transferase enzyme assay and immunological membrane markers in the diagnosis of leukemia: a multiparameter analysis of 300 cases. *Br J Haematol* 1980;44:221–234.
150. McGraw TP, Folds JD, Bollum FJ, et al. Terminal deoxynucleotidyl transferase-positive acute myeloblastic leukemia. *Am J Hematol* 1981;10:251–258.
151. Catovsky D, Cardullo L, O'Brien M, et al. Cytochemical markers of differentiation in acute leukemia. *Cancer Res* 1981;41:4824–4832.
152. Bradstock KF, Hoffbrand AV, Ganeshaguru K, et al. Terminal deoxynucleotidyl transferase expression in acute non-lymphoid leukemia: an analysis by immunofluorescence. *Br J Haematol* 1981;47: 133–143.
153. Bradstock KF, Pizzolo G, Papageorgiou ES, et al. Terminal transferase expression in relapsed acute myeloid leukaemia. *Br J Haematol* 1981;49:621–627.
154. Bradstock KF, Hewson J, Kerr A, et al. Expression of terminal deoxynucleotidyl transferase in malignant myeloblasts. *Am J Clin Pathol* 1983;80:800–805.
155. Benedetto P, Mertelsmann R , Szatrowski TH, et al. Prognostic significance of terminal deoxynucleotidyl transferase activity in acute nonlymphoblastic leukemia. *J Clin Oncol* 1986;4:489–495.
156. Parreira A, Pombo de Oliveira MS, Matutes E, et al. Terminal deoxynucleotidyl transferase positive acute myeloid leukemia: an association with immature myeloblastic leukemia. *Br J Haematol* 1988;69: 219–224.
157. Drexler HG, Sperling C, Wolf-Dieter L. Terminal deoxynucleotidyl transferase (TdT) expression in acute myeloid leukemia: review. *Leukemia* 1993;7:1142–1150.
158. Bradstock KF, Janossy G, Tidman N, et al. Immunological monitoring of residual disease in treated thymic acute lymphoblastic leukaemia. *Leuk Res* 1981;5:301–309.
159. Van Dongen JJM, Hooijkaas H, Adriaansen HJ, et al. Detection of minimal residual acute lymphoblastic leukemia by immunological marker analysis: possibilities and limitations. In: Hagenbeek A, Lowenberg B, eds. *Minimal residual disease in acute leukemia*. Dordecht: M. Nijhoff, 1986;113–121.
160. Campana D, Coustan-Smith E, Janossy G. The immunological detection of minimal residual disease in acute leukemia. *Blood* 1990;76: 163–171.
161. Campana D, Coustan-Smith E, Behm FG. The definition of remission in acute leukemia with immunologic techniques. *Bone Marrow Transplant* 1991;8:429–437.
162. Drach J, Drach D, Glassl H, et al. Flow cytometric determination of atypical antigen expression in acute leukemia for the study of minimal residual disease. *Cytometry* 1992;13:893–901.
163. Campana D. Monitoring minimal residual disease in acute leukemia: expectations, possibilities and initial clinical results. *Int J Clin Lab Res* 1994;24:47–59.
164. Hooijkaas H, Hahlen K, Adriaansen HJ, et al. Terminal deoxynucleotidyl transferase (TdT)-positive cells in cerebrospinal fluid and development of overt CNS leukemia: a 5-year follow-up study in 113 children with a TdT-positive leukemia or non-Hodgkin's lymphoma. *Blood* 1989;74:416–422.
165. Thomas JA, Janossy G, Eden OB, et al. Nuclear terminal deoxynucleotidyl transferase in leukaemic infiltrates of testicular tissue. *Br J Cancer* 1982;45:709–717.
166. Greaves MF. Differentiation-linked leukemogenesis in lymphocyte. *Science* 1986;234:697–704.
167. Beutler E, Kuhl W. An assay for terminal deoxynucleotidyl transferase in leukocytes and bone marrow. *Am J Clin Pathol* 1978;70: 733–737.
168. Stass SA, Schumacher HR, Keneklis TP, et al. Terminal deoxynucleotidyl transferase immunofluorescence of bone marrow smears: experience in 156 cases. *Am J Clin Pathol* 1979;72:898–903.
169. Janossy G, Thomas JA, Pizzolo G, et al. Immuno-histological diagnosis of lymphoproliferative diseases by selected combinations of antisera and monoclonal antibodies. *Br J Cancer* 1980;42:224–242.
170. Tidman N, Janossy G, Bodger M, et al. Delineation of human thymocyte differentiation pathways utilizing double-staining techniques with monoclonal antibodies. *Clin Exp Immunol* 1981;45:457–467.
171. Slaper-Cortenbach ICM, Admiraal LG, Kerr JM, et al. Flow-cytometric detection of terminal deoxynucleotidyl transferase and other intracellular antigens in combination with membrane antigens in acute lymphatic leukemias. *Blood* 1988;72:1639–1644.
172. Almasri NM, Iturraspe JA, Benson NA, et al. Flow cytometric analy-

sis of terminal deoxynucleotidyl transferase. *Am J Clin Pathol* 1991; 95:376–380.

173. Drach J, Gattringer C, Huber H. Combined flow cytometric assessment of cell surface antigens and nuclear TdT for the detection of minimal residual disease in acute leukaemia. *Br J Haematol* 1991; 77:37–42.
174. Syrjala MT, Tiirikainen M, Jansson SE, et al. Flow cytometric analysis of terminal deoxynucleotidyl transferase: a simplified method. *Am J Clin Pathol* 1993;99:298–303.
175. Pizzolo G, Vincenzi C, Nadali G, et al. Detection of membrane and intracellular antigens by flow cytometry following ORTHO Permeafix fixation. *Leukemia* 1994;8:672–676.
176. Fetterhoff TJ, McCarthy RC. Avidin-biotin amplification procedures for the detection of human terminal deoxynucleotidyl transferase in cell smears. *Am J Clin Pathol* 1985;83:565–570.
177. Stass SA, Dean L, Peiper SC, et al. Determination of terminal deoxynucleotidyl transferase on bone marrow smears by immunoperoxidase. *Am J Clin Pathol* 1982;77:174–176.
178. Erber WN, Mason DY. Immunoalkaline phosphatase labeling of terminal transferase in hematologic samples. *Am J Clin Pathol* 1987; 88:43–50.
179. Folds JD, Bollum FJ, Dean L, et al. Simultaneous evaluation for terminal deoxynucleotidyl transferase and myeloperoxidase in leukemia. *Am J Hematol* 1982;12:391–396.
180. Tavares de Castro J, San Miguel JF, et al. Method for the simultaneous labelling of terminal deoxynucleotidyl transferase (TdT) and membrane antigens. *J Clin Pathol* 1984;37:628–632.
181. Racklin B, Bearman R, Sheibani K, et al. The demonstration of terminal deoxynucleotidyl transferase on frozen tissue sections and smears by the avidin-biotin complex (ABC) method. *Leuk Res* 1983; 7:431–437.
182. Halverson CA, Falini B, Taylor CR, et al. Detection of terminal transferase in paraffin sections with the immunoperoxidase technique. *Am J Pathol* 1981;105:241–254.
183. Said JW, Shintaku IP, Pinkus GS. Immunohistochemical staining for terminal deoxynucleotidyl transferase (TdT): an enhanced method in routinely processed formalin-fixed tissue sections. *Am J Clin Pathol* 1988;89:649–652.
184. Leong AS-Y, Milios J. An assessment of the efficacy of the microwave antigen-retrieval procedure on a range of tissue antigens. *Appl Immunohistochem* 1993;1:267–274.
185. Orazi A, Cattoretti G, John K, et al. Terminal deoxynucleotidyl transferase staining of malignant lymphomas in paraffin sections. *Mod Pathol* 1994;7:582–586.
186. Greaves MF, Brown G, Rapson NT, et al. Antisera to acute lymphoblastic leukemia cells. *Clin Immunol Immunopathol* 1975;4:67–84.
187. Clavell LA, Lipton JM, Blast RC, et al. Absence of common ALL antigen on normal bipotent myeloid, erythroid and granulocytic progenitors. *Blood* 1981;58:333–336.
188. Ritz J, Nadler LM, Ghan AK, et al. Expression of common acute lymphoblastic leukemia antigen (cALLa) by lymphomas of B-cell and T-cell lineage. *Blood* 1981;58:648–652.
189. Greaves MF, Hariri G, Newman RA, et al. Selective expression of the common acute lymphoblastic leukemia (gp100) antigen on immature lymphoid cells and their malignant counterparts. *Blood* 1983;61:628–639.
190. Roberts M, Greaves M, Janossy G, et al. Acute lymphoblastic leukaemia (ALL) associated antigen: I. Expression in different haematopoietic malignancies. *Leuk Res* 1978;2:105–114.
191. Ritz J, Pesandro JM, Motis-McConarty J, et al. A monoclonal antibody to human acute lymphoblastic leukemia antigen. *Nature* 1980; 283:583–585.
192. LeBien TW, Boue DR, Bradley G, et al. Antibody affinity may influence antigenic modulation of the common acute lymphoblastic leukemia antigen in vitro. *J Immunol* 1982;129:2287–2292.
193. Knapp W, Majdic O, Bettelheim P, et al. VIL-A1, a monoclonal antibody reactive with common acute lymphatic leukemia cells. *Leuk Res* 1982;6:137–147.
194. Male D, Champion B, Cooke A. Class I and II molecules of the major histocompatibility complex. In: Male D, Champion B, Cooke A, eds. *Advanced immunology.* Philadelphia: JB Lippincott, 1987: 5.1–5.14.
195. Mann DL, Abelson L, Harris S, et al. Detection of antigens specific for B-lymphoid cultured cell lines with human alloantisera. *J Exp Med* 1975;142:84–89.
196. Winchester RJ, Wang CY, Halper JP, et al. Studies with B-cell allo- and heteroantisera: parallel reactivity and special properties. *Scand J Immunol* 1976;5:745–757.
197. Lampson LA, Levy R. Two populations of Ia-like molecules on a human B cell line. *J Immunol* 1980;125:293–299.
198. Nadler LM, Stashenko P, Hardy R, et al. Monoclonal antibody identifies a new Ia-like (p29,34) polymorphic system linked to the HLA-D/DR region. *Nature* 1981;290:591–593.
199. Natali PG, De Martino C, Quaranta V, et al. Expression of Ia-like antigens in normal human nonlymphoid tissues. *Transplantation* 1981;31:75–78.
200. Rowden G, Lewis MG, Sullivan AK. Ia antigen expression on human epidermal Langerhans cells. *Nature* 1977;268:247–248.
201. Klareskog L, Tjeinlund UM, Forsum U, et al. Epidermal Langerhans cells express Ia antigens. *Nature* 1977;268:248–250.
202. Hoffman T, Wang CY, Winchester RJ, et al. Human lymphocytes bearing "Ia-like" antigens; absence in patients with infantile agammaglobulinemia. *J Immunol* 1977;119:1520–1524.
203. Winchester RJ, Ross GD, Jarowski CI, et al. Expression of Ia-like antigen molecules on human granulocytes during early phases of differentiation. *Proc Natl Acad Sci USA* 1977;74:4012–4016.
204. Van Dongen JJM, Hooijkaas H, Comans-Bitter M, et al. Human bone marrow cells positive for terminal deoxynucleotidyl transferase (TdT), HLA-DR, and a T cell marker may represent prothymocytes. *J Immunol* 1985;135:3144–3150.
205. Halper J, Fu SM, Wang CY, et al. Patterns of expression of human "Ia-like" antigens during the terminal stages of B cell development. *J Immunol* 1978;120:1480–1484.
206. Winchester RJ, Meyers PA, Broxmeyer HE, et al. Inhibition of human erythropoietic colony formation in culture by treatment with Ia antisera. *J Exp Med* 1978;148:613–618.
207. Rabellino EM, Nachman RL, Williams W, et al. Human megakaryocytes: I. Characterization of the membrane and cytoplasmic components of isolated bone marrow megakaryocytes. *J Exp Med* 1979; 149:1273–1287.
208. Moore MAS, Broxmeyer HE, Sheridan APC, et al. Continuous human bone marrow culture: Ia antigen characterization of probable pluripotential stem cells. *Blood* 1980;55:682–690.
209. Belzer MB, Fitchen JH, Ferrone S, et al. Expression of Ia-like antigens on human erythroid progenitor cells as determined by monoclonal antibodies and heteroantiserum to Ia-like antigens. *Clin Immunol Immunopath* 1981;20:111–115.
210. Robinson J, Sieff C, Delia D, et al. Expression of cell-surface HLA-DR, HLA-ABC and glycophorin during erythroid differentiation. *Nature* 1981;289:68–71.
211. Fitchen JH, LeFevre C, Ferrone S, et al. Expression of Ia-like and HLA-A,B antigens on human multipotential hematopoietic progenitor cells. *Blood* 1982;59:188–190.
212. Foucar K, Foucar E. The mononuclear phagocyte and immunoregulatory effector (M-PIRE) system: evolving concepts. *Semin Diagn Pathol* 1990;7:4–18.
213. Steinman RM. The dendritic cell system and its role in immunogenicity. *Annu Rev Immunol* 1991;9:271–296.
214. Halper JP, Knowles DM, Wang CY. Ia antigen expression by human malignant lymphomas: correlation with conventional lymphoid markers. *Blood* 1980;55:373–382.
215. Evans RL, Faldetta TJ, Humphreys RE, et al. Peripheral human T cells sensitized in mixed leukocyte culture synthesize and express Ia-like antigens. *J Exp Med* 1978;148:1440–1445.
216. Fu SM, Chiorazzi N, Wang CY, et al. Ia–bearing T lymphocytes in man: their identification and role in the generation of allogeneic helper activity. *J Exp Med* 1978;148:1423–1428.
217. Yu DTY, Winchester RJ, Fu SM, et al. Peripheral blood Ia-positive T cells. Increases in certain diseases and after immunization. *J Exp Med* 1980;151:91–100.
218. Anderson KC, Bates MP, Slaughenhoupt BL, et al. Expression of human B cell-associated antigens on leukemias and lymphomas: a model of human B cell differentiation. *Blood* 1984;63:1424–1433.
219. Knowles DM, Dodson L, Burke JS, et al. sIg^{-} E^{-} ("null-cell") non-Hodgkin's lymphomas: multiparametric determination of their B- or T-cell lineage. *Am J Pathol* 1985;120:356–370.
220. Knowles DM, Inghirami G, Ubriaco A, et al. Molecular genetic

analysis of three AIDS-associated neoplasms of uncertain lineage demonstrates their B-cell derivation and the possible pathogenetic role of the Epstein-Barr virus. *Blood* 1989;73:792–799.
221. Pittaluga S, Raffeld M, Lipford EH, Cossman J. 3A1 (CD7) expression precedes T_β gene rearrangements in precursor T (lymphoblastic) neoplasms. *Blood* 1986;68:134–139.
222. Feller AC, Parwaresch MR, Stein H, et al. Immunophenotyping of T-lymphoblastic lymphoma/leukemia: correlation with normal T-cell maturation. *Leuk Res* 1986;10:1025–1031.
223. Haynes BF, Hensley LL, Jegasothy BV. Phenotypic characterization of skin-infiltrating T cells in cutaneous T cell lymphoma: comparison with benign cutaneous T cell infiltrates. *Blood* 1982;60:463–473.
224. Willemze R, De Graaff-Reitsma CB, Cnossen J, et al. Characterization of T cell subpopulations in skin and peripheral blood of patients with cutaneous T cell lymphomas and benign inflammatory dermatoses. *J Invest Dermatol* 1983;80:60–66.
225. Ralfkiaer E, Saati TA, Bosq J, et al. Immunocytochemical characterization of cutaneous lymphomas other than mycosis fungoides. *J Clin Pathol* 1986;39:553–563.
226. Salhany KE, Cousar JB, Greer JP, et al. Transformation of cutaneous T cell lymphoma to large cell lymphoma: a clinicopathologic and immunologic study. *Am J Pathol* 1988;132:265–277.
227. Borowitz MJ, Reichert TA, Byrnes RK, et al. The phenotypic diversity of peripheral T-cell lymphomas: the Southeastern Cancer Study Group experience. *Hum Pathol* 1986;17:567–574.
228. Jones DB, Wright DH, Paul F, et al. Phenotypic heterogeneity displayed by T-non Hodgkin's lymphoma (T-NHL) cells dispersed from diagnostic lymph node biopsies. *Hematol Oncol* 1986;4:219–226.
229. Tobinai K, Minato K, Ohtsu T, et al. Clinicopathologic, immunophenotypic and immunogenotypic analyses of immunoblastic lymphadenopathy-like T-cell lymphoma. *Blood* 1988;72:1000–1006.
230. Morimoto C, Matsuyama T, Oshige C, et al. Functional and phenotypic studies of Japanese adult T cell leukemia cells. *J Clin Invest* 1985;75:836–843.
231. Chadburn A, Athan E, Wieczorek R, et al. Detection and characterization of human T-cell lymphotropic virus type I (HTLV-I) associated T-cell neoplasms in an HTLV-I nonendemic region by polymerase chain reaction. *Blood* 1991;77:2419–2430.
232. Griffin JD, Linch D, Sabbath K, et al. A monoclonal antibody reactive with normal and leukemic human myeloid progenitor cells. *Leuk Res* 1984;8:521–534.
233. Hanson CA, Gajl-Peczalska J, Parkin JL, et al. Immunophenotyping of acute myeloid leukemia using monoclonal antibodies and the alkaline phosphatase-antialkaline phosphatase technique. *Blood* 1987; 70:83–89.
234. Merle-Beral H, Cong Duc LN, LeBlond V. Diagnostic and prognostic significance of myelomonocytic cell surface antigens in acute myeloid leukaemia. *Br J Haematol* 1989;73:323–330.
235. Ortuno F, Soler J, Vilella R, et al. Immunophenotype of blast cells in acute myelofibrosis. *Leuk Res* 1990;14:849–856.
236. Griffin JD, Todd RF, Ritz J, et al. Differentiation patterns in the blastic phase of chronic myeloid leukemia. *Blood* 1983;61:85–91.
237. Bettelheim P, Lutz D, Majdic O, et al. Cell lineage heterogeneity in blast crisis of chronic myeloid leukaemia. *Br J Haematol* 1985;59: 395–409.
238. Wilson BS, Indiveri F, Pellegrino AM, et al. DR (Ia-like) antigens on human melanoma cells: serological detection and immunochemical characterization. *J Exp Med* 1979;149:658–668.
239. Thompson JJ, Herlyn M, Elder DE, et al. Expression of DR antigen in freshly frozen human tumors. *Hybridoma* 1982;1:161–168.
240. Wilson BS, Herzig MA, Lloyd RV. Immunoperoxidase staining for Ia-like antigens in paraffin-embedded tissue from human melanoma and lung carcinoma. *Am J Pathol* 1984;115:102–108.
241. Kohler G, Milstein C. Continuous cultures of fused cells secreting antibody of predefined specificity. *Nature* 1975;256:495–497.
242. Kung PC, Goldstein G, Reinherz EL, et al. Monoclonal antibodies defining distinctive human T-cell surface antigens. *Science* 1979; 206:347–349.
243. Reinherz EL, Schlossman SF. The differentiation and function of human T lymphocytes. *Cell* 1980;19:821–827.
244. Reinherz EL, Schlossman SF. Regulation of the immune response-inducer and suppressor T lymphocyte subsets in human beings. *N Engl J Med* 1980;303:370–373.
245. Cobbold S, Hale G, Waldmann H. Non-lineage, LFA-1 family, and leucocyte common antigens: new and previously defined clusters. In: McMichael AJ, Beverley PCL, Cobbolds S, et al, eds. *Leucocyte typing III: white cell differentiation antigens*. Oxford: Oxford University Press, 1987;788–804.
246. Scheid MP, Triglia D. Further description of the Ly-5 system. *Immunogenetics* 1979;9:423–433.
247. Trowbridge IS. CD45: A prototype for transmembrane protein tyrosine phosphatases. *J Biol Chem* 1991;266:23517–23520.
248. Thomas ML, Lefrancois L. Differential expression of the leucocyte common antigen family. *Immunol Today* 1988;9:320–326.
249. Weiss LM, Arber DA, Chang KL. CD45: a review. *Appl Immunohistochem* 1993;1:166–181.
250. Ralph SJ, Thomas ML, Morton CC, et al: Structural variants of human T200 glycoprotein (leukocyte-common antigen). *EMBO J* 1987;6:1251–1257.
251. Hall LR, Streuli M, Schlossman SF, et al. Complete exon-intron organization of the human leukocyte common antigen (CD45) gene. *J Immunol* 1988;141:2781–2787.
252. Woollett GR, Williams AF, Shotton DM. Visualization by low-angle shadowing of the leucocyte-common antigen: a major cell surface glycoprotein of lymphocytes. *EMBO J* 1985;4:2827–2830.
253. Thomas ML. The leukocyte common antigen family. *Annu Rev Immunol* 1987;7:339–369.
254. Charbonneau H, Tonks NK, Walsh KA, et al. The leukocyte common antigen (CD45): a putative receptor-linked protein tyrosine phosphatase. *Proc Natl Acad Sci USA* 1988;85:7182–7186.
255. Tonks NK, Charbonneau H, Diltz CD, et al. Demonstration that the leukocyte common antigen is a protein tyrosine phosphatase. *Biochemistry* 1988;27:8695–8701.
256. Streuli M, Hall LR, Saga Y, et al. Differential usage of three exons generates at least five different mRNAs encoding human leukocyte common antigens. *J Exp Med* 1987;166:1548–1566.
257. Saga Y, Tung JS, Shen FS, et al. Alternative use of 5′ exons in the specification of Ly 5 isoforms distinguishing hematopoietic cell lineages. *Proc Natl Acad Sci USA* 1987;84:5364–5368.
258. Saga Y, Furukawa K, Rogers P, et al. Further data on the selective expression of Ly-5 isoforms. *Immunogenetics* 1990;31:296–306.
259. Omary MB, Trowbridge IS, Battifora HA. Human homologue of murine T200 glycoprotein. *J Exp Med* 1980;152:842–852.
260. Dalchau R, Kirkley J, Fabre JW. Monoclonal antibody to a human leukocyte-specific membrane glycoprotein probably homologous to the leukocyte-common (L-C) antigen of the rat. *Eur J Immunol* 1980; 10:737–744.
261. Newman W, Targan SR, Fast LD. Immunobiological and immunochemical aspects of the T-200 family of glycoproteins. *Mol Immunol* 1984;21:1113–1121.
262. Woollett GR, Barclay AN, Puklavec M, et al. Molecular and antigenic heterogeneity of the rat leukocyte-common antigen from thymocytes and T and B lymphocytes. *Eur J Immunol* 1985;15: 168–173.
263. Maddox JF, Mackay CR, Brandon MR. The sheep analogue of leucocyte common antigen (LCA). *Immunology* 1985;55:347–353.
264. Pingel JT, Thomas ML. Evidence that the leukocyte-common antigen is required for antigen-induced T lymphocyte proliferation. *Cell* 1989;58:1055–1065.
265. Koretzsky GA, Picus J, Schultz T, et al. Tyrosine phosphatase CD45 is required for T-cell antigen receptor and CD2-mediated activation of a protein tyrosine kinase and interleukin 2 production. *Proc Natl Acad Sci USA* 1991;88:2037–2041.
266. Weaver CT, Pingel JT, Nelson JO, et al. $CD8^+$ T-cell clones deficient in the expression of the CD45 protein tyrosine phosphatase have impaired responses to T-cell receptor stimuli. *Mol Cell Biol* 1991;11:4415–4422.
267. Schraven B, Samstag Y, Alterogt P, et al. Association of CD2 and CD45 on human T lymphocytes. *Nature* 1990;345:71–74.
268. Volarevic S, Burns C, Sussman JJ, et al. Intimate association of Thy-1 and the T-cell antigen receptor with the CD45 tyrosine phosphatase. *Proc Natl Acad Sci USA* 1990;87:7085–7089.
269. Dianzani U, Redoglia V, Molavasi F, et al. Isoform-specific associations of CD45 with accessory molecules in human T lymphocytes. *Eur J Immunol* 1987;22:365–371.
270. Seaman WE, Talal N, Herzenberg LA, et al. Surface antigens on mouse natural killer cells: use of monoclonal antibodies to inhibit or to enrich cytotoxic activity. *J Immunol* 1981;127:982–986.

271. Gilbert CW, Zaroukian MH, Esselman WJ. Poly-N-acetyl-lactosamine structures on murine cell surface T200 glycoprotein participate in natural killer cell bindings to YAC-1 targets. *J Immunol* 1988; 140:2821–2828.
272. Schwinzer R. Cluster report: CD45/CD45R. In: Knapp W, Dorken B, Gilks WE, et al, eds. *Leucocyte typing IV: white cell differentiation antigens.* New York: Oxford University Press, 1989:628–634.
273. Streuli M, Morimoto C, Schrieber M, et al. Characterization of CD45 and CD45R monoclonal antibodies using transfected mouse cell lines that express individual human leukocyte common antigens. *J Immunol* 1988;141:3910–3914.
274. Smith SH, Brown MH, Rowe D, et al. Functional subsets of human helper-inducer cells defined by a new monoclonal antibody, UCHL1. *Immunology* 1986;58:63–69.
275. Cebian M, Carrera AC, DeLandazuri MO, et al. Three different antigen specificities within the leukocyte common antigen or T200 complex: a biochemical, cell distribution, and functional comparative study. In: McMichael AJ, Beverley PCL, Cobbold S, et al, eds. *Leukocyte typing III: white cell differentiation antigens.* Oxford: Oxford University Press, 1987;823–826.
276. Poppema S, Lai R, Visser L. Antibody MT3 is reactive with a novel exon B associated 190 kd carbohydrate epitope of the leucocyte common antigen complex. *J Immunol* 1991;147:218–223.
277. Lefrancois L, Puddington L, Machamer CE, et al. Acquisition of cytotoxic T lymphocyte-specific carbohydrate differentiation antigens. *J Exp Med* 1985;162:1275–1293.
278. Kurtin PJ, Pinkus GS. Leukocyte common antigen: a diagnostic discriminant between hematopoietic and nonhematopoietic neoplasms in paraffin sections using monoclonal antibodies. Correlation with immunologic studies and ultrastructural localization. *Hum Pathol* 1985;16:353–365.
279. Michels S, Swanson PE, Frizzera G, et al. Immunostaining for leukocyte common antigen using an amplified avidin-biotin-peroxidase complex method and paraffin sections. *Arch Pathol Lab Med* 1987; 111:1035–1039.
280. Lai R, Visser L, Poppema S. Tissue distribution of restricted leukocyte common antigens: a comparative study with protein- and carbohydrate-specific CD45R antibodies. *Lab Invest* 1991;64:844–854.
281. Jensen GS, Poppema S, Mant MJ, et al. Transition in CD45 isoform expression during differentiation of normal and abnormal B cells. *Int Immunol* 1989;1:229–236.
282. Hathcock KS, Hirano H, Murakami S, et al. CD45 expression by B cells. Expression of different CD45 isoforms by subpopulations of activated B cells. *J Immunol* 1992;149:2286–2294.
283. Poppema S, Visser L, Lai R, et al. Antibody MT3 is reactive with a predominant 190 kd band of the leukocyte common antigen in plasmacytomas. In Knapp W, Dörken B, Gilks WR, et al, eds. *Leukocyte typing IV: white cell differentiation antigens.* Oxford: Oxford University Press, 1989;637–639.
284. Lefrancois L, Bevan MJ. Novel antigenic determinants of the T200 glycoprotein expressed preferentially by activated cytotoxic T lymphocytes. *J Immunol* 1985;135:374–383.
285. Lefrancois L, Thomas ML, Bevan MJ, et al. Different classes of T lymphocytes have different mRNAs for the leukocyte-common antigen, T200. *J Exp Med* 1986;163:1337–1342.
286. Lefrancois L, Goodman T. Developmental sequence of T200 antigen modification in murine T cells. *J Immunol* 1987;139:3718–3724.
287. Beverley PCL. Functional analysis of human T cell subsets defined by CD45 isoform expression. *Semin Immunol* 1992;4:35–41.
288. Janossy G, Bofill M, Rowe D, et al. The tissue distribution of T lymphocytes expressing different CD45 polypeptides. *Immunology* 1989;66:517–525.
289. Spickett GP, Brandon MR, Mason DW, et al. MRC OX-22, a monoclonal antibody that labels a new subset of T lymphocytes and reacts with the high molecular weight form of the leukocyte-common antigen. *J Exp Med* 1983;158:795–810.
290. Akbar AN, Terry L, Timms A, et al. Loss of CD45R and gain of UCHL1 reactivity is a feature of primed T cells. *J Immunol* 1988; 140:2171–2178.
291. Michie CA, McLean A, Alcock C, et al. Lifespan of human lymphocyte subsets defined by CD45 isoforms. *Nature* 1992;360:264–265.
292. Lansdorp PM, Sutherland HJ, Eaves CJ. Selective expression of CD45 isoforms on functional subpopulations of CD34$^+$ hemopoietic cells from human bone marrow. *J Exp Med* 1990;172:363–366.
293. Wood GS, Link M, Warnke RA, et al. Panleukocyte monoclonal L3B12: characterization and application to research and diagnostic problems. *Am J Clin Pathol* 1984;81:176–183.
294. Wood GS, Beckstead JH, Medeiros LJ, et al. The cells of giant cell tumor of tendon sheath resemble osteoclasts. *Am J Surg Pathol* 1988; 12:444–452.
295. Harris NL, Demirjian Z. Plasmacytoid T-zone proliferation in a patient with chronic myelomonocytic leukemia: histologic and immunohistologic characterization. *Am J Surg Pathol* 1991;15:87–95.
296. Wood GS, Freudenthal PS, Edinger A, et al. CD45 epitope mapping of human CD1a $^+$ dendritic cells and peripheral blood dendritic cells. *Am J Pathol* 1991;138:1451–1459.
297. Wood GS, Turner RR, Shiurba RA, et al. Human dendritic cells and macrophages: in situ immunophenotypic definition of subsets that exhibit specific morphologic and microenvironmental characteristics. *Am J Pathol* 1985;119:73–82.
298. Pulford KAF, Falini B, Heryet A, et al. 4KB5, a new monoclonal anti-B-cell antibody for the routine diagnosis of lymphoid tissue biopsies. In: McMichael AJ, Beverley PCL, Cobbold S, et al, eds. *Leuocyte typing III: white cell differentiation antigens.* Oxford: Oxford University Press, 1987:82.
299. Pulido R, Cebrian M, Acevedo A, et al. Comparative biochemical and tissue distribution study of four distinct CD45 antigen specificities. *J Immunol* 1988:140;3851–3857.
300. Dörken B, Moller P, Pezzutto A, et al. B-Cell antigens: CD45-like group. In: Knapp W, Dorken B, Gilks WR, et al, eds. *Leucocyte typing IV: white cell differentiation antigens.* New York: Oxford University Press, 1989:128–129.
301. Norton AJ, Ramsay AD, Smith SH, et al. Monoclonal antibody (UCHL1) that recognises normal and neoplastic T cells in routinely fixed tissues. *J Clin Pathol* 1986;39:399–405.
302. Terry LA, Brown MH, Beverley PCL. The monoclonal antibody, UCHL1, recognizes a 180,000 MW component of the human leucocyte-common antigen, CD45. *Immunology* 1988;64:331–336.
303. Berti E, Aversa GG, Soligo D, et al. A6: a new 45RO monoclonal antibody for immunostaining of paraffin-embedded tissues. *Am J Clin Pathol* 1991;95:188–193.
304. Poppema S, Hollema H, Visser L, et al. Monoclonal antibodies (MT1, MT2, MB1, MB2, MB3) reactive with leukocyte subsets in paraffin-embedded tissue sections. *Am J Pathol* 1987;127:418–429.
305. Butler MG, Wells C, D'Ardenne AJ, et al. Ultrastructural localization of antigens recognized by the monoclonal antibodies MB1, MB2, MT1, UCHL1, and TAL 1B5. *Ultrastruct Pathol* 1988;12:301–305.
306. Yoshino T, Mukuzono H, Aoki H, et al. A novel monoclonal antibody (OPD4) recognizing a helper/inducer T cell subset: its application to paraffin-embedded tissues. *Am J Pathol* 1989;134: 1339–1346.
307. Chadburn A, Husain S, Knowles DM. Monoclonal antibody OPD4 detects neoplastic T cells but does not distinguish between CD4 and CD8 neoplastic T cells in paraffin tissue sections. *Hum Pathol* 1992; 23:940–947.
308. Norton AJ, Isaacson PG. Lymphoma phenotyping in formalin-fixed and paraffin wax-embedded tissues: I. Range of antibodies and staining patterns. *Histopathology* 1989;14:437–446.
309. Salter DM, Krajewski AS, Dewar AE. Immunohistochemical staining of non-Hodgkin's lymphoma with monoclonal antibodies specific for the leucocyte common antigen. *J Pathol* 1985;146:345–353.
310. Pizzolo G, Sloane J, Beverley P, et al. Differential diagnosis of malignant lymphoma and nonlymphoid tumors using monoclonal antileucocyte antibody. *Cancer* 1980;46:2640–2647.
311. Battifora H, Trowbridge IS. A monoclonal antibody useful for the differential diagnosis between malignant lymphoma and nonhematopoietic neoplasms. *Cancer* 1983;51:816–821.
312. Gatter KC, Alcock C, Heryet A, et al. The differential diagnosis of routinely processed anaplastic tumors using monoclonal antibodies. *Am J Clin Pathol* 1984;82:33–43.
313. Norton AJ, Isaacson PG. An immunocytochemical study of T-cell lymphomas using monoclonal and polyclonal antibodies effective in routinely fixed wax embedded tissues. *Histopathology* 1986;10: 1243–1260.
314. Strickler JG, Weiss LM, Copenhaver CM, et al. Monoclonal antibodies reactive in routinely processed tissue sections of malignant lymphoma, with emphasis on T-cell lymphomas. *Hum Pathol* 1987;18: 808–814.

315. Hall PA, D'Ardenne AJ, Stansfeld AG. Paraffin section immunohistochemistry: II. Hodgkin's disease and large cell anaplastic (Ki1) lymphoma. *Histopathology* 1988;13:161-169.
316. Noorduyn LA, van der Valk P, van Heerde P, et al. Stage is a better prognostic indicator than morphologic subtype in primary noncutaneous T-cell lymphoma. *Am J Clin Pathol* 1990;93:49–57.
317. Elghetany MT, Kurec AS, Schuehler K, et al. Immunophenotyping of non-Hodgkin's lymphomas in paraffin-embedded tissue sections: a comparison with genotypic analysis. *Am J Clin Pathol* 1991;95: 517–525.
318. Harris NL, Bhan AK. Distribution of leukocyte common antigen (T-200) in B cell neoplasia: T200 is lost in terminal B cell differentiation. *Lab Invest* 1985;52:28A.
319. Wieczorek R, Buck D, Bindl J, et al. Monoclonal antibody Leu-22 (L60) permits the demonstration of some neoplastic T cells in routinely fixed and paraffin-embedded tissue sections. *Hum Pathol* 1988;19:1434–1443.
320. Hall PA, d'Ardenne AJ, Stansfeld AG. Paraffin section immunohistochemistry: I. Non-Hodgkin's lymphoma. *Histopathology* 1988;13: 149–160.
321. Behm FG, Raimondi SC, Schell MJ, et al. Lack of CD45 antigen on blast cells in childhood acute lymphoblastic leukemia is associated with chromosomal hyperdiploidy and other favorable prognostic features. *Blood* 1992;79:1011–1016.
322. Davey FR, Gatter KC, Ralfkiaer E, et al. Immunophenotyping of non-Hodgkin's lymphomas using a panel of antibodies on paraffin-embedded tissues. *Am J Pathol* 1987;129:54–63.
323. Norton AJ, Isaacson PG. Detailed phenotypic analysis of B-cell lymphoma using a panel of antibodies reactive in routinely fixed wax-embedded tissue. *Am J Pathol* 1987; 128:225–240.
324. Martin JME, Boras VF, Houwen B, et al. Hairy cell leukemia and anti-leukocyte common antigen. *Am J Clin Pathol* 1988;90:412–420.
325. Clark JR, Williams ME, Swerdlow SH. Detection of B- and T cells in paraffin-embedded tissue sections: diagnostic utility of commercially obtained 4KB5 and UCHL-1. *Am J Clin Pathol* 1990;93: 58–69.
326. Strickler JG, Audeh MW, Copenhaver CM, et al. Immunophenotypic differences between plasmacytoma/multiple myeloma and immunoblastic lymphoma. *Cancer* 1988;61:1782–1786.
327. Delsol G, Al Saati T, Gatter KC, et al. Coexpression of epithelial membrane antigen (EMA), Ki-1, and interleukin-2 receptor by anaplastic large cell lymphomas: diagnostic value in so-called malignant histiocytosis. *Am J Pathol* 1988;130:59–70.
328. Norton J, Isaacson PG. Lymphoma phenotyping in formalin-fixed and paraffin wax-embedded tissues: II. Profiles of reactivity in the various tumour types. *Histopathology* 1989;14:557–579.
329. Chott A, Kaserer K, Augustin I, et al. Ki-1-positive large cell lymphoma: a clinicopathologic study of 41 cases. *Am J Surg Pathol* 1990;14:439–448.
330. Leoncini L, Del Vecchio MT, Kraft R, et al. Hodgkin's disease and CD30-positive anaplastic large cell lymphomas-a continuous spectrum of malignant disorders: a quantitative morphometric and immunohistologic study. *Am J Pathol* 1990;137:1047–1057.
331. Falini B, Pileri S, Stein H, et al. Variable expression of leucocyte-common (CD45) antigen in CD30 (Ki-1)-positive anaplastic large-cell lymphoma: implications for the differential diagnosis between lymphoid and nonlymphoid malignancies. *Hum Pathol* 1990;21: 624–629.
332. Pinkus GS, Said JW. Hodgkin's disease, lymphocyte predominance type, nodular-a distinct entity? Unique staining profile for L & H variants of Reed-Sternberg cells defined by monoclonal antibodies to leukocyte common antigen, granulocyte-specific antigen, and B-cell-specific antigen. *Am J Pathol* 1985;118:1–6.
333. Dorfman RF, Gatter KC, Pulford KAF, et al. An evaluation of the utility of antigranulocyte and antileukocyte monoclonal antibodies in the diagnosis of Hodgkin's disease. *Am J Pathol* 1986;123:508–519.
334. Chittal SM, Caveriviere P, Schwarting R, et al. Monoclonal antibodies in the diagnosis of Hodgkin's disease: the search for a rational panel. *Am J Surg Pathol* 1988;12:9–21.
335. Medeiros LJ, Weiss LM, Warnke RA, et al. Utility of antigranulocyte and anti-leukocyte antibodies in differentiating Hodgkin's disease from non-Hodgkin's lymphoma. *Cancer* 1988;62:2475–2481.
336. Hsu SM, Yang K, Jaffe ES. Phenotypic expression of Hodgkin's and Reed-Sternberg cells in Hodgkin's disease. *Am J Pathol* 1985; 118:209–217.
337. Casey TT, Olson SJ, Cousar JB, et al. Immunophenotypes of Reed-Sternberg cells: a study of 19 cases of Hodgkin's disease in plastic-embedded sections. *Blood* 1989;74:2624–2628.
338. Myskow MW, Krajewski AS. Immunoreactivity of Reed-Sternberg cells in paraffin and frozen sections [Letter]. *J Clin Pathol* 1986;39: 1043–1045.
339. Andrade RE, Wick MR, Frizzera G, et al. Immunophenotyping of hematopoietic malignancies in paraffin sections. *Hum Pathol* 1988; 19:394–402.
340. Kurec AS, Cruz VE, Barrett D, et al. Immunophenotyping of acute leukemias using paraffin-embedded tissue sections. *Am J Clin Pathol* 1990;93;502–509.
341. Horny HP, Campbell M, Steinke B, et al. Acute myeloid leukemia: immunohistologic findings in paraffin-embedded bone marrow biopsy specimens. *Hum Pathol* 1990;21:648–655.
342. Caldwell CW, Patterson WP, Toalson BD, et al. Surface and cytoplasmic expression of CD45 antigen isoforms in normal and malignant myeloid cell differentiation. *Am J Clin Pathol* 1991;95: 180–187.
343. Traweek ST. Immunophenotypic analysis of acute leukemia. *Am J Clin Pathol* 1993;99:504–512.
344. Traweek ST, Arber DA, Rappaport H, et al. Extramedullary myeloid cell tumors: an immunohistochemical and morphologic study of 28 cases. *Am J Surg Pathol* 1993;17:1011–1019.
345. Beckstead JH, Wood GS, Turner RR. Histiocytosis X cells and Langerhans cells: enzyme histochemical and immunologic similarities. *Hum Pathol* 1984;15:826–833.
346. Monda L, Warnke R, Rosai J. A primary lymph node malignancy with features suggestive of dendritic reticulum cell differentiation. *Am J Pathol* 1986;122:562–572.
347. Pallesen G, Myhre-Jensen O. Immunophenotypic analysis of neoplastic cells in follicular dendritic cell sarcoma. *Leukemia* 1987;1: 549–557.
348. Franchino C, Reich C, Distenfeld A, et al. A clinicopathologically distinctive primary splenic histiocytic neoplasm: demonstration of its histiocytic derivation by immunophenotypic and molecular genetic analysis. *Am J Surg Pathol* 1988;12:398–404.
349. Weiss LM, Berry GJ, Dorfman RF, et al. Spindle cell neoplasms of lymph nodes of probable reticulum cell lineage: true reticulum cell sarcoma? *Am J Surg Pathol* 1990;14:405–414.
350. Nickoloff BJ, Wood GS, Chu M, et al. Disseminated dermal dendrocytomas: a new cutaneous fibrohistocytic disorder? *Am J Surg Pathol* 1990;14:867–871.
351. Van Eyken P, De Wolf-Peeters C, Van den Oord J, et al. Expression of leukocyte common antigen in lymphoblastic lymphoma and small noncleaved undifferentiated non-Burkitt's lymphoma: an immunohistochemical study. *J Pathol* 1987;151:257–261.
352. Yoshino T, Hoshida Y, Murakami I, et al. Comparison of monoclonal antibodies reactive with lymphocyte subsets in routinely fixed paraffin-embedded material: flow cytometric analyses, immunoperoxidase staining and influence of fixatives. *Acta Med Okayama* 1990; 44:243–250.
353. Cerroni L, Smolle J, Soyer P, et al. Immunophenotyping of cutaneous lymphoid infiltrates in frozen and paraffin-embedded tissue sections: a comparative study. *J Am Acad Dermatol* 1990;22:405–413.
354. Myskow MW, Krajewski AS, Salter DM, et al. Paraffin section immunophenotyping of non-Hodgkin's lymphoma, using a panel of monoclonal antibodies. *Am J Clin Pathol* 1988;90:564–574.
355. Moldenhauer G, Schwartz-Albiez R. Immunochemistry and epitope analysis using CD72, CD73, CD74, CDw75, CD76, CD77, CDw78, and unclustered mAb. In: Knapp W, Dorken B, Gilks WR, et al, eds. *Leucocyte typing IV: white cell differentiation antigens.* Oxford: Oxford University Press, 1989:154–164.
356. Ling NR, Maclennan ICM, Mason DY. B cell and plasma cell antigens new and previously defined clusters. In McMichael AJ, Beverley PCL, Cobbold S, et al, eds. *Leukocyte typing III: white cell differentiation antigens.* Oxford: Oxford University Press, 1989: 302–335.
357. Hauschild A, Sterry W . Formalin-resistant leukocyte surface antigens in the diagnosis of cutaneous malignant lymphomas. *Am J Pathol* 1989;135:177–184.
358. Ng CS, Chan JKC, Hui PK, et al. Monoclonal antibodies reactive

with normal and neoplastic T cells in paraffin sections. *Hum Pathol* 1988;19:295–303.
359. Poppema S, Lai R, Visser L. Monoclonal antibody OPD4 is reactive with CD45RO, but differs from UCHL1 by the absence of monocyte reactivity. *Am J Pathol* 1991;139:725–729.
360. Linder J, Ye Y, Harrington DS, et al. Monoclonal antibodies marking T lymphocytes in paraffin-embedded tissue. *Am J Pathol* 1987;127: 1–8.
361. Macon WR, Casey TT, Kinney MC, et al. Leu-22 (L60). A more sensitive marker than UCHL1 for peripheral T-cell lymphomas, particularly large-cell types. *Am J Clin Pathol* 1991;95:696–701.
362. Wilson MS, Weiss LM, Gatter KC, et al. Malignant histiocytosis: a reassessment of cases previously reported in 1975 based on paraffin section immunophenotyping studies. *Cancer* 1990;66:530–536.
363. Borowitz MJ, Stevanovic G, Gottfried M. Differential diagnosis of undifferentiated malignant tumors with monoclonal antibody T29/33. *Hum Pathol* 1984;15:928–934.
364. Warnke RA, Rouse RV. Limitations encountered in the application of tissue section immunodiagnosis to the study of lymphoma and related disorders. *Hum Pathol* 1985;16:326–331.
365. McDonnell JM, Beschorner WE, Kuhajda FP, et al. Common leukocyte antigen staining of a primitive sarcoma. *Cancer* 1987;59: 1438–1441.
366. Arber DA, Weiss LM. CD10: a review. *Appl Immunohistochem* 1997;5:125–140.
367. Dörken B, Moller P, Pezzutto A, et al. B cell antigens: section report. In: Knapp W, Dorken B, Gilks WR, et al, eds. *Leucocyte typing IV: white cell differentiation antigens.* New York: Oxford University Press, 1989:17–32.
368. Tedder, TF, Wagner N, Engel P. B cell antigens: section report. In Schlossman SF, Boumsell L, Gilks WR, et al, eds. *Leukocyte typing V: white cell differentiation antigens.* New York: Oxford University Press, 1995:483–504.
369. Letarte M, Vera S, Tran R, et al. Common acute lymphocytic leukemia antigen is identical to neutral endopeptidase. *J Exp Med* 1988; 168:1247–1253.
370. Shipp MA, Vijayaraghavan J, Schmidt EV, et al. Common acute lymphoblastic leukemia antigen (CALLA) is active neutral endopeptidase 24.11 (''enkephalinase''): direct evidence by cDNA transfection analysis. *Proc Natl Acad Sci USA* 1989;86:297–301.
371. LeBien TW, McCormack RT. The common acute lymphoblastic leukemia antigen (CD10): emancipation from a functional enigma. *Blood* 1989;73:625–635.
372. Barker PE, Shipp MA, D'Adamio L, et al. The common acute lymphoblastic leukemia antigen gene maps to chromosomal region 3 (q21-q27). *J Immunol* 1989;142:283–287.
373. D'Adamio L, Shipp MA, Masteller EL, et al. Organization of the gene encoding common acute lymphoblastic leukemia antigen (neutral endopeptidase 24.11): multiple miniexons and separate 5′ untranslated regions. *Proc Natl Acad Sci USA* 1989;86:7103–7107.
374. Haouas H, Morello D, Lavenu A, et al. Characterization of the 5′ region of the CD10/neutral endopeptidase 24.11 gene. *Biochem Biophys Res Commun* 1995;207:933–942.
375. Ishimaru F, Shipp MA. Analysis of the human CD10/neutral endopeptidase 24.11 promoter region: two separate regulatory elements. *Blood* 1995;85:3199–3207.
376. Metzgar RS, Borowitz MJ, Jones NJ, et al. Distribution of common acute lymphoblastic leukemia antigen in nonhematopoietic tissues. *J Exp Med* 1981;154:1249–1254.
377. Braun MP, Martin PJ, Ledbetter JA, et al. Granulocytes and cultured human fibroblasts express common acute lymphoblastic leukemia-associated antigens. *Blood* 1983;61:718–725.
378. Shipp MA, Richardson NE, Sayre PH, et al. Molecular cloning of the common acute lymphoblastic leukemia antigen (CALLA) identifies a type II integral membrane protein. *Proc Natl Acad Sci USA* 1988;85:4819–4823.
379. Shipp MA, Look AT. Hematopoietic differentiation antigens that are membrane-associated enzymes: cutting is the key! *Blood* 1993; 82:1052–1070.
380. Ganju RK, Shpektor RG, Brenner DG, et al. CD10/Neutral endopeptidase 24.11 is phosphorylated by casein kinase II and coassociates with other phosphoproteins including the lyn src-related kinase. *Blood* 1996;88:4159–4165.
381. Gafford JT, Skidgel RA, Erdös EG, et al. Human kidney ''enkephalinase,'' a neutral metalloendopeptidase that cleaves active peptides. *Biochemistry* 1983;22:3265–3271.
382. Shipp MA, Stefano GB, D'Adamio L, et al. Downregulation of enkephalin-mediated inflammatory responses by CD10/neutral endopeptidase 24.11. *Nature* 1990;347:394–396.
383. Salles G, Chen C-Y, Reinherz EL, et al. CD10 NEP is expressed on Thy-1low B220$^+$ murine B-cell progenitors and functions to regulate stromal cell-dependent lymphopoiesis. *Blood* 1992;80:2021–2029.
384. Borson DB, Gruenert DC. Glucocorticoids induce neutral endopeptidase in transformed human tracheal epithelial cells. *Am J Physiol* 1991;260:L83–89.
385. Pesando JM, Tomaselli KJ, Lazarus H, et al. Distribution and modulation of a human leukemia-associated antigen (CALLA). *J Immunol* 1983;131:2038–2045.
386. Werb Z, Clark EJ. Phorbol diesters regulate expression of the membrane neutral metalloendopeptidase (EC 3.4.24.11) in rabbit synovial fibroblasts and mammary epithelial cells. *J Biol Chem* 1989;264: 9111–9113.
387. Erdös KG, Wagner B, Harbury CB, et al. Down-regulation and inactivation of neutral endopeptidase 24.11 (enkephalinase) in human neutrophils. *J Biol Chem* 1989;264:14519–14523.
388. Benayahu D, Fried A, Shamay A, et al. Differential effects of retinoic acid and growth factors on osteoblastic markers and CD10/NEP activity in stromal-derived osteoblasts. *J Cell Biochem* 1994;56:62–73.
389. Cossman J, Neckers LM, Leonard WJ, et al. Polymorphonuclear neutrophils express the common acute lymphoblastic leukemia antigen. *J Exp Med* 1983;157:1064–1069.
390. McCormack RT, Nelson RD, LeBien TW. Structure/function studies of the common acute lymphoblastic leukemia antigen (CALLA/CD10) expressed on human neutrophils. *J Immunol* 1986;137: 1075–1082.
391. Tran-Paterson R, Boileau G, Giguère V, et al. Comparative levels of CALLA/neutral endopeptidase on normal granulocytes, leukemic cells, and transfected COS-1 cells. *Blood* 1990;76:775–782.
392. Hokland P, Nadler LM, Griffin JD, et al. Purification of common acute lymphoblastic leukemia antigen positive cells from normal human bone marrow. *Blood* 1984;64:662–666.
393. Caldwell CW, Poje E, Helikson MA. B-cell precursors in normal pediatric bone marrow. *Am J Clin Pathol* 1991;95:816–823.
394. Terstappen LWMM, Huang S, Picker LJ. Flow cytometric assessment of human T-cell differentiation in thymus and bone marrow. *Blood* 1992;79:666–677.
395. Delia D, Cattoretti G, Bonati A, et al. Detection of the common acute lymphoblastic leukaemia antigen (CALLA) on B cells from human fetal tissues: a multiple phenotypic characterization. *Clin Exp Immunol* 1985;59:305–314.
396. Longacre TA, Foucar K, Crago S, et al. Hematogones: a multiparameter analysis of bone marrow precursor cells. *Blood* 1989;73: 543–552.
397. Loken MR, Shah VO, Dattilio KL, et al. Flow cytometric analysis of human bone marrow: II. Normal B lymphocyte development. *Blood* 1987;70:1316–1324.
398. LeBien TW, Wörmann B, Villablanca JG, et al. Multiparameter flow cytometric analysis of human fetal bone marrow B cells. *Leukemia* 1990;4:354–358.
399. Gore SD, Kastan MB, Civin CI. Normal human bone marrow precursors that express terminal deoxynucleotidyl transferase include T-cell precursors and possible lymphoid stem cells. *Blood* 1991;77: 1681–1690.
400. Clark P, Normansell DE, Innes DJ, et al. Lymphocyte subsets in normal bone marrow. *Blood* 1986;67:1600–1606.
401. Shin SS, Sheibani K, Kezirian J, et al. Immunoarchitecture of normal human bone marrow: a study of frozen and fixed tissue sections. *Hum Pathol* 1992;23:686–694.
402. Punnonen J, Aversa GG, Vandekerckhove B, et al. Induction of isotype switching and Ig production by CD5$^+$ and CD10$^+$ human fetal B cells. *J Immunol* 1992;148:3398–3404.
403. Caldwell CW, Patterson WP. Relationship between T200 antigen expression and stages of B cell differentiation in resurgent hyperplasia of bone marrow. *Blood* 1989;70:1165–1172.
404. Kobayashi SD, Seki K, Suwa N, et al. The transient appearance of small blastoid cells in the marrow after bone marrow transplantation. *Am J Clin Pathol* 1991;96: 191–195.
405. Sandhaus LM, Chen TL, Ettinger LJ, et al. Significance of increased

proportions of CD10-positive cells in nonmalignant bone marrow of children. *Am J Pediatr Hematol Oncol* 1993;15:65–70.
406. Greaves M, Delia D, Janossy G, et al. Acute lymphoblastic leukemia associated antigen: IV. Expression on non-leukemiac "lymphoid" cells. *Leuk Res* 1980;4:15–32.
407. Mari B, Breittmayer J-P, Guerin S, et al. High levels of functional endopeptidase 24.11 (CD10) activity on human thymocytes: preferential expression on immature subsets. *Immunology* 1994;82: 433–438.
408. Hsu S-M, Jaffe ES. Phenotypic expression of B-lymphocytes: I. Identification with monoclonal antibodies in normal lymphoid tissues. *Am J Pathol* 1984;114:387–395.
409. Gregory CD, Tursz T, Edwards CF, et al. Identification of a subset of normal B cells with a Burkitt's lymphoma (BL)-like phenotype. *J Immunol* 1987;139:313–318.
410. Kiyokawa N, Kokai Y, Ishimoto K, et al. Characterization of the common acute lymphoblastic leukaemia antigen (CD10) as an activation molecule on mature human B cells. *Clin Exp Immunol* 1990; 79:322–327.
411. Dowell BL, Borowitz MJ, Boyett JM, et al. Immunologic and clinicopathologic features of common acute lymphoblastic leukemia antigen-positive childhood T-cell leukemia: a pediatric oncology group study. *Cancer* 1987;59:2020–2026.
412. Hurwitz CA, Loken MR, Graham ML, et al. Asynchronous antigen expression in B lineage acute lymphoblastic leukemia. *Blood* 1988; 72:299–307.
413. Kaplan SS, Penchansky L, Stoic V, et al. Immunophenotyping in the classification of acute leukemia in adults: interpretation of multiple lineage reactivity. *Cancer* 1989;63:1520–1527.
414. Kurec AS, Belair P, Stefanu C, et al. Significance of aberrant immunophenotypes in childhood acute lymphoid leukemia. *Cancer* 1991; 67:3081–3086.
415. Rosanda C, Cantù-Rajnoldi A, Ivernizzi R, et al. B cell acute lymphoblastic leukemia (B-ALL): a report of 17 pediatric cases. *Haematologica* 1992;77:151–155.
416. Pui C, Rivera GK, Hancock ML, et al. Clinical significance of CD10 expression in childhood acute lymphoblastic leukemia. *Leukemia* 1993;7:35–40.
417. Creutzig U, Harbott J, Sperling C, et al. Clinical significance of surface antigen expression in children with acute myeloid leukemia: results of study AML-BFM-87. *Blood* 1995;86:3097–3108.
418. Reading CL, Estey EH, Huh YO, et al. Expression of unusual immunophenotype combinations in acute myelogenous leukemia. *Blood* 1993;81:3083–3090.
419. Del Poeta G, Stasi R, Venditti A, et al. Prognostic value of cell marker analysis in de novo acute myeloid leukemia. *Leukemia* 1994; 8:388–394.
420. Bradstock K, Matthews J, Benson E, et al, Australian Leukaemia Study Group. Prognostic value of immunophenotyping in acute myeloid leukemia. *Blood* 1994;84:1220–1225.
421. Basso G, Putti MC, Cantù-Rajnoldi A, et al. The immunophenotype in infant acute lymphoblastic leukaemia: correlation with clinical outcome. An Italian multicentre study (AIEOP). *Br J Haematol* 1992;81:184–191.
422. Kersey J, Goldman A, Abramson C, et al. Clinical usefulness of monoclonal-antibody phenotyping in childhood acute lymphoblastic leukaemia. *Lancet* 1982;ii:1419–1423.
423. Vannier JP, Bene MC, Faure GC, et al. Investigation of the CD10 (cALLA) negative acute lymphoblastic leukaemia: further description of a group with a poor prognosis. *Br J Haematol* 1989;72: 156–160.
424. Glencross DK, Adam F, Poole J, et al. CD10 antigen density in childhood common acute lymphoblastic leukaemia: comparisons of race and sex. *Leuk Res* 1992;16: 1197–1201.
425. Lavabre-Bertrand T, Janossy G, Ivory K, et al. Leukemia-associated changes identified by quantitative flow cytometry: I. CD10 expression. *Cytometry* 1994;18: 209–217.
426. Boucheix C, David B, Sebban C, et al. Immunophenotype of adult acute lymphoblastic leukemia, clinical parameters, and outcome: an analysis of a prospective trial including 562 tested patients. (LALA87). *Blood* 1994;84:1603–1612.
427. Shuster JJ, Falletta JM, Pullen J, et al. Prognostic factors in childhood T-cell acute lymphoblastic leukemia: a Pediatric Oncology Group study. *Blood* 1990;75: 166–173.
428. Gómez E, San Miguel JF, González M, et al. The value of the immunological subtypes and individual markers compared to classical parameters in the prognosis of acute lymphoblastic leukemia. *Hematol Oncol* 1991;9:33–42.
429. Robbins BA, Ellison DJ, Spinosa JC, et al. Diagnostic application of two-color flow cytometry in 161 cases of hairy cell leukemia. *Blood* 1993;82:1277–1287.
430. Durie BGM, Grogan TM. CALLA-positive myeloma: an aggressive subtype with poor survival. *Blood* 1985;66:229–232.
431. Kurabayashi H, Kubota K, Murakami H, et al. Ultrastructure of myeloma cells in patients with common acute lymphoblastic leukemia antigen (CALLA)-positive myeloma. *Cancer Res* 1988;48: 6234–6237.
432. Tamura J, Kurabayashi H, Sawamura M, et al. Clinical features of common acute lymphoblastic leukemia antigen (CALLA)-positive myeloma: a report of four cases. *Blut* 1989;58:229–233.
433. Efremidis AP, Bekesi JG. Anti-common acute lymphoblastic leukemia antibody (CALLA) (J5) reactivity by small cell lung cancer (SCLS) cells. *Blood* 1986;67:252–253.
434. Bunn PA Jr, Jewett PB, Gazdar AF, et al. Anti-common acute lymphoblastic leukemia antibody (CALLA) (J5) reactivity by small cell lung cancer (SLCL) cells-reply. *Blood* 1986;67:253.
435. Ganju RK, Sunday M, Tsarwhas DG, et al. CD10/NEP in non-small cell lung carcinomas: relationship to cellular proliferation. *J Clin Invest* 1994;94:1784–1791.
436. Cohen AJ, Bunn PA, Franklin W, et al. Neutral endopeptidase: variable expression in human lung, inactivation in lung cancer, and modulation of peptide-induced calcium flux. *Cancer Res* 1996;56: 831–839.
437. Hishima T, Fukayama M, Fujisawa M, et al. CD5 expression in thymic carcinoma. *Am J Pathol* 1994;145:268–275.
438. Carrel S, Schmidt-Kessen A, Mach J-P, et al. Expression of common acute lymphoblastic leukemia antigen (CALLA) on human malignant melanoma cell lines. *J Immunol* 1983;130:2456–2460.
439. Carrel S, Zografos L, Schreyer M, et al. Expression of CALLA/CD10 on human melanoma cells. *Melanoma Res* 1993;3:319–323.
440. Tedder TF, Zhou L-J, Engel P. The CD19/CD21 signal transduction complex of B lymphocytes. *Immunol Today* 1994;15:437–442.
441. Schriever F, Freedman AS, Freeman G, et al. Isolation and phenotypic characterization of dendritic cells from human tonsil. In: Knapp W, Dörken G, Gilks WR, et al, eds. *Leukocyte typing IV: white cell differentiation antigens.* New York: Oxford University Press, 1989; 185.
442. Nadler LM, Anderson KC, Marti G, et al. B4, a human B lymphocyte-associated antigen expressed on normal, mitogen-activated, and malignant B lymphocytes. *J Immunol* 1983;131:244–250.
443. Meeker TC, Miller RA, Link MP, et al. A unique human B lymphocyte antigen defined by a monoclonal antibody. *Hybridoma* 1984; 3:305–320.
444. Moldenhauer G, Dorken B, Schwartz R, et al. Analysis of ten B lymphocyte specific workshop monoclonal antibodies. In: Reinherz EL, Haynes BF, Nadler LM, eds. *Leukocyte typing*, vol 2. New York: Springer-Verlag, 1986:61–67.
445. Sato S, Tedder TF. CD19 workshop panel report. In Kishimoto T, Kikutani H, von dem Borne AEGK, et al, eds. *Leukocyte typing VI: white cell differentiation antigens.* New York: Garland Publishing, 1998;133–135.
446. Ord DC, Edelhoff S, Dushkin H, et al. CD19 maps to a region of conservation between human chromosome 16 and mouse chromosome 7. *Immunogenetics* 1994;39:322–328.
447. Zhou L-J, Ord DC, Omori SA, et al. Structure of the genes encoding the CD19 antigen of human and mouse B lymphocytes. *Immunogenetics* 1992;35:102–111.
448. Tedder TF, Isaacs CM. Isolation of cDNAs encoding the CD19 antigen of human and mouse B lymphocytes: a new member of the immunoglobulin superfamily. *J Immunol* 1989;143:712–717.
449. Zhou L-J, Ord DC, Hughes AL, et al. Structure and domain organization of the CD19 antigen of human, mouse, and guinea pig B lymphocytes: conservation of the extensive cytoplasmic domain. *J Immunol* 1991;147:1424–1432.
450. Matumoto AK, Kopicky-Burd J, Carter RH, et al. Intersection of the complement and immune systems: a signal transduction complex of the B lymphocyte-containing complement receptor type 2 and CD19. *J Exp Med* 1991;173:55–64.

451. Bradbury L, Kansas GS, Levy S, et al. The CD19/CD21 signal transducing complex of human B lymphocytes includes the target of antiproliferatice antibody-1 and Leu-13 molecules. *J Immunol* 1992;149: 2841–2850.
452. van Noesel CJM, Lankester AC, van Lier RA. Dual antigen recognition by B cells. *Immunol Today* 1993;14:8–11.
453. Uckun FM, Ledbetter JA. Immunobiologic differences between normal and leukemic human B-cell precursors. *Proc Natl Acad Sci USA* 1988;85:8603–8607.
454. Uckun FM, Burkhardt AL, Jarvis L, et al. Signal transduction through the CD19 receptor during discrete developmental stages of human B-cell ontogeny. *J Biol Chem* 1993;268:21172–21184.
455. Chalupny NJ, Kanner SB, Schieven GL, et al. Tyrosine phosphorylation of CD19 in pre-B and mature B cells. *EMBO J* 1993;12: 2891–2896.
456. Zhou L-J, Smith HM, Waldschmidt TJ, et al. Tissue-specific expression of the human CD19 gene in transgenic mice inhibits antigen-independent B-lymphocyte development. *Mol Cell Biol* 1994;14: 3884–3894.
457. Engel P, Zhou L-J, Ord DC, et al. Abnormal B lymphocyte development, activation, and differentiation in mice that lack or overexpress the CD19 signal transduction molecule. *Immunity* 1995;3:39–50.
458. Rickert RC, Rajewsky K, Roes J. Impairment of T-cell-dependent B-cell responses and B-1 cell development in CD19-deficient mice. *Nature* 1995;376:352–355.
459. Sato S, Steeber DA, Tedder TF. The CD19 signal transduction molecule is a response regulator of B-lymphocyte differentiation. *Proc Natl Acad Sci USA* 1995;92:11558–11562.
460. Sato S, Ono N, Steeber DA, et al. CD19 regulates B lymphocyte signaling thresholds critical for the development of B-1 lineage cells and autoimmunity. *J Immunol* 1996;157:4371–4378.
461. Nadler LM, Korsmeyer SJ, Anderson KC, et al. B cell origin of non-T cell acute lymphoblastic leukemia: a model for discrete stages of neoplastic and normal pre-B cell differentiation. *J Clin Invest* 1984; 74:332–340.
462. Jennings CD, Foon KA. Recent advances in flow cytometry: Application to the diagnosis of hematologic malignancy. *Blood* 1997;90: 2863-2892.
463. Cuneo A, Michaux JL, Ferrant A, et al. Correlation of cytogenetic patterns and clinicobiological features in adult acute myeloid leukemia expressing lymphoid markers. *Blood* 1992;79:720–727.
464. Zhou L-J, Tedder TF. CD20 workshop panel report. In Schlossman SF, Boumsell L, Gilks WR, et al, eds. *Leukocyte typing V: white cell differentiation antigens.* New York: Oxford University Press, 1995:511–514.
465. Ono N, Sato S, Tedder TF. CD20 workshop panel report. In Kishimoto T, Kikutani H, von dem Borne AEGK, et al, eds. *Leukocyte typing VI: white cell differentiation antigens.* New York: Garland Publishing, 1998:135–137.
466. Ishii Y, Takami T, Yuasa H, et al. Two distinct antigen systems in human B lymphocytes: identification of cell surface and intracellular antigens using monclonal antibodies. *Clin Exp Immunol* 1984;58: 183–192.
467. Mason DY, Comans-Bitter WM, Cordell JL, et al. Antibody L26 recognizes an intracellular epitope on the B-cell-associated CD20 antigen. *Am J Pathol* 1990;136:1215–1222.
468. Dörken B, Moller P, Pezzutto A, et al. B-cell antigens: unclustered mAb. In: Knapp W, Dörken B, Gilks WR, et al, eds. *Leucocyte typing IV: white cell differentiation antigens.* New York: Oxford University Press, 1989:129–131.
469. Norton AJ, Isaacson PG. Monoclonal antibody L26: an antibody that is reactive with normal and neoplastic B lymphocytes in routinely fixed and paraffin wax embedded tissues. *J Clin Pathol* 1987;40: 1405–1412.
470. Chang KL, Arber DA, Weiss LM. CD20: A review. *Appl Immunohistochem* 1996;4:1–15.
471. Tedder TF, Disteche CM, Louie E, et al. The gene that encodes the human CD20 (B1) differentiation antigen is located on chromosome 11 near the t(11;14)(q13;q32) translocation site. *J Immunol* 1989; 142:2555–2559.
472. Tedder TF, Klejman F, Schlossman SF, et al. Structure of the gene encoding the human B lymphocyte differentiation antigen CD20 (B1). *J Immunol* 1989;142:2560–2568.
473. Thθvenin C, Lucas BP, Kozlow EJ, et al. Cell type- and stage-specific expression of the CD20/B1 antigen correlates with the activity of a diverged octamer DNA motif present in its promoter. *J Biol Chem* 1991;268:5949–5956.
474. Einfeld DA, Brown JP, Valentine MA, et al. Molecular cloning of the human B cell CD20 receptor predicts a hydrophobic protein with multiple transmembrane domains. *EMBO J* 1988;7:711–717.
475. Stamenkovic I, Seed B. Analysis of two cDNA clones encoding the B lymphocyte antigen CD20 (B1,Bp35), a type III integral membrane protein. *J Exp Med* 1988;167:1975–1980.
476. Tedder TF, Streuli M, Schlossman SF, et al. Isolation and structure of a cDNA encoding the B1 (CD20) cell-surface antigen of human B lymphocytes. *Proc Natl Acad Sci USA* 1988;85:208–212.
477. Clark EA, Shu G, Ledbetter JA. Role of the Bp35 cell surface polypeptide in human B-cell activation. *Proc Natl Acad Sci USA* 1985; 82:1766–1770.
478. Clark EA, Shu G. Activation of human B cell proliferation through surface Bp35 (CD20) polypeptides or immunoglobulin receptors. *J Immunol* 1987;138:720–725.
479. Valentine MA, Meier KE, Rossie S, et al. Phosphorylation of the CD20 phosphoprotein in resting B lymphocytes. *J Biol Chem* 1989; 264:11282–11287.
480. Tedder TF, Penta A. Structure of the CD20 antigen and gene of human and mouse B-cells: use of transfected cell lines to examine the Workshop panel of antibodies. In: Knapp W, Dörken B, Gilks WR, et al, eds. *Leukocyte typing IV: white cell differentiation antigens.* Oxford: Oxford University Press, 1989:48–50.
481. Clark EA, Shu GL, Luscher B, et al. Activation of human B cells: comparison of the signal transduced by IL-4 to four different competence signals. *J Immunol* 1989;143:3873–3880.
482. Golay JT, Clark E, Beverley PCL. The CD20 (Bp35) antigen is involved in activation of B cells from the G_0 to the G_1 phase of the cell cycle. *J Immunol* 1985;135:3795–3801.
483. Smeland E, Godal T, Ruud E, et al. The specific induction of myc protooncogene expression in normal human B cells is not a sufficient event for acquisition of competence to proliferate. *Proc Natl Acad Sci USA* 1985;82:6255–6259.
484. Tedder TF, Forsgren A, Boyd AW, et al. Antibodies reactive with the B1 molecule inhibit cell cycle progression but not activation of human B lymphocytes. *Eur J Immunol* 1986;16:881–887.
485. Bubien JK, Zhou LJ, Bell PD, et al. Transfection of the CD20 cell surface molecule into ectopic cell types generates a $Ca^{+}2$ conductance found constitutively in B lymphocytes. *J Cell Biol* 1993;121: 1121–1132.
486. Tedder TF, Zhou LJ, Bell PD, et al. The CD20 surface molecule of B lymphocytes function as a calcium channel. *J Cell Biochem* 1990; 14D:195–205.
487. Bubien JK, Bell PD, Frizzell RA, et al. CD20 directly regulates transmembrane ion flux in B-lymphocytes. In: Knapp W, Dörken B, Gilks WR, et al, eds. *Leucocyte typing IV: white cell differentiation antigens.* Oxford: Oxford University Press, 1989;51–54.
488. Hokland P, Ritz J, Schlossman SF, et al. Orderly expression of B cell antigens during the in vitro differentiation of non-malignant human pre-B cells. *J Immunol* 1985;135:1746–1751.
489. Uckun FM, Haissig S, Ledbetter JA, et al. Developmental hierarchy during early human B-cell ontogeny after autologous bone marrow transplantation using autografts depleted of $CD19^{+}$ B-cell precursors by an anti-CD19 pan-B-cell immunotoxin containing pokeweed antiviral protein. *Blood* 1992;79:3369–3379.
490. Moreau I, Duivert V, Banchereau J, et al. Culture of human fetal B-cell precursors on bone marrow stroma maintains highly proliferative CD20dim cells. *Blood* 1993;81:1170–1178.
491. Stashenko P, Nadler LM, Hardy R, et al. Expression of cell surface markers after human B lymphocyte activation. *Proc Natl Acad Sci USA* 1981;78:3848–3852.
492. Boyd A, Freedman AS, Anderson KC, et al. Phenotypic changes occurring during in vitro activation of human splenic B lymphocytes. In: Reinherz EL, Haynes BF, Nadler LM, et al, eds. *Leukocyte typing II.* Berlin: Springer Verlag, 1986;429–442.
493. Ledbetter JA, Clark EA. Surface phenotype and function of tonsillar germinal center and mantle zone B cell subsets. *Hum Immunol* 1986; 15:30–43.
494. Fend F, Nachbaur D, Oberwasserlechner F, et al. Phenotype and topography of human thymic B cells: an immunohistologic study. *Virchows Arch* 1991;60:381–388.

495. Staal FJT, Roederer M, Bubp J, et al. CD20 expression is increased on B lymphocytes from HIV-infected individuals. *J AIDS* 1992;5: 627–632.
496. Lane HC, Depper JM, Greene WC, et al. Qualitative analysis of immune function in patients with AIDS: evidence for a selective defect in soluble antigen recognition. *N Engl J Med* 1985;313:79–83.
497. Hutlin LE, Hausner MA, Hutlin PM, et al. CD20 (pan-B cell) antigen is expressed at a low level on a subpopulation of human T lymphocytes. *Cytometry* 1993;14:196–204.
498. Quintanilla-Martinez L, Preffer F, Rubin D, et al. CD20$^+$ T-cell lymphoma: neoplastic transformation of a normal T-cell subset. *Am J Clin Pathol* 1994;102:483–489.
499. Said JW, Sassoon AF, Shintaku IP, et al. Immuno-ultrastructural localization of B-cell-specific monoclonal antibodies B1 and B2. *J Histochem Cytochem* 1986;34:607–611.
500. Hall PA, D'Ardenne AJ, Richards MA, et al. Lymphoplasmacytoid lymphoma: an immunohistological study. *J Pathol* 1987;153: 213–223.
501. Linder J, Ye Y, Armitage JO, et al. Monoclonal antibodies marking B-cell non-Hodgkin's lymphoma in paraffin-embedded tissue. *Mod Pathol* 1988;1:29–34.
502. Chadburn A, Knowles DM. Paraffin-resistant antigens detectable by antibodies L26 and polyclonal CD3 predict the B- or T-cell lineage of 95% of diffuse aggressive non-Hodgkin's lymphomas. *Am J Clin Pathol* 1994;102:284–291.
503. San Miguel JF, González M, Gascón A, et al. Immunophenotypic heterogeneity of multiple myeloma: influence on the biology and clinical course of the disease. *Br J Haematol* 1991;77:185–190.
504. Leo R, Boecker M, Peest D, et al. Multiparameter analyses of normal and malignant human plasma cells: CD38$^+$, CD56$^+$, CD54$^+$, cIg$^+$ is the common phenotype of myeloma cells. *Ann Hematol* 1992;64: 132–139.
505. Harada H, Kawano MM, Huang N, et al. Phenotypic difference of normal plasma cells from mature myeloma cells. *Blood* 1993;81: 2658–2663.
506. Ruiz-Argüelles GJ, San Miguel JF. Cell surface markers in multiple myeloma. *Mayo Clin Proc* 1994;69:684–690.
507. Strauchen JA, Dimitriu-Bona A. Immunopathology of Hodgkin's disease: characterization of Reed-Sternberg cells with monoclonal antibodies. *Am J Pathol* 1986;123:293–300.
508. Pinkus GS, Said JW. Hodgkin's disease, lymphocyte predominance type, nodular-further evidence for a B cell derivation: L & H variants of Reed-Sternberg cells express L26, a pan B cell marker. *Am J Pathol* 1988;133:211–217.
509. Coles FB, Cartun RW, Pastuszak WT. Hodgkin's disease, lymphocyte-predominant type: immunoreactivity with B-cell antibodies. *Mod Pathol* 1988;1:274–278.
510. Agnarsson B, Kadin ME. The immunophenotype of Reed-Sternberg cells: a study of 50 cases of Hodgkin's disease using fixed frozen tissues. *Cancer* 1989;63:2083–2087.
511. Chittal SM, Alard C, Rossi R-F, et al. Further phenotypic evidence that nodular, lymphocyte-predominant Hodgkin's disease is a large B-cell lymphoma in evolution. *Am J Surg Pathol* 1990;14: 1024–1035.
512. Nicholas DS, Harris S, Wright DH. Lymphocyte predominance Hodgkin's disease-an immunohistochemical study. *Histopathology* 1990;16:157–165.
513. Chu W-S, Abbondanzo SL, Frizzera G. Inconsistency of the immunophenotype of Reed-Sternberg cells in simultaneous and consecutive specimens from the same patients: a paraffin section evaluation in 56 patients. *Am J Pathol* 1992;141:11–17.
514. Enblad G, Sundström C, Glimelius B. Immunohistochemical characteristics of Hodgkin and Reed-Sternberg cells in relation to age and clinical outcome. *Histopathology* 1993;22:535–541.
515. Stoler MH, Nichols GE, Symbula M, et al. Lymphocyte predominance Hodgkin's disease: evidence for a κ light chain-restricted monotypic B cell neoplasm. *Am J Pathol* 1995;146:812–818.
516. Zukerberg LR, Collins AB, Ferry JA, et al. Coexpression of CD15 and CD20 by Reed-Sternberg cells in Hodgkin's disease. *Am J Pathol* 1991;139:475–483.
517. Schmid C, Pan L, Diss T, et al. Expression of B-cell antigens by Hodgkin's and Reed-Sternberg cells. *Am J Pathol* 1991;139: 701–707.
518. Carbone A, Gloghini A, Volpe R. Paraffin section immunohistochemistry in the diagnosis of Hodgkin's disease and anaplastic large cell (CD30$^+$) lymphomas. *Virchows Arch* 1992;420:527–532.
519. Bai MC, Jiwa NM, Horstman A, et al. Decreased expression of cellular markers in Epstein-Barr virus-positive Hodgkin's disease. *J Pathol* 1994;174:49–55.
520. Macon WR, Williams ME, Greer JP, et al. T-cell-rich B-cell lymphomas: a clinicopathologic study of 19 cases. *Am J Surg Pathol* 1992;16:351–363.
521. Warzynski MJ, Graham DM, Axtell RA, et al. Low level CD20 expression on T cell malignancies. *Cytometry* 1994; 18:88–92.
522. Hansmann M-L, Fellbaum C, Bohm A. Large cell anaplastic lymphoma: evaluation of immunophenotype on paraffin and frozen sections in comparison with ultrastructural features. *Virchows Arch* 1991;418:427–433.
523. Kurtin PJ, Roche PC. Immunoperoxidase staining on non-Hodgkin's lymphomas for T-cell lineage associated antigens in paraffin sections: comparison of the performance characteristics of four commercially available antibody preparations. *Am J Surg Pathol* 1993;17: 898–904.
524. Drexler H, Thiel E, Ludwig W-D. Acute myeloid leukemias expressing lymphoid-associated antigens: diagnostic incidence and prognostic significance. *Leukemia* 1993;7:489–498.
525. Hanson CA, Abaza M, Sheldon S, et al. Acute biphenotypic leukaemia: immunophenotypic and cytogenetic analysis. *Br J Haematol* 1993;84:49–60.
526. Hudock J, Chatten J, Miettinen M. Immunohistochemical evaluation of myeloid leukemia infiltrates (granulocytic sarcomas) in formaldehyde-fixed, paraffin-embedded tissue. *Am J Clin Pathol* 1994;102: 55–60.
527. Ornvold K, Ralfkiaer E, Carstensen H. Immunohistochemical study of the abnormal cells in Langerhans' cell histiocytosis (histiocytosis X). *Virchows Arch* 1990;416:403–410.
528. Chilosi M, Castelli P, Martignoni G, et al. Neoplastic epithelial cells in a subset of human thymomas express the B cell-associated CD20 antigen. *Am J Surg Pathol* 1992;16:988–997.
529. Timens W. CD21 workshop panel report. In: Schlossman SF, Boumsell L, Gilks WR, et al, eds. *Leukocyte typing V: white cell differentiation antigens.* New York: Oxford University Press, 1995: 516–518.
530. Timens W. CD21 workshop panel report. In Kishimoto T, Kikutani H, von dem Borne AEGK, et al, eds. *Leukocyte typing VI: white cell differentiation antigens.* New York: Garland Publishing, 1998: 140–142.
531. Carel JC, Myones BL, Frazier B, et al. Structural requirements for C3d,g/Epstein-Barr virus receptor (CR2/CD21) ligand binding, internalization, and viral infection. *J Biol Chem* 1990;265: 12293–12299.
532. Ling NR, Brown B, Hardie D. Synergy test for recognition of epitopes on soluble proteins: its application in the study of CD21 and CD23 antigens and their respective antibodies. *J Immunol Methods* 1994;173:11–17.
533. Cooper NR, Moore MD, Nemerow GR. Immunobiology of CR2, the B lymphocyte receptor for Epstein-Barr virus and the C3d complement fragment. *Ann Rev Immunol* 1988;6:85–113.
534. Timens W, Boes A, Rozeboom-Uiterwijk T, et al. Immaturity of the human splenic marginal zone in infancy: possible contribution to the deficient infant immune response. *J Immunol* 1989;143:3200–3206.
535. Weis JJ, Toothaker LE, Smith JA, et al. Structure of the human B lymphocyte receptor for C3d and the Epstein-Barr virus and relatedness to other members of the family of C3/C4 binding proteins. *J Exp Med* 1988;167:1047–1066.
536. Aubry J-P, Pochon S, Gauchat JF, et al. CD23 interacts with a new functional extracytoplasmic domain involving N-linked oligosaccharides on CD21. *J Immunol* 1994;152:5806–5813.
537. Bradbury LE, Goldmacher VS, Tedder TF. The CD19 signal transduction complex of B lymphocytes: deletion of the CD19 cytoplasmic domain alters signal transduction but not complex formation with TAPA-1 and Leu 13. *J Immunol* 1993;151:2915–2927.
538. Luxembourg AT, Cooper NR. Modulation of signaling via the B cell antigen receptor by CD21, the receptor for C3dg and EBV. *J Immunol* 1994;153:4448–4457.
539. Aubry JP, Pochon S, Graber P, et al. CD21 is a ligand for CD23 and regulates IgE production. *Nature* 1992;358:505–507.
540. Gagro A, Rabatic S. Allergen-induced CD23 on CD4$^+$ T lympho-

cytes and CD21 on B lymphocytes in patients with allergic asthma: evidence and regulation. *Eur J Immunol* 1994;24:1109–1114.
541. Henchoz S, Gauchat J-F, Aubry J-P, et al. Stimulation of human IgE production by a subset of anti-CD21 monoclonal antibodies: requirement of a co-signal to modulate epsilon transcripts. *Immunol* 1994;81:285–290.
542. Kalli KR, Ahearn JM, Fearon DT. Interaction of iC3b with recombinant isotypic and chimeric forms of CR2. *J Immunol* 1991;147: 590–594.
543. Kroese FGM, Timens W, Nieuwenhuis P. Reaction patterns of the lymph node 1: cell types and functions. In Grundmann E, Vollner E, eds. *Current topics in pathology*. Berlin: Springer-Verlag, 1990; 103–148.
544. Bonnefoy J-Y, Henchoz S, Hardie D, et al. A subset of anti-CD21 antibodies promote the rescue of germinal center B cells from apoptosis. *Eur J Immunol* 1993;23:969–972.
545. Gerdes J, Stein H. Complement (C3) receptors on dendritic reticulum cells of normal and malignant lymphoid tissues. *Clin Exp Immunol* 1982;48:348–352.
546. Schriever F, Freedman AS, Freeman G, et al. Isolated human follicular dendritic cells display a unique antigenic phenotype. *J Exp Med* 1989;169:2043–2058.
547. Fisher E, Delibrias C, Kazatchkine MD. Expression of CR2 (the C3dg/EBV receptor, CD21) on normal human peripheral blood T lymphocytes. *J Immunol* 1991;146:865–869.
548. Tsoukas CD, Lambris JD. Expression of EBV/C3d receptors on T cells: biological significance. *Immunol Today* 1993;14:56–59.
549. Young LS, Dawson CW, Brown KW, et al. Identification of a human epithelial cell surface protein sharing an epitope with the C3d/Epstein-Barr virus receptor molecule of B lymphocytes. *Int J Cancer* 1989;43:786–794.
550. Timens W, Boes A, Vos H, et al. Tissue distribution of the C3d/EBV-receptor: CD21 monoclonal antibodies reactive with a variety of epithelial cells, medullary thymocytes, and peripheral T-cells. *Histochemistry* 1991;95:605–611.
551. Birkenbach M, Tong X, Bradbury LE, et al. Characterization of an Epstein-Barr virus receptor on human epithelial cells. *J Exp Med* 1992;176:1405–1414.
552. Fingeroth JD, Clabby ML, Strominger JD. Characterization of a T-lymphocyte Epstein-Barr virus/C3d receptor (CD21). *J Virol* 1988; 62:1442–1447.
553. Behm FG, Fitzgerald TJ, Patton DF, et al. CD21 (CR2) is frequently expressed on the blasts of childhood T cell acute lymphoblastic leukemia (T-ALL). In: Knapp W, Dörken B, Gilks WR, et al, eds. *Leukocyte typing IV: white cell differentiation antigens*. New York: Oxford University Press, 1989:61–62.
554. Dörken B, Moldenhauer G, Pezzutto A, et al. HD39 (B3), a B lineage-restricted antigen whose cell surface expression is limited to resting and activated human B lymphocytes. *J Immunol* 1986;136: 4470–4479.
555. Schwarting R, Stein H, Wang CY. The monoclonal antibodies α-S-HCL1 (α-Leu-14) and α-S-HCL3 (α-LeuM5) allow the diagnosis of hairy cell leukemia. *Blood* 1985;65:974–983.
556. Mason DY, Cordell JL, Pulford KAF. Production of monoclonal antibodies for immunocytochemical use. In: Bullock GR, Petrusz P, eds. *Techniques in immunocytochemistry*, vol 2. London: Academic Press, 1983:175–216.
557. Kehrl JH. The CD22 workshop panel report. In Schlossman SF, Boumsell L, Gilks WR, et al, eds. *Leukocyte typing V: white cell differentiation antigens*. New York: Oxford University Press, 1995: 523–525.
558. Wilson GL, Najfield V, Kozlow E, et al. Genomic structure and chromosomal mapping of the human CD22 gene. *J Immunol* 1993; 150:5013–5024.
559. Wilson GL, Fox CH, Fauci AS, et al. cDNA cloning of the B cell membrane protein CD22: a mediator of B-B cell interactions. *J Exp Med* 1991;173:137–146.
560. Engel P. CD22 workshop panel report. In: Kishimoto T, Kikutani H, von dem Borne AEGK, et al, eds. *Leukocyte typing VI: white cell differentiation antigens*. New York: Garland Publishing, 1998: 142–144.
561. Leprince C, Draves KE, Geahlen RC, et al. CD22 associates with the human surface IgM-B-cell antigen receptor complex. *Proc Natl Acad Sci USA* 1993;90:3236–3240.
562. Engel P, Wagner N, Miller A, et al. Identification of the ligand-binding domains of CD22, a member of the immunoglobulin superfamily that uniquely binds a sialic acid-dependent ligand. *J Exp Med* 1995;181:1581–1586.
563. Engel P, Wagner N, Smith H, et al. Structure/function analysis of CD22: domains that mediate adhesion. In: Schlossman SF, Boumsell L, Gilks WR, et al, eds. *Leukocyte typing V: white cell differentiation antigens*. New York: Oxford University Press, 1995;526–527.
564. Stamenkovic I, Seed B. The B-cell antigen CD22 mediates monocyte and erythrocyte adhesion. *Nature* 1990;345:74–77.
565. Tuscano J, Engel P, Tedder TF, et al. Engagement of the adhesion receptor CD22 triggers a potent stimulatory signal for B cells and blocking CD22/CD22L interactions impairs T-cell proliferation. *Blood* 1996;26:1246–1252.
566. Doody GM, Justement LB, Delibrias CC, et al. A role in B cell activation for CD22 and the protein tyrosine phosphatase SHP. *Science* 1995;269:242–244.
567. Campbell MA, Klinman NR. Phosphotyrosine-dependent association between CD22 and protein tyrosine phosphatase 1C. *Eur J Immunol* 1995;25:1573–1579.
568. Campana D, Janossy G, Bofill M, et al. Human B cell development: I. Phenotypic differences of B lymphocytes in the bone marrow and peripheral lymphoid tissue. *J Immunol* 1985;134:1524–1530.
569. Dörken B, Pezzutto M, Kohler M, et al. Expression of cytoplasmic CD22 in B-cell ontogeny. In: McMichael AJ, Beverley PCL, Cobbold S, et al, eds. *Leukocyte typing III: white cell differentiation antigens*. Oxford: Oxford University Press, 1987:474–476.
570. Loken MR, Shah VO, Dattilio KL, et al. Flow cytometric analysis of human bone marrow: II. normal B lymphocyte development. *Blood* 1987;70:1316–1324.
571. Mason DY, Stein H, Gerdes J, et al. Value of monoclonal anti-CD22 (p135) antibodies for the detection of normal and neoplastic B lymphoid cells. *Blood* 1987;69:836–840.
572. Boue DR, LeBein TW. Expression and structure of CD22 in acute leukemia. *Blood* 1988;71:1480–1486.
573. Thorley-Lawson DA, Nadler LM, Bhan AK, et al. BLAST-2 [EBVCS], an early surface marker of human B cell activation, is superinduced by Epstein Barr virus. *J Immunol* 1985;134: 3007–3012.
574. Rowe M, Hildreth JEK, Rickinson AB, et al. Monoclonal antibodies to Epstein-Barr virus-induced, transformation-associated cell surface antigens: binding patterns and effect upon virus-specific T-cell cytotoxicity. *Int J Cancer* 1982;29:373–381.
575. Dörken B, Moller P, Pezzutto A, et al. B cell antigens: CD23. In Knapp W, Dörken B, Gilks WR, et al, eds. *Leukocyte typing IV: white cell differentiation antigens*. New York: Oxford University Press, 1989:67–70.
576. Sarfati M, Ishihara H, Delespesse G. CD23 workshop panel report. In: Schlossman SF, Boumsell L, Gilks WR, et al, eds. *Leukocyte typing V: white cell differentiation antigens*. New York: Oxford University Press, 1995:530–533.
577. Kinter C, Sugden B. Identification of antigenic determinants unique to the surfaces of cells transformed by Epstein-Barr virus. *Nature* 1981;294:458–460.
578. Kikutani H, Inui S, Sato R, et al. Molecular structure of human lymphocyte receptor for immunoglobulin E. *Cell* 1986;47:657–665.
579. Yukawa K, Kikutani H, Owaki H, et al. A B cell-specific differentiation antigen, CD23, is a receptor for IgE (FcϵR) on lymphocytes. *J Immunol* 1987;138:2576–2580.
580. Wendel-Hansen V, Riviere M, Uno M, et al. The gene encoding CD23 leukocyte antigen. *Somat Cell Mol Genet* 1990;16:283–289.
581. Sarfati M. CD23 workshop panel report. In: Kishimoto T, Kikutani H, von dem Borne AEGK, et al, eds. *Leukocyte typing VI: white blood cell differentiation antigens*. New York: Garland Publishing, 1998;144–147.
582. Delespesse G, Sarfati M, Wu CY, et al. The low-affinity receptor for IgE. *Immunol Rev* 1992;125:77–97.
583. Letellier M, Sarfati M, Delespesse G. Mechanisms of formation of IgE-binding factors (soluble CD23): I. Fc epsilon RII bearing B cells generate IgE-binding factors of different molecular weights. *Mol Immunol* 1989;26:1105–1112.
584. Yokota A, Kikutani H, Tanaka T, et al. Two species of human Fc epsilon receptor II (Fc epsilon RII/CD23): tissue-specific and IL-4-specific regulation of gene expression. *Cell* 1988;55:611–618.

585. Sarfati M, Rector E, Wong K, et al. In vitro synthesis of IgE by human lymphocytes: II. Enhancement of the spontaneous IgE synthesis by IgE-binding factors secreted by RPMI 8866 lymphoblastoid B cells. *Immunology* 1984;53:197–205.
586. Sarfati M, Delespesse G. Possible role of human lymphocyte receptor for IgE (CD23) or its soluble fragments in the in vitro synthesis of human IgE. *J Immunol* 1988;141:2195–2199.
587. Flores-Romo L, Shields J, Humbert Y, et al. Inhibition of an in vivo antigen-specific IgE response by antibodies to CD23. *Science* 1993; 261:1038–1041.
588. Bonnefoy JY, Lecoanet-Henchoz S, Aubry JP, et al. CD23 and B-cell activation. *Curr Opin Immunol* 1995;7:355–359.
589. Armant M, Ishihara H, Rubio M, et al. Regulation of cytokine production by soluble CD23: costimulation of interferon gamma secretion and triggering of tumor necrosis factor alpha release. *J Exp Med* 1994;180:1005–1011.
590. Lecoanet-Henchoz S, Gauchat JF, Aubry JP, et al. CD23 regulates monocyte activation through a novel interaction with the adhesion molecules CD11b-CD18 and CD11c-CD18. *Immunity* 1995;3: 119–125.
591. Kikutani H, Suemura M, Owaki H, et al. Fcϵ receptor, a specific differentiation marker transiently expressed on mature B cells before isotype switching. *J Exp Med* 1986;164:1455–1469.
592. Pallesen G. The distribution of CD23 in normal human tissues and in malignant lymphomas. In McMichael AJ, Beverley PCL, Cobbold S, et al, eds. *Leukocyte typing III: white cell differentiation antigens.* Oxford: Oxford University Press, 1987:383–386.
593. Swendeman S, Thorley-Lawson DA. The activation antigen BLAST-2, when shed, is an autocrine BCGF for normal and transformed B cells. *EMBO J* 1987;167:1637–1642.
594. Gordon J, Cairns JA, Millsum MJ, et al. Interleukin 4 and soluble CD23 as progression factors for human B lymphocytes: analysis of their interactions with agonists of the phosphoinositide "dual pathway" of signaling. *Eur J Immunol* 1988;18:1561–1565.
595. Capron M, Jouault T, Prin L, et al. Functional study of a monoclonal antibody to IgE Fc receptor (FcϵR2) of eosinophils, platelets, and macrophages. *J Exp Med* 1986;164:72–89.
596. Hardie DL, Johnson GD, Khan M, et al. Quantitative analysis of molecules which distinguish functional compartments within germinal centers. *Eur J Immunol* 1993;23:997–1004.
597. Yamaoka KA, Arock M, Issaly F, et al. Granulocyte macrophage colony stimulating factor induces Fc epsilon RII/CD23 expression on normal human polymorphonuclear neutrophils. *Int Immunol* 1996;8: 479–490.
598. Sarfati M, Chevret S, Chastang C, et al. Prognostic importance of serum soluble CD23 level in chronic lymphocytic leukemia. *Blood* 1996;88:4259–4264.
599. Banks PM, Chan J, Cleary ML, et al. Mantle cell lymphoma: a proposal for unification of morphologic, immunologic, and molecular data. *Am J Surg Pathol* 1992;16:637–640.
600. Harris NL, Jaffe ES, Stein H, et al. A revised European-American classification of lymphoid neoplasms: A proposal from the International Lymphoma Study Group. *Blood* 1994;84:1361–1392.
601. Abramson CS, Kersey JH, LeBien TW. A monoclonal antibody (BA-1) reactive with cells of human B lymphocyte lineage. *J Immunol* 1981;126:83–88.
602. Le Bien T. CD24 workshop panel report. In Schlossman SF, Boumsell L, GilksWR, et al, eds. *Leukocyte typing V: white cell differentiation antigens.* New York: Oxford University Press, 1995;539–541.
603. Hough MR, Rosten PM, Sexton TL, et al. Mapping of CD24 and homologous sequences to multiple chromosomal loci. *Genomics* 1994;22:154–161.
604. Fischer GF, Majdic O, Gadd S, et al. Signal transduction in lymphocytic and myeloid cells via CD24, a new member of phosphoinositol-anchored membrane molecules. *J Immunol* 1990;144:638–641.
605. Pirruccello SJ, LeBien TW. The human B cell-associated antigen CD24 is a single chain sialoglycoprotein. *J Immunol* 1986;136: 3779–3784.
606. Kay R, Rosten PM, Humphries RK. CD24, a signal transducer modulating B cell activation responses, is a very short peptide with a glycosyl phophatidylinositol membrane anchor. *J Immunol* 1991; 147:1412–1416.
607. Engel P, Ingles J, Gallart T, et al. Changes in the expression of B cell surface antigen detected by the Workshop CD24 monoclonal antibodies (mAbs) following in vitro activation. In: McMichael AJ, Beverley PCL, Cobbold S, et al, eds. *Leukocyte typing III: white cell differentiation antigens.* Oxford: Oxford University Press, 1987: 368–369.
608. Mehmet H, Larkin M, Tang PW, et al. Monoclonal antibody BA-1 to the human B lymphocyte marker CD24 recognizes a sialic acid (N-acetylneuraminic acid) dependent epitope in multivalent display on peptide. *Clin Exp Immunol* 1990;81:489–495.
609. Chappel S, Kay R, Humphries RK. CD24 workshop panel report. In Kishimoto T, Kikutani H, von dem Borne AEGK, et al., *eds, Leukocyte typing VI: white cell differentiation antigens.* New York: Garland Publishing, 1998:147–149.
610. Melink GB, LeBien TW. Construction of an antigenic map for human B cell precursors. *J Clin Immunol* 1983;3:260–267.
611. Duperray C, Boiron JM, Boucheix C, et al. The CD24 antigen discriminates between pre-B and B cells in human bone marrow. *J Immunol* 1990;145:3678–3683.
612. Solvason N, Kearney JF. The human fetal omentum: a site of B cell generation. *J Exp Med* 1992;175:397–404.
613. Kemshead JT, Fritschy J, Asser U, et al. Monoclonal antibodies defining markers with apparent selectivity for particular haemopoietic cell types may also detect antigens on cells of neural crest origin. *Hybridoma* 1982;1:109–123.
614. Platt JL, LeBien TW, Michael AF. Stages of renal ontogenesis identified by monoclonal antibodies reactive with lymphohematopoietic differentiation antigens. *J Exp Med* 1983;157:155–172.
615. Kersey J, Abramson C, Perry G, et al. Clinical usefulness of monoclonal antibody phenotyping in childhood acute lymphoblastic leukemia. *Lancet* 1982;ii:1419–1423.
616. Schiavone EM, Luciano L, LoPardo C, et al. CD24 identifies an early myeloid subset in chronic myelogenous leukemia. In: Schlossman SF, Boumsell L, Gilks WR, et al, eds. *Leukocyte typing V: white cell differentiation antigens.* New York: Oxford University Press, 1995:542–543.
617. Engel P, Wagner N, Tedder TF. CD79 workshop report. In: Schlossman SF, Boumsell L, Gilks WR, et al, eds. *Leukocyte typing V: white cell differentiation antigens.* New York: Oxford University Press, 1995;667–670.
618. Mason DY, van Noesel CJM, Cordell JL, et al. The B29 and mb-1 polypeptides are differentially expressed during human B cell differentiation. *Eur J Immunol* 1992;22:2753–2756.
619. Borst J, Brouns GS, deVries E, et al. Antigen receptors on T and B lymphocytes: parallels in organization and function. *Immunol Rev* 1993;132:49–84.
620. Venkitaraman AR, Williams GT, Dariavich P, et al. The B-cell antigen receptor of the five immunoglobulin classes. *Nature* 1997;352: 777–781.
621. Nakamura T. CD79 workshop panel report. In Kishimoto T, Kikutani H, von dem Borne AEGK, et al, eds. *Leukocyte typing VI: white cell differentiation antigens.* New York: Garland Publishing, 1998: 180–182.
622. Mason DY, Cordell JL, Tse AG, et al. The IgM-associated protein mb-1 as a marker of normal and neoplastic B cells. *J Immunol* 1991; 147:2474–2482.
623. Okazaki M, Luo Y, Han T, et al. Three new monoclonal antibodies that define a unique antigen associated with prolymphocytic leukemia/non-Hodgkin's lymphoma and are effectively internalized after binding to the cell surface antigen. *Blood* 1993;81:84–94.
624. Mason DY, Cordell JL, Brown MH, et al. CD79a: a novel marker for B-cell neoplasms in routinely processed tissue samples. *Blood* 1995;86:1453–1459.
625. Nakamura T, Kubagawa H, Cooper MD. Heterogeneity of immunoglobulin-associated molecules on human B cells identified by monoclonal antibodies. *Proc Natl Acad Sci USA* 1992;89:8522–8526.
626. Comans-Bitter WM, de Bruin-Versteig S, Broe MK, et al. CD79 workshop: Intracellular CD79 expression in precursor B cells tested with the CD79 panel of monoclonal antibodies. In Kishimoto T, Kikutani H, von dem Borne AEGK, et al, eds. *Leukocyte typing VI: white cell differentiation antigens.* New York: Garland Publishing, 1998:182–184.
627. Hashimoto S, Mohrenweiser HW, Gregersen PK, et al. Chromosomal localization, genomic structure, and allelic polymorphism of the human CD79 alpha (Ig-alpha/mb-1) gene. *Immunogenetics* 1994; 40:287–295.

628. Ha H, Kubagawa H, Burrows PD. Molecular cloning and expression pattern of a human gene homologous to the murine mb-1 gene. *J Immunol* 1992;148:1526–1531.
629. Wood WJ, Thompson AA, Korenberg J, et al. Isolation and chromosomal mapping of the human immunoglobulin-associated B29 gene (IgB). *Genomics* 1993;16:187–192.
630. Hashimoto S, Chiorazzi N, Gregersen PK. The complete sequence of the human CD79b (Ig beta/B29) gene: identification of a conserved exon/intron organization, immunoglobulin-like regulatory regions, and allelic polymorphism. *Immunogenetics* 1994;40:145–149.
631. Kerner JD, Appleby MW, Mohn RN, et al. Impaired expansion of mouse B cell progenitors lacking Btk. *Immunity* 1995;3:301–312.
632. Cheng AM, Rowley B, Pao W, et al. Syk tyrosine kinase required for mouse viability and B-cell development. *Nature* 1995;378:303–306.
633. Kim KM, Alber G, Weiser P, et al. Differential signaling through the Ig-alpha and Ig-beta components of the B cell antigen receptor. *Eur J Immunol* 1993;23:911–916.
634. Takata M, Sabe H, Hata A, et al. Tyrosine kinases Lyn and Syk regulate B cell receptor-coupled $Ca2^+$ mobilization through distinct pathways. *EMBO J* 1994;13:1341–1349.
635. Torres RM, Flaswinkel H, Reth M, et al. Aberrant B cell development and immune response in mice with a compromised BCR complex. *Science* 1996;272:1804–1808.
636. Gong S, Nussenzweig MC. Regulation of an early developmental checkpoint in the B cell pathway by Ig beta. *Science* 1996;272:411–416.
637. Nakamura T, Koyama M, Koike Y, et al. Suppression of humoral immunity by monoclonal antibody to CD79b, an invariant component of antigen receptors on B lymphocytes. *Int J Hematol* 1996;64:39–46.
638. Buccheri V, Mihaljevic B, Matutes E, et al. mb-1: a new marker for B-lineage lymphoblastic leukemia. *Blood* 1993;82:853–857.
639. Kanavaros P, Gaulard P, Charlotte F, et al. Discordant expression of immunoglobulin and its associated molecule mb-1/CD79a is frequently found in mediastinal large B cell lymphomas. *Am J Pathol* 1995;146:735–741.
640. Arber DA, Jenkins KA, Slovak ML. $CD79_{\alpha}$ expression in acute myeloid leukemia. High frequency of expression in acute promyelocytic leukemia. *Am J Pathol* 1996;149:1105–1110.
641. Korkolopoulou P, Cordell J, Jones M, et al. The expression of the B cell marker mb-1 (CD79a) in Hodgkin's disease. *Histopathology* 1994;24:511–515.
642. Clément C, Vouijs WC, Klein B, et al. B-B2 and B-B4, two new mAb against secreting plasma cells. In Schlossman SF, Boumsell L, Gilks WR, et al, eds. *Leukocyte typing V: white cell differentiation antigens.* New York: Oxford University Press, 1995:714–715.
643. Horvathova M, Gaillard JP, Liautard J, et al. Identification of novel and specific antigens of human plasma cells by mAb. In: Schlossman SF, Boumsell L, Gilks WR, et al, eds. *Leukocyte typing V: white cell differentiation antigens.* New York: Oxford University Press, 1995:713–714.
644. Wijdenes J, Clément C, Klein B, et al. CD138 (syndecan-1) workshop panel report. In: Kishimoto T, Kikutani H, von dem Borne AEGKr, et al, eds. *Leukocyte typing VI: white cell differentiation antigens.* New York: Garland Publishing, 1998:249–252.
645. Mali M, Jaakkola P, Arvilommi A-M, et al. Sequence of human syndecan indicates a novel gene family of integral membrane proteoglycans. *J Biol Chem* 1990;265:6884–6889.
646. Bernfield M, Kokenyesi R, Kato M, et al. Biology of the syndecans: a family of transmembrane heparan sulfate proteoglycans. *Annu Rev Cell Biol* 1992;8:365–393.
647. Bernfield M, Hinkes MT, Gallo RL. Developmental expression of the syndecans: possible function and regulation. *Dev Suppl* 1993;205–212.
648. Elenius K, Jalkanen M. Function of the syndecans: a family of cell surface proteoglycans. *J Cell Sci* 1994;107:2975–2982.
649. Leppa S, Mali M, Miettinen HM, et al. Syndecan expression regulates cell morphology and growth of mouse mammary epithelial tumor cells. *Proc Natl Acad Sci USA* 1992;89:932–936.
650. Sanderson RD, Turnbull JE, Gallagher JT, et al. Fine structure of heparan sulfate regulates syndecan-1 function and cell behavior. *J Biol Chem* 1994;269:13100–13106.
651. Sanderson RD, Lalor P, Bernfield M. B lymphocytes express and lose syndecan at specific stages of differentiation. *Cell Regul* 1989;1:27–35.
652. Ridley RC, Xiao H, Hata H, et al. Expression of syndecan regulates human myeloma plasma cell adhesion to type 1 collagen. *Blood* 1993;81:767–774.
653. Wijdenes J, Vouijs WC, Clement C, et al. A plasmocyte selective monoclonal antibody (B-B4) recognizes syndecan-1. *Br J Hematol* 1996;94:318–323.
654. Gaidano G, Gloghini A, Gattai V, et al. Association of Kaposi's sarcoma-associated herpesvirus-positive primary effusion lymphoma with expression of the CD138/syndecan-1 antigen. *Blood* 1997;90:4894–4900.
655. Inki P, Larjava H, Haapasalmi K, et al. Expression of syndecan-1 is induced by differentiation and suppressed by malignant transformation of human keratinocytes. *Eur J Cell Biol* 1994;63:43–51.
656. Inki P, Joensuu H, Grenman R, et al. Association between syndecan-1 expression and clinical outcome in squamous cell carcinoma of the head and neck. *Br J Cancer* 1994;70:319–323.
657. McMichael AJ, Pilch JR, Galfre G, et al. A human thymocyte antigen defined by a hybrid myeloma monoclonal antibody. *Eur J Immunol* 1979;9:205–210.
658. Van Agthoven A, Terhorst C. Further biochemical characterization of the human thymocyte differentiation antigen T6. *J Immunol* 1982;128:426–432.
659. Boumsell L, Amiot M, Raynal B, et al. Epitopic groups of CD1 molecules. In Reinherz EL, Haynes BF, Nadler LM, et al, eds. *Leukocyte typing II, vol 1: Human T lymphocytes.* New York: Springer-Verlag, 1986:289–302.
660. Amiot M, Bernard A, Raynal B, et al. Heterogeneity of the first cluster of differentiation: characterization and epitopic mapping of three CD1 molecules on normal human thymus cells. *J Immunol* 1986;136:1752–1758.
661. Amoit M, Dastot H, Degos L, et al. Study of the CD1 monoclonal antibodies from the Workshop panel. In: McMichael AJ, Beverley PCL, Cobbold S, et al, eds. *Leucocyte typing III: white cell differentiation antigens.* Oxford: Oxford University Press, 1987:80–81.
662. Balk SP, Bleicher PA, Terhorst C. Isolation and characterization of a cDNA and gene coding for a fourth CD1 molecule. *Proc Natl Acad Sci USA* 1989;86:252–256.
663. Wood GS, Warner NL, Warnke RA. Anti-Leu-3/T4 antibodies react with cells of monocyte/macrophage and Langerhans lineage. *J Immunol* 1983;131:212–216.
664. Olive D, Dubreuil P, Mawas C. Two distinct TL-like molecular subsets defined by monoclonal antibodies on the surface of human thymocytes with different expression on leukemia lines. *Immunogenetics* 1984;20:253–264.
665. Knowles RW, Bodmer WF. A monoclonal antibody recognizing a human TL-like antigen. *Eur J Immunol* 1982;12:676–681.
666. Boumsell L. T cell antigens: section report. In: Schlossman SF, Boumsell L, Gilks WR, et al, eds. *Leukocyte typing V: white cell differentiation antigens.* New York: Oxford University Press, 1995;241–279.
667. Fainboim L, Salamone MC. CD1 workshop panel report. In: Kishimoto T, Kikutani H, von dem Borne AEGK, et al, eds. *Leukocyte typing VI: white cell differentiation antigens.* New York: Garland Publishing, 1998:33–37.
668. Boumsell L. Cluster report CD1. In: Knapp W, Dörken B, Gilks WR, et al, eds. *Leucocyte typing IV: white cell differentiation antigens.* New York: Oxford University Press, 1989:251–254.
669. Krenacs L, Tiszalvicz L, Krenacs T, et al. Immunohistochemical detection of CD1a antigen in formalin-fixed and paraffin-embedded tissue sections with monoclonal antibody O10. *J Pathol* 1993;171:99–104.
670. Emile JF, Wechsler J, Brousse N, et al. Langerhans' cell histiocytosis: definitive diagnosis with the use of monoclonal antibody O10 on routinely paraffin-embedded samples. *Am J Surg Pathol* 1995;19:636–641.
671. Terhorst C, van Agthoven A, LeClair K, et al. Biochemical studies of the human thymocyte cell-surface antigens T6, T9 and T10. *Cell* 1981;23:771–780.
672. Van de Rijn M, Lerch P, Knowles RW, et al. The thymic differentiation markers T6 and M241 are two unusual MHC class I antigens. *J Immunol* 1983;131:851–855.
673. Kefford RF, Calabi F, Fearnley IM, et al. Serum beta 2-microglobulin

binds to a T-cell differentiation antigen and increases its expression. *Nature* 1984;308:641–642.

674. Calabi F, Yung Yu C, Bilsland CAG, et al. In deSrivastava R, Ram B, Tyle P, eds. *Immunogenetics of the major histocompatability complex.* New York: VCH Publishers, 1991:215–243.
675. Yu CY, Milstein C. A physical map linking the five CD1 human thymocyte differentiation antigen genes. *EMBO J* 1989;8: 3727–3732.
676. Martin LH, Calabi F, Milstein C. Isolation of CD1 genes: a family of major histocompatibility complex-related differentiation antigens. *Proc Natl Acad Sci USA* 1986;83:9154–9158.
677. Calabi F, Milstein C. A novel family of human major histocompatibility complex-related genes not mapping to chromosome 6. *Nature* 1986;323:540–543.
678. Martin LH, Calabi F, Lefebvre FA, et al. Structure and expression of the human thymocyte antigens CD1a, CD1b, and CD1c. *Proc Natl Acad Sci USA* 1987;84:9189–9193.
679. Melian A, Beckman EM, Porcelli SA, et al. Antigen presentation by CD1 and MHC-encoded class I-like molecules. *Curr Opin Immunol* 1996;8:82–88.
680. Mooney N, Zilber M-T, Charron D, et al. CD1 workshop: The CD1a molecule participates in superantigen-induced activation of human thymocytes and peripheral blood T cells. In: Kishimoto T, Kikutani H, von dem Borne AEGK, et al, eds. *Leukocyte typing VI: white cell differentiation antigens.* New York: Garland Publishing, 1998: 38–39.
681. Porcelli S, Brenner MB, Greenstein JL, et al. Recognition of cluster of differentiation I antigens by human $CD4^-CD8^-$ cytolytic T lymphocytes. *Nature* 1989;341:447–450.
682. Cattoretti G, Berti E, Mancuso A, et al. A MHC class 1 related family of antigens with widespread distribution on resting and activated cells. In: McMichael AJ, Beverley PCL, Cobbold S, et al, eds. *Leukocyte typing III: white cell differentiation antigens.* Oxford: Oxford University Press, 1987;89–92.
683. Salamone MC, Fainboim L. Intracellular expression of CD1 molecules on PHA-activated normal T lymphocytes. *Immunol Lett* 1992; 33:61–66.
684. Picozzi VJ, Coleman CN. Lymphoblastic lymphoma. *Semin Oncol* 1990;17:96–103.
685. Fithian E, Kung P, Goldstein G, et al. Reactivity of Langerhans cells with hybridoma antibody. *Proc Natl Acad Sci USA* 1981;78: 2541–2544.
686. Ray A, Schmitt D, Dezutter-Dambuyant C, et al. Reappearance of CD1a antigenic sites after endocytosis on human Langerhans cells evidenced by immunogold relabeling. *J Invest Dermatol* 1989;92: 217–224.
687. Van de Rijn M, Lerch PG, Bronstein BR, et al. Human cutaneous dendritic cells express two glycoproteins T6 and M241 which are biochemically identical to those found on cortical thymocytes. *Hum Immunol* 1984;9:201–210.
688. Bujdoso R, Hopkins J, Dutia BM, et al. Characterization of sheep afferent lymph dendritic cells and their role in antigen carriage. *J Exp Med* 1989; 170:1285–1302.
689. Favera BE, McCarthy RC, Mierau GW. Histiocytosis X. *Hum Pathol* 1983;14:663–676.
690. Schuler G, Stingl G, Aberer W, et al. Histiocytosis X cells in esoinphilic granuloma express Ia and T6 antigens. *J Invest Dermatol* 1983; 80:405–409.
691. Turner RR, Wood GS, Beckstead JH, et al. Histiocytic malignancies: morphologic, immunologic, and enzymatic heterogeneity. *Am J Surg Pathol* 1984;8:485–500.
692. Franklin WA, Mason DY, Pulford K, et al. Immunohistological analysis of human mononuclear phagocytes and dendritic cells by using monoclonal antibodies. *Lab Invest* 1986;54:322–335.
693. Roholl PJM, Kleyne J, Prins MEF, et al. Immunologic marker analysis of normal and malignant histiocytes: a comparative study of monoclonal antibodies for diagnostic purposes. *Am J Clin Pathol* 1988;89:187–194.
694. Salamone MC, Roisman FR, Morelli AE, et al. Analysis of CD1 molecules on haematological malignancies of myeloid and lymphoid origin: II. Intracellular detection of CD1 antigens. *Dis Markers* 1990; 8:275–281.
695. Small TN, Knowles RW, Keever C, et al. M241 (CD1) expression on B lymphocytes. *J Immunol* 1987;138:2864–2868.
696. Delia D, Cattoretti G, Polli N, et al. CD1c but neither CD1a nor CD1b molecules are expressed on normal, activated, and malignant human B cells: identification of a new B-cell subset. *Blood* 1988; 72:241–247.
697. Small TN, Keever CA, Knowles RW, et al. CD1c expression during normal B cell ontogeny. In: Knapp W, Dörken B, Gilks WR, et al, eds. *Leucocyte typing IV: white cell differentiation antigens.* New York: Oxford University Press, 1989:265–266.
698. Reinherz EL. A molecular basis for thymic selection: regulation of T11 induced thymocyte expansion by the T3-Ti antigen/MHC receptor pathway. *Immunol Today* 1985;6:75–79.
699. Moingeon P, Chang HC, Sayre PH, et al. The structural biology of CD2. *Immunol Rev* 1989;111:111–144.
700. Bierer BE, Sleckman BP, Ratnofsky SE, et al. The biologic roles of CD2, CD4, and CD8 in T-cell activation. *Annu Rev Immunol* 1989; 7:579–599.
701. McMichael AJ, Gotch FM. T cell antigens: new and previously defined clusters. In: McMichael AJ, Beverley PCL, Cobbold S, et al, eds. *Leucocyte typing III: white cell differentiation antigens.* Oxford: Oxford University Press, 1987;31–62.
702. Meuer SC. Cluster report: CD2. In: Knapp W, Dörken B, Gilks WR, et al, eds. *Leukocyte typing IV: white cell differentiation antigens.* Oxford: Oxford University Press, 1989:270–272.
703. Denning SM. CD2 cluster report. In: Schlossman SF, Boumsell L, Gilks WR, et al, eds. *Leukocyte typing V: white cell differentiation antigens.* New York: Oxford University Press, 1995:342–343.
704. Kato K. CD2 workshop panel report. In: Kishimoto T, Kikutani H, von dem Borne AEGK, et al, eds. *Leukocyte typing VI: white cell differentiation antigens.* New York: Garland Publishing, 1998: 39–43.
705. Sewell WA, Palmer RW, Spurr NK, et al. The human LFA-3 gene is located at the same chromosome band as the gene for its receptor CD2. *Immunogenetics* 1988;28:278–282.
706. Sewell WA, Brown MH, Dunne J, et al. Molecular cloning of the human T-lymphocyte surface CD2 (T11) antigen. *Proc Natl Acad Sci USA* 1986;83:8711–8722.
707. Meuer SC, Hussey RE, Fabbi M, et al. An alternative pathway of T-cell activation: a functional role for the 50 kd T11 sheep erythrocyte receptor protein. *Cell* 1984; 36:897–906.
708. Kabelitz D. Do CD2 and CD3-TCR T-cell activation pathways function independently? *Immunol Today* 1990; 11:44–46.
709. Yang SY, Chouaib S, Dupont B. A common pathway for T lymphocyte activation involving both the CD3-Ti complex and CD2 sheep erythrocyte receptor determinants. *J Immunol* 1986;137:1097–1100.
710. Yang SY, Rhee S, Angelos G, et al. Functional analysis of CD2 (T,p50) epitopes detected by 24 CD2 antibodies. In: McMichael AJ, Beverley PCL, Cobbold S, et al, eds. *Leukocyte typing III: white cell differentiation antigens.* Oxford: Oxford University Press, 1987: 113–115.
711. Meuer SC, Fitzgerald KA, Hussey RE, et al. Clonotypic structures involved in antigen-specific human T cell function: Relationship to the T3 molecular complex. *J Exp Med* 1983;157:705–719.
712. Haskins K, Kubo R, White J, et al. The major histocompatibility complex-restricted antigen receptor on T cells: I. Isolation with a monoclonal antibody. *J Exp Med* 1983;157:1149–1169.
713. Meuer SC, Acuto O, Hussey RE, et al. Evidence for the T3-associated 90K heterodimer as the T-cell antigen receptor. *Nature* 1983;303: 808–810.
714. Kanner SB, Damle NK, Blake J, et al. CD2/LFA-3 ligation induces phospholipase-C gamma 1 tyrosine phosphorylation and regulates CD3 signaling. *J Immunol* 1992;148:2023–2029.
715. Howard FD, Moingeon P, Moebius U, et al. The CD3 zeta cytoplasmic domain mediates CD2-induced T cell activation. *J Exp Med* 1992;176:139–145.
716. Bowden G, Diaz LA, Li LL, et al. Epitopes and functional responses defined by workshop anti-CD2 mAb. In: Schlossman SF, Boumsell L, Gilks WR, et al, eds. *Leukocyte typing V: white cell differentiation antigens.* New York: Oxford University Press, 1995:346–347.
717. Shaw S, Luce GE, Quinones R, et al. Two antigen-independent adhesion pathways used by human cytotoxic T-cell clones. *Nature* 1986; 323:262–264.
718. Wallner BP, Frey AZ, Tizard R, et al. Primary structure of lymphocyte function-associated antigen 3 (LFA-3): the ligand of the T lymphocyte CD2 glycoprotein. *J Exp Med* 1987;166:923–932.

719. Hahn WC, Menu E, Bothwell AL, et al. Overlapping but nonidentical binding sites on CD2 for CD58 and a second ligand CD59. *Science* 1992;256:1805–1807.
720. Arulanandam ARN, Moingeon P, Concino MF, et al. A soluble multimeric recombinant CD2 protein identifies CD48 as a low affinity ligand for human CD2: divergence of CD2 ligands during the evolution of humans and mice. *J Exp Med* 1993;177:1439–1450.
721. Warren HS, Altin JG, Waldron JC, et al. A carbohydrate structure associated with CD15 (Lewis x) on myeloid cells is a novel ligand for human CD2. *J Immunol* 1996;156:2866–2873.
722. Bierer BE, Peterson A, Barbosa J, et al. Expression of the T-cell surface molecule CD2 and an epitope-loss CD2 mutant to define the role of lymphocyte function-associated antigen 3 (LFA-3) in T-cell activation. *Proc Natl Acad Sci USA* 1988;85:1194–1198.
723. Dustin ML, Sanders ME, Shaw S, et al. Purified lymphocyte function-associated antigen 3 binds to CD2 and mediates T lymphocyte adhesion. *J Exp Med* 1987;165:677–692.
724. Vollger LW, Tuck DT, Springer TA, et al. Thymocyte binding to human thymic epithelial cells is inhibited by monoclonal antibodies to CD-2 and LFA-3 antigens. *J Immunol* 1987;138:358–363.
725. Lanier LL, Phillips JH. A map of the cell surface antigens expressed on resting and activated human natural killer cells. In: Reinherz El, Haynes BF, Nadler LM, et al, eds. *Leucocyte typing II: human, myeloid and hematopoietic cells.* New York: Springer-Verlag, 1986: 157–170.
726. Picker LJ, Weiss LM, Medeiros JL, et al. Immunophenotypic criteria for the diagnosis of non-Hodgkin's lymphoma. *Am J Pathol* 1987; 128:181–201.
727. Weiss LM, Crabtree GS, Rouse RV, et al. Morphologic and immunologic characterization of 50 peripheral T cell lymphomas. *Am J Pathol* 1985;118:316–324.
728. Uckun FM, Muraguchi A, Ledbetter JA, et al. Biphenotypic leukemic lymphocyte precursors in $CD2^+CD19^+$ acute lymphoblastic leukemia and their putative normal counterparts in human fetal hematopoietic tissues. *Blood* 1989;73:1000–1015.
729. Mirro J, Antouin GR, Zipf TF, et al. The E-rosette associated antigen of T cells can be identified on blasts from patients with acute myeloblastic leukemia. *Blood* 1985;65:363–367.
730. Venditti A, Del Poeta G, Buccisano F, et al. Minimally differentiated acute myeloid leukemia (AML-M0): comparison of 25 cases with other French-American-British subtypes. *Blood* 1997;89:621–629.
731. Rovelli A, Biondi A, Rajnoldi AC, et al. Microgranular variant of acute promyelocytic leukemia in children. *J Clin Oncol* 1992;10: 1413–1418.
732. Claxton DF, Reading CL, Nagarajan L, et al. Correlation of CD2 expression with PML gene breakpoints in patients with acute promyelocytic leukemia. *Blood* 1992;80:582–586.
733. Adriaansen HJ, te Boekhorst PAW, Hagemeijer AM, et al. Acute myeloid leukemia M4 with bone marrow eosinophilia (M4Eo) and inv(16) (p13q22) exhibits a specific immunophenotype with CD2 expression. *Blood* 1993;81:3043–3051.
734. Paietta E, Wiernik PH, Andersen J, et al. Acute myeloid leukemia M4 with inv(16) (p13q22) exhibits a specific immunophenotype with CD2 expression, correspondence. *Blood* 1993;82:2595.
735. Larson RA, Williams SF, Le Beau MM, et al. Acute myelomonocytic leukemia with abnormal eosinophils and inv (16) or t(16;16) has a favorable prognosis. *Blood* 1986;68:1242–1249.
736. Haferlach T, Gassmann W, Loffler H, et al. The AML Cooperative Group: clinical aspects of acute myeloid leukemias of the FAB types M3 and M4Eo. *Ann Hematol* 1993;66:165–170.
737. Reinherz E, Hussey RE, Schlossman SF. A monoclonal antibody blocking human T cell function. *Eur J Immunol* 1980;10:758–762.
738. Burns GF, Boyd AW, Beverley PCL. Two monoclonal anti-human T lymphocyte antibodies have similar biologic effects and recognize the same cell surface antigen. *J Immunol* 1982;129:1451–1457.
739. Ledbetter JA, Evans RL, Lipinski M, et al. Evolutionary conservation of surface molecules that distinguish T lymphocyte helper/inducer and cytotoxic/suppressor subpopulations in mouse and man. *J Exp Med* 1981;153:310–323.
740. Saito T, Yamazaki T. CD3 workshop panel report. In: Kishimoto T, Kikutani H, von dem Borne AEGK, et al, eds. *Leukocyte typing VI: white cell differentiation antigens.* New York: Garland Publishing, 1998:44–48.
741. Mason DY, Cordell J, Brown M, et al. Detection of T cells in paraffin wax embedded tissue using antibodies against a peptide sequence from the CD3 antigen. *J Clin Pathol* 1989;42:1194–1200.
742. Mason DY, Krissansen GW, Davey FR, et al. Antisera against epitopes resistant to denaturation on T3 (CD3) antigen can detect reactive and neoplastic T cells in paraffin embedded tissue biopsy specimens. *J Clin Pathol* 1988;41:121–127.
743. Anderson C, Rezuke WN, Kosciol CM, et al. Identification of T-cell lymphomas in paraffin-embedded tissues using polyclonal anti-CD3 antibody: comparison with frozen section immunophenotyping and genotypic analysis. *Mod Pathol* 1991;4:358–362.
744. Steward M, Bishop R, Piggott NH, et al. Production and characterization of a new monoclonal antibody effective in recognizing the CD3 T cell associated antigen in formalin-fixed embedded tissue. *Histopathology* 1997;30:16–22.
745. Evans GA, Lewis KA, Lawless GM. Molecular organization of the human CD3 gene family on chromosome 11q23. *Immunogenetics* 1988;28:365–373.
746. Tunnacliffe A, Olsson C, Buluwela L, et al. Organization of the human CD3 locus on chromosome 11. *Eur J Immunol* 1988;18: 1639–1642.
747. Nanni L, Poggi A. CD3 ζ workshop panel report. In Kishimoto T, Kikutani H, von dem Borne AEGK, et al, eds. *Leukocyte typing VI: white cell differentiation antigens.* New York: Garland Publishing, 1998:268–269.
748. Mercep M, Bonifacino JS, Garcia-Morales P, et al. T cell CD3-zeta eta heterodimer expression and coupling to phosphoinositide hydrolysis. *Science* 1988;242:571–574.
749. Samelson LE, Phillips AF, Luong ET, et al. Association of the fyn protein-tyrosine kinase with the T-cell antigen receptor. *Proc Natl Acad Sci USA* 1990;87:4358–4362.
750. Weisman AM, Hou D, Orloff DG, et al. Molecular cloning and chromosomal localization of the human T-cell receptor zeta chain: distinction from the molecular CD3 complex. *Proc Natl Acad Sci USA* 1988;85:9709–9713.
751. Ashwell JD, Klausner RD. Genetic and mutational analysis of the T-cell antigen receptor. *Annu Rev Immunol* 1990;8:139–167.
752. Van Wauwe JP, De Mey JR, Goossens JG. OKT3: a monoclonal anti-human T lymphocyte antibody with potent mitogenic properties. *J Immunol* 1980;124:2708–2713.
753. Von Wussow P, Platsoukas CD, Wiranowska-Stewart M, et al. Human gamma interferon production by leukocytes induced with monoclonal antibodies recognizing T cells. *J Immunol* 1981;127: 1197–1200.
754. Platzer E, Rubin BY, Lu L, et al. OKT3 monoclonal antibody induces production of colonly-stimulating factor(s) for granulocytes and macrophages in cultures of human T lymphocytes and adherent cells. *J Immunol* 1985:134:265–271.
755. Tsoukas CD, Valentine MA, Lotz M, et al. The role of the T3 molecular complex on human T lymphocyte-mediated cytotoxicity. *Adv Exp Med Biol* 1985;184:365–385.
756. Spits H, Yssel H, Leeuwenberg J, et al. Antigen specific cytotoxic T cell and antigen-specific proliferating T cell clones can be induced to cytolytic activity by monoclonal antibodies against T3. *Eur J Immunol* 1985;15:88–91.
757. Tax WJ, Willems HW, Reekers PP, et al. Polymorphism in mitogenic effect of IgG1 monoclonal antibodies against T3 antigen on human T cells. *Nature* 1983;304:445–447.
758. Kaneoka H, Preez-Rojas G, Sasasuki T, et al. Human T lymphocyte proliferation induced by a pan-T monoclonal antibody (anti-Leu4): heterogeneity of response is a function of monocytes. *J Immunol* 1983;131:158–164.
759. Looney RJ, Abraham GN. The Fc portion of intact IgG blocks stimulation of human PBMC by anti-T3. *J Immunol* 1984;133:154–156.
760. Smith KG, Austyn JM, Hariri G, et al. T cell activation by anti-T3 antibodies: comparison of IgG1 and IgG2b switch variants and direct evidence for accessory function of macrophage Fc receptors. *Eur J Immunol* 1986;16:478–486.
761. Goldsmith MA, Weiss A. New clues about T-cell antigen receptor complex function. *Immunol Today* 1988;9:220–222.
762. Irving BA, Weiss A. The cytoplasmic domain of the T cell receptor zeta chain is sufficient to couple to receptor-associated signal transduction pathways. *Cell* 1991;64:891–901.
763. Reth M. Antigen receptor tail clue. *Nature* 1989;333:383–384.
764. Osman N, Turner H, Lucas S, et al. The protein interactions of the

immunoglobulin receptor family tyrosine-based activation motifs present in the T cell receptor zeta subunits and the CD3 gamma, delta and epsilon chains. *Eur J Immunol* 1996;26:1063–1068.
765. Bernard A, Boumsell L, Reinherz EL, et al. Cell surface characterization of malignant T cells from lymphoblastic lymphoma using monoclonal antibodies: evidence for phenotypic differences between malignant T cells from patients with acute lymphoblastic leukemia and lymphoblastic lymphoma. *Blood* 1981;57:1105–1110.
766. Roper M, Crist WM, Metzgar R, et al. Monoclonal antibody characterization of surface antigens in childhood T-cell lymphoid malignancies. *Blood* 1983;61:830–837.
767. Link MP, Stewart SJ, Warnke RA, et al. Discordance between surface and cytoplasmic expression of the Leu-4 (T3) antigen in thymocytes and in blast cells from childhood T lymphoblastic malignancies. *J Clin Invest* 1985;76:248–253.
768. Campana D, Thompson JS, Amlot P, et al. The cytoplasmic expression of CD3 antigens in normal and malignant cells of the T lymphoid lineage. *J Immunol* 1987;138:648–655.
769. van Dongen JJM, Krissansen GW, Wolvers-Tettero ILM, et al. Cytoplasmic expression of the CD3 antigen as a diagnostic marker for immature T-cell malignancies. *Blood* 1988;71:603–612.
770. van Dongen JJM, Quertermous T, Bartram CR, et al. T cell receptor-CD3 complex during early T cell differentiation: analysis of immature T cell acute lymphoblastic leukemias (T-ALL) at DNA, RNA, and cell membrane level. *J Immunol* 1987;138:1260–1269.
771. Campana D, Janossy G, Coustan-Smith E, et al. The expression of T cell receptor-associated proteins during T cell ontogeny in man. *J Immunol* 1989;142;57–66
772. Haynes BF, Martin ME, Kay HH, et al. Early events in human T cell ontogeny: phenotypic characterization and immunohistologic localization of T cell precursors in early human fetal tissues. *J Exp Med* 1988;168:1061–1080.
773. Biassoni R, Ferrini S, Prigione I, et al. CD3-negative lymphokine-activated cytotoxic cells express the CD3 epsilon gene. *J Immunol* 1988;140:1685–1689.
774. Garson JA, Beverley PCL, Coakham HB, et al. Monoclonal antibodies against human T lymphocytes label Purkinje neurons of many species. *Nature* 1982;298:375–377.
775. Transy C, Moingeon PE, Marshall B, et al. Most murine anti-human CD3 mAb recognize the human CD3ϵ subunit. In: Knapp W, Dorken B, Gilks WR, et al, eds. *Leukocyte typing IV: white cell differentiation antigens.* New York: Oxford University Press, 1989:293–295.
776. Scott CS, Richards SJ. Classification of large granular lymphocyte (LGL) and NK-associated (NKa) disorders. *Blood Rev* 1992;6: 220–233.
777. Rambaldi A, Pelicci PG, Allavena P, et al. T cell receptor β chain gene rearrangements in lymphoproliferative disorders of large granular lymphocytes/natural killer cells. *J Exp Med* 1985;162: 2156–2162.
778. Loughran TP Jr. Clonal diseases of large granular lymphocytes. *Blood* 1993;82:1–14.
779. Otsuki T, Kumar S, Ensoli B, et al. Detection of HHV-8/KSHV DNA sequences in AIDS-associated extranodal lymphoid malignancies. *Leukemia* 1996;10:1358–1362.
780. Cantor H, Boyse EA. Regulation of cellular and humoral immune responses by T-cell subclasses. *Cold Spring Harbour Symp Quant Biol* 1977;41:23–32.
781. Evans RL, Breard JM, Lazarus H, et al. Detection, isolation and functional characterization of two human T cell subclasses bearing unique differentiation antigens. *J Exp Med* 1977;145:221–233.
782. Reinherz EL, Moretta L, Roper M, et al. Human T lymphocyte subpopulations defined by Fc receptors and monoclonal antibodies: a comparison. *J Exp Med* 1980;151:969–974.
783. Reinherz EL, Kung PC, Goldstein G, et al. Separation of functional subsets of human T cells by a monoclonal antibody. *Proc Natl Acad Sci USA* 1979;76:4061–4065.
784. Evans RL, Wall DW, Platsoucas CD, et al. Thymus-dependent membrane antigens in man: inhibition of cell-mediated lympholysis by monoclonal antibodies to the TH2 antigen. *Proc Natl Acad Sci USA* 1981;78:544–548.
785. Reinherz EL, Kung PC, Goldstein G, et al. A monoclonal antibody reactive with the human cytotoxic/suppressor T cell subset previously defined by a heteroantiserum termed TH2. *J Immunol* 1980; 124:1301–1307.
786. Moebius U. Cluster report: CD4. In: Knapp W, Dörken B, Gilks WR, et al, eds. *Leukocyte typing IV: white cell differentiation antigens.* Oxford: Oxford University Press, 1989:314–316.
787. Moebius U. Cluster report: CD8. In: Knapp W, Dörken B, Gilks WR, et al, eds. *Leukocyte typing IV: white cell differentiation antigens.* Oxford: Oxford University Press, 1989:342–343.
788. Piatier-Tonneau D. CD4 workshop panel report. In: Kishimoto T, Kikutani H, von dem Borne AEGK, et al, eds. *Leukocyte typing VI: white cell differentiation antigens.* New York: Garland Publishing, 1998:49–54.
789. Nakauchi H. CD8 workshop panel report. In: Kishimoto T, Kikutani H, von dem Borne AEGK, et al, eds. *Leukocyte typing VI: white cell differentiation antigens.* New York: Garland Publishing, 1998: 65–67.
790. Williamson SLH, Steward M, Milton I, et al. New monoclonal antibodies to the T cell antigens CD4 and CD8: production and characterization in formalin-fixed paraffin-embedded tissue. *Am J Pathol* 1998;152:1421–1426.
791. Littman DR. The structure of the CD4 and CD8 genes. *Annu Rev Immunol* 1987;5:561–584.
792. Maddon PJ, Littman DR, Godfrey M, et al. The isolation and nucleotide sequence of a cDNA encoding the T cell surface protein T4: a new member of the immunoglobulin gene family. *Cell* 1985;42: 93–104.
793. Littman DR, Gettner SN. Unusual intron in the Ig-like domain of the newly isolated mouse CD4 (L3T4) gene. *Nature* 1987;325:453–455.
794. Isobe M, Huebner K, Maddon PJ, et al. The gene encoding the T-cell surface protein T4 is located on human chromosome 12. *Proc Natl Acad Sci USA* 1986;83:4399–4402.
795. Littman DR, Thomas Y, Maddon PJ, et al. The isolation and sequence of the gene encoding T8: a molecule defining functional classes of T lymphocytes. *Cell* 1985;40:237–246.
796. Terry LA, DiSanto JP, Small TN, et al. Differential expression of the CD8 and Lyt-3 antigens on a subset of human T cell receptor γ/δ-bearing lymphocytes. In: Knapp W, Dörken B, Gilks WR, et al, eds. *Leukocyte typing IV: white cell differentiation antigens.* Oxford: Oxford University Press, 1989:345–346.
797. DiSanto JP, Knowles RW, Flomenberg N. The human Lyt-3 molecule requires CD8 for cell surface expression. *EMBO J* 1988;7: 3465–3470.
798. Sukhatme VP, Sizer KC, Vollmer AC, et al. The T cell differentiation antigen Leu2/T8 is homologous to immunoglobulin and T cell receptor variable regions. *Cell* 1985;40:591–597.
799. Norment AM, Littman DR. A second subunit of CD8 is expressed in human T cells. *EMBO J* 1988;7:3433–3439.
800. Shiue L, Gorman SD, Parnes JR. A second chain of human CD8 is expressed on peripheral blood lymphocytes. *J Exp Med* 1988;168: 1993–2005.
801. Sukhatme VP, Vollmer A, Erikson J, et al. Gene for the human T cell differentiation antigen Leu-2/T8 is closely linked to the κ light chain locus on chromosome 2. *J Exp Med* 1985;161:429–434.
802. Nakayama K-I, Tokito S, Okumura K, et al. Structure and expression of the gene encoding CD8 alpha chain (Leu-2/T8). *Immunogenetics* 1989;30:393–397.
803. Nakayama K-I, Kawachi Y, Tokito S, et al. Recent duplication of the two human CD8 beta-chain genes. *J Immunol* 1992;148:1919–1927.
804. Giblin P, Ledbetter JA, Kavathas P. A secreted form of the human lymphocyte cell surface molecule CD8 arises from alternative splicing. *Proc Natl Acad Sci USA* 1989;86:998–1002.
805. Fujimoto J, Levy S, Levy R. Spontaneous release of the Leu-2 (T8) molecule from human T cells. *J Exp Med* 1983;159:752–766.
806. Agostini C, Semenzato G, Vinante F, et al. Increased levels of soluble CD8 molecule in the serum of patients with acquired immunodeficiency syndrome (AIDS) and AIDS-related disorders. *Clin Immunol Immunopathol* 1989;50:146–153.
807. Swain SL. T cell subsets and the recognition of MHC class. *Immunol Rev* 1983;74:129–142.
808. Doyle C, Strominger JL. Interaction between CD4 and class II MHC molecules mediates cell adhesion. *Nature* 1987;330:256–259.
809. Ratnofsky SE, Peterson A, Greenstein JL, et al. Expression and function of CD8 in a murine T cell hybridoma. *J Exp Med* 1987;166: 1747–1757.
810. König R, Huang LY, Germain RN. MHC class II interaction with

CD4 mediated by a region analogous to the MHC class I binding site for CD8. *Nature* 1992;356:796–798.
811. Cammarota G, Scheirle A, Takacs B, et al. Identification of a CD4 binding site on the beta 2 domain of HLA-DR molecules. *Nature* 1992;356:799–801.
812. Newell MK, Haughn LJ, Maroun CR, et al. Death of mature T cells by separate ligation of CD4 and the T-cell receptor for antigen. *Nature* 1990;347:286–289.
813. Mazerolles F, Auffray C, Fischer A. Down regulation of T-cell adhesion by CD4. *Hum Immunol* 1991;31:40–46.
814. Salter RD, Benjamin RJ, Wesley PK, et al. A binding site for the T-cell co-receptor CD8 on the alpha 3 domain of HLA-A2. *Nature* 1990;345:41–46.
815. Dalgleish AG, Beverley PCL, Clapham PR, et al. The CD4 (T4) antigen is an essential component of the receptor for the AIDS retrovirus. *Nature* 1984;312:763–766.
816. Klatzmann D, Champagne E, Chamaret S, et al. T-lymphocyte T4 molecule behaves as the receptor for human retrovirus LAV. *Nature* 1984;312:767–768.
817. Moore JP, Koup RA. Chemoattractants attract HIV researchers [Comment]. *J Exp Med* 1996;184:311–313.
818. Lapham CK, Ouyang J, Chandrasekhar B, et al. Evidence for cell-surface association between fusin and the CD4-gp120 complex in human cell lines. *Science* 1996;274:602–605.
819. Center DM, Kornfeld H, Cruikshank WW. Interleukin 16 and its function as a CD4 ligand. *Immunol Today* 1996;17:476–481.
820. Autiero M, Cammarota G, Friedlein A, et al. A 17-kda CD4-binding glycoprotein present in human seminal plasma and in breast tumor cells. *Eur J Immunol* 1995;25:1461–1464.
821. Veillette A, Bookman MA, Horak EM, et al. The CD4 and CD8 T cell surface antigens are associated with the internal membrane tyrosine-protein kinase p56lck. *Cell* 1988;55:301–308.
822. Rudd CE, Trevellyan JM, Dasgupta JD, et al. The CD4 receptor is complexed in detergent lysates to a protein-tyrosine kinase (pp58) from human T lymphocytes. *Proc Natl Acad Sci USA* 1988;85:5190–5194.
823. Barber EK, Dasgupta JD, Schlossman SF, et al. The CD4 and CD8 antigens are coupled to a protein-tyrosine kinase (p56lck) that phosphorylates the CD3 complex. *Proc Natl Acad Sci USA* 1989;86:3277–3281.
824. Yarden Y, Escobedo JA, Kuang W-J, et al. Structure of the receptor for platelet-derived growth factor helps define a family of closely related growth factor receptors. *Nature* 1986;323:226–232.
825. Kisielow P, von Boehmer H. Development and selection of T cells: facts and puzzles. *Adv Immunol* 1995;58:87–209.
826. Gaubin M, Autiero M, Houlgatte R, et al. Molecular basis of T lymphocyte CD4 antigen functions. *Eur J Clin Chem Clin Biochem* 1996;34:723–728.
827. Baldari CT, Milia E, DiSomma MM, et al. Distinct signaling properties identify functionally different CD4 epitopes. *Eur J Immunol* 1995;25:1843–1850.
828. Sakihama T, Smolyar A, Reinherz EL. Oligomerization of CD4 is required for stable binding to class II major histocompatibility complex proteins but not for interaction with human immunodeficiency virus gp120. *Proc Natl Acad Sci USA* 1995;92:6444–6448.
829. Zhang X, Piatier-Tonneau D, Auffray C, et al. Synthetic CD4 exocyclic peptides antagonize CD4 holoreceptor binding and T cell activation. *Nature Biotechnol* 1996;14:472–475.
830. Fung-Leung WP, Schilham MW, Rahemtulla A, et al. CD8 is needed for development of cytotoxic T cells but not helper T cells. *Cell* 1991;65:443–449.
831. Nakayama K, Nakayama K, Negishi I, et al. Requirement for CD8 beta chain in positive selection of CD8-lineage T cells. *Science* 1994;263:1131–1133.
832. Van Dongen JJ, Comans-Bitter WM, Wolvers-Tettero IL, et al. Development of human T lymphocytes and their thymus-dependency. *Thymus* 1990;16:207–234.
833. Thomas Y, Rogozinski L, Chess L. Relationship between human T cell functional heterogeneity and human T cell surface molecules. *Immunol Rev* 1983;74:113–128.
834. Biddison WE, Shaw S. CD4 expression and function in HLA class II-specific T cells. *Immunol Rev* 1989;109:5–15.
835. Morimoto C, Letvin NL, Distaso JA, et al. The isolation and characterization of the human suppressor inducer T cell subset. *J Immunol* 1985;134:1508–1515.
836. Tedder TF, Cooper MD, Clement LT. Human lymphocyte differentiation antigens HB-10 and HB-11: II. Differential production of B cell growth and differentiation factors by distinct helper T cell subpopulations. *J Immunol* 1985;134:2989–2994.
837. Morimoto C, Letvin NL, Boyd AW, et al. The isolation and characterization of the human helper inducer T cell subset. *J Immunol* 1985;134:3762–3769.
838. Sanders ME, Makgoba MW, Shaw S. Human naive and memory T cells: reinterpretation of helper-inducer and suppressor-inducer subsets. *Immunol Today* 1988;9:195–199.
839. Morimoto C, Torimoto Y, Levinson G, et al. 1F7, a novel cell surface molecule, involved in helper function of CD4 cells. *J Immunol* 1989;143:3430–3439.
840. Rao PE, Talle MA, Kung PC, et al. Five epitopes of a differentiation antigen on human inducer T cells distinguished by monoclonal antibodies. *Cell Immunol* 1983;80:310–319.
841. Negoro T, Tanigaki N. Serological and functional analysis of the epitope clusters on Leu3/T4 antigen. *Hum Immunol* 1986;15:137–149.
842. Stohl W, Kunkel HG. Heterogeneity in expression of the T4 epitope in black individuals. *Scand J Immunol* 1984;20:273–278.
843. Stohl W. Deficient OKT4 epitope on helper T cells in a patient with SLE: confusion with AIDS. *N Engl J Med* 1984;310:1531.
844. Janossy G, Tidman N, Selby WS, et al. Subpopulations of human T lymphocytes occupy different microenvironments. *Nature* 1980;288:81–84.
845. Centers for Disease Control. 1993 Revised classification system for HIV infection and expanded surveillance case definition for AIDS among adolescents and adults. *MMWR* 1992;41:1–19.
846. Centers for Disease Control. 1994 Revised classification system for human immunodeficiency virus infection in children less than 13 years of age. *MMWR* 1994;43:1–10.
847. Haynes FR, Metzgar RS, Minna JD, et al. Phenotypic characterization of cutaneous T-cell lymphoma: use of monoclonal antibodies to compare with other malignant T cells. *N Engl J Med* 1981;304:1319–1323.
848. Haynes BF, Bunn P, Mann D, et al. Cell surface differentiation antigens of the malignant T cell in Sezary syndrome and mycosis fungoides. *J Clin Invest* 1981;67:523–530.
849. Reinherz EL, Kung PC, Goldstein G, et al. A monoclonal antibody with selective reactivity with functionally mature human thymocytes and all peripheral human T cells. *J Immunol* 1979;123:1312–1317.
850. Wang CY, Good RA, Ammirati P, et al. Identification of a p69,71 complex expressed on human T cells sharing determinants with B-type chronic lymphatic leukemic cells. *J Exp Med* 1980;151:1539–1544.
851. Engleman EG, Warnke R, Fox RI, et al. Studies of a human T lymphocyte antigen recognized by a monoclonal antibody. *Proc Natl Acad Sci USA* 1981;78:1791–1795.
852. Royston I, Majda JA, Baird SM, et al. Human T cell antigens defined by monoclonal antibodies: the 65,000-dalton antigen of T cells (T65) is also found on chronic lymphocytic leukemia cells bearing surface immunoglobulins. *J Immunol* 1980;125:725–731.
853. Arber DA, Weiss LM. CD5: a review. *Appl Immunohistochem* 1995;3:1–22.
854. Ben-Ezra JM, Kornstein MJ. Antibody NCL-CD5 fails to detect neoplastic $CD5^+$ cells in paraffin sections. *Am J Clin Pathol* 1996;106:370–373.
855. Dorfman DM, Shaksafaei A. Usefulness of a new CD5 antibody for the diagnosis of T cell and B cell lymphoproliferative disorders in paraffin tissue sections. *Mod Pathol* 1997;10:859–863.
856. Jones NH, Clabby ML, Dialynas DP, et al. Isolation of complementary DNA clones encoding the human lymphocyte glycoprotein T1/Leu-1. *Nature* 1986;323:346–349.
857. Lozano F, Calvo J, Roca A, et al. CD5 workshop panel report. In: Kishimoto T, Kikutani H, von dem Borne AEGK, et al, eds. *Leukocyte typing VI: white cell differentiation antigens.* New York: Garland Publishing, 1998:56–58.
858. Huang H-JS, Jones NH, Strominger JL, et al. Molecular cloning of Ly-1, a membrane glycoprotein of mouse T lymphocytes and a subset of B cells: molecular homology to its human counterpart Leu-1/T1 (CD5). *Proc Natl Acad Sci USA* 1987;84:204–208.

859. Martin PJ, Hansen JA, Nowinski RC, et al. A new human T-cell differentiation antigen: unexpected expression on chronic lymphocytic leukemia cells. *Immunogenetics* 1980;11:429–439.
860. Boumsell L, Coppin J, Pham D, et al. An antigen shared by a human T cell subset and B cell chronic lymphocytic leukemic cells: distribution on normal and malignant lymphoid cells. *J Exp Med* 1980;152: 229–234.
861. Caligaris-Cappio F, Gobbi M, Bonfill M, et al. Infrequent normal B lymphocyte express features of B chronic lymphocytic leukemia. *J Exp Med* 1982;155:623–628.
862. Gadol N, Ault KA. Phenotypic and functional characterization of human Leu1 (CD5) B cells. *Immunol Rev* 1986;93:23–34.
863. Hardy RR, Hayakawa K. Development and physiology of Ly-1 B and its human homolog, Leu-1 B. *Immunol Rev* 1986;93:53–79.
864. Mayer R, Logtenberg T, Strauchen J, et al. CD5 and immunoglobulin V gene expression in B-cell lymphomas and chronic lymphocytic leukemia. *Blood* 1990;75:1518–1524.
865. Wood GS, Freudenthal PS. CD5 monoclonal antibodies react with human peripheral blood dendritic cells. *Am J Pathol* 1992;141: 789–795.
866. Bárcena A, Muench MA, Galey AHM, et al. Phenotypic and functional analysis of T-cell precursors in the human fetal liver and thymus: CD7 expression in the early stages of T- and myeloid-cell development. *Blood* 1993;82:3401–3414.
867. Sánchez MJ, Spits H, Lanier LL, et al. Human natural killer cell committed thymocytes and their relation to the T cell lineage. *J Exp Med* 1993;178:1857–1866.
868. Terstappen LWMM, Huang S, Picker LJ. Flow cytometric assessment of human T-cell differentiation in thymus and bone marrow. *Blood* 1992;79:666–677.
869. Brierer BE, Nishimura Y, Burakoff SJ, et al. Phenotypic and functional characterization of human cytolytic T cells lacking expression of CD5. *J Clin Invest* 1988;81:1390–1397.
870. Brierer BE, Burakoff SJ, Smith BR. A large proportion of T lymphocytes lack CD5 expression after bone marrow transplantation. *Blood* 1989;73:1359–1366.
871. McKay PJ, Kyle B, McLaren A, et al. CD5-T lymphocytes in renal transplant recipients. *Clin Lab Haematol* 1991;13:335–340.
872. Srour EF, Leemus T, Jenski L, et al. Characterization of normal human $CD3^+$ $CD5^-$ and $\gamma\delta$ T cell receptor positive T lymphocytes. *Clin Exp Immunol* 1990;80:114–121.
873. Ueno Y, Hays EF, Hultin L, et al. Human thymocytes do not respond to interleukin-2 after removal of mature "bright" CD5 positive cells. *Cell Immunol* 1989;124:239–251.
874. Beyers AD, Spruyt LL, Williams AF. Molecular associations between the T-lymphocyte antigen receptor complex and the surface antigens CD2, CD4, or CD8 and CD5. *Proc Natl Acad Sci USA* 1992;89:2945–2949.
875. Lankester AC, van Schijndel GMW, Cordell JL, et al. CD5 is associated with the human B cell antigen receptor complex. *Eur J Immunol* 1994;24:812–816.
876. Ledbetter JA, Martin PJ, Spooner CE, et al. Antibodies to Tp67 and Tp44 augment and sustain proliferative responses of activated T cells. *J Immunol* 1985;135:2331–2336.
877. Tarakhovsky A, Kanner SB, Hombach J, et al. A role for CD5 in TCR-mediated signal transduction and thymocyte selection. *Science* 1995;269:535–537.
878. Burgess KE, Yamamoto M, Prasad KVS, et al. CD5 acts as a tyrosine kinase substrate within a receptor complex comprising T-cell receptor ζ chain/CD3 and protein-tyrosine kinases $p56^{lck}$ and $p56^{fyn}$. *Proc Natl Acad Sci USA* 1992;89:9311–9315.
879. Spertini F, Stohl W, Ramesh N, et al. Induction of human T cell proliferation by a monoclonal antibody to CD5. *J Immunol* 1991; 146:47–52.
880. Vandenberghe P, Ceuppens JL. Immobilized anti-CD5 together with prolonged activation of protein kinase C induce interleukin 2-dependent T cell growth: evidence for signal transduction through CD5. *Eur J Immunol* 1988;18:747–753.
881. Alberola-Ila J, Places L, Cantrell DA, et al. Intracellular events involved in CD5-induced human T cell activation and proliferation. *J Immunol* 1992;148:1287–1293.
882. Verwilghen J, Vandesande R, Vandeberghe P, et al. Crosslinking of the CD5 antigen on human T cells induces functional IL2 receptors. *Cell Immunol* 1990;131:109–119.
883. Verwilghen J, Vandenberghe P, Wallays G, et al. Simultaneous ligation of CD5 and CD28 on resting T lymphocytes induces T cell activation in the absence of T cell receptor/CD3 occupancy. *J Immunol* 1993;150:835–846.
884. Nishimura Y, Bierer BE, Burakoff SJ. Expression of CD5 regulates responsiveness to IL-1. *J Immunol* 1988;141:3438–3444.
885. Van de Velde H, von Hoegen I, Luo W, et al. The B-cell surface protein CD72/Lyb-2 is the ligand for CD5. *Nature* 1991;351: 662–665.
886. Biancone L, Bowen MA, Lim A, et al. Identification of a novel inducible cell-surface ligand of CD5 on activated lymphocytes. *J Exp Med* 1996;184:811–819.
887. Solvason N, Kearney JF. The human fetal omentum: a site of B cell generation. *J Exp Med* 1992;175:397–404.
888. Bofill M, Janossy G , Janossa M, et al. Human B cell development: II. Subpopulations in the human fetus. *J Immunol* 1985;134: 1531–1538.
889. Antin JH, Emerson SG, Martin P, et al. Leu-1^+ ($CD5^+$) B cells: a major lymphoid subpopulation in human fetal spleen. Phenotypic and functional studies. *J Immunol* 1986;136:505–510.
890. Timens W, Rozeboom T, Poppema S. Fetal and neonatal development of human spleen: an immunohistological study. *Immunology* 1987;60:603–609.
891. Waddick KG, Uckun FM. CD5 antigen-positive B lymphocytes in human B cell ontogeny during fetal development and after autologous bone marrow transplantation. *Exp Hematol* 1993;21:791–798.
892. Thilaganathan B, Nicolaides KH, Mansur CA, et al. Fetal B lymphocyte subpopulations in normal pregnancies. *Fetal Diagn Ther* 1993; 8:15–21.
893. Durandy A, Thuillier L, Forvielle M, et al. Phenotypic and functional characteristics of human newborns' B lymphocytes. *J Immunol* 1990; 144:60–65.
894. Rabian-Herzog C, Lesage S, Gluckman E. Characterization of lymphocyte subpopulations in cord blood. *Bone Marrow Transplant* 1992;9[Suppl 1]:64–67.
895. Ibegbu CC, Nahmias AJ, Spira TJ, et al. $CD5^+$ B cells in normal newborns and infants, and in those with HIV and intrauterine infections. *Ann NY Acad Sci* 1992;651:572–575.
896. Kipps TJ, Vaughan JH. Genetic influences on the levels of circulating CD5 B lymphocytes. *J Immunol* 1987;139:1060–1064.
897. Valente G, Geuna M, Novero D, et al. CD5-positive B-cells of the fetal and adult spleen lymphoid tissue: an immunophenotypical study. *Verh Dtsch Ges Pathol* 1990;74:155–158.
898. Kumamoto T, Inaba M, Imamura H, et al. Characterization of B cells in human thymus. *Immunobiology* 1991;183:88–93.
899. Peakman M, Buggins AGS, Nicolaides KH, et al. Analysis of lymphocyte phenotypes in cord blood from early gestational fetuses. *Clin Exp Immunol* 1992;90:345–350.
900. Werner-Favre C, Vischer TL, Wohlwend D, et al. Cell surface antigen CD5 is a marker for activated human B cells. *Eur J Immunol* 1989;19:1209–1213.
901. Vernino LA, Pisetsky DS, Lipsky PE. Analysis of the expression of CD5 by human B cells and correlation with functional activity. *Cell Immunol* 1992;139:185–197.
902. Casali P, Notkins AL. $CD5^+$ B lymphocytes, polyreactive antibodies and the human B-cell repertoire. *Immunol Today* 1989;10:364–368.
903. UytdeHaag F, van der Heijden R, Osterhaus A. Maintenance of immunological memory: a role for $CD5^+$ B cells. *Immunol Today* 1991; 12:439–442.
904. Hardy RR. Variable gene usage, physiology and development of Ly-1^+ ($CD5^+$) B cells. *Curr Opin Immunol* 1992;4:181–185.
905. Hardy RR, Hayakawa K. CD5 B cells, a fetal B cell lineage. *Adv Immunol* 1994;55:297–339.
906. Kipps TJ, Tomhave E, Chen PP, et al. Autoantibody-associated K light chain variable region gene expressed in chronic lymphocytic leukemia with little or no somatic mutation: implications for etiology and immunotherapy. *J Exp Med* 1988;167:840–852.
907. Sanz I, Dang H, Takei M, et al. VH sequence of a human anti-Sm autoantibody: evidence that autoantibodies can be unmutated copies of germline genes. *J Immunol* 1989;142:883–887.
908. Burastero SE, Casali P. Characterization of human CD5 (Leu-1, OKT $1)^+$ B lymphocytes and the antibodies they produce. *Contrib Microbiol Immunol* 1989;11:231–262.
909. Inghirami G, Foitl DR, Sabichi A, et al. Autoantibody-associated

cross-reactive idiotype-bearing human B lymphocytes: distribution and characterization, including Ig VH gene and CD5 antigen expression. *Blood* 1991;78:1503–1515.
910. Kasaian MT, Ikematsu H, Casali P. CD5+ B lymphocytes. *Proc Soc Exp Biol Med* 1991;197:226–241.
911. Kantor A. A new nomenclature for B cells. *Immunol Today* 1991; 12:338.
912. Kasaian MT, Ikematsu H, Casali P. Identification and analysis of a novel human surface CD5+ B lymphocyte subset producing natural antibodies. *J Immunol* 1992;148:2690–2702.
913. Herzenberg LA, Kantor AB. B-cell lineages exist in the mouse. *Immunol Today* 1993;14:79–83.
914. Haughton G, Arnold LW, Whitemore AC, et al. B-1 cells are made and not born. *Immunol Today* 1993;14:87–91.
915. Kasaian MT, Casali P. Autoimmunity-prone B-1 (CD5 B) cells, natural antibodies and self recognition. *Autoimmunity* 1993;15:315–329.
916. Kuerbitz SJ, Civin CI, Krischer JP, et al. Expression of myeloid-associated and lymphoid-associated cell-surface antigens in acute myeloid leukemia of childhood: a pediatric oncology group study. *J Clin Oncol* 1992;10:1419–1429.
917. Smith FO, Lampkin BC, Versteeg C, et al. Expression of lymphoid-associated cell surface antigens by childhood acute myeloid leukemia cells lacks prognostic significance. *Blood* 1992;79:2415–2422.
918. Knowles DM, Halper JP, Azzo W, et al: Reactivity of monoclonal antibodies Leu1 and OKT1 with malignant human lymphoid cells: correlation with conventional cell markers. *Cancer* 1983;52: 1369–1377.
919. Matolcsy A, Inghirami G, Knowles DM. Molecular genetic demonstration of the diverse evolution of Richter's syndrome (chronic lymphocytic leukemia and subsequent large cell lymphoma). *Blood* 1994;83:1363–1372.
920. Zukerberg LR, Medeiros JL, Ferry JA, et al. Diffuse low-grade B-cell lymphomas: four clinically distinct subtypes defined by a combination of morphologic and immunophenotypic features. *Am J Clin Pathol* 1993;100:373–385.
921. Bataille R, Duperray C, Zhang XG, et al. CD5 B lymphocyte antigen in monoclonal gammopathy. *Am J Hematol* 1992;41:102–106.
922. Gonzalez M, San Miguel JF, Gascon A, et al. Increased expression of natural-killer-associated and activation antigens in multiple myeloma. *Am J Hematol* 1992;39:84–89.
923. Hishima T, Fukayama M, Fujisawa M, et al. CD5 expression in thymic carcinoma. *Am J Pathol* 1994;145:268–275.
924. Haynes B, Eisenbarth G, Fauci A. Human lymphocyte antigens: production of a monoclonal antibody that defines functional thymus-derived lymphocyte subsets. *Proc Natl Acad Sci USA* 1979;76: 5829–5833.
925. Morishima Y, Kobayashi M, Yang SY, et al. Functionally different T lymphocyte subpopulations determined by their sensitivity to complement-dependent cell lysis with the monoclonal antibody 4A. *J Immunol* 1982;129:1091–1098.
926. Vodinelich W, Tax W, Bai Y, et al. A monoclonal antibody (WT1) for detecting leukemias of T-cell precursors (T-ALL). *Blood* 1983; 62:1108–1113.
927. Link M, Warnke R, Finlay J, et al. A single monoclonal antibody identifies T-cell lineage of childhood lymphoid malignancies. *Blood* 1983;62:722–728.
928. Palker TJ, Scearce RM, Hensley LL, et al. Comparison of the CD7 (3A1) group of T cell workshop antibodies. In: Reinherz EL, Haynes BF, Nadler LM, et al, eds. *Leucocyte typing II: human T lymphocytes,* vol 1. New York: Springer-Verlag, 1986:303–313.
929. Bowen MA. CD7 workshop panel report. In: Kishimoto T, Kikutani H, von dem Borne AEGK, et al, eds. *Leukocyte typing VI: white cell differentiation antigens.* New York: Garland Publishing, 1998: 62–63.
930. Chang KL, Weiss LM. CD7: a review. *Appl Immunohistochem* 1994; 2:146–156.
931. Osada S, Utsami KR, Ueda R, et al. Assignment of a gene coding for a human T-cell antigen with a molecular weight of 40,000 daltons to chromosome 17. *Cytogenet Cell Genet* 1998;47:8–10.
932. Aruffo A, Seed B. Molecular cloning of two CD7 (T-cell leukemia antigen) cDNAs by a COS cell expression system. *EMBO J* 1987: 6:3313–3316.
933. Schanberg LE, Fleenor DE, Kurtzberg J, et al. Isolation and characterization of the genomic human CD7 gene: structural similarity with the murine Thy-1 gene. *Proc Natl Acad Sci USA* 1991;88:603–607.
934. Yoshikawa K, Seto M, Ueda R, et al. Molecular cloning of the gene coding for the human T cell differentiation antigen CD7. *Immunogenetics* 1991;33:352–360.
935. Emara M, Baldwin WM III, Finn OJ, et al. A human suppressor T-cell factor that inhibits T-cell replication by interaction with the IgM-Fc receptor (CD7). *Hum Immunol* 1989;25:87–102.
936. Pricop L, Rabinowich H, Morel PA, et al. Characterization of the Fcμ receptor of human natural killer cells. *J Immunol* 1993;151: 3018–3029.
937. Haynes BF, Denning SM, Singer KH, et al. Ontogeny of T-cell precursors: a model for the initial stages of human T-cell development. *Immunol Today* 1989;10:87–91.
938. Ware RE, Haynes BF. T cell CD7 mRNA expression is regulated by both transcriptional and post-transcriptional mechanisms. *Int Immunol* 1992;5:179–187.
939. Ware RE, Hart MK, Haynes BF. Induction of T cell CD7 gene transcription by nonmitogenic ionomycin-induced transmembrane calcium flux. *J Biol Chem* 1992;147:2787–2794.
940. Costantinides Y, Kingsley G, Pitzalis C, et al. Inhibition of lymphocyte proliferation by a monoclonal antibody (RFT2) against CD7. *Clin Exp Immunol* 1991;85:164–167.
941. Chatila TA, Geha RS. Phosphorylation of T cell membrane proteins by activators of protein kinase C. *J Immunol* 1988;140:4308–4314.
942. Jung LKL, Fu SM. Effect of tumor promoter 12-O-tetra-decanoyl-phorbol 13-acetate on CD7 expression by T lineage cells. *Eur J Immunol* 1988;18:711–715.
943. Lazarovits AI, Karsh J. A monoclonal antibody, 7G5 (CD7), induces modulation of Tp40 and inhibits proliferation in the allogeneic and autologous mixed lymphocyte reactions. *Transplant Proc* 1988;20: 1253–1257.
944. Lobach DF, Hensley LL, Ho W, et al. Human T cell antigen expression during the early stages of fetal thymic maturation. *J Immunol* 1985;135:1752–1759.
945. Bertho JM, Mossalayi MD, Dalloul AH, et al. Isolation of an early T-cell precursor (CFU-TL) from human bone marrow. *Blood* 1990; 75:1064–1068.
946. Haynes B, Mann D, Hemler M, et al. Characterization of a monoclonal antibody that defines an immunoregulatory T cell subset for immunoglobulin synthesis in humans. *Proc Natl Acad Sci USA* 1980; 77:2914–2918.
947. Haynes B. Human T lymphocyte antigens as defined by monoclonal antibodies. *Immunol Rev* 1981;57:127–161.
948. Jung LK, Fu SM, Hara T, et al. Defective expression of T cell-associated glycoprotein in severe combined immuno-deficiency. *J Clin Invest* 1986;77:940–946.
949. Garand R , Vannier JP, Béné MC, et al. Comparison of outcome, clinical, laboratory and immunological features in 164 children and adults with T-ALL. *Leukemia* 1990;4:739–744.
950. Thiel E, Kranz BR, Raghavachar A, et al. Prethymic phenotype and genotype of pre-T ($CD7^+/ER^-$) cell leukemia and its clinical significance within adult acute lymphoblastic leukemia. *Blood* 1989;73: 1247–1258.
951. Garand R, Voisin S, Papin S, et al. Characteristics of pro-T ALL subgroups: comparison with late T-ALL. *Leukemia* 1992;7:161–167.
952. Ben-Ezra J, Winberg CD, Wu A, et al. Leu-9 (CD7) positivity in acute leukemias: a marker of T-cell lineage? *Hematol Pathol* 1987; 1:147–156.
953. Lo Coco F, de Rossi G, Pasqualetti D, et al. CD7 positive acute myeloid leukaemia: a subtype associated with cell immaturity. *Br J Haematol* 1989;73:480–485.
954. Zutter MM, Martin PJ, Janke D, et al. CD7+ acute non-lymphocytic leukemia: evidence for an early multipotential progenitor. *Leuk Res* 1990;14:23–26.
955. Tien HF, Wang CH, Su IJ, et al. A subset of acute non-lymphocytic leukemia with expression of surface antigen CD7-morphologic, cytochemical, immunocytochemical and T cell receptor gene analysis on 13 patients. *Leuk Res* 1990;14:515–523.
956. Osada H, Emi N, Ueda R, et al. Genuine CD7 expression in acute leukemia and lymphoblastic lymphoma. Leuk Res 1990;14: 869–877.
957. Eto T, Akashi K, Harada M, et al. Biological characteristics of CD7

positive acute myelogenous leukaemia. *Br J Haematol* 1992;82: 508–514.
958. Ribrag V, Bayle C, Brault P, et al. Acute myelogenous leukemia with T-cell features. *Bull Cancer (Paris)* 1992;79:1165–1171.
959. Kondo S, Okamura S, Harada N, et al. CD7-positive acute myeloid leukemia: further evidence of cellular immaturity. *J Cancer Res Clin Oncol* 1992;118:386–388.
960. Buccheri V, Matutes E, Dyer MJS, et al. Lineage commitment in biphenotypic acute leukemia. *Leukemia* 1993;9:919–927.
961. Kita K, Miwa H, Nakase K, et al. Clinical importance of CD7 expression in acute myelocytic leukemia. *Blood* 1993;81:2399–2405.
962. Tien HF, Wang CH, Chen YC, et al. Characterization of acute myeloid leukemia (AML) coexpressing lymphoid markers: different biologic features between T-cell antigen positive and B-cell antigen positive AML. *Leukemia* 1993;7:688–695.
963. Kasparu H, Koller U, Krieger O, et al. Significance of gp40/CD7 or TdT positivity in AML patients. In: Knapp W, Dorken B, Gilks WR, et al, eds. *Leucocyte typing IV: white cell differentiation antigens.* New York: Oxford University Press, 1989;936–937.
964. Schwonzen M, Kuehn N, Vetten B, et al. Phenotyping of acute myelomonocytic (AMMOL) and monocytic leukemia (AMOL): association of T-cell-related antigens and skin-infiltration in AMOL. *Leuk Res* 1989;13:893–898.
965. Seremetis SV, Pelicci PG, Tabilio A, et al. High frequency of clonal immunoglobulin or T cell receptor gene rearrangements in acute myelogenous leukemia expressing terminal deoxyribonucleotidyl transferase. *J Exp Med* 1987;165:1703–1712.
966. Jensen AW, Hokland M, Jørgensen H, et al. Solitary expression of CD7 among T-cell antigens in acute myeloid leukemia: correlations with morphology and immunophenotype. *Br J Haematol* 1991;78: 494–499.
967. Kurtzberg J, Waldmann TA, Davey MP, et al. $CD7^+$, $CD4^-$, $CD8^-$ acute leukemia: a syndrome of malignant pluripotent lymphohematopoietic cells. *Blood* 1989;73: 381–390.
968. Yumura-Yagi K, Hara J, Kurahashi H, et al. Clinical significance of CD7-positive stem cell leukemia: a distinct subtype of mixed lineage leukemia. *Cancer* 1991;68:2273–2280.
969. Ferrara F, Cimino R, Antinolfi I, et al. Clinical relevance of immunological dissection in T-ALL: a report on 20 cases with stem cell ($CD7^+$, $CD4^-$, $CD8^-$, $CD1^-$) phenotype. *Am J Hematol* 1992;40: 98–102.
970. Medeiros LJ, Picker LJ, Abel A, et al. Cutaneous lymphoid hyperplasia: immunologic characteristics and assessment of criteria recently proposed as diagnostic of malignant lymphoma. *J Am Acad Dermatol* 1989;21:929–942.
971. Lazarovits AI, Karsh J. Decreased expression of CD7 occurs in rheumatoid arthritis. *Clin Exp Immunol* 1988;72:470–475.
972. Marrack P, Kappler J. The T-cell receptor. *Science* 1987;238: 1073–1079.
973. Acuto O, Meuer SC, Hodgdon JC, et al. Peptide variability exists within α and β subunits of T cell receptor for antigen. *J Exp Med* 1983;158:1368–1373.
974. Brenner MB, McLean J, Scheft H, et al. Two forms of the T-cell receptor γ protein found on peripheral blood cytotoxic T lymphocytes. *Nature* 1987;325:689–694.
975. Borst J, Van Dongen JJM, Bolhuis RLH, et al. Distinct molecular forms of human T-cell receptor γ/δ detected on viable T cells by a monoclonal antibody. *J Exp Med* 1988;167:1625–1644.
976. Spits H, Borst J, Tax W, et al. Characteristics of a monoclonal antibody (WT31) that recognizes a common epitope on the human T cell receptor for antigen. *J Immunol* 1985;135:1922–1928.
977. Lanier LL, Weiss A. Presence of Ti (WT31) negative T lymphocytes in normal blood and thymus. *Nature* 1986;324:268–270.
978. Brenner MB, McLean J, Scheft H, et al. Characterization and expression of the human γ/δ T cell receptor using a framework monoclonal antibody. *J Immunol* 1987;138:1502–1509.
979. Inghirami G, Zhu BY, Chess L, et al. Flow cytometric and immunohistochemical characterization of the γ/δ T lymphocyte population in normal human lymphoid tissue and peripheral blood. *Am J Pathol* 1990;136:357–367.
980. Brenner MB, Groh V, Porcelli SA, et al. Structure and distribution of the human $\gamma\delta$ T cell receptor. In: Knapp W, Dörken B, Gilks WR, et al, eds. *Leukocyte typing IV: white cell differentiation antigens.* Oxford: Oxford University Press, 1989:1049–1053.
981. Chan WC, Borowitz MJ, Hammami A, et al. T cell receptor antibodies in the immunohistochemical studies of normal and malignant lymphoid cells. *Cancer* 1988;62:2118–2124.
982. Picker LJ, Brenner MB, Weiss LM, et al. Discordant expression of CD3 and T-cell receptor beta-chain antigens in T lineage lymphomas. *Am J Pathol* 1987;129:434–440.
983. Ng CS, Chan JKC, Jui PK, et al. Application of a T cell receptor antibody βF_1 for immunophenotypic analysis of malignant lymphomas. *Am J Pathol* 1988;132:365–371.
984. Band H, Hochstenbach F, McLean J, et al. Immunochemical proof that a novel rearranging gene encodes the T cell receptor delta subunit. *Science* 1987;238:682–684.
985. Hochstenbach F, Parker C, McLean J, et al. Characterization of a third form of the human T cell receptor gamma/delta. *J Exp Med* 1988;168:761–776.
986. Groh V, Porcelli S, Fabbi M, et al. Human lymphocytes bearing T cell receptor gamma/delta are phenotypically diverse and evenly distributed throughout the lymphoid system. *J Exp Med* 1989;169: 1277–1294.
987. Picker LJ, Brenner MB, Michie S, et al. Expression of T cell receptor delta chains in benign and malignant T lineage lymphoproliferations. *Am J Pathol* 1988;132:401–405.
988. Gouttenfangeas C, Bensussan A, Boumsell L. Study of the CD3 associated T cell receptors reveals further differences between T cell acute lymphoblastic lymphoma and leukemia. *Blood* 1990;75: 931–934.
989. Unkeless JC, Scigliano E, Freedman V. Structure and function of human and murine receptors of IgG. *Annu Rev Immunol* 1988;6: 251–281.
990. Ravetch JV, Perussia G. Alternative membrane forms of Fc gamma RIII (CD16) on human natural killer cells and neutrophils: cell type-specific expression of two genes that differ in single nucleotide substitutions. *J Exp Med* 1989;170:481–497.
991. Gessner JE, Grussenmeyer T, Schmidt RE. Differentially regulated expression of human IgG Fc receptor class III genes. *Immunobiology* 1995;193:341–355.
992. Schmidt RE, Perussia B. Cluster report: CD16. In: Knapp W, Dörken B, Gilks WR, et al, eds. *Leukocyte typing IV: white cell differentiation antigens.* New York: Oxford University Press, 1989:574–578.
993. Klaassen RJL, Ouwehand WH, Huizinga TWJ, et al. The Fc-receptor III of cultured human monocytes: structural similarity with FcRIII of natural killer cells and role in the extracellular lysis of sensitized erythrocytes. *J Immunol* 1990;144:599–606.
994. Huizinga TW, van der Schoot CE, Jost C, et al. The PI-linked receptor FcRIII is released on stimulation of neutrophils. *Nature* 1988; 333:667–669.
995. Huizinga TWJ, Kleijer M, Tetteroo PAT, et al. Biallelic neutrophil NA-antigen system is associated with a polymorphism on the phospho-inositol-linked Fc gamma receptor III (CD16). *Blood* 1990;75: 213–217.
996. Huizinga TWJ, Kleijer M, Roos D, et al. Differences between FcRIII of human neutrophils and human K/NK lymphocytes in relation to the NA antigen system. In: Knapp W, Dörken B, Gilks WR, et al, eds. *Leukocyte typing IV: white cell differentiation antigens.* New York: Oxford University Press, 1989:582–585.
997. Edberg JC, Barinsky M, Redecha PB, et al. Fc gamma RIII expressed on cultured monocytes is a N-glycosylated transmembrane protein distinct from Fc gamma RIII expressed on natural killer cells. *J Immunol* 1990;144:4729–4734.
998. Tetteroo PAT, Visser F-J, Bos MJE, et al. Serological, biochemical, and cytogenetic studies with the granulocyte monoclonal antibodies of the "M Protocol". In: Reinherz EL, Haynes BF, Nadler LM, et al, eds. *Leukocyte typing II, vol 3: human myeloid and hematopoietic cells.* New York: Springer-Verlag, 1986:27–45.
999. Perussia B, Starr S, Abraham S, et al. Human natural killer cells analyzed by B73.1, a monoclonal antibody blocking Fc receptor functions: I. Characterization of the lymphocyte subset reactive with B73.1. *J Immunol* 1983;130:2133–2141.
1000. Perussia B, Acuto O, Terhorst C, et al. Human natural killer cells analyzed by B73.1, a monoclonal antibody blocking Fc receptor functions: II. Studies of B73.1 antibody-antigen interaction on the lymphocyte membrane. *J Immunol* 1983;130:2142–2148.
1001. Rumpold JH, Kraft D, Obexer G, et al. A monoclonal antibody

against a surface antigen shared by human large granular lymphocytes and granulocytes. *J Immunol* 1982;129:1458–1464.
1002. Kleijer M, de Haas M, Roos D, et al. PEN1, a novel FcγRIII mAb with a unique specificity for neutrophil NA2-FcγRIIIb carrying a small N-linked oligosaccharide. In: Schlossman SF, Boumsell L, Gilks WR, et al, eds. *Leukocyte typing V: white cell differentiation antigens.* New York: Oxford University Press, 1995;814–817.
1003. Schmidt RE. CD16 cluster workshop report. In: Schlossman SF, Boumsell L, Gilks WR, et al, eds. *Leukocyte typing V: white cell differentiation antigens.* New York: Oxford University Press, 1995: 805–806.
1004. Schmidt RE. Non-lineage/natural killer section report: new and previously defined clusters. In: Knapp W, Dörken B, Gilks WR, et al, eds. *Leukocyte typing IV: white cell differentiation antigens.* New York: Oxford University Press, 1989:517–542.
1005. Tomasello E, Revello V, Poggi A. CD16 workshop panel report. In: Kishimoto T, Kikutani H, von dem Borne AEGK, et al, eds. *Leukocyte typing VI: white cell differentiation antigens.* New York: Garland Publishing, 1998:269–271.
1006. Perussia B, Trinchieri G, Jackson A, et al. The Fc receptor for IgG on human natural killer cells: phenotypic, functional, and comparative studies with monoclonal antibodies. *J Immunol* 1984;133:180–189.
1007. Perussia B, Trinchieri G. Antibody 3G8, specific for the human neutrophil Fc receptor, reacts with natural killer cells. *J Immunol* 1984; 132:1410–1415.
1008. deHaas M, Kleijer M, Roos D, et al. Characterization of mAb of the CD16 cluster and six newly generated CD16 mAb. In: Schlossman SF, Boumsell L, Gilks WR, et al, eds. *Leukocyte typing V: white cell differentiation antigens.* New York: Oxford University Press, 1995:811–814.
1009. Perussia B, Ravetch JV. Fc gamma RIII (CD16) on human macrophages is a functional product of the Fc gamma RIII-2gene. *Eur J Immunol* 1991;21:425–429.
1010. Tetteroo PAT, von der Schoot CE, Visser FJ, et al. Three different types of Fcγ receptor on human leukocytes defined by workshop antibodies: FcγR_{low} of neutrophils, FcγR_{low} of K/NK lymphocytes, and FcγRII. In: McMichael AJ, Beverley PCL, Cobbold S, et al, eds. *Leukocyte typing III: white cell differentiation antigens.* Oxford: Oxford University Press, 1987:702–706.
1011. Lanier LL, Ruitenberg JJ, Phillips JH. Functional and biochemical analysis of CD16 antigen on natural killer cells and granulocytes. *J Immunol* 1988;141:3478–3485.
1012. Graziano RF, Fanger MW. Fc gamma RI and Fc gamma RII on monocytes and granulocytes are cytotoxic trigger molecules for tumor cells. *J Immunol* 1987;139:3536–3541.
1013. Werfel TH, Uciechowski P, Tetteroo PAT, et al. Activation of cloned human natural killer cells via Fc gamma RIII. *J Immunol* 1989;142: 1102–1106.
1014. Anegon I, Cuturi MC, Trinchieri G, et al. Interaction of Fc receptor (CD16) ligands induces transcription of interleukin 2 receptor (CD25) and lymphokine genes and expression of their products in human natural killer cells. *J Exp Med* 1988;167:452–472.
1015. Stahls A, Liwszyc GE, Couture C, et al. Triggering of human natural killer cells through CD16 induces tyrosine phosphorylation of the p72syk kinase. *Eur J Immunol* 1994;24:2491–2496.
1016. Galandrini R, Palmieri G, Piccoli M, et al. CD16-mediated p21 ras activation is associated with Shc and p36 tyrosine phosphorylation and their binding with Grb2 in human natural killer cells. *J Exp Med* 1996;183:179–186.
1017. Cone JC, Lu Y, Trevillyan JM, et al. Association of the p56lck protein tyrosine kinase with the Fc gamma RIIIA/CD16 complex in human natural killer cells. *Eur J Immunol* 1993;23:2488–2497.
1018. Ortaldo JR, Mason AT, O'Shea JJ. Receptor-induced death in human natural killer cells: involvement of CD16. *J Exp Med* 1995;181: 339–344.
1019. Robertson MJ, Ritz J. Biology and clinical relevance of human natural killer cells. *Blood* 1990;76:2421–2438.
1020. Nagler A, Lanier LL, Cwirla S, et al. Comparative studies of human FcRIII-positive and negative natural killer cells. *J Immunol* 1989; 143:3183–3191.
1021. Bulmer JN, Lunny DP, Hagin SV. Immunohistochemical characterization of stromal leucocytes in nonpregnant human endometrium. *Am J Reprod Immunol Microbiol* 1988;17:83–90.
1022. King A, Wellings V, Garner L, et al. Immunocytochemical characterization of the unusual large granular lymphocytes in human endometrium throughout the menstrual cycle. *Hum Immunol* 1989;24: 195–205.
1023. King A, Balendran N, Wooding P, et al. CD3-leukocytes present in the human uterus during early placentation: phenotypic and morphologic characterization of the CD56^{++} population. *Dev Immunol* 1991;1:169–190.
1024. King A, Loke YW. On the nature and function of human uterine granular lymphocytes. *Immunol Today* 1991;12:432–435.
1025. Passlick B, Flieger D, Ziegler-Heitbrock L. Identification and characterization of a novel monocyte subpopulation in human peripheral blood. *Blood* 1989;74:2527–2534.
1026. Pulford K, Micklem K, Tse A, et al. The immunocytochemical distribution of the CD16, CD32 and CD64 antigens. In: Schlossman SF, Boumsell L, Gilks WR, et al, eds. *Leukocyte typing V: white cell differentiation antigens.* New York: Oxford University Press, 1995: 817–821.
1027. Stain C, Jager U, Majdic O, et al. The phenotyping of human basophils with the myeloid workshop panel. In: McMichael AJ, Beverley PCL, Cobbold S, et al, eds. *Leukocyte typing III: white cell differentiation antigens.* Oxford: Oxford University Press, 1987:720–722.
1028. Lanier LL, Kipps TJ, Phillips JH. Functional properties of a unique subset of cytotoxic CD3$^+$ T lymphocytes that express Fc receptors for IgG (CD16/Leu-11 antigen). *J Exp Med* 1985;162:2089–2106.
1029. McDaniel HL, MacPherson BR, Tindle BH, et al. Lymphoproliferative disorder of granular lymphocytes: a heterogeneous disease. *Arch Pathol Lab Med* 1992;116:242–248.
1030. Wong KF, Chan JKC, Ng CS, et al. CD56 (NKH1)-positive hematolymphoid malignancies: an aggressive neoplasm featuring frequent cutaneous/mucosal involvement, cytoplasmic azurophilic granules, and angiocentricity. *Hum Pathol* 1992;23:798–804.
1031. Kern WF, Spier CM, Miller TP, et al. NCAM (CD56) positive malignant lymphoma. *Leuk Lymphoma* 1993;12:1–10.
1032. Wong KF, Chan JKC, Ng CS. CD56 (NCAM) positive malignant lymphoma. *Leuk Lymphoma* 1994;14:29–36.
1033. Jaffe ES, Chan JKC, Su I-J, et al. Report of the workshop on nasal and related extranodal angiocentric T/natural killer cell lymphomas: definitions, differential diagnosis and epidemiology. *Am J Surg Pathol* 1996;20:103–111.
1034. Swerdlow SH, Habeshaw JA, Richards MA, et al. T lymphoblastic lymphoma with Leu-7 positive phenotype and unusual clinical course: a multiparameter study. *Leuk Res* 1985;9:167–173.
1035. Kaplan J, Ravindranath Y, Inoue S: T cell acute lymphoblastic leukemia with natural killer cell phenotype. *Am J Hematol* 1986;22: 355–364.
1036. Pizzolo G, Trentin L, Vinante F, et al. Rearrangement for the T cell receptor gene and co-expression of immature T cell markers and natural killer cell phenotype in a patient with acute lymphoblastic leukemia. *Br J Haematol* 1987;65:17–22.
1037. Sheibani K, Winberg CD, Burke JS, et al. Lymphoblastic lymphoma expressing natural killer cell-associated antigens: a clinicopathologic study of six cases. *Leuk Res* 1987;11:371–377.
1038. Ichinohasama R, Endoh K, Ishizawa K, et al. Thymic lymphoblastic lymphoma of committed natural killer cell precursor origin: a case report. *Cancer* 1996;77:2592–2603.
1039. Lanier LL, Le AM, Civin CI, et al. The relationship of CD16 (Leu-11) and Leu-19 (NKH-1) antigen expression on human peripheral blood NK cells and cytotoxic T lymphocytes. *J Immunol* 1986;136: 4480–4486.
1040. Hercend T, Griffin JD, Bensussan A, et al. Generation of monoclonal antibodies to a human natural killer clone: characterization of two natural killer-associated antigens, NKH1A and NKH2, expressed on subsets of large granular lymphocytes. *J Clin Invest* 1985;75: 932–943.
1041. Thiery J-P, Brackenbury R, Rutishauser U, et al. Adhesion among neural cells of the chick embryo. *J Biol Chem* 1977;252:6841–6845.
1042. Lanier LL, Testi R, Bindl J, et al. Identity of Leu-19 (CD56) leukocyte differentiation antigen and neural cell adhesion molecule. *J Exp Med* 1989;169:2233–2238.
1043. Schubert J, Lanier LL, Schmidt RE. Cluster report: CD56. In: Knapp W, Dörken B, Gilks WR, et al, eds. *Leukocyte typing IV: white cell differentiation antigens.* Oxford: Oxford University Press, 1989: 699–702.
1044. Griffin JD, Hercend T, Beveridge RP, et al. Characterization of an

antigen expressed by human natural killer cells. *J Immunol* 1983; 130:2947–2951.
1045. Edelman GM. Cell adhesion molecules in the regulation of animal form and tissue pattern. *Ann Rev Cell Biol* 1986;2:81–116.
1046. Cunningham BA, Hemperly JJ, Murray BA, et al. Neural cell adhesion molecule: structure, immunoglobulin-like domains, cell surface modulation, and alternative RNA splicing. *Science* 1987;236: 799–806.
1047. Edelman GM. Morphoregulatory molecules. *Biochemistry* 1988;27: 3533–3543.
1048. Edelman GM. Cell adhesion molecules. *Science* 1983;219:450–457.
1049. Robertson MJ. Natural killer cell clinical studies: surface antigens of human natural killer cells in health and disease. In: Kishimoto T, Kikutani H, von dem Borne AEGK, et al, eds. *Leukocyte typing VI: white cell differentiation antigens.* New York: Garland Publishing, 1998:327–329.
1050. Lanier LL, Hemperly JJ. CD56 and CD57 cluster workshop report. In: Schlossman SF, Boumsell L, Gilks WR, et al, eds. *Leukocyte typing V: white cell differentiation antigens.* New York: Oxford University Press, 1995:1398–1400.
1051. Santoni MJ, Barthels D, Vopper G, et al. Differential exon usage involving an unusual splicing mechanism generates at least eight types of NCAM cDNA in mouse brain. *EMBO J* 1989;8:385–392.
1052. Dickson G, Gower HJ, Barton CH, et al. Human muscle neural cell adhesion molecule (N-CAM): identification of a muscle-specific sequence in the extracellular domain. *Cell* 1987;50:1119–1130.
1053. Barton CH, Dickson G, Gower HJ, et al. Complete sequence and in vitro expression of a tissue-specific phosphatidylinositol-linked N-CAM isoform from skeletal muscle. *Development* 1988;104: 165–173.
1054. Gower HJ, Barton CH, Elsom VL, et al. Alternative splicing generates a secreted form of N-CAM in muscle and brain. *Cell* 1988;55: 955–964.
1055. Small SJ, Shull GE, Santoni MJ, et al. Identification of a cDNA clone that contains the complete coding sequence for a 140-kd rat NCAM polypeptide. *J Cell Biol* 1987;105:2335–2345.
1056. Hemperly JJ, DeGuglielmo JK, Reid RA. Characterization of cDNA clones defining variant forms of human neural cell adhesion molecule N-CAM. *J Mol Neurosci* 1990;2:71–78.
1057. Edelman GM, Crossin KL. Cell adhesion molecules: implications for a molecular histology. *Annu Rev Biochem* 1991;60:155–190.
1058. Tsang WYW, Chan JKC, Ng CS, et al. Utility of a paraffin section reactive CD56 antibody (123C3) for characterization and diagnosis of lymphomas. *Am J Surg Pathol* 1996;20:202–210.
1059. Pang G, Buret A, Batey RT, et al. Morphological, phenotypic and functional characteristics of a pure population of $CD56^+CD16^-CD3^-$ large granular lymphocytes generated from human duodenal mucosa. *Immunol* 1993;79:498–505.
1060. Ellis TM, Creekmore SP, McMannis JD, et al. Appearance and phenotypic characterization of circulating Leu 19^+ cells in cancer patients receiving recombinant interleukin 2. *Cancer Res* 1988;48: 6597–6602.
1061. Robertson MJ, Caligiuri MA, Manley TJ, et al. Human natural killer cell adhesion molecules. *J Immunol* 1990;145:3194–3201.
1062. Schmidt RE, Murray C, Daley JF, et al. A subset of natural killer cells in peripheral blood displays a mature T cell phenotype. *J Exp Med* 1986;164:351–356.
1063. Lanier LL, Le AM, Ding A, et al. Expression of Leu-19 (NKH-1) antigen on IL 2-dependent cytotoxic and non-cytotoxic T cell lines. *J Immunol* 1987;138:2019–2023.
1064. Van Camp B, Durie BGM, Spier C, et al. Plasma cells in multiple myelomas express a natural killer cell-associated antigen: CD56 (NKH-1;Leu-19). *Blood* 1990;76:377–382.
1065. Van Riet I, De Waele M, Remels L, et al. Expression of cytoadhesion molecules (CD56,CD54,CD18 and CD29) by myeloma plasma cells. *Br J Haematol* 1991;79:421–427.
1066. Crossin KL, Chuong CM, Edelman GM. Expression sequencies of cell adhesion molecules. *Proc Natl Acad Sci USA* 1985;82: 6942–6946.
1067. Akeson RA, Wujek JR, Roe S, et al. Smooth muscle cells transiently express NCAM. *Brain Res* 1988;4:107–120.
1068. Mechtersheimer G, Staudter M, Moller P. Expression of the natural killer cell-associated antigens CD56 and CD57 in human neural and striated muscle cells and in their tumors. *Cancer Res* 1991;51: 1300–1307.
1069. Feichert H-J, Pietsch T, Hadam MR, et al. NK cell marker: mAb T-109 detects a new antigenic determinant distinct from the N901, Leu 19 and Leu 7 antigens or antigen epitopes expressed on NK cells. In: Knapp W, Dörken B, Gilks WR, et al, eds. *Leukocyte typing IV: white cell differentiation antigens.* Oxford: Oxford University Press, 1989:705–708.
1070. Gentile TC, Uner AH, Hutchison RE, et al. $CD3^+CD56^+$ aggressive variant of large granular lymphocyte leukemia. *Blood* 1994;84: 2315–2321.
1071. Chan JKC, Sin VC, Wong KF, et al. Non-nasal lymphoma expressing the natural killer cell marker CD56: a clinicopathologic study of 49 cases of an uncommon aggressive neoplasm. *Blood* 1997;89: 4501–4513.
1072. Wong KF, Chan JKC, Matutes E, et al. Hepatosplenic $\gamma\delta$ T cell lymphoma: a distinctive aggressive lymphoma type. *Am J Surg Pathol* 1995;19:718–726.
1073. Macon WR, Williams ME, Greer JP, et al. Natural killer-like T-cell lymphomas: aggressive lymphomas of T-large granular lymphocytes. *Blood* 1996;87:1474–1483.
1074. Kaiser U, Jaques G, Havemann K. Serum NCAM: a potential new prognostic marker for multiple myeloma. *Blood* 1994;83:871–873.
1075. Hammer RD, Vnencak-Jones CL, Manning SS, et al. Microvillous lymphomas are B cell neoplasms that frequently express CD56. *Mod Pathol* 1998;11:239–246.
1076. Scott AA, Head DR, Kopecky KJ, et al. HLA-DR-$CD33^+$ $CD56^+CD16^-$ myeloid/natural killer cell acute leukemia: a recently unrecognized form of acute leukemia potentially misdiagnosed as French-American-British acute myeloid leukemia-M3. *Blood* 1994; 84:244–255.
1077. Patel K, Moore SE, Dickson G, et al. Neural cell adhesion molecule (NCAM) is the antigen recognized by monoclonal antibodies of similar specificity in small-cell lung carcinoma and neuroblastoma. *Int J Cancer* 1989;44:573–578.
1078. Komminoth P, Roth J, Lackie PM, et al. Polysialic acid of the neural cell adhesion molecule distinguishes small cell lung carcinoma from carcinoids. *Am J Pathol* 1991;139:297–304.
1079. Michalides R, Kwa B, Springall D, et al. NCAM and lung cancer. *Int J Cancer* 1994;8[Suppl]: 34–37.
1080. Roth J, Zuber C, Wagner P, et al. Re-expression of poly(sialic acid) units of the neural cell adhesion molecule in Wilms tumor. *Proc Natl Acad Sci USA* 1988;85:2999–3003.
1081. Kaufmann O, Georgi T, Dietel M. Utility of 123C3 monoclonal antibody against CD56 (NCAM) for the diagnosis of small cell carcinomas on paraffin sections. *Hum Pathol* 1997;28:1373–1378.
1082. Schubart J, Lanier LL, Schmidt RE. Cluster report: CD57. In: Knapp W, Dorken B, Gilks WE, et al, eds. *Leucocyte typing IV: white cell differentiation antigens.* New York: Oxford University Press, 1989: 711–714.
1083. Abo T, Balch CM. A differentiation antigen of human NK and K cells identified by a monoclonal antibody (HNK-1). *J Immunol* 1981; 127:1024–1029.
1084. Abo T, Balch CM. Characterization of HNK-1 (Leu-7) human killer cells from activated NK-like cells. *J Immunol* 1982;129:1758–1761.
1085. Abo T, Cooper MD, Balch CM. Characterization of HNK-1 (Leu-7) human lymphocytes: I. Two distinct phenotypes of human NK cells with different cytotoxic capacities. *J Immunol* 1982;129: 1752–1757.
1086. Arber DA, Weiss LM. CD57: a review. *Appl Immunohistochem* 1995;3:137–152.
1087. Kubagawa H, Abo T, Balch CM, et al. Biochemical analysis of antigenic determinants on human natural killer cells by HNK-1 (Leu7) antibody. *Federal Proceedings* 1983;42:1219.
1088. McGarry RC, Helfand SL, Quarles RH, et al. Recognition of myelin-associated glycoprotein by the monoclonal antibody HNK-1. *Nature* 1983;306:376–378.
1089. Schröder J, Nikinmaa B, Kavathas P, et al. Fluorescence-activated cell sorting of mouse-human hybrid cells aids in locating the gene for the Leu 7 (HNK-1) antigen to human chromosome 11. *Proc Natl Acad Sci USA* 1983;80:3421–3424.
1090. Kay HD, Horwitz DA. Evidence by reactivity with hybridoma antibodies for a probable myeloid origin of peripheral blood cells active

in natural cytotoxicity and antibody-dependent cell-mediated cytotoxicity. *J Clin Invest* 1980;66:847–851.
1091. Lanier LL, Le AM, Phillips JH, et al. Subpopulations of human natural killer cells defined by expression of the Leu-7 (HNK-1) and Leu-11 (NK-15) antigens. *J Immunol* 1983;131:1789–1796.
1092. Lanier LL, Engleman EG, Gatenby P, et al. Correlation of functional properties of human lymphoid cell subsets and surface marker phenotypes using multiparameter analysis and flow cytometry. *Immunol Rev* 1983;74:143–160.
1093. Berry SM, Fine N, Bichalski JA, et al. Circulating lymphocytes in second-and-third trimester fetuses: comparison with newborns and adults. *Am J Obstet Gynecol* 1992;167:895–900.
1094. Rabian-Herzog C, Lesage S, Gluckman E. Characterization of lymphocyte subpopulations in cord blood. *Bone Marrow Transplant* 1992;9[Suppl 1]:64–67.
1095. Abo T, Cooper MD, Balch CM. Postnatal expansion of the natural killer and killer cell population in humans identified by the monoclonal HNK-1 antibody. *J Exp Med* 1982;155:321–326.
1096. Slukvin II, Chernishow VP. Two-color cytometric analysis of natural killer and cytotoxic T-lymphocyte subsets in peripheral blood of normal human neonates. *Biol Neonate* 1992;61:156–161.
1097. Yamashiki M, Nishimura A, Kosaka Y, et al. Two-color analysis of peripheral lymphocyte surface antigens in inherently healthy adults. *J Clin Lab Anal* 1994;8:22–26.
1098. Ligthart GJ, van Vlokhoven PC, Schuit HRE, et al. The expanded null cell compartment in aging: increase in the number of natural killer cells and changes in T-cell and NK-cell subsets in human blood. *Immunology* 1986;59:353–357.
1099. Clement LT, Grossi CE, Gartland GL. Morphologic and phenotypic features of the subpopulation of Leu-2$^+$ cells that suppresses B cell differentiation. *J Immunol* 1984;133:2461–2468.
1100. Wang ECY, Taylor-Wiedeman J, Perera P, et al. Subsets of CD8$^+$, CD57$^+$ cells in normal, healthy individuals: correlations with human cytomegalovirus (HCMV) carrier status, phenotype and functional analyses. *Clin Exp Immunol* 1993;94:297–305.
1101. Phillips JH, Lanier LL. Lectin-dependent and anti-CD3 induced cytotoxicity are preferentially mediated by peripheral blood cytotoxic T lymphocytes expressing Leu-7 antigen. *J Immunol* 1986;136: 1579–1585.
1102. Yamashita N, Nguyen L, Fahey JL, et al. Phenotypic properties of cytotoxic functions of human CD8$^+$ cells expressing the CD57 antigen. *Nat Immun* 1993;12:79–91.
1103. Rüthlein J, James SP, Strober W. Role of CD2 in activation and cytotoxic function of CD8/Leu-7-positive T cells. *J Immunol* 1988; 141:3791–3797.
1104. Wang ECY, Lehner PJ, Graham S, et al. CD8high (CD57$^+$) T cells in normal, healthy individuals specifically suppress the generation of cytotoxic T lymphocytes to Epstein-Barr virus-transformed B cell lines. *Eur J Immunol* 1994;24:2903–2909.
1105. Rouleau M, Bernard A, Lantz O, et al. Apoptosis of activated CD8$^+$/CD57$^+$ T cells is induced by some combination of anti-CD2 mAb. *J Immunol* 1993;151:3547–3556.
1106. Gupta S . Abnormality of Leu 2-7$^+$ cells in acquired immune deficiency syndrome (AIDS), AIDS-related complex, and asymptomatic homosexuals. *J Clin Immunol* 1986;6:502–509.
1107. d'Angeac AD, Monier S, Jorgensen C, et al. Increased percentage of CD3$^+$CD57$^+$ lymphocytes in patients with rheumatoid arthritis: correlation with duration of disease. *Arthritis Rheum* 1993;36: 608–612.
1108. Bowman SJ, Sivakumaran M, Snowden N, et al. The large granular lymphocyte syndrome with rheumatoid arthritis: immunogenetic evidence for a broader definition of Felty's syndrome. *Arthritis Rheum* 1994;37:1326–1330.
1109. James SP, Neckers LM, Graeff AS, et al. Suppression of immunoglobulin synthesis by lymphocyte subpopulations in patients with Crohn's disease. *Gastroenterology* 1984;86:1510–1518.
1110. Mizuno S-I, Morishima Y, Kodera Y, et al. Gamma-interferon production capacity and T lymphocyte subpopulation after allogeneic bone marrow transplantation. *Transplantation* 1986;41:311–315.
1111. Leroy E, Calvo CF, Divine M, et al. Persistence of T8$^+$/HNK-1$^+$ suppressor lymphocytes in the blood of long-term surviving patients after allogeneic bone marrow transplantation. *J Immunol* 1986;137: 2180–2189.
1112. Reipert B, Scheuch CH, Lukowsky A, et al. CD3$^+$ CD57$^+$ lymphocytes are not likely to be involved in antigen specific rejection processes in long-term allograft recipients. *Clin Exp Immunol* 1992;89: 143–147.
1113. Loughran TP, Starkebaum G, Kidd P, et al. Clonal proliferation of large granular lymphocytes in rheumatoid arthritis. *Arthritis Rheum* 1988;31:31–36.
1114. Ritichie AWS, James K, Micklem HS. The distribution and possible significance of cells identified in human lymphoid tissue by the monoclonal antibody HNK-1. *Clin Exp Immunol* 1983;51:439–447.
1115. Si L, Whiteside TL. Tissue distribution of human NK cells studied with anti-Leu-7 monoclonal antibody. *J Immunol* 1983;130: 2149–2155.
1116. Swerdlow SH, Murray LJ. Natural killer (Leu 7$^+$) cells in reactive lymphoid tissues and malignant lymphomas. *Am J Clin Pathol* 1984; 81:459–463.
1117. Miller ML, Tubbs RR, Fishleder AJ, et al. Immunoregulatory Leu-7$^+$ and T8$^+$ lymphocytes in B-cell follicular lymphomas. *Hum Pathol* 1984;15:810–817.
1118. Poppema S, Visser L, De Leij L. Reactivity of presumed anti-natural killer cell antibody Leu 7 with intrafollicular T lymphocytes. *Clin Exp Immunol* 1983;54:834–837.
1119. Velardi A, Tilden AB, Millo R, et al. Isolation and characterization of Leu 7$^+$ germinal-center cells with the T helper-cell phenotype and granular lymphocyte morphology. *J Clin Immunol* 1986;6:205–215.
1120. Schuller-Petrovic S, Gebhart W, Lassmann H, et al. A shared antigenic determinant between natural killer cells and nervous tissue. *Nature* 1983;306:179–181.
1121. Nobile-Orazio E, Hays AP, Latov N, et al. Specificity of mouse and human monoclonal antibodies to myelin-associated glycoprotein. *Neurology* 1984;34:1336–1342.
1122. Doberson MJ, Gascon P, Trost S, et al. Murine monoclonal antibodies to the myelin-associated glycoprotein react with large granular lymphocytes of human blood. *Proc Natl Acad Sci USA* 1985;82: 552–555.
1123. Murray N, Steck AJ. Indication of a possible role in a demyelinating neuropathy for an antigen shared between myelin and NK cells. *Lancet* 1984;i:711–713.
1124. Kruse J, Mailhammer, R, Wernecke H, et al. Neural cell adhesion molecules and myelin-associated glycoprotein share a common carbohydrate moiety recognized by monoclonal antibodies L2 and HNK-1. *Nature* 1984;311:153–155.
1125. Kruse J, Keilhauer G, Faissner A, et al. The J1 glycoprotein-a novel nervous system cell adhesion molecule of the L2/HNK-1 family. *Nature* 1985;316:146–148.
1126. Inuzuka T, Quarles RH, Noronha AB, et al. A human lymphocyte antigen is shared with a group of glycoproteins in peripheral nerve. *Neurosci Lett* 1984;51:105–111.
1127. Ilyas AA, Quarles RH, Brady RO. The monoclonal antibody HNK-1 reacts with a human peripheral nerve ganglioside. *Biochem Biophys Res Commun* 1984;122:1206–1211.
1128. McGarry RC, Riopelle RJ, Frail DE, et al. The characterization and cellular distribution of a family of antigens related to myelin associated glycoprotein in the developing nervous system. *J Neuroimmunol* 1985;10:101–104.
1129. Hoffman S, Edelman GE. A proteoglycan with HNK-1 antigenic determinants is a neuron-associated ligand for cytotactin. *Proc Natl Acad Sci USA* 1987;84:2523–2527.
1130. Chou DKH, Ilyas AA, Evans JE, et al. Structure of sulfated glucuronyl glycolipids in the nervous system reacting with HNK-1 antibody and some IgM paraproteins in neuropathy. *J Biol Chem* 1986;261: 11717–11725.
1131. Chou DKH, Schwarting GA, Jungalwala FB. Sulfated glucuronyl glycolipids in the nervous system. *Trans Am Soc Neurochem* 1986; 17:146.
1132. Shashoua VE, Jungalwala RB, Chou DKH, et al. Sulfated glucuronyl glycoconjugates in ependymins of fish and human CSF. *Trans Am Soc Neurochem* 1986;17:148.
1133. Lipinski M, Braham K, Caillaud JM, et al. HNK-1 antibody detects an antigen expressed on neuroctodermal cells. *J Exp Med* 1983;158: 1775–1780.
1134. Bunn PA, Linnoila I, Minna JD, et al. Small cell lung cancer, endocrine cells of the fetal bronchus, and other neuroendocrine cells express the Leu-7 antigenic determinant present on natural killer cells. *Blood* 1985;65:764–768.

1135. Wahab ZA, Wright GL. Monoclonal antibody (anti-Leu 7) directed against natural killer cells reacts with normal, benign and malignant prostate tissues. *Int J Cancer* 1985;36:677–683.
1136. Kodoma T, Watanabe S, Sato Y, et al. An immunohistochemical study of thymic epithelial tumors: I. Epithelial component. *Am J Surg Pathol* 1986;10:26-33.
1137. Pandolfi F, Loughran TP, Starkebaum G, et al. Clinical course of prognosis of the lymphoproliferative disease of granular lymphocytes: a multicenter study. *Cancer* 1990;65:341–348.
1138. Chan JKC, Ng CS, Tsang WYW. Nasal/nasopharyngeal lymphomas: an immunohistochemical analysis of 57 cases on frozen tissues. *Mod Pathol* 1993;6:87A.
1139. Poppema S. The nature of the lymphocytes surrounding Reed-Sternberg cells in nodular lymphocyte predominance and in other types of Hodgkin's disease. *Am J Pathol* 1989;135:351–357.
1140. Kamel OW, Gelb AB, Shibuya RB, et al. Leu 7 (CD57) reactivity distinguishes nodular lymphocyte predominance Hodgkin's disease from nodular sclerosing Hodgkin's disease, T-cell-rich B-cell lymphoma and follicular lymphoma. *Am J Pathol* 1993;142:541–546.
1141. Springer T, Galfre G, Secher DS, et al. Mac-1: a macrophage differentiation antigen identified by monoclonal antibody. *Eur J Immunol* 1979;9:301–306.
1142. Ault KA, Springer TA: Cross-reaction of a rat-anti-mouse phagocyte-specific monoclonal antibody (anti-Mac-1) with human monocytes and natural killer cells. *J Immunol* 1981;126:359–364.
1143. Hynes RO. Integrins, a family of cell surface receptors. *Cell* 1987; 48:549–555.
1144. Ruoslahti E, Pierschbacher MD. New perspectives in cell adhesion: RGD and integrins. *Science* 1987;238:491–497.
1145. Springer TA, Dustin ML, Kishimoto TK, et al. The lymphocyte function-associated LFA-1, CD2, and LFA-3 molecules: cell adhesion receptors of the immune system. *Annu Rev Immunol* 1987;5: 223–252.
1146. Stewart M, Thiel M, Hogg N. Leukocyte integrins. *Curr Opin Cell Biol* 1995;7:690–696.
1147. Springer TA. Adhesion receptors of the immune system. *Nature* 1990;346:425–434.
1148. Kishimoto TK, Hollander N, Roberts TM, et al. Heterogeneous mutations in the beta subunit common to the LFA-1, Mac-1, and p150, 95 glycoproteins cause leukocyte adhesion deficiency. *Cell* 1987; 50:193–202.
1149. Anderson DC, Springer TA. Leukocyte adhesion deficiency: an inherited defect in the Mac-1, LFA-1 and p150,95 glycoproteins. *Annu Rev Med* 1987;38:175–194.
1150. Todd RF, Freyer DR. The CD11/CD18 leukocyte glycoprotein deficiency. *Hematol Oncol Clin North Am* 1988;2:13–31.
1151. Dana N, Styrt B, Griffin JD, et al. Two functional domains in the phagocyte membrane glycoprotein Mo1 identified with monoclonal antibodies. *J Immunol* 1986;136:3259–3263.
1152. Corbi AL, Larson RS, Kishimoto TK, et al. Chromosomal location of the genes encoding the leukocyte adhesion receptors LFA-1, Mac-1 and p150, 95: identification of a gene cluster involved in cell adhesion. *J Exp Med* 1988;167:1597–1607.
1153. Corbi AL, Larson RS, Kishimoto TK, et al. The human leukocyte adhesion glycoprotein Mac-1 (complement receptor type 3, CD11b) alpha subunit: cloning, primary structure, and relation to the integrins, von Willebrand factor and factor B. *J Biol Chem* 1988;263: 12403–12411.
1154. Michishita M, Videm V, Arnaout MA. A novel divalent cation-binding site in the A domain of the beta 2 integrin CR3 (CD11b/CD18) is essential for ligand binding. *Cell* 1993;72:857–867.
1155. Diamond MS, Garcia-Agular J, Bickford JK, et al. The I domain is a major recognition site on the leukocyte integrin Mac-1 (CD11b/CD18) for four distinct adhesion ligands. *J Cell Biol* 1993;120: 1031–1043.
1156. Luk J, Springer TA. CD11b cluster report. In: Schlossman SF, Boumsell L, Gilks WR, et al, eds. *Leukocyte typing V: white cell differentiation antigens.* New York: Oxford University Press, 1995:1588–1590.
1157. Kishimoto TK, Larson RS, Corbi AL, et al. The leukocytic integrins. *Adv Immunol* 1989;46:149–182.
1158. Carlos TM, Harlan JM. Membrane proteins involved in phagocyte adherence to endothelium. *Immunol Rev* 1990;114:5–28.
1159. Arnaout MA. Leukocyte adhesion molecules deficiency: its structural basis, pathophysiology and implications for modulating the inflammatory response. *Immunol Rev* 1990;114:145–180.
1160. Petty HR, Todd RF. Integrins as promiscuous signal transduction devices. *Immunol Today* 1996;5:209–212.
1161. Köller U. Summary of immunohistology studies. In: Knapp W, Dörken B, Gilks WR, et al, eds. *Leukocyte typing IV: white cell differentiation antigens.* Oxford: Oxford University Press, 1989:862–867.
1162. Landay A, Gartland GL, Clement LT. Characterization of a phenotypically distinct subpopulation of Leu-2 cells that suppresses T cell proliferative responses. *J Immunol* 1983;131:2757–2761.
1163. Clement LT, Grossi CE, Gartland GL. Morphologic and phenotypic features of the subpopulation of Leu-2^+ cells that suppresses B cell differentiation. *J Immunol* 1984; 133:2461–2468.
1164. Van der Reijden HJ, Van Rhenen DJ, Lansdorp PM, et al. A comparison of surface marker analysis and FAB classification in acute myeloid leukemia. *Blood* 1983;61:443–448.
1165. Linch DC, Allen C, Beverley PCL, et al. Monoclonal antibodies differentiating between monocytic and nonmonocytic variants of AML. *Blood* 1984;63:566–573.
1166. Drexler HG, Minowada J. The use of monoclonal antibodies for the identification and classification of acute myeloid leukemias. *Leuk Res* 1986;10:279–290.
1167. Matutes E, Rodriguez B, Polli N, et al. Characterization of myeloid leukemias with monoclonal antibodies 3C5 and MY9. *Hematol Oncol* 1985;3:179–186.
1168. Drexler HG, Sagawa K, Menon M, et al. Phenotyping of malignant hematopoietic cells: II. Reactivity pattern of myeloid monoclonal antibodies with emphasis on MCS-2. *Leuk Res* 1986;10:17–23.
1169. Nichols GE, Normansell DE, Williams ME. Lymphoproliferative disorder of granular lymphocytes: nine cases including one with features of CD56 (NKH1)-positive aggressive natural killer cell lymphoma. *Mod Pathol* 1994;7:819–824.
1170. Lanier LL, Arnaout MA, Schwarting R, et al. p150/95, Third member of the LFA-1/CR3 polypeptide family identified by anti-Leu M5 monoclonal antibody. *Eur J Immunol* 1985;15:713–718.
1171. Springer TA, Miller LJ, Anderson DC. P150,95, the third member of the Mac-1, LFA-1 human leukocyte adhesion glycoprotein family. *J Immunol* 1986;136:240–245.
1172. Miller LJ, Springer TA. Biosynthesis and glycosylation of p150,95 and related leukocyte adhesion proteins. *J Immunol* 1987;139: 842–847.
1173. Corbi AL, Garcia-Aguilar J, Springer TA. Genomic structure of an integrin alpha subunit, the leukocyte p150,95 molecule. *J Biol Chem* 1990;265:2782–2788.
1174. Micklem KJ, Sim RB. Isolation of complement-fragment iC3b-binding proteins by affinity chromatography: the identification of p150,95 as an iC3b-binding protein. *Biochem J* 1985;231:233–236.
1175. Malhotra V, Hogg N, Sim RB. Ligand binding by the p150,95 antigen of U937 monocytic cells: properties in common with complement receptor type 3 (CR3). *Eur J Immunol* 1986;16:1117–1123.
1176. Myones BL, Dalzell JG, Hogg N, et al. Neutrophil and monocyte cell surface p150,95 has iC3b-receptor (CR4) activity resembling CR3. *J Clin Invest* 1988;82:640–651.
1177. Stacker SA, Springer TA. Leukocyte integrin p150,95 (CD11c/CD18) functions as an adhesion molecule binding to a counter-receptor on stimulated endothelium. *J Immunol* 1991;146:648–655.
1178. Loike JD, Sodeik B, Cao L, et al. CD11c/CD18 on neutrophils recognizes a domain at the N terminus of the A alpha chain of fibrinogen. *Proc Natl Acad Sci USA* 1991;88:1044–1048.
1179. Keizer GD, Te Velde AA, Schwarting R, et al. Role of p150,95 in adhesion, migration, chemotaxis and phagocytosis of human monocytes. *Eur J Immunol* 1987;17:1317–1322.
1180. TeVelde AA, Keizer GD, Figdor CG. Differential function of LFA-1 family molecules (CD11 and CD18) in adhesion of human monocytes to melanoma and endothelial cells. *Immunology* 1987;61: 261–267.
1181. Arnaout MA, Lanier LL, Faller DV. Relative contribution of the leukocyte molecules Mo1, LFA-1 and p150,95 (LeuM5) in adhesion of granulocytes and monocytes to vascular endothelium is tissue-and stimulus-specific. *J Cell Physiol* 1988;137:305–309.
1182. Keizer GD, Borst J, Visser W, et al. Membrane glycoprotein p150,95 of human cytotoxic T cell clone is involved in conjugate formation with target cells. *J Immunol* 1987;138:3130–3136.
1183. Postigo AA, Corbi AL, Sanchez-Madrid F, et al. Regulated expres-

sion and function of CD11c/CD18 integrin on human B lymphocytes: relation between attachment to fibrinogen and triggering of proliferation through CD11c/CD18. *J Exp Med* 1991;174:1313–1322.

1184. Berton G, Laudanna C, Sorio C, et al. Generation of signals activating neutrophil functions by leukocyte integrins: LFA-1 and gp150/95, but not CR3, are able to stimulate the respiratory burst of human neutrophils. *J Cell Biol* 1992;116:1007–1017.

1185. Giorno R. Immunohistochemical analysis of human peripheral blood and lymphoid tissues using monoclonal antibodies immunoreactive with non-lymphoid cells. *Histochemistry* 1986;84:241–245.

1186. Cabanas D, Sanches-Madrid F, Acevedo A, et al. Characterization of a CD11c-reactive monoclonal antibody (HC1/1) obtained by immunizing with phorbol ester differentiated U937 cells. *Hybridoma* 1988;7:167–176.

1187. Hogg N, Takacs L, Palmer DG, et al. The p150,95 molecule is a marker of human mononuclear phagocytes: comparison with expression of class II molecules. *Eur J Immunol* 1986;16:240–248.

1188. Miller LJ, Schwarting R, Springer TA. Regulated expression of the Mac-1, LFA-1, p150,95 glycoprotein family during leukocyte differentiation. *J Immunol* 1986;137:2891–2900.

1189. Akiyama H, McGeer PL. Brain microglia constitutively express beta-2 integrins. *J Neuroimmunol* 1990;30:81–93.

1190. Miller LJ, Bainton DF, Borregaard N, et al. Stimulated mobilization of monocyte Mac-1 and p150,95 adhesion proteins from an intracellular vesicular compartment to the cell surface. *J Clin Invest* 1987; 80:535–544.

1191. Chadburn A, Inghirami G, Knowles DM. Hairy cell leukemia-associated antigen LeuM5 (CD11c) is preferentially expressed by benign activated and neoplastic CD8 T cells. *Am J Pathol* 1990;136:29–37.

1192. Falini B, Pulford K, Erber WN, et al. Use of a panel of monoclonal antibodies for the diagnosis of hairy cell leukemia: an immunocytochemical study of 36 cases. *Histopathology* 1986;10:671–687.

1193. Sainati L, Matutes E, Mulligan S, et al. A variant form of hairy cell leukemia resistant to α-interferon: clinical and phenotypic characteristics of 17 patients. *Blood* 1990;76:157–162.

1194. Wormsley SB, Baird SM, Gadol N, et al. Characteristics of $CD11c^{+}CD5^{+}$ chronic B cell leukemias and the identification of novel peripheral blood B cell subsets with chronic lymphoid leukemia immunophenotypes. *Blood* 1990;76:123–130.

1195. Hanson CA, Gribbin TE, Schnitzer B, et al. CD11c (LeuM5) expression characterizes a B cell chronic lymphoproliferative disorder with features of both chronic lymphocyte leukemia and hairy cell leukemia. *Blood* 1990;76:2360–2367.

1196. Caligaris-Cappio F, Pizzolo G, Chilosi M, et al. Phorbol ester induces abnormal chronic lymphocytic leukemia cells to express features of hairy cell leukemia. *Blood* 1985;66:1035–1042.

1197. Matutes E, Morilla R, Owusu-Ankomah K, et al. The immunophenotype of splenic lymphoma with villous lymphocytes and its relevance to the differential diagnosis with other B cell disorders. *Blood* 1994; 83:1558–1562.

1198. Inghirami G, Wieczorek R, Zhu B, et al. Differential expression of LFA-1 molecules in non-Hodgkin's lymphoma and lymphoid leukemia. *Blood* 1988;72:1431–1434.

1199. Weiss LM, Picker LJ, Copenhaver CM, et al. Large-cell hematolymphoid neoplasms of uncertain lineage. *Hum Pathol* 1988;19: 967–973.

1200. Scott CS, Richards SJ, Master PS, et al. Flow cytometric analysis of membrane CD11b, CD11c and CD14 expression in acute myeloid leukaemia: relationships with monocytic subtypes and the concept of relative antigen expression. *Eur J Haematol* 1990;44:24–29.

1201. Drexler HG, Sagawa K, Menon M, et al. Pan-myeloid reagent: the monoclonal antibody MCS2 in the routine immunodiagnostic service of leukemia phenotyping. *Gann* 1985;76:235–239.

1202. Gadd S. Cluster report: CD13. In: Knapp W, Dörken B, Gilks WR, et al, eds. *Leukocyte typing IV: white cell differentiation antigens.* New York: Oxford University Press, 1989:782–784.

1203. Ashmun RA, Holmes KV, Shapiro LH, et al. CD13 (aminopeptidase N) cluster workshop report. In: Schlossman SF, Boumsell L, Gilks WR, et al, eds. *Leukocyte typing V: white cell differentiation antigens.* New York: Oxford University Press, 1995:771–775.

1204. Look AT, Ashmun RA, Shapiro LH, et al. Human myeloid plasma membrane glycoprotein CD13 (gp150) is identical to aminopeptidase N. *J Clin Invest* 1989;83:932–941.

1205. Olsen J, Cowell GM, Konishofer E, et al. Complete amino acid sequence of human intestinal aminopeptidase N as deduced from cloned cDNA. *FEBS Lett* 1988;238:307–314.

1206. Look AT, Peiper SC, Rebentisch MB, et al. Molecular cloning, expression, and chromosomal localization of the gene encoding a human myeloid membrane antigen (gp150). *J Clin Invest* 1986;78: 914–921.

1207. Jongeneel CV, Bouvier J, Bairoch A. A unique signature identifies a family of zinc-dependent metallopeptidases. *FEBS Lett* 1989;242: 211–214.

1208. Vallee BL, Auld DS. Zinc coordination, function, and structure of zinc enzymes and other proteins. *Biochemistry* 1990;29:5647–5659.

1209. O'Connell PJ, Gerkis V, d'Apice AJF. Variable O-glycosylation of CD13 (aminopeptidase N). *J Biol Chem* 1991;266:4593–4597.

1210. Ashmun RA, Shapiro LH, Look AT. Deletion of the zinc-binding motif of CD13/aminopeptidase N molecules results in loss of epitopes that mediate binding of inhibitory antibodies. *Blood* 1992;79: 3344–3349.

1211. Look AT, Peiper SC, Rebentisch MB, et al. Transfer and expression of the gene encoding a human myeloid membrane antigen (gp150). *J Clin Invest* 1985;75:569–579.

1212. Semenza G. Anchoring and biosynthesis of stalked brush border membrane proteins: glycosidases and peptidases of enterocytes and renal tubuli. *Annu Rev Cell Biol* 1986;2:255–313.

1213. Larsen SL, Petersen LO, Buus S, et al. T cell responses affected by aminopeptidase N (CD13)-mediated trimming of major histocompatibility complex class II-bound peptides. *J Exp Med* 1996;184: 183–189.

1214. Connelly JC, Skidgel RA, Schulz WW, et al. Neutral ndopeptidase 24.11 in human neutrophils: cleavage of chemotactic peptide. *Proc Natl Acad Sci USA* 1985;82:8737–8741.

1215. Painter RG, Dukes R, Sullivan J, et al. Function of neutral endopeptidase on the cell membrane of human neutrophils. *J Biol Chem* 1988; 263:9456–9461.

1216. Najjar VA. Tuftsin, a natural activator of phagocyte cells: an overview. *Ann NY Acad Sci* 1983;419:1–11.

1217. Matsas R, Stephenson SL, Hryszko J, et al. The metabolism of neuropeptides: phase separation of synaptic membrane preparations with Triton X-114 reveals the presence of aminopeptidase N. *Biochem J* 1985;231:445–449.

1218. Yeager CL, Ashmun RA, Williams RK, et al. Human aminopeptidase N is a receptor for human coronavirus 229E. *Nature* 1992;357: 420–422.

1219. Griffin JD, Ritz J, Beveridge RP, et al. Expression of MY7 antigens on myeloid precursor cells. *Int J Cell Cloning* 1983;1:33–48.

1220. Pombo de Oliveira MS, Matutes E, et al. Early expression of MCS2 (CD13) in the cytoplasm of blast cells from acute myeloid leukemia. *Acta Haemat* 1988;80:61–64.

1221. Cuneo A, Van Orshoven A, Michaus JL, et al. Morphologic, immunologic, and cytogenetic studies in erythroleukemia: evidence for multilineage involvement and identification of two distinct cytogenetic-clinicopathological types. *Br J Haematol* 1990;75:346–354.

1222. Stasi R, Del Poeta G, Venditti A, et al. Analysis of treatment failure in patients with minimally differentiated acute myeloid leukemia (AML-M0). *Blood* 1994;83:1619–1625.

1223. Sobol RE, Royston I, Lebien TW, et al. Adult acute lymphoblastic leukemia phenotypes defined by monoclonal antibodies. *Blood* 1985; 65:730–735.

1224. Griffin JD, Davis R, Nelson DA, et al. Use of surface marker analysis to predict outcome of adult acute myeloblastic leukemia. *Blood* 1986; 68:1232–1241.

1225. Schwarzinger I, Valent P, Koller U, et al. Prognostic significance of surface marker expression on blasts of patients with de novo acute myeloblastic leukemia. *J Clin Oncol* 1990;8:423–430.

1226. Mechtersheimer G, Moller P. Expression of aminopeptidase N (CD13) in mesenchymal tumors. *Am J Pathol* 1990;137:1215–1222.

1227. Favaloro EJ, Moraitis N, Bradstock K, et al. Co-expression of haemopoietic antigens on vascular endothelial cells: a detailed phenotypic analysis. *Br J Haematol* 1990;74:385–394.

1228. Look AT, Ashmun RA, Shapiro LH, et al. Report on the CD13 (aminopeptidase N) cluster workshop. In: Knapp W, Dorken B, Gilks WR, et al, eds. *Leucocyte typing IV: white cell differentiation antigens.* New York: Oxford University Press, 1989:784–787.

1229. Finstad CL, Cordon-Cardo C, Bander NH, et al. Specificity analysis

of mouse monoclonal antibodies defining cell surface antigens of human renal cancer. *Proc Natl Acad Sci USA* 1985;82:2955–2959.
1230. Dimitriu-Bona A, Burmester GR, Waters SJ, et al. Human mononuclear phagocyte differentiation antigens: I. Patterns of antigenic expression on the surface of human monocytes and macrophages defined by monoclonal antibodies. *J Immunol* 1983;130:145–152.
1231. Goyert SM, Tesio L, Ashman LK, et al. Report on the CD14 cluster workshop. In: Knapp W, Dörken B, Gilks WR, et al, eds. *Leukocyte typing IV: white cell differentiation antigens.* Oxford: Oxford University Press, 1989:789–794.
1232. Goyert SM, Haziot A, Jiao D, et al. CD14 cluster workshop report. In Schlossman SF, Boumsell L, Gilks WR, et al, eds. *Leukocyte typing V: white cell differentiation antigens.* New York: Oxford University Press, 1995:777–782.
1233. Goyert SM, Cohen L, Gangloff SC, et al. CD14 workshop panel report. In Kishimoto T, Kikutani H, von dem Borne AEGK, et al, eds. *Leukocyte typing VI: white cell differentiation antigens.* New York: Garland Publishing, 1998:963–965.
1234. Maliszewski CR, Currier J, Fisher J, et al. Monoclonal antibodies that bind to the My23 human myeloid cell surface molecule: epitope analysis and antigen modulation studies. *Mol Immunol* 1987;24: 17–25.
1235. Schutt C, Witt S, Grunwald U, et al. Epitope mapping of CD14 glycoprotein. In: Schlossman SF, Boumsell L, Gilks WR, et al, eds. *Leukocyte typing V: white cell differentiation antigens.* New York: Oxford University Press, 1995:785–789.
1236. Haziot A, Chen S, Ferrero EM, et al. The monocyte differentiation antigen, CD14, is anchored to the cell membrane by a phosphatidylinositol linkage. *J Immunol* 1988;141:547–552.
1237. Simmons DL, Tan S, Tenen DG, et al. Monocyte antigen CD14 is a phospholipid anchored membrane protein. *Blood* 1989;73:284–289.
1238. Low MG, Saltiel AR. Structural and functional roles of glycosylphosphatidylinositol in membranes. *Science* 1988;239:268–275.
1239. Maliszewski CR, Ball ED, Graziano RF, et al. Isolation and characterization of My23, a myeloid cell-derived antigen reactive with the monoclonal antibody AML-2-23. *J Immunol* 1985;135:1929–1936.
1240. Goyert SM, Ferrero EM, Seremetis SV, et al. Biochemistry and expression of myelomonocytic antigens. *J Immunol* 1986;137: 3909–3914.
1241. Kinoshita T, Medof ME, Silber R, et al. Distribution of decay-accelerating factor in the peripheral blood of normal individuals and patients with paroxysmal nocturnal hemoglobinuria. *J Exp Med* 1985; 162:75–92.
1242. Grunwald U, Kruger C, Westermann J, et al. An enzyme-linked immunosorbent assay for the quantification of solubilized CD14 in biological fluids. *J Immunol Methods* 1992;155:225–232.
1243. Bazil V, Horejsi V, Baudys M, et al. Biochemical characterization of a soluble form of the 53-kda monocyte surface antigen. *Eur J Immunol* 1986;16:1583–1589.
1244. Bazil V, Strominger JL. Shedding as a mechanism of down-modulation of CD14 on stimulated human monocytes. *J Immunol* 1991; 147:1567–1574.
1245. Haziot A, Tsuberi BZ, Goyert SM. Neutrophil CD14: biochemical properties and role in the secretion of tumor necrosis factor-alpha in response to lipopolysaccharide. *J Immunol* 1993;150:5556–5565.
1246. Labeta MO, Durieux JJ, Fernandez N, et al. Release from a human monocyte-like cell line of two different soluble forms of the lipopolysaccharide receptor, CD14. *Eur J Immunol* 1993;23:2144–2151.
1247. Bufler P, Stiegler G, Schuchmann M, et al. Soluble lipopolysaccha ride receptor (CD14) is released via two different mechanisms from human monocytes and CD14 transfectants. *Eur J Immunol* 1995;25: 604–610.
1248. Goyert SM, Ferrero E, Rettig WJ, et al. The CD14 monocyte differentiation antigen maps to a region encoding growth factors and receptors. *Science* 1988;239:497–500.
1249. LeBeau MM, Albain KS, Larson RA, et al. Clinical and cytogenetic correlations in 63 patients with therapy-related myelodysplastic syndromes and acute non-lymphocytic leukemia: further evidence for characteristic abnormalities of chromosomes no. 5 and 7. *J Clin Oncol* 1986;4:325–345.
1250. Schumann RR, Leong SR, Flaggs GW, et al. Structure and function of lipopolysaccharide binding protein. *Science* 1990;249: 1429–1431.
1251. Wright SD, Ramos RA, Tobias PS, et al. CD14, a receptor for complexes of lipopolysaccharide (LPS) and LPS binding protein. *Science* 1990;249:1431–1433.
1252. Ferrero E, Jiao D, Tsuberi BZ, et al. Transgenic mice expressing human CD14 are hypersensitive to lipopolysaccharide. *Proc Natl Acad Sci USA* 1993;90:2380–2384.
1253. Haziot A, Rong GW, Silver J, et al. Recombinant soluble CD14 mediates the activation of endothelial cells by lipopolysaccharide. *J Immunol* 1993;151:1500–1507.
1254. Pugin J, Schürer-Maly CC, Leturcq D, et al. Lipopolysacccharide activation of human endothelial and epithelial cells is mediated by lipopolysaccharide-binding protein and soluble CD14. *Proc Natl Acad Sci USA* 1993;90:2744–2748.
1255. Haziot A, Katz I, Jiao D, et al. Functional epitopes of CD14. In: Schlossman SF, Boumsell L, Gilks WR, et al, eds. *Leukocyte typing V: white cell differentiation antigens.* New York: Oxford University Press, 1995:782–784.
1256. Van Voorhis WC, Steinman RM, Hair LS, et al. Specific antimononuclear phagocyte monoclonal antibodies: application to the purification of dendritic cells and the tissue localization of macrophages. *J Exp Med* 1983;158:126–145.
1257. Ziegler-Heitbrock HWL, Passlick B, Flieger D. The monoclonal antimonocyte antibody My4 stains B lymphocytes and two distinct monocyte subsets in human peripheral blood. *Hybridoma* 1988;7: 521–527.
1258. Medeiros LJ, Herrington RD, Gonzalez CL, et al. My4 antibody staining of non-Hodgkin's lymphomas. *Am J Clin Pathol* 1991;95: 363–368.
1259. Morabito F, Prasthofer EF, Dunlap NE, et al. Expression of myelomonocytic antigens on chronic lymphocytic leukemia B cells correlates with their ability to produce interleukin 1. *Blood* 1987;70: 1750–1757.
1260. Andrews RG, Torok-Storb B, Bernstein ID. Myeloid-associated differentiation antigens on stem cells and their progeny identified by monoclonal antibodies. *Blood* 1983;62:124–132.
1261. Knapp W. Myeloid section report. In: Knapp W, Dörken B, Gilks WR, et al, eds. *Leukocyte typing IV: white cell differentiation antigens.* Oxford: Oxford University Press, 1989:812–813.
1262. Peiper SC, Andrews RG. CD33 cluster workshop report. In: Schlossman SF, Boumsell L, Gilks WR, et al, eds. *Leukocyte typing V: white cell differentation antigens.* New York: Oxford University Press, 1995:837–840.
1263. Peiper SC, Guo H-H. CD33 workshop panel report. In: Kishimoto T, Kikutani H, von dem Borne AEGK, et al, eds. *Leukocyte typing VI: white cell differentiation antigens.* New York: Garland Publishing, 1998:972–974.
1264. Favaloro EJ, Bradstock KF, Kabral A, et al. Characterization of monoclonal antibodies to the human myeloid-differentiation antigen, gp67 (CD-33). *Dis Markers* 1987;5:215–225.
1265. Peiper SC, Ashmun RA, Look AT. Molecular cloning, expression, and chromosomal localization of a human gene encoding the CD33 myeloid differentiation antigen. *Blood* 1988;72:314–321.
1266. Simmons D, Seed BJ. Isolation of a cDNA encoding CD33, a differentiation antigen of myeloid progenitor cells. *J Immunol* 1988;141: 2797–2800.
1267. Sabbath KD, Griffin JD. Differentiation-associated states of clonogenic cells in acute myeloblastic leukemia using monoclonal antibodies. In: Reinherz EL, Haynes BF, Nadler LM, et al, eds. *Leukocyte typing II: human myeloid and hematopoietic cells*, vol 3. New York: Springer-Verlag, 1986:261–265.
1268. Valen P, Ashman LK, Hinterberger W, et al. Mast cell typing: demonstration of a distinct hematopoietic cell type and evidence for immunophenotypic relationship to mononuclear phagocytes. *Blood* 1989;73:1778–1785.
1269. Andrews RG, Singer JW, Bernstein ID. Precursors of colony-forming cells in humans can be distinguished from colony-forming cells by expression of the CD33 and CD34 antigens and light scatter properties. *J Exp Med* 1989;169:1721–1731.
1270. Berti E, Paindelli MG, Parravicini C, et al. Immunohistochemical reactivity of anti-myeloid/stem cell workshop monoclonal antibodies in thymus, lymph node, lung, liver and normal skin. In: Reinherz EL, Haynes BF, Nadler LM, et al, eds. *Leukocyte typing II: human myeloid and hematopoietic cells*, vol 3. New York: Springer-Verlag, 1986:237–247.

1271. Hancock WW, Kraft N, Atkins RC. Immunohistochemical studies of anti-myeloid monoclonal antibodies. In: Reinherz EL, Haynes BF, Nadler LM, et al, eds. *Leukocyte typing II: human myeloid and hematopoietic cells*, vol 3. New York: Springer-Verlag, 1986: 249–253.
1272. De Fraissinette A, Dezutter-Dambuyant C, Schmitt D, et al. Ontogeny of Langerhans cells: phenotypic differentiation from the bone marrow to the skin. *Dev Comp Immunol* 1990;14:335–346.
1273. Goordyal P, Isaacson PG. Immunocytochemical characterization of monocyte colonies of human bone marrow: a clue to the origin of Langerhans cells and interdigitating reticulum cells. *J Pathol* 1985; 146:189–195.
1274. Ritz J, Takvorian T, Sallan SE, et al. In vitro applications of monoclonal antibodies for bone marrow transplantation. In: McMichael AJ, ed. *Leukocyte typing III: proceeding of the third International Workshop on human leukocyte differentiation antigens*. Oxford: Oxford University Press, 1987:938–942.
1275. Robertson MJ, Soiffer RJ, Freedman AS, et al. Human bone marrow depleted of CD33-positive cells mediates delayed but durable reconstitution of hematopoiesis: clinical trial of MY9 monoclonal antibody-purged autografts for the treatment of acute myeloid leukemia. *Blood* 1992;79:2229–2236.
1276. Caron PC, Jurcic JG, Scott AM, et al. A phase 1B trial of humanized monoclonal antibody M195 (anti-CD33) in myeloid leukemia: specific targeting without immunogenicity. *Blood* 1994;83:1760–1768.
1277. Parwaresch MR, Radzun HJ, Kreipe H, et al. Monocyte/macrophage-reactive monoclonal antibody Ki-M6 recognizes an intracytoplasmic antigen. *Am J Pathol* 1986;125:141–151.
1278. Kreipe H, Radzun HF, Parwaresch MR, et al. Ki-M7 monoclonal antibody specific for myelomonocytic cell lineage and macrophages in human. *J Histochem Cytochem* 1987;35:1117–1126.
1279. Kelly PMA, Bliss E, Morton JA, et al. Monoclonal antibody EBM/11: high cellular specificity for human macrophages. *J Clin Pathol* 1988;41:510–515.
1280. Davey FR, Cordell JL, Erber WN, et al. Monoclonal antibody (Y1/82A) with specificity towards peripheral blood monocytes and tissue macrophages. *J Clin Pathol* 1988;41:753–758.
1281. Pulford KAF, Rigney EM, Micklem KF, et al. KP1: a new monoclonal antibody that detects a monocyte/macrophage associated antigen in routinely processed tissue sections. *J Clin Pathol* 1989;42: 414–421.
1282. Stockinger H. Cluster report: CD68. In: Knapp W, Dorken B, Gilks WR, et al, eds. *Leucocyte typing IV: white cell differentiation antigens*. New York: Oxford University Press, 1989:841–843.
1283. Falini T, Flenghi L, Pileri S, et al. PG-M1: a new monoclonal antibody directed against a fixative-resistant epitope on the macrophage-restricted form of the CD68 molecule. *Am J Pathol* 1993;142: 1359–1372.
1284. Cordell JL, Falini B, Flenghi L, et al. CD68 cluster workshop report. In: Schlossman SF, Boumsell L, Gilks WR, et al, eds. *Leukocyte typing V: white cell differentiation antigens*. New York: Oxford University Press, 1995:925–927.
1285. Micklem K, Rigney E, Cordell J, et al. A human macrophage-associated antigen (CD68) detected by six different monoclonal antibodies. *Br J Haematol* 1989;73:6–11.
1286. Micklem K, Cordell J, Rigney E, et al. A macrophage-associated antigen defined by five mAb. In: Knapp W, Dorken B, Gilks WR, et al, eds. *Leucocyte typing IV: white cell differentiation antigens*. New York: Oxford University Press, 1989:843–846.
1287. Weiss LM, Arber DA, Chang KL. CD68: a review. *Appl Immunohistochem* 1994;2:2–8.
1288. Fukuda M. Lysosomal membrane glycoproteins: structure, biosynthesis, and intracellular trafficking. *J Biol Chem* 1991;266: 21327–21330.
1289. Rabinowitz SS, Gordon S. Macrosialin, a macrophage-restricted membrane sialoprotein differentially glycosylated in response to inflammatory stimuli. *J Exp Med* 1991;174:827–836.
1290. Pulford KAF, Sipos A, Cordell JL, et al. Distribution of the CD68 macrophage/myeloid-associated antigen. *Int Immunol* 1990;2: 973–980.
1291. Saito N, Pulford KAF, Breton-Gorius J, et al. Ultrastructural localization of the CD68 macrophage-associated antigen in human blood neutrophils and monocytes. *Am J Pathol* 1991;139:1053–1059.
1292. Greywoode GIN, McCarthy SP, McGee JO. Labelling of cells of the mononuclear phagocyte system in routinely processed archival biopsy specimens with monoclonal antibody EBM/11. *J Clin Pathol* 1990;43:992–996.
1293. Gloghini A, Volpe R, Carbone A. Ki-M6 immunostaining in routinely processed sections of human lymphoid tissue. *Am J Clin Pathol* 1990;94:734–741.
1294. Gloghini A, Volpe R, Canzonieri V, et al. Immunohistochemical characterization of Ki-M6 monoclonal antibody in Bouin-fixed, paraffin-embedded sections of normal and neoplastic human tissues. *Virchows Arch* 1991;418:355–360.
1295. Dooper IM, Bogman MJ, Hoitsma AJ, et al. Detection of interstitial increase in macrophages, characteristic of acute interstitial rejection, in routinely processed renal allograft biopsies using the monoclonal antibody KP1. *Transpl Int* 1992;5:209–213.
1296. Horny H-P, Schaumburg-Lever G, Bolz S, et al. Use of monoclonal antibody KP1 for identifying normal and neoplastic human mast cells. *J Clin Pathol* 1990;43:719–722.
1297. Thiele J, Braeckel C, Wagner S, et al. Macrophages in normal human bone marrow and in chronic myeloproliferative disorders: an immunohistochemical and morphometric study by a new monoclonal antibody (PG-M1) on trephine biopsies. *Virchows Arch* 1992;421: 33–39.
1298. Hulette CM, Downey BT, Burger PC. Macrophage markers in diagnostic neuropathology. *Am J Surg Pathol* 1992;16:493–499.
1299. Facchetti F, De Wolf-Peeters C, Van den Oord JJ, et al. Plasmacytoid monocytes (so-called plasmacytoid T-cells) in Kikuchi's lymphadenitis: an immunohistologic study. *Am J Clin Pathol* 1989;92:42–50.
1300. Strobl H, Scheinecker C, Csmarits B, et al. Flow cytometric analysis of intracellular CD68 molecule expression in normal and malignant haemopoiesis. *Br J Haematol* 1995;90:774–782.
1301. Warnke RA, Pulford KAF, Pallesen G, et al. Diagnosis of myelomonocytic and macrophage neoplasms in routinely processed tissue biopsies with monoclonal antibody KP1. *Am J Pathol* 1989;135: 1089–1095.1299.
1302. Hanson CA, Jaszca W, Kersey JH. True histiocytic lymphoma: histopathologic, immunophenotypic and genotypic analysis. *Br J Haematol* 1989;73:187–198.
1303. Ralfkiaer E, Delsol G, O'Connor NTJ, et al. Malignant lymphomas of true histiocytic origin: a clinical, histological, immunophenotypic and genotypic study. *J Pathol* 1990;160:9–17.
1304. Milchgrub S, Kamel OW, Wiley E, et al. Malignant histiocytic neoplasms of the small intestine. *Am J Surg Pathol* 1992;16:11–20.
1305. Ruco LP, Pulford KAF, Mason DY, et al. Expression of macrophage-associated antigens in tissues involved by Langerhans' cell histiocytosis (histiocytosis X). *Am J Clin Pathol* 1989;92:273–279.
1306. Carbone A, Gloghini A, Volpe R, et al. KP1 (CD68)-positive large cell lymphomas: a histopathologic and immunophenotypic characterization of 12 cases. *Hum Pathol* 1993;24:886–896.
1307. Tsang WYW, Chan JKC. KP1 (CD68) staining of granular cell neoplasms: is KP1 a marker for lysosomes rather than the histiocytic lineage? *Histopathology* 1992;21:84–86.
1308. Dei Tos AP, Doglioni C, Laurino L, et al. PK1 (CD68) expression in benign neural tumors: further evidence of its low specificity as a histiocytic/myeloid marker. *Histopathology* 1993;23:185–187.
1309. Longacre TA, Smoller BR, Rouse RV. Atypical fibroxanthoma: multiple immunohistologic profiles. *Am J Surg Pathol* 1993:17: 1199–1209.
1310. Smith MEF, Costa MJ, Weiss SW. Evaluation of CD68 and other histiocytic antigens in angiomatoid malignant fibrous histiocytoma. *Am J Surg Pathol* 1991;15:757–763.
1311. Binder SW, Said JW, Shintaku IP, et al. A histiocyte-specific marker in the diagnosis of malignant fibrous histiocytoma: use of monoclonal antibody KP-1 (CD68). *Am J Clin Pathol* 1992;97:759–763.
1312. Kaiser U, Hansmann M-L, Papadopoulos I, et al. Monocyte/macrophage-directed antibodies Ki-M3 and Ki-M7 detect renal-cell carcinomas. *Int J Cancer* 1988;3:45–49.
1313. Facchetti F, Bartalot G, Grigolato PG. KP1 (CD68) staining of malignant melanomas. *Histopathology* 1991;19:141–145.
1314. Civin CI, Strauss LC, Brovall C, et al. Antigenic analysis of hematopoiesis: III. A hematopoeitic progenitor cell surface antigen defined by a monoclonal antibody raised against KG-Ia cells. *J Immunol* 1984;133:157–165.
1315. Tindle RW, Nichols RAB, Chan L, et al. A novel monoclonal antibody BI-3C5 recognises myeloblasts and non-B non-T lymphoblasts

in acute leukaemias and CGL blast crises, and reacts with immature cells in normal bone marrow. *Leuk Res* 1985;9:1–9.

1316. Greaves MF, Titley I, Colman SM, et al. CD34 cluster workshop report. In: Schlossman SF, Boumsell L, Gilks WR, et al, eds. *Leukocyte typing V: white cell differentiation antigens.* New York: Oxford University Press, 1995:840–846.
1317. Fina L, Molgaard HV, Robertson D, et al. Expression of the CD34 gene in vascular endothelial cells. *Blood* 1990;75:2417–2426.
1318. Schlingemann RO, Rietveld FJR, deWaal RMW, et al. Leukocyte antigen CD34 is expressed by a subset of cultured endothelial cells and on endothelial abluminal microprocesses in the tumor stroma. *Lab Invest* 1990;62:690–696.
1319. Sutherland DR, Marsh JC, Davidson J, et al. Differential sensitivity of CD34 epitopes to cleavage by Pasteurella haemolytica glycoprotease: implications for purification of CD34-positive progenitor cells. *Exp Hematol* 1992;20:590–599.
1320. van de Rijn M, Rouse RV. CD34: a review. *Appl Immunohistochem* 1994;2:71–80.
1321. Howell SM, Molgaard HV, Greaves MF, et al. Localization of the gene coding for the haemopoietic stem cell antigen CD34 to chromosome 1q32. *Hum Genet* 1991;87:625–627.
1322. Greaves MF, Brown J, Molgaard HV, et al. Molecular features of CD34: a hematopoietic progenitor cell-associated molecule. *Leukemia* 1992;1:31–36.
1323. Simmons DL, Satterthwaite AB, Tenen DG, et al. Molecular cloning of a cDNA encoding CD34, a sialomucin of human hematopoietic stem cells. *J Immunol* 1992;148:267–271.
1324. Suda J, Sudo T, Ito M, et al. Two types of murine CD34 mRNA generated by alternative splicing. *Blood* 1992;79:2288–2295.
1325. Nakamura Y, Komano H, Nakauchi H. Two alternative forms of cDNA encoding CD34. Exp Haematol 1993;21:236–242.
1326. Baumheuter S, Singer MS, Henzel W, et al. Binding of L-selectin to the vascular sialomucin CD34. *Science* 1993;262:436–438.
1327. Delia D, Lampugnani MG, Resnati M, et al. CD34 expression is regulated reciprocally with adhesion molecules in vascular endothelial cells in vitro. *Blood* 1993;81:1001–1008.
1328. Fackler MJ, Givin CI, Sutherland DR, et al. Activated protein kinase C directly phosphorylates the CD34 antigen on hematopoietic cells. *J Biol Chem* 1990;265:11056–11061.
1329. Sutherland DR, Fackler MJ, May WS, et al. Activated protein kinase C directly phosphorylates the CD34 antigen in acute lymphoblastic leukemia cells. *Leuk Lymphoma* 1992;8:337–344.
1330. Civin CI, Banquerigo ML, Strauss LC, et al. Antigenic analysis of hematopoiesis: VI. Flow cytometric characterization of My-10-positive progenitor cells in normal human bone marrow. *Exp Hematol* 1987;15:10–17.
1331. Soligo D, Delia D, Oriani A, et al. Identification of CD34$^+$ cells in normal and pathological bone marrow biopsies by QBEND10 monoclonal antibody. *Leukemia* 1991;5:1026–1030.
1332. Hanson CA, Ross CW, Schnitzer B. Anti-CD34 immunoperoxidase staining in paraffin sections of acute leukemia: comparison with flow cytometric immunophenotyping. *Hum Pathol* 1992;23:26–32.
1333. Leary AG, Ogawa M, Strauss LC, et al. Single cell origin of multilineage colonies in culture: evidence that differentiation of multipotent progenitors and restriction of proliferative potential of monopotent progenitors are stochastic processes. *J Clin Invest* 1984;74: 2193–2197.
1334. Leary AG, Strauss LC, Civin CI, et al. Disparate differentiation in hematopoietic colonies derived from human paired progenitors. *Blood* 1985;66:327–332.
1335. Strauss LC, Rowley SD, La Russa VF, et al. Antigenic analysis of hematopoiesis: V. Characterization of My-10 antigen expression by normal lymphohematopoietic progenitor cells. *Exp Hematol* 1986; 14:878–886.
1336. Lu L, Walker D, Broxmeyer HE, et al. Characterization of adult human marrow hematopoietic progenitors highly enriched by two-color cell sorting with MY10 and major histocompatibility class II monoclonal antibodies. *J Immunol* 1987;139:1823–1829.
1337. Briddell RA, Brandt JE, Straneva JE, et al. Characterization of the human burst-forming unit-megakaryocyte. *Blood* 1989;74:145–151.
1338. Berenson RJ, Andrews RG, Bensinger WI, et al. Antigen CD34$^+$ marrow cells engraft lethally irradiated baboons. *J Clin Invest* 1988; 81:951–955.
1339. Andrews RG, Bryant EM, Bartelmez SH, et al. CD34$^+$ marrow cells, devoid of T and B lymphocytes, reconstitute stable lymphopoiesis and myelopoiesis in lethally irradiated allogeneic baboons. *Blood* 1992;80:1693–1701.
1340. Berenson RJ, Bensinger WI, Hill RS, et al. Engraftment after infusion of CD34$^+$ marrow cells in patients with breast cancer or neuroblastoma. *Blood* 1991;77:1717–1722.
1341. Ryan D, Kossover S, Mitchell S, et al. Subpopulations of common acute lymphoblastic leukemia antigen-positive lymphoid cells in normal bone marrow identified by hematopoietic differentiation antigens. *Blood* 1986;68:417–425.
1342. Simmons PJ, Torok-Storb B. CD34 expression by stromal precursors in normal human adult bone marrow. *Blood* 1991;78:2848–2853.
1343. Huang S, Terstappen LW. Formation of haematopoietic microenvironment and haematopoietic stem cells from single human bone marrow stem cells. *Nature* 1992;360:745–749.
1344. Siena S, Bregni M, Brando B, et al. Flow cytometry for clinical estimation of circulating hematopoietic progenitors for autologous transplantation in cancer patients. *Blood* 1991;77:400–409.
1345. Siena S, Bregni M, Brando B, et al. Circulation of CD34$^+$ hematopoietic stem cells in the peripheral blood of high-dose cyclophosphamide-treated patients: enhancement by intravenous recombinant human granulocyte-macrophage colony-stimulating factor. *Blood* 1989;74:1904–1914.
1346. Emminger W, Fritsch G, Emminger SW, et al. Recovery kinetics after chemotherapy and circulating mononuclear cells expressing the CD34 antigen in pediatric cancer patients. *Blood* 1991;64:181–184.
1347. Beschorner WE, Civin CI, Strauss LC. Localization of hematopoietic progenitor cells in tissue with the anti-MY-10 monoclonal antibody. *Am J Pathol* 1985;119:1–4.
1348. Terstappen LW, Huang S, Picker LJ. Flow cytometric assessment of human T-cell differentiation in thymus and bone marrow. *Blood* 1992;79:666–677.
1349. Borowitz MJ, Gockerman JP, Moore JO, et al. Clinicopathologic and cytogenic features of CD34 (My10)-positive acute nonlymphocytic leukemia. *Am J Clin Pathol* 1989;91:265–270.
1350. Koike T, Aoki S, Maruyama S, et al. Cell surface phenotyping of megakaryoblasts. *Blood* 1987;69:957–960.
1351. Guyotat D, Campos L, Thomas X, et al. Myelodysplastic syndromes: a study of surface markers and in vitro growth patterns. *Am J Hematol* 1990;34:26–31.
1352. Borowitz MJ, Shuster JJ, Civin CI, et al. Prognostic significance of CD34 expression in childhood B-precursor acute lymphocytic leukemia: a Pediatric Oncology Group study. *J Clin Oncol* 1990;8: 1389–1398.
1353. Pui CH, Hancock ML, Head DR, et al. Clinical significance of CD34 expression in childhood acute lymphoblastic leukemia. *Blood* 1993; 82:889–894.
1354. Civin CI, Trischman TM, Fackler MJ, et al. Report on the CD34 cluster workshop. In: Knapp W, Dörken B, Gilks WR, et al, eds. *Leukocyte typing IV: white cell differentiation antigens.* New York: Oxford University Press, 1989:818–825.
1355. Rowley JD, Golomb H, Vardiman J. Non-random chromosome abnormalities in acute leukemic and dysmyelopoietic syndromes in patients with previously treated malignant disease. *Blood* 1981;58: 759–767.
1356. Koeffler HP. Preleukaemia. *Clin Haematol* 1986;15:829–850.
1357. Vaughan WP, Civin CI, Weisenburger DD, et al. Acute leukemia expressing the normal human hematopoietic stem cell membrane glycoprotein CD34 (MY10). *Leukemia* 1988;2:661–666.
1358. Geller RB, Zahurak M, Hurwitz CA, et al. Prognostic importance of immunophenotyping in adults with acute myelocytic leukemia: the significance of the stem cell glycoprotein CD34 (MY10). *Br J Haematol* 1990;76:340–347.
1359. Myint H, Lucie NP. The prognostic significance of the CD34 antigen in acute myeloid leukaemia. *Leuk Lymphoma* 1992;7:425–429.
1360. Kuzu I, Bicknell R, Harris AL, et al. Heterogeneity of vascular endothelial cells with relevance to diagnosis of vascular tumours. *J Clin Pathol* 1992;45:143–148.
1361. Sankey EA, More L, Dhillon AP. QBEnd/10: a new immunostain for the routine diagnosis of Kaposi's sarcoma. *J Pathol* 1990;161: 267–271.
1362. Nickoloff BJ. The human progenitor cell antigen (CD34) is localized on endothelial cells, dermal dendritic cells, and perifollicular cells

and stromal spindle-shaped cells in Kaposi's sarcoma. *Arch Dermatol* 1991;127:523–529.
1363. Cohen PR, Rapini RP, Farhood AI. Expression of the human hematopoietic progenitor cell antigen CD34 in vascular and spindle cell tumors. *J Cutan Pathol* 1993;20:15–20.
1364. Aziza J, Mazerolles C, Selves J, et al. Comparison of the reactivities of monoclonal antibodies QBEND10 (CD34) and BNH9 in vascular tumors. *Appl Immunohistochem* 1993;1:51–57.
1365. Traweek ST, Kandalaft PL, Mehta P, et al. The human hematopoietic progenitor cell antigen (CD34) in vascular neoplasia. *Am J Clin Pathol* 1991;96:25–31.
1366. Hanjan SNS, Kearney JF, Cooper MD. A monoclonal antibody (MMA) that identifies a differentiation antigen on human myelomonocytic cells. *Clin Immunol Immunopathol* 1982;23:172–188.
1367. Civin CI, Mirro J, Banquerigo ML. My-1, a new myeloid-specific antigen identified by a mouse monoclonal antibody. *Blood* 1981;57:842–845.
1368. Bernstein ID, Andrews RG, Cohen SF, et al. Normal and malignant human myelocytic and monocytic cells identified by monoclonal antibodies. *J Immunol* 1982;128:876–881.
1369. Majdic O, Liszka K, Dieter L, et al. Myeloid differentiation antigen defined by a monoclonal antibody. *Blood* 1981;58:1127–1133.
1370. Arber DA, Weiss LM. CD15: a review. *Appl Immunohistochem* 1993;1:17–30.
1371. Solter D, Knowles BB. Monoclonal antibody defining a stage-specific mouse embryonic antigen. (SSEA-1). *Proc Natl Acad Sci USA* 1978;75:5565–5569.
1372. Huang LC, Civin CI, Magnani JL, et al. My-1, the human myeloid-specific antigen detected by mouse monoclonal antibodies, is a sugar sequence found in lacto-N-fucopentaose III. *Blood* 1983;61:1020–1023.
1373. Urdal DL, Brentnall TA, Bernstein ID, et al. A granulocyte reactive monoclonal antibody, 1G10, identifies the Gal(1-4(Fuc(1-3)GlcNAc (X determinant) expressed in HL-60 cells on both glycolipid and glycoprotein molecules. *Blood* 1983;62:1022–1026.
1374. Hakomori S-I, Nudelman E, Kannagi R, et al. The common structure in fucosyllactosaminolipids accumulating in human adenocarcinomas, and its possible absence in normal tissue. *Biochem Biophys Res Commun* 1982;109:36–44.
1375. Kannagi R, Nudelman E, Levery SB, et al. A series of human erythrocyte glycosphingolipids reacting to the monoclonal antibody directed to a developmentally regulated antigen, SSEA-1. *J Biol Chem* 1982;257:14865–14874.
1376. Skubitz K, Balke J, Ball E, et al. Report on the CD15 cluster workshop. In: Knapp W, Dorken B, Gilks WR, et al, eds. *Leucocyte typing IV: white cell differentiation antigens.* New York: Oxford University Press, 1989:800–805.
1377. Kannagi R. CD15s workshop panel report. In: Kishimoto T, Kikutani H, von dem Borne AEGK, et al, eds. *Leukocyte typing VI: white cell differentiation antigens.* New York: Garland Publishing, 1998:352–355.
1378. Yang H-J, Hakomori S-I. A sphingolipid having a novel type of ceramide and lacto-N-fucopentaose III. *J Biol Chem* 1971;246:1192–1200.
1379. Strauss LC, Stuart RK, Civin CI. Antigenic analysis of hematopoiesis: I. Expression of the My-1 granulocyte surface antigen on human marrow cells and leukemic cell lines. *Blood* 1983;61:1222–1231.
1380. Hsu SM, Jaffe ES. LeuM1 and peanut agglutinin stain the neoplastic cells of Hodgkin's disease. *Am J Clin Pathol* 1984;82:29–32.
1381. Norton AJ, Isaacson PG. Granulocytic and HLA-D region specific monoclonal antibodies in the diagnosis of Hodgkin's disease. *J Clin Pathol* 1985;38:1241–1246.
1382. Hsu SM, Ho YS, Li PJ, et al. L & H variants of Reed-Sternberg cells express sialylated Leu M1 antigen. *Am J Pathol* 1986;122:199–203.
1383. Pinkus GS, Said JW. Leu-M1 immunoreactivity in non-hematopoietic neoplasms and myeloproliferative disorders: an immunoperoxidase study of paraffin sections. *Am J Clin Pathol* 1986;85:278–282.
1384. West KP, Warford A, Fray L, et al. The demonstration of B-cell, T-cell and myeloid antigens in paraffin sections. *J Pathol* 1986;150:89–101.
1385. Pinkus GS, Thomas P, Said JW. Leu-M1: a marker for Reed-Sternberg cells in Hodgkin's disease. An immunoperoxidase study of paraffin-embedded tissues. *Am J Pathol* 1985;119:244–252.
1386. Swerdlow SH, Wright SA. The spectrum of Leu-M1 staining in lymphoid and hematopoietic proliferations. *Am J Clin Pathol* 1986;85:283–288.
1387. Schienle HW, Stein H, Muller-Ruchholtz W. Neutrophil granulocytic cell antigen defined by a monoclonal antibody: its distribution within normal haemic and non-haemic tissue. *J Clin Pathol* 1982;35:959–966.
1388. Combs SG, Marder RJ, Minna JD, et al. Immunohistochemical localization of the immunodominant differentiation antigen lacto-N-fucopentaose III in normal adult and fetal tissues. *J Histochem Cytochem* 1984;32:982–988.
1389. Sheibani K, Battifora H, Burke JS, et al. Leu-M1 antigen in human neoplasms: an immunohistologic study of 400 cases. *Am J Surg Pathol* 1986;10:227–236.
1390. Sewell HF, Jaffray B, Thompson WD. Reaction of monoclonal anti Leu M1—a myelomonocytic marker (CD15)—with normal and neoplastic epithelia. *J Pathol* 1987;151:279–284.
1391. Holowiecki J, Lutz D, Krzemien S, et al. CD-15 antigen detected by the VIM-D5 monoclonal antibody for prediction of ability to achieve complete remission in acute non-lymphocytic leukemia. *Acta Haematol* 1986;76:16–19.
1392. Campos L, Guyotat D, Archimbaud E, et al. Surface marker expression in adult acute myeloid leukaemia: correlations with initial characteristics, morphology and response to therapy. *Br J Haematol* 1989;72:161–166.
1393. Davey FR, Olson S, Kurec AS, et al. The immunophenotyping of extramedullary myeloid cell tumors in paraffin-embedded tissue sections. *Am J Surg Pathol* 1988;12:699–707.
1394. van der Schoot CE, von dem Borne AEGKr, Tetteroo PAT. Characterization of myeloid leukemia by monoclonal antibodies, with an emphasis on antibodies against myeloperoxidase. *Acta Haematol* 1987;78:32–40.
1395. Ball ED, Schwarz LM, Bloomfield CD. Expression of the CD15 antigen on normal and leukemic myeloid cells: effects of neuraminidase and variable detection with a panel of monoclonal antibodies. *Mol Immunol* 1991;28:951–958.
1396. Weiner M, Borowitz, Boyett J, et al. Clinical pathologic aspects of myeloid antigen positivity in pediatric patients with acute lymphoblastic leukemia (ALL). *Proc Am Soc Clin Oncol* 1985;4:172.
1397. Pui C-H, Behm FG, Singh B, et al. Myeloid-associated antigen expression lacks prognostic value in childhood acute lymphoblastic leukemia treated with intensive multiagent chemotherapy. *Blood* 1990;75:198–202.
1398. Cantu-Rajnoldi A, Putti C, Saitta M, et al. Co-expression of myeloid antigens in childhood acute lymphoblastic leukaemia: relationship with the stage of differentiation and clinical significance. *Br J Haematol* 1991;79:40–43.
1399. Kornstein MJ, Bonner H, Gee B, et al. Leu M1 and S100 in Hodgkin's disease and non-Hodgkin's lymphomas. *Am J Clin Pathol* 1986;85:433–437.
1400. Frierson HF, Innes DJ. Sensitivity of anti-Leu M1 as a marker in Hodgkin's disease. *Arch Pathol Lab Med* 1985;109:1024–1028.
1401. Jack AS, Cunningham D, Soukop M, et al. Use of Leu M1 and antiepithelial membrane antigen monoclonal antibodies for diagnosing Hodgkin's disease. *J Clin Pathol* 1986;39:267–270.
1402. Warhol MJ, Pinkus GS, Said JW. Ultrastructural localization of Leu M1 in Reed-Sternberg cells and normal myeloid cells. *Hum Pathol* 1987;18:824–829.
1403. Hall PA, D'Ardenne AJ. Value of CD15 immunostaining in diagnosing Hodgkin's disease: a review of published literature. *J Clin Pathol* 1987;18:808–814.
1404. Oka K, Mori N, Kojima M. Anti-Leu-3a antibody reactivity with Reed-Sternberg cells of Hodgkin's disease. *Arch Pathol Lab Med* 1988;112:139–142.
1405. Fellbaum C, Hansmann M-L, Parwaresch MR, et al. Monoclonal antibodies Ki-B3 and Leu-M1 discriminate giant cells of infectious mononucleosis and of Hodgkin's disease. *Hum Pathol* 1988;19:1168–1173.
1406. De Mascarel I, Trojani M, Eghbali H, et al. Prognostic value of phenotyping by Ber-H2, Leu-M1, EMA in Hodgkin's disease. *Arch Pathol Lab Med* 1990;114:953–955.
1407. Della Croce DR, Imam A, Brynes RK, et al. Anti-BLA.36 monoclonal antibody shows reactivity with Hodgkin's cells and B lympho-

cytes in frozen and paraffin-embedded tissues. *Hematol Oncol* 1991; 9:103–114.
1408. Stein H, Uchanska-Ziegler B, Gerdes J, et al. Hodgkin and Sternberg-Reed cells contain antigens specific to late cells of granulopoiesis. *Int J Cancer* 1982;29:283–290.
1409. Stein H, Gerdes J, Schwab U, et al. Identification of Hodgkin and Sternberg-Reed cells as a unique cell type derived from a newly-detected small-cell population. *Int J Cancer* 1982;30:445–459.
1410. Hyder DM, Schnitzer B. Utility of Leu M1 monoclonal antibody in the differential diagnosis of Hodgkin's disease. *Arch Pathol Lab Med* 1986;110:416–419.
1411. Stein H, Hansmann M-L, Lennert K, et al. Reed-Sternberg and Hodgkin's cells in lymphocyte-predominant Hodgkin's disease of nodular subtype contain J chain. *Am J Clin Pathol* 1986;86:292–297.
1412. Wieczorek R, Burke JS, Knowles DM. Leu-M1 antigen expression in T-cell neoplasia. *Am J Pathol* 1985;121:374–380.
1413. Meis JM, Osborne BM, Butler JJ. A comparative marker study of large cell lymphoma, Hodgkin's disease, and true histiocytic lymphoma in paraffin-embedded tissue. *Am J Clin Pathol* 1986;86: 591–599.
1414. Caveriviere P, Mallem O, Al Saati T, et al. Reed-Sternberg-like cells in Richter's syndrome express granulocytic associated antigen (Leu-M1). *Am J Clin Pathol* 1986;85:755–756.
1415. De Mascarel A, Coindre JM, De Mascarel I, et al. Leu-M1 antigen expression in acute leukaemias. *J Pathol* 1987;153:225–232.
1416. Kubic VL, Brunning RD. Immunohistochemical evaluation of neoplasms in bone marrow biopsies using monoclonal antibodies reactive in paraffin-embedded tissue. *Mod Pathol* 1989;2:618–629.
1417. Wieczorek R, Suhrland M, Ramsay D, et al. Leu-M1 antigen expression in advanced (tumor) stage mycosis fungoides. *Am J Clin Pathol* 1986; 86:25–32.
1418. Rosso R, Paulli M, Magrini U, et al. Anaplastic large cell lymphoma: CD30/Ki-1 positive, expressing the CD15/Leu-M1 antigen. Immunohistochemical and morphologic relationships to Hodgkin's disease. *Virchows Arch* 1990;416:229–235.
1419. Greer JP, Kinney MC, Collins RD, et al. Clinical features of 31 patients with Ki-1 anaplastic large-cell lymphoma. *J Clin Oncol* 1991;9:539–547.
1420. Wick MR, Swanson PE, Manivel JC. Immunohistochemical findings in tumors of the skin. In: DeLellis RA, ed. *Advances in immunohistochemistry.* New York: Raven Press, 1988:395–430.
1421. Parham DM, Morton K, Coghill G, et al. Expression of CD15 antigen in urinary bladder transitional cell carcinoma. *J Clin Pathol* 1990; 43:541–543.
1422. Schwab U, Stein H, Gerdes J, et al. Production of a monoclonal antibody specific for Hodgkin and Sternberg-Reed cells of Hodgkin's disease and a subset of normal lymphoid cells. *Nature* 1982; 299:65–67.
1423. Schwarting R, Gerdes J, Dürkop H, et al. Ber-H2: a new anti-Ki-1 (CD30) monoclonal antibody directed at a formol-resistant epitope. *Blood* 1989; 74:1678–1689.
1424. Schwarting R, Stein H. Cluster report: CD30. In: Knapp W, Dorken B, Gilks WR, et al, eds. *Leukocyte typing IV: white cell differentiation antigens.* New York: Oxford University Press, 1989:419–422.
1425. Davey FR, Elghetany MT, Kurec AS. Immunophenotyping of hematologic neoplasms in paraffin-embedded tissue sections. *Am J Clin Pathol* 1990;93[Suppl 1]:S17–S26.
1426. Chang KL, Arber DA, Weiss LM. CD30: a review. *Appl Immunohistochem* 1993:1:244–255.
1427. Fonatsch C , Diehl V, Dürkop H, et al. Assignment of the human CD30 (Ki-1) gene to 1p36. *Genomics* 1992;14:825–826.
1428. Fonatsch C, Diehl V, Schaadt M, et al. Cytogenetic investigations in Hodgkin's disease: I. Involvement of specific chromosomes in marker formation. *Cancer Genet Cytogenet* 1986;20:39–52.
1429. van den Berghe E, de Wolf-Peeters C, Louwagie A, et al. Chromosome 1p abnormalities in B non-Hodgkin's lymphoma. *Leuk Lymphoma* 1991;5:193–199.
1430. Kemper O, Derré J, Cherif D, et al. The gene for the type II (p75) tumor necrosis factor receptor (TNF-RII) is localized on band 1p36.2-p36.3. *Hum Genet* 1991;87:623–624.
1431. Lawrence JB, Villnave CA, Singer RH. Sensitive, high-resolution chromatin and chromosome mapping in situ: presence and orientation of two closely integrated copies of EBV in a lymphoma line. *Cell* 1988;52:51–61.
1432. Dürkop H, Latza U, Hummel M, et al. Molecular cloning and expression of a new member of the nerve growth factor receptor family that is characteristic for Hodgkin's disease. *Cell* 1992;68:421–427.
1433. Mallett S, Barclay AN. A new superfamily of cell surface proteins related to the nerve growth factor receptor. *Immunol Today* 1991; 12:220–223.
1434. Hansen H, Lemke H, Bredfeldt G, et al. The Hodgkin-associated Ki-1 antigen exists in an intracellular and a membrane-bound form. *Biol Chem Hoppe Seyler* 1989;370:409–416.
1435. Rohde D, Hansen H, Hafner M, et al. Cellular localizations and processing of the two molecular forms of the Hodgkin-associated Ki-1 (CD30) antigen: the protein kinase Ki-1/57 occurs in the nucleus. *Am J Pathol* 1992;140:473–482.
1436. Hansen H, Bredfeldt G, Havsteen B, et al. Protein kinase activity of the intracellular but not of the membrane-associated form of the Ki-1 antigen (CD30). *Res Immunol* 1990;141:13–31.
1437. Froese P, Lemke H, Gerdes J, et al. Biochemical characterization and biosynthesis of the Ki-1 antigen in Hodgkin-derived and virus-transformed human B and T lymphoid cell lines. *J Immunol* 1987; 139:2081–2087.
1438. Berenbeck C, Schroeder J, da Costa L, et al. Detection of soluble Hodgkin-associated CD30 antigen in the sera of patients with Hodgkin's lymphoma. In: Knapp W, Dorken B, Gilks WR, eds. *Leucocyte typing IV: white cell differentiation antigens.* New York: Oxford University Press, 1989:425.
1439. Josimovic-Alasevic O, Dürkop H, Schwarting R, et al. Ki-1 (CD30) antigen is released by Ki-1-positive tumor cells in vitro and in vivo: I. Partial characterization of soluble Ki-1 antigen and detection of the antigen in cell culture supernatants and in serum by an enzyme-linked immunosorbent assay. *Eur J Immunol* 1989;19:157–162.
1440. Gause A, Pohl C, Tschiersch A, et al. Clinical significance of soluble CD30 antigen in the sera of patients with untreated Hodgkin's disease. *Blood* 1991;77:1983–1988.
1441. Fattovich G, Vinante F, Guistina G, et al. Serum levels of soluble CD30 in chronic hepatitis B virus infection. *Clin Exp Immunol* 1996; 103:105–110.
1442. Dürkop H, Latza U, Stein H. Overview of CD30. In: Schlossman SF, Boumsell L, Gilks WR, et al, eds. *Leukocyte typing V: white cell differentiation antigens.* New York: Oxford University Press, 1995:1115–1116.
1443. Smith CA, Gruss H-J, Davis T, et al. CD30 antigen, a marker for Hodgkin's lymphoma, is a receptor whose ligand defines an emerging family of cytokines with homology to TNF. *Cell* 1993;73: 1349–1360.
1444. Armitage RJ. CD153 (CD30 ligand) workshop panel report. In: Kishimoto T, Kikutani H, von dem Borne AEGK, et al, eds. *Leukocyte typing VI: white cell differentiation antigens.* New York: Garland Publishing, 1998:98–100.
1445. Gedrich RW, Gilfillan MC, Duckett CS, et al. CD30 contains two binding sites with different specificities for members of the tumor necrosis factor receptor-associated factor family of signal transducing proteins. *J Biol Chem* 1996;271:12852–12858.
1446. Lee SY, Park CG, Choi Y. T cell receptor-dependent cell death of T cell hybridomas mediated by the CD30 cytoplasmic domain in association with tumor necrosis factor receptor-associated factors. *J Exp Med* 1996;183:669–674.
1447. Amakawa R, Hakem A, Kundig TM, et al. Impaired negative selection of T cells in Hodgkin's disease antigen CD30-deficient mice. *Cell* 1996;84:551–562.
1448. Andreesen R, Osterholz J, Lohr GW, et al. The Hodgkin cell specific antigen is expressed on a subset of auto-and alloactivated T (helper) lymphoblasts. *Blood* 1984;63:1299–1302.
1449. Stein H, Mason DY, Gerdes J, et al. The expression of the Hodgkin's disease associated antigen Ki-1 in reactive and neoplastic lymphoid tissues: evidence that Reed-Sternberg cells and histiocytic malignancies are derived from activated lymphoid cells. *Blood* 1985;66: 848–858.
1450. Chadburn A, Inghirami G, Knowles DM. The kinetics and temporal expression of T-cell activation-associated antigens CD15 (LeuM1), CD30 (Ki-1), EMA and CD11c (LeuM5) by benign activated T cells. *Hematol Pathol* 1992;6:193–202.
1451. Gerdes J, Schwarting R, Stein H. High proliferative activity of Reed Sternberg associated antigen Ki-1 positive cells in normal lymphoid tissue. *J Clin Pathol* 1986;39:993–997.

1452. Abbondanzo SL, Sato N, Straus SE, et al. Acute infectious mononucleosis. CD30 (Ki-1) antigen expression and histologic correlations. *Am J Clin Pathol* 1990;93:698–702.
1453. Andreesen R, Brugger W, Löhr GW, et al. Human macrophages can express the Hodgkin's cell-associated antigen Ki-1 (CD30). *Am J Pathol* 1989;134:187–192.
1454. Epstein ML, Windebank KP, Burt AD, et al. CD30 expression by peripheral blood monocytes and hepatic macrophages in a child with miliary tuberculosis. *J Clin Pathol* 1992;45:638–639.
1455. Herlin T, Pallesen G, Kristensen T, et al. Unusual immunophenotype displayed by histiocytes in haemophagocytic lymphohistiocytosis. *J Clin Pathol* 1987;40:1413–1417.
1456. Van der Valk P, Mullink H, Huijgens PC, et al. Immunohistochemistry in bone marrow diagnosis: value of a panel of monoclonal antibodies on routinely processed bone marrow biopsies. *Am J Surg Pathol* 1989;13:97–106.
1457. Ree HJ, Neiman RS, Martin AW, et al. Paraffin section markers for Reed-Sternberg cells: a comparative study of peanut agglutinin, Leu-M1, LN-2, and Ber-H2. *Cancer* 1989;63:2030–2036.
1458. Miettinen M. CD30 distribution: immunohistochemical study on formaldehyde-fixed, paraffin-embedded Hodgkin's and non-Hodgkin's lymphomas. *Arch Pathol Lab Med* 1992;116:1197–1201.
1459. Kinney MC, Greer JP, Glick AD, et al. Anaplastic large-cell Ki-1 malignant lymphomas: recognition, biological and clinical implications. *Pathol Annu* 1991;26:1–24.
1460. Nador RG, Cesarman E, Chadburn A, et al. Primary effusion lymphoma: a distinct clinicopathologic entity associated with the Kaposi's sarcoma-associated herpesvirus. *Blood* 1996;88:645–656.
1461. Piris M, Gatter KC, Mason DY. CD30 expression in follicular lymphoma. *Histopathology* 1990;18:25–29.
1462. Piris M, Brown DC, Gatter KC, et al. CD30 expression in non-Hodgkin's lymphoma. *Histopathology* 1990;17:211–218.
1463. Kaudewitz P, Stein H, Burg G, et al. Atypical cells in lymphomatoid papulosis express the Hodgkin cell-associated antigen Ki-1. *J Invest Dermatol* 1986;86:350–354.
1464. Möller P, Matthaei-Maurer DU, Moldenhauer G. CD30 (Ki-1) antigen expression in a subset of gastric mucosal plasma cells and in a primary gastric plasmacytoma. *Am J Clin Pathol* 1989;91:18–23.
1465. Pallesen G, Hamilton-Dutoit SJ. Ki-1 (CD30) antigen is regularly expressed by tumor cells of embryonal carcinoma. *Am J Pathol* 1988; 133:446–450.
1466. Stross WP, Flavell DJ, Gatter KC, et al. Monoclonal antibody Leu22 [Letter]. *Am J Clin Pathol* 1990;93:299.
1467. Stross WP, Warnke RA, Flavell DJ, et al. Molecule detected in formalin fixed tissue by antibodies MT1, DF-T1, and L60 (Leu-22) corresponds to CD43 antigen. *J Clin Pathol* 1989;42:953–961.
1468. Stoll M, Dalchau R, Schmidt R. Cluster report: CD43. In: Knapp W, Dorken G, Gilks WR, et al, eds. *Leucocyte typing IV: white cell differentiation antigens.* Oxford: Oxford University Press, 1989: 604–608.
1469. Remold-O'Donnell E. CD43 cluster report. In: Schlossman SF, Boumsell L, Gilks WR, et al, eds. *Leukocyte typing V: white cell differentiation antigens.* New York: Oxford University Press, 1995; 1697–1701.
1470. Horejsi V, Stockinger H. CD43 workshop panel report. In: Kishimoto T, Kikutani H, von dem Borne AEGK, et al, eds. *Leukocyte typing VI: white cell differentiation antigens.* New York: Garland Publishing, 1998:494–497.
1471. Arber DA, Weiss LM. CD43: a review. *Appl Immunohistochem* 1993;1:88–96.
1472. Said JW, Stoll PN, Shintaku P, et al. Leu-22: a preferential marker for T-lymphocytes in paraffin sections. *Am J Clin Pathol* 1989;91: 542–549.
1473. Remold-O'Donnell E, Kenney DM, Parkman R, et al. Characterization of a human lymphocyte surface sialoglycoprotein that is defective in Wiskott-Aldrich syndrome. *J Exp Med* 1984;159:1705–1723.
1474. Piller F, Le Deist F, Weinberg KI, et al. Altered O-glycan synthesis in lymphocytes from patients with Wiskott-Aldrich syndrome. *J Exp Med* 1991;173:1501–1510.
1475. Pallant A, Eskenazi A, Mattei M-G, et al. Characterization of cDNAs encoding human leukosialin and localization of the leukosialin gene to chromosome 16. *Proc Natl Acad Sci USA* 1989;86:1328–1332.
1476. Shelley CS, Remold-O'Donnell E, David AE III, et al. Molecular characterization of sialoglycoprotein (CD43), the lymphocyte surface sialoglycoprotein defective in Wiskott-Aldrich syndrome. *Proc Natl Acad Sci USA* 1989;86:2819–2823.
1477. Gahmberg CG, Autero M, Hermonen J. Major O-glycosylated sialoglycoproteins of human hematopoietic cells: differentiation antigens with poorly understood functions. *J Cell Biochem* 1988;37:91–105.
1478. Bierer BE, Peterson A, Park J, et al. T-cell activation: the T-cell erythrocyte receptor (CD2) and sialophorin (CD43). *Immunol Allergy Clin North Am* 1988;8:51–67.
1479. Piller V, Piller F, Fukuda M. Phosphorylation of the major leukocyte surface sialoglycoprotein, leukosialin, is increased by phorbol 12-myristate 13-acetate. *J Biol Chem* 1989;264:18824–18831.
1480. Carlsson SR, Sasaki H, Fukuda M. Structural variations of O-linked oligosaccharides present in leukosialin isolated from erythroid, myeloid, and T-lymphoid cell lines. *J Biol Chem* 1986;261: 12787–12795.
1481. Remold-O'Donnell E, Zimmerman C, Kenney D, et al. Expression on blood cells of sialophorin, the surface glycoprotein that is defective in Wiskott-Aldrich syndrome. *Blood* 1987;70:104–109.
1482. Remold-O'Donnell E, Kenney D, Rosen FS. Biosynthesis of human sialophorins and analysis of the polypeptide core. *Biochemistry* 1987; 26:3908–3913.
1483. Bazil V, Strominger L. CD43, the major sialoglycoprotein of human leukocytes, is proteolytically cleaved from the surface of stimulated lymphocytes and granulocytes. *Proc Natl Acad Sci USA* 1993;90: 3792–3796.
1484. Schmid K, Hediger MA, Brossmer R, et al. Amino acid sequence of human plasma galactoglycoprotein: identity with the extracellular reigon of CD43 (sialophorin). *Proc Natl Acad Sci USA* 1992;89: 663–667.
1485. Sperling AI, Green JM, Mosley RL, et al. CD43 is a murine T cell costimulatory receptor that functions independently of CD28. *J Exp Med* 1995;182:139–146.
1486. Alvarado M, Klassen C, Cerny J, et al. MEM-59 monoclonal antibody detects a CD43 epitope involved in lymphocyte activation. *Eur J Immunol* 1995;25:1051–1055.
1487. Ardman B, Sikorski MA, Staunton DE. CD43 interferes with T-lymphocyte adhesion. *Proc Natl Acad Sci USA* 1992;89:5001–5005.
1488. Manjunath N, Johnson RS, Staunton DE, et al. Targeted disruption of CD43 gene enhances T lymphocyte adhesion. *J Immunol* 1993; 151:1528–1534.
1489. Manjunath N, Correa M, Ardman M, et al. Negative regulation of T-cell adhesion and activation by CD43. *Nature* 1995;377:535–538.
1490. Nathan C, Xie QW, Halbwachs-Mecarelli L, et al. Albumin inhibits neutrophil spreading and hydrogen peroxide release by blocking the shedding of CD43 (sialophorin, leukosialin). *J Cell Biol* 1993;122: 243–256.
1491. Mentzer SJ, Remold-O'Donnell E, Crimmins MAV, et al. Sialophorin, a surface sialoglycoprotein defective in the Wiskott-Aldrich syndrome, is involved in human T lymphocyte proliferation. *J Exp Med* 1987;165:1383–1392.
1492. Nong Y-H, Remold-O'Donnell E, LeBien TW, et al. A monoclonal antibody to sialophorin (CD43) induces homotypic adhesion and activation of human monocytes. *J Exp Med* 1989;170:259–267.
1493. Vargas-Cortes M, Axelsson B, Larsson A, et al. Enchancement of human spontaneous cell-mediated cytotoxicity by a monoclonal antibody against the large sialoglycoprotein (CD43) on peripheral blood lymphocytes. *Scand J Immunol* 1988;27:661–671.
1494. de Smet W, Walter H, de Baetselier P. Workshop adhesion structure subpanel 9 (CD43) mAb define at least four different epitopes on human leukosialin. In: Schlossman SF, Boumsell L, Gilks WR, et al, eds. *Leukocyte typing V: white cell differentiation antigens.* New York: Oxford University Press, 1995:1706–1707.
1495. Remold-O'Donnell E, Rosen FS. Sialophorin (CD43) and the Wiskott-Aldrich syndrome. *Immunodeficiency Rev* 1990;2:151–174.
1496. Bettaieb A, Farace F, Mitjavila MT, et al. Use of a monoclonal antibody (GA3) to demonstrate lineage restricted O-glycosylation on leukosialin during terminal erythroid differentiation. *Blood* 1988; 71:1226–1233.
1497. Gunji Y, Nakamura M, Hagiwara T, et al. Expression and function of adhesion molecules on human hematopoietic stem cells: $CD34^+$ LFA-1-cells are more primitive than $CD34^+$ $LFA\text{-}1^+$ cells. *Blood* 1992;80:429–436.
1498. Wiken M, Bjork P, Axelsson B, et al. Studies on the role of CD43

in human B-cell activation and differentiation. *Scand J Immunol* 1989;29:353–361.
1499. Facchetti F, de Wolf-Peeters C, Mason DY, et al. Plasmacytoid T cells: immunohistochemical evidence for their monocyte/macrophage origin. *Am J Pathol* 1988;133:15–21.
1500. Fellbaum C, Hansmann M-L. Immunohistochemical differential diagnosis of granulocytic sarcomas and malignant lymphomas on formalin-fixed material. *Virchows Arch* 1990;416:351–355.
1501. Segal GH, Stoler MH, Tubbs RR. The "CD43 only" phenotype: an aberrant, nonspecific immunophenotype requiring comprehensive analysis for lineage resolution. *Am J Clin Pathol* 1992;97:861–865.
1502. Contos MJ, Kornstein MJ, Innes DJ, et al. The utility of CD20 and CD43 in subclassification of low-grade B-cell lymphoma on paraffin sections. *Mod Pathol* 1992;5:631–633.
1503. Ngan BY, Picker LJ, Medeiros LJ, et al. Immunophenotypic diagnosis of non-Hodgkin's lymphoma in paraffin sections. *Am J Clin Pathol* 1989;91:579
1504. Aisenberg AC, Wilkes B. Unusual human lymphoma phenotype defined by monoclonal antibody. *J Exp Med* 1980;152:1126–1131.
1505. Goding JW, Burns GF. Monoclonal antibody OKT-9 recognizes the receptor for transferrin on human acute lymphoctyic leukemia cells. *J Immunol* 1981:127:1256–1258.
1506. Sutherland R, Della D, Schneider C, et al. Ubiquitous, cell surface glycoprotein on tumor cells is proliferation-associated receptor for transferrin. *Proc Natl Acad Sci USA* 1981;78:4515–4519.
1507. Newman R, Schneider C, Sutherland R, et al. The transferrin receptor. *Trends Biochem* Sci 1982;1:397.
1508. Schwarting R, Stein H. Cluster report: CD71. In: Knapp W, Dorken B, Gilks WR, et al, eds. *Leucocyte typing IV: white cell differentiation antigens.* New York: Oxford University Press, 1989:455–460.
1509. Trowbridge IS. Overview of CD71. In: Schlossman SF, Boumsell L, Gilks WR, et al, eds. *Leukocyte typing V: white cell differentiation antigens.* New York: Oxford University Press, 1995;1139–1141.
1510. Goding JW, Dubljevic V, Sali A. CD71 workshop panel report. In: Kishimoto T, Kikutani H, von dem Borne AEGK, et al, eds. *Leukocyte typing VI: white cell differentiation antigens.* New York: Garland Publishing, 1998:524–529.
1511. Trowbridge IS, Collawn JF, Hopkins CR. Signal-dependent membrane protein trafficking in the endocytic pathway. *Annu Rev Cell Biol* 1993;9:129–161.
1512. Casey JL, Hentze MW, Koeller DM, et al. Iron-responsive elements: regulatory RNA sequences that control mRNA levels and translation. *Science* 1988;240:924–928.
1513. Friden PM, Walus LR, Musso GF, et al. Anti-transferrin receptor antibody and antibody-drug conjugates cross the blood brain barrier. *Proc Natl Acad Sci USA* 1991;88:4771–4775.
1514. Friden PM, Walus LR, Watson P, et al. Blood-brain barrier penetration and in vivo activity of an NGF conjugate. *Science* 1993;259: 373–377.
1515. Batra J, Jinno Y, Chaudhary VK, et al. Cytoxic activity of a recombinant fusion protein between interleukin 4 and Pseudomonas exotoxin. *Proc Natl Acad Sci USA* 1989;86:8545–8549.
1516. Kohgo Y, Niitsu Y, Kondo H, et al. Serum transferrin receptor as a new index of erythropoiesis. *Blood* 1987;70:1955–1958.
1517. Cook JD, Skikne BS, Baynes RD. Serum transferrin receptor. *Annu Rev Med* 1993;44:63–74.
1518. Judd W, Poodry CA, Strominger JL. Novel surface antigen expressed on dividing cells but absent from nondividing cells. *J Exp Med* 1980; 152:1430–1435.
1519. Omary MB, Trobridge IS, Minowada J. Human cell-surface glycoprotein with unusual properties. *Nature* 1980;286:888–891.
1520. Trowbridge IS, Omary MB. Human cell surface glycoprotein related to cell proliferation is the receptor for transferrin. *Proc Natl Acad Sci USA* 1981;78:3039–3043.
1521. Pileri S, Gobbi M, Rivano MT, et al. Immunohistological study of transferrin receptor expression in non-Hodgkin's lymphoma. *Br J Haematol* 1984;58:501–508.
1522. Habeshaw JA, Lister TA, Greaves MF. Correlation of transferrin receptor expression with histologic class and outcome in non-Hodgkin's lymphoma. *Lancet* 1983;i:498–500.
1523. Kersey JH, LeBien TW, Abramson CS, et al. p24: A human leukemia-associated and lymphohemopoeitic progenitor cell surface structure identified with monoclonal antibody. *J Exp Med* 1981;153: 726–731.
1524. Jones NH, Borowitz MJ, Metzgar RS. Characterization and distribution of a 24,000 molecular weight antigen defined by a monoclonal antibody (DU-ALL-1) elicited to common acute lymphoblastic leukemia (cALL) cells. *Leuk Res* 1982;6:449–464.
1525. Horton MA, Hogg N. Platelet antigens: new and previously defined clusters. In: McMichael AJ, Beverley PCL, Cobbold S, et al, eds. *Leukocyte typing III: white cell differentiation antigens.* Oxford: Oxford University Press, 1987:733–746.
1526. von dem Borne AEGK, Modderman PW. Cluster report: CD9. In: Knapp W, Dörken B, Gilks WR, et al, eds. *Leukocyte typing IV: white cell differentiation antigens.* New York: Oxford University Press, 1989;989–990.
1527. Jennings LK, Crossno Jr JT, White MM. CD9 cluster workshop report: cell surface binding and functional analysis. In: Schlossman SF, Boumsell L, Gilks WR, et al, eds. *Leukocyte typing V: white cell differentiation antigens.* New York: Oxford University Press, 1995;1249–1251.
1528. de Haas, von dem Borne AEGK. CD9 workshop panel report. In: Kishimoto T, Kikutani H, von dem Borne AEGK, et al, eds. *Leukocyte typing VI: white cell differentiation antigens.* New York: Garland Publishing, 1998:629–631.
1529. Wright MD, Tomlinson MG. The ins and outs of the transmembrane 4 superfamily. *Immunol Today* 1994;15:588–594.
1530. Katz F, Povey S, Parkar M, et al. Chromosome assignment of monoclonal antibody-defined determinants on human leukemic cells. *Eur J Immunol* 1983;13:1008–1013.
1531. Hercend T, Nadler LM, Pesando JM, et al. Expression of a 26,000-dalton glycoprotein on activated human T cells. *Cell Immunol* 1981; 64:192–199.
1532. Ash RC, Jansen J, Kersey JH, et al. Normal human pluripotential and committed hematopoietic progenitors do not express the p24 antigen detected by monoclonal antibody BA-2: implication for immunotherapy of lymphocytic leukemia. *Blood* 1982;60:1310–1316.
1533. Flug F, Dodson L, Wolff J, et al. B-lymphocyte associated differentiation antigen expression by "non-B, non-T" acute lymphoblastic leukemia. *Leuk Res* 1985;9:1051–1058.
1534. San Miguel JF, Caballero MD, Gonzalez M, et al. Immunological phenotype of neoplasms involving the B cell in the last step of differentiation. *Br J Haematol* 1986;62:75–83.
1535. Ashman LK, White D, Zola H, et al. Expression of the non-T ALL-associated p24 antigen on leukaemic blasts from patients with ANLL. *Leuk Res* 1987;11:97–101.
1536. Komada Y, Peiper SC, Melvin SL, et al. A monoclonal antibody (SJ-9A4) to P24 present on common ALLs, neuroblastomas and platelets: I. Characterization and development of a unique radioimmunometric assay. *Leuk Res* 1983;7:487–498.
1537. Marx JL. The trials of conducting AIDS drug trials. *Science* 1988; 244:916–918.
1538. Rose DSC, Maddox PH, Brown DC. Which proliferation markers for routine immunohistology? A comparison of five antibodies. *J Clin Pathol* 1994;47:1010–1014.
1539. Gerdes J, Schwab U, Lemke H, et al. Production of a monoclonal antibody reactive with a human nuclear antigen associated with cell proliferation. *Int J Cancer* 1983;31:13–20.
1540. Gerdes J, Li L, Schlueter C, et al. Immunohistochemical and molecular biologic characterization of the cell proliferation-associated nuclear antigen that is defined by monoclonal antibody Ki-67. *Am J Pathol* 1991;138:867–873.
1541. Fonatsch C, Duchrow M, Rieder H, et al. Assignment of the human Ki-67 gene (MKI-67) to 10q25-qter. *Genomics* 1991;11:476–477.
1542. Gerdes J, Lemke H, Baisch H, et al. Cell cycle analysis of a cell proliferation-associated human nuclear antigen defined by the monoclonal antibody Ki-67. *J Immunol* 1984;133:1710–1715.
1543. Lopez F, Belloc F, Lacombe F, et al. Modalities of synthesis of Ki-67 antigen during the stimulation of lymphocytes. *Cytometry* 1991; 12:42–49.
1544. Bruno S, Dazynkiewicz Z. Cell cycle dependent expression and stability of the nuclear antigen detected by Ki-67 antibody in HL-60 cells. *Cell Prolif* 1992;25:31–40.
1545. Verheijen R, Kuijpers HJH, Schlingemann RO, et al. Ki-67 detects a nuclear matrix-associated proliferation-related antigen: I. Intracellular localization during interphase. *J Cell Sci* 1989;92:123–130.
1546. Verheijen R, Kuijpers HJH, Van Driel R, et al. Ki-67 detects a nuclear matrix-associated proliferation-related antigen: localization in

mitotic cells and association with chromosomes. *J Cell Sci* 1989; 92:531–540.

1547. Gerdes J, Duchrow M, Schlueter C, et al. Molecular cloning of the human Ki-67 gene (MKI-67). *Anal Cell Pathol* 1992;4:159.
1548. Sawhney N, Hall PA. Ki-67 structure, function and new antibodies. *J Clin Pathol* 1992;168:161–162.
1549. Schwarting R, Gerdes J, Niehus J, et al. Determination of the growth fraction in cell suspensions by flow cytometry using the monoclonal antibody Ki-67. *J Immunol Methods* 1986;90:65–70.
1550. Cattoretti G, Becker MHG, Key G, et al. Monoclonal antibodies against recombinant parts of the Ki-67 antigen (MIB 1 and MIB 3) detect proliferating cells in microwave-processed formalin-fixed paraffin sections. *J Pathol* 1992;168:357–363.
1551. Key G, Becker MHG, Duchrow M, et al. New Ki-67 equivalent murine monoclonal antibodies (MIB1-3) prepared against recombinant parts of the Ki-67 antigen. *Anal Cell Pathol* 1992;4:181.
1552. Key G, Petersen JL, Becker MHG, et al. New antiserum against Ki-67 antigen suitable for double immunostaining of paraffin wax sections. *J Clin Pathol* 1993;46:1080–1084.
1553. Reynolds GM, Rowlands DC, Mead GP. Detection of Ki-67 antigen by a new sheep polyclonal antiserum. *J Clin Pathol* 1995;48: 1138–1140.
1554. Scott RJ, Hall PA, Haldane JS, et al. A comparison of immunohistochemical markers of cell proliferation with experimentally determined growth fraction. *J Pathol* 1991;165:173-178.
1555. Brown DC, Gatter KC. Monoclonal antibody Ki-67: its use in histopathology. *Histopathology* 1990;17:489–523.
1556. Garrido MC, Cordell JL, Becker MHG, et al. Monoclonal antibody JC1: new reagent for studying cell proliferation. *J Clin Pathol* 1992; 45:860–865.
1557. Hall PA, Levison DA, Woods AL, et al. Proliferating cell nuclear antigen (PCNA) immunolocalization in paraffin sections: an index of cell proliferation with evidence of deregulated expression in some neoplasms. *J Pathol* 1990;162:285–294.
1558. Ogata K, Kurki P, Celis JE, et al. Monoclonal antibodies to a nuclear protein (PCNA/cyclin) associated with DNA replication. *Exp Cell Res* 1987;168:475–486.
1559. Bravo R, Frank R, Blundell PA, et al. Cyclin/PCNA is the auxillary protein of DNA polymerase δ. *Nature* 1987;326:515–517.
1560. Prelich G, Tan C-K, Kostura M, et al. Functional identity of proliferating cell nuclear antigen and a DNA polymerase δ auxillary protein. *Nature* 1987;326:517–520.
1561. Diebold J, Dopfer K, Lai M, et al. Comparison of different monoclonal antibodies for the immunohistochemical assessment of cell proliferation in routine colorectal biopsy specimens. *Scand J Gastroenterol* 1994;29:47–53.
1562. Lynch DAF, Clarke AMT, Jackson P, et al. Comparison of labelling by bromodeoxyuridine, MIB 1, and proliferating cell nuclear antigen in gastric mucosal biopsy specimens. *J Clin Pathol* 1994;47: 122–125.
1563. Gatter KC, Dunnill MS, Gerdes J, et al. New approach to assessing lung tumours in man. *J Clin Pathol* 1986;39:590–593.
1564. Gerdes J, Lelle RJ, Pickartz H, et al. Growth fractions in breast cancers determined in situ with monoclonal antibody Ki-67. *J Clin Pathol* 1986;39:977–980.
1565. Burger PC, Shibata T, Kleihues P. The use of the monoclonal antibody Ki-67 in the identification of proliferating cells: application to neuropathology. *Am J Surg Pathol* 1986;10:611–617.
1566. Barnard NJ, Hall PA, Lemoine NR, et al. Proliferative index in breast carcinoma determined in situ by Ki-67 immunostaining and its relationship to pathological and clinical variables. *J Pathol* 1987;152: 287–295.
1567. Locker AP, Birrell K, Bell JA, et al. Ki-67 immunoreactivity in breast carcinoma: relationships to prognostic variables and short term survival. *Eur J Surg Oncol* 1992;18:224–229.
1568. Michie BA, Black C, Reid RP, et al. Image analysis derived ploidy and proliferation indices in soft tissue sarcomas: comparison with clinical outcome. *J Clin Pathol* 1994;47:443–447.
1569. Kruger S, Muller H. Correlation of morphometry, nucleolar organizing regions, proliferating cell nuclear antigen and Ki-67 antigen expression with grading and staging in urinary bladder carcinomas. *Br J Urol* 1995;75:480–484.
1570. Garzetti GG, Liavattini A, Goteni G, et al. Ki-67 antigen immunostaining (MIB 1 monoclonal antibody) in serous ovarian tumors: index of proliferative activity with prognostic significance. *Gynecol Oncol* 1995;56:169–174.
1571. Resnick M, Lester S, Tate JE, et al. Viral and histopathologic correlates of MN and MIB 1 expression in cervical intraepithelial neoplasia. *Hum Pathol* 1996;27:234–239.
1572. Bubendorf L, Sauter G, Moch H, et al. Ki-67 labelling index: An independent predictor of progression in prostate cancer treated by radical prostatectomy. *J Pathol* 1996;178:437–441.
1573. Gerdes J, Dallenbach F, Lennert K. Growth fractions in malignant non-Hodgkin's lymphomas (NHL) as determined in situ with the monoclonal antibody Ki-67. *Hematol Oncol* 1984;2:365–371.
1574. Weiss LM, Strickler JG, Medeiros LJ, et al. Proliferative rates of non-Hodgkin's lymphomas as assessed by Ki-67 antibody. *Hum Pathol* 1987;18:1155–1159.
1575. Hall PA, Richards MA, Gregory WM, et al. The prognostic value of Ki-67 immunostaining in non-Hodgkin's lymphoma. *J Pathol* 1988;154:223–235.
1576. Grogan TM, Lippman SM, Spier C, et al. Independent prognostic significance of a nuclear proliferation antigen in diffuse large cell lymphomas as determined by the monoclonal antibody Ki-67. *Blood* 1988;71:1157–1160.
1577. Rosenberg N, Kincade PW. B-lineage differentation in normal and transformed cells and the microenvironment that supports it. *Curr Opin Immunol* 1994;6:203–11.
1578. Boismenu R, Havran WL. An innate view of gamma delta T cells. *Curr Opin Immunol* 1997;9:57–63.
1579. Spits H, Lanier LL, Phillips JH. Development of human T and natural killer cells. *Blood* 1995;85:2654–2670.
1580. Wu L, Kincade PW, Shortman K. The CD44 expressed on the earliest intrathymic precursor population functions as a thymus homing molecule but does not bind to hyaluronate. *Immunol Lett* 1993;38:69–75.
1581. Mojcik CF, Salomon DR, Chang AC, et al. Differential expression of integrins on human thymocyte subpopulations. *Blood* 1995;86: 4206–4217.
1582. van Ewijk W. T-cell differentiation is influenced by thymic microenvironments. *Annu Rev Immunol* 1991;9:591–615.
1583. Anderson G, Moore NC, Owen JJ, et al. Cellular interactions in thymocyte development. *Annu Rev Immunol* 1996;14:73–99.
1584. von Boehmer H. The developmental biology of T lymphocytes. *Annu Rev Immunol* 1988;6:309–326.
1585. Phagocytes [Editorial]. JAMA 1989;261:2555.
1586. Lasser A. The mononuclear phagocytic system: a review. *Hum Pathol* 1983;14:108–126.
1587. Johnston RB, Zucker-Franklin D. The mononuclear phagocyte system: monocytes and macrophages. In: Zucker-Franklin D, Greaves MF, Grossi CE, et al, eds. *Atlas of blood cells, function and pathology*, ed. 2. Philadelphia: Lea & Febiger, 1988.
1588. Murphy GF, Messadi D, Fonferko E, et al. Phenotypic transformation of macrophages to Langherhans cells in the skin. *Am J Pathol* 1986; 123:401–406.
1589. Meuret G, Baumert J, Hoffman G. Kinetics of human monocytopoiesis. *Blood* 1974;44:801–810.
1590. Johnston RB. Monocytes and macrophages. *N Engl J Med* 1988; 318:747–752.
1591. Isaacson PG. Commentary: histiocytic malignancy. *Histopathology* 1985;9:1007–1011.
1592. Hsu SM. Phenotypic expression of cells of stationary elements in human lymphoid tissues: a histochemical and immunohistochemical study. *Hematol Pathol* 1987;1:45–46.
1593. Radzun HJ, Kreipe H, Zavazava N, et al. Diversity of the human monocyte/macrophage system as detected by monoclonal antibodies. *J Leuk Biol* 1988;43:41–50.
1594. Hsu SM, Zhang HZ, Jaffe ES. Utility of monoclonal antibodies directed against B and T lymphocytes and monocytes in paraffin-embedded sections. *Am J Clin Pathol* 1983;80:415–420.
1595. Hofman FM, Lopez D, Husmann L, et al. Heterogeneity of macrophage populations in human lymphoid tissue and peripheral blood. *Cell Immunol* 1984;88:61–74.
1596. Hall PA, O'Doherty CJ, Levison DA. Langherhans cell histiocytosis: an unusual case illustrating the value of immunohistochemistry in diagnosis. *Histopathology* 1987;11:1181–1191.
1597. Baroni CD, Vitolo D, Remotti D, et al. Immunohistochemical heterogeneity of macrophage subpopulations in human lymphoid tissues. *Histopathology* 1987;11:1029–1042.

1598. Langerhans P. Ueber die Nerven der menochlichen Haut: *Virchows Arch* 1868;44:325–337.
1599. Birbeck MS, Breathnach AS, Everall JD. An electron microscopic study of basal melanocytes and high level clear cells (Langerhans cells) in vitiligo. *J Invest Dermatol* 1961;37:51–64.
1600. Thorbecke GJ, Silverberg-Sinakin I, Flotte TJ. Langerhans cells as macrophages in skin and lymphoid organs. *J Invest Dermatol* 1980; 75:32–43.
1601. Tew JG, Thorbecke J, Steinman RM. Dendritic cells in the immune response: characteristics and recommended nomenclature (a report from the Reticuloendothelial Society Committee on nomenclature). *J Reticuloendothel Soc* 1982;31:371–380.
1602. Haines KA, Flotte TJ, Springer TA, et al. Staining of Langerhans cells with monoclonal antibodies to macrophages and lymphoid cells. *Proc Natl Acad Sci USA* 1983;80:3448–3451.
1603. Katz SI, Tamaki K, Sach DH. Epidermal Langerhans cells are derived from cells originating in bone marrow. *Nature* 1979;282: 321–323.
1604. Tamaki K, Stingl G, Katz SI. The origin of Langerhans cells. *J Invest Dermatol* 1980;74:309–311.
1605. Cocchia D, Michetti F, Donato R. Immunochemical and immunocytochemical localization of S-100 antigen in normal human skin. *Nature* 1981;294:85–87.
1606. Takashi K, Yamaguchi H, Ishizeki J, et al. Immunohistochemical and immunoelectron microscopic localization of S-100 protein in the interdigitating reticulum cells of the human lymph node. *Virchows Arch* 1981;37:125–135.
1607. Stingl G, Tamaki K, Katz SJ. Origin and function of epidermal Langerhans cells. *Immunol Rev* 1980;53:149–174.
1608. Romani N, Koide S, Crowley M, et al. Presentation of exogenous protein antigens by dendritic cells to T cell clones: intact protein is presented best by immature, epidermal Langerhans cells. *J Exp Med* 1989;169:1169–1178.
1609. Silverberg-Sinakin I, Thorbecke GJ, Baer RL, et al. Antigen bearing Langerhans cells in skin, dermal lymphatics and lymph nodes. *Cell Immunol* 1976;25:137–151.
1610. Vernon ML, Fountain L, Krebs HM, et al. Birbeck granules (Langerhans' cell granules) in human lymph nodes. *Am J Clin Pathol* 1973;60:771–779.
1611. Hoefsmit ECM, Duijvestijn AM, Kamperdijk WA. Relation between Langerhans cells, veiled cells, and interdigitating cells. *Immunobiology* 1982;161:255–265.
1612. Rausch E, Kaiserling E, Goos M. Langerhans cells and interdigitating reticulum cells in the thymus-dependent region in human dermatopathic lymphadenitis. *Virchows Arch* 1977;25:327–343.
1613. Romani N, Lenz A, Glassl H, et al. Cultured human Langerhans cells resemble lymphoid dendritic cells in phenotype and function. *J Invest Dermatol* 1989;93:600–609.
1614. Teunissen MBM, Wormmeester J, Krieg SR, et al. Human epidermal Langerhans cells undergo profound morphologic and phenotypical changes during in vitro culture. *J Invest Dermatol* 1990;94:166–173.
1615. Schuler G, Steinman RM. Murine epidermal Langerhans cells mature into potent immunostimulatory dendritic cells in vitro. *J Exp Med* 1985;161:526–546.
1616. Silverberg-Sinakin I, Baer RL, Thorbecke GJ. Langerhans cells: a review of their nature with emphasis on their immunologic functions. *Progress Allergy* 1978;24:268–294.
1617. Harrist TJ, Muhlbauer JE, Murphy GF, et al. T6 is superior to Ia (HLA-DR) as a marker for Langerhans cells and indeterminate cells in normal epidermis: a monoclonal antibody study. *J Invest Dermatol* 1983;80:100–103.
1618. Breathnach AS. Development and differentiation of dermal cells in man. *J Invest Dermatol* 1978;71:2–8.
1619. Murphy GF, Bhan AK, Sato S, et al. A new immunologic marker for Langerhans cells. *N Engl J Med* 1981;34:791–792.
1620. Murphy GF, Bhan AK, Harrist TJ, et al. Identification of indeterminate cells in normal human dermis by the use of monoclonal anti-T6 antibody. *Lab Invest* 1982;46:60A.
1621. Daniels TE. Human mucosal Langerhans cells: postmortem identification of regional variations in oral mucosa. *J Invest Dermatol* 1984; 82:21–24.
1622. Gothelf Y, Hanau D, Tsur H, et al. T6 positive cells in the peripheral blood of burn patients: are they Langerhans cells precursors? *J Invest Dermatol* 1988;90:142–148.
1623. Weinberg DS, Pinkus GS, Murphy GF. Tonsillar epithelial dendritic cells: demonstration by lectin binding, immunohistochemical characterization, and ultrastructure. *Lab Invest* 1987;56:622–628.
1624. Spry CJF, Pflug AJ, Janossy G, et al. Large mononuclear (veiled) cells with "Ia-like" membrane antigens in human afferent lymph. *Clin Exp Immunol* 1980;39:750–755.
1625. Lampert IA, Pizzolo G, Thomas A, et al. Immunohistochemical characterization of cells involved in dermatopathic lymphadenopathy. *J Pathol* 1980;131:145–156.
1626. Weiss LM, Beckstead JH, Warnke RA, et al. Leu-6-expressing cells in lymph nodes: dendritic cells phenotypically similar to interdigitating cells. *Pathology* 1986;17:179–184.
1627. Freudenthal P, Steinman RM. The distinct surface of human dendritic cells, as observed after an improved isolation technique. *Proc Natl Acad Sci USA* 1990;87:7698–7702.
1628. Dijkstra CD. Characterization of nonlymphoid cells in rat spleen, with special reference to strongly Ia positive branched cells in T-cell areas. *J Reticuloendothel Soc* 1982;32:167–178.
1629. Witmer MD, Steinman RM. The anatomy of peripheral lymphoid organs with emphasis on accessory cells: light microscopic, immunocytochemical studies of mouse spleen, lymph node and Peyer's patch. *Am J Anat* 1984;170:465–481.
1630. Veldman JE, Kaiserling E. Interdigitating cells. In: Carr I, Daems WT, eds. *The reticuloendothelial system: a comprehensive treatise.* New York: Plenum Press, 1980:381–416.
1631. Barclay AN, Mayrhofer G. Bone marrow origin of Ia-positive cells in the medulla of rat thymus. *J Exp Med* 1981;153:1666–1671.
1632. Pelletier M, Tautu C, Landry D, et al. Characterization of human thymic dendritic cells in culture. *Immunology* 1986;58:263–270.
1633. Barthelemy H, Pelletier M, Landry D, et al. Demonstration of OKT6 antigen on human thymic dendritic cells in culture. *Lab Invest* 1986; 55:540–545.
1634. Pure E, Inaba K, Crowley MT, et al. Antigen processing by epidermal Langerhans' cells correlates with the level of biosynthesis of MHC class II molecules and expression of invariant chain. *J Exp Med* 1990;172:1459–1469.
1635. Boog CJP, Boes J, Melief CJM. Role of dendritic cells in the regulation of class I restricted cytotoxic T lymphocyte responses. *J Immunol* 1988;140:3331–3337.
1636. Murphy GF, Bhan AK, Sato S, et al. Characterization of Langerhans cells by the use of monoclonal antibodies. *Lab Invest* 1981;45: 465–468.
1637. Metlay JP, Witmer-Pack MD, Agger R, et al. The distinct leukocyte integrins of mouse spleen dendritic cells as identified with new hamster monoclonal antibodies. *J Exp Med* 1990;171:1753–1772.
1638. Bancherau J, Steinman RM. Dendritic cells and the control of immunity. *Nature* 1998;392:245–252.
1639. Schmitt DA, Hanau D, Bieber T, et al. Human epidermal Langerhans cells express only the 40-kilodalton Fc gamma receptor (FcγRII). *J Immunol* 1990;144:4284–4290.
1640. Bieber T, Rieger A, Neuchrist C, et al. Induction of FcR/CD23 on human epidermal Langerhans cells by human recombinant interleukin-4 and interferon-gamma. *J Exp Med* 1989;170:309–314.
1641. Stein H, Gerdes J, Mason DY. The normal and malignant germinal center. *Clin Haematol* 1982;11:531–559.
1642. Tew JG, Kosco MH, Burton GF, et al. Follicular dendritic cells as accessory cells. *Immunol Rev* 1990;117:185–211.
1643. Gerdes JH, Stein H, Mason DY, et al. Human dendritic reticulum cells of lymphoid follicles: their antigenic profile and their identification as multinucleated giant cells. *Virchows Arch* 1983:42:161–172.
1644. Naiem M, Gerdes J, Abdulaziz Z, et al. Production of a monoclonal antibody reactive with human dendritic reticulum cells and its use in the immunohistochemical analysis of lymphoid tissue. *J Clin Pathol* 1983;36:167–175.
1645. Peters JPJ, Rademakers LHPM, Roelofs JMM, et al. Distribution of dendritic reticulum cells in follicular lymphoma and reactive hyperplasia: light microscopic identification and general morphology. *Virchows Arch* 1984;46:215–228.
1646. Van der Valk P, Van der Loo EM, Janser J, et al. Analysis of lymphoid and dendritic cells in human lymph node, tonsil and spleen: a study using monoclonal and heterologous antibodies. *Virchows Arch* 1984;45:169–185.
1647. Dijkstra CD, Van den Berg TK. The follicular dendritic cell: possible

regulatory roles of associated molecules. *Res Immunol* 1991;142: 227–231.
1648. Serrate SA, Vose BM, Timonen T, et al. Association of human natural killer activity against human primary tumors with large granular lymphocytes. In: Herberman RB, ed. *NK cells and other natural effector cells.* New York: Academic Press, 1982:1055–1060.
1649. Trinchieri G, Santoli D. Antiviral activity induced by culturing lymphocytes with tumor-derived or virus-transformed cells: enhancement of human natural killer cell activity by interferon and antagonistic inhibition of susceptibility of target cells to lysis. *J Exp Med* 1978;147:1314–1333.
1650. Trinchieri G. Biology of natural killer cells. *Adv Immunol* 1989;47: 187–376.
1651. Lanier LL, Phillips J, Hackett J, et al. Natural killer cells: definition of a cell type rather than a function. *J Immunol* 1986;137:2735–2739.
1652. Hackett J, Bennett M, Kumar V. Origin and differentiation of natural killer cells: I. Characteristics of a transplantable NK cell precursor. *J Immunol* 1985;134:3731–3738.
1653. Hackett J, Bosma GC, Bosma MJ, et al. Transplantable progenitors of natural killer cells are distinct from those of T and B lymphocytes. *Proc Natl Acad Sci USA* 1986;83:3427–3431.
1654. Young JD-E, Cohn ZA. Cellular and humoral mechanisms of cytotoxicity: structural and functional analogies. *Adv Immunol* 1987;41: 269–332.
1655. Young JD-E, Hengartner H, Podack ER, et al. Purification and characterization of a cytolytic pore-forming protein from granules of cloned lymphocytes with natural killer activity. *Cell* 1986;44: 849–859.
1656. Trinchieri G, Matsumoto-Kobayashi M, Clark SC, et al. Response of resting human peripheral blood natural killer cells to interleukin-2. *J Exp Med* 1984;160:1147–1169.
1657. Cuturi MC, Anegon I, Sherman F, et al. Production of hematopoietic colony-stimulating factors by human natural killer cells. *J Exp Med* 1989;169:569–583.
1658. Perussia B, Fanning V, Trinchieri G. Phenotype characterization of human natural killer and antibody-dependent killer cells as an homogeneous and discrete cell subset. In: Herberman RB, ed. *NK cells and other natural effector cells.* New York: Academic Press, 1982: 47.
1659. Knowles DM, Halper JP, Jakobiec FA. T lymphocyte subpopulations in B cell derived non-Hodgkin's lymphomas and Hodgkin's disease. *Cancer* 1984;54:633–651.
1660. Lanier LL, Ruitenberg JJ, Phillips JH. Human $CD3^+$ T lymphocytes that express neither CD4 nor CD8 antigens. *J Exp Med* 1986;164: 339–344.
1661. Taylor CR. Results of multiparameter studies of B cell lymphomas. *Am J Clin Pathol* 1979;72[Suppl]:687–697.
1662. Levy N, Nelson J, Meyer P, et al. Reactive lymphoid hyperplasia with single class (monoclonal) surface immunoglobulin. *Am J Clin Pathol* 1983;80:300–308.
1663. Palutke M, Schnitzer B, Mirchandani I, et al. Increased numbers of lymphocytes with single class surface immunoglobulins in reactive hyperplasia of lymphoid tissue. *Am J Clin Pathol* 1982;78:316–323.
1664. Arnold A, Cossman J, Bakhski A, et al. Immunoglobulin gene rearrangements as unique clonal markers in human lymphoid neoplasms. *N Engl J Med* 1983;309:1593–1599.
1665. Cleary ML, Chao J, Warnke R, et al. Immunoglobulin gene rearrangement as a diagnostic criterion of B-cell lymphoma. *Proc Natl Acad Sci USA* 1984;81:593–597.
1666. Knowles DM, Athan E, Ubriaco A, et al. Extranodal non-cutaneous lymphoid hyperplasias represent a continuous spectrum of B-cell neoplasia: demonstration by molecular genetic analysis. *Blood* 1989; 73:1635–1645.
1667. Knowles DM, Neri A, Pelicci PG, et al. Immunoglobulin and T cell receptor beta chain gene rearrangement analysis of Hodgkin's disease: clinical and biological implications. *Proc Natl Acad Sci USA* 1986;83:7942–7946.
1668. Marcos MR, Gaspar ML, De la Hear A, et al. Selective expansion of a $CD3^+$ $CD4^-$ $CD8^-$ subpopulation in clinical groups associated with human immunodeficiency virus infection. *Scand J Immunol* 1987;25:321–333.
1669. Kadin ME, Nasu K, Sako D, et al. Lymphomatoid papulosis: a cutaneous proliferation of activated helper T cells expressing Hodgkin's disease associated antigens. *Am J Pathol* 1985;119:315–325.
1670. Wood GS, Strickler JG, Deneau DG, et al. Lymphomatoid papulosis expresses immunophenotypes associated with T cell lymphoma but not inflammation. *J Am Acad Dermatol* 1986;15:444–458.
1671. Macaulay WL. Lymphomatoid papulosis: a continuing self-healing eruption, clinically benign, histologically malignant. *Arch Dermatol* 1968;97:23–30.
1672. Willemze R, Meyer CJLM, Van Vloten WA, et al. The clinical and histological spectrum of lymphomatoid papulosis. *Br J Dermatol* 1982;107:131–144.
1673. Barth RK, Kim BS, Lon NC, et al. The murine T cell receptor uses a limited repertoire of expressed V beta gene segments. *Nature* 1985; 316:517–523.
1674. Clark DM, Hall PA, Boylston AW, et al. Antibodies to T cell antigen receptor beta chain families detect monoclonal T cell proliferation. *Lancet* 1986;ii:835–836.
1675. Lukes RJ, Butler JJ. The pathology and nomenclature of Hodgkin's disease. *Cancer Res* 1966;26:1063–1081.
1676. Lukes RJ, Butler JJ, Hicks EB. Natural history of Hodgkin's disease as related to its pathologic picture. *Cancer* 1966;19:317–344.
1677. Colby TV, Hoppe RT, Warnke RA. Hodgkin's disease: a clinicopathologic study of 659 cases. *Cancer* 1982;49:1848–1858.
1678. Aisenberg AC, Wilkes BM. Lymph node T-cells in Hodgkin's disease: analysis of suspensions with monoclonal antibody and rosetting techniques. *Blood* 1982;59:522–527.
1679. Poppema S, Bhan AK, Reinherz EL, et al. In situ immunologic characterization of cellular constituents in lymph nodes and spleens involved by Hodgkin's disease. *Blood* 1982;59:226–232.
1680. Timens W, Visser L, Poppema S. Nodular lymphocyte predominance type of Hodgkin's disease is a germinal center lymphoma. *Lab Invest* 1986;54:457–461.

CHAPTER 4

Immunohistochemical Analysis of Lymphoid Tissue

Roger A. Warnke and Peter G. Isaacson

Since the first edition of *Neoplastic Hematopathology*, there have been exciting and ongoing developments in the generation of antibodies that react with antigenic determinants (i.e., epitopes) that are preserved in routinely fixed paraffin-embedded tissues. Although it is still important for definitive phenotypic or genotypic studies to snap freeze portions of diagnostic lymph node biopsies or samples from any specimen in which the clinical or gross findings suggest lymphoma, most diagnostic problems for lymphoid tissues may be addressed by panels of antibodies applied to routine sections. Our approach to these diagnostic problems is emphasized in this chapter.

Important advances have occurred in the molecular methods that address the clonality of T-cell and B-cell proliferations and in those that detect chromosomal translocations and other molecular abnormalities. Certain diagnostic problems may be addressed by a small panel of markers applied to routine sections, followed by molecular studies on routinely fixed, paraffin-embedded tissue; the molecular studies may be rendered more timely and cost-effective as a result of phenotypic findings. Careful integration of the clinical, histologic, phenotypic and other findings is critical to optimal patient management.

Remarkable developments have also occurred in the technical aspects of immunohistology. Although enzyme digestion is still used for the detection of some cellular antigens, heat-induced antigen retrieval by microwaving, steaming, pressure cooking, or other methods has improved detection of many epitopes and is a necessary pretreatment for some of the new and important markers. An overview of some of the technical aspects of immunohistochemistry is provided at the end of this chapter.

R. A. Warnke: Department of Pathology, Stanford University Medical Center, Stanford, California 94305

P. G. Isaacson: Department of Histopathology, Royal Free and University College Medical School, London, United Kingdom

EVALUATION OF FOLLICULAR LESIONS

Follicular Lymphoma versus Follicular Hyperplasia

The most useful panel for differentiating follicular lymphoma from follicular hyperplasia includes antibodies to the BCL-2 protein and to immunoglobulin light chains (Table 4.1). Polymerase chain reaction (PCR) studies for rearrangement at the immunoglobulin heavy-chain locus or the *BCL2* locus are less sensitive than these protein markers (1). Some investigators find MT2 to be a useful marker in this setting (2–4), but others find it less useful (1,5–7). Preliminary information suggests that antibodies to fascin may also prove useful in this diagnostic setting (8).

BCL-2 Protein

Approximately 90% of follicular small cleaved cell, 80% of follicular mixed small cleaved and large cell, and 70% of follicular large cell lymphomas stain for BCL-2 protein (1,9–11). Because the germinal center cells of secondary follicles do not express the BCL-2 protein, detection of this protein is the most useful tool for distinguishing reactive from neoplastic follicles (Fig. 4.1). Different patterns of BCL-2 protein expression occur in follicular lymphoma, and their identification requires careful correlation with morphologic features and other markers (9).

Small cleaved cells or centrocytes often stain more intensely than large lymphoid cells or centroblasts and typically stain more intensely than normal B and T cells; there is overexpression of the BCL-2 protein as a consequence of the t(14;18) translocation. Nevertheless, intense labeling may be seen in cases in which a t(14;18) cannot be documented and any degree of expression in follicle center cells is abnormal, because this protein is not expressed by germinal center B cells (Fig. 4.1). In some cases, a large number of T cells or plasma cells may lead to an erroneous impression

TABLE 4.1. *Evaluation of follicular lesions in paraffin sections*

Differential diagnosis	Panel antibodies	Comment
Follicular lymphoma versus follicular hyperplasia	BCL-2 (Fig. 4.1)	About 80% of follicular lymphomas stain for BCL-2, whereas germinal center B cells do not (1,9–11).
	Kappa (polyclonal), lambda (polyclonal)	Light chain restriction (deviation from the normal kappa to lambda ratio of 2–3 : 1) may be detected in about 30–80% of cases (1,10).
	CD3 (polyclonal) ± VS38 or CD138/syndecan	A T-cell marker such as CD3 and a plasma cell marker such as VS38 or CD138 can facilitate evaluation of BCL-2 expression on B cells in follicle centers.
	± MT2 and/or fascin	In contrast to the lack of MT2 staining in germinal centers, MT2 stains >50% of cells in >50% of cases of follicular lymphoma (better in B5 than formalin-fixed tissues, and there are borderline cases, particularly with heat pretreatment) (1–7); fascin-reactive germinal center dendritic cells are decreased in follicular lymphomas compared with reactive follicles (8).
Follicular versus diffuse pattern	CD20, CD3 (polyclonal)	CD3 is better than CD20 at highlighting a follicular pattern when there are large numbers of interfollicular lymphoma cells.
	CD21	CD21 and other follicular dendritic cell (FDC) markers highlight the FDC networks of follicular lymphoma (181).
	Ki-67 (polyclonal)	A follicular or diffuse component is often highlighted by proliferation markers such as Ki-67.
Follicular versus other lymphomas with a follicular growth pattern	CD10	About 60% of follicular lymphomas stain, whereas other lymphomas with a follicular pattern rarely stain (6); small numbers of germinal center cells in mantle cell lymphomas and in marginal zone lymphomas with follicular colonization may be highlighted.
	CD43 ± CD5	In contrast to follicular lymphoma, SLL/CLL and mantle cell lymphoma often express CD43 and/or CD5 (10,16).
	CD23	The large cells in the pseudofollicles of SLL/CLL often stain for CD23.
	CyclinD1/BCL-1 (Fig. 4.2)	Present in the nuclei of the cells in mantle cell lymphoma
	CD21	CD21 and other FDC markers highlight the FDC meshworks in follicular, mantle cell, and marginal zone lymphomas; in contrast, pseudofollicles contain few or no FDCs.
	BCL-2	Often decreased in the pseudofollicles of SLL/CLL (182); residual germinal center cells may be highlighted by their lack of staining in some mantle cell and marginal zone lymphomas.
Confirm follicle lysis	CD21	CD21 and other FDC markers highlight the breakup of the FDC networks (183).

SLL/CLL, small lymphocytic lymphoma/chronic lymphocytic leukemia.

of BCL-2 positivity, which can be avoided by careful correlation with T-cell and plasma cell markers. Normal primary follicles, the mantle zones of secondary follicles, and interfollicular T cells stain for BCL-2, and they can serve as excellent internal positive controls. Immunostaining for BCL-2 is of no value for distinguishing follicular lymphoma from other types of lymphoma, because a wide variety of indolent and aggressive B-cell and T-cell lymphomas may express this apoptosis-related protein.

Ki-67 in Follicular Lymphomas

Ki-67 is another useful reagent for distinguishing between follicular lymphoma and follicular hyperplasia. In reactive follicles, this antibody reveals a high growth fraction and accentuates the division of the follicle center into dark and light zones. In most follicular lymphomas, there is a much lower growth fraction, and zonation or polarization is not observed.

Immunoglobulin Light Chains

Identification of a markedly predominant κ-expressing or λ-expressing B-lineage population (e.g., 90% or greater predominance of one light chain over the other) provides strong support for malignancy (12,13). Optimal fixation and processing and meticulous attention to the details of staining procedures are essential to the identification of immunoglobulin in paraffin sections. The aim should be to achieve satisfactory staining of immunoglobulin light chains in mantle

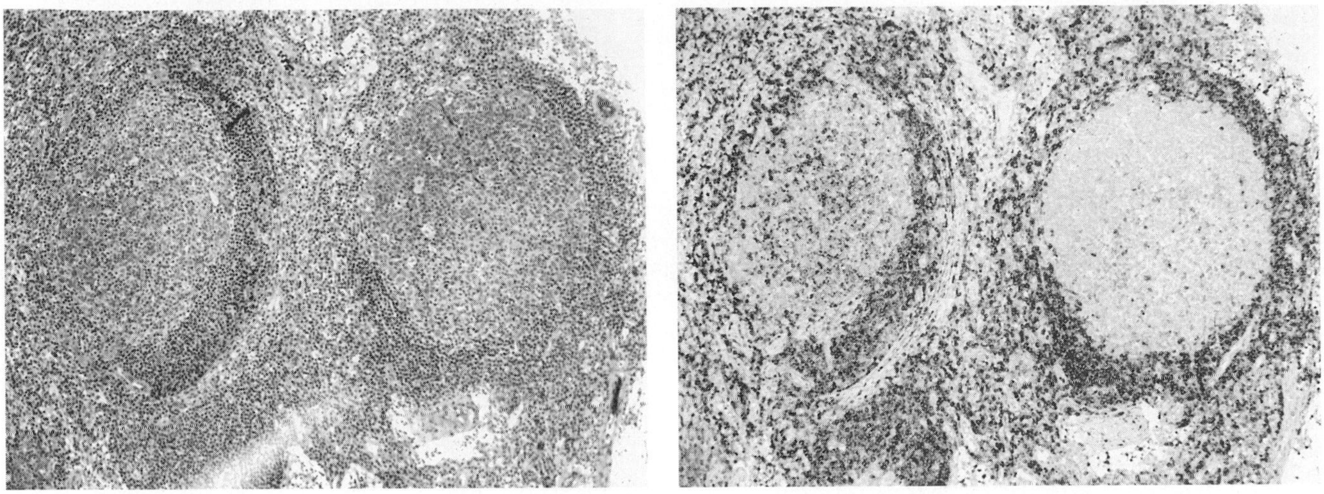

FIG. 4.1. BCL-2 in follicular lymphoma and in follicular hyperplasia. **A:** The follicle center at right shows polarization with a dark zone containing tingible body macrophages, and the follicle at the left shows admixed follicle center cells without tingible body macrophages (hematoxylin and eosin stain, original magnification: 40× magnification). **B:** The BCL-2 stain shows a lack of staining of the follicle center cells at right, consistent with a germinal center, whereas the follicle on the left contains many labeled, atypical cells, supporting the idea of partial involvement by follicular lymphoma. Staining was performed on the Ventana ES after antigen retrieval in citrate buffer (immunoperoxidase stain, original magnification: 40× magnification).

zone small lymphocytes in control sections. Nevertheless, the alteration or destruction of immunoglobulin by fixation and processing or the presence of too much immunoglobulin in the form of interstitial deposits or immunoglobulin within macrophages or other cell types may complicate the identification of a monotypic B-cell population in paraffin sections (14).

Although the pattern of staining in small lymphocytes may appear membranous and approximate that seen in cryostat sections, the staining is perinuclear. In larger transformed B cells, immunoglobulin staining is strongest in the Golgi region or cytoplasm. Careful comparison of both light-chain stains in the identical areas of the sections is essential for correct interpretation. Moreover, because the μ and δ chains are the most frequently expressed heavy chains in lymphomas and are less prevalent in serum than the other heavy chains and light chains, correlation with these markers may facilitate the interpretation of the κ and λ stains. In some cases, light-chain monotypia of a plasmacytoid subpopulation may indicate the neoplastic nature of a largely unstained predominant B-cell population. Normal plasma cells provide convenient internal positive controls for immunoglobulin stains.

Interfollicular B Cells in Follicular Lymphoma

A significant interfollicular population of neoplastic cells may be present between the follicles. These cells are often smaller than the intrafollicular lymphoma cells and can be highlighted by B-cell markers such as CD20 or more specifically by CD10, a marker of reactive and neoplastic follicle center cells.

Follicular versus Diffuse Pattern

A panel of antibodies that includes lineage markers, a follicular dendritic cell (FDC) marker, and a proliferation marker is useful for confirming a follicular component in an otherwise diffuse lymphoma (Table 4.1). When there are large numbers of interfollicular lymphoma cells, a follicular component may be revealed only by markers of FDCs and proliferation. Identification of a follicular component increases the likelihood of widespread disease, including marrow involvement, and diminishes the likelihood of cure.

Follicular Lymphoma versus Other Lymphoma with a Follicular Growth Pattern

If a follicle is defined as a group of B cells bound together by the FDC meshwork, several lymphomas in addition to classic follicular lymphoma may be considered to have a follicular growth pattern. The follicles in some of these lymphomas most closely resemble primary unstimulated follicles, but in others, they resemble reactive secondary follicles with germinal centers. The lymphomas that most often assume a follicular growth pattern include mantle cell lymphoma, marginal zone or mucosa-associated lymphoid tissue (MALT) lymphoma with follicular colonization, and splenic marginal zone lymphoma. Nodular lymphocyte predominance Hodgkin's disease (NLPHD) and a subtype of classic Hodgkin's disease, follicular Hodgkin's disease (15), may also simulate non-Hodgkin's lymphomas manifesting a follicular pattern. The proliferation centers of small lymphocytic lymphoma/chronic lymphocytic leukemia (SLL/CLL) are sometimes so prominent that they resemble the follicles of follicular lymphoma. A panel of antibodies that includes

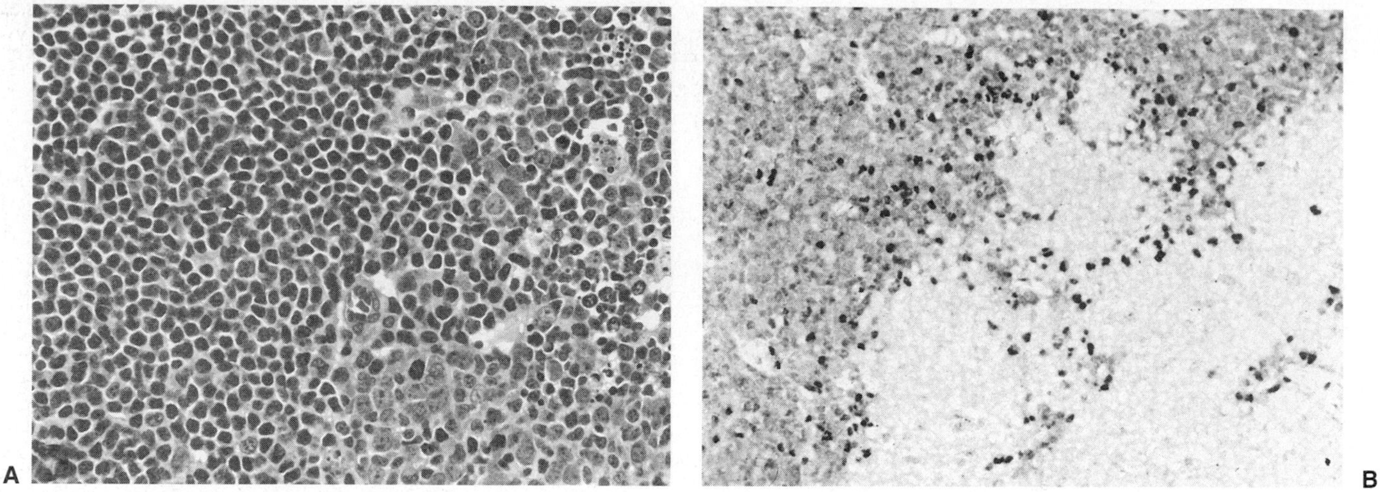

FIG. 4.2. Cyclin D1/BCL-1 in mantle cell lymphoma. **A:** The residual germinal center surrounded by atypical, small to medium-sized lymphoid cells with clumped nuclear chromatin suggests mantle cell lymphoma (hematoxylin and eosin stain, original magnification: 200× magnification). **B:** The largely unstained germinal center is focally infiltrated and surrounded by lymphoma cells that demonstrate nuclear labeling for cyclin D1/BCL-1. There is variable intensity of the labeling after antigen retrieval in Tris buffer and staining on the Ventana Nexes (immunoperoxidase stain, original magnification: 200× magnification).

those against CD10, CD43 or CD5 (or both), CD23, cyclin D1/BCL-1, CD21 (or other FDC markers), and BCL-2 are useful in this setting (Table 4.1).

Aberrant expression of the T-cell–associated marker CD43 occurs in a variety of B-cell neoplasms. However, this marker is frequently expressed in SLL/CLL and mantle cell lymphoma and is seldom expressed in follicular lymphomas (10). Although CD5 is even more discriminating in this problem area, its staining pattern in paraffin sections in some laboratories is less reliable than CD43 despite amplification methods employing biotinylated tyramine (16). In contrast, this amplification method does improve the detection of CD23 in SLL/CLL (16). Cyclin D1/BCL-1 is the most sensitive and specific marker for mantle cell lymphoma (17–20), but it requires optimized methods for detection (Fig. 4.2) One approach was reported by Brynes and colleagues (21). CD10 expression is common in follicular lymphomas and rarely observed in other diffuse small cell neoplasms such as mantle cell lymphoma, marginal zone lymphoma, or SLL/CLL. CD21 or another marker of FDCs is useful for highlighting a true follicular pattern; in contrast, the pseudofollicles of SLL/CLL contain few or no FDCs but do stain for BCL-2 (often weakly) and typically share the immunophenotype of the surrounding small cell component. Antibodies to IgM and IgD may sometimes be useful for highlighting residual or infiltrated mantle zones.

Confirmation of Follicle Lysis

Markers of FDCs such as CD21 highlight the breakup and dissolution of the floridly reactive follicles in the lymph nodes of patients infected with the human immunodeficiency virus (HIV).

EVALUATION OF DIFFUSE SMALL LYMPHOCYTIC PROLIFERATIONS

In the past, confirmation of a diagnosis of lymphoma or leukemia composed of small lymphocytes required identification of immunoglobulin light-chain restriction in a B-cell population in cell suspensions or in cryostat sections (22,23) (Table 4.2). Most of these problem cases now are resolved by studies using paraffin sections. Unlike cryostat sections, for which the immunoglobulin staining may be weak, expression of immunoglobulin may be strong in paraffin sections of small lymphocytic proliferations. Some markers such as CD23 that formerly worked only on fresh material can work after antigen retrieval on routine sections and allow a more specific diagnosis of SLL/CLL (16,24). Moreover, the most sensitive and specific marker of mantle cell lymphoma, cyclin D1/BCL-1, works best on routine sections (17–21) (Fig. 4.2).

Lymphoma versus Hyperplasia

A panel of markers that includes CD20, CD43, CD3, and polyclonal antibodies to the κ and λ light chains can be used to confirm the diagnosis in lymphomas composed predominantly of small lymphocytes (Table 4.2). Identification of sheets of extrafollicular small B lymphocytes strongly suggests a diagnosis of lymphoma, which can often be confirmed by identification of immunoglobulin light-chain restriction or of anomalous expression of the T-cell–associated marker CD43 on B cells (10,25–28). This aberrant expression of a normal T-cell marker on neoplastic B cells is most frequently detected with antibodies against CD43, less often with antibodies against CD5, occasionally with antibodies against CD45RO, but not with antibodies against CD3. We

TABLE 4.2. *Evaluation of diffuse small lymphocytic proliferations in paraffin sections*

Differential diagnosis	Panel antibodies	Comment
Lymphoma versus hyperplasia	CD20 ± CD79a	Large numbers of extrafollicular B cells are typical of lymphoma; some SLL/CLL cases stain better for CD79a than CD20.
	CD43	About 70% of SLL/CLL and mantle cell lymphomas and about 30% of marginal zone lymphomas express CD43, whereas normal small B cells do not (10,25–28).
	CD3 (polyclonal)	Because this marker is not expressed on B-cell lymphomas, it can be used to highlight reactive T cells to facilitate the identification of anomalous CD43 expression.
	Kappa (polyclonal), lambda (polyclonal)	About 70% of lymphoplasmacytoid, about 50% of SLL/CLL and mantle cell lymphomas, and about 40% of marginal zone lymphomas show light-chain restriction (10,184).
Subtyping diffuse small B-cell lymphoma/leukemia		
Mantle cell lymphoma	CD43 ± CD5	About 70% of mantle cell lymphomas express CD43 (10,25–28) and/or CD5 (16).
	Cyclin D1/BCL-1 (Fig. 4.2)	About 95% of mantle cell lymphomas stain for cyclin D1/BCL-1, whereas other diffuse small cell lymphomas do not (17–20); blastic or large cell variants often stain intensely (29).
SLL/CLL	CD43 ± CD5	About 70% of SLL/CLL cases express CD43 (10,25–28) and/or CD5 (16).
	CD23	About 90% of SLL/CLL cases express CD23 (24); use of biotinylated tyramine may be necessary (16).

SLL/CLL, small lymphocytic lymphoma/chronic lymphocytic leukemia.

have observed that some antibodies to CD43 such as Leu-22 more commonly stain splenic marginal zone B-cell lymphoma than others such as MT1 (unpublished observations).

Subtyping Diffuse Small B-Cell Lymphomas and Leukemias

Mantle Cell Lymphoma

The identification of CD43 or CD5 expression on B cells makes a diagnosis of SLL/CLL or mantle cell lymphoma likely. The distinction between these two lymphomas is aided by antibodies to cyclin D1/BCL-1, which are invaluable for confirming a diagnosis of mantle cell lymphoma (17–21) (Fig. 4.2). Although polyclonal antibodies worked better than monoclonal antibodies in initial studies (18,19,29), some reports showed excellent results that depended on the use of single or multiple clones (21,30), selection of a particular method or buffer for heat-induced antigen retrieval (e.g., Tris at pH 10.0), and benefit from automated staining methods, including incubations at 37°C and swirling of the reaction mixtures (21,30). Blastic or large cell variants often show strong cyclin D1/BCL-1 expression (29). Only rare cyclin D1/BCL-1–reactive cells are seen in normal lymphoid tissues; labeling of the nuclei of occasional endothelial cells provides a convenient positive internal control (see Chapter 22).

Small Lymphocytic Lymphoma and Chronic Lymphocytic Leukemia

Although identification of CD43, CD5, or both together with the lack of cyclin D1/BCL-1 suggests SLL/CLL, expression of CD23 is useful for confirmation. Some investigators report excellent results with particular antibody clones and automated staining methods (24), but others report better results with detection methods that employ biotinylated tyramine (16). Follicular dendritic cells typically stain more intensely for CD23 than SLL/CLL cells and provide an excellent positive internal control (see Chapters 21 and 40).

EVALUATION OF DIFFUSE LARGE LYMPHOCYTIC PROLIFERATIONS

Lymphoma versus Hyperplasia

The problem of diagnosing lymphoma or hyperplasia is more prevalent in small than in large lymphoid cell proliferations; nevertheless, the immunohistochemical approach to the problem is the same (Table 4.3). A panel of antibodies that includes CD20, CD43, and polyclonal antibodies to the κ and λ light chains is used. Because large lymphoid cells are often admixed with a variety of cell types, many of which stain for CD43 and immunoglobulin (e.g., macrophages and plasma cells in lymphoid organs, myeloid cells in bone marrow), T-cell markers such as CD3, a plasma cell marker such as VS38 or CD138 (i.e., syndecan), and a myelomonocytic marker such as CD68 may be essential for the identification of anomalous CD43 expression or monotypic immunoglobulin light-chain staining in large B cells.

When an interfollicular large B-cell proliferation raises suspicion for a T-cell–rich large B-cell lymphoma but is found to comprise an admixture of κ-bearing and λ-bearing cells, an antibody to the latent membrane protein (LMP) of Epstein-Barr virus (EBV) or *in situ* hybridization for EBV-

TABLE 4.3. *Evaluation of diffuse large lymphocytic proliferations in paraffin sections*

Differential diagnosis	Panel antibodies	Comment
Lymphoma versus hyperplasia	CD20 ± CD79a, CD43	Large numbers of extrafollicular B cells suggest lymphoma; about 30% of large B-cell lymphomas express CD43 (25–27); rarely, the B cells in infectious mononucleosis may express CD43 (31).
	CD3 (polyclonal) ± CD68, VS38 or CD138/syndecan	T-cell and other markers may be essential to the interpretation of possible CD43 coexpression by neoplastic B cells, because CD43 may be expressed by macrophages, plasma cells, and red blood cell and white blood cell precursors (185).
	Kappa (polyclonal), lambda (polyclonal), ± other (Epstein-Barr virus [EBV], CD68, myeloperoxidase)	Light-chain restriction may be detected in about 30–80% of cases (10,184); large numbers of kappa- and lambda-reactive large B cells may be encountered in EBV-associated lymphoid proliferations; CD68 and myeloperoxidase highlight the plasmacytoid monocytes in Kikuchi's disease.
Determining the lineage	CD20 ± CD79a, CD3 (polyclonal), ± CD45RO and/or CD43	Antibodies to CD20 and CD3 may identify the lineage of about 95% of aggressive B- and T-cell lineage lymphomas (186–188); CD79a is an excellent backup or alternative to CD20, and either can stain >95% of B-cell lineage cases (33); CD79a is preferable to CD20 for identifying precursor and plasmacytic lesions; although CD3 is the most specific marker for T-cell lineage (38) and stains about 80% of cases; other less specific (T-associated) markers such as CD43 and CD45RO may be more sensitive and stain about 90% of cases (39–41); CD43 stains significantly more B-cell lymphomas than CD45RO except in the setting of HIV (189).
	± Other (CD30, CD56, cyclin D1/BCL-1)	Lymphomas that do not stain for lineage markers or stain only for T-cell lineage markers should be stained for CD30 to address anaplastic large cell lymphoma and for CD56 to address natural killer (NK) cell lymphoma; large B-cell proliferations that show nuclear or other features of mantle cell lymphoma may stain for cyclin D1/BCL-1 (37).
Determining the growth fraction	Ki-67 (polyclonal) or MIB-1	Antibodies to Ki-67 or other proliferation markers are used to identify a high growth fraction, which is associated with a worse prognosis in B-cell and T-cell lymphomas (45,46).

encoded RNA (EBER) is useful for determining EBV infection. A rare example of apparent infectious mononucleosis that showed anomalous expression of CD43 on large B cells has been reported (31). EBV often is seen in the lymphoid proliferations that complicate the immunodeficiency after transplantation or HIV infection. A polyclonal or monoclonal EBV-associated lymphoid proliferation may complicate T-cell lymphomas, particularly of the angioimmunoblastic type (32).

Kikuchi's disease may be mistaken for large cell lymphoma, particularly in its early phase, before apoptosis is well established, because sheets of $CD3^+$ large cells may dominate the histologic picture. These large lymphoid cells are invariably accompanied by numerous so-called plasmacytoid monocytes that can be identified by their reactivity for myeloperoxidase [MPO] (S. Pileri, personal communication, 1998) and their typical reactivity for CD68. The combination of large T cells and these MPO-containing mononuclear cells should prevent an erroneous diagnosis of lymphoma.

Determining the Lineage

Antibodies to CD20 and CD3 identify the lineage of most aggressive B-cell and T-cell lymphomas (Table 4.3). Antibodies to the immunoglobulin-associated molecule CD79a may be helpful for determining the B-cell lineage of $CD20^-$ precursor B-cell tumors (33), but the results should be interpreted with caution, because a small number of precursor T-cell tumors may also express CD79a (K. C. Gatter and B. Falini, personal communication, 1998). CD79a is also useful as a marker for lymphomas with plasmacytic differentiation that often lack CD20 expression (33). Some B-cell lymphomas show partial expression of CD20, CD79a, or both. Occasionally, other B-lineage lymphomas may show a $CD20^-/CD79a^+$ phenotype. Rare T-cell lymphomas stain for CD20 (34,35). Other B-lineage markers are less sensitive or less specific for B-cell lineage (e.g., antibodies to CD45RA react with naive or virgin T lymphocytes) (36). Some large B-cell lymphomas, particularly those that express CD43, may show nuclear or other features of mantle cell lymphoma; some of these cases can be stained for cyclin D1/BCL-1 to confirm an aggressive variant of mantle cell lymphoma (37).

Polyclonal antibodies to CD3 are the most specific for identifying a lymphoma of T-cell lineage (38). Nevertheless, some lymphomas, particularly those of activated T cells, lack expression of CD3 but stain for less specific T-cell–associated markers such as CD45RO and CD43 (39–41). Nonspecific cytoplasmic labeling of macrophages and megakaryocytes may be encountered with polyclonal anti-CD3. If the lineage of a lymphoma remains unclear after using a panel of B- and T-cell markers or if only T-lineage markers are reactive, antibody stains for CD30 and CD56 should be performed; some reports indicate that anaplastic large cell lymphomas (ALCLs) of T and null types are more curable than other T-lineage lymphomas (42), whereas natural killer (NK) or T-cell lymphomas are unusually aggressive in their behavior (43,44).

Determining the Growth Fraction

Because the growth fraction in aggressive B- and T-lineage lymphomas affects clinical outcome (45,46), proliferation markers such as Ki-67 are important for estimating the fraction of proliferating lymphoma cells. Studies have generally focused on the most proliferative area of a lymphoma. This approach minimizes the problem of admixed nonproliferating host T cells and macrophages. Nevertheless, the most accurate approaches for assessing proliferation employ double-label immunohistochemistry (47), combining Ki-67 with a B- or T-cell marker. When estimating the number of proliferating cells, weakly and strongly labeled nuclei should be evaluated. Exclusive labeling of mitotic figures may be a clue to artifactually low labeling as a consequence of delay in fixation, processing, or technical problems in the staining.

UNUSUAL LARGE CELL LYMPHOMAS OF B-CELL LINEAGE

Body Cavity Based Lymphomas

The rare primary effusion or body cavity lymphomas most often occur in the setting of HIV infection, and they harbor the Kaposi sarcoma–associated herpesvirus (human herpesvirus-8) and EBV (48–50) (Table 4.4). These lymphomas typically stain for leukocyte common antigen but lack expression of the usual B- and T-lineage markers, except those associated with plasma cells (48–50). Nevertheless, immunoglobulins are seldom detected (48–50). Cases typically stain for CD30 and epithelial membrane antigen (EMA) (48–50) (see Chapter 28).

ALK-1–Positive Lymphomas

Lymphomas of B-cell lineage can simulate ALCLs by their cytologic appearance and their involvement of lymphatic sinuses. These rare cases lack CD30 expression and do not have t(2;5); they express cytoplasmic but not nuclear ALK kinase (51). These lymphomas have an unusual constellation of immunophenotypic findings, with similarities to plasma cells ($CD20^-VS38^+EMA^+IgA^+$), but they often stain for leukocyte common antigen (CD45), lack CD79a, and surprisingly express T-cell–associated markers CD4 and CD57.

FURTHER EVALUATION OF PERIPHERAL NATURAL KILLER/T-CELL–LINEAGE LYMPHOMAS

Anaplastic Large Cell Lymphoma

ALCLs (i.e., primary systemic or ALK lymphomas), a category now restricted to T and null phenotypes, have a much better prognosis than other peripheral T-cell lymphomas (42) (Table 4.5). Antibodies to CD30, EMA, and the ALK protein highlight the involvement of lymphatic sinuses and perivascular areas typical of this lymphoma (52). Because CD30 and EMA are expressed by a variety of normal and neoplastic lymphoid and nonlymphoid cells (53,54), antibodies to the ALK protein (Fig 4.3) can prove extremely useful in diagnosis because reactivity for this marker is largely restricted to lymphomas with a t(2;5) translocation (52). Because the size of the cells may not be large (i.e., in the small cell variant) and because the cells may not be anaplastic (i.e., many cases are monomorphic), some investi-

TABLE 4.4. *Unusual large cell lymphomas of B-lineage in paraffin sections*

Differential diagnosis	Panel antibodies	Comment
Body cavity based lymphoma (48–50)	CD45	More than 95% stain for leukocyte common antigen.
	CD79a, VS38	CD79a and VS38 are much better than CD20 for identifying B-lineage lines.
	CD30	About 60% stain for CD30.
	EMA	About 70% stain for EMA.
	EBV	About 80% harbor EBV (nearly all of the data is based on *in situ* hybridization for EBER).
$ALK-1^+$ lymphoma (51)	ALK-1	Cytoplasmic granular plus Golgi area staining in most cases.
	VS38	All cases reactive.
	CD79	All cases unreactive.
	IgA	Five of 7 cases reactive.
	EMA	All cases were reactive.
	CD4	All tested cases were reactive.
	CD57	Five of 7 cases were partially reactive.

EBV, Epstein-Barr virus; EMA, epithelial membrane antigen.

TABLE 4.5. *Subtyping peripheral T-cell and natural killer cell lymphomas in paraffin sections*

Differential diagnosis	Panel antibodies	Comment
Anaplastic large cell, (primary systemic, "ALK lymphoma")	CD30	About 100% express CD30 (especially high in formalin-fixed tissue, lower in B5) (54,55,190).
	EMA	About 85% stain for EMA (52,114).
	ALK-1 (Fig. 4.3)	About 85% stain for ALK-1 (usually cytoplasmic and nuclear) (52).
Angioimmunoblastic	CD30	CD30 highlights small to large numbers of clear cells around arborizing venules (55).
	CD21	About 60% show an expanded network of FDCs far beyond the confines of remnant B zones adjacent to vessels (56,57,191).
	EBV	More than 85% show increased numbers of EBV containing cells (*in situ* hybridization for EBER better than detection of latent membrane protein/LMP-1 of EBV) (32,59–61,120).
Hepatosplenic gamma/delta	Beta chain of the TCR (βF1)	Most of these lymphomas lack staining for the beta chain of the TCR complex because they derive from $\gamma\delta$ T cells (62–65).
	CD4, CD8	Cases lack staining for CD4 and CD8 (62,63,65,66) or are $CD4^-CD8^+$ (65).
	CD56	About 80% express CD56 (62,65,66).
	Cytotoxic granule proteins (e.g., TIA-1)	About 100% stain for TIA-1 (64,65).
Enteropathy-type intestinal	CD4, CD8	About 40% express CD8, and the remainder lack expression of T subset antigens (67,68).
	Cytotoxic granule proteins (e.g., TIA-1, granzyme B)	About 100% stain for TIA-1 (64,68), and about 75% stain for granzyme B (68).
	CD30	About 50% express CD30 (67,68,70).
	± CD103	About 100% express CD103, an integrin that is a human mucosa-associated T-cell marker (71,72); detectable only on fresh cells or frozen tissue.
Extranodal NK/T, nasal ("angiocentric")	CD43, CD3 (polyclonal)	About 95% stain for CD43 (80,82,192), and about 70% stain for CD3 (polyclonal) (80,82).
	CD56 (Fig. 4.4)	About 80% stain for CD56 (80,82).
	CD30	About 25% express CD30 (81).
	EBV	About 90% contain EBV mRNA (77–82).
	Cytotoxic granule proteins (e.g., TIA-1, granzyme B)	About 90% stain for TIA-1 (64), and about 60% stain for granzyme B (82).
Subcutaneous, panniculitis-like	CD4, CD8	About 80% express CD8, about 10% are $CD4^+CD8^+$, about 10% are $CD4^-CD8^-$ (may derive from $\gamma\delta$ T cells and express CD56) (85,86).
	Cytotoxic granule proteins (e.g., TIA-1, perforin)	Almost 100% stain for these markers (85,86).

EBV, Epstein-Barr virus; EMA, epithelial membrane antigen; EBER, Epstein-Barr virus encoded RNA; LMP-1, latent membrane protein-1; FDC, follicular dendritic cells.

gators recommend the term *ALK lymphoma* in place of ALCL (52) (see Chapter 25).

Angioimmunoblastic T-Cell Lymphoma

A panel of antibodies, including those against CD30 and FDCs, may aid the diagnosis of angioimmunoblastic T-cell lymphoma, a rare but distinctive lymphoma (Table 4.5). Although one or both of these markers may suggest a T-cell lymphoma (55–57), gene rearrangement studies by PCR or by the Southern blot procedure are often indicated. These results usually confirm a clonal T-cell proliferation (57,58), but a significant number of cases also show clonal immunoglobulin heavy-chain gene rearrangement (57). This finding may be caused by clonal populations of EBV-infected B cells (32,59,60), and it has been associated with distinctive clinical features (57). Increased numbers of EBV-infected B cells are typically found in this special variant of peripheral T-cell lymphoma (32,59,60). *In situ* hybridization for EBER is more sensitive than antibody staining for EBV LMP-1 for identifying EBV-infected B cells (32,59–61). EBV-infected T cells can also be identified (59).

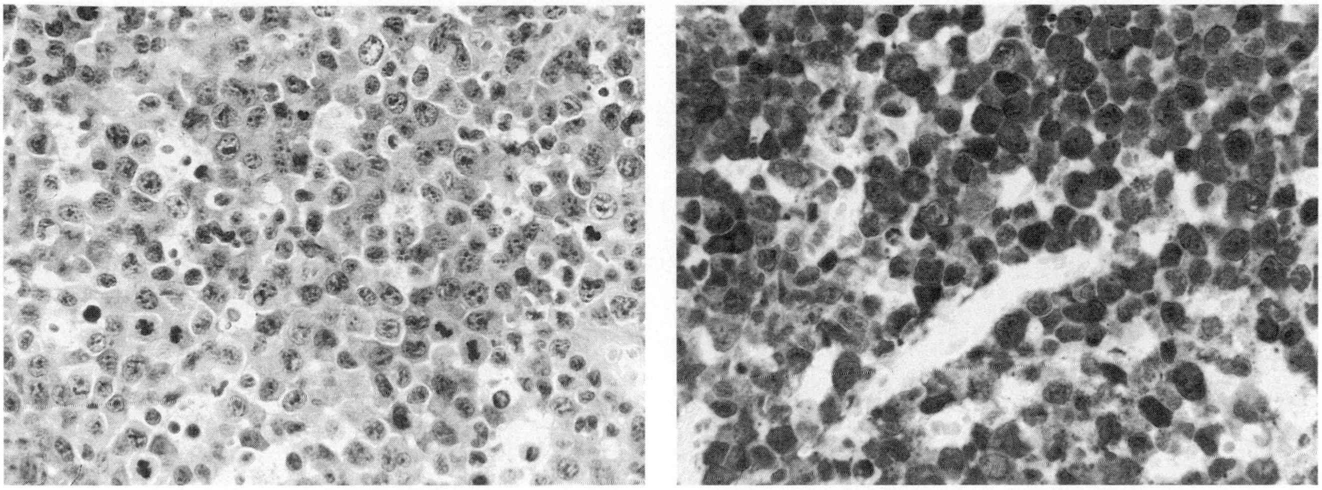

FIG. 4.3. ALK-1 in anaplastic large cell lymphoma. **A:** The lymphoma cells are large and relatively monomorphic, with a high mitotic rate (hematoxylin and eosin stain, original magnification: 400× magnification). **B:** There is strong nuclear and cytoplasmic labeling of the ALK protein. Staining was performed on the Ventana Nexes after antigen retrieval in Tris buffer (immunoperoxidase stain, original magnification: 400× magnification).

Hepatosplenic $\gamma\delta$ T-Cell Lymphoma

Hepatosplenic $\gamma\delta$ T-cell lymphomas are rare and aggressive. Their distinctive phenotype can be detected by a panel of markers that includes antibodies to the β chain of the T-cell receptor (TCR), to the T-cell subsets CD4 and CD8, to the neural cell adhesion molecule (NCAM [CD56]) and to cytotoxic granule proteins such as TIA-1 (Table 4.5). Nearly all of these lymphomas lack staining for the β chain of the TCR because they derive from $\gamma\delta$ T cells(62–65). Biotinylated tyramine may enhance the staining with antibodies such as βF1. These lymphomas lack staining for CD4 and CD8 or stain only for CD8 (62,63,65,66). Although these lymphomas stain for the cytotoxic granule protein TIA-1 (64,65), they lack staining for perforin (65).

Enteropathy-Type Intestinal T-Cell Lymphoma

A panel of antibodies that includes those to the T-subset markers CD4 and CD8, to the activation marker CD30, and to cytotoxic granule proteins such as TIA-1 aids the diagnosis of enteropathy-type intestinal T-cell lymphoma (Table 4.5). Cases lack T-subset markers or less frequently express CD8 (67,68). A subset of cases has been described in which the tumor cells express CD56 (69). CD30 is commonly expressed by these lymphomas (67,70). Reports indicate that these lymphomas have a cytotoxic T-cell phenotype (64,68) that is better detected by antibodies to TIA-1 than by those to granzyme B (68). If fresh tissue is available, antibodies to CD103 (an integrin involved in the homing of T cells to mucosal sites) can be used to verify the relation of this lymphoma to mucosal T cells (71,72). EBV has been implicated in these lymphomas by some groups (73,74) but not by others (70,75).

Nasal-Type Extranodal Natural Killer or T-Cell Lymphoma

A paraffin-reactive anti-CD56 antibody is extremely useful for identifying this rare, highly aggressive lymphoma (43,76) (Fig. 4.4). Because EBV mRNA is almost always present in these nasal-type, extranodal NK/T-cell lymphomas (77–82), *in situ* hybridization is a valuable tool for diagnosis and for monitoring recurrences. For the detection of EBV in this setting, *in situ* hybridization for EBER is much more sensitive than immunostaining for LMP (61). Approximately 25% of these lymphomas stain for CD30 (81). More of these lymphomas stain for CD43 than CD3 (80,82). In contrast to the limited reactivity of these lymphomas with monoclonal antibodies to CD3 in cryostat sections, polyclonal antibodies to CD3 stain most cases in paraffin sections (83). Most samples stain for the cytotoxic granule protein TIA-1, and fewer stain for granzyme B (64,82). Because aggressive CD56^{+} myeloid leukemias often present with extramedullary disease, evaluation of these cases with myeloid markers is indicated (84).

Subcutaneous Panniculitis-like T-Cell Lymphoma

All examples of subcutaneous panniculitis-like T-cell lymphoma, a rare lymphoma, have expressed cytotoxic granule proteins TIA-1 and perforin (85,86). At least 70% of cases appear to derive from $\alpha\beta$ T cells and typically stain for CD8, although cases may express both subset markers (85,86). Approximately 10% of cases appear to derive from $\gamma\delta$ T cells; these examples most often lack T-cell subset marker expression and may stain for CD56 (86). Despite the presence of a hemophagocytic syndrome in some of these

A 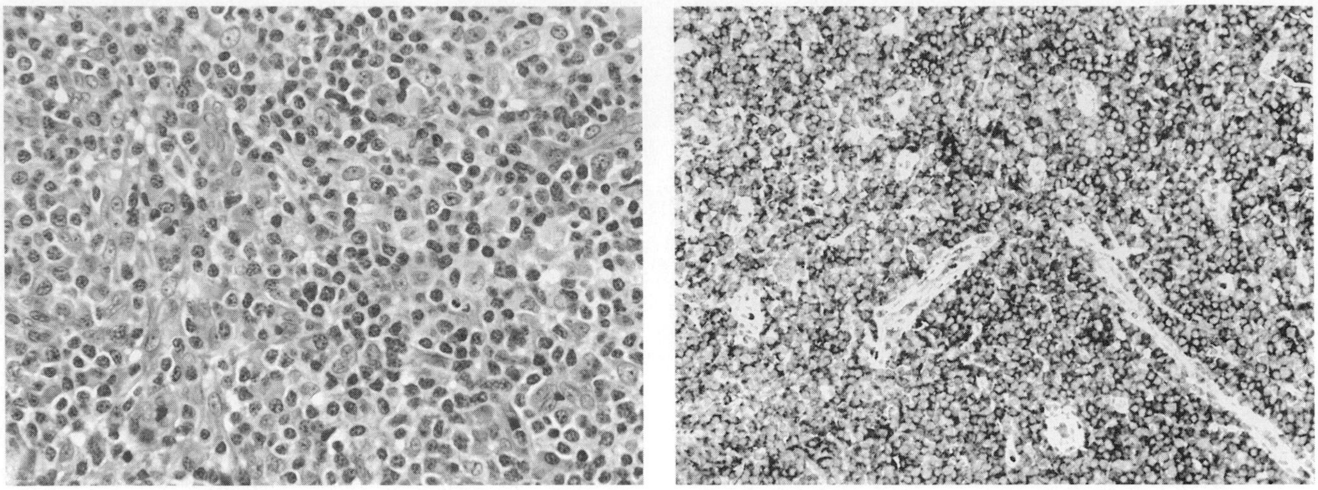 B

FIG. 4.4. CD56 in natural killer (NK)/T-cell lymphomas. **A:** The oropharyngeal biopsy shows an atypical lymphoid infiltrate composed of small to medium-sized cells associated with numerous plasma cells. The number of plasma cells suggested an extranodal marginal zone or MALT-type lymphoma (hematoxylin and eosin stain, original magnification: 200× magnification). **B:** The lymphoid component shows strong membrane labeling for CD56. The plasma cells represented an admixture of kappa and lambda stained cells, and the lymphoid cells contained EBV-encoded mRNA (EBER-1) (not shown). Detection of CD56 binding was achieved by biotin and streptavidin reagents in Coplin jars (Appendix 2) after antigen retrieval in citrate buffer (immunoperoxidase stain, original magnification: 200× magnification).

patients (87), EBV has not been identified in these lymphomas (85,86).

PAN-T-CELL ANTIGEN LOSS IN FROZEN SECTIONS

The lack of expression of one or more pan-T-cell antigens may be seen in approximately 80% of peripheral T-cell lymphomas and is a finding seldom observed in reactive disorders except those in the skin (23,88,89) (Table 4.6). Reactive T cells provide important and convenient internal positive controls for each of the pan-T-cell markers. Nevertheless, the development of PCR methods for detecting rearrangement of the γ gene of the T-cell receptor in formalin- or alcohol-fixed, paraffin-embedded tissue has obviated the need for frozen section phenotypic studies in most instances (90,91). If molecular studies of paraffin-embedded tissue are unsuccessful, TCR gene rearrangement studies may be performed on fresh or fresh frozen tissue by PCR or Southern blot methods.

EVALUATION OF BLASTIC LYMPHOMAS AND LEUKEMIAS

Lymphoblastic and myeloblastic tumors, whether arising in the marrow or presenting at extramedullary sites, can be reliably identified and differentiated from peripheral B- and T-lineage lymphomas and leukemias by a combination of markers on precursor cells (i.e., terminal deoxynucleotidyl transferase [TdT], CD99, CD1a, and CD34) and broadly reactive lineage-specific markers (i.e., CD79a, CD3, MPO, and CD68) (Table 4.7). With the exception of CD1a, the precursor cell markers are not lineage specific and should not be used alone. Polyclonal antibodies to MPO are the most sensitive and specific for myeloid leukemia (92–95), but cases with a monocytic component may only stain with

TABLE 4.6. *Pan T-cell antigen loss in peripheral T-cell lymphomas in frozen sections*

Differential diagnosis	Panel antibodies	Comment
Peripheral T-cell lymphoma versus hyperplasia (23,89)	CD2	About 15% lack expression.
	CD3	About 10% lack expression.
	CD5	About 25% lack expression.
	CD7	About 50% of non–mycosis fungoides cases and about 70% of mycosis fungoides cases lack expression.
	Beta chain of T-cell receptor	About 25% lack expression.

TABLE 4.7. *Evaluation of blastic lymphomas and leukemias in paraffin sections*

Differential diagnosis	Panel antibodies	Comment
Blastic lymphoma/leukemia versus other types	TdT	More than 90% of B-cell lineage, >90% of T-cell lineage, and about 40% of myeloid neoplasms stain, whereas peripheral B- and T-cell neoplasms do not (193–195); among myeloid malignancies, labeling for TdT may be more common in those with monocytic differentiation (196).
	CD99	More than 90% of T-cell lineage (195,197), >50% of B-cell lineage (195,197), and about 80% of myeloid neoplasms stain (198), whereas few peripheral B- and T-cell neoplasms stain in our experience; the incidence of staining is controversial (195,197–199).
	CD79a	More than 90% of B-cell lineage cases stain (33); about 90% of acute promyelocytic leukemias also stain (200).
	CD3 (polyclonal) ± CD1a	More than 90% of T-cell lineage cases stain (38,201); about 50% of T-cell lineage cases stain for CD1a (202).
	CD34	About 50% of B-cell lineage cases, about 15% of T-cell lineage cases, and about 33% of acute myeloid leukemias stain (195,203).
	MPO (polyclonal) ± elastase	About 95% of acute myeloid leukemias stain for MPO (92–95); about 40% of acute myeloid leukemias stain for elastase (204).
	CD68 ± lysozyme (polyclonal)	More than 80% of acute myeloid leukemias stain for CD68 or lysozyme (92,94,96,97); these markers are especially important for labeling cases that have a monocytic component.
	BCL-1	Almost 100% of blastic mantle cell lymphomas stain (29).
	± Other (CD56, CD31, CD61, factor VIII, and glycophorin C)	Aggressive CD56⁺ myeloid leukemias often manifest with extramedullary disease (84); markers reactive with megakaryocytes such as CD31, CD61, and factor VIII may be used to support M7 leukemia, and antibodies to glycophorin C may be used to support M6 leukemia.

markers such as CD68 and lysozyme (lysozyme staining is discussed later), which stain myeloid and monocytic cells (92–97). Mantle cell lymphomas that have blastic features can be reliably identified by antibodies to cyclin D1/BCL-1 (29). Aggressive CD56$^+$ myeloid leukemias often present with extramedullary disease (84). Megakaryocytic or erythroid differentiation may be supported by reactivity with their respective markers (Table 4.7).

LYMPHOID VERSUS PLASMA CELL PROLIFERATIONS

One of the earliest immunohistochemical studies using routinely fixed and paraffin-embedded tissues investigated the staining of plasma cells (Table 4.8). Most plasma cell neoplasms were found to stain for a single immunoglobulin heavy chain (usually γ or α) and a single light chain (κ or λ) (98). Studies of plasmacytomas and recurrences of myeloma after bone marrow transplantation have confirmed the specificity of light-chain staining (99,100). The broad B-lineage reactivity of CD79a makes it a useful plasma cell marker (33), but VS38 is an even better marker of plasmacytoid lymphoid cells and plasma cells (101). VS38 must be used judiciously because a significant number of nonhematolymphoid neoplasms may stain with this marker (102). Approximately one third of plasma cell neoplasms may show reactivity with one or more cytokeratin antibodies (103),

TABLE 4.8. *Evaluation of plasmacytoid lymphoid and plasma cell proliferations in paraffin sections*

Differential diagnosis	Panel antibodies	Comment
Lymphoid and plasma cell proliferations	Kappa (polyclonal), lambda (polyclonal)	About 95% of plasma cell neoplasms show a monotypic pattern of light-chain staining (98–100,104).
	VS38 or CD138/syndecan, CD79a	Almost 100% of plasma cell neoplasms stain for VS38 (101) or CD138 (205); about 50% stain for CD79a (33).
	CD20	Less than 5% show a majority of plasma cells that stain (104).
	CD45	About 15% show a majority of plasma cells that stain (104).
	IgG, IgA, and IgM	The identification of IgG or IgA favors a plasma cell neoplasm, but IgM favors plasmacytoid lymphoma, which is also favored if there is staining for CD20 and/or CD45RB.

and many react for EMA (104). In contrast to plasma cell neoplasms, lymphomas with plasmacytic or plasmacytoid differentiation typically express μ heavy chains (105) and often express CD20, leukocyte common antigen (CD45), or both (106).

HODGKIN'S VERSUS NON-HODGKIN'S LYMPHOMA

Many cases of Hodgkin's and non-Hodgkin's lymphomas may simulate each other histologically (Table 4.9). An accurate diagnosis is essential because optimal treatments are often different for each disease. This is such a common and difficult problem that it was chosen as the topic for the first slide workshop sponsored by the Society for Hematopathology: The Interrelationship of Hodgkin's Disease and Non-Hodgkin's Lymphoma (107). The panel of antibodies chosen depends on the particular diagnostic question. Some of the more common differential diagnostic problems are addressed in the following sections.

Classic Hodgkin's Disease

Nodular Sclerosis versus Diffuse Large B-Cell Lymphoma

Differentiating between nodular sclerosis (syncytial, grade II) and diffuse large B-cell lymphoma is a problem often encountered in mediastinal biopsies. The neoplastic cells in Hodgkin's disease typically have a $CD45^-/CD15^+$ phenotype, whereas those in diffuse large B-cell lymphoma express $CD45^+/CD15^-$ (108–110). It is common within each specimen that only a minority of Hodgkin's cells stains for CD15; technical factors play a role in at least some cases (111). For example, most anti-CD15 antibodies are mouse antibodies with a μ heavy chain; detection systems that employ anti-mouse μ antibodies stain more cases of Hodgkin's disease and stain more cells in a given case (112). Because Hodgkin's cells are typically surrounded by $CD45^+$ T cells, assessing reactivity with this marker often requires identifying an area where neoplastic cells abut one another so that the cell membranes of the malignant cells can be visualized. Although CD20 reactivity is found in at least 20% of Hodgkin's cases, reactivity is seldom seen in most of the cells, as occurs in cases of diffuse large B-cell lymphoma. CD30 may not be a useful marker in this setting because approximately two thirds of primary mediastinal large B-cell lymphomas express CD30 when heat-induced antigen retrieval methods are used (J. P. Higgins and R. A. Warnke, unpublished data).

Grade II Nodular Sclerosis versus Anaplastic Large Cell Lymphoma

Although the neoplastic cells in Hodgkin's disease and ALCL (i.e., primary systemic or ALK lymphoma) stain for CD30, this marker may highlight sinus or perivascular infiltration that is common in ALCL and rare in Hodgkin's disease. Because a significant number of cases of ALCL lack leukocyte common antigen expression (113) and some may express CD15 (114), lineage markers are especially important in this differential diagnosis. Expression of a B-cell marker supports Hodgkin's disease, and expression of a T-cell marker supports ALCL. Application of additional markers is often useful. EBV expression favors Hodgkin's disease (outside the setting of HIV), and expression of EMA favors ALCL (114). ALK protein expression is seen in most ALCLs but not in Hodgkin's disease (115). Nevertheless, the cases of ALCL that simulate Hodgkin's disease seldom stain for the ALK protein (115), and there remain a small number of cases that cannot be diagnosed as Hodgkin's disease or ALCL with confidence.

Mixed Cellularity or Lymphocyte-Rich versus T-Cell–Rich Diffuse Large B-Cell Lymphoma

A $CD45^-CD15^+CD30^+CD20^-$ phenotype supports Hodgkin's disease over a T-cell– or macrophage-rich diffuse large B-cell lymphoma (116,117), but additional markers are often useful. For example, the neoplastic cells in Hodgkin's cases typically stain for κ and λ light chains because of passive uptake of immunoglobulin (118), and neoplastic large B cells often show light-chain restriction. Most mixed-cellularity cases contain EBV (119), and most examples of T-cell–rich large B-cell lymphomas have not contained EBV (120). It is possible that the cases reported from Hong Kong of T-cell–rich large B-cell lymphoma with EBV represented EBV-related lymphoproliferative disorders complicating T-cell lymphomas (121), because two of the four cases were originally interpreted as angioimmunoblastic T-cell lymphoma. EBV may not be a useful discriminant in the lung, where angiocentric T-cell–rich large B-cell lymphomas typically contain EBV (so-called lymphomatoid granulomatosis) (122).

Mixed Cellularity or Lymphocyte-Rich versus Peripheral T-Cell Lymphoma

Expression of CD45 by atypical large cells supports the diagnosis of peripheral T-cell lymphoma over Hodgkin's disease. The Reed-Sternberg or Hodgkin cell–associated markers CD15 and CD30 are less helpful because isolated, pleomorphic lymphoma T cells may express CD15, CD30, or both markers (54,111). The expression of CD20 supports Hodgkin's disease, and the expression of a T-cell marker by pleomorphic large cells supports T-cell lymphoma. Although EBV expression is seen in most mixed cellularity cases, it is also seen in T-cell lymphomas complicated by an EBV-associated B-lymphoproliferative disorder. Molecular studies to confirm a clonal T-cell proliferation are often helpful in this setting.

Nodular Lymphocyte Predominance

When a panel of experts used morphologic assessment alone to identify NLPHD (i.e., nodular paragranuloma), ap-

TABLE 4.9. *Hodgkin's versus non-Hodgin's lymphomas in paraffin sections*

Differential diagnosis	Panel antibodies	Comment
Classic Hodgkin's disease (HD) versus other lymphomas	CD15	About 85% of classic HD stains (111,206), whereas <5% of NLPHD stains (123); anti-mouse IgM detection increases the number of reactive cases (112); about 5% of B-cell and about 20% of T-cell lymphomas stain (111,207).
	CD30	About 95% of classic HD stains (54,206,208), whereas about 5% of NLPHD stains (123); about 15% of diffuse aggressive B-cell and about 20% of nonanaplastic peripheral T-cell lymphomas show varied numbers of CD30+ cells (54).
	CD45	About 5% of classic HD stains for CD45, whereas about 65% of NLPHD stains (209); in contrast, about 95% of diffuse aggressive B-cell and 90% of peripheral T-cell lymphomas stain (209).
	CD20 ± CD79a	About 25% of classic HD stains for CD20, but typically only a minority of the atypical cells stain (187); about 95% of NLPHD stains (187); about 20% of classic HD stains for CD79a, but only about 1% of cases show labeling of most atypical cells (210); labeling of a minority of the neoplastic cells for CD20 and/or CD79a contrasts with the extensive labeling usually seen in diffuse aggressive B-cell lymphomas (187).
	CD3 (polyclonal)	Although about 10% of classic HD cases have been reported to stain (211), definite membrane staining is rare in our experience; the atypical cells in classical HD and NLPHD are ringed by CD3+ T cells (212), which can erroneously be interpreted as staining of the atypical cells.
	± EBV, EMA, fascin	Less than 5% of NLPHD cases, about 20% of nodular sclerosis cases, about 70% of mixed cellularity cases, and about 95% of HIV-associated cases stain for the latent membrane protein (LMP) of EBV (119,213–216); about 70% of NLPHD cases and about 5% of classic HD cases show membrane and/or paranuclear staining for EMA (about 20% of cases show focal cytoplasmic staining) (110); antibodies to fascin label the atypical cells in cases of classic HD but not in cases of NLPHD (217).
Nodular lymphocyte predominance Hodgkin's disease (NLPHD) versus other lymphomas	CD20 ± CD79a	About 95% of NLPHD stains for CD20 and CD79a (in contrast to cases of classic HD, most atypical cells stain) (187,210); B-cell markers highlight the large nodules of B cells in the background.
	CD3	The atypical cells in NLPHD and classic HD are ringed by T cells (212).
	CD45	About 65% of NLPHD stains, whereas less than 5% of classic HD stains (209).
	CD57	In contrast to cases of classic HD and large B-cell lymphomas rich in T cells, many of the T cells that surround the atypical cells in NLPHD express CD57 (125,126).
	EMA	About 70% of NLPHD cases but only about 5% of classic HD cases show membrane and/or paranuclear staining (110).
	± EBV, J chain, BCL-2	In contrast to classic HD cases in which about 50% stain for the LMP of EBV, less than 5% of NLPHD cases stain (119,213–216); about 60% of cases express J chain (218); cases do not stain for the BCL-2 protein (133,134).

EBV, Epstein-Barr virus; EMA, epithelial membrane antigen; HIV, human immunodeficiency virus.

proximately 25% of cases were misclassified. More than 10% of cases that were thought to represent classic Hodgkin's disease had immunophenotypic findings indicative of NLPHD (123). Cases of NLPHD may be confused with cases of follicular or diffuse B-cell lymphoma, and an approach to these problems is outlined in the following sections.

Nodular Lymphocyte Predominance versus the Cellular Phase of Nodular Sclerosis or Follicular Hodgkin's Disease

Although expression of CD45 by the neoplastic ''popcorn'' cells supports the diagnosis of NLPHD over nodular forms of classic Hodgkin's disease, ringing of the neoplastic cells by T cells and the infrequent occurrence of tumor cells bordering on one another makes this marker of limited utility (123). Because neoplastic cells in some cases that appear to represent NLPHD may stain for CD15 or CD30 (123), other markers are helpful in this problem area. Although extensive staining for a B-lineage marker supports NLPHD, this finding may be observed in so-called follicular Hodgkin's disease (15). The J chain and BCL-6 protein are almost always present in popcorn cells and never in classic Hodgkin's cells (124). The presence of EMA favors NLPHD, although classic Hodgkin's cells can sometimes express this antigen. Rosetting of neoplastic cells by $CD3^+$ T cells that are often also $CD57^+$ supports NLPHD (123,125,126). Immunoglobulin light-chain restriction in the popcorn cells, particularly the κ type, is a feature of NLPHD (127); this finding has been confirmed by studies of immunoglobulin mRNA and DNA (128–132).

Nodular Lymphocyte Predominance versus Follicular Lymphoma

A problem in discriminating between nodular lymphocyte predominance and follicular lymphoma may arise in cases of NLPHD when there are very few atypical cells or in follicular lymphomas composed principally of small cleaved cells or centrocytes with only few large cells or centroblasts. Expression of EMA or J chain by popcorn cells or their ringing by $CD57^+$ T cells supports NLPHD. Although atypical large cells in both lymphomas may show immunoglobulin light-chain restriction, the background small lymphocytes are monoclonal in follicular lymphoma and polyclonal in NLPHD. Follicular lymphoma cells are often $CD10^+$, and those comprising the nodules of NLPHD show the $IgM^+IgD^+CD10^-$ phenotype of primary follicle B cells. BCL-2 expression is typically seen in follicular lymphoma but not reported in the lymphocytic and histiocytic (L&H) cells of NLPHD (133,134).

Nodular and Diffuse Lymphocyte Predominance versus Diffuse Large B-Cell Lymphoma

Because evidence suggests that a subset of diffuse large cell lymphomas rich in T cells or macrophages represents progression of NLPHD, it is not surprising that there are not good immunophenotypic criteria for separating diffuse areas of NLPHD from T-cell– or macrophage-rich B-cell lymphomas (135–137). The utility of antibody stains rests on the identification of nodular areas that may be difficult to perceive without the aid of a B-cell marker such as CD20. The ringing of L&H or popcorn cells by $CD57^+$ T cells is seen in the nodules of NLPHD but not when these cells are in internodular or diffuse areas (R. A. Warnke, unpublished observations). EMA may be present in NLPHD with diffuse areas and in the diffuse large B-cell lymphomas that are derived from NLPHD (135–137). Identification of a t(14; 18) translocation in a T-cell– or macrophage-rich large B-cell lymphoma mitigates against an association with NLPHD (135,138).

EVALUATION OF MACROPHAGE AND ACCESSORY CELL PROLIFERATIONS

Rosai-Dorfman Disease

Staining for S-100 protein is useful for identifying the atypical histiocytes in sinus histiocytosis with massive lymphadenopathy (SHML), also called Rosai-Dorfman disease (139–141). Although examples of Langerhans cell histiocytosis and interdigitating dendritic cell tumors and some examples of follicular dendritic cell tumors also express the S-100 protein, the staining highlights the abundant cytoplasm, which often contains lymphocytes, plasma cells, neutrophils, or red blood cells in cases of SHML (Table 4.10). Subtle extranodal examples of Rosai-Dorfman disease often benefit from S-100 staining.

Langerhans Cell Histiocytosis

S-100 protein is a sensitive marker for Langerhans cell histiocytosis (142,143). The paraffin-reactive antibody to CD1a is a valuable adjunct, because it seldom reacts with other neoplasms in the differential diagnosis (143,144) (see Chapter 51).

Follicular Dendritic Cell Tumors

Follicular dendritic cell tumors are rare. Identification requires markers for complement receptor proteins such as CD21 and CD35 (145,146) or newer markers such as CNA.42 (147). If tissue is available for ultrastructural examination, desmosomes may be identified; an immunohistochemical alternative is the identification of desmoplakin in about one half of cases (145). A subset of these neoplasms stains for S-100 protein (145,146). In one series, most neoplasms expressed EMA; however, keratin staining has not been reported. These neoplasms lack expression of CD45 (146). Rare proliferations of follicular dendritic cells in extranodal sites such as the liver have been labeled inflammatory pseudotumor and have contained EBV (148).

Interdigitating Dendritic Cell Tumors

Interdigitating dendritic cell tumors are rare. Identification by their reactivity for S-100 protein and CD68 (144,149) is compromised by the reactivity of many other tumor types for these markers (150–152). A large panel of markers to a variety of hematopoietic and nonhematopoietic cell antigens is usually required to support the diagnosis of an interdigitating dendritic cell neoplasm, which typically stains for CD45 and for additional hematopoietic cell markers such as CD43 and CD45RO (144,149).

Malignant Tumors of Histiocytes

Most true histiocytic neoplasms of the past (e.g., cases of malignant histiocytosis) represent ALCLs or other T- or B-

TABLE 4.10. *Evaluation of macrophage and accessory cell proliferations in paraffin sections*

Differential diagnosis	Panel antibodies	Comment
Rosai-Dorfman disease	S-100	About 100% stain (139–141).
Langerhans cell histiocytosis	S-100	About 100% stain (142,143).
	CD1A	About 100% stain (143).
Follicular dendritic cell tumor	CD21 ± CNA.42	About 95% stain (145–147).
	EMA	About 70% stain (145,146).
	S-100	About 40% stain (145,146).
Interdigitating dendritic cell tumor	S-100	About 100% stain (144,149).
	CD68	About 100% stain (144,149).
	CD45 ± CD43 and other markers	About 70% stain (144,149).
Malignant tumors of histiocytes	CD68 ± lysozyme	About 100% stain (154,155).
	CD45 ± CD43 and other markers	About 70% stain (154,155).

cell lymphomas, and rare examples represent infection-associated hemophagocytic syndromes (153). The current definition requires cytologic evidence of malignancy and expression of markers specific for hematopoietic cells (e.g., CD45, CD43, CD45RO) together with expression of histiocytic markers such as CD68 and lysozyme (154,155). Lysozyme is an important marker in this context, but the interpretation of positive staining may be difficult because lysozyme is easily taken up by cells from the surrounding interstitial fluid. This results in a diffuse cytoplasmic stain that often overlaps into the nucleus. In contrast, when lysozyme is synthesized by cells, the cytoplasmic staining has a granular quality, often with concentration in the Golgi region, and the nucleus is unstained. Valid examples of histiocytic neoplasms lack expression of T- and B-cell–specific markers or CD30.

Many tumors of histiocytic lineage exhibit phenotypic characteristics of interdigitating dendritic cells and monocyte-macrophages. This is not surprising, because both are derived from the same bone marrow–derived progenitor cell.

EVALUATION OF UNDIFFERENTIATED MALIGNANT NEOPLASMS

A panel of antibodies that includes those against leukocyte common antigen, low-molecular-weight cytokeratin, and S-100 protein can identify most lymphomas, carcinomas, and melanomas that masquerade as undifferentiated malignant neoplasms (156) (Table 4.11). The lymphomas that are identified by this approach have the behavior of diffuse large cell lymphoma (157). The lineage markers CD20 and CD3 may be used in place of CD45. Additional markers may be needed to confirm a diagnosis of carcinoma, melanoma, or a specific sarcoma. Diagnosis of an undifferentiated malignant neoplasm in a pediatric patient may require antibodies against muscle markers, neuroendocrine markers, and CD99,

TABLE 4.11. *Evaluation of undifferentiated malignant neoplasms in paraffin sections and the reaction patterns expected in lymphomas*

Differential diagnosis	Panel antibodies	Comment
Lymphoma versus other neoplasm	CD45 and/or CD20 plus CD3	About 95% of diffuse, aggressive B-cell lymphomas, about 90% of peripheral T-cell lymphomas, and about 95% of extramedullary myeloid tumors stain for CD45, whereas nonhematopoietic tumors rarely stain (96,209,219); the lineage markers CD20 and CD3 are as sensitive and more specific for lymphoma.
	Cytokeratins	About 35% of plasma cell neoplasms (103), about 30% of anaplastic large cell lymphomas (220), and rare large B-cell lymphomas stain (220,221).
	S-100	Rare T-cell lymphoproliferative disorders express S-100 protein (222).
	± CD30	CD30 may be added to the panel to identify an anaplastic large cell lymphoma, because about 40% of anaplastic large cell lymphomas lack CD45 expression and less than 50% express CD3 (113,201).
	± CD79, VS38 or CD138/ syndecan	These markers may be useful to identify plasma cell neoplasms because these tumors typically lack expression of CD45 and CD20 (104).
	± MPO and CD68	Because about 95% of extramedullary myeloid tumors stain for CD45, the addition of one or more myeloid markers to the panel prevents the erroneous diagnosis of lymphoma in a case of myeloid leukemia.

as well as markers for lymphoblastic and myeloblastic disease. Modification of this approach is necessary for identifying ALCLs, anaplastic plasma cell neoplasms, and extramedullary myeloid tumors (Table 4.11) (see Chapter 30).

TECHNICAL ASPECTS

Immunohistochemical methods continue to evolve; for example, the field of antigen retrieval has seen many changes in the past few years. It is beyond the scope of this chapter to cover the numerous and ever-changing technical aspects of the immunohistochemical methods that are applied to frozen and paraffin tissue sections. A brief overview with selected references is provided in the following sections, and more information can be found in Chapters 11 and 12.

Freezing, Transport, and Storage of Fresh or Frozen Tissue

Any specimen suspected of harboring lymphoma should be submitted to the pathologist intact in saline or culture medium in a Petri dish or other specimen container to avoid desiccation of the tissue (158–160). Most lymph node and other tissue biopsies yield sufficient tissue for routine histologic analysis such that fresh cells or frozen tissue can be reserved for phenotypic and genotypic studies. Storage of a lymph node at 4°C for 24 hours or occasionally longer is often satisfactory for morphologic assessment, and a surprising number of cellular antigens are also preserved. Cooling a specimen to 4°C delays autolysis, and slicing lymph nodes at 2- to 3-mm intervals can enhance cellular preservation for optimal fixation. Ammonium sulfate–based transport medium such as Michel's medium may not preserve some antigens and the morphologic preservation is often suboptimal.

Representative tissue should be frozen whenever lymphoma is a reasonable possibility because most of the ancillary studies in hematopathology are best performed on frozen tissue. Frozen tissue can be used for several immunostains that do not work on paraffin-embedded tissue, and the same frozen tissue can be used for molecular studies such as VDJ or T γ PCR to determine B- or T-cell clonality (the success rate is often higher with frozen than with paraffin-embedded tissue, and confirmatory studies may be performed by the Southern blot method). Snap freezing in liquid nitrogen or in an isopentane and dry ice mixture is ideal, but satisfactory results may also be obtained if a slice less than 2 mm thick is frozen on a rapid-freeze chuck accessory in a cryotome. Tissue can be frozen in embedding medium in electron microscopy embedding capsules (Appendix 1) or on a cryostat chuck. The use of plastic capsules permits easy storage and avoids desiccation of specimens. Tissue frozen in OCT, a hyperviscous mounting medium, on a chuck or on a solid block of OCT must be wrapped in foil or plastic for storage to avoid desiccation. A surgical pathologist often is requested to perform frozen sections during surgery to assess adequacy of a specimen for diagnosis. Frozen sections are also performed to determine the optimal allocation of tissue for routine and special studies. When the amount of tissue is limited, the frozen section remnant can be left frozen and retained for possible phenotypic or genotypic studies, if the cut surface is covered with additional freezing medium and refrozen.

Frozen tissue is ideally stored at −70°C, but storage at −20°C is probably suitable for many antigens. Because many microtomes and refrigerator freezing compartments feature automatic defrost cycles, it is critical to transfer frozen tissue to a noncycling freezer for safekeeping. An alternative is to freeze and perform short-term storage in an automatic cryobath. When the frozen tissue is transported, it must be packaged in sufficient dry ice to prevent thawing in transit. Many antigens may survive improper freezing or thawing, but the accurate detection of some antigens such as immunoglobulins usually requires optimally frozen tissue.

Fixation in Formalin, Mercuric Chloride, Bouin's Solution, or Alcohol

The most critical factors in the preparation of optimal histologic sections include fixation and technical precision. Lymph nodes should be sliced completely at 2- to 3-mm intervals. Many laboratories employ two fixatives in the routine fixation of lymph nodes. One is generally a metal-based fixative, and the second is usually neutral-buffered formaldehyde. The particular metal fixative varies according to the preference of the surgical pathologist but is commonly B5, neutral Zenker's solution, Bouin's solution, or zinc sulfate. Although B5 yields excellent nuclear detail, it has several disadvantages. Close attention must be paid to time of fixation, mercuric chloride crystals must be removed from sections, the cost is relatively high, and mercury presents an environmental hazard. Nonspecific staining may be encountered with immunologic stains on tissues overfixed in B5 or in Zenker's fixative (see Fig. 4.5). Zinc sulfate is an attractive second fixative because it often yields good nuclear detail, is low in cost, and requires no special precautions for disposal.

Alcohol-based fixatives have been promoted for enhanced preservation of some antigens and for enhanced preservation of RNA and DNA for a variety of molecular studies. However, morphology may be suboptimal after alcohol fixation, particularly in small biopsy specimens. As a general rule, formalin, preferably buffered, is the most satisfactory fixative for immunohistochemistry. A more detailed discussion of different fixatives is provided by Banks (161). Plastic embedding may be used to enhance cytologic detail; technical modifications have been made to preserve immunoreactivity for many antigens (162,163). Methods employing cold acetone fixation followed by methyl benzoate and xylene treatment before paraffin embedding (AMEX and ModAMEX) have also been used to preserve morphology and enhance antigenicity (164,165).

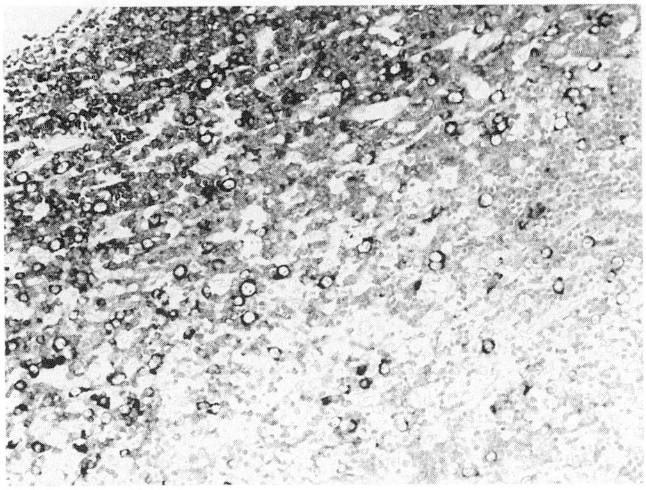

FIG. 4.5. Nonspecific labeling of small and large lymphoid cells for the latent membrane protein of Epstein-Barr virus (EBV LMP). A peripheral band of nonspecific staining of small and large lymphoid cells may be seen with this antibody cocktail, particularly when tissue is fixed in mercury-based fixatives such as B5. Staining was performed on the Ventana ES (immunoperoxidase stain, original magnification: 200× magnification).

Heat-induced antigen retrieval methods have improved the detectability of many antigens in variously fixed and processed tissues, giving the pathologist more freedom in choosing a fixative. For example, the detection of CD20 is markedly enhanced in Bouin-fixed, acid-decalcified bone marrows by heat-induced antigen retrieval.

Preparation, Handling, and Storage of Slides

Frozen Sections

Adherence of tissue to glass slides is enhanced by overnight storage of the frozen section in a dry environment at room temperature or in a freezer. Tissues prone to detachment such as skin or bone marrow should be placed on specially treated slides (e.g., poly-L-lysine coated, sialinized). Slides must be kept dry before staining. For example, slides fixed in acetone before storage may be wrapped individually in foil if stored in a freezer before staining. Unfixed slides stored in the freezer in a dry environment should be immediately transferred to fixative before staining so that moisture does not develop on the slides and alter antigenicity.

Paraffin Sections

Adherence of paraffin sections to glass slides is enhanced by placement on poly-L-lysine–coated or sialinized slides. Use of pretreated glass slides has become more important, because antigen retrieval methods may employ ''harsh'' buffers such as EDTA and Tris (Figs. 4.2 and 4.3); moreover, heating methods such as the use of a pressure cooker or microwave oven may promote alteration or disintegration of the sections. Although some antigens may be detected in sections that are baked at high temperatures, it is preferable not to bake sections at a temperature higher than 60°C. Although some antigens may be detected in paraffin sections that have been stored at room temperature for prolonged periods, some antigens are rendered undetectable after variable periods of storage. Such antigens are best detected on fresh sections from the paraffin block.

Antigen Retrieval Using Enzymes and Heat

Enzyme digestion has been used since the early days of paraffin section immunohistochemistry to enhance the detectability of a variety of cellular antigens such as immunoglobulin (166). The development of antigen unmasking methods that employ heat through microwaving, steaming, pressure cooking, or other techniques has improved the detection of many epitopes and is a necessary pretreatment for some of the new and important markers (Figs. 4.1 through 4.4) (167,168). A large and growing body of information compares different enzymes, buffers, and heat delivery systems (167,169,170) that are applied to the detection of a wide variety of cellular antigens.

Unfortunately, there are no simple rules for antigen detection, and the antigen retrieval technique needs to be individualized for each antibody. A few markers such as neutrophil elastase as detected by clone NP57 only work on paraffin sections that have not been pretreated with enzyme or heat (169). Other markers such as CD21 (clone 1F8) only work with enzyme or a proprietary antigen retrieval solution (Dako, Carpinteria, CA) as opposed to no pretreatment or conventional heat pretreatment (169). Some markers such as CD23 are best detected after enzyme pretreatment if one clone (BU38) is used (167), whereas only heat is efficacious if a different clone (MHM6) is used (169). The data in the literature are not entirely consistent, and a variety of factors probably are important, including fixation and processing variables, the particular target antigenic determinant, antigen retrieval techniques, and detection methods. Antigen retrieval methods often need to be optimized for individual antibodies in particular laboratories.

Many cellular antigens may be detected after no pretreatment or after multiple different pretreatments. Sometimes, a particular pretreatment but not another may work on a particular case (e.g., detection of CD30 with antibody BerH2 after protease pretreatment but not after microwaving in citrate buffer). Material fixed briefly allows detection of CD20 by L26 without antigen retrieval; when a specimen has been fixed only briefly, microwave treatment in citrate buffer may even abolish the reaction of L26 with CD20. After prolonged fixation, heat-induced antigen retrieval may be necessary to detect CD20. Morphology may be adversely affected by some pretreatments (e.g., pressure cooking in Tris buffer at pH 10.0); this may lead to the selection of a buffer and heat delivery method that gives less intense immunolabeling with a higher concentration of antibody to allow better preservation of morphology. Double-label immunohistochemistry re-

TABLE 4.12. *Principal antibodies used in the immunohistochemical analysis of paraffin–embedded lymphoid tissues*

Antigen	Antibody (clone or polyclonal)	Treatment	Source
ALK kinase (Fig. 4.3)	ALK-1	H	Dako
BCL-2 (Fig. 4.1)	124	H	Dako
CD1a	010	H	AMAC
CD3	Polyclonal	H,[a] E	Dako
CD4	1F6	H	Novocastra
CD5	4C7	H	Novocastra
CD8	C8/144B	H	Dako
CD10	56C6	H	Novocastra
CD15	LeuM1	N,[b] E, H	Becton-Dickinson
CD20	L26	N, E, H[a]	Dako
CD21	1F8	E	Dako
CD23	BU38	E	Binding Site
CD30	BerH2	E, H[a]	Dako
CD31	JC/70A	E	Dako
CD34	My10	N,[a] H	Becton-Dickinson
CD43	L60/Leu22	N, E, H[a]	Becton-Dickinson
CD45RA	4KB5	N,[a] H	Dako
CD45	PD7/26 (anti-CD45RB)	N, E, H[a]	Dako
CD45RO	A6	N, E, H[a]	Zymed
CD56 (Fig. 4.4)	123C3	H	Monosan
CD57	HNK-1	N[b]	Becton-Dickinson
CD61	Y2/51	E,[a] H	Dako
CD68	KP1	N, E, H[a]	Dako
CD79a	JCB117	H	Dako
CD99 (MIC-2)	12E7	N, H[a]	Dako
CNA.42	CNA.42	E[b]	Dako
Cyclin D1 (BCL-1) (Fig. 4.2)	DCS-6	H	Dako
Elastase	NP57	N	Dako
EBV-LMP	CS1–4	N,[a] H	Dako
EMA	E29	N,[a] H	Dako
Factor VIII	F8/86	H	Dako
Glycophorin C	Ret40f	E	Dako
Immunoglobulins			
Alpha chains	Polyclonal	N, E,[a] H	Dako
Delta chains	Polyclonal	H	Dako
Gamma chains	Polyclonal	N, E,[a] H	Dako
Kappa chains	Polyclonal	N, E,[a] H	Dako
Lambda chains	Polyclonal	N, E,[a] H	Dako
Mu chains	Polyclonal	E,[a] H	Dako
Ki-67	Ki-67 (polyclonal)	H	Dako
	MIB-1	H	AMAC
Lysozyme	Polyclonal	E	Dako
Myeloperoxidase	Polyclonal	N	Dako
S-100	Polyclonal	N, E,[a] H	Dako
TCR beta chains	BF-1	E[c]	T-cell Diagnostics
TIA-1	NS/1-AG4	H	Coulter
TdT	Polyclonal	H	Supertechs
VS38	VS38	H	Dako

N, none; E, enzyme; H, heat.
[a] Preferred.
[b] Anti-mu detection.
[c] Tyramide.

quires selection of a pretreatment suitable for both of the markers that are being labeled. Our preferences for many of the common leukocyte markers are included in Table 4.12.

Monoclonal and Polyclonal Antibodies

Table 4.12 lists the principal antibodies that we use in routinely fixed and paraffin-embedded tissue sections. For monoclonal antibodies, we include the clone designation. Although a common source for each antibody is provided, many antibodies can be obtained from more than one source. New markers reactive with fixation-resistant epitopes continue to be produced, and advances in the unmasking of antigenic determinants after routine fixation will continue to modify the list of antibodies that can be used in clinical immunodiagnosis.

With few exceptions, monoclonal antibodies that stain well in paraffin sections stain as well or better in acetone-fixed frozen sections. Antigenic determinants embedded in the cell membrane or within the cytoplasm or nucleus are more easily detected in cell monolayers or tissue sections than in cells in suspension, which requires permeabilization of the cell membrane. Cytoplasmic or nuclear antigens may be preferentially detectable in paraffin rather than frozen sections (e.g., immunoglobulins in plasma cells, cyclin D1/BCL-1 protein in mantle cell lymphomas) (Fig. 4.2). Polyclonal antisera often contain a significant number of unwanted reactivities that may lead to nonspecific staining in paraffin sections and limit their application to fresh cells in suspension or to cryostat sections. Nevertheless, those generated by immunization with highly purified antigens may work well in fresh and fixed tissues (12,38).

Detection Methods

It is beyond the scope of this chapter to discuss the many methods for detection that have been addressed in several articles (158,159,171,172). A variety of indirect three-stage methods can be used successfully to label a wide range of leukocyte markers. For example, several methods may be used to detect the binding of a mouse monoclonal antibody: goat anti-mouse followed by fluorochrome-labeled or enzyme-labeled swine anti-goat; biotin-labeled goat anti-mouse followed by enzyme labeled streptavidin (Fig. 4.4) or enzyme-labeled avidin-biotin complexes (ABC); or goat anti-mouse followed by labeled enzyme anti-enzyme complexes (generated in the same species as the primary antibody— PAP for horseradish peroxidase or APAAP for alkaline phosphatase). Occasionally, a more specific method, such as using immunoglobulin heavy-chain–specific conjugates to detect the μ chain of certain mouse monoclonal antibodies such as Leu-M1 and Leu-7, may be useful (112).

Some extremely sensitive methods employ biotinylated tyramine (173,174). With the use of these amplification methods, some monoclonal antibodies that only work on cryostat sections with conventional detection methods may work on paraffin sections and at extremely low antibody concentrations. Nevertheless, not all antibodies benefit from these enhanced detection methods. Nonspecific fine granular background staining may occur, particularly when buffers such as EDTA and Tris are employed with heat-induced antigen retrieval.

Selected Pitfalls in Immunohistochemical Staining

Background Staining

The advent of monoclonal antibodies has resulted in a very low level of background staining, which usually was unobtainable with polyclonal antisera. However, in some cases, undesirable background staining may result if detection reagents are suboptimal. Some monoclonal antibodies are supplied in the form of ascites or purified monoclonal antibodies. These should be diluted with a sufficient quantity of nonspecific protein (e.g., bovine serum albumin, normal serum), or they may yield high background staining. This problem is not generally encountered when using hybridoma culture supernatants.

A second type of background staining arises when attempting to detect a cellular antigen present at substantial concentration in the extracellular environment. The best examples are immunoglobulin chains that are found in highest concentration in extracellular fluid (i.e., γ and α heavy chains and κ and λ light chains). The presence of these immunoglobulin classes may obscure a monoclonal pattern of immunoglobulin expressed by a population of lymphoma cells. Tissue washing procedures may diminish the amount of extracellular immunoglobulin in tissues but usually are applied only in research protocols.

A third type of background or nonspecific staining may be encountered at the edge of the tissue on sections. The cause of this ''edge artifact'' is unknown, but it can be particularly pronounced in small samples. Care must be taken to distinguish this artifact from true staining in the center of the specimen. We have also encountered a broader band of nonspecific edge staining, particularly in certain specimens fixed in mercury-based fixatives; sometimes, the nonspecific staining is restricted to certain antibodies (e.g., EBV LMP) (see Fig. 4.5).

Endogenous Peroxidase and Pseudoperoxidase

Endogenous peroxidase activity in cryostat sections is mainly seen in eosinophils, mast cells, and erythrocytes (i.e., pseudoperoxidase). Because these cells are easily recognized by their morphology and by intense granular cytoplasmic staining and because blocking procedures frequently diminish or destroy various antigenic reactivities, we rarely use blocking procedures for cryostat sections. To avoid these unwanted reactivities, the investigator may use a different enzyme label such as alkaline phosphatase. Most antigenic determinants that survive fixation and processing are resistant to alteration by blocking procedures. Although fixation and processing may diminish or destroy endogenous peroxidase activity, we usually incubate paraffin sections in 3% hydrogen peroxide in distilled water for 8 minutes.

Endogenous Alkaline Phosphatase

Alkaline phosphatase labeling is ideally suited to the study of tissues such as bone marrow that are rich in endogenous peroxidase or preparations with many erythrocytes containing pseudoperoxidase. In contrast to the antigenic destruction that occurs in cryostat sections subjected to blocking of endogenous peroxidase or pseudoperoxidase, such destruction does not occur when blocking endogenous alkaline phosphatase by adding levamisole to the enzyme substrate (this inhibitor selectively blocks tissue alkaline phosphatase activity, for example, in endothelial cells, bladder epithelium, kidney) without affecting the intestinal alkaline phosphatase used for antibody or streptavidin labeling.

Endogenous Biotin

Endogenous avidin binding activity usually results from high levels of tissue biotin, as in hepatocytes and renal tubules. Formerly, this pitfall was encountered only in cryostat sections, but newer heat-induced antigen retrieval techniques reveal endogenous biotin in paraffin sections (175–177). Such binding may be circumvented by use of a detection system that does not employ avidin or streptavidin or by sequential incubation with free avidin (or egg whites) followed by free biotin because biotin is univalent (175–177).

Automated Staining

High-quality and cost-effective manual labeling of cellular antigens in tissue sections may depend on considerable technical and mental dexterity in the performance of arduous multistep staining procedures. When less than optimally applied, these procedures may result in considerable variations among technologists and laboratories. The technical demands of manual staining and consequent labor costs, as well as the increasing number and variety of antibody tests, have generated several approaches to the automation of immunohistochemical staining.

An early approach to large-volume staining used detection reagents in Coplin jars (Fig. 4.4) (178). Some automated approaches have employed robotic arms to deliver slides to reagent containers (e.g., BioTek/Ventana Medical Systems, Tucson, AZ) or to deliver a reagent-containing pipette to an array of glass slides (e.g., Dako Autostainer, Carpinteria, CA). Those based on capillary action required pairing of customized slides (179). Those based on robotic delivery of reagents from a pipette mimic manual staining. Although the machines that employ robotic arms may have a considerable setup time to computer-match slides with reagents, they often provide flexibility by running several different detection protocols at the same time.

Other machines use menus stored in a computer that match bar-coded reagent dispensers with bar-coded slides (Ventana ES and Nexes, Tucson, AZ) (Figs. 4.1, 4.2, 4.3, and 4.5) (180). By optimizing reaction kinetics by air jets that swirl reagents and by incubations at up to 40°C, the staining time may be reduced twofold to threefold. Some of these systems employ standardized detection reagents that are U>.S. Food and Drug Administration approved. The increased amounts or costs of reagents with many of the machines may be offset by lowered technical costs. Automation can produce more standardized, high-quality immunohistochemical stains, ultimately leading to more accurate diagnoses and treatments.

Controls

Because most hematopoietic cell markers are normally present in tonsils or bone marrow, these tissues are ideal for titering antibodies and for serving as external positive control tissues. Many of these hematopoietic antigens are at least focally present in many tissues, and most diagnostic problem cases contain built-in positive controls (e.g., normal $CD20^+$ B cells in T-cell lymphomas, normal $CD3^+$ T cells in B-cell lymphomas, $CD15^+$ granulocytes in Hodgkin's disease). Such internal positive controls are the best indicator of the integrity of a particular antigenic determinant in a given tissue section. When panels of antibodies are constructed to include positive and negative markers for each diagnostic possibility (e.g., a keratin and a leukocyte marker for an undifferentiated malignant neoplasm), the slide with the unreactive marker may serve as a negative control. Preferably, each of the antibodies are from the same species, of the same isotype, and require the same pretreatment. If small panels of antibodies or antibodies from multiple species are employed, more attention must be paid to negative and positive controls.

SUMMARY AND CONCLUSIONS

The immunohistochemical analysis of lymphoid tissue begins with a careful evaluation of the histologic findings in conjunction with any pertinent clinical and laboratory findings. The diagnostic problem determines which antibodies are most useful to address the different diagnostic possibilities. By judicious selection of a particular panel of antibodies, the investigator is most likely to answer the diagnostic question in a timely and cost-effective manner. High-quality immunohistochemical stains are essential to facilitate interpretation of cellular reactivities. The cellular reactivities and patterns must be carefully correlated with the morphologic features. The remarkable and ongoing advances in reagents and methods allow most diagnostic problems in hematopathology to be addressed by studies in routine paraffin sections.

ACKNOWLEDGMENTS

We are indebted to the innumerable pathologists who have shared their diagnostic problems with us. They have provided the cases that have formed the foundation for our approach to diagnostic problems with lymphoid tissues. We have also benefited from stimulation by numerous technologists, residents, fellows, and colleagues. We are indebted to Matt van de Rijn for his critical review of the chapter.

APPENDIX 1. REPRESENTATIVE TISSUE FREEZING PROTOCOL

1. Cut two to four tissue blocks of approximately 5 × 5 × 3 mm. It is usually possible to freeze at least two capsules (i.e., electron microscopy embedding capsules).
2. Fill plastic capsules approximately three-fourths full with Tissue Tek O.C.T. embedding compound.
3. Insert one tissue block into the middle of each of two to four capsules. Make sure the tissue is placed about

halfway down into the O.C.T. so that it does not dry out.

4. If specimen is tiny (e.g., skin biopsy, bone marrow), mark the outside of the capsule with black permanent ink to show the location of the tissue. Bone marrow cores should be placed horizontally. For skin biopsies, standardize the orientation of the specimen so that well-oriented sections can be obtained.
5. Write the patient's name and date of specimen freezing on the front of the stringed tag; write the site and the specimen number, if available, on the back of the tag *in pencil*. Lay the string over the capsule tops, and seal the capsules.
6. Use one tag per patient, but all capsules from the same specimen may be strung along one tag.
7. Drop the capsules with the tag into the histobath or other freezing bath for rapid freezing and short-term storage.

APPENDIX 2. REPRESENTATIVE BIOTIN-AVIDIN HORSERADISH PEROXIDASE METHOD FOR FROZEN SECTION STAINING

Preparation

1. Cut the frozen specimens at 5 μm, and place three sections on a poly-L-lysine–coated slide.
2. Air dry overnight in a dry chamber.
3. The samples can be stored long term at $-70°C$ in an airtight slide box with Drierite.

Staining Procedure

1. Place in cold acetone for 10 minutes, and air dry.
2. Incubate primary antibodies at room temperature for 30 minutes.
3. Rinse in phosphate-buffered saline (PBS) $\times$ 2.
4. Incubate with biotin-conjugated goat anti-mouse IgG for 40 minutes.
5. Rinse in PBS $\times$ 2.
6. Incubate with streptavidin conjugated to horseradish peroxidase for 40 minutes.
7. Rinse in PBS $\times$ 2.
8. Prepare diaminobenzidene (DAB) according to the number of slides, and stain for 5 minutes.
9. Rinse with PBS; then rinse with water.
10. Incubate with 0.5% copper sulfate (0.5 gm cupric sulfate in 180 ml 1 N NaCL) for 5 minutes.
11. Rinse in water.
12. Counterstain in 2% methylene blue for 10 minutes.
13. Rinse and dehydrate through three changes of 100% ethanol, clear in three changes of Hemo De, and apply a coverslip.

APPENDIX 3. HEAT-INDUCED ANTIGEN RETRIEVAL BY MICROWAVE TREATMENT

Process

1. Deparaffinize slides through two changes of Hemo De, 10 minutes each. Hydrate slides to water: 10 dips each in two 100% ethanol vats, 95% ethanol, 80% ethanol, 70% ethanol, and two water changes.
2. Treat for endogenous peroxidase with 3% H_2O_2 in distilled water for 8 minutes.
3. Rinse in water.
4. Put into a black plastic staining dish (holds 25 slides, Shandon, Inc., Pittsburgh, PA, catalog #195, with slide rack, catalog #196). Immerse slides in appropriate buffer and cover with lid.
5. Microwave for a total of 15 minutes for one slide box and 20 minutes for two slide boxes. With 12 minutes remaining, reduce the power level to 80%. Microwave ovens vary in wattage, and the power levels often are different. Our microwave oven is 1.25 kW.
6. Make sure the liquid level does not go below the tissue; because the mixture boils, refill with warm buffer as needed.
7. Remove from microwave oven and uncover. Cool slides in the dish at room temperature for at least 30 minutes. Cooling time is critical!
8. After cooling, rinse the slides in water and then in PBS.
9. You are ready to start staining.

Buffers We Use

1. 10 mM citric acid monohydrate, pH 6 (Figs. 4.1 and 4.4)
2. 0.5M Tris base, pH 10 (Figs. 4.2 and 4.3)
3. 1 mM EDTA (Sigma #E4884), pH 8

APPENDIX 4. REPRESENTATIVE BIOTIN-AVIDIN HORSERADISH PEROXIDASE METHOD FOR PARAFFIN SECTION STAINING

1. Deparaffinize slides through two changes of Hemo De, 10 minutes each. Hydrate slides to water: 10 dips each in two 100% ethanol vats, 95% ethanol, 80% ethanol, 70% ethanol, and two water changes (Fig. 4.4).
2. Treat for endogenous peroxidase with 3% H_2O_2 in distilled water for 8 minutes.
3. Block endogenous peroxidase activity using 3% H_2O_2 in distilled water for 8 minutes.
4. Rinse in PBS.
5. Incubate with the primary antibody at room temperature for 30 minutes.
6. Rinse in PBS $\times$ 2.
7. Incubate with biotin-conjugated goat anti-mouse IgG or other appropriate secondary reagent (to detect binding of a mouse primary, we use goat anti-mouse IgG from Jackson ImmunoResearch, West Grove, PA, catalog #115-065-062, at 1:400 in Coplin jars [178]) for 40 minutes.
8. Rinse in PBS $\times$ 2.
9. Incubate with streptavidin conjugated to horseradish

peroxidase (Jackson ImmunoResearch, West Grove, PA, catalog #016-030-984; we use at 1:400 in Coplin jars) for 40 minutes.
10. Rinse in PBS × 2.
11. Prepare DAB (30 mg/mL of 3.3 DAB [Sigma #D5637] in 0.01% H_2O_2 in PBS) according to the number of slides. Stain for 5 minutes.
12. Rinse with PBS, and then rinse with water.
13. Incubate with 0.5% copper sulfate for 5 minutes.
14. Rinse in water × 2.
15. Counterstain in hematoxylin for 30 seconds, rinse, and blue in ammonia water.
16. Rinse in water.
17. Dehydrate through three changes of 95% ethanol and three changes of 100% ethanol. Clear in three changes of Hemo De, and apply a coverslip.

APPENDIX 5. REPRESENTATIVE TYRAMIDE AMPLIFICATION OF A BIOTIN-AVIDIN HORSERADISH PEROXIDASE METHOD IN PARAFFIN SECTIONS

1. Deparaffinize slides through two changes of Hemo De, 10 minutes each.
2. Hydrate slides to water: 10 dips each twice in 100% ethanol, 95% ethanol, 80% ethanol, 70% ethanol, and twice in water.
3. Block endogenous peroxidase activity using 3% H_2O_2 in distilled water for 8 minutes.
4. Rinse in water.
5. If needed, treat with the appropriate enzyme or heat treat for antigen retrieval.
6. Rinse in PBS.
7. Incubate with mouse monoclonal antibody at room temperature in a humidified box for 30 to 60 minutes.
8. Rinse in PBS.
9. Incubate with biotin-conjugated goat anti-mouse IgG for 40 minutes.
10. Rinse in PBS.
11. Incubate with streptavidin-conjugated to horseradish peroxidase for 40 minutes.
12. Rinse in PBS.
13. Incubate with biotinylated tyramine (500 μL of biotinylated tyramine plus 50 mL of Tris/HCl at pH 8.0 plus 100 μL of 30% H_2O_2) for 40 minutes. Biotinylated tyramine was prepared as described by Kerstens and colleagues (173).
14. Rinse in PBS.
15. Incubate with streptavidin-conjugated to horseradish peroxidase for 30 minutes.
16. Rinse in PBS.
17. Incubate in DAB for 5 minutes.
18. Rinse in water.
19. Incubate in 0.5% copper sulfate for 5 minutes.
20. Rinse in water.
21. Counterstain in hematoxylin for 30 seconds, rinse, and blue in ammonia water.
22. Rinse in water.
23. Dehydrate through three changes of 95% ethanol and three changes of 100% ethanol. Clear in three changes of Hemo De, and apply a coverslip.

REFERENCES

1. Ashton-Key M, Diss TC, Isaacson PG, et al. A comparative study of the value of immunohistochemistry and the polymerase chain reaction in the diagnosis of follicular lymphoma [See comments]. *Histopathology* 1995;27:501–508.
2. Browne G, Tobin B, Carney DN, et al. Aberrant MT2 positivity distinguishes follicular lymphoma from reactive follicular hyperplasia in B5- and formalin-fixed paraffin sections. *Am J Clin Pathol* 1991;96: 90–94.
3. Chilosi M, Mombello A, Menestrina F, et al. Immunohistochemical differentiation of follicular lymphoma from florid reactive follicular hyperplasia with monoclonal antibodies reactive on paraffin sections. *Cancer* 1990;65:1562–1569.
4. Veloso J, Rezuke W, Cartun R, et al. Immunohistochemical distinction of follicular lymphoma from follicular hyperplasia in formalin-fixed tissues using monoclonal antibodies MT2 and bcl-2. *Appl Immunohistochem* 1995;3:153–159.
5. Norton AJ, Rivas C, Isaacson PG. A comparison between monoclonal antibody MT2 and immunoglobulin staining in the differential diagnosis of follicular lymphoid proliferations in routinely fixed wax-embedded biopsies. *Am J Pathol* 1989;134:63–70.
6. Utz GL, Swerdlow SH. Distinction of follicular hyperplasia from follicular lymphoma in B5-fixed tissues: comparison of MT2 and bcl-2 antibodies [See comments]. *Hum Pathol* 1993;24:1155–1158.
7. Wood B, Bacchi M, Bacchi C, et al. Immunocytochemical differentiation of reactive hyperplasia from follicular lymphoma using monoclonal antibodies to cell surface and proliferation-related markers. *Appl Immunohistochem* 1994;2:48–53.
8. Said JW, Pinkus JL, Shintaku IP, et al. Alterations in fascin-expressing germinal center dendritic cells in neoplastic follicles of B-cell lymphomas. *Mod Pathol* 1998;11:1–5.
9. Gaulard P, d'Agay MF, Peuchmaur M, et al. Expression of the bcl-2 gene product in follicular lymphoma. *Am J Pathol* 1992;140: 1089–1095.
10. Gelb AB, Rouse RV, Dorfman RF, et al. Detection of immunophenotypic abnormalities in paraffin-embedded B-lineage non-Hodgkin's lymphomas. *Am J Clin Pathol* 1994;102:825–834.
11. LeBrun DP, Kamel OW, Cleary ML, et al. Follicular lymphomas of the gastrointestinal tract. Pathologic features in 31 cases and bcl-2 oncogenic protein expression. *Am J Pathol* 1992;140:1327–1335.
12. Levy R, Warnke R, Dorfman RF, et al. The monoclonality of human B-cell lymphomas. *J Exp Med* 1977;145:1014–1028.
13. Warnke R, Levy R. Immunopathology of follicular lymphomas: a model of B-lymphocyte homing. *N Engl J Med* 1978;298:481–486.
14. Ho J, Shintaku I, Preston M, et al. Can microwave antigen retrieval replace frozen section immunohistochemistry in the phenotyping of lymphoid neoplasms? A comparative study of kappa and lambda light chain staining in frozen sections, B5-fixed paraffin sections, and microwave urea antigen retrieval. *Appl Immunohistochem* 1994;2: 282–286.
15. Ashton-Key M, Thorpe PA, Allen JP, et al. Follicular Hodgkin's disease. *Am J Surg Pathol* 1995;19:1294–1299.
16. Butmarc JR, Kourea HP, Levi E, et al. Improved detection of CD5 epitope in formalin-fixed paraffin-embedded sections of benign and neoplastic lymphoid tissues by using biotinylated tyramine enhancement after antigen retrieval. *Am J Clin Pathol* 1998;109:682–688.
17. Swerdlow SH, Yang WI, Zukerberg LR, et al. Expression of cyclin
18. Yang WI, Zukerberg LR, Motokura T, et al. Cyclin D1 (Bcl-1, PRAD1) protein expression in low-grade B-cell lymphomas and reactive hyperplasia. *Am J Pathol* 1994;145:86–96.
19. Zukerberg LR, Yang WI, Arnold A, et al. Cyclin D1 expression in non-Hodgkin's lymphomas: detection by immunohistochemistry. *Am J Clin Pathol* 1995;103:756–760.

20. de Boer CJ, Schuuring E, Dreef E, et al. Cyclin D1 protein analysis in the diagnosis of mantle cell lymphoma. *Blood* 1995;86:2715–2723.
21. Brynes R, McCourty A, Tamayo R, et al. Demonstration of cyclin D1/bcl-1 in mantle cell lymphoma. *Appl Immunohistochem* 1997;5: 45–48.
22. Foon KA, Todd RFD. Immunologic classification of leukemia and lymphoma. *Blood* 1986;68:1–31.
23. Picker LJ, Weiss LM, Medeiros LJ, et al. Immunophenotypic criteria for the diagnosis of non-Hodgkin's lymphoma. *Am J Pathol* 1987; 128:181–201.
24. Kumar S, Green GA, Teruya-Feldstein J, et al. Use of CD23 (BU38) on paraffin sections in the diagnosis of small lymphocytic lymphoma and mantle cell lymphoma. *Mod Pathol* 1996;9:925–929.
25. Ngan BY, Picker LJ, Medeiros LJ, et al. Immunophenotypic diagnosis of non-Hodgkin's lymphoma in paraffin sections: co-expression of L60 (Leu-22) and L26 antigens correlates with malignant histologic findings. *Am J Clin Pathol* 1989;91:579–583.
26. Said JW, Stoll PN, Shintaku P, et al. Leu-22: a preferential marker for T-lymphocytes in paraffin sections. Staining profile in T- and B-cell lymphomas, Hodgkin's disease, other lymphoproliferative disorders, myeloproliferative diseases, and various neoplastic processes. *Am J Clin Pathol* 1989;91:542–549.
27. Poppema S, Hollema H, Visser L, et al. Monoclonal antibodies (MT1, MT2, MB1, MB2, MB3) reactive with leukocyte subsets in paraffin-embedded tissue sections. *Am J Pathol* 1987;127:418–429.
28. Arber D, Weiss L. CD43—a review. *Appl Immunohistochem* 1993; 1:88–96.
29. Soslow RA, Zukerberg LR, Harris NL, et al. BCL-1 (PRAD-1/cyclin D-1) overexpression distinguishes the blastoid variant of mantle cell lymphoma from B-lineage lymphoblastic lymphoma. *Mod Pathol* 1997;10:810–817.
30. Kumar S, Krenacs L, Otsuki T, et al. Bcl-1 rearrangement and cyclin D1 protein expression in multiple lymphomatous polyposis. *Am J Clin Pathol* 1996;105:737–743.
31. Shin S, Berry G, Weiss L. Infectious mononucleosis: diagnosis by in situ hybridization in two cases with atypical features. *Am J Surg Pathol* 1991;15:625–631.
32. Ohshima K, Takeo H, Kikuchi M, et al. Heterogeneity of Epstein-Barr virus infection in angioimmunoblastic lymphadenopathy type T-cell lymphoma. *Histopathology* 1994;25:569–579.
33. Mason DY, Cordell JL, Brown MH, et al. CD79A: a novel marker for B-cell neoplasms in routinely processed tissue samples. *Blood* 1995;86:1453–1459.
34. Algino KM, Thomason RW, King DE, et al. CD20 (pan-B cell antigen) expression on bone marrow-derived T cells. *Am J Clin Pathol* 1996;106:78–81.
35. Quintanilla-Martinez L, Preffer F, Rubin D, et al. CD20$^+$ T-cell lymphoma. Neoplastic transformation of a normal T-cell subset. *Am J Clin Pathol* 1994;102:483–489.
36. Beverley PC. Functional analysis of human T cell subsets defined by CD45 isoform expression. *Semin Immunol* 1992;4:35–41.
37. Ott MM, Ott G, Kuse R, et al. The anaplastic variant of centrocytic lymphoma is marked by frequent rearrangements of the bcl-1 gene and high proliferation indices. *Histopathology* 1994;24:329–334.
38. Mason DY, Krissansen GW, Davey FR, et al. Antisera against epitopes resistant to denaturation on T3 (CD3) antigen can detect reactive and neoplastic T cells in paraffin embedded tissue biopsy specimens. *J Clin Pathol* 1988;41:121–127.
39. Macon WR, Casey TT, Kinney MC, et al. Leu-22 (L60). A more sensitive marker than UCHL1 for peripheral T-cell lymphomas, particularly large-cell types. *Am J Clin Pathol* 1991;95:696–701.
40. Kurtin PJ, Roche PC. Immunoperoxidase staining of non-Hodgkin's lymphomas for T-cell lineage associated antigens in paraffin sections: comparison of the performance characteristics of four commercially available antibody preparations. *Am J Surg Pathol* 1993;17:898–904.
41. Cabecadas JM, Isaacson PG. Phenotyping of T-cell lymphomas in paraffin sections—which antibodies? *Histopathology* 1991;19: 419–424.
42. A clinical evaluation of the International Lymphoma Study Group classification of non-Hodgkin's lymphoma: the Non-Hodgkin's Lymphoma Classification Project. *Blood* 1997;89:3909–3918.
43. Cheung MM, Chan JK, Lau WH, et al. Primary non-Hodgkin's lymphoma of the nose and nasopharynx: clinical features, tumor immunophenotype, and treatment outcome in 113 patients. *J Clin Oncol* 1998; 16:70–77.
44. Chan JK, Sin VC, Wong KF, et al. Nonnasal lymphoma expressing the natural killer cell marker CD56: a clinicopathologic study of 49 cases of an uncommon aggressive neoplasm. *Blood* 1997;89: 4501–4513.
45. Miller TP, Grogan TM, Dahlberg S, et al. Prognostic significance of the Ki-67–associated proliferative antigen in aggressive non-Hodgkin's lymphomas: a prospective Southwest Oncology Group trial. *Blood* 1994;83:1460–1466.
46. Grierson HL, Wooldridge TN, Purtilo DT, et al. Low proliferative activity is associated with a favorable prognosis in peripheral T-cell lymphoma. *Cancer Res* 1990;50:4845–4848.
47. Namikawa R, Takeshita M. Proliferating cell population in angioimmunoblastic lymphadenopathy with dysproteinemia (AILD) lesions analyzed by double immunoenzymatic staining and immunomolecular markers. *Nippon Ketsueki Gakkai Zasshi* 1987;50:1644–1651.
48. Ansari MQ, Dawson DB, Nador R, et al. Primary body cavity-based AIDS-related lymphomas [See comments]. *Am J Clin Pathol* 1996; 105:221–229.
49. Karcher DS, Alkan S. Human herpesvirus-8–associated body cavity-based lymphoma in human immunodeficiency virus-infected patients: a unique B-cell neoplasm. *Hum Pathol* 1997;28:801–808.
50. Nador RG, Cesarman E, Chadburn A, et al. Primary effusion lymphoma: a distinct clinicopathologic entity associated with the Kaposi's sarcoma-associated herpesvirus. *Blood* 1996;88:645–656.
51. Delsol G, Lamant L, Mariame B, et al. A new subtype of large B-cell lymphoma expressing the ALK kinase and lacking the 2;5 translocation. *Blood* 1997;89:1483–1490.
52. Benharroch D, Meguerian-Bedoyan Z, Lamant L, et al. ALK-positive lymphoma: a single disease with a broad spectrum of morphology. *Blood* 1998;91:2076–2084.
53. Pinkus GS, Kurtin PJ. Epithelial membrane antigen—a diagnostic discriminant in surgical pathology: immunohistochemical profile in epithelial, mesenchymal, and hematopoietic neoplasms using paraffin sections and monoclonal antibodies. *Hum Pathol* 1985;16:929–940.
54. Chang K, Arber D, Weiss L. CD30: A review. *Appl Immunohistochem* 1993;1:244–255.
55. Stein H, Mason DY, Gerdes J, et al. The expression of the Hodgkin's disease associated antigen Ki-1 in reactive and neoplastic lymphoid tissue: evidence that Reed-Sternberg cells and histiocytic malignancies are derived from activated lymphoid cells. *Blood* 1985;66: 848–858.
56. Leung CY, Ho FC, Srivastava G, et al. Usefulness of follicular dendritic cell pattern in classification of peripheral T-cell lymphomas. *Histopathology* 1993;23:433–437.
57. Feller AC, Griesser H, Schilling CV, et al. Clonal gene rearrangement patterns correlate with immunophenotype and clinical parameters in patients with angioimmunoblastic lymphadenopathy. *Am J Pathol* 1988;133:549–556.
58. Weiss LM, Strickler JG, Dorfman RF, et al. Clonal T-cell populations in angioimmunoblastic lymphadenopathy and angioimmunoblastic lymphadenopathy-like lymphoma. *Am J Pathol* 1986;122:392–397.
59. Anagnostopoulos I, Hummel M, Finn T, et al. Heterogeneous Epstein-Barr virus infection patterns in peripheral T-cell lymphoma of angioimmunoblastic lymphadenopathy type. *Blood* 1992;80:1804–1812.
60. Weiss LM, Jaffe ES, Liu XF, et al. Detection and localization of Epstein-Barr viral genomes in angioimmunoblastic lymphadenopathy and angioimmunoblastic lymphadenopathy-like lymphoma. *Blood* 1992;79:1789–1795.
61. Hamilton-Dutoit SJ, Pallesen G. A survey of Epstein-Barr virus gene expression in sporadic non-Hodgkin's lymphomas. Detection of Epstein-Barr virus in a subset of peripheral T-cell lymphomas. *Am J Pathol* 1992;140:1315–1325.
62. Salhany KE, Feldman M, Kahn MJ, et al. Hepatosplenic gamma delta T-cell lymphoma: ultrastructural, immunophenotypic, and functional evidence for cytotoxic T lymphocyte differentiation. *Hum Pathol* 1997;28:674–685.
63. Farcet JP, Gaulard P, Marolleau JP, et al. Hepatosplenic T-cell lymphoma: sinusal/sinusoidal localization of malignant cells expressing the T-cell receptor gamma delta. *Blood* 1990;75:2213–2219.
64. Felgar RE, Macon WR, Kinney MC, et al. TIA-1 expression in lymphoid neoplasms: identification of subsets with cytotoxic T lym-

phocyte or natural killer cell differentiation. *Am J Pathol* 1997;150: 1893–1900.
65. Cooke CB, Krenacs L, Stetler-Stevenson M, et al. Hepatosplenic T-cell lymphoma: a distinct clinicopathologic entity of cytotoxic gamma delta T-cell origin [See comments]. *Blood* 1996;88:4265–4274.
66. Macon WR, Williams ME, Greer JP, et al. Natural killer–like T-cell lymphomas: aggressive lymphomas of T-large granular lymphocytes [See comments]. *Blood* 1996;87:1474–1483.
67. Murray A, Cuevas EC, Jones DB, et al. Study of the immunohistochemistry and T cell clonality of enteropathy-associated T cell lymphoma. *Am J Pathol* 1995;146:509–519.
68. de Bruin PC, Connolly CE, Oudejans JJ, et al. Enteropathy-associated T-cell lymphomas have a cytotoxic T-cell phenotype [published erratum appears in *Histopathology* 1997;31:578]. *Histopathology* 1997; 31:313–317.
69. Chott A, Haedicke W, Mosberger I, et al. Most CD56$^+$ intestinal lymphomas are CD8$^+$CD5$^-$ T-cell lymphomas of monomorphic small to medium size histology. *Am J Pathol* 1998;153:1483–1490.
70. Walsh SV, Egan LJ, Connolly CE, et al. Enteropathy-associated T-cell lymphoma in the west of Ireland: low-frequency of Epstein-Barr virus in these tumors. *Mod Pathol* 1995;8:753–757.
71. Micklem KJ, Dong Y, Willis A, et al. HML-1 antigen on mucosa-associated T cells, activated cells, and hairy leukemic cells is a new integrin containing the beta 7 subunit. *Am J Pathol* 1991;139: 1297–1301.
72. Spencer J, Cerf-Bensussan N, Jarry A, et al. Enteropathy-associated T cell lymphoma (malignant histiocytosis of the intestine) is recognized by a monoclonal antibody (HML-1) that defines a membrane molecule on human mucosal lymphocytes. *Am J Pathol* 1988;132: 1–5.
73. Quintanilla-Martinez L, Lome-Maldonado C, Ott G, et al. Primary intestinal non-Hodgkin's lymphoma and Epstein-Barr virus: high frequency of EBV-infection in T-cell lymphomas of Mexican origin. *Leuk Lymphoma* 1998;30:111–121.
74. Pan L, Diss TC, Peng H, et al. Epstein-Barr virus (EBV) in enteropathy-associated T-cell lymphoma (EATL). *J Pathol* 1993;170: 137–143.
75. de Bruin PC, Jiwa NM, Oudejans JJ, et al. Epstein-Barr virus in primary gastrointestinal T cell lymphomas: association with gluten-sensitive enteropathy, pathological features, and immunophenotype. *Am J Pathol* 1995;146:861–867.
76. Tsang WY, Chan JK, Ng CS, et al. Utility of a paraffin section-reactive CD56 antibody (123C3) for characterization and diagnosis of lymphomas. *Am J Surg Pathol* 1996;20:202–210.
77. Arber DA, Weiss LM, Albujar PF, et al. Nasal lymphomas in Peru. High incidence of T-cell immunophenotype and Epstein-Barr virus infection [See comments]. *Am J Surg Pathol* 1993;17:392–399.
78. Chan JK, Yip TT, Tsang WY, et al. Detection of Epstein-Barr viral RNA in malignant lymphomas of the upper aerodigestive tract [published erratum appears in *Am J Surg Pathol* 1994;18:1274]. *Am J Surg Pathol* 1994;18:938–946.
79. Strickler JG, Meneses MF, Habermann TM, et al. Polymorphic reticulosis: a reappraisal. *Hum Pathol* 1994;25:659–665.
80. van de Rijn M, Bhargava V, Molina-Kirsch H, et al. Extranodal head and neck lymphomas in Guatemala: high frequency of Epstein-Barr virus-associated sinonasal lymphomas. *Hum Pathol* 1997;28: 834–839.
81. van Gorp J, Weiping L, Jacobse K, et al. Epstein-Barr virus in nasal T-cell lymphomas (polymorphic reticulosis/midline malignant reticulosis) in western China. *J Pathol* 1994;173:81–87.
82. Van Gorp J, De Bruin PC, Sie-Go DM, et al. Nasal T-cell lymphoma: a clinicopathological and immunophenotypic analysis of 13 cases [See comments]. *Histopathology* 1995;27:139–148.
83. Chan JK, Tsang WY, Pau MY. Discordant CD3 expression in lymphomas when studied on frozen and paraffin sections. *Hum Pathol* 1995;26:1139–1143.
84. Suzuki R, Yamamoto K, Seto M, et al. CD7$^+$ and CD56$^+$ myeloid/natural killer cell precursor acute leukemia: a distinct hematolymphoid disease entity. *Blood* 1997;90:2417–2428.
85. Kumar S, Krenacs L, Medeiros J, et al. Subcutaneous panniculitic T-cell lymphoma is a tumor of cytotoxic T lymphocytes. *Hum Pathol* 1998;29:397–403.
86. Salhany KE, Macon WR, Choi JK, et al. Subcutaneous panniculitis-like T-cell lymphoma: clinicopathologic, immunophenotypic, and genotypic analysis of alpha/beta and gamma/delta subtypes. *Am J Surg Pathol* 1998;22:881–893.
87. Gonzalez CL, Medeiros LJ, Braziel RM, et al. T-cell lymphoma involving subcutaneous tissue. A clinicopathologic entity commonly associated with hemophagocytic syndrome. *Am J Surg Pathol* 1991; 15:17–27.
88. Smoller B, Bishop K, Glusac E, et al. Reassessment of lymphocyte immunophenotyping in the diagnosis of patch and plaque stage lesions of mycosis fungoides. *Appl Immunohistochem* 1995;3:32–36.
89. Hastrup N, Ralfkiaer E, Pallesen G. Aberrant phenotypes in peripheral T cell lymphomas. *J Clin Pathol* 1989;42:398–402.
90. Ashton-Key M, Diss TC, Du MQ, et al. The value of the polymerase chain reaction in the diagnosis of cutaneous T-cell infiltrates. *Am J Surg Pathol* 1997;21:743–747.
91. Chhanabhai M, Adomat SA, Gascoyne RD, et al. Clinical utility of heteroduplex analysis of TCR gamma gene rearrangements in the diagnosis of T-cell lymphoproliferative disorders. *Am J Clin Pathol* 1997;108:295–301.
92. Wong K, Chan J. Antimyeloperoxidase: antibody of choice for labeling of myeloid cells including diagnosis of granulocytic sarcoma. *Adv Anat Pathol* 1995;2:65–68.
93. Pinkus GS, Pinkus JL. Myeloperoxidase: a specific marker for myeloid cells in paraffin sections. *Mod Pathol* 1991;4:733–741.
94. Arber DA, Jenkins KA. Paraffin section immunophenotyping of acute leukemias in bone marrow specimens [See comments]. *Am J Clin Pathol* 1996;106:462–468.
95. Traweek ST, Arber DA, Rappaport H, et al. Extramedullary myeloid cell tumors: an immunohistochemical and morphologic study of 28 cases. *Am J Surg Pathol* 1993;17:1011–1019.
96. Hudock J, Chatten J, Miettinen M. Immunohistochemical evaluation of myeloid leukemia infiltrates (granulocytic sarcomas) in formaldehyde-fixed, paraffin-embedded tissue. *Am J Clin Pathol* 1994;102: 55–60.
97. Warnke RA, Pulford KA, Pallesen G, et al. Diagnosis of myelomonocytic and macrophage neoplasms in routinely processed tissue biopsies with monoclonal antibody KP1. *Am J Pathol* 1989;135: 1089–1095.
98. Taylor CR, Mason DY. The immunohistological detection of intracellular immunoglobulin in formalin-paraffin sections from multiple myeloma and related conditions using the immunoperoxidase technique. *Clin Exp Immunol* 1974;18:417–429.
99. Maia DM, Kell DL, Goates JJ, et al. The significance of light chain–restricted bone marrow plasma cells after peripheral blood stem cell transplantation for multiple myeloma. *Am J Clin Pathol* 1997; 107:643–652.
100. Aguilera NS, Kapadia SB, Nalesnik MA, et al. Extramedullary plasmacytoma of the head and neck: use of paraffin sections to assess clonality with in situ hybridization, growth fraction, and the presence of Epstein-Barr virus. *Mod Pathol* 1995;8:503–508.
101. Turley H, Jones M, Erber W, et al. VS38: a new monoclonal antibody for detecting plasma cell differentiation in routine sections. *J Clin Pathol* 1994;47:418–422.
102. Thomas G, Kay E, Nyhan B, et al. VS38c shows lack of specificity as a marker of plasma cells. *Appl Immunohistochem* 1997;5:185–188.
103. Wotherspoon AC, Norton AJ, Isaacson PG. Immunoreactive cytokeratins in plasmacytomas [See comments]. *Histopathology* 1989;14: 141–150.
104. Petruch UR, Horny HP, Kaiserling E. Frequent expression of haemopoietic and non-haemopoietic antigens by neoplastic plasma cells: an immunohistochemical study using formalin-fixed, paraffin-embedded tissue. *Histopathology* 1992;20:35–40.
105. Patsouris E, Noel H, Lennert K. Lymphoplasmacytic/lymphoplasmacytoid immunocytoma with a high content of epithelioid cells: histologic and immunohistochemical findings. *Am J Surg Pathol* 1990;14: 660–670.
106. Feiner HD, Rizk CC, Finfer MD, et al. IgM monoclonal gammopathy/Waldenstrom's macroglobulinemia: a morphological and immunophenotypic study of the bone marrow. *Mod Pathol* 1990;3:348–356.
107. Banks PMGE. The Interrelationship of Hodgkin's disease and non-Hodgkin's lymphoma. *Semin Diagn Pathol* 1992;9:249–314.
108. Dorfman RF, Gatter KC, et al. An evaluation of the utility of anti-granulocyte and anti-leukocyte monoclonal antibodies in the diagnosis of Hodgkin's disease. *Am J Pathol* 1986;123:508–519.
109. Medeiros LJ, Weiss LM, Warnke RA, et al. Utility of combining

antigranulocyte with antileukocyte antibodies in differentiating Hodgkin's disease from non-Hodgkin's lymphoma. *Cancer* 1988;62: 2475–2481.

110. Chittal SM, Caveriviere P, Schwarting R, et al. Monoclonal antibodies in the diagnosis of Hodgkin's disease: the search for a rational panel. *Am J Surg Pathol* 1988;12:9–21.
111. Arber D, Weiss L. CD15: a review. *Appl Immunohistochem* 1993;1: 17–30.
112. LeBrun DP, Kamel OW, Dorfman RF, et al. Enhanced staining for Leu M1 (CD15) in Hodgkin's disease using a secondary antibody specific for immunoglobulin M. *Am J Clin Pathol* 1992;97:135–138.
113. Falini B, Pileri S, Stein H, et al. Variable expression of leucocyte-common (CD45) antigen in CD30 (Ki-1)–positive anaplastic large-cell lymphoma: implications for the differential diagnosis between lymphoid and nonlymphoid malignancies. *Hum Pathol* 1990;21: 624–629.
114. Delsol G, Al ST, Gatter KC, et al. Coexpression of epithelial membrane antigen (EMA), Ki-1, and interleukin-2 receptor by anaplastic large cell lymphomas: diagnostic value in so-called malignant histiocytosis. *Am J Pathol* 1988;130:59–70.
115. Chittal SM, Delsol G. The interface of Hodgkin's disease and anaplastic large cell lymphoma. *Cancer Surv* 1997;30:87–105.
116. Macon WR, Williams ME, Greer JP, et al. T-cell–rich B-cell lymphomas: a clinicopathologic study of 19 cases [See comments]. *Am J Surg Pathol* 1992;16:351–363.
117. McBride JA, Rodriguez J, Luthra R, et al. T-cell–rich B large-cell lymphoma simulating lymphocyte-rich Hodgkin's disease [See comments]. *Am J Surg Pathol* 1996;20:193–201.
118. Kadin ME, Stites DP, Levy R, et al. Exogenous immunoglobulin and the macrophage origin of Reed-Sternberg cells in Hodgkin's disease. *N Engl J Med* 1978;299:1208–1214.
119. Delsol G, Brousset P, Chittal S, et al. Correlation of the expression of Epstein-Barr virus latent membrane protein and in situ hybridization with biotinylated *Bam*HI-W probes in Hodgkin's disease. *Am J Pathol* 1992;140:247–253.
120. d'Amore F, Johansen P, Houmand A, et al. Epstein-Barr virus genome in non-Hodgkin's lymphomas occurring in immunocompetent patients: highest prevalence in nonlymphoblastic T-cell lymphoma and correlation with a poor prognosis: Danish Lymphoma Study Group, LYFO. *Blood* 1996;87:1045–1055.
121. Loke SL, Ho F, Srivastava G, et al. Clonal Epstein-Barr virus genome in T-cell–rich lymphomas of B or probable B lineage. *Am J Pathol* 1992;140:981–989.
122. Myers JL, Kurtin PJ, Katzenstein AL, et al. Lymphomatoid granulomatosis: evidence of immunophenotypic diversity and relationship to Epstein-Barr virus infection. *Am J Surg Pathol* 1995;19:1300–1312.
123. von Wasielewski R, Werner M, Fischer R, et al. Lymphocyte-predominant Hodgkin's disease: an immunohistochemical analysis of 208 reviewed Hodgkin's disease cases from the German Hodgkin Study Group. *Am J Pathol* 1997;150:793–803.
124. Carbone A, Gloghini A, Gaidano G, et al. Expression status of BCL-6 and syndecan-1 identifies distinct histogenetic subtypes of Hodgkin's disease. *Blood* 1998;92:2220–2228.
125. Hansmann ML, Fellbaum C, Hui PK, et al. Correlation of content of B cells and Leu7-positive cells with subtype and stage in lymphocyte predominance type Hodgkin's disease. *J Cancer Res Clin Oncol* 1988; 114:405–410.
126. Kamel OW, Gelb AB, Shibuya RB, et al. Leu7 (CD57) reactivity distinguishes nodular lymphocyte Hodgkin's disease, T cell rich B cell lymphoma and follicular lymphoma. *Am J Pathol* 1993;142:541–546.
127. Schmid C, Sargent C, Isaacson PG. L and H cells of nodular lymphocyte predominant Hodgkin's disease show immunoglobulin light-chain restriction. *Am J Pathol* 1991;139:1281–1289.
128. Delabie J, Tierens A, Wu G, et al. Lymphocyte predominance Hodgkin's disease: lineage and clonality determination using a single-cell assay. *Blood* 1994;84:3291–3298.
129. Marafioti T, Hummel M, Anagnostopoulos I, et al. Origin of nodular lymphocyte-predominant Hodgkin's disease from a clonal expansion of highly mutated germinal-center B cells [See comments]. *N Engl J Med* 1997;337:453–458.
130. Stoler MH, Nichols GE, Symbula M, et al. Lymphocyte predominance Hodgkin's disease: evidence for a kappa light chain–restricted monotypic B-cell neoplasm. *Am J Pathol* 1995;146:812–818.
131. Braeuninger A, Kuppers R, Strickler JG, et al. Hodgkin and Reed-Sternberg cells in lymphocyte predominant Hodgkin disease represent clonal populations of germinal center–derived tumor B cells [published erratum appears in *Proc Natl Acad Sci USA* 1997;94:14211]. *Proc Natl Acad Sci USA* 1997;94:9337–9342.
132. von Wasielewski R, Wilkens L, Nolte M, et al. Light-chain mRNA in lymphocyte-predominant and mixed-cellularity Hodgkin's disease. *Mod Pathol* 1996;9:334–338.
133. Algara P, Martinez P, Sanchez L, et al. Lymphocyte predominance Hodgkin's disease (nodular paragranuloma)—a bcl-2 negative germinal centre lymphoma. *Histopathology* 1991;19:69–75.
134. Alkan S, Ross CW, Hanson CA, et al. Epstein-Barr virus and bcl-2 protein overexpression are not detected in the neoplastic cells of nodular lymphocyte predominance Hodgkin's disease. *Mod Pathol* 1995; 8:544–577.
135. De Jong D, Van Gorp J, Sie-Go D, et al. T-cell rich b-cell non-Hodgkin's lymphoma: a progressed form of follicle centre cell lymphoma and lymphocyte predominance Hodgkin's disease [See comments]. *Histopathology* 1996;28:15–24.
136. Delabie J, Vandenberghe E, Kennes C, et al. Histiocyte-rich B-cell lymphoma: a distinct clinicopathologic entity possibly related to lymphocyte predominant Hodgkin's disease, paragranuloma subtype. *Am J Surg Pathol* 1992;16:37–48.
137. Chittal SM, Brousset P, Voigt JJ, et al. Large B-cell lymphoma rich in T-cells and simulating Hodgkin's disease. *Histopathology* 1991; 19:211–220.
138. Hansmann ML, Shibata D, Lorenzen J, et al. Incidence of Epstein-Barr virus bcl-2 expression and chromosomal translocation t(14;18) in large cell lymphoma associated with paragranuloma (lymphocyte-predominant Hodgkin's disease). *Hum Pathol* 1994;25:240–243.
139. Eisen RN, Buckley PJ, Rosai J. Immunophenotypic characterization of sinus histiocytosis with massive lymphadenopathy (Rosai-Dorfman disease). *Semin Diagn Pathol* 1990;7:74–82.
140. Miettinen M, Paljakka P, Haveri P, et al. Sinus histiocytosis with massive lymphadenopathy: a nodal and extranodal proliferation of S-100 protein positive histiocytes? *Am J Clin Pathol* 1987;88:270–277.
141. Paulli M, Rosso R, Kindl S, et al. Immunophenotypic characterization of the cell infiltrate in five cases of sinus histiocytosis with massive lymphadenopathy (Rosai-Dorfman disease). *Hum Pathol* 1992;23: 647–654.
142. Azumi N, Sheibani K, Swartz WG, et al. Antigenic phenotype of Langerhans cell histiocytosis: an immunohistochemical study demonstrating the value of LN-2, LN-3, and vimentin. *Hum Pathol* 1988; 19:1376–1382.
143. Emile JF, Wechsler J, Brousse N, et al. Langerhans' cell histiocytosis: definitive diagnosis with the use of monoclonal antibody O10 on routinely paraffin-embedded samples. *Am J Surg Pathol* 1995;19: 636–641.
144. Weiss LM, Berry GJ, Dorfman RF, et al. Spindle cell neoplasms of lymph nodes of probable reticulum cell lineage: true reticulum cell sarcoma? *Am J Surg Pathol* 1990;14:405–414.
145. Chan JK, Fletcher CD, Nayler SJ, et al. Follicular dendritic cell sarcoma: clinicopathologic analysis of 17 cases suggesting a malignant potential higher than currently recognized. *Cancer* 1997;79:294–313.
146. Perez-Ordonez B, Erlandson RA, Rosai J. Follicular dendritic cell tumor: report of 13 additional cases of a distinctive entity. *Am J Surg Pathol* 1996;20:944–955.
147. Raymond I, Al Saati T, Tkaczuk J, et al. CNA.42, a new monoclonal antibody directed against a fixative-resistant antigen of follicular dendritic reticulum cells. *Am J Pathol* 1997;151:1577–1585.
148. Selves J, Meggetto F, Brousset P, et al. Inflammatory pseudotumor of the liver: evidence for follicular dendritic reticulum cell proliferation associated with clonal Epstein-Barr virus. *Am J Surg Pathol* 1996; 20:747–753.
149. Nakamura S, Koshikawa T, Kitoh K, et al. Interdigitating cell sarcoma: a morphologic and immunologic study of lymph node lesions in four cases. *Pathol Int* 1994;44:374–386.
150. McHugh M, Meittinen M. KP1 (CD68): its limited specificity for histiocytic tumors. *Appl Immunohistochem* 1994;2:186–190.
151. Tsang WY, Chan JK. KP1 (CD68) staining of granular cell neoplasms: is KP1 a marker for lysosomes rather than the histiocytic lineage? *Histopathology* 1992;21:84–86.
152. Gloghini A, Rizzo A, Zanette I, et al. KP1/CD68 expression in malignant neoplasms including lymphomas, sarcomas, and carcinomas. *Am J Clin Pathol* 1995;103:425–431.

153. Wilson MS, Weiss LM, Gatter KC, et al. Malignant histiocytosis: a reassessment of cases previously reported in 1975 based on paraffin section immunophenotyping studies. *Cancer* 1990;66:530–536.
154. Kamel OW, Gocke CD, Kell DL, et al. True histiocytic lymphoma: a study of 12 cases based on current definition. *Leuk Lymphoma* 1995; 18:81–86.
155. Lauritzen AF, Delsol G, Hansen NE, et al. Histiocytic sarcomas and monoblastic leukemias: a clinical, histologic, and immunophenotypical study. *Am J Clin Pathol* 1994;102:45–54.
156. Michie SA, Spagnolo DV, Dunn KA, et al. A panel approach to the evaluation of the sensitivity and specificity of antibodies for the diagnosis of routinely processed histologically undifferentiated human neoplasms. *Am J Clin Pathol* 1987;88:457–462.
157. Horning SJ, Carrier EK, Rouse RV, et al. Lymphomas presenting as histologically unclassified neoplasms: characteristics and response to treatment. *J Clin Oncol* 1989;7:1281–1287.
158. Rouse RV, Warnke RA. Special application of tissue section immunologic staining in the characterization of monoclonal antibodies and in the study of normal and neoplastic tissues. In: Weir DM, Herzenberg LA, Blackwell CC, Herzenberg LA, eds. *Handbook of experimental immunology*, 4th ed. Edinburgh: Blackwell, 1986:116.1–116.10.
159. Sheibani K. Immunohistochemical analysis of lymphoid tissue. In: Knowles DM, ed. *Neoplastic hematopathology*. Baltimore: Williams & Wilkins, 1992:197–213.
160. Weiss LM, Dorfman RF, Warnke RA. Lymph node work-up. In: Fenoglio-Preiser C, ed. *Advances in pathology*, vol 1. Chicago: Year Book Medical Publishers, 1988:111–130.
161. Banks PM. Technical factors in the preparation and evaluation of lymph node biopsies. In: Knowles DM, ed. *Neoplastic hematopathology*. Baltimore: Williams & Wilkins, 1992:367–384.
162. Casey TT, Olson SJ, Cousar JB, et al. Plastic section immunohistochemistry in the diagnosis of hematopoietic and lymphoid neoplasms. Clin Lab Med 1990;10:199–213.
163. Beckstead JH. Optimal antigen localization in human tissues using aldehyde-fixed plastic-embedded sections. *J Histochem Cytochem* 1985;33:954–958.
164. Delsol G, Chittal S, Brousset P, et al. Immunohistochemical demonstration of leucocyte differentiation antigens on paraffin sections using a modified AMeX (ModAMeX) method. *Histopathology* 1989;15: 461–471.
165. Sato Y, Mukai K, Watanabe S, et al. The AMeX method: a simplified technique of tissue processing and paraffin embedding with improved preservation of antigens for immunostaining. *Am J Pathol* 1986;125: 431–435.
166. Curran RC, Gregory J. Demonstration of immunoglobulin in cryostat and paraffin sections of human tonsil by immunofluorescence and immunoperoxidase techniques: effects of processing on immunohistochemical performance of tissues and on the use of proteolytic enzymes to unmask antigens in sections. *J Clin Pathol* 1978;31:974–983.
167. Cattoretti G, Pileri S, Parravicini C, et al. Antigen unmasking on formalin-fixed, paraffin embedded tissue sections. *J Pathol* 1993;171: 83–98.
168. Shi SR, Key ME, Kalra KL. Antigen retrieval in formalin-fixed, paraffin-embedded tissues: an enhancement method for immunohistochemical staining based on microwave oven heating of tissue sections. *J Histochem Cytochem* 1991;39:741–748.
169. Pileri SA, Roncador G, Ceccarelli C, et al. Antigen retrieval techniques in immunohistochemistry: comparison of different methods. *J Pathol* 1997;183:116–123.
170. Taylor CR, Shi SR, Chen C, et al. Comparative study of antigen retrieval heating methods: microwave, microwave and pressure cooker, autoclave, and steamer. *Biotech Histochem* 1996;71:263–270.
171. Gatter KC, Cordell JL, Falini B, et al. Monoclonal antibodies in diagnostic pathology: techniques and applications. *J Biol Res Mod* 1983; 2:369–395.
172. Hancock WH, Atkins RC. Immunohistological studies with monoclonal antibodies. In: Langone JJ, Van Vunakis H, ed. *Methods in enzymology*, vol 121 Orlando: Academic Press, 1986:828–848.
173. Kerstens HM, Poddighe PJ, Hanselaar AG. A novel in situ hybridization signal amplification method based on the deposition of biotinylated tyramine. *J Histochem Cytochem* 1995;43:347–352.
174. Jacobs W, Dhaene K, Van Marck E. Tyramine-amplified immunohistochemical testing using "homemade" biotinylated tyramine is highly sensitive and cost-effective [See comments]. *Arch Pathol Lab Med* 1998;122:642–643.
175. Miller R, Kubier P. Blocking of endogenous avidin-binding activity in immunohistochemistry: the use of egg whites. *Appl Immunohistochem* 1997;5:63–66.
176. Rodriquez-Soto J, Warnke R, Rouse R. Endogenous avidin-binding activity in paraffin-embedded tissue revealed after microwave treatment. *Appl Immunohistochem* 1997;5:59–62.
177. Wood GS, Warnke R. Suppression of endogenous avidin-binding activity in tissues and its relevance to biotin-avidin detection systems. *J Histochem Cytochem* 1981;29:1196–1204.
178. Bindl JM, Warnke RA. Advantages of detecting monoclonal antibody binding to tissue sections with biotin and avidin reagents in Coplin jars. *Am J Clin Pathol* 1986;85:490–493.
179. Brigati D, Budgeon LR, Unger ER, et al. Immunocytochemistry is automated: development of a robotic workstation based upon the capillary action principle. *J Histotechnol* 1988;11:165–183.
180. Grogan TM, Casey TT, Miller PC, et al. Automation of immunohistochemistry. In: Weinstein RS, ed. *Advances in pathology and laboratory medicine*, vol 6. St Louis: CV Mosby, 1993:253–283.
181. Gloghini A, Carbone A. The nonlymphoid microenvironment of reactive follicles and lymphomas of follicular origin as defined by immunohistology on paraffin-embedded tissues. *Hum Pathol* 1993;24: 67–76.
182. Schmid C, Isaacson PG. Proliferation centres in B-cell malignant lymphoma, lymphocytic (B-CLL): an immunophenotypic study. *Histopathology* 1994;24:445–451.
183. Said JW, Pinkus JL, Yamashita J, et al. The role of follicular and interdigitating dendritic cells in HIV-related lymphoid hyperplasia: localization of fascin. *Mod Pathol* 1997;10:421–427.
184. Norton AJ, Isaacson PG. Detailed phenotypic analysis of B-cell lymphoma using a panel of antibodies reactive in routinely fixed wax-embedded tissue. *Am J Pathol* 1987;128:225–240.
185. Segal GH, Stoler MH, Tubbs RR. The "CD43 only" phenotype: an aberrant, nonspecific immunophenotype requiring comprehensive analysis for lineage resolution. *Am J Clin Pathol* 1992;97:861–865.
186. Chadburn A, Knowles D. Paraffin-resistant antigens detectable by antibodies L26 and polyclonal CD3 predict the B or T cell lineage of 95% of diffuse aggressive non-Hodgkin's lymphomas. *Am J Clin Pathol* 1994;102:284–291.
187. Chang K, Arber D, Weiss L. CD20: A review. *Appl Immunohistochem* 1996;4:1–15.
188. Cartun RW, Coles FB, Pastuszak WT. Utilization of monoclonal antibody L26 in the identification and confirmation of B-cell lymphomas: a sensitive and specific marker applicable to formalin- and B5-fixed, paraffin-embedded tissues. *Am J Pathol* 1987;129:415–421.
189. Gloghini A, De Paoli P, Gaidano G, et al. High frequency of CD45RO expression in AIDS-related B-cell non-Hodgkin's lymphomas. *Am J Clin Pathol* 1995;104:680–688.
190. Falini B, Pileri S, Pizzolo G, et al. CD30 (Ki-1) molecule: a new cytokine receptor of the tumor necrosis factor receptor superfamily as a tool for diagnosis and immunotherapy. *Blood* 1995;85:1–14.
191. Jones D, Jorgensen JL, Shahsafaei A, et al. Characteristic proliferations of reticular and dendritic cells in angioimmunoblastic lymphoma. *Am J Surg Pathol* 1998;22:956–964.
192. Chott A, Rappersberger K, Schlossarek W, et al. Peripheral T cell lymphoma presenting primarily as lethal midline granuloma. *Hum Pathol* 1988;19:1093–1101.
193. Orazi A, Cotton J, Cattoretti G, et al. Terminal deoxynucleotidyl transferase staining in acute leukemia and normal bone marrow in routinely processed paraffin sections. *Am J Clin Pathol* 1994;102:640–645.
194. Orazi A, Cattoretti G, John K, et al. Terminal deoxynucleotidyl transferase staining of malignant lymphomas in paraffin sections. *Mod Pathol* 1994;7:582–586.
195. Soslow RA, Bhargava V, Warnke RA. MIC2, TdT, bcl-2, and CD34 expression in paraffin-embedded high-grade lymphoma/acute lymphoblastic leukemia distinguishes between distinct clinicopathologic entities. *Hum Pathol* 1997;28:1158–1165.
196. McCurley TL, Greer JP, Glick AD. Terminal deoxynucleotidyl transferase (TdT) in acute nonlymphocytic leukemia: a clinical, morphologic, cytochemical, immunologic, and ultrastructural study. *Am J Clin Pathol* 1988;90:421–430.
197. Robertson PB, Neiman RS, Worapongpaiboon S, et al. O13 (CD99)

positivity in hematologic proliferations correlates with TdT positivity. *Mod Pathol* 1997;10:277–282.

198. Dorfman DM, Kraus M, Perez-Atayde AR, et al. CD99 (p30/32MIC2) immunoreactivity in the diagnosis of leukemia cutis. *Mod Pathol* 1997;10:283–288.
199. Vartanian RK, Sudilovsky D, Weidner N. Immunostaining of monoclonal antibody O13 (anti-MIC2 gene product/CD99) in lymphomas. Impact of heat-induced epitope retrieval. *Appl Immunohistochem* 1996;4:43–55.
200. Arber DA, Jenkins KA, Slovak ML. CD79 alpha expression in acute myeloid leukemia: high frequency of expression in acute promyelocytic leukemia. *Am J Pathol* 1996;149:1105–1110.
201. Mason DY, Cordell J, Brown M, et al. Detection of T cells in paraffin wax embedded tissue using antibodies against a peptide sequence from the CD3 antigen. *J Clin Pathol* 1989;42:1194–1200.
202. Krenacs L, Tiszalvicz L, Krenacs T, et al. Immunohistochemical detection of CD1A antigen in formalin-fixed and paraffin-embedded tissue sections with monoclonal antibody 010. *J Pathol* 1993;171: 99–104.
203. Hanson CA, Ross CW, Schnitzer B. Anti-CD34 immunoperoxidase staining in paraffin sections of acute leukemia: comparison with flow cytometric immunophenotyping. *Hum Pathol* 1992;23:26–32.
204. Kurec AS, Cruz VE, Barrett D, et al. Immunophenotyping of acute leukemias using paraffin-embedded tissue sections. *Am J Clin Pathol* 1990;93:502–509.
205. Wijdenes J, Vooijs WC, Clement C, et al. A plasmocyte selective monoclonal antibody (B-B4) recognizes syndecan-1 [See comments]. *Br J Haematol* 1996;94:318–323.
206. von Wasielewski R, Mengel M, Fischer R, et al. Classical Hodgkin's disease: clinical impact of the immunophenotype. *Am J Pathol* 1997; 151:1123–1130.
207. Hall PA, d'Ardenne AJ, Stansfeld AG. Paraffin section immunohistochemistry. I. Non-Hodgkin's lymphoma. *Histopathology* 1988;13: 149–160.
208. Schwarting R, Gerdes J, Durkop H, et al. BER-H2: a new anti-Ki-1 (CD30) monoclonal antibody directed at a formol-resistant epitope. *Blood* 1989;74:1678–1689.
209. Weiss L, Arber D, Chang K. CD45: a review. *Appl Immunohistochem* 1993;1:166–181.
210. Korkolopoulou P, Cordell J, Jones M, et al. The expression of the B-cell marker mb-1 (CD79a) in Hodgkin's disease. *Histopathology* 1994;24:511–515.
211. Enblad G, Sundstrom C, Glimelius B. Immunohistochemical characteristics of Hodgkin and Reed-Sternberg cells in relation to age and clinical outcome. *Histopathology* 1993;22:535–541.
212. Poppema S. The nature of the lymphocytes surrounding Reed-Sternberg cells in nodular lymphocyte predominance and in other types of Hodgkin's disease. *Am J Pathol* 1989;135:351–357.
213. Pallesen G, Hamilton DS, Rowe M, et al. Expression of Epstein-Barr virus latent gene products in tumour cells of Hodgkin's disease [See comments]. *Lancet* 1991;337:320–322.
214. Pinkus GS, Lones M, Shintaku IP, et al. Immunohistochemical detection of Epstein-Barr virus-encoded latent membrane protein in Reed-Sternberg cells and variants of Hodgkin's disease. *Mod Pathol* 1994; 7:454–461.
215. Siebert JD, Ambinder RF, Napoli VM, et al. Human immunodeficiency virus-associated Hodgkin's disease contains latent, not replicative, Epstein-Barr virus [See comments]. *Hum Pathol* 1995;26: 1191–1195.
216. Bellas C, Santon A, Manzanal A, et al. Pathological, immunological, and molecular features of Hodgkin's disease associated with HIV infection: comparison with ordinary Hodgkin's disease. *Am J Surg Pathol* 1996;20:1520–1524.
217. Pinkus GS, Pinkus JL, Langhoff E, et al. Fascin, a sensitive new marker for Reed-Sternberg cells of Hodgkin's disease: evidence for a dendritic or B cell derivation? *Am J Pathol* 1997;150:543–562.
218. Stein H, Hansmann ML, Lennert K, et al. Reed-Sternberg and Hodgkin cells in lymphocyte-predominant Hodgkin's disease of nodular subtype contain J chain. *Am J Clin Pathol* 1986;86:292–297.
219. Davey FR, Olson S, Kurec AS, et al. The immunophenotyping of extramedullary myeloid cell tumors in paraffin-embedded tissue sections. *Am J Surg Pathol* 1988;12:699–707.
220. Gustmann C, Altmannsberger M, Osborn M, et al. Cytokeratin expression and vimentin content in large cell anaplastic lymphomas and other non-Hodgkin's lymphomas. *Am J Pathol* 1991;138:1413–1422.
221. Lasota J, Hyjek E, Koo CH, et al. Cytokeratin-positive large-cell lymphomas of B-cell lineage: a study of five phenotypically unusual cases verified by polymerase chain reaction. *Am J Surg Pathol* 1996;20: 346–354.
222. Zarate-Osorno A, Raffeld M, Berman EL, et al. S-100–positive T-cell lymphoproliferative disorder: a case report and review of the literature. *Am J Clin Pathol* 1994;102:478–482.

CHAPTER 5

Flow Cytometric Analysis of Hematologic Specimens

Catherine P. Leith and Cheryl L. Willman

Flow cytometry is a powerful technology that allows the simultaneous measurement of multiple different characteristics of cells moving in a fluid stream (1–4). In the flow cytometer, cells pass one by one through a laser light beam. As each cell passes through the light beam, light is scattered in different directions, depending on the physical characteristics (i.e., size and internal complexity) of the cell. Simultaneously, the laser light source excites fluorochrome-conjugated probes bound to the cell and endogenous fluorescent material. The light emitted from these excited fluorochromes is simultaneously detected and measured. Depending on the flow cytometer used, fluorescence emissions of two, three, or more wavelengths can be simultaneously detected. As a result, cellular physical characteristics and binding of multiple fluorochrome-labeled probes, such as monoclonal antibodies, can be rapidly measured on thousands of cells.

Compared with more traditional microscopic methods of cellular analysis, the flow cytometer provides a more rapid, sensitive, and quantitative means to measure multiple biologic properties of individual cells in a heterogeneous cell suspension (5). As a result, flow cytometry is a powerful method for classifying and counting subsets of normal and neoplastic hematopoietic cells. Flow cytometry is routinely used to determine the immunophenotype of benign and neoplastic cells, allowing the hematopathologist to diagnose hematologic disorders much more precisely and to predict prognosis and monitor therapeutic responsiveness more effectively (5–8). Flow cytometry can also be used for functional measurements in living cells, such as measurements of efflux-mediated multidrug resistance and cellular apoptosis in response to different pharmacologic agents.

This chapter focuses largely on the use of flow cytometry for the immunophenotyping of hematopoietic neoplasms. The chapter also reviews the general principles of flow cytometry, flow cytometric measurements, uses of flow cytometry in the analysis of hematologic specimens, the handling and preparation of hematologic specimens for flow cytometric analysis, reagents used in flow cytometry, principles of staining of cells for immunophenotypic analysis, and the principles and methods of analysis of flow cytometric data.

GENERAL PRINCIPLES OF FLOW CYTOMETRY

Background

The general principles behind flow cytometry involve making optical and fluorescence measurements on cells suspended in a liquid flow stream as they pass in single file by a source of monochromatic light. A highly simplified flow cytometer schematic that emphasizes the basic components of the instrument is shown in Figure 5.1. The physical and fluorescence parameters that may be assessed on individual cells are listed in Table 5.1.

In flow cytometry, intrinsic physical properties of the cell, such as size and cytoplasmic granularity, can be measured on unstained cells according to how the cells scatter the incident laser light beam. Cells also may be tagged with fluorochrome-conjugated antibodies directed toward cell surface, cytoplasmic, or nuclear antigens or with specific fluorescent dyes that stain DNA, RNA, or protein. As fluorochrome-tagged cells pass through the flow cytometer in single file and are individually illuminated by the laser light source for approximately 10^{-6} seconds, the fluorescent dye bound to each cell is excited to a higher energy state by absorbing photons of light of the particular wavelength or ''color'' emitted by the light source (Fig. 5.1). As the excited fluorochrome rapidly returns to its relaxed lower energy state within 10^{-9} seconds, it emits photons of light; this is the fluorescent signal. The energy of the photons emitted by a

C. P. Leith and C. L. Willman: Department of Pathology, University of New Mexico School of Medicine, Albuquerque, New Mexico 87131

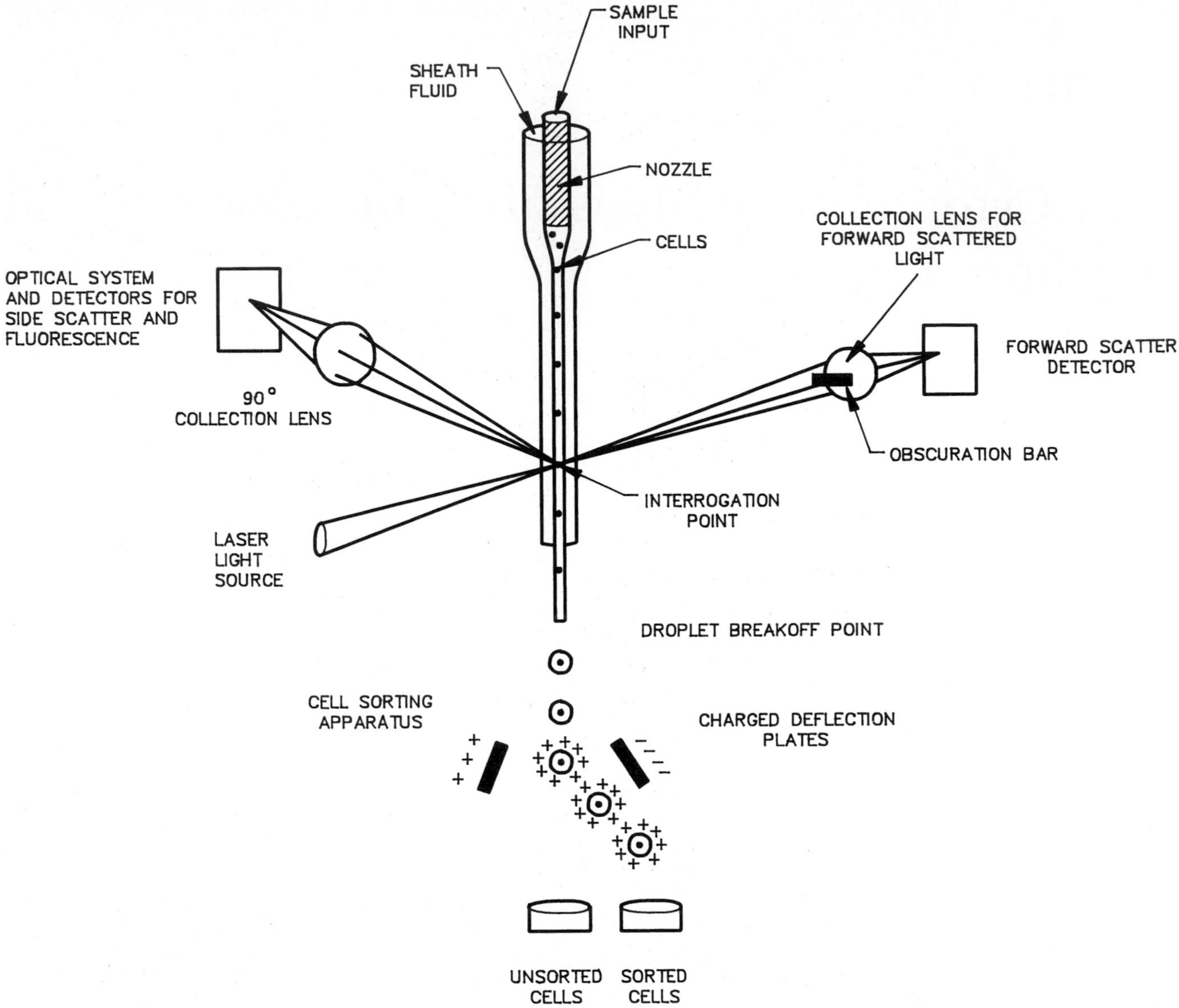

FIG. 5.1. A simplified schematic of the component systems of a flow cytometer.

TABLE 5.1. *Cellular parameters that may be assessed using flow cytometry*

Biologic parameter	Flow cytometric measurement
Intrinsic parameters	
Cell size or cell shape	Forward angle light scatter (FALS)
Cytoplasmic granularity	Right angle light scatter; 90-degree side scatter (SSC)
Extrinsic parameters	
Cell viability or membrane integrity	Exclusion of fluorescent dyes
Total protein content	Emission of fluorescein isothiocyanate
DNA content or cell cycle distributions	Fluorescence emission of DNA-binding dyes
DNA synthesis	Fluorescence emission of DNA-binding dyes Fluoresceinated antibodies to bromodeoxyuridine Fluoresceinated antibodies to nuclear cell cycle-dependent proteins
Total RNA content reticulocyte counting	Emission of RNA-binding fluorochromes pyronin Y, thioflavin T
Cell membrane and intracellular antigens	Emission of fluorochrome-conjugated antibodies
Cellular activation	Emission of fluorescent probes measuring ion fluxes, pH, and membrane potential
Cellular drug resistance	Efflux of fluorescent dyes and drugs

fluorochrome are always of a lower energy (and hence of a longer wavelength and different color) than those absorbed, because energy is lost during emission through internal conversion and nonradiative mechanisms (5,9). Fluorescence emissions and scattered laser light are detected by photodetectors, and the optical signals generated are converted to electronic signals that can be analyzed by computer.

Flow cytometers used for clinical applications have four basic component systems:

1. A sample chamber
2. A light source and illumination optics
3. A light collection and detection system that collects light (photons) emitted by the cells and directs the photons to photodetectors that convert photons to proportional electronic signals
4. A computer that receives these electronic signals, performs data analysis, and controls operation of the instrument

Flow Cytometric Sample Chambers

Within the sample chamber, the cell suspension to be analyzed is aspirated and then injected through a specially designed nozzle into the center of a flowing stream of isotonic sheath fluid. The geometry of the nozzle and the equal velocities of the sample stream containing the cells and the sheath fluid surrounding the cells ensure laminar flow so the cells pass single file by the light source, much like beads on a string (Fig. 5.1). Correct positioning of the sample stream within the sheath fluid is critical to ensure the cells accurately bisect the light source. The velocity of the sample stream must also be kept constant during analysis so that each cell spends an equal amount of time in the illumination and analysis region (5,9).

Flow Cytometric Light Sources and Illumination Optics

A cell passing through a flow cytometer is usually illuminated for only 10^{-6} seconds (9). Flow cytometers require more intense light sources than traditional light microscopes to make measurements. Most flow cytometers used in clinical diagnostics are equipped with small, low-power, air-cooled argon lasers as a light source. The argon lasers used in clinical flow cytometers put out 20 to 25 milliwatts (mW) of monochromatic blue-green light at a wavelength of 488 nm and are ideal for exciting many fluorochromes used in immunofluorescence and DNA content measurements (Table 5.2). These small argon lasers have tube lifetimes of more than 6,000 hours when run at 20 to 25 mW and have excellent sensitivity for fluorescence measurements (9). Some clinical flow cytometers have, in addition to an argon laser, one or two other lasers, which emit light of a longer wavelength (e.g., a helium-neon [HeNe] laser, which emits at 633 nm, a red diode laser emitting at 614 nm). Additional

TABLE 5.2. *Fluorochromes used for extrinsic flow cytometric measurements*

Dye	Laser used for excitation	Dye excitation/ absorption wavelength	Dye emission wavelength
Protein-staining fluorochromes[a]			
Fluorescein (FITC)	Argon	488 nm (blue-green)	525 nm (green)
Phycoerythrin (PE)	Argon	488 nm (blue-green; peak, 514 nm)	575 nm (orange-red)
Peridinin chlorophyll protein (PerCP)	Argon	488 nm	672 nm (red)
PE-Texas red tandem (RED 613)	Argon	488 nm (blue-green)	620
PE-Cy5 tandem conjugate (RED 670)	Argon	488 nm	667 nm
Allophycocyanin (APC)	Helium-neon/red diode	633 nm	660 nm (red)
Cy-5	Helium neon/red diode	633	667
DNA-staining fluorochromes			
Hoechst 33342	Argon helium-cadmium	325–355 nm (UV)	450 nm (blue)
Propidium iodide (PI)	Argon	342–514 nm (UV to yellow)	615 nm (orange-red)
Ethidium bromide	Argon	342–514 nm (UV to yellow)	615 nm (orange-red)
RNA-staining fluorochromes			
Pyronin Y	Argon	480–550 nm (blue-green)	570–600 nm (orange-red)
Acridine orange (AO)	Argon	480–550 nm (blue-green)	570–600 nm (orange-red)
Thioflavin T	Argon	480–550 nm (blue-green)	570–600 nm (orange-red)
Cellular function dyes			
Rhodamine 123	Argon	507	526
Calcein-AM	Argon	494	517
$Di(OC)_2$	Argon		

[a] May be conjugated to antibody molecules.
[b] See text for full discussion of tandem conjugate reagents.

lasers mean that cells can be stained with fluorochromes that are excited at these longer wavelengths and with fluorochromes excited at 488 nm.

The laser beam is focused by the computer system to a round or elliptical shape such that the narrowest portion of the beam (i.e., beam waist) bisects the cells in the sample stream. The point at which the finely focused laser beam illuminates the cells flowing in the sample stream is referred to as the *interrogation point* of the flow cytometer. Past the interrogation point, an obscuration bar blocks further axial transmission of the laser beam but allows light scattered by the cells at small angles to reach the forward light scatter detector, a photomultiplier tube that converts these scattered photons to electronic signals (Fig. 5.1). The amount of laser light scattered by the cell at small angles in the forward direction is roughly proportional to cell size (5,9).

Flow Cytometric Light Collection and Detection Systems

The optical system used in clinical flow cytometers to collect scattered light and fluorescence signals emitted by various fluorochromes consists of a series of filters and mirrors. These collection systems are arranged at a 90-degree angle to the laser light source and the forward scatter detector (i.e., orthogonal geometry) (Fig. 5.1). Between the lens that collects photons and the detectors that convert these photons to electronic signals are optical components that limit the bandwidth, or wavelength of light, that reaches each detector. Optical filters may absorb (i.e., colored glass filters) or reflect (i.e., dichroic filters) light outside the wavelength that they normally transmit. These mirrors and filters separate light beams of different wavelengths, directing the light beams to the appropriate detector. Figure 5.2 illustrates the light collection and detection system of the Becton-Dickinson FACScan Flow Cytometer, a single-laser instrument, showing how light of different wavelengths is transmitted to the relevant detectors. A forward-scatter detector placed just off the axis of the laser light detects laser light scattered by cells in the forward direction. All light scattered by cells at 90 degrees (a rough measurement of cytoplasmic granularity) and all fluorescence signals are collected by a lens placed 90 degrees from the laser light source (Figs. 5.1, 5.2).

Between this collection lens and the various detectors are a series of mirrors and filters that direct light of particular wavelengths to the appropriate detectors (Fig. 5.2). A dichroic mirror (DM) and a 560 nm short pass (SP) filter allow light of 560 nm or less to pass upward to a Brewster window (Fig. 5.2). The Brewster window reflects light to a side scatter detector (SSC), which detects and records the photons of light scattered by cells at 90 degrees. The Brewster window simultaneously allows light of 560 nm or less to pass upward to a 530-nm bandpass filter. This filter allows only photons of this wavelength (i.e., wavelength of photons emitted by the fluorochrome fluorescein isothiocyanate [FITC]) to pass to the first fluorescence detector (FL1). The dichroic mirror reflects light greater than 560 nm to a 640-nm long pass (LP) filter. The 640-nm LP filter reflects photons between 640 nm and 560 nm to a bandpass filter of 585 nm, which allows only photons of this wavelength (usually emitted by the fluorochrome phycoerythrin [PE]) to the second fluorescence detector (FL2). Light greater than 640 nm passes through the 640-nm LP filter to a second 650-nm LP filter. This allows photons of these longer wavelengths to reach the third fluorescence detector (FL3).

All detectors are photomultiplier tubes (PMTs) that convert photons of particular wavelengths (energies) to proportional electrical impulses. These electrical currents are then transmitted to the computer system. These measurements can be expanded still further if the flow cytometer is equipped with a second laser light source, which can be used to excite additional fluorochromes with longer absorption wavelengths, allowing simultaneous measurement of four, five, or more colors simultaneously (10–13). Through this complex optical system, clinical flow cytometers can simultaneously activate, detect, and record the emissions from multiple different fluorochromes, allowing the clinical laboratory to perform simultaneous multiparameter flow cytometric measurements on individual cells.

Flow Cytometric Computer Systems

As cells pass through the interrogation point of the flow cytometer and scatter laser light or emit fluorescent signals, the photons of scattered and emitted light are converted by transducers (PMTs) in the various detectors to discrete electrical pulses (Figs. 5.1, 5.2). These pulses are then amplified, integrated, and converted to digital form for acceptance by a computer. A continuum of fluorescence intensity or some physical characteristic such as cell size (forward angle light scatter [FALS]) or cytoplasmic granularity (SSC) is converted into discrete digital steps or channels. Each cell is then regarded as an event of a particular intensity and is placed in an appropriate channel proportional to intensity.

The computer systems on flow cytometers have become increasingly powerful over the years, allowing rapid storage and analysis of increased amounts of data collected. As a result, it is practical to collect all the raw data on the cells run through the instrument (i.e., list mode data) rather than collecting only selected data as determined by the operator. Collecting and storing all data ensures that data on abnormal populations are gathered, whereas selective collection of specific cell subsets (e.g., setting a lymphocyte collection gate) may result in abnormal populations being missed in the data collection process. Data can be readily collected on tens of thousands of cells from each staining tube, which is useful if the abnormal cells in a population are rare, as in minimal residual disease detection. In addition to the development of powerful computer systems that can store large amounts of data, there are numerous data analysis software

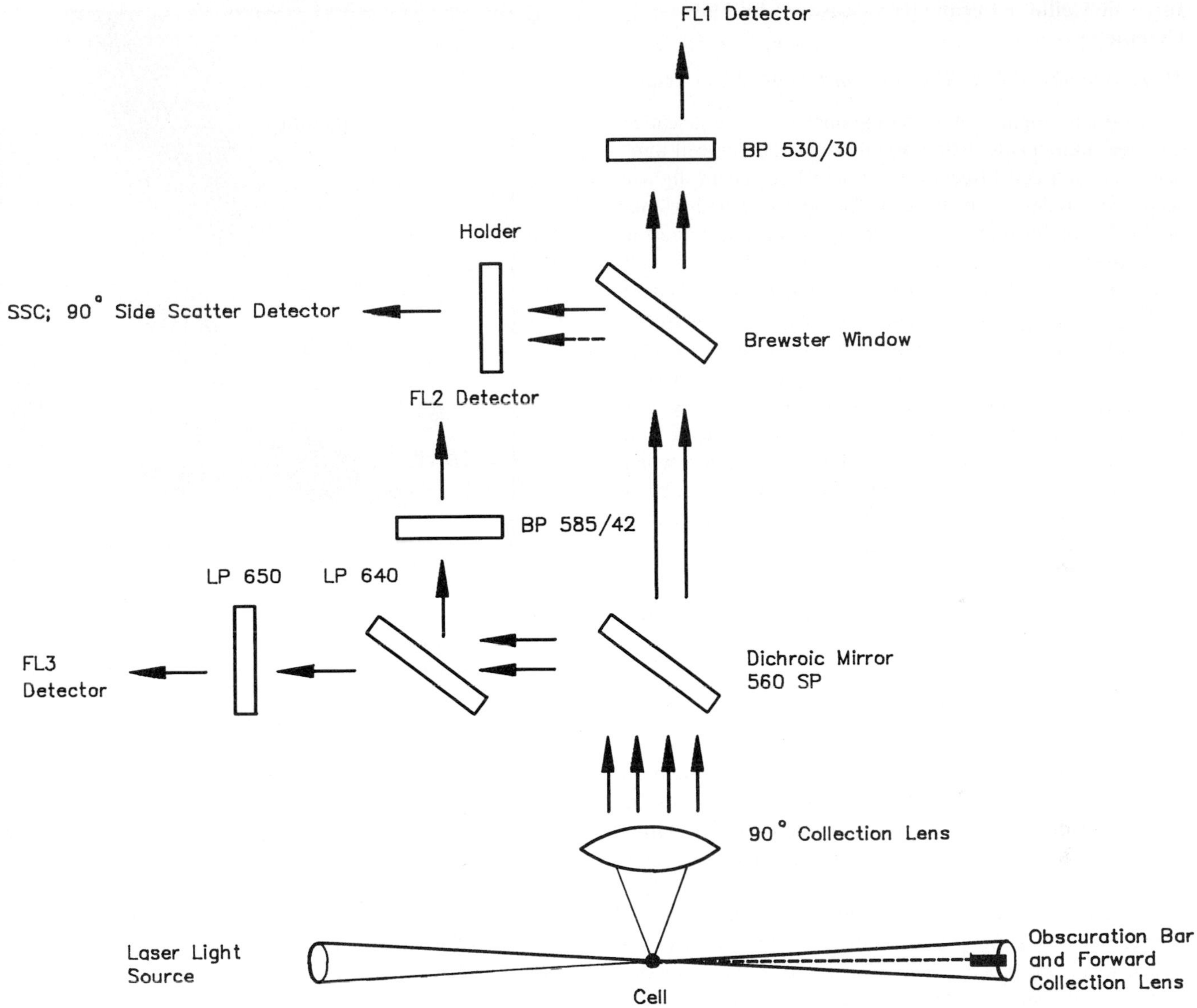

FIG. 5.2. A schematic of the collection optics and detection systems in the Becton-Dickinson FACScan Flow Cytometer.

packages that enable much easier and more powerful multiparameter data analysis (9,12).

In addition to accurately measuring multiple parameters on a cell, flow cytometers can be used to sort and purify specific cell populations with precisely defined characteristics. Flow cytometers can sort cells by droplet sorting or by mechanical sorting. The latter method is preferred for clinical samples that may have infectious agents because the process does not have the risk of aerosol formation that exists with droplet sorters. Cells may be positively selected by any combination of physical or fluorescence parameters that may be measured by a flow cytometer. Viable sorted cells may be collected directly into tissue culture medium. Alternatively, cells may be collected directly onto nitrocellulose filters for molecular or biochemical studies or onto glass slides for morphologic, histochemical, or *in situ* hybridization analysis.

FLOW CYTOMETRIC MEASUREMENTS

Flow cytometry can measure intrinsic properties of the cell (i.e., those that can be detected on unstained cells because of cell size or features attributable to intrinsic autofluorescence) and extrinsic parameters that require addition of fluorescent probes for their detection. The intrinsic parameters that may be measured on unstained cells in a flow cytometer and the extrinsic parameters that may be assessed using fluorescent probes directed to cellular constituents and probes for cellular function are listed in Table 5.1.

Intrinsic Cellular Parameters Measured by Flow Cytometry

Measurements of Cell Size: Forward Angle Light Scatter

Modern multiparameter flow cytometers use light-scattering measurements to estimate cell size and count cell numbers. As each cell bisects the incident laser beam, light is scattered 360 degrees by the cell. The light scattered at small or "low" angles (0.5 to 2.0 degrees) by the cell in the forward direction, referred to as low angle or FALS, is roughly proportional to cell size, if the cell is a homogeneous sphere. FALS measurements are made by placing an obscuration bar between the cell at its point of interrogation by the incident laser beam and the forward light scatter detector (Fig. 5.1). The obscuration bar prevents directly oncoming laser light from reaching the detector, and the amount of light scattered at low angles is measured by the detector, which is placed a few degrees off the axis of the incident laser beam (Fig. 5.1). FALS is only an estimate of cell size because most cells are not homogeneous spheres (9).

Measurements of Cytoplasmic Granularity: 90 Degrees or Side Scatter

The amount of incident laser light scattered orthogonally by a cell 90 degrees from the axis of the incident laser beam depends on the refractile properties of the cell, particularly the granularity of the cytoplasm (Figs. 5.1, 5.2). This measurement, referred to as 90-degree scatter or SSC, is useful in distinguishing granulated from nongranulated cells. Granulocytes, with their cytoplasmic granules, have the highest degree of side scatter while monocytes have an intermediate degree and lymphocytes have the lowest degree.

FALS versus SSC characteristics can be plotted as a two-dimensional dot plot, in which each dot represents a cell with particular size and granularity characteristics (Fig. 5.3). These two-dimensional dot plots allow distinction of smaller, less granular lymphocytes from larger monocytes and highly granular cells such as granulocytes, eosinophils, and basophils (Fig. 5.3). Dot plots of FALS versus SSC can be useful for identification of populations of interest based on cell size and granularity. Selective analysis (i.e., gating) of a particular population of cells based on their light-scattering characteristics is frequently a useful first step in the analysis of a population of interest in a heterogeneous specimen.

Extrinsic Cellular Parameters Measured by Flow Cytometry

Flow cytometers are ideal for quantifying extrinsic properties of cells, particularly cellular constituents that can be detected by the binding of particular fluorochrome probes (Table 5.2). As each cell under analysis bisects the incident laser beam, the particular fluorochromes bound to a cell are activated to a higher energy state (Fig. 5.1). As these activated fluorochromes rapidly return to their lower energy state, they emit photons of light within 10^{-9} seconds. As energy is lost during fluorescence emission, the photons emitted by each fluorochrome are of lower energy and therefore of longer wavelength (hence a different color) than those absorbed. Each fluorochrome used for fluorescence measurements has an ideal wavelength for excitation or absorption and a characteristic emission spectrum.

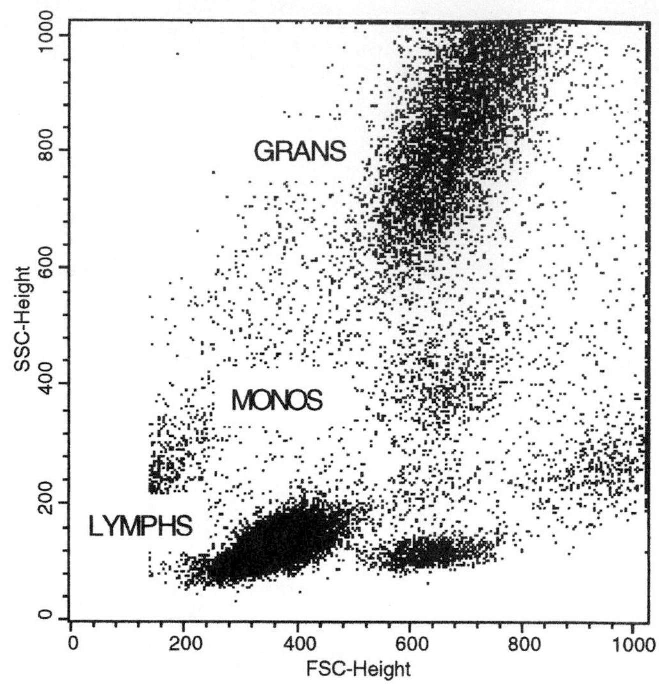

FIG. 5.3. Two-dimensional dot plot obtained by correlating the forward angle light scatter (FALS) (linear scale) and side scatter (SSC) (log scale) measurements on unstained peripheral blood cells. Correlated measurements of FALS versus SSC resolve different hematopoietic cell subsets for further detailed analysis.

Because each fluorochrome is activated by light of a specific wavelength, fluorochromes used for flow cytometric analysis must be matched to the excitation capabilities of the available light sources. The 488-nm monochromatic blue-green light produced by an argon laser is ideal for the excitation of numerous fluorochromes used in measurements of immunofluorescence and DNA content (Table 5.2). Fluorochromes routinely used in clinical flow cytometry include FITC and PE. Because FITC and PE absorb at 488 nm, a single argon laser can activate them. However, their different emission wavelengths (FITC at 530 nm and PE at 585 to 590 nm) (Table 5.2) can be distinguished by appropriate collection and detection systems (Fig. 5.2), allowing excellent simultaneous two-color immunofluorescence measurements. A variety of third-color reagents are available that can also be activated by an argon laser but that emit in the far red wavelengths. These include Peridinin Chlorophyll Protein (PerCP), excited at 490 nm with peak emissions at 680 nm and a variety of tandem conjugate reagents (Table 5.2). Tandem conjugates consist of pairs of fluorochromes that have been chemically coupled. An argon laser excites the donor fluorochrome (usually PE). Through nonradiative energy transfer, the PE molecule activates a second fluorochrome, such as Texas red or Cy-5, which then emits photons of longer wavelength (Table 5.2) detected by detector 3 on the flow cytometer (9,12).

Although each fluorochrome has its own particular peak emission wavelength, each fluorochrome produces a spectrum of emissions of various wavelengths, generally with a long "tail" of emissions at longer wavelength. There is often some overlap in the emission spectra between fluorochromes; FITC, for example, emits maximally at about 525 nm (detectable on detector 1 of the flow cytometer), but the tail of its emission spectrum extends beyond 600 nm and into the range of detector 2. As a result, a cell with strong staining with a FITC-labeled antibody shows some weak fluorescence on the PE detector (i.e., detector 2). These cells would be falsely positive for the PE-labeled antibody. This overlap in fluorescence emissions spectra can be compensated for electronically in the flow cytometer by instructing the instrument to essentially disregard these low-intensity signals. Undercompensation results in false-positive staining because of detection of "bleed-over" of fluorescence from one detector to another, whereas overcompensation can result in false-negative results, because weak but real staining is discounted by the computer (9,12). Optimal compensation is essential for the correct interpretation of flow cytometric results and is particularly important in the analysis of neoplastic hematologic specimens in which particular antigens may be expressed at low antigen density and therefore show only dim fluorescence. Figure 5.4 illustrates the effects of undercompensation and overcompensation on the analysis of CD45 and CD3 staining on leukemic blasts.

In addition to fluorochrome-conjugated antibodies being used to determine the immunophenotype of cells, fluorochromes can be used to measure a wide variety of intracellular parameters by flow cytometry. DNA and RNA content, for example, can be measured using fluorescent dyes that directly intercalate with nucleic acid. DNA content is particularly useful in the assessment of pediatric acute lymphoblastic leukemia (ALL), because DNA index is one measure used to stratify patients into different risk groups. All normal, nondividing eukaryotic cells in the G_0/G_1 phase of the cell cycle have the same 2N (diploid) DNA content. During the synthetic (S) phase of the cell cycle, each chromosome replicates, and the cellular DNA content gradually increases from 2N to 4N. DNA content remains 4N throughout the G_2 and mitotic (M) phases of the cell. Using fluorescent dyes that bind stoichiometrically to DNA, flow cytometry can be used to determine the percentage of cells in each phase of the cell cycle and to detect abnormalities in DNA content in neoplastic cells. RNA content can also be measured by flow cytometry using dyes such as acridine orange and its homologue pyronin Y. RNA content determination is used for flow cytometric detection and counting of reticulocytes.

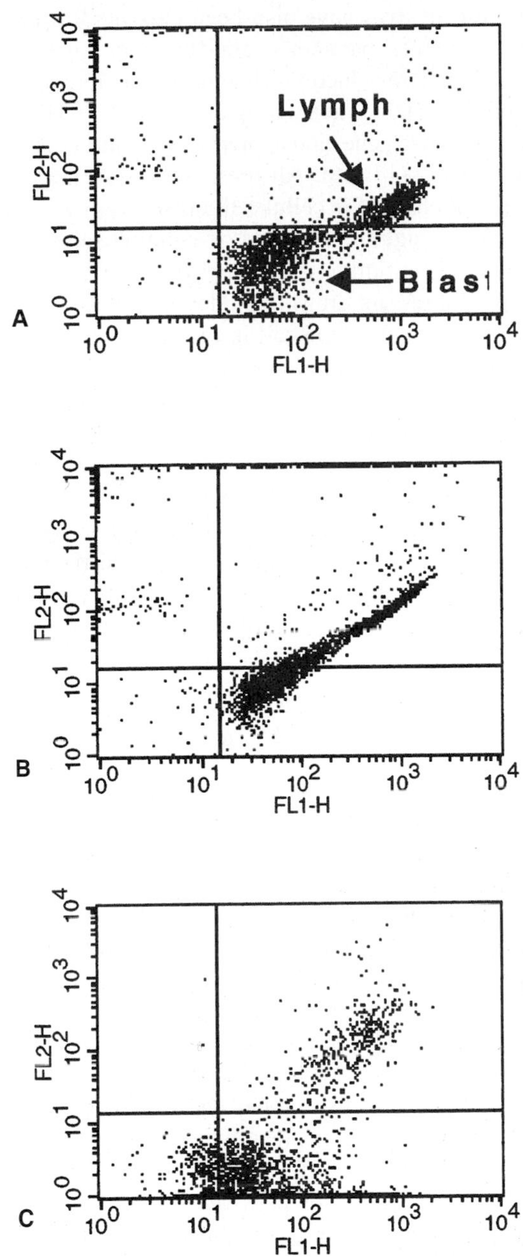

FIG. 5.4. The effects of electronic compensation on flow cytometric measurements. Leukemic blast cells from a patient with acute myeloid leukemia (AML) have been stained for CD45 (FL1, x axis) and CD3 (FL2, y axis). **A:** Correct compensation: a large cluster of leukemic blasts is weakly positive for CD45 and is negative for CD3. A small cluster of residual lymphocytes is also present, showing bright CD45 and CD3 expression. **B**: Undercompensation: the fluorescent signals bleeding over from the CD45 FITC-labeled blasts into FL2 (the PE detector) result in apparent weak expression of CD3 by the leukemic blasts. **C**: Overcompensation: the computer has been instructed to disregard the low-intensity signal in FL1. As a result, the weak fluorescence of the blasts with CD45 is not readily detected, and a discrete cluster of blasts can no longer be seen.

Fluorescent dyes have also been exploited to measure a variety of cellular parameters and functions, such as assessment of signal transduction, changes in membrane potential, intracellular pH, functional drug efflux mediated by the multidrug resistance gene, and apoptotic response to chemotherapeutic agents (14–16). All these assays are based on the detection of changes in cellular fluorescence associated with particular cellular functions. For example, the functional ability of the multidrug resistance-1 protein (P-glycoprotein) to efflux fluorescent drugs (e.g., daunomycin) or dyes (e.g., rhodamine 123) from the cell in the presence or absence of P-glycoprotein modulators such as cyclosporine or PSC 633 (15). Functional measurements of apoptosis are also readily made by flow cytometry by measuring, for example, the binding of fluorescently labeled annexin V or by analyzing DNA fragmentation using fluorochrome-labeled nucleotide probes. As the clinical significance of these assays is determined in large studies on uniformly treated patients, some of these functional assays will likely become integrated into the routine analysis of hematologic specimens.

USES OF FLOW CYTOMETRY IN THE ANALYSIS OF HEMATOLOGIC SPECIMENS

Flow cytometry is widely used in the diagnosis and monitoring of patients with leukemia and lymphoma. Flow cytometric immunophenotyping has proved a powerful adjunct to morphology in the diagnosis and classification of a wide variety of hematologic neoplasms, including low-grade B-cell lymphoproliferative disorders, large granular lymphocyte disorders, malignant lymphomas, and acute leukemias (6–8,17). For example, in a patient with a mild absolute lymphocytosis and a suspected B-cell lymphoproliferative disorder, flow cytometric immunophenotyping can establish whether the B cells are clonal and whether they express the characteristic immunophenotype of chronic lymphocytic leukemia (CLL) ($CD5^+/CD23^+$). Flow cytometry can be used in the evaluation of peripheral blood, bone marrow, and fresh tissue specimens; for assessment of hematopoietic cells in body fluids such as cerebral spinal fluid and pleural or peritoneal effusions; and for evaluation of fine needle aspirates (FNA) of tissue masses. Flow cytometric evaluation of FNA material is used increasingly to evaluate patients with lymphadenopathy without the need for an open biopsy (18).

In addition to being useful in the accurate diagnosis of patients with suspected hematologic malignancies, flow cytometric studies can also provide useful biologic and prognostic information regarding the patient's disease, such as DNA ploidy, S-phase analysis, and assessment of a drug-resistant phenotype. Flow cytometry has proven a highly sensitive method to detect expression and functional activity of the multidrug resistance protein, MDR-1. Expression of MDR-1 has been associated with decreased remission rates and, in some studies, survival of patients with acute myeloid leukemia (AML) (19,20). New therapies that incorporate MDR-1 modulators have been used in clinical trials, and initial results indicate that such therapies may significantly improve clinical response (21). If these results are corroborated in subsequent studies, assessment of the drug-resistant phenotype may move from the research to the clinical flow cytometry laboratory.

Flow cytometric immunophenotyping can also be used in the follow-up evaluation of patients diagnosed with hematopoietic malignancies. With multiparameter flow cytometry, assays can detect 1 in 10^3 to 10^4 cells and are much more sensitive than morphologic assessment. The role of minimal residual disease testing for chronic lymphoproliferative disorders is not entirely clear and awaits large studies of uniformly treated patients. However, for patients with acute leukemia, studies indicate that monitoring of minimal residual disease is useful for predicting relapse in AML and ALL patients (22,23). If these results are confirmed in large multi-institutional trials, minimal residual disease testing may become an important part of the flow cytometric evaluation and follow-up evaluation of patients with acute leukemias.

HANDLING AND PREPARATION OF HEMATOLOGIC SPECIMENS FOR FLOW CYTOMETRIC ANALYSIS

Sample Collection and Transportation

Hematopoietic cells lend themselves readily to analysis by flow cytometry because they are already in cell suspension (i.e., blood and bone marrow) or are often quite easily disaggregated (i.e., lymph node and other solid tissues). Peripheral blood and bone marrow specimens need to be carefully anticoagulated immediately on collection. Blood can be collected directly into EDTA or sodium heparin tubes, and bone marrow can be aspirated into syringes that have been rinsed with sodium heparin. Excess heparin can interfere with staining because the strongly negatively charged heparin anticoagulant may interfere with immunofluorescence staining protocols. Sodium heparin is preferred over lithium heparin, which can result in the loss of cell viability.

Blood and bone marrow specimens are best transported at room temperature because temperature extremes can jeopardize specimen integrity. Very high temperatures result in cell death and specimen degradation, whereas cold temperatures can result in staining artifacts, such as increased nonspecific binding of immunoglobulins to Fc receptors, and in preferential loss of certain cell surface antigens, such as CD4. Because specimen overheating can be a more serious problem than specimen cooling, particularly in the summer months and southern climates, transport of the specimen with a cool pack is preferable to exposing it to excess heat. If significant time is likely to elapse before the specimen is processed (e.g., if transported by overnight courier), addition of sterile tissue culture media helps to preserve cell viability. With the addition of media, blood and marrow specimens can be reliably analyzed after a delay of 24 to 36 hours (5), and metabolically inactive cells (such as CLL cells) frequently are preserved for analysis even after several days. However, rapid transportation and processing ensures optimal specimen integrity.

Solid tissue specimens should be thinly sliced and transported in culture media. Unlike liquid specimens, specimen degradation can be more of a problem because the cells are not all equally bathed in any added culture media. These specimens are better kept cool at 4°C and processed as rapidly as possible.

Separation and Purification of Hematopoietic Samples

The method of specimen processing depends on the specimen type, the population of interest (e.g., white blood cells, red blood cells), and whether preservation of the sample for future use or immediate flow cytometric analysis is desired. In general, a minimum of sample preparation is recommended to ensure that cell populations are not altered by the processing method (12). For white blood cell analysis of blood and bone marrow specimens, it is highly desirable to remove unwanted platelets and red blood cells from the specimen. Red blood cell lysis is a recommended method (12). Ammonium chloride solution can lyse red cells without compromising cell viability, and several proprietary reagents are available that lyse red cells and simultaneously fix white cells. Red cell lysis is simple, and because all white cells are preserved, it is useful for quantifying cellular subsets in blood or bone marrow. In some circumstances, erythrocytes may insufficiently lyse, resulting in erythrocyte ghosts that lead to spurious flow cytometric data (5). Another issue to be aware of is that different proprietary and in-house solutions may result in the selective loss of different types of white cells (12,24). Each laboratory needs to be familiar with the particular reagents it uses for red cell lysis.

Cells can also be separated using discontinuous Ficoll-Hypaque density-gradient centrifugation. This method can be useful if the specimen is to be cryopreserved for future studies. Anticoagulated blood or bone marrow is usually diluted with tissue culture medium before being layered onto Ficoll-Hypaque. After centrifugation, the mononuclear cells suspended as a layer at the interface are harvested for subsequent staining, and most dead cells, erythrocytes, and granulocytes are centrifuged through the gradient and can be discarded as a cell pellet. Because discontinuous density gradient centrifugation removes mature granulocytes, red cells, and dead cells, the neoplastic cell population is enriched. One disadvantage of density centrifugation is the selective loss of certain mononuclear cells, such as CD8-positive ($CD8^+$) T cells (25,26). A second disadvantage is that estimates of the percentage of the population of interest within the specimen (e.g., $CD34^+$ blasts) cannot be made, because the specimen has been selectively depleted of cells such as granulocytes. The neoplastic cell population may separate into another layer of the gradient, and different layers may need to be tested to ensure that a neoplastic population is not mistakenly overlooked (12).

For processing of solid tissue specimens, mechanical disaggregation using scalpel and forceps, wire mesh screen, needle, and syringe or a mechanical disaggregation device is generally preferred (27,28). This method generally works well if there is little connective tissue. When connective tissue is present, the yield of cells often is more variable and difficult to predict. Body fluids such as pleural fluids or cerebral spinal fluid frequently require concentration of the cells by centrifugation (29).

Viability Testing

When the specimen is processed for flow cytometric analysis, it is important to test the cellular integrity of the cells by assessing cellular viability. This is essential in samples older than 24 hours or when there is a suspicion that the sample may have been damaged, such as by excessively high temperatures, and it is a good idea to test all samples regardless of age (12). Microscopic assessment of viability can be made by staining cells with dyes such as Trypan blue and by calculating the percentage of cells that exclude the dye (i.e., viable cells) compared with those that take up the dye (i.e., dead cells). Viability can also be assessed by flow cytometry by staining cells with dyes such as propidium iodide (PI) or 7-AAD (12,30). Dead but not viable cells take up PI, and the percentage of fluorescent cells identified gives a measure of the percent of dead cells present. Dyes such as 7-AAD can be incorporated into multicolor flow cytometry panels so that dead cells specifically can be excluded from immunophenotypic analysis.

Because specimens sent for flow cytometric analysis are often irretrievable or difficult to recollect (e.g., solid tissue biopsies, bone marrows), poor cellular viability on its own should not be an indication to cancel analysis of a specimen. However, the low viability must be taken into account in the analysis and interpretation of the flow cytometric data and may lead to the operator performing the flow cytometric analysis somewhat differently (e.g., adding PI/7-AAD in all the staining tubes to exclude dead cells) (12,30). Low viability can lead to spurious results because the population of interest has been selectively lost, because of loss of cellular staining or nonspecific staining with reagents. The data produced must be viewed with more skepticism and needs to be integrated with clinical and morphologic features of the case to determine its significance.

Staining Methods

A large number of monoclonal antibodies directed toward cell surface, cytoplasmic, and nuclear antigens are available to distinguish the lineage and function of hematopoietic cells (see Chapter 3). For most clinical purposes, cells are stained with antibodies that are directly conjugated to a fluorochrome (i.e., direct immunofluorescence). Less often, indirect immunofluorescence may be used. In this case, cells are stained with unlabeled antibody, and that antibody is subsequently labeled in a second step with fluorochrome-conjugated antibody. This latter method is particularly used in research when novel antibodies are being tested. When amplification of cell signal is required (e.g., in multidrug-resistance testing in which P-glycoprotein is often expressed at low antigen density), indirect labeling techniques may be useful (15). For most clinical purposes, labeling with directly conjugated monoclonal antibodies is preferable, because the technique is much more rapid and easier to use, particularly in multicolor flow cytometric analysis.

For direct labeling of cell surface antigens, a known number of cells (generally 0.5 to 1.0×10^6, in accordance with the manufacturer's recommendations) are dispensed into each staining tube. The cells are then incubated with directly labeled antibodies according to the manufacturer's recommendations. After staining, lysing reagent is added (whole blood and marrow specimens). After red cell lysis, cells are washed and resuspended in phosphate-buffered saline with 0.2% azide and kept cold until running. The κ and λ staining can be particularly tricky because of nonspecific staining due to Fc receptor binding. For detection of heavy or light chains, cells should be washed in isotonic buffer before staining to remove serum and reduce nonspecific staining. If Fc receptor binding of antibody is a particular problem, a 1-hour 37°C incubation in isotonic buffer can help to reduce nonspecific binding. Fc receptor binding of light chains by non-B cells (mainly monocytes) can be a particular problem. Incorporation of a pan-B-cell marker such as CD19 into the κ or λ staining tube allows specific gating on the $CD19^+$ B-cell population and helps to discriminate between light chain staining on B cells and nonspecific staining often detected on monocytes (12).

Intracellular Staining Methods

In addition to detecting the expression of cell surface markers, a number of intracellular parameters can also be measured by flow cytometry, including DNA and RNA content and the expression of intracellular antigens. Staining for cytoplasmic CD3, CD22, myeloperoxidase, and intranuclear terminal deoxynucleotidyl transferase (TdT) are of particular use in the assessment of acute leukemias. Similarly, staining for cytoplasmic κ and λ chains is useful in the assessment of plasma cell clonality (17,31).

Staining of intracellular components with fluorescent-labeled antibody requires cellular permeabilization before staining. Depending on the antigen to be analyzed, cells may be fixed in various fixatives or may be permeabilized with various detergents, followed by labeling with specific antibodies and appropriate controls. Several permeabilization methods have been described, including proprietary kits specifically manufactured to detect intracellular antigens and commercial lysing reagents that fix and permeabilize white blood cells and lyse red blood cells. The type of permeabilization method to use depends in part on the antigen to be detected, because specific permeabilization methods may be excellent for detection of some but not other intracellular antigens. Each laboratory should determine the optimal methods to detect particular intracellular antigens.

As with surface marker staining, the staining for intracellular antigens can be combined with staining for surface or other markers simultaneously. This multiparameter approach can better identify the population of interest and its phenotype. For example, monoclonal plasma cells can be detected using CD45 and CD38 surface markers and cytoplasmic immunoglobulin, and B lymphoblasts and hematogones can be detected using CD45 and CD19 surface markers with nuclear TdT.

Morphologic Assessment of the Specimen

Proper interpretation of flow cytometric data relies on the fact that the specimen submitted for flow cytometry is representative of the tissue of interest. Making a smear or cytospin preparation of the specimen for flow cytometry is essential in all cases so the material submitted for flow cytometry can be assessed for the cells of interest. In some cases, the cells of interest are not represented in the flow specimen. For example, a bone marrow biopsy may contain suspicious lymphoid aggregates, but these may not be represented on the material submitted for flow cytometry. A negative finding for clonality in this instance could well be a sampling artifact. In another circumstance, the specimen for flow may contain very few cells of interest. For example, the cell suspension from a lymph node suspicious for large cell lymphoma may contain very few large cells and a predominance of small lymphocytes. The presence of this very small population of large cells should be recognized so that they can be selectively analyzed, because they probably represent the malignant cells and should not be overlooked.

REAGENTS USED IN FLOW CYTOMETRY AND PRINCIPLES OF STAINING OF CELLS FOR IMMUNOPHENOTYPIC ANALYSIS

A huge number of monoclonal antibodies, many of them directly conjugated to a fluorochrome, are available for use in flow cytometry. The choice of antibodies to use to examine any particular case depends on the case particulars (e.g., clinical history, morphologic impressions) and on the information required. To correctly assign lineage and differentiation stage to a hematopoietic process and to identify normal cellular elements, it is important to include sufficient antibodies of different lineages in the panel, because many antigens are not completely lineage specific. For example, many T-cell antigens, particularly CD7 and CD4 but also CD2 and CD5, can be expressed by the blasts in AML, and the myeloid antigens CD13 and CD33 may be expressed in T-lineage ALL. Correct discrimination between T-lineage ALL and

AML requires a panel of several anti-T-cell and anti-myeloid antibodies.

A variety of approaches can be taken to antibody panel design, depending on the clinical circumstances and the optimal work flow in the laboratory. Some laboratories favor performing short screening panels to determine the likely lineage of the cells of interest and then performing a second, more comprehensive panel focusing on the lineage in question. In other laboratories, initial use of broader, more comprehensive panels may be more efficient. Regardless of the strategy employed, antibody panels must clearly include a sufficient repertoire of antibodies to determine the cell lineage and stage of maturation and to answer any other clinically relevant questions. The panel must be designed with knowledge of the reactivity patterns of the antibodies used with cells of different lineages and stages of differentiation and of the staining patterns observed in neoplastic cells, including loss of antigens (7,8,12,17,32,33). The reactivity of the antibody combinations devised for use by any particular laboratory needs to be validated by the laboratory before being used in clinical diagnosis.

Besides taking into account the likely reactivity of different cell types with different antibodies, panel design should also take into account the likely level of intensity of staining with various antibodies. The different physicochemical properties of different fluorochromes result in differences in sensitivity of detection of fluorescence when they are conjugated to the same antigen. For example, one to three molecules of FITC can be conjugated to each antibody molecule without decreasing the binding specificity or the quantum yield, in contrast to up to 34 PE chromophores, each with an absorbency and quantum yield roughly equivalent to FITC per antibody molecule (9). PE-conjugated monoclonal antibodies tend to generate much larger fluorescence shifts when bound to their cell-associated antigens than FITC-associated antibodies, and therefore weak staining is more readily detected with PE than FITC-labeled antibody. This is important when the level of antigen expression may be low. Leukemic blasts, for example, may only weakly stain with CD34, and expression of CD34 is therefore more readily detected with PE- than FITC-labeled antibodies. Expression of the myeloid antigens CD33 and CD13 is likewise easier to detect with PE-labeled than with FITC-labeled antibodies. Similarly, for some of the third-color reagents, including tandem reagent products, different manufacturers may produce antibodies with different fluorochromes, which may show different levels of sensitivity for detection.

All laboratories need to ensure that reagents with suitable sensitivity are used for their assays (12). Proper identification of cell phenotype requires the use of antibodies conjugated to the optimal fluorochrome for their detection. This difference in sensitivity of detection of staining depending on the fluorochrome used also means that direct comparisons between results where different fluorochromes were used for labeling cannot be made.

The use of multiparameter analysis has greatly facilitated the accurate identification of even small populations of cells in a heterogeneous cell mixture. Historically, when single-color immunofluorescence measurements were used, distinction of different cell populations depended on the ability to distinguish them by their light-scattering (size and granularity) characteristics. This limited sensitivity in the detection, as for small monoclonal B-lymphoid populations when the specimen contained numerous similarly sized reactive T cells. With the advent of multiparameter analysis, accurate electronic gating has become much more sophisticated; the cells of interest can be identified by light-scattering characteristics and by their phenotype. B cells can be readily distinguished from reactive T cells if a pan-B-cell marker such as CD19 is included and the analysis gate is set to include only $CD19^+$ cells. These gated B cells can then be more accurately assessed for surface light chain expression. Five-parameter (i.e., FALS, SSC, and three-color fluorescence staining) analysis is generally the minimum recommended for the examination of hematopoietic processes (12).

To optimize the utility of such a multiparameter approach, the panel should be designed with the likely phenotype of the cells of interest in mind. For B-cell analysis, inclusion of a pan-B-cell marker in each staining tube optimizes identification of the B-cell population. For example, a tube containing CD20, CD5, and CD23 can reliably determine whether circulating B-lymphoid cells ($CD20^+$) coexpress CD5 and CD23, as seen in CLL. Table 5.3 shows a panel that could be used for the workup of B-lymphoproliferative disorders. Using a similar principle, leukemic blasts can be accurately identified using CD45/SSC gating, because blasts characteristically show low CD45 expression and low SSC characteristics. Inclusion of CD45 in each staining tube and specific analysis of the CD45 low/low SSC population can be helpful in phenotyping blast populations, especially when the total blast percentage is low (10,33).

When examining the staining pattern of a suspected neoplastic population, it is important to exclude nonspecific staining with antibody (i.e., background staining). Different antibodies have different inherent abilities to nonspecifically bind to hematopoietic cells. Such binding results in these cells giving a false-positive signal with that particular fluorochrome-conjugated antibody. Antigens that are a particular

TABLE 5.3. *Antibody panel for identification and categorization of B-lymphoproliferative disorders*

Population to identify	Three-color antibody combination[a]
Clonal B-cells	Kappa/lambda/CD19
Chronic lymphocytic leukemia phenotype	CD20/CD5/CD23
Hairy cell phenotype	CD19/CD11c/CD103
Circulating lymphoma	CD20/FMC7/CD10
Identification of normal T cells	CD3/CD4/CD8

[a] In all cases, a pan-B-cell antibody is included with markers used to subcategorize the B-cell process.

problem include κ and λ chains, for which nonspecific binding to Fc receptors can lead to false-positive signals (including dual staining for κ and λ, as in monocytes). Antibodies of certain subclasses such as IgG2 antibodies tend to be inherently stickier than IgG class 1 antibodies and show more background staining. Historically, isotype control tubes have been used to control for this background staining. Optimally, the control should be not just the same isotype but should also be labeled with the same fluorochrome (e.g., nonspecific binding with a PE-labeled antibody may be much more easily detected and therefore much more of a problem than similar binding with a FITC-labeled antibody). However, constructing an antibody panel that includes all the correct controls (isotype and fluorochrome specific) entails incorporation of a large number of controls in the experiment, and this may not always be technically feasible.

An alternative method, one that is recommended for use in the analysis of hematopoietic neoplasms, is to use the background normal cells that are always present in hematopoietic specimens as internal control cells in each tube. For example, T cells ($CD19^-$) can be used for the background control in the CD19 B-cell tube (12).

PRINCIPLES AND METHODS OF ANALYSIS OF IMMUNOPHENOTYPIC DATA

Analysis of Immunophenotype Using Electronic Gating

One of the most powerful capabilities of the flow cytometer is the ability to identify and analyze individual cell populations through their size and fluorescence characteristics, even in a very heterogeneous specimen. The ability to do this resides in being able to draw an electronic bit map or gate around the population of interest and in instructing the analysis program to examine that population alone and ignore the other cell populations present. This is a particularly useful tool when the cells of interest are only a subset of the cells under evaluation. For example, the cell surface immunophenotype of leukemic myeloid cells in a bone marrow aspirate may be difficult to determine if the blast cell percentage is low. Moreover, the leukemic blasts may share cell surface antigens with many normal residual myeloid elements in the bone marrow aspirate. The selective identification of the blast cell population is greatly facilitated by using CD45 staining and SSC light-scattering characteristics to identify the leukemic blasts. Blasts characteristically have low SSC and, in contrast to contaminating CD45 bright lymphocytes, have dim CD45 expression (10,33). The operator can then instruct the computer to draw an electronic gate around this blast cell population. In this fashion, the cell surface immunophenotype of the gated blast cell population can be precisely determined. Optimization of gating on the cells of interest requires that the panel contain suitable reagent combinations that allow the best gating strategies to be applied.

Gating is also extremely useful in removing dead cells from flow cytometric analysis. Removal of dead cells and debris is essential in immunofluorescence analysis, because dead cells can avidly and nonspecifically bind many monoclonal antibodies. Exclusion of nonviable from viable cells can be achieved using light scattering characteristics, because cells with damaged membranes have a lower refractive index and hence appear smaller in FALS measurements. However, this discrimination is not perfect when the cells under analysis are heterogeneous in size; dead large cells may fall in the same channels as viable small cells. In this setting, the DNA-binding fluorochrome PI or 7-AAD (Table 5.2) may be used to gate out nonviable cells from immunofluorescence analysis (12).

Analysis of DNA Content

Measurements of the DNA content of a cell may be performed rapidly and precisely using a variety of fluorochromes that bind to DNA (Table 5.2). Because DNA fluorochromes bind to nuclei and chromosomes in a stoichiometric fashion, the fluorescence emission from each cell is proportional to the DNA content of each cell. Flow cytometric measurements of DNA content (i.e., ploidy) can be used to detect and analyze abnormalities in DNA content (e.g., aneuploidy). This can be particularly useful, for example, in the analysis of pediatric ALL cases. Leukemic blasts that have hyperdiploid DNA content can be distinguished from normal diploid cells by differences in cellular fluorescence after staining with PI. The DNA content or ploidy status of tumor cell nuclei is assessed relative to normal control cells and is expressed as the DNA index (DI):

$$DI = \frac{\text{Peak channel of the aneuploid } G_0/G_1 \text{ peak}}{\text{Peak channel of the normal diploid control } G_0/G_1 \text{ peak}}$$

A normal diploid population would have a DI of 1.0. Hyperdiploid ALL cases have DI values greater than 1.0. Because most ALL cases include some residual normal cells, analysis of a hyperdiploid ALL generally identifies two peaks, one of normal cells and one of the leukemic blasts (Fig. 5.5A). To determine which peak corresponds to the normal or to the neoplastic cells, a normal control sample is run independently to determine the peak fluorescence channel for normal diploid cells. A mixing experiment in which fresh normal lymphocytes are added to the tumor specimen in a 3:1 ratio before analysis (Fig. 5.5B) is useful to confirm which peak is that of the normal cells. After adding normal diploid cells to the sample, the most proximal peak in the histogram has an increased number of cells, confirming this peak to contain normal cells. The second peak is the neoplastic peak and has an increased or hyperdiploid DNA content.

Data Interpretation

The method of data interpretation, whether descriptive or numeric, depends on the question asked in each case. In

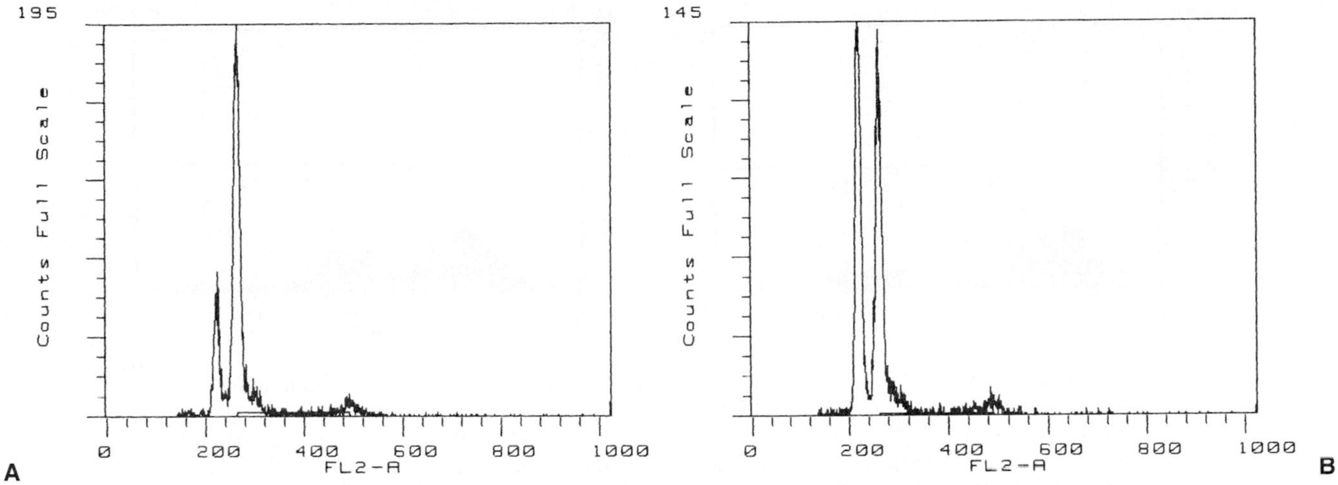

FIG. 5.5. A: The flow cytometric DNA histogram is generated by plotting the number of cells (counts full scale) against propidium iodide (PI) fluorescence intensity on a myeloid leukemia sample. Two G_0/G_1 peaks are present in the specimen. **B:** Addition of normal peripheral blood mononuclear cells to the sample results in an increase in the height of the first G_0/G_1 peak compared with **A**, identifying this peak as containing cells with normal DNA content, presumably residual normal marrow cells. The second G_0/G_1 peak contains leukemic cells with an abnormal hyperdiploid DNA content.

certain situations, enumeration of actual numbers of cells is required, as in the measurement of percent and absolute numbers of $CD34^+$ cells in leukapheresis specimens or $CD3^+$/$CD4^+$ cells in the setting of human immunodeficiency virus (HIV) infection. However, when flow cytometry is used to define and analyze a malignant population, as in hematopathology studies, a qualitative description of the phenotype of the malignant population is most valuable and is generally recommended (34).

There are several reasons why a qualitative description of the population of interest is more valuable. Qualitative descriptions of phenotype can focus on the cells of interest, and residual normal cells can be ignored. For example, in the examination of a probable chronic lymphocytic leukemia case, a qualitative report can focus on expression of CD5 on circulating B cells and ignore CD5 expression by normal T cells. Qualitative descriptions can also include comments about the level of intensity of staining with particular antigens that are not apparent if only numeric data are reported. Such a description can include whether an entire population or only a subset of cells is positive for a particular antigen. In contrast, numeric reporting does not differentiate between subsets of cells expressing an antigen brightly and the entire population of interest expressing the antigen dimly. Figure 5.6 illustrates a case of AML in which the leukemic blasts were stained for CD38 and CD34 in a multicolor experiment. As can be seen from the histograms, CD38 shows a spectrum of staining from dim to bright in the leukemic blasts, whereas CD34 staining shows a distinct subset of brightly positive cells. When the same data were analyzed numerically, about 40% of the cells were positive for each antigen tested. Such a numeric reporting system misses differences in antigen expression pattern that are readily identifiable on histograms or dot plots and that could be reported in a qualitative fashion.

In some cases, particularly when expression of an antigen may be very low on the cell surface, a more precise method to quantify antigen expression may be useful. The Kolmogorov-Smirnov (KS) statistic may be helpful in this regard. The KS statistic, denoted as D, measures the difference between two distribution functions and generates a value ranging from 0 to 1.0 (35). The KS statistic may be used to compare antibody-stained cells with cells stained with isotype control. Because the KS statistic sensitively identifies even small differences in fluorescence, it is useful in the detection of low-level antigen expression, as occurs frequently with MDR-1 expression in primary patient samples (15,36).

Optimal interpretation of flow cytometric results lies in the correlation of the flow cytometric studies with clinical information and with morphologic impressions. In some cases, the flow cytometric immunophenotype generated may be essentially diagnostic for a particular disorder. For example, some diseases such as precursor-B ALL or B-cell chronic lymphocytic leukemia have very well defined characteristic phenotypes. In other diseases, such as follicle center cell lymphomas or peripheral T-cell lymphomas, flow cytometry can greatly aid in the diagnosis, but exact categorization of the disease process requires incorporation of other clinical, morphologic, and laboratory parameters. Even in cases with characteristic phenotypes, detection of the appropriate immunophenotype alone may not always ensure a diagnosis of that disease. For example, regenerating normal marrow B-cell precursors (i.e., hematogones) have a phenotype very similar to precursor-B ALL. Identification of small numbers of B precursors in the marrow of an ALL patient

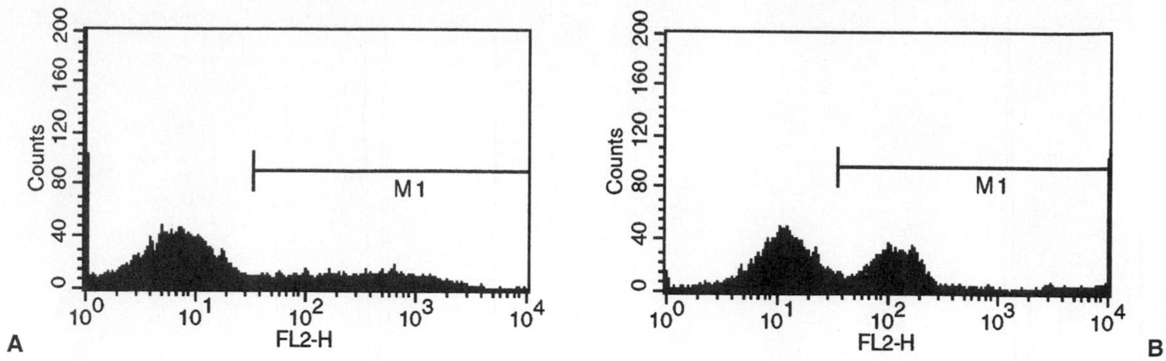

FIG. 5.6. Comparison of data reporting using qualitative or quantitative analysis. A bone marrow specimen from a patient with acute myeloid leukemia (AML) was analyzed. The data are from a gate drawn round the blasts based on light-scattering characteristics. Blasts were stained in three color experiments. Staining with individual antibodies (CD38 in **A** and CD34 in **B**) is displayed in histograms plotting increasing fluorescence (x axis) against cell number (y axis). By quantitative reporting, approximately 40% of the blasts were positive for these markers. However, comparison of the fluorescent histograms shows marked differences in the expression patterns of these two antigens. CD38 **(A)** shows weak expression in a large proportion of the blasts, whereas CD34 **(B)** is brightly expressed in a discrete subset of blasts; the remainder of the blast population is CD34$^-$.

on therapy does not necessarily indicate that the patient has minimal residual disease, but it could indicate that the patient's marrow contains normal regenerating B cells. Differentiation of such cells may require further immunophenotypic characterization (37).

In each case, the results of flow cytometric testing should be incorporated with other clinical, morphologic, and laboratory data for correct interpretation. This requires the expertise of physicians or scientists knowledgeable in flow cytometry and in hematopathology (34).

SUMMARY AND CONCLUSIONS

The development of flow cytometric instruments that are compatible with the clinical laboratory setting has provided an important diagnostic tool for hematopathologists. Flow cytometry is a highly sensitive, quantitative, and high-speed technology that may be used to measure simultaneously multiple biologic properties of viable and fixed cells in suspension. One of the most powerful features of flow cytometric analysis is gating, allowing selective analysis of individual cell populations identified by physical or staining characteristics in a heterogeneous suspension. This approach enables selective analysis of populations of interest even when they constitute only a small fraction of a heterogeneous cell mixture.

The continued development of new monoclonal antibodies and fluorochromes with different emission spectra has allowed increasing sophistication in clinical flow cytometric measurements. Multiple cell surface antigens may be simultaneously assessed and correlated on each hematopoietic cell under analysis. The ability to perform sophisticated flow cytometric measurements of cellular immunofluorescence and cellular function in the clinical laboratory is improving clinical diagnosis and prediction of prognosis for neoplastic and nonneoplastic hematopoietic disorders and is helping follow-up evaluations of patients with hematologic malignancies.

REFERENCES

1. Van Dilla MA, Trujillo TT, Mullaney PF, et al. Cell microfluorometry: a method for rapid fluorescence measurement. *Science* 1969;163: 1213–1214.
2. Kamentsky LA. Cytology automation. *Adv Biol Med Phys* 1973;14: 93–161.
3. Hernzenberg LA, Sweet RG, Herzenberg LA. Fluorescence activated cell sorting. *Sci Am* 1976;234:108–117.
4. Horan PK, Wheeless LL. Quantitative single cell analysis and sorting. *Science* 1977;198:149–157.
5. Melamed MR, Lindmo T, Mendelsohn ML. *Flow cytometry and sorting,* 2nd ed. New York: Wiley-Liss, 1990.
6. Davis BH, Foucar K, Szczarkowski W, et al. U.S.-Canadian consensus recommendations on the immunophenotypic analysis of hematologic neoplasia by flow cytometry: medical indications. *Cytometry* 1997;30: 249–263.
7. Jennings CD, Foon KA. Recent advances in flow cytometry: application to the diagnosis of hematologic malignancy. *Blood* 1997;90: 2863–2892.
8. Jennings CD, Foon KA. Flow cytometry: recent advances in diagnosis and monitoring of leukemia. *Cancer Invest* 1997;15:384–399.
9. Shapiro HM. *Practical flow cytometry,* 3rd ed. New York: Wiley-Liss, 1995.
10. Lacombe F, Durrieu F, Briais A, et al. Flow cytometry CD45 gating for immunophenotyping of acute myeloid leukemia. *Leukemia* 1997; 11:1878–1886.
11. DeMaria MA, Johnson RP, Rosenzweig M. Four color immunofluorescence detection using two 488-nm lasers on a Becton Dickinson FACS Vantage flow cytometer. *Cytometry* 1997;29:178–181.
12. Stelzer GT, Marti G, Hurley A, et al. U.S.-Canadian consensus recommendations on the immunophenotypic analysis of hematologic neoplasia by flow cytometry: standardization and validation of laboratory procedures. *Cytometry* 1997;30:214–230.
13. Roederer M, De Rosa S, Gerstein R, et al. Eight color, 10-parameter flow cytometry to elucidate complex leukocyte heterogeneity. *Cytometry* 1997;29:328–339.
14. Gorman AM, Samali A, McGowen AJ, et al. Use of flow cytometry

techniques in studying mechanisms of apoptosis in leukemia cells. *Cytometry* 1997;29:97–105.

15. Leith CP, Chen IM, Kopecky KJ, et al. Correlation of multidrug resistance (MDR1) protein expression with functional dye-drug efflux in acute myeloid leukemia by multiparameter flow cytometry: identification of discordant $CD34^{+}/MDR1^{-}$ $Efflux^{+}$ and $MDR1^{+}/Efflux^{-}$ cases. *Blood* 1995;86:2329–2342.
16. Lybarger L, Dempsey D, Patterson GH, et al. Dual-color flow cytometric detection of fluorescent proteins using single-laser (488-nm) excitation. *Cytometry* 1998;31:147–152.
17. Rothe G, Schmitz G. Consensus protocol for the flow cytometric immunophenotyping of hematopoietic malignancies. *Leukemia* 1996;10: 877–895.
18. Robins DB, Katz RL, Swan F, et al. Immunophenotyping of lymphoma by fine-needle aspiration: a comparative study of cytospin preparations and flow cytometry. *Am J Clin Pathol* 1994;101:569–576.
19. Leith CP, Kopecky KJ, Godwin JE, et al. Acute myeloid leukemia in the elderly: assessment of multidrug resistance (MDR1) and cytogenetics distinguishes biologic subgroups with remarkably distinct responses to standard chemotherapy. A Southwest Oncology Group study. *Blood* 1997;89:3323–3329.
20. Leith CP, Kopecky KJ, Chen IM, et al. Frequency and clinical significance of expression of the multidrug resistance proteins, MDR1/P-glycoprotein, MRP1 and LRP in acute myeloid leukemia. A Southwest Oncology Group study. *Blood* 1999;94:1086–1099.
21. List AF, Kopecky KJ, Willman CL, et al. Benefit of cyclosporine (CsA) modulation of anthracyline resistance in high-risk AML: a Southwest Oncology Group (SWOG) study. *Blood* 1999;92:312(abst).
22. San Miguel JF, Martinez A, Macedo A, et al. Immunophenotyping investigation of minimal residual disease is a useful approach for predicting relapse in acute myeloid leukemia patients. *Blood* 1997;90: 2465–2470.
23. Coustan-Smith E, Behm FG, Sanchez J, et al. Immunological detection of minimal residual disease in children with acute lymphoblastic leukaemia. *Lancet* 1998;550–554.
24. Carter P, Resto-Ruiz S, Washington G, et al. Flow cytometric analysis of whole blood lysis, three anticoagulants, and five cell preparations. *Cytometry* 1992;13:68–74.
25. De Paoli P, Villalta D, Battistin S, et al. Selective loss of OKT8 lymphocytes on density gradient centrifugation separation of blood mononuclear cells. *J Immunol Methods* 1983;61:259–260.
26. Renzi P, Ginns L. Analysis of T-cell subsets in normal adults: comparison of whole blood lysis technique to Ficoll-Hypaque separation by flow cytometry. *J Immunol Methods* 1987;98:53–56.
27. Wovzynski MJ, Podgurski AE, Boldt DM, et al. An automated method to prepare cell suspensions from human biopsy samples for immunophenotyping by flow cytometry. *Am J Clin Pathol* 1990;93:104–108.
28. Duque R, Andreeff M, Braylan RC, et al. Consensus review of the clinical utility of DNA flow cytometric in neoplastic hematopathology. *Cytometry* 1993;14:492–496.
29. Finn WJ, Peterson LC, James CMT, et al. Enhanced detection of malignant lymphoma in cerebrospinal fluid by multiparameter flow cytometry. *Am J Clin Pathol* 1998;110:341–346.
30. Schmid I, Krall W, Uittenbogaart C, et al. Dead cell discrimination with 7-amino actinomycin D in combination with dual color immunofluorescence in single laser flow cytometry. *Cytometry* 1992;13: 204–208.
31. Groeneveld, te Marvelde JG, van den Beemd MWM, et al. Flow cytometric detection of intracellular antigens for immunophenotyping of normal and malignant leukocytes. *Leukemia* 1996;10:1383–1389.
32. Stewart CC, Behm FG, Carey JL, et al. U.S.-Canadian consensus recommendations on the immunophenotypic analysis of hematologic neoplasia by flow cytometry: selection of antibody combinations. *Cytometry* 1997;30:231–235.
33. Borowitz MJ, Guenther L, Shults KE, et al. Immunophenotyping of acute leukemia by flow cytometric analysis. *Am J Clin Pathol* 1993; 100:534–540.
34. Braylan RC, Atwater SK, Diamond L, et al. US-Canadian consensus recommendations on the immunophenotypic analysis of hematologic neoplasia by flow cytometry: data reporting. *Cytometry* 1997;30: 245–248.
35. Young IT. Proof without prejudice: use of the Kolmogorov-Smirnov test for the analysis of histograms from flow systems and other sources. *J Histochem Cytochem* 1997;25:935–941.
36. Beck WT, Grogan TM, Willman CL, et al. Methods to detect P-glycoprotein-associated multidrug resistance in patient tumors: consensus recommendations. *Cancer Res* 1996;56:3010–3020.
37. Weir EG, Cowan K, Borowitz MJ. A limited antibody panel can distinguish B-precursor acute lymphoblastic leukemia from normal B precursors with four color flow cytometry: implications for residual disease detection. *Leukemia* 1999;13:558–567.

CHAPTER 6

Normal Histology and Immunoarchitecture of the Lymphohematopoietic System

Chris De Wolf-Peeters, Anna Tierens, and Ruth Achten

Lymphoid tissue is found all over the body. It occurs in well-organized lymphoid organs, such as the lymph nodes and the spleen, or as extranodal lymphoid tissue as part of the gut, skin, and lung. It may develop in any part of the body under specific conditions.

Classic histology divides the lymphoid organs into central and peripheral organs. The bone marrow and the thymus comprise the central lymphoid organs, and the lymph nodes, the spleen, and extranodal lymphoid tissues constitute the peripheral lymphoid organs. The bone marrow is the site of lymphopoiesis. Some lymphocytic precursors develop into B cells, but most become T cells. The generation of a diversity of effector B cells requires a two-step maturation process. The first step occurs in the bone marrow and results in the development of virgin or naive B cells. The second step takes place in the peripheral lymphoid organs, where affinity maturation of the naive B cells takes place on encounter with a specific antigen, resulting in the formation of plasma cells and memory B cells. The generation of T cells occurs exclusively in the thymus, where T-cell precursors develop into a variety of mature CD4-positive ($CD4^+$) and $CD8^+$ T cells through a process of positive and negative selection. No evidence is available that T cells require further affinity maturation in secondary lymphoid tissues. In contrast to B cells, T cells are activated only in secondary lymphoid organs and start to proliferate on appropriate antigen stimulation.

The architecture of the thymus and of the peripheral lymphoid organs offers the ideal microenvironment for these processes. Knowledge of these structures and the immunophenotype of their cellular components within their natural microanatomic environment has been improved significantly by the introduction of immunohistochemistry to the morphologic studies on lymphoid tissues. As for lymphoid cells, immunophenotyping allows identification of cell lineage and provides information on the stage of maturation, activation, and differentiation of these cells. Immunohistochemistry has offered the opportunity to identify and distinguish more precisely the nonlymphoid components of these tissues, including the monocyte-derived antigen-presenting cells and macrophages. Using antibodies against adhesion molecules expressed by endothelial lining cells and by lymphocytes, data on lymphocyte trafficking and homing have been generated.

Together with molecular techniques performed on tissue fragments and particularly experiments carried out on selected and defined areas, on cell clusters, or on single cells dissected from tissue sections, a new approach to the histologic investigation of these tissues has been developed. Data generated with these techniques have been confronted with information obtained from *in vitro* experiments and from knockout and transgenic animal experiments. The latter approach has profoundly changed our understanding of the structure of lymphoid tissues and has resulted in new views and concepts of the functional microanatomy of these tissues as the morphologic substrate of the immune response. This knowledge is essential in the analysis of lymphoid tissues in pathologic conditions, because it is helpful to recognize underlying pathogenic mechanisms.

This chapter discusses the histology and the immunohistology of the thymus, lymph node, and spleen. The historical description of the microanatomy of these organs, as reported by classic histology and electron microscopy, is presented first. This information is complemented by the results obtained by immunohistologic analysis. The functional significance of the various compartments identified by morphology is discussed. We consider the thymus as the microenviron-

C. De Wolf-Peeters and R. Achten: Department of Pathology, University Hospitals K. U. Leuven, Leuven, Belgium

A. Tierens: Department of Pathology, The Norwegian Radiumhospital and Institution for Cancer Research, Montebello, Oslo, Norway ment in which prothymocytes develop into mature T cells and show how it represents the structure providing a tridimensional framework for the selection of T cells by means of positive and negative interactions with major histocompatibility complex (MHC) products presented by thymic stromal cells. Similarly, we discuss the functional significance of the B follicle and the adjacent T-cell area or the "composite nodule" in the lymph node and in the spleen. This microanatomic unit provides an architectural construct for T-cell–controlled B-cell activation and selection by antigens, carried along with the lymph stream in the lymph node and arriving through the blood flow in the spleen.

The bone marrow, which is the site of lymphopoiesis in postnatal life and represents an additional microenvironment for B-cell maturation, is discussed in Chapter 1. Particular features of extranodal lymphoid tissues are the subject of Chapters 33 and 35.

THE THYMUS

General Comments

The thymus is a completely encapsulated, pyramid-shaped organ located in the anterosuperior mediastinum. It is composed of two lobes that join at their lower poles, which may reach the level of the fourth costal cartilage. The upper poles extend into the neck. The gray color of the thymus during infancy turns yellow with increasing age because of accumulation of fat tissue. Because this fat merely takes the place of normal thymus parenchyma, the organ's shape and volume remain unchanged (1).

In relation to body weight, thymic weight is maximal at birth, and its absolute weight peaks at puberty. Even after excluding age-related differences in the weight of this organ, large interindividual variations exist. These concepts are based on autopsy findings showing a thymus weighing 12 to 15 g at birth and 30 to 40 g at puberty. This prominent increase in absolute mass is followed by a gradual decrease, or "age-related thymic involution," leaving a thymus weighing no more than 10 to 15 g at the age of 60 years. Involution is accompanied by a gradual replacement of the thymic parenchyma by fat tissue until 40 to 50 years of age, after which little changes (1,2).

Sonographic evaluation of the thymic volume reveals somewhat different data. Using this technique, the thymus is visualized under normal conditions, allowing longitudinal studies on the evolution of the thymic volume during life. Data generated by this technique are only available for normal children between the ages of 2 and 8 years (3) and for the size evolution from birth to 12 months (4,5). These investigations demonstrate that the thymus increases in size from birth up to 8 months of age, after which its volume starts to decrease continuously, at least until the age of 8 years. The same studies also demonstrate that thymic measurements are strictly correlated with body weight and length of the child. This relationship appears to be the major factor determining individual variations. Another important factor responsible for individual size variation is the breast-feeding status of the child; breast-feeding is associated with a larger thymic size. Illness has not been proven to exert any significant influence on thymic size during infancy (4). The first signs of age-related thymic involution appear shortly before the age of 1 year and progress throughout life, although at a nearly undetectable rate after 40 to 50 years of age.

Despite of its notable decrease in size, the thymus never disappears completely, and it remains functionally active even after puberty (1). Remnants of the thymus with residual epithelium and cortical thymocytes are preserved, permitting the thymus to act as a site of T-cell differentiation and maturation throughout the entire life (6).

Although the mechanisms leading to age-related involution of the thymus remain to be unraveled, the phenomenon has been extensively studied at the histologic level. Microscopically, the process results from an atrophy of the parenchyma and a concomitant accumulation of subcapsular fat tissue. This insidious and gradual decrease in lymphoid cells and epithelial cells is accompanied by an accentuation of Hassall's corpuscles. Some of the corpuscles calcify, but others transform into thymic cysts (2). The morphology of the residual epithelial cells does not show any significant changes, which probably implies that they remain biologically active. Later studies using immunohistochemistry demonstrated that this persistent decrease in the number of epithelial cells and thymocytes is not the only event responsible for age-related thymic involution. An even more pronounced decrease in medullary interdigitating dendritic cells occurs (7).

Age-induced regression of thymic parenchyma differs considerably from the "acute accidental thymus atrophy" occurring in severely diseased patients or in association with trauma. This reversible atrophy is characterized by massive thymocyte death associated with an increase in macrophages. Age-related thymic atrophy must also be distinguished from human immunodeficiency virus (HIV)–induced thymic atrophy. In the latter condition, epithelial cell damage leading to lysis is superimposed on a prominent dearth of thymocytes (8).

Embryology

The thymus, together with the thyroid and the parathyroid glands, develops from the pharyngeal region. At 4 weeks of gestation, the thymic rudiment is formed by ectoderm of the third pharyngeal cleft and by endoderm from the third pharyngeal pouch. Consequently, postnatal thymic epithelium, particularly in the subcapsular and the medullary region, consists of ectodermal derived cells. Cortical epithelial cells are of endodermal origin. By 8 weeks of gestation, the right and the left thymic rudiment have moved caudally and eventually fuse at the midline. Subsequently, the connection with the branchial cleft is broken, and T-cell precursors begin to colonize the thymic rudiment. In the 10-week-old fetus, mesoderm-derived connective tissue surrounding the vessels invades the primitive thymus (9).

At the beginning of the second trimester of pregnancy, a configuration similar to the postnatal structure of the thymic microenvironment, is obtained. The thymus becomes identifiable as such because the distinction between the cortex and the medulla appears and Hassall's corpuscles are formed (6,10). In the course of the seventh and eighth week of gestation, multipotent hematopoietic progenitor cells derived from the yolk sac, the fetal liver, and the bone marrow seed the fetal thymus and colonize the thymic primordia. These cells are identical to the aforementioned T-cell precursors. They give rise to natural killer (NK) cells (9,11,12). Despite initial evolution of the thymic primordia independent of other influences at a specific developmental stage, the homing of T-cell precursors is a prerequisite for the normal maturation of the thymic microenvironment. In patients with severe combined immunodeficiency (SCID), a syndrome characterized by the absence of normal T-cell development, the rudimentary thymus is devoid of a medulla and consists entirely of a monotonous population of reticuloepithelial cells (13).

Macrophages, interdigitating dendritic cells, and B cells appear in the fetal thymus only from the 12th week of gestation onward (12,14). These cells invade the mesenchymal septa and the perivascular spaces of the thymic rudiment, resulting in large numbers of interdigitating dendritic cells in the medulla at the time this inner part is separated from the cortex. B cells appear initially at the corticomedullary junction, but with increasing age of gestation, they migrate toward the medulla. B lymphocytes preferentially occupy the area surrounding Hassall's corpuscles (15).

Developmental Anomalies

Aberrantly located thymic nodules are found in about 20% of humans, and occasionally, the thymus is entirely situated in the neck. This ectopic localization usually is caused by failed descent of the organ during embryogenesis. Thymuses in this abnormal position carry an increased risk of cystic alteration. The presence of ectopic parathyroid glands within the thymic capsule is also a common finding. An acceptable explanation for this phenomenon is the closely related embryogenesis of both organs (2).

Structural abnormalities of the thymus are invariably found in association with congenital immune deficiencies related to T-cell defects. These diseases encompass the DiGeorge syndrome (i.e., congenital absence of the thymus and the parathyroid glands), Nezelof's disease (i.e., congenital dysplasia of the thymus), and combined immunodeficiencies. In the latter two conditions, the thymus is thin and almost exclusively composed of epithelial cells with blurring of the distinction between cortex and medulla. Combined immunodeficiency associated with adenosine deaminase deficiency is not really characterized by dysplasia. Rather, it displays features reminiscent of acute thymic atrophy. In DiGeorge's syndrome, the thymus can be completely absent. However, several isolated cases of the latter condition have been described in which a hypoplastic thymus was observed. This thymic rudiment showed a preserved architecture colonized by normal cellular constituents (2).

True thymic hyperplasia, characterized by a concurrent increase in size and weight of the thymus, is a rare condition that should be distinguished from lymphofollicular hyperplasia. Although in the latter type of thymic enlargement lymphoid follicles with genuine germinal centers are clearly identifiable, the diagnosis of true thymic hyperplasia is restricted to cases presenting with a normal microscopic appearance for the age of the patient. Three distinct subtypes of this pathology have been recognized: thymic hyperplasia with massive enlargement of the gland; thymic rebound, which has been observed in children in a variety of conditions, especially after the treatment of childhood tumors; and true thymic hyperplasia in association with other diseases, particularly endocrinopathies, sarcoidosis, and Beckwith-Wiedemann syndrome (16).

Histology and Immunohistology

Because the fibrous capsule that surrounds the thymus extends into the thymic parenchyma as loose septa, the organ is incompletely subdivided into various lobules measuring 0.5 to 2 mm. These lobules represent the basic structural units of the thymus, which comprises two morphologically distinct areas, a cortex and a medulla (Fig. 6.1). Epithelial cells with a dendritic morphology, as seen by electron microscopy, and T lymphocytes or thymocytes constitute the major components of both regions. The subcapsular area of the cortex is occupied by somewhat larger thymocytes with a blastlike nucleus and a high number of mitotic figures. The distinction between cortex and medulla at the light microscopic level is evident because the amount of lymphocytes in the cortex far outnumbers those in the medulla. The medulla is much less intensely stained than the cortex. Alternatively, this mediastinal organ can be divided into two other morphologically distinct portions: an intraparenchymal compartment comprised of cortex and medulla and an extraparenchymal compartment that corresponds to the fibrous septa with the blood vessels and their perivascular spaces.

Thymic Epithelium

The epithelial cells, which may be difficult to recognize by routine light microscopy, are a heterogeneous population of round to spindle-shaped cells. Ultrastructurally, six different subtypes have been identified and described, of which four variants are localized to the cortex and two are confined to the medulla (9). As a whole, epithelial cells provide the appropriate microenvironment for T-cell maturation. However, because the development of T lymphocytes is an extremely complex process, each of the epithelial cell variants

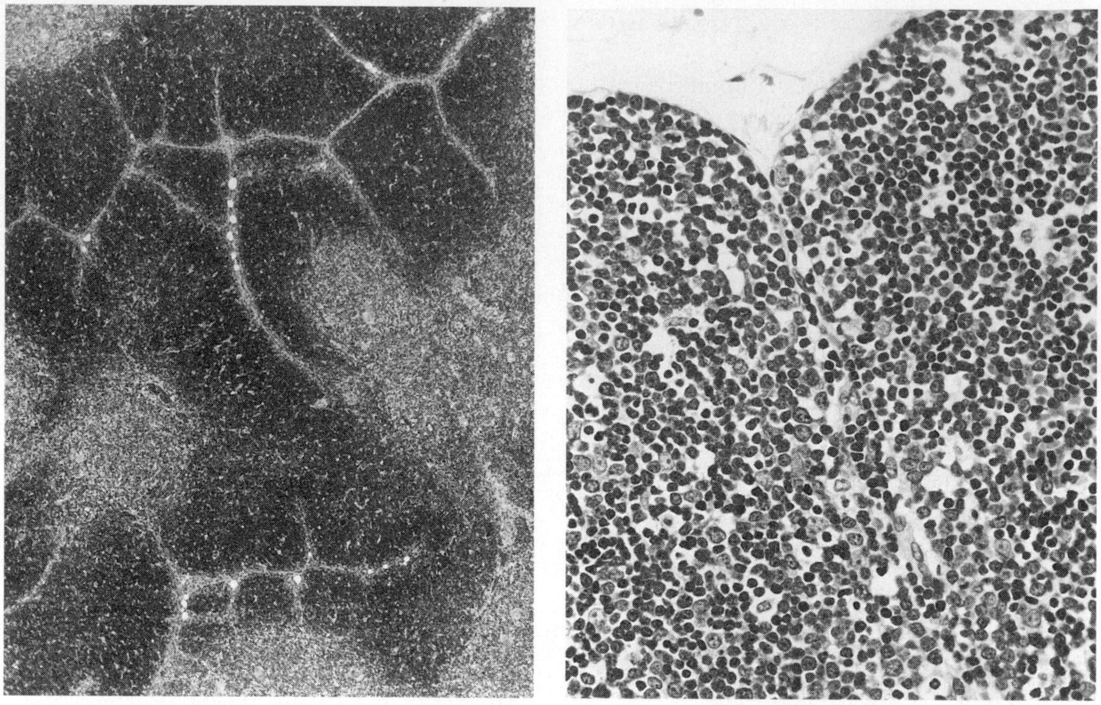

A B

FIG. 6.1. Hematoxylin and eosin–stained, paraffin-embedded thymic tissue of a child. **A:** Lobulation of the thymic parenchyma and clear delineation between the dark-stained cortex and the lighter medulla are shown (hematoxylin and eosin stain, original magnification: 20× magnification). **B:** Detail of the cortex shows the thymocytic variability with blast-like cells in the subcapsular area (hematoxylin and eosin stain, original magnification: 200× magnification).

exercises its own specific function in the establishment of an effective T-cell compartment.

In addition to its presence in the cortex underneath the thymic surface, type 1 epithelium is also found lining the perivascular spaces. These epithelial cells, together with their basal membrane, constitute the epithelial barrier separating the thymic parenchyma from the extraparenchymal compartment, as it was defined comprising the mesenchymal tissues of the thymus, including the perivascular spaces. The structural basis for the *blood-thymus barrier,* a functional concept that is discussed in detail later, is completed by the endothelial lining of the blood vessels and numerous perivascular macrophages (17).

The epithelial network of the middle and deep cortex consists of type 2 and 3 cells, both characterized by their long cytoplasmic processes embracing thymocytes. These cortical epithelial cells represent the *in vivo* equivalent of thymic nurse cells, a cell population that has been extensively studied *in vitro* (18). The results of these *in vitro* experiments, using cell lines derived from murine thymic nurse cells, suggest that they could be involved in the negative selection process of thymocytes by inducing thymocytic apoptosis (19). An analysis of the thymus dissected from cyclophosphamide-treated mice demonstrated pronounced thymocytic apoptosis concentrated around the thymic nurse cells. The latter cells function as phagocytes, clearing the cortical parenchyma from the apoptotic debris (20). Whether the minor structural differences that distinguish type 2 from type 3 medullary epithelial cells correlate with functional dissimilarities remains to be elucidated. Type 4 epithelial cells are restricted to the medullary region, and type 5 epithelial cells predominantly occupy the corticomedullary junction but can also be found in small clusters in the medulla. Hassall's corpuscles, the hallmark of the thymic medulla, represent the sixth type of epithelial cells in the thymus (14) (Fig. 6.2A).

Despite the marked differences in the appearance of the various epithelial cell types, striking similarities in their morphology, accentuating their common origin, are evident. First, every thymic epithelial cell displays slender cytoplasmic processes, which explains the term *dendritic cell.* These dendrites exhibit well-developed desmosomes at their ends through which the epithelial cells are connected with one another. The whole of thymic epithelial cells creates a firm meshwork throughout the entire parenchyma in which the other cell types are embedded. The epithelial origin of these cells is further confirmed by the presence of a supporting basement membrane. Nevertheless, the basal lamina surrounding medullary epithelial cells shows important focal gaps, and only cortical epithelial cells lining mesenchymal spaces have a continuous basal membrane to separate them from the neighboring fibrous tissue (6). Immunohistochemistry and electron microscopy of thymic epithelial cells have shown the presence of intermediate and thin filaments within the cytoplasm of these cells. The intermediate filaments, which correspond to tonofilaments, are clustered in

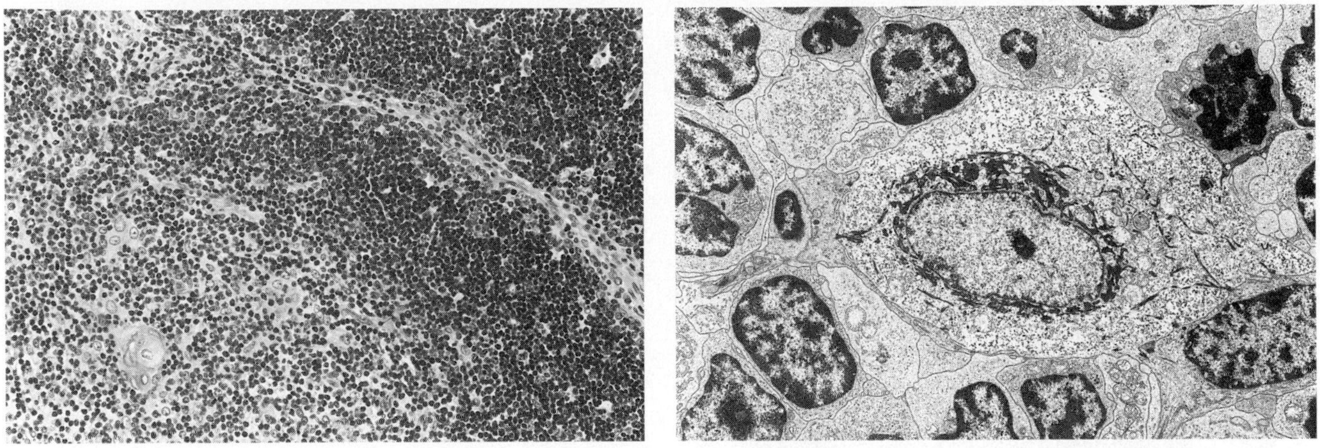

A B

FIG. 6.2. A: Light microscopy shows the morphology of Hassall's corpuscles (hematoxylin and eosin stain, original magnification: 200× magnification). **B:** Electron microscopy shows the well-developed framework of tonofilaments characteristic of type 6 epithelial cells composing Hassall's corpuscles (original magnification: 25,000× magnification).

thick bundles attached to the desmosomes. They form an extensive filamentous network within the cell body and the cytoplasmic processes of the cortical and the medullary epithelial cells. Bundles of thin actin-like filaments, located immediately underneath the plasma membrane, complete the filamentous cytoskeleton of the epithelial cells. Subcortical epithelial cells typically show an abundance of thin filaments, but this portion of the cytoskeleton is nearly undetectable in medullary epithelial cells (21).

Type 6 epithelial cells, composing Hassall's corpuscles are provided with a particularly well-developed framework of tonofilaments (21) (Fig. 6.2B). These thymic corpuscles do not constitute isolated epithelial islets within the thymic medulla. Together with the other epithelial components of the inner part of the thymic parenchyma, they establish an uninterrupted epithelial structure, supporting admixed lymphocytic elements. Hassall's corpuscles are clusters of concentrically arranged epithelial cells, but in addition to their thymic epithelial cell features, they acquire characteristics of squamous epithelium by exhibiting a variable degree of keratinization. Their precise function or significance is unresolved. Although interpreted in the past as a terminal phase of a degenerative process, they are considered a dynamic structure that is involved in the intrathymic maturation of T cells (22).

Subcapsular epithelial cells, a minority of cortical epithelial cells, and almost all medullary epithelial cells can be considered as a functionally distinct group of neuroendocrine cells. These cells strongly express oxytocin, vasopressin, and neurophysin-like peptides (23). These peptides are synthesized within these cells, where the proteins can be demonstrated and the corresponding mRNA is found (24). It has been suggested that, analogous to neurosecretory cells found elsewhere, neuroendocrine cells of the thymus convert neuronal signals into neuropeptide secretion. Accepting this hypothesis, thymic oxytocin and vasopressin, secreted as a result of yet undefined neuronal influences, are expected to exert a direct immunomodulation on T-cell maturation (23).

Antibodies against other substances involved in intercellular signaling—the thymic hormones thymuline, members of the thymosin family, and thymopoietin—immunoreact with a subpopulation of these neuroendocrine cells, particularly subcapsular and medullary epithelial cells (25). These hormones also affect the maturation of T-cell precursors and the expression of T-cell antigens.

The entire cortical epithelium, including the nurse cells, reacts with Mab-MR6, recognizing a component of the interleukin-4 (IL-4) receptor complex. Consequently, these cells may act as an IL-4 reservoir for the surrounding immature cortical thymocytes (14). Antibodies against MHC class II molecules (e.g., HLA-DR) stain a fine meshwork of cytoplasmic processes originating from the epithelial cells in the outer cortex that embrace nonreactive thymocytes, arranged singly or in small clusters (Fig. 6.3). Considerable parts of the inner cortex are found to be devoid of positively stained cells.

T Lymphocytes

T lymphocytes (i.e., thymocytes) displaying heterogeneous features corresponding to the various stages of thymocyte maturation predominate in the thymic cortex. Large lymphoid cells resembling lymphoblasts are found in the subcapsular region. Medium-sized thymocytes occur throughout the cortex and at the corticomedullary junction, whereas small lymphocytes are scattered among the epithelial cells in the medulla. In other words, immature thymocytes are found in the subcapsular region and the cortex, whereas well-differentiated thymocytes migrate to the medulla and leave the thymus to enter the circulation. The details of this complex process of thymocyte development are explained in a separate section.

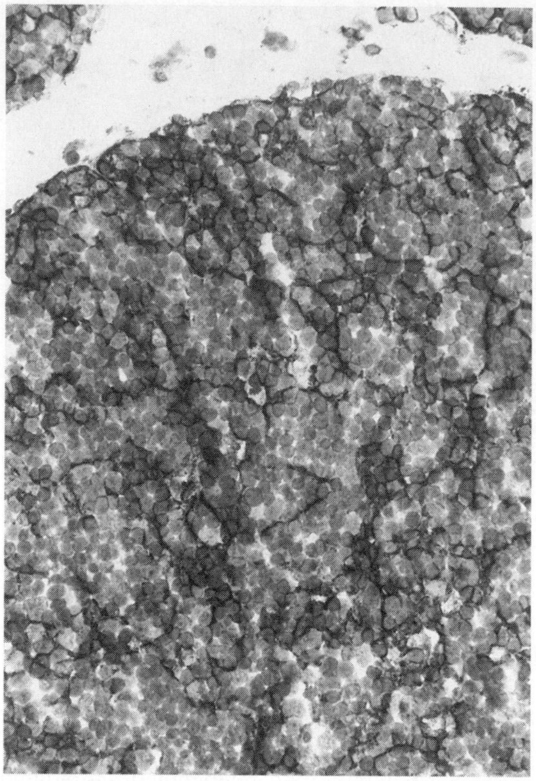

FIG. 6.3. Fresh frozen tissue section from the thymus stained for HLA-DR. Antibodies directed against this surface marker highlight the epithelial network in the subcapsular area embracing nonreactive thymocytes. Cortical epithelial cells probably correspond to thymic nurse cells (immunostaining of HLA-DR, original magnification: 200× magnification).

B Lymphocytes

The presence of B cells as a consistent component of the human thymus is well proven (15,26–28). Like T cells, B lymphocytes exist as a heterogeneous population with a distinct B-cell subset found in the intraparenchymal compartment, preferentially in the neighborhood of Hassall's corpuscles. These B cells are occasionally found in the adult thymic cortex as scattered single elements. In the fetal thymus, they are observed preferentially at the corticomedullary junction (15).

In contrast with B cells localized in the perivascular area, thymic intraparenchymal B lymphocytes are morphologically and phenotypically distinct from the B cells composing the lymphocytic corona and the germinal center of the B follicle of the lymph node, but they do express most pan-B-cell markers, including CD19, CD20, CD22, CD37, CD72, CD76, and they weakly express IgM and IgD (15).

An important subset of human thymic B cells is $CD2^+$ and $CD40^+$, markers that are invariably present on T lymphocytes but only occasionally found on B cells (28). Whether CD2 expression on these B cells is induced by the thymic environment or, alternatively, favors homing of this particular B-cell subset in the thymus has not been elucidated. CD2 may mediate the interaction of the B cells with the surrounding thymocytes and epithelial cells through its ligand LFA-3, which is expressed on the latter cells. B and T cells would benefit from this CD2 interaction through the acquisition of improved self-antigen recognition capacity (28,29).

Among the intraparenchymal B lymphocytes, a subpopulation of somewhat larger cells displaying dendritic cytoplasmic extensions is seen near Hassall's corpuscles. These peculiar cells, also designated *asteroid cells*, consistently lack IgD but do express an additional marker, CD23, pointing out their activated status (15).

As a whole, the B cells of the thymic parenchyma belong to the microenvironment of the medulla and do not represent mere passengers derived from the perivascular space, which also comprises a B-lymphocytic population, including B follicles. Whether the B follicles occasionally found in the medulla are delineated from the surrounding T-cell microenvironment by a continuous layer of epithelial cells supported by a basal membrane is subject to debate (15). Although some immunohistologic and electron microscopic studies demonstrated the presence of an intact layer of epithelial cells separating lymphoid follicles from the thymic medulla, other investigators indicated that this separation is not always continuous and that this leaky barrier might allow B-cell traffic between the periphery of the follicle and the thymic medullary parenchyma (15). During fetal development, B lymphocytes initially are restricted to the perivascular compartment while progressively increasing numbers of these cells are observed within the thymic parenchyma, and it seems likely that thymic medullary B lymphocytes are acquired by migration from the extraparenchymal area. The number of B cells in the thymic medulla is related to the number of individual B lymphocytes and B follicles present in the extraparenchymal compartment, which supports the hypothesis that the intramedullary and extramedullary B-cell compartments do not constitute entirely separate regions but that they are at least subject to similar influences (15).

B follicles become much more numerous in persons with myasthenia gravis. These B follicles are accompanied by a T-cell area, resembling the paracortex of peripheral lymph node. The features of the thymic medulla become reminiscent of those displayed by a peripheral lymph node (30). Because thymectomy in myasthenia gravis reduces the level of antibodies against the acetylcholine receptor (31,32), thymic $CD2^+$ B cells could play a role in this disease. Although engagement of the CD2 receptor does not directly trigger B-cell antibody production, it does promote cell adhesions and antigen recognition and might therefore contribute indirectly through enhanced T-cell stimulation to the production of autoantibody in this condition.

Based on topographic, morphologic, and immunohistochemical similarities, it has been suggested that intrathymic B cells represent a specific type of marginal zone B cell intrinsic to the thymic parenchyma. Nevertheless, important immunophenotypic differences exist between B lymphocytes of the thymic parenchyma and marginal zone cells as they are observed in the spleen, peripheral lymph, nodes, and mucosa-associated lymphoid tissues (15). This particular subset of B cells awaits further examination to elucidate its precise stage in B-lymphocytic differentiation.

Similar investigations may help to define the normal cellular counterpart of the neoplastic cells composing mediastinal large B-cell lymphomas. This malignancy, listed in the Revised European-American Lymphoma (REAL) classification as a large B-cell lymphoma subtype, is characterized by its presentation as a locally invasive anterior mediastinal mass originating in the thymus (33). Because the atypical cells of this mediastinal tumor are unmistakably of B-cell type, it was postulated that they originate from the B lymphocytes that are normally found in the thymic parenchyma. However, because the neoplasm is composed of large cells with variable nuclear features, no clear morphologic indications link these cells to constituents of nonneoplastic extrathymic lymphoid tissues.

Küppers and colleagues demonstrated that, like other diffuse large B-cell lymphomas, mediastinal large B cell lymphoma cells harbor mutated V region genes, which indicates derivation from postgerminal center B lymphocytes (34). From the point of view of the stage of development of the tumor precursor, an integration of mediastinal large B-cell lymphomas in the larger entity represented by all diffuse large B-cell lymphomas seems therefore arguable. Nevertheless, these malignancies show a distinct clinical image, and their molecular genetic pattern, in particular the rarity of structural alterations of the *BCL6* gene (35), bears little resemblance to that known for diffuse large B-cell lymphomas in general. Mediastinal large B-cell lymphomas and their hypothetical normal counterpart merit further consideration, probably resulting in the recognition of this tumor as a distinct clinicopathologic entity (see Chapter 25).

Other Cell Types

Besides thymic epithelial cells and lymphocytes, several other cells have been identified in the thymus. This minor population is comprised of various cell types, including macrophages, interdigitating dendritic cells, and myoid cells. Macrophages are mainly found in the cortex, but they also occur in the medulla. As regular phagocytic cells, they are characterized by their α-naphthol esterase and acid phosphatase activity. Being devoid of HLA-DR antigens, these macrophages are not expected to function as genuine antigen-presenting cells. Together with the thymic nurse cells, they eliminate dying thymocytes that have been negatively selected during maturation processes (14).

Interdigitating dendritic cells are exclusively localized in the medulla. These cells stand out by their irregularly shaped and folded nucleus and by their long cytoplasmic processes that embrace the surrounding T cells. Because of this intimate contact and the expression of HLA-DR antigens by interdigitating dendritic cells, investigators have speculated that these cells contribute to the final maturation of medullary T lymphocytes. Although Langerhans cells with characteristic Birbeck granules do occur in the thymus of animals, these cells are consistently lacking in human thymuses (6).

Myoid cells have been identified in adult and fetal thymuses. These cells are unevenly distributed throughout the thymus, with a preferential occurrence in small clusters, predominantly located in the medullary parenchyma. These cells display the ultrastructural features of degenerating striated muscle cells, typically containing myosin and actin filaments in their cytoplasm (21). The presence of acetylcholine receptor-like material (22) has been demonstrated on the surface of thymic myoid cells, a finding that might explain the link between myasthenia gravis and the thymus. Although the number of myoid cells showed no significant increase in this condition, the occupancy of the myoid cell membrane by this substance might trigger intrathymic B cells, probably stimulated by self-reactive T cells, to produce acetylcholine receptor-specific antibodies (30). Such a scenario in which lymphocytes develop autoreactivity rather than self-tolerance in the thymus would explain the symptoms of myasthenia gravis, which are brought about by autoantibodies to the acetylcholine receptor of skeletal muscles. Because the number and size of B follicles are markedly increased in the thymic medulla of myasthenia gravis patients, these antibodies may be generated by the germinal center cells of the thymic B follicles (36).

Blood vessels and the associated perivascular spaces belong to the extraparenchymal compartment of the thymus. The perivascular space, its macrophages, vascular endothelium, and type 1 thymic epithelium represent the blood-thymus barrier, which was thought to guarantee an antigen-free environment in the thymic cortex, protecting thymocytes from inappropriate stimulation. Nieuwenhuis and associates demonstrated the existence of a transcapsular pathway by which antigens may bypass the thymic-blood barrier (37). Since these results were published, the functional significance of the blood-thymic barrier was seriously questioned. Nevertheless, cortical thymocytes are undoubtedly efficiently protected against bloodborne antigens, whether this shelter is entirely provided for by the described structures or not. Morphologically, the perivascular space is based on an extensive reticulin meshwork that surrounds the complete vascular system of the thymus. On either side, this specialized region is bordered by a basement membrane, with the one produced by the endothelium on the vascular side and the one lining the type 1 epithelial cells on the other. The overall appearance and the cellular composition of the perivascular area shows considerable variation among the two components of the thymic parenchyma. Whereas the medulla generally is poorer in lymphocytes, its wide perivascular spaces contain many of these cells. The cortex is provided with narrow perivascular areas, mostly devoid of lymphocytes.

The vascular network embedded in this fibrous tissue is derived from interlobular arteries, in particular the arterioles at the corticomedullary junction and a capillary network located in the cortex. In the subcapsular area, they unite in an anastomosing arcade that drains in postcapillary venules. The extraparenchymal compartment contains lymphatics and nerves. Whereas afferent lymphatic vessels are consistently absent, efferent ones, arising from the medulla and the corticomedullary junction, run along with arteries and veins. Eventually, they leave the organ also by perforating the capsule, particularly in the clefts formed by the interlobular septa, meanwhile having drained the perivascular spaces (38). The thymus is innervated by autonomic nerves that are derived from the sympathetic chain and the vagus and are mainly restricted to the capsule and its septa. A neural plexus is formed along the corticomedullary junction by closely interwoven sympathetic and vagal fibers. This autonomic innervation is crucial to vasomotor control but probably also serves other purposes. The overall function of the nervous system and the aforementioned neuroendocrine cells remains to be elucidated (38).

T-Cell Development within the Microenvironment of the Thymus

The most immature thymic T cells (i.e., T-cell precursors) are identified by the expression of CD34, CD33, CD45RA, and CD38^{low}, typically lacking surface CD2, CD5, CD1, and CD3 (39). They express the integrins very late activation (VLA) antigen-4 (VLA-4, $\alpha_4\beta_1$, CD49d/CD29), VLA-5 ($\alpha_5\beta_1$, CD49e/CD29), and PGP-1 (CD44), which potentially mediate homing of the precursors to the thymus (40,41). T-cell receptor (TCR) genes are still in the germline configuration. These multipotent progenitor cells have the capacity to develop into T cells and NK cells (42).

Unlike their predecessors, the earliest committed T-cell progenitors have acquired surface CD1, CD2, CD5, CD7, and cytoplasmic CD3, but they are still devoid of surface CD3, CD8, and CD4. These triple-negative thymocytes show an intense proliferative activity, which depends on IL-7 (43–45) and stem cell factor (46,47). BCL-2, an anti-apoptosis protein, may add to the prolonged cell survival of these early thymocytes (48). Precisely during this stage of thymocyte development, the TCR β chain is rearranged. After this pivotal event in T-cell maturation, TCR β is expressed on the cell surface in a complex with gp33 and the pre-TCR α chain. The resultant primitive TCR complex occurs in association with CD3, which was already present on the cell's surface (49–51). Signaling through this pre-TCR complex is crucial for the next step in the generation of mature T lymphocytes, which comprises three molecular biologic events: the concomitant upregulation of CD4 and CD8 resulting in double-positive thymocytes, rearrangement of the TCR α locus, and allelic exclusion of the TCR β locus (49,52,53). There is some evidence that signal transduction through the pre-TCR complex may involve the lymphocyte-specific tyrosine kinases p56^{lck} and p59^{fyn} (54,55), as well as p21^{ras} protein activity (56). However, among the abundance of signaling molecules present in the thymic microenvironment, the ligands specifically involved in the triggering of the pre-TCR complex remain to be identified (57). As a consequence of this complex event, CD4$^+$CD8$^+$TCR^{low} cortical thymocytes are brought about, representing the first thymic T-cell population to express the definitive TCR $\alpha\beta$ chain (42).

Subsequently, these CD3^{low}, double-positive thymocytes are positively or negatively selected by thymic stromal cells. Many factors, such as the density of the MHC molecules and co-receptors expressed on the auxiliary thymic cells and the nature and concentration of peptides presented on their surface determine the ultimate fate of the T cells subject to this selection process (58–60). However, the level of avidity between TCR and MHC-peptide complexes is the main factor mediating survival signals or deletion by apoptosis. High-affinity binding of the TCR to peptides, derived from autoantigen, superantigens, or both, presented in the context of self-MHC results in clonal deletion of autoreactive T cells (61,62). In contrast, low or intermediate avidity confers to positive selection, which is indispensable for the final maturation of double-positive thymocytes to CD4 or CD8 single-positive T cells. It is still a matter of debate how the engagement of the TCR with an MHC class I or II molecule forces the double-positive thymocyte to specifically downregulate one of these two main lineage markers. Two alternative models have been proposed: the instructive and the stochastic or selection hypothesis.

The instructive model implies that lineage commitment and positive selection occur simultaneously (63,64). From this point of view, engagement of MHC class I molecules during positive selection dictates an uncommitted precursor to become a CD8$^+$ T cell, whereas the recognition of class II MHC molecules instructs a double-positive T-cell to become a CD4 single-positive T cell.

In contrast, the stochastic or selection model regards lineage commitment, established by the downregulation of one of the coreceptors, as the primary event occurring independently of TCR specificity (58,63,65,66). Thymocytes bearing class I–specific TCRs undergo positive selection on the condition that they have turned off CD4, meanwhile maintaining CD8 as a surface marker. Likewise, positive selection of thymocytes with class II–specific TCRs requires the expression of CD4 without CD8 interference.

Positive selection *in vivo* is mediated predominantly by cortical epithelial cells that express MHC class I or class II molecules (67), whereas *in vitro* experiments suggest that negative selection comes about most efficiently when the antigen is presented by medullary dendritic cells (68). The signal transduction pathways involved in positive and negative selection are only partially elucidated. Increasing evidence emerges supporting the hypothesis that positive and negative selection are mediated through distinct biochemical pathways. The greater part of the information regarding TCR-mediated signaling processes was obtained from studies with mature T cells. The development of gene-manipulated animals and the availability of specific inhibitors of signal transduction molecules were particularly valuable in the elucidation of the various signaling pathways involved in T-cell development. The TCR signal transduction pathways leading to positive selection encompass a myriad of intracellular substances, including the CD45 phosphatase (69), $p21^{ras}$ and the downstream effector MAP kinase (70,71), the T-cell tyrosine kinase ZAP-70 (72–74), and the calcium-, calmodulin-dependent phosphatase calcineurin (75). The signaling pathways involved in negative selection and the accessory molecules involved in defining the final function of the T cells, as determined by their phenotype, remain to be unraveled.

Most thymocytes, unable to pass through the selection process because of defective TCR/MHC interaction, die of neglect. All thymocytes triggered to die, whether apoptosis is a result of negative selection or caused by lack of stimulation, are thoroughly eliminated by the numerous phagocytes in the cortex and medulla, among which are the aforementioned cortical epithelial nurse cells.

THE LYMPH NODE AND THE SPLEEN

The lymph node and the spleen offer a specialized microenvironment that is extremely well suited to allow the occurrence of immune responses through the interaction between blood-borne and lymph-borne antigens, accessory cells and lymphocytes.

The Lymph Node

Lymph nodes are small, bean-shaped lymphoid organs, generally measuring only a few millimeters in the longest dimension. In an activated state, however, they enlarge to reach a size of more than 1 cm. These encapsulated organs occur throughout the entire body, invariably intercalated in the lymph stream. They are most frequently found in the axillary, cervical, and inguinal regions, in the mediastinum, and in the retroperitoneum. They serve innate and specific immunity. Their macrophages ingest the bulk of invading, lymph-borne microorganisms, reducing the load of foreign antigens that is carried along with the lymphatics. Lymphocytes may continuously enter the lymph node parenchyma through the highly specialized postcapillary venules, allowing a recruitment of specific lymphocytes from a large circulating pool. In this way, a system capable of generating an adequate immune response to nearly all lymph-borne antigens is created (76).

Embryology

The development of human lymph nodes occurs during fetal life with primitive follicles emerging from the 16th gestational week on. At first, a network of follicular dendritic cells is formed, which is subsequently seeded by small, mainly round lymphocytes of B- and T-cell lineage. The B cells uniformly express CD20, CD21, CD24, IgM, and IgD. A considerable proportion of these B cells is also immunoreactive with antibodies directed against epitopes on the CD5 molecule, which is an antigen normally present on mature T cells only. It is noteworthy that the neoplastic B cells in chronic lymphocytic leukemia and mantle cell lymphoma express this surface marker too (see Chapters 21, 22, and 40). The T cells present are CD3, CD5, and $CD4^+$ or $CD8^+$ (77). These rudimentary follicles are similar in appearance to the primary B follicles found in postnatal life, except for the peculiar B lymphocytic population expressing CD5. Although the follicular structures of the fetal lymph node do increase in size, genuine germinal centers only appear after birth (77).

In mice, the development of the lymph nodes starts with the nearly exclusive accumulation of a particular $CD4^+CD3^-$ progenitor cell population that can develop into NK cells, dendritic antigen-presenting cells, and not further characterized "follicular cells" (78). The developmentally controlled expression of lymphocyte homing receptors and vascular addressins regulates lymphocyte entrance to the lymph nodes, allowing only $CD4^+CD3^-$ cells to colonize lymph nodes during fetal life (79). In fetal mice, nodal high endothelial venules express mucosal addressin cell adhesion molecule-1 (MAdCAM-1), resulting in a selective attraction of $\alpha_4\beta_7$ integrin-positive cells, although this population accounts for only 1% to 2% of the entire lymphocytic pool, with most circulating lymphocytes expressing the homing receptor L-selectin. This allows seeding of the initial lymph node structure by two unusual lymphocyte populations expressing Peyer's patch homing receptor or the $\alpha_4\beta_7$ integrin: the $CD4^+CD3^-$ cells and the TCR $\gamma\delta$ T cells.

As early as 1 to 2 days after birth, the classic lymph node addressin, peripheral lymph node vascular addressin (PNAd), appears on the endothelial lining of the high endothelial venules, resulting in a dramatic substitution of the $CD4^+CD3^-$ cell recruitment by ordinary lymphocytes expressing L-selectin (79).

Histology and Immunohistology

The lymph node is surrounded by a fibrous capsule from which fibrous septa derive, resulting in an incomplete subdivision of the parenchyma into segments. Several afferent lymphatics reach the lymph node at its convex margin to end into the subcapsular or marginal sinus, which can be regarded as a huge lymph reservoir located immediately underneath the lymph node capsule. Subsequently, the lymph percolates through the cortical sinuses that communicate with the medullary sinuses and eventually converge to give rise to only one efferent lymphatic that leaves the lymph node at its hilus. The sinus network does not randomly drain the lymph node. Instead, it constitutes an ingenious irrigation system, relating each afferent lymphatic to a well-defined functional compartment (80).

The sinuses form a labyrinth of wide, irregular spaces that

resemble thin-walled blood vessels (81). The sinus lacework is bordered by a discontinuous monolayer of sinus lining cells to which delicate collagen fibers are attached. This supportive fibrous skeleton stretches out in the lumen, preventing the sinus walls from collapsing. Broad intercellular gaps in the sinus lining allow unimpeded contact between the luminal contents and the surrounding tissue. The absence of a basal membrane promotes direct interaction between the circulating lymph and the lymph node parenchyma. Although most nodal sinuses lack such a structure, an authentic basal membrane is found underlying the cellular monolayer, lining the capsular side of the marginal sinus (82).

In normal lymph nodes, sinus lining cells are inconspicuous and can hardly be distinguished from the macrophages and other mononuclear cells abundantly present in the sinus lumen. Sinus lining cells should be discriminated from ordinary macrophages, like the ones piled up in the lumen, for they show no evidence of phagocytosis. They are provided with long dendrites that connect the cell with its neighbors through well-developed desmosomes. Consequently, another wide-meshed network is built up traversing the sinus lumen. This network may function as a cellular sieve and facilitate the capture and neutralization of lymph-borne antigens. Another peculiar ultrastructural feature of sinus lining cells is their intimate association with reticulin fibers from the sinus cavity. These components of the fibrous network supporting the sinuses, typically composed of type IV collagen, are engulfed by slender protrusions extending from the cell's body (82,83) (Fig. 6.4).

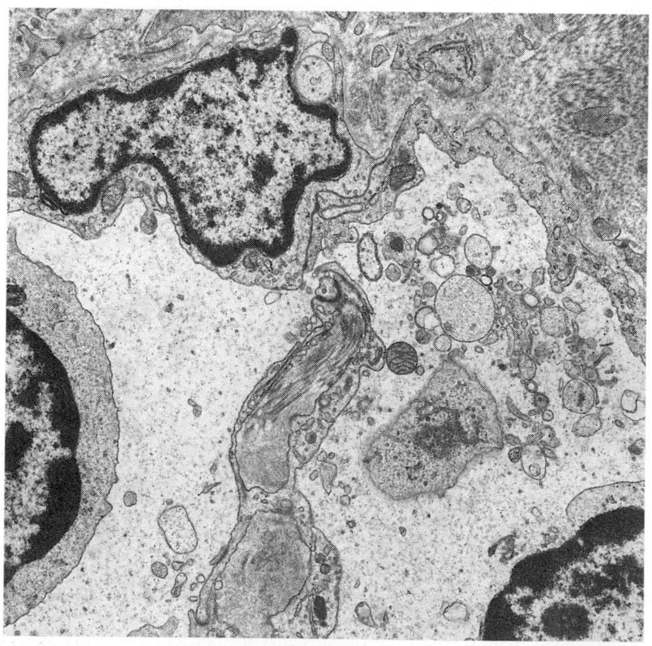

FIG. 6.4. Ultrastructural image of a lymph node sinus. Electron microscopy shows the filamentous network supporting the sinus, which is composed of type IV collagen. This material is engulfed by slender protrusions of the sinus lining cells (original magnification: 72,500× magnification).

Based on marked morphologic similarities, it has been suggested that the sinus lining cells originate from dendritic cells. However, unlike follicular dendritic cells and interdigitating dendritic cells, they do not display any phagocytic activity. Moreover, they consistently lack S-100 protein and CD1a, molecules frequently present on interdigitating dendritic cells. In contrast, they do react with antibodies directed against the highly restricted antigens Ki-M9 and Ki-M4, which have only been identified on the surface of follicular dendritic cells. The latter finding, together with the demonstration of IL-6 production by sinus lining cells (84), strongly suggests that these cells really function as genuine antigen-binding and -presenting cells (83).

Occasionally, lymph node sinuses transform into or are replaced with blood vessels. This rare pathologic condition has been described as "vascular transformation of the lymph node" and is usually confined to one lymph node region (85). More frequently, an accumulation of impressive numbers of histiocytes is found within markedly dilated sinuses. This reactive condition is known as sinus histiocytosis or sinus catarrh (85,86) (see Chapter 15).

The nodal arteries enter the lymph node through the hilus and give rise to arterioles that follow the fibrous trabeculae. From these small vessels, extensive capillary networks branch off that are connected with postcapillary venules. Most of these highly specialized vessels, also called high endothelial venules because of their unusual morphology, are situated in the paracortex (82). After its passage through the high endothelial venules (discussed later), the blood is drained by the nodal veins, which leave the node together with the efferent lymphatic. In humans, no communications exist between the sinuses and the vascular system.

The lymph node parenchyma is subdivided by classic histology into the cortex, comprised of nodular aggregates of B cells or B follicles; the deep cortex or paracortex, underlying the entire cortex and commonly regarded as a uniform layer; and the medulla, the innermost region. In addition to these three domains, orientated parallel to the capsule, a fourth microanatomic area has been described. This domain is directed perpendicular to the other regions and comprises the sinuses with their numerous macrophages (82,87,88).

These anatomic areas do not correspond to the functional domains recognized by tridimensional studies (80) and by immunohistology (89). Visualization of the lymph flow through the sinus system has demonstrated that the various afferent lymphatics ending in the subcapsular sinus delineate functional lymph node compartments (80). Each compartment is comprised of the terminal part of an afferent lymphatic and the adjacent part of the subcapsular sinus. Oddly enough, the lymph received from that particular lymphatic does not circulate through the marginal sinus, but remaining strictly confined to a well-delineated portion, it immediately continues its passage through the other parts of the functional unit: the underlying region of the cortex, a deep cortical fraction, and the medullary cords contiguous with these cortical elements. At the periphery of each compartment, medullary sinuses may connect directly with the subcapsular sinus. Although this functional topography of the lymph node was initially described and extensively studied in rats, especially focusing on the deep cortical unit, the lymph nodes of other species show a similar architecture (90).

The lymph node compartments as described in these tridimensional studies correspond roughly to the concept of the composite nodule as it was identified by combined enzyme chemistry and immunohistochemistry in human lymph nodes (89). Application of these techniques on nonspecific, reactive lymph nodes reveals the presence of nodular aggregates rich in T cells that are preferentially located in the paracortex. Moreover, these T nodules frequently occur in strict association with adjacent B follicles. In its most characteristic presentation, an ovoid structure comprising two portions, a classic B domain or B follicle, located at the periphery, in combination with a central T region can be identified (Fig. 6.5). This composite nodule represents a dynamic microanatomic structure, continuously changing and remodeling in answer to the type of antigen challenge and the course of the immune response, that fades away with decreasing antigenic stimulation. The impressive variation in the appearance of a lymph node as a reflection of different pathologic conditions merely represents alternative presentations of its composite nodules that can adapt to the specific type of antigen. In follicular hyperplasia, for example, the T compartment of the composite nodule is reduced to a narrow crescent, while in dermatopathic lymphadenitis adjacent T nodules fuse to give rise to a semicircular structure associated with several B follicles. The latter morphologic variant, in which individual composite nodules join in one larger entity, in particular shows striking similarities to the structures described by Sainte-Marie (80).

Using a combined enzyme chemistry and immunohistochemical approach to investigate extranodal lymphoid tissues, including the spleen, the composite nodule appears to be the universal structural entity of the entire lymphoid system. Moreover, it displays an identical architecture and cellular composition, regardless of the anatomic site in which it is identified (91). Because the composite nodule represents the morphologic equivalent of the pivotal functional entity of the lymphoid system as a whole, its characteristics are discussed in a separate section.

Nevertheless, human reactive lymph nodes present a unique microenvironment especially suited to eliminate antigens carried along by lymphatics. For this reason, the obser-

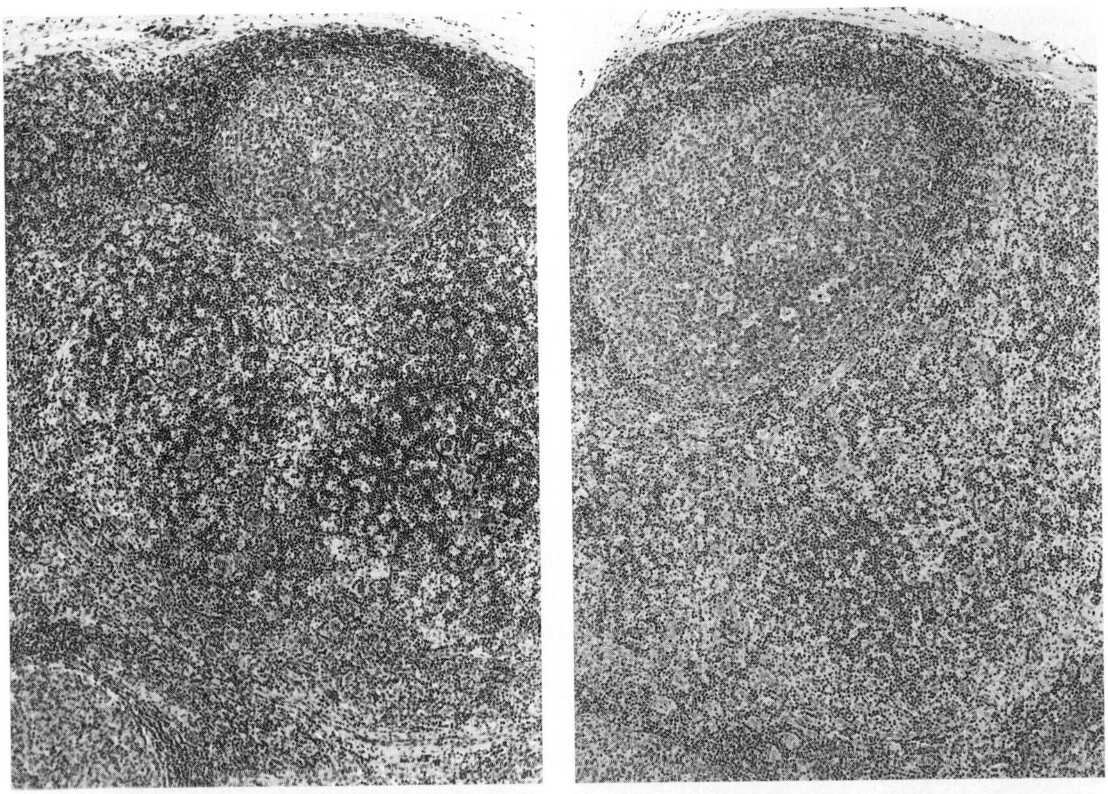

A B

FIG. 6.5. Hematoxylin and eosin–stained, paraffin-embedded sections of two reactive lymph nodes. In both nodes, a composite nodule is easily recognized, with a B follicle in the upper part and the adjacent T nodule in the lower part; the morphology of the latter is variable in **A** and **B**. **A:** A primary T-cell nodule is typically surrounded by a rim of interdigitating dendritic cells (hematoxylin and eosin stain, original magnification: 50× magnification). **B:** The same cells are admixed with T lymphocytes, resulting in a less well demarcated T-cell area, characteristic for the secondary T-cell nodule (hematoxylin and eosin stain, original magnification: 50× magnification).

vation of some specific features of B follicles and T nodules in the reactive lymph node hardly comes as a surprise. The remainder of this discussion focuses on these structural peculiarities.

The typical B follicle of the lymph node is comprised of two distinct compartments: the germinal center and the follicle mantle. Although in other sites, including the spleen and Peyer's patches, two different regions can be distinguished in the follicle mantle (i.e., lymphocytic corona and a marginal zone), a clear-cut marginal zone is only occasionally demarcated in the lymph node (Fig. 6.6). Mesenteric lymph nodes are exceptions to this rule, because they regularly show a well-developed marginal zone that may be confused with a marginal zone lymphoma. In other lymph nodes, marginal zone B cells usually occur as a minor population, inconspicuously intermingled with the small lymphocytes of the outer part of the lymphocytic corona (92,93).

Because of their striking morphologic and phenotypic resemblance to splenic marginal zone B cells, examiners have been able to identify these scarce cells, which are also described as monocytoid B cells. The number of marginal zone cells in the lymph node may increase dramatically in certain inflammatory conditions such as toxoplasmosis or HIV infections (see Chapters 15 and 28). This marginal zone cell hyperplasia was first described as immature sinus histiocytosis (94), but because the proliferating cells were identified as B lymphocytes, this condition is referred to as monocytoid B-cell hyperplasia (95), postulating that they represent the nodal counterpart of the marginal zone cells of the spleen (92,95). The finding of these monocytoid B cells admixed with granulocytes, macrophages, small lymphocytes, occasional plasma cells, and blast cells underscores this hypothesis because a similar cellular heterogeneity is observed in the spleen (96).

The morphology of the T nodules in human lymph nodes ranges from clearly delineated nodules to ill-defined structures (91,97). The framework of these nodules is composed of interdigitating dendritic cells, uniformly characterized by distinct morphologic features, and by S-100 β expression. A variable number of interdigitating dendritic cell–related cells have been identified as Langerhans cells, which typically express CD1a on their surface and contain racquet-shaped Birbeck granules in their cytoplasm (Fig. 6.7). In this lacework, numerous T lymphocytes, predominantly of the $CD4^+$ phenotype, are embedded.

Based on their architectural composition and cellular components, three types of T nodule can be identified. Well-delineated nodules, called primary T nodules, constitute clearly distinct structures, consisting of a rim of concentrically arranged interdigitating dendritic cells, surrounding a

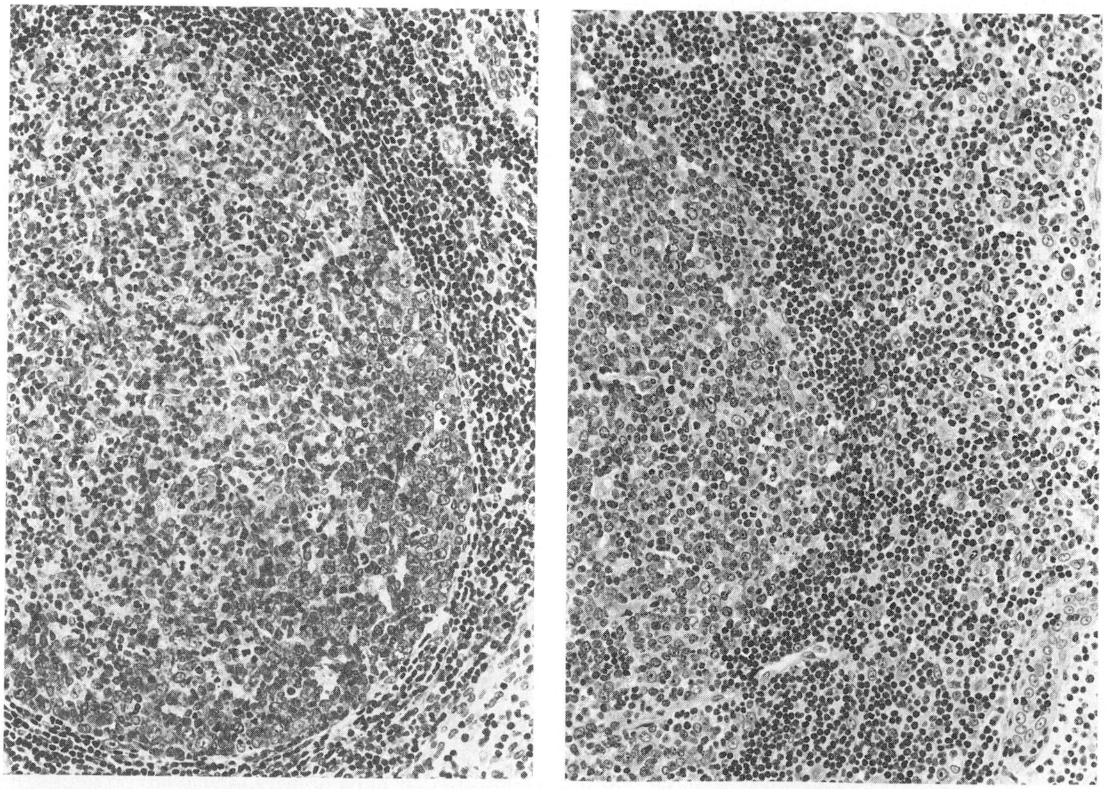

A B

FIG. 6.6. Hematoxylin and eosin–stained paraffin sections of two reactive lymph nodes illustrate the B follicle, showing the follicle mantle and the follicle center. **A:** No marginal zone can be identified (hematoxylin and eosin stain, original magnification: 200× magnification). **B:** The mantle is composed of a lymphocytic corona, presenting as a compact layer of small lymphocytes, progressively extending in a marginal zone comprising somewhat larger cells with more abundant cytoplasm (hematoxylin and eosin stain, original magnification: 200× magnification).

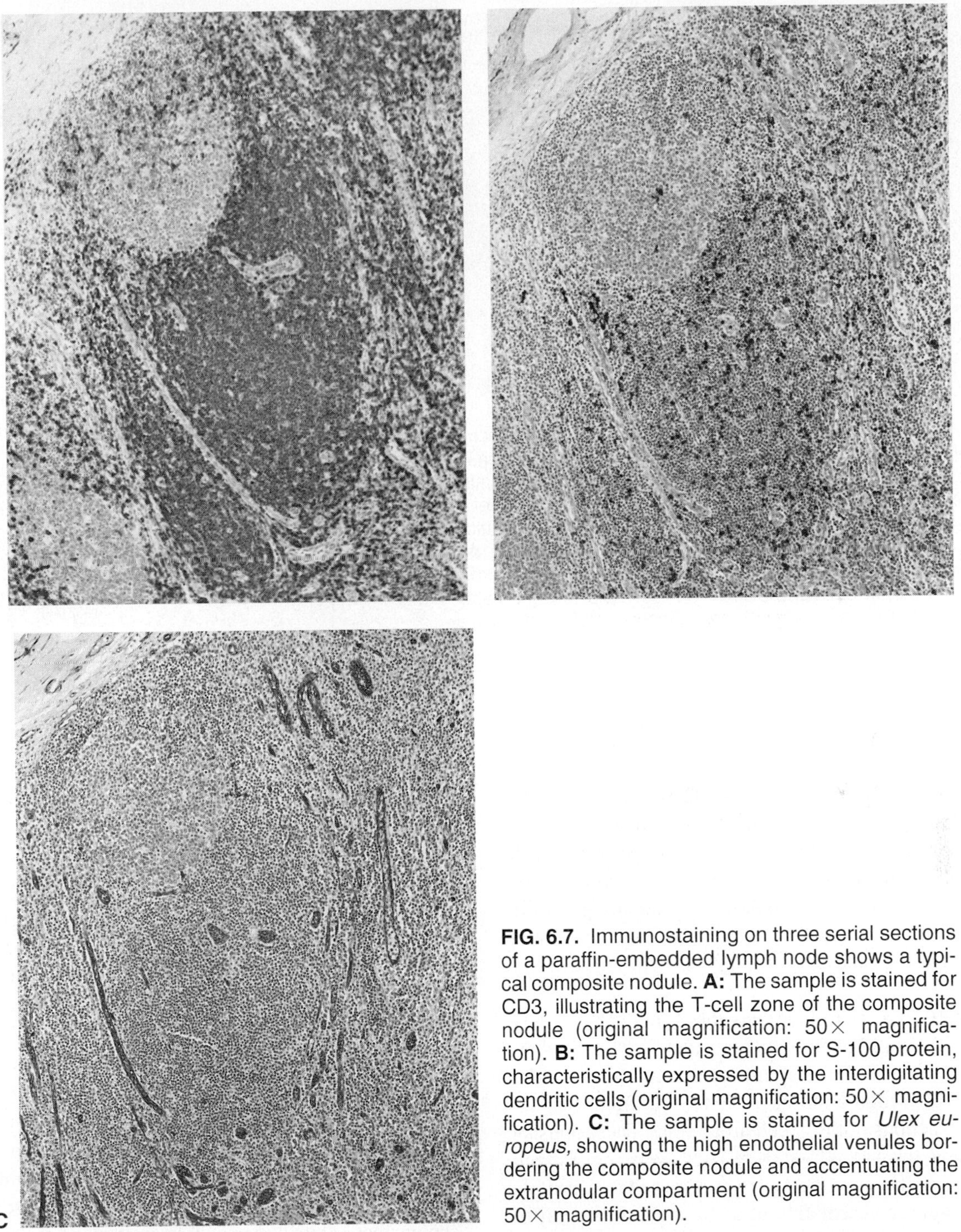

FIG. 6.7. Immunostaining on three serial sections of a paraffin-embedded lymph node shows a typical composite nodule. **A:** The sample is stained for CD3, illustrating the T-cell zone of the composite nodule (original magnification: 50× magnification). **B:** The sample is stained for S-100 protein, characteristically expressed by the interdigitating dendritic cells (original magnification: 50× magnification). **C:** The sample is stained for *Ulex europeus,* showing the high endothelial venules bordering the composite nodule and accentuating the extranodular compartment (original magnification: 50× magnification).

central core of small, almost exclusively $CD4^+$ T cells. Secondary nodules, considerably less well demarcated, show a typical starry-sky appearance because of the presence of scattered interdigitating dendritic cells within an impressive collection of $CD4^+$ T cells admixed with some $CD8^+$ T lymphocytes. Moreover, although high endothelial venules border primary T nodules, separating them from the adjacent area, these vessels occur scattered throughout the secondary T nodule. Primary and secondary T nodules are considered to represent the morphologic substrate of the interactions, demonstrated *in vitro*, among an antigen, interdigitating dendritic cells acting as antigen-presenting cell, and T cells. This complex phenomenon, taking place in the appropriate microenvironment provided by the T nodule, results in local activation and proliferation of antigen-specific T cells (91,97). The third variant of the paracortical T nodule, the tertiary nodule, is found in lymph nodes affected by dermatopathic lymphadenitis, of which they are considered to be the morphologic hallmark (Fig. 6.8A). The latter condition affects superficial lymph nodes of patients suffering from

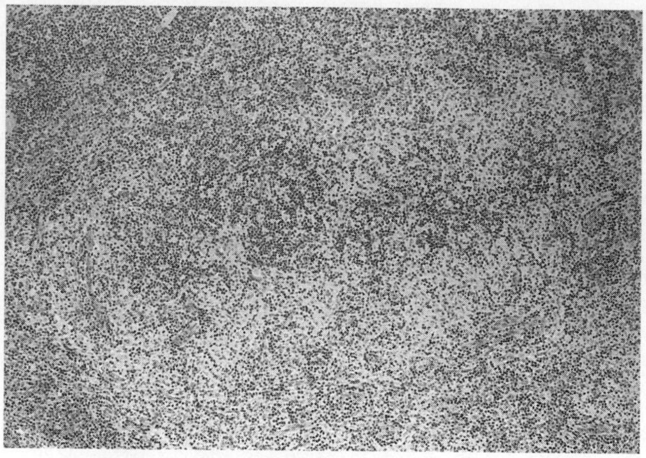

A

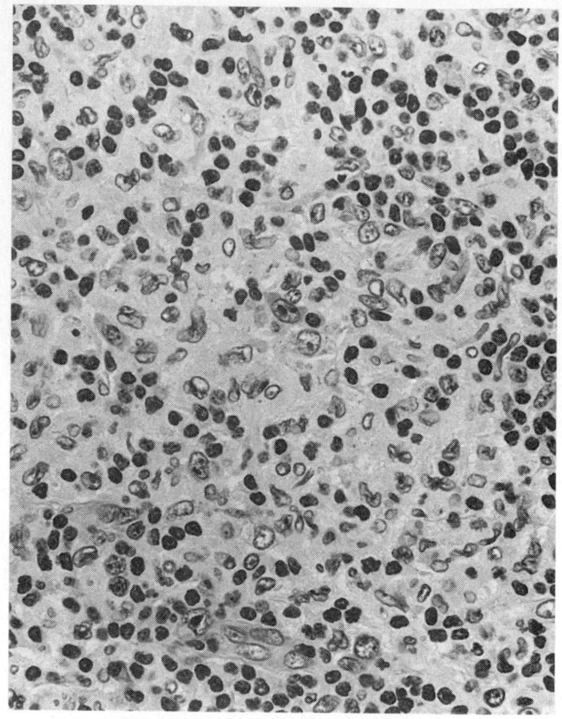

B

FIG. 6.8. **A:** Hematoxylin and eosin–stained paraffin section of a lymph node shows a tertiary T-cell nodule, characteristic of dermatopathic lymphadenitis. Notice the overwhelming number of dendritic cells compared with the low number of T cells (hematoxylin and eosin stain, original magnification: 50× magnification). **B:** Detail of the dendritic cells, which may be subdivided immunohistochemically into CD1a$^-$ interdigitating dendritic cells and CD1a$^+$ Langerhans cells (hematoxylin and eosin stain, original magnification: 200× magnification).

long-standing and severely pruritic skin diseases (98–101). These tertiary T nodules, compared with primary and secondary T nodules, are very large and extremely rich in CD1a- and S-100 β-positive cells (97,98,102,103) (Fig. 6.8B). Lymph nodes with this morphology may be difficult to distinguish from lymph nodes involved by cutaneous T-cell lymphoma, in particular by mycosis fungoides and by Sezary's syndrome. However, neoplastic T nodules generally harbor a more extensive population of T cells that display an atypical morphology and an aberrant phenotype (see Chapter 15).

Occasionally, the B follicle and the T nodule not only fuse to form a simple ovoid structure, identified as a clear-cut composite nodule, but they merge in a massive nodular structure, composed of a mosaic of B-follicle fragments admixed with fractions of the T-cell area (104). These unusual structures have been identified as progressively transformed germinal centers because they were considered to constitute the morphologic representation of a late event in a derailed immune response. The nodular lymphocyte predominance variant of Hodgkin's disease, also indicated as nodular paragranuloma, may be particularly difficult to distinguish from progressively transformed germinal centers. Moreover, both entities seem to be related, because they are occasionally observed within the same lymph node. Nevertheless, it has not been possible to document convincingly the postulated relationship between progressively transformed follicle centers and nodular paragranuloma (105,106) (see Chapter 15).

Another condition associated with the presence of aberrantly organized composite nodules showing typical alterations in the B-cell area is Castleman's disease. The pathologic features of this entity are discussed in Chapter 16.

The remaining lymph node parenchyma represents the extranodular compartment, which largely corresponds to the lymph node pulp described by Lennert (107). This part of the lymph node comprises a mixture of B and T cells, macrophages, plasma cells, plasmacytoid monocytes, specialized postcapillary venules called high endothelial venules, and lymphatics. Extending from the subcapsular sinus to the corticomedullary junction, this compartment is highlighted by the monoclonal antibody HECA-452. This antibody specifically reacts with two distinct structures characterizing this section of the lymph node: high endothelial venules and plasmacytoid monocytes (88).

High endothelial venules, also designated as epithelioid venules, are found throughout the full extranodular compartment. These particular vessels are easily distinguished by their plump, cuboidal to cylindrical endothelial cell lining and typically display a large, round nucleus and abundant cytoplasm (Fig. 6.9). Scanning electron microscopy has shown that the tridimensional structure of these vessels is unique. Extensive portions of the high endothelial venules show a cobblestone surface with lymphocytes located in the crevices separating adjacent endothelial cells. The remaining parts of these vessels are bordered by interlacing plates that are formed by cytoplasmic processes arising from the endothelium (108). Because of these peculiar features, turbulent blood flow is brought about along the high endothelial venules, which may account for an important improvement of the interactions between circulating lymphocytes and the endothelial surface. These specialized postcapillary vessels play a crucial part in the recruitment of circulating lymphocytes into the lymph node parenchyma, for this process is

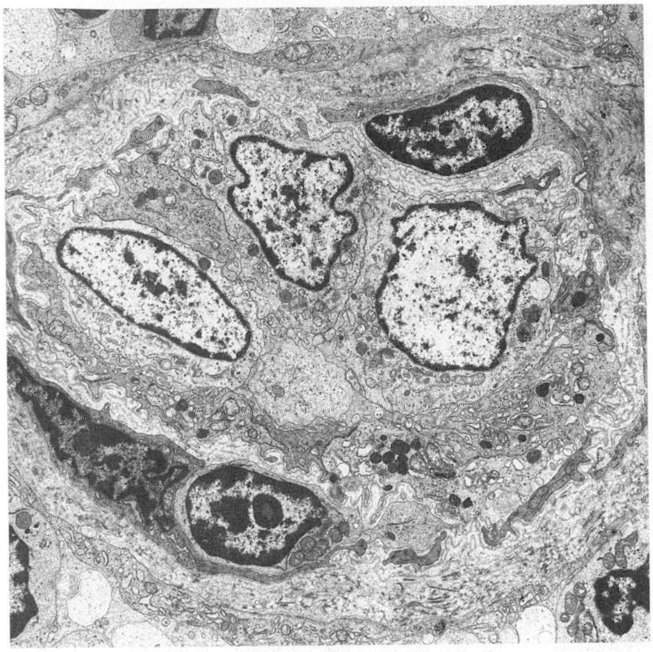

FIG. 6.9. Electron microscopic picture of a high endothelial venule. Notice the cuboidal aspect of the endothelial cells, with each typically displaying a large, round nucleus (original magnification: 36,250× magnification).

essentially based on cell-cell interactions between endothelial cells and lymphocytes.

Lymphocyte migration out of the vascular system comprises several stages. The process is initiated by a pronounced deceleration of the blood flow during its passage through the high endothelial venules, allowing lymphocytes to marginate. Subsequently, the lymphocytes interact loosely with the endothelial cell lining so that they roll over the vascular surface until they become firmly attached to the vessel wall. This adhesion is generally followed by diapedesis, which implies penetration through the intercellular junctions. Alternatively, lymphocytes can emigrate through emperipolesis, which means that they cross the vessel wall through the endothelial cell body. Eventually, after extravasation, the cells move away from the high endothelial venules into the lymph node parenchyma (108).

Specific adhesion molecules expressed by the lymphocytes that interact with their ligands, present on the endothelial lining, are undoubtedly the main mediators of the entire transendothelial pathway of lymphocyte trafficking. To elucidate the exact interactions on the molecular level, the expression of these regulatory structures has been documented by immunohistochemistry at the light microscopic and the ultrastructural level. The latter studies have demonstrated that the luminal and the intercellular portion of the endothelial cell surface are prominently decorated with ligands, whereas the basal part of the membrane is completely devoid of these components (109–111).

Leukocyte migration in general and lymphocyte trafficking through the wall of high endothelial venules in particular, is a multistep process. Each and every phase in this multistep process is controlled by the upregulation of the appropriate receptor on a distinct subpopulation of leukocytes, followed by an activation-induced increase in the receptor affinity for the ligand and is completed by shedding of the receptor from the cell surface when its expression has become superfluous (112–115).

The initial *rolling* of the lymphocytes along the vessel wall, a transient and rather weak interaction, is mediated by a member of the selectin family expressed by the adhering lymphocyte and its ligands, which are present on the endothelium. These complex carbohydrates connected to surface proteins are indicated as vascular addressins. Peripheral node addressins include GlyCAM-1 and CD34 (115). The selectin family of adhesion molecules, also involved in the rolling event, comprises three members: L-selectin (leukocyte adhesion molecule, LECAM-1 or Lam-1, Leu-8, TQ-1, DREG-56), E-selectin (ELAM-1), and P-selectin (platelet–endothelial cell adhesion molecule such as PADGEM, GMP-140, CD62P). These molecules show striking structural similarities, invariably containing a calcium-dependent carbohydrate-binding lectin domain, which accounts for their designation (116). L-selectin is highly expressed on most circulating T cells. After they have acquired entrance to peripheral lymphoid organs, T lymphocytes lose this surface marker almost completely. Reentry to the circulation is accompanied by an immediate upregulation of L-selectin, allowing the T cell to adhere to endothelial cells expressing the proper ligand, wherever lymphocytic extravasation might be required. In the spleen, a peculiar subset of stable, noncirculating L-selectin–negative cells is found. This lymphocyte subset comprises mucosal lymphocyte antigen-positive T cells and TCR $\gamma\delta$ T cells. By their phenotype and their morphology, these cells seem to correspond to the T lymphocytes present in the lamina propria and in the epithelial lining of the gut (117).

To penetrate the vessel wall, lymphocytes need to establish firm contacts with the underlying endothelium. This high-affinity interaction, also referred to as *sticking,* is brought about by members of the integrin family present on the lymphocyte surface. Integrins are heterodimeric proteins composed of an α and a β chain through which they interact with adhesion molecules such as ICAM-1, ICAM-2, ICAM-3, VCAM-1, PECAM-1, and MAdCAM-1, all belonging to the immunoglobulin gene superfamily (114).

This description presents an oversimplified version of the highly complex interactions that are taking place. Several other molecules are involved in lymphocyte trafficking, including chemoattractants secreted by high endothelial venules and their receptors expressed by naive lymphocytes. These substances are responsible for the upregulation of the adhesion molecules mediating high-affinity binding. Several other surface molecules are known to reinforce the basic interactions between selectins and addressins on one hand and integrins and immunoglobulin gene superfamily members on the other, but unraveling this molecular tangle would exceed the purpose of this chapter.

Another fascinating phenomenon characterizing lymphocyte trafficking is the preferential recirculation of memory lymphocytes to the organ site where the antigen in question was initially encountered. This specificity appears to be based on the expression of a particular subset of homing receptors. In accordance with this hypothesis, it has been demonstrated that the adhesion receptors expressed on memory cells have been profoundly modified compared with those present on naive lymphocytes. These alterations may contribute to a different or preferential recirculation pathway used by naive and memory lymphocytes and to the organ-specific homing of memory lymphocytes (118).

The other HECA-425–positive population intimately associated with the high endothelial venules of the extranodular compartment, the plasmacytoid monocytes, was originally referred to as T-associated plasma cells (119). Later, the same cells were identified as plasmacytoid T cells, and eventually immunophenotypic studies demonstrated that they belong to the histiocytic lineage. Plasmacytoid monocytes express several myelomonocytic markers and most highly selective monocyte-macrophage–specific surface molecules. Morphologically, they are medium-sized cells with a faintly stained oval nucleus displaying an inconspicuous nucleolus. Similar to plasma cells, this nucleus is eccentrically located within a moderate amount of intense basophilic cytoplasm (Fig. 6.10B). These staining properties can be explained by the presence of an abundant rough endoplasmic reticulum arranged in parallel cisternae (Fig. 6.10C). When clustered in small groups, mimicking germinal centers of the B follicle, they are readily recognized (Fig. 6.10A).

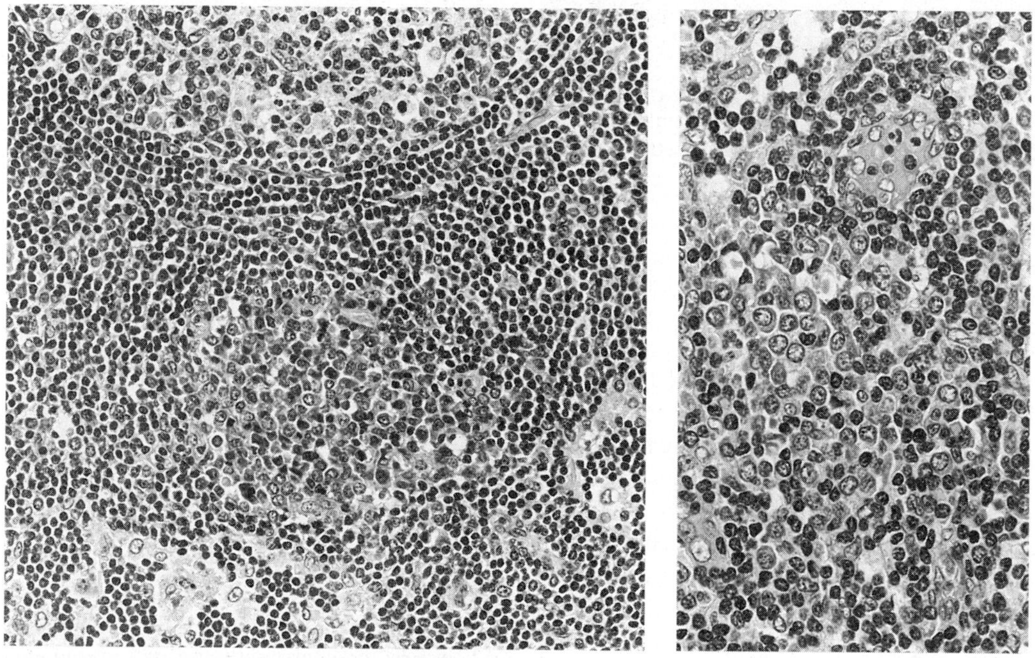

A B

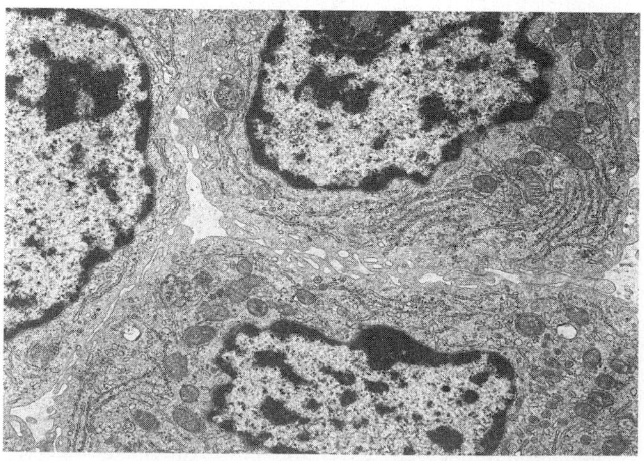

C

FIG. 6.10. Optical and ultrastructural features of plasmacytoid monocytes. **A:** A cluster of stained cells from a reactive lymph node embedded in a paraffin section is shown near a germinal center to demonstrate the morphologic resemblance of both structures. Within the group of plasmacytoid monocytes, several apoptotic cells are found (hematoxylin and eosin stain, original magnification: 125× magnification). **B:** Several plasmacytoid monocytes taken from stained paraffin sections of a reactive lymph node are visualized at a higher magnification, showing the eccentrically located nucleus with a clear rim of cytoplasm at the opposite side of the cells, mimicking plasma cells. The nuclear characteristics also can be evaluated; the nuclear chromatin is open, and inconspicuous nucleoli can be seen (hematoxylin and eosin stain, original magnification: 200× magnification). **C:** Ultrastructural features of the same cell. At this level, the characteristic aspect of the well-developed rough endoplasmic reticulum, organized in parallel arranged cisternae reminiscent of plasma cells, is also revealed in the electron micrograph (original magnification: 63,000× magnification).

However, occasionally occurring in loose aggregates or even as single cells, their identification is not always evident. Plasmacytoid monocytes do not display an impressive proliferative activity, although a mitotic figure can be noticed sporadically. Single-cell death is a frequent finding, especially in cell clusters. Apoptotic plasmacytoid monocytes are invariably accompanied by tingible body macrophages responsible for the rapid elimination of the karyorrhectic debris.

When examined carefully, every reactive lymph node reveals the presence of these peculiar cells, and even extranodal lymphoid tissues, such as the skin, uncommonly contain plasmacytoid monocytes (120,121). In Kikuchi's lymphadenitis, they become particularly numerous, arranged in large sheets, bordering a central area of necrotic cells (122).

Rarely, plasmacytoid monocytes give rise to a malignant clone. In the few cases reported, this neoplastic proliferation was associated with or developed in the course of a chronic myelomonocytic leukemia (123).

Plasmacytoid monocytes have been isolated from tonsil tissue, using centrifugation and cell sorting (124). The $CD4^+CD11c^-$ isolated cells displayed the light microscopic and ultrastructural features of plasmacytoid monocytes, which suggests that the investigators separated the correct population. Moreover, the phenotype of these isolated cells is similar to that reported for plasmacytoid monocytes using immunohistochemical staining on tissue sections. They express CD45RA, confirming their hematopoietic origin, but they lack lineage markers for B and T lymphocytes, NK cells, and myeloid cells. The isolated plasmacytoid monocytes are immunoreactive with antibodies directed against MHC class II antigens, several adhesion molecules, CD40, and $CD38^{low}$. The presence of other surface markers, such as CD80, CD86, CD14, and CD11b, could not be demonstrated. The absence of the latter two molecules on the surface of the isolated cells is noteworthy, because these monocytic markers have been demonstrated on the membrane of plasmacytoid monocytes in tissue sections (124). The reported phenotype of the extracted monocytes is identical to the one carried by a particular subset of circulating mononuclear cells that differentiate into dendritic cells when cultured *in vitro* (125). The preferential localization of plasmacytoid monocytes near high endothelial venules and even within their lumen suggests that they are derived from circulating $CD4^+CD11c^-$ dendritic cell precursors that enter the lymph node through the high endothelial venules (121,124).

Cultured $CD4^+CD11c^-$ cells extracted from tonsils show an impressive apoptotic rate, similar to plasmacytoid monocyte clusters *in vivo*. However, in the former condition, programmed cell death may be prevented by adding IL-3 to the culture medium, while the subsequent addition of CD40 ligand to the medium stimulates the rescued cells to differentiate into dendritic cells expressing CD13, CD33, and $CD1a^{low}$. These findings further support the assumption that plasmacytoid monocytes merely represent an intermediate stage in the differentiation of circulating precursors to well-developed dendritic cells *in loco*.

When Facchetti and colleagues indisputably demonstrated that plasmacytoid monocytes are essential participants in T-cell–dependent immune responses, they speculated that these cells acted by recruiting T cells in the paracortex, allowing them to penetrate the high endothelial venules (119,121). The data collected by Grouard and her group, however, favor an alternative hypothesis. According to the latter presumption, the plasmacytoid monocyte precursors produced in the bone marrow migrate to the peripheral lymphoid tissues. In this site, they are eliminated immediately by apoptosis unless IL-3 and CD40 ligand, generated by an ongoing T-cell–dependent immune response, rescue them and provide the appropriate signal to complete their differentiation process. In conclusion, plasmacytoid monocytes and their circulating precursors represent a comprehensive reservoir with the capacity to differentiate into mature dendritic cells when recruited by IL-3 and CD40 ligand as products of an active immune response (124).

The Spleen

The spleen is an abdominal organ, situated in the left hypochondrium beneath the diaphragm. The weight of the spleen may vary considerably depending on the age, sex, size, and weight of the individual. In general, a weight of 150 g is considered normal.

Embryology

The primordium of the spleen appears in human embryos of 8 to 9 mm as a small thickening of the dorsal mesogastrium, consisting of a closely aggregated mass of mesenchymal elements. The constituents of this mesenchymal primordium form the reticular network of the white and red pulp. In the meshes of this framework, primitive basophilic elements can be identified, which give rise to red corpuscles, granular myelocytes, leukocytes, and megakaryocytes. In contrast to earlier suggestions that they represent mesenchymal cells that have become isolated from the rest, it has been demonstrated that these wandering cells arise from stem cell precursors of yolk sac, liver or bone marrow origin.

The white pulp of the spleen can be detected after 15 weeks of gestation. It is composed of B and T lymphocytes, which arise from the bone marrow and the thymus, respectively, and of dendritic cells. At this stage, the splenic lymphoid tissue exists as a homogeneous mass in which not a single compartment can be distinguished.

During ontogeny, the number of B cells increases gradually (126). Meanwhile, these cells, many of which display CD5 positivity at 15 weeks of gestation, lose this surface marker, leaving only very few $CD5^+$ B lymphocytes at 25 weeks of gestation (127). Immunohistologic studies at 23 weeks of gestation have indicated that, at this time of fetal life, as much as one third of the cells within the B follicles express autoantibody associated cross-reactive idiotypes (128).

T lymphocytes originating from the thymus reach the

spleen between the 12th and the 16th gestational week (129). Most $CD3^+$ cells display the TCR $\alpha\beta$ complex, indicating that their maturation was completed inside the thymus. However, at 28 weeks of gestation, a significant portion still lacks the important T-cell markers CD4, CD8, and CD5. At birth, all splenic T lymphocytes have acquired CD3, CD5, TCR $\alpha\beta$, and the lineage marker CD4, indicating helper T-cell properties, or have acquired CD8, indicating suppressor or cytotoxic activity (126).

In humans, there seems to be very little hemopoiesis, even in the embryonal spleen (130). The organ may be involved in erythropoiesis, because it captures nucleated erythroid cells and promotes their terminal differentiation. Lymphopoiesis is restricted to the omentum, the liver, and the bone marrow (130).

Histology and Immunohistology

On its freshly sectioned surface, the two components of the spleen can be distinguished even with the naked eye. Elongated or rounded gray areas, measuring 0.2 to 0.7 cm in diameter and called the white pulp, correspond microscopically to accumulations of lymphoid tissue. The reddish, soft mass that they are embedded in, the red pulp, represents merely the entire vascular labyrinth that carries the cellular constituents of the blood along the splenic parenchyma. This network comprises the arterial branches, the red pulp cords, the sinusoids, and the draining veins. The spleen functions as an ingenious filter, intercalated in the bloodstream. Its entire structure is therefore based on the vascular supply provided by the splenic artery. This branch of the truncus celiacus perforates the splenic capsule that completely surrounds the spleen at the hilus to give rise to two smaller vessels, which further subdivide into segmental arteries, each supplying one splenic segment.

The arterial branches, which together with their concomitant vein and lymphatics, form a vascular triad embedded in fibrous, mainly collagenous tissue (131). The arteries end up as smaller arterioles, which are no longer accompanied by venules and collagenous fibers but are surrounded by a cuff of lymphoid tissue. Subsequently, capillaries, oriented perpendicularly to the arterioles, branch off and terminate in a specialized vascular structure highly characteristic for the spleen: the sheathed capillaries or periarteriolar macrophage sheaths.

At this level of the splenic vascularization, the endothelium of the capillaries is replaced by concentrically arranged macrophages. Blood is forced through these sheathed capillaries and may reach the sinuses through the cordal stroma of the red pulp after having crossed the basal membrane lining the sinus endothelium. Alternatively, blood can enter the perifollicular zone, a distinct part of the red pulp immediately adjacent to the white pulp that directly gives entrance to the sinuses (132). The sinusoidal channels, covered by a flattened, elongated endothelial lining, form a blind ending system that debouch into the veins, which parallel the arteries (131). As a whole, the sinuses constitute a complex meshwork with many interconnections and bulblike extensions inside the intersinus reticular tissue, which are known as the cords of Billroth. These cords contain reticulum cells, macrophages, and plasma cells, and together with the sinus labyrinth, they account for the main mass of the red pulp, representing 75% of the splenic weight.

Most blood cells pass through the region bordering the white pulp, including its outermost portion, the marginal zone. Microanatomic data on this region caused confusion because they resulted from studies on spleens from various species or from humans with different pathologic conditions (132–134). Nevertheless, these studies did demonstrate the occurrence of arteriolar-capillary bundles within the white pulp that show extensive ramifications in the marginal zone. Whether a human equivalent of the marginal sinus, bordering the marginal zone in rats, exists is still debated. The perifollicular zone (132), largely similar to the perimarginal cavernous sinus previously described (133,134), may be accepted as the corresponding structure in humans. This perifollicular zone appears to be part of the red pulp and comprises sheathed capillaries; blood-filled, large flattened spaces; terminal sinuses; and scattered B cells, T cells, and macrophages (132). Because the perifollicular zone drains directly into the venous sinuses, most of the splenic blood flow is found bypassing the filtration beds of the red pulp cords.

Another controversial issue regarding the splenic circulation is the existence of direct connections between capillaries and venous sinuses, which would result in a closed circulation. Although data supporting this hypothesis have been published, other investigators were able to demonstrate that most capillaries end into the reticular meshwork of the red pulp cords or terminate in the marginal zone, creating an open circulation (134).

The white pulp of the spleen is comprised of primary and secondary B follicles and periarteriolar T-cell areas (Fig. 6.11). The lymphoid tissue is organized into well-developed composite nodules, which are completely surrounded by a marginal zone in rats. In humans, however, the periarteriolar area is nearly devoid of an identifiable marginal zone (132). It harbors intermediate-sized B cells or marginal zone B cells, dendritic cells or so-called metallophilic macrophages, and marginal zone macrophages. The latter cells, provided with long cytoplasmic extensions, display close contacts with the surrounding marginal zone B lymphocytes. Human splenic macrophages are also provided with slender cellular protrusions and mainly occupy the perifollicular zone, but B lymphocytes are preferentially located in the marginal zone, completely separated from the macrophages. Similar to the interdigitating dendritic cells of the T-cell area of the white pulp, these dendritic cells of the perifollicular zone express CD11c and CD13. Apart from this resemblance, no phenotypic similarities to these antigen-presenting cells have been demonstrated. Moreover, splenic macrophages do display phagocytic activity (135).

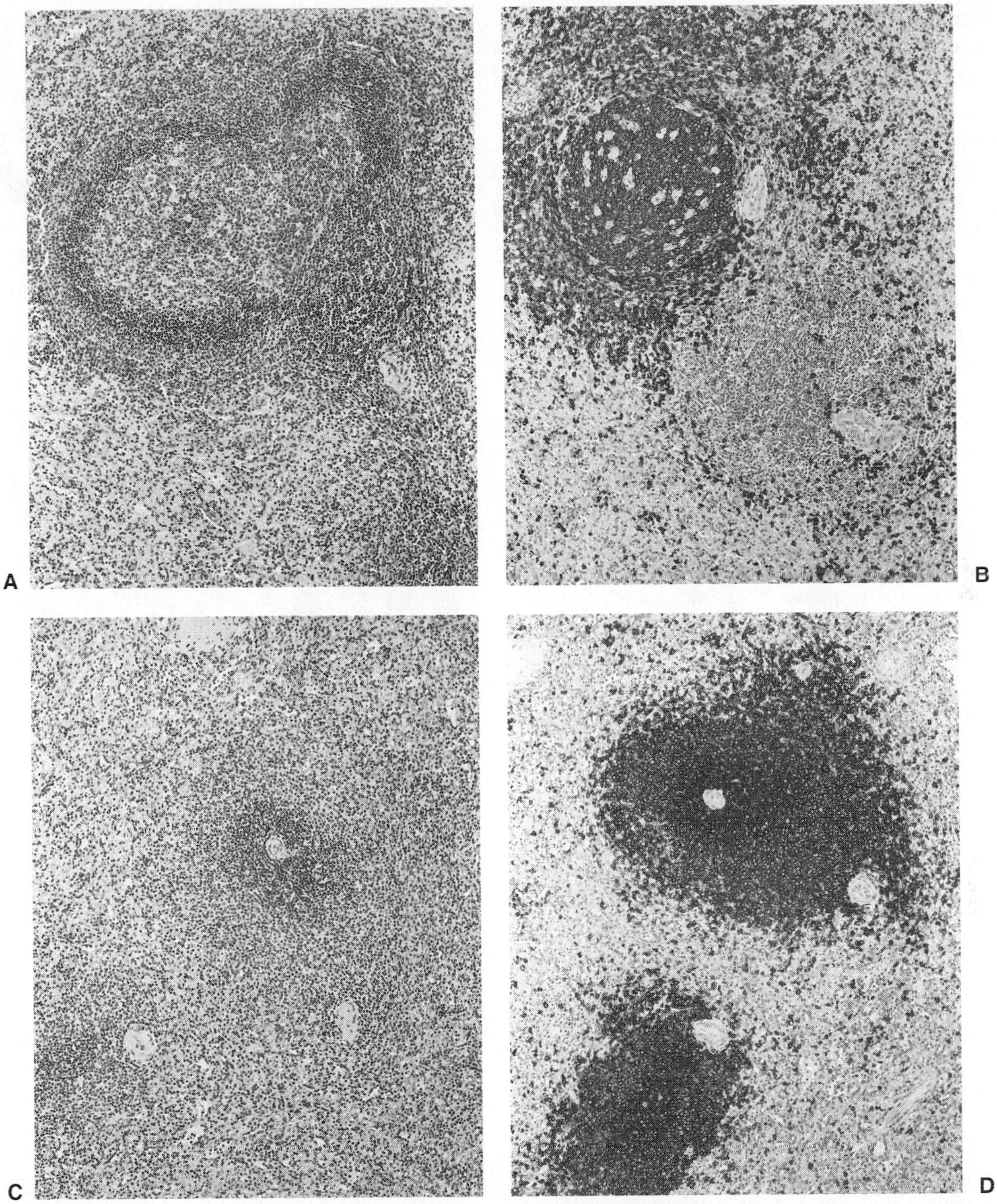

FIG. 6.11. The white pulp of the spleen is comprised of B follicles and adjacent T-cell areas, resulting in the formation of composite nodules similar to the ones observed in other lymphoid tissues, including the lymph node. **A:** The sample is from hematoxylin and eosin–stained paraffin sections of a normal spleen (original magnification: 50× magnification). In a young adult, the B follicles have a well-developed germinal center. **B:** In elderly people, these germinal centers are less obvious, and the greater part of the B-cell area is composed of small lymphocytic cells. This is particularly illustrative of an accentuated marginal zone. This serial section was stained for CD20 (original magnification: 50× magnification). **C:** The sample is from hematoxylin and eosin–stained paraffin sections of a normal spleen (50× magnification). **D:** This serial section was stained for CD20 (original magnification: 50× magnification). This staining highlights the B part of the white pulp, and it shows the marginal zone, which extends around the T-cell part of the composite nodule.

Many other cells present in the marginal zone, including small lymphocytes, NK cells, granulocytes, and monocytes, must be regarded as incidental passengers.

HISTOLOGY AND IMMUNOHISTOLOGY OF THE COMPOSITE NODULE AS THE MICROANATOMIC AND FUNCTIONAL SUBUNIT OF SECONDARY LYMPHOID TISSUES

The lymph node and the spleen provide by their structure and by their cellular composition a tridimensional framework that particularly favors an adequate immune response. Reduced to its essence, this framework comprises two major components: a B follicle, responsible for humoral immunity–related events, and a T nodule, accounting for cellular immunity. Immunoglobulin-secreting plasma cells, together with long-lived, antigen-specific memory B cells, are generated in the former area, and in the latter region, antigen-specific T lymphocytes become activated, which results in an impressive clonal expansion of these cells.

During the immune response, T nodules and B follicles unify in an ovoid structure designated the composite nodule. This microanatomic structure should be regarded as the functional unit of lymphoid tissues because it provides an appropriate environment in which antigens, accessory cells, and B and T lymphocytes cooperate to protect the body adequately against various antigenic threats. In addition to its occurrence in the lymph nodes and the spleen, the composite nodule is almost universally present throughout the entire body, concentrated in the extranodal lymphoid tissues, underscoring the ubiquitous need for a refined defense system (89).

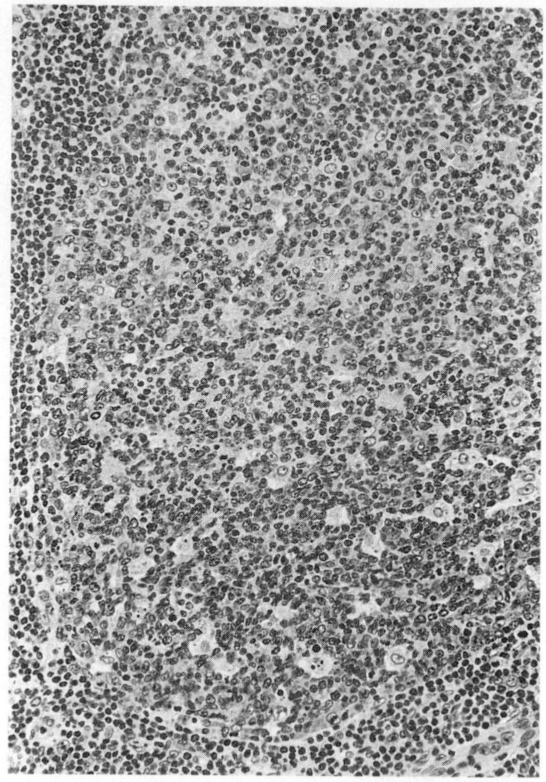

FIG. 6.12. Hematoxylin and eosin–stained paraffin section shows the germinal center of a B follicle of a reactive lymph node (original magnification: 125× magnification). The darkly stained lower part is comprised of the centroblasts admixed with tingible body macrophages. The lighter stained upper part harbors the centrocytes.

B-Cell Area of the Composite Nodule

The B-cell area essentially consists of a framework of follicular dendritic cells colonized by B cells, a specific subpopulation of T cells, and tingible body macrophages. In nonstimulated lymphoid tissue, only small, mainly round lymphocytes are embedded in this underlying follicular dendritic cell network. These elementary B follicles are designated primary B follicles. Secondary B follicles arise as the result of antigenic stimulation and can be distinguished from their unstimulated counterparts by the presence of a well-developed germinal center or follicle center, surrounded by a follicle mantle, comprised of the lymphocytic corona and the marginal zone. In the germinal center at least two B-cell types are recognized morphologically: small irregular cells (i.e., centrocytes or cleaved cells) and large cells (i.e., centroblasts) (Fig. 6.12).

Centrocytes are identified by an ample amount of clear cytoplasm and an irregular, somewhat elongated nucleus with rather dense nuclear chromatin and inconspicuous nucleoli. Classically, these cleaved cells are found preferentially in the paler staining upper half of the germinal center, immediately underneath the thickened cuff of the corona facing the source of antigenic challenge. Centroblasts occupy the opposite side of the follicle center, which stains considerably more intensely because its large cellular constituents are packed together in a small area. The latter cells have a small rim of cytoplasm and a round nucleus with less condensed chromatin and several nucleoli located along the nuclear membrane. In contrast to the cells homing in the mantle, germinal center B cells do not express BCL-2. Centroblasts and centrocytes, typically lacking this cytoplasmic protein involved in the protection against apoptosis, are programmed to die, unless they are rescued by high-affinity interaction between their antigen receptor and a given antigen. Germinal center cells can be recognized by their highly specific binding of a lectin, peanut agglutinin (136), and their expression of the nuclear phosphoprotein BCL-6 (137–139). With its expression strictly confined to the follicle center, at least in nonneoplastic lymphoid tissues, it has been speculated that this transcription factor controls the proliferation and differentiation of B cells within the germinal center (140–142).

Although the lymphocytic corona is mainly composed of morphologically similar small lymphoid cells, it is heterogeneous with respect to phenotype and function of the lymphoid cells. In anatomic sites where an abundant influx of antigens is known to occur, a third and distinct region, encompassing the lymphocytic corona and part of the follicle mantle, designated the marginal zone, is recognized. It is composed predominantly of typical marginal zone B cells, somewhat larger cells with abundant clear cytoplasm, and an irregular bean-shaped nucleus containing vesicular chromatin and an inconspicuous nucleolus. By pure morphology, marginal zone B cells resemble monocytoid cells and centrocytes of the germinal center. They were previously designated immature sinus histiocytes in the lymph node and centrocyte-like cells in Peyer's patches of the small intestine. Nevertheless, marginal zone B cells have a distinct phenotype. Studies demonstrating Ki-67 expression in marginal zone cells (143) indicate that, in contrast with the traditional point of view (144), they display proliferative activity.

In addition to the characteristic marginal zone cell population, a variable number of different B lymphocytes is observed, among which larger cells with immunoblast-like features and plasma cells expressing cytoplasmic IgM can be recognized. The diversity characterizing the cellular composition of the marginal zone is reflected in the heterogeneity of marginal zone cell lymphomas of the lymph node, the spleen, and extranodal sites (143). Admixed with these peculiar lymphocytic elements, other cells such as macrophages, granulocytes, and ordinary small lymphocytes are also detected (96).

B-Cell Subsets of the B Follicle

The composite nodule represents the universal morphologic unit, characteristic of all secondary lymphoid tissues, because it offers the perfect microenvironment for every aspect of the specific immune response, including T-cell–dependent B-cell development. Human tonsils subject to repeated antigen-stimulation because of their strategic position at the entrance of the respiratory and digestive tract, represent an ideal working model for the study of the various B-cell subsets.

Using immunohistochemistry on tonsillar tissue and multicolor flow cytometric analysis on isolated cells extracted from these samples, the peripheral B-cell subsets that give rise to the secondary B-cell repertoire have been isolated, identified, and extensively characterized. Molecular genetic studies and functional experiments yielded additional data, allowing the determination of the exact position of each cell type in the maturation process of the naive B cell.

IgD^+CD38^- B cells found in the follicle mantle are small resting B cells expressing IgM, CD5, CD44, and BCL-2 protein. They correspond to naive B cells as they have not yet undergone somatic mutation. Based on the differential expression of CD23, two subpopulations of these mantle cells can be distinguished. The $CD23^-$ subset, designated as Bm1, probably represents recently generated naive B cells, and the acquisition of this surface marker by the remainder of these B lymphocytes, Bm2, could reflect their selection by a particular ligand.

IgD^+ B lymphocytes that also express CD38 are the first ones to show the features of a genuine germinal center cell. They are immunoreactive with antibodies directed against CD10, CD71, and FAS, but they lack BCL-2, implying that they are not constitutively protected against programmed cell death. In cell culture, these BCL-2–negative elements undergo spontaneous apoptosis. The demonstration of Ki-67 expression, a well-known proliferation-associated nuclear antigen, denotes that these cells are mitotically active. Two subpopulations of these IgD^+CD38^+ B lymphocytes are recognized. An IgM^+ subset, called Bm2′, may correspond to germinal center founder cells, because their immunoglobulin variable genes (V_H) carry few or no mutations. The other IgD^+CD38^+ cells, which show no IgM expression, display an extraordinarily high number of somatic mutations in their V_H genes. The mutation frequency of these genes, averaging 40 mutations per sequence, is threefold higher than the one detected in the IgV γ sequences of regular germinal center B cells extracted from the same tonsil. Cells belonging to this peculiar subpopulation demonstrate a remarkable clonal relatedness, predominant expression of the immunoglobulin light chain λ, cytoplasmic μ to cytoplasmic δ switch, and a single IgD isotype. The functional significance of these $IgD^+CD38^+IgM^-$ cells, carrying hypermutated IgV_H genes, remains elusive. Most of the IgD^+CD38^+ cells with a high number of mutations are deleted within the tonsils, leaving only a small portion of IgD^+ germinal center cells provided with low to intermediate numbers of mutations. The latter cells eventually differentiate into mature plasma cells or long-lived memory B cells.

IgD^-CD38^+ cells represent the traditional germinal center cell population, consistently expressing CD10, CD71, and FAS and demonstrating intense proliferative activity, as indicated by Ki-67. Lacking BCL-2, these germinal center cells are programmed to die, unless they are selected by an appropriate signal, which can be provided by a specific antigen or by CD40 ligand. The two characteristic properties of these follicle center cells—their impressive mitotic rate and their propensity to undergo apoptosis—should both be conferred by their elevated levels of P53, MYC, BAX, and FAS.

Even by pure morphology, two subgroups can clearly be separated: smaller centrocytes, with a dense, cleaved nucleus, and larger centroblasts, showing a nucleus with a regular outline containing vesicular chromatin. Immunohistochemically, this distinction can be highlighted by the surface marker CD77: centroblasts, or Bm3, being $CD77^+$ and centrocytes, Bm4, lacking this surface marker. Molecular genetic studies confirmed that both cell types are subject to antigen selection because sequence analysis of their V_H genes demonstrated the presence of a considerable, though variable, number of somatic mutations. Sterile transcripts, a marker for the initiation of isotype switch, and switch circles, which indicate switching deletion, were exclusively detected within the centrocytes, which strongly suggests that the onset of somatic mutation taking place in centroblasts also precedes the initiation of somatic mutation during B-cell maturation within the germinal center.

An IgD^-CD38^- B-lymphocytic population was identified. Because they are not stained with antibodies directed against typical germinal center cell markers nor with antisera recognizing follicle mantle cell antigens, they are supposed to represent resting memory B cells, expressing CD20, CD44, CD39, and BCL-2. Besides their capacity to rapidly induce an immune response on recognition of a specific antigen and potentially even one of the effector mechanisms in the establishment of this activity, IgD^-CD38^- B cells can trigger proliferation of allo-$CD4^+$ T cells, which is associated with a rapid upregulation of CD80 and CD86.

Marginal zone B lymphocytes constitute a distinct B-cell subset, undoubtedly present in all secondary lymphoid tissues as demonstrated by immunohistochemistry. However, only in those organs challenged by an abundant antigenic influx, such as the spleen, Peyer's patches, and mesenteric lymph nodes, are they readily identified as somewhat larger cells, characterized by abundant, clear cytoplasm (Fig. 6.13). Marginal zone cells express pan-B-cell markers and surface IgM but little or no IgD (Fig. 6.14). They are not reactive with antibodies against surface CD5, CD10, and CD23. Phenotypic features frequently used to accentuate these cells include their alkaline phosphatase positivity and their expression of CD21 and CD25. It is not hard to detect marginal zone cells in the spleen because they are grouped together in a distinct area near the perimarginal cavernous sinus identified as the perifollicular zone. This unique positioning at the entrance of the antigenic influx, highly similar to their localization in the lymphocytic corona and the dome or crypt epithelium in Waldeyer's ring and Peyer's patches, respectively, considerably facilitates their exposure to and interaction with foreign antigens. In peripheral lymph nodes, marginal zone cells are much less conspicuous, but the isolated collections of these cells that can be demonstrated do appear in the same strategic position underneath the subcapsular sinus and along the cortical and paracortical sinuses (92).

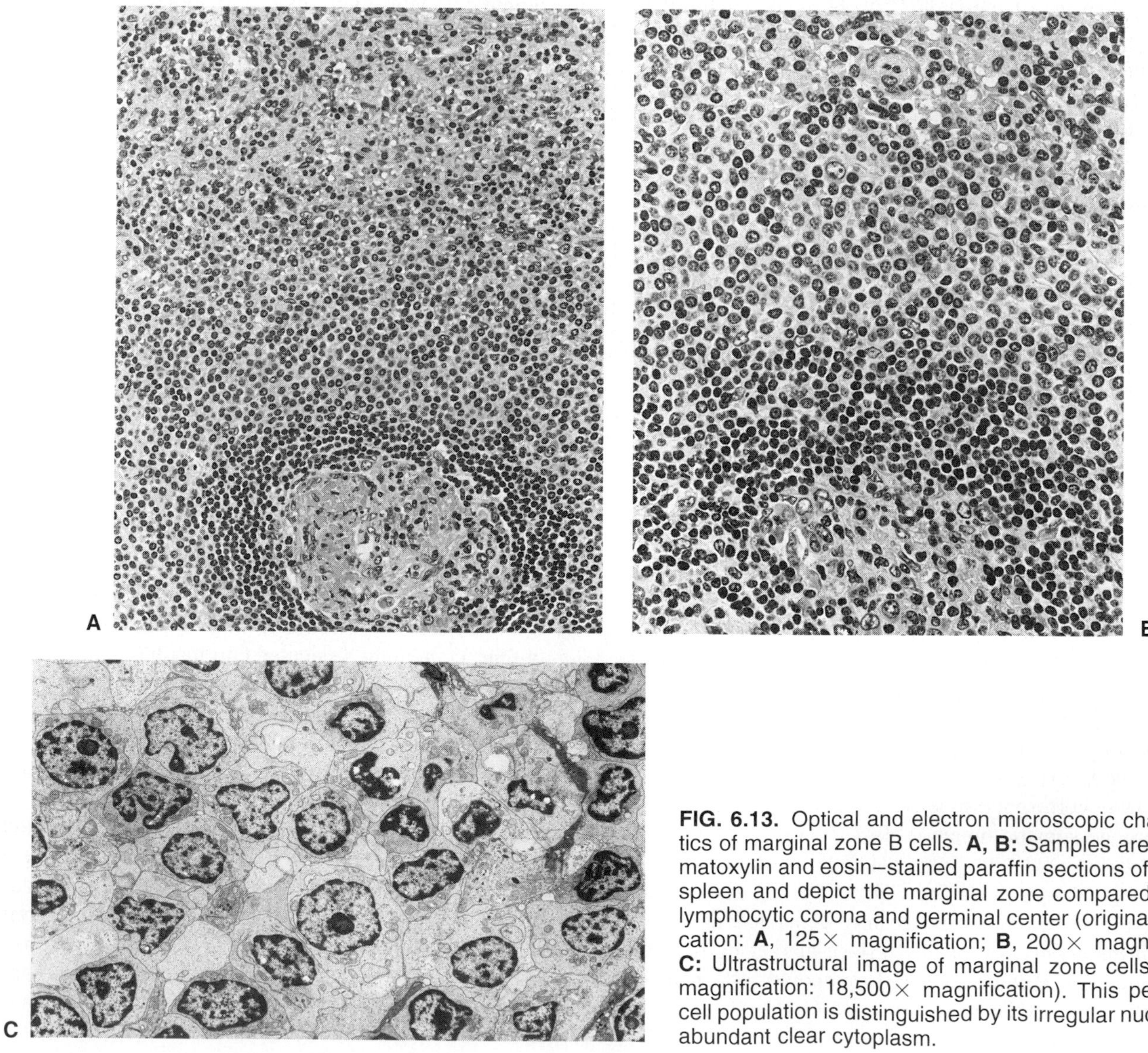

FIG. 6.13. Optical and electron microscopic characteristics of marginal zone B cells. **A, B:** Samples are from hematoxylin and eosin–stained paraffin sections of a normal spleen and depict the marginal zone compared with the lymphocytic corona and germinal center (original magnification: **A**, 125× magnification; **B**, 200× magnification). **C:** Ultrastructural image of marginal zone cells (original magnification: 18,500× magnification). This peculiar B-cell population is distinguished by its irregular nucleus and abundant clear cytoplasm.

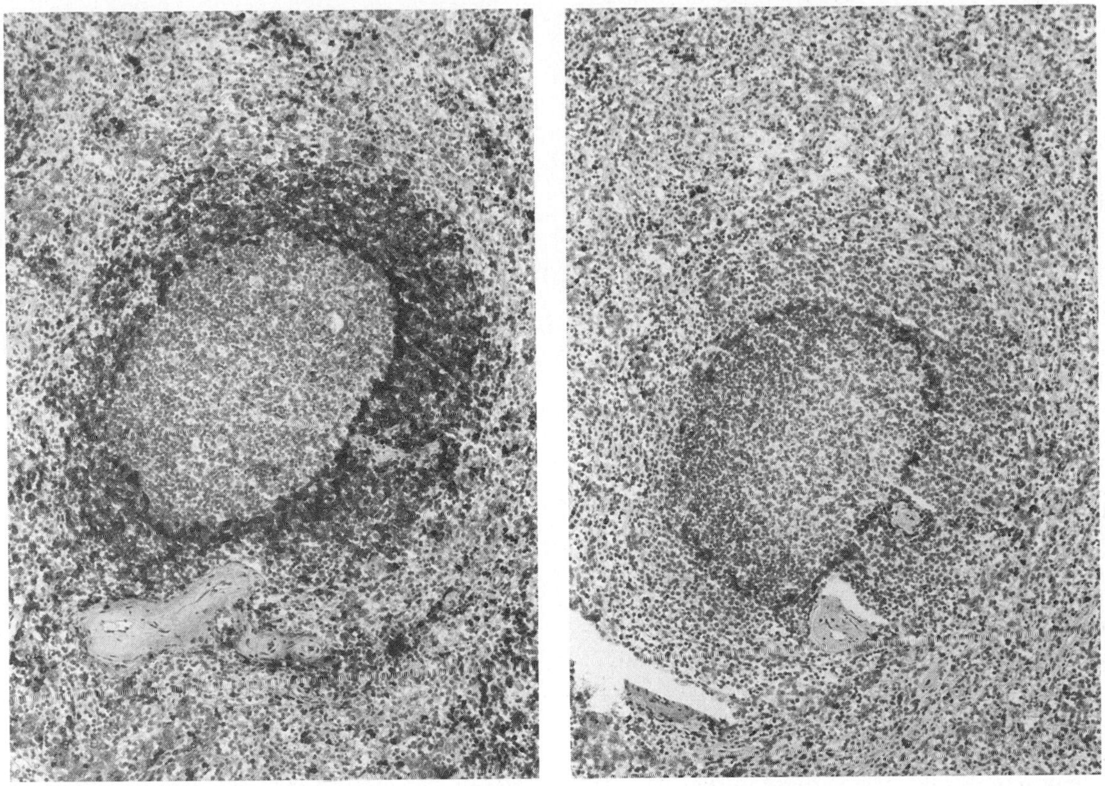

FIG. 6.14. Two serial sections taken from freshly frozen normal spleen and stained for IgM **(A)** and for IgD **(B)** (hematoxylin and eosin stain, original magnification: 50× magnification). The IgM^+, IgD^+ lymphocytic corona is near the germinal center, surrounded by the IgM^+, IgD^- marginal zone. When the germinal center is less well developed, the full inner part of the B domain reacts with anti-IgM and anti-IgD antibodies.

Germinal Center T Cells

Germinal centers harbor a significant number of $CD2^+$, $CD3^+$, and $CD4^+$-only T cells. These granular lymphocytes coexpress CD57 (Leu-7) (145) and are $CD45RA^-$ and $CD45RO^+$. Although the specific activation marker CD69 can be demonstrated on this particular subset of helper T cells, other surface molecules indicating cellular activation, such as CD25 (IL-2 receptor) and CD71 (transferrin receptor), are consistently absent. This unusual phenotype correlates with the observation that, on activation, these $CD57^+$ T cells produce various cytokines but never secrete IL-2, IL-4, interferon-γ, and tumor necrosis factor (145,146). This peculiar T-cell population may reach its activated state through stimulation by antigen-presenting B lymphocytes, because complex bidirectional interactions take place between T lymphocytes on one hand and centroblasts and centrocytes on the other. Various adhesive and costimulatory receptor-counterreceptor systems are involved, particularly CD80/CD86, CD40, LFA-1, and LFA-3 expressed on B cells and CD28, CD40 ligand, CD54, and CD2 on the T-cell surface.

Extensive *in vitro* studies have suggested that a reciprocal yin-yang effect dominates the interactions between B and T cells in the follicle center, whereby CD80/CD86, upregulated after crosslinking of surface immunoglobulin on the B lymphocyte surface, induces the expression of CD40 ligand on the T-cell membrane. Subsequently, the latter activation marker binds to its counterreceptor, CD40, expressed by the B lymphocyte, an event that is pivotal in the process of affinity maturation (147–151). *In vivo* experiments with knockout animals have substantiated the critical roles of CD40, CD40 ligand, and CD80/CD86 in the development of humoral immunity (152–154).

The specialized T lymphocyte subset of the germinal center also expresses cytotoxic T-lymphocyte–associated molecule-4 (CTLA-4), which is strongly related to the CD28 molecule identified on the B-cell membrane (155,156). However, as indicated by studies in mice, its role in T-cell responses is inhibitory rather than costimulatory (157–159). Expression of CTLA-4 shows a strong predilection for the germinal center, in particular its dark zone; only low numbers of scattered T cells in the paracortex of lymph nodes, displaying well-developed T-cell areas, additionally react with anti-CTLA-4 antibodies. This highly restricted pattern of CTLA-4 expression suggests that this surface marker is also directly or indirectly involved in feedback mechanisms controlling the expansion of follicle centers or in the transition of its cells into antibody-producing plasma cells or memory B cells (155).

An alternative way for T lymphocytes to acquire the appropriate signals for activation may occur through interaction with $CD11c^+$ germinal center dendritic cells. The latter cells carry immune complexes and may act as potent memory T-cell activators (160). The presence of this particular subset of T cells, which is characteristic of follicle centers, is considered to indicate the follicular origin of some pathologic conditions such as Hodgkin's paragranuloma (161).

Follicular Dendritic Cells

B cells lay embedded in a cellular lacework built up by follicular dendritic cells, a unique cell population exclusively found in primary and secondary lymphoid follicles. These cells stand out by their ability to retain antigens integrated in large immune complexes on their surface for a prolonged period (162–164). By routine light microscopy alone, it takes a considerable effort to identify these cells, because only by their nucleus, which displays a very open chromatin pattern in contrast with the rather condensed one observed in the surrounding lymphoid cells, can they be distinguished from the surrounding cells. Nevertheless, immunohistologic and ultrastructural examinations of the B follicle allowed unequivocal detection of these peculiar cells and comprehensible description of their unique features.

Electron microscopy demonstrates that follicular dendritic cells have one or more large, irregularly shaped nuclei with vesicular chromatin and long cytoplasmic dendrites connected by desmosomes, which together form an intricate network of delicate processes seeded with lymphocytes (Fig. 6.15). Along the slender cellular protrusions, small globular structures or iccosomes, representing immune complex–coated bodies, are observed. Except for some mitochondria and well-developed Golgi regions, remarkably few organelles are detected in the cytoplasm of follicular dendritic cells.

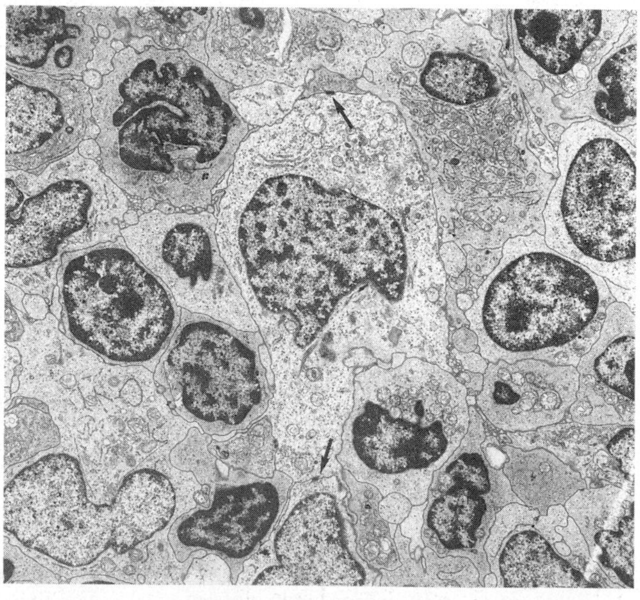

FIG. 6.15. Although follicular dendritic cells are hardly recognized by light microscopy, their distinct features are easily identified at the electron microscopic level (original magnification: 25,000× magnification). These large cells have a round nucleus with vesicular chromatin, and their cytoplasm contains sparse organelles. They are provided with plump cytoplasmic dendrites, which are connected with each other by desmosomes *(arrow).*

In contrast with ultrastructural studies that usually focus on individual cells, immunohistochemistry yields an overall picture of the cellular meshwork created by follicular dendritic cells and of their interrelationship with admixed lymphocytes. By visualizing the immune complexes bound on their surface, phenotyping of follicular dendritic cells highlights the network they form. However, because follicular dendritic cells acquire these complexes only after they have been confronted with foreign antigens, these particular cell markers are not useful during intrauterine life.

All follicular dendritic cells express the monocytic marker CD14, the three types of complement receptors—CD35 (CR-1), the long isoform of CD21 (CR-2), and CD11b (CR-3)—and the immunoglobulin Fc receptor CD32 (165,166). Displaying the latter receptors on their plasma membrane, the entire population of follicular dendritic cells is provided with an efficient mechanism to trap passing antigen-antibody-C3 (Ag-Ab-C3) complexes. A subset of the follicular dendritic cells in the light zone of the germinal center additionally expresses CD23, which is the low-affinity receptor for IgE, and one of the ligands for CD21, allowing them to bind complexes containing CD21 with higher affinity and to interact with IgE. Numerous adhesion molecules, including ICAM-1, VCAM-1, VLA-3, VLA-4, VLA-5, VLA-6, and VLA β chain, reinforce the primary connections between the antigen-presenting cells and initially loosely attached lymphocytes (167). Adhesion between follicular dendritic cells and B cells is mediated by ICAM-1/LFA-1 (CD11a) and VCAM-1/VLA-4 (168,169), whereas CD40–CD40 ligand interaction, CD3-TCR complexes, and MHC class II molecules strengthen interactions with T lymphocytes (170). The latter HLA molecules appear on the follicular dendritic cell surface as a result of entrapment of MHC molecules shed by neighboring B cells. Whether follicular dendritic cells express B-cell markers such as CD19, CD20, and CD24 or the pan-leukocyte antigen CD45 constitutionally or as the result of passive adherence remains controversial.

Follicular dendritic cells are essential participants in the antigen-triggered development of B cells within the selective microenvironment of the germinal center, regardless of the occurrence of additional T-cell help. During the early stages of every immune response, antigen-antibody (Ag-Ab) complexes are formed that activate the complement system, on which C3 fragments covalently bind to the immune complexes which had previously initiated their production (171,172). Subsequently, the Ag-Ab-C3 complexes are scavenged by the follicular dendritic cells through their Fc and complement receptors and may persist on the cell surface for up to 18 months (173). The mechanism that prevents follicular dendritic cells from internalizing antigens, allowing them to retain these molecules in their native form on the cell surface, remains elusive. Nevertheless, the precise function of this phenomenon in the overall immune response seems obvious. The Ag-Ab-C3 complexes probably contribute to the positive selection of high-affinity mutant B cells and influence the subsequent process of clonal expansion in the light zone of the germinal center. It has been demonstrated in rats that blocking follicular antigen trapping through irradiation or through C3 depletion after administration of cobra venom factor causes a significant decrease in average germinal center size, which supports the hypothesis that continuous antigen-stimulation provided by follicular dendritic cells is essential for the regular maturation of memory B cells in full-fledged germinal centers (174).

Gray and colleagues showed that memory B cells transferred into irradiated congenic animals are lost within 4 weeks if no antigen is provided by follicular dendritic cells, whereas the same cell population, inevitably dying in the former animals, can be transferred indefinitely into congenic animals that have been challenged with the appropriate antigen (175). It seems likely that besides promoting germinal center formation, the long-term retention of the Ag-Ab complexes is also essential for the maintenance of memory B-cell clones and for a sustained antibody response.

In the earliest stages of the immune response, during the induction phase of germinal center reactions, the proliferation of antigen-specific B cells within the follicles may elapse independent of Ag-Ab-C3 complexes, because evidence of ongoing follicular B-cell proliferation was observed before clear signs of follicular antigen trapping could be identified (176). Although germinal center T cells probably obtain sufficient antigen-presenting signals from the surrounding B lymphocytes (177), a subset of follicular dendritic cells may also contribute to T-cell activation, because it has been demonstrated that highly purified follicular dendritic cells are able to induce the proliferation of allogeneic T cells or T-cell lines (178).

Keeping these data in mind, it may be of interest to reconsider the findings of Grouard and coworkers that were based on extensive immunohistochemical analysis of human tonsil sections. These investigators detected a previously ignored subpopulation of dendritic cells within the germinal centers that are potentially involved in the activation of $CD4^+$ T cells and are characterized by their $CD4^+CD3^-$ phenotype (160). As these $CD4^+CD3^-$ cells are further typed as $CD1a^-CD40^{low}$, $CD80/CD86^{low}$, and $DRC1^-$, they could not possibly represent Langerhans cells ($CD1a^+$), interdigitating dendritic cells ($CD40^{high}$, $CD80^{high}$, $CD86^{high}$), or follicular dendritic cells ($DRC\text{-}1^+$, $Ki\text{-}M4^+$). Isolation of these specialized cells yielded additional information. They have the morphology of a classic monocytic-dendritic cell, are characterized by intense reactivity with antibodies directed against MHC class II molecules, and display potent stimulatory activity on $CD4^+$ T cells. *In situ* hybridization studies revealed that this subset of dendritic cells expresses high levels of a bacteria-like metalloproteinase on CD40 activation (179). Considering that identical metalloproteinases are known to regulate the activity of tumor necrosis factor-α and that these substances are also involved in FAS ligand processing, the metalloproteinases may be of particular importance in dendritic cell function and in their interactions with germinal center T cells (179).

It is still a matter of debate whether follicular dendritic cells are derived from mesenchymal reticular fibroblasts or from hematopoietic progenitors. Several experimental findings favor the former assumption, including the demonstration of expression of the fibroblast marker 1B10 (180), associated with a consistent absence of the leukocyte common antigen CD45 (181) on freshly isolated human tonsillar follicular dendritic cells. Second, the transfer of bone marrow or splenic cells into SCID mice does not result in the generation of a follicular dendritic cell progeny of donor origin, but only follicular dendritic cells of host origin were brought about (182). However, the shared expression of Ki-M4 by human follicular dendritic cells and a subset of circulating monocytes suggests a hematopoietic cell origin of follicular dendritic cells. Supporting the latter hypothesis, ultrastructurally, antigen-transporting cells have been observed migrating from the subcapsular sinus of the lymph node into the germinal center, where they developed into genuine follicular dendritic cells (183). Alternatively, and in keeping with the identification of a novel type of dendritic cell in the germinal centers (160), two dendritic cell types, one derived from primitive fibroblasts and the other originating from hematopoietic stem cells, may coexist within the follicles.

To complete this discussion on follicular dendritic cells, it is useful to stress their functional significance by setting forth some clinicopathologic conditions in which their usual morphologic features are severely altered, pointing to a pivotal role in the etiopathogenesis of these entities. Follicular dendritic cells presumably contribute to the unique features of HIV pathology that seriously affects the germinal centers. Secondary lymphoid organs of HIV-infected patients are characterized by an initial follicular hyperplasia, followed by a dramatic follicular involution because of dissolution of the entire supporting follicular dendritic cell network (184–186). In the first hypertrophic stage of the disease, HIV bound to follicular dendritic cells induces clonal overexpansion of HIV-specific B cells, thereby severely restricting the diversity of the B-cell repertoire (187,188). The HIV gp120 protein functions as a potent B-cell superantigen, stimulating IgV_{H3}-expressing B cells to undergo early clonal expansion until this proliferation is interrupted abruptly by apoptosis, resulting in deletion of the clone (189). Follicular dendritic cells are also involved in the mechanisms that augment the virulence and the pathogenic capacity of the virus, because it captures CD59 expressed on the surface of follicular dendritic cells (178). In a similar way, antibodies and immune complexes attached to the latter cells are fetched by the infectious agent, allowing it to enter its target cells more efficiently (190,191). Progression of the disease is accompanied by a gradual destruction of the follicular dendritic cell network, resulting in follicular involution (see Chapter

28). The exact mechanisms implicated in the progressive destruction of the framework provided by the follicular dendritic cells remain to be elucidated. However, as the disease process advances and virtually all $CD4^+$ T lymphocytes are eliminated, the survival signals provided by the remaining helper T cells may no longer suffice to protect the follicular dendritic cells from cell death.

In typical low-grade follicular lymphomas, a well-established network of follicular dendritic cells is observed in close association with malignant B cells (192), and some T-cell lymphomas display a similar dense dendritic cell meshwork. The phenotype of follicular dendritic cells in these lymphomas shows no alterations compared with the one observed in normal germinal centers (192). *In vitro* studies suggest that follicular dendritic cells may provide signals that favor the growth of follicular lymphoma cells (193), and analogous to the situation in normal follicles, malignant B cells and follicular dendritic cells do adhere by their surface markers VLA-4 and VCAM-1 (194). However, direct evidence for ongoing interactions between the neoplastic cells of T-cell lymphomas and follicular dendritic cells is still lacking.

Macrophages

The last cell population invariably detectable within the germinal center is represented by the tingible body macrophages, displaying the classic phenotype of macrophages as they express neuron-specific enolase, acid phosphatase, CD11b, CD14, CD68, and HLA-DR (76,195). They owe their name to the presence of cellular debris in their cytoplasm, which underscores their phagocytic activity and is probably used to eliminate the remnants of apoptotic B cells.

T-Cell Area

The second major component of the composite nodule, intimately related to the B follicle, is the T nodule. In contrast to the extensive studies that succeeded in unraveling almost the entire microarchitecture of its B-cell counterpart, the architecture of the T-cell area is less well appreciated. Moreover, depending on the stage of the immune response or the particular features of the antigen involved, the morphology of the T-cell area may vary from a well-delineated nodule with dendritic cells at the periphery to a less well-defined aggregate composed of a variable number of interdigitating dendritic cells, with or without an admixture of Langerhans cells, and T cells. Several investigators did focus on the T nodule and subsequently reported some interesting data elucidating its structure, but the exact microanatomy of the T nodule remains elusive. To a great extent, this lack of detailed information is caused by the variable features of the T-cell area. Although the B follicle invariably shows a clearly recognizable architecture, regardless of the challenging antigen or the stage of the immune response, the morphology of the T nodule may vary from a well-delineated nodule with dendritic cells at its periphery to an ill-defined aggregate. The latter accumulations are composed of interdigitating dendritic cells and T cells, potentially admixed with Langerhans cells, and represent the specific type of T nodule that generally occurs in association with a B-cell area, creating the classic composite nodule (89). Demarcation of the T-cell area is subject to considerable variation, and its precise cellular composition shows even greater fluctuations, depending on the particular features of the antigen involved and on the stage of the immune response.

In contrast with B lymphocytes, T cells cannot be activated by soluble antigen; they require contact of their TCR with antigenic peptide presented on autologous MHC molecules—MHC class I for $CD8^+$ T cells and MHC class II for $CD4^+$ T cells. At the time of antigen recognition, numerous other cognate interactions occur, many of which serve to stabilize the interaction between the antigen-presenting cell and the T lymphocyte. A minority of these accessory interactions are coupled to distinct and sometimes unique intracellular signal transduction cascades within the T cell. Among the latter group, association between CD28 on the T cell and CD80 (B7-1) and CD86 (B7-2) on the antigen-presenting cell has emerged as a crucial checkpoint in pathways leading to T lymphocyte activation (196–198). The type of the ensuing immune response is critically determined by CD28. If this receptor is engaged by CD80 or CD86, the T cell begins to secrete IL-2 and subsequently enters successive rounds of clonal expansion. In the absence of these costimulatory signals, anergy, ignorance, tolerance, or apoptosis follows (197–199).

Immunohistochemical studies have demonstrated that CD80 and CD86 are expressed in the T domain of the composite nodule, which harbors a specific dendritic cell population, the interdigitating dendritic cells. By means of the numerous cytoplasmic processes they are provided with, these cells establish a tridimensional network that envelops T lymphocytes and creates a unique microenvironment for T-cell activation and proliferation (200). In contrast with follicular dendritic cells, for which well-developed desmosomes serve as connection between the dendritic protrusions of different cells, the cellular extensions of interdigitating dendritic cells join, as their name indicates, by forming *interdigitations*. These cells have abundant, pale-staining cytoplasm encompassing a large, elongated, bizarre, but very characteristic nucleus. Its outline is provided with several deep clefts and folds, and it contains very delicate chromatin and inconspicuous nucleoli (87) (Fig. 6.16). These dendritic cells derive from bone marrow monocytes and display quite similar light microscopic, ultrastructural, and phenotypic features to Langerhans cells of the epidermis but lack Birbeck granules, a specific, racquet-shaped cell organelle. Langerhans cells are known to migrate to the lymph node. The resultant image of Langerhans cells and interdigitating dendritic cells occurring side by side in an extended paracortex is particularly prominent in dermatopathic lymphadenitis (97,98,201) (see Chapter 15).

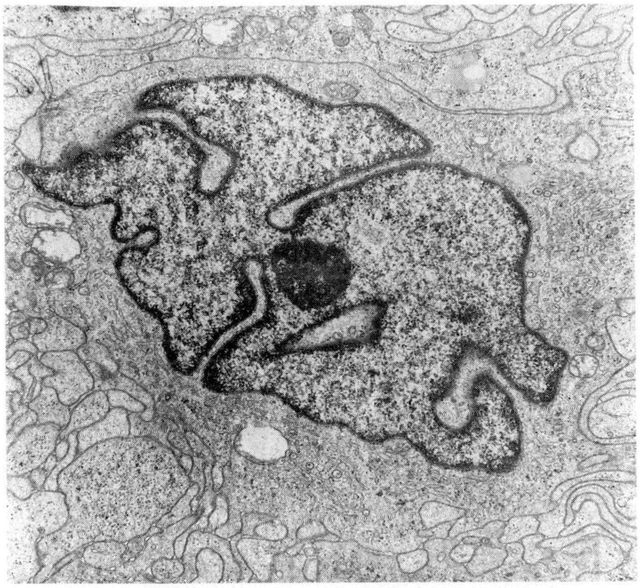

FIG. 6.16. Electron microscopic picture of a typical interdigitating dendritic cell of the T-cell domain of the composite nodule (original magnification: 40,000× magnification). Unlike follicular dendritic cells, which are typically joined by desmosomes, the cytoplasmic processes of interdigitating dendritic cells contact by forming "interdigitations." Notice the irregular outline of the nucleus, also identified with optical microscopy as a distinct feature of this dendritic cell.

Because dendritic cells can be successfully generated from bone marrow precursors, a detailed analysis of this intriguing cell population has become feasible. These *in vitro* studies indicate that dendritic cells function as very potent antigen-presenting cells, able to capture antigens and, in a second phase, to stimulate T cells. Consequently, the latter cells acquire the capacity to interact with B cells to form antibodies, with macrophages to release cytokines, or with target cells for lysis.

An *in vivo* equivalent of this immune response occurs in lymphoid tissues. The T-cell area of the composite nodule, where dendritic cells and T lymphocytes are found in close association, probably represents the exact microanatomic site for this process of T-cell triggering, although this hypothesis remains to be proven (202).

Dendritic cells express CD11c leukocyte integrin, the DEC-205 multilectin receptor for antigen-presentation, very high levels of MHC class I and MHC class II products, and many accessory molecules such as CD40, CD54, and CD86 (203). Moreover, they synthesize high levels of IL-2 (202). The dendritic cells are particularly well equipped to stimulate the growth and activation of a variety of T lymphocytes, including $CD8^+$ cytotoxic T cells and $CD4^+$ helper T cells.

Most dendritic cells detectable outside the secondary lymphoid organs display an incompletely differentiated phenotype, which means that they lack accessory surface markers involved in T-cell stimulation. Nevertheless, they do express the molecular machinery required to capture antigens, an interaction that induces their full maturation. Similarly, "immature" dendritic cells of the skin (i.e., Langerhans cells) only become fully developed antigen-presenting cells when, on contact with an antigen penetrating the cutaneous barrier, they migrate along dermal lymphatics and reach a regional lymph node in search of antigen-specific T cells.

Westerman and his group demonstrated that, at least in rats, memory T cells migrate through the T-cell area at a very high rate, and as they continuously recirculate, meanwhile surveying the surface of the interdigitating dendritic cells, they could eventually encounter their specific antigen (204). Because mature interdigitating dendritic cells and completely differentiated Langerhans cells have acquired the appropriate accessory surface molecules on encounter with their specific antigen presented by the aforementioned cells, selected T lymphocytes undergo activation and eventually proliferate intensely.

A study provided additional data on the dendritic cells harbored in the T nodule, grossly confirming the speculations explained previously regarding ongoing maturation processes during the establishment of their function. As a result of comprehensive investigations comprising morphologic and immunohistochemical techniques applied to tissue sections, cell suspensions, and cell cultures, three distinct subpopulations of these dendritic cells were defined. The first population, outnumbering the other two by far, is characterized by the expression of CD1a and the absence or very weak expression of CD86 and CD83. These cells represent an immature population, closely related to dermal dendritic cells and preferentially located within the sinus lumen. When cultured in an appropriate medium, they differentiate into mature interdigitating dendritic cells. The second subtype of T-cell area–related dendritic cells does react with antibodies directed to CD86 and CD83 but lacks CD1a. CD86 has been identified as one of the costimulatory markers expressed on professional antigen-presenting cells particularly involved in T-cell activation as an accessory molecule. The exact functions mediated by CD83, also detectable on epidermal Langerhans cells, still require clarification. This second cell type corresponds to well-differentiated interdigitating dendritic cells and is seldom observed in the studied cell suspensions, which confirms previous indications that fully developed elements constitute only a small fraction of the entire dendritic cell population. A third subset reacts avidly with antibodies against the three surface markers, CD1a, CD86, and CD83. This strong expression of CD1a, which together with CD1b and CD1c constitutes the CD1 family, showing some structural similarities to the HLA molecules, is of special interest. Although the precise significance of CD1 expression is not fully elucidated, convincing evidence suggests that the CD1 family groups a number of antigen-presenting molecules engaged in the presentation of nonpeptide antigens, such as lipids and glycolipids, to a selected subpopulation of T cells. This last type of dendritic cell represents activated interdigitating dendritic cells, which occur in small clusters in the T nodule and become particularly prominent in dermatopathic lymphadenitis. On stimulation with granulocyte-macrophage colony-stimulating factor, this population can be generated from cultured immature dendritic cells (205).

In conclusion, the T-cell area of the lymph node contains a diverse population of dendritic cells reflecting different stages in their development from immature cells to potent, well-equipped professional antigen-presenting cells. However, by pure morphology, distinct variants of dendritic cells residing in the T-cell area were previously described, including interdigitating dendritic cells, Langerhans cells, and the peculiar population that is brought about by plasmacytoid monocytes. All these cells display the unique propensity to activate resting T cells and to initiate their proliferation, a capacity that they only acquire after termination of a strict maturation process. Because they apparently perform almost identical functions, one could speculate about a certain relatedness between these three dendritic cell types, but the exact nature of such a relationship remains elusive.

Final B-Cell Maturation within the Composite Nodule

The hallmark of B lymphocytes is their production of a multitude of antibodies with extremely diverse antigen-binding specificities. During B-cell ontogeny, the compilation of B cells secreting antibodies with unique binding specificities is created at two distinct stages. The primitive B-cell repertoire is shaped in the bone marrow through immunoglobulin gene rearrangements, resulting in naive B lymphocytes (206). Generation of a far more diverse and highly specific collection of B cells takes place in the secondary lymphoid organs after antigen-stimulation through somatic hypermutation (207). In humans and in mice, this somatic hypermutation mechanism seems to occur exclusively in the specialized microenvironment provided by the germinal center of the B follicle during a T-cell–dependent immune response. However, in other species, somatic hypermutations have been demonstrated to occur independently of the antigen selection process. For example, in sheep and in the toad *Xenopus,* somatic mutations contribute to the diversification of the primary B-cell repertoire, defined as the naive B-cell repertoire, as it emerges in Peyer's patches in the complete absence of external antigens (208–210).

The microanatomic localization and the kinetics of secondary B-cell development during T-cell–dependent (211–216) and T-cell–independent immune responses (217) have been thoroughly studied in animal models. In these experiments, immunohistology again demonstrated its inestimable value, representing an adequate tool to identify antigen-specific B cells on tissue sections.

Integration of the data provided by these studies yields a clarified view on the complex microenvironment of the germinal center, which accounts for the developmentally regulated proliferation of B lymphocytes, for the subsequent occurrence of somatic hypermutations within their immunoglobulin genes and for the eventual selection of newly generated B cells, based on their superior specificity for the challenging antigen, giving rise to the secondary B-cell repertoire. The various stages in the maturation of uncommitted B lymphocytes as they are produced within the bone marrow through simple rearrangement of their immunoglobulin genes, resulting in the expression of a functionally active, although not very potent antigen receptor, into antibody-secreting plasma cells or long-lived memory cells, are discussed in the following section.

As they are recruited by high endothelial venules in the paracortex of the lymph node, naive B cells are eliminated, join the recirculating B-cell pool, or are confronted with an antigen they recognize. On such an antigen encounter, naive B cells bearing specific antigen receptors are inevitably activated, whether this recognition event occurs with the assistance of antigen-presenting cells or stimulated T lymphocytes or not. These activated B blasts may follow two different pathways. Although a portion of these cells proliferates *in loco,* more precisely within the marginal zone, and differentiates into plasma cells responsible for the early production of antibodies, a subpopulation migrates into the primary follicle and begins to proliferate at a high rate, embraced by the extensive cytoplasmic processes of follicular dendritic cells. These germinal center founder cells, characterized by antigen receptors with a relatively high affinity to the presented antigen, are solely selected to undergo clonal expansion and differentiation into centroblasts. Afterward, the germinal center polarizes into a dark zone, proximal to the T-cell area of the composite nodule or the periarteriolar T lymphocyte sheath in the spleen, and a distal or upper light zone. The dark zone contains rapidly dividing B blasts or centroblasts that accumulate somatic hypermutations within their immunoglobulin V_H genes in a stepwise fashion, resulting in a mixture of three types of mutants: those displaying low or high affinity for the challenging antigen and autoreactive mutants, the generation of which could not be prevented by this randomly occurring process. These mutants migrate to the distal light zone, which is particularly rich in follicular dendritic cells and $CD4^+$ T cells. The survival of the newly formed centrocytes in this area depends entirely on their binding to antigen-antibody immune complexes present on the surface of follicular dendritic cells. Only high-affinity mutants are able to retrieve antigen from follicular dendritic cells, which saves them from a certain death because, completely devoid of protective BCL-2, they are predestined to die. Subsequently, rescued centroblasts that have come to demonstrate the features of a centrocyte process the given antigen and present it to T cells. After this interaction, the T lymphocytes are activated to express CD40 ligand and to secrete high levels of IL-4 and IL-10, cytokines that induce clonal expansion and isotype switch of high-affinity centrocytes.

Erroneously generated autoreactive clones are confronted with impressive concentrations of soluble antigens. However, because only their antigen receptor is activated, in the absence of costimulatory signals from follicular dendritic cells, helper T cells, or FAS ligand–expressing T cells, these self-reactive B cells are relentlessly deleted. Alternatively, these autoreactive clones may undergo secondary VDJ gene rearrangements, also called receptor editing, to eliminate their autoreactivity and to rescue them from apoptotic death (218). In this respect, germinal centers should be regarded as primary lymphoid organs, confirming previously acquired data pointing out that the follicle center potentially engages more primitive mechanisms to generate diversity to establish an even more specific progeny. Germinal center B cells may reexpress RAG-1 and RAG-2 proteins after immunization, and similar to immature B cells, they are responsive to IL-7 (219,220).

A germinal center B cell that has successfully passed all the selection processes cited earlier, meanwhile accomplishing affinity maturation and isotype switch, may eventually differentiate into an antibody-secreting plasma cell or become a well-developed memory B cell. The key molecule in determining the final faith of the centrocyte is CD40, which preferentially directs germinal center B cells toward the memory B-cell pathway. A third option represents migrating back into the dark zone to reinitiate proliferation.

Newly formed germinal center B cells represent oligoclonal B-cell populations (151,213,221,222), because on average each mature germinal center is derived from only one to three B-cell clones. The germinal center reaction reaches its maximum by day 10 to 12 of primary immune responses. Without further antigenic stimulation, germinal centers wane by 21 days after immunization.

An intriguing population composes the marginal zone. B cells of this area represent a functionally heterogeneous population, regardless of the anatomic site in which they are detected (223–225). Mutation analysis of the rearranged immunoglobulin heavy chain variable genes provided evidence that the marginal zone B-cell compartment of all secondary lymphoid organs is comprised of naive and memory B cells. The relative number of these subsets does vary substantially according to the exact anatomic site they reside in, which probably results from differences in antigen exposure. We and others have demonstrated that marginal zone B cells show a variable pattern of somatic hypermutations in their rearranged immunoglobulin heavy chain genes (223–225).

Three patterns could be observed: cells lacking somatic hypermutations, cells with somatic hypermutations but without evidence of antigen selection, and cells displaying somatic hypermutations characteristic of antigen selection. A minority of the marginal zone B cells represent naive B cells carrying unmutated immunoglobulin variable genes (223–225). B cells with a distribution of somatic hypermutations in their rearranged immunoglobulin heavy chain variable genes, compatible with affinity maturation or antigen selection, are typically generated in the T-cell–dependent immune reactions that take place in the germinal center, extensively described earlier. Afterward, not all generated memory B cells are released in the circulation, but a minority remains inside the secondary lymphoid organ after migration from the follicle center to the lymphocytic corona or the marginal zone.

It is not clear which type of immune response gives rise to the specific marginal zone B-cell subset with a random pattern of somatic hypermutations in their rearranged immunoglobulin variable genes. The presence of somatic hypermutations in the absence of apparent antigen selection may be characteristic of an early memory B-cell generated during the primary stages of the T-cell–dependent immune response (i.e., a cell that has not undergone multiple rounds of antigen selection in the germinal center) (223,226). Alternatively, these cells with a low level of somatic hypermutations in their rearranged immunoglobulin variable genes may represent memory B cells of the T-cell–independent immune response, brought about in the marginal zone proper. Marginal zone B cells may be cycling, because clones of B cells, clearly distinct from those belonging to the nearby germinal center, are identified in the marginal zone (225). These data strongly indicate that clonal expansion with resultant generation of memory cells may take place in the marginal zone itself, independent of the germinal center. It is tempting to speculate that the somatic hypermutations that are present in marginal zone cells are acquired during clonal expansion in the marginal zone itself, but this speculation awaits further confirmation.

In addition to their role in T-cell–dependent immune responses, circumstantial evidence indicates that human marginal zone B cells are also involved in T-cell–independent type 2 immune responses. For example, newborns and infants up to the age of 2 years show limited response to T-cell–independent type 2 antigens, which corresponds to the age at which a fully developed marginal zone is seen (227). The involvement of marginal zone B cells in the T-cell–independent type 2 immune response has not been proven in adults, but it has been suggested based on the impaired antibody response to T-cell–independent type 2 antigens in splenectomized patients (228).

The potential relationship between marginal zone cells and a particular subpopulation of circulating B lymphocytes merits further consideration. Splenic and nodal marginal zone B cells preferentially rearrange a restricted set of V_{H3} genes such as DP47, DP49, DP54, and DP58 (225). Rearrangements of these genes have also been demonstrated in circulating IgM^+ B cells (229). The preferential use of the D21-9, J_{H4}, and J_{H6} genes is a striking characteristic of the marginal zone B cells and the peripheral blood IgM^+ B cells. Both cell types probably represent memory B cells, because they carry somatically mutated immunoglobulin variable genes (225,229,230). Taken together, these data indicate that the marginal zone B cells and the circulating IgM^+ B cells belong to the same B-cell compartment (230).

The composite nodule is the morphologic expression of the immune response. Based on the data discussed earlier, a functional significance can be assigned to the various compartments and components of the composite nodule. Figure

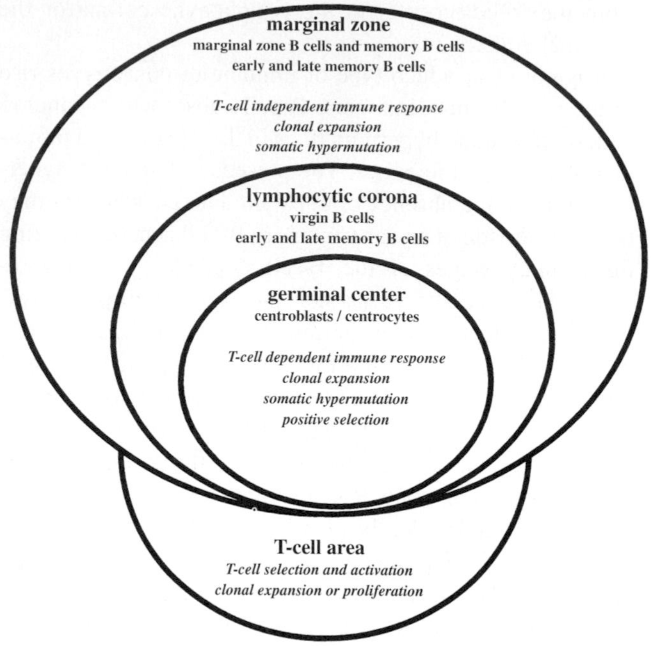

FIG. 6.17. Schematic representation of the composite nodule as the morphologic expression of the immune response.

6.17. illustrates the microarchitecture of the composite nodule, indicating the localization of the various steps of the immune response.

SUMMARY AND CONCLUSIONS

The introduction of more sophisticated morphologic techniques, including immunohistochemistry and molecular genetics, has profoundly altered the classic histologic concepts of the lymphoid system as a whole and of the thymus, the lymph nodes, and the spleen in particular. Histologic descriptions related to the established or speculated function of the various components of the lymphoid organs are preferred to notions merely based on the morphologic appearance of the structure under consideration.

The thymus can be regarded as a central or primary lymphoid organ, because it is responsible for the generation of mature T cells. Similarly, the bone marrow, representing the unique microenvironment for the development of mature though naive B cells, functions as the second primary lymphoid organ. T cells derived from the thymus only require activation of their specific antigen receptor through recognition of the appropriate antigen. This process of selected activation, followed by proliferation of the activated T cells, occurs in the secondary or peripheral lymphoid tissues without any further affinity maturation requirement. In contrast, naive B cells leaving the bone marrow demand additional affinity maturation to become effector cells, an event also evolving in the highly adapted settings of the secondary lymphoid organs, including the lymph nodes and the spleen.

The universal microanatomic unit recognized in all secondary lymphoid organs, the composite nodule, is composed of a B-cell domain adjacent to a T-cell area. It identifies the exact site of selected T-cell activation and proliferation, and B-cell affinity maturation with generation of memory B cells and plasma cells also occurs within its boundaries. The surrounding parenchyma or traffic area accounts for the recruitment of specific subgroups of lymphocytes from the large circulating pool, an activity that hinges on the high endothelial venules and their adhesion molecule expression.

For efficient progress of their activation, interaction, and proliferation, B and T lymphocytes depend on the integrity of the entire microenvironment provided by the lymphoid organs. Although for initial B-cell activation, sole interaction with antigen-specific T lymphocytes can suffice, this process is remarkably enhanced by additional contact with the professional antigen-presenting cells of the germinal center, the follicular dendritic cells. Subsequent steps in T-cell–dependent B-cell maturation, such as positive selection and further proliferation of high-affinity mutants in the germinal center, as well as the survival of memory B cells, are potentiated in a similar way by these dendritic cells, providing the appropriate antigenic stimulus.

In the T-cell area, a comparable population of antigen-presenting cells, also displaying a dendritic cell morphology, contributes to the primary activation of T cells. Although most of the cells present are in an immature differentiation stage lacking the surface markers involved in T-cell signaling, on encounter with a foreign antigen, these dendritic cells reach a fully mature status, highly convenient for efficient T-cell triggering. The interdigitating dendritic cell was the first cell type displaying these activities to be identified and fully characterized. Soon, these cells were correlated with epidermal Langerhans cells, which showed a nearly identical morphology and performed similar antigen-presenting functions. Plasmacytoid monocytes, which can be detected in every reactive peripheral lymph node after careful examination, may represent an intermediate stage in the maturation of circulating precursors into cells also capable of providing a potent antigenic stimulus to specific T lymphocytes.

Tingible body macrophages are required to eliminate the remnants of the multitude of lymphocytes generated in the course of the immune response that underwent apoptosis because of insufficient affinity of their receptor for the challenging antigen. Nevertheless, B and T lymphocytes play the leading part in the complex phenomena occurring in the lymph node during specific immune response. As a result of their activation by a challenging antigen, T cells belonging to the helper T or to the cytotoxic or suppressor T subset gain the capacity to stimulate antigen-specific B lymphocytes, to kill their target, or to exert negative feedback control on the ongoing immune reaction, respectively.

On encounter with an appropriate antigen, B cells undergo affinity maturation that results in the creation of a panel of highly antigen-specific effector cells, the antibody-secreting plasma cells and long-lived memory B cells. In the course of this process, most generated B lymphocytes are eliminated because of insufficient specificity or autoreactivity.

Until recently, it was assumed that affinity maturation exclusively occurred within the specialized microenvironment of the germinal center. However, the detection of somatic mutations with evidence for ongoing mutations in the V_H genes of marginal zone cells suggests that similar reactions also take place in this area of lymphoid tissues.

Unfortunately, part of the functional interpretation of the morphology of the thymus, the lymph node, and the spleen is still speculative, because it is based on data obtained exclusively by *in vitro* analysis of the cellular components of these lymphoid tissues. Further improvement of morphologic investigative techniques, including *in situ* hybridization and molecular analysis carried out on well-defined areas or on isolated cells picked from tissue sections, is imperative to confirm these preliminary interpretations. Moreover, these techniques may provide additional data that can improve our understanding of the immune response and its morphologic substrate, the histology of lymphoid tissues.

ACKNOWLEDGMENTS

We thank J. J. van den Oord, whose critical comments have been of inestimable value for the clarity and structuring of this chapter. We also are indebted to R. de Vos, who most kindly provided us with exquisite electron microscopic pictures.

REFERENCES

1. Kendall MD, Johnson HR, Singh J. The weight of the human thymus gland at necropsy. *J Anat* 1980;131:483–497.
2. Rosai J, Levine GD. Nonneoplastic conditions of the thymus. In: Rosai J, Levine G, eds. *Tumors of the thymus,* vol 13. Washington, DC: Armed Forces Institute of Pathology, 1976:22–33.
3. Adam EJ, Ignotus PI. Sonography of the thymus in healthy children: frequency of visualization, size, and appearance. *Am J Roentgenol* 1993;161:153–155.
4. Hasselbalch H, Nielsen MB, Jeppesen D, et al. Sonographic measurement of the thymus in infants. *Eur Radiol* 1996;6:700–703.
5. Hasselbalch H, Jeppesen DL, Ersboll AK, et al. Thymus size evaluated by sonography: a longitudinal study on infants during the first year of life. *Acta Radiol* 1997;38:222–227.
6. von Gaudecker B, Muller Hermelink HK. Ontogeny and organization of the stationary non-lymphoid cells in the human thymus. *Cell Tissue Res* 1980;207:287–306.
7. Nakahama M, Mohri N, Mori S, et al. Immunohistochemical and histometrical studies of the human thymus with special emphasis on age-related changes in medullary epithelial and dendritic cells. *Virchows Arch* 1990;58:245–251.
8. Muller JG, Krenn V, Czub S, et al. The thymic epithelial reticulum and interdigitating cells in SIV-induced thymus atrophy and its comparison with other forms of thymus involution. *Res Virol* 1993;144: 93–98.
9. von Gaudecker B. The development of the human thymus microenvironment. *Curr Top Pathol* 1986;75:1–41.
10. Lobach DF, Haynes BF, Hiramine C, et al. Ontogeny of the human thymus during fetal development: thymic nurse cells as the site of thymocyte apoptosis and apoptotic cell clearance in the thymus of cyclophosphamide-treated mice. *J Clin Immunol* 1987;7:81–97.
11. Haynes BF, Heinly CS. Early human T cell development: analysis of the human thymus at the time of initial entry of hematopoietic stem cells into the fetal thymic microenvironment. *J Exp Med* 1995;181: 1445–1458.
12. Haynes BF. Human thymic epithelium and T cell development: current issues and future directions. *Thymus* 1990;16:143–157.
13. Nezelof C. Thymic pathology in primary and secondary immunodeficiencies. *Histopathology* 1992;21:499–511.
14. von Gaudecker B. Functional histology of the human thymus. *Anat Embryol (Berl)* 1991;183:1–15.
15. Fend F, Nachbaur D, Oberwasserlechner F, et al. Phenotype and topography of human thymic B cells: an immunohistologic study. *Virchows Arch* 1991;60:381–388.
16. Hofmann WJ, Moller P, Otto HF. Thymic hyperplasia. I. True thymic hyperplasia: review of the literature. *Klin Wochenschr* 1987;65: 49–52.
17. Raviola E, Karnovsky MJ. Evidence for a blood-thymus barrier using electron-opaque tracers. *J Exp Med* 1972;136:466–498.
18. Wekerle H, Ketelsen UP, Ernst M. Thymic nurse cells. Lymphoepithelial cell complexes in murine thymuses: morphological and serological characterization. *J Exp Med* 1980;151:925–944.
19. Hiramine C, Nakagawa T, Hojo K. Murine nursing thymic epithelial cell lines capable of inducing thymocyte apoptosis express the self-superantigen Mls-1a. *Cell Immunol* 1995;160:157–162.
20. Hiramine C, Nakagawa T, Miyauchi A, et al. Thymic nurse cells as the site of thymocyte apoptosis and apoptotic cell clearance in the thymus of cyclophosphamide-treated mice. *Lab Invest* 1996;75: 185–201.
21. Drenckhahn D, von Gaudecker B, Muller Hermelink HK, et al. Myosin and actin containing cells in the human postnatal thymus. Ultrastructural and immunohistochemical findings in normal thymus and in myasthenia gravis. *Virchows Arch* 1979;32:33–45.
22. Kao I, Drachman DB. Thymic muscle cells bear acetylcholine receptors: possible relation to myasthenia gravis. *Science* 1977;195:74–75.
23. Moll UM, Lane BL, Robert F, et al. The neuroendocrine thymus. Abundant occurrence of oxytocin-, vasopressin-, and neurophysin-like peptides in epithelial cells. *Histochemistry* 1988;89:385–390.
24. Geenen V, Legros JJ, Franchimont P, et al. The neuroendocrine thymus: coexistence of oxytocin and neurophysin in the human thymus. *Science* 1986;232:508–511.
25. Schmitt D, Monier JC, Dardenne M, et al. Location of FTS (facteur thymique serique) in the thymus of normal and auto-immune mice. *Thymus* 1982;4:221–231.
26. Isaacson PG, Norton AJ, Addis BJ. The human thymus contains a novel population of B lymphocytes. *Lancet* 1987;2:1488–491.
27. Spencer J, Choy M, Hussell T, et al. Properties of human thymic B cells. *Immunology* 1992;75:596–600.
28. Punnonen J, de Vries JE. Characterization of a novel $CD2^+$ human thymic B cell subset. *J Immunol* 1993;151:100–110.
29. Vollger LW, Tuck DT, Springer TA, et al. Thymocyte binding to human thymic epithelial cells is inhibited by monoclonal antibodies to CD-2 and LFA-3 antigens. *J Immunol* 1987;138:358–363.
30. Bofill M, Janossy G, Willcox N, et al. Microenvironments in the normal thymus and the thymus in myasthenia gravis. *Am J Pathol* 1985;119:462–473.
31. Staber FG, Fink U, Sack W. B lymphocytes in the thymus of patients with myasthenia gravis [Letter]. *N Engl J Med* 1975;292:1032–1033.
32. Berrih Aknin S, Morel E, Raimond F, et al. The role of the thymus in myasthenia gravis: immunohistological and immunological studies in 115 cases. *Ann N Y Acad Sci* 1987;505:50–70.
33. Harris NL, Jaffe ES, Stein H, et al. A revised European-American classification of lymphoid neoplasms: a proposal from the International Lymphoma Study Group. *Blood* 1994;84:1361–1392.
34. Kuppers R, Rajewsky K, Hansmann ML. Diffuse large cell lymphomas are derived from mature B cells carrying V region genes with a high load of somatic mutation and evidence of selection for antibody expression. *Eur J Immunol* 1997;27:1398–1405.
35. Tsang P, Cesarman E, Chadburn A, et al. Molecular characterization of primary mediastinal B cell lymphoma. *Am J Pathol* 1996;148: 2017–2025.
36. Willcox HNA, Newsom-Davis J, Calder LR. Greatly increased auto-antibody production in myasthenia gravis by thymocyte suspensions prepared with proteolytic enzymes. *Clin Exp Immunol* 1983;54: 378–386.
37. Nieuwenhuis P, Stet RJ, Wagenaar JP, et al. The transcapsular route:

a new way for (self-) antigens to bypass the blood-thymus barrier? *Immunol Today* 1988;9:372–375.
38. Bannister L, Kendall M. Lymphoid cells and tissues: thymus. In: Williams PL, Bannister LH, Berry MM, et al, eds. *Gray's anatomy,* 38th ed. New York: Churchill Livingstone 1995:1423–1431.
39. Res P, Martinez Caceres E, Cristina Jaleco A, et al. $CD34^+CD38^{dim}$ cells in the human thymus can differentiate into T, natural killer, and dendritic cells but are distinct from pluripotent stem cells. *Blood* 1996; 87:5196–5206.
40. Wu L, Kincade PW, Shortman K. The CD44 expressed on the earliest intrathymic precursor population functions as a thymus homing molecule but does not bind to hyaluronate. *Immunol Lett* 1993;38:69–75.
41. Mojcik CF, Salomon DR, Chang AC, et al. Differential expression of integrins on human thymocyte subpopulations. *Blood* 1995;86: 4206–4217.
42. Spits H, Lanier LL, Phillips JH. Development of human T and natural killer cells. *Blood* 1995;85:2654–2670.
43. Peschon JJ, Morrissey PJ, Grabstein KH, et al. Early lymphocyte expansion is severely impaired in interleukin 7 receptor-deficient mice. *J Exp Med* 1994;180:1955–1960.
44. Conlon PJ, Morrissey PJ, Nordan RP, et al. Murine thymocytes proliferate in direct response to interleukin-7. *Blood* 1989;74:1368–1373.
45. Watson JD, Morrissey PJ, Namen AE, et al. Effect of IL-7 on the growth of fetal thymocytes in culture. *J Immunol* 1989;143: 1215–1222.
46. Matsuzaki Y, Gyotoku J, Ogawa M, et al. Characterization of c-kit positive intrathymic stem cells that are restricted to lymphoid differentiation. *J Exp Med* 1993;178:1283–1292.
47. Rodewald HR, Kretzschmar K, Swat W, et al. Intrathymically expressed c-kit ligand (stem cell factor) is a major factor driving expansion of very immature thymocytes in vivo. *Immunity* 1995;3:313–319.
48. Veis DJ, Sentman CL, Bach EA, et al. Expression of the Bcl-2 protein in murine and human thymocytes and in peripheral T lymphocytes. *J Immunol* 1993;151:2546–2554.
49. Raulet DH, Garman RD, Saito H, et al. Developmental regulation of T cell receptor gene expression. *Nature* 1985;314:103–107.
50. Groettrup M, Ungewiss K, Azogui O, et al. A novel disulfide-linked heterodimer on pre-T cells consists of the T cell receptor beta chain and a 33 kd glycoprotein. *Cell* 1993;75:283–294.
51. Saint Ruf C, Ungewiss K, Groettrup M, et al. Analysis and expression of a cloned pre-T cell receptor gene. *Science* 1994;266:1208–1212.
52. Philpott KL, Viney JL, Kay G, et al. Lymphoid development in mice congenitally lacking T cell receptor alpha beta-expressing cells. *Science* 1992;256:1448–1452.
53. Uematsu Y, Ryser S, Dembic Z, et al. In transgenic mice the introduced functional T cell receptor beta gene prevents expression of endogenous beta genes. *Cell* 1988;52:831–841.
54. Molina TJ, Kishihara K, Siderovski DP, et al. Profound block in thymocyte development in mice lacking p56lck. *Nature* 1992;357: 161–164.
55. van Oers NS, Lowin Kropf B, Finlay D, et al. The alpha beta T cell development is abolished in mice lacking both Lck and Fyn protein tyrosine kinases. *Immunity* 1996;5:429–436.
56. Izquierdo Pastor M, Reif K, Cantrell D. The regulation and function of p21ras during T cell activation and growth. *Immunol Today* 1995; 16:159–164.
57. Owen MJ, Venkitaraman AR. Signalling in lymphocyte development. *Curr Opin Immunol* 1996;8:191–198.
58. Crump AL, Grusby MJ, Glimcher LH, et al. Thymocyte development in major histocompatibility complex–deficient mice: evidence for stochastic commitment to the CD4 and CD8 lineages. *Proc Natl Acad Sci USA* 1993;90:10739–10743.
59. von Boehmer H. Positive selection of lymphocytes. *Cell* 1994;76: 219–228.
60. Nossal GJ. Negative selection of lymphocytes. *Cell* 1994;76:229–239.
61. Allen PM. Peptides in positive and negative selection: a delicate balance. *Cell* 1994;76:593–596.
62. Ashton Rickardt PG, Tonegawa S. A differential-avidity model for T cell selection. *Immunol Today* 1994;15:362–366.
63. Borgulya P, Kishi H, Muller U, et al. Development of the CD4 and CD8 lineage of T cells: instruction versus selection. *EMBO J* 1991; 10:913–918.
64. Robey EA, Fowlkes BJ, Gordon JW, et al. Thymic selection in CD8 transgenic mice supports an instructive model for commitment to a CD4 or CD8 lineage. *Cell* 1991;64:99–107.
65. Davis CB, Killeen N, Crooks ME, et al. Evidence for a stochastic mechanism in the differentiation of mature subsets of T lymphocytes. *Cell* 1993;73:237–247.
66. van Meerwijk JP, Germain RN. Development of mature $CD8^+$ thymocytes: selection rather than instruction? *Science* 1993;261:911–915.
67. Anderson G, Owen JJ, Moore NC, et al. Thymic epithelial cells provide unique signals for positive selection of $CD4^+CD8^+$ thymocytes in vitro. *J Exp Med* 1994;179:2027–2031.
68. Mazda O, Watanabe Y, Gyotoku J, et al. Requirement of dendritic cells and B cells in the clonal deletion of Mls-reactive T cells in the thymus. *J Exp Med* 1991;173:539–547.
69. Kishihara K, Penninger J, Wallace VA, et al. Normal B lymphocyte development but impaired T cell maturation in CD45-exon 6 protein tyrosine phosphatase-deficient mice. *Cell* 1993;74:143–156.
70. Swan KA, Alberola IJ, Gross JA, et al. Involvement of p21ras distinguishes positive and negative selection in thymocytes. *EMBO J* 1995; 14:276–285.
71. Alberola IJ, Forbush KA, Seger R, et al. Selective requirement for MAP kinase activation in thymocyte differentiation. *Nature* 1995; 373:620–623.
72. Arpaia E, Shahar M, Dadi H, et al. Defective T cell receptor signaling and $CD8^+$ thymic selection in humans lacking ZAP-70 kinase. *Cell* 1994;76:947–958.
73. Chan AC, Kadlecek TA, Elder ME, et al. ZAP-70 deficiency in an autosomal recessive form of severe combined immunodeficiency. *Science* 1994;264:1599–1601.
74. Elder ME, Lin D, Clever J, et al. Human severe combined immunodeficiency due to a defect in ZAP-70, a T cell tyrosine kinase. *Science* 1994;264:1596–1599.
75. Wang CR, Hashimoto K, Kubo S, et al. T cell receptor–mediated signaling events in $CD4^+CD8^+$ thymocytes undergoing thymic selection: requirement of calcineurin activation for thymic positive selection but not negative selection. *J Exp Med* 1995;181:927–941.
76. Fossum S, Ford WL. The organization of cell populations within lymph nodes: their origin, life history and functional relationships. *Histopathology* 1985;9:469–499.
77. Asano S, Akaike Y, Muramatsu T, et al. Immunohistologic detection of the primary follicle (PF) in human fetal and newborn lymph node anlages. *Pathol Res Pract* 1993;189:921–927.
78. Mebius RE, Rennert P, Weissmann IL. Developing lymph nodes collect $CD4^+CD3^-$ $LTbeta^+$ cells that can differentiate to APC, NK cells, and follicular cells but not T or B cells. *Immunity* 1997;7: 493–504.
79. Mebius RE, Streeter PR, Michie S, et al. A developmental switch in lymphocyte homing receptor and endothelial vascular addressin expression regulates lymphocyte homing and permits $CD4^+CD3^-$ cells to colonize lymph nodes. *Proc Natl Acad Sci USA* 1996;93: 11019–11024.
80. Sainte-Marie G, Peng FS, Belisle, C. Overall architecture and pattern of lymph flow in the rat lymph node. *Am J Anat* 1982;164:275–309.
81. Kurokawa T, Ogata T. A scanning electron microscopic study on the lymphatic microcirculation of the rabbit mesenteric lymph node: a corrosion cast study. *Acta Anat* 1980;107:439–466.
82. Castenholz A. Architecture of the lymph node with regard to its function. In: Grundmann E, Vollmer E, eds. *Reaction patterns of the lymph node,* vol 1. Berlin: Springer-Verlag, 1990:1–32.
83. Wacker HH, Frahm SO, Heidebrecht HJ, et al. Sinus-lining cells of the lymph nodes recognized as a dendritic cell type by the new monoclonal antibody Ki-M9. *Am J Pathol* 1997;151:423–434.
84. Peters J, Krams M, Wacker HH, et al. Detection of rare RNA sequences by single enzyme in situ RT-PCR: high resolution analysis of interleukin-6 mRNA in paraffin sections of lymph nodes. *Am J Pathol* 1996;150:469–476.
85. Haferkamp O, Rosenau W, Lennert K. Vascular transformation of lymph node sinuses due to venous obstruction. *Arch Pathol* 1971;92: 81–83.
86. Lennert K. *Handbuch der Speziellen Pathologishen Anatomie und Histologie.* Berlin: Springer, 1961.
87. van der Valk P, Meijer CJ. The histology of reactive lymph nodes. *Am J Surg Pathol* 1987;11:866–882.
88. Facchetti F, De Wolf-Peeters C, van den Oord JJ, et al. Anti-high endothelial venule monoclonal antibody HECA-452 recognizes plas-

macytoid T cells and delineates an "extranodular" compartment in the reactive lymph node. *Immunol Lett* 1989;20:277–282.
89. van den Oord JJ, De Wolf-Peeters C, Desmet VJ. The composite nodule: a structural and functional unit of the reactive human lymph node. *Am J Pathol* 1986;122:83–91.
90. Bélisle C, Sainte-Marie G. Topography of the deep cortex of the lymph nodes of various mammalian species. *Anat Rec* 1981;201: 553–561.
91. van den Oord JJ, Facchetti F, Delabie J, et al. T lymphocytes in Non-neoplastic lymph nodes. In: Grundmann E, Vollmer E, eds. *Reaction patterns of the lymph node,* vol 1. Berlin: Springer-Verlag, 1990: 149–78.
92. van den Oord JJ, de Wolf Peeters C, Desmet VJ. The marginal zone in the human reactive lymph node. *Am J Clin Pathol* 1986;86:475–479.
93. van Krieken JH, von Schilling C, Kluin PM, et al. Splenic marginal zone lymphocytes and related cells in the lymph node: a morphologic and immunohistochemical study. *Hum Pathol* 1989;20:320–362.
94. Lennert K. Diagnose und aetiologie der Piringerschen lymphadenitis. *Verh Dtsch Ges Pathol* 1959;42:203–208.
95. van den Oord JJ, de Wolf Peeters C, de Vos R, et al. Immature sinus histiocytosis: light- and electron-microscopic features, immunologic phenotype, and relationship with marginal zone lymphocytes. *Am J Pathol* 1985;118:266–277.
96. Kraal G. Cells in the marginal zone of the spleen. *Int Rev Cytol* 1992; 132:31–74.
97. van den Oord JJ, de Wolf-Peeters C, Desmet VJ, et al. Nodular alteration of the paracortical area. An in situ immunohistochemical analysis of primary, secondary, and tertiary T nodules. *Am J Pathol* 1985; 120:55–66.
98. van den Oord JJ, de Wolf Peeters C, de Vos R, et al. The paracortical area in dermatopathic lymphadenitis and other reactive conditions of the lymph node. *Virchows Arch* 1984;45:289–299.
99. Weiss LM, Wood GS, Warnke RA. Immunophenotypic differences between dermatopathic lymphadenopathy and lymph node involvement in mycosis fungoides. *Am J Pathol* 1985;120:179–185.
100. Weiss LM, Beckstead JH, Warnke RA, et al. Leu-6–expressing cells in lymph nodes: dendritic cells phenotypically similar to interdigitating dendritic cells. *Hum Pathol* 1986;17:179–184.
101. Burke JS, Sheibani K, Rappaport H. Dermatopathic lymphadenopathy: an immunophenotypic comparison of cases associated and unassociated with mycosis fungoides. *Am J Pathol* 1986;123:256–263.
102. Gould E, Porto R, Albores Saavedra J, et al. Dermatopathic lymphadenitis: the spectrum and significance of its morphologic features. *Arch Pathol Lab Med* 1988;112:1145–1150.
103. Herrera GA. Light microscopic, S-100 immunostaining, and ultrastructural analysis of dermatopathic lymphadenopathy, with and without associated mycosis fungoides. *Am J Clin Pathol* 1987;87: 187–195.
104. van den Oord JJ, de Wolf-Peeters C, Desmet VJ. Immunohistochemical analysis of progressively transformed follicular centers. *Am J Clin Pathol* 1985;83:560–564.
105. Poppema S. Lymphocyte-predominance Hodgkin's disease. *Semin Diagn Pathol* 1992;9:257–264.
106. Ferry JA, Zukerberg LR, Harris NL. Florid progressive transformation of germinal centers: a syndrome affecting young men, without early progression to nodular lymphocyte predominance Hodgkin's disease. *Am J Surg Pathol* 1992;16:252–258.
107. Lennert K. *Handbuch der Speziellen Pathologishen Anatomie und Histologie.* Berlin: Springer-Verlag, 1961.
108. Cho Y, De Bruyn PP. The endothelial structure of the postcapillary venules of the lymph node and the passage of lymphocytes across the venule wall. *J Ultrastruct Res* 1979;69:13–21.
109. Perry ME, Brown KA, von Gaudecker B. Ultrastructural identification and distribution of the adhesion molecules ICAM-1 and LFA-1 in the vascular and extravascular compartments of the human palatine tonsil. *Cell Tissue Res* 1992;268:317–326.
110. Kikuta A, Rosen SD. Localization of ligands for L-selectin in mouse peripheral lymph node high endothelial cells by colloidal gold conjugates. *Blood* 1994;84:3766–3775.
111. Tanaka H, Saito S, Sasaki H, et al. Morphological aspects of LFA-1/ICAM-1 and VLA4/VCAM-1 adhesion pathways in human lymph nodes. *Pathol Int* 1994;44:268–279.
112. Shimizu Y, Newman W, Tanaka Y, et al. Lymphocyte interactions with endothelial cells. *Immunol Today* 1992;13:106–112.
113. Picker LJ. Mechanisms of lymphocyte homing. *Curr Opin Immunol* 1992;4:277–286.
114. Springer TA. Traffic signals for lymphocyte recirculation and leukocyte emigration: the multistep paradigm. *Cell* 1994;76:301–314.
115. Carlos TM, Harlan JM. Leukocyte-endothelial adhesion molecules. *Blood* 1994;84:2068–2101.
116. Springer TA. Adhesion receptors of the immune system. *Nature* 1990; 346:425–434.
117. Wallace DL, Beverley PC. Characterization of a novel subset of T cells from human spleen that lacks L-selectin. *Immunology* 1993;78: 623–628.
118. Sprent J. T and B memory cells. *Cell* 1994;76:315–322.
119. Facchetti F, de Wolf-Peeters C, Mason DY, et al. Plasmacytoid T cells: immunohistochemical evidence for their monocyte/macrophage origin. *Am J Pathol* 1988;133:15–21.
120. Facchetti F, de Wolf Peeters C, van den Oord JJ, et al. Plasmacytoid T cells in a case of lymphocytic infiltration of skin: a component of the skin-associated lymphoid tissue? *J Pathol* 1988;155:295–300.
121. Facchetti F, de Wolf-Peeters C, van den Oord JJ, et al. Plasmacytoid T cells—a cell population normally present in the reactive lymph node: an immunohistochemical and electron microscopic study. *Hum Pathol* 1988;19:1085–1092.
122. Facchetti F, de Wolf-Peeters C, de Vos R, et al. Plasmacytoid monocytes (so-called plasmacytoid T cells) in granulomatous lymphadenitis. *Hum Pathol* 1989;20:588–593.
123. Facchetti F, de Wolf-Peeters C, Kennes C, et al. Leukemia-associated lymph node infiltrates of plasmacytoid monocytes (so-called plasmacytoid T cells): evidence for two distinct histological and immunophenotypical patterns. *Am J Surg Pathol* 1990;14:101–112.
124. Grouard G, Rissoan MC, Filgueira L, et al. The enigmatic plasmacytoid T cells develop into dendritic cells with interleukin (IL)-3 and CD40-ligand. *J Exp Med* 1997;185:1101–1111.
125. O'Doherty U, Peng M, Gezelter S, et al. Human blood contains two subsets of dendritic cells, one immunologically mature and the other immature. *Immunology* 1994;82:487–493.
126. Settmacher U, Volk HD, Jahn S, et al. Characterization of human lymphocytes separated from fetal liver and spleen at different stages of ontogeny. *Immunobiology* 1991;182:256–265.
127. Timens W, Rozeboom T, Poppema S. Fetal and neonatal development of human spleen: an immunohistological study. *Immunology* 1987; 60:603–609.
128. Kipps TJ, Robbins BA, Carson DA. Uniform high frequency expression of autoantibody-associated crossreactive idiotypes in the primary B cell follicles of human fetal spleen. *J Exp Med* 1990;171:189–196.
129. Royo C, Touraine JL, de Bouteiller O. Ontogeny of T lymphocyte differentiation in the human fetus: acquisition of phenotype and functions. *Thymus* 1987;10:57–73.
130. Wilkins BS, Green A, Wild AE, et al. Extramedullary haemopoiesis in fetal and adult human spleen: a quantitative immunohistological study. *Histopathology* 1994;24:241–247.
131. van Krieken JH, te Velde J. Normal histology of the human spleen. *Am J Surg Pathol* 1988;12:777–785.
132. Steiniger B, Barth P, Herbst B, et al. The species-specific structure of miroanatomical compartments in the human spleen: strongly sialoadhesin-positive macrophages occur in the perifollicular zone, but not in the marginal zone. *Immunology* 1997;92:307–316.
133. Schmidt EE, MacDonald IC, Groom AC. Comparative aspects of splenic microcirculatoty pathways in mammals: the region bordering the white pulp. *Scanning Microsc* 1993;7:613–628.
134. Schmidt EE, MacDonald I, Groom AC. Microcirculatory pathways in normal human spleen, demonstrated by scanning electron microscopy of corrosion casts. *Am J Anat* 1988;181:253–266.
135. Leenen PJ, Radosevic K, Voerman JS, et al. Heterogeneity of mouse spleen dendritic cells: in vivo phagocytic activity, expression of macrophage markers, and subpopulation turnover. *J Immunol* 1998; 160:2166–2173.
136. Rose ML, Birbeck MS, Wallis VJ, et al. Peanut lectin binding properties of germinal centers of mouse lymphoid tissue. *Nature* 1980;284: 364–366.
137. Allman D, Jain A, Dent A, et al. BCL-6 expression during B cell activation. *Blood* 1996;87:5257–5268.
138. Cattoretti G, Chang CC, Cechova K, et al. BCL-6 protein is expressed in germinal-center B cells. *Blood* 1995;86:45–53.
139. Onizuka T, Moriyama M, Yamochi T, et al. BCL-6 gene product, a

92- to 98-kD nuclear phosphoprotein, is highly expressed in germinal center B cells and their neoplastic counterparts. *Blood* 1995;86:28–37.
140. Ye BH, Cattoretti G, Shen Q, et al. The BCL-6 proto-oncogene controls germinal-center formation and Th2-type inflammation. *Nat Genet* 1997;16:161–170.
141. Dent AL, Shaffer AL, Yu X, et al. Control of inflammation, cytokine expression, and germinal center formation by BCL-6. *Science* 1997; 276:589–592.
142. Pittaluga S, Ayoubi TA, Wlodarska I, et al. BCL-6 expression in reactive lymphoid tissue and in B cell non-Hodgkin's lymphomas. *J Pathol* 1996;179:145–150.
143. Tierens A, Delabie J, Michiels L, et al. Marginal zone B cells in the human lymph node and spleen show somatic hypermutation and display clonal expansion. *Blood* 1999;93:226–234.
144. Liu YJ, Oldfield S, MacLennan IC. Memory B cells in T cell–dependent antibody responses colonize the splenic marginal zones. *Eur J Immunol* 1988;18:355–362.
145. Velardi A, Mingari MC, Moretta L, et al. Functional analysis of cloned germinal center $CD4^+$ cells with natural killer cell–related features: divergence from typical T helper cells. *J Immunol* 1986;137: 2808–2813.
146. Bowen MB, Butch A, Parvin CA, et al. Germinal center T cells are distinct helper-inducer T cells. *Hum Immunol* 1991;31:67–75.
147. Vandenberghe P, Delabie J, de Boer M, et al. In situ expression of B7/BB1 on antigen-presenting cells and activated B cells: an immunohistochemical study. *Int Immunol* 1993;5:317–321.
148. Vyth Dreese FA, Dellemijn TA, Majoor D, et al. Localization in situ of the co-stimulatory molecules B7.1, B7.2, CD40 and their ligands in normal human lymphoid tissue. *Eur J Immunol* 1995;25:3023–3029.
149. Munro JM, Freedman AS, Aster JC, et al. In vivo expression of the B7 costimulatory molecule by subsets of antigen-presenting cells and the malignant cells of Hodgkin's disease. *Blood* 1994;83:793–798.
150. Nozawa Y, Wachi E, Tominaga K, et al. A novel monoclonal antibody (FUN-1) identifies an activation antigen in cells of the B cell lineage and Reed-Sternberg cells. *J Pathol* 1993;169:309–315.
151. Liu YJ, Johnson GD, Gordon J, et al. Germinal centers in T cell–dependent antibody responses. *Immunol Today* 1992;13:17–21.
152. Borriello F, Sethna MP, Boyd SD, et al. B7-1 and B7-2 have overlapping, critical roles in immunoglobulin class switching and germinal center formation. *Immunity* 1997;6:303–313.
153. Grewal IS, Flavell RA. The CD40 ligand: at the center of the immune universe? *Immunol Res* 1997;16:59–70.
154. Shahinian A, Pfeffer K, Lee KP, et al. Differential T cell costimulatory requirements in CD28-deficient mice. *Science* 1993;261:609–612.
155. Vandenborre K, Delabie J, Boogaerts MA, et al. Human CTLA-4 is expressed in situ on T lymphocytes in germinal centers, in cutaneous graft-versus-host disease, and in Hodgkin's disease. *Am J Pathol* 1998;152:963–973.
156. Xerri L, Devilard E, Hassoun J, et al. In vivo expression of the CTLA4 inhibitory receptor in malignant and reactive cells from human lymphomas. *J Pathol* 1997;183:182–187.
157. Linsley PS. Distinct roles for CD28 and cytotoxic T lymphocyte-associated molecule-4 receptors during T cell activation? *J Exp Med* 1995;182:289–292.
158. Tivol EA, Borriello F, Schweitzer AN, et al. Loss of CTLA-4 leads to massive lymphoproliferation and fatal multiorgan tissue destruction, revealing a critical negative regulatory role of CTLA-4. *Immunity* 1995;3:541–547.
159. Waterhouse P, Penninger JM, Timms E, et al. Lymphoproliferative disorders with early lethality in mice deficient in CTLA-4. *Science* 1995;270:985–988.
160. Grouard G, Durand I, Filgueira L, et al. Dendritic cells capable of stimulating T cells in germinal centers. *Nature* 1996;384:364–367.
161. Braeuninger A, Kuppers R, Strickler JG, et al. Hodgkin and Reed-Sternberg cells in lymphocyte predominant Hodgkin disease represent clonal populations of germinal center–derived tumor B cells. *Proc Natl Acad Sci USA* 1997;94:9337–9342.
162. Kaplan MH, Coons AH, Deane HW. Localization of antigen in tissue cells. III. Cellular distribution of pneumococcal polysaccharides types II and III in the mouse. *J Exp Med* 1950;91:15–29.
163. Szakal AK, Gieringer RL, Kosco MH, et al. Isolated follicular dendritic cells: cytochemical antigen localization, Nomarski, SEM, and TEM morphology. *J Immunol* 1985;134:1349–1359.
164. Nossal GJ, Abbot A, Mitchell J, et al. Antigens in immunity. XV. Ultrastructural features of antigen capture in primary and secondary lymphoid follicles. *J Exp Med* 1968;127:277–290.
165. Tew JG, Kosco MH, Burton GF, et al. Follicular dendritic cells as accessory cells. *Immunol Rev* 1990;117:185–211.
166. Dijkstra CD, Van den Berg TK. The follicular dendritic cell: possible regulatory roles of associated molecules. *Res Immunol* 1991;142: 227–231.
167. Liu YJ, Grouard G, de Bouteiller O, et al. Follicular dendritic cells and germinal centers. *Int Rev Cytol* 1996;166:139–179.
168. Freedman AS, Munro JM, Rice GE, et al. Adhesion of human B cells to germinal centers in vitro involves VLA-4 and INCAM-110. *Science* 1990;249:1030–1033.
169. Koopman G, Parmentier HK, Schuurman HJ, et al. Adhesion of human B cells to follicular dendritic cells involves both the lymphocyte function-associated antigen 1/intercellular adhesion molecule 1 and very late antigen 4/vascular cell adhesion molecule 1 pathways. *J Exp Med* 1991;173:1297–1304.
170. Banchereau J, Bazan F, Blanchard D, et al. The CD40 antigen and its ligand. *Annu Rev Immunol* 1994;12:881–922.
171. Pryjma J, Humphrey JH. Prolonged C3 depletion by cobra venom factor in thymus-deprived mice and its implication for the role of C3 as an essential second signal for B cell triggering. *Immunology* 1975; 28:569–576.
172. van den Berg TK, Dopp EA, Daha MR, et al. Selective inhibition of immune complex trapping by follicular dendritic cells with monoclonal antibodies against rat C3. *Eur J Immunol* 1992;22:957–962.
173. Tew JG, Phipps RP, Mandel TE. The maintenance and regulation of the humoral immune response: persisting antigen and the role of follicular antigen-binding dendritic cells as accessory cells. *Immunol Rev* 1980;53:175–201.
174. Kroese FG, Wubbena AS, Nieuwenhuis P. Germinal center formation and follicular antigen trapping in the spleen of lethally x-irradiated and reconstituted rats. *Immunology* 1986;57:99–104.
175. Gray D, Skarvall H. B cell memory is short-lived in the absence of antigen. *Nature* 1988;336:70–73.
176. Rooijen NV. Antigens in the spleen: the non-specificity of the follicles in the process of antigen trapping and the role of antibody. *Immunology* 1972;22:757–765.
177. Liu YJ, Barthelemy C, de Bouteiller O, et al. Memory B cells from human tonsils colonize mucosal epithelium and directly present antigen to T cells by rapid up-regulation of B7-1 and B7-2. *Immunity* 1995;2:239–248.
178. Butch AW, Hug BA, Nahm MH. Properties of human follicular dendritic cells purified with HJ2, a new monoclonal antibody. *Cell Immunol* 1994;155:27–41.
179. Mueller CG, Rissoan MC, Salinas B, et al. Polymerase chain reaction selects a novel disintegrin proteinase from CD40-activated germinal center dendritic cells. *J Exp Med* 1997;186:655–663.
180. Kim HS, Zhang X, Choi YS. Activation and proliferation of follicular dendritic cell-like cells by activated T lymphocytes. *J Immunol* 1994; 153:2951–2961.
181. Schriever F, Freeman G, Nadler LM. Follicular dendritic cells contain a unique gene repertoire demonstrated by single-cell polymerase chain reaction. *Blood* 1991;77:787–791.
182. Yoshida K, Kaji M, Takahashi T, et al. Host origin of follicular dendritic cells induced in the spleen of SCID mice after transfer of allogeneic lymphocytes. *Immunology* 1995;84:117–126.
183. Kapasi ZF, Kosco Vilbois MH, Shultz LD, et al. Cellular origin of follicular dendritic cells. *Adv Exp Med Biol* 1994;355:231–235.
184. Armstrong JA, Horne R. Follicular dendritic cells and virus-like particles in AIDS-related lymphadenopathy. *Lancet* 1984;2:370–372.
185. Heath SL, Tew JG, Tew JG, et al. Follicular dendritic cells and human immunodeficiency virus infectivity. *Nature* 1995;377:740–744.
186. Pantaleo G, Graziosi C, Demarest JF, et al. Role of lymphoid organs in the pathogenesis of human immunodeficiency virus (HIV) infection. *Immunol Rev* 1994;140:105–130.
187. Muller S, Nara P, D'Amelio R, et al. Clonal patterns in the human immune response to HIV-1 infection. *Int Rev Immunol* 1992;9:1–13.
188. D'Amelio R, Biselli R, Nisini R, et al. Spectrotype of anti-gp120 antibodies remains stable during the course of HIV disease. *J Acquir Immune Defic Syndr* 1992;5:930–935.
189. Berberian L, Goodglick L, Kipps TJ, et al. Immunoglobulin V_{H3} gene products: natural ligands for HIV gp120. *Science* 1993;261: 1588–1591.

190. van de Wiel BA, Bakker LJ, de Graaf L, et al. Complement and antibody enhance binding and uptake of HIV-1 by bone marrow cells. *Adv Exp Med Biol* 1994;355:159–163.
191. Schwartz DH. Potential pitfalls on the road to an effective HIV vaccine. *Immunol Today* 1994;15:54–57.
192. Stein H, Gerdes J, Mason DY. The normal and malignant germinal center. *Clin Haematol* 1982;11:531–559.
193. Petrasch SG, Kosco MH, Perez Alvarez CJ, et al. Proliferation of germinal center B lymphocytes in vitro by direct membrane contact with follicular dendritic cells. *Immunobiology* 1991;183:451–462.
194. Freedman AS, Munro JM, Rhynhart K, et al. Follicular dendritic cells inhibit human B lymphocyte proliferation. *Blood* 1992;80: 1284–1288.
195. Kroese FGM, Timens W, Niewenhuis P. Germinal center reaction and B lymphocytes: morphology and function. In: Grundmann E, Vollmer E, eds. *Reaction patterns of the lymph node,* vol 1, part 1. Berlin: Springer-Verlag, 1990:116–117.
196. June CH, Ledbetter JA, Gillespie MM, et al. T cell proliferation involving the CD28 pathway is associated with cyclosporine-resistant interleukin 2 gene expression. *Mol Cell Biol* 1987;7:4472–4481.
197. June CH, Bluestone JA, Nadler LM, et al. The B7 and CD28 receptor families. *Immunol Today* 1994;15:321–331.
198. Reiser H, Stadecker MJ. Costimulatory B7 molecules in the pathogenesis of infectious and autoimmune diseases. *N Engl J Med* 1996;335: 1369–1377.
199. Schwartz RH. A cell culture model for T lymphocyte clonal anergy. *Science* 1990;248:1349–1356.
200. Crivellato E, Baldini G, Basa M, et al. The three-dimensional structure of interdigitating cells. *Ital J Anat Embryol* 1993;98:243–258.
201. Thorbecke GJ, Silberberg Sinakin I, Flotte TJ. Langerhans' cells as macrophages in skin and lymphoid organs. *J Invest Dermatol* 1980; 75:32–43.
202. Banchereau J, Steinman RM. Dendritic cells and the control of immunity. *Nature* 1998;392:245–252.
203. Inaba K, Pack M, Inaba M, et al. High levels of a major histocompatibility complex II–self peptide complex on dendritic cells from the T cell areas of lymph nodes. *J Exp Med* 1997;186:665–672.
204. Westermann J, Geismar U, Sponholz A, et al. $CD4^+$ T cells of both the naive and the memory phenotype enter rat lymph nodes and Peyer's patches via high endothelial venules: within the tissue their migratory behavior differs. *Eur J Immunol* 1997;27:3174–3181.
205. Takahashi K, Asagoe K, Zaishun J, et al. Heterogeneity of dendritic cells in human superficial lymph node: in vitro maturation of immature dendritic cells into mature or activated interdigitating dendritic cells. *Am J Pathol* 1998;153:745–755.
206. Stewart AK, Schwartz RS. Immunoglobulin V regions and the B cell. *Blood* 1994;83:1717–1730.
207. Tonegawa S. Somatic generation of antibody diversity. *Nature* 1983; 302:575–581.
208. Wilson M, Hsu E, Marcuz A, et al. What limits affinity maturation of antibodies in *Xenopus*—the rate of somatic mutation or the ability to select mutants? *EMBO J* 1992;11:4337–4347.
209. Reynaud CA, Mackay CR, Muller RG, et al. Somatic generation of diversity in a mammalian primary lymphoid organ: the sheep ileal Peyer's patches. *Cell* 1991;64:995–1005.
210. Reynaud CA, Garcia C, Hein WR, et al. Hypermutation generating the sheep immunoglobulin repertoire is an antigen-independent process. *Cell* 1995;80:115–125.
211. Berek C, Berger A, Apel M. Maturation of the immune response in germinal centers. *Cell* 1991;67:1121–1129.
212. Berek C. Somatic mutation and memory. *Curr Opin Immunol* 1993; 5:218–222.
213. Jacob J, Kassir R, Kelsoe G. In situ studies of the primary immune response to (4-hydroxy-3-nitrophenyl)acetyl. I. The architecture and dynamics of responding cell populations. *J Exp Med* 1991;173: 1165–1175.
214. Kelsoe G. In situ studies of the germinal center reaction. *Adv Immunol* 1995;60:267–288.
215. MacLennan IC. Germinal centers. *Annu Rev Immunol* 1994;12: 117–139.
216. MacLennan IC, Gulbranson Judge A, Toellner KM, et al. The changing preference of T and B cells for partners as T-dependent antibody responses develop. *Immunol Rev* 1997;156:53–66.
217. Liu YJ, Zhang J, Lane PJ, et al. Sites of specific B cell activation in primary and secondary responses to T cell–dependent and T cell–independent antigens. *Eur J Immunol* 1991;21:2951–2962.
218. Ohmori H, Hikida M. Expression and function of recombination activating genes in mature B cells. *Crit Rev Immunol* 1998;18:221–235.
219. Hikida M, Mori M, Takai T, et al. Reexpression of RAG-1 and RAG-2 genes in activated mature mouse B cells. *Science* 1996;274: 2092–2094.
220. Han S, Zheng B, Schatz DG, et al. Neoteny in lymphocytes: Rag1 and Rag2 expression in germinal center B cells. *Science* 1996;274: 2094–2097.
221. Jacob J, Miller C, Kelsoe G. In situ studies of the antigen-driven somatic hypermutation of immunoglobulin genes. *Immunol Cell Biol* 1992;70:145–152.
222. Jacob J, Kelsoe G. In situ studies of the primary immune response to (4-hydroxy-3-nitrophenyl)acetyl. II. A common clonal origin for periarteriolar lymphoid sheath-associated foci and germinal centers. *J Exp Med* 1992;176:679–687.
223. Dunn-Walters DK, Isaacson PG, Spencer J. Analysis of mutations in immunoglobulin heavy chain variable region genes of microdissected marginal zone (MGZ) B cells suggests that the MGZ of human spleen is a reservoir of memory B cells. *J Exp Med* 1995;182:559–566.
224. Dunn-Walters DK, Isaacson PG, Spencer J. Sequence analysis of rearranged IgV_H genes from microdissected human Peyer's patch marginal zone B cells. *Immunology* 1996;88:618–624.
225. Tierens A, Delabie J, Pittaluga S, et al. Mutation analysis of the rearranged immunoglobulin heavy chain genes of marginal zone cell lymphomas indicates an origin from different marginal zone B lymphocyte subsets. *Blood* 1998;91:2381–2386.
226. Kepler TB, Perelson AS. Cyclic re-entry of germinal center B cells and the efficiency of affinity maturation. *Immunol Today* 1993;14: 412–415.
227. Timens W, Boes A, Rozeboom-Uiterwijk T, et al. Immaturity of the human splenic marginal zone in infancy: possible contribution to the deficient infant immune response. *J Immunol* 1989;143:3200–3206.
228. Amlot PL, Hayes AE. Impaired human antibody response to the thymus-independent antigen, DNP-Ficoll, after splenectomy. implications for post-splenectomy infections. *Lancet* 1985;1:1008–1011.
229. Brezinschek HP, Foster SJ, Brezinschek RI, et al. Analysis of the human V_H gene repertoire. Differential effects of selection and somatic hypermutation on human peripheral $CD5(^+)/IgM^+$ and $CD5(^-)/IgM^+$ B cells. *J Clin Invest* 1997;99:2488–2501.
230. Klein U, Kuppers R, Rajewsky K. Evidence for a large compartment of IgM-expressing memory B cells in humans. *Blood* 1997;89: 1288–1298.

CHAPTER 7

Antigen Receptor Genes: Structure, Function, and Genetic Analysis of Their Rearrangements

Langxing Pan, Ethel Cesarman, and Daniel M. Knowles

The primary effector molecules of the adaptive immune system are the antigen receptors: immunoglobulin (Ig) and T-cell receptor (TCR). These are members of the Ig gene superfamily that encompasses large numbers of related gene families with diverse functions in separate cell lineages (1–3). The structure and functional evolution of Ig and TCR are unique and remarkably complex. The genes encoding these molecules undergo variable, diversity, and joining or V-(D)-J segment recombination to become functional during lymphocyte development. In B lymphocytes, rearranged Ig genes are further remodeled, and antigen affinity is refined by somatic hypermutation. These complex rearrangement and refining processes form the basis of extensive diversity of antigen receptors, allowing the human body to combat pathogens with the greatest possible flexibility and efficiency.

Antigen receptor molecules have been used in diagnostic pathology for many years as valuable markers for the cell lineage of lymphoid malignancies. Molecular detection of Ig and TCR gene rearrangements has been used widely to document the clonality of malignant lymphoid proliferations. Studies have revealed that the nucleotide sequences of rearranged antigen receptor genes, particularly rearranged Ig genes, harbor important information concerning the biology of tumor clones, such as the developmental stage of the cells of origin, and the influence of antigen and tumor progression. In this chapter, we describe the structure and products of antigen receptor genes, the genetic basis of their diversity, and molecular analyses of their rearrangements for use in the diagnosis and investigation of lymphoid malignancies.

L. Pan, E. Cesarman, and D. M. Knowles: Department of Pathology, Weill Medical College of Cornell University, New York, New York 10021

PRODUCTS OF ANTIGEN RECEPTOR GENES

Immunoglobulins

Basic Structure

Ig molecules of all classes share a similar basic Y-shaped structure consisting of four polypeptide chains: two identical heavy (H) chains of about 50 to 60 kd and two identical light (L) chains of 23 to 25 kd. The IgH and IgL chains comprise domains of about 110 amino acids held together in a loop by a disulfide bond between two cysteine residues in the chain (Fig. 7.1). The amino acid sequences of the N-terminal domains of the IgH and IgL chains vary among different Ig molecules. These sequences are known as variable (V) regions composed of one domain. Variable region amino acid variability is further localized into three clusters known as the complementarity-determining regions (CDRs). The CDRs of the IgH and IgL chains make up the actual antigen-binding sites. Each Ig molecule has two antigen-binding sites and is therefore bivalent. The structure of the antigen-binding site is unique to that Ig molecule and is referred to as an *idiotypic determinant.* In any individual, there may be 106 to 107 different Ig molecules made up by 103 different IgV_H regions associating with 103 different IgV_L regions. Conserved amino acid sequences in the V regions that do not form antigen-binding sites are known as *framework regions* (FRs).

The portion of the Ig molecule next to the V region is the constant (C) region. The IgL C regions contain a single domain (C_L). There are two alternative types of C_L chain, known as kappa (κ) and lambda (λ). Generally, an Ig molecule has two κ or two λ chains with a proportion of 6:4. However, about 0.2% to 0.5% of peripheral B cells express antigen receptors with both light chains (4). The IgH C regions consist of three or four domains (C_H1, C_H2, C_H3, C_H4) with a hinge region lying between C_H1 and C_H2. When bind-

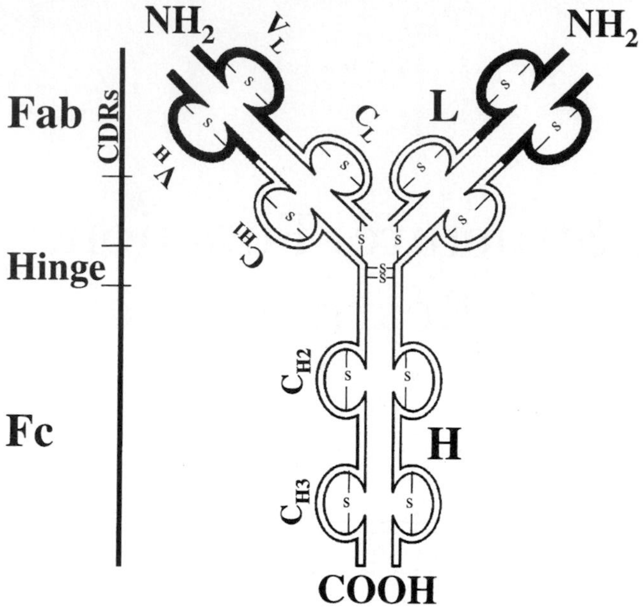

FIG. 7.1. Within the basic Y-shape structure of immunoglobulin, the molecule contains intrachain and interchain disulfide bonds (-s-). H and L, heavy and light chains; NH_2 and COOH, amino- and carboxyl-terminal ends; V_H and VL, variable domains of the heavy and light chains; C_H1, C_H2, C_H3, and C_L, constant domains of the heavy and light chains; Fab, antigen binding fragment; Hinge, hinge region; Fc, Fc fragment; CDRs, complementarity-determining regions.

ing with antigens with multiple antigenic determinants, Ig molecules can form large immune complexes and precipitate out of solution. The efficiency of antigen binding and cross-linking is greatly enhanced by the flexible hinge region, which allows bivalent recognition of variably spaced antigenic determinants.

The proteolytic enzymes papain and pepsin digest Ig molecules into characteristic fragments. Papain produces two identical fragment antigen binding (Fab) fragments, each with one antigen-binding site, and one Fc fragment (so called because it readily crystallizes). Pepsin generates one $F(ab')_2$ fragment consisting of two covalently linked F(ab′) fragments; the remainder of the molecule is broken down into small fragments. Because $F(ab')_2$ fragments are bivalent, they can still cross-link antigens and form precipitates, unlike the univalent Fab fragments.

Immunoglobulin Classes

There are no known functional differences between κ and λ light chains. However, there are several types of heavy chains that determine the classes (isotype) and physiologic functions of Ig molecules. The Ig classes include IgA, IgD, IgE, IgG, and IgM, each with its own class of H chain: α, δ, ϵ, γ, and μ, respectively.

IgM appears during the early phase of the immune response and provides the first protection against invading microorganisms. It consists of five basic units (with 10 antigen-binding sites) held by a joining (J) chain and penetrates poorly into tissues because of its large size. Because of the multiplicity of its combining sites, IgM is very efficient in agglutination and cytolytic reactions.

IgG consists of a single basic unit and is the only Ig that crosses the placenta to provide immune protection to the neonate. It is the major class of immunoglobulins, which is produced in large quantities during secondary immune responses. There are four subclasses of IgG (IgG1 through IgG4). Besides activating the complement system, the Fc regions of IgG molecules bind to specific receptors on the surface of macrophages and some other cells, allowing these cells to destroy infecting microorganisms.

IgA is the major mucosal immunoglobulin. In mucosal secretions, it consists of two basic units joined by a J chain. On mucosal surfaces, IgA molecules react with microorganisms that try to penetrate the mucosa and prevent their invasion into the body.

IgD consists of one basic unit. It mainly exists on the surface of mature B cells serving as an antigen-specific part of the B-cell receptor (BCR).

IgE also consists of one basic unit. It is produced by plasma cells but taken up by specific IgE receptors on the surfaces of mast cells and basophils. The surface membrane-bound IgE molecules trigger the release of chemically active substances that initiate allergic and inflammatory reactions and serve as chemoattractants for other cells. IgE molecules therefore are important participants in allergic reactions and reactions against infecting parasites.

Membrane Form of Immunoglobulin and B-Cell Receptors

B cells produce secreted and membrane-bound forms of Ig. Although secreted Igs act as essential soluble mediators of adaptive immunity, membrane-bound Ig molecules serve as an important part of the BCR (5). The BCR has a complex hetero-oligomeric structure in which ligand binding and signal transduction are compartmentalized into distinct receptor subunits. The ligand-binding portion of this receptor is membrane-bound Ig, which is a tetrameric complex of two IgH and two IgL chains; the signal transduction component comprises a disulfide-bonded heterodimer of the Igα (CD79α) and Igβ (CD79β) molecules. Antigen-binding of membrane-bound Ig generates signals that are subsequently transmitted by an immunoreceptor tyrosine-based activation motif (ITAM) in the cytoplasmic portions of Igα and Igβ to an array of intracellular signaling molecules (6). These molecules amplify or dampen the signals, leading to proliferation, survival, death, anergy, or receptor editing of B cells (5).

T-Cell Receptors

Basic Structure

Four TCR subunits are recognized: α, β, γ, and δ chains. Each TCR chain is about 300 amino acids long and consists

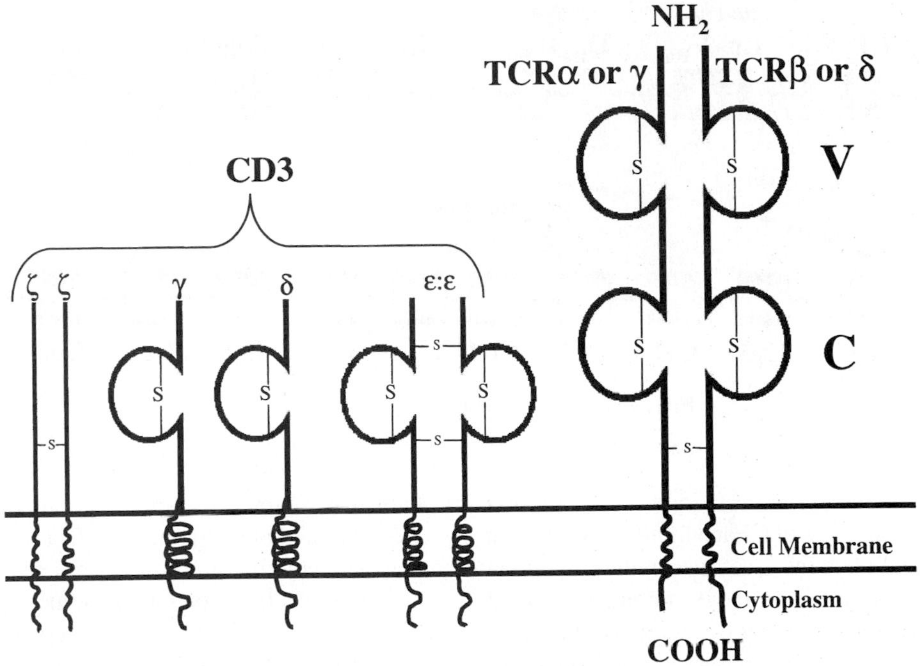

FIG. 7.2. Basic structures of the T-cell receptor (TCR) and CD3 molecules. The TCR is closely associated with the CD3 molecule, although the exact arrangements of both molecules are not reflected in the diagram. The TCR and CD3 molecules contain intrachain and interchain disulfide bonds (-s-). NH_2 and COOH, amino- and carboxyl-terminal ends; V and C, variable and constant domains of the TCR.

of two domains: a variable (V) domain, which is an extracellular N-terminal portion with highly variable sequences, and a constant (C) domain, which is a charged transmembrane portion with a short cytoplasmic tail (Fig. 7.2). Similar to Ig molecules, amino acid variability in the TCR V region mainly falls within three CDRs and an additional fourth hypervariable region (HV4). These CDRs and HV4 regions determine the specific antigen recognition of TCRs.

Unlike Ig subunits, the four TCR chains do not randomly pair with each other. TCR molecules only exist in membrane-bound form as $\alpha\beta$ and $\gamma\delta$ heterodimers on the surface of normal T cells. These two types of TCRs characterize two fundamental groups of T cells (7). T cells bearing $\alpha\beta$ TCRs predominate in adults and are further divisible into those expressing the transmembrane co-receptor CD4 (helper T cells) or CD8 (suppressor or cytotoxic T cells). Helper T cells recognize peptide antigen bound to class II molecules and use coreceptor CD4 to enhance binding and intracellular signaling. Suppressor or cytotoxic T cells recognize antigen bound to class I molecules and similarly use co-receptor CD8 to increase binding and signaling.

The $\gamma\delta$ T cells account for a small proportion (1% to 2%) of total T cells, although about 10% of intraepithelial T cells have $\gamma\delta$ TCR. These $\gamma\delta$ T cells do not appear to rely on co-receptor molecules and possess a less stringent mode of antigen recognition; they are not necessarily restricted to "seeing" only those antigens that are bound in the form of peptides to class I or class II molecules (8,9).

Signal Transduction Through T-Cell Receptors

TCR-ligand interactions, in the presence of certain soluble interleukins and costimulators, induce a complex series of protein modifications and signal transduction events that can lead to T-cell death or activation (10,11). These events, although triggered by the antigen receptor heterodimer, are closely associated with several transmembrane peptides that make up the CD3 molecule (Fig. 7.2). Signal transduction through the CD3 complex occurs under the influence of a group of intracellular tyrosine kinases (i.e., p56 [LCK], p59 [FYN], ZAP-70) that associate with the ITAMs within the cytosolic tails of the CD3 molecule (12). Blocks may occur at several stages of the T-cell signaling pathway, ranging from defective expression of the CD3-TCR complex on the cell surface to absence of intracellular tyrosine kinases, and result in marked immunodeficiency.

STRUCTURE OF ANTIGEN RECEPTOR GENES

Immunoglobulin Heavy-Chain Gene

The inherited Ig heavy-chain gene consists of clusters of variable (V_H), diversity (D), joining (J_H), and constant (C_H) regions, which are located near the telomere of the long arm of chromosome 14 in band 14q32 in the order of 5′-V_H-D-J_H-C_H-3′ (Fig. 7.3). There are more than 100 V_H segments that are interspersed throughout a region over 1 Mbp of 14q32 (13,14). These V_H segments are categorized into seven families that contain various numbers of members.

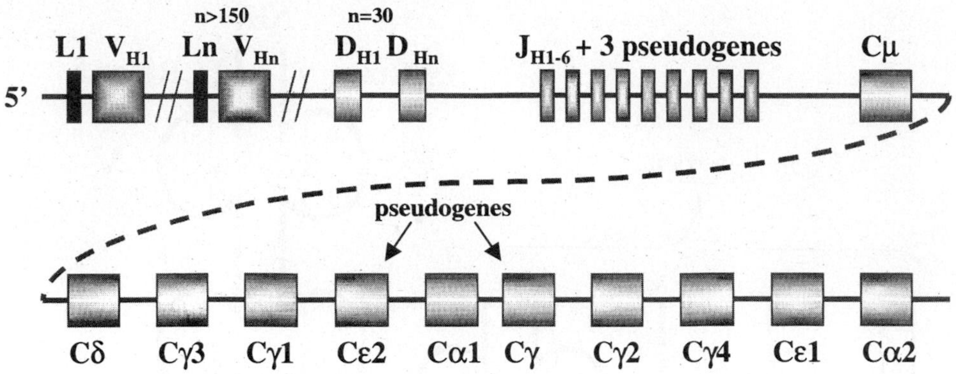

FIG. 7.3. Immunoglobulin heavy-chain gene.

The largest families are V_H3 and V_H1, and the smallest is V_H6, containing only one segment. Each family has a unique 5′ flanking region and contains a consensus nucleotide sequence with 80% or greater homology among individual family members. Sequences among different families have less than 70% homology. The conserved nucleotide sequences are often those encoding the three FRs of IgV_H molecules. The V_H segments are not necessarily clustered in family groups, but are often mixed with members of different families and dispersed across the entire V_H complex. Among all the V_H segments identified, approximately 50, have been found to be functional (13). Other V_H segments are referred to as nonfunctional segments or pseudogenes. Clusters of nonfunctional V_H segments (i.e., orphans) have also been mapped to chromosomes 15 and 16 (15,16).

There are about 30 estimated functional D segments on chromosome 14. At least 27 of them have been completely mapped and sequenced (17). They can be grouped into six families that are arranged in four tandem clusters. Nine J_H segments have been identified at a position about 700 bp 3′ to the last D segments. Six are functional, and the remaining three are nonfunctional or pseudo-J_H fragments. There are 11 C_H segments located about 8 kb downstream of the last J_H fragment and organized as 5′-C_μ-(5 kb)-C_δ-(60 kb)-$C_\gamma3$-(26 kb)-$C_\gamma1$-(19 kb)-$\phi C_{\epsilon 2}$-(13 kb)-$C_\alpha1$-(35 kb)-ϕC_γ-(40 kb)-$C_\gamma2$-(18 kb)-$C_\gamma4$-(23 kb)-$C_{\epsilon 1}$-(10 kb)-$C_\alpha2$-3′ (Fig. 7.3).

Immunoglobulin Light-Chain Genes

κ Light Chain

The human κ light-chain locus is located on chromosome 2 at band p11-12, occupying about 1.8 Mbp of DNA (Fig. 7.4). It is composed of 50 to 100 V_κ segments, five J_κ segments, and one C_κ gene (18–20). The V_κ segments are grouped into four families (V_κI through V_κIV). From the known V_κ segments, about 32 are functional, and the others are nonfunctional with minor defects and referred to as pseudogenes. Nonfunctional V_κ segments (i.e., orphans) have also been identified on chromosomes 1, 22, and others (21). Compared with other antigen receptor genes, Igκ is one of the least complicated. The limited number of V_κ families may increase the recombination efficiency, which, together with speculated bias in antigen-driven selection, may be the basis for the dominant κ chain expression observed in human B cells (22,23).

λ Light Chain

The human λ light-chain locus is located on chromosome 22 at band p11, covering about 0.8 to 3 Mbp of DNA (24) (Fig. 7.5). It consists of a V_λ segment region and seven J_λ-C_λ clusters. The presence of alternating pairs of J_λ-C_λ is unique among Ig loci. It has been found that four J_λ-C_λ (J_λ-C_λ 1, 2, 3, 7) clusters are functional and encode four serologically different J_λ-C_λ isotypes (Mcg, Ke^-Oz^-, Ke^-Oz^+, Ke^+Oz^-). Three others are pseudogenes ($\phi C_\lambda4$, $\phi C_\lambda5$, and $\phi C_\lambda6$). There are about 20 to 70 functional V_λ segments that are localized 14 kb upstream from the J_λ-C_λ region and grouped into 10 families (25,26). Members of different V_λ families are grouped into three clusters (A, B, C) (27). The most frequently used V_λ segments, which are within A cluster, are located closest to the J_λ-C_λ region, accounting for 62% of the expressed V_λ segments. Two orphan V_λ genes have also been found on chromosome 8q11 (28). The λ light-chain locus also includes two genes encoding surrogate λ chains ($V_{pre\text{-}B}$ and $V_\lambda5$) (29,30).

T-Cell Receptor Genes

T-Cell Receptor α

The TCRα locus is located on chromosome 14 at band q11, covering more than 1 Mbp of DNA (31,32) (Fig. 7.6).

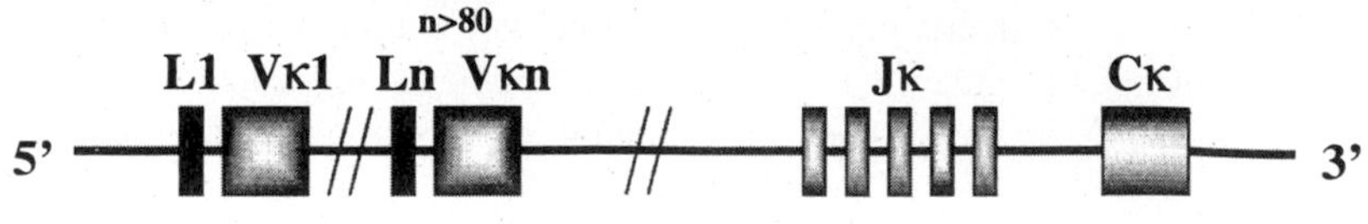

FIG. 7.4. Immunoglobulin κ light-chain gene.

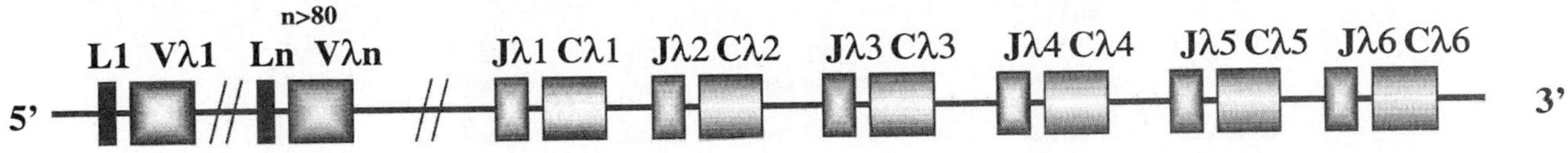

FIG. 7.5. Immunoglobulin λ light-chain gene.

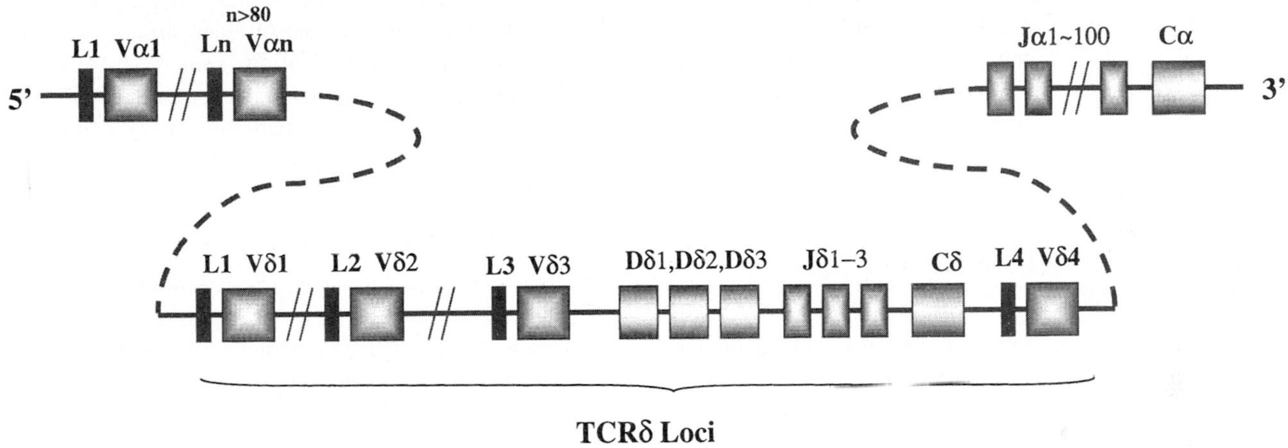

FIG. 7.6. T-cell receptor α- and δ-chain genes.

It consists of 50 to 100 V segments, 50 to 100 J segments and one C region. The V_α segments can be grouped into 22 families, with 15 families containing only one member. Members of V_α families spread widely over more than 600 kb of DNA. There are no known D segments for TCRα. The known J segments cover an 80-kb region separated by about 100 kb from the 3′ end of the last V segment. The C_α region is located about 5 kb from the 3′-most J segment.

T-Cell Receptor β

The TCRβ locus is located on chromosome 7 at band q35, occupying about 700 kb of DNA (33) (Fig. 7.7). It has 75 to 100 V segments, 2 D segments, 13 J segments, and 2 C regions (31). The V_β segments have been categorized into 34 different families that share about 75% nucleotide sequence homology. The two C_β regions form clusters with upstream D_β and J_β segments: $C_\beta1$ rearranges only with $D_\beta1/J_\beta1$ segments, whereas $C_\beta2$ can rearrange with $D_\beta1/J_\beta1$ and $D_\beta2/J_\beta2$ segments (Fig. 7.7). The two C_β genes are highly homologous. As a result, there is no known functional difference between these two β isotypes.

T-Cell Receptor γ

The TCRγ locus is located at band p15 of chromosome 7 spreading over 150 kb of DNA (31) (Fig. 7.8). It has 14 V segments grouped into six families, with five families containing a single member. Six of the V_γ segments are functional, and the remainder are pseudogenes (9,34). There is no known D segment in the TCRγ locus. The V_γ segments are followed at the 3′ end by five $_\gamma$ and two C_γ genes. Nucleotide sequences of $C_\gamma1$ and $C_\gamma2$ share high homology. However, the $C_\gamma2$ gene lacks the cysteine residue that forms an interchain disulfide bridge for all other TCR heterodimeric pairs. C_β and C_γ are structurally more similar to one another than to the C_α or C_β genes.

T-Cell Receptor δ

The TCR-δ is located within the TCRα locus on chromosome 14 and has the same transcriptional orientation as the TCRα locus (31,32,35). It consists of at least 10 V segments, three D segments, three J segments, and one C region. All D, J, C_δ, and perhaps all V_δ sequences are localized between the 3′-most V_α and 5′-most J_α gene segments (Fig. 7.6).

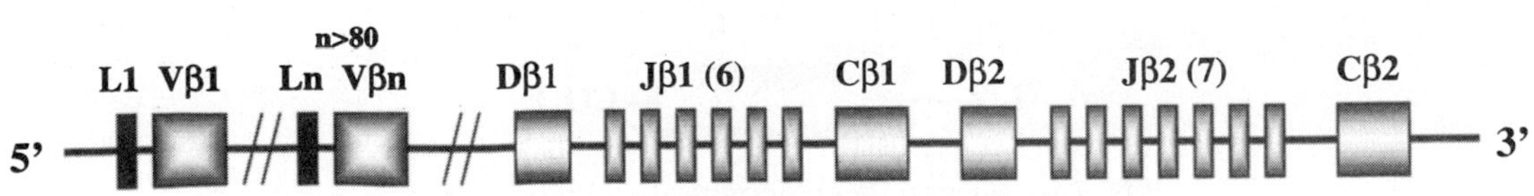

FIG. 7.7. T-cell receptor β-chain gene.

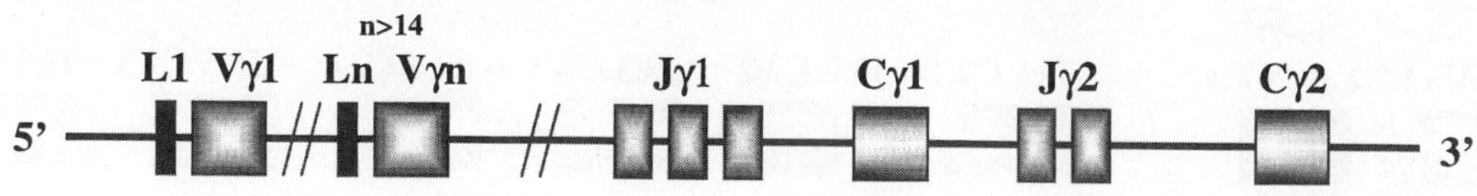

FIG. 7.8. T-cell receptor γ-chain gene.

The interspersion of these two structurally and functionally related loci is in support of the suggestion that one locus evolves from the other by gene duplication. The unique organization of the TCRα and TCRδ loci results in deletion of the δ locus on rearrangement of the V_α and J_α segments. The single C_δ gene is located about 80 kb upstream of the C_α gene.

DIVERSITY GENERATION OF ANTIGEN RECEPTOR GENES

Effective immune responses in humans depend on the generation of a vast repertoire of specific Ig and TCR molecules by individual B and T cells. The extent of the whole repertoire of the antigen receptors is determined by the diversity of the germline genome (i.e., number of V, D, and J segments), the combinatorial diversity (i.e., number of possible V-(D)-J combinations) and the junctional diversity (i.e., diversity from the imprecise joining of the V, D, and J segments). In B cells during immune responses, further diversification and refinement of the Ig repertoire are achieved by isotype switching recombination, somatic hypermutation, and receptor editing or revision. In T cells, the diversity of TCR remains largely unmodified after the selection process in the thymus.

V-(D)-J Recombination

All seven loci encoding the Ig heavy and light (κ, λ) chains and the TCR (α, β, γ, δ) chains undergo somatic DNA rearrangements to form a complete variable domain from V, (D), and J segments during lymphocyte development in the bone marrow (B cells) or in the thymus (T cells) (36–40). This process occurs in a highly ordered fashion to generate proteins that interact with a membrane-signaling complex (Fig. 7.9). For example, the first step of Ig gene rearrangement is the D to J_H joining, which takes place in pro-B lymphocytes. The second step occurs in pre-B lymphocytes

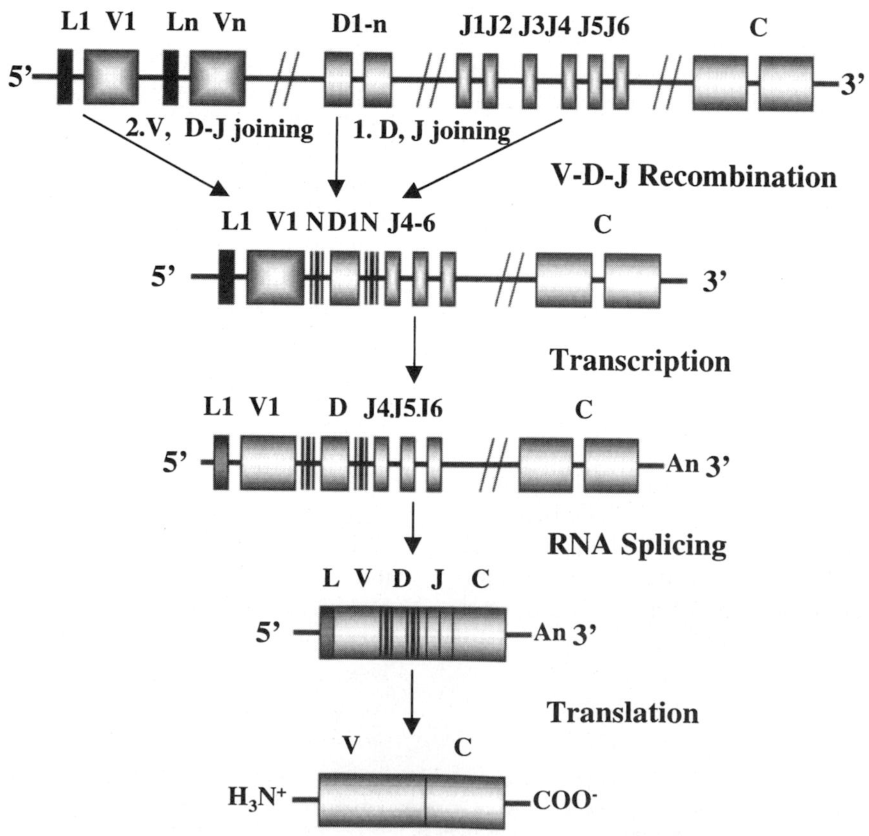

FIG. 7.9. Antigen receptor gene V-D-J recombination.

and involves the joining between V_H and DJ_H. After the joining of V_HDJ_H with the C_μ region, the complete μ chain is expressed on the surface of B lymphocytes as a complex with the surrogate light chains. Expression of this protein complex triggers further differentiation of early pre-B cells into late pre-B cells in which the Ig light-chain locus rearrangements (κ preceding λ) occur.

Successful completion of IgH and IgL gene rearrangements results in production of surface-expressed Ig. This signal triggers repression of the recombination machinery and differentiation of pre-B cells into immature (i.e., virgin) B cells (41). V-(D)-J rearrangement generates the major part of the antigen receptor diversity and can produce critical mediators that drive cellular expansion and differentiation and deliver survival or death signals that shape the composition of the immune system (5,12).

In the arrays of V, (D), J segments, recombination is accurately targeted by characteristic recognition signal sequences (RSS) that flank each of the coding regions, even when these sites are separated by distances of 1 to 2 Mbp (36). An RSS consists of conserved palindromic heptamer and AT-rich nonamer sequences separated by a nonconserved 12 or 23 nucleotide spacer. The consensus form of an RSS is 5′-(coding sequences)-CACAGTG-(12- or 23-bp spacer)-ACAAAAACC-3′. V-(D)-J recombination can be considered as a sequential process comprised of DNA cleavage, synapses and rejoining. The cleavages are carried out by the lymphoid-specific recombinase components RAG-1 and RAG-2, which require an open or accessible conformation of the target locus and occur precisely at the border between RSS and coding segment (42–44). The rearrangement is restricted to the proper pairs of sites (V to J or V to D to J regions) between an RSS with a 12-bp spacer and one with a 23-bp spacer (i.e., the 12/23 rule). This property prevents nonproductive V to V or J to J rearrangements. Moreover, TCR genes do not rearrange in B cells, and Ig genes (except $D\text{-}J_H$) do not rearrange in T cells. Because development of the immune system relies on recombination, it is not surprising that deregulation of the RAG genes accounts for some immunodeficiencies in humans. For example, Omenn syndrome, a combined B- and T-cell immunodeficiency, has been shown to result from point mutations of *RAG1* or *RAG2* genes (45,46).

After the cleavage step, a complete V-(D)-J fragment results from the rejoining of the two coding elements (coding joints) and the two heptamers of the RSS (signal joints), respectively (39). There is reciprocal rejoining of coding and signal ends. Rejoining between two genes flanked by RSS with opposite orientation, located in the chromosome between the two recombining segments, results in excision of the intervening sequences as a circle (47). However, rejoining between gene segments flanked by two similarly orientated RSS results in inversion of the intervening sequences between the recombining gene segments (48). Most rearrangements are associated with deletions. Inversions have been mainly noticed at the TCRβ, TCRδ, and IgLκ loci (39).

Signal joints are recombined precisely, without gain or loss of germline sequence (49). In contrast, coding joints are generally inaccurate, with base losses and insertions (39). Base losses at the open coding ends result from nuclease activity during the recombination process. Base additions are caused by templated and nontemplated mechanisms. Templated insertions arise from off-center opening of the sealed hairpin structure, which generates short complementary sequences (generally shorter than 4 bp) at coding joints recognized as palindromic (P) nucleotides (50,51). Insertions of nontemplated nucleotides (N nucleotides, up to 15 bp) at the coding junctions occur through the mediation of terminal deoxynuclotidyl transferase (TdT) (52). These properties produce extreme sequence diversity at the site of V-(D)-J joints, which correspond to the antigen contact residues of TCR and Ig molecules (i.e., CDRs). The base losses and insertions help greatly to diversify the receptor repertoire and introduce the risk of nonfunctional genes because of out-of-frame joining and creation of stop codons.

The machinery required for rejoining overlaps with general cellular pathways responsible for repairing double-strand DNA breaks (42,53–55). The key component of the rejoining process is the DNA-dependent protein kinase (DNA-PK) complex, which includes the DNA-PK catalytic subunit (DNA-PKcs), along with the KU nuclear protein (56,57). KU, originally isolated as an autoantigen in human autoimmune disorders, is a dimer consisting of 70- and 80-kd subunits (i.e., KU70, also called G22P1, and KU80, also called XRCC5). This nuclear protein exhibits DNA end-binding activity and, in concert with DNA, activates the kinase function of the DNA-PKcs (56,58). The final step in V-(D)-J rejoining involves ligation of DNA ends. Two essential components are found to participate in this process. They are XRCC4 and DNA ligase IV. XRCC4 appears to facilitate recruitment of the ligase to the rejoining complex (59–61).

Immunoglobulin Isotype Switching Recombination

Before immune stimulation, the IgH locus contains a V-D-J segment just upstream of the C_μ C region, and B cells at this stage express IgM (62). The B cells can also simultaneously express IgD. This coexpression of IgM and IgD is governed by the mechanisms of alternative RNA processing and termination of transcription (63). After immune stimulation, antigen-reactive B cells frequently undergo isotype class switching, a process whereby a B-cell changes the constant region of its IgH locus and produces new Ig molecules with the same light chain and IgV_H but with a different IgH isotype (62). The Ig isotype switch does not affect antigenic specificity but permits a more diverse immunologic response by altering the effector function of the Ig molecules.

The Ig class switch is a regulated nonhomologous recombination process (64). Because the constant region clusters for different IgH isotypes are located 3′ of C_μ and C_δ within the IgH locus, switching recombination results in deletion of DNA sequences (65). The recombination involves characteristic DNA regions, called switch (S) regions, that span 2 to 10 kb and are located in the introns upstream of each C region (except for C_δ). Switch regions contain characteristic tandem arrays of short repetitive sequences that are G rich on the nontemplate strand. Although the repeats in all the S regions are G rich, the S regions are not homologous to one another (63,66). Of the hundreds of switch recombination junctions examined, there is no sequence specificity identified in switch region breakpoints. Switch recombination is different from V-(D)-J recombination in many aspects. It involves C regions but not V regions. It is region specific but not sequence specific. The recombination does not require the two proteins, RAG-1 and RAG-2, which are essential for V-(D)-J recombination.

It is not known how switch recombination is initiated. Studies have shown that B cells carry out class switching in response to T-cell signals, including a variety of cytokines, which stimulate antigen-specific B cells to initiate a signaling cascade (63,64). Essential to this cascade is interaction between the B-cell surface receptor and the T-cell CD40 ligand, CD40L (67). The effects of these interactions are mediated in part through regulation of germline transcription, which is controlled by upstream promoter regions and enhancer/locus control region (LCR) elements in the IgH locus (68–70). Studies suggest that germline transcription alone is not sufficient for activation of class switching and that RNA splicing and the processed transcript are involved in this process (67,71–73). The last step of switch recombination, rejoining of DNA breaks, shares the same pathway with V-(D)-J recombination, requiring the presence of DNA-PKcs, KU70, KU86, DNA ligase IV, and XRCC4 (65,74–76).

Somatic Hypermutation

Mature B cells further diversify their Ig molecules during immune responses by the induction of somatic hypermutation in the V regions of IgH and IgL genes (77,78). In germinal center B cells, mutations in the V regions increase dramatically at a rate of up to 1 in 1,000 bp per division. This process, together with stringent antigen-driven selection, results in the production of antibodies with much improved affinity and specificity for target antigens in a secondary immune response. Somatic hypermutation of Ig genes is confined to a region within about 1.5 kb downstream of the promoter (79). The mutations are primarily point mutations, mostly single nucleotide substitutions, although nucleotide insertions or deletions may occur occasionally (80,81). In general, single nucleotide transitions occur more often than transversions. There is a predominance of mutations of A versus T and G versus C bases (82). This bias indicates that mutations modify only one DNA strand of the double helix. However, studies also indicate that both DNA strands are targeted (83). Some studies have identified certain sequences as potential hot spots for hypermutation. For example, codons containing RGYW (R = purine; G, guanine; Y, pyrimidine; W, A or T) motif are frequently targeted for mutations (83,84). Although somatic hypermutation is considered to be a feature of B cells, hypermutation of TCRα and TCRβ genes has also been reported in germinal center T cells (85,86). However, this finding is still controversial, because other laboratories have not been able to identify mutations in TCR genes in T cells (87).

The molecular mechanism of somatic hypermutation remains largely unknown. Studies using transgenic mice indicate that Ig gene hypermutation is closely linked to transcription. It has been suggested that transcriptional enhancers and *cis*-acting DNA sequences play a crucial role in hypermutation (88–90). In the past few years, as genes critical to DNA repair, replication, and recombination have been identified, many studies have focused on the role of these genes in hypermutation (91,92). Studies in mice deficient in DNA mismatch repair components PMS2 and MSH2 have produced some interesting results. PMS2 deficiency alters hypermutation levels (93–95), and MSH2 deficiency alters the spectrum of hypermutation (96). Based on these results, it is still unclear whether these gene products play an active role in somatic hypermutation. The close association of somatic hypermutation with transcription strongly indicates a role for nucleotide excision repair (NER) and transcription-coupled repair in the hypermutation process. However, this role has been largely excluded by the finding that somatic hypermutation is normal in humans and mice with deficient genes responsible for NER- and transcription-coupled repair system (97–100).

Base excision repair (BER) is another crucial process for DNA repair. This involves removal of damaged and mispaired bases by glycosylase and subsequent repair by DNA polymerase β (92,101). Possible involvement of BER in somatic hypermutation is consistent with the observation of overexpressed glycosylase levels in human tonsil germinal centers (102) and the error-prone nature of DNA polymerase β (103,104). However, studies of these two enzymes in mouse models have not generated evidence supporting the involvement of BER in hypermutation (100,105). A DNA polymerase, called polymerase ζ, may be a testable candidate for the role of error-prone DNA synthesis in hypermutation (92).

Because insertions or deletions can also occur in hypermutation, it is possible that somatic hypermutation involves DNA strand breaks. This possibility has been supported by experiments using a Burkitt lymphoma cell line. It has been found that by artificially expressing TdT in the tumor cells, a substantial fraction of acquired mutations in IgH V regions exhibit nontemplated base additions (106). These nucleotide insertions indicate that the mutation mechanism involves free DNA ends. It would be interesting and important to find out whether rejoining of these presumed free DNA ends involves any of the elements shared between V-(D)-J and class switch recombinations.

Receptor Editing and Revision

In the past few years, several studies have demonstrated that V regions of functional IgL and IgH genes can be replaced by newly rearranged Ig V region gene segments (107–109). These studies have provided novel insights into molecular mechanisms generating antigen receptor diversity and pathways leading to B-cell tolerance. This secondary Ig gene rearrangement was first detected in the bone marrow of transgenic mice that carry self-reactive antibody (110–112). Instead of finding the expected clonal deletion of all self-reactive cells in these mice, investigators found that some B cells had deleted their autoreactive receptors and developed entirely new receptors. This phenomenon, known as *receptor editing,* is considered a crucial mechanism to prevent the emergence of autoreactive Ig specificities. One interpretation for this editing process is that immature B cells with self-reactive receptors are induced to undergo secondary V-(D)-J recombination by interacting with antigen (109).

Receptor editing was originally thought to be restricted to immature B cells in the bone marrow. However, some studies have indicated that secondary rearrangements of functional antigen receptors can occur in mature B and T cells (113,114). These secondary rearrangements are referred to as *receptor revision* to distinguish them from those occurring in immature bone marrow B cells. Receptor revision was suggested by the finding that germinal center B cells express RAG-1 and RAG-2, which are required for V-(D)-J recombination (109). Receptor revision has been confirmed in studies showing that mature B cells contain intermediates of V-(D)-J recombination and that mature B cells with induced RAG expression can change their Ig genes. Receptor revision has also been demonstrated on the normal allele in mice with gene-targeted V-D-J rearrangements of the other allele (113). However, studies have also questioned reexpression of *RAG* genes in RAG-negative mature B cells (115,116). The origin, regulation and function of receptor revision in mature B cells in response to antigen signals remain largely unknown. Receptor revision by V-(D)-J recombination has also been identified in mature T cells (108), but its role in regulating the peripheral T-cell repertoire is unclear.

GENETIC ANALYSIS OF ANTIGEN RECEPTOR GENE REARRANGEMENTS

The molecular genetic rearrangements that result in the generation of antigen receptor diversity are not of purely academic interest. They can be applied to answer certain crucial questions concerning the origin and nature of lymphoproliferative disorders, such as their clonal nature and their B- and T-cell lineage (117,118). The fundamental basis for these clinical applications is that these gene rearrangements distinguish one clonal lymphoid population from another. Sequence analyses further reveal that the structural diversity created by recombination and refinement of individual V, (D), and J antigen receptor gene segments forms a unique ''molecular fingerprint'' that records the developmental process and the biologic behavior of a particular lymphocyte or lymphoid clone (119). These findings also have profound clinical implications. In the following sections, we review the techniques commonly employed in the genetic analysis of antigen receptor gene rearrangements and their application in the diagnosis and investigation of lymphoproliferative disorders.

Southern Blot Analysis of Immunoglobulin and T-Cell Receptor Gene Rearrangements

Southern blot analysis (named after its inventor, Edwin Southern) represents one of the first important advances in the development of techniques to accurately characterize the configuration of gene segments. This analysis has two key components: separation of restriction endonuclease-digested DNA fragments by high-resolution gel electrophoresis and the hybridization of these fragments with specific DNA probes (120). The hybridized probes are usually localized by autoradiography. Stable genes exhibit bands on the autoradiograph with characteristic size for a given gene and restriction enzyme (or a range of sizes in different individuals if the locus is polymorphic). These bands are designated *germline bands.* Genes that contain deletions, insertions, rearrangements, or point mutations in restriction sites yield bands of different sizes as the relative positions of restriction sites are altered. These bands of different sizes are referred to as rearranged bands.

DNA Sampling

Southern blot analysis requires DNA with relatively high molecular weight. Formalin-fixed or autolyzed tissues are not good sources for this technique. A single Southern blot analysis with one restriction endonuclease can be carried out on 5 to 10 μg of DNA, roughly the amount obtained from about 4×10^5 cells or 0.4 mm^3 of fresh or frozen tissue. The standard method for DNA extraction uses phenol and chloroform to remove cell lipid and protein contaminants, followed by precipitation of high-molecular-weight DNA in cold ethanol and salt (121). Other protocols, including commercial kits, are also available for DNA extraction.

Restriction Endonucleases

Restriction endonucleases, mainly purified from bacteria, cut double stranded DNA at specific, short nucleotide sequences, usually 4 to 8 bp long. The property of purified restriction endonucleases to cleave specific sequences in genomic DNA is retained *in vitro.* The most useful ones for Southern blot analysis are those that recognize specific sequences that are 6 bp long. These hexameric sequences exist across, on average, every 4,096 bp in the human genome (3.3×10^9 bp in total per haploid genome).

To avoid alterations of enzyme cutting sites by polymorphisms or mutations in antigen receptor genes, it is necessary to digest each sample with at least three restriction endonucleases. The common endonucleases used for antigen receptor gene analysis by Southern blot include *Eco*RI, *Hin*dIII and *Bam*HI (118).

Probes

Probes refer to nucleic acid sequences, usually molecularly cloned DNA fragments, that are complementary to the target DNA sequences. A probe binds to its target sequence through the formation of hydrogen bonds between complementary bases in the single strands of the target and the probe. This binding is achieved through a process called hybridization in which probe and target double-stranded DNAs are separated into single strands (i.e., denatured) and complementary single DNA strands of probe and target are reannealed. The annealing of one strand of nucleic acid to another is affected by a number of factors, including temperature, ionic strength of the hybridization solution, pH, and the presence of certain chemicals such as formamide that can weaken the hydrogen binding between complementary bases. Increase in temperature and decrease in ionic strength favor the separation of double strands and *vice versa.* For diagnostic purposes, a probe complementary to IgJ_H fragment is commonly used for the detection of Ig gene rearrangements, and a probe to TCRβ fragment ($J_{\beta}2$ or C_{β}) is frequently used for the detection of TCR gene rearrangements (118). In complicated cases, probes to IgL and TCRγ genes may be necessary. Probes to TCRα and TCRγ genes are rarely used because blotting of the TCRα gene results in complex germline patterns and the TCRδ gene is often deleted by rearrangement of the TCRα gene (122,123).

Probe Labeling

Southern blot analysis commonly uses a radioactive tag for probe labeling. This tag usually is ^{32}P that is joined to the sugar phosphate backbone of the nucleic acid, such as $\alpha^{32}P$-dCTP. The tag is commonly incorporated into the probe through two protocols called nick translation and random oligonucleotide priming (121,124). Nick translation uses the action of *Escherichia coli* DNA polymerase I to extend a single-stranded nick in double-stranded DNA in a 5′ to 3′ direction. The nicks are introduced by the simultaneous action of pancreatic deoxyribonuclease I (DNase I). If one or more appropriately radioactive tags are introduced in the reaction mixture, radioactively labeled DNA (probe) results. In random priming, the probe is denatured and a mixture of short oligonucleotides containing random sequences (normally hexamers) is allowed to anneal to the single strands of the probe. These random hexamers serve as primers for copying single stranded templates in the presence of DNA polymerase. If radioactive tags are added during the process, all copies of the probe become radiolabeled.

Methods of nonradioactive Southern blot hybridization have also been developed using biotin or digoxigenin as tag. Biotinylated- or digoxigenin-labeled probes are localized on the hybridized membrane by avidin or appropriate antibodies conjugated with certain enzymes such as peroxidase or alkaline phosphatase (125,126). Substrates of the enzymes are added to generate insoluble, colored reaction products *in situ.* Alkaline phosphatase can catalyze certain chemilumi-

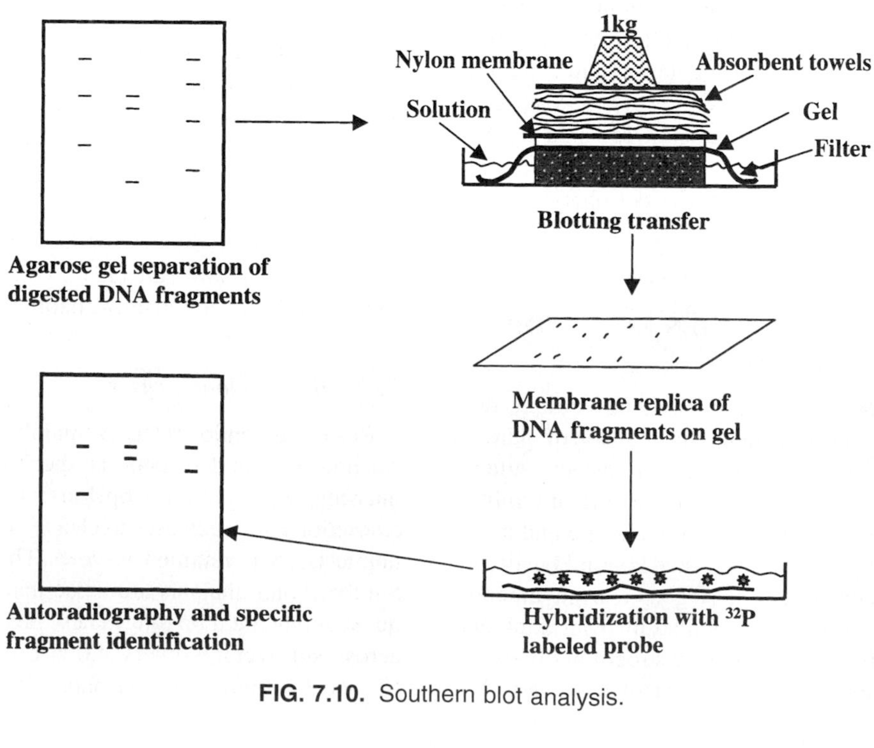

FIG. 7.10. Southern blot analysis.

nescent substrates. Dephosphorylation of these substrates yields weak visible light that can be exposed on x-ray film. Detection of probes by this and other chemiluminescent systems seems to be as sensitive as radioactivity but requires much less exposure time than radioactive probes (127,128).

Basic Procedures

Southern blot analysis consists of several basic steps. The DNA samples are digested with restriction enzymes, and the DNA fragments are size separated on agarose gels. The DNA fragments in the gel are then denatured to separate the strands, neutralized, and faithfully transferred to nylon or nitrocellulose membrane (121). The most common method for DNA transfer is to place a membrane between the gel and a stack of absorbent towels and allow the flow of fluid through the gel and the membrane to move the DNA fragments out of the gel (Fig. 7.10). The DNA fragments bind to the membrane and form a replica of the DNA pattern of the gel. After fixing or ultraviolet (UV) light crossing, the membranes are hybridized to radioactive DNA probes. The membranes are washed under stringent conditions so that the probes bind specifically, and exposed to x-ray films that are developed to reveal the sites of hybridization. The probe can be stripped off the membrane by boiling in water, and the membrane can be reused for a new hybridization.

Interpretation of Results and Clinical Application

During antigen receptor gene rearrangement certain DNA segments are deleted, and others are relocated. These processes change the distances between the specific cutting sites of restriction endonucleases, generating restriction fragments of different sizes. In a monoclonal lymphoid proliferation, all the lymphocytes carry identical Ig gene (in B cells) or TCR gene (in T cells) rearrangements, and in a reactive polyclonal lymphoid proliferation, different lymphocytes carry different Ig and TCR gene rearrangements. Southern blot analysis allows visualization of the uniform antigen receptor gene rearrangements in monoclonal lymphoid proliferation as one discrete band (or two bands if both alleles are rearranged) of a size different from the germline band. In polyclonal lymphoid proliferations, Southern blot analysis demonstrates the antigen receptor gene germline as a discrete band (or more than one band in the situation of polymorphism) of expected size. The individual rearrangements of an antigen receptor gene in individual lymphocytes comprising a large population are too weak to be visualized within the smear of the other heterogeneous rearrangements (Figs. 7.11, 7.12). Because malignancies are considered as monoclonal proliferations and antigen receptor gene rearrangements are cell type specific, Southern blot analysis of antigen receptor gene rearrangements provides a valuable tool to distinguish malignant monoclonal lymphoid proliferations from reactive polyclonal lymphoid lesions and to verify the cell lineage of lymphoproliferative disorders (118,129,130).

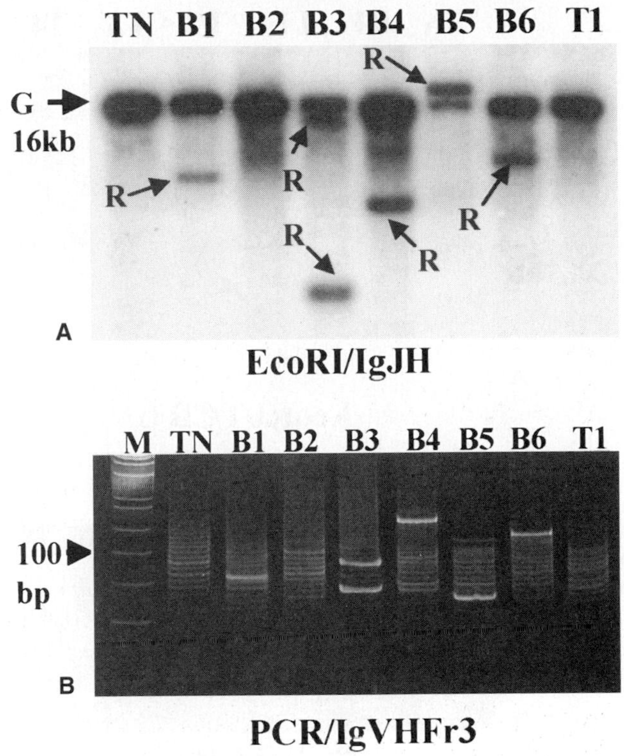

FIG. 7.11. Immunoglobulin gene rearrangement–based clonality analyses. **A:** Southern blot analysis with probe to IgJ_H fragment. TN, tonsil; B1, monoclonal B cell line (10% diluted with tonsil DNA as positive and sensitivity control); B2 to B6, B-cell lymphomas; T1, T-cell lymphoma; G, germline; R, rearrangement. **B:** Polymerase chain reaction (PCR) analysis with primers to IgV_HFR3/J_H region. For comparison, the same cases analyzed in **A** were examined. All cases that showed rearranged immunoglobulin gene bands in the Southern blot analysis exhibited discrete monoclonal IgV_HFR3/J_H bands in the PCR analysis, whereas only the cases that showed a germline band in Southern blot analysis showed polyclonal ladder or smear products. M, marker; TN, tonsil; B1, control B-cell line (10% diluted with tonsil DNA as positive and sensitivity control); B2 to B6, B-cell lymphomas; T1, T-cell lymphoma.

Limitations

Although clonality analysis by Southern blot has proved an important diagnostic tool, there are several limitations. The method is time consuming, expensive, usually requires radioactive isotopes, and may be difficult to interpret. False-negative results may occur because of degradation of a DNA sample, low tumor cell numbers (>5% tumor cells in a sample) (129,131,132), comigration of a rearranged band with the germline band or because the tumor cells have deleted antigen receptor genes. False-positive results may occur because of polymorphisms that yield apparently nongermline fragments, partial restriction digest of DNA that may cause spurious bands, or contaminating DNA in the probe or sample that may result in the appearance on the autoradiograph of nonantigen receptor-related bands. Occasional B-cell neoplasms may demonstrate rearranged TCR genes and *vice*

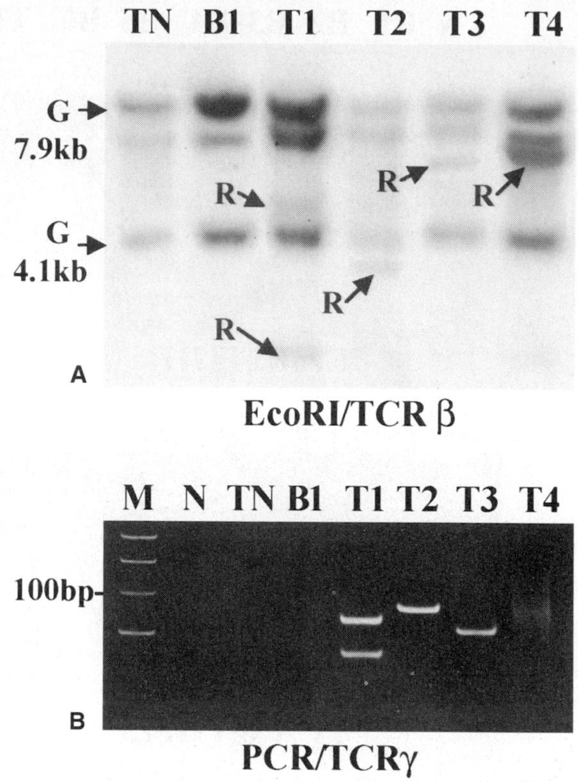

FIG. 7.12. T-cell receptor gene rearrangement–based clonality analyses. **A:** Southern blot analysis of the T-cell receptor (TCR) β gene rearrangement. TN, tonsil; B1, B-cell lymphoma; T1, T-cell lymphoma with known monoclonal TCRβ gene rearrangement (10% diluted with tonsil DNA as positive and sensitivity control); T2 to T4, T-cell lymphomas; G, germline; R, rearrangement. **B:** Polymerase chain reaction (PCR) analysis of TCR γ gene rearrangement. For comparison, the same cases analyzed in **A** were examined. Three of the four cases that showed rearranged TCRβ gene bands in Southern blot analysis exhibited discrete monoclonal TCR γ bands in the PCR analysis. M, marker; N, negative control without template DNA; TN, tonsil; B1, B-cell lymphoma; T1, T-cell lymphoma with known monoclonal TCR gene rearrangement (10% diluted with tonsil DNA as positive and sensitivity control); T2 to T4, T-cell lymphomas.

versa (133). Some myeloid tumors may also display antigen receptor gene rearrangements (133). However, the most important limitation of Southern blot analysis in diagnostic pathology is the requirement of fresh or frozen tissue samples that are often not available in many cases. Attempts have been made to use DNA extracted from formalin-fixed, paraffin-embedded tissues, but the results have been unreliable (134,135).

Polymerase Chain Reaction Analysis of Antigen Receptor Gene Rearrangements

The most important advance in molecular biologic methods probably has been the development of polymerase chain reaction (PCR) and its application for rapid and massive amplification of any known nucleic acid sequence (136). With this technique, it is possible to carry out genetic analysis on almost any pathologic specimen, including fresh cells and tissues, archival formalin-fixed and paraffin-embedded tissues, and even cells microdissected from stained tissue sections (137). PCR has provided a powerful alternative to many traditional molecular genetic analytical methods, including Southern blot analysis, and has revolutionized the way in which molecular genetic studies are conducted.

Polymerase Chain Reaction

PCR is a single-tube reaction (138). The reaction mixture is composed of sample DNA (template), two short oligonucleotides (primers), a thermostable DNA polymerase, the four nucleotides (dNTPs) and a buffer containing magnesium chloride. The tube is placed in a heating block that is programmed to alter temperature in repetitive, three-step cycles. In the first step, double-stranded sample DNA is separated into single strands (denatured) at 93°C to 95°C. In the second step, primers bind to their specific sites within the target sequence (annealing) at 50°C to 60°C. In the final step, DNA polymerase recognizes the bound primers and initiates copying of the sequence between the primers (extension) at 72°C (Fig. 7.13). Because each new strand can serve as a template for the complementary primer, each cycle doubles the amount of the specific DNA fragment. After 25 to 40 cycles, a several million-fold increase of specific DNA occurs in a few hours, yielding sufficient DNA products that are readily analyzed using gel electrophoresis or are used as templates for sequencing reactions.

Sources of DNA

Reliable PCR amplification can be achieved using DNA extracted from almost all specimen sources in the clinical laboratory, including blood, urine, effusions, fine needle aspirates, fresh or frozen solid tissue, formalin-fixed, paraffin-embedded tissue, previously stained tissue sections and blood films, and even decalcified tissue (139–141). Standard phenol/chloroform methods can be used to extract DNA from fresh tissue. The preparation of DNA from paraffin-embedded tissue samples can be achieved by simply boiling the sections in distilled water (142), but this method has a high failure rate. The most popular method involves removal of the wax, overnight digestion with a proteinase enzyme to release the DNA, and heat treatment to inactivate the enzyme (143). This approach produces a relatively impure extract containing a high proportion of proteins but is usually adequate for PCR. Large fragments, up to several kilobases, can be amplified from high-molecular-weight DNA, though only smaller segments (e.g., up to 250 bp) are efficiently amplifiable from fixed, processed samples. Some fixatives, such as Bouin's and mercuric solutions, inhibit amplification and are best avoided, if at all possible (143). The ability to examine DNA extracted from stained sections permits microdis-

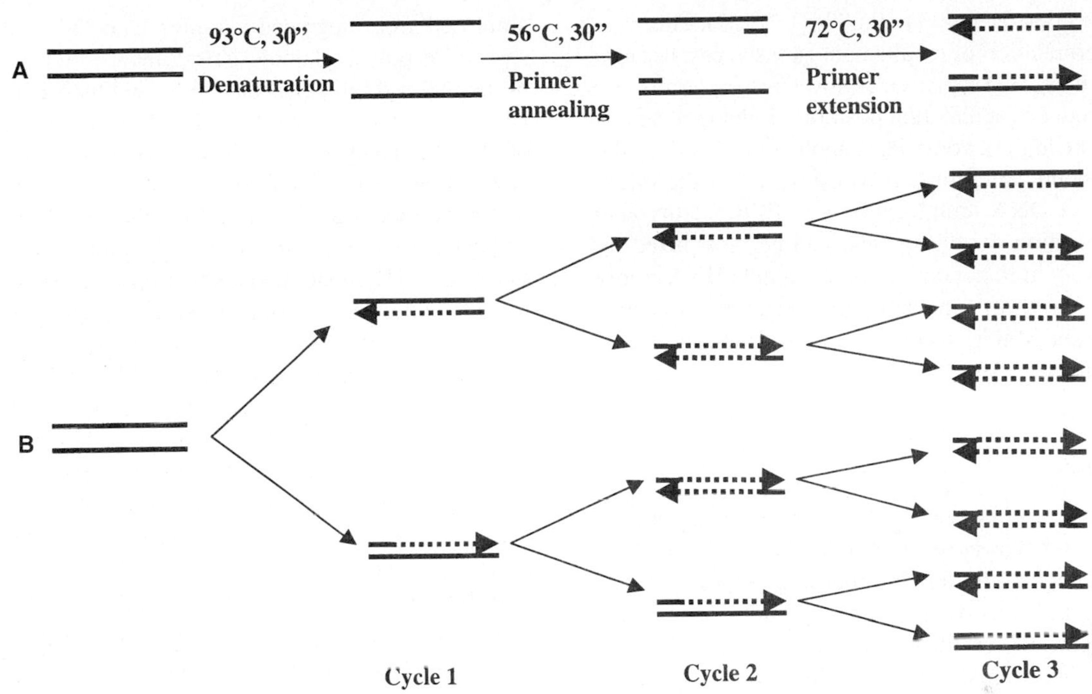

FIG. 7.13. Polymerase chain reaction (PCR). **A:** Three steps of a typical PCR cycle. **B:** Theoretical results of DNA amplification after three cycles of PCR.

section of selected cells or areas and more precise correlation of PCR with morphology (144).

Primer Design

The sequence of the primers determines the specificity of PCR amplification. Two oligonucleotide primers, about 20 bases long and complementary to opposite ends of the target sequence, are usually commercially synthesized for each reaction. Ideally, they are less than 500 bp apart or about 200 bp apart for amplification from paraffin-embedded material. They may have precise homology to their target sequence, or they may be closely related consensus sequences with some mismatches, if the target sequence cannot be predicted precisely (145). Sequences at the 3′ ends of primers should match the template precisely, because any mismatch prevents primer extension by DNA polymerase. However, mismatches at the 5′ ends of the primers do not significantly affect the efficiency of PCR amplification, allowing the addition of DNA sequences, such as restriction enzyme sites to facilitate cloning (146). Target gene sequence information can be acquired from the extensive and ever-expanding genomic databases, such as GenBank and EMBL, and primers designed with the help of widely available software packages, such as the Primer program (Whitehead Institute for Biomedical Research, Cambridge, MS).

Sensitivity and Specificity

PCR conditions and cycling parameters must be optimized for each primer set to maximize the yield of specific product and minimize amplification of nontarget sequences. The magnesium chloride concentration and annealing temperature are critical and usually have to be adjusted empirically. When these factors are optimized, the required sensitivity can be achieved by altering cycle number or enzyme concentration. If problems of sensitivity or specificity occur, "nested" PCR may be employed (145,147). This technique involves a second round of PCR in which internal primers are used to amplify products from the first round. Nonspecific products may result as a consequence of annealing primers to nontarget regions at room temperature during setup. This can be solved by using "hot start" PCR in which the reaction is heated to about 70°C before addition of the Taq polymerase, dNTPs, or template (148,149). The sensitivity and specificity of PCR can also be enhanced by "touchdown" PCR, a method in which sequential reduction of the annealing temperature is used (150), and by "heat-soaked" PCR, a method in which the DNA sample is heated at 94°C for 30 minutes before addition of the Taq polymerase, dNTPs, and primers (151). The specificity of amplification can be confirmed by the size and sequence of the product.

Fidelity

Errors are inevitably introduced at a low rate into the sequences of PCR products. The number of errors produced per nucleotide synthesized is known as the fidelity of amplification and is a function of the polymerase enzyme used. The most commonly used polymerase, Taq, has a relatively high error rate (1 error in 400 to 9,000) (152,153). This does not affect interpretation of results in most instances, because the proportion of altered bases is low and the errors are randomly introduced at different positions. Fidelity of amplification must be high in some PCR applications, such as the detection of point mutations, particularly when the initial copy number of DNA templates is low. PCR fidelity also depends on reaction conditions and can be maximized by using a relatively high concentration of sample DNA, a low number of cycles, short extension times, and low concentrations of dNTP and $MgCl_2$ in combination with an appropriate polymerase enzyme (154,155).

Product Analysis

PCR products may be analyzed by size using agarose or, for smaller fragments, polyacrylamide gel electrophoresis. Gels are stained with ethidium bromide and visualized under UV light. This indicates whether specific amplification has occurred, which shows if the target sequence is present, and may reveal polymorphisms or abnormalities that result in alterations of fragment size. Alternative means of analysis, which depend on the sequence of the product, can be used to detect point mutations. These include single-strand conformational polymorphism (SSCP) analysis (156) and denaturing or temperature gradient gel electrophoresis (DGGE or TGGE) (157). Direct sequencing of products permits rapid determination of nucleotide sequence that confirms specificity and reveals any point mutations (158).

Results Interpretation, and Clinical Application

The basis for PCR detection of antigen receptor gene rearrangements is that the rearrangements bring V, (D), and J segments into proximity, allowing PCR to amplify across these segments (117,130). In the germline configuration, these segments are too far away to be amplified by PCR. The cells comprising a monoclonal lymphoid proliferation contain uniform rearrangements of the antigen receptor genes. PCR amplification generates one dominant band or two dominant bands if two alleles are rearranged. In polyclonal proliferations, each cell or clone carries a distinct gene rearrangement. PCR amplification produces heterogeneous products of different sizes, appearing in a gel as a ladder or smear pattern (Figs. 7.11, 7.12). PCR has been used widely to determine the clonal nature and cell lineage of lymphoproliferative diseases, helping clinicians tremendously in the diagnosis and management of these diseases.

Immunoglobulin gene-based PCR clonality analysis can be carried out by amplification of the highly variable V-D-J junction (CDRIII), followed by polyacrylamide gel analysis of the products. Primers have been designed to amplify from FR1, FR2, or FR3 to the joining region (FR/J_H) (159–162). However, amplification of $FR3/J_H$ has been preferred because the products are small and are more readily amplified from degraded samples, and they are better resolved on polyacrylamide gels. Methods for amplification of the IgK and IgL genes have been published (163,164) but have not been widely used for clonality analysis. Evaluations of clonality analysis by PCR amplification of the IgH gene have shown that PCR offers sensitivity similar to that of Southern blot analysis, that formalin-fixed and paraffin-embedded tissue samples can be used, and that a high proportion of B-cell lymphomas can be amplified. However, false-negative rates may be high in some lymphoma types, and false-positive results have occasionally been reported. In general, PCR amplification of $FR3/J_H$ can demonstrate monoclonality in 70% to 80% of B-cell lymphomas (145,165,166). The detection rate can be improved by using multiple primers (167,168). The high sensitivity of PCR may permit early detection of malignant lymphoma and help to define poorly understood lymphoproliferative disorders that may or may not be malignant.

PCR approaches for T-cell clonality analysis have been mainly devised to target TCRβ and TCRγ because of the complexity of the TCRα gene and frequent deletion of the TCRδ gene in mature T cells. Six sets of primers are used to cover TCRβ gene rearrangements (169). PCR analysis for TCRγ rearrangements commonly uses two sets of primers (170). The TCRγ gene is theoretically the most informative as the locus is less frequently involved in chromosome translocations with oncogenes in lymphomas and leukemias than TCRα, TCRβ, and TCRδ loci and because biallelic TCRγ gene rearrangements are common. The TCRγ locus is simpler than TCRβ, because there are no D regions and only small numbers of V segments, permitting the design of primers with near perfect fit to all target sequences. Results suggest that clonality analysis by amplification of TCRβ and TCRγ genes is reliable with a clonality detection rate of about 70% in T-cell malignancies and offers comparable sensitivities to Southern blot (1% tumor cells in a lymphoid background) (169,171–173). PCR analysis of TCR genes is applicable generally to problematic T-cell proliferations, especially those occurring in extranodal sites such as skin and gastrointestinal tract. However, false-negative results occur in a significant proportion of malignant lymphomas, especially using TCRβ primers. The TCRγ locus is preferred by most, although amplification of TCRβ is useful when TCRγ PCR is unhelpful. Amplification of the TCRδ gene may be employed when precursor T-cell proliferations are studied (174).

Limitations

False-positive results have occasionally been reported in PCR studies of clonality using amplification of IgH or TCR genes. For example, dominant clonal populations of B cells have been demonstrated in apparently reactive, *Helicobacter pylori*–associated gastritis specimens (175,176). However, in most studies, false-positive results are rare. It is possible that differences in methodologies or criteria for interpretation account for variations in the reported false-positive results or that dominant bands do not represent true monoclonality in some instances, particularly when small lymphocyte populations are analyzed.

False-negative results have been a frequent problem when analyzing the clonality of B- and T-cell lymphomas, even when high-molecular-weight DNA samples have been analyzed (166,173). Apart from samples containing inadequate DNA, the false-negative findings are thought to result from failure of binding of primers to tumor sequences. This may be the result of somatic mutations or deletion of the specific region, use of a germline segment not targeted by the primers, or translocation or inversion causing loss of or incorrect orientation of target sequences. False-negative rates can reach 20% to 30%, depending on primers used and lymphoma type, in low-grade B-cell lymphomas (159,165,166). Higher false-negative rates (about 50%) have been reported for high-grade B-cell lymphomas (177,178). Although false-negative rates may be reduced by the use of multiple primer sets (167,168), primer sets that amplify larger fragments have proved to be of minimal use in analyzing paraffin-embedded tissue samples (140). Some B-cell lymphoma types that are associated with frequent somatic mutations or deletions in the IgH gene are less amenable to amplification than others, notably follicular and mucosa-associated lymphoid tissue (MALT) lymphomas and immunoproliferative small intestinal disease (166,167,179). Polyclonal patterns do not always reflect the absence of an expanded clone.

It is important to optimize methodology and to adhere to strict criteria for the definition of monoclonality to minimize the probability of false positive and negative results. Sufficient cells should be analyzed to permit a statistically valid size analysis. Because PCR is sufficiently sensitive to amplify rare B or T cells, a single or apparently oligoclonal pattern of amplification may be seen after amplification of a poor DNA sample. It is essential to ensure that DNA samples are of adequate quality and, in all samples, to amplify duplicate aliquots, to run the products side by side on the gel, and to interpret as monoclonal only those cases that yield clearly visible dominant bands of identical size in both repeats. Cases in which nonreproducible or weakly amplifying bands are seen should be repeated or disregarded as evidence of monoclonality.

Appropriate controls are essential to confirm specificity of amplification and to identify contamination, which is a potentially serious problem. Each experiment should be accompanied by a positive control to ensure that amplification is specific, a negative reaction with no DNA to control for contamination before or during setup, and a blank extraction procedure control to control for contamination during the DNA extraction process. Because DNA degradation is difficult to assess in paraffin-embedded tissue extracts, most workers employ a control amplification of a nonrearranging gene (e.g., β-globin) to confirm the presence of amplifiable DNA). However, lymphoid samples containing reactive lymphocytes should yield polyclonal products that, in the presence or absence of an amplifiable tumor rearrangement, confirm the presence of adequate DNA.

To precisely define a dominant band, most workers prefer to analyze products on polyacrylamide minigels or high-resolution gels. Agarose gel electrophoresis is generally inadequate for accurate clonality analysis of small PCR products (180), although high-percentage NuSieve/agarose gels are sometimes used. TGGE, DGGE, or SSCP analysis, which separates DNA fragments on the basis of sequence rather than size alone, may offer increased sensitivity (181,182). However, these methods may give rise to complex patterns, especially if the tumor that is amplified exhibits intraclonal sequence variation. Analysis of fluorescent-labeled PCR products on automated sequencing gels with dedicated software provides graphic data that permits application of objective criteria to define monoclonality (175). All of these approaches have different sensitivities and capacity for introducing artifacts, which have not yet been fully assessed or directly compared. Further cooperative studies are necessary to improve current methodologies, particularly with respect to primer design and product analysis.

Sequence Analysis of Antigen Receptor Gene Rearrangements

Nucleotide sequencing analysis is the most precise way to characterize the DNA region of interest. In the past, information generated by sequence analysis of antigen receptor genes has been used to confirm clonality and to demonstrate clonal link between different components and disseminated lesions of a malignant lymphoid proliferation. Clone-specific sequences revealed by sequence analysis have been used as specific primers that greatly increase PCR sensitivity and permit the reliable detection of minimal residual disease in B- or T-cell malignancies. The study of the nucleotide sequences of the variable regions of rearranged Ig genes has also revealed much concerning the biology of malignant B-cell clones. The developmental stage of the cells of origin, the biologic behaviors of lymphoid tumors, and the influence of antigen can readily be evaluated using PCR amplification and sequencing of Ig variable regions (119).

DNA Sequencing

Two fundamental methods are used for DNA sequencing. These are the chemical method of Maxam and Gilbert (183) and the chain-termination method of Sanger (184), both of which have three basic features: base specificity, partial reaction, and accurate size discrimination from a fixed end by gel electrophoresis. Most methods employed are based on the chain-termination method, which uses enzymatic synthesis to produce a ladder of products terminating at a specific base. The terminating bases are nucleotide analogues, dideoxynucleotide triphosphates (ddNTP), that stop nucleotide extension in sequencing reaction on incorporation because they lack the 3′-OH group on the sugar for subsequent elongation. In chain-termination–based protocols, single-stranded target DNA (or denatured double-stranded DNA) is used as the template for a DNA polymerase. A specific oligonucleotide primer is then annealed to the template. DNA synthesis is performed in four separate reactions, each containing the four normal deoxyribonucleotide triphosphates (dNTPs) and a relevant ddNTP in appropriate proportion. In each reaction, incorporation of a terminating base occurs from the primer through the sequence, generating a series of single-stranded DNA molecules, each with one base longer than the last. Usually, a ^{32}P- or ^{35}S-labeled dNTP is included in the reaction or is incorporated as a 5′-end label on the primer. This radiolabel allows detection for newly synthesized DNA molecules. The reaction products are then separated by high-resolution denaturing acrylamide gel electrophoresis, yielding a ladder of autoradiographic signals (Fig. 7.14). The sequence of a target can be easily read from this ladder.

Many modifications of the original chain-termination method have been made. For example, PCR has been used to generate single-stranded DNA template and even been used to perform directly chain-termination reaction (i.e., cycle sequencing) (158,185). These so-called direct sequencing methods have replaced the time-consuming and complex cloning template generation step, and cycle sequencing combines the template generation and sequencing reactions into one step. The most important modification is the development of an automated sequencer, such as ABI 377 (PE Biosystems, Foster City, CA), in which fluorescent-labeled products of the four termination reactions can be analyzed simultaneously in the same lane of a gel. This machine greatly speeds up the sequencing process.

Clone-Specific Sequences

Antigen receptor gene rearrangements are clone specific. Comparison of sequences derived from rearranged Ig genes can determine clonal identity. Using this strategy, it has been found that follicle center cell lymphomas contain two clonally linked but phenotypically distinct tumor populations in the tumor follicles and interfollicular zones, respectively (186). Analysis of clonal identity provides a powerful tool

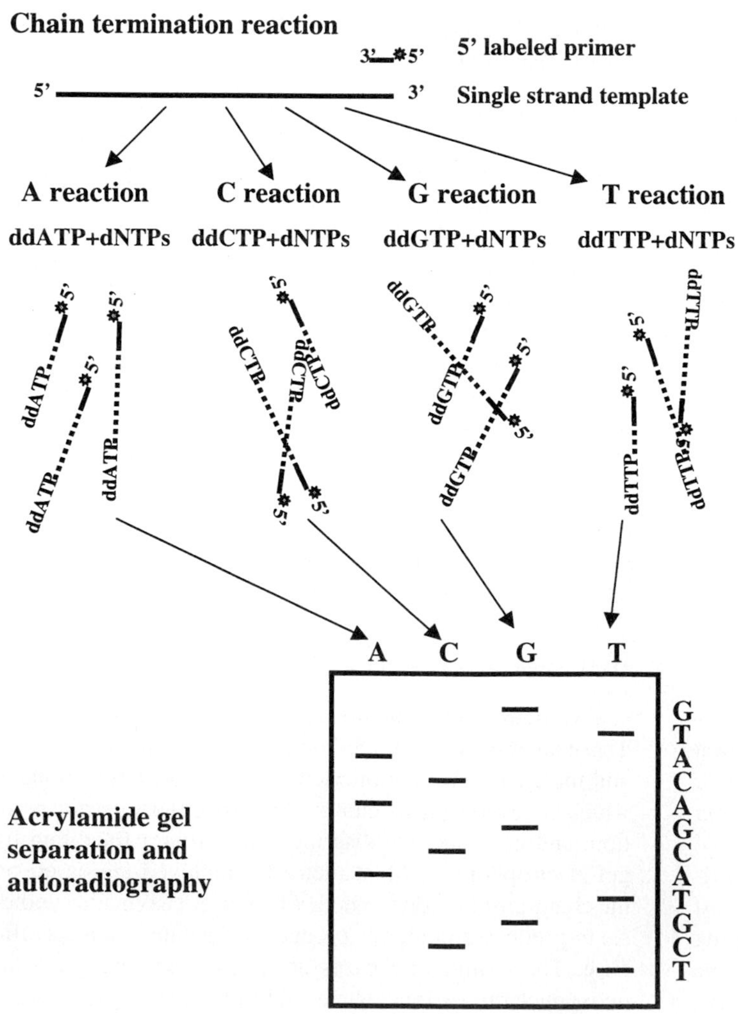

FIG. 7.14. Chain-termination (dideoxy) sequencing method of Sanger.

for studying the clonal origin of certain complex lymphomas, such as composite lymphomas. Based on clone-specific sequences, it has been shown that composite mantle cell and follicle center cell lymphoma may be derived from the same clone (187) or from separate clones (188). The pattern of accumulation of somatic mutations together with clone-specific sequences can determine the sequence of clonal evolution in different lesions.

Analysis of the Ig gene mutation pattern and clone-specific sequences allowed investigators to demonstrate that concurrent MALT lymphomas of the stomach and small intestine originated from a single clone and that the gastric lesion preceded the intestinal lesion in each case (189). Clone-specific sequences of rearranged Ig genes have also been used as valuable markers in studying the progression of B-cell lymphomas. By analyzing clone-specific sequences in sequential biopsies, it was found that a low-grade B-cell gastric MALT lymphoma clone disseminated to lip and bone marrow and recurred in the stomach over a 13-year period (190). In another study of B-cell lymphomas with late relapse, it was demonstrated that two of five cases had different clones at relapse (191). By comparison of IgH clone-specific sequences it has been shown that morphologic transformation from low- to high-grade disease in follicle center cell and MALT lymphomas represents the evolution of single clones (192,193). These studies are essential for the understanding of the biology of lymphoma heterogeneity, progression, and relapse and have important implications for disease monitoring.

Ig gene clone-specific sequences obtained from a B-cell tumor permit the design of primers that selectively amplify the specific tumor clone. The use of such clone-specific primers improves the PCR sensitivity by a factor of up to 1,000 compared with consensus primers for IgV_H gene rearrangements, because the reactive B cells present in the tissue samples do not compete with and obscure the products of amplification from the specific lymphoma clone (194). This approach has been used to improve the detection of minimal residual disease in leukemia patients (195) and to study the relationship between nodular lymphocyte predominance Hodgkin's disease and large B-cell lymphomas that occurred sequentially in some patients (194). PCR analysis of microdissected components of the immune system with clone-specific primers has shown that gastric MALT lymphoma cells preferentially disseminate to the splenic marginal zone, supporting the notion that MALT lymphomas are of marginal zone cell origin (196). Clone-specific primers similarly can be designed for T-cell tumors, based on the sequence of rearranged TCR genes. This approach has been used to detect minimal residual disease (197) and to trace a dominant T-cell clone in ulcerative jejunitis lesions (198). It was shown that the abnormal clone was widespread throughout the ulcerated mucosa, despite being undetectable using consensus primers.

Cell Lineage and Developmental Stage

Sequence analysis data reveal that the patterns of IgV gene mutation correlate strongly with specific stages of B-cell differentiation and maturation (78). Pregerminal center B cells commonly lack IgV gene somatic hypermutations. Cells undergoing the germinal center reaction exhibit high frequency of mutation with sequence variations within each clone (ongoing mutation), and post–germinal center B cells such as memory cells or plasma cells have mutations but without obvious ongoing mutations. Comparison of IgV gene mutation patterns of B-cell malignancies with those of normal B-cell subsets has provided clues to the progenitor cells of these tumors in terms of their maturation stages.

IgV gene mutation patterns can be used as a novel means for categorizing B-cell tumors (78,119,199). In this new category, B-lineage chronic lymphocytic leukemia and mantle cell lymphomas that show infrequent mutations are considered to be derived from pre–germinal center B cells. Follicle center cell lymphomas have a high degree of mutation (about 10%) and ongoing mutations and therefore show the features of germinal center B cells. Splenic marginal zone B-cell lymphomas, MALT lymphomas and some hairy cell leukemias show an average of 4% mutations, mimicking the features of post–germinal center memory B cells. Plasmacytomas and multiple myelomas exhibit a low frequency of mutations with no ongoing mutations in keeping with their phenotypic characteristics of post–germinal center plasma cells. In addition to the link to cell lineage, IgV gene mutation status can also serve as an important prognostic indicator of certain B-cell tumors (200). For example, two studies showed that CLL patients with IgV gene mutations have a much better response to treatment and a more promising prognosis than those without IgV mutations (201,202).

Influence of Antigenic Stimulation

Antigen binding to the Ig receptor forms the basis of a recurring selection process for clonal survival of developing and mature B cells. This selection process, resulting from antigen availability and binding affinity, leads to relative overrepresentation or underrepresentation of distinctive V_H families and V_H genes in the receptor repertoire of B cells. This biased usage of V_H genes has been demonstrated in normal lymphocytes and in certain B-cell tumors (203,204). Sequence analysis of rearranged IgV_H genes can provide clues to the immunologic signals that drive lymphoma development. For example, studies of IgH V region germline segment usage have suggested that follicle center cell and MALT lymphoma clones are frequently associated with autoimmunity (204–206). The role of antigenic stimulation in tumors can also be deduced by IgV gene mutation patterns. Positive selection for enhanced Ig binding to antigen is indicated by high ratios of replacement to silent mutations within the CDRs compared with the FRs (119). This feature has been found in follicle center cell and Burkitt's lymphomas, and the selection pressure is present throughout clonal expansion of follicular lymphomas (207,208). The accumulation of excess silent mutations above an expected random value, especially in the CDRs, is referred to as negative selection and is thought to be associated with the preservation of primary antibody structures in the antigen-driven selection process (119,199). Evidence of positive and negative selections has been found in some lymphomas, such as MALT lymphomas in the stomach, and in multiple myeloma (206,209,210). The presence of ongoing mutations indicates that follicle center cell and low-grade MALT lymphomas are subject to persistent antigen drive during expansion of the tumor clones (206,207). The absence of ongoing mutation in high-grade MALT lymphomas and diffuse large B-cell lymphomas indicates that these tumors are no longer subject to antigen stimulation or somatic hypermutation (199,206). These studies have greatly helped our understanding of the role of antigenic stimulation and the associations between autoimmunity and B-cell malignancy.

SUMMARY AND CONCLUSIONS

Antigen receptors are the primary effector molecules to combat pathogens in adaptive immune responses and are critical mediators that drive cellular expansion and differentiation and that deliver survival or death signals that shape the composition of the immune system. The basis for these important functions of antigen receptors is their enormous diversity, which enables them to accommodate a universe of antigens with strict discrimination of self from nonself. This diversity is achieved by V-(D)-J rearrangements of the antigen receptor genes during lymphocyte development. In B cells, the diversity of Ig molecules is further refined through isotype switching recombination, somatic hypermutation, and receptor editing or revision of the Ig genes.

The rearrangements of antigen receptor genes are cell type specific and unique to individual lymphocytes or lymphoid clones. For these reasons, gene rearrangements are used widely as genetic markers for determination of the cell lineage and clonality of lymphoproliferative disorders. The commonly used approaches for determination of these gene rearrangements include Southern blot, PCR, and sequence analysis. Southern blot analysis provides accurate configuration of rearranged gene segments in lymphocytes using high-molecular-weight DNA. PCR amplifies the junctional sequences of the rearranged V-(D)-J segments and provides rapid means for clonality analysis of lymphocytes in almost any type of pathologic specimen. Sequence analysis is the most precise way to analyze gene rearrangements and provides definite confirmation of lymphocyte clonality and clonal link of different components of individual lymphoid malignancies. It also reveals clone-specific sequences that can be used to design clone-specific PCR for the detection of minimal residual disease and monitoring of lymphoid tumors.

Studies of the nucleotide sequences of rearranged antigen receptor genes, particularly rearranged Ig genes, have generated crucial information concerning the biology of lymphocytes and lymphoid malignancies. Sequence analysis has demonstrated that the hypermutation patterns of rearranged Ig genes correlate well with the developmental stage of the cells of origin and biologic behaviors of neoplastic B cells and has confirmed the influence of antigen on their clonal expansion. These findings have greatly facilitated our understanding of the pathogenesis of B-cell malignancies and helped to design effective treatment and management regimens for these tumors.

REFERENCES

1. Williams AF. The immunoglobulin superfamily takes shape. *Nature* 1984;308:12–913.
2. Hood L, Kronenberg M, Hunkapiller T. T cell antigen receptors and the immunoglobulin supergene family. *Cell* 1985;40:225–229.
3. Williams AF, Davis SJ, He Q, et al. Structural diversity in domains of the immunoglobulin superfamily. *Cold Spring Harb Symp Quant Biol* 1989;54[Pt 2]:637–647.
4. Giachino C, Padovan E, Lanzavecchia A. Kappa^{+}lambda^{+} dual receptor B cells are present in the human peripheral repertoire. *J Exp Med* 1995;181:1245–1250.
5. Kurosaki T. Genetic analysis of B cell antigen receptor signaling. *Annu Rev Immunol* 1999;17:555–592.
6. Reth M, Hombach J, Wienands J, et al. The B-cell antigen receptor complex. *Immunol Today* 1991;12:196–201.
7. Davis MM, Bjorkman PJ. T-cell antigen receptor genes and T-cell recognition. *Nature* 1988;334:395–402.
8. Brenner MB, Strominger JL, Krangel MS. The gamma delta T cell receptor. *Adv Immunol* 1988;43:133–192.
9. Raulet DH. The structure, function, and molecular genetics of the gamma/delta T cell receptor. *Annu Rev Immunol* 1989;7:175–207.
10. Rudd CE. Adaptors and molecular scaffolds in immune cell signaling. *Cell* 1999;96:5–8.
11. Lanzavecchia A, Lezzi G, Viola A. From TCR engagement to T cell activation: a kinetic view of T cell behavior. *Cell* 1999;96:1–4.
12. Clements JL, Boerth NJ, Lee JR, et al. Integration of T cell receptor–dependent signaling pathways by adapter proteins. *Annu Rev Immunol* 1999;17:89–108.
13. Cook GP, Tomlinson IM, Walter G, et al. A map of the human immunoglobulin V_H locus completed by analysis of the telomeric region of chromosome 14q. *Nat Genet* 1994;7:162–168.
14. Matsuda F, Ishii K, Bourvagnet P, et al. The complete nucleotide sequence of the human immunoglobulin heavy chain variable region locus. *J Exp Med* 1998;188:2151–2162.
15. Tomlinson IM, Cook GP, Carter NP, et al. Human immunoglobulin V_H and D segments on chromosomes 15q11.2 and 16p11.2. *Hum Mol Genet* 1994;3:853–860.
16. Nagaoka H, Ozawa K, Matsuda F, et al. Recent translocation of variable and diversity segments of the human immunoglobulin heavy chain from chromosome 14 to chromosomes 15 and 16. *Genomics* 1994;22:189–197.
17. Corbett SJ, Tomlinson IM, Sonnhammer EL, et al. Sequence of the human immunoglobulin diversity (D) segment locus: a systematic analysis provides no evidence for the use of DIR segments, inverted D segments, "minor" D segments or D-D recombination. *J Mol Biol* 1997;270:587–597.
18. Zachau HG. The immunoglobulin kappa locus—or what has been learned from looking closely at one-tenth of a percent of the human genome. *Gene* 1993;135:167–173.
19. Malcolm S, Barton P, Murphy C, et al. Localization of human immunoglobulin kappa light chain variable region genes to the short arm of chromosome 2 by *in situ* hybridization. *Proc Natl Acad Sci U S A* 1982;79:4957–4961.
20. McBride OW, Hieter PA, Hollis GF, et al. Chromosomal location of human kappa and lambda immunoglobulin light chain constant region genes. *J Exp Med* 1982;155:1480–1490.

21. Arnold N, Wienberg J, Ermert K, et al. Comparative mapping of DNA probes derived from the V kappa immunoglobulin gene regions on human and great ape chromosomes by fluorescence *in situ* hybridization. *Genomics* 1995;26:147–150.
22. Ramsden DA, Wu GE. Mouse kappa light-chain recombination signal sequences mediate recombination more frequently than do those of lambda light chain. *Proc Natl Acad Sci U S A* 1991;88:10721–10725.
23. Cohn M, Langman RE. The protection: the unit of humoral immunity selected by evolution. *Immunol Rev* 1990;115:11–147.
24. Vasicek TJ, Leder P. Structure and expression of the human immunoglobulin lambda genes. *J Exp Med* 1990;172:609–620.
25. Chuchana P, Blancher A, Brockly F, et al. Definition of the human immunoglobulin variable lambda (IGLV) gene subgroups. *Eur J Immunol* 1990;20:1317–1325.
26. Williams SC, Winter G. Cloning and sequencing of human immunoglobulin V lambda gene segments. *Eur J Immunol* 1993;23:1456–1461.
27. Frippiat JP, Williams SC, Tomlinson IM, et al. Organization of the human immunoglobulin lambda light-chain locus on chromosome 22q11.2. *Hum Mol Genet* 1995;4:983–991.
28. Frippiat JP, Dard P, Marsh S, et al. Immunoglobulin lambda light chain orphons on human chromosome 8q11.2. *Eur J Immunol* 1997;27:1260–1265.
29. Sakaguchi N, Melchers F. Lambda 5, a new light-chain–related locus selectively expressed in pre-B lymphocytes. *Nature* 1986;324:579–582.
30. Melchers F, Karasuyama H, Haasner D, et al. The surrogate light chain in B-cell development. *Immunol Today* 1993;14:60–68.
31. Arden B, Clark SP, Kabelitz D, Mak TW. Human T-cell receptor variable gene segment families. *Immunogenetics* 1995;42:455–500.
32. Koop BF, Rowen L, Wang K, et al. The human T-cell receptor TCRAC/TCRDC (C alpha/C delta) region: organization, sequence, and evolution of 97.6 kb of DNA. *Genomics* 1994;19:478–493.
33. Rowen L, Koop BF, Hood L. The complete 685-kilobase DNA sequence of the human beta T cell receptor locus. *Science* 1996;272:1755–1762.
34. Lefranc MP, Rabbitts TH. The human T-cell receptor gamma (TRG) genes. *Trends Biochem Sci* 1989;14:214–218.
35. Chien YH, Iwashima M, Kaplan KB, et al. A new T-cell receptor gene located within the alpha locus and expressed early in T-cell differentiation. *Nature* 1987;327:677–682.
36. Tonegawa S. Somatic generation of antibody diversity. *Nature* 1983;302:575–581.
37. von Boehmer H, Fehling HJ. Structure and function of the pre-T cell receptor. *Annu Rev Immunol* 1997;15:433–452.
38. Krangel MS, Hernandez-Munain C, Lauzurica P, et al. Developmental regulation of V(D)J recombination at the TCR alpha/delta locus. *Immunol Rev* 1998;165:131–147.
39. Gellert M. A new view of V(D)J recombination. *Genes Cells* 1996;1:269–275.
40. Alt FW, Oltz EM, Young F, et al. VDJ recombination. *Immunol Today* 1992;13:306–314.
41. Willerford DM, Swat W, Alt FW. Developmental regulation of V(D)J recombination and lymphocyte differentiation. *Curr Opin Genet* Dev 1996;6:603–609.
42. Oettinger MA, Schatz DG, Gorka C, et al. RAG-1 and RAG-2, adjacent genes that synergistically activate V(D)J recombination. *Science* 1990;248:1517–1523.
43. McBlane JF, van Gent DC, Ramsden DA, et al. Cleavage at a V(D)J recombination signal requires only RAG1 and RAG2 proteins and occurs in two steps. *Cell* 1995;83:387–395.
44. Stanhope-Baker P, Hudson KM, Shaffer AL, et al. Cell type-specific chromatin structure determines the targeting of V(D)J recombinase activity in vitro. *Cell* 1996;85:887–897.
45. Villa A, Santagata S, Bozzi F, et al. Partial V(D)J recombination activity leads to Omenn syndrome. *Cell* 1998;93:885–896.
46. Villa A, Santagata S, Bozzi F, et al. Omenn syndrome: a disorder of Rag1 and Rag2 genes. *J Clin Immunol* 1999;19:87–97.
47. Shimizu T, Iwasato T, Yamagishi H. Deletions of immunoglobulin C kappa region characterized by the circular excision products in mouse splenocytes. *J Exp Med* 1991;173:1065–1072.
48. Weichhold GM, Klobeck HG, Ohnheiser R, et al. Megabase inversions in the human genome as physiological events. *Nature* 1990;347:90–92.
49. Lieber MR, Hesse JE, Mizuuchi K, et al. Lymphoid V(D)J recombination: nucleotide insertion at signal joints as well as coding joints. *Proc Natl Acad Sci U S A* 1988;85:8588–8592.
50. Lafaille JJ, De Cloux A, Bonneville M, et al. Junctional sequences of T cell receptor gamma delta genes: implications for gamma delta T cell lineages and for a novel intermediate of V-(D)-J joining. *Cell* 1989;59:859–870.
51. McCormack WT, Tjoelker LW, Carlson LM, et al. Chicken IgL gene rearrangement involves deletion of a circular episome and addition of single nonrandom nucleotides to both coding segments. *Cell* 1989;56:785–791.
52. Kallenbach S, Doyen N, Fanton dA, et al. Three lymphoid-specific factors account for all junctional diversity characteristic of somatic assembly of T-cell receptor and immunoglobulin genes. *Proc Natl Acad Sci U S A* 1992;89:2799–2803.
53. Taccioli GE, Rathbun G, Shinkai Y, et al. Activities involved in V(D)J recombination. *Curr Top Microbiol Immunol* 1992;182:107–114.
54. Taccioli GE, Rathbun G, Oltz E, et al. Impairment of V(D)J recombination in double-strand break repair mutants. *Science* 1993;260:207–210.
55. Roth DB, Lindahl T, Gellert M. Repair and recombination: how to make ends meet. *Curr Biol* 1995;5:496–499.
56. Gottlieb TM, Jackson SP. The DNA-dependent protein kinase: requirement for DNA ends and association with Ku antigen. *Cell* 1993;72:131–142.
57. Taccioli GE, Gottlieb TM, Blunt T, et al. Ku80: product of the XRCC5 gene and its role in DNA repair and V(D)J recombination. *Science* 1994;265:1442–1445.
58. Dvir A, Peterson SR, Knuth MW, et al. Ku autoantigen is the regulatory component of a template-associated protein kinase that phosphorylates RNA polymerase II. *Proc Natl Acad Sci U S A* 1992;89:11920–11924.
59. Li Z, Otevrel T, Gao Y, et al. The XRCC4 gene encodes a novel protein involved in DNA double-strand break repair and V(D)J recombination. *Cell* 1995;83:1079–1089.
60. Grawunder U, Wilm M, Wu X, et al. Activity of DNA ligase IV stimulated by complex formation with XRCC4 protein in mammalian cells. *Nature* 1997;388:492–495.
61. Grawunder U, Zimmer D, Fugmann S, et al. DNA ligase IV is essential for V(D)J recombination and DNA double-strand break repair in human precursor lymphocytes. *Mol Cell* 1998;2:477–484.
62. Stavnezer J. Antibody class switching. *Adv Immunol* 1996;61:79–146.
63. Stavnezer J. Immunoglobulin class switching. *Curr Opin Immunol* 1996;8:199–205.
64. Stavnezer J. Molecular processes that regulate class switching. *Curr Top Microbiol Immunol* 2000;245:127–168.
65. Iwasato T, Shimizu A, Honjo T, et al. Circular DNA is excised by immunoglobulin class switch recombination. *Cell* 1990;62:143–149.
66. Kinoshita K, Tashiro J, Tomita S, et al. Target specificity of immunoglobulin class switch recombination is not determined by nucleotide sequences of S regions. *Immunity* 1998;9:849–858.
67. Snapper CM, Marcu KB, Zelazowski P. The immunoglobulin class switch: beyond "accessibility." *Immunity* 1997;6:217–223.
68. Madisen L, Groudine M. Identification of a locus control region in the immunoglobulin heavy-chain locus that deregulates c-myc expression in plasmacytoma and Burkitt's lymphoma cells. *Genes Dev* 1994;8:2212–2226.
69. Cogne M, Lansford R, Bottaro A, et al. A class switch control region at the 3′ end of the immunoglobulin heavy chain locus. *Cell* 1994;77:737–747.
70. Manis JP, van der Stoep N, Tian M, et al. Class switching in B cells lacking 3′ immunoglobulin heavy chain enhancers. *J Exp Med* 1998;188:1421–1431.
71. Jung S, Rajewsky K, Radbruch A. Shutdown of class switch recombination by deletion of a switch region control element. *Science* 1993;259:984–987.
72. Bottaro A, Lansford R, Xu L, et al. S region transcription per se promotes basal IgE class switch recombination but additional factors regulate the efficiency of the process. *EMBO J* 1994;13:665–674.
73. Hein K, Lorenz MG, Siebenkotten G, et al. Processing of switch transcripts is required for targeting of antibody class switch recombination. *J Exp Med* 1998;188:2369–2374.
74. Rolink A, Melchers F, Andersson J. The SCID but not the RAG-2 gene

product is required for S mu–S epsilon heavy chain class switching. *Immunity* 1996;5:319–330.
75. Manis JP, Gu Y, Lansford R, et al. Ku70 is required for late B cell development and immunoglobulin heavy chain class switching. *J Exp Med* 1998;187:2081–2089.
76. Casellas R, Nussenzweig A, Wuerffel R, et al. Ku80 is required for immunoglobulin isotype switching. *EMBO J* 1998;17:2404–2411.
77. Storb U. The molecular basis of somatic hypermutation of immunoglobulin genes. *Curr Opin Immunol* 1996;8:206–214.
78. Klein U, Goossens T, Fischer M, et al. Somatic hypermutation in normal and transformed human B cells. *Immunol Rev* 1998;162: 261–280.
79. Storb U. Progress in understanding the mechanism and consequences of somatic hypermutation. *Immunol Rev* 1998;162:5–11.
80. Goossens T, Klein U, Kuppers R. Frequent occurrence of deletions and duplications during somatic hypermutation: implications for oncogene translocations and heavy chain disease. *Proc Natl Acad Sci U S A* 1998;95:2463–2468.
81. Wilson PC, de Bouteiller O, Liu YJ, et al. Somatic hypermutation introduces insertions and deletions into immunoglobulin V genes. *J Exp Med* 1998;187:59–70.
82. Padlan EA. Does base composition help predispose the complementarity-determining regions of antibodies to hypermutation? *Mol Immunol* 1997;34:765–770.
83. Dorner T, Foster SJ, Farner NL, et al. Somatic hypermutation of human immunoglobulin heavy chain genes: targeting of RGYW motifs on both DNA strands. *Eur J Immunol* 1998;28:3384–3396.
84. Dorner T, Foster SJ, Brezinschek HP, et al. Analysis of the targeting of the hypermutational machinery and the impact of subsequent selection on the distribution of nucleotide changes in human V_HDJ_H rearrangements. *Immunol Rev* 1998;162:161–171.
85. Zheng B, Xue W, Kelsoe G. Locus-specific somatic hypermutation in germinal centre T cells. *Nature* 1994;372:556–559.
86. Cheynier R, Henrichwark S, Wain-Hobson S. Somatic hypermutation of the T cell receptor V beta gene in microdissected splenic white pulps from HIV-1–positive patients. *Eur J Immunol* 1998;28: 1604–1610.
87. McHeyzer-Williams MG, Davis MM. Antigen-specific development of primary and memory T cells in vivo. *Science* 1995;268:106–111.
88. Storb U, Peters A, Klotz E, et al. *Cis*-acting sequences that affect somatic hypermutation of Ig genes. *Immunol Rev* 1998;162:153–160.
89. Winter DB, Sattar N, Gearhart PJ. The role of promoter-intron interactions in directing hypermutation. *Curr Top Microbiol Immunol* 1998; 229:1–10.
90. Neuberger MS, Ehrenstein MR, Klix N, et al. Monitoring and interpreting the intrinsic features of somatic hypermutation. *Immunol Rev* 1998;162:107–116.
91. Wiesendanger M, Scharff MD, Edelmann W. Somatic hypermutation, transcription, and DNA mismatch repair [Comment]. *Cell* 1998;94: 415–418.
92. Harris RS, Kong Q, Maizels N. Somatic hypermutation and the three R's: repair, replication and recombination. *Mutat Res* 1999;436: 157–178.
93. Cascalho M, Wong J, Steinberg C, et al. Mismatch repair co-opted by hypermutation. *Science* 1998;279:1207–1210.
94. Winter DB, Gearhart PJ. Dual enigma of somatic hypermutation of immunoglobulin variable genes: targeting and mechanism. *Immunol Rev* 1998;162:89–96.
95. Frey S, Bertocci B, Delbos F, et al. Mismatch repair deficiency interferes with the accumulation of mutations in chronically stimulated B cells and not with the hypermutation process. *Immunity* 1998;9: 127–134.
96. Phung QH, Winter DB, Cranston A, et al. Increased hypermutation at G and C nucleotides in immunoglobulin variable genes from mice deficient in the MSH2 mismatch repair protein. *J Exp Med* 1998;187: 1745–1751.
97. Kim N, Kage K, Matsuda F, et al. B lymphocytes of xeroderma pigmentosum or Cockayne syndrome patients with inherited defects in nucleotide excision repair are fully capable of somatic hypermutation of immunoglobulin genes. *J Exp Med* 1997;186:413–419.
98. Kim N, Storb U. The role of DNA repair in somatic hypermutation of immunoglobulin genes. *J Exp Med* 1998;187:1729–1733.
99. Wagner SD, Elvin JG, Norris P, et al.Somatic hypermutation of Ig genes in patients with xeroderma pigmentosum (XP-D). *Int Immunol* 1996;8:701–705.
100. Jacobs H, Fukita Y, van der Horst GT, et al. Hypermutation of immunoglobulin genes in memory B cells of DNA repair-deficient mice. *J Exp Med* 1998;187:1735–1743.
101. Sobol RW, Horton JK, Kuhn R, et al. Requirement of mammalian DNA polymerase-beta in base-excision repair. *Nature* 1996;379: 183–186.
102. Kuo FC, Sklar J. Augmented expression of a human gene for 8-oxoguanine DNA glycosylase (MutM) in B lymphocytes of the dark zone in lymph node germinal centers. *J Exp Med* 1997;186:1547–1556.
103. Kunkel TA, Alexander PS. The base substitution fidelity of eucaryotic DNA polymerases: mispairing frequencies, site preferences, insertion preferences, and base substitution by dislocation. *J Biol Chem* 1986; 261:160–166.
104. Clairmont CA, Narayanan L, Sun KW, et al. The Tyr-265-to-Cys mutator mutant of DNA polymerase beta induces a mutator phenotype in mouse LN12 cells. *Proc Natl Acad Sci U S A* 1999;96:9580–9585.
105. Esposito G, Texido G, Betz UA, et al. Mice reconstituted with DNA polymerase β-deficient fetal liver cells are able to mount a T cell–dependent immune response and mutate their Ig genes normally. *Proc Natl Acad Sci U S A* 2000;97:1166–1171.
106. Sale JE, Neuberger MS. TdT-accessible breaks are scattered over the immunoglobulin V domain in a constitutively hypermutating B cell line. *Immunity* 1998;9:859–869.
107. Fanning L, Bertrand FE, Steinberg C, et al. Molecular mechanisms involved in receptor editing at the Ig heavy chain locus. *Int Immunol* 1998;10:241–246.
108. Nussenzweig MC. Immune receptor editing: revise and select. *Cell* 1998;95:875–878.
109. Nemazee D. Receptor editing in B cells. *Adv Immunol* 2000;74: 89–126.
110. Tiegs SL, Russell DM, Nemazee D. Receptor editing in self-reactive bone marrow B cells. *J Exp Med* 1993;177:1009–1020.
111. Gay D, Saunders T, Camper S, et al. Receptor editing: an approach by autoreactive B cells to escape tolerance. *J Exp Med* 1993;177: 999–1008.
112. Chen C, Radic MZ, Erikson J, et al. Deletion and editing of B cells that express antibodies to DNA. *J Immunol* 1994;152:1970–1982.
113. Papavasiliou F, Casellas R, Suh H, et al. V(D)J recombination in mature B cells: a mechanism for altering antibody responses. *Science* 1997;278:298–301.
114. McMahan CJ, Fink PJ. RAG reexpression and DNA recombination at T cell receptor loci in peripheral $CD4^+$ T cells. *Immunity* 1998;9: 637–647.
115. Yu W, Nagaoka H, Jankovic M, et al. Continued RAG expression in late stages of B cell development and no apparent re-induction after immunization. *Nature* 1999;400:682–687.
116. Monroe RJ, Seidl KJ, Gaertner F, et al. RAG2: GFP knockin mice reveal novel aspects of RAG2 expression in primary and peripheral lymphoid tissues. *Immunity* 1999;11:201–212.
117. Diss TC, Pan L. Polymerase chain reaction in the assessment of lymphomas. In: Tooze J, Franks LM, eds. *Cancer surveys.* New York: Cold Spring Harbor Laboratory Press, 1997.
118. Medeiros LJ, Carr J. Overview of the role of molecular methods in the diagnosis of malignant lymphomas. *Arch Pathol Lab Med* 1999; 123:1189–1207.
119. Muller-Hermelink HK, Greiner A. Molecular analysis of human immunoglobulin heavy chain variable genes (IgV_H) in normal and malignant B cells [Comment]. *Am J Pathol* 1998;153:1341–1346.
120. Southern EM. Detection of specific sequences among DNA fragments separated by gel electrophoresis. *J Mol Biol* 1975;98:503–517.
121. Sambrook J, Fritsch EF, Maniatis T, et al, eds. *Molecular cloning: a laboratory manual,* 2nd ed. New York: Cold Spring Harbor Laboratory Press, 1989.
122. Cossman J, Uppenkamp M. T-cell gene rearrangements and the diagnosis of T-cell neoplasms. *Clin Lab Med* 1988;8:31–44.
123. Hockett RD, de Villartay JP, Pollock K, et al. Human T-cell antigen receptor (TCR) delta-chain locus and elements responsible for its deletion are within the TCR alpha-chain locus. *Proc Natl Acad Sci U S A* 1988;85:9694–9698.
124. Feinberg AP, Vogelstein B. A technique for radiolabeling DNA restriction endonuclease fragments to high specific activity [Addendum]. *Anal Biochem* 1984;137:266–267.

125. McCreery T, Helentjaris T. Hybridization of digoxigenin-labeled probes to Southern blots and detection by chemoluminescence. *Methods Mol Biol* 1994;28:107–112.
126. Solanas M, Escrich E. An improved protocol to increase sensitivity of Southern blot using dig-labelled DNA probes. *J Biochem Biophys Methods* 1997;35:153–159.
127. Badenes ML, Parfitt DE. Reducing background interference on Southern blots probed with nonradioactive chemiluminescent probes. *Biotechniques* 1994;17:622–624.
128. Hodges KA, Kosciol CM, Rezuke WN, et al. Chemiluminescent detection of gene rearrangements in hematologic malignancy. *Ann Clin Lab Sci* 1996;26:114–118.
129. Arnold A, Cossman J, Bakhshi A, et al. Immunoglobulin-gene rearrangements as unique clonal markers in human lymphoid neoplasms. *N Engl J Med* 1983;309:1593–1599.
130. Cossman J, Zehnbauer B, Garrett CT, et al. *Gene* rearrangements in the diagnosis of lymphoma/leukemia. Guidelines for use based on a multiinstitutional study. *Am J Clin Pathol* 1991;95:347–354.
131. Cleary ML, Chao J, Warnke R, et al. Immunoglobulin gene rearrangement as a diagnostic criterion of B-cell lymphoma. *Proc Natl Acad Sci U S A* 1984;81:593–597.
132. Bertness V, Kirsch I, Hollis G, et al. T-cell receptor gene rearrangements as clinical markers of human T-cell lymphomas. *N Engl J Med* 1985;313:534–538.
133. van Dongen JJ, Wolvers-Tettero IL. Analysis of immunoglobulin and T cell receptor genes. Part I: Basic and technical aspects. *Clin Chim Acta* 1991;198:1–91.
134. Warford A, Pringle JH, Hay J, et al. Southern blot analysis of DNA extracted from formal-saline fixed and paraffin wax embedded tissue. *J Pathol* 1988;154:313–320.
135. Gledhill S, Krajewski AS, Jarrett RF. Demonstration of Epstein-Barr viral DNA in formalin-fixed, paraffin-embedded samples of Hodgkin's disease [Letter; comment]. *J Pathol* 1991;163:149–151.
136. Saiki RK, Scharf S, Faloona F, et al. Enzymatic amplification of beta-globin genomic sequences and restriction site analysis for diagnosis of sickle cell anemia. *Science* 1985;230:1350–1354.
137. Pan LX, Diss TC, Isaacson PG. The polymerase chain reaction in histopathology [Invited review]. *Histopathology* 1995;26:201–217.
138. Saiki RK, Gelfand DH, Stoffel S, et al. Primer-directed enzymatic amplification of DNA with a thermostable DNA polymerase. *Science* 1988;239:487–491.
139. Kuppers R, Rajewsky K, Zhao M, et al. Hodgkin's disease: clonal Ig gene rearrangements in Hodgkin and Reed-Sternberg cells picked from histological sections. *Ann N Y Acad Sci* 1995;764:523–524.
140. Diss TC, Pan LX, Peng HZ, et al. Sources of DNA for detecting B cell monoclonality using PCR. *J Clin Pathol* 1994;47:493–496.
141. Weirich G, Funk A, Hoepner I, et al. PCR-based assays for the detection of monoclonality in non-Hodgkin's lymphoma: application to formalin-fixed, paraffin-embedded tissue and decalcified bone marrow samples. *J Mol Med* 1995;73:235–241.
142. Coates PJ, d'Ardenne AJ, Khan G, et al. Simplified procedures for applying the polymerase chain reaction to routinely fixed paraffin wax sections. *J Clin Pathol* 1991;44:115–118.
143. Greer CE, Lund JK, Manos MM. PCR amplification from paraffin-embedded tissues: recommendations on fixatives for long-term storage and prospective studies. *PCR Methods Appl* 1991;1:46–50.
144. Pan LX, Diss TC, Peng HZ, et al. Clonality analysis of defined B-cell populations in archival tissue sections using microdissection and the polymerase chain reaction. *Histopathology* 1994;24:323–327.
145. Wan JH, Trainor KJ, Brisco MJ, et al. Monoclonality in B cell lymphoma detected in paraffin wax embedded sections using the polymerase chain reaction. *J Clin Pathol* 1990;43:888–890.
146. Ludecke HJ, Senger G, Claussen SU, et al. Cloning defined regions of the human genome by microdissection of banded chromosomes and enzymatic amplification. *Nature* 1989;338:348–350.
147. Wakefield AJ, Fox JD, Sawyerr AM, et al. Detection of herpesvirus DNA in the large intestine of patients with ulcerative colitis and Crohn's disease using the nested polymerase chain reaction. *J Med Virol* 1992;38:183–190.
148. D'Aquila RT, Bechtel LJ, Videler JA, et al. Maximizing sensitivity and specificity of PCR by pre-amplification heating. *Nucleic Acids Res* 1991;19:3749–3749.
149. Chou Q, Russell M, Birch DE, et al. Prevention of pre-PCR mispriming and primer dimerization improves low-copy-number amplifications. *Nucleic Acids Res* 1992;20:1717–1723.
150. Don RH, Cox PT, Wainwright BJ, et al. "Touchdown" PCR to circumvent spurious priming during gene amplification. *Nucleic Acids Res* 1991;19:4008–4008.
151. Ruano G, Pagliaro EM, Schwartz TR, et al. Heat-soaked PCR: an efficient method for DNA amplification with applications to forensic analysis. *Biotechniques* 1992;13:266–274.
152. Dunning AM, Talmud P, Humphries SE. Errors in the polymerase chain reaction. *Nucleic Acids Res* 1988;16:10393–10393.
153. Krawczak M, Reiss J, Schmidtke J, et al. Polymerase chain reaction: replication errors and reliability of gene diagnosis. *Nucleic Acids Res* 1989;17:2197–2201.
154. Eckert KA, Kunkel TA. High fidelity DNA synthesis by the *Thermus aquaticus* DNA polymerase. *Nucleic Acids Res* 1990;18:3739–3744.
155. Eckert KA, Kunkel TA. DNA polymerase fidelity and the polymerase chain reaction. *PCR Methods Appl* 1991;1:17–24.
156. Orita M, Suzuki Y, Sekiya T, et al. Rapid and sensitive detection of point mutations and DNA polymorphisms using the polymerase chain reaction. *Genomics* 1989;5:874–879.
157. Bourguin A, Tung R, Galili N, et al. Rapid, nonradioactive detection of clonal T-cell receptor gene rearrangements in lymphoid neoplasms. *Proc Natl Acad Sci U S A* 1990;87:8536–8540.
158. Rao VB. Direct sequencing of polymerase chain reaction–amplified DNA. *Anal Biochem* 1994;216:1–14.
159. Trainor KJ, Brisco MJ, Story CJ, et al. Monoclonality in B lymphoproliferative disorders detected at the DNA level. *Blood* 1990;75:2220–2222.
160. Deane M, McCarthy KP, Wiedemann LM, et al. An improved method for detection of B-lymphoid clonality by polymerase chain reaction. *Leukemia* 1991;5:726–730.
161. Ramasamy I, Brisco M, Morley A. Improved PCR method for detecting monoclonal immunoglobulin heavy chain rearrangement in B cell neoplasms. *J Clin Pathol* 1992;45:770–775.
162. Derksen PW, Langerak AW, Kerkhof E, et al. Comparison of different polymerase chain reaction-based approaches for clonality assessment of immunoglobulin heavy-chain gene rearrangements in B-cell neoplasia. *Mod Pathol* 1999;12:794–805.
163. Kuppers R, Zhao M, Rajewsky K, et al. Detection of clonal B cell populations in paraffin-embedded tissues by polymerase chain reaction. *Am J Pathol* 1993;143:230–239.
164. Gong JZ, Zheng S, Chiarle R, et al. Detection of immunoglobulin kappa light chain rearrangements by polymerase chain reaction: an improved method for detecting clonal B-cell lymphoproliferative disorders. *Am J Pathol* 1999;155:355–363.
165. McCarthy KP, Sloane JP, Wiedemann LM. Rapid method for distinguishing clonal from polyclonal B cell populations in surgical biopsy specimens. *J Clin Pathol* 1990;43:429–432.
166. Diss TC, Peng HZ, Wotherspoon AC, et al. Detection of monoclonality in low-grade B-cell lymphomas using the polymerase chain reaction is dependent on primer selection and lymphoma type. *J Pathol* 1993;169:291–295.
167. Segal GH, Jorgensen T, Scott M, et al. Optimal primer selection for clonality assessment by polymerase chain reaction analysis: II. Follicular lymphomas. *Hum Pathol* 1994;25:1276–1282.
168. Lombardo JF, Hwang TS, Maiese RL, et al. Optimal primer selection for clonality assessment by polymerase chain reaction analysis. III. Intermediate and high-grade B-cell neoplasms. *Hum Pathol* 1996;27:373–380.
169. McCarthy KP, Sloane JP, Kabarowski JH, et al. The rapid detection of clonal T-cell proliferations in patients with lymphoid disorders. *Am J Pathol* 1991;138:821–828.
170. McCarthy KP, Sloane JP, Kabarowski JH, et al. A simplified method of detection of clonal rearrangements of the T-cell receptor-gamma chain gene. *Diagn Mol Pathol* 1992;1:173–179.
171. Slack DN, McCarthy KP, Wiedemann LM, et al. Evaluation of sensitivity, specificity, and reproducibility of an optimized method for detecting clonal rearrangements of immunoglobulin and T-cell receptor genes in formalin-fixed, paraffin-embedded sections. *Diagn Mol Pathol* 1993;2:223–232.
172. Lorenzen J, Jux G, Zhao Hohn M, et al. Detection of T-cell clonality in paraffin-embedded tissues. *Diagn Mol Pathol* 1994;3:93–99.
173. Diss TC, Watts M, Pan L, et al. The polymerase chain reaction in the

demonstration of monoclonality in T cell lymphomas. *J Clin Pathol* 1995;48:1045–1050.
174. Langlands K, Craig JI, Anthony RS, et al. Clonal selection in acute lymphoblastic leukaemia demonstrated by polymerase chain reaction analysis of immunoglobulin heavy chain and T-cell receptor delta chain rearrangements. *Leukemia* 1993;7:1066–1070.
175. Calvert R, Randerson J, Evans P, et al. Genetic abnormalities during transition from *Helicobacter pylori*–associated gastritis to low-grade MALToma. *Lancet* 1995;345:26–27.
176. Hsi ED, Greenson JK, Singleton TP, et al. Detection of immunoglobulin heavy chain gene rearrangement by polymerase chain reaction in chronic active gastritis associated with *Helicobacter pylori. Hum Pathol* 1996;27:290–296.
177. Ben Ezra J. Variable rate of detection of immunoglobulin heavy chain V-D-J rearrangement by PCR: a systematic study of 41 B-cell non-Hodgkin's lymphomas and leukemias. *Leuk Lymphoma* 1992;7: 289–295.
178. Diss TC, Wotherspoon AC, Pan LX, et al. PCR analysis of clonality in high grade B cell lymphomas. *J Pathol* 1994;172[Suppl]:90(abst).
179. Pan LX, Diss TC, Mathan M, et al. Configuration and expression of immunoglobulin genes in immunoproliferative small intestinal disease. *J Pathol* 1994;173[Suppl]:211(abst).
180. Pollard P, Owen G, Worwood M. PCR-based immunogenotyping at the Ig heavy chain CDR3 locus: improvements in resolution. *Br J Haematol* 1993;84:169–171.
181. Yelamos J, Klix N, Lozano F, et al. Targeting of non-Ig sequences in place of the V segment by somatic hypermutation. *Nature* 1995; 376:225–229.
182. Signoretti S, Murphy M, Cangi MG, et al. Detection of clonal T-cell receptor gamma gene rearrangements in paraffin-embedded tissue by polymerase chain reaction and nonradioactive single-strand conformational polymorphism analysis. *Am J Pathol* 1999;154:67–75.
183. Maxam AM, Gilbert W. A new method for sequencing DNA. *Proc Natl Acad Sci U S A* 1977;74:560–564.
184. Sanger F, Nicklen S, Coulson AR. DNA sequencing with chain-terminating inhibitors. *Proc Natl Acad Sci U S A* 1977;74:5463–5467.
185. Gyllensten UB, Erlich HA. Generation of single-stranded DNA by the polymerase chain reaction and its application to direct sequencing of the HLA-DQA locus. *Proc Natl Acad Sci U S A* 1988;85: 7652–7656.
186. Dogan A, Du MQ, Aiello A, et al. Follicular lymphomas contains a clonally linked but phenotypically distinct neoplastic B-cell population in the interfollicular zone. *Blood* 1998;91:4708–4714.
187. Tsang P, Pan L, Cesarman E, et al. A distinctive composite lymphoma consisting of clonally related mantle cell lymphoma and follicle center cell lymphoma. *Hum Pathol* 1999;30:988–992.
188. Fend F, Quintanilla-Martinez L, Kumar S, et al. Composite low grade B-cell lymphomas with two immunophenotypically distinct cell populations are true biclonal lymphomas: a molecular analysis using laser capture microdissection. *Am J Pathol* 1999;154:1857–1866.
189. Du MQ, Xu CF, Diss TC, et al. Intestinal dissemination of gastric mucosa-associated lymphoid tissue lymphoma. *Blood* 1996;88: 4445–4451.
190. Diss TC, Peng HZ, Wotherspoon AC, et al. Brief report: a single neoplastic clone in sequential biopsy specimens from a patient with primary gastric-mucosa-associated lymphoid-tissue lymphoma and Sjogren's syndrome. *N Engl J Med* 1993;329:172–175.
191. Nishiuchi R, Yoshino T, Matsuo Y, et al. The Fas antigen is detected on immature B cells and the representative cell lines show Fas-mediated apoptosis. *Br J Haematol* 1996;92:302–307.
192. Zelenetz AD, Chen TT, Levy R. Histologic transformation of follicular lymphoma to diffuse lymphoma represents tumor progression by a single malignant B cell. *J Exp Med* 1991;173:197–207.
193. Peng H, Du M, Diss TC, et al. Genetic evidence for a clonal link between low and high-grade components in gastric MALT B-cell lymphoma. *Histopathology* 1997;30:425–429.
194. Pan LX, Diss TC, Peng HZ, et al. Nodular lymphocyte predominance Hodgkin's disease: a monoclonal or polyclonal B-cell disorder? *Blood* 1996;87:2428–2434.
195. Yamada M, Hudson S, Tournay O, et al. Detection of minimal disease in hematopoietic malignancies of the B-cell lineage by using third-complementarity–determining region (CDR-III)–specific probes. *Proc Natl Acad Sci U S A* 1989;86:5123–5127.
196. Du MQ, Peng HZ, Dogan A, et al. Preferential dissemination of B-cell gastric mucosa–associated lymphoid tissue (MALT) lymphoma to the splenic marginal zone. *Blood* 1997;90:4071–4077.
197. Kuang S, Gu L, Dong S, et al. Long-term follow-up of minimal residual disease in childhood acute lymphoblastic leukemia patients by polymerase chain reaction analysis of multiple clone-specific or malignancy-specific gene markers. *Cancer Genet Cytogenet* 1996;88: 110–117.
198. Ashton-Key M, Diss TC, Pan L, et al. Molecular analysis of T-cell clonality in ulcerative jejunitis and enteropathy-associated T-cell lymphoma. *Am J Pathol* 1997;151:493–498.
199. Stevenson F, Sahota S, Zhu D, et al. Insight into the origin and clonal history of B-cell tumors as revealed by analysis of immunoglobulin variable region genes. *Immunol Rev* 1998;162:247–259.
200. Naylor M, Capra JD. Mutational status of Ig V(H) genes provides clinically valuable information in B-cell chronic lymphocytic leukemia [Comment]. *Blood* 1999;94:1837–1839.
201. Damle RN, Wasil T, Fais F, et al. Ig V gene mutation status and CD38 expression as novel prognostic indicators in chronic lymphocytic leukemia. *Blood* 1999;94:1840–1847.
202. Hamblin TJ, Davis Z, Gardiner A, et al. Unmutated Ig V(H) genes are associated with a more aggressive form of chronic lymphocytic leukemia. *Blood* 1999;94:1848–1854.
203. Brezinschek HP, Foster SJ, Brezinschek RI, et al. Analysis of the human V_H gene repertoire: differential effects of selection and somatic hypermutation on human peripheral CD5(+)/IgM$^+$ and CD5(−)/ IgM$^+$ B cells. *J Clin Invest* 1997;99:2488–2501.
204. Stevenson FK, Spellerberg MB, Chapman CJ, et al. Differential usage of an autoantibody-associated V_H gene, V_H4-21, by human B-cell tumors. *Leuk Lymphoma* 1995;16:379–384.
205. Chapman CJ, Dunn Walters DK, Stevenson FK, et al. Sequence analysis of immunoglobulin variable region genes which encode autoantigenes expressed by lymphomas of mucosa-asociated lymphoid tissue. *J Clin Pathol* 1996;49:M29–M32
206. Du MQ, Diss TC, Xu CF, et al. Ongoing mutation in MALT lymphoma immunoglobulin V_H gene suggests that antigen stimulation plays a role in the clonal expansion. *Leukemia* 1996;10:1190–1197.
207. Bahler DW, Levy R. Clonal evolution of a follicular lymphoma: evidence for antigen selection. *Proc Natl Acad Sci U S A* 1992;89: 6770–6774.
208. Tamaru J, Hummel M, Marafioti T, et al. Burkitt's lymphomas express V_H genes with a moderate number of antigen-selected somatic mutations. *Am J Pathol* 1995;147:1398–1407.
209. Rettig MB, Vescio RA, Cao J, et al. V_H gene usage is multiple myeloma: complete absence of the V_H4.21 (V_H4-34) gene. *Blood* 1996; 87:2846–2852.
210. Qin Y, Greiner A, Hallas C, et al. Intraclonal offspring expansion of gastric low-grade MALT-type lymphoma: evidence for the role of antigen-driven high-affinity mutation in lymphomagenesis. *Lab Invest* 1997;76:477–485.

CHAPTER 8

Protooncogenes and Tumor Suppressor Genes in Hematopoietic Malignancies

Wayne Tam and Riccardo Dalla-Favera

Cancer derives from alterations of the cellular genome (1). The breakthrough in the identification of specific cellular genes involved in carcinogenesis took place nearly three decades ago with the development of recombinant DNA technology. Eukaryotic genes related to the viral oncogenes carried by acute transforming retroviruses were discovered (2,3). At about the same time, biologically active cellular oncogenes were identified by the ability of tumor DNA, but not normal cellular DNA, to induce transformation in gene transfer assays (1,4–9). Viral and cellular oncogenes were later shown to be genetically altered, or "activated," versions of normal cellular genes called *protooncogenes* (1). This finding implicates cellular oncogene activation in the pathogenesis of human cancers.

Malignant cells often are characterized by the loss of specific genetic material. This finding led to the concept and demonstration of the existence of tumor suppressor genes, the inactivation of which is involved in tumorigenesis (10,11).

Studies of the normal and oncogenic functions of protooncogenes and tumor suppressor genes in hematopoietic neoplasms are critical to the understanding of their pathogenesis. In this chapter, we begin with an introduction of the concept of protooncogenes and tumor suppressor genes, with particular reference to hematopoietic neoplasms. The next section outlines the mechanisms of their activation and inactivation. This is followed by a discussion of the specific protooncogenes and tumor suppressor genes involved in the pathogenesis of hematologic neoplasms of myeloid and lymphoid origin: acute leukemia of B and T lineage, chronic myelogenous leukemia, B- and T-cell non-Hodgkin's lymphoma (NHL), multiple myeloma (MM), and Hodgkin's lymphoma.

W. Tam: Department of Pathology, Weill Medical College of Cornell University, New York, New York 10021

R. Dalla-Favera: Department of Pathology, Institute of Cancer Genetics, Columbia University, New York, New York 10032

Emphasis is placed on how these genes become activated or inactivated and on the mechanisms by which alterations of these genes result in transformation of hematopoietic cells. Additional information regarding the specific roles of these genetic alterations can be found in the chapters focusing on specific tumor types.

PROTOONCOGENES

Protooncogenes can be defined as normal cellular genes that have the potential to contribute to tumorigenesis when their expression or structure is altered, resulting in aberrant function. They represent a heterogeneous family of genes that play a critical role in many cellular processes, including cell proliferation, growth, differentiation, and apoptosis. Some of these genes are involved specifically in subtypes of lymphoid or myeloid neoplasms; others are implicated in other human cancers. The protooncogenes involved in hematopoietic neoplasms can generally be classified as encoding transcription factors, signal transducers, and cell death regulators.

Transcription Factors

The class of protooncogenes that produces transcription factors is particularly important in the pathogenesis of hematopoietic neoplasms because they are frequently the targets of chromosomal translocations (12–15). Transcription factors include nuclear proteins with functional domains that mediate specific DNA binding and protein-protein interactions, as well as components of the transcription machinery that interact with other transcription factors but do not contact DNA directly (i.e., coactivators and corepressors). Transcription factors can be classified into different families based on the presence of specific functional domains. On receiving signals from the cytoplasm of the cells conveyed through the signal transduction pathways, activation of transcription factors results in an increase (activation) or decrease (repression) of transcription of the target genes. In this way, transcription factors play a pivotal role in regulating cellular processes, including cell proliferation, cell differentiation and apoptosis (16–18). Oncogenic conversion of transcription factors by chromosomal translocations occurs by two mechanisms: deregulated expression due to heterologous regulatory sequences or alteration of function due to fusion with another protein (14).

Signal Transducers

Signal transducers are a class of proteins that play central roles in transmitting extracellular signals through essential signal transduction pathways to their terminal components: transcription factors within the nucleus. Through this signal-transducing function, they control many important cellular processes, including cell cycle entry and apoptosis (19–21). The signal transducers that are involved in hematologic malignancies include three groups: tyrosine kinase (receptor and nonreceptor type), serine/threonine protein kinase, and guanine nucleotide (GTP)-binding protein. Tyrosine kinase and serine/threonine protein kinase are protein kinases that relay signals by phosphorylating intracellular signaling molecules at the tyrosine or serine/threonine residues, respectively. Receptor tyrosine kinase include proteins that possess an extracellular ligand-binding domain linked to a membrane-spanning segment and an intracellular effector kinase domain. Binding of the ligand to the extracellular domain results in oligomerization of the receptor and activation of the kinase activity. An example of receptor tyrosine kinase involved in hematopoietic neoplasms is the orphan receptor tyrosine kinase ALK, a target of chromosomal translocation t(2;5) (22,23). ABL, activated by chromosomal translocation in chronic myelogenous leukemia, encodes a nonreceptor tyrosine kinase (24,25). It is present in the nucleus and cytoplasm, where it has distinct cellular functions. Its biologic activity depends on multiple protein-protein interactions, protein-DNA interactions, and its kinase activity (26–28). An example of serine/threonine kinase is BCR, the fusion partner for ABL in t(9;22) translocations (29).

Among the GTP-binding proteins, one subclass that is involved in hematopoietic malignancies is RAS, whose role in cancer has been well established. There are three members of the RAS family: HRAS, KRAS, and NRAS. Mutations in the RAS family occur in about 30% of human cancers, although with heterogenous frequency among different types (30). RAS is a plasma membrane protein that is active in the GTP-bound state but inactive in the GDP-bound state. Regulation of GTP binding and hydrolysis is mediated by positive and negative regulators (21,31). In general, the conversion of these signal transducers to oncogenes occurs by a variety of structural alterations, the result of which is increased deregulated catalytic activity (20,31,32).

Cell Death Regulators

Regulation of programmed cell death, called *apoptosis,* is essential for maintaining homeostasis of the hematopoietic cell population and is mediated by positive and negative regulators. Ineffective apoptosis can lead to disturbance of homeostasis of hematopoietic cells and consequently to tumorigenesis (33–35). Negative regulators of apoptosis can act as protooncogenes (36). The prototype of an antiapoptotic gene is *BCL2,* the target of the chromosomal translocation t(14;18) in follicular lymphoma. *BCL2* encodes an integral membrane protein localized to the inner mitochondrial membrane, endoplasmic reticulum, and nuclear membranes. It belongs to a family of BCL-2–related apoptosis regulators, which include BAX, BAD, and BCL-X (37,38). BCL-2 functions through heterodimerization with BAX, which also can form homodimers. The functional activity of BCL-2 can be determined by the ratio of antiapoptotic BCL-2/BAX heterodimers and proapoptotic BAX/BAX homodimers (37,39). Deregulation of BCL-2 leads to a predominance of BCL-2/BAX heterodimers and inhibition of apoptosis. The antiapoptotic function of BCL-2 appears to be related to its biochemical role in preventing oxidative damage by free oxygen radicals at their sites of production (40,41). Activation of negative regulators of apoptosis is likely to be the early step in the pathogenesis of hematologic lesions in which the neoplastic cells are long-lived and nonproliferative, such as in chronic lymphocytic leukemia and follicular lymphoma. Acquisition of antiapoptotic lesions can also be an important event in tumor progression in hematopoietic malignancies composed of highly proliferative cells (34).

MECHANISMS OF ONCOGENE ACTIVATION IN HEMATOPOIETIC NEOPLASMS

The type and nature of genetic alterations associated with hematologic malignancies and solid tumors are in part different. Tumors of epithelial origin are associated with general random genomic instability, characterized by marked aneuploidy, nonreciprocal translocations, large deletions, and a significant number of nonclonal alterations. In contrast, the genome of leukemias and lymphomas are relatively stable during most stages of the disease with few, occasionally single, clonal alterations, including balanced reciprocal translocations, as well as deletions and amplifications (42). Each of these nonrandom chromosomal aberrations is predominantly associated with a specific subtype of hematologic malignancy. The relatively "simple" nature of chromosomal abnormalities in hematologic neoplasms provides ample opportunities for identification and characterization of protoonocogenes.

Activation by Chromosomal Translocation

The major mechanism by which oncogenes are activated in hematopoietic malignancies is chromosomal translocation. Chromosomal translocations are detected in virtually all types of hematologic malignancies of lymphoid and myeloid lineages, except chronic lymphocytic leukemia (43). The chromosomal translocations associated with activation of protooncogenes in leukemias and lymphomas are recurrent, reciprocal, balanced translocations that involve exchange of portions of chromosome between two chromosomes without apparent loss of chromosomal material. These translocations often are associated with a specific type of leukemia or lymphoma and are clonally represented in the tumors. The translocations usually involve exchange between two specific chromosomes in most cases of a particular tumor type. An example is t(14;18), which involves *BCL2* and the immunoglobulin heavy chain (IgH) locus in follicular lymphoma. In a few cases, however, a chromosomal site may be translocated to multiple various partner chromosomal sites among different cases of a certain tumor type. Examples of promiscuous translocations include translocations affecting the *MLL* gene at chromosomal band 11q23 in acute myelogenous (AML) and lymphoblastic leukemias (ALL) and those affecting *BCL6* at 3q27 in diffuse large cell lymphoma (43,44).

The precise mechanisms leading to chromosomal translocations in hematopoietic neoplasms are not clearly understood. However, data suggest that the translocation process occurs most likely during immunoglobulin (Ig) gene and T-cell receptor (TCR) gene rearrangements in B and T cells, respectively, as a consequence of errors of the VDJ recombination machinery or the class switch machinery. This idea is supported by several observations. First, a significant fraction of translocations involve chromosomal breakpoints within the Ig or TCR loci. Second, in B-cell NHL, breakpoints within the Ig loci are often located precisely within sequences that normally mediate Ig gene rearrangement in B cells, such as the J and switch (S) sequences (45). Moreover, N-nucleotides, which are template-independent nucleotide additions generated at the site of VDJ recombination by terminal deoxynucleotidyl transferase (TdT), can be detected at certain breakpoint junctions, suggesting the action of the recombinase (46). Third, similarity has been shown between the sequences surrounding the breakpoints and recombination targeting motifs, such as the heptamers or nonamers and the bp45 nuclease binding sequence (47).

Not all the chromosomal translocations are caused by errors of the recombination machinery of the immune system. A defect in DNA damage repair mechanism may be responsible in at least some translocations (48). For example, based on sequence analysis of reciprocal chromosomal breakpoints, the chromosomal translocation t(4;11), seen in acute leukemias of B lineage, appears to be initiated by several DNA strand breaks on participating chromosomes and subsequent DNA repair by an "error-prone" DNA repair mechanism. Similarly, analysis of the breakpoint junction sequence at *TEL* (also called *ETV6*) in t(12;21)(p13;q22) support the occurrence of staggered DNA double-strand breaks followed by DNA repair (49). The generation of DNA double-strand breaks by exogenous and endogenous sources (e.g., chemicals, oxygen free radicals) or faulty DNA repair can lead to chromosomal rearrangements (50,51). These models have been validated by mouse models but have yet to be proven in humans (52).

It has also been suggested that translocations occurring in lymphoid malignancies derived from germinal center B cells, such as Burkitt's lymphoma and diffuse large B-cell lymphoma, may be a result of somatic hypermutation that takes place in the germinal center B cells (53). It has been shown that deletions and duplications can be introduced to the rearranged V_H genes in a substantial portion of germinal center cells during somatic hypermutation. Because the formation of these deletions and duplications is intrinsically associated with DNA double-strand breaks, they may provide a potential source for chromosomal translocations in the germinal center B cells. Somatic hypermutation may be the underlying mechanism of the chromosomal translocations between the IgH locus and *MYC* in the endemic form of Burkitt's lymphoma, which are thought to result from errors of the VDJ recombination machinery (54). This idea is supported by the observation that the breakpoints at the IgH loci in endemic Burkitt's lymphoma are not usually directly adjacent to the recombination signal sequence that mediates VDJ recombination but are located in the J intron or within rearranged VJ genes (i.e., the target region for hypermutation) (53). It remains to be seen whether somatic hypermutation also plays a role in the generation of chromosomal translocations at the *BCL6* locus, which is also a target for somatic hypermutation in diffuse large B-cell lymphomas (see Diffuse Large B-Cell Lymphoma Section) (43).

The common feature of all chromosomal translocations associated with hematopoietic malignancy is the presence of protooncogenes in proximity to the chromosomal breakpoints. Because of the translocations, the protooncogene can be altered in the pattern or degree of expression, with preservation of the structure of the coding domain, by the regulatory sequences of a heterologous gene juxtaposed by the translocation. This mechanism of activation is consistently seen in most types of B-NHL. Alternatively, chromosomal translocations can result in juxtaposition of two genes to form a chimeric gene coding for a fusion protein with novel function (15). This mechanism is common in acute leukemias but rare in NHLs, except for the t(2;5)(p23;q35) of anaplastic large cell lymphoma and t(11;18)(p21;q21) of extranodal marginal zone B-cell lymphoma of the mucosa-associated lymphoid tissues (MALT).

Activation by Point Mutation

A protooncogene can be converted to an oncogene by a DNA base pair mutation in the coding sequence, causing a change in the amino acid sequence that alters the structure of the protein. Oncogene activation by point mutation is best demonstrated by the RAS family. *RAS* mutations are found in a variety of human neoplasms at three specific codons:

12, 13, and 61. The genetic mutations result in amino acid substitutions leading to constitutive activation of the signal-transducing function of RAS. *NRAS* mutations are the most frequent and occur in approximately 10% to 30% of some types of hematologic malignancies, including AML, ALL, MM, and myelodysplastic syndromes (55–57). *RAS* mutations result in constitutive activation of RAS, which remains in the GTP-bound state regardless of regulatory signals. This results in deregulated activity of multiple signal transduction pathways, including the mitogen-activated protein kinase pathway, which leads to abnormal activation of transcription factors and gene deregulation (31).

Activation by Gene Amplification

Gene amplification is defined as an excess copy number of a given oncogene, and it is one of the molecular mechanisms by which gene expression can be deregulated. A number of examples of amplification that involve protooncogenes have been characterized in various human cancers. This alteration can be detected at different levels of gene specificity by conventional cytogenetics, comparative genomic hybridization, fluorescence *in situ* hybridization (FISH), and Southern blot analysis. The best-characterized examples of oncogene amplification in human cancers are the amplification of the *MYCN* gene in neuroblastoma, *NEU* gene amplification in breast and ovarian carcinoma, and *ERBB1* gene amplification in glioblastoma (58).

In hematologic neoplasms, protooncogene amplification is a rather frequent phenomenon in B-cell NHL, particularly in diffuse large B-cell lymphoma (DLCL) (59,60). The detection of these gene amplifications is initially facilitated by the use of comparative genomic hybridization, which is a sensitive technique for the detection of high-level amplifications in chromosomal regions. The protooncogenes that are amplified in DLCL include *REL, MYC, BCL2, GLI1, CDK4,* and *MDM2* (60–62). The frequency of involvement of these genes ranges from 10% to 20% of DLCL cases. *REL* amplification is associated with extranodal presentation (62). Further characterization of the highly amplified DNA regions and the genes contained in the amplicons will provide information on the genetic mechanism of pathogenesis of DLCL.

TUMOR SUPPRESSOR GENES AND THEIR INACTIVATION IN HEMATOPOIETIC NEOPLASMS

Several tumor suppressor genes are involved in the pathogenesis of leukemias and lymphomas, including those for p53 *(TP53),* cyclin-dependent kinase *(CDK)* inhibitors, retinoblastoma *(RB1)*, ataxia-telangiectasia mutated *(ATM)*, and several DNA repair genes. Conventionally, these tumor suppressor genes belong to two groups: *gatekeepers* and *caretakers* (63). *TP53, CDK, RB1,* and *ATM* are gatekeepers. Gatekeepers are genes, such as *TP53*, that control the cell cycle, apoptosis, or both. Inactivation of these genes leads to deregulation in cell cycle control and continued cell survival despite the appropriate signals, for example, on DNA damage. Caretakers are DNA repair genes that play an important role in the maintenance of genomic stability.

The mechanisms by which tumor suppressor genes are inactivated include point mutations, gross deletion, and hypermethylation. Point mutations are mostly nucleotide substitutions present in the coding region that result in nonsense and missense mutations. Infrequently, they affect the splicing sites or regulatory sequences. Small deletions and insertions in the coding region that lead to frameshift mutations can also occur. Gross deletion results in removal of the entire gene locus. Hypermethylation occurs at the CG island of the gene promoter and can lead to transcriptional silencing of the gene without any structural alterations (64). Inactivation of tumor suppressor genes usually occurs through gross deletion of one allele and nonsense/missense mutation in the other allele. Less frequently, homozygous deletions occur. Alternatively, hypermethylation of promoters can lead to gene inactivation by affecting intact alleles or by silencing the remaining allele when the other allele has been deleted.

The *TP53* tumor suppressor gene is the most frequently mutated gene in human cancers. An extensive review on the structure and function of p53 is beyond the scope of this chapter but can be found elsewhere (65). In brief, p53 is a 393–amino acid sequence-specific transcription factor that plays a critical role in activating expression of genes involved in cell cycle arrest and apoptosis (e.g., p21, BAX) on DNA damage (66,67). Through this transactivating activity, p53 functions to maintain genomic integrity by preventing propagation of cells containing genetic alterations. Inactivation of p53 leads to continual survival and cell cycling despite the presence of damaged DNA, which results in genomic instability (68). P53 may exert a caretaker DNA repair function by virtue of its exonuclease activity (69).

The mechanism of inactivation of p53 in hematopoietic neoplasms is similar to that in solid tumors and occurs predominantly through point mutation in one allele and deletion of the other allele (70). In addition to this classic mechanism of p53 inactivation, mutant p53 can lead to formation of dominant-negative p53 mutants that transform by acting as inhibitory proteins interfering with the normal functions of the wild-type p53 protein (65). Similar to solid tumors, *TP53* mutations in leukemias and lymphomas are mostly clustered from exon 5 to 10 (amino acids 120 to 290), which corresponds to the DNA-binding domain (70). These mutations are mostly missense mutations. Alterations of *TP53* are present in different types of hematopoietic neoplasms at variable frequencies. In general, they are less common (10% to 15%) in hematologic malignancies than in solid tumors. *TP53* gene alterations have been found in 20% of chronic myelogenous leukemia (CML) blast crisis; 15% of AML, 2% of ALL (up to 50% of L3 ALL); 10% of chronic lymphocytic leukemia (CLL) and 40% in Richter's transformation; 30% to 40% of adult T-cell leukemia; 5% to 10% of MM, and 30% of high grade B-cell NHL (rare in low-grade NHL) (71).

P15, p16, p18, p19, and p21 are cyclin-dependent kinase inhibitors that are altered at variable frequency in hematopoietic malignancies. The most frequent alterations are inactivation of p15 and p16 because of deletions (usually biallelic) or 5′ CG island methylation of the p15 and p16 promoters (72). Homozygous deletions and hypermethylation represent an alternate mode of inactivation of tumor suppressor genes, in contrast to the classic inactivation mechanism of a prototypic tumor suppressor gene such as *TP53*. Homozygous deletions in p15 and p16 are most frequent in ALL (precursor B and T) but much less frequent in B- and T-cell NHLs, AML, and CML. Deletions and hypermethylation of p18 and p19 occur infrequently (72).

The *RB1* gene is one of the first tumor suppressor genes identified by virtue of its role in hereditary retinoblastoma (73). The retinoblastoma protein (RB) encodes a 107-kd nuclear phosphoprotein that acts as a cell cycle control checkpoint in the G_1 phase (74). RB can interact with many cellular proteins, including E2F, a transcription factor. RB suppresses the G_1/S transition in the cell cycle by binding to E2F and inhibiting E2F-mediated transactivation of a variety of genes involved in initiating DNA synthesis, such as *MYC, MYB,* and *CDC2* and those for dihydrofolate reductase and thymidine kinase. RB function is regulated by phosphorylation mediated by the cyclin-dependent kinase, the activity of which is regulated by the cyclin-dependent kinase inhibitors such as p16. Hypophosphorylated or dephosphorylated RB is activated, and it binds E2F, thereby inducing cell-cycle arrest; in contrast, phosphorylated RB is inactivated, and it cannot bind E2F, thereby promoting entry of cells into S phase. RB can be inactivated by point mutations, deletions, or binding to transforming viral proteins encoded by SV40, adenovirus, and human papillomavirus (75). Inactivation of RB can lead to deregulation of cell cycle control and eventually to neoplasia (76,77).

The *ATM* (ataxia-telangiectasia mutated) gene is consistently inactivated in patients with ataxia telangiectasia, who have strong predisposition to lymphoid malignancies among other phenotypes (78). This suggests that *ATM* can act as a tumor suppressor gene. Consistent with this, ATM-deficient mice develop thymic lymphomas with a relatively short latency (79,80). ATM is a member of a family of protein kinases acting as a key regulator of multiple signaling cascades that respond to DNA strand breaks induced by damaging agents or by normal processes, such as meiotic or V(D)J recombination. These responses involve the activation of cell cycle checkpoints, DNA repair, and apoptosis (81–83). ATM also has a caretaker role, because it can suppress tumorigenesis in specific T-cell lineages by suppressing aberrant V-D-J recombination (84). Deletion and point mutation of *ATM* can frequently be detected in mantle cell lymphoma, implicating an important role of ATM in its pathogenesis (85–87).

Emerging evidence implicates defects in the DNA repair system in hematopoietic malignancies. Inactivation of DNA repair genes can contribute to the neoplastic process by causing genomic instability (88). Mutations in DNA mismatch repair genes have been detected in sporadic and hereditary tumors of colon, endometrium, and ovary (89). One study showed that microsatellite instability, a manifestation of an underlying defect of DNA mismatch repair genes (90), is found in approximately 33% of B-lineage ALL, 50% of T-lineage ALL, and 10% of AML (91). The frequency of microsatellite instability in B-NHL varies among studies, ranging from 0% to 20% (91,92). This suggests that inactivation of DNA mismatch repair genes may be present in hematopoietic neoplasms, particularly in acute leukemia of the lymphoid lineage.

Apart from DNA mismatch repair genes, other DNA repair genes are also implicated in the pathogenesis of hematopoietic neoplasms. For example, loss of p53 and Ku80, a subunit of DNA-dependent protein kinase, can synergize in the development of pre-B-cell lymphomas in mice, suggesting cooperativity between a gatekeeper and a caretaker in tumorigenesis. These lymphomas are associated with chromosomal abnormalities, including *MYC* translocations (52). Double-strand break DNA repair genes may have a tumor suppressor role in hematopoietic malignancies by maintaining genomic stability and suppressing chromosomal rearrangement. Although this model has been suggested by mouse studies, it needs to be confirmed in human tumors by additional studies.

Specific chromosomal deletions are associated with hematopoietic malignancies, suggesting the presence of unknown tumor suppressor genes. The most frequent chromosomal deletion associated with the pathogenesis of B-NHL is the deletion of the long arm of chromosome 6 at regions 6q21-q23 and 6q25-q27 (93). Moreover, deletion of chromosome 13q14 represents the most frequent lesion in B-CLL/small lymphocytic leukemia (SLL), occurring in more than 50% of cases (94,95). Characterization of the candidate genes located at these deletion regions should lead to identification of new tumor suppressor genes involved in the pathogenesis of hematopoietic malignancies.

ACUTE MYELOID LEUKEMIA

There is a great degree of heterogeneity in the genetic lesions associated with AML. Some molecular lesions are specific for or are predominantly associated with a defined AML subtype according to the French-American-British classification. These are generally balanced, reciprocal chromosomal translocations that result in the fusion of two protooncogenes (Table 8.1). Others are more equally distributed among the different subtypes. These are usually monosomies (e.g., −7, −5), trisomies (e.g., +8), or complex chromosomal defects (96). Moreover, inactivation of *TP53* is also associated with different AML subtypes, albeit at a low frequency (7% of AML) (97).

PML-RARA in t(15;17) or *X-RARA* in t(X;17)

Acute promyelocytic leukemia (APL) is characterized by a malignant proliferation of myeloid cells blocked at the

TABLE 8.1. *Protooncogenes and tumor suppressor genes in acute leukemia*

Genes	Chromosomal translocation	Biologic function	Mechanism of activation or inactivation	Leukemia type
Protooncogenes				
AML1 *ETO*	t(8;21)(q22;q22)	CBF transcription factor α subunit, transcriptional corepressor	Protein fusion	AML-M2
BCR *ABL*	t(9;22)(q34;q11)	Serine/threoine protein kinase; GTPase activation, non–receptor tyrosine kinase (nuclear and cytoplasmic)	Protein fusion	Precursor B-ALL
CBFB *MYH11*	Inv(16)(p13q22)	CBF transcription factor β subunit, smooth muscle myosin heavy chain	Protein fusion	AML-M4E0
DEK *CAN*	t(6;9)(p23;q34)	Transcription regulator? (autoantigen), nuceloporin/nucleocytoplasmic transport	Protein fusion	TdT^+ AML
E2A *HLF*	t(17;19)(q22;p13)	Transcription factor (helix-loop-helix family), transcription factor (basic zipper family)	Protein fusion	Precursor B-ALL
E2A *PBX1*	t(1;19)(q23;p13)	Transcription factor (helix-loop-helix family), transcription factor (homeobox family)	Protein fusion	Precursor B-ALL
HOX11	t(10;14)(q24;q11)	Transcription factor (homeobox family)	Transcription, deregulation	Precursor T-ALL
MLL V[b]	t(v;11)(v:q23)	Transcription factor, variable	Protein fusion	AML-M5, M4, M1 precursor B-ALL
PML[a] *RAR*	t(15;17)(q22;q21)	Component of PML nuclear bodies, transcription factor (nuclear hormone receptor family)	Protein fusion	AML-M3 (APL)
TAL1	t(1;14)(p32;q11) 5′ small deletion[c]	Transcription factor (helix-loop-helix-family)	Transcription, deregulation	Precursor T-ALL
TAN1	t(7;9)(q34;q34)	Transmembrane receptor (Notch family)	Transcription, deregulation, protein truncation	Precursor T-ALL
TEL *AML1*	t(12;21)(p12;q22)	Transcription factor (ETS family), CBF transcription factor alpha subunit	Protein fusion	Precursor B-ALL
TTG1	t(11;14)(p15;q11)	Transcription factor (rhombotin gene family)	Transcription, deregulation	Precursor T-ALL
TTG2	t(11;14)(p13;q11)	Transcription regulator (rhombotin gene family)	Transcription, deregulation	Precursor T-ALL
Tumor suppressor genes				
TP53 (p53)		Transcription factor/maintains genomic stability	Point mutation; deletion	AML, CML(blast crisis) precursor B and T-ALL
CDKN2B (p15)		Cell cycle regulator (cdk inhibitor)	Deletion; hypermethylation	Precursor B and T-ALL
CDKN2A (p16)		Cell cycle regulator (cdk inhibitor)	Deletion; hypermethylation	CML (lymphoid blast crisis) precursor B- and T-ALL

[a] Other partner genes of *RARA* are *PLZF, NPM,* and *NUMA.*
[b] More than 30 chromosomal sites are involved.
[c] 90-kb submicroscopic deletion that juxtaposes *TAL* to *SIL,* creating a SIL-TAL fusion transcript.

promyelocytic stage of differentiation. It is invariably associated with four related reciprocal chromosomal translocations involving the gene *(RARA)* for the retinoic acid receptor-α (RARα) on chromosome 17. RARα belongs to the nuclear ligand-activated transcription factor family (98). It contains several functional domains, including a DNA-binding domain, a ligand-binding domain, and a heterodimerization domain with RXRα. In more than 99% of APL cases, t(15; 17)(q22;q21) results in translocation of *RARA* to a gene called promyelocytic leukemia *(PML)* on chromosome 15 (99–101), which encodes a component of a marcomolecular organelle called PML oncogenic domains (or PML nuclear bodies) (102,103). In less than 1% of cases, *RARA* translocates to *PLZF* on chromosome 11, which codes for a transcription factor. Translocations of *RARA* to the *NUMA1* gene (coding for an essential component for the function of mitotic spindles) on chromosome 11 and *NPM* gene (coding for a RNA-binding nucleolar phosphoprotein) on chromosome 5 are rare, and only one or two such cases are well documented (104,105). All these protein products of the partner genes contain dimerization domains at their N-terminal portions. The result of the translocations is the production of fusion proteins between RARα and the proteins encoded by partner genes (X), creating RARα-X and X-RARα proteins (106–108). Most of the studies have focused on X-RARα, which is therefore the main subject of this discussion. The X-RARα proteins are identical in their RARα-derived sequence and retain the domains for DNA and ligand (retinoic acid) binding, as well as the region for heterodimerization with retinoic X-receptor (RXRα). They also contain the homodimerization domain of the partner proteins X (Fig. 8.1).

PML-RARα, PLZF-RARα, and NPM-RARα play crucial

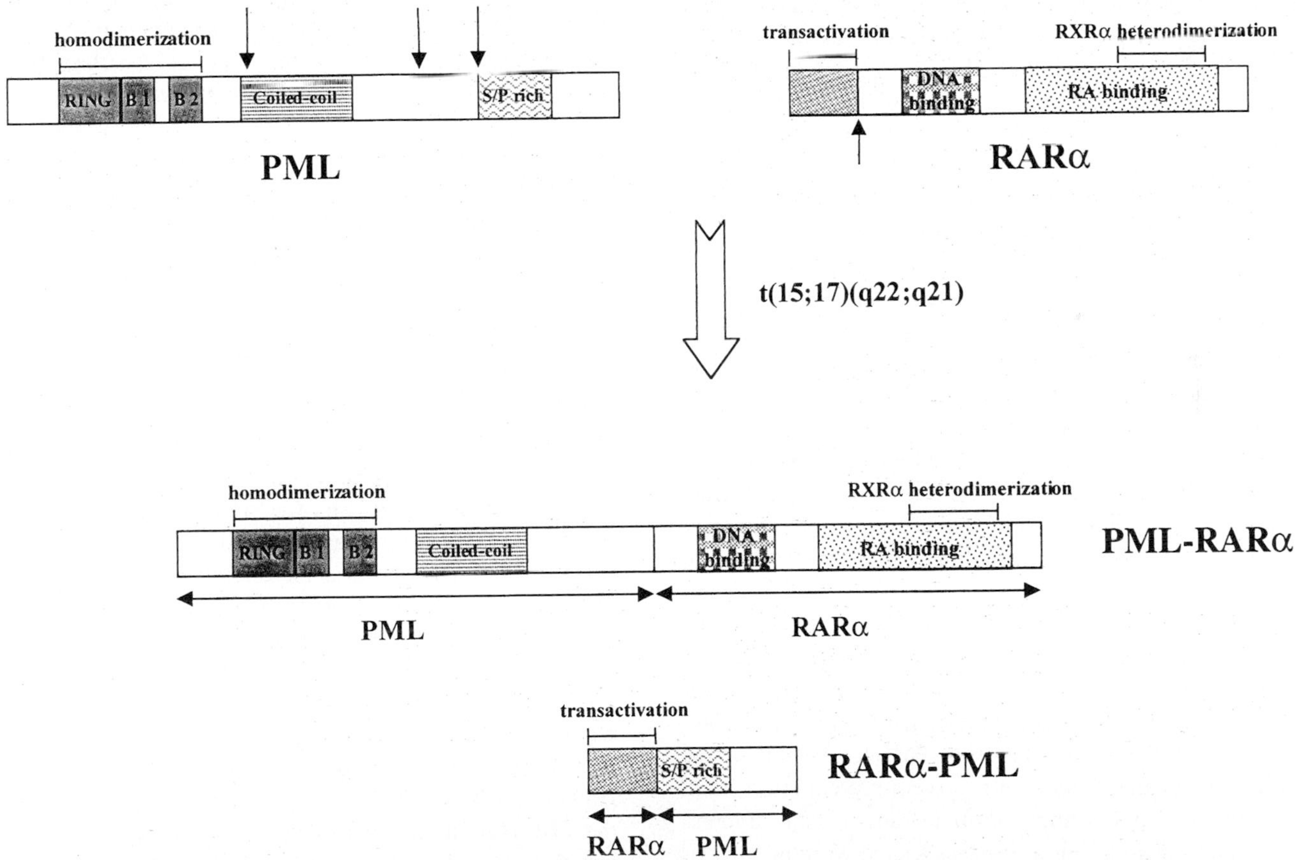

FIG. 8.1. Schematic representation of the wild-type *RARA, PML,* and their fusion proteins resulting from t(15;17). The modular configurations of RARα and PML with their distinct functional domains are indicated at the top panel. RARα contains a transactivation domain and a DNA-binding domain at its N-terminal portion and a retinoic acid (RA) binding domain and RXRα dimerization domain at its C-terminal portion. PML contains at its N-terminal part a RING finger-B Box domain, which represents the homodimerization interface for PML. The breakpoints where the proteins are fused are indicated by vertical arrows. PML-RARα contains the RING and B-box (with or without the coiled-coil region) of PML fused to almost the entire RARα. Because of the functional domains contributed by the partner proteins, PML-RARα can interfere with the retinoic acid–mediated transactivation pathway and the normal function of the wild-type PML. The reciprocal fusion protein RARα-PML consists of the transactivation domain of RARα fused to the C-terminal portion of PML. No definite biochemical functions have been attributed to RARα-PML.

roles in the pathogenesis of APL. Transgenic mice carrying *PML-RARA, PLZF-RARA,* or *NPM-RARA* fusion genes develop leukemias ranging from typical APL to CML-like leukemia preceded by a preleukemic phase, indicating that the *X-RARA* fusion genes are necessary but not sufficient for leukemogenicity (106,109,110). The oncogenicity of the fusion protein appears to rely on the interference of retinoic acid–mediated transactivation in the RARα/RXRα pathway and on disruption of normal function of the RARα partner proteins (106).

In the absence of RA, RARα is a transcription repressor (111). On binding to retinoic acid, RARα activates the transcription of genes required for cellular differentiation and growth inhibition (106). X-RARα, which can also heterodimerize with RXRα, binds DNA and retinoic acid. However, X-RARα are potent transcriptional repressors despite the presence of physiologic amounts of retinoic acid because of the inability of RXRα/RARα to dissociate from the corepressor complex (110). The sensitivity of these corepressor interactions to retinoic acid also determines the responsiveness of APL to pharmacologic doses of retinoic acid. High-dose retinoic acid can induce differentiation of malignant cells to mature granulocytes resulting in complete, albeit transient, remission in most cases of APL. However, APL associated with translocation between *RARA* and *PLZF* has a worse prognosis and a poor response to retinoic acid. Consistent with this, PML-RARα and NPM-RARα transgenic mice develop retinoic acid–sensitive leukemia, whereas PLZF-RARα transgenic mice develop retinoic acid–resistant leukemia (106,110,112). Corepressors can be dissociated from the complexes formed by PML-RARα or NPM-RARα by high-dose retinoic acid, but PLZF forms corepressor complexes that are insensitive to high-dose retinoic acid (110,112). These findings indicate a crucial role for interactions of these fusion proteins with corepressors and transcriptional silencing in APL pathogenesis and resistance to retinoic acid in APL.

The X-RARα fusion proteins can also interfere with the normal functions of the partner proteins through heterodimerization with the native partner proteins and inhibit their normal function in a dominant-negative fashion (106). Among the RARα partner proteins, PML has been the most studied. It contains domains for protein-protein interaction, including the RING finger domain, and it can suppress growth and transformation. It is associated with the nuclear matrix and is responsible for the formation of PML nuclear bodies, the presence of which are essential for the growth and tumor suppressor potential of PML (113,114). PML is a mediator of apoptosis by multiple signals, including FAS, tumor necrosis factor, and interferons (115). In APL with t(15;17) translocation, expression of PML-RARα leads to disruption of the nuclear bodies (114,116) and resistance of apoptosis in hematopoietic progenitor cells (115) presumably by a dominant-negative manner. This implicates a critical role for disruption of the growth- or tumor-suppressing and apoptosis inducing function of PML in the pathogenesis of APL.

The reciprocal RARα-PML fusion transcripts are detected in 70% to 80% of APL cases with t(15;17) (101,117,118), and the RARα-PLZF fusion transcripts are consistently found in all the cases with t(11;17) (114). The RARα-X fusion protein consists of the N-terminal transactivation domain of RARα and the C-terminal portion of the partner proteins. Preliminary transgenic mice studies show RARα-X fusion proteins alone do not lead to leukemia, although they can contribute to its development in the presence of X-RARα (106). However, little is known about the biochemical functions of X-RARα fusion proteins.

AML1-ETO in t(8;21)

The t(8;21)(q22;q22.3) translocation is present in approximately 10% to 15% of AMLs. It is predominantly, but not exclusively, associated with the AML subtype M2 (about 25% of M2 AML) and involves rearrangement of the *AML1* gene on chromosome 21 and the *ETO* gene on chromosome 8 (119,120). AML1 is a widely expressed transcription factor with approximately 70% homology to the *Drosophila* pair-rule gene, called *runt*, at its 5′ part (121,122). It forms the α subunit of the heterodimeric core-binding factor (CBF). The runt homology protein mediates specific DNA-binding and protein-protein interactions of AML1. The C-terminal end of AML contains a transactivation domain and nuclear-matrix–targeting signal that direct the protein to the appropriate nuclear matrix-associated foci. Based on the analysis of knockout mice, AML is an important regulator for hematopoiesis and regulates many hematopoietic genes (123,124). ETO, originally thought of as a DNA-binding transcription factor (125), was found to be a corepressor for the PLZF protein (126). Its C-terminal end was shown to interact with other corepressors, such as SMRT and N-CoR. Like AML1, it is also associated with the nuclear matrix (127). ETO itself has transforming properties *in vitro* (128).

The t(8;21) translocation fuses the N terminus of AML containing the DNA-binding runt domain to near full-length ETO (119,127,129,130). The C-terminal portion of AML1, which contains the transactivation domain and the nuclear-matrix–targeting signal, is not retained in the fusion protein. However, AML1-ETO can bind to DNA and dimerize with the CBP β subunit. Consequently, this fusion with ETO alters the intranuclear targeting and transcriptional activity of AML1. First, AML1-ETO is misrouted by the ETO component to alternate nuclear-matrix–associated foci, leading AML1 away from its native foci that support gene expression (131). Second, the substitution of the C-terminal portion of AML1 by the C-terminal part of ETO generates an aberrant transcriptional regulator because of the ability of ETO to recruit the transcriptional corepressors SMRT and N-CoR (126). AML-ETO therefore can antagonize the normal AML1 in a dominant-negative fashion. Both of these mechanisms can result in deregulation of AML effector genes, which is likely to be important for the pathogenesis of AML (132). Transgenic mice with a knockin *AML1-ETO* allele have impaired hematopoiesis similar to AML1-deficient mice, demonstrating the dominant-negative action of AML-ETO (133–135). Also seen in the AML1-ETO transgenic mice are dysplasia and increased renewal capacity of progenitors, properties that may be important in leukemogenesis (133).

MLL in Translocations Affecting 11q23

Chromosomal translocations affecting 11q23 are seen in approximately 9% of AMLs and in 5% of childhood precursor B-ALLs (96). Among the AML cases with 11q23 rearrangements, 50% are M5a, 20% are M4, 10% are M1 or M5b, and 5% are M2 (136,137). These chromosomal translocations are promiscuous (see Chromosomal Translocations section), resulting in fusion of the *MLL* gene (also called *ALL1* or *HRX*) on chromosome 11q23 to many alternative (>30) partner genes in different cases (44,137,138). The breakpoints at 11q23 span a genomic region of 8 kb between exons 5 and 11 of MLL, whereas the breakpoints at the partner genes are more variable (137,138). Based on molecular and cytogenetic data, the crucial chimeric gene is the 5′*MLL*-3′-partner fusion, which is consistently obtained in tumor cells (139).

The *MLL* gene encodes a putative transcription factor that shares homology with the Drosophila trithorax protein (140). It contains multiple DNA-binding structures: a centrally located zinc finger–like DNA-binding domain similar to trithorax, a domain with homology to DNA methyltransferase, and an N-terminal AT-hook DNA-binding motif of high mobility group proteins. Another domain with homology to trithorax that interacts with the chromatin remodeling system is located at the C terminus (141). The 11q23 translocations result in the formation of chimeric proteins that contain the N-terminal portion of MLL, including the AT-hook domain, the DNA methyltransferase domain, and the zinc finger–like domain fused to the partner protein (44).

More than 10 chimeric genes formed by translocations involving *MLL* have been identified (44), but no common features of the fusion partner genes can be found that can definitely explain the leukemogenicity of these fusion genes. The partner genes that fuse to *MLL* are heterogeneous, and their products can be generally classified into the following groups:

1. *Bona fide* transcription factors: AF4 (142); AF9 (143); ENL (144); AFX and AF6q21, forkhead transcription factors (145,146)
2. Factors related to transcription: CBP (CREB-binding protein), transcriptional coactivator (147); ELL, RNA polymerase elongation factor (148)
3. Cytoplasmic signaling proteins: EEN, a novel protein with SRC homology-3 (SH3) domain (149); AbI-1 (ABL-interacting protein) (150); AF6, an RAS-binding protein (151)
4. Septin family (cytoskeleton-associated GTPase): MSF (MLL septin-like fusion) (152); hCDCrel-1 (153); AF17q25 (154)
5. Others: AF1q (155), MEN (156), FEL (157), MLLT1, and MLLT3 (158).

The leukemogenicity of the fusion proteins is directly demonstrated by transgenic mice carrying the fusion gene *MLL-AF9*. These mice develop AML preceded by a nonmalignant myeloproliferation, indicating that *MLL-AF9* is necessary but not sufficient for the development of acute leukemia (159,160). Introduction of *MLL-ENL* into myeloid progenitors by retroviral gene transfer leads to their immortalization (161). The mechanism by which MLL fusion proteins lead to leukemogenesis is not clear, although a few reports have attempted to shed light on the mechanism of pathogenesis. It has been shown that MLL-ENL fusion protein is a potent transcriptional activator and that the DNA binding motifs present in the N terminus of MLL and transcriptional transactivation domain of ENL are indispensable for the transforming activity of MLL-ENL (162). This observation supports a model of AML pathogenesis in which the fusion protein induces transformation by deregulating subordinate genes through a gain-of-function mechanism. However, the N-terminal portion of *MLL* fused to the bacterial *LacZ* gene can cause acute leukemia in transgenic mice, although the disease is of long latency compared with that in the MLL-AF9 mice (163). This indicates that truncation and fusion of MLL to any partner protein *per se* can be leukemogenic. The importance of the N-terminal portion of MLL in leukemogenicity is supported by the observations that the N terminus of MLL itself can regulate myelomonocytic differentiation (164). MLL-ENL, MLL-ELL, and MLL-AF9 have also been shown to be negative regulators of post-DNA-damage–induced apoptosis (165). Inhibition of apoptosis of myeloid progenitors can be one of the pathogenic mechanisms of these fusion proteins.

CBFβ in Inv(16)(p13q22)

Inv(16)(p13q22) and its variants, t(16;16)(p13;q22) and del(16)(q22), are detected in 5% to 10% of AMLs. The 16q22 anomaly is present in all M4Eo cases and is rare in other AML subtypes (166,167). The gene involved is the heterodimeric core-binding factor (CBF) βa subunit gene on 16q, which becomes rearranged to the smooth muscle myosin heavy chain gene *(MYH11)* on 16p. This rearrangement generates a CBFβ-MYH11 fusion protein (168,169). This chimeric protein has transforming properties (170) and functions as a transcriptional corepressor for AML-1 (171), thereby interfering with normal transcriptional regulation by the AML1/CBFβ complex. The observation that both subunits of CBF (i.e., AML1 [CBFα] and CBFβ) are the targets of chromosomal translocations in AML underscores the importance of the CBF complex in myeloid differentiation.

DEK-CAN in t(6;9)

The translocation t(6;9)(p23;q34) is detected at a low frequency (about 1% of cases) (172). Although it is not associated with a specific subtype of AML according to the French-American-British classification, it appears to be associated with TdT-positive AML and an unfavorable prognosis (173). In this translocation, the 3′ portion of the gene *CAN* on chromosome 9q34 is fused to the 5′ part of the gene *DEK* on chromosome 6p23. The breakpoints at *CAN* and *DEK* occur at a specific intron. This results in the generation of an invariable fusion transcript that encodes a DEK-CAN fusion protein (174–178). DEK has been demonstrated to be an autoantigen in a subtype of juvenile rheumatoid arthritis (179). Moreover, it has been shown to bind to human immunodeficiency virus (HIV) enhancer, suggesting that it may function as a transcriptional regulator (180). CAN is a nucleoporin associated with the nuclear pore complex and plays a crucial role in nucleocytoplasmic transport processes (181). Although CAN is normally associated with the nuclear envelope, the fusion protein DEK-CAN is located in the nucleus (182). The significance of this relocation and the oncogenic function of DEK-CAN remain to be determined.

CHRONIC MYELOGENOUS LEUKEMIA

A pathognomonic feature of CML is the juxtaposition of the *BCR* gene on chromosome 22 and the *ABL* gene on chromosome 9 to form the chimeric *BCR-ABL* gene because of the chromosomal translocation t(9;22)(q34;q11) (96,183,184). In more than 95% of the cases, the translocation can be detected as the Philadelphia (Ph1) chromosome by standard cytogenetic analysis. In the rest of the cases, the translocation is masked karyotypically and can only be detected by other more sensitive molecular techniques.

ABL is a tyrosine kinase that is predominantly in the nucleus but is also present in the cytoplasm. It has three SH (SRC homology) domains (SH1, SH2, and SH3) at its N-terminal portion, as well as DNA and actin binding domains at the C-terminal portion. The SH3 domain is able to negatively regulate the SH1 domain, which has tyrosine kinase activity (29). BCR is a ubiquitously expressed cytoplasmic protein that possesses serine/threonine kinase activity at the N-terminal portion (185). It also contains an N-terminal SH2 binding domain and GTPase activating domain within the C-terminal portion (186,187). Depending on the precise breakpoint within the *BCR* gene, fusion proteins of two different molecular masses, 210 kd (BCR-ABL p210) or 190 kd (BCR-ABL p190), can be produced (Fig. 8.2). Both p190 and p210 contain the same *ABL*-derived coding sequence, but they differ in the number of *BCR*-derived amino acids. In almost all cases of CML, the breakpoint in the *BCR* gene is grouped in the major breakpoint cluster region (188). This results in the production of the larger chimeric protein p210 (183,188,189). In rare cases of CML, the breakpoint occurs 40 kb upstream of the major breakpoint cluster region in the *BCR* gene (i.e., minor breakpoint cluster region) (190,191). This leads to the production of the smaller chimeric protein p190, which is mainly associated with precursor B-ALL (192–196). In both p210 and p190, the N-terminal serine/threonine kinase domain and SH2 domain of BCR is fused to almost the entire coding domain of ABL (Fig. 8.2).

The oncogenic potential of BCR-ABL has been demonstrated using *in vitro* transformation assays and *in vivo* mouse models. In several *in vivo* mouse models, expression of BCR-ABL p210 in bone marrow cells by retroviral transduction or by transgenic method efficiently induces a myeloproliferative disease similar to CML (197,198). These mouse models would be most useful for the study of the pathogenesis and treatment of CML and to investigate the functional domains of BCR-ABL that are necessary for the pathogenesis of CML. However, mice carrying the *BCR-ABL* transgene expressing p190 develop acute leukemia of the B-cell lineage, analogous to precursor B-ALL in humans (199–203). The difference in phenotypes of these transgenic mice demonstrates the difference in biologic activities of the p210 and p190 proteins.

The ABL kinase domain and the BCR sequences have been shown to be essential for the ability of BCR-ABL to cause myeloproliferative disease *in vivo* (186). Unlike ABL, BCR-ABL is cytoplasmic in location, which may contribute to its oncogenicity. BCR-ABL shows activated ABL kinase activity. This results from binding of the N-terminal portion of BCR to the SH2 domain of ABL, which inhibits the negative regulatory activity of the SH3 domain on the tyrosine kinase activity (29,186). Through protein-protein interactions mediated by multiple functional domains, BCR-ABL can bind to and phosphorylate different effectors, activating signal transduction pathways important for regulating many cellular functions (20,25). The oncogenicity of BCR-ABL probably results from its ability to stimulate proliferation by activating the RAS signal transduction pathway, PI3-K (phosphatidyl inositol 3′ kinase) pathway, and MYC; to inhibit apoptosis; and to increase cell adhesive abnormalities, which may play a role in the dissemination of the tumor cells (29). Further research is necessary to fully understand the role played by these pathways and cellular functions affected by BCR-ABL.

CML can progress from an indolent phase to a fatal blast crisis. This disease progression is associated with additional genetic alterations, which are largely unknown. Accumulating evidence shows that mutations in *TP53* are associated with 15% to 20% of blast crises but rarely with the chronic phase (204–206). *TP53* mutations in these cases are closely associated with the loss of chromosome 17p, the site of p53, through the formation of isochromosome i(17)q and, less frequently, through unbalanced translocations (207). The importance of p53 inactivation in the blast crisis is directly demonstrated by a study that shows that *BCR-ABL* (p210) transgenic, $TP53^{-}$ heterozygous ($p53^{+/-}$) mice develop in a short latency blastic crisis preceded by a chronic myeloproliferative phase. The residual *TP53* allele is frequently inactivated in the tumor tissues (208).

Another genetic lesion associated with blast crisis is the

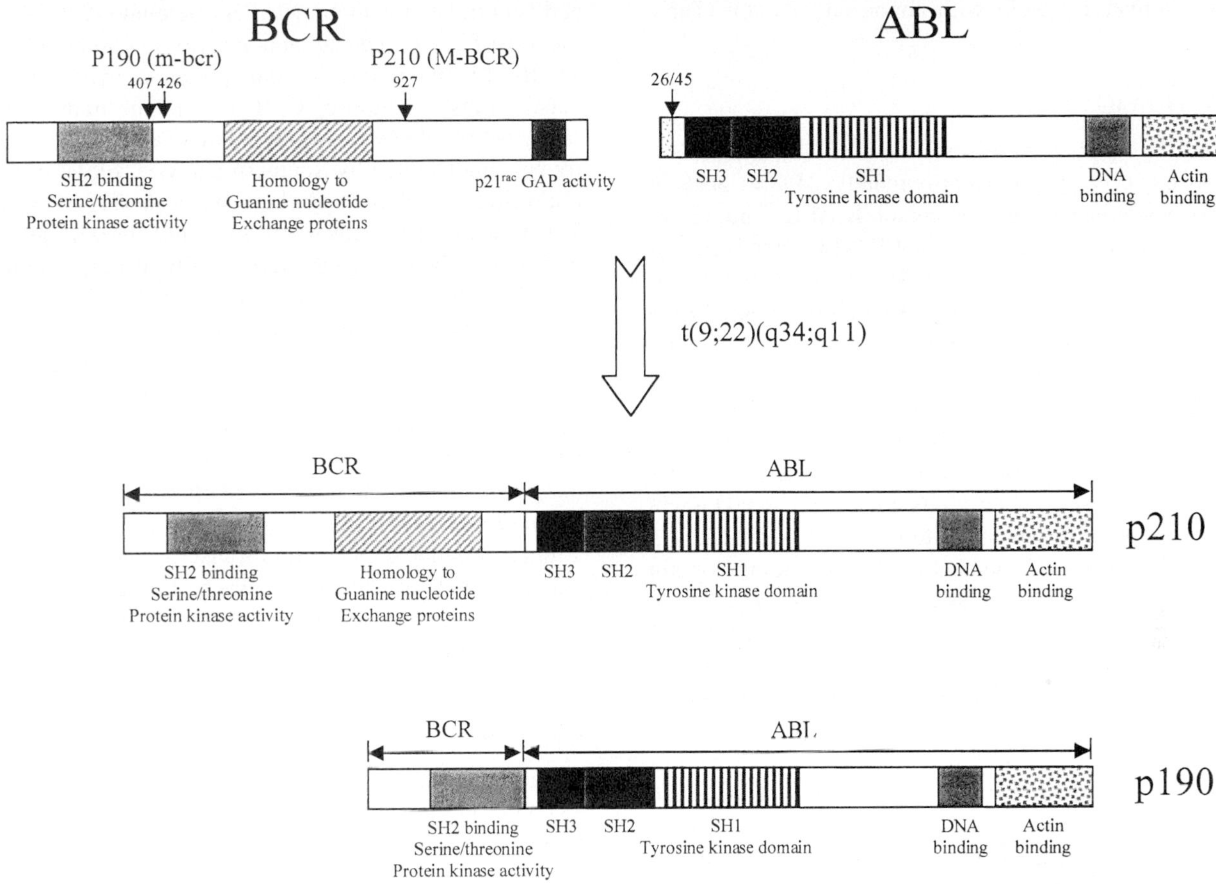

FIG. 8.2. Schematic representation of protein fusion between BCR and ABL in t(9;22)(q34;q11). The modular organizations of BCR and ABL are shown in the top panel. BCR contains an N-terminal SH2 binding domain, which overlaps with a region with serine/threonine kinase activity, a central domain with homology to proteins with guanine nucleotide exchange activity, and a C terminus with GTPase-activating protein (GAP) activity for $p21^{rac}$, a member of the RAS-related small GTPase family. ABL contains three SRC homology (SH) domains: SH1, which has tyrosine kinase activity; SH2; and SH3, which negatively regulates SH1. ABL possesses DNA- and actin-binding domains at the C terminus. The first 26 or 45 amino acids of ABL are encoded by alternative exons 1a or 1b, respectively. The breakpoints where the proteins are fused are indicated by vertical arrows. The number corresponds to the amino acid number where the breakpoints occur. The point of fusion at the carboxyl terminus of BCR depends on whether the translocation breakpoints are located at the major breakpoint cluster region (M-BCR) or minor breakpoint cluster region (m-bcr). The point of fusion at the amino terminus of ABL is located at amino acid 26 of type 1a ABL, which corresponds to amino acid 45 of type 1b ABL. BCR-ABL p210 produced by t(9;22) involving the M-BCR consists of 927 BCR-derived amino acids fused to ABL. BCR-ABL p190 produced by t(9;22) involving the m-bcr consists of 407 or 426 amino acids (depending on the exact location of the breakpoint at m-bcr) fused to ABL. In both p210 and p190, the ABL-derived sequence is the same and represents the near full-length product (amino acids encoded by *ABL* exon 1 are not present). The SH2-binding domain of BCR interacts with the SH2 domain of ABL in BCR-ABL and constitutively activates ABL kinase activity.

fusion between *AML* gene and *EVI1* gene because of chromosomal translocation t(3;21)(q26;q22), which can be detected up to 1% of AML cases (130). This translocation results in the formation of a chimeric transcription factor consisting of the *runt* homology domain of AML1 and the zinc finger DNA-binding and acidic transactivation domains of EVI-1. This fusion protein may contribute to tumor progression in CML by blocking cell differentiation and stimulation of proliferation (209).

Other genetic alterations involved in blast crisis include inactivation of p16. Homozygous deletions of p16 occur in up to 40% to 50% of blast crises of the lymphoid type but are not present in blast crises of the myeloid type (210,211).

ACUTE LEUKEMIA OF B-CELL LINEAGE

The clinical heterogeneity of acute leukemia of the B lineage is reflected at the molecular level by the presence of specific chromosomal translocations, which often have prognostic significance. These translocations predominantly involve fusion of two protooncogenes, resulting in the formation of a chimeric protein with abnormal function (Table 8.1).

E2A-PBX1 in t(1;19)

The t(1:19)(q23;p13) translocation is common in precursor B-ALLs, occurring in approximately 25% to 30% of childhood cytoplasmic Ig^+ precursor B-ALLs and 1% of childhood cytoplasmic Ig^- precursor B-ALLs, and is associated with a poor prognosis (212). This translocation juxtaposes a transcription factor *E2A* gene on chromosome 19p13 with a homeobox gene *PBX1* on 1q23, leading to the formation of a fusion gene that encodes a chimeric transcription factor (213,214). The E2A protein is widely expressed in human tissues and contains the transcriptional activation domain at the N-terminal portion and a basic helix-loop-helix DNA binding site at the C terminus. PBX is a homeodomain transcription factor that is ubiquitously expressed except in the B and T lineages. It contains the DNA-binding domain and the adjacent HOX-cooperativity domain (for interaction with other homeodomain proteins). The fusion E2A-PBX1 fusion protein contains the N-terminal transactivation domain of E2A fused to the C-terminal DNA-binding homeodomain and HOX cooperativity motif of PBX1 (213–215).

The E2A-PBX1 fusion transcription factor has been demonstrated to have oncogenic potential by *in vitro* and *in vivo* experiments. E2A-PBX1 causes T-cell lymphomas and myeloid leukemia in mice, transforms fibroblasts, and blocks differentiation of cultured myeloid progenitors (216–219). These observations demonstrate directly the leukemogenicity of E2A-PBX1 and strongly support the involvement of E2A-PBX1 in the pathogenesis of ALL of B lineage.

The oncogenicity of E2A-PBX1 appears to depend on dimeric interaction of the fusion protein with other homeodomain proteins mediated by the HOX cooperativity motif and on the conversion of a DNA-binding nonactivator to a constitutive transcriptional activator because of the E2A transactivation domain (217,220). The ectopic expression of E2A-PBX1 in the B lineage (PBX1 is not normally expressed in B cells) can lead to aberrant activation of tissue- and developmental-specific genes normally regulated by the dimers formed between PBX and its partner homeodomain proteins (221).

Studies on the target genes of E2A-PBX1 have provided insights into the mechanism of transformation by E2A-PBX1. Several genes have been shown to be upregulated by E2A-PBX1. These include those for granulocyte colony-stimulating factor (222); *EB1,* a tyrosine kinase signal transduction gene not normally expressed in B-cell precursors (223); *WNT16,* a member of the *WNT* gene family (224); and the gene for angiogenin-3, a new member of the angiogenin family (225).

TEL-AML1 in t(12;21)

The t(12;21)(p12;q22) translocation is specifically observed in approximately 25% of pediatric precursor B-ALLs and is correlated with an excellent outcome (226,227). It is the most frequent genetic abnormality in childhood precursor B-ALL but is rare in adult precursor ALL and in the blastic transformation of CML (228). The translocation is rarely detectable by conventional cytogenetics but can readily be demonstrated by Southern analysis, FISH, or reverse transcriptase–polymerase chain reaction (RT-PCR) (226). This translocation leads to the fusion of the *TEL* gene with *AML1.* TEL belongs to the ETS family of transcription factors (229). It contains an N-terminal "pointed" domain that has transcriptional repression activity (230). The ETS domain at its C terminus mediates specific DNA binding. AML1 is a transcription factor that constitutes the α subunit of the heterodimeric CBF (see *AML1-ETO* in t(8;21) section). Chromosomal translocations result in the fusion of the pointed domain to nearly the entire AML1 transcription factor (231,232). This fusion appears to convert AML1 from a transcriptional activator to a transcriptional repressor and may contribute to leukemogenesis by the specific inhibition of AML-1–dependent activation of normal target genes (230,233,234).

BCR-ABL in t(9;22)

The *BCR-ABL* rearrangements that result from t(9;22)(q34;q11) are present in precursor B-ALL at different frequencies, according to the age of onset (children, 2% to 5%; adults, 25% to 40%) (235–237). In about 50% of the cases, breakpoints on chromosome 22 differ from those detected in CML and occur 40 kb upstream of the site involved in CML, resulting in the production of a fusion protein p190 (192–196). In the remaining cases, t(9;22) chromosomal translocation results in the production of p210, similar to that of CML. Independent of the type of BCR-ABL protein produced, t(9;22)-positive ALL signifies a very poor prognosis (238).

MLL in Translocations Affecting 11q23

The 11q23 rearrangements can be detected in approximately 5% of childhood precursor B-ALLs. Among the promiscuous translocations involving 11q23, the t(4;11)(q21;q23) is predominantly (95% of t(4;11) cases) associated with precursor B-ALL. One half of these occur in childhood, with one third present in infants (>1 year) (137,239). The t(4;11) results in fusion of MLL with AF4, a transcription factor.

E2A-HLF in t(17;19)

E2A can also be fused to the partner gene *HLF* in the chromosomal translocation t(17;19)(q22;p13), which occurs in 1% of childhood precursor B-ALLs (215). HLF is a transcription factor that possesses a PAR (proline- and acidic amino acid–rich region) domain at its amino-terminal portion and a basic leucine zipper (bZIP) domain at the carboxyl terminus for DNA-binding and heterodimerization. It is normally expressed in liver but is not expressed in hematopoietic cells. The t(17;19) translocation generates a fusion protein composed of the N-terminal transactivation domain of E2A and the C-terminal bZIP domain of HLF (240). The transforming function of E2A-HLF depends on its ability to alter transcription of effector genes through a gain-of-function mechanism (241).

MYC in t(8;14), t(2;8), or t(8;22)

MYC rearrangements due to chromosomal translocations involving 8q24 to one of the immunoglobulin gene loci on chromosomes 14, 2, or 8 are associated with B-cell ALL (ALL L3), which is considered a leukemic form of Burkitt's lymphoma. Details of the molecular architecture of the breakpoint and the role of *MYC* in tumorigenesis are discussed in the section on Burkitt's lymphoma.

P16 and P15

Inactivation of cell cycle inhibitors may also play a role in the pathogenesis of ALL. Homozygous deletion of p16, mostly with co-deletion of p15, can be seen in 6.5% to 36% of precursor B-ALLs in different studies, suggesting a pathogenetic role of p16 and p15 in this malignancy (242). Point mutations of the genes for p15 and p16 are rare (242).

NRAS

Mutations in *NRAS* have been reported in 15% to 20% of precursor B-ALLs (57). However, other reports find only infrequent *NRAS* mutations in precursor B-ALL (243,244).

TP53 and *TP73*

TP53 point mutations are rare (about 2%) in precursor B-ALL and is more frequent (up to 50%) in ALL L3 (245). *TP73,* a new putative tumor suppressor gene related to *TP53,* is inactivated by hypermethylation in approximately 30% of precursor B-ALLs, suggesting a role for p73 in the development of pre-B-ALL (246).

ACUTE LEUKEMIA OF THE T-CELL LINEAGE

Precursor T-ALL is a relatively uncommon disease and accounts for only 15% of the newly diagnosed ALL cases in the United States. Oncogene activation in precursor T-ALL can occur as a result of transcriptional deregulation, or rarely, protein fusion resulting from chromosomal translocations. The most specific and frequent genetic lesions involved in the pathogenesis of precursor T-ALL are described subsequently (Table 8.1).

TAL1 in t(1;14)

The *TAL1* gene is located on chromosome 1p32 and is the most frequently rearranged gene in precursor T-lymphoblastic leukemia (approximately 30%) (247). It encodes a protein of the basic helix-loop-helix (bHLH) transcription family with marked homology to LYL-1 and TAL-2, two other bHLH proteins involved in chromosomal translocations in precursor T-ALL (248). TAL binds to E-box enhancers as heterodimers with the E-Box HLH proteins, suggesting that TAL may function as a transcriptional regulator that influences cell-type determination in hematopoiesis (248,249). In about 3% to 5% of T-ALL cases, the 5′ portion of the *TAL1* gene is altered as a consequence of the t(1; 14)(p32; q11) translocation. Consequently, the entire TAL coding sequence is juxtaposed to the gene for TCR-δ. In about 25% of cases, however, TAL is altered at its 5′ portion by cytogenetically undetectable site-specific deletions of approximately 90 kb, which juxtapose the coding exons of TAL to the noncoding exon of SIL, a gene located centromeric to TAL and actively transcribed during T-cell development (250,251). This rearrangement results in the production of a chimeric SIL-TAL transcript, which codes for a full-length TAL protein. Whereas TAL is not expressed in normal T cells, the t(1;14) translocation and submicroscopic deletions lead to the ectopic expression of TAL in T cells by the regulatory elements of TCR-δ and SIL, respectively (251,252).

Based on the homology between the breakpoint junction sequences and the recombination signal sequence of immunoglobulin/TCR, the rearrangement between *TAL* and *SIL* is thought to be mediated by aberrant V-D-J recombinase (252) (see Chromosomal Translocation section). These site-specific deletions are restricted to T cells of the TCR $\alpha\beta$ lineage, suggesting that they may be mediated by the same deletion mechanism as TCR-δ gene deletion (252). The oncogenicity of *TAL1* has been directly demonstrated by *in vitro* and transgenic mice studies. Transgenic mice carrying *TAL1* gene driven by a T-cell specific promoter develop T-cell malignancies (249,253).

The mechanism by which TAL-1 exerts its oncogenicity is unknown. It is proposed that TAL-1 may compete with other tissue-specific HLH proteins for binding to common E-box HLH proteins, thereby interfering with the formation of heterodimeric bHLH complexes that drive cellular differentiation (254,255).

HOX11 in t(10;14)

The chromosomal translocation t(10;14)(q24;q11) is observed in 4% to 7% of precursor T-ALLs (255) and involves the *HOX11* gene. *HOX11* codes for a homeobox-containing transcription factor important for controlling expression of developmentally important genes related to the genesis of the spleen (256,257). In this translocation, the *HOX11* gene on chromosome 10 is juxtaposed to the TCR-δ gene, resulting in ectopic expression of HOX11 in thymocytes (256,258,259). Deregulation of *HOX11* in precursor T-ALL may represent the first example of involvement of homeobox genes in human cancer.

Several observations demonstrate that deregulation of *HOX11* may play an important role in the development of precursor T-ALL. First, HOX11 can immortalize murine hematopoietic precursors *in vitro* (257). Moreover, mice transplanted with bone marrow cell lines containing HOX-11–expressing retrovirus develop precursor T-cell leukemia–like malignancy after a long latency (260). Mice expressing the *HOX11* transgene in the thymus develop T-cell lymphoma (261). The leukemogenicity of HOX11 may depend on its ability to promote cell survival (262) or to abrogate the G_2/M cell cycle checkpoint (261).

TTG1/rhombotin-1/*LMO1* and *TTG2*/rhombotin-2/*LMO2* in t(11;14)(p15;q11) and t(11;14)(p13;q11)

TTG1 and *TTG2* (also designated *LMO1* and *LMO2*) are two members of the rhombotin gene family that are the targets of chromosomal translocations t(11;14)(p15;q11) and t(11;14)(p13;q11), respectively. The t(11;14)(p15;q11) translocation is rarely found in precursor T-ALL, whereas t(11;14)(p13;q11) is found in 5% to 10% of precursor T-ALLs (263,264). *TTG1* and *TTG2* encode non–DNA-binding transcription regulators that possess the cysteine-rich LIM domains that mediate protein-protein interactions (265–267). TTG-1 is expressed in neural linage cells but not in T cells (268). TTG-2 is strongly expressed in hematopoietic progenitors of the myeloid and erythroid lineages and is expressed at a very low level in the thymus during early development (264,269). TTG-2 can interact with TAL and GATA-1 in an erythroid transcriptional complex (270) and plays a central role in early hematopoiesis, probably at the level of the pluripotent stem cells (271). As a result of chromosomal translocations, *TTG1* or *TTG2* is associated with the $\alpha\delta$ T-cell receptor gene locus, leading to deregulated or ectopic expression (263,264). In the case of *TTG2,* the breakpoints occur upstream of the gene (265,266).

Deregulated expression of TTG-1 or TTG-2 in transgenic mice results in immature T-cell acute lymphoblastic leukemia, which demonstrates directly their leukemogenicity (272,273). They may help cause tumors by disturbing T-cell differentiation through gene deregulation (274).

NOTCH1 in t(7;9)

NOTCH1 (formerly designated *TAN1*) is located on chromosome 7 and is translocated to the TCR-β locus on chromosome 9. This t(7;9) translocation is rarely detected in precursor T-ALL. *NOTCH1* is the human homologue of the *Drosophila notch* gene that encodes a transmembrane receptor that helps determine cell fate during development (275). The breakpoints occur within 100 bp of an intron in *NOTCH1*, resulting in the formation of a truncated transcript and truncated protein consisting only of the intracellular domain (276). Truncated NOTCH-1 protein in precursor T-ALL has been shown to be transforming. This truncated protein is located in the nucleus instead of the cell surface and is believed to be constitutively active (277). Truncated NOTCH-1 can bind to CBF-1 (also called RBPJk), a transcriptional repressor, through its N-terminal region and activates transcription of *CBF1* target genes (278,279).

Other Genetic Lesions

Chromosomal translocations t(8;14)(q24;q21) can be detected in about 2% of precursor T-ALL. In these translocations, the TCR-α locus at 14q21 is juxtaposed 3′ to the *MYC* gene at 8q24, resulting in its transcriptional deregulation. This configuration of translocations is similar to the variant translocations involving immunoglobulin light chain loci in Burkitt's lymphoma. Fusion of *MLL* with *ENL* in t(11;19)(q23;p13.3) is also rarely observed in precursor T-ALL (137). Mutations in *TP53* are infrequent (5%) in childhood precursor T-ALL but tend to be associated with poor clinical outcome. *RAS* mutations are also infrequently (4%) found (280). P15 and p16 appear to be frequently altered by homozygous deletions of their genes in T-ALL, with a frequency of up to 83% for p16 (242,281). The genes for p15 and p16 may also be inactivated by hypermethylation in precursor T-ALL, with hypermethylation of *TP15* occurring more frequently (280,282). Point mutations in *TP15* and *TP16* are rare (242).

B-CELL NON-HODGKIN'S LYMPHOMAS

The Revised European-American Lymphoma (REAL) classification and the most recent World Health Organization (WHO) classification separate NHLs into distinct categories based on morphology, immunophenotype, and molecular genetics (283,284). In B-cell NHL, these distinct entities are often associated with specific genetic lesions (Table 8.2). Each of these lesions is critical to the transformation process of mature B cells at a specific stage of differentiation (Fig. 8.3). Almost all types of B-cell NHL have reciprocal chromosomal translocations leading to transcriptional deregulation of protooncogenes. An exception is chronic lymphocytic leukemia, which does not possess translocations, suggesting a biologically different mechanism of pathogenesis. The following section describes the genes involved in the pathogenesis of the main types of B-cell lymphomas.

B-Cell Chronic Lymphocytic Leukemia

Using interphase cytogenetics, the most frequent chromosomal aberrations in B-cell chronic lymphocytic leukemia/small lymphocytic lymphoma (CLL/SLL) are deletions involving chromosome band 13q14, followed by deletions of the genomic region 11q22.3-q23.1, trisomy 12, deletions of 6q21-q23, and deletions at 17p13 (94,95). Except for *TP53* at the 17p13 locus, the candidate genes for these chromosomal aberrations are yet to be identified. Because B-CLL is a disease of clonal expansion of mature B cells, most of which are not proliferating, it is possible that these chromosomal

TABLE 8.2. *Protooncogenes and tumor suppressor genes in non-Hodgkin's lymphoma*

Genes	Chromosomal translocation	Biologic function	Mechanism of activation or inactivation	Lymphoma type
Protooncogenes				
API2	t(11;18)(q21;q21)	Regulator of apoptosis?	Protein fusion	MALT
MLT				
BCL1	t(11;14)(q13;q32)	Cyclin D1/cell cycle regulator	Transcription, deregulation	MCL
BCL2	t(14;18)(q32;q21)	Inner mitochondrial membrane protein, regulator of apoptosis	Transcription, deregulation	FL, a subset of DLCL
BCL6	t(3;v)(q27;v)[a]	Transcription factor	Transcription, deregulation	DLCL
BCL10	t(1;14)(p22;q32)	Regulator of apoptosis	Protein truncation, transcription, deregulation	MALT
LYT10	t(10;14)(q24;q32)	Transcription factor/NF-κB family	Protein truncation	CTCL
MYC	t(8;14)(q24;q32) t(2;8)(p11;q24) t(8;22)(q24;q11)	Transcription factor	Transcription, deregulation	BL
NPM	t(2;5)(p23;q35)	Nucleolar phosphoprotein, receptor tyrosine kinase	Protein fusion	ALCL
ALK				
PAX5	t(9;14)(p13;q32)	Transcription factor	Transcription, deregulation	LPL
Tumor suppressor genes				
TP53 (p53)		Transcription factor, maintains genomic stability	Point mutation;deletion	B-CLL;BL;ATLL;Transformed FL and MCL
CDKN2B (p15)		Cell cycle regulator (cdk inhibitor)	Deletion; hypermethylation	Transformed NHL
CDKN2A (p16)		Cell cycle regulator (cdk inhibitor)	Deletion; hypermethylation	Transformed NHL
CDKN1A (p21)		Cell cycle regulator (cdk inhibitor)	Deletion	Transformed NHL
ATM		Protein kinase, maintains genomic stability	Point mutation, deletion	MCL

ALCL, anaplastic large cell lymphoma; ATLL, adult T-cell leukemia/lymphoma; BL, Burkitt's lymphoma; CLL, B-cell chronic lymphocytic leukemia; CTCL, cutaneous T-cell lymphoma; DLCL, diffuse large B-cell lymphoma; FL, follicular lymphoma; LPL, lymphoplasmacytoid lymphoma; MALT, extranodal marginal zone B-cell lymphoma of mucosa-associated lymphoid tissue; MCL, mantle cell lymphoma; NHL, non-Hodgkin's lymphoma.

[a] More than 10 different partner chromosomal sites, including IgH, are identified.

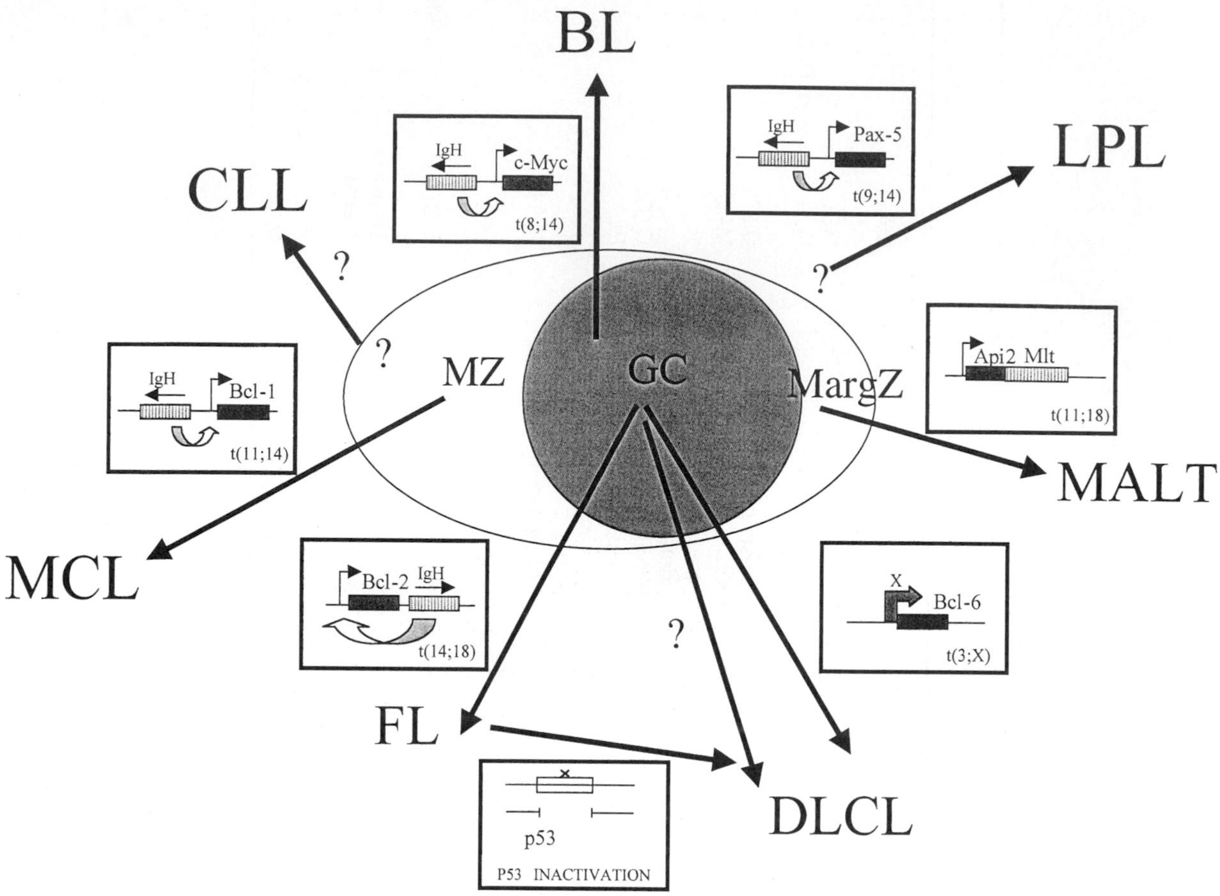

FIG. 8.3. Genetic pathways in B-cell lymphomagenesis. The categories of B-cell non-Hodgkin's lymphoma (CLL, B-cell chronic lymphocytic leukemia; LPL, lymphoplasmacytoid lymphoma; MCL, mantle cell lymphoma; FL, follicular lymphoma; DLCL, diffuse large B-cell lymphoma; BL, Burkitt's lymphoma; and MALT, extranodal marginal zone B-cell lymphoma of the MALT type) are shown with the mature B-cell compartments from which they are postulated to be derived (MZ, mantle zone; GC, germinal center; and MargZ, marginal zone). The normal counterparts of CLL and LPL are controversial. The protooncogenes activated by the typical chromosomal translocations in B-NHL are schematically depicted in boxes. *BCL1, BCL2, MYC,* and *PAX5* are deregulated by enhancer elements of the IgH locus *(curved arrows). BCL6* is deregulated through promoter substitution *(bold arrow)* by different partner genes (X). *AMPI2-MLT* in MALT lymphoma is a fusion gene. *TP53* with its classic inactivation pattern (point mutation, indicated by cross, of one allele and deletion of the other allele) is also shown in the progression of follicular lymphomas to DLCL. The genetic lesions involved in CLL and a subset of DLCL remain to be determined.

abnormalities generate genetic lesions that facilitate evasion of apoptosis of the CLL cells (285). Deletion of 13q14.3 is seen in approximately 50% of cases, suggesting the existence of one or more tumor suppressor genes in this locus. The identity of the genes is unknown.

Deletion in 11q22-q23 is detected in 20% of B-CLL cases and is associated with extensive nodal involvement and inferior prognosis (286). A candidate gene in this chromosomal site is *ATM,* which is found to be disrupted at both alleles by deletion and point mutation in approximately 20% of cases with deletion in 11q22-q23 (287).

Trisomy 12 is detected in 10% to 20% of B-CLL cases. It is rarely found in typical CLL (288) but is associated with a subgroup of B-CLL with atypical morphology and immunophenotype, including CLL/PL, stronger surface immunoglobulin and FMC-7 expression, expression of CD11a, and adverse prognosis (289–291). The mechanism of transformation by trisomy 12 is unknown, but it is postulated that extra copies of one of more genes on chromosome 12 may lead to lymphomagenesis.

TP53 mutations are found in approximately 10% of cases and are associated with an increased number of prolymphocytes, advanced clinical stage, and poor prognosis (292,293). *TP53* mutations may also play a role in Richter's transformation (294).

Lymphoplasmacytoid Lymphoma

Lymphoplasmacytoid lymphoma (LPL) is a low-grade lymphoma composed of small lymphocytes, plasmacytoid lymphocytes, and plasma cells (283). The t(9;14)(p13;q32) translocation is found in approximately 50% of LPL cases. The target of this translocation is *PAX5* (295), which encodes a B-cell–specific transcription factor of the paired box family that plays a critical role in commitment to the B-cell lineage (296). Molecular cloning of the t(9;14) breakpoints in a LPL case shows that the breakpoints are located at the 5′ noncoding portion of the *PAX5* gene and the switch region of the IgH locus, which is juxtaposed in an opposite transcriptional orientation to *PAX5*. This rearrangement results in transcriptional deregulation of *PAX5*. Further experiments are required to demonstrate directly the lymphomagenic potential of *PAX5*.

Mantle Cell Lymphoma

Mantle cell lymphoma (MCL) is characterized cytogenetically by the chromosomal translocation t(11;14)(q13;q32) (297). The 11q13 breakpoints are dispersed over a genomic region of more than 100 kb. However, in approximately 50% of cases, the breakpoints are tightly clustered in the major translocation cluster (MTC) region at the *BCL1 (PRAD1)* locus (298–302). *BCL1* encodes cyclin D1, a member of the G1 cyclins, which is not normally expressed in lymphocytes. Its expression is related to the cell cycle, levels are highest in the G1 phase and lowest in S phase (303). The t(11;14) translocation results in deregulation of the *BCL1* gene by regulatory elements of the IgH locus (304–307). *BCL1* gene overexpression is a highly sensitive and specific marker of mantle cell lymphoma. Although *BCL1* gene rearrangement can be detected only in approximately 50% of cases, overexpression of cyclin D1 can be detected in most MCLs and is only rarely present in other benign or malignant lymphoproliferative disorders (308–312).

Cyclin D1 is important for triggering cells to progress from G_0/G_1 to S phase of the cell cycle and promoting cell proliferation. Its function depends on formation of a complex with the cyclin-dependent kinase CDK-4, which binds to and phosphorylate RB, resulting in G_0/S phase transition (313–315). Overexpression of cyclin D1 in the B-cell compartment of transgenic mice leads to B-cell lymphomas in cooperation with MYC, demonstrating directly the lymphomagenicity of cyclin D1 (316,317). However, despite the established biochemical role of cyclin D1 in cell cycle control and the increase in cellular proliferation observed on constitutive cyclin D1 expression in murine epithelial tissues (318–320), enforced expression of cyclin D1 alone in the B-cell compartment of transgenic mice does not cause significant cell-cycle abnormalities (316,317). The precise role of cyclin D1 in the pathogenesis of MCL needs to be further defined.

Besides t(11;14), deletion of the chromosomal region 11q22-q23 is a frequent chromosomal aberration in MCL (85). The *ATM* tumor suppressor gene located at this chromosomal site is inactivated in about 75% of MCL cases by deletion and deleterious point mutations (86). This finding implicates an important role for ATM in the pathogenesis of MCL.

Aggressive variants of mantle cell lymphoma are associated with additional genetic alterations besides BCL1 overexpression. These include *TP53* gene mutations and protein overexpression (321–323) and deletions or loss of expression of genes for cell cycle inhibitors p15, p16, and p21 (324,325). Deletions and loss of expression of p16 and p21 appear to occur in a subset of aggressive variants of mantle cell lymphoma with a wild-type p53, suggesting that these genetic alterations may represent alternate pathways in the pathogenesis of these aggressive variants of MCL (325).

Follicular Lymphoma

Chromosomal translocation t(14;18)(q32;q21) is present in 80% to 90% of follicular lymphomas and involves the *BCL2* gene at the 18q21 locus. The protein product of the *BCL2* gene is an integral membrane protein that acts as a negative regulator of apoptosis (see the Protooncogenes section). The t(14;18) translocation juxtaposes the 3′ portion of the *BCL2* gene to the IgH locus (326–330) (Fig. 8.4). Approximately 70% of the breakpoints are in the major breakpoint region (MBR), joining the *BCL2* 3′UTR with the J_H segment. The remaining breakpoints are clustered within the minor cluster region (mcr) located 3′ of the MBR (330). Novel t(14;18) breakpoints have been found approximately 800 bp downstream of MBR in the 3′ untranslated region of BCL-2 (331). The t(14;18) translocation results in overexpression of a normal BCL-2, mainly through transcriptional activation by the Ig regulatory elements (332,333). In those follicular lymphomas with t(14;18) breakpoints located at the MBR region, BCL-2–Ig fusion mRNAs with J_H and $C\mu$ 3′ end can also be produced. These fusion mRNAs have a posttranscriptional processing advantage, possibly related to RNA splicing or nucleocytoplasmic transport (334).

In the B-cell compartment, BCL-2 appears to be important for the emergence of long-living memory cells by promoting survival of antigen-selected germinal center cells (335). Deregulation of BCL-2 expression can contribute to the pathogenesis of follicular lymphoma by preventing apoptosis of germinal center cells that are normally destined to die (336). The role of this mechanism in follicular lymphomagenesis is supported by the studies of transgenic mice with enforced expression of BCL-2 in B cells, which develop follicular lymphoproliferative disease composed of long-lived B cells analogous to human follicular lymphoma (337). Like human follicular lymphomas, a fraction of these indolent follicular lymphomas can progress to large cell lymphoma. In mice, this histologic transformation is frequently associated with *MYC* gene rearrangements (338).

In addition to *BCL2* gene rearrangement, deletions in 6q27 occur in approximately 20% of cases of follicular lymphoma (93). Additional genetic alterations are associated with histologic transformation of follicular lymphoma. These include *TP53* mutations (80% of cases) (339,340), *TP16* inactivation due to deletion or hypermethylation (100% of cases) (341),

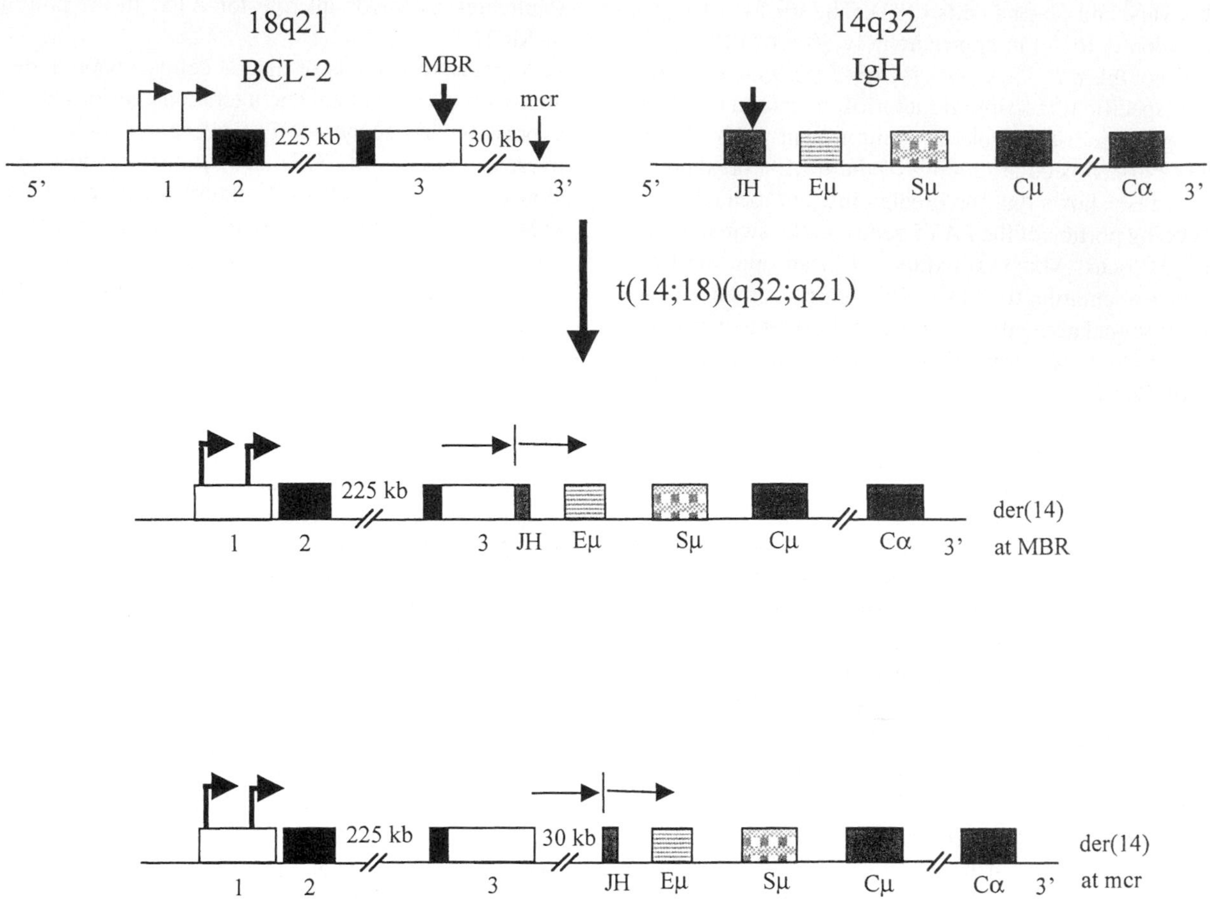

FIG. 8.4. Schematic representation of t(14;18) translocations involving the *BCL2* gene. The germline configuration of the human *BCL2* gene is shown in the top left panel. It consists of three exons with a large intron 2. The coding region is indicated in black and the noncoding region in white. The major breakpoint region (MBR) and the minor cluster region (mcr) are indicated by vertical arrows. The promoters of *BCL2* within *BCL2* exon 1 are marked by arrows. MBR is located in the 3′ untranslated region of *BCL2*, and mcr is located approximately 30 kb 3′ of exon 3. The immunoglobulin heavy chain (IgH) locus with the J_H region, the IgH core enhancer (Eμ), the switch recombination region (Sμ), and the constant region (Cμ to Cα) are shown in the top right panel. Breakpoints at IgH are located at the J_H region *(vertical arrow)*. The t(14;18) translocation results in the juxtaposition of the IgH locus to *BCL2* in a head to tail fashion, resulting in transcriptional deregulation of *BCL2* by the IgH regulatory elements, including Eμ. A translocated *BCL2* allele at der(14) involving the MBR or the mcr is represented in the bottom panel. Transcripts generated from the translocated *BCL2* allele involving MBR consists of fusion between *BCL2* exon 3 and JH-Cμ sequence derived from IgH. Normal BCL-2 transcripts are generated from the translocated *BCL2* allele involving mcr. Both types of transcripts give rise to a normal BCL-2 protein.

and rarely, *MYC* gene rearrangement (342). These genetic alterations may provide additional growth advantage to the cells that have been protected from apoptosis by deregulation of BCL-2. The genetic pathways that lead to transformation of follicular lymphoma to diffuse large cell lymphoma need to be further dissected.

Extranodal Marginal Zone B-Cell Lymphoma of the Mucosa-Associated Lymphoid Tissues

Little was known about the molecular genetics of MALT lymphoma until the t(11;18)(q21;q21) translocation was identified as a recurrent genetic lesion in MALT lymphoma, occurring in approximately 50% of low-grade MALT lymphomas with cytogenetic abnormalities (343–346). This translocation is associated with rearrangements of the *API2* gene on chromosome 11 and the *MALT1* gene on chromosome 18, generating abnormal chimeric mRNAs that code for an API2-MLT fusion protein (347–351). API2, also known as cIAP2, is a member of the inhibitors of apoptosis (IAP) protein family that consist of suppressors of apoptosis that act by inhibiting caspases, the integral components of many cell-death programs. It contains three baculovirus IAP repeats at its N-terminal portion and the caspase recruitment domain (CARD) at its C-terminal region (352,353). MLT is a novel protein with immunoglobulin-like C2 domains and partial homology to capases, suggesting its role in apoptosis (349). Breakpoints at the *API2* occur in an intron that separates the exons coding for the IAP domains and the CARD domain. The API2-MLT fusion protein contains the IAP domains fused to the C-terminal portion of MLT, which contains the immunoglobulin C2 domains. The function of API2-MLT is unclear but is probably related to apoptosis in view of the structure and function of the normal counterparts.

Another recurrent but infrequent chromosomal abnormality in MALT lymphoma is t(1;14)(p22;q32) (354). The breakpoint at chromosome 1 is located upstream of the promoter of a novel gene *BCL10* (355,356). *BCL10,* a cellular homologue of the equine herpesvirus-2 E10 gene, contains the CARD domain at its amino terminus. It activates NF-κB and induces apoptosis in B-cell lines. In MALT lymphomas with the t(1;14) translocation, mutant BCL-10 proteins with frameshift mutations producing truncations in or distal to the CARD domain are overexpressed. These truncated BCL-10 proteins lose their apoptotic activity and may show gain-of-function transforming activity with retained ability to activate NF-κB (355,356). The role of BCL-10 in the pathogenesis of MALT lymphoma may be twofold: loss of the wild-type BCL-10 may decrease apoptosis of B cells, and overexpression of the mutant BCL-10 may provide anti-apoptotic and proliferative signals mediated by NF-κB activation. MALT can transform from a low-grade lymphoma to a high-grade lymphoma. This progression can be associated with homozygous deletions or hypermethylation of the *TP16* gene in about 80% of cases (341,357). *TP53* does not appear to play an important role in MALT lymphomas (358).

Diffuse Large B-Cell Lymphoma

DLCL accounts for approximately 40% of NHL in adulthood and is a clinically heterogeneous disease (283,359). Its clinical heterogeneity is likely to be determined by its genetic heterogeneity rather than simply by its histologic appearance, which does not appear to have clinical significance. The recurrent chromosomal aberrations detected by cytogenetics in DLCL are heterogeneous, which include t(14; 18)(q32;q21) (17%), t(8;14)(q24;q32) (19%), translocations affecting 3q27 (12%) and 1q21-23 (16%), trisomy 7 (16%), trisomy 12 (13%), and deletions of the long arm of chromosome 6 (6q−) (14%) (360). Except for 3q27 translocations, which are found predominantly in DLCL, most of these chromosomal aberrations are also seen with other NHL types at comparable frequency.

Chromosomal alterations affecting band 3q27 involve reciprocal translocations between the 3q27 region and various alternative chromosomal partner sites, including the Ig heavy (14q32) or light (2p12, 22q11) chain loci (promiscuous translocations). Cloning of the breakpoints at the 3q27 region led to the identification of a putative protooncogene *BCL6* (361–365). *BCL6* encodes a 95-kd nuclear phosphoprotein belonging to the POZ/zinc finger family of transcription factors. It has transcriptional repressor activities (366–368). It shows a very restricted pattern of expression in normal tissues. In the B-cell lineage, BCL-6 protein is expressed only in germinal center cells, but not in pre–germinal center cells such as the mantle zone cells or post–germinal center cells such as immunoblasts and plasma cells (369–371). Mice deficient for BCL-6 are not capable of forming germinal centers and show a complete lack of affinity maturation (372,373). BCL-6 appears to be a pivotal regulator of germinal center development.

BCL-6 may act as a transcriptional switch for germinal center (GC) formation and differentiation by integrating various signals important for GC development (43,374). Antigen-receptor and CD40 signaling, which takes place during differentiation of GC cells, results in downregulation of BCL-6 (43,375). BCL-6 can modulate interleukin-4 activity by antagonizing STAT-6 induced transcription (376). The mechanisms by which BCL-6 is induced during GC induction and downregulated on GC cell differentiation warrant further studies.

Rearrangement of the *BCL6* gene can be detected in approximately 35% of DLCLs and in a minority (5% to 10%) of follicular lymphomas (377). Chromosomal translocation at the *BCL6* locus results in juxtaposition of *BCL6* to various chromosomal sites, including IgH (14q23), Igκ (2p12), Igλ (22q11), and at least 10 other chromosomal sites unrelated to the immunoglobulin loci (378,379). Many genes in these other chromosomal sites have been identified and include TTF (small GTPase of the RAS superfamily associated with cytoskeleton) (380), BOB1 (B-cell coactivator) (381), L-plastin (actin-binding protein) (382), H4 (histone) (378), IKAROS (383), HSP89A (heat shock protein) (384), major histocompatibility complex (MHC) class II transactivator (CIITA), PIM-1, eukaryotic initiation factor 4AII (translation factors), and a transferrin receptor (385). This marked degree of promiscuity of 3q27 translocations is apparently unique among B-NHL. Most of these translocations give rise to a fusion transcript in which exon 1 and the promoter of BCL-6 is replaced by the partner gene sequences (378,384) (Fig. 8.5). These fusion transcripts are initiated from the heterologous promoters and they contain the intact coding exons of BCL-6 (i.e., promoter substitution). Compared with the BCL-6 promoter, these promoters demonstrate a broader spectrum of activity in B-cell development, including expression in the post–germinal center differentiation stage such as immunoblasts and plasma cells (378). Consequently, they can prevent the normal downregulation of BCL-6 expression that occurs during differentiation into post–germinal center cells. The lymphomagenicity of BCL-6 may be related to its normal function in germinal center formation. It is hypothesized that this deregulated expression of a normal *BCL6* gene product may play a critical role in the pathogenesis of DLCL by blocking the normal exit of germinal center cells and triggering an uncontrolled proliferation of the ger-

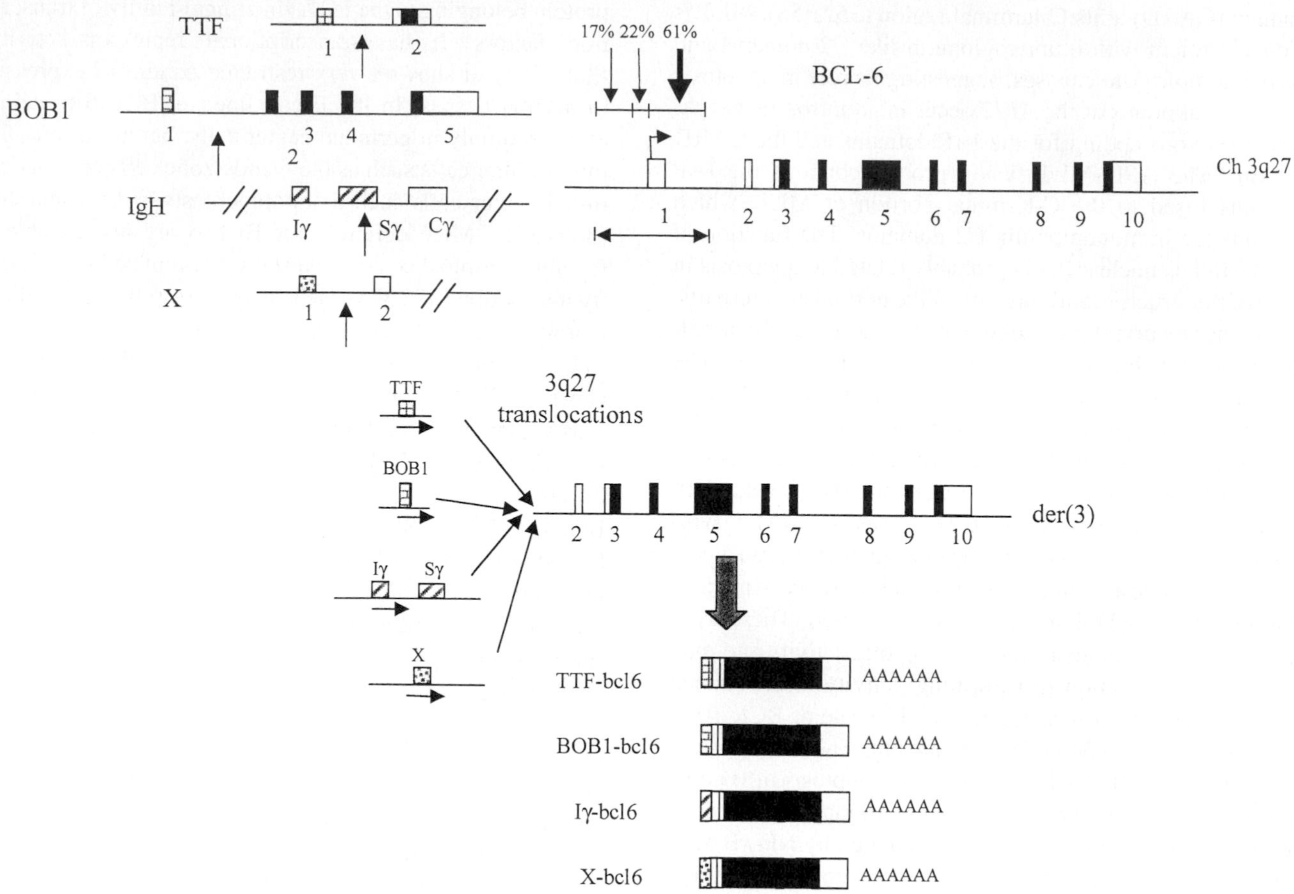

FIG. 8.5. Promoter substitution of *BCL6* in promiscuous translocations affecting 3q27. The top right panel is a schematic representation of the human *BCL6* gene, showing the clusters of chromosomal breakpoints with their respective frequency among diffuse large B-cell lymphoma (DLCL) cases carrying rearranged *BCL6 (vertical arrows)* and the region of somatic hypermutations *(horizontal double arrows)*. The coding and noncoding exons are indicated by filled and empty boxes, respectively. Most breakpoints at *BCL6* are located in intron 1, but they can also occur within exon 1 or 5′ of exon 1. The top left panel shows the exon-intron structures of the partner genes (e.g., *TTF*, *BOB1*, IgH, others [X]) involved in 3q27 translocations. Only the 5′ region of partner gene X is schematically represented. The breakpoints at the partner chromosomes are indicated by arrows. In the translocations shown here, the promoter and exon 1 of *BCL6* are replaced by the sequences derived from the partner genes. These sequences provide a heterologous promoter to *BCL6,* leading to transcriptional deregulation (i.e., promoter substitution). The bottom panel represents the fusion transcripts (i.e., TTF/BCL-6; BOB1/BCL-6; Iγ/BCL-6, and X/BCL-6) generated from the translocated alleles. These fusion transcripts contain a heterologous exon spliced to exon 2 of *BCL6.* The entire coding region of *BCL6* is retained, which translates into a normal BCL-6 protein.

minal center cells. *In vivo* studies are necessary to confirm this hypothesis.

Besides promoter substitution, the *BCL6* gene can also be altered by somatic hypermutation at its 5′ noncoding region. Hypermutation of *BCL6* can be found in normal germinal center cells (386,387). It is also found in many NHLs, most frequently in DLCL (73%), independently of *BCL6* rearrangement (388,389). Functional analysis of *BCL6* promoter-containing mutations indicates that some mutations derived from DLCL, but not from normal germinal center cells, may deregulate the basal level of BCL-6 transcription (unpublished results). This indicates that *BCL6* can also be deregulated by somatic hypermutation of its promoter and further supports the role of *BCL6* deregulation in the pathogenesis of DLCL.

Rearrangement of *BCL6* in DLCL may carry prognostic significance. Some studies have suggested that cases associated with *BCL6* rearrangement have the most favorable prognosis, whereas those with *BCL2* rearrangement but without *BCL6* have the worst outcome (390–392). DLCL with rearrangement of *BCL6* may have a biologic behavior distinct from those with other genetic lesions. Based on the genetic configuration of *BCL6* and *BCL2,* DLCL can be separated into three categories. The first type, accounting for approximately 40% of the cases, associates with rearrangement of *BCL6* without other known genetic lesions. The second type contains *BCL2* rearrangement with or without the presence of *TP53* alterations. This type probably presents DLCL evolving from clinical or subclinical follicular lymphoma. The third type contains germline *BCL2* and *BCL6*. These categories should provide a framework for further studies in the pathogenesis of DLCL.

Burkitt's Lymphoma

Burkitt's lymphomas can be divided into sporadic, endemic, and AIDS-associated types. All cases are characterized by chromosomal translocations involving region 8q24 and one of the immunoglobulin loci on chromosomes 2, 14, or 22 (393–397). In 80% of the cases, chromosomal translocation t(8;14)(q24;q32) involving IgH is present. The remaining 20% have t(2;8)(p11;q24) involving the Igκ locus (15%) and t(8;22)(q24;q11) involving the Igλ locus (5%).

The *MYC* protooncogene is the target of the translocation on 8q24. It encodes a transcription factor that contains an N-terminal transactivation domain and a C-terminal basic helix-loop-helix leucine zipper (bHLHLZ) domain. MYC controls different aspects of cellular processes, including cell cycle progression, differentiation, and apoptosis, through gene regulation (398,399). Many target genes of MYC have been identified. These genes have diverse roles in cell cycle, apoptosis, DNA metabolism and dynamics, energy metabolism, and protein synthesis, all of which can be regulated by MYC to regulate cell growth (400–402). Mechanistically, MYC functions by binding to specific DNA sequences when heterodimerized with a partner protein, called MAX. Specific DNA binding and protein-protein interaction by MYC is mediated through its C-terminal basic helix-loop-helix leucine zipper region. MAX heterodimerizes with MAD and antagonizes MYC function. This MYC/MAX/MAD network provides an intricate way to regulate MYC function through protein-protein interaction and specific DNA binding (403). There is growing evidence that MYC, through the N-terminal transactivation domain and the C-terminal bHLHLZ domain, can interact with other proteins, such as p107, Bin1, PAM, YY1, MIZ1, TFII-1, and TRRAP (400). These protein-protein interactions can modulate the ability of MYC to interact with the transcriptional machinery, providing additional complexity in the regulation of MYC function (404).

Because of the chromosomal translocations, *MYC* becomes juxtaposed to the Ig locus. The t(8;14), t(2;8) and t(8;22) translocations are somewhat different in the precise locations of the breakpoints. The t(8;14) breakpoints are located 5′ and centromeric to *MYC,* whereas the breakpoints map 3′ and telomeric to *MYC* in t(2;8) and t(8;22) (393–397). Within the t(8;14), the molecular architecture of the translocation region vary between different subtypes. The endemic form of Burkitt's lymphoma is associated predominantly with breakpoints at an undefined distance (>100 kb) 5′ to the *MYC* locus on chromosome 8 and within or in proximity to Ig J_H region on chromosome 14. In contrast, the t(8;14) translocation in sporadic and in AIDS-associated Burkitt's lymphomas involves sequences within or immediately 5′ (<3 kb) to *MYC* on chromosome 8 and sequences within the IgH switch region on chromosome 14 (405–407) (Fig. 8.6). The difference in location of the breakpoints between the endemic and sporadic forms of Burkitt's lymphoma suggest that chromosomal translocations associated with the endemic form occur during VDJ joining in pre-B cells in the bone marrow, whereas those associated with the sporadic form take place at a later stage of B-cell differentiation, most likely during isotype switching in the germinal center (54). However, in Burkitt's lymphoma, *MYC* chromosomal translocations may be a result of somatic hypermutation that takes place in the germinal center (53) (see the section on mechanisms of oncogene activation by chromosomal translocation).

The common effect of t(8;14), t(2;8), and t(8;22) is that *MYC* becomes transcriptionally deregulated by at least two mechanisms: juxtaposition of heterologous regulatory elements in the Ig loci to *MYC* (393–397) and removal or mutations in the 5′ regulatory region, including exon 1, of *MYC* (408). In all forms of Burkitt's lymphoma, the full-length MYC protein is constitutively expressed. In addition to transcriptional activation, the oncogenicity of MYC is thought to be enhanced by amino acid substitutions in the N-terminal transactivation domain of MYC (409,410). These mutations abolish the physiologic ability of p107, a protein related to RB, to modulate MYC transcriptional activation activity (411).

The pathogenic role of a deregulated *MYC* in Burkitt's lymphoma is directly demonstrated by *in vitro* and *in vivo* experiments. *In vitro,* constitutive expression of MYC in Epstein-Barr virus (EBV)-immortalized human B-cell lines results in their malignant transformation (412). *In vivo,* mice transgenic for *MYC* driven by the immunoglobulin enhancer develop pre-B and B-cell lymphomas at relatively high frequency (413,414). Constitutive expression of MYC can promote cell cycle entry, increase cellular metabolism, block differentiation and in the absence of adequate growth support, induce apoptosis (415). The oncogenicity of *MYC* in Burkitt's lymphoma is most likely related to its ability to stimulate cell proliferation and increase cellular metabolism.

Other Genetic Lesions

In addition to *MYC* rearrangement in 100% of Burkitt's lymphoma cases, disruption of *TP53* occurs in 30% of sporadic and endemic Burkitt's lymphomas (294). The 6q deletion is present in approximately 30% of Burkitt's lymphoma cases (93). Another important lesion that contributes to the development of Burkitt's lymphoma is monoclonal EBV infection, which is present in virtually all cases of endemic Burkitt's lymphoma and in approximately 30% of sporadic cases (416). EBV infection in Burkitt's lymphoma displays a type I latency, characterized by a restricted set of EBV gene expression (417). *LMP1* and *EBNA2,* which are shown to have oncogenic potential, are not expressed in Burkitt's

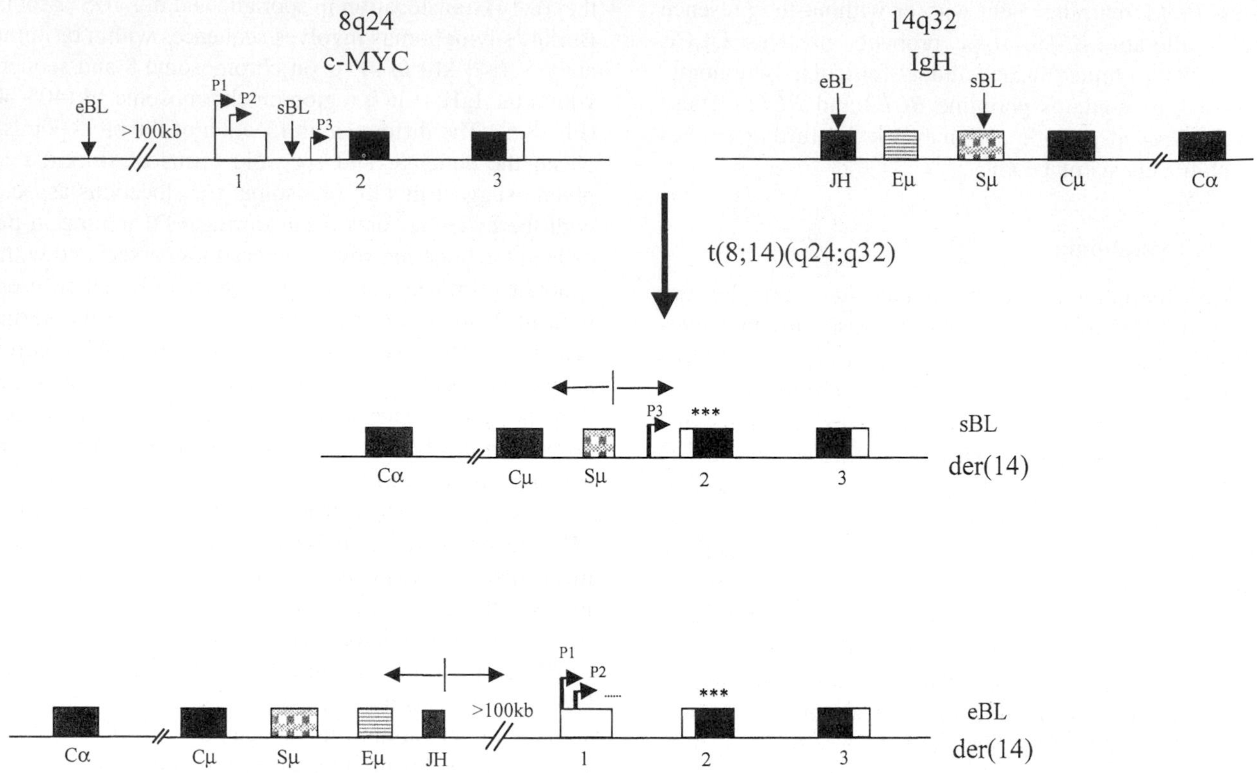

FIG. 8.6. Schematic diagram of t(8;14) in sporadic and endemic Burkitt's lymphomas. The germline configuration of human *MYC* is shown in the top left panel. It consists of three exons. The coding region is indicated in black and the noncoding region in white. The two major promoters of *MYC,* P1 and P2, and the minor intronic promoter P3, are marked by arrows. The top right panel represents the germline configuration of the immunoglobulin heavy chain (IgH) locus, including the J_H region, the core enhancer ($E\mu$), the switch recombination region ($S\mu$), and the constant region ($C\mu$ to $C\alpha$). The breakpoint regions in sporadic Burkitt's lymphoma (sBL) and endemic Burkitt's lymphoma (eBL) are indicated by vertical arrows. The configurations of the translocated *MYC* alleles in sBL and eBL are represented in the bottom panel. In the case of t(8;14) in sBL, the breakpoints tend to cluster in intron 1 of *MYC* and the $S\mu$ region of IgH. The exon 1, including the major promoters of *MYC,* is deleted. Translocation results in deregulation of *MYC* transcription initiated near the intronic promoter P3 by immunoglobulin regulatory elements. Because the coding domain is structurally intact, a normal-sized MYC protein is generated. In the case of t(8;14) in eBL, the breakpoints are located more than 100 kb 5′ of the first exon of *MYC* and at the J_H region of IgH. As a result of the translocation, *MYC* transcription initiated from P1 and P2 is deregulated by regulatory elements of the IgH locus, including $E\mu$. Mutations can be detected in exon 1–intron 1 border *(dots)*, where *MYC* transcriptional regulatory sequences are located. As in the case of sBL, a normal-sized MYC protein is produced. In both types of translocated *MYC* alleles, the coding region in exon 2 frequently harbor point mutations that result in amino acid substitutions at the N-terminal transactivation domain of *MYC (asterisks).* These mutations contribute to the oncogenicity of *MYC.*

lymphoma. The role of these two EBV-coded oncogenes in the pathogenesis of Burkitt's lymphoma is unknown.

MULTIPLE MYELOMA

MM is a malignant clonal expansion of terminally differentiated B cells (i.e., plasma cells). Based on Southern blot analysis, most MMs (mostly cell lines) harbor chromosomal translocations involving the IgH locus or one of the IgL loci, despite the relatively low incidence of karyotypically detectable chromosomal translocations involving the Ig loci (418). These translocations mainly occur at the IgH switch regions, suggesting that they are a byproduct of isotype switching and may represent an early event in the pathogenesis of MM (419). They involve a promiscuous array of partner chromosomes (420). The protooncogenes deregulated by recurrent IgH translocations in MM are described in the following sections.

BCL1

The *BCL1* locus at 11q13 is translocated to the IgH locus at 14q23 in 25% of cases. However, unlike mantle cell lymphoma in which the 11q13 breakpoints are predominantly clustered in one region (major cluster region), the 11q13 breakpoints in myeloma are located approximately 120 kb centromeric to the *BCL1* gene and do not involve the major cluster region (419,421). Moreover, the breakpoints at IgH locus involve the switch region instead of the J_H region (see Mantle Cell Lymphoma section). Despite the difference in locations of the breakpoints, *BCL1* is upregulated in myelomas with t(11;14) translocations, suggesting the importance of *BCL1* deregulation in the pathogenesis of MM (421).

Fibroblast Growth Receptor-3

Twenty-five percent (25%) of MMs have been found to have a karyotypically silent chromosomal translocation t(4; 14)(p16;q32), which results in deregulation of the fibroblast growth factor receptor-3 gene *(FGFR3)* (422). Activating mutations in the coding region of *FGFR3* are also detected in 33% to 50% of MMs (422). The same mutations are also present in the germline of patients with the most severe form of dwarfism (423,424). The mutated allele is always selectively deregulated by the chromosomal translocation (420), suggesting deregulated expression of a mutated *FGFR3* confers further growth advantage to MM cells. It is postulated that deregulated expression of *FGFR3* results in continuous FGF-mediated signals from the stromal cells of the bone marrow, resulting in increased growth, block in differentiation, or apoptosis. Subsequent activating mutation may confer the tumor cells with FGF-independent growth or survival (420).

MUM1/IRF4

MUM1/IRF4 was cloned from a t(6;14) translocation breakpoint on 6p25 in a myeloma cell line using Southern blot assay that detects translocations involving IgH switch sequences (425). This translocation cannot be detected by conventional cytogenetics, but it is found in approximately 20% of MM cell lines using FISH (426). *MUM1/IRF4* is a member of the interferon regulatory factors (IRF) family of transcription factors important for the transcriptional regulation of interferon-stimulated genes (427). *IRF4* is a lymphoid specific gene expressed in a subset of germinal center cells, plasma cells, and activated T cells (428). Its expression is deregulated as a result of the translocation to IgH (425). Transgenic mice deficient in IRF-4 are hypogammaglobulinemic and unable to mount a detectable antibody response, suggesting that IRF-4 plays a critical role in plasma cell development (429). Its precise role in the pathogenesis of MM remains to be determined.

Other Lesions

Deregulation of the aforementioned protooncogenes by chromosomal translocations is thought to represent early events in the pathogenesis of MM (420). Genetic lesions that may play a role in tumor progression in MM include *MYC* deregulation, *RAS* mutations; mutations in *TP53* and *RB1*; deletions in the cyclin-dependent kinase *(CDK)* inhibitors p15, p16, and p18; and overexpression of *MDM2.*

MYC

Using FISH, the *MYC* locus is found to be affected by chromosomal abnormalities in 95% of MM cell lines and approximately 50% of advanced primary MM tumors (430). About 20% of these chromosomal abnormalities are classic or variant t(8;14) translocations. The rest are mostly complex and unusual translocations and insertions that juxtapose *MYC* to the IgH or IgL locus. It is thought that chromosomal aberrations affecting the *MYC* locus in MM occur during tumor progression, instead of as a result of errors in switch recombination or somatic hypermutation (430,431). Chromosomal aberrations are usually associated with deregulation of MYC expression and selective expression of the one *MYC* allele (430–432).

RAS

Mutations in *RAS* occur in about 40% of newly diagnosed MM patients. *RAS* mutations are correlated with disease progression. Although mutations in *NRAS* or *KRAS* are rarely detected in monoclonal gammopathy of unknown significance (MGUS), they occur in 9% to 30% of MM and in 63% to 70% of terminal disease or plasma cell leukemia (55,433–435). The most frequent *RAS* mutation is the *NRAS* codon 61 mutation (55,433,434). It is postulated that *RAS* mutations contribute to tumor progression in MM by allowing interleukin-6–independent tumor expansion and dissemination outside the bone marrow (420).

TP53

The *TP53* mutations are uncommon in MM and are likely to be a late event. Although *TP53* mutations occur in only about 5% of early MM, they are present in 20% to 40% of plasma cell leukemia (435–439). *TP53* mutations may block apoptosis of tumor cells, thereby facilitating tumor progression.

RB1

Inactivation of the *RB1* gene has been found in approximately 35% of MMs (437), and deletions of *RB1* are detected in up to 70% of MMs (440,441). However, biallelic deletion of *RB1* is found in only 1% to 10% of MM. Although monoallelic loss of the *RB1* gene is found in a high percentage of MM cases, it is not associated with inactivation of *RB1* (441). This finding suggests that another tumor suppressor gene may be present in the region 13q12-14 deleted in MM.

Cyclin-Dependent Kinase Inhibitors

Homozygous deletions of the genes for the CDK inhibitors p15, p16, and p18 can be found in about 5% to 10% of

MM patients (442). Hypermethylation of *TP15* and *TP16* occurs in 70% of MM cases (443). This hypermethylation appears to correlate with disease progression (443).

MDM2

The product of *MDM2* can inactivate *TP53* (65). In a limited study, overexpression of MDM2 was detected in three MM cell lines and cells isolated from two plasma cell leukemia cases, suggesting its involvement in tumor progression of MM (444).

T-CELL PROLYMPHOCYTIC LEUKEMIA AND T-CELL NON-HODGKIN'S LYMPHOMA

The molecular genetics of lymphoid malignancies of mature T cells is less well characterized than for B-NHL and acute leukemia. The most consistent genetic abnormalities associated with these neoplasms are those associated with T-cell prolymphocytic leukemia (T-PLL), anaplastic large cell lymphoma (ALCL), cutaneous T-cell lymphoma (CTCL), and adult T-cell leukemia/lymphoma (ATLL).

T-Cell Prolymphocytic Leukemia

The *TCL1* locus at 14q32.1 is rearranged in 75% of T-PLLs, a disease that occurs frequently in patients with ataxia telangiectasia, with chromosomal translocations t(14; 14)(q11;q32.1) and inversions inv(14)(q11;q32.1) with the TCR $\alpha\delta$ loci (445–446). *TCL1* encodes a 14-kd protein with homology to a protein encoded by *MTCP1,* a gene on Xq28 that is associated with t(X;14) translocations found also in T-PLL (447), suggesting that *TCL* and *MTCP1* may be members of a new gene family. TCL is normally expressed in pre-B cells, in immature thymocytes, and at low levels, in activated T cells. It is not expressed in normal peripheral B and T cells (445). TCL has been shown to enhance the kinase activity and nuclear transport of *AKT,* a protooncogene whose retroviral homologue, *akt*, can induce T-cell lymphomas in mice (448). In t(14:14)(q11;q32.1) and inv(14)(q11;q32.1), the *TCL1* gene is juxtaposed under the regulatory control of the TCR locus, which is located 5′ or 3′ to *TAL1,* respectively (445). This leads to transcriptional deregulation of *TCL1* (445,449). Transgenic mice expressing a *TCL1* transgene under a T-cell specific promoter develop mature T-cell leukemias (450), indicating that deregulated *TCL1* is oncogenic. The mechanism of oncogenesis by TAL is unknown but is probably related to its ability to activate AKT.

Anaplastic Large Cell Lymphoma

The t(2;5)(p23;q35) chromosomal translocation occurs frequently in anaplastic large cell lymphoma (ALCL) (451). The percentage of cases positive for the t(2;5) translocation, as measured with excellent correlation by cytogenetics, FISH, RT-PCR, or immunohistochemistry using antibodies (p80 and ALK-1) directed against the fusion protein, varies from 25% to 30% to approximately 70% (452–455). This spectrum probably reflects the types of ALCL cases examined in the different studies. The t(2;5) translocation is associated with specific clinical characteristics in ALCL. It occurs in a younger patient population and is associated with a better survival rate (456,457).

Molecular characterization of the breakpoint shows that the t(2;5) translocation causes the fusion of two genes, the nucleophosmin *(NPM)* gene encoding for a nucleolar phosphoprotein on chromosome 5 and the anaplastic lymphoma kinase *(ALK)* gene encoding for a novel orphan receptor tyrosine kinase on chromosome 2. This creates an 80-kd fusion protein that contains the amino-terminal portion of NPM joined to the entire cytoplasmic catalytic portion of ALK (22,23). NPM-ALK has transforming ability *in vitro* (458,459). Moreover, it can cause B-cell lymphoma in mice on transplantation of bone marrow cells infected with retrovirus expressing NPM-ALK, demonstrating a direct causative role for NPM-ALK in human lymphoma (460).

The fusion of *NPM* to *ALK* has two distinct consequences, both of which are important in the oncogenicity of their fusion protein. First, it leads to the ectopic expression of NPM-ALK in T cells (459). Second, it results in the constitutive activation of ALK kinase activity because of oligomerization mediated by the NPM segment. This activated kinase function activates the mitogenic signal transduction pathway through phospholipase Cγ (458,459).

Between 10% and 20% of ALK-positive ALCLs express ALK-fusion proteins other than NPM-ALK (461). An example is the TRK-fused gene *(TFG)* (462). The ALK breakpoints in these other translocations involving TRK are the same as in the classic t(2;5) translocation. Like NPM-ALK, TFG-ALK fusion proteins have functional tyrosine kinase activity (462).

Adult T-Cell Leukemia/Lymphoma

ATLL is associated with human T-cell lymphotrophic virus type 1 (HTLV-1) infection of the tumor clone in 100% of cases (463). A viral gene *tax* is shown to have a critical role for the pathogenesis of ATLL. TAX can transform T cells in cultured cell systems and in transgenic animals by regulating cellular gene expression, including interleukin-2 (IL-2) and IL-2 receptor genes through the NF-κB and CREB pathways (463–465). However, based on the observation of the low incidence of ATLL in HTLV-1–infected patients and the long latency (10 to 30 years) of the disease, it is clear that TAX alone is not sufficient for full-blown malignancy and additional genetic lesions are required (463). The hypothesis is supported by the observation that *TP53* is inactivated in 40% of ATLL cases, representing the most frequent lesion of a cellular gene identified in ATLL (466).

Cutaneous T-Cell Lymphoma

CTCL is one of the most common types of extranodal NHL. The most frequent known genetic lesion associated with CTCL is rearrangement of the gene for NFκB-2/Lyt-10, which occurs in approximately 15% of cases (467). The NFκB-2 gene *(NFKB2)* encodes a component of the NF-κB transcription factor complex, which is involved in regulating cell proliferation, differentiation, activation, and apoptosis in response to a variety of extracellular signals (468,469). Rearrangements cluster within the 3′ terminal ankyrin-coding domain of *NFKB2,* resulting in the generation of a protein truncated at its C terminus, which occasionally is fused to heterologous proteins (470). These alterations convert NF-κB-2 from a repressor to a constitutive transcriptional activator, leading to abnormal expression of effector genes that are normally repressed (471).

HODGKIN'S LYMPHOMA

Biologic studies of classic Hodgkin's lymphoma (HL) have been hampered for many years mainly by the paucity of Hodgkin and Reed-Sternberg (HRS) cells, which are the neoplastic cells of HL, in the tissue samples affected by HL (472). The development of sophisticated microdissection techniques and PCR technology has allowed the isolation and enrichment of HRS cells, permitting studies of the origin and genetic alterations of these cells (473).

Cytogenetic investigations, studies of EBV genome in the HRS cells, and analyses of Ig gene rearrangements show that HRS cells represent a clonal outgrowth of a single cell. Approximately 95% of HL cases originate from a B-cell based on the detection of Ig gene rearrangements (474,475) and genome-based analysis of gene expression (476). The presence and pattern of somatic mutations in the rearranged Ig gene indicate that the cellular precursors of HRS are germinal center cells (472,474,477). The lymphocytic and histiocytic cells in lymphocyte predominance HL are probably derived from antigen-selected germinal center cells. In classic HL, the HRS cells often have "crippled" mutations and nonfunctional Ig genes, suggesting that they are derived from negatively selected germinal center cells that are destined to undergo apoptosis but rescued by a transforming event (477).

The transforming events that lead to HL from the normal cellular precursors are unknown. Analysis of micromanipulated HRS cells has revealed a recurrent genetic abnormality in a subset of HL: deleterious mutations in the IκBα gene, which is an inhibitor for NF-κB transcription factor complex (478–481) (see T-Cell Non-Hodgkin's Lymphoma section). The exact frequency of this mutation in HL is unknown, because the number of studies and primary cases analyzed is still limited. This finding, however, may account for the constitutive activation of NF-κB observed in HRS (482). The mechanism by which constitutively activated NF-κB leads to transformation of HRS cell precursors is unknown. Considering that HRS cells may be derived from negatively selected germinal center cells, one hypothesis is that aberrant NF-κB activity may rescue the HRS precursors from apoptosis (482).

EBV infection is detected frequently in HL. Notably, the EBV infection of HRS cells is monoclonal, suggesting that infection precedes clonal expansion (483,484). Of the two B-cell–transforming antigens encoded by the EBV genome, infected HRS cells most commonly express LMP-1 but not EBNA-2 (485,486). This expression profile is different from that of EBV-infected lymphoblastoid cell lines (LMP-1 and EBNA-2 positive) and Burkitt's lymphoma (LMP-1 and EBNA-2 negative). The role of LMP-1 in the pathogenesis of HL is unknown. It is likely to be related to its ability to activate different signal transduction pathways, including NF-κB and Jun activation (487).

SUMMARY AND CONCLUSIONS

Similar to other human cancers, hematopoietic malignancies occur through activation of protooncogenes and inactivation of tumor suppressor genes. The genome of hematopoietic neoplasms is characterized by the preponderance of reciprocal balanced chromosomal translocations. The molecular dissection of these alterations has led to the identification of protooncogenes that have been shown to contribute to the pathogenesis of these tumors. Although some of these genes are also involved in solid tumors, many of them are specific to lymphoid or myeloid tumors. Alterations of these genes lead to subversion of the normal cellular processes that control growth, proliferation, apoptosis, and differentiation of the hematopoietic cell, resulting in neoplastic transformation.

From a clinical standpoint, the identification and characterization of protooncogenes and tumor suppressor genes are important in several aspects. First, because many protooncogenes in hematopoietic malignancies are specific to certain subtypes, they can be used as diagnostic adjuncts for routine histopathologic analysis. This is exemplified by the utility of the detection of *BCL1* and *BCL2* gene rearrangements in the diagnosis of mantle cell lymphoma and follicular lymphoma, respectively. Second, studies of genes involved in leukemias and lymphomas may help refine the classification of hematologic tumors and allow the identification of subsets within each subtype, which may not be possible based on histologic analysis alone. Third, rearrangements and fusions involving protooncogenes provide sensitive and specific parameters for the detection of minimal residual disease, particularly in acute leukemia. The protooncogenes and tumor suppressor genes involved in hematopoietic malignancies may serve as targets for development of specific therapeutic strategies.

REFERENCES

1. Bishop JM. Molecular themes in oncogenesis. *Cell* 1991;64:235–248.
2. Stehelin D, Varmus HE, Bishop JM, et al. DNA related to the trans-

forming gene(s) of avian sarcoma viruses is present in normal avian DNA. *Nature* 1976;260:170–173.
3. Stehelin D, Guntaka RV, Varmus HE, et al. Purification of DNA complementary to nucleotide sequences required for neoplastic transformation of fibroblasts by avian sarcoma viruses. *J Mol Biol* 1976; 101:349–365.
4. Shih C, Padhy LC, Murray M, et al. Transforming genes of carcinomas and neuroblastomas introduced into mouse fibroblasts. *Nature* 1981; 290:261–264.
5. Krontiris TG, Cooper GM. Transforming activity of human tumor DNAs. *Proc Natl Acad Sci USA* 1981;78:1181–1184.
6. Perucho M, Goldfarb M, Shimizu K, et al. Human-tumor–derived cell lines contain common and different transforming genes. *Cell* 1981;27: 467–476.
7. Pulciani S, Santos E, Lauver AV, et al. Oncogenes in human tumor cell lines: molecular cloning of a transforming gene from human bladder carcinoma cells. *Proc Natl Acad Sci USA* 1982;79:2845–2849.
8. Shimizu K, Goldfarb M, Suard Y, et al. Three human transforming genes are related to the viral ras oncogenes. *Proc Natl Acad Sci USA* 1983;80:2112–2116.
9. Hall A, Marshall CJ, Spurr NK, et al. Identification of transforming gene in two human sarcoma cell lines as a new member of the ras gene family located on chromosome 1. *Nature* 1983;303:396–400.
10. Stanbridge EJ. Human tumor suppressor genes. *Annu Rev Genet* 1990; 24:615–657.
11. Marshall CJ. Tumor suppressor genes. *Cell* 1991;64:313–326.
12. Barr FG. Chromosomal translocations involving paired box transcription factors in human cancer. *Int J Biochem Cell Biol* 1997;29: 1449–1461.
13. Cleary ML. Oncogenic conversion of transcription factors by chromosomal translocations. *Cell* 1991;66:619–622.
14. Nichols J, Nimer SD. Transcription factors, translocations, and leukemia. *Blood* 1992;80:2953–2963.
15. Rabbitts TH. Perspective: chromosomal translocations can affect genes controlling gene expression and differentiation—why are these functions targeted? *J Pathol* 1999;187:39–42.
16. Kehrl JH. Hematopoietic lineage commitment: role of transcription factors. *Stem Cells* 1995;13:223–241.
17. Orkin SH. Transcription factors and hematopoietic development. *J Biol Chem* 1995;270:4955–4958.
18. Tenen DG, Hromas R, Licht JD, et al. Transcription factors, normal myeloid development, and leukemia. *Blood* 1997;90:489–519.
19. Joneson T, Bar-Sagi D. Ras effectors and their role in mitogenesis and oncogenesis. *J Mol Med* 1997;75:587–593.
20. Sawyers CL. Signal transduction pathways involved in BCR-ABL transformation. *Baillieres Clin Haematol* 1997;10:223–231.
21. Rebollo A, Martinez AC. Ras proteins: recent advances and new functions. *Blood* 1999;94:2971–2980.
22. Morris SW, Kirstein MN, Valentine MB, et al. Fusion of a kinase gene, ALK, to a nucleolar protein gene, NPM, in non-Hodgkin's lymphoma [published erratum appears in *Science* 1995;267:316–37]. *Science* 1994;263:1281–1284.
23. Ladanyi M. The NPM/ALK gene fusion in the pathogenesis of anaplastic large cell lymphoma. *Cancer Surv* 1997;30:59–75.
24. Warmuth M, Danhauser-Riedl S, Hallek M. Molecular pathogenesis of chronic myeloid leukemia: implications for new therapeutic strategies. *Ann Hematol* 1999;78:49–64.
25. Gishizky ML. Molecular mechanisms of Bcr-Abl–induced oncogenesis. *Cytokines Mol Ther* 1996;2:251–261.
26. Laneuville P. Abl tyrosine protein kinase. *Semin Immunol* 1995;7: 255–266.
27. Shaul Y. C-abl: activation and nuclear targets [in process citation]. *Cell Death Differ* 2000;7:10–16.
28. Wang JY. Abl tyrosine kinase in signal transduction and cell-cycle regulation. *Curr Opin Genet Dev* 1993;3:35–43.
29. Gotoh A, Broxmeyer HE. The function of BCR/ABL and related proto-oncogenes. *Curr Opin Hematol* 1997;4:3–11.
30. Bos JL. Ras oncogenes in human cancer: a review [published erratum appears in *Cancer Res* 1990;50:1352]. *Cancer Res* 1989;49: 4682–4689.
31. Maruta H, Burgess AW. Regulation of the Ras signalling network. *Bioessays* 1994;16:489–496.
32. Cantley LC, Auger KR, Carpenter C, et al. Oncogenes and signal transduction [published erratum appears in *Cell* 1991;65:following 914]. *Cell* 1991;64:281–302.
33. Wickremasinghe RG, Hoffbrand AV. Biochemical and genetic control of apoptosis: relevance to normal hematopoiesis and hematological malignancies. *Blood* 1999;93:3587–3600.
34. McKenna SL, Cotter TG. Functional aspects of apoptosis in hematopoiesis and consequences of failure. *Adv Cancer Res* 1997;71: 121–164.
35. Yoshida Y, Anzai N, Kawabata H. Apoptosis in normal and neoplastic hematopoiesis. *Crit Rev Oncol Hematol* 1996;24:185–211.
36. Korsmeyer SJ. Bcl-2 initiates a new category of oncogenes: regulators of cell death. *Blood* 1992;80:879–886.
37. Chao DT, Korsmeyer SJ. BCL-2 family: regulators of cell death. *Annu Rev Immunol* 1998;16:395–419.
38. Korsmeyer SJ. BCL-2 gene family and the regulation of programmed cell death. *Cancer Res* 1999;59:1693s–1700s.
39. Oltvai ZN, Milliman CL, Korsmeyer SJ. Bcl-2 heterodimerizes in vivo with a conserved homolog, Bax, that accelerates programmed cell death. *Cell* 1993;74:609–619.
40. Korsmeyer SJ, Yin XM, Oltvai ZN, et al. Reactive oxygen species and the regulation of cell death by the Bcl-2 gene family. *Biochim Biophys Acta* 1995;1271:63–66.
41. Gross A, McDonnell JM, Korsmeyer SJ. BCL-2 family members and the mitochondria in apoptosis. *Genes Dev* 1999;13:1899–1911.
42. Johansson B, Mertens F, Mitelman F. Primary vs. secondary neoplasia-associated chromosomal abnormalities—balanced rearrangements vs. genomic imbalances? *Genes Chromosomes Cancer* 1996; 16:155–163.
43. Dalla-Favera R, Migliazza A, Chang CC, et al. Molecular pathogenesis of B cell malignancy: the role of BCL-6. *Curr Top Microbiol Immunol* 1999;246:257–263.
44. Downing JR, Look AT. MLL fusion genes in the 11q23 acute leukemias. *Cancer Treat Res* 1996;84:73–92.
45. Tycko B, Sklar J. Chromosomal translocations in lymphoid neoplasia: a reappraisal of the recombinase model. *Cancer Cells* 1990;2:1–8.
46. Tycko B, Reynolds TC, Smith SD, et al. Consistent breakage between consensus recombinase heptamers of chromosome 9 DNA in a recurrent chromosomal translocation of human T cell leukemia. *J Exp Med* 1989;169:369–377.
47. Jaeger U, Karth GD, Knapp S, et al. Molecular mechanism of the t(14;18)—a model for lymphoid-specific chromosomal translocations. *Leuk Lymphoma* 1994;14:197–202.
48. Gillert E, Leis T, Repp R, et al. A DNA damage repair mechanism is involved in the origin of chromosomal translocations t(4;11) in primary leukemic cells. *Oncogene* 1999;18:4663–4671.
49. Romana S, Poirel H, Della Valle V, et al. Molecular analysis of chromosomal breakpoints in three examples of chromosomal translocation involving the TEL gene. *Leukemia* 1999;13:1754–1759.
50. Richardson C, Moynahan ME, Jasin M. Homologous recombination between heterologs during repair of a double-strand break. Suppression of translocations in normal cells. *Ann NY Acad Sci* 1999;886: 183–186.
51. Morgan WF, Corcoran J, Hartmann A, et al. DNA double-strand breaks, chromosomal rearrangements, and genomic instability. *Mutat Res* 1998;404:125–128.
52. Difilippantonio MJ, Zhu J, Chen HT, et al. DNA repair protein Ku80 suppresses chromosomal aberrations and malignant transformation. *Nature* 2000;404:510–514.
53. Goossens T, Klein U, Kuppers R. Frequent occurrence of deletions and duplications during somatic hypermutation: implications for oncogene translocations and heavy chain disease. *Proc Natl Acad Sci USA* 1998;95:2463–2468.
54. Magrath I. The pathogenesis of Burkitt's lymphoma. *Adv Cancer Res* 1990;55:133–270.
55. Neri A, Murphy JP, Cro L, et al. Ras oncogene mutation in multiple myeloma. *J Exp Med* 1989;170:1715–1725.
56. Ahuja HG, Foti A, Bar-Eli M, et al. The pattern of mutational involvement of RAS genes in human hematologic malignancies determined by DNA amplification and direct sequencing. *Blood* 1990;75: 1684–1690.
57. Neri A, Knowles DM, Greco A, et al. Analysis of RAS oncogene mutations in human lymphoid malignancies. *Proc Natl Acad Sci USA* 1988;85:9268–9272.

58. Schwab M. Oncogene amplification in solid tumors. *Semin Cancer Biol* 1999;9:319–325.
59. Werner CA, Dohner H, Joos S, et al. High-level DNA amplifications are common genetic aberrations in B-cell neoplasms. *Am J Pathol* 1997;151:335–342.
60. Rao PH, Houldsworth J, Dyomina K, et al. Chromosomal and gene amplification in diffuse large B-cell lymphoma. *Blood* 1998;92: 234–240.
61. Monni O, Joensuu H, Franssila K, et al. BCL2 overexpression associated with chromosomal amplification in diffuse large B-cell lymphoma. *Blood* 1997;90:1168–1174.
62. Houldsworth J, Mathew S, Rao PH, et al. REL proto-oncogene is frequently amplified in extranodal diffuse large cell lymphoma. *Blood* 1996;87:25–29.
63. Kinzler KW, Vogelstein B. Cancer-susceptibility genes. Gatekeepers and caretakers [news, comment]. *Nature* 1997;386:761, 763.
64. Herman JG. Hypermethylation of tumor suppressor genes in cancer. *Semin Cancer Biol* 1999;9:359–367.
65. May P, May E. Twenty years of p53 research: structural and functional aspects of the p53 protein. *Oncogene* 1999;18:7621–7636.
66. Bates S, Vousden KH. P53 in signaling checkpoint arrest or apoptosis. *Curr Opin Genet Dev* 1996;6:12–18.
67. Amundson SA, Myers TG, Fornace AJ Jr. Roles for p53 in growth arrest and apoptosis: putting on the brakes after genotoxic stress. *Oncogene* 1998;17:3287–3299.
68. Wahl GM, Linke SP, Paulson TG, et al. Maintaining genetic stability through *TP53* mediated checkpoint control. *Cancer Surv* 1997;29: 183–219.
69. Albrechtsen N, Dornreiter I, Grosse F, et al. Maintenance of genomic integrity by p53: complementary roles for activated and non-activated p53. *Oncogene* 1999;18:7706–7717.
70. Hollstein M, Sidransky D, Vogelstein B, et al. P53 mutations in human cancers. *Science* 1991;253:49–53.
71. Imamura J, Miyoshi I, Koeffler HP. P53 in hematologic malignancies. *Blood* 1994;84:2412–2421.
72. Drexler HG. Review of alterations of the cyclin-dependent kinase inhibitor INK4 family genes p15, p16, p18 and p19 in human leukemia-lymphoma cells. *Leukemia* 1998;12:845–859.
73. Weinberg RA. The Rb gene and the negative regulation of cell growth. *Blood* 1989;74:529–532.
74. Hatakeyama M, Weinberg RA. The role of RB in cell cycle control. *Prog Cell Cycle Res* 1995;1:9–19.
75. Nevins JR, Leone G, DeGregori J, et al. Role of the Rb/E2F pathway in cell growth control. *J Cell Physiol* 1997;173:233–236.
76. Benedict WF, Xu HJ, Takahashi R. The retinoblastoma gene: its role in human malignancies. *Cancer Invest* 1990;8:535–540.
77. Vooijs M, Berns A. Developmental defects and tumor predisposition in Rb mutant mice. *Oncogene* 1999;18:5293–5303.
78. Shiloh Y, Rotman G. Ataxia-telangiectasia and the ATM gene: linking neurodegeneration, immunodeficiency, and cancer to cell cycle checkpoints. *J Clin Immunol* 1996;16:254–260.
79. Xu Y, Ashley T, Brainerd EE, et al. Targeted disruption of ATM leads to growth retardation, chromosomal fragmentation during meiosis, immune defects, and thymic lymphoma [see comments]. *Genes Dev* 1996;10:2411–2422.
80. Barlow C, Hirotsune S, Paylor R, et al. Atm-deficient mice: a paradigm of ataxia telangiectasia. *Cell* 1996;86:159–171.
81. Xu Y. ATM in lymphoid development and tumorigenesis. *Adv Immunol* 1999;72:179–189.
82. Rotman G, Shiloh Y. ATM: from gene to function. *Hum Mol Genet* 1998;7:1555–1563.
83. Rotman G, Shiloh Y. ATM: a mediator of multiple responses to genotoxic stress. *Oncogene* 1999;18:6135–6144.
84. Liao MJ, Van Dyke T. Critical role for Atm in suppressing V(D)J recombination-driven thymic lymphoma. *Genes Dev* 1999;13: 1246–1250.
85. Stilgenbauer S, Schaffner C, Winkler D, et al. The ATM gene in the pathogenesis of mantle-cell lymphoma. *Ann Oncol* 2000;11:127–130.
86. Schaffner C, Idler I, Stilgenbauer S, et al. Mantle cell lymphoma is characterized by inactivation of the ATM gene [In Process Citation]. *Proc Natl Acad Sci USA* 2000;97:2773–2778.
87. Stilgenbauer S, Winkler D, Ott G, et al. Molecular characterization of 11q deletions points to a pathogenic role of the ATM gene in mantle cell lymphoma. *Blood* 1999;94:3262–3264.
88. Schmutte C, Fishel R. Genomic instability: first step to carcinogenesis. *Anticancer Res* 1999;19:4665–4696.
89. Peltomaki P. DNA mismatch repair gene mutations in human cancer. *Environ Health Perspect* 1997;105[Suppl 4]:775–780.
90. Honchel R, Halling KC, Thibodeau SN. Genomic instability in neoplasia. *Semin Cell Biol* 1995;6:45–52.
91. Indraccolo S, Minuzzo S, Nicoletti L, et al. Mutator phenotype in human hematopoietic neoplasms and its association with deletions disabling DNA repair genes and bcl-2 rearrangements. *Blood* 1999; 94:2424–2432.
92. Gamberi B, Gaidano G, Parsa N, et al. Microsatellite instability is rare in B-cell non-Hodgkin's lymphomas. *Blood* 1997;89:975–979.
93. Gaidano G, Hauptschein RS, Parsa NZ, et al. Deletions involving two distinct regions of 6q in B-cell non-Hodgkin lymphoma. *Blood* 1992; 80:1781–1787.
94. Dohner H, Stilgenbauer S, Dohner K, et al. Chromosome aberrations in B-cell chronic lymphocytic leukemia: reassessment based on molecular cytogenetic analysis. *J Mol Med* 1999;77:266–281.
95. Stilgenbauer S, Dohner K, Bentz M, et al. Molecular cytogenetic analysis of B-cell chronic lymphocytic leukemia. *Ann Hematol* 1998; 76:101–110.
96. Rowley JD. Recurring chromosome abnormalities in leukemia and lymphoma. *Semin Hematol* 1990;27:122–136.
97. Trecca D, Longo L, Biondi A, et al. Analysis of p53 gene mutations in acute myeloid leukemia. *Am J Hematol* 1994;46:304–309.
98. Chambon P. A decade of molecular biology of retinoic acid receptors. *FASEB J* 1996;10:940–954.
99. Borrow J, Goddard AD, Sheer D, et al. Molecular analysis of acute promyelocytic leukemia breakpoint cluster region on chromosome 17. *Science* 1990;249:1577–1580.
100. de The H, Chomienne C, Lanotte M, et al. The t(15;17) translocation of acute promyelocytic leukaemia fuses the retinoic acid receptor alpha gene to a novel transcribed locus. *Nature* 1990;347:558–561.
101. Alcalay M, Zangrilli D, Fagioli M, et al. Expression pattern of the RAR alpha-PML fusion gene in acute promyelocytic leukemia. *Proc Natl Acad Sci USA* 1992;89:4840–4844.
102. Dyck JA, Maul GG, Miller WH Jr, et al. A novel macromolecular structure is a target of the promyelocyte–retinoic acid receptor oncoprotein. *Cell* 1994;76:333–343.
103. Hodges M, Tissot C, Howe K, et al. Structure, organization, and dynamics of promyelocytic leukemia protein nuclear bodies. *Am J Hum Genet* 1998;63:297–304.
104. Redner RL, Rush EA, Faas S, et al. The t(5;17) variant of acute promyelocytic leukemia expresses a nucleophosmin-retinoic acid receptor fusion. *Blood* 1996;87:882–886.
105. Wells RA, Catzavelos C, Kamel-Reid S. Fusion of retinoic acid receptor alpha to NuMA, the nuclear mitotic apparatus protein, by a variant translocation in acute promyelocytic leukaemia. *Nat Genet* 1997;17: 109–113.
106. He LZ, Merghoub T, Pandolfi PP. In vivo analysis of the molecular pathogenesis of acute promyelocytic leukemia in the mouse and its therapeutic implications. *Oncogene* 1999;18:5278–5292.
107. Lin RJ, Egan DA, Evans RM. Molecular genetics of acute promyelocytic leukemia. *Trends Genet* 1999;15:179–184.
108. Pandolfi PP. PML, PLZF and NPM genes in the molecular pathogenesis of acute promyelocytic leukemia. *Haematologica* 1996;81: 472–482.
109. He LZ, Tribioli C, Rivi R, et al. Acute leukemia with promyelocytic features in PML/RARalpha transgenic mice. *Proc Natl Acad Sci USA* 1997;94:5302–5307.
110. Cheng GX, Zhu XH, Men XQ, et al. Distinct leukemia phenotypes in transgenic mice and different corepressor interactions generated by promyelocytic leukemia variant fusion genes PLZF-RARalpha and NPM-RARalpha. *Proc Natl Acad Sci USA* 1999;96:6318–6323.
111. Hong SH, David G, Wong CW, et al. SMRT corepressor interacts with PLZF and with the PML-retinoic acid receptor alpha (RARalpha) and PLZF-RARalpha oncoproteins associated with acute promyelocytic leukemia. *Proc Natl Acad Sci USA* 1997;94:9028–9033.
112. He LZ, Guidez F, Tribioli C, et al. Distinct interactions of PML-RARalpha and PLZF-RARalpha with co-repressors determine differential responses to RA in APL. *Nat Genet* 1998;18:126–135.
113. Mu ZM, Le XF, Glassman AB, et al. The biologic function of PML and its role in acute promyelocytic leukemia. *Leuk Lymphoma* 1996; 23:277–285.

114. Grimwade D, Solomon E. Characterisation of the PML/RAR alpha rearrangement associated with t(15;17) acute promyelocytic leukaemia. *Curr Top Microbiol Immunol* 1997;220:81–112.
115. Wang ZG, Ruggero D, Ronchetti S, et al. PML is essential for multiple apoptotic pathways [see comments]. *Nat Genet* 1998;20:266–272.
116. Seeler JS, Dejean A. The PML nuclear bodies: actors or extras? *Curr Opin Genet Dev* 1999;9:362–367.
117. Grimwade D, Howe K, Langabeer S, et al. Establishing the presence of the t(15;17) in suspected acute promyelocytic leukaemia: cytogenetic, molecular and PML immunofluorescence assessment of patients entered into the M.R.C. ATRA trial. M.R.C. Adult Leukaemia Working Party. *Br J Haematol* 1996;94:557–573.
118. Chang KS, Stass SA, Chu DT, et al. Characterization of a fusion cDNA (RARA/myl) transcribed from the t(15;17) translocation breakpoint in acute promyelocytic leukemia. *Mol Cell Biol* 1992;12: 800–810.
119. Ohki M. Molecular basis of the t(8;21) translocation in acute myeloid leukaemia. *Semin Cancer Biol* 1993;4:369–375.
120. Andrieu V, Radford-Weiss I, Troussard X, et al. Molecular detection of t(8;21)/AML1-ETO in AML M1/M2: correlation with cytogenetics, morphology and immunophenotype. *Br J Haematol* 1996;92: 855–865.
121. Lo Coco F, Pisegna S, Diverio D. The AML1 gene: a transcription factor involved in the pathogenesis of myeloid and lymphoid leukemias. *Haematologica* 1997;82:364–370.
122. Meyers S, Downing JR, Hiebert SW. Identification of AML-1 and the (8;21) translocation protein (AML-1/ETO) as sequence-specific DNA-binding proteins: the runt homology domain is required for DNA binding and protein-protein interactions. *Mol Cell Biol* 1993; 13:6336–6345.
123. Okuda T, van Deursen J, Hiebert SW, et al. AML1, the target of multiple chromosomal translocations in human leukemia, is essential for normal fetal liver hematopoiesis. *Cell* 1996;84:321–330.
124. Wang Q, Stacy T, Binder M, et al. Disruption of the Cbfa2 gene causes necrosis and hemorrhaging in the central nervous system and blocks definitive hematopoiesis. *Proc Natl Acad Sci USA* 1996;93: 3444–3449.
125. Erickson PF, Robinson M, Owens G, et al. The ETO portion of acute myeloid leukemia t(8;21) fusion transcript encodes a highly evolutionarily conserved, putative transcription factor. *Cancer Res* 1994;54: 1782–1786.
126. Melnick AM, Westendorf JJ, Polinger A, et al. The ETO protein disrupted in t(8;21)-associated acute myeloid leukemia is a corepressor for the promyelocytic leukemia zinc finger protein [in process citation]. *Mol Cell Biol* 2000;20:2075–2086.
127. Le XF, Claxton D, Kornblau S, et al. Characterization of the ETO and AML1-ETO proteins involved in 8;21 translocation in acute myelogenous leukemia. *Eur J Haematol* 1998;60:217–225.
128. Wang J, Wang M, Liu JM. Transformation properties of the ETO gene, fusion partner in t(8:21) leukemias. *Cancer Res* 1997;57: 2951–2955.
129. Erickson P, Gao J, Chang KS, et al. Identification of breakpoints in t(8; 21) acute myelogenous leukemia and isolation of a fusion transcript, AML1/ETO, with similarity to *Drosophila* segmentation gene, *runt*. *Blood* 1992;80:1825–1831.
130. Nucifora G, Rowley JD. AML1 and the 8;21 and 3;21 translocations in acute and chronic myeloid leukemia. *Blood* 1995;86:1–14.
131. McNeil S, Zeng C, Harrington KS, et al. The t(8;21) chromosomal translocation in acute myelogenous leukemia modifies intranuclear targeting of the AML1/CBFalpha2 transcription factor. *Proc Natl Acad Sci USA* 1999;96:14882–14887.
132. Hiebert SW, Downing JR, Lenny N, et al. Transcriptional regulation by the t(8;21) fusion protein, AML-1/ETO. *Curr Top Microbiol Immunol* 1996;211:253–258.
133. Okuda T, Cai Z, Yang S, et al. Expression of a knocked-in AML1-ETO leukemia gene inhibits the establishment of normal definitive hematopoiesis and directly generates dysplastic hematopoietic progenitors. *Blood* 1998;91:3134–3143.
134. Yergeau DA, Hetherington CJ, Wang Q, et al. Embryonic lethality and impairment of haematopoiesis in mice heterozygous for an AML1-ETO fusion gene. *Nat Genet* 1997;15:303–306.
135. Castilla LH, Wijmenga C, Wang Q, et al. Failure of embryonic hematopoiesis and lethal hemorrhages in mouse embryos heterozygous for a knocked-in leukemia gene CBFB-MYH11. *Cell* 1996;87:687–696.
136. Poirel H, Rack K, Delabesse E, et al. Incidence and characterization of MLL gene (11q23) rearrangements in acute myeloid leukemia M1 and M5. *Blood* 1996;87:2496–2505.
137. Bernard OA, Berger R. Molecular basis of 11q23 rearrangements in hematopoietic malignant proliferations. *Genes Chromosomes Cancer* 1995;13:75–85.
138. Rubnitz JE, Behm FG, Downing JR. 11q23 rearrangements in acute leukemia. *Leukemia* 1996;10:74–82.
139. Johansson B, Moorman AV, Secker-Walker LM. Derivative chromosomes of 11q23–translocations in hematologic malignancies. European 11q23 Workshop participants. *Leukemia* 1998;12:828–833.
140. Mbangkollo D, Burnett R, McCabe N, et al. The human MLL gene: nucleotide sequence, homology to the *Drosophila* trx zinc-finger domain, and alternative splicing. *DNA Cell Biol* 1995;14:475–483.
141. Broeker PL, Harden A, Rowley JD, et al. The mixed lineage leukemia (MLL) protein involved in 11q23 translocations contains a domain that binds cruciform DNA and scaffold attachment region (SAR) DNA. *Curr Top Microbiol Immunol* 1996;211:259–268.
142. Domer PH, Fakharzadeh SS, Chen CS, et al. Acute mixed-lineage leukemia t(4;11)(q21;q23) generates an MLL-AF4 fusion product. *Proc Natl Acad Sci USA* 1993;90:7884–7888.
143. Super HJ, Martinez-Climent J, Rowley JD. Molecular analysis of the Mono Mac 6 cell line: detection of an MLL-AF9 fusion transcript [Letter, comment]. *Blood* 1995;85:855–856.
144. Rubnitz JE, Morrissey J, Savage PA, et al. ENL, the gene fused with HRX in t(11;19) leukemias, encodes a nuclear protein with transcriptional activation potential in lymphoid and myeloid cells. *Blood* 1994; 84:1747–1752.
145. Borkhardt A, Repp R, Haas OA, et al. Cloning and characterization of AFX, the gene that fuses to MLL in acute leukemias with a t(X; 11)(q13;q23). *Oncogene* 1997;14:195–202.
146. Hillion J, Le Coniat M, Jonveaux P, et al. AF6q21, a novel partner of the MLL gene in t(6;11)(q21;q23), defines a forkhead transcriptional factor subfamily. *Blood* 1997;90:3714–3719.
147. Sobulo OM, Borrow J, Tomek R, et al. MLL is fused to CBP, a histone acetyltransferase, in therapy-related acute myeloid leukemia with a t(11;16)(q23;p13.3). *Proc Natl Acad Sci USA* 1997;94: 8732–8737.
148. Thirman MJ, Levitan DA, Kobayashi H, et al. Cloning of ELL, a gene that fuses to MLL in a t(11;19)(q23;p13.1) in acute myeloid leukemia. *Proc Natl Acad Sci USA* 1994;91:12110–12114.
149. So CW, Caldas C, Liu MM, et al. EEN encodes for a member of a new family of proteins containing an Src homology 3 domain and is the third gene located on chromosome 19p13 that fuses to MLL in human leukemia. *Proc Natl Acad Sci USA* 1997;94:2563–2568.
150. Taki T, Shibuya N, Taniwaki M, et al. ABI-1, a human homolog to mouse Abl-interactor 1, fuses the MLL gene in acute myeloid leukemia with t(10;11)(p11.2;q23). *Blood* 1998;92:1125–1130.
151. Joh T, Yamamoto K, Kagami Y, et al. Chimeric MLL products with a Ras binding cytoplasmic protein AF6 involved in t(6;11) (q27;q23) leukemia localize in the nucleus. *Oncogene* 1997;15:1681–1687.
152. Osaka M, Rowley JD, Zeleznik-Le NJ. MSF (MLL septin-like fusion), a fusion partner gene of MLL, in a therapy-related acute myeloid leukemia with a t(11;17)(q23;q25). *Proc Natl Acad Sci USA* 1999; 96:6428–6433.
153. Megonigal MD, Rappaport EF, Jones DH, et al. t(11;22)(q23;q11.2) In acute myeloid leukemia of infant twins fuses MLL with hCDCrel, a cell division cycle gene in the genomic region of deletion in Di-George and velocardiofacial syndromes. *Proc Natl Acad Sci USA* 1998;95:6413–6418.
154. Taki T, Ohnishi H, Shinohara K, et al. AF17q25, a putative septin family gene, fuses the MLL gene in acute myeloid leukemia with t(11;17)(q23;q25). *Cancer Res* 1999;59:4261–4265.
155. Tse W, Zhu W, Chen HS, et al. A novel gene, AF1q, fused to MLL in t(1;11) (q21;q23), is specifically expressed in leukemic and immature hematopoietic cells. *Blood* 1995;85:650–656.
156. Mitani K, Kanda Y, Ogawa S, et al. Cloning of several species of MLL/MEN chimeric cDNAs in myeloid leukemia with t(11;19)(q23; p13.1) translocation. *Blood* 1995;85:2017–2024.
157. Griesinger F, Elfers H, Ludwig WD, et al. Detection of HRX-FEL fusion transcripts in pre-pre-B-ALL with and without cytogenetic demonstration of t(4;11). *Leukemia* 1994;8:542–548.
158. Iida S, Seto M, Yamamoto K, et al. MLLT3 gene on 9p22 involved

in t(9;11) leukemia encodes a serine/proline rich protein homologous to MLLT1 on 19p13. *Oncogene* 1993;8:3085–3092.
159. Corral J, Lavenir I, Impey H, et al. An Mll-AF9 fusion gene made by homologous recombination causes acute leukemia in chimeric mice: a method to create fusion oncogenes. *Cell* 1996;85:853–861.
160. Dobson CL, Warren AJ, Pannell R, et al. The mll-AF9 gene fusion in mice controls myeloproliferation and specifies acute myeloid leukaemogenesis. *EMBO J* 1999;18:3564–3574.
161. Lavau C, Szilvassy SJ, Slany R, et al. Immortalization and leukemic transformation of a myelomonocytic precursor by retrovirally transduced HRX-ENL. *EMBO J* 1997;16:4226–4237.
162. Slany RK, Lavau C, Cleary ML. The oncogenic capacity of HRX-ENL requires the transcriptional transactivation activity of ENL and the DNA binding motifs of HRX. *Mol Cell Biol* 1998;18:122–129.
163. Dobson CL, Warren AJ, Pannell R, et al. Tumorigenesis in mice with a fusion of the leukaemia oncogene mll and the bacterial lacZ gene [in process citation]. *EMBO J* 2000;19:843–851.
164. Caslini C, Shilatifard A, Yang L, et al. The amino terminus of the mixed lineage leukemia protein (MLL) promotes cell cycle arrest and monocytic differentiation [in process citation]. *Proc Natl Acad Sci USA* 2000;97:2797–2802.
165. Adler HT, Chinery R, Wu DY, et al. Leukemic HRX fusion proteins inhibit GADD34-induced apoptosis and associate with the GADD34 and hSNF5/INI1 proteins. *Mol Cell Biol* 1999;19:7050–7060.
166. Betts DR, Rohatiner AZ, Evans ML, et al. Abnormalities of chromosome 16q in myeloid malignancy: 14 new cases and a review of the literature. *Leukemia* 1992;6:1250–1256.
167. Bitter MA, Le Beau MM, Larson RA, et al. A morphologic and cytochemical study of acute myelomonocytic leukemia with abnormal marrow eosinophils associated with inv(16)(p13q22). *Am J Clin Pathol* 1984;81:733–741.
168. Liu P, Seidel N, Bodine D, et al. Acute myeloid leukemia with Inv (16) produces a chimeric transcription factor with a myosin heavy chain tail. *Cold Spring Harb Symp Quant Biol* 1994;59:547–553.
169. Liu PP, Hajra A, Wijmenga C, et al. Molecular pathogenesis of the chromosome 16 inversion in the M4Eo subtype of acute myeloid leukemia [see comments] [published erratum appears in *Blood* 1997; 89:1842]. *Blood* 1995;85:2289–2302.
170. Hajra A, Liu PP, Collins FS. Transforming properties of the leukemic inv(16) fusion gene CBFB-MYH11. *Curr Top Microbiol Immunol* 1996;211:289–298.
171. Lutterbach B, Hou Y, Durst KL, et al. The inv(16) encodes an acute myeloid leukemia 1 transcriptional corepressor. *Proc Natl Acad Sci USA* 1999;96:12822–12827.
172. Soekarman D, von Lindern M, van der Plas DC, et al. Dek-can rearrangement in translocation (6;9)(p23;q34). *Leukemia* 1992;6: 489–494.
173. Adriaansen HJ, van Dongen JJ, Hooijkaas H, et al. Translocation (6; 9) may be associated with a specific TdT-positive immunological phenotype in ANLL. *Leukemia* 1988;2:136–140.
174. von Lindern M, Breems D, van Baal S, et al. Characterization of the translocation breakpoint sequences of two DEK-CAN fusion genes present in t(6;9) acute myeloid leukemia and a SET-CAN fusion gene found in a case of acute undifferentiated leukemia. *Genes Chromosomes Cancer* 1992;5:227–234.
175. von Lindern M, Fornerod M, Soekarman N, et al. Translocation t(6; 9) in acute non-lymphocytic leukaemia results in the formation of a DEK-CAN fusion gene. *Baillieres Clin Haematol* 1992;5:857–879.
176. von Lindern M, Fornerod M, van Baal S, et al. The translocation (6; 9), associated with a specific subtype of acute myeloid leukemia, results in the fusion of two genes, dek and can, and the expression of a chimeric, leukemia-specific dek-can mRNA. *Mol Cell Biol* 1992; 12:1687–1697.
177. Soekarman D, von Lindern M, Daenen S, et al. The translocation (6; 9) (p23;q34) shows consistent rearrangement of two genes and defines a myeloproliferative disorder with specific clinical features. *Blood* 1992;79:2990–2997.
178. Sierakowska H, Williams KR, Szer IS, et al. The putative oncoprotein DEK, part of a chimera protein associated with acute myeloid leukaemia, is an autoantigen in juvenile rheumatoid arthritis [published erratum appears in *Clin Exp Immunol* 1994;96:177]. *Clin Exp Immunol* 1993;94:435–439.
179. Murray KJ, Szer W, Grom AA, et al. Antibodies to the 45 kDa DEK nuclear antigen in pauciarticular onset juvenile rheumatoid arthritis and iridocyclitis: selective association with MHC gene. *J Rheumatol* 1997;24:560–567.
180. Fu GK, Grosveld G, Markovitz DM. DEK, an autoantigen involved in a chromosomal translocation in acute myelogenous leukemia, binds to the HIV-2 enhancer. *Proc Natl Acad Sci USA* 1997;94:1811–1815.
181. Fornerod M, Boer J, van Baal S, et al. Interaction of cellular proteins with the leukemia specific fusion proteins DEK-CAN and SET-CAN and their normal counterpart, the nucleoporin CAN. *Oncogene* 1996; 13:1801–1808.
182. Fornerod M, Boer J, van Baal S, et al. Relocation of the carboxyterminal part of CAN from the nuclear envelope to the nucleus as a result of leukemia-specific chromosome rearrangements. *Oncogene* 1995;10:1739–1748.
183. Shtivelman E, Lifshitz B, Gale RP, et al. Fused transcript of abl and bcr genes in chronic myelogenous leukaemia. *Nature* 1985;315:550–554.
184. Rowley JD. The Philadelphia chromosome translocation: a paradigm for understanding leukemia. *Cancer* 1990;65:2178–2184.
185. Maru Y, Witte ON. The BCR gene encodes a novel serine/threonine kinase activity within a single exon. *Cell* 1991;67:459–468.
186. Pendergast AM, Muller AJ, Havlik MH, et al. BCR sequences essential for transformation by the BCR-ABL oncogene bind to the ABL SH2 regulatory domain in a non-phosphotyrosine-dependent manner. *Cell* 1991;66:161–171.
187. Diekmann D, Brill S, Garrett MD, et al. Bcr encodes a GTPase-activating protein for p21rac. *Nature* 1991;351:400–402.
188. Groffen J, Stephenson JR, Heisterkamp N, et al. Philadelphia chromosomal breakpoints are clustered within a limited region, bcr, on chromosome 22. *Cell* 1984;36:93–99.
189. Ben-Neriah Y, Daley GQ, Mes-Masson AM, et al. The chronic myelogenous leukemia-specific P210 protein is the product of the bcr/abl hybrid gene. *Science* 1986;233:212–214.
190. Melo JV, Myint H, Galton DA, et al. P190BCR-ABL chronic myeloid leukaemia: the missing link with chronic myelomonocytic leukaemia? [see comments]. *Leukemia* 1994;8:208–211.
191. Kunieda Y, Okabe M, Kurosawa M, et al. Chronic myeloid leukemia presenting ALL-type BCR/ABL transcript. *Ann Hematol* 1994;69: 189–193.
192. Chan LC, Karhi KK, Rayter SI, et al. A novel abl protein expressed in Philadelphia chromosome positive acute lymphoblastic leukaemia. *Nature* 1987;325:635–637.
193. Hermans A, Heisterkamp N, von Linden M, et al. Unique fusion of bcr and c-abl genes in Philadelphia chromosome positive acute lymphoblastic leukemia. *Cell* 1987;51:33–40.
194. Clark SS, McLaughlin J, Crist WM, et al. Unique forms of the abl tyrosine kinase distinguish Ph1-positive CML from Ph1-positive ALL. *Science* 1987;235:85–88.
195. Kurzrock R, Shtalrid M, Romero P, et al. A novel c-abl protein product in Philadelphia-positive acute lymphoblastic leukaemia. *Nature* 1987; 325:631–635.
196. Walker LC, Ganesan TS, Dhut S, et al. Novel chimaeric protein expressed in Philadelphia positive acute lymphoblastic leukaemia. *Nature* 1987;329:851–853.
197. Pear WS, Miller JP, Xu L, et al. Efficient and rapid induction of a chronic myelogenous leukemia-like myeloproliferative disease in mice receiving P210 bcr/abl-transduced bone marrow. *Blood* 1998; 92:3780–3792.
198. Daley GQ, Van Etten RA, Baltimore D. Induction of chronic myelogenous leukemia in mice by the P210bcr/abl gene of the Philadelphia chromosome. *Science* 1990;247:824–830.
199. Huettner CS, Zhang P, Van Etten RA, et al. Reversibility of acute B-cell leukaemia induced by BCR-ABL1. *Nat Genet* 2000;24:57–60.
200. Castellanos A, Pintado B, Weruaga E, et al. A BCR-ABL(p190) fusion gene made by homologous recombination causes B-cell acute lymphoblastic leukemias in chimeric mice with independence of the endogenous bcr product. *Blood* 1997;90:2168–2174.
201. Voncken JW, Kaartinen V, Pattengale PK, et al. BCR/ABL P210 and P190 cause distinct leukemia in transgenic mice. *Blood* 1995;86: 4603–4611.
202. Voncken JW, Griffiths S, Greaves MF, et al. Restricted oncogenicity of BCR/ABL p190 in transgenic mice. *Cancer Res* 1992;52: 4534–4539.
203. Heisterkamp N, Jenster G, ten Hoeve J, et al. Acute leukaemia in bcr/abl transgenic mice. *Nature* 1990;344:251–253.

204. Stuppia L, Calabrese G, Peila R, et al. P53 loss and point mutations are associated with suppression of apoptosis and progression of CML into myeloid blastic crisis. *Cancer Genet Cytogenet* 1997;98:28–35.
205. Marasca R, Luppi M, Barozzi P, et al. P53 gene mutations in chronic myelogenous leukemia medullary and extramedullary blast crisis. *Leuk Lymphoma* 1996;24:175–182.
206. Lanza F, Bi S. Role of p53 in leukemogenesis of chronic myeloid leukemia. *Stem Cells* 1995;13:445–452.
207. Nakai H, Misawa S, Toguchida J, et al. Frequent p53 gene mutations in blast crisis of chronic myelogenous leukemia, especially in myeloid crisis harboring loss of a chromosome 17p. *Cancer Res* 1992;52:6588–6593.
208. Honda H, Ushijima T, Wakazono K, et al. Acquired loss of p53 induces blastic transformation in p210(bcr/abl)-expressing hematopoietic cells: a transgenic study for blast crisis of human CML. *Blood* 2000;95:1144–1150.
209. Mitani K. Molecular mechanism of blastic crisis in chronic myelocytic leukemia. *Leukemia* 1997;11 Suppl 3:503–505.
210. Serra A, Gottardi E, Della Ragione F, et al. Involvement of the cyclin-dependent kinase-4 inhibitor (CDKN2) gene in the pathogenesis of lymphoid blast crisis of chronic myelogenous leukaemia. *Br J Haematol* 1995;91:625–629.
211. Sill H, Aguiar CT, Schmidt H, et al. Mutational analysis of the p15 and p16 genes in acute leukaemias. *Br J Haematol* 1996;92:681–683.
212. Troussard X, Rimokh R, Valensi F, et al. Heterogeneity of t(1;19)(q23; p13) acute leukaemias: French Haematological Cytology Group. *Br J Haematol* 1995;89:516–526.
213. Nourse J, Mellentin JD, Galili N, et al. Chromosomal translocation t(1;19) results in synthesis of a homeobox fusion mRNA that codes for a potential chimeric transcription factor. *Cell* 1990;60:535–545.
214. Kamps MP, Murre C, Sun XH, et al. A new homeobox gene contributes the DNA binding domain of the t(1;19) translocation protein in pre-B ALL. *Cell* 1990;60:547–555.
215. Hunger SP. Chromosomal translocations involving the E2A gene in acute lymphoblastic leukemia: clinical features and molecular pathogenesis. *Blood* 1996;87:1211–1224.
216. Kamps MP, Wright DD. Oncoprotein E2A-Pbx1 immortalizes a myeloid progenitor in primary marrow cultures without abrogating its factor-dependence. *Oncogene* 1994;9:3159–3166.
217. Kamps MP. E2A-Pbx1 induces growth, blocks differentiation, and interacts with other homeodomain proteins regulating normal differentiation. *Curr Top Microbiol Immunol* 1997;220:25–43.
218. Kamps MP, Baltimore D. E2A-Pbx1, the t(1;19) translocation protein of human pre-B-cell acute lymphocytic leukemia, causes acute myeloid leukemia in mice. *Mol Cell Biol* 1993;13:351–357.
219. Dedera DA, Waller EK, LeBrun DP, et al. Chimeric homeobox gene E2A-PBX1 induces proliferation, apoptosis, and malignant lymphomas in transgenic mice [published erratum appears in *Cell* 1993; 75:826]. *Cell* 1993;74:833–843.
220. Chang CP, de Vivo I, Cleary ML. The Hox cooperativity motif of the chimeric oncoprotein E2a-Pbx1 is necessary and sufficient for oncogenesis. *Mol Cell Biol* 1997;17:81–88.
221. Fu X, Kamps MP. E2a-Pbx1 induces aberrant expression of tissue-specific and developmentally regulated genes when expressed in NIH 3T3 fibroblasts. *Mol Cell Biol* 1997;17:1503–1512.
222. de Lau WB, Hurenkamp J, Berendes P, et al. The gene encoding the granulocyte colony-stimulating factor receptor is a target for deregulation in pre-B ALL by the t(1;19)-specific oncoprotein E2A-Pbx1. *Oncogene* 1998;17:503–510.
223. Fu X, McGrath S, Pasillas M, et al. EB-1, a tyrosine kinase signal transduction gene, is transcriptionally activated in the t(1;19) subset of pre-B ALL, which express oncoprotein E2a-Pbx1. *Oncogene* 1999; 18:4920–4929.
224. McWhirter JR, Neuteboom ST, Wancewicz EV, et al. Oncogenic homeodomain transcription factor E2A-Pbx1 activates a novel WNT gene in pre-B acute lymphoblastoid leukemia. *Proc Natl Acad Sci USA* 1999;96:11464–11469.
225. Fu X, Roberts WG, Nobile V, et al. Angiogenin-3, a target gene of oncoprotein E2a-Pbx1, encodes a new angiogenic member of the angiogenin family. *Growth Factors* 1999;17:125–137.
226. Romana SP, Poirel H, Leconiat M, et al. High frequency of t(12;21) in childhood B-lineage acute lymphoblastic leukemia. *Blood* 1995; 86:4263–4269.
227. Loh ML, McLean TW, Buckley JD, et al. Lack of TEL/AML1 fusion in pediatric AML: further evidence for lineage specificity of TEL/AML1. *Leuk Res* 1998;22:461–464.
228. Hoshino K, Asou N, Suzushima H, et al. TEL/AML1 fusion gene resulting from a cryptic t(12;21) is uncommon in adult patients with B-cell lineage ALL and CML lymphoblastic transformation. *Int J Hematol* 1997;66:213–218.
229. Dittmer J, Nordheim A. Ets transcription factors and human disease. *Biochim Biophys Acta* 1998;1377:F1–11.
230. Fenrick R, Amann JM, Lutterbach B, et al. Both TEL and AML-1 contribute repression domains to the t(12;21) fusion protein. *Mol Cell Biol* 1999;19:6566–6574.
231. Golub TR, Barker GF, Bohlander SK, et al. Fusion of the TEL gene on 12p13 to the AML1 gene on 21q22 in acute lymphoblastic leukemia. *Proc Natl Acad Sci USA* 1995;92:4917–4921.
232. Romana SP, Mauchauffe M, Le Coniat M, et al. The t(12;21) of acute lymphoblastic leukemia results in a tel-AML1 gene fusion. *Blood* 1995;85:3662–3670.
233. Uchida H, Downing JR, Miyazaki Y, et al. Three distinct domains in TEL-AML1 are required for transcriptional repression of the IL-3 promoter. *Oncogene* 1999;18:1015–1022.
234. Song H, Kim JH, Rho JK, et al. Functional characterization of TEL/AML1 fusion protein in the regulation of human CR1 gene promoter. *Mol Cells* 1999;9:560–563.
235. Schlieben S, Borkhardt A, Reinisch I, et al. Incidence and clinical outcome of children with BCR/ABL-positive acute lymphoblastic leukemia (ALL): a prospective RT-PCR study based on 673 patients enrolled in the German pediatric multicenter therapy trials ALL-BFM-90 and CoALL-05-92. *Leukemia* 1996;10:957–963.
236. Radich JP, Kopecky KJ, Boldt DH, et al. Detection of BCR-ABL fusion genes in adult acute lymphoblastic leukemia by the polymerase chain reaction. *Leukemia* 1994;8:1688–1695.
237. Westbrook CA, Hooberman AL, Spino C, et al. Clinical significance of the BCR-ABL fusion gene in adult acute lymphoblastic leukemia: a Cancer and Leukemia Group B study (8762). *Blood* 1992;80: 2983–2990.
238. Fletcher JA, Tu N, Tantravahi R, et al. Extremely poor prognosis of pediatric acute lymphoblastic leukemia with translocation (9;22): updated experience. *Leuk Lymphoma* 1992;8:75–79.
239. Pui CH, Carroll LAJ, Raimondi SC, et al. Childhood acute lymphoblastic leukemia with the t(4;11)(q21;q23): an update [Letter]. *Blood* 1994;83:2384–2385.
240. Inaba T, Roberts WM, Shapiro LH, et al. Fusion of the leucine zipper gene HLF to the E2A gene in human acute B-lineage leukemia. *Science* 1992;257:531–534.
241. Inukai T, Inaba T, Yoshihara T, et al. Cell transformation mediated by homodimeric E2A-HLF transcription factors. *Mol Cell Biol* 1997; 17:1417–1424.
242. Quesnel B, Preudhomme C, Fenaux P. P16ink4a gene and hematological malignancies. *Leuk Lymphoma* 1996;22:11–24.
243. Yokota S, Nakao M, Horiike S, et al. Mutational analysis of the N-ras gene in acute lymphoblastic leukemia: a study of 125 Japanese pediatric cases. *Int J Hematol* 1998;67:379–387.
244. Kawamura M, Kikuchi A, Kobayashi S, et al. Mutations of the p53 and ras genes in childhood t(1;19)-acute lymphoblastic leukemia. *Blood* 1995;85:2546–2552.
245. Fenaux P, Jonveaux P, Quiquandon I, et al. Mutations of the p53 gene in B-cell lymphoblastic acute leukemia: a report on 60 cases. *Leukemia* 1992;6:42–46.
246. Kawano S, Miller CW, Gombart AF, et al. Loss of p73 gene expression in leukemias/lymphomas due to hypermethylation. *Blood* 1999; 94:1113–1120.
247. Goldfarb AN, Greenberg JM. T-cell acute lymphoblastic leukemia and the associated basic helix-loop-helix gene SCL/tal. *Leuk Lymphoma* 1994;12:157–166.
248. Goldfarb AN, Goueli S, Mickelson D, et al. T-cell acute lymphoblastic leukemia—the associated gene SCL/tal codes for a 42–Kd nuclear phosphoprotein. *Blood* 1992;80:2858–2866.
249. Kelliher MA, Seldin DC, Leder P. Tal-1 induces T cell acute lymphoblastic leukemia accelerated by casein kinase II alpha. *EMBO J* 1996; 15:5160–5166.
250. Bernard O, Lecointe N, Jonveaux P, et al. Two site-specific deletions and t(1;14) translocation restricted to human T-cell acute leukemias disrupt the 5′ part of the tal-1 gene. *Oncogene* 1991;6:1477–1488.
251. Brown L, Cheng JT, Chen Q, et al. Site-specific recombination of the

tal-1 gene is a common occurrence in human T cell leukemia. *EMBO J* 1990;9:3343–3351.
252. Pulford K, Lecointe N, Leroy-Viard K, et al. Expression of TAL-1 proteins in human tissues. *Blood* 1995;85:675–684.
253. Condorelli GL, Facchiano F, Valtieri M, et al. T-cell–directed TAL-1 expression induces T-cell malignancies in transgenic mice. *Cancer Res* 1996;56:5113–5119.
254. Valtieri M, Tocci A, Gabbianelli M, et al. Enforced TAL-1 expression stimulates primitive, erythroid and megakaryocytic progenitors but blocks the granulopoietic differentiation program. *Cancer Res* 1998; 58:562–569.
255. Goldfarb AN, Lewandowska K. Inhibition of cellular differentiation by the SCL/tal oncoprotein: transcriptional repression by an Id-like mechanism. *Blood* 1995;85:465–471.
256. Dube ID, Kamel-Reid S, Yuan CC, et al. A novel human homeobox gene lies at the chromosome 10 breakpoint in lymphoid neoplasias with chromosomal translocation t(10;14). *Blood* 1991;78:2996–3003.
257. Hawley RG, Fong AZ, Lu M, et al.. The HOX11 homeobox-containing gene of human leukemia immortalizes murine hematopoietic precursors. *Oncogene* 1994;9:1–12.
258. Hatano M, Roberts CW, Minden M, et al. Deregulation of a homeobox gene, HOX11, by the t(10;14) in T cell leukemia. *Science* 1991;253: 79–82.
259. Kennedy MA, Gonzalez-Sarmiento R, Kees UR, et al. HOX11, a homeobox-containing T-cell oncogene on human chromosome 10q24. *Proc Natl Acad Sci USA* 1991;88:8900–8904.
260. Hawley RG, Fong AZ, Reis MD, et al. Transforming function of the HOX11/TCL3 homeobox gene. *Cancer Res* 1997;57:337–345.
261. Kawabe T, Muslin AJ, Korsmeyer SJ. HOX11 interacts with protein phosphatases PP2A and PP1 and disrupts a G2/M cell-cycle checkpoint. *Nature* 1997;385:454–458.
262. Dear TN, Colledge WH, Carlton MB, et al. The Hox11 gene is essential for cell survival during spleen development. *Development* 1995; 121:2909–2915.
263. McGuire EA, Hockett RD, Pollock KM, et al. The t(11;14)(p15;q11) in a T-cell acute lymphoblastic leukemia cell line activates multiple transcripts, including Ttg-1, a gene encoding a potential zinc finger protein. *Mol Cell Biol* 1989;9:2124–2132.
264. Boehm T, Foroni L, Kaneko Y, et al. The rhombotin family of cysteine-rich LIM-domain oncogenes: distinct members are involved in T-cell translocations to human chromosomes 11p15 and 11p13. *Proc Natl Acad Sci USA* 1991;88:4367–4371.
265. Royer-Pokora B, Loos U, Ludwig WD. TTG-2, a new gene encoding a cysteine-rich protein with the LIM motif, is overexpressed in acute T-cell leukaemia with the t(11;14)(p13;q11). *Oncogene* 1991;6: 1887–1893.
266. Boehm T, Foroni L, Kennedy M, et al. The rhombotin gene belongs to a class of transcriptional regulators with a potential novel protein dimerization motif. *Oncogene* 1990;5:1103–1105.
267. Mao S, Neale GA, Goorha RM. T-cell proto-oncogene rhombotin-2 is a complex transcription regulator containing multiple activation and repression domains. *J Biol Chem* 1997;272:5594–5599.
268. McGuire EA, Davis AR, Korsmeyer SJ. T-cell translocation gene 1 (Ttg-1) encodes a nuclear protein normally expressed in neural lineage cells. *Blood* 1991;77:599–606.
269. Dong WF, Billia F, Atkins HL, et al. Expression of rhombotin 2 in normal and leukaemic haemopoietic cells. *Br J Haematol* 1996;93: 280–286.
270. Wadman IA, Osada H, Grutz GG, et al. The LIM-only protein Lmo2 is a bridging molecule assembling an erythroid, DNA-binding complex which includes the TAL1, E47, GATA-1 and Ldb1/NLI proteins. *EMBO J* 1997;16:3145–3157.
271. Yamada Y, Warren AJ, Dobson C, et al. The T cell leukemia LIM protein LMO2 is necessary for adult mouse hematopoiesis. *Proc Natl Acad Sci USA* 1998;95:3890–3895.
272. Fisch P, Boehm T, Lavenir I, et al. T-cell acute lymphoblastic lymphoma induced in transgenic mice by the RBTN1 and RBTN2 LIM-domain genes. *Oncogene* 1992;7:2389–2397.
273. McGuire EA, Rintoul CE, Sclar GM, et al. Thymic overexpression of Ttg-1 in transgenic mice results in T-cell acute lymphoblastic leukemia/lymphoma. *Mol Cell Biol* 1992;12:4186–4196.
274. Neale GA, Rehg JE, Goorha RM. Disruption of T-cell differentiation precedes T-cell tumor formation in LMO-2 (rhombotin-2) transgenic mice. *Leukemia* 1997;11[Suppl 3]:289–290.
275. Joutel A, Tournier-Lasserve E. Notch signalling pathway and human diseases. *Semin Cell Dev Biol* 1998;9:619–625.
276. Ellisen LW, Bird J, West DC, et al. TAN-1, the human homolog of the Drosophila notch gene, is broken by chromosomal translocations in T lymphoblastic neoplasms. *Cell* 1991;66:649–661.
277. Capobianco AJ, Zagouras P, Blaumueller CM, et al. Neoplastic transformation by truncated alleles of human NOTCH1/TAN1 and NOTCH2. *Mol Cell Biol* 1997;17:6265–6273.
278. Lu FM, Lux SE. Constitutively active human Notch1 binds to the transcription factor CBF1 and stimulates transcription through a promoter containing a CBF1-responsive element. *Proc Natl Acad Sci USA* 1996;93:5663–5667.
279. Hsieh JJ, Henkel T, Salmon P, et al. Truncated mammalian Notch1 activates CBF1/RBPJk-repressed genes by a mechanism resembling that of Epstein-Barr virus EBNA2. *Mol Cell Biol* 1996;16:952–959.
280. Ohnishi H, Kawamura M, Ida K, et al. Homozygous deletions of p16/MTS1 gene are frequent but mutations are infrequent in childhood T-cell acute lymphoblastic leukemia. *Blood* 1995;86:1269–1275.
281. Ogawa S, Hirano N, Sato N, et al. Homozygous loss of the cyclin-dependent kinase 4-inhibitor (p16) gene in human leukemias. *Blood* 1994;84:2431–2435.
282. Kawamura M, Ohnishi H, Guo SX, et al. Alterations of the p53, p21, p16, p15 and RAS genes in childhood T-cell acute lymphoblastic leukemia. *Leuk Res* 1999;23:115–126.
283. Harris NL, Jaffe ES, Stein H, et al. A revised European-American classification of lymphoid neoplasms: a proposal from the International Lymphoma Study Group [see comments]. *Blood* 1994;84: 1361–1392.
284. Harris NL, Jaffe ES, Diebold J, et al. The World Health Organization classification of hematological malignancies report of the Clinical Advisory Committee Meeting, Airlie House, Virginia, November 1997. *Mod Pathol* 2000;13:193–207.
285. Reed JC. Molecular biology of chronic lymphocytic leukemia. *Semin Oncol* 1998;25:11–18.
286. Dohner H, Stilgenbauer S, James MR, et al. 11q Deletions identify a new subset of B-cell chronic lymphocytic leukemia characterized by extensive nodal involvement and inferior prognosis. *Blood* 1997; 89:2516–2522.
287. Schaffner C, Stilgenbauer S, Rappold GA, et al. Somatic ATM mutations indicate a pathogenic role of ATM in B-cell chronic lymphocytic leukemia. *Blood* 1999;94:748–753.
288. Woessner S, Sole F, Perez-Losada A, et al. Trisomy 12 is a rare cytogenetic finding in typical chronic lymphocytic leukemia [see comments]. *Leuk Res* 1996;20:369–374.
289. Matutes E, Oscier D, Garcia-Marco J, et al. Trisomy 12 defines a group of CLL with atypical morphology: correlation between cytogenetic, clinical and laboratory features in 544 patients. *Br J Haematol* 1996;92:382–388.
290. Su'ut L, O'Connor SJ, Richards SJ, et al. Trisomy 12 is seen within a specific subtype of B-cell chronic lymphoproliferative disease affecting the peripheral blood/bone marrow and co-segregates with elevated expression of CD11a. *Br J Haematol* 1998;101:165–170.
291. Tefferi A, Bartholmai BJ, Witzig TE, et al. Clinical correlations of immunophenotypic variations and the presence of trisomy 12 in B-cell chronic lymphocytic leukemia. *Cancer Genet* Cytogenet 1997; 95:173–177.
292. Cordone I, Masi S, Mauro FR, et al. P53 expression in B-cell chronic lymphocytic leukemia: a marker of disease progression and poor prognosis. *Blood* 1998;91:4342–4349.
293. Lens D, Dyer MJ, Garcia-Marco JM, et al. P53 abnormalities in CLL are associated with excess of prolymphocytes and poor prognosis. *Br J Haematol* 1997;99:848–857.
294. Gaidano G, Ballerini P, Gong JZ, et al. P53 mutations in human lymphoid malignancies: association with Burkitt lymphoma and chronic lymphocytic leukemia. *Proc Natl Acad Sci USA* 1991;88: 5413–5417.
295. Iida S, Rao PH, Nallasivam P, et al. The t(9;14)(p13;q32) chromosomal translocation associated with lymphoplasmacytoid lymphoma involves the PAX-5 gene. *Blood* 1996;88:4110–4117.
296. Enver T. B-cell commitment: Pax5 is the deciding factor. *Curr Biol* 1999;9:R933–935.
297. Raffeld M, Jaffe ES. Bcl-1, t(11;14), and mantle cell-derived lymphomas [editorial]. *Blood* 1991;78:259–263.
298. Tsujimoto Y, Yunis J, Onorato-Showe L, et al. Molecular cloning of

the chromosomal breakpoint of B-cell lymphomas and leukemias with the t(11;14) chromosome translocation. *Science* 1984;224: 1403–1406.

299. Tsujimoto Y, Jaffe E, Cossman J, et al. Clustering of breakpoints on chromosome 11 in human B-cell neoplasms with the t(11;14) chromosome translocation. *Nature* 1985;315:340–343.
300. Erikson J, Finan J, Tsujimoto Y, et al. The chromosome 14 breakpoint in neoplastic B cells with the t(11;14) translocation involves the immunoglobulin heavy chain locus. *Proc Natl Acad Sci USA* 1984;81: 4144–4148.
301. Williams ME, Meeker TC, Swerdlow SH. Rearrangement of the chromosome 11 bcl-1 locus in centrocytic lymphoma: analysis with multiple breakpoint probes. *Blood* 1991;78:493–498.
302. Williams ME, Swerdlow SH, Meeker TC. Chromosome t(11;14)(q13; q32) breakpoints in centrocytic lymphoma are highly localized at the bcl-1 major translocation cluster. *Leukemia* 1993;7:1437–1440.
303. Bartkova J, Lukas J, Strauss M, et al. Cell cycle-related variation and tissue-restricted expression of human cyclin D1 protein. *J Pathol* 1994;172:237–245.
304. Withers DA, Harvey RC, Faust JB, et al. Characterization of a candidate bcl-1 gene. *Mol Cell Biol* 1991;11:4846–4853.
305. Rimokh R, Berger F, Delsol G, et al. Rearrangement and overexpression of the BCL-1/PRAD-1 gene in intermediate lymphocytic lymphomas and in t(11q13)-bearing leukemias. *Blood* 1993;81: 3063–3067.
306. Rosenberg CL, Wong E, Petty EM, et al. PRAD1, a candidate BCL1 oncogene: mapping and expression in centrocytic lymphoma. *Proc Natl Acad Sci USA* 1991;88:9638–9642.
307. Seto M, Yamamoto K, Iida S, et al. Gene rearrangement and overexpression of PRAD1 in lymphoid malignancy with t(11;14)(q13;q32) translocation. *Oncogene* 1992;7:1401–1406.
308. Bosch F, Jares P, Campo E, et al. PRAD-1/cyclin D1 gene overexpression in chronic lymphoproliferative disorders: a highly specific marker of mantle cell lymphoma. *Blood* 1994;84:2726–2732.
309. Chibbar R, Leung K, McCormick S, et al. Bcl-1 gene rearrangements in mantle cell lymphoma: a comprehensive analysis of 118 cases, including B-5–fixed tissue, by polymerase chain reaction and Southern transfer analysis. *Mod Pathol* 1998;11:1089–1097.
310. Yang WI, Zukerberg LR, Motokura T, et al. Cyclin D1 (Bcl-1, PRAD1) protein expression in low-grade B-cell lymphomas and reactive hyperplasia. *Am J Pathol* 1994;145:86–96.
311. de Boer CJ, van Krieken JH, Schuuring E, et al. Bcl-1/cyclin D1 in malignant lymphoma. *Ann Oncol* 1997;8:109–117.
312. Swerdlow SH, Yang WI, Zukerberg LR, et al. Expression of cyclin D1 protein in centrocytic/mantle cell lymphomas with and without rearrangement of the BCL1/cyclin D1 gene. *Hum Pathol* 1995;26: 999–1004.
313. Bates S, Peters G. Cyclin D1 as a cellular proto-oncogene. *Semin Cancer Biol* 1995;6:73–82.
314. Callanan M, Leroux D, Magaud JP, et al. Implication of cyclin D1 in malignant lymphoma. *Crit Rev Oncol* 1996;7:191–203.
315. Garcia-Conde J, Cabanillas F. Mantle cell lymphoma: a lymphoproliferative disorder associated with aberrant function of the cell cycle. *Leukemia* 1996;10[Suppl 2]:s78–83.
316. Bodrug SE, Warner BJ, Bath ML, et al. Cyclin D1 transgene impedes lymphocyte maturation and collaborates in lymphomagenesis with the myc gene. *EMBO J* 1994;13:2124–2130.
317. Lovec H, Grzeschiczek A, Kowalski MB, et al. Cyclin D1/bcl-1 cooperates with myc genes in the generation of B-cell lymphoma in transgenic mice. *EMBO J* 1994;13:3487–3495.
318. Mueller A, Odze R, Jenkins TD, et al. A transgenic mouse model with cyclin D1 overexpression results in cell cycle, epidermal growth factor receptor, and p53 abnormalities. *Cancer Res* 1997;57: 5542–5549.
319. Robles AI, Larcher F, Whalin RB, et al. Expression of cyclin D1 in epithelial tissues of transgenic mice results in epidermal hyperproliferation and severe thymic hyperplasia. *Proc Natl Acad Sci USA* 1996; 93:7634–7638.
320. Wang TC, Cardiff RD, Zukerberg L, et al. Mammary hyperplasia and carcinoma in MMTV-cyclin D1 transgenic mice. *Nature* 1994;369: 669–671.
321. Greiner TC, Moynihan MJ, Chan WC, et al. P53 mutations in mantle cell lymphoma are associated with variant cytology and predict a poor prognosis. *Blood* 1996;87:4302–4310.
322. Zoldan MC, Inghirami G, Masuda Y, et al. Large-cell variants of mantle cell lymphoma: cytologic characteristics and p53 anomalies may predict poor outcome. *Br J Haematol* 1996;93:475–486.
323. Hernandez L, Fest T, Cazorla M, et al. P53 gene mutations and protein overexpression are associated with aggressive variants of mantle cell lymphomas. *Blood* 1996;87:3351–3359.
324. Gronbaek K, Nedergaard T, Andersen MK, et al. Concurrent disruption of cell cycle associated genes in mantle cell lymphoma: a genotypic and phenotypic study of cyclin D1, p16, p15, p53 and pRb. *Leukemia* 1998;12:1266–1271.
325. Pinyol M, Hernandez L, Cazorla M, et al. Deletions and loss of expression of p16INK4a and p21Waf1 genes are associated with aggressive variants of mantle cell lymphomas. *Blood* 1997;89:272–280.
326. Bakhshi A, Jensen JP, Goldman P, et al. Cloning the chromosomal breakpoint of t(14;18) human lymphomas: clustering around JH on chromosome 14 and near a transcriptional unit on 18. *Cell* 1985;41: 899–906.
327. Tsujimoto Y, Finger LR, Yunis J, et al. Cloning of the chromosome breakpoint of neoplastic B cells with the t(14;18) chromosome translocation. *Science* 1984;226:1097–1099.
328. Cleary ML, Smith SD, Sklar J. Cloning and structural analysis of cDNAs for bcl-2 and a hybrid bcl-2/immunoglobulin transcript resulting from the t(14;18) translocation. *Cell* 1986;47:19–28.
329. Cleary ML, Sklar J. Nucleotide sequence of a t(14;18) chromosomal breakpoint in follicular lymphoma and demonstration of a breakpoint-cluster region near a transcriptionally active locus on chromosome 18. *Proc Natl Acad Sci USA* 1985;82:7439–7443.
330. Cleary ML, Galili N, Sklar J. Detection of a second t(14;18) breakpoint cluster region in human follicular lymphomas. *J Exp Med* 1986; 164:315–320.
331. Wang YL, Addya K, Edwards RH, et al. Novel bcl-2 breakpoints in patients with follicular lymphoma. *Diagn Mol Pathol* 1998;7:85–89.
332. Graninger WB, Seto M, Boutain B, et al. Expression of Bcl-2 and Bcl-2–Ig fusion transcripts in normal and neoplastic cells. *J Clin Invest* 1987;80:1512–1515.
333. Ngan BY, Chen-Levy Z, Weiss LM, et al. Expression in non-Hodgkin's lymphoma of the bcl-2 protein associated with the t(14;18) chromosomal translocation. *N Engl J Med* 1988;318:1638–1644.
334. Petrovic AS, Young RL, Hilgarth B, et al. The Ig heavy chain 3′ end confers a posttranscriptional processing advantage to Bcl-2–IgH fusion RNA in t(14;18) lymphoma. *Blood* 1998;91:3952–3961.
335. Nunez G, Hockenbery D, McDonnell TJ, et al. Bcl-2 maintains B cell memory. *Nature* 1991;353:71–73.
336. Smith KG, Light A, O'Reilly LA, et al. Bcl-2 transgene expression inhibits apoptosis in the germinal center and reveals differences in the selection of memory B cells and bone marrow antibody-forming cells. *J Exp Med* 2000;191:475–484.
337. McDonnell TJ, Deane N, Platt FM, et al. Bcl-2–immunoglobulin transgenic mice demonstrate extended B cell survival and follicular lymphoproliferation. *Cell* 1989;57:79–88.
338. McDonnell TJ, Korsmeyer SJ. Progression from lymphoid hyperplasia to high-grade malignant lymphoma in mice transgenic for the t(14; 18). *Nature* 1991;349:254–256.
339. Lo Coco F, Gaidano G, Louie DC, et al. P53 mutations are associated with histologic transformation of follicular lymphoma. *Blood* 1993; 82:2289–2295.
340. Sander CA, Yano T, Clark HM, et al. P53 mutation is associated with progression in follicular lymphomas. *Blood* 1993;82:1994–2004.
341. Villuendas R, Sanchez-Beato M, Martinez JC, et al. Loss of p16/INK4A protein expression in non-Hodgkin's lymphomas is a frequent finding associated with tumor progression. *Am J Pathol* 1998;153: 887–897.
342. Yano T, Jaffe ES, Longo DL, et al. MYC rearrangements in histologically progressed follicular lymphomas. *Blood* 1992;80:758–767.
343. Bertoni F, Cotter FE, Zucca E. Molecular genetics of extranodal marginal zone (MALT-type) B-cell lymphoma. *Leuk Lymphoma* 1999; 35:57–68.
344. Horsman D, Gascoyne R, Klasa R, et al. T(11;18)(q21;q21.1): a recurring translocation in lymphomas of mucosa-associated lymphoid tissue (MALT)? *Genes Chromosomes Cancer* 1992;4:183–187.
345. Auer IA, Gascoyne RD, Connors JM, et al. T(11;18)(q21;q21) is the most common translocation in MALT lymphomas. *Ann Oncol* 1997; 8:979–985.
346. Ott G, Katzenberger T, Greiner A, et al. The t(11;18)(q21;q21) chro-

mosome translocation is a frequent and specific aberration in low-grade but not high-grade malignant non-Hodgkin's lymphomas of the mucosa-associated lymphoid tissue (MALT) type. *Cancer Res* 1997; 57:3944–3948.
347. Dierlamm J, Baens M, Wlodarska I, et al. The apoptosis inhibitor gene API2 and a novel 18q gene, MLT, are recurrently rearranged in the t(11;18)(q21;q21) p6 associated with mucosa-associated lymphoid tissue lymphomas [see comments]. *Blood* 1999;93:3601–3609.
348. Morgan JA, Yin Y, Borowsky AD, et al. Breakpoints of the t(11; 18)(q21;q21) in mucosa-associated lymphoid tissue (MALT) lymphoma lie within or near the previously undescribed gene MALT1 in chromosome 18. *Cancer Res* 1999;59:6205–6213.
349. Suzuki H, Motegi M, Akagi T, et al. API1-MALT1-MLT is involved in mucosa-associated lymphoid tissue lymphoma with t(11;18)(q21; q21) [Letter; comment]. *Blood* 1999;94:3270–3271.
350. Akagi T, Motegi M, Tamura A, et al. A novel gene, MALT1 at 18q21, is involved in t(11;18) (q21;q21) found in low-grade B-cell lymphoma of mucosa-associated lymphoid tissue. *Oncogene* 1999;18: 5785–5794.
351. Akagi T, Tamura A, Motegi M, et al. Molecular cytogenetic delineation of the breakpoint at 18q21.1 in low-grade B-cell lymphoma of mucosa-associated lymphoid tissue. *Genes Chromosomes Cancer* 1999;24:315–321.
352. Deveraux QL, Reed JC. IAP family proteins—suppressors of apoptosis. *Genes Dev* 1999;13:239–252.
353. Deveraux QL, Stennicke HR, Salvesen GS, et al. Endogenous inhibitors of caspases. *J Clin Immunol* 1999;19:388–398.
354. Wotherspoon AC, Pan LX, Diss TC, et al. Cytogenetic study of B-cell lymphoma of mucosa-associated lymphoid tissue. *Cancer Genet Cytogenet* 1992;58:35–38.
355. Zhang Q, Siebert R, Yan M, et al. Inactivating mutations and overexpression of BCL10, a caspase recruitment domain-containing gene, in MALT lymphoma with t(1;14)(p22;q32). *Nat Genet* 1999;22:63–68.
356. Willis TG, Jadayel DM, Du MQ, et al. Bcl10 is involved in t(1; 14)(p22;q32) of MALT B cell lymphoma and mutated in multiple tumor types [see comments]. *Cell* 1999;96:35–45.
357. Neumeister P, Hoefler G, Beham-Schmid C, et al. Deletion analysis of the p16 tumor suppressor gene in gastrointestinal mucosa-associated lymphoid tissue lymphomas. *Gastroenterology* 1997;112:1871–1875.
358. Levy V, Miller C, Koeffler HP, et al. P53 in lymphomas of mucosal-associated lymphoid tissues. *Mod Pathol* 1996;9:245–248.
359. Armitage JO, Weisenburger DD. New approach to classifying non-Hodgkin's lymphomas: clinical features of the major histologic subtypes. Non-Hodgkin's Lymphoma Classification Project. *J Clin Oncol* 1998;16:2780–2795.
360. Offit K, Wong G, Filippa DA, et al. Cytogenetic analysis of 434 consecutively ascertained specimens of non-Hodgkin's lymphoma: clinical correlations. *Blood* 1991;77:1508–1515.
361. Ye BH, Lista F, Lo Coco F, et al. Alterations of a zinc finger-encoding gene, BCL-6, in diffuse large-cell lymphoma. *Science* 1993;262: 747–750.
362. Ye BH, Rao PH, Chaganti RS, et al. Cloning of bcl-6, the locus involved in chromosome translocations affecting band 3q27 in B-cell lymphoma. *Cancer Res* 1993;53:2732–2735.
363. Miki T, Kawamata N, Hirosawa S, et al. Gene involved in the 3q27 translocation associated with B-cell lymphoma, BCL5, encodes a Kruppel-like zinc-finger protein. *Blood* 1994;83:26–32.
364. Kerckaert JP, Deweindt C, Tilly H, et al. LAZ3, a novel zinc-finger encoding gene, is disrupted by recurring chromosome 3q27 translocations in human lymphomas. *Nat Genet* 1993;5:66–70.
365. Baron BW, Nucifora G, McCabe N, et al. Identification of the gene associated with the recurring chromosomal translocations t(3;14)(q27; q32) and t(3;22)(q27;q11) in B-cell lymphomas. *Proc Natl Acad Sci USA* 1993;90:5262–5266.
366. Deweindt C, Albagli O, Bernardin F, et al. The LAZ3/BCL6 oncogene encodes a sequence-specific transcriptional inhibitor: a novel function for the BTB/POZ domain as an autonomous repressing domain. *Cell Growth Differ* 1995;6:1495–1503.
367. Seyfert VL, Allman D, He Y, et al. Transcriptional repression by the proto-oncogene BCL-6. *Oncogene* 1996;12:2331–2342.
368. Chang CC, Ye BH, Chaganti RS, et al. BCL-6, a POZ/zinc-finger protein, is a sequence-specific transcriptional repressor. *Proc Natl Acad Sci USA* 1996;93:6947–6952.
369. Cattoretti G, Chang CC, Cechova K, et al. BCL-6 protein is expressed in germinal-center B cells. *Blood* 1995;86:45–53.
370. Dalla-Favera R, Ye BH, Lo Coco F, et al. BCL-6 and the molecular pathogenesis of B-cell lymphoma. *Cold Spring Harb Symp Quant Biol* 1994;59:117–123.
371. Allman D, Jain A, Dent A, et al. BCL-6 expression during B-cell activation. *Blood* 1996;87:5257–5268.
372. Ye BH, Cattoretti G, Shen Q, et al. The BCL-6 proto-oncogene controls germinal-centre formation and Th2-type inflammation. *Nat Genet* 1997;16:161–170.
373. Dent AL, Shaffer AL, Yu X, et al. Control of inflammation, cytokine expression, and germinal center formation by BCL-6. *Science* 1997; 276:589–592.
374. Staudt LM, Dent AL, Shaffer AL, Yu X. Regulation of lymphocyte cell fate decisions and lymphomagenesis by BCL-6. *Int Rev Immunol* 1999;18:381–403.
375. Niu H, Ye BH, Dalla-Favera R. Antigen receptor signaling induces MAP kinase-mediated phosphorylation and degradation of the BCL-6 transcription factor. *Genes Dev* 1998;12:1953–1961.
376. Harris MB, Chang CC, Berton MT, et al. Transcriptional repression of Stat6-dependent interleukin-4–induced genes by BCL-6: specific regulation of epsilon transcription and immunoglobulin E switching. *Mol Cell Biol* 1999;19:7264–7275.
377. Lo Coco F, Ye BH, Lista F, et al. Rearrangements of the BCL6 gene in diffuse large cell non-Hodgkin's lymphoma. *Blood* 1994;83: 1757–1759.
378. Chen W, Iida S, Louie DC, et al. Heterologous promoters fused to BCL6 by chromosomal translocations affecting band 3q27 cause its deregulated expression during B-cell differentiation. *Blood* 1998;91: 603–607.
379. Ye BH, Chaganti S, Chang CC, et al. Chromosomal translocations cause deregulated BCL6 expression by promoter substitution in B cell lymphoma. *EMBO J* 1995;14:6209–6217.
380. Dallery E, Galiegue-Zouitina S, Collyn-d'Hooghe M, et al. TTF, a gene encoding a novel small G protein, fuses to the lymphoma-associated LAZ3 gene by t(3;4) chromosomal translocation. *Oncogene* 1995;10:2171–2178.
381. Galiegue-Zouitina S, Quief S, Hildebrand MP, et al. Fusion of the LAZ3/BCL6 and BOB1/OBF1 genes by t(3; 11) (q27; q23) chromosomal translocation. *C R Acad Sci III* 1995;318:1125–1131.
382. Galiegue-Zouitina S, Quief S, Hildebrand MP, et al. Nonrandom fusion of L-plastin (LCP1) and LAZ3 (BCL6) genes by t(3;13)(q27; q14) chromosome translocation in two cases of B-cell non-Hodgkin lymphoma. *Genes Chromosomes Cancer* 1999;26:97–105.
383. Hosokawa Y, Maeda Y, Ichinohasama R, et al. The Ikaros gene, a central regulator of lymphoid differentiation, fuses to the BCL6 gene as a result of t(3;7)(q27;p12) translocation in a patient with diffuse large B-cell lymphoma. *Blood* 2000;95:2719–2721.
384. Xu WS, Liang RH, Srivastava G. Identification and characterization of BCL6 translocation partner genes in primary gastric high-grade B-cell lymphoma: heat shock protein 89 alpha is a novel fusion partner gene of BCL6. *Genes Chromosomes Cancer* 2000;27:69–75.
385. Yoshida S, Kaneita Y, Aoki Y, et al. Identification of heterologous translocation partner genes fused to the BCL6 gene in diffuse large B-cell lymphomas: 5M′-RACE and LA-PCR analyses of biopsy samples. *Oncogene* 1999;18:7994–7999.
386. Pasqualucci L, Migliazza A, Fracchiolla N, et al. BCL-6 mutations in normal germinal center B cells: evidence of somatic hypermutation acting outside Ig loci. *Proc Natl Acad Sci USA* 1998;95:11816–11821.
387. Shen HM, Peters A, Baron B, et al. Mutation of BCL-6 gene in normal B cells by the process of somatic hypermutation of Ig genes. *Science* 1998;280:1750–1752.
388. Migliazza A, Martinotti S, Chen W, et al. Frequent somatic hypermutation of the 5′ noncoding region of the BCL6 gene in B-cell lymphoma. *Proc Natl Acad Sci USA* 1995;92:12520–12524.
389. Capello D, Vitolo U, Pasqualucci L, et al. Distribution and pattern of BCL-6 mutations throughout the spectrum of B-cell neoplasia. *Blood* 2000;95:651–659.
390. Yunis JJ, Mayer MG, Arnesen MA, et al. Bcl-2 and other genomic alterations in the prognosis of large-cell lymphoma [see comments]. *N Engl J Med* 1989;320:1047–1054.
391. Offit K, Lo Coco F, Louie DC, et al. Rearrangement of the bcl-6 gene as a prognostic marker in diffuse large-cell lymphoma [see comments]. *N Engl J Med* 1994;331:74–80.
392. Tang SC, Visser L, Hepperle B, et al. Clinical significance of bcl-2–MBR gene rearrangement and protein expression in diffuse large-

cell non-Hodgkin's lymphoma: an analysis of 83 cases. *J Clin Oncol* 1994;12:149–154.
393. Dalla-Favera R, Bregni M, Erikson J, et al. Human c-myc oncogene is located on the region of chromosome 8 that is translocated in Burkitt lymphoma cells. *Proc Natl Acad Sci USA* 1982;79:7824–7827.
394. Dalla-Favera R, Martinotti S, Gallo RC, et al. Translocation and rearrangements of the c-myc oncogene locus in human undifferentiated B-cell lymphomas. *Science* 1983;219:963–967.
395. Taub R, Kirsch I, Morton C, et al. Translocation of the c-myc gene into the immunoglobulin heavy chain locus in human Burkitt lymphoma and murine plasmacytoma cells. *Proc Natl Acad Sci USA* 1982; 79:7837–7841.
396. Davis M, Malcolm S, Rabbitts TH. Chromosome translocation can occur on either side of the c-myc oncogene in Burkitt lymphoma cells. *Nature* 1984;308:286–288.
397. Hollis GF, Mitchell KF, Battey J, et al. A variant translocation places the lambda immunoglobulin genes 3′ to the c-myc oncogene in Burkitt's lymphoma. *Nature* 1984;307:752–755.
398. Schmidt EV. The role of c-myc in cellular growth control. *Oncogene* 1999;18:2988–2996.
399. Obaya AJ, Mateyak MK, Sedivy JM. Mysterious liaisons: the relationship between c-Myc and the cell cycle. *Oncogene* 1999;18: 2934–2941.
400. Dang CV. c-Myc target genes involved in cell growth, apoptosis, and metabolism. *Mol Cell Biol* 1999;19:1–11.
401. Wu KJ, Grandori C, Amacker M, et al. Direct activation of TERT transcription by c-MYC. *Nat Genet* 1999;21:220–224.
402. Wu KJ, Polack A, Dalla-Favera R. Coordinated regulation of iron-controlling genes, H-ferritin and IRP2, by c-MYC. *Science* 1999;283: 676–679.
403. Luscher B, Larsson LG. The basic region/helix-loop-helix/leucine zipper domain of Myc proto-oncoproteins: function and regulation. *Oncogene* 1999;18:2955–2966.
404. Sakamuro D, Prendergast GC. New Myc-interacting proteins: a second Myc network emerges. *Oncogene* 1999;18:2942–2954.
405. Pelicci PG, Knowles DMd, Magrath I, et al. Chromosomal breakpoints and structural alterations of the c-myc locus differ in endemic and sporadic forms of Burkitt lymphoma. *Proc Natl Acad Sci USA* 1986; 83:2984–2988.
406. Neri A, Barriga F, Knowles DM, et al. Different regions of the immunoglobulin heavy-chain locus are involved in chromosomal translocations in distinct pathogenetic forms of Burkitt lymphoma. *Proc Natl Acad Sci USA* 1988;85:2748–2752.
407. Shiramizu B, Barriga F, Neequaye J, et al. Patterns of chromosomal breakpoint locations in Burkitt's lymphoma: relevance to geography and Epstein-Barr virus association. *Blood* 1991;77:1516–1526.
408. Cesarman E, Dalla-Favera R, Bentley D, et al. Mutations in the first exon are associated with altered transcription of c-myc in Burkitt lymphoma. *Science* 1987;238:1272–1275.
409. Bhatia K, Spangler G, Hamdy N, et al. Mutations in the coding region of c-myc occur independently of mutations in the regulatory regions and are predominantly associated with myc/Ig translocation. *Curr Top Microbiol Immunol* 1995;194:389–398.
410. Bhatia K, Huppi K, Spangler G, et al. Point mutations in the c-Myc transactivation domain are common in Burkitt's lymphoma and mouse plasmacytomas. *Nat Genet* 1993;5:56–61.
411. Gu W, Bhatia K, Magrath IT, et al. Binding and suppression of the Myc transcriptional activation domain by p107. *Science* 1994;264: 251–254.
412. Lombardi L, Newcomb EW, Dalla-Favera R. Pathogenesis of Burkitt lymphoma: expression of an activated c-myc oncogene causes the tumorigenic conversion of EBV-infected human B lymphoblasts. *Cell* 1987;49:161–170.
413. Adams JM, Harris AW, Pinkert CA, et al. The c-myc oncogene driven by immunoglobulin enhancers induces lymphoid malignancy in transgenic mice. *Nature* 1985;318:533–538.
414. Butzler C, Zou X, Popov AV, et al. Rapid induction of B-cell lymphomas in mice carrying a human IgH/c-mycYAC. *Oncogene* 1997; 14:1383–1388.
415. Cole MD, McMahon SB. The Myc oncoprotein: a critical evaluation of transactivation and target gene regulation. *Oncogene* 1999;18: 2916–2924.
416. Neri A, Barriga F, Inghirami G, et al. Epstein-Barr virus infection precedes clonal expansion in Burkitt's and acquired immunodeficiency syndrome-associated lymphoma [see comments]. *Blood* 1991; 77:1092–1095.
417. Hamilton-Dutoit SJ, Pallesen G. A survey of Epstein-Barr virus gene expression in sporadic non-Hodgkin's lymphomas: detection of Epstein-Barr virus in a subset of peripheral T-cell lymphomas. *Am J Pathol* 1992;140:1315–1325.
418. Bergsagel PL, Nardini E, Brents L, et al. IgH translocations in multiple myeloma: a nearly universal event that rarely involves c-myc. *Curr Top Microbiol Immunol* 1997;224:283–287.
419. Bergsagel PL, Chesi M, Nardini E, et al. Promiscuous translocations into immunoglobulin heavy chain switch regions in multiple myeloma. *Proc Natl Acad Sci USA* 1996;93:13931–13936.
420. Hallek M, Leif Bergsagel P, Anderson KC. Multiple myeloma: increasing evidence for a multistep transformation process. *Blood* 1998; 91:3–21.
421. Chesi M, Bergsagel PL, Brents LA, et al. Dysregulation of cyclin D1 by translocation into an IgH gamma switch region in two multiple myeloma cell lines [see comments]. *Blood* 1996;88:674–681.
422. Chesi M, Nardini E, Brents LA, et al. Frequent translocation t(4; 14)(p16.3;q32.3) in multiple myeloma is associated with increased expression and activating mutations of fibroblast growth factor receptor 3. *Nat Genet* 1997;16:260–264.
423. Naski MC, Wang Q, Xu J, et al. Graded activation of fibroblast growth factor receptor 3 by mutations causing achondroplasia and thanatophoric dysplasia. *Nat Genet* 1996;13:233–237.
424. Rousseau F, el Ghouzzi V, Delezoide AL, et al. Missense FGFR3 mutations create cysteine residues in thanatophoric dwarfism type I (TD1). *Hum Mol Genet* 1996;5:509–512.
425. Iida S, Rao PH, Butler M, et al. Deregulation of MUM1/IRF4 by chromosomal translocation in multiple myeloma. *Nat Genet* 1997;17: 226–230.
426. Yoshida S, Nakazawa N, Iida S, et al. Detection of MUM1/IRF4–IgH fusion in multiple myeloma. *Leukemia* 1999;13:1812–1816.
427. Grossman A, Mittrucker HW, Nicholl J, et al. Cloning of human lymphocyte-specific interferon regulatory factor (hLSIRF/hIRF4) and mapping of the gene to 6p23-p25. *Genomics* 1996;37:229–233.
428. Falini B, Fizzotti M, Pucciarini A, et al. A monoclonal antibody (MUM1p) detects expression of the MUM1/IRF4 protein in a subset of germinal center B cells, plasma cells, and activated T cells [in process citation]. *Blood* 2000;95:2084–2092.
429. Mittrucker HW, Matsuyama T, Grossman A, et al. Requirement for the transcription factor LSIRF/IRF4 for mature B and T lymphocyte function. *Science* 1997;275:540–543.
430. Shou Y, Martelli ML, Gabrea A, et al. Diverse karyotypic abnormalities of the c-myc locus associated with c-myc dysregulation and tumor progression in multiple myeloma. *Proc Natl Acad Sci USA* 2000;97: 228–233.
431. Kuehl WM, Brents LA, Chesi M, et al. Dysregulation of c-myc in multiple myeloma. *Curr Top Microbiol Immunol* 1997;224:277–282.
432. Selvanayagam P, Blick M, Narni F, et al. Alteration and abnormal expression of the c-myc oncogene in human multiple myeloma. *Blood* 1988;71:30–35.
433. Corradini P, Ladetto M, Voena C, et al. Mutational activation of N- and K-ras oncogenes in plasma cell dyscrasias. *Blood* 1993;81: 2708–2713.
434. Tanaka K, Takechi M, Asaoku H, et al. A high frequency of N-RAS oncogene mutations in multiple myeloma. *Int J Hematol* 1992;56: 119–127.
435. Portier M, Moles JP, Mazars GR, et al. P53 and RAS gene mutations in multiple myeloma. *Oncogene* 1992;7:2539–2543.
436. Yasuga Y, Hirosawa S, Yamamoto K, et al. N-ras and p53 gene mutations are very rare events in multiple myeloma. *Int J Hematol* 1995; 62:91–97.
437. Corradini P, Inghirami G, Astolfi M, et al. Inactivation of tumor suppressor genes, p53 and Rb1, in plasma cell dyscrasias. *Leukemia* 1994; 8:758–767.
438. Neri A, Baldini L, Trecca D, et al. P53 gene mutations in multiple myeloma are associated with advanced forms of malignancy. *Blood* 1993;81:128–135.
439. Preudhomme C, Facon T, Zandecki M, et al. Rare occurrence of P53 gene mutations in multiple myeloma. *Br J Haematol* 1992;81: 440–443.
440. Dao DD, Sawyer JR, Epstein J, et al. Deletion of the retinoblastoma gene in multiple myeloma. *Leukemia* 1994;8:1280–1284.

441. Juge-Morineau N, Mellerin MP, Francois S, et al. High incidence of deletions but infrequent inactivation of the retinoblastoma gene in human myeloma cells. *Br J Haematol* 1995;91:664–667.
442. Tasaka T, Berenson J, Vescio R, et al. Analysis of the p16INK4A, p15INK4B and p18INK4C genes in multiple myeloma. *Br J Haematol* 1997;96:98–102.
443. Ng MH, Chung YF, Lo KW, et al. Frequent hypermethylation of p16 and p15 genes in multiple myeloma. *Blood* 1997;89:2500–2506.
444. Teoh G, Urashima M, Ogata A, et al. MDM2 protein overexpression promotes proliferation and survival of multiple myeloma cells. *Blood* 1997;90:1982–1992.
445. Virgilio L, Narducci MG, Isobe M, et al. Identification of the TCL1 gene involved in T-cell malignancies. *Proc Natl Acad Sci USA* 1994; 91:12530–12534.
446. Virgilio L, Isobe M, Narducci MG, et al. Chromosome walking on the TCL1 locus involved in T-cell neoplasia. *Proc Natl Acad Sci USA* 1993;90:9275–9279.
447. Stern MH, Soulier J, Rosenzwajg M, et al. MTCP-1: a novel gene on the human chromosome Xq28 translocated to the T cell receptor alpha/delta locus in mature T cell proliferations. *Oncogene* 1993;8: 2475–2483.
448. Pekarsky Y, Koval A, Hallas C, et al. Tcl1 enhances akt kinase activity and mediates its nuclear translocation [In Process Citation]. *Proc Natl Acad Sci USA* 2000;97:3028–3033.
449. Narducci MG, Virgilio L, Isobe M, et al. TCL1 oncogene activation in preleukemic T cells from a case of ataxia-telangiectasia. *Blood* 1995;86:2358–2364.
450. Virgilio L, Lazzeri C, Bichi R, et al. Deregulated expression of TCL1 causes T cell leukemia in mice. *Proc Natl Acad Sci USA* 1998;95: 3885–3889.
451. Kadin ME, Morris SW. The t(2;5) in human lymphomas. *Leuk Lymphoma* 1998;29:249–256.
452. Lamant L, Meggetto F, al Saati T, et al. High incidence of the t(2; 5)(p23;q35) translocation in anaplastic large cell lymphoma and its lack of detection in Hodgkin's disease: comparison of cytogenetic analysis, reverse transcriptase-polymerase chain reaction, and P-80 immunostaining. *Blood* 1996;87:284–291.
453. Cataldo KA, Jalal SM, Law ME, et al. Detection of t(2;5) in anaplastic large cell lymphoma: comparison of immunohistochemical studies, FISH, and RT-PCR in paraffin-embedded tissue. *Am J Surg Pathol* 1999;23:1386–1392.
454. Mathew P, Sanger WG, Weisenburger DD, et al. Detection of the t(2; 5)(p23;q35) and NPM-ALK fusion in non-Hodgkin's lymphoma by two-color fluorescence in situ hybridization. *Blood* 1997;89: 1678–1685.
455. Pulford K, Lamant L, Morris SW, et al. Detection of anaplastic lymphoma kinase (ALK) and nucleolar protein nucleophosmin (NPM)-ALK proteins in normal and neoplastic cells with the monoclonal antibody ALK1. *Blood* 1997;89:1394–1404.
456. Shiota M, Nakamura S, Ichinohasama R, et al. Anaplastic large cell lymphomas expressing the novel chimeric protein p80NPM/ALK: a distinct clinicopathologic entity. *Blood* 1995;86:1954–1960.
457. Shiota M, Mori S. Anaplastic large cell lymphomas expressing the novel chimeric protein p80NPM/ALK: a distinct clinicopathologic entity. *Leukemia* 1997;11[Suppl 3]:538–540.
458. Bai RY, Dieter P, Peschel C, et al. Nucleophosmin-anaplastic lymphoma kinase of large-cell anaplastic lymphoma is a constitutively active tyrosine kinase that utilizes phospholipase C-gamma to mediate its mitogenicity. *Mol Cell Biol* 1998;18:6951–6961.
459. Bischof D, Pulford K, Mason DY, et al. Role of the nucleophosmin (NPM) portion of the non-Hodgkin's lymphoma–associated NPM-anaplastic lymphoma kinase fusion protein in oncogenesis. *Mol Cell Biol* 1997;17:2312–2325.
460. Kuefer MU, Look AT, Pulford K, et al. Retrovirus-mediated gene transfer of NPM-ALK causes lymphoid malignancy in mice. *Blood* 1997;90:2901–2910.
461. Falini B, Pulford K, Pucciarini A, et al. Lymphomas expressing ALK fusion protein(s) other than NPM-ALK. *Blood* 1999;94:3509–3515.
462. Hernandez L, Pinyol M, Hernandez S, et al. TRK-fused gene (TFG) is a new partner of ALK in anaplastic large cell lymphoma producing two structurally different TFG-ALK translocations. *Blood* 1999;94: 3265–3268.
463. Smith MR, Greene WC. Molecular biology of the type I human T-cell leukemia virus (HTLV-I) and adult T-cell leukemia. *J Clin Invest* 1991;87:761–766.
464. Bex F, Gaynor RB. Regulation of gene expression by HTLV-I Tax protein. *Methods* 1998;16:83–94.
465. Li XH, Gaynor RB. Regulation of NF-kappaB by the HTLV-1 Tax protein. *Gene Exp* 1999;7:233–245.
466. Cesarman E, Chadburn A, Inghirami G, et al. Structural and functional analysis of oncogenes and tumor suppressor genes in adult T-cell leukemia/lymphoma shows frequent p53 mutations. *Blood* 1992;80: 3205–3216.
467. Neri A, Fracchiolla NS, Roscetti E, et al. Molecular analysis of cutaneous B- and T-cell lymphomas. *Blood* 1995;86:3160–3172.
468. Siebenlist U, Franzoso G, Brown K. Structure, regulation and function of NF-kappa B. *Annu Rev Cell Biol* 1994;10:405–455.
469. de Martin R, Schmid JA, Hofer-Warbinek R. The NF-kappaB/Rel family of transcription factors in oncogenic transformation and apoptosis. *Mutat Res* 1999;437:231–243.
470. Neri A, Chang CC, Lombardi L, et al. B cell lymphoma-associated chromosomal translocation involves candidate oncogene lyt-10, homologous to NF-kappa B p50. *Cell* 1991;67:1075–1087.
471. Chang CC, Zhang J, Lombardi L, et al. Rearranged NFKB-2 genes in lymphoid neoplasms code for constitutively active nuclear transactivators. *Mol Cell Biol* 1995;15:5180–5187.
472. Stein H, Hummel M. Cellular origin and clonality of classic Hodgkin's lymphoma: immunophenotypic and molecular studies. *Semin Hematol* 1999;36:233–241.
473. Kuppers R, Hansmann ML, Diehl V, et al. Molecular single-cell analysis of Hodgkin and Reed-Sternberg cells. *Mol Med Today* 1995;1: 26–30.
474. Kuppers R, Hansmann ML, Rajewsky K. Clonality and germinal centre B-cell derivation of Hodgkin/Reed-Sternberg cells in Hodgkin's disease. *Ann Oncol* 1998;9:S17–20.
475. Kuppers R, Rajewsky K, Zhao M, et al. Hodgkin disease: Hodgkin and Reed-Sternberg cells picked from histological sections show clonal immunoglobulin gene rearrangements and appear to be derived from B cells at various stages of development. *Proc Natl Acad Sci USA* 1994;91:10962–10966.
476. Cossman J, Annunziata CM, Barash S, et al. Reed-Sternberg cell genome expression supports a B-cell lineage. *Blood* 1999;94: 411–416.
477. Kuppers R, Rajewsky K. The origin of Hodgkin and Reed/Sternberg cells in Hodgkin's disease. *Annu Rev Immunol* 1998;16:471–493.
478. Jungnickel B, Staratschek-Jox A, Brauninger A, et al. Clonal deleterious mutations in the IkappaBalpha gene in the malignant cells in Hodgkin's lymphoma [in process Citation]. *J Exp Med* 2000;191: 395–402.
479. Krappmann D, Emmerich F, Kordes U, et al. Molecular mechanisms of constitutive NF-kappaB/Rel activation in Hodgkin/Reed-Sternberg cells. *Oncogene* 1999;18:943–953.
480. Wood KM, Roff M, Hay RT. Defective IkappaBalpha in Hodgkin cell lines with constitutively active NF-kappaB. *Oncogene* 1998;16: 2131–2139.
481. Emmerich F, Meiser M, Hummel M, et al. Overexpression of I kappa B alpha without inhibition of NF-kappaB activity and mutations in the I kappa B alpha gene in Reed-Sternberg cells. *Blood* 1999;94: 3129–3134.
482. Bargou RC, Emmerich F, Krappmann D, et al. Constitutive nuclear factor-kappaB-RelA activation is required for proliferation and survival of Hodgkin's disease tumor cells. *J Clin Invest* 1997;100: 2961–2969.
483. Weiss LM, Strickler JG, Warnke RA, et al. Epstein-Barr viral DNA in tissues of Hodgkin's disease. *Am J Pathol* 1987;129:86–91.
484. Weiss LM, Movahed LA, Warnke RA, et al. Detection of Epstein-Barr viral genomes in Reed-Sternberg cells of Hodgkin's disease. *N Engl J Med* 1989;320:502–506.
485. Pallesen G, Hamilton-Dutoit SJ, Rowe M, et al. Expression of Epstein-Barr virus latent gene products in tumour cells of Hodgkin's disease [see comments]. *Lancet* 1991;337:320–322.
486. Herbst H, Dallenbach F, Hummel M, et al. Epstein-Barr virus latent membrane protein expression in Hodgkin and Reed-Sternberg cells. *Proc Natl Acad Sci USA* 1991;88:4766–4770.
487. Farrell PJ. Signal transduction from the Epstein-Barr virus LMP-1 transforming protein. *Trends Microbiol* 1998;6:175–177, discussion 177–178.

CHAPTER 9

Application of Molecular Genetics to the Diagnosis and Classification of Malignant Lymphoma

Jeffrey Cossman, Falko Fend, Louis Staudt, and Mark Raffeld

Molecular genetics has revealed much about the normal development of the immune system and the pathogenesis of neoplasms arising from it. In this chapter, we demonstrate how basic principles of molecular genetics are directly applied to the detection, classification, and monitoring of human malignant lymphoma. Using standard tools of molecular biology, it is possible to accurately detect most malignant lymphomas using routinely obtained diagnostic samples. Molecular genetics provides unique tumor markers that serve to subclassify the neoplasm, provide prognostic information, guide therapy, and detect minimal disease long before it is apparent by conventional means.

Genomic DNA rearrangements in neoplastic cells that are not carried by accompanying normal cells distinguish neoplastic cells from normal cells and provide a unique tumor marker. In most lymphomas, DNA rearrangements occur before clonal expansion. A lymphoma consists of genetically identical progeny of a single cell wherein the daughter cells contain at least one identical genetic marker not seen in normal cells (Fig. 9.1). In the case of malignant lymphomas, which are neoplasms of T and B lymphocytes, the rearrangements may actually be the normal, physiologic antigen receptor gene rearrangements occurring in the immunoglobulin (Ig) or T-cell receptor (TCR) genes.

These are normal gene rearrangements and are exploited as diagnostic markers because their sequence and configuration differs from that of nonlymphoid cells and even from other lymphocytes. A second major class of genomic DNA

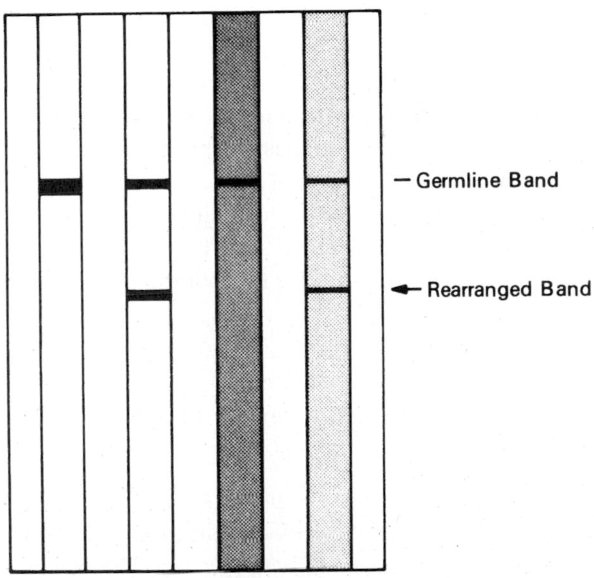

FIG. 9.1. Southern blot analysis. Immunoglobulin gene rearrangement appears as a nongermline band in monoclonal B cells. Two nongermline bands usually result from rearrangement of both alleles or a split by chromosomal translocation. Highly polyclonal B cells exhibit many different types of rearrangements whose restriction fragments are dispersed throughout the lane and theoretically give rise to a smear without distinct bands being evident. If monoclonal B cells are present within a background of polyclonal B cells, the band contributed by the monoclonal B cells is apparent when these cells reach approximately 1% to 5% of the total cell population.

J. Cossman: Department of Pathology, Georgetown University Medical Center, Washington, D.C. 20007
F. Fend: Technical University, Munich, Germany
L. Staudt and M. Raffeld: National Cancer Institute, National Institutes of Health, Bethesda, Maryland

rearrangements occurs in malignant lymphomas as a consequence of chromosomal aberrations, such as translocations. Translocations are not only important in the pathogenesis of lymphoma but have provided an assortment of diagnostic DNA rearrangement markers and potential targets for intervention and therapy. The tools of molecular genetics are more than just a diagnostic test to distinguish benign from malignant lymphoproliferative processes. They have the potential to produce highly specific and clinically valuable information to guide and monitor the choice of therapy. Genetic errors, which are the root cause of malignant lymphoma, also tell us about the expected behavior of the neoplasm and where its vulnerabilities to chemotherapy may lie. Molecular genetic techniques, using DNA amplifications such as polymerase chain reaction (PCR), are being used to monitor the success of chemotherapy and bone marrow transplantation as early sentinel hallmarks of the onset of recurrent disease.

BACKGROUND

Molecular Genetic Methods

As with any other complex diagnostic laboratory test, interpretation of genotyping for the diagnosis of lymphoma requires an understanding of the basic principles of the assay. It is particularly important to guard against false-positive interpretations, which may lead to the erroneous conclusion that a clone or malignant neoplasm is present although none exists. The techniques described here are *in vitro* laboratory tests. They should be used only in conjunction with conventional diagnostic pathology tests, such as histopathology and immunohistochemistry, to place the molecular result in context.

Application of Molecular Biology to Lymphoma Diagnosis

The molecular genetic diagnostics of malignant lymphoma had its beginnings with the discovery of the rearrangement of Ig genes in B lymphocytes. The cloning of the human Ig genes and discovery of their rearrangement in normal and neoplastic human B lymphocytes, by Stanley Korsmeyer, Philip Leder, and colleagues (1), prompted hematopathologists to consider ways in which this discovery might be applicable to the clinical diagnosis of lymphoma. The first principle revealed by the early application of Ig gene rearrangement was that it was cell lineage specific. Rearrangement of Ig genes occurred in B lymphocytes but not in other cell types. Ig gene rearrangement had potential value as a lineage marker for B-cell neoplasms. This was particularly important early on because no specific phenotypic markers of B lymphocytes, other than Igs, were available. If the Ig genes were not expressed at the protein level and therefore were not detectable by immunohistochemistry or immunofluorescence using antibodies, an investigator could not be certain that the neoplasm was of B-cell lineage.

The first applications of Ig gene rearrangement analysis to human clinical samples was in acute lymphoblastic leukemia (ALL). ALL was studied because approximately 80% of cases were so-called common or ''non-B, non-T'' type. They were known to be lymphoid, but it was not known whether they were of B- or T-cell origin. Korsmeyer and colleagues convincingly demonstrated by Southern blotting that virtually all cases of common ALL contained Ig heavy-chain gene rearrangements and were of B-cell lineage derivation (1). This has subsequently been confirmed and corroborated through many studies, including those with the monoclonal antibodies to B-lineage markers, such as CD19 and CD20. The ALL studies were quickly followed by applications of Ig gene rearrangement analysis to other B-cell neoplasms (2,3).

A Unique, Clonal Lymphoma Marker

A second and arguably even more valuable application of the Ig gene rearrangement test became apparent. By Southern blot analysis (the technique is explained later), it was clear that malignant B-cell neoplasms and cloned B-cell lines harbor one or two rearranged Ig genes that appear as one or two distinct bands by Southern analysis. In contrast, polyclonal B-cell lymphocytes, although containing B cells with Ig gene rearrangements, do not show single bands but rather smears. These smears are a manifestation of the many thousands of different rearrangements among polyclonal B cells, which generate different restriction fragment sizes of the rearranged Ig genes. Ig gene rearrangement was also a clonal marker of B-cell neoplasia and possibly could distinguish benign, polyclonal B-cell lymphoid proliferations from monoclonal, malignant lymphomas and leukemias. A technique was born that simultaneously determined B-cell lineage and clonality in lymphoproliferative processes (4).

Within a few years, the human TCR genes were discovered. The first of these was the TCR β-chain gene cloned by Mak and his associates (5), who also found that, like Ig genes, TCR genes rearrange before their expression (6). The rearrangement of TCR genes serves as lineage and clonality markers of T-cell neoplasms when tested by Southern blot analysis (4,7).

Molecular Cytogenetics Emerges from Antigen Receptor Genes

After the Ig and TCR genes were cloned, probes of these genes were used to map the chromosomal locations of the genes (8). The fascinating result of these chromosomal studies was that the antigen receptor (Ig and TCR) genes were located on chromosomal bands frequently involved in translocations in lymphomas and leukemias (9–14). This discovery set off an intense search for genes located at the breakpoint of the partner chromosomes, which became joined to the region of the antigen receptor genes as a consequence of translocation. The search was well rewarded as investigators prospecting at the sites of translocation discovered partner genes, many of which were previously unknown. In their new location, the expression of the genes was altered, often overexpressed, and probably candidates contributing to the neoplastic process itself. Examples such as *MYC* (8), *BCL1* (11), *BCL2* (13), and many others became useful as diagnostic probes to detect the presence of translocation without the need to perform conventional cytogenetic analysis. In addition to their value as diagnostic markers, the discovery of the translocated genes has led researchers into a productive direction toward the development of specific therapeutic interventions for the management of lymphoid neoplasms.

Polymerase Chain Reaction Replaces Southern Blotting

Southern blot analysis has largely been supplanted by the simpler, faster, less expensive, and more sensitive method of PCR. PCR has enabled the broad application of lymphoma molecular genetic testing far beyond research laboratories. It is the same method used elsewhere in the clinical laboratory (e.g., microbiology, tissue typing) and works effectively on virtually any type of tissue sample, whether fixed or fresh. Southern blot analysis is reserved for the study of larger genomic fragments when the precise location of the marker sequence is unknown. Because the Southern blot method is sometimes still used in hematopathology, we describe it in the next section.

Techniques

Southern Blot Analysis

Although it is a slow process, Southern blot analysis (Fig. 9.1) examines a larger segment of the genome, and its results are reproducible when strict guidelines are followed (15). Southern blot analysis begins with the extraction of high-molecular-weight, relatively intact DNA. The DNA is digested with restriction enzymes that recognize 6 base pair (bp) sequences scattered randomly throughout the genomic DNA. These sequences should be, on average, separated by 4^6 (4,096) bp. Because they are randomly distributed throughout the genome, the digested fragments of DNA (i.e., restriction fragments) vary in size, with a presumed binomial distribution spread around a median of approximately 4,000 bp. The digested DNA is electrophoresed through a gel to separate the digested fragments by size. The separated fragments are then blotted onto a piece of filter paper in their fixed, electrophoresed location.

To detect the position of a specific gene, such as the Ig heavy-chain gene, a cloned probe containing a portion of the human Ig heavy-chain gene is used. The probe is radiolabeled, usually with radioactive phosphorous (^{32}P), which is denatured into single-stranded probes of DNA in a hybridizing salt solution, and the filter is soaked within this solution. The probe hybridizes to the spot on the filter where its single strands find their corresponding opposing strand containing human Ig gene sequence. Unbound DNA fragments are washed away, and the filter is then exposed to photographic film. The film reveals the location of the hybridization of the probe and the position of the electrophoresed fragment containing the Ig heavy-chain gene. This location is compared with unrearranged (germline) Ig heavy-chain genes, derived from a control source devoid of B lymphocytes. Molecular weight markers help to measure the size of the band of interest.

In a sense, the technique examines the entire genome and should find virtually any rearrangement if it is present. However, it is a slow, labor-intensive process, which can take 1 to 2 weeks to complete. It also requires a substantial amount of nondegraded DNA, usually from fresh or fresh-frozen tissue.

Probes for Immunoglobulin Gene Rearrangement by Southern Blotting

Initially, rearrangements of the Ig genes were analyzed with probes of the constant (C) regions of the heavy-chain (C_μ) genes and (C_κ) and (C_λ) light-chain genes (1) (Fig. 9.2). Although useful, these probes have certain limitations not encountered with joining (J) region probes. The physiologic heavy-chain switch of B cells deletes the C_μ locus but not J_H so that rearrangements that are not detected with a C_μ probe in a switched Ig heavy-chain gene can still be seen with a J_H probe (4). The κ light-chain genes rearrange before λ light-chain genes. If the κ light-chain gene rearrangements are nonproductive (i.e., a functional κ light-chain protein is not encoded), the cell proceeds to rearrange its λ light-chain genes (16). In many cases, cells that have λ light-chain gene rearrangements have deleted one or both of their κ light-chain gene alleles. This process holds true in neoplasms of B cells as well, in which κ light-chain gene rearrangements or deletions occur in virtually all mature B-cell neoplasms and λ light-chain gene rearrangements occur only in a fraction of cases.

For Southern blot analysis, the most effective probe for κ light-chain gene rearrangement is J_κ, which is less frequently deleted than C_κ in λ-expressing B cells. Probing for λ light-chain gene rearrangements is usually unnecessary because a rearrangement marker can usually be detected with J_H or J_κ. However, if λ light-chain gene rearrangements are

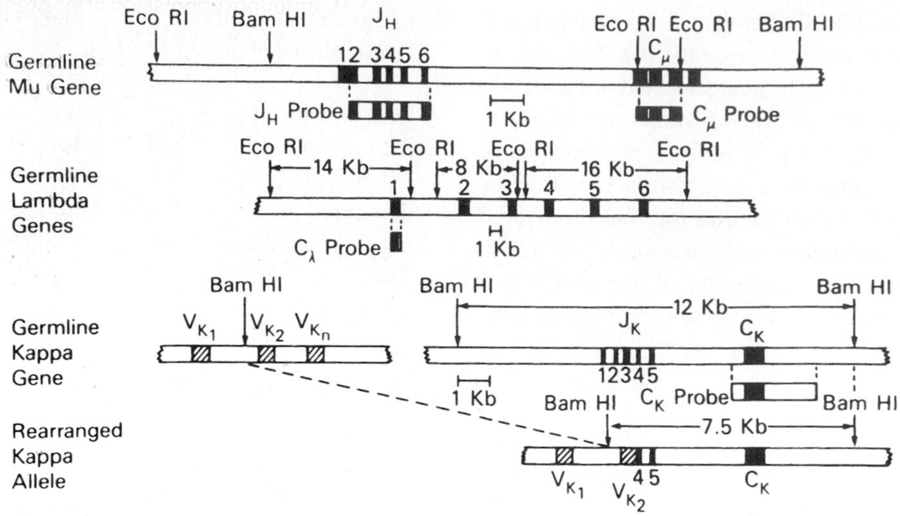

FIG. 9.2. Human immunoglobulin genes. The germline (unrearranged) configurations of each of the three immunoglobulin genes are shown and one example of a rearrangement of a κ light-chain gene is demonstrated at the bottom. Only *Eco*RI and *Bam*HI restriction enzyme sites are shown. Probes of the joining (J) regions of the heavy and κ light-chain genes are the most useful for detection of rearrangement, because this region usually is involved in conventional V_H-D_H-J_H and V_κ-J_κ joinings. Because a single J_λ is paired with each of the C_λ loci and significant homology exists among the C_λ loci, hybridization with a single C_λ probe can reveal V_λ-J_λ rearrangement. As shown for the κ light-chain gene, rearrangement displaces restriction enzyme sites, creating a *Bam*HI fragment, which in this case is smaller in the rearranged allele than in the germline.

sought, they are usually detected by digestion of genomic DNA with *Eco*RI and probing with C_λ (17). Occasionally, in B-cell lymphomas, rearrangements of the Ig heavy-chain gene are not identified using a J_H probe, whereas κ or λ light-chain gene rearrangements are present. This may occur because the light-chain gene probes may be more sensitive in detecting rearrangements in a minor clone. Alternatively, neoplastic B cells may not always follow the hierarchy of gene rearrangements.

T-Cell Receptor Genes

The TCR α-chain gene has been difficult to study. As a consequence of the enormous size of its J region, it is not amenable to standard restriction enzyme digestion and Southern blot analysis. It is more straightforward to analyze the TCR β-chain gene using probes of the J_β (Fig. 9.3). Polymorphisms of restriction enzyme sites occur in this region and one must be aware of the known restriction fragment length polymorphisms that have been observed (4).

Rearrangements of the TCR γ-chain gene can be detected in Southern blot analysis using conventional restriction enzymes. However, the presence of polyclonal T cells complicates the interpretation of TCRγ gene rearrangements (Fig. 9.4). There are only a limited number (7,8) of potentially productive V_γ genes so that only a few restriction sizes of TCRγ rearrangements may occur (5). A population of polyclonal T cells yields a pattern of seven or eight bands with various intensities (18). If approximately 10% of a cell sample is composed of polyclonal T cells, an array of bands attributable to the polyclonal T cells are seen and mask the presence of a clone. Conversely, the presence of multiple rearrangements of various intensities can be misinterpreted as a clone when only polyclonal T cells exist (i.e., pseudoclonality).

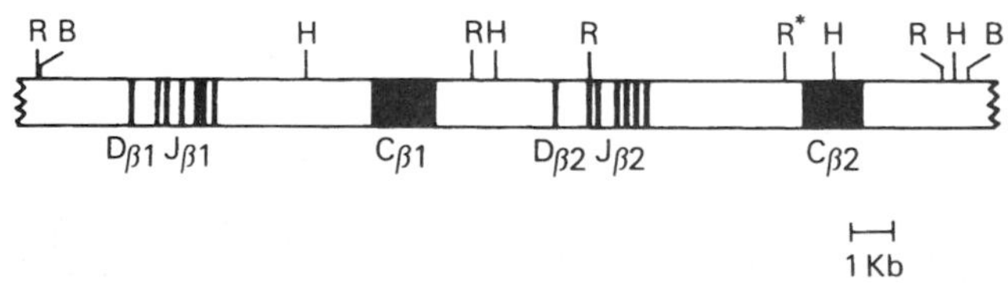

FIG. 9.3. Human T-cell receptor (TCR) β-chain gene: genomic restriction map. The V_β regions, which are 5′ *(left)* of the region demonstrated, are not shown. Probes of the $J_\beta1$ and $J_\beta2$ regions are useful for detecting TCR β-chain gene rearrangements. C region probes may also be used, and a single probe can hybridize to the highly homologous C1 and $C_\beta2$ loci. However, a *Hind*III (H) restriction enzyme site between $J_\beta1$ and $C_\beta1$ prevents detection of $J_\beta1$ rearrangements using this enzyme and a $C_\beta1$ probe. In a parallel fashion, an *Eco*RI restriction site (R) between $C_\beta2$ and $J_\beta2$ prevents detection of rearrangements to $J_\beta2$ using a C_β probe. A relatively resistant *Eco*RI restriction site (R*) may give rise to partially digested DNA, resulting in an additional 8.5-kb band. R, *Eco*RI; B, *Bam*HI; H, *Hind*III.

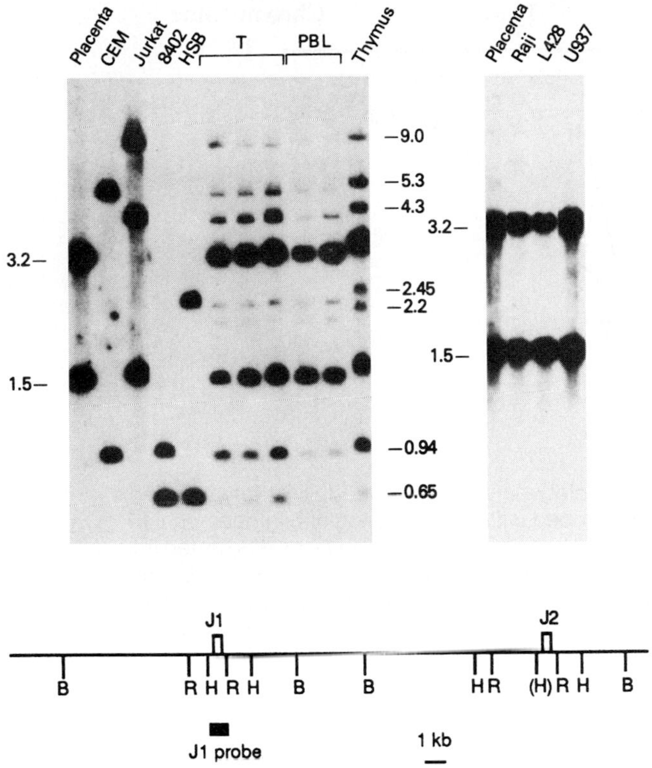

FIG. 9.4. T-cell receptor γ-chain gene: pseudoclonality. The limited number of V_γ genes permits only 8 or 9 V_γ-J_γ restriction fragments, which depend on the V_γ gene used. In polyclonal T cells, distinct bands contributed by rearrangements can be seen. When digested with the restriction enzyme *Eco*RI (R), two germline bands of 3.2 and 1.5 kb are seen (in placenta). Seven different rearrangements are seen among purified polyclonal T cells (T) or peripheral blood lymphocytes (PBL). These same rearrangements can be seen in normal thymus. Clonal T cells, such as in the T-cell leukemia cell lines CEM, Jurkat, 8402, and HSB, each show distinct rearrangements but not the multiple band pattern of polyclonal T cells. Non-T-cell hematopoietic neoplasms, such as the Burkitt's lymphoma cell line, Raji, the Hodgkin's cell line L428, and the histiocytic cell line U937, show only germline patterns of the TCR γ-chain gene. A partial restriction map of the $J_\gamma1$ and $J_\gamma2$ regions is shown below. B, *Bam*HI; R, *Eco*RI; H, *Hind*III.

CLINICAL IMPLICATIONS OF CLONALITY: BENIGN CLONAL LYMPHADENOPATHY

When applying genotypic analysis to assist in the differential diagnosis of benign versus malignant, is monoclonality tantamount to a diagnosis of malignancy? There is a significant correlation between clonality at the level of the rearranged antigen receptor genes and malignant lymphoma, but it is important to be aware of the status of the host immune system when relying on molecular genetic analysis. For example, clones of lymphoid cells without evidence of malignant lymphoma have been detected by molecular genetic analysis in patients with congenital immune deficiency, autoimmune disease, angioimmunoblastic lymphadenopathy (AILD), immunosuppression after organ transplantation, and in acquired immunodeficiency syndrome (AIDS) (2,4,19). Patients with any of these immunologic disorders are at heightened risk of developing an overt, high-grade malignant lymphoma. It appears that, as a consequence of a dysregulated immune system, lymphoid cells are permitted to repeatedly divide beyond their normal constraints in the setting of antigenic challenge or by mitogenesis induced by host Epstein-Barr virus (EBV). The expanded, dividing cell population represents a pool of cells at risk for secondary genetic damage, perhaps in the form of chromosomal translocation that could transform a cell to undergo independent growth, such as in lymphoma. An early manifestation of this phenomenon is oligoclonal lymphoid expansion with subsequent spontaneous regression as may occur in AILD (20). Later, a clone emerges and grows as the lymphoma. As may also be seen in AIDS, the lymphoma, but not the precursor lymphoid proliferation, carries a rearranged *MYC* oncogene (21).

Chromosomal Translocations

Chromosomal translocations can also be detected by Southern blot analysis. For example, the t(14;18) translocation of follicular lymphoma (Fig. 9.5) involves the fusion of a portion of the Ig heavy-chain gene from chromosome 14 with the *BCL2* gene of chromosome 18 (12) (Fig. 9.6). In this position, the *BCL2* gene becomes constitutively activated while under the influence of the Ig heavy-chain promoter system, which is turned on in the context of the B lymphocyte (22). The translocation event alters the DNA sequences flanking the region of the breakpoint and replaces certain restriction enzyme sites. Southern blot analysis can reveal the rearrangement of the Ig heavy-chain and *BCL2* gene in follicular lymphoma by using probes of the two genes. The two probes are hybridized to the same band when

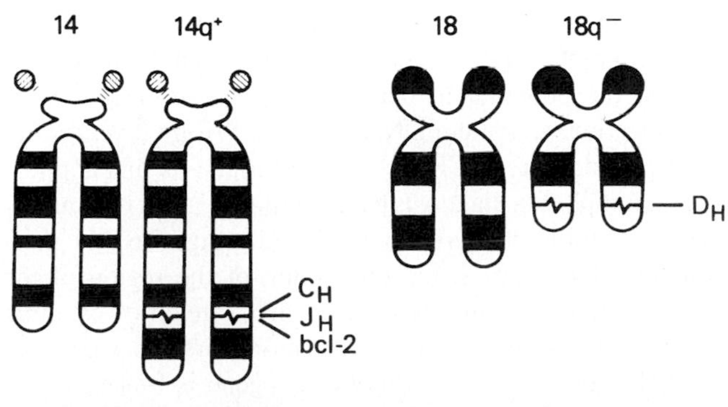

FIG. 9.5. Chromosomal translocation t(14;18) in follicular lymphoma. The balanced translocation between chromosomes 14 and 18 juxtaposes the *BCL2* gene from chromosome 18 to a position adjacent to the immunoglobulin heavy-chain gene on chromosome 14. Diversity (D_H) sequences from the immunoglobulin heavy-chain gene are transposed to the derivative chromosome 18.

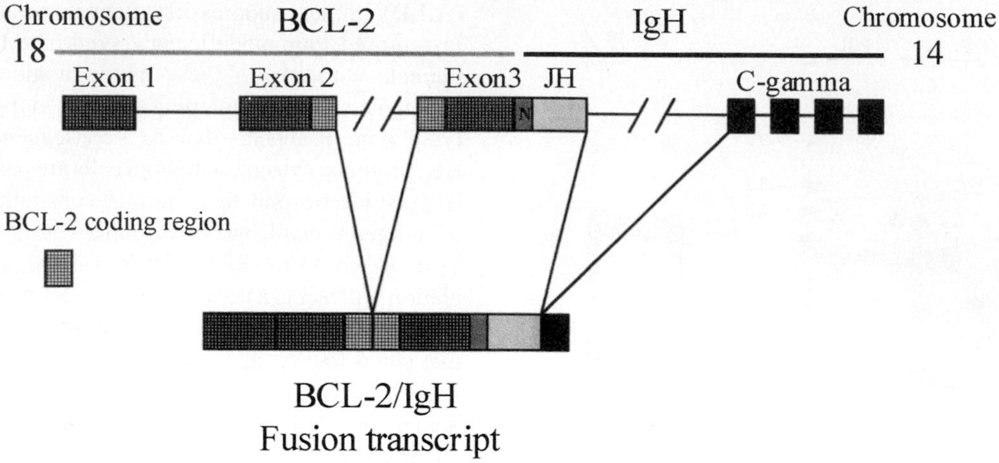

FIG. 9.6. The t(14;18) translocation detected by Southern blot analysis. DNA of a follicular lymphoma was analyzed by digestion with *Hind*III and successively probed with the immunoglobulin heavy-chain gene probe J_H and a BCL-2 major breakpoint region (mbr) probe. Germline bands are indicated by dashes and rearrangements by arrows. Comigration of the single rearrangement detected by J_H and BCL-2 indicates that these two loci co-occupy the same restriction fragment, a consequence of chromosomal joining that demonstrates the t(14;18) translocation.

the t(14;18) translocation was present (12), because fusion of the two genes and hybridized probes of J_H and *BCL2* co-occupy the same restriction fragment (Fig. 9.7). Southern blot analysis can diagnose t(14;18) without microscopy of a metaphase spread. In a similar way, chromosomal translocations can be detected with probes of other genes known to translocate in a B-cell neoplasm (i.e., *BCL1*, *BCL3*, *BCL6*, and *MYC*) and in T-cell neoplasms with probes of TCR genes to detect partner chromosomes.

Polymerase Chain Reaction

The invention of the DNA amplification technique, PCR, in the mid-1980s by Mullis and colleagues (23) provided scientists with a means to detect specific DNA sequences rapidly and inexpensively. To those who were conducting Southern blot studies of human malignant lymphomas, PCR offered the potential to detect specific rearrangements or translocations in patient DNA samples. Within 2 years after the reporting of the PCR technique, it found its first application in lymphoma diagnosis by detecting the t(14;18) translocation of follicular lymphoma (24,25) (Fig. 9.6). In most follicular lymphomas, the breakpoint of the region of the *BCL2* gene occurs in a relatively small stretch of genomic DNA spanning only a few hundred base pairs. An even more refined region of the Ig heavy-chain gene is broken in the translocation. In nearly all cases, this break occurs at one of the J_H segments. Although the J_H segments vary from one another in their primary genomic DNA sequence, there are conserved regions such that only one oligonucleotide primer is needed to hybridize to any of the six human J_H segments. A single primer of the opposite strand, *BCL2*, flanking the major breakpoint region is used to complete the primer pair.

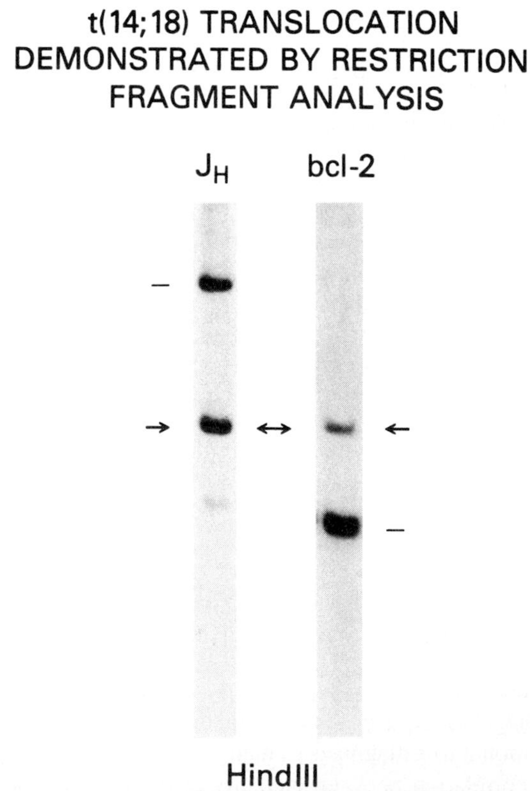

FIG. 9.7. The t(14;18) chromosomal translocation joins *BCL2* and the immunoglobulin heavy chain (IgH) gene to create a fusion gene. The joining is usually within the 3′-untranslated region of *BCL2* and one of J_H segments of IgH. The transcript of this gene includes sequences from both chromosomes. The BCL-2 protein coding region is not directly affected by the translocation event. For polymerase chain reaction, opposing primers corresponding to *BCL2* exon 3 and J_H consensus amplify most BCL-2/IgH joinings.

In PCR, a genomic DNA sample, heat denatured into single strands of DNA, is mixed with synthetically generated oligonucleotides (short sequences of, for example, 25 nucleotides) to hybridize to their corresponding sequence in the test genomic DNA and amplified through repeated rounds of polymerization and denaturation.

For the detection of t(14;18), the opposing primers are J_H and *BCL2*. If the two primers extend by polymerization, the copied strand extends into the sequence corresponding to the opposite primer. In the example of t(14;18), the first primer, J_H, copies the genomic DNA into the region of *BCL2*, and the *BCL2* primed copy is extended into the region of J_H. After this first copying, the DNA is heat denatured to release single strands of DNA. Using a heat-stable DNA polymerase such as Taq, an automated thermocycler, and 40 cycles of copying and polymerization, theoretically, 2^{40} (10^{12}) copies of the original single copy of the joined J_H-BCL-2 segment can be generated. This highly amplified specific sequence can readily be detected by electrophoresis of the amplified DNA in an agarose gel and visualization of the DNA by use of a DNA dye that can be seen under ultraviolet light. Alternatively, the amplified DNA can be directly sequenced in an automated sequencer to determine the primary DNA sequence.

Because the amplification process is exponential, only a tiny amount of starting DNA is necessary. In contrast to Southern blotting, the DNA can be degraded because only a short segment, usually in the range of 50 to 1,000 bp, is amplified, which is why PCR is applicable to virtually any type of tissue sample, including archived tissue.

Immunoglobulin and T-Cell Receptor Gene Rearrangements and Polymerase Chain Reaction Methods

The application of PCR to lymphoma diagnosis was greatly expanded by 1990, when it was shown that rearrangements of the antigen receptor genes are also amenable to PCR (26). Although the Ig heavy-chain gene contains many V_H segments (V or variable because of the differences of primary DNA sequence among them), they also contain relatively conserved stretches or framework regions. The framework regions serve as useful targets for oligonucleotide primers in PCR. About 85% of the V_H segments productively used in the heavy-chain gene can be detected by hybridization with a single 25-base primer (27). If Ig heavy-chain gene rearrangement occurs, it brings a V_H segment close enough to a J_H segment that a single primer pair of V_H and J_H can (theoretically) detect 85% of Ig heavy-chain gene rearrangements. However, in practical experience, fewer rearrangements are found than expected, presumably as a consequence of somatic mutation and infrequency of the target sequence. Rearrangements and their PCR products vary from one B cell to the next in primary sequence and in length. The length differences are caused by differences in size of the intervening D_H segments and variability in the number of nontemplated (N) nucleotides, which are inserted between V_H-D_H-J_H. The primer pairs often used for Ig heavy-chain gene rearrangement are a single pair, with each primer of about 20 to 25 bases long. The κ light-chain gene can also be detected in some circumstances using PCR, but this is not widely applied because primer sets have not been generally applicable to most rearrangements, in contrast to heavy-chain rearrangements, which are detected in nearly every B-cell neoplasm. However, detection of κ gene rearrangements by PCR has been improved with the use of multiple degenerate primers, which permit detection of κ gene rearrangement in most B-cell lymphomas (28). However, not all B-cell lymphomas have Ig gene rearrangements demonstrable by PCR using any combination of primer pair, and false-negative results can be expected in at least 15% of cases.

TCR gene rearrangements can also be detected by PCR. The simplest gene for detection by PCR is TCR γ where a limited number or even a single pair of V_γ and J_γ primers can be used to detect rearrangements (29,30). Specialized electrophoretic techniques to detect TCR gene rearrangements are described elsewhere in the sections on Technology of the Future and T-Cell Lymphomas. The same caution described above for Southern blot analysis of the TCR γ gene also applies to PCR because of the limited number of V γ genes available (18). Careful interpretation is needed because of the possibility of polyclonal T cells when evaluating TCRγ rearrangements.

Chromosomal Translocations and Polymerase Chain Reaction

A number of chromosomal translocations can be detected by PCR among malignant lymphomas (described under specific disease sections in this chapter). Breakpoints in some of the genes involved in translocation are scattered along the oncogene involved. A single primer of, for example, *BCL2* cannot detect all *BCL2* gene translocations in t(14;18)–carrying lymphoma. The addition of more primers flanking other breakpoint regions is advisable in pursuing most breakpoints.

Interpretation of Polymerase Chain Reaction Results

PCR is an extraordinarily sensitive method. Accompanying this sensitivity is the risk of false-positive results, which can be caused by contamination wherein a positive sample, even a very limited amount, contaminates an otherwise negative sample. In the case of antigen receptor gene rearrangements and translocations, this can usually be identified because of the differences in size of the amplified fragments that vary from one B cell or neoplasm to another. A second type of false-positive result is a consequence of the presence of small numbers of cells that carry translocations, such as t(14;18), in otherwise normal individuals (31). Rearranged and translocated Ig heavy chain or *BCL2* genes can be found in normal individuals, including the peripheral blood of normal blood donors, hyperplastic lymph nodes, and tonsils. Most individuals carrying *BCL2* gene rearrangements do not have follicular lymphoma, and few ever develop it. Such translocations must occur at a low frequency in many individuals and are not sufficient to cause neoplastic transformation. Other genetic events must occur to evoke the development of a full-fledged clinical lymphoma. The presence of small numbers of cells with translocations containing "lymphoma markers" can foil attempts to predict the development of lymphoma in presymptomatic individuals or complicate diagnostic interpretation in those suspected of having lymphoma. The interpreter should be aware of the situations and interpret the data in the context of the clinical and pathologic information available.

Minimal Disease Detection

PCR is capable of detecting clonal cells carrying a DNA marker even when they are as rare as 1 in 1,000,000 cells (24). Even with the possibility of a false-positive result, what does this mean to an individual when so few cells are present in a lymph node, peripheral blood, or bone marrow? The power of this sensitivity has begun to be fully revealed in the monitoring of minimal residual disease after therapy. In some settings, the presence of residual cells detectable only by PCR and unseen by microscopy portends subsequent clinical relapse (32). The prediction of relapse can be made by PCR many months before it would otherwise have been apparent clinically. Some treated patients in apparent long-term remission have residual disease detected by sensitive PCR (see the Follicular Lymphoma section). In some circumstances, periodic monitoring of the treated patient can help in monitoring the effectiveness of therapy or autologous bone marrow transplantation during remission and prompt early, perhaps lifesaving, intervention (33). Minimal disease detection has been shown to be effective on easily accessible samples, such as peripheral blood.

TECHNOLOGY OF THE FUTURE

Substantial improvements in the techniques of gene sequencing and mapping have rapidly accelerated the pace with which the human genome is being deciphered. Estimates from the public and private sector of the Human Genome Project agree that the sequencing of the human genome will be substantially completed by 2001 (34). Fragments of most expressed human genes, estimated to be more than 100,000, have been sequenced. With this vast database, medicine is faced with the daunting task of deciphering the role of genes, genetic alterations, and gene expression in human disease. In the case of malignant lymphoma, the new tools of molecular biology and bioinformatics can help point the way to genetic markers that may predict susceptibility to lymphoma, enable a precise diagnostic profile, and provide targets for therapy and sensitive methods for monitoring the success of treatment.

It is possible to envision a diagnostic marker panel of genes or gene expression that directs clinical management to highly specific, effective therapies. This concept is analogous to the traditional use of microscopy-based classification systems of lymphoma to help guide the therapist in the selection of regimens (i.e., histologic chemosensitivity assay). The classification of neoplasms for clinical use will be driven by the advent of successful therapies. Treatments based on the expression of a particular receptor, such as the use of anti-CD20 monoclonal antibody for immunotherapy of B-cell lymphoma, may be a critical datapoint for the selection of therapy (35).

The new generation of therapeutics, based on functional genomics (i.e., sequencing of expressed genes and their association with diseases) will provide an abundant database for hematopathologists to prospect for biologically and clinically relevant molecular markers. Molecular diagnostic hematopathology will be an enabling approach for the development of targeted, highly specific therapies to attack molecular pathways linked to the pathogenesis and progression of lymphoma. Innovative applications of powerful molecular technologies are being tested in hematopathology studies (Table 9.1). Only time will tell what future lymphoma classification technologies will be. The nucleic acid–based technologies and protein detection by immunohistochemistry or flow cytometry are already shaping clinical strategies for the management of lymphoma. In the following sections, we describe some emerging research methods that could be adapted as the basis for future clinical molecular diagnostics of lymphoma.

Quantitative Polymerase Chain Reaction Methods

The precise measurement of tumor burden is a highly significant prognostic indicator, particularly of relapse after chemotherapy or bone marrow transplantation in leukemia. An improvement in the ability to compare the relative proportion of neoplastic cells has been improved by the use of real-time PCR (36) (Fig. 9.8). This technique is based on the 5′-exonuclease enzymatic activity of Taq polymerase. When Taq catalyzes the linear polymerization of DNA from the point of a PCR primer, it also removes DNA on the same strand that it encounters during the polymerization process. Real-time PCR exploits this property by adding a fluorochrome to the 5′ primer and a quencher of the fluorochrome to a 3′ probe. If polymerization occurs, the probe containing the quencher is digested and removed, thereby releasing a fluorescent signal. The intensity of the fluorescent signal is proportionate to the amount of DNA copies and ultimately to the number of cells that contain them. The readout can be automatically determined by a fluorescence analyzer, such as a DNA sequencer.

TABLE 9.1. *Emerging molecular technology in diagnostic hematopathology*

Technique	Example	Internet resource	Reference
High-throughout sequencing	All expressed genes	www.hodgkins.georgetown.edu, www.ncbi.nlm.nih.gov/ncicgap//	37, 38
Serial analysis of gene expression (SAGE)	All expressed genes	http://www.sagenet.org/	63
Microarrays	Selected genes: (DNA, or RNA)	www.ncbi.nlm.nih.gov/ncicgap// cgapdeliv.cgi?title = Expression + Technology& ins__file = expression__tech__info.html__frag	39–42, 62
Comparative genomic hybridization (CGH)	All chromosomal regions	http://biochem.boehringer.com/prod__inf/manuals/ pcr__man/p148-152.pdf	45, 46
Spectral karyotyping (SKY)	All translocations	www.spectral-imaging.com/website/webpages/ aboutSKY.html	47, 48
Real-time polymerase chain reaction (PCR)	IgH, *BCL2* DNA	http://www2.perkin-elmer.com/ab/about/pcr/sds/ white.html	36
Automated sequence analysis	IgH, *BCL2* DNA	www2.perkin-elmer.com/ab/about/dna/genotyping/ GeneScan/	64, 65
Heteroduplex analysis	TCR-β	www.bioproducts.com/technical/heterodupl exanalysiswithmdegelsolution.shtml	66
Rapid amplification of cDNA ends (RACE)	IgH cDNA	www.clontech.co.uk/archive/JAN99UPD/ smartrace.html	67
LightCycler	*BCL2* DNA	www.biochem.boehringer-mannheim.com/ lightcycler/monito00.htm	68
Microdissection	Any tissue. DNA or RNA (cDNA)	www.ncbi.nlm.nih.gov/ncicgap//, www.hodgkins.georgetown.edu	38, 53–59

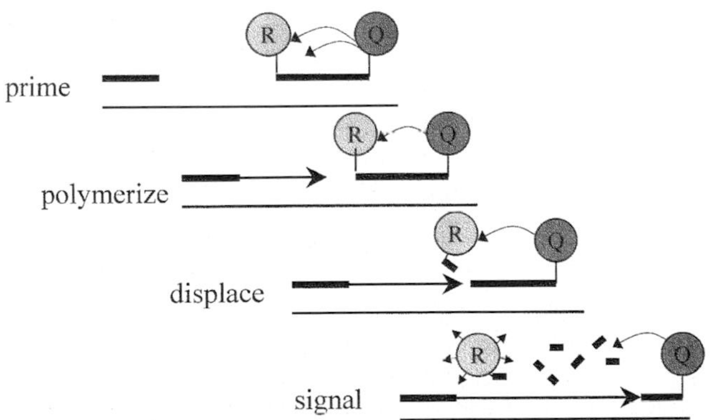

FIG. 9.8. Real-time polymerase chain reaction (PCR), which exploits the 5′ exonuclease activity of *Taq* polymerase, achieves quantitative PCR. A probe is prepared that hybridizes to the target nucleic acid sequence. The probe contains a fluorescent reporter (R) and a nearby quencher (Q). When intact, the quencher suppresses fluorescence from the reporter. A primer corresponding to a sequence 5′ of the reporter is synthesized and hybridized to the target (i.e., prime). The primer is extended by polymerization catalyzed by *Taq* (i.e., polymerize). When the extended primer sequence reaches the hybridized reporter, the 5′ exonuclease activity of *Taq* "displaces" the reporter. Freed, the reporter is no longer suppressed by the quencher, and a fluorescent signal is emitted. The signal intensity is measured as it is emitted and computed as a quantitative unit of target molecules (36).

High-Throughput Sequencing

In the past, malignant lymphomas and other neoplasms were studied for the expression of only a few genes at a time. This has largely been done by gene expression at the protein level using monoclonal antibodies and immunohistochemistry or flow cytometry. However, high-throughput, automated sequencing of portions of the complementary DNAs (cDNAs) of expressed sequences (i.e., expressed sequence tags) (37), determines the expression of a very large number of genes in a single experiment. It is estimated that perhaps more than 80% of all expressed human genes have had some portion of their sequence determined by this method. Cancers can also be studied in this way (see http://www.ncbi.nlm.nih.gov/ncicgap//), even at the single cell level for the study of Hodgkin's disease (38) (http://www.hodgkins.georgetown.edu). The data can be analyzed by matching the expressed genes of one cell to another. In this way, the investigator can determine what is similar or different between the malignant cell and a normal cell or one malignant cell and another, such as during clinical progression.

High-throughput sequencing can also be applied to any cells removed from tissue in which the RNA remains intact. Messenger RNA extracted from whole tumor tissue would contain messages derived from many cell types in addition to the neoplastic cell, including fibroblasts, endothelial cells, and inflammatory cells. To look at the neoplastic cells more precisely, microdissection has been developed to collect small numbers of homogeneous neoplastic cells. Under the microscope, the pathologist selects cells for microdissection, and these are removed through a process of laser light activation and adherence to a film or from viable cell suspensions by micropipette. Then, cDNA libraries can be prepared and sequenced, as with the single Hodgkin's disease cells. High-throughput sequencing is beginning to provide a massive data set of the expressed genes of cancers (http://www.ncbi.nlm.nih.gov/ncicgap//), and such sets also will be developed for lymphomas. The entire gene expression profile of the various lymphomas can be searched to determine which pathways are active and what the critical differences are between normal and neoplastic cells and one neoplastic type from another.

Microarrays

Another approach to broadly examine the gene expression profile of lymphoma cells in a single experiment is the use of microarrays, which promises to dramatically enhance the molecular diagnosis of lymphoid malignancies (39). Whereas most current technologies analyze one gene or protein at a time, the genomics revolution has made it possible to quantify the expression of thousands of genes simultaneously. This new method can therefore define a molecular fingerprint of a cell in unprecedented detail.

Genomic-scale gene expression analysis begins with the creation of an ordered array of cDNA fragments or oligonucleotides deposited on a solid substrate, with each element in the array derived from a distinct gene (39–44). Robotic fabrication techniques can create high-density microarrays representing thousands of genes on a single glass microscope slide or microchip. Radioactive or fluorescent cDNA or RNA probes are then prepared from total mRNA from the cell to be analyzed and hybridized to the microarray under standard Southern blotting conditions. High-throughput scanners are used to quantify the amount of cDNA probe hybridized to each microarray element. The amount of cDNA probe hybridizing to a microarray element is proportional to the expression of mRNA for the corresponding gene in the cell. In one version of this technology, the gene expression in two samples is directly compared by labeling the cDNA probes from the two samples with different fluorochromes and hybridizing the two probes to the same cDNA microarray (37–40).

In one experiment, the gene expression in two different diffuse large B-cell lymphoma samples was compared using a microarray containing 6,500 cDNAs. Most genes are expressed equivalently in both lymphoma samples, and the corresponding microarray elements are seen as yellow. Nonetheless, this example illustrates that a large number of striking gene expression differences exists between lymphoma samples within the same diagnostic category. Molecular fingerprints obtained using cDNA microarrays have begun to divide existing large cell lymphoma into new subtypes that are associated with different survival times after treatment. Gene expression microarray analyses have been performed in non-Hodgkin's lymphoma (NHL) and Hodgkin's disease.

Comparative Genomic Hybridization

Comparative genomic hybridization (CGH) is a fluorescence chromosome technique that demonstrates chromosomal regions that are lost or amplified (45). Most cancers, including malignant lymphomas (46), have regions of chromosomal loss and amplification that presumably contain genes whose overexpression or loss are important to the pathogenesis and progression of the disease. By determining the specific regions of gain or loss, molecular biologists can potentially clone genes from the critical regions, which can then be tested as diagnostic markers, as therapeutic targets, and as having a possible role in the pathogenesis of disease.

To perform CGH, DNA is extracted from neoplastic tissue or cells and is globally amplified with random PCR primers. As few as five Reed-Sternberg cells have been successfully used for CGH. The amplified DNA is labeled with a fluorochrome and then applied as a probe to normal cell metaphase spreads. All chromosomes within the metaphase spreads are hybridized with fluorescent probes if the probes are from normal cells. However, if the probes were derived from cells that have lost or gained chromosomal material, they appear as dimmer or brighter fluorescent signals, respectively, along the length of the normal chromosomes. The intensity of fluorescence can be measured by image analysis and the relative gain or loss within the regions of chromosomes can be determined.

Multicolor Spectral Karyotyping

Spectral karyotyping (SKY) is a fluorescence *in situ* hybridization technique that examines the chromosomes of cancer cells to identify the presence of any chromosomal translocation (47). In this method, normal chromosomes are flow-sorted into separate groups of each individual chromosome. The chromosomal DNA is amplified by PCR, and each chromosome is labeled with a different combination of fluorochrome dyes to generate a distinctly labeled probe set for each of the 22 autosomes and the 2 sex chromosomes. The dye combinations are designed so that they can be distinguished under the microscope using a specialized imaging system employing an interferometer. In this method, metaphase spreads are prepared from tumor cells and then hybridized with the mix of chromosomal SKY probes.

Each chromosome appears as a distinct and homogeneous color. If a translocation event has occurred, the chromosome appears as at least two colors, with an abrupt change in color exactly at the band where the chromosomal joining has taken place. This technique has revealed many new chromosomal translocations and corrected previously misinterpreted translocations observed by conventional G banding. SKY has a resolution of detection of a chromosomal break of approximately 1 million bases (1 Mb), which permits cloning of the breakpoint region. This technique is useful in the discovery of recurring translocations in cancers and has begun to identify chromosomal aberrations in malignant lymphoma (48).

The cloning of DNA sequences at the points of aberration probably will generate diagnostic probes in the future.

Polymorphisms

The molecular genetic abnormalities described so far in this chapter are somatic. Somatic changes in DNA sequence occur during the lifetime of the individual, and only some cells are affected while all other cells of the body remain unchanged or do not contain the same genetic lesion. These genetic abnormalities usually are neither inherited nor passed through the germline. Somatic genetic changes have been readily observed and widely described for cancers, but descriptions of germline cancer genes are relatively rare. However, the evolution of the great diversity of life forms, including humans, is accounted for by germline genetic sequence differences.

The role of germline genetics in cancer development is just beginning to unfold. Individuals are not equally susceptible to the development of cancer, suggesting that genetic polymorphisms contribute to cancer. Environmental factors account for much of this and probably cause or select for some somatic genetic lesions in cancers, including lymphoma. Even so, there are strong examples of individuals who are highly susceptible to the development of certain cancers on an inherited basis (including malignant lymphoma) (19). For example, children born with congenital immunodeficiency disorders, such as ataxia telangiectasia, severe combined immunodeficiency (SCID), adenosine deaminase deficiency (ADA), and others, are at risk for the development of malignant lymphoma that is several orders of magnitude higher than the general population. In many inherited syndromes, the genetic changes cripple the cellular immune system and disable its capacity to control the proliferation of mitogenically stimulated lymphocytes. In addition to the congenital immunodeficiencies, there may be individuals whose immune systems are entirely or substantially intact but have inherited an increased risk of the development of malignant lymphoma, in a manner analogous to individuals who inherit mutated *BRCA1* genes who are at risk of developing breast and other cancers. Inheritance of a mutation in the death domain of the CD95 (FAS) gene is associated with the autoimmune lymphoproliferative syndrome, also called Canale-Smith syndrome, and a heightened risk of NHL and Hodgkin's disease (49). An inheritance pattern has been described in monozygous twin pairs such that if one sibling is affected by Hodgkin's disease the twin has a 100-fold increased risk of developing Hodgkin's disease compared with a dizygous twin with an affected sibling (50). Familial patterns of NHL also occur. Lymphoma genes of this type presumably are awaiting discovery.

What are the genetic polymorphisms that account for disease susceptibility in presymptomatic individuals? The human genome is riddled with single nucleotide polymorphisms (SNPs) that occur, on average, every 300 bp. A base substitution encoding a critical functional region, transcription factor binding site, or gene regulatory region may be responsible for disease susceptibility. As the entire human genome sequence is determined, SNPs will be identified and a massive database generated (51). A major challenge to genetics and medical science will be to find links between SNPs and clinically important manifestations, such as disease susceptibility and responsiveness or refractoriness to therapy. As these associations are determined, they will become important prognostic markers in clinical management of patients, surveillance of presymptomatic individuals, and selection of therapy based on genetic profile or pharmacogenetics. The completion of the sequence of the entire human genome will generate a database of perhaps 300,000 SNPs and enable identification of the associations between SNPs and disease (52).

Microdissection

The detection of genetic alterations with molecular techniques critically depends on the representation of target (tumor) cells present in the sample used for the extraction of nucleic acids. In particular, the determination of clonality or genetic alteration by Southern blotting or by PCR analysis can yield false-negative results in the presence of a predominant nonneoplastic cell population. In addition to techniques such as flow cytometry and PCR for the detection of minimal residual disease, microdissection technology has gained importance for enrichment of the cell population in question. With new, easy to perform techniques of laser capture and laser microbeam microdissection (53,54), microdissection promises to enter molecular diagnostics. The unveiling of the gene expression (38), lineage (38,55,56), and clonality (55,56) of the Reed-Sternberg cell; the correlation of anatomic structures of lymphoid tissues with somatic mutation in B cells (57); and the confirmation of separate malignant clones in composite lymphomas (58) are early examples of the impact of microdissection on hematopathology. For genomic DNA, conventional single-step or nested PCR assays can be performed on cells isolated from fresh or fixed, paraffin-embedded tissues (59). Because neither conventional stains nor immunohistochemistry interfere with PCR, cell populations can be isolated according to morphology and according to immunophenotype (9).

Microdissected cells can be used for genomic DNA amplification by PCR directly or after a proteinase digestion step but without other purification. From genomic DNA, it is possible to determine B- and T-cell clonality, loss of heterozygosity (LOH), or tumor-specific translocations using microdissection. However, the analysis of small numbers of cells requires special caution with regard to PCR artifacts, such as the appearance of seemingly clonal bands because of the scarcity of templates for amplification, identification of biologically irrelevant clones, or contamination. With these precautions in mind, microdissection can provide an excellent tool for the analysis of molecular heterogeneity of tissues.

Gene expression can be broadly determined after microdissection. For example, Reed-Sternberg cells released into viable cell suspensions have been singly collected by micropipette to create readily analyzed cDNA libraries (38,60,61). The single cell cDNA libraries can be probed (60), tested by specific reverse transcriptase–PCR (RT-PCR) (61), subjected to high-throughput sequencing (38), or applied to microarrays (62). The genome-wide gene expression profile of a single lymphoma cell can be determined. This provides a basis to discover any diagnostic marker and also a method to diagnose the presence of an expressed gene or panel of genes in any cell (63–68).

APPLICATION OF MOLECULAR GENETICS TO LYMPHOMA DIAGNOSIS

Follicular Lymphoma

Follicle center cell lymphomas (FCLs) are B-cell tumors that originate from germinal center cells and have a characteristic immunophenotype (i.e., $CD20^+$, $CD19^+$, $CD22^+$, $CD10^+$, $CD5^-$, BCL-2^+, and BCL-6^+) that distinguish them from most other low-grade B-cell neoplasms (see Chapter 24). All cases show clonal Ig gene rearrangements by Southern blot analysis (4,69–71), and most express surface Ig, most commonly IgM (71). A smaller percentage of cases express IgG, and rare IgA^+ cases have also been reported (71). These immunophenotypic features are consistent for cells originating from the germinal center. FCLs also show a high frequency of somatic mutations of their Ig genes, and most reveal evidence of antigen selection (72–74). This is not surprising, because the follicle center is the site in which somatic mutation and antigen selection normally take place.

Like most lymphomas derived from mature B cells, rearrangements of TCR genes are not expected. Infiltrating T cells, commonly present in FCLs, may give rise to pseudoclonal TCRγ restriction patterns in Southern blot analysis (4,18), and the presence of rearranged bands should not be attributed by the interpreter as derived from the neoplastic cell population. Nonetheless, rare cases of FCL having rearrangements of the TCRβ gene have been reported in the literature (69,70).

Although all FCLs show rearrangement of Ig genes by Southern blotting, only 50% to 60% of cases have rearrangement by PCR using common consensus primers to framework 3 (FR3) (74), probably because of the high rate of somatic mutation of the Ig genes that results in template mismatches with the usual consensus primers used for FR3-PCR. A second factor is that the FR3 variable region gene primer commonly used in Ig heavy-chain PCR analyses may not be sufficiently homologous to the more than 50 productive variable region gene sequences so that efficient annealing does not take place for some V_H segments. A final consideration is that there is only one rearranged VDJ allele for targeting in FCLs, because the sister allele is involved in a characteristic translocation involving the Ig gene and the anti-apoptosis gene, *BCL2*.

By adding a second consensus primer set, homologous to FR2 and J_H, it is possible to increase the rate of clonal detection to approximately 80% (74,75). A further increase in the rate of clonal detection—up to 90%—can be achieved by using a set of V_H family specific primers homologous to FR1 sequences or leader sequences (76,77). However, the use of V_H family specific primers is not amenable to analysis of the usually degraded DNA in fixed paraffin-embedded tissue samples because of the relatively large size of the DNA template required.

The cytogenetic hallmark of FCL is the reciprocal translocation, t(14;18) involving the *BCL2* gene at chromosome 18q21 and an IgH joining region on chromosome 14q32 (12,13,22,78) (Table 9.2 and Figs. 9.5, 9.6). The *BCL2* gene

TABLE 9.2. *Molecular genetics of non-Hodgkin's lymphomas*

Lymphoma	Cytogenetics	Incidence (%)	Gene
Follicular	t(14;8)(q32;q21)	>90	*BCL2*
	t(2;18)(p12;q21)	<5	*BCL2*
	t(3;14)(q27;q32)	10	*BCL6*
Mantle cell	t(11;14)(q13;q32)	90	*BCL1, CCND1*(cyclin D1)
Marginal zone/MALT	t(11;18)(q21;q21)	20–50	*API2/MLT*
	t(1;14)(p22;q21)		*BCL10*/CARD
	trisomy 3	20–50	
Lymphoplasmacytoid	t(9;14)(p13;q32)	50	*PAX5* (BSAP)
Diffuse large B cell	t(14;18)(q32;q21)	25	*BCL2*
	t(3;14)(q27;q32)	30	*BCL6*
	t(3;22)(q27;q11)	5	*BCL6*
	t(10;14)(q24;q32)	<5	*NFK32* (NF-κB2, LYT-10)
	t(14;15)(q32;q11-13)	<5	*BCL8*
Burkitt	t(8;24)(q24;q32)	85	*MYC*
	t(2;8)(p12;q24)	10	*MYC*
	t(8;22)(p24;q11)	5	*MYC*
Burkitt-like	t(14;18)(q32;q21)	30	*BCL2*
Anaplastic large cell	t(2;5)(p23;q35)	30–70	*ALK*
Cutaneous T cell	t(10;14)(q24;q32)	?	*NFKB2* (NF-κB,2 LYT-10)

consists of one 5′ nontranslated exon and two 3′ coding exons that are separated by a long intron of 225 kb. Approximately 50% to 60% of the translocation breakpoints on chromosome 18 cluster within a 150 base pair major breakpoint region (mbr) located in the 3′ untranslated region of exon III (79). Another 20% to 25% of the breakpoints occur within a second minor cluster region (mcr) located 20 kb downstream of the mbr (80). A small percentage of FCLs show breakpoints 5′ to the *BCL2* gene (81). The remainder are scattered between the major and minor breakpoints (82). Regardless of the location of the breakpoint on chromosome 18, the chromosome 14 breakpoints always involve an Ig heavy-chain joining segment, and only rare exceptions involve an Ig light-chain gene (83). Molecular probes to the *BCL2* mbr and mcr are commercially available, and in combination with an Ig heavy-chain gene probe, they can be used to identify lymphomas with t(14;18) translocations. Such cases show comigrating *BCL2* and J_H restriction fragments in serial Southern blot analyses of tumor DNA, evidence of a fusion between the Ig gene on chromosome 14 and the *BCL2* gene on chromosome 18 (4,13) (Fig. 9.6).

The focused locations of the breakpoints within the *BCL2* and Ig heavy-chain genes have made possible the development of PCR-based assays for amplification of the genomic breakpoint sequences (24,84,85). PCR assays using consensus primer sets targeting the mbr and mcr can identify rearrangements in up to 60% to 70% of FCLs (86) and can be performed on DNA extracted from fixed, paraffin-embedded tissues or from fresh or frozen-banked tissues (87). These translocation-specific assays have a sensitivity of between 10^{-4} and 10^{-5} cells. Because the BCL-2/IgH joinings vary from case to case, the translocation amplicons can serve as a specific marker for an individual's lymphoma. Long distance (LD) PCR assays have been developed that are capable of detecting nearly 100% of BCL-2–rearranged FCLs (82). However, the application of LD-PCR is restricted to fresh tumor specimens, because the assay requires high-molecular-weight DNA template.

Fluorescent *in situ* hybridization (FISH) assays using probes flanking the *BCL2* or Ig genes (or both) have also been used to detect the neoplastic cells in paraffin and frozen sections, but these are more time consuming and technically demanding (88).

In addition to its use in the primary diagnosis of FCL, PCR assays for BCL-2/IgH junctional sequences have been particularly useful for the detection of minimal residual disease of t(14;18)-carrying tumors (32,33,89–93). Studies from several centers have provided data indicating that the detection of molecular disease after ablative chemotherapy and autologous bone marrow transplant is predictive for recurrence, and molecular remission is highly predictive of clinical remission (89,90). Results such as these imply that it may be desirable to continue treatment in patients who have not achieved complete molecular eradication of their clone.

Other studies, however, raise some cautions about the usefulness of PCR for analyzing minimal residual disease in other situations. Several investigators have reported the detection of tumor specific BCL-2/J_H joining sequences in the peripheral blood of previously treated patients with follicular lymphomas who had achieved sustained clinical remissions using conventional therapies or anti-idiotypic antibody and vaccine therapy (91–94). Despite molecular evidence of persistence of the tumor clone, most patients had no evidence of recurrent clinical disease. The presence of BCL-2/J_H joining sequences may have less predictive value for late relapse in patients who have attained a sustained remission. In such patients, it may be more helpful to examine bone marrow biopsies or blood samples serially over time to obtain a clear picture of whether the tumor specific signal is increasing or stable (95).

Inappropriate expression of the BCL-2 gene product occurs as a result of the activity of juxtaposed Ig gene regulatory sequences. The BCL-2 protein is a constituent of the membrane systems of mitochondria, nuclei, and endoplasmic reticulum and functions as an antagonist of apoptosis (96,97). In cells containing t(14;18), elevated levels of BCL-2 protein interfere with normal B-cell turnover, leading to a pool of long-lived cells that are at risk for generating a lymphoma. The fact that BCL-2/J_H junctional sequences have been found in hyperplastic lymph nodes, tonsils and peripheral blood in otherwise normal individuals suggests that the translocation alone is insufficient for the development of lymphoma and that additional genetic abnormalities are necessary (31). Consistent with this interpretation are studies from BCL-2 transgenic mice. Such mice develop B-cell hyperplasias but do not develop lymphomas until they acquire secondary genetic lesions, such as *MYC* gene rearrangements (98). From the diagnostic viewpoint, identification of BCL-2/J_H sequences in normal individuals poses a theoretical concern, but their detection requires very sensitive assay conditions, and in practice, these molecules are not sufficiently numerous to be detected in standard clinical PCR assays (99).

Excellent antibodies to BCL-2 protein have been commercially available for several years. Using these antibodies, about 90% of cases of FCL can be shown to express high levels of BCL-2 (100). However, antibodies do not distinguish a BCL-2 protein encoded by a fusion gene of t(14;18) from BCL-2 encoded by a normal chromosome 18. Some non-t(14;18) translocated lymphomas, particularly other low-grade lymphomas, express high levels of BCL-2. BCL-2 expression cannot be used to distinguish the various forms of low-grade lymphoma.

Low-grade FCLs undergo histologic progression to an aggressive higher-grade lymphoma in as many as 70% of cases. Approximately one third of these transformed cases acquire a mutation of the *TP53* tumor suppressor gene at the time of histologic progression, implicating p53 inactivation in follicular lymphoma progression (101,102). Inactivation of the p16 *(INK4A)* tumor suppressor gene has also been implicated in up to 50% of transformed cases (103). Transformed follicular lymphomas may also acquire *MYC* gene rearrangements, but this occurs in less than 10% of transformed cases (104). Other candidate progression-related genes include one or more undefined tumor suppressor genes believed to be located on chromosome 6q23-27 (105). The transformation of low-grade FCL to an aggressive, high-grade lymphoma appears to involve a limited number of secondary genetic events that most frequently involve the inactivation of tumor suppressor genes. In the future, it should be possible to monitor patients for acquisition of these genetic abnormalities and institute appropriate interventive measures.

Mantle Cell Lymphoma

Mantle cell lymphoma (MCL) is a B-cell neoplasm in which the putative precursor cell is an unmutated, $CD5^+$ virgin B cell of the follicle mantle with unmutated Ig genes (see Chapter 22). Mantle cell lymphoma usually shows clonally rearranged Ig heavy and light chains by Southern blot and by PCR assays using conventional family-specific or consensus Ig heavy-chain primers (106–108). The rearranged Ig heavy-chain genes of MCL show a very low rate of somatic mutation without evidence for antigen-driven selection, consistent with a pre–germinal center cell origin, although more heterogeneous results have been found in the blastic variant of MCL (109,110).

The t(11;14)(q13;q32) translocation is the cytogenetic hallmark of MCL, occurring in about 50% to 70% of cases (107,111–113) (Table 9.2). The breakpoint on chromosome 11 was originally called *BCL1*. As in other translocations of B-cell NHL, the site on chromosome 14 is in the Ig heavy-chain joining region (114–116). This translocation leads to the deregulation of the *PRAD1/CCND1* gene located approximately 200 kb from the *BCL1* locus, which encodes for the cell cycle–regulating protein cyclin D1 (117,118). By Southern blot analysis, translocations of the *BCL1* locus can be identified in 35% to 70% of cases of MCL, in part depending on the number of probes used (112,119,120). About 80% of the breakpoints detected by Southern blotting occur in a tightly clustered region designated as the major translocation cluster (MTC) (121), whereas the remaining breakpoints are dispersed over approximately 120 kb, making their detection with the commonly used probes difficult. PCR amplification using primers flanking the MTC detects *BCL1* rearrangements in approximately 40% to 50% of MCLs and can be applied to paraffin-embedded archival tissue (121–123).

Deregulation of the *PRAD1/CCND1* gene leads to overexpression of cyclin D1 mRNA and protein detectable by Northern blot analysis and by Western blot methods or immunohistochemistry on paraffin sections, respectively, and is a highly specific marker of MCL (124). Cyclin D1 overexpression is found in most cases of MCL, regardless of the presence or absence of a *BCL1* translocation, suggesting additional mechanisms of deregulation (125). The overexpression of cyclin D1 probably leads to deregulation of the cell cycle by overcoming the suppressive effects of retinoblastoma (RB) protein and p27 (106,126–128). The occurrence of t(11;14) or *BCL1* rearrangements has also been reported in a small percentage of multiple myeloma, prolymphocytic leukemia, and chronic lymphocytic leukemia/small lymphocytic lymphoma (CLL/SLL) cases. However, most previously reported cases of CLL with t(11;14) probably represent leukemic MCL (112). Hairy cell leukemia is the only other B-cell neoplasm exhibiting overexpression of cyclin D1 mRNA and protein, albeit at much lower levels and without detectable *BCL1* translocation.

Rearrangements characteristic for other lymphoma subtypes, such as the *BCL2* gene rearrangement of follicular lymphoma, are not found in MCL. Similar to CLL/SLL, deletions at 13q14 and at 11q21-23 occur frequently as secondary aberrations. As in CLL, the 13q14 deletion is not associated with a loss of RB1 protein expression, suggesting involvement of another tumor suppressor gene at this locus (127,129).

Although transformation to a conventional diffuse large cell morphology does not occur in MCL, histologic progression to or initial presentation as so-called blastic or anaplastic variants of MCL is well recognized and is associated with a worse prognosis (108,130). In contrast to typical MCL, these cases frequently show secondary genetic alterations, especially *TP53* gene mutations or deletions of other cell cycle-regulating genes such as p16 *(INK4A)* or p21 *(WAF1)* (131–134).

Marginal Zone B-Cell Lymphoma

The broad category of marginal zone B-cell lymphoma (MZL) contains nodal and extranodal neoplastic proliferations thought to arise from B cells of the marginal zone of lymphoid follicles. Extranodal MZL of the mucosa-associated lymphoid tissue (MALT) type, or MALT lymphoma, has been described in most extranodal sites, but most cases arise in the gastrointestinal tract (mainly in the stomach), salivary glands, skin, and thyroid (135). These lymphomas frequently arise in the background of autoimmune disease, such as Hashimoto's thyroiditis or Sjögren's syndrome, and in chronic infections, notably *Helicobacter pylori* gastritis. Because of their frequently indolent clinical evolution, MZLs often were diagnosed as pseudolymphoma before the advent of molecular determination of clonality. It is still controversial whether the detection of clonality in an extranodal lymphoid proliferation should be equated with malignancy (136–141). The nodal counterpart of extranodal MZL, morphologically indistinguishable from lymph node involvement by MALT lymphoma, is monocytoid B-cell lymphoma (MCBL) or nodal MZL (142,143). Both tumors express surface Ig and, in part, cytoplasmic Ig and pan-B-cell markers but lack CD5 and CD23 (see Chapter 23).

All subtypes of MZL have rearranged Ig genes but usually lack TCR gene rearrangements. Most cases from different extranodal sites analyzed show a high load of somatic mutations of the Ig genes, most with evidence of antigen selection, indicating an origin from post–germinal center B cells (144,145). Ongoing mutations in some cases suggest a role of antigen in the evolution of the clone. The dependence of lymphoma growth on stimulation by antigen or antigen-specific T cells has been demonstrated for gastric MALT lymphoma, which can regress after eradication of *H. pylori* (146,147).

Since the advent of the PCR, a multitude of studies have tried to establish the utility of PCR for the diagnosis and follow-up of MALT lymphoma on endoscopic, especially gastric, biopsies. Although most MALT lymphomas show clonal rearrangements by PCR and the persistence or recurrence of the malignant clone can be demonstrated during follow-up, the clinical utility of PCR surveillance is limited by an inherent risk to detect clonal populations of questionable clinical significance. Most investigators have encountered occasional patterns suggesting clonality in control biopsies without lymphoma. A prolonged persistence of the malignant clone can be demonstrated by PCR in some patients who show complete histologic regression of lymphoma after treatment (148–152). Southern blot analysis of gastric biopsy specimens, although cumbersome and therefore restricted in its practical application, is less likely to lead to false-positive results, probably because of its lower sensitivity and the absence of PCR artifacts such as irreproducible clonal bands due to a low number of available templates from an already restricted B-cell population (152–154). Molecular determination of clonality in biopsy specimens can be a helpful adjunct for the diagnosis of extranodal lymphoma, but PCR results should always be interpreted carefully in conjunction with the histologic findings.

MALT lymphomas differ from nodal lymphomas in their cytogenetics. Rearrangements of *BCL1, BCL2,* and *MYC* are generally absent (155). The most frequently described cytogenetic anomalies are t(11;18)(q21;q21) and trisomy 3, occurring in approximately 20% to 50% each (156–160) (Table 9.2). In two cases of MALT lymphoma carrying a t(11;18), rearrangement of the apoptosis inhibitor gene *API2* and a novel gene, designated *MLT*, has been demonstrated, leading to the expression of a fusion mRNA lacking the amino-terminal caspase recruitment domain (CARD) of API1 (161). Another recurrent anomaly is the t(1;14)(p22; q21), involving a novel gene designated *BCL10* (162–164). *BCL10* is an apoptotic signaling gene also encoding a CARD. Cases carrying the translocation show a variety of mutations, most resulting in truncations of the protein (164). Mutations of *BCL10* have also been found in a variety of other lymphoma subtypes and were initially reported as mutated in other nonhematologic tumors (162), although subsequent studies have not confirmed mutations of *BCL10* in cancers other than lymphomas (165). The mutated protein retains the ability to activate NF-κB but is unable to induce cell death. These findings suggest that in MALT lymphoma, similar to some other low-grade B-cell NHLs, the inhibition of programmed cell death through translocations or mutations of genes involved in apoptotic pathways play an important role in the pathogenesis of these neoplasms.

In contrast to most other lymphoma subtypes studied, a replication error (RER^+) phenotype as an indicator of genetic instability is relatively frequent and seems to be positively associated with secondary alterations such as mutations of the *TP53* gene (166).

Transformation to high-grade lymphomas can occur in MZL, and neoplasms containing low- and high-grade components are frequent (165). Except for *TP53* mutations, no specific genetic alterations associated with tumor progression have been identified (166). Whether diffuse large cell lymphomas at extranodal sites represent the high-grade end of the spectrum of MALT lymphoma, however, has remained controversial. Data suggest that at least some of these cases without evidence of a low-grade component show different molecular alterations, indicating a distinct histogenesis (158,167–169).

A particularly virulent form of follicular lymphoma has been described that contains substantial numbers of monocytoid B cells whose cytology is the same as that seen in MCBL/nodal MZL (170). The monocytoid B cells are clonally related to the follicular lymphoma cells and may represent neoplastic counterparts of normal post–germinal center monocytoid cells found in the lymphoid marginal zone (171,172). As a testament to their germinal center origin, the monocytoid B cells seen in follicular lymphoma have a t(14;18) by PCR (173). This molecular feature should be useful in distinguishing the aggressive follicular lymphoma with monocytoid B cells from MCBL.

Splenic marginal zone lymphoma (SMZL) is distinct from MALT lymphoma and MCBL clinically, pathologically, and phenotypically. SMZL overlaps with splenic lymphoma with villous lymphocytes (174–176). SMZL shows rearranged Ig genes and the pattern of somatic mutation indicates an origin from post–germinal center cells (11,177). Trisomy 3 is a frequent finding in SMZL, although at a lower rate than in MALT lymphomas, whereas the translocations t(1; 14) and t(11;18) seen in MALT lymphomas have not been described in SMZLs. Whether cases of splenic lymphoma with villous lymphocytes carrying a t(11;14) with *BCL1* translocation belong to the category of SMZL or are variants of MCL remains to be determined (178–181).

Lymphoplasmacytic Lymphoma

Lymphoplasmacytoid (lymphoplasmacytic) lymphoma, also called immunocytoma, shows a range of differentiation from small lymphocytes to lymphoplasmacytoid cells and plasma cells and lacks defining features of other small B-cell neoplasms. The neoplastic cells have rearranged Ig heavy and light-chain genes and express surface and cytoplasmic Ig, frequently IgM, and lack CD5 and CD10. Most patients have a monoclonal paraprotein in the serum, commonly IgM; these cases correspond to Waldenström's macroglobulinemia.

Despite the expression of IgM, the lymphoplasmacytoid cells of Waldenstrom's macroglobulinemia are like germinal center B cells in that they have somatic mutations of their rearranged Ig genes. This evidence of antigenic selection suggests an origin from post–germinal center cells that did not undergo class switching (182,183). Low-grade B-cell lymphomas, predominantly lymphoplasmacytic lymphoma and monocytoid B-cell lymphomas have an increased prevalence of chronic hepatitis C virus (HCV) infection. Many patients also have mixed cryoglobulinemia (184–186). An analysis of the expressed Ig genes in HCV-associated immunocytomas revealed a predominant expression of V_H 51p1 and kv325 V_L genes, pointing to a derivation from a highly selected, antigen-driven B-cell population (187).

The t(9;14)(p13;q32) translocation is a recurrent chromosomal anomaly associated with approximately 50% of lymphoplasmacytic lymphomas (188) (Table 9.2). It juxtaposes the *PAX5* gene, encoding a B-cell–specific transcription factor (BSAP), to the Ig heavy-chain gene locus (189). The translocation leads to an enhanced transcription of an unmutated *PAX5* gene and increased BSAP expression. By definition, genetic alterations characteristic for other small B-cell lymphoma subtypes, such as *BCL1* or *BCL2* translocations, should be absent in lymphoplasmacytic lymphoma.

Diffuse Large B-Cell Lymphoma

The Revised European-American Lymphoma (REAL) classification scheme calls diffuse large B-cell lymphoma (DLBCL) a single entity by combining diffuse large cell lymphoma and diffuse large cell immunoblastic lymphoma subtypes from the Working Formulation (143) (see Chapter 25). In keeping with a B-cell origin of DLBCL, the Ig heavy-chain gene loci are rearranged on one or both chromosomes (detectable by PCR or Southern blotting), and the TCR gene loci are in germline configurations. The rearranged Ig genes from DLBCLs contain a large number of somatic point mutations (190,191). Because hypermutation of Ig genes is a characteristic feature of normal germinal center B lymphocytes, DLBCLs most likely originate from germinal center B cells or their descendants. The pattern of Ig somatic mutations in DLBCLs suggests that antigen stimulation and selection was active for some time after malignant transformation (191). Some cases of DLBCL exhibit intraclonal variation in Ig sequences (190), suggesting that Ig somatic hypermutation continued after malignant transformation. These observations indicate that the germinal center B-cell is most likely the cell that is transformed in DLBCL.

One of the key molecular events in the pathogenesis of many DLBCLs is translocation of the *BCL6* gene, located at 3q27, which encodes a zinc finger transcriptional repressor (192–197) (Table 9.2). The incidence of *BCL6* translocations in DLBCLs ranges from 18% to 45% in various reports (192,196–198) and is the most frequent genetic alteration in this malignancy. The translocations typically break the *BCL6* gene within or immediately downstream of its first noncoding exon, removing the *BCL6* promoter. Most or all *BCL6* translocations can be detected by Southern blotting using a probe derived from the *BCL6* gene just downstream of this major translocation cluster region. In some instances, a chimeric BCL-6–IgH transcript is formed that can be detected by RT-PCR (199). The diverse translocation partner genes are derived from more than 10 different chromosomes and invariably provide a promoter that drives the expression of the wild-type coding exons of *BCL6.* Malignant transformation by *BCL6* presumably results from dysregulation of its expression during B-cell differentiation.

Critical insights into the function of *BCL6* as an oncogene came from an analysis of its role in normal lymphocyte differentiation (200). The BCL-6 protein is selectively expressed in germinal center B cells and is reduced or absent at other stages of B-cell differentiation (201,202). Targeted disruption of the *BCL6* gene in mice results in failure of B cells to form germinal centers (203–205). It would seem likely that the ability of BCL-6 to transform germinal center B cells is intertwined with its role as a regulator of normal germinal center differentiation (206–208). Terminal differentiation of B cells into plasma cells is accompanied by the loss of BCL-6 expression. Translocations of the *BCL6* gene may prevent this physiologic silencing of BCL-6 expression and potentially prevent terminal differentiation of a germinal center B cell. Prolonged residence within the germinal center stage may allow second oncogenic hits to accumulate. *BCL6* translocations may be very early events in transformation toward DLBCL because they occur as the sole detectable chromosomal abnormality in some cases (209). However, most DLBCLs with *BCL6* translocations harbor multiple other chromosomal abnormalities, which may profoundly influence the clinical behavior of the lymphoma. In keeping with this notion, no consistent association has been found between *BCL6* translocations and clinical prognosis: one study found that *BCL6* translocations correlated with improved prognosis (210), but other studies did not find correlations with clinical end points (194,211,212).

The t(14;18) involving the *BCL2* gene is another common chromosomal abnormality in DLBCL, which is found in roughly 25% of cases (213–218) (Table 9.2). The t(14;18) translocation is found in cases that have progressed from follicular lymphoma and in *de novo* cases. In the *de novo* cases, t(14;18) may suggest the presence of a preexisting occult follicular lymphoma. Conflicting evidence has been presented regarding the association of t(14;18) with clinical parameters; studies have correlated t(14;18) with decreased responsiveness to therapy or shorter disease-free survival (219,220) or have found no prognostic value of t(14;18) (221). Another recurrent abnormality in DLBCL is deletion or inactivation of the genes for p15 and p16 that encode inhibitors of the cyclin-dependent protein kinases (103,222–226). These tumor suppressors target cyclin D/CDK4 (cyclin-dependent protein kinase-4), a critical regulator of the G_1 checkpoint that controls cell cycle progression to S phase. The molecular mechanisms that lead to the loss of p16 protein expression include allelic loss or, infrequently, nonsense mutations in the p16 gene and methylation of a CpG island in the 5′ region of the gene. Deletions in this chromosomal locus would also eliminate another tumor suppressor, p19 *(ARF)*, which is encoded in an alternate reading frame of the p16 gene (227,228). Inactivation of the p16 gene *(CDKN2A)* accompanied progression from follicular lymphoma to DLBCL in 44% of cases studied (224,225). The tumor suppressor gene, *TP53,* is mutated in a smaller number of DLBCLs (229), but the gene mutations may accompany histologic progression of follicular lymphoma (101,102). The oncogene *REL* on chromosome 2p13 is amplified in some cases of DLBCL, particularly those that are extranodal and associated with tumor progression (230).

Burkitt's Lymphoma

Burkitt's lymphoma (BL) is a cytogenetically homogeneous disease characterized by translocations involving the *MYC* gene at chromosome 8q24. Burkitt-like, small non–cleaved cell lymphomas generally do not have *MYC* involvement, are genetically heterogeneous, and overlap with the large B-cell lymphomas (231) (see Chapter 27). The following discussion is specifically focussed on Burkitt's lymphoma.

Burkitt's lymphoma is divided into the endemic African type, and the sporadic form, which occurs more commonly in non-African countries including the United States and Europe (232). The Burkitt's lymphoma variants are morphologically identical and have translocations involving the *MYC* gene on chromosome 8q24 and one of the Ig gene loci (233) (Table 9.2). However, the two are epidemiologically and clinically distinct. One of the more biologically interesting differences between the two variants is the 100% association of the EBV with the endemic form of Burkitt's lymphoma, but EBV is found in only 10% to 20% of sporadic variants (232).

Burkitt's lymphoma is a B-cell neoplasm of follicle center cell origin and is $CD20^+$, $CD19^+$, $CD22^+$, $CD5^-$, $CD10^{+/-}$, $BCL\text{-}2^-$, and $BCL\text{-}6^+$ (204,234,235). The Ig heavy and light-chain genes are always rearranged and most cases express cell surface IgM and IgD, suggesting an early germinal center stage of B-cell differentiation (3,236). The Ig genes are usually somatically mutated indicating antigen selection (237–240). TCR gene rearrangements do not occur in classic Burkitt's lymphoma (231,232).

Approximately 85% of Burkitt's lymphomas have a t(8; 14)(q24;q32) translocation that joins the *MYC* gene on chromosome 8q24 and the Ig heavy-chain gene from chromosome 14q32 (233). The remaining 15% of Burkitt's lymphomas have variant translocations, either t(2;8)(p12;q24) or t(8;22)(q24;q11), involving the κ and λ light-chain genes, respectively. The coding region of the *MYC* gene (exons 2 and 3) is never disrupted, and the major consequence of the classic t(8;14) and the variant translocations is altered MYC expression. Deregulation of MYC expression is presumably central to the cellular proliferation, differentiation, and inhibited apoptosis underlying neoplastic transformation (241,242).

Molecular features of translocation and its consequent diagnostic implications are different in endemic and sporadic Burkitt's lymphoma (243,244). In sporadic Burkitt's lymphoma, the t(8;14) generally has breakpoints located within the first exon or intron of the *MYC* gene and within an Ig heavy-chain switch region rather than an Ig heavy-chain joining region and is often detectable by Southern blotting. In endemic Burkitt's lymphoma, the chromosome 8 breakpoints are located much further, even hundreds of kilobases 5′ of the *MYC* gene, and chromosome 14 breakpoints are in an Ig heavy-chain joining region. As a result of the long distance of the breakpoint from *MYC*, gene rearrangements of *MYC* in sporadic Burkitt's lymphomas are undetectable by routine Southern blotting.

Variant translocations often occur 3′ of exon 3 of *MYC*. The Ig light-chain genes break upstream of the joining regions (245,246) and are too distant from *MYC* to be detected by Southern blot analysis.

PCR analysis is not commonly used diagnostically because of the breakpoints on chromosome 8, which are not focused in one or two sites so that detection requires many primers or long distance PCR assays (247,248). The latter method requires intact, nondegraded DNA and is not suitable for paraffin-embedded tissue. FISH analysis overcomes these limitations by its ability to reveal translocations regardless of the breakpoint location. It can be applied to interphase nuclei or metaphase nuclei and is therefore suited for routinely prepared cells (249–251).

A small percentage of large B-cell lymphomas, but no low-grade lymphomas, have *MYC* gene translocations. Rare cases of T-cell lymphoma have translocations of *MYC* involving one of the TCR genes (252). Burkitt-like, small non–cleaved cell lymphomas do not have *MYC* gene translocations, but about 30% have *BCL2* gene rearrangements, something that never occurs in Burkitt's lymphoma (253). Burkitt lymphomas also have a relatively high frequency of *TP53* gene mutation, which is thought to predict a poorer response to treatment (254,255).

Hodgkin's Disease

The elusive origin of the Reed-Sternberg cell has been substantially solved since the first edition of this textbook. Through the combined power of two technologies, microdissection and ultra-high-throughput expressed gene sequencing, it is evident that the Reed-Sternberg cell is an aberrant form of a germinal center B cell (38,256). The Reed-Sternberg cell in classic Hodgkin's disease is clonal and has suffered numerous somatic mutations in its rearranged Ig heavy-chain variable region (V_H) genes that disable its capacity to productively synthesize Ig protein (256,257). Reed-Sternberg cell variants in nodular lymphocyte predominance Hodgkin's disease have mutated Ig heavy-chain genes with noncrippling somatic mutations, indicative of antigen selection of a germinal center B cell (258). Reed-Sternberg cells of many cases of Hodgkin's disease contain EBV genomic DNA, express EBV RNA (EBER) and protein (latent membrane protein, LMP1), and sometimes have partial deletions of the EBV LMP1 gene (259,260). EBV is more often associated with the extremes of ages (i.e., children and older adults) and occurs less frequently in most young adult cases, suggesting the possibility of an undiscovered virus in the disease (260).

The molecular findings have not produced a specific and sensitive molecular diagnostic marker for the differential diagnosis and clinical monitoring of Hodgkin's disease. The rearranged Ig genes are generally not detectable by routine Southern blotting or even PCR but require microdissection of few or even single Reed-Sternberg cells. EBV genes and their expressions are not specific for Hodgkin's disease because they are found in many other benign and malignant conditions and are not present in all cases of Hodgkin's disease. No consistent cytogenetic abnormalities have been found in Hodgkin's disease. However, if Hodgkin's disease is similar to other hematopoietic neoplasms, it remains a distinct possibility that genetic lesions will be found that may be useful for molecular cytogenetics and diagnosis. Discovery of such genetic abnormalities awaits further technical refinements based on some earlier studies using comparative genomic hybridization (261,262) and future analyses with multicolor *in situ* hybridization such as SKY.

The complete profile of genes expressed by a malignant cell defines the cell type, provides clues to its origin, and is a resource for potential diagnostic markers and therapeutic targets. To better understand the genome-wide gene expression profile of the Reed-Sternberg cell, we performed ultra-high-throughput sequencing of the expressed genes of single Reed-Sternberg cells and cell lines derived from Hodgkin's disease. In all, more than 27,000 gene sequences were determined that provided 2666 distinct, named genes expressed in Hodgkin's disease (38). In one sequencing study, the number of named genes or proteins known to be expressed in Hodgkin's disease was increased by approximately 20-fold. Approximately the same number of to-be-named genes was also found in Hodgkin's cells in this study. This nearly complete profile of the expressed genes of Reed-Sternberg cells provides a resource for investigators to identify genes whose expression is highly associated with Hodgkin's disease and clinical outcome. By isolating the rare Reed-Sternberg cell and analyzing its genome-wide gene expression, the technologies of microdissection and molecular gene expression have been pushed to their limits to demonstrate the enormous power of the technology to provide leads for diagnosis and, ultimately, therapy. Accordingly, many other cancers, including other types of lymphoma and leukemia, are being analyzed in this way. The gene expression profile of Reed-Sternberg cells from the high-throughput gene sequencing study can be found on the Internet (http://www.hodgkins.georgetown.edu).

T-Cell Lymphomas

The mature (peripheral) T-cell lymphomas are nearly always clonal and, like their B-cell lymphoma counterparts, have undergone antigen receptor gene rearrangements before clonal expansion (4,6,7,263,264), although no rearrangements are seen in some (265). In most cases, rearrangement involves the TCR α, β, and γ genes and deletion of the TCR δ gene. About 95% of T cells and T-cell lymphomas are of $\alpha\beta$ type and have undergone rearrangement of the α and β loci (4,6,7,263,264). The rarer $\gamma\delta$ T cells and T-cell lymphomas have rearrangements of the TCR γ- and δ-chain genes that encode their surface TCR $\gamma\delta$ receptor. Common to the TCR $\alpha\beta$ and TCR $\gamma\delta$ cells is rearrangement of the TCR γ-chain gene. TCR γ-chain gene rearrangement analysis can be universally applied to all T-cell neoplasms whether they are of TCR $\alpha\beta$ or TCR $\gamma\delta$. The Ig heavy-chain and light-chain genes are not rearranged. In addition to TCR gene rearrangements, in precursor T-cell lymphoblastic lymphoma, Ig heavy-chain rearrangements frequently occur, in parallel to its leukemic counterpart, precursor T-cell acute lymphoblastic leukemia (see Chapters 7 and 26).

The genomic configuration and sequence of the TCR gene family complicate detection of TCR gene rearrangements in T-cell lymphomas. For practical purposes, the TCRγ gene is the best suited for routine diagnostics (4). This is a consequence of its rearrangement in all types of T-cell lymphoma and its small number of V_γ and J_γ genes, permitting the use of a modest number of consensus primers for amplification of all possible TCRγ V-J rearrangements (262,266). By contrast, the enormous size of the TCRα locus with its many V and J segments renders it unusable for Southern blot analysis or PCR (267). Restriction fragment analysis and Southern blotting (5,6) can readily analyze the TCRβ gene. It has generally been thought that the TCRβ locus is impractical for PCR analysis. However, through the use of highly degenerate J_β primers and a consensus V_β primer, it is possible to amplify virtually all TCRβ gene rearrangements (268,269). For detection of the TCRγ gene, sets of primers have been successfully and routinely applied to amplify the rearranged V-J segments (29,30,262,266). These can be visualized as electrophoretically separated fragments in routine agarose gels. Others have shown improvements in the precision of separating and revealing rearranged fragments through the use of PCR followed by single-stranded conformational polymorphism (270), denaturing gradient gel electrophoresis (271–273), or heteroduplex strand formation (66). Whether any of these or other techniques will replace agarose gel electrophoresis for detection of TCRγPCR products remains to be determined. The most practical approach for detection of clonality in T-cell lymphomas is the use of TCRγ gene rearrangements.

The mature T-cell lymphomas that contain TCR α-, β-, and γ-chain rearrangements are peripheral T-cell lymphoma, AILD-like T-cell lymphoma, enteropathy-associated T-cell lymphoma, and cutaneous T-cell lymphomas such as mycosis fungoides. In each of these, clonality can be detected through the use of TCR γ chain PCR, and this technique is also useful in staging the extent of disease and monitoring relapse after therapy (263,274,275). A distinct clinical pathologic type of T-cell lymphoma is hepatosplenic T-cell lymphoma that originates from a cytotoxic $\gamma\delta$ T cell. This lymphoma, like $\alpha\beta$ T-cell lymphomas, also contains γ-chain rearrangements, which can be detected by PCR (276). It frequently has an isochromosome 7q (276), but no molecular set of genetic markers has been reported. Another unusual type of mature T-cell lymphoma is subcutaneous panniculitic T-cell lymphoma, another type of cytotoxic T-cell lymphoma, and it contains TCRγ gene rearrangements detectable by PCR (277). Lymphomas of natural killer cell type, such as those that occur in the nasal tract do not generally contain TCR gene rearrangements, although they frequently contain EBV (278,279).

Compared with B-cell lymphomas, molecular cytogenetic markers have not been as forthcoming for T-cell lymphomas (14,15), although markers have been identified for the T-cell lymphoblastic leukemias (see Chapter 29). One example of a T-cell lymphoma translocation is t(10;14)(q24;q32), found in some cases of cutaneous T-cell lymphoma and sometimes in large B-cell lymphoma (Table 9.2). It involves rearrangement and 3′ truncation of the NF-κB transcription factor, LYT-10 (NF-κB2) at 10q24 and presumably deregulates NF-κB (280–282). Detection of LYT-10 rearrangement is achieved by Southern blotting and has not yet been extended to widespread application as a diagnostic test.

Anaplastic Large Cell Lymphoma

Although relatively few diagnostic molecular genetic markers have been reported for mature T-cell neoplasms, experience with other lymphoid neoplasms suggests that as yet undiscovered diagnostic markers and therapeutic targets will emerge from molecular genetic investigations of peripheral T-cell lymphomas. One example is anaplastic large cell lymphoma (ALCL) (see Chapter 25).

TCR gene rearrangement analysis by PCR indicates that more than 90% of ALCLs have TCR gene rearrangements (283). Early studies using Southern blot analysis had indicated that about two thirds of ALCLs have TCRβ or TCRγ gene rearrangements, and one third of cases had neither TCR gene rearrangements nor Ig gene rearrangements (284). By definition, Ig gene rearrangements are not found in ALCL.

A high percentage of ALCLs are characterized by a specific translocation involving chromosomes 2 and 5 (285–287) that results in the juxtaposition of a novel tyrosine kinase gene *(ALK)* on chromosome 2p23 to the nucleophosmin gene *(NPM)* on chromosome 5q35 (288) (Table 9.2). Although the breakpoints on chromosomes 2 and 5 are widely dispersed, they occur within a single intron of the *ALK* and *NPM* genes, and splicing out of the fused intronic sequences generates a single mRNA species consisting of 5′ sequences from *NPM* and 3′ sequences of *ALK* (288,289). The translocation leads to the inappropriate expression of an NPM/ALK fusion protein with constitutive kinase activity, which is thought to play a central role in the pathogenesis of ALCL (290). In addition to the classic t(2;5) translocation, a variant translocation involving chromosome 1q25 and an inversion (2)(p23q35) have been described (291,292). These variant abnormalities also result in inappropriate ALK kinase activity. Cases with the t(2;5) translocation or variants have been recognized as a distinct subset of ALCL (293–295). These ALCL forms occur in children and young adults and have a much better prognosis than ALK$^-$ ALCLs, which tend to occur in older individuals.

Genomic restriction fragment analysis (296), LD-PCR (289,297), and RT-PCR (298,299) have been used to identify cases containing the t(2;5) translocation. From a diagnostic point of view, RT-PCR is the method of choice because of its speed and the ability to perform the assay on RNA extracted from formalin-fixed, paraffin-embedded tissues. With RT-PCR, 40% to 70% of primary ALCLs can be shown to possess the fusion transcript (298–301). LD-PCR is sensitive and easy to perform but cannot be performed on paraffin-embedded tissue because the fragment sizes generated range from approximately 700 bp to several thousand base pairs. LD-PCR and RT-PCR can be used for minimal residual disease monitoring, because each is capable of identifying 1 in 10^4 to 10^5 tumor cells. FISH using specific probes flanking the breakpoint sequences can also be used diagnostically (302), but it is not suitable for minimal residual disease monitoring.

Two excellent commercially available antibodies react with the ALK portion of the fusion protein (303,304). These stain all cases of ALCL with evidence of ALK rearrangement but do not mark the ALK$^-$ cases. These antibodies mark a rare group of large B-cell lymphomas that express the ALK kinase but that show no evidence of the t(2;5) translocation (305).

NPM/ALK transcripts have also been reported in occasional cases of peripheral T-cell lymphoma (PTCL) (300) and in Hodgkin's disease (306). The identification of NPM/ALK transcripts in PTCLs may reflect differences in histologic diagnostic criteria. However, the identification of NPM/ALK transcripts in Hodgkin's disease is more difficult to explain and has not been confirmed by other groups (307).

SUMMARY AND CONCLUSIONS

Somatic mutation, antigen receptor gene rearrangements, and chromosomal translocations are the genetic basis of lymphoma pathogenesis. Collectively, these genetic changes have been exploited for more than a decade as unique molecular markers for diagnosis, prognosis, and monitoring of malignant lymphoma. The Human Genome Project is providing a new set of efficient, high-throughput technologies and a genome-wide database that can be channeled into clinical laboratory practice. Automated expressed gene sequencing, the completed human genome sequence, massively parallel gene expression microarrays, and deep understanding of cellular pathways are changing the way we see malignant lymphoma cells. The coordinate expression of tens of thousands of genes can be determined from a single, clinical lymphoma specimen and electronically searched for markers of pathogenesis and prognosis. The success of therapy can be monitored by sensitive molecular detection of even a single residual cell. With these tools, we can anticipate a new era of diagnostic precision, patient stratification, and therapeutic targets in lymphoma oncology. Selection of therapy will increasingly shift from the results of interpretive morphology to molecular markers as the ''chemosensitivity assay.'' Reproducible, specific diagnostic markers will naturally evolve as precise, new medicines are developed to correct the molecular lesions of lymphoma.

ACKNOWLEDGMENTS

The authors of this chapter wish to thank Loesje Troglia for editorial assistance and Drs. Kenneth Carter, Douglas Dolginow, and David Cooper for collaboration and insightful discussions.

REFERENCES

1. Korsmeyer SJ, Hieter PA, Ravetch JV, et al. Developmental hierarchy of immunoglobulin gene rearrangements in human leukemic pre-B-cells. *Proc Natl Acad Sci U S A* 1981;78:7096–7100.
2. Arnold A, Cossman J, Bakhshi A, et al. Immunoglobulin-gene rearrangements as unique clonal markers in human lymphoid neoplasms. *N Engl J Med* 1984;309:1593–1599.
3. Cleary ML, Chao J, Warnke R, et al. Immunoglobulin gene rearrangement as a diagnostic criterion of B-cell lymphoma. *Proc Natl Acad Sci U S A* 1984;81:593–597.
4. Cossman J, Uppenkamp M, Sundeen J, et al. Molecular genetics and the diagnosis of lymphoma. *Arch Pathol Lab Med* 1988;112:117–127.
5. Toyonaga B, Yoshikai Y, Vadasz V, et al. Organization and sequences of the diversity, joining, and constant region genes of the human T-cell receptor γ chain. *Proc Natl Acad Sci U S A* 1985;82:8624–8628.
6. Griesser H, Tkachuk D, Reis MD, et al. Gene rearrangements and translocations in lymphoproliferative diseases. *Blood* 1989;73:1402–1415.
7. Flug F, Pelicci P-G, Bonetti F, et al. T-cell receptor gene rearrangements as markers of lineage and clonality in human T-cell malignancies. *Proc Natl Acad Sci U S A* 1985;82:3460–3464.
8. Leder P, Battey J, Lenoir G, et al. Translocations among antibody genes in human cancer. *Science* 1983;222:765–771.
9. Dalla-Favera R, Bregni M, Erikson J, et al. Human c-myc oncogene is located on the region of chromosome 8 that is translocated in Burkitt lymphoma cells. *Proc Natl Acad Sci U S A* 1982; 79:7824–7827.
10. Taub R, Kirsch I, Morton C, et al. Translocation of the c-myc gene into the immunoglobulin heavy chain locus in human Burkitt lymphoma and murine plasmacytoma cells. *Proc Natl Acad Sci U S A* 1982; 79:7837–7841.
11. Tsujimoto Y, Yunis J, Onorato-Showe L, et al. Molecular cloning of the chromosome breakpoint of B-cell lymphoma and leukemias with the t(11;14) chromosome translocation. *Science* 1984; 224:1403–1406.
12. Tsujimoto Y, Finger LR, Yunis J, et al. Cloning of the chromosome breakpoint of neoplastic B cells with the t(14;18) chromosome translocation. *Science* 1984;226:1097–1099.
13. Tsujimoto Y, Cossman J, Jaffe E, et al. Involvement of the bcl-2 gene in human follicular lymphoma. *Science* 1985;228:1440–1443.
14. Haluska FG, Finger LR, Kagan J, et al. Molecular genetics of chromosomal translocations in B- and T-lymphoid malignancies. In: Cossman J, ed. *Molecular genetics in cancer diagnosis.* New York: Elsevier, 1990:154–158.
15. Cossman J, Zehnbauer B, Garrett CT, et al. Gene rearrangements in the diagnosis of lymphoma/leukemia: guidelines for use based on a multi-institutional study. *Am J Clin Pathol* 1991;95:347–354.
16. Siminovitch KA, Bakhshi A, Goldman P, et al. A uniform deleting element mediates the loss of K genes in human B cells. *Nature* 1985; 316:260–262.
17. Taub RA, Hollis GF, Hieter PA, et al. Variable amplification of immunoglobulin lambda light-chain genes in human populations. *Nature* 1983;304:172–174.
18. Uppenkamp M, Andrade R, Sundeen J, et al. Diagnostic interpretation of T gamma gene rearrangement: effect of polyclonal T cells. *Hematol Oncol* 1988;2:15–24.
19. Knowles DM. Immunodeficiency-associated lymphoproliferative disorders. *Mod Pathol* 1999;12:200–217.
20. Lipford EH, Smith HR, Pittaluga S, et al. Clonality of angioimmunoblastic lymphadenopathy and implications for its evolution to malignant lymphoma. *J Clin Invest* 1987;79:637–642.
21. Pelicci PG, Knowles DM, Arlin Z, et al. Multiple monoclonal B cell expansions and c-myc oncogene rearrangements in acquired immune deficiency syndrome-related lymphoproliferative disorders: implications for lymphomagenesis. *J Exp Med* 1986;164:2049–2076.
22. Cleary ML, Smith SD, Sklar J. Cloning and structural analysis of cDNAs for bcl-2 and a hybrid bcl-2/immunoglobulin transcript resulting from the t(14;18) translocation. *Cell* 1986;47:19–28.
23. Saiki RK, Bugawan TL, Horn GT, et al. Analysis of enzymatically amplified beta-globin and HLA-DQ alpha DNA with allele-specific oligonucleotide probes. *Nature* 1986;24:163–166.
24. Stetler-Stevenson M, Raffeld M, Cohen P, et al. Detection of occult follicular lymphoma by specific DNA amplification. *Blood* 1988;72:1822–1825.
25. Lee MS, Chang KS, Cabanillas F, et al. Detection of minimal residual cells carrying the t(14;18) by DNA sequence amplification. *Science* 1987;237:175–178.
26. Deane M, Norton JD. Detection of immunoglobulin gene rearrangement in B lymphoid malignancies by polymerase chain reaction gene amplification. *Br J Haematol* 1990;74:251–256.
27. Sioutos N, Bagg A, Michaud GY, et al. Polymerase chain reaction versus Southern blot hybridization: detection of immunoglobulin heavy-chain gene rearrangements. *Diagn Mol Pathol* 1995;4:8–13.
28. McCarthy KP, Sloane JP, Kabarowski JH, et al. A simplified method of detection of clonal rearrangements of the T-cell receptor-gamma chain gene. *Diagn Mol Pathol* 1992;1:173–179.
29. Gong JZ, Zheng S, Chiarle R, et al. Detection of immunoglobulin kappa light chain rearrangements by polymerase chain reaction: an improved method for detecting clonal B-cell lymphoproliferative disorders. *Am J Pathol* 1999;155:355–363.
30. Dippel E, Assaf C, Hummel M, et al. T-cell receptor gamma-chain gene rearrangement by PCR-based GeneScan analysis in advanced cutaneous T-cell lymphoma: a critical evaluation. *J Pathol* 1999;188:146–154.
31. Limpens J, de Jong D, van Krieken JH, et al. Bcl-2/J_H rearrangements in benign lymphoid tissues with follicular hyperplasia. *Oncogene* 1991;6:2271–2276.
32. Lopez-Guillermo A, Cabanillas F, McLaughlin, et al. The clinical significance of molecular response in indolent follicular lymphomas. *Blood* 1998;91:2955–2960.
33. Gribben JG, Neuberg D, Freedman AS, et al. Detection by polymerase chain reaction of residual cells with the bcl-2 translocation is associated with increased risk of relapse after autologous bone marrow transplantation for B-cell lymphoma. *Blood* 1993;81:3449–3457.
34. Marshall E. Sequencers endorse plan for a draft in 1 year. *Science* 1999;84:1439–1441.
35. Maloney DG, Grillo-Lopez AJ, White CA, et al. IDEC-C2B8 (Rituximab) anti-CD20 monoclonal antibody therapy in patients with relapsed low-grade non-Hodgkin's lymphoma. *Blood* 1997;90:2188–2195.
36. Luthra R, McBride JA, Cabanillas F, et al. Novel 5′ exonuclease-based real-time PCR assay for the detection of t(14;18)(q32;q21) in patients with follicular lymphoma. *Am J Pathol* 1998;153:63–68.
37. Adams MD, Kerlavage AR, Fleischmann RD, et al. Initial assessment of human gene diversity and expression patterns based upon 83 million nucleotides of cDNA sequence. *Nature* 1995;377[Suppl]:3–174.

38. Cossman J, Annunziata CM, Barash S, et al. Reed-Sternberg cell genome expression supports a B-cell lineage. *Blood* 1999;94: 411–416.
39. Alizadeh A, Eisen M, Botstein D, et al. Probing lymphocyte biology by genomic-scale gene expression analysis. *J Clin Immunol* 1998;18: 373–379.
40. DeRisi J, Penland L, Brown PO, et al. Use of a cDNA microarray to analyse gene expression patterns in human cancer. *Nat Genet* 1996; 14:457–460.
41. Schena M, Shalon D, Davis RW, et al. Quantitative monitoring of gene expression patterns with a complementary DNA microarray. *Science* 1995;270:467–470.
42. Schena M, Shalon D, Heller R, et al. Parallel human genome analysis: microarray-based expression monitoring of 1000 genes. *Proc Natl Acad Sci U S A* 1996;93:10614–10619.
43. Lockhart DJ, Dong H, Byrne MC, et al. Expression monitoring by hybridization to high-density oligonucleotide arrays. *Nat Biotechnol* 1996;14:1675–1680.
44. Brown PO, Botstein D. Exploring the new world of the genome with DNA microarrays. *Nat Genet* 1999;21[Suppl]:33–37.
45. du Manoir S, Schrock E, Bentz M, et al. Quantitative analysis of comparative genomic hybridization. *Cytometry* 1995;19:27–41.
46. Bea S, Ribas M, Hernandez JM, et al. Increased number of chromosomal imbalances and high-level DNA amplifications in mantle cell lymphoma are associated with blastoid variants. *Blood* 1999;93: 4365–4374.
47. Schrock E, du Manoir S, Veldman T, et al. Multicolor spectral karyotyping of human chromosomes. *Science* 1996;273:494–497.
48. Hilgenfeld E, Padilla-Nash H, Schrock E, et al. Analysis of B-cell neoplasias by spectral karyotyping. *Curr Top Microbiol Immunol* 1999;246:169–174.
49. Peters AM, Kohfink B, Martin H, et al. Defective apoptosis due to a point mutation in the death domain of CD95 associated with autoimmune lymphoproliferative syndrome, T-cell lymphoma, and Hodgkin's disease. *J Exp Hematol* 1999;27:868–874.
50. Mak TM, Cozen W, Shibata DK, et al. Concordance for Hodgkin's disease in identical twins suggesting genetic susceptibility to the young-adult form of the disease. *N Engl J Med* 1995;332:413.
51. Wang DG, Fan JB, Siao CJ, et al. Identification, mapping, and genotyping of single-nucleotide polymorphisms in the human genome. *Science* 1998;280:1077–1082.
52. Venter JC, Adams MD, Sutton GG, et al. Shotgun sequencing of the human genome. *Science* 1998;280:1540–1542.
53. Emmert-Buck MR, Bonner RF, Smith PD, et al. Laser capture microdissection. *Science* 1996;274:998–1001.
54. Böhm M, Wieland I, Schütze K, et al. Microbeam MOMenT: noncontact laser microdissection of membrane-mounted native tissue. *Am J Pathol* 1997;151:63–67.
55. Küppers R, Rajewsky K, Zhao M, et al. Hodgkin's disease: Hodgkin and Reed-Sternberg cells picked from histological sections show clonal immunoglobulin gene rearrangements and appear to be derived from B cells at various stages of development. *Proc Natl Acad Sci U S A* 1994;91:10962–10966.
56. Kanzler H, Küppers R, Hansmann ML, et al. Hodgkin and Reed-Sternberg cells in Hodgkin's disease represent the outgrowth of a dominant tumor clone derived from (crippled) germinal center B cells. *J Exp Med* 1996;184:1495–1505.
57. Küppers R, Zhao M, Hansmann ML, et al. Tracing B cell development in human germinal centres by molecular analysis of single cells picked from histological sections. *EMBO J* 1993;12:4955–4967.
58. Fend F, Quintanilla-Martinez L, Kumar S, et al. Composite low grade B-cell lymphomas with two immunophenotypically distinct cell populations are true biclonal lymphomas: a molecular analysis using laser capture microdissection. *Am J Pathol* 1999;154:1857–1866.
59. Fend F, Emmert Buck MR, Chaqui R, et al. Laser capture microdissection of immunostained frozen sections for mRNA analysis. *Am J Pathol* 1999;154:61–66.
60. Trumper LH, Brady G, Loke SL, et al. Single-cell analysis of Hodgkin and Reed-Sternberg cells: molecular heterogeneity of gene expression and p53 mutations. *Blood* 1993;81:3097–3115.
61. Messineo C, Jamerson MH, Hunter E, et al. Gene expression by single Reed-Sternberg cells: pathways of apoptosis and activation. *Blood* 1998;91:2443–2451.
62. Cossman J, Vockley J, Carter K, et al. Genome-wide gene expression of the rare, malignant Reed-Sternberg cell of Hodgkin's lymphoma. *Nat Genet* 1999;23:40(abst).
63. Zhang L, Zhou W, Velculescu VE, et al. Gene expression profiles in normal and cancer cells. *Science* 1997;276:1268–1272.
64. Ruschenburg I, Schlott T, Linke B, et al. Automated molecular genetic DNA analysis for detecting B-cell non-Hodgkin's lymphoma in cytologic specimens. *Anal Quant Cytol Histol* 1997;19:255–263.
65. Luthra R, McBride JA, Hai S, et al. The application of fluorescence-based PCR and PCR-SSCP to monitor the clonal relationship of cells bearing the t(14;18)(q32;q21) in sequential biopsy specimens from patients with follicle center cell lymphoma. *Diagn Mol Pathol* 1997; 6:71–77.
66. Chhanabhai M, Adomat SA, Gascoyne RD, et al. Clinical utility of heteroduplex analysis of TCR gamma gene rearrangements in the diagnosis of T-cell lymphoproliferative disorders. *Am J Clin Pathol* 1997;108:295–301.
67. Doenecke A, Winnacker EL, Hallek M. Rapid amplification of cDNA ends (RACE) improves the PCR-based isolation of immunoglobulin variable region genes from murine and human lymphoma cells and cell lines. *Leukemia* 1997;11:1787–1792.
68. Bohling SD, King TC, Wittwer CT, et al. Rapid simultaneous amplification and detection of the MBR/J_H chromosomal translocation by fluorescence melting curve analysis. *Am J Pathol* 1999;154:97–103.
69. Williams ME, Innes DJ, Borowitz MJ, et al. Immunoglobulin and T cell receptor gene rearrangements in human lymphoma and leukemia. *Blood* 1987;69:79–86.
70. Aisenberg AC, Wilkes BM, Jacobson JO, et al. Immunoglobulin gene rearrangements in adult non-Hodgkin's lymphoma. *Am J Med* 1987; 82:738–744.
71. Harris NL, Data RE. The distribution of neoplastic and normal B-lymphoid cells in nodular lymphomas: use of an immunoperoxidase technique on frozen sections. *Hum Pathol* 1982;13:610–617.
72. Levy S, Mendel E, Kon S, et al. Mutational hot spots in Ig V region genes of human follicular lymphomas. *J Exp Med* 1988;168:475–489.
73. Zelenetz AD, Chen TT, Levy R, et al. Clonal expansion in follicular lymphoma occurs subsequent to antigenic selection. *J Exp Med* 1992; 176:1137–1148.
74. Segal GH, Jorgensen T, Scott M, et al. Optimal primer selection for clonality assessment by polymerase chain reaction analysis: II. Follicular lymphomas. *Hum Pathol* 1994;25:1276–1282.
75. Miettinen M, Lasota J. Polymerase chain reaction based gene rearrangement studies in the diagnosis of follicular lymphoma—performance in formaldehyde-fixed tissue and application in clinical problem cases. *Pathol Res Pract* 1997;193:9–19.
76. Deane M, McCarthy KP, Wiedemann LM, et al. An improved method for detection of B-lymphoid clonality by polymerase chain reaction. *Leukemia* 1991,5:726–730.
77. Campbell MJ, Zelenetz AD, Levy S, et al. Use of family specific leader region primers for PCR amplification of the human heavy chain variable region gene repertoire. *Mol Immunol* 1992;29:193–203.
78. Cleary ML, Sklar J. Nucleotide sequence of a t(14;18) chromosomal breakpoint in follicular lymphoma and demonstration of a breakpoint-cluster region near a transcriptionally active locus on chromosome 18. *Proc Natl Acad Sci U S A* 1985;82:7439–7443.
79. Weiss LM, Warnke RA, Sklar J, et al. Molecular analysis of the t(14; 18) chromosomal translocation in malignant lymphomas. *N Engl J Med* 1987;317:1185–1189.
80. Cleary ML, Galili N, Sklar J. Detection of a second t(14;18) breakpoint cluster region in human follicular lymphomas. *J Exp Med* 1986; 164:315–320.
81. Tsujimoto Y, Bashir MM, Givol I, et al. DNA rearrangements in human follicular lymphoma can involve the 5′ or the 3′ region of the bcl-2 gene. *Proc Natl Acad Sci U S A* 1987;84:1329–1333.
82. Akasaka T, Akasaka H, Yonetani N, et al. Refinement of the BCL2/immunoglobulin heavy chain fusion gene in t(14;18)(q32;q21) by polymerase chain reaction amplification for long targets. *Genes Chromosomes Cancer* 1998;21:17–29.
83. Hillion J, Mecucci C, Aventin A, et al. A variant translocation t(2; 18) in follicular lymphoma involves the 5′ end of bcl-2 and Ig kappa light chain gene. *Oncogene* 1991;6:169–172.
84. Lee MS, Chang KS, Cabanillas F, et al. Detection of minimal residual cells carrying the t(14;18) by DNA sequence amplification. *Science* 1987;237:175–178.
85. Crescenzi M, Seto M, Herzig GP, et al. Thermostable DNA polymer-

ase chain amplification of t(14;18) chromosome breakpoints and detection of minimal residual disease. *Proc Natl Acad Sci U S A* 1988; 85:4869–4873.
86. Horsman DE, Gascoyne RD, Coupland RW, et al. Comparison of cytogenetic analysis, Southern analysis, and polymerase chain reaction for the detection of t(14;18) in follicular lymphoma. *Am J Clin Pathol* 1995;103:472–478.
87. Shibata D, Hu E, Weiss LM, et al. Detection of specific t(14;18) chromosomal translocations in fixed tissues. *Hum Pathol* 1990;21: 199–203.
88. Rack KA, Salomon-Nguyen F, Radford-Weiss I, et al. FISH detection of chromosome 14q32/IgH translocations: evaluation in follicular lymphoma. *Br J Haematol* 1998;103:495–504.
89. Gribben JG, Freedman A, Woo SD, et al. All advanced stage non-Hodgkin's lymphomas with a polymerase chain reaction amplifiable breakpoint of bcl-2 have residual cells containing the bcl-2 rearrangement at evaluation and after treatment. *Blood* 1991;78:3275–3280.
90. Hardingham JE, Kotasek D, Sage RE, et al. Significance of molecular marker-positive cells after autologous peripheral-blood stem-cell transplantation for non-Hodgkin's lymphoma. *J Clin Oncol* 1995;13: 1073–1079.
91. Price CG, Meerabux J, Murtagh S, et al. The significance of circulating cells carrying t(14;18) in long remission from follicular lymphoma. *J Clin Oncol* 1991;9:1527–1532.
92. Lambrechts AC, Hupkes PE, Dorssers LC, et al. Clinical significance of t(14;18)-positive cells in the circulation of patients with stage III or IV follicular non-Hodgkin's lymphoma during first remission. *J Clin Oncol* 1994;12:1541–1546.
93. Finke J, Slanina J, Lange W, et al. Persistence of circulating t(14; 18)-positive cells in long-term remission after radiation therapy for localized-stage follicular lymphoma. *J Clin Oncol* 1993;11: 1668–1673.
94. Davis TA, Maloney DG, Czerwinski DK, et al. Anti-idiotype antibodies can induce long-term complete remissions in non-Hodgkin's lymphoma without eradicating the malignant clone. *Blood* 1998;92: 1184–1190.
95. Lopez-Guillermo A, Cabanillas F, McLaughlin P, et al. The clinical significance of molecular response in indolent follicular lymphomas. *Blood* 1998;91:2955–2960.
96. Hockenbery D, Nunez G, Milliman C, et al. Bcl-2 is an inner mitochondrial membrane protein that blocks programmed cell death. *Nature* 1990;348:334–336.
97. Korsmeyer SJ. Bcl-2: an antidote to programmed cell death. *Cancer Surv* 1992;15:105–118.
98. McDonnell TJ, Korsmeyer SJ. Progression from lymphoid hyperplasia to high-grade malignant lymphoma in mice transgenic for the t(14; 18). *Nature* 1991;349:254–256.
99. Segal GH, Scott M, Jorgensen T, et al. Standard polymerase chain reaction analysis does not detect t(14;18) in reactive lymphoid hyperplasia. *Arch Pathol Lab Med* 1994;118:791–794.
100. Pezzella F, Tse AG, Cordell JL, et al. Expression of the bcl-2 oncogene protein is not specific for the 14;18 chromosomal translocation. *Am J Pathol* 1990;137:225–232.
101. Lo Coco F, Gaidano G, Louie DC, et al. P53 mutations are associated with histologic transformation of follicular lymphoma. *Blood* 1993; 82:2289–2295.
102. Sander CA, Yano T, Clark HM, et al. P53 mutation is associated with progression in follicular lymphomas. *Blood* 1993;82:1994–2004.
103. Elenitoba-Johnson KS, Gascoyne RD, Lim MS, et al. Homozygous deletions at chromosome 9p21 involving p16 and p15 are associated with histologic progression in follicle center lymphoma. *Blood* 1998; 91:4677–4685.
104. Yano T, Jaffe ES, Longo DL, et al. MYC rearrangements in histologically progressed follicular lymphomas. *Blood* 199;80:758–767.
105. Gaidano G, Hauptschein RS, Parsa NZ, et al. Deletions involving two distinct regions of 6q in B-cell non-Hodgkin lymphoma. *Blood* 1992; 80:1781–1787.
106. Campo E, Raffeld M, Jaffe ES. Mantle cell lymphoma. *Semin Hematol* 1999;36:115–127.
107. Weisenburger DD, Sanger WG, Armitage JO, et al. Intermediate lymphocytic lymphoma: immunophenotypic and cytogenetic findings. *Blood* 1987;69:1617–1621.
108. Lardelli P, Bookman M, Sundeen J, et al. Lymphocytic lymphoma of intermediate differentiation: morphologic and immunophenotypic spectrum and clinical correlations. *Am J Surg Pathol* 1990;14: 752–762.
109. Hummel M, Tamaru J, Kalvelage B, et al. Mantle cell lymphoma (previously centrocytic) lymphomas express V_H genes with no or very little somatic mutations like the physiologic cells of the follicle mantle. *Blood* 1994;84:403–407.
110. Pittaluga S, Tierens A, Pinyol M, et al. Blastic variant of mantle cell lymphoma shows a heterogeneous pattern of somatic mutations of the rearranged immunoglobulin heavy chain variable genes. *Br J Haematol* 1998;102:1301–1306.
111. Leroux D, Le Marc'Hadour F, Gressin R, et al. Non-Hodgkin's lymphomas with the t(11;14)(q13;q32): a subset of mantle zone/intermediate lymphocytic lymphoma? *Br J Haematol* 1991;77:346–353.
112. Raffeld M, Jaffe ES. Bcl-1, t(11;14) and mantle cell-derived lymphomas. *Blood* 1991;78:259–263.
113. Vandenberghe E, de Wolf-Peeters C, van den Oord J, et al. Translocation t(11;14): a cytogenetic anomaly associated with B-cell lymphomas of non-follicle centre cell lineage. *J Pathol* 1991;163:13–18.
114. Tsujimoto Y, Yunis Y, Onorato-Showe L, et al. Molecular cloning of the chromosomal breakpoint of B-cell lymphomas and leukemias with the t(11;14) chromosome translocation. *Science* 1984;224: 1403–1406.
115. Tsujimoto Y, Jaffe ES, Cossman J, et al. Clustering of breakpoints on chromosome 11 in human B-cell neoplasms with the t(11;14) chromosome translocation. *Nature* 1985;315:343–345.
116. Erikson J, Finan J, Tsujimoto Y, et al. The chromosome 14 breakpoint in neoplastic B cells with the t(11;14) translocation involves the immunoglobulin heavy chain locus. *Proc Natl Acad Sci U S A* 1984;81: 4144–4149.
117. Motokura T, Bloom T, Kim H, et al. A novel cyclin encoded by a bcl-1–linked candidate oncogene. *Nature* 1991;350:512–515.
118. Rosenberg CL, Wong E, Petty EM, et al. PRAD1, a candidate BCL1 oncogene: mapping and expression in centrocytic lymphoma. *Proc Natl Acad Sci U S A* 1991;88:9638–9642.
119. Medeiros J, van Krieken JH, Jaffe ES, et al. Association of bcl-1 rearrangements with lymphocytic lymphoma of intermediate differentiation. *Blood* 1990;76:2086–2090.
120. Williams ME, Meeker TC, Swerdlow SH. Rearrangement of the chromosome 11 bcl-1 locus in centrocytic lymphoma: analysis with multiple breakpoint probes. *Blood* 1991;78:493–498.
121. Williams ME, Swerdlow SH, Meeker TC. Chromosome t(11;14)(q13; q32) breakpoints in centrocytic lymphoma are highly localized at the bcl-1 major translocation cluster. *Leukemia* 1993;7:1437–1440.
122. Rimokh R, Berger F, Delsol G, et al. Detection of the chromosomal translocation t(11;14) by polymerase chain reaction in mantle cell lymphomas. *Blood* 1994;83:1871–1875.
123. Kumar S, Krenacs L, Otsuki T, et al. Bcl-1 rearrangement and cyclin D1 protein expression in multiple lymphomatous polyposis. *Am J Clin Pathol* 1996;105:737–743.
124. Bosch F, Jares P, Campo E, et al. PRAD-1/cyclin D1 gene overexpression in chronic lymphoproliferative disorders: a highly specific marker of mantle cell lymphoma. *Blood* 1994;84:2726–2732.
125. Yang W, Zukerberg L, Motokura T, et al. Cyclin D1 (BCL-1, PRAD1) protein expression in low-grade B-cell lymphomas and reactive hyperplasia. *Am J Pathol* 1994;145:86–96.
126. Quintanilla-Martinez L, Thieblemont C, Fend F, et al. Mantle cell lymphomas lack expression of p27kip1, a cyclin-dependent kinase inhibitor. *Am J Pathol* 1998;153:175–182.
127. Jares P, Campo E, Pinyol M, et al. Expression of retinoblastoma gene product (pRB) in mantle cell lymphomas: correlation with cyclin D1 (PRAD1/CCND1) mRNA levels and proliferative activity. *Am J Pathol* 1996;148:1591–1600.
128. Dreyling MH, Bullinger L, Ott G, et al. Alterations of the cyclin D1/ p16–pRB pathway in mantle cell lymphoma. *Cancer Res* 1997;57: 4608–4614.
129. Monni O, Zhu Y, Franssila K, et al. Molecular characterization of deletion 11q22.1-23.3 in mantle cell lymphoma. *Br J Haematol* 1999; 104:665–671.
130. Ott G, Kalla J, Ott MM, et al. Blastoid variants of mantle cell lymphoma: frequent bcl-1 rearrangements at the major translocation cluster region and tetraploid chromosome clones. *Blood* 1997;89: 1421–1429.
131. Greiner TC, Moynihan MJ, Chan WC, et al. P53 mutations in mantle

cell lymphoma are associated with variant cytology and predict a poor prognosis. *Blood* 1996;87:4302–4310.

132. Hernandez L, Fest T, Cazorla M, et al. P53 gene mutations and protein overexpression are associated with aggressive variants of mantle cell lymphoma. *Blood* 1996;87:3351–3359.
133. Louie DC, Offit K, Jaslow R, et al. P53 overexpression as a marker of poor prognosis in mantle cell lymphomas with the t(11;14)(q13; q32). *Blood* 1995;86:2892–2899.
134. Pinyol M, Hernandez L, Cazorla M, et al. Deletions and loss of expression of p16INK4a and p21Waf1 genes are associated with aggressive variants of mantle cell lymphoma. *Blood* 1997;89:272–280.
135. Isaacson PG, Norton AJ. *Extranodal lymphomas,* 1st ed. Edinburgh: Churchill Livingstone, 1994.
136. Fishleder A, Tubbs R, Hesse B, et al. Uniform detection of immunoglobulin-gene rearrangement in benign lymphoepithelial lesions. *N Engl J Med* 1987;316:1118–1121.
137. Knowles DM, Jakobiec FA, McNally L, et al. Lymphoid hyperplasia and malignant lymphoma occurring in the ocular adnexa (orbit, conjunctiva, and eyelids): a prospective multiparametric analysis of 108 cases during 1977–1987. *Hum Pathol* 1989;21:959–973.
138. Knowles DM, Athan E, Ubriaco A, et al. Extranodal noncutaneous lymphoid hyperplasias represent a continuous spectrum of B-cell neoplasia: demonstration by molecular genetic analysis. *Blood* 1989;73: 1635–1645.
139. Neri A, Jakobiec FA, Pelicci P-G, et al. Immunoglobulin and T cell receptor β chain gene rearrangement analysis of ocular adnexal lymphoid neoplasms: clinical and biologic implications. *Blood* 1989; 70:1519–1529.
140. Spencer J, Diss TC, Isaacson PG. Primary B cell gastric lymphoma: a genotypic analysis. *Am J Pathol* 1989;135:557–564.
141. Sigal SH, Saul SH, Auerbach HE, et al. Gastric small lymphocytic proliferation with immunoglobulin gene rearrangement in pseudolymphoma versus lymphoma. *Gastroenterology* 1989;97:195–201.
142. Sheibani K, Sohn CC, Burke JS, et al. Monocytoid B-cell lymphoma: a novel B-cell neoplasm. *Am J Pathol* 1986;124:310–318.
143. Harris NL, Jaffe ES, Stein H, et al. A revised European-American classification of lymphoid neoplasms: a proposal from the International Lymphoma Study Group. *Blood* 1994;84:1361–1392.
144. Qin Y, Greiner A, Trunk MJ, et al. Somatic hypermutation in low-grade mucosa-associated lymphoid tissue-type B-cell lymphoma. *Blood* 1995;86:3528–3534.
145. Tierens A, Delabie J, Pittaluga S, et al. Mutation analysis of the rearranged immunoglobulin heavy chain genes of marginal zone cell lymphomas indicates an origin from different marginal zone B lymphocyte subsets. *Blood* 1998;91:2381–2386.
146. Wotherspoon AC, Doglioni C, Diss TC, et al. Regression of primary low-grade B-cell gastric lymphoma of mucosa-associated lymphoid tissue type after eradication of *Helicobacter pylori*. *Lancet* 1993;342: 575–577.
147. Savio A, Franzin G, Wotherspoon AC, et al. Diagnosis and posttreatment follow-up of *Helicobacter pylori*–positive gastric lymphoma of mucosa-associated lymphoid tissue: histology, polymerase chain reaction, or both? *Blood* 1996;87:1255–1260.
148. de Mascarel A, Dubus P, Belleannee G, et al. Low prevalence of monoclonal B cells in *Helicobacter pylori* gastritis patients with duodenal ulcer. *Hum Pathol* 1998;29:784–790.
149. Nakamura S, Azoyagi K, Furuse M, et al. B-cell monoclonality precedes the development of gastric MALT lymphoma in *Helicobacter pylori*–associated chronic gastritis. *Am J Pathol* 1998;152: 1271–1279.
150. Thiede C, Alpen B, Morgner A, et al. Ongoing somatic mutations and clonal expansions after cure of *Helicobacter pylori* infection in gastric mucosa–associated lymphoid tissue B-cell lymphoma. *J Clin Oncol* 1998;16:3822–3831.
151. Torlakovic E, Cherwitz DL, Jessurun J, et al. B-cell gene rearrangement in benign and malignant lymphoid proliferations of mucosa-associated lymphoid tissue and lymph nodes. *Hum Pathol* 1997;28: 166–173.
152. Weston AP, Banerjee SK, Horvat RT, et al. Specificity of polymerase chain reaction monoclonality for diagnosis of gastric mucosa-associated lymphoid tissue (MALT) lymphoma: direct comparison to Southern blot gene rearrangement. *Dig Dis Sci* 1998;43:290–299.
153. Osborne BM, Pugh WC. Practicality of molecular studies to evaluate small lymphocytic proliferations in endoscopic gastric biopsies. *Am J Surg Pathol* 1992;16:838–844.
154. Fend F, Schwaiger A, Weyrer K, et al. Early diagnosis of gastric lymphoma: gene rearrangement analysis of endoscopic biopsy samples. *Leukemia* 1994;8:35–39.
155. Pan L, Diss TC, Cunningham D, et al. The bcl-2 gene in primary B cell lymphoma of mucosa-associated lymphoid tissue (MALT). *Am J Pathol* 1989;135:7–11.
156. Auer IA, Gascoyne RD, Connors JM, et al. t(11;18)(q21;q21) is the most common translocation in MALT lymphomas. *Ann Oncol* 1997; 8:979–985.
157. Horsman D, Gascoyne R, Klasa R, et al. t(11;18)(q21;q21.1): a recurring translocation in lymphomas of mucosa-associated lymphoid tissue (MALT)? *Genes Chromosomes Cancer* 1992;4:183–187.
158. Ott G, Katzenberger T, Greiner A, et al. The t(11;18)(q21;q21) chromosome translocation is a frequent and specific aberration in low-grade but not high-grade malignant non-Hodgkin's lymphomas of the mucosa-associated lymphoid tissue (MALT) type. *Cancer Res* 1997; 57:3944–3948.
159. Ott G, Kalla J, Steinhoff A, et al. Trisomy 3 is not a common feature in malignant lymphomas of mucosa-associated lymphoid tissue type. *Am J Pathol* 1998;153:689–694.
160. Wotherspoon AC, Finn TM, Isaacson PG. Trisomy 3 in low-grade B-cell lymphomas of mucosa-associated lymphoid tissue. *Blood* 1995; 85:2000–2004.
161. Dierlamm J, Baens M, Wlodarska I, et al. The apoptosis inhibitor gene API1 and a novel 18q gene, MLT, are recurrently rearranged in the t(11;18)(q21;q21) associated with mucosa-associated lymphoid tissue lymphomas. *Blood* 1999;93:3601–3609.
162. Willis TG, Jadayel DM, Du MQ, et al. Bcl-10 is involved in t(1; 14)(p22;q32) of MALT B cell lymphoma and mutated in multiple tumor types. *Cell* 1999;96:35–45.
163. Wotherspoon AC, Pan LX, Diss DC, et al. Cytogenetic study of B-cell lymphoma of mucosa-associated lymphoid tissue. *Cancer Genet Cytogenet* 1992;58:35–38.
164. Zhang Q, Siebert R, Yan M, et al. Inactivating mutations and overexpression of BCL-10, a caspase recruitment domain-containing gene, in MALT lymphoma with t(1;14)(p22;q32). *Nat Genet* 1999;22:63–68.
165. Lambers AR, Gumbs C, Ali S, et al. Bcl-10 is not a target for frequent mutation in human carcinomas. *Br J Cancer* 1999;80:1575–1576.
166. Peng H, Chen G, Du M, et al. Replication error phenotype and p53 gene mutation in lymphomas of mucosa-associated lymphoid tissue. *Am J Pathol* 1996;148:643–648.
167. Chan JKC, Ng CS, Isaacson PG. Relationship between high-grade lymphoma and low-grade B-cell mucosa-associated lymphoid tissue lymphoma (MALToma). *Am J Pathol* 1990;136:1153–1164.
168. Du M, Peng H, Singh N, et al. The accumulation of p53 abnormalities is associated with progression of mucosa-associated tissue lymphoma. *Blood* 1995;86:4587–4593.
169. De Wolf-Peeters C, Achten R. The histogenesis of gastric large cell lymphomas. *Histopathology* 1999;34:71–75.
170. Nathwani BN, Anderson JR, Armitage JO, et al. Clinical significance of follicular lymphoma with monocytoid B cells: non-Hodgkin's Lymphoma Classification Project. *Hum Pathol* 1999;30:263–268.
171. Tierens A, Delabie J, Michiels L, et al. Marginal-zone B cells in the human lymph node and spleen show somatic hypermutations and display clonal expansion. *Blood* 1999;93:226–234.
172. Cossman J. A new, lethal form of follicular lymphoma? *Hum Pathol* 1999;30:249–250.
173. Hernandez AM, Nathwani BN, Nguyen D, et al. Nodal benign and malignant monocytoid B cells with and without follicular lymphomas: a comparative study of follicular colonization, light chain restriction, bcl-2, and t(14;18) in 39 cases. *Hum Pathol* 1995;26:625–632.
174. Melo J, Hedge U, Parreira A, et al. Splenic B cell lymphoma with circulating villous lymphocytes: differential diagnosis of B cell leukemias with large spleens. *J Clin Pathol* 1987;40:642–651.
175. Mollejo M, Menarguez J, Lloret E, et al. Splenic marginal zone lymphoma: a distinctive type of low-grade B-cell lymphoma. A clinicopathological study of 13 cases. *Am J Surg Pathol* 1995;19:1146–1157.
176. Schmid C, Kirkham N, Diss T, et al. Splenic marginal zone lymphoma. *Am J Surg Pathol* 1992;16:455–466.
177. Dunn-Walters DK, Boursier L, Spencer J, et al. Analysis of immunoglobulin genes in splenic marginal zone lymphoma suggests ongoing mutation. *Hum Pathol* 1998;29:585–593.

178. Jadayel D, Matutes E, Dyer MJ, et al. Splenic lymphoma with villous lymphocytes: analysis of BCL-1 rearrangements and expression of the cyclin D1 gene. *Blood* 1994;83:3664–3671.
179. Gruzka-Westwood AM, Matutes E, Coignet LJ, et al. The incidence of trisomy 3 in splenic lymphoma with villous lymphocytes: a study by FISH. *Br J Haematol* 1999;104:600–604.
180. Oscier DG, Matutes E, Gardiner A, et al. Cytogenetic studies in splenic lymphoma with villous lymphocytes. *Br J Haematol* 1993;85: 487–491.
181. Sole F, Woessner S, Florensa L, et al. Frequent involvement of chromosomes 1,3,7 and 8 in splenic marginal zone lymphoma. *Br J Haematol* 1997;98:446–449.
182. Wagner SD, Martinelli V, Luzzatto L. Similar patterns of Vκ gene usage but different degrees of somatic mutation in hairy cell leukemia, prolymphocytic leukemia, Waldenstrom's macroglobulinemia, and myeloma. *Blood* 1994;83:3647–3653.
183. Aoki H, Takishita M, Kosaka M, et al. Frequent somatic mutations in D and/or J_H segments of Ig gene in Waldenstrom's macroglobulinemia and chronic lymphocytic leukemia (CLL) with Richter's syndrome, but not in common CLL. *Blood* 1995;85:1913–1919.
184. Zuckerman E, Zuckerman T, Levine AM, et al. Hepatitis C virus infection in patients with B-cell non-Hodgkin lymphoma. *Ann Intern Med* 1997;127:423–428.
185. Silvestri F, Pipan C, Barillari G, et al. Prevalence of hepatitis C virus infection in patients with lymphoproliferative disorders. *Blood* 1996; 87:4296–4301.
186. Pozzato G, Mazzaro C, Crovatto M, et al. Low-grade malignant lymphoma, hepatitis C virus infection, and mixed cryoglobulinemia. *Blood* 1994;84:3047–3053.
187. Ivanovski M, Silvestri F, Pozzato G, et al. Somatic hypermutation, clonal diversity, and preferential expression of the V_H 51p1/VL kv325 immunoglobulin gene combination in hepatitis C virus-associated immunocytomas. *Blood* 1998;91:2433–2442.
188. Offit K, Parsa NZ, Filippa D, et al. t(9;14)(p13;q32) denotes a subset of low-grade non-Hodgkin's lymphoma with plasmacytoid differentiation. *Blood* 1992;80:2594–2599.
189. Iida S, Rao PH, Nallasivam P, et al. The t(9;14)(p13;q32) chromosomal translocation associated with lymphoplasmacytoid lymphoma involves the PAX-5 gene. *Blood* 1996;88:4110–4117.
190. Kume M, Suzuki R, Yatabe Y, et al. Somatic hypermutations in the V_H segment of immunoglobulin genes of CD5-positive diffuse large B-cell lymphomas. *Jpn J Cancer Res* 1997;88:1087–1093.
191. Kuppers R, Rajewsky K, Hansmann ML. Diffuse large cell lymphomas are derived from mature B cells carrying V region genes with a high load of somatic mutation and evidence of selection for antibody expression. *Eur J Immunol* 1997;27:1398–1405.
192. Ye BH, Lista F, Lo Coco F, et al. Alterations of a zinc finger–encoding gene, BCL-6, in diffuse large-cell lymphoma. *Science* 1993;262: 747–750.
193. Miki T, Kawamata N, Arai A, et al. Molecular cloning of the breakpoint for 3q27 translocation in B-cell lymphomas and leukemias. *Blood* 1994;83:217–222.
194. Bastard C, Deweindt C, Kerckaert JP, et al. LAZ3 rearrangements in non-Hodgkin's lymphoma: correlation with histology, immunophenotype, karyotype, and clinical outcome in 217 patients. *Blood* 1994; 83:2423–2427.
195. Chang CC, Ye BH, Chaganti RS, et al. BCL-6, a POZ/zinc-finger protein, is a sequence-specific transcriptional repressor. *Proc Natl Acad Sci U S A* 1996;93:6947–6952.
196. Otsuki, T, Yano T, Clark HM, et al. Analysis of LAZ3 (BCL-6) status in B-cell non-Hodgkin's lymphomas: results of rearrangement and gene expression studies and a mutational analysis of coding region sequences. *Blood* 1995;85:2877–2884.
197. Ohno H, Kerckaert JP, Bastard C, et al. Heterogeneity in B-cell neoplasms associated with rearrangement of the LAZ3 gene on chromosome band 3q27. *Jpn J Cancer Res* 1994;85:592–600.
198. Lo Coco F, Ye BH, Lista F, et al. Rearrangements of the BCL6 gene in diffuse large cell non-Hodgkin's lymphoma. *Blood* 1994;83: 1757–1759.
199. Kawamata N, Nakamura Y, Miki T, et al. Detection of chimaeric transcripts of the immunoglobulin heavy chain and BCL6 genes by reverse transcriptase–polymerase chain reaction in B-cell non-Hodgkin's lymphomas. *Br J Haematol* 1998;100:484–489.
200. Seyfert VL, Allman D, He Y, et al. Transcriptional repression by the proto-oncogene BCL-6. *Oncogene* 1996;12:2331–2342.
201. Deweindt, C, Albagil O, Bernardin F, et al. The LAZ3/BCL6 oncogene encodes a sequence-specific transcriptional inhibitor: a novel function for the BTB/POZ domain as an autonomous repressing domain. *Cell Growth Differ* 1995;6:1495–1503.
202. Staudt LM, Dent AL, Shaffer AL, et al. Regulation of Lymphocyte cell fate decisions and lymphomagenesis by BCL-6. *Int Rev Immunol* 1999;18:381–403.
203. Cattoretti G, Chang CC, Cechova K, et al. Bcl-6 protein is expressed in germinal-center B cells. *Blood* 1995;86:45–53.
204. Onizuka T, Moriyama M, Yamochi T, et al. Bcl-6 gene product, a 92- to 98-kD nuclear phosphoprotein, is highly expressed in germinal center B cells and their neoplastic counterparts. *Blood* 1995;86:28–37.
205. Allman D, Jain A, Dent A, et al. BCL-6 expression during B-cell activation. *Blood* 1996;87:5257–5268.
206. Dent AL, Shaffer AL, Yu X, et al. Control of inflammation, cytokine expression, and germinal center formation by BCL-6. *Science* 1997; 276:589–592.
207. Ye BH, Cattoretti G, Shen Q, et al. The BCL-6 proto-oncogene controls germinal-centre formation and Th2-type inflammation. *Nat Genet* 1997;16:161–710.
208. Fukuda T, Yoshida T, Okada S, et al. Disruption of the Bcl-6 gene results in an impaired germinal center formation. *J Exp Med* 1997; 186:439–448.
209. Mitelman F. *Catalog of chromosomal aberrations in cancer,* 5th ed. New York: Wiley-Liss, 1994.
210. Offit K, Lo Coco F, Louie DC, et al. Rearrangement of the bcl-6 gene as a prognostic marker in diffuse large-cell lymphoma [see comments]. *N Engl J Med* 1994;331:74–80.
211. Pescarmona E, De Sanctis V, Pistilli A, et al. Pathogenetic and clinical implications of Bcl-6 and Bcl-2 gene configuration in nodal diffuse large B-cell lymphomas. *J Pathol* 1997;183:281–286.
212. Vitolo U, Gaidano G, Botto B, et al. Rearrangements of bcl-6, bcl-2, c-myc and 6q deletion in B-diffuse large-cell lymphoma: clinical relevance in 71 patients. *Ann Oncol* 1998;9:55–61.
213. Yunis JJ, Oken MM, Kaplan ME, et al. Distinctive chromosomal abnormalities in histologic subtypes of non-Hodgkin's lymphoma. *N Engl J Med* 1982;307:1231–1236.
214. Levine EG, Arthur DC, Frizzera G, et al. There are differences in cytogenetic abnormalities among histologic subtypes of the non-Hodgkin's lymphomas. *Blood* 1985;66:1414–1422.
215. Bloomfield CD, Arthur DC, Frizzera G, et al. Nonrandom chromosome abnormalities in lymphoma. *Cancer Res* 1983;43:2975–2984.
216. Offit K, Jhanwar SC, Ladanyi M, et al. Cytogenetic analysis of 434 consecutively ascertained specimens of non-Hodgkin's lymphoma: correlations between recurrent aberrations, histology, and exposure to cytotoxic treatment. *Genes Chromosomes Cancer* 1991;3:189–201.
217. Juneja S, Lukeis R, Tan L, et al. Cytogenetic analysis of 147 cases of non-Hodgkin's lymphoma: non-random chromosomal abnormalities and histological correlations. *Br J Haematol* 1990;76:231–237.
218. Schouten HC, Sanger WG, Weisenburger DD, et al. Chromosomal abnormalities in untreated patients with non-Hodgkin's lymphoma: associations with histology, clinical characteristics, and treatment outcome. The Nebraska Lymphoma Study Group. *Blood* 1990;75: 1841–1847.
219. Yunis JJ, Mayer MG, Arnesen MA, et al. Bcl-2 and other genomic alterations in the prognosis of large-cell lymphoma [see comments]. *N Engl J Med* 1989;320:1047–1054.
220. Offit K, Koduru PR, Hollis R, et al. 18q21 rearrangement in diffuse large cell lymphoma: incidence and clinical significance. *Br J Haematol* 1989;72:178–183.
221. Romaguera JE, Pugh W, Luthra R, et al. The clinical relevance of t(14;18)/BCL-2 rearrangement and del 6q in diffuse large cell lymphoma and immunoblastic lymphoma. *Ann Oncol* 1993;4:51–54.
222. Gombart AF, Morosetti R, Miller CW, et al. Deletions of the cyclin-dependent kinase inhibitor genes p16INK4A and p15INK4B in non-Hodgkin's lymphomas. *Blood* 1995;86:1534–1539.
223. Pinyol M, Cobo F, Bea S, et al. P16(INK4a) gene inactivation by deletions, mutations, and hypermethylation is associated with transformed and aggressive variants of non-Hodgkin's lymphomas. *Blood* 1998;91:2977–2984.
224. Dreyling MH, Roulston D, Bohlander SK, et al. Codeletion of CDKN2 and MTAP genes in a subset of non-Hodgkin's lymphoma may be

associated with histologic transformation from low-grade to diffuse large-cell lymphoma. *Genes Chromosomes Cancer* 1998;22:72–78.
225. Villuendas R, Sanchez-Beato M, Martinez JC, et al. Loss of p16/INK4A protein expression in non-Hodgkin's lymphomas is a frequent finding associated with tumor progression. *Am J Pathol* 1998;153: 887–897.
226. Koduru PR, Zariwala M, Soni M, et al. Deletion of cyclin-dependent kinase 4 inhibitor genes P15 and P16 in non-Hodgkin's lymphoma. *Blood* 1995;86:2900–2905.
227. Quelle DE, Zindy F, Ashmun RA, et al. Alternative reading frames of the INK4a tumor suppressor gene encode two unrelated proteins capable of inducing cell cycle arrest. *Cell* 1995;83:993–1000.
228. Kamijo T, Zindy F, Roussel MF, et al. Tumor suppression at the mouse INK4a locus mediated by the alternative reading frame product p19ARF. *Cell* 1997;91:649–659.
229. Volpe G, Vitolo U, Carbone A, et al. Molecular heterogeneity of B-lineage diffuse large cell lymphoma. *Genes Chromosomes Cancer* 1996;16:21–30.
230. Houldsworth J, Mathew S, Rao PH, et al. REL proto-oncogene is frequently amplified in extranodal diffuse large cell lymphoma. *Blood* 1996;87:25–29.
231. Yano T, van Krieken JH, Magrath IT, et al. Histogenetic correlations between subcategories of small noncleaved cell lymphomas. *Blood* 1992;79:1282–1290.
232. Magrath I. The pathogenesis of Burkitt's lymphoma. *Adv Cancer Res* 1990;55:133–270.
233. Leder P, Battey J, Lenoir G, et al. Translocations among antibody genes in human cancer. *Science* 1983;222:765–771.
234. Garcia CF, Weiss LM, Warnke RA. Small noncleaved cell lymphoma: an immunophenotypic study of 18 cases and comparison with large cell lymphoma. *Hum Pathol* 1986;17:454–461.
235. Spina D, Leoncini L, Megha T, et al. Cellular kinetic and phenotypic heterogeneity in and among Burkitt's and Burkitt-like lymphomas. *J Pathol* 1997;182:145–150.
236. Williams ME, Innes DJ, Borowitz MJ, et al. Immunoglobulin and T cell receptor gene rearrangements in human lymphoma and leukemia. *Blood* 1987;69:79–86.
237. Chapman CJ, Mockridge CI, Rowe M, et al. Analysis of V_H genes used by neoplastic B cells in endemic Burkitt's lymphoma shows somatic hypermutation and intraclonal heterogeneity. *Blood* 1995;85: 2176–2181.
238. Klein U, Klein G, Ehlin-Henriksson B, et al. Burkitt's lymphoma is a malignancy of mature B cells expressing somatically mutated V region genes. *Mol Med* 1995;1:495–505.
239. Chapman CJ, Zhou JX, Gregory C, et al. V_H and V_L gene analysis in sporadic Burkitt's lymphoma shows somatic hypermutation, intraclonal heterogeneity, and a role for antigen selection. *Blood* 1996; 88:3562–3568.
240. Tamaru J, Hummel M, Marafioti T, et al. Burkitt's lymphomas express V_H genes with a moderate number of antigen-selected somatic mutations. *Am J Pathol* 1995;147:1398–1407.
241. Steiner P, Rudolph B, Muller D, Eilers M. The functions of Myc in cell cycle progression and apoptosis. *Prog Cell Cycle Res* 1996;2: 73–82.
242. Dang CV. C-Myc target genes involved in cell growth, apoptosis, and metabolism. *Mol Cell Biol* 1999;19:1–11.
243. Pelicci PG, Knowles DM, Magrath I, et al. Chromosomal breakpoints and structural alterations of the c-myc locus differ in endemic and sporadic forms of Burkitt lymphoma. *Proc Natl Acad Sci U S A* 1986; 83:2984–2988.
244. Neri A, Barriga F, Knowles DM, et al. Different regions of the immunoglobulin heavy-chain locus are involved in chromosomal translocations in distinct pathogenetic forms of Burkitt lymphoma. *Proc Natl Acad Sci U S A* 1988;85:2748–2752.
245. Henglein B, Synovzik H, Groitl P, et al. Three breakpoints of variant t(2;8) translocations in Burkitt's lymphoma cells fall within a region 140 kilobases distal from c-myc. *Mol Cell Biol* 1989;9:2105–2113.
246. Zeidler R, Joos S, Delecluse HJ, et al. Breakpoints of Burkitt's lymphoma t(8;22) translocations map within a distance of 300 kb downstream of MYC. *Genes Chromosomes Cancer* 1994;9:282–287.
247. Akasaka T, Muramatsu M, Ohno H, et al. Application of long-distance polymerase chain reaction to detection of junctional sequences created by chromosomal translocation in mature B-cell neoplasms. *Blood* 1996;88:985–994.
248. Joos S, Haluska FG, Falk MH, et al. Mapping chromosomal breakpoints of Burkitt's t(8;14) translocations far upstream of c-myc. *Cancer Res* 1992;52:6547–6552.
249. Lishner M, Kenet G, Lalkin A, et al. Fluorescent in situ hybridization for the detection of t(8:14) in Burkitt's lymphoma. *Acta Haematol* 1993;90:186–189.
250. Veronese ML, Ohta M, Finan J, et al. Detection of myc translocations in lymphoma cells by fluorescence in situ hybridization with yeast artificial chromosomes. *Blood* 1995;85:2132–2138.
251. Siebert R, Matthiesen P, Harder S, et al. Application of interphase fluorescence in situ hybridization for the detection of the Burkitt translocation t(8;14)(q24;q32) in B-cell lymphomas. *Blood* 1998;91: 984–990.
252. McKeithan TW, Shima EA, Le Beau MM, et al. Molecular cloning of the breakpoint junction of a human chromosomal 8;14 translocation involving the T-cell receptor alpha-chain gene and sequences on the 3′ side of MYC. *Proc Natl Acad Sci U S A* 1986;83:6636–6640.
253. Lipford E, Wright JJ, Urba W, et al. Refinement of lymphoma cytogenetics by the chromosome 18q21 major breakpoint region. *Blood* 1987;70:1816–1823.
254. Gaidano G, Ballerini P, Gong JZ, et al. P53 mutations in human lymphoid malignancies: association with Burkitt lymphoma and chronic lymphocytic leukemia. *Proc Natl Acad Sci U S A* 1991;88: 5413–5417.
255. Gutierrez MI, Bhatia K, Diez B, et al. Prognostic significance of p53 mutations in small non-cleaved cell lymphomas. *Int J Oncol* 1994;4: 567–571.
256. Kuppers R, Rajewsky K. The origin of Hodgkin and Reed/Sternberg cells in Hodgkin's disease. *Annu Rev Immunol* 1998;16:471–493.
257. Kanzler H, Kuppers R, Hansmann ML, et al. Hodgkin and Reed-Sternberg cells in Hodgkin's disease represent the outgrowth of a dominant tumor clone derived from (crippled) germinal center B cells. *J Exp Med* 1996;184:1495–505.
258. Braeuninger A, Kuppers R, Strickler JG, et al. Hodgkin and Reed-Sternberg cells in lymphocyte predominant Hodgkin disease represent clonal populations of germinal center-derived tumor B cells. *Proc Natl Acad Sci U S A* 1997;94:9337–9342.
259. Cossman J, Messineo C, Bagg A. Reed-Sternberg cell: survival in a hostile sea. *Lab Invest* 1998;78:229–236.
260. Jarrett RF, MacKenzie J. Epstein-Barr virus and other candidate viruses in the pathogenesis of Hodgkin's disease. *Semin Hematol* 1999; 36:260–269.
261. Riley C, Messineo C, Bagg A, et al. Comparative genome hybridization (CGH) of single Reed-Sternberg cells. *Lab Invest* 1997;76:131.
262. Ohshima K, Ishiguro M, Ohgami A, et al. Genetic analysis of sorted Hodgkin and Reed-Sternberg cells using comparative genomic hybridization. *Int J Cancer* 1999;82:250–255.
263. Waldmann TA, Davis MM, Bongiovanni K, et al. Rearrangements of genes for the antigen receptor on T cells as markers of lineage and clonality in human lymphoid neoplasms. *N Engl J Med* 1985;313: 776–783.
264. Bertness V, Kirsch I, Hollis G, et al. T-cell receptor gene rearrangements as clinical markers of human T-cell lymphomas. *N Engl J Med* 1985;313:534–538.
265. Weiss LM, Picker LJ, Grogan TM, et al. Absence of clonal beta and gamma T-cell receptor gene rearrangements in a subset of peripheral T cell lymphomas. *Am J Pathol* 1988;130:436–442.
266. Fodinger M, Winkler K, Mannhalter C, et al. Combined polymerase chain reaction approach for clonality detection in lymphoid neoplasms. *Diagn Mol Pathol* 1999;8:80–91.
267. Isobe M, Sadamori N, Russo G, et al. Rearrangements in the human T-cell-receptor alpha-chain locus in patients with adult T-cell leukemia carrying translocations involving chromosome 14q11. *Cancer Res* 1990;50:6171–6175.
268. Kneba M, Bolz I, Linke B, et al. Analysis of rearranged T-cell receptor beta-chain genes by polymerase chain reaction (PCR) DNA sequencing and automated high resolution PCR fragment analysis. *Blood* 1995;86:3930–3937.
269. Lue C, Mitani Y, Crew MD, et al. An automated method for the analysis of T-cell receptor repertoires: rapid RT-PCR fragment length analysis of the T-cell receptor beta chain complementarity-determining region 3. *Am J Clin Pathol* 1999;111:683–690.
270. Signoretti S, Murphy M, Cangi MG, et al. Detection of clonal T-cell receptor gamma gene rearrangements in paraffin-embedded tissue by

polymerase chain reaction and nonradioactive single-strand conformational polymorphism analysis. *Am J Pathol* 1999;154:67–75.

271. Theodorou I, Bigorgne C, Delfau MH, et al. VJ rearrangements of the TCR gamma locus in peripheral T-cell lymphomas: analysis by polymerase chain reaction and denaturing gradient gel electrophoresis. *J Pathol* 1996;178:303–310.
272. Meyer JC, Hassam S, Dummer R, et al. Realistic approach to the sensitivity of PCR-DGGE and its application as a sensitive tool for the detection of clonality in cutaneous T-cell proliferations. *Exp Dermatol* 1997;6:122–127.
273. Greiner TC. Advances in molecular hematopathology: T-cell receptor and bcl-2 genes. *Am J Pathol* 1999;154:7–9.
274. Ashton-Key M, Diss TC, Pan L, et al. Molecular analysis of T-cell clonality in ulcerative jejunitis and enteropathy-associated T-cell lymphoma. *Am J Pathol* 1997;151:493–498.
275. Delfau-Larue MH, Petrella T, Lahet C, et al. Value of clonality studies of cutaneous T lymphocytes in the diagnosis and follow-up of patients with mycosis fungoides. *J Pathol* 1998;184:185–190.
276. Cooke CB, Krenacs L, Stetler-Stevenson M, et al. Hepatosplenic T-cell lymphoma: a distinct clinicopathologic entity of cytotoxic gamma delta T-cell origin. *Blood* 1996;88:4265–4274.
277. Kumar S, Krenacs L, Medeiros J, et al. Subcutaneous panniculitic T-cell lymphoma is a tumor of cytotoxic T lymphocytes. *Hum Pathol* 1998;29:397–403.
278. Zhang Y, Wong KF, Siebert R, et al. Chromosome aberrations are restricted to the $CD56^{+}$, $CD3^{-}$ tumour cell population in natural killer cell lymphomas: a combined immunophenotyping and FISH study. *Br J Haematol* 1999;105:737–742.
279. Kwong YL, Chan AC, Liang RH. Natural killer cell lymphoma/leukemia: pathology and treatment. *Hematol Oncol* 1997;15:71–79.
280. Fracchiolla NS, Lombardi L, Salina M, et al. Structural alterations of the NF-kappa B transcription factor lyt-10 in lymphoid malignancies. *Oncogene* 1993;8:2839–2845.
281. Migliazza A, Lombardi L, Rocchi M, et al. Heterogeneous chromosomal aberrations generate 3′ truncations of the NFKB2/lyt-10 gene in lymphoid malignancies *Blood* 1994;84:3850–3860.
282. Thakur S, Lin HC, Tseng WT, et al. Rearrangement and altered expression of the NFKB-2 gene in human cutaneous T-lymphoma cells. *Oncogene* 1994;9:2335–2344.
283. Foss HD, Anagnostopoulos I, Araujo I, et al. Anaplastic large-cell lymphomas of T-cell and null-cell phenotype express cytotoxic molecules. *Blood* 1996;88:4005–4011.
284. O'Connor NT, Stein H, Gatter KC, et al. Genotypic analysis of large cell lymphomas which express the Ki-1 antigen. *Histopathology* 1987; 11:733–740.
285. Rimokh R, Magaud JP, Berger F, et al. A translocation involving a specific breakpoint (q35) on chromosome 5 is characteristic of anaplastic large cell lymphoma (''Ki-1 lymphoma''). *Br J Haematol* 1989;71:31–36.
286. Le Beau MM, Bitter MA, Larson RA, et al. The t(2;5)(p23;q35): a recurring chromosomal abnormality in Ki-1–positive anaplastic large cell lymphoma. *Leukemia* 1989;3:866–870.
287. Mason DY, Bastard C, Rimokh R, et al. CD30-positive large cell lymphomas (''Ki-1 lymphoma'') are associated with a chromosomal translocation involving 5q35. *Br J Haematol* 1990;74:161–168.
288. Morris SW, Kirstein MN, Valentine MB, et al. Fusion of a kinase gene, ALK, to a nucleolar protein gene, NPM, in non-Hodgkin's lymphoma. *Science* 1994;263:1281–1284.
289. Ladanyi M, Cavalchire G. Detection of the NPM-ALK genomic rearrangement of Ki-1 lymphoma and isolation of the involved NPM and ALK introns. *Diagn Mol Pathol* 1996;5:154–158.
290. Kuefer MU, Look AT, Pulford K, et al. Retrovirus-mediated gene transfer of NPM-ALK causes lymphoid malignancy in mice. *Blood* 1997;90:2901–2910.
291. Lamant L, Dastugue N, Pulford K, et al. A new fusion gene TPM3-ALK in anaplastic large cell lymphoma created by a (1;2)(q25;p23) translocation. *Blood* 1999;93:3088–3095
292. Wlodarska I, De Wolf-Peeters C, Falini B, et al. The cryptic inv(2)(p23q35) defines a new molecular genetic subtype of ALK-positive anaplastic large-cell lymphoma. *Blood* 1998;92:2688–2695.
293. Suzuki R, Kagami Y, Ogura M, et al. Anaplastic large cell lymphoma: a distinct molecular pathologic entity: a reappraisal with special reference to p80 (NPM/ALK) expression. *Am J Surg Pathol* 1997;21: 1420–1432.
294. Falini B, Pileri S, Zinzani PL, et al. ALK^{+} lymphoma: clinicopathological findings and outcome. *Blood* 1999;93:2697–2706.
295. Gascoyne RD, Aoun P, Wu D, et al. Prognostic significance of anaplastic lymphoma kinase (ALK) protein expression in adults with anaplastic large cell lymphoma. *Blood* 1999;93:3913–3921.
296. Bullrich F, Morris SW, Hummel M, et al. Nucleophosmin (NPM) gene rearrangements in Ki-1–positive lymphomas. *Cancer Res* 1994; 54:2873–2877.
297. Waggott W, Lo YM, Bastard C, et al. Detection of NPM-ALK DNA rearrangement in CD30 positive anaplastic large cell lymphoma. *Br J Haematol* 1995;89:905–907.
298. Wellmann A, Otsuki T, Vogelbruch M, et al. Analysis of the t(2; 5)(p23;q35) translocation by reverse transcription–polymerase chain reaction in $CD30^{+}$ anaplastic large-cell lymphomas, in other non-Hodgkin's lymphomas of T-cell phenotype, and in Hodgkin's disease. *Blood* 1995;86:2321–2328.
299. Ladanyi M, Cavalchire G, Morris SW, et al. Reverse transcriptase polymerase chain reaction for the Ki-1 anaplastic large cell lymphoma-associated t(2;5) translocation in Hodgkin's disease. *Am J Pathol* 1994;145:1296–1300.
300. Downing JR, Shurtleff SA, Zielenska M, et al. Molecular detection of the (2;5) translocation of non-Hodgkin's lymphoma by reverse transcriptase–polymerase chain reaction. *Blood* 1995;85:3416–3422.
301. Elmberger PG, Lozano MD, Weisenburger DD, et al. Transcripts of the npm-alk fusion gene in anaplastic large cell lymphoma, Hodgkin's disease, and reactive lymphoid lesions. *Blood* 1995;86:3517–3521.
302. Mathew P, Sanger WG, Weisenburger DD, et al. Detection of the t(2; 5)(p23;q35) and NPM-ALK fusion in non-Hodgkin's lymphoma by two-color fluorescence in situ hybridization. *Blood* 1997;89: 1678–1685.
303. Pulford K, Lamant L, Morris SW, et al. Detection of anaplastic lymphoma kinase (ALK) and nucleolar protein nucleophosmin (NPM)-ALK proteins in normal and neoplastic cells with the monoclonal antibody ALK1. *Blood* 1997;89:1394–1404.
304. Shiota M, Nakamura S, Ichinohasama R, et al. Anaplastic large cell lymphomas expressing the novel chimeric protein p80NPM/ALK: a distinct clinicopathologic entity. *Blood* 1995;86:1954–1960.
305. Delsol G, Lamant L, Mariame B, et al. A new subtype of large B-cell lymphoma expressing the ALK kinase and lacking the 2;5 translocation. *Blood* 1997;89:1483–1490.
306. Orscheschek K, Merz H, Hell J, et al. Large-cell anaplastic lymphoma-specific translocation (t[2;5] [p23;q35]) in Hodgkin's disease: indication of a common pathogenesis? *Lancet* 1995;345:87–90.
307. Downing JR, Ladanyi M, Raffeld M, et al. Large-cell anaplastic lymphoma-specific translocation in Hodgkin's disease. *Lancet* 1995;345: 918–920.

CHAPTER 10

Role of Cytogenetics in the Diagnosis and Classification of Hematopoietic Neoplasms

Michelle M. Le Beau

The malignant cells in many patients who have leukemia, lymphoma, or another hematologic neoplasm have acquired clonal chromosomal abnormalities. In many cases, they represent specific cytogenetic abnormalities that are closely and sometimes uniquely associated with morphologically and clinically distinct subsets of leukemia or lymphoma (1–3). The detection of one of these recurring abnormalities can establish the correct diagnosis and can add information of prognostic importance. Moreover, the detection of a cytogenetic abnormality clearly distinguishes between benign reactive lymphoid or myeloid hyperplasia and a malignant proliferation. This chapter focuses on the genetics of the leukemias and lymphomas from primarily a cytogenetic perspective.

GENETIC CONSEQUENCES OF CHROMOSOMAL REARRANGEMENTS

During the past few years, the genes that are located at the breakpoints of a number of the recurring chromosomal translocations have been identified (Table 10.1); many of these genes proved to be novel, previously unrecognized genes. Alterations in the expression of the genes or in the properties of the encoded proteins resulting from the rearrangement play an integral role in the process of malignant transformation (4,5). The transforming genes that are involved in chromosomal translocations fall into several functional classes, including tyrosine or serine protein kinases, cell surface receptors and growth factors (Table 10.1). However, the largest class of genes encodes transcriptional regulating factors (4,5). Transcription factors are proteins that are involved in the initiation of gene transcription; they recognize and bind to target sequences located in the regulatory elements of genes or to other DNA-binding proteins, often functioning in a tissue-specific fashion. In this way, they play critical roles in differentiation and development as well as maintaining the function of differentiated cells.

There are two general mechanisms by which chromosomal translocations result in altered gene function. The first is deregulation of gene expression. This mechanism is characteristic of the translocations in lymphoid neoplasms that involve the immunoglobulin genes in B-lineage tumors and the T-cell receptor genes in T-lineage tumors. These rearrangements result in inappropriate expression of an oncogene (overexpression or aberrant expression in a tissue that does not normally express the gene), with no alteration in its protein structure.

The second mechanism is the expression of a novel fusion protein, resulting from the juxtaposition of coding sequences from two genes that are normally located on different chromosomes. Such chimeric proteins are "tumor specific" in that the fusion gene does not exist in nonmalignant cells; the detection of such a fusion gene or protein can be important in the diagnosis or in the detection of residual disease or early relapse. They may also be appropriate targets for tumor-specific therapies. An example is the chimeric BCR/ABL protein resulting from the t(9;22) in chronic myelogenous leukemia. All of the translocations cloned in the myeloid leukemias result in a fusion protein (Tables 10.1, 10.2).

Chromosomal translocations result in the activation of genes in a dominant fashion. A number of human tumors, including retinoblastoma, Wilms' tumor, and colon carcinoma, are believed to result from homozygous, recessive mutations (6). These mutations lead to the absence of a functional protein product, suggesting that these genes function as "suppressor" genes whose normal roles are to limit cellular proliferation. The hallmark of tumor suppressor genes is the loss of genetic material in malignant cells. Such a loss may result from chromosomal loss or deletion, as well as by other genetic mechanisms, such as mitotic recombination.

M. M. Le Beau: Section of Hematology/Oncology, Department of Medicine, University of Chicago, Chicago, Illinois 60637

TABLE 10.1. *Functional classification of transforming genes at translocation junctions*

Gene	Location	Translocation	Consequence	Disease
SRC family (TYR protein kinases)				
ABL	9q34	t(9;22)	Fusion protein	CML/ALL
LCK	1p34	t(1;7)	Deregulated expression	T-ALL
Serine protein kinase				
BCR[a]	22q11	t(9;22)	Fusion protein	CML/ALL
Cell surface receptor				
TAN1[a]	9q34	t(7;9)	Deregulated expression	T-ALL
Growth factor				
IL3	5q31	t(5;14)	Deregulated expression	Pre-B-ALL
Inner mitochondrial membrane protein				
BCL2[a]	18q21	t(14;18)	Deregulated expression	NHL
Transcriptional regulating factors[b]				
BCL3[a]	19q13	t(14;19)	Deregulated expression	B-CLL
LYT10	10q24	t(10;14)	Deregulated expression	B-NHL
PBX1[a]	1q23	t(1;19)	Fusion protein	Pre-B-ALL
E2A	19p13	t(1;19)	Fusion protein	Pre-B-ALL
CAN[a]	9q34	t(6;9)	Fusion protein	AML
HOX11[a]	10q24	t(10;14)/t(7;10)	Deregulated expression	T-ALL
LYL1[a]	19p13	t(7;19)	Deregulated expression	T-ALL
MYC	8q24	t(8;14)	Deregulated expression	B-ALL/NHL
PML[a]	15q22	t(15;17)	Fusion protein	APL
RARA	17q11.2	t(15;17)	Fusion protein	APL
AML1(RUNX1)[a]	21q22	t(8;21)/t(3;21)	Fusion protein	AML
		t(12;21)	Fusion protein	ALL
TEL(CETV6)[a]	12p12	t(12;21)	Fusion protein	ALL
TAL1(SCL)[a]	1p32	t(1;14)	Deregulated expression	T-ALL
TAL2[a]	9q32	t(7;9)	Deregulated expression	T-ALL
RBTN1(TTG1)[a]	11p15	t(11;14)	Deregulated expression	T-ALL
RBTN2[a]	11p13	t(11;14)	Deregulated expression	T-ALL

ALL, acute lymphoblastic leukemia; AML, acute myeloid leukemias; APL, acute promyelocytic leukemia; CLL, chronic lymphocytic leukemia; CML, chronic myelogenous leukemia; NHL, non-hodgkin's lymphoma.
[a] Gene first identified by cloning breakpoints.
[b] Partial list of transcription factors.

TABLE 10.2. *Recurring chromosome abnormalities in malignant myeloid diseases*

Disease	Chromosome abnormality	Frequency[a]	Involved Genes[b]	
CML	t(9;22)(q34;q11)	~98% (100%)[c]	*ABL*	*BCR*
CML blast phase	t(9;22) with +8, +Ph, +19, or i(17q)	~70%	*ABL*	*BCR*
AML-M2	t(8;21)(q22;q22)	18% (30%)	*ETO*	*AML1*
AML-M3, M3V	t(15;17)(q22;q11–12)	14% (98%)	*PML*	*RARA*
AMMoL-M4Eo	inv(16)(p13q22) or t(16;16)(p13;q22)	8% (~100%)	*MYH11*	*CBFB*
AMMoL-M4, AMoL-M5	t(9;11)(p22;q23)	11% (30%) for	*AF9*	*MLL*
	t(10;11)(p11–p15;q23)	All t(11q23)	*AF10*	*MLL*
	t(11;17)(q23;q25)		*MLL*	*AF17*
	t(11;19)(q23;p13.3)		*MLL*	*ENL*
	t(11;19)(q23;p13.1)		*MLL*	*ELL*
	t(6;11)(q27;q23)		*AF6*	*MLL*
	Other t(11q23)		*MLL*	
	del(11)(q23)			
AML	+8	10%		
	+11	1–2%	*MLL*	
	−7 or del(7q)	10%		
	−5 or del(5q)	10%		
	t(6;9)(p23;q34)	1%	*DEK*	*CAN*
	t(3;3)(q21;q26) or inv (3)(q21q26)	2%	*EVII*	
	del (20q)	5%		
	t(12p) or del(12p)	2%		
Therapy related	−7 or del(7q) and/or −5 or del(5q)	75%		
	der(1;7)(q10;p10)	2%		

(continued)

TABLE 10.2. *Continued.*

Disease	Chromosome abnormality	Frequency[a]	Involved Genes[b]	
AML	t(9;11)(p22;q23)/t(11q23)	3%	*MLL*	
	t(21q22)	2%	*AML1*	
CMMoL	t(5;12)(q33;p12)	2–5%	*PDGFRB*	*TEL*

AML-M2, acute myeloblastic leukemia with maturation; AMMOL, acute myelomonocytic leukemia; AMMoL-M4Eo, acute myelomonocytic leukemia with abnormal eosinophils; AMoL, acute monoblastic leukemia; AML, acute myeloid leukemia; APL-M3, M3V, hypergranular (M3) and micrograpular (M3V) acute promyelocytic leukemia; CML, chronic myelogenous leukemia; CMMoL, chronic myelomonocytic leukemia.

[a] The percentage refers to the frequency within the disease overall. The numbers in the parentheses refer to the frequency within the morphologic or immunologic subtype of the disease (2).

[b] Genes are listed in order of citation in the karyotype, such as for CML, *ABL* is at 9q34 and *BCR* at 22q11.

[c] Some patients with CML have an insertion of *ABL* adjacent to *BCR* in a normal appearing chromosome 22.

The identification of recurring chromosomal loss or deletions in the leukemias and lymphomas suggests that, as for a number of solid tumors, tumor suppressor genes may be involved in the pathogenesis of some hematologic malignant diseases (3,6).

METHODS

Cytogenetic analyses of malignant diseases must be based on the study of the tumor cells themselves. In leukemia, the specimen is usually obtained by bone marrow aspiration and is processed immediately (direct preparation) or cultured for 24 to 72 hours. When a bone marrow aspirate cannot be obtained, a bone marrow biopsy (bone core specimen) can often be processed successfully. Alternatively, for patients who have a white blood cell (WBC) count higher than 10,000/μL with more than 10% immature myeloid or lymphoid cells, a sample of peripheral blood can be cultured. The karyotype of the dividing cells is similar to that obtained from the bone marrow. Mitogens are not added routinely to peripheral blood cultures in acute leukemia, because stimulation of division of normal lymphocytes may interfere with the analysis of spontaneously dividing malignant cells. An involved lymph node or tumor mass specimen or malignant effusion may be processed similarly for the analysis of lymphomas. The use of amethopterin to synchronize dividing cells, combined with brief exposures to mitotic inhibitors such as colchicine, or DNA-binding agents (ethidium bromide) are used by some laboratories to obtain elongated chromosomes that have an increased number of bands.

Cytogenetic studies are feasible only for specimens that contain viable dividing cells. For this reason, it is critical that the specimen be transported to the laboratory without delay. In some cases, analyses may be performed on specimens that have been transported by overnight delivery services; however, the shipment of specimens frequently results in loss of cell viability, and most laboratories experience a high proportion of inadequate analyses using such specimens. For optimally handled specimens, 95% to 98% of all cases should be adequate for cytogenetic analysis.

Chromosomal abnormalities are described according to the International System for Human Cytogenetic Nomenclature (7) (Appendix 1 and 2). The observation of at least two cells with the same structural rearrangement (e.g., translocations, deletions, inversions) or gain of the same chromosome or of three cells with each showing loss of the same chromosome is considered evidence for the presence of an abnormal clone. However, one cell with a normal karyotype is considered evidence for the presence of a normal cell line. Patients whose cells show no alteration or nonclonal (single cell) abnormalities are considered to be normal. An exception to this is a single cell characterized by a recurring structural abnormality. In such instances, it is likely that this represents the karyotype of the malignant cells in that particular patient.

Many laboratories have incorporated the technique of fluorescence *in situ* hybridization (FISH) in their diagnostic services. Using FISH, labeled probes are hybridized to chromosomes or nuclei, and the probe is detected with fluorochromes. This technique is a rapid and sensitive means of detecting recurring numerical and structural abnormalities.

CHRONIC MYELOPROLIFERATIVE DISORDERS

Chronic Myelogenous Leukemia

Chronic Phase

Chronic myelogenous leukemia (CML) is a particularly important subtype of leukemia because it was in this disease that the first consistent chromosomal abnormality in a malignant disease was noted (Table 10.2). This abnormality, the Philadelphia or Ph chromosome, was first described in 1960 by Nowell and Hungerford as a deletion of part of the long arm of a G-group chromosome, and later with the use of fluorescence banding techniques as a 22q−. The nature of the chromosomal aberration was clarified in 1973, when Rowley reported that the Ph chromosome resulted from a reciprocal translocation involving chromosomes 9 (break at band q34) and 22 (break at band q11) (Fig. 10.1A). The t(9;22) also represents the first rearrangement shown to result in a fusion protein.

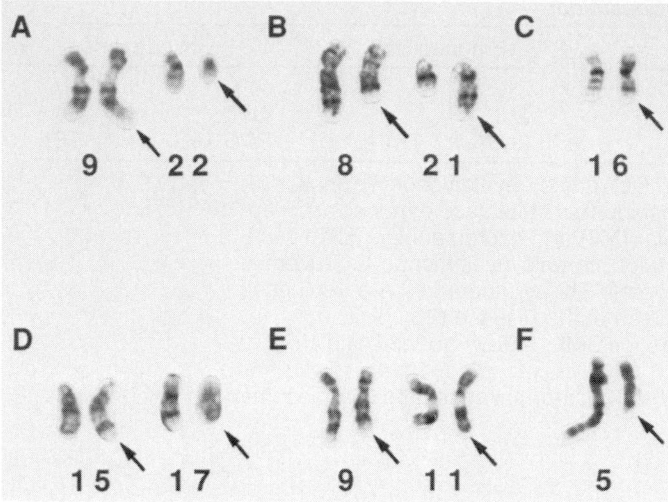

FIG. 10.1. Partial karyotypes from trypsin-Giemsa-banded metaphase cells depicting nonrandom chromosomal rearrangements observed in myeloid malignant diseases. **A:** t(9;22)(q34;q11), chronic myelogenous leukemia (CML). **B:** t(8;21)(q22;q22), acute myeloblastic leukemia with maturation (AML-M2). **C:** inv(16)(p13q22), acute myelomonocytic leukemia with abnormal eosinophils (AMoL-M4Eo). **D:** t(15;17)(q22;q11-12), acute promyelocytic leukemia (APL). **E:** t(9;11)(p22;q23) in acute monoblastic leukemia AMoL-M5. **F:** del(5)(q13q33) in therapy-related AML (t-AML). The rearranged chromosomes are identified with arrows.

It is generally accepted that CML is defined by the presence of the Ph chromosome or its molecular consequence, the *BCR/ABL* fusion gene, and that patients without this abnormality should be considered to have a different disorder. It is critical that *BCR/ABL*+ patients be distinguished from those that lack this rearrangement because of the use of different treatment approaches and different survival (8). Pugh and colleagues reviewed 25 patients initially diagnosed with CML but whose cells lacked the Ph chromosome and showed that most of these patients had a myelodysplastic syndrome (MDS), most commonly chronic myelomonocytic leukemia (CMMoL) or refractory anemia with excess blasts (RAEB) or the poorly understood disorder of atypical CML (9). The most common abnormality in these patients was trisomy 8. These observations have been confirmed by others. However, the leukemia cells in occasional cases that lack the Ph chromosome contain a DNA rearrangement in which the molecular consequences are identical to that of the t(9;22), and the term Ph-negative (Ph−) CML should be reserved for these rare cases of typical CML.

About 92% of Ph-positive (Ph+) patients have the standard t(9;22). The remaining patients have variant translocations, such as three-way translocations involving chromosomes 9, and 22, and a third chromosome (10). In a variant translocation, material from chromosome 9 translocates to chromosome 22, material from 22q translocates to a third chromosome, and material from the third chromosome translocates to 9q. In the standard and variant rearrangements, the *ABL* oncogene (9q34) is relocated adjacent to the *BCR* gene on chromosome 22 (q11) (11–13). Analysis of leukemia cells from rare patients with typical CML who lack the Ph chromosome has revealed a rearrangement involving *ABL* and *BCR* that is detectable only at the molecular level (1% to 2% of cases) (14). However, this rearrangement is not present in most patients who have been diagnosed as having Ph− CML, providing further evidence that the t(9;22) and subsequent *BCR/ABL* fusion is characteristic of all CML cases (15).

On chromosome 22, most breaks cluster in a small, 5.8-kilobase (kb) region between exons b2 and b3 or between b3 and b4, known as the breakpoint cluster region (bcr) (12,13). In contrast, the breaks on chromosome 9 occur over more than 200 kb, usually upstream (5′) of exon II, and the *ABL* coding sequences are translocated to chromosome 22 and fused in frame with the *BCR* gene. A novel chimeric 8.5 kb mRNA is produced, which is translated into a chimeric protein ($p210^{BCR\text{-}ABL}$) (13). Analysis of mice transplanted with bone marrow cells transfected with the fusion gene, or *BCR/ABL* transgenic mice has clearly shown that the fusion gene leads to leukemia (16). The ABL protein is normally a nuclear protein and may function as a transcription factor that is regulated by the retinoblastoma protein, RB1. The BCR/ABL protein is located on the cytoplasmic surface of the cell membrane and acquires a novel function in transmitting growth-regulatory signals from cell surface receptors to the nucleus through the RAS signal transduction pathway (17). The *BCR/ABL* fusion gene can be detected with standard Southern blot analysis of DNA or polymerase chain reaction (PCR) analysis of mRNA by reverse transcription (RT-PCR) (18) for diagnosis and detection of residual disease. FISH can also be used to detect the Ph chromosome in both metaphase and interphase cells (19).

When patients with CML are treated with busulfan or hydroxyurea and a hematologic remission is achieved, the bone marrow morphology and leukocyte alkaline phosphatase score may return to normal. However, the percentage of Ph+ cells in the bone marrow usually remains unchanged (the Ph chromosome is typically found in 100% of cells examined). Attempts have been made to eradicate the Ph+ clone with aggressive cytotoxic therapy, but only rarely can this be achieved, and even then, the benefit is transient. Intensive chemoradiotherapy followed by allogeneic bone marrow transplantation has been successful in eradicating the Ph+ cell line and restoring normal hematopoiesis of donor origin. The daily use of interferon-alfa can induce complete cytogenetic remission in approximately 20% of patients with CML in the chronic phase (20). The reappearance of cytogenetically normal marrow cells requires several months of treatment. In most cases, molecular methods can still detect cells with the *BCR/ABL* fusion transcript. However, patients who have a cytogenetic complete response to interferon therapy have a longer survival than nonresponders or those treated only with hydroxyurea.

Acute Phase

As they enter the terminal acute phase (i.e., blast crisis of CML), 80% of patients show karyotypic evolution with the appearance of new chromosomal abnormalities in very distinct patterns in addition to the Ph chromosome (10,21). For this reason, cytogenetic studies may be useful in confirming the clinical impression of the accelerated or acute phase of the disease. A change in the karyotype is considered to be a grave prognostic sign (10,21). The available data suggest that with the exception of an isochromosome of the long arm of chromosome 17 [i(17)(q10)], which is usually associated with a myeloid type of blast transformation, there is no association of a particular karyotype with the lymphoid or with the myeloid type of blast transformation, and that these additional abnormalities are not correlated with the response to therapy during the acute phase (10,21). The most common changes, a gain of chromosomes 8 or 19, or a second Ph (by gain of the first), or an i(17q), frequently occur in combination to produce modal chromosome numbers of 47 through 50 (10). Taken together, these changes occur in 70% of cases with secondary abnormalities. Less common abnormalities include −7, −17, +17, + 21, −Y, and the t(3;21)(q26;q22); these occur in about 15% of cases with additional changes. Rarely, one of the recurring abnormalities in acute myeloid leukemia (AML) can be seen with the t(9;22), such as an inv(16) in myelomonocytic blast crisis.

The t(9;22) can be observed in acute lymphoblastic leukemia (ALL); patients who present with lymphoblastoid blast phase but who have no prior history suggestive of CML can be difficult to differentiate from Ph+ ALL. In CML patients, the Ph chromosome is present in granulocytic, erythroid, and megakaryocytic cells, and in some B cells (22). Moreover, Ph+ ALL is a lymphoblast-restricted disease and often involves a different breakpoint in *BCR*, whereas lymphoid blast phase of CML is a multilineage disease always involving a break in the bcr of the *BCR* gene (23,24). The overall survival of patients with multilineage disease is significantly better than that of patients with lymphoblast-restricted disease (23,24).

Polycythemia Vera

Cytogenetic abnormalities are relatively uncommon in untreated polycythemia vera (PV) patients (~14%), but occur at a higher frequency in those who have been treated with cytotoxic agents (39%), or who have progressed to acute leukemia (85%) (10). The presence of cytogenetic abnormalities at diagnosis does not necessarily predict a short survival or the development of leukemia (10,25). An evolutionary change in the karyotype during the disease course, however, may be an ominous sign.

In the polycythemic phase of PV, a gain of chromosomes, which usually involves chromosomes 8 (15%) or 9 (20%), is frequently observed. A number of patients with PV show gains of chromosomes 8 and 9; clones containing both +8 and +9 are seldom observed in other hematologic diseases and may be unique to PV. Structural rearrangements most often involve a deletion of chromosome 20 [del(20q) (30%)] or a duplication of 1q (20%), especially bands 1q25 to 1q32. A del(20q) is not specific for PV, and has been noted in other malignant myeloid diseases; a duplication of 1q has been observed in other hematologic diseases as well as in solid tumors (1–3).

The cytogenetic pattern of the malignant cells in PV patients who have developed AML show some similarities to those observed in the polycythemic phase, e.g., +8, +9, del(20q), but there are certain striking differences as well. For example, loss of chromosome 7 is rarely observed in the polycythemic phase but is seen in 20% of patients in the leukemic phase. Rearrangements of chromosome 5, particularly a del(5q), are the most frequent changes noted in advanced disease (40% of patients) (1,10,25). Abnormalities of chromosomes 5 and 7 are the most common abnormalities observed in therapy-related leukemia, suggesting that the leukemia in some patients with PV may have a similar cause. It has been shown that the chronic use of oral alkylating agents such as chlorambucil or the use of ^{32}P during the chronic phase of PV significantly increases the rate of transformation to leukemia.

Essential Thrombocythemia and Myeloid Metaplasia with Myelofibrosis

During the Third International Workshop on Chromosomes in Leukemia, 170 cases of essential thrombocythemia were analyzed, and only 5% had a chromosomal abnormality (26). Moreover, no recurring abnormality could be identified in these patients.

Cytogenetic analysis of bone marrow cells of patients with myeloid metaplasia with myelofibrosis has revealed the presence of clonal abnormalities in 35% of patients (27). In general, these abnormalities are similar to those noted in other myeloid disorders. The most common anomalies are +8, −7 or a del(7q), del(11q), del(13q), and del(20q) (1,2,27,28). Similar to CML and PV, a change in the karyotype may signal evolution to acute leukemia.

PRIMARY MYELODYSPLASTIC SYNDROMES

The myelodysplastic syndromes (MDS) are a heterogeneous group of hematopoietic stem cell disorders characterized by anemia, neutropenia, or thrombocytopenia in various combinations (29). A number of studies on large series of patients have reported that clonal chromosomal abnormalities can be detected in bone marrow cells in 40% to 70% of patients with primary MDS at the time of diagnosis (30–32). The frequency of chromosomal abnormalities correlates with the severity of the disease. Only 25% to 30% of low-grade MDS cases (refractory anemia (RA), or RA with ringed sideroblasts (RARS)) have clonal abnormalities, whereas about 70% of the high-grade cases (RAEB and RAEB in transformation, RAEB-T) have abnormal karyotypes. In CMMoL, the frequency is 30% to 40%. This contrasts with the approximately 85% incidence of cytogenetic abnormalities detected in patients with AML *de novo*. Although +8, −5/del(5q), −7/del(7q), and del(20q) are common in both disorders, the specific structural rearrangements that are closely associated with distinct morphologic subsets of AML *de novo* (Table 10.2) are almost never seen in MDS.

TABLE 10.3. *Single chromosome changes in primary myelodyplastic syndrome*

−7 or del(7q)
+8
del(5)(q13q33) and translocations involving 5q[a]
del(11q)[b]
del(12)(p11p13)
del(13q)[c]
del(20)(q11q13)
t(1;3)(p36;q21.2)
der(1;7)(q10;p10)
t(2;11)(p21;q23)
t(6;9)(p23;q34)

[a] Chromosomal breakpoints of the interstitial deletions of 5q are variable, but band q31 is invariably deleted; proximal breakpoints frequently occur in bands 5q13-15 and distal breakpoints frequently occur in bands q33-35.

[b] q23.1 is always involved in interstitial or terminal deletions.

[c] q14 is always involved in interstitial deletions of variable size.

With several exceptions (e.g., 5q− syndrome), chromosomal abnormalities in MDS have not correlated with specific clinical or morphologic subsets using the criteria of the French-American-British (FAB) group; however, there are some morphologic associations. These include the association of sideroblastosis with deletions of 11q, ringed sideroblasts with Xq13 abnormalities, and prominent dyserythropoiesis with a del(20q).

Patients with MDS may have single or multiple chromosome changes (Table 10.3). A single chromosome change is a single numerical change, a structural abnormality involving only one chromosome, or a balanced translocation involving two chromosomes. Occasionally, several unrelated clones may be detected (5% of cases), one of which is often characterized by +8; the frequency of such unrelated clones is higher than that observed in AML (<1%). Additional aberrations may evolve during the course of MDS or an abnormal clone may emerge in a patient with a previously normal karyotype; these changes typically portend transformation to leukemia.

The ability of cytogenetic analysis to predict the outcome of any individual patient with MDS is made more difficult because MDS is a life-threatening disorder because of persistent and profound pancytopenia. Nonetheless, several studies have demonstrated the prognostic significance of cytogenetic abnormalities in MDS for predicting survival and progression to AML. Patients with abnormal karyotypes (particularly those with complex abnormalities) were found to have a shorter survival and a higher incidence of progression to AML than patients with normal karyotypes (30–32). The International MDS Risk Analysis Workshop combined cytogenetic, morphologic, and clinical data for 816 patients from seven large, previously reported risk-based studies (32). The major variables predictive of evolution to AML were cytogenetic abnormalities, percentage of bone marrow blasts, and number of cytopenias; variables predictive for survival included those mentioned previously as well as age and gender. Patients with a "good outcome" had normal karyotypes, −Y alone, del(5q) alone, or del(20q) alone, those with a "intermediate outcome" had other abnormalities, and those with a "poor outcome" had complex karyotypes (three abnormalities, typically with abnormalities of chromosome 5, 7, or both), or chromosome 7 abnormalities. The median survival of patients within these three groups were 3.8, 2.4, and 0.8 years, respectively, and the times for 25% of the patients to undergo evolution to AML were 5.6, 1.6, and 0.9 years.

Hypocellular MDS is relatively common, and can be difficult to differentiate from aplastic anemia. The presence of a recurring abnormality typical of myeloid disorders, such as −7 or del(7q), +8, supports the diagnosis of MDS (33,34). However, the finding of any abnormality may not be sufficient, because diseases associated with a +6 or t(1;20) have been reported to show a clinicopathologic picture that is more typical of aplastic anemia than MDS (35).

The 5q− syndrome is a distinctive hematologic disorder that occurs primarily in older women (36,37). In contrast to other MDS where males predominate, the male : female ratio here is 0.5. Eighty percent of patients are older than 50 years. Patients present with a refractory macrocytic anemia and normal or elevated platelet counts. The marrow is characterized by the presence of micromegakaryocytes with monolobulated or bilobulated nuclei. Approximately two thirds of patients have less than 5% blasts (RA or RARS), and the remainder have RAEB. Although 75% of cases have a del(5)(q13q33), other interstitial deletions, such as del(5)(q15q33), may be present. These patients typically have a relatively benign course that extends over several years. The molecular features of the del(5q) are described in a later section.

ACUTE MYELOID LEUKEMIA *DE NOVO*

There have now been numerous reports describing cytogenetic analyses of relatively large series of unselected patients with AML; citations for a number of later studies are included here (38–45). In earlier series, abnormal karyotypes were reported in approximately 50% of patients whose bone marrow cells were examined with banding techniques (44). The detection of cytogenetic abnormalities increases markedly when techniques for culturing leukemia cells and for obtaining prophase and prometaphase chromosomes are used. Currently, the investigators are detecting an abnormal clone in 85% of AML patients. Initially, it appeared that AML patients with a normal karyotype had a significantly longer survival than those with any chromosomal abnormality. It has become clear that the prognostic importance resides within specific chromosome changes, several of which are associated with higher response rates and longer survival than the medians observed in AML patients who have no detectable abnormality (44,45). This discussion emphasizes certain aberrations that occur frequently or appear to be of exceptional biologic interest (Table 10.2).

Chromosomal Gain and Loss

Although the karyotypes of patients with AML may be variable, the recurring gain and loss of chromosomes and the involvement in structural rearrangements are evident. The number of chromosomes gained or lost in 354 patients with a clonal abnormality was examined at the Fourth International Workshop on Chromosomes in Leukemia (44). With the exceptions of chromosome 16, which was never observed as a gain, and chromosome 1, which was never lost, each of the autosomes and sex chromosomes contributed to the numerical changes.

Trisomy 8

Trisomy 8 is the most frequent trisomy in malignant myeloid diseases and can occur as a sole abnormality or as a secondary change. The overall frequency of +8 in AML is about 10%; as a sole abnormality, the frequency may vary among the FAB subtypes: M5, 10.4%; M7, 7.3%; M2, 6.2%; M4 and M1, 4.7% each (46). Trisomy 8 is observed as a secondary abnormality in AML in 31% of cases with a der(1; 7), 17% of cases with a t(9;11), and 10% of cases with an inv(16) or t(15;17). In MDS, it occurs most frequently in RARS and CMMoL. In CML, +8 is the most frequent secondary change in the acute phase (20% of cases). When AML patients with +8 as a sole abnormality were evaluated, the complete remission (CR) rate was 51%, with an overall survival of 9 to 11 months (45). In MDS, +8 is associated with an intermediate outcome (32). The molecular basis by which trisomy 8 is involved in transformation is unknown, but a dosage effect of a wild-type allele, such as *MYC* on 8q, or amplification of a mutated oncogene, resulting from gain of a chromosome containing a mutated allele, have been proposed.

Trisomy 11

Trisomy 11 is a rare abnormality, identified as a sole aberration in 1% to 2% of all AML or MDS cases (45,47). There is no association of +11 with any particular subtype of MDS; AML cases are typically M1 or M2 or, less commonly, M4. In AML, a +11 is associated with dysplasia, and an unfavorable outcome (CR, 60%; median survival is unknown) (47). Although rare, trisomy 11 is notable in that duplications of the *MLL* gene are detected in 90% of AMLs with +11 as the sole abnormality but in only 30% of cases in which trisomy 11 is part of a complex karyotype; *MLL* duplications have also been identified in 10% of AML cases with an apparently normal karyotype (48,49). *MLL* is involved in a number of recurring translocations in AML and ALL. The rearrangement is the result of a partial tandem duplication of *MLL* exons 2 through 6 or 2 through 8 mediated by recombination between Alu repetitive elements (48). Analysis of the transcripts revealed that the duplication is in frame, suggesting that the mRNA is capable of encoding a partially duplicated protein. The association of *MLL* duplications with trisomy 11 represents the first identification of a specific gene rearrangement associated with a recurring trisomy in human cancer. Whether other trisomies are associated with specific gene rearrangements or a more general gene dosage effect is unknown.

−5/del(5q) and −7/del(7q)

Loss of a whole chromosome 5, or a deletion of the long arm of this chromosome, del(5q), are noted in 10% of patients MDS or AML arising *de novo*; their frequency is substantially higher in therapy-related MDS or AML (t-MDS/t-AML, ~42%) (1–3,44,45,50). In MDS, −5/del(5q) is typically observed in the advanced stages (i.e., RAEB or RAEB-T), and is usually associated with a complex karyotype often with abnormalities of chromosome 7 (30). A distinct subset of MDS, called the 5q− syndrome, was described earlier (36,37). Monosomy 5/del(5q) may be seen in all FAB subtypes, but the frequency is higher in AML-M6 (~60%) (50). Many of the patients with MDS or AML *de novo* and abnormalities of chromosomes 5, 7, or both have had significant occupational exposure to potential carcinogens, suggesting that abnormalities of these chromosomes may be a marker of mutagen-induced leukemia. The molecular biology of leukemias with abnormalities of chromosomes 5 and 7 is described in the section on t-AML.

Monosomy 7 and del(7q) are also among the most common cytogenetic alterations found in MDS/AML and occur in three general contexts: *de novo* MDS and AML (10% to 12%); leukemia associated with a constitutional predisposition or with aplastic anemia; and t-MDS/t-AML (50%) (51). The similar clinical and biologic features of the myeloid disorders associated with monosomy 7 or del(7q) suggest that the same genes are altered in patients with different antecedent risk factors. As described earlier for chromosome 5, abnormalities of chromosome 7 in MDS typically occur in the advanced stages (RAEB and RAEB-T); they occur in all subtypes of AML with the highest frequency noted in AML-M6 (~45%) (1–3,44,45). Monosomy 7/del(7q) are the most common cytogenetic abnormalities identified in patients with t-MDS/t-AML (50%), and are associated with prior therapy with alkylating agents.

Monosomy 7/del(7q) is the most common cytogenetic abnormality detected in the bone marrows of patients with constitutional predispositions to myeloid leukemia including Fanconi's anemia (42%), neurofibromatosis type 1 (25%), severe congenital neutropenia (73%), and familial monosomy 7 syndrome (100%) (51). Monosomy 7 or del(7q) is usually identified as an isolated cytogenetic abnormality in the bone marrow of some subsets of patients, e.g., pediatric patients with MDS or juvenile myelomonocytic leukemia, JMML (previously known as juvenile chronic myelogenous leukemia), whereas it is generally associated with additional alterations in adults with MDS or AML *de novo*, patients with t-MDS/t-AML or occupational exposures, and congenital neutropenia.

Although there is spectrum of diseases associated with −5/del(5q) and −7/del(7q), trilineage dysplasia is a common morphologic feature. Abnormalities of chromosomes 5, 7, or both are associated with a poor response to therapy and poor survival (for chromosome 5, CR of 50% and median survival of 5 months; for chromosome 7, CR of 80% and median survival of 12 months) (45). In AML, −7 is associated with increased incidence of fever and infection.

Monosomy 7 Syndrome

An entity called monosomy 7 syndrome has been described in young children, and is characterized by a preponderance of affected males, hepatosplenomegaly, leukocytosis, thrombocytopenia, absence of the Philadelphia chromosome, and poor prognosis (51). In these patients, monosomy 7 is usually the only cytogenetic abnormality. Monosomy 7 syndrome shares many features with JMML and some children with JMML have monosomy at diagnosis (20%) or as a new cytogenetic finding with disease acceleration (51).

Loss of the Y Chromosome

Loss of the Y chromosome or loss of the X chromosome is associated with the t(8;21) in 80% to 90% of cases (44). Loss of a Y chromosome as the sole abnormality is also observed, but the significance of this abnormality is uncertain because a missing Y chromosome has been reported in bone marrow cells of hematologically normal males, particularly those over 60 years old (2,10). In contrast, the t(8;21) in AML is usually observed in younger adults (10,38–44).

Specific Structural Rearrangements

8;21 Translocation in M2 Acute Myeloblastic Leukemia

In 1973, Rowley first described a balanced translocation between chromosomes 8 and 21 (t(8;21)(q22;q22), Fig. 10.1B). The t(8;21) is common and is observed in 18% of all AML cases with an abnormal karyotype, and 30% of the M2 patients (44,52). This translocation is the most frequent abnormality in children with AML, and occurs in 15% to 20% of karyotypically abnormal cases. Most cases with the t(8;21) are classified as AML with maturation (M2), but some cases have been diagnosed as M4 leukemia.

Although AML-M2 is heterogeneous, the presence of the t(8;21) identifies a morphologically and clinically distinct subset. In this disorder, blasts tend to have indented nuclei, and the cytoplasm is generally basophilic with a prominent paranuclear hof that may contain a few azurophilic granules (53). Promyelocytes, myelocytes, and metamyelocytes are often quite prominent and may be large. Their cytoplasm has a waxy, orange appearance and lacks a granular texture in Romanowski-stained specimens. Auer rods are easily identified, and several may be seen in a single cell. Bone marrow eosinophilia is also common (53). Malignant cells in rare patients may be cytogenetically normal or contain only a −Y or del(9q). However, FISH or RT-PCR methods can demonstrate the *AML1/ETO* rearrangement.

AML-M2 with the t(8;21) has a favorable prognosis in adults, but the outcome in children is poor (44,45,54). The median age of affected adults is 25 to 30 years, significantly younger than that of AML patients overall (44,45). Rare patients have less than 30% blasts at diagnosis and are therefore classified as having MDS. There is an increased incidence of extramedullary disease (granulocytic sarcoma) associated with this anomaly. The CR rate is uniformly high (93%), and with intensive postremission consolidation chemotherapy, the expected disease-free survival exceeds 2 years, after which time relapses are uncommon (45). Remarkably, however, some patients in remission for as long as 10 years have the fusion AML1/ETO mRNA detectable in circulating leukocytes (55). The cell reservoir of the persistent AML1/ETO transcripts has not been identified, but may be a primitive hematopoietic progenitor.

At the molecular level, the t(8;21) is important because it involves a transcription factor pathway that is critical in hematopoiesis. In the t(8;21), the *AML1*/RUNX1 gene on chromosome 21 is fused to the *ETO* gene on chromosome 8 and results in an AML1/ETO chimeric protein (52) (Fig. 10.2). The AML1 protein (also known as core binding factor-α [CBFA2]) heterodimerizes with another protein, CBFB, to form a transcription factor. The *CBFB* gene is located at 16q22, at the breakpoint in the inv(16)(16;16) associated with AML-M4 with abnormal eosinophils. The AML1/CBFB transcription factor binds directly to an enhancer core motif that is present in the regulatory regions of a number of genes that are critical to myeloid cell differentiation, and thereby regulates expression of the genes (56). The target genes include the genes encoding IL3, GM-CSF, the CSF1 receptor, myeloperoxidase, and neutrophil elastase (56). Mutant mice with loss of *AML1* or *CBFB* gene function are deficient in definitive hematopoiesis, and die during embryogenesis, indicating that the AML1/CBFB-regulated target genes are essential for hematopoiesis of all lineages. By using gene targeting, Okuda and colleagues found that mouse embryos with an *AML1/ETO* knockin allele that mimics the t(8;21) have complete absence of normal fetal liver–derived definitive hematopoiesis. Before death at embryonic day 13.5, the fetal livers contained dysplastic multilineage hematopoietic progenitors that had abnormally high self-renewal capacity *in vitro* (57).

AML1/ETO interferes with normal activation of gene expression by the normal AML1/CBFB transcription factor (56). Moreover, AML1/ETO has gained a new function within the cell, and is capable of activating expression of the *BCL2* gene, an antiapoptosis gene, and possibly other genes. Transformation by AML1/ETO likely results from altered transcriptional regulation of normal AML1 target

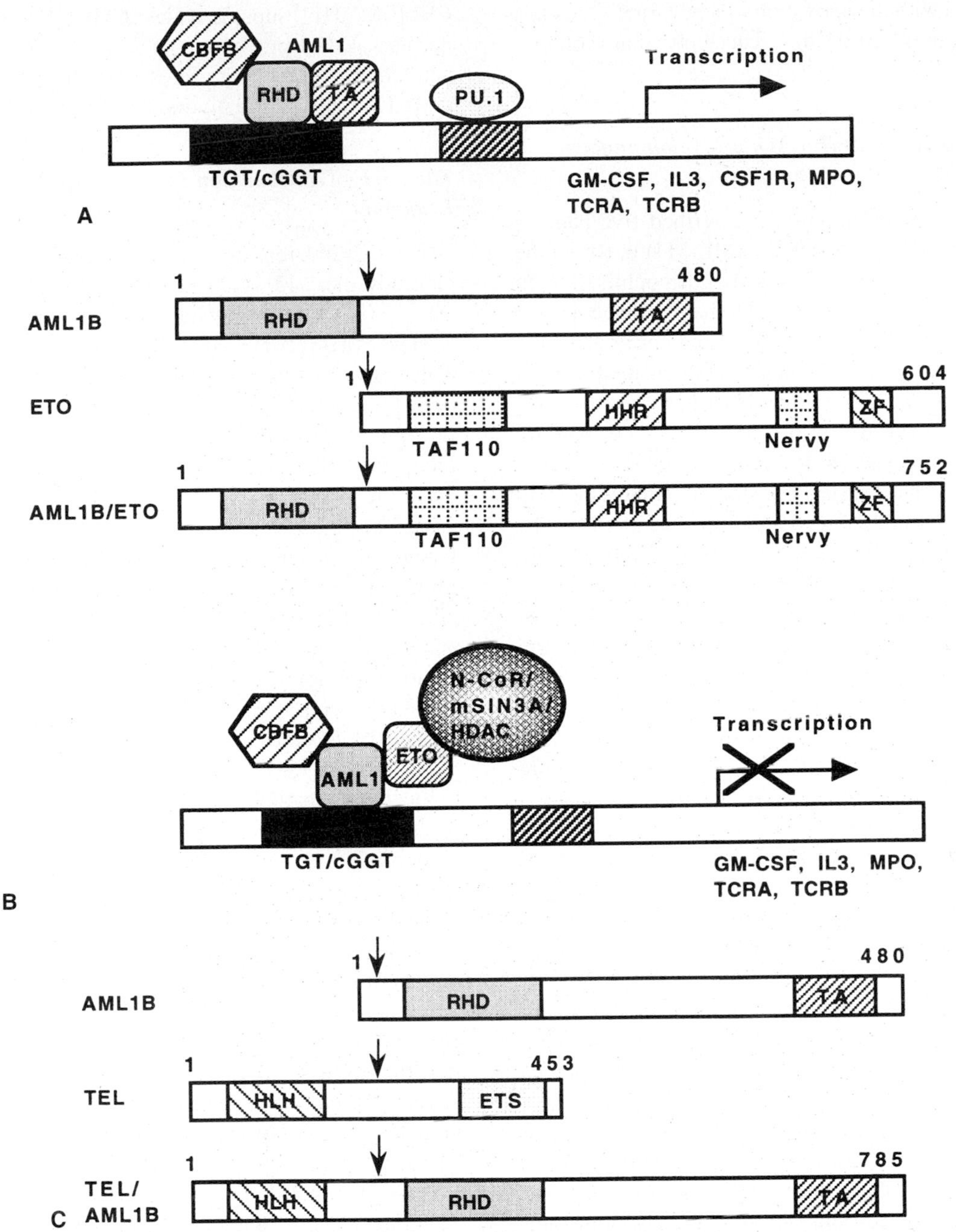

FIG. 10.2. Schematic diagram of the normal AML1B, ETO, and TEL proteins, and the AML1/ETO and TEL/AML1 fusion proteins. **A:** Diagram of the heterodimeric AML1/CBFB transcription factor. The transcription factor binds by means of the DNA binding domain of AML1 (runt homology domain [RHD]) directly to a specific core motif present in the regulatory region of a number of genes that are involved in myeloid cell growth and thereby regulates their expression. **B:** Schematic diagram of the normal AML1B and ETO proteins and the AML1/ETO fusion protein, with a schematic model for the role of AML1/ETO in the pathogenesis of myeloid leukemias. For AML1, RHD refers to the runt homology domain and TA refers to transactivation domain. The ETO protein contains three domains characteristic of transcription factors: TAF110 refers to a domain with homology to the *Drosophila* TAF110 transcriptional coactivator; HHR refers to a leucine zipper–like hydrophobic heptad repeat; and ZF refers to a zinc finger domain. Nervy refers to a domain homologous to the *Drosophila* gene, *nervy*. AML1/ETO represses transcription of AML1 target genes. **C:** Schematic diagram of the normal AML1B and TEL proteins and the TEL/AML1 fusion protein. For TEL, HLH refers to a helix-loop-helix domain and ETS refers to an ETS DNA binding domain.

genes, combined with the activation of new target genes that prevent programmed cell death or cause aberrant proliferation.

Inv(16) and t(16;16) in M4Eo Acute Myelomonocytic Leukemia with Abnormal Eosinophils

In 1983, Arthur and Bloomfield described five patients (three with AML-M2 and two with AML-M4) in whom the bone marrow contained an excess of eosinophils (8% to 54%); all five patients were reported to have a deleted chromosome 16. Le Beau reported on a related entity in 18 patients, all of whom had M4 leukemia with eosinophils that showed alterations of morphology, cytochemical reactions, and ultrastructure (58). All of the patients had a pericentric inversion of chromosome 16, inv(16)(p13q22) (Fig. 10.1C) or, less commonly, a reciprocal translocation involving both chromosome 16 homologues, t(16;16)(p13;q22) (58). The inv(16)/t(16;16) occurs in virtually all cases of M4Eo leukemia, and accounts for 8% of all AML cases. Additional abnormalities noted in one third of cases include +22, +8, and +21, in order of decreasing frequency (58). Trisomy 22 is not observed as a recurring abnormality in any other subtype of AML. Leukemias with the inv(16)/t(16;16) have a number of similarities to those with the t(8;21). At the molecular level, both involve the genes encoding the core binding factor, a heterodimeric transcription factor that is required for hematopoiesis. Second, they both have distinctive morphologic phenotypes. Third, they both have a good overall prognosis.

The inv(16)/t(16;16) occurs in a distinctive subset of acute myelomonocytic leukemia (AMMoL) in which the eosinophils are variable in number, but consistently abnormal (59). Eosinophil abnormalities include the presence of large and irregular basophilic granules, and positive reactions with periodic acid–Schiff and chloroacetate esterase. These features may be best appreciated in eosinophils at immature stages of maturation. Patients with an inv(16)/t(16;16) have central nervous system (CNS) involvement at presentation or relapse more frequently than other AML cases (45). Despite this, they have a good response to intensive chemotherapy with a CR rate of about 90% and an overall 5-year survival rate of about 75% (45,58).

The inversion breakpoint at 16q22 occurs within the *CBFB* gene (also known as *PEBP2B*), which encodes one subunit of the heterodimeric AML1/CBFB transcription factor (60,61). A smooth muscle myosin heavy-chain gene *(MYH11)* is interrupted by the breakpoint on 16p. A fusion protein containing the 5′ region of *CBFB* (165 of 182 amino acids), including the domain that heterodimerizes with *AML1*, fused to the 3′ portion of *MYH11* is produced. This portion of MYH11 contains a repeated α helical structure involved in myosin filament interactions and may cause multimerization of the fusion protein. The precise mechanism by which the fusion protein mediates transformation is not known, but several models have been proposed: multimeric CBFB/MYH11 superactivates AML1; CBFB/MYH11 sequesters AML1 preventing its access to DNA binding sites; and CBFB/MYH11 interferes with the normal function of AML1 through steric hindrance (60,61).

The 15;17 Translocation in M3 Acute Promyelocytic Leukemia

A structural rearrangement involving the long arms of chromosomes 15 and 17, t(15;17)(q22;q11.2-12) (Fig. 10.1D), in acute promyelocytic leukemia (APL or AML-M3) was first recognized by Rowley and associates in 1977. This rearrangement is highly specific for APL and has not been found in any other disease. Although t(15;17) was believed to be present in all cases of APL initially, it is now recognized that there are rare variant translocations that occur in less than 2% of cases. These include the t(11;17)(q23;q11.2-12) and t(5;17)(q34;q11.2-12) (62). Establishing the diagnosis of APL with the typical t(15;17) is important, because this disease is sensitive to therapy with all-*trans* retinoic acid (ATRA), whereas other cases of AML, and the APL-like disorders associated with the variant translocations do not respond to this treatment (63). The t(15;17) is usually seen alone, but may be seen with trisomy 8 in about 10% of cases (1,2).

Acute promyelocytic leukemia is widely recognized as a unique clinicopathologic entity characterized by infiltration of the bone marrow by promyelocytes in association with a hemorrhagic diathesis. The characteristic folded, reniform (kidney-shaped), or bilobed nucleus is invariably found in some of the promyelocytes. Coarse azurophilic granules and multiple Auer rods are common (53). The microgranular variant of APL differs from the more frequent hypergranular type only in that the cytoplasmic granules of the leukemia cells are smaller and sometimes beyond the limit of resolution of the light microscope (53). Auer rods may also be fewer in number and the WBC count higher in the microgranular variant, but the t(15;17) is similarly present.

Patients with APL are younger than other individuals who have AML (44,45). They have a favorable prognosis with a CR rate of about 70% and an overall 5-year survival of 30% to 40% (45). Clinical or laboratory evidence of disseminated intravascular coagulation (DIC) is almost invariably present at diagnosis and may worsen during the initial cytolytic response to chemotherapy. Acute promyelocytic leukemia cells are exquisitely sensitive to the differentiating effect of ATRA, and evidence of DIC rapidly resolves after starting this treatment (64). Cases that lack the t(15;17) do not respond to ATRA. Patients with APL may enter CR without experiencing a period of marrow hypoplasia; the malignant promyelocytes are often slow to clear from the marrow even as normal hematopoiesis recovers.

The breakpoint on chromosome 17 occurs within the first intron of the α retinoic acid receptor gene *(RARA)* in most patients, whereas the break on chromosome 15 occurs within the *PML* gene (65). The variant translocations involve *RARA* and the *PLZF* gene at 11q23, or the *NPM* (nucleophosmin) gene at 5q34 (62). The RARA protein is a member of a superfamily of nuclear hormone receptors. These proteins have a ligand binding domain that mediates binding to steroid hormones, including retinoic acid (RA), a DNA-binding domain that mediates binding to regulatory elements of target genes, and a dimerization domain that permits heterodimerization with retinoid X receptors (RXRs), a second class of nuclear retinoid receptors. The retinoic acid–receptor complex acts as a transcription factor to induce other genes and thereby induces cellular differentiation of myeloid progenitors. The translocation results in a fusion *PML/RARA* gene that contains most of the *PML* coding sequences, and the DNA-binding and ligand-binding domains of the *RARA* gene (65). *PML* is an interferon-inducible gene. The PML RING-finger protein is a critical component of the RA pathway and its absence results in failure of myeloid precursor cells to undergo terminal differentiation (66). Through its ability to heterodimerize with PML and RXR, the PML/RARA fusion protein is thought to interfere with PML and RAR/RXR-RA pathways, acting as a double dominant negative oncogenic protein (65,66).

Rearrangements of the Long Arm of Chromosome 11 in M5 Acute Monoblastic Leukemia

In 1980, Berger and coworkers reported a high frequency of abnormalities of chromosome 11, band q23, in patients with acute monoblastic leukemia, particularly the poorly differentiated form (M5a). This association was confirmed at the Fourth International Workshop on Chromosomes in Leukemia (44). Abnormalities of 11q23 are seen in about 35% of M5 patients and in slightly less than half of the patients with M5a (2,67–69).

Recurring translocations involving 11q23 are of great interest in human acute leukemia for at least three reasons. First, there are more than 30 different recurring rearrangements that involve 11q23, and along with band 14q32, 11q23 is one of the bands most frequently involved in rearrangements in human tumor cells (1,3,68,69). The breakpoints in the translocation partners include 1p32, 4q21, and 19p13.3 in ALL, and 1q21, 2q21, 6q27, 9p22, 10p11, 17q25, 19p13.3, and 19p13.1 in AML. Second, these translocations occur in lymphoid and myeloid leukemias. One common translocation in infants, t(4;11)(q21;q23), usually has a lymphoblastic phenotype, whereas other translocations, such as the t(9;11), (p22;q23) (Fig. 10.1E) and t(11;19)(q23; p13.1), are common in monoblastic leukemias. These data suggest that a gene at 11q23 may be involved in determining the differentiation of primitive hematopoietic stem cells into lymphoblasts or monoblasts, or that it may be a gene which is active in both cell lineages. Translocations involving 11q23 have a very unusual age distribution; they comprise about three fourths of the chromosome abnormalities in leukemia cells of children under one year of age (67,69). With the exception of the t(9;11) which may have an intermediate outcome, translocations of 11q23 are associated with a poor outcome (43,45).

Translocations of 11q23 involve the *MLL* gene (also called *ALL1* or *HRX*). The *MLL* gene is a very large gene (>100 Kb) with multiple transcripts of 12-15 kb (70). All breakpoints fall within an 8.3 kb breakpoint cluster region encompassing exons 5 through 11; *MLL* translocations can be detected by Southern blot analysis of DNA using a small cDNA probe containing these exons (71). The MLL protein contains two potential DNA-binding motifs (zinc fingers and AT hooks), a transcriptional activation domain in the COOH-terminus, and a repression domain in the N-terminal portion (72). This protein has homology to the *Drosophila* trithorax gene product, a transcription factor that regulates *HOX* gene expression and embryonic development. *MLL* also regulates expression of *HOX* genes, which play important roles in embryogenesis and hematopoiesis. Mice with a homozygous mutation of *MLL* (*Mll* $-/-$) die at embryonic day 11.5 to 14.5 and have a reduction in the number of hematopoietic precursors, whereas heterozygous mutant mice (*Mll* $+/-$) show homeotic transformations of the axial skeleton, and hematologic abnormalities, including anemia and thrombocytopenia (73).

Translocations of *MLL* result in the formation of a chimeric gene on the derivative 11 chromosome, consisting of the 5′ region of *MLL* and the 3′ region of the partner gene from the other chromosome, with subsequent expression of fusion mRNAs. The AT hook and repression domain are retained in the fusion protein; however, the strong activation domain is lost (72). The splitting of these domains may alter the function of *MLL* and contribute to leukemogenesis. Chimeric mice containing an *MLL/AF9* fusion gene from the t(9;11) develop AML, whereas leukemia is not observed in mice with a disrupted *MLL* gene (74). These results suggest that the fusion gene itself plays a role in leukemogenesis and that the partner gene is required for this process. Although a number of the partner genes have been cloned, the function of these genes is largely unknown. An exception is the *ELL* gene at 19p13.1 that encodes an elongin, which increases the catalytic rate of gene transcription by RNA polymerase II by suppressing transient pausing. Whether the genes on the partner chromosomes interact with *MLL* to affect the myeloid or lymphoid phenotype of the corresponding leukemias, or whether the cell lineage and stage at which the translocation occurs dictates the phenotype is unknown.

The t(3;3) and inv(3) in Acute Myelogenous Leukemia with Thrombocytosis

Several groups of investigators have identified an association of the inv(3)(q21q26), and t(3;3)(q21;q26) with thrombocytosis in AML patients (45,75). The t(3;3) and inv(3) comprise about 2% of AML cases and have been identified in all AML subtypes except M3, and in a few patients with MDS (usually RAEB or RAEB-T). Although most patients have increased platelets, this is not invariably present. A specific feature is the presence of abnormal megakaryocytes in the bone marrow (75). The megakaryocytes are typically quite prominent and markedly dysplastic with tiny micromegakaryocytic forms. Multilineage dysplasia is observed in many cases, but this may be because of the coexistence of −7/del(7q) in about 75% of cases. The inv(3)/t(3;3) is associated with a poor outcome (CR rate, 33%; median survival, 9 months) (45).

The *EVI1* gene, located at 3q26, is activated by chromosomal rearrangements 5′ of the gene in the t(3;3) or 3′ of the gene in the inv(3) by juxtaposition of the gene to enhancer elements of the ribophorin gene located at 3q21 (76). Activation of *EVI1* can also occur in the t(3;21)(q26;q22) as part of the fusion mRNA, *AML1/EVI1,* that is transcribed from the der(3) chromosome. Abnormal expression of EVI1 has also been detected in patients with AML and a normal karyotype, suggesting that inappropriate activation of this gene occurs through various mechanisms (77). EVI1 is a zinc finger transcription factor and may mediate malignant transformation by inducing inappropriate gene expression.

Del(20q)

A deletion of an F group chromosome was described initially in PV; however, the rearrangement was identified subsequently as a del(20q) (78,79). The deletion is observed in about 10% of PV patients, and in 5% of patients with AML or MDS (2,79). The deletion may occur as the sole abnormality, but is frequently observed with additional changes, particularly del(5q) and +8 (1). The prognostic significance of the del(20q) in MDS and AML is variable. The International MDS Risk Analysis Workshop found that patients with a del(20q) alone fell into a ''good-risk'' group with a median survival of 48 months, whereas a del(20q) observed in association with a complex karyotype identified a poor-risk group (median survival for the entire poor-risk group, 9.6 months) (32). In another study, AML patients with a del(20q) had a poor response to treatment and short survival (5 months); however, the majority had complex karyotypes, often with abnormalities of chromosomes 5 and 7 (80). Taken together, these data suggest that the del(20q) in MDS or AML may be associated with a favorable outcome when noted as a sole abnormality, but with a less favorable prognosis in the setting of a complex karyotype.

Disorders with a del(20q) are believed to arise in a primitive hematopoietic cell with myeloid and lymphoid potential (78). Although B lymphocytes may be involved in some cases, the abnormality is rarely seen in lymphoid neoplasms. The loss or inactivation of one or more genes on 20q alters the regulation of multipotent progenitors. By cytogenetic and molecular analysis using microsatellite markers, the commonly deleted segment of 20q has been defined as an approximately 8-Mb interval within 20q12; however, the involved gene has not yet been identified (78,81).

Other Less Common Structural Abnormalities

The t(6;9)(p23;q34) is a rare abnormality observed in about 1% of AML patients, and rare cases of MDS, and is associated with basophilia (82). Bodger and colleagues demonstrated that the translocation is present in the basophils (83). Most cases have been categorized as M1, M2, or M4 (1). These leukemias usually have dysplasia in at least the granulocytic and erythroid series. Because relatively few patients with the t(6;9) have been reported, the clinical features are poorly defined; most patients have been younger, and have had a poor outcome. The rearrangement fuses the *CAN* gene (9q34) with the 3′ end of the *DEK* gene (6p23), and a fusion transcript and protein are produced (82). The normal CAN protein (also know as NUP214) is a component of the nuclear pore complex that faces the cytoplasm. The consequence of the fusion is the relocation of the C terminus of CAN into the nucleus; however, the mechanism by which the fusion protein mediates transformation is unknown (84).

The t(1;22)(p13;q13) is restricted to AML-M7 occurring in infants less than 12 months of age (85,86). The rearrangement is observed in about 30% of infants with this type of leukemia, and is a useful marker for this disorder in cases that are otherwise difficult to diagnose (86). Frequently, the blast cells appear primitive, and may resemble metastatic carcinoma, neuroblastoma, or even sarcoma. Clinically, the patients present with hepatosplenomegaly and cytopenias, although the platelet count can be normal or elevated (85). The outcome is variable. The molecular consequences of the translocation are unknown.

The t(8;16)(p11;p13) is observed in 1% to 2% of patients with AML and t-AML; however, this rare abnormality is of interest because of advances at the molecular level, and an unusual morphologic phenotype (1,87). The disease is typically M4 or M5; erythrophagocytosis or hemophagocytosis is reported as a distinctive feature in most cases. Many patients (40%) are young (<17 years), and hepatosplenomegaly is common. The involved genes on 8p and 16p are *MOZ* and *CBP* (core binding protein), respectively, and a MOZ/CBP fusion protein is produced (88). The MOZ protein is a histone acetyltransferase, which transfers acetyl groups to the charged residues on the tails of the histone proteins, thereby relaxing the nucleosome structure and facilitating gene transcription. The CBP protein is a transcriptional coactivator that facilitates transcriptional activation of many target genes. Moreover, CBP also has histone acetyltransferase activity. Leukemogenesis is believed to occur through a heretofore unrecognized mechanism, namely, altered transcriptional regulation resulting from aberrant chromatin acetylation. Other rearrangements involving 8p11 that are associated with similar pathologic features include the t(8;22)(p11;q13) and t(8;19)(p11)(q13) (87). The t(8;22) involves the *P300* gene at 22q13, which encodes a protein related to CBP.

THERAPY-RELATED MYELODYSPLASTIC SYNDROME AND ACUTE MYELOID LEUKEMIA

Of increasing interest are the characteristic chromosomal abnormalities found in patients who develop t-MDS or t-AML after chemotherapy, radiation therapy, or both for an earlier disorder, such as Hodgkin's disease, non-Hodgkin's lymphoma (NHL), carcinoma, rheumatoid arthritis, or renal transplantation (89). Several clinical and biologic subsets of t-MDS or t-AML have been recognized; distinct subsets have correlated with the specific therapy administered for the primary disease (Table 10.4). The most common type typically presents after a latency period of about 5 years in patients who received alkylating agents. Two thirds of these patients are first recognized by evidence of myelodysplasia (usually trilineage dysplasia), marrow failure, and pancytopenia. Often, the initial disease is still present at the time of secondary bone marrow dysfunction. One half of the patients diagnosed with t-MDS (<30% marrow blasts) evolve to t-AML within a median of 6 months, but the other half die of infectious or hemorrhagic complications of pancytopenia. Survival times are usually short (median, 8 months). Abnormalities of chromosomes 5, 7, or both are characteristic of this subtype of t-MDS/t-AML, and the karyotypes are often complex (89–92). The detection of a clonal abnormality in a pancytopenic patient is convincing evidence of the existence of a secondary neoplasm even though the percentage of blasts in the marrow is not yet elevated.

A second subtype of t-AML has been identified that is distinctly different from the more common leukemia that follows alkylating agents or irradiation. This type of t-AML was first observed among patients receiving extremely high cumulative doses of etoposide for lung cancer, but has also been seen in patients receiving other drugs known to inhibit topoisomerase II, such as teniposide and doxorubicin (89,92,93). Clinically, these patients have a shorter latency period (1 to 2 years), present with overt leukemia, usually with monocytic features (they rarely present with MDS), and have a favorable response to intensive remission induction therapy (Table 10.4). Balanced translocations involving the *MLL* gene at 11q23 or the *AML1* gene at 21q22 are common in this subgroup (89,92,93). A third subtype of t-AML is therapy-related APL characterized by the t(15;17) after treatment for psoriasis with bimolane, a dioxopiperazine derivative that also interacts with topoisomerase II (89).

The following section summarizes the findings in the updated University of Chicago series of 270 patients with t-MDS/t-AML (90 and unpublished data). Seventy-two had Hodgkin's disease, 61 had NHL, 22 had multiple myeloma or another hematologic malignant disease, 101 had various solid tumors, and 14 had nonmalignant disease, primarily an autoimmune disease or an organ transplant. One hundred eighteen of the patients had received prior radiotherapy and chemotherapy, and 112 patients had only chemotherapy. Thirty-eight patients had had only radiotherapy. The median time between the original diagnosis and the diagnosis of secondary bone marrow dysfunction was 62 months.

TABLE 10.4. *Contrasting features of therapy-related myeloid leukemia from alkylating agents or topoisomerase II inhibitors*

Therapy agent	Chromosome abnormality	Preleukemia phase	FAB	Age	Latency	Response to induction chemotherapy	Long-term survival	Chemotherapy drugs
Alkylating agents	−5/del(5q) −7/del(7q)	MDS	Not classifiable by current criteria	Typically older patients	5–7 yr	Poor	Poor	Melphalan, mechlorethamine, chlorambucil, cyclophosphamide, carmustine, lomustine, semustine, procarbazine, dacarbazine, mitolactol
Topoisomerase II inhibitor	t(11q23) t(21q22)	None	Usually M4, M5; some M1, M2 and ALL-L1	Younger patients	6 mo–5 yr	Good	Poor	Etoposide, teniposide actinomycin D, doxorubicin, 4 epi-doxorubicin, mitoxantrone
	inv(16)	None	M4Eo	Younger patients	<3 yr	Good	Good	
Various agents	t(15;17)	None	M3	Younger patients	2–3 yr	Good	Good	Bimolane

FAB, French-American-British classification; MDS, myelodysplastic syndrome.
Adapted from Thirman M, Larson RA. Therapy-related myeloid leukemia. *Hematol Oncol Clin North Am* 1996;10:293–320.

Ninety-three percent (252 of 270) had chromosomal abnormalities, and 70% (191 of 270) had abnormalities of chromosome 5, 7, or both (90, unpublished data). Among these 191 patients, 35 had −5, 55 had a del(5q), 25 had loss of 5q after unbalanced translocations, 96 had −7, 26 had a del(7q), 15 had loss of 7q as a result of an unbalanced translocation, and 1 patient had a balanced translocation of 7q22. Sixty-two patients had abnormalities of chromosomes 5 and 7. Overall, 115 patients (43%) had loss of 5q, and 138 (51%) had loss of 7q. A del (5q) was the most common structural aberration (Fig. 10.1F).

By analogy to the deletions observed in solid tumors, such as retinoblastoma, one can propose that there are critical genes located on 5q that are related to leukemogenesis. By cytogenetic analysis of 177 patients with malignant myeloid diseases and a del (5q), we identified a small segment of 5q, consisting of band 5q31, that was deleted in each patient (94). This segment has been called the commonly deleted segment. Distal 5q contains a number of genes encoding growth factors, hormone receptors, and proteins involved in signal transduction or transcriptional regulation (94). These include the genes encoding five hematopoietic growth factors (i.e., GM-CSF, IL3, IL4, IL5, and IL9). By FISH of probes to metaphase cells with overlapping deletions involving 5q31, we have narrowed the commonly deleted segment to a region of approximately 1 Mb, flanked by the D5S479 and D5S500 markers, and containing the *EGR1* tumor suppressor gene and *CDC25C* G_2 checkpoint gene (94). The five hematopoietic growth factor genes, and seven other genes are excluded from this region. A larger, overlapping commonly detected segment has been identified by other investigators (95). We have detected no mutations of the remaining *EGR1* or *CDC25C* alleles, suggesting that a novel tumor suppressor gene in 5q31 is involved in the pathogenesis of t-AML characterized by a del(5q) (94).

Boultwood and coworkers examined three patients with the 5q− syndrome who had small deletions extending from q31-q33 and identified a commonly deleted segment of about 3 Mb between *ADRB2* and *NKSF1,* which included the gene encoding the receptor for CSF1 (FMS) (96). This region is distal to that identified in other studies (94,95), suggesting that there is probably more than one region and gene involved in the pathogenesis of myeloid disorders associated with abnormalities of chromosome 5. Whether the putative tumor suppressor gene in 5q33 is involved in myeloid leukemias or is restricted to the 5q− syndrome is unknown.

Molecular analysis of the deletions of 7q has revealed that the deletions are interstitial, and that there may be two distinct deleted segments of chromosome 7. Eighty percent of patients have a commonly deleted segment within q22; however, a smaller group have a distal deletion with loss of q32-33. By using probes from 7q for FISH analysis, the commonly deleted segment at 7q22 has been narrowed to 2 to 3 Mb flanked by the markers D7S1503 and D7S1841 (97). Using similar techniques, Fischer and colleagues identified a slightly more distal, but overlapping, commonly deleted segment on 7q (98). Mutations of candidate tumor suppressor genes in this interval have not been found; thus, 7q22 may contain a novel gene involved in myeloid leukemogenesis.

ACUTE LYMPHOBLASTIC LEUKEMIA

The most useful prognostic indicators in ALL, which is the most common leukemia in children, are age, WBC count, immunophenotype, karyotype (including ploidy), and CNS status (26,99). Children who are between 2 and 10 years old, who have a WBC count of less than 10,000/μL, and whose leukemia cells express the common ALL antigen (CALLA, CD10) have the best prognosis (see Chapter 46). A number of recurring cytogenetic abnormalities are associated with distinct immunologic phenotypes of ALL (Table 10.5) with distinct outcomes (26,99–102).

This review includes data on the chromosomal patterns of 330 patients evaluated at the Third International Workshop (26,103), as well as four other large series of 443 adults (104) and 547 children (105–107). A high proportion (~85%) of ALL patients have clonal abnormalities. There are notable differences in the frequency of the t(9;22) and hyperdiploidy (>50 chromosomes) between children and adults. The t(9; 22) is observed in 5% of children and in 30% of adults with ALL, whereas a hyperdiploid karyotype is found in 30% of children but rarely in adults (2% to 5%). The presence of the t(4;11) or t(9;22) are associated with treatment failure, whereas the t(12;21) and hyperdiploidy are associated with a favorable outcome.

Specific Abnormalities

The 8;14 Translocation

A reciprocal translocation involving the long arms of chromosomes 8 and 14 [t(8;14)(q24;q32)] is observed in a high proportion of Burkitt's tumors of African and non-African origin (Fig. 10.3C). An identical translocation is found in patients with B-cell ALL (L3), indicating that Burkitt's lymphoma and B-cell ALL are probably different manifestations of the same disease (Table 10.5). This group of patients has a high incidence of CNS involvement and of abdominal nodal involvement at diagnosis. Although the outcome for children with the t(8;14) has been poor, event-free survival (EFS) of 80% is possible now with intensive chemotherapy (108). A poor outcome was observed in a series of 21 adult patients with a t(8;14) (62% CR; median EFS, 2 months) (104); however, the use of short duration, high intensity chemotherapy programs has markedly improved the outcomes of patients with B-cell ALL (109).

Variant translocations have been reported in Burkitt's lymphoma and B-cell ALL [t(2;8)(p12;q24) and t(8;22)(q24; q11)]. The first chromosomal abnormalities to be analyzed at the molecular level were the three translocations characteristic of L3 leukemia and Burkitt's lymphoma (described in the later section on lymphomas).

TABLE 10.5. *Cytogenetic-imunophenotypic correlations in malignant lymphoid diseases*

Phenotype	Chromosome abnormality	Frequency[a]	Involved genes[b]	
Acute lymphoblastic leukemia				
Precursor B	t(12;21)(p12;q22)	25%	*TEL*	*AML1*
	t(9;22)(q34;q11)	10%[c]	*ABL*	*BCR*
	t(4;11)(q21;q23)	5%	*AF4*	*MLL*
	t(17;19)(q21–22;p13)	1%	*HLF*	*E2A*
	t(11;19)(q23;p13.3)	1%	*MLL*	*ENL*
Pre-B	t(1;19)(q23;p13)	6% (30%)	*PBX1*	*TCF3 (E2A)*
B (sIg⁺)	t(8;14)(q24;q32)	5% (95%)	*MYC*	*IGH*
	t(2;8)(p12;q24)	<1% (1%)	*IGK*	*MYC*
	t(8;22)(q24;q11)	<1% (4%)	*MYC*	*IGL*
	dic(9;12)(p11;p12)	1%		
Other	hyperdiploidy (50–60 chromosomes)	10%		
	del(9p),t(9p)	10%		
	del(12p),t(12p)	10%		
T	t(11;14)(p15;q11)	1%	*RBTN1*	*TCRA*
	t(11;14)(p13;q11)	3%	*RBTN2*	*TCRA*
	t(8;14)(q24;q11)	<1%	*MYC*	*TCRA*
	inv(14)(q11q32)	<1%	*TCRA*	*IGH*
	inv(14)(q11q32)	<1%	*TCRA*	*TCL1*
	t(10;14)(q24;q11)	3%	*HOX11*	*TCRA*
	t(1;14)(p34;q11)	<1%	*LCK*	*TCRD*
	t(1;14)(p32;q11)	1%	*TAL1*	*TCRD*
	t(7;9)(q34–35;q32)		*TCRB*	*TAL2*
	t(7;9)(q34–35;q34)	2%	*TCRB*	*TAN1*
	t(7;7)(p15;q11)		*TCRG*	
	t(14;14)(q11;q32)	*<1%*	*TCRA*	*IGH*
	t(7;14)(q34–35;q11)	<1%	*TCRB*	*TCRD*
	t(7;14)(p15;q11)	<1%		
	t(7;19)(q34–35;p13)	<1%		
	del(9p),t(9p)	<1% (10%)	*CDKN2A*	
Non-Hodgkin's lymphoma				
B-cell NHL				
Burkitt	t(8;14)(q24;q32)	95%	*MYC*	*IGH*
	t(2;8)(p12;q24)	1%	*IGK*	*MYC*
	t(8;22)(q24;q11)	4%	*MYC*	*IGL*
Follicular SNCL	t(14;18)(q32;q21)	80%	*IGH*	*BCL2*
DLCL		20%		
DLCL	t(3;22)(q27;q11)	45% for all	*BCL6*	*IGL*
	t(3;14)(q27;q32)	t(3q27)	*BCL6*	*IGH*
	t(3q27)		*BCL6*	
MCL	t(11;14)(q13;q32)		*CCND1*	*IGH*
LPL	t(9;14)(p13;q32)		*PAX5*	*IGH*
SLL	t(14;19)(q32;q13.3)		*IGH*	*BCL3*
MALT	t(11;18)(q21;q21)		*API2*	*MALT1*
T-cell NHL				
(CD30⁺) NHL ALCL	t(2;5)(p23;q35)	75%	*ALK*	*NPM*
Other	see T-cell ALL			
	t(4;16)(q26;p13.1)	>1%	*IL2*	*BCM*
CTCL	t(10q24)		*LYT10*	
Chronic lymphocytic leukemia				
B	t(11;14)(q13;q32)	10%	*CCND1*	*IGH*
	t(14;19)(q32;q13)	10%	*IGH*	*BCL3*
	t(2;14)(p13;q32)	5%		*IGH*
	t(14q32)	20%		
	del(13q)	30%		
	+12	30%		

(continued)

TABLE 10.5. *Continued.*

Phenotype	Chromosome abnormality	Frequency[a]	Involved genes[b]	
T	t(8;14)(q24;q11)	5%	*MYC*	*TCRA*
	inv(14)(q11q32)	5%	*TCRA/D*	*IGH*
	inv(14)(q11q32)	5%	*TCRA/D*	*TCL1*
Multiple myeloma				
B	t(11;14)(q13;q32)	10%	*CCND1*	*IGH*
	t(14q32)			
Adult T-cell leukemia/lymphoma				
	t(14;14)(q11;q32)		*TCRA*	*IGH*
	inv(14)(q11q32)		*TCRA/D*	*IGH*
	+3			

ALCL, anaplastic large cell lymphoma; CTCL, cutaneous T-cell lymphoma; DLCL, diffuse large B-cell lymphomas; Ki-1, anti-CD30 antibody; LPL, lymphoplasmacytoid lymphoma; MALT, mucosa-associated lymphoid tumor; MCL, mantle cell lymphoma; sIg, surface immunoglobulin; SLL, small lymphocytic lymphoma; SNCL, small noncleaved cell lymphoma.

[a] The percentage refers to the frequency within the disease overall. The number in the parentheses refers to the frequency within the morphological or immunological subtype of the disease.

[b] Genes are listed in order of citation in karyotype; for example, for precursor B ALL, *TEL* is at 12p12 and *AML1* at 21q22.

[c] By cytogenetic analysis, the frequency in children is about 5%, and in adults is about 25%; using molecular probes this frequency is 30% in adults.

The 4;11 Translocation

Translocations involving 11q23 are observed in 5% to 7% of ALL patients (26,104,105). Of these, the most common is the t(4;11)(q21;q23) (Fig. 10.3A). The t(11;19)(q23; p13.3) is second in frequency; however, this rearrangement is not limited to ALL in that about 50% of these cases have AML, usually AML-M5. Patients with the t(4;11) have high leukocyte counts (median WBC, 183,000/μL), L1 or L2 morphology, an immature precursor B phenotype (CD10−CD19+), with coexpression of monocytic or, less commonly, T-cell markers (99,104,110–112). Clinically, they have aggressive features with hyperleukocytosis, extramedullary disease, and a poor response to conventional chemotherapy. In one series, adults with the t(4;11) had a CR rate of 75% but a median EFS of only 7 months (104). Children with the t(4;11) have a similarly poor outcome (26,105–107,110–112).

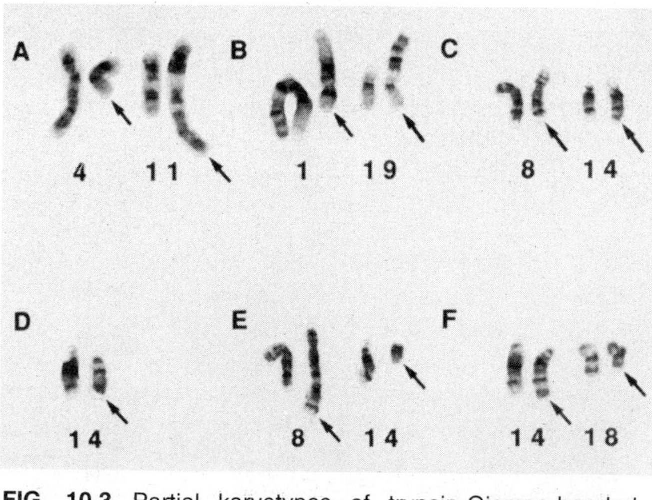

FIG. 10.3. Partial karyotypes of trypsin-Giemsa-banded metaphase cells depicting nonrandom chromosomal rearrangements *(arrows)* observed in lymphoid malignant diseases. **A:** t(4;11) (q21;q23) in acute myeloid leukemia (ALL). **B:** t(1;19) (q23;p13) in pre-B-cell ALL. **C:** t(8;14) (q24;q32) in B-cell ALL and Burkitt's lymphoma. **D:** inv(14) (q11q32) in T-cell leukemia/lymphoma. **E:** t(8;14) (q24;q11) in T-cell leukemia/lymphoma. **F:** t(14;18) (q32;q21) in B-cell non-Hodgkin's lymphoma (NHL).

Acute leukemia with the t(4;11) may express myeloid antigens (~50% of cases). In most cases, blasts have been described as lymphoid in appearance, but occasional blasts may appear monocytic, and in some patients, populations of lymphoid and monocytoid blasts may occur in approximately equal proportion. Positive staining for myeloperoxidase or with Sudan black B may be present in some cases, and the nonspecific esterase reaction may be positive in variable numbers of cells (53). These leukemia cells are generally terminal deoxynucleotidyl transferase (TdT) positive, and they have expressed pan-B-cell antigens in most cases studied (53). CD10 is positive in some instances.

Between 60% and 80% of translocations involve 11q23 in infant ALL; this association is particularly interesting in view of the low incidence of ALL in this age group (acute leukemias in this very young age group are usually of the myeloid type) (26,110). As described earlier, the breakpoint on 11q23 involves the *MLL* gene. Several studies have examined the frequency of *MLL* rearrangements in infant ALL using Southern blot analysis (110,111) or RT-PCR (112) to detect the t(4;11). These studies revealed *MLL* rearrangements in 70% and 81%, respectively, including some cases that were normal or inadequate by cytogenetic analysis. Abnormalities of *MLL* were associated with early treatment failure and a very poor outcome (111,112); in one series, the estimated EFS for patients with *MLL* rearrangements was 19% at 3 years, compared with 46% for patients with germline *MLL* (111). Among patients with *MLL* rearrangements, the t(4;11) may confer a particularly poor prognosis, and some investigators have recommended intensified therapy, including bone marrow transplantation, for this group of patients (112). Rearrangements affecting *MLL* represent a major class of mutations in acute leukemia, and identify patients with a poor outcome.

The 9;22 Translocation in Acute Lymphoblastic Leukemia

Ph+ leukemia occurs in two major forms, CML (described in an earlier section) and ALL. The incidence of Ph+ patients with ALL is 30% in adults and 5% in children. The Ph chromosome is the most frequent rearrangement in adult ALL. The incidence of three-way translocations is 8%, which is similar to that observed in CML patients. About one half of the patients show abnormalities in addition to the Ph chromosome, a frequency that is substantially higher than that observed in CML in the chronic phase. With the exception of trisomy 8 which is seen occasionally, these abnormalities differ from those observed in the acute phase of CML. Monosomy 7 is a common secondary abnormality in Ph+ ALL and is associated with a poorer outcome (113). A chromosomally normal cell line is frequently noted in the bone marrow of Ph+ ALL patients (70%), whereas normal cells are rarely observed in untreated CML patients.

The results of studies using newer immunophenotyping techniques have suggested that Ph+ ALL is of precursor B lineage; however, some cases have had B-cell and myeloid markers (102,114). The disease in adults and children is characterized by high WBC counts, a high percentage of circulating blasts, and a poor prognosis. In a prospective Cancer and Leukemia Group B study, the median age of Ph+ and Ph− patients was similar (39 versus 37 years). The CR rate did not differ (71% versus 77%); however, median remission duration (10 versus 18 months) and survival (11 versus 22 months) were considerably shorter for Ph+ patients (114).

Molecular studies of Ph+ ALL have revealed that there are two distinct subgroups of patients. In the first group (~30% of adult cases), the molecular rearrangement is identical to that observed in CML, in that the breaks occur within the *ABL* gene and within the bcr of the *BCR* gene, giving rise to a chimeric 8.5-kb message and a 210 kilodalton (kd) fusion protein. In the remaining patients, the breakpoint occurs upstream (5′) of bcr but still within the *BCR* gene, giving rise to smaller fusion messages (6.5 to 7.4 kb) and smaller proteins (185 to 190 kd) (115). The clinical outcomes for both groups of patients appear to be similar. We do not know whether the structural difference in the 210- and 185-kd proteins correspond to functional differences in the leukemia cells. Both proteins are involved in constitutive signaling through the RAS pathway of signal transduction. Mice transplanted with cells transfected with $p185^{BCR/ABL}$ develop tumors more rapidly than those transplanted with $p210^{BCR/ABL}$ containing bone marrow cells. Such a functional difference might account for the biologic and clinical differences of Ph+ ALL which, although characterized by the same chromosomal abnormality, is distinct from CML. Patients in whom the Ph chromosome is restricted to lymphoblasts have shorter survivals than those with multilineage involvement (23,24).

The 1;19 Translocation

In 1978, pre-B-cell ALL was recognized as a distinct immunologic subtype of ALL, which can be distinguished from null-cell and B-cell ALL by the presence of cytoplasmic immunoglobulin μ-chain (C_μ) expression. A reciprocal translocation involving chromosomes 1 and 19 [t(1;19)(q23;p13)] is associated with pre-B-cell ALL (30% of pre-B-cell ALL cases and 6% of all ALL cases) (Fig. 10.3B). A characteristic surface antigen profile is CD19+, CD10+, CD22+, CD34−, and CD20+/−. Patients with the t(1;19) have low WBC counts, but experience early treatment failure; this translocation distinguishes a subgroup of patients with pre-B-cell ALL who have a poor prognosis (116,117). In one large study, the adverse outcome of patients with the t(1;19) remained significant even after adjustment for recognized adverse clinical features, indicating that it is an independent risk factor (117). The t(1;19) occurs in two forms: a reciprocal translocation, t(1;19)(q23;p13) noted in 25% of cases and an unbalanced form characterized by two normal chromosome 1 and 19 homologues, and a rearranged chromosome 19, der(19)t(1;19)(q23;p13) (75%). Presenting clinical and laboratory features as well as EFS appear to be the same for these two subtypes (116,117).

The t(1;19) involves the *E2A* gene at 19p13, which encodes two transcription factors (E12 and E47), which bind to enhancer elements in the *IGK* gene, as well as the regulatory elements of other genes (118,119). The breakpoint on 1q occurs within *PBX1*, a homeobox *(HOX)* gene. *HOX* genes encode DNA-binding transcription factors that regulate developmental processes. *E2A/PBX1* fusion mRNAs are formed and code for a chimeric protein that consists of the transcriptional activating domain of E12/E47 and the DNA-binding and protein dimerization domains of PBX1 (118,119). The *E2A* and *PBX1* genes are expressed in multiple tissues, but PBX1 is not expressed in lymphoid cells. PBX1 normally forms complexes with select HOX proteins, which then regulate transcription of target genes in a positive or negative manner (118,119). The E2A/PBX1 fusion protein is a potent transactivator and may directly activate gene transcription of PBX1-HOX complex target genes or of E2A target genes. Alternatively, PBX-HOX complexes formed with other ubiquitously expressed PBX family members, PBX2 and PBX3, may normally inhibit transcription, whereas E2A/PBX1/HOX complexes may induce transcription of genes normally repressed in lymphoid cells. In each of these scenarios, the presence of the E2A/PBX1 fusion protein may result in the transactivation of a cadre of genes that are not normally expressed in lymphoid tissues.

The 12;21 Translocation in Precursor B-Cell Acute Lymphoblastic Leukemia

A recurring translocation, t(12;21)(p12;q22), has been identified in a high proportion (~25%) of childhood B-lineage ALL cases, specifically precursor B leukemia (120,121). The translocation is not easily detected by cytogenetic analysis because of the similarity in size and banding pattern of 12p and 21q. However, the rearrangement can be detected reliably using RT-PCR or FISH analysis (121). The t(12;21) defines a distinct subgroup of patients characterized by an age between 1 and 10 years, B-lineage immunophenotype (CD10+CD19+), and a favorable outcome (120,122). It is not seen in T-cell ALL and is uncommon in adults (~4% of ALL cases). In one series, patients with the t(12;21) had a 5-year EFS of 91%, compared with 65% for patients without this rearrangement (122). One half of these patients would have fallen into a high-risk group using standard risk factors; the presence of this rearrangement therefore may identify a subset of patients within the high-risk group who would benefit from well-tolerated, less toxic, antimetabolite therapy.

The t(12;21) fuses the *TEL* gene at 12p12 with the *AML1* gene at 21q22, and results in the production of a fusion protein (Fig. 10.2) (123). TEL is a ubiquitously expressed 453 amino acid protein that contains two domains found in other ETS family transcription factors: a helix-loop-helix (HLH) protein dimerization domain and an ETS DNA binding domain. The consequence of the translocation is fusion of the 5′ HLH domain of TEL with the 3′ DNA-binding and transactivation domain of the AML1 transcription factor (123). By means of the HLH domain, TEL/AML1 can form homodimers as well as heterodimers with the TEL protein (123). Moreover, TEL/AML1 inhibits transactivation of genes by the normal AML1 protein. In most ALL cases with the t(12;21), the *TEL* allele on the other chromosome 12 homologue is deleted. Alteration of both *TEL* alleles suggests that TEL may be a negative regulator of cell proliferation, i.e., a tumor suppressor gene. The *TEL* gene is also involved in several other recurring translocations, t(5;12)(q33;p12) in CMMoL, t(9;12)(q34;p12) in AML, ALL, and CML, and t(12;22)(p12;q11) in myeloproliferative disorders, suggesting that interference with the regulation of TEL target genes plays a significant role in leukemogenesis.

Hyperdiploidy with 50 to 60 Chromosomes

The leukemia cells of some patients with ALL are characterized by a gain of many chromosomes. Two distinct subgroups are recognized: a group with one to four extra chromosomes (47–50) and the more common group with more than 50 chromosomes. Chromosome numbers usually range from 51 to 60, and a few patients may have up to 65 chromosomes. Hyperdiploidy (>50 chromosomes) is common in children (~30%) but is rarely observed in adults (<5%). Certain additional chromosomes are common (X chromosome, and chromosomes 4,6,10,14,17,18, and 21) (124,125). Chromosome 21 is gained most frequently (100% of cases), and multiple additional copies of this chromosome are common (26,124,125).

Patients who have hyperdiploidy with more than 50 chromosomes have all of the previously recognized clinical factors that indicate a good prognosis, including age between 1 and 9 years, low WBC count (median, 6,700/μL), and favorable immunophenotype (i.e., early pre-B or pre-B) (26,99). In an analysis of 186 children with hyperdiploid ALL, Raimondi and colleagues suggested that ALL defined by 51 to 55 compared with 56 to 65 chromosomes may be distinct clinical entities (126). The 105 patients in the first group (51 to 55 chromosomes) had an EFS at 5 years of 72% compared with 86% ($p = 0.04$) for patients with more than 56 chromosomes (63 patients). Structural rearrangements occur in hyperdiploid ALL cells more frequently than was previously recognized, perhaps in as many as 50% of cases (126). The most common are duplication of 1q (15%) and an i(17q) (5%) (126). The t(9;22) and t(1;19) have also been observed. Overall, the presence of structural abnormalities does not appear to influence EFS; however, specific recurring abnormalities, such as the t(9;22), have a poor prognosis (126). The cellular mechanisms giving rise to hyperdiploidy and the molecular consequences are unknown.

T-Cell Acute Lymphoblastic Leukemia

A distinct pattern of recurring karyotypic abnormalities in T-cell neoplasms has emerged (102). Rearrangements involving 14q11 (Fig. 10.3D,E) and two regions of chromosome 7 (7q34-35 and 7q15) are particularly frequent in T-cell malignancies (Table 10.5). The most common are the t(11;14) (p13;q11) (~3%), t(10;11)(q24;q11) (~3%), and t(7;9)(q34-35;q34) (~2%) (1,102). In addition to their occurrence in T-cell leukemia, these T-cell–specific abnormalities have been observed in lymphomas of T-cell origin. The genes that are located at the breakpoints of a number of these abnormalities have been identified and are described in a later section (Table 10.5). Patients with T-cell ALL are most often young males and often have a mediastinal tumor mass, high WBC count, and leukemia cells in the cerebrospinal fluid. These same clinical characteristics are associated with lymphoblastic lymphoma, another T-cell malignancy (see Chapters 26 and 46).

MALIGNANT LYMPHOPROLIFERATIVE DISORDERS

Cytogenetic analyses of NHL have been reported in a number of large series (127–134). These investigations have demonstrated that a high proportion of cases (>90%) are characterized by clonal chromosomal abnormalities and, more importantly, many of the recurring abnormalities correlate with histology and immunophenotype (Table 10.5). For example, the t(14;18) is observed in a high proportion of follicular small cleaved cell lymphomas (70% to 90%), most patients with a t(3;22)(q27;q11) or t(3;14)(q27;q32) have diffuse large B-cell lymphomas, and patients with a t(8;14)(q24;q32) have Burkitt's or diffuse large B-cell lymphomas (DLCLs). Band 14q32, the location of the Ig heavy-chain gene *(IGH)* is frequently involved in translocations in B-cell neoplasms (~70%). In contrast, a large proportion of neoplasms of T-cell origin are characterized by rearrangements that involve 14q11,7q34-35, or 7p15, the locations of the T-cell receptor genes, *TCRA/D, TCRB,* and *TCRG,* respectively.

Burkitt's Lymphoma

In 1972, Manolov and Manolova identified a consistent abnormality (14q+) in the cells of fresh Burkitt's lymphomas and in cultured cell lines. Several years later, Zech and associates suggested that the rearrangement was a reciprocal translocation involving chromosomes 8 and 14, t(8;14)(q24;q32). The t(8;14) is characteristic of endemic and nonendemic Burkitt tumors, as well as Epstein-Barr virus (EBV)–negative (EBV^-) and EBV^+ tumors. The t(8;14) has also been observed in other B-cell lymphomas, particularly small noncleaved cell (non-Burkitt) and large cell immunoblastic lymphomas, acquired immunodeficiency syndrome (AIDS)–associated Burkitt's lymphomas (100%), and AIDS-related DLCLs (30%) (128,131–136,137). As additional Burkitt tumors were examined, it became apparent that at least two other related translocations occur: t(2;8)(p12;q24) and t(8;22)(q24;q11). All three translocations involve chromosome band 8q24. These same translocations have been seen in some patients with B-cell ALL.

The t(8;14) involves a break within the *IGH* locus on chromosome 14 and a break 5′ or within *MYC* on chromosome 8 and relocates the *MYC*-coding exons to chromosome 14 in a "head to head" orientation. The translocations correlate roughly with the two forms of Burkitt's lymphomas: endemic Burkitt's lymphomas usually have breaks upstream of *MYC,* whereas sporadic or AIDS-related Burkitt's lymphomas usually contain breaks within *MYC* (137). *MYC* plays a role in a number of cellular processes, including proliferation, and apoptosis, and its oncogenic properties result from its constitutive expression. *In vitro* and *in vivo* studies have demonstrated its transforming abilities: expression of *MYC* results in the transformation of EBV-immortalized B-cell lines, whereas Eμ-*Myc* transgenic mice frequently develop lymphoblastic lymphoma (138). The biologic function of MYC resides in two regions. The amino terminus is important in activating gene transcription, whereas the carboxyl terminus contains a basic-HLH-leucine zipper domain that promotes interaction with a related protein, MAX. Binding to MAX appears to be essential for the transforming activity of MYC. MAX has been shown to have two other partners that are important in regulating its function: MAD and MXI1. Both of these proteins are thought to influence MYC-mediated activation of target genes by binding to MAX and sequestering it from forming complexes with MYC, or by competing with MYC-MAX heterodimers for binding to common target sites (139).

The 14;18 Translocation

Between 70% and 90% of follicular lymphomas and 20% of diffuse B-cell lymphomas have the t(14;18) (Fig. 10.3F) in which the *BCL2* gene at 18q21 is juxtaposed to the *IGH* J segment (127,137), leading to the deregulated expression of *BCL2* (127,140). Other lymphocytic malignancies that overexpress *BCL2* but do not harbor the t(14;18) include hairy cell leukemia and chronic lymphocytic leukemia (CLL). The cloning of this gene led to the discovery of a new class of oncogenes, which instead of promoting proliferation, contribute to development of a neoplastic state by preventing programmed cell death (141).

The *BCL2* gene encodes a 26-kd membrane protein that functions to increase cell survival (141). For example, BCL2 protects lymphoid cells against a number of apoptotic stimuli including γ-irradiation, glucocorticoids, and the cross linking of cell surface receptors. Targeted gene disruption studies have shown that BCL2 is required for survival beyond the first few weeks of life. *Bcl2* −/− mice develop polycystic kidney disease, hair hypopigmentation, and immunodeficiency as a result of massive B- and T-lymphocyte death (141). Transgenic mice containing a *Bcl2-Ig* minigene develop polyclonal follicular hyperplasia, and some, after a long latency, develop high-grade lymphomas, many of which possessed translocations involving Myc (142). Many normal individuals harbor the t(14;18) in tonsils and peripheral blood lymphocytes (143). These findings suggest that the t(14;18) occurs as an early event in the multistep process of lymphomagenesis. Moreover, *BCL2* overexpression is not transforming per se but requires the presence of other transforming events, such as *MYC* or *TP53* mutations. Such mutations may accumulate in those cells that fail to undergo cell death.

BCL2 interacts with other proteins, specifically BAX and BAD, which regulate its function (144). BAX dimerizes with itself and with BCL2, and the ratio of BCL2 to BAX determines the likelihood of a cell undergoing apoptosis on exposure to a given stimulus. In cells in which BAX is overexpressed, apoptosis is accelerated, whereas in cells in which BCL2 is overexpressed, heterodimers with BAX predominate, and cell death is repressed.

The prognostic significance of having the t(14;18) or overexpressing *BCL2* is unclear. One study suggested that rearrangements in the major breakpoint region of the *BCL2* gene were associated with a shorter disease-free period in extranodal lymphomas but this remains to be confirmed (145). Another study examining DLCL showed that high levels of *BCL2* expression predicted for a shorter disease-free survival

(146). The biologic basis for the poorer prognosis may be that such cells have increased resistance to chemotherapeutic drugs.

The 11;14 Translocation

The t(11;14) (q13;q32) is observed in mantle cell lymphoma (147). In most series, the percentages of cases having the t(11;14) by molecular analysis have varied between 30% to 55% of cases, but these may be underestimates as only the major breakpoint cluster regions have been looked for. Besides mantle cell lymphomas, the t(11;14) has also been reported in 3% of multiple myeloma, and up to 20% of prolymphocytic leukemias (147). Mantle cell lymphomas are currently regarded as a poor prognostic group with a median survival from diagnosis of 3 years (see Chapter 22).

This translocation results in the activation of the cyclin D1 *(CCND1)* gene by the *IGH* gene (148). The *CCND1* gene is located 100 to 130 kb away from the breakpoint on 11q13. The D-type cyclins act as growth factor sensors, causing cells to go through the restriction start point of the cell cycle at G_1 and committing them to divide. CCND1 together with activated cyclin dependent kinase 4 (CDK4) phosphorylates and inactivates RB1, releasing from it E2F, a transcription factor responsible for activating a series of genes required for cell division (149). The ectopic expression of *CCND1* under the control of the Eμ promoter in mice is not transforming per se, because Eμ-CCND1 mice do not develop lymphoma. In lymphoid cells, the oncogenic ability of *CCND1* appears to depend on synergy with other oncogenes, specifically *MYC* (150). Circumstantial evidence of its involvement in other tumors are the frequent amplifications of 11q13 and overexpression of *CCND1* in solid tumors, including head and neck, esophageal, bladder, breast, small cell lung, and hepatocellular carcinomas (149).

Translocations of 3q27

The *BCL6* gene was cloned from the recurring breakpoint at 3q27 in cells characterized by a t(3;22)(q27;q11), t(3; 14)(q27;q32) or, rarely, t(2;3)(p12;q27) (151,152). *BCL6* rearrangements occur in 40% of DLCLs and, in some series, up to 10% of follicular lymphomas. Two retrospective studies have assessed the clinical significance of *BCL6* rearrangements. One found a more favorable outcome in terms of survival and freedom from progression among diffuse lymphomas with a large cell component (153), whereas the other failed to confirm these findings (154). The prognostic significance of *BCL6* rearrangements is unclear.

The translocations lead to the truncation of the *BCL6* gene within the first exon or the first intron, substitution of its promoter sequences with an *IG* promoter, and deregulated expression. The *BCL6* gene product is a 96-kd nuclear protein that is predominantly expressed in the B-cell lineage, particularly in mature B cells, but not in immature bone marrow precursors or the more mature plasma cell. The protein contains six zinc-finger motifs and an N-terminal POZ domain, which in related proteins have been shown to regulate the DNA binding of zinc-finger proteins. BCL6 has been shown to be a potent transcriptional repressor. A role in germinal center formation is suggested by topographic restriction of *BCL6* expression to germinal centers in normal human lymphoid tissue and the fact that mice with targeted disruptions of *Bcl6* are incapable of forming germinal centers (155).

T-Cell Non-Hodgkin's Lymphoma

A number of recurring chromosomal abnormalities have been recognized in T-cell leukemias and lymphomas (Table 10.5). Similar to B-cell neoplasms, in which rearrangements frequently involve the chromosomal bands containing the immunoglobulin gene loci, T-cell neoplasms often have rearrangements involving band q11 of chromosome 14, the site of the T-cell receptor α-chain and δ-chain genes *(TCRA, TCRD)* (127,137) or, less often, one of two regions of chromosome 7 (7q34-35 and 7p15) to which the T-cell receptor β-chain *(TCRB)* and γ-chain *(TCRG)* genes have been localized, respectively (1,2) (Table 10.5). With few exceptions, the involved gene on the partner chromosome encodes a transcription factor, whose expression is deregulated or activated as a result of the rearrangement (3,4) (Table 10.5). These studies indicate that, perhaps as a result of their capacity to be specifically rearranged, transcribed, and mutated in B cells or in T cells, the immunoglobulin and T-cell receptor gene loci are appropriate DNA sequences to mediate the activation of cellular oncogenes. A chromosomal rearrangement which brings an oncogene under the controlling influence of promoters or enhancers that are active for immunoglobulin synthesis in B cells or T-cell receptor synthesis in T cells may as a consequence impart a proliferative advantage to that cell and result in malignant clonal expansion. These translocations are believed to result from aberrant recombination events during V-D-J recombination.

CD30-Positive Anaplastic Large Cell Lymphomas

A distinctive subtype of NHL, namely, $CD30^+$ anaplastic large cell lymphoma (ALCL) has been characterized during the past few years. CD30 is observed in nearly all cases of Hodgkin's disease; however, this antigen is also expressed by a variable proportion of lymphoma cells in a variety of NHL subtypes. A subset of NHL with distinctive clinical and morphologic features is strongly $CD30^+$. These patients tend to be young, and they present with skin or lymph node infiltration (or both) by large, often bizarre lymphoma cells, which preferentially involve the paracortical areas and lymph node sinuses (156). Most such tumors express one or more T-cell antigens, a minority express B-cell antigens, and some express T- and B-cell antigens (i.e., null phenotype) (see Chapter 25).

A reciprocal translocation, t(2;5)(p23;q35), appears to be

restricted to ALCL of T-cell or null phenotype and is present in a high percentage of these cases (157). Since its initial description in ALCL, this translocation has also been found in the CD30+ primary cutaneous lymphomas and the related entity of lymphomatoid papulosis, suggesting a common pathogenesis of these cutaneous disorders with ALCL. The initial report that the fusion transcript resulting from the t(2;5) was also present in the Reed-Sternberg (RS) cells of some Hodgkin's disease cases has not been confirmed, and the consensus is that, at the cytogenetic and molecular level, the t(2;5) and resultant fusion gene are absent in RS cells (158). The molecular consequence of the translocation is the production of a unique fusion protein, resulting from the fusion of the nucleophosmin *(NPM)* gene on 5q35 to a tyrosine protein kinase gene *(ALK)* on 2p23. *ALK* encodes a tyrosine kinase that is normally expressed in intestine, testis, and brain but not in normal lymphoid cells (159). The NPM/ALK fusion protein is localized to the cytoplasm and is able to transform NIH 3T3 cells, suggesting that the translocation is the primary transforming event in ALCL (160). The intracellular targets for phosphorylation by normal ALK and for the fusion protein have yet to be elucidated.

Other Lymphoproliferative Disorders

Our understanding of the cytogenetic pattern of malignant lymphoproliferative disorders other than those already discussed is poor. In part, this results from the low proliferative rate and the inability to stimulate mitoses in the malignant lymphoid cells without also stimulating cell division in the residual normal T or B lymphocytes. Karyotypes have most often been reported to be normal in patients with CLL, multiple myeloma, or hairy cell leukemia.

Trisomy 12 is the most common cytogenetic abnormality reported in patients with B-cell CLL; it is found in 20% to 60% of those with a cytogenetic abnormality (161). Abnormalities involving band 14q32 are also common, such as t(14;19)(q32;q13) (162) (Table 10.5). Unfortunately, only one half of patients with B-CLL have an adequate number of metaphase cells in unstimulated cultures for thorough evaluation. Several groups have shown that FISH is a simple and sensitive method for detecting trisomy 12 in interphase CLL cells; 30% of patients have trisomy 12, and this abnormality is associated with a poorer survival (163). Similarly, a del(13q) can be detected in 30% of CLL cases using FISH.

Chronic T-cell leukemia (T-CLL) and large granular lymphocytic leukemia are uncommon disorders in which the malignant mature lymphocytes have a T-cell immunophenotype. Rearrangements involving band 14q11 with or without an accompanying break in 14q32 have been reported in T-CLL as well as other T-cell lymphomas (1–3) (Table 10.5). The most common is an inv(14)(q11q32).

NEW TECHNIQUES TO DETECT CHROMOSOMAL ABNORMALITIES

Cytogenetic analysis of human tumors is often technically difficult because of the presence of multiple abnormal cell lines and the complexity of the chromosomal pattern, and requires highly skilled personnel. These factors have led investigators to seek alternative methods for identifying chromosomal abnormalities, such as Southern blot analysis of DNA, RT-PCR analysis of RNA from tumor cells, or FISH (164).

The technique of FISH is based on the same principle as Southern blot analysis, namely, the ability of single stranded DNA to anneal to complementary DNA. In the case of FISH, the target DNA is the nuclear DNA of interphase cells, or the DNA of metaphase chromosomes that are affixed to a glass microscope slide. FISH can also be accomplished with bone marrow or peripheral blood smears, or fixed and sectioned tissue. The test probe is labeled with biotin- or digoxigenin-labeled nucleotides, and detected with fluorescein isothiocyanate- or CY3-conjugated avidin or rhodamine-labeled anti-digoxigenin antibodies. Probes that are directly labeled with fluorochrome are also available for hybridization, thereby simplifying the technique by eliminating the probe detection steps. With the development of dual- and triple-pass filters, most laboratories now have the capacity to detect two or three probes simultaneously.

Several types of probes can be used to detect chromosomal abnormalities by FISH. Hybridization of centromere-specific probes has been used to detect monosomy, trisomy and other aneuploidies in leukemias and solid tumors (Fig. 10.4; see also Color Plate 1, between pp. 1446–1447). Chromosome-specific libraries, which paint the chromosomes, are particularly useful in identifying marker chromosomes (rearranged chromosomes of unidentified origin), or structural rearrangements, such as translocations. Translocations and deletions can also be identified in interphase or metaphase cells by using genomic probes that are derived from the breakpoints of recurring translocations or within the deleted segment. The newest innovation in FISH technology is spectral karyotyping, or multiplex FISH (165). Using this approach, 24 differentially labeled painting probes representing each chromosome are cohybridized; Fourier spectroscopy is used to distinguish each spectrally overlapping probe, and imaging software assigns a unique color to each chromosome. Often referred to as "color karyotyping," this method is applicable to the identification of numeric abnormalities and to many structural abnormalities.

FISH techniques have a number of applications (Table 10.6). In some cases, FISH analysis provides more sensitivity in that cytogenetic abnormalities have been identified by FISH in samples that appeared to be normal by morphology and conventional cytogenetic analyses. FISH is most powerful when the analysis is targeted toward those abnormalities that are known to be associated with a particular tumor or disease. Cytogenetic analysis could be performed at the time of diagnosis to identify the chromosomal abnormalities in an individual patient's malignant cells. Thereafter, FISH with the appropriate probes could be used to detect residual disease or early relapse, and to assess the efficacy of therapeutic regimens. For example, the use of FISH to detect the

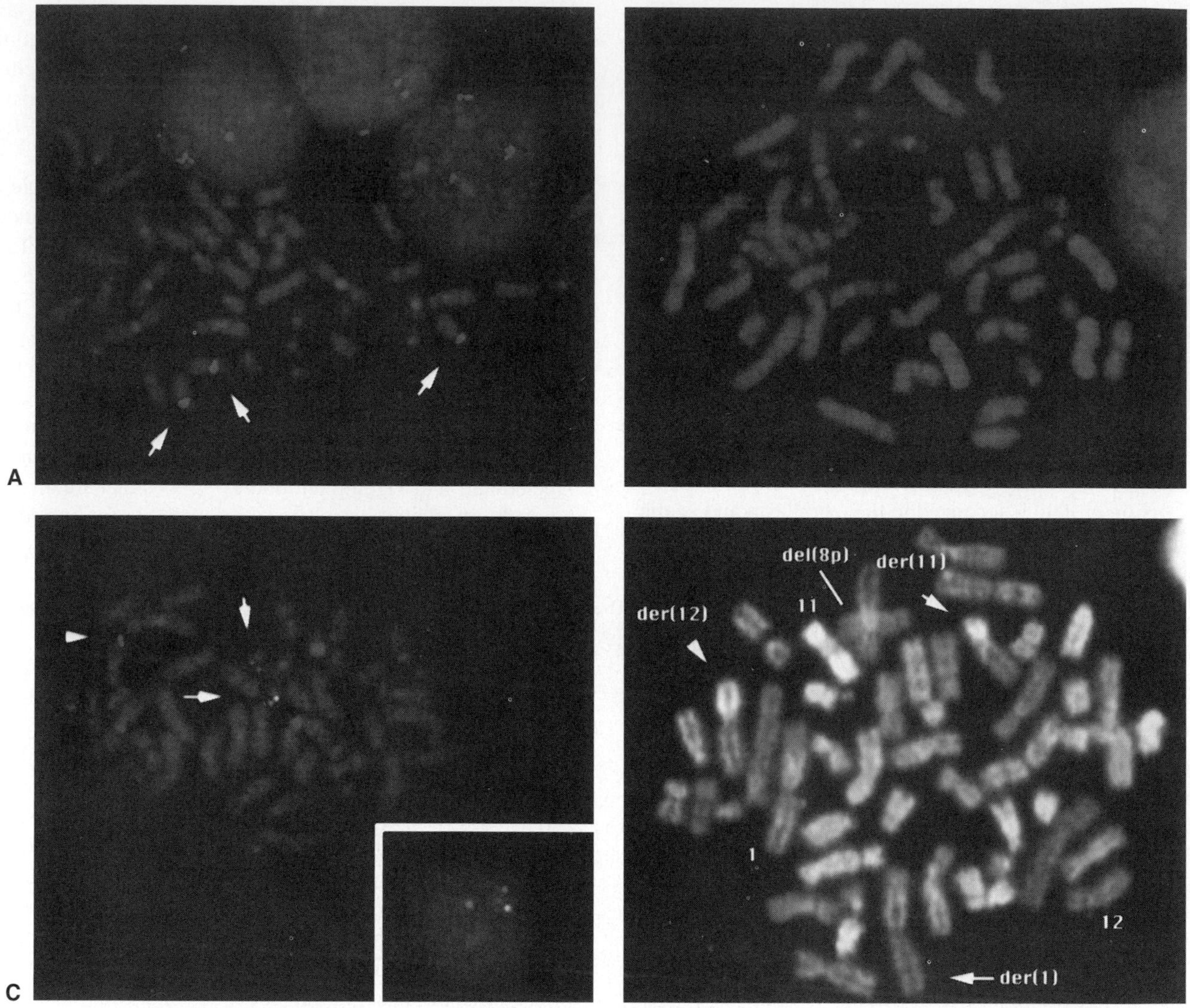

FIG. 10.4. Photomicrographs of metaphase and interphase cells after fluorescence *in situ* hybridization (FISH). In **A** through **C**, the cells are counterstained with 4,6-diamidino-2-phenylindole-dihydrochloride (DAPI). **A:** Hybridization of a directly labeled centromere-specific probe for chromosome 8 (CEP8 Spectrum Green, Vysis, Inc., Downers Grove, IL) to metaphase and interphase cells with trisomy 8 from a bone marrow aspirate of a patient with acute myeloid leukemia (AML). Centromere-specific probes hybridize to the repetitive DNA sequences that are present at the centromeres of human chromosomes. The chromosome 8 homologues are identified with arrows. **B:** Hybridization of a directly labeled chromosome 8–specific painting probe (WCP8 Spectrum Green, Vysis, Inc.) to a metaphase cell with trisomy 8 from a bone marrow aspirate of a patient with AML. **C:** Hybridization of a locus-specific probe for the detection of a recurring translocation, the t(9;22)(q34;q11.2) in chronic myelogenous leukemia (CML). The probe is a mixture of digoxigenin-labeled DNA probes (detected with rhodamine-labeled antibodies) for the major breakpoint cluster region of the *BCR* gene at 22q11.2 and biotin-labeled probes (detected with fluorescein-labeled avidin) for the *ABL* gene at 9q34 (M-bcr/abl probe, Ventana Medical Systems, Tucson, AZ). In cells with the t(9;22), only one green signal *(arrowhead)* and one red signal *(short arrow)* are observed on the normal 9 and 22 homologues, and a yellow fusion signal *(long arrow)* is observed on the Ph chromosome as a result of the juxtaposition of the *ABL* and *BCR* sequences. **D:** Spectral karyotyping analysis of a metaphase cell from a case of AML-M7. Twenty-four differentially labeled probes representing each human chromosome were cohybridized, and imaging analysis software assigned a unique color to each. A complex karyotype was identified by conventional cytogenetic analysis, including a derivative chromosome 1 with additional material of unknown origin on 1p, a deletion of 8p, a derivative chromosome 11 resulting from an unbalanced translocation involving 1 and 11, and a derivative chromosome 12 consisting of 11q and 12q. The results of spectral karyotyping confirmed the identity of the rearranged chromosome 12 *(arrowhead)* but clarified the other abnormalities. The additional material on 1p was derived from chromosome 8 (*long arrow*, blue signal), and the der(11) actually consisted of material from chromosomes 1, 11, and 12 (*short arrow,* 11p white signal; chromosome 12, brown signal; 1p, blue-pink signal). See Color Plate 1, between pp. 1446–1447.

TABLE 10.6. *Applications and Advantages of FISH*

Applications
- Detection of numerical and structural chromosomal abnormalities
- Identification of marker chromosomes (rearranged chromosomes of uncertain origin)
- Monitoring the effects of therapy and detection of minimal residual disease or early relapse
- Identification of the origin of bone marrow cells after bone marrow transplantation
- Identification of the lineage of neoplastic cells
- Examination of the karyotypic pattern of nondividing or interphase cells
- Detection of gene amplification

Advantages
- Rapid technique
- The efficiency of hybridization and detection is high.
- The sensitivity and specificity are very high.
- Large numbers of cells can be analyzed in a short time.
- Cytogenetic data can be obtained from nondividing or terminally differentiated cells, from tumors with a low mitotic index (e.g., chronic lymphocytic leukemia), or from poor samples that contain too few cells for routine cytogenetic studies.
- Direct correlation of cytogenetic and cytologic or morphologic features enables pathologists to differentiate malignant from benign conditions in equivocal cases.
- Automated systems for analysis of hybridized slides are available.

t(9;22) in CML patients after transplantation or interferon therapy, or sex chromosome determination after a sex-mismatched transplantation have become widespread.

Our new sophistication regarding the genetic changes in hematologic malignant diseases provides us with some very critical new diagnostic tools. Standard Southern blot analysis of tumor DNA can reveal clonal rearrangements of genes, such as immunoglobulin or T-cell receptor genes, as well as a number of recurring translocations. PCR can increase the sensitivity of detection of these aberrations; sometimes the sensitivity is too great to be clinically applicable. Translocations that result in fusion genes are especially suited for RT-PCR, a technique in which the fusion mRNA is copied into cDNA and then with appropriate primers from each gene, the fusion transcript is amplified by PCR. We and others have used this strategy to detect the rearranged genes in the t(8;21) (55). Using probes from *AML1* and *ETO* on standard Southern blot analysis, rearrangements can usually be detected in DNA from about 80% of patients known to have a t(8;21). With RT-PCR, the detection rate is 100%. A caveat is that several groups have identified the *AML1/ETO* fusion transcript by RT-PCR in patients in CR who were negative on cytogenetic analysis and standard Southern blotting. However, the translocation can be detected in peripheral blood cells from patients in unmaintained remission for more than 5 years (55). This indicates that these patients have circulating t(8;21)-positive cells even though they appear to be "cured" of their leukemia. The biologic significance of these observations remains to be determined; it seems clear, however, that decisions on whether to continue therapy cannot be based solely on a positive signal with RT-PCR methods.

This increasing precision in identifying the genetic changes in malignant cells comes at a most opportune time, because physicians may soon be in a position to use targeted therapy aimed at the specific genetic defects. Although a number of genes are involved with various genetic changes, those reflected in chromosomal changes may be among the easiest to monitor.

SUMMARY AND CONCLUSIONS

Cytogenetic analysis provides pathologists and clinicians with a powerful tool for the diagnosis and classification of hematologic malignant diseases. The detection of an acquired, somatic mutation establishes the diagnosis of a neoplastic disorder and excludes a reactive hyperplasia or morphologic changes caused by toxic injury or vitamin deficiency. Given an equivocal pathologic diagnosis, the detection of a clonal chromosomal abnormality in a bone marrow specimen or in lymph node tissue provides sufficient justification to institute cytotoxic treatment with radiation therapy or chemotherapy.

Specific cytogenetic abnormalities identify homogeneous subsets of various malignant diseases and enable clinicians to predict their clinical course and their likelihood of responding to particular treatments. In many cases, the prognostic information derived from cytogenetic analysis is independent of that provided by other clinical features. Patients with favorable prognostic features benefit from standard therapies with well-known spectra of toxicities, whereas those with less favorable clinical or cytogenetic characteristics may be better treated with more intensive or investigational therapies. The disappearance of a chromosomal abnormality present at diagnosis is an important indicator of CR after treatment, and its reappearance invariably heralds relapse of the disease. Pretreatment cytogenetic analysis can be useful in choosing between postremission therapies that differ widely in cost, acute and chronic morbidity, and effectiveness.

The presence of the Ph chromosome differentiates CML from other myeloproliferative disorders or myelodysplastic syndromes and also serves as an important marker of persistent disease during interferon therapy or after allogeneic bone marrow transplantation. Karyotypic evolution in a patient with CML portends transformation to the acute phase and provides a useful signal to proceed, if possible, with transplantation in higher risk groups, such as older patients or those without HLA-identical sibling donors.

The delineation of recurring chromosomal abnormalities has had an important impact on molecular biologic studies of human tumors. Recurring chromosomal abnormalities represent genetic mutations that are highly involved in the process of malignant transformation. The molecular analysis of recurring translocations has led to the identification of a number of novel genes, and to insights into the processes that regulate normal cell growth and differentiation as well as malignant transformation.

APPENDIX 1. GLOSSARY OF CYTOGENETIC TERMINOLOGY

Aneuploidy. An abnormal chromosome number resulting from the gain or loss of chromosomes.

Banded chromosomes. Chromosomes with alternating dark and light segments because of special stains or pretreatment of metaphase cells with enzymes before staining. Each chromosome pair has a unique pattern of bands.

Breakpoint. A specific site on a chromosome containing a DNA break that is involved in a structural rearrangement, such as a translocation or deletion.

Centromere. The constriction along the length of the chromosome that is the site of the spindle fiber attachment. The position of the centromere determines whether chromosomes are metacentric (X-shaped, such as chromosomes 1–3, 6–12, X, 16, 19, and 20) or acrocentric (inverted V-shaped, such as chromosomes 13–15, 21, 22, and Y). During mitosis, the two exact copies of the DNA in each chromosome are separated by shortening of the spindle fibers attached to opposite sides of the dividing cell.

Clone. In the cytogenetic sense, this is defined as two cells with the same additional or structurally rearranged chromosome or three cells with loss of the same chromosome.

Deletion. A segment of a chromosome is missing as the result of two breaks and loss of the intervening piece (interstitial deletion). Molecular studies of many recurring chromosomal deletions have shown that, in each case, the deletions were interstitial rather than terminal (i.e., single break with loss of the terminal segment).

Diploid. Normal chromosome number and composition of chromosomes.

FISH. Fluorescence *in situ* hybridization.

Haploid. Only one half the normal complement (i.e., 23 chromosomes for humans).

Hyperdiploid. Additional chromosomes; therefore, the modal number is 47 or greater.

Hypodiploid. Loss of chromosomes with a modal number of 45 or less.

Inversion. Two breaks occur in the same chromosome with rotation of the intervening segment. If both the breaks are on the same side of the centromere, it is called a paracentric inversion. If they are on opposite sides, it is called a pericentric inversion.

Isochromosome. A chromosome that consists of identical copies of one chromosome arm with loss of the other arm. For example, an isochromosome for the long arm of chromosome 17 [i(17q)] contains two copies of the long arm (separated by the centromere) with loss of the short arm of the chromosome.

Karyotype. Arrangement of chromosomes from a particular cell according to a well-established system such that the largest chromosomes are first and the smallest ones are last. A normal female karyotype is described as 46,XX and a normal male karyotype is 46,XY. An idiogram is an idealized diagram of the chromosomes.

Pseudodiploid. A diploid number of chromosomes accompanied by structural chromosomal abnormalities.

Recurring abnormality. A numerical or structural abnormality seen in multiple patients who have a similar neoplasm. Such abnormalities are characteristic or diagnostic of distinct subtypes of leukemia and lymphoma that have unique morphologic or immunophenotypic features. Recurring abnormalities represent genetic mutations that are involved in the pathogenesis of the corresponding diseases; many recurring abnormalities have prognostic significance.

RT-PCR. Reverse transcription–polymerase chain reaction.

Translocation. A break in at least two chromosomes with exchange of material. In a reciprocal translocation, there is no obvious loss of chromosomal material. Translocations are indicated by t; the chromosomes involved are noted in the first set of parentheses and the breakpoints in the second set of parentheses. The Ph translocation is t(9;22)(q34;q11).

Nomenclature Symbols

p—short arm
q—long arm
+ —if before the chromosome, indicates a gain of a whole chromosome (e.g., +8).
− —if before the chromosome, indicates a loss of a whole chromosome (e.g., −7), and if after the chromosome, indicates loss of part of the chromosome (e.g., 5q−, loss of part of the long arm of chromosome 5)
?—indicates uncertainty about the identity of the chromosome or band listed just after the ?.
t—translocation
del—deletion
inv—inversion
i—isochromosome
mar—marker chromosome
r—ring chromosome

Modified from Rowley JD: Chromosome abnormalities in human cancer. In: De Vita VT, Hellman S, Rosenberg S, eds. *Principles and Practice of Oncology,* 3rd ed. Philadelphia, JB Lippincott, 1991.

APPENDIX 2. EXAMPLES OF CYTOGENETIC NOMENCLATURE

46,XX or 46,XY. Nomenclature description of a normal female or male karyotype, respectively.

47,XX, + 8,t(9;22)(q34;q11). Female with an extra chromosome 8 and a translocation affecting chromosome 9 with a break in the long arm, band q34, and chromosome 22 with a break in the long arm, band q11. The latter is the usual translocation seen in chronic myelogenous leukemia. The abnormal chromosome 22 is known as the Philadelphia (Ph) chromosome.

46,XX,t(9;22;10)(q34;q11;q24). Female with a variant (complex) Philadelphia translocation affecting chromosome 9 with a break in band q34, chromosome 22 with a break in band q11, and chromosome 10 with a break in the long arm at band q24. Chromosomal material from 9q is translocated to 22q, material from 22q is translocated to 10q, and material from 10q is translocated to 9q.

46,XY,inv(16)(p13q22). Male with a pericentric inversion of chromosome 16 resulting from breaks in the short arm in band p13, and in the long arm in band q22. The inv(16) is a recurring chromosomal abnormality that is associated with acute myelomonocytic leukemia with abnormal eosinophils.

46,XY,del(5)(q13q33). Deletion of part of the long arm of chromosome 5 including bands q13-33.

REFERENCES

1. Mitelman F. *Catalog of chromosome aberrations in cancer*, 5th ed. New York: Wiley-Liss, 1994.
2. Heim S, Mitelman F. *Cancer cytogenetics*, 2nd ed. New York: Wiley-Liss, 1995.
3. Mitelman F, Mertens F, Johansson B. A breakpoint map of recurrent chromosomal rearrangements in human neoplasia. *Nat Genet* 1997;15:417–474.
4. Rabbitts T. Chromosomal translocations in human cancer. *Nature* 1994;372:143–149.
5. Look AT. Oncogenic transcription factors in the human acute leukemias. *Science* 1997;278:1059–1064.
6. Brown MA. Tumor suppressor genes and human cancer. *Adv Hum Genet* 1997;36:45–135.
7. Mitelman F, ed. *ISCN: an international system for human cytogenetic nomenclature.* Basel: Karger, 1995.
8. Kantarjian HM, Smith TL, McCredie KB, et al. Chronic myelogenous leukemia: a multivariate analysis of the associations of patient characteristics and therapy with survival. *Blood* 1985;66:1326–1335.
9. Pugh WC, Pearson M, Vardiman JW, et al. Philadelphia chromosome-negative chronic myelogenous leukaemia: a morphological reassessment. *Br J Haematol* 1985;60:457–467.
10. Rowley JD, Testa JR. Chromosome abnormalities in malignant hematologic diseases. *Adv Cancer Res* 1982;36:103–148.
11. Hagemeijer A, Bartram CR, Smit EME, et al. Is the chromosomal region 9q34 always involved in variants of the Ph[1] translocation? *Cancer Genet Cytogenet* 1984;13:1–16.
12. Groffen J, Stephenson JR, Heisterkamp N, et al. Philadelphia chromosomal breakpoints are clustered within a limited region, bcr, on chromosome 22. *Cell* 1984;36:93–99.
13. Witte ON. Role of the BCR/ABL oncogene in human leukemia. *Cancer Res* 1993;53:485–489.
14. Ganesan TS, Rassool F, Guo A-P, et al. Rearrangement of the bcr gene in Philadelphia chromosome-negative chronic myeloid leukemia. *Blood* 1986;68:957–960.
15. Gordon MY, Goldman JM. Cellular and molecular mechanisms in chronic myeloid leukemia. *Br J Haematol* 1996;95:10–20.
16. Daley GQ, van Etten RA, Baltimore D. Induction of chronic myelogenous leukemia in mice by the P210bcr/abl gene of the Philadelphia chromosome. *Science* 1990;247:824–830.
17. Sawyers CL, McLaughlin J, Witte ON. Genetic requirements for Ras in the transformation of fibroblasts and hematopoietic cells by the Bcr-Abl oncogene. *J Exp Med* 1995;181:307–313.
18. Kawasaki ES, Clark SS, Coyne MY, et al. Diagnosis of chronic myeloid and acute lymphocytic leukemias by detection of leukemia-specific mRNA sequences amplified *in vitro*. *Proc Natl Acad Sci USA* 1988;85:5698–5702.
19. Tkachuk DC, Westbrook CA, Andreeff M, et al. Detection of bcr-abl fusion in chronic myelogenous leukemia by in situ hybridization. *Science* 1990;250:559–562.
20. Fialkow PJ, Jacobson RJ, Papayannopoulou T. Chronic myelocytic leukemia: clonal origin in a stem cell common to the granulocyte, erythrocyte, platelet and monocyte/macrophage. *Am J Med* 1977;63:125–130.
21. Guilhot F, Chastang C, Michallet M, et al. Interferon alfa-2b combined with cytarabine versus interferon alone in chronic myelogenous leukemia. *N Engl J Med* 1997;337:270.
22. Mitelman F. The cytogenetic scenario of chronic myeloid leukemia. *Leuk Lymphoma* 1993;11[Suppl 1]:11–13.
23. Secker-Walker L, Craig JM. Prognostic implications of breakpoint and lineage heterogeneity in Philadelphia-positive acute lymphoblastic leukemia: a review. *Leukemia* 1993;7:147–151.
24. Anastasi J, Feng JJ, Dickstein JD, et al. Lineage involvement by BCR/ABL in Ph+ lymphoblastic leukemias: chronic myelogenous leukemia presenting in lymphoid blast phase versus Ph+ acute lymphoblastic leukemia. *Leukemia* 1996;10:795–802.
25. Dewald GW, Wright PI. Chromosome abnormalities in the myeloproliferative disorders. *Semin Oncol* 1995;22:341–354.
26. Third International Workshop on Chromosomes in Leukemia. *Cancer Genet Cytogenet* 1981;4:95–142.
27. Demory JL, Dupriez B, Fenaux P, et al. Cytogenetic studies and their prognostic significance in agnogenic myeloid metaplasia: a report on 47 cases. *Blood* 1988;72:855–859.
28. Johnson DD, Dewald GW, Pierre RV, et al. Deletions of chromosome 13 in malignant hematologic disorders. *Cancer Genet Cytogenet* 1985;18:235–241.
29. Bennett JM, Catovsky D, Daniel MT, et al. Proposals for the classification of the myelodysplastic syndromes. *Br J Haematol* 1982;51:189–199.
30. Morel P, Hebbar M, Lai JL, et al. Cytogenetic analysis has strong prognostic value in *de novo* myelodysplastic syndromes and can be incorporated in a new scoring system: a report on 408 cases. *Leukemia* 1993;7:1315–1323.
31. Toyama K, Ohyashiki K, Yoshida Y, et al. Clinical implications of chromosomal abnormalities in 401 patients with MDS: a multicentric study in Japan. *Leukemia* 1993;7:499–508.
32. Greenberg P, Cox C, Le Beau MM, et al. International scoring system for evaluating prognosis in myelodysplastic syndromes. *Blood* 1997;89:2079–2088.
33. Applebaum FR, Barrall J, Storb R, et al. Clonal cytogenetic abnormalities in patients with otherwise typical aplastic anemia. *Br J Haematol* 1987;15:1134–1139.
34. Rosati S, Anastasi J, Vardiman JW. Recurring diagnostic problems in the pathology of the myelodysplastic syndromes. *Semin Hematol* 1996;33:111–126.
35. Moormeier JA, Rubin CM, LeBeau MM, et al. Trisomy 6: a recurrent cytogenetic abnormality associated with marrow hypoplasia. *Blood* 1991;77:1397–1398.
36. Boultwood J, Lewis S, Wainsoat JS. The 5q− syndrome. *Blood* 1994;84:3253–3260.
37. Van den Berghe H, Michaux L. 5q−: Twenty-five years later. *Cancer Genet Cytogenet* 1997;94:1–7.
38. Keating MJ, Smith TL, Kantarjian H, et al. Cytogenetic patterns in acute myelogenous leukemia: a major reproducible determination of outcome. *Leukemia* 1988;2:403–412.
39. Schiffer CA, Lee EJ, Tomiyasu T, et al. Prognostic impact of cytogenetic abnormalities in patients with *de novo* acute nonlymphocytic leukemia. *Blood* 1989;73:263–270.
40. Fenaux P, Preudhomme C, Lai JL, et al. Cytogenetics and their prognostic value in *de novo* acute myeloid leukaemia: a report on 283 cases. *Br J Haematol* 1989;73:61–67.
41. Marosi C, Köller U, Koller-Weber E, et al. Prognostic impact of karyotype and immunologic phenotype in 125 adult patients with *de novo* AML. *Cancer Genet Cytogenet* 1992;61:14–25.
42. Dastugue N, Payen C, Lafage-Pochitaloff M, et al. Prognostic significance of karyotype in *de novo* adult acute myeloid leukemia. *Leukemia* 1995;9:1491–1498.

43. Joventino LP, Stock W, Lane NJ, et al. Certain HLA antigens are associated with specific morphologic and cytogenetic subsets of acute myeloid leukemia. *Leukemia* 1995;9:433–439.
44. Fourth International Workshop on Chromosomes in Leukemia. *Cancer Genet Cytogenet* 1984;71:249–360.
45. Mrózek K, Heinonen K, de la Chapelle A, et al. Clinical significance of cytogenetics in acute myeloid leukemia. *Semin Oncol* 1997;24: 17–31.
46. Secker-Walker LM, Fitchett M. Constitutional and acquired trisomy 8. *Leuk Res* 1995;19:737–740.
47. Caligiuri MA, Strout MP, Gilliland DG. Molecular biology of acute myeloid leukemia. *Semin Oncol* 1997;24:32–44.
48. Schichman SA, Caligiuri MA, Strout MP, et al. ALL-1 tandem duplication in acute myeloid leukemia with a normal karyotype involves homologous recombination between Alu elements. *Cancer Res* 1994; 54:4277–4280.
49. Caligiuri MA, Strout MP, Schichman SA, et al. Partial tandem duplication of ALL1 as a recurrent molecular defect in acute myeloid leukemia with trisomy 11. *Cancer Res* 1996;56:1418–1425.
50. Olopade OI, Thangavelu M, Larson RA, et al. Clinical, morphologic, and cytogenetic characteristics of 26 patients with acute erythroblastic leukemia. *Blood* 1992;80:2873–2882.
51. Luna-Fineman S, Shannon K, Lange BJ. Childhood monosomy 7: epidemiology, biology, and mechanistic implications. *Blood* 1995;85: 1985–1999.
52. Nucifora G, Rowley JD. *AML1* and the 8;21 and 3;21 translocations in acute and chronic myeloid leukemia. *Blood* 1995;86:1–14.
53. Bitter MA, Le Beau MM, Rowley JD, et al. Associations between morphology, karyotype, and clinical features in myeloid leukemias. *Hum Pathol* 1987;18:211–225.
54. Martinez-Climent JA, Lane NJ, Rubin CM, et al. Clinical and prognostic significance of chromosomal abnormalities in childhood acute myeloid leukemia *de novo*. *Leukemia* 1995;9:95–101.
55. Nucifora G, Larson RA, Rowley JD. Persistence of the 8;21 translocation in patients with AML-M2 in long-term remission. *Blood* 1993; 82:712–715.
56. Meyers S, Lenny N, Hiebert SW. The t(8;21) fusion protein interferes with AML-1B dependent transcriptional activation. *Mol Cell Biol* 1995;15:1974–1982.
57. Okuda T, Cai Z, Yang S, et al. Expression of a knocked-in *AML1-ETO* leukemia gene inhibits the establishment of normal definitive hematopoiesis and directly generates dysplastic hematopoietic progenitors. *Blood* 1998;91:3134–3143.
58. Larson RA, Williams SF, Le Beau MM, et al. Acute myelomonocytic leukemia with abnormal eosinophils and inv(16) or t(16;16) has a favorable prognosis. *Blood* 1986;68:1242–1249.
59. Bitter MA, Le Beau MM, Larson RA, et al. A morphologic and cytochemical study of acute myelomonocytic leukemia with abnormal marrow eosinophils associated with inv(16)(p13q22). *Am J Clin Pathol* 1984;81:733–741.
60. Liu P, Tarlé S, Hajra A, et al. A fusion between transcription factor CBFβ and a myosin heavy chain is generated by the chromosome 16 inversion in acute myelomonocytic leukemia M4E0. *Science* 1993; 261:1041–1044.
61. Hajra A, Liu PP, Collins FS. Transforming properties of the leukemia inv(16) fusion gene CBFb-MYH11. *Curr Top Microbiol Immunol* 1996;211:289–298.
62. Pandolfi PP. *PML, PLZF,* and *NPM* genes in the molecular pathogenesis of acute promyelocytic leukemia. *Haematologica* 1996;81: 472–482.
63. Grignani F, Fagioli M, Alcalay M, et al. Acute promyelocytic leukemia: from genetics to treatment. *Blood* 1994;83:10–25.
64. Castaigne S, Chomienne C, Daniel MT, et al. All-trans retinoic acid as differentiation therapy for acute promyelocytic leukemia: clinical results. *Blood* 1990;76:1704–1709.
65. De Thé H, Chomienne C, Lanotte M, et al. The t(15;17) translocation of acute promyelocytic leukaemia fuses the retinoic acid receptor α gene to a novel transcribed locus. *Nature* 1990;347:558–561.
66. Wang ZG, Delva L, Gaboli M, et al. Role of PML in cell growth and the retinoic acid pathway. *Science* 1998;279:1547–1551.
67. Kaneko Y, Maseki N, Takasaki N, et al. Clinical and hematologic characteristics in acute leukemia with 11q23 translocations. *Blood* 1986;67:484–491.
68. Rowley JD. Rearrangements involving chromosome band 11q23 in acute leukemia. *Semin Cancer Biol* 1993;4:377–385.
69. Bernard O, Berger R. Molecular basis of 11q23 rearrangements in hematopoietic malignant proliferations. *Genes Chromosomes Cancer* 1995;13:75–85.
70. Djabali M, Selleri L, Parry P, et al. A trithorax-like gene is interrupted by chromosome 11q23 translocations in acute leukaemias. *Nat Genet* 1992;2:113–118.
71. Thirman MJ, Gill HJ, Burnett RC, et al. A cDNA probe detects all rearrangements of the MLL gene in leukemias with common and rare 11q23 translocations. *N Engl J Med* 1993;329:909–914.
72. Zeleznik-Le, Harden AM, Rowley JD. 11q23 Translocations split the ''AT-hook'' cruciform DNA-binding region and the transcriptional repression domain from the activation domain of the mixed-lineage leukemia *(MLL)* gene. *Proc Natl Acad Sci USA* 1994;91: 10610–10614.
73. Yagi H, Deguchi K, Aono A, et al. Growth disturbance in fetal liver hematopoiesis of *Mll*-mutant mice. *Blood* 1998;92:108–117.
74. Corral J, Lavenir I, Impey H, et al. An *MLL-AF9* fusion gene made by homologous recombination causes acute leukemia in chimeric mice: a method to create fusion oncogenes. *Cell* 1996;85:853–861.
75. Bitter MA, Neilly ME, Le Beau MM, et al. Rearrangements of chromosome 3 involving bands 3q21 and 3q26 are associated with normal or elevated platelet counts in acute nonlymphocytic leukemia. *Blood* 1985;66:1362–1370.
76. Morishita K, Parganas E, Willman CL, et al. Activation of EVI1 gene expression in human acute myelogenous luekemias by translocations spanning 300–400 kilobases on chromosome band 3q26. *Proc Natl Acad Sci USA* 1992;89:3937–3941.
77. Russel M, List M, Greenberg P, et al. Expression of EVI1 in myelodysplastic syndromes and other hematologic malignancies without 3q26 translocations. *Blood* 1994;84:1243–1248.
78. Asimakopoulos FA, Green AR. Deletions of 20q and the pathogenesis of myeloproliferative disorders. *Br J Haematol* 1996;95:219–226.
79. Davis MP, Dewald GW, Pierre RV, et al. Hematologic manifestations associated with deletions of the long arm of chromosome 20. *Cancer Genet Cytogenet* 1984;12:63–71.
80. Campbell LJ, Garson OM. The prognostic significance of deletions of the long arm of chromosome 20 in myeloid disorders. *Leukemia* 1994;8:67–71.
81. Wang PW, Iannantuoni K, Davis EM, et al. Refinement of the commonly deleted segment in myeloid leukemias with del(20q). *Genes Chromosomes Cancer* 1998;21:75–81.
82. Soekarman D, von Lindern M, Daenen S, et al. The translocation (6; 9)(p23;q34) shows consistent rearrangement of two genes and defines a myeloproliferative disorder with specific clinical features. *Blood* 1992;79:2990–2997.
83. Bodger MP, Morris CM, Kennedy MA, et al. Basophils of (Bsp-1+) derive from the leukemia clone in human myeloid leukemias involving the chromosome breakpoint 9q34. *Blood* 1989;73:777–781.
84. Fornerod M, Boer J, van Baal S, et al. Relocation of the carboxy terminal part of CAN from the nuclear envelope to the nucleus as a result of leukemia-specific chromosome rearrangements. *Oncogene* 1995;10:1739–1748.
85. Lion T, Haas OA. Acute megakaryoblastic leukemia with the t(1; 22)(p13;q13). *Leuk Lymphoma* 1993;11:15–20.
86. Carroll A, Civin C, Schneider N, et al. The t(1;22)(p13;q13) is nonrandom and restricted to infants with acute megakaryoblastic leukemia: a Pediatric Oncology Group study. *Blood* 1991;78:748–752.
87. Stark B, Resnitzky P, Jeison M, et al. A distinct subtype of M4/M5 acute myeloblastic leukemia (AML) associated with t(8;16)(p11;p13) in a patient with the variant t(8;19)(p11;q13): Case report and review of the literature. *Leuk Res* 1995;19:367–379.
88. Borrow J, Stanton VP Jr, Andresen JM, et al. The translocation t(8; 16)(p11;p13) of acute myeloid leukemia fuses a putative acetyltransferase to the CREB-binding protein. *Nat Genet* 1996;14:33–41.
89. Thirman M, Larson RA. Therapy-related myeloid leukemia. *Hematol Oncol Clin North Am* 1996;10:293–320.
90. Le Beau MM, Albain KS, Larson RA, et al. Clinical and cytogenetic correlations in 63 patients with therapy-related myelodysplastic syndromes and acute nonlymphocytic leukemia: further evidence for characteristic abnormalities of chromosomes no. 5 and 7. *J Clin Oncol* 1986;4:325–345.
91. Pedersen-Bjergaard J, Philip P. Cytogenetic characteristics of therapy-

related acute non-lymphocytic leukemia, preleukemia, and acute myeloproliferative syndrome: correlation with clinical data in 61 consecutive cases. *Br J Haematol* 1987;66:199–207.
92. Pedersen-Bjergaard, Rowley JD. The balanced and the unbalanced chromosome aberrations of acute myeloid leukemia may develop in different ways and may contribute differently to malignant transformation. *Blood* 1994;83:2780–2786.
93. Ratain MJ, Rowley JD. Therapy-related acute myeloid leukemia secondary to inhibitors of topoisomerase II: from the bedside to the target genes. *Ann Oncol* 1992;3:107–111.
94. Zhao N, Stoffel A, Wang PW, et al. Molecular delineation of the smallest commonly deleted region of chromosome 5 in malignant myeloid diseases to 1–1.5 Mb and preparation of a PAC-based physical map. *Proc Natl Acad Sci USA* 1997;94:6948–6953.
95. Fairman J, Chumakov I, Chinault AC, et al. Physical mapping of the minimal region of loss in 5q− chromosome. *Proc Natl Acad Sci USA* 1995;92:7406–7410.
96. Boultwood J, Fidler C, Lewis S, et al. Molecular mapping of uncharacteristically small 5q deletions in two patients with the 5q− syndrome: delineation of the critical region on 5q − breakpoint. *Genomics* 1994; 19:425–432.
97. Le Beau MM, Espinosa R II, Davis EM, et al. Cytogenetic and molecular delineation of a region of chromosome 7 commonly deleted in malignant myeloid diseases. *Blood* 1996;88:1930–1935.
98. Fischer K, Fröhling S, Scherer SW, et al. Molecular cytogenetic delineation of deletions and translocations involving chromosome band 7q22 in myeloid leukemias. *Blood* 1997;89:2036–2041.
99. Camitta BM, Pullen J, Murphy S. Biology and treatment of acute lymphoblastic leukemia in children. *Semin Oncol* 1997;24:83–91.
100. Raimondi SC. Current status of cytogenetic research in childhood acute lymphoblastic leukemia. *Blood* 1993;81:2237–2251.
101. Pui CH. Childhood leukemias. *N Engl J Med* 1995;332:1618–1630.
102. Thandla S, Aplan PD. Molecular biology of acute lymphocytic leukemia. *Semin Oncol* 1997;24:45–56.
103. Bloomfield CD, Goldman AI, Alimena G, et al. Chromosomal abnormalities identify high-risk and low-risk patients with acute lymphoblastic leukemia. *Blood* 1986;67:415–420.
104. Groupe Francais de Cytogenetique Hematologique. Cytogenetic abnormalities in adult acute lymphoblastic leukemia: correlations with hematologic findings and outcome. *Blood* 1996;87:3135–3142.
105. Williams DL, Harber J, Murphy SB, et al. Chromosomal translocations play a unique role in influencing prognosis in childhood acute lymphoblastic leukemia. *Blood* 1986;68:205–212.
106. Rubin CM, Le Beau MM, Mick R, et al. Impact of chromosomal translocations on prognosis in childhood acute lymphoblastic leukemia. *J Clin Oncol* 1991;9:2183–2190.
107. Kobayashi H, Maseki N, Homma C, et al. Clinical significance of chromosome abnormalities in childhood acute lymphoblastic leukemia in Japan. *Leukemia* 1994;8:1944–1950.
108. Bowman WP, Shuster JJ, Cook B, et al. Improved survival for children with B-cell acute lymphoblastic leukemia and stage IV small noncleaved cell lymphoma: a Pediatric Oncology Group study. *J Clin Oncol* 1996; 14:1252–1261.
109. Laport GF, Larson RA. Treatment of adult ALL. *Semin Oncol* 1997; 24:70–82.
110. Chen C-S, Sorenson PHB, Domer PH, et al. Molecular rearrangements on chromosome 11q23 predominate in infant acute lymphoblastic leukemia and are associated with specific biologic variables and poor outcome. *Blood* 1993;81:2386–2393.
111. Rubnitz JE, Link MP, Shuster JJ, et al. Frequency and prognostic significance of HRX rearrangements in infant acute lymphoblastic leukemia: a Pediatric Oncology Group study. *Blood* 1994;84: 570–573.
112. Hilden JM, Frestedt JL, Moore RO, et al. Molecular analysis of infant acute lymphoblastic leukemia: MLL gene rearrangement and reverse transcriptase-polymerase chain reaction for t(4;11)(q21;q23). *Blood* 1995;86:3876–3882.
113. Russo R, Carroll A, Kohler S, et al. Philadelphia chromosome and monosomy 7 in childhood acute lymphoblastic leukemia: a Pediatric Oncology Group study. *Blood* 1991;77:1050–1056.
114. Westbook CA, Hooberman AL, Spino C, et al. Clinical significance of the BCR-ABL fusion gene in adult acute lymphoblastic leukemia: a Cancer and Leukemia Group B study (8762). *Blood* 1992;80: 2983–2990.
115. Clark SS, McLaughlin J, Crist WM, et al. Unique forms of the *abl* tyrosine kinase distinguish Ph[1]-positive CML from Ph[1]-positive ALL. *Science* 1987;235:85–88.
116. Pui C-H, Raimondi SC, Hancock ML, et al. Immunologic, cytogenetic, and clinical characterization of childhood acute lymphoblastic leukemia with the t(1;19)(q23;p13) or its derivative. *J Clin Oncol* 1994;12:2601–2606.
117. Crist WM, Carroll AJ, Shuster JJ, et al. Poor prognosis of children with pre-B acute lymphoblastic leukemia is associated with the t(1; 19)(q23;p13): a Pediatric Oncology Group study. *Blood* 1990;76: 117–122.
118. Hunger SP. Chromosomal translocations involving the *E2A* gene in acute lymphoblastic leukemia: clinical features and molecular pathogenesis. *Blood* 1996;87:1211–1224.
119. Kamps MP. E2A-PBX1 induces growth, blocks differentiation, and interacts with other homeodomain proteins regulating normal differentiation. *Curr Top Microbiol Immunol* 1997;220:25–41.
120. Shurtleff SA, Buijs A, Behm FG, et al. *TEL/AML1* fusion resulting from a cryptic t(12;21) is the most common genetic lesion in pediatric ALL and defines a subgroup of patients with an excellent prognosis. *Leukemia* 1995;9:1985–1989.
121. Romana SP, Poirel H, Leconiat M, et al. High frequency of t(12;21) in childhood B lineage acute lymphoblastic leukemia. *Blood* 1995; 86:4263–4269.
122. Rubnitz JE, Downing JR, Pui C-H, et al. *TEL* gene rearrangement in acute lymphoblastic leukemia: a new genetic marker with prognostic significance. *J Clin Oncol* 1997;15:1150–1157.
123. Golub TR, Barker GF, Bohlander SK, et al. Fusion of the *TEL* gene on 12p13 to the *AML1* gene on 21q22 in acute lymphoblastic leukemia. *Proc Natl Acad Sci USA* 1995;92:4917–4921.
124. Mertens F, Johansson B, Mitelman F, et al. Dichotomy of hyperdiploid acute lymphoblastic leukemia on the basis of the distribution of gained chromosomes. *Cancer Genet Cytogenet* 1996;92:8–10.
125. Moorman AV, Clark R, Farrell DM, et al. Probes for hidden hyperdiploidy in acute lymphoblastic leukaemia. *Genes Chromosomes Cancer* 1996;16:40–45.
126. Raimondi SC, Pui C-H, Hancock ML, et al. Heterogeneity of hyperdiploid (51-67) childhood acute lymphoblastic leukemia. *Leukemia* 1996;10:213–224.
127. Ong ST, Le Beau MM. Chromosomal abnormalities and molecular genetics of non-Hodgkin's lymphoma. *Semin Oncol*, in press.
128. Bloomfield CD, Arthur DC, Frizzera G, et al. Nonrandom chromosome abnormalities in lymphoma. *Cancer Res* 1983;43:2975–2984.
129. Levine EG, Arthur DA, Frizzera G, et al. There are differences in cytogenetic abnormalities among histological subtypes of the non-Hodgkin's lymphomas. *Blood* 1985;66:1414–1422.
130. Yunis JJ, Frizzera G, Oken MM, et al. Multiple recurrent genomic defects in follicular lymphoma: a possible model for cancer. *N Engl J Med* 1987;316:79–84.
131. Fifth International Workshop on Chromosomes in Leukemia-Lymphoma. Correlation of chromosome abnormalities in non-Hodgkin's lymphoma and adult T-cell leukemia lymphoma. *Blood* 1987;70: 1554–1564.
132. Kristoffersson U, Heim S, Mandahl N, et al. Prognostic implications of cytogenetic findings in 106 patients with non-Hodgkin's lymphoma. *Cancer Genet Cytogenet* 1987;25:55–64.
133. Offit K, Jhanwar SC, Ladanyi M, et al. Cytogenetic analysis of 434 consecutively ascertained specimens of non-Hodgkin's lymphoma: correlations between recurrent aberrations, histology, and exposure to cytotoxic treatment. *Genes Chromosomes Cancer* 1991;3:189–201.
134. Hammond DW, Goepel JR, Aitken M, et al. Cytogenetic analysis of a United Kingdom series of non-Hodgkin's lymphoma. *Cancer Genet Cytogenet* 1992;61:31–38.
135. Offit K, Wong G, Filippa DA, et al. Cytogenetic analysis of 434 consecutively ascertained specimens of non-Hodgkin's lymphoma: clinical correlations. *Blood* 1991;77:1508–1515.
136. Gaidano G, Dalla Favera R. Molecular pathogenesis of AIDS-related lymphomas. *Antibiot Chemother* 1994;46:117–124.
137. Gaidano G, Dalla Favera R. Lymphomas. In: DeVita VT, Hellman S, Rosenberg SA, eds. *Cancer: principles and practice of oncology*, 5th ed. New York: Lippincott-Raven, 1997:2131–2145.
138. Adams JM, Harris AW, Pinkert CA, et al. The c-*myc* oncogene driven by immunoglobulin enhancers induces lymphoid malignancy in transgenic mice. *Nature* 1985;318:533–538.

139. Amati B, Brooks MW, Levy N, et al. Oncogenic activity of the c-Myc protein requires dimerization with Max. *Cell* 1993;72:233–245.
140. Bakhshi A, Jensen JP, Goldman P, et al. Cloning the chromosomal breakpoint of t(14;18) human lymphomas: clustering around JH on chromosome 14 and near a transcriptional unit on 18. *Cell* 1985;41: 899–906.
141. Yang E, Korsmeyer SJ. Molecular thanatopsis: a discourse on the *BCL2* family and cell death. *Blood* 1996;88:386–401.
142. McDonnell TJ, Korsmeyer SJ. Progression from lymphoid hyperplasia to high grade malignant lymphoma in mice transgenic for the t(14; 18). *Nature* 1991;349:254–256.
143. Limpens J, Stad R, Vos C, et al. Lymphoma-associated translocation t(14;18) in blood B cells of normal individuals. *Blood* 1995;85: 2528–2536.
144. Yang E, Zha J, Jockel J, et al. Bad, a heterodimeric partner for Bcl-XL and Bcl-2, displaces Bax and promotes cell death. *Cell* 1995;80: 285–291.
145. Tang SC, Visser L, Hepperle B, et al. Clinical significance of *bcl-2*-MBR gene rearrangement and protein expression in diffuse large-cell non-Hodgkin's lymphoma: an analysis of 83 cases. *J Clin Oncol* 1994; 12:149–154.
146. Kramer MH, Hermans J, Parker J, et al. Clinical significance of bcl2 and p53 protein expression in diffuse large B-cell lymphoma: a population-based study. *J Clin Oncol* 1996;14:2131–2138.
147. Raffeld M, Jaffe ES. *Bcl-1*, t(11;14), and mantle cell–derived lymphomas. *Blood* 1991;78:259–263.
148. Motokura T, Bloom T, Kim HG, et al. A novel cyclin encoded by a *bcl1*-linked candidate oncogene. *Nature* 1991;350:512–515.
149. Hall M, Peters G. Genetic alterations of cyclins, cyclin-dependent kinases, and Cdk inhibitors in human cancer. *Adv Cancer Res* 1996; 68:67–108.
150. Bodrug SE, Warner BJ, Bath ML, et al. Cyclin D1 transgene impedes lymphocyte maturation and collaborates in lymphomagenesis with the *myc* gene. *EMBO J* 1994;13:2124–2130.
151. Baron BW, Nucifora G, McCabe N, et al. Identification of the gene associated with the recurring chromosomal translocations t(3;14)(q27; q32) and t(3;22)(q27;q11) in B-cell lymphomas. *Proc Natl Acad Sci USA* 1993;90:5262–5266.
152. Ye BH, Lista F, Lo CF, et al. Alterations of a zinc finger-encoding gene, *BCL-6*, in diffuse large-cell lymphoma. *Science* 1993;262: 747–750.
153. Offit K, Lo CF, Louie DC, et al. Rearrangement of the *bcl-6* gene as a prognostic marker in diffuse large-cell lymphoma. *N Engl J Med* 1994;331:74–80.
154. Bastard C, Deweindt C, Kerckaert JP, et al. *LAZ3* rearrangements in non-Hodgkin's lymphoma: correlation with histology, immunophenotype, karyotype, and clinical outcome in 217 patients. *Blood* 1994; 83:2423–2427.
155. Dent AL, Shaffer AL, Yu X, et al. Control of inflammation, cytokine expression, and germinal center formation by bcl-6. *Science* 1997; 276:589–592.
156. Agnarsson B, Kadin ME. Ki-1 positive large cell lymphoma: a morphologic and immunologic study of 19 cases. *Am J Surg Pathol* 1988; 12:264–274.
157. Rimokh R, Magaud J-P, Berger F, et al. A translocation involving a specific breakpoint (q35) on chromosome 5 is characteristic of anaplastic large cell lymphoma (''Ki-1 lymphoma''). *Br J Haematol* 1989;71:31–36.
158. Sarris AH, Luthra R, Papadimitracopoulou V, et al. Amplification of genomic DNA demonstrates the presence of the t(2;5) (p23;q35) in anaplastic large cell lymphoma, but not in other non-Hodgkin's lymphomas, Hodgkin's disease, or lymphomatoid papulosis. *Blood* 1996; 88:1771–1779.
159. Morris SW, Kirstein MN, Valentine MB, et al. Fusion of a kinase gene, *ALK,* to a nucleolar protein gene, *NPM,* in non-Hodgkin's lymphoma. *Science* 1994;263:1281–1284.
160. Fujimoto J, Shiota M, Iwahara T, et al. Characterization of the transforming activity of p80, a hyperphosphorylated protein in a Ki-1 lymphoma cell line with chromosomal translocation t(2;5). *Proc Natl Acad Sci USA* 1996;93:4181–4186.
161. Döhner H, Stilgenbauer S, Fischer K, et al. Cytogenetic and molecular cytogenetic analysis of B cell chronic lymphocytic leukemia: specific chromosome aberrations identify prognostic subgroups of patients and point to loci of candidate genes. *Leukemia* 1997;11:S19–S24.
162. McKeithan TW, Rowley JD, Shows TB, et al. Cloning of the chromosome translocation breakpoint junction of the t(14;19) in chronic lymphocytic leukemia. *Proc Natl Acad Sci USA* 1987;84:9257–9260.
163. Anastasi J, Le Beau MM, Vardiman JW, et al. Detection of trisomy 12 in chronic lymphocytic leukemia by fluorescence *in situ* hybridization to interphase cells: a simple and sensitive method. *Blood* 1992; 79:1796–1801.
164. Le Beau MM. Fluorescence *in situ* hybridization in cancer diagnosis. In: De Vita VT, Hellman S, Rosenberg SA, eds. *Important advances in oncology.* Philadelphia: Lippincott, 1993:29–45.
165. Le Beau MM. One FISH, two FISH, red FISH, blue FISH. *Nat Genet* 1996;12:341–344.

CHAPTER 11

Organization and Operation of a Hematopathology Laboratory

Daniel M. Knowles, Angela Murray, and Amy Chadburn

Multiple diagnostic dilemmas are commonly encountered in the routine diagnosis and classification of hematopoietic neoplasms. Examples include the differential diagnosis of non-Hodgkin's lymphoma versus undifferentiated carcinoma, lymphoid hyperplasia versus non-Hodgkin's lymphoma in lymphatic and in extralymphatic tissues, Hodgkin's disease versus non-Hodgkin's lymphoma, acute leukemias of lymphoid versus myeloid origin, and chronic leukemias of B-cell versus T-cell origin. The application of solely morphologic criteria in these situations is fraught with difficulties. The purely cytomorphologic detection of minimal neoplastic disease, such as partial involvement of lymph nodes by non-Hodgkin's lymphoma and the presence of small numbers of lymphoma/leukemia cells in peripheral blood, bone marrow, effusions, and cerebrospinal fluid (CSF) is often difficult. Morphologic criteria are frequently incapable of correctly forecasting the lineage of diffuse aggressive hematologic neoplasms (1–5).

Immunophenotypic analysis is capable of determining the polyclonal or monoclonal B-cell or T-cell nature of a lymphoid proliferation, thereby often distinguishing benign from malignant lymphoid proliferations; determining the lineage, subset, and approximate stage of differentiation of neoplastic hematopoietic cells; and detecting minimal neoplastic disease (6–10). Immunogenotypic analysis, the evaluation of clonal rearrangements of the antigen recognition molecules of B and T cells (immunoglobulin and T-cell receptors, respectively), is capable of determining the lineage and clonality of B- and T-cell proliferations at the molecular level (11–17) and of detecting clonal B- and T-cell populations that escape detection by morphologic examination and immunophenotypic analysis (18–23). Immunogenotypic analysis may help when immunophenotypic analysis is incapable of resolving a diagnostic dilemma. Immunophenotypic analysis and immunogenotypic analysis have become invaluable adjuncts to morphology in the differential diagnosis and classification of hematopoietic neoplasms.

For this reason, physicians providing care to patients who have hematopoietic neoplasms require access to a hematopathology laboratory capable of performing these studies on all solid tissue and fluid pathologic specimens. Unfortunately, some clinical pathologists accustomed to handling high-volume clinical testing with sophisticated automated instrumentation prefer performing cytofluorometric analysis of isolated cells in suspension and fail to correlate their results with the histopathology of the pathologic specimens from which the cells were isolated. Many anatomic pathologists accustomed to evaluating tissue sections prefer performing immunohistochemical staining of tissue sections and ignore ''wet'' hematologic samples. Even worse, many of these individuals extol the virtues of their approach and ignore and remain biased against the other approach, refusing to recognize the advantages as well as the disadvantages of both methodologies. Too few ''full-service'' hematopathology laboratories exist; many large institutions remain in need of a hematopathologist capable of establishing and operating such a facility.

The hematopathology laboratory, whose organization and operation is described here, is now based at the New York Weill–Cornell campus of New York Presbyterian Hospital and is directed by Drs. Daniel Knowles and Amy Chadburn and managed by Ms. Angela Murray. This laboratory was initially established at the Columbia-Presbyterian Medical Center by Dr. Daniel Knowles in 1978. Initially, immunofluorescent analysis of isolated cells in suspension was routinely performed on all specimens because it was believed at that time that this was the best all-around approach for handling the greatest number and variety of pathologic speci-

D. M. Knowles, A Murray, and A. Chadburn: Department of Pathology, Weill Medical College of Cornell University, New York, New York, 10021 mens. Since then, the assays performed in the hematopathology laboratory have been continually improved as each new significant technologic advance (i.e., monoclonal antibodies, flow cytometry, immunohistochemistry, antigen retrieval, automated immunohistochemistry, Southern blotting, and polymerase chain reaction [PCR]) has been incorporated into the laboratory, which has been continuously reorganized to accommodate the changes. The result today is a full-service hematopathology laboratory capable of routinely performing the entire array of immunophenotypic, immunogenotypic, and molecular biologic analyses currently available on a large number of solid and fluid pathologic specimens. In this chapter, the organization and daily operation of this laboratory, including the handling and processing of pathologic specimens, reagent maintenance, and our approach to immunophenotypic evaluation and diagnosis, are described. Synopses of 13 cases are provided to illustrate the role of these studies in the diagnosis and management of patients with hematopoietic neoplasms. An appendix provides the recipes for performing many of the laboratory's procedures. Many other excellent hematopathology laboratories offering alternative but equally reliable approaches exist, but the intent of this chapter is to provide an overview of the daily routine operation of one laboratory.

LABORATORY ORGANIZATION AND DAILY OPERATION

Immunophenotypic analysis can be performed on virtually any pathologic specimen, including all solid tissues, peripheral blood, aspirated bone marrow, pleural and abdominal effusions, and CSF. A hematopathology laboratory should be capable of effectively analyzing all these different types of samples on any given day. This can be readily accomplished if the laboratory establishes appropriate guidelines for the correct handling and processing of each of these different types of pathologic specimens; is capable of performing cytofluorometric analysis of isolated cells in suspension, and immunohistochemical analysis of cytospin preparations and frozen and paraffin tissue sections; is cognizant of the utility and reactivity of the many monoclonal antibodies currently available in cell suspensions, cytospins, and frozen and paraffin tissue sections and the immunophenotypic profiles of the various hematopoietic neoplasms; is capable of performing antigen receptor gene rearrangement analysis and other molecular genetic assays as an adjunct to immunophenotypic analysis; and tailors the methodologic approach of the analysis to the individual requirements of each pathologic specimen and the specific diagnostic problem requiring resolution. Under these circumstances, the only factors limiting the successful outcome of immunophenotypic analysis are adequacy of sample size, technical difficulties inherent in the various phenotyping techniques, and the limits of immunophenotypic criteria applied to the diagnosis and classification of hematopoietic neoplasms. However, the large volume and diverse nature of the specimens submitted to the hematopathology laboratory and the labor-intensive nature of the assays performed on them dictate that each specimen be handled rapidly and efficiently and that all assays be performed expeditiously but accurately. We have adopted a specific operational approach to the immunophenotypic analysis of pathologic specimens, which is described later. Based on this correlative clinical, morphologic, and immunophenotypic approach, a definitive diagnosis can be made in most cases within 48 hours.

HANDLING AND PROCESSING OF PATHOLOGIC SPECIMENS

Accessioning Specimens and Tracking Data

Peripheral blood samples submitted to the laboratory for T-cell subset (CD4/CD8) analysis are accessioned into the hospital laboratory information system by personnel on the hospital floors, by accession clerks in outpatient laboratory services, or by the hematopathology laboratory technicians. All the remaining specimens submitted to the laboratory for diagnostic leukemia/lymphoma evaluation are accompanied by a New York Presbyterian Hospital requisition form or paperwork submitted by the referring hospital or physician. Specimen accessioning and data tracking are performed manually. The specimen is logged in the accession book and assigned a laboratory identification number. A laboratory data sheet is prepared and stapled to the front of the submitted requisition or paperwork so that all the information and paperwork concerning each specimen are together and are available when needed. The technician accessioning the specimen completes the front sheet by filling in the patient's name and location, age, sex, hospital number, physician's name and location, referring institution, a summary of the pertinent clinical information, the hematopathology laboratory number, date, time of arrival, and the nature of the specimen. The front sheet with the attached requisition or paperwork remains in the laboratory during the entire workup of the specimen. Notations concerning specimen handling and ongoing laboratory findings are continuously added to the front sheet during the evaluation of the specimen. In this way, the front sheet becomes a complete summary of the case when the evaluation process is completed, at which time a final hematopathology laboratory report is generated. The laboratory is in the process of being computerized, and once the computer system is fully operational, each specimen arriving in the laboratory will be assigned a unique identifying number and accessioned into the computer system accompanied by the patient's demographics as outlined previously. The results of hematopathology laboratory evaluation are entered on an ongoing basis. After a final report is generated, all the information concerning each specimen is stored in the mainframe computer. The specimen data archives are retrievable by patient name, laboratory identification number, patient history number, ICD9 diagnosis code, or SNOMED diagnosis code.

Specimen Collection

Peripheral blood samples obtained from immunodeficient patients and transplant recipients for T-cell subset (CD4/CD8) analysis and all peripheral venous blood and aspirated bone marrow samples submitted for the diagnosis and classification of leukemia/lymphoma must be anticoagulated with sodium or lithium heparin to prevent clotting. In general, peripheral blood samples are drawn and submitted in green-top tubes (i.e., sterile and preheparinized), and bone marrow samples are drawn and submitted in a sterile syringe prerinsed with and containing a small residual amount (<1 mL) of heparin or in a green-top tube. Inadequate anticoagulation results in clots that interfere with mononuclear cell isolation by Ficoll-Hypaque density gradient centrifugation and with accurate analysis by the whole blood lysis technique. Over-anticoagulation with unnecessarily large volumes of heparin can alter the results of immunophenotypic analysis.

The quantity of peripheral blood necessary to perform immunophenotypic analysis depends on the patient's white blood cell (WBC) count, the proportion of lymphocytes or other mononuclear cells whose analysis is desired, and the number and type of assays to be performed. For example, only 2 mL of heparinized peripheral blood is required to perform T-cell subset analysis in an immunodeficient individual with a normal WBC count using the whole blood lysis technique. However, approximately 10 mL of peripheral blood from the same individual is required to perform a comparable analysis on isolated mononuclear cells. Approximately 1×10^7 mononuclear cells can be isolated by Ficoll-Hypaque density gradient centrifugation from every 10 mL of peripheral blood obtained from an individual with a normal WBC count. This represents a sufficient number of mononuclear cells for examination with approximately 10 monoclonal antibodies (1×10^6 cells per reagent). Very large numbers of mononuclear cells, sufficient to perform extensive immunophenotypic analysis, can be obtained even when only 10 mL of peripheral blood is taken from a leukemic patient with a high leukocyte count. In these instances, all cells in excess of that needed for immunodiagnosis are cryopreserved for future studies.

In general, 1 to 3 mL of aspirated bone marrow yields sufficient numbers of cells, usually between 10 and 20×10^6, to permit adequate cytofluorometric analysis. Attempts to aspirate large amounts of bone marrow frequently result in peripheral blood contamination of the bone marrow sample by normal peripheral blood B and T cells. Introducing this artifact may make the immunophenotypic identification and analysis of neoplastic cells from the bone marrow considerably more difficult.

Ideally, the physician desiring immunophenotypic analysis of an effusion should submit a fresh specimen obtained from a recent-onset effusion. Chronic, long-standing effusions may lack sufficient numbers of viable cells for analysis. The physician should submit the entire effusion to the hematopathology laboratory in a sterile container, anticoagulated with heparin and without fixatives, minus the relatively small portions necessary for the microbiology and cytopathology laboratories, so that the maximum number of viable cells can be isolated for immunophenotypic analysis.

Unfortunately, in our experience, this ideal situation is not always achieved. In some instances, physicians fail to heparinize the collection container, which can result in fibrin clots or large blood clots if the effusion is bloody. These clots interfere significantly with cell isolation. Because cells become entrapped within these clots, the number of cells available for analysis is reduced and the sample may be rendered nonrepresentative. However, because most effusions represent an excellent physiologic medium and support cell viability very well, immunophenotypic analysis can be performed on most of these specimens, even if they have not been submitted under ideal conditions.

Immunophenotypic analysis can be performed on CSF samples; the limiting factor is the number of cells necessary to perform the analyses required to resolve the particular diagnostic problem. In our experience, CSF samples containing fewer than 50 cells/mm^3 are often inadequate for diagnostic immunophenotypic analysis. One exception is immunostaining for terminal deoxynucleotidyl transferase (TdT); even if positive on only a few cells, it is diagnostic of involvement by acute leukemia. The physician should submit the largest volume of CSF that can be safely obtained from the patient in a sterile collection tube without fixative. Heparinization is unnecessary.

Peripheral blood, aspirated bone marrow, and effusions contain single cells in suspension that continue to be bathed in their natural physiologic environment even after removal from the body. In contrast, lymph nodes and other solid tissues generally contain tightly packed clusters and sheets of cells, sometimes surrounded by dense connective tissue, whose nutrient support is wholly dependent on continuous and appropriate vascular perfusion. Removal from the body results in the interruption of blood flow to these cells, alters their physiologic environment, and consequently places their viability at risk almost immediately. All lymph node and other solid tissue specimens must be handled carefully and expeditiously to maximize cell viability and antigen preservation.

The entire lymph node or other solid tissue biopsy specimen should be submitted in sterile RPMI 1640 (preferable) or sterile physiologic saline (if more accessible to the surgeon) in a sterile container immediately after its removal from the patient, transported immediately to the laboratory and be evaluated, handled, and processed without delay on arrival in the laboratory. One factor that unavoidably delays appropriate processing is a request for intraoperative frozen section consultation. Cell viability can decrease rapidly and markedly if the solid tissue is allowed to dry out on a laboratory counter top at room temperature for even 10 minutes. The entire biopsy, or representative portions in the case of large resection specimens, should be floated in tissue culture media or saline during the intraoperative consultation to maximize cell viability.

In general, the typical lymph node biopsy specimen is sufficient in size to permit the preparation of histologic sections, the cryopreservation of tissue blocks for immunohistochemical staining, and the preparation of a cell suspension for cytofluorometric analysis. A representative cell suspension totalling about 5 $\times$ 10^7 cells can be prepared from a a 0.5 to 0.7 cm^2 piece of lymphoid cell–rich tissue devoid of necrosis and fibrous connective tissue. In the case of smaller biopsy specimens, representative portions are taken for histology, cryopreservation, and cell suspension in that order of priority. For example, 3- to 6-mm cutaneous punch biopsies are always divided in half for histology and cryopreservation. Cell suspensions are not usually prepared from densely fibrotic or extensively necrotic tissues because this is usually unsuccessful or the resultant cell suspensions are nonrepresentative.

Specimen Transport

Rapid specimen transport and processing are recommended because this maximizes cell viability and antigen preservation. CSF samples should always be transported immediately because these specimens usually contain very few cells and their analysis is often crucial for diagnosis. In general, peripheral blood, aspirated bone marrow, and effusion specimens should be delivered to the laboratory within 3 hours of being obtained from the patient. However, we and others (24) have found that the mononuclear cells present in most unseparated whole peripheral blood, aspirated bone marrow, and effusion samples, with the possible exception of CD4 T cells, remain viable, without antigen loss, for 24 hours or longer after collection. These specimens should be maintained at room temperature during unavoidable delays in processing. Even specimens obtained in the late evening after the laboratory is closed should be stored overnight at room temperature until they can be processed the next day.

One notable exception is peripheral blood samples submitted for T-cell subset analysis, because CD4 T cells often do not remain viable if left overnight in unseparated whole blood, whether stored at room temperature or at 4°C. For this reason, immunophenotypic analysis of peripheral blood mononuclear cells that have remained unseparated for longer than 24 hours before isolation and analysis often results in artificially low CD4:CD8 ratios. However, antigen preservation is somewhat dependent on the type of anticoagulant. Whole blood specimens anticoagulated with heparin can remain unseparated for up to 48 hours with only minimal antigen loss, but specimens anticoagulated with EDTA exhibit significant antigen loss after 30 hours. The unseparated specimens should be maintained at room temperature, on a rocker if possible, until processing. This includes those specimens obtained in the late evening after the laboratory is closed.

All solid tissue specimens, especially resection specimens too large to be floated in tissue culture media or saline, should be delivered to the laboratory immediately after removal from the patient because cell viability is most difficult to maintain in these specimens. Tissue specimens procured from within the medical center that are delivered promptly to the laboratory and processed immediately on their arrival may be maintained at room temperature. Tissue specimens procured from outside the medical center or that must be in transit for 2 hours or more should be kept cool on ice but not allowed to freeze. This is especially important on hot summer days, when cell viability may be severely compromised by the excessive heat. However, maintaining tissue samples on ice does not ensure cell viability and antigen preservation if the cells are not also floated in sterile tissue culture media or physiologic saline.

Handling Cell Suspensions

Peripheral blood samples collected from immune deficient patients and transplant recipients are submitted to the laboratory for T-cell subset analysis. The mononuclear cells in these samples are isolated and immunostained using the whole blood lysis technique, which disrupts the erythrocytes and leaves all the other cells intact (see Appendix 1). The immunostained cells are then analyzed by three color cytofluorometry on a FACSCaliber flow cytometer (Becton-Dickinson, Mountain View, CA). These specimens are always studied the same day they are obtained from the patient; analyses are never postponed until the following day. The results are reported directly into the hospital laboratory computer system with absolute CD4, CD8, and other cell counts calculated on the basis of a complete blood count with differential. The evaluation and monitoring of the immune system in immune deficient and transplant patients by analyzing their peripheral blood mononuclear cell distribution have been extensively reviewed elsewhere (25–27) and are not discussed further in this chapter.

All other specimens arriving in the laboratory are examined and handled in a sterile, laminar flow tissue culture hood (Sterilgard Hood, Baker Instrument Co., Baker, ME). Specimen containers are never opened to room air and are never casually examined on a laboratory bench top. All physicians and laboratory personnel handling specimens wear gloves and take appropriate safety precautions. Moreover, all manipulations, including cell isolation, cryopreservation, and thawing of cells, are performed under sterile conditions in a sterile laminar flow tissue culture hood. This approach provides maximum protection to the entire laboratory staff and permits the preparation of sterile cell suspensions useful for a variety of research programs.

All peripheral blood samples, other than those for T-cell subset analysis, are submitted for immunophenotypic analysis to aid in the diagnosis and classification of leukemia/lymphoma. These samples are not subjected to whole blood lysis unless the samples are small or contain large numbers of erythrocytes that cannot be removed by Ficoll-Hypaque density centrifugation without endangering the mononuclear cell population under study. In most instances the mononuclear cells are isolated from these samples by Ficoll-Hypaque density gradient centrifugation, which eliminates erythrocytes, granulocytes, and dead cells (see Appendix 2). This approach provides the maximum number of viable cells for immunophenotypic analysis and for cryopreservation for future studies. These specimens are accessioned as they arrive, maintained briefly at room temperature, appropriately diluted, placed over Ficoll-Hypaque, and centrifuged throughout the day along with cell suspensions prepared from other pathologic specimens arriving on the same day. All peripheral blood and other samples requiring Ficoll separation are processed the same day; specimens are never left unprocessed overnight.

Peripheral blood samples are placed into Nunc 260-mL (80-cm^2) flasks and diluted with sterile phosphate-buffered saline (PBS, Gibco, Grand Island, NY) according to the WBC count before Ficoll-Hypaque density gradient centrifugation. This approach provides post-Ficoll mononuclear cell layers of ideal size and maximum yields of recovery. Overdilution results in thin post-Ficoll cell layers that are difficult to visualize and harvest. Underdilution results in thick, oversized post-Ficoll cell layers and decreases cell recovery. Peripheral blood samples with a normal WBC count of 5,000 to 10,000/mm^3 are diluted 1:3 (i.e., 50 mL of blood and 100 mL of PBS). Peripheral blood samples having a WBC greater than normal are diluted with PBS until the WBC is within the normal range. The sample is then further diluted 1:3. For example, a blood sample with a WBC count of 30,000/mm^3 is diluted 1:4 (e.g., 50 mL of blood and 150 mL of PBS) to bring the WBC to approximately 7,500/mm^3. This is then diluted again by 1:3 for a total dilution of 1:12. The diluted sample is then placed over Ficoll-Hypaque.

Aspirated bone marrow samples are placed into sterile Falcon #1029 Petri dishes for easy handling. The bone marrow spicules are mechanically disrupted to liberate the bone marrow cells by grinding them for about 15 minutes with the flat rubber bottom of a plunger removed from a sterile 10-mL syringe. The specimen is gradually thinned out during this process by diluting it approximately 1:10 with sterile PBS. Thick specimens, often encountered when marrows are packed with leukemic cells, may be further diluted but not by more than 1:20. The diluted sample is then placed over Ficoll-Hypaque.

In the case of solid tissues, we require that the surgeon submit the entire tissue specimen to the laboratory intact in sterile tissue culture media RPMI 1640 (Gibco, Grand Island, NY) or physiologic saline. The only exceptions are cases submitted in consultation from outside institutions. In these instances, we prefer that the local referring pathologist divide the specimen, submit a representative portion of the biopsy fresh and unfixed in RPMI 1640 to the laboratory, process the remainder for histopathology in his or her own laboratory, and send us representative recut histologic slides to review and keep in our files. In our institution, a pathologist examines all gross specimens immediately on their arrival in the laboratory and, after examination of a Diff-Quick (modified Wright-Giemsa)–stained touch preparation (see Appendix 3), determines those portions that are suitable for routine histopathology, cell suspension preparation, and snap-freezing. These samples are always handled expeditiously to maximize cell viability and antigen preservation. If a cell suspension is prepared, cell viability and the degree of contamination by erythrocytes, dead cells, and debris are assessed immediately, and a decision to Ficoll or not is made.

Examination of a touch preparation of a solid tissue specimen is important for several reasons. The touch preparation gives the pathologist insight into the type of lesion he or she is dealing with, which influences how the tissue should be handled. For example, if a lymph node touch prep shows a mixed cell population containing many eosinophils and large binucleated cells with prominent nucleoli suggestive of Reed-Sternberg cells, the pathologist may choose to freeze tissue blocks and submit tissue for routine histology and not prepare a cell suspension because cytofluorometric analysis is not useful in arriving at a diagnosis of Hodgkin's disease. Alternatively, the pathologist may identify metastatic carcinoma, obviating the need to prepare a cell suspension. A touch preparation may suggest that the tissue is largely fibrotic and that it is likely that only a small number of cells will be obtained if an attempt is made to prepare a cell suspension. The touch preparation also gives the pathologist a general idea of the viability of the cells within the specimen. If most cells in the touch prep are not viable, it is often more useful to save the specimen as frozen tissue blocks that can be used for DNA studies rather than place the dying cells in suspension only to lose them during Ficoll separation.

That portion of a lymph node or other tissue specimen used to prepare a cell suspension is placed in a Falcon #1029 Petri dish and covered with a small volume of RPMI 1640 containing 1% penicillin and 1% streptomycin. The cells are isolated from the tissue by a combination of cutting, teasing, and scraping manipulations. However, before placing the entire specimen into suspension, a small number of cells are isolated and their viability checked by trypan blue dye exclusion (see Appendix 4). If the viability is poor, (<50%), it is often preferable to preserve the remainder of the specimen as frozen tissue blocks. If the viability is greater than 50%, the tissue is cut into small pieces that are more workable; this also ensures maximum perfusion by the tissue culture media. Each piece is held at the bottom of the Petri dish by a sterile forceps held in one hand and alternately sliced and scraped with a sterile scalpel blade held in the other hand. The maximum number of cells are drawn out of the tissue in the shortest period of time when only a small amount of fluid is maintained around the piece of tissue being teased apart. The media becomes progressively cloudier as cells are scraped out of the tissue and into the fluid. Every few minutes, the cloudy cell-rich supernatant is drawn off with a Pasteur pipette and collected into a Falcon #2070 50-mL tube and a comparable volume of fresh media is added to the Petri dish. This process is continued until all the tissue pieces have been chopped, the fluid is clear, and only white fibrous connective tissue fragments remain. These tissue fragments are then ground to a white fibrous pulp using the flat rubber bottom of a plunger removed from a 60-mL syringe to ensure that the maximum number of cells is collected. In our experience, this approach results in higher cell yields, better viability, and more representative cell suspensions than the commonly used approach of forcing tissue through a nylon mesh.

The 50-mL tube is capped and shaken, the tissue debris is allowed to settle toward the bottom for about 30 to 60 seconds, and the cell-rich supernatant is then drawn off with a Pasteur pipette and placed in another 50 mL tube; the debris remaining at the bottom of the tube is discarded. The cells are examined and counted in a hemocytometer and their viability is assessed by trypan blue dye exclusion (see Appendix 4). Cell suspensions of less than 80% viability or containing erythrocytes and cellular debris require Ficoll-Hypaque density gradient centrifugation. The cells should be suspended to a final concentration of 5 to 10 $\times$ 10^6 cells/mL before adding Ficoll to produce optimum post-Ficoll mononuclear cell layers and maximum cell recovery. Cell suspensions not requiring Ficoll separation are stored overnight, as described later.

Bloody effusion specimens are treated like peripheral blood samples. They are diluted 1:2 to 1:4 with PBS and then placed over Ficoll-Hypaque. Nonbloody effusion specimens are handled like cell suspensions prepared from lymph nodes. The cells are examined and counted on a hemocytometer and their viability is assessed by trypan blue dye exclusion. Cell suspensions of less than 80% viability or containing erythrocytes and cellular debris are suspended to a concentration of 5 to 10 $\times$ 10^6 cells/mL and placed over Ficoll-Hypaque. Cell suspensions not requiring Ficoll-Hypaque separation are stored overnight.

CSF samples are transferred to a sterile 15-mL Falcon #2097 conical tube and pelleted in a Sorvall RT 6000 centrifuge at 1,000 rpm for 8 minutes at room temperature. The supernatant is discarded, and the cells are resuspended in a small volume (0.5 to 1.0 mL) of RPMI 1640 and counted. In our experience, these samples never require Ficoll separation and nearly always contain too few cells to do so anyway.

The mononuclear cells isolated and collected from each specimen are counted, their viability is reassessed, and they are resuspended in sterile RPMI 1640 containing 10% heat-inactivated fetal or newborn calf serum (Flow Laboratories, McClean VA), 1% penicillin, and 1% streptomycin (overnight solution). Diff-Quik (modified Wright-Giemsa)–stained cytocentrifuge slides (cytospins) of each cell suspension are prepared (see Appendix 3) to evaluate the morphologic features of the cells and determine the approximate percentage of neoplastic cells in the sample before cytofluorometric analysis. These slides also provide a permanent morphologic record of the cell suspension prepared from each specimen. At the end of the day, the laboratory physician staff examine these cytocentrifuge slides, as well as Diff-Quik–stained frozen tissue sections, in conjunction with the clinical information, formulate a differential diagnosis, and develop an appropriate immunostaining panel for each specimen. When acute leukemia is suspected, additional cytocentrifuge slides may be prepared for immunostaining for TdT (see Appendix 5) and cytoplasmic μ (see Appendix 6). When multiple myeloma or plasmacytoma is suspected, additional cytocentrifuge slides may be prepared for immunostaining for cytoplasmic immunoglobulin (see Appendix 6). Alternatively, TdT, cytoplasmic μ, and cytoplasmic immunoglobulin may be determined by flow cytometry (24,28,29). The residual resuspended cells are then stored in overnight solution at 4°C. In our experience, viable mononuclear cell suspensions stored in this manner are nearly always as viable the next day and even over the weekend in most cases. The principal exceptions are some high-grade lymphomas, especially Burkitt's lymphoma, immunoblastic lymphomas, and plasmacytoma or multiple myeloma. The viability of the cell suspensions prepared from these neoplasms often continue to decrease, even after the harvesting of only viable cells by Ficoll-Hypaque. When possible, these neoplastic cells are analyzed the same day that the specimens are obtained from the patient. The next morning, a technician counts and reassesses the viability of the multiple cell suspensions collected the previous day. After direct and indirect immunofluorescent staining and cytofluorometric analysis based on the staining key developed the prior evening, the residual cells are cryopreserved in liquid nitrogen at −170°C. The proper handling of cell suspensions for cytofluorometric analysis and immunohistochemical analysis of cytospins are discussed in Chapters 5 and 38, respectively.

Handling Frozen and Paraffin-Embedded Tissues

A representative portion of every tissue specimen submitted to the laboratory is snap-frozen and cryopreserved except for exceedingly small biopsies that are entirely submitted for histopathology. A freshly prepared mixture of isopentane and dry ice is used to snap-freeze each tissue specimen. In general, a minimum of one, usually two, but sometimes as many as 10 tissue blocks ranging in size from 0.1 cm^3 to 1.0 $\times$ 1.0 $\times$ 0.3 cm are taken from each pathologic specimen and snap-frozen.

Round 2.2-cm cork disks (Superior Technologies, Pittsburgh PA) are covered with OCT embedding compound (Tissue-Tek, Naperville, IL). The tissue block is firmly placed in the middle of the OCT-covered disc and covered with additional OCT. The specimen is then held in the isopentane–dry ice mixture with forceps for about 1 to 2 minutes or until thoroughly frozen. The frozen blocks belonging to each specimen are placed in a zip-lock bag inscribed in indelible ink with the laboratory identification number of the specimen, the tissue type, the number of frozen blocks, and the date. The bag is stored in a −80°C freezer until needed. Tissue blocks cryopreserved in this manner may be used to prepare frozen tissue sections for immunohistochemical staining for many years if they are not allowed to thaw. DNA may be extracted from these cryopreserved tissue blocks and used for immunogenotypic analysis even if the blocks thaw.

Two factors that are critical in achieving optimal frozen tissue sections for immunohistochemical staining are rapidity in handling and processing tissue specimens once they are removed from the patient and the speed of the actual freezing process. The first factor is important for preserving cell surface antigens and reducing diffusion artifact during immunostaining. The second factor is important for preventing ice crystal formation, which results in suboptimal tissue sections that often cannot be interpreted accurately after immunostaining. These and other considerations in handling frozen tissue are discussed in Chapter 4.

Referring institutions sometimes submit frozen blocks of tissue that have been improperly handled. In some instances, the tissue has been frozen slowly by allowing it to sit in a −30°C cryostat overnight. In other instances, the tissue may have been frozen properly initially but partially thawed during transport. In these situations, we have found that rapidly thawing and snap-freezing the specimen according to the procedure outlined above often enhances the immunohistochemical staining results.

When immunohistochemical staining is required, the cryopreserved tissue block is removed from the freezer and mounted in a cryostat, and a sufficient number of 4 to 6 μm thick serial sections are prepared. The sections are air dried at room temperature for 1 hour to overnight, depending on when the immunostaining is to be performed, fixed in room temperature acetone for 10 minutes, and then air dried for 5 minutes (see Appendix 7). One or two of the sections are stained with Diff-Quik (see Appendix 3) to review the morphology of the lesion being analyzed and to help determine the immunostaining panel. The remaining sections are then placed in 0.05% TTBS (Tween-Tris buffered saline) for 5 minutes after which they are loaded onto the Tech Mate 500 Automated Immunostaining System (Ventana, Tuscon, AZ).

Paraffin tissue sections are baked overnight in a 56°C oven and are deparaffinized by four serial 5-minute washes in xylene the following morning. The sections are then serially immersed for 5 minutes each in 100% ethanol and 95% ethanol and placed into 0.45% H_2O_2 in methanol (3 mL of 30% H_2O_2 in 200 mL of methanol) for 20 minutes. The sections are then transferred into room temperature distilled water to await antigen retrieval. Tissues that have been fixed in Bouin's solution must be debouinized before immunostaining to remove the yellow background color, which may interfere with interpretation. This is accomplished by placing the paraffin tissue sections in a freshly prepared supersaturated solution of lithium carbonate in 70% ethanol for 30 to 60 seconds between the 100% and 95% ethanol steps in the hydration procedure. Tissues fixed in B5 have pigment that must be removed, because it may interfere with interpretation. Before counterstaining, the B5-fixed tissues are immersed in 100 mL of H_2O containing 1 g of iodine and 2 g of potassium iodide for 5 minutes, after which the sections are placed in 0.2% sodium thiosulfate for 8 minutes to remove the pigment (see Appendix 7). Because the type of fixative and the duration of fixation affect antigen detection, the fixation used for each specimen (i.e., formalin, Bouin's, B5) is always recorded and the monoclonal antibody used to detect a particular antigen is used at the titer appropriate for the particular fixative and detection system employed (see Chapters 4 and 30). Visualization of specific antigens in paraffin tissue sections frequently requires antigen retrieval. The antigen retrieval techniques used in our laboratory include proteolytic digestion with trypsin or protease and special heating procedures involving microwave or pressure cooker techniques. After these preparatory steps, the paraffin tissue sections are loaded onto the TechMate 500 Automated Immunostaining System (Ventana, Tucson, AZ).

Banking Cryopreserved Cells and Tissues for Future Studies

All excess cells isolated from pathologic specimens submitted to the laboratory for immunophenotypic analysis are cryopreserved in a viable state in fetal calf serum and dimethylsulfoxide and are stored in liquid nitrogen at −170°C (see Appendix 8). The laboratory has continuously stored vials of cryopreserved cells in this manner on a daily basis since 1978. Approximately 20,000 vials of lymphoma and leukemia cells have been accumulated since then. These cells may be stored indefinitely and thawed in the distant future (see Appendix 9) to perform additional studies. Similarly, all excess snap-frozen tissue blocks have been collected and stored since 1982 in −85°C freezers. These excess cells and tissues are never discarded.

These banks of cryopreserved cells and tissues are an important clinical resource because they permit additional evaluations of the pathologic specimens in the future. They have allowed many hematopoietic neoplasms that were previously evaluated but incompletely understood or unsuccessfully diagnosed to be reevaluated with new monoclonal antibodies and by new technologies (i.e., molecular biologic assays for protooncogene and tumor suppressor gene alterations) that were unavailable when the neoplasms were initially accessioned. These banks also permit reevaluation of the initial diagnostic specimens in patients who return in relapse or with a second neoplasm in parallel with the new pathologic sample. The availability of these banks of cryopreserved cells and tissues contributes significantly to the diagnosis and management of patients who have hematopoietic neoplasms.

These cell and tissue banks have formed the basis for the clinical and basic science research programs of the hematopathology laboratory. Cryopreserved cells and tissues have frequently been employed to prepare, screen, and characterize new monoclonal antibodies (30–35) or to further characterize existing monoclonal antibodies (36,37). They have been frequently employed in immunophenotypic analyses of interesting and unusual hematopoietic neoplasms (38–46) and in large clinicopathologic studies (3,47–55). *In vitro* functional studies have even been successfully performed on lymphoma/leukemia cells cryopreserved in this manner for as long as 10 years (56). DNA and RNA can be extracted from these cryopreserved cells and tissues for use in a variety of molecular biologic assays. This has enabled the laboratory to perform or participate in numerous original molecular genetic investigations of hematopoietic neoplasia (3,14, 16–19,22,57–100), including studies aimed at detecting Epstein-Barr virus (EBV), human T-cell lymphotropic virus type 1 (HTLV-1), and other viruses in hematopoietic neoplasms (101–103). Cryopreserved cells and tissues from this laboratory were used in the initial discovery and characterization of the Kaposi's sarcoma–associated herpesvirus (KSHV) (104), its presence in a subset of acquired immunodeficiency syndrome (AIDS)–related lymphomas (105), and the subsequent characterization of these lymphomas as a distinct clinicopathologic entity (106).

ESTABLISHING AND MAINTAINING LABORATORY STANDARDS

Handling Monoclonal Antibodies and Other Reagents

The efficient daily operation of the laboratory requires the establishment and maintenance of a large inventory of commercially available and privately generated monoclonal antibodies, heteroantisera, and other reagents. The laboratory supervisor oversees the maintenance of this inventory, including the replacement of exhausted reagents. As each monoclonal antibody or other reagent is received in the laboratory, its source, identifying lot number, and date of arrival are recorded in a reagent inventory log book. The entries provide a running historical account since the laboratory's inception of every reagent used in the laboratory and its specific period of use for purposes of quality control.

Commercially available monoclonal antibodies are of generally high quality and of reliable concentration and composition. Nonetheless, we do not take the integrity of these reagents and their stated optimal working dilutions for granted, and they are not simply thrown into refrigerators and freezers undiluted and awaiting use. All monoclonal antibodies are stored under the appropriate conditions (usually 4°C) to ensure their reliability and to maximize their shelf life. Before routine use, an aliquot is removed from storage and titered on the appropriate cells or tissue to determine the ideal working dilution of that particular ''lot'' of antibody for daily use, which is recorded in the reagent inventory log book. The optimal working dilution of each antibody differs in flow cytometry and in frozen and paraffin tissue section immunohistochemistry. The optimal working dilutions of monoclonal antibodies that detect paraffin-resistant antigens vary with the fixative (e.g., formalin, Bouin's solution, B5) and with the sensitivity of the detection system used. Each antibody reagent must be titered on the appropriate cells or tissue in each detection system in which it is to be employed.

Quality Control in the Laboratory

Rigorous quality control must be employed in handling and processing specimens, establishing and maintaining reagent panels, and performing cytofluorometric and immunohistochemical analysis of pathologic specimens. Processing normal tissues in conjunction with pathologic specimens in an analogous manner contributes significantly to monitoring the consistency and quality of the laboratory. This approach may also be used to establish the normal values of the laboratory and is an important source of material for positive and negative controls. For example, a normal peripheral blood sample should be immunostained in conjunction with peripheral blood samples obtained from immunodeficient and transplant patients using the whole blood lysis technique. Commercially available, stabilized, normal peripheral blood leukocytes expressing surface antigens detectable with monoclonal antibodies (CD-Chex, Streck Laboratories, Inc., Omaha, NE) are used as controls. These cells, when stained with monoclonal antibodies, provide reference values for a wide range of leukocyte antigen expression, including those of T cell, B cell, Natural killer (NK) cell, and myeloid or monocytic cells. Mononuclear cells isolated from normal peripheral blood or the commercially available CD-Chexs are used in evaluating new antibodies or new lots of antibodies to ensure quality control. Fresh tonsils are an excellent source of ''normal tissue'' for preparing cell suspensions, cryopreserved tissue blocks, and formalin-fixed, paraffin-embedded tissue blocks for use as positive and negative controls. The cells may be cryopreserved in aliquots of 5×10^7 cells and thawed for use as future controls. Similarly, a viable cell suspension can be prepared from fresh thymus, cryopreserved in aliquots of 1×10^7 cells, and the aliquots thawed in the future for use as positive TdT controls in the evaluation of acute leukemias. Alternatively, acute lymphoblastic leukemia cell lines may be used as controls for TdT expression.

All labeled and unlabeled monoclonal antibodies and heteroantisera must be carefully evaluated continuously to ensure their specificity and sensitivity. All reagents should be titered on the appropriate benign or neoplastic cells or tissues using a minimum of six serial dilutions that encompass the range of strong positivity to virtual negativity. The proper dilution is the one giving the highest acceptable level of brightness in conjunction with the lowest background. Retitering with additional, more appropriate serial dilutions may be necessary to arrive at the optimal working dilution.

The flow cytometer must be properly aligned, appropriately calibrated, and its settings optimally adjusted daily to consistently perform accurate cytofluorometric analysis. Isotype-matched, murine monoclonal antibodies with irrelevant specificity (e.g., IgG1, IgG2a) are used to establish the background noise level and the zero point of the analysis. Immunostaining for CD45 and CD14 indicates the purity of the analysis gate based on cellular composition with respect to lymphocytes and monocytes. The laboratory participates in the New York State proficiency testing program (New York State Department of Health, Albany, NY). Quality control procedures in flow cytometry are discussed in more detail in Chapter 5.

Positive and negative controls must be routinely employed in immunohistochemical staining as well. For example, immunostaining of paraffin tissue sections of a diffuse large cell lymphoma with monoclonal antibodies L26 (CD20) and Leu-22 (CD43) should be accompanied by parallel immunostaining of paraffin sections of a normal tonsil. Immunostaining of paraffin tissue sections of a suspected case of Hodgkin's disease with monoclonal antibodies Leu-M1 (CD15) and Ber-H2 (CD30) should be accompanied by parallel immunostaining of paraffin sections of a known case of Hodgkin's disease expressing those antigens. The diagnostic case slides should be evaluated in light of the results obtained with the known positive control slides. If, for example, the Reed-Sternberg cells in the known positive control sections are $CD30^-$ or only very weakly positive, $CD30^-$ diagnostic case slides are probably invalid, and the immunostaining should be repeated. Negative controls should include sections stained with isotype-matched, irrelevant murine monoclonal antibodies followed by the appropriate labeled secondary antibody and sections stained only with the labeled secondary antibody. Quality control procedures in immunohistochemical staining are discussed in Chapter 4.

APPROACH TO IMMUNOPHENOTYPIC ANALYSIS OF LYMPHOMA AND LEUKEMIA

General Comments

Laboratories approach immunophenotypic analysis differently, often depending on the philosophical biases and the methodologic preferences of the director. Unfortunately, some of the approaches that are commonly chosen fail to achieve a precise immunodiagnosis or do so only after a needless expenditure of time, effort, and money because they are not targeted to the specific diagnostic problem.

The limited screening approach most often results in failure to achieve a precise immunodiagnosis and, worse, sometimes results in an incorrect diagnosis. In this case, the pathologist tends to screen all cell suspensions and frozen tissue sections with the same limited panel of monoclonal antibody reagents. This panel may include, for example, anti-B-cell antibody B1 (CD20), anti-T-cell antibody Leu-4 (CD3), anti-monocyte antibody Leu-M3 (CD14), anti-T-cell subset antibodies Leu-3a (CD4) and Leu2a (CD8), and antibodies recognizing κ and λ light chains and an anti-TdT antibody in the case of acute leukemia. However, this approach fails to take into account several facts:

1. CD20 is an excellent pan-B-cell marker in flow cytometry, but CD22 is a better pan-B-cell marker in frozen tissue sections (personal observation).
2. CD20 is expressed by only about 50%, but CD19 is expressed by almost 95% of precursor B-cell lymphoblastic lymphomas/leukemias (7,9).
3. CD3 is detectable in most precursor T-cell lymphoblastic lymphomas/leukemias by frozen tissue immunohistochemistry but not by flow cytometry (107).
4. Some peripheral T-cell lymphomas lack CD3 but express some combination of pan-T-cell antigens CD2, CD7, and CD5 (8,108).
5. The immunodiagnosis of peripheral T-cell lymphoma is often dependent on demonstrating the deletion of one or more pan-T-cell antigens (8,108).

This approach fails to consider the special immunophenotypic profiles of chronic lymphocytic leukemia, hairy cell leukemia, mantle cell lymphoma, and other lymphoproliferative disorders whose precise immunodiagnosis can only be made by employing additional monoclonal antibodies (6,7,9, 10).

In contrast, the "shot-gun" approach nearly always arrives at a correct immunodiagnosis but at a price. In this case, the pathologist routinely employs a large panel of monoclonal antibodies that detect a wide array of B-cell, T-cell, monocyte-macrophage, myeloid, leukemia-associated and other antigens to arrive at the correct immunodiagnosis. The price of this approach is an unnecessary expenditure of time, effort, and money.

The other reasons investigators sometimes have difficulty achieving a correct immunodiagnosis are failure to recognize the pitfalls and disadvantages inherent in each immunophenotypic approach; failure or inability to employ an alternative approach when the initial approach fails; and failure to correlate the immunophenotypic results with the clinical information and careful examination of the histopathologic sections. For example, some pathologists exclusively perform flow cytometric analysis of cells in suspension and report their results without correlating their findings with the histopathology. Pitfalls exist in the cytofluorometric analysis of cell suspensions, however. For example, the poor viability of some cell suspensions may result in preferential loss of the neoplastic cells accompanied by selective enrichment of the residual benign T cells. In these instances, the pathologist may report the immunophenotypic profile of the normal and not the neoplastic cells, resulting in misdiagnosis. Review of the viability data and the histopathologic sections should alert the pathologist to the discrepant results and the obvious reason for them. The pathologist should reanalyze this case by immunohistochemical staining of frozen or paraffin tissue sections. Unfortunately, the failure of some laboratories to recognize and rectify such problems has led some hematopathologists to question the validity of performing cytofluorometric analysis of lymph nodes and other tissue specimens.

However, pathologists who exclusively analyze lymph nodes by frozen section immunohistochemistry sometimes may be unable, for example, to detect partial nodal involvement by a B-cell lymphoma or identify a T-cell–rich B-cell lymphoma. In these instances, preferential gated cytofluorometric analysis of the different constituent cell populations comprising a lymph node or other tissue specimen may detect a monoclonal B-cell population that evades detection in tissue sections.

We believe that a laboratory requires four attributes to routinely perform immunophenotypic analyses of pathologic specimens reliably and reproducibly:

1. Knowledge of the distribution of reactivity of the numerous available monoclonal antibody reagents with benign and malignant hematopoietic cells in cell suspensions and frozen and paraffin tissue sections (Table 11.1) (see Chapter 3)
2. Knowledge of the immunophenotypic profiles of the principal hematopoietic neoplasms (Tables 11.2–11.5)
3. Knowledge of the different methodologic approaches to immunophenotypic analysis and an appreciation of the advantages, disadvantages, and pitfalls intrinsic to each (see Chapter 3)
4. The ability to implement the appropriate combination of immunophenotypic methodology and monoclonal antibodies and other reagents to resolve the diagnostic dilemma posed by each individual case.

Our Approach

Immunophenotypic analyses of all peripheral blood, bone marrow aspiration, and effusion specimens, as well as all solid tissue specimens, obtained fresh and adequate in size to prepare a representative viable cell suspension are performed by direct and indirect immunofluorescent staining of the cells in suspension followed by cytofluorometric analysis of the immunostained cells (see Appendix 10). In general, single-color analysis (168) is performed using unlabeled primary murine monoclonal antibodies followed by affinity-purified, solid-phase human immunoglobulin-absorbed, fluorescein isothiocyanate (FITC)–conjugated $F(ab')_2$ fragments of sheep anti-mouse immunoglobulin (ICN Biomedicals, Costa Mesa, CA). Total surface immunoglobulin and the individual immunoglobulin heavy- and light-chain classes are detected with fluoroscein-labeled $F(ab')_2$ fragments of goat anti-human immunoglobulin (BioSource International, Camarillo, CA). Two-color and three-color analysis are used to determine if two or more antigens are expressed by the same cell population (168). This is helpful, for example, in clarifying occasional ambiguous results obtained by one-color analysis and in diagnosing acute mixed lineage (biphenotypic) leukemias. This approach is also useful when only limited numbers of cells are available for analysis, because two or three antigens can be detected using the number of cells normally assayed for one antigen. Cell suspension analysis of tissue specimens is preferred because it permits nearly all the specimens arriving each day to be batched and analyzed using the same methodology. This allows all the analyses to be performed rapidly in the least labor-intensive and the most time-efficient and cost-effective manner. This approach is objective and provides precise quantitative data while simultaneously measuring cell size and cytoplasmic granularity (24). The technical aspects of cytofluorometric analysis are discussed in detail in Chapter 5.

CSF samples often contain too few cells to be analyzed in this manner. In these cases, the cells are placed onto glass microscope slides by cytocentrifugation and are then immunostained by avidin-biotin complex (ABC) immunoperoxidase (see Appendix 7), by alkaline phosphatase–anti-alkaline phosphatase (APAAP) (see Appendix 7), or by indirect immunofluorescence modified for cytospin preparations (see Appendix 10).

Immunohistochemical staining of frozen or paraffin-embedded tissue sections is performed on solid tissue specimens in which a representative viable cell suspension cannot be prepared for technical reasons or because only fixed tissue is available and when the results of cell suspension analysis are equivocal or do not correlate with the histopathologic sections. One of the major advantages of immunohistochemical staining of frozen and especially paraffin tissue sections is architectural preservation, which permits precise topographic localization of the positively stained cells and their cytomorphologic evaluation. Most monoclonal antibodies used in flow cytometry also may be used in the immunohistochemical staining of frozen tissue sections (Table 11.1). Immunohistochemical staining of paraffin tissue sections requires a separate panel of reagents capable of detecting antigens that are resistant to formalin fixation and paraffin embedding. However, the new antigen retrieval techniques allow a wide range of antigens to be detected in routinely fixed and paraffin-embedded tissues, including many antigens that traditionally have been considered identifiable only in frozen tissue sections.

In most cases, frozen and paraffin tissue sections are immunostained by an ABC immunoperoxidase technique (see Appendix 7) because this method is highly sensitive and rapid. One technician can easily perform one and sometimes even two immunostaining "runs" of 120 slides each day using the Tech Mate 500 Automated Immunostaining System. Because the pseudoperoxidase activity of erythrocytes and the myeloperoxidase activity of neutrophils and other myeloid cells can make interpretation of immunoperoxidase-stained sections difficult, endogenous peroxidase activity is blocked in paraffin tissue sections before immunoperoxidase staining. An endogenous peroxidase blocking step is not included in the case of frozen sections or cytospin preparations because this can be damaging to the antigen to be demonstrated. The use of a negative control for the identification

TABLE 11.1. *Principal monoclonal antibodies employed in immunophenotypic analysis*

General category	CD no. or antigen	Principal antibodies	Antigen recognized (kd)	Principal pattern of reactivity	Comments
Hematopoietic	CD45	PD7/26/16 and 2B11 (P), HLe-1	gp180-220	Panhematopoietic cell	Leukocyte common antigen (LCA)
T lineage	CD1	OKT6, T6, Leu6, NA1/34,010 (P)	gp43-49	Cortical thymocytes, Langerhan cells, B cell subset	Now designated CD1a, CD1b, and CD1c
	CD2	OKT11, T11, Leu5, 9.6, MT910 (P)	gp50	Pan-T lymphocyte, natural killer cells	Sheep erythrocyte (E) rosette receptor
	CD3	OKT3, T3, Leu4, UCHT1, polyclonal CD3 (P)	gp/p 26, 20, 20, 16, 28	Pan-T lymphocyte, natural killer cells	CD3 complex of 5 chains; most antibodies detect ϵ chain
	CD4	OKT4, T4, Leu3a, 1F6 (P)	gp59	Cortical thymocytes, helper/inducer T cells, monocytes-macrophages	MHC class II receptor, HIV receptor
	CD5	OKT1, T1, Leu1, T101, UCHT2, 4C7 (P)	gp67	Pan-T lymphocyte, B-lymphocyte subset	
	CD7	Leu9, 3A1, WT1, OKT16	gp40	Pan-T lymphocyte, natural killer cells	Earliest appearing T lymphocyte antigen
	CD8	OKT8, T8, Leu2a, UCHT4, C8/144B (P)	gp32	Cortical thymocytes, suppressor/cytotoxic T cells, natural killer cell subset	MHC class I receptor
	CD43	Leu22 (L60) (P), MT1 (P)	gp95–135	Stem cells, erythroblasts, megakaryocytes, myeloid cells, macrophages, pan-T cell, all mature white blood cells except resting B cells	Sialophorin, leukosialin
	CD45RO	UCHL-1 (P), A6 (P), OPD4 (P)	gp180	T-cell subset, granulocytes, monocytes-macrophages	LCA isoform without A, B or C exons
	TCR $\alpha\beta$	WT31, βF1	gp47–49, 40	T lymphocytes expressing $\alpha\beta$ T-cell receptor	Use WT31 in flow cytometry and βF1 on frozen tissue sections
	TCR $\gamma\delta$	Anti-TCR $\gamma\delta$	gp40, 43	T lymphocytes expressing $\gamma\delta$ T-cell receptor	$<$5% normal T cells
B lineage	CD19	B4, Leu12,HD37	gp95	Pan-B lymphocyte	Earliest appearing B-lymphocyte antigen
	CD20	B1, Leu16, L26 (P)	p33	Pan-B lymphocyte	Appears after CD19 and CD22 in B cell ontogeny
	CD21	B2, OKB7, HB-5, 1F8 (P)	gp145	Mature B lymphocyte subset, follicular dendritic cells	C3d/Epstein-Barr virus receptor (CR2)
	CD22	Leu14, To15	gp130/140	Pan-B lymphocyte	Appears early in B cell ontogeny, after CD19
	CD45RA	4KB5 (P)	gp205–220	Pan-B lymphocyte, natural killer cells	LCA isoforms containing exon A

(continued)

TABLE 11.1. *Continued.*

General category	CD no. or antigen	Principal antibodies	Antigen recognized (kd)	Principal pattern of reactivity	Comments
B lineage	CD79a	HM57 (P), JCB117 (P)	gp33	Pan-B lymphocyte	Surface Ig receptor complex
	NA	Immunoglobulin (Ig) μ, δ, γ, α, κ, λ		B lymphocytes	Precursor B cells contain cytoplasmic μ, mature B cells express surface Ig, plasma cells contain cytoplasmic Ig
Myeloid/monocytic lineages	CD11b	Mo1, OKM1, Leu15	gp165	Monocytes-macrophages, granulocytes, natural killer cells	iC3b receptor (CR3)
	CD11c	LeuM5 (S-HCL3)	gp150	Granulocytes, monocytes-macrophages, natural killer cells, activated T and B cells	Hairy cell leukemia associated
	CD13	MY7, MCS-2, LeuM7	gp130–150	Myeloid cells, monocytes-macrophages	Aminopeptidase N, coronavirus receptor
	CD14	MY4, LeuM3, 63D3, Mo2	gp55	Monocytes-macrophages, granulocytes	Expressed by some B-cell lymphomas
	CD15	LeuM1 (P), Tu9 (P), VIM-D5 (P), IG10 (P)	X-hapten, Lewis antigen	Granulocytes, eosinophils, activated T cells, monocytes-macrophages, Langerhan cells	Expressed by Reed-Sternberg cells of Hodgkin's disease
	CD33	MY9, L4F3, LeuM9	gp67	Immature myeloid cells, granulocytes, monocytes-macrophages	Function unknown
	CD41	PBM 6.4, 5B12	gp120/23	Megakaryocytes, platelets	Glycoprotein IIb Forms complex with GPIIIa (CD61)
	CD61	Y2/51	gp105	Megakaryocytes, platelets	Glycoprotein IIIa
	CD68	KP-1 (P), PG-M1 (P)	gp110	Monocytes-macrophages, granulocytes, mast cells	KP-1 and PG-M1 exhibit differential reactivities with benign and malignant cells
	Glycophorin A	JC159	Sialoglycoprotein	Erythroid precursors excluding BFU-E and CFU-E	M, N blood group antigens
Natural killer	CD16	Leu11c, VEP-13, B73.1, 3G8	gp50–80	Natural killer cells, granulocytes, macrophages	FcγRIII
	CD56	Leu19, NKH-1, 123C3 (P)	gp180	Natural killer cells	Neural cell adhesion molecule (NCAM)
	CD57	Leu7 (HNK-1) (P)	gp110	Natural killer cell subset, T-cell subset	Expressed by various carcinomas, function unknown
Leukemia associated					
	CD10	J5, BA-3, CALLA	gp100	Precursor B cells, mature B-cell subset, granulocytes	Neutral endopeptidase

(continued)

TABLE 11.1. *Continued.*

General category	CD no. or antigen	Principal antibodies	Antigen recognized (kd)	Principal pattern of reactivity	Comments
Proliferation associated	CD71	OKT9, 5E9, T9	gp95	Thymocytes, activated B and T cells	Transferrin receptor
	NA	Ki-67, MIB-1 (P)	NR	Proliferating cells	Nuclear proliferation antigen
Activation associated	CD23	Leu20 (BLAST-2), Tu1, Bu38 (P), 1B12 (P)	gp45	Follicle mantle B cells, activated B cells, follicular dendritic cells, monocytes, platelets	FcϵRII
	CD25	Tac, 2A3, Tu69 (P)	gp55	Activated T cells, B cells and monocytes	Interleukin-2 receptor
	CD30	Ki-1, Ber-H2 (P)	gp105–120	Activated B and T cells	Expressed by Reed-Sternberg cells of Hodgkin's disease and anaplastic large cell lymphoma
	CD38	OKT10, Leu17, T16	gp46	Thymocytes, activated B and T cells, plasma cells	
	NA	HLA-DR, 1B5 (P), LN3 (P)	gp29, 34	B Lymphocytes, monocytes-macrophages, activated T cells and immature cells of many lineages	MHC class II molecule
Precursor	CD34	HPCA-1, MY10 (P), BI-3C5 (P), QBend/10 (P)	gp110	Myeloid, lymphoid and stromal progenitor cells, vascular endothelial cells	Earliest stem cell antigen
	TdT	Anti-TdT (P)	p60	Precursor B and T cells	Intranuclear DNA polymerase involved in formation of nucleotide (N) regions
Oncogene and tumor suppressor gene products	BCL-1	DCS-6 (P), p19 (P), Cyclin D1 (P)	p36	Absent in normal lymphoid tissue	Mantle cell lymphoma associated
	BCL-2	124 (P)	p24–26	Medullary thymocytes, T and non–germinal center B cells	Useful in distinguishing follicular lymphoma and hyperplasia
	p53	D01 (P), D07 (P), 1801 (P)	p53	Absent in normal lymphoid tissue	p53 protein overexpression and gene mutations do not necessarily correlate

NA, not available; NR, not reported; gp, glycoprotein; p, protein; kd, kilodaltons; (P), paraffin.
Compiled from references 6, 7, 9, 10, 24, 109–161, and personal observations.

TABLE 11.2. *Immunophenotypic profiles of subcategories of acute lymphoblastic leukemia and lymphoblastic lymphoma*

Category	Common immunophenotypic profile	Comments
Precursor B cell		~80% of ALLs ~20% of LBLs
Pre-pre-B cell	TdT(+), HLA-DR(+), CD19(±)	~10% of precursor B-ALLs
Common type	TdT(+), HLA-DR(+), CD19(+), CD10(+), CD20(±)	~70% of precursor B-ALLs
Pre-B cell	TdT(+), HLA-DR(+), CD19(+), CD10(+), CD20(+), cytoplasmic μ(+)	~20% of precursor B-ALLs
B cell	TdT(−), HLA-DR(+), CD19(+), CD20(+), sIg(+)	FAB-L3 morphology (Burkitt's leukemia)
Precursor T cell		~20% of ALLs ~80% of LBLs
Prothymocyte	TdT(+), CD7(+), CD2(±), cCD3(+), CD38(+), CD71(+)	~70% of precursor T-ALLs and ~30% of precursor T-LBLs express prothymocyte and immature thymocyte phenotypes.
Immature (early) thymocyte	TdT(+), CD7(+), CD5(+), CD2(±), cCD3(+), CD38(+), CD71(±)	
Common thymocyte	TdT(+), CD7(+), CD5(+), CD2(±), cCD3(+), sCD3(+), CD38(+), CD1(+), CD4(±), CD8(±)	~30% of precursor T-ALLs and ~70% of precursor T-LBLs express common and mature thymocyte phenotypes
Mature (medullary) thymocyte	TdT(+), CD7(+), CD5(+), CD2(+),cCD3(±), sCD3(+), CD38(±), CD4(±), CD8(±)	~1% of precursor T-ALLs

ALL, acute lymphoblastic leukemia; LBL, lymphoblastic lymphoma, FAB, French-American-British Classification (162); cCD3, cytoplasmic CD3; sCD3, surface CD3.

Compiled from references 6, 7, 9, 10, 24, 108, and personal observations.

TABLE 11.3. *Immunophenotypic profiles of subcategories of acute myeloid leukemia*

Category	FAB classification	Common immunophenotypic profile
Acute myeloblastic leukemia	M1, M2	HLA-DR(+), CD11b(±), CD13(+), CD14(±), CD15(±), CD33(+)
Acute promyelocytic leukemia	M3	HLA-DR(−), CD11b(±), CD13(+), CD14(−), CD15(±), CD33(+)
Acute myelomonocytic leukemia	M4	HLA-DR(+), CD11b(+), CD13(+), CD14(+), CD15(±), CD33(+)
Acute monocytic leukemia	M5	HLA-DR(+), CD11b(+), CD13(±), CD14(+), CD15(+), CD33(+)
Acute erythroblastic leukemia	M6	Glycophorin A(+)
Acute megakaryoblastic leukemia	M7	Platelet glycoprotein IIb/IIIa(+), Ib(±)
Chronic myelogenous leukemia in blast crisis		Blast crisis cell phenotype comparable to that of corresponding type of acute leukemia

FAB, French-American-British classification (162).

Compiled from references 7, 9, 24, 111, 163, and personal observations.

TABLE 11.4. *Immunophenotypic profiles of principal categories of mature B cell lymphoma and lymphoid leukemia*

Category	Common immunophenotypic profile
Small lymphocytic lymphoma; chronic lymphocytic leukemia	HLA-DR(+), CD19(+), CD20(+), CD22(±), CD5(+), CD23(+), CD10(−), low-density surface Ig(+)
Small lymphocytic lymphoma, plasmacytoid; Waldenström's macroglobulinemia	HLA-DR(+), CD19(+), CD20(+), CD22(±), CD5(−), CD10(−), CD23(±), CD38(+), surface and cytoplasmic Ig(+)
Mantle cell lymphoma	HLA-DR(+), CD19(+), CD20(+), CD22(+), CD5(+), BCL-1(+), CD10(−), CD23(−), surface Ig(+)
Small cleaved cell; mixed small cleaved and large cell lymphoma (follicular and diffuse)	HLA-DR(+), CD19(+), CD20(+), CD22(+), CD5(−), CD21(±), CD10(±), surface Ig(±)
Large cell lymphoma	HLA-DR(+), CD19(+), CD20(+), CD22(+), CD10(±), CD21(±), surface Ig(±)
Burkitt's lymphoma	HLA-DR(+), CD19(+), CD20(+), CD22(+), CD10(+), CD21(−), surface Ig(+)
Prolymphocytic leukemia	HLA-DR(+), CD19(+), CD20(+), CD22(+), CD21(±), high-density surface Ig(+)
Hairy cell leukemia	HLA-DR(+), CD19(+), CD20(+), CD11c(+), CD25(+), CD11b(+), CD5(−), surface Ig(+)
Plasmacytoma; multiple myeloma	HLA-DR(−), CD19(−), CD20(−), CD10(±), CD38(+), cytoplasmic Ig(+), surface Ig(±)

Ig, immunoglobulin.
Compiled from references 6, 7, 9, 10, 24, 153, 157, 164–166, and personal observations.

TABLE 11.5. *Immunophenotypic profiles of principal categories of postthymic T-cell non-Hodgkin's lymphoma and lymphoid leukemia*

Category	Common immunophenotypic profile[a]	Comments
Mycosis fungoides; Sézary syndrome	CD2(+), CD3(+), CD5(+), CD7(±), CD4(+), CD8(−), HLA-DR(±)	Two thirds of cases CD7(−), occasionally CD4(−) CD8(+), rarely CD4(+) CD8(+) or CD4(−) CD8(−)
Peripheral T-cell lymphoma	CD2/CD3/CD5 and/or CD7(±), CD4(±), CD8(±), HLA-DR(+), CD25(±)	~75% lack one or more pan-T-cell antigens, ~60% CD4(+) CD8(−), ~20% CD4(−) CD8(+); variably express multiple activation antigens
Chronic lymphocytic leukemia; prolymphocytic leukemia	CD2(+), CD3(+), CD5(+), CD7(+), CD4(+), CD8(−), HLA-DR(±)	Occasionally CD4(+) CD8(+) or CD4(−) CD8(+)
Adult T-cell leukemia/lymphoma	CD2(+), CD3(+), CD5(+), CD7(−), CD4(+), CD8(−), CD25(+), HLA-DR(±)	Usually exhibit suppressor function despite helper T-cell phenotype
Tγ-lymphoproliferative disease	CD2(+), CD3(+), CD5(±), CD7(±), CD4(−), CD8(+), CD11b(±), CD16(+), CD57(+), HLA-DR(±)	Express a multiplicity of immunophenotypes, rarely CD3(−)

[a] Postthymic T-cell neoplasms are uniformly CD1 and TdT negative.
Compiled from references 6–10, 24, 108, 167, and personal observations.

of endogenous peroxidase activity on frozen sections or the APAAP technique (see Appendix 7) on cytospin preparations are preferred.

Our approach to the immunophenotypic analysis of the acute leukemias, chronic lymphoid leukemias, and non-Hodgkin's lymphomas is broadly outlined. This approach is illustrated in a variety of specific diagnostic situations using synopses of 14 cases studied in this laboratory. These cases also provide an overview of the role of immunophenotypic and, in some instances, immunogenotypic analysis in the diagnosis and management of patients with hematopoietic neoplasms.

Acute Leukemia

In most cases, the diagnosis of acute leukemia has already been made or is strongly suspected clinically. In these instances, samples of involved peripheral blood or aspirated bone marrow are usually submitted to determine the immunophenotypic profile and thereby the nature of the leukemic cells. Often, most cells isolated from these specimens are malignant, and only a small number of residual benign cells are present, making analysis of these cases relatively straightforward. However, the results of cytofluorometric analysis of some acute myeloid leukemias can be confusing because of high background staining due to Fc binding. In most instances, this problem can be resolved by using conjugated monoclonal antibodies.

Acute leukemias are analyzed in cell suspension with an antibody panel (i.e., leukemia screen) (Table 11.6) chosen to permit their broad subclassification as precursor B-cell acute lymphoblastic leukemia (ALL), precursor T-cell ALL, or acute myeloid leukemia (AML), as well as to detect acute mixed lineage (biphenotypic) and chronic lymphoid leukemias. Additional expanded immunophenotypic profiles (Table 11.7) are then performed based on the results of this initial screening to further clarify the nature of the leukemia. Using this approach, definitive immunophenotypic analysis sometimes becomes a two-step process. However, the clinical information and morphologic examination of Diff-Quik–stained cytospin preparations are helpful in narrowing the differential diagnosis and planning a definitive one-step immunophenotypic analysis. For example, a 12-year-old boy presenting with a large mediastinal mass and a WBC count of 75,000/mm^3 probably has precursor T-cell ALL. In this case, an expanded T-cell screen (Table 11.7) should be performed initially in conjunction with the leukemia screen in the interest of time and efficiency. A carefully planned immunophenotypic analysis based on review of all of the available information and material is always strongly recommended.

Occasionally, a patient has a near normal peripheral blood

TABLE 11.6. *Monoclonal antibodies employed in the immunophenotypic analysis of acute leukemia (leukemia screen) and their reactivity with neoplastic cells*

Antigen or CD no.	Monoclonal antibody	Reactivity with neoplastic cells		
		B cells	T cells	Myeloid cells
TdT	Anti-TdT	~100% precursor B-ALL/LBL, absent from mature B-NHLs/LLs	~100% precursor T-ALL/LBL Absent from postthymic T-NHLs/LLs	~20% AMLs
HLA-DR	Anti-HLA-DR	~100% precursor B-ALL/LBL ~100% mature B-NHLs/LLs	~5% precursor B-ALL/LBL ~50% postthymic T-NHLs/LLs	~75% AMLs
CD10	J5	~60% precursor B-ALL/LBL, variable among B-NHLs/LLs	~20% precursor T-ALL/LBL Absent from postthymic T-NHLs/LLs	Absent
CD19	B4	~95% precursor B- ALL/LBL ~95% mature B-NHLs/LLs	Absent	~5% AMLs
CD20	B1	~50% precursor B- ALL/LBL ~95% mature B-NHLs/LLs	Absent	Absent
CD7	Leu9	Absent	~100% precursor T-cell ALL/LBL ~60% postthymic T-NHLs/LLs	~20% AMLs
CD5	Leu1	Variable among mature B-NHLs/LLs	~90% precursor T-ALL/LBL ~60% postthymic T-NHLs/LLs	Absent
CD13	MY7	Absent	Absent, may be expressed on mixed lineage leukemias	~80% AMLs
CD33	MY9	Absent	Absent, may be expressed on mixed lineage leukemias	~80% AMLs
CD34	MY10	~75% precursor B-ALL/LBL	~30% precursor T-ALL/LBL	~50% AMLs

TdT, terminal deoxynucleotidyl transferase; ALL, acute lymphoblastic leukemia; LBL, lymphoblastic lymphoma; AML, acute myeloid leukemia; NHL, non-Hodgkin's lymphoma; LL, lymphoid leukemia.

Compiled from references 6–10, 24, 108, 163, 167, 169–172, and personal observations.

TABLE 11.7. *Diagnostic implications and expanded immunophenotypic profiles performed based on the results of the leukemia screen*

Results of leukemia screen	Diagnostic implications	Expanded immunophenotypic profiles
TdT(+), HLA-DR(+), CD19(+), CD20(±), CD10(±), others (−)	Precursor B cell ALL; chronic myelogenous leukemia in lymphoid blast crisis	Cytoplasmic μ
TdT(+), CD7(+), CD5(±), CD10(±), others (−)	Precursor T-cell ALL	CD1, CD2, CD3, CD4, CD8, CD38, CD71
TdT(−), CD13 and/or CD33(+), HLA-DR(±), others (−)	Acute myeloid leukemia; chronic myelogenous leukemia in myeloid blast crisis	CD11b, CD11c, CD14, CD34, others as desired or necessary for precise classification
TdT(−), CD7 and/or CD5(+), HLA-DR(±), others (−)	Postthymic T-cell leukemia/lymphoma	CD1, CD2, CD3, CD4, CD8, CD25, CD38, CD71
TdT(−), CD19(+), CD20(+), HLA-DR(+), CD10(±), others (−)	Mature B-cell leukemia/lymphoma	Surface immmunoglobulin μ, δ, γ, α, κ, λ; others as necessary or desired for precise classification
TdT(+), CD19(+), CD20(±), CD13 and/or CD33(+), HLA-DR(+), CD10(±), others (−)	Acute mixed-lineage (biphenotypic) leukemia	Cytoplasmic μ, CD11b, CD11c, CD14, CD34
TdT(+), CD7,[a] and/or CD5(+), CD13 and/or CD33(+), others (−)	Acute mixed-lineage (biphenotypic) leukemia	CD1, CD2, CD3, CD4, CD8, Cd11b, CD11c, CD14, CD15, CD34, CD38, CD71

[a] CD7 is expressed by a small proportion of AMLs that otherwise express a pure myeloid phenotype.
Compiled from references 6, 7, 9, 10, 24, 108, 163, 167, and personal observations.

WBC count and differential count and a bone marrow packed with leukemic cells but that cannot be aspirated. In these cases, immunophenotypic analysis can be performed on paraffin tissue sections prepared from a bone marrow biopsy core. The hematopoietic cell antigens that are most helpful in the diagnosis of acute leukemia in routinely processed paraffin tissue sections are listed in Table 11.1 (see Chapters 4 and 38).

In some instances, other types of pathologic specimens (e.g., cutaneous punch biopsies, testicular and liver needle biopsies, effusions, CSF) are submitted for identification and analysis of leukemic cells. The same leukemia antibody panels may be employed in these situations. However, it is sometimes more difficult to analyze these specimens because of the small size of the tissue biopsy, the limited numbers of cells that can be harvested from the specimen, and the presence of many residual normal cells. In these instances, it is important to employ the immunodiagnostic reagents in order of diagnostic priority, such as TdT before κ or λ. If flow cytometry is employed, it is important to preferentially gate the neoplastic cells, thereby eliminating the normal cells from analysis and avoiding confusion in determining the immunophenotype of the leukemic cells.

B-Cell and T-Cell Non-Hodgkin's Lymphomas and Chronic Lymphoid Leukemias

Cell suspensions and frozen tissue sections prepared from pathologic specimens are analyzed with an antibody panel (i.e., lymphoma screen) (Table 11.8) chosen to broadly classify lymphoid proliferations as polyclonal or monoclonal B cell or T cell, and in the case of frozen tissue sections, to detect nonhematopoietic neoplasms as well. Additional expanded immunophenotypic profiles (Table 11.8) aimed at further classifying the nature of the process are then performed based on the results of this initial screen. The comments made about acute leukemia apply here as well. Careful consideration of the clinical information and morphologic examination of Diff-Quik–stained cytospin preparations and frozen tissue sections nearly always narrows the differential diagnosis significantly. A single-step definitive immunophenotypic analysis is possible in most cases if these factors are carefully evaluated before analysis. The immunodiagnostic reagents should always be used in order of diagnostic priority when the number of cells or the amount of tissue is severely limited. For example, if a B-cell lymphoma/leukemia is strongly suspected, immunostaining for κ and λ light chains, a pan-B-cell antigen (CD19, CD20, or CD22), and a pan-T-cell antigen (CD3) should be performed in that order. Preferential gated analysis should be performed in the case of flow cytometry.

In the case of lymph nodes and other solid tissue specimens, the results of cell suspension analysis are always correlated immediately with the histopathologic sections. Additional cell suspension studies are performed if it is believed that they will contribute to the further understanding of the case or if the results of morphologic examination and immunophenotypic analysis fail to correlate with one another or are equivocal. Immunostaining of frozen or paraffin tissue sections may be performed, depending on the specific diagnostic problem. If the results of all these additional studies are still nondiagnostic, it may be necessary to perform anti-

TABLE 11.8. *Monoclonal antibodies employed in the immunophenotypic analysis of nonlymphoblastic B- and T-cell non-Hodgkin's lymphoma and the diagnostic implications and expanded immunophenotypic profiles performed based on the results of the lymphoma screen*

Antibodies	Suspect benign/reactive initial panel	Suspect B-NHL/LL initial panel	Suspect T-NHL/LL initial panel
HLA-DR	•	•	•
Kappa	•	•	•
Lambda	•	•	•
CD19	•	•	•
CD5	•	•	•
CD3	•	•	•
CD4	•		•
CD8	•	•	•
CD10		•	•
CD23		•	•
IgM		•	
IgD		•	
IgG		•	
IgA		•	
CD2			•
CD7			•

	Suspect benign/reactive initial panel				Suspect B-NHL/LL initial panel				Suspect T-NHL/LL initial panel		
Findings	Polyclonal B cells; mixture of CD4 and CD8 cells	Polyclonal B cells; Reversed CD4:CD8 ratio	Elevated CD4:CD8 ratio	Monoclonal B cells	Monoclonal B cells; faint Ig^+, $CD5^+$, $CD23^+$	Monoclonal B cells; bright Ig^+, $CD5^+$, $CD23^-$	Monoclonal B cells; $CD5^-$, $CD23^-$	Polyclonal B cells or sIg^-, but clinical/morphogic suspicion of B-NHL/LL	Loss of pan-T-cell antigens	No pan-T-cell antigen loss; increased CD8 cells	Normal or increased CD4:CD8 ratio; no loss of pan-T-cell antigens
Immunodiagnosis	? Benign ? Hodgkin's disease	? Benign ? T-NHL/LL	? Benign ? T-NHL/LL ? Hodgkin's disease	B-NHL/LL	B-CLL	B-NHL/LL ? mantle cell	B-NHL/LL ? type	? Benign ? B-NHL/LL	T-NHL/LL	? Benign ? T-NHL/LL ? NK tumor	? Benign ? Hodgkin's disease
Additional Immunostaining	CD15, CD30 in paraffin tissue sections if necessary	CD2, CD3, CD7; If ? NK tumor then CD16, CD56, CD57	CD2, CD3, CD7; CD15, CD30 in paraffin tissue sections	Ig heavy chains		BCL-1 if necessary	CD11c, CD25 if necessary	Coexpression of CD5 and CD19; BCL-2 expression	CD25 if necessary	CD16, CD56, CD57	CD15, CD30 in paraffin tissue sections if necessary
Additional studies (if necessary)		Ig/TCR gene rearrangements	Ig/TCR gene rearrangements	BCL-1, CD11c, CD23, CD25; *BCL1, BCL2* gene rearrangements		*BCL1, BCL2* gene rearrangements		Ig/TCR, *BCL-1* or *BCL-2* gene rearrangements		Ig/TCR gene rearrangements	Ig/TCR gene rearrangements

gen receptor gene rearrangement analysis and possibly other molecular genetic studies on DNA extracted from the residual cells or cryopreserved tissue block.

Role of Antigen Receptor Gene Rearrangement Analysis

This laboratory has contributed significantly to the general understanding of the role of antigen receptor gene rearrangement analysis in the diagnosis and classification of hematopoietic neoplasia (3,14,16–19,22,46,57–59,61–64,67,89, 90,108). Nonetheless, most hematopoietic neoplasms encountered in daily practice can be accurately diagnosed and classified on the basis of morphologic examination and immunophenotypic analysis alone. Antigen receptor gene rearrangement analysis is laborious, time consuming, and costly. The routine application of this technology to lymphoma and leukemia samples often delays diagnosis unnecessarily. This laboratory therefore reserves the performance of antigen receptor gene rearrangement analysis for diagnostic dilemmas unresolvable by morphologic and immunophenotypic analysis and those occasional situations where such analyses may provide additional useful information.

For example, approximately 30% of follicular, mixed small cleaved, and large cell lymphomas and a smaller proportion of follicular, predominantly small cleaved cell lymphomas lack surface immunoglobulin (6,7,9). Immunophenotypic analysis sometimes cannot confirm the morphologic diagnosis of follicular lymphoma in these instances. Follicular and diffuse B-cell lymphomas sometimes only partially involve lymphatic and extralymphatic tissues or are surrounded by a significant inflammatory response. In these instances, it may be impossible to demonstrate a monotypic surface immunoglobulin-positive cell population and thereby confirm the morphologic diagnosis of B-cell lymphoma. The demonstration of clonal immunoglobulin heavy and light chain gene rearrangements can be very helpful in confirming the diagnosis of B-cell lymphoma in all these situations.

Similarly, even with the benefit of immunophenotypic analysis, it is sometimes difficult to make a definitive diagnosis of peripheral T-cell lymphoma or distinguish it from mixed cellularity Hodgkin's disease. Immunophenotypic analysis of T-cell leukemias and lymphomas contaminated by the presence of many benign T cells often leads to ambiguous results. Unlike B cells, for which monotypic surface immunoglobulin can be used to infer clonality, no phenotypic markers of T-cell clonality exist. The demonstration of clonal T-cell receptor gene rearrangements is extremely helpful in confirming the morphologic diagnosis of T-cell lymphoma and leukemia.

However, employing antigen receptor gene rearrangement analysis in the diagnosis of hematopoietic neoplasia is not without complication. First, clonal immunoglobulin and T-cell receptor gene rearrangements are not entirely lineage specific. Approximately 10% of B- and T-cell leukemias/lymphomas are bigenotypic (57), and rare T-cell malignancies have been reported to display clonal light chain gene rearrangements (173,174). Some acute myeloid leukemias exhibit clonal immunoglobulin and T-cell receptor gene rearrangements (61). Second, the demonstration of clonality does not necessarily indicate malignancy. Clonal immunoglobulin gene rearrangements have been demonstrated in hyperplastic lymph nodes from human immunodeficiency virus (HIV)–infected patients (18), in extranodal lymphoid hyperplasias (19,22,23), in the benign lymphoepithelial lesions of Sjögren's syndrome (20,22), and in systemic Castleman's disease (21). Clonal T-cell receptor gene rearrangements have been demonstrated in lymphomatoid papulosis (175,176) and in a variety of cutaneous lymphoproliferative disorders (108). Considerable caution should be exercised in interpreting the results of antigen receptor gene rearrangement analysis. This is discussed in Chapter 9.

ANALYSIS AND INTERPRETATION OF IMMUNOPHENOTYPIC DATA

The accurate morphologic evaluation of hematopoietic neoplasms ranges from easy to difficult, depending on the knowledge, expertise, and experience of the pathologist. The same holds true for the accurate immunophenotypic evaluation of hematopoietic neoplasms. Ideally, the person analyzing, interpreting, and reporting the results of immunophenotypic analysis should have knowledge of the clinical characteristics and be expert in the morphologic evaluation of hematopoietic neoplasia, as well as have considerable experience in performing immunophenotypic analysis and analyzing and interpreting the results. If such a person is not available to perform these diagnostic studies, two or more individuals possessing these skills in combination should coordinate the diagnostic activities.

In the late afternoon in our laboratory, the entire physician staff review the results of all cytofluorometric and immunohistochemical studies in conjunction with the clinical information, morphologic review of the histopathologic sections, and any other available information and renders a definitive diagnosis or requests additional studies in each case under study. The correlative morphologic examination and immunophenotypic analysis of each specimen is usually completed within 48 hours, unless extensive additional studies are necessary.

The two most important factors to be considered in the analysis and interpretation of immunophenotypic data are the clinical characteristics of the patient and the results of morphologic evaluation of the pathologic specimen. Immunophenotypic data should always be interpreted in light of, and never reported without considering, this information. Failure to do so may result in erroneous conclusions with grave consequences for the patient.

In general, it is best to approach each case systematically, taking all the available information into consideration and asking yourself the critical questions as you proceed. First, the clinical characteristics of the patient and the results of other pertinent laboratory tests that have been performed should be reviewed. Based on this information, what is the most likely diagnosis? What are the other diagnostic possibilities? Second, the morphology of the histopathologic sections, peripheral blood, bone marrow smears, and other pathologic material should be carefully evaluated. Is a hematopoietic neoplasm present? If so, can it be definitively diagnosed and classified? If diagnosis and classification are not possible, what is the diagnostic dilemma--benign versus malignant, Hodgkin's disease versus non-Hodgkin's lymphoma, B cell versus T cell, or lymphoid versus myeloid? Third, the Diff-Quik–stained cytocentrifuge slides prepared from the cell suspension or the Diff-Quik–stained frozen tissue sections should be reviewed. Are the cells or tissue present in these slide preparations the same as those in the histopathologic sections? In other words, are these preparations representative? What is the proportion of neoplastic cells or tissue in these preparations? Fourth, the immunophenotypic results should be reviewed. Do these results correlate with the histopathologic interpretation? If a hematopoietic neoplasm is present, does the immunophenotypic profile clearly indicate its lineage and classification? If the results do not correlate with the morphologic interpretation, why not? Is this because of technical problems encountered during immunophenotypic analysis? Is the initial morphologic interpretation incorrect? What additional studies can be performed to resolve this discrepancy? If the morphologic evaluation of the pathologic specimen did not lead to a definitive diagnosis, do the results of the immunophenotypic analysis resolve the diagnostic dilemma? Will the performance of additional studies provide additional important diagnostic or prognostic information? Does the final morphologic and immunophenotypic diagnosis in this case correlate with the clinical scenario? If so, a definitive diagnosis is rendered.

EXAMPLES OF IMMUNOPHENOTYPIC ANALYSIS

The remainder of this chapter consists of a brief discussion of 13 illustrative examples of hematopoietic neoplasms diagnosed and classified with the assistance of flow cytometry, frozen and paraffin tissue section immunohistochemistry, and antigen receptor gene rearrangement analysis.

Case 1

This 65-year-old woman had undergone a mastectomy for an infiltrating lobular carcinoma of the breast several years earlier. She presented with anemia and an elevated erythrocyte sedimentation rate. Radiologic studies demonstrated lytic bone lesions. A bone marrow biopsy showed diffuse replacement by neoplastic cells. The referring pathologist thought that the neoplastic cells most closely resembled those of multiple myeloma but, in view of the history, also included metastatic breast carcinoma in the differential.

Immunohistochemical staining of paraffin tissue sections from this biopsy can be used to confirm the correct diagnosis of multiple myeloma. However, the improper use of immunohistochemical stains in this case can also be used to support the erroneous diagnosis of metastatic breast carcinoma. Figure 11.1 illustrates the results of immunohistochemical staining of paraffin tissue sections of the bone marrow biopsy for CD45 (leukocyte common antigen; *top left*), epithelial membrane antigen (*top right*), κ light chains (*bottom left*) and λ light chains (*bottom right*; immunoperoxidase stain, original magnification: 400× magnification). These studies demonstrate that only residual normal hematopoietic elements in the bone marrow are $CD45^+$; the neoplastic cells are $CD45^-$. Many of the neoplastic cells are epithelial membrane antigen positive. The results of these two immunostains could be used to support the incorrect diagnosis of metastatic breast carcinoma. However, neoplasms related to the terminal stages of B-cell differentiation, such as immunoblastic lymphoma and multiple myeloma, are often $CD45^-$. Myeloma plasma cells may be epithelial membrane antigen positive. Additional immunostains for κ and λ light chains unequivocally demonstrate that most neoplastic cells contain κ light chains and lack λ light chains, consistent with a clonal plasma cell proliferation, confirming the correct morphologic diagnosis of multiple myeloma in this case.

Case 2

A 54-year-old asymptomatic woman presented with left cervical lymphadenopathy, which was subsequently biopsied (Fig. 11.2). The histopathologic sections (*top left*, hematoxylin and eosin stain, original magnification: 40× magnification) show that the lymph node architecture is effaced. Numerous small, benign-appearing germinal centers are present. Most of these are surrounded by thick mantle zones. Immunostaining demonstrates that the germinal center and the surrounding mantle zone lymphocytes are predominantly B cells based on the expression of CD22 (*top right*, immunoperoxidase stain, original magnification: 40× magnification). Immunostaining for CD3 (*middle and bottom left*, immunoperoxidase stain, original magnifications: 40× and 100× magnification) show that only small numbers of scattered T cells are present within the germinal centers and mantle zones. Immunostaining for CD5 (*middle and bottom right*, immunoperoxidase stain, original magnifications: 40× and 100× magnification) helps to distinguish the benign and the malignant B-cell populations in this case. The only $CD5^+$ cells present within the germinal centers are benign T cells that strongly express CD5; most germinal center B cells are $CD5^-$. However, most mantle zone B cells, which are $CD22^+CD3^-$, weakly express CD5. The mantle zone lymphocytes in this case coexpress B-lineage–associated antigen CD22 and the CD5 antigen. Normally, $CD5^+$ B cells are present only in small numbers in lymph nodes and are not readily identifiable by single-color immunohistochemical staining. The presence of a conspicu-

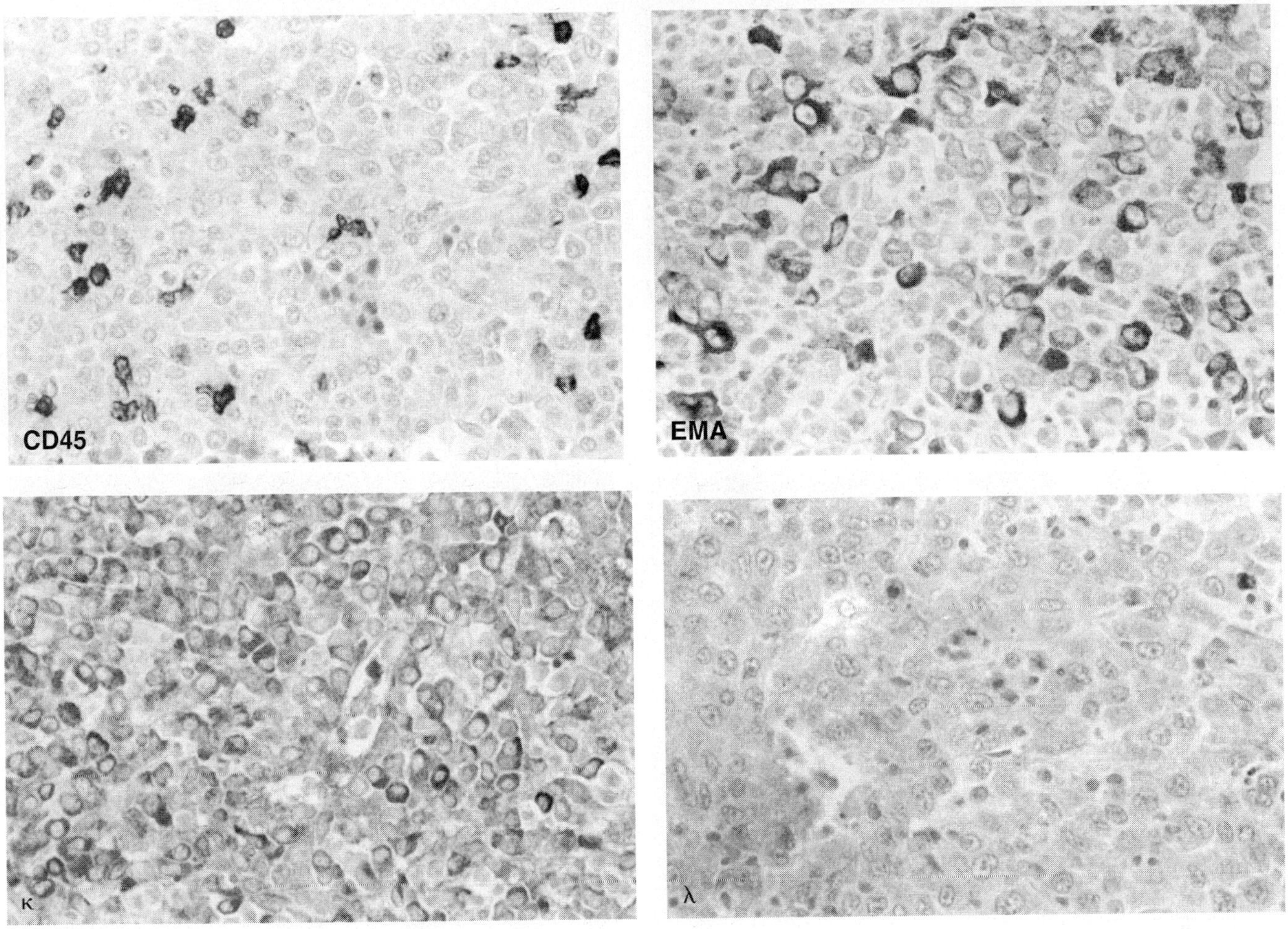

FIG. 11.1.

ous lymphocyte proliferation coexpressing B-lineage–associated antigens and CD5 is one of the principal immunophenotypic criteria for B-cell neoplasia. The immunophenotypic findings in this case, in conjunction with the histopathology, are consistent with a mantle cell lymphoma.

Case 3

This 62-year-old woman presented with a mass in the right breast that was biopsied and subsequently studied morphologically, immunophenotypically in frozen tissue sections, and by immunoglobulin gene rearrangement analysis (Fig. 11.3). The histopathologic sections (*top left*, hematoxylin and eosin stain, original magnification: 40× magnification) show that the breast parenchyma and associated fibrofatty tissue contain nodules of lymphoid tissue. Higher power magnification examination of these cells (*top right*, hematoxylin and eosin stain, original magnification: 630× magnification) shows that these nodules are predominantly composed of small lymphoid cells possessing irregularly shaped and cleaved nuclei, suggesting a follicular, predominantly small cleaved cell lymphoma. However, extensive evaluation of the patient failed to reveal any additional evidence of malignant lymphoma. Because the hematologist desired additional evidence that this lesion represented a malignant lymphoma and not merely an extranodal lymphoid hyperplasia, frozen tissue section immunohistochemistry was performed. These studies demonstrate that the central portions of each of the nodules contains predominantly B cells and that the surrounding lymphocytes are predominantly T cells (data not shown). However, immunostaining for κ light chains (*middle left*, immunoperoxidase stain, original magnification: 100× magnification) and λ light chains (*middle right*, immunoperoxidase stain, original magnification: 100× magnification) showed only small numbers of immunoglobulin-positive B cells, which predominantly surround the follicles and do not lie within them. The immunophenotypic results demonstrate that these follicles are largely composed of surface immunoglobulin-negative B cells. The monoclonal B-cell nature of these follicles cannot be definitively demonstrated by immunophenotypic analysis. Approximately 30% of follicular lymphomas are surface immunoglobulin negative and can conceivably present this diagnostic dilemma. In this case, DNA was extracted from the remaining cryopreserved tissue, and antigen receptor gene rearrangement analysis was performed *(bottom)*. These

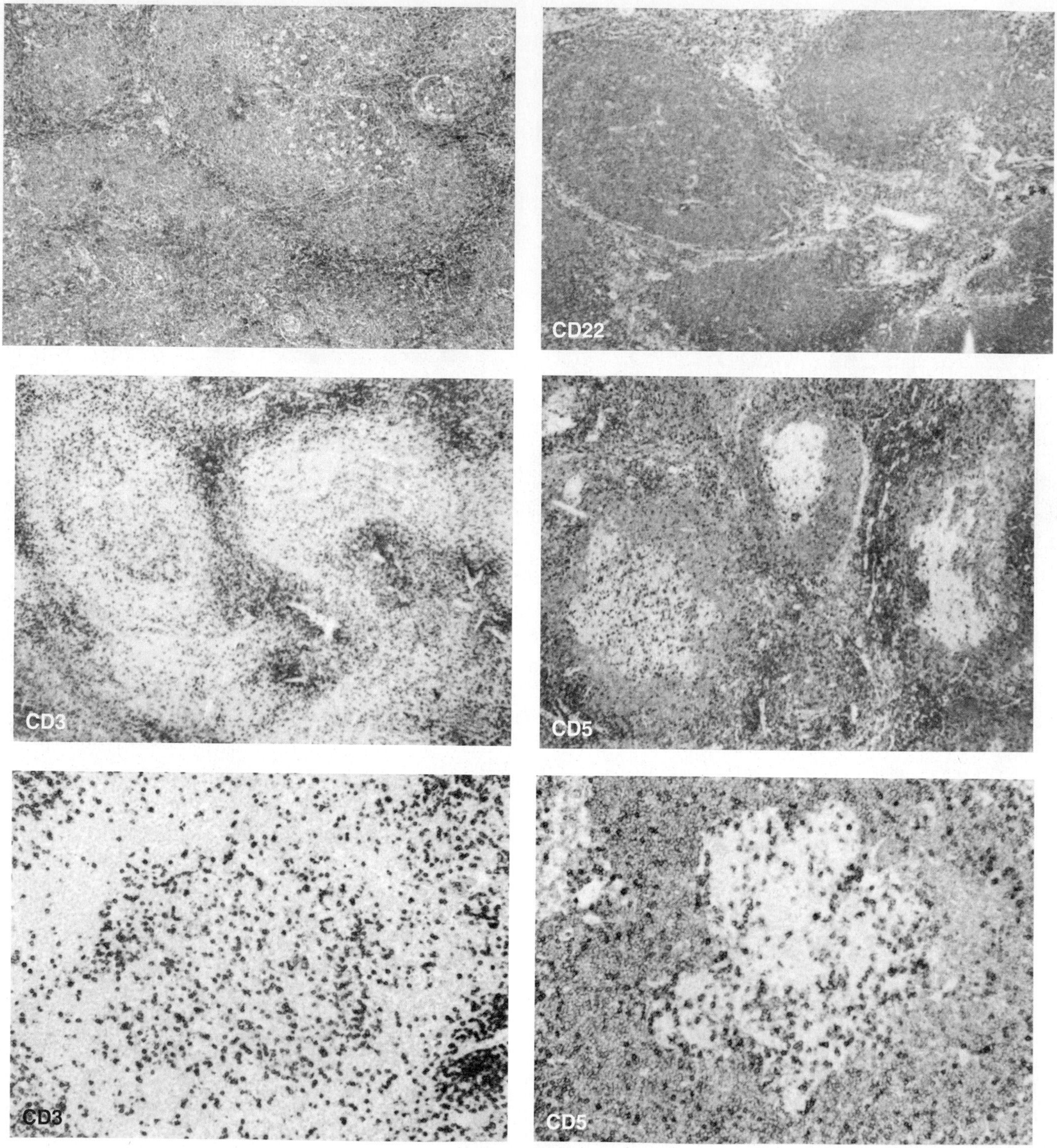

FIG. 11.2.

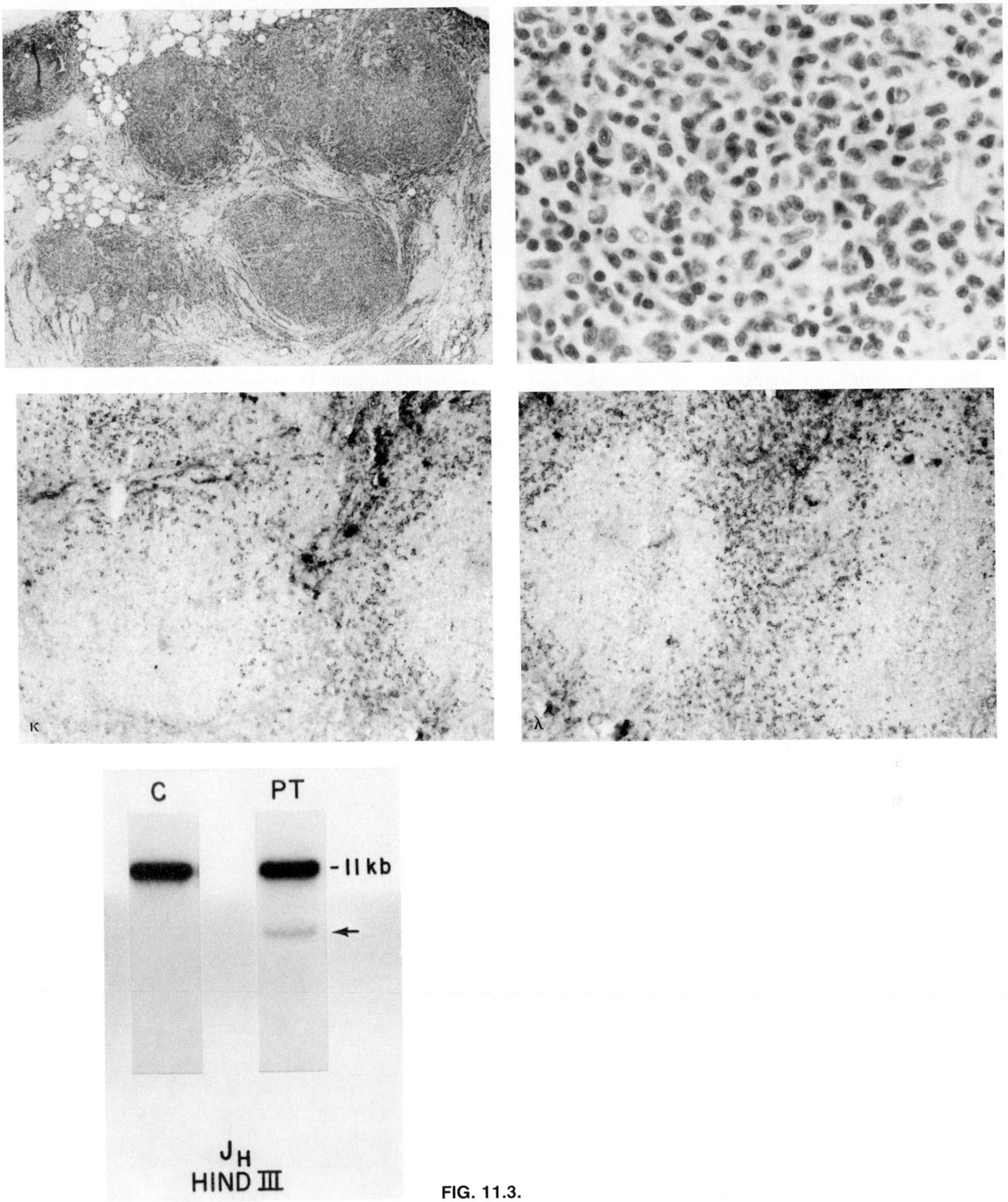

FIG. 11.3.

studies demonstrate the presence of a clonal immunoglobulin heavy-chain gene rearrangement *(arrow)* on hybridization of *Hin*dIII-digested DNA to an immunoglobulin heavy-chain joining region (J_H) DNA probe. The T-cell receptor gene is in the germline configuration (not shown). Immunogenotypic analysis confirms the morphologic impression of malignant lymphoma by demonstrating the clonal nature of the proliferation. In summary, this patient has a stage IE follicular, predominantly small cleaved cell lymphoma, which is negative for surface immunoglobulin but can be shown to be a monoclonal B-cell proliferation by antigen receptor gene rearrangement analysis.

Case 4

This 73-year-old woman presented with meningeal signs and symptoms. A CSF examination revealed the presence of 540 WBCs/mm^3, most of which were cytomorphologically malignant. A subsequent CSF sample was submitted to the hematopathology laboratory for immunophenotypic analysis. The cells were isolated from this sample and placed onto glass microscope slides by cytocentrifugation, and immunophenotypic analysis was performed by immunoperoxidase staining (Fig. 11.4). These studies demonstrate that virtually all of the cytomorphologically malignant cells are T cells based on the expression of CD7 (*top left*, immunoperoxidase stain, original magnification: 400× magnification) and of CD3 and CD2 (not shown). However, these cells lack pan-T-cell antigen CD5 (*top right*, immunoperoxidase stain, original magnification: 400× magnification), exclusively express CD4, and lack CD8 (not shown) and express a variety of activation-associated antigens including HLA-DR (*bottom left*, immunoperoxidase stain, original magnification: 400× magnification). These cytomorphologically malignant cells express an anomalous T-cell immunophenotype, subset antigen restriction, and various activation-associated antigens. This constellation of findings led to the diagnosis of CSF involvement by a peripheral T-cell lymphoma. Subsequently, the patient's past medical history was obtained from another hospital, and it was learned that the patient had been diagnosed with malignant lymphoma several years earlier. Retrieval of the archival pathologic mate-

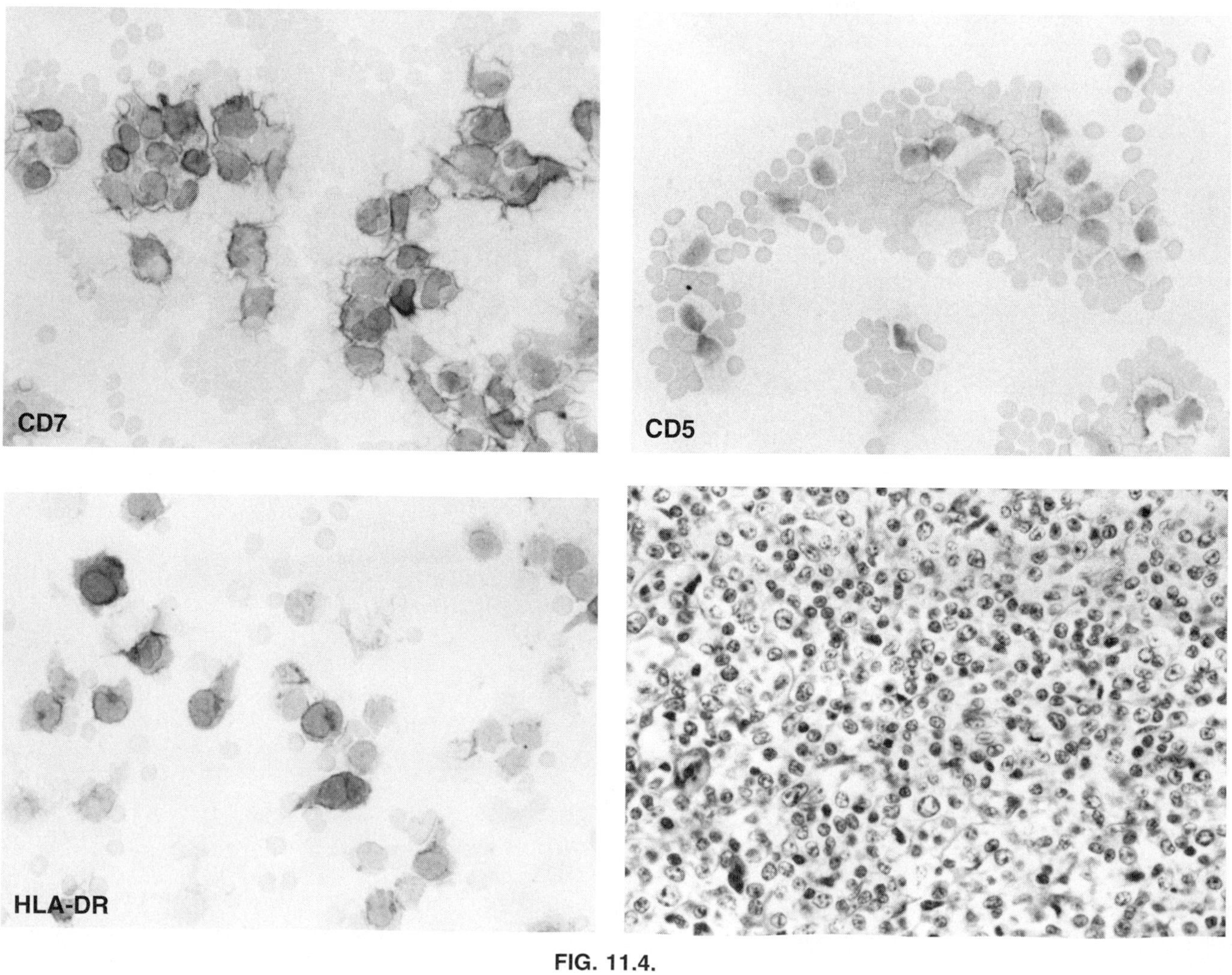

FIG. 11.4.

rial from that institution revealed that the patient's previous malignant lymphoma was a peripheral T-cell lymphoma (*bottom right*, hematoxylin and eosin stain, original magnification: 400× magnification).

Case 5

This 38-year-old man presented complaining of increasing weakness. Clinical evaluation revealed splenomegaly containing multiple solid hypoechoic regions and a decrease in the WBC and platelet counts. There was no evidence of lymphadenopathy and bone marrow aspiration and biopsy were negative. The patient subsequently underwent diagnostic splenectomy (Fig. 11.5). The spleen weighed 264 g and contained multiple, variably sized, well-circumscribed nodules, some of which were subdivided by collagen septa (*top*, hematoxylin and eosin stain, original magnification: 5× magnification). Higher-power examination of the nodules (*middle*, hematoxylin and eosin stain, original magnification: 630× magnification) reveals that they contain loosely aggregated large neoplastic cells lying singly and in small clusters and lacking cohesiveness. The neoplastic cells exhibit distinct cytoplasmic borders and contain abundant acidophilic cytoplasm and large round to ovoid vesicular and occasionally pleomorphic nuclei, often containing prominent nucleoli. Many binucleate and occasional multinucleate cells are present. Phagocytosed erythrocytes, hemosiderin, and leukocytes are readily identified in numerous tumor cells. Immunophenotypic analysis demonstrates that the large erythrophagocytic tumor cells exhibit a phenotype consistent with a tissue macrophage derivation. Specifically, the neoplastic cells contain α_1-antichymotrypsin (*bottom*, immunoperoxidase stain, original magnification: 630× magnification), monocyte-associated antigen CD14, and myeloid/monocyte–associated antigens CD13 and CD33. The cells lack B- and T-lineage–associated antigens and lack CD45, CD1, CD30, and S-100 protein (not shown). The neoplastic cells also lack clonal immunoglobulin and T-cell receptor gene rearrangements, further confirmation of a non-B-cell, non-T-cell lineage derivation for these neoplastic cells. Immunophenotypic and genotypic analyses have demonstrated that most neoplasms once believed to be derived from histiocytes or monocytes-macrophages are derived from B-lineage or T-lineage cells. However, immunophenotypic and immunogenotypic analysis in this particular case were instrumental in documenting the macrophage derivation of this hematopoietic neoplasm. (From Franchino C, Reich C, Distenfeld A, et al. A clinicopathologically distinctive primary splenic histiocytic neoplasm: demonstration of its histiocytic derivation by immunophenotypic and molecular genetic analysis. *Am J Surg Pathol* 1988;12:398–404, with permission.)

Case 6

This 62-year-old woman presented with nausea, vomiting, and abdominal cramps associated with a 30-lb weight loss over 2 months. After extensive evaluation, she was diagnosed as having the nephrotic syndrome. Lymphadenopathy and organomegaly were absent. Extensive radiologic examination and bone marrow biopsy failed to reveal evidence of malignancy. A renal biopsy was subsequently performed (Fig. 11.6). This biopsy was interpreted as minimal change disease. However, the glomerular capillary lumina contain large neoplastic cells that appear to be circulating in the glomerular capillaries (*top left*, hematoxylin and eosin stain, original magnification: 320× magnification). These neoplastic cells have indistinct cytoplasm and contain large, irregular hyperchromatic nuclei with prominent nucleoli *(arrows)*. Electron microscopic examination shows the glomerular capillary lumina to be frequently occluded by marginated neoplastic cells with irregularly folded nuclei, numerous polyribosomes, and scattered mitochondria (*bottom left*, original magnification: 5,460× magnification). Immunophenotypic analysis was performed by immunohistochemical staining of paraffin tissue sections. Immunohistochemical staining for factor VIII–related antigen (*top right*, immunoperoxidase stain, original magnification: 320× magnification) reveals staining of the glomerular endothelium, highlighting the intraluminal neoplastic cells, which are factor VIII–related antigen negative. Additional immunostains show that the neoplastic cells express CD45 (*middle right*, immunoperoxidase stain, original magnification: 320× magnification) and B-lineage–restricted antigen CD20 (*bottom right*, immunoperoxidase stain, original magnification: 320× magnification). These paraffin tissue section immunohistochemical studies of the renal biopsy permitted diagnosis of an angiotropic or intravascular B-cell large cell lymphoma. (From D'Agati V, Sablay LB, Knowles DM, et al. Angiotropic large cell lymphoma (intravascular malignant lymphomatosis) of the kidney: presentation as minimal change disease. *Hum Pathol* 1989;20:263–268, with permission.)

Case 7

This 49-year-old man presented with a variety of constitutional symptoms, generalized lymphadenopathy, and organomegaly. A lymph node biopsy was performed (Fig. 11.7). The histopathologic sections (*top left*, hematoxylin and eosin stain, original magnification: 100× magnification) show diffuse infiltration of the lymph node by large anaplastic tumor cells. Many of the neoplastic cells form clusters in the interfollicular and paracortical regions and display a propensity for sinusoidal distribution. The neoplastic cells are exceptionally large, often contain abundant cytoplasm, and frequently contain one or more nuclei with prominent nucleoli. Wreath-like nuclei are often identified. Binucleated cells with prominent nucleoli sometimes resemble the Reed-Sternberg cells of Hodgkin's disease (*top right*, hematoxylin and eosin stain, original magnification: 400× magnification). The referring pathologist considered several clinicopathologic entities in the differential diagnosis, including

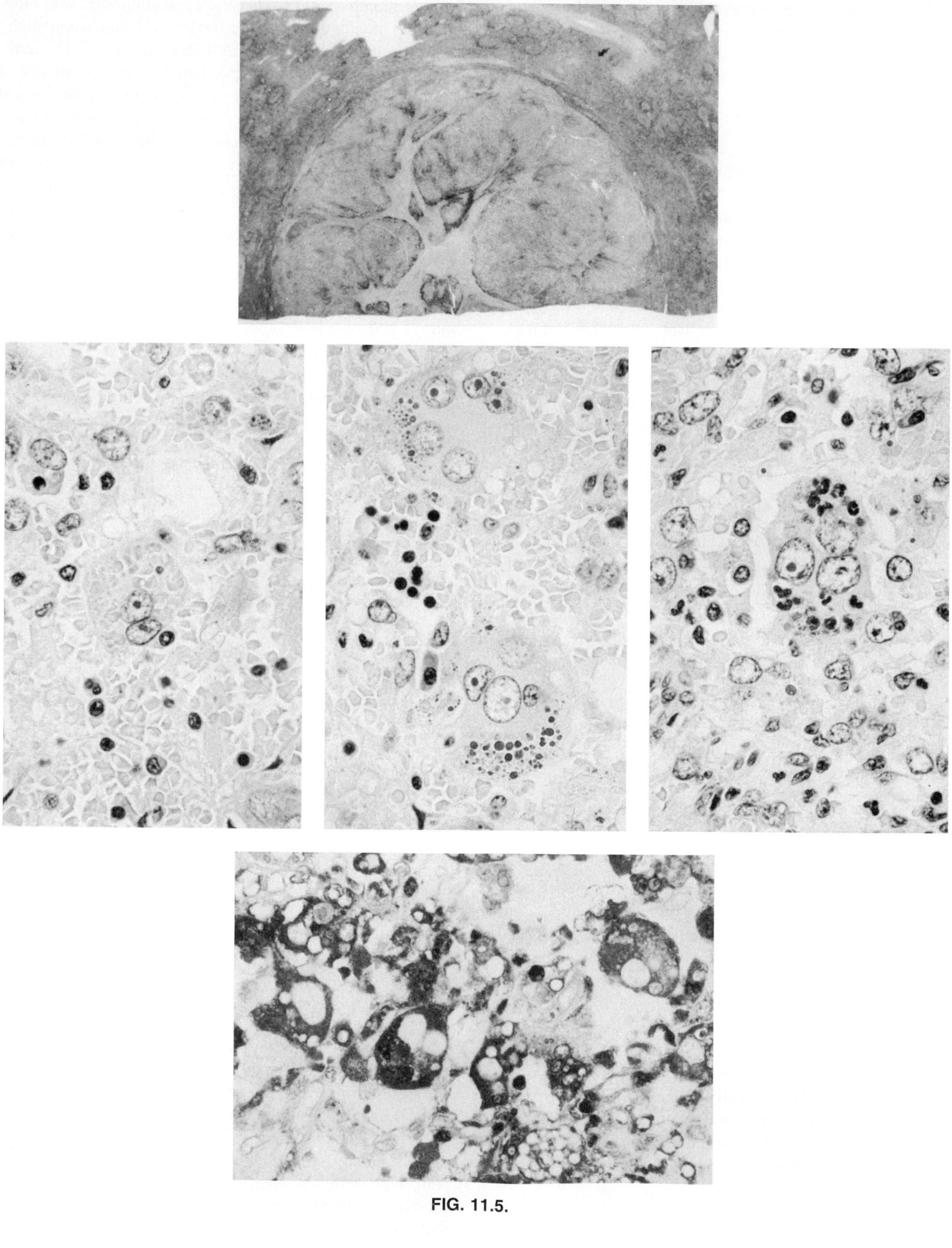

FIG. 11.5.

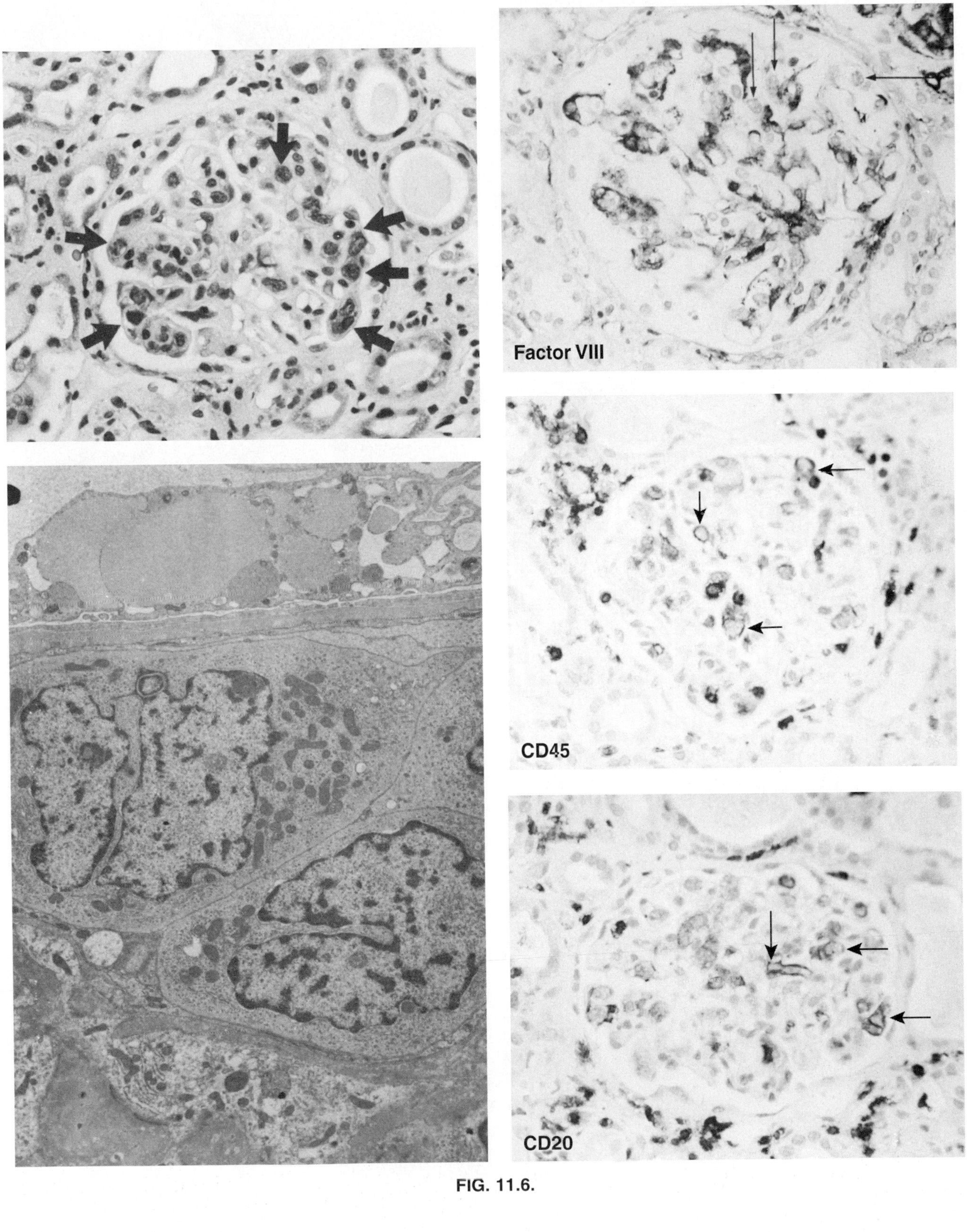

FIG. 11.6.

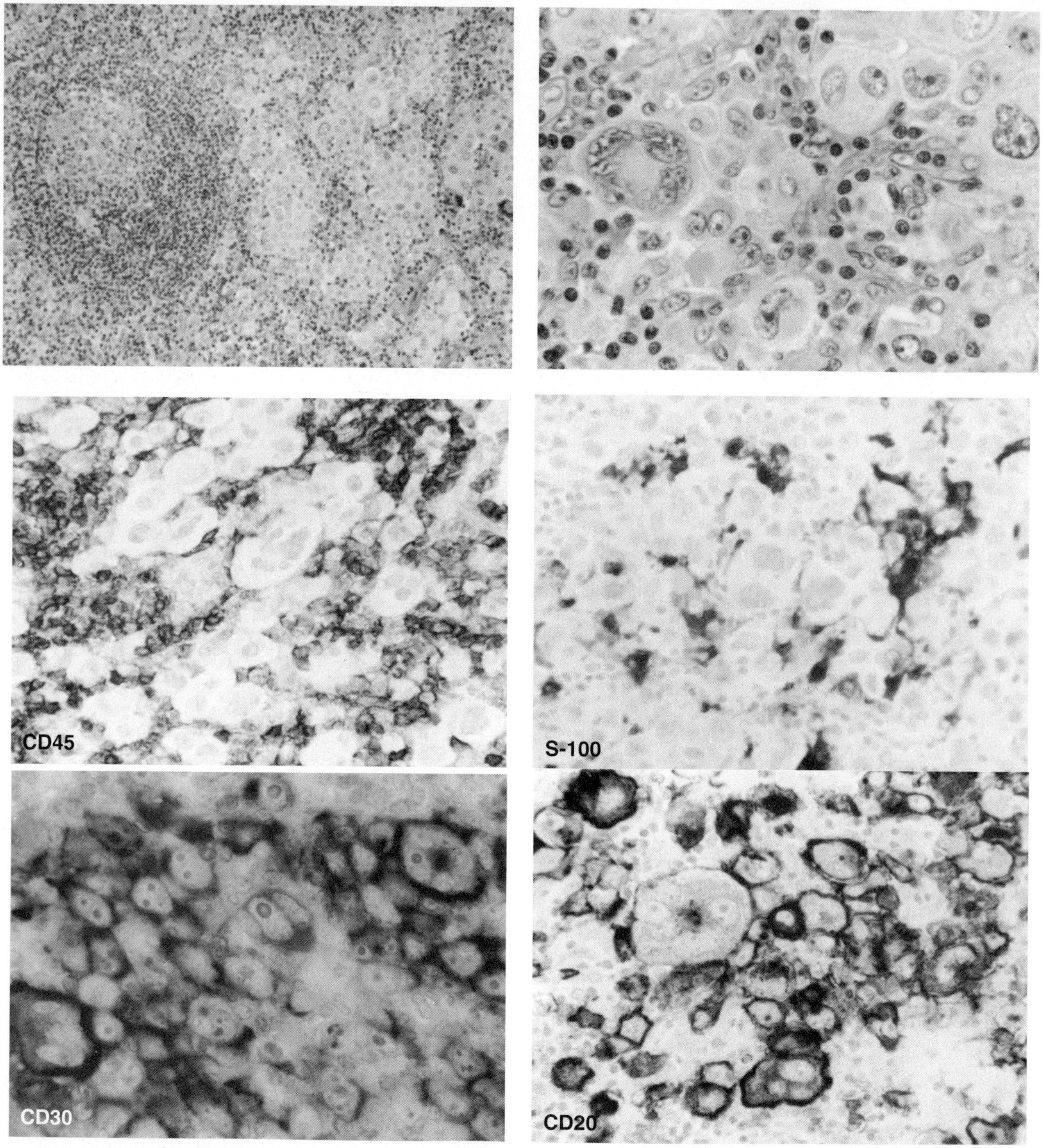

FIG. 11.7.

disseminated amelanotic melanoma and CD30$^+$ anaplastic large cell lymphoma. Immunohistochemical staining (*middle left*, immunoperoxidase stain, original magnification: 400× magnification) demonstrates that the large anaplastic tumor cells are CD45$^-$. Small residual benign lymphocytes are strongly CD45$^+$ and thereby serve as an internal positive control. However, approximately 30% of CD30$^+$ anaplastic large cell lymphomas are CD45$^-$ when evaluated in paraffin tissue sections. The absence of CD45 expression does not exclude malignant lymphoma in this case. The anaplastic tumor cells are S-100 protein negative (*middle right*, immunoperoxidase stain, original magnification: 250× magnification). Dendritic cells strongly positive for S-100 protein serve as an internal positive control. Virtually all of the anaplastic tumor cells show abundant and strong membrane, cytoplasmic, and Golgi region staining for the CD30 antigen (*bottom left*, alkaline phosphatase–anti-alkaline phosphatase, original magnification: 400× magnification). Approximately 95% of anaplastic large cell lymphomas are CD30$^+$. The anaplastic tumor cells express B-lineage–restricted antigen CD20 (*bottom right*, immunoperoxidase stain, original magnification: 400× magnification). Most CD30$^+$ anaplastic large cell lymphomas express T-lineage–associated antigens and only a minority express B-lineage–associated antigens, as in this case. These immunophenotypic findings confirm the morphologic impression of anaplastic large cell lymphoma and rule out malignant melanoma, metastatic carcinoma, and other clinicopathologic entities from diagnostic consideration in this case (see Chapter 25).

Case 8

This 6-year-old girl presented with a several-week history of subcutaneous lumps about the head and neck that were increasing in size. One of the lesions was biopsied and submitted for histopathologic evaluation (Fig. 11.8). The dermatopathologist reviewing the slides recognized the probable neoplastic nature of the diffuse, dense dermal infiltrate of predominantly small lymphoid cells (*top left*, hematoxylin and eosin stain, original magnification: 100× magnification) but commented that he had not seen a comparable case previously. Consequently, the case was submitted to the hematopathology laboratory in consultation, where the histopathologic sections were reviewed and immunohistochemical staining of paraffin tissue sections was performed. The clinical presentation raised the possibility of a lymphoblastic lymphoma/acute lymphoblastic leukemia in our minds because these entities are known to occur preferentially in young children and sometimes have a primarily cutaneous presentation. The histopathologic sections show diffuse infiltration by a monotonous population of intermediate-sized lymphoid cells having scanty cytoplasm and predominantly round nuclei with finely dispersed chromatin, highly suggestive of lymphoblastic lymphoma. Immunohistochemical staining demonstrates that only very small numbers of the cells in the lesion, presumably residual benign B cells, express B-lineage–restricted antigen CD20 (*top right*, immunoperoxidase stain, original magnification: 100× magnification). In contrast, essentially all of the infiltrating lymphoid cells express T-cell–associated antigen CD43 (*bottom left*, immunoperoxidase stain, original magnification: 100× magnification). The results of these immunohistochemical studies, in conjunction with the clinical presentation and histopathologic findings, might initially suggest a precursor T-cell lymphoblastic lymphoma/leukemia based on the absence of B-cell–associated antigen CD20 and the presence of T-cell–associated antigen CD43. However, CD20 appears relatively late in B-cell ontogeny, and only approximately 50% of precursor B-cell lymphoblastic lymphomas/leukemias are CD20$^+$. Moreover, as many as 40% of immature and mature B-cell lymphomas/leukemias express CD43. Additional immunohistochemical stains were performed. These studies demonstrate that only very small numbers of lymphoid cells within the infiltrate, presumably benign residual T cells, express T-lineage–associated antigen CD45RO (*bottom right*, immunoperoxidase stain, original magnification: 100× magnification). We concluded that this lesion represents a precursor B-cell lymphoblastic lymphoma/leukemia that is too immature to express B-cell–associated antigen CD20 and exhibits anomalous expression of T-cell–associated antigen CD43. That conclusion is in agreement with the clinical presentation and histopathologic findings in that a small number of children with lymphoblastic lymphoma, generally younger than 6 years of age and often girls, present with primarily cutaneous disease. These lesions are almost invariably precursor B-cell neoplasms, especially if the patient does not have a mediastinal mass. Subsequently, the patient was further evaluated and discovered to have small numbers of malignant lymphoblasts in the bone marrow and peripheral blood. In both instances, flow cytometric studies demonstrated that the malignant lymphoblasts were TdT$^+$ and expressed a precursor B-cell immunophenotype, including CD19, CD10, and cytoplasmic μ, but lacked CD20 (see Chapter 26).

Case 9

In 1990, this 46-year-old HIV-seropositive homosexual man was admitted to the hospital with fever, dyspnea and abdominal distention. He did not have a history of severe opportunistic infections or Kaposi's sarcoma and did not carry a diagnosis of AIDS. One month before admission, his absolute CD4 count was 561 cells/mm^3, and his lactate dehydrogenase (LDH) level was normal. On admission, an abdominal computed tomography scan showed abdominal and pleural effusions. His laboratory studies were remarkable for an LDH level of 1925 U/L. Paracentesis was performed, which removed 800 mL of straw-colored fluid containing 22,000 WBCs/mm^3 with 65% lymphocytes. A Wright-Giemsa–stained cytospin preparation of the ascitic fluid showed large, pleomorphic, malignant cells possessing abundant basophilic cytoplasm and large round to ovoid nu-

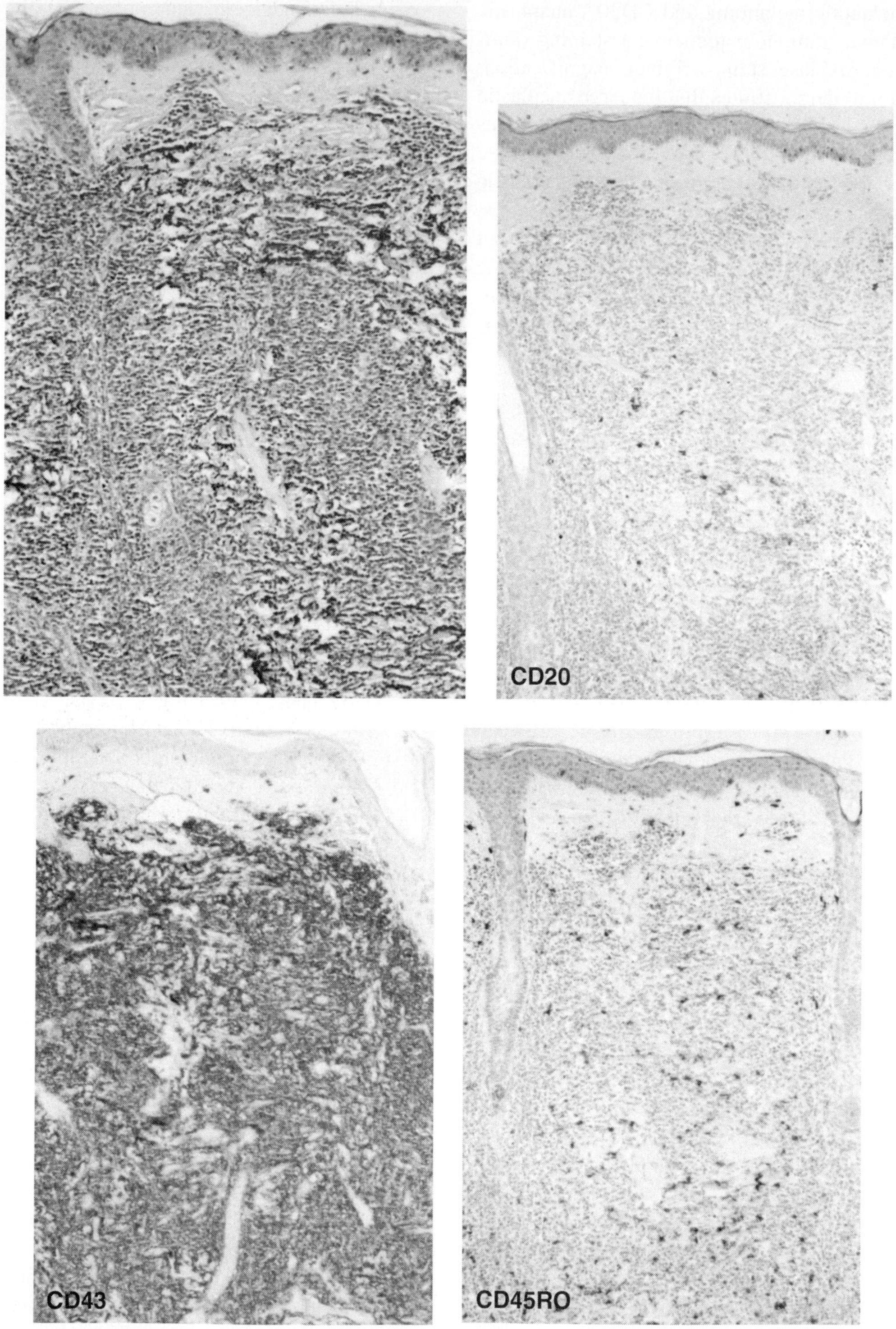

FIG. 11.8.

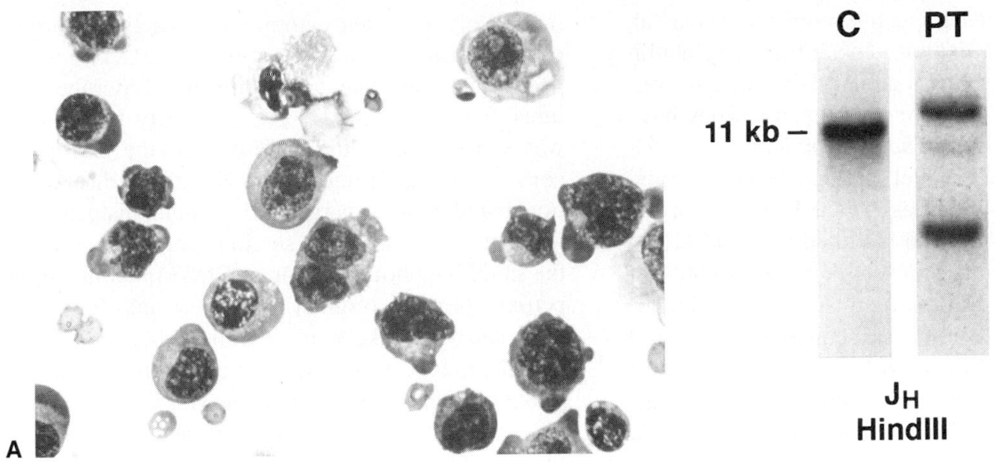

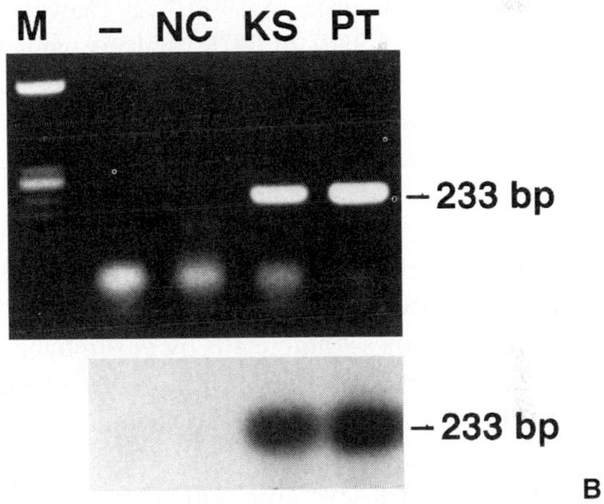

FIG. 11.9.

clei containing one or more large, prominent nucleoli. Some of the cells exhibited a jellyfish-like nuclear configuration (i.e., a large polylobate nucleus surrounding a prominent clear Golgi zone). Other cells resembled Reed-Sternberg cells. Mitotic figures were numerous (Fig. 11.9A) (Wright-Giemsa stain, original magnification: 630× magnification) (from Chadburn A, Cesarman E, Jagirdar J, et al. CD30 (Ki-1) positive anaplastic large cell lymphomas in individuals infected with the human immunodeficiency virus. *Cancer* 1993;72:3078–3090). A number of entities, including immunoblastic large cell lymphoma, lymphocyte depleted Hodgkin's disease and undifferentiated carcinoma were considered in the differential diagnosis. Immunophenotypic analysis was performed by cytofluorometric analysis of cells in suspension and immunohistochemical staining of cytospin preparations. These studies showed that the large neoplastic cells expressed CD45, indicating their hematopoietic origin, but lacked B-cell, T-cell, myeloid, and macrophage lineage-associated antigens, although they expressed several activation-associated antigens, including CD30, CD38, CD71, and HLA-DR. The cells also expressed epithelial membrane antigen, which is expressed by epithelial cells and by activated lymphoid cells. Immunostaining of cytospin preparations showed the absence of cytoplasmic κ and λ immunoglobulin light chains. Precise lineage assignment was not possible by immunophenotypic analysis. For this reason, DNA was extracted from a representative aliquot of these cells and investigated for antigen receptor gene rearrangements. These studies demonstrated the presence of clonal immunoglobulin heavy- and light-chain gene rearrangements (Fig. 11.9B, *top*), whereas the T-cell receptor β chain gene remained in the germline configuration (not shown), indicative of a clonal B-cell neoplasm. The tumor cells contained a single form of EBV, further confirming the clonal nature of the tumor. Taken together, these studies demonstrated that this case was strikingly similar to an unusual subset of uncommonly occurring AIDS-related lymphomas that we had previously described (67). These lymphomas are unusual in that they arise in the body cavities in the absence of an identifiable tumor mass, exhibit morphologic features bridging immunoblastic and anaplastic large cell lymphoma, display an indeterminate phenotype, exhibit clonal immunoglobulin gene rearrangements indicating a clonal B-cell origin, contain EBV, and lack *MYC* gene rearrangements. They have been referred to as *body cavity–based lymphomas*.

In 1994, we discovered a novel, previously unidentified human herpesvirus, which we designated KSHV, in a KS lesion of a homosexual man who had died of AIDS (104). We now know that this virus is present in more than 90% of KS lesions in more than 90% of individuals with all clinical-epidemiologic forms of KS. We subsequently discovered KSHV in a subset of AIDS-related lymphomas associated with an effusion and exhibiting the immunophenotypic, molecular, and viral characteristics described previously (105). We designated these KSHV-containing lymphomas *primary effusion lymphomas* to emphasize their unique origination as effusions and to avoid their confusion with solid lymphomas occurring in the body cavities. These lymphomas represent a newly discovered distinct clinicopathologic entity (106). In light of these discoveries, a vial of cryopreserved cells from this case, accessioned in 1990, was thawed in 1997 and investigated for KSHV by PCR analysis using primers to a KSHV 233-bp fragment from the KS330 Bam region (Fig. 11.9B, *bottom*). In this figure, lane PT represents the patient, M is a molecular weight marker, lane—is a negative water control, lane NC is a negative tissue control, and lane KS is a positive Kaposi's sarcoma tissue control. Lanes KS and PT display a prominent amplification product confirmed by an internal oligonucleotide control. KSHV was also directly visualized in these tumor cells by *in situ* hybridization using a probe against the KSHV cyclin D homologue (not shown). This case represents a KSHV-containing primary effusion lymphoma.

This case illustrates several important points. First, antigen receptor gene rearrangement analysis is often valuable in determining the clonal origin and lineage derivation of hematopoietic neoplasms that are not definable by immunophenotypic analysis. Second, cryopreserved cells and tissues are an invaluable resource for clinical and basic science research. Third, careful observation in conjunction with appropriate investigative studies may lead to the recognition of new clinicopathologic entities possessing biologic significance.

Case 10

A 33-year-old woman presented with massive lymphadenopathy for which she underwent diagnostic biopsy evaluation (Fig. 11.10). The histopathologic sections (*top left*, hematoxylin and eosin stain, original magnification: 400× magnification) show a polymorphic infiltrate predominantly composed of small lymphocytes but also containing histiocytes, plasma cells, and occasional large obviously neoplastic cells. Closer examination of the large malignant-appearing cells (*top right*, hematoxylin and eosin stain, original magnification: 630× magnification) shows them to possess moderately abundant cytoplasm and a single large nucleus often containing a prominent nucleolus. Occasional cells appear to be binucleate and exhibit Reed-Sternberg–like features. For this reason, mixed cellularity Hodgkin's disease was seriously considered. However, the presentation was considered slightly unusual for Hodgkin's disease, and additional studies were performed. Immunohistochemical studies of the paraffin tissue sections demonstrate that most of the small lymphocytes express CD43 (*middle left*, immunoperoxidase stain, original magnification: 400× magnification) and most likely are T cells, whereas the very large malignant-appearing cells strongly express CD20 but not CD43 (*middle right*, immunoperoxidase stain, original magnification: 400× magnification) and therefore are most likely of B-cell origin. These large neoplastic cells are $CD15^-$ and $CD30^-$ (not shown). These results raise the alternative possibility of a T-cell–rich B-cell lymphoma. Additional immunohistochemical staining demonstrates that the large neoplastic cells contain abundant intracytoplasmic immunoglobulin κ light chains (*bottom left*, immunoperoxidase stain, original magnification: 400× magnification) but not immunoglobulin λ light chains (*bottom right*, immunoperoxidase stain, original magnification: 400× magnification). In summary, the large neoplastic cells within this lesion express B-lineage–restricted antigen CD20, lack T-cell–associated antigens, and contain clonal intracytoplasmic immunoglobulin. These findings support the diagnosis of a T-cell–rich B-cell non-Hodgkin's lymphoma. The immunohistochemical studies performed in this case played a key role in arriving at the correct diagnosis, which has an impact on the therapy, management, and prognosis of this patient.

Case 11

This 33-year-old Hispanic woman from Santo Domingo initially presented with generalized lymphadenopathy, was diagnosed as having malignant lymphoma based on morphologic evaluation of hematoxylin and eosin–stained histologic sections of a lymph node biopsy, and was treated with chemotherapy. The patient initially responded to therapy but returned 1 year later with recurrent lymphadenopathy, cutaneous involvement, hypercalcemia, lytic bone lesions, and circulating neoplastic cells. The patient did not respond to further therapy and died 2 months later, 14 months after the initial presentation (Fig. 11.11A). The histologic sections of the biopsy of the recurrent lymphadenopathy (*top left*, hematoxylin and eosin stain, original magnification: 400× magnification) show diffuse replacement of a lymph node by a predominantly large lymphoid cell proliferation in which the cells show slight variability in size and shape. Most large lymphoid cells contain generally round nuclei and prominent nucleoli. Occasional very large lymphoid cells with a centrally placed prominent nucleolus are identified. Numerous mitotic figures are present. A skin biopsy obtained at the time of recurrence shows diffuse dermal infiltration by large variably sized and shaped malignant

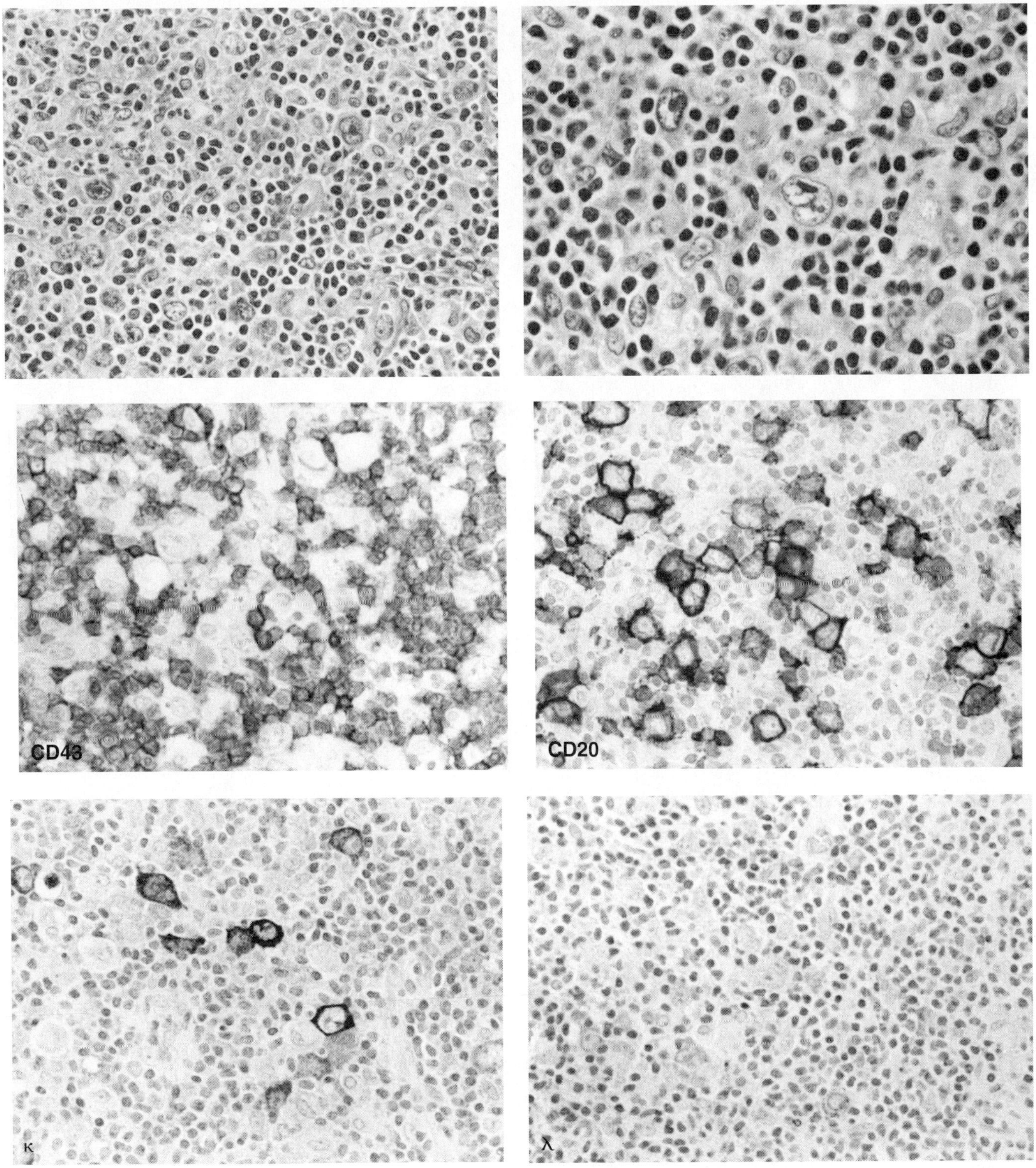

FIG. 11.10.

lymphoid cells, some of which infiltrate the overlying epidermis (*top right*, hematoxylin and eosin stain, original magnification: 400× magnification). Immunohistochemical staining of frozen tissue sections of a biopsy of the recurrent lymphadenopathy shows that virtually all the neoplastic cells express CD4 (*middle left*, immunoperoxidase stain, original magnification: 400× magnification), whereas virtually none expresses CD8 (*bottom left*, immunoperoxidase stain, original magnification: 400× magnification). In addition to subset antigen restriction, the malignant cells also show conspic-

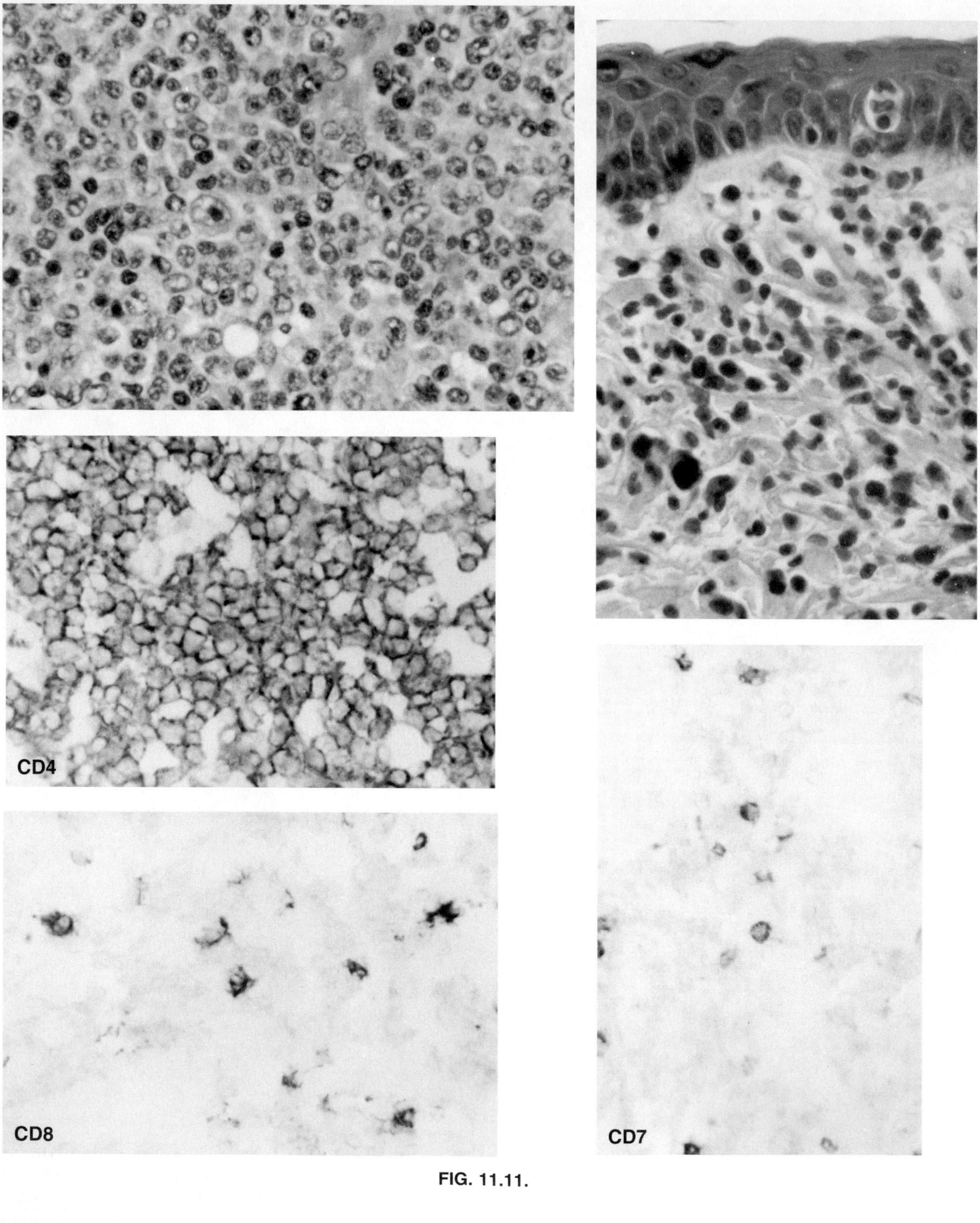

FIG. 11.11.

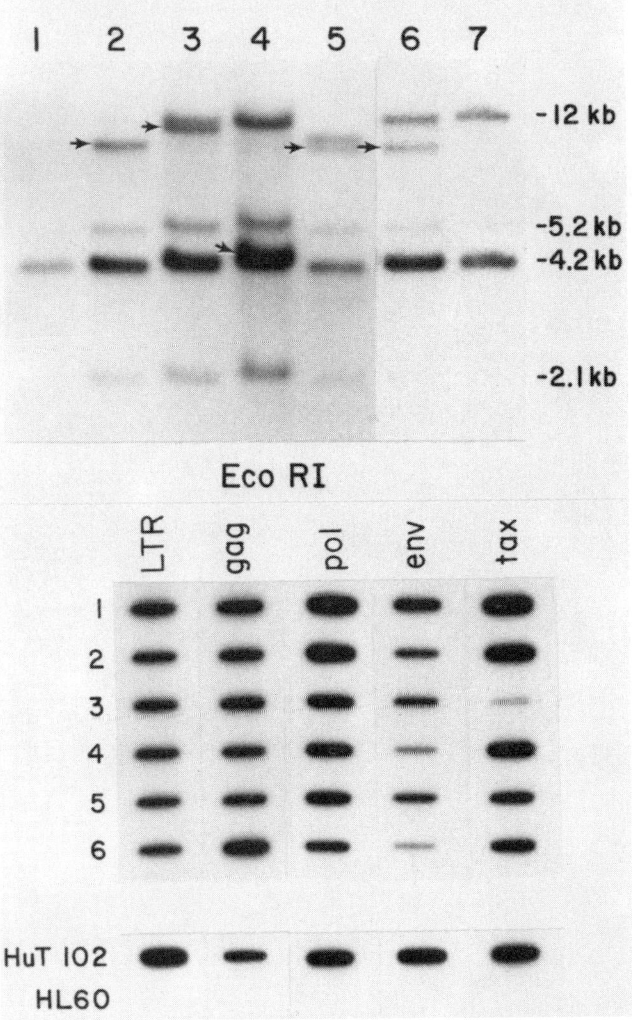

FIG. 11.11. *Continued.*

uous deletion of pan-T-cell antigen CD7 (*bottom right*, immunoperoxidase stain, original magnification: 400× magnification).

This T-cell lymphoma was among the 75 postthymic T-cell neoplasms that we screened for the presence of human T-cell lymphotropic virus type 1 (HTLV-1) by PCR. This T-cell neoplasm and five others among the entire cohort of 75 postthymic T-cell neoplasms contained evidence of HTLV-1 by PCR. All six HTLV-1–associated T-cell neoplasms were analyzed by gene rearrangement analysis (Fig. 11.11B, *top*). In this figure, numbers 1 through 6 above each lane correspond to the case numbers, and number 7 is the negative control (HL60 cell line). Case number 3 is the case under discussion here. Dashes indicate germline bands, and arrows indicate clonal rearrangement bands. All six HTLV-1–associated T-cell neoplasms were shown to be clonal T-cell proliferations based on this analysis. Representative data of slot-blot hybridization analysis of PCR-amplified genomic DNAs for the presence of HTLV-1 LTR and *gag, pol, env,* and *tax* gene regions in the six positive cases are illustrated in Figure 11.11B *(bottom)*. Numbers 1 through 6 correspond to the case numbers. The HUT-102 cell line contains integrated HTLV-1 proviruses and serves as a positive control, and the HL60 cell line is negative for HTLV-1 and serves as a negative control. All six cases contain evidence of HTLV-1 genomic sequences by PCR. (From Chadburn A, Athan E, Wieczorek R, et al. Detection and characterization of human T-cell lymphotropic virus type I [HTLV-I] associated T-cell neoplasms in an HTLV-I nonendemic region by polymerase chain reaction. *Blood* 1991; 77:2419–2430, with permission.)

Five of the six patients discovered to have an HLTV-1–associated T-cell neoplasm had immigrated from HTLV-1–endemic regions: five were black, five were women, and five were younger than 45 years of age. The incidence of hypercalcemia and lytic bone lesions was significantly more common among these patients than among patients with HTLV-1$^-$ T-cell neoplasms. Moreover, all six HTLV-1$^+$ neoplasms were CD7 negative. In summary, the use of ancillary techniques such as immunohistochemistry, antigen receptor gene rearrangement, and PCR analysis for viral sequences provides considerable additional information about hematopoietic neoplasms that has clinical and biologic implications.

Case 12

This 25-year-old man presented to his physician with cervical lymphadenopathy. He was asymptomatic and had a normal chest radiograph, serum electrolyte determinations, complete blood cell count, and peripheral blood smear. A lymph node biopsy was performed and interpreted histologically as malignant lymphoma, most likely mantle cell lymphoma, at an outside institution. However, because the cell morphology suggested a blastic appearance to the outside observer and numerous mitotic figures were present, the specimen was referred to our laboratory for histopathologic review and immunophenotypic analysis (Fig. 11.12). The histologic sections showed diffuse replacement of the lymph node by a monotonous, intermediate-sized mononuclear cell population possessing a small rim of acidophilic cytoplasm, and round to slightly irregular nuclei containing dispersed nuclear chromatin and occasional small nucleoli (*top left*, hematoxylin and eosin stain, original magnification: 630× magnification). Our differential diagnosis included lymphoblastic lymphoma and the lymphoblastic variant of mantle cell lymphoma, but we also considered granulocytic sarcoma. Immunohistochemical staining of paraffin tissue sections showed that the malignant cells lacked B-cell–associated antigens CD20 (*top right*, immunoperoxidase stain, original magnification: 40× magnification), CD79a, and CD45RA (not shown), effectively excluding a B-cell lymphoma, and expressed T-cell–associated antigen CD43 (*middle left*, immunoperoxidase stain, original magnifica-

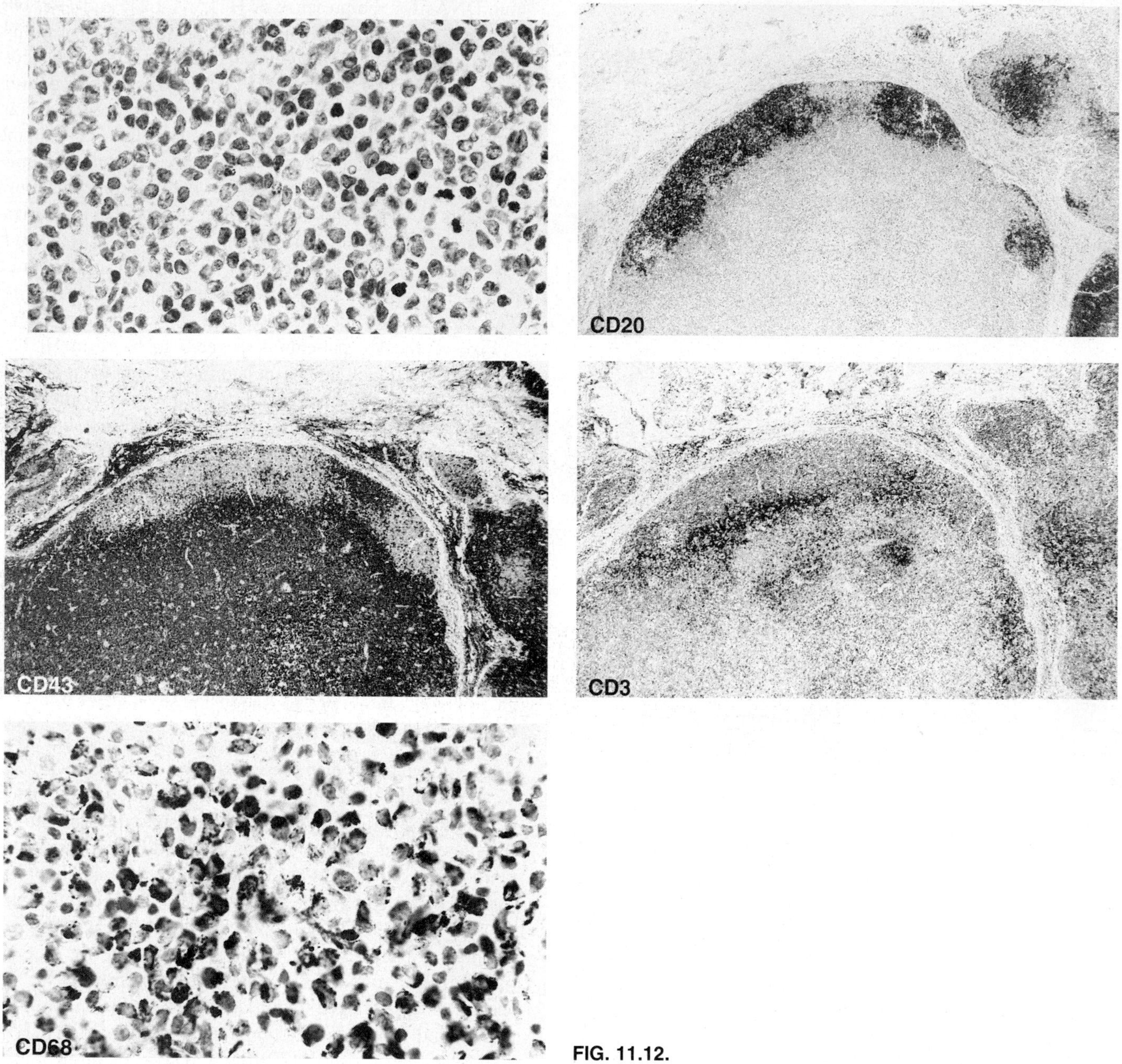

FIG. 11.12.

tion: 40× magnification) in the absence of CD3 (*middle right*, immunoperoxidase stain, original magnification: 40× magnification). Based on this immunophenotypic profile some observers concluded that the lesion represented a T-cell lymphoma, perhaps precursor T-cell lymphoblastic lymphoma. However, one clue that this lesion was not of T-cell origin is the lack of CD3 expression. We have found that CD3 is expressed by 95% of diffuse, aggressive T-cell lymphomas, including all precursor T-cell lymphoblastic lymphomas, when evaluated in paraffin tissue sections with the polyclonal CD3 antibody (177). The lack of polyclonal CD3 antibody reactivity with this lesion strongly suggests that it is not a T-cell neoplasm. CD43 has a wide spectrum of expression, and although routinely considered a pan-T-cell marker, CD43 (i.e., leukosialin or sialophorin) is also expressed by macrophages, plasma cells, some malignant B cells, and benign and malignant myeloid cells (Table 11.1). A lesion that is only $CD43^+$ based on a small immunostaining panel should be further characterized using additional antibodies, including those directed against myeloid cells. One study examining tumors with the CD43 only immunophenotype, based on immunostaining for CD20, CD45RO, and CD43, showed that more extensive immunophenotyping revealed that most such lesions are of myeloid origin and many of the remainder are of B-cell origin (178). Because we suspected granulocytic sarcoma, we performed additional immunostaining with monoclonal antibody KP1, which detects the myeloid-associated antigen CD68. Virtually all the tumor cells expressed CD68 (*bottom*, immunoperoxidase stain, original magnification: 630× magnification), confirming our morphologic impression of a myeloid proliferation. The patient subsequently underwent bone marrow biopsy and aspiration. The bone marrow contained small collections of malignant cells cytomorphologically identical to those seen in the lymph node. Flow cytometric analysis of the aspirated bone marrow showed that these malignant cells were TdT^+, $HLA\text{-}DR^+$, $CD14^+$, and $My8^+$, consistent with a TdT^+ acute myeloid leukemia.

This case illustrates two important points. First, granulocytic sarcoma should be considered in the differential diagnosis of diffuse aggressive lymphomas. Granulocytic sarcomas display a broad morphologic spectrum that can mimic lymphoblastic lymphoma, large cell lymphoma, and even Burkitt's lymphoma. Second, significant errors in diagnosis may occur when only a limited number of antibodies are employed to immunophenotype a neoplasm of questionable histogenesis or the results are misinterpreted because all the diagnostic implications of the immunophenotypic profile are not appreciated.

Case 13

This 20-year-old woman was discovered to have cervical lymphadenopathy on routine physical examination. Excisional biopsy of a superficial cervical lymph node was performed (Fig.11.13). Review of the histologic sections

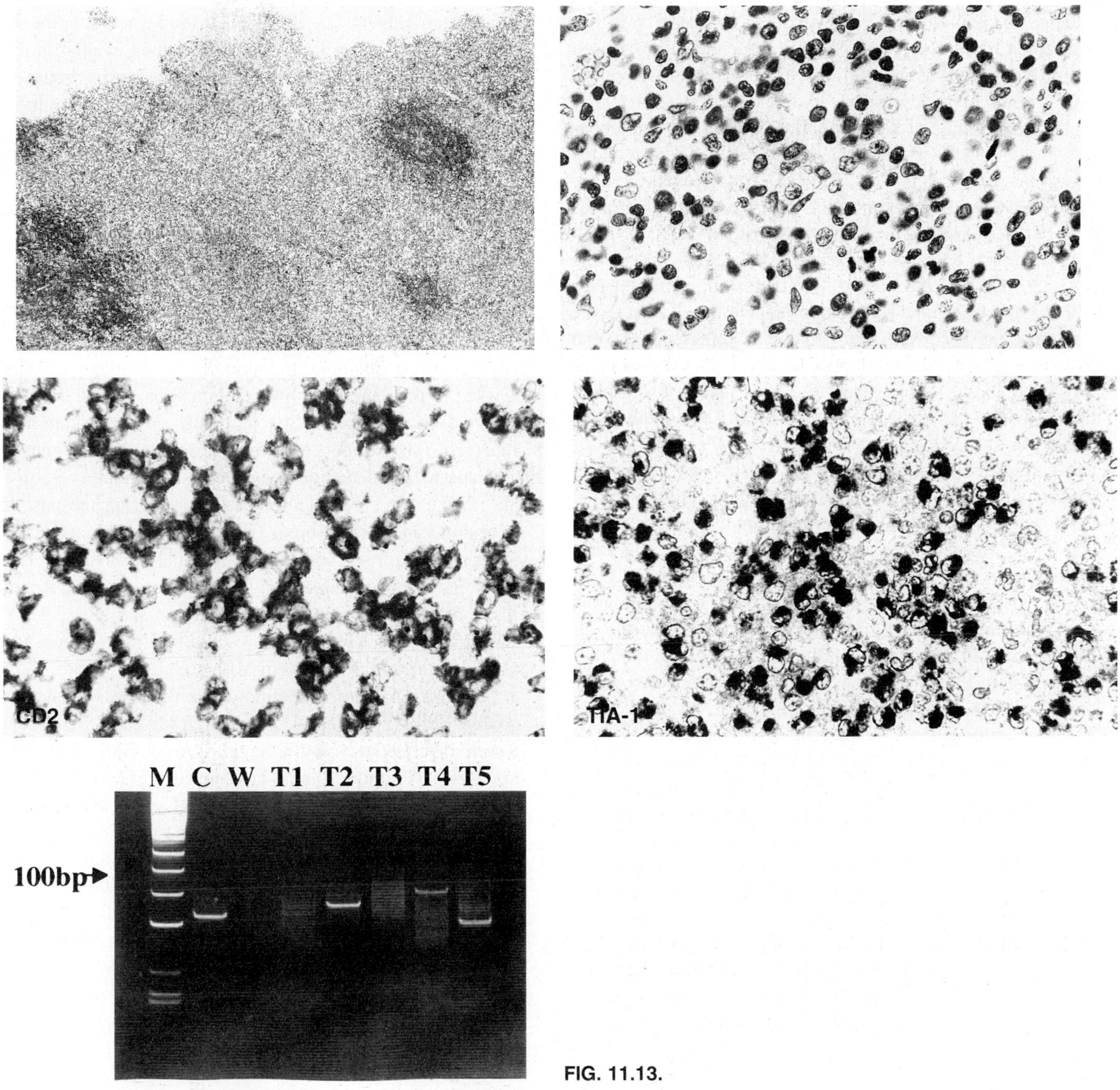

FIG. 11.13.

showed that the internal lymph node architecture was markedly altered by the presence of clusters and sheets of large, apparently lymphoid cells containing abundant clear cytoplasm and by variably sized, round to moderately irregular nuclei. These cells replaced most of the lymph node, leaving behind several small areas of residual benign lymphoid tissue (*top left and right*, hematoxylin and eosin stain, original magnifications: 40× and 630× magnification). Some observers concluded that these cells represented clear cell immunoblasts and that this lesion represented a peripheral T-cell lymphoma. However, the patient was young, and further clinical evaluation failed to disclose any evidence of additional lymphadenopathy. In view of the young age of the patient and the lack of additional disease, the hematologist-oncologist desired additional evidence to support the diagnosis of peripheral T-cell lymphoma before committing the patient to chemotherapy. However, fresh tissue was not available for immunophenotyping because the entire excised lymph node had been submitted in fixative, and a second biopsy could not be performed to obtain fresh tissue because additional lymph nodes could not be palpated. Immunophenotypic analysis was performed in paraffin tissue sections using antigen retrieval techniques. These studies demonstrated that the large clear cells expressed pan-T-cell antigens CD2 (*middle left*, immunoperoxidase stain, original magnification: 630× magnification), CD3, and CD43 in the absence of CD5 (not shown). Immunostaining for pan-T-cell antigen CD7 could not be performed in paraffin tissue sections. These cells lacked CD4 but expressed CD8 and TIA-1 (*middle right*, immunoperoxidase stain, original magnification: 630× magnification). These cells also lacked CD15, CD30, CD56, CD57, and B-cell–, myeloid-, and monocyte-associated antigens (not shown). *In situ* hybridization studies for EBV-encoded RNA (EBER) were negative. In summary, these immunophenotypic studies suggested that the large clear cells were of T-cell origin, lacked at least one pan-T-cell antigen consistent with an anomalous immunophenotype, and exclusively belonged to the $CD4^-CD8^+$ subset. These immunophenotypic findings support the morphologic impression of peripheral T-cell lymphoma, although they do not provide information about the clonality of the lesion. For this reason, DNA was extracted from the paraffin block and investigated for the presence of clonal T-cell receptor gamma chain gene rearrangements by PCR (*bottom*). In this figure, lanes T1 through T5 represent five lesions suspected of being peripheral T-cell lymphomas. Lane T2 is the case under discussion here, lane M is a molecular weight marker, lane C is a peripheral T-cell lymphoma–positive control, and lane W is a negative water control. A distinct band was identified, indicating the presence of a clonal T-cell population and validating the morphologic impression of peripheral T-cell lymphoma. This case illustrates the value of immunophenotypic and molecular genetic analyses in the diagnosis and classification of hematopoietic neoplasms when morphologic evaluation alone is inconclusive or insufficient.

SUMMARY AND CONCLUSIONS

Multiple diagnostic dilemmas are commonly encountered in the routine diagnosis and classification of hematopoietic neoplasms. Immunophenotypic analysis is a useful adjunct to histopathology and can be of considerable assistance in resolving many of these diagnostic dilemmas. Immunophenotypic analysis can be performed on virtually any pathologic specimen using flow cytometric cell suspension or frozen and paraffin tissue section immunohistochemistry. Each of these methodologic approaches has distinct advantages and disadvantages. Attention must be paid to the manner in which pathologic specimens are handled during transportation and on arrival within the laboratory, cell suspensions are prepared and their viability and suitably for analysis assessed, tissues are snap-frozen or fixed and routinely processed, and reagents are chosen and used, including the determination of appropriate antibody dilutions, evaluation and storage. Moreover, immunophenotypic analysis should be tailored to the nature of the pathologic specimen and individualized according to the particular diagnostic problem. Results of immunophenotypic analysis should always be correlated with the clinical findings and histopathologic examination of the pathologic specimen under analysis.

ACKNOWLEDGMENTS

The senior author expresses his sincere gratitude and appreciation to each one of the numerous individuals who has worked in this laboratory in a technical or clerical capacity during the past 12 years. Special thanks go to the laboratory supervisor Mrs. Angela Murray, whose intelligence, energy, enthusiasm, and dedication have been substantially responsible for the successes of this laboratory during the past 15 years, and to Maria Abreu, Claudine Alexis, Mary Azzo, Sherry Lynn Burney, Elizabeth Cochrane, Lisa Dodson, Erin Early, Tonya Florestal, Susan Fox, Rebecca Gaston, Robert Koch, Shaiju Kuruvilla, Nilda Inghirami, Ji Guang Liu, Yi Fang Liu, Teresa Marcotrigiano, Julia Martinez, Donna McCarthy, Laurie McFall, Robin Miller, Christie Moore, Katherine Morrison, Jaime Paladino, Ryne Paulose, Melissa Ragovoy, Edy Restrepo, Jessica Rodriguez, Christine Rosenvinge Dellet, Cynthia Sagullo, Anjali Saqi, Tom Taylor, Betty Tolidjian, Sanya Tomsic, Sirike Trumees, Margaret Walden, Lenore Weingarten, Liang Ying, Gloria Young, Mei Zheng, and Bang Ying Zhu for their outstanding work and support. The author thanks Dr. Kathy Foucar, whose excellent article (*Semin Diagn Pathol* 1989;6:13–36) concerning the organization and operation of a flow cytometry laboratory served as the inspiration for this chapter. The author also wishes to thank Mrs. Awilda Melendez-Cruz for assistance in preparing the manuscript and Al Lamme, FBPA, and Scientific Photographic Services (Edgewater, NJ) for the excellent photomicrographs and figures.

APPENDIX 1. T-CELL SUBSET ANALYSIS BY WHOLE BLOOD LYSIS

The wash solution is phosphate-buffered saline (PBS) containing 0.1% sodium azide.

1. Place 100 μL of the heparinized whole peripheral blood sample into an appropriately labeled Falcon #2052 12 × 75 mm tube for each monoclonal antibody to be tested and for each corresponding control.
2. Add the labeled monoclonal antibodies to the appropriate tubes, vortex gently, and incubate the cell and antibody reaction mixtures for 10 minutes at room temperature. Examples of monoclonal antibody combinations used in T-cell subset analysis are CD45/CD14, CD3/CD19, CD3/CD4, CD3/CD8, CD3/CD16 and CD56, and corresponding murine isotype-matched irrelevant (control) antibodies (e.g., IgG1, IgG2a).
3. Add 2 mL of FACS lysing solution (Becton-Dickinson, San Jose, CA) diluted 1:10 with distilled water to each tube, vortex gently, and incubate for 10 minutes at room temperature.
4. Centrifuge at 1,100 rpm for 5 minutes at room temperature.
5. Wash the reaction mixtures with 2 mL of wash solution and centrifuge at 1,100 rpm in a Sorvall RT 6000 centrifuge for 5 minutes at room temperature. Decant the supernatant and wash the cells with 2 mL of wash solution.
6. Centrifuge at 1,100 rpm for 5 minutes at room temperature.
7. Remove the supernatant, resuspend the cells in 0.5 mL of wash solution and 100 μL of 1% paraformaldehyde, and analyze them on a FACSCalibur flow cytometer (Becton-Dickinson, Mountain View, CA).

APPENDIX 2. FICOLL-HYPAQUE DENSITY GRADIENT CENTRIFUGATION

All samples should be processed under sterile conditions using aseptic techniques and reagents in a Sterilgard laminar flow hood (Baker Co., Sanford, ME).

1. Place 15 mL of room-temperature Ficoll-Hypaque (Pharmacia, Piscataway, NJ) into a Falcon #2070 screw-cap 50-mL tube.
2. Hold the 50-mL tube at a 45-degree angle, and slowly but steadily overlay the Ficoll-Hypaque with up to 30 mL of the appropriately diluted sample using a 10- or 25-mL disposable serologic pipette.
3. Recap the tube and centrifuge at 1,900 rpm (400 *g*) in a Sorvall RC3B centrifuge for 30 minutes at room temperature without applying a brake.
4. After centrifugation, using a Pasteur pipette or a disposable transfer pipette, carefully remove the supernatant to within 1 cm above the mononuclear cell layer and discard.
5. Carefully remove the mononuclear cell layer with a Pasteur pipette and transfer the cells to a Falcon #2070 50-mL tube. Up to 30 mL of cell-rich fluid may be combined into each 50-mL tube. Be careful not to place the Pasteur pipette too far below the mononuclear cell layer because this draws in Ficoll and neutrophils.
6. Fill the tubes containing the harvested cells to 50 mL with PBS.
7. Discard the original tubes containing residual Ficoll and pellets composed of erythrocytes, dead cells, and debris.
8. Centrifuge the 50-mL tubes at 1,900 rpm in a Sorvall RC3B centrifuge for 10 minutes at room temperature. The brake may now be applied.
9. Decant the supernatant from each of the tubes, resuspend the cells in small volumes of PBS, combine the cells from each tube into one 50-mL tube, and fill the tube with PBS.
10. Centrifuge the cells at 1,100 rpm in a Sorvall RC3B centrifuge for 10 minutes at room temperature.
11. Decant the supernatant and resuspend the cells in RPMI 1640 containing 10% heat-inactivated fetal calf serum, 1% penicillin, and 1% streptomycin (overnight media).
12. Count the cells, assess their viability by trypan blue dye exclusion (see Appendix 4), prepare Diff-Quik–stained cytocentrifuge slides for morphologic examination (see Appendix 3), and adjust the final concentration to 5×10^6 cells/mL.

In the case of smaller sample volumes, Falcon #2097 tubes may be filled with 4 mL of Ficoll-Hypaque and overlaid with 8 mL of sample. The second wash (step 10) may be eliminated to reduce cell loss if the cell pellet is observed to be very small after the first wash (step 8).

APPENDIX 3. DIFF-QUIK (MODIFIED WRIGHT-GIEMSA) STAIN OF CYTOCENTRIFUGE SLIDE PREPARATIONS, TOUCH PREPARATIONS, AND FROZEN TISSUE SECTIONS

Diff-Quik stain is a modification of Wright stain (Dade Diagnostics of P.R., Inc., Aguada, Puerto Rico).

1. Prepare cytocentrifuge slides, touch preparations, and frozen tissue sections.
2. Dip the slide in fixative solution five times, 1 second each time. Allow the excess to drain off.
3. Dip the slide in solution I five times, 1 second each time. Allow the excess to drain off.
4. Dip the slide in solution II five times, 1 second each time. Allow the excess to drain off.
5. Rinse the slide with distilled or deionized water.
6. Allow the slide to dry, dip in xylene, coverslip with Permount, and examine with a light microscope.

The intensity of staining can be changed by increasing or decreasing the number of dips in solutions I and II, but do not go below 3 dips of 1 full second each each time.

APPENDIX 4. MANUAL CELL COUNTING AND VIABILITY ASSESSMENT

1. Clean a hemocytometer with alcohol before use.
2. Place a clean coverslip over the counting chamber of the hemocytometer.
3. Combine a 50-μL representative aliquot of the cell suspension with 50 μL of 0.4% trypan blue dye (Gibco, Grand Island, NY) and allow to sit for 30 to 60 seconds.
4. Load one side of the hemocytometer with about 50 μL of a representative aliquot of the cell suspension (do not overfill).
5. Load the other side of the hemocytometer with about 50 μL of the cell suspension treated with trypan blue dye (do not overfill).
6. Allow the cells to settle on the hemocytometer for 30 to 60 seconds before counting.
7. Place the loaded hemocytometer on the light microscope stage, focus on the counting chamber filled with non–trypan blue dye–treated cells with the 10× objective, and then focus with the 40× objective.
8. Count all the leukocytes (excluding any contaminant erythrocytes) present in one row of five squares comprising one 4 × 4 grid. Multiply this number by 5 to obtain the total field count and then by 10^4 to obtain the cell count per milliliter.
9. Focus the 40× objective on the other side of the counting chamber containing the cells treated with trypan blue dye. The clear cells are viable, and the blue cells are dead. Count a total of 200 consecutive cells (clear and blue), and calculate the viability as follows: live (clear) cells/total of live (clear) and dead (blue) cells × 100 = percent (%) viability.
10. The number of viable cells per milliliter is calculated by multiplying the cell count/mL by the percent viability.

APPENDIX 5. INDIRECT IMMUNOFLUORESCENT IMMUNOCYTOCHEMICAL ASSAY FOR TERMINAL DEOXYNUCLEOTIDYL TRANSFERASE

1. Prepare a minimum of two cytocentrifuge slides from each cell suspension sample to be tested. One or two slides can serve as the test slides, and one can serve as a negative control slide. A cytocentrifuge slide of normal thymocytes may be used as a positive control slide.
2. The cytocentrifuge slides should be freshly prepared and immediately fixed in cold methanol for 30 minutes at 4°C.
3. Hydrate the slides for 5 minutes at room temperature in a beaker containing PBS and a stirring bar, placed on top of a magnetic stirrer.
4. Remove the slides and quickly but carefully wipe off the excess PBS from around the cell pellets. Do not allow the pellets to dry out.
5. Immediately place the slides in a moist chamber, and overlay each slide with 20 μL of normal goat serum (Supertechs, Bethesda, MD).
6. Incubate the slides for 5 minutes at room temperature in a moist chamber.
7. Wash the slides for 10 minutes at room temperature in a beaker containing PBS, stirring as in step 3.
8. Wipe the excess PBS from the slides as in step 4, and return them to the moist chamber.
9. Overlay the test and the positive control slides with 20 μL of unlabeled rabbit anti-TdT antibody (Supertechs, Bethesda, MD). Overlay the negative control slide with 20 μL of normal rabbit immunoglobulin (Supertechs).
10. Incubate the slides for 30 minutes at room temperature in the moist chamber.
11. Remove the slides from the moist chamber, and wash them twice in PBS for 10 minutes each with stirring, as in step 3.
12. Wipe off the excess PBS from around the cell pellets as in step 4, and return the slides to the moist chamber.
13. Overlay the slides with 20 μL of fluorescein isothiocyanate labeled $F(ab')_2$ goat anti-rabbit immunoglobulin (Supertechs).
14. Incubate the slides for 30 minutes at room temperature in the moist chamber.
15. Repeat step 12.
16. Repeat step 4.
17. Place one drop of Vectashield mounting media for fluorescence (Vector Laboratories, Inc., Burlingame, CA) on top of the cell pellet, coverslip, and seal the cell pellet with clear nail polish.
18. Store the slides in a moist chamber at 4°C until ready to be examined.
19. Examine with an appropriate immunofluorescent microscope.

APPENDIX 6. IMMUNOFLUORESCENT IMMUNOCYTOCHEMCAL ASSAY FOR CYTOPLASMIC (INTRACELLULAR) IMMUNOGLOBULIN

1. Prepare cytocentrifuge slides of the cell suspension sample to be tested, label with the patient's name, and allow them to air dry for 5 to 10 minutes before fixation.
2. Fix the slides in absolute ethanol containing 5% glacial acetic acid for 15 minutes at room temperature.
3. Wash the slides at room temperature in a beaker of PBS containing a stirring bar, placed on top of a magnetic stirrer. Change the PBS several times, and then allow the slides to continue to wash overnight in PBS at room temperature.
4. The next morning, discard the PBS in the beaker, and wash the slides in fresh PBS for an additional 30 minutes at room temperature.
5. Remove the slides one at a time, and quickly but care-

fully wipe off all excess PBS from around the cell pellets. Do not allow the cell pellets to dry out.

6. Immediately place each slide in a moist chamber, labeling the frosted end of each slide with the antibody to be applied. Overlay the entire cell pellet with 100 to 150 μL of the appropriate fluorescein isothiocyanate conjugated anti-human heteroantiserum (anti-total Ig, κ, λ, μ, γ, δ, and α) (Biosource International, Camariallo, CA).
7. Incubate the slides in a moist chamber for 30 minutes at room temperature.
8. Wash the slides three times in PBS, 10 minutes for each wash, at room temperature.
9. Repeat step 5.
10. Place 1 drop of Vectashield mounting media (Vector Laboratories, Inc., Burlingame, CA) on top of each cell pellet, coverslip, and seal the pellet with clear nail polish.
11. Store the slides in a moist chamber at 4°C until ready to be examined.
12. Examine the slides with an appropriate immunofluorescent microscope.

APPENDIX 7. IMMUNOHISTOCHEMICAL STAINING OF CYTOSPIN PREPARATIONS AND FROZEN AND PARAFFIN TISSUE SECTIONS

All immunohistochemical staining is performed using the Tech Mate 500 Automated Immunohistochemical System (Ventana Medical Systems, Tuscon, AZ).

Preparation of Cytospins for Immunostaining

1. Prepare cytocentrifuge slides of the cell suspension sample to be tested (50,000 to 100,000 cells per slide) using ChemMate Capillary Gap Plus blue slides (Ventana Medical Systems, Tuscon, AZ).
2. Allow the slides to air dry for a minimum of 30 minutes at room temperature. Alternatively, the slides may be left to air dry overnight for immunostaining the following morning.
3. Fix the slides in acetone for 10 minutes at room temperature, and then air dry the slides for 5 minutes at room temperature. At this point, the slides may be immunostained or stored at −20°C to −80°C in a sealed plastic slide container for up to 3 months.
4. When the stored slides are needed, remove the sealed container from the freezer, and allow it to warm to room temperature before removing the slides.
5. Remove the stored slides from the container, and allow them to air dry for 5 minutes at room temperature. The slides are then ready to be immunostained.

Preparation of Frozen Tissue Sections for Immunostaining

1. Cut frozen tissue sections 5 μm thick, and place onto TechMate Capillary Gap Plus blue slides (Ventana Medical Systems, Tuscon, AZ).
2. Allow the slides to air dry for a minimum of 1 hour at room temperature. Alternatively, the slides may be left to air day overnight for immunostaining the following morning.
3. Fix the slides in acetone for 10 minutes at room temperature, and then air dry the slides for 5 minutes at room temperature. At this point, the slides may be immunostained or stored at −20°C to −80°C in a sealed plastic slide container for up to 3 months.
4. When the stored slides are needed, remove the sealed container from the freezer, and allow it to warm to room temperature before removing the slides.
5. Remove the stored slides from the container, and allow them to air dry for 5 minutes at room temperature. The slides are then ready to be immunostained.

Preparation of Paraffin Tissue Sections for Immunostaining

1. Cut paraffin tissue sections 2 to 3 μm thick, and place onto Tech Mate Capillary Gap Plus gray slides (Ventana Medical Systems, Tuscon, AZ).
2. Place the slides in a rack, and bake overnight in a 56°C oven.
3. Remove the slides from the oven the following morning. The slides are ready to be immunostained.

Immunostaining of Cytospin Preparations and Frozen Tissue Sections

Tris-buffered saline (TBS) is 10 L of distilled H_2O, 80 g of NaCl, 6.05 g of Tris [hydroxymethyl] aminomethane (Sigma, St. Louis, MO). Adjust the pH to 7.4 with 40 mL of 1 N HCl.

1. After the slides have air dried for 5 minutes after fixation, the slides are ready to be immunostained.
2. Prewet the slides in TBS containing 0.05% Tween 20 (Sigma, St. Louis, MO) for 5 minutes.
3. The slides are then ready to be loaded onto the TechMate 500 Automated Immunohistochemical System. Primary antibodies are diluted in ChemMate antibody dilution buffer (Ventana Medical Systems, Tuscon, AZ) in appropriately determined titers. We use the ChemMate Secondary Detection Kit Alkaline Phosphatase (Ventana Medical Systems, Tuscon, AZ) as the secondary detection system for cytospin preparations. The secondary detection system for frozen tissue sections is the ChemMate Secondary Detection Kit Peroxidase/DAB.

We exclude the endogenous peroxidase blocking step of the Techmate staining procedure in the case of frozen tissue sections because this step can damage antigens to be demonstrated. If endogenous peroxidase activity is excessive, the ChemMate Secondary Detection Kit Alkaline Phosphatase is used.

4. When the staining run is completed, remove the slides from the TechMate instrument.
5. Wash the slides gently in running tap water for 5 minutes.
6. Transfer the slides to 0.5% ammonia water for 1 minute.
7. Wash the slides briefly and gently in running tap water.
8. Dehydrate the slides by serial immersion in 95% alcohol (once), in 100% alcohol (twice), and in xylene (twice).
9. Mount the slides with Permount and coverslip.

Immunostaining of Paraffin Tissue Sections

Tris-buffered saline (TBS) is 10 L of distilled H_2O, 80 g of NaCl, 6.05 g of Tris [hydroxymethyl] aminomethane (Sigma, St. Louis, MO). Adjust the pH to 7.4 with 40 mL of 1 N HCl.

1. Deparaffinize the slides with four 5-minute washes in xylene. Then serially immerse the slides in 100% ethanol and 95% ethanol for 5 minutes each. Bouin's solution–fixed tissue sections may be debouinized after the 100% ethanol wash by placing the sections in a supersaturated solution of lithium carbonate in 70% ethanol for 30 to 60 seconds.
2. Place the slides in a mixture of 3 mL of 30% H_2O_2 in 200 mL of methanol for 20 minutes. Then transfer the slides into room-temperature distilled H_2O until antigen retrieval is performed. A variety of antigen retrieval methods are used depending on the antibody being employed. These include heating methods (i.e., microwave and pressure cooker techniques) and enzymatic digestion methods (i.e., trypsin and protease treatments).
3. After antigen retrieval is completed, prewet the slides in TBS containing 0.05% Tween 20 (Sigma, St. Louis, MO) for 10 minutes.
4. The slides are ready to be loaded onto the TechMate 500 Automated Immunostaining System (Ventana Medical Systems, Tuscon, AZ). Primary antibodies are diluted in ChemMate antibody dilution buffer (Ventana Medical Systems, Tuscon, AZ) in appropriately determined titers. The ChemMate Secondary Detection Kit Peroxidase/DAB (Ventana Medical Systems, Tuscon, AZ) is used as the secondary detection system. See the manufacturer's operating manual for information regarding complete specifications for running individual protocols.
5. When the staining run is completed, remove the slides from the TechMate instrument.
6. Wash the slides in running tap water for 5 minutes.

Immerse the B5-fixed slides in 1 g of iodine with 2 g of potassium iodide in 100 mL of H_2O for 5 minutes, and then place them in 0.2% sodium thiosulfate for 8 minutes to remove the pigment. Transfer the slides into distilled water, and counterstain with Mayer's Modified Hematoxylin (Ventana Medical Systems, Tuscon, AZ) for 2 to 3 minutes.

7. Wash the slides in running tap water for 5 minutes.
8. Transfer the slides to 0.5% ammonia water for 1 minute.
9. Wash the slides briefly in running tap water.
10. Dehydrate the slides by serial immersions in 95% alcohol (once), 100% alcohol (twice), and in xylene (twice).
11. Mount the slides with Permount and coverslip.

APPENDIX 8. CELL CRYOPRESERVATION USING METHANOL FREEZING METHOD

Freezing Solution

1. Slowly add (drop by drop) 1 volume of dimethylsulfoxide (DMSO) to 9 volumes of heat-inactivated fetal bovine serum (FBS). For example, add 5 mL of DMSO to 45 mL of FBS.
2. Filter the solution through a 0.22-μm syringe or bottle transfer system and then transfer the filtered solution to a Falcon #2070 screw-cap 50-mL tube. This freezing solution can be used fresh or stored at -20°C for up to 2 weeks for later use.

Freezing Procedure

1. Determine the total number of cells to be cryopreserved; this determines the total number of vials and the cell concentration per vial. The best cell viability is achieved when the number of cells per vial lies in the range of 20 to 50 $\times$ 10^6 cells.
2. Write the patient's name, freeze number, specimen, and number of cells on each 1.8-mL cryotube (Nunc #368632).
3. Prepare fresh freezing solution, or thaw previously prepared freezing solution in a 37°C water bath. Determine the total number of vials to be cryopreserved and the total volume of freezing solution needed; 1.5 mL of freezing solution is required for each vial to be frozen. Place the freezing solution on ice until ready to use.
4. Pellet the cells by centrifugation at 1,500 rpm in a Sorvall RT 6000 centrifuge for 10 minutes at 4°C, and decant the supernatant.
5. Remove the caps from the vials carefully under sterile conditions, and place them into a sterile Petri dish screw side down.
6. With a serologic pipette, add the calculated volume of cold freezing solution to the pellet. Resuspend the cells well. Carefully distribute the suspended cells among the

vials (1.5 mL per vial) using a serologic pipette, and place immediately on ice. Recap the vials, and transfer quickly to a Styrofoam container. Cover with another Styrofoam container, and tape in place to create a protected environment. Store at −80°C for 24 hours, and then transfer to a liquid nitrogen storage tank (−170°C). Note the location of the vials in the cell cryopreservation log.

APPENDIX 9. RECONSTITUTING CRYOPRESERVED CELLS

Thawing media consists of RPMI 1640 and 20% fetal calf serum.

1. Place 30 mL of thawing media in a Falcon #2070 screw-cap 50-mL tube labeled with the patient's name.
2. Remove a vial of cryopreserved cells from the liquid nitrogen storage tank and thaw quickly by immersion in a 37°C water bath.
3. After the vial of cells is thawed, carefully open the vial under sterile conditions. Using a sterile transfer pipette, carefully add 100 to 200 μL of thawing media, and gently resuspend the cells.
4. Transfer 0.5 mL of suspended cells to the Falcon tube containing the thawing media. Repeat this procedure until all the cells in the vial have been transferred to the Falcon tube.
5. Centrifuge the cells at 600 rpm in a Sorvall RT6000 centrifuge for 10 minutes at 4°C.
6. Decant the supernatant, and resuspend the cells in thawing media to a final concentration of 5×10^6 cells/mL.
7. Assess the viability of the cells by trypan blue dye exclusion (see Appendix 4).

APPENDIX 10. DIRECT AND INDIRECT IMMUNOFLUORESCENCE FOR CELL SURFACE ANTIGENS

The wash solution consists of phosphate-buffered saline (PBS), 10% fetal calf serum, and 0.1% sodium azide. The overnight solution is RPMI 1640, 10% fetal calf serum, 1% L-glutamine, 1% penicillin, and 1% streptomycin.

1. Prepare specimens according to protocols, and resuspend final cell suspensions to 5×10^6 cells/mL in overnight solution.
2. Label each Falcon #2052 12 × 75 mm capless tube with the patient's name and the antibody to be tested. Prepare the wash solution and refrigerate. Be certain that the centrifuge is adjusted to 4°C and that a water bath is adjusted to 37°C. Have all antibodies appropriately titered, diluted, and ready for use.
3. Add 1×10^6 cells to each labeled tube.
4. Add 1 mL of RPMI 1640 with 20% fetal calf serum to each tube that will receive labeled anti-immunoglobulin antibodies (anti-total Ig, κ, λ, μ, γ, δ, and α) and place them in a 37°C water bath for 1 to 2 hours. This allows cells to shed cytophilic immunoglobulin.
5. Add 2 mL of wash solution to tubes receiving directly labeled antibodies other than anti-immunoglobulins, and store at 4°C.
6. Add 2 mL of wash solution to each of the remaining tubes that will receive unlabeled primary antibodies, and spin the tubes at 1,100 rpm in a Sorvall RT 6000 centrifuge for 5 minutes at 4°C.
7. Decant, vortex, and place the tubes in a test tube rack in order by antibody to be received (e.g., all "CD19" tubes together, all "CD3" tubes together).
8. Add the appropriate amount of titered unlabeled primary antibody to the corresponding tube, and incubate for 30 minutes at 4°C.
9. After incubation, wash twice with 2 mL of wash solution, spinning between washes as in step 6, and decant and vortex as in step 7.
10. During the first wash, remove "directly labelled anti-immunoglobulin" tubes from the 37°C water bath, and add 2 mL of wash solution to each tube.
11. Add all the other "directly labelled" tubes (i.e., those that were stored at 4°C) to the second wash of the "indirect" tubes, and spin them all together as in step 6.
12. Decant and vortex.
13. Separate "indirect" from "direct" stained tubes.
14. Add appropriate amount of titered labeled secondary antibody to all "indirect" tubes.
15. Add the appropriate amount of labeled primary antibody to all "direct" tubes.
16. Incubate all tubes for 30 minutes at 4°C.
17. Wash all tubes twice with wash solution, as in step 6.
18. After the second wash, decant and resuspend the cells in 0.2 to 0.5 mL of wash solution and analyze them on a FACS Scan flow cytometer (Becton-Dickinson, Mountain View, CA).

REFERENCES

1. Jaffe ES, Strauchen JA, Berard CW. Predictability of immunologic phenotype by morphologic criteria in diffuse aggressive non-Hodgkin's lymphomas. *Am J Clin Pathol* 1982;77:46–49.
2. Wood GS, Burke JS, Horning S, et al. The immunologic and clinicopathologic heterogeneity of cutaneous lymphomas other than mycosis fungoides. *Blood* 1983;62:464–472.
3. Knowles DM, Dodson LG, Burke JS, et al. SIg^- E^- ("null cell") non-Hodgkin's lymphomas: multiparametric determination of their B- or T-cell lineage. *Am J Pathol* 1985; 120:356–370.
4. Chan LC, Pegram SM, Greaves MF. Contribution of immunophenotype to the classification and differential diagnosis of acute leukaemia. *Lancet* 1985;1:475–479.
5. Krause JR, Penchansky L, Contis L, et al. Flow cytometry in the diagnosis of acute leukemia. *Am J Clin Pathol* 1988;89:341–346.
6. Knowles DM. Lymphoid cell markers: their distribution and usefulness in the immunophenotypic analysis of lymphoid neoplasms. *Am J Surg Pathol* 1985;9[Suppl]:85–108.
7. Foon KA, Todd RF. Immunologic classification of leukemia and lymphoma. *Blood* 1986;68:1–31.
8. Picker LJ, Weiss LM, Medeiros JL, et al. Immunophenotypic criteria

for the diagnosis of non-Hodgkin's lymphoma. *Am J Pathol* 1987; 128:181–201.
9. Freedman AS, Nadler LM. Cell surface markers in hematologic malignancies. *Semin Oncol* 1987;14:193–212.
10. Deegan MJ. Membrane antigen analysis in the diagnosis of lymphoid leukemias and lymphomas. *Arch Pathol Lab Med* 1989;113:606–618.
11. Korsmeyer SJ, Arnold A, Bakhshi A, et al. Immunoglobulin gene rearrangement and cell surface antigen expression in acute lymphocytic leukemias of T-cell and B-cell precursor origins. *J Clin Invest* 1983;71:301–313.
12. Arnold A, Cossman J, Bakhski A, et al. Immunoglobulin gene rearrangements as unique clonal markers in human lymphoid neoplasms. *N Engl J Med* 1983;309:1593–1599.
13. Cleary ML, Chao J, Warnke R, et al. Immunoglobulin gene rearrangement as a diagnostic criterion of B-cell lymphoma. *Proc Natl Acad Sci USA* 1984;81:593–597.
14. Flug F, Pelicci PG, Bonetti F, et al. T cell receptor gene rearrangements as markers of lineage and clonality in T cell neoplasms. *Proc Natl Acad Sci USA* 1985;82:3460–3464.
15. Waldmann TA, Davis MM, Bongiovanni KF, et al. Rearrangements of gene for the antigen receptor on T cells as markers of lineage and clonality in human lymphoid neoplasms. *N Engl J Med* 1985;313: 776–783.
16. Rambaldi A, Pelicci PG, Allavena P, et al. T cell receptor β chain gene rearrangements in lymphoproliferative disorders of large granular lymphocytes/natural killer cells. *J Exp Med* 1985;162:2156–2162.
17. Knowles DM, Neri A, Pelicci PG, et al. Immunoglobulin and T cell receptor beta chain gene rearrangement analysis of Hodgkin's disease: implications for lineage determination and differential diagnosis. *Proc Natl Acad Sci USA* 1986;83:7942–7946.
18. Pelicci PG, Knowles DM, Arlin Z, et al. Multiple monoclonal B cell expansions and c-myc oncogene rearrangements in acquired immune deficiency syndrome-related lymphoproliferative disorders: implications for lymphomagenesis. *J Exp Med* 1986;164:2049–2060.
19. Neri A, Jakobiec FA, Pelicci PG, et al. Immunoglobulin and T cell receptor β chain gene rearrangement analysis of ocular adnexal lymphoid neoplasms: clinical and biologic implications. *Blood* 1987; 70:1519–1529.
20. Fishleder A, Tubbs R, Hessie B, et al. Uniform detection of immunoglobulin gene rearrangement in benign lymphoepithelial lesions. *N Engl J Med* 1987;316:1118–1121.
21. Hanson CA, Frizzera G, Patton DF, et al. Clonal rearrangement of immunoglobulin and T-cell receptor genes in systemic Castleman's disease: association with Epstein-Barr virus. *Am J Pathol* 1988;131: 84–91.
22. Knowles DM, Athan E, Ubriaco A, et al. Extranodal noncutaneous lymphoid hyperplasias represent a continuous spectrum of B-cell neoplasia: demonstration by molecular genetic analysis. *Blood* 1989;73: 1635–1645.
23. Wood GS, Ngan BY, Tung R, et al. Clonal rearrangements of immunoglobulin genes and progression to B cell lymphoma in cutaneous lymphoid hyperplasia. *Am J Pathol* 1989;135:13–19.
24. Foucar K, Chen IM, Crago S. Organization and operation of a flow cytometric immunophenotyping laboratory. *Semin Diagn Pathol* 1989;6:13–36.
25. Buckley RH. Immunodeficiency disorders. *JAMA* 1987;258: 2841–2851.
26. Auti F, Luzig G. Clinical immunology of immunodeficiency diseases: symptoms and signs of primary immunodeficiencies. *Ann Clin Res* 1987;19:230–247.
27. Garner RJ, Springgate C, Hoyt T. Immune monitoring of blood in heart transplant recipients: application of flow cytometry. *Semin Diagn Pathol* 1989;6:83–90.
28. Little JV, Foucar K, Horvath A, et al. Flow cytometric analysis of lymphoma and lymphoma-like disorders. *Semin Diagn Pathol* 1989; 6:37–54.
29. Zipf TF, Bryant LD, Koskowich GN, et al. Enumeration of cytoplasmic mu immunoglobulin positive acute lymphoblastic leukemia cells by flow cytometry: comparison with fluorescence microscopy. *Cytometry* 1984;5:610–613.
30. Knowles DM, Tolidjian B, Marboe CC, et al. A new human B lymphocyte surface antigen (BL2) detectable by a hybridoma monoclonal antibody: distribution on benign and malignant lymphoid cells. *Blood* 1983;62:191–198.
31. Knowles DM, Tolidjian B, Marboe CC, et al. Distribution of antigens defined by OKB monoclonal antibodies on benign and malignant lymphoid cells and nonlymphoid tissues. *Blood* 1984;63: 886–896.
32. Wang CY, Azzo W, Al-Katib A, et al. Preparation and characterization of monoclonal antibodies recognizing three distinct differentiation antigens (BL1, BL2, BL3) on human B lymphocytes. *J Immunol* 1984; 133:684–691.
33. Peng R, Al-Katib A, Knowles DM, et al. Preparation and characterization of monoclonal antibodies recognizing two distinct differentiation antigens (Pro-Im1, Pro-Im2) on early hematopoietic cells. *Blood* 1984; 64:1169–1178.
34. Knowles DM, Tolidjian B, Marboe CC, et al. Monoclonal anti-human monocyte antibodies OKM1 and OKM5 possess distinctive tissue distributions including differential reactivity with vascular endothelium. *J Immunol* 1984;132:2170–2173.
35. Posnett DN, Marboe CC, Knowles DM, et al. A membrane antigen (HC1) selectively present on hairy cell leukemia cells, endothelial cells and epidermal basal cells. *J Immunol* 1984;132:2700–2702.
36. Knowles DM, Halper JP, Azzo W, et al. The expression and distribution of Leu1 on benign and malignant human lymphoid cells: correlation with conventional cell markers and with monoclonal antibody OKT1. *Cancer* 1983;52:1369–1377.
37. Chadburn A, Inghirami G, Knowles DM. Hairy cell leukemia-associated antigen LeuM5 (CD11c) is preferentially expressed by benign activated and neoplastic CD8 T cells. *Am J Pathol* 1990;136:29–37.
38. Friedman SM, Thompson G, Halper JP, et al. OT-CLL: a human chronic lymphocytic leukemia that produces IL2 in high titer. *J Immunol* 1982;128:935–940.
39. Bonetti F, Knowles DM, Chilosi M, et al. A distinctive cutaneous malignant neoplasm expressing the Langerhans cell phenotype: synchronous occurrence with B-chronic lymphocytic leukemia. *Cancer* 1985;55:2417–2425.
40. Wieczorek R, Greco MA, McCarthy K, et al. Familial erythrophagocytic lymphohistiocytosis: immunophenotypic, immunohistochemical and ultrastructural demonstration of its relationship to sinus histiocytes. *Hum Pathol* 1986;17:55–63.
41. Wieczorek R, Suhrland M, Ramsay D, et al. LeuM1 antigen expression in advanced (tumor) stage mycosis fungoides. *Am J Clin Pathol* 1986;86:25–32.
42. Bonetti F, Chilosi M, Menestrina F, et al. Immunohistological analysis of Rosai-Dorfman histiocytosis: a disease of S-100^{+} CD1^{-} histiocytes. *Virchows Arch A* 1987;411:129–135.
43. Franchino C, Reich C, Distenfeld A, et al. A clinicopathologically distinctive primary splenic histiocytic neoplasm: demonstration of its histiocytic derivation by immunophenotypic and molecular genetic analysis. *Am J Surg Pathol* 1988;12:398–404.
44. Thomas FP, Vallejos U, Foitl DR, et al. B-cell small lymphocytic lymphoma and chronic lymphocytic leukemia with peripheral neuropathy; two cases with neuropathological findings and lymphocyte marker analysis. *Acta Neuropathol* 1990;80:198–203.
45. Wisniewski T, Sisti M, Inghirami G, et al. Intracerebral solitary plasmacytoma. *Neurosurgery* 1990;27:826–829.
46. Gold JE, Louis-Charles A, Ghali V, et al. T-cell chronic lymphocytic leukemia with unusual morphologic, phenotypic, and karyotypic features in association with light-chain amyloidosis. *Cancer* 1992;70: 86–93.
47. Knowles DM, Halper JP. Human T cell malignancies: correlative clinical, histopathologic, immunologic and cytochemical analysis of 23 cases. *Am J Pathol* 1982;106:197–203.
48. Wieczorek R, Burke JS, Knowles DM. Leu M1 antigen expression in T cell neoplasia. *Am J Pathol* 1985;121:374–380.
49. Flug F, Dodson L, Wolff J, et al. B lymphocyte associated differentiation antigen expression by "non-B, non-T" acute lymphoblastic leukemia. *Leuk Res* 1985;9:1051–1058.
50. McNally L, Jakobiec FA, Knowles DM. Clinical, morphologic, immunophenotypic and molecular genetic analysis of bilateral ocular adnexal lymphoid neoplasms: clinical and biological implications. *Am J Ophthalmol* 1987;103:555–568.
51. Inghirami G, Wieczorek R, Zhu BY, et al. Differential expression of LFA-1 molecules in non-Hodgkin's lymphoma and lymphoid leukemia. *Blood* 1988;72:11431–1434.
52. Knowles DM, Chamulak G, Subar M, et al. Clinicopathologic, immunophenotypic and molecular genetic analysis of AIDS-associated

lymphoid neoplasia: clinical and biological implications. *Pathol Ann* 1988;23:33–67.
53. Knowles DM, Chamulak GA, Subar M, et al. Lymphoid neoplasia associated with AIDS: the New York University Medical Center experience with 105 cases (1981–1986). *Ann Intern Med* 1988;108: 744–753.
54. Knowles DM, Jakobiec FA, McNally L, et al. Lymphoid hyperplasia and malignant lymphoma occurring in the ocular adnexa (orbit, conjunctiva, and eyelids): a prospective multiparametric analysis of 108 cases during 1977–1987. *Hum Pathol* 1990;21:959–973.
55. Inghirami G, Lederman S, Yellin MJ, et al. Phenotypic and functional characterization of T-BAM (CD40 ligand) positive T cell non-Hodgkin's lymphomas. *Blood* 1994:84:866–872.
56. Harrington W, Ubriaco AR, Knowles DM. Phenotypic-functional disassociation and functional heterogeneity of T cell malignancies. *Lab Invest* 1986;54:25A(abst).
57. Pelicci PG, Knowles DM, Dalla-Favera R. Lymphoid tumors displaying rearrangements of both immunoglobulin and T-cell receptor genes. *J Exp Med* 1985;162:1015–1024.
58. Foa R, Migone N, Lauria F, et al. Analysis of T-cell receptor gene rearrangements demonstrates the monoclonal nature of T-cell chronic lymphoproliferative disorders. *Blood* 1986;67:247–250.
59. Knowles DM, Pelicci PG, Dalla-Favera R. T-cell receptor beta chain gene rearrangements: genetic markers of T cell lineage and clonality. *Hum Pathol* 1986;17:546–551.
60. Pelicci PG, Knowles DM, Magrath I, et al. Chromosomal breakpoints and structural alterations of the c-myc locus differ in endemic and sporadic forms of Burkitt lymphoma. *Proc Natl Acad Sci USA* 1986; 83:2984–2988.
61. Seremetis SV, Pelicci PG, Tabilio A, et al. High frequency of clonal immunoglobulin or T-cell receptor gene rearrangements in the subset of acute myelogenous leukemia expressing terminal deoxynucleotidyl transferase. *J Exp Med* 1987;165:1703–1712.
62. Pelicci P, Allavena P, Alessandro R, et al. T-cell receptor (α, β, γ) gene rearrangements and expression distinguish large granular lymphocyte/natural killer cells. *Blood* 1987;70:1500–1508.
63. Subar M, Pelicci PG, Neri A, et al. T-gamma gene rearrangements: different patterns in T- and B-cell neoplasms. *Leukemia* 1988;2: 19–26.
64. Neri A, Knowles DM, Magrath IT, et al. Different regions of the immunoglobulin heavy chain locus are involved in chromosomal translocations in endemic and sporadic forms of Burkitt lymphoma. *Proc Natl Acad Sci USA* 1988;85:2748–2752.
65. Subar M, Neri A, Inghirami G, et al. Frequent c-myc oncogene activation and infrequent presence of Epstein-Barr virus genome in AIDS-associated lymphoma. *Blood* 1988;7:667–671.
66. Neri A, Knowles DM, McCormick F, et al. Analysis of RAS oncogene in human lymphoid malignancies. *Proc Natl Acad Sci USA* 1988;85: 9268–9272.
67. Knowles DM, Inghirami G, Ubriaco A, et al. Molecular genetic analysis of three AIDS-associated neoplasms of uncertain lineage demonstrates their B-cell derivation and the possible pathogenetic role of the Epstein-Barr virus. *Blood* 1989;73:792–799.
68. Logtenberg T, Schutte MEM, Inghirami G, et al. Immunoglobulin V_H gene expression in human B cell lines and tumors: biased V_H gene expression in chronic lymphocytic leukemia. *Int Immunol* 1989;1: 362–366.
69. Neri A, Barriga F, Inghirami G, et al. Epstein-Barr virus infection precedes clonal expansion in Burkitt's and AIDS-associated lymphoma. *Blood* 1991;77:1092–1095.
70. Athan E, Foitl DR, Knowles DM. Bcl-1 gene rearrangement: frequency and clinical significance among B cell chronic lymphocytic leukemias and non-Hodgkin's lymphomas. *Am J Pathol* 1991;138: 591–597.
71. Gaidano G, Ballerini P, Gong JZ, et al. P53 mutations in human lymphoid malignancies: association with Burkitt's lymphoma and chronic lymphocytic leukemia. *Proc Natl Acad Sci USA* 1991;88: 5413–5417.
72. Berman JE, Nickerson KG, Pollock RR, et al. V_H gene usage in humans: biased usage of the V_H6 gene in immature B lymphoid cells. *Eur J Immunol* 1991;21:1311–1314.
73. Athan E, Chadburn A, Knowles DM. The bcl-2 gene translocation is undetectable in Hodgkin's disease by Southern blot hybridization and polymerase chain reaction. *Am J Pathol* 1992;141:193–201.
74. Gaidano G, Hauptschein RS, Parsar NZ, et al. Deletions involving two distinct regions of 6q in B-cell non-Hodgkin lymphoma. *Blood* 1992;80:1781–1787.
75. Cesarman E, Chadburn A, Inghirami G, et al. Structural and functional analysis of oncogenes and tumor suppressor genes in adult T-cell leukemia/lymphoma (ATLL) reveals frequent p53 mutations. *Blood* 1992;80:3205–3216.
76. Gaidano G, Parsa NZ, Tassi V, et al. In vitro establishment of AIDS-related lymphoma cell lines: phenotypic characterization, oncogene and tumor suppressor gene lesions, an heterogeneity in Epstein-Barr virus infection. *Leukemia* 1993;7:1621–1629.
77. Cesarman E, Inghirami G, Chadburn A, et al. High levels of p53 protein expression do not correlate with p53 gene mutations in anaplastic large cell lymphoma. *Am J Pathol* 1993;143:1–12.
78. Ballerini P, Gaidano G, Gong JZ, et al. Multiple genetic lesions in AIDS-related non-Hodgkin lymphoma. *Blood* 1993;81:166–176.
79. Ye BH, Lista F, LoCoco F, et al. Alterations of a zinc-finger encoding gene, BCL-6, in diffuse large cell lymphoma. *Science* 1993;262: 747–750.
80. Corradini P, Ladetto M, Voena C, et al. Mutational activation of N- and K-ras oncogenes in plasma cell dyscrasias. *Blood* 1993;81: 2708–2714.
81. Cesarman E, Liu YF, Knowles DM. The MDM2 oncogene is rarely amplified in human lymphoid tumors and does not correlate with p53 gene expression [Letter]. *Int J Cancer* 1994;56:457–458.
82. Matsushima AY, Cesarman E, Chadburn A, et al. Post-thymic T cell lymphomas frequently overexpress p53 protein but infrequently exhibit p53 gene mutations. *Am J Pathol* 1994;144:573–584.
83. Gaidano G, Lo Coco F, Ye BH, et al. Rearrangements of the BCL-6 gene in AIDS-associated non-Hodgkin's lymphoma: association with diffuse large-cell subtype. *Blood* 1994;84:397–402.
84. Matolcsy A, Inghirami G, Knowles DM. Molecular genetic demonstration of the diverse evolution of Richter's syndrome (chronic lymphocytic leukemia and subsequent large cell lymphoma). *Blood* 1994;83:1363–1372.
85. Lo Coco F, Ye BH, Lista F, et al. Rearrangements of the BCL6 gene in diffuse large-cell non Hodgkin's lymphoma. *Blood* 1994;83: 1757–1759.
86. Riboldi P, Gaidano G, Schettino EW, et al. Two AIDS-associated Burkitt's lymphomas produce specific anti-i IgM cold agglutinins utilizing somatically mutated V_H4-21 segments. *Blood* 1994;83: 2952–2961.
87. Inghirami G, Macri L, Cesarman E, et al. Molecular characterization of CD30 positive anaplastic large cell lymphoma: high frequency of c-myc proto-oncogene activation. *Blood* 1994;83:3581–3590.
88. Corradini P, Inghirami G, Astolfi M, et al. Inactivation of tumor suppressor genes, p53 and RB1, in plasma cell dyscrasias. *Leukemia* 1994;8:758–767.
89. Knowles DM, Cesarman E, Chadburn A, et al. Correlative morphologic and molecular genetic analysis demonstrates three distinct categories of post-transplantation lymphoproliferative disorders. *Blood* 1995;85:552–565.
90. Chadburn A, Cesarman E, Liu YF, et al. Molecular genetic analysis demonstrates that multiple post-transplantation lymphoproliferative disorders occurring in one anatomic site in a single patient represent distinct primary lymphoid neoplasms. *Cancer* 1995;75:2747–2756.
91. Matolcsy A, Chadburn A, Knowles DM. De novo CD5 positive and Richter's syndrome associated diffuse large B cell lymphomas are genotypically distinct. *Am J Pathol* 1995;147:207–216.
92. Chadburn A, Suciu-Foca N, Cesarman E, et al. Post-transplantation lymphoproliferative disorders (PT-LPDs) arising in solid organ transplant recipients are usually of recipient origin. *Am J Pathol* 1995;174: 1862–1870.
93. Matolcsy A, Casali P, Knowles DM. Different clonal origin of B cell populations of chronic lymphocytic leukemia and large cell lymphoma in Richter's syndrome. *Ann N Y Acad Sci* 1995;764:496–503.
94. Migliazza A, Martinotti S, Chen W, et al. Frequent somatic hypermutation of the 5′ non-coding region of the BCL6 gene in B cell lymphoma. *Proc Natl Acad Sci USA* 1995;92: 12520–12524.
95. Tsang P, Cesarman E, Chadburn A, et al. Molecular characterization of primary mediastinal B cell lymphoma. *Am J Pathol* 1996;148: 2017–2025.
96. Gamberi B, Gaidano G, Parsa N, et al. Microsatellite instability is rare in B-cell non-Hodgkin's lymphomas. *Blood* 1997;89:975–979.

97. Matolcsy A, Casali P, Liu Y, et al. Molecular characterization of IgA- and/or IgG-switched chronic lymphocytic leukemia B cells. *Blood* 1997;89:1732–1739.
98. Matolcsy A, Warnke RA, Knowles DM. Somatic mutations of the translocated bcl-2 gene are associated with morphologic transformation of follicular lymphoma to diffuse large cell lymphoma. *Ann Oncol* 1997;8[Suppl 2]:119–122.
99. Horenstein MG, Nador RG, Chadburn A, et al. Epstein-Barr virus latent gene expression in primary effusion lymphomas containing Kaposi's sarcoma-associated herpesvirus/human herpesvirus-8. *Blood* 1997;90:1186–1191.
100. Scheinfeld AG, Nador RG, Cesarman E, et al. Epstein-Barr virus latent membrane protein-1 oncogene deletion in post-transplantation lymphoproliferative disorders. *Am J Pathol* 1997;151:805–812.
101. Inghirami G, Chilosi M, Knowles DM. Western thymomas lack Epstein-Barr virus by Southern blotting analysis and by polymerase chain reaction. *Am J Pathol* 1990;136: 1429–1436.
102. Chadburn A, Athan E, Wieczorek R, et al. Detection and characterization of HTLV-I associated T cell neoplasms in an HTLV-I non-endemic region by polymerase chain reaction. *Blood* 1991;77: 2419–2430.
103. Frank D, Cesarman E, Liu YF, et al. Post-transplantation lymphoproliferative disorders frequently contain type A and not type B Epstein-Barr virus. *Blood* 1995;85:1396–1403.
104. Chang Y, Cesarman E, Pessin MS, et al. Kaposi's sarcoma-associated DNA sequences of nonhuman origin: evidence for a new human herpes virus. *Science* 1994;266:1865–1869.
105. Cesarman E, Chang Y, Moore PS, et al. Kaposi's sarcoma-associated herpesvirus-like DNA sequences in AIDS-related body-cavity based lymphomas. *N Engl J Med* 1995;332:1186–1191.
106. Nador RG, Cesarman E, Chadburn A, et al. Primary effusion lymphoma: a distinct clinicopathologic entity associated with the Kaposi's sarcoma-associated herpesvirus. *Blood* 1996;88:645–656.
107. Link MP, Stewart SJ, Warnke RA, et al. Discordance between surface and cytoplasmic expression of the Leu-4 (T3) antigen in thymocytes and in blast cells from childhood T lymphoblastic malignancies. *J Clin Invest* 1985;76:248–253.
108. Knowles DM. Immunophenotypic and antigen receptor gene rearrangement analysis in T cell neoplasia. *Am J Pathol* 1989;134: 761–785.
109. Gahmberg CG, Jokinen M, Andersson LC. Expression of the major sialoglycoprotein (glycophorin) on erythroid cells in human bone marrow. *Blood* 1978;52:379–387.
110. Robinson J, Sieff C, Delia D, et al. Expression of cell-surface HLA-DR, HLA-ABC and glycophorin during erythroid differentiation. *Nature* 1981;289:68–71.
111. Greaves MF, Sieff C, Edwards PAW. Monoclonal antiglycophorin as a probe for erythroleukemias. *Blood* 1983;61:645–651.
112. Warnke RA, Gatter KC, Falini B, et al. Diagnosis of human lymphoma with monoclonal antileukocyte antibodies. *N Engl J Med* 1983;309: 1275–1281.
113. Civin CI, Strauss IC, Brovall C, et al. Antigenic analysis of hematopoiesis. III. A hematopoietic progenitor cell surface antigen defined by a monoclonal antibody raised against KG la cells. *J Immunol* 1984; 133:157–165.
114. Pinkus GS, Thomas P, Said J. Leu M1—a marker for Reed-Sternberg cells in Hodgkin's disease. *Am J Pathol* 1985;119:244–252.
115. Sheibani K, Battifora H, Burke JS, et al. Leu-M1 antigen in human neoplasms: an immunohistologic study of 400 cases. *Am J Surg Pathol* 1986;10:227–236.
116. Banks L, Matlashewski G, Crawford L. Isolation of human p53-specific monoclonal antibodies and their use in the studies of human p53 expression. *Eur J Biochem* 1986;159:529–534.
117. Andrews RG, Singer JW, Bernstein ID. Monoclonal antibody 12-8 recognizes a 115-kd molecule present on both unipotent and multipotent hematopoietic colony-forming cells. *Blood* 1986;67:842–845.
118. Norton AJ, Ramsay AD, Smith SA, et al. Monoclonal antibody (UCHL1) that recognizes normal and neoplastic T cells in routinely fixed tissues. *J Clin Pathol* 1986;39:399–405.
119. Brenner MB, McLean J, Scheft H, et al. Characterization and expression of the human $\alpha\beta$ T cell receptor using a framework monoclonal antibody. *Immunology* 1987;138:1502–1509.
120. Linder J, Ye Y, Harrington DS, et al. Monoclonal antibodies marking T lymphocytes in paraffin-embedded tissue. *Am J Pathol* 1987;127: 1–8.
121. Cartun RW, Coles FB, Pastuszak WT. Utilization of monoclonal antibody L26 in the identification and confirmation of B-cell lymphomas: a sensitive and specific marker applicable to formalin and B5-fixed, paraffin-embedded tissues. *Am J Pathol* 1987;129:415–421.
122. Dobson CM, Myskow MW, Krajewski AS, et al. Immunohistochemical staining of non-Hodgkin's lymphoma in paraffin sections using the MB1 and MT1 monoclonal antibodies. *J Pathol* 1987;153:203–212.
123. Hall PA, Lindeman R, Butler MG, et al. Demonstration of lymphoid antigens in decalcified bone marrow trephines. *J Clin Pathol* 1987; 40:870–873.
124. Norton AJ, Isaacson PG. Monoclonal antibodies (MT1, MT2, MB1, MB2, MB3) reactive with leukocyte subsets in paraffin embedded tissue sections. *Am J Pathol* 1987;127:418–429.
125. Schwarting R, Gerdes J, Stein H. Ber H-2: a new monoclonal antibody of the Ki-1 family for the detection of Hodgkin's disease in formaldehyde fixed tissue. In: McMichael AJ, Beverley PCL, Cobbold S, et al, eds. *Leucocyte typing, III. White cell differentiation antigens.* Oxford: Oxford University Press, 1987:574–575.
126. Band H, Hochstenbach F, McLean J, et al. Immunochemical proof that a novel rearranging gene encodes the T cell receptor δ subunit. *Science* 1987;238:682–684.
127. Chittal SM, Caveriviere P, Schwarting R, et al. Monoclonal antibodies in the diagnosis of Hodgkin's disease: the search for a rational panel. *Am J Surg Pathol* 1988;12:9–21.
128. Pinkus GS, Said JW. Hodgkin's disease, lymphocyte predominance type, nodular.Further evidence for a B cell derivation: L & H variants of Reed-Sternberg cells express L26, a pan B cell marker. *Am J Pathol* 1988;133:211–217.
129. Pallesen G, Hamilton-Dutoit SJ. Ki-1 (CD30) antigen is regularly expressed by tumor cells of embryonal carcinoma. *Am J Pathol* 1988; 133:446–450.
130. Ng CS, Chan JKC, Hui PK, et al. Monoclonal antibodies reactive with normal and neoplastic T cells in paraffin sections. *Hum Pathol* 1988;19:295–303.
131. Wieczorek R, Buck D, Bindl J, et al. Monoclonal antibody Leu-22 (L60) permits the demonstration of some neoplastic T cells in routinely fixed and paraffin-embedded tissue sections. *Hum Pathol* 1988; 19:1434–1443.
132. Mason DY, Krissansen GW, Davey FR, et al. Antisera against epitopes resistant to denaturation on T3 (CD3) antigen can detect reactive and neoplastic T cells in paraffin embedded tissue biopsy specimens. *J Clin Pathol* 1988;41:121–127.
133. Borst J, van Dongen JJM, Bolhuis RLH, et al. Distinct molecular forms of human T cell receptor γ/δ detected on viable T cells by a monoclonal antibody. *J Exp Med* 1988;167:1625–1644.
134. Pulford K, Rigney E, Jones M, et al. KP1 (CD68)—a new monoclonal antibody detecting a monocyte/macrophage associated antigen in routinely processed tissue sections. *J Clin Pathol* 1989;42:414–421.
135. Mason DY, Cordell J, Brown M, et al. Detection of T cells in paraffin wax embedded tissue using antibodies against a peptide sequence from the CD3 antigen. *J Clin Pathol* 1989;42:1194–1200.
136. Ngan BY, Picker LJ, Medeiros J, et al. Immunophenotypic diagnosis of non-Hodgkin's lymphoma in paraffin sections: co-expression of L60 (Leu-22) and L26 antigens correlates with malignant histologic findings. *Am J Clin Pathol* 1989;91:579–583.
137. Clark JR, Williams ME, Swerdlow SH. Detection of B- and T-cells in paraffin-embedded tissue sections: diagnostic utility of commercially obtained 4KB5 and UCHL-1. *Am J Clin Pathol* 1990;93:58–69.
138. Fina L, Molgaard HV, Robertson D, et al. Expression of the CD34 gene in vascular endothelial cells. *Blood* 1990;75:2417–2426.
139. Pezzella F, Tse AGD, Cordell JL, et al. Expression of the bcl-2 oncogene protein is not specific for the 14;18 chromosomal translocation. *Am J Pathol* 1990;137:225–232.
140. Hockenbery D, Nunez G, Milliman C, et al. Bcl-2 is an inner mitochondrial membrane protein that blocks programmed cell death. *Nature* 1990;348:334–336.
141. Zutter M, Hockenbery D, Silverman GA, et al. Immunolocalization of the Bcl-2 protein within hematopoietic neoplasms. *Blood* 1991;78: 1062–1068.
142. van Noesel CJM, van Lier RAW, Cordell JL, et al. The membrane IgM-associated heterodimer on human B cells is a newly defined B

cell antigen that contains the protein product of the mb-1 gene. *J Immunol* 1991;146:3881–3888.
143. Simmons PJ, Torok-Storb B. CD34 expression by stromal precursors in normal human adult bone marrow. *Blood* 1991;78:2848–2853.
144. Vojtesck B, Bartek J, Midgley CA, et al. An immunohistochemical analysis of the human nuclear phosphoprotein p53: new monoclonal antibodies and epitope mapping using recombinant p53. *J Immunol Methods* 1992;151:237–244.
145. Chadburn A, Husain S, Knowles DM. Monoclonal antibody OPD4 detects neoplastic T cells but does not distinguish between CD4 and CD8 neoplastic T cells in paraffin tissue sections. *Hum Pathol* 1992; 23:940–947.
146. Cattoretti G, Pileri S, Parravicini C, et al. Antigen unmasking on formalin-fixed paraffin-embedded tissue sections. *J Pathol* 1993;171: 83–98.
147. Falini B, Flenghi L, Pileri S, et al. PG-M1: a new monoclonal antibody directed against a fixative-resistant epitope on the macrophage-restricted form of the CD68 molecule. *Am J Pathol* 1993;142: 1359–1372.
148. Jiang W, Zhang YJ, Kahn SM, et al. Altered expression of the cyclin D1 and retinoblastoma genes in human esophageal cancer. *Proc Natl Acad Sci USA* 1993;90:9026–9030.
149. Cesarman E, Inghirami G, Chadburn A, et al. High levels of p53 expression do not correlate with p53 gene mutations in anaplastic large cell lymphoma. *Am J Pathol* 1993;43:845–846.
150. Matsushima AY, Cesarman E, Chadburn A, et al. Post-thymic T cell lymphomas frequently overexpress p53 protein but infrequently exhibit p53 gene mutations. *Am J Pathol* 1994;144:573–584.
151. Bartkova J, Lukas J, Strauss M, et al. Cell cycle-related variation and tissue-restricted expression of human cyclin D1 protein. *J Pathol* 1994;172:237–245.
152. Yang WI, Zukerberg LR, Motokura T, et al. Cyclin D1 (Bcl-1, PRAD1) protein expression in low-grade B-cell lymphomas and reactive hyperplasia. *Am J Pathol* 1994;145:86–96.
153. Cuevas EC, Bateman AC, Wilkins BS, et al. Microwave antigen retrieval in immunocytochemistry: a study of 80 antibodies. *J Clin Pathol* 1994;47:448–452.
154. Norton AJ, Jordan S, Yeomans P. Brief, high-temperature heat denaturation (pressure cooking): a simple and effective method of antigen retrieval for routinely processed tissues. *J Pathol* 1994;173:371–379.
155. Pezzella F, Gatter K. What is the value of bcl-2 protein detection for histopathologists? *Histopathology* 1995;26:89–93.
156. Zukerberg LR, Yang WI, Arnold A, et al. Cyclin D1 expression in non-Hodgkin's lymphomas. *Am J Clin Pathol* 1995;103:756–760.
157. Mason DY, Cordell JL, Brown MH, et al. CD79a: a novel marker for B-cell neoplasms in routinely processed tissue samples. *Blood* 1995;86:1453–1459.
158. Shi SR, Gu J, Kalra KL, et al. Antigen retrieval technique: a novel approach to immunohistochemistry on routinely processed tissue sections. *Cell Vision* 1995;2:7–22.
159. Schlossman SF, Boumsell L, Gilks W, et al, eds. *Leukocyte typing, V: White cell differentiation antigens.* New York, Oxford University Press, 1995.
160. Tsang WYW, Chan JKC, Pau MY. Utility of a paraffin section-reactive CD56 antibody (123C3) for characterization and diagnosis of lymphomas. *Am J Surg Pathol* 1996;20:202–210.
161. Bonsing BA, Corver WE, Gorsira MCB, et al. Specificity of seven monoclonal antibodies against p53 evaluated with Western blotting, immunohistochemistry, confocal laser scanning microscopy, and flow cytometry. *Cytometry* 1997;28:11–24.
162. Bennett JM, Catovsky D, Daniel MT, et al. Proposals for the classification of the acute leukemias: French-American-British (FAB) cooperative Group. *Br J Haematol* 1976;33:451–458.
163. Griffin JD. The use of monoclonal antibodies in the characterization of myeloid leukemias. *Hematol Pathol* 1987;1:81–91.
164. Zukerberg LR, Medeiros LJ, Ferry JA, et al. Diffuse low-grade B-cell lymphomas: four clinically distinct subtypes defined by a combination of morphologic and immunophenotypic features. *Am J Clin Pathol* 1993;100:373–385.
165. Dorfman DM, Pinkus GS. Distinction between small lymphocytic and mantle cell lymphoma by immunoreactivity for CD23. *Mod Pathol* 1994;7:326–331.
166. Matutes E, Owusu-Ankomah K, Morilla R, et al. The immunological profile of B-cell disorders and proposal of a scoring system for the diagnosis of CLL. *Leukemia* 1994;8:1640–1650.
167. Knowles DM. The human T-cell leukemias: clinical, cytomorphologic, immunophenotypic,and genotypic characteristics. *Hum Pathol* 1986;17:14–33.
168. Inghirami G, Zhu BY, Chess L, et al. Flow cytometric and Immunohistochemical characterization of the γ/δ T-lymphocyte population in normal human lymphoid tissue and peripheral blood. *Am J Pathol* 1990;136:357–367.
169. Borowitz MJ, Shuster JJ, Civin CI, et al. Prognostic significance of CD34 expression in childhood B-precursor acute lymphocytic leukemia: a Pediatric Oncology Group study. *J Clin Oncol* 1990;8: 1389–1398.
170. Pui CH, Hancock ML, Head DR, et al. Clinical significance of CD34 expression in childhood acute lymphoblastic leukemia. *Blood* 1993; 82:889–894.
171. Thomas X, Archimbaud E, Charrin C, et al. CD34 expression is associated with major adverse prognostic factors in adult acute lymphoblastic leukemia. *Leukemia* 1995;9:249–253.
172. Sperling C, Buchner T, Creutzig U, et al. Clinical, morphologic, cytogenetic and prognostic implications of CD34 expression in childhood and adult de novo AML. *Leuk Lymphoma* 1994;17:417–426.
173. Ha-Kawa K, Hara J, Keiko Y, et al. Kappa-chain gene rearrangement in an apparent T-lineage lymphoma. *J Clin Invest* 1986;78: 1439–1442.
174. Sheibani K, Wu A, Ben-Ezra J, et al. Rearrangement of κ-chain and T-cell receptor β-chain genes in malignant lymphomas of "T-cell" phenotype. *Am J Pathol* 1987;129:201–206.
175. Weiss LM, Wood GS, Trela M, et al. Clonal T-cell population in lymphomatoid papulosis: evidence of a lymphoproliferative origin for a clinically benign disease. *N Engl J Med* 1986;315:475–479.
176. Kadin ME, Vonderheid ED, Sako D, et al. Clonal composition of T cells in lymphomatoid papulosis. *Am J Pathol* 1987;126:13–17.
177. Chadburn A, Knowles DM. Paraffin resistant antigens detectable by antibodies L26 and polyclonal CD3 predict the B or T cell lineage of 95% of diffuse aggressive non-Hodgkin's lymphomas. *Am J Surg Pathol* 1994;102:284–291.
178. Segal GH, Stoler MH, Tubbs RR. The "CD43 only" phenotype. An aberrant, nonspecific immunophenotype requiring comprehensive analysis for lineage resolution. *Am J Clin Pathol* 1992;97:861–865.

CHAPTER 12

Technical Factors in the Preparation and Evaluation of Lymph Node Biopsies

Peter M. Banks

The most underrepresented aspect of hematopathology in publications is that of specimen preparation. This belies the subject's importance, because high-quality conventional paraffin section preparations are the essential starting point for accurate diagnosis (1,2).

The pathologist's charge has grown considerably over the past two decades as ancillary studies of diagnostic importance have become a part of established practice, requiring special tissue allocations. It is sobering to realize that in modern practice the failure to allocate biopsied tissue appropriately may represent a greater failure than the erroneous interpretation of paraffin tissue sections. Although the latter error can often be corrected by consultative review, the former may oblige the patient to an additional surgical procedure. The task is made all the more difficult by current trends toward ever smaller biopsy samples.

Pathologists should regularly reevaluate and update the quality of their stock in trade, the conventional paraffin tissue section products of their laboratory, and their practices in tissue allocation of lymph node and related tissue biopsy specimens.

CONVENTIONAL PARAFFIN TISSUE SECTIONS

The importance of consistently high-quality paraffin tissue sections to the hematopathologist cannot be exaggerated. Conventional microscopy remains the gold standard and starting point for our understanding of lymphoid proliferations. It is always a top priority, at least in initial samplings, that representative tissue blocks be submitted for conventional paraffin processing. Plastic embedding techniques have been improved and provide outstanding cytologic detail (3,4). Although these methods offer substantive advantages over conventional paraffin embedding for some applications, such as for preparation of undecalcified bone marrow biopsy sections, they remain less practical in handling large tissue blocks than those for paraffin processing. Plastic blocks are still less versatile than paraffin blocks in most applications, and their security for long-term storage is unproved. The quality of the paraffin used for conventional processing has improved greatly with the addition of plastic polymers, which enhance its physical characteristics for sectioning. The commercial availability of useful antibodies that can identify antigens in paraffin preparations makes high-quality sections all the more valuable.

Because of the long sequence involved in the production of paraffin tissue sections, potential shortcomings are many and diverse. The critical reviews of slide preparations by the pathologist and technologist allow recognition of telltale deficiencies specific to particular steps in processing (Table 12.1). A chronology of routine processing with reference to morphologic artifacts follows; it can be used as a guide for troubleshooting.

Specimen Delivery

Even when the laboratory receives biopsy specimens directly from the operating rooms, irreversible drying artifacts can be introduced if transport is in dry towels or surgical sponges (Fig. 12.1). The surface tissue is desiccated, resulting in dehydrational denaturation of cellular proteins, commonly recognizable as a dark edge in hematoxylin and eosin (H&E)–stained sections (Fig. 12.2). This can be a serious problem with small samples, such as needle biopsies, especially if delivered on gauze pads in which the delicate tissue adheres to the dry interstices and may be damaged in an attempt to remove it or even be effectively inextricable. To avoid such catastrophes, the investigator should instruct sur-

P. M. Banks: Department of Hematopathology, Carolinas Medical Center, Charlotte, North Carolina 28203 and Department of Pathology, University of North Carolina, Chapel Hill, North Carolina 27599

TABLE 12.1. *Common errors in routine tissue processing and their consequences*

Step	Error	Result
Delivery	Specimen on dry towel	"Edge" artifact due to desiccation of surface tissue (Figs. 12.1 and 12.2)
Blocking	Tissue blocks too thick	"Soft" central core of block that fragments in sections (Figs. 12.4 and 12.5)
Fixation	Inadequate time for fixation; overfixation in mercuric solutions (B5, Zenker's solution)	Uniform fragmentation of sections; brittle tissue blocks with cracking in sections
Dehydration	Aqueous contamination of alcohols or inadequate time in alcohols in processor	Sections show small, irregular cracks with faint staining, blurred nuclear chromatin
Clearing	Excessive time in xylenes; alcohols contaminating xylenes with poor paraffin infiltration	Tissue hard and brittle; sections compressed and wrinkled; do not ribbon
Infiltration	Paraffin too hot	Cellular shrinkage and retraction; collagen basophilic (Fig. 12.8)
Embedding	Delay in embedding after removal from paraffin bath	Air spaces around tissue, poor connection to surrounding paraffin disrupts sections
Sectioning	Improper knife angle; defective knife edge	"Venetian blind" shutter effect lines across sections (Fig. 12.11)
Floating section	Inadequate attention to teasing sections flat on water bath	Folds and/or tears in sections (Fig. 12.9)
Drying	Oven temperature set too high	Nuclear "bubbling" in large, delicate nuclei
Staining	Inadequate rinse after eosin stain	Sections have overall red hue; even nucleoli in immunoblasts are eosinophilic.

Data from Beard C, Nabers K, Bowling MC, et al. Achieving technical excellence in lymph node specimens: an update. Lab Med 1985;16:468–475.

geons and nurse circulators to submit all specimens on paper or fine-mesh polyvinyl alcohol pads moistened with sterile saline. Transport and short-term storage within sealed jars containing saline or tissue culture media are also satisfactory, and cooling the specimen to 4°C delays autolysis, a problem related to the kinetic activity of the sampled process. For morphologic purposes, storage at 4°C for up to 24 hours is usually satisfactory, and the preservation of immunoreactivity is surprisingly durable for most antigens (5) (see Chapter 11).

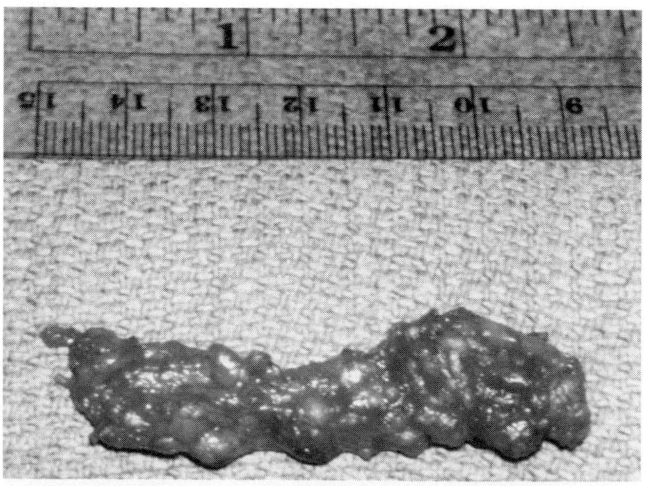

FIG. 12.1. Biopsy specimen delivery from the operating room on a dry towel produces an "edge" drying artifact (see Fig. 12.2). This artifact can be avoided by soaking the carriers in sterile saline.

Tissue Blocking

Representation of the biopsy specimen in paraffin tissue sections should never be jeopardized, and in fashioning tissue blocks, the pathologist frames the image of the sampling as it ultimately will appear on the microscope stage. A large, sweeping cut through the long axis of a small lymph node ensures assessment of nodal architecture. The block should be no more than 3 mm thick to allow adequate diffusion of liquids during fixation and processing. Today's thin-profile tissue cassettes, serving doubly as labels for storage as well, require an especially thin block to allow circulation of fluid within the interior space (Fig. 12.3). If too thick a block is submitted, the result is a paraffin-embedded block that is soft in the center (Fig. 12.4). Adequate sections simply cannot be made from such a preparation, because the central portion retracts from the microtome knife, and in the paraffin ribbons, these areas crack and disintegrate on contact with the water bath (Fig. 12.5) (blocking procedures are discussed under Allocation of Tissue Specimens).

Fixation

Fixatives are substances that denature cellular and extracellular tissue constituents to preserve them and render them suitable for treatments such as dehydration, infiltration by a supporting medium, and staining. There is no one fixative that is best for all purposes, and the examiner must select a fixative or combination of fixatives for each purpose (Table 12.2).

The most universal fixative in hospital pathology is 10% formalin (3.7% aqueous formaldehyde solution). This fixa-

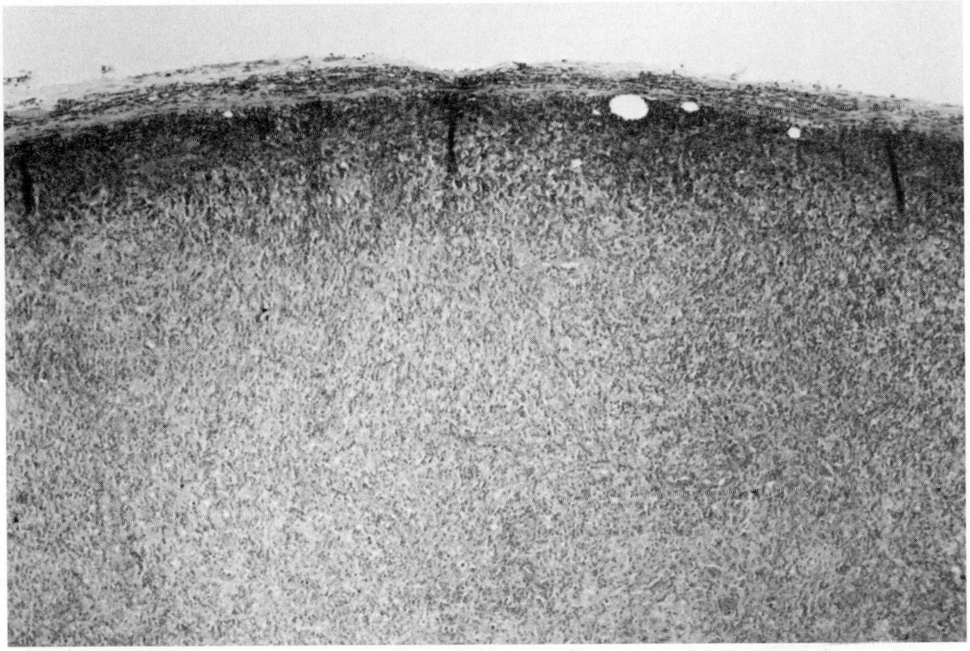

FIG. 12.2. An edge artifact in a lymph node biopsy section (paraffin section) is introduced by carriage of the specimen in a dry cloth substance (hematoxylin and eosin stain, original magnification: 4× magnification).

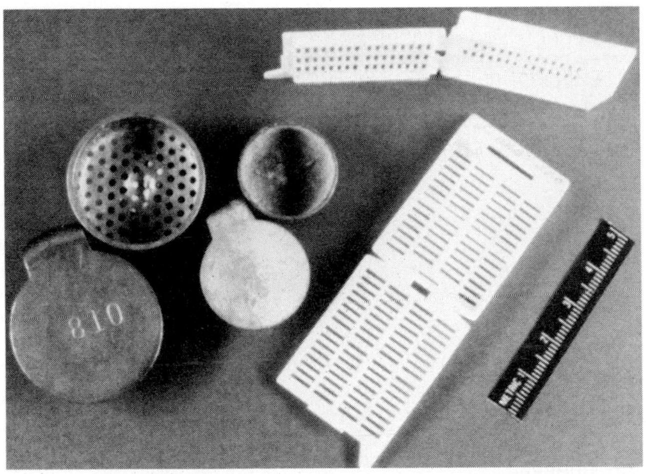

FIG. 12.3. Comparison of old-fashioned, deep-profile metal tissue carriers with modern, shallow-profile plastic cassettes. The small inner diameter of the cassettes requires thin tissue blocks (<3 mm) for adequate circulation of fixing and processing fluids.

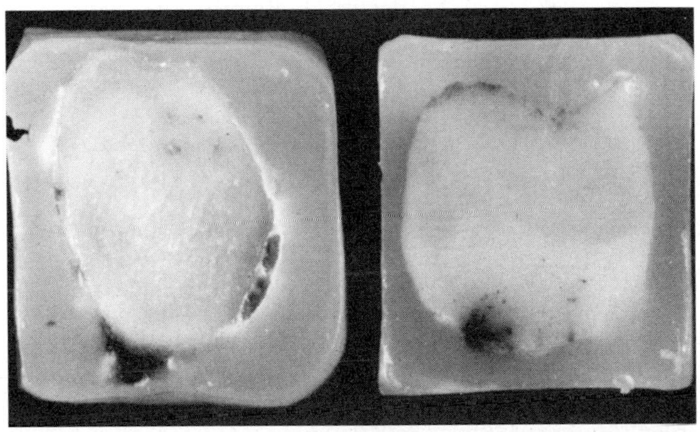

FIG. 12.4. Comparison of sectioning faces of poorly and well-processed lymph node tissue blocks. The poorly processed block *(left)* is inadequately infiltrated by paraffin, resulting in a soft central region that retracts from the cutting surface and producing disrupted sections (see Fig. 12.5).

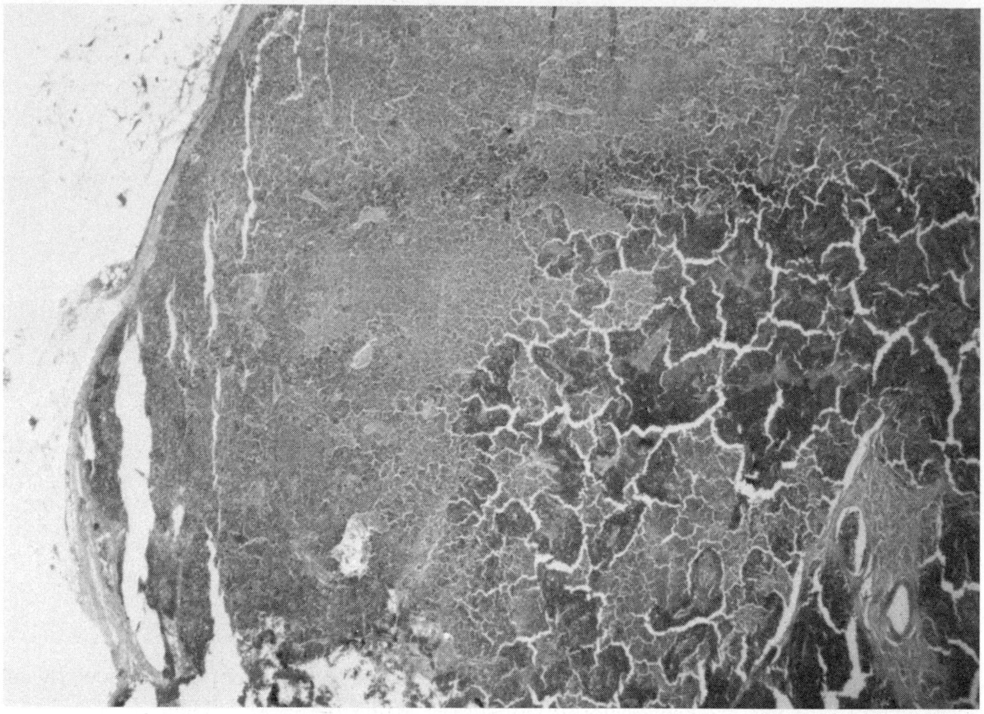

FIG. 12.5. Section resulting from poorly processed tissue block displays fragmentation in the central regions. This type of problem can result from a too-thick block or from inadequacy of any of the steps in the sequence of fixation, dehydration, clearing, and paraffin infiltration (hematoxylin and eosin stain, original magnification: 4× magnification).

TABLE 12.2. *Comparison of commonly used fixatives*

Characteristic	Neutral buffered formalin	B5	Zinc formalin (e.g., B plus)	Bouin's solution	Alcohols (e.g., Pennfix)
Nuclear detail	Bubbling artifact in large nuclei	Sharp	Sharper than formalin	Sharp	Sharp but shrunken
Immunopreservation	Moderate	Variable	Strong	Strong	Strong
Used on processor	Yes	No	Yes	Yes, but messy	Yes
Stability	Long	Very short (hours)	Short (days)	Short (days)	Long
Cost	Low	High	Low	Low	Moderate
Work exposure hazard	Slight	Moderate	Slight	Slight	Minimal
Environmental pollution	No	Yes	No	No	No
Electron microscopy	Good	Poor	Adequate	Poor	Poor
Additional comments	Best for storage of tissue	Sections must be decrystallized with hypo	Good trade-off for overall utility; good for all antigens in immunostaining	Messy to work with	Very small samples can be "burned"

tive is relatively safe, is inexpensive, rapidly diffuses into tissues, and is not an environmental disposal problem. For storage of specimens, a slightly alkaline buffer is added to retard the formation of formene pigment, a black, insoluble polymeric product of formaldehyde. The formation of formene is catalyzed at acidic pH. Aldehyde fixatives, such as formalin solution, act chemically by producing methylene or longer carbon chain bridges between sterically apposed amino groups of proteins. This is a very delicate quality of fixation, ideal, for example, for ultrastructural studies, as with glutaraldehyde. However, for the purposes of paraffin section cytomorphology, this type of fixation predisposes to the common nuclear bubbling artifact (Fig. 12.6A). Large nuclei with dispersed chromatin are disrupted by sectioning.

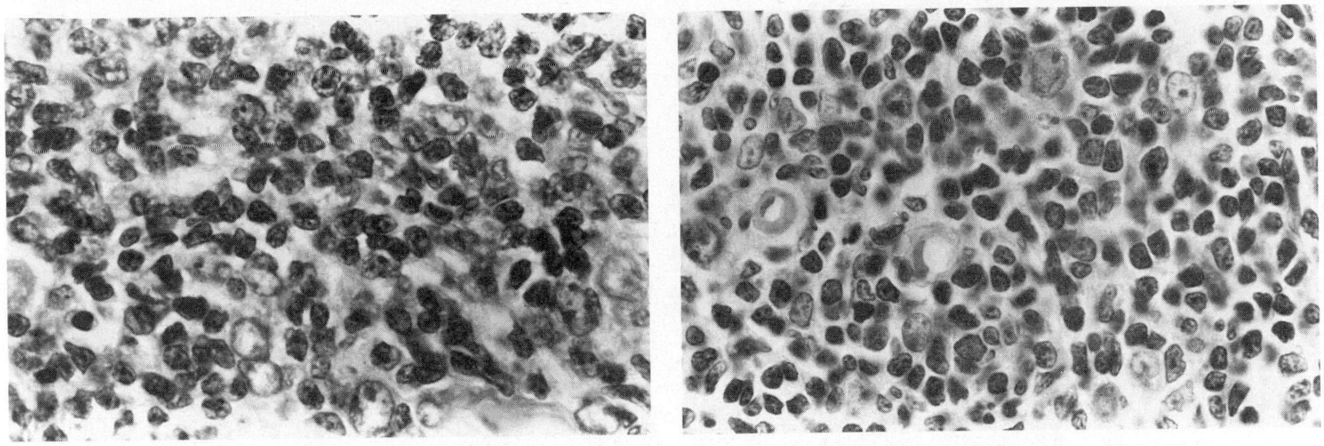

A B

FIG. 12.6. Comparison of neutral buffered formalin with a protein-precipitating, zinc-containing fixative (B-Plus) on nuclear detail. **A:** With formalin fixation of paraffin sections, there is a nuclear "bubbling" artifact caused by coalescence of delicate nucleoproteins into strands, which is most noticeable in the large vesicular nuclei of this follicle center lymphoma (hematoxylin and eosin stain, original magnification: 400× magnification). **B:** With zinc-precipitating fixative of the paraffin sections, the nucleoproteins are more rigidly denatured, resulting in sharper nuclear detail (hematoxylin and eosin stain, original magnification: 400× magnification).

At the moment of deparaffinization, if physical rigidity is insufficient, there is coalescence into strands of chromatin with clearing of chromatin.

A variety of fixatives can be used instead of formalin or after initial formalin fixation to avoid nuclear bubbling artifact. These are all protein-precipitating agents that produce physically rigid denaturation of nucleoproteins. Some of these are acids, which denature proteins by taking them away from their isoelectric points (i.e., acetic acid and picric acid [Bouin's solution]). Others are metallic cationic solutions, which form large, insoluble coordination complexes with the organic groups that extend out from the amino acid chains of proteins (i.e., mercuric chloride [B5 solution, Zenker's solution] and zinc chloride solution). Many fixatives consist of a mixture of formaldehyde solution with a protein precipitating agent (i.e., B5, Bouin's solution, zinc chloride, formalin) (6) (Table 12.3).

Protein-precipitating agents afford sharper nuclear detail in H&E sections (Fig. 12.6B) and they enhance immunoreactivity. Surprisingly, the cytomorphologic and immunoreactive limitations of formalin fixation are improved by ''run-back'' procedures in which paraffin-embedded tissue is sequenced back to aqueous solution and then refixed in a protein precipitant. The refixed block is then forward processed in standard sequence to paraffin (7) (Fig. 12.7).

Alcohol mixtures are good for immunopreservation and genetic probe analysis (8,9). However, conventional H&E histology is often suboptimal, with cellular shrinkage and drying artifact in small biopsy specimens.

In our laboratory, we choose to fix most surgical specimens alike, initially in neutral buffered formalin and thereafter for several hours in a solution of zinc chloride in 10% formalin (B-Plus) (Table 12.3). When tissue of any type is exposed for 3 or more hours to this fixative, an adequate degree of protein precipitation is added to the aldehyde fixation effect, allowing crisp nuclear detail and strong immunoreactivity (6).

Automated Processing

Automated sequence processing is carried out in laboratories using a variety of commercially available processors. Later equipment offers the option of rapid sequencing, with heat and vacuum applied to accelerate diffusion and reactivity of the reagents. Minimal time required for adequate fixa-

TABLE 12.3. *Formulations for some popular fixatives*

Neutral buffered formalin (10)	
37–40% formalin	100 mL
Distilled water	900 mL
Sodium phosphate monobasic, monohydrate	4 g
Sodium phosphate dibasic, anhydrous	6.5 g
Zinc chloride-formalin	
37–40% formalin	100mL
Distilled water	900 mL
$ZnCl \cdot 7\ H_2O$	10 g
B5 fixative (10)	
Stock solution:	
Murcuric chloride	12 g
Sodium acetate	2.5 g
Distilled water	200 mL
Working solution:	
Stock B5 solution	20 mL
Add 2 mL 40% formalin immediately before use	
Alcohol fixative	
Absolute isopropanol	700 mL
Absolute ethanol	200 mL
Absolute methanol	100 mL

A

B

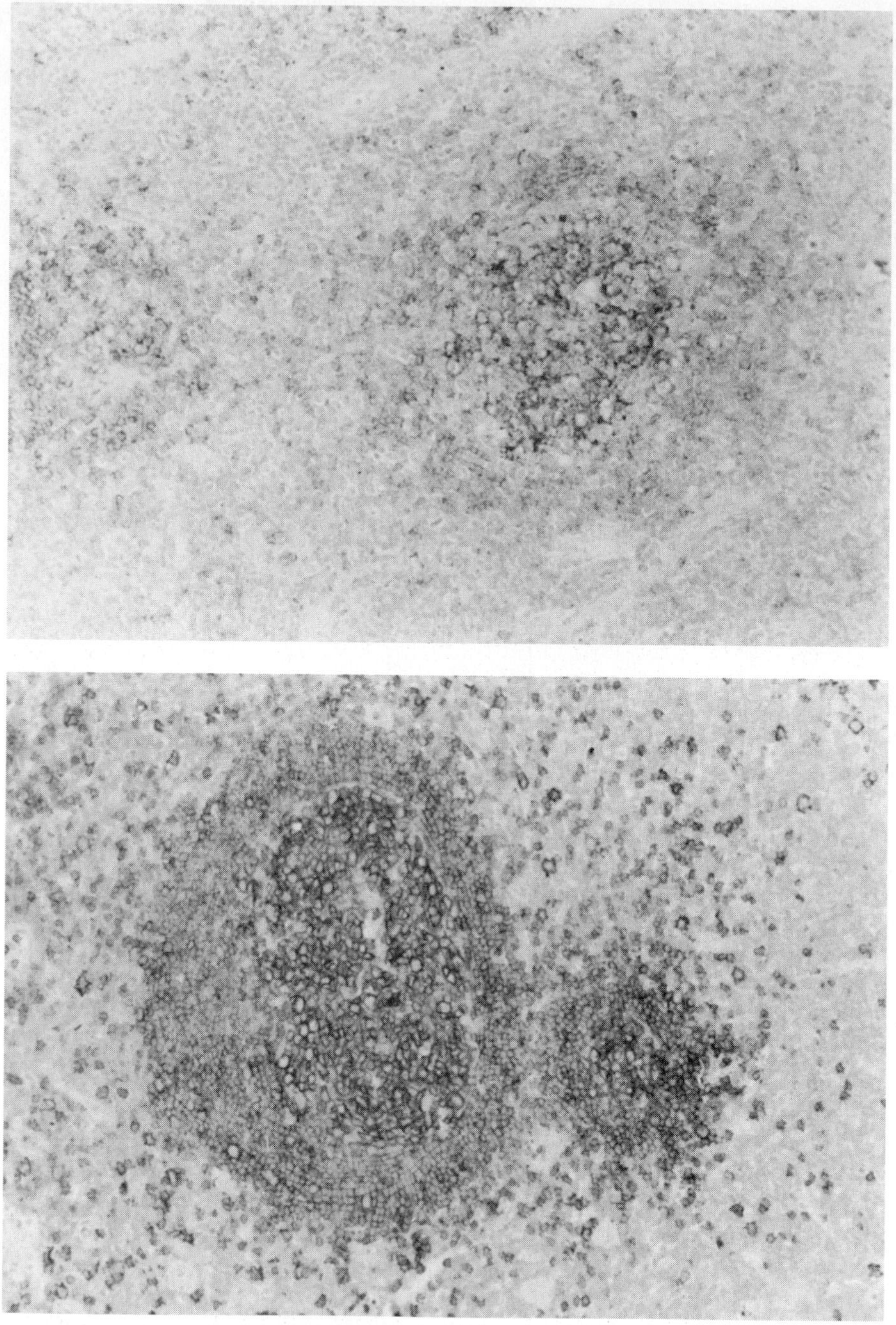

FIG. 12.7. Retrieval of immunoreactivity in paraffin-embedded tissue by "runback" refixation is demonstrated. **A:** Immunohistochemistry demonstrates only faint reactivity in a follicular structure for monoclonal antibody L26 (i.e., pan-B-cell antigen CD20) (original fixation in neutral buffered formalin). **B:** The identical immunohistochemical method demonstrates strong reactivity with antibody L26 after runback of the original block in aqueous solution and refixation in zinc sulfate formalin solution (ethylcarbazole color reagent and hematoxylin counterstain, original magnification: 20× magnification).

tion, dehydration, clearing, and paraffin infiltration depends on the size and quality of the specimens; a very thin block of porous tissue such as lung is adequately processed much more rapidly than a thick block of an impervious tissue such as muscle. Fixation and subsequent processing of bloody tissues such as spleen can be enhanced by initially agitating thin cut blocks in a jar of buffered formalin. In general, perfectly satisfactory processing can be carried out with an overnight schedule (total of 12 hours), as long as the tissue blocks are less than 3 mm thick. At least 4 hours of fixation should be allowed, and heating to 45°C accelerates the process without risking the introduction of artifact or reduction of immunoreactivity.

It is important to replace the fluids in the processor regularly, and this can be done in part with a ''forward shift'' of identical reagent sequence; yesterday's second 95% ethanol becomes today's first 95% ethanol bath. The alcohol sequence used for dehydration should be graded, starting with 70% or 80% ethanol, and absolute ethanol should not be used more than a total time of 2 hours (10). Initial exposure to concentrated alcohol or prolonged time in absolute alcohol can produce a ''burned'' effect, in which sections show contracted nuclei and a pale gray refractile hematoxylin tint with excessive eosin staining.

The temperature of the molten paraffin should be checked periodically. Excessive heat (>70°C) leads to ''cooking,''

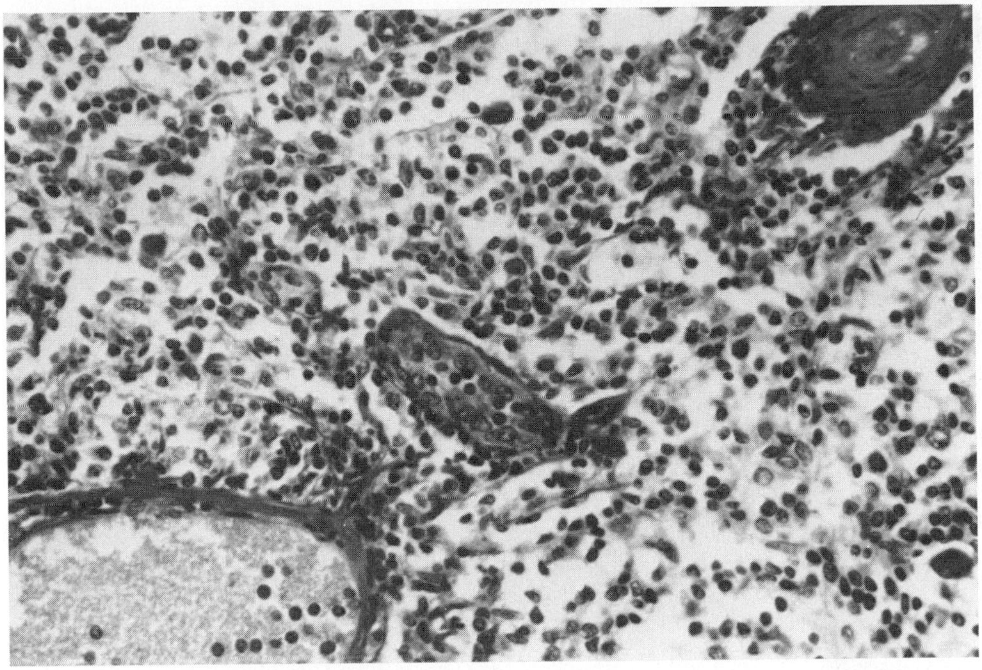

FIG. 12.8. Excessively hot paraffin (75°C) results in cellular shrinkage and denaturation of collagen. The vascular *(upper right and lower left)* structures in the paraffin section stained hematoxyphilic rather than eosinophilic because of thermally induced changes in the collagen structure (hematoxylin and eosin stain, original magnification: 20× magnification).

or the thermal denaturation of proteins, with shrunken cells and collagen that stains more hematoxyphilic than is normally seen (Fig. 12.8). For the purpose of preserving antigens for immunostaining, it is best to maintain molten paraffin below 62°C.

Embedding

Processed tissue blocks infiltrated with molten paraffin must be aligned in position for sectioning under the cassette base, a process known as *embedding*. This often overlooked hands-on step is crucial because, if tissue is not correctly oriented in relation to the cutting surface, the plane of section cannot allow optimal microscopic interpretation of tissue architecture and much of the tissue block is wasted in an attempt to cut down into the block adequately. For lymph nodes, it is best to carefully orient the largest, flattest tissue surface against the bottom of the embedding mold so that minimal tissue need be cut away to reach a complete sectioning face.

Sectioning

The most difficult and most laborious step in the production of conventional slides is sectioning. Pathologists should regularly review slides with histotechnologists to maintain high-quality sectioning techniques. Sloppy sectioning results in tears and folds in the tissue ribbon, precluding low-magnification assessment of lymphoid architecture (Fig. 12.9). Such problems are related to poor cutting techniques and to mounting (i.e., when the section ribbons are teased out smoothly on the surface of the water bath). Proper temperature and the addition to the water bath of proteins, detergents, or both augment section mounting, because they reduce tension along the interface, adhering the sections to the glass more perfectly.

Because many hematolymphoid cells are relatively small in diameter, thin sections (3 or 4 μm) are needed for cytomorphologic assessment (Fig. 12.10). However, the thinner the sections, the more difficult is the task of producing large, undisrupted preparations free of imperfections. It is particularly important that microtome knives be sharpened flawlessly, and in most laboratories, disposable blade systems are used to encourage frequent switching to a new, perfect edge (Fig. 12.11). To avoid ''shuttering'' or the ''Venetian blind'' effect, the knife cutting angle must be maintained sufficiently acute to the sectioning surface (Fig. 12.11).

Proper sectioning can be carried out only if the tissue block has been adequately fixed and processed (Fig. 12.5). Minor shortcomings can sometimes be remedied with trick methods, such as smearing glycerol on the cutting surface when tissue has been excessively dehydrated in alcohols or applying an ice cube to the block face when insufficient fixation has led to a soft tissue core.

Section Drying

Wet mounted sections are annealed to the underlying glass slides by oven drying. The temperature should not exceed 55°C to avoid the production of disruptions in the chromatin

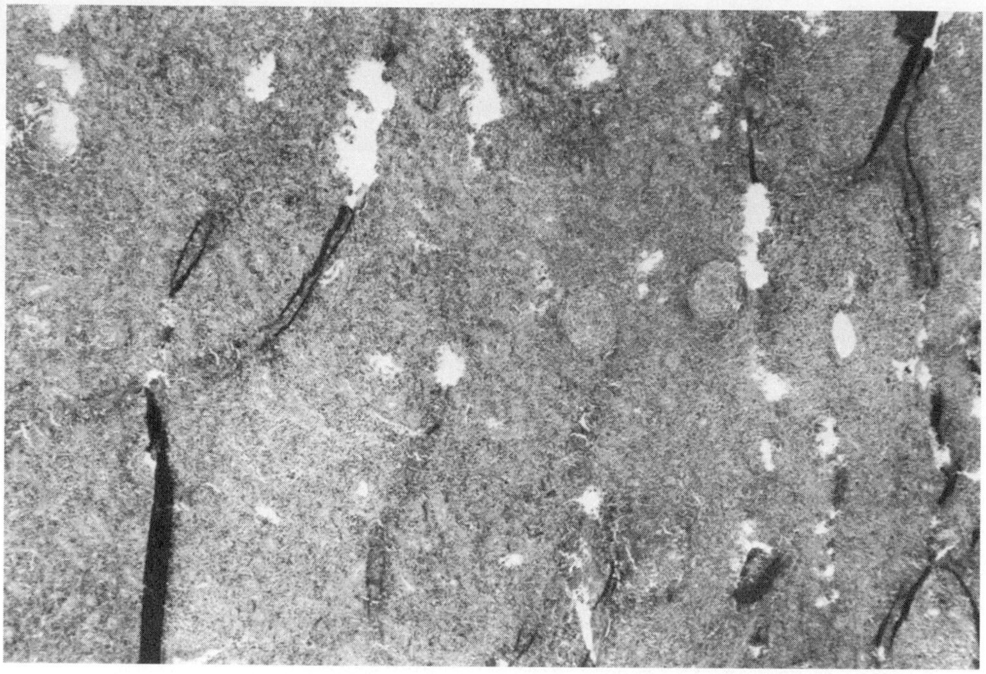

FIG. 12.9. Poor sectioning technique renders architectural interpretation difficult. Notice the tears and folds in this example (hematoxylin and eosin stain, original magnification: 4× magnification).

A 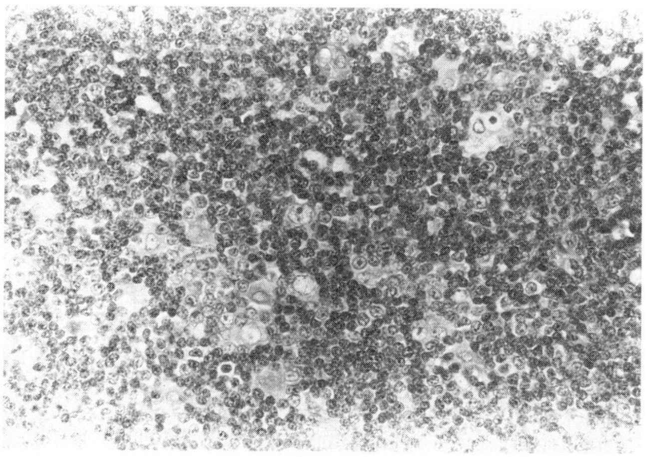

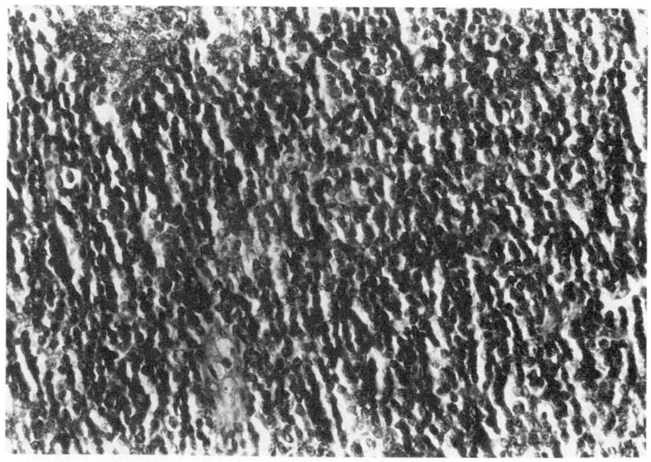 B

FIG. 12.10. The importance of preparing adequately thin paraffin sections for cytomorphologic evaluation is demonstrated in this comparison of thick and thin sections from the same paraffin block in a case of paracortical hyperplasia simulating early "interfollicular" Hodgkin's disease. **A:** This sample was sectioned at 3 μm, enabling recognition of delicate immunoblasts (hematoxylin and eosin stain, original magnification: 40× magnification). **B:** This sample was sectioned at 6 μm, resulting in obscuration of even large cells by superimposition of cell nuclei (hematoxylin and eosin stain, original magnification: 40× magnification).

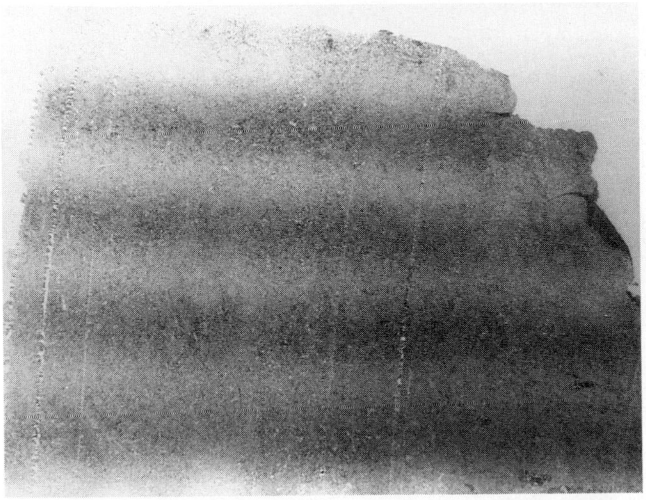

FIG. 12.11. Two common sectioning artifacts in the same paraffin section: horizontal zones of pallor represent a "Venetian blind" effect from improper blade angle or positioning, and vertical scoring tears result from imperfections in knife edge (hematoxylin and eosin stain, original magnification: 2× magnification).

of large, delicate vesicular nuclei. With excessive heat, the supportive paraffin medium becomes so soft that water vapor penetrates through the section selectively at points of least physical resistance. Usually 2 hours at 45°C is adequate for drying, depending on ambient humidity.

Staining

Thorough deparaffinization in xylenes is necessary before the sections can be gradually hydrated in graded alcohols, making regular rotation and replacement of the xylenes mandatory. In general, the progressive type of hematoxylin solution (Mayer, Schmitt) is superior to the regressive type (Harris) because the variability from slide to slide with the extra decolorization step is not a problem (11). Progressive hematoxylins do not form precipitates requiring daily filtration, as do the regressive types.

The balance between hematoxylin and eosin is important for distinguishing cell types in hematopathology and not merely an arbitrary or subjective matter of esthetic preference. For example, the nucleoli of large transformed follicle center cells and of reactive immunoblasts should be hematoxyphilic and not eosinophilic, while those in Reed-Sternberg cells should be eosinophilic. To avoid overstaining with eosin, the technologist should thoroughly rinse the slides in 95% alcohol before dehydrating, clearing, and coverslipping.

Coverslipping

Although shortcomings in coverslipping are usually not serious and can be repaired, they are nonetheless inconvenient and can obscure sections. Mounting medium should not be diluted by too much xylene remaining on slides, because this leads to air bubbles forming underneath the coverslip. Even very old slides can be recoverslipped as long as the investigator is patient enough to allow release of the old coverslip by soaking in xylene. When this method fails, the slide can be pressed against a hot plate for a few seconds. Such heat usually quickly releases the coverslip. Then the preparation can be rinsed in xylene and coverslipped afresh.

Strict adherence to all these recommended procedural guidelines results in production of high-quality H&E paraffin tissue sections. Such preparations provide large, intact tissue architecture and fine cytologic detail for microscopic evaluation (Fig. 12.12).

A

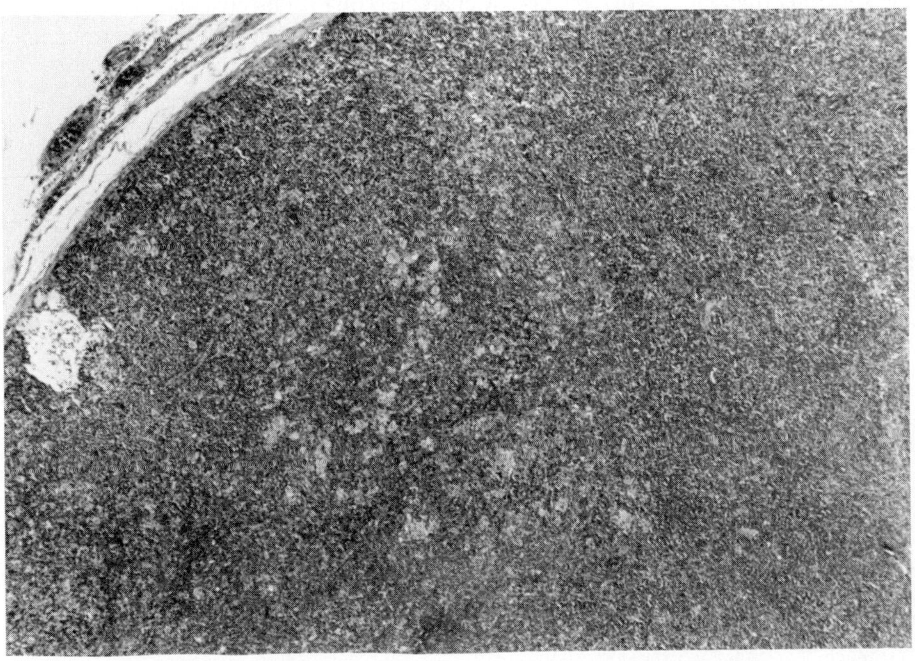

FIG. 12.12. A well-processed block correctly sectioned allows evaluation of architecture under low magnification and cytologic detail under high magnification. **A:** In a paraffin section, faint nodularity with mottling suggests nodular variant lymphocyte predominance Hodgkin's disease (hematoxylin and eosin stain, B5 fixative, original magnification: 4× magnification). *(continued)*

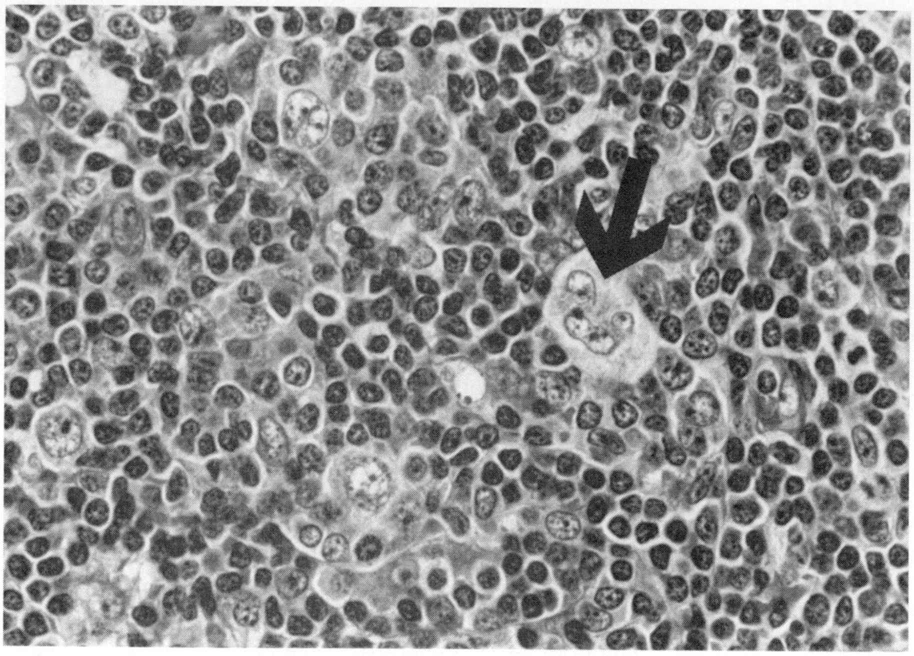

B

FIG. 12.12. *Continued.* **B:** High-quality cytologic detail (original magnification: 1,000× magnification) permits confirmation of the diagnosis, because delicate multilobated lymphocytic and histiocytic variant tumor giant cells *(arrow)* can be identified in a background of benign-appearing small lymphocytes. Large nuclei with dispersed chromatin are vulnerable to "bubbling" artifact (Fig. 12.6).

ALLOCATION OF TISSUE SPECIMENS

Intraoperative Interpretations

There is a common fallacy among pathologists and surgeons that intraoperative microscopic interpretations should not be attempted on lymph nodes biopsied for suspected lymphoma. Although it is true that accurate diagnosis and classification of lymphoma should not be attempted by this means, such on-the-spot interpretations are beneficial for confirmation of adequate sampling and for selection of tissue allocations (Table 12.4). Although frozen tissue section interpretation results in a portion of the tissue suffering freeze-thaw artifact, the frozen tissue block can be stored as a valuable resource for potential ancillary studies. It is far better to inform the surgeon during surgery that the sampling is inadequate for diagnosis than to do so 1 or 2 days postoperatively! Imprints or scrape smear preparations can be used to augment or even replace frozen tissue sections for intraoperative microscopy.

As is always good practice, pathologists should communicate fully with the managing physician and surgeon before the biopsy to render the best possible interpretation of the observations. If there is evidence of inflammation (e.g., suppuration or granuloma formation, especially in a patient with signs or symptoms of infection), fresh sterile tissue should be sent for microbial cultures. Similarly, if frozen tissue sections or imprints show cohesive sheets of anaplastic large cells, flow cytometric phenotyping is unlikely to be an effective means for characterizing such cells, and allocation of a small shaving of tissue for electron microscopy attains a relatively higher priority.

Pathologists should recognize their role as stewards of the sampled tissue. They are responsible for its proper handling and division for appropriate special studies. It is essential

TABLE 12.4. *Tissue allocation requirements for ancillary studies*

	Allocations				
Studies	Fresh, sterile tissue	Fresh tissue	Air-dried cell monolayers	Frozen tissue	Paraffin sections
Immunostains for cytoplasmic and some surface antigens[a]			X	X	X
Immunostains for cell surface Ig and other antigens			X[b]	X	
Automated flow cytometric phenotyping		X			
Genetic probe analysis (Southern blot)				X	X[c]
Chromosomal analysis	X				
Microbial culture	X				

[a] Highly dependent on antigen and fixative.
[b] Direct imprint is not optimal for surface Ig; cytocentrifuge preparations are better.
[c] Only alcohol-fixed tissues are suitable (9).

that the strengths and weaknesses of the various available ancillary studies be understood in order that tissue allocations and the subsequent studies themselves be selected appropriately, in a manner that most directly affords a definitive diagnosis and is least wasteful. Unnecessary tissue allocations and special studies are to be avoided (Table 12.4).

Blocking for Conventional Processing

Selection and production of the portion of tissue to be submitted for conventional processing is critical. Optimal plane of section and representation of the pathologic process must be obtained. It is usually best to stabilize the lymph node on a dry, rough-surfaced base, such as a paper towel. A large scalpel or sharp knife is then used to cut away the encapsulated deep aspect of the specimen. The fresh cut deep surface of the upper portion is then quickly stabilized on another dry surface, and with a decisive slice parallel to and about 3 to 4 mm away from the paper towel, a large, thin block is produced. Imprints can then be produced from any of the cut tissue surfaces. It is best to use pieces of node with adherent capsule for purposes other than conventional processing. These are not suitable for paraffin blocks because the capsule serves as a barrier to fluid diffusion.

Immediately after division of the specimen, the portions are immersed in one sort of fluid or another, according to the type of allocation, to avoid drying artifact. Although ideally the pathologist could submit some tissue sampling for all possible ancillary studies (12), in practice this is neither affordable nor, with small specimens, feasible. Based on the combination of preoperative clinical differential diagnosis and intraoperative histopathologic or cytomorphologic interpretation, tissue is allocated according to priority of anticipated importance of the respective ancillary studies that can derive from these (see Chapter 11).

Imprints and Smears

Monolayers of cells can be obtained by direct touch preparations of lymph nodes, offering preparations similar to those of fine needle aspiration cytology or cytocentrifuge methods for detailed single cell analysis. The allocation is simple, inexpensive, and effectively consumes no tissue. It should not be attempted on very small specimens that may suffer cellular crush artifact from such maneuvers. Densely sclerotic processes do not yield intact cells.

Slides should be labeled ahead of time, usually 6 to 8, depending on the needs of the individual case. Anchoring one end of the slide face down against the cutting surface (i.e., towel) adjacent to a fresh cut specimen surface, the slide is gently levered down into contact with the tissue surface and then pulled away, avoiding any sideways shearing motion. The first two preparations, carrying the thickest layer of cells, are immediately placed in a Coplin jar containing formalin or 95% alcohol solution; the remaining imprints are allowed to air dry. Alternatively, cells can be extruded from the fresh-cut surface by gently scraping with the edge of a slide. The wet cellular material is then quickly smeared over the surface of another slide and fixed or air dried. Such preparations can be stained immediately for intraoperative cytomorphologic interpretation. Compared with frozen tissue section methods, imprints can be produced faster, conserve sampled tissue, and can be produced from bony tissues.

To avoid infectious disease contamination problems, all imprint preparations can be fixed; those initially air dried can be placed in a 50:50 mixture of acetone and methanol for 1 minute. This retains immunoreactivity and cytochemical properties (see Chapter 38).

Wet-fixed imprints can be stained with H&E for cytomorphology equivalent to that in H&E-stained paraffin tissue sections, with clear nuclear detail provided (Fig. 12.13A). Air-dried preparations show less cellular shrinkage than those wet-fixed, and Romanovsky-type stains, such as Wright-Giemsa or Diff-Quik, can be used to achieve cytoplasmic staining, as is favored in hematology (Fig. 12.13B). Cytochemical (13) and immunocytochemical (14) preparations of imprints are typically of outstanding clarity, in contrast to corresponding frozen tissue section preparations (Fig. 12.13C, D). Only immunostaining for immunoglobulin light chains is less suited to imprints and smears because of the dense coating of the cellular monolayers by interstitial plasma proteins. In this application, cytocentrifuge preparations deriving from washed, suspended cells are usually preferable.

Fixation of air-dried imprints should be in accord with the type of study to be done. Thoroughly dried preparations stored at 20°C retain most antigens for about 1 week (14); however, nuclear terminal deoxynucleotidyl transferase, a nuclear antigen useful for marking lymphoblastic malignancies (see Chapter 3), is exceptionally labile, lasting only 3 to 4 days. Maintaining air-dried imprints at −70°C allows immunocytochemical analysis months or even years later. It is necessary to store such imprints in sealed five-slide plastic containers so that warming to 20°C can be done without direct exposure to ambient air, because this results in wet, runny-appearing preparations. Anhydrous acetone is generally the gentlest fixative; however, brief (1 minute) fixation in a 50:50 mixture of absolute methanol and anhydrous acetone at 20°C is superior for diminished nonspecific background staining. Enzyme cytochemical studies often require formol-acetone fixation (13).

Frozen Tissue

Tissue representative of the pathologic process should be frozen away whenever possible because this represents an insurance policy for some of the most powerful ancillary studies in hematopathology. Virtually all antigenically defined markers and enzyme cytochemical activities are preserved indefinitely at −70°C (see Chapters 3, 4, and 38), and genetic probes are best applied to cryopreserved tissues and homogenates (see Chapters 7, 8, and 9).

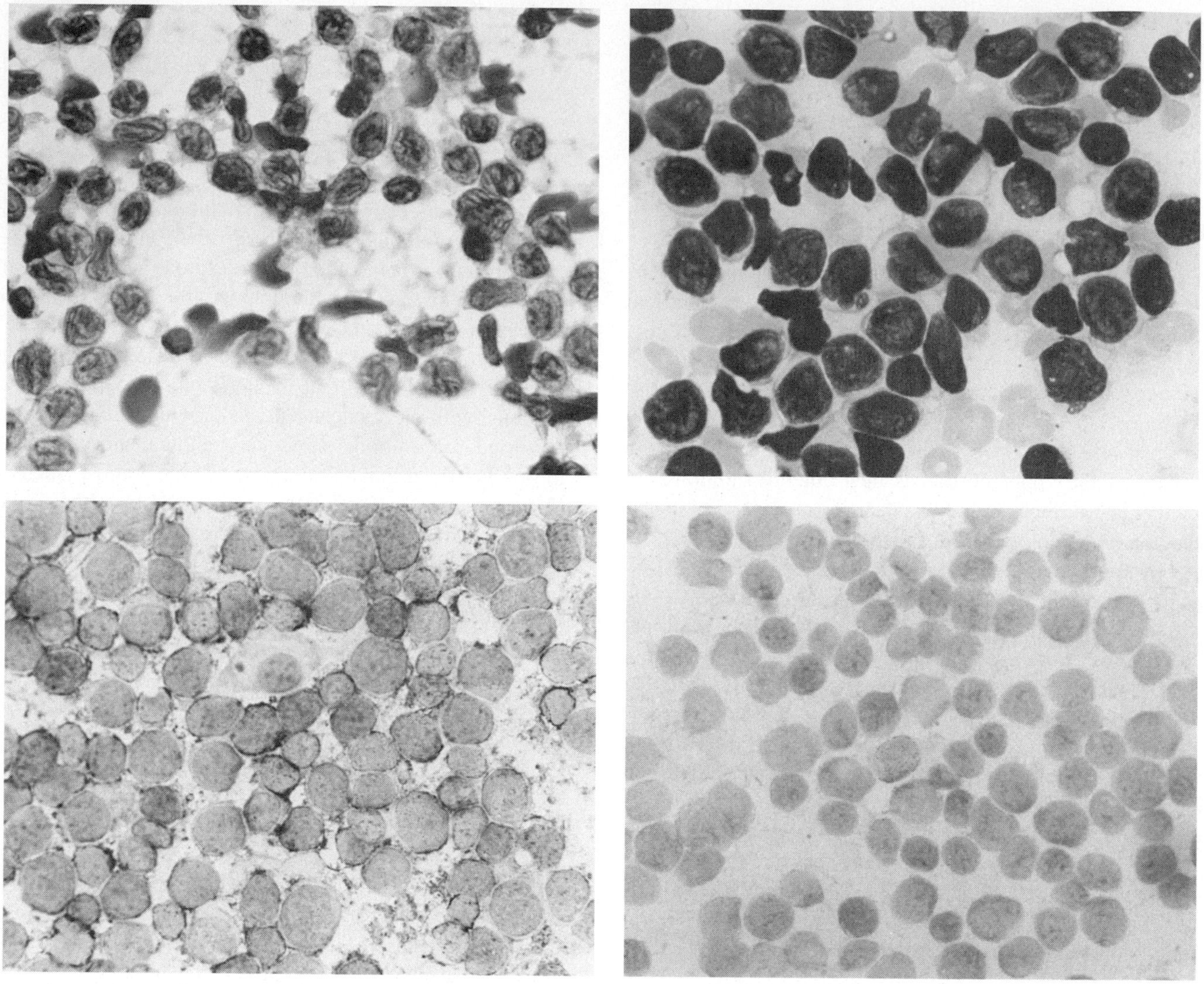

A B C D

FIG. 12.13. Imprint preparations from a lymph node involved by a cutaneous T-cell lymphoma show versatility in different methods of study. **A:** In a hematoxylin and eosin–stained, alcohol-fixed imprint, notice the nuclear membrane and chromatin detail. **B:** In an air-dried, Giemsa-stained imprint, notice the large cell size without fixation shrinkage, lack of nuclear detail, and distinct staining of cytoplasm. Air-dried, acetone-fixed immunocytochemical preparations are positive **(C)** for pan-T-cell antigen CD43 and negative **(D)** for pan-B-cell antigen CD22 (ethylcarbazole color reagent, hematoxylin counterstain, original magnification: 1,000× magnification).

The faster tissue is frozen, the more intact the cellular structures. Although ideally supercooled liquids such as liquid nitrogen or isopentane are used, for practical diagnostic purposes, the rapid freeze chuck accessory in a cryotome is perfectly suitable. However, it is imperative that the block of tissue for freezing be thin (<2 mm). When intraoperative frozen tissue sections are to be rendered, the tissue should be rapidly frozen and stored afterward for the potential ancillary studies mentioned. The production of "frozen section control" paraffin blocks is seldom useful diagnostically anyway. Because most cryotomes feature automatic defrost cycles, it is necessary to transfer the frozen block to a −70°C freezer for safekeeping. If long-term storage is a possibility, covering the tissue with a hyperviscous mounting medium such as OCT is necessary to prevent desiccation.

Fresh Tissue Allocations

No morphologist can surrender fresh tissue to other laboratories without some apprehension regarding its disappearance. However, some such studies are definitely indicated in many cases. A common situation is automated flow cytometry for immunophenotyping. Compared with frozen or paraffin tissue section immunohistochemistry, the method is complementary (15). It is very rapid, safely handles infectious tissues, and is particularly sensitive for the detection of surface antigens, which can be compared two or even three at a time with multiple channel analysis (see Chapter 5). However, the method is less convenient than immunohistochemistry because it must be carried out rapidly on fresh samples. Small compartments of cells, especially large, cohesive tumor cells, may not be detectable or even survive into the suspension to be analyzed. Some degree of reassurance can be given the anxious morphologist by using a small portion of the cell suspension to produce cytocentrifuge slides, stained ones for cytomorphologic correlation and unstained ones for potential immunocytochemical studies (Fig. 12.14).

The most fastidious allocation requirements are those for microbial culture or cytogenetics, because sterile fresh tissue is needed (see Chapter 10). Logistically, it is often easier to have the surgeon divide the specimen under sterile conditions in the operating room. The sealed sterile container can then be sent directly to the appropriate laboratories without

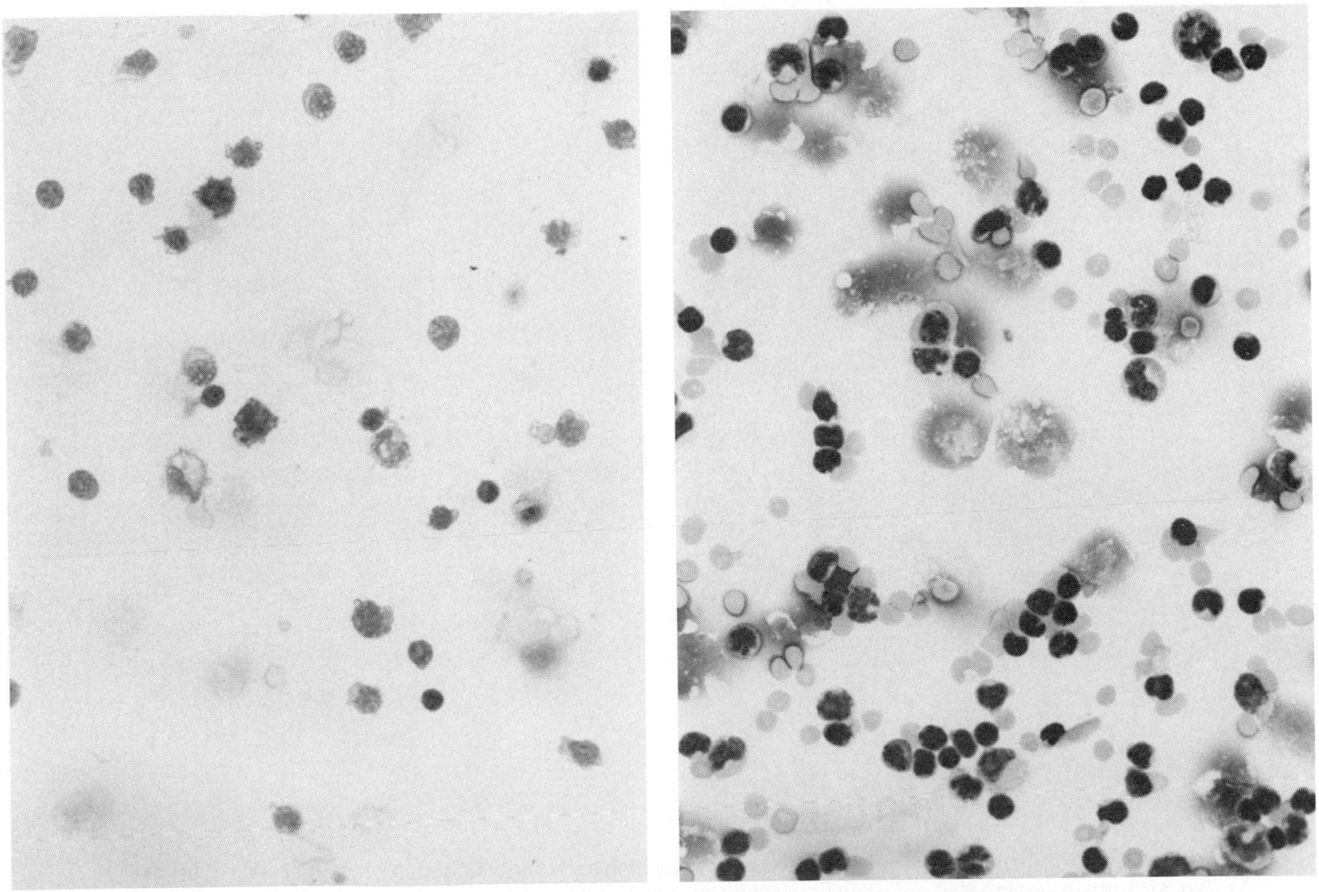

A B

FIG. 12.14. Comparison of poor-quality and good-quality cytocentrifuge preparations from a lymph node suspension for automated flow cytometry. **A:** Disruption and distortion of lymphoid cells is caused by excessive centrifugation and by acid lysis for destruction of erythrocytes. **B:** Intact lymphoid cells are associated with erythrocytes left unlysed (Diff-Quik, original magnification: 400× magnification).

contamination in the pathology gross room, where it is possible to envision a microbial veneer covering all surfaces.

Electron Microscopy

Because paraffin section immunostaining has become such an effective means for determining tumor histogenesis, ultrastructure has been largely bypassed (16). Nevertheless, in some cases, electron microscopy remains definitive, and more importantly, it is a modality independent from cell markers, which can then be used to verify or refute equivocal immunologic results (Fig. 12.15). When dealing with an anaplastic neoplasm, as recognized during intraoperative study, the pathologist should allocate a small portion of tissue to buffered glutaraldehyde solution. It is not necessary to finely dice tissue at the time of initial fixation. Rather, a very thin shaving of representative tissue (<1 mm thick) from a fresh cut face should be placed in glutaraldehyde solution and agitated for maximal diffusion. For diagnostic purposes, tissues fixed initially in buffered formalin are usually satisfactory for ultrastructural study as long as one carefully selects a shave sample off a face of tissue first fixed in formalin. Obtaining tissue from central portions of the block is to be avoided, because diffusion of fixative is retarded there, allowing autolytic alterations.

Conventional Special Stains

Stains that have been available for many decades as adjuncts to H&E in paraffin tissue sections are sometimes very informative, extremely fast, convenient, and low cost, but today they are often overlooked. Giemsa staining of sections is recommended by Lennert as a primary stain for paraffin sections because of its differential cytoplasmic tinctorial qualities, which are superior to those of H&E (17) (Fig. 12.16). However, a bad Giemsa stain is definitely worse than a good H&E stain. Careful alcoholic differentiation is necessary with microscopic monitoring of stain balance. Conventional histochemical methods such as periodic acid–Schiff (PAS), mucicarmine, and reticulin silver im-

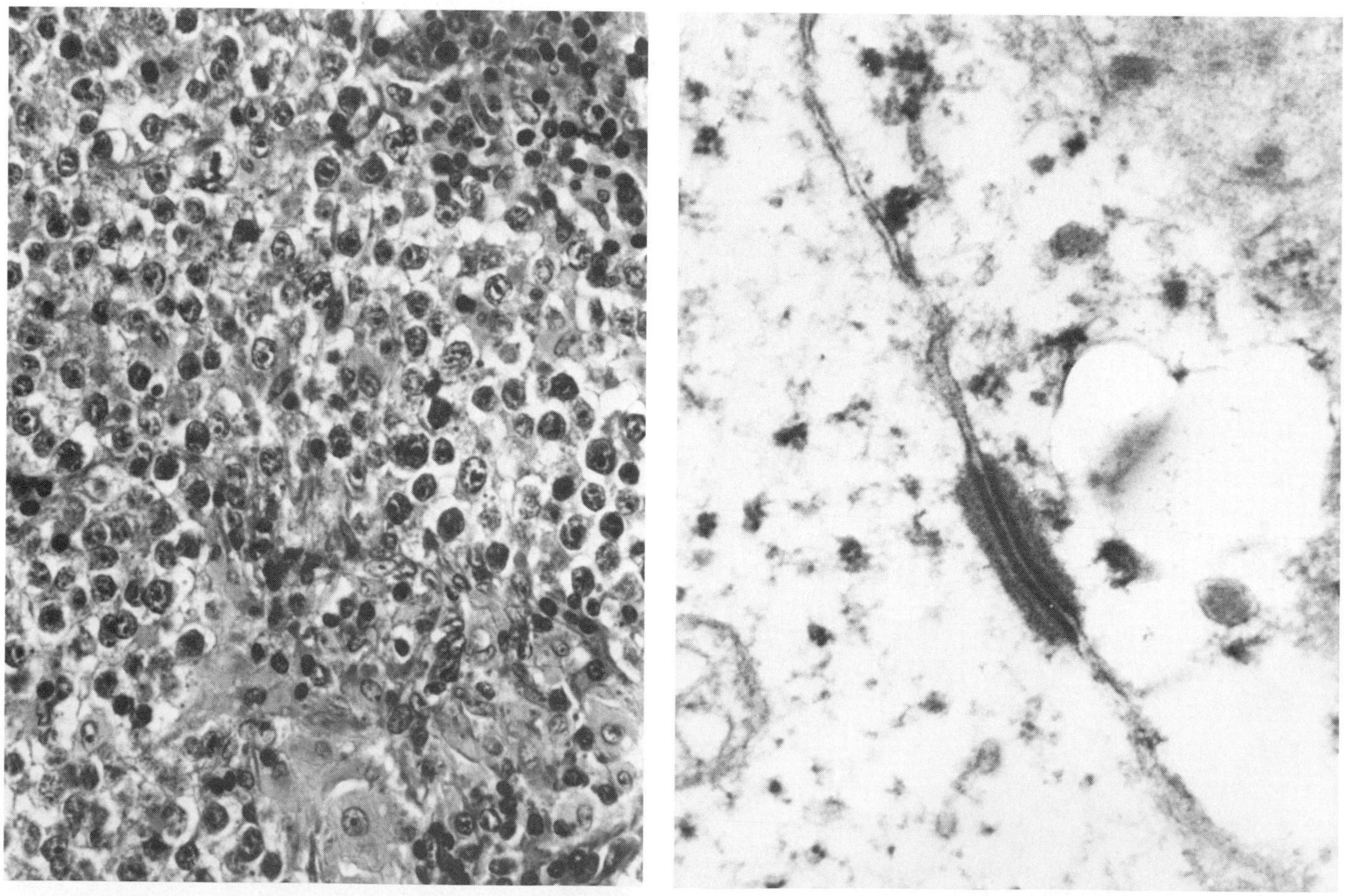

A B

FIG. 12.15. Utility of electron microscopy in distinguishing a germinoma from a lymphoma. **A:** Hematoxylin and eosin–stained paraffin tissue section in which cytomorphology suggests lymphoma (original magnification: 400× magnification). **B:** An electron micrograph of formalin-fixed tissue from this same tissue biopsy, in which junctional complexes between the tumor cells indicate a nonlymphomatous process (uranyl acetate lead citrate stain, original magnification: 7,300× magnification). (Courtesy of Dr. Cliff Richmond, Santa Rosa Northwest Hospital, San Antonio, TX.)

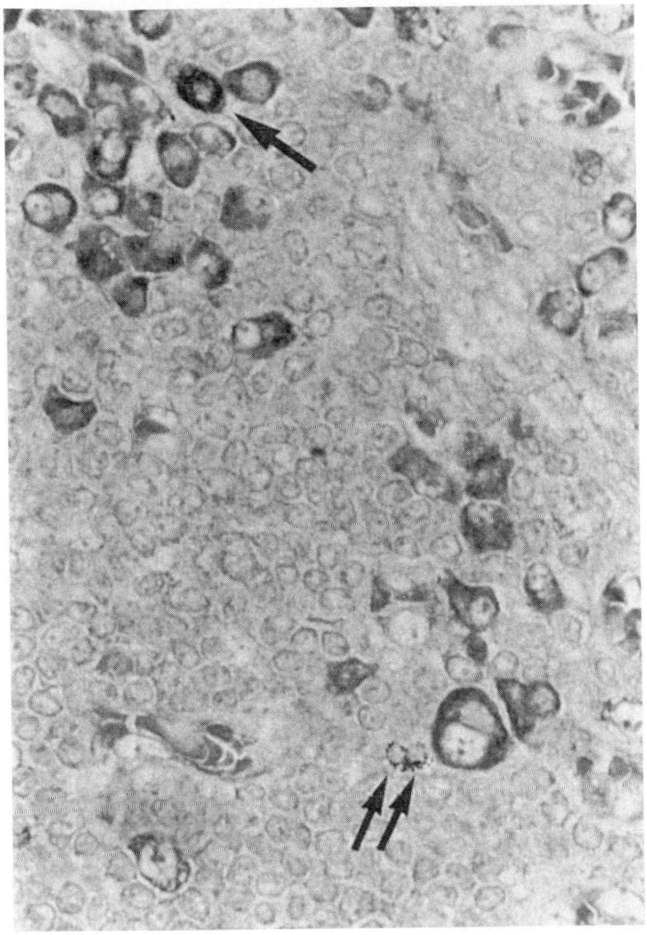

FIG. 12.16. Giemsa stain of paraffin tissue section illustrates differential cytoplasmic reactivity superior to that of hematoxylin and eosin stain. Plasmacytic and immunoblastic cells show darkly staining cytoplasm. Cytoplasmic granules are seen in mast cells *(arrow)* and eosinophil *(double arrow)* (original magnification: 400× magnification).

pregnation should not be forgotten in hematopathology. At least one useful enzyme cytochemical marker, chloroacetate esterase, is preserved in paraffin sections. This is a practical means to detect granulocytic and mast cell differentiation in conventional preparations (1,13) (see Chapter 38).

It is a mark of mastery to employ simple, rapid methods rather than more sophisticated and expensive ones to solve a diagnostic problem (Fig. 12.17). Special stains for microor-

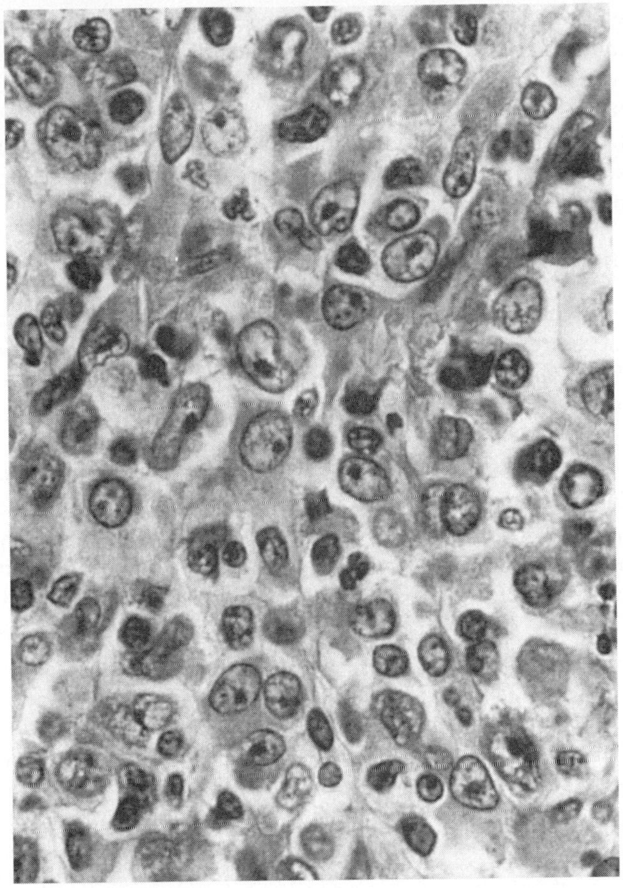

A

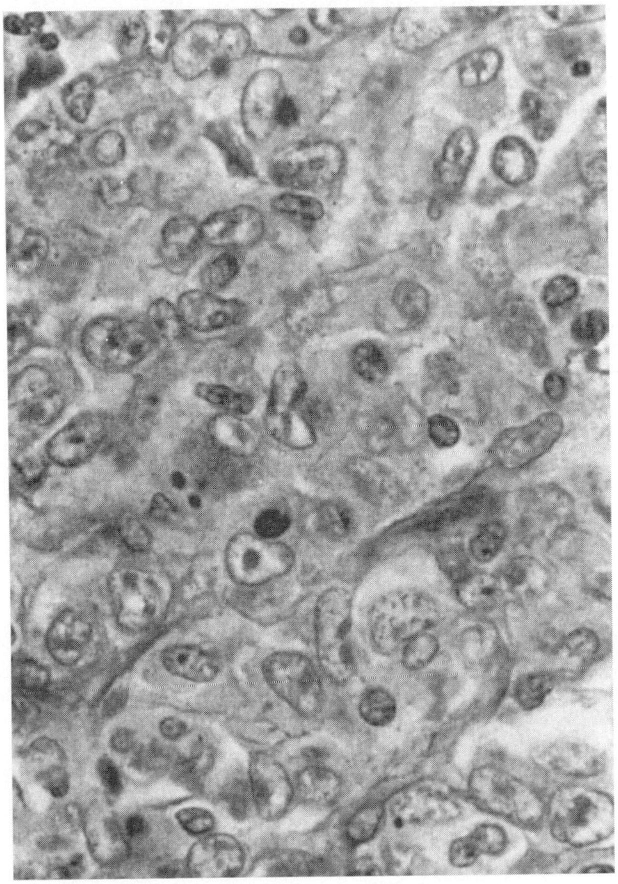

B

FIG. 12.17. Utility of conventional special stain is demonstrated in this case of anaplastic large cell gastric malignancy. **A:** In hematoxylin and eosin–stained sections, this neoplasm appears to be a large cell lymphoma (original magnification: 1,000× magnification). **B:** However, periodic acid–Schiff stain and mucicarmine stain show strong staining of intracytoplasmic lumens, indicative of a particularly poorly differentiated adenocarcinoma (original magnification: 1,000× magnification). (Courtesy of Dr. Randall Harper, St. Luke's Lutheran Hospital, San Antonio, TX.)

ganisms are an important and necessary everyday tool for modern hematopathology. Spontaneous and acquired immunodeficiencies can result in the presence of opportunistic infectious agents without an inflammatory response recognizable in H&E sections alone. Stains such as acid-fast and silver methods for fungi, *Pneumocystis,* and even cat-scratch bacilli are used on a regular basis in hematopathology.

SUMMARY AND CONCLUSIONS

Technical factors in the preparation of lymph node specimens are of critical importance for accurate interpretation. The pathologist should work with the laboratory's technologists to constantly monitor the quality of conventional paraffin section slides, troubleshooting avoidable problems.

Intraoperative interpretation is appropriate for cases of suspected lymphoproliferative disease. This ensures adequacy of sampling and can be used to determine appropriate allocation of tissue for ancillary studies. Such interpretations can be based on frozen tissue sections, imprints, or both. For initial biopsy specimens, top priority in allocation must always be given to adequate representation in conventionally processed paraffin section material. Imprints are usually a no-risk method of preparation suitable for diverse special staining purposes. A frozen tissue block, stored after intraoperative frozen section interpretation, serves as an insurance policy for powerful ancillary studies, including frozen tissue section immunohistochemistry and genetic probe analysis.

ACKNOWLEDGMENTS

Linda Streckfus and Faye Blakeney assisted in the production of this manuscript. Coranelle Shelton provided valuable technical consultation.

REFERENCES

1. Beard C, Nabers K, Bowling MC, et al. Achieving technical excellence in lymph node specimens: an update. *Lab Med* 1985;16:468–475.
2. Banks PM, Long JC, Howard CA. Preparation of lymph node biopsy specimens. *Hum Pathol* 1979;10:617–621.
3. Casey TT, Cousar JB, Collins RD. A simplified plastic embedding and immunohistologic technique for the immunophenotypic analysis of human hematopoietic and lymphoid tissues. *Am J Pathol* 1988;131:183.
4. Block MH, Trenner L, Ruegg P, et al. Glycol methacrylate embedding technique emphasizing cost containment, ultra-rapid processing, and adaptability to a variety of staining techniques. *Lab Med* 1982;13:290–298.
5. Pelstring RJ, Allred DC, Esther RJ, et al. Differential antigen preservation during tissue autolysis. *Hum Pathol* 1991;22:237–241.
6. Herman GE, Chlipala E, Bochenski G, et al. Zinc formalin fixative for automated tissue processing. *J Histotechnol* 1988;11:85–89.
7. Abbondanzo SL, Allred DC, Lampkin S, et al. Enhancement of immunoreactivity among lymphoid malignant neoplasms in paraffin-embedded tissues by refixation in zinc sulfate formalin. *Arch Pathol Lab Med* 1991;115:31–33.
8. Bostwick D, AlAnnouf N, Choi C, et al. Establishment of the formalin free surgical pathology laboratory. *Mod Pathol* 1991;4:126(abst).
9. Smith LJ, Braylan RC, Nutkis JE, et al. Extraction of cellular DNA from human cells and tissues fixed in ethanol. *Anal Biochem* 1987;160: 135–138.
10. Gordon KC. Tissue processing. In: Bancroft JD, Stevens A, eds. *Theory and practice of histological techniques.* New York: Churchill Livingstone, 1990:43–59.
11. Sheehan DC, Hrapchak BB, eds. *Theory and practice of histotechnology,* 2nd ed. St Louis: CV Mosby, 1980:139–144.
12. Collins RD. Lymph node examination. What is an adequate workup? *Arch Pathol Lab Med* 1985;109:796–799.
13. Sun T, Li CY, Yam LT, eds. *Atlas of cytochemistry and immunocytochemistry of hematologic neoplasms.* Chicago: American Society of Clinical Pathologists Press, 1985:22–33.
14. Banks PM, Caron BL, Morgan TW. Use of imprints for monoclonal antibody studies: suitability of air-dried preparations from lymphoid tissues with an immunohistochemical method. *Am J Clin Pathol* 1983;79:438–442.
15. Witzig TE, Banks PM, Stenson MJ, et al. Rapid immunotyping of B cell non-Hodgkin's lymphomas by flow cytometry: a comparison with the standard frozen section methods. *Am J Clin Pathol* 1990;94:280–286.
16. Gatter KC, Alcock C, Heryet A, et al. The differential diagnosis of routinely processed anaplastic tumors using monoclonal antibodies. *Am J Clin Pathol* 1984;82:33–43.
17. Lennert K, ed. *Histopathology of non-Hodgkin's lymphomas (based on the Kiel classification).* New York: Springer-Verlag, 1981:119.

CHAPTER 13

The Role of Fine Needle Aspiration Biopsy in the Diagnosis and Management of Hematopoietic Neoplasms

Lawrence M. Weiss and William C. Pitts

Fine needle aspiration biopsy (FNAB) is a rapid, minimally invasive technique for the cytologic evaluation of mass lesions and for many years has been an accepted diagnostic procedure in Europe (1–3). Koss (4) speculates that its acceptance in Europe in the 1950s resulted largely from the relative lack of skilled European surgical pathologists at that time. Despite its introduction earlier in this century for the diagnosis of tumors at the Memorial Center for Cancer and Allied Diseases (5), needle aspiration biopsy until recently largely was neglected by pathologists in the United States. Most American pathologists have been reluctant to adopt this technique for the evaluation of disease processes, particularly if they involve superficial lymph nodes (6). This reluctance to use FNAB in the evaluation of superficial lymphadenopathy may stem from several factors. The aspiration studies reported 25 to 30 years ago were performed at a time at which there was great confusion and difficulty in the recognition and classification of malignant lymphoma in tissue sections (7–9). These studies, therefore, are difficult to reconcile with the current concepts and terminologies of the malignant lymphomas. Furthermore, until recently, there have been relatively few well-illustrated articles demonstrating the fixed and air-dried cytologic appearances of malignant lymphomas (10). Many pathologists trained in the United States have had little formal training in interpretation of needle aspiration biopsies and are not as familiar with air-dried aspirate smears as they are with Papanicolaou-stained slides. Pathologists have been justifiably skeptical and reluctant to interpret cytologic smears from lymph node aspirations, because a surgeon easily could excise a superficial enlarged lymph node.

The utility of FNAB of enlarged lymph nodes varies depending on the clinical situation. Frequently it is performed in a setting of presumed reactive hyperplasia or infection to reassure anxious patients or to obtain material for bacterial or fungal cultures, respectively. In large series composed of more than 100 cases each, anywhere from 25% to 60% of aspirated enlarged lymph nodes yielded a reactive pattern that was confirmed by subsequent excisional biopsy or a benign clinical outcome on close follow-up (11–15). The percentage of reactive cases is even higher in children, in whom malignancies are seen in less than 5% of cases (16). FNAB may be particularly useful in the setting of human immunodeficiency virus (HN) infection, in which infection, benign lymphadenopathy, and neoplasm are possibilities (17–19). FNAB is also a useful tool in the evaluation of lymphadenopathy in the clinical setting of known or suspected epithelial malignancy (20,21). In patients with carcinoma or malignant melanoma, FNAB can be used to document suspected nodal involvement of the tumor. In this situation nonlymphoid cells can be identified readily in FNAB specimens from lymph nodes, and these results can be used to optimize further investigative procedures (22). Patients with malignant lymphoma diagnosed by FNAB constitute a small subset of those with malignant diagnoses in large series. For example, several large studies have demonstrated that malignant lymphomas comprise approximately 10% of the malignant cases diagnosed by FNAB (11–13,23).

In the initial evaluation of lymphadenopathy, FNAB can provide clinical confirmation of presumed reactive conditions, provided that adequate clinical follow-up is available to provide a diagnosis in patients who are poor candidates for excisional biopsy. In histologically documented cases of

L. M. Weiss: Division of Pathology, City of Hope National Medical Center, Duarte, California 91010
W. C. Pitts: Department of Anatomic Pathology, Community Hospitals of Central California, Fresno, California 93701

hematolymphoid malignancy involving lymph nodes, FNAB has a role in the clinical management of the patient, including documentation of disease extent, relapse, progression, or transformation and gauging of the effects of therapy (24,25). For the primary diagnosis of malignant lymphoma, the role of FNAB is potentially controversial, given the frequent use of immunophenotyping and other ancillary studies for diagnosis and the importance of the diagnosis on therapy selection. FNAB can aid, however, in the identification of nodal groups that may prove more productive for the diagnosis of malignant lymphoma through open biopsy. FNAB of lymph nodes may lead to open biopsy sooner in cases of falsely presumed reactive nodal enlargement. Furthermore, FNAB material is amenable to immunophenotyping studies (26–31), augmenting careful cytomorphologic assessment of properly obtained and prepared needle aspiration smears. One also can aspirate sufficient cells to perform morphometric studies (32), to obtain flow cytometric results (33), and to extract DNA for molecular analysis (34,35).

GENERAL CONSIDERATIONS

The advantages of FNAB include patient acceptance and tolerance of a minimally invasive, simple, and rapid technique; low cost; and accuracy of diagnosis. Potential pitfalls or misdiagnoses primarily involve sampling error (poor biopsy technique, partial involvement of the lymph node by the tumor, extensive necrosis, marked nodal sclerosis) or failure to properly interpret the cellular findings.

BIOPSY TECHNIQUE

Optimal diagnostic results are achieved if the cytopathologist performs the aspiration biopsy and interprets the cytologic smears (1,36,37). Correlation of the clinical setting with the cytologic findings of the aspirate material is best achieved in this fashion. Diagnostic accuracy and maintenance of aspiration skills are directly related to volume of cases handled by (38) and the experience of the examiner (39). A commonly used technique of aspiration biopsy is that described by Zajicek (3) and others (1,11). A thin (21- to 25-gauge) needle most commonly is used; infrequently an 18-gauge needle is employed. The use of thin needles rarely results in complications such as small hematomas and has not been associated with needle track tumor seeding. The syringe is placed in a pistol-like holding device, allowing the examiner to use the other hand to palpate and stabilize the palpable mass. Local anesthesia (1% xylocaine or lidocaine) is used in several centers in the United States; in many European clinics no form of anesthesia is used. If cutaneous anesthesia is used, it is important not to inject the anesthesia into the lesion because this has the potential to dilute the aspiration sample. Use of too much anesthesia in the overlying skin may make it difficult to palpate small superficial masses.

The skin is cleansed with an alcohol wipe, and the needle on the aspirating syringe is inserted quickly through the skin into the mass. Often a difference in resistance can be appreciated as the needle passes through the subcutaneous tissue and into the target lesion. The needle should enter but not extend beyond the target mass. Once the needle has entered the mass, full suction in the aspirating syringe is created by drawing back on the sliding pistol handle. The needle is repositioned rapidly back and forth in the mass, sometimes at slightly different angles, with negative pressure or suction maintained. Six to 12 samples can be obtained in this fashion during a 1- to 2-second time interval. At the end of this time, or if any blood or fluid is seen in the syringe hub, the aspiration procedure is concluded by releasing the sliding pistol handle, which removes the vacuum created in the syringe. Once the syringe plunger is returned to the original position, the needle and syringe are removed from the target lesion. The syringe alternatively can be removed from the needle at the conclusion of the aspiration segment of the biopsy. This helps to minimize the amount of material that is drawn into the hub of the needle. The fine needle biopsy procedure also can be performed without the use of aspiration (40). A needle is placed in the palpable mass and passed back and forth through the lesion. The capillary action draws a sample into the needle. This technique is a satisfactory alternative or complement to the aspiration technique, especially in younger patients and those who are easily alarmed by the large syringe and holding device. The patient, or preferably an assistant, subsequently applies light pressure to the puncture site to minimize local hemorrhage.

SMEAR TECHNIQUE

The second step in aspiration biopsy cytology is the proper preparation of the smear slides (Figs. 13.1, 13.2). The techniques used in Sweden have been well outlined by Abele and colleagues (41). Their work illustrates various techniques for

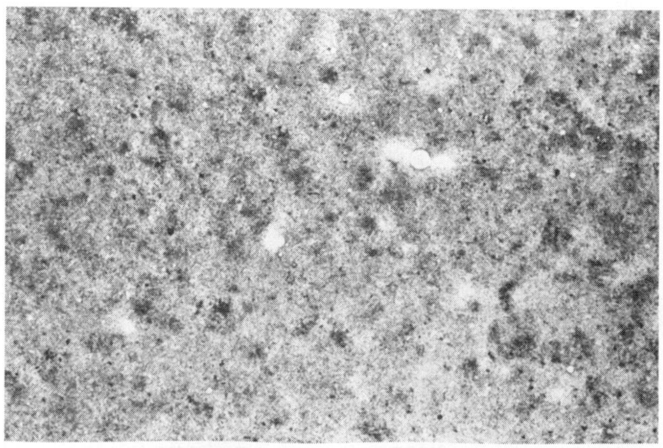

FIG. 13.1. Nodal involvement by malignant melanoma. The properly prepared direct smear shows a uniform distribution of the aspirate material (May-Grünwald-Giemsa stain, original magnification: 4× magnification).

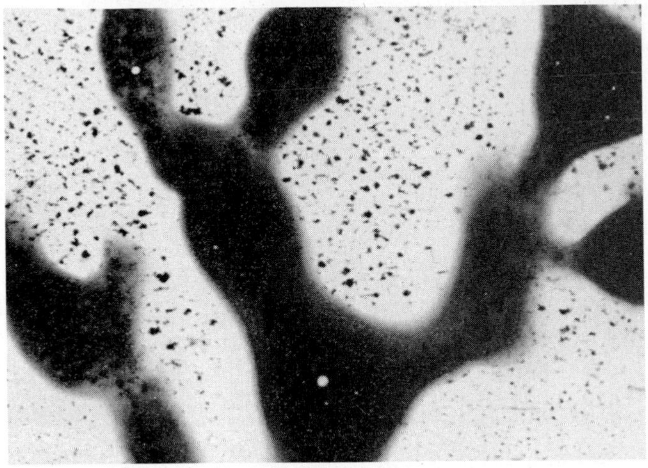

FIG. 13.2. Lymph node aspirate. This smear was prepared using a "pull apart" method, resulting in material that is unevenly distributed on the slide and thus too concentrated for proper staining (Papanicolaou stain, original magnification: 4× magnification).

preparing direct smears, depending on the consistency of the aspirated material. Using these techniques, one can concentrate the material and optimize cytologic interpretation. In most cases, the one-step smearing technique suffices. Alcohol-fixed smears stained by the Papanicolaou or hematoxylin and eosin method provide excellent and familiar nuclear detail; air-dried smears stained by the Wright-Giemsa or May-Grunwald-Giemsa method emphasize cytoplasmic features.

STRATEGIES OF FNAB INTERPRETATION

A strategy for the evaluation of FNAB of lymph nodes is outlined in Figures 13.3 and 13.4. Improper aspiration biopsy technique fails to yield smears that are sufficiently cellular for confident evaluation and reliable results. Large, centrally necrotic masses are best sampled at the periphery. Some lymphoid neoplasms are associated with marked sclerosis, such as nodular sclerosing Hodgkin's disease and sclerosing large cell lymphoma, often yielding paucicellular samples. In some clinical conditions, a paucicellular or acellular smear is the result of a nonhematolymphoid process that clinically mimics enlarged lymph nodes. These clinical settings in the head and neck include cystic squamous cell carcinoma involving lymph nodes, benign stromal processes such as nodular fasciitis and scars, salivary gland tumors, and branchial cleft cysts. Faulty smearing techniques can result in marked dilution or inappropriate concentration of the cellular material, resulting in poorly stained smears that are difficult to interpret (Fig. 13.2). Useful interpretation of smears of fine needle aspirate can be made only if the aspiration procedure and smearing of the material are carried out properly.

The architectural pattern and cytologic features of lymphoid processes provide the surgical pathologist with important clues in the evaluation of lymph node processes (41,42). Adopting the histopathologic approach to the evaluation of lymph nodes, the pathologist similarly can note cell patterns on scanning magnification of the lymph node aspirate smears. In this way one can differentiate small cellular aggregates or nodules (Fig. 13.5) from discohesive or dispersed cell patterns (Fig. 13.6). The examination of nuclear and chromatin patterns at high magnification allows further separation into monomorphous and polymorphous lymphoid cell populations. Lymph nodes that display an admixture of small, medium-sized, and large lymphocytes (polymorphous

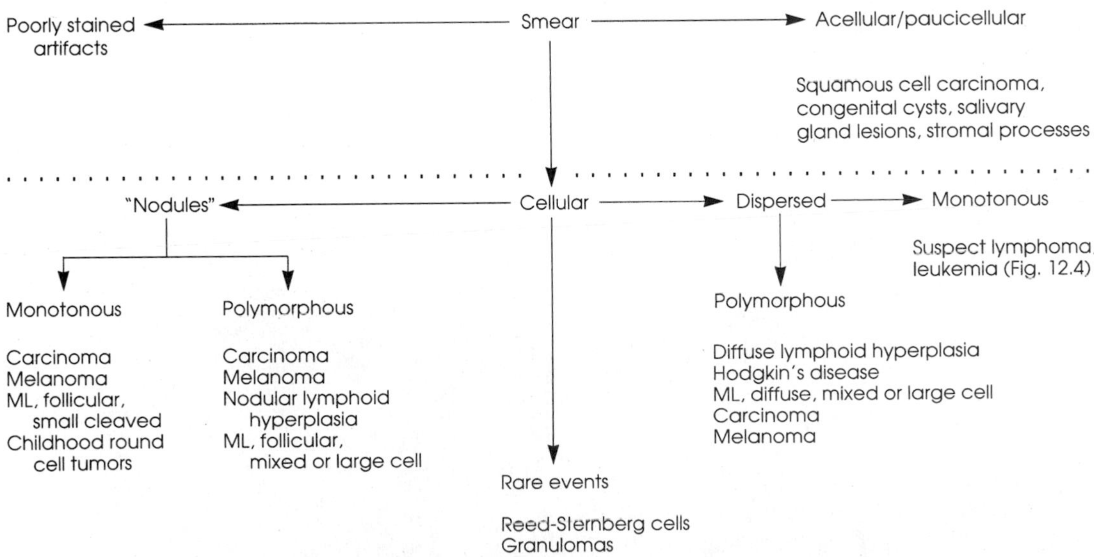

FIG. 13.3. Flow chart for the morphologic evaluation of lymph node aspirations. Findings above the dotted line frequently are associated with nonhematolymphoid processes or are indications of inadequate samples. Cellular and well-stained aspirates allow for further interpretation as explained in the text. *ML*, malignant lymphoma. (From *Pathology Annual 1988*, part 2. Norwalk: Appleton and Lange, 1988, with permission.)

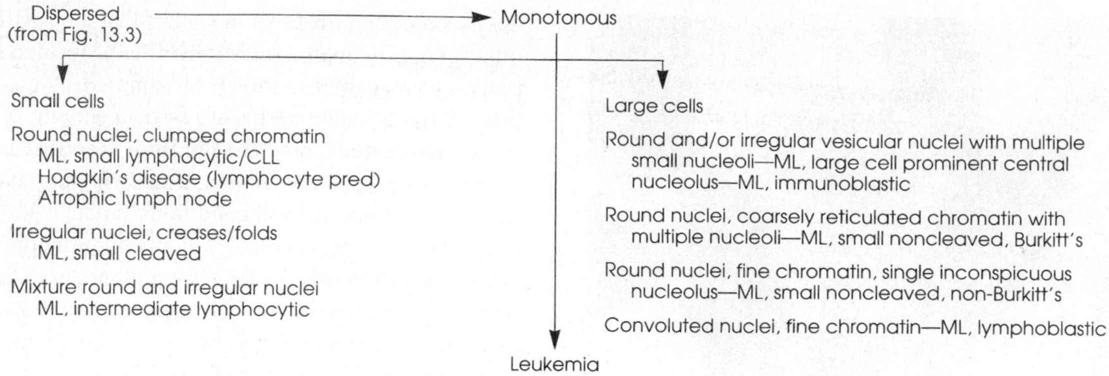

FIG. 13.4. Flow chart for the morphologic evaluation of lymph node aspirates (continued). *CLL*, chronic lymphocytic leukemia; *Pred*, predominant. (From Pitts WC, Weiss LM. *Pathology Annual 1988*, part 2. Norwalk: Appleton and Lange, 1988, with permission.)

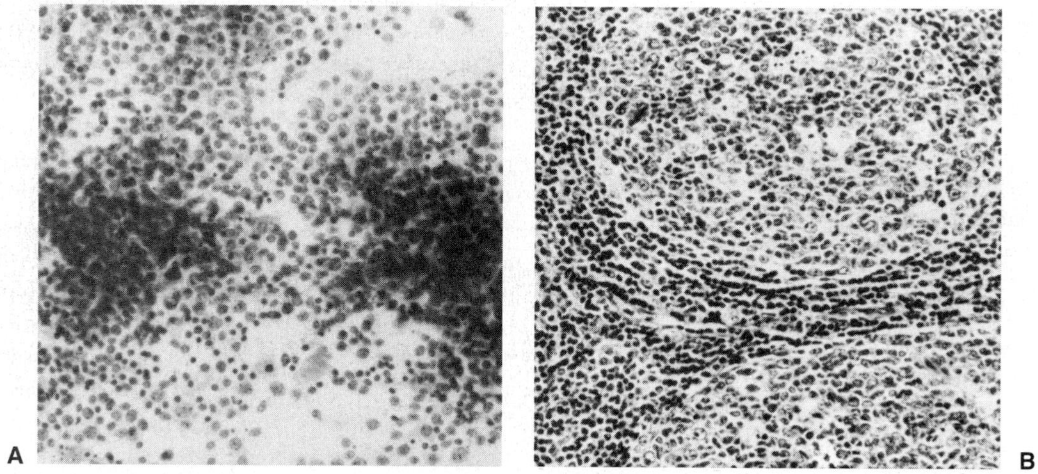

FIG. 13.5. Reactive follicular hyperplasia. **A:** Nodular aggregates of polymorphous lymphoid cells with scattered tingible body macrophages are seen on direct smears (Papanicolaou stain, original magnification: 100× magnification). **B:** A histologic section from the patient in *A* reveals a comparable admixture of small and large lymphoid cells and tingible body macrophages (hematoxylin and eosin, original magnification: 100× magnification).

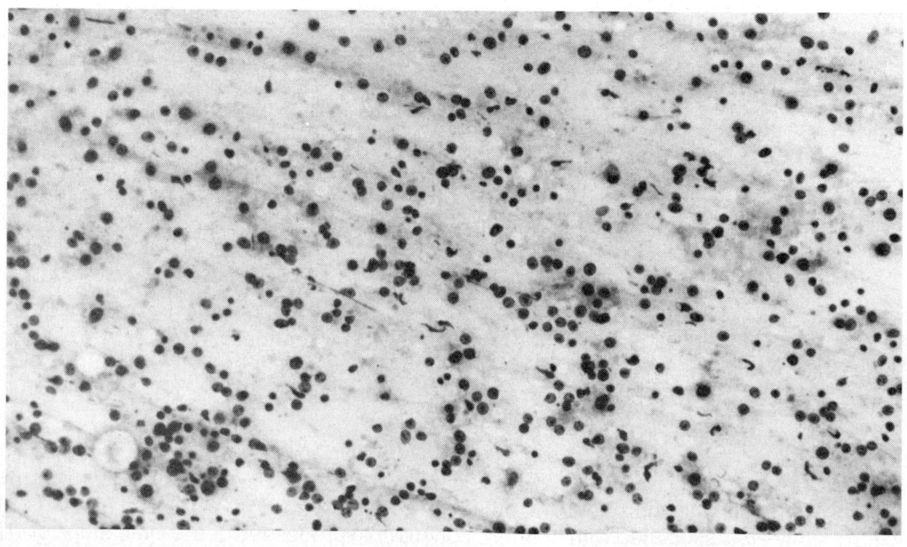

FIG. 13.6. Immunoblastic lymphoma. A dispersed pattern is encountered in nodes involved by high grade and many forms of intermediate grade lymphoma (hematoxylin and eosin stain, original magnification: 200× magnification).

population) in addition to tingible body macrophages and histiocytes usually are associated with benign or reactive conditions. Several exceptions to this rule exist: Hodgkin's disease, mixed small and large cell lymphomas including peripheral T-cell lymphoma, malignant lymphoma with a high content of epithelioid histiocytes, or mycosis fungoides involving the lymph node can exhibit a polymorphous lymphoid population. In contrast, a monotonous or monomorphous cell population generally implies that one is dealing with a malignant condition. Monotony in a cellular lymph node aspirate does not always indicate malignant lymphoma. Many carcinomas appear extremely discohesive and monotonous on FNAB smears.

ANCILLARY METHODS OF DIAGNOSIS

The application of immunophenotyping has enhanced our ability to diagnose and classify malignant lymphomas in tissue (43,44). Several medical centers routinely correlate the FNAB morphologic smear findings with immunophenotyping and immunogenotyping results (27–31,45). A simple antibody panel including, for example, leukocyte common antigen (CD45), cytokeratin, and the S-100 protein can be useful with direct aspirate smears, cytospin preparations, or cell block preparations in narrowing the differential diagnosis of non-Hodgkin's lymphoma, carcinoma, or malignant melanoma (46–48). Once a lesion is determined to be lymphoid, an expanded battery of monoclonal antibodies can be employed. The presence of light-chain restriction is the most useful criterion for determining B-cell malignancy in the immunologic evaluation of FNAB smears; the evaluation of such restriction in FNAB may be superior to that in frozen sections, because good correlation with cytologic features is afforded (Fig. 13.7). There has been limited success using the monoclonal antibody to dendritic reticulum cells R4/23 (DAKO DRC1) (49), in conjunction with other monoclonal antibodies, to distinguish between follicular and diffuse lymphomas in needle aspirate fluid. The identification of DRC1-positive cells alone does not separate benign from malignant lymph nodes, because similar clusters of DRC1-positive cells can be seen in reactive lymph nodes, most likely corresponding to the "lymphohistiocytic aggregates" described by morphologists. Evaluation of antigen loss, crucial to the immunologic diagnosis of peripheral T-cell lymphoma, may be more difficult to perform in FNAB smears than in frozen sections, because assessment of antigen expression within specific regions of the lymph node architecture is not possible. Immunophenotyping by flow cytometry is also possible with FNAB specimens (50). Some investigators have proposed that determining the ratio of CD4-positive : CD8-positive cells may be an important tool in staging patients clinically and assessing response to therapy in patients infected with HIV (51–53).

Sufficient DNA may be obtained by FNAB for analysis by flow cytometry, Southern blotting, the polymerase chain reaction, or *in situ* hybridization. One study demonstrated that the results obtained from DNA-flow cytometric analysis of fine needle aspiration–derived material was comparable in most cases to those obtained from surgical specimens (54). Similarly, in one prospective study, adequate DNA for

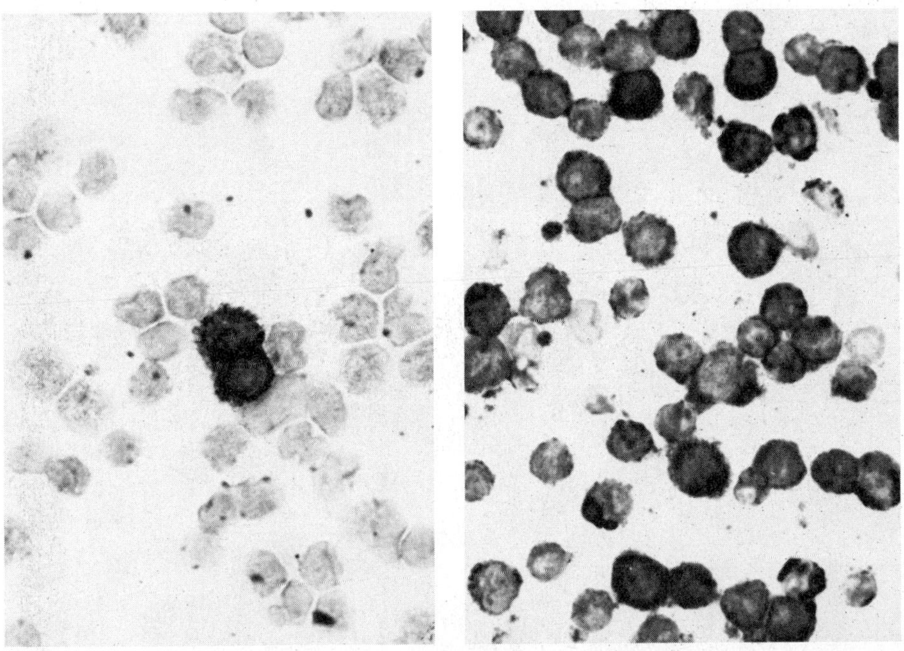

A B

FIG. 13.7. Nodal involvement by chronic lymphocytic leukemia. Immunoperoxidase studies carried out on cytospin preparations can demonstrate light-chain restriction (cytospin preparations, immunoperoxidase stain, original magnification: 640× magnification). **A:** Kappa light chain. **B:** Lambda light chain. (From *Pathology Annual 1988*, part 2. Norwalk: Appleton and Lange, 1988, with permission.)

molecular studies was obtained in 20 (74%) of 27 cases (35). The pattern of gene rearrangements obtained on analysis of aspiration specimens has been shown to correlate precisely with the pattern of gene rearrangements obtained on analysis of DNA from the excised lymph node (34). In addition to assessment of the status of the antigen receptor genes, DNA obtained from FNAB samples may be analyzed for the presence of specific chromosomal translocations, viral genomes, and activated or amplified oncogenes (35). For example, determination of the presence of a 14;18 translocation, by Southern blotting or by the polymerase chain reaction, may provide conclusive evidence of lymphoid malignancy (55). In addition, polymerase chain reaction studies on FNAB specimens may be used to determine viral load in patients infected with the human immunodeficiency virus (51,53). The identification of specific molecular lesions by polymerase chain reaction may provide a highly sensitive technique to identify cytologically or even histologically occult disease. Epstein-Barr virus detection by *in situ* hybridization may be performed in FNAB specimens and has been used to demonstrate origin of carcinoma from the nasopharynx (56,57). Immunoglobulin light-chain mRNA also may be detected by *in situ* hybridization in FNAB specimens and may be more sensitive than immunocytochemistry in the diagnosis of B-cell lymphoma (58).

SPECIFIC CONSIDERATIONS

Reactive Lymphoid Hyperplasia

The cause of reactive lymphoid hyperplasia is frequently unknown. In some cases the adenopathy is presumed to be secondary to viral, bacterial, or fungal infection. In the clinical setting of persistent or increasing adenopathy, FNAB may be warranted to exclude a malignant lymphoma and possibly implicate a cause of the nodal enlargement. In most cases lymphoid hyperplasia histologically assumes a follicular, diffuse, sinus, or mixed architectural pattern (42). The histologic distinction from malignant lymphoma is also based on the polymorphous nature of the lymphoid cells. In FNAB smears, the presence of small round mature-appearing lymphocytes, plasma cells, transformed lymphocytes including immunoblasts, histiocytes, and tingible body macrophages implies a benign or reactive condition (Fig. 13.8).

A relative preponderance of a nodular cell pattern is seen in reactive conditions involving lymph nodes that have a prominent follicular component on aspiration. Follicular lymphoid hyperplasia frequently produces small cellular aggregates (nodules). *Lymphohistiocytic aggregates* is the term applied to these nodules of mixed small and large lymphoid cells in a report by O'Dowd and colleagues (59) (Fig. 13.9). These were seen most frequently in their examples of follicular hyperplasia. Similar nodules were seen in other reactive lymphoid conditions. The finding of lymphoid aggregates does not ensure that one is dealing with a reactive lymphoid condition, because similar loose aggregates of lymphoid cells may be seen in examples of low-grade follicular small cleaved cell lymphoma (Fig. 13.10) or follicular mixed small cleaved and large cell lymphoma (60). Thus, proper identification of the cell pattern and the cell type is important in the recognition of reactive conditions. In addition to the clusters of mixed small and large cells, the background of the typical reactive lymphoid smear contains a similar admixture of small, medium-sized, and large lymphocytes with scattered plasma cells and tingible body macrophages. It is rea-

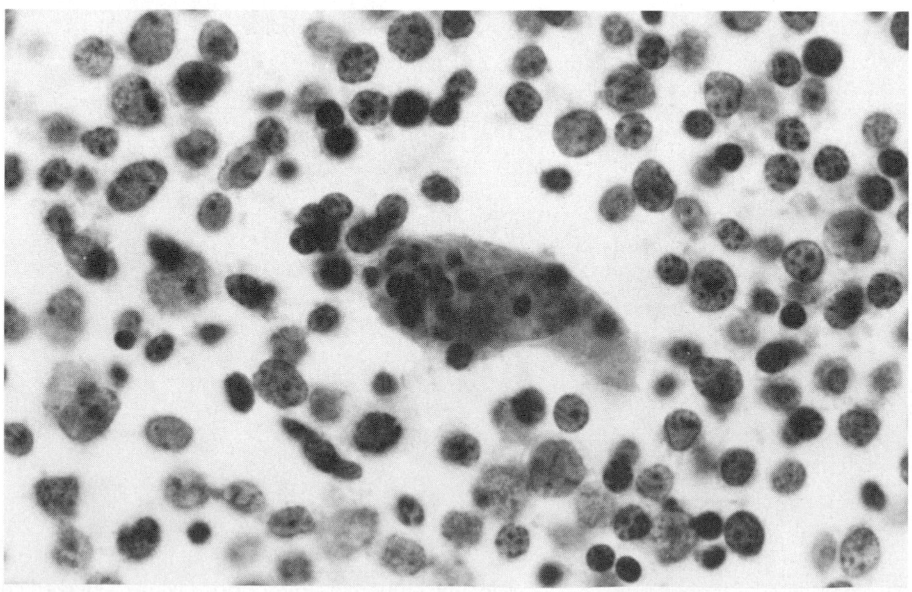

FIG. 13.8. Reactive lymphoid hyperplasia. The background lymphoid cells show a mixture of small, medium-sized, and large nuclei along with a tingible body macrophage (hematoxylin and eosin stain, original magnification: 1,000× magnification).

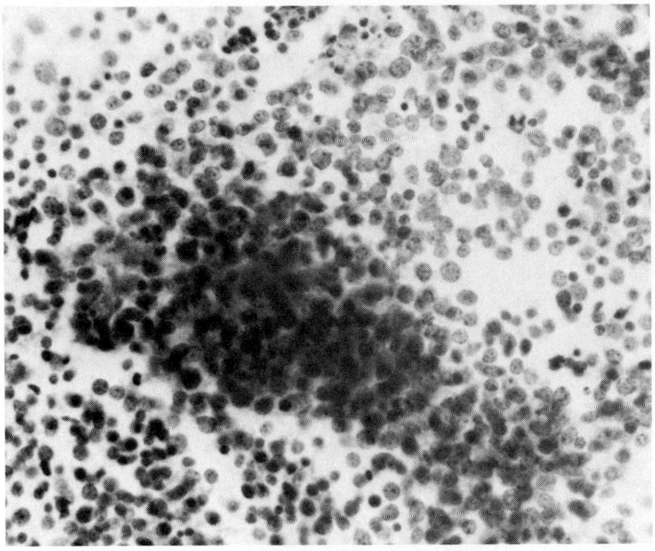

FIG. 13.9. Reactive lymphoid hyperplasia. Intact or fragmented germinal centers may be encountered on needle aspiration biopsy. Tingible body macrophages (TBMs) may be seen within these aggregates of small and large lymphoid cells and at the periphery of these nodules (hematoxylin and eosin stain, original magnification: 200× magnification).

sonable to conclude that the lymph node aspirate represents a benign or hyperplastic state if uncommon cytologic findings such as Reed-Sternberg cells and granulomas are lacking. A diagnosis of toxoplasmic lymphadenitis may be suggested if monocytoid B cells and epithelioid histiocytes are seen in a reactive background; confirmation through serologic studies is mandatory (61). A diagnosis of Kimura's disease may be suggested if dissociated and clustered endothelial cells, eosinophils, and Warthin-Finkeldey giant cells are seen (62).

Some forms of lymph node hyperplasia are characterized in tissue sections by an expansion of the interfollicular zones resulting from a polymorphous population of lymphoid cells. Germinal centers are generally lacking or inconspicuous. In this setting the recognition of the admixed nature of the lymphoid cells in FNAB specimens supports a reactive lymphadenopathy. Occasionally, Langerhans cells and melanin-laden macrophages may be seen (Fig. 13.11). This may suggest a specific diagnosis of dermatopathic lymphadenopathy. Gene rearrangement studies performed on DNA extracted from an FNAB sample may help to distinguish dermatopathic lymphadenopathy with subtle involvement by mycosis fungoides from that associated with benign dermatologic disorders (63).

It must be emphasized again that FNAB can be used to diagnose reactive lymphoid conditions if adequate clinical follow-up is available. If adenopathy persists or further nodal enlargement occurs after a reactive lymphoid process is diagnosed based on FNAB, there must be an opportunity to perform repeat FNAB or an open biopsy.

Granulomatous Processes

Clusters of epithelioid histiocytes and multinucleated giant cells can be seen in a variety of benign (64–66) and malignant (67,68) conditions affecting the lymph node (Fig. 13.12). Histiocytes typically have moderately abundant, frequently finely vacuolated cytoplasm and oval to elongated nuclei with fine, evenly dispersed chromatin. The nuclear

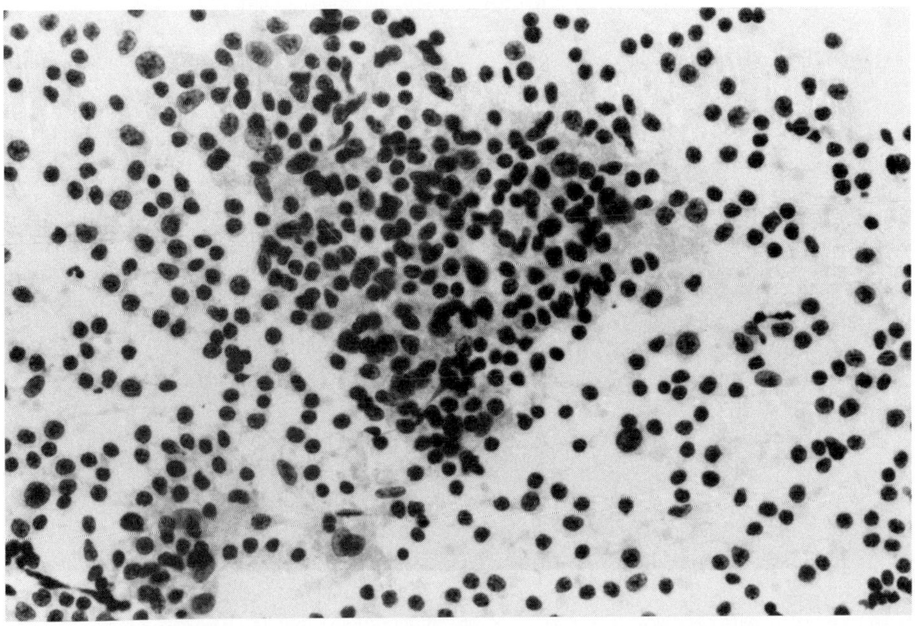

FIG. 13.10. Malignant lymphoma of the follicular small cleaved cell type. A "nodular" aggregate of atypical small cleaved lymphoid cells is present in this low-grade lymphoma (Papanicoloau stain, original magnification: 400× magnification).

A

B

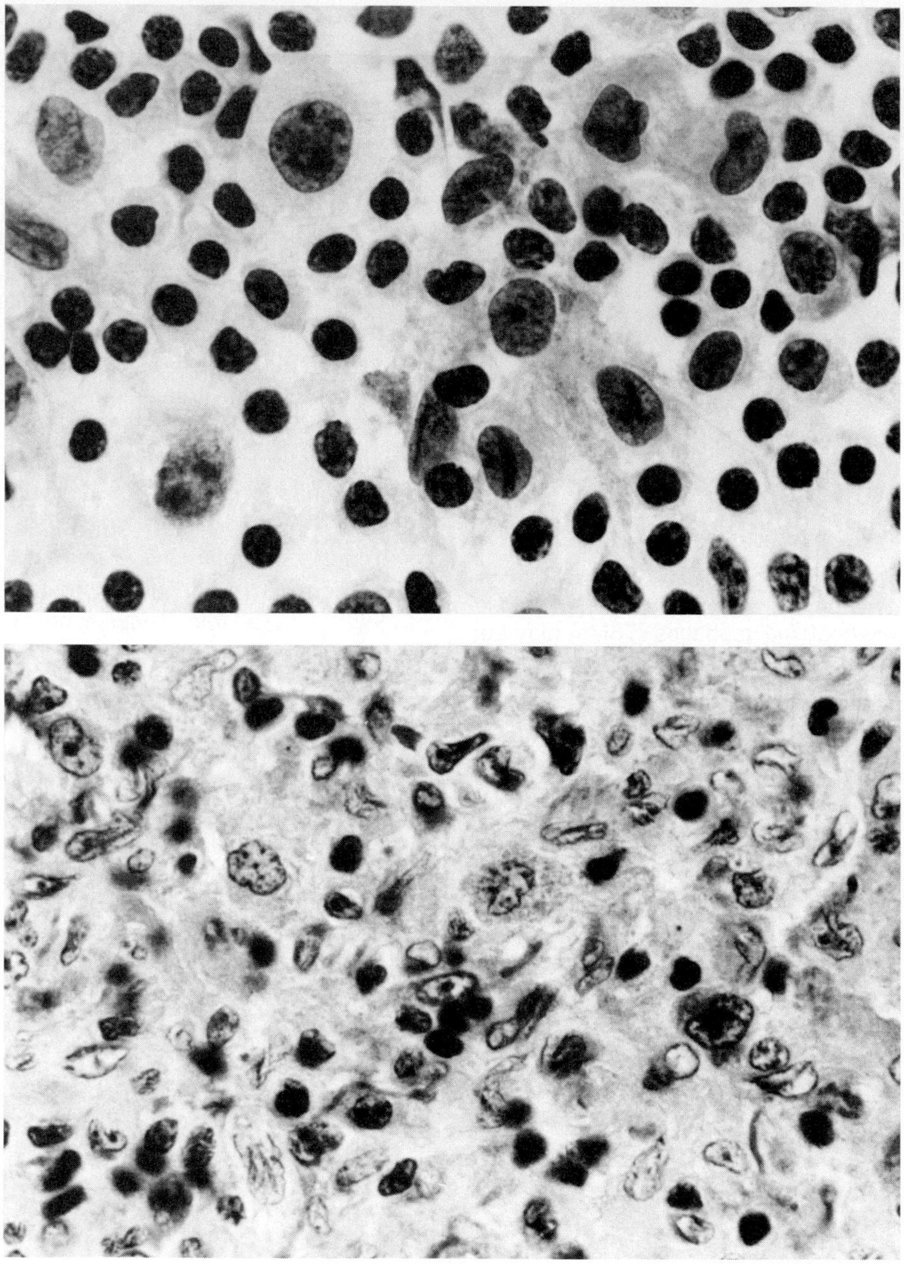

FIG. 13.11. Dermatopathic lymphadenopathy. **A:** Several Langerhans' cells are seen with a mixture of small and large lymphoid cells in this aspirate biopsy smear. The linear nuclear folds or grooves of Langerhans cells can be identified (Papanicoloau stain, original magnification: 1,000× magnification). **B:** A histologic section from the patient in **A** reveals a mixture of lymphoid cells and many Langerhans cells (hematoxylin and eosin stain, original magnification: 1,000× magnification).

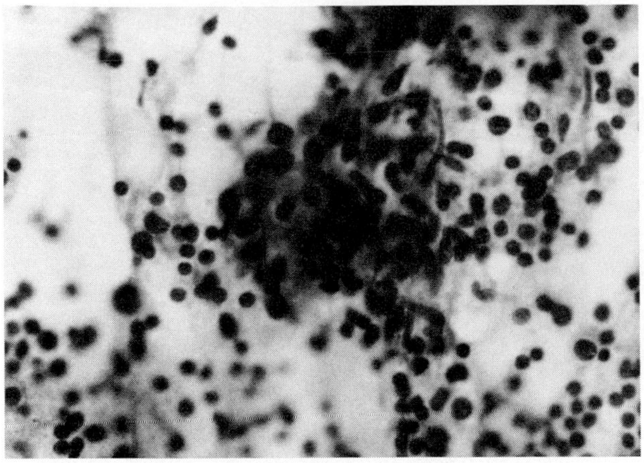

FIG. 13.12. Granulomatous lymphadenitis, secondary to sarcoid. A loose aggregate of epithelioid cells is seen (Papanicoloau stain, original magnification: 200× magnification).

borders are generally thin. Small but readily identifiable nucleoli may be seen. Occasionally the elongated nuclei display central linear nuclear grooves or creases. Multinucleated histiocytic giant cells are easily recognized by virtue of their large size and the monotonous, uniform appearance of their many nuclei.

Infectious Granulomatous Conditions

Infection is suggested strongly in the setting of abundant karyorrhectic and cytoplasmic debris (Fig. 13.13) and in the absence of lymphoid monotony. However, the combination of randomly activated lymphoid cells, necrotic debris, karyorrhectic cells, and prominent histiocytes also should suggest the possibility of Kikuchi's histiocytic necrotizing lymphadenitis (69). Concern for tuberculosis is appropriate if numerous epithelioid histiocytes are present. In tuberculosis the most common finding, seen in about 50% of cases, is the presence of epithelioid clusters with or without Langhans giant cells with necrosis; necrosis is absent in about one third of cases (70). FNAB shows a sensitivity of about 75% in the detection of tuberculous lymphadenitis (71). Reaspiration of the node for cultures (72) is indicated in these situations. Alternatively, appropriate special stains can be used on decolorized alcohol-fixed and air-dried slides (73); special stains are most useful in cases with extensive necrosis (70).

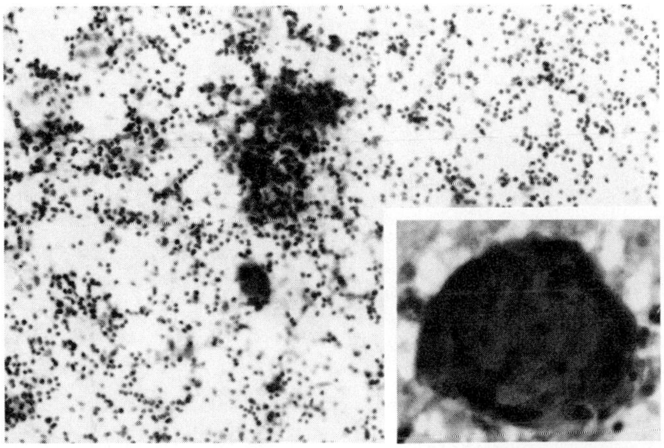

FIG. 13.13. Necrotizing granulomatous lymphadenitis, secondary to tuberculosis. A large, loose aggregate of epithelioid cells is accompanied by two multinucleated giant cells and mixture of background lymphocytes (Papanicoloau stain, original magnification: 100× magnification). **Insert:** A large multinucleated giant cell (Papanicoloau stain, original magnification: 1,000× magnification).

Noninfectious Granulomatous Conditions

Aspirate smears from lymph nodes showing lymphangiogram effect may contain multinucleated giant cells with scalloped cytoplasmic borders (Fig. 13.14). Nodular aggregates of epithelioid histiocytes in FNAB samples may suggest sarcoidosis (65) (Fig. 13.12). If a granulomatous process is recognized in FNAB specimens from lymph nodes, one must inspect the background cells for evidence of coexistent malignancy, because Hodgkin's disease, non-Hodgkin's lymphoma, and carcinoma may be accompanied by clusters of epithelioid histiocytes or granulomas.

Non-Hodgkin's Lymphoma

Important in the recognition of most non-Hodgkin's lymphomas on FNAB is the identification of a monotonous lymphoid cell population (Fig. 13.15) in properly prepared smear material. The monomorphous feature of the suspect neoplastic lymphoid cells is reflected not so much in their nuclear size but in the essentially uniform appearance of the chromatin pattern from cell to cell. Once the monotony of the lymphoid population is appreciated, the initial subclassification into small and large lymphoid cells requires the comparison of the suspect neoplastic lymphoid cells to typical small mature lymphocytes, plasma cells, or histiocytes (Fig. 13.15). The tingible body macrophage is recognized easily in smear preparations. By using the nuclei of these cells as an internal reference, one can assess the relative size of the lymphoid cells and separate them into small and large. Careful evaluation of the chromatin pattern aids in further subclassifying the type of lymphoid cell. In this manner, one frequently can diagnose monotonous cell populations, especially if confronted with higher-grade lymphoid malignancies.

Low-Grade Non-Hodgkin's Lymphoma

Chronic Lymphocytic Leukemia or Small Lymphocytic Lymphoma

In aspirate smears obtained from lymph nodes involved in chronic lymphocytic leukemia or small lymphocytic lymphoma, there is a predominantly dispersed cell pattern at scanning magnification. These smears show a preponderance of small lymphoid cells with round regular nuclear membranes and clumped chromatin patterns (Figs. 13.15,

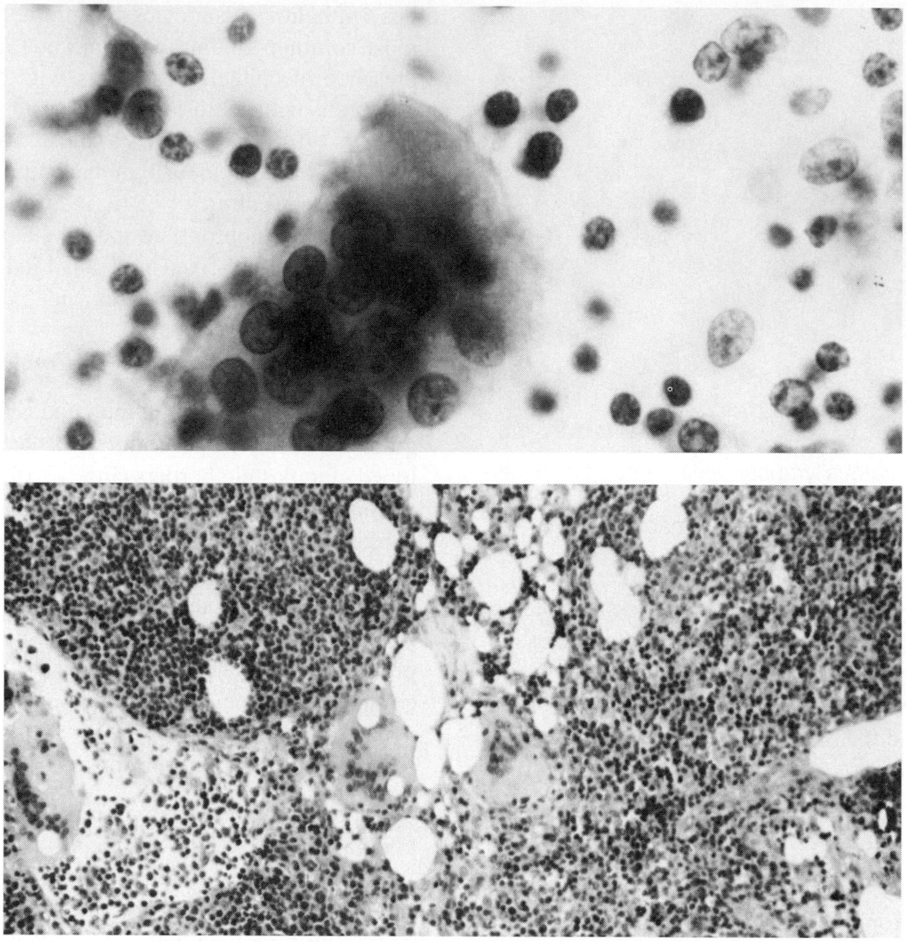

A

B

FIG. 13.14. Lymphangiogram effect. **A:** Aspirate biopsies display an admixture of small, medium and large lymphoid cells with multinucleated giant cells. The latter can have scalloped or concave cytoplasmic borders (Papanicolau stain, original magnification: 1,000× magnification). **B:** A histologic section from **A** demonstrates these cytologic features. Several giant cells next to lipid vacuoles have scalloped or concave borders (hematoxylin and eosin stain, original magnification: 200× magnification).

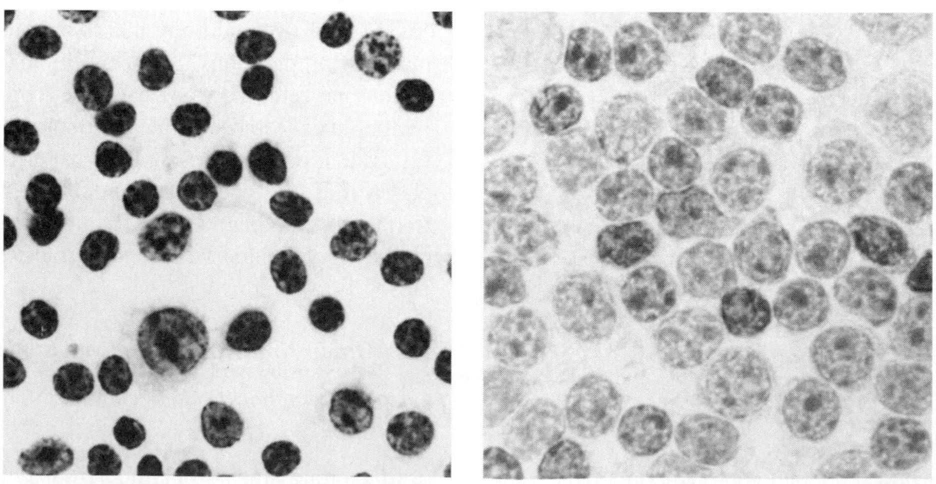

A B

FIG. 13.15. Nodal involvement by chronic lymphocytic leukemia. A dispersed pattern of predominantly small round, mature lymphocytes is commonly seen on needle aspiration. A clumped chromatin pattern distributed along the nuclear membranes can be seen in fixed and air-dried material. (**A:** Papanicoloau stain, original magnification: 100× magnification; **B:** May-Grünwald-Giemsa stain, original magnification: 1,000× magnification).

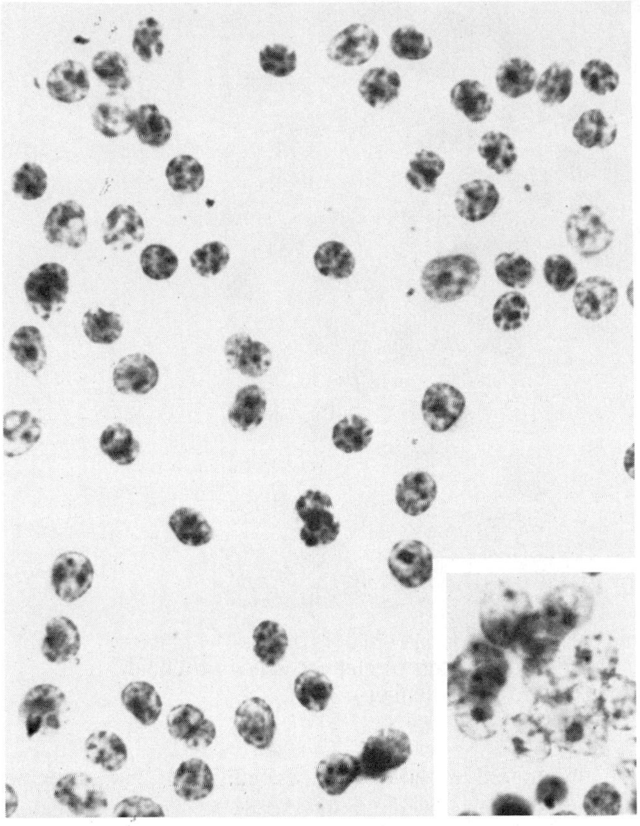

FIG. 13.16. Nodal involvement by chronic lymphocytic leukemia. In addition to a dispersed background population of small mature-appearing lymphoid cells, occasional loose clusters of prolymphocytes may be noted. These have somewhat enlarged nuclei that often contain small but accentuated nucleoli in addition to their typical blocked chromatin pattern. **Insert:** Loose aggregate of prolymphocytes (Papanicoloau stain, original magnification: 1,000× magnification). (From *Pathology Annual 1988*, part 2. Norwalk: Appleton and Lange, 1988, with permission.)

13.16). Relative to the nuclear size of the histiocyte, these nuclei are small. These cells have very scant pale- to lightly basophilic-staining cytoplasm. Occasionally, cells of similar size show an open chromatin pattern and a prominent nucleolus; these are prolymphocytes (Fig. 13.16, **insert**). One easily can compare a peripheral blood smear or a bone marrow aspirate to note the similarities in an aspirated lymph node in cases of known chronic lymphocytic leukemia with presumed lymph node involvement. Patients with chronic lymphocytic leukemia or small lymphocytic leukemia occasionally develop adenopathy as a result of transformation to a large cell lymphoma. On aspiration biopsy, the small rounded nuclear contours and clumped chromatin pattern of the small lymphocytic cells serve to distinguish nodes involved with low-grade lymphoma from nodal involvement by a large cell lymphoma.

Marginal Zone B-Cell Lymphoma

The cytologic features of marginal zone B-cell lymphoma of mucosa-associated lymphoid tissue and the primary nodal marginal zone monocytoid B-cell lymphoma are indistinguishable; these lymphomas also may be very difficult to distinguish from chronic lymphocytic leukemia or small lymphocytic lymphoma. At low magnification, a dispersed cell pattern is seen. The nuclei generally are small and the chromatin clumped, although the nuclear outlines are often more irregular than those seen in chronic lymphocytic leukemia or small lymphocytic lymphoma, with bean-shaped or indented monocytoid chromatin. The most clear distinguishing feature is that a distinct moderate rim of pale or clear cytoplasm may be discerned (Fig. 13.17). There also may be a variable number of cells showing plasmacytoid differentiation. Scattered large cells with prominent nucleoli also may be seen and if large in number may suggest transformation to a higher-grade neoplasm.

Follicular Lymphoma

The same nuclear membrane abnormalities that are identified in histologic sections of small cleaved cell lymphoma can be appreciated in aspirate biopsy smears. In addition to the small nuclear size, the nuclear contours are noticeably wrinkled or indented. The chromatin pattern is similarly coarsely clumped and consequently hyperchromatic (Fig. 13.18). The lightly basophilic cytoplasm is scant, and cytoplasmic borders are poorly defined. In aspirates from pa-

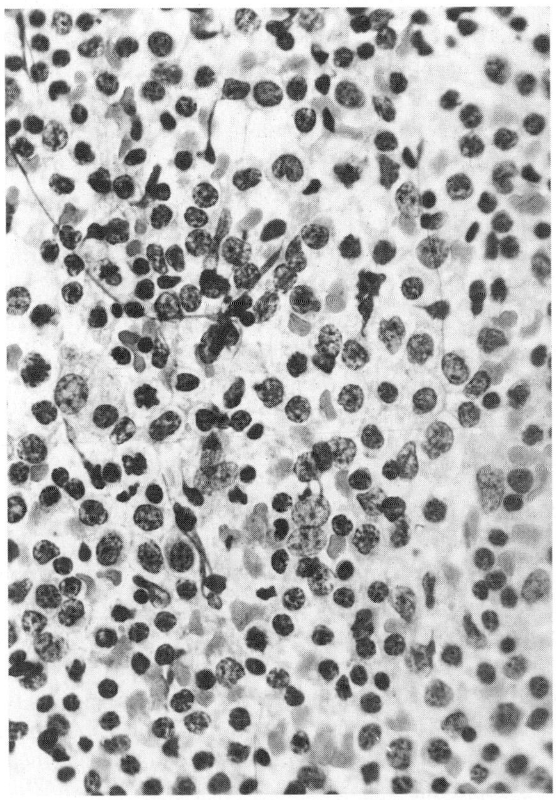

FIG. 13.17. Malignant lymphoma of the nodal marginal zone monocytoid B-cell type. The nuclei are slightly atypical, and the cytoplasm is pale and moderately abundant (hematoxylin and eosin stain, original magnification: 1,000× magnification).

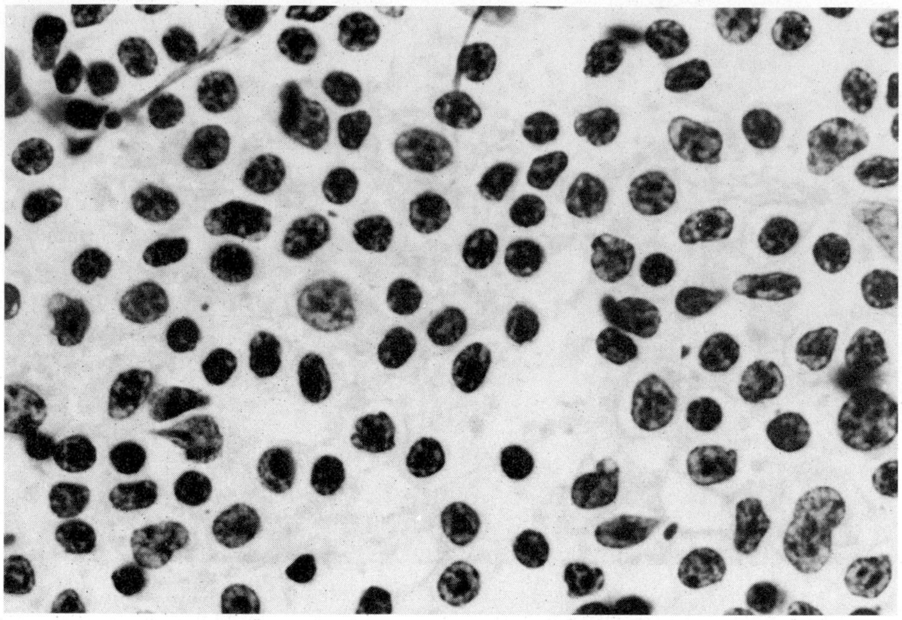

FIG. 13.18. Malignant lymphoma, follicular, small cleaved cell type. The loose clusters of small lymphoid cells seen on low magnification in Figure 13.9 are composed of angulated or cleaved small lymphoid cells (hematoxylin and eosin stain, original magnification: 1,000× magnification).

tients with follicular lymphoma of the small cleaved or mixed cell type, vague aggregates of these lymphoid cells are present, imparting a nodular pattern at low magnification (Fig. 13.10). If small lymphoid cells with wrinkled nuclear contours are approximately equally mixed with larger lymphoid cells having vesicular nuclei, a diagnosis of mixed small and large cell lymphoma is suggested. The presence of nodular aggregates supports inclusion in the category of low-grade lymphomas. One would expect that the cytologic recognition of a mixed small and large cell lymphoma, follicular or diffuse, would be somewhat difficult. This distinction between reactive hyperplasia and low-grade follicular mixed lymphoma frequently is cited as a serious obstacle to the use of fine needle aspiration biopsy in the diagnosis of malignant lymphoma. The application of immunophenotypic or immunogenotypic studies, however, can clarify diagnoses in many borderline cases.

Follicular large cell lymphoma may present vague aggregates if seen with low magnification; at high magnification the constituent cells display nuclear features typical of a diffuse large cell lymphoma (10). These cells and those seen in diffuse large cell lymphoma have scant to moderately abundant cytoplasm ranging from pale-staining to deeply basophilic on air-dried smears. Some cells display cytoplasmic vacuoles. The distinction between diffuse and follicular large cell lymphoma may be difficult on FNAB but may not be important clinically, because each is an intermediate-grade lymphoma.

Intermediate- to High-grade Lymphomas

Monomorphous large cell lymphoid neoplasms are more easily identified than small cell lymphomas. Just as with the low-grade lymphomas, the recognition of a monotonous appearance of the large lymphoid cells is based on an evaluation of their nuclear size relative to a histiocyte nucleus, and on the chromatin pattern. A subset of intermediate- to high-grade lymphomas, particularly the peripheral T-cell lymphomas, has a polymorphous appearance; such lymphomas may be very difficult to recognize. Some large B-cell lymphomas may show a heterogeneous lymphoid population (diffuse mixed small and large cell– or T-cell-rich B-cell lymphoma) and also are difficult to recognize cytologically. Most intermediate- to high-grade lymphomas present with dispersed cellular patterns.

Mantle Cell Lymphoma

As would be expected from the histologic appearance of mantle cell lymphoma, needle aspiration smears show a relatively homogeneous population of small to medium-sized lymphoid cells with irregular and scant to moderately abundant basophilic-staining cytoplasm (Fig. 13.19). The chromatin pattern is less clumped or coarse than that seen in small lymphocytic or small cleaved cell lymphoma (10). The proliferation is highly homogeneous, without the presence of larger cells with prominent nucleoli, although occasional epithelioid histiocytes may be identified and even may be helpful in determining the diagnosis.

Diffuse Large B-Cell Lymphoma

Typically, large cell lymphomas have rounded or cleaved vesicular nuclei with irregularly thick and thin nuclear membranes (Fig. 13.20). There are usually multiple small nu-

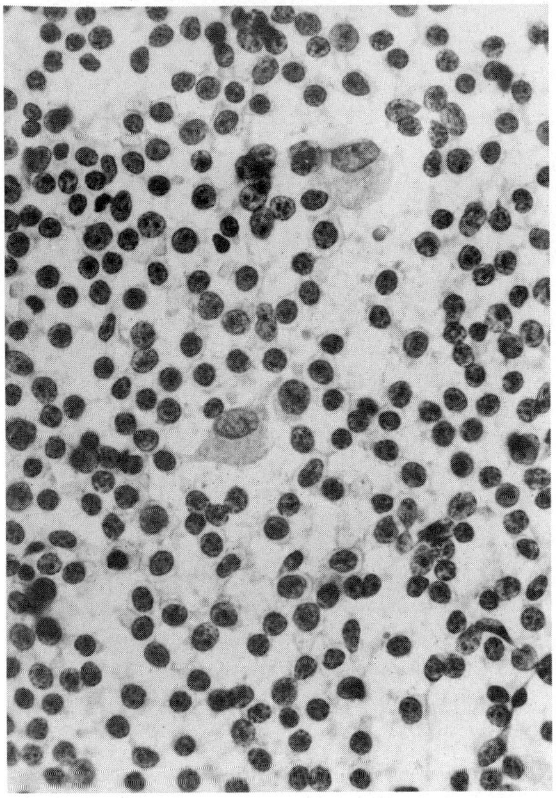

FIG. 13.19. Malignant lymphoma, mantle cell type. There is a homogeneous population of relatively small lymphoid cells. Note the scattered epithelioid histiocytes (hematoxylin and eosin stain, original magnification: 1,000× magnification).

cleoli, many of which are situated peripherally on the nuclear membrane. The faintly pale- to basophilic-staining cytoplasm varies from scant to abundant and may show cytoplasmic vacuoles. Smears of diffuse large cell lymphoma show a dispersed pattern if viewed at low magnification. Often there is necrosis, and mitoses can be seen easily. Generally, immunoblastic lymphomas have nuclear features quite similar to those seen in large cell lymphomas. Large cell lymphoma and immunoblastic lymphoma are distinguished by the number and the character of the nucleoli. A central prominent nucleolus is characteristic of an immunoblastic lymphoma (Fig. 13.21). These lymphomas may show abundant pale or clear to intensely basophilic cytoplasm, which may displace the nucleus eccentrically, imparting a plasmacytoid appearance. The distinction between large cell lymphoma and immunoblastic lymphoma is often difficult on aspirate biopsy. This is not dissimilar to the difficulty sometimes encountered in histologic sections, in which there is frequent interobserver disagreement as to the classification of a particular case as large cell lymphoma or immunoblastic lymphoma (74). Fortunately, these distinctions may not have clinical or even biologic importance (Chapter 25).

A mixture of small cleaved and large lymphoid cells displaying a dispersed pattern raises the possibility of an intermediate lymphoma or reactive lymphoid hyperplasia. This problem is even more difficult in T-cell-rich B-cell lymphoma, in which there is a marked predominance of small, mature lymphocytes, with only scattered large cells; in this case, Hodgkin's disease may be simulated. In the absence of a prior diagnosis of malignant lymphoma or results of

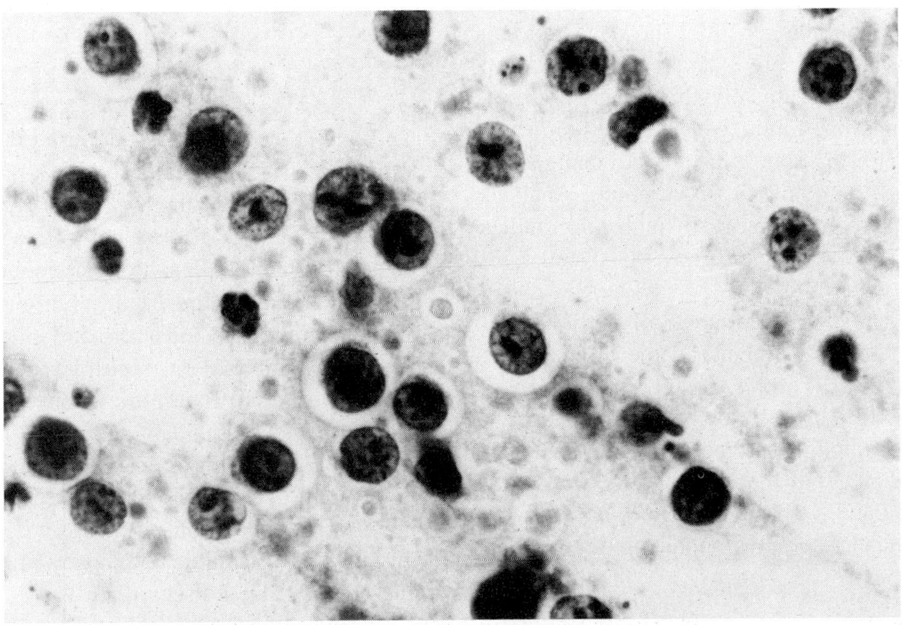

FIG. 13.20. Malignant lymphoma, large cell type. Aspirated material from a large cell lymphoma frequently yields a dispersed population of large lymphoid cells with multiple nucleoli and clear chromatin. The smear background also shows fragments of lymphoid cytoplasm representing so-called lymphoglandular bodies. These are light gray on Papanicolaou stains and blue on May-Grünwald-Giemsa stains (hematoxylin and eosin stain, original magnification: 1,000× magnification).

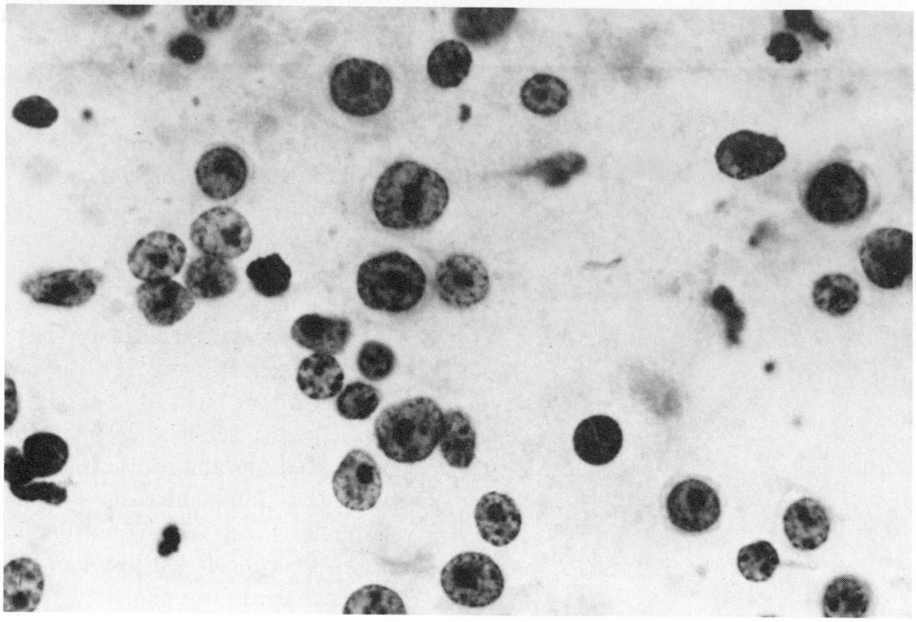

FIG. 13.21. Immunoblastic lymphoma. Prominent central single nucleoli occur in most of these medium to large lymphoid cells. Occasional cells resemble large cell lymphoma (Fig. 13.18) (Papanicoloau stain, original magnification: 1,000× magnification).

additional studies such as immunophenotyping and immunogenotyping, caution should be exercised in the interpretation of such smears. Some cases may remain suspicious clinically and cytologically and may require open biopsy.

Peripheral T-Cell Lymphoma

Peripheral T-cell lymphoma generally shows a heterogeneous population of lymphoid cells and may be very difficult to recognize cytologically; fortunately, this category of lymphoma is very uncommon. Immunostains may confirm a proliferation with a T lineage, but a diagnosis of malignancy is difficult to establish on cytologic preparations. Analysis of T-cell receptor gene rearrangements by molecular studies may be very useful in making a diagnosis of T-cell lymphoma.

Sometimes, one can identify a subset of cytologically highly atypical cells; this is particularly true in anaplastic large cell lymphoma (75,76). In this variant of peripheral T-cell lymphoma, cohesive clusters of cytologically malignant cells may be present, mimicking carcinoma or malignant melanoma. Expression of CD30 by the atypical cells, along with the absence of keratin and S-100 protein, may establish the diagnosis of anaplastic large cell lymphoma in this setting.

Lymphoblastic Lymphoma

Needle aspirates of lymphoblastic lymphoma usually show a dispersed monomorphous population of lymphoid cells with a nuclear size slightly larger than that of small lymphocytes (Fig. 13.22). The fine, dusty, or delicate chromatin pattern is identical to that seen in acute lymphoblastic leukemia in bone marrow aspirates or peripheral blood smears. Convoluted or nonconvoluted nuclear outlines may be seen. Nucleoli are usually inconspicuous. Cytoplasm is generally scant in this lymphoma and lightly basophilic on air-dried smears (Chapter 26).

Burkitt's Lymphoma

The term *small, noncleaved*, used in the Working Formulation to describe Burkitt's and Burkitt's-like (non-Burkitt's, atypical Burkitt's) lymphoma, is somewhat of a misnomer, because the nuclei of these cells are actually larger than the nuclei of small lymphocytic lymphoma or small cleaved cell lymphoma. Nuclei in Burkitt's lymphoma tend to be round and uniform in size and shape and display a coarsely reticulated chromatin pattern. Multiple nucleoli, ranging in number from three to five, are evident (Fig. 13.23). The cytoplasm is usually abundant and deeply basophilic on Wright stain, because of the high RNA content of the cytoplasm. Fine, small cytoplasmic vacuoles often can be appreciated in air-dried smears, but these are not absolutely specific to this diagnosis. Tingible body macrophages are often present, and mitoses may be seen readily.

Burkitt's-like (non-Burkitt's, atypical Burkitt's) lymphoma cells (Fig. 13.24) contain similar round nuclei, usually with a single, conspicuous nucleolus along with a fine delicate chromatin pattern. These lymphomas may be more similar biologically to large cell lymphoma (Chapter 27).

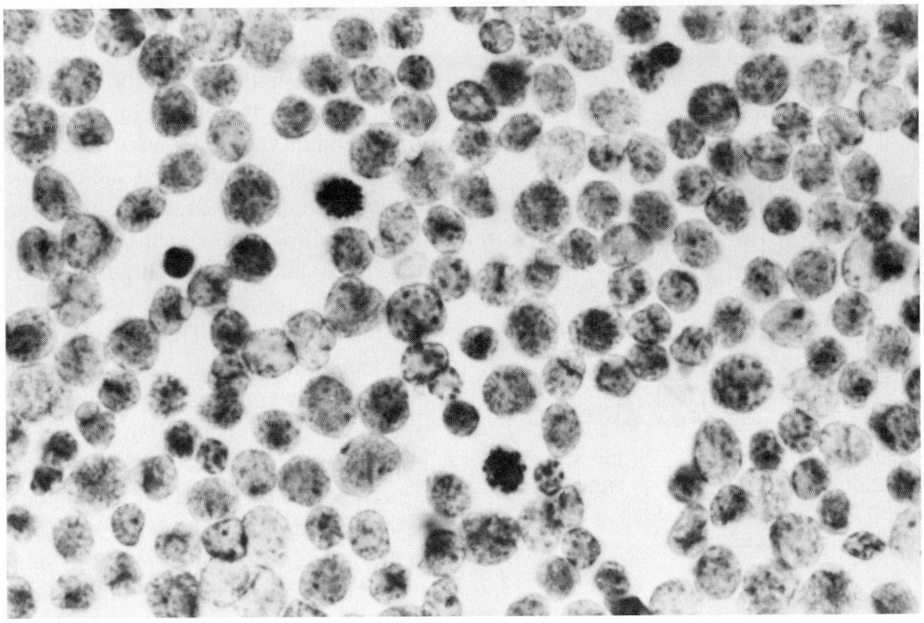

FIG. 13.22. Lymphoblastic lymphoma. Aspirates from lymphoblastic lymphoma typically contain cells with uniform appearing nuclei, finely distributed chromatin and many mitoses (hematoxylin and eosin stain, original magnification: 1,000× magnification).

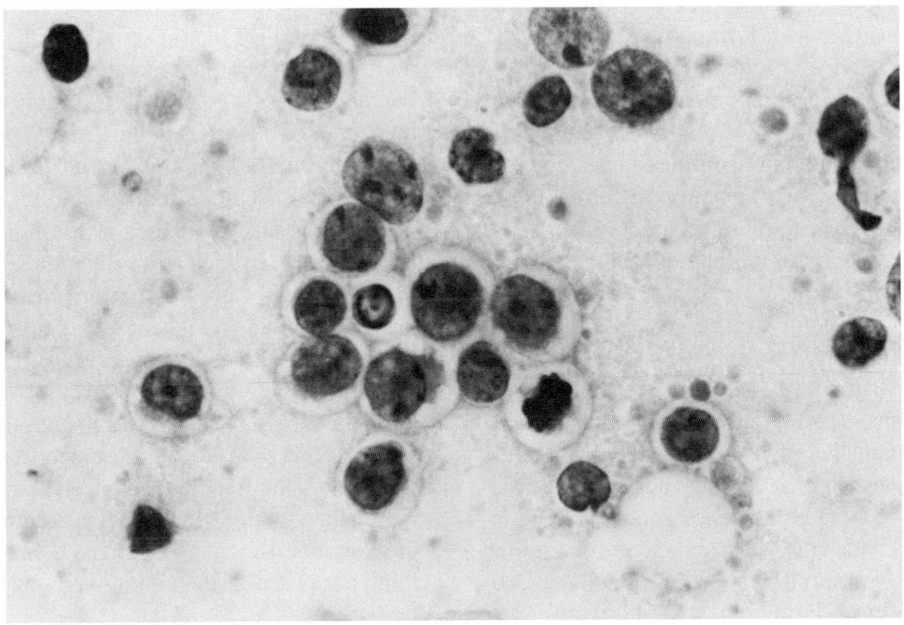

FIG. 13.23. Small noncleaved, Burkitt's lymphoma. The nuclei appear round, uniform in size and typically have many small inconspicuous nucleoli. Mitoses are readily seen (Papanicoloau stain, original magnification: 1,000× magnification).

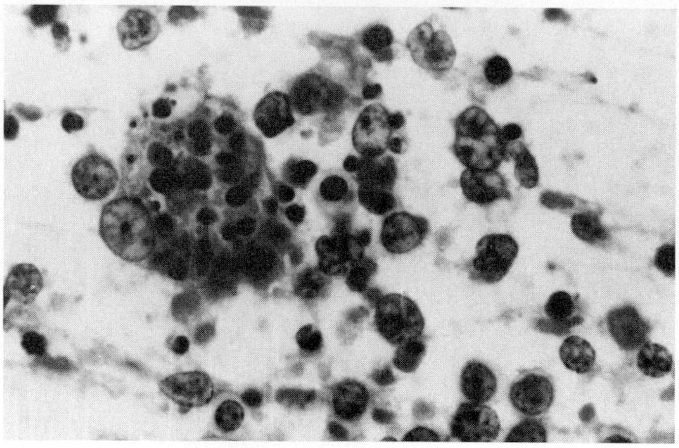

FIG. 13.24. Small noncleaved, non-Burkitt's lymphoma. The nuclei show some variation from cell to cell. A tingible body macrophage is also seen (hematoxylin and eosin stain, original magnification: 1,000× magnification).

Summary of Non-Hodgkin's Lymphomas

There may be limited utility for FNAB in the evaluation of lymphoid neoplasms, in light of the importance of architectural pattern and individual cell morphology in the current classifications of non-Hodgkin's lymphomas (77,78). In addition, many pathologists find it difficult to apply the older literature on FNAB of lymph nodes to their practice.

The results of most FNAB studies of malignant lymphoma have been reported using not the Working Formulation or the Revised European American Lymphoma classification, but rather one of the preexisting schemes (e.g., the Kiel classification) (60,79–81), no classification at all (11–13,23), or a separate cytologic classification of malignant lymphomas (82). Some of these are limited in usefulness, because clinically important distinctions and translation to current terminology cannot be achieved with these schemes. Older series on the cytologic classification of lymph node punctures used outdated descriptions of lymphoid cell types, making it difficult to identify cytomorphologic criteria needed to accurately predict malignant lymphoma subtypes based on FNAB (7–9). Finally, many of the older and some recent studies fail to emphasize the clinically important distinctions that FNAB of malignant lymphoma can offer, such as the distinction between low-grade and high-grade lymphoid malignancies. Exceptions include the series from Australia reported by Russell and colleagues (80) and the series reported by Pilotti and coworkers from Italy (81). In Russell's experience (80), non-Hodgkin's lymphoma was correctly diagnosed in 53 of 59 patients. The cytologic material was deemed to be inadequate in five of the remaining six patients. The remaining patient had cytologic material that was interpreted as being normal or reactive. An important conclusion of this study is that FNAB can separate high- from low-grade lymphoid malignancies; no high-grade non-Hodgkin's lymphoma was misclassified as a low-grade lymphoma. In 15 of 16 cases, the cytologic diagnoses correlated with the histologic diagnoses as to the subtype of high-grade non-Hodgkin's lymphoma (15 of 16 cases). Some difficulty was encountered in diagnosing the specific subtype of low-grade non-Hodgkin's lymphoma in this study. Of 27 cases of low-grade lymphoma, the most difficult subtype to recognize and correctly diagnose was the centrocytic or centroblastic (which includes mixed, small, and large cell lymphoma). Of the 22 centrocytic or centroblastic cases, three were diagnosed as unclassified, high-grade non-Hodgkin's lymphoma, one as centrocytic (small cleaved cell lymphoma), and one as reactive. The remaining examples of low-grade non-Hodgkin's lymphoma in this series were correctly subclassified. Even in light of the difficulty in recognizing centrocytic or centroblastic lymphoma, 17 of 22 cases of low-grade lymphoma were classified correctly. Similar results were reported by Pilotti and colleagues (81). All 16 of their cases of high-grade lymphoma were recognized as such. Difficulty was encountered in establishing a malignant diagnosis in cases of low-grade lymphoma, particularly follicular lymphoma. However, no low-grade lymphomas were misclassified as high-grade.

The morphologic appearance of low-grade lymphomas on FNAB may be mistaken easily for benign, reactive lymphoid processes; this difficulty has major implications for patient care. In many series (13,14,60,80–82) patients who were determined mistakenly to have reactive adenopathy subsequently were shown to have low-grade lymphomas. Despite this morphologic limitation of the aspirate technique in the evaluation of low-grade non-Hodgkin's lymphomas, it is important to realize that in some clinical settings of low-grade non-Hodgkin's lymphoma, therapy is withheld until the patient becomes symptomatic or shows transformation to a higher grade lymphoma. In a study performed at Stanford (83), minimally symptomatic untreated patients with low-grade non-Hodgkin's lymphoma did as well as the cohort of patients that was treated after tissue diagnosis. Some of the untreated patients showed spontaneous regression, and the incidence of progression or transformation to a higher-grade lymphoid malignancy was no different between the treated and untreated groups. Thus, a false negative result based solely on morphology of a low grade non-Hodgkin's lymphoma seen in FNAB specimens is not likely to affect the patient's outcome adversely or significantly alter therapeutic decision making. If confronted with persistent or progressive lymphadenopathy after FNAB evaluation suggests a reactive process, one should recommend a surgical biopsy to determine the cause of the continued nodal enlargement.

Hodgkin's Disease

Diagnostic Reed-Sternberg cells may be easy or difficult to identify on FNAB, depending on the histopathologic type of Hodgkin's disease. Hodgkin's disease not otherwise specified was diagnosed with 91.8% accuracy in one study (84), but the accuracy of subtyping Hodgkin's disease was only 83.1%. The typical aspirate smear contains a dispersed popu-

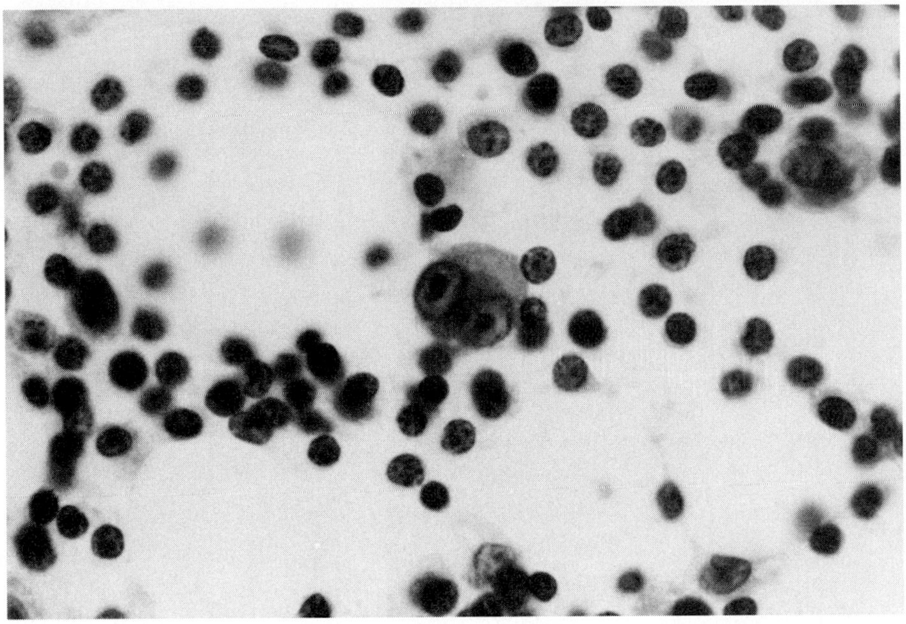

FIG. 13.25. Hodgkin's disease. Aspirates frequently display a mixture of small and large lymphoid cells with scattered Reed-Sternberg cells (Papanicoloau stain, original magnification: 600× magnification).

lation of admixed small, medium-sized, and large lymphoid cells, in which there are scattered, markedly enlarged, atypical cells. The latter usually are apparent on low-power with scanning magnification (Fig. 13.25). These large atypical cells have moderately abundant cytoplasm and frequently bilobed or polylobated nuclei that contain prominent round nucleoli. Often the nucleoli have smooth contours and occupy 25% or more of the lobated nucleus diameter. Classic Reed-Sternberg cells seen in alcohol-fixed and air-dried stained material are illustrated in Figure 13.26. If diagnostic Reed-Sternberg cells are identified in the appropriate polymorphous, dispersed population, the diagnosis of Hodgkin's disease should be made. Reed-Sternberg–like cells mimicking Hodgkin's disease may be seen in other diseases (85), but with lymph node FNAB, the background pathologic processes rarely should be mistaken for Hodgkin's disease. Examples of malignant melanoma and carcinoma as described by Strum and colleagues (85) should be recognized as nonhematolymphoid neoplasms with FNAB, for the reasons described subsequently.

A,B

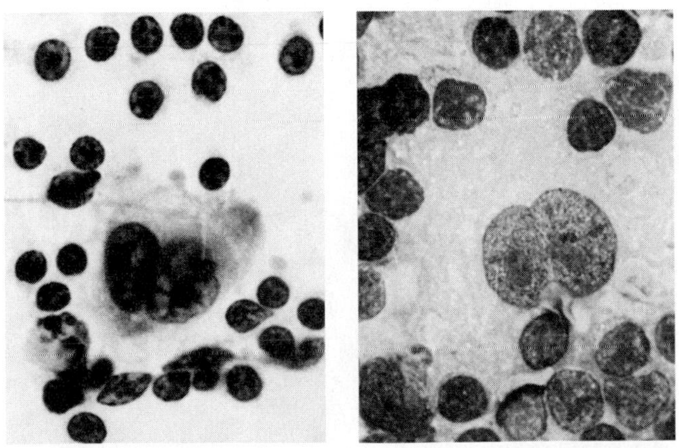

FIG. 13.26. Hodgkin's disease. Diagnostic Reed-Sternberg cells are seen (**A:** Papanicoloau stain, original magnification: 1,000× magnification; **B:** May-Grünwald-Giemsa stain, original magnification: 1,000× magnification).

Cytospin preparations from FNAB specimens in some cases allow the identification of Hodgkin's disease–associated antigens on the large atypical cells, as recognized by anti-CD15 and -CD30 antibodies (Fig. 13.27). In nodular lymphocyte predominance Hodgkin's disease, so-called popcorn or L and H cells may be recognized on FNAB (Fig. 13.28); however, it may be significantly more difficult to recognize nodular lymphocyte predominance Hodgkin's disease than classic forms of Hodgkin's disease (81).

In addition to diagnosing Hodgkin's disease in the initial evaluation of lymphadenopathy, FNAB can be helpful in establishing the stage of disease and recognizing unusual tumor distribution within a given stage or recurrent disease after therapy. Friedman and colleagues (24) found the technique useful in the management of their patients with known Hodgkin's disease. Hodgkin's disease was correctly diagnosed in 161 (88%) of 182 cases. The relative proportion of diagnostic Reed-Sternberg cells present in the four histopathologic subtypes may have influenced the percentages of false negative cases seen in their series. Specifically, although two of eight (25%) cases of lymphocyte predominance Hodgkin's disease were misdiagnosed as reactive, only 2 (4%) of 48 cases of Hodgkin's disease with mixed cellularity were not recognized properly. At the time of a relapse, the yield of Reed-Sternberg cells might be expected to be increased; Colby and Warnke (86) showed that in about

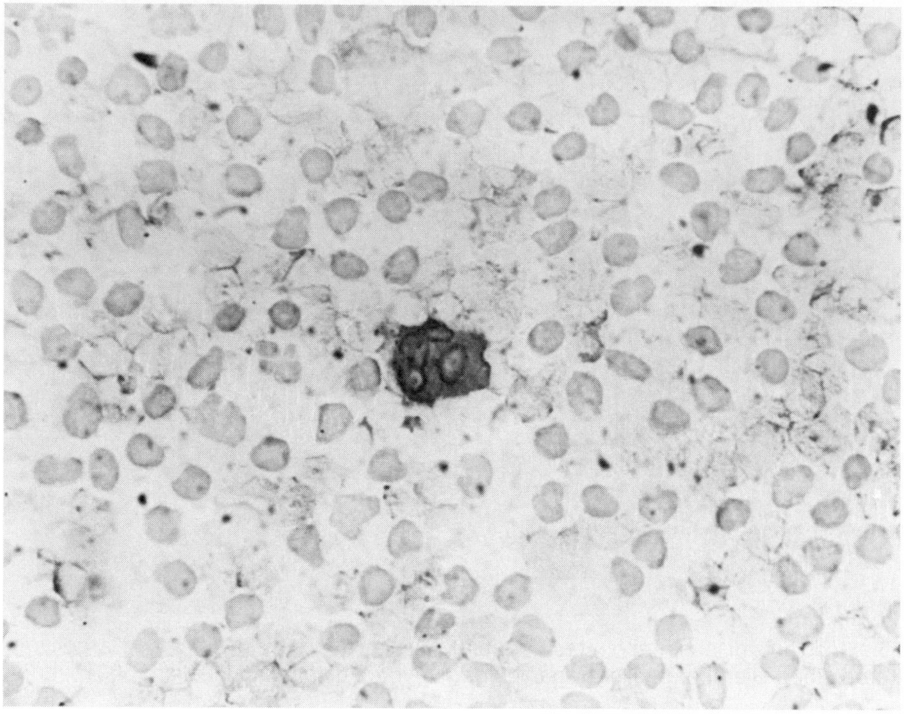

FIG. 13.27. Hodgkin's disease. The antigranulocyte marker CD15 is expressed by this polylobated variant of the Reed-Sternberg cell (cytospin preparation, immunoperoxidase stain, original magnification: 640× magnification). (From *Pathology Annual 1988*, part 2. Norwalk: Appleton and Lange, 1988, with permission.)

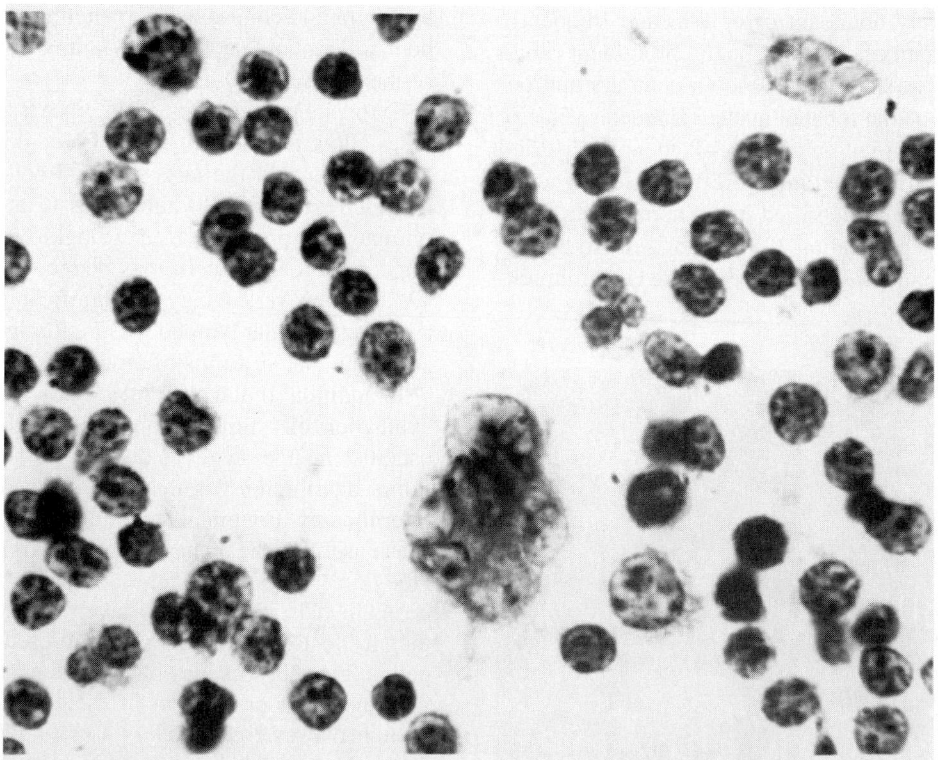

FIG. 13.28. Hodgkin's disease, nodular lymphocyte predominance type. In addition to numerous, small, mature-appearing lymphocytes and occasional histiocytes (*upper right corner*), a "popcorn" cell or L and H Hodgkin's cell is noted in the low center (hematoxylin and eosin stain, original magnification: 1,000× magnification). (From *Pathology Annual 1988*, part 2. Norwalk: Appleton and Lange, 1988, with permission.)

50% of relapses of Hodgkin's disease an increase in the number of atypical cells on histologic examination is seen. The likelihood of recognizing Reed-Sternberg cells in FNAB specimens in recurrent Hodgkin's disease may be even greater; approximately 40% of the cases studied by Colby and Warnke (86) showed a decrease in the number of background normal-appearing lymphocytes. Insufficient material was obtained through needle aspiration of lymph nodes in 20% of patients with Hodgkin's disease in another series (24). About half of the unsatisfactory aspirations were in minimally enlarged (less than 1 cm) lymph nodes. Other factors contributing to the inability to aspirate sufficient material included locations that were difficult to reach (e.g., high axillary), nodular sclerosing histologic subtype, and postradiation residue. The latter masses generally are formed by nodules of hyalinized connective tissue, in which only scattered lymphoid cells are present (87) (Chapter 17). In view of the histopathology of these residual treated masses, it is not surprising that FNAB would yield insufficient cells for satisfactory cytomorphologic examination.

Histiocytic and Dendritic Cell Neoplasms

The key to diagnosing Langerhans cell histiocytosis is the identification of the characteristic nuclear features of Langerhans cells, which usually are admixed with numerous eosinophils. Langerhans cell nuclei have a folded, indented, or grooved appearance, generally with a fine chromatin pattern, inconspicuous nucleoli, and a thin nuclear membrane. One must keep in mind that dermatopathic lymph nodes may contain numerous Langerhans cells and eosinophils; therefore, one must consider dermatopathic lymphadenitis in the cytologic differential diagnosis. FNAB in sinus histiocytosis with massive lymphadenopathy shows large histiocyte-like cells with abundant pale, eosinophilic cytoplasm containing well-preserved lymphocytes and occasional plasma cells and granulocytes. The diagnosis can be supported by the demonstration of S-100 protein in the large cells (88).

There is only scant information on FNAB findings in dendritic cell tumors. In one study of two cases of follicular dendritic cell tumors, cellular smears showed cells forming syncytia of varying size, in addition to a prominent single-cell population (89). The cell borders were poorly defined with the syncytia, and the cytoplasm was abundant, eosinophlic, and focally fibrillary in nature. The nuclei were round to oval and moderately pleomorphic, with a spindle cell component. Mature lymphocytes were present, intimately associated with the cells forming the syncytia and scattered among the single-cell population. As in the tissue diagnosis of follicular dendritic cell tumor, immunostains are essential to establish a definitive diagnosis, particularly a specific dendritic cell marker such as DRC1 or the complement markers CD21 or CD35.

TABLE 13.1.

Series	Total cases no.	Reactive cases,[a] %
Frable (11)	173	30
Frable and Frable (12)	649	38
Ramzy et al. (13)	350	27
Kline et al. (14)	340	35
Gertner et al. (15)	138	58

[a] Corrected for false negative cases.

Adapted from Pitts WC, Weiss LM. Fine needle aspiration biopsy of lymph nodes. In: Rosen PP, Fechner RE, eds. *Pathology Annual* 1988, part 2. Norwalk, CT: Appleton & Lange, 1988:329–360, with permission.

Metastatic Neoplasms

Undifferentiated Carcinomas

The evaluation of enlarged lymph nodes by FNAB in the setting of suspected metastatic carcinoma is clinically useful. In several large series of FNAB of lymph nodes, metastatic cancer represented about 50% of the reported cases (Table 13.1). In addition to low cost and rapidity of diagnosis (12), FNAB of lymph nodes can tailor further clinical decision making regarding the investigation for potential primary sites if an initial FNAB reveals metastatic carcinoma (22). Metastatic carcinoma can yield both nodular and dispersed cell patterns composed of monomorphous or polymorphous cells. Key features to identify include cohesive cell groupings (Fig. 13.29), common cell borders, epithelial cytoplasmic differentiation (mucin vacuoles on air-dried preparations, squamous differentiation on Papanicolaou stains) and nuclear molding. The latter is an important feature in recog-

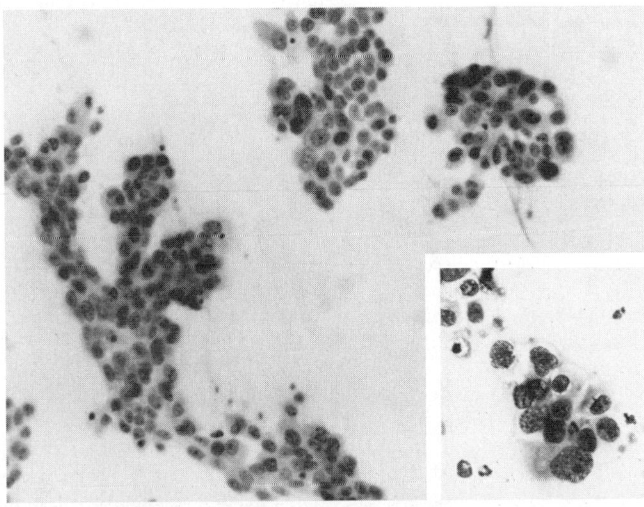

FIG. 13.29. Metastatic carcinoma. Intact, cohesive cell groupings composed of cells with relatively abundant cytoplasm characterize many metastatic carcinomas (hematoxylin and eosin stain, original magnification: 100× magnification; **Insert:** May-Grünwald-Giemsa, original magnification: 100× magnification). (From *Pathology Annual 1988*, part 2. Norwalk: Appleton and Lange, 1988, with permission.)

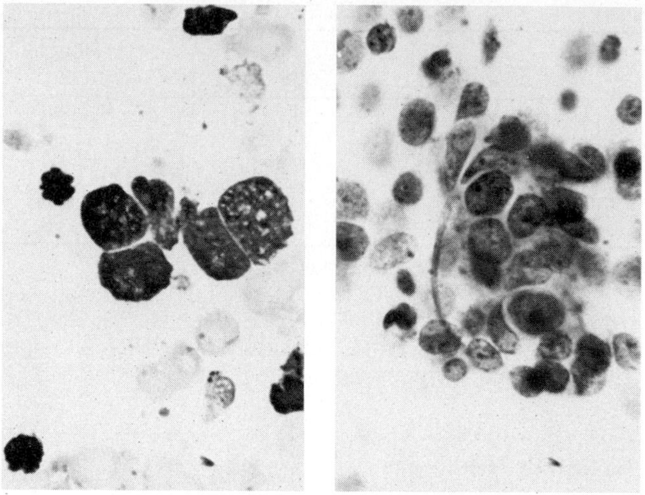

A,B

FIG. 13.30. Metastatic small cell undifferentiated carcinoma of the lung. Nuclear molding is easily identified in PAP (**A**) and May-Grünwald-Giemsa stains (**B**). The neoplastic cells have fine to coarse, evenly dispersed chromatin and scanty cytoplasm. Aggregates of cohesive tumor cells are a helpful feature in recognizing metastatic oat cell carcinoma (original magnification: 1,000× magnification). (From *Pathology Annual 1988*, part 2. Norwalk: Appleton and Lange, 1988, with permission.)

nizing metastatic small cell undifferentiated carcinoma (Fig. 13.30). In a study of fine needle aspiration cytology performed on neck lymph node metastases, a presumption of primary sites could be achieved for the thyroid (monolayered papillary fronds with intranuclear cytoplasmic inclusions), perioral (large, polygonal, keratinized cells with a low nuclear : cytoplasmic ratio and anucleated squames), and nasopharyngeal carcinomas (numerous naked and destroyed nuclei and marked lymphocytic infiltrates) (90). Epithelial markers, such as cytokeratin, and tumor-specific markers, such as prostate-specific antigen, can be applied easily to direct aspirate smears or cytospin samples.

Malignant Melanoma

Fine needle aspiration biopsy is a very accurate, rapid, and cost-efficient way to establish the diagnosis of malignant melanoma metastatic to lymph nodes (91). A detailed description of the cytomorphologic features of malignant melanoma is available (92). The cell pattern on scanning magnification in malignant melanoma involving lymph nodes may be dispersed or nodular and similarly monomorphous or polymorphous in cell type. Most melanoma cells have a polygonal or fusiform shape and contain moderately abundant cytoplasm. Nuclei are rounded or oblong and often show intranuclear cytoplasmic invaginations and prominent nucleoli (Fig. 13.31). The cytoplasm may appear dusty brown in alcohol-fixed material; in the air-dried preparations it stains blue to dark purple. One also may see small vacuoles in air-dried material. Occasionally tumor cells may contain bizarre, giant nuclei, a feature not seen in lymphoid cells. Antibodies directed against the S-100 protein or melanoma-specific antigen also may aid in documenting cases of metastatic malignant melanoma.

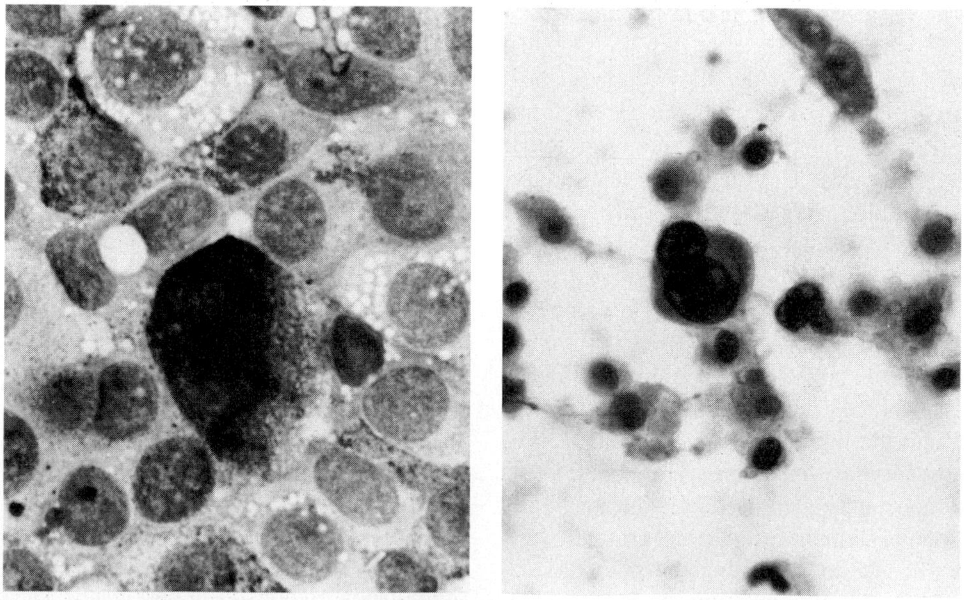

A B

FIG. 13.31. Metastatic melanoma. There is generally a marked tendency toward cellular dispersion in aspirates from metastatic melanoma. Air-dried smears may show a granular blue to purple staining of the cytoplasm with May-Grünwald-Giemsa staining (**A**), and intranuclear cytoplasmic invaginations may be seen in fixed material on a Papanicoloau stain (**B**). (**A:** Original magnification: 1,000× magnification; **B:** Original magnification: 200× magnification).

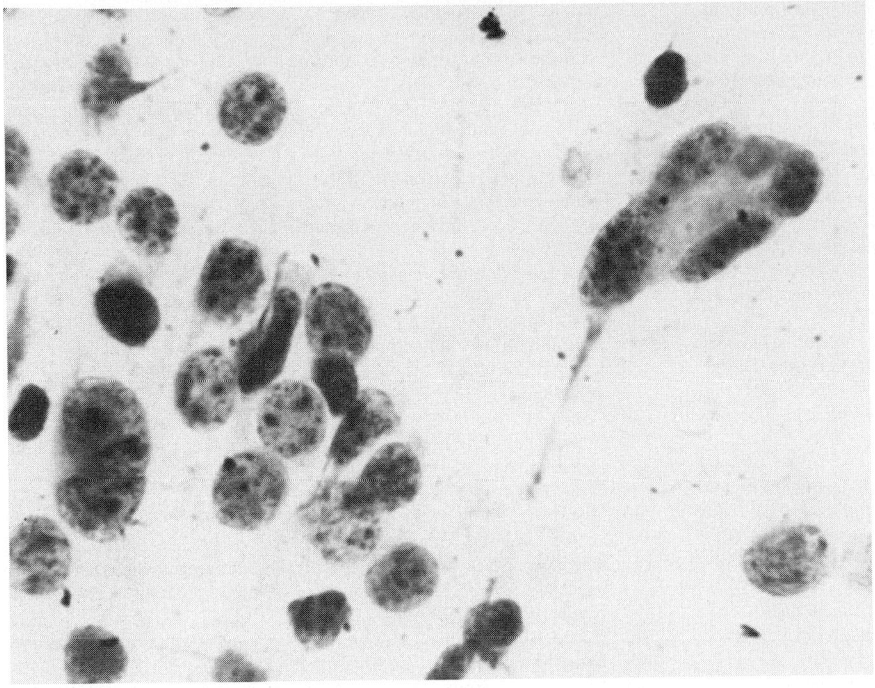

FIG. 13.32. Metastatic neuroblastoma. In addition to loosely aggregated neoplastic cells, a Homer-Wright rosette is present in the *upper right corner* (hematoxylin and eosin stain, 1,000× magnification). (From *Pathology Annual 1988*, part 2. Norwalk: Appleton and Lange, 1988, with permission.)

Small Round Cell Tumors of Childhood

Occasionally, FNAB specimens from enlarged lymph nodes in children who have nonlymphoid small cell malignancies are obtained for interpretation. In these malignancies, such as neuroblastoma, rhabdomyosarcoma, and Ewing's sarcoma, the tumor cells frequently form small cellular aggregates in addition to discohesive cells (Fig. 13.32). The nuclear features of these malignancies help to separate them from malignant lymphoma. The nuclei of neuroblastoma often are round and have a densely speckled chromatin pattern. Rhabdomyosarcoma nuclei tend to be round or oval and have a somewhat vesicular chromatin pattern, occasionally with prominent nucleoli. Additional clues for the separation from malignant lymphoma include the relatively abundant cytoplasm seen in many cases of rhabdomyosarcoma. Ewing's sarcoma tends to have spherical to ellipsoid nuclei with small nucleoli. The chromatin pattern is often faintly stippled. Accurate assessment of nodal involvement is possible with FNAB, prior open biopsy material, and sufficient cytoplasmic differentiation.

CHANGES IN LYMPH NODES ATTRIBUTABLE TO FINE NEEDLE ASPIRATION

Fine needle aspiration of lymph nodes is not a "passive" process and in itself may cause histologic changes that affect subsequent assessment; fortunately, such changes are rare. In one study of 230 cases, changes attributable to FNAB were identified in 10 cases (4.3%) (93). In four cases hemorrhage accompanied by various stages of organization was seen, three cases showed segmental infarction of the nodal parenchyma, and three cases showed total coagulative necrosis. The authors concluded that the FNAB procedure affects histologic assessment of lymph nodes in rare cases if there is florid myofibroblastic proliferation or total infarction; the latter is most likely to occur in lymph nodes involved by malignant lymphoma.

SUMMARY AND CONCLUSIONS

Fine needle aspiration biopsy of lymph nodes is a rapid, relatively inexpensive, and efficient technique for the evaluation of peripheral lymphadenopathy. It is useful in evaluating patients with primary unexplained lymphadenopathy and in patients who have a known malignancy. Although it is not currently the procedure of choice in the primary documentation of malignant lymphoma, this area is undergoing considerable change. The widespread application of lymphoid markers and DNA studies to aspirated material may obviate the necessity to obtain a surgical biopsy in many cases of suspected malignant lymphoma.

REFERENCES

1. Soderstrom N. *Fine-needle aspiration biopsy used as a direct adjunct in clinical diagnostic work.* New York: Grune & Stratton 1966.
2. Zajicek J. Part I: Cytology of supradiaphragmatic organs. In: *Monographs in clinical cytology: aspiration biopsy cytology,* vol. 4. Basel: Karger, 1974.
3. Zajicek J. Part 2: Cytology of infradiaphragmatic organs. In: *Monographs in clinical cytology: aspiration biopsy cytology,* vol. 7. Basel: Karger, 1979.
4. Koss L. On the history of cytology [Editorial]. *Acta Cytol* 1980;24:1–3.
5. Martin HE, Ellis EB. Biopsy by needle puncture and aspiration. *Ann Surg* 1930;92:169–181.
6. Hajdu SI, Melamed MR. Limitations of aspiration cytology in the diagnosis of primary neoplasm. *Acta Cytol* 1984;28:337–345.

7. Morrison M, Samwick AA, Rubinstein J, et al. Lymph node aspiration: clinical and hematologic observations in 101 patients. *Am J Clin Pathol* 1952;2:255–262.
8. Lopes CP. The cytologic diagnosis of lymph node punctures. *Acta Cytol* 1964;8:194–205.
9. Bloch M. Comparative study of lymph node cytology by puncture and histopathology. *Acta Cytol* 1967;11:139–144.
10. Koo CH, Rappaport H, Sheibani K, et al. Imprint cytology of non-Hodgkin's lymphomas: based on a study of 212 immunologically characterized cases. *Hum Pathol* 1989;20(suppl):1–137.
11. Frable WJ. Thin-needle aspiration biopsy: personal experience with 469 cases. *Am J Clin Pathol* 1976;65:168–182.
12. Frable MAS, Frable WJ. Fine-needle aspiration biopsy revisited. *Laryngoscope* 1982;92:1414–1418.
13. Ramzy I, Rone R, Schultenover SJ, et al. Lymph node aspiration biopsy: diagnostic reliability and limitations. An analysis of 350 cases. *Diagn Cytopathol* 1985;1:39–45.
14. Kline TS, Kannan V, Kline IK. Lymphadenopathy and aspiration biopsy cytology: review of 376 superficial nodes. *Cancer* 1984;54: 1076–1081.
15. Gertner R, Podoshin L, Fradis M. Accuracy of fine needle aspiration biopsy in neck masses. *Laryngoscope* 1984;94:1370–1371.
16. Buchino JJ, Jones VF. Fine needle aspiration in the evaluation of children with lymphadenopathy. *Arch Pediatr Adolesc Med* 1994;148: 1327–1330.
17. Oertel J, Oertel B, Lobeck H, et al. Immunocytochemical analysis of lymph node aspirates in patients with human immunodeficiency virus infection. *J Clin Pathol* 1990;43:844–846.
18. Martin-Bates E, Tanner A, Suvarna SK, et al.. Use of fine needle aspiration cytology for investigating lymphadenopathy in HIV positive patients. *J Clin Pathol* 1993;43:564–566.
19. Shapiro AL, Pincus RL. Fine-needle aspiration of diffuse cervical lymphadenopathy in patients with acquired immunodeficiency syndrome. *Otolaryngol Head Neck Surg* 1991;105:419–421.
20. Wolf JS, Cher M, Dall'era M, et al. The use and accuracy of cross-sectional imaging and fine needle aspiration cytology for detection of pelvic lymph node metastases before radical prostatectomy. *J Urol* 1995;153:993–999.
21. Oyen RH, Van Poppel HP, Ameye FE, et al.. Lymph node staging of localized prostatic carcinoma with CT and CT-guided fine-needle aspiration biopsy: prospective study of 285 patients. *Radiology* 1994; 190:315–322.
22. Schultenover SJ, Ramzy I, Page CP, et al. Needle aspiration biopsy: role and limitations in surgical decision making. *Am J Clin Pathol* 1984;82:405–410.
23. Betsill WL, Hajdu SI. Percutaneous aspiration biopsy of lymph nodes. *Am J Clin Pathol* 1980;73:471–479.
24. Friedman M, Kim U, Shimaoka K, et al. Appraisal of aspiration cytology in management of Hodgkin's disease. *Cancer* 1980;45.
25. Carrasco CH, Richli WR, Lawrence D, et al. Fine needle aspiration biopsy in lymphoma. *Radiol Clin North Am* 1990;28:879–883.
26. Martin SE, Zhang H, Magyarosy E, et al. Immunologic methods in cytology: definitive diagnosis of non-Hodgkin's lymphoma using immunologic markers for T-and B-cells. *Am J Clin Pathol* 1984;82: 666–673.
27. Oertel J, Oertel B, Kastner M, et al. The value of immunocytochemical staining of lymph node aspirates in diagnostic cytology. *Br J Haematol* 1988;70:307–316.
28. Tani EM, Christensson B, Porwit A, et al. Immunocytochemical analysis and cytomorphologic diagnosis on fine needle aspiriates of lymphoproliferative disease. *Acta Cytol* 1988;32:209–2152.
29. Cafferty LL, Katz RL, Ordonez NG, et al. Fine needle aspiration diagnosis of intraabdominal and retroperitoneal lymphomas by morphologic and immunocytochemical approach. *Cancer* 1990;65:72–77.
30. Kornstein MJ, Wakely PE, Kardos TF, et al. Dendritic reticulum cell and immunophenotype in aspiration biopsies of lymph nodes: value in the subclassification of non-Hodgkin's lymphomas. *Am J Clin Pathol* 1990;94:165–169.
31. Sneige N, Dekmezian RH, Katz RL, et al. Morphologic and immunocytochemical evaluation of 220 fine needle aspirates of malignant lymphoma and lymphoid hyperplasia. *Acta Cytol* 1990;34:311–322.
32. Dawsey SM, Korn EL, Layfield LJ. Morphometric analysis of the homogeneity of lymphoid cell populations in fine needle aspiration cytology smears. *Am J Clin Pathol* 1989;92:458–464.
33. Witzig TE, Banks PM, Stenson MJ, et al. Rapid immunophenotyping of B-cell non-Hodgkin's lymphomas by flow cytometry. A comparison with the standard frozen-section method. *Am J Clin Pathol* 1990;94: 280–286.
34. Hu E, Horning S, Flynn S, et al. Diagnosis of B cell lymphoma by analysis of immunoglobulin gene rearrangements in biopsy specimens obtained by fine needle aspiration. *J Clin Oncol* 1986;4:278–283.
35. Williams ME, Frierson HF, Tabbarah S, et al. Fine-needle aspiration of non-Hodgkin's lymphoma: Southern blot analysis for antigen receptor, bcl-2, and c-myc gene rearrangements. *Am J Clin Pathol* 1990;93: 754–759.
36. Koss LG. Thin needle aspiration biopsy [Editorial]. *Acta Cytol* 1980; 24:1–3.
37. Christopherson WM. Cytologic detection and diagnosis of cancer: its contribution and limitations. *Cancer* 1983;51:1201–1208.
38. Ljung B. Fine-needle aspiration of the thyroid nodule. *Ann Intern Med* 1982;96:221–232.
39. Cohen MB, Rodgers RPC, Hales MS, et al. Influence of training and experience in fine-needle aspiration biopsy of breast: receiver operating characteristics curve analysis. *Arch Pathol Lab Med* 1987;111: 518–520.
40. Zajdela A, Zillhardt P, Voillemot N. Cytological diagnosis by fine needle sampling without aspiration. *Cancer* 1987;59:1201–1205.
41. Abele JS, Miller TR, King EB, et al. Smearing techniques for the concentration of particles from fine needle aspiration biopsy. *Diagn Cytopathol* 1985;1:59–65.
42. Dorfman RF, Warnke RA. Lymphadenopathy simulating the malignant lymphomas. *Hum Pathol* 1974;5:519–550.
43. Warnke RA, Rouse RV. Limitations encountered in the application of tissue section immunodiagnosis to the study of lymphomas and related disorders. *Hum Pathol* 1985;16:326–331.
44. Picker LJ, Weiss LM, Medeiros LJ, et al. Immunophenotypic criteria for the diagnosis of non-Hodgkin's lymphma. *Am J Pathol* 1987;128: 181–201.
45. Kung ITM, Yuen RWS. Fine needle aspiration of the thyroid: Distinction between colloid nodules and follicular neoplasms using cell blocks and 21-gauge needles. *Acta Cytol* 1989;33:56–60.
46. Warnke RA, Gatter KC, Falini B, et al. Diagnosis of human lymphoma with monoclonal antileukocyte antibodies. *N Engl J Med* 1983;309: 1275–1281.
47. Spagnolo DV, Michie SA, Crabtree GS, et al. Monoclonal antikeratin (AE1) reactivity in routinely-processed tissue from 166 human neoplasms. *Am J Pathol* 1985;84:697–704.
48. Michie SA, Spagnolo DV, Dunn KA, et al. A panel approach to the evaluation of the sensitivity and specificity of antibodies for the diagnosis of routinely processed histologically undifferentiated human neoplasms. *Am J Pathol* 1987;88:457–462.
49. Naiem M, Gerdes J, Abdulaziz A, et al. Production of a monoclonal antibody reactive with human dendritic cells and its use in the immunohistological analysis of lymphoid tissue. *J Clin Pathol* 1983;36: 167–175.
50. Saddik M, El Dabbagh L, Mourad WA. Ex vivo fine-needle aspiration cytology and flow cytometric phenotyping in the diagnosis of lymphoproliferative disorders: a proposed algorithm for maximum resource utilization. *Diagn Cytopathol* 1997;16:126–131.
51. Meylan PRA, Burgisser P, Weyrich-Suter C, et al. Viral load and immunophenotype of cells obtained from lymph nodes by fine needle aspiration as compared with peripheral blood cells in HIV-infected patients. *J Acquir Immune Defic Syndr Hum Retrovirol* 1996;13:39–47.
52. Cajigas A, Suhrland M, Harris C, et al. Correlation of the ratio of CD4 + /CD8 + cells in lymph node fine needle aspiration biopsies with HIV clinical status: a preliminary study. *Acta Cytol* 1997;41: 1762–1768.
53. Burgisser P, Spertini F, Weyrich-Suter C, et al. Monitoring responses to antiretroviral treatment in human immunodeficiency virus type 1 (HIV-1)–infected patients by serial lymph node aspiration. *J Infect Dis* 1997;175:1202–1205.
54. Sneige N, Dekmezian R, El Naggar A, et al. Cytomorphologic, immunocytochemical and nucleic acid flow cytometric study of 50 lymph nodes by fine needle aspiration: comparison with results obtained by subsequent excisional biopsy. *Cancer* 1991;67:1003–1007.
55. Weiss LM, Warnke RA, Sklar J, et al. Molecular analysis of the t(14; 18) chromosomal translocation in malignant lymphomas. *N Engl J Med* 1987;317:1185–1189.

56. Smith SS, Fowler LJ, Hausenfluke L, et al. Diagnosis of Epstein-Barr virus associated nasopharyngeal carcinoma using fine-needle aspiration biopsy and molecular diagnostics. *Diagn Cytopathol* 1995;13: 155–159.
57. Pacchioni D, Negro F, Valente G, et al. Epstein-Barr virus detection by in situ hybridization in fine-needle aspiration biopsies. *Diagn Mol Pathol* 1994;3(2):100–104.
58. Stewart CJR, Farquharson MA, Kerr T, et al. Immunoglobulin light chain mRNA detected by in situ hybridisation in diagnostic fine needle aspiration cytology specimens. *J Clin Pathol* 1996;49:749–754.
59. O'Dowd GJ, Frable WF, Behm FG. Fine needle aspiration cytology of benign lymph node hyperplasias: diagnostic significance of lympho-histiocytic aggregates. *Acta Cytol* 1985;29:554–558.
60. Orell SR, Skinner JM. The typing of non-Hodgkin's lymphomas using fine needle aspiration cytology. *Pathology* 1982;14:389–394.
61. Jayaram N, Ramaprasad AV, Chethan M, et al. Toxoplasma lymphadenitis: analysis of cytologic and histopathologic criteria and correlation with serologic tests. *Acta Cytol* 1997;41:653–658.
62. Jayaram G, Boo Peh K. Fine-needle aspiration cytology in Kimura's disease. *Diagn Cytopathol* 1995;13:295–299.
63. Weiss LM, Hu E, Wood GS, et al. Clonal rearrangements of the T cell receptor gene in mycosis fungoides and dermatopathic lymphadenopathy. *N Engl J Med* 1985;313:539–544.
64. Christ ML, Feltes-Kennedy M. Fine needle aspiration cytology of toxoplasmic lymphadenitis. *Acta Cytol* 1982;26:425–428.
65. Frable MAS, Frable WJ. Fine needle aspiration biopsy: efficacy in the diagnosis of head and neck sarcoidosis. *Laryngoscope* 1984;94: 1281–1283.
66. Silverman JF. Fine needle aspiration cytlogy of cat scratch disease. *Acta Cytol* 1985;29:542–547.
67. Sacks EL, Donaldson SS, Gordon J, et al. Epithelioid granulomas associated with Hodgkin's disease: clinical correlations in 55 previously untreated patients. *Cancer* 1978;41:562–567.
68. Kim H, Jacobs C, Warnke R, et al. Malignant lymphoma with a high content of epithelioid histiocytes: a distinct clinicopathologic entity and a form of so-called "Lennert's lymphoma." *Cancer* 1978;41:620–635.
69. Kung ITM, Ng W, Yuen RWS, et al. Kikuchi's histiocytic necrotizing lymphadenitis: diagnosis by fine needle aspiration. *Acta Cytol* 1990; 34:323–328.
70. Gupta AK, Nayar M, Chandra M. Critical appraisal of fine needle aspiration cytology in tuberculous lymphadenitis. *Acta Cytol* 1992;36: 391–394.
71. Hsu C, Leung BSY, Lau S, et al. Efficacy of fine-needle aspiration and sampling of lymph nodes in 1,484 chinese patients. *Diagn Cytopathol* 1990;6:154–159.
72. Layfield LJ, Glasgow BJ, DuPuis MH. Fine needle aspiration of lymphadenopathy of suspected infectious etiology. *Arch Pathol Lab Med* 1985;109:810–812.
73. Bottles K, Cohen MB, Brodie H, et al. Fine needle aspiration cytology of lymphadenopathy in homosecual males. *Diagn Cytopathol* 1986;2: 31–35.
74. Warnke RA, Strauchen JA, Burke JS, et al. Morphologic types of diffuse large-cell lymphoma. *Cancer* 1982;50:690–695.
75. Yazdi HM, Burns BF. Fine needle aspiration biopsy of Ki-1-positive large-cell "anaplastic" lymphoma. *Acta Cytol* 1991;35:306–310.
76. McCluggage WG, Anderson N, Herron B, et al. Fine needle aspiration cytology, histology and immunohistochemistry of anaplastic large cell Ki-1-positive lymphoma. *Acta Cytol* 1996;40:779–785.
77. Non-Hodgkin's Lymphoma Pathologic Classification Project. National Cancer Institute sponsored study of classifications of non-Hodgkin's lymphomas: summary and description of a Working Formulation for clinical usage. *Cancer* 1982;49:2112–2135.
78. Harris NL, Jaffe ES, Stein H, et al. A revised European-American classification of lymphoid neoplasms: proposal from the International Lymphoma Study Group. *Blood* 1994;84:1361–1392.
79. Lopes Cardozo P. The significance of fine needle aspiration cytology for the diagnosis and treatment of malignant lymphomas. *Folia Haematolog (Leipzig)* 1980;107:601–620.
80. Russell J, Skinner J, Orell S, et al. Fine needle aspiration cytology in the management of lymphoma. *Aust N Z J Med* 1983;13:365–368.
81. Pilotti S, Di Palma S, Alasio L, et al. Diagnostic assessment of enlarged superficial lymph nodes by fine needle aspiration. *Acta Cytol* 1993;37: 853–866.
82. Qizilbash AH, Elavathil LJ, Chen V, et al. Aspiration biopsy cytology of lymph nodes in malignant lymphoma. *Diagn Cytopathol* 1985;1: 18–22.
83. Horning SJ, Rosenberg SA. The natural history of initially untreated low grade non-Hodgkin's lymphomas. *N Engl J Med* 1984;311: 1471–1475.
84. Das DK, Gupta SK, Datta BM, et al. Fine needle aspiration cytodiagnosis of Hodgkin's disease and its subtypes: I. Scope and limitations. *Acta Cytol* 1989;34:329–336.
85. Strum SB, Park JK, Rappaport H. Observation of cells resembling Sternberg-Reed cells in conditions other than Hodgkins disease. *Cancer* 1970;26:176–190.
86. Colby TV, Warnke RA. The histology of the initial relapse of Hodgkin's disease. *Cancer* 1980;45:289–292.
87. Chen JL, Osborne BM, Butler JJ. Residual fibrous masses in treated Hodgkin's disease. *Cancer* 1987;60:407–413.
88. Pettinato G, Manivel JC, d'Amore ESG, et al. Fine needle aspiration cytology and immunocytochemical characterization of histiocytes in sinus histiocytosis with massive lymphadenopathy (Rosai-Dorfman syndrome). *Acta Cytol* 1990;34:771–777.
89. Wright CA, Nayler SJ, Leiman G. Cytopathology of follicular dendritic cell tumors. *Diagn Cytopathol* 1997;17:138–142.
90. Liu YJ, Lee YT, Hsieh SW, et al. Presumption of primary sites of neck lymph node metastases on fine needle aspiration cytology. *Acta Cytol* 1997;41:1477–1482.
91. Basler GC, Fader DJ, Yahanda S, et al. The utility of fine needle aspiration in the diagnosis of melamona metastatic to lymph nodes. *J Am Acad Dermatol* 1997;36:403–408.
92. Layfield LJ, Ostrzega N. Fine needle aspirate morphology in metastatic melanoma. *Acta Cytol* 1989;33:606–612.
93. Tsang WYW, Chan JKC. Spectrum of morphologic changes in lymph nodes attributable to fine needle aspiration. *Hum Pathol* 1992;23: 562–65.

CHAPTER 14

Diagnostic Significance of Morphologic Patterns of Lymphoid Proliferations in Lymph Nodes

Bharat N. Nathwani, Antonio M. Hernandez, and Milton R. Drachenberg

In this era of immunology and molecular biology (1–7) and with the impending advent of gene chips as diagnostic tools (8), it is necessary periodically to question the value of microscopic morphology. Proponents of gene chips have suggested that, in the near future, because these DNA biochips will consist of arrays of specific molecular codes for various infectious microbes and different types of leukemias and lymphomas, cells obtained by fine needle aspiration will be sufficient to make an accurate diagnosis (8). The profound implications of this for pathologists are that morphology rapidly will lose its value and eventually may not be required. We believe, however, that it will take 5 to 20 years or more for these DNA biochips to become a part of the routine practice of pathology. It is necessary that pathologists maintain their microscopic diagnostic skills, because morphology is the first and most important step toward making an accurate diagnosis (9–11). There are many problems with morphology, however, that we discuss in this chapter. We also discuss solutions to some of these problems, which consist of using cytologic and low-magnification approaches to diagnosis. After emphasizing the practicality and importance of the evaluation of architectural features, patterns, and colors, we define types of patterns in lymph node pathology and their differential diagnoses.

PROBLEMS IN ANATOMIC PATHOLOGY

The effective practice of surgical and lymph node pathology requires that the pathologist recognize the limitations and inherent problems of morphology.

B. N. Nathwani: Department of Pathology, University of Southern California, Los Angeles, California 90033

A. M. Hernandez and M. R. Drachenberg: Long Beach Memorial Medical Center, Long Beach, California 90801-1428

Surgical Pathology

Too Many Diseases and Features

There are more than 5,000 diseases dealt with in surgical pathology, and their recognition depends on the identification of 10,000 features (12). It is almost impossible for any pathologist to remember the diagnostic criteria for all these diseases or the images of every histologic feature. Moreover, each disease has different stages and can have a wide spectrum of features, further compounding the diagnostic difficulties (12,13).

Lack of Dictionary and Vocabulary for Features

Pathologists make diagnoses on the basis of histologic features, but systematically organized definitions of histologic features are generally lacking in surgical pathology. Moreover, there are very few books or atlases organized according to histologic features (14–19).

Explosion and Complexity of New Knowledge

The diagnostic difficulties encountered by pathologists are compounded by the explosion of new knowledge in the fields of immunology, molecular biology, and cell kinetics. Pathologists feel overwhelmed by the sheer volume and complexity of new information. The rate at which new knowledge is becoming available outstrips our ability to comprehend it and to utilize it effectively in our practices. This is aggravated by a lack of correlation with histopathology in many published papers.

Evolving and Changing Concepts

Experience suggests that what we see is influenced greatly by what we know. In addition, the terminology and the classification system that we use are influenced by what we have learned, by our individual and prevailing concepts, and also by our pride and prejudices.

"Sensitization" Factor for Recognizing Features

Recognizing features accurately, to a great extent, depends on a phenomenon for which we use the term *sensitization*. We believe that for an image of a feature to be imprinted permanently in memory, it is necessary that it be seen many times, probably from five to several hundred, depending on how frequently the image is seen and for how long, and on what types of other images have been imprinted in the memory.

Lymph Node Pathology

Artifacts and Fixatives Used (e.g., B5, Formalin, Zinc Formalin)

One of the most important factors influencing diagnostic accuracy is the set of changes produced in cells as a result of different fixatives and artifacts. Without knowledge of these important changes, it is easy to misinterpret cytologic features and patterns, which can lead to errors (20–22).

Dynamic Nature of the Lymph Node

In the examination of histologic sections of different organs, it is apparent that for some organs such as those in the gastrointestinal tract or genitourinary tract, it is relatively easy to evaluate the different tissue compartments or layers sequentially, because these compartments are very well demarcated and very different from each other in appearance. This evaluation often is difficult for lymph node sections. The lymph node is a dynamic organ, the seat of many immune functions intimately supported by an intricate architecture (23,24). The normal lymphoid cells dramatically change their size and nuclear and cytoplasmic appearance in response to stimuli or because of neoplastic transformation. The changes in the cells are also dependent on their location, activation status, and phase in the cell cycle (25,26). As a consequence, the different compartments in the lymph node also increase and decrease in size and change appearance. Moreover, cells of different types migrate throughout, which often results in blurring of the boundaries of the compartments (10,11). A lack of familiarity with these dynamic events can lead to difficulties in rationalizing the different changes occurring in lymphoid tissue at both nodal and extranodal sites.

Inability to Accurately Quantitate Cells

Quantification of cells of different types is very important in differential diagnosis but impossible to achieve with great accuracy. In one of our studies, we counted the total number of cells in one high-power field from a case of small cleaved follicular lymphoma and found that there were 1,314. It took us 22 minutes to count these cells in this field, and by the time we finished we were exhausted and knew that our error was at least ± 200 cells (27).

Spectrum of Histologic Features

Many benign and malignant lymphoid cells have wide cytologic spectra. For example, lacunar cells can vary in size from 30 to 200 μm or more (28). Moreover, their appearance varies depending on the fixative used (28). In addition, differences in the duration of fixation and processing also induce variations in the appearance of many types of cells.

Limited Experience and Knowledge

The ability to distinguish different patterns and cells with accuracy and to quantify them with some degree of confidence is entirely a function of experience. To do this well probably requires the study of thousands of lymph node biopsy sections at a rate of 5 to 10 per day. Only the few lymph node pathologists see a large volume of lymph node biopsies. General pathologists deal with a few lymph nodes each year and also have to do surgical and autopsy pathology, microbiology, virology, and chemistry.

Inadequate Sampling

In this era of fine needle aspiration and needle biopsy, inadequate sampling is a problem for pathologists, especially because of the demand for immunologic and genetic analysis for diagnostic and research purposes, which further reduces the amount of material available for study. Pathologic lesions are often focal, especially in patients who are infected with HIV or otherwise immunocompromised. Neoplastic conditions can coexist with reactive elements in a lymph node. The presence or progression of lymphoma is often focal, and metastases also may be focal.

SOLUTIONS TO PROBLEMS

We have made errors in our practice, and we are aware of why mistakes are made in lymph node pathology by other pathologists and by residents. To minimize the problems and the inherent difficulties, many investigators have suggested solutions to some of these problems. We built a highly interactive "expert system" for lymph node pathology, with a videodisc including a systematic dictionary for histologic features (12,13). We also have found that automated extraction of histologic features by robot microscopes can be useful (29–31). In addition, several authors have written about recognizing different types of artifacts, their causes, and prevention (20–22). There are innumerable publications on immunology and molecular biology, which have assisted pathologists in making accurate diagnoses; the numerous chapters in this book dealing with these topics are a testament to this. Many pathologists intuitively have adopted an approach that places great emphasis on evaluating cytologic features. We discuss in the next section the advantages and limitations of using the cytologic approach for diagnosing lymph node diseases. Subsequently, we discuss the use of low magnification to evaluate architectural features, patterns, compartments, and colors in lymph node pathology.

CYTOLOGIC APPROACH TO DIAGNOSIS

Young pathologists feel particularly comfortable using the cytologic approach to diagnosis because the area examined cytologically at high magnification (40×, 60×, and 100× objective lenses) is very small compared with the surface area seen with a 2× or 4× objective lens (Table 14.1). The relative smallness of the area inspires confidence because the number of cells examined cytologically in one high-power field is small, and it can be done readily with little effort or training. In addition, at high magnification the cells appear much closer to the eye, larger, and sharper (Table 14.1). Because benign and malignant lymphoid cells of different types are much smaller than the cells and compartments seen in other organs, it seems easier to study lymph nodes at high rather than at low magnification. Because cancer is an abnormality of the cell, conceptually it is much easier to pay attention to cytologic features than to architectural features or patterns. In addition, because all molecular and immunologic research is done at the cellular level, it would seem natural that only cells are important. For these and other reasons, cytologic evaluation is very useful.

On the other hand, as we gained more experience, we gradually realized that we made diagnostic mistakes if we paid too much attention to cytologic features, and we came to the conclusion that relying on cytology alone is like having a car in Seattle without wipers. For example, if the pattern in a lymph node biopsy specimen is completely diffuse, the study of cytologic features is most useful and the only microscopic evaluation possible. A completely diffuse pattern, however, is seen in only 10% of lymph node biopsies. The majority (60%) of non-Hodgkin's lymphomas do not have diffuse patterns but rather have distinctive patterns such as follicular, mantle zone, marginal zone, inverse follicular, follicular colonization, pseudofollicular, interfollicular, and sinus patterns; a completely diffuse pattern is present in only 20% of patients with Hodgkin's lymphoma, with distinctive patterns such as fibrous nodular, lymphocytic and histiocytic (L&H) nodular, interfollicular, and Lennert's patterns seen in the remaining cases. Moreover, benign diseases, which are more common than malignant lymphomas, rarely show a completely diffuse pattern; the hallmark of benign diseases is the presence of multiple small focal pathologies in different compartments. In addition, lymph node slides from patients with carcinoma or sarcoma usually do not exhibit a completely diffuse pattern: In the regional lymph nodes there is evidence of either no metastasis (sinus histiocytosis is most common) or focal or multifocal metastases. Thus, in our estimation, pathologists encounter a completely diffuse pattern in only 10% of the lymph node biopsies that they see in their practices.

Lymphoid cells are fragile and very prone to significant cytologic distortions in their size, nuclear chromatin appearance, staining, and amount of cytoplasm caused by differences in fixation and by artifacts, compared with cells from other organs (20–22). The cells in B5-fixed sections appear to be about 15% to 20% smaller than those in formalin-fixed sections and have finer chromatin structure and sharper nuclear and cytoplasmic membranes. In formalin-fixed sections, on the other hand, the cells appear to be larger, the nuclei appear to be vesicular because of ballooning, and the cytoplasmic borders are poorly defined. In tissues that are not fixed adequately, shrinkage of nuclei is a consistent find-

TABLE 14.1. *Utility of low-magnification and high-magnification evaluations*

Morphology	Low magnification	High magnification
How much surface area is evaluated?	Large	Small
How sharp is the area evaluated?	Not sharp	Very sharp
Can multiple compartments be compared and	Yes	No
transition between compartments be recognized?	Yes (mostly)	Difficult
Can migration (trafficking) of cells be evaluated?	Yes (mostly)	No
Can pathologic processes be found?	Yes	Very difficult
Can patterns be recognized?	Yes	No
Can cells of different types be recognized and how?	Based on colors	Direct study
How accurate are the observations?	Accurate	Accurate
Is it necessary?	Yes	Yes
What is the speed of evaluation per unit area?	Fast	Slow
Can mistakes be made without realizing them?	Occasionally	Commonly
Which artifacts can be recognized?	Venetian blind, chilling, moth-eaten, shatter, dry-earth effect, wrinkled, dark smudgy rim	Bubbly nuclei, nuclear shrinkage, waxy collagen, thick sections, formalin pigment
How easy is it?	Difficult	Easy
Does it require experience?	Much	Little
Can it be reproducibly learned and taught?	Yes	Yes

ing and results in an artifactual increase in the amount of cytoplasm, which is often clear and occasionally eosinophilic and thus appears plasmacytoid. Because of shrinkage and condensation, the nuclear chromatin stains darkly and is obscured. Lymphoblasts or blastic mantle cells can lose their fine chromatin structure and appear like lymphocytes. In some instances less than 5% of the lymph node may present technically optimal areas for cytologic evaluation, and the remainder of the node may not be adequate for evaluation of cytologic features. It is very difficult for young pathologists, without knowledge and familiarity with these changes, to distinguish cytologic artifacts from real findings; this often results in errors in diagnosis (20–22) (Chapter 12).

Diagnostic accuracy can be compromised further if cytologic features are reviewed in smears from fine needle aspiration and sections from needle biopsy of lymph nodes, because the material available for study is very limited in these specimens.

LOW-MAGNIFICATION APPROACH TO DIAGNOSIS

Before we had experience, we placed great emphasis on evaluating cytologic features. As we accumulated significant experience in lymph node pathology, however, we found that our diagnostic approach evolved subconsciously. We spent less time viewing slides at high magnification and more and more at low magnification, studying architectural features, size and shape of different compartments, their relationship to each other, and patterns (9–11). We also began comparing the colors of different compartments, because different colors closely correlate with cells of different types, and this type of comparison allows us to identify cells of certain types rapidly at low magnification (9–11). Using this approach, we can quickly and accurately identify pathologic processes, which in turn allows us to form a diagnosis or a differential diagnosis. We then search carefully at low magnification for specific histologic features of each disease in the differential diagnosis, which further narrows it. We proceed to high magnification with the sole purpose of evaluating specific cytologic features, and we switch back and forth between high and low magnification with specific purposes until we reach a diagnosis. We also slowly have learned in which situations to give precedence to patterns over cytologic features and vice-versa. Both low- and high-magnification evaluations are absolutely necessary to reach a correct diagnosis (Table 14.1). Although we initially review the slides without the clinical history to be unbiased, we subsequently correlate our diagnosis with the clinical history to avoid errors. We judiciously order, if needed, immunostains or molecular studies that resolve a specific differential diagnosis or confirm a diagnosis. This methodical approach has served us well over the years in arriving at an accurate diagnosis and preventing errors.

The value of low magnification evaluation is also apparent in an expert system of lymph node pathology wherein 80% of the histologic features that are used to arrive at a diagnosis deal with architectural features, patterns, and locations of cells in specific compartments (13). The value of low magnification in lymph node pathology has been known for a long time (32–35), and surgical pathologists always have paid great attention to architectural features and patterns (15–19). We also have discussed and tested our approach while teaching and while acquiring knowledge in order to build expert systems for various organ systems (12). During these endeavors we have found that our approach, in fact, is similar to those used by pathologists expert in other organ systems (15–19). Because there are multiple ways of teaching and learning, and our approach to diagnoses is one of several used by pathologists, we urge readers to try other approaches that may help them in their diagnostic practice.

We have considered the specific reasons for the evolution of our approach from cytologic to pattern-based. This switch is directly related to the amount of our experience and has had very little to do with intelligence, hard work, or other abilities. As more and more experience accumulated, we began to recognize features instantly and accurately as soon as we saw them, because they were permanently imprinted in the brains; that is, we became sensitized to the images. Permanent imprinting of images does not take place unless very specific features have been seen over and over again at very frequent intervals. If thousands of images of different types have been imprinted and correlated with diseases, an instantaneous and accurate diagnosis often can be made. When we discovered our ability to make rapid diagnoses at low magnification, we sought additional reasons to explain our "new abilities" or progress. We rationalized that we diagnose (or "see") what we know, and as we know more, we see more. Moreover, what we see also is influenced greatly by our personal, and the prevailing, concepts and also by the criteria we use and our approach to diagnosis. Our reasoning can be appreciated better if one takes into consideration that we do not know or cannot appreciate the value of what we have yet to learn.

Before we explain in detail what we do at low magnification, we must emphasize the need for a microscope equipped to perform two important functions.

Microscope Prerequisites

A microscope must have an objective scanning lens and a continuous rheostat for modulating the intensity of light, because these two features facilitate accurate identification of different types of patterns and the relationship of compartments to one another.

Using a 2× or 2.5× Objective Scanning Lens

The examiner's microscope must have a scanning lens (2× or 2.5× objective) (9). A microscope equipped with a 4× objective is inadequate, because the area examined with this lens is much smaller than a 2× objective lens, and it is difficult to quantify the percentage area of the section occupied by each of the compartments of the lymph node and to recognize different types of patterns.

Creating Optimum Contrast by Modulating Light Intensity

At 2× or 2.5× scanning magnification, numerous histopathologic features of a lymph node may be enhanced or accentuated dramatically by an increase in contrast (9). This is achieved by manipulation of the intensity of the light passing through the microscope condenser. Histopathologic patterns associated with lymphoid diseases are often subtle and easily may be overlooked if there is low contrast, resulting from light of normal intensity passing through the condenser. Contrast should be increased by a gradual decrease in the intensity of light passing through the condenser, until an optimal level is achieved. This requires minimal practice. Once the eye has adjusted to the low level of light, features that previously were not apparent, such as a pseudofollicular pattern or spherical structures, become obvious. Modulating the light intensity in the study of lymph nodes is important, because different histopathologic features and different sections require different intensities of light for optimal enhancement.

Although a decrease in light intensity allows ready recognition of most patterns, if Hodgkin's lymphoma is suspected on the basis of the pattern observed at low light intensity, it is necessary to restore a normal light intensity in order to recognize Sternberg-Reed cells and variants. Increasing the light intensity to normal also allows the recognition of different colors, and thus a correlation between colors and different cell types can be made at low magnification (9).

Recognizing Cells Based on Colors

For accurate recognition of colors, the light passing through the condenser must be of normal intensity. Fine cellular details are visualized best at high magnification. If cells of different types (lymphocytes, transformed lymphoid cells, blast cells, mummified cells, plasma cells, eosinophils, histiocytes, epithelioid cells) occur in *compact groups*, they can be recognized at low magnification on the basis of their colors (Table 14.2) or their locations (e.g., follicles, mantle zones, marginal zones, interfollicular areas, sinuses, medulla).

TABLE 14.2. *Identification of cells based on colors at low magnification*

Cell type	Color or shade
Small lymphoid cells	Black to dark blue
Plasma cells	Purple
"Mummified" cells	Dark purple
Blast cells	Bluish
Large lymphoid (transformed) cells	Pale blue
Eosinophils	Brick red
Epithelioid cells and histiocytes	Pink
Mitotic figures	Black with a surrounding clear space

From Nathwani BN, Burke JS, Winberg CD. Architectural features of normal, neoplastic, and non-neoplastic-lymph nodes: a practical diagnostic approach. In: Murphy GF, Mihm MC, eds. *Lymphoproliferative disorders of the skin.* Boston: Butterworth, 1986.

Assessing Cellularity

As we gained more experience, we realized that one of the reasons why we were able to make rapid diagnoses, at low magnification, was the fact that we intuitively assessed the cellularity of the lymphoid proliferation (number of cells per unit area), which allowed us to come to a quick decision as to whether or not the proliferation was likely to be a non-Hodgkin's lymphoma or some other disease. For example, it is well known that most malignant proliferations, regardless of their cellular origin, exhibit an increased number of cells per unit area (hypercellularity) or an increase in the number of structures, such as glands, per unit area. The same principle applies in lymphoid diseases. It is essential to provide a very brief description of the factors that influence the cellularity of a lymphoid proliferation both at nodal and extranodal sites (Table 14.3).

Factors Influencing Cellularity

Table 14.3 shows that hypercellularity (a great increase in the number of cells per unit area) is dependent on the presence of one or more of the following histologic features: obliterated sinuses, an increase in the number of structures (follicles, pseudofollicles, and mantle cell nodules) present, or an increase in the number of cells per unit area. If cells of similar size have scant cytoplasm and are packed closely together, they appear hypercellular. This is particularly true of small and medium-sized lymphoid cells, because they have more compact chromatins than transformed large lymphoid cells. Per unit area, more small and medium-sized cells can be packed together. Histologic features that cause a proliferation to appear normocellular or hypocellular are preserved follicles, patent or empty sinuses, epithelioid cells, histiocytes, necrosis, fibrocollagenous bands, vascular proliferation, and fatty infiltration of the lymph node. In essence, the smaller the number of nuclei per unit area, the more likely that the proliferation is hypocellular.

Differential Diagnoses Based on Cellularity

Most non-Hodgkin's lymphomas, with the exceptions of angioimmunoblastic T-cell lymphoma, histiocyte-rich large B-cell lymphoma, and histiocyte-rich anaplastic large cell lymphoma, appear very hypercellular (9) (Table 14.4). This is especially true of lymphomas of small to medium cell

TABLE 14.3. *Histologic features affecting cellularity*

Hypercellularity	Normocellularity	Hypocellularity

Sinus obliteration
Pericapsular infiltration
Increase in number of structures per unit area
  Follicles
  Pseudofollicles
  Mantle cell nodules
Increase in number of cells per unit area; cells with darkly staining or hyperchromatic nuclei and scanty cytoplasm
Proliferation of cells of one type (monomorphism)
	Few scattered follicles
	Patent sinuses with histiocytes
		Patent empty sinuses
		Presence of many epithelioid cells, histiocytes, "clear" cells
		Dendritic reticulum cells in follicles
		Vascular proliferation
		Necrosis
		Eosinophilic background
		Presence of fibrosclerosis/hyalization/amyloid
		Infiltration by fat

size, such as mantle cell lymphoma, lymphoblastic lymphoma, and Burkitt's lymphoma. These lymphomas appear hypercellular because the proliferating cells are monomorphic with respect to size (small or medium) and chromatin structure, and they have scant cytoplasm. Follicular lymphomas and small lymphocytic lymphoma with proliferation centers often appear to be hypercellular at low magnification because they show great increases in the number of follicles or "proliferation centers" per unit area (Table 14.4). Lymphocyte depletion Hodgkin's disease shows a preponderance of many large, pleomorphic malignant cells, and grade II nodular sclerosis Hodgkin's lymphoma appears to have hypercellular areas because of the presence of compact clusters and islands of lacunar cells. In leukemia and carcinoma, involved portions appear hypercellular because the proliferating cells have very similar size and chromatin structure. In viral lymphadenitis of various types there is often an exuberant proliferation of monomorphic large cells in multifocal places, and these foci often appear hypercellular at low magnification (Table 14.4).

Benign diseases of many types, especially those showing necrosis or vascular proliferation and many histiocytes or epithelioid cells, appear to be hypocellular or normocellular (Table 14.4). Hodgkin's lymphoma of the mixed cell, L&H nodular, or L&H diffuse type and occasionally marginal zone lymphoma and Kaposi's sarcoma also can appear normocellular, because of the presence of histiocytes in the first two and because involved areas can be focal or multifocal in the last two (Table 14.4).

Identifying Pathologic Processes (Predominant and Focal)

Formation of a differential diagnosis does not begin until the pathologic process has been identified. In many non-

TABLE 14.4. *Differential diagnosis based on cellularity*

Hypercellularity	Normocellularity	Hypocellularity

Mantle cell lymphoma
Lymphoblastic lymphoma
Burkitt's lymphoma
Diffuse large B-cell lymphoma
Follicular lymphoma
Peripheral T-cell lymphoma
Small lymphocytic lymphoma
Lymphoplasmacytoid lymphoma
Anaplastic large cell lymphoma
Plasmacytoma
Hodgkin's lymphocyte depletion
Hodgkin's, nodular sclerosis, grade II
Adult T-cell leukemia/lymphoma
Leukemia
Carcinoma
Viral lymphadenitis
Systemic lupus erythematosus
Dilantin hypersensitivity
Abnormal immune response
	Dermatopathic lymphadenitis
	Follicular hyperplasia
	Rheumatoid arthritis
	Giant lymph node hyperplasia
	  Plasma cell type
	  Hyaline vascular type
	Marginal zone lymphoma
	Kaposi's sarcoma
	Mast cell disease
	Sinus histiocytosis
	Angioimmunoblastic T-cell lymphoma
		Angioimmunoblastic T-cell lymphoma
		AIDS, involutionary
		Cat-scratch disease
		Granulomatous lymphadenitis
		Necrotizing lymphadenitis
		  Kikuchi
		  Non-Kikuchi
		Histiocytosis
		  Sinus
		  Mycobacterial
		Sinus histiocytosis with massive lymphadenopathy
		Sarcoidosis
		Postlymphangiography
		Tuberculosis
		Whipple's disease
		Syphilis
		Hodgkin's disease
		  Mixed cellularity
		  Lymphocytic and histiocytic diffuse
		  Diffuse fibrosis
		T-cell/histiocytic large B-cell lymphoma
		Histiocytic rich anaplastic large cell lymphoma

Hodgkin's lymphomas, the pathologic process is the predominant finding and therefore is obvious. For most benign diseases, Hodgkin's lymphoma, and some non-Hodgkin's lymphomas, the pathologic foci are focal or multifocal, and unless they are recognized a correct diagnosis cannot be reached.

Therefore, in diagnostic pathology one must learn to recognize the location of the pathologic process, whether it is focal or multifocal, and the relationship of the cellular constituents to one another. For a young pathologist, a safe and methodical approach to identifying pathologic processes is to evaluate, sequentially at scanning magnification, the capsule, subcapsular and medullary sinuses, follicles, mantle zones, marginal zones, interfollicular areas, and medulla for abnormalities (9). The abnormalities that occur in these compartments are listed in Table 14.5; their recognition permits formulation of a differential diagnosis. The recognition of abnormalities in each compartment is facilitated by comparing the same compartments with each other. For example, comparison of adjacent follicle center cell compartments with one another and with distant counterparts as to size and shape, whether they are well or poorly defined, and whether one contains particular cell types that are not apparent in another aids in identification of abnormalities. The same is true for comparison of a mantle zone with adjacent mantle zones and those throughout the lymph node with respect to size, shape, thickness, infiltration of the follicle center cell compartment, fusion with adjacent mantle cells, and so forth. With experience, several pathologic processes can be recognized immediately.

The pathologic foci can be recognized because they are well demarcated, and also because their color is different from the neighboring areas; a comparison of subtle differences in color is a useful aid in the identification of focal pathology (9). It is also important to be aware of what constitutes ''normal'' and how it differs from pathologic areas. Many benign diseases produce pathologic lesions in the interfollicular areas that may be focal, multifocal, or present throughout, uniformly (Table 14.6). Normally the interfollicular areas contain a preponderance of small round T lympho-

TABLE 14.5. *Abnormal or pathologic findings in different compartments*

Follicular centers	Mantle zones Marginal zones	Interfollicular	Sinuses	Other
Absent or markedly increased Back-to-back or closely packed Poorly defined Prominent polarity Starry-sky pattern without polarity Atrophic or burnt out Surrounded by mantle zones Radially penetrating blood vessels Hemorrhages or lymphocytic infiltration Marked preponderance of centrocytes or centroblasts Similar cells inside and outside of follicles Colonization by: Benign mantle cells leading to progressively transformed germinal center nodules Malignant mantle cells Malignant monocytoid B cells/ marginal zone B cells Lymphocytic and histiocytic nodules	Mantle zones Mantle zone lymphocytes forming concentric rims Thick mantle zones Mantle cell nodules with or without fusion Irregular or blastic mantle lymphocytes Marginal zones Marginal zone pattern Inverse follicular pattern Confluence Invasion of follicular centers	Interfollicular areas expansion, focal, multifocal, uniform Starry-sky pattern Mottling Epithelioid cell clusters Clusters of monocytoid B cells Intravascular or extravascular clusters of lymphoid cells Overt necrosis Sternberg–Reed (SR) cells and variants Foreign body or Langhans' giant cells Lipid or lipid-like vacuoles Foamy histiocytes Benign histiocytes Langerhans' cells Increased eosinophils Increased neutrophils Increased or immature plasma cells Russell or Dutcher bodies Clusters of plasmacytoid monocytes High mitotic activity Metastatic or leukemic cells	Sinuses distended or completely obliterated Vascular transformation of sinuses	Patterns Psuedofollicles Lymphocytic and histiocytic nodules Progressively transformed germinal center nodules Mass effect Crush artifacts Single-file arrangement Alveolar, organoid, perivascular, rosettes, storiform, herringbone, etc. Capsule, stroma, and vessels Collagenous bands or sclerosis with or without nodule formation Pericapsular infiltration Capsule thickening Marked vascular proliferation Slit-like Non–slit-like Hyalinization of walls of vessels Obliterated lumens Endothelial proliferation

TABLE 14.6. *Differential diagnosis for interfollicular pattern (expansion of interfollicular areas)*

Focal	Multifocal	Throughout
Benign	Benign	Benign
Necrotizing lymphadenitis	Necrotizing lymphadenitis	Interfollicular hyperplasia
Kikuchi–Fujimoto	Kikuchi–Fujimoto disease	AIDS, involutionary
Cat-scratch disease	Cat-scratch disease	Lymphogranuloma venerum
Dermatopathic lymphadenitis	AIDS, involutionary	Dermatopathic lymphadenitis
Paracortical nodular hyperplasia	Toxoplasmosis	Paracortical nodular hyperplasia
Malignant	Lymphogranuloma venerum	Viral lymphadenitis
Interfollicular Hodgkin's disease	Syphilis	Giant lymph node hyperplasia
Carcinoma	Dermatopathic lymphadenitis	Malignant
Kaposi's sarcoma	Paracortical nodular hyperplasia	Interfollicular Hodgkin's disease
Mycosis fungoides	Viral lymphadenitis	Carcinoma
Langerhans' cell histiocytosis	Giant lymph node hyperplasia	Leukemia
	Malignant	Kaposi's sarcoma
	Interfollicular Hodgkin's disease	Mycosis fungoides
	Carcinoma	Langerhans' cell histiocytosis
	Leukemia	Mast cell disease
	Kaposi's sarcoma	Anaplastic large cell lymphoma
	Mycosis fungoides	Plasmacytoma
	Langerhans' cell histiocytosis	Hodgkin's disease, mixed cellularity
	Mast cell disease	Monocytoid B-cell lymphoma
	Anaplastic large cell lymphoma	Hodgkin's nodular sclerosis
	Monocytoid B-cell lymphoma	Small lymphocytic lymphoma
	Hodgkin's nodular sclerosis	Lymphoplasmacytic lymphoma
	Small lymphocytic lymphoma	Peripheral T-cell lymphoma

cytes with some vascular proliferation and very few plasma cells; anything other than this is abnormal. Similarly, normal sinuses are patent and show benign histiocytes; otherwise, a sinus should be considered abnormal.

In summary, we strongly believe that making diagnoses is not a ''gestalt'' but a very well-defined process, involving systematic study of architectural features and patterns and the relationship of one compartment to another, tracking the migratory pathways of cells, and comparing colors. This methodical approach facilitates identification of the pathologic processes, which in most instances constitute distinctive patterns, which in turn have major diagnostic relevance.

Patterns, Their Formation, and Their Utility

To further understand patterns, we must discuss how they are formed. Patterns are formed in lymph nodes because cells of different types (a few hundred to several thousand) are organized and distributed in a very specific manner in different locations. These cells of different types can be recognized accurately at low magnification because they are well demarcated (compartmentalized), and also because they have subtle but significant differences in their colors. For example, if hundreds of cells of only one type, small lymphoid cells with scant cytoplasm, aggregate together and are distributed in a specific way in a specific location, they appear monotonous and can be recognized as small lymphoid cells because they have a dark blue color at low magnification. They can be identified accurately, for instance as mantle cells, if they are well demarcated and arranged in well-defined complete rings around aggregates of hundreds of other cells such as follicle center cells, which have a lighter color at low magnification. The example in the above instance was of follicles; if many follicles are seen in a lymph node, the term *follicular pattern* is used, and a differential diagnosis can be formulated. Many patterns result from an exaggeration of the normal compartment (e.g., follicular centers, mantle zones, marginal zones, sinuses, interfollicular areas) or a marked proliferation of certain cell types, such as starry-sky phagocytes (starry-sky pattern) or epithelioid histiocytes (Lennert's pattern). Other distinctive patterns (e.g., fibrous nodular, pseudofollicular) have no preexisting normal compartments.

The designation of patterns of different types serves as a language that succinctly summarizes some of the most important findings in a lymph node. Table 14.7 shows that for many common lymphoid diseases, there are a few selected histologic features or patterns that are pathognomonic for each disease, and these are always recognizable at low magnification. For example, although clusters of epithelioid cells are seen in toxoplasmosis, Hodgkin's lymphomas, T-cell lymphomas, and other diseases, their presence *within follicles* is characteristic of toxoplasmosis, and such cells can be recognized readily at low magnification. Clusters of monocytoid B cells, which always are seen in toxoplasmosis, also are identifiable at low magnification. Using cytology alone, one would have difficulty recognizing these two features or any other feature or pattern shown in Table 14.7,

TABLE 14.7. *Diagnostic significance of patterns*

Disease	Features/patterns seen at low magnification
Benign	
Giant lymph node hyperplasia, hyaline vascular type	Radially penetrating blood vessels, very thick mantle zones with concentric rimming, marked vascular proliferation (hyalinization) in interfollicular areas *(mantle zone, mottling, and vascular patterns)*
Infectious mononucleosis/viral lymphadenitis	Reactive follicles, mottling by transformed cells, intravascular or extravascular clusters of transformed cells, clusters of monocytoid B cells and epithelioid cells *(interfollicular and mottling patterns)*
Sinus histiocytosis with massive lymphadenopathy	Distended sinuses with histiocytosis and emperipolesis, interfollicular plasmacytosis *(sinus pattern)*
Toxoplasmosis	Reactive follicles, clusters of epithelioid cells encroaching upon and present within follicles, clusters of monocytoid B cells *(follicular and interfollicular patterns)*
Cat-scratch disease	Reactive follicles, multiple foci of interfollicular necrosis and microabscesses, clusters of epithelioid cells *(interfollicular and necrosis patterns)*
HIV early	Numerous reactive follicles with polarity and starry-sky histiocytes, clusters of monocytoid B cells *(follicular pattern)*
Langerhans' cell histiocytosis	Reactive follicles, clusters of Langerhans' cells admixed with eosinophils in sinuses and interfollicular areas *(sinus and interfollicular patterns)*
Kikuchi–Fujimoto disease	Reactive follicles, circumscribed pathologic areas with or without necrosis containing crescent histiocytes and transformed cells, clusters of "immature monocytes," mottling *(interfollicular mottling, necrosis pattern)*
Lymphoma	
Follicular	Back-to-back poorly defined follicles throughout usually without mantle zones *(follicular pattern)*
Mantle cell	Small reactive follicle centers with very thick mantle zones, nodules of mantle cell lymphocytes, and fusion of mantle zones
Marginal zone	Benign follicles surrounded by confluent monocytoid B cells in the marginal zones, interfollicular areas, and sinuses *(marginal zone, inverse follicular, interfollicular, sinus patterns)*
Small lymphocytic lymphoma	Poorly defined, one-layer ball-like structures that contain "prolymphocytes and paraimmunoblasts" *(pseudofollicular pattern)*
Hodgkin's disease L&H nodular	Large, closely packed spherical ball-like structures that have dark blue color (small lymphocytes) that is well demarcated from a lighter color (L&H cells often admixed with histiocytes and epithelioid cells *(L&H nodular pattern)*
Nodular sclerosis	Fibrous bands produce a nodular appearance and mottled appearance produced by lacunar cells *(fibrous nodular pattern)*
Mixed	Reactive follicles, interfollicular areas with well-defined clusters of epithelioid cells, mummified cells, and Hodgkin's cells *(interfollicular and Lennert's patterns)*

L&H, lymphocytic and histiocytic.

and the process would be slow and prone to error. Study at high magnification should not be ''aimless wandering'' and ''stumbling on to'' cytologic features; it should be a directed process with the sole purpose of evaluating specific and reliable features.

Based on our long experience in learning and teaching about patterns, we can state confidently that pattern recognition can be taught and learned, and patterns can be very helpful in making accurate diagnoses.

PATTERNS: SPHERICAL STRUCTURES

Recognizing Spherical Structures Accurately

We have learned through experience and discussions with other pathologists that identification and definition of spherical or ball-like structures seen in lymph nodes is an area of great confusion and misunderstanding. To promote standardization, enhance communication and understanding, and increase diagnostic accuracy, it is necessary to have precise definitions of the different types of spheres. The terms *follicular*, *inverse follicular*, *mantle zone*, *marginal zone*, *pseudofollicular*, and *nodular* should not be used interchangeably, because each, if used precisely, has diagnostic utility. We provide definitions, schematic representation, pictures, and a systematic approach to the identification of spherical structures (Fig. 14.1, Table 14.8). The first step in the systematic approach is to determine whether the spherical structure is composed of one layer (or compartment), two layers, or three layers. If there are two layers, the second step is to determine whether the structure has a normal arrangement of colors at low magnification or an inverse arrangement or intermingling of colors. The third step is to determine which layer is expanding (proliferating). This should be followed by a careful study of the cells proliferating in each layer to determine whether they are centrocytes, centroblasts, mantle

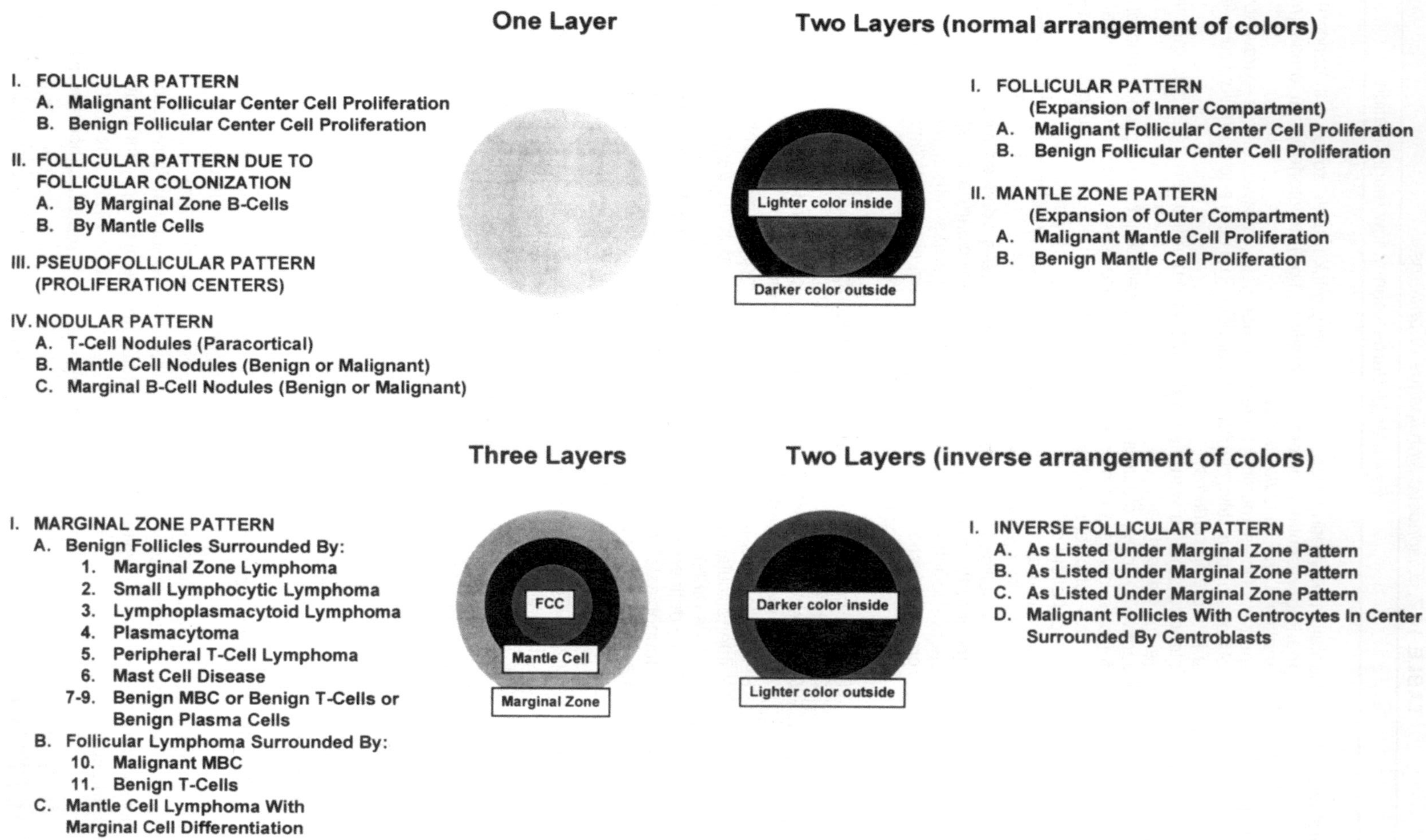

One Layer
I. FOLLICULAR PATTERN
A. Malignant Follicular Center Cell Proliferation
B. Benign Follicular Center Cell Proliferation
II. FOLLICULAR PATTERN DUE TO FOLLICULAR COLONIZATION
A. By Marginal Zone B-Cells
B. By Mantle Cells
III. PSEUDOFOLLICULAR PATTERN (PROLIFERATION CENTERS)
IV. NODULAR PATTERN
A. T-Cell Nodules (Paracortical)
B. Mantle Cell Nodules (Benign or Malignant)
C. Marginal B-Cell Nodules (Benign or Malignant)
Two Layers (normal arrangement of colors)
Lighter color inside
Darker color outside
I. FOLLICULAR PATTERN
(Expansion of Inner Compartment)
A. Malignant Follicular Center Cell Proliferation
B. Benign Follicular Center Cell Proliferation
II. MANTLE ZONE PATTERN
(Expansion of Outer Compartment)
A. Malignant Mantle Cell Proliferation
B. Benign Mantle Cell Proliferation
Three Layers
I. MARGINAL ZONE PATTERN
A. Benign Follicles Surrounded By:
1. Marginal Zone Lymphoma
2. Small Lymphocytic Lymphoma
3. Lymphoplasmacytoid Lymphoma
4. Plasmacytoma
5. Peripheral T-Cell Lymphoma
6. Mast Cell Disease
7-9. Benign MBC or Benign T-Cells or Benign Plasma Cells
B. Follicular Lymphoma Surrounded By:
10. Malignant MBC
11. Benign T-Cells
C. Mantle Cell Lymphoma With Marginal Cell Differentiation
FCC
Mantle Cell
Marginal Zone
Two Layers (inverse arrangement of colors)
Darker color inside
Lighter color outside
I. INVERSE FOLLICULAR PATTERN
A. As Listed Under Marginal Zone Pattern
B. As Listed Under Marginal Zone Pattern
C. As Listed Under Marginal Zone Pattern
D. Malignant Follicles With Centrocytes In Center Surrounded By Centroblasts

FIG. 14.1. A schematic showing similarities and differences among the main types of spherical (ball-like) structures that are seen at low magnification. The main criteria used at low magnification are whether the spheres have one, two, or three layers and whether the arrangement of colors is normal or inverse.

TABLE 14.8. *Approach for accurate identification of spherical structures*

I. Morphology
  A. Layers or compartments
    1. Number: 1, 2, or 3
    2. Arrangement: normal, inverse, or intermingling
    3. Expansion: follicle center cell, mantle cell, marginal zone
  B. Cytology in each layer: centrocytes, centroblasts, immunoblasts, mantle cells, monocytoid/marginal zone B cells, small lymphocytes, prolymphocytes, plasma cells
II. Immunohistochemical staining in each layer: CD3, CD5, CD10, CD20, CD21, CD23, CD43, cyclin D1, bcl-2
III. Molecular biology: t(14;18), t(11;14)

cells, monocytoid or marginal zone B cells, ''prolymphocytes,'' plasma cells, or immunoblasts. It also should be determined whether or not these cells are present in the compartments in which they should be present. If the expected correlation between pattern and cytologic features is not present, a reappraisal of the pattern should be done. In this setting, cytologic features are most useful in accurately identifying a spherical structure. For example, if prolymphocytes and paraimmunoblasts are seen in a one-layer spherical structure, it is a proliferation center (pseudofollicle) and not a true follicle or any other type of spherical structure. Similarly, if centrocytes and centroblasts are seen in a one-layer sphere, it is a true follicle and not any other type of sphere. Also, if in a one-layer spherical structure there are only small lymphoid cells with scant cytoplasm and without histiocytes, Langerhans cells, centrocytes, centroblasts, prolymphocytes, or paraimmunoblasts, it is most likely a mantle cell nodule. The next step, if required, is to perform appropriate immunohistochemical studies (CD20, CD3, CD43, CD5, cyclin D1, BCL-2, CD23) on paraffin sections to correlate their results with morphology and establish the identity of the sphere. The staining of cells in each compartment (layer) is different, and cells move from one compartment to another. Again, if the expected immunologic correlation is not present, a careful reexamination of morphology should be done. The final step is to perform molecular studies, if necessary. The differential diagnosis for spherical structures is provided in Tables 14.9 through 14.12.

Because some spheres are much more common than others, we list here the spheres or patterns in decreasing frequency, regardless of the disease process causing them: follicular pattern, mantle zone pattern, mantle cell nodules, nodular paracortical T-cell or zone hyperplasia, fibrous nodular pattern, pseudofollicular pattern, marginal zone pattern, marginal zone B-cell nodules, follicular colonization, inverse follicular pattern, progressively transformed germinal centers, and L&H nodules.

Although different types of spherical structures can coexist, and some spherical structures may be present only focally, they should be recognized, because their presence has diagnostic significance. The designation of sphere or pattern is given even though it presents focally.

Structure of Follicle (Follicle Center Zone, Mantle Zone, and Marginal Zone)

The normal secondary follicle in a peripheral lymph node consists of two zones (compartments or layers) (Fig. 14.2). The inner zone (compartment) contains mainly follicle center cells and appears lightly stained at low magnification. This zone is completely surrounded by the mantle zone layer (outer layer), which consists of small, round, densely packed mantle lymphocytes and is dark blue at low magnification. On the other hand, in the spleen, the normal follicle usually consists of three zones (Fig. 14.3): an inner (first or central) compartment consisting of follicle center cells, a middle (second) layer composed of mantle cells, and an outer (third) layer consisting of lightly staining lymphoid cells with an appearance similar to monocytoid B cells (36). This third layer is called the *marginal zone*. It usually is seen in the splenic follicle but can be present in peripheral lymph nodes (37). Mesenteric lymph nodes and extranodal mucosa-associated lymphoid tissue may exhibit marginal zones (partial or complete) focally or multifocally (38).

A secondary follicle in a lymph node may display a marked proliferation of follicle center cells or a marked proliferation of mantle lymphocytes. If the predominating

TABLE 14.9. *Differential diagnosis of two-layered spherical structures having a normal arrangement of colors*

Proliferation	Cytology	Immunology and molecular abnormalities
Follicle pattern		
Malignant follicle center cell proliferation	Centrocytes and centroblasts	bcl2$^+$, CD20$^+$, CD10$^+$, CD5$^-$, CD43$^-$, CD23$^-$, t(14;18)
Benign follicle center cell proliferation	Centrocytes and centroblasts	bcl2$^-$, CD20$^+$, CD43$^-$, CD3$^-$, CD10$^+$, CD23$^-$
Mantle zone pattern		
Malignant mantle cell proliferation	Small lymphoid cells with nuclear irregularities; no centroblasts	bcl2$^+$, CD20$^+$, CD5$^+$, CD43$^+$, cyclin D1$^+$, CD10$^-$, CD23$^-$, t(11;14)
Benign mantle cell proliferation	Small lymphoid cells with round nuclei; no centroblasts	bcl2$^+$, CD20$^+$, CD5$^-$, CD43$^-$, CD3$^-$, cyclin D1$^-$, CD10$^-$, CD23$^-$

All benign B-cell proliferations are polyclonal and do not show immunoglobulin gene rearrangements. All malignant B-cell proliferations are monoclonal B and show immunoglobulin gene rearrangements.

TABLE 14.10. *Differential diagnosis of marginal-zone pattern*

Diseases/cells producing marginal-zone pattern	Probability, %	Immunology and molecular biology of cells in the third pattern
Benign follicles surrounded by:		
MZL	40	bcl2⁺, CD20⁺, CD3⁻, CD43;⁻/⁺, CD5⁻, CD23⁻, monoclonal plasma cells in 35%, trisomy 3, t(11;18)
Small lymphocytic lymphoma	5	bcl2⁺, CD20⁺, CD43⁺, CD5⁺, CD23⁺, trisomy 12
Mastocytosis	5	bcl2⁻, CD20⁻, CD3⁻, CD43⁻, CD5⁻, tryptase⁺
Mantle cells appearing like MZL	2	bcl2⁺, CD20⁺, CD5⁺, cyclin D1⁺
Plasmacytoma	1	Bcl2⁻, CD20⁺/⁻, CD43⁺/⁻, CD5⁻, monoclonal plasma cells
Benign monocytoid B cells	1	bcl2⁻, CD20⁺, CD3⁻, CD43⁻, CD5⁻, CD23⁻, cyclin D1⁻
Lymphoplasmacytoid lymphoma	<1	Monoclonal lymphoplasmacytoid cells
Peripheral T cell lymphoma	<1	bcl2⁺, CD20⁻, CD3⁺, CD43⁺, CD5⁺
Benign small T cells	<1	bcl2⁺, CD20⁻, CD3⁺, CD43⁺, CD5⁺
Benign plasma cells	<1	bcl2⁻, CD20⁻, CD43⁺, CD5⁻
Metastatic carcinoma	<1	
Follicular lymphomas surrounded by:		
Benign T cells	1	bcl2⁺, CD20⁻, CD3⁺, CD43⁺, CD5⁺
MZL	5	bcl2⁺, CD20⁺, CD43⁻/⁺, CD5⁻

All benign B-cell proliferations are polyclonal and do not show immunoglobulin gene rearrangements. All malignant B-cell proliferations are monoclonal B and show immunoglobulin gene rearrangements. All malignant T-cell proliferations show T-cell receptor gene rearrangements.

MZL, marginal zone lymphoma.

TABLE 14.11. *Differential diagnosis of inverse follicular pattern*

Diseases/cells producing inverse follicular pattern	Probability, %	Immunology and molecular biology of cells in the second layer
Naked follicular center surrounded by:		
MZL	80	bcl2⁺, CD20⁺, CD3⁻, CD43⁻/⁺, CD5⁻, CD23⁻, monoclonal plasma cells in 35%, trisomy 3, t(11;18)
Small lymphocytic lymphoma	5	bcl2⁺, CD20⁺, CD43⁺, CD5⁺, CD23⁺, trisomy 12
Mastocytosis	5	bcl2⁻, CD20⁻, CD3⁻, CD43⁻, CD5⁻, tryptase⁺
Mantle cells appearing like MZL	2	bcl2⁺, CD20⁺, CD5⁺, cyclin D1⁺
Plasmacytoma	1	Bcl2⁻, CD20⁺/⁻, CD43⁺/⁻, CD5⁻, monoclonal plasma cells
Benign monocytoid B cells	1	bcl2⁻, CD20⁺, CD3⁻, CD43⁻, CD5⁻, CD23⁻, cyclin D1⁻
Lymphoplasmacytoid lymphoma	<1	Monoclonal lymphoplasmacytoid cells
Peripheral T-cell lymphoma	<1	bcl2⁺, CD20⁻, CD3⁺, CD43⁺, CD5⁺
Benign small T cells	<1	bcl2⁺, CD20⁻, CD3⁺, CD43⁺, CD5⁺
Benign plasma cells	<1	bcl2⁻, CD20⁻, CD43⁺, CD5⁻
Follicular lymphomas surrounded by:		
Benign T cells	1	bcl2⁺, CD20⁻, CD3⁺, CD43⁺, CD5⁺
MZL	5	bcl2⁺, CD20⁺, CD43⁻/⁺, CD5⁻
Follicular lymphoma: centrocytes in center surrounded by centroblasts	2	bcl2⁺, CD20⁺, CD43⁻, CD5⁻, CD23⁻, CD10⁺, t(14;18)

All benign B-cell proliferations are polyclonal and do not show immunoglobulin gene rearrangements. All malignant B-cell proliferations are monoclonal B and show immunoglobulin gene rearrangements. All malignant T-cell proliferations show T-cell receptor gene rearrangements.

MZL, marginal-zone lymphoma.

TABLE 14.12. *Differential diagnosis of one-layered spherical structures*

Proliferations	Cytology	Immunology and molecular abnormalities
Follicular pattern		
Malignant follicle center cell proliferation	Centrocytes and centroblasts	bcl2⁺, CD20⁺, CD10⁺, CD5⁻, CD43⁻, CD23⁻, t(14;18)
Benign follicle center cell proliferation	Centrocytes and centroblasts	bcl2⁻, CD20⁺, CD43⁻, CD3⁻, CD10⁺, CD23⁻
Follicular colonization by:		
Mantle cells	Small lymphoid cells with nuclear irregularities; no centroblasts	bcl2⁺, CD20⁺, CD5⁺, CD43⁺, cyclin D1⁺, CD10⁻, CD23⁻, t(11;14)
Marginal zone B cells	Monocytoid B cells	bcl2⁺, CD20⁺, CD5⁻, CD43⁺, cyclin D1⁻, CD10⁻, CD23⁻, trisomy 3, t(11;18)
Pseudofollicular pattern (proliferation centers)	Prolymphocytes and paraimmunoblasts	bcl2⁺, CD20⁺, CD5⁺, CD43⁺, CD23⁺, CD10⁻, cyclin D1⁻, trisomy 12
Paracortical T-cell nodules (small T-cell proliferation)	Small lymphoid cells with mottling by interdigitating dendritic cells, Langerhans' cells, histiocytes	bcl2⁺, CD20⁻, CD3⁺, CD43⁺
Mantle cell nodules		
Malignant	Small lymphoid cells with nuclear irregularities; no centroblasts	bcl2⁺, CD20⁺, CD5⁺, CD43⁺, cyclin D1⁺, CD10⁻, CD23⁻, t(11;14)
Benign	Small lymphoid cells; no centroblasts	bcl2⁺, CD20⁺, CD5⁻, CD43⁻, CD3⁻, cyclin D1⁻, CD10⁻, CD23⁻
Marginal B-cell nodules (marginal B-cell proliferation)	Monocytoid B cells	bcl2⁻, CD20⁺, CD5⁻, CD3⁻, CD43⁻, CD23⁻, cyclin D1⁻

All benign B-cell proliferations are polyclonal and do not show immunoglobulin gene rearrangements.
All malignant B-cell proliferations are monoclonal B and show immunoglobulin gene rearrangements.

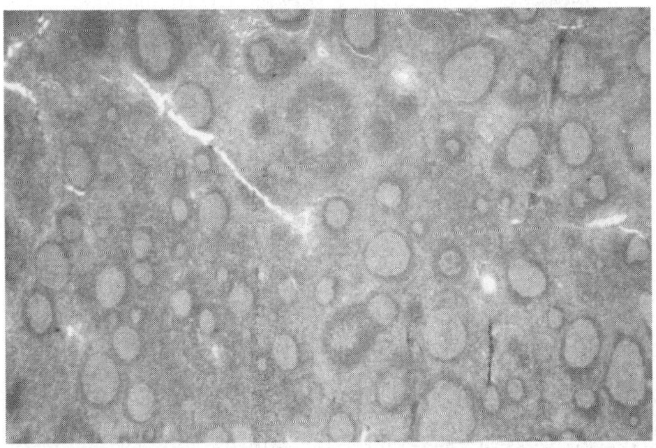

FIG. 14.2. Follicular pattern. This lymph node is from a patient with follicular hyperplasia. Note that most benign follicles show two layers (compartments), with the normal arrangement of colors. The inner follicle center cell compartment is lightly stained, whereas the outer mantle cell compartment consists of more darkly stained small lymphocytes (hematoxylin and eosin stain, original magnification: 20× magnification).

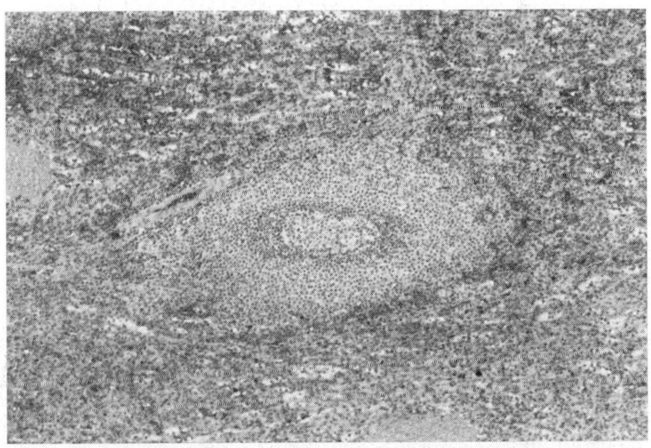

FIG. 14.3. Marginal zone pattern in normal spleen. The white pulp of spleen has three distinct compartments. The inner compartment is composed of lightly stained follicle center cells. This zone is surrounded by the mantle cell compartment, which is composed of darkly stained small lymphocytes. The marginal zone (outer third layer) is composed of lightly stained lymphoid cells (hematoxylin and eosin stain, original magnification: 100× magnification).

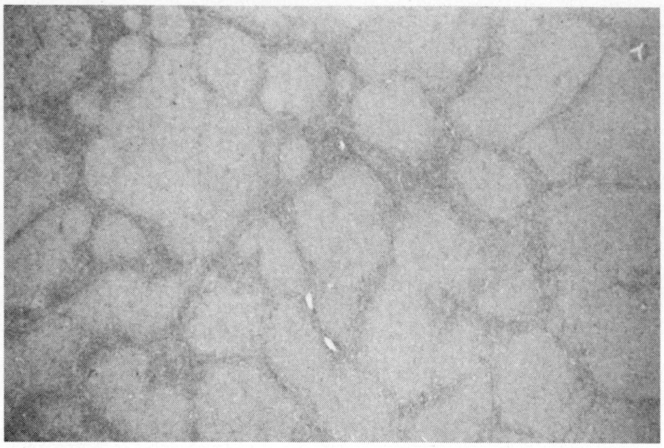

FIG. 14.4. Follicular pattern. This lymph node is from a patient with follicular lymphoma. The neoplastic follicles have a back-to-back arrangement and are not surrounded by mantle zones (hematoxylin and eosin stain, original magnification: 40× magnification).

proliferation is one of follicle center cells (Fig. 14.4), we use the term *follicular pattern*. If there is a substantial proliferation of mantle cells in one or more follicles, we use the term *mantle zone pattern* (Fig. 14.5). Occasionally in lymph nodes, a variety of cell types is found in the marginal (third) zone, and they produce a distinctive ring (Fig. 14.6). The term *marginal zone pattern* is used if one or more follicles exhibit a third layer, which may be thin or thick (11,39).

At low magnification, we use the term *inverse follicular pattern* because the arrangement of colors in a two-layer spherical structure is reversed (11). Normally, at low magnification, follicle center cells are present in the center of the follicle (the inner layer), which is lightly staining, and these cells are surrounded by the outer mantle cell layer, which

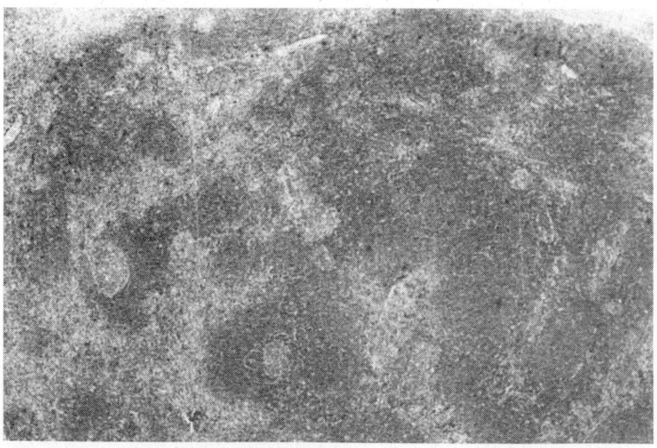

FIG. 14.5. Mantle zone pattern. In this mantle cell lymphoma, a few follicles are seen in which the follicular centers are small and surrounded by thick and expansile mantle zones (mantle zone pattern). In addition, there are other one-layer spherical structures, nodules composed of only mantle cell lymphocytes (mantle cell nodular pattern) (hematoxylin and eosin stain, original magnification: 40× magnification).

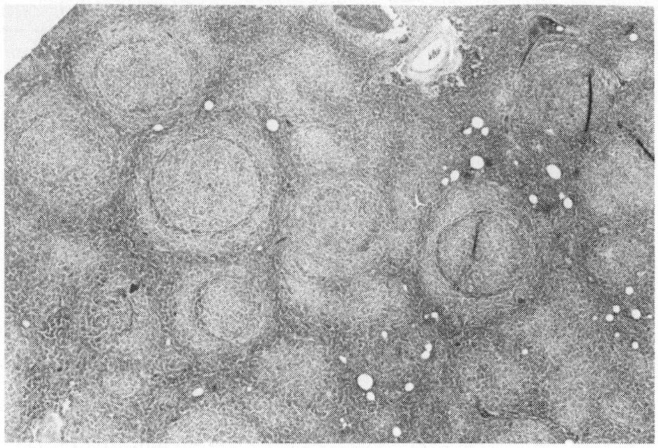

FIG. 14.6. Marginal zone pattern. In this case of small lymphocytic lymphoma, a marginal zone pattern is evident in several follicles. The marginal zone pattern is characterized by follicles with three distinct zones. The inner zone is the follicular center cell zone (lightly stained). The middle zone is composed of darkly stained mantle cell lymphocytes. The outer zone is the "marginal zone" that is lightly stained and composed of malignant cells that, in this instance, are those seen within the pseudofollicles of a small lymphocytic lymphoma. The pseudofollicles completely surround the reactive follicles. Note that in between the follicles there are a few pseudofollicles, which are present mainly in the lower righthand portion of the figure (hematoxylin and eosin stain, original magnification: 40× magnification).

is darkly staining. In an inverse arrangement, darkly staining cells are in the center and are surrounded by an outer layer of pale-staining cells (Fig. 14.7). The term inverse follicular pattern is used as long as there is at least one spherical structure exhibiting this inverse arrangement. The diseases in which an inverse arrangement can be seen are listed in Table 14.11.

Follicular Pattern

If a ball-like structure of one or two layers shows a proliferation of follicle center cells (centroblasts and centrocytes), it is said to display a follicular pattern. The centroblasts (noncleaved cells or transformed cells) have multiple small nucleoli, often located on the nuclear membranes, and have scant cytoplasm. The centrocytes are usually small and exhibit scant cytoplasm, and their twisted, folded, or angulated nuclei do not have distinct nucleoli. In addition, admixed within the follicles are both nonneoplastic small T cells, which vary in number from few to many, and follicular dendritic cells. The follicular dendritic cells differ from benign histiocytes and centroblasts because they have round, oval, or spindle-shaped nuclei that appear bland, with one or no small nucleolus and scant cytoplasm. These cells often occur in tight pairs. The follicular dendritic cells express CD21 and CD35. By definition, follicular lymphoma excludes those conditions wherein "follicular colonization" or invasion of

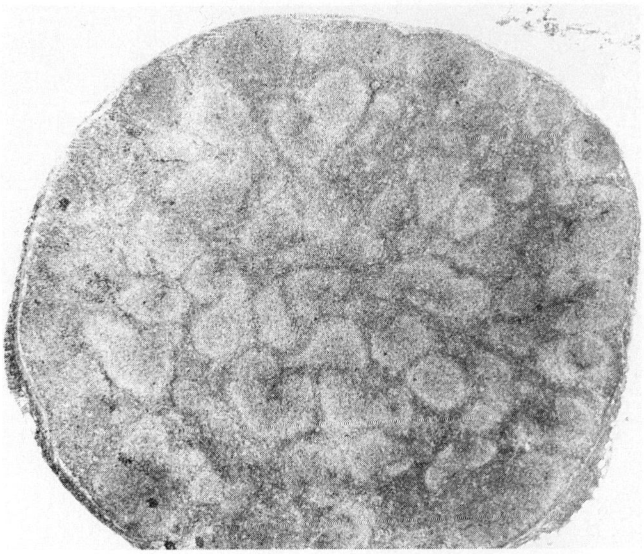

FIG. 14.7. Inverse follicular pattern. In this follicular lymphoma, the central portions of these follicles are darkly stained and contain mainly centrocytes (Fig. 14.12), whereas the peripheral portions are lightly stained and contain mainly centroblasts (Fig. 14.13). This pattern is the reverse (inverse) of that seen in a normal reactive follicle, in which the darker color is on the outside (in the mantle cell layer) and the lightly stained compartment (follicle center cells) is in the center (hematoxylin and eosin stain, original magnification: 40× magnification).

follicular centers is produced by mantle cells or marginal zone B cells.

Malignant Follicles (One or Two Layers)

Malignant follicles usually are poorly defined; they either are closely packed together or have a back-to-back arrangement (Fig. 14.4). Neoplastic follicles usually are not surrounded by a rim of mantle cell lymphocytes. If mantle zones are present, they are usually thin and incompletely encircle the follicle. Within the follicles there usually is a marked preponderance of either centrocytes or centroblasts. Malignant follicle center cells of a follicular lymphoma show light chain restriction and express CD20, CD10, and BCL-2 (FL grade I, 99%; grade II, 85%; grade III, 75%) but not CD5, CD43, or cyclin D1.

Benign Follicles (One or Two Layers)

The characteristics of benign follicles are the presence of polarity, high amounts of mitotic and phagocytic activity, a mixed proliferation of follicle center cells, and a thin to thick mantle zone completely surrounding most follicles (Fig. 14.2). Benign follicles usually do not show a back-to-back arrangement, although in the early stages of the progressive generalized lymphadenopathy seen in patients with HIV infection such a pattern can be seen in a few cases. Benign follicular pattern is seen in follicular hyperplasia, early phases of HIV infection, rheumatoid arthritis, giant lymph node hyperplasia of the plasma cell type, toxoplasmosis, and syphilis.

Mantle Zone Pattern

In the mantle zone pattern, one to many follicles show an exuberant proliferation of mantle lymphocytes, resulting in broad and expansile mantle zones (40) (Fig. 14.5). The diameters of the mantle zones are often greater than the diameter of the follicle center cell compartment (Fig. 14.5).

Malignant Mantle Cell Proliferation

If the mantle lymphocytes are neoplastic (as in mantle cell lymphoma), they exhibit the features of a malignant proliferation. Because of the massive proliferation of lymphocytes in the mantle zones, these zones become broad and expansile and often fuse with adjacent mantle zones (Fig. 14.5). In addition, the mantle lymphocytes form round compact islands (mantle cell nodules) (Fig. 14.8). The lymphocytes in the mantle zones exhibit nuclear irregularities. In some instances, however, they may be round (41). Among the mantle cells, centroblasts are absent. The best method of establishing the malignant nature of the lymphocytes in the mantle zones and mantle cell nodules seen in a mantle cell lymphoma is to demonstrate light chain restriction in the mantle cells, which also express CD20, CD5, CD43, and cyclin D1 but not CD23 or CD10; the follicle center cells are polyclonal.

Benign Mantle Cell Proliferation

If the mantle zones are benign, confluence of the adjacent mantle zones is usually absent. However, one can see nodules consisting of only mantle cells. In hyperplasia of mantle zones, the lymphocytes are round and, in rare cases, show slight nuclear irregularities. Benign mantle zone pattern is seen in giant lymph node hyperplasia of the hyaline vascular type, mantle zone hyperplasia, and lymphocyte-rich classic Hodgkin's lymphoma. In unstimulated lymph nodes, follicular centers are small and mantle zones are very thick.

Marginal Zone Pattern

The marginal zone in the spleen forms the third (outer) layer of the follicle and is composed of cells that are 1.5 to three times the size of the mantle lymphocytes. These cells have moderate to abundant quantities of lightly staining to clear cytoplasm and have an appearance similiar to monocytoid B cells. This third zone rarely is seen in normal peripheral lymph nodes (36,37). We use the term marginal zone pattern if one or more three-layer spherical structures are seen in a node (11,39). In the third (outer) layer, which forms a distinct ring, we see a population of either benign or neoplastic cells of different types (42) (Fig. 14.6). The differential diagnosis

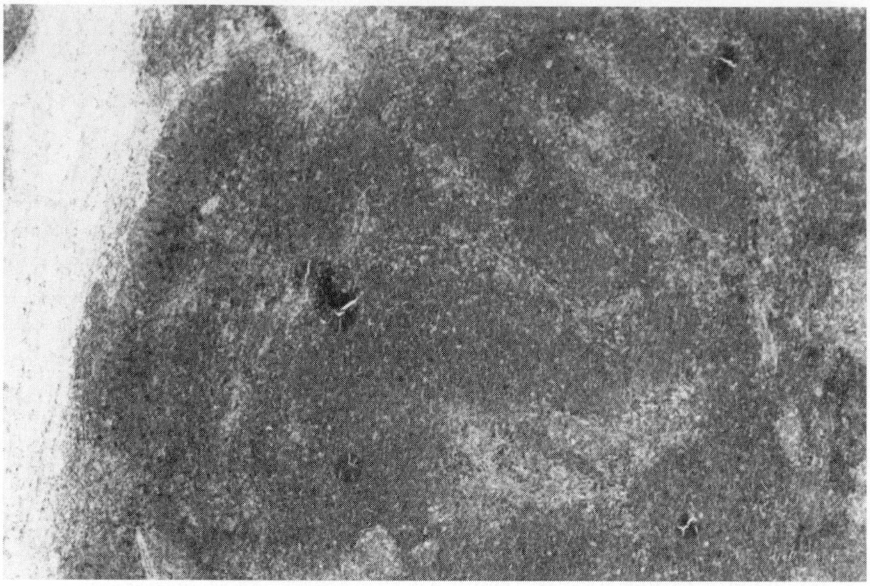

FIG. 14.8. Mantle cell nodular pattern. In this mantle cell lymphoma, there are many one-layer spherical ball-like structures (nodules), which are dark blue and composed of mantle cell lymphocytes (hematoxylin and eosin stain, original magnification: 100× magnification).

of a marginal zone pattern can be rationalized because of the fact that the marginal zone is also the *margin* between the B- and T-cell zones of a lymph node. In view of this, B-cell and T-cell diseases of different types that arise of the interfollicular compartment can surround a follicle completely and produce a marginal zone pattern (Table 14.10). Diseases shown in Table 14.10 are ranked according to their frequency from the most common to the rarest. *Virtually all conditions that produce a marginal zone pattern also can produce an inverse follicular pattern if the mantle cell layer is absent.*

Benign Follicles Surrounded by Malignant Monocytoid B Cells, as Seen in Marginal Zone or Monocytoid B-cell Lymphoma

In approximately 30% of cases of nodal or extranodal marginal zone B-cell lymphoma, the malignant cells completely surround one or more reactive follicles and form a distinct third layer or ring (39,43–45). Monocytoid or marginal zone B cells also are seen in the interfollicular areas in the form of sheets, and often within and around sinuses in the lymph node.

In primary splenic marginal zone B-cell lymphoma, according to some investigators, there are few to many benign follicles surrounded by a third (marginal) zone, which contains cells having features of monocytoid B cells (46–48). Others have suggested that there is another type of B-cell lymphoma that has been identified mistakenly as marginal zone B-cell lymphoma of the spleen (49–51); this lymphoma is said to have a biphasic cytology and distinctive immunophenotype. In this lymphoma, there are few to many *neoplastic* two-layer spherical structures with an inverse follicular pattern (Fig. 14.9); the inner layer contains small B lymphoid cells with round to slightly irregular nuclear membranes and scant cytoplasm (mantle cell–like) (Fig. 14.10), which are surrounded by an outer layer of cells that appear like marginal zone or monocytoid B cells (49,50) (Fig. 14.11). The populations are part of the same neoplastic B-cell clone, and

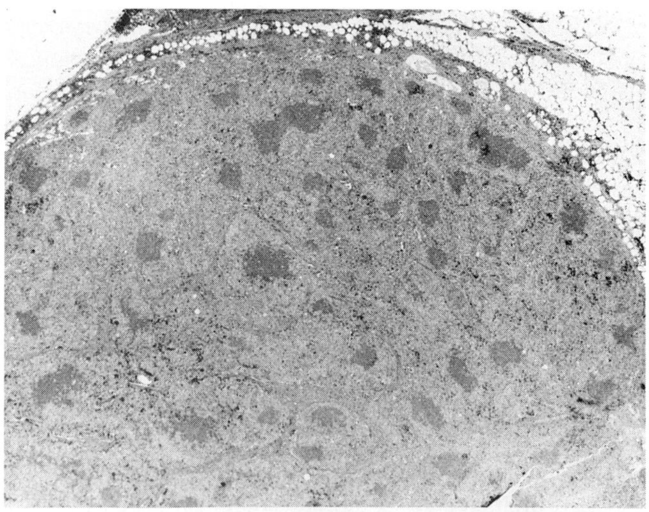

FIG. 14.9. Inverse follicular pattern. This is a splenic hilar node from a patient with splenic marginal zone B-cell lymphoma with biphasic cytology. The darkly stained centers of the spheres are composed of small round lymphoid cells (see Figure 14.10), and the lightly stained outer ring is composed of cells that appear like monocytoid B cells (Fig. 14.11). The populations show identical light chain restriction (hematoxylin and eosin stain, original magnification: 40× magnification).

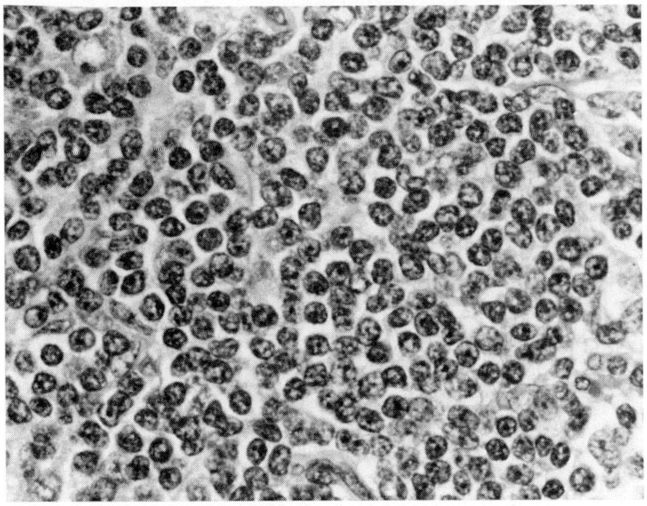

FIG. 14.10. High-magnification view of the darkly staining central portion of the inverse spherical structure in Figure 14.9, which contains B cells with round nuclei and scant cytoplasm. These are monoclonal B cells (hematoxylin and eosin stain, original magnification: 400× magnification).

the neoplastic cells are IgM-positive (IgM^+) and IgD^+ but CD43-negative ($CD43^-$) (49,50).

Malignant Follicles Surrounded by Malignant Monocytoid B Cells, as Seen in Follicular or Monocytoid B-Cell Lymphoma

In about 9% of follicular lymphomas, malignant monocytoid B cells surround several malignant follicles in a marginal zone pattern (39,52,53). Monocytoid B cells in such cases often form sheets, islands, clusters in the interfollicular areas, resulting in an interfollicular pattern. Monocytoid B cells also often are seen in the sinuses.

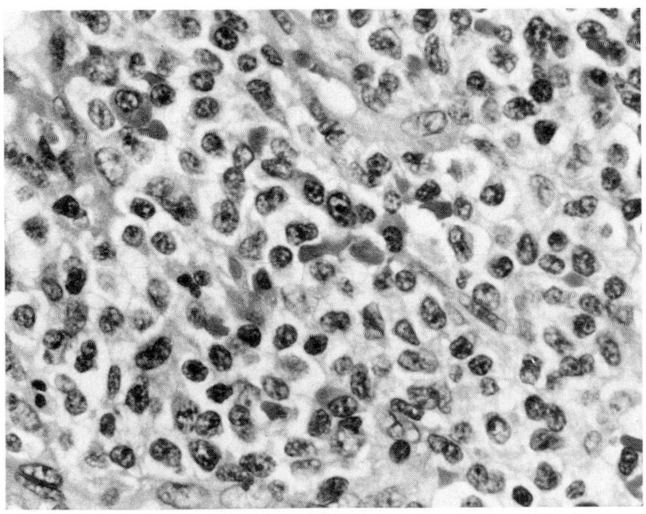

FIG. 14.11. High-magnification view of the peripheral portion (light staining) of the inverse spherical structure (Fig. 14.9), which contains cells with features of marginal zone or monocytoid B cells. These cells have abundant quantities of pale-staining cytoplasm and are monoclonal B cells with the same light chain restriction as the small round cells shown in Figure 14.10 (hematoxylin and eosin stain, original magnification: 400× magnification).

Benign Follicles Surrounded by Pseudofollicles, as Seen in Small Lymphocytic Lymphoma

In the early stages of small lymphocytic lymphoma, pseudofollicles (proliferation centers or pseudofollicular proliferation growth centers) are evident between many reactive follicles (54) (Fig. 14.6). Some pseudofollicles may surround one or more reactive follicles completely and produce a marginal zone pattern (third layer) (54) (Fig. 14.6). This third layer is composed of cells that are identical to those seen within the pseudofollicles present in the interfollicular areas; small, medium, and large cells with round nuclei, in varying proportions, are present in this marginal zone. Most importantly, many medium-sized and larger cells have features of prolymphocytes (cells with a centrally placed, prominent nucleolus) (55).

Benign Follicles Surrounded by Malignant T Cells, as Seen in Peripheral T-cell Lymphoma

In rare cases of peripheral T-cell lymphoma of the mixed-cell type and in so-called T-zone lymphomas in which there are scattered reactive follicles, malignant T cells of small, medium, and large sizes are present in interfollicular areas; in these rare cases, they can surround one or more benign follicles and form distinctive rings, resulting in a marginal zone pattern (11,56). The T cells are $CD3^+$ and $CD20^-$.

Malignant Follicles Surrounded by Benign T Cells, as Seen in Follicular Lymphoma

In rare cases of follicular lymphoma, one or more malignant follicles are surrounded by thin mantle zones, which in turn are surrounded by thin rims of benign T cells forming a marginal zone pattern. It is important to distinguish benign T cells from monocytoid B cells; CD20 and CD3 stains are useful.

Benign Follicles Surrounded by Benign Monocytoid B Cells, as Seen in Benign Diseases

In the early phase of HIV infection, monocytoid B cells usually are seen in the sinuses and adjacent to follicles in the form of small clusters; in rare instances, reactive monocytoid B cells may completely surround a rare reactive follicle and form a third layer.

Benign Follicles Surrounded by Benign T Cells, as Seen in Benign Diseases

Benign T cells are seen within follicular centers and are usually few in number. Occasionally T cells are present also in the mantle zones admixed with the mantle cells, and in rare instances they form a thin distinctive ring (a third layer) around one or more mantle zones. The T cells are small in size and have moderate to abundant quantities of pale-staining cytoplasm, and they can resemble monocytoid B cells. They are $CD3^+$ but $CD20^-$.

Benign Follicles Surrounded by Benign Plasma Cells, as Seen in Benign Diseases

Benign plasma cells can surround the mantle zones of one or more follicles in the form of a third ring (a marginal zone) in those diseases in which there is marked proliferation of benign plasma cells in the interfollicular areas.

Benign Follicles Surrounded by Malignant Plasma Cells, as Seen in Plasmacytoma

In a plasmacytoma, sheets of plasma cells are seen in interfollicular areas. They can completely surround one or more benign follicles and produce a marginal zone pattern.

Benign Follicles Surrounded by Neoplastic Lymphoplasmacytoid Cells, as Seen in Lymphoplasmacytoid Lymphoma

We have seen rare examples of lymphoplasmacytoid lymphoma, in its early stages, in which the neoplastic lymphoplasmacytoid cells completely surround a reactive follicle as a third zone and produce a marginal zone pattern.

Benign Follicles Surrounded By Mast Cells, as Seen in Mast Cell Disease

In mast cell disease or systemic mastocytosis, mast cell clusters and islands are seen in multiple locations; sometimes these cells form distinct rings around one or more benign follicles and produce a marginal zone pattern. The mast cells are positive with tryptase, toluidine blue, and naphthol-ASD-chloroacetate esterase stains (57). The mast cells are of medium size, with coffee bean–shaped nuclei, and have abundant quantities of lightly eosinophilic cytoplasm.

Mantle Cell Lymphoma with Marginal Cell Differentiation

In rare cases of mantle cell lymphoma, a few follicles may be surrounded completely by a thin layer of small cells that have moderate to abundant pale-staining cytoplasm, creating an appearance similar to marginal zone or monocytoid B-cells (58); such cells may represent true marginal cell differentiation, or variants of mantle cells with clear cytoplasm. In the spleen, however, a marginal zone pattern is more common in mantle cell lymphoma and follicular lymphoma (59,60). Mantle cells would be cyclin D1–positive, and B cells would coexpress CD5 and CD43. Marginal zone B cells would be cyclin $D1^-$ and $CD5^-$.

Inverse Follicular Pattern

Virtually all conditions that produce a marginal zone pattern can also produce an inverse follicular pattern if the mantle cell layer is absent (Table 14.11). An inverse follicular pattern also is produced if mantle cell nodules are surrounded by cells of different types that produce the marginal zone pattern (third layer shown in Table 14.10). Below, we list those lymphomas which are not listed under marginal zone pattern in Table 14.10.

Malignant Follicles with Centrocytes in the Center Surrounded by Centroblastsm as Seen in Follicular Lymphoma

In approximately 2% of follicular lymphomas, a few to many follicles display darkly staining neoplastic centrocytes (small cleaved cells) in the center of the follicle (Fig. 14.12), with the neoplastic centroblasts (transformed cells), which are lightly staining, in the periphery of the follicle (11) (Fig. 14.13).

Follicular Pattern Resulting from Follicular Colonization

Follicular Colonization by Mantle Cells

In mantle cell lymphoma, the neoplastic mantle cells rapidly proliferate and grow outward as well as inward into the follicle center (colonization). If they grow outward they produce mantle zone and mantle cell nodular patterns. If they grow inward into the benign follicle centers, they replace the benign follicle center cells either partially or completely, which can result in a pattern that can be indistinguishable from a true follicular pattern (61). In such instances, however, these follicles can be recognized as massive follicular colonization because the neoplastic mantle cells do not have twisted, angulated, wrinkled, folded, or spindle-shaped nuclei like follicle center cells but rather relatively more roundish nuclei with irregular contours. Among the neoplastic mantle cells, there are no admixed centroblasts, unless they happen to be surviving residual benign centroblasts of the benign follicle. The B cells in such cases have the phenotype of neoplastic mantle cells ($CD20^+$, $CD5^+$, $CD43^+$, and cyclin D1–positive).

Follicular Colonization by Marginal Zone B Cells

In marginal zone (44,45) or monocytoid (39) B-cell lymphomas, the malignant B cells can invade the follicle center cell compartment (colonization) and either partially or completely replace the benign follicle center cells, with a pattern resulting that may appear to be indistinguishable from a true

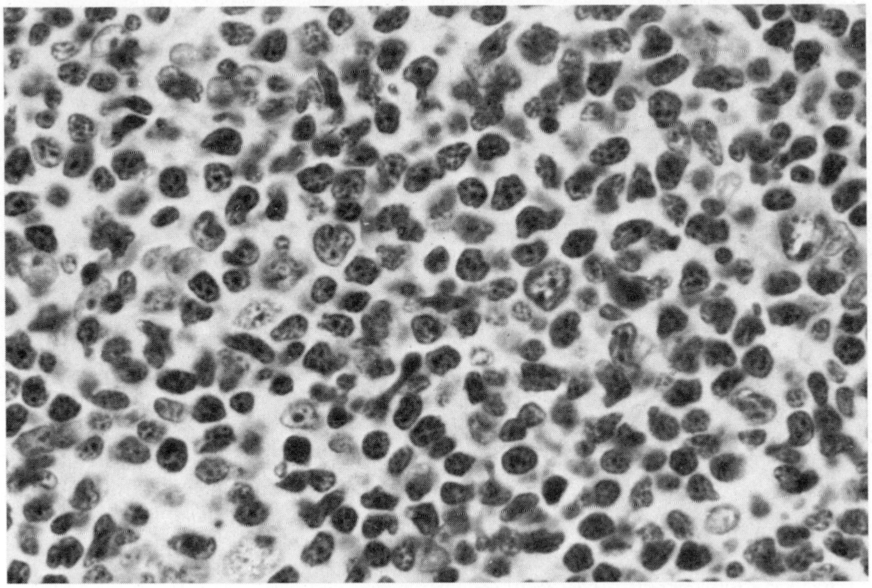

FIG. 14.12. Higher-magnification view of the central portions of the neoplastic follicles shown in Figure 14.7. The darkly stained center of the sphere shows centrocytes (small, cleaved cells) (hematoxylin and eosin stain, original magnification: 400× magnification).

follicular pattern (62) (Fig. 14.14). The marginal zone or monocytoid B cells are of medium size and have abundant quantities of pale-staining to clear cytoplasm, and they are $CD10^-$ and may be $CD43^+$. Follicle center cells (centrocytes and centroblasts) typically have scant cytoplasm and are $CD10^+$ and $CD43^-$.

Pseudofollicular Pattern (Proliferation Centers)

To recognize pseudofollicles, one must decrease the intensity of the light passing through the condenser and create optimum contrast. Pseudofollicles are one-layer ball-like structures that are very vague and pale-staining and are never surrounded by mantle zones (Fig. 14.15). Pseudofollicles may be few or many, and they may be far apart or closely packed together. Moreover, they are usually of small size and contain small round lymphoid cells (55). Admixed among them there are other cells of small, medium, and large size that have features of prolymphocytes (one centrally placed, prominent nucleolus) (Fig. 14.16). A pseudofollicular pattern is seen in approximately 95% of small lympho-

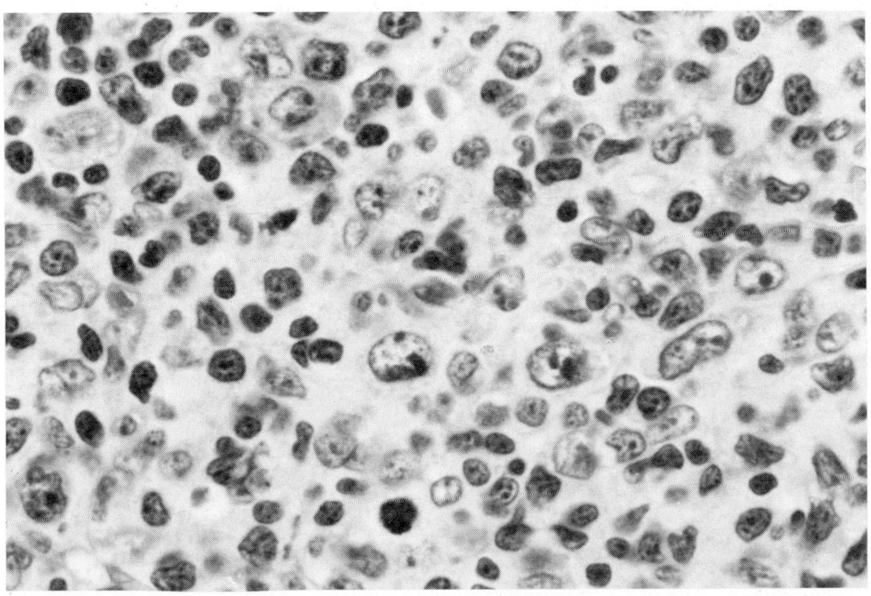

FIG. 14.13. Higher-magnification view of the peripheral portions of the neoplastic follicles shown in Figure 14.7. The lightly stained periphery of the sphere is largely composed of centroblasts (noncleaved cells) (hematoxylin and eosin stain, original magnification: 400× magnification).

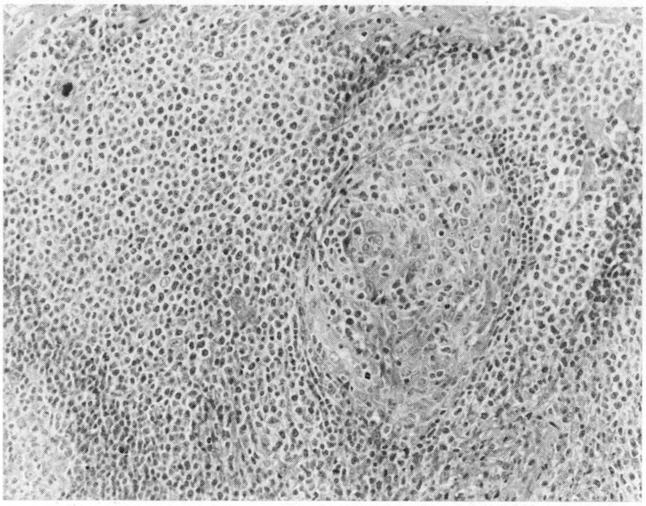

FIG. 14.14. Follicular colonization in marginal zone B-cell lymphoma. The large benign follicle center is surrounded by a thick layer of marginal zone B cells, which have features of monocytoid B cells. The latter cells have abundant clear cytoplasm and are present as a large island to the left of the follicle. These monocytoid B cells invade (colonize) the benign follicle center in the form of clusters (6 to 9 o'clock in the follicle and also 12 to 1 o'clock) (hematoxylin and eosin stain, original magnification: 400× magnification).

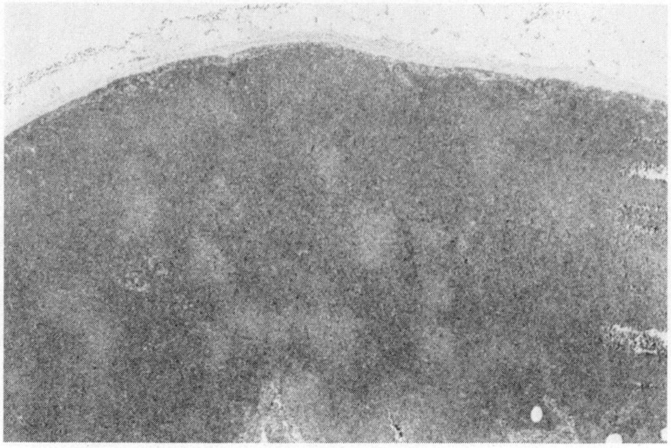

FIG. 14.15. Pseudofollicular pattern. The term *pseudofollicular pattern* is used synonymously with the term *proliferation centers* or *pseudofollicular proliferation growth centers*. In this small lymphocytic lymphoma, the pseudofollicles are small and poorly defined. They are lightly stained because the lymphoid cells within them are loosely packed and contain a mixture of small, medium-sized, and large lymphoid cells (Figure 14.16) (hematoxylin and eosin stain, original magnification: 20× magnification).

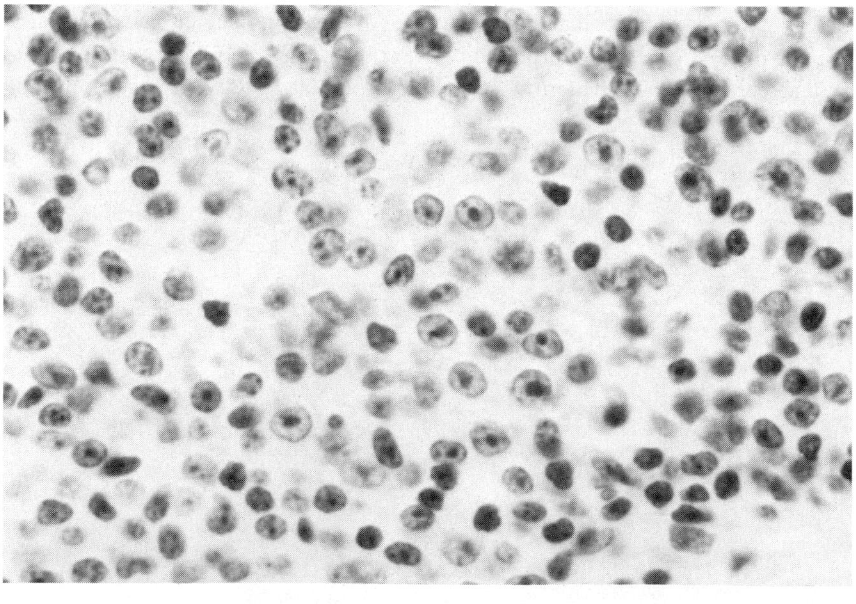

FIG. 14.16. High magnification of one pseudofollicular proliferation growth center. Note that the cells are loosely packed together and there are clear spaces separating them. There are many medium and large cells with a centrally placed prominent nucleolus (prolymphocytes) (hematoxylin and eosin stain, original magnification: 400× magnification).

TABLE 14.13. *Differences between pseudofollicles and true follicles*

Spherical structure	Pseudofollicles	Malignant (true) follicles
How are they arranged?	Difficult to recognize; usually separated	Easily recognized; often closely packed
Are they sharply defined?	No	Rarely
What is their size?	Small or large	Small or large
Are they surrounded by mantle zones?	No	Sometimes
Are the cells within loosely packed together?	Yes	No
Are the cells within separated by clear spaces?	Yes	No
Are all cells within round?	Yes (90%)	No
Do the small cells within resemble centrocytes?	No	Yes
Do the transformed cells within have features of centroblasts?	No	Yes
Do the medium-sized and large cells within have a centrally placed, prominent nucleolus?	Yes	No
Are mitotic figures seen within?	Rarely	Yes
Are benign histiocytes seen within?	Rarely	Yes

cytic lymphomas or chronic lymphocytic leukemias and in less than 5% of lymphoplasmacytoid lymphomas, but not in any benign disease. The characteristic features of pseudofollicles and the criteria for distinguishing them from true follicles are presented in Table 14.13 (55).

In the early stages of small lymphocytic lymphoma, because the disease process starts in the interfollicular areas, pseudofollicular proliferation growth centers (pseudofollicular pattern or proliferation centers) are seen in the interfollicular areas (Fig. 14.17). In addition, reactive follicles are identified readily. Pseudofollicles may surround a few reactive follicles completely and produce a marginal zone pattern (Fig. 14.6), or they may surround naked benign follicle centers and produce an inverse follicular pattern.

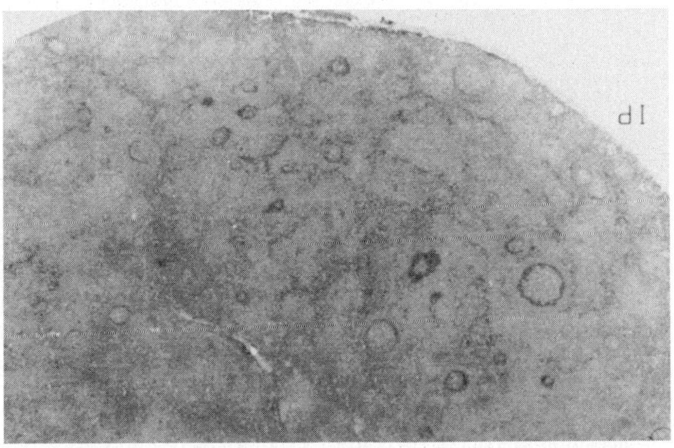

FIG. 14.17. Pseudofollicular pattern in interfollicular areas. The lymph node shows approximately 20 benign follicles that have two zones: follicle center cells, which are lightly stained, and mantle lymphocytes, which are darkly stained. The major finding in this picture is the presence of numerous, poorly defined pseudofollicles in the interfollicular areas (hematoxylin and eosin stain, original magnification: 20× magnification).

One-Layer Nodular Pattern (Table 14.12)

Nodular Paracortical T-Cell Hyperplasia (T-Cell Nodules with Mottling)

In dermatopathic lymphadenitis (Fig. 14.18) and so-called paracortical nodular T-zone hyperplasia (63) (Figs. 14.19, 14.20), in between follicles, there are subtle nodules of small, medium, or large size that contain mainly small round T

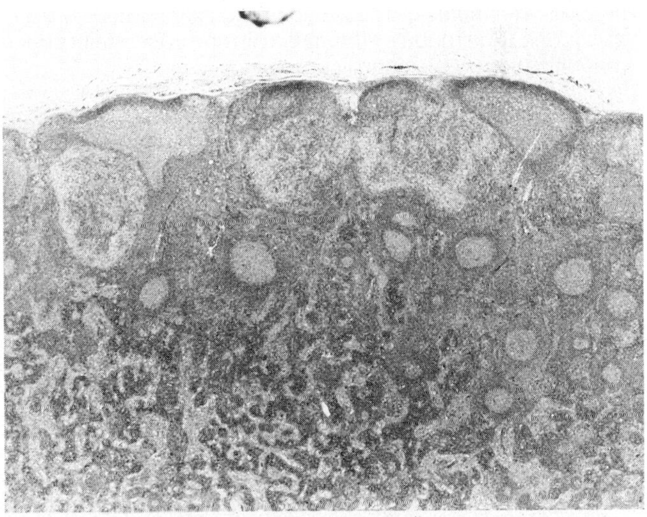

FIG. 14.18. Nodular pattern produced by paracortical nodular expansion in a patient with dermatopathic lymphadenitis. There are many reactive follicles in the cortex, and in the medullary region the sinuses are distended by benign histiocytes. In between the follicles, there are four large nodular areas that are well demarcated (pathologic foci) and represent foci of dermatopathic lymphadenitis that contain many histiocytes and Langerhans cells (pale-staining) and small lymphocytes (darkly staining), as well as melanin pigment that is not visible at this magnification. The histiocytes often contain phagocytic material, which may be debris or melanin pigment (hematoxylin and eosin stain, original magnification: 40× magnification).

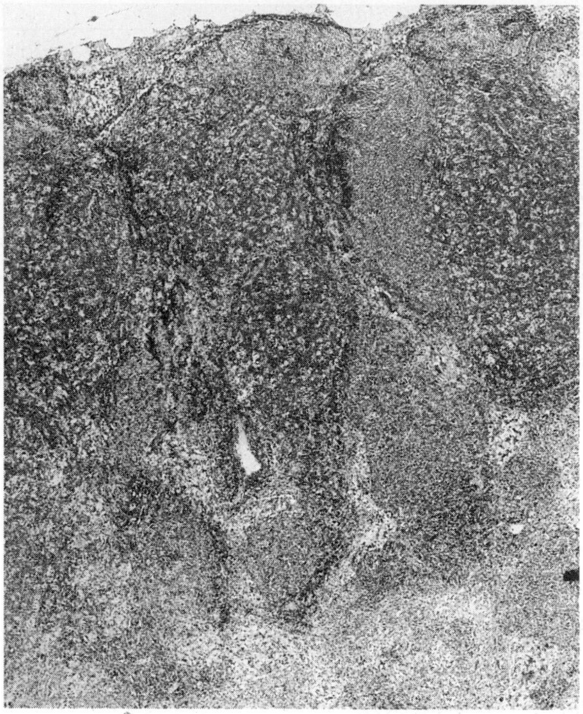

FIG. 14.19. Nodular pattern produced by paracortical nodular T-zone hyperplasia and marginal zone B-cell nodules. There are three large, darkly staining nodules with small lymphocytes in which there is prominent mottling produced by interdigitating dendritic cells. The small lymphocytes in these nodules are T lymphocytes. There are five other nodules that are smaller and do not show any mottling; they also stain more lightly than the nodules with mottling. These lighter-staining nodules are marginal zone B-cell nodules (hematoxylin and eosin stain, original magnification: 40× magnification).

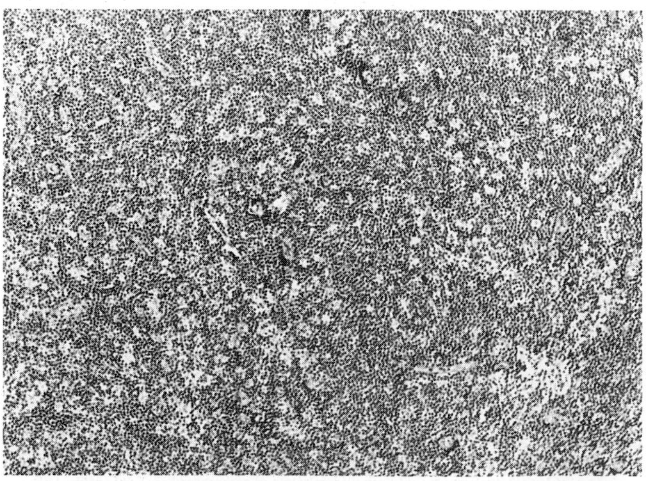

FIG. 14.20. Paracortical nodular T-zone hyperplasia. Higher-magnification view of the T-cell nodule showing mottling (Fig. 14.19). The mottling is produced by interdigitating dendritic cells, which are morphologically indistinguishable from Langerhans cells. These cells, unlike benign histiocytes, never show any phagocytic material in their cytoplasm. There is no melanin pigment in these T-cell areas, unlike in those seen in dermatopathic lymphadenitis (hematoxylin and eosin stain, original magnification: 400× magnification).

cells; they can be identified because scattered among them are Langerhans cells or interdigitating dendritic cells and histiocytes, which produce characteristic mottling. These mottled nodules must be recognized, because they commonly are seen in a variety of benign and malignant diseases. They are often numerous and can be large and cause diagnostic difficulties (Fig. 14.18).

Nodules of Mantle Cells

In mantle cell hyperplasia and mantle cell lymphoma, one can find monomorphic nodules composed only of mantle cell lymphocytes (Fig. 14.8). The only confirmation that these nodules are mantle lymphocytic in origin is the presence of an accompanying mantle zone pattern (Fig. 14.5). If such a pattern is not present, immunologic studies show that malignant mantle cells are $CD20^+$, $CD5^+$, $CD43^+$, and cyclin D1–positive; however, benign mantle cells do not have a distinctive phenotype.

Nodules of Marginal Cells (Marginal B-Cell Proliferation)

In marginal zone hyperplasia and marginal zone lymphoma, because of expansion of the marginal zones, there is a marginal zone pattern and also nodules in which there are only marginal zone B-cells; these nodules usually are present in the cortex and adjacent to follicles; however, they may be seen in the medulla (Fig. 14.21). If there is no adjacent marginal zone pattern present, the marginal cell nodules

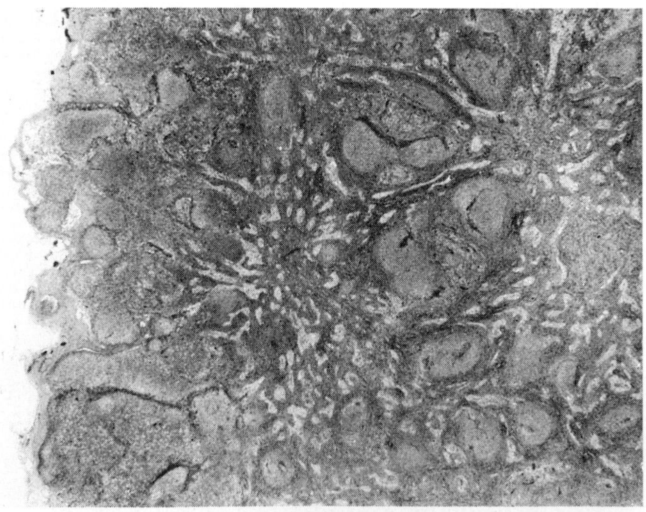

FIG. 14.21. Nodular pattern produced by marginal zone B-cell nodules. This node is from a patient with a primary, nodal marginal zone B-cell lymphoma. The capsule is on the left, and immediately beneath it there are many small, closely packed, uniform nodules. In the medullary portions there also are many small nodules. In this case, the marginal zone cell nodules are strongly monoclonal kappa. Also present are numerous sinuses that are distended by benign histiocytes (hematoxylin and eosin stain, original magnification: 20× magnification).

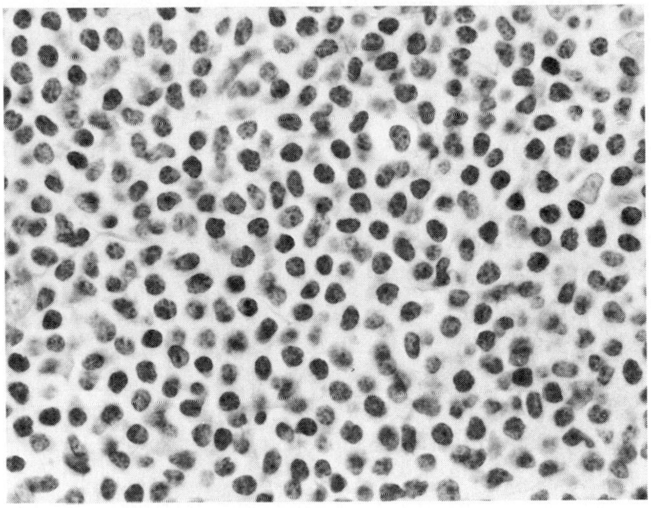

FIG. 14.22. High-magnification view of marginal zone B-cell nodules. Note that there is monomorphic proliferation of small lymphoid cells, which have round to very slightly irregular nuclei and moderate quantities of pale to clear cytoplasm. There is one follicular dendritic cell, but no centroblast or any other type of transformed lymphoid cell (hematoxylin and eosin stain, original magnification: 400× magnification).

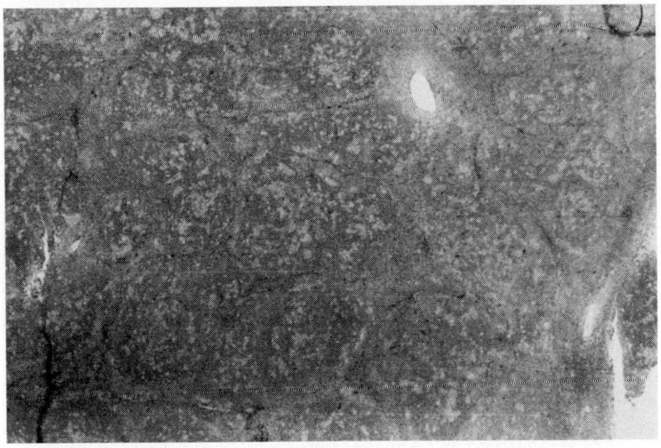

FIG. 14.23. Lymphocytic and histiocytic nodular pattern of Hodgkin's lymphoma. Numerous closely packed large spherical structures are present throughout the lymph node. These ball-like structures contain many darkly stained areas consisting of small lymphocytes; the lightly stained areas contain lymphocytic and histiocytic variants of Sternberg-Reed cells and histiocytes. These two colors are well demarcated and separated from each other without any transition. This combination of pattern and colors within the ball-like structures is pathognomonic of nodular lymphocytic and histiocytic Hodgkin's lymphoma (hematoxylin and eosin stain, original magnification: 20× magnification).

have to be distinguished from the other types of nodules. The marginal zone B-cells in such cases can be recognized because they are larger than small lymphocytes, and they usually have moderate to abundant lightly staining cytoplasm (Fig. 14.22).

Nodules with Intermingling of Layers

Nodular Lymphocytic and Histiocytic Hodgkin's Lymphoma

In nodular L&H Hodgkin's lymphoma, there are many large, closely packed spherical structures (L&H nodules) that show a preponderance of small, dark blue lymphocytes (28). These small cells are admixed with epithelioid histiocytes or histiocytes, and L&H variants of Sternberg-Reed cells, which are much larger and pale staining. Therefore, at low magnification, one sees within these nodules, side-by-side, two distinct colors with no transition between the two colors (dark blue small lymphocytes and pale epithelioid histiocytes or L&H variants of Sternberg-Reed cells) (Fig. 14.23). This pattern is distinctive and is pathognomonic of L&H Hodgkin's lymphoma.

Progressively Transformed Germinal Center Pattern

Progressively transformed germinal centers, as their name suggests, are abnormal follicles; they are large, with irregular outlines (64). The center of a progressively transformed germinal center becomes small because the follicle center cell compartment is invaded (colonized) extensively by benign mantle lymphocytes from a thickened mantle zone (Fig. 14.24). Progressively transformed germinal centers may precede, coexist with, or follow L&H Hodgkin's lymphoma (64,65). Progressively transformed germinal centers also may be seen in nonspecific lymphadenitis.

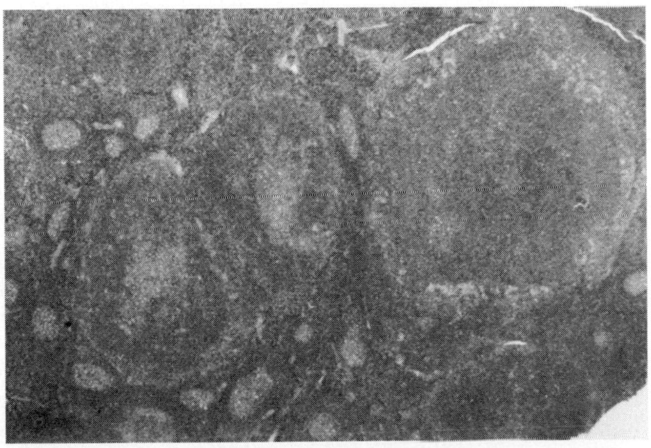

FIG. 14.24. Progressively transformed germinal centers. This is a reactive lymph node in which there are many small reactive follicles, but the striking feature is the presence of three very large ball-like structures, which are progressively transformed germinal centers. These have small follicle centers because they are heavily infiltrated by mantle lymphocyte. The mantle zones are thick (hematoxylin and eosin stain, original magnification: 40× magnification).

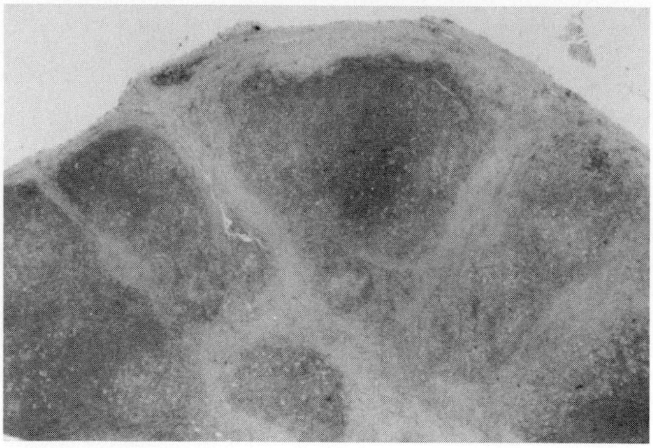

FIG. 14.25. Fibrous nodular pattern produced by thick fibrocollagenous bands. This is a case of nodular sclerosis Hodgkin's lymphoma, in which numerous fibrocollagenous bands produce compartmentalization (large spherical appearance). Note that the lacunar cells (cells with clear cytoplasm) can be seen at this low magnification (hematoxylin and eosin stain, original magnification: 20× magnification).

Nodularity Produced by Thin or Thick Fibrocollagenous Bands

Thin or thick fibrocollagenous bands, a characteristic feature of nodular sclerosing Hodgkin's lymphoma, produce a distinctive nodular pattern (28) (Fig. 14.25). This nodular pattern is a nonspecific feature and can be seen in a variety of benign and malignant diseases.

ADDITIONAL PATTERNS

Sinus Pattern

If cells present in the sinuses cause their distention, the designation *sinus pattern* is used. This pattern can be seen focally, multifocally, or throughout the node (Fig. 14.26).

TABLE 14.14. *Differential diagnosis for sinus pattern*

Benign	Malignant
Sinus histiocytosis with massive lymphadenopathy	Anaplastic large cell lymphoma
Lymphangiography effect	Marginal-zone/monocytoid B-cell lymphoma
Whipple's disease	Mycosis fungoides
Vascular transformation of sinuses	Carcinoma
Sinus histiocytosis	Leukemia
	Kaposi's sarcoma
	Langerhans' cell histiocytosis

The diseases in which a sinus pattern is seen are listed in Table 14.14.

Interfollicular Pattern

The term *interfollicular pattern* implies that the lymph nodes contain several benign follicles or mantle cell nodules, but the interfollicular regions are expanded by the pathologic process. The interfollicular areas may be expanded uniformly by the pathologic process, with no normal intervening regions, as seen in involvement by leukemias, T-cell lymphomas, or viral lymphadenitis. In interfollicular Hodgkin's lymphoma and many benign diseases, the pathologic processes are separated from each other by normal intervening regions (Fig. 14.27). The diseases in which an interfollicular pattern is noted are summarized in Table 14.6.

Lennert's Pattern

We refer to an epithelioid cell population diffusely scattered throughout the lymph node as *Lennert's pattern* (Fig. 14.28). The presence of a diffuse epithelioid cell proliferation is a nonspecific phenomenon seen in a variety of benign

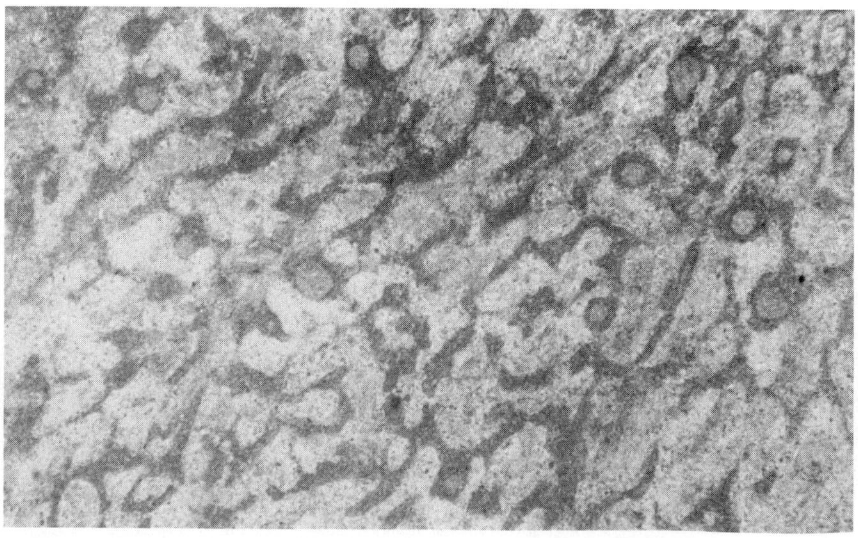

FIG. 14.26. Sinus pattern. This node is from a patient with sinus histiocytosis with massive lymphadenopathy. The sinuses are expanded markedly and show distention by benign histiocytes (hematoxylin and eosin stain, original magnification: 20× magnification).

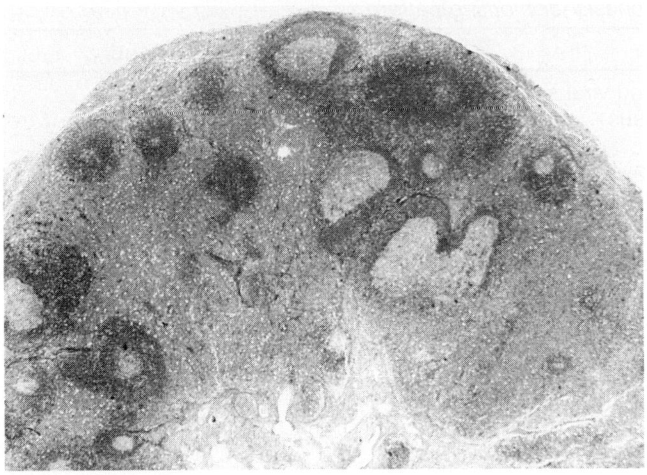

FIG. 14.27. Interfollicular pattern. This node is from a patient with myelomonocytic leukemia. Note that there are several reactive follicles and a few benign mantle cell nodules. The interfollicular areas are expanded by a pathologic process consisting of leukemic blasts. There are no normal areas in the interfollicular regions of the lymph node. The myelomonoblasts are much larger than small mantle lymphocytes (darkly staining) and therefore have a lighter appearance. Note that there is also a starry-sky pattern in the areas of leukemic infiltration (hematoxylin and eosin stain, original magnification: 40× magnification).

and malignant diseases of lymph nodes (66,67). The diseases in which such an epithelioid cell proliferation commonly is observed are listed in Table 14.15.

TABLE 14.15. *Differential diagnosis for Lennert's pattern (diffuse, epithelioid cell proliferation)*

Benign	Malignant
Granulomatous lymphadenitis[a]	Peripheral T-cell lymphomas
Abnormal immune response	T cell–rich large B-cell lymphoma
Abnormal diffuse, lymphoplasmacytic and immunoblastic proliferation	Mixed cellularity Hodgkin's lymphoma
Tuberculosis	Nodular lymphocytic and histiocytic Hodgkin's lymphoma
Sarcoidosis	Rarely other lymphomas

[a] Can be due to different types of infectious diseases

Mottling Pattern

At low magnification, the term *mottling* conventionally is used for scattered, transformed lymphoid cells, among a predominating population of small lymphocytes as seen in cases of viral lymphadenitis. Mottling can be focal or multifocal. We have extended the use of the term to include, besides transformed cells, histiocytes (non–starry sky) (Figs. 14.19, 14.20) and Langerhans' cells and interdigitating dendritic cells, as seen in paracortical nodular T-zone hyperplasia and dermatopathic lymphadenitis. Mottling patterns should be distinguished from the starry-sky pattern (discussed in a subsequent section). The diseases in which mottling is present are listed in Table 14.16.

Vascular Pattern

Marked vascular proliferation, of different types, is seen in many diseases, which can be divided into two main groups: lymphoid diseases and nonlymphoid diseases (22,63) (Table 14.17). The common lymphoid diseases in which marked vascular proliferation is seen include angioimmunoblastic T-cell lymphoma, the hyaline vascular type of giant lymphoid hyperplasia, and angioimmunoblastic lymphadenopathy. In all three conditions, the walls of the vessels show overt hyalinization. The vessels are lined by plump endothelial cells

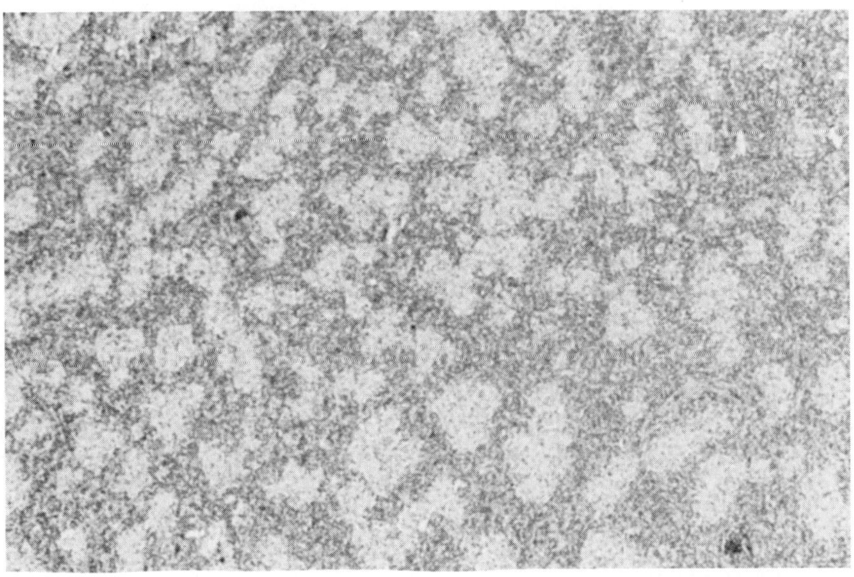

FIG. 14.28. Lennert's pattern. This node is from a patient with Hodgkin's lymphoma of mixed cellularity. There are numerous well-defined clusters of epithelioid histiocytes of varying sizes throughout the lymph node (hematoxylin and eosin stain, original magnification: 40× magnification).

TABLE 14.16. *Differential diagnosis for mottling pattern*

Dominant pathologic feature	Benign	Malignant
Transformed large lymphoid cells	Infectious mononucleosis and viral lymphadenitis Systemic lupus erythematosus Dilantin hypersensitivity	Mycosis fungoides Non-Hodgkin's lymphoma (rare)
Langerhans' cell, interdigitating dendritic cells, histiocytes	Paracortical nodular T-cell hyperplasia[a] Dermatopathic lymphadenitis[a] AIDS, florid and involutionary Kikuchi–Fujimoto disease	

[a] Can be seen in many diseases, both focally and multifocally.

that obliterate their lumen, and the lymphoid cells show proliferation or abnormalities. In all other diseases listed in Table 14.17, except for bacillary angiomatosis, the vascular abnormality is the main pathologic finding, and the lymphoid tissue itself (cells and compartments) is not abnormal.

Necrotic Pattern

The term *necrosis pattern* is used if necrosis can be identified readily (at one large focus or multiple small foci) in a lymph node (63,68) (Table 14.18). Careful study of the areas immediately surrounding the necrotic foci often reveals the most important findings. For example, in nodular sclerosing Hodgkin's lymphoma, Hodgkin's cells in variable numbers almost always are present in the areas immediately adjacent to the necrotic foci.

TABLE 14.17. *Differential diagnosis for vascular pattern*

Benign	Malignant
Hyaline vascular type of giant lymph node hyperplasia	Angioimmunoblastic T-cell lymphoma
Angioimmunoblastic lymphadenopathy[a]	Kaposi's sarcoma
Angiolipomatous hamartoma[b]	
Vascular transformation of sinuses	
Bacillary angiomatosis	
Hemangioma	
Epithelioid hemangioma[c]	
Hemangioendothelioma	
Epithelioid	
Spindle and Epithelioid	
Polymorphous	
Lymphangioma	
Kimura's disease	

[a] May be malignant.
[b] In hyaline vascular type of giant lymph node hyperplasia.
[c] Also known as angiolymphoid hyperplasia with eosinophilia.

TABLE 14.18. *Differential diagnosis for necrosis pattern*

Benign	Malignant
Cat-scratch disease	Nodular sclerosis Hodgkin's lymphoma
Kikuchi–Fujimoto disease	Other lymphomas
Necrotizing lymphadenitis	Nasopharyngeal carcinoma
Lymph node infarction	

Diffuse Pattern

If there are no follicles in the lymph node, and if the proliferation diffusely infiltrates the lymph node or obliterates the lymph node architecture, the term *diffuse pattern* is used (Fig. 14.29). The benign diseases in which a diffuse pattern can be seen are infectious mononucleosis, systemic lupus erythematosus, phenytoin hypersensitivity, angioimmunoblastic lymphadenopathy, and abnormal lymphoplasmacytic and immunoblastic proliferation. All non-Hodgkin's lymphomas other than the follicular type can have a diffuse pattern. Similarly, mixed cellularity and lymphocyte-depletion Hodgkin's lymphomas can have diffuse patterns. Finally, all metastatic processes in the lymph node can have diffuse patterns.

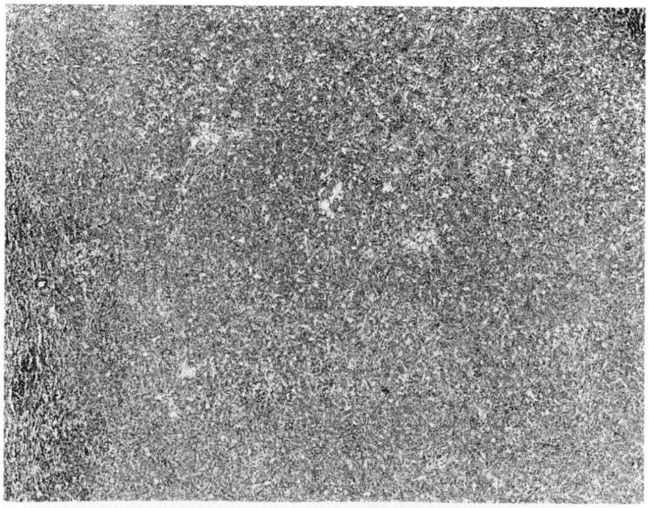

FIG. 14.29. Diffuse pattern. This node is from a patient with large cell lymphoma. There is a great increase in the number of cells per unit area, and the population is lightly stained, which suggests that the proliferating cells are likely to be large cells (hematoxylin and eosin stain, original magnification: 40× magnification).

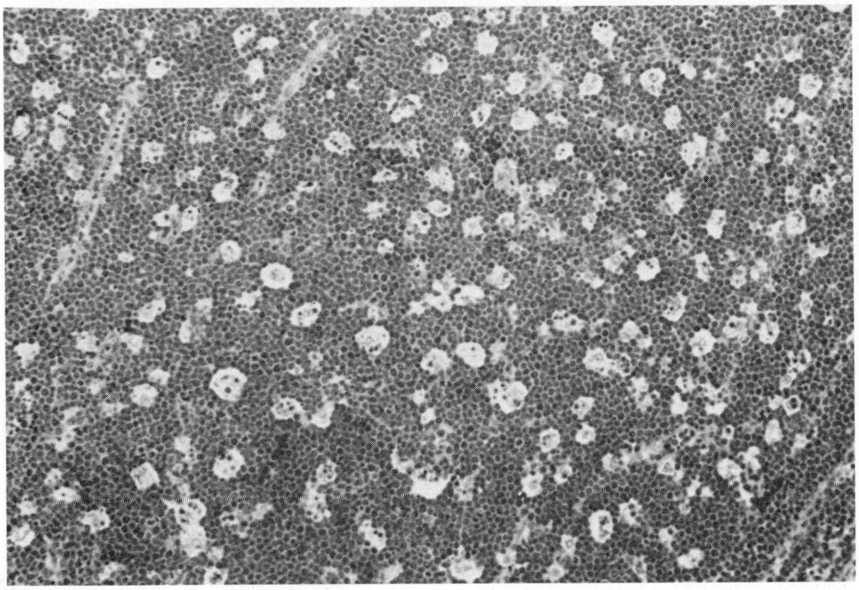

FIG. 14.30. Starry-sky pattern. The lymph node is from a patient with Burkitt's lymphoma, which has a diffuse pattern. In addition, however, there is a very prominent starry-sky pattern at low magnification. Note that there is extensive debris within the cytoplasm of many of the histiocytes. Also, there is a great increase in the number of cells per unit area (hematoxylin and eosin stain, original magnification: 40× magnification).

Starry-Sky Pattern in Diffuse Areas

The presence of numerous benign histiocytes with abundant clear cytoplasm and phagocytosis is termed a *starry-sky pattern*; such a pattern can be seen focally, multifocally, or throughout the node (Fig. 14.30). Because lacunar cells have abundant clear cytoplasm, in nodular sclerosing Hodgkin's lymphoma they produce an appearance that resembles a starry-sky pattern on low-magnification viewing. The diseases in which a starry-sky pattern can be seen include infectious mononucleosis, benign lymphocyte-rich epithelial thymoma, all intermediate and high grade non-Hodgkin's lymphomas, and acute myeloid leukemias.

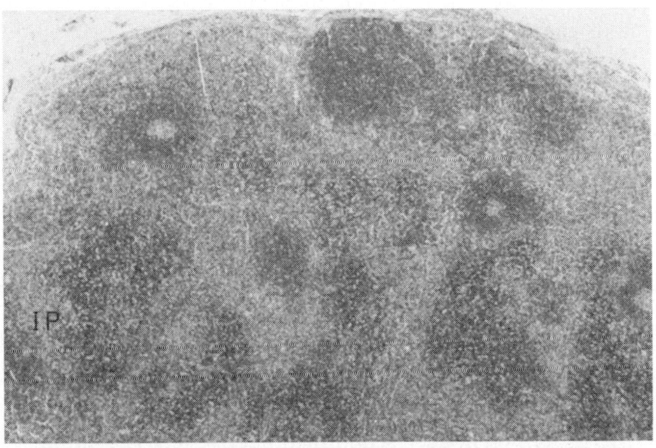

FIG. 14.31. Mixed patterns. This node is from a patient with viral lymphadenitis in which the following are present: sinus, interfollicular, and mantle zone patterns and nodular paracortical T-cell hyperplasia with mottling. The transformed lymphoid cells are seen in subcapsular and medullary sinuses and the interfollicular (pale-staining) areas. Note that the sinuses and the interfollicular areas have the same color, suggesting the location of the pathology. There are at least eight nodules of paracortical nodular T-cell hyperplasia in which there is mottling. Other examples of mixed patterns (with multiple pathologies) are seen in Figures 14.5, 14.6, 14.17, 14.18, and 14.19 (hematoxylin and eosin stain, original magnification: 40× magnification).

Mixed Patterns

If pathologic processes are found in two or more compartments, the term *mixed* is used. Spherical structures and patterns of different types commonly coexist, and they have to be correlated with each other to establish a correct diagnosis. Moreover, multiple pathologic processes or patterns are commonly seen in benign diseases (Fig. 14.31). Figures 14.5, 14.6, 14.17, 14.19, and 14.27 show the presence of multiple patterns.

Miscellaneous

Diseases that can show extensive infiltration of pericapsular fat are listed in Table 14.19. Although pericapsular infil-

TABLE 14.19. *Differential diagnosis for infiltration of pericapsular fat*

Benign	Malignant
Giant lymph node hyperplasia	Non-Hodgkin's lymphoma (common)
Florid reactive follicular hyperplasia	Angioimmunoblastic lymphadenopathy
Kikuchi–Fujimoto disease	Rare except in nodular sclerosing Hodgkin's lymphoma
Necrotizing lymphadenitis	Carcinoma (rare)
Systemic lupus erythematosus	Leukemia (common)
Cat-scratch disease	
Lymphogranuloma venereum	
Infectious mononucleosis	
Abnormal lymphoplasmacytic and immunoblastic proliferation	

tration is very common in non-Hodgkin's lymphomas, it also is seen in several benign diseases (Table 14.19).

Marked thickening of the capsule is common in giant lymph node hyperplasia, syphilis, other chronic infectious diseases, nodular sclerosing Hodgkin's lymphoma, and metastatic nasopharyngeal carcinoma. It sometimes can be seen in other malignant lymphomas.

HIGH MAGNIFICATION

Cytologic features should be evaluated at high magnification only after the lymph node has been carefully examined at low magnification. Because malignant lymphomas are neoplasms of individual cells, it is very important to study the different cellular constituents carefully. Every effort should be made to recognize and quantify cells of different types, because this helps to make an accurate diagnosis.

Changes Produced by Different Fixatives, and Recognition of Artifacts

Recognizing fixation artifacts and subtle changes produced by different fixatives is one of the most important aspects of lymph node pathology (20,21). This is discussed in detail in Chapter 12.

Assessing Cellularity

Assessment of cellularity requires considerable experience but provides a parameter useful in distinguishing between benign and malignant proliferations. For example, in most non-Hodgkin's lymphomas there is a great increase in the number of cells per unit area (hypercellularity). In most Hodgkin's lymphomas and most benign diseases, the lymph node is normocellular or hypocellular.

Predominating Population

The concept of a predominating cell population, determined at low magnification based on colors or patterns, is also very useful at high magnification. The presence of an exclusive population, in one or multiple compartments, usually indicates a diagnosis of non-Hodgkin's lymphoma.

Mitotic Figures in Nonfollicular Areas

We have found that determination of the number of mitotic figures in nonfollicular areas, which is a reproducible morphologic parameter, is useful for arriving at a precise diagnosis. In most non-Hodgkin's lymphomas, many mitotic figures are readily identified; in Hodgkin's lymphoma, there is less mitotic activity (69). In most benign diseases, mitotic figures are few, although in various types of viral lymphadenitis, Kikuchi's disease, and systemic lupus erythematosus, many mitotic figures are seen, as in non-Hodgkin's lymphoma.

CORRELATING HISTOLOGIC DIAGNOSIS WITH CLINICAL INFORMATION

Before one orders immunostains or molecular studies, a careful review of the clinical history is necessary, because many diseases have characteristic clinical findings at presentation. For example, if sheets of large cells are seen in a lymph node or tonsil in a young person who has acute onset of cervical lymphadenopathy or tonsillar enlargement, the cause is most likely to be infectious mononucleosis rather than a large cell or Hodgkin's lymphoma. Follicular lymphomas are very rare in the first two decades of life. Other low-grade B-cell lymphomas also are rare in children. A large mediastinal mass in a boy is strongly suggestive of lymphoblastic lymphoma. A large mediastinal mass in a young female is strongly suggestive of nodular sclerosing Hodgkin's lymphoma or primary mediastinal large B-cell lymphoma. Mediastinal mass is also typical of giant lymph node hyperplasia of the hyaline vascular type. In elderly patients (older than 75 years), lymph node enlargement is more likely to result from malignant than from benign diseases. Most lymphomas in the stomach are mucosa-associated lymphoid tumors. Primary Hodgkin's lymphoma in the skin or at extranodal sites is very rare. Awareness of clinicopathologic correlations helps in establishing a diagnosis. If expected clinical correlations are not present, slides must be studied again carefully, to determine whether any significant pathologic findings were overlooked.

SUMMARY AND CONCLUSIONS

The cardinal rules for making accurate diagnoses of lymph node diseases are as follows:

- The lymph node should be received in a fresh state, several touch imprints should be made, and one should be stained immediately so that cytologic features can be evaluated. Slices 3 mm in thickness should be placed in B5 fixative and 10% neutral buffered formalin, and a slice should be frozen for immunologic and molecular biologic studies. For polymerase chain reaction–based studies, a formalin-fixed paraffin block is required. Awareness of the changes produced by different fixatives and of artifacts is essential.
- To distinguish different patterns and quantify the percentage of the total area occupied by each of the compartments of the lymph node, a scanning objective lens (2× or 2.5×) is absolutely necessary. To enhance pattern recognition, optimal contrast is needed. To achieve this, the microscope should be equipped with a continuous rheostat, with which the intensity of light passing through the condenser can be modulated. Both low and high magnifications are absolutely essential to make an accurate diagnosis (Tables 14.1, 14.5, 14.7). Smears obtained through fine needle aspiration should be discouraged, because they have many limitations (Tables 14.1, 14.3–14.8).
- The best morphologic approach is to evaluate the lymph node extensively at low magnification with a scanning

lens, in order to study the colors in the different compartments, the architectural features, and the patterns and assess the cellularity of the proliferation. Non-Hodgkin's lymphomas, like other cancers, exhibit an increase in the number of cells per unit area (hypercellularity); benign proliferations, with a few exceptions, do not (Tables 14.3, 14.4). A correlation between colors and cells should be made by switching between low and high magnifications (Table 14.2). This method permits identification of cells of certain types at low magnification.

- At low magnification, the pathologic process or processes must be identified so that a differential diagnosis can be formed. In most benign diseases and some Hodgkin's lymphomas, the pathologic changes are focal or multifocal, and methods to identify these should be learned and practiced. Complete familiarity with the pathologic abnormalities occurring in different compartments is essential (Table 14.5). The pathologic process in most non-Hodgkin's lymphomas displays a distinctive pattern, and recognition of this pattern is necessary to form a proper differential diagnosis (Tables 14.5–14.7). Many patterns are formed as a result of an exaggeration of the normal compartments or a marked proliferation of certain cell types. Spherical structures should be identified accurately because most lymphomas exhibit this pattern (Fig. 14.1, Tables 14.8–14.13). All patterns are defined in detail and illustrated in this chapter (Figs. 14.2–14.31), and for each pattern a differential diagnosis is presented (Tables 14.6, 14.8–14.19).
- After lymph node sections have been evaluated thoroughly at low magnification, cytologic features should be studied carefully at high magnification. The presence of a predominant population in different compartments should be observed, and the number of mitotic figures in nonfollicular areas should be counted. The cellularity of the lymph node should be assessed at high magnification.
- Clinical history must be carefully correlated with morphologic findings before doing immunologic or molecular studies.
- Immunologic or molecular biologic studies, if required, should be performed on B5- or formalin-fixed or frozen sections. If after these studies have been performed a definitive diagnosis cannot be reached, a repeat biopsy should be undertaken, and further consultation should be sought with an expert.

REFERENCES

1. Rowley JD, Fukuhara S. Chromosome studies in non-Hodgkin's lymphomas. *Semin Oncol* 1980;7:255–266.
2. Sandberg AA. Chromosome changes in the lymphomas. *Hum Pathol* 1981;12:531–540.
3. Yunis JJ. The chromosomal basis of human neoplasia. *Science* 1983; 221:227–235.
4. Levine EG, Arthur DC, Frizzera G, et al. There are differences in cytogenetic abnormalities among histologic subtypes of non-Hodgkin's lymphomas. *Blood* 1985;66:1414–1422.
5. Cleary ML, Warnke R, Sklar J. Immunoglobulin gene rearrangement studies as a diagnostic criterion of B-cell lymphoma. *Proc Natl Acad Sci USA* 1981;81:593–597.
6. Sklar J. DNA hybridization in diagnostic pathology. *Hum Pathol* 1985; 16:654–658.
7. Cleary ML, Trela MJ, Weiss LM, et al. Most null large cell lymphomas are B-lineage neoplasms. *Lab Invest* 1985;53:521–525.
8. Vardiman JW. Acute leukemias and myeloid disorders. *Am J Surg Pathol* 1997;21:114–121(abst).
9. Nathwani BN, Burke JS, Winberg CD. Architectural features of normal, neoplastic, and non-neoplastic lymph nodes: a practical diagnostic approach. In: Murphy GF, Martin MC, eds. *Lymphoproliferative disorders of the skin.* Boston: Butterworth, 1986:73–119.
10. Nathwani BN. Classifying non-Hodgkin's lymphomas. In: Berard CW, Dorfman RF, eds. *Malignant lymphomas.* IAP Monograph no. 29. Baltimore: Williams & Wilkins, 1987:18–80.
11. Nathwani BN. Diagnostic significance of morphologic patterns in lymph node proliferations. In: Knowles DM, ed. *Neoplastic hematopathology.* Baltimore: Williams & Wilkins, 1992;407–425.
12. Nathwani BN, Heckerman DE, Horvitz EJ, et al. Integrated expert systems and videodisc in surgical pathology: an overview. *Hum Pathol* 1990;21:11–27.
13. Nathwani B, Clarke K, Lincoln T, et al. Evaluation of an expert system on lymph node pathology. *Hum Pathol* 1997;28:1097–1110.
14. Ackerman AB, Niven J, Grant-Kels JM. *Differential diagnosis in dermatopathology.* Philadelphia: Lea & Febiger, 1982.
15. Toker C. *Tumors: an atlas of differential diagnosis.* Baltimore: University Park Press, 1983.
16. Hajdu S. *Differential diagnosis of soft tissue and bone tumors.* Philadelphia: Lea & Febiger, 1986.
17. Ackerman A, Jacobson M, Vitale P. *Clues to diagnosis in dermatopathology.* Chicago: ASCP Press, 1991.
18. Gal AG, Koss MN. *Differential diagnosis in pathology: pulmonary disorders.* Baltimore: Williams & Wilkins, 1997.
19. Al-Nafussi AW, Atif I, Hughes D. *Differential diagnosis in pathology: two different approaches. Histological diagnosis of tumors by pattern analysis. An A-Z guide.* London: Arnold, 1997.
20. Bowling MC. Lymph node specimens: achieving technical excellence. *Lab Med* 1979;10:467–476.
21. Beard C, Nabers K, Bowling MC, et al. Achieving technical excellence in lymph node specimens: an update. *Lab Med* 1985;16:468–475.
22. Warnke RA, Weiss LM, Chan JKC, et al. *Atlas of tumor pathology: tumors of the lymph nodes and spleen.* Washington, DC: Armed Forces Institute of Pathology, 1995.
23. Gretz JE, Kaldjian EP, Anderson AO, et al. Sophisticated strategies for information encounter in the lymph node: the reticular network as a conduit of soluble information and a highway for cell traffic. *J Immunol* 1996;157:495–499.
24. Gretz JE, Anderson AO, Shaw S. Cords, channels, corridors and conduits: critical architectural elements facilitating cell interactions in the lymph node cortex. *Immunol Rev* 1997;156:11–24.
25. Lukes RF, Collins RD. New observations on follicular lymphoma. In: Akazaki K, Rappaport H, Berard CW, et al, eds. *Malignant diseases of the hematopoietic system.* GANN Monograph on Cancer Research No. 15. Tokyo: University of Tokyo Press, 1973:209–215.
26. Lennert K, Mohri N, Stein H, et al. The histopathology of malignant lymphoma. *Br J Haematol* 1975;31[Suppl]:193–203.
27. Metter GE, Nathwani BN, Burke JS, et al. Morphological subclassification of follicular lymphoma: variability of diagnoses among hematopathologists, a collaborative study between the Repository Center and Pathology Panel for Lymphoma Clinical Studies. *J Clin Oncol* 1985; 3:25–38.
28. Lukes RJ, Butler JJ. The pathology and nomenclature of Hodgkin's disease. *Cancer Res* 1966;26:1–63.
29. Kaufman AG, Nathwani BN, Preston K Jr. Subclassification of follicular lymphomas by computerized microscopy. *Hum Pathol* 1987;18: 226–231.
30. Link N, Nathwani BN, Preston K. Subclassification of follicular lymphoma by computerized image processing. *Anal Quant Cytol* 1989;11: 119–130.
31. Preston K Jr, Firestone LM, Nathwani BN. Use of three-dimensional mathematical morphology in analyzing histologic images with applications in subtyping follicular lymphomas. *Anal Quant Cytol Histol* 1990; 12:399–416.

32. Robb-Smith AHT. The lymph node biopsy. In: Dyke SC, ed. Recent advances in clinical pathology. London: Churchill, 1947:350.
33. Butler JJ. Non-neoplastic lesions of lymph nodes of man to be differentiated from lymphomas. *Natl Cancer Inst Monogr* 1969;32:233–255.
34. Dorfman RF, Warnke R. Lymphadenopathy simulating the malignant lymphomas. *Hum Pathol* 1974;5:519–550.
35. Robb-Smith AHT, Taylor CR. A diagnostic atlas. New York: Oxford University Press, 1981.
36. Van Krieken JHJM, von Schilling C, Kluin PM, et al. Splenic marginal zone lymphocytes and related cells in the lymph node: a morphologic and immunohistochemical study. *Hum Pathol* 1989;20:320–325.
37. Van den Oord JJ, de Wolf-Peeters C, Desmet VJ. The marginal zone in the human reactive lymph node. *Am J Clin Pathol* 1986;86:475–479.
38. Spencer J, Finn T, Pulford KAF, et al. The human gut contains a novel population of B lymphocytes which resemble marginal zone cells. *Clin Exp Immunol* 1985;62:607–612.
39. Nathwani BN, Mohrmann RL, Brynes RK, et al. Monocytoid B-cell lymphomas: an assessment of diagnostic criteria and a perspective on histogenesis. *Hum Pathol* 1992;23:1061–1071.
40. Weisenburger DD, Kim H, Rappaport H. Mantle-zone lymphoma: a follicular variant of intermediate lymphocytic lymphoma. *Cancer* 1982; 49:1429–1438.
41. Samoszuk MK, Epstein AL, Said J, et al. Sensitivity and specificity of immunostaining in the diagnosis of mantle zone lymphoma. *Am J Clin Pathol* 1986;85:557–563.
42. Nathwani BN, Drachenberg MR, Hernandez AM, et al. Nodal monocytoid B-cell lymphoma (nodal marginal-zone B-cell lymphoma). *Semin Hematol* 1999;36:128–138.
43. Nathwani BN, Hernandez AM, Deol I, et al. Marginal zone B-cell lymphomas: an appraisal. *Hum Pathol* 1997;28:42–46.
44. Harris NL, Jaffe ES, Stein H, et al. A revised European-American Classification of lymphoid neoplasms: a proposal from the International Lymphoma Study Group. *Blood* 1994;84:1361–1392.
45. Isaacson PG, Spencer J. Monocytoid B-cell lymphomas [letter]. *Am J Surg Pathol* 1990;14:888–890.
46. Dierlamm J, Pittaluga S, Wlodarska I, et al. Marginal zone B-cell lymphomas of different sites share similar cytogenetic and morphologic features. *Blood* 1996;87:299–307.
47. Pittaluga S, Verhoef G, Criel A, et al. ''Small'' B-cell non-Hodgkin's lymphomas with splenomegaly at presentation are either mantle cell lymphoma or marginal zone cell lymphoma: a study based on histology, cytology, immunohistochemistry, and cytogenetic analysis. *Am J Surg Pathol* 1996:20:211–223.
48. Hammer RD, Glick AD, Greer JP, et al. Splenic marginal zone lymphoma: a distinct B-cell neoplasm. *Am J Surg Pathol* 1996;20:613–626.
49. Isaacson PG. Splenic marginal zone lymphoma [Letter]. *Blood* 1996; 88:751.
50. Mollejo M, Lloret E, Men*β*rguez J, et al. Lymph node involvement by splenic marginal zone lymphoma: morphological and immunohistochemical features. *Am J Surg Pathol* 1997;21:772–780.
51. Dierlamm J, Pittaluga S, Wlodarska I, et al. Response to ''Letter to the Editor'' on splenic marginal zone lymphoma. *Blood* 1996;88:751–752.
52. Hernandez AM, Nathwani BN, Nguyen D, et al. Nodal benign and malignant monocytoid B cells with and without follicular lymphomas: a comparative study of follicular colonization, light chain restriction, Bcl-2 and t(14:18) in 39 Cases. *Hum Pathol* 1995;26:625–632.
53. Nathwani BN, Anderson JR, Armitage JO, et al. Clinical significance of follicular lymphoma with monocytoid B-cells. *Hum Pathol* 1999; 30:263–268.
54. Ellison DJ, Nathwani BN, Cho SY, et al. Interfollicular small lymphocytic lymphoma: the diagnostic significance of pseudofollicles. *Hum Pathol* 1989;20:1108–1118.
55. Nathwani BN, Winberg CD. Non-Hodgkin's lymphomas: an appraisal of the ''working formulation'' of non-Hodgkin's lymphomas for clinical usage. In: Sommers SC, Rosen PP, eds. *Malignant lymphomas: a pathology annual monograph.* Norwalk, CT: Appleton–Century–Crofts, 1983:1–64.
56. Ott G, Rüdiger TH, Ichinohasama R, et al. Peripheral T-cell lymphomas with peri-follicular growth pattern. Presented at the ninth meeting of the European Association for Haematopathology, Leiden, Netherlands, 1998 (abst O-14).
57. Horny H-P, Sillaber C, Menke D, et al. Diagnostic value of immunostaining for tryptase in patients with mastocytosis. *Am J Surg Pathol* 1998;22:1132–1140.
58. Swerdlow SH, Zukerberg LR, Yang W-I, et al. The morphologic spectrum of non-Hodgkin's lymphomas with BCL1/cyclin D1 gene rearrangements. *Am J Surg Pathol* 1996;20:627–640.
59. Dunn-Walters DK, Boursier L, Spencer J, et al. Analysis of immunoglobulin genes in splenic marginal zone lymphoma suggests ongoing mutation. *Hum Pathol* 1998;29:585–593.
60. Alkan S, Ross CW, Hanson CA, et al. Follicular lymphoma with involvement of the splenic marginal zone: a pitfall in the differential diagnosis of splenic marginal zone cell lymphoma. *Hum Pathol* 1996; 27:503–506.
61. Isaacson PG, MacLennan KA, Subbuswamy SG. Multiple lymphomatous polyposis of the gastrointestinal tract. *Histopathology* 1984;8: 641–656.
62. Isaacson PG, Wotherspoon AC, Diss T, et al. Follicular colonization in B-cell lymphoma of mucosa-associated lymphoid tissue. *Am J Surg Pathol* 1991;15:819–828.
63. Chan JKC, Tsang WYW. Reactive lymphadenopathies. In: Weiss LM, ed. *Contemporary issues in surgical pathology: pathology of lymph nodes.* New York: Churchill Livingstone, 1996;81–168.
64. Poppema S, Kaiserling E, Lennert K. Hodgkin's disease with lymphocytic predominance, nodular type (nodular paragranuloma) and progressively transformed germinal centers: cytohistological study. *Histopathology* 1979;3:295–308.
65. Burns BF, Colby TV, Dorfman RF. Differential diagnostic features of nodular L & H Hodgkin's disease, including progressive transformation of germinal centers. *Am J Surg Pathol* 1984;8:253–261.
66. Lennert K, Metsdagh J. Lymphogranulomatosen mit konstant hohem epithelioid-Zellgehalt. *Virchows Arch A* 1968;344:1–20.
67. Kim H, Nathwani BN, Rappaport H. So-called ''Lennert's Lymphoma:'' Is it a clinico-pathologic entity? *Cancer* 1980;45:1379–1399.
68. Schnitzer B. Reactive lymphoid hyperplasias. In: Jaffe ES, ed. *Surgical pathology of the lymph nodes and related organs.* Philadelphia: WB Saunders, 1995;98–132.
69. Nguyen D, Nathwani BN, Ellison DJ, et al. Differential diagnosis between T-cell lymphoma and Hodgkin's disease: the value of mitotic counts and pericapsular infiltration. *Hematol Pathol* 1989;3:63–71.

CHAPTER 15

The Reactive Lymphadenopathies

Bertram Schnitzer

Pathologists must be thoroughly familiar with the many different types of benign lymphadenopathies (reactive hyperplasias), because a substantial number of lymph nodes reveal benign rather than malignant lymphoproliferations if biopsy is performed. Paradoxically, the amount of published literature about benign reactive lymphadenopathies is far exceeded by the number of publications about malignant lymphomas. Recognition of reactive hyperplasias permits the pathologist to suggest a cause of the lymphoproliferation in a limited number of cases and, more importantly, aids in the differential diagnosis with Hodgkin's disease and non-Hodgkin's lymphomas, which hyperplastic lymph nodes sometimes mimic closely. If the distinction between benign lymphoproliferations and lymphoma cannot be established clearly on morphologic grounds alone, the pathologist must correlate morphologic findings with those of such ancillary techniques as immunophenotyping (which can be carried out readily on paraffin-embedded sections), immunogenotypic analysis, and *in situ* hybridization, in order to differentiate polyclonal from monoclonal (presumably, but not invariably, malignant) proliferations (1). If such techniques are not readily available or fresh or cryopreserved tissue is lacking, the pathologist must rely on the gold standard of diagnosis, his morphologic acumen, to make an interpretation. If a definitive diagnosis cannot be established, a repeat lymph node biopsy should be undertaken.

Because the cause of reactive lymphadenopathies is usually unknown, an etiologic classification is impractical. Therefore, reactive hyperplasias, which may be defined as polyclonal proliferations of B and T lymphocytes, are classified according to the structural and immunologic compartments from which they arise, or according to a composite scheme of nodal abnormalities (2–6). These hyperplasias may involve the follicles, which are B-cell areas, the paracortical or interfollicular (T-cell) regions, or the cells of the sinuses, which belong to the monocyte–macrophage system (6). Plasmacytosis of medullary cords, which may accompany follicular hyperplasia, is also morphologic evidence of a B-cell response. The B-cell response is indicative of humoral antibody production, whereas hyperplasia of paracortical T cells is associated with cell-mediated immune reactions. Expansions of the paracortical regions may result from a proliferation of indigenous T cells or may be secondary to the accumulation of B cells that have migrated from stimulated germinal centers. Simultaneous proliferations of cells of several compartments, such as follicles and paracortical areas, or sinus cells, or a combination of paracortical cells and sinus cells, may be present. Although the cause of proliferation of cells of the various compartments of the lymph nodes is not known, this expansion probably results in part from bacterial and viral agents, or their products, and the cytokines produced by the stimulated lymphoid cells. The many varied types of hyperplasia may differ somewhat from one another because the immunologic makeup of individuals differs. The morphologic appearance of the hyperplasia varies even if the stimulating agent is the same, depending on the age of the patient, past experience with the offending agent, the time period following exposure to the stimulus, and the duration of the exposure. Although the causes of the majority of cases of reactive lymphadenopathies is not known, some agents produce characteristic histologic changes, enabling the pathologist to suggest a specific diagnosis or a differential diagnosis that may be confirmed by histochemical stains, additional cultures, serologic tests, or molecular methods (e.g., polymerase chain reaction). For example, the histologic changes in lymph nodes of patients with rheumatoid arthritis and syphilis may be characteristic but not specific, and the clinical history and serologic or genotypic studies may be used to confirm the histologic impression (7–9). Acute acquired toxoplasmosis may show characteristic lymph node changes, and the suggested diagnosis must be verified by appropriate serologic studies (10). HIV infection may be suspected from histologic findings, and appropriate testing can be suggested (11). Systemic

B. Schnitzer: Department of Pathology, University of Michigan, Ann Arbor, Michigan 48109-0602

TABLE 15.1. *Patterns of lymph node hyperplasia*

Follicular pattern
Reactive follicular hyperplasia (nonspecific)
AIDS-related (Chapter 28)
Rheumatoid arthritis
Syphilis
Castleman's disease
Progressive transformation of germinal centers
Sinus pattern
Sinus histiocytosis
Sinus histiocytosis with massive lymphadenopathy
Monocytoid B-cell hyperplasia
Hemophagocytic syndrome
Whipple's disease
Lymphangiographic changes
Langerhans' cell histiocytosis
Vascular transformation of sinuses
Kaposi's sarcoma
Diffuse pattern
Infectious mononucleosis
Herpes zoster and herpes simplex lymphadenitis
Postvaccinial lymphadenitis
Drug-induced hypersensitivity reactions
Angioimmunoblastic lymphadenopathy (Chapter 16)
Mixed pattern
Toxoplasmic lymphadenitis
Dermatopathic lymphadenitis
Granulomatous lymphadenitis
Nonnecrotizing: sarcoidosis
Necrotizing: cat-scratch disease, lymphogranuloma venereum, yersinia
Histiocytic necrotizing lymphadenitis (Kikuchi's disease)
Systemic lupus erythematosus
Mucocutaneous lymph node syndrome (Kawasaki disease)

lupus erythematosus and Kikuchi's disease may be inseparable on morphologic grounds, but clinical history and immunologic studies differentiate between these entities (12). The histologic pictures of cat-scratch disease and lymphogranuloma venereum may be similar or identical; however, the Warthin-Starry stain demonstrates characteristic filamentous pleomorphic organisms in the former but not in the latter disorder (13,14). Polymerase chain reaction studies also differentiate between these infectious diseases (14).

Four categories of hyperplasia are discussed and illustrated here: follicular, diffuse, sinus, and mixed (Table 15.1).

FOLLICULAR HYPERPLASIA

Follicular hyperplasia may be defined as an increase in the number and size of follicles contributing to the enlargement of the lymph node. It is usually secondary to enlargement of the germinal center, often at the expense of the mantle zone, although in some instances the mantle zone also is increased in size. Mantle zones are usually intact but may be attenuated around large germinal centers. The follicles generally vary not only in size but also in shape. Follicular hyperplasia commonly is seen in children and adolescents, and its cause generally is unknown. In these age groups the hyperplasia may be exuberant, with follicles composed predominantly of large germinal centers occupying cortical, paracortical, and even medullary zones. Such a florid follicular hyperplasia is uncommonly seen in adults, except in patients with rheumatoid arthritis or, less commonly, other autoimmune disorders (7,15,16). In recent years, a severe florid or ''explosive'' reactive follicular hyperplasia has been reported in patients with AIDS or AIDS-related complex (17) (Chapter 28).

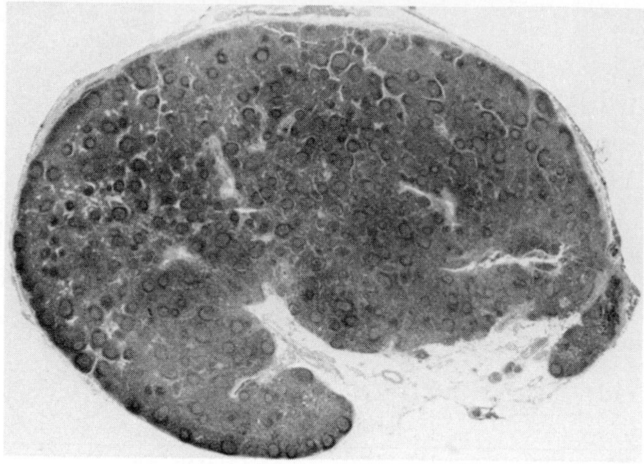

FIG. 15.1. Lymph node from a patient with rheumatoid arthritis showing follicular hyperplasia. The enlarged follicles with prominent germinal centers vary in size and shape and are seen throughout both cortex and medulla (hematoxylin and eosin stain, original magnification: 5× magnification).

In addition to an increase in the size and number of follicles (Figs. 15.1, 15.2), the enlarged germinal center is characterized by a mixture of follicle center lymphocytes, ranging from small (centrocytes) to large (centroblasts), some cells having cleaved and others noncleaved nuclei (Fig. 15.3). Plasma cells, occasionally in substantial numbers, may be present among the follicle center cells (Fig. 15.4).

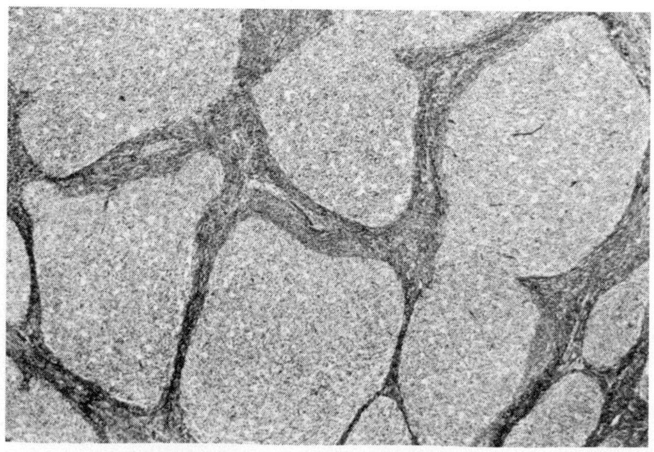

FIG. 15.2. Nonspecific follicular hyperplasia. The follicles vary in size and shape and contain many tingible body macrophages imparting a starry-sky appearance (hematoxylin and eosin stain, original magnification: 120× magnification).

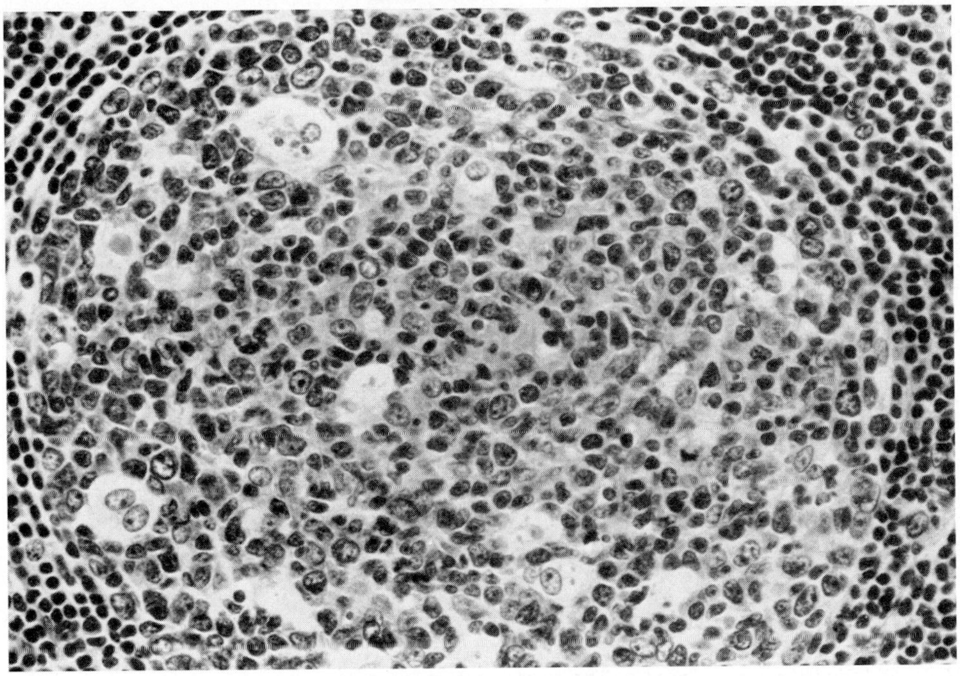

FIG. 15.3. Hyperplastic germinal center is sharply demarcated from the surrounding mantle zone lymphocytes and contains a mixture of small and large cleaved and noncleaved cells interspersed with tingible body macrophages (hematoxylin and eosin stain, original magnification: 500× magnification).

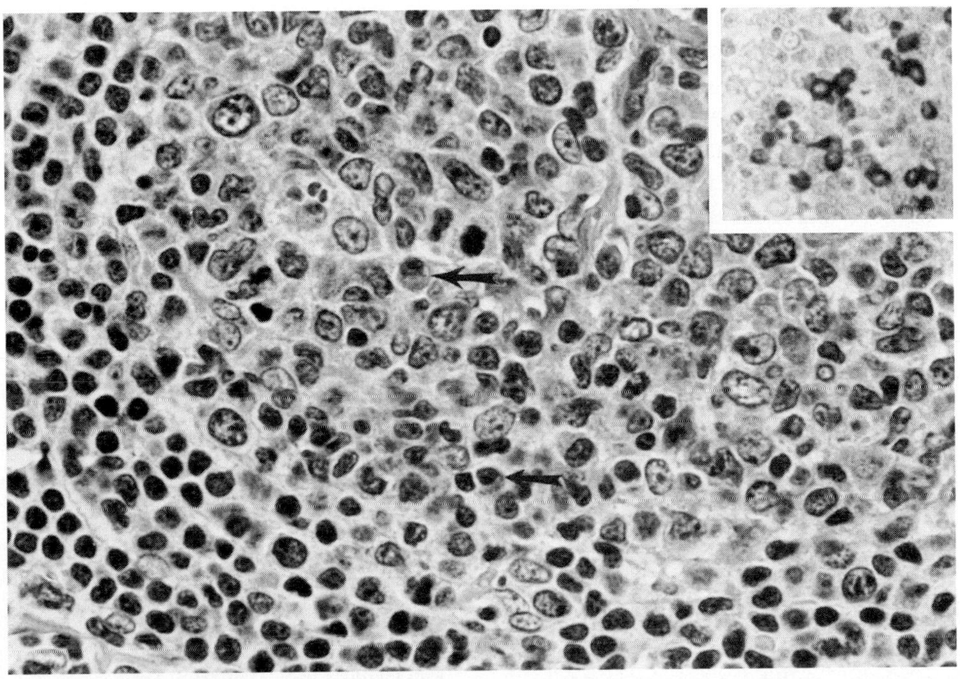

FIG. 15.4. Occasional plasma cells (*arrows*) are seen among the germinal center cells in a reactive germinal center (hematoxylin and eosin stain, original magnification: 625× magnification). **Inset:** Plasma cells are easily detected by staining for immunoglobulin light chains (hematoxylin and eosin stain, original magnification: 500× magnification).

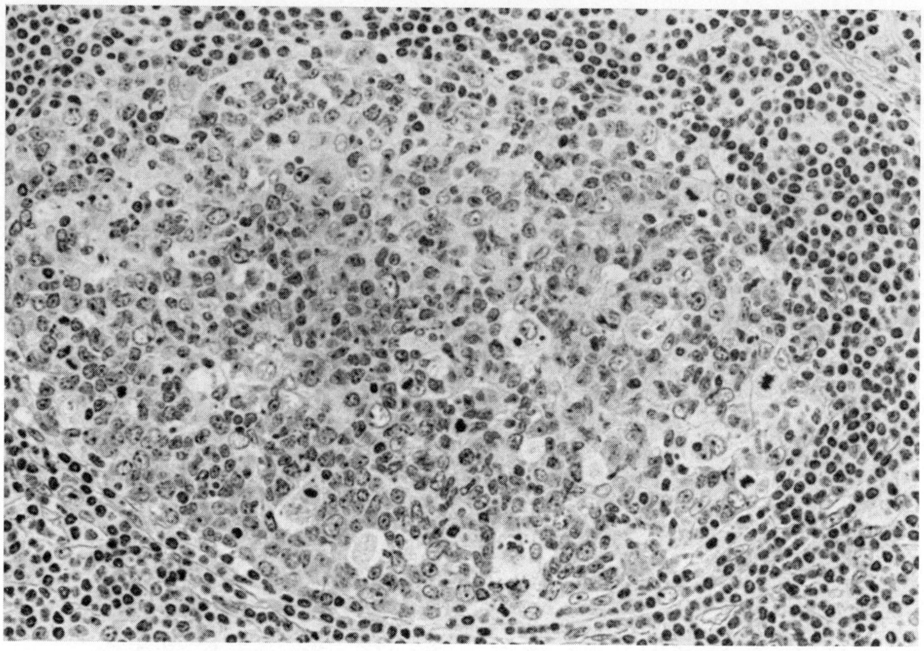

FIG. 15.5. Polarized germinal center. The lower part of the germinal center consists predominantly of large transformed lymphoid cells interspersed with tingible body macrophages, and there is a high rate of mitosis. The remainder of the germinal center is composed of a mixture of small and large cells and lacks evidence of a high proliferative rate (hematoxylin and eosin stain, original magnification: 500× magnification).

A prominent feature that is usually but not invariably present is a starry-sky pattern caused by the presence of histiocytes (macrophages) containing phagocytosed debris (apoptotic cells) among the proliferating cells, which exhibit a moderate to high proliferative rate as evidenced by many mitotic figures (Figs. 15.2–15.5). Apoptotic bodies usually can be seen easily among the proliferating cells. A minority of follicles show germinal centers organized or polarized into two zones: a light-staining zone that faces the sinus, the site of antigen entry into the node, composed predominantly of small cleaved cells and antigen-presenting dendritic cells; and a dark-staining zone at the opposite pole of the follicle and farthest from the sinus, composed of noncleaved large lymphocytes. A high rate of mitosis, apoptotic cells, and tingible body macrophages are present in the dark zone (Fig 15.5). The mantle zone is often wider around the light than the dark zone (Fig. 15.5). Demarcation of the germinal center from the mantle zone lymphocytes is sharp in most but not all instances, as is the border between the mantle zone and paracortical areas. If follicles become very large, the mantle zone may become attenuated or may be completely replaced by the expanded germinal center (Fig. 15.6), thus compressing the sinuses. In explosive follicular hyperplasia, which may be seen in lymph nodes of HIV-positive patients, sinuses are dilated and are filled with monocytoid B cells, which also may infiltrate the paracortical areas (Fig. 15.7). Another feature of a more explosive follicular hyperplasia is the fusion of two or more neighboring germinal centers, resulting in oddly shaped geographic outlines (Fig. 15.8).

The interfollicular regions may be compressed by the expanded follicles, or there may be a concomitant proliferation of a variety of cells in these areas. The cellular composition varies but usually consists of mixtures of small lymphocytes, plasma cells, immunoblasts, and, occasionally, histiocytes and eosinophils. A vascular proliferation is often present. Plasmacytosis of medullary cords usually accompanies follicular hyperplasia.

Differential Diagnosis

Follicular hyperplasias must be differentiated from follicular lymphomas, especially from those of the mixed small

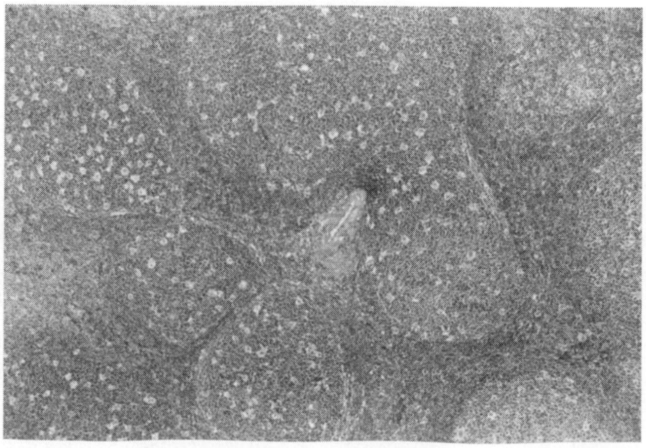

FIG. 15.6. Explosive follicular hyperplasia with absent mantle zones in a patient who has tested positive for HIV (hematoxylin and eosin stain, original magnification: 200× magnification).

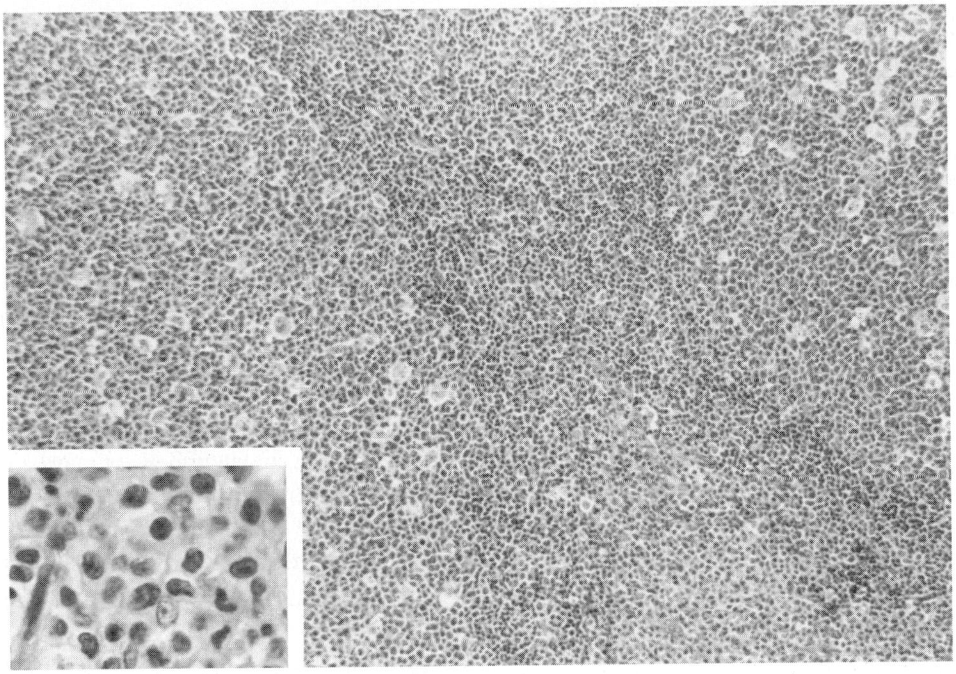

FIG. 15.7. Parts of two huge hyperplastic germinal centers with many tingible body macrophages, absent mantle zones, and paracortical monocytoid B cells in an HIV-positive male (hematoxylin and eosin stain, original magnification: 400× magnification). **Inset:** Higher-magnification view of monocytoid B cells (original magnification: 500× magnification).

cleaved and large cell type, the large cell type, and less often the small cleaved cell type, in which the population of cells is much more uniform than in hyperplastic follicles (Table 15.2) (Chapter 24). Mantle cell lymphoma, small lymphocytic lymphoma or chronic lymphocytic leukemia with proliferation centers, and even the nodular form of lymphocyte predominance Hodgkin's disease are considered occasionally in the differential diagnosis (Chapters 17, 21, 22). The difficulties encountered in differentiating follicular hyperplasia from these lymphomas are compounded by having to make a diagnosis from suboptimal sections. The criteria useful in differentiating reactive follicular hyperplasia origi-

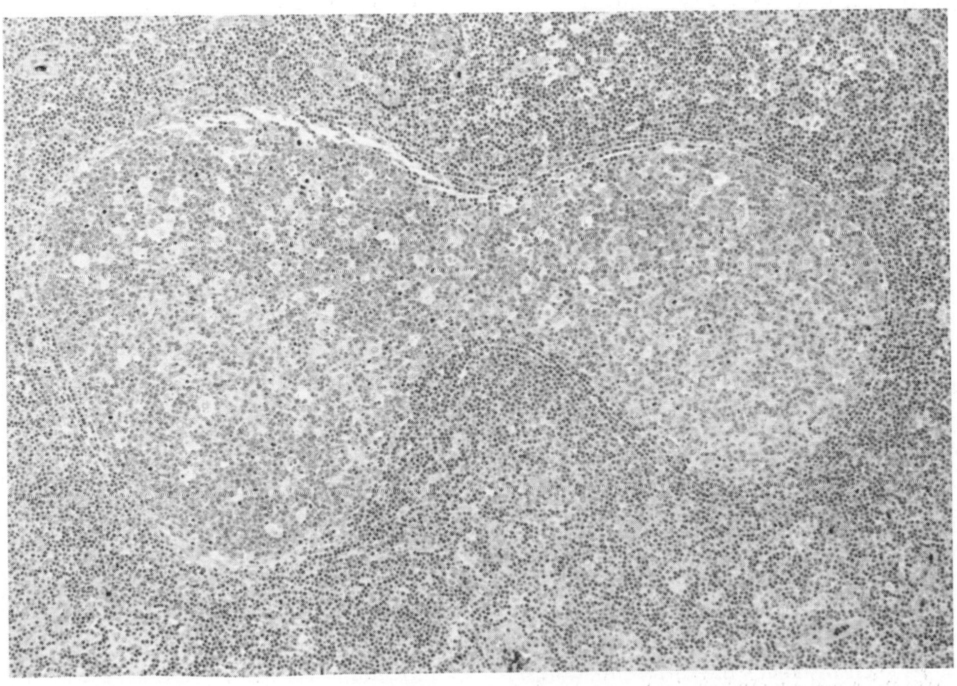

FIG. 15.8. Fusion of two adjacent germinal centers resulting in a dumbbell-shaped structure (hematoxylin and eosin stain, original magnification: 300× magnification).

TABLE 15.2. *Architecture and cytologic features of follicular hyperplasia and follicular lymphoma*

Follicular hyperplasia	Follicular lymphoma
Preservation of nodal architecture	Effacement of nodal architecture
Variation in size and shape of germinal centers	Uniformity of follicles
Density of follicles low	Density of follicles high
Ample interfollicular tissue containing inflammatory cells	Sparse interfollicular tissue that may contain neoplastic cells
Sharp demarcation of germinal centers from mantle zone lymphocytes	Borders of follicles not well defined; mantle zones incomplete or breached
Polarization of large transformed cells in germinal centers	Absence of polarization in follicles
Moderate to high mitotic rate in germinal centers	Few mitotic figures in neoplastic follicles
Tingible body macrophages in germinal centers	Absence of tingible body macrophages in neoplastic follicles

nally devised by Rappaport et al. (18) are listed in Table 15.2. No single criterion should be used to distinguish between benign or neoplastic follicular proliferation in an individual case: All of the morphologic features must be scrutinized to arrive at a correct diagnosis.

Perhaps the most reliable morphologic feature in differentiating benign from neoplastic follicular proliferations is the density of follicles per unit area and their even distribution throughout the lymph node, best noted by examining sections under very low magnification (19). In the vast majority of cases, the neoplastic follicles are apposed closely to their neighboring follicles (back-to-back) and show less variation in size and shape than the follicles in hyperplastic nodes. An equally reliable and useful feature that aids in differentiating follicular hyperplasia from lymphoma is polarity, which is absent in neoplastic follicles; however, polarization of follicles is not always present in follicular hyperplasia and, if found, may be confined to a minority of germinal centers. The amount of residual interfollicular space is smaller in the nodes of follicular lymphoma. Intrafollicular plasma cells are much more frequently present in nodes of follicular hyperplasia, although they rarely are reported within neoplastic follicles in follicular lymphomas (20). The numbers of mitotic figures, tingible body macrophages, and apoptotic cells are greater in benign than in neoplastic follicles, and such greater numbers almost always point to a benign diagnosis. Occasionally, follicular small cleaved cell lymphomas contain tingible body macrophages. The presence of a vast majority of small cleaved cells, however, strongly suggests the neoplastic nature of the lesion, whereas reactive follicles contain many more large cells. The mantle zone in follicular hyperplasia is usually intact; in follicular lymphoma it is often, but not invariably, incomplete, absent, or breached by malignant cells that may be seen in the interfollicular areas, a feature diagnostic of lymphoma. In follicular hyperplasia, the interfollicular areas contain predominantly small lymphocytes or a polymorphous population of cells, including plasma cells and sometimes varying numbers of immunoblasts. Although interfollicular plasma cells commonly are seen in hyperplastic nodes, it is not unusual to find some in nodes involved by follicular lymphoma (19,20).

The characteristic features listed in Table 15.2 are sometimes missing, and in such instances the differentiation between hyperplasia and neoplasia becomes difficult. For example, the germinal centers in follicular hyperplasia may be quite uniform, and their density may be as high as in follicular lymphoma, in which the neoplastic follicles are not always back-to-back (19). Sharp demarcation of neoplastic follicular centers from the mantle zone lymphocytes may be seen, and the mantle zone may be completely intact. With the exception of follicular large cell lymphoma, which is the least common type of follicular lymphoma, the rate of mitosis and the number of tingible body macrophages within follicles are much higher in benign proliferations. In follicular large cell lymphomas, there are often areas of diffuse involvement that aid in differentiation from benign proliferations.

In cases in which a clear-cut distinction between follicular hyperplasia and follicular lymphoma cannot be established, ancillary procedures may suggest a diagnosis of either benignity or lymphoma (21,22). Immunohistochemical staining for BCL-2 protein in paraffin sections resolves the diagnostic dilemma in most but not all instances. The follicle center cells in the vast majority of cases of follicular lymphoma express BCL-2 protein, whereas the cells in benign germinal centers do not. A potential pitfall in interpretation is the presence of BCL-2–positive T cells, which sometimes are seen in substantial numbers in benign germinal centers. To avoid such a problem, a corresponding section should be stained with a pan T-cell antibody. Frozen-section immunophenotyping or genotypic analysis may be needed in rare instances to determine whether or not a monoclonal proliferation (presumably malignant) is present. If a clear-cut diagnosis still cannot be established, bilateral iliac crest bone marrow biopsy may show the presence of lymphoma, because a high percentage of follicular lymphomas involve the bone marrow. If the bone marrow does not contain lymphoma, repeat lymph node biopsy is indicated.

The possibility of interfollicular Hodgkin's disease should be considered if one examines lymph nodes with prominent follicular hyperplasia (23). The large reactive follicles may overshadow the focal, often inconspicuous, interfollicular expansion by Hodgkin's disease. The polymorphous infiltrate, often containing histiocytes, is best found on low magnification, and Reed-Sternberg cells or their variants then should be sought under higher magnification. Immunostaining with CD15 and CD30 may be helpful in highlighting Reed-Sternberg cells.

Rheumatoid Arthritis

Patients with rheumatoid arthritis often develop lymphadenopathy, either localized or generalized, at some time during the course of their disease (7,24). Because these patients are at a slightly increased risk for the development of non-Hodgkin's lymphoma, lymph node biopsies commonly are carried out, especially if enlarged nodes are found in several sites.

Histologically, findings include follicular hyperplasia, which in its fully developed stage may be striking, involving both cortex and medullary areas (7,24,25) (Fig. 15.1). The follicles vary in size and shape, and their enlargement results from an expansion of the germinal centers at the expense of the mantle zone, which often is reduced in size. The germinal centers are demarcated sharply from the mantle zones. In some germinal centers, a mixture of small and large cleaved and noncleaved cells is present; in others there may be a predominance of large transformed cells. As in nonspecific follicular hyperplasia, a high rate of mitosis, apoptotic cells, tingible body macrophages, and polarization of large cells often are present. Variable numbers of polytypic plasma cells are found within germinal centers. The interfollicular areas are compressed by the expanding follicles and contain sheets of polytypic plasma cells, a moderate vascular proliferation, and scattered immunoblasts (Fig 15.9). The sinuses also are compressed and may contain varying numbers of polymorphonuclear leukocytes. Changes similar to those seen in lymph nodes of rheumatoid arthritis may be found in patients with related disorders such as Sjögren's syndrome and Felty's syndrome (16,26).

Syphilis

Regional enlarged lymph nodes developing in association with primary syphilis rarely undergo biopsy; however, the generalized lymphadenopathy usually found in patients with secondary syphilis often results in biopsy because lymphoma is suspected clinically. The pathologist should be acquainted with the characteristic, although not specific, histologic changes of secondary syphilis, especially because its incidence is increasing. Some of the changes, including follicular hyperplasia and interfollicular plasmacytosis, are similar to those seen in rheumatoid arthritis (8,15,27). In contrast to the changes in the latter disease, however, the nodal fibrous capsule and trabeculae in syphilis are thickened and infiltrated by lymphocytes and plasma cells, usually in a perivascular distribution. Sarcoidal-type granulomas and clusters of epithelioid cells may be seen in the interfollicular areas (15), and fibrosing endarteritis, periarteritis, and venulitis may be evident. Spirochetes may be demonstrated with the Warthin-Starry stain, especially within the walls of blood vessels and occasionally among epithelioid histiocytes (8).

Progressive Transformation of Germinal Centers

Progressively transformed germinal centers are large nodules composed predominantly of small lymphocytes, which

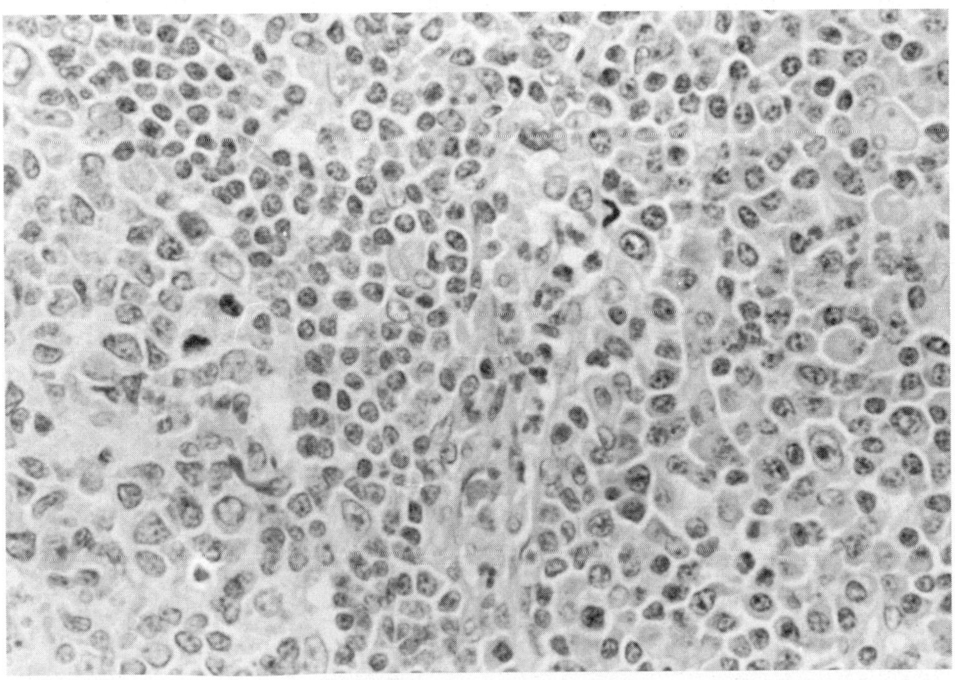

FIG. 15.9. Rheumatoid arthritis. Part of a germinal center with attenuated mantle zone adjacent to a compressed sinus containing histiocytes and neutrophils next to an interfollicular dense plasma cell infiltrate (hematoxylin and eosin stain, original magnification: 575× magnification).

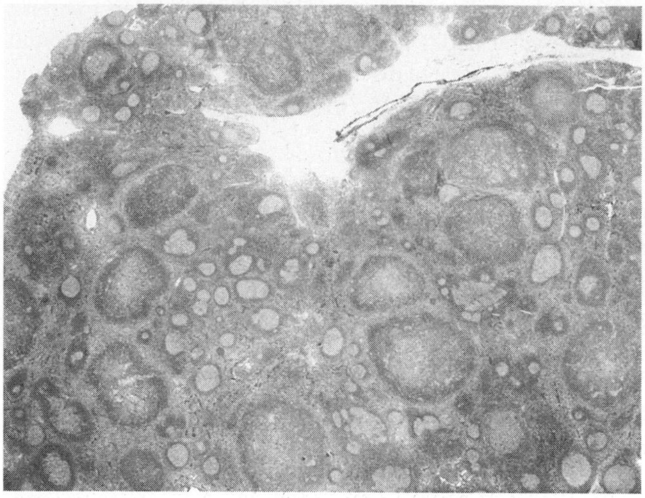

FIG. 15.10. Lymph node with follicular hyperplasia and a number of progressively transformed germinal centers readily recognized by their large size (hematoxylin and eosin stain, original magnification: 80× magnification).

are differentiated from primary and secondary follicles by their size and cellular content (28). In most instances these transformed germinal centers are seen in lymph nodes with follicular hyperplasia. A single or several progressively transformed germinal centers are scattered among the germinal centers or occasionally in small clusters (Fig. 15.10). Rarely, florid progressive transformation of germinal centers has been reported, especially in young males; in such cases it may resemble nodular lymphocyte predominance Hodgkin's disease, because of the unusually large numbers of these structures within the node (29). Progressively transformed germinal centers are occasionally present in lymph nodes along with, before, or after a diagnosis of nodular lymphocyte predominance Hodgkin's disease (28–33). A relationship between progressively transformed germinal centers and nodular lymphocyte predominance Hodgkin's disease has been proposed, and evidence has been presented that this type of Hodgkin's disease arises from or preferentially involves these altered B-cell germinal centers (28–33).

Progressively transformed germinal centers usually are confined to a solitary lymph node, most often in the cervical region, predominantly in young persons and in males. As in the case of nodular lymphocyte predominance Hodgkin's disease, lymph nodes with progressively transformed germinal centers tend to recur in the same site. Although the risk of developing nodular lymphocyte predominance Hodgkin's disease is very low, repeat biopsy is indicated if lymphadenopathy recurs, especially if florid progressive transformation of germinal centers is present. Histologically, the progressively transformed germinal centers are spotted easily under low magnification (Fig. 15.10). They are at least three to four times larger than most reactive follicles, which usually accompany these large structures, and their cellular composition is completely different. The predominant cells in the fully developed large nodule are small polytypic IgM^+IgD^+ mantle zone lymphocytes and scattered T cells ($CD4^+CD57^+$) with some residual germinal center cells and follicular dendritic cells among them (30, 32, 33) (Fig. 15.11). The mantle zone is obscured, and the interfollicular areas usually contain small lymphocytes. Transition between reactive and transformed germinal centers may be seen. In such structures, varying numbers of follicle center cells are still visible, sometimes in clusters, and an occasional residual starry-sky macrophage may be present. Sometimes, the large transformed germinal centers are surrounded by epithelioid histiocytes.

Differentiation of progressively transformed germinal centers from nodular lymphocyte predominance Hodgkin's disease occasionally can be difficult. Although the presence of typical polylobulated lymphocytic and histiocytic variant Reed-Sternberg cells (popcorn cells) within the nodules is diagnostic of Hodgkin's disease, these variant cells occasionally are mimicked by residual large germinal center cells. Epithelioid histiocytes surrounding and within progressively transformed germinal centers are seen occasionally but not nearly as frequently as in Hodgkin's disease. Immunostaining may or may not be helpful in differentiating between this type of Hodgkin's disease and progressively transformed germinal centers. The small lymphocytes are B cells in the follicular structures of both disorders, and the Reed-Sternberg variants and the residual germinal center cells, which may occasionally mimic them (Fig. 15.12), both stain with B cell–associated antibodies and leukocyte common antigen, and they are both for $CD15^-$ and $CD30^-$ (28,34). The lymphocytes immediately surrounding Reed-Sternberg cell variants in nodular lymphocyte predominance Hodgkin's disease, however, are $CD4^+CD57^+$ T cells, and the Reed-Sternberg variants are often epithelial membrane antigen–positive; residual germinal center cells are negative and not surrounded by T cells (34). In addition, the T cells in Hodgkin's disease often are in clusters, imparting a mottled or moth-eaten appearance to the nodule; in the progressively transformed germinal center, the T and $CD57^+$ cells are scattered throughout the nodule. These staining characteristics, and the presence of interspersed reactive hyperplastic follicles in nodes containing progressively transformed germinal centers and their absence in nodular lymphocyte predominance Hodgkin's disease, are helpful differential diagnostic features. In lymphocyte predominance Hodgkin's disease, any residual follicles present almost always are found compressed in a rim around the area involved by Hodgkin's disease. In rare instances, part of a lymph node shows follicular hyperplasia, and another area contains a focus of lymphocyte predominance Hodgkin's disease.

Differentiation of progressively transformed germinal centers from follicular non-Hodgkin's lymphomas should not be a major problem, because the nodules of small round but not cleaved lymphocytes are inconsistent with a diagnosis of follicular lymphoma (35,36). The neoplastic follicles usually do not attain the size of the follicular structures seen

FIG. 15.11. Lymph node with a hyperplastic follicle and a much larger, poorly defined, progressively transformed germinal center that consists predominantly of small lymphocytes and scattered residual follicle center cells (hematoxylin and eosin stain, original magnification: 200× magnification).

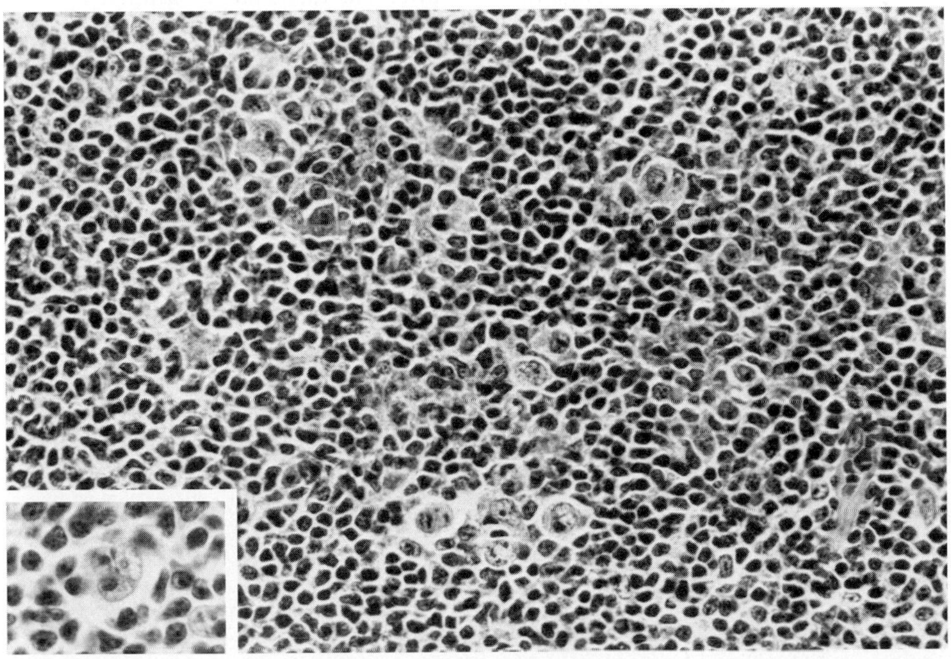

FIG. 15.12. Higher magnification of a progressively transformed germinal center containing scattered residual follicle center cells (hematoxylin and eosin stain, original magnification: 500× magnification). **Inset:** follicular center cell resembling the polylobulated Reed-Sternberg cell variant of nodular lymphocyte predominant Hodgkin's disease (original magnification: 625× magnification).

in progressive transformation of germinal centers, with the exception of the floral variant of follicular lymphoma (35,36). This distinctive lymphoma is characterized by prominent mantle zone lymphocytes surrounding as well as infiltrating the large neoplastic follicles, creating a scalloped or ''floral'' appearance and mimicking a partially transformed germinal center. In contrast to lymph nodes with progressively transformed germinal centers, follicular lymphomas generally are not associated with follicular hyperplasia in the same node.

Castleman's Disease

Castleman's disease, also referred to as angiofollicular or giant lymph node hyperplasia, initially was described as a solitary lesion in the mediastinum, which still is the most frequent site of involvement (37), although it has been reported in many other locations, among the more common being the abdominal cavity. Other locations include the pulmonary parenchyma, neck, axillary regions, and skeletal muscle (38). There are two forms of Castleman's disease, the much more common localized type and the less common multicentric type (38–40). The potentially more aggressive multicentric form of Castleman's disease is discussed in detail in Chapter 16.

The localized or solitary lesions of Castleman's disease are usually rounded masses varying in size from 1.5 to 16 cm (38). Histologically, two major types have been described (38,40). These include the more frequently seen hyaline vascular form and the much less common plasma cell type. A transitional type with features of both has been described (38). The two major types differ considerably, not only in their histologic appearance but also in their clinical presentations. Patients with the hyaline vascular type are mostly asymptomatic unless the mass abuts or partially compresses a neighboring structure, such as a bronchus; patients with the plasma cell type often present with a variety of symptoms or abnormal laboratory test results (38). After total excision of the solitary mass, these patients become asymptomatic, and their abnormal laboratory test results return to normal.

Hyaline Vascular Type

This type is by far the more common, comprising more than 90% of cases reported in one large series (38). The ages of patients with this type of Castleman's disease ranged from 8 to 66 years in one study and 12 to 69 (median 33) years in another report, and there was no predilection for either sex (38,40). Grossly, the lesion most often consists of a single mass. The main histologic features include abnormal follicles and a striking interfollicular vascularity (Fig. 15.13). The latter feature accounts for the profuse bleeding experienced if the lesion is incised during the surgical procedure. The proportions of the follicular and interfollicular components may vary considerably from case to case, resulting in different appearances of the lesions. The follicles often have expanded mantle zones composed of small lymphocytes with round nuclei surrounding abnormal germinal cen-

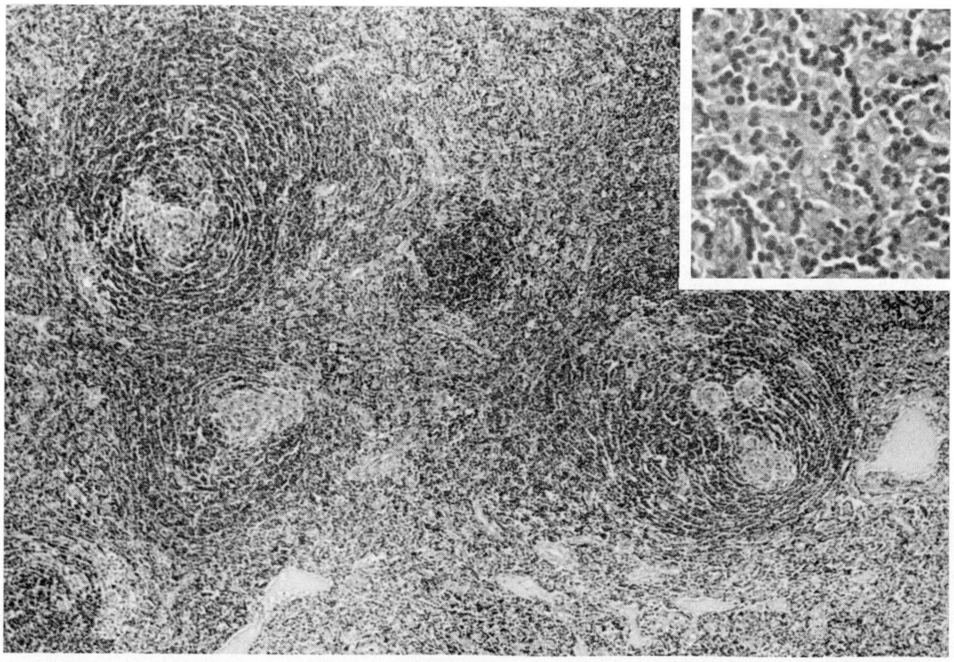

FIG. 15.13. Hyaline vascular Castleman's disease. The follicles consist of large, concentrically arranged mantle zone lymphocytes surrounding atrophic germinal centers. The interfollicular areas contain a network of small vessels (hematoxylin and eosin stain, original magnification: 200× magnification). **Inset:** Small vessels with thickened walls in the interfollicular regions (original magnification: 400× magnification).

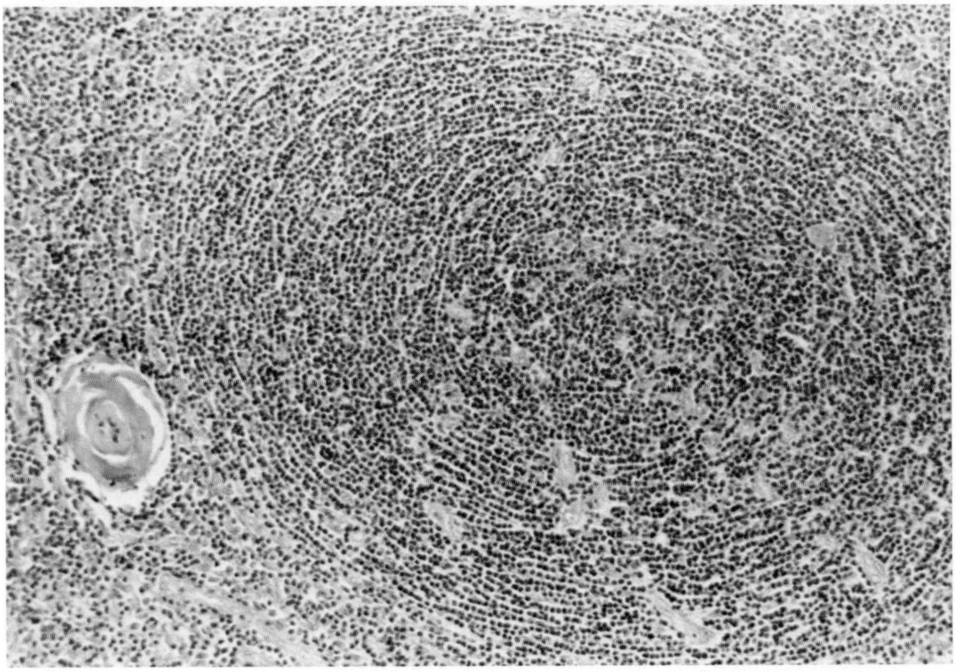

FIG. 15.14. Hyaline vascular Castleman's disease, lymphoid variant. The follicle is composed entirely of concentrically arranged small lymphocytes penetrated by a number of small vessels. Perivascular fibrosis is present in the interfollicular area (hematoxylin and eosin stain, original magnification: 320× magnification).

ters, which range in size from medium to barely perceptible. Most of the germinal centers are small. They are composed predominantly of follicular dendritic cells and endothelial cells of penetrating vessels. Some large, bizarre, dystrophic cells are believed to be abnormal follicular dendritic cells. The larger germinal centers are also abnormal. Many of the follicles contain one or more small blood vessels entering from the vascular perifollicular tissue. Some of these vessels have thickened walls, resulting in small hyalinized germinal centers that superficially resemble Hassall's corpuscles (37,38). Some vessels within the germinal centers have many endothelial cells, and thus the germinal centers are more cellular. Other germinal centers may be surrounded by greatly expanded, concentrically arranged (''onion skin'') small mantle zone lymphocytes, which also may obscure the germinal center completely. If these histologic features predominate, the lesion may be referred to as the *lymphoid variant* of the hyaline vascular type (38) (Fig. 15.14). An aberrant immunophenotype of the mantle zone lymphocytes that may be helpful in confirming a diagnosis in small biopsy sections and difficult cases has been demonstrated in both types of Castleman's disease (41). Another characteristic finding is the presence of more than one small germinal center within a single follicle (40) (Fig. 15.15). The interfollicular areas contain varying numbers of small blood vessels, which may be extremely numerous (Fig. 15.13). Most are lined by a flattened endothelium, but some have prominent endothelial cells and resemble postcapillary venules. Small lymphocytes are the predominant cells between the vessels and occasional plasma cells, and rare immunoblasts may be present. Large fibrotic masses, which often surround larger vessels, as well as sclerotic bands may be scattered in the interfollicular areas (Fig 15.14). Lymph node architecture, such as sinuses, often is seen at the periphery of the lesion. Clusters of plasmacytoid monocytes may be present in the interfollicular region. Stromal cell overgrowths (myoid cells, follicular dendritic cells, or dendritic histiocytes) and neoplasms rarely are associated with this type of Castleman's disease (42).

The hyaline vascular type of germinal center is not specific for Castleman's disease. It is seen occasionally as a single follicle in nonspecific reactive lymph nodes, and it also has been reported in lymph nodes of patients with HIV-associated lymphadenopathy and in those with angioimmunoblastic lymphadenopathy (40). These small remnants of germinal centers also are called ''regressively transformed'' or ''burnt out'' follicles (40).

In summary, the diagnostic features, as the name of the disorder implies, are small hyalinized germinal centers (one or more) within an expanded mantle zone, as well as a highly vascularized interfollicular network.

Differential Diagnosis

The differential diagnosis includes the lymphoid depletion type of lymph node from patients infected with HIV, and mantle cell lymphoma, which may resemble in particular the lymphoid variant of Castleman's disease (4,40,43). The lymph nodes from patients with HIV-related lymphadenopathy and those with mantle cell lymphoma do not have the

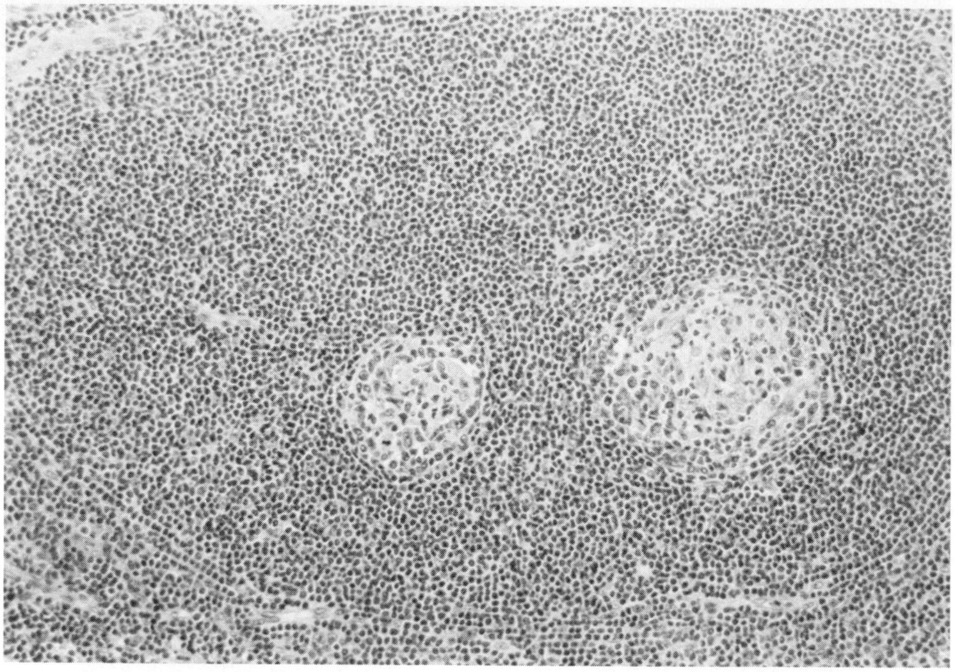

FIG. 15.15. Hyaline vascular Castleman's disease showing a single large follicle containing two small germinal centers (hematoxylin and eosin stain, original magnification: 320× magnification).

interfollicular vascular network of the hyaline vascular type of Castleman's disease. In mantle cell lymphoma, there is considerably more variation in nuclear contour of the small lymphocytes, which also show a distinctive immunophenotype and light chain restriction (43), in contrast to the polytypic surface markers of the lymphocytes in Castleman's disease. An increase in plasma cells often is seen in the lymph nodes of patients in the advanced stages of AIDS with lymphocyte involution and depletion, whereas plasma cells generally are not prominent in hyaline vascular Castleman's disease (Chapter 28).

Plasma Cell Type

The ages of patients with the plasma cell type of Castleman's disease reported in the literature range from 8 to 62 (median 22) years, and no predilection for either sex has been found (40). The lesions range in size from 3 to 15 cm and are composed of several discrete, matted nodes or a mass with adjacent smaller nodes. Clinically, patients differ from those with the hyaline vascular type of this disorder in that there are constitutional symptoms and abnormal laboratory test results including anemia, which is most often hypochromic; a polyclonal increase in gamma globulin; an elevated erythrocyte sedimentation rate (ESR); bone marrow plasmacytosis; thrombocytosis; and a variety of other abnormalities. Some of the symptoms are caused by secretion of such cytokines as interleukin-6 by germinal center cells (44). Most patients with this type of Castleman's disease have increased serum levels of interleukin-6, and alleviation of the systemic manifestations by monoclonal antibodies against this cytokine has been reported (45). Following excision of the mass, the symptoms disappear, and laboratory test results return to normal. There are also differences in location of the lesions of the hyaline vascular and plasma cell types. More of the plasma cell lesions are found in the abdomen, usually in the small bowel mesentery; fewer are located in the mediastinum (all anterior); and fewer still are found in peripheral lymph nodes.

Approximately 10% of patients with localized Castleman's disease have the plasma cell type (40). Characterized by hyperplastic follicles and a dense interfollicular plasmacytosis (Fig. 15.16), it is histologically completely different from the hyaline vascular type. In contrast to the small vascularized germinal centers of the hyaline vascular type, the germinal centers in the plasma cell type are identical to those in cases of follicular hyperplasia. The latter are composed of a mixture of cleaved and noncleaved small and large cells and have varying numbers of tingible body macrophages and readily recognizable mitotic figures. The mantle zone is usually intact and surrounded by sheets of mature-appearing plasma cells. Scattered immunoblasts may be present among the plasma cells, but they are not prominent. The vascular proliferation characteristic of the hyaline vascular type is usually inconspicuous or absent. Sinuses may or may not be identified. The plasma cells in the majority of cases are polytypic, but in close to 40% of cases, they are monotypic, almost always lambda light chain restricted (46).

Differential Diagnosis

The plasma cell type of Castleman's disease may resemble cases of follicular hyperplasia with interfollicular plas-

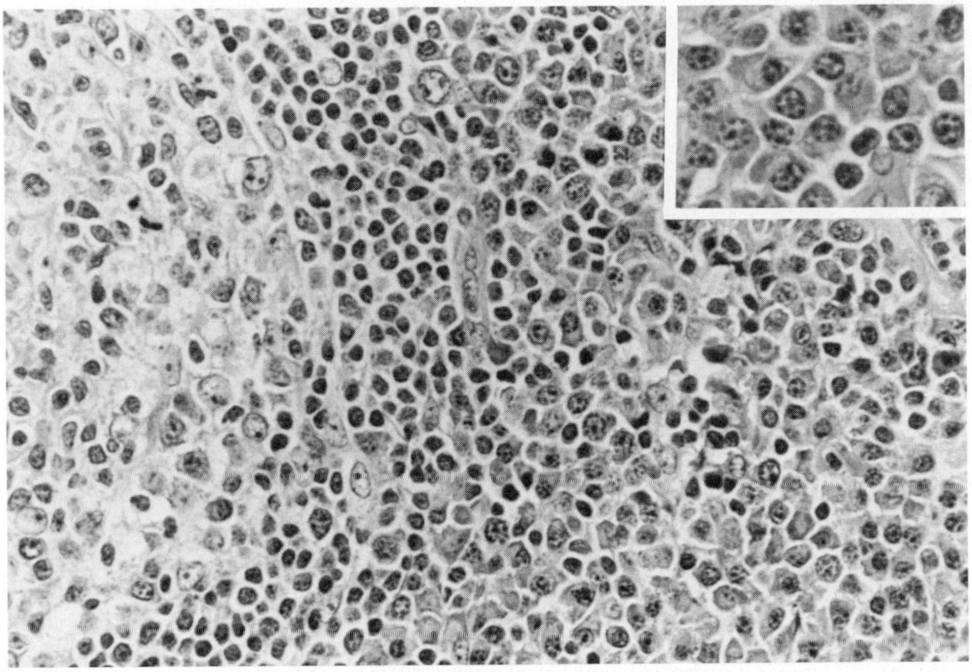

FIG. 15.16. Castleman's disease, plasma cell type. Part of a hyperplastic follicle surrounded by a thin mantle of small lymphocytes adjacent to a solid area composed of plasma cells (hematoxylin and eosin stain, original magnification: 500× magnification). **Inset:** Higher-magnification view of mature plasma cells (original magnification: 625× magnification).

macytosis, with features that are seen in lymph nodes of patients with rheumatoid arthritis, such other autoimmune disorders as systemic lupus erythematosus, or syphilis and in nodes draining carcinomas (40). Sinuses are obscured more often by the plasma cell proliferation in Castleman's disease than in other benign proliferations. Because there are other reactive hyperplasias with plasmacytosis, a diagnosis of Castleman's disease should be made with certainty only if other diseases causing such plasmacytic proliferations have been excluded (40). Cases of Castleman's disease with light chain restriction in plasma cells must be differentiated from the rare case of primary plasmacytoma of lymph nodes (47). In the latter disorder, the follicular hyperplasia seen in Castleman's disease is usually absent, although residual follicles may remain.

SINUS PATTERN

Sinus Histiocytosis

Sinus hyperplasia, usually referred to as *sinus histiocytosis*, is a nonspecific finding in many lymph node biopsies. It may be the only or the most prominent finding, or it may be associated with follicular hyperplasia or paracortical expansion. It is sometimes seen in nodes draining neoplasms or infectious processes, but usually the cause of sinus histiocytosis is obscure. The histiocytes are indigenous to sinuses, derived from monocytes. The histologic appearance is characterized by dilated sinuses containing increased numbers of histiocytes (macrophages) (Fig. 15.17). Cytologically, the sinus histiocytes are uniform in size and have ample cytoplasm with round or oval and sometimes indented nuclei with inconspicuous nucleoli (Fig. 15.17). Within the thorax of adults, the histiocytes in lymph nodes often contain carbon pigment, which, if present in large amounts, may show a dark discoloration on gross examination resembling metastatic melanoma. Erythrophagocytosis and hemosiderin deposition may be seen in the cytoplasm of patients with hemolytic anemia or after transfusion. Pigment from tattoos also is seen in sinus histiocytes of regional lymph nodes. Sinus histiocytosis also is observed in lymph nodes after hip arthroplasty, silicone arthroplasty, and mammaplasty (48,49). Signet-ring sinus histiocytosis is an uncommon but distinctive proliferation of histiocytes in lymph nodes of the axilla and pelvis in patients with carcinoma of the breast and prostate, respectively. The signet-ring appearance of the histiocytes resembles metastatic carcinoma and signet-ring cell lymphoma but is differentiated from these malignancies by appropriate immunostains (50).

Sinus Histiocytosis with Massive Lymphadenopathy

In 1969, Rosai and Dorfman (51) described four cases of this entity that now bears their name (Rosai-Dorfman disease). An additional 30 cases were described in detail by these authors in 1972, confirming that this idiopathic disorder is a distinct clinicopathologic entity (52). Although a specific cause of this disorder has not been documented, some cases have been associated with human herpesvirus-

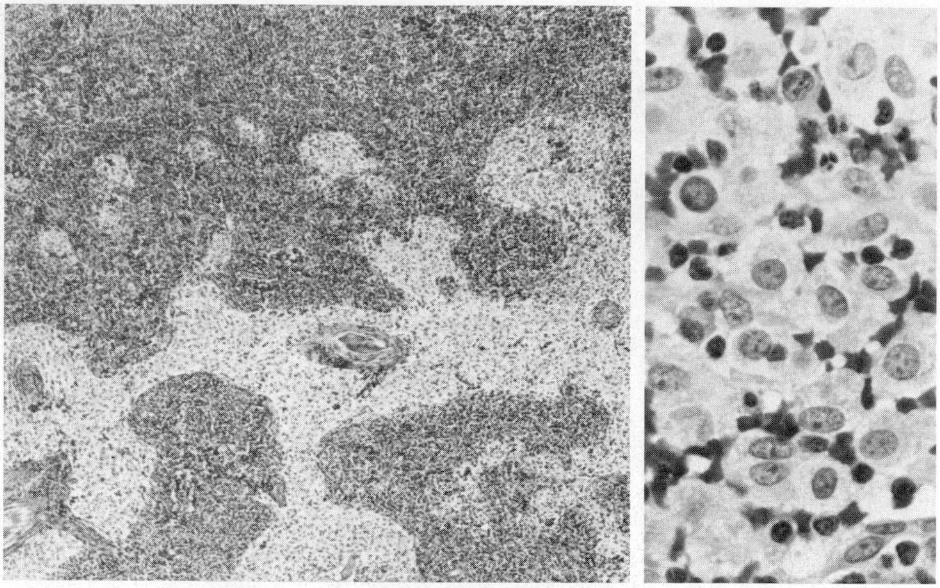

FIG. 15.17. Sinus histiocytosis. **A:** Sinuses are dilated and filled with histiocytes (hematoxylin and eosin stain, original magnification: 120× magnification). **B:** Higher magnification. The histiocytes have ample cytoplasm, and the bland nuclei have inconspicuous small nucleoli (hematoxylin and eosin stain, original magnification: 500× magnification).

6 (53). In addition, the histiocytes have been shown to be polytypic (54).

The most consistent and predominant finding is bilateral, painless cervical lymphadenopathy, which may progress slowly to reach voluminous proportions. This adenopathy may or may not be accompanied by fever, but most patients are otherwise in good health. The disease most often affects individuals in the first or second decades of life, but it may be seen at any age. Males are affected slightly more often than females, and the distribution of the disease is worldwide (55). The disorder generally runs a benign course with spontaneous resolution, but the lymphadenopathy may persist for a period of years, or the condition may improve but later reappear. Leukocytosis caused by neutrophilia, polyclonal hypergammaglobulinemia, and an elevated erythrocyte sedimentation rate are common laboratory findings.

The excised lesion consists of a multinodular mass of lymph nodes separated by bands of fibrous tissues. The cut surface has a yellow-white appearance. The histologic findings are distinctive. There is marked fibrous thickening of the capsule with pericapsular fibrosis, often infiltrated by small lymphocytes and plasma cells. There is a conspicuous dilatation of all sinuses, which contain a predominance of large histiocytes with ample clear or sometimes foamy cytoplasm, a vesicular nucleus, and often a distinct nucleolus (52–55) (Fig. 15.18). A minority of histiocytes may have an atypical appearance with hyperchromatic nuclei and prominent nucleoli. Occasional multinucleated cells are sometimes present. Mitoses rarely are seen. Characteristic of this disorder is the presence of lymphocytes within the cytoplasm of the histiocytes and, less commonly, other hematopoietic cells (e.g., plasma cells, erythrocytes, neutrophils) (Fig. 15.18). The intracytoplasmic lymphocytes appear viable and show no evidence of degradation (emperipolesis), as is seen in phagocytosed cells. Some of the cytoplasm of the histiocytes is filled with lymphocytes. Scattered lymphocytes, plasma cells, and rare neutrophils are also present in the sinuses. Only remnants of intersinusoidal tissue containing scattered follicles and lymphocytes are seen; the medullary cords contain predominantly plasma cells. Immunostaining of the histiocytes show them to be S-100^+ and $CD1^-$ (56,57). In contrast, the cells of Langerhans cell histiocytosis (histiocytosis X) are S-100^- and $CD1^+$ (57). The histiocytes in each disorder are placental alkaline phosphatase–positive (57). Monocyte-, macrophage-, or granulocyte-associated antigens CD11c, CD14, CD33, and CD68 are expressed by the histiocytes in sinus histiocytosis with massive lymphadenopathy (58). Sinus histiocytosis with massive lymphadenopathy also can be diagnosed by cytology, in conjunction with immunohistochemistry and clinical history (59).

In recent years, reports of this disorder involving extranodal sites in about 25% of cases have appeared in the literature (55,60–62). These extranodal sites may be the initial and only manifestations of the disease, and lymphadenopathy may be inconspicuous or entirely absent. The most commonly affected extranodal sites include the skin, ocular adnexa, skeletal system, upper respiratory tract, and breast (55,60–62). The histologic appearance is similar to that in lymph nodes. Sinus histiocytosis with massive lymphadenopathy is regarded as an indolent disease that may affect

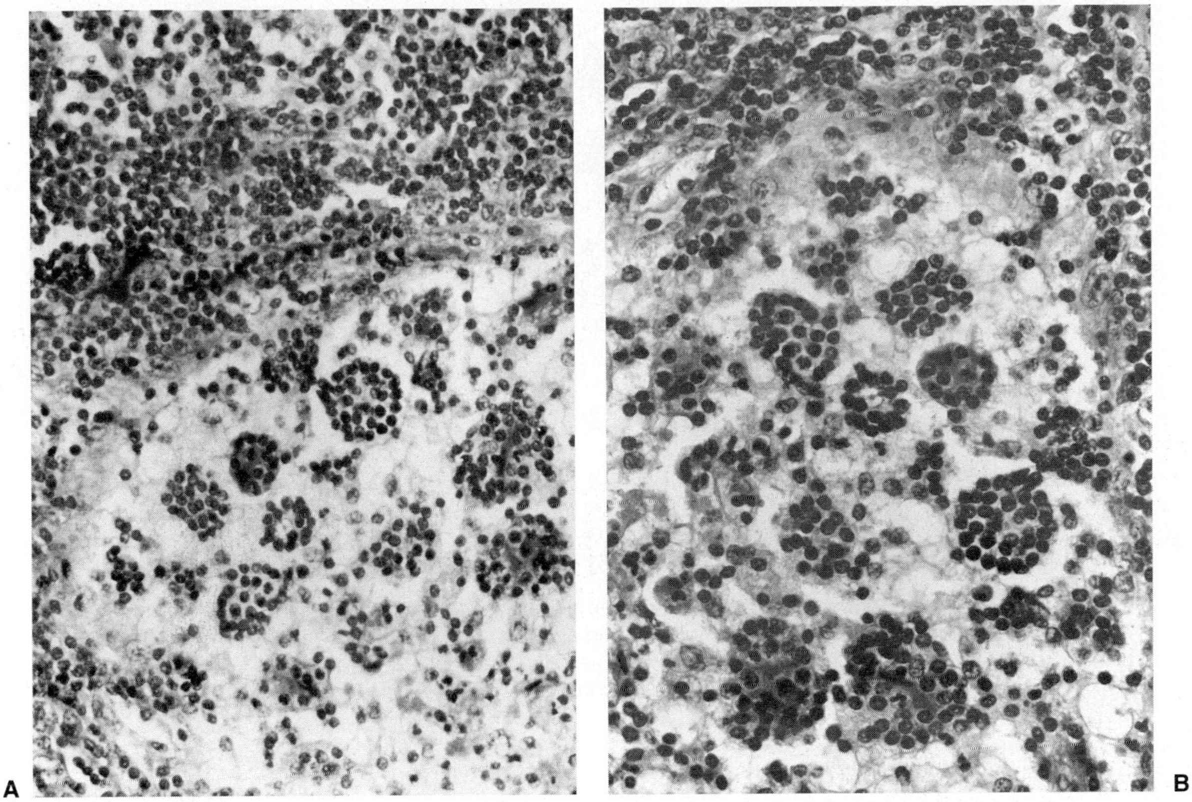

FIG. 15.18. Sinus histiocytosis with massive lymphadenopathy. **A:** Dilated sinuses are filled with histiocytes containing lymphocytes in their cytoplasm (hematoxylin and eosin stain, original magnification: 500× magnification). **B:** Higher-magnification view (hematoxylin and eosin stain, original magnification: 625× magnification).

individuals of any age and involve virtually any organ (Chapter 51).

Monocytoid B-Cell Hyperplasia

Monocytoid B-cell hyperplasia that has a predominant sinusoidal and paracortical pattern is seen in lymph nodes of toxoplasmosis lymphadenitis, viral disorders such as infectious mononucleosis, HIV infections, cytomegalovirus lymphadenitis, cat-scratch disease, lymphogranuloma venereum, and nonspecific hyperplasias (2,10,11,13,14). It also occasionally is associated with lymphomas (63). The proliferation is characterized by focal or occasionally widespread expansion of sinuses that are filled with large cells with ample pale to clear cytoplasm and centrally placed, round or kidney-shaped nuclei with moderately clumped to fine chromatin and inconspicuous nucleoli (Fig. 15.7). Segmented neutrophils usually are scattered among the monocytoid cells. In most instances, the proliferation of these cells is associated with prominent follicular hyperplasia. Cytologic features of benign or neoplastic monocytoid B cells (marginal zone cells) and their pattern of lymph nodal involvement may be mimicked by infiltration by cells of hairy cell leukemia or peripheral T-cell lymphoma or mast cells in mastocytosis (64,65). These disorders may be distinguished from monocytoid B-cell proliferations by immunophenotypic analysis. Mast cells are identified by Giemsa and chloracetate esterase (Leder) staining, or by sensitive immunohistochemical staining with tryptase. In some cases, it may be difficult to differentiation benign proliferations of monocytoid cells from monocytoid B-cell (marginal zone) lymphoma (64,65).

Lymphangiography Effect

The radiopaque lipid-based material utilized for lymphangiography is associated with sinus histiocytosis (66). The medium, which is dissolved during tissue processing, leaves behind large vacuoles within the sinuses; numerous multinucleated giant cells, some stretched around vacuoles, also are noted (Fig. 15.19). Eosinophils sometimes are seen within sinuses and medullary cords.

Lipophagic vacuolization of histiocytes and a multinucleated giant cell reaction usually are present in the sinuses of lymph nodes in the region of the porta hepatis and celiac axis. These vacuoles generally are considerably smaller than those associated with lymphangiography. In cases of pneumatosis intestinalis, large gas vacuoles surrounded by a granulomatous reaction are seen within sinuses. Silicone lymphadenopathy secondary to augmentation mammaplasty also

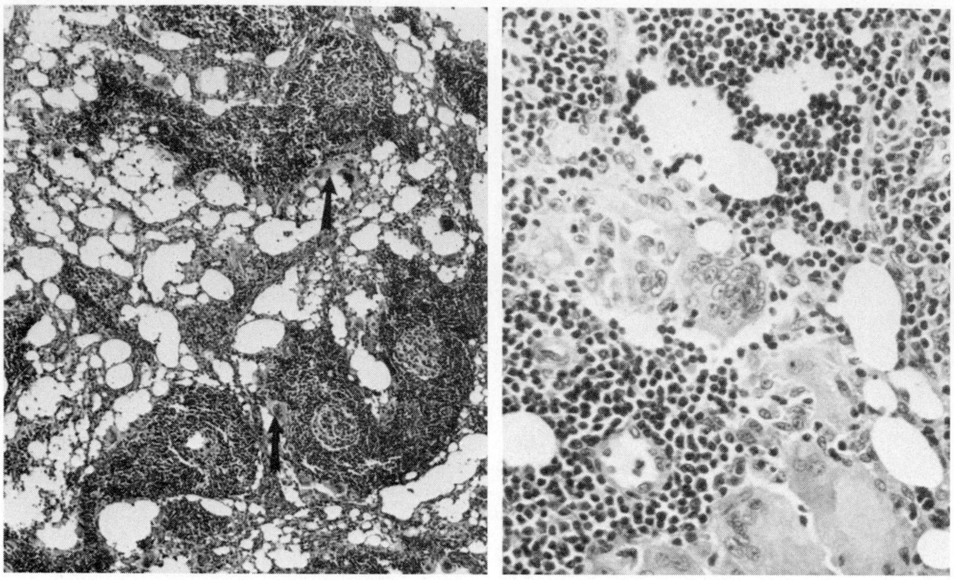

FIG. 15.19. Lymphangiography effect. **A:** Sinuses are dilated and contain large vacuoles associated with multinucleated giant cells (*arrows*) (hematoxylin and eosin stain, original magnification: 120× magnification). **B:** Higher magnification showing vacuoles and multinucleated giant cells (hematoxylin and eosin stain, original magnification: 400× magnification).

may show large sinusoidal vacuoles and sinus histiocytosis (48,49).

Whipple's Disease

Whipple's disease is a multisystem bacterial infection most often involving the small bowel. It most frequently affects middle-aged males. Clinically, symptoms vary considerably and include fever, weight loss, diarrhea, lymphadenopathy, and arthralgias; sometimes patients may have no specific complaints (67–71).

Abdominal lymph nodes frequently are involved in gastrointestinal Whipple's disease, but peripheral and even mediastinal nodes also may become enlarged; occasionally this is the initial manifestation of the disease (68–71). The sinuses generally are dilated and contain large vacuoles resulting from loss of lipid material during processing. Large histiocytic cells with abundant vacuolated cytoplasm are present within sinuses, which also may contain nonnecrotizing granulomas. These histologic changes may resemble lymph nodes after lymphangiography. Evidence that these are not lymphangiographic changes is the presence of diastase-resistant, periodic acid Schiff (PAS) stain–-positive, sickle-form particles in the cytoplasm of the histiocytes, which are characteristic of Whipple's disease (68–73) (Fig. 15.20). The disorder is caused by these PAS stain–positive structures, which represent the bacillary organisms that can be demonstrated by electron microscopy. The organism responsible for this disease is *Tropheryma whippeli*, which can be identified by polymerase chain reaction of species-specific sequences of the 16S recombinant RNA of the organism from tissue and in some cases from peripheral blood (72,73). This polymerase chain reaction method is useful not only in confirming a diagnosis but also in monitoring therapy (72,73). *Mycobacterium avium* complex infection in HIV-positive individuals may mimic Whipple's disease in lymph nodes. The former organisms are also PAS stain–positive, but in contrast to *T. whippeli* they are acid-fast stain–positive (2,4). Acid-fast stains should be carried out in cases of suspected Whipple's disease to exclude *M. avium* complex infection, which also may involve the small bowel. Occasionally, Whipple's disease mimics sarcoidosis in lymph nodes, in that well-formed granulomas are found.

Hemophagocytic Syndromes

The disorder described today as *hemophagocytic syndrome* or *virus-associated hemophagocytic syndrome* (74) is probably the same as or at least similar to the disease reported in 1939 as "histiocytic medullary reticulosis" (75). The virus-associated hemophagocytic syndrome is usually but not invariably seen in immunocompromised hosts and initially was thought to occur only in patients with viral infections, particularly cytomegalovirus and other herpesviruses. It was found subsequently in association with bacterial, fungal, and parasitic infections, and its name was changed to *infection-associated hemophagocytic syndrome* (76). The immunodeficiency associated with this disorder may be secondary to immunosuppression in transplant patients, or to neoplasms, or to therapy, or this immunodeficiency may be primary in individuals with congenital immunodeficiency (76). It also has been reported in association with acute lymphoblastic leukemia, usually of T-cell type, and with T- or natural killer cell lymphomas, particularly subcutaneous panniculitic T-cell lymphoma, in which the hemophagocytic syndrome is the most frequent cause of

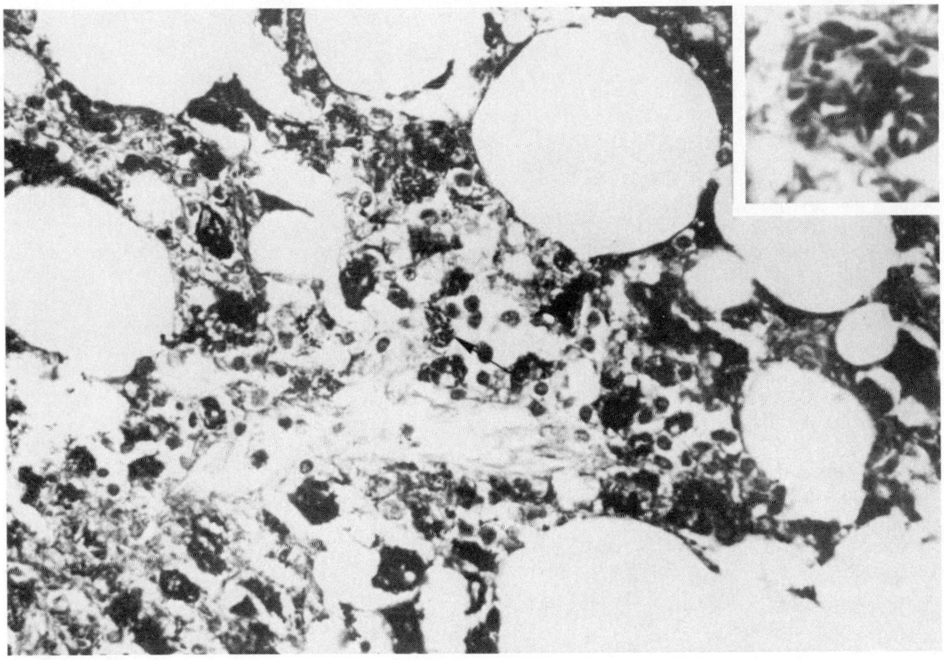

FIG. 15.20. Whipple's disease. Large vacuoles and histiocytes containing periodic acid–Schiff stain–positive, sickle-form particles are present within sinuses (original magnification: 400× magnification). **Inset:** A histiocyte containing sickle-form particles in the cytoplasm (original magnification: 700× magnification). (From Schnitzer B. The pathology of lymph nodes: A differential diagnosis of non-lymphomatous lesions. *University of Michigan Medical Center Journal* 1970:36:179–187, with permission.)

death (77–79). Clinically, there is evidence of multisystem involvement including fever, splenomegaly, hepatomegaly, anemia, leukopenia, coagulopathy, and abnormal liver function test results.

Histologically, bland-appearing histiocytes containing phagocytosed red blood cells and often platelets and other cellular elements may be seen in bone marrow aspirates, from which a diagnosis is usually made. In lymph nodes, the histiocytes fill sinuses, which often are dilated (Fig. 15.21). In addition to erythrocytes, neutrophils, lymphocytes, and platelets may be present within the cytoplasm of the histiocytes. These phagocytic histiocytes greatly expand the red pulp of the spleen and are noted in hepatic sinuses. The proliferation of histiocytes apparently is caused by lymphokines produced by T cells, which may be benign, malignant, or associated with infections (80).

The differential diagnosis includes neoplasms of true histiocytes such as malignant histiocytes, anaplastic large cell lymphomas, large cell lymphomas with a sinusoidal pattern, monocytoid B-cell proliferations, hairy cell leukemia, and metastatic nonhematolymphoid tumors.

Malignant histiocytosis or "true histiocytic neoplasms" (81,82) rarely are diagnosed today. Many cases of these disorders were examples of viral-associated hemophagocytic syndrome or, in those cases in which the cells were atypical or had frankly malignant features, most likely large cell lymphomas, especially of the anaplastic large cell type. In such obviously malignant proliferations, phagocytosis, usually erythrophagocytosis, by the malignant cells, occasionally was noted but usually was present in benign histiocytes among the neoplastic cells (80,83). These large cell lymphomas and monocytoid B-cell proliferations, which may be benign or malignant; the rare case of hairy cell leukemia involving lymph nodes; and metastatic nonhematolymphoid neoplasms may resemble the hemophagocytic syndrome only by virtue of their sinusoidal pattern of lymph node involvement (84,85). Metastatic nonlymphoid neoplasms, including undifferentiated carcinomas and melanoma, may resemble malignant histocytosis and anaplastic large cell lymphoma but should be differentiated from the benign-appearing, avidly phagocytic histiocyte of hemophagocytic syndromes. Immunostaining may aid in differentiation among the various sinusoidal proliferations. The degree of phagocytosis of blood cells and the benign appearance of the histiocytes usually do not cause problems in differential diagnosis from malignant proliferations (Chapter 51). Familial hemophagocytic lymphohistiocytosis may resemble or be clinically and morphologically indistinguishable from infection-associated hemophagocytic syndrome. It occurs in infants and young children and is usually fatal (86) (Chapter 51).

Langerhans Cell Histiocytosis

Langerhans cell histiocytosis is found predominantly in children and young adults and is another disorder characteristically involving lymph node sinuses. It has been shown recently to be a clonal proliferative disease, indicating that

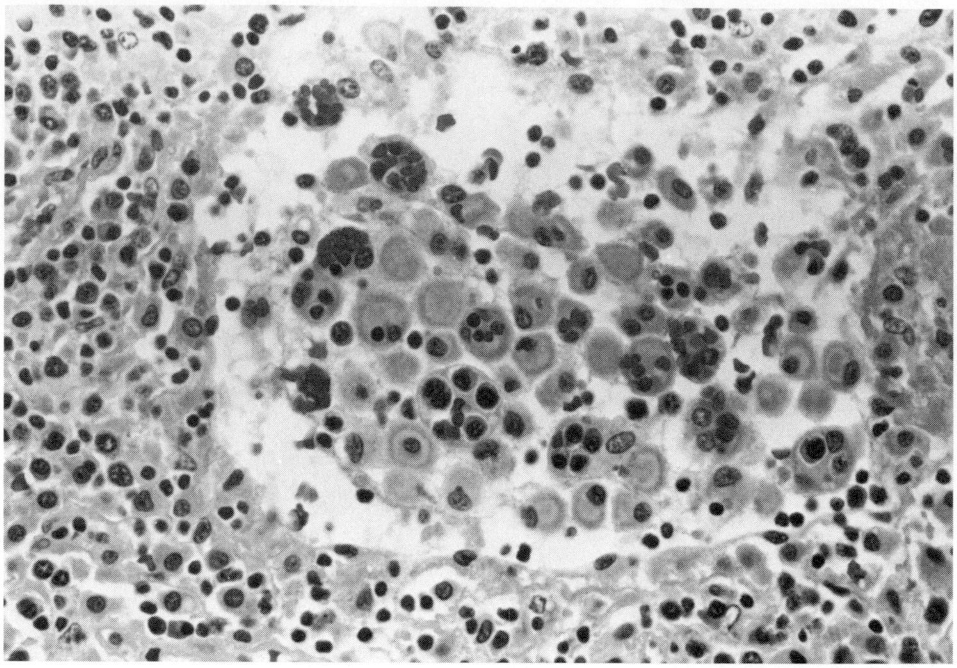

FIG. 15.21. Infection-associated hemophagocytic syndrome. Sinus histiocytes contain phagocytosed erythrocytes and lymphocytes (hematoxylin and eosin stain, original magnification: 500× magnification).

it is probably neoplastic despite its highly variable clinical behavior (87). The cells have distinctive light- and electron-microscopic as well as immunophenotypic findings (57,87–90). They are large mononuclear cells with delicate, folded, grooved nuclei and usually small, inconspicuous nucleoli. Rare multinucleated giant cells are present, varying numbers of eosinophils are seen among the Langerhans cells, and eosinophilic abscesses also may be seen. The cells are classically positive for CD1, S-100 protein in a diffuse nuclear and cytoplasmic pattern, CD68 in some cases, and, surprisingly, placental alkaline phosphatase (57). Ultrastructurally, Langerhans cells contain characteristic cytoplasmic Birbeck granules, which are specific for these cells (57,87,88,90). Lymph node involvement is usually a sign of disease elsewhere, but lesions confined to lymph nodes have been described (89) (Chapter 51). Included in the differential diagnosis of Langerhans cell histiocytosis are sinus histiocytosis, sinus histiocytosis with massive lymphadenopathy, and metastatic tumors. These disorders are differentiated from Langerhans cell histiocytosis on the basis of morphologic and immunohistochemical features.

Vascular Transformation of Lymph Node Sinuses

Vascular transformation of sinuses is a benign vasoproliferative process in which lymph node sinuses are converted into vascular channels (91–93). It is a rare condition seen in children as well as adults. Although its cause is unknown, it often is associated with tumors and lymphomas in the vicinity of the affected node, which may cause extranodal obstruction of veins or efferent lymphatics (91,92). Common sites of involvement include intraabdominal nodes sampled during staging laparotomy for lymphomas and regional nodes removed for cancer operations of breast, colon, and testes (15,93).

Histologically, the vasoproliferative process is present in expanded sinuses (Fig. 15.22). The subcapsular sinus most often is involved together with the intermediate or medullary sinuses. Sinusoidal sclerosis often accompanies the vascular proliferation. The fibrous capsule of the node is never involved. Four patterns of vascular proliferation have been described: cleft-like spaces, which are the most common; rounded vascular channels, which are most often found in the subcapsular sinus and may be empty or filled with erythrocytes; solid foci of spindled cells interspersed with collagen, accompanied by transition to ectatic vascular channels toward the subcapsular sinus; and a plexiform pattern (92). The more cellular areas of vascular transformation may resemble Kaposi's sarcoma, from which vascular proliferation is differentiated primarily by the absence of the capsular and trabecular involvement that commonly is seen in Kaposi's sarcoma. In addition, the spindle cell fascicles seen in well-developed Kaposi's sarcoma are never present in vascular transformation of sinuses. Also, the ectatic, rounded vascular spaces often seen in subcapsular sinuses and the sinusoidal sclerosis usually present in vascular transformation are absent in Kaposi's sarcoma (92). Nodular spindle cell vascular transformation of lymph nodes occurring mostly in abdominal lymph nodes draining cancer also can simulate Kaposi's sarcoma (93) (Chapter 30).

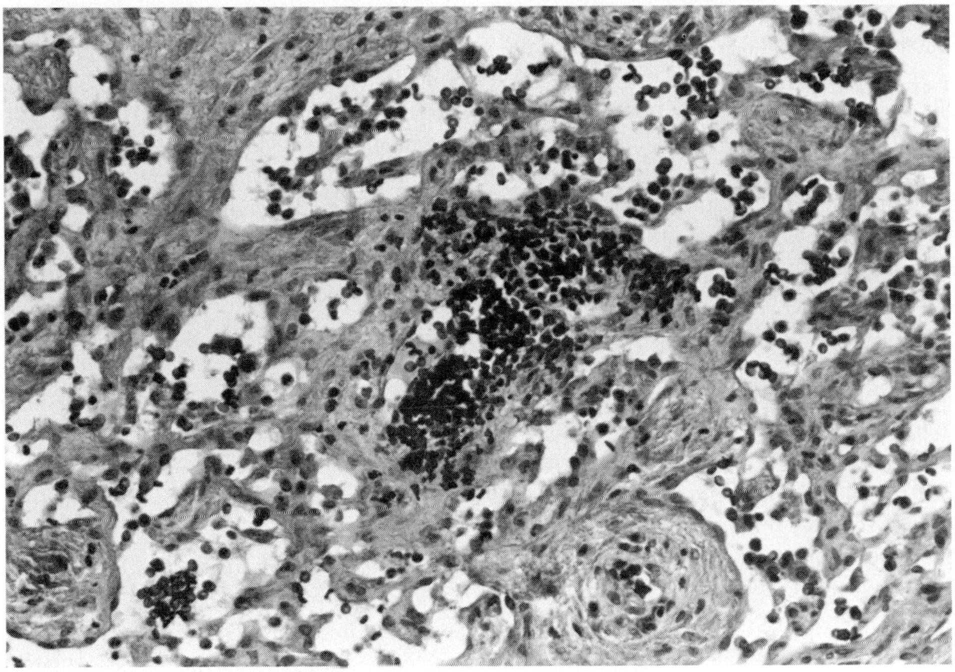

FIG. 15.22. Vascular transformation of sinuses. A subcapsular sinus with endothelium-lined spaces containing red blood cells (hematoxylin and eosin stain, original magnification: 400× magnification).

Kaposi's Sarcoma

Prior to the AIDS epidemic, Kaposi's sarcoma was a very rare and indolent tumor that, in North America, was seen almost exclusively in elderly males (94). Since 1979, there has been a dramatic increase in the incidence of this disorder (94–96). The vast majority of cases today are found in young homosexual males with AIDS, and the clinical course in these individuals resembles the lymphadenopathic form of the disease seen in children in Africa (94–96). In patients with HIV infections, early nodal involvement may or may not be associated with skin involvement. In the early stages of nodal involvement, Kaposi's sarcoma may be limited to the capsule or subcapsular or trabecular sinuses; subsequently, single or multiple confluent nodules may be present, or the entire lymph node may be replaced, with extension of the lesion into the perinodal tissue. Well-developed Kaposi's sarcoma is characterized by a proliferation of well-formed, criss-crossing spindle cell fascicles, which are separated by cleft-like spaces containing red blood cells (Fig. 15.23). Extravasated red cells are usually present, and eosinophilic PAS stain–positive globules may be found either within macrophages or spindle cells or extracellularly (94). Recognition of the early lesion may be difficult or, at times, impossible. In lymph nodes of patients with HIV infection, Kaposi's sarcoma may coexist with the benign lymphocyte-depletion stage of the disease, including nodes showing changes similar to those of Castleman's disease, and as a rare complication of multicentric Castleman's disease (39,94). The differential diagnosis of Kaposi's sarcoma is discussed in the previous section.

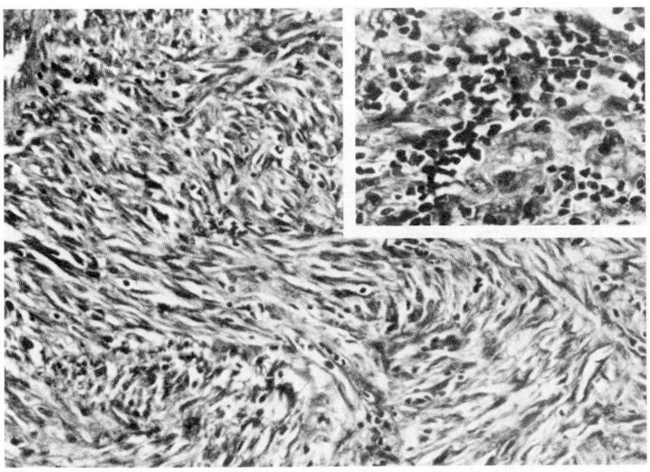

FIG. 15.23. Lymph node with Kaposi's sarcoma characterized by spindle cells that are separated by cleft-like spaces containing erythrocytes, some of which are extravasated (hematoxylin and eosin stain, original magnification: 300× magnification). **Inset:** Higher-magnification view of extravasated red cells (original magnification: 500× magnification).

DIFFUSE PATTERN

Paracortical (Interfollicular) Hyperplasia

The paracortical region of an unstimulated lymph node is less conspicuous than the circumscribed polymorphous germinal center. It is populated predominantly by small T lymphocytes and contains postcapillary venules, which bring circulating lymphocytes into this region.

Hyperplasia of this zone is noted easily on low-magnification examination. The follicles are spread apart, and the cellular composition depends on the stimulus and its duration. There may be a predominance of small lymphocytes or varying mixtures of small lymphocytes and lymphocytes in various stages of transformation to immunoblasts, usually associated with increased high endothelial vessels. The transformed cells are usually mixtures of T or B cells. T immunoblasts arise from the indigenous population of small cells; prolonged stimulation of B-cell areas may result in the presence of B immunoblasts migrating from the germinal centers. The degree of interfollicular expansion varies. It may be so slight as to be hardly perceptible, or it may be so severe that only small follicles remain or that even those are obliterated. These severe paracortical hyperplasias cause the pathologist the greatest difficulty in differentiating benign proliferations from Hodgkin's disease or from non-Hodgkin's lymphomas.

The most common causes of paracortical hyperplasia are viral infections, drug-induced hypersensitivity reactions, and, less frequent today, the aftereffects of vaccinations.

Infectious Mononucleosis

In classic cases of infectious mononucleosis, a lymph node biopsy is not indicated. In fact, it has been stated with more truth than humor that a complication of infectious mononucleosis is a lymph node biopsy. There are cases, however, in which the presentation of the illness is not characteristic or the lymphadenopathy is prolonged, and the surgical pathologist is presented with a lymph node or a tonsil from such a patient. Although a definitive diagnosis of infectious mononucleosis cannot be established on morphologic grounds alone, the pathologist might suggest carrying out appropriate studies to confirm the diagnosis.

As in most reactive lymphadenopathies, the histiologic picture varies from a completely nonspecific follicular hyperplasia to a proliferation suggesting non-Hodgkin's lymphoma or Hodgkin's disease (97–101). Most of the virus-associated disorders are characterized by an immunoblastic proliferation of varying severity, which imparts a characteristic mottled appearance to a variably expanded paracortex (Fig. 15.24). The mottled appearance results from the presence of large immunoblasts (transformed lymphocytes) among the small paracortical T cells. Mitotic figures are not uncommon among transformed lymphocytes. Varying numbers of plasma cells and plasmacytoid cells are admixed with lymphocytes and immunoblasts, resulting in a polymorphous picture. Patchy necrosis and single cell necrosis are not unusual. This proliferative process may extend into the capsule and trabeculae. Vascular proliferation with prominent endothelial cells is always present. The sinuses usually are patent, contain immunoblasts and small lymphocytes, and are compressed or focally dilated and filled with monocytoid B cells.

The differential diagnosis of infectious mononucleosis includes non-Hodgkin's lymphomas, particularly large cell lymphomas; Hodgkin's disease; and such benign prolifera-

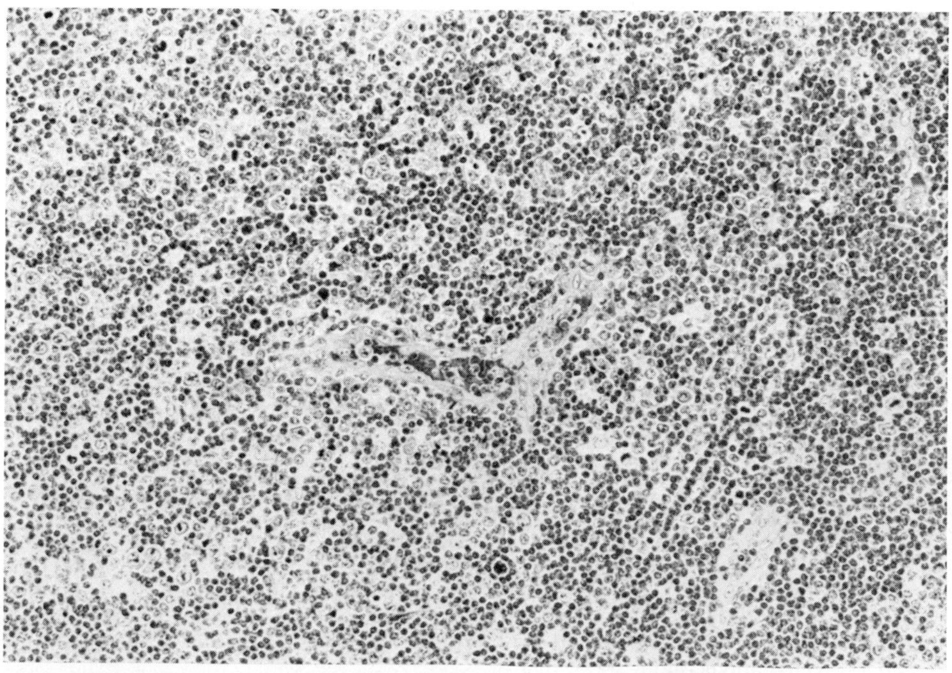

FIG. 15.24. Infectious mononucleosis. The mottled appearance of the paracortex is the result of large transformed lymphocytes (immunoblasts) among small lymphocytes. A vessel with prominent endothelial cells is present (hematoxylin and eosin stain, original magnification: 400× magnification).

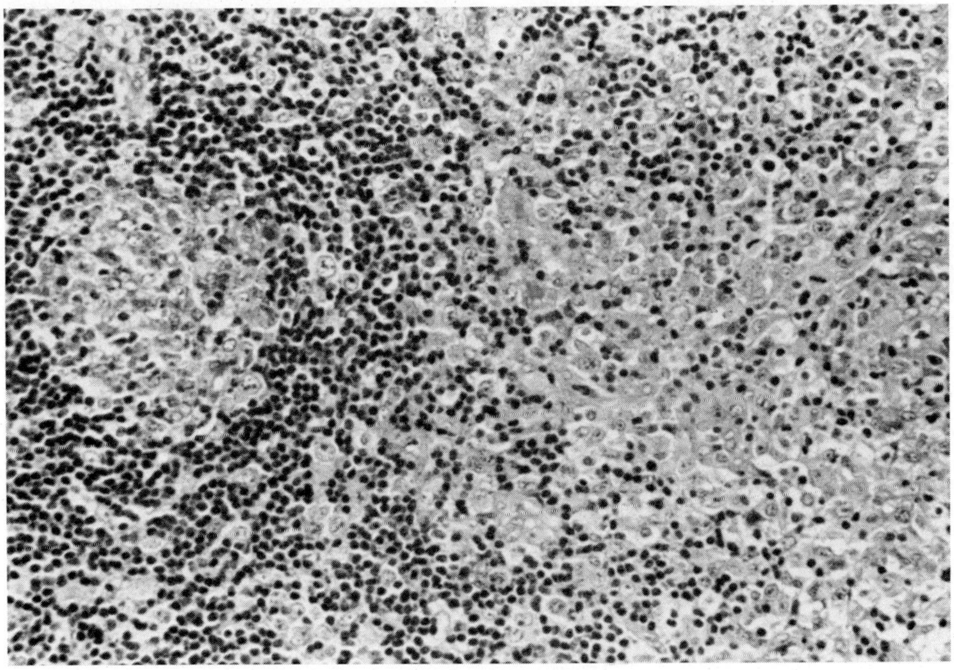

FIG. 15.25. Lymph node from a patient with infectious mononucleosis showing a small follicle and a sheet of immunoblasts in the paracortex (hematoxylin and eosin stain, original magnification: 475× magnification).

tions as other viral infections and hypersensitivity reactions to medications. In some instances of infectious mononucleosis, immunoblasts are present in clusters, or they may form sheets, effacing portions of the node (Figs. 15.24, 15.25). Such accumulations of large cells may be difficult or at times impossible to differentiate from large cell (immunoblastic) lymphomas. It is important to not focus solely on these areas of monomorphous proliferations but view the entire node and look for the more characteristic polymorphous infiltrate and the mottled areas described previously. If the lymph node biopsy is fragmented and architectural relationships are lost, differentiation of benign from malignant proliferation may be difficult. If such a diagnostic dilemma cannot be resolved, immunohistochemistry or, rarely, genotyping may be required to determine whether the proliferation is clonal. Generally, large cell immunoblastic lymphomas replace the entire node, or portions of uninvolved node do not show the polymorphous infiltrate, mottled appearance, and follicles that usually are seen in infectious mononucleosis. In addition, large cell lymphomas are composed exclusively of either B or T cells, whereas the immunoblasts of infectious mononucleosis are mixtures of Epstein-Barr virus--infected B cells expressing latent membrane protein and Epstein-Barr virus–encoded RNA and $CD8^+$ T cells (101). In rare cases, the B-cell immunoblasts may coexpress CD43. Anaplastic large cell lymphoma rarely may be confused with the lymph node changes of infectious mononucleosis. The resemblance of these two disorders is further intensified by the $CD30^+$ staining of the large cells in both, although the intensity of staining and the number of cells stained are greater in anaplastic large cell lymphoma. In contrast to the large cells in infectious mononucleosis, which are predominantly B cells, anaplastic large cells have a T- or null-cell phenotype and in addition are often EMA-positive.

Occasionally, some of the immunoblasts are binucleate and closely resemble or are indistinguishable from Reed-Sternberg cells (Fig. 15.26), and the proliferation may resemble Hodgkin's disease (97–101). We have seen this Hodgkin's disease–like proliferation in lymph nodes and especially the tonsils of individuals with infectious mononucleosis. As described in Chapter 17, the presence of Reed-Sternberg--like cells alone is insufficient grounds for a diagnosis of Hodgkin's disease. These giant cells must be found in an appropriate cellular environment characteristic of one of the subtypes of Hodgkin's disease. If one looks at the entire node, the characteristically mottled appearance is seen, and although this mottled appearance occasionally is mimicked by scattered lacunar variants of Reed-Sternberg cells, the sclerosis of nodular sclerosis Hodgkin's disease is lacking, and most immunoblasts do not have the cytologic features of even mononuclear lacunar cells. The nucleoli of the latter cells are usually much smaller. Intact sinuses also point to a benign disorder, and immunoblasts within sinuses are not seen in Hodgkin's disease. The presence of follicles does not help in the differentiation from Hodgkin's disease, because partial involvement of the lymph node by this lymphoma is not unusual. Immunostaining for CD15 with Leu M1 aids in differentiating true Reed-Sternberg cells from the imposter giant cells in viral disorders, which do not react with this antibody; however, the Reed-Sternberg–like cells in infectious mononucleosis may stain for CD30 (99–101).

In summary, it is essential to correlate the histologic find-

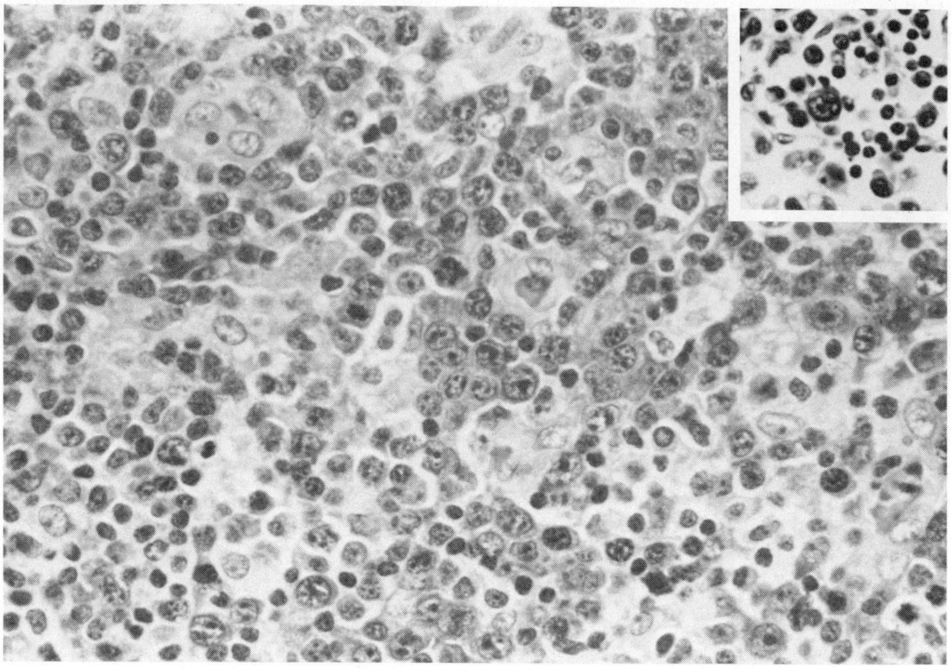

FIG. 15.26. Infectious mononucleosis. Single and clusters of immunoblasts are present among small lymphocytes and vessels with prominent endothelial cells (hematoxylin and eosin stain, original magnification: 625× magnification). **Inset:** Binucleate immunoblast that is indistinguishable from a Reed-Sternberg cell (original magnification: 625× magnification).

ings with the clinical history and the results of hematologic and serologic studies in order to make a diagnosis of infectious mononucleosis in lymph nodes.

Cytomegalovirus infections may produce lymph nodal changes similar to those of Epstein-Barr virus infections. Another distinctive histologic pattern of nodal involvement that usually presents with localized lymphadenopathy has been described (2). It is characterized by follicular hyperplasia and a prominent paracortical monocytoid B-cell proliferation. Careful examination may reveal rare lymphoid cells with cytomegalovirus inclusions, especially within areas of monocytoid B cells. These inclusion-containing cells have a T-cell phenotype (either $CD4^+$ or $CD8^+$) and are often $CD15^+$, which occasionally causes confusion with Reed-Sternberg cells. In contrast to Reed-Sternberg cells, cytomegalovirus-infected cells show Golgi or diffuse cytoplasmic staining with CD15; membranous staining is absent. A diagnosis of cytomegalovirus lymphadenitis can be confirmed by immunohistochemical staining for cytomegalovirus antigen or *in situ* hybridization for cytomegalovirus sequences (2,102,103).

The histologic picture of infectious mononucleosis is not specific and is similar to or indistinguishable from lymph nodes draining sites of vaccinations or herpes simplex or zoster infections (104,105). Herpes simplex infections may cause enlargement of regional lymph nodes. Biopsies usually are not done, because the diagnosis of herpes simplex infection is established by the characteristic skin or mucous membrane lesions. The histologic changes are similar to those described in other viral disorders involving a polymorphous interfollicular infiltrate in which immunoblasts may be prominent. Necrosis, which may be fairly extensive, multinucleated giant cells, and ground-glass intranuclear inclusions may be seen (104). The various types of virus-associated lymphadenopathies often can be distinguished from one another by immunohistochemical and DNA hybridization techniques (104). Similar to the changes found in infectious mononucleosis are hypersensitivity reactions to certain medications, the classic example of which is the anticonvulsant diphenylhydantoin (106). Eosinophils among the polymorphous infiltrate are more often evident in hypersensitivity reactions than in viral disorders. Other medications such as carbamazepine, another anticonvulsant, also may produce virus-like syndromes with lymphadenopathy (106,107). Non-Hodgkin's lymphomas, some of them Epstein-Barr virus–positive, have been reported after long-term diphenylhydantoin or carbamazepine therapy preceded by benign lymphadenopathy (108).

Postvaccinial Lymphadenitis

The typical immunoblastic proliferation following vaccination against smallpox is seen infrequently today, because such vaccination no longer is required routinely for travel through most parts of the world. The histologic picture of this disorder is similar to that associated with other viral infections, and it may resemble Hodgkin's disease or non-Hodgkin's lymphoma. Almost 50% of the cases of postvaccinial lymphadenitis reported by Hartsock (109) previously had been misdiagnosed as lymphoma. The majority of patients complained of painful enlargement of the left supraclavicular lymph nodes, which drained the site of vaccination. Seven to 15 days after inoculation these lymph nodes underwent biopsy; for unknown reasons, a history of vaccination was not elicited.

The histologic findings in postvaccinial lymphadenitis include follicular or diffuse hyperplasia, proliferation of immunoblasts with a mottled appearance of the paracortex, vascular and sinusoidal changes, and a polymorphous cellular infiltrate composed of lymphocytes, eosinophils, plasma cells, and mast cells. The basic nodal architecture remains intact, although it usually is distorted. The mottled appearance described in other viral infections is the most characteristic finding. Immunoblasts resembling Reed-Sternberg cells with a polymorphous infiltrate may simulate Hodgkin's disease (109). Lymph nodes undergoing biopsy 15 days after vaccination usually showed a prominent follicular hyperplasia, whereas diffuse hyperplasia characterized lymph nodes undergoing biopsy earlier. As in other viral disorders with paracortical immunoblasts, vascular proliferation with prominent endothelial cells is present in this disorder.

A histologic picture of lymph nodes resembling that in postvaccinial lymphadenitis has been reported after subcutaneous or intramuscular inoculation of live attenuated measles virus (110). Regional nodes enlarge within several days to 2 weeks, and the nodes show an immunoblastic proliferation, an increase in numbers of plasma cells, and variable numbers of Warthin-Finkeldey giant cells characteristic of measles.

MIXED PATTERN

Toxoplasmic Lymphadenopathy

Toxoplasma gondii has a worldwide distribution; approximately 50% of adults in the United States are infected by the organism (111). Individuals with acute acquired toxoplasmosis may be asymptomatic, or they may experience an infectious mononucleosis–like illness with reactive lymphocytes found in smears of peripheral blood. The mode of transmission of the organism to humans is through exposure to cat feces containing oocysts or through handling or ingestion of uncooked meat (112,113). Clinical or subclinical lymphadenopathy may develop and involve either a solitary node, especially a posterior cervical node, or many nodes. In contrast to the self-limiting course of the infection in immunocompetent individuals, immunodeficient patients, particularly those with AIDS, are at great risk for developing encephalitis. Also, infection during pregnancy may have devastating consequences for the fetus.

The histologic picture of toxoplasmic lymphadenitis is quite distinctive. The lymph nodes show an intact architecture and a pronounced follicular hyperplasia. The germinal centers are large with ragged, indistinct margins and contain numerous tingible body macrophages and many mitotic figures. Multiple small aggregates of epithelioid histiocytes are present in the paracortical regions, and they encroach on and are present within germinal centers (10,114–116) (Fig. 15.27, 15.28). The clusters of histiocytes usually do not exceed 20 in number, and they do not form well-defined granu-

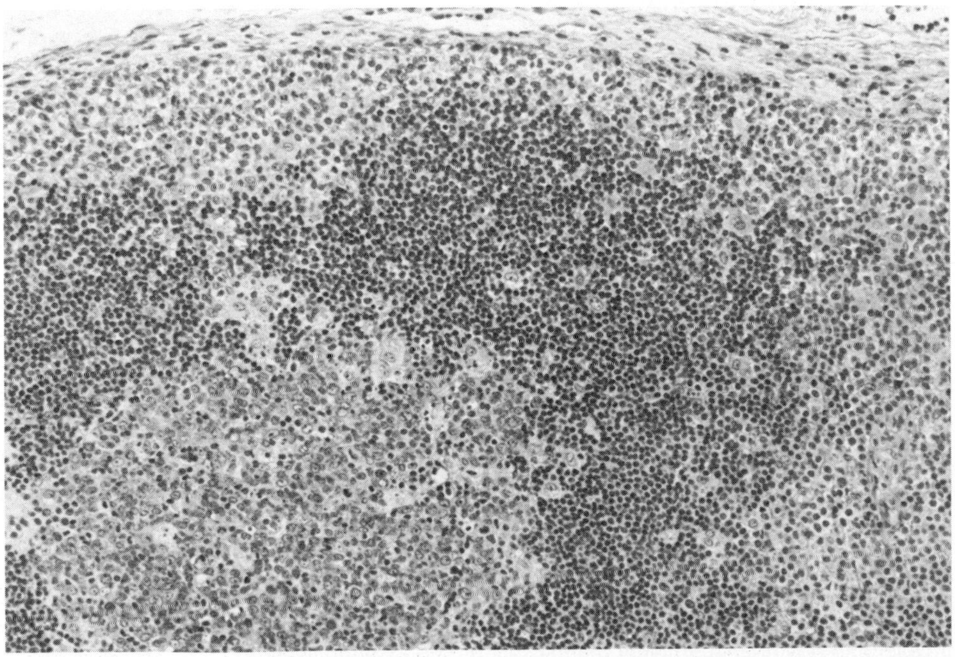

FIG. 15.27. Toxoplasmic lymphadenitis. A large germinal center with irregular, indistinct borders contains numerous tingible body macrophages. Clusters of epithelioid histiocytes encroach on and are present within the germinal center. The subcapsular and trabecular sinuses are dilated and filled with monocytoid B cells (hematoxylin and eosin stain, original magnification: 250× magnification).

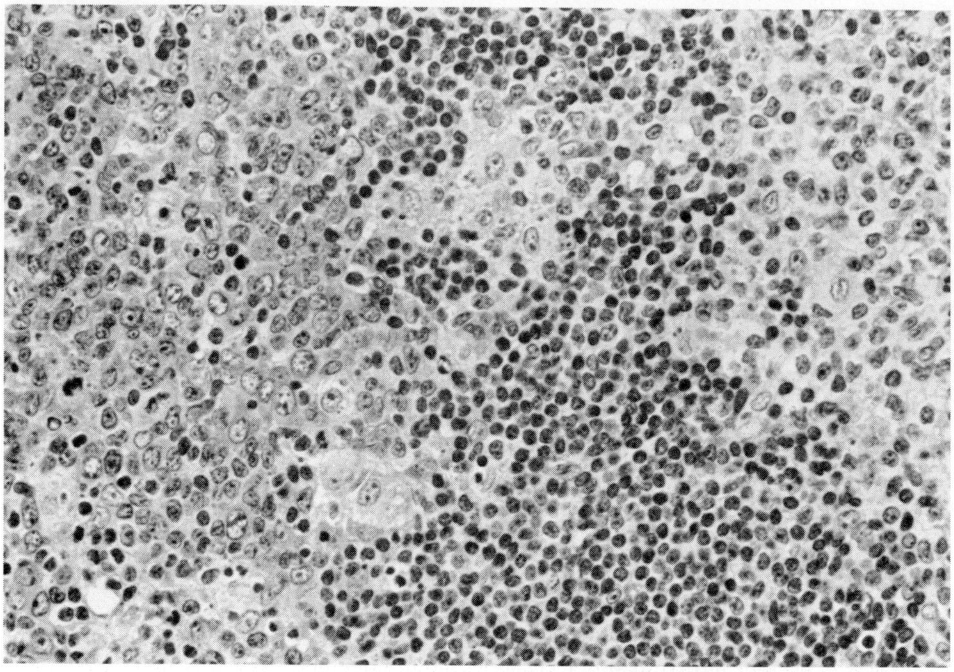

FIG. 15.28. Toxoplasmic lymphadenitis. Part of a germinal center (**left**). The interfollicular area with small clusters of histiocytes encroaches on and within the follicle center and is part of a dilated sinus filled with monocytoid B cells (**right**) (hematoxylin and eosin stain, original magnification: 500× magnification).

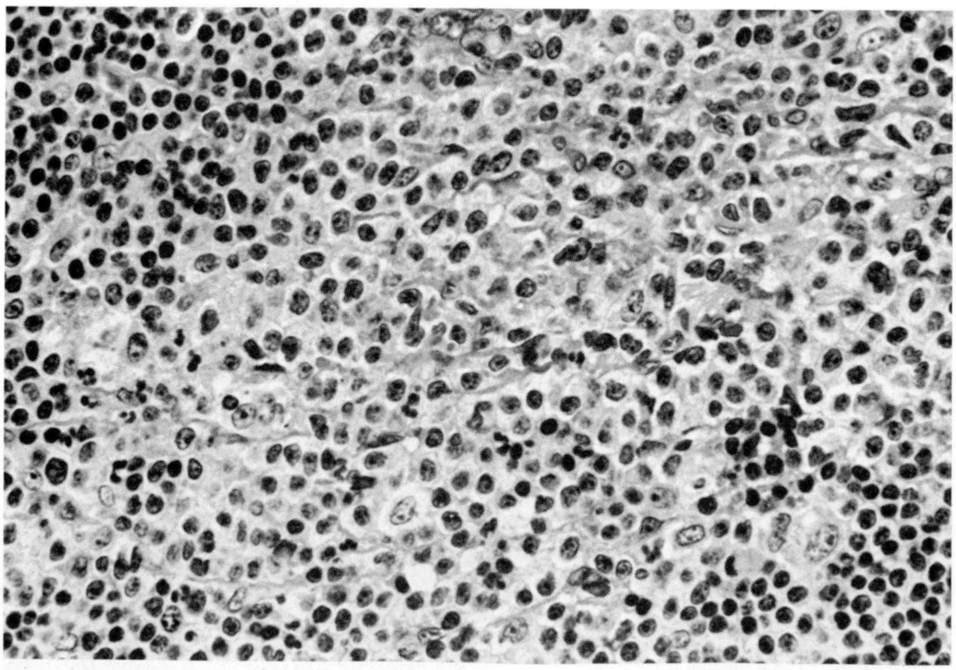

FIG. 15.29. Higher-magnification view of monocytoid B cells that have ample cytoplasm and large, irregularly contoured, bland nuclei. Scattered neutrophils are present among the monocytoid B cells (hematoxylin and eosin stain, original magnification: 500× magnification).

lomas, nor do they contain multinucleated giant cells or necrosis. Another feature is focal dilatation of the subcapsular or trabecular sinuses, which are filled with monocytoid B cells (Figs. 15.27–15.29). Parasitic cysts in lymph nodes rarely have been reported, and toxoplasmic genomes only rarely are detected by polymerase chain reaction (116,117). These findings indicate that the changes in the lymph nodes do not result directly from the effects of contact with the organism but rather represent a reaction to its products (117). Many plasma cells and some immunoblasts are present in the medullary cords.

Although a definitive diagnosis cannot be established on histologic grounds alone, the pathologist may suggest the diagnosis of toxoplasmic lymphadenitis, which must be confirmed by the appropriate serologic tests (10).

A histologic picture similar to that of toxoplasmic lymphadenitis may be seen in lymph nodes from HIV-infected patients. A florid or explosive follicular hyperplasia and a sinusoidal and paracortical monocytoid B-cell proliferation may be seen in these nodes (11). The epithelioid histiocytes usually are missing. Leishmanial lymphadenitis is included in the differential diagnosis of toxoplasmic lymphadenitis. The histiocytes in the paracortex and germinal centers contain the diagnostic Leishman-Donovan bodies that are seen in hematoxylin and eosin–stained sections.

Dermatopathic Lymphadenitis

The histologic picture of dermatopathic lymphadenitis may be associated with a variety of benign skin disorders, and occasionally lesions similar to dermatopathic lymphadenitis are noted in patients without apparent skin lesions (118). In cases of mycosis fungoides, enlargement of lymph nodes showing the histologic picture of dermatopathic lymphadenitis often is seen (119). Dermatopathic changes in lymph nodes of homosexual males without evidence of dermatitis has been reported (120).

Histologically, the fully developed lesion has a characteristic appearance under low magnification (Fig. 15.30). The paracortex shows varying degrees of a nodular expansion by pale-staining cells, some of which may contain melanin and occasionally hemosiderin. The pale-staining cells consist of histiocytes that contain the pigment, Langerhans cells, and interdigitating dendritic cells (118). Varying numbers of eosinophils and plasma cells often are admixed among the pale-staining cells. Langerhans cells are characterized by their complex and delicately folded nuclear membranes (Fig. 15.31) and their expression of S-100 protein, HLA-DR, and CD1 (118). Small lymphocytes with markedly irregular nuclear contours, resembling or indistinguishable from cells of mycosis fungoides, often are seen on careful examination of the paracortex. Because these cells are present in patients without evidence of mycosis fungoides, it is not possible to detect early nodal involvement by this cutaneous T-cell lymphoma in lymph nodes unless at least partial architectural effacement of the node is present (119). Clonal rearrangement of the β T-cell receptor gene, however, is capable of detecting only as little as 1% to 5% of malignant cells in these lymph nodes (121). The germinal centers may show varying degrees of hyperplasia and, depending on the degree of paracortical expansion, they often are compressed in the outer cortex (Fig. 15.29). Sinus histiocytosis in the medullary areas is usually present. The sinus histiocytes have round or oval nuclei, lack the nuclear complexity of the paracortical Langerhans cells, and are S-100^-.

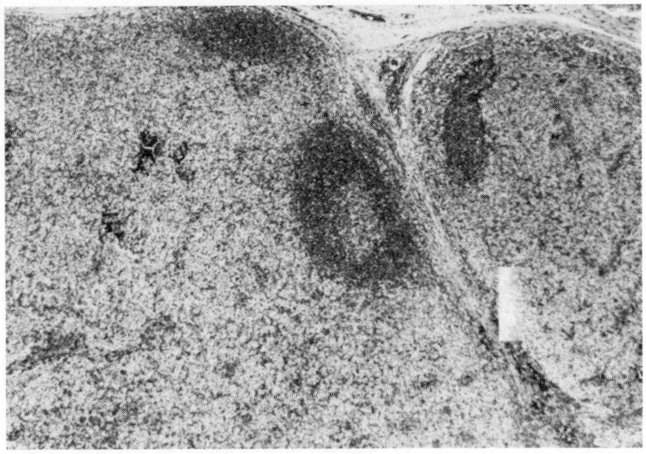

FIG. 15.30. Dermatopathic lymphadenitis showing massive expansion of the paracortex by large, pale-staining cells that include Langerhans cells and histiocytes. A germinal center is compressed in the outer cortex (hematoxylin and eosin stain, original magnification: 80× magnification).

Granulomatous Inflammation

There are many causes of infective or noninfective granulomatous inflammation involving lymph nodes (122). The granulomas may be of the epithelioid type, such as those associated with sarcoidosis, or they may be necrotizing granulomas, characterized by caseous necrosis of tuberculosis. Suppurative granulomas classically are seen in cat-scratch disease, lymphogranuloma venereum, chronic granulomatous disease, atypical mycobacterial infection, and infections with *Yersinia* species (13,14,123–125).

Sarcoidosis

Sarcoidosis is a multisystem granulomatous disease in which there is no clearly defined causative agent or known pathogenetic mechanism. The course of the disease, clinical presentation, and laboratory and pathologic features, are well known (126). Histologically, sarcoidosis is characterized by discrete, nonnecrotizing epithelioid granulomas, in which Langhans giant cells may or may not be present (Fig. 15.32). Occasionally granulomas have small central foci of fibrinoid necrosis. The granulomas are surrounded by lymphocytes and plasma cells and sometimes fibrosis. Asteroid bodies, Schaumann's bodies, and crystals of calcium oxalate rarely are seen in the giant cells but are not specific for sarcoidosis.

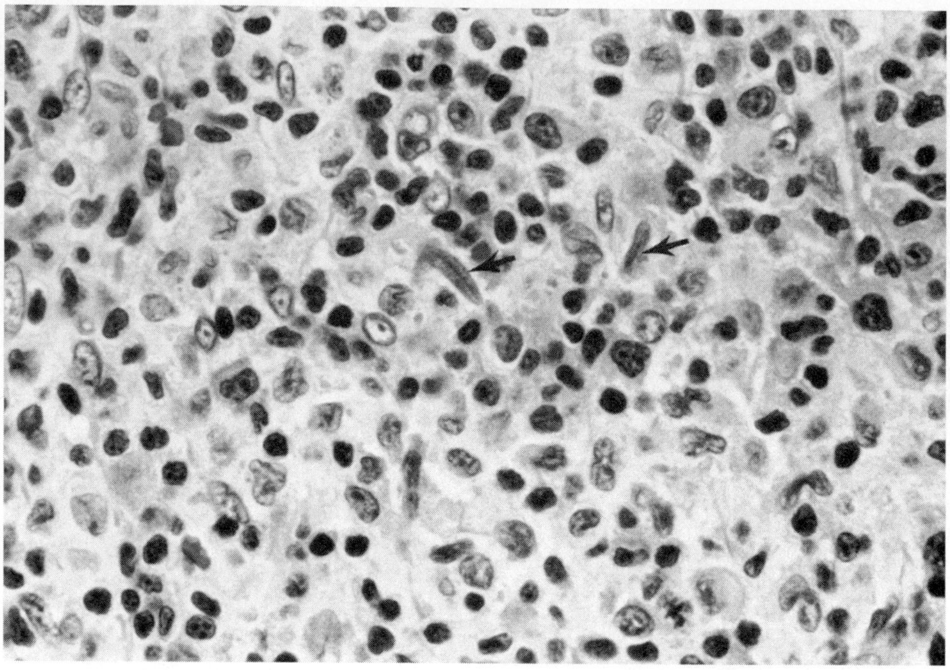

FIG. 15.31. Higher-magnification view of the section in Figure 15.30, showing a polymorphous infiltrate including small lymphocytes, histiocytes, occasional immunoblasts, and cells with delicate nuclear membrane folds characteristic of Langerhans cells (*arrows*) (hematoxylin and eosin stain, original magnification: 500× magnification).

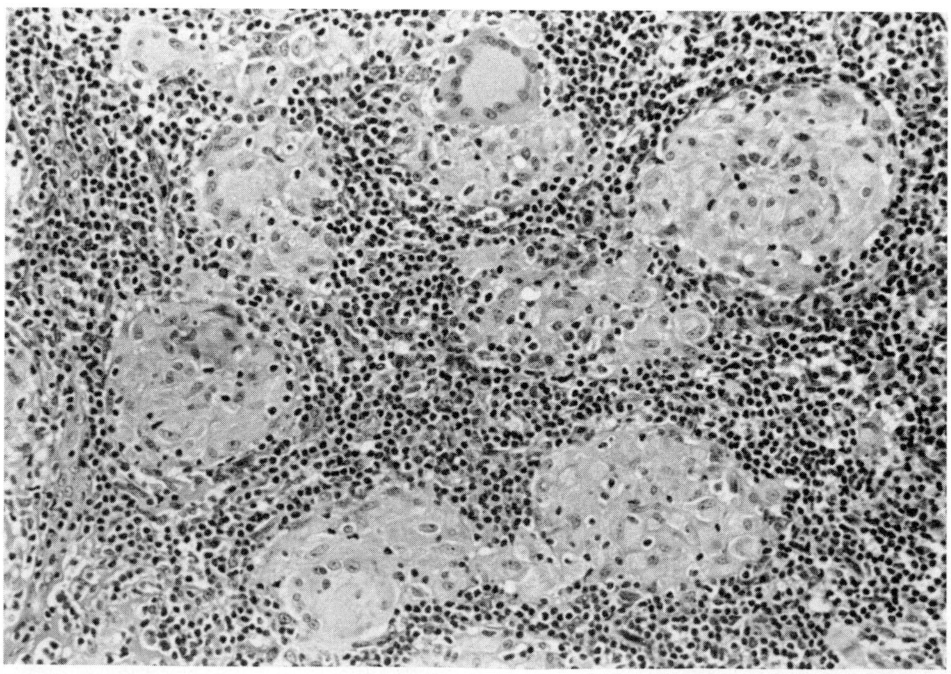

FIG. 15.32. Lymph node from a patient with sarcoidosis containing multiple small, well-circumscribed epithelioid granulomas, some with multinucleated giant cells (hematoxylin and eosin stain, original magnification: 400× magnification).

Hamazaki-Wesenberg bodies, which are small needle-like or oval PAS stain–positive and acid-fast structures, also may be found in the cytoplasm of the giant cells (127). Because there are numerous other causes of sarcoid-like granulomas, the diagnosis of sarcoidosis is one of exclusion. Sarcoid-type granulomas may be seen in lymph nodes in patients with Hodgkin's disease; small epithelioid granulomas are also seen in mesenteric lymph nodes of patients with Crohn's disease and in nodes draining carcinomas (128). Staining for acid-fast bacilli and fungi should be carried out to exclude these organisms as causative agents. Granulomas in tuberculosis may be indistinguishable from those in sarcoidosis, but more commonly they contain central areas of necrosis surrounded by epithelioid histiocytes and Langhans giant cells. Fungal infections may show similar necrotizing granulomas or suppurative lesions. Rarely, Whipple's disease may resemble sarcoidosis in lymph nodes; a PAS stain is helpful in establishing a diagnosis of Whipple's disease in such cases.

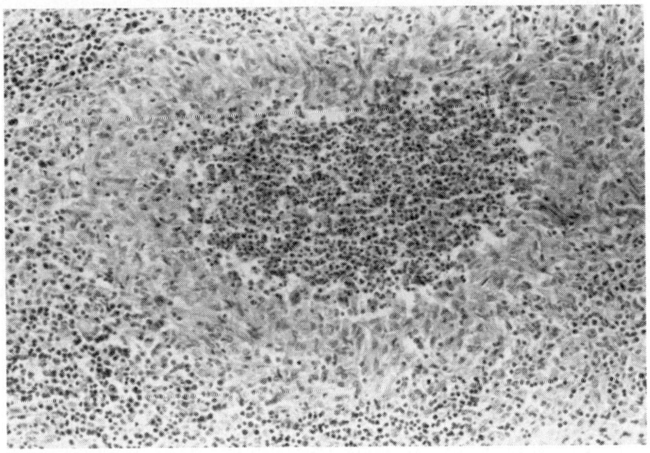

FIG. 15.33. Cat-scratch disease. Suppurative necrosis surrounded by palisading histiocytes in a lymph node of a child with a history of being scratched by a cat (hematoxylin and eosin stain, original magnification: 400× magnification).

Cat-scratch Disease and Lymphogranuloma Venereum

Cat-scratch disease is a zoonotic infection recently reported to be caused by a small pleomorphic, gram-negative bacterium, *Bartonella henselae*, which also causes bacillary angiomatosis; lymphogranuloma venereum is a sexually transmitted disease caused by chlamydia (13,14,124,129). Cat-scratch disease is characterized by tender regional lymph node enlargement, a primary inoculation site in the skin, and a history of contact with a cat, often a kitten. The disease usually resolves spontaneously, in 2 to 4 months. Although in the past the histologic features of the nodal lesion only suggested the possibility of cat-scratch disease, we now can establish the diagnosis firmly by identifying the gram-negative, Warthin-Starry stain–positive, pleomorphic bacteria in tissue sections (13,123) and with a recently developed serologic test (130), as well as by using polymerase chain reaction–based detection of the causative agent in formalin-fixed tissue (131). Furthermore, demonstration of the organisms aids in the differential diagnosis of other disorders, which may show identical histologic changes.

Cat-scratch disease, which most often affects children, usually is found in cervical and axillary nodes; lymphogranuloma venereum is more likely to involve inguinal nodes. This regional nodal involvement, however, no longer can be used to differentiate definitively between these two infectious disorders, because inguinal lymph nodes also have been reported to be involved in cat-scratch disease, and coincidental involvement of inguinal and supraclavicular nodes has been noted in lymphogranuloma venereum (123,124).

Histologically, the fully developed suppurative granuloma is quite distinctive (Fig. 15.33). The histologic features, however, vary with time (122,123). The early lesions show small focal areas of necrosis, and small clusters of neutrophils surrounded by histiocytes are seen beneath the subcapsular sinus. The small developing abscesses may involve germinal centers, which usually show a marked degree of hyperplasia containing many tingible body macrophages and numerous mitotic figures. It is in this stage that the organisms are demonstrated most readily within areas of microabscesses or within walls of capillaries. The sinuses may be distended with monocytoid B cells, immunoblasts, and neutrophils. In later stages, the areas of suppuration increase in size and extend deeper into the node, and the surrounding rim of macrophages that have an epithelioid appearance becomes larger. All stages of development from a granulomatous appearance with very small foci of suppuration to the fully developed lesion may be seen within the same node.

Lymphogranuloma venereum is caused by *Chlamydia trachomatis* serotypes L1, L2, and L3 (14). It most often involves inguinal nodes and is preceded by a papule or intraepidermal or subdermal vesicle in the skin of the penis or the mucous membrane of the vagina, vulva, or rectum. The disease generally is unsuspected prior to histologic examinations of the lymph node, and it is considered in the differential diagnosis of cat-scratch disease, tularemia, and fungal and mycobacterial infection, only after histologic examination. The sand-like organisms are identified within vacuolated macrophages as intravacuolar particles (14). The vacuolated histiocytes are most prominent at the margin of suppuration, and the organisms may be identified on hematoxylin and eosin–stained sections and with Brown-Hopps and Warthin-Starry stains. The organisms can be confirmed to be chlamydia by utilizing the polymerase chain reaction (14).

Mesenteric lymphadenitis is a self-limited disorder caused by the gram-negative organisms *Yersinia pseudotuberculosis* and *Y. enterocolitica* (125). Patients may present with a clinical picture of appendicitis. Histologically, there is capsular thickening, an immunoblastic proliferation in the paracortical and cortical regions, follicular hyperplasia, dilated sinuses containing lymphocytes, and in the case of *Y. pseudotuberculosis* infection, small granulomas and abscesses may be present. The diagnosis should be confirmed by culture of organisms. Chronic granulomatous disease of childhood should also be considered in the differential diagnosis of suppurative granulomas.

Kikuchi's Disease

Kikuchi's histiocytic necrotizing lymphadenitis was described in 1972 (132,133) and initially was not well known outside of Japan. It is now recognized as a distinct clinicopathologic entity throughout the world (12,134,135). The disease typically affects young adults, mostly women, especially of Asian descent. It is usually a benign and self-limiting disorder characterized by isolated lymphadenopathy, most often of cervical lymph nodes. The disease usually resolves in several months. Fever may accompany the adenopathy, or the presenting symptom may be fever of unknown origin. It is important to recognize the lesion histologically, because it is not infrequently misdiagnosed as lymphoma, most often as non-Hodgkin's lymphoma but occasionally also as Hodgkin's disease (12,132–136). Kikuchi's disease may represent a *forme fruste* of systemic lupus erythematosus. A small number of patients with this disorder have developed lupus erythematosus, and histologically the lesions are similar (12). Although its cause is unknown, a viral or autoimmune pathogenesis for Kikuchi's disease currently is favored (12,137).

The histologic findings in Kikuchi's disease are quite distinctive (Chapter 51): localized, patchy areas of necrosis with prominent karyorrhectic nuclear debris, usually confined to paracortical and cortical areas (132–139) (Fig. 15.34). In contrast to necrotic lesions in most other diseases, there is an absence of polymorphonuclear leukocytes (Fig. 15.35). Surrounding the necrotic areas and accounting for the misdiagnosis of lymphoma are large mononuclear cells of atypical appearance. These mononuclear cells consist of mixtures of immunoblasts, predominantly at the periphery of the necrosis, and cells with atypical, irregularly twisted nuclei and histiocytes, often with crescentic nuclei and many containing phagocytosed karyorrhectic debris. Also present are varying numbers of plasmacytoid monocytes, with their characteristic appearance of nuclei with dispersed chromatin, absence of nucleoli, and eccentric rim of amphophilic cytoplasm without the Golgi zone of plasma cells. Foamy histiocytes occasionally are present immediately around the necrotic areas. Plasma cells usually are absent. In some cases of Kikuchi's disease, necrosis is absent and the focal lesions consist only of immunoblasts, plasmacytoid monocytes, and a few apoptotic bodies and histiocytes. It may be especially difficult to differentiate such lesions from large cell lymphoma (135). Recently, Kikuchi's disease has been divided into three types: proliferative, necrotizing (the most common), and xanthomatous (139). These patterns probably represent the various stages of evolution of the disease. In the adjacent uninvolved areas, immunoblasts are scattered among the small lymphocytes, producing a mottled appearance of the paracortex. Immunophenotypic analysis has demonstrated a vast predominance of T cells, mostly $CD8^+$. Recent studies have shown that apoptotic cell death mediated by cytolytic T lymphocytes is the principal mechanism of cellular destruction in Kikuchi's disease (137).

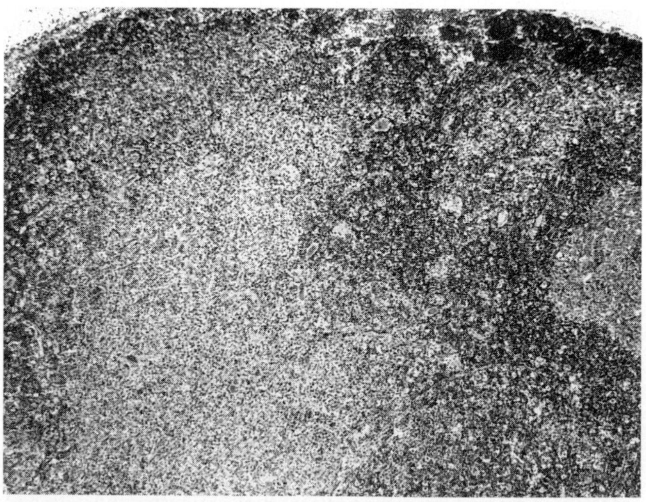

FIG. 15.34. Kikuchi's disease. A focus of cortical and paracortical necrosis is surrounded by a prominent rim of large, pale-staining cells. A hyperplastic follicle is present in the uninvolved part of the node (hematoxylin and eosin stain, original magnification: 200× magnification).

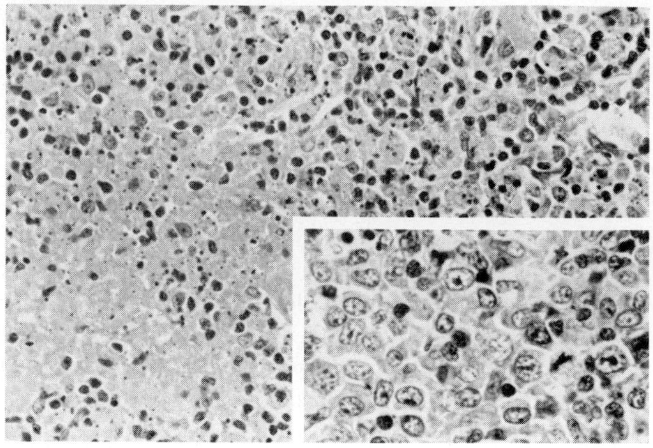

FIG. 15.35. Kikuchi's disease. An area of necrosis surrounded by large cells including immunoblasts and histiocytes. Neutrophils are not seen, but karyorrhectic debris is present within the necrotic area (original magnification: 500× magnification). **Inset:** Higher magnification of immunoblasts and histiocytes (original magnification: 625× magnification).

Differential diagnosis of Kikuchi's disease includes systemic lupus erythematosus, herpes simplex lymphadenitis, non-Hodgkin's lymphoma, and Hodgkin's disease (12,135). Although the necrosis-containing karyorrhectic nuclear debris may be identical in both systemic lupus and Kikuchi's disease, hematoxylin bodies, if present, and plasma cells are characteristic of the former disorder (12). Areas of necrosis tend to be more extensive in lupus. Necrosis may be extensive in herpes simplex lymphadenitis, and some histiocytes may surround the necrosis. The histiocytic infiltrate is never as pronounced as in Kikuchi's disease; some neutrophils may be present, and viral inclusions are found only in herpes simplex (104). In addition, skin or mucous membrane lesions are usually present in areas drained by the lymph nodes. Necrosis associated with Hodgkin's disease, especially the syncytial variant of nodular sclerosis, usually contains segmented neutrophils. Surrounding masses of lacunar variants of Reed-Sternberg cells may resemble superficially the mononuclear cells seen in Kikuchi's disease. Reed-Sternberg cells, in contrast to the large cells in Kikuchi's disease, are $CD15^+$ and $CD30^+$ and $CD45^-$. Other necrotizing lesions, such as cat-scratch disease (13,123), lymphogranuloma venereum (14,124), Kawasaki disease (140), and *Yersinia* infection (125), contain numerous polymorphonuclear leukocytes.

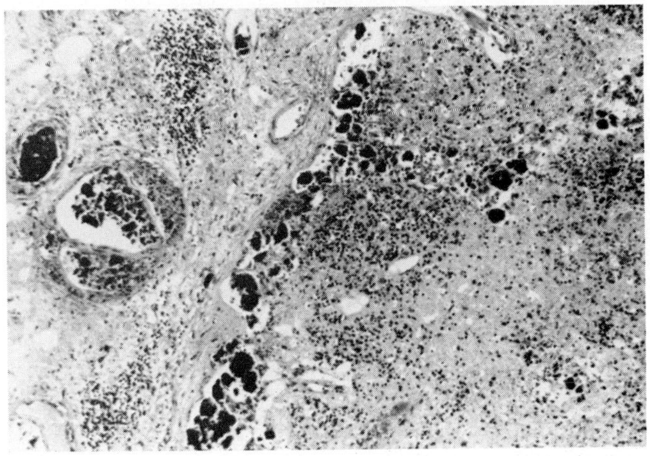

FIG. 15.36. Lymph node from a patient with disseminated systemic lupus erythematosus showing extensive necrosis without neutrophil reaction and numerous hematoxylin bodies, especially prominent within sinuses and vessels in the perinodal tissues (hematoxylin and eosin stain, original magnification: 200× magnification).

Systemic Lupus Erythematosus

Lymph node enlargement is not uncommon in systemic lupus erythematosus, occurring in 30% to 60% of cases (141–143). Lymph nodes in the cervical region are most likely to be involved, and occasionally their enlargement is the first clinical manifestation of the disease. Because patients with lupus are at risk to develop lymphomas, lymph node biopsy is indicated.

Microscopically, the lymph nodes may show completely nonspecific follicular hyperplasia and varying degrees of plasmacytosis. The characteristic findings include varying amounts of necrosis and nonspecific lymphoid hyperplasia (15,141–143). The necrotic foci may be similar or identical to those seen in Kikuchi's disease, consisting of eosinophilic amorphous material; if the necrosis is more extensive than that usually seen in Kikuchi's disease, it is of the coagulative type, devoid of viable cells. As in Kikuchi's disease, there is an absence of segmented neutrophils associated with the necrosis, and karyorrhectic debris is always present. There are usually, but not invariably, more plasma cells present in systemic lupus than in Kikuchi's disease (15,141). Immunostaining of frozen sections does not help in differentiating between the two disorders (142). Diagnostic of lupus erythematosus and absent in Kikuchi's disease are hematoxylin bodies (Fig. 15.36), which are found in necrotic areas, especially at their edges and within sinuses. Altered DNA, which probably represents degenerated nuclei that have reacted with antinuclear antibodies, also may be seen within the walls of blood vessels (the Azzopardi phenomenon) (141–143). These hematoxylin bodies consist of amorphous material that stains intensely with hematoxylin, Feulgen methods, and periodic acid--Schiff. However, hematoxylin bodies are not always present in the lymph nodes of patients with lupus erythematosus, and thus this diagnosis cannot be made on morphologic grounds alone. Appropriate serologic tests are required to confirm the morphologic impression of lupus lymphadenitis.

Kawasaki Disease

Kawasaki disease, also known as *mucocutaneous lymph node syndrome*, is a self-limited, acute exanthematous disease of childhood of obscure etiology (140,144). Most cases of the disease occur in Japan, and the disease is uncommon in the United States. Approximately 1.5% of affected children die during the acute phase of the disease or later, usually secondary to coronary arteritis and its complications. Included in the criteria for establishing a clinical diagnosis is the presence of acute nonsuppurative cervical adenopathy. Few lymph node biopsies in cases of Kawasaki disease have been reported (144). The most characteristic histologic findings include multiple foci of necrosis and fibrin thrombi in small vessels (144). Initially, the necrosis resembles small infarcts without neutrophils; later many neutrophils are present. Concentric infiltrates of the adventitia of vessels by transformed lymphocytes and histiocytes are seen occasionally. Histologically, the presence of fibrin thrombi in microvasculature may resemble that in thrombotic thrombocytopenic purpura, but the latter disorder can be excluded clinically. The bland necrosis seen in the early phases may resemble that in systemic lupus, which also can be excluded from the differential diagnosis on clinical grounds.

SUMMARY AND CONCLUSIONS

In this chapter the histologic features of many of the benign lymphadenopathies are described and depicted, and their differential diagnoses have been discussed. Because many lymph nodes show one of the many types of benign proliferations on biopsy, the surgical pathologist should be thoroughly familiar with them, not only to differentiate benign from malignant lymphadenopathies but also to suggest a specific cause if possible.

The benign lymphoproliferative disorders have been placed in four categories according to the compartments from which they arise: follicles, sinuses, or paracortex or a mixed pattern of more than one compartment. In most cases, the cause of the lymphoid proliferations is not known, but in a number of instances a specific cause may be suggested or a different diagnosis formulated on morphologic grounds. Correlation of the morphologic features with the clinical history and results of ancillary studies such as histochemistry, cultures, serologic tests, immunohistochemistry, *in situ* hybridization, and genotypic analysis may be helpful in selected cases in establishing a specific diagnosis and in differentiating benign lymphadenopathies from lymphomas.

REFERENCES

1. Knowles DM. Immunophenotypic and immunogenotypic approaches useful in distinguishing benign and malignant lymphoid proliferations. *Semin Oncol* 1993;20:583–610.
2. Swerdlow SH. Reactive lymph node hyperplasia. In: *Biopsy interpretation series: biopsy interpretation of lymph nodes.* New York: Raven Press, 1992:39–124.
3. Krishnan J, Danon AD, Frizzera G. Reactive lymphadenopathies and atypical lymphoproliferative disorders. *Am J Clin Pathol* 1993;99: 385–396.
4. Weiss LM, Chan WC, Schnitzer B. Lymph nodes. In: Damjanov I, Lindner J, eds. *Anderson's pathology,* vol 1, 10th ed. St. Louis: Mosby, 1996:1115–1200.
5. Chan JKC, Tsang WYW. Reactive lymphadenopathies. In: Weiss L, ed. *Contemporary issues in surgical pathology: pathology of lymph nodes.* New York: Churchill Livingstone, 1996:81–168.
6. DeWolf-Peeters C, Delabie J. Anatomy and histophysiology of lymphoid tissue. *Semin Oncol* 1993;20:555–569.
7. Nosanchuk JS, Schnitzer B. Follicular hyperplasia in lymph nodes from patients with rheumatoid arthritis. *Cancer* 1969;24:343–354.
8. Hartsock RJ, Halling LW, King FM. Luetic lymphadentitis: a clinical and histologic study of 20 cases. *Am J Clin Pathol* 1970;53:304–314.
9. Inagaki H, Kawai T, Miyata M, et al. Gastric syphilis: Polymerase chain reaction detection of treponemal DNA in pseudolymphomatous lesions. *Hum Pathol* 1996;27:761–761.
10. Dorfman RF, Remington JS. Value of lymph node biopsy in the diagnosis of acute acquired toxoplasmosis. *N Engl J Med* 1973;289: 878–881.
11. Butler JJ, Osborne BM. Lymph node enlargement in patients with unsuspected human immunodeficiency virus infections. *Hum Pathol* 1988;19:849–854.
12. Dorfman RF, Berry GJ. Kikuchi's histiocytic necrotizing lymphadenitis: an analysis of 108 cases with emphasis on differential diagnosis. *Semin Diagn Pathol* 1988;5:329–345.
13. Wear DJ, Margileth AM, Hadfield TL, et al. Cat scratch disease: a bacterial infection. *Science* 1983;221:1403–1405.
14. Hadfield TL, Lamy Y, Wear DJ. Demonstration of Chlamydia trachomatis in inguinal lymphadenitis of lymphogranuloma venereum: a light microscopy, electron microscopy, and polymerase chain reaction study. *Mod Pathol* 1995;8:924–929.
15. Dorfman RF, Warnke R. Lymphadenopathy simulating the malignant lymphomas. *Hum Pathol* 1974;5:519–550.
16. Burke JS. Reactive lymphadenopathies. *Semin Diagn Pathol* 1988;5: 312–316.
17. Ioachim HL, Lerner CW, Tapper ML. The lymphoid lesions associated with the acquired immunodeficiency syndrome. *Am J Surg Pathol* 1983;7:543–553.
18. Rappaport H, Winter WJ, Hicks EB. Follicular lymphoma: a re-evaluation of its position in the scheme of malignant lymphoma, based on a survey of 253 cases. *Cancer* 1956;9:792–821.
19. Nathwani BN, Winberg CD, Diamond LW, et al. Morphologic criteria for the differentiation of follicular lymphoma from florid reactive follicular hyperplasia: a study of 80 cases. *Cancer* 1981;48: 1794–1806.
20. Keith TA, Cousar JB, Glick AD, et al. Plasmacytic differentiation in follicular center cell (FCC) lymphoma. *Am J Clin Pathol* 1985;84: 283–290.
21. Utz GL, Swerdlow SH. Distinction of follicular hyperplasia from follicular lymphoma in B5-fixed tissues: comparison of MT2 and bcl-2 antibodies. *Hum Pathol* 1993;24:1155–1158.
22. Ashton-Key M, Diss TC, Isaacson PG, et al. A comparative study of the value of immunohistochemistry and the polymerase chain reaction in the diagnosis of follicular lymphoma. *Histopathology* 1995;27: 501–508.
23. Doggett RS, Colby TV, Dorfman RF. Interfollicular Hodgkin's disease. *Am J Surg Pathol* 1983;7:145–149.
24. Schnitzer B. Pathology of lymphoid tissue in rheumatoid arthritis and allied disorders. In: Glynn LE, Schlumberger HD, eds. *Bayer Symposium VI: Experimental models of chronic inflammatory diseases.* New York: Springer-Verlag, 1977:331–348.
25. Kondratowicz GM, Symmons DP, Bacon PA, et al. Rheumatoid lymphadenopathy: A morphological and immunohistochemical study. *J Clin Pathol* 1990;43:106–113.
26. Talal N, Schnitzer B. Lymphadenopathy and Sjoegren's syndrome. *Clin Rheum Dis* 1977;3:421–432.
27. Turner DR, Wright DJM. Lymphadenopathy in early syphilis. *J Pathol* 1973;110:305–308.
28. Burns EB, Colby TV, Dorfman RF. Differential diagnostic features of nodular L&H Hodgkin's disease, including progressive transformation of germinal centers. *Am J Surg Pathol* 1984;8:253–261.
29. Ferry JA, Zukerberg LR, Harris NL. Florid progressive transformation of germinal centers: a syndrome affecting young men, without early progression to nodular lymphocyte predominance Hodgkin's disease. *Am J Surg Pathol* 1992;16:252–258.
30. Osborne BM, Butler JJ. Clinical implications of progressive transformation of germinal centers. *Am J Surg Pathol* 1984;8:725–733.
31. Timens W, Visser L, Poppema S. Nodular lymphocyte predominance type of Hodgkin's disease is a germinal center lymphoma. *Lab Invest* 1986;54:457–461.
32. Crossley B, Heryet A, Gatter KC. Does nodular lymphocyte predominant Hodgkin's disease arise from progressively transformed germinal centers? A case report with an unusually prolonged history. *Histopathology* 1987;11:621–630.
33. Hansmann ML, Fellbaum C, Hui PK, et al. Progressive transformation of germinal centers with and without association to Hodgkin's disease. *Am J Clin Pathol* 1990;93:219–226.
34. Mason DY, Banks P, Chan J, et al. Nodular lymphocyte predominance Hodgkin's disease: a distinct clinicopathological entity. *Am J Surg Pathol* 1994;18:520–530.
35. Osborne BM, Butler JJ. Follicular lymphoma mimicking progressive transformation of germinal centers. *Am J Clin Pathol* 1987;88: 264–269.
36. Goates JJ, Kamel OW, LeBrun DP, et al. The floral variant of follicular lymphoma, immunologic and molecular studies support a neoplastic process. *Am J Surg Pathol* 1994;18:37–47.
37. Castleman B, Iverson I, Menendez VP. Localized mediastinal lymph node hyperplasia resembling thymoma. *Cancer* 1956;9:822–830.
38. Keller AR, Hochholzer L, Castleman B. hyaline vascular and plasmacell types of giant lymph node hyperplasia of mediastinum and other locations. *Cancer* 1972;29:670–683.
39. Peterson BA, Frizzera G. Multicentric Castleman's disease. *Semin Oncol* 1993;20:636–647.
40. Frizzera G. Castleman's disease and related disorders. *Semin Diagn Pathol* 1988;5:346–364.
41. Menke DM,Tiemann M, Camoriano JK, et al. Diagnosis of Castleman's disease by identification of an immunophenotypically aberrant population of mantle zone B lymphocytes in paraffin-embedded lymph node biopsies. *Am J Clin Pathol* 1996;105:268–276.
42. Lin O, Frizzera G, Angiomyoid and follicular dendritic cell proliferative lesions in Castleman's disease of hyaline vascular type: a study of 10 cases. *Am J Surg Pathol* 1997;21:1295–1306.
43. Banks P, Chan J, Cleary M, et al. Mantle cell lymphoma: a proposal for unification of morphologic, immunologic and molecular data. *Am J Surg Pathol* 1994;18:526–530.

44. Hsu SM, Waldron JA, Xie SS, et al. Expression of interleukin-6 in Castleman's disease. *Hum Pathol* 1993;24:833–839.
45. Beck JT, Hsu SM, Wijdenes J, et al. Brief report: Alleviation of systemic manifestations of Castleman's disease by monoclonal anti-interleukin-6 antibody. *N Engl J Med* 1994;330:602–605.
46. Hall PA, Donaghy M, Cotter FE, et al. An immunohistochemical and genotypic study of the plasma cell form of Castleman's disease. *Histopathology* 1989;14:333–346.
47. Bryan T-Y, Weiss L. Primary plasmacytoma of lymph nodes. *Hum Pathol* 1997;28:1083–1090.
48. Albores-Saavedra J, Vuitch F, Delgado R, et al. Sinus histiocytosis of pelvic lymph nodes after hip replacement: a histiocytic proliferation induced by cobalt-chromium and titanium. *Am J Surg Pathol* 1994; 81:83–90.
49. Truong L, Cartwright J, Goodman D, et al. Silicone lymphadenopathy associated with augmentation mammoplasty: morphologic features of nine cases. *Am J Surg Pathol* 1988;12:484–495.
50. Guerrero-Medrano J, Delgado R, Albores-Saaveda J. Signet-ring sinus histiocytosis: a reactive disorder that mimics metastatic adenocarcinoma. *Cancer* 1997;80:277–285.
51. Rosai J, Dorfman RF. Sinus histiocytosis with massive lymphadenopathy: a newly recognized benign clinicopathologic entity. *Arch Pathol* 1969;87:63–70.
52. Rosai J, Dorfman RF. Sinus histiocytosis with massive lymphadenopathy: a pseudolymphomatous benign disorder. Analysis of 34 cases. *Cancer* 1972;30:1174–1188.
53. Levine PH, Jahan N, Murari P, et al. Detection of human herpesvirus 6 in tissues involved by sinus histiocytosis with massive lymphadenopathy (Rosai-Dorfman disease). *J Infect Dis* 1992;166:291–295.
54. Paulli M, Bergmaschi G, Tonon L, et al. Evidence for the polyclonal nature of the cell infiltrate in sinus histiocytosis with massive lymphadenopathy (Rosai-Dorfmann disease). *Br J Haematol* 1995;91: 415–418.
55. Foucar E, Rosai J, Dorfman RF. Sinus histiocytosis with massive lymphadenopathy (Rosai-Dorfman disease): review of the entity. *Semin Diagn Pathol* 1990;7:19–73.
56. Paulli M, Rosso R, Kindl S, et al. Immunophenotypic characterization of the cell infiltrate in five cases of sinus histiocytosis with massive lymphadenopathy. *Hum Pathol* 1992;23:647–654.
57. Hage C, Willman C, Favara BE, et al. Langerhans cell histiocytosis (histiocytosis X): immunophenotype and growth fraction. *Hum Pathol* 1993;28:840–845.
58. Eisen RN, Buckley PJ, Rosai J. Immunophenotypic characterization of sinus histiocytosis with massive lymphadenopathy (Rosai-Dorfman disease). *Semin Diagn Pathol* 1990;7:74–82.
59. Stastny JF, Wilkerson ML, Hamati HF, et al. Cytologic features of sinus histiocytosis with massive lymphadenopathy: a report of three cases. *Acta Cytol* 1997;41:871–876.
60. Heidelberger KP, Schnitzer B, Tilford D, et al. Sinus histiocytosis with massive lymphadenopathy and gross skeletal involvement. *Skeletal Radiol* 1980;5:42–46.
61. Leighton SEJ, Gallimore AP. Extranodal sinus histiocytosis with massive lymphadenopathy affecting the subglottis and trachea. *Histopathology* 1994;24:393–394.
62. Green I, Dorfman RF, Rosai J. Breast involvement by extranodal Rosai-Dorfman disease. Report of seven cases. *Am J Surg Pathol* 1997;21:664–668.
63. Nathwani BN, Mohrmann RL, Brynes RK. Monocytoid B-cell lymphomas: an assessment of diagnostic criteria and a perspective on histogenesis. *Hum Pathol* 1992;23:1061–1071.
64. Sheibani K, Burke JS, Swartz WG, et al. Monocytoid B-cell lymphoma: clinicopathologic study of 21 cases of a unique type of low-grade lymphoma. *Cancer* 1988;62:1531–1538.
65. Plank L, Hell K, Hansmann ML, et al. Reactive versus neoplastic monocytoid B-cell proliferations: in situ hybridization study of immunoglobulin light chain mRNA. *Am J Clin Pathol* 1995;103:330–337.
66. Ravel R. Histopathology of lymph nodes after lymphangiography. *Am J Clin Pathol* 1966;46:335–340.
67. Sieracki JC. Whipple's disease: observations on systemic involvement: I. Cytologic observations. *Arch Pathol* 1958;66:464–467.
68. Sieracki JC, Fine G. Whipple's disease: observations on systemic involvement: II. Gross and histologic observations. *Arch Pathol* 1959; 67:81–93.
69. Eck M, Kreipe H, Harmsen D, et al. Invasion and destruction of mucosal plasma cells by *Tropheryma whippelii*. *Hum Pathol* 1997; 28:1424–1428.
70. Fleming JL, Wiesner RH, Shorter RG. Whipple's disease: Clinical, biochemical, and histopathologic features and assessment of treatment in 29 patients. *Mayo Clin Proc* 1988;63:539–551.
71. Ereno C, Lopez JI, Ellizalde JM, et al. A case of Whipple's disease presenting as supraclavicular lymphadenopathy. *Acta Pathol Microbiol Immunol Scand* 1993;101:865–868.
72. Mueller C, Petermann D, Stain C, et al. Whipple's disease: comparison of histology with diagnosis based on polymerase chain reaction in four consecutive cases. *Gut* 1997;40:425–427.
73. Lowsky R, Archer GI, Fyles G, et al. Brief report: diagnosis of Whipple's disease by molecular analysis of peripheral blood. *N Engl J Med* 1994;20:1343–1346.
74. Risdall RJ, McKenna RW, Nesbit ME, et al. Virus-associated hemophagocytic syndrome: a benign histiocytic proliferation distinct from malignant histiocytosis. *Cancer* 1979;44:993–1002.
75. Scott RB, Robb-Smith AHT. Histiocytic medullary reticulosis. *Lancet* 1939:194–198.
76. Risdall RJ, Brunning RD, Hernandez JI, et al. Bacteria-associated hemophagocytic syndrome. *Cancer* 1984;54:2968–2972.
77. Gaffey MJ, Frierson HF Jr, Medeiros LJ, et al. The relationship of Epstein-Barr virus to infection-related (sporadic) and familial hemophagocytic syndrome and secondary (lymphoma related) hemophagocytosis: an in situ hybridization study. *Hum Pathol* 1993;24:657–667.
78. Yao M, Cheng A-L, Su I-J, et al. Clinicopathological spectrum of haemophagocytic syndrome in Epstein-Barr virus-associated peripheral T-cell lymphoma. *Br J Haematol* 1994;87:535–543.
79. Wang CY, Su WP, Kurtin PJ. Subcutaneous panniculitic T-cell lymphoma. *Int J Dermatol* 1996;35:1–8.
80. Simrell CR, Margolick JB, Crabtree GR, et al. Lymphokine-induced phagocytosis in angiocentric immunoproliferative lesions (AIL) and malignant lymphoma arising in AIL. *Blood* 1985;65:1469–1476.
81. Weiss LM, Trela MJ, Cleary ML, et al. Frequent immunoglobulin and T-cell receptor rearrangements in "histiocytic" neoplasms. *Am J Pathol* 1985;121:369–373, 1985.
82. Weiss LM, Picker LJ, Copenhaver CM, et al. Large-cell hematolymphoid neoplasms of uncertain lineage. *Hum Pathol* 1988;19:967–973.
83. Falini B, Pileri S, DeSolas I, et al. Peripheral T-cell lymphoma associated with hemophagocytic syndrome. *Blood* 1990;75:434–444.
84. Schnitzer B, Roth MS, Hyder DM, et al. Ki-1 lymphomas in children. *Cancer* 1988;61:1213–1221.
85. Osborne BM, Butler JJ, McKay B. Sinusoidal large cell (histiocytic) lymphoma. *Cancer* 1980;46:2484–2491.
86. Favara BE. Hemophagocytic lymphohistiocytosis: A hemophagocytic syndrome. *Semin Diagn Pathol* 1992;9:63–74.
87. Willman CL, Busque L, Griffith BB, et al. Langerhans'-cell histiocytosis (histiocytosis X): A clonal proliferative disease. *N Engl J Med* 1994;331:154–160.
88. Writing Group of the Histiocyte Society. Histiocytosis syndromes in children. *Lancet* 1987:208–209.
89. Motoi M, Helbron D, Kaiserling E, et al. Eosinophilic granuloma of lymph nodes: a variant of histiocytosis X. *Histopathology* 1980;4: 585–606.
90. Lieberman PH, Jones CR, Steinman RM, et al. Langerhans cell (eosinophilic) granulomatosis: a clinicopathologic study encompassing 50 years. *Am J Surg Pathol* 1996;20:519–552.
91. Haferkamp O, Rosenau W, Lennert K. Vascular transformation of lymph node sinuses due to venous obstruction. *Arch Pathol* 1971;92: 81–83.
92. Chan JKC, Warnke RA, Dorfman R. Vascular transformation of sinuses in lymph nodes: a study of its morphological spectrum and distinction from Kaposi's sarcoma. *Am J Surg Pathol* 1991;15: 732–743.
93. Cook PD, Czerniak B, Chan JK, et al. Nodular spindle cell vascular transformation of lymph nodes: a benign process occurring predominantly in retroperitoneal lymph nodes draining carcinomas that can simulate Kaposi's sarcoma or metastatic tumor. *Am J Surg Pathol* 1995;19:1010–1020.
94. Ziegler JL, Dorfman RF. Overview of Kaposi's sarcoma: history, epidemiology, and biomedical features. In: Ziegler JL, Dorfman RF, eds. *Kaposi's sarcoma, pathology, physiology and clinical management.* New York: Marcel Dekker, 1988:1–22.

95. Krigel RL, Friedman-Kien AE. Epidemic Kaposi's sarcoma. *Semin Oncol* 1990;17:350–360.
96. Finkbeiner WE, Egbert BM, Groundwater JR, et al. Kaposi's sarcoma in young homosexual men: A histopathologic study with particular reference to lymph node involvement. *Arch Pathol Lab Med* 1982; 106:261–264.
97. Tindle BH, Parker JW, Lukes RJ. "Reed-Sternberg cells" in infectious mononucleosis. *Am J Clin Pathol* 1972;58:607–617.
98. Childs CC, Parham DM, Berard CW. Infectious mononucleosis: The spectrum of morphologic changes simulating lymphoma in lymph nodes and tonsils. *Am J Surg Pathol* 1987;11:122–132.
99. Abbondanzo SL, Sato N, Straus SE, et al. Acute infectious mononucleosis: (CD30) (Ki-1) antigen expression and histologic correlations. *Am J Clin Pathol* 1990;93:698–702.
100. Segal GH, Kjeldsberg CR, Smith GP, et al. CD30 antigen expression in florid immunoblastic proliferations: a clinicopathologic study of 14 cases. *Am J Clin Pathol* 1994;102:292–298.
101. Isaacson PG, Schmid CR, Pan L, et al. Epstein-Barr virus latent membrane protein expression by Hodgkin and Reed-Sternberg-like cells in acute infectious mononucleosis. *J Pathol* 1992;167:267–271.
102. Younes M, Podesta A, Helie M, et al. Infection of T but not B lymphocytes by cytomegalovirus in lymph node: an immunophenotypic study. *Am J Surg Pathol* 1991;15:75–80.
103. Rushin JM, Riordan GP, Heaton RB, et al. Cytomegalovirus-infected cells express Leu-M1 antigen: a potential source of diagnostic error. *Am J Pathol* 1990;136:989–995.
104. Gaffey MJ, Ben-Ezra JM, Weiss LM. Herpes simplex lymphadenopathies. *Am J Clin Pathol* 1991;95:709–714.
105. Patterson SD, Larson EB, Corey L. Atypical generalized zoster with lymphadenitis mimicking lymphoma. *N Engl J Med* 1980;302: 848–851.
106. Abbondanzo SL, Irey NS, Frizzera G. Dilantin-associated lymphadenopathy: spectrum of histopathologic patterns. *Am J Surg Pathol* 1995; 19:675–686.
107. Katzin WE, Julius CJ, Tubbs RR, et al. Lymphoproliferative disorders associated with carbamazepine. *Arch Pathol Lab Med* 1990;114: 1244–1248.
108. Garcia-Suarez J, Dominguez-Franjo P, Del Campo F, et al. EBV-positive non-Hodgkin's lymphoma developing after phenytoin therapy. *Br J Haematol* 1996;95:376–379.
109. Hartsock RJ. Postvaccinial lymphadenitis: hyperplasia of lymphoid tissue that simulates malignant lymphomas. *Cancer* 1968;21: 632–649.
110. Dorfman RF, Herweg J. Live attenuated measles virus vaccine: Inguinal lymphadenopathy complicating administration. *JAMA* 1966;198: 320–321.
111. Richardson EP Jr. Toxoplasmosis: the time has come. *N Engl J Med* 1988;318:313–316.
112. Kean BH, Kimball AC, Christenson WN. An epidemic of acute toxoplasmosis. *JAMA* 1969;208:1002–1004.
113. Bowie WR, King AS, Werker DH, et al. Outbreak of toxoplasmosis associated with municipal drinking water. *Lancet* 1997;350:173–177.
114. Saxen L, Saxen E, Tenhunen A. The significance of histologic diagnosis in glandular toxoplasmosis. *Acta Pathol Microbiol Scan* 1962;56: 284.
115. Stansfeld AG. The histologic diagnosis of toxoplasmic lymphadenitis. *J Clin Pathol* 1961;14:565–573.
116. Aisner SC, Aisner J, Moravec C, et al. Acquired toxoplasmic lymphadenitis with demonstration of the cyst form. *Am J Clin Pathol* 1983;79:125–127.
117. Weiss LM, Chen YY, Berry GJ, et al. Infrequent detection of Toxoplasma gondii genome in toxoplasmic lymphadenitis: a polymerase chain reaction study. *Hum Pathol* 1992;23:154–158.
118. Gould E, Porto R, Albores-Saavedra J, et al. Dermatopathic lymphadenitis: the spectrum and significance of its morphologic features. *Arch Pathol Lab Med* 1988;112:1145–1150.
119. Burke JS, Sheibani K, Rappaport H. Dermatopathic lymphadenopathy: an immunophenotypic comparison of cases associated and unassociated with mycosis fungoides. *Am J Pathol* 1986,123:256–263.
120. Burns BF, Wood GS, Dorfman RF. The varied histopathology of lymphadenopathy in the homosexual male. *Am J Surg Pathol* 1985; 9:287–297.
121. Weiss LM, Hu E, Wood GS, et al. Clonal rearrangements of the T-cell receptor genes in mycosis fungoides and dermatopathic lymphadenopathy. *N Engl J Med* 1985;313:539–544.
122. Symmers W St C. Sarcoidosis and other varieties of granulomatous lymphadenitis of reactive cause. In: Henry K, Symmers W St C, eds. *Thymus lymph nodes, spleen, lymphatics: systemic pathology,* vol 7, 3rd ed. Edinburgh: Churchill Livingstone, 1992:493–543.
123. Miller-Catchpole R, Variakojis D, Vardiman JW, et al. Cat scratch disease: identification of bacteria in seven cases of lymphadenitis. *Am J Surg Pathol* 1986;10:276–281.
124. Walzer PD, Armstrong D. Lymphogranuloma venereum presenting as supraclavicular and inguinal lymphadenopathy. *Sex Transm Dis* 1977;4:12–14.
125. Schapers RFM, Reif R, Lennert K, et al. Mesenteric lymphadenitis due to Yersinia enterocolitica. *Virchows Arch* 1981;390:127–138.
126. Bascom R, Johns CJ. The natural history and management of sarcoidosis. *Adv Intern Med* 1986;31:213–241.
127. Sieracki JC, Fisher E. The ceroid nature of the so-called "Hamazaki-Wesenberg bodies." *Am J Clin Pathol* 1973;59:248–253.
128. Kadin ME, Donaldson SS, Dorfman RF. Isolated granulomas in Hodgkin's disease. *N Engl J Med* 1970;283:859–861.
129. Chan JK, Lewin KJ, Lombard CM, et al. The histopathology of bacillary angiomatosis of lymph node. *Am J Surg Pathol* 1991;15:430–437.
130. Zangwill UM, Hamilton DH, Perkins BA, et al. Cat scratch disease in Connecticut: epidemiology, risk factors, and evaluation of a new diagnostic test. *N Engl J Med* 1993;329:8–13.
131. Mouritsen CL, Litwin CM, Maiese RL, et al. Rapid polymerase chain reaction-based detection of the causative agent of cat scratch disease (Bartonella henselae) in formalin-fixed, paraffin-embedded samples. *Hum Pathol* 1997;28:820–826.
132. Kikuchi M. Lymphadenitis showing focal reticulum cell hyperplasia with nuclear debris and phagocytosis. *Nippon Ketsueki Gakkai Zasshi* 1972;35:379–380.
133. Fujimoto Y, Kozima Y, Yamaguchi K. Cervical subacute necrotizing lymphadenitis: a new clinicopathologic entity. *Naika* 1972;20: 920–927.
134. Pileri S, Kikuchi M, Helbron D. Histologic necrotizing lymphadenitis without granulocytic infiltration. *Virchows Arch* 1982;395:257–271.
135. Chamulak GA, Brynes RK, Nathwani BN. Kikuchi-Fujimoto disease mimicking malignant lymphoma. *Am J Surg Pathol* 1990;14: 514–523.
136. Case Records of the Massachusetts General Hospital: Case 5-1997. *N Engl J Med* 1997;336:492–499.
137. Felgar RE, Furth EE, Wasik MA, et al. Histiocytic necrotizing lymphadenitis (Kikuchi's disease): In situ end-labeling, immunocytochemical and serologic evidence supporting cytotoxic lymphocyte-mediated apoptotic cell death. *Mod Pathol* 1997;10:231–241.
138. Tsang WYN, Chan JKC, Ng CS. Kikuchi's lymphadenitis: a morphologic analysis of 75 cases with special reference to unusual features. *Am J Surg Pathol* 1994;18:219–231.
139. Kuo T. Kikuchi's disease (histiocytic necrotizing lymphadenitis): a clinicopathologic study of 79 cases with an analysis of histologic subtypes, immunohistology, and DNA ploidy. *Am J Surg Pathol* 1995; 20:798–809.
140. Kawasaki T. Acute febrile mucocutaneous syndrome with lymphoid involvement with specific desquamation of the fingers and toes in children. *Jpn J Allerg* 1967;16:178–222.
141. Schnitzer B. Reactive lymphoid hyperplasia in surgical pathology of the lymph nodes and related organs. In: Jaffe ES, ed. *Surgical pathology of the lymph nodes and related organs.* Major Problems in Pathology Series, vol 16. Philadelphia: WB Saunders, 1995;123–124.
142. Medeiros LJ, Kaynor B, Harris NL. Lupus lymphadenitis: report of a case with immunohistologic studies on frozen sections. *Hum Pathol* 1989;20:295–299.
143. Eisner MD, Amory J, Mullaney B, et al. Necrotizing lymphadenitis associated with systemic lupus erythematosus. *Semin Arthr Rheumatol* 1996;26:477–482.
144. Giesker DW, Pastuszak WT, Forouhar FA, et al. Lymph node biopsy for early diagnosis in Kawasaki disease. *Am J Surg Pathol* 1982;6: 493–501.

CHAPTER 16

Atypical Lymphoproliferative Disorders

Glauco Frizzera

The term *atypical lymphoproliferative disorders* (ALPDs) is used in this chapter to indicate a pathologically and clinically heterogeneous group of diseases at the border between reactive lymphoid proliferations and *bona fide* lymphomas, which are discussed in other chapters. The histopathologic manifestations of these disorders are often florid enough to suggest a neoplastic lymphoid process, but they also involve a variable risk of developing into one. An excessive lymphoid proliferation is associated with an increased risk of genetic errors, resulting in the emergence of clones with a selective proliferative advantage.

Because of their heterogeneity, the ALPDs are perhaps best defined pathogenetically as varied forms of abnormal immune response that progress unchecked because of some dysfunction of immune regulatory mechanisms. Such dysfunction is well established in LPDs developing in patients iatrogenically immunosuppressed for organ or bone marrow transplantation and in immunodeficiency states, either genetically determined or acquired, as in acquired immunodeficiency syndrome (AIDS). However, the role and specific characteristics of immune system abnormalities are less well defined in other LPDs, such as those arising after prolonged chemotherapy for neoplastic or nonneoplastic diseases, or in autoimmune diseases, as well as in ALPDs of unknown origin, such as angioimmunoblastic lymphadenopathy-like lesions and multicentric Castleman's disease.

It is only recently that negative control mechanisms of the immune response have begun to be analyzed, along with those involved in the stimulation and activation of immune cells (1). These inhibitory mechanisms include effector cells, such as regulatory T cells (2); inhibitory cytokines, such as interferon (IFN)-α, -β, and -γ and transforming growth factor-β (TGF-β); and the expression by activated cells of surface molecules (i.e., CTLA-4, FAS/CD95, and tumor necrosis factor receptor [TNFR]) that, on binding with the appropriate ligands, leads to their death by means of apoptosis (i.e., activation-induced cell death) (3–5). Defects of these homeostatic mechanisms may lead to a harmful prolongation of the proliferation and effector functions of immune cells in response to a nonself antigen or to the development of autoreactive clones resulting in autoimmune disease (1). The relevance of these defects to lymphoid proliferation and autoimmunity has become evident in a newly described disease, the autoimmune lymphoproliferative syndrome, whose basis is in abnormal lymphocyte apoptosis (6–8). These data support the essential and unifying role of a dysfunction of immune regulation in the pathogenesis of ''atypical'' lymphoid proliferations. Other elements, however, play a role in the development of ALPDs: the types of cells involved, the occurrence of genomic abnormalities, and the activity of cellular and viral genes. The variability and diverse relevance of these factors in different ALPDs, along with largely undefined differences in the specific immune abnormalities at play in each, account for the variety of these processes.

The discussion that follows is limited to a group of three prototypical, well-characterized clinicopathologic entities: angioimmunoblastic lymphoproliferations, the LPDs that develop in transplant recipients, and multicentric Castleman's disease. LPDs that arise in congenital immunodeficiencies and in iatrogenic (nontransplantation) settings have been reviewed in detail (9,10), and those developing in the course of autoimmune diseases and AIDS are discussed in Chapters 15 and 28, respectively.

ANGIOIMMUNOBLASTIC LYMPHADENOPATHY

Background

In the early 1970s, similar lymphoma-like clinical syndromes, characterized by generalized lymphadenopathy, hepatosplenomegaly, anemia, and hypergammaglobulinemia, were independently described by several groups under different terms: *diffuse sarcomatosis with plasmacytic differentiation* (11), *chronic pluripotential immunoproliferative syndrome* (12), *lymphogranulomatosis X (LgX)* (13),

G. Frizzera: Department of Pathology, Weill Medical College of Cornell University, New York, New York 10021 *immunoblastic lymphadenopathy (IBL)* (14,15), *immunodysplastic disease* (16), and *angioimmunoblastic lymphadenopathy with dysproteinemia (AIL)* (17,18). Three of these, LgX (13,19,20), IBL (14,15), and AIL (17,18), are histopathologically similar and most probably represent one entity, here discussed as AIL.

Strong pathologic and clinical similarities also exist between this disorder and a variant of T-cell lymphoma, originally described by a Japanese group as IBL-like (21,22) and today referred to as *angioimmunoblastic T-cell lymphoma* (AITCL) (23), so much so that the distinction between the original AIL and AITCL and the very existence of AIL as a reactive process has become controversial. There are in the literature two quite opposite views. According to one, all lesions with the histologic features of AIL are neoplastic (23–25). In another more nuanced view, AIL and AITCL are considered part of a spectrum of diseases whose pathologic and clinical similarities are accounted for by a common pathogenesis (26–30). This second position is based on multiple lines of evidence but can be summarized as follows. The clinical evolution is variable and includes a substantial number of cases that undergo spontaneous remission or are relatively indolent; the histology, despite many similarities, is heterogeneous, as attested by several attempts at classification; a good proportion of cases does not show at presentation evidence of clonality by molecular or cytogenetic criteria; and transitions have been reported between nonclonal AIL and AITCL. Strong, although indirect, support for this latter view comes from the recognition that lymphomas of the AITCL type differ significantly from other non-Hodgkin's lymphomas in their clinical and laboratory characteristics (31), precisely, it can be argued, because of the unique pathogenesis they share with AIL. Acceptance of one or the other of these positions is more than a theoretical issue, as, according to the former, all ''histologically satisfactory cases . . . should be treated as outright malignant lymphomas'' (24), while, according to the latter, it is recognized that ''cytotoxic treatment is clearly not curative'' (32) and innovative therapeutic approaches are being attempted (28,30,33–40).

In this situation of uncertainty about the categorization of AIL-like processes, it is very difficult in a retrospective review of the literature to separate AIL from AITCL and determine characteristics that can differentiate them. However, this is attempted throughout this section at the cost of some overlap with the discussion of the *bona fide* AITCLs in Chapter 29.

Histopathologic Features

Angioimmunoblastic lymphadenopathy is recognized by a combination of characteristic features in involved lymph nodes: a pronounced disarray of the nodal architecture; a very prominent increase in vascularity; and polymorphic cell infiltration, including abundant immunoblasts (17,18). At low power, the pattern is diffuse, with loss of most normal topographic markings in the lymph node and frequent pronounced infiltration of the capsule (Fig. 16.1). Sinuses are frequently recognizable, however, and abnormal reactive germinal centers may be found in many cases. These may take several forms: loose aggregates of large lymphoid cells scattered among small lymphocytes, pale histiocytes, and small blood vessels; focal areas of cellular depletion, often associated with eosinophilic amorphous material; or aggregates of spindle eosinophilic cells (follicular dendritic cells [FDCs]) and blood vessels, associated with sparse lymphoid cells. These may form tight, almost granulomatous, clusters (i.e., burned-out or regressively transformed [41] germinal centers) or, more commonly, ill-defined, stretched, and ramified pale cellular collections (Fig. 16.2) located along the

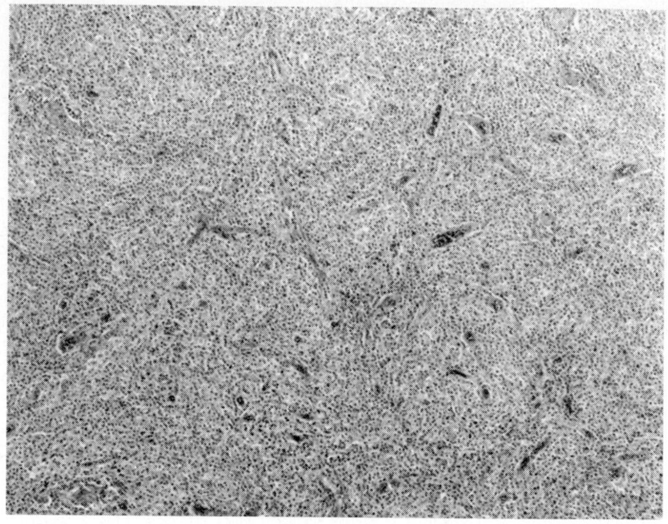

FIG. 16.1. Angioimmunoblastic lymphadenopathy. Abundance of high endothelial (postcapillary) venules (hematoxylin and eosin stain, original magnification: 75× magnification).

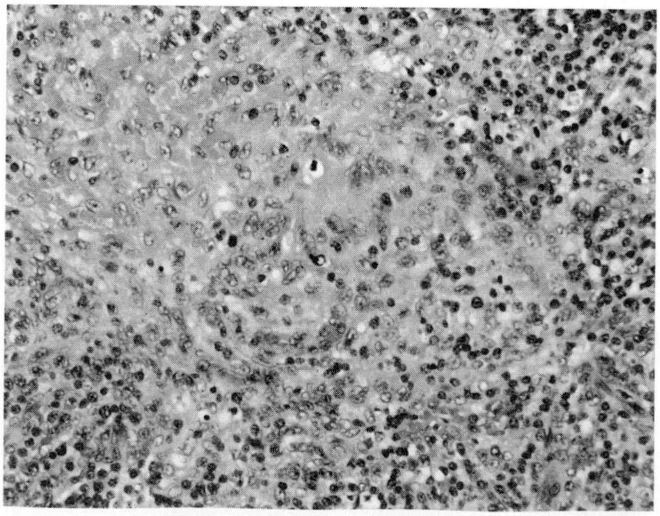

FIG. 16.2. Angioimmunoblastic lymphadenopathy. Ill-defined collections of follicular dendritic cells (hematoxylin and eosin stain, original magnification: 300× magnification).

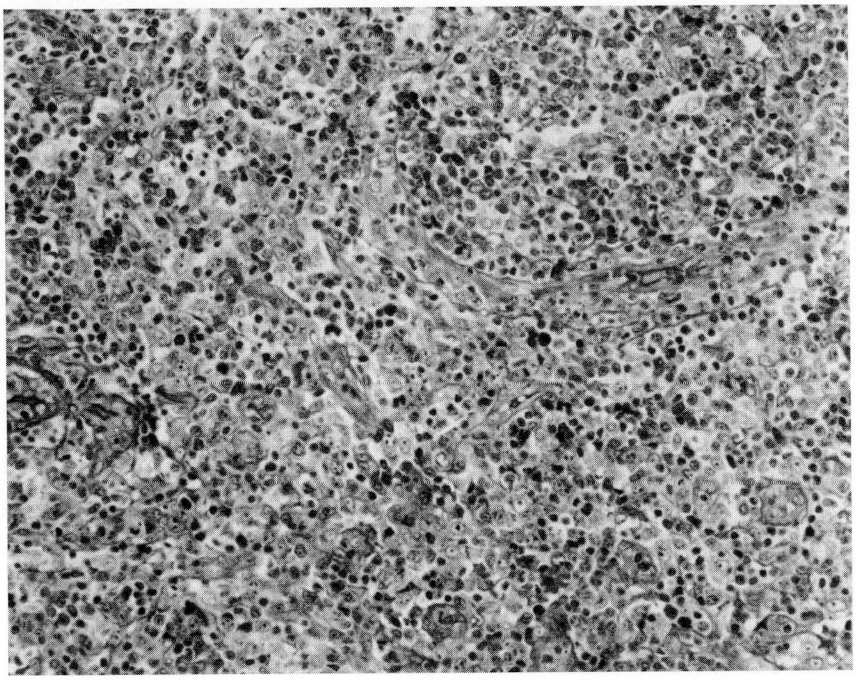

FIG. 16.3. Angioimmunoblastic lymphadenopathy. The cellular infiltrate is polymorphic, with abundant transformed lymphocytes (hematoxylin and eosin stain, original magnification: 240× magnification).

capsule or the trabeculae (42). Whether the usual hyperplastic germinal centers are seen is a moot point. In one group's opinion, with which we and others (29) agree, their presence would exclude a diagnosis of AIL and fit that of an "hyperimmune reaction" (19,20). However, cases with these features (i.e., AIL and hyperplastic germinal centers with ill-defined borders) have been interpreted on the basis of molecular studies and clinical evolution as a variant of AITCL (43).

At medium power, the rich vascularity results from an increased number of high endothelial venules that frequently show very thick endothelium and lymphocytes traversing the wall. The polymorphic cell component (Fig. 16.3) includes small lymphocytes with regular nuclear contours, sparse plasma cells, and abundant immunoblasts, the cytoplasm of which may be pale basophilic or homogeneous and amphophilic as in adjacent plasma cells. Additional cell types, such as eosinophils, frequently in large numbers, or epithelioid histiocytes, scattered or in loose small aggregates, may be observed. In less than half the cases, sparse deposits of intercellular amorphous eosinophilic material can be seen. Because many of these characteristic features relate to the architecture of the lymph nodes, and because other features are shared by any florid immune response, a diagnosis of AIL cannot be made with certainty in an extranodal location.

The criteria that we proposed for the diagnosis of AIL largely overlap those required for the diagnosis of IBL and LgX (Table 16.1). All these processes feature a diffuse obliteration of the architecture, increased vascularity, and polymorphic cytologic composition. The criteria for IBL are more restrictive, however, because, in addition, a diffuse hypocellularity of the lymph node and the presence of interstitial material are required for diagnosis. In contrast, LgX clearly appears to be the most extensive category, as indicated by the description of five histologic subtypes (immunoblastic, plasma cell, epithelioid cell, lymphocytic, and mixed cell).

As any pathologist knows, having well-defined criteria for a disease does not make its diagnosis easy. In the case of AIL, considerable diagnostic acumen is needed to distinguish it from other atypical lymphoid hyperplasias and from lymphoid malignancies. In the former group, two processes appear to us to be distinct from AIL. Multicentric Castleman's disease (44) and LgX with excessive plasma cells (20), which appears to be identical to it, share with AIL an abundance of high endothelial venules and the presence of regressively transformed germinal centers. The low-power

TABLE 16.1. *Histopathologic criteria for the diagnosis of angioimmunoblastic lymphadenopathies*

Criteria	AIL	IBL	Lgx
Obliteration of the architecture	Yes	Yes[a]	Yes
Burned-out germinal centers	33%	Rare	Yes
Increase in epithelioid venules	Yes	Yes	Yes
Polymorphic cytology	Yes	Yes	Yes
Abundance of IB and PC	Yes	Yes	5 cell subtypes
Interstitial material	25%	100%	50%

AIL, angioimmunoblastic lymphadenopathy with dysproteinemia; IB, immunoblasts; IBL, immunoblastic lymphadenopathy; LgX, lymphogranulomatosis X; PC, plasma cells.
[a] Hypocellularity.
Data from references 15, 18, 107.

pattern tends to be nodular, however, because of the prominence of ill-defined follicular areas and the tissue between the nodules shows a massive plasmacytosis that we have not seen in AIL. The disorder described by Flandrin and colleagues as *plasmacytic sarcomatosis* (11) and considered by them to be synonymous with AIL (45) is, in our opinion, similar to cases reported as "*extramedullary leukemic plasmacytoma*" (46) and "*systemic polyclonal immunoblastic proliferations*" (47,48). These are distinguished from AIL, however, by a diffuse, marked proliferation of immunoblasts and immature plasma cells and a less prominent vascularity. The distinction of AIL from AITCL is a difficult one because of a morphologic continuum between them and appears to rest on the presence of nuclear atypicalities and clusters of clear cells in AITCL, but not in AIL (22,26,49,50) (Figs. 16.4, 16.5). In some attempts at subtyping lesions classified as AITCLs, cases at the lower end of the spectrum (i.e., those without clear or convoluted cells [51] or those with mild atypia, fewer immunoblasts, and no or few clear cells [24]), may correspond to what others would call AIL proper. In the final analysis, the distinction between AIL and AITCL requires a combination of histologic, immunophenotypic, molecular, and cytogenetic data.

Histologic transformation or progression of AIL has been reported. In 43% of a large series, lymph nodes with AIL also contained collections of immunoblasts within or outside the sinuses, which were interpreted as representing immunoblastic lymphoma arising in AIL (52). In one long-term follow-up study, progression to lymphoma was recorded in 18% of patients (53). Because of the limited immunophenotypic evaluation possible at that time, it is unclear which of two possible phenomena was being described: the evolution to a T-cell lymphoma or the development of a large B-cell lymphoma. The former was reported in 21% of a series of AIL and described as resulting in a T-zone lymphoma or immunoblastic T-cell lymphoma (32): the interpretation of these and similar cases (30,34,54) depends on the definition of AIL versus AITCL. There is instead clear evidence that large B-cell lymphomas may also develop in AIL (20, 55–63) between a few months (60,62) and several years (61,63) from the diagnosis of AIL and possibly in relation to an intercurrent Epstein-Barr virus (EBV) infection (60,61,63). In one patient with AIL, the development of a plasma cell neoplasm with biclonal paraproteinemia has also been reported (64).

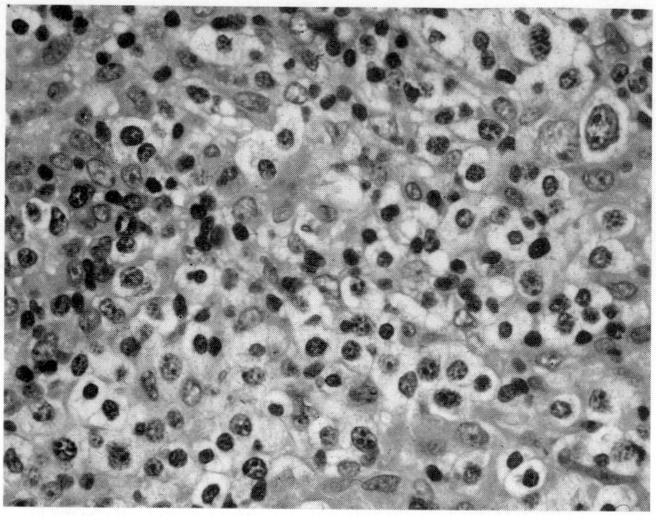

FIG. 16.5. Angioimmunoblastic T-cell lymphoma. Neoplastic cells with round nucleus and clear cytoplasm are observed in clusters or isolated (hematoxylin and eosin stain, original magnification: 300× magnification).

FIG. 16.4. Angioimmunoblastic T-cell lymphoma. Numerous isolated or confluent foci of pale cells stand out in a background of prominent high endothelial venules and reactive cells (hematoxylin and eosin stain, original magnification: 200× magnification).

Immunophenotypic Findings

In studies that used monoclonal antibodies applied to fresh-frozen tissue, there appears to be a general consensus that most lesions with histopathologic features of AIL (IBL, LgX) are predominantly T-cell proliferations (22,26,27,29, 42,50,65–69). With the exception of one study (22), in which cytotoxic/suppressor cells were found to predominate in all cases, all other studies have reported a distinct predominance of the helper/inducer subset (29,67), various ratios of the two subsets (26,27,42,66), or either situation in different cases (50,68). By double staining of cell membrane antigens and nuclear proliferation antigens, such as Ki-67 or DNA polymerase, it was determined that, in most cases, the proliferating cells were predominantly CD4 positive ($CD4^+$) and, in smaller proportions, $CD8^+$ (42,50). This variability of the cell composition is a distinctive feature also of AITCLs (70–72) a result of the mixture of neoplastic and reactive T cells, leading to an indeterminate CD4/CD8 subset definition in up to 76% of cases (72). Expression of activation antigens (22,66,67), including CD30 on immunoblasts and Reed-

Sternberg–like cells (69,73) and loss of pan-T-cell antigens on T cells (26,66,67), as occurs characteristically in *bona fide* T-cell lymphomas, has been reported only in some cases of AIL. Loss of pan-T-cell antigens is uncommon also in AITCLs, as opposed to T-cell lymphomas of other types (27,70,72).

A second consistent feature of AIL (and AITCLs) is a variable admixed component of polyclonal B cells and plasma cells (22,27,42,50,66–69). The B cells are mainly small and are collected within the remnants of follicles and scattered about. However, increasing numbers of large transformed B cells have been reported in AITCLs, which may be Reed-Sternberg–like in appearance, express CD30, and contain EBV (73).

Germinal center remnants are also identified by the presence of follicular dendritic cells, visualized by monoclonal antibodies such as Ki-M4, Tü 1, or R4/23 (27,42,69,74), or antibodies against the human low-affinity nerve growth factor receptor (75) (Fig. 16.6). These cells are thought to be proliferating beyond the confines of the follicles (42) and produce coarse networks that occupy 20% to 40% (27) and even 50% to 90% of the section area of the node (42). Whether this proliferation accounts for the alterations of germinal centers in AIL (and what its cause is) is unclear. In AITCL with hyperplastic germinal centers, thought to precede classic AITCL, the germinal centers—detected by their reactivity with an anti-BCL-6 antibody—are said to have ill-defined borders and to be disintegrating because of an outward migration of BCL-6–positive intrafollicular T cells (76). In any case, the characteristic pattern of follicular dendritic cell networks in AIL (42) is so specific of AITCLs, unlike other types of peripheral T-cell lymphomas, as to be a useful aid in diagnosis (75,77). ''Zonated,'' rather than diffuse, networks of desmin-positive fibroblastic reticulum cells associated with areas of greatest vascularity were also characteristically seen in AITCL but not in other non-Hodgkin's lymphomas (75).

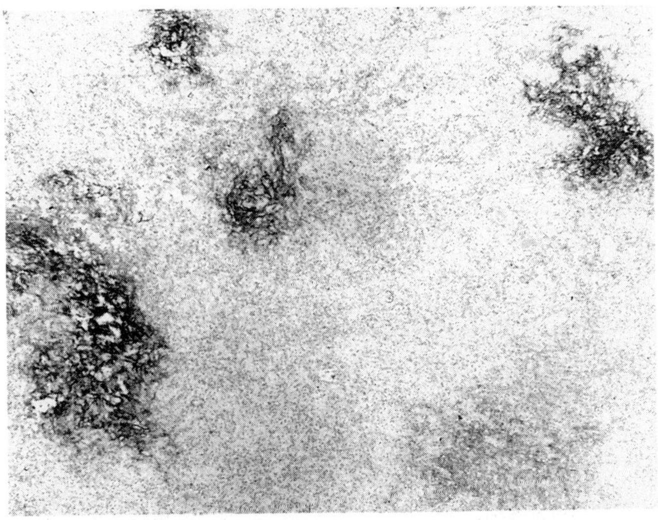

FIG. 16.6. Angioimmunoblastic lymphadenopathy. Irregularly shaped, disorganized clusters of $CD21^+$ follicular dendritic cells (immunoperoxidase stain, original magnification: 75× magnification).

DNA Hybridization Studies

The analysis of antigen receptor genes has demonstrated that the lymphoid lesions diagnosed as AIL (IBL, LgX) are genomically heterogeneous. In a review of the literature for the previous edition of this textbook (78), we evaluated the incidence of clonality in lymph node biopsies diagnosed as AIL (IBL, LgX) at presentation of disease (26,32,42,66, 79–83). Seventy three per cent of these, studied by Southern blotting, had a monoclonal pattern. A literature review confirms and expands these findings, as shown in Table 16.2. Monoclonal rearrangements within AIL lesions (AIL and AITCL) were found at presentation in 70% (48 of 69) of new cases evaluated by Southern blotting (24,28,29,33,34, 36,43,68,70,84–89) and in 66% (22 of 33) of those studied with the polymerase chain reaction (PCR) (29,30,43,69,86, 90,91). Conversely, no evidence of rearrangements could be found in approximately 30% of cases at presentation. Sampling problems or the small size of a clone (below the threshold of detection by the Southern blot technique) can be a plausible explanation for some, but not all, of these cases. These negative findings support the notion that at least some of the lesions with morphologic features of AIL represent initially a reactive process.

Most of the rearrangements detected in AIL lesions (Table 16.2) involve the T-cell receptor (TCR) genes, confirming the primary involvement of T cells in this process. Among all nodal specimens with a clonal pattern studied by Southern blotting, 81% showed rearrangement of the TCR-β chain gene alone in the old series (78), or 92% rearrangement of the TCR-β and TCR-γ chain genes alone in the newly reviewed cases. In studies using PCR, 73% of the total clonal cases had rearrangements of the TCR-β or TCR-γ genes alone. Often, the rearrangement bands have been observed to be significantly lighter in intensity than usual or multiple (24,29,42,79,81,86,88). The oligoclonal, rather than monoclonal pattern, has been stressed in some studies (29,30,91). In one case, the products at each immunoglobulin (Ig) heavy-chain clonal band were cloned and sequenced, revealing different VH3 clonal sequences, data supporting oligoclonality over somatic mutations occurring within a single neoplastic population (91). These T-cell oligoclones ''suggest reactive rather than malignant T-cell infiltrates,'' because they are also found in autoimmune disease, in response to superantigens and among CD3/$CD8^+$ populations in the elderly (91). Different oligoclones were detected in a lymph node and a skin lesion, both with features of AIL, obtained at the same time in one patient (30), reminiscent of the situation observed in the posttransplantation LPDs. Disappearance of several clones with time has been observed in one study, in which consecutive biopsies were examined in the same patients (81).

TABLE 16.2. *DNA analysis of tissues in angioimmunoblastic lymphadenopathies and related disorders*

Studies	With clonal rearrangement (%)	Cell lineage of clonal cases[a]		
		T alone	T and B	B alone
Previous review (78)	73[b]	81[c]	12[c]	7[c]
By Southern[b] (24, 28, 29, 33, 34, 36, 43, 68, 70, 84–89)	70	92	6	2
By PCR[b] (29, 30, 43, 69, 86, 90, 91)	66	73	18	9

[a] T, rearrangement (R) of TCR-β and/or TCR-γ genes alone; T and B, coexisting R of TCR-β and/or TCR-γ genes and Ig heavy- or light-chain genes; B, R of Ig heavy- and light-chain genes.
[b] At presentation.
[c] At presentation and during the course of the disease.

In a substantial proportion of AIL-like lesions, rearrangements of the Ig heavy- or light-chain genes (these also are occasionally oligoclonal [29,91]) have been found to coexist with rearrangements of the TCR-β or TCR-γ genes; this occurred in 6% to 12% of the lesions studied by Southern blotting and in 18% of those studied by PCR (Table 16.2) (26,29,34,42,69,81,91,92). This finding might indicate the existence of two separate, T- and B-cell, clonal populations (i.e., a true bilineage lymphoma) (92) or of one clone that carries both rearrangements (26,42,81). The latter case may be explained as an "an illegitimate Ig gene rearrangement in mature T-cell neoplasms," which arises "by aberrant activation of the recombinase machinery or as part of chromosomal abnormalities involving immune receptor gene loci" (92). A small group of cases diagnosed as AIL lesions demonstrates clonal abnormalities of the Ig (heavy and light chain) genes alone (42,69,79,81,84) or along with a TCR-β rearrangement (24). These cases may represent a misdiagnosis of a B-cell atypical lymphoid proliferation as AIL or the development of a large B-cell lymphoma within AIL.

There are different interpretations of such data. Weiss and colleagues (26) concluded that the lesions they studied included *bona fide* lymphomas; lymphoid proliferations histologically interpreted as AIL that "contain clonal T-cell populations and probably represent peripheral T-cell lymphomas"; and cases that lacked detectable clonal TCR-β gene rearrangements "consistent with the existence of a separate nonneoplastic entity of AILD." They thought it "reasonable to propose that lymphomas may arise in a preexisting condition of AILD, rather than that all cases diagnosed as AILD are actually *ab initio* T-cell lymphomas." From their data, O'Connor and associates (80) could not decide whether the polytypic proliferation characteristic of AIL was a secondary reaction to an underlying monoclonal (B- or T-cell) population or a primary hyperreactive disorder that affects T and B cells, from which T- or B-cell clones might arise. The latter seemed to Lipford and associates (81) to be the best explanation for their data. They stressed, however, that clonality is not synonymous with malignancy.

Chromosomal Findings

Cytogenetic studies have demonstrated a unique chromosomal pattern in AIL lesions (27,93–95). First, cytogenetic changes are found in the majority, but not all, of the cases. In a review of the older literature and personal cases by Gödde-Salz and colleagues (93), 17% of cases diagnosed as AIL (IBL, LgX) had a normal karyotype. A similar figure of 20% is arrived at from a review of later reports, totalling 59 cases evaluated at presentation (27,29,33,34,87,96), including our study of 10 T-cell lesions (hyperplasias and lymphomas) histologically characterized by "reactive (AIL-type) features" (94). By combining classic metaphase cytogenetics and interphase cytogenetics, 11% of cases with a diagnosis of AITCL had a normal karyotype (95). These figures, like those of approximately 30% obtained from studies with DNA hybridization techniques, again confirm the existence of a hyperplastic process within the spectrum of AIL-like lesions. Second, in most if not all cases evaluated, a large proportion (up to 98%) of normal mitoses is present (27,94), suggesting a sizable polyclonal background.

Third, only 31% of the total series contained monoclonal chromosomal changes (i.e., two or more metaphase cells with identical extra chromosomes or identical structural rearrangements, or three or more metaphase cells with loss of identical chromosomes); all others were multiple unrelated chromosomal changes, such as unrelated clones, one clone and single-cell abnormalities, or only single-cell abnormalities (27,94). "This means that nearly half of the cases of AILD-type T-cell lymphomas are polyclonal (or oligoclonal) from a cytogenetic point of view" (27). This is a unique phenomenon, because unrelated clones are otherwise an exceptional finding among lymphomas in general (0.6%) (97). The high incidence of single-cell abnormalities is characteristic of AITCL compared with the high-grade T-cell lymphomas (94,98). The most frequent alterations are trisomy 3 (often seen as the sole abnormality), trisomy 5, and trisomy X, whereas structural abnormalities involving the sites of TCR genes (i.e., 7q35, 14q11, and 7p13) are uncommon (27,95,96,99). By interphase cytogenetics, which evaluates the proportion of abnormal versus normal cells better than metaphase cytogenetics, the incidence of cells with abnormalities is low (e.g., cells with +3 represent only 4.5% of all mitotic cells), corresponding to the histologic picture of a mixed infiltrate, in which only a few neoplastic cells are present in a very rich reactive background (95).

Sequential cytogenetic evaluation of one half of the patients in our study of AIL-type T-cell lesions (94) found that, in some instances, some of the clonal or nonclonal abnormalities appeared not to progress, even after a long time, and some disappeared; in other instances, some clones became predominant in subsequent lymphoid tissue or bone marrow specimens. We concluded that AIL-like lesions "appear to arise from a hyperplastic (hyperreactive) background, mainly involving T cells; while some of them may subside, most manifest an unstable coexistence of a very large population of normal cells and small numbers of abnormal clonal and nonclonal cells, which in turn may or may not selectively proliferate and develop into a full-blown malignancy." Similar conclusions were later reached by Schlegelberger and colleagues, who suggested a stepwise development of chromosomal changes in AIL: starting within chronic T-cell proliferations with normal metaphases, unrelated clones may appear "because of increased genetic instability and because of an immune defect resulting in impaired elimination of aberrant cells"; trisomy 3 may be the key event that provides a clone with a selective proliferative advantage leading to monoclonal +3 proliferation; and "during tumor progression more malignant clones or subclones occur, determining the clinical course of the disease" (27,95). This sequence has been verified in other patients (29,34). Our study (94) and the sequential molecular data in some patients already mentioned (81,100) prove that such an evolution is not obligatory and can be reversed.

Clinical Features

Any attempt to describe the clinical picture and evolution, prognostic factors, and the best management of AIL (IBL, LgX) versus AITCL is defeated by the heterogeneity of the cases included in most studies. It has to be accepted therefore that most of the information discussed here and in other reviews (100–103) refers to the entire group of AIL-like lesions, without any possibility of distinguishing the reactive forms from the *bona fide* lymphomas.

Angioimmunoblastic lymphadenopathy occurs with no gender predilection in advanced adulthood, with peak onset in the sixth and seventh decades of life; the median reported age varies from 53 (32) to 64 (51) years. Rare questionable cases have been reported in young adults and children (32,104). Tables 16.3 and 16.4 summarize the main clinical and laboratory findings at presentation, as compiled from the 10 earlier largest series (15,52,105–112). These findings and figures are not different from those obtained in patients with AITCLs in three of the recent largest studies (31,113,114) (Tables 16.3, 16.4).

The clinical presentation is usually acute, with prominent constitutional symptoms, generalized lymphadenopathy,

TABLE 16.3. *Main clinical findings in patients with angioimmunoblastic lymphadenopathy and angioimmunoblastic T-cell lymphoma*

Finding	AIL patients (%)	AITCL patients (%)
B symptoms		68–85
Fever	71	
Night sweats	40	
Pruritus	36	
Loss of weight	59	
Lymphadenopathy, diffuse	85	97
Splenomegaly	65	59–73
Hepatomegaly	60	31–52
Rash	44	48–49
Pulmonary involvement	38	
Arthralgias	17	18

AIL, angioimmunoblastic lymphadenopathy with dysproteinemia; AITCL, angioimmunoblastic T-cell lymphoma.
Data for AIL from references 15, 52, and 105–112 and for AITCL from references 31, 113, and 114.

TABLE 16.4. *Main laboratory findings in patients with angioimmunoblastic lymphadenopathy and angioimmunoblastic T-cell lymphoma*

Finding	AIL patients (%)	AITCL patients (%)
Anemia	71	33–40 (<10)–57 (<12)
(positive Coombs' tests)	53	32–43
Leukocytosis	34	25
Leukopenia	17	3
Eosinophilia	30	26–39
Atypical circulating PCs	27	
Lymphopenia	47	
Thrombocytosis	26	12
Thrombocytopenia	25	20
Polyclonal hyper-γ-globulinemia	66	24–51
Autoantibodies	18	66 31 RF, 33 SMA

AIL, angioimmunoblastic lymphadenopathy with dysproteinemia; AITCL, angioimmunoblastic T-cell lymphoma; PC, plasma cells; RF, rheumatoid factor; SMA, smooth muscle antibodies.
Data for AIL from references 15, 52, and 105–112 and for AITCL from references 31, 113, and 114.

hepatosplenomegaly, and frequently, cutaneous rash. In some cases, however, this picture may develop over a longer period or may be incomplete. The cutaneous manifestations are clinically and histopathologically diverse and nonspecific (115) (i.e., ''lymphocytoma cutis'' [54]), although they may bear a striking similarity to the nodal lesions (28,30,60, 84). Their incidence vary from as little as 15% (69) or 57% (68) to 96% (32) of AIL lesions and from 49% (31) to 58% (70) of AITCLs. Arthritis is present in 17% to 21% of cases (31,32,116). The presence of edema, ascites, and pleural effusions, observed in up to one third of patients with AIL (32), has been stressed, along with skin manifestations and arthritis, as a special feature of AITCLs compared with other non-Hodgkin's lymphomas (31).

The laboratory manifestations are equally variegated (Table 16.4). Polyclonal hypergammaglobulinemia, although characteristic of AIL, may be absent in the quiescent phases of the disease. Uncommonly (3% to 10%), hypogammaglobulinemia (31,32,117,118) or, in rare cases, monoclonal gammopathy may occur (31,119). Serum autoantibodies are less common findings, except for anti-erythrocyte antibodies; the Coombs' test result is positive in 32% to 45% of cases (31,32,70,118). Autoantibodies, however, have been found more frequently in another series of AIL (one third of patients [32]) and—along with the high incidence of cold agglutinins, cryoglobulins, circulating immune complexes, positive Coombs' test results, and hypergammaglobulinemia—have been identified as distinct laboratory findings of AITCLs versus other non-Hodgkin's lymphomas (31). The presence of autoantibodies directed against vimentin seems to be a characteristic serologic marker of AIL (120). Hypocomplementemia has been observed in most cases of a series of AITCL and paralleled the state of disease activity (121). Abnormalities of lymphocyte subsets (101,122,123), lymphopenia (32,118) and skin anergy (118) are frequent. Increased serum levels of various cytokines have been found in patients with AIL (33,100,124,125). Elevated serum levels of soluble FAS/CD95 were detected in AITCL but not in other types of non-Hodgkin's lymphoma, and it was suggested that, by blocking apoptosis of activated cells, they may explain the autoimmune manifestations in this disease (126). Bone marrow involvement, represented in biopsies by infiltrates of plasma cells and immunoblasts associated with fibrosis and vascular proliferation (127) or by granuloma-like foci (128,129), has been identified in 60% to 70% of patients. In addition to the previously described reported features, many clinical associations and laboratory abnormalities have been described in isolated cases of AIL, such as synovitis (84), peripheral neuropathy (130), nodular regenerative hyperplasia of the liver (131), pure red cell aplasia (132), aplastic anemia (38), myelofibrosis (133), myelodysplastic syndrome (134), amyloidosis (135), and hypercalcemia (136).

The evolution of AIL lesions is usually aggressive, with one or a few episodes, only partially controlled by, or refractory to, therapy. The clinical course, however, may vary in individual patients. Some die in the very first weeks after diagnosis. However, spontaneous remissions may occur (32,34,53,118,137). The evolution of the disease is complicated by intercurrent, often severe, infections with conventional and opportunistic organisms: mycobacteria, cytomegalovirus (CMV), *Aspergillus,* and *Pneumocystis carinii* are among the most frequent (31). Infections were the direct cause of death in 62% of the evaluable cases in older series of AIL (15,52,105–112), and in 54% of a large series of AITCL (31). These occur during cytostatic treatments otherwise well tolerated in patients with other lymphomas (31) and in the absence of cytopenias to explain them. Processes that were morphologically interpreted as malignant lymphomas developed in a total of 11% of the evaluable patients in the major series, with figures varying from 0% (17) to 35% (52) in separate studies. Only a few of these cases, however, have been documented immunophenotypically to be *bona fide* malignant lymphomas (20,55–59,138), especially immunoblastic lymphomas (60,61,63). Other types of neoplasms reported to develop in patients with AIL include Hodgkin's lymphoma (19,139,140), Kaposi's sarcoma (KS) (141–143), glioblastoma (31), melanoma (118), and carcinomas (24,144).

In a long-term (5 or more years) follow-up study of 41 patients with AIL, 30 (73%) died; the median survival was 30 months (53). In earlier series, this ranged from 2.5 to 15 months for patients who died and from 13 to 61 months for surviving patients (15,52,105–112). The figures for overall median survival vary from 12 (69) to 24 months (68) in later series that included patients with AIL and AITCL, 52 months for patients with initial diagnosis of ''atypical AIL'' (29), and 13 to 20 months for those with AITCL (24,25,31,43,70, 117,137). To counterbalance this dismal picture, there is in the literature some evidence for a subset of AIL-like lesions with a better outlook. Of a total of 46 such patients who survived 20 months or longer, 76% were alive 20 to 192 or more months from diagnosis (median, 36 + months), and the rest died at 21 to 150 months (median, 43 months) (25,27–30,32,34,36,38,43,54,63,68,96,137,139,145–148). We found nothing distinct in these cases as to clinical presentation or pathologic features, including genotypic or cytogenetic data, when given; however, more patients were alive among those treated with prednisone alone or chemotherapy than among those who received no therapy at all.

The therapeutic approach to patients with AIL lesions has not been consistent nor is there any consensus about which course is the best. A clinical review of the earlier published data (102) concluded that prednisone, given as a single agent, resulted in complete remission in approximately one half of the patients. The data on the efficacy of single-agent chemotherapy (mainly cyclophosphamide with or without prednisone) are discordant. Somewhat better results than with either of the two previous approaches have been obtained with multiple-agent chemotherapy, with an overall complete remission rate of 58%. In most studies, combination chemotherapy, usually including doxorubicin, has been used

(24,43,68,69,117,145), with resulting median survivals of 12 to 24 months. In others, to avoid overtreatment, a subset of patients was initially treated with prednisone alone; most of them (89%), however, after partial or complete remission, required subsequent chemotherapy (25,31). It was concluded that ''prednisone with or without COPBLAM/IMVP-16 treatment in AILD-type lymphoma leads to complete remissions in about half of the patients and to long-term disease-free survival for one third'' (25). In another study ''therapy-induced remission'' was obtained in almost all patients with any treatment (i.e., prednisone alone, ''nonaggressive,'' and ''aggressive'' chemotherapy) and median survival was 14, 7.5, and 21 months, respectively, in these three groups. The conclusions reached in this 1996 study, that ''new treatment strategies are needed'' for these patients (137) echo those of a 1987 study, which stated that ''cytotoxic treatment is clearly not curative and may be inappropriate for elderly patients'' (32). The most promising among the new approaches are immunomodulating therapies and purine analogues. IFN-α has been used in several single cases (34,38,149–152) and in one small series of 12 patients (153); it has produced remissions, usually of short duration, but no cures. Remissions, one of which is continuing after 2.5 years (28), have been obtained also with cyclosporine (33,35), an effect thought to be caused by the inhibition of cytokines involved in the expansion of T cells (i.e., interleukin-2 [IL-2]) and in the stimulation of B cells (IL-6) (28,33). Fludarabine has produced complete remissions of 22+ months in one patient (36) and 10+ and 32+ months in two others, one of whom had been resistant to CHOP therapy (40). The 2-chlorodeoxyadenosine, which had produced a partial durable response of 9+ months in one patient (89), was used later in seven patients with refractory or relapsed AIL. The overall response rate was 57%, and two patients (28.5%) achieved complete and sustained responses of 19 and 21 months, respectively, with minimal toxicity (37).

Of the several clinical prognostic factors that have been considered, the one that appears most consistently useful is achievement of a complete remission (or not) with any therapy; complete responders have significantly longer median survival rates than patients who have a partial or no response (25,32,52,53,118,145). Patients with rashes (118), drug-related onset of disease, or an allergic history have statistically worse survival rates (111,118,154). In a study of AITCL, the simultaneous occurrence at presentation of more than one of three clinical symptoms (i.e., rash or pruritus, edema, ascites) was correlated with poor survival (31). Other unfavorable prognostic parameters appear to be the presence of hematologic abnormalities, hypoalbuminemia, hypergammaglobulinemia (154), or elevated serum lactate dehydrogenase (118). Involvement of the bone marrow was associated with worse survival in some studies (128,129), but had no prognostic value in others (118,127). In several studies, the type of therapy used (prednisone, aggressive or nonaggressive chemotherapy) had no influence on survival (25,70,137). Among histologic criteria, the occurrence of clusters of immunoblasts in the sinuses or paracortex was shown to be a predictor of poor outcome (52). Absence of clear or convoluted cells was associated with a more favorable prognosis in one study (51), but not in another (145). A high proliferative index, expressed as reactivity in more than 25% of lymph node cells for monoclonal antibody Ki-67 was an ominous sign (74). Immunogenotypic patterns (absence of clonal TCR-β gene rearrangement or clonal rearrangement of the TCR-β without rearrangement of the Ig gene) had favorable prognostic implications in some studies (42,71), but not in another (69). Cytogenetic findings may prove valuable. In one large study, trisomy 3 correlated with more frequent spontaneous remissions, and there was a better survival, in multivariate analysis, for patients without aberrant metaphases, a +X clone, structural changes in 1p, or complex aberrant clones (137).

Pathogenesis

The immunogenotypic and cytogenetic studies and many clinical findings presented earlier support the concept that the lesions with morphologic features of AIL (IBL, LgX) represent a spectrum of disorders, from reactive lymphoid proliferations to malignant lymphomas (26–30,34,49,54,60, 63,68,81,92,94,95,100,155,156), which are unique among LPDs and distinctly different from other T-cell lymphoid proliferations (Table 16.5). Angioimmunoblastic lymphadenopathy begins as ''a deregulated response to antigenic stimulation'' (157), which involves T and B lymphocytes and may lead to multiple proliferating clones (oligoclones). Some of these may regress spontaneously. However, ''expanding clones would be susceptible to genetic errors during the repeating cell division process''; these errors might ''produce malignant transformation and selective proliferation of the malignant clone'' (81). The special theme running through this continuum and explaining its uniqueness in terms of other T-cell LPDs is immune dysregulation, which led some investigators to define AIL tout court as a *disorder of cellular immunoregulation* (29,34,60,100).

Immunologic abnormalities have been reported frequently in AIL (IBL, LgX) (101,122). They include, in different studies, a decrease in circulating T cells, an altered CD4:CD8 ratio, altered absolute numbers of $CD4^-$ or $CD8^+$ cells, defective responsiveness of lymphocytes *in vitro*, reduced helper and enhanced suppressor functions *in vitro*, monocytic suppressor effect, and high levels of NK cells. It has also been suggested that T-cell inducer effects on B cells may be characteristic of the early stages of disease, followed later by potent suppressor-inducer effects (123). Lymphopenia is seen in 50% (118) to 62% (32) of patients with AIL and skin test anergy in 68% (118). The high incidence of autoimmune phenomena in AITCLs, versus other lymphomas, indicates an abnormality of humoral immunity (31) and ''the high incidence of fatal infectious complications during and after cytostatic treatment regimens otherwise relatively well tolerated in lymphoma'' (31) and in the

TABLE 16.5. *Differences between angioimmunoblastic lymphadenopathy-like proliferations and non–angioimmunoblastic lymphadenopathy posttransplantation T-cell lymphomas*

Feature	AIL-like proliferations	Non-AIL PTCLs
Autoimmune manifestations	Very common	Uncommon
Intercurrent infections	Very common	Uncommon
Histology		
Reactive features	Characteristic	Uncommon
Cellular atypia	Unusual	Common
IHC		
Definite subset predominance	Inconstant	Common
Pan-T-cell antigen loss	Inconstant	Common
Prominent B-cell component	Common	Rare
FDC proliferation	Characteristic	No
DNA		
Oligoclonality	Common	No
Coexistent B and T-cell clones	Common	No
Cytogenetics		
Unrelated clones	70%	Rare
Many mitotic cells	Characteristic	Rare
Disappearance of clones	Yes	No
EBV infection of B and T cells	Characteristic	No

AIL, angioimmunoblastic lymphadenopathy with dysproteinemia; EBV, Epstein-Barr virus; FDC, follicular dendritic cell; PTCLs, posttransplantation T-cell lymphomas.

absence of cytopenias, ''is suggestive of a disturbance also of the cellular immunity quite unique in AILD'' (31). On the basis of these data and the poor success of all lymphoma chemotherapy regimens, ''the question arises whether new treatment strategies are needed'' (137), directed to ameliorating the patients' abnormal immune system rather than to killing the proliferating cells.

The abnormal immune response in AIL-like lesions involves T and B lymphocytes, as well as follicular dendritic cells. It is characterized by ''a status of enhanced immunoactivation,''expressed in high serum levels of soluble molecules related to cell activation, such as sIL-2, sCD30, sCD8, and IFN-γ (124,125). Increased levels of serum IL-6 (33,100,124) and spontaneous *in vitro* production of IL-6 by lymph node mononuclear cells (33) were reported in patients with AIL and correlated with clinical disease (33). Increased expression of various cytokines (TNF-α, LT, IL-6, and IL-1β) has been detected by ISH, using specific RNA probes (158), or by immunohistochemistry (159), in lymph nodes involved by AITCLs, suggesting a pivotal role for cytokines in the excessive proliferation of lymphoid cells, including the possible development of B-cell lymphomas (158). Cytokines may also contribute to the clinical manifestations of the disease, such as fever, loss of weight, hypergammaglobulinemia (158), or suppression of hematopoiesis (38). Aberrant lymphocyte activation and lymphokine synthesis might involve B7, an antigen that provides a costimulatory signal for T-cell activation and whose gene has been mapped to chromosome 3 (160). Trisomy 3 may not only provide a proliferative advantage to the cell, but ''disturb the cellular interactions that induce the characteristic cellular composition of AILD-type T-cell lymphoma'' (95).

The initial stimulus for the lymphoid proliferation remains undetermined. Two categories of etiologic factors have been considered. In a variable proportion of cases in series of AIL (8% to 37%) (51,105,106,118) and of AITCLs (22%) (70), and in single case reports (87,161,162), exposure to drugs, most commonly antibiotics and rarely anticonvulsants, preceded the onset of the disease. In other case reports, a host of infectious agents have been implicated, based on temporal association with an infectious disease, on serology or detection of the possible agents in the tissues of AIL lesions: *Mycobacterium tuberculosis* (88), *Yersinia* (163), *Eskenella* (164), *Listeria* (165), cryptococcus (146,166), herpes zoster (124), hepatitis C virus (167), rubella (168), and human immunodeficiency virus (HIV) (142,169–171). It remains unclear, however, whether these infections are the cause of the disease, directly or producing an immune dysfunction (34), or rather a consequence of the immune compromise observed in these patients. Most commonly, it is viruses that have been detected in the tissues of AIL lesions: the rubella virus by immunofluorescence (172), CMV by immunohistochemistry and DNA dot hybridization (173), HHV-6 by PCR in two studies (174,175) but not by ISH in another (148), HHV-8 by PCR in one study (176) but not in another (177), and especially EBV. The incidence of positive cases for EBV varies from 36% by Southern blotting alone (29) and 42% to 96% with PCR or ISH alone (148,155,174,178), to 97%

to 100% when a combination of these techniques is used (29,85,157,179). The pattern of involvement in ISH varies in different cases, from a signal limited to sparse small lymphocytes to positivity of many immunoblasts (29,157,178). Latent membrane protein-1 (LMP-1) is expressed in a smaller number of cells than observed by ISH and only in the larger activated lymphoid cells (29,148,179). With double staining techniques, most of the infected cells are B cells (29,157,178), but a diffuse pattern of positive neoplastic T cells has also been detected in a large number (42%) of cases (157). EBV infection of both lymphoid lineages is unique to AIL lesions (157) and the heterogeneous pattern of EBV infection in AIL lesions may depend on genetic alterations and the T-cell reactions to EBV-infected cells; on these bases, certain EBV^{+} or EBV^{-} clones may expand or disappear (157). Predominantly strain A (29) or both A and B (179) were detected. In a study that evaluated the EBV termini by Southern blot, there was no clonality of the cellular population harboring EBV in most cases (180), in contrast to the findings in posttransplantation lymphoproliferative disorders (PT-LPDs). Opposite conclusions have been drawn from these studies: that EBV infection is an indication and a consequence of decreased immunocompetence in these patients (34,148,178,179) or that EBV is a strong etiologic factor in AIL-like lesions, by infecting B and T cells (155,157). EBV has been detected in and is therefore strongly suspected to be the cause of large B-cell lymphomas that develop in AIL lesions (60,61,63). The EBV in this last study showed a specific deletion in the *LMP1* gene, which might have allowed escape from cytotoxic T cells or enhanced the oncogenicity of LMP-1 (63).

POSTTRANSPLANTATION LYMPHOPROLIFERATIVE DISORDERS

Background

Since the original reports of McKhann (181) and Penn and coworkers (182) in 1969, it has been well established that there is an increased incidence of neoplasms, especially skin and lip carcinomas and lymphoid lesions, in transplant recipients (183,184). The other key relationship between PT-LPDs and EBV infection became evident shortly thereafter (185,186). The PT-LPDs were initially thought of as malignancies associated with high mortality (187). In 1981, however, we presented evidence that these lesions represent a more complex group of B-cell proliferations, covering a spectrum from reactive lymphoid hyperplasias to lymphoma, had a unique morphology that we referred to as *polymorphic* and that were different from sporadic non-Hodgkin's lymphomas (188,189).

The existence of a pathologic spectrum fitted well the pathogenetic scenario proposed by Purtilo in 1980 and since then generally accepted: "Defective immune responses to EBV permit persistence of polyclonal proliferation of B cells. Conversion from polyclonal to monoclonal proliferation is probably the result of a cytogenetic error in a B cell" (190). The Pittsburgh group later showed that some of these lesions are reversible with reduction of immunosuppression and therefore arguably nonneoplastic (191). This concept opened the way to modern therapeutic strategies, which aim at restoring the patient's immune response to the EBV-driven proliferation. It also presents pathologists with a double challenge. The first is to provide as precise as possible a set of criteria that guide early recognition of these disorders in terms of other unrelated inflammatory responses; underdiagnosis or delay in diagnosis allows the proliferation to progress, and overdiagnosis can lead to unnecessary or excessive therapy. The second is to establish criteria to discern which lesions are likely to regress with immunologic intervention and which are likely to progress as *bona fide* lymphomas.

TABLE 16.6. *Epstein-Barr virus–related posttransplantation lymphoproliferative disorders*

Infectious mononucleosis-like (atypical) lymphoid hyperplasia
Plasmacytic hyperplasia
Polymorphic lymphoproliferative disorders
Monomorphic lymphomas
Plasmacytoma/multiple myeloma
T-cell lymphomas
Hodgkin's-like lymphoproliferative disorders
Others (e.g., composite)

Reserving to a later section more detailed definitions, suffice it to say at this point that the term PT-LPD is used in this review, and in many studies, to include all the varied lymphoid proliferations that arise as a direct consequence of organ or bone marrow transplantation (Table 16.6). For clarity, the most common EBV-related B-cell PT-LPDs are reviewed first, followed by posttransplantation T-cell lymphomas, Hodgkin's lymphoma, and the EBV^{-} PT-LPDs.

Incidence and Risk Factors

The incidence of lymphoid lesions, as reported in the literature, varies depending on the type of organ transplanted, the age of the recipient and the immunosuppressive regimen used. In cases of solid organ transplantation, the overall incidence of PT-LPDs is 1.4% to 1.7% of all patients transplanted (192,193). The variable figures given for the various organs (as number of cases per number of patients transplanted) are 0.6% for pancreas (194); 1% to 2% for liver (194–196); 0.3% to 3% for kidney (193,194,196–202); 1.8% to 9.8% for heart (193,195–197,199,203,204); 3.7% to 7.9% for lung (193,197,204,205); 4.6% to 12.5% for heart and lung (195,197,206); and 32% for transplantation of pancreas alone and with other viscera (207).

Comparison within the same institution (University of Pittsburgh) of the experience with pediatric and adult transplantation reveals consistently a higher frequency of PT-LPD among children: 4% (versus 0.8%, $p < 0.005$) among all organ transplants (208) and 9.7% (versus 3.5%) among all thoracic organ transplants (204,209). This is probably because children are more often EBV seronegative (EBV^-) before transplantation and seroconvert after transplantation (208,209).

For bone marrow transplantation, the overall frequency of PT-LPD in recipients of allogeneic grafts varies from 0.4% up to 7.4% (210–217). The striking differences in incidence depend on the type of bone marrow grafted: 0% to 0.4% for recipients of unmanipulated marrow (215–217) but 6% to 9% for those with T-cell–depleted marrow (213,215,217) and 16% to 24% for those with mismatched and T-cell–depleted marrow (213,215,216,218). Among recipients of autologous bone marrow, there are no cases of LPDs reported in several studies (210,213,219), but two cases have been described in a small series of T-cell–depleted autologous grafts (14%) (220) in addition to other sporadic reports (221,222). A unique case of PT-LPD was reported in a patient who underwent autologous peripheral stem cell transplantation (219).

The variations in the incidence of PT-LPDs in relation to the diverse immunosuppressive regimens used has received much attention; the risk is related to the aggressiveness of the regimen (199,223,224). The incidence of LPDs in patients treated with conventional immunosuppression (such as antilymphocyte globulin, steroids, and azathioprine [AZT]) was from about 1% (196,225) to 4.9% (226). Initial reports on patients treated with cyclosporine A (CSA) suggested a much higher incidence of LPDs (9% to 13%) (227,228), but later figures are between 0% and 1.5% (199,229–231) as a result of dose reduction and careful monitoring of serum levels of the drug. There has been also an increase in PT-LPDs reported in patients treated with FK506 (tacrolimus), an immunosuppressant that is about 100 times more potent than CSA (201,207,232). There is mounting evidence about the risk of using multiple agents. A significantly increased incidence of PT-LPDs has been associated with the use of triple therapy (CSA in combination with AZT and prednisone) in several studies (199,200,233,234), and an even higher incidence with the further addition of OKT3 (i.e., "quadruple therapy") (235).

The statistics given for the overall incidence of PT-LPD are only a general indication of the risk of this complication in transplantation. In addition to the influence of the different immunosuppressive regimens, other very important risk factors have been reported. A first encounter with EBV after transplantation has emerged as the major risk factor for the development of PT-LPD. The incidence of this complication is many times higher among seronegative than seropositive patients, such as 33% versus less than 2% among recipients of lung transplants (205); 50% versus 0.8% among adult recipients of nonrenal organs (236); or 25% versus 0% among children receiving transplantation of solid organs (237). Unrelated to EBV, and contributing additional significant immune dysregulation (223), a CMV infection adds to the risk of PT-LPD. A history of symptomatic CMV disease in a recipient (223) and a CMV seromismatch ($host^-$/$donor^+$) (238) are important risk factors for this complication in two studies.

In bone marrow transplantation (BMT), several risk factors are consistently detected by multivariate analysis, although not in the same order of statistical relevance: T-cell depletion of the grafted marrow, human leukocyte antigen (HLA) disparity between donor and host, use of anti-CD3 (or ATG), and primary immune deficiency in the host and acute graft-versus-host disease grades 3 or 4 (210,214,239). The methods used for T-cell depletion of the donor marrow have been found to be very relevant. Although the incidence of PT-LPD using unmanipulated bone marrow is 0.45% when HLA-identical and 1.4% when HLA-mismatched (217), the incidence remains similar (1.3%) with marrows treated with the CAMPATH (CD52) antibodies or elutriation, which also remove B cells (240), but it rises up to 8%, 11%, 14%, and 26% with other protocols for T-cell depletion (222,240). The conclusion was reached that "The simplest way of preventing EBV lymphoproliferation . . . may be to deplete B cells from the donor marrow prior to infusion to prevent the transmission of EBV-infected B cells" (222). A detailed evaluation of these risk factors can be found in several excellent reviews (222,241).

Pathologic Features

Grossly, PT-LPDs form tumoral masses or infiltrate the organ diffusely (189,195). Multiple lesions are common in the same patient and in the same organ, especially in lymph nodes, lungs (206), central nervous system (CNS), and the gastrointestinal tract, where several small ulcers leading to perforation are often observed (242).

Histologically, the lymphoid proliferations observed in transplant recipients are quite heterogeneous. This spectrum has been clarified through the efforts of many in the past 20 years (243) (Table 16.6). However, the distinctions between these forms are not always sharp, because overlapping patterns may be observed, and characteristically, more than one of these patterns may be observed simultaneously at different sites (189,195,216,244,245) or consecutively in the same patient (246–248).

The most common of the PT-LPDs are the lesions we described as polymorphic (189) and those reported, in contrast, as monomorphic (195). The former account for 46% to 69%, and the latter for 16% to 48%, of the lymphoid proliferations reported in different series of organ transplant patients (193,194,247,249–251). In BMT recipients, 68% to 70% of the lesions have been classified as polymorphic and 14% to 30% as monomorphic (215,216).

Polymorphic B-cell lesions (189) are recognized by a characteristic variable mixture of cells of different sizes and types (Fig. 16.7): lymphoplasmacytoid forms, plasma cells, large transformed cells of centroblastic or immunoblastic morphology, as well as small lymphocytes with an irregular, angulated nucleus that resemble cleaved follicle center cells

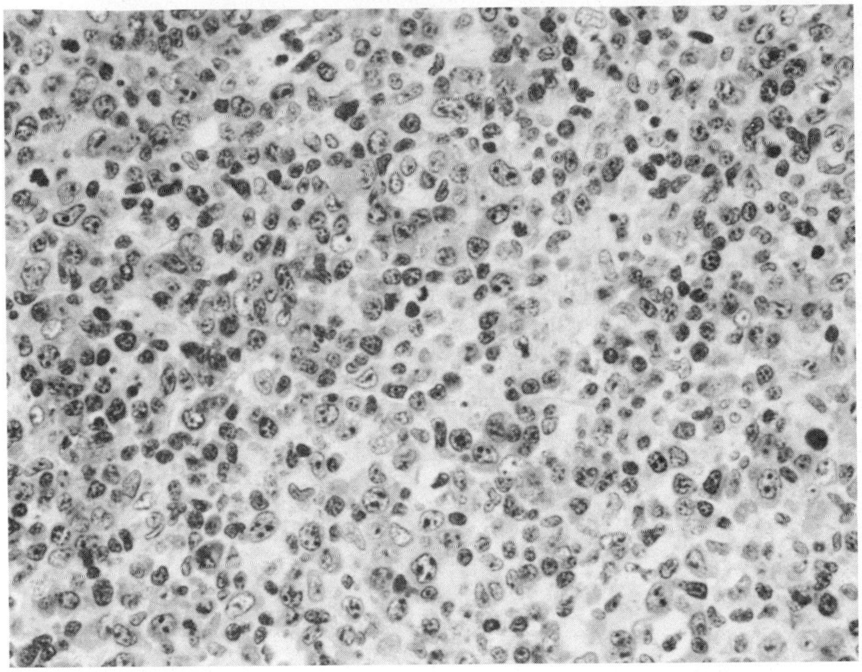

FIG. 16.7. Polymorphic B-cell lymphoproliferative disorder (LPD) in a renal transplant recipient. Characteristic mixture of cells of various size, some with plasmacytoid morphology and others with angulated nuclei (hematoxylin and eosin stain, original magnification: 400× magnification).

but may be mostly T cells (252). As a second main characteristic, the lesions display histologic evidence of aggressiveness, i.e., disruption of the architecture of the organ involved and invasion of blood vessels, nerves, or other organ structures. Within the polymorphic category so defined, we recognized at one extreme lesions with prominent plasmacytic differentiation, no cytologic atypia, and necrosis of single-cell type or limited to small foci (polymorphic B-cell hyperplasia [PBCH]) (Fig. 16.8) and, at the other extreme, lesions with less obvious plasmacytic differentiation, prominent cytologic atypia, and large confluent and ramified areas of coagulative necrosis (polymorphic B-cell lymphoma [PBCL]) (Fig. 16.9). Intermediate patterns may be seen between these extremes (PBCH with occasional atypical cells) (216). The presence of small cells with an irregular, angulated nucleus in a diffuse distribution differentiates PBCH and PBCL from, respectively, other atypical lymphoid hyperplasias and immunoblastic lymphoma (plasmacytoid).

Monomorphic PT-LPDs include all processes that morphologically resemble those observed in the general population: large B-cell lymphoma of centroblastic or immunoblastic type and small noncleaved cell lymphomas, Burkitt's or Burkitt-like. The term does not imply "a completely monotonous population of cells" but requires "a marked predominance of transformed cells" (243). Monomorphic tumors do not display the mixed composition, with abundant, but dispersed large cells, multinucleated neoplastic cells, and small cells with an irregular, angulated nucleus, characteristic of PBCL. Uncommonly, PT-LPDs have the purely plasmacytic composition of plasma cell neoplasms. Some of these cases fulfill the classic clinical and laboratory criteria of multiple myeloma (247,253–256); others have been reported in the literature as extramedullary plasmacytomas (196,253,257,258). In some of the latter, however, a definitive distinction from polymorphic lesions with a prominent plasmacytic differentiation (259–262) and even from plasmacytic hyperplasia (208) is not possible from the information provided.

In two studies of LPDs, arising in BMT (216) and after cardiac transplantation (249), we described a somewhat different histologic form of lymphoid proliferation, which accounted for 18% to 26% of the lesions observed in those series and we referred to as "*atypical lymphoid hyperplasia-infectious mononucleosis-like.*" This process, later also recognized by others (248,263), may be difficult to distinguish from PBCH, with which it shares the polymorphic composition, but differs from it in the overall retention of the organ architecture (germinal centers are often recognizable if the lesion is in the lymph node) and lack of invasion of normal tissue structures. It is indistinguishable from (and probably does represent) infectious mononucleosis (IM); it may be a manifestation of "uncomplicated" IM, which may occasionally occur in transplant recipients (264), but it may also be followed in the same patient by classic polymorphic lesions (248). Similarly, the distinctive histologic features of EBV hepatitis may be followed by more aggressive lymphoid proliferations (265). Recognition of these processes as belonging to the spectrum of PT-LPDs is important for correct therapy (reduction of immunosuppression) and to avoid further progression of the process (248,265).

Some PT-LPDs are composed of a diffuse plasmacytic hyperplasia intermixed with lymphocytes and only sparse immunoblasts, which spares the organ architecture. This was originally observed by Nalesnick and colleagues (195) in many organs and referred to as *minimally polymorphic,* and it represented 29% of the PT lesions in their series. The same

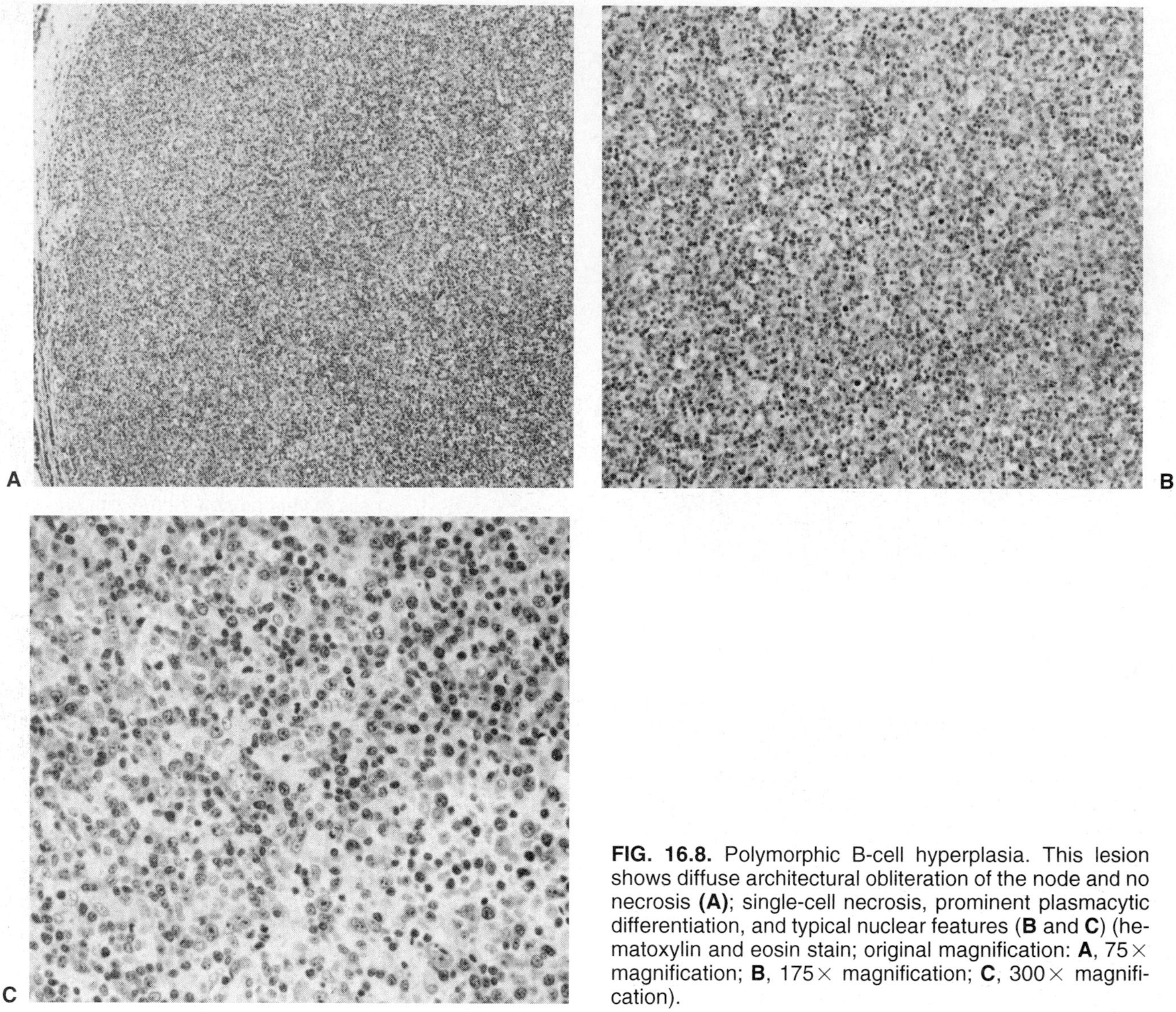

FIG. 16.8. Polymorphic B-cell hyperplasia. This lesion shows diffuse architectural obliteration of the node and no necrosis **(A)**; single-cell necrosis, prominent plasmacytic differentiation, and typical nuclear features (**B** and **C**) (hematoxylin and eosin stain; original magnification: **A**, 75× magnification; **B**, 175× magnification; **C**, 300× magnification).

process was identified by us and referred to as *plasmacytic hyperplasia* (PH) (247,266) and identified by others (244,250,251,267); its incidence in these series varied from 4% (250,251) to 37% (247,266) or 61.5% in a series of pediatric heart transplant recipients (267). In this last study (267), as in ours (247,266), PH was localized predominantly in the tonsils or adenoids. The relationship of this type of PT-LPD to the others is unclear. It may not even belong among the PT-LPDs, and it is unknown how it differs from a nonspecific inflammatory response (i.e., infection, autoimmune or allergic response). We and others believe it to be part of the spectrum of PT lymphoid proliferations because it has the same relation to EBV, clinical presentation, organ distribution, and response to therapy as all the other forms. Some investigators favor considering PH as a variant of IM-like hyperplasia (248), and others have listed it as an ''early'' lesion (268), which it is not, because it may occur at any time after transplantation and is common at autopsy (195). To us, it appears to be an exaggeration of the characteristic tendency to plasmacytic differentiation of all PT-LPDs (especially PBCH)—also documented in experimental conditions (269,270)—and probably represents a burned-out stage of a more active proliferation or a less florid or indolent form of EBV-driven response.

The presence of plasmacytic elements is considered a hallmark of a PT-LPD with regard to rejection in biopsies of grafted liver (271) and pancreas (272), or in cytology specimens of PT-LPDs (273). In a transplant recipient, the predominance of these cells within an infiltrate, along with the detection of EBV in it, should suggest a PT-LPD rather than a nonspecific inflammation of other cause and lead to the appropriate therapeutic response. Somewhat stricter ''minimal criteria'' for a diagnosis of PT-LPD have been used in the grading of EBV-related proliferations in gastrointestinal and other tissue biopsies from children with transplantation of small intestine (207). In bone marrow biopsies from pa-

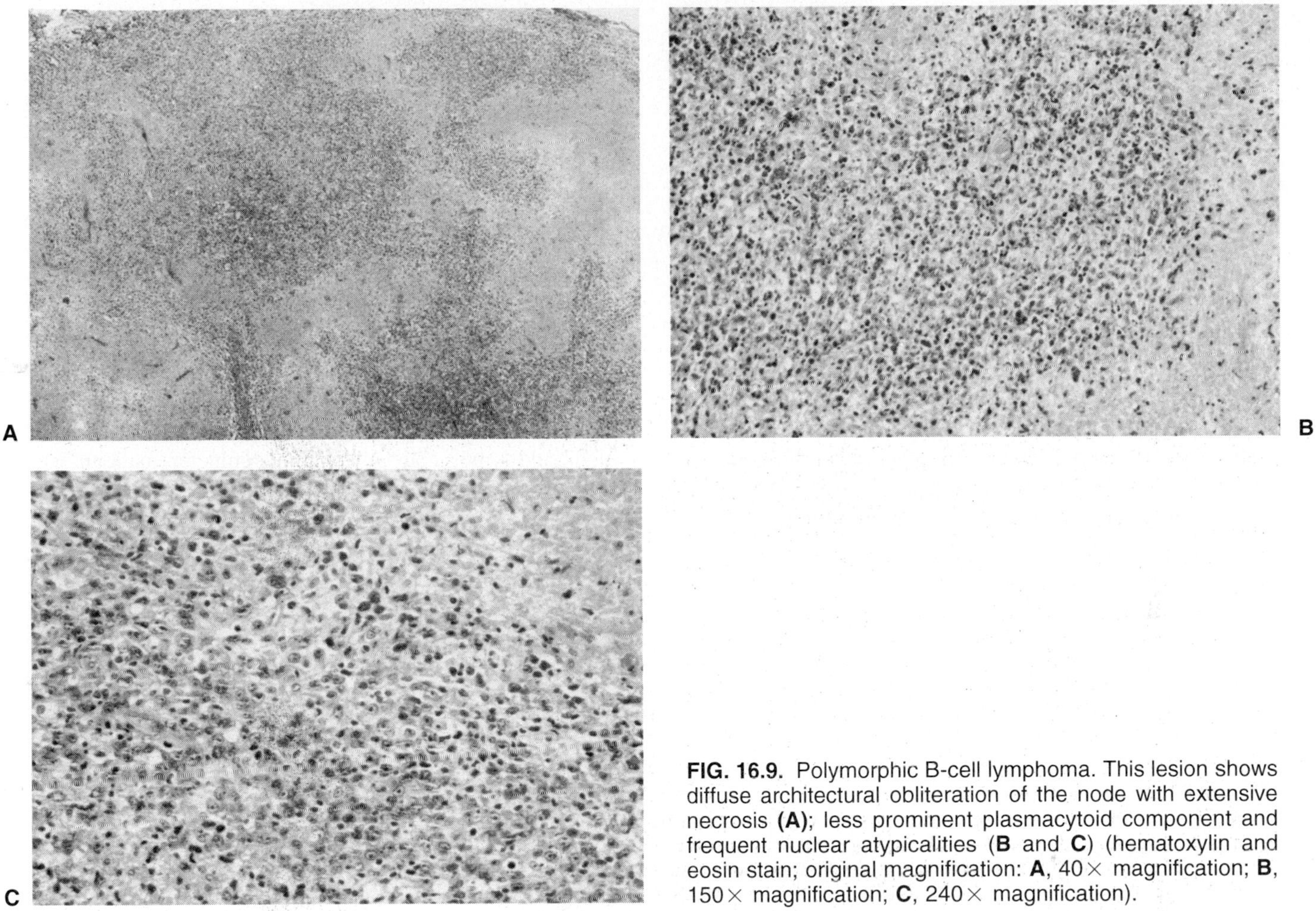

FIG. 16.9. Polymorphic B-cell lymphoma. This lesion shows diffuse architectural obliteration of the node with extensive necrosis **(A)**; less prominent plasmacytoid component and frequent nuclear atypicalities (**B** and **C**) (hematoxylin and eosin stain; original magnification: **A**, 40× magnification; **B**, 150× magnification; **C**, 240× magnification).

tients with solid organ PT-LPD, the presence of lymphoid aggregates of variable size and atypia or clusters of plasma cells was considered evidence of involvement by PT-LPD, because these were not found in any marrow biopsy from transplant recipients without LPD: EBER$^+$ cells were detected in 69% of the involved bone marrow biopsies but in none of the biopsies of uninvolved marrow from patients with PT-LPD and in none of those from transplant recipients without LPDs (250).

The determination of minimal criteria for the diagnosis of PT-LPD is particularly important in biopsies of grafted organs, where this issue overlaps with the issue of distinguishing PT-LPD from rejection, two diagnoses that lead to opposite therapeutic choices. From a review of many studies confronting this issue, and granting that the two processes may coexist (207,272,274), a consistent set of features emerges that favor PT-LPD over rejection in the liver (271,275,276), kidney (274,277) and pancreas (272). These constitute the expansile, nodular (versus diffuse) appearance of the infiltrate: its polymorphic composition, with large transformed cells, numerous plasmacytic or plasmacytoid elements, nuclear atypia, and absence or paucity of neutrophils and eosinophils; absence or paucity of vasculitis or damage of specific organ structures (e.g., bile ducts, pancreatic acini); definite predominance of B cells over T cells; and detection of EBV.

The last criterion needs to be better defined, because different techniques have been used in these studies (e.g., EBER-ISH, NotI-ISH, PCR, immunohistochemistry of LMP-1) and different conclusions proposed with regard to inflammatory infiltrates of other origin. In most studies, evidence of EBV was considered by itself a sign of PT-LPD, as none was otherwise found in tissues without PT-LPD (250,272,275,277–280), suggesting that EBV-infected cells are not recruited in sites of inflammation (280). However, in other studies, EBV was found in inflammatory conditions/rejection of kidney (274) and liver (271,276), in 20% of routine tonsillectomy specimens in children (224) and commonly in biopsies of the intestine and other tissues from recipients of small intestinal transplants (207). EBV was detected by ISH in 10% to 12% of sites without PT-LPD evaluated in two series of transplant recipients (244,281) and by PCR in 7% of grafted kidneys without PT-LPD (282) and 40% of patients without PT-LPD who had graft lung biopsies (283). EBER$^+$ cells in excess of 15 per field in biopsies from patients with intestinal graft (207) and in excess of 50% in grafted kidney biopsies (274) are required by some investigators to support a diagnosis of PT-LPD. In this context, it has been suggested that PCR might be too sensitive and detect EBV "even in cases in which the virus is clinically irrelevant" (224). For the diagnosis of PT-LPD in grafted lung, one study relied on the recognition of a central nodule of monomorphic B cells, but the distinction from rejection was considered impossible on a small transbronchial biopsy that only showed the polymorphic periphery of such a mass unless LMP-1–positive cells were found (284). Whether or not it may be applicable to all grafted organs, a scoring system has been proposed to evaluate these biopsies (285): grade 0, EBV$^+$ cells and predominance of polyclonal B cells = consistent with, but not diagnostic of, PT-LPD; grade I, EBV$^+$ cells and predominance of plasma cells = PH; grade II, EBV$^+$ cells and polymorphic composition = polymorphic LPD; and grade III, EBV$^+$ cells and monomorphic composition = monomorphic LPD.

Immunophenotypic Features

The EBV-induced LPDs that occur in transplant recipients are mostly B-cell proliferations and express variable clonality patterns (189,195,196,206,211,215–217,263, 286–289). Some of them express polyclonal surface or cytoplasmic Ig; others are monoclonal; others, the majority in the Stanford series (287), are composed of Ig$^-$ B cells that bear HLA-DR and pan-B-cell antigens. Polyclonal and monoclonal lesions may be found at different sites in the same patient (195,216,225,244) and clones might be identical or different at different sites (244). In a review of the literature (196), these four phenotypic patterns accounted for 36%, 29%, 20%, and 15%, respectively, of 55 reported cases. The LPDs that occurred in patients treated with CSA, compared with those after conventional immune suppression, more often bear monoclonal Ig (35% versus 8%) and are less often Ig$^-$ (14% versus 42%). In a compilation of other, later studies, 63% of PT-LPDs were immunophenotypically monoclonal, 28% were polyclonal, and 9% were Ig$^-$ (193,215,244,286,288).

The expression of the classic B-cell–associated antigens (e.g., CD19, CD20, CD21, CD22) by these cells is heterogeneous (286,288); CD21, in particular, is expressed uncommonly (286) or in a small proportion of cells (215,263). The cells variably express antigens suggestive of germinal center cells, such as CD38 and CD10, and activation antigens, such as CD23, CD30, CD39, and CDw70 (215,263,286, 288–290), and cell adhesion molecules, such as CD11a, CD54, and CD58 (263,286,288,290). They express major histocompatibility complex (MHC) class I and II antigens and strongly immunoregulatory markers (CD80, CD86) (263). All or most cases of PT-LPD strongly express BCL-2 (291,292). P53 expression was detected in a variable proportion of cells in 50% of cases of PT-LPD in one study (215) and 86% of cases in another (293). In the latter, an inverse pattern of p53 and BCL-2 expression was also observed in PT-LPDs with "high-grade" histology; they strongly express BCL-2, whereas p53 was downregulated.

The proliferating B lymphocytes are associated with a variable proportion of mature T cells, usually limited (196,286), but at times prominent (252,294). These cells may be more numerous in polymorphic than in monomorphic lesions (224), raising the intriguing possibility that "some polymorphic PT-LPDs are monoclonal B-cell proliferations (i.e., lymphomas) that are associated with a marked host immune response" and conversely that "some monomorphic PT-LPDs may represent a subset of lymphomas which fails to elicit this response" (295). The T cells are a mixture of CD4$^+$ and CD8$^+$ cells (196,263,286). The ratio of the two subsets in the tissue of PT-LPD is 2:1, in contrast to the predominant CD8$^+$ response to EBV in the peripheral blood and lymph nodes of immunocompetent patients with IM (263). Although CD4$^+$ cells may have cytolytic functions, they "may also encourage tumor proliferation by providing inappropriate signals for B-cell activation and growth by the production of cytokines" (263). The T-cell microenvironment in PT-LPDs is poor in cells efficient in killing EBV-infected cells and rich in cells that facilitate B-cell growth. However, in that study, there was no correlation between the degree of T-cell infiltration and clinical outcome (263). No CD56$^+$ cells were detected within PT-LPDs, in contrast to the tissues of IM (296).

Epstein-Barr Virus Studies

Many different methods, molecular and immunohistochemical, have documented the presence of EBV in the tissue of PT-LPDs, the former including the detection of viral DNA by slot-blot (297,298), Southern blot (193,279,299–304), polymerase chain reaction (PCR) (215,282,283,303,305,306), or *in situ* hybridization (ISH) techniques (244,279,280,307–309); EBER by ISH (193, 288,298,303,310,311); viral mRNA by reverse transcriptase (RT)–PCR (310,311); or proteins by Western blot (304). With one or more of these techniques EBV has been detected in all cases of PT-LPD (279,280,292,304,310,311) or in most of them, from a low of 68% to 75% (193,306) to 87% to 90% (196,215,298,303,305,309) or 94% to 97% (244,303).

Two main types (1 and 2) of EBV are distinguished on the basis of sequence variations in the EBNA-2 proteins and, in the West, more than 90% of people carry type 1 (312). In up to 33% of transplant recipients and other immunosuppressed individuals (versus 3% of the general population), the peripheral blood lymphocytes are infected with EBV of type 2 (305). Despite this, it is type 1 EBV that is most often detected in the tissues of PT-LPD by molecular techniques, with an incidence of 83% (251), 98% (313) and 100% (305,314), or by immunohistochemistry (100%, with monoclonal antibodies R3 and 3E9) (310). This is thought to reflect the greater efficiency of type 1 in transforming B cells (312). Special variants of EBV that carry a specific 30-base pair deletion of the *LMP1* gene (del-LMP1 variants) and have been previously reported in Hodgkin's lymphoma, undifferentiated nasopharyngeal carcinoma, peripheral T-cell lymphomas and other lymphomas, as well as in benign EBV-driven lesions (251), were also found initially in the aggressive, but not in the ''reactive,'' histologic forms of PT-LPD and were thought to contribute to the lymphomatous process (314). However, such variants were later detected in 41% to 44% (251,313) of PT-LPDs and in a similar proportion of reactive EBV lesions (251). No correlation was found between the presence of the 30-bp deletion (or point mutations [251]) of *LMP1* and the histologic type of the lesions or patients' survival in these two studies (251,313). The wild or deleted type of LMP-1 was the same in the same patient, in multiple lesions, and in tissues not involved by PT-LPD (313). These data lead to the conclusion that the EBV strain in a PT-LPD depends on the one that the patient is carrying (313).

Most EBV-encoded proteins expressed in infected tissues can be detected by immunohistochemistry in frozen and paraffin-embedded material (215,286,288,290,292,293,304, 306,310,311,315). There are 10 main products of the latent cycle genes (two RNA species, EBER-1 and EBER-2; six EBV nuclear antigens [EBNA-1 through EBNA-6]; and three latent membrane proteins [LMP-1, LMP-2A, LMP-2B]), as well as several products of the lytic cycle genes. It is the former that are relevant to the transformation of B cells and they are differently expressed in cell lines and human EBV-related proliferations (312). Three ''latency patterns'' are distinguished (EBNA1 and the EBERs are a feature in all of them): latency I (only EBNA1$^+$ and EBER$^+$), characteristic of Burkitt's lymphoma; latency II (LMP1$^+$ and LMP2$^+$), observed in nasopharyngeal carcinoma and Hodgkin's lymphoma; and latency III (all latent gene products), typical of lymphoblastoid cell lines (LCLs) (312).

In the PT-LPDs, the infected B cells express EBV gene products characteristic of the latent type of infection, but much less lytic cycle antigens. Overall, EBNA1 is expressed by a variable proportion of small and large cells in 95% to 100% of cases (286,292,310,311); EBNA2 in 22% to 100% of cases (286,288,292,310,311), depending strongly on the type of antibody used (310); EBNA3 in 50% (286); and LMP-1, in very different proportions of cases in different studies, from 37% to 55% (286,288,310) to 75% to 100% (215,292,293,306,311,315). The reactivity with LMP-1 is observed in the cytoplasm and on the membranes of large cells, but also of intermediate and small cells. It is positively correlated with the expression of BCL-2, consistent with the idea that LMP-1 upregulates BCL2 (292,293), and is colocalized with that of TNF receptor–associated factor (TRAF1), through which LMP-1 is thought to transmit growth signals to the nucleus, contributing to the pathogenesis of the PT-LPDs (306). EBER (Fig. 16.10) is detected by ISH in all PT-LPDs (288,310,311).

The expression of these latent cycle proteins in PT-LPDs

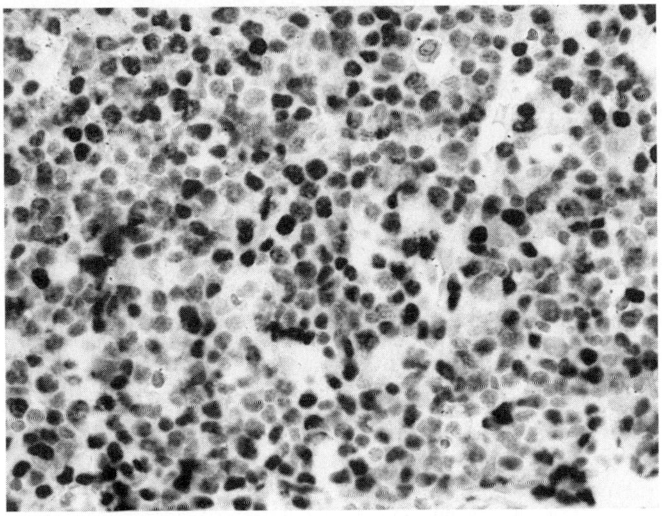

FIG. 16.10. Posttransplantation lymphoproliferative disorders (LPDs). A large number of lymphoid cells in this polymorphic lesion express strong nuclear signal for EBER (*in situ* hybridization, original magnification: 450× magnification).

is very heterogeneous, reflecting different virus:host cell interactions in different lesions (292,304,310–312,316). Evaluation of these phenotypic subsets not only contributes to an understanding of the pathogenesis of these lesions, but may have practical implications as well, as these subsets ''may emerge as an important diagnostic parameter and also account for differences in the response of individual tumours to treatment'' (316). Initial studies of PT-LPD identified a latency III type of infection, similar to that of LCLs (290). However, it has now become clear that pattern III is variably detected in 22% to 64% (286,288,317) of lesions, largely depending on the antibody used, and that other latency patterns may be expressed as well: latency I in 22% to 55% and latency II in 14% to 22% of cases (288,317). Double-staining methods have shown heterogeneity even within single lesions, with a pattern III expressed in only 5% to 30% of the cells in one study (310) and patterns I, II, and III detected in more than 60%, 10%, and less than 1%, respectively, of three cases (311). Another novel pattern of expression has emerged in some studies: EBNA-1$^+$, EBER$^+$, EBNA-2$^+$, but LMP-1$^-$ cells (286,311). It is unclear whether this represents a stable fourth type of EBV latency or a transitory phenomenon (312), such as an instance of the possible drifts that may occur within PT-LPDs, as they occur *in vitro*, along a continuum of latency types (310–312).

In one study, this continuum correlated with distinct cytologic types within the PT-LPD, the smaller lymphoid cells expressing latency pattern I or II, large cells (at times resembling mononuclear Reed-Sternberg cells), pattern II (as in Hodgkin's lymphoma), and cells of intermediate size, pattern III (310). In other studies, correlations have been found between latency types and histologic types of PT-LPD (288,317–319). Although PH mostly expressed a partially restricted pattern (type II) (319), polymorphic lesions expressed mostly pattern III (317,319), and monomorphic lesions (288,318) or immunoblastic plasmacytoid lymphomas/multiple myelomas (317,319) tended to express pattern I (EBNA-2, LMP-1). The expression of a pattern III versus a pattern I has been interpreted as a reflection of the immune status of the host under different transplantation regimens: severe immune suppression would allow the growth of cells expressing an unrestricted form of latency (III), while persistent immune response may select clones "with the minimal amount of host cytotoxic recognition" (type I) (224,304). Proliferation is mainly driven by the immortalizing function of EBNA2 in the former situation and requires genetic abnormalities in the latter (304), as supported by such abnormalities in the immunoblastic plasmacytoid lymphomas/multiple myelomas but not in polymorphic lesions (266). The complementary conclusion, that it is the lesions with unrestricted pattern of latency that could mostly benefit from immunomodulatory therapeutic approaches (290), has been challenged in a study (319).

In addition to proteins of the latent cycle, lytic cycle products can be detected immunohistochemically in PT-LPDs (as well as by RT-PCR (311), by ISH (309), and by Southern blot (312). The immediately early BZLF1 gene was found to be expressed in 55% to 95% (288,292,309) of cases; EA-D in 54%, and EA-R in 52% of cases (309); MA and VCA were found in 33% of cases (288). In one of these studies, 92% of all cases expressed at least one of three proteins (BZLF1, EA-D, EA-R) and 29% all three (309). However, the proportion of cells entering the lytic cycle is very small (<5%) (311). Although this has raised questions about the relevance of EBV replication in the pathogenesis of PT-LPDs (312), the presence of active EBV infection may explain why some patients benefit from treatment with acyclovir (202,246,309), which inhibits EBV DNA replication. It has been commented that, although the number of cells in replicative cycle at any given time might be small, "the additional viral burden produced during the lifetime of LPD" might be considerable and pathogenetically important (202).

Molecular Genetic Features

B-cell PT-LPDs are heterogenous at the genomic level (193,195,203,215,217,251,287–289,299,313,317,320,321) (Fig. 16.11A). In some of these lesions, no rearrangement of the Ig genes is detected (polyclonal lesions). In others, clonal Ig gene rearrangement bands are found, which may be weakly or strongly hybridizing (monoclonal lesions) (195,299). Rarely, multiple rearrangement bands have been observed, which are interpreted as representing multiple minor emerging clones (oligoclonal lesions) (251,289,311, 322). In a compilation of cases (193,203,215,217,251,288, 289,311,313,317,321), 76% (132 of 174) of cases were monoclonal, 21% (22 of 105) were polyclonal, and 12% (4 of 34) were oligoclonal. There appears to be poor correlation between histologic type and Ig genomic pattern in some studies (195,251). This is true, however, of the polymorphic lesions; of 64 evaluable in five studies, 72% were monoclonal, 26.5% were polyclonal, and 1.5% were oligoclonal (193,251,288,311,313). However, 90% to 92% of PH are polyclonal (266,313), and 80% to 100% of monomorphic lesions (193,195,251,288) or immunoblastic lymphoma/multiple myeloma (313) are monoclonal.

In studies in which multiple lesions in the same patient were evaluated, different clonal bands can be found (up to 24 clones in 24 separate tumor masses [242]), indicating the presence of multiclonal proliferations (266,287,320,321), or the same band is observed, suggesting the metastatic dissemination of one clone from one to another site (266,321,323, 324). Similarly, different genomic patterns can be detected in consecutive lesions of the same patient (224,248,266): a germline pattern followed by a clonal lesion, same clone, or different clones in consecutive lesions. Clinical "recurrence" of PT-LPD "cannot be assumed to represent pathologic recurrence of the original tumor" (224). There are occasional reports of PT-LPDs in which T-cell clones were found, in addition to B-cell clones (251,325–327), with one case showing a predominance of the T-cell clone in an early lesion and of the B-cell clone in a later one (327). It is unclear whether this phenomenon represents the coexistence of two neoplastic populations or "a dual genotype in a single tumor cell population" (326).

Clonality patterns of PT-LPD have also been studied by using the molecular configuration of the fused termini of the EBV genome in its circular (or episomal) form within latently infected cells (251,299–301,313,321). This configuration is unique for each episome and is transmitted by the infected cell to its progeny. Southern blot analyses of PT-LPDs using probes for the fused termini demonstrated, as for the Ig genes, polyclonal (smear), monoclonal, or oligoclonal patterns; the latter were observed in isolation or coexistent with a smear, indicative of the emergence of clones from a polyclonal B-cell proliferation (251,300,313,321) (Fig. 16.11B). In the same patients, different or identical bands can be found at different sites (300,321). Consecutive lesions in two patients demonstrated the same EBV clonal band but different rearrangement bands of the Ig gene, suggesting that the pattern of EBV termini is a more stable marker of clonality, because "additional rearrangement or somatic hypermutation of Ig genes following primary rearrangement" is possible (321). As is the case for Ig genes, the correlation between histologic type and EBV genomic pattern is poor, with PH being polyclonal or monoclonal and polymorphic lesions showing a smear with one clonal band or definite clonal bands; however, all monomorphic lesions had a monoclonal pattern (313).

Genomic abnormalities have been looked for in PT-LPDs in an attempt to better understand the pathogenesis of these disorders. In a pivotal study, alterations of one or more oncogenes or tumor suppressor genes (i.e., *NRAS* gene codon 61 point mutation, *TP53* gene mutation, or *MYC* gene rearrangement) were found only in the immunoblastic lym-

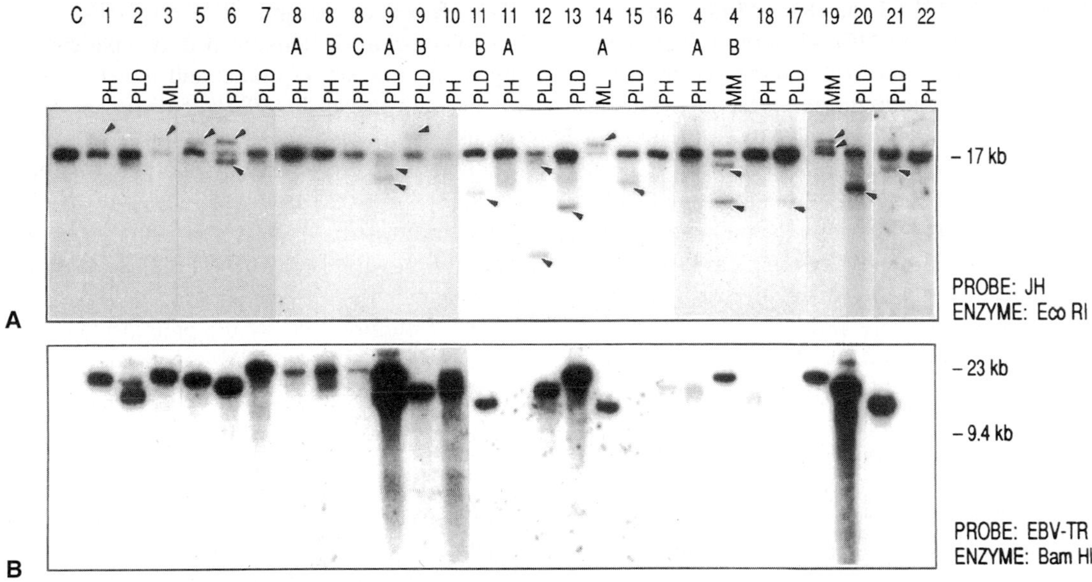

FIG. 16.11. Posttransplantation lymphoproliferative disorders (LPDs). Southern blot hybridization analysis for immunoglobulin (Ig) heavy-chain gene rearrangements **(A)** and for Epstein-Barr virus (EBV) termini heterogeneity **(B)**. DNAs were digested with *Eco*RI and hybridized to an Ig heavy-chain joining region (J_H) probe and with *Bam*HI and hybridized to a DNA probe specific for the fused termini of the EBV genome. Numbers 1 through 22 above each lane correspond to the case number, and the letters under these numbers denote different specimens from the same patient. C indicates the germline or negative control (HL60 cell line). The histologic classification of each case is indicated above each lane as follows: PH, plasmacytic hyperplasia; PLD, polymorphic B-cell hyperplasia; PLD, polymorphic B-cell lymphoma; ML, pleomorphic immunoblastic lymphoma; ML, plasmacytoid immunoblastic lymphoma or multiple myeloma. **A:** All of the cases show the germline band at 17 kb; additional clonal rearrangement bands are marked by arrowheads. Of the 10 cases of plasmacytic hyperplasia (PH), 9 lacked clonal Ig gene rearrangements, and the tenth (case 1) exhibited a solitary faint clonal Ig heavy-chain gene rearrangement band. All of the polymorphic B-cell hyperplasia (PLD), polymorphic B-cell lymphoma (PLP), immunoblastic lymphoma (ML), and multiple myeloma (MM) cases exhibited one or two, generally strong, Ig heavy-chain gene rearrangement bands, indicating the presence of a significant clonal B-cell population in each of these specimens. **B:** The locations of the 23-kb and 9.4-kb size markers are shown *(dashes).* Of 10 cases of plasmacytic hyperplasia (PH), 8 exhibited hybridization smears and/or a solitary, usually faint, band indicative of multiple EBV infection events and/or a minor cell population infected by a single form of EBV. Three of five polymorphic B-cell hyperplasia (PLD) cases and all of the 12 cases of polymorphic B-cell lymphoma (PLD), immunoblastic lymphoma (ML), and multiple myeloma (MM) exhibited solitary strong bands, sometimes accompanied by one of more additional faint bands, indicative of clonal EBV infection, sometimes in conjunction with a second or third EBV infection event. (From Knowles DM, Cesarman E, Chadburn A, et al. Correlative morphologic and molecular genetic analysis demonstrates three distinct categories of posttransplantation lymphoproliferative disorders. *Blood* 1995; 85:552–565, with permission).

phoma/multiple myeloma histologic category and therefore were taken as indicating the emergence of a fully neoplastic clone (266). These data are in agreement with the finding of *MYC* gene rearrangement in monomorphic lymphomas (299) and one of three PT plasmacytomas (317), but in contrast to the lack of *TP53* gene mutations in the PT-LPD of another study (328). Deletions of a region on chromosome 9p, which codes for IFN-α, were found in 44% of PT-LPDs, in contrast to 1.7% of intermediate and high-grade non-Hodgkin's lymphomas, and in the two cases studied, a very close region on 9p21, which codes for the tumor suppressor gene p16, was also deleted, which is deleted in 15% of diffuse large cell lymphomas (329). This information led to the suggestion that PT-LPDs "may represent a distinct pathologic entity with high incidence of 9p deletion" (329). Other important genomic abnormalities of PT-LPD are those of the *BCL6* gene, located on 3q27. Clonal rearrangements of *BCL6,* which are found in about 40% of diffuse large B-cell lymphoma and 20% of AIDS-related large B-cell lymphomas, are rare (7%) (330) or lacking (245) in PT-LPDs. However, *BCL6* point mutations are detected in these disorders, by single-strand conformation polymorphism and sequence analysis, in 44% of cases, as frequently as in large cell lymphomas of AIDS patients or the general population (245). In patients with multiple lesions, the same or different mutations of the gene are present (245). Importantly, there is a statistically significant difference in the incidence of *BCL6* gene mutations in different histologic types: 0% of

PH, 37% of PBCH, 48% of PBCL, and 87% of monomorphic lymphomas/multiple myeloma (245). The presence of mutations correlates with shorter survival and resistance of the lesions to discontinuation of immunosuppression or surgical excision (245). In this study it is concluded that, as the *BCL6* gene appears to control the formation of germinal centers, it is likely that PT-LPDs derive from germinal center cells. Whether *BCL6* mutations are a cause in the pathogenesis of PT-LPD or reflect a genetic instability secondary to malignant transformation is unclear: however, they may be the first genetic abnormality in these processes, because they precede mutations or rearrangements of other genes (245).

With the use of many different molecular techniques (331,332), among which the most common are PCR amplification of various polymorphic loci of the human genome and ISH for the Y chromosome in sex-mismatched transplants, most LPDs after organ transplantation have been of recipient origin. This is probably a reflection of the disproportionate predominance of the preserved recipient (versus donor) B lymphocytes (333). Only 13 cases have been shown to be of donor origin (331,332,334–338), and these are accounted for by the presence of circulating donor ''passenger'' lymphocytes, which has been reported in the graft (339,340), as well as in the recipient native organs (334,339). Even in one case of PT-LPD of host origin, a proportion of infiltrating cells was of donor origin, leading to genomic chimerism (198). The PT-LPDs of donor origin appear to be distinct in many regards. As a rule, they are localized to the allograft (six liver, five kidney, and two lung) or immediately adjacent areas, are of histologically aggressive types, and despite that, allow long-lasting freedom from disease after various therapies. This good prognosis may be a result of their being localized, or both features may result from a more effective immune response provoked by ''antigenically rich'' proliferations (which bear alloantigens in addition to EBV antigens) (334).

In contrast, most PT-LPDs arising in recipients of BMT are of donor origin (216,217,303,337,341–344), because the immune system of these patients is disproportionately of foreign origin (333), including B cells that are not removed by many T-cell depletion methods. Only occasional cases of recipient origin have been reported (217,303,343), which represent 14% to 17% of three series of post-BMT-LPDs (217,303,345) and 28.5% of our Minnesota series (216). These cases demonstrate that recipient B cells can survive the pretransplantation conditioning regimen (343). No special clinical characteristics have been suggested for these cases in the two series, but in one case report the lesion was an EBV^- immunoblastic lymphoma, arising nine years after the BMT (343).

These studies on the origin of PT-LPD prove that EBV can transform the recipient's and donor's B cells (339). A study of heart/lung transplant patients showed that the EBV driving the transformation might also be of different origin: donor origin in the PT-LPD of two seronegative patients and recipient origin in the PT-LPD of two seropositive patients (346). B-cell origin and EBV origin in a PT-LPD might not coincide, as demonstrated in two patients who received organs from a single donor and developed LPDs of host origin, both driven by EBV of donor origin (347). These results are explained by studies of EBV isolates in donor/host pairs. In seronegative organ transplant recipients, EBV is acquired from exogenous sources or from virus contained in the graft (in a cell-free state or in B cells or epithelia in lytic cycle), while seropositive patients maintain their pretransplantation isolate (346); in BMT recipients, EBV host isolates are eliminated by the pretransplantation conditioning regimens and donor EBV isolates might be acquired with the BM graft (346,348).

Cytogenetic Features

There are only sparse cytogenetic data on the PT-LPDs and they show no specific karyotypic pattern. From a compilation of the reported findings (189,208,215,216,225,235, 325,345,349–353), the most common changes (each occurring 8 times) are two of the classic translocations of Burkitt's lymphoma [(t(8;14) and t(8;22)], observed mostly in neoplasms with Burkitt's morphology; and abnormalities of chromosome 11 (trisomy 11 or dup11q). These latter changes, as well as monosomy 21 and a break at 1q21, which have been observed in two cases of PT-LPD (345,349), are rare in primary non-Hodgkin's lymphomas and have been thought to be characteristic chromosomal alterations of secondary (posttherapy) lymphomas (349,350). Less common recurrent abnormalities in PT-LPDs are trisomy 9 (occurring five times); translocations involving chromosome 1, 3 (each, four times), or 14 (three times); and monosomy 6 (three times). Most often, these changes occur as part of very complex karyotypes. The occurrence of unrelated clones (216,350) and nonclonal abnormalities (349–352,354) has also been reported, supporting the multiclonal origin of these processes, as well as the presence of many normal metaphases associated with abnormal clones (215). Some cases of PT-LPD have shown a normal karyotype (215,352,355).

The correlation of histologic or immunologic types and cytogenetic pattern is poor. In our original studies, all PBCH were cytogenetically normal, but so were 6 of 10 PBCLs (301,320) and, in another study, two additional cases of PBCL (215). In two other series, however, clonal abnormalities were detected in 83% of the monomorphic, but in none of the 10 polymorphic (oligoclonal or polyclonal) cases (352) and in all four immunohistochemically monoclonal cases, but in none of the five polyclonal lesions (345).

Cytokines

Several studies have addressed the role of cytokines and chemokines in the development of PT-LPDs (356,357). Most of the evidence, both at the level of involved tissues and in the patients' serum, seems to indicate the predominance of a T_H2 over a T_H1 environment (198,224,358,359).

The former, characterized by high levels of IL-4, IL-6, and IL-10, is geared to provide help to B cells and favors B-cell growth (360). In particular, IL-6 is a B-cell growth factor; suppresses natural killer (NK) cell cytotoxicity; promotes the EBV lytic cycle, increasing the number of infected cells; and promotes neovascularization, helping local tumor growth (356,361). IL-10, produced by EBV-infected cells, promotes proliferation and differentiation of B cells and inhibits T_H1 cytokines (202,356). The T_H1 environment, characterized by high levels of IFN-γ and IL-2, provides help for cytotoxic T cells and NK cells (360). In particular, IL-2 is the main autocrine factor for T cells and stimulates growth and cytotoxic activity of NK cells. IFN-α is the first cytokine released by B and NK cells, in response to EBV infection and favors the production of T_H1 cytokines (357). As Faro states about EBV infection, "EBV induces B cells to secrete cytokines that produce an environment that the virus can thrive in, a T_H2 environment. The immune system's response is for T cells to release IL-2 and IFN-γ and NK cells to release IFN-α and establish a T_H1 environment that will allow CTLs and NK cells to thrive and successfully combat the virus" (357).

An alteration of this equilibrium, expressed in an imbalance of circulating cytokines that favors B-cell proliferation, has been demonstrated in many studies of patients with PT-LPD. These show an increase in serum levels of IL-4 (358,362), IL-6 (363,364), and IL-10 (202,363), as well as a decrease of serum levels of IL-2 (362) and IFN-α (358). Similar findings have been reported in the tissues involved by PT-LPDs. In an evaluation by semiquantitave RT-PCR, a pattern of increased mRNA expression of IL-4 and IL-10 and decreased expression of IFN-γ and IL-2 was found in these tissues that was not detected in tissues of transplant recipients without LPDs or normal lymph nodes (359). That pattern was also present in the normal spleen of one patient with PT-LPD, indicating a systemic phenomenon, and it disappeared, in two patients, with resolution of their PT-LPD (359). In a later study (296) using the same technique, IFN-γ and another lymphokine, IL-18 (known to promote the expression of IFN-γ) were found significantly reduced in the tissues of PT-LPD compared with lymphoid tissues of patients with IM, suggesting again that T_H1 factors important in an effective response to EBV are missing in PT-LPDs. In this study, however, the level of expression of IL-10 was actually decreased as compared with tissues of IM.

Clinical Presentation and Course

The clinical heterogeneity of PT-LPDs is as great as their pathologic heterogeneity, largely because of the type and degree of immunosuppression and partially because of the organ grafted. At one extreme, the development of LPD can be clinically so subtle that, in approximately 8% to 14% of cases in organ transplant recipients (193,195,365) and in an even greater proportion of BMT recipients (20% to 53%) (211,214–217), it might go clinically unrecognized and the diagnosis could be made only at autopsy.

The interval between transplantation and diagnosis of PT-LPD in organ transplant recipients varies widely in different studies. For all transplants in general and for each organ, the interval is always shorter in patients treated with CSA or FK506 than in those treated with conventional immunosuppression with AZT (224,366–368). In a review of older studies, LPDs developed 23 to 32 months from transplantation of different organs (368). With modern regimens, those in renal, heart and liver transplantation develop at medians of 1.5 to 17 months (193,197,230) and at even shorter intervals (medians of 2 to 5 months) in lung or heart/lung transplantation. In renal transplant recipients treated with conventional immune suppression at the University of Minnesota, two primary clinical groups were identified (355) in relation to the time of occurrence. In one, at a short interval after transplantation or anti-rejection therapy (mean, 9 months) young patients (mean, 21 years) manifested an IM-like syndrome. In the other group, at a longer interval from transplantation (mean, 5.3 years), older patients (mean, 47 years), developed localized extranodal tumor masses, most of them fatal. Several more studies in the CSA era correlated early or late onset of PT-LPD with clinical presentation, although with contradictory findings (203,204,249).

Five somewhat distinct clinical patterns can be observed in adult and pediatric organ transplant recipients. One is the IM-like picture (208,264,267,355,369) that is most common in young patients (369,370). Also common is the presentation with one or several localized tumor masses in one or more organs (i.e., lymph nodes or extranodal, including the allograft) (193,208,209,223,224,267,298,370). Third, disseminated involvement can be seen at presentation, soon associated with multiorgan failure and often with multiple opportunistic infections (208,209,224,370). In other cases, the predominant or exclusive signs and symptoms are those pointing to allograft dysfunction (274,371,372). There remains a group of patients in whom PT-LPD has presented with persistent fever, malaise, leukopenia, without any localizing signs or symptoms (223).

The heterogeneity of the clinical picture of PT-LPDs is further compounded by the variety of sites involved by the process. Isolated involvement of the lymph nodes is seen less commonly than in usual lymphomas (16% to 27%) (194,249). One or more extranodal sites usually are involved; the most common sites are the lungs (193,194,247, 249,298), gastrointestinal tract (193,224,249,373), and liver (193). The incidence of CNS involvement (24% to 27%) in some studies (193,194,374) is similar to that of 28% quoted for the era before CSA (223). Involvement of the allograft overall is found in approximately 20% of PT-LPDs (230), but the figures given vary for different allografts: from 0% to 16% in cardiac (204,298) to 80% to 100% in lung transplantation (198,204,365). Bone marrow was considered to be negative in all cases (298) or involved in only 14% of the patients with PT-LPD in one study (194). In another series, however, lymphoid aggregates or simply clusters of plasma cells were found in 54% of patients with PT-LPD, but not in organ transplant patients without PT-LPD (250).

Despite great progress in treatment, PT-LPDs are still a serious complication of transplantation, with variable survival rates in different series, from 21% (194) up to 63% (193,209,247,249,298). The mortality rate for LPD (rather than for surgical complications or infections) varies from 19% to 21% in two series of patients with different types of organ transplants (247,298) to 36% in a series of pediatric heart-lung transplants (209).

The LPDs in bone marrow transplant recipients are distinctly different clinically from those that arise in solid organ transplantation (211,213–217,303,345). First, they develop very early after transplantation; the median intervals reported are between 52 and 101 days (213–217,303,345) and correspond to the period of defective T-cell function from the beginning of engraftment (30 days after transplantation) to 6 to 8 months after BMT (218,375). Second, most LPDs (211,214–217) manifest as disseminated disease with early and rapid organ dysfunction (215,303), although some may manifest with IM-like illness (216,217) or tumor masses (214,216,217) or may be clinically subtle enough as to be detected only at postmortem. In contrast to the organ distribution observed in organ transplantation LPDs, the "lymphoreticular system" (lymph nodes, spleen and liver) is involved predominantly (71% to 82%, 64% to 71%, and 86% to 93%, respectively) and extranodal organs less commonly (303,345). These PT-LPDs are distinct in their rapid clinical course and high mortality rate (213–217,376). Overall survival was dismal in most series (8% to 12.5%) (213–216), except for one study of patients treated with anti-B-cell monoclonal antibody, 35% of whom were alive at one year (303).

A detailed discussion of the many different therapies employed in patients with PT-LPDs and evaluation of their efficacy is beyond the scope of this chapter. A brief review, however, is important insofar as it helps shed light on the nature of these disorders. The treatment strategy has dramatically changed with the demonstration, by the Pittsburgh group, that some PT-LPDs are reversible with reduction of immunosuppression (191) or, as shown later by others, with other methods of boosting the patients' immune response. Reduction of immunosuppression (RIS) is recognized almost universally as the first step in treating organ transplant LPDs, although the complete response rate varied from 31% (247) up to 75% to 83% (202,232,238,377,378) in different series. This approach, however, is usually ineffective in recipients of BMT (222). Surgery, with or without RIS, has a definite role in resectable lesions (249,298,370,379), as does radiation therapy in unresectable limited lesions (202,238, 247,298,370,379). There are conflicting views in the literature about the efficacy of antiviral agents in PT-LPDs (380), but they are commonly used, alone (286,320) or in combination with RIS (202,232,238,249,286,370,379) to prevent additional B cells from being infected (202,224,320). Standard antineoplastic chemotherapy has not been successful in some series, producing a complete response rate of only 28% to 33% (194,247) and being associated with high mortality (193). It is, however, widely considered the appropriate treatment for patients who have failed other approaches (247,298,370,379,381) or for those with multiple myeloma/ monomorphic lymphoma (247) and late onset, monomorphic monoclonal lesions (224). The findings summarized here seem to have fostered a wide consensus for a sequential approach to the treatment of organ transplant LPDs (224,232,247,298,379), which in its most detailed form proposes the following order: RIS with surgery or radiotherapy of localized lesions; IFN-α; and systemic chemotherapy (298,379).

In addition to these classic therapies, newer exciting ones have been proposed. Some aim at reducing the proliferation of EBV-infected cells, such as gene therapy with modified EBV vectors that target these cells (382,383) or anti-B-cell monoclonal antibodies (anti-CD21 and anti-CD24). The latter have been used in three French studies of PT-LPDs (193,303,345) and are considered an approach of special promise for LPDs developing in BMT recipients (241,377). Other strategies (222) have focused instead on boosting the patients' immune response to the EBV-infected cells. In an attempt to restore the imbalance of circulating cytokines (high levels of IL-4 and low levels of IFN-α), which favors B-cell proliferation, administration of IFN-α has been proposed (358,384) and used in several studies (357) of organ and bone marrow PT-LPDs. To favor a T_H1 microenvironment that facilitates the cytotoxic response, the use of anti-IL-4 or anti-IL-6 has been advocated (241,359). Arguably the most promising immunomodulatory approach, so far tested only in BMT-LPDs, is adoptive immunotherapy (or prophylaxis) with infusion of donor unprimed or EBV-specific cytotoxic T cells (375,385–387).

Clinicopathologic Correlations

The striking heterogeneity of PT-LPDs at all levels (histologic, immunophenotypic, genomic, EBV expression patterns) presents pathologists with the difficult challenge of determining which pathologic features are relevant in helping oncologists with the treatment of these patients. In reviewing the literature, as well as in dealing with a specific patient's disease, it is important to consider the variations in any pathologic parameters that are common at different sites of involvement; in either situation, the evaluation of the disease based on a single lesion "may lead to failure to assess accurately the pathobiologic nature and clinical aggressiveness of the patient's disease" and helps explain, in part, the lack of correlation between pathologic parameters and outcome in some cases (388).

In the original Pittsburgh series, there was no correlation between the histologic subdivision of the lesions into minimally polymorphic, polymorphic and monomorphic and response to therapy (195). However, in our latest experience at this institution, there was a striking correlation between histologic and clinical aggressiveness, with a mortality rate of 0% for PH, 13% for polymorphic lesions, and 67% for monomorphic tumors (247). Correlation of molecular clonality of the PT-LPD and outcome is considered poor (195,303). Other genomic changes, however, have been shown to be important in predicting outcome. Abnormalities of oncogenes and tumor suppressor genes are poor prognostic factors (245,247,299). The presence of *NRAS* or *TP53* gene mutations or *MYC* gene rearrangement was associated with 67% mortality (247), and *BCL6* gene mutations were correlated with shorter survival and refractoriness to therapy (245).

Among clinical parameters, the extent of disease at presentation (localized versus disseminated) has long been recognized as an important prognostic factor in PT-LPD; localization to a single organ is associated with a good prognosis (366,368), and mortality is higher for patients with disseminated disease (249,377). The correlation of time of onset of the PT-LPD with outcome is a disputed issue. Although in most studies late-onset PT-LPDs have a worse prognosis than those of early onset (193,204,249,355,368,389), the difference, when evaluated statistically, is not significant (193,249).

Correlating this wealth and variety of pathologic and clinical features with outcome to provide meaningful categorization to guide oncologists in the management of PT-LPDs has proven difficult. However, one picture is emerging that may begin clarifying some of this complexity. The Pittsburgh group has proposed the existence of three categories in this continuum: nonclonal polymorphic lesions that regress with RIS; polymorphic lesions with different clonality patterns (i.e., polyclonal, oligoclonal, or monoclonal), which have different responses to RIS, perhaps depending on the strength of the clonal bands; and monomorphic monoclonal lesions with *MYC* gene rearrangement, which showed progression despite RIS (299). A similar, but more complex, pathologic categorization has resulted from studies at this institution (Table 16.7), that correlates well with clinical behavior. Three groups of lesions are recognized in it: PHs are nearly always polyclonal and contain multiple EBV infection events or only a minor cell population infected by a single form of EBV and lack alterations of oncogenes or tumor suppressor genes (e.g., (*MYC*, *BCL6*, *NRAS*, *TP53*); polymorphic lesions (PBCH and PBCL) are nearly always monoclonal, usually contain a single form of EBV, and lack alterations of oncogenes or tumor suppressor genes (except for *BCL6* mutations, detected in one half of them); and monomorphic lymphomas or multiple myeloma, which are monoclonal, contain a single form of EBV, and show alterations of oncogenes or tumor suppressor genes (266,313). Clinically, PH corresponds to a localized (stage I) lesion, usually in the tonsils and lymph nodes of younger patients; it is controlled by RIS or surgical excision, without any fatality in this series (247). At the opposite extreme, monomorphic lymphoma/multiple myeloma are disseminated lesions (stages III and IV) that develop in older people, do not respond to RIS and respond poorly to medical treatment, and are associated with a high mortality. The polymorphic lesions remain a somewhat heterogeneous category presenting at different sites and in different stages and have a relatively unpredictable clinical course. In this last group, the detection of the wild or mutant type of *BCL6* gene may be able to separate those patients who respond to RIS or surgical excision from those who require aggressive medical treatment (245,388).

Pathogenesis

It has been said that PT-LPDs "straddle the borderland between infection and neoplasia" (224) and evidence has been presented throughout this section indicating that EBV infection of B cells is the starting point, that the proliferation of the infected cells is not controlled by an inefficient immune response, and that genomic changes may occur within such proliferations that give rise to *bona fide* neoplasms.

The role of EBV in these disorders, suspected initially on the basis of clinical and serologic evidence of primary or secondary EBV infection (390,391) and increased oropharyngeal shedding of the virus in transplant recipients (392–394), was proven by the immunohistochemical demonstration of EBNA in PT-LPDs (185) and by EBV-DNA hybridization studies (188) and confirmed by a wealth of molecular and immunohistochemical data that have been al-

TABLE 16.7. *Posttransplantation lymphoproliferative disorders: relation of pathologic parameters with response to reduced immunosuppression*

Pathologic parameter	PH	PBCH/L	IBL/MM
Involved sites	Oropharynx or lymph nodes	Lymph nodes or extranodal	Disseminated
Immunoglobulin genes	Polyclonal	Monoclonal	Monoclonal
Oncogene or tumor suppressor gene alterations	No	No	Yes
Response to RIS	Regress	Mostly regress	Progress

PH, plasmacytic hyperplasia; PBCH/L, polymorphic B-cell hyperplasia/lymphoma; IBL/MM, immunoblastic lymphoma/multiple myeloma; RIS, reduced immunosuppression.

From Knowles DM, Cesarman E, Chadburn A, et al. Correlative morphologic and molecular genetic analysis demonstrates three distinct categories of posttransplantation lymphoproliferative disorders. *Blood* 1995;85:552–565.

ready discussed. EBV is a potent polyclonal stimulator of B-cell proliferation (395). To summarize some exhaustive reviews (396–399), several genes are required for such proliferation *in vitro,* that act at different points of the cell cycle: EBNA-2, EBNA-3A, EBNA-3C, and LMP-1 (398). LMP-1, in particular, has been shown to be oncogenic in rodent fibroblasts (356) and in LMP-1 transgenic mice (400). LMP-1 acts as a constitutively activated membrane receptor (398) and, by direct interaction with TNF-receptor–associated factor (TRAF), mediates activation of the nuclear factor (NF)-κB transcription factor and so promotes cell growth (356,396). Such direct interaction has been demonstrated in PT-LPDs (306). Other mechanisms of LMP-1 transformation include the upregulation of other cellular genes, such as the *BCL2* gene and its viral lytic cycle homologue (i.e., BHRF-1) (397), resulting in prevention of apoptosis (397), and of the genes of lymphokines (e.g., IL-1, IL-2, IL-6, IL-10) and chemokines (i.e., IL-8, IP-10, MIG), supporting B-cell growth in an autocrine fashion (222,356). In addition to this ''transforming'' role, LMP-1 has ''immunomodulating'' properties. It upregulates cellular adhesion molecules (i.e., ICAM-1, LFA-1, and LFA-3) and activation markers (i.e., CD21, CD23, and CD40), which promote B-cell growth (396,397). All these factors create a T_H2 type of environment which initially favors B-cell growth (357).

This proliferation, however, is tightly regulated in the normal host by a complex set of immune mechanisms, both cellular and humoral, the latter including neutralizing and nonneutralizing antibodies to virally encoded proteins which results in the typical serologic pattern of IM (223). There is an MCH-unrestricted response that creates a T_H1 type of environment (i.e., IL-2 and IFN-γ), resulting in autocrine stimulation of the T cells and in the growth and enhanced cytolytic function of NK cells (357,375). There follows the main, MHC class I–restricted cytotoxic T-lymphocyte (CTL) response (401). With the exception of EBNA-1, all other latent proteins elicit an HLA-restricted response (397), but the immunodominant target antigens are EBNA-3A, EBNA-3B, EBNA-3C (312,399), and EBNA-2 (397). ''The precise target antigen choice is clearly influenced by the host HLA class I haplotype,'' each of which recognizes and targets preferentially different epitopes (397). In IM, the CTL response is reflected in the predominance of $CD8^+$ cells in both tissues (263,402) and peripheral blood (''atypical lymphocytosis''), where they have been shown to be oligoclonal (402). In conclusion, in the normal host, the EBV's attempt to survive, producing a T_H2 type of environment favorable to the proliferation of infected B cells, is defeated by a T_H1 type immune response (357). The infected cells that display a latency III pattern (LMP-1^+, EBNA-2^+, EBNA-3^+) are recognized and lysed by EBV-specific CTLs, and in more than 90% of adults worldwide, a latent infection follows characterized by a small subset of B cells which only display a latency I pattern, silent to EBV-specific CTLs (223,312,397). These resting memory cells might be reactivated should the individual's immune status change.

In recipients of organ transplants, the virus to host equilibrium is shifted in favor of EBV, initially and largely because of the immunosuppressive regimens used to facilitate acceptance of the graft. In a follow-up of EBV-seropositive heart transplant recipients, it was shown that in the 6 months after cardiothoracic transplantation there is a complete loss of EBV-specific CTLs and an increase in circulating EBV^+ lymphocytes, and that both of these parameters return to normal after that period (346). The number of circulating infected cells is high in pretransplantation seropositive patients, higher still in seronegative patients, and highest in those who develop PT-LPD (222,237,403). In contrast to the tissues of IM, in those of PT-LPDs, $CD4^+$ cells predominate, which can inappropriately stimulate B-cell growth (263), and no $CD56^+$ NK cells are detected (296). The studies of cytokines in patients with PT-LPDs all demonstrate the predominance of a T_H2 type of environment (IL-4^+, IL-6^+, IL-10^+) favoring B-cell growth, and a decrease of those factors (IFN-α, IFN-γ, IL-2) which antagonize it.

The role of each immunosuppressive drug in the different facets of these immune abnormalities is not always clear (224). Glucocorticoids inhibit lymphocyte proliferation and downregulate the production of IL-1 and IL-2 (224). Patients treated with AZT and prednisone lack EBV-specific cytotoxic T-cell function (404) and manifest a decrease in the number of NK effector cells (405). Monoclonal antibody OKT3 strongly reduces the number of circulating $CD3^+$ cells (406) and has been shown to block the cytotoxic T-cell killing of EBV-transformed lymphocytes *in vitro* (407). Although CSA has a pleiotropic effect on the immune response (408), its major role in the pathogenesis of PT-LPDs is probably in the inhibition of T-cell responses by a block of antigen-induced IL-2 gene activation (361). It promotes the secretion of IL-6 by T cells and macrophages and of IL-13 (409), favoring EBV-driven B-cell proliferation, and activates the lytic cycle in EBV-infected cells (361,410). Like CSA, FK506 interferes with the activation of T cells (224).

The pathogenetic factors operative in the development of LPDs in BMT recipients are in part similar to and in part different from those discussed for solid organ PT-LPDs (222,375). As in solid organ recipients, an increased EBV load is associated with an increased risk of post-BMT-LPD (222,411), and these processes develop when CTLs are insufficient, such as during the first 6 months after transplantation (215,218,222,375). Specific to BMT recipients, most PT-LPDs arise from donor infected B cells, and B-cell depletion of the graft has been shown to be essential in reducing the risk of LPDs (222). T-cell depletion of the graft also is an important factor; the emerging cells in the recipients may not be effective because of prolonged deficits in IL-2 production (375). Mismatched BM graft or GVHD may cause a chronic antigenic stimulation of B cells and perhaps lead to the activation of other viruses, such as human herpes virus (HHV)-6, which may interact with EBV (216,217).

Because the pathogenetic mechanisms of EBV infection

and immunosuppression are operative in all transplant recipients, different combinations of contributing factors may be relevant in different patients and help explain why PT-LPDs develop only in a minority of them. It is widely accepted that the type of conditioning regimen and the degree of immunosuppression obtained in each patient is of paramount importance. A primary EBV infection after transplantation (versus reactivation infection) was discussed as a major risk factor for the development of LPDs. The route of this infection (e.g., aspiration of oropharyngeal secretions in heart-lung transplant recipients) (412) or the abundance of EBV-infected cells in the epithelium and lymphoid tissue of the grafted lung (346) that infect host B cells may account for the 80% to 100% incidence of PT-LPDs arising in the graft (198,204,365). An additional state of immunodeficiency in the host, which is genetically determined (210,213) or the result of CMV infection (223,238), increases the risk of PT-LPD. Because the host HLA class I haplotype influences the normal response to EBV, it may also explain a diverse response to EBV-infected cells in different individuals and different propensities for the development of PT-LPDs (397).

What has been discussed up to this point are the reasons for the alterations of the normal host: virus equilibrium and the uncontrolled proliferation of EBV-infected B cells that ensues in PT-LPD. This proliferation is heterogeneous and includes populations of cells "differing in their level of permissiveness for EBV gene expression . . . . It is at this step that immunologic parameters (produced by the immunosuppressive regimens used) are critical and will determine the selective advantage *in vivo*" of different B-cell populations (224,304). Extreme immunosuppression allows the emergence of populations of B cells with unrestricted EBV-antigen expression (latency type III), whose growth is driven by the transforming properties of EBNA-2 and LMP-1. In contrast, a residual efficient immune response in the transplant recipient may favor the growth of B-cell populations that downregulate EBNA-2 and LMP-1 (latency type I) and so escape recognition by the host CTLs, a situation similar to that of Burkitt's lymphoma (413,414). In this second situation, the proliferative advantage depends, as in Burkitt's lymphoma, on a different mechanism, the acquisition of genomic alterations of oncogenes (e.g., *BCL6, MYC, NRAS*) or tumor suppressor genes (i.e., *TP53*), which parallels the propensity for EBNA-2 and LMP-1 expression to diminish with the progression from polyclonal lesions to monomorphic lymphoma (312). These EBV immunologically silent clones are not responsive to immunomodulation (247,266). This scenario, now supported by many (224,266,312,397), is concordant with the one proposed by the Minnesota group (355) and concludes that some PT-LPDs, independent of their clonal status, should be regarded as an exaggerated response to EBV infection and treated as such, while others are true neoplasms capable of autonomous growth (388).

Posttransplantation T-Cell Lymphomas

Although uncommon, a total of 62 cases of posttransplantation T-cell lymphoma have been reported in the literature (193,194,248,251,415–429) and have been the subject of several reviews (415,416,425,426). With the exception of three cases observed in BMT (430), they all developed in organ transplant recipients, and span the entire spectrum of these disorders in the general population: peripheral T-cell lymphoma (26 cases), NK cell lymphoma/leukemia (16 cases), $\gamma\delta$ lymphoid proliferations (6 cases), cutaneous T-cell lymphoma (5 cases), lymphoblastic lymphoma (5 cases), adult T-cell lymphoma/leukemia (2 cases), and (one case each) enteropathy-associated T-cell lymphoma (431) and intravascular large cell lymphoma (416).

The first and most numerous group, peripheral T-cell lymphoma, includes a variety of histologic types, most frequently reported as large cell or "diffuse, mixed cell." Of 18 cases in which the information was provided half were EBV^+ and half were EBV^-. The lymphomas presented equally in males and females, and in a wide range of ages (2 to 67 years; median, 42 years). The patients were overwhelmingly recipients of kidney, rather than heart or other organs (16, 6, and 4 cases, respectively), and were diagnosed with lymphoma at intervals of days to 221 months (median, 60 months) from transplantation. The interval was shorter in patients with EBV^- than EBV^+ lesions (medians of 35 and 69 months, respectively). The most common presentation was with involvement of multiple organs (9 cases) or with localized tumor in the small or large intestine (5 cases). Seventy-six per cent of the patients died in a matter of days or a few months (1 to 12; median, 3 months) from diagnosis. The longest survivals (19, 24, and 48 months) were in patients with an unspecified lymphoma of the brain (432), a $CD30^+$ anaplastic large cell lymphoma localized to the colon (433), and an unspecified EBV^+ lymphoma of the lung (434), respectively. As suggested by others (426), there might be a relation between EBV status of the LPD and survival, because all patients with EBV^- lesions died (in days or a few months, except for one death at 138 months), whereas 4 (44%) of 9 patients with EBV^+ lesions were alive (4 to 48 months), and 5 died (days to 7 months).

The next most common category is represented by NK cell proliferations (419–421,425,427,428). Of these, only two are of true NK cell type: one that presented as an EBV^- renal allograft tumor 8 years after transplantation (425) and another that had otherwise all features of a hepatosplenic $\gamma\delta$ T-cell lymphoma but showed no evidence of T-cell receptor gene rearrangement (421). The remaining cases fall into either of the two classic categories of NK-like T-cell disorders. Four cases, which developed at various intervals from transplantation (4 to 132 months) and were all EBV^-, were clinically indolent, chronic T–large granular cell leukemias and all patients were alive 19 + to 36 + months after diagnosis (419,427). The other 10 (420,421,428) are disproportionately frequent examples of aggressive T–large granular cell lymphoma/leukemia (435), a rare type of neoplasm in the general population. They all developed late after transplantation (4 to 26 years; median, 15 years) and were equally EBV^+ or EBV^-, with no relationship between the EBV status of the tumor and the interval from transplantation. They developed in patients 31 to 64 years of age, mostly renal transplant recipients (6 of 10), and involved lung, bone marrow, peripheral blood, and uncommonly, the lymph nodes. The course was rapidly fatal in all, with survival of days to 20 months (median, 2.5 months). All tumors studied were monoclonal T-cell proliferations with a $CD3^+CD8^+CD56^+CD57^-$ phenotype.

The six cases of $\gamma\delta$ T-cell lymphoproliferation (417,418,422,423,429) developed 2 to 5 years after transplantation (all but one in kidney recipients) and all were EBV^-. They include classic hepatosplenic neoplasms (422,423) and others that primarily involved the spleen (417,418). Like those observed in the general population, they were aggressive disorders of clonally rearranged $\alpha\beta^-$, $\gamma\delta^+$ T cells, with the $CD4^-CD8^-CD56^+$ or $CD4^-CD8^+CD56^+$ phenotype, and two showed the classic cytogenetic changes of hepatosplenic $\gamma\delta$ T-cell lymphoma, isochrome 7q, and trisomy 8 (422,423). Unusual features, however, were the very young age of one patient (a 5-year-old child in whom an EBV^- hepatosplenic $\gamma\delta$ T-cell lymphoma developed four months after an EBV-related atypical LPD in a tonsil) (423); the association with HHV-6 in one case (429); and in four cases, the high-grade cytology of the proliferation, which was described as intermediate to large cell (418,423), medium-sized undifferentiated blast cell (422), or immunoblastic (417).

The primary cutaneous PT T-cell lymphomas (436–438), exclusive of two HTLV-1–positive cases (439,440), developed at variable intervals from transplantation (1.5 to 11 years) in men 52 to 86 years of age, who were all renal graft recipients. The neoplasms manifested with localized or disseminated disease (Sezary syndrome), the latter associated with very short survivals. The only case in which this information was available was EBV^-. The five lymphoblastic lymphomas (415,430,441) developed at various intervals (21 to 120 months) from renal (three cases) or bone marrow (two cases) transplantation and, in the three cases in which the information is available, were all EBV^-. Clinical presentation and immunophenotypic characteristics were no different from those observed in the general population. In the four cases with follow-up, survival was short (1 to 28 months).

Posttransplantation Hodgkin's Lymphoma

The definition and the very existence of HL as a complication of transplantation are still disputed. Atypical mononuclear and multinucleated cells resembling Reed-Sternberg cells are common in PT-LPDs (189,291,442). Like those observed in IM (443), they are a form of activated B cells that, in addition to leukocyte common antigen (LCA) and B-cell antigens, express CD30, but not CD15 (291,442). Characteristically, also, they contain EBV and consistently coexpress LMP-1 and BCL-2 (291,442). In several reported cases, they are clearly monoclonal by analysis of the immunoglobulin genes and EBV termini (256,444,445). For all of these reasons, these cells are thought to differ from true Reed-Sternberg cells and processes in which they are observed have been referred to by several investigators as Hodgkin's disease–like lymphomas, rather than true HL (243,248,444,445).

However, as in the case of Reed-Sternberg cells developing in the context of chronic lymphocytic leukemia (which are EBV^+) (446,447), also in reported cases of PT-LPD there appears to be a spectrum of immunophenotypic expressions by Reed-Sternberg–like cells, with intermediate stages showing progressive loss of LCA and B-cell markers and acquisition of CD15 and a final null, $CD15^+$, and $CD30^+$ phenotype classic of HL. This phenomenon has a parallel in the ''modulation'' of antigen expression described in HL, in which the loss of CD20 and the acquisition of CD15 were found to be related to the presence of neutrophils and eosinophils (448). Although a ''transformation'' from B-cell PT-LPD to true HL may be hypothesized and has been reported in the same patient several times (248,444,449,450), it is still unclear where the line between the two is to be drawn in this spectrum. In addition to the immunophenotypic characteristics, other features have been reported that may help distinguish HL from B-cell PT-LPDs within this spectrum. These include a background of small lymphocytes and increased fibrosis (444,445); the presence of neutrophils and eosinophils, which are uncommon in PT-LPDs (291); and in the liver, the presence of Reed-Sternberg cells in the sinusoids (444); the predominant or exclusive localization of EBER to the Reed-Sternberg cells (rather than its diffuse expression by immunoblasts) (444,445); and the lack of coexpression of LMP-1 and BCL-2 by the Reed-Sternberg–like cells (291,442).

Given the uncertainties in the definition of HL arising in transplant recipients, many literature cases reported as such, but without an immunophenotypic support of this diagnosis, cannot be evaluated (202,249,251,451–457). Among organ transplant recipients, there are 11 immunohistochemically documented cases of HL (449,450,458–460). Proven cases represented an incidence of 0.13% of 2267 organ transplant recipients studied in one institution (459). In these cases, the neoplastic cells expressed CD15 and CD30 and, in the cases so evaluated, were $CD45^-$ (6 of 6) and B- and T-cell antigen negative (4 of 4). Nine of 11 cases were EBV^+ and expressed LMP-1 and EBER but not (in one case) EBNA-2 (460). All these patients were males, and their ages at diagnosis of HL were between 6 and 47 years (median, 26). These were recipients of kidney (7), heart (2), or liver (2) transplants, treated usually with triple immunosuppressive regimens. The HL developed late after transplantation (26 to 88 months; median, 60 years), with the exception of an unusual case diagnosed as lymphocyte predominance in the grafted kidney 9 months PT (458). The disease presented equally in early or advanced stage, with or without symptoms, and was localized consistently (with the exception mentioned) in lymph nodes, as in classic HL. All patients responded well to standard HL therapy, and all are alive in complete remission 9 to 72 months (median, 12) after diagnosis, except for a patient who died at 7 months of "iatrogenic complications" (459). In contrast to the data from the Cincinnati Transplant Tumor Registry (461), which suggests a disseminated presentation, and literature data (449) suggesting a high frequency of systemic symptoms, advanced-stage disease, and extranodal involvement, these patients have a clinical presentation and response to therapy that is similar to that observed in HL arising in immunocompetent patients (449,459). This behavior is also in striking contrast to that of HL developing in HIV$^+$ patients (462).

There are three reports of HL developing in allogeneic BMT recipients, for a total of 10 cases (210,463,464), of which only one is documented by immunohistochemistry (463). In the study from the International BMT Registry describing eight such cases (464), the incidence was higher than expected in the general population (observed/expected ratio of 6.2), amounting to an increased risk of 1.6 cases per 10.000 person-years, with both values similar to those arrived at in a series from the University of Minnesota (210). These cases were classified as mixed cellularity (5), nodular sclerosis (2) or lymphocyte depletion (1) and 5 of 6 were EBV$^+$. The disease developed late PT (2.9 to 9.1 years; median, 4.2 years), and the patient had a good response to therapy and outcome. In addition to their late onset, these cases also differed from B-cell PT-LPDs because they were not associated with the established risk factors of T-cell depletion and HLA disparity (464).

Epstein-Barr Virus–Negative Posttransplantation Lymphoproliferative Disorders

EBV is not detected in a variable percentage (3% to 32%) of B-cell PT-LPDs. These EBV$^-$ cases are described in sparse case reports (343,465,466), and were specifically studied in two large series, from Pittsburgh (243,467) and from Paris, France (256). In both series, in which they represented, respectively, 8% and 28.5% of all B-cell PT-LPDs occurring in adults, it is suggested that they may represent a distinct entity. They are mainly characterized by their occurrence at long intervals from transplantation; the range is 38 to 146 months in the former series and 6 to 115 months in the latter (after excluding cases of T-cell lymphoma and multiple myeloma), and the medians are 62 and 30 months, respectively. With the increasing experience in the management of PT-LPDs and the longer survivals obtained, the incidence of EBV$^-$ lesions appears to be increasing with time (243,256). Extranodal involvement was present in 71% of the EBV$^-$ compared with 100% of the EBV$^+$ cases (256). Reduction of immunosuppression failed to prevent disease progression in one series (256), but was successful in some cases of the other series (243). In the former, most patients were treated with aggressive chemotherapy and died of complications (256); in the latter, 86% of patients (only half of whom underwent chemotherapy) were alive (at 7 to 28 months) (467). Histologically, EBV$^-$ cases were all (256) or largely (67%) (467) monomorphic (343,465,466), rather than polymorphic lesions. Despite this common histologic feature, the clinical findings suggest that, rather than being a distinct entity, the EBV$^-$ PT-LPDs may be heterogeneous. Some appear similar to the usual EBV$^+$ cases, and others behave as conventional lymphomas in the immunocompetent patients (243) and could represent sporadic lymphomas developing independently of immunosuppression (224,312). Different and multiple causes may be at play in different cases; chronic antigenic stimulation and deficient immune surveillance may produce mutations in critical genes (256), or alternative viral causes can be considered (346), such as HHV-8 documented in two patients with PT-primary effusion lymphoma (466,468).

Among the less common forms of PT-LPDs (i.e., PTCL, NK-like T-cell lymphomas, plasmacytic neoplasms, and HD-like proliferations), the incidence of EBV$^-$ cases varies. They are as common as the EBV positive cases in most of these forms, except for the NK-like T-cell chronic disorders and the $\gamma\delta$ T-cell proliferations, all reported cases of which were EBV$^-$, and the HLs, of which instead only a minority (18%) was EBV$^-$. There appears to be no relationship between the EBV$^-$ status and late development PT, or vice versa. The median interval was shorter for the EBV$^-$ than the EBV$^+$ cases of PTCL, and most of the HL, a typically "late" complication, were EBV$^+$. However, all $\gamma\delta$ T-cell proliferations were EBV$^-$ and late occurrences.

MULTICENTRIC CASTLEMAN'S DISEASE: INTERLEUKIN-6 SYNDROME

Background and Definition

Three different disorders are usually incorporated under the term of *Castleman's disease* (CD) (i.e., *giant or angiofollicular lymph node hyperplasia*). The disease originally described by Castleman and colleagues (469) consisted of a localized lymph node hyperplasia characterized by abnormal follicles, with small germinal centers simulating the Hassall corpuscles of the thymus, and marked capillary proliferation. Later, another lesion was reported, characterized by hyperplastic germinal centers, abundant plasma cells in the interfollicular areas, persistence of sinuses, and associated systemic clinical and laboratory changes (470–472). The two lesions were combined as variants—hyaline-vascular (HV) and plasma cell (PC) —of one disease, although the only common denominator mentioned was that "numerous lymph follicles were present in all cases" (472). A third disorder, with histologic features similar to those of this composite CD but with more extensive lymphadenopathy and systemic clinical manifestations (e.g., B symptoms, increased levels of acute-phase reactants, hypergammaglobulinemia, autoimmune manifestations), was originally described by Leibetseder and Thurner in 1973 (473) and by Gaba and associates in 1978 (474) and then reported in the literature under various terms: *multicentric angiofollicular lymphoid hyperplasia* (475), *angiofollicular and plasmacytic polyadenopathy* (476), *systemic lymphoproliferative disorder with morphologic features of Castleman's disease* (CD) (44,477), *idiopathic plasmacytic lymphadenopathy with polyclonal hypergammaglobulinemia* (478), *plasma cell dyscrasia* (479,480), *lymphogranulomatosis X with excessive plasmacytosis* (20), and most commonly, *multicentric CD* (MCD).

From additional experience, the HV form of CD appears to be a well-defined entity, whose diagnosis is independent of clinical findings and totally reliant on a characteristic histopathologic triad of abnormal hypervascular follicles, with one or more atrophic germinal centers; hypervascular interfollicular lymphoid tissue; and absence of sinuses within the lesion (481). In contrast, the nodal histologic changes of the PC variant in its localized and multicentric expressions are similar to those of a nonspecific nodal reaction (44,482); the differences, if any, are purely quantitative (483). The clinical and laboratory manifestations of this disorder are common to many inflammatory and lymphoproliferative disorders. It is therefore not surprising that a clinicopathologic complex similar to that described in MCD has been reported in many different clinical situations (482) (Table 16.8), making CD one of the most ubiquitous associations in the literature. Several lines of evidence strongly suggest that these clinicopathologic similarities are mediated by a common mechanism—the overproduction of IL-6, probably in association with other cytokines—that occurs (484) in all of these situations. What is commonly referred to as MCD should more correctly be indicated as IL-6 syndrome or, when referring specifically to its pathologic changes, as IL-6 lymphadenopathy (LNA).

Within this large and heterogeneous category, it is useful to separate cases that are associated with or ''secondary'' to other diseases (Table 16.9) to identify a distinct, autonomous disease (''primary'' MCD) and try to determine its pathologic and clinical characteristics and its cause. A solid description of such disease emerges from cases reported in six series in the literature (475,477,485–488), as well as in numerous case reports (489). These fit a combined clinicopathologic definition that includes the following criteria (477,489): histopathology of CD, usually the PC type; predominantly lymphadenopathic disease, consistently involving multiple sites; and exclusion of associated diseases. Evidence suggests that, in a subset of patients, ''primary'' MCD is related to the Kaposi's sarcoma–associated human herpesvirus (KSHV/HHV-8), joining KS and primary effusion lymphoma (PEL) as disorders directly caused by HHV-8 (490). The genome of this virus contains a gene homologue of the human IL-6 gene (491) and this protein (rather than, or in concert with, human IL-6) may account for the clinicopathologic manifestations of IL-6 syndrome in these patients.

TABLE 16.8. *Disorders associated with the histology or the clinicopathologic complex of interleukin–6 syndrome*

Autoimmune diseases
Rheumatoid arthritis (564)
Sjögren's syndrome (565)
Systemic lupus erythematosus
Mixed connective tissue disease (566)
Human immunodeficiency virus (HIV) infection (633–641)
Human herpes virus (HHV)-8 infection (176,177,501,525, 544,546–548)
Kaposi's sarcoma (177,475,477,500,525,541,581,642–644, 646,647,682)
Plasma cell dyscrasias, especially the POEMS syndrome (480,499,614,648,649,651,654–656,658–662)
Other neoplasms, especially Hodgkin's lymphoma (502, 524,630,671–678)
Others: primary immunodeficiencies, glomerulopathy, skin diseases (482)

TABLE 16.9. *Forms of interleukin-6 syndrome*

Primary
Non-HHV-8–related
HHV-8–related
Secondary[a]
In HIV infection (with or without KS)
In Kaposi's sarcoma
In plasma cell dyscrasias
In malignant lymphomas
In autoimmune diseases
In other clinical situations

HHV, human herpesvirus; HIV, human immunodeficiency virus; KS, Kaposi's sarcoma.
[a] May be related to HHV-8.

Histopathologic Features

The histologic findings of ''MCD'' in lymph nodes are in most cases similar to those described in localized CD-type PC, and include relative preservation of the nodal architecture, abundance and prominent alterations of the germinal centers, and marked plasmacytic infiltration. The first feature is frequently emphasized by the dilatation of the sinuses, which are filled with hyperchromatic lymph (44,476,480, 483,492). The germinal centers are numerous, giving the process a distinctly follicular pattern (Fig. 16.12). Although some show the usual hyperplastic features, with sharp borders and minimal vascularity, most are markedly abnormal. They may show poorly defined borders, increased vascularity, decreased number of follicular center cells, and prominence of paler, eosinophilic cells that represent follicular dendritic cells and histiocytes. Other germinal centers are small, penetrated by several vessels, frequently with hyaline walls, and constituted predominantly by pale eosinophilic cells (Fig. 16.13) that may be surrounded by concentric (i.e., ''onion skin'') layers of lymphocytes. The latter alterations

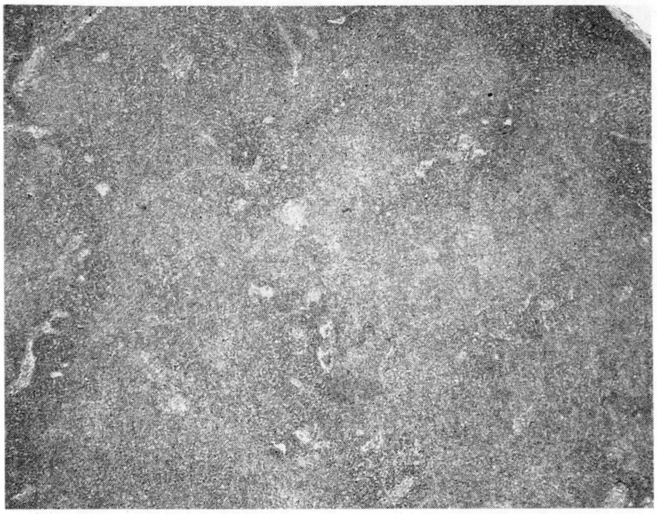

FIG. 16.12. Multicentric Castleman's disease. The pattern is follicular, and much of the nodal architecture is preserved (hematoxylin and eosin stain, original magnification: 30× magnification).

have been reported under such terms as *epithelioid* (493), *HV* (472), *burned-out* (17,18), *regressively transformed* (41), or *angiosclerotic germinal centers* (480). One group has described as a consistent feature within the germinal centers the presence of large, multilobated, dystrophic follicular dendritic cells (494); however, these, in our experience, are only common in the HV form of CD (481,495). The interfollicular tissue shows a prominent infiltration of plasma cells.

One can see variations on this basic theme. In some of the cases, there is an abundance of high endothelial venules, and the plasma cells are associated with immature forms and immunoblasts, as well as many mitoses (Fig. 16.14A). In these cases, a "starry-sky" pattern is quite common, with contracted, miniature plasma cells lying free or within the cytoplasm of macrophages. In other instances, there is little or no evidence of increased vascularity, plasma cell immaturity, immunoblasts, or mitoses (Fig. 16.14B). By examining multiple biopsies in the same patients, we demonstrated that these two patterns are successive phases, proliferative and accumulative, in the evolution of the same process (44). Other patterns that we observed at one time or another in our patients before or after a nodal biopsy with one of the more characteristic histologic features are a nonspecific reactive hyperplasia or a burned-out stage, with abundant hyaline-vascular germinal centers, interfollicular sclerotic blood vessels, and a minor component of plasma cells. This last aspect of the disorder may be easily misinterpreted as a HV or "mixed" form of CD if the persistence of the normal architecture, in particular of the sinuses, is overlooked. We tend to believe that most or all of the cases of MCD of the HV or mixed type reported in the literature, especially those associated with the clinical syndrome characteristic of this disorder (475,483,494,496–502), are cases of the PC type caught in a burned-out phase. A new variant of MCD has been described by the term *plasmablastic* (503); it is characterized by the presence of medium-sized to large plasmablastic cells scattered in the mantle zones of the follicles. This variant is linked to HHV-8 (503).

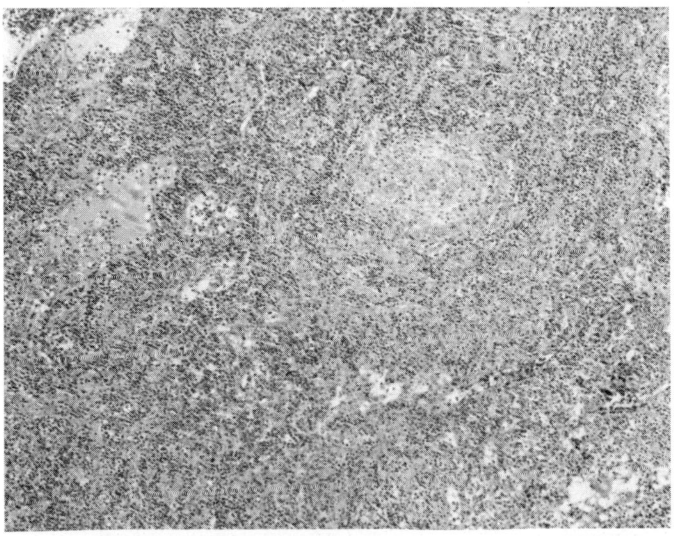

FIG. 16.13. Multicentric Castleman's disease. Hyaline-vascular germinal center and diffuse interfollicular plasmacytosis (hematoxylin and eosin stain, original magnification: 75× magnification).

The separation of MCD from other atypical lymphoid hyperplasias that manifest with marked plasmacytosis in the lymph nodes can be difficult. Cases of MCD with abundant vascularity and immunoblasts (proliferative pattern) may simulate AIL (17); they differ from it because of the follicular pattern, the abundance of abnormal germinal centers (rare in AIL) and the diffuse dense plasmacytosis (not a feature of AIL). Similar cases may also resemble plasmacytic sarcomatosis (11) or systemic polyclonal immunoblastic proliferation (47,48). However, this entity is distinguished histopathologically by a near total effacement of the nodal architecture by B immunoblasts and mature and immature plasma cells and by a paucity of germinal centers and high endothelial venules. It also typically features marked plasmacytosis of blood and bone marrow, prominent autoimmune phenomena, and a rapid response to steroids. An MCD with a proliferative pattern may need to be distinguished from a lymphoplasmacytoid lymphoma with abundant large cells (polymorphic immunocytoma) (504). The latter usually obliterates the nodal architecture and is not accompanied by prominent vascularization, and its predominant cell type is lymphoplasmacytoid rather than the mature plasma cell. The morphologic distinction of MCD with an accumulative pattern from nodal plasmacytoma is based on the even interplay of follicular and plasma cellular components in the former or on the displacement of the follicles and disruption of the nodal architecture by and possibly the cytologic atypia of the plasma cell component in the latter. In difficult cases, determination of Ig light-chain restriction may be necessary.

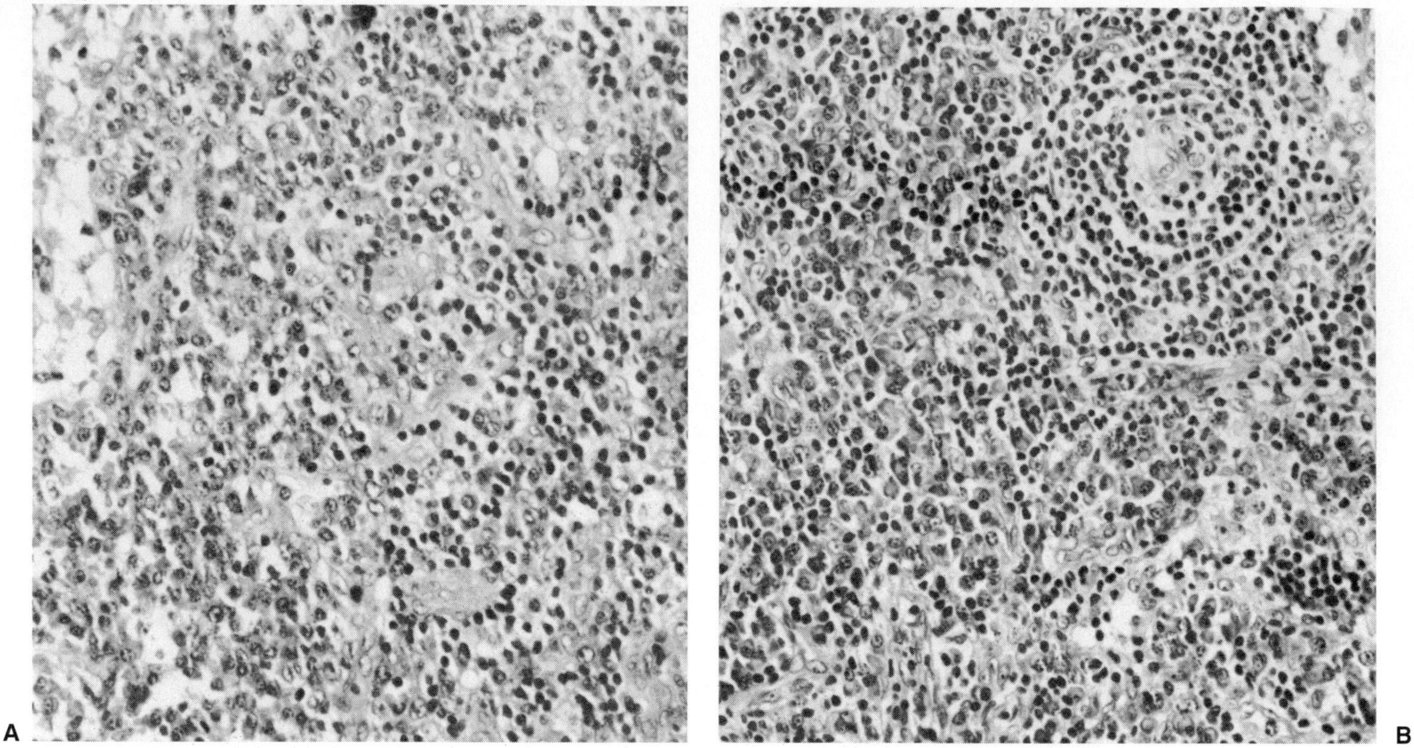

FIG. 16.14. Multicentric Castleman's disease. **A:** "Proliferative" pattern, with abundant blood vessels and immunoblasts. **B:** "Accumulative" pattern, with inconspicuous vascularity and mature plasma cells (hematoxylin and eosin stain, original magnification: 300× magnification).

The extranodal pathology of MCD is also nonspecific and, as for AIL, does not permit in our opinion a definitive diagnosis of this disorder because similar changes can be seen in other inflammatory conditions and ALPs (44). We and others have observed variable abnormalities in the spleen of germinal centers and prominent plasmacytosis; fibrosis, hemosiderin deposits, and lymphoid depletion of the periarteriolar lymphoid sheaths; increased reticulin formation and accumulation of plasma cells in the marginal zones; and foci of plasma cells in the red pulp, especially in the paratrabecular areas (44,505). Bone marrow biopsies may show focal infiltrates of plasma cells and, in the lung, thickening of the alveolar walls, because of diffuse infiltration by immunoblasts, plasma cells, and fibroblasts was seen in one case (44). In Japanese case reports (506,507) and a series of cases (508) the changes in the lung biopsies were those of lymphocytic interstitial pneumonia and included a lymphocytic and plasma cellular infiltrate around the bronchioles and in the interlobular septa and adjacent alveolar septa. One case interpreted as MCD in a child showed an enlarged thymus with an increase in HV germinal centers, plasma cells and medullary epithelium (509). There are occasional reports in the literature of a disorder characterized by multiple reddish brown skin nodules, associated (510–512) or not (513,514) with CD-like lymphadenopathy (LNA) and laboratory abnormalities; based on the presence of hyperplastic follicles and intervening increased vascularity and plasmacytosis, these cases too have been interpreted as MCD or idiopathic plasmacytic lymphadenopathy with polyclonal hypergammaglobulinemia (478).

Immunophenotypic, Genotypic, and Cytogenetic Findings

The immunohistochemical findings in the lymph node lesions of MCD are similar to those described in the localized form of CD. The peripheral areas of the abnormal follicles are composed of small B cells that express the phenotype of mantle zone lymphocytes (515). However, in contrast to normal mantle cells, these lymphocytes have been shown to be $CD5^+$ (515) and Ki-B3/$CD45RA^-$ and to preferentially express λ light chain, a phenotype corresponding to that of a normal small lymphocyte subset in mice referred to as Ly-1 sister B lymphocytes (494). The central regions of the follicles display an abundance of follicular dendritic cells associated with sparse T cells (515,516). The dendritic cell network, in our experience, but not in others' (492), is irregular, with intermingled tighter and looser areas, and without the distinction that exists in normal germinal centers between a dark and a light zone (44). The germinal centers have been said to show a decreased proliferation rate with the Ki-S5 antibody and decreased numbers of macrophages with CD68 (494) and the stains for factor VIII–related antigen and *Ulex europaeus*-1 lectin demonstrate an abundance of blood ves-

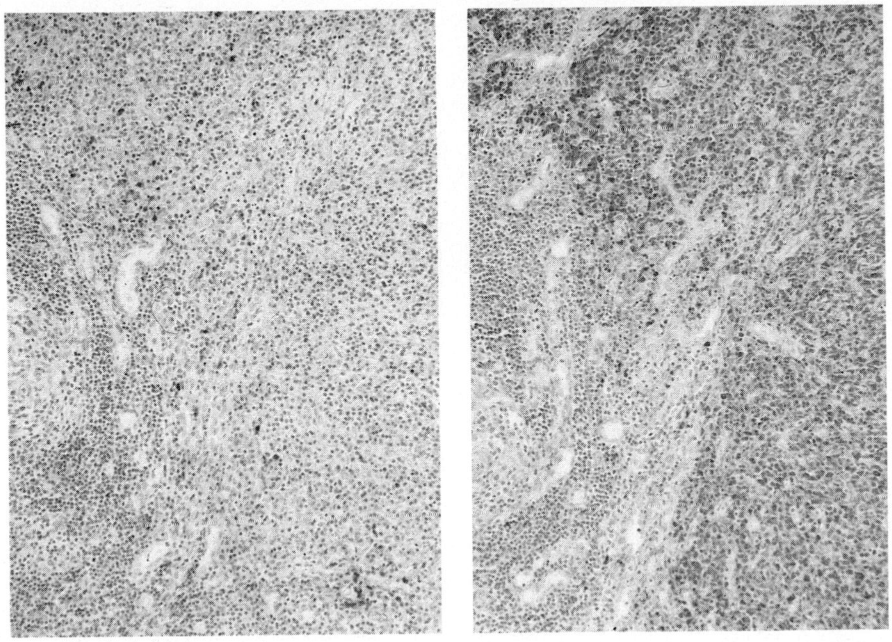

FIG. 16.15. Multicentric Castleman's disease. In two serial sections a focus of plasma cells that bear λ **(B)** but not κ **(A)**, immunoglobulin (Ig) light chains is seen within a polyclonal background (immunoperoxidase stain, original magnification: 120× magnification).

sels (515). We and others (505,517,518) have found no abnormality of the ratio of $CD4^+$ to $CD8^+$ cells in the follicles. However, the abnormal germinal centers lack the characteristic T-cell zoning (515) and any number of $CD57^+$ (Leu-7) cells (515,517).

The interfollicular tissue contains T-cell subsets in normal proportions (515,517,518) and a predominant population of plasma cells, which in most cases is polyclonal. Several reports in the literature, however, have documented within this polyclonal proliferation the development of a monoclonal plasma cell component, diffusely replacing the interfollicular areas or forming recognizable nodules (480,494,502,515, 519–522) (Fig. 16.15). These focal proliferations were mostly of IgGλ or IgAλ type and were often associated with a serum paraprotein. The phenomenon of a clonal plasma cell proliferation that arises within lymph node lesions with the morphology of CD, PC type, is particularly common (29%) in the cases associated with the POEMS (polyneuropathy, organomegaly, endocrinopathy, M proteins, skin lesions) syndrome (480). It has been stated several times that the presence of such a monoclonal component does not predict a worse survival (494,520,522).

Molecular genetic analysis of the antigen receptor genes in MCD has been done only in a small number of cases (502,515,518,521–523). A clonal rearrangement of the Ig heavy-chain gene was detected in 8 of 24 cases (33%) studied by Southern blotting and in 1 of 14 cases (7%) studied by PCR (excluding those associated with a lymphoma or osteosclerotic myeloma). One band on a polyclonal background (502,518) can also be present. In a study of PC-type CD, including unicentric and multicentric cases, 21% showed monoclonal Ig heavy-chain rearrangement by PCR, as did 36% of those of the HV type (494). This latter finding, when compared with the absence of such rearrangement in 8 cases of localized HV-type CD evaluated by Southern blotting in two other studies (502,518), supports our contention that cases diagnosed as MCD of the HV type may be burned-out PC lesions. A minor T-cell clone, mostly on a polyclonal background, was reported in 6 (25%) of 24 specimens studied by Southern blotting, and in one of our cases, it was associated with clonal rearrangements of the Ig heavy- and light-chain genes (518) (Fig. 16.16). Molecular techniques have occasionally detected EBV in the tissues of MCD, in 2 of 6 cases by Southern blotting (518,521) and in 2 of 8 cases by ISH for EBER (524,525), arguing for the irrelevance of this virus in the pathogenesis of the disease. Two reports have described cytogenetic abnormalities in MCD: ins(1)(1pter→1cen::?::1cen→1qter) in one case (521) and t(7;14)(p22;q22) (526) in another. The latter case is particularly interesting because the patient had high IL-6 serum levels, a phenomenon that was thought perhaps to be related to the involvement of the IL-6 gene, located at 7p21-22 (526).

Interleukin-6 and Human Herpesvirus-8 Studies

A role for IL-6 in CD was first suggested by Yoshizaki and colleagues in 1989 (527), who reported an increase in serum levels of this lymphokine in two such cases, one localized, the other multicentric, and the disappearance of all symptoms and laboratory abnormalities after the excision of a lymph node in the former, but not in the latter. This finding

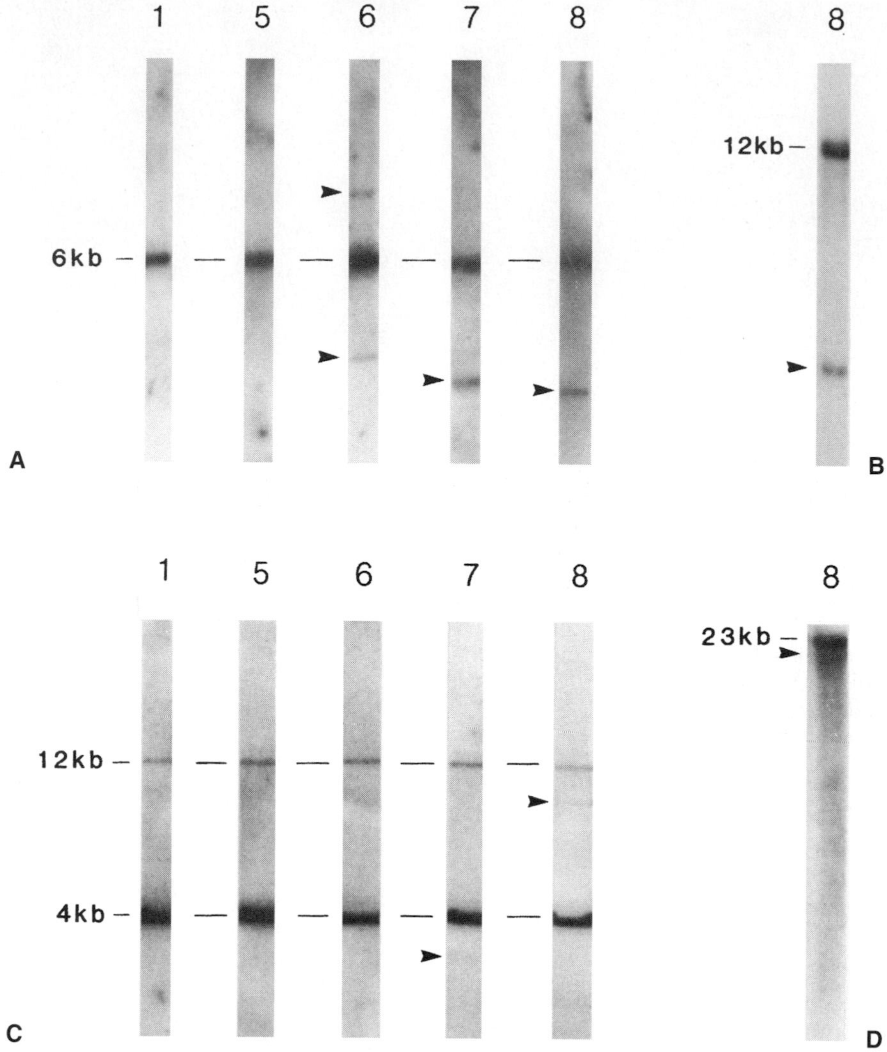

FIG. 16.16. Multicentric Castleman's disease. Southern blot hybridization analysis of immunoglobulin (Ig) and T-cell receptor-β (TCR-β) genes in DNA extracted from lymph nodes of four patients (numbers 5 through 8). **A:** Selected analysis of DNA samples with the heavy-chain joining region (JH) probe after digestion with *Bam*H1 and *Hin*dIII restriction enzymes. **B:** DNA analysis after *Bam*H1 digestion and hybridization with the κ light-chain probe. **C** and **D**: Selected DNA analysis with the TCR-β chain gene probe and digestion with *Eco*R1 and *Bam*H1, respectively. The 7.2-kb rearranged band in case 8 **(C)** is a smaller fragment than the 8- to 9-kb fragment occasionally seen with *Eco*R1 digestions. Restriction fragments characteristic of the germline configuration are denoted by dashes along with the size in kilobases. Arrows denote rearranged bands. (From Hanson CA, Frizzera G, Patton DF, et al. Clonal rearrangement for immunoglobulin and T-cell receptor genes in systemic Castleman's disease: association with Epstein-Barr virus. *Am J Pathol* 1988;131:84–91, with permission.)

has been confirmed many times (528–539). It was also shown that cultured cells from the involved tissues produce human (hu) IL-6 (527,530), but the distribution of such cells as determined by immunohistochemistry or mRNA ISH is somewhat disputed. Hu-IL-6–positive cells have been detected by some in MCD (530,531,535) and the PC type in general (525,527,529) but only in localized PC-type CD associated with symptoms and not in localized PC-type CD without symptoms or in MCD by others (540); in the HV type by some (525) but not by others (529); and in normal controls by some (525,540) but not others (527). The positive cells have been found in the germinal centers and considered to be germinal center cells (527,529,535) or follicular dendritic cells (525,540), as well as sparsely in the marginal zone (531) and in the interfollicular areas (525, ,529–531,540), and interpreted as immunoblasts (529,535), macrophages (530,540) or other cells (interdigitating, lymphoid, endothelial) (540). Viral v-IL-6–producing cells have been detected by immunohistochemistry (503,525,541, 542), mRNA-ISH (543) or reverse-transcriptase PCR (544) in cases of CD associated with HHV-8. These cells are located in the mantle zone, where they represent a minority

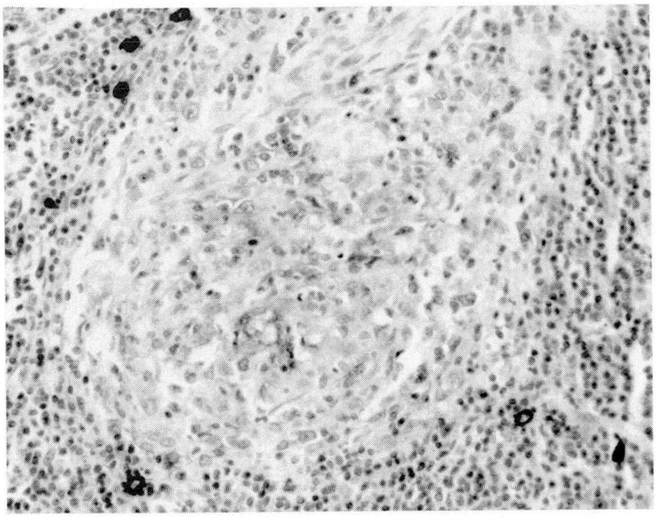

FIG. 16.17. Multicentric Castleman's disease. Numerous plasmacytoid cells in the mantle zone strongly express viral interleukin-6 (IL-6) (immunoperoxidase stain, original magnification: 250× magnification).

of the resident cells (503,525,541–543) (Fig. 16.17). They have the appearance of large plasmacytoid cells (503,541,542), which in one study did not express CD20, CD3, CD45RO, CD30, CD68, or EMA (525) and in another corresponded to λ-bearing plasma cells, rarely to CD3$^+$ cells, or often were negative for B- or T-cell antigens (543). Other HHV-8 genes, homologous to human cyclin D, BCL-2, and IL-8 receptor genes, were also found expressed in one case of MCD by reverse transcriptase PCR (545).

Genomic sequences of HHV-8 have been detected in lymph nodes and spleen with MCD by several groups (176,177,501,525,544,546–548). HHV-8 was also detected by PCR and ISH in a lung biopsy showing lymphocytic interstitial pneumonia in one case of MCD (506). HHV-8 has also been detected by PCR in peripheral blood mononuclear cells of HIV$^-$, KS$^-$ (549), and HIV$^+$ MCD (550,551). The infected cells were B and T lymphocytes (549) and the viral DNA load appeared to vary in parallel with the clinical activity of the disease (551). Once, according to the criteria proposed at the start of this section, one excludes those cases that were associated with KS and other diseases, 16 of 34 cases of ''primary'' MCD (47%) contained, in their tissues or peripheral blood mononuclear cells, HHV-8 sequences by PCR. This is in contrast to 7% of non-CD-like reactive lymph nodes so studied (176,177,541,547,552,553).

The morphology and localization of HHV-8–infected cells, in a study of HIV$^+$ ''MCD'' that used a monoclonal antibody to a latent nuclear antigen of the virus (548), are very much like those of the v-IL-6$^+$ cells mentioned in other studies of HIV$^-$ MCD (503,525,541,542). They had immunoblastic features and were found in small number in the mantle zone of follicles. They were CD20$^+$ and CD79a$^-$ and negative for T-cell and activation antigens (548). In another study (543), using mRNA-ISH for the latent or lytic gene TO.7 and the lytic gene nut-1, the signal for these viral antigens colocalized in the same few cells that contained high copy level of v-IL-6 and corresponded, as mentioned, to λ-bearing plasma cells, rare CD3$^+$ cells or cells negative for B- or T-cell markers (543). From these combined studies, it is apparent that, in a proportion of cases of MCD, mantle zone B cells are latently infected by HHV-8 and may produce v-IL-6. Whether all of these cases correspond histologically to the ''plasmablastic variant'' (503) remains to be determined.

TABLE 16.10. *Main clinical findings in 44 patients with primary interleukin-6 syndrome*

Findings	Patients (%)
Symptoms	98
Lymphadenopathy	100
Peripheral	100
Abdominal	33
Mediastinal	9.5
Splenomegaly	69
Hepatomegaly	54
Edema or effusions	23
Rash	20
Neurologic changes	11

Data from references 475, 477, 485, 487, and 683.

Clinical Findings

The clinical characteristics of ''primary'' MCD have been well defined by numerous case reports (489) and by six series (475,477,485–488). The data from the latter, totalling 44 cases, are the basis for the following summary (Tables 16.10, 16.11). This is a disease of older age groups (range, 19 to 85 years; median, 55.5 years), and affects more often male than female individuals (1.4:1). Only rare cases has been reported in children (509,531,554), which have been reviewed elsewhere (555); some of these are possibly MCD-like manifestations in the context of primary immunodeficiencies. The disease presents with systemic symptoms and multiple lymphadenopathies, consistently at peripheral sites. Involvement of deeper nodal regions is uncommon at presentation, although it occurs with increasing frequency with

TABLE 16.11. *Main laboratory findings in 44 patients with primary interleukin-6 syndrome*

Findings	Patients (%)
Elevated erythrocyte sedimentation rate	90
Anemia	88
Hyper-γ-globulinemia	82
Hypoalbuminemia	67
Thrombocytopenia	62.5
Proteinuria	16

Data from references 475, 477, 485, 487, and 683.

progression of the disease (477). Hepatomegaly and splenomegaly are quite common. Skin manifestations include unspecified rashes, as well as a host of other nonspecific changes (556). In the East, the disease has been associated rarely with characteristic multiple violaceous nodules, histologically represented by dermal plasma cell infiltration (510–512), and more recently, skin lesions with an unusual histology (i.e., glomeruloid hemangioma) have been described in a few patients (557,558).

Neurologic manifestations are relatively uncommon in MCD as defined previously. In our review of 44 cases, they were mentioned only in 5 cases and included undefined CNS changes (477,485), persistent seizures (475), and peripheral neuropathy (475,488). Other isolated cases of peripheral neuropathy, usually of sensory-motor type, have been reported (474,519,559) and reviewed (559), along with a small, interesting series describing peripheral neuropathy and pseudotumor cerebri (560). Particularly these last cases raise the issue of the overlapping of MCD and the POEMS syndrome (561), to be discussed later.

A wide variety of rheumatologic symptoms and signs can accompany MCD. They include arthralgia and myalgia, joint effusions, keratoconjunctivitis sicca, xerostomia, and Raynaud's phenomenon (475–477,562). It may be difficult to distinguish MCD from an autoimmune disease (563). These overlaps have been reported as an association of MCD with rheumatoid arthritis (564), Sjögren's syndrome (565), or mixed connective tissue disease (566); as MCD presenting with findings of an autoimmune disease (562,563,567); or as an autoimmune disease (SLE) presenting with histopathologic features of MCD (568). In our own series, we used as criteria favoring MCD the predominance of lymphoproliferative over autoimmune phenomena (44) and that the pattern of clinical and serologic findings is insufficient to permit the definitive diagnosis of a rheumatologic entity (569).

The most common laboratory findings are listed in Table 16.11 and indicate the involvement of multiple systems in this disorder. Anemia is found in most patients and is often autoimmune in origin (475–477,570–574). Thrombocytopenia is common and again may be autoimmune in type (570). The bone marrow often shows mild plasmacytosis. Erythrocyte sedimentation rate is often elevated, as is gammaglobulinemia, which is usually polyclonal, although monoclonal gammopathy at presentation (519) or developing on a polyclonal background (485) has also been reported. Antinuclear antibodies, rheumatoid factor, inhibitors of factors VII and VIII, and cryoglobulins have been reported in these 44 cases and other literature cases, as well as anti-smooth muscle, anti-gastric, and anti-salivary gland antibodies (476,496); antiphospholipid antibodies (572); and cold agglutinins (474,575). Lymphocyte function studies have demonstrated various abnormalities, such as low numbers of T cells, inversion of the CD4:CD8 ratio, and T-cell unresponsiveness to mitogens (487,511,576,577), as well as cell-mediated immunodeficiency (577,578) and reduced NK cell activity (576). In a study of four HIV$^-$ patients with MCD, a set of alterations was found that was similar to those of AIDS (530). These included anergy (possibly because of a decreased expression of CD28 on T cells [579]), decreased IL-2 production, decreased T-cell colony formation, reduced numbers and activity of NK cells, an increased soluble IL-2 receptor, and a reduced CD4:CD8 ratio. Increased serum levels of IL-6 and other cytokines seems to be a consistent feature of these patients.

Renal dysfunction occurred relatively uncommonly in our review of 44 cases. Proteinuria is mentioned in 16% and hematuria in 7% of these cases, although these signs and evidence of renal insufficiency are also described in many single case reports (533,572,580,581–582). In cases in which a renal biopsy was obtained, the pathology was very heterogenous and included no specific abnormalities; membranous, mesangioproliferative, or membranoproliferative glomerulonephropathy patterns; interstitial nephritis (533, 572,581); and amyloidosis (583,584). There are rare reports of renal thrombotic microangiopathy, thought to result from autoantibodies (572) and, in two cases, from a unique combination of mesangial proliferation, plasma cell infiltration of the interstitium and negative immunofluorescence. This was attributed to the hyperproduction of IL-6, a known growth factor for mesangial cells, by the plasma cells (533).

Multicentric CD has been associated with a variety of syndromes. Amyloidosis is most common in localized CD. It may involve the lymphoid mass or single organs or be systemic in distribution, is characteristically of AA type (585–588), and is thought to be related to an excess of the acute-phase reactant, serum amyloid A (SAA), caused by hyperproduction of IL-6 (585,586,588). However, MCD also has been associated with amyloidosis, which was systemic (589), renal (583,584) or intestinal (590) and also of AA type (584,589,590). This appears to be a different situation from that of "MCD" associated with the POEMS syndrome and amyloidosis of AL (λ) type (591). Other reported associations include thrombotic thrombocytopenic purpura (575), myelofibrosis (580), pure red cell aplasia (584), γ-heavy-chain disease (592), vasculitis (475), pulmonary hyalinizing granuloma (593), myasthenia gravis (594), Behçet's disease (537), and peliosis hepatis (556,595).

Multicentric CD follows three possible patterns of clinical evolution: an aggressive, rapidly fatal course; a chronic course with sustained clinical manifestations; or one with recurrent exacerbations and remissions. These were seen in 18.5%, 37%, and 44.5%, respectively, of a total of 27 patients, for whom this information can be obtained (475, 477,487). Forty-five percent of 44 literature patients evaluated (once those with lymphomas or myeloproliferative disorder are excluded) died; infections were by far the most common cause of death (60%), and lymphoproliferative disorder was mentioned as the sole cause in 20% of patients. The overall median survival time in this series (excluding the patients that developed neoplastic complications) was 34 months. However, the median survival was 14 months for the patients who died and 46 + months for those who survived. In our series (477), we found that male gender, presence of enlarged mediastinal lymph nodes, and an episodic pattern of disease were the three clinical features that together best predicted a fatal outcome ($p = 0.002$). Only one morphologic feature (i.e., the finding of only the proliferative pattern in multiple biopsies) was associated significantly with fatal outcome ($p = 0.005$).

It is difficult to draw conclusions on the management of MCD from our data or those presented in the literature, given the multiplicity of treatments used, the variability of the clinical situations, and the difficulty of exactly defining response retrospectively (477,569). Most commonly, steroids alone or chemotherapy (with single or multiple agents) have been used. It appears that all treatment modalities were able to produce at least transient symptomatic improvement in some patients, including (in unique cases) surgery alone (i.e., splenectomy or excision of the main nodal mass) (477,574) and radiation therapy alone (487). Overall, steroids had apparently greater success than chemotherapy, with 69% of patients alive at the end of the study with the former compared with 36% with the latter approach. Death from infectious complications was equally frequent in patients treated with either approach. New treatments reported to have favorable response in MCD include IFN-γ (537,596), 2-chloro-deoxyadenosine (597), cimetidine (598), and autologous bone marrow transplantation in a refractory case (599). The systemic symptoms of the disease may be alleviated by the administration of monoclonal anti-human IL-6 (535,600).

From accrued experience, a stepwise strategy has been proposed (569). Some patients may have spontaneous remission or not require therapeutic intervention. Otherwise, corticosteroids might be employed as a first line treatment, as they appear to have less toxicity and can result in long-term remissions. Chemotherapy may need to be used in the steroid-refractory cases.

Pathogenesis

Much of the evidence presented points to an essential role for IL-6 in the pathogenesis of the pathologic and clinical manifestations that are often loosely referred to as MCD. In addition to the already mentioned high levels of IL-6, these patients' peripheral blood B cells have been shown to express higher density IL-6 receptors (CD126) and to be hyperresponsive to IL-6 (601). Treatment with an anti-IL-6 antibody in one patient with localized CD, PC type (535), and one (HIV^+) with MCD (600) lead to normalization of IL-6 serum levels and reversal of symptoms and laboratory abnormalities. Other supportive evidence for the role of IL-6 is experimental. In congenitally anemic mice, reconstitution with bone marrow cells transduced with a retroviral vector carrying the coding sequences of this cytokine produced clinical and pathologic changes similar to those of CD (602). Mice lacking a negative transcriptional regulator of IL-6, C/EBPβ, develop pathologic traits similar to MCD, including high levels of IL-6, and the simultaneous inactivation of IL-6 and the C/EBPβ genes, by the generation of a IL-6$-/-$, C/EBP$\beta-/-$ double mutant mouse, prevents the development of such traits (603,604). Local overexpression of IL-6 and IL-6 receptor genes, by introducing expression vectors in Wistar rats through the trachea, induces changes of lymphocytic interstitial pneumonia (605), as observed in a group of patients with MCD (508).

IL-6 is a pleiotropic lymphokine produced by various types of normal cells: B and T lymphocytes, monocytes/macrophages, fibroblasts, endothelial cells, epidermal keratinocytes, mesangial cells, and syncytiotrophoblasts (484, 606). Among other functions, it is an important factor in the terminal differentiation of activated B cells to plasma cells (601), stimulates myeloma cell growth *in vitro*, possibly through an antiapoptotic mechanism (607) and regulates T-cell activation (606). It stimulates hematopoiesis, and is a potent inducer of terminal macrophage differentiation and platelet differentiation. It is an endogenous pyrogen and stimulates the production of acute-phase reactants (C-reactive protein, fibrinogen, haptoglobin, etc) from hepatocytes, but inhibits the secretion of albumin (602,608). The production of IL-6 may explain many of the manifestations of MCD: the B-cell hyperreactivity and plasmacytosis in the lymphoid tissues; the presence of B symptoms; the elevated erythrocyte sedimentation rate, acute-phase reactants, and gammaglobulinemia; and the hypoalbuminemia. It does not, however, explain all manifestations of this disease, particularly the thrombocytopenia rather than the expected thrombocytosis, and it has been shown that, in addition to it (527,528,532,536,538,539,606), other factors are produced in excess in these patients: TNF-α (528,532), TNF-β (539), IFN-γ (539), macrophage colony-stimulating factor (M-CSF) (532), IL-1 (528), and vascular endothelial growth factor (VEGF) (609,610). These may act synergistically in inducing systemic manifestations (528,539) or have a pathogenetic role in other facets of the disease, such as VEGF in the angiogenesis observed in the lymph nodes of MCD patients (609,610) or perhaps in the development of the characteristic glomeruloid hemangioma (557).

IL-6 is thought to play a pathogenetic role in many disorders: autoimmune diseases (484,536,606), HIV infection (536,611), other infections (612,613), and plasma cell dyscrasias (484), including the POEMS syndrome (614). It is produced and has an autocrine effect on KS cells (615). No production of IL-6 in culture has been detected in a series of B-cell lymphomas, mostly low grade, in one study (616), but IL-6 production by ISH and immunohistochemistry was found in all 24 high grade B-cell lymphomas (most of them from HIV^+ patients), in another (617). Reed-Sternberg cells have been shown, by immunohistochemistry and molecular techniques, to produce IL-6 (618–622) and elevated serum levels of this cytokine are detected in more than one half of patients with Hodgkin's lymphoma (618). All of these are the disorders in which ''secondary'' MCD is so often described.

The origin of IL-6 overproduction in cases of "primary" MCD is an open issue, except for those related to HHV-8. The virus codes for a homologue of the human IL-6 (491,623) and v-IL-6 has been found in the same tissues in which HHV-8 was detected by PCR (525,543,544) and actually co-localized with the virus in the same mantle zone cells (543). This combination was reported in HIV$^-$ (525,544) and HIV$^+$ (543) patients. HHV-8 codes for a protein that has functional similarities to, but also some differences in structural and receptor binding properties from, human IL-6 (624); viral IL-6 mimics *in vitro* the effects of human IL-6 (600) and may serve as an autocrine growth factor in MCD, as it does in PEL (625,626). In this subgroup of patients, the clinicopathologic manifestations of MCD may be the result of an infection of the lymphoid tissue by HHV-8 and expression of v-IL-6, while lymphoid tissue HHV-8 infection per se is not associated with the histologic or the clinical features of MCD and may result in several other histologic patterns (176,177,501,552,627). Although this scenario is attractive, it may be premature or incomplete. In one HIV$^+$ patient with MCD, it was shown that hu-IL-6, not v-IL-6, was responsible for the systemic symptoms, because these were alleviated by neutralizing anti-hu-IL-6 monoclonal antibodies (600). HHV-8 may not necessarily act through viral homologues of human proteins, but by deregulating *in vivo* the production of human cytokines (600) or HHV-8–infected cells, it may also produce human cytokines, as observed *in vitro* with PEL cell lines, which released v-IL-6, hu-IL-6, and hu-IL-10 (626). Other HHV-8 genes may be at play. Viral-IL-6, v-cyclin-D, v-bcl-2, and v-IL-8 receptor genes were all found to be expressed in the case of MCD already mentioned, but only the first two were expressed in cases of florid follicular hyperplasia (545), suggesting that other genes may be essential to the MCD phenotype.

Although most of the pathologic and clinical manifestations of MCD can be accounted for by an excess of IL-6, other facets of this disorder remain to be explained. Autoimmune manifestations are quite frequent, sometimes making it difficult to separate it from a *bona fide* autoimmune disease. One explanation given for them centers on the antiapoptotic role of this lymphokine and proposes that the increased production of IL-6 in the germinal centers affects the normal elimination of B cells that "have undergone inappropriate Ig gene mutations," favoring the emergence of autoreactive clones (536). A somewhat different explanation emerges from the evidence discussed previously—that the lymphocytes of the abnormal lymphoid follicles of CD express CD5 (515) and lack Ki-B3/CD45RA, in contrast to the lymphocytes of the normal mantle zone (494,628), and have a propensity for rearranging the Ig λ chain gene. They may correspond to the long-lived memory B-cell subset Ly-1 in the mouse and the human CD5$^+$ subset, which naturally produce autoantibodies (629). These data complement those already discussed and suggests a general pathogenetic picture of MCD as a lymphoproliferation of a specific autoantibody-producing B-cell subset, driven by IL-6 and resulting in the sustained production and accumulation of plasma cells. This may explain the area of overlap between MCD and autoimmune diseases and supports the statement that MCD "should be considered an autoimmune disease with unremitting or progressive lymphadenopathy" (567).

There is some evidence that may implicate underlying abnormalities of immune regulation as an additional pathogenetic factor in MCD (477): the occurrence of the disease in older age groups, with senescent immune system; the high frequency of intercurrent infections; and the demonstration of abnormal lymphoid subsets and functions in some cases (see Clinical Findings section).

Secondary Multicentric Castleman's Disease

With this practical term, one can identify all the cases in which the clinicopathologic complex of MCD occurs in association with another well-recognized disease, such as HIV and other infections, specific autoimmune diseases, plasma cell dyscrasias, and Hodgkin's and non-Hodgkin's lymphoma. In none of these situations, we and others believe (475,477,482,486,569,630), the associated histologic or clinicopathologic complex deserves the term of MCD, because it does not represent a disease but rather is the identical end point of a cytokine environment (i.e., IL-6 syndrome). This term applies even less properly to CD-like features that may occur in lymph nodes in response to the most varied adjacent inflammatory and neoplastic lesions: lymphoid interstitial pneumonia (507), pulmonary hyalinizing granuloma (593), skin diseases, or glomerulopathy (482). These cases represent a paracrine effect of the IL-6 produced by the main disorder.

As in primary MCD, an infection by HHV-8 is the cause of a portion of the secondary MCD (Table 16.12). The presence of the virus has been documented in most cases associated with HIV infection or KS (501,503,546,548) and the POEMS syndrome (501,525,631,632). The contribution of the human or viral cytokine to the IL-6 syndrome in these cases (600) remains to be explored.

It is well established that, among the various histologic forms of HIV-related LNA, one manifests the "angiofollicular changes" (hyperplastic or hyaline-vascular germinal centers, hypervascular paracortex and plasmacytosis) considered characteristic of CD (633–641). This form accounted for 2% or less of the HIV-associated lymph nodes evaluated in three large series (636,638,641). This association (MCD and HIV infection) may represent "a distinct clinicopathologic entity that can be differentiated from other types of HIV-associated systemic lymphoproliferative disorders" (638). The clinical presentation and laboratory findings in these patients are very similar to those of MCD in HIV$^-$ patients, except for a younger age at presentation (median, 39 years), predominance of men (M:F of 19:1), a high prevalence (65%) of pulmonary symptoms (e.g., cough, dyspnea, interstitial infiltrates) and pancytopenia (35%), as well as a

TABLE 16.12. *Causes of interleukin-6 syndrome*

Disease forms	HHV-8(+) (%)	HHV-8(−) (%)
Primary	47	53
Secondary, associated with		
Kaposi's sarcoma	87.5	12.5
HIV infection and Kaposi's sarcoma	100	
HIV infection only	95.6	4.4
POEMS syndrome	90	10
Lymphoma		
Non-Hodgkin's	"Plasmablastic"	"Late" lymphomas
Hodgkin's		Paracrine IL-6 disease
Autoimmune disease	?	Most cases?

HHV-8, human herpesvirus-8; HIV, human immunodeficiency virus; POEMS, polyneuropathy, organomegaly, endocrinopathy, M proteins, and skin lesions;

stronger association with KS (75%). Mortality was found to be high (70%), with a median survival of 9.5 months in the entire series and 12.5 months among those who survived (638). However, this poor prognosis may result from the added KS (i.e., a "triple hit") rather than HIV infection alone. Considering only the reported cases of MCD in HIV^+ patients without KS, the mortality rate is 50% (503,550,638, 639), and considering only the HIV^- MCD with KS, the mortality rate is 81% (177,475,477,500,525,541,581, 642–647).

POEMS syndrome (648) is a multisystem disorder that is also referred to as Crow-Fukase's (649) or Takatsuki's (650) syndrome. It is characterized by the combination of peripheral polyneuropathy, organomegaly (i.e., lymphadenopathy and hepatosplenomegaly), endocrine abnormalities (i.e., diabetes mellitus, hypogonadism, and hypothyroidism), serum monoclonal peak (i.e., IgG or IgA λ) associated with various forms of plasma cell dyscrasia (but especially osteosclerotic myeloma), and skin lesions. It is generally accepted that the antitissue effects of Igs (651), especially anti-nerve antibodies (652,653), and one or more soluble factors produced by the plasma cells are responsible for most of such varied manifestations (654). Lymphadenopathy is a feature of 42% to 73% of patients with POEMS syndrome (614,649,654–656) and the nodal histologic findings are varied, including plasmacytoma, nonspecific abnormalities and even normal histology, but most often (63%) Castleman's-like changes (649,654). This last observation was first made by Japanese pathologists, who also found that 29% of these lymph nodes contain sheetlike or nodular accumulations of monoclonal plasma cells within a polyclonal background, blurring somewhat the distinction between MCD with a monoclonal component and nodal plasmacytoma (480). These observations were later confirmed in the West (499,648,651,657–662).

Along with the histologic nodal lesions of CD, patients with POEMS may present with clinical and laboratory features characteristic of MCD: weight loss, splenomegaly, edema and effusions, nephropathy, autoimmune manifestations (566,663), and cutaneous glomeruloid hemangiomas (661). In large series of POEMS patients, the incidence of the MCD clinicopathologic complex was 38% to 50% (614,631,632). In many POEMS patients (654), there is a serum increase of the same cytokines detected in MCD (566,614,662,664), more specifically, IL-6 and TNF-α in 67% and IL-1β in 93% of patients (614). Although it has been suggested that the activation of these proinflammatory cytokines, coupled with a decreased antagonistic reaction by TGF-β1, accounts for the manifestations of POEMS syndrome, it is most likely that IL-6 accounts rather for those of MCD: no IL-6 increase has been found in a series of POEMS patients without MCD (665).

There is a definite overlap between POEMS syndrome and MCD, which is explained by the production of IL-6 in a subset of POEMS patients. PCR has demonstrated that tissues from 90% of POEMS patients with MCD (501,525,632), but only 17% of those without MCD (632), contained DNA sequences of HHV-8. This evidence is strong enough to support the concept that a subset of patients with the POEMS syndrome (most of them with osteosclerotic myeloma) are associated with HHV-8 driven MCD (632). It has been suggested that in this subset of POEMS patients an immunodeficiency state or an unknown cofactor induces the reactivation of the virus latent in the lymphoid tissues, resulting in an increased systemic virus load, production of lymphokines and MCD (632). The pathogenesis of MCD in the remaining $HHV\text{-}8^-$ POEMS patients (15% [632] or 80% [631]) is unclear, but may involve human, rather than viral, IL-6 produced by the plasma cells.

Several types of neoplasms, in addition to those of the plasma cells discussed, occasionally are diagnosed in patients with CD of the localized or multicentric type. They appear to fall into different categories. Some have been discovered simultaneously and usually in close topographic association, with a LNA showing CD. These include cases of nonlymphoid tumors, such as rectal carcinoma (666), neurofibromatosis and pheochromocytoma (667), renal cell carcinoma (668) and a double carcinoma (thyroid and kidney) (669); non-Hodgkin's lymphoma (NHLs) of peripheral T-cell type (475,670); but, most commonly (a total of 30 cases), Hodgkin's lymphoma (HL) (502,524,630,671–678). A case of this type is illustrated in Fig. 16.12. The CD component is described as PC or HV in type and HL as interfollicular, nodular sclerosis, mixed cellularity, or rarely, lymphocyte predominance in type (630,675,677). The unanimous interpretation of the association of HL and CD is that the lesion of "CD" is a nonspecific pathologic finding (619,630, 672–676), the result of the production of cytokines by HL. Reed-Sternberg cells produce IL-6, and they express IL-6 receptors, suggesting that IL-6 is involved in the pathogenesis of HL by an autocrine or paracrine mechanism (618). This explanation may also be true for the NHLs, although their capability to produce IL-6 is more controversial (616,617) and has been offered in the cases of nonlymphoid tumors (667,668). This does not exclude the possibility that, for other patients in this first group, other explanations may apply, such as a coincidental occurrence (679,680) or the development of either disease on the basis of an immunodeficient state associated with the other (668,672,674–676,681).

A second group of neoplasms is represented by NHLs also reported to occur simultaneously with the clinicopathologic syndrome of "MCD" (640,644) or to develop rapidly (2 to 9 months) during its course (475,485,502,503), but represented by diffuse large cell lymphomas (475), immunoblastic lymphomas (638) and a specific variant referred to as "plasmablastic lymphomas" (503). These are composed of cells of medium size with amphophilic cytoplasm and prominent nucleoli and that express λ light chain. They may be similar to other cases reported as composed of "large primitive cells with prominent nucleoli" (640) or as lymphoplasmacytoid (485), which were also λ light chain restricted. Some of these plasmablastic lymphomas were shown to contain HHV-8 and were proposed as a new HHV-8–linked disease entity, au pair with KS, PEL, and some cases of MCD (503). Other cases in this second group were observed in HHV-8–infected patients (HIV$^+$ or HIV$^-$), who had KS (638,640,644) or HHV-8–positive MCD (501,502). In some patients with lymphomas detected simultaneously with or early in the development of MCD, both diseases may be etiologically related to HHV-8 (503).

A third group of neoplasms develop as a late complication of MCD and include rare cases of nonlymphoid neoplasms, such as carcinomas (477,681), myeloproliferative disorder and thymoma (475), and cases of NHLs. In our review of 44 cases of "primary" MCD, five patients developed NHLs (11%) (475,477,485,486), to which other rare single case reports can be added (483,494,513,544,578,681). These neoplasms occurred usually several years after the diagnosis of MCD and were classified as diffuse mixed or large cell. Only rarely is there any immunophenotypic (513), and in none genotypic, documentation of clonality and cell lineage. The pathogenesis of these lymphomas is unclear, and perhaps diverse. One such lymphoma was proven to be HHV-8–related (544). A coincidental occurrence of two diseases, development of both in an immunodeficient state, or the MCD to hu-IL-6 to lymphoma sequence may be considered as possible explanations for others.

SUMMARY AND CONCLUSIONS

Despite the various clinical situations in which they arise, the ALPDs described in this chapter manifest many pathologic similarities and a common thread in their pathogenesis.

The diagnosis of ALPD starts with the recognition of common histopathologic characteristics that, in most cases, allow their distinction from malignant lymphoma at the microscopic level. In my view, all ALPDs manifest all or most of the following features: an extensive disturbance of the nodal architecture that permits the recognition of some basic topographic markings of the lymph node (pseudo-obliterative pattern). The impression is produced that the LPDs evolve by expanding the architectural components of the lymph node rather than by destroying them, as malignant lymphomas with similar aggressiveness do; by a prominent interfollicular activation, caused by immunoblastic transformation; and by marked increase in vascularity. Although this is associated with high mitotic activity, as in lymphomas, there is little or no nuclear atypicality in the small and large transformed cells; and concurrent abnormalities of the germinal centers. The simultaneous involvement of the main functional compartments of the lymph node, cortex, and paracortex, suggests a physiologic response, albeit poorly regulated. This contrasts with the malignant lymphomas (except, of course, the follicular lymphomas), in which the germinal centers, if recognizable, are morphologically normal.

The immunophenotyping of ALPDs most commonly provides evidence of polyclonality or conflicting findings rather than definite evidence of monotypism, as in lymphoid malignancies. In the LPDs of B-cell type, the proliferation is most often polyclonal, or a monoclonal component may be evident within the polyclonal background. In AIL, the proliferation is polytypic (B and T cells, the latter with various ratios of CD4$^+$ to CD8$^+$ cells), as in a reactive process, but, in some cases, loss of pan-T-cell antigens may be observed, as in peripheral T-cell lymphomas.

In those ALPDs in which cytogenetic studies have been done, such as AIL-like lesions, a large background of normal mitotic cells has been detected, as well as the presence of nonclonal abnormalities or multiple unrelated clones. This contrasts with malignant lymphomas, which are characterized by a paucity of normal mitoses and the presence of clonal and related abnormalities.

The presence of one or multiple clones in association with a polyclonal background is also a common theme in gene rearrangement studies of ALPDs, such as those that occur in transplant recipients, AIL, and MCD. Multiple and faint rearrangement bands or a diffuse smearing are characteristic of these disorders, in contrast to the sharply defined and mostly single bands in malignant lymphomas.

Although the clinical presentation and settings may be different, these processes share in common an extensive involvement of lymphoid tissue and other organs (a reflection of the ubiquity of lymphoid cells), the frequency of systemic symptoms (evidence of a hyperactive cytokine environment) and often aggressive course, in some cases consistent with a medical emergency. A high prevalence of autoimmune phenomena is also shared by AIL-like lesions and MCD, which is accounted for by the commonality of an underlying dysfunction of immunoregulatory mechanisms in their pathogenesis. On this basis also, all of these ALPDs share a high frequency of intercurrent infections, which are a common cause of death. All of them appear responsive, in different degrees, to therapeutic interventions directed at restoring the patient's immune system.

In all the processes described in this chapter, a recurring theme is evident despite the differences in histologic and clinical findings. Rather than a sharp separation between purely reactive and definitely malignant lymphoid proliferations, there is a spectrum of lesions that represents all intermediate stages between these two extremes. The ALPDs are processes somehow intermediate between reactive, self-limited growths (hyperplasias) and autonomous, clonal proliferations (neoplasias). They are reactive in origin, but not properly downregulated by a defective immune system and therefore are prone to chromosomal errors. These lead to the emergence of one or more unrelated clones, some of which may develop into *bona fide* clinical malignancies.

However, the common pathogenetic factors that play a role in this evolution—abnormalities of immunoregulation, a resulting hyperactive lymphokine environment, stepwise genomic alterations, and activation of cellular and viral genes—have different relevance in different ALPDs and result in specific characteristics. In angioimmunoblastic proliferations, a variety of immunologic defects is central to the prominent autoimmune manifestations and intercurrent infections that characterize these ALPDs. In the predominant proliferation of mature $CD4^+$ T cells, characteristic chromosomal changes may occur (e.g., single-cell abnormalities, unrelated clones, +3, +5) that may lead to AITCL. However, molecular and cytogenetic regression has also been documented. In PT-LPDs, viral genes are pivotal in driving cell proliferation and in establishing a T_H2 lymphokine environment that favors B-cell growth. These proliferations evolve from polyclonal to monoclonal processes (plasmacytic hyperplasia, ''polymorphic'' B-cell lesions) that can regress with immune manipulation, to *bona fide* neoplasms (large B-cell lymphomas and multiple myeloma), which are characterized by additional genomic changes (e.g., *BCL6* and *TP53* mutations, *MYC* rearrangements) and have become unresponsive to immune manipulation. In MCD, the clinicopathologic findings are the result of IL-6 excess, which putatively acts on a $CD45RA^-$ mantle cell population, contributing to the development of autoimmune manifestations that are common in this disorder. The fact that IL-6 drives the lymphoid proliferation to plasma cell differentiation may explain why only focal monoclonal plasma cell lesions, rather than lymphomas, develop in this disease. However, in the subset of MCD (47% of patients studied), which is related to HHV-8, viral genes play the pivotal role; viral IL-6 accounts for the clinical and pathologic manifestations of the disease and other, still undefined, genes for the progression to an $HHV\text{-}8^+$ lymphoma.

In these unstable lymphoproliferative states (i.e., ALPDs), no single gold standard exists at this time to define a malignancy. The search for definite pathologic criteria that characterize their stages of progression is a challenge for future prospective studies. Until these become available, the appropriate management of these patients remains undetermined. However, if one lesson has been learned in the study of these disorders, it is that restoration of the patient's immune system is the first step to their treatment.

REFERENCES

1. Sinclair NR, Anderson CC. Co-stimulation and co-inhibition: equal partners in regulation. *Scand J Immunol* 1996;43:597–603.
2. Mason D, Powrie F. Control of immune pathology by regulatory T cells. *Curr Opin Immunol* 1998;10:649–655.
3. Saito T. Negative regulation of T cell activation. *Curr Opin Immunol* 1998;10:313–321.
4. Winoto A. Cell death in the regulation of immune responses. *Curr Opin Immunol* 1997;9:365–370.
5. Van Parijs L, Abbas AK. Role of Fas-mediated cell death in the regulation of immune responses. *Curr Opin Immunol* 1996;8:355–361.
6. Straus SE, Sneller M, Lenardo MJ, et al. An inherited disorder of lymphocyte apoptosis: the autoimmune lymphoproliferative syndrome. *Ann Intern Med* 1999;130:591–601.
7. Jackson CE, Puck JM. Autoimmune lymphoproliferative syndrome, a disorder of apoptosis. *Curr Opin Pediatr* 1999;11:521–527.
8. Sneller MC, Straus SE, Jaffe ES, et al. A novel lymphoproliferative/autoimmune syndrome resembling murine lpr/gld disease. *J Clin Invest* 1992;90:334–341.
9. Elenitoba-Johnson KS, Jaffe ES. Lymphoproliferative disorders associated with congenital immunodeficiencies. *Semin Diagn Pathol* 1997;14:35–47.
10. Kamel OW. Iatrogenic lymphoproliferative disorders in nontransplantation settings. *Semin Diagn Pathol* 1997;14:27–34.
11. Flandrin G, Daniel MY, EL Yafi G, et al. Sarcomatoses ganglionnaires diffuse è différenciation plasmocytaire avec anémie hémolytique autoimmune. *Actual Hematol* 1972;6:25–41.
12. Westerhausen M, Oehlert W. Chronische pluripotentielles immunproliferatives Syndrom. *Dtsch Med Wochenschr* 1972;97:1407–1413 passim.
13. Lennert K. Pathologisch-histologische Klassifizierung der malignen Lymphome. In: Stacher A, ed. *Leukaemien und maligne Lymphome.* Munich: Urban & Schwarzenberg, 1973:181–194.
14. Lukes RJ. Immunoblastic lymphadenopathy. In: *Workshop on the classification of non-Hodgkin's lymphomas, 1973.* Chicago: University of Chicago, 1973.
15. Lukes RJ, Tindle BH. Immunoblastic lymphadenopathy: a hyperimmune entity resembling Hodgkin's disease. *N Engl J Med* 1975;292:1–8.
16. Suchi T. Atypical lymph node hyperplasia with fatal outcome: a report on the histopathological, immunological and clinical investigations of the cases. *Recent Adv Res* 1974;14:13–34.
17. Frizzera G, Moran EM, Rappaport H. Angio-immunoblastic lymphadenopathy: diagnosis and clinical course. *Am J Med* 1975;59:803–818.
18. Frizzera G, Moran EM, Rappaport H. Angio-immunoblastic lymphadenopathy with dysproteinaemia. *Lancet* 1974;1:1070–1073.
19. Knecht H, Lennert K. Vorgeschichte und klinisches Bild der Lymphogranulomatosis X (einschliesslich (angio)immunoblastischer Lymphadenopathie). *Schweiz Med Wochenschr* 1981;111:1108–1121.
20. Knecht H, Schwarze EW, Lennert K. Histological, immunohistological and autopsy findings in lymphogranulomatosis X (including angioimmunoblastic lymphadenopathy). *Virchows Arch A Pathol Anat Histopathol* 1985;406:105–124.
21. Shimoyama M, Minato K, Saito H, et al. Immunoblastic lymphadenopathy (IBL)–like T-cell lymphoma. *Jpn J Clin Oncol* 1979; 9[Suppl]:347–356.

22. Watanabe S, Sato Y, Shimoyama M, et al. Immunoblastic lymphadenopathy, angioimmunoblastic lymphadenopathy, and IBL-like T-cell lymphoma: a spectrum of T-cell neoplasia. *Cancer* 1986;58: 2224–2232.
23. Harris NL, Jaffe ES, Stein H, et al. A revised European-American classification of lymphoid neoplasms: a proposal from the International Lymphoma Study Group [see comments]. *Blood* 1994;84: 1361–1392.
24. Nakamura S, Suchi T. A clinicopathologic study of node-based, low-grade, peripheral T-cell lymphoma: angioimmunoblastic lymphoma, T–zone lymphoma, and lymphoepithelioid lymphoma. *Cancer* 1991; 67:2566–2578.
25. Siegert W, Agthe A, Griesser H, et al. Treatment of angioimmunoblastic lymphadenopathy (AILD)-type T-cell lymphoma using prednisone with or without the COPBLAM/IMVP-16 regimen: a multicenter study. Kiel Lymphoma Study Group. *Ann Intern Med* 1992;117: 364–370.
26. Weiss LM, Strickler JG, Dorfman RF, et al. Clonal T-cell populations in angioimmunoblastic lymphadenopathy and angioimmunoblastic lymphadenopathy-like lymphoma. *Am J Pathol* 1986;122:392–397.
27. Schlegelberger B, Feller A, Godde E, et al. Stepwise development of chromosomal abnormalities in angioimmunoblastic lymphadenopathy. *Cancer Genet Cytogenet* 1990;50:15–29.
28. Advani R, Warnke R, Sikic BI, et al. Treatment of angioimmunoblastic T-cell lymphoma with cyclosporine. *Ann Oncol* 1997;8:601–603.
29. Ohshima K, Kikuchi M, Hashimoto M, et al. Genetic changes in atypical hyperplasia and lymphoma with angioimmunoblastic lymphadenopathy and dysproteinaemia in the same patients. *Virchows Arch* 1994;425:25–32.
30. Schmuth M, Ramaker J, Trautmann C, et al. Cutaneous involvement in prelymphomatous angioimmunoblastic lymphadenopathy. *J Am Acad Dermatol* 1997;36:290–295.
31. Siegert W, Nerl C, Agthe A, et al. Angioimmunoblastic lymphadenopathy (AILD)-type T-cell lymphoma: prognostic impact of clinical observations and laboratory findings at presentation. The Kiel Lymphoma Study Group. *Ann Oncol* 1995;6:659–664.
32. Ganesan TS, Dhaliwal HS, Dorreen MS, et al. Angio-immunoblastic lymphadenopathy: a clinical, immunological and molecular study. *Br J Cancer* 1987;55:437–442.
33. Yamamura M, Honda M, Yamada Y, et al. Increased levels of interleukin-6 (IL-6) in serum and spontaneous *in vitro* production of IL-6 by lymph node mononuclear cells of patients with angio-immunoblastic lymphadenopathy with dysproteinemia (AILD), and clinical effectiveness of cyclosporin A. *Leukemia* 1996;10:1504–1508.
34. Kozuru M, Hashimoto M, Takahira H, et al. AILD-like dysplasia transformed in AILD-type T cell lymphoma in an HTLV-1 carrier: usefulness of interferon-alpha. *Acta Haematol* 1996;96:92–98.
35. Murayama T, Imoto S, Takahashi T, et al. Successful treatment of angioimmunoblastic lymphadenopathy with dysproteinemia with cyclosporin A. *Cancer* 1992;69:2567–2570.
36. Ong ST, Koeppen H, Larson RA, et al. Successful treatment of angioimmunoblastic lymphadenopathy with dysproteinemia with fludarabine [Letter]. *Blood* 1996;88:2354–2355.
37. Sallah S, Wehbie R, Lepera P, et al. The role of 2-chlorodeoxyadenosine in the treatment of patients with refractory angioimmunoblastic lymphadenopathy with dysproteinemia. *Br J Haematol* 1999;104: 163–165.
38. Schwarzmeier JD, Reinisch WW, Kurkciyan IE, et al. Interferon-alpha induces complete remission in angioimmunoblastic lymphadenopathy (AILD): late development of aplastic anaemia with cytokine abnormalities. *Br J Haematol* 1991;79:336–337.
39. Hast R, Gustafsson B. Improved response to chemotherapy after interferon alpha-2b in angioimmunoblastic lymphadenopathy (AILD) [Letter]. *Eur J Haematol* 1991;46:51–52.
40. Hast R, Jacobsson B, Petrescu A, et al. Successful treatment with fludarabine in two cases of angioimmunoblastic lymphadenopathy with dysproteinemia. *Leuk Lymphoma* 1999;34:597–601.
41. Müller-Hermelink HK, Lennert K. *The cytologic, histologic, and functional basis for a modern classification of lymphomas.* Berlin: Springer-Verlag, 1978.
42. Feller AC, Griesser H, Schilling CV, et al. Clonal gene rearrangement patterns correlate with immunophenotype and clinical parameters in patients with angioimmunoblastic lymphadenopathy. *Am J Pathol* 1988;133:549–556.
43. Ree HJ, Kadin ME, Kikuchi M, et al. Angioimmunoblastic lymphoma (AILD-type T-cell lymphoma) with hyperplastic germinal centers. *Am J Surg Pathol* 1998;22:643–655.
44. Frizzera G, Banks PM, Massarelli G, et al. A systemic lymphoproliferative disorder with morphologic features of Castleman's disease: pathological findings in 15 patients. *Am J Surg Pathol* 1983;7:211–231.
45. Flandrin G. Angioimmunoblastic lymphadenopathy: clinical, biologic, and follow-up study of 14 cases. *Recent Results Cancer Res* 1978;64:247–262.
46. Forster G, Moeschlin S. Extramedullaeres, leukaemisches Plasmacytom mit Dysproteinaemie und erworbener haemolytischer Anaemie. *Schweiz Med Wochenschr* 1954;84:1106–1110.
47. Peterson LC, Kueck B, Arthur DC, et al. Systemic polyclonal immunoblastic proliferations. *Cancer* 1988;61:1350–1358.
48. Peterson L, Marcelli A, Arthur D, et al. Systemic polyclonal immunoblastic proliferation: a distinct atypical lymphoproliferative disorder. *Mod Pathol* 1998;11:138A(abst).
49. Frizzera G, Kaneko Y, Sakurai M. Angioimmunoblastic lymphadenopathy and related disorders: a retrospective look in search of definitions. *Leukemia* 1989;3:1–5.
50. Namikawa R, Suchi T, Ueda R, et al. Phenotyping of proliferating lymphocytes in angioimmunoblastic lymphadenopathy and related lesions by the double immunoenzymatic staining technique. *Am J Pathol* 1987;127:279–287.
51. Aozasa K, Ohsawa M, Fujita MQ, et al. Angioimmunoblastic lymphadenopathy: review of 44 patients with emphasis on prognostic behavior. *Cancer* 1989;63:1625–1629.
52. Nathwani BN, Rappaport H, Moran EM, et al. Malignant lymphoma arising in angioimmunoblastic lymphadenopathy. *Cancer* 1978;41: 578–606.
53. Pangalis GA, Moran EM, Nathwani BN, et al. Angioimmunoblastic lymphadenopathy: long-term follow-up study. *Cancer* 1983;52: 318–321.
54. Yu RC, Schofield J, Alaibac M, et al. Angioimmunoblastic lymphadenopathy with dysproteinemia and dermal T-cell lymphoma. *Cancer* 1994;74:1801–1807.
55. Boros L, Bhaskar AG, D'Souza JP. Monoclonal evolution of angioimmunoblastic lymphadenopathy. *Am J Clin Pathol* 1981;75:856–860.
56. Aizawa Y, Zawadzki ZA, Micolonghi TS, et al. Vasculitis and Sjögren's syndrome with IgA-IgG cryoglobulinemia terminating in immunoblastic sarcoma. *Am J Med* 1979;67:160–166.
57. Bauer TW, Mendelsohn G, Humphrey RL, et al. Angioimmunoblastic lymphadenopathy progressing to immunoblastic lymphoma with prominent gastric involvement. *Cancer* 1982;50:2089–2098.
58. Krugliak L, Zimlichman RR, Schlaeffer F, et al. Immunoblastic lymphoma and thymic epithelial hyperplasia in angioimmunoblastic lymphadenopathy following gold therapy. *Isr J Med Sci* 1985;21: 381–385.
59. Pirker R, Schwarzmeier JD, Radaszkiewicz T, et al. B-immunoblastic lymphoma arising in angioimmunoblastic lymphadenopathy. *Acta Haematol* 1986;75:105–109.
60. Abruzzo LV, Schmidt K, Weiss LM, et al. B-cell lymphoma after angioimmunoblastic lymphadenopathy: a case with oligoclonal gene rearrangements associated with Epstein-Barr virus. *Blood* 1993;82: 241–246.
61. Matsue K, Itoh M, Tsukuda K, et al. Development of Epstein-Barr virus-associated B cell lymphoma after intensive treatment of patients with angioimmunoblastic lymphadenopathy with dysproteinemia. *Int J Hematol* 1998;67:319–329.
62. Viraben R, Brousset P, Lamant L. Cutaneous B-cell lymphoma associated with angioimmunoblastic lymphadenopathy. *J Am Acad Dermatol* 1998;38:992–994.
63. Knecht H, Martius F, Bachmann E, et al. A deletion mutant of the LMP1 oncogene of Epstein-Barr virus is associated with evolution of angioimmunoblastic lymphadenopathy into B immunoblastic lymphoma. *Leukemia* 1995;9:458–465.
64. Higuchi T, Tada J, Mori H, et al. Immunoblastic lymphadenopathy-like T cell lymphoma evolving into a massive plasma cell proliferation with biclonal paraproteinemia. *Acta Haematol* 1998;100:151–155.
65. Suchi T, Lennert K, Tu LY, et al. Histopathology and immunohistochemistry of peripheral T cell lymphomas: a proposal for their classification. *J Clin Pathol* 1987;40:995–1015.
66. Ohno T, Kita K, Miwa H, et al. Immunophenotypical and molecular

genetical examination of angioimmunoblastic lymphadenopathy. *Nippon Ketsueki Gakkai Zasshi* 1987;50:1657–1667.
67. Jaffe ES. Morphologic features. In: Steinberg AD, ed. *Angioimmunoblastic lymphadenopathy with dysproteinemia*: *Ann Intern Med* 1988: 577–579.
68. Ohsaka A, Saito K, Sakai T, et al. Clinicopathologic and therapeutic aspects of angioimmunoblastic lymphadenopathy-related lesions. *Cancer* 1992;69:1259–1267.
69. Lorenzen J, Li G, Zhao-Hohn M, et al. Angioimmunoblastic lymphadenopathy type of T-cell lymphoma and angioimmunoblastic lymphadenopathy: a clinicopathological and molecular biological study of 13 Chinese patients using polymerase chain reaction and paraffin-embedded tissues. *Virchows Arch* 1994;424:593–600.
70. Tobinai K, Minato K, Ohtsu T, et al. Clinicopathologic, immunophenotypic, and immunogenotypic analyses of immunoblastic lymphadenopathy-like T-cell lymphoma. *Blood* 1988;72:1000–1006.
71. Takagi N, Nakamura S, Ueda R, et al. A phenotypic and genotypic study of three node-based, low-grade peripheral T-cell lymphomas: angioimmunoblastic lymphoma, T-zone lymphoma, and lymphoepithelioid lymphoma. *Cancer* 1992;69:2571–2582.
72. Nakamura S, Koshikawa T, Koike K, et al. Phenotypic analysis of peripheral T cell lymphoma among the Japanese. *Acta Pathol Jpn* 1993;43:396–412.
73. Quintanilla-Martinez L, Fend F, Moguel LR, et al. Peripheral T-cell lymphoma with Reed-Sternberg–like cells of B-cell phenotype and genotype associated with Epstein-Barr virus infection. *Am J Surg Pathol* 1999;23:1233–1240.
74. Knecht H, Odermatt BF, Maurer R, et al. Diagnostic and prognostic value of monoclonal antibodies in immunophenotyping of angioimmunoblastic lymphadenopathy/lymphogranulomatosis X. *Br J Haematol* 1987;67:19–24.
75. Jones D, Jorgensen JL, Shahsafael A, et al. Characteristic proliferations of reticular and dendritic cells in angioimmunoblastic lymphoma. *Am J Surg Pathol* 1998;22:956–964.
76. Ree HJ, Kadin ME, Kikuchi M, et al. Bcl-6 expression in reactive follicular hyperplasia, follicular lymphoma, and angioimmunoblastic T-cell lymphoma with hyperplastic germinal centers: heterogeneity of intrafollicular T-cells and their altered distribution in the pathogenesis of angioimmunoblastic T-cell lymphoma. *Hum Pathol* 1999;30: 403–411.
77. Leung CY, Ho FC, Srivastava G, et al. Usefulness of follicular dendritic cell pattern in classification of peripheral T-cell lymphomas. *Histopathology* 1993;23:433–437.
78. Frizzera G. Atypical lymphoproliferative disorders. In: Knowles DM, ed. *Neoplastic hematopathology,* 1st ed. Baltimore: Williams & Wilkins, 1992:459–495.
79. Griesser H, Feller A, Lennert K, et al. Rearrangement of the beta chain of the T cell antigen receptor and immunoglobulin genes in lymphoproliferative disorders. *J Clin Invest* 1986;78:1179–1184.
80. O'Connor NT, Crick JA, Wainscoat JS, et al. Evidence for monoclonal T lymphocyte proliferation in angioimmunoblastic lymphadenopathy. *J Clin Pathol* 1986;39:1229–1232.
81. Lipford EH, Smith HR, Pittaluga S, et al. Clonality of angioimmunoblastic lymphadenopathy and implications for its evolution to malignant lymphoma. *J Clin Invest* 1987;79:637–642.
82. Suzuki H, Namikawa R, Ueda R, et al. Clonal T cell population in angioimmunoblastic lymphadenopathy and related lesions. *Jpn J Cancer Res* 1987;78:712–720.
83. Knecht H, Odermatt BF, Hayoz D, et al. Polyclonal rearrangements of the T-cell receptor beta-chain in fatal angioimmunoblastic lymphadenopathy. *Br J Haematol* 1989;73:491–496.
84. Boumpas DT, Wheby MS, Jaffe ES, et al. Synovitis in angioimmunoblastic lymphadenopathy with dysproteinemia simulating rheumatoid arthritis. *Arthritis Rheum* 1990;33:578–582.
85. Kon S, Sato T, Onodera K, et al. Detection of Epstein-Barr virus DNA and EBV-determined nuclear antigen in angioimmunoblastic lymphadenopathy with dysproteinemia type T cell lymphoma. *Pathol Res Pract* 1993;189:1137–1144.
86. Araki A, Taniguchi M, Mikata A. T cell receptor V beta repertoires of angioimmunoblastic lymphadenopathy-like T cell lymphoma. *Leuk Lymphoma* 1994;16:135–140.
87. Nakano A, Hatta K, Kobashi Y, et al. Salazosulfapyridine-induced angioimmunoblastic lymphadenopathy. *Intern Med* 1996;35: 894–897.
88. Rho R, Laddis T, McQuain C, et al. Miliary tuberculosis in a patient with Epstein-Barr virus-associated angioimmunoblastic lymphadenopathy. *Ann Hematol* 1996;72:333–335.
89. Sallah AS, Bernard S. Treatment of angioimmunoblastic lymphadenopathy with dysproteinemia using 2-chlorodeoxyadenosine. *Ann Hematol* 1996;73:295–296.
90. Knecht H, Joske DJ, Bachmann E, et al. Expression of human recombination activating genes (RAG-1 and RAG-2) in angioimmunoblastic lymphadenopathy and anaplastic large cell lymphoma of T-type. *Br J Haematol* 1993;83:655–659.
91. Hodges E, Quin CT, Wright DH, et al. Oligoclonal populations of T and B cells in a case of angioimmunoblastic T-cell lymphoma predominantly infiltrated by T cells of the VB5.1 family. *Mol Pathol* 1997; 50:15–17.
92. Griesser DH. [Analyses of the rearrangement of T-cell receptor and immunoglobulin genes in the diagnosis of lymphoproliferative disorders]. *Veroff Pathol* 1995;144:1–109.
93. Göde-Salz E, Feller AC, Lennert K. Chromosomal abnormalities in lymphogranulomatosis X (LgrX)/angioimmunoblastic lymphadenopathy (AILD). *Leuk Res* 1987;11:181–190.
94. Kaneko Y, Maseki N, Sakurai M, et al. Characteristic karyotypic pattern in T-cell lymphoproliferative disorders with reactive "angioimmunoblastic lymphadenopathy with dysproteinemia-type" features. *Blood* 1988;72:413–421.
95. Schlegelberger B, Zhang Y, Weber-Matthiesen K, et al. Detection of aberrant clones in nearly all cases of angioimmunoblastic lymphadenopathy with dysproteinemia-type T-cell lymphoma by combined interphase and metaphase cytogenetics. *Blood* 1994;84:2640–2648.
96. Schlegelberger B, Feller A, Himmler A, et al. Inv(14)(q11;q32) in one of four different clones in a case of angioimmunoblastic lymphadenopathy. *Cancer Genet Cytogenet* 1990;44:77–81.
97. Heim S, Mitelman F. Cytogenetically unrelated clones in hematological neoplasms. *Leukemia* 1989;3:6–8.
98. Schlegelberger B, Himmler A, Godde E, et al. Cytogenetic findings in peripheral T-cell lymphomas as a basis for distinguishing low-grade and high-grade lymphomas. *Blood* 1994;83:505–511.
99. Cosimi MF, Casagranda I, Ghiazza G, et al. Rearrangements on chromosomes 7 and 14 with breakpoints at 7q35 and 14q11 in angioimmunoblastic lymphadenopathy and IBL-like T-cell lymphoma. *Pathologica* 1990;82:391–397.
100. Freter CE, Cossman J. Angioimmunoblastic lymphadenopathy with dysproteinemia. *Semin Oncol* 1993;20:627–635.
101. Azevedo SJ, Yunis AA. Angioimmunoblastic lymphadenopathy. *Am J Hematol* 1985;20:301–312.
102. Knecht H. Angioimmunoblastic lymphadenopathy: ten years' experience and state of current knowledge. *Semin Hematol* 1989;26: 208–215.
103. Sallah S, Gagnon GA. Angioimmunoblastic lymphadenopathy with dysproteinemia: emphasis on pathogenesis and treatment. *Acta Haematol* 1998;99:57–64.
104. de Terlizzi M, Toma MG, Santostasi T, et al. Angioimmunoblastic lymphadenopathy with dysproteinemia: report of a case in infancy with review of literature. *Pediatr Hematol Oncol* 1989;6:37–44.
105. Schauer PK, Straus DJ, Bagley CM Jr, et al. Angioimmunoblastic lymphadenopathy: clinical spectrum of disease. *Cancer* 1981;48: 2493–2498.
106. Ironside P, Cornell FN. Immunoblastic lymphadenopathy: a clinicopathological study of 16 cases. *Pathology* 1979;11:27–37.
107. Radaszkiewicz T, Lennert K. Lymphogranulomatosis X: Klinisches Bild, Therapie und Prognose. *Dtsch Med Wochenschr* 1975;100: 1157–1163.
108. Moor SB, Harrison EG Jr, Weiland LH. Angioimmunoblastic lymphadenopathy. *Mayo Clin Proc* 1976;51:273–280.
109. Meuge C, de Mascarel A. Lymphadénopathie angioimmunoblastique. Revue de la littærature et réflexions è propos de 13 cas. *Arch Anat Cytol Pathol* 1977;25:187–199.
110. Cullen MH, Stansfeld AG, Oliver RT, et al. Angio-immunoblastic lymphadenopathy: report of ten cases and review of the literature. *Q J Med* 1979;48:151–177.
111. Coupland RW, Pontifex AH, Salinas FA. Angioimmunoblastic lymphadenopathy with dysproteinemia: circulating immune complexes and the review of 18 cases. *Cancer* 1985;55:1902–1906.
112. Debray J, Hervouet D, Krulik M, et al. Étude clinique, anatomopathologique et évolutive de la lymphadénopathie angio-immunoblas-

tique: À propos de 25 observations personnelles. *Rev Med Interne* 1982;3:85–92.
113. Pautier P, Devidas A, Delmer A, et al. Angioimmunoblastic-like T-cell non Hodgkin's lymphoma: outcome after chemotherapy in 33 patients and review of the literature. *Leuk Lymphoma* 1999;32: 545–552.
114. Gisselbrecht C, Gaulard P, Lepage E, et al. Prognostic significance of T-cell phenotype in aggressive non-Hodgkin's lymphomas: Groupe d'Etudes des Lymphomes de l'Adulte (GELA). *Blood* 1998;92: 76–82.
115. Frizzera G. Angioimmunoblastic lymphadenopathy. In: Demis DJ, ed. *Clinical dermatology*. Philadelphia: Harper & Row. 1987, 1–6.
116. Layton MA, Musgrove C, Dawes PT. Polyarthritis, rash and lymphadenopathy: case reports of two patients with angioimmunoblastic lymphadenopathy presenting to a rheumatology clinic. *Clin Rheumatol* 1998;17:148–151.
117. Nakamura S, Suchi T, Koshikawa T, et al. Clinicopathologic study of 212 cases of peripheral T-cell lymphoma among the Japanese. *Cancer* 1993;72:1762–1772.
118. Archimbaud E, Coiffier B, Bryon PA, et al. Prognostic factors in angioimmunoblastic lymphadenopathy. *Cancer* 1987;59:208–212.
119. Offit K, Macris NT, Finkbeiner JA. Monoclonal hypergammaglobulinemia without malignant transformation in angioimmunoblastic lymphadenopathy with dysproteinemia. *Am J Med* 1986;80:292–294.
120. Dellagi K, Brouet JC, Seligmann M. Antivimentin autoantibodies in angioimmunoblastic lymphadenopathy. *N Engl J Med* 1984;310: 215–218.
121. Higuchi T, Mori H, Niikura H, et al. Hypocomplementemia and hematological abnormalities in immunoblastic lymphadenopathy and immunoblastic lymphadenopathy-like T cell lymphoma. *Acta Haematol* 1996;96:68–72.
122. Pizzolo G, Vinante F, Agostini C, et al. Immunologic abnormalities in angioimmunoblastic lymphadenopathy. *Cancer* 1987;60:2412–2418.
123. Steinberg AD, Seldin MF, Jaffe ES, et al. Cellular immunology. In: Steinberg AD, ed. *Angioimmunoblastic lymphadenopathy with dysproteinemia: Ann Intern Med* 1988:579–580.
124. Boni R, Dummer R, Dommann-Scherrer C, et al. Necrotizing herpes zoster mimicking relapse of vasculitis in angioimmunoblastic lymphadenopathy with dysproteinaemia. *Br J Dermatol* 1995;133: 978–982.
125. Pizzolo G, Stein H, Josimovic-Alasevic O, et al. Increased serum levels of soluble IL-2 receptor, CD30 and CD8 molecules, and gamma-interferon in angioimmunoblastic lymphadenopathy: possible pathogenetic role of immunoactivation mechanisms. *Br J Haematol* 1990;75:485–488.
126. Yufu Y, Choi I, Hirase N, et al. Soluble Fas in the serum of patients with non-Hodgkin's lymphoma: higher concentrations in angioimmunoblastic T-cell lymphoma. *Am J Hematol* 1998;58:334–336.
127. Pangalis GA, Moran EM, Rappaport H. Blood and bone marrow findings in angioimmunoblastic lymphadenopathy. *Blood* 1978;51:71–83.
128. Ghani AM, Krause JR. Bone marrow biopsy findings in angioimmunoblastic lymphadenopathy. *Br J Haematol* 1985;61:203–213.
129. Schnaidt U, Vykoupil KF, Thiele J, et al. Angioimmunoblastic lymphadenopathy: histopathology of bone marrow involvement. *Virchows Arch [Pathol Anat]* 1980;389:369–380.
130. Ferrer I, Vidaller A, Fernandez de Sevilla A, et al. Peripheral neuropathy associated with angioimmunoblastic lymphadenopathy. *Clin Neurol Neurosurg* 1988;90:159–162.
131. Cadranel JF, Cadranel J, Buffet C, et al. Nodular regenerative hyperplasia of the liver, peliosis hepatis, and perisinusoidal fibrosis: association with angioimmunoblastic lymphadenopathy and severe hypoxemia. *Gastroenterology* 1990;99:268–273.
132. Lynch JW, Elfenbein GJ, Noyes WD, et al. Pure red cell aplasia associated with angioimmunoblastic lymphadenopathy with dysproteinemia. *Am J Hematol* 1994;46:72–78.
133. Orth T, Treichel U, Mayet WJ, et al. [Reversible myelofibrosis in angioimmunoblastic lymphadenopathy]. *Dtsch Med Wochenschr* 1994;119:694–698.
134. Anzai T, Hirose W, Nakane H, et al. Myelodysplastic syndrome associated with immunoblastic lymphadenopathy-like T-cell lymphoma: simultaneous clinical improvement with chemotherapy. *Jpn J Clin Oncol* 1994;24:106–110.
135. Lim AK, Ferreira MA, Majumdar A, et al. Renal amyloidosis and angioimmunoblastic lymphadenopathy. *Nephrol Dial Transplant* 1998;13:453–454.
136. Wasser WG, Bockman RS, Alderete M, et al. Immunoblastic lymphadenopathy with hypercalcemia. *Mt Sinai J Med* 1980;47:13–16.
137. Schlegelberger B, Zwingers T, Hohenadel K, et al. Significance of cytogenetic findings for the clinical outcome in patients with T-cell lymphoma of angioimmunoblastic lymphadenopathy type [see comments]. *J Clin Oncol* 1996;14:593–599.
138. Rubinstein A, Dauber LG. Lymphoma of cytotoxic/suppressor T cell phenotype (T8) following angioimmunoblastic lymphadenopathy. *Oncology* 1983;40:195–199.
139. Nakamura S, Sasajima Y, Koshikawa T, et al. Angioimmunoblastic T-cell lymphoma (angioimmunoblastic lymphadenopathy with dysproteinemia [AILD]-type T-cell lymphoma) followed by Hodgkin's disease associated with Epstein-Barr virus. *Pathol Int* 1995;45: 958–964.
140. Yataganas X, Papadimitriou C, Pangalis G, et al. Angio-immunoblastic lymphadenopathy terminating as Hodgkin's disease. *Cancer* 1977; 39:2183–2189.
141. Friedman-Birnbaum R, Gilhar A, Carter A. Coexistence of Kaposi's sarcoma and angioimmunoblastic lymphadenopathy. *J Dermatol Surg Oncol* 1985;11:76–79.
142. Helm TN, Steck WD, Proffitt MR, et al. Kaposi's sarcoma, angioimmunoblastic lymphadenopathy, and antibody to HIV-1 p24 antigen in a patient nonreactive for HIV-1 with use of ELISA. *J Am Acad Dermatol* 1990;23:317–318.
143. Varsano S, Manor Y, Steiner Z, et al. Kaposi's sarcoma and angioimmunoblastic lymphadenopathy. *Cancer* 1984;54:1582–1585.
144. Cavanna L, Di Stasi M, Paties C, et al. Angioimmunoblastic lymphadenopathy with disproteinemia associated with carcinoma: case report and review of the literature. *Oncology* 1988;45:318–321.
145. Ch'ang HJ, Su IJ, Chen CL, et al. Angioimmunoblastic lymphadenopathy with dysproteinemia: lack of a prognostic value of clear cell morphology. *Oncology* 1997;54:193–198.
146. Konig M, Grunder K, Nilles M, et al. Cutaneous cryptococcosis as the first symptom of a disseminated cryptococcosis in a patient with lymphogranulomatosis X. *Mycoses* 1991;34:309–311.
147. Mihaljevic B, Donfrid M, Jancic-Nedeljkov R, et al. Angioimmunoblastic lymphadenopathy (AILD) with benign course. *Haematologia (Budap)* 1996;28:21–25.
148. Khan G, Norton AJ, Slavin G. Epstein-Barr virus in angioimmunoblastic T-cell lymphomas. *Histopathology* 1993;22:145–149.
149. Rossi JF, Fegueux N, Calvet B, et al. Alpha-interferon in angioimmunoblastic lymphadenopathy [Letter]. *Ann Intern Med* 1988;109: 512–513.
150. Meuthen I, Lennert K, Siegert W. Lymphogranulomatosis X: complete remission by low dose interferon-alpha. *Br J Haematol* 1990; 75:438–439.
151. Imoto S, Ito M, Nakagawa T. [A remarkable effect of alpha-interferon in a case of angioimmunoblastic lymphadenopathy with dysproteinaemia (AILD) refractory to steroids and combination chemotherapies]. *Rinsho Ketsueki* 1991;32:681–685.
152. Milone G, Guglielmo P, Cacciola E, et al. Alpha interferon as first line therapy for angioimmunoblastic lymphadenopathy: Possible value of DR^+ cells in monitoring therapeutical response [Letter]. *Haematologica* 1992;77:524–525.
153. Siegert W, Nerl C, Meuthen I, et al. Recombinant human interferon-alpha in the treatment of angioimmunoblastic lymphadenopathy: results in 12 patients. *Leukemia* 1991;5:892–895.
154. Blanchard F, Briancon S, Bethevenot G, et al. Reécherche de facteurs pronostiques dans la L.A.I.D. *Agressologie* 1982;23:63–64.
155. Knecht H, Sahli R, Shaw P, et al. Detection of Epstein-Barr virus DNA by polymerase chain reaction in lymph node biopsies from patients with angioimmunoblastic lymphadenopathy [published erratum appears in *Br J Haematol* 1990;76:450]. *Br J Haematol* 1990;75: 610–614.
156. Fest T, Angonin R, Dupond JL, et al. [Angioimmunoblastic lymphadenopathy: a pathogenetic intersection between dysimmune, viral and lymphomatous diseases]. *Rev Med Interne* 1991;12:383–388.
157. Anagnostopoulos I, Hummel M, Finn T, et al. Heterogeneous Epstein-Barr virus infection patterns in peripheral T-cell lymphoma of angioimmunoblastic lymphadenopathy type. *Blood* 1992;80:1804–1812.
158. Foss HD, Anagnostopoulos I, Herbst H, et al. Patterns of cytokine

gene expression in peripheral T-cell lymphoma of angioimmunoblastic lymphadenopathy type. *Blood* 1995;85:2862–2869.

159. Hsu SM, Waldron JA Jr, Fink L, et al. Pathogenic significance of interleukin-6 in angioimmunoblastic lymphadenopathy-type T-cell lymphoma. *Hum Pathol* 1993;24:126–131.
160. Freeman GJ, Disteche CM, Gribben JG, et al. The gene for B7, a costimulatory signal for T-cell activation, maps to chromosomal region 3q13.3-3q21. *Blood* 1992;79:489–494.
161. Lau CP, Wong KL, Wong CK, et al. Acute lymphadenopathy complicating quinidine therapy. *Postgrad Med J* 1990;66:406–407.
162. De Ponti F, Lecchini S, Cosentino M, et al. Immunological adverse effects of anticonvulsants: what is their clinical relevance? *Drug Saf* 1993;8:235–250.
163. Baert F, Knockaert D, Bobbaers H. Bilateral hilar lymphadenopathy associated with *Yersinia enterocolitica* infection [Letter]. *Clin Infect Dis* 1994;19:197–198.
164. Monkemuller KE, Bronze MS. Immunoblastic lymphadenopathy presenting as an acute abdomen and mixed bacteremia with *Eikenella corrodens* and group C streptococci. *Am J Gastroenterol* 1998;93:652–653.
165. Gerl A, Mittermuller J, Bise K, et al. [Listeriosis in malignant diseases]. *Dtsch Med Wochenschr* 1991;116:1144–1148.
166. Ghezzo F, Romano S, Gorzegno G, et al. [Cryptococcosis in a female patient with angioimmunoblastic lymphadenopathy and dysproteinemia]. *Ann Ital Med Int* 1992;7:111–113.
167. Ozyilkan O, Ozyilkan E, Karagoz F, et al. Hepatitis C virus infection and angioimmunoblastic lymphadenopathy [Letter]. *Am J Gastroenterol* 1995;90:1029–1030.
168. Kondo H, Okagawa K, Takeichi T, et al. [IBL-type lymphadenopathy after infection of rubella virus]. *Rinsho Ketsueki* 1991;32:976–980.
169. Hernandez DE, Da Costa O, Rodriguez A. [Angioimmunoblastic lymphadenopathy: comparison of 2 clinical cases, one of them with antibodies against human immunodeficiency virus (HIV)] [Letter]. *Sangre (Barc)* 1996;41:72.
170. Sahuquillo JC, Moysset I. [Fever, adenopathies, hepatosplenomegaly and cutaneous lesions in a 31-year-old woman with human immunodeficiency virus infection (clinical conference)]. *Med Clin (Barc)* 1995;104:188–195.
171. Closs F, Oksenhendler E, Prophette B, et al. [Hemophagocytosis syndrome: angioimmunoblastic lymphadenitis developing into T-lymphoma in a HIV-positive female patient] [Letter]. *Presse Med* 1995;24:371.
172. Krueger GR, Bergholz M, Bartsch HH, et al. Rubella virus antigen in lymphocytes of patients with angioimmunoblastic lymphadenopathy (AIL). *J Cancer Res Clin Oncol* 1979;95:87–91.
173. Yu AM, Song RL, Yu Z, et al. Detection of human cytomegalovirus antigen and DNA in lymph nodes and peripheral blood mononuclear cells of patients with angioimmunoblastic lymphadenopathy with dysproteinemia. *Arch Pathol Lab Med* 1992;116:490–494.
174. Luppi M, Marasca R, Barozzi P, et al. Frequent detection of human herpesvirus-6 sequences by polymerase chain reaction in paraffin-embedded lymph nodes from patients with angioimmunoblastic lymphadenopathy and angioimmunoblastic lymphadenopathy-like lymphoma. *Leuk Res* 1993;17:1003–1011.
175. Daibata M, Ido E, Murakami K, et al. Angioimmunoblastic lymphadenopathy with disseminated human herpesvirus 6 infection in a patient with acute myeloblastic leukemia. *Leukemia* 1997;11:882–885.
176. Luppi M, Barozzi P, Maiorana A, et al. Human herpesvirus-8 DNA sequences in human immunodeficiency virus–negative angioimmunoblastic lymphadenopathy and benign lymphadenopathy with giant germinal center hyperplasia and increased vascularity. *Blood* 1996;87:3903–3909.
177. Chadburn A, Cesarman E, Nador RG, et al. Kaposi's sarcoma-associated herpesvirus sequences in benign lymphoid proliferations not associated with human immunodeficiency virus. *Cancer* 1997;80:788–797.
178. Weiss LM, Jaffe ES, Liu XF, et al. Detection and localization of Epstein-Barr viral genomes in angioimmunoblastic lymphadenopathy and angioimmunoblastic lymphadenopathy-like lymphoma. *Blood* 1992;79:1789–1795.
179. Borisch B, Caioni M, Hurwitz N, et al. Epstein-Barr virus subtype distribution in angioimmunoblastic lymphadenopathy. *Int J Cancer* 1993;55:748–752.
180. Ohshima K, Takeo H, Kikuchi M, et al. Heterogeneity of Epstein-Barr virus infection in angioimmunoblastic lymphadenopathy type T-cell lymphoma. *Histopathology* 1994;25:569–579.
181. McKhann CF. Primary malignancy in patients undergoing immunosuppression for renal transplantation. *Transplantation* 1969;8:209–212.
182. Penn I, Hammond W, Brettschneider L, et al. Malignant lymphomas in transplantation patients. *Transplant Proc* 1969;1:106–112.
183. Hoover R, Fraumeni JF Jr. Risk of cancer in renal-transplant recipients. *Lancet* 1973;2:55–57.
184. Penn I. *Cancer* is a complication of severe immunosuppression. *Surg Gynecol Obstet* 1986;162:603–610.
185. Crawford DH, Thomas JA, Janossy G, et al. Epstein Barr virus nuclear antigen positive lymphoma after cyclosporin A treatment in patient with renal allograft [Letter]. *Lancet* 1980;1:1355–1356.
186. Nagington J, Gray J. Cyclosporin A immunosuppression, Epstein-Barr antibody, and lymphoma [Letter]. *Lancet* 1980;1:536–537.
187. Penn I. Malignancies associated with immunosuppressive or cytotoxic therapy. *Surgery* 1978;83:492–502.
188. Hanto DW, Frizzera G, Purtilo DT, et al. Clinical spectrum of lymphoproliferative disorders in renal transplant recipients and evidence for the role of Epstein-Barr virus. *Cancer Res* 1981;41:4253–4261.
189. Frizzera G, Hanto DW, Gajl-Peczalska KJ, et al. Polymorphic diffuse B-cell hyperplasias and lymphomas in renal transplant recipients. *Cancer Res* 1981;41:4262–4279.
190. Purtilo DT. Epstein-Barr-virus-induced oncogenesis in immune-deficient individuals. *Lancet* 1980;1:300–303.
191. Starzl TE, Nalesnik MA, Porter KA, et al. Reversibility of lymphomas and lymphoproliferative lesions developing under cyclosporin-steroid therapy. *Lancet* 1984;1:583–587.
192. Penn I. The problem of cancer in organ transplant recipients: an overview. *Transplant Sci* 1994;4:23–32.
193. Leblond V, Sutton L, Dorent R, et al. Lymphoproliferative disorders after organ transplantation: a report of 24 cases observed in a single center. *J Clin Oncol* 1995;13:961–968.
194. Morrison VA, Dunn DL, Manivel JC, et al. Clinical characteristics of post-transplant lymphoproliferative disorders. *Am J Med* 1994;97:14–24.
195. Nalesnik MA, Jaffe R, Starzl TE, et al. The pathology of posttransplant lymphoproliferative disorders occurring in the setting of cyclosporine A-prednisone immunosuppression. *Am J Pathol* 1988;133:173–192.
196. Ferry JA, Jacobson JO, Conti D, et al. Lymphoproliferative disorders and hematologic malignancies following organ transplantation. *Mod Pathol* 1989;2:583–592.
197. Mihalov ML, Gattuso P, Abraham K, et al. Incidence of post-transplant malignancy among 674 solid-organ-transplant recipients at a single center. *Clin Transplant* 1996;10:248–255.
198. Nalesnik MA. Clinical and pathological features of post-transplant lymphoproliferative disorders (PTLD). *Springer Semin Immunopathol* 1998;20:325–342.
199. Opelz G, Henderson R. Incidence of non-Hodgkin lymphoma in kidney and heart transplant recipients [see comments]. *Lancet* 1993;342:1514–1516.
200. Melosky B, Karim M, Chui A, et al. Lymphoproliferative disorders after renal transplantation in patients receiving triple or quadruple immunosuppression. *J Am Soc Nephrol* 1992;2:S290–S294.
201. Ciancio G, Siquijor AP, Burke GW, et al. Post-transplant lymphoproliferative disease in kidney transplant patients in the new immunosuppressive era. *Clin Transplant* 1997;11:243–249.
202. Birkeland SA, Bendtzen K, Moller B, et al. Interleukin-10 and post-transplant lymphoproliferative disorder after kidney transplantation. *Transplantation* 1999;67:876–881.
203. Swinnen LJ, Mullen GM, Carr TJ, et al. Aggressive treatment for postcardiac transplant lymphoproliferation. *Blood* 1995;86:3333–3340.
204. Armitage JM, Kormos RL, Stuart RS, et al. Posttransplant lymphoproliferative disease in thoracic organ transplant patients: ten years of cyclosporine-based immunosuppression. *J Heart Lung Transplant* 1991;10:877–886; discussion, 886–877.
205. Aris RM, Maia DM, Neuringer IP, et al. Post-transplantation lymphoproliferative disorder in the Epstein-Barr virus-naive lung transplant recipient. *Am J Respir Crit Care Med* 1996;154:1712–1717.
206. Randhawa PS, Yousem SA, Paradis IL, et al. The clinical spectrum, pathology, and clonal analysis of Epstein-Barr virus-associated

lymphoproliferative disorders in heart-lung transplant recipients. *Am J Clin Pathol* 1989;92:177–185.
207. Finn L, Reyes J, Bueno J, et al. Epstein-Barr virus infections in children after transplantation of the small intestine. *Am J Surg Pathol* 1998;22:299–309.
208. Ho M, Jaffe R, Miller G, et al. The frequency of Epstein-Barr virus infection and associated lymphoproliferative syndrome after transplantation and its manifestations in children. *Transplantation* 1988; 45:719–727.
209. Boyle GJ, Michaels MG, Webber SA, et al. Posttransplantation lymphoproliferative disorders in pediatric thoracic organ recipients. *J Pediatr* 1997;131:309–313.
210. Bhatia S, Ramsay NK, Steinbuch M, et al. Malignant neoplasms following bone marrow transplantation. *Blood* 1996;87:3633–3639.
211. Davey DD, Kamat D, Laszewski M, et al. Epstein-Barr virus-related lymphoproliferative disorders following bone marrow transplantation: an immunologic and genotypic analysis. *Mod Pathol* 1989;2:27–34.
212. Deeg HJ, Socie G, Schoch G, et al. Malignancies after marrow transplantation for aplastic anemia and Fanconi anemia: a joint Seattle and Paris analysis of results in 700 patients. *Blood* 1996;87:386–392.
213. Gross TG, Steinbuch M, DeFor T, et al. B cell lymphoproliferative disorders following hematopoietic stem cell transplantation: risk factors, treatment and outcome. *Bone Marrow Transplant* 1999;23: 251–258.
214. Micallef IN, Chhanabhai M, Gascoyne RD, et al. Lymphoproliferative disorders following allogeneic bone marrow transplantation: the Vancouver experience. *Bone Marrow Transplant* 1998;22:981–987.
215. Orazi A, Hromas RA, Neiman RS, et al. Posttransplantation lymphoproliferative disorders in bone marrow transplant recipients are aggressive diseases with a high incidence of adverse histologic and immunobiologic features. *Am J Clin Pathol* 1997;107:419–429.
216. Shapiro RS, McClain K, Frizzera G, et al. Epstein-Barr virus associated B cell lymphoproliferative disorders following bone marrow transplantation. *Blood* 1988;71:1234–1243.
217. Zutter MM, Martin PJ, Sale GE, et al. Epstein-Barr virus lymphoproliferation after bone marrow transplantation. *Blood* 1988;72:520–529.
218. Lucas KG, Small TN, Heller G, et al. The development of cellular immunity to Epstein-Barr virus after allogeneic bone marrow transplantation. *Blood* 1996;87:2594–2603.
219. Peniket AJ, Perry AR, Williams CD, et al. A case of EBV-associated lymphoproliferative disease following high-dose therapy and CD34-purified autologous peripheral blood progenitor cell transplantation. *Bone Marrow Transplant* 1998;22:307–309.
220. Anderson KC, Soiffer R, DeLage R, et al. T-cell-depleted autologous bone marrow transplantation therapy: analysis of immune deficiency and late complications. *Blood* 1990;76:235–244.
221. Shepherd JD, Gascoyne RD, Barnett MJ, et al. Polyclonal Epstein-Barr virus-associated lymphoproliferative disorder following autografting for chronic myeloid leukemia. *Bone Marrow Transplant* 1995;15:639–641.
222. Aguilar LK, Rooney CM, Heslop HE. Lymphoproliferative disorders involving Epstein-Barr virus after hemopoietic stem cell transplantation. *Curr Opin Oncol* 1999;11:96–101.
223. Basgoz N, Preiksaitis JK. Post-transplant lymphoproliferative disorder. *Infect Dis Clin North Am* 1995;9:901–923.
224. Nalesnik MA, Starzl TE. Epstein-Barr virus, infectious mononucleosis, and posttransplant lymphoproliferative disorders. *Transplant Sci* 1994;4:61–79.
225. Hanto DW, Gajl-Peczalska KJ, Frizzera G, et al. Epstein-Barr virus (EBV) induced polyclonal and monoclonal B-cell lymphoproliferative diseases occurring after renal transplantation: clinical, pathologic, and virologic findings and implications for therapy. *Ann Surg* 1983;198: 356–369.
226. Weintraub J, Warnke RA. Lymphoma in cardiac allotransplant recipients: clinical and histological features and immunological phenotype. *Transplantation* 1982;33:347–351.
227. Calne RY, Rolles K, White DJ, et al. Cyclosporin A initially as the only immunosuppressant in 34 recipients of cadaveric organs: 32 kidneys, 2 pancreases, and 2 livers. *Lancet* 1979;2:1033–1036.
228. Bieber CP, Heberling RL, Jamieson SW, et al. Lymphoma in cardiac transplant recipients: associated with the use of cyclosporine A, prednisone and antithymocyte globulin. In: Purtilo DT, ed. *Immune deficiency and cancer: Epstein-Barr virus and lymphoproliferative malignancies.* New York: Plenum Press, 1983:309–320.
229. Cockburn I. Assessment of the risks of malignancy and lymphomas developing in patients using Sandimmune. *Transplant Proc* 1987;19: 1804–1807.
230. Boubenider S, Hiesse C, Goupy C, et al. Incidence and consequences of post-transplantation lymphoproliferative disorders. *J Nephrol* 1997; 10:136–145.
231. Kahan BD, Flechner SM, Lorber MI, et al. Complications of cyclosporin therapy. *World J Surg* 1986;10:348–360.
232. Praghakaran K, Wise B, Chen A, et al. Rational management of posttransplant lymphoproliferative disorder in pediatric recipients. *J Pediatr Surg* 1999;34:112–115; discussion, 115–116.
233. Wilkinson AH, Smith JL, Hunsicker LG, et al. Increased frequency of posttransplant lymphomas in patients treated with cyclosporine, azathioprine, and prednisone. *Transplantation* 1989;47:293–296.
234. Smith JL, Wilkinson AH, Hunsicker LG, et al. Increased frequency of posttransplant lymphomas in patients treated with cyclosporin, azathioprine, and prednisone. *Transplant Proc* 1989;21:3199–3200.
235. Swinnen LJ, Costanzo-Nordin MR, Fisher SG, et al. Increased incidence of lymphoproliferative disorder after immunosuppression with the monoclonal antibody OKT3 in cardiac-transplant recipients [see comments]. *N Engl J Med* 1990;323:1723–1728.
236. Walker RC, Paya CV, Marshall WF, et al. Pretransplantation seronegative Epstein-Barr virus status is the primary risk factor for posttransplantation lymphoproliferative disorder in adult heart, lung, and other solid organ transplantations. *J Heart Lung Transplant* 1995;14: 214–221.
237. Savoie A, Perpete C, Carpentier L, et al. Direct correlation between the load of Epstein-Barr virus-infected lymphocytes in the peripheral blood of pediatric transplant patients and risk of lymphoproliferative disease. *Blood* 1994;83:2715–2722.
238. Walker RC, Marshall WF, Strickler JG, et al. Pretransplantation assessment of the risk of lymphoproliferative disorder. *Clin Infect Dis* 1995;20:1346–1353.
239. Witherspoon RP, Fisher LD, Schoch G, et al. Secondary cancers after bone marrow transplantation for leukemia or aplastic anemia [see comments]. *N Engl J Med* 1989;321:784–789.
240. Hale G, Waldmann H. Risks of developing Epstein-Barr virus-related lymphoproliferative disorders after T-cell-depleted marrow transplants. CAMPATH Users. *Blood* 1998;91:3079–3083.
241. Deeg HJ, Socie G. Malignancies after hematopoietic stem cell transplantation: many questions, some answers. *Blood* 1998;91: 1833–1844.
242. Chadburn A, Cesarman E, Liu YF, et al. Molecular genetic analysis demonstrates that multiple posttransplantation lymphoproliferative disorders occurring in one anatomic site in a single patient represent distinct primary lymphoid neoplasms. *Cancer* 1995;75:2747–2756.
243. Swerdlow SH. Classification of the posttransplant lymphoproliferative disorders: from the past to the present. *Semin Diagn Pathol* 1997; 14:2–7.
244. d'Amore ES, Manivel JC, Gajl-Peczalska KJ, et al. B-cell lymphoproliferative disorders after bone marrow transplant: an analysis of ten cases with emphasis on Epstein-Barr virus detection by in situ hybridization. *Cancer* 1991;68:1285–1295.
245. Cesarman E, Chadburn A, Liu YF, et al. BCL-6 gene mutations in posttransplantation lymphoproliferative disorders predict response to therapy and clinical outcome. *Blood* 1998;92:2294–2302.
246. Hanto DW, Frizzera G, Gajl-Peczalska KJ, et al. Epstein-Barr virus-induced B-cell lymphoma after renal transplantation: acyclovir therapy and transition from polyclonal to monoclonal B-cell proliferation. *N Engl J Med* 1982;306:913–918.
247. Chadburn A, Chen JM, Hsu DT, et al. The morphologic and molecular genetic categories of posttransplantation lymphoproliferative disorders are clinically relevant. *Cancer* 1998;82:1978–1987.
248. Wu TT, Swerdlow SH, Locker J, et al. Recurrent Epstein-Barr virus-associated lesions in organ transplant recipients. *Hum Pathol* 1996; 27:157–164.
249. Chen JM, Barr ML, Chadburn A, et al. Management of lymphoproliferative disorders after cardiac transplantation. *Ann Thorac Surg* 1993; 56:527–538.
250. Koeppen H, Newell K, Baunoch DA, et al. Morphologic bone marrow changes in patients with posttransplantation lymphoproliferative disorders. *Am J Surg Pathol* 1998;22:208–214.
251. Smir BN, Hauke RJ, Bierman PJ, et al. Molecular epidemiology of deletions and mutations of the latent membrane protein 1 oncogene of

the Epstein-Barr virus in posttransplant lymphoproliferative disorders [published erratum appears in *Lab Invest* 1997;76:439]. *Lab Invest* 1996;75:575–588.

252. Minervini MI, Swerdlow SH, Zeevi A, et al. Polymorphic posttransplant disorders (PLTD) are B cell tumors with numerous infiltrating T cells. *Mod Pathol* 1998;11:136A(abst).
253. Joseph G, Barker RL, Yuan B, et al. Posttransplantation plasma cell dyscrasias. *Cancer* 1994;74:1959–1964.
254. Fischer T, Miller M, Bott-Silverman C, et al. Posttransplant lymphoproliferative disease after cardiac transplantation: two unusual variants with predominantly plasmacytoid features. *Transplantation* 1996;62:1687–1690.
255. Chucrallah AE, Crow MK, Rice LE, et al. Multiple myeloma after cardiac transplantation: an unusual form of posttransplant lymphoproliferative disorder. *Hum Pathol* 1994;25:541–545.
256. Leblond V, Davi F, Charlotte F, et al. Posttransplant lymphoproliferative disorders not associated with Epstein-Barr virus: a distinct entity? *J Clin Oncol* 1998;16:2052–2059.
257. Shustik C, Jamison BM, Alfieri C, et al. A solitary plasmacytoma of donor origin arising 14 years after kidney allotransplantation. *Br J Haematol* 1995;91:167–168.
258. Rees L, Thomas A, Amlot PL. Disappearance of an Epstein-Barr virus-positive post-transplant plasmacytoma with reduction of immunosuppression [Letter]. *Lancet* 1998;352:789.
259. Kuster G, Woods JE, Anderson CF, et al. Plasma cell lymphoma after renal transplantation. *Am J Surg* 1972;123:585–587.
260. Melato M, Paladini G. Multiple myeloma following reactivated Epstein-Barr virus infection in a renal-transplant recipient. *Haematologica* 1986;71:241–243.
261. Sabido O, Alamartine E, Barthelemy JC, et al. Over-expression of c-myc oncoprotein in B lymphocytes of renal transplant recipients with lymphoproliferative disorders. *Transplantation* 1993;56:467–470.
262. Schemankewitz E, Hammami A, Stahl R, et al. Multiple extramedullary plasmacytomas following orthotopic liver transplantation in a patient on cyclosporine therapy. *Transplantation* 1990;49:1019–1022.
263. Perera SM, Thomas JA, Burke M, et al. Analysis of the T-cell microenvironment in Epstein-Barr virus-related post-transplantation B lymphoproliferative disease. *J Pathol* 1998;184:177–184.
264. Billiar TR, Hanto DW, Simmons RL. Inclusion of uncomplicated infectious mononucleosis in the spectrum of Epstein-Barr virus infections in transplant recipients. *Transplantation* 1988;46:159–161.
265. Randhawa PS, Markin RS, Starzl TE, et al. Epstein-Barr virus-associated syndromes in immunosuppressed liver transplant recipients: clinical profile and recognition on routine allograft biopsy. *Am J Surg Pathol* 1990;14:538–547.
266. Knowles DM, Cesarman E, Chadburn A, et al. Correlative morphologic and molecular genetic analysis demonstrates three distinct categories of posttransplantation lymphoproliferative disorders. *Blood* 1995;85:552–565.
267. Zangwill SD, Hsu DT, Kichuk MR, et al. Incidence and outcome of primary Epstein-Barr virus infection and lymphoproliferative disease in pediatric heart transplant recipients. *J Heart Lung Transplant* 1998;17:1161–1166.
268. Harris NL, Ferry JA, Swerdlow SH. Posttransplant lymphoproliferative disorders: summary of Society for Hematopathology Workshop. *Semin Diagn Pathol* 1997;14:8–14.
269. Scala G, Quinto I, Ruocco MR, et al. Induction of tumorigenicity and plasmacytoid differentiation in EBV-B cells by expression of exogenous interleukin-6 or IL-6 receptor genes. *Leukemia* 1992;6:26S–29S.
270. Rochford R, Hobbs MV, Garnier JL, et al. Plasmacytoid differentiation of Epstein-Barr virus-transformed B cells *in vivo* is associated with reduced expression of viral latent genes. *Proc Natl Acad Sci USA* 1993;90:352–356.
271. Rizkalla KS, Asfar SK, McLean CA, et al. Key features distinguishing post-transplantation lymphoproliferative disorders and acute liver rejection. *Mod Pathol* 1997;10:708–715.
272. Drachenberg CB, Abruzzo LV, Klassen DK, et al. Epstein-Barr virus-related posttransplantation lymphoproliferative disorder involving pancreas allografts: histological differential diagnosis from acute allograft rejection. *Hum Pathol* 1998;29:569–577.
273. Dusenbery D, Nalesnik MA, Locker J, et al. Cytologic features of post-transplant lymphoproliferative disorder. *Diagn Cytopathol* 1997;16:489–496.
274. Randhawa PS, Magnone M, Jordan M, et al. Renal allograft involvement by Epstein-Barr virus associated post-transplant lymphoproliferative disease. *Am J Surg Pathol* 1996;20:563–571.
275. Alshak NS, Jiminez AM, Gedebou M, et al. Epstein-Barr virus infection in liver transplantation patients: correlation of histopathology and semiquantitative Epstein-Barr virus-DNA recovery using polymerase chain reaction. *Hum Pathol* 1993;24:1306–1312.
276. Lones MA, Shintaku IP, Weiss LM, et al. Posttransplant lymphoproliferative disorder in liver allograft biopsies: a comparison of three methods for the demonstration of Epstein-Barr virus. *Hum Pathol* 1997;28:533–539.
277. Randhawa P, Demetris AJ, Pietrzak B, et al. Histopathology of renal posttransplant lymphoproliferation: comparison with rejection using the Banff schema. *Am J Kidney Dis* 1996;28:578–584.
278. Montone KT, Friedman H, Hodinka RL, et al. In situ hybridization for Epstein-Barr virus NotI repeats in posttransplant lymphoproliferative disorder. *Mod Pathol* 1992;5:292–302.
279. Berg LC, Copenhaver CM, Morrison VA, et al. B-cell lymphoproliferative disorders in solid-organ transplant patients: detection of Epstein-Barr virus by in situ hybridization. *Hum Pathol* 1992;23:159–163.
280. Randhawa PS, Jaffe R, Demetris AJ, et al. The systemic distribution of Epstein-Barr virus genomes in fatal post-transplantation lymphoproliferative disorders: an in situ hybridization study. *Am J Pathol* 1991;138:1027–1033.
281. Randhawa PS, Jaffe R, Demetris AJ, et al. Expression of Epstein-Barr virus-encoded small RNA (by the EBER-1 gene) in liver specimens from transplant recipients with post-transplantation lymphoproliferative disease [see comments]. *N Engl J Med* 1992;327:1710–1714.
282. Lager DJ, Burgart LJ, Slagel DD. Epstein-Barr virus detection in sequential biopsies from patients with a posttransplant lymphoproliferative disorder. *Mod Pathol* 1993;6:42–47.
283. Hoffmann DG, Gedebou M, Jimenez A, et al. Detection of Epstein-Barr virus by polymerase chain reaction in transbronchial biopsies of lung transplant recipients: evidence of infection? *Mod Pathol* 1993;6:555–559.
284. Rosendale B, Yousem SA. Discrimination of Epstein-Barr virus-related posttransplant lymphoproliferations from acute rejection in lung allograft recipients. *Arch Pathol Lab Med* 1995;119:418–423.
285. Dietze O. Post-transplantation lymphoproliferative disorder versus acute liver rejection: do we need a scoring system? *Adv Anat Pathol* 1998;5:30–35.
286. Thomas JA, Hotchin NA, Allday MJ, et al. Immunohistology of Epstein-Barr virus-associated antigens in B cell disorders from immunocompromised individuals. *Transplantation* 1990;49:944–953.
287. Cleary ML, Warnke R, Sklar J. Monoclonality of lymphoproliferative lesions in cardiac-transplant recipients: clonal analysis based on immunoglobulin-gene rearrangements. *N Engl J Med* 1984;310:477–482.
288. Rea D, Fourcade C, Leblond V, et al. Patterns of Epstein-Barr virus latent and replicative gene expression in Epstein-Barr virus B cell lymphoproliferative disorders after organ transplantation. *Transplantation* 1994;58:317–324.
289. Quintanilla-Martinez L, Lome-Maldonado C, Schwarzmann F, et al. Post-transplantation lymphoproliferative disorders in Mexico: an aggressive clonal disease associated with Epstein-Barr virus type A. *Mod Pathol* 1998;11:200–208.
290. Young L, Alfieri C, Hennessy K, et al. Expression of Epstein-Barr virus transformation-associated genes in tissues of patients with EBV lymphoproliferative disease. *N Engl J Med* 1989;321:1080–1085.
291. Chetty R, Biddolph S, Gatter K. An immunohistochemical analysis of Reed-Sternberg–like cells in posttransplantation lymphoproliferative disorders: the possible pathogenetic relationship to Reed-Sternberg cells in Hodgkin's disease and Reed-Sternberg–like cells in non-Hodgkin's lymphomas and reactive conditions. *Hum Pathol* 1997;28:493–498.
292. Murray PG, Swinnen LJ, Constandinou CM, et al. BCL-2 but not its Epstein-Barr virus-encoded homologue, BHRF1, is commonly expressed in posttransplantation lymphoproliferative disorders [see comments]. *Blood* 1996;87:706–711.
293. Chetty R, Biddolph S, Kaklamanis L, et al. Bcl-2 protein is strongly expressed in post-transplant lymphoproliferative disorders. *J Pathol* 1996;180:254–258.

294. Kowal-Vern A, Swinnen L, Pyle J, et al. Characterization of post-cardiac transplant lymphomas: histology, immunophenotyping, immunohistochemistry, and gene rearrangement. *Arch Pathol Lab Med* 1996;120:41–48.
295. Nalesnik MA. Clinicopathologic features of posttransplant lymphoproliferative disorders. *Ann Transplant* 1997;2:33–40.
296. Setsuda J, Teruya-Feldstein J, Harris NL, et al. Interleukin-18, interferon-gamma, IP-10, and Mig expression in Epstein-Barr virus-induced infectious mononucleosis and posttransplant lymphoproliferative disease. *Am J Pathol* 1999;155:257–265.
297. Tlsty TD, Brown PC, Johnston R, et al. Enhanced frequency of generation of methotrexate resistance and gene amplification in cultured mouse and hamster cell lines. In: Schimke, RT, ed. *Gene amplification.* Cold Spring Harbor, NY: Cold Spring Harbor Laboratory, 1982: 231–238.
298. Davis CL, Wood BL, Sabath DE, et al. Interferon-alpha treatment of posttransplant lymphoproliferative disorder in recipients of solid organ transplants. *Transplantation* 1998;66:1770–1779.
299. Locker J, Nalesnik M. Molecular genetic analysis of lymphoid tumors arising after organ transplantation. *Am J Pathol* 1989;135:977–987.
300. Cleary ML, Nalesnik MA, Shearer WT, et al. Clonal analysis of transplant-associated lymphoproliferations based on the structure of the genomic termini of the Epstein-Barr virus. *Blood* 1988;72:349–352.
301. Patton DF, Wilkowski CW, Hanson CA, et al. Epstein-Barr virus—determined clonality in posttransplant lymphoproliferative disease. *Transplantation* 1990;49:1080–1084.
302. Ho M, Miller G, Atchison RW, et al. Epstein-Barr virus infections and DNA hybridization studies in posttransplantation lymphoma and lymphoproliferative lesions: the role of primary infection. *J Infect Dis* 1985;152:876–886.
303. Benkerrou M, Jais JP, Leblond V, et al. Anti-B-cell monoclonal antibody treatment of severe posttransplant B-lymphoproliferative disorder: prognostic factors and long-term outcome. *Blood* 1998;92: 3137–3147.
304. Cen H, Williams PA, McWilliams HP, et al. Evidence for restricted Epstein-Barr virus latent gene expression and anti-EBNA antibody response in solid organ transplant recipients with posttransplant lymphoproliferative disorders. *Blood* 1993;81:1393–1403.
305. Frank D, Cesarman E, Liu YF, et al. Posttransplantation lymphoproliferative disorders frequently contain type A and not type B Epstein-Barr virus. *Blood* 1995;85:1396–1403.
306. Liebowitz D. Epstein-Barr virus and a cellular signaling pathway in lymphomas from immunosuppressed patients [see comments]. *N Engl J Med* 1998;338:1413–1421.
307. Weiss LM, Movahed LA. In situ demonstration of Epstein-Barr viral genomes in viral-associated B cell lymphoproliferations. *Am J Pathol* 1989;134:651–659.
308. Borisch-Chappuis B, Nezelof C, Müller H, et al. Different Epstein-Barr virus expression in lymphomas from immunocompromised and immunocompetent patients. *Am J Pathol* 1990;136:751–758.
309. Montone KT, Hodinka RL, Salhany KE, et al. Identification of Epstein-Barr virus lytic activity in post-transplantation lymphoproliferative disease. *Mod Pathol* 1996;9:621–630.
310. Brink AA, Dukers DF, van den Brule AJ, et al. Presence of Epstein-Barr virus latency type III at the single cell level in post-transplantation lymphoproliferative disorders and AIDS related lymphomas. *J Clin Pathol* 1997;50:911–918.
311. Oudejans JJ, Jiwa M, van den Brule AJ, et al. Detection of heterogeneous Epstein-Barr virus gene expression patterns within individual post-transplantation lymphoproliferative disorders. *Am J Pathol* 1995; 147:923–933.
312. Rowe M, Niedobitek G, Young LS. Epstein-Barr virus gene expression in post-transplant lymphoproliferative disorders. *Springer Semin Immunopathol* 1998;20:389–403.
313. Scheinfeld AG, Nador RG, Cesarman E, et al. Epstein-Barr virus latent membrane protein-1 oncogene deletion in post-transplantation lymphoproliferative disorders. *Am J Pathol* 1997;151:805–812.
314. Kingma DW, Weiss WB, Jaffe ES, et al. Epstein-Barr virus latent membrane protein-1 oncogene deletions: correlations with malignancy in Epstein-Barr virus-associated lymphoproliferative disorders and malignant lymphomas. *Blood* 1996;88:242–251.
315. Dhir RJ, Nalesnik MA, Demetris AJ, et al. Latent membrane protein expression in posttransplant lymphoproliferative disease. *Appl Immunohistochem* 1995;3:123–126.
316. Thomas JA, Crawford DH, Burke M. Clinicopathologic implications of Epstein-Barr virus related B cell lymphoma in immunocompromised patients. *J Clin Pathol* 1995;48:287–290.
317. Delecluse HJ, Kremmer E, Rouault JP, et al. The expression of Epstein-Barr virus latent proteins is related to the pathological features of post-transplant lymphoproliferative disorders. *Am J Pathol* 1995; 146:1113–1120.
318. Niedobitek G, Mutimer DJ, Williams A, et al. Epstein-Barr virus infection and malignant lymphomas in liver transplant recipients. *Int J Cancer* 1997;73:514–520.
319. Chadburn A, Hyjeck E, Ying L, et al. Expression of Epstein-Barr virus (EBV) genes in posttransplant lymphoproliferative disorders (PTLPDs). *J Acquir Immune Defic Syndr* 1999;21:A30(abst)
320. Hanto DW, Birkenbach M, Frizzera G, et al. Confirmation of the heterogeneity of posttransplant Epstein-Barr virus-associated B cell proliferations by immunoglobulin gene rearrangement analyses. *Transplantation* 1989;47:458–464.
321. Kaplan MA, Ferry JA, Harris NL, et al. Clonal analysis of posttransplant lymphoproliferative disorders, using both episomal Epstein-Barr virus and immunoglobulin genes as markers. *Am J Clin Pathol* 1994; 101:590–596.
322. Shearer WT, Ritz J, Finegold MJ, et al. Epstein-Barr virus-associated B-cell proliferations of diverse clonal origins after bone marrow transplantation in a 12-year-old patient with severe combined immunodeficiency. *N Engl J Med* 1985;312:1151–1159.
323. Brown NA, Liu C, Garcia CR, et al. Clonal origins of lymphoproliferative disease induced by Epstein-Barr virus. *J Virol* 1986;58:975–978.
324. Cleary ML, Dorfman RF, Sklar J. Failure in immunological control of the virus infection: post-transplant lymphomas. In: Epstein MA, Achong BG, eds. *The Epstein-Barr: recent advances.* New York: Wiley & Sons; 1986:163–181.
325. Dror Y, Greenberg M, Taylor G, et al. Lymphoproliferative disorders after organ transplantation in children. *Transplantation* 1999;67: 990–998.
326. Hollingsworth HC, Stetler-Stevenson M, Gagneten D, et al. Immunodeficiency-associated malignant lymphoma: three cases showing genotypic evidence of both T- and B-cell lineages. *Am J Surg Pathol* 1994;18:1092–1101.
327. Nelson BP, Locker J, Nalesnik MA, et al. Clonal and morphological variation in a posttransplant lymphoproliferative disorder: evolution from clonal T-cell to clonal B-cell predominance. *Hum Pathol* 1998; 29:416–421.
328. Edwards RH, Raab-Traub N. Alterations of the p53 gene in Epstein-Barr virus-associated immunodeficiency-related lymphomas. *J Virol* 1994;68:1309–1315.
329. Wood A, Angus B, Kestevan P, et al. Alpha interferon gene deletions in post-transplant lymphoma. *Br J Haematol* 1997;98:1002–1003.
330. Delecluse HJ, Rouault JP, Jeammot B, et al. Bcl6/Laz3 rearrangements in post-transplant lymphoproliferative disorders. *Br J Haematol* 1995;91:101–103.
331. Lones MA, Lopez-Terrada D, Weiss LM, et al. Donor origin of post-transplant lymphoproliferative disorder localized to a liver allograft: demonstration by fluorescence in situ hybridization [see comments]. *Arch Pathol Lab Med* 1997;121:701–706.
332. Wood BL, Sabath D, Broudy VC, et al. The recipient origin of post-transplant lymphoproliferative disorders in pulmonary transplant patients: a report of three cases. *Cancer* 1996;78:2223–2228.
333. Chadburn A, Suciu-Foca N, Cesarman E, et al. Post-transplantation lymphoproliferative disorders arising in solid organ transplant recipients are usually of recipient origin. *Am J Pathol* 1995;147:1862–1870.
334. Weissmann DJ, Ferry JA, Harris NL, et al. Posttransplantation lymphoproliferative disorders in solid organ recipients are predominantly aggressive tumors of host origin. *Am J Clin Pathol* 1995;103: 748–755.
335. Armes JE, Angus P, Southey MC, et al. Lymphoproliferative disease of donor origin arising in patients after orthotopic liver transplantation. *Cancer* 1994;74:2436–2441.
336. Mentzer SJ, Longtine J, Fingeroth J, et al. Immunoblastic lymphoma of donor origin in the allograft after lung transplantation. *Transplantation* 1996;61:1720–1725.
337. Le Frere-Belda MA, Martin N, Gaulard P, et al. Donor or recipient origin of post-transplantation lymphoproliferative disorders: evaluation by in situ hybridization. *Mod Pathol* 1997;10:701–707.
338. Cheung AN, Chan AC, Chung LP, et al. Post-transplantation lympho-

proliferative disorder of donor origin in a sex-mismatched renal allograft as proven by chromosome in situ hybridization. *Mod Pathol* 1998;11:99–102.

339. Godyn JJ, Hicks DG, Hsu SH, et al. Demonstration of passenger leukocytes in a case of Epstein-Barr virus posttransplant lymphoproliferative disorder using restriction fragment length polymorphism analysis. *Arch Pathol Lab Med* 1992;116:249–252.
340. Hruban RH, Long PP, Perlman EJ, et al. Fluorescence in situ hybridization for the Y-chromosome can be used to detect cells of recipient origin in allografted hearts following cardiac transplantation. *Am J Pathol* 1993;142:975–980.
341. Lones MA, Lopez-Terrada D, Shintaku IP, et al. Posttransplant lymphoproliferative disorder in pediatric bone marrow transplant recipients: disseminated disease of donor origin demonstrated by fluorescence in situ hybridization. *Arch Pathol Lab Med* 1998;122:708–714.
342. Schouten HC, Hopman AH, Haesevoets AM, et al. Large-cell anaplastic non-Hodgkin's lymphoma originating in donor cells after allogenic bone marrow transplantation. *Br J Haematol* 1995;91:162–166.
343. Trimble MS, Waye JS, Walker IR, et al. B-cell lymphoma of recipient origin 9 years after allogeneic bone marrow transplantation for T-cell acute lymphoblastic leukaemia. *Br J Haematol* 1993;85:99–102.
344. O'Riordan JM, Molloy K, O'Briain DS, et al. Localized, late-onset, high-grade lymphoma following bone marrow transplantation: response to combination chemotherapy. *Br J Haematol* 1994;86: 183–186.
345. Fischer A, Blanche S, Le Bidois J, et al. Anti-B-cell monoclonal antibodies in the treatment of severe B-cell lymphoproliferative syndrome following bone marrow and organ transplantation. *N Engl J Med* 1991;324:1451–1456.
346. Haque T, Crawford DH. Role of donor versus recipient type Epstein-Barr virus in post-transplant lymphoproliferative disorders. *Springer Semin Immunopathol* 1998;20:375–387.
347. Cen H, Breinig MC, Atchison RW, et al. Epstein-Barr virus transmission via the donor organs in solid organ transplantation: polymerase chain reaction and restriction fragment length polymorphism analysis of IR2, IR3, and IR4. *J Virol* 1991;65:976–980.
348. Gratama JW, Oosterveer MA, Zwaan FE, et al. Eradication of Epstein-Barr virus by allogeneic bone marrow transplantation: implications for sites of viral latency. *Proc Natl Acad Sci USA* 1988;85:8693–8696.
349. Cabanillas F, Pathak S, Zander A, et al. Monosomy 21, partial duplication of chromosome 11, and structural abnormality of chromosome 1q21 in a case of lymphoma developing in a transplant recipient: characteristic abnormalities of secondary lymphoma? *Cancer Genet Cytogenet* 1987;24:7–10.
350. Olopade OL, Anastasi J, Thangavelu M, et al. Cytogenetic abnormalities in a secondary lymphoma complicating cardiac transplantation. *Leukemia* 1989;3:303–304.
351. Forman SJ, Sullivan JL, Wright C, et al. Epstein-Barr-virus-related malignant B cell lymphoplasmacytic lymphoma following allogeneic bone marrow transplantation for aplastic anemia. *Transplantation* 1987;44:244–249.
352. Lyons SF, Liebowitz DN. The roles of human viruses in the pathogenesis of lymphoma. *Semin Oncol* 1998;25:461–475.
353. Delecluse HJ, Rouault JP, Ffrench M, et al. Post-transplant lymphoproliferative disorders with genetic abnormalities commonly found in malignant tumours. *Br J Haematol* 1995;89:90–97.
354. Gollin SM, Cen H, Storto PD, et al. Consistent nonclonal cytogenetic abnormalities in post-transplant lymphoproliferative disease. *Am J Hum Genet* 1990;47:A7(abst).
355. Hanto DW, Frizzera G, Gajl-Peczalska KJ, et al. Epstein-Barr virus, immunodeficiency, and B cell lymphoproliferation. *Transplantation* 1985;39:461–472.
356. Tosato G, Teruya-Feldstein J, Setsuda J, et al. Post-transplant lymphoproliferative disease (PTLD): lymphokine production and PTLD. *Springer Semin Immunopathol* 1998;20:405–423.
357. Faro A. Interferon-alpha and its effects on post-transplant lymphoproliferative disorders. *Springer Semin Immunopathol* 1998;20:425–436.
358. Mathur A, Kamat DM, Filipovich AH, et al. Immunoregulatory abnormalities in patients with Epstein-Barr virus-associated B cell lymphoproliferative disorders. *Transplantation* 1994;57:1042–1045.
359. Nalesnik MA, Zeevi A, Randhawa PS, et al. Cytokine mRNA profiles in Epstein-Barr virus-associated post-transplant lymphoproliferative disorders. *Clin Transplant* 1999;13:39–44.
360. Morel PA, Oriss TB. Crossregulation between Th1 and Th2 cells. *Crit Rev Immunol* 1998;18:275–303.
361. Tanner JE, Alfieri C. Interactions involving cyclosporine A, interleukin-6, and Epstein-Barr virus lead to the promotion of B-cell lymphoproliferative disease. *Leuk Lymphoma* 1996;21:379–390.
362. Burke GW, Cirocco R, Hensley G, et al. The rapid development of a fatal, disseminated B cell lymphoma following liver transplantation: serial changes in levels of soluble serum interleukin 2 and interleukin 4 (B cell growth factor). *Transplantation* 1992;53:1148–1150.
363. Birkeland SA, Hamilton-Dutoit S, Sandvej K, et al. EBV-induced post-transplant lymphoproliferative disorder (PTLD). *Transplant Proc* 1995;27:3467–3472.
364. Tosato G, Jones K, Breinig MK, et al. Interleukin-6 production in posttransplant lymphoproliferative disease. *J Clin Invest* 1993;91: 2806–2814.
365. Montone KT, Litzky LA, Wurster A, et al. Analysis of Epstein-Barr virus-associated posttransplantation lymphoproliferative disorder after lung transplantation. *Surgery* 1996;119:544–551.
366. Penn I. *Cancers* following cyclosporine therapy. *Transplantation* 1987;43:32–35.
367. Penn I. The changing pattern of posttransplant malignancies. *Transplant Proc* 1991;23:1101–1103.
368. Cohen JI. Epstein-Barr virus lymphoproliferative disease associated with acquired immunodeficiency. *Medicine (Baltimore)* 1991;70: 137–160.
369. Hanto DW. Classification of Epstein-Barr virus-associated posttransplant lymphoproliferative diseases: implications for understanding their pathogenesis and developing rational treatment strategies. *Annu Rev Med* 1995;46:381–394.
370. Swinnen LJ. Transplant immunosuppression-related malignant lymphomas. *Cancer Treat Res* 1993;66:95–110.
371. Renoult E, Kessler M. [Lymphoproliferative lesions localized in the renal graft: a French multicenter study]. *J Radiol* 1994;75:53–56.
372. Raymond E, Tricottet V, Samuel D, et al. Epstein-Barr virus-related localized hepatic lymphoproliferative disorders after liver transplantation. *Cancer* 1995;76:1344–1351.
373. Younes BS, Ament ME, McDiarmid SV, et al. The involvement of the gastrointestinal tract in posttransplant lymphoproliferative disease in pediatric liver transplantation [see comments]. *J Pediatr Gastroenterol Nutr* 1999;28:380–385.
374. Martinez AJ, Ahdab-Barmada M. The neuropathology of liver transplantation: comparison of main complications in children and adults. *Mod Pathol* 1993;6:25–32.
375. Lucas KG, Pollok KE, Emanuel DJ. Post-transplant EBV induced lymphoproliferative disorders. *Leuk Lymphoma* 1997;25:1–8.
376. Cavazzana-Calvo M, Bensoussan D, Jabado N, et al. Prevention of EBV-induced B-lymphoproliferative disorder by ex vivo marrow B-cell depletion in HLA-phenoidentical or non-identical T-depleted bone marrow transplantation. *Br J Haematol* 1998;103:543–551.
377. Benkerrou M, Durandy A, Fischer A. Therapy for transplant-related lymphoproliferative diseases. *Hematol Oncol Clin North Am* 1993;7: 467–475.
378. Vogl M, Griesmacher A, Grimm M, et al. Tissue polypeptide specific antigen for the detection of lymphoproliferative diseases induced by cyclosporin [published erratum appears in *J Clin Pathol* 1996;49: 190]. *J Clin Pathol* 1995;48:1039–1044.
379. Swinnen LJ. Treatment of organ transplant-related lymphoma. *Hematol Oncol Clin North Am* 1997;11:963–973.
380. Darenkov IA, Marcarelli MA, Basadonna GP, et al. Reduced incidence of Epstein-Barr virus-associated posttransplant lymphoproliferative disorder using preemptive antiviral therapy. *Transplantation* 1997;64:848–852.
381. Garrett TJ, Chadburn A, Barr ML, et al. Posttransplantation lymphoproliferative disorders treated with cyclophosphamide-doxorubicin-vincristine-prednisone chemotherapy. *Cancer* 1993;72:2782–2785.
382. Franken M, Estabrooks A, Cavacini L, et al. Epstein-Barr virus-driven gene therapy for EBV-related lymphomas. *Nat Med* 1996;2: 1379–1382.
383. Kenney S, Ge JQ, Westphal EM, et al. Gene therapy strategies for treating Epstein-Barr virus-associated lymphomas: comparison of two different Epstein-Barr virus-based vectors [see comments]. *Hum Gene Ther* 1998;9:1131–1141.
384. Shapiro RS, Chauvenet A, McGuire W, et al. Treatment of B-cell

lymphoproliferative disorders with interferon alfa and intravenous gamma globulin [Letter]. *N Engl J Med* 1988;318:1334.
385. Heslop HE, Rooney CM. Adoptive cellular immunotherapy for EBV lymphoproliferative disease. *Immunol Rev* 1997;157:217–222.
386. Rooney CM, Smith CA, Ng CY, et al. Infusion of cytotoxic T cells for the prevention and treatment of Epstein-Barr virus-induced lymphoma in allogeneic transplant recipients. *Blood* 1998;92:1549–1555.
387. O'Reilly RJ, Small TN, Papadopoulos E, et al. Biology and adoptive cell therapy of Epstein-Barr virus-associated lymphoproliferative disorders in recipients of marrow allografts. *Immunol Rev* 1997;157: 195–216.
388. Knowles DM. The molecular genetics of post-transplantation lymphoproliferative disorders. *Springer Semin Immunopathol* 1998;20: 357–373.
389. Alfrey EJ, Friedman AL, Grossman RA, et al. A recent decrease in the time to development of monomorphous and polymorphous post-transplant lymphoproliferative disorder. *Transplantation* 1992;54: 250–253.
390. Spencer ES, Andersen HK. Antibodies to the Epstein-Barr virus in kidney transplant recipients. *Acta Med Scand* 1972;191:107–110.
391. Marker SC, Ascher NL, Kalis JM, et al. Epstein-Barr virus antibody responses and clinical illness in renal transplant recipients. *Surgery* 1979;85:433–440.
392. Chang RS, Lewis JP, Abildgaard CF. Prevalence of oropharyngeal excreters of leukocyte-transforming agents among a human population. *N Engl J Med* 1973;289:1325–1329.
393. Chang RS, Lewis JP, Reynolds RD, et al. Oropharyngeal excretion of Epstein-Barr virus by patients with lymphoproliferative disorders and by recipients of renal homografts. *Ann Intern Med* 1978;88: 34–40.
394. Strauch B, Andrews LL, Siegel N, et al. Oropharyngeal excretion of Epstein-Barr virus by renal transplant recipients and other patients treated with immunosuppressive drugs. *Lancet* 1974;1:234–237.
395. Tosato G, Blaese RM. Epstein-Barr virus infection and immunoregulation in man. *Adv Immunol* 1985;37:99–149.
396. Knecht H, Berger C, al-Homsi AS, et al. Epstein-Barr virus oncogenesis. *Crit Rev Oncol Hematol* 1997;26:117–135.
397. Su IJ, Chen JY. The role of Epstein-Barr virus in lymphoid malignancies. *Crit Rev Oncol Hematol* 1997;26:25–41.
398. Manet E, Bourillot PY, Waltzer L, et al. EBV genes and B cell proliferation. *Crit Rev Oncol Hematol* 1998;28:129–137.
399. Ambinder RF, Lemas MV, Moore S, et al. Epstein-Barr virus and lymphoma. *Cancer Treat Res* 1999;99:27–45.
400. Kulwichit W, Edwards RH, Davenport EM, et al. Expression of the Epstein-Barr virus latent membrane protein 1 induces B cell lymphoma in transgenic mice. *Proc Natl Acad Sci USA* 1998;95: 11963–11968.
401. Rickinson AB, Lee SP, Steven NM. Cytotoxic T lymphocyte responses to Epstein-Barr virus. *Curr Opin Immunol* 1996;8:492–497.
402. Callan MF, Steven N, Krausa P, et al. Large clonal expansions of $CD8^+$ T cells in acute infectious mononucleosis. *Nat Med* 1996;2: 906–911.
403. Riddler SA, Breinig MC, McKnight JL. Increased levels of circulating Epstein-Barr virus (EBV)-infected lymphocytes and decreased EBV nuclear antigen antibody responses are associated with the development of posttransplant lymphoproliferative disease in solid-organ transplant recipients. *Blood* 1994;84:972–984.
404. Gaston JS, Rickinson AB, Epstein MA. Epstein-Barr-virus-specific T-cell memory in renal-allograft recipients under long-term immunosuppression. *Lancet* 1982;1:923–925.
405. Legendre CM, Guttmann RD, Yip GH. Natural killer cell subsets in long-term renal allograft recipients: a phenotypic and functional study. *Transplantation* 1986;42:347–352.
406. Swinnen LJ, Fisher RI. OKT3 monoclonal antibodies induce interleukin-6 and interleukin-10: a possible cause of lymphoproliferative disorders associated with transplantation. *Curr Opin Nephrol Hypertens* 1993;2:670–678.
407. Ren EC, Chan SH. Possible enhancement of Epstein-Barr virus infections by the use of OKT3 in transplant recipients. *Transplantation* 1988;45:988–989.
408. Kahan BD. Cyclosporine [see comments]. *N Engl J Med* 1989;321: 1725–1738.
409. Nazaruk RA, Rochford R, Hobbs MV, et al. Functional diversity of the CD8(+) T-cell response to Epstein-Barr virus (EBV): implications for the pathogenesis of EBV-associated lymphoproliferative disorders. *Blood* 1998;91:3875–3883.
410. Savage P, Waxman J. Post-transplantation lymphoproliferative disease. *Q J Med* 1997;90:497–503.
411. Lucas KG, Burton RL, Zimmerman SE, et al. Semiquantitative Epstein-Barr virus (EBV) polymerase chain reaction for the determination of patients at risk for EBV-induced lymphoproliferative disease after stem cell transplantation. *Blood* 1998;91:3654–3661.
412. Randhawa PS, Yousem SA. Epstein-Barr virus-associated lymphoproliferative disease in a heart-lung allograft: demonstration of host origin by restriction fragment-length polymorphism analysis. *Transplantation* 1990;49:126–130.
413. Rowe DT, Rowe M, Evan GI, et al. Restricted expression of EBV latent genes and T-lymphocyte–detected membrane antigen in Burkitt's lymphoma cells. *EMBO J* 1986;5:2599–2607.
414. Gregory CD, Murray RJ, Edwards CF, et al. Downregulation of cell adhesion molecules LFA-3 and ICAM-1 in Epstein-Barr virus-positive Burkitt's lymphoma underlies tumor cell escape from virus-specific T cell surveillance. *J Exp Med* 1988;167:1811–1824.
415. van Gorp J, Doornewaard H, Verdonck LF, et al. Posttransplant T-cell lymphoma: report of three cases and a review of the literature. *Cancer* 1994;73:3064–3072.
416. Ghorbani RP, Shokouh-Amiri H, Gaber LW. Intragraft angiotropic large-cell lymphoma of T cell-type in a long-term renal allograft recipient [see comments]. *Mod Pathol* 1996;9:671–676.
417. Rostaing L, Tkaczuk J, Rigal-Huguet F, et al. T-cell gamma-delta lymphoproliferative disorders after renal transplantation. *Transplant Proc* 1995;27:1774–1775.
418. Ross CW, Schnitzer B, Sheldon S, et al. Gamma/delta T-cell posttransplantation lymphoproliferative disorder primarily in the spleen. *Am J Clin Pathol* 1994;102:310–315.
419. Feher O, Barilla D, Locker J, et al. T-cell large granular lymphocytic leukemia following orthotopic liver transplantation. *Am J Hematol* 1995;49:216–220.
420. Hanson MN, Morrison VA, Peterson BA, et al. Posttransplant T-cell lymphoproliferative disorders: an aggressive, late complication of solid-organ transplantation [see comments]. *Blood* 1996;88: 3626–3633.
421. Macon WR, Williams ME, Greer JP, et al. Natural killer–like T-cell lymphomas: aggressive lymphomas of T–large granular lymphocytes [see comments]. *Blood* 1996;87:1474–1483.
422. Francois A, Lesesve JF, Stamatoullas A, et al. Hepatosplenic gamma/delta T-cell lymphoma: a report of two cases in immunocompromised patients, associated with isochromosome 7q. *Am J Surg Pathol* 1997; 21:781–790.
423. Kraus MD, Crawford DF, Kaleem Z, et al. T gamma/delta hepatosplenic lymphoma in a heart transplant patient after an Epstein-Barr virus positive lymphoproliferative disorder: a case report. *Cancer* 1998;82:983–992.
424. Yasunaga C, Kasai T, Nishihara G, et al. Early development of Epstein-Barr virus-associated T-cell lymphoma after a living-related renal transplantation. *Transplantation* 1998;65:1642–1644.
425. Hsi ED, Picken MM, Alkan S. Post-transplantation lymphoproliferative disorder of the NK-cell type: a case report and review of the literature. *Mod Pathol* 1998;11:479–484.
426. Dockrell DH, Strickler JG, Paya CV. Epstein-Barr virus-induced T cell lymphoma in solid organ transplant recipients. *Clin Infect Dis* 1998;26:180–182.
427. Gentile TC, Hadlock KG, Uner AH, et al. Large granular lymphocyte leukaemia occurring after renal transplantation. *Br J Haematol* 1998; 101:507–512.
428. Natkunam Y, Warnke RA, Zehnder JL, et al. Aggressive natural killer–like T-cell malignancy with leukemic presentation following solid organ transplantation. *Am J Clin Pathol* 1999;111:663–671.
429. Lin WC, Moore JO, Mann KP, et al. Post transplant $CD8^+$ gamma delta T-cell lymphoma associated with human herpes virus-6 infection. *Leuk Lymphoma* 1999;33:377–384.
430. Zutter MM, Durnam DM, Hackman RC, et al. Secondary T-cell lymphoproliferation after marrow transplantation. *Am J Clin Pathol* 1990;94:714–721.
431. Borisch B, Hennig I, Horber F, et al. Enteropathy-associated T-cell lymphoma in a renal transplant patient with evidence of Epstein-Barr virus involvement. *Virchows Arch A Pathol Anat Histopathol* 1992; 421:443–447.

432. Hacker SM, Knight BP, Lunde NM, et al. A primary central nervous system T cell lymphoma in a renal transplant patient. *Transplantation* 1992;53:691–692.
433. Ng K, Trotter J, Metcalf C, et al. Extranodal Ki-1 lymphoma in a renal transplant patient. *Aust N Z J Med* 1992;22:51–53.
434. Waller EK, Ziemianska M, Bangs CD, et al. Characterization of posttransplant lymphomas that express T-cell-associated markers: immunophenotypes, molecular genetics, cytogenetics, and heterotransplantation in severe combined immunodeficient mice. *Blood* 1993;82: 247–261.
435. Jaffe ES. Classification of natural killer (NK) cell and NK-like T-cell malignancies [Editorial; comment]. *Blood* 1996;87:1207–1210.
436. Raftery MJ, Tidman MJ, Koffman G, et al. Posttransplantation T cell lymphoma of the skin. *Transplantation* 1988;46:475–477.
437. Euvrard S, Noble CP, Kanitakis J, et al. Brief report: successive occurrence of T-cell and B-cell lymphomas after renal transplantation in a patient with multiple cutaneous squamous-cell carcinomas. *N Engl J Med* 1992;327:1924–1926.
438. Pascual J, Torrelo A, Teruel JL, et al. Cutaneous T cell lymphomas after renal transplantation. *Transplantation* 1992;53:1143–1145.
439. Zanke BW, Rush DN, Jeffery JR, et al. HTLV-1 T cell lymphoma in a cyclosporine-treated renal transplant patient. *Transplantation* 1989;48:695–697.
440. Tsurumi H, Tani K, Tsuruta T, et al. Adult T-cell leukemia developing during immunosuppressive treatment in a renal transplant recipient. *Am J Hematol* 1992;41:292–294.
441. Lippman SM, Grogan TM, Carry P, et al. Post-transplantation T cell lymphoblastic lymphoma. *Am J Med* 1987;82:814–816.
442. Chetty R, Biddolph SC, Kaklamanis L, et al. EBV latent membrane protein (LMP-1) and bcl-2 protein expression in Reed-Sternberg–like cells in post-transplant lymphoproliferative disorders. *Histopathology* 1996;28:257–260.
443. Reynolds DJ, Banks PM, Gulley ML. New characterization of infectious mononucleosis and a phenotypic comparison with Hodgkin's disease. *Am J Pathol* 1995;146:379–388.
444. Nalesnik MA, Randhawa P, Demetris AJ, et al. Lymphoma resembling Hodgkin disease after posttransplant lymphoproliferative disorder in a liver transplant recipient. *Cancer* 1993;72:2568–2573.
445. Tinguely M, Vonlanthen R, Muller E, et al. Hodgkin's disease–like lymphoproliferative disorders in patients with different underlying immunodeficiency states. *Mod Pathol* 1998;11:307–312.
446. Tsang WY, Chan JK, Sing C. The nature of Reed-Sternberg–like cells in chronic lymphocytic leukemia. *Am J Clin Pathol* 1993;99:317–323.
447. Momose H, Jaffe ES, Shin SS, et al. Chronic lymphocytic leukemia/small lymphocytic lymphoma with Reed-Sternberg–like cells and possible transformation to Hodgkin's disease: mediation by Epstein-Barr virus [see comments]. *Am J Surg Pathol* 1992;16:859–867.
448. Zukerberg LR, Collins AB, Ferry JA, et al. Coexpression of CD15 and CD20 by Reed-Sternberg cells in Hodgkin's disease. *Am J Pathol* 1991;139:475–483.
449. Bierman PJ, Vose JM, Langnas AN, et al. Hodgkin's disease following solid organ transplantation. *Ann Oncol* 1996;7:265–270.
450. Goyal RK, McEvoy L, Wilson DB. Hodgkin disease after renal transplantation in childhood. *J Pediatr Hematol Oncol* 1996;18:392–395.
451. Sterling WA, Wu LY, Dowling EA, et al. Hodgkin's disease in a renal transplant recipient: a case report. *Transplantation* 1974;17:315–317.
452. Cerilli J, Rynasiewicz JJ, Lemos LB, et al. Hodgkin's disease in human renal transplantation. *Am J Surg* 1977;133:182–184.
453. Doyle TJ, Venkatachalam KK, Maeda K, et al. Hodgkin's disease in renal transplant recipients. *Cancer* 1983;51:245–247.
454. Bedrossian J, Metivier F, Jaccard A, et al. Hodgkin's disease and cadaveric renal transplantation. *Transplant Proc* 1995;27:1783–1784.
455. Garnier JL, Lebranchu Y, Lefrancois N, et al. Hodgkin's disease after renal transplantation. *Transplant Proc* 1995;27:1785.
456. Garnier JL, Lebranchu Y, Dantal J, et al. Hodgkin's disease after transplantation. *Transplantation* 1996;61:71–76.
457. Hood IM, Mahendra P, McNeil K, et al. Hodgkin's disease after cardiac transplant: a report of two cases. *Clin Lab Haematol* 1996;18: 115–116.
458. Oldhafer KJ, Bunzendahl H, Frei U, et al. Primary Hodgkin's lymphoma: an unusual cause of graft dysfunction after kidney transplantation. *Am J Med* 1989;87:218–220.
459. Moreau A, Dantal J, Heymann MF, et al. [Post-transplantation of Hodgkin's disease: clinico-pathologic study of 3 cases]. *Ann Pathol* 1996;16:124–127.
460. Conter V, Tschumperlin B, Gridelli B, et al. Hodgkin's disease occurring in a child after liver transplantation. *Ann Oncol* 1998;9:673–676.
461. Penn I. Lymphomas complicating organ transplantation. *Transplant Proc* 1983;15:2790–2797.
462. Tirelli U, Errante D, Dolcetti R, et al. Hodgkin's disease and human immunodeficiency virus infection: clinicopathologic and virologic features of 114 patients from the Italian Cooperative Group on AIDS and Tumors. *J Clin Oncol* 1995;13:1758–1767.
463. Meignin V, Devergie A, Brice P, et al. Hodgkin's disease of donor origin after allogeneic bone marrow transplantation for myelogenous chronic leukemia. *Transplantation* 1998;65:595–597.
464. Rowlings PA, Curtis RE, Passweg JR, et al. Increased incidence of Hodgkin's disease after allogeneic bone marrow transplantation. *J Clin Oncol* 1999;17:3122–3127.
465. Hjelle B, Evans-Holm M, Yen TS, et al. A poorly differentiated lymphoma of donor origin in a renal allograft recipient. *Transplantation* 1989;47:945–948.
466. Jones D, Ballestas ME, Kaye KM, et al. Primary-effusion lymphoma and Kaposi's sarcoma in a cardiac-transplant recipient [see comments]. *N Engl J Med* 1998;339:444–449.
467. Nelson BP, Nalesnik MA, Locker JD, et al. EBV negative posttransplant lymphoproliferative disorders: a distinct entity? *Lab Invest* 1996; 74:118A(abst).
468. Dotti G, Fiocchi R, Motta T, et al. Primary effusion lymphoma after heart transplantation: a new entity associated with human herpesvirus-8. *Leukemia* 1999;13:664–670.
469. Castleman B, Iverson L, Menendez VP. Localized mediastinal lymph node hyperplasia resembling thymoma. *Cancer* 1956;9:822–830.
470. Flendrig JA, Schillings PHM. Benign giant lymphoma: the clinical signs and symptoms. *Folia Med Neerl* 1969;12:119–120.
471. Flendrig JA. *Benign giant lymphoma: clinicopathologic correlation study.* Chicago: Year Book Medical, 1970.
472. Keller AR, Hochholzer L, Castleman B. Hyaline-vascular and plasma-cell types of giant lymph node hyperplasia of the mediastinum and other locations. *Cancer* 1972;29:670–683.
473. Leibetseder F, Thurner J. Angiofollikulare Lymphknotenhyperplasie (Zwiebelschalenlymphom). *Med Klin* 1973;68:817–820.
474. Gaba AR, Stein RS, Sweet DL, et al. Multicentric giant lymph node hyperplasia. *Am J Clin Pathol* 1978;69:86–90.
475. Weisenburger DD, Nathwani BN, Winberg CD, et al. Multicentric angiofollicular lymph node hyperplasia: a clinicopathologic study of 16 cases. *Hum Pathol* 1985;16:162–172.
476. Diebold J, Tulliez M, Bernadou A, et al. Angiofollicular and plasmacytic polyadenopathy: a pseudotumorous syndrome with dysimmunity. *J Clin Pathol* 1980;33:1068–1076.
477. Frizzera G, Peterson BA, Bayrd ED, et al. A systemic lymphoproliferative disorder with morphologic features of Castleman's disease: clinical findings and clinicopathologic correlations in 15 patients. *J Clin Oncol* 1985;3:1202–1216.
478. Mori S, Mohri N, Uchida T, et al. Idiopathic plasmacytic lymphadenopathy with polyclonal hyperimmunoglobulinemia: a syndrome related to giant lymph node hyperplasia of plasma cell type. *J Jpn Soc Res* 1981;20[Suppl]:85–94.
479. Mori N, Tsunoda R, Kojima K. Multicentric lymphadenopathy histologically simulating Castleman's disease. *J Jpn Soc Res* 1981; 20[Suppl]:55–66.
480. Kojima M, Sakuma H, Mori N. Histopathological features of plasma cell dyscrasia with polyneuropathy and endocrine disturbances, with special reference to germinal center lesions. *Jpn J Clin Oncol* 1983; 13:557–575.
481. Danon AD, Krishnan J, Frizzera G. Morpho-immunophenotypic diversity of Castleman's disease, hyaline-vascular type: with emphasis on a stroma-rich variant and a new pathogenetic hypothesis. *Virchows Arch A Pathol Anat Histopathol* 1993;423:369–382.
482. Frizzera G. Castleman's disease: more questions than answers. *Hum Pathol* 1985;16:202–205.
483. Menke DM, Camoriano JK, Banks PM. Angiofollicular lymph node hyperplasia: a comparison of unicentric, multicentric, hyaline vascular, and plasma cell types of disease by morphometric and clinical analysis. *Mod Pathol* 1992;5:525–530.
484. Akira S, Taga T, Kishimoto T. Interleukin-6 in biology and medicine. *Adv Immunol* 1993;54:1–78.

485. Kessler E. Multicentric giant lymph node hyperplasia: a report of seven cases. *Cancer* 1985;56:2446–2451.
486. Herrada J, Cabanillas F, Rice L, et al. The clinical behavior of localized and multicentric Castleman disease. *Ann Intern Med* 1998;128: 657–662.
487. Artusi T, Bonacorsi G, Saragoni A, et al. Castleman's lymphadenopathy: twenty years of observation. II: generalized form. *Haematologica* 1982;67:124–142.
488. Bowne WB, Lewis JJ, Filippa DA, et al. The management of unicentric and multicentric Castleman's disease: a report of 16 cases and a review of the literature. *Cancer* 1999;85:706–717.
489. Frizzera G. Castleman's disease and related disorders. *Semin Diagn Pathol* 1988;5:346–364.
490. Cesarman E, Knowles DM. Kaposi's sarcoma-associated herpesvirus: a lymphotropic human herpesvirus associated with Kaposi's sarcoma, primary effusion lymphoma, and multicentric Castleman's disease [published erratum appears in *Semin Diagn Pathol* 1997;14:161–162]. *Semin Diagn Pathol* 1997;14:54–66.
491. Neipel F, Albrecht JC, Ensser A, et al. Human herpesvirus 8 encodes a homolog of interleukin-6. *J Virol* 1997;71:839–842.
492. Nguyen DT, Diamond LW, Hansmann ML, et al. Castleman's disease: differences in follicular dendritic network in the hyaline vascular and plasma cell variants. *Histopathology* 1994;24:437–443.
493. Millikin PD. Epitheloid germinal centers in the human spleen. *Arch Pathol* 1970;89:314–320.
494. Menke DM, Tiemann M, Camoriano JK, et al. Diagnosis of Castleman's disease by identification of an immunophenotypically aberrant population of mantle zone B lymphocytes in paraffin-embedded lymph node biopsies. *Am J Clin Pathol* 1996;105:268–276.
495. Ruco LP, Gearing AJ, Pigott R, et al. Expression of ICAM-1, VCAM-1 and ELAM-1 in angiofollicular lymph node hyperplasia (Castleman's disease): evidence for dysplasia of follicular dendritic reticulum cells. *Histopathology* 1991;19:523–528.
496. Summerfield GP, Taylor W, Bellingham AJ, et al. Hyaline-vascular variant of angiofollicular lymph node hyperplasia with systemic manifestations and response to corticosteroids. *J Clin Pathol* 1983;36: 1005–1011.
497. Rosen LB, Robinson MJ, Rywlin AM. Familial multicentric angiofollicular lymphoid hyperplasia. *South Med J* 1983;76:1183–1184.
498. Cousineau S, Beauchamp G, Boileau J. Extramedullary plasmacytoma associated with angiofollicular lymph node hyperplasia. *Arch Pathol Lab Med* 1986;110:157–158.
499. Gould SJ, Diss T, Isaacson PG. Multicentric Castleman's disease in association with a solitary plasmacytoma: a case report. *Histopathology* 1990;17:135–140.
500. Leoncini L, del Vecchio MT, Minacci C, et al. Kaposi's sarcoma of lymph nodes associated with multicentric angiofollicular hyperplasia. *Appl Pathol* 1989;7:329–332.
501. Soulier J, Grollet L, Oksenhendler E, et al. Kaposi's sarcoma-associated herpesvirus-like DNA sequences in multicentric Castleman's disease [see comments]. *Blood* 1995;86:1276–1280.
502. Soulier J, Grollet L, Oksenhendler E, et al. Molecular analysis of clonality in Castleman's disease. *Blood* 1995;86:1131–1138.
503. Dupin N, Diss TL, Kellam P, et al. HHV-8 is associated with a plasmablastic variant of Castleman's disease that is linked to HHV-8-positive plasmablastic lymphoma. *Blood* 2000;95:1406–1412.
504. Lennert K, Mohri N. Histopathology and diagnosis of non-Hodgkin's lymphomas. In: Lennert K, ed. *Malignant lymphomas other than Hodgkin's disease.* Berlin: Springer-Verlag, 1978:111–469.
505. Weisenburger DD. Multicentric angiofollicular lymph node hyperplasia: pathology of the spleen. *Am J Surg Pathol* 1988;12:176–181.
506. Hayashi M, Aoshiba K, Shimada M, et al. Kaposi's sarcoma-associated herpesvirus infection in the lung in multicentric Castleman's disease [see comments]. *Intern Med* 1999;38:279–282.
507. Torii K, Ogawa K, Kawabata Y, et al. Lymphoid interstitial pneumonia as a pulmonary lesion of idiopathic plasmacytic lymphadenopathy with hyperimmunoglobulinemia. *Intern Med* 1994;33:237–241.
508. Johkoh T, Muller NL, Ichikado K, et al. Intrathoracic multicentric Castleman disease: CT findings in 12 patients. *Radiology* 1998;209: 477–481.
509. O'Reilly PE Jr, Joshi VV, Holbrook CT, et al. Multicentric Castleman's disease in a child with prominent thymic involvement: a case report and brief review of the literature. *Mod Pathol* 1993;6:776–780.
510. Watanabe S, Ohara K, Kukita A, et al. Systemic plasmacytosis: a syndrome of peculiar multiple skin eruptions, generalized lymphadenopathy, and polyclonal hypergammaglobulinemia. *Arch Dermatol* 1986;122:1314–1320.
511. Kitamura K, Tamura N, Hatano H, et al. A case of plasmacytosis with multiple peculiar eruptions. *J Dermatol* 1980;7:341–349.
512. Kubota Y, Noto S, Takakuwa T, et al. Skin involvement in giant lymph node hyperplasia (Castleman's disease). *J Am Acad Dermatol* 1993;29:778–780.
513. Nitta Y. Case of malignant lymphoma associated with primary systemic plasmacytosis with polyclonal hypergammaglobulinemia. *Am J Dermatopathol* 1997;19:289–293.
514. Skelton HG, Smith KJ. Extranodal multicentric Castleman's disease with cutaneous involvement. *Mod Pathol* 1998;11:93–98.
515. Hall PA, Donaghy M, Cotter FE, et al. An immunohistological and genotypic study of the plasma cell form of Castleman's disease. *Histopathology* 1989;14:333–346; discussion, 429–332.
516. Weisenburger DD, Lipscomb Grierson H, Purtilo D. Immunologic studies of multicentric (M) and unicentric (U) angiofollicular lymphoid hyperplasia (AFH). *Lab Invest* 1986;54:68A(abst).
517. Martin JM, Bell B, Ruether BA. Giant lymph node hyperplasia (Castleman's disease) of hyaline vascular type: clinical heterogeneity with immunohistologic uniformity. *Am J Clin Pathol* 1985;84:439–446.
518. Hanson CA, Frizzera G, Patton DF, et al. Clonal rearrangement for immunoglobulin and T-cell receptor genes in systemic Castleman's disease: association with Epstein-Barr virus. *Am J Pathol* 1988;131: 84–91.
519. Hineman VL, Phyliky RL, Banks PM. Angiofollicular lymph node hyperplasia and peripheral neuropathy: association with monoclonal gammopathy. *Mayo Clin Proc* 1982;57:379–382.
520. Radaszkiewicz T, Hansmann ML, Lennert K. Monoclonality and polyclonality of plasma cells in Castleman's disease of the plasma cell variant. *Histopathology* 1989;14:11–24.
521. Ohyashiki JH, Ohyashiki K, Kawakubo K, et al. Molecular genetic, cytogenetic, and immunophenotypic analyses in Castleman's disease of the plasma cell type. *Am J Clin Pathol* 1994;101:290–295.
522. Liu K, Liu J, Mann KP, et al. B-cell clonality in Castleman's disease, plasma cell type. *Mol Pathol* 1997;10.
523. Nagai M, Irino S, Uda H, et al. Molecular genetic and immunohistochemical analyses of a case of multicentric Castleman's disease. *Jpn J Clin Oncol* 1988;18:149–157.
524. Murray PG, Deacon E, Young LS, et al. Localization of Epstein-Barr virus in Castleman's disease by in situ hybridization and immunohistochemistry. *Hematol Pathol* 1995;9:17–26.
525. Parravicini C, Corbellino M, Paulli M, et al. Expression of a virus-derived cytokine, KSHV vIL-6, in HIV-seronegative Castleman's disease. *Am J Pathol* 1997;151:1517–1522.
526. Nakamura H, Nakaseko C, Ishii A, et al. [Chromosomal abnormalities in Castleman's disease with high levels of serum interleukin-6]. *Rinsho Ketsueki* 1993;34:212–217.
527. Yoshizaki K, Matsuda T, Nishimoto N, et al. Pathogenic significance of interleukin-6 (IL-6/BSF-2) in Castleman's disease. *Blood* 1989;74: 1360–1367.
528. Herbelin C, Roux-Lombard P, Herbelin A, et al. Inflammation: ''a natural experiment'' for the systemic pathogenicity of cytokines. *Eur Cytokine Netw* 1998;9:57–60.
529. Hsu SM, Waldron JA, Xie SS, et al. Expression of interleukin-6 in Castleman's disease. *Hum Pathol* 1993;24:833–839.
530. Ishiyama T, Nakamura S, Akimoto Y, et al. Immunodeficiency and IL-6 production by peripheral blood monocytes in multicentric Castleman's disease. *Br J Haematol* 1994;86:483–489.
531. Kinney MC, Hummell DS, Villiger PM, et al. Increased interleukin-6 (IL-6) production in a young child with clinical and pathologic features of multicentric Castleman's disease. *J Clin Immunol* 1994; 14:382–390.
532. Lee M, Hirokawa M, Matuoka S, et al. Multicentric Castleman's disease with an increased serum level of macrophage colony-stimulating factor. *Am J Hematol* 1997;54:321–323.
533. Lui SL, Chan KW, Li FK, et al. Castleman's disease and mesangial proliferative glomerulonephritis: the role of interleukin-6. *Nephron* 1998;78:323–327.
534. Mandler RN, Kerrigan DP, Smart J, et al. Castleman's disease in POEMS syndrome with elevated interleukin-6 [see comments]. *Cancer* 1992;69:2697–2703.
535. Beck JT, Hsu SM, Wijdenes J, et al. Brief report: alleviation of sys-

temic manifestations of Castleman's disease by monoclonal anti-interleukin-6 antibody. *N Engl J Med* 1994;330:602–605.
536. Emilie D, Zou W, Fior R, et al. Production and roles of IL-6, IL-10, and IL-13 in B-lymphocyte malignancies and in B-lymphocyte hyperactivity of HIV infection and autoimmunity. *Methods* 1997;11:133–142.
537. Strohal R, Tschachler E, Breyer S, et al. Reactivation of Behçet's disease in the course of multicentric HHV8-positive Castleman's disease: long-term complete remission by a combined chemo/radiation and interferon-alpha therapy regimen. *Br J Haematol* 1998;103:788–790.
538. Veldhuis GJ, van der Leest AH, de Wolf JT, et al. A case of localized Castleman's disease with systemic involvement: treatment and pathogenetic aspects. *Ann Hematol* 1996;73:47–50.
539. Winter SS, Howard TA, Ritchey AK, et al. Elevated levels of tumor necrosis factor-beta, gamma-interferon, and IL-6 mRNA in Castleman's disease. *Med Pediatr Oncol* 1996;26:48–53.
540. Leger-Ravet MB, Peuchmaur M, Devergne O, et al. Interleukin-6 gene expression in Castleman's disease. *Blood* 1991;78:2923–2930.
541. Matsushima AY, Strauchen JA, Lee G, et al. Posttransplantation plasmacytic proliferations related to Kaposi's sarcoma-associated herpesvirus. *Am J Surg Pathol* 1999;23:1393–1400.
542. Cannon JS, Nicholas J, Orenstein JM, et al. Heterogeneity of viral IL-6 expression in HHV-8-associated diseases. *J Infect Dis* 1999;180:824–828.
543. Staskus KA, Sun R, Miller G, et al. Cellular tropism and viral interleukin-6 expression distinguish human herpesvirus 8 involvement in Kaposi's sarcoma, primary effusion lymphoma, and multicentric Castleman's disease. *J Virol* 1999;73:4181–4187.
544. Teruya-Feldstein J, Zauber P, Setsuda JE, et al. Expression of human herpesvirus-8 oncogene and cytokine homologues in an HIV-seronegative patient with multicentric Castleman's disease and primary effusion lymphoma. *Lab Invest* 1998;78:1637–1642.
545. Luppi M, Barozzi P, Maiorana A, et al. Expression of cell-homologous genes of human herpesvirus-8 in human immunodeficiency virus-negative lymphoproliferative diseases. *Blood* 1999;94:2931–2933.
546. Gessain A, Sudaka A, Briere J, et al. Kaposi sarcoma-associated herpes-like virus (human herpesvirus type 8) DNA sequences in multicentric Castleman's disease: is there any relevant association in non-human immunodeficiency virus-infected patients? [Letter; comment]. *Blood* 1996;87:414–416.
547. Corbellino M, Poirel L, Aubin JT, et al. The role of human herpesvirus 8 and Epstein-Barr virus in the pathogenesis of giant lymph node hyperplasia (Castleman's disease). *Clin Infect Dis* 1996;22:1120–1121.
548. Dupin N, Fisher C, Kellam P, et al. Distribution of human herpesvirus-8 latently infected cells in Kaposi's sarcoma, multicentric Castleman's disease, and primary effusion lymphoma. *Proc Natl Acad Sci USA* 1999;96:4546–4551.
549. Kikuta H, Itakura O, Taneichi K, et al. Tropism of human herpesvirus 8 for peripheral blood lymphocytes in patients with Castleman's disease. *Br J Haematol* 1997;99:790–793.
550. Dupin N, Gorin I, Deleuze J, et al. Herpes-like DNA sequences, AIDS-related tumors, and Castleman's disease [Letter; comment]. *N Engl J Med* 1995;333:798; discussion, 798–799.
551. Grandadam M, Dupin N, Calvez V, et al. Exacerbations of clinical symptoms in human immunodeficiency virus type 1-infected patients with multicentric Castleman's disease are associated with a high increase in Kaposi's sarcoma herpesvirus DNA load in peripheral blood mononuclear cells. *J Infect Dis* 1997;175:1198–1201.
552. Huh J, Kang GH, Gong G, et al. Kaposi's sarcoma-associated herpesvirus in Kikuchi's disease. *Hum Pathol* 1998;29:1091–1096.
553. Chang Y, Cesarman E, Pessin MS, et al. Identification of herpesvirus-like DNA sequences in AIDS-associated Kaposi's sarcoma [see comments]. *Science* 1994;266:1865–1869.
554. Smir BN, Greiner TC, Weisenburger DD. Multicentric angiofollicular lymph node hyperplasia in children: a clinicopathologic study of eight patients. *Mod Pathol* 1996;9:1135–1142.
555. Parez N, Bader-Meunier B, Roy CC, et al. Paediatric Castleman disease: report of seven cases and review of the literature. *Eur J Pediatr* 1999;158:631–637.
556. Sherman D, Ramsay B, Theodorou NA, et al. Reversible plane xanthoma, vasculitis, and peliosis hepatis in giant lymph node hyperplasia (Castleman's disease): a case report and review of the cutaneous manifestations of giant lymph node hyperplasia. *J Am Acad Dermatol* 1992, 26:105–109.
557. Chan JK, Fletcher CD, Hicklin GA, et al. Glomeruloid hemangioma: a distinctive cutaneous lesion of multicentric Castleman's disease associated with POEMS syndrome. *Am J Surg Pathol* 1990;14:1036–1046.
558. Yang SG, Cho KH, Bang YJ, et al. A case of glomeruloid hemangioma associated with multicentric Castleman's disease. *Am J Dermatopathol* 1998;20:266–270.
559. Scherokman B, Vukelja SJ, May E. Angiofollicular lymph node hyperplasia and peripheral neuropathy: case report and literature review. *Arch Intern Med* 1991;151:789–790.
560. Feigert JM, Sweet DL, Coleman M, et al. Multicentric angiofollicular lymph node hyperplasia with peripheral neuropathy, pseudotumor cerebri, IgA dysproteinemia, and thrombocytosis in women: a distinct syndrome [see comments]. *Ann Intern Med* 1990;113:362–367.
561. Gherardi RK, Malapert D, Degos JD. Castleman disease-POEMS syndrome overlap [Letter; comment]. *Ann Intern Med* 1991;114:520–521.
562. Kingsmore SF, Silva OE, Hall BD, et al. Presentation of multicentric Castleman's disease with sicca syndrome, cardiomyopathy, palmar and plantar rash. *J Rheumatol* 1993;20:1588–1591.
563. Gohlke F, Marker-Hermann E, Kanzler S, et al. Autoimmune findings resembling connective tissue disease in a patient with Castleman's disease. *Clin Rheumatol* 1997;16:87–92.
564. Ben-Chetrit E, Flusser D, Okon E, et al. Multicentric Castleman's disease associated with rheumatoid arthritis: a possible role of hepatitis B antigen. *Ann Rheum Dis* 1989;48:326–330.
565. Tavoni A, Vitali C, Baglioni P, et al. Multicentric Castleman's disease in a patient with primary Sjögren's syndrome. *Rheumatol Int* 1993;12:251–253.
566. Nanki T, Tomiyama J, Arai S. Mixed connective tissue disease associated with multicentric Castleman's disease. *Scand J Rheumatol* 1994;23:215–217.
567. Suwannaroj S, Elkins SL, McMurray RW. Systemic lupus erythematosus and Castleman's disease. *J Rheumatol* 1999;26:1400–1403.
568. Kojima M, Nakamura S, Itoh H, et al. Systemic lupus erythematosus (SLE) lymphadenopathy presenting with histopathologic features of Castleman' disease: a clinicopathologic study of five cases. *Pathol Res Pract* 1997;193:565–571.
569. Peterson BA, Frizzera G. Multicentric Castleman's disease. *Semin Oncol* 1993;20:636–647.
570. Carrington PA, Anderson H, Harris M, et al. Autoimmune cytopenias in Castleman's disease. *Am J Clin Pathol* 1990;94:101–104.
571. Marsh JH, Colbourn DS, Donovan V, et al. Systemic Castleman's disease in association with Evan's syndrome and vitiligo. *Med Pediatr Oncol* 1990;18:169–172.
572. Lajoie G, Kumar S, Min KW, et al. Renal thrombotic microangiopathy associated with multicentric Castleman's disease: report of two cases. *Am J Surg Pathol* 1995;19:1021–1028.
573. Liberato NL, Bollati P, Chiofalo F, et al. Autoimmune hemolytic anemia in multicentric Castleman's disease. *Haematologica* 1996;81:40–43.
574. Lerza R, Castello G, Truini M, et al. Splenectomy induced complete remission in a patient with multicentric Castleman's disease and autoimmune hemolytic anemia. *Ann Hematol* 1999;78:193–196.
575. Couch WD. Giant lymph node hyperplasia associated with thrombotic thrombocytopenic purpura. *Am J Clin Pathol* 1980;74:340–344.
576. Massey GV, Kornstein MJ, Wahl D, et al. Angiofollicular lymph node hyperplasia (Castleman's disease) in an adolescent female: clinical and immunologic findings. *Cancer* 1991;68:1365–1372.
577. Shohat B, Cohen I, Fogel R, et al. Suppressor mononuclear cells in giant lymph node hyperplasia and thymoma. *Cancer* 1981;48:923–926.
578. Perez Pena F, Tejero Lamarca J, Martin Rodilla C, et al. Enfermedad de Castleman: linfoma difuso histiocitico en la evolucion de la hiperplasia linfonodular hialinovascular es una entidad benigna? *Rev Clin Esp* 1980;158:83–86.
579. Ishiyama T, Koike M, Kakimoto T, et al. The presence of CD28-negative T cells in a patient with multicentric Castleman's disease. *Ann Hematol* 1996;73:199–200.
580. Karcher DS, Pearson CE, Butler WM, et al. Giant lymph node hyperplasia involving the thymus with associated nephrotic syndrome and myelofibrosis. *Am J Clin Pathol* 1982;77:100–104.

581. Chim CS, Lam KY, Chan KW. Castleman's disease with Kaposi's sarcoma and glomerulonephritis [Letter]. *Am J Med* 1999;107: 186–188.
582. Said R, Tarawneh M. Membranoproliferative glomerulonephritis associated with multicentric angiofollicular lymph node hyperplasia: case report and review of the literature. *Am J Nephrol* 1992;12: 466–470.
583. Moon WK, Kim SH, Im JG, et al. Castleman disease with renal amyloidosis: imaging findings and clinical significance. *Abdom Imaging* 1995;20:376–378.
584. Hattori K, Irie S, Isobe Y, et al. Multicentric Castleman's disease associated with renal amyloidosis and pure red cell aplasia. *Ann Hematol* 1998;77:179–181.
585. Ordi J, Grau JM, Junque A, et al. Secondary (AA) amyloidosis associated with Castleman's disease: report of two cases and review of the literature. *Am J Clin Pathol* 1993;100:394–397.
586. Ikeda S, Chisuwa H, Kawasaki S, et al. Systemic reactive amyloidosis associated with Castleman's disease: serial changes of the concentrations of acute phase serum amyloid A and interleukin 6 in serum. *J Clin Pathol* 1997;50:965–967.
587. Tanaka K, Horita M, Shibayama H, et al. Secondary amyloidosis associated with Castleman's disease. *Intern Med* 1995;34:122–126.
588. Perfetti V, Bellotti V, Maggi A, et al. Reversal of nephrotic syndrome due to reactive amyloidosis (AA-type) after excision of localized Castleman's disease. *Am J Hematol* 1994;46:189–193.
589. Kanoh T, Shimada H, Uchino H, et al. Amyloid goiter with hypothyroidism. *Arch Pathol Lab Med* 1989;113:542–544.
590. Miura A, Sato I, Suzuki C. Fatal diarrhea in a patient with Castleman's disease associated with intestinal amyloidosis. *Intern Med* 1995;34: 1106–1109.
591. West KP, Morgan DR, Lauder I. Angiofollicular lymph node hyperplasia with amyloidosis. *Postgrad Med J* 1989;65:108–111.
592. Okuda K, Himeno Y, Toyama T, et al. Gamma heavy chain disease and giant lymph node hyperplasia in a patient with impaired T cell function. *Jpn J Med* 1982;21:109–114.
593. Atagi S, Sakatani M, Akira M, et al. Pulmonary hyalinizing granuloma with Castleman's disease. *Intern Med* 1994;33:689–691.
594. Pasaoglu I, Dogan R, Topcu M, et al. Multicentric angiofollicular lymph-node hyperplasia associated with myasthenia gravis. *Thorac Cardiovasc Surg* 1994;42:253–256.
595. Molina T, Delmer A, Le Tourneau A, et al. Hepatic lesions of vascular origin in multicentric Castleman's disease, plasma cell type: report of one case with peliosis hepatis and another with perisinusoidal fibrosis and nodular regenerative hyperplasia. *Pathol Res Pract* 1995;191: 1159–1164.
596. Pavlidis NA, Briassoulis E, Klouvas G, et al. Is interferon-α an active agent in Castleman's disease? *Ann Oncol* 1992;3:85–86.
597. Bordeleau L, Bredeson C, Markman S. 2-Chloro-deoxyadenosine therapy for giant lymph node hyperplasia. *Br J Haematol* 1995;91: 668–670.
598. Barbounis V, Efremidis A. A plasma cell variant of Castleman's disease treated successfully with cimetidine: case report and review of the literature. *Anticancer Res* 1996;16:545–547.
599. Repetto L, Jaiprakash MP, Selby PJ, et al. Aggressive angiofollicular lymph node hyperplasia (Castleman's disease) treated with high dose melphalan and autologous bone marrow transplantation. *Hematol Oncol* 1986;4:213–217.
600. Foussat A, Fior R, Girard T, et al. Involvement of human interleukin-6 in systemic manifestations of human herpesvirus type 8-associated multicentric Castleman's disease [Letter]. *AIDS* 1999;13:150–152.
601. Ishiyama T, Koike M, Nakamura S, et al. Interleukin-6 receptor expression in the peripheral B cells of patients with multicentric Castleman's disease. *Ann Hematol* 1996;73:179–182.
602. Brandt SJ, Bodine DM, Dunbar CE, et al. Dysregulated interleukin 6 expression produces a syndrome resembling Castleman's disease in mice. *J Clin Invest* 1990;86:592–599.
603. Screpanti I, Musiani P, Bellavia D, et al. Inactivation of the IL-6 gene prevents development of multicentric Castleman's disease in C/EBP beta-deficient mice. *J Exp Med* 1996;184:1561–1566.
604. Screpanti I, Romani L, Musiani P, et al. Lymphoproliferative disorder and imbalanced T-helper response in C/EBP beta-deficient mice [published erratum appears in *EMBO J* 1995;14:3596]. *EMBO J* 1995;14: 1932–1941.
605. Yoshida M, Sakuma J, Hayashi S, et al. A histologically distinctive interstitial pneumonia induced by overexpression of the interleukin 6, transforming growth factor beta 1, or platelet-derived growth factor B gene. *Proc Natl Acad Sci USA* 1995;92:9570–9574.
606. Yoshizaki K, Kuritani T, Kishimoto T. Interleukin-6 in autoimmune disorders. *Semin Immunol* 1992;4:155–166.
607. Kawano MM, Mihara K, Huang N, et al. Differentiation of early plasma cells on bone marrow stromal cells requires interleukin-6 for escaping from apoptosis. *Blood* 1995;85:487–494.
608. Ramadori G, Christ B. Cytokines and the hepatic acute-phase response. *Semin Liver Dis* 1999;19:141–155.
609. Foss HD, Araujo I, Demel G, et al. Expression of vascular endothelial growth factor in lymphomas and Castleman's disease. *J Pathol* 1997; 183:44–50.
610. Nishi J, Arimura K, Utsunomiya A, et al. Expression of vascular endothelial growth factor in sera and lymph nodes of the plasma cell type of Castleman's disease. *Br J Haematol* 1999;104:482–485.
611. Marfaing-Koka A, Aubin JT, Grangeot-Keros L, et al. *In vivo* role of IL-6 on the viral load and on immunological abnormalities of HIV-infected patients. *J Acquir Immune Defic Syndr Hum Retrovirol* 1996; 11:59–68.
612. Suffredini AF, Fantuzzi G, Badolato R, et al. New insights into the biology of the acute phase response. *J Clin Immunol* 1999;19: 203–214.
613. Presterl E, Lassnigg A, Mueller-Uri P, et al. Cytokines in sepsis due to *Candida albicans* and in bacterial sepsis. *Eur Cytokine Netw* 1999; 10:423–430.
614. Gherardi RK, Belec L, Soubrier M, et al. Overproduction of proinflammatory cytokines imbalanced by their antagonists in POEMS syndrome. *Blood* 1996;87:1458–1465.
615. Miles SA, Rezai AR, Salazar-Gonzalez JF, et al. AIDS Kaposi sarcoma-derived cells produce and respond to interleukin 6. *Proc Natl Acad Sci USA* 1990;87:4068–4072.
616. Burger R, Wendler J, Antoni K, et al. Interleukin-6 production in B-cell neoplasias and Castleman's disease: evidence for an additional paracrine loop. *Ann Hematol* 1994;69:25–31.
617. Emilie D, Coumbaras J, Raphael M, et al. Interleukin-6 production in high-grade B lymphomas: correlation with the presence of malignant immunoblasts in acquired immunodeficiency syndrome and in human immunodeficiency virus-seronegative patients. *Blood* 1992;80: 498–504.
618. Tesch H, Jucker M, Klein S, et al. Hodgkin and Reed-Sternberg cells express interleukin 6 and interleukin 6 receptors. *Leuk Lymphoma* 1992;7:297–303.
619. Hsu SM, Xie SS, Hsu PL, et al. Interleukin-6, but not interleukin-4, is expressed by Reed-Sternberg cells in Hodgkin's disease with or without histologic features of Castleman's disease. *Am J Pathol* 1992; 141:129–138.
620. Hsu SM, Hsu PL. Autocrine and paracrine functions of cytokines in malignant lymphomas. *Biomed Pharmacother* 1994;48:433–444.
621. Foss HD, Herbst H, Oelmann E, et al. Lymphotoxin, tumour necrosis factor and interleukin-6 gene transcripts are present in Hodgkin and Reed-Sternberg cells of most Hodgkin's disease cases. *Br J Haematol* 1993;84:627–635.
622. Jucker M, Abts H, Li W, et al. Expression of interleukin-6 and interleukin-6 receptor in Hodgkin's disease. *Blood* 1991;77:2413–2418.
623. Nicholas J, Ruvolo VR, Burns WH, et al. Kaposi's sarcoma-associated human herpesvirus-8 encodes homologues of macrophage inflammatory protein-1 and interleukin-6. *Nat Med* 1997;3:287–292.
624. Wan X, Wang H, Nicholas J. Human herpesvirus 8 interleukin-6 (vIL-6) signals through gp130 but has structural and receptor-binding properties distinct from those of human IL-6. *J Virol* 1999;73:8268–8278.
625. Gillison ML, Ambinder RF. Human herpesvirus-8. *Curr Opin Oncol* 1997;9:440–449.
626. Jones KD, Aoki Y, Chang Y, et al. Involvement of interleukin-10 (IL-10) and viral IL-6 in the spontaneous growth of Kaposi's sarcoma herpesvirus-associated infected primary effusion lymphoma cells. *Blood* 1999;94:2871–2879.
627. Trovato R, Luppi M, Barozzi P, et al. Cellular localization of human herpesvirus 8 in nonneoplastic lymphadenopathies and chronic interstitial pneumonitis by in situ polymerase chain reaction studies. *J Hum Virol* 1999;2:38–44.
628. Isaacson PG. Castleman's disease [Commentary]. *Histopathology* 1989;14:429–432.

629. Kasaian MT, Casali P. Autoimmunity-prone B-1 (CD5 B) cells, natu ral antibodies and self recognition. *Autoimmunity* 1993;15:315–329.
630. Molinie V, Perie G, Melo I, et al. [Association of Castleman's disease and Hodgkin's disease: eight cases and review of the literature]. *Ann Pathol* 1994;14:384–391.
631. Papo T, Soubrier M, Marcelin AG, et al. Human herpesvirus 8 infection, Castleman's disease and POEMS syndrome [Letter]. *Br J Haematol* 1999;104:932–933.
632. Belec L, Mohamed AS, Authier FJ, et al. Human herpesvirus 8 infection in patients with POEMS syndrome-associated multicentric Castleman's disease. *Blood* 1999;93:3643–3653.
633. Harris NL. Hypervascular follicular hyperplasia and Kaposi's sarcoma in patients at risk for AIDS [Letter]. *N Engl J Med* 1984;310:462–463.
634. Lachant NA, Sun NC, Leong LA, et al. Multicentric angiofollicular lymph node hyperplasia (Castleman's disease) followed by Kaposi's sarcoma in two homosexual males with the acquired immunodeficiency syndrome (AIDS). *Am J Clin Pathol* 1985;83:27–33.
635. Lowenthal DA, Filippa DA, Richardson ME, et al. Generalized lymphadenopathy with morphologic features of Castleman's disease in an HIV-positive man. *Cancer* 1987;60:2454–2458.
636. Ost A, Baroni CD, Biberfeld P, et al. Lymphadenopathy in HIV infection: histological classification and staging. *APMIS Suppl* 1989;8: 7–15.
637. Racz P, Tenner-Racz K, van Vloten F, et al. Classification of histopathological changes of lymph nodes in HIV-1 infection: significance of Castleman's disease–like lymph node lesion concerning the diagnosis of HIV-1-related Kaposi's sarcoma. *Antibiot Chemother* 1991; 43:201–213.
638. Oksenhendler E, Duarte M, Soulier J, et al. Multicentric Castleman's disease in HIV infection: a clinical and pathological study of 20 patients. *AIDS* 1996;10:61–67.
639. Revuelta MP, Nord JA. Successful treatment of multicentric Castleman's disease in a patient with human immunodeficiency virus infection. *Clin Infect Dis* 1998;26:527.
640. Perlow LS, Taff ML, Orsini JM, et al. Kaposi's sarcoma in a young homosexual man: association with angiofollicular lymphoid hyperplasia and a malignant lymphoproliferative disorder. *Arch Pathol Lab Med* 1983;107:510 513.
641. Diebold J, Audouin J, Le Tourneau A, et al. Lymph node reaction patterns in patients with AIDS or AIDS-related complex. *Curr Top Pathol* 1991;84:189–221.
642. Rywlin AM, Recher L, Hoffman EP. Lymphoma-like presentation of Kaposi's sarcoma: three cases without characteristic skin lesions. *Arch Dermatol* 1966;93:554–561.
643. Chen KT. Multicentric Castleman's disease and Kaposi's sarcoma. *Am J Surg Pathol* 1984;8:287–293.
644. Dickson D, Ben-Ezra JM, Reed J, et al. Multicentric giant lymph node hyperplasia, Kaposi's sarcoma, and lymphoma. *Arch Pathol Lab Med* 1985;109:1013–1018.
645. Kwong YL, Chan AC. Absence of Kaposi's sarcoma associated herpesvirus-like DNA sequences (KSHV) in HIV-negative multicentric Castleman's disease complicated by KSHV-positive Kaposi's sarcoma [Letter]. *Br J Haematol* 1997;96:881–882.
646. Zeidman A, Fradin Z, Cohen AM, et al. Kaposi's sarcoma associated with Castleman's disease [Letter]. *Eur J Haematol* 1999;63:67–70.
647. Kessler E, Beer R. Multicentric giant lymph node hyperplasia clinically simulating angioimmunoblastic lymphadenopathy: associated Kaposi's sarcoma in two of three cases. *Isr J Med Sci* 1983;19: 230–234.
648. Bardwick PA, Zvaifler NJ, Gill GN, et al. Plasma cell dyscrasia with polyneuropathy, organomegaly, endocrinopathy, M protein, and skin changes: the POEMS syndrome: report on two cases and a review of the literature. *Medicine (Baltimore)* 1980;59:311–322.
649. Nakanishi T, Sobue I, Toyokura Y, et al. The Crow-Fukase syndrome: a study of 102 cases in Japan. *Neurology* 1984;34:712–720.
650. Pruzanski W. Takatsuki syndrome: a reversible multisystem plasma cell dyscrasia [Letter]. *Arthritis Rheum* 1986;29:1534–1535.
651. Farhangi M, Merlini G. The clinical implications of monoclonal immunoglobulins. *Semin Oncol* 1986;13:366–379.
652. Adams D, Said G. Ultrastructural characterisation of the M protein in nerve biopsy of patients with POEMS syndrome. *J Neurol Neurosurg Psychiatry* 1998;64:809–812.
653. Ropper AH, Gorson KC. Neuropathies associated with paraproteinemia. *N Engl J Med* 1998;338:1601–1607.
654. Soubrier MJ, Dubost JJ, Sauvezie BJ. POEMS syndrome: a study of 25 cases and a review of the literature. French Study Group on POEMS Syndrome. *Am J Med* 1994;97:543–553.
655. Takatsuki K, Sanada I. Plasma cell dyscrasia with polyneuropathy and endocrine disorder: clinical and laboratory features of 109 reported cases. *Jpn J Clin Oncol* 1983;13:543–555.
656. Miralles GD, O'Fallon JR, Talley NJ. Plasma-cell dyscrasia with polyneuropathy: the spectrum of POEMS syndrome. *N Engl J Med* 1992; 327:1919–1923.
657. Case records of the Massachusetts General Hospital: weekly clinicopathological exercises. Case 10-1987: a 59-year-old woman with progressive polyneuropathy and monoclonal gammopathy. *N Engl J Med* 1987;316:606–618.
658. Bitter MA, Komaiko W, Franklin WA. Giant lymph node hyperplasia with osteoblastic bone lesions and the POEMS (Takatsuki's) syndrome. *Cancer* 1985;56:188–194.
659. Rolon PG, Audouin J, Diebold J, et al. Multicentric angiofollicular lymph node hyperplasia associated with a solitary osteolytic costal IgG lambda myeloma: POEMS syndrome in a South American (Paraguayan) patient. *Pathol Res Pract* 1989;185:468–475; discussion 476–469.
660. Muñoz G, Geijo P, Moldenhauer F, et al. Plasmacellular Castleman's disease and POEMS syndrome. *Histopathology* 1990;17:172–174.
661. Judge MR, McGibbon DH, Thompson RP. Angioendotheliomatosis associated with Castleman's lymphoma and POEMS syndrome. *Clin Exp Dermatol* 1993;18:360–362.
662. Rose C, Zandecki M, Copin MC, et al. POEMS syndrome: report on six patients with unusual clinical signs, elevated levels of cytokines, macrophage involvement and chromosomal aberrations of bone marrow plasma cells. *Leukemia* 1997;11:1318–1323.
663. Murphy N, Schumacher HR Jr. POEMS syndrome in systemic lupus erythematosus. *J Rheumatol* 1992;19:796–799.
664. Pasqui AL, Bova G, Saletti M, et al. POEMS syndrome with vascular lesions and renal carcinoma: Possible role of cytokines. *Eur J Med Res* 1998;3:304–306.
665. Emile C, Danon F, Fermand JP, et al. Castleman disease in POEMS syndrome with elevated interleukin-6 [Letter; comment]. *Cancer* 1993;71:874.
666. Wengrower D, Libson E, Okon E, et al. Gastrointestinal manifestations in Castleman's disease. *Am J Gastroenterol* 1990;85: 1179–1181.
667. Stelfox HT, Stewart AK, Bailey D, et al. Castleman's disease in a 44-year-old male with neurofibromatosis and pheochromocytoma. *Leuk Lymphoma* 1997;27:551–556.
668. Tissier F, de Pinieux G, Thiounn N, et al. [Castleman's disease and chromophobe carcinoma of the kidney: an incidental association? *Ann Pathol* 1998;18:429–431.
669. Mizutani N, Okada S, Tanaka J, et al. Multicentric giant lymph node hyperplasia with ascites and double cancers: an autopsy case. *Tohoku J Exp Med* 1989;158:1–7.
670. Hanchard B, Williams N, Green M. Concurrent multicentric angiofollicular lymph node hyperplasia and peripheral T-cell lymphoma. *West Indian Med J* 1987;36:104–107.
671. Brice P, Marolleau JP, D'Agay MF, et al. Autoimmune hemolytic anemia disclosing Hodgkin's disease associated with Castleman's disease. *Nouv Rev Fr Hematol* 1991;33:273–274.
672. Drut R, Larregina A. Angiofollicular lymph node transformation in Hodgkin's lymphoma. *Pediatr Pathol* 1991;11:903–908.
673. Maheswaran PR, Ramsay AD, Norton AJ, et al. Hodgkin's disease presenting with the histological features of Castleman's disease. *Histopathology* 1991;18:249–253.
674. Pettit C, Ferry JA, Harris NL. Simultaneous occurrence of Hodgkin's disease and angiofollicular hyperplasia (Castleman's disease): report of 3 cases. *Mod Pathol* 1990;4:81A(abst).
675. Zarate-Osorno A, Medeiros LJ, Danon AD, et al. Hodgkin's disease with coexistent Castleman-like histologic features: a report of three cases [see comments]. *Arch Pathol Lab Med* 1994;118:270–274.
676. Abdel-Reheim FA, Koss W, Rappaport ES, et al. Coexistence of

Hodgkin's disease and giant lymph node hyperplasia of the plasma-cell type (Castleman's disease). *Arch Pathol Lab Med* 1996;120: 91–96.
677. McAloon EJ. Hodgkin's disease in a patient with Castleman's disease [Letter]. *N Engl J Med* 1985;313:758.
678. Doggett RS, Colby TV, Dorfman RF. Interfollicular Hodgkin's disease. *Am J Surg Pathol* 1983;7:145–149.
679. Franco V. Report of a case of localized Castleman's disease with progression to malignant lymphoma [Letter; comment]. *Am J Clin Pathol* 1993;100:707–708.
680. Buijs L, Wijermans PW, van Groningen K, et al. Hyaline-vascular type Castleman's disease with concomitant malignant B-cell lymphoma. *Acta Haematol* 1992;87:160–162.
681. Baker WJ, Vukelja SJ, Weiss RB, et al. Multicentric angiofollicular lymph node hyperplasia and associated carcinoma. *Med Pediatr Oncol* 1994;22:384–388.

CHAPTER 17

Hodgkin's Disease: Histopathology and Differential Diagnosis

Jerome S. Burke

In 1832, Thomas Hodgkin (1) described seven patients with an unusual disease of lymph nodes that became known by his name more than 30 years later (2). The latter half of the 19th century also saw the first descriptions of the characteristic giant cell of Hodgkin's disease, but it is Sternberg and Reed (3–5) who are recognized as having provided the first detailed descriptions and illustrations of the giant cells and the other histopathologic characteristics that define Hodgkin's disease. During the period in which Sternberg and Reed defined the pathologic aspects of Hodgkin's disease, and until very recently, the precise nature of the disorder was controversial. There were some who considered Hodgkin's disease a form of granulomatous infection or inflammation, like tuberculosis; others suggested that it was a type of chronic immunologic disorder; and still others concluded that Hodgkin's disease was a malignant neoplasm (6). Today, the malignant nature of Hodgkin's disease is established. The past 40 years have witnessed remarkable achievements in the understanding of the clinical patterns of Hodgkin's disease both at the onset of the disorder and during progression, in the development of new diagnostic techniques for accurate staging, in the illumination of the pathologic characteristics, and in the establishment of successful therapeutic protocols (6–9). Despite the current relative stability of the understanding of Hodgkin's disease in terms of overall pathologic characteristics and therapy, especially viewed in contrast with the non-Hodgkin's lymphomas, Hodgkin's disease remains a subject of intense investigation. The sustained interest in Hodgkin's disease results not only from of the continuous refinement in the pathologic criteria and therapeutic regimens, but also because the germinal center B-cell derivation of the neoplastic cells in both the classic and lymphocyte predominance forms, as well as other molecular and biologic aspects of the disease, only now is becoming clear (10–12).

This chapter concentrates on the current histopathologic concepts and characteristics of Hodgkin's disease, including the differential diagnosis, and emphasizes the salient clinicopathologic correlations at the time of initial biopsy, staging, and relapse. The immunobiology and pathogenesis of Hodgkin's disease, as well as the origin of the Reed-Sternberg cell, are not stressed, because these subjects are discussed in Chapter 18. Nor is any attempt made to recapitulate all details concerning the history, epidemiology, clinical characteristics, and therapeutic aspects of Hodgkin's disease, which are described in several superb reviews (6,8,9,13–15).

HISTOPATHOLOGIC CLASSIFICATION AND DEFINITION

More than 30 years have elapsed since Lukes and Butler (16,17) proposed their histopathologic classification of Hodgkin's disease. This classification was based on the predominant histologic features seen in pretherapy lymph node biopsies and was an attempt to further the earlier concepts of Jackson and Parker (18) in the identification of histologic groups of Hodgkin's disease that were prognostically significant. Lukes and Butler introduced the concept of nodular sclerosis and identified a nodular variant of the former paragranuloma group of Jackson and Parker, resulting in a classification containing six categories (Table 17.1). The histopathologic categories in the Lukes and Butler classification reflect the significance of lymphocytic proliferation, the inverse relationship between the number of lymphocytes and that of Reed-Sternberg cells, and the presence of two distinctly different types of connective tissue proliferation found in nodular sclerosis and diffuse fibrosis (16,17).

The original Lukes and Butler classification persists as

J. S. Burke: Department of Anatomic Pathology, Alta Bates Medical Center, Berkeley, California 94705

TABLE 17.1. *Comparison of histologic classifications of Hodgkin's disease*

Lukes and Butler	Rye	REAL	World Health Organization (Hodgkin's *lymphoma*)
Lymphocytic and histiocytic			
Nodular	Lymphocyte predominance	Lymphocyte predominance	Nodular lymphocyte predominance
Diffuse		Lymphocyte-rich classic	Lymphocyte-rich classic
Nodular sclerosis	Nodular sclerosis	Nodular sclerosis	Nodular sclerosis (grades I and II)
Mixed cellularity	Mixed cellularity	Mixed cellularity	Mixed cellularity
Diffuse fibrosis reticular	Lymphocytic depletion	Lymphocytic depletion	Lymphocytic depletion

REAL, revised European–American lymphoma.

the foundation for the modern classification of Hodgkin's disease, despite the popular simplification of the six categories of Lukes and Butler to four groups at the Rye Conference, and the recent addition of a lymphocyte-rich classic form in the Revised European-American Lymphoma (REAL) and proposed World Health Organization (WHO) classifications (19–23). In both the REAL classification and the most recent version of the WHO scheme, the categories of nodular sclerosis, mixed cellularity, and lymphocytic depletion are combined under the designation *classic Hodgkin's disease*, in order to underscore the tight bond among these histologic types, and their distinction from lymphocyte predominance (20–23). The WHO classification also emphasizes that lymphocyte predominance is essentially nodular and formally divides nodular sclerosis into two grades based mainly on European data showing that cases of nodular sclerosis with significant nuclear pleomorphism and lymphocyte depletion (grade II) are associated with a poorer prognosis (22–25). The lymphocytic depletion subtype is retained in both the REAL classification and the current WHO proposal, but in the WHO classification this category includes some cases that provisionally were denoted in the REAL classification

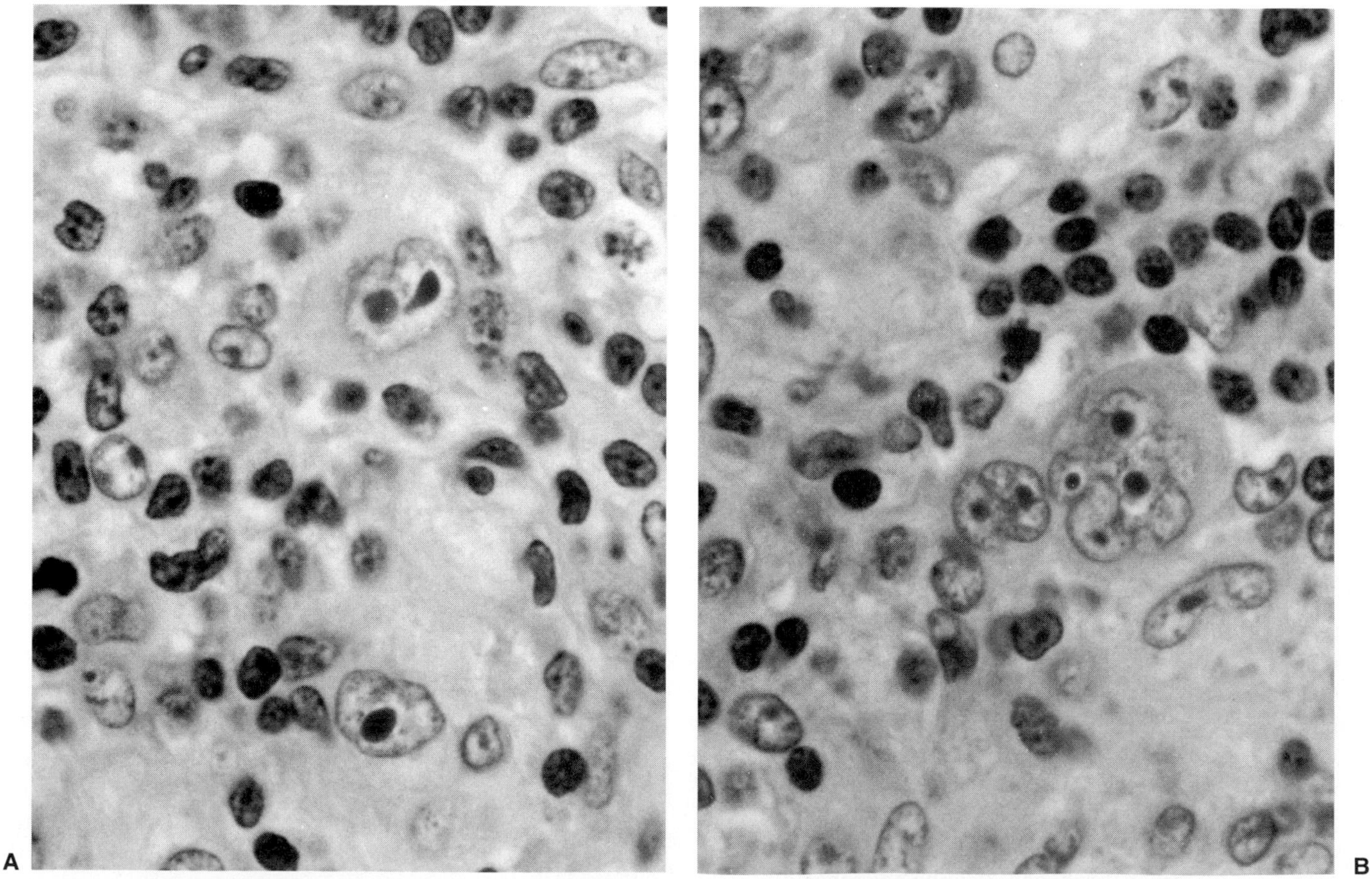

FIG. 17.1. A: Lobated Reed-Sternberg cell with characteristic large acidophilic nucleoli. A mononuclear variant also is present (hematoxylin and eosin stain, original magnification: 1,200× magnification). **B:** Binucleated and multinucleated types of Reed-Sternberg cells. Note the heterogeneous cell background (hematoxylin and eosin stain, original magnification: 1,200× magnification).

as *anaplastic large cell lymphoma Hodgkin's-like* (20–23). Recent studies have demonstrated that almost all cases so classified probably are related biologically to classic Hodgkin's disease, of either the lymphocytic depletion or nodular sclerosis with lymphocytic depletion type (grade II) (21–23). Similar to Hodgkin's disease, most specimens in the Hodgkin's-like anaplastic large cell group fail to express anaplastic large cell lymphoma kinase as a consequence of the translocation t(2;5), which is in contrast to cases of systemic anaplastic large cell lymphoma (26–29). The WHO classification also suggests that the idiom *Hodgkin's disease* be altered to *Hodgkin lymphoma* in order to lend credence to the fact that this disorder is actually neoplastic (21,22).

Notwithstanding these new proposals, the pathologist should continue to be familiar with the criteria and terminology of the original Lukes and Butler classification. The original classification provides specific criteria and descriptive histologic categories that aid in the pathologic diagnosis and in the differentiation from benign and malignant conditions that may simulate Hodgkin's disease (30–32). Although modern therapy has reduced the differences in prognosis and survival traditionally found among the histologic groups of Hodgkin's disease, pathologic classification of Hodgkin's disease remains important, because the various histologic groups correlate with specific clinical parameters including stage and sites of involvement (33–35).

The definition of Hodgkin's disease that unifies the different histologic types is the *identification of diagnostic Reed-Sternberg cells in the appropriate cellular environment.* Both parts of this definition are essential. The diagnostic Reed-Sternberg cell is a large cell that may be lobated, binucleated, or multinucleated and contains homogeneous, acidophilic, inclusion-like nucleoli that are approximately one quarter of the size of the nucleus (17,30) (Fig. 17.1); the cytoplasm is usually abundant and amphophilic. Variants of Reed-Sternberg cells which aid in the diagnosis include a mononuclear variant, the folded and lobated ("popcorn") cell of the lymphocyte predominance type, and the lacunar cell of nodular sclerosis (30) (Fig. 17.2). Because cells similar to Reed-Sternberg cells and its variants are found in conditions other than Hodgkin's disease, including infectious mononucleosis and non-Hodgkin's lymphomas, the identification of only a Reed-Sternberg cell is insufficient for an absolute diagnosis of Hodgkin's disease (36,37). Reed-Sternberg cells must be viewed in the context of one of the described histologic types of Hodgkin's disease. The cellular

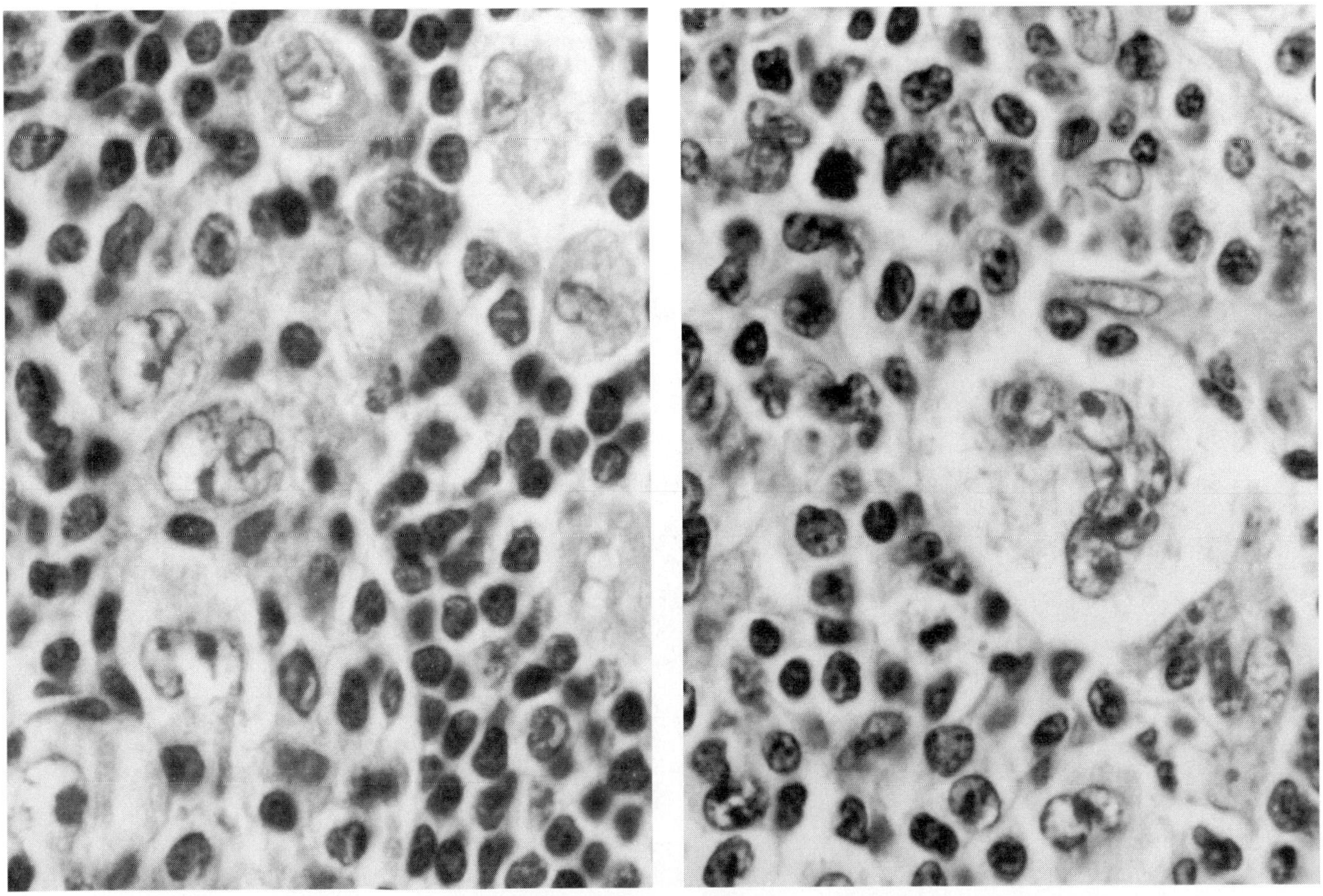

A B

FIG. 17.2. A: Folded and lobated ("popcorn") L&H variants of Reed-Sternberg cells are typical of lymphocyte predominance (hematoxylin and eosin stain, original magnification: 1,200× magnification). **B:** Hyperlobated lacunar cells are another variant of cells characteristically found in nodular sclerosis (hematoxylin and eosin stain, original magnification: 1,200× magnification).

TABLE 17.2. *Predominant cellular composition of the histologic types of Hodgkin's disease*

Histologic categories	Small lymphocytes	Reactive histiocytes	Eosinophils	Plasma cells	Collagen	Noncollagenous fibrous tissue	Classic Reed–Sternberg cells
Lymphocyte predominance	5+	+ to 3+	0	0	0	0	0
Lymphocyte-rich classical	4+	+ to 3+	0 to +	0 to +	0	0	+
Nodular sclerosis	+ to 4+	+ to 2+	+	+	+ to 4+	+	+
Mixed cellularity	2 to 3+	+ to 3+	2+	+	0	2+	2 to 3+
Lymphocytic depletion	0 to +	0 to +	+ to 2+	+	0	+ to 4+	2 to 5+

Adapted from Lukes RJ, Butler JJ. The pathology and nomenclature of Hodgkin's disease. *Cancer Res* 1966;26:1063–1081, with permission.

background is usually heterogeneous in Hodgkin's disease, particularly in the nodular sclerosis and mixed cellularity types (Table 17.2). In these classic types of Hodgkin's disease, the heterogeneous cell population includes diverse mixtures of small lymphocytes devoid of significant nuclear membrane irregularities, plasma cells, large lymphoid cells, histiocytes, and varying mixtures of inflammatory cells including eosinophils and polymorphonuclear leukocytes, with or without necrosis (Fig. 17.3). The definition of an *appropriate* cellular environment, however, is somewhat vague, because this environment is mutable, and similar heterogenous cell populations including Reed-Sternberg–like cells may be observed in a variety of non-Hodgkin's lymphomas, especially peripheral T-cell lymphomas, T cell–rich B-cell lymphomas, and anaplastic large cell or anaplastic large cell lymphoma kinase–positive lymphomas (28,29,38–42).

A modern definition of Hodgkin's disease, therefore, requires expansion, with the incorporation of immunologic criteria in order to differentiate Hodgkin's disease and the Reed-Sternberg cell from those non-Hodgkin's lymphomas that histologically simulate, and are frequently indistinguishable from, Hodgkin's disease (43–48) (Fig. 17.4, Table 17.3). In patients with classic Hodgkin's disease (nodular sclerosis and mixed cellularity types), moreover, the immunophenotype appears to have a direct impact on clinical

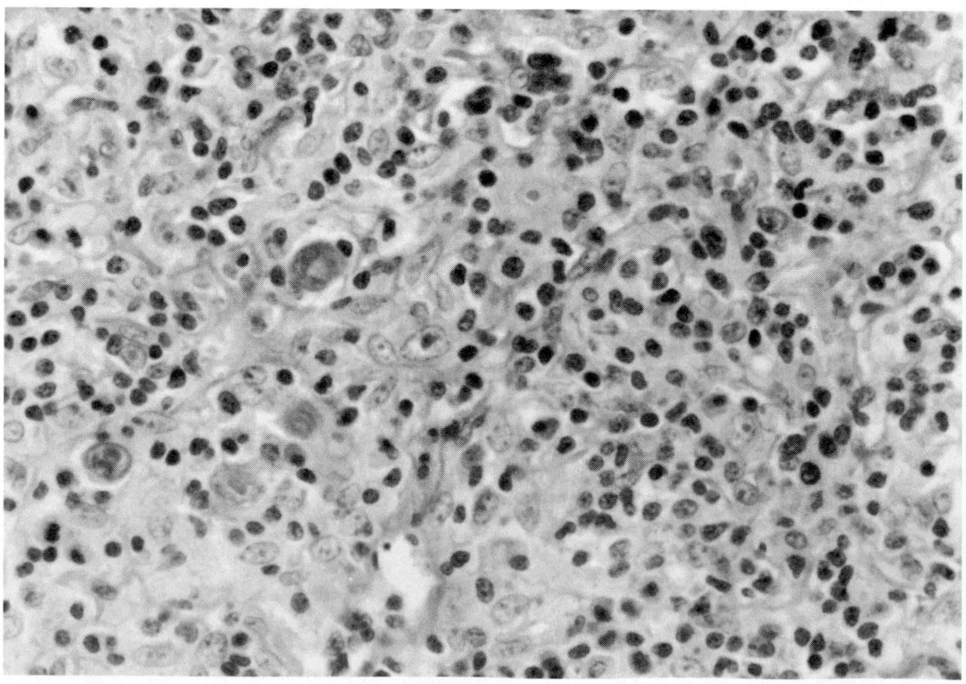

FIG. 17.3. A heterogeneous cell population is characteristic of most types of Hodgkin's disease and includes varying numbers of small lymphocytes, plasma cells, histiocytes, eosinophils, and polymorphonuclear leukocytes as well as Reed-Sternberg cells (hematoxylin and eosin stain, original magnification: 480× magnification).

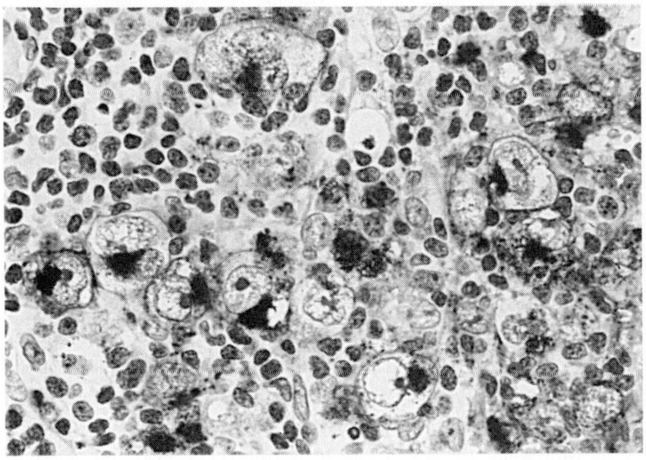

FIG. 17.4. Positive reactivity for CD15 is characteristic, but not pathognomonic, of the Reed-Sternberg cells in classic Hodgkin's disease. This image is from a patient with the syncytial variant of nodular sclerosis (immunoperoxidase stain, original magnification: 600× magnification).

TABLE 17.3. *Histopathologic and immunologic definition of classic Hodgkin's disease*

Histopathologic criterion: Diagnostic Reed–Sternberg cells in the appropriate cellular environment	
Immunologic criteria	
Reed–Sternberg Cells	
CD15	+
CD30	+
Vimentin	+
Fascin	+
CD40	+
CD45	−
CD20	−/+
CD3	−
EMA	−
ALK	−
Surrounding cells: T cells, predominantly CD4+, TIA-1+	

prognosis (49). In contrast to patients with a classic immunophenotype, patients who lack CD15 have a significantly worse freedom from treatment failure and survival; by multivariate analysis, the absence of CD15 expression is an independent negative prognostic factor for relapses and survival (49) (Chapters 18, 25, 29).

GENERAL CLINICAL CHARACTERISTICS INCLUDING PATTERNS OF DISSEMINATION, STAGING, AND THERAPY

Hodgkin's disease has a characteristic bimodal age curve with one peak in early adult life (15–35 years) and a second increase in incidence at 50 years of age or older (50). The younger group has an approximately equal male:female ratio, with a predominance of the nodular sclerosis type, and a more favorable clinical course. The male:female ratio is higher in the older group, with a greater incidence of mixed cellularity Hodgkin's disease, and a more aggressive clinical course (50). An analysis of both unadjusted survival and adjusted survival rates concluded that the prognosis of older patients with Hodgkin's disease has been obscured in previous studies by the inclusion of deaths resulting from other causes, and that Hodgkin's disease in the elderly does not have a different natural history from that in younger patients (51). Curiously, the incidence of Hodgkin's disease is declining in older adults, but there has been a persistent increase in young adults with nodular sclerosis (52,53). Part of the falling incidence of Hodgkin's disease in older patients likely is related to earlier overdiagnosis of lymphocytic depletion Hodgkin's disease and underdiagnosis of non-Hodgkin's lymphomas (53).

In the United States, Hodgkin's disease accounts for 14% of malignant lymphomas and 0.5% of all malignancies (54). The age-adjusted incidence rate of Hodgkin's disease in whites in the United States between 1973 and 1977 and 1983 and 1987 was stable at 3.1 and 3.0 cases per 100,000, respectively; there was a decrease in the age-adjusted rate for blacks between the same periods from 2.1 to 1.8 per 100,000 (53). The epidemiologic pattern of Hodgkin's disease differs according to the socioeconomic level of a region; for example, in Third World countries and in referral medical centers serving populations at lower socioeconomic levels in the United States, there is an increased incidence of symptomatic, advanced disease, often in children, with a higher rate of the mixed cellularity and lymphocytic depletion types (55,56); this pattern may be related to Epstein-Barr virus (EBV) infection (57). In contrast, patients from relatively affluent areas present with asymptomatic, low-stage disease and nodular sclerosis histology. The risk of Hodgkin's disease is increased significantly by 7.6-fold among patients with the AIDS (58). The incidence of Hodgkin's disease is especially high in regions with populations at increased risk for HIV infection (53), and the natural history and biologic features of Hodgkin's disease associated with HIV appear altered, with an increased incidence of advanced-stage disease, involvement of extranodal sites including skin at presentation, increased proportions of the mixed cellularity histologic type, a high frequency of EBV infection in the Reed-Sternberg cells, and a more aggressive clinical course compared with Hodgkin's disease in the general population (53,59–61) (Chapter 28).

Constitutional symptoms, age, and histopathologic type classically are the most important factors influencing the clinical evaluation of Hodgkin's disease (6). Patients with night sweats, fever, or significant weight loss are more likely to have an accelerated pace of disease and more widespread dissemination. Traditionally, patients older than 50 years of age also are reported to have more advanced disease compared with children and young adults (62). At one extreme, lymphocyte predominance histology is associated with an overall indolent course; at the other, lymphocytic depletion Hodgkin's disease is associated with constitutional symptoms, wide dissemination, and usually a rapidly fatal course (6,13,63,64). Nodular sclerosis and mixed cellularity Hodgkin's disease tend to have intermediate rates of evolution. Modern therapy is diminishing the differences in survival rates and the prognoses of the histopathologic types of Hodgkin's disease (8,13–15).

Many of the accomplishments in the treatment of Hodgkin's disease in the past 40 years are directly attributable to the development of superior diagnostic methods to quantitate the extent of disease. The advent of bipedal lymphangiography, staging laparotomy with splenectomy and selective biopsies, computed tomography, and magnetic resonance imaging has allowed critical assessment of the spleen and retroperitoneal lymph nodes and accurate staging of patients (6–8,13–15). Lymphangiography led to the observation that the spread of Hodgkin's disease is nonrandom, and that there is an orderly progression of disease, with dissemination to contiguous lymph node groups including the spleen (14,65). *Contiguity* refers to the existence of direct connections between pairs of lymph node chains by way of lymphatic channels that do not have to pass through, and be filtered by, intervening lymph nodes or other lymphatic tissue barriers (6). As a result, paraaortic or celiac lymph node involvement is associated with a high probability of splenic involvement, and splenic involvement commonly is followed by involvement of the liver and bone marrow. In the chest, the sequence of spread appears to be from the mediastinal to the hilar lymph nodes and then to the pulmonary parenchyma. Another important association is between involvement of the lower cervical or supraclavicular lymph nodes and the occurrence of relapse in the upper lumbar paraaortic nodes (6,14). Vascular invasion and hematogeneous dissemination of Hodgkin's disease are less clear. Vascular invasion appears more common in patients with lymphocytic depletion but also may occur in lymph nodes and spleens from patients with nodular sclerosis and mixed cellularity Hodgkin's disease (66–68). These studies demonstrate an association between vascular invasion and extranodal involvement; however, a review of the original lymph node biopsies from 11 patients who had localized Hodgkin's disease, and who later developed extranodal dissemination, failed to identify vascular invasion (69).

Staging laparotomy with splenectomy and selective biopsies also greatly contributed to the understanding of the patterns of Hodgkin's disease (70–72). Staging laparotomy is the most accurate diagnostic procedure for determining involvement of the spleen and clarifying involvement of the paraaortic, celiac, and portahepatic lymph nodes (8). This procedure was employed not only to define the extent of Hodgkin's disease but also to select patients primarily for radiation therapy. Currently, the role of staging laparotomy in the management of early-stage Hodgkin's disease is controversial, despite decision-analytic models that predict a gain in life expectancy for younger patients undergoing this procedure (73). Staging laparotomy has become uncommon because of the increased diagnostic accuracy of computed tomography in identifying involvement of abdominal lymph nodes in Hodgkin's disease, and the widespread employment of multiagent chemotherapy for specific clinical settings, such as patients with large mediastinal masses and even patients with nonbulky early-stage disease (8,14,15,74,75). Staging laparotomies also have been abandoned because of the expense and risk of morbidity, given the known association of splenectomy with subsequent bacterial sepsis, especially in children, and the discovery that splenectomy is a predisposing risk factor for acute leukemia, particularly in patients older than 40 years of age (14,74–77).

The development of more accurate diagnostic techniques for determining the extent and pattern of Hodgkin's disease at presentation resulted in the adoption of the Ann Arbor staging classification in 1971; this system is the basis for the curent staging classification of Hodgkin's disease (14,15,78) (Table 17.4). The Ann Arbor scheme divides Hodgkin's disease into four stages depending on the extent of nodal or extranodal disease: *E* denotes extranodal disease by direct extension from lymph nodes and is distinguished from stage IV disseminated extranodal Hodgkin's disease. The absence (*A*) or presence (*B*) of specific clinical symptoms is affixed to each stage, and the scheme also distinguishes between the clinical stage (*CS*) and the pathologic stage (*PS*) (14). There are newer recommendations, referred to as the *Cotswolds classification*, to formally revise the Ann Arbor system by adding computed tomographic results, modifying the criteria for clinical involvement of the spleen and liver to include evidence of focal defects on two imaging techniques, designating bulky disease (greater than 10 cm) with *X*, and introducing a new category of response to therapy, unconfirmed or uncertain complete remission—*CR(u)*—in order to accommodate the difficulty of persistent radiologic abnormalities of uncertain significance (8,14,79).

It is beyond the scope of this chapter to provide a detailed account of the remarkable progress in the therapy of Hodgkin's disease. Highlights include the development of the linear accelerator and the standardization of the mantle, inverted Y, and total nodal lymphoid fields for radiotherapy,

TABLE 17.4. *Ann Arbor staging classification of Hodgkin's disease*

Stage I	Involvement of a single lymph node region (I) or a single extralymphatic organ or site (I_E)
Stage II	Involvement of two or more lymph node regions on the same side of the diaphragm (II) or localized involvement of an extralymphatic organ or site (II_E)
Stage III	Involvement of lymph node regions on both sides of the diaphragm (III) or localized involvement of an extralymphatic organ or site (III_E) or spleen (III_S) or both (III_{ES})
Stage IV	Diffuse or disseminated involvement of one or more extralymphatic organs with or without associated lymph node involvement

A, asymptomatic; B, fever, sweats, or weight loss >10% of body weight; CS, clinical stage that denotes the stage as determined by all diagnostic examinations and a single diagnostic biopsy only (if a second biopsy of any sort is obtained, whether negative or positive, the term *pathologic stage* [PS] is used).

the use of combination chemotherapy regimens such as mechlorethamine, vincristine, procarbazine, and prednisone; doxorubicin, bleomycin, vinblastine, and decarbazine; and more recently bleomycin, etoposide, doxorubicine, cyclophosphamide, vincristine, procarbazine, and prednisone for patients with stage IIIB or IV disease, and the strategy of employing combined modality therapy (8,9,13–15,77). For example, the actuarial disease-specific survival rate of patients with pathologic stage I, II, or IIIA disease after initial treatment at Stanford University Medical Center between 1980 and 1993 is 96.5% at 10 years; the 10-year survival rate for patients with stage IIIB or IV disease also is impressive, at 81.2% (14). Therapy continues to be refined, with protocols designed to determine the chemotherapy regimen that is the least toxic or most successful, the best treatment options for patients with both early- and advanced-stage disease, and the most effective salvage treatment including the use of autologous bone marrow or peripheral stem cell transplantation for patients who experience relapses (7–9,14,15, 75,77,80,81). There also is a concerted effort to reduce many of the late complications of therapy, such as thyroid, cardiovascular, and pulmonary dysfunction induced by radiation therapy; gonadal dysfunction as a result of chemotherapy; and secondary malignancies, specifically acute myeloid leukemias, non-Hodgkin's lymphomas, and solid tumors (8,14,15,82). Secondary malignancies are the most important cause of death, apart from Hodgkin's disease (15). Depending on the center, the relative risk of any secondary malignancy is from 3.5 to 5.6, and in pediatric patients the risk is even greater, at 15.4 (83–85); the highest relative risk is for the development of acute leukemia. The extent of treatment of Hodgkin's disease emerges as the most significant risk factor for the evolution to secondary malignancies, and survivors of Hodgkin's disease, particularly pediatric patients, require lifelong observation (84,85).

PATHOLOGIC FEATURES, CLINICOPATHOLOGIC CORRELATIONS, AND DIFFERENTIAL DIAGNOSIS

Lymphocyte Predominance

The lymphocyte predominance type comprises approximately 5% of cases of Hodgkin's disease (86). Despite its relative rarity, lymphocyte predominance has generated considerable interest since the recent demonstration that this form of Hodgkin's disease has not only unique morphologic features but also clinical, immunophenotypic, and molecular characteristics that differ from those of classic Hodgkin's disease (11–15,43,47,63,87,88). Although the lymphocyte predominance category traditionally included both the nodular and diffuse lymphocytic and histiocytic (L&H) types noted by Lukes and Butler, the pure diffuse type is uncommon, comprising less than 10% of cases (16,17,19,89). In effect, lymphocyte predominance is considered virtually synonomous with the nodular type (21–23) (Fig. 17.5). Paradoxically, the studies by Lukes and Butler included more diffuse than nodular cases of L&H Hodgkin's disease (16,17). The majority of diffuse cases in those studies likely would be incorporated into the nodular type today, because the nodular pattern may be subtle or focal, masked in thick sections, and sometimes evident only with a reticulin stain or the demonstration of a follicular dendritic cell meshwork by immunohistochemistry (30,87,90) (Fig. 17.6). Other cases of diffuse lymphocyte predominance could be examples of lymphocyte-rich classic Hodgkin's disease or T cell or histiocyte-rich B-cell lymphoma (20,40,41,91,92).

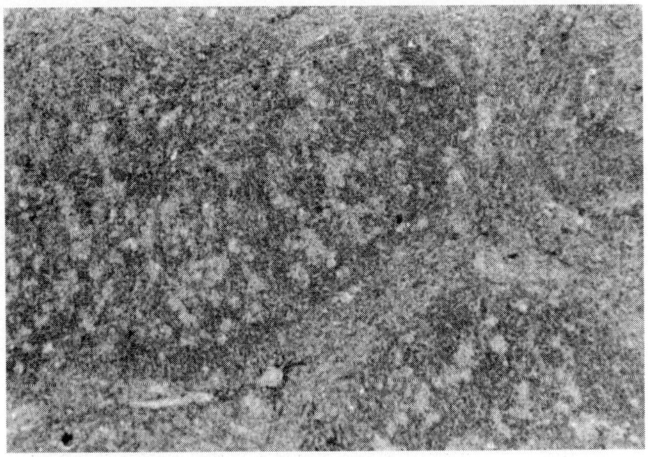

FIG. 17.5. In nodular lymphocyte predominance, the nodules vary in size and frequently are poorly defined (hematoxylin and eosin stain, original magnification: 48× magnification).

Nodular lymphocyte predominance is composed of a diverse mixture of small lymphocytes with round nuclear contours and reactive histiocytes (Fig. 17.7). The histiocytes may be single or clustered, suggesting epithelioid or sarcoid

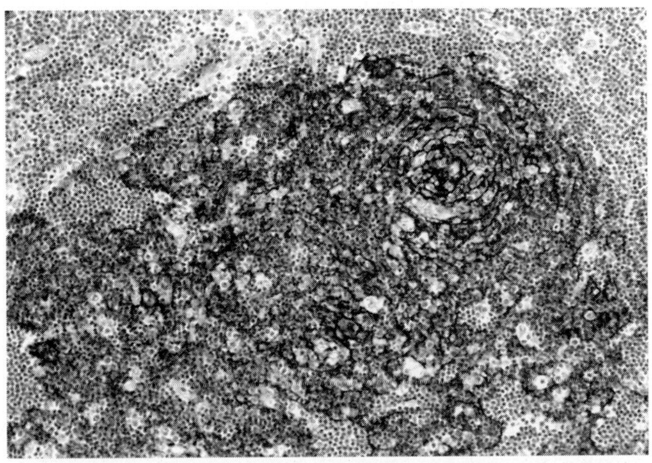

FIG. 17.6. A stain for CD21 highlights the large spherical follicular dendritic cell meshwork in nodular lymphocyte predominance. A similar dendritic cell pattern is found in progressive transformation of germinal centers (immunoperoxidase stain, original magnification: 150× magnification).

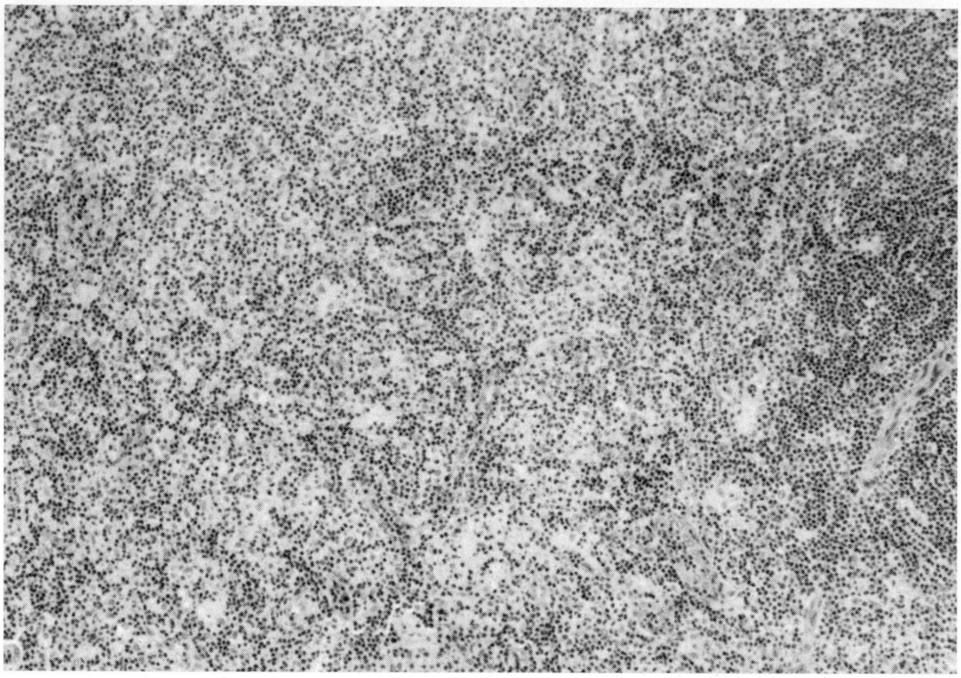

FIG. 17.7. The cell population in lymphocyte predominance mainly is composed of a mixture of small lymphocytes and reactive histiocytes (hematoxylin and eosin stain, original magnification: 120× magnification).

granulomas (16,30,87). The nodal architecture almost always is effaced, and residual germinal centers, if present, usually are confined to a subcapsular position; the capsule is characteristically intact, and there usually is no capsular thickening (30). Eosinophils, plasma cells, and necrosis are rare. The nodules are variable in size and often poorly defined, with vague borders that may be accentuated by the use of a reticulin stain or by immunohistochemistry employing CD21 to illustrate an expanded follicular dendritic cell meshwork (47,87,90). The nodules often exhibit increased numbers of small lymphocytes and only a few histiocytes; any diffuse areas more likely contain a predominance of histiocytes and smaller numbers of lymphocytes. The most pathognomonic characteristic of lymphocyte predominance is the proliferation of so-called L&H variants of Reed-Sternberg cells, which represent up to 10% of the cell population (17,30). These cells have a polyploid shape with abundant pale-staining cytoplasm and large folded, twisted, or even lobated or multilobated ''popcorn-like'' nuclei with lacy chromatin, thin nuclear membranes, and small nucleoli (17,87) (Fig. 17.8). The L&H cells frequently concentrate in the center of the nodules but are not cohesive (16). Most significant, Reed-Sternberg cells, including mononuclear variants, usually are rare and difficult to identify and may not be present in lymphocyte predominance Hodgkin's disease (88). The paucity of Reed-Sternberg cells is as important for the classification of lymphocyte predominance as is the surfeit of lymphocytes. If classic Reed-Sternberg cells can be identified readily, then the classification of lymphocyte predominance is incorrect and the correct classification is more likely lymphocyte-rich classic Hodgkin's disease or mixed cellularity Hodgkin's disease (20,30). Historically, a diagnostic Reed-Sternberg cell was mandatory for the diagnosis of Hodgkin's disease, but it has been suggested that diagnostic classic Reed-Sternberg cells are not required, and they are no longer essential for the diagnosis in cases that otherwise have the characteristic morphologic features of lymphocyte predominance (88,89,93).

Nodular lymphocyte predominance expresses immunophenotypic characteristics that are distinct from the other types of Hodgkin's disease, leading to the suggestion that it be classified as a non-Hodgkin's lymphoma (23,43,47,87,88,94). As is detailed in Chapter 18, the L&H cells in nodular lymphocyte predominance Hodgkin's disease consistently express B-cell lineage-restricted antigens, such as CD20. They also express CD45 (leukocyte common antigen) and frequently epithelial membrane antigen as well. Despite the B-cell phenotype, immunoglobulin light chain restriction usually is not demonstrable by standard immunohistochemical methods but may be shown by *in situ* hybridization for light chain messenger RNA (mRNA) (95); this is in contrast to classic Hodgkin's disease, in which such RNA is not detectable in Reed-Sternberg cells (96). Most significant and unlike classic Hodgkin's disease, the L&H cells of lymphocyte predominance do not express CD15 and almost never express CD30; vimentin similarly is not expressed by L&H cells (47). The nodular type differs from the uncommon diffuse type of lymphocyte predominance by the presence of a large, spherical follicular dendritic cell meshwork that is either absent or poorly defined and small in the diffuse variety (90). At least 50% of the small lymphocytes in the nodular areas are B cells. The T cells present frequently express

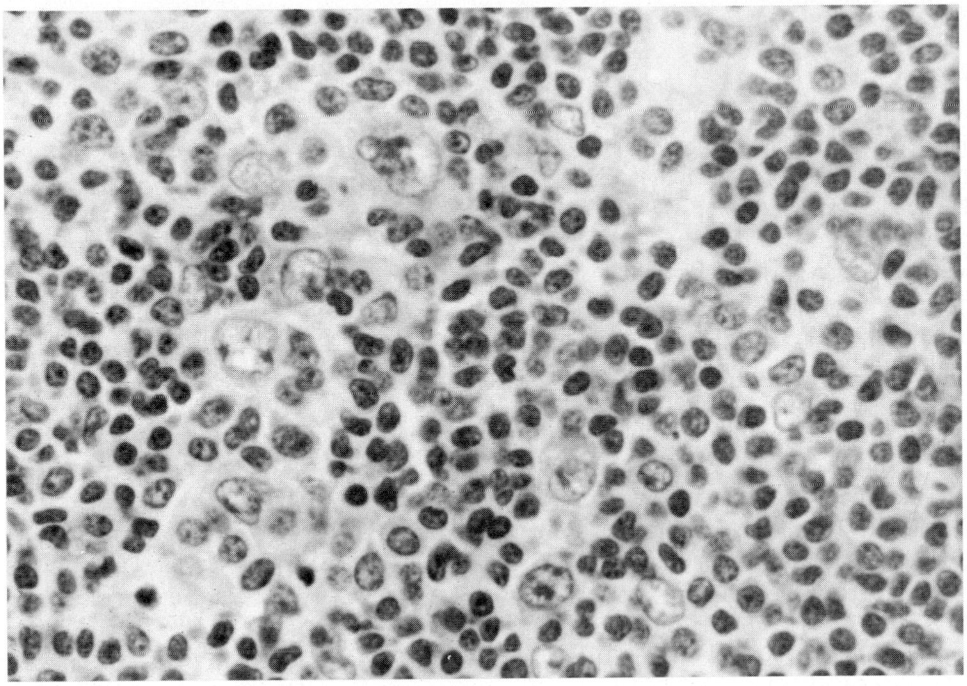

FIG. 17.8. The lymphocytic and histiocytic variants of Reed-Sternberg cells are typical of lymphocyte predominance and have a polyploid shape with folded, twisted, and often lobated nuclei and inconspicuous nucleoli. Note the absence of classic Reed-Sternberg cells (hematoxylin and eosin stain, original magnification: 720× magnification).

CD57 and form rosettes around the L&H cells (97); the CD57-positive ($CD57^+$) rosetting pattern is an important diagnostic aid in differentiating lymphocyte predominance from lymphocyte-rich classic Hodgkin's disease and T cell– or histiocyte-rich B-cell lymphoma (92,98).

The discovery that nodular lymphocyte predominance is composed of B cells correlates with the proposal that this form of Hodgkin's disease is a germinal center–derived lymphoma (11,12). This proposal coincides with earlier suggestions that nodular lymphocyte predominance Hodgkin's disease is related to an unusual form of reactive hyperplasia found in 3.5% to 10% of lymph nodes with chronic nonspecific lymphadenitis and referred to as *progressive transformation of germinal centers* (PTGC) (99–101). This is a condition in which the follicles become enlarged as a result of the infiltration by small B lymphocytes, leading to distortion of the germinal centers and sometimes completely masking them (99) (Fig. 17.9). The small lymphocytes of PTGC exhibit the immunologic characteristics of mantle zone lymphocytes, and it has been suggested that they represent early, transient stages in the transformation of primary into secondary lymphoid follicles (100,102). There is a remarkable similarity between the patterns of PTGC and nodular lymphocyte predominance, and epithelioid histiocyte clusters even may be found in pediatric patients with PTGC (101); however, L&H cells are absent in PTGC (103). Moreover, the lymph node usually is not replaced totally in PTGC, and there is associated, frequently florid reactive follicular hyperplasia. This is in contrast to nodular lymphocyte predominance, in which the architecture generally is effaced completely, and any residual germinal centers are compressed and confined to the subcapsular region (16,30,89). Nonetheless, the histologic similarity between PTGC and nodular lymphocyte predominance, coupled with the discovery of an association between the two conditions in some cases, led to the proposal

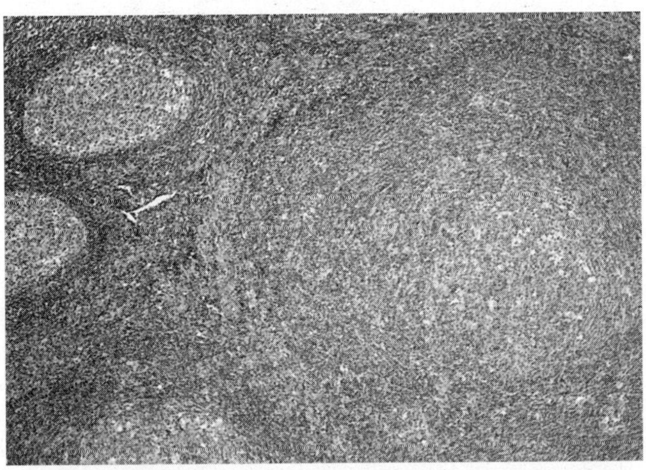

FIG. 17.9. A large progressively transformed germinal center is seen in association with smaller, usual reactive follicles. Progressive transformation of germinal centers resembles nodular lymphocyte predominance, but in lymphocyte predominance, reactive follicles usually are absent or limited to the subcapsular region of the lymph node (hematoxylin and eosin stain, original magnification: 60× magnification).

that PTGC represents a prelymphomatous disorder (99). In one study, 18% of 171 cases of nodular L&H Hodgkin's disease coexisted with PTGC in the same lymph node (104); two additional patients had PTGC in lymph node biopsies prior to developing nodular lymphocyte predominance, and three patients with histologically proven Hodgkin's disease were found on subsequent lymph node biopsy to have PTGC. The association between these two disorders, however, is tenuous. Independent studies have shown that in most cases PTGC arises in patients, especially pediatric patients and young adults, who have not had and will not develop Hodgkin's disease (100,101,103,105); a minority of patients who have associated PTGC and Hodgkin's disease develop mixed-cell and nodular sclerosis as well as lymphocyte predominance types (100).

Most patients who have lymphocyte predominance Hodgkin's disease are men in the fourth decade of life and present with localized, persistent lymph node enlargement (13–16). They usually have clinical stage I or IIA disease with few risk factors, rare involvement of the mediastinum, and relatively indolent clinical courses (13–16,86,106,107); only a minority of patients have advanced disease, and some may present in extranodal sites (108,109). Clinical studies usually include patients with both nodular and diffuse variants of lymphocyte predominance. In at least two studies, patients with the nodular type of lymphocyte predominance had a different clinical course than those with the diffuse type (63,110). Patients with the diffuse type had an excellent clinical prognosis, but their course was similar to that of other types of Hodgkin's disease (63); they had a significantly greater rate of freedom relapse rate than patients with nodular histology (110). Patients with the nodular type had significantly more relapses, which were independent of stage or treatment and were distributed equally in time of occurrence across 10 to 12 years after initial therapy. Despite the frequent relapses, patients with nodular lymphocyte predominance still had an indolent course, with only a few deaths resulting from Hodgkin's disease (63,110). Other clinical studies have not verified these reports and have found that patients with the nodular and diffuse types of lymphocyte predominance have similar natural histories, both in terms of extent and distribution of disease and persistent patterns of multiple relapses (111–113). Although late but salvageable relapses are associated with lymphocyte predominance, patients respond to therapy that is standard for classic forms of Hodgkin's disease and survive these relapses better than

A

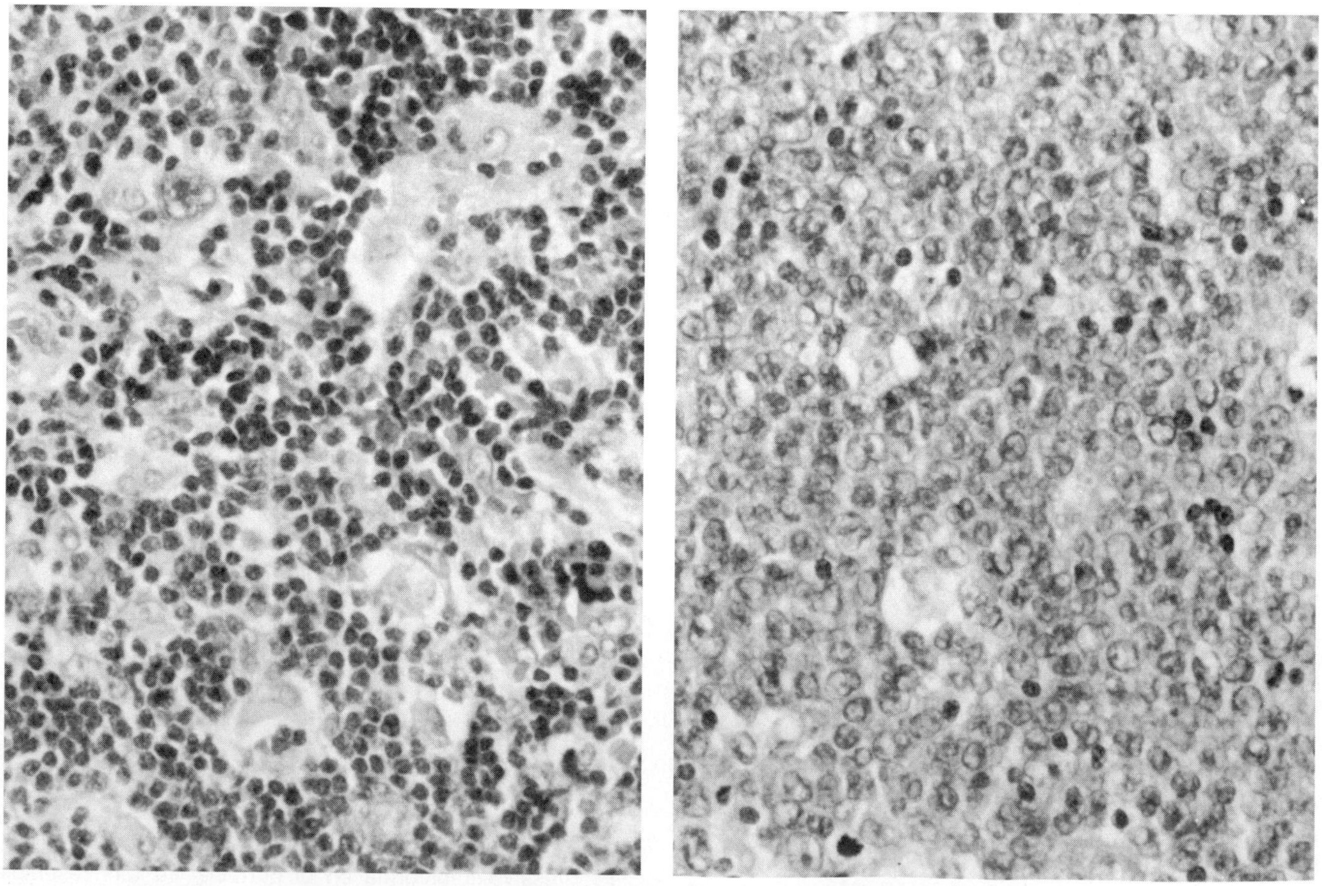

B

FIG. 17.10. A: Nodular lymphocyte predominance was found in one portion of this biopsy specimen (hematoxylin and eosin stain, original magnification: 480× magnification). **B:** Diffuse large B-cell lymphoma also was present in the same specimen. Large B-cell lymphoma is found in 2% to 3% of patients with nodular lymphocyte predominance (hematoxylin and eosin stain, original magnification: 480× magnification).

patients with such forms (113). The current strategy is to find less intensive treatment protocols for patients with lymphocyte predominance Hodgkin's disease, including a "watch and wait" approach, as a means of reducing treatment toxicities that are a major cause of death (113).

Some reports, mainly earlier ones, indicate that relapse in the lymphocytic predominance type of Hodgkin's disease usually is associated with histologic progression toward morphologically more classic forms, including rare cases of composite nodular lymphocyte predominance and classic Hodgkin's disease (16,114,115). More recent studies suggest that the majority of patients with nodular lymphocyte predominance who experience relapse have histologic persistence of nodular lymphocyte predominance (116). Approximately 2% to 3% of patients with nodular lymphocyte predominance evolve to large B-cell lymphoma, coexisting in the same biopsy specimen, distant from the presenting site, or occurring as a later relapse (110,117–121) (Fig. 17.10). The large cells frequently are multilobated, similar to L&H cells, or noncleaved (119,122). In some patients, in whom the condition is termed *L&H cell–rich*, the large cells appear to arise from clustering and aggregation of the L&H cells but do not fulfill criteria for frank large cell lymphoma (118,122) (Fig. 17.11). The L&H cell–rich cases do not exhibit clonal immunoglobulin heavy chain gene rearrangements on polymerase chain reaction analysis, suggesting that such cases represent merely nodular lymphocyte predominance with increased numbers of L&H cells (122). In contrast, cases of unequivocal large B-cell lymphoma are found to be clonal with either immunoglobulin heavy chain gene rearrangements on polymerase chain reaction or *in situ* hybridization for light chain messenger RNA (122–125). Despite evident clonality in the large cell component, a clonal link between the large B-cell lymphoma and the preceding nodular lymphocyte predominance Hodgkin's disease usually is not detectable or is found only in a small minority of cases (122–124). Although the clonal link between the nodular lymphocyte predominance and large B-cell lymphoma constituents is tenuous, the large B-cell lymphomas associated with nodular lymphocyte predominance differ clinically from the usual cases of diffuse large B-cell lymphoma. Patients with large B-cell lymphoma associated with nodular lymphocyte predominance have indolent clinical courses with a favorable prognosis similar to that of lymphocyte predominance, rather than the typically aggressive course of most large B-cell lymphomas (118–121). The large B-cell lymphomas arising in patients with nodular lymphocyte predominance result from the natural history of the

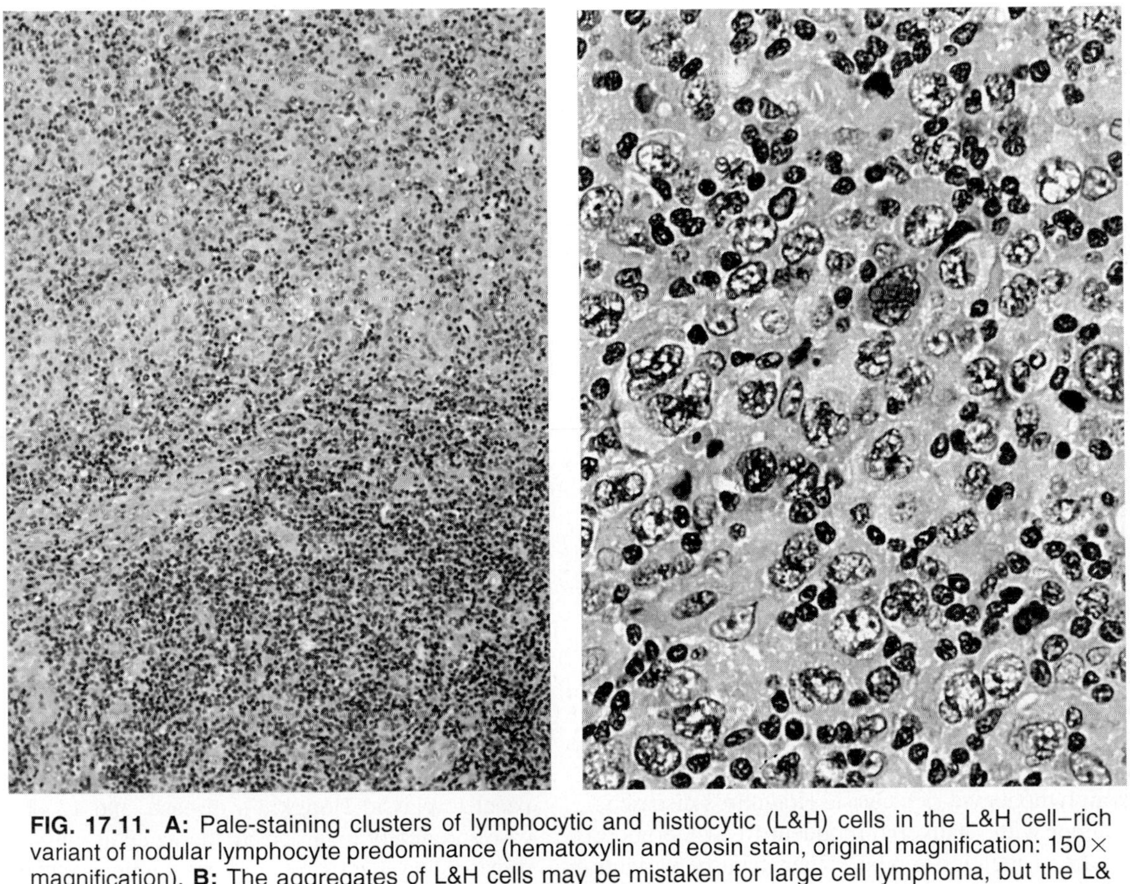

A B

FIG. 17.11. A: Pale-staining clusters of lymphocytic and histiocytic (L&H) cells in the L&H cell–rich variant of nodular lymphocyte predominance (hematoxylin and eosin stain, original magnification: 150× magnification). **B:** The aggregates of L&H cells may be mistaken for large cell lymphoma, but the L&H cell–rich cases do not have clonal immunoglobulin heavy chain rearrangements (hematoxylin and eosin stain, original magnification: 600× magnification).

disease rather than induced by therapy (117). Rare cases of concurrent lymphocyte predominance and T-cell lymphomas are described, but like the large B-cell lymphoma cases, the T-cell cases are not therapy-related (126); the pathogenetic relationship between the synchronous lymphocyte predominance Hodgkin's disease and T-cell lymphomas is enigmatic.

The differential diagnosis of lymphocyte predominance depends on whether the pattern is nodular or the uncommon diffuse type. For the nodular variety, the main differential diagnosis concerns PTGC. The distinction from PTGC is related directly to both pattern and cytologic characteristics. In nodular lymphocyte predominance, the nodules are poorly defined, closely approximated, and coalescent and blend into diffuse areas. Reactive follicles are either not present or are limited to the periphery of the node (16,30,89). In PTGC, the nodules are sharply circumscribed, discrete, and set amid a score of reactive follicles (103). Cytologically, the conditions have many small lymphocytes and variable numbers of epithelioid histiocytes, but in nodular lymphocyte predominance L&H cells are appreciated readily, whereas in PTGC L&H cells are absent and there are only scattered follicle center cells. Immunohistochemical stains are of marginal utility in distinguishing nodular lymphocyte predominance from PTGC (127). Both conditions contain identical CD21$^+$ follicular dendritic cell meshworks. B and T cells are found in the nodules of nodular lymphocyte predominance and PTGC, but there are distributional differences. In nodular lymphocyte predominance, B cells are dispersed irregularly with a mottled pattern, whereas in PTGC B cells form well-circumscribed confluent nodules. T cells in nodular lymphocyte predominance aggregate and surround L&H cells; in contrast, T cells in PTGC are scattered but may form rings around transformed lymphocytes (127). One distinct immunophenotypic difference is the presence of CD57 rosettes around L&H cells in nodular lymphocyte predominance; CD57 rosettes are not found in PTGC. Reactivity for epithelial membrane antigen also is seen in nodular lymphocyte predominance, but not in PTGC.

The differential diagnosis of the rare, pure diffuse variety of lymphocyte predominance mainly concerns classic types of Hodgkin's disease, particularly lymphocyte-rich classic Hodgkin's disease and T cell– or histiocyte-rich B-cell lymphoma. This differential diagnosis is discussed in the next section.

Lymphocyte-Rich Classic Hodgkin's Disease

Lymphocyte-rich classic Hodgkin's disease is a newly described subtype that originally was proposed as a provisional entity by the proponents of the REAL classification and now has been incorporated into the WHO classification (20–22). By definition, lymphocyte-rich classic Hodgkin's disease is "a diffuse tumor with relatively infrequent Reed-Sternberg cells, which are of the classic type, rather than the variants seen in nodular lymphocyte predominance; some lacunar cells may be present, in a background of lymphocytes, with

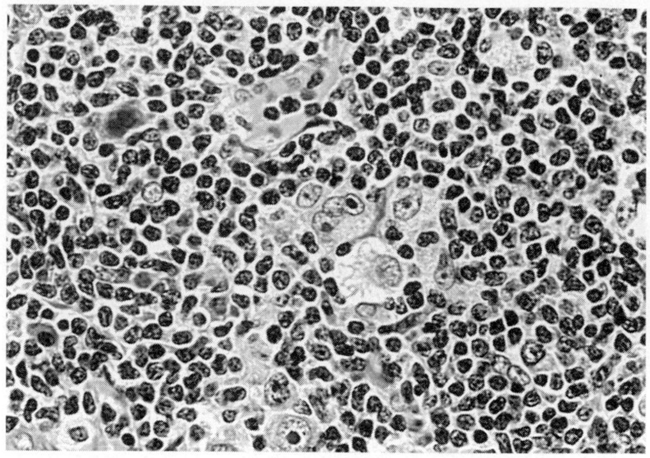

FIG. 17.12. A classic Reed-Sternberg cell can be identified in lymphocyte-rich classic Hodgkin's disease, as opposed to the virtual absence of such cells in lymphocyte predominance (hematoxylin and eosin stain, original magnification: 600× magnification).

infrequent eosinophils or plasma cells. There is morphologic overlap with diffuse lymphocyte predominance, the cellular phase of nodular sclerosis, and mixed cellularity. In contrast to diffuse lymphocyte predominance, the Reed-Sternberg cells have the morphology and immunophenotype of classic Reed-Sternberg cells" (20) (Fig. 17.12). A nodular or follicular variant also occurs (128) (Fig. 17.13). The nodules are composed of mantle zone lymphocytes with a loose CD21$^+$ follicular dendritic cell meshwork. The nodules may contain eccentrically located, atrophic-appearing germinal centers. Diagnostic classic and lacunar variants of Reed-Sternberg cells are scattered and usually found at the periphery of the mantle zone nodules (128). The Reed-Sternberg cells in both the diffuse and nodular forms of lymphocyte-rich classic Hodgkin's disease express the classic Hodgkin's disease-associated antigens CD15 and CD30 and also may be CD20$^+$ (20,128).

The immunophenotype is essential for the diagnosis of lymphocyte-rich classic Hodgkin's disease and its distinction from lymphocyte predominance Hodgkin's disease. For example, in an immunohistochemical analysis from the German Hodgkin Study Group, 104 morphologically confirmed cases of lymphocyte predominance were compared with 104 classic Hodgkin's disease cases that originally had been classified as lymphocyte predominance and were revised by a panel of pathologists. In most cases, immunoperoxidase revealed either a lymphocyte predominance phenotype (CD20$^+$CD15$^-$CD30$^-$CD45$^+$) or a classic Hodgkin's disease phenotype (CD15$^+$CD30$^+$CD20$^-$CD45$^-$). In 25 (24%) of 104 cases, immunohistochemistry altered the morphologic diagnosis of lymphocyte predominance by the panel to classic Hodgkin's disease, and 13 (12%) of 104 cases originally regarded by the panel as classic Hodgkin's disease showed a lymphocyte predominance phenotype. Immunophenotypic confirmation had an impact on clinical outcome: Patients with lymphocyte predominance had a signifi-

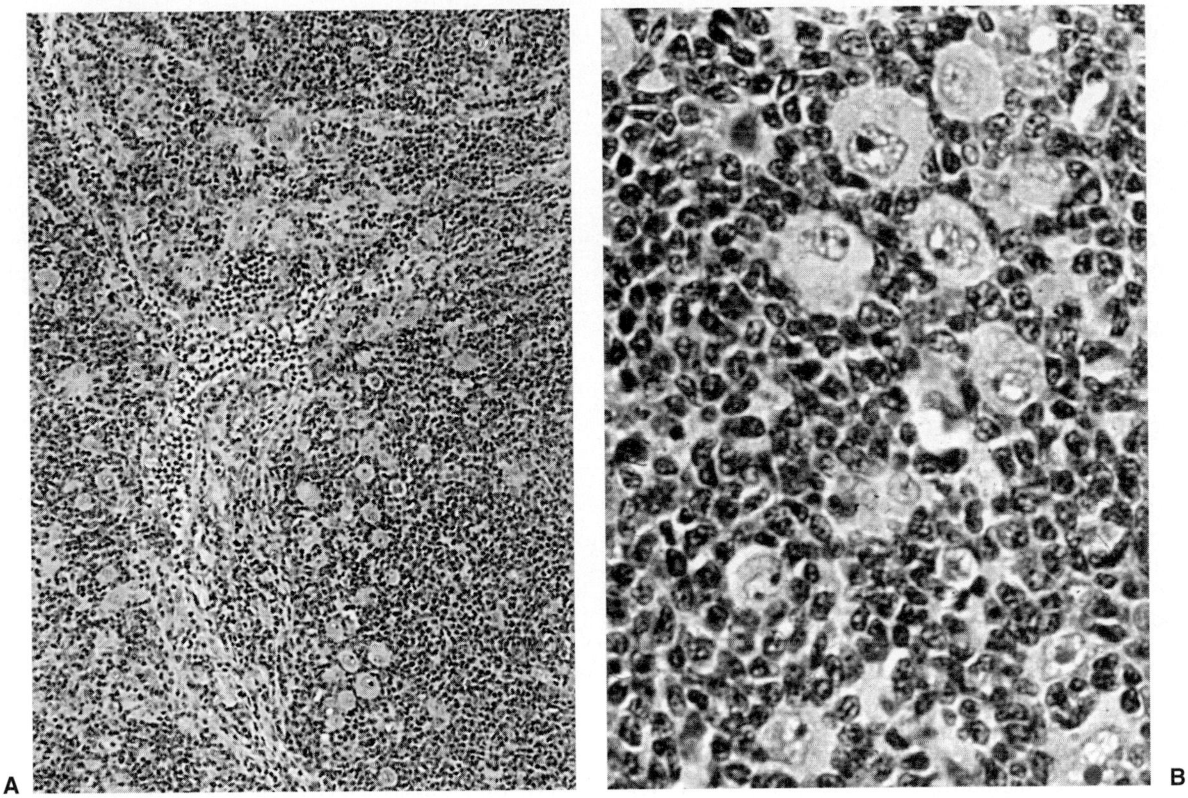

FIG. 17.13. A: The nodular variant of lymphocyte-rich classic Hodgkin's disease is a result of expanded mantle zones. Germinal centers (not shown) often are eccentrically located and atrophic (hematoxylin and eosin stain, original magnification: 150× magnification). B: Lacunar Reed-Sternberg cells are at the periphery of the nodules. This type of case may represent an early form of nodular sclerosis, cellular phase (hematoxylin and eosin stain, original magnification: 600× magnification).

cantly better rate of freedom from treatment failure than those with classic Hodgkin's disease; this finding could not be demonstrated in the original study group based solely upon morphology (129). Another study demonstrated the value of employing immunohistochemical criteria to aid in the classification of lymphocyte predominance and lymphocyte-rich classic Hodgkin's disease (113). Of 426 cases that initially were interpreted as lymphocyte predominance morphologically, only 219 cases (51%) were classified as lymphocyte predominance after histologic review and immunohistochemical studies. Lymphocyte-rich classic Hodgkin's disease comprised 115 cases (27%), and the remainder were a mixture of other forms of classic Hodgkin's disease, non-Hodgkin's lymphomas and reactive lesions or were considered technically inadequate (113).

The clinical features of lymphocyte-rich classic Hodgkin's disease have been studied recently and compared with lymphocyte predominance (113,130). In one review of 1,339 cases of Hodgkin's disease with followup information, 4.1% were classified as lymphocyte-rich classic type and 5.2% as lymphocyte predominance (130). Similar to patients with lymphocyte predominance, patients who have lymphocyte-rich classic Hodgkin's disease are predominantly male and have early-stage disease and few risk factors; however, the patients who have lymphocyte-rich classic Hodgkin's disease tend to be older (113,130). Survival and failure-free survival rates are similar for both groups and comparable to those for stage-matched patients with other forms of classic Hodgkin's disease (nodular sclerosis and mixed cellularity). The patients with lymphocyte-rich classic Hodgkin's disease have significantly fewer multiple relapses compared with those with the lymphocyte predominance type (113); however, patients who have lymphocyte predominance exhibit a significantly superior survival rate after relapse in comparison with those with lymphocyte-rich or other types of classic Hodgkin's disease. The clinical data, particularly the mode of presentation, suggest that lymphocyte rich classic Hodgkin's disease is more closely related to lymphocyte predominance, in spite of its distinct immunophenotype (113,130).

The main differential diagnosis of lymphocyte-rich classic Hodgkin's disease includes not only lymphocyte predominance but also T cell– or histiocyte-rich B-cell lymphoma. Although T cell– or histiocyte-rich B-cell lymphoma lacks precise diagnostic criteria, the cases associated with a diffuse small lymphocytic milieu mimic both lymphocyte-rich classic and diffuse lymphocyte predominance Hodgkin's disease (40,41,91,92). In T cell– or histiocyte-rich B-cell lymphoma, the lymph node architecture is effaced by a prolifera-

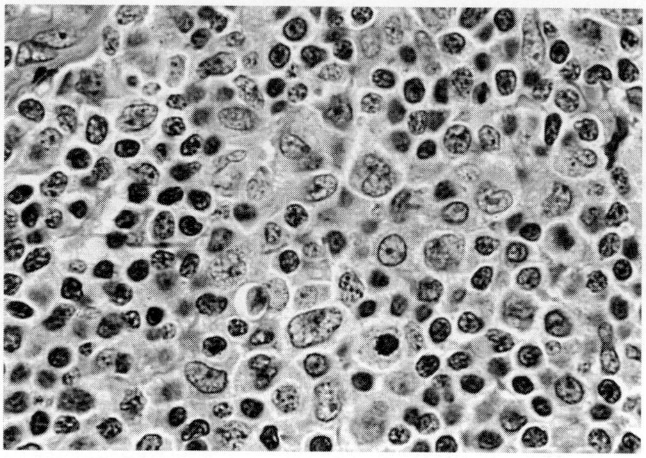

FIG. 17.14. The cellular constituents of T cell– or histiocyte-rich B-cell lymphoma are confused easily with those of lymphocytic-predominant and lymphocyte-rich classic Hodgkin's disease. Immunophenotypic analysis is mandatory to diffentiate these entities accurately. (Hematoxylin and eosin stain, 600× magnification.)

tion of small, mainly round lymphocytes and varying numbers of histiocytes (Fig.17.14). The histiocytes may obscure atypical large cells, including cells resembling L&H cells and even classic Reed-Sternberg–type cells. Similar to lymphocyte predominance, patients are mainly male and in their forties. The patients with T cell– or histiocyte-rich B-cell lymphoma, however, mainly have advanced disease, stage III or IV, with frequent splenomegaly, liver, and bone marrow involvement (40,41,91,92). Patients with T cell– or histiocyte-rich B-cell lymphoma do not respond to standard Hodgkin's disease protocols and have a reported 5-year survival rate of 20% (92). Immunophenotypic analysis is essential and is the most practical means of separating both lymphocyte-rich classic and lymphocyte predominance Hodgkin's disease from T cell– or histiocyte-rich B-cell lymphoma (47) (Table 17.5). CD15 and CD30, as well as vimentin, clearly distinguish lymphocyte-rich classic from lymphocyte predominance cases and T cell– or histiocyte-rich B-cell lymphoma. In contrast, there is considerable immunohistochemical and morphologic overlap between the latter two disorders. Although clonal immunoglobulin heavy chain gene rearrangements are detectable in cases of T cell– or histiocyte-rich B-cell lymphoma, important differences between both entities are found in the background cell population (47,91). In lymphocyte predominance, the small lymphocytes include many B cells, as well as T cells; the T cells are often $CD57^+$, form rosettes, but do not express TIA-1 (47). In contrast, the background lymphocytes in T cell– or histiocyte-rich B-cell lymphoma are virtually exclusively $CD3^+$ T cells that are also TIA-1^+ but lack CD57 reactivity (47,92). The similar morphologic and immunophenotypic features, as well as the reports of T cell– or histiocyte-rich B-cell lymphomas developing in patients with documented prior histories of lymphocyte predominance, suggest a histogenetic relationship between the two disorders (91,92,131, 132). T cell– or histiocyte-rich B-cell lymphomas conceivably are an aggressive, advanced stage of lymphocyte predominance (23) (see Chapter 25).

In addition to T cell– or histiocyte-rich B-cell lymphoma, lymphocyte-rich classic Hodgkin's disease must be distinguished from small lymphocytic lymphoma and related lymphoproliferative disorders, such as chronic lymphocytic leukemia. The differential diagnosis is especially pertinent in cases of small lymphocytic lymphoma or chronic lymphocytic leukemia containing epithelioid histiocytes and even blasts with Reed-Sternberg cell-like features (133,134). One

TABLE 17.5. *Immunohistochemical panel to distinguish lymphocyte-rich classic Hodgkin's disease from lymphocyte predominance and T-cell/histiocyte-rich B-cell lymphoma*

	Lymphocyte-rich classic Hodgkin's disease (Reed-Sternberg cells)	Lymphocyte predominance (lymphocytic and histiocytic cells)	T-cell/histiocyte-rich B-cell lymphoma (large cells)
CD15	+	−	−
CD30	+	−	−
CD20	−	+	+
J-chain	−	+/−	−/+
Vimentin	+	−	−
CD45	−	+	+
EMA	−/+	+/−	+/−
CD3 background	+	−/+	+
TIA-1 background	+	−	+
CD57 background	−	+	−
CD20 background	−/+	+/−	−

* Adapted from Rüdiger T, Ott G, Ott MM, et al. Differential diagnosis between classic Hodgkin's lymphoma, T-cell-rich B-cell lymphoma, and paragranuloma by paraffin immunohistochemistry. *Am J Surg Pathol* 1998;22:1184–1191, with permission.

morphologic aid is the fact that capsular invasion is common in small lymphocytic lymphoma and chronic lymphocytic leukemia but usually does not occur in Hodgkin's disease. Studies to determine clonality are important in differentiating between these two conditions, as well as determining whether any Reed-Sternberg–like cells express CD15 or CD30. Compounding the diagnostic difficulty, cases of chronic lymphocytic leukemia may coexist with genuine Hodgkin's disease, including cases of lymphocyte predominance (135–137); in most instances, the Hodgkin's disease develops after an initial diagnosis of chronic lymphocytic leukemia, similar to Richter's syndrome and frequently is of the nodular sclerosis or mixed cellularity type. Composite chronic lymphocytic leukemia and Hodgkin's disease, however, including cases of lymphocyte predominance, may occur at presentation, and in these cases the classic Reed-Sternberg cells or L&H cells have their usual immunophenotypic characteristics of Hodgkin's disease, in contrast to the clonal B-cell immunophenotype of the surrounding neoplastic small lymphocytes (136–138). The typical Reed-Sternberg cells in such cases contain EBV RNA, but the surrounding chronic lymphocytic leukemia cells do not have EBV RNA (139). With the use of polymerase chain reaction on isolated single cells, a clonal relationship recently was established between the cells of chronic lymphocytic leukemia and the Reed-Sternberg cells in cases of Hodgkin's-type Richter's syndrome (140) (Chapters 21 and 40).

Because of the nodular pattern in some cases, lymphocyte-rich classic Hodgkin's disease may be mistaken for follicular lymphoma. In follicular lymphomas, the follicles typically are small, uniform, and sharply demarcated in contrast to the macronodules seen in lymphocyte-rich classic Hodgkin's disease; the lymphocytes in follicular lymphomas are atypical and cleaved, in contrast to the usual round nuclear contours of the benign mantle cells found in nodular lymphocyte-rich classic Hodgkin's disease (128). Reed-Sternberg–like cells, however, occasionally can be observed in follicular lymphomas (37). The Reed-Sternberg–like cells usually are in the center of the neoplastic follicles, in which case they probably represent transformed follicle center cells (Fig. 17.15), but occasionally they are located in the interfollicular regions or even are associated with epithelioid histiocytes (141). In addition to histologic features, these cases are differentiated from nodular lymphocyte-rich classic Hodgkin's disease by immunologic studies that demonstrate reactivity of the Reed-Sternberg–like cells with antibodies directed against B-cell antigens and CD45, but not those against CD15 or CD30; immunogenetic studies may reveal *BCL2* gene rearrangements (141) (Chapter 24).

Nodular Sclerosis

Nodular sclerosis is the most common type of Hodgkin's disease, comprising more than 60% of cases, and provides the best levels of agreement in review by different pathologists (86,130,142). This type of Hodgkin's disease is more common in females and less common in patients older than 50 years of age (33,34). Nodular sclerosis tends to involve

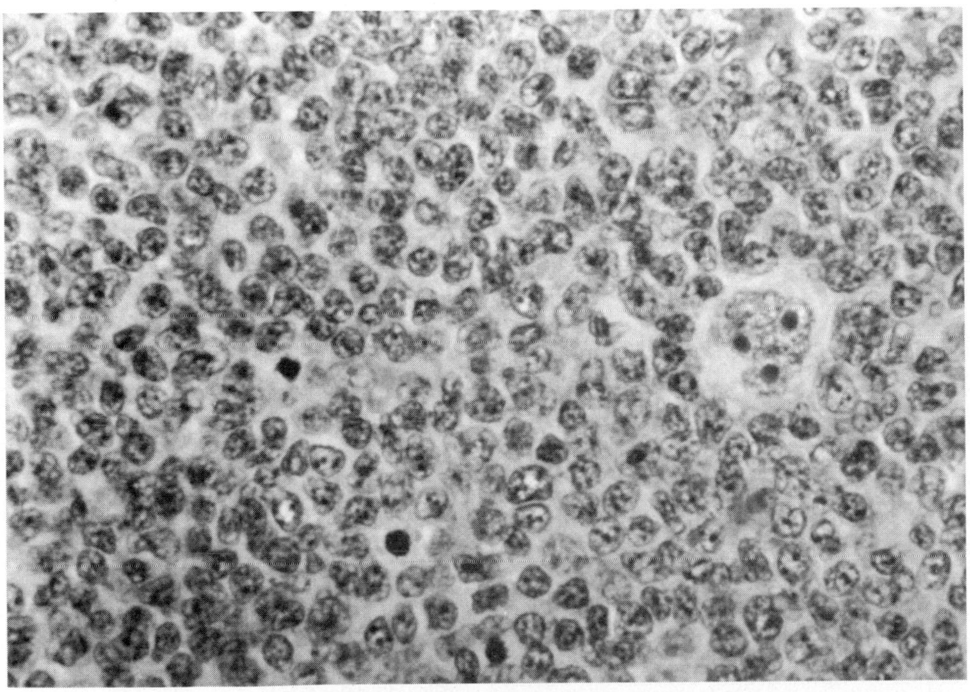

FIG. 17.15. A giant cell indistinguishable from a Reed-Sternberg cell is found in the center of a follicular small cleaved cell lymphoma. This Reed-Sternberg–like cell is interpreted as a transformed follicle center B cell (hematoxylin and eosin stain, original magnification: 720× magnification).

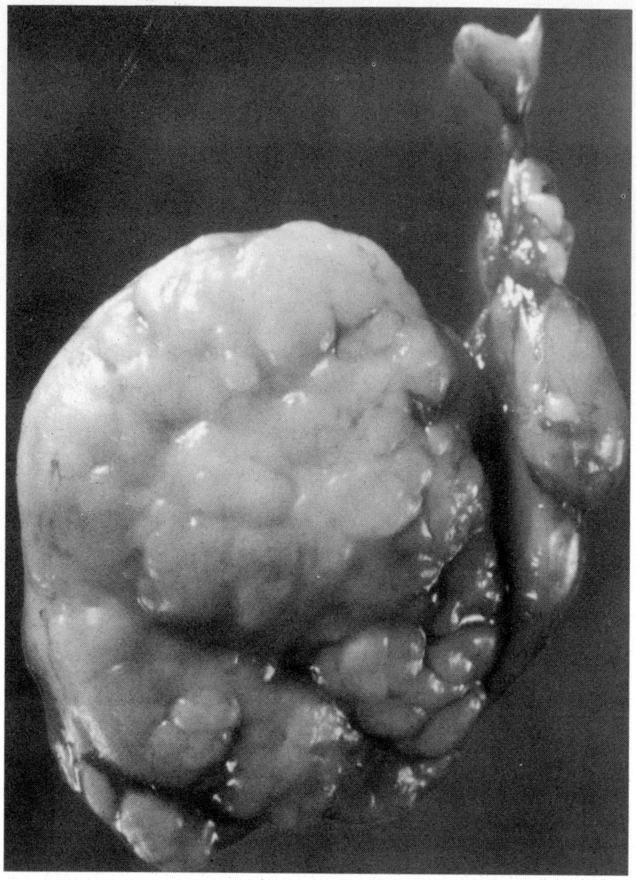

FIG. 17.16. The distinct nodules on the cut surface of this lymph node strongly suggest the nodular sclerosis type of Hodgkin's disease.

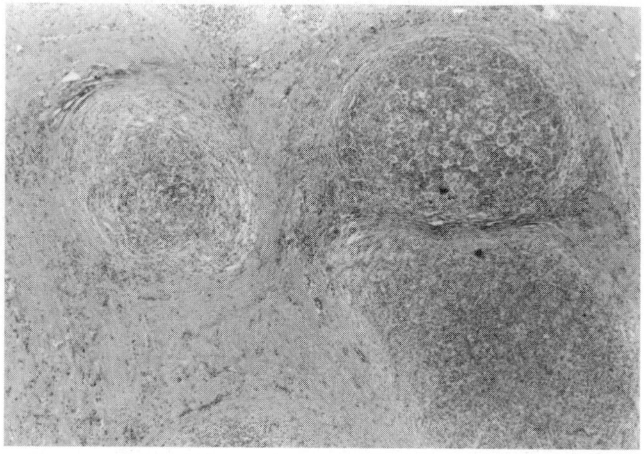

FIG. 17.17. In typical nodular sclerosis, bands of fibrous connective tissue subdivide the lymph node into a series of nodules. Lacunar cells are evident within the abnormal lymphoid nodules (hematoxylin and eosin stain, original magnification: 48× magnification).

the lower cervical and supraclavicular lymph nodes, mediastinal lymph nodes, and contiguous structures (16,34); the majority of patients have stage II disease at presentation and have an excellent prognosis.

The diagnosis of nodular sclerosis can be suspected at the time of gross examination by the delineation of distinct nodules defined by retracted gray-white interconnecting bands on the cut surface of a lymph node (16) (Fig. 17.16). This histologic type of Hodgkin's disease is characterized by orderly bands of interconnecting collagenous connective tissue that partially or entirely subdivide abnormal lymphoid tissue into isolated cellular nodules (16,17) (Fig. 17.17). The degree of collagen and the character of the cellular proliferation vary widely even within the same specimen. The connective tissue bands are identified as collagen by their birefringent character as seen under polarized light (Fig. 17.18). In some cases, the entire lymph node undergoes spontaneous sclerosis. At the opposite extreme, the process may be predominantly cellular and the formation of collagen bands and isolation of nodules limited to only a small portion of the specimen (16). Minimal alteration usually is related to focal thickening of the lymph node capsule, from which a collagen band extends into the cortex but does not produce distinctive nodules (30,32) (Fig. 17.19).

The cellular proliferation within the abnormal lymphoid nodules is highly variable, but the distinctive feature is the presence of the lacunar variants of Reed-Sternberg cells. These cells occur in clusters and are characterized by abundant and water-clear to slightly eosinophilic cytoplasm with sharply defined cellular borders situated in a lacuna-like space (16,17) (Fig. 17.20); the lacuna-like spaces are artifacts of formalin fixation and are less prominent in tissues fixed in a Zenker's-type fixative, such as B5. The nuclei of the lacunar cells usually are hyperlobated, with delicate nuclear chromatin, and contain small nucleoli. Paradoxically, classic diagnostic Reed-Sternberg cells may be difficult to identify in nodular sclerosis despite the presence of numerous lacunar variants (89). The cellular constituents associated with lacunar cells and Reed-Sternberg cells are variable. They may be predominantly lymphocytic or of

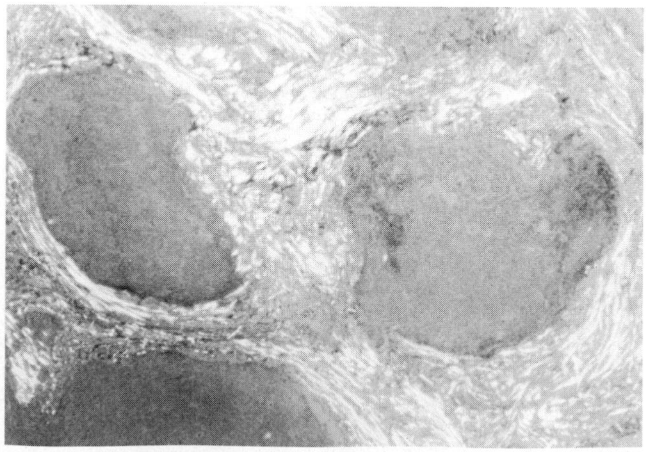

FIG. 17.18. The bands of fibrous connective tissue in nodular sclerosis appear characteristically birefringent in examination under polarized light (hematoxylin and eosin stain, original magnification: 48× magnification).

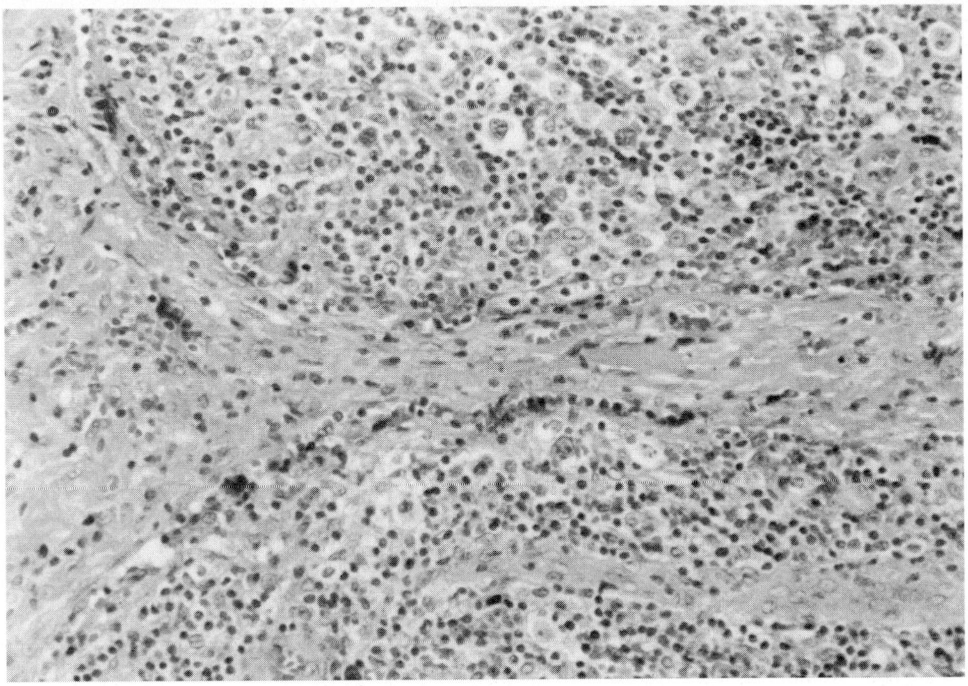

FIG. 17.19. In minimal nodular sclerosis, there is thickening of the capsule and formation of an early collagen band extending into the cortex. Lacunar cells are evident. This pattern has been termed by some the *cellular phase* of nodular sclerosis (hematoxylin and eosin stain, original magnification: 240× magnification).

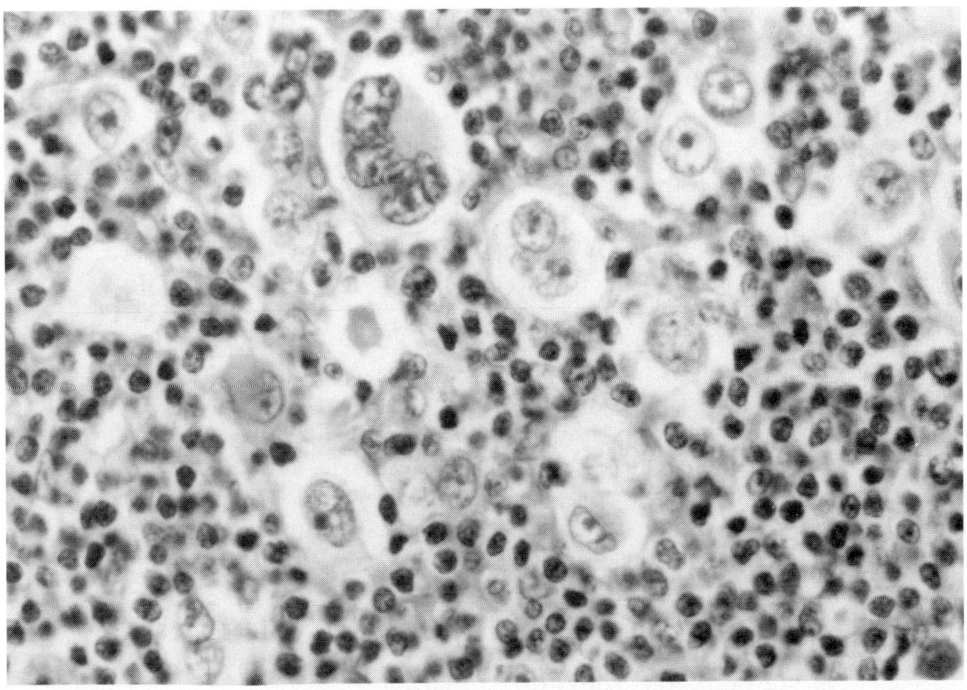

FIG. 17.20. Clusters of lacunar cells are characteristic of the lymphoid islands in nodular sclerosis. The nuclei frequently are hyperlobated, and the nucleoli generally are smaller than those seen in classic Reed-Sternberg cells (hematoxylin and eosin stain, original magnification: 720× magnification).

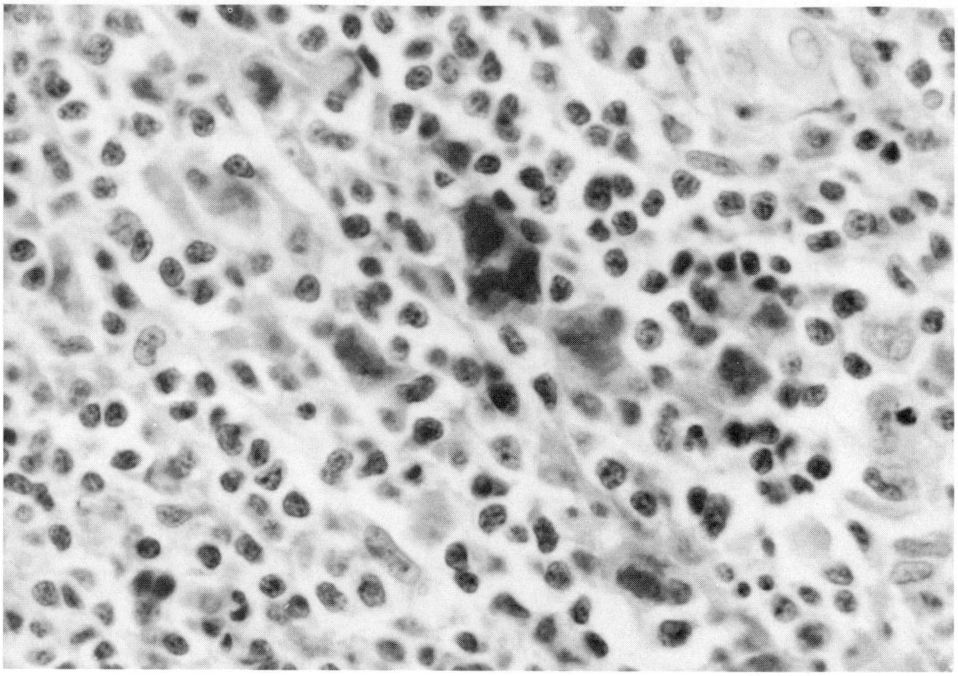

FIG. 17.21. Degenerating Reed-Sternberg cells commonly are found in nodular sclerosis and mixed cellularity Hodgkin's disease. These cells have been called "mummified" or "zombie" cells. (Hematoxylin and eosin stain, 720× magnification.)

mixed composition, with the addition of mature granulocytes and numerous eosinophils as well as increased small blood vessels. Eosinophilic abscesses and areas of central necrosis may occur (86). Necrosis often is associated with a predominance of Reed-Sternberg cells, which form cohesive clusters and sheets (17). The Reed-Sternberg cells frequently appear degenerated and shrunken to impart a ''mummified'' appearance; these cells sometimes are referred to as ''zombie'' cells (32) (Fig. 17.21). In some cases, the areas of necrosis may be accompanied by foamy macrophages, which may mask Hodgkin's disease and lead to a misdiagnosis of a lipid storage disease or even sinus histiocytosis with massive lymphadenopathy (86,143) (Fig. 17.22).

The presence of both lacunar cells and collagen bands, usually in association with a thickened capsule, is required for an absolute diagnosis of nodular sclerosis, and the diagnosis is more reproducible if both criteria are used (30,32). The finding of lacunar cells without fibrous septa raises the question of the so-called cellular phase of nodular sclerosis (30). Definitions of nodular sclerosis vary from one requiring only the identification of cellular nodules containing clusters of lacunar cells but without demonstrable fibrosis (Fig. 17.23), to another in which there must be at least a single band of collagen extending from a thickened capsule in association with the characteristic cellular proliferation containing lacunar cells (16,17,114,144,145). Both Lukes (30) and Butler and Pugh (32) acknowledge that occasional cases may exhibit a true cellular phase without collagen bands, but in order to achieve diagnostic consistency, these cases should be classified with the mixed cellularity type. Their proposal has been supported by a large clinicopathologic study in which their original criteria were used to define the cellular phase, in that cases were required to have at least one sclerotic band (86). Ten percent of cases were categorized as nodular sclerosis, cellular phase, and the patients with that classification exhibited clinical features and an overall survival that was more like those with mixed cellularity Hodgkin's disease than those with nodular sclerosis (86).

The same study also demonstrated that sclerosis was a significant factor in survival. By separately tabulating the amount of collagen or acellular sclerosis from the number of visible, plump, spindled fibroblasts, patients with increased numbers of fibroblasts were determined to have a shorter duration of relapse-free survival (86) (Fig. 17.24). Some cases with the ''fibroblastic variant'' of nodular sclerosis may have a spindle and storiform pattern reminiscent of malignant fibrous histiocytoma (86,146).

A case should be classified as nodular sclerosis even if typical nodular sclerosis is limited to only a portion of the lymph node biopsy specimen and the remaining tissue contains neither nodularity nor bands (145). The classification of nodular sclerosis takes precedence over other histologic types that appear to be present in the same section, even if the area of nodular sclerosis is small (32,145). Lymph node involvement by nodular sclerosis may exhibit wide architectural variations from total sclerosis to partial or even focal involvement (30). Focal involvement of the lymph node by Hodgkin's disease is observed with the mixed cellularity and nodular sclerosis types. Focal involvement by Hodgkin's disease, also referred to as *interfollicular Hodgkin's disease*,

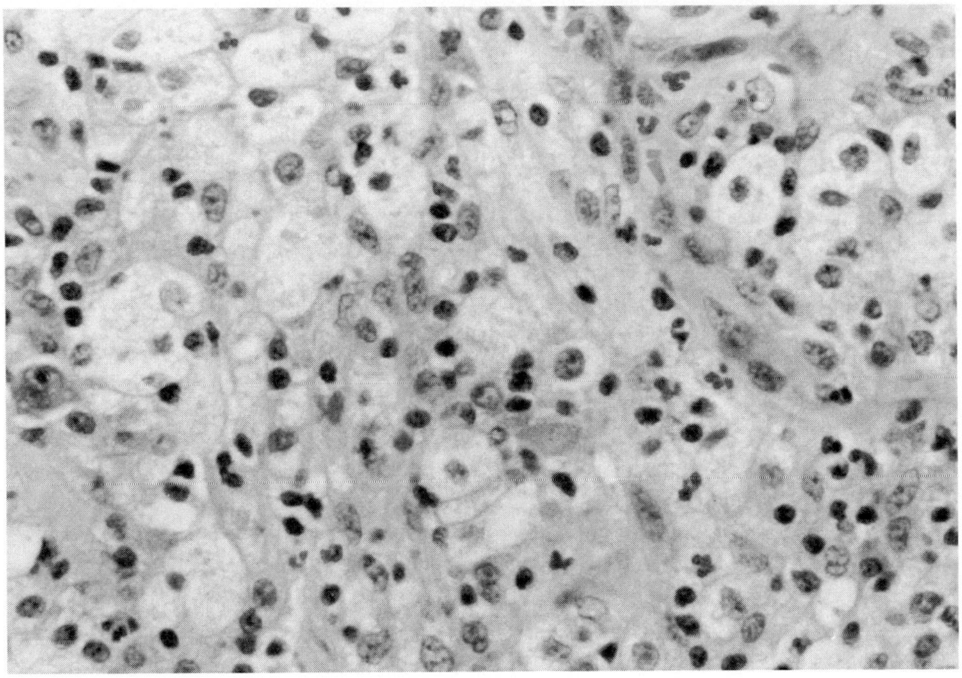

FIG. 17.22. In nodular sclerosis, areas of necrosis and degeneration may occur associated with a proliferation of foamy macrophages. The macrophages may obscure the diagnosis of Hodgkin's disease (hematoxylin and eosin stain, original magnification: 480× magnification).

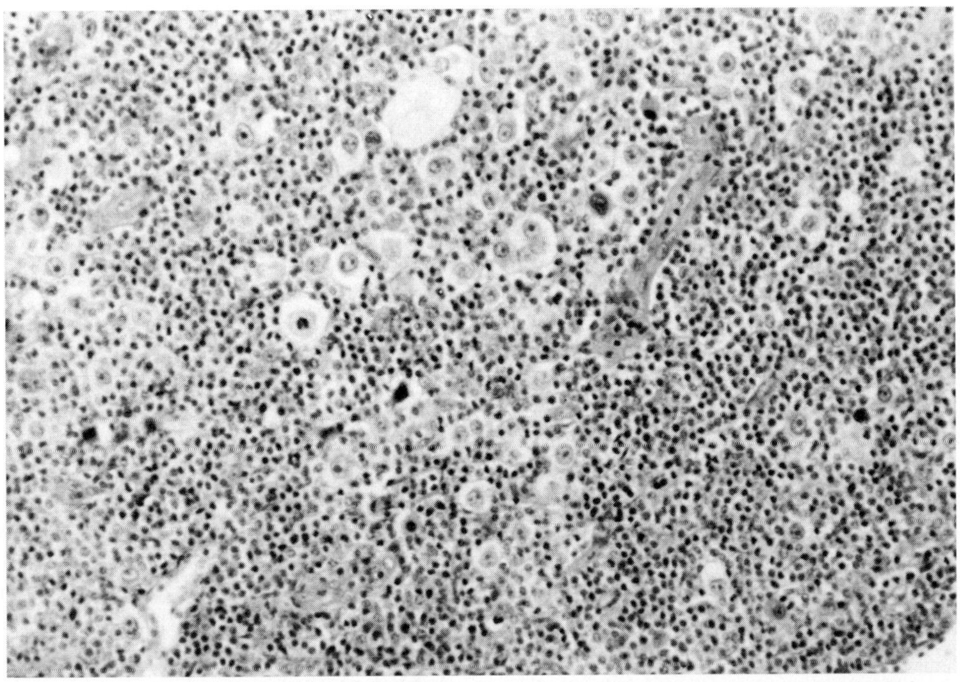

FIG. 17.23. Clusters of lacunar cells found within cellular nodules, but without fibrous bands, probably represent the true cellular phase of nodular sclerosis; however, in the absence of fibrous bands, it probably is more prudent to classify this type of case as mixed cellularity (hematoxylin and eosin stain, original magnification: 240× magnification).

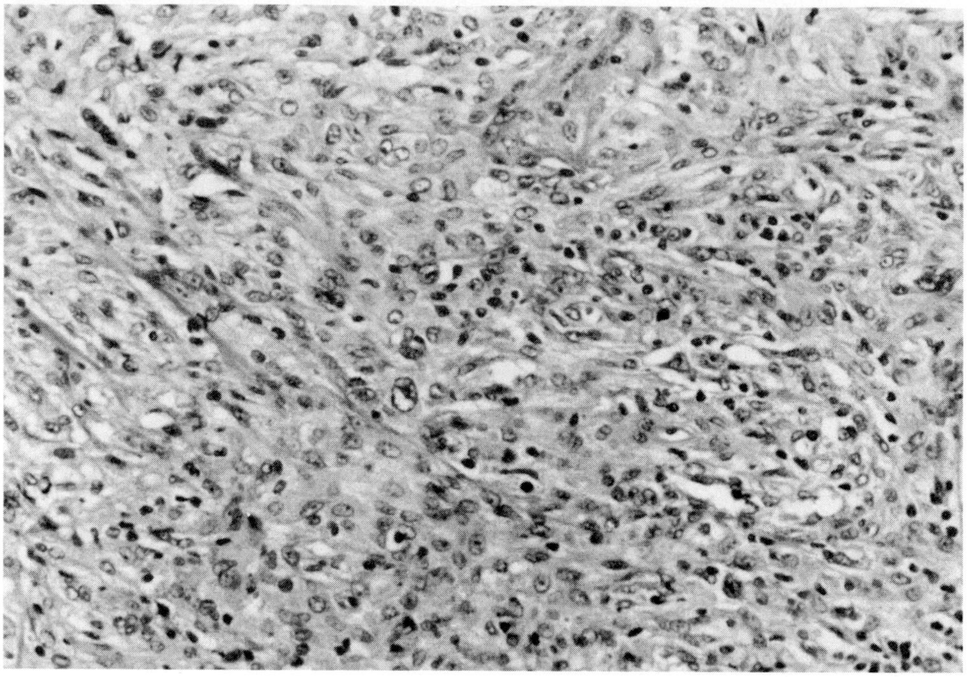

FIG. 17.24. The "fibroblastic variant" of nodular sclerosis is associated with a shorter duration of relapse-free survival and may be confused with malignant fibrous histiocytoma (hematoxylin and eosin stain, original magnification: 240× magnification).

usually is characterized by an essentially preserved lymph node architecture associated with reactive follicular hyperplasia (30,147,148) (Fig. 17.25). There is usually vague expansion of the interfollicular region as a result of a heterogeneous proliferation of small lymphocytes, plasma cells, eosinophils, epithelioid histiocytes, and diagnostic Reed-Sternberg cells that frequently are difficult to identify (30,147,148). In some cases, plasma cells are prominent; these cases easily can be confused with the plasma cell variant of Castleman's disease (148,149). Cases may be mistaken for benign reactive follicular hyperplasia, including toxoplasmic lymphadenitis, especially if interfollicular epithelioid histiocytes are prominent. Focal Hodgkin's disease also has been reported to occur in monocytoid B-cell clusters within lymph nodes, and monocytoid B cells have been described at the periphery of the nodules of nodular sclerosis (150,151). Because focal involvement of the lymph node by Hodgkin's disease is of limited size, accurate classification according to the Rye classification is not possible, but often deeper sections or a second biopsy specimen reveal nodular sclerosis or mixed cellularity (30,148). The pattern of focal or interfollicular Hodgkin's disease has no bearing on prognosis (86).

Because the cellular composition of nodular sclerosis is so variable, there have been several attempts to determine whether subdividing nodular sclerosis according to the predominant histologic type has any prognostic significance. The results are inconsistent. One early study was unable to detect any statistical differences in survival rate if Hodgkin's disease of the nodular sclerosis type was subdivided into lymphocyte predominance, mixed cellularity, and lymphocytic depletion types (152). In another early study, increased numbers of small lymphocytes significantly improved the predictability of prognosis in nodular sclerosis (153). Colby and associates (86) also demonstrated that the number of lymphocytes independently affects prognosis for all cases of Hodgkin's disease but not in patients with nodular sclerosis. Later studies, mainly in Europe, demonstrated that there is a relationship between the histopathologic composition in nodular sclerosis and both survival and relapse rates (24,25,154,155). Cases of nodular sclerosis were classified as grade I or II. For grade II, more than 25% of the cellular nodules were required to contain areas of pleomorphic lymphocyte depletion or numerous bizarre and anaplastic-appearing lacunar cells without lymphocyte depletion, or 80% or more of the cellular nodules had to have a fibrohistiocytic variant of lymphocytic depletion (24) (Fig. 17.26); grade I included all other types of nodular sclerosis, comprising approximately 73% to 83% of cases. These studies concluded that nodular sclerosis with extensive areas of lymphocytic depletion or pleomorphic lacunar cells is associated with a statistically significant poor response to initial therapy, an increased relapse rate, and a decreased survival rate compared with other forms of nodular sclerosis (24,25,154, 155). A recent German Hodgkin Study Group report of the grading of nodular sclerosis found no differences in clinical outcome between grades I and II nodular sclerosis among patients with early and intermediate stages of Hodgkin's disease (156). In advanced stage, however, with multivariate analysis significant differences were found in rates of treatment failure between the histologic grades. Most American

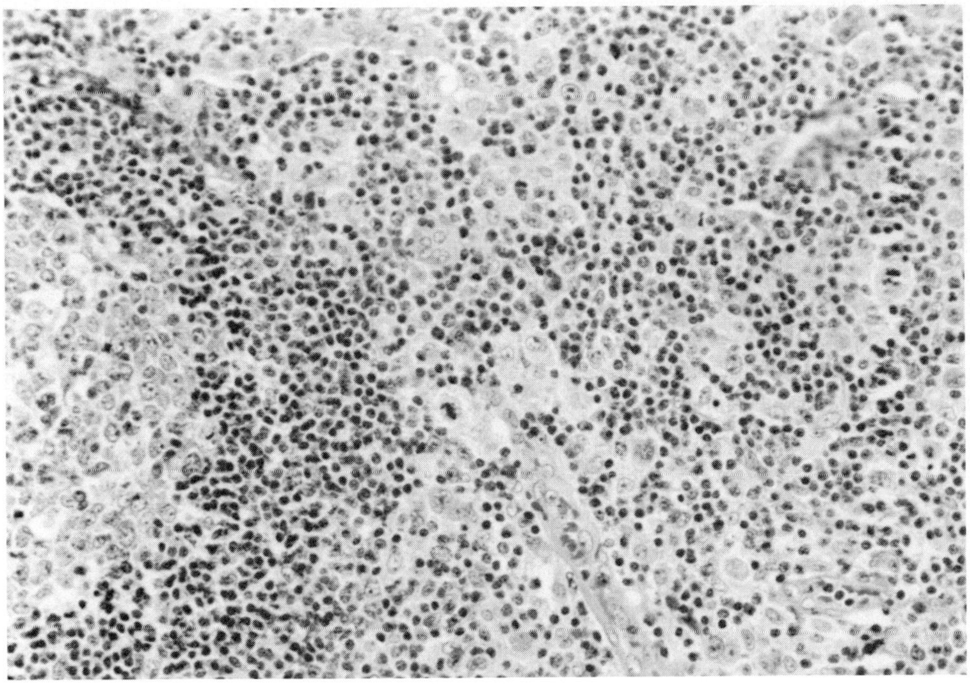

FIG. 17.25. Adjacent to a germinal center with its surrounding mantle zone on the left, the interfollicular region is expanded because of focal involvement by Hodgkin's disease (hematoxylin and eosin stain, original magnification: 240× magnification).

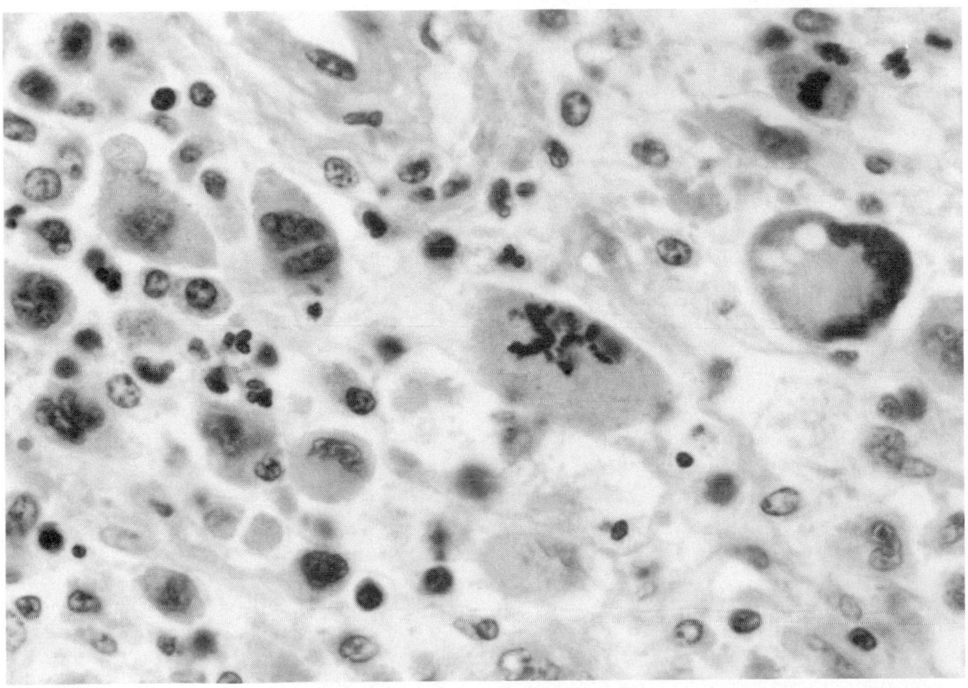

FIG. 17.26. Cases of nodular sclerosis may have areas of lymphocytic depletion containing bizarre and pleomorphic lacunar cells. In some studies, these cases have been associated with a worse prognosis (hematoxylin and eosin stain, original magnification: 720× magnification).

studies conclude that grading of either advanced or limited stage nodular sclerosis, including uniformly staged and treated patients, has no predictive clinical value (157–159). Because there are data indicating that the presence of follicular dendritic cells has positive prognostic relevance in Hodgkin's disease, one study found that combining the follicular dendritic cell status with nodular sclerosis grades defined the best survival group (160,161); patients with many well-delineated follicle-like structures as determined by immunohistochemistry and grade I nodular sclerosis morphology had the best survival rate. Despite the controversy and the complex variability in results on the grading of nodular sclerosis, pathologists should continue to grade nodular sclerosis, or at least acknowledge the more pleomorphic grade II type if present, so that additional data can be accumulated and clinicians can have the grading results to possibly employ as another parameter in guiding treatment. The grading scheme for nodular sclerosis has been adopted by the WHO classification (22).

Cases of nodular sclerosis that are composed predominantly of clusters and sheets of pleomorphic lacunar cells and mononuclear Reed-Sternberg cells also have been termed the *syncytial variant* (89,162,163) (Fig. 17.27). The atypical-appearing lacunar cells and mononuclear Reed-Sternberg cells often concentrate around areas of necrosis; because they form cohesive aggregates with only a few lymphocytes, such cases frequently are misdiagnosed as large cell lymphoma, metastatic carcinoma, seminoma, or melanoma (32,163). The syncytial variant of nodular sclerosis is diagnosed by recognizing the lacunar-like spaces associated with the proliferating cells, the discovery of more typical areas of nodular sclerosis in other parts of the biopsy specimen, and the employment of immunologic studies to verify the Reed-Sternberg nature of the large cells and exclude other malignancies.

The pattern of classic nodular sclerosis with broad, birefringent collagen bands outlining lymphoid nodules may be mimicked by a number of disorders. Similar patterns are

A

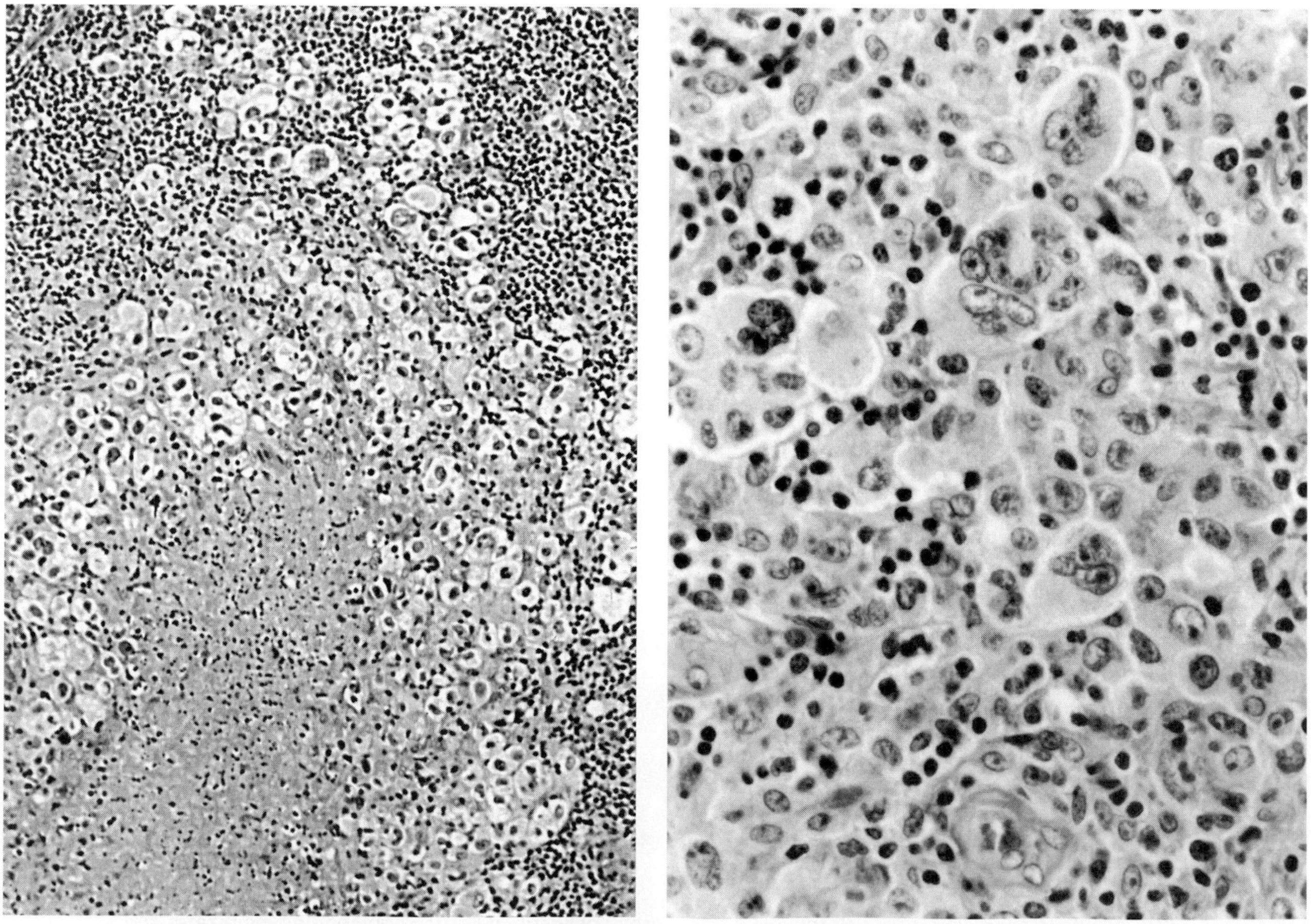

B

FIG. 17.27. A: Clusters of lacunar cells concentrate around a zone of necrosis in the "syncytial variant" of nodular sclerosis (hematoxylin and eosin stain, original magnification: 150× magnification). **B:** The syncytial variant is characterized by sheets or clusters of lacunar cells and mononuclear Reed-Sternberg–type cells. These cases often are misdiagnosed as large cell lymphoma, metastatic carcinoma, or malignant melanoma (hematoxylin and eosin stain, original magnification: 480× magnification).

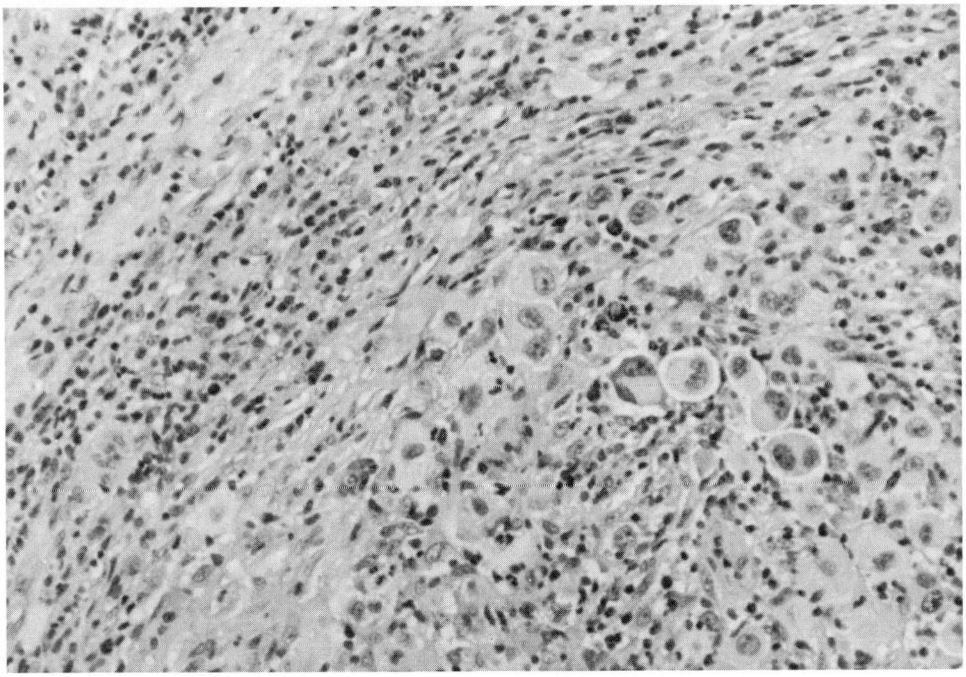

FIG. 17.28. This retroperitoneal mass contains both fibrous connective tissue bands and nodules with many giant cells similar to Reed-Sternberg cells. Unlike in Hodgkin's disease, the giant cells did not express any Hodgkin's disease–associated antigens or any hematopoietic antigens; however, they did express vimentin and muscle-specific actin, indicating that the mass is likely an epithelioid leiomyosarcoma (hematoxylin and eosin stain, original magnification: 240× magnification).

observed in some cases of reactive lymphadenitis, carcinomatous metastases, sarcomas, and large cell lymphomas with sclerosis. Reactive lymphadenitis with an infectious etiology frequently leads to thickening of the fibrous capsule and intranodal fibrosis. Although occasionally double-nucleated immunoblasts may resemble Reed-Sternberg cells, lacunar cells and true Reed-Sternberg cells are absent in these reactive lesions. Metastases, such as metastatic lymphoepithelial carcinoma of nasopharyngeal origin, may evoke a desmoplastic response and form islands in lymphoid tissue; however, the metastatic lesions are distinguished from nodular sclerosis, including the syncytial variant, through identification of cohesive aggregates of malignant epithelial cells and the use of immunohistochemical stains employing a panel of antibodies directed against cytokeratin, CD45, CD15, and CD30 (163–165). Occasionally, the giant and atypical cells in various sarcomas and mesenchymal tumors, notably those with inflammatory and lymphocytic infiltrates, may resemble Reed-Sternberg cells and be confused with Hodgkin's disease (166–168) (Fig. 17.28). Complicating matters, a storiform pattern may be present in the fibroblastic variant of nodular sclerosis (86). A sarcoma is distinguished from Hodgkin's disease by the absence of true lacunar cells in the sarcoma, coupled with the use of appropriate immunohistochemical or molecular studies.

Lacunar- and Reed-Sternberg–like cells cause special difficulty in distinguishing nodular sclerosis from large cell lymphoma with sclerosis in the mediastinum; this difficulty is compounded in small needle biopsy specimens. In mediastinal large B-cell lymphomas, the large cells often have clear cytoplasm and simulate lacunar cells, and they also may exhibit considerable nuclear pleomorphism and resemble classic Reed-Sternberg cells (169–171). Despite this difficulty, in large cell lymphoma the sclerosis tends to compartmentalize small groups of lymphoma cells rather than produce true lymphoid islands (169). Immunologic studies almost always substantiate the non-Hodgkin's nature of mediastinal large cell lymphomas by demonstrating a B-cell lineage, but with needle biopsy specimens appropriate caution is required in the interpretation of immunophenotypic studies because, like nodular sclerosis, mediastinal large B-cell lymphomas often express CD30 (172) (Chapter 25).

Occasionally, patients have composite lymphomas in which Hodgkin's disease (including nodular sclerosis) and non-Hodgkin's lymphoma coexist in the same anatomic site (173,174). The most common combination is nodular sclerosis and large cell lymphoma, most frequently with a diffuse pattern. Unlike cases in which Reed-Sternberg–like or true Reed-Sternberg cells are admixed intimately with non-Hodgkin's lymphoma, in true composite lymphoma with both Hodgkin's disease and a non-Hodgkin's lymphoma there generally is some demarcation between the different histologic types (134–138,141,173,174). In some respects, the pattern is analogous to that seen in the cases of lymphocyte predominance Hodgkin's disease associated with large cell lymphoma (118–125); however, in composite lymphomas in which the Hodgkin's disease component has a nodular sclerosis or mixed cellularity appearance, the Reed-Sternberg cells are $CD15^+$ and $CD30^+$ but $CD45^-$, reflecting an immunophenotype that is typical of nonlymphocyte predominance (174). This is in contrast to the non-Hodgkin's lymphoma component, which invariably has a B-cell phenotype. In addition to composite lymphoma, Hodgkin's disease, most frequently nodular sclerosis, may develop in patients with known non-Hodgkin's lymphomas of B-cell lineage (175,176). Patients with non-Hodgkin's lymphomas are at an almost threefold risk of developing subsequent Hodgkin's disease (175).

Mixed Cellularity

The mixed cellularity type of Hodgkin's disease follows the nodular sclerosis type in frequency (86,130). It is slightly more common in males and often is associated with systemic symptoms. Mixed cellularity occurs in all clinical stages and traditionally has a prognosis intermediate between those of the lymphocyte predominance and lymphocytic depletion types (13,16,86).

Histologically, mixed cellularity Hodgkin's disease also occupies an intermediate position between the lymphocyte predominance and lymphocytic depletion groups (16,17,30). The mixed cellularity type is a repository for cases that do not fit into the other types in the original Lukes and Butler classification (16,17,30,89). It usually is characterized by a heterogeneous cell population composed of variable numbers of small lymphocytes with either no or minimal nuclear membrane irregularities, plasma cells, neutrophils, and eosinophils (Fig. 17.29); the degree of tissue eosinophilia may be related to the immunophenotype of the T lymphocytes present in the affected lymph nodes (177). In mixed cellularity, there generally is also a variable number of reactive histiocytes, which often form small clusters (Fig. 17.30), and an inconsistent degree of disorderly fibrosis without collagen formation. Necrosis also may be present, but this is usually not overly conspicuous. Reed-Sternberg cells usually can be detected easily (16,17). The nodal architecture often is effaced completely in mixed cellularity Hodgkin's disease, but focal or interfollicular involvement is observed occasionally (16,17,30,89,147,148).

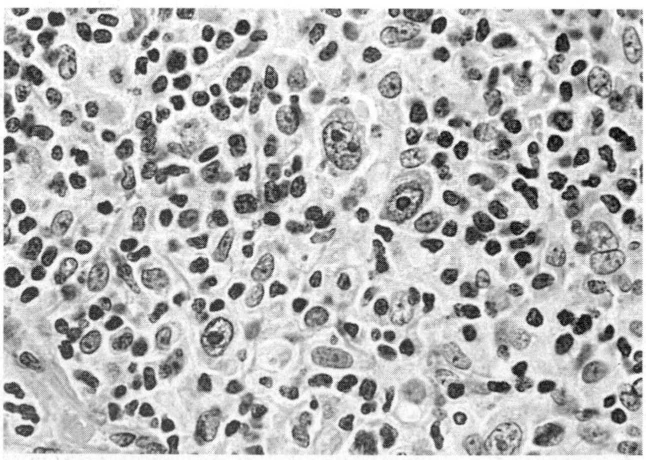

FIG. 17.29. Mixed cellularity Hodgkin's disease typically is composed of a polymorphous cell population with small lymphocytes, plasma cells, eosinophils, neutrophils, histiocytes, and diagnostic Reed-Sternberg cells (hematoxylin and eosin stain, original magnification: 600× magnification).

Because mixed cellularity occupies a central position in the spectrum from lymphocyte predominance to lymphocytic depletion, there is considerable overlap (30,86). For example, cases that otherwise fulfill the criteria for lymphocyte predominance but in which classic diagnostic Reed-Sternberg cells can be identified with minimal search are classified as the lymphocyte-rich classic or mixed cellularity type. Also, cases containing numerous variants of Reed-Sternberg cells but few absolutely diagnostic Reed-Sternberg cells with characteristic large nucleoli are not included in the reticular form of lymphocytic depletion but qualify for the mixed cellularity group (30). The mixed cellularity group also comprises cases with lacunar cells in which there is an absence of sclerosis (86,89).

The differential diagnosis of mixed cellularity Hodgkin's disease is broad and includes viruses, angioimmunoblastic lymphadenopathy (AILD), and non-Hodgkin's lymphomas, specifically the peripheral T-cell lymphomas of the mixed medium and large cell type, including those with epithelioid histiocytes (lymphoepithelioid cell or Lennert's lymphoma). Virus-induced lymphadenopathies frequently lead to a proliferation of immunoblasts, and the binucleated forms may resemble Reed-Sternberg cells, such as in infectious mononucleosis (36,37) (Fig. 17.31). These lesions are distinguished from Hodgkin's disease by the recognition of immunoblasts with their characteristic strongly amphophilic and pyroninophilic cytoplasm; the immunoblasts almost always display a mottled pattern if seen on low-power microscopy. AILD also contains immunoblasts but lacks a mottled pattern. In AILD, there is marked arborizing vascularity, deposition of periodic acid–Schiff stain–positive interstitial material, and a clinical history that differs from Hodgkin's disease (178,179). Unlike mixed cellularity Hodgkin's disease, most cases of AILD are a form of T-cell lymphoma, which can be verified by immunologic, cytogenetic, and molecular genetic studies (180–184) (Chapter 16).

Other types of peripheral T-cell lymphomas, such as those with a mixed cellular composition including cases of Lennert's lymphoma, also may be difficult to distinguish objectively from mixed cellularity Hodgkin's disease (38,39,185–188). In Lennert's lymphoma, for example, the architectural characteristics and cellular composition often are identical to the mixed cellularity type, with many epithelioid histiocytes, but in contrast to the small, generally round lymphocytes found in Hodgkin's disease, the lymphocytes in Lennert's lymphoma are atypical, with nuclear membrane irregularities (Fig. 17.32). Other features that distinguish lymphomas of peripheral T-cell origin from Hodgkin's dis-

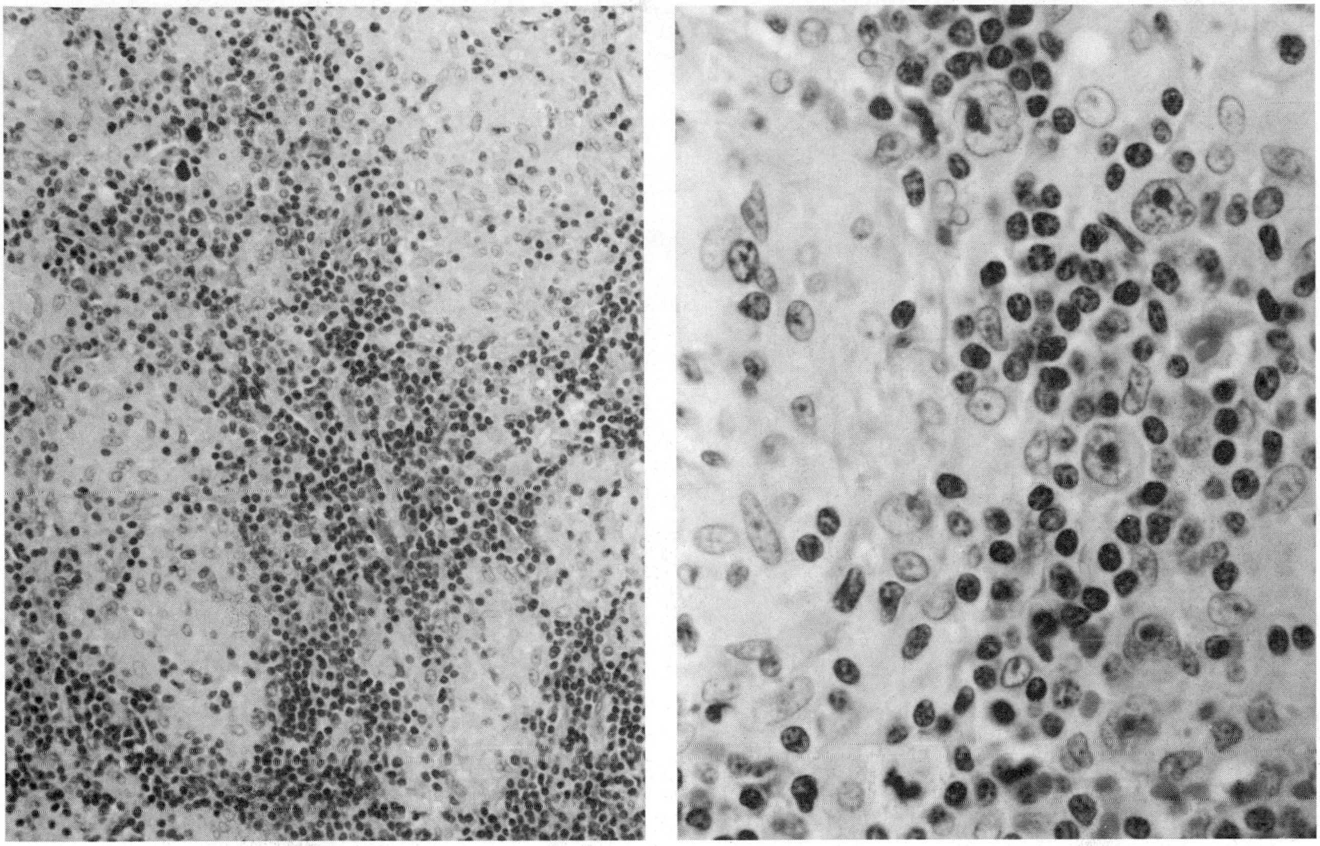

FIG. 17.30. **A:** Some cases of mixed cellularity Hodgkin's disease contain numerous clusters of epithelioid histiocytes and have a pattern indistinguishable from a non-Hodgkin's lymphoma of Lennert's type (hematoxylin and eosin stain, original magnification: 240× magnification). **B:** Unlike Lennert's lymphoma, mixed cellularity Hodgkin's disease has readily identifiable Reed-Sternberg cells and variants. Note that the small lymphocytes are not atypical (hematoxylin and eosin stain, original magnification: 720× magnification).

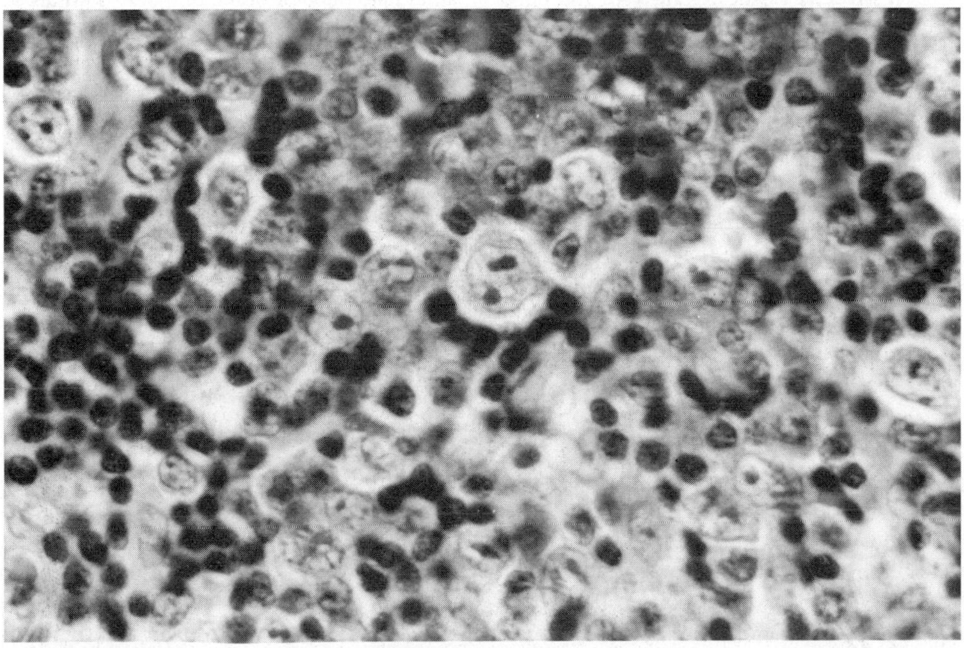

FIG. 17.31. A binucleated immunoblast in infectious mononucleosis resembles a Reed-Sternberg cell. A mottled pattern and recognition of the proliferating cells as immunoblasts help to differentiate virus-induced lymphadenopathies from Hodgkin's disease (hematoxylin and eosin stain, original magnification: 720× magnification).

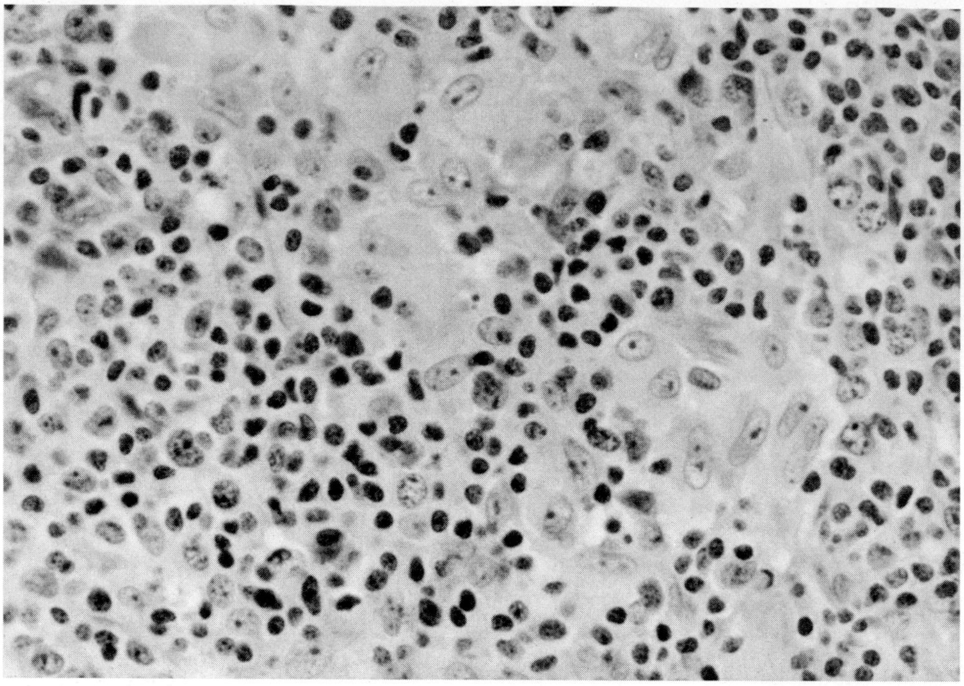

FIG. 17.32. The small lymphocytes in this non-Hodgkin's lymphoma with epithelioid histiocytes (Lennert's lymphoma) have irregular nuclear contours. Compare with Figure 17.30. These small lymphocytes are T cells, but unlike in most cases of Lennert's lymphoma, the large cells expressed B cell lineage–associated antigens. The case was interpreted as an example of a T cell– or histiocyte-rich B-cell lymphoma (hematoxylin and eosin stain, original magnification: 480× magnification).

ease are capsular invasion and a lack of sufficient numbers of diagnostic Reed-Sternberg cells (185–188). Peripheral T-cell lymphomas also show significantly higher rates of proliferative activity, as demonstrated by higher rates of mitotis and a higher proportion of cells in the S phase of the cell cycle (189,190). In many cases the histologic differences are subtle, and differentiation of mixed cellularity Hodgkin's disease from a non-Hodgkin's lymphoma of T-cell type or even a T cell– or histiocyte-rich B-cell lymphoma may not be possible or objectively reliable (38–41,191). Immunohistologic studies are almost mandatory for diagnostic verification, with the qualification that a panel of antibodies must be employed because of the observation that the CD15 antigen often is expressed in the pleomorphic large cells, including the Reed-Sternberg–like cells, of peripheral T-cell lymphomas, as well as in the diagnostic Reed-Sternberg cells of Hodgkin's disease (43,47,48,192–195) (Chapter 29).

Lymphocytic Depletion

Lymphocytic depletion is the least common form of Hodgkin's disease, found in approximately 1% of cases (86,130). It is the Hodgkin's disease type causing the most contention, which is reflected by the various proposals in the WHO classification as to whether lymphocytic depletion should be a category of anaplastic large cell lymphoma (21,22). Lymphocytic depletion is retained in the latest WHO classification proposal and includes cases that formerly were considered Hodgkin's-like anaplastic large cell lymphoma but that currently are reinterpreted as anaplastic large cell lymphoma-like Hodgkin's disease (20,22,23,28, 196). The latter is an aggressive form of Hodgkin's disease that also may embrace cases of nodular sclerosis, of grade II or the syncytial variant, and cases of lymphocytic depletion.

Lymphocytic depletion traditionally comprises the diffuse fibrosis and reticular types of Lukes and Butler (16,17). The diffuse fibrosis type is characterized by a disordered proliferation of nonbirefringent connective tissue of noncollagenous type (Fig. 17.33). The fibrous connective tissue often is fibrillar, loosely cellular, and random in distribution (16,17). It occasionally has a fibroblastic appearance or resembles amorphous proteinaceous material. In addition to the connective tissue, this type of Hodgkin's disease overall is depleted of cells, particularly of lymphocytes, but rare cellular areas may be observed, with increased numbers of Reed-Sternberg cells. The reticular type of lymphocytic depletion is characterized by two essential patterns. One pattern may resemble mixed cellularity Hodgkin's disease, but with a predominance of Reed-Sternberg cells. In the other pattern, there also are increased numbers of Reed-Sternberg cells, but these appear pleomorphic and almost sarcomatous (16,17) (Fig. 17.34). The presence of Reed-Sternberg cells in almost every high-power microscopic field is the main characteristic of the reticular type of lymphocytic depletion (30). In some biopsy specimens, areas with diffuse fibrosis and reticular patterns may coexist (17).

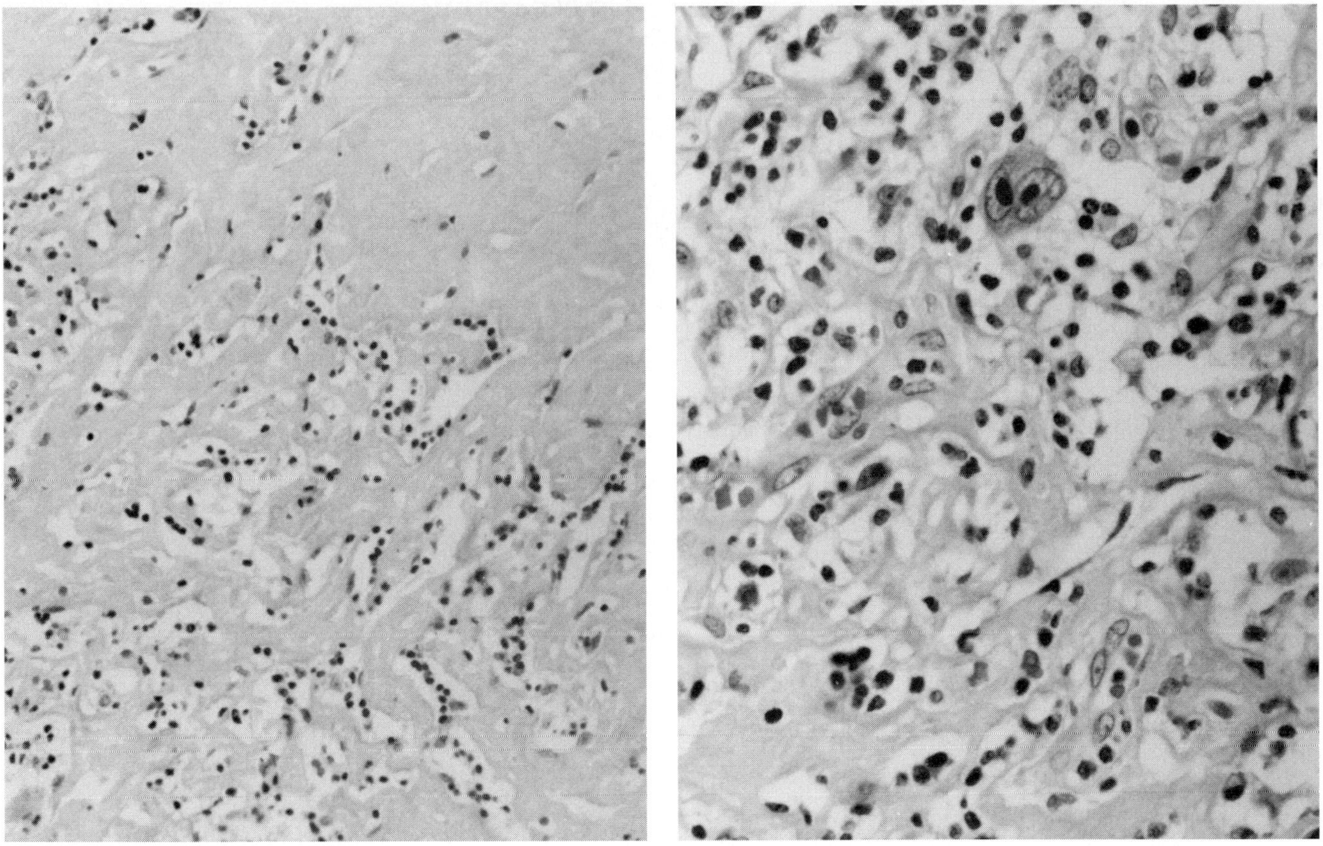

A B

FIG. 17.33. A: The diffuse fibrosis type of lymphocytic depletion typically has broad areas of amorphous nonbirefringent connective tissue of noncollagenous type (hematoxylin and eosin stain, original magnification: 240× magnification). **B:** In addition to a paucity of lymphocytes, Reed-Sternberg cells also may be few (hematoxylin and eosin stain, original magnification: 480× magnification).

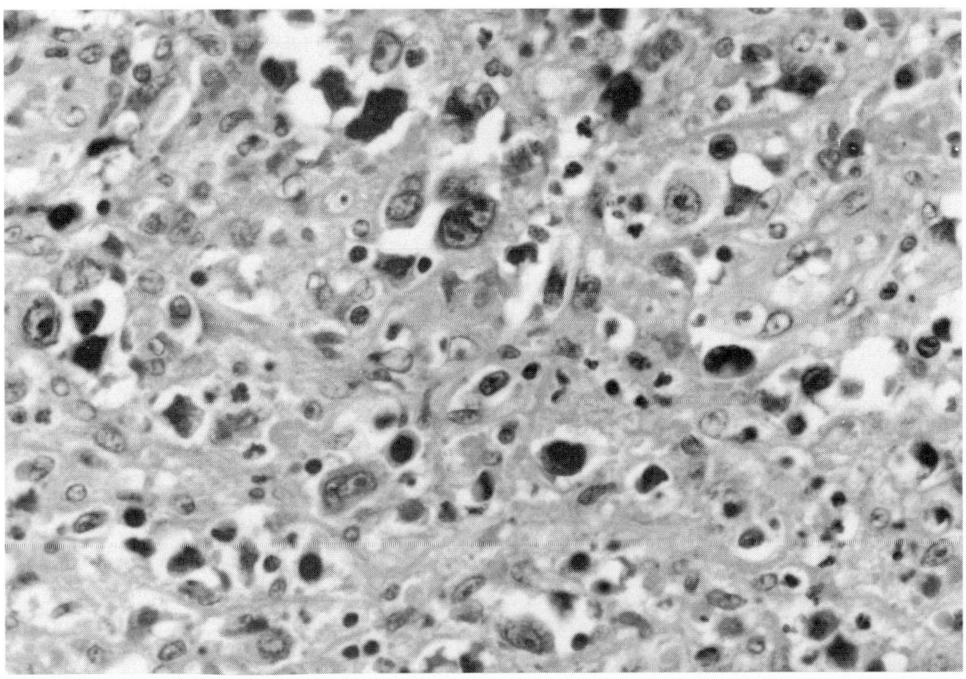

FIG. 17.34. In the reticular type of lymphocytic depletion, pleomorphic Reed-Sternberg cells are evident in virtually every high-power microscopic field (hematoxylin and eosin stain, original magnification: 480× magnification).

Lymphocytic depletion generally occurs in elderly patients with constitutional symptoms and stage III or IV disease at the time of diagnosis (13,64). Historically, the lymphocytic depletion type of Hodgkin's disease has been the most aggressive, with the shortest median length of survival (13,17,33,152,153). In one study, lymphocytic depletion appeared to define a syndrome in which the patients were older (median age, 51 years) and presented with fevers, wasting, and hepatic dysfunction (64); peripheral lymphadenopathy was uncommon, but there was extensive subdiaphragmatic disease, with involvement of liver, spleen, retroperitoneal lymph nodes and bone marrow. It has been suggested, however, that peripheral lymph node enlargement is common in lymphocytic depletion and that most patients adhere to the characteristic clinical presentation of Hodgkin's disease, albeit with more aggressive clinical features (197). Yet another series, describing 25 patients with lymphocytic depletion Hodgkin's disease, concluded that some patients conform to the syndrome described, including constitutional symptoms, subdiaphragmatic disease, frequent marrow involvement, and advanced-stage disease, but others had clinical symptoms paralleling those found in other patients with Hodgkin's disease, including the mixed cellularity type (198). In this latter study, the median survival was longer in the diffuse fibrosis subtype (39 months) than in the reticular subtype (10 months). There is a general consensus that most patients with lymphocytic depletion can be treated with systemic chemotherapy, similar to patients with other histologic types of Hodgkin's disease (8,13,197,198).

The differential diagnosis of lymphocytic depletion Hodgkin's disease includes, in addition to anaplastic large cell lymphoma, other forms of Hodgkin's disease, particularly nodular sclerosis grade II together with the syncytial variant, and the mixed cellularity type with increased numbers of mononuclear cells rather than true diagnostic Reed-Sternberg cells (26–30,42,163). In fact, most historical cases of the lymphocytic-depletion type of Hodgkin's disease do not represent that entity. In one histologic review of 39 cases considered originally to reflect lymphocytic depletion, only nine (23%) were regarded as morphologically acceptable for that entity (199); the remaining cases were examples of nodular sclerosis with lymphocytic depletion (grade II) and probably included the syncytial variant, other forms of Hodgkin's disease, and non-Hodgkin's large cell lymphomas (Table 17.6). Other studies combining both morphologic and immunologic assessment confirmed that a variety of large cell malignant neoplasms, including metastatic carcinomas as well as other varieties of Hodgkin's disease and non-Hodgkin's lymphomas, may be confused with lymphocytic depletion (89,200).

Anaplastic large cell lymphomas are the most difficult cases to differentiate from lymphocytic depletion Hodgkin's disease, because there appears to be a continuous spectrum between these disorders with clinical, morphologic, and immunologic overlap (Fig. 17.35). Cases of anaplastic large cell lymphoma tend to have sinusoidal and perivascular patterns of infiltration with sheets of pleomorphic, cohesive large cells associated with active mitotic figures (28,196). The large cells of anaplastic large cell lymphoma characteristically have eccentric, frequently kidney-shaped nuclei with small nucleoli, which are less conspicuous than in classic Reed-Sternberg cells (28). The paranuclear region tends to be eosinophilic. This morphologic appearance, however, is inconsistent, and there may be morphologic ambiguity, with cells indistinguishable from Reed-Sternberg cells, together with an inflammatory background, fibrous bands, and a thickened capsule (20,23,26,28,29,196,201,202). An immunohistochemical panel is paramount in attempting to resolve such cryptic cases, and although generally successful, a panel may not always settle the ambiguity. For example, cases of lymphocytic depletion tend to be $CD15^+$, $CD45^-$, and T cell– and epithelial membrane antigen–negative; the

TABLE 17.6. *Morphologic review of 39 patients originally classified as lymphocytic depletion*

Diagnosis	Number of patients
Hodgkin's disease	29
Lymphocytic depletion	9 (23%)
Nodular sclerosis with lymphocytic depletion (grade II)	13
Nodular sclerosis	3
Mixed cellularity	1
Composite	1
Unclassified	2
Non-Hodgkin's lymphoma large-cell	10
Immunoblastic	8
Noncleaved	2

From Kant JA, Hubbard SM, Longo DL, et al. The pathologic and clinical heterogeneity of lymphocyte-depleted Hodgkin's disease. *J Clin Oncol* 1986;4:284–294, with permission.

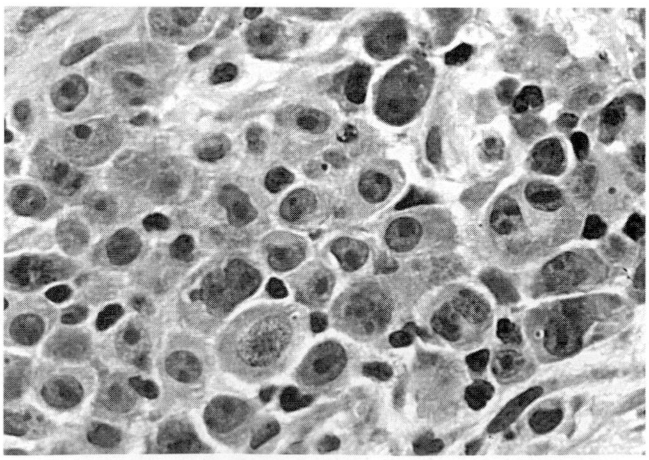

FIG. 17.35. Pleomorphic large cells, including some Reed-Sternberg–like cells, infiltrate a peripheral lymph node sinus in anaplastic large cell lymphoma. This type of non-Hodgkin's lymphoma is difficult to distinguish from Hodgkin's disease, including the lymphocytic depletion type, because of both morphologic and immunologic overlap (hematoxylin and eosin stain, original magnification: 900× magnification).

opposite usually is found in anaplastic large cell lymphoma (42,46,48,201,202). Nonetheless, CD15 expression is lacking in approximately 15% of patients with classic Hodgkin's disease, and the other markers also are mutable with a range of reactivities (49,201,202). Fascin is a sensitive marker for classic Hodgkin's disease, but fascin also may be expressed in anaplastic large cell lymphoma (45,203). The follicular dendritic cell marker CD21 is reactive in the Reed-Sternberg cells of a small number of patients with classic Hodgkin's disease, including the lymphocytic depletion type (204); however, there are too few positive cases to regard CD21 as a valid discriminator. Tumor expression of the translocation t(2;5) or anaplastic large cell lymphoma kinase supports anaplastic large cell lymphoma, but most cases with features of anaplastic large cell lymphoma and Hodgkin's disease are anaplastic large cell lymphoma kinase–negative (26,27). Thus, despite evaluation of the growth pattern, cytology, immunophenotype, and molecular genetics, there are a persistent small number of borderline, unclassifiable, or ''gray zone'' cases that are not strictly either anaplastic large cell lymphoma or classic Hodgkin's disease, particularly the lymphocytic depletion type (196,202,205); these cases remain unresolvable. Fortunately, patients who have these unusual lymphomas respond to chemotherapy for high-grade non-Hodgkin's lymphomas and to conventional Hodgkin's disease treatment (206) (Chapters 18, 25).

PATHOLOGY OF STAGING

Laparotomy for the pathologic staging of Hodgkin's disease has become rare and occurs today only in special circumstances, if it is felt that pathologic staging will alter therapy (74,76). The era of staging laparotomies for Hodgkin's disease provided considerable knowledge concerning the patterns of spread and the pathologic nuances of Hodgkin's disease in various abdominal sites. The criteria for involvement of spleen, abdominal lymph nodes, liver, and bone marrow essentially remain those proposed at the Ann Arbor conference of 1971 (145). Splenic involvement of Hodgkin's disease is discovered in 39% of patients at staging laparotomy, but the weight of the spleen has no bearing on predicting involvement (144). Typically, there are multiple, single or coalescent, white, discrete nodules scattered throughout the spleen in a miliary-type distribution (207) (Fig. 17.36) (Chapter 53). Because of the demonstration that five or more splenic nodules of Hodgkin's disease are associated with a relatively unfavorable prognosis, the number of macroscopic nodules in the spleen should be recorded (208). Many spleens removed at laparotomy, however, manifest tumor involvement by only a solitary nodule measuring from 1 to 3 mm in diameter (144). Unless the spleen is sectioned meticulously and examined at 2- to 3-mm intervals, these isolated small nodules may be overlooked (31,207). Solitary splenic nodules often are limited to the T zones of the spleen in the periarteriolar lymphoid sheaths or marginal zones

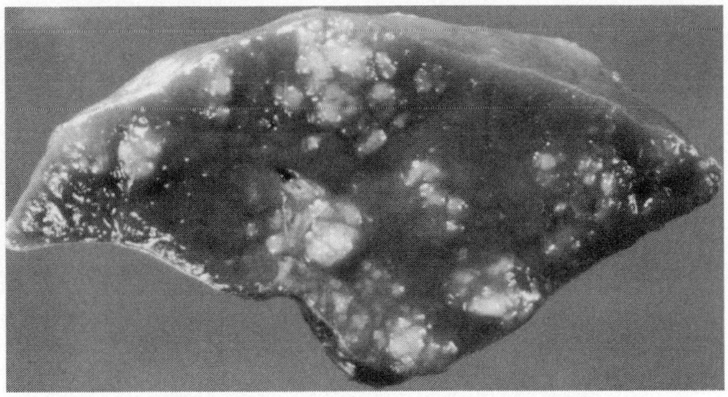

FIG. 17.36. Multiple, random, pale tumor nodules are characteristic of Hodgkin's disease in the spleen.

(Fig. 17.37). The cytologic criteria for the diagnosis of Hodgkin's disease in the spleen are identical to those employed in lymph nodes. All histologic types of disease may be found in the spleen and may be so designated (30,108,109); however, in many cases the distinction between nodular sclerosis and mixed cellularity Hodgkin's disease is not possible. Classification is not mandatory, because the type of Hodgkin's disease generally is known prior to laparotomy and is not a crucial factor in therapy (13). There may be confusion in the diagnosis of Hodgkin's disease in the spleen because of the presence of clusters of histiocytes forming epithelioid or sarcoid-like granulomas (209). Granulomas are observed in up to 9% of cases of Hodgkin's disease and may even form visible nodules on the splenic cut surface (210). The finding of granulomas in the spleen or other organs does not indicate involvement of these organs by Hodgkin's disease. Rarely, spleens contain isolated tumor-like nodules on the splenic cut surface that are not the result of Hodgkin's disease but rather an unusual, localized type of reactive lymphoid hyperplasia (211). These nodules are a result of either localized coalescence of germinal centers from contiguous segments of white pulp or a tumorous proliferation of lymphocytes, immunoblasts, plasma cells, and other inflammatory cells indicative of an inflammatory pseudotumor (212).

In most cases, abdominal lymph node involvement by Hodgkin's disease produces a histologic classification identical to an original diagnostic lymph node biopsy specimen. The diagnosis of Hodgkin's disease in paraaortic nodes is possible despite distortion induced by lymphangiography (144). Focal involvement often is found together with the lymphangiogram effect, but depending on the size of the focus, classification as to the type of Hodgkin's disease may not be possible. In many instances, the involved lymph nodes at staging laparotomy are found to be unenlarged, particularly splenic hilar lymph nodes (144). Mesenteric lymph node involvement is very uncommon in Hodgkin's disease. As in the spleen, sarcoid-like granulomas can be observed in abdominal lymph nodes.

The criteria for the diagnosis of Hodgkin's disease in liver and bone marrow biopsy specimens are identical for patients

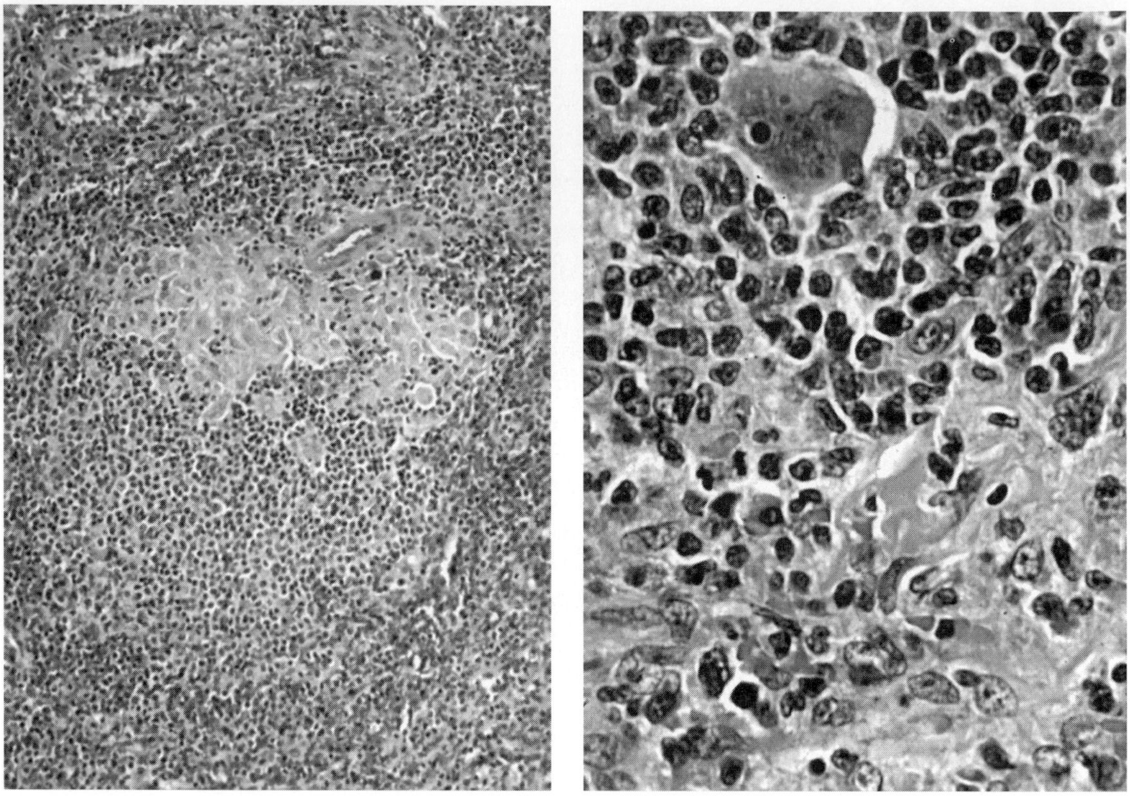

A B

FIG. 17.37. A: Hodgkin's disease in the spleen usually concentrates in the T zones, such as the periarteriolar lymphoid sheaths (hematoxylin and eosin stain, original magnification: 150× magnification). **B:** A Reed-Sternberg cell is found adjacent to epithelioid histiocytes. Epithelioid histiocytes may form sarcoid-type granulomas in the spleen but are not an indication of Hodgkin's disease unless an appropriate Reed-Sternberg cell is identified (hematoxylin and eosin stain, original magnification: 600× magnification).

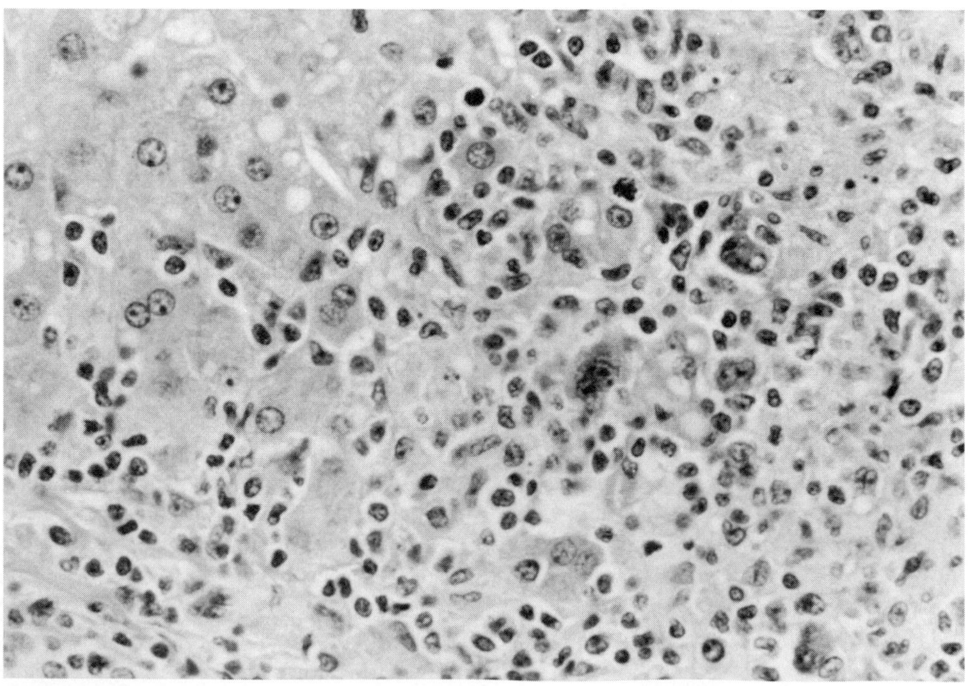

FIG. 17.38. Hodgkin's disease in the liver is manifested by infiltrates in the portal areas containing Reed-Sternberg cells and mononuclear variants. The small lymphocytes frequently appear atypical in the liver (hematoxylin and eosin stain, original magnification: 480× magnification).

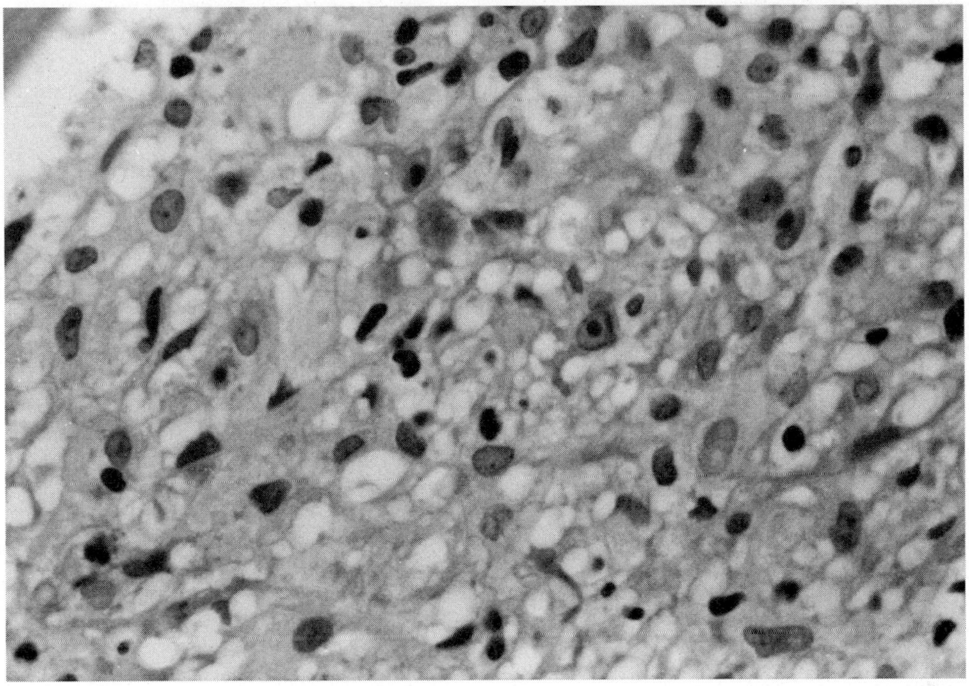

FIG. 17.39. A mononuclear variant of a Reed-Sternberg cell in an area of fibrosis is sufficient for a diagnosis of Hodgkin's disease in the bone marrow in a patient with established Hodgkin's disease (hematoxylin and eosin stain, original magnification: 720× magnification).

with biopsy-proven Hodgkin's disease (145). Because the amount of tissue available for histologic examination is relatively small, however, classic Reed-Sternberg cells may not be discovered. Multiple sections should be obtained to search for the cells; if none are found, however, proof of involvement of these sites is not as rigorous as that required for an initial diagnosis of Hodgkin's disease. A mononuclear cell with a single large nucleolus found in a cellular environment appropriate for Hodgkin's disease suffices for an absolute diagnosis. In the liver, lymphocytic infiltrates in the portal areas frequently are observed, but these have no definite relationship to Hodgkin's disease (30,213). Patients with hepatic involvement of Hodgkin's disease are much more likely to have histologic evidence of large portal infiltrates, with a predominance of atypical lymphocytes, and also may exhibit changes of acute cholangitis and portal edema (214) (Fig. 17.38). In the bone marrow, foci of fibrosis should lead to serial sectioning in the search for diagnostic Reed-Sternberg cells or the mononuclear variants (145) (Fig. 17.39). Bone marrow involvement of Hodgkin's disease is found in 3.5% to 14% of patients, with the greatest risk to patients with the mixed cellularity and lymphocytic depletion types (64,144,215–218). The uninvolved bone marrow frequently exhibits a variety of nonspecific reactions including stromal edema, hypocellularity, myeloid hyperplasia, and benign lymphoid nodules (215–217). In the bone marrow and liver, epithelioid granulomas may be prominent and are similar to those noted in the spleen. Bone marrow involvement by Hodgkin's disease does not define a special high-risk group, necessitating a different therapeutic strategy, because the prognosis of patients with Hodgkin's disease in the bone marrow is not worse than that of other advanced stage Hodgkin's disease patients (218) (Chapter 39).

EXTRANODAL HODGKIN'S DISEASE

Primary stage IE extranodal Hodgkin's disease is very rare, except in patients with AIDS (53,59) (Chapter 28). Before the AIDS epidemic, Wood and Coltman (219) estimated the incidence to be 0.025% of the overall incidence of Hodgkin's disease. In most extranodal sites, an initial diagnosis of Hodgkin's disease should be viewed with skepticism, because most cases likely represent other malignancies, particularly large cell lymphoma, including pleomorphic lymphomas with Reed-Sternberg–like cells. To unequivocally establish a diagnosis of extranodal Hodgkin's disease, the diagnostic requisites are the same as in lymph nodes, and immunologic verification should be sought (30).

The lung is perhaps the most common extralymphatic site for Hodgkin's disease apart from the liver, but even in the lung Hodgkin's disease is rare; one review found only 61 documented cases (220). Most cases of pulmonary Hodgkin's disease are of the nodular sclerosis type and are a result of contiguous spread from the mediastinum (30) (Fig. 17.40). The criteria for the diagnosis of primary pulmonary Hodgkin's disease are restriction of the disease to the lung with minimal or no hilar lymph node involvement, exclusion of disease at distant sites, and documentation of the typical

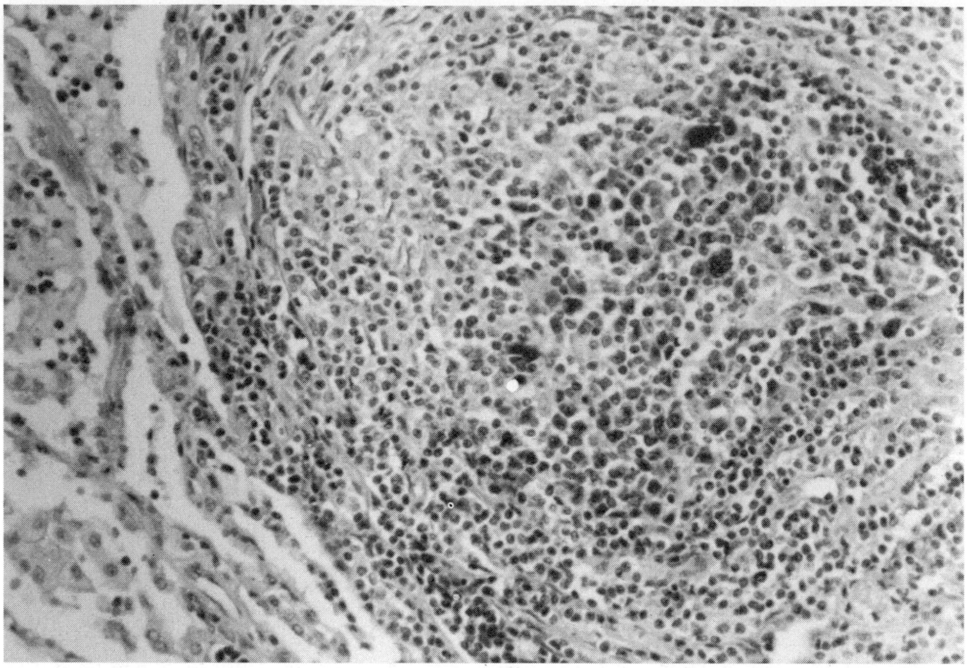

FIG. 17.40. Hodgkin's disease in the lung usually is of the nodular sclerosis type and often is a consequence of contiguous spread from the mediastinum (hematoxylin and eosin stain, original magnification: 240× magnification).

histologic features of Hodgkin's disease (221,222). Hodgkin's disease of the lung occurs more frequently in women and radiologically appears as a solitary nodule or multinodular disease, frequently with cavitation (220,221). Nodular sclerosis predominates in the lung, and all cases must be differentiated from Wegener's granulomatosis and non-Hodgkin's lymphomas, specifically the mixed medium and large cell peripheral T cell type (222).

Primary extranodal Hodgkin's disease in other sites is even less common than in lung, with many descriptions limited to single anecdotal case reports and with only the contemporary cases validated by appropriate immunohistochemical studies. For example, of 2,185 patients with Hodgkin's disease evaluated at Stanford University, none had intracranial disease at presentation, and only 12 patients (0.5%) later developed documented intracranial disease (223). Most patients with central nervous system Hodgkin's disease present with cranial nerve palsy, motor deficits, headache, and seizures, with predominant involvement of brain cortex and meninges. The nodular sclerosis type predominates in these cases, and similar histology has been reported in the rare cases of primary solitary intracranial Hodgkin's disease (224). Extradural nodular sclerosis leading to spinal cord compression also is uncommon but is a well-recognized clinical presentation of Hodgkin's disease (13,225). Patients with Hodgkin's disease in the spinal epidural space respond to radiation therapy, chemotherapy, or therapy combining modalities.

An incidence of 0.5% also has been cited for cutaneous involvement of Hodgkin's disease (226). Skin involvement in Hodgkin's disease generally manifests in the formation of small papules and nodules, as a result of retrograde lymphatic spread of regionally involved lymph nodes. The majority of patients with cutaneous Hodgkin's disease have a rapid clinical course, and skin involvement is regarded as a symptom of stage IV disease (226). Bona fide cases of primary cutaneous Hodgkin's disease are exceedingly rare. The most convincing reports describe patients presenting with disease in the skin, with later development of node-based Hodgkin's disease, usually mixed cellularity type (227,228). In fact, most case reports of primary cutaneous Hodgkin's disease likely represent cases of lymphomatoid papulosis (Fig. 17.41) or anaplastic large cell lymphoma with Reed-Sternberg–like cells (226–228); both lymphomatoid papulosis and cutaneous anaplastic large cell lymphoma ($CD30^+$ cutaneous large T-cell lymphoma) are thought to fall on a clinical and morphologic continuum of closely related skin lesions (229–231). Although immunophenotypic studies aid in differentiating cutaneous Hodgkin's disease from lymphomatoid papulosis and anaplastic large cell lymphoma (the latter lesions are usually $CD15^-$, $CD45^+$, T cell–positive, and EBV-negative), there may be immunophenotypic overlap with Hodgkin's disease (227,228). Under this circumstance, the clinical history is paramount. A history of periodic recurrence and regression of crops of skin lesions at different stages of development without evidence of other disease should signal that the disorder is likely lymphomatoid papulosis, even in the setting of an immunophenotype of Hodgkin's disease (226,228–231) (Chapter 32). Breast involvement of Hodgkin's disease also is uncommon. In a series from the M.D . Anderson Hospital and Tumor Institute, only six cases of Hodgkin's disease of the breast were

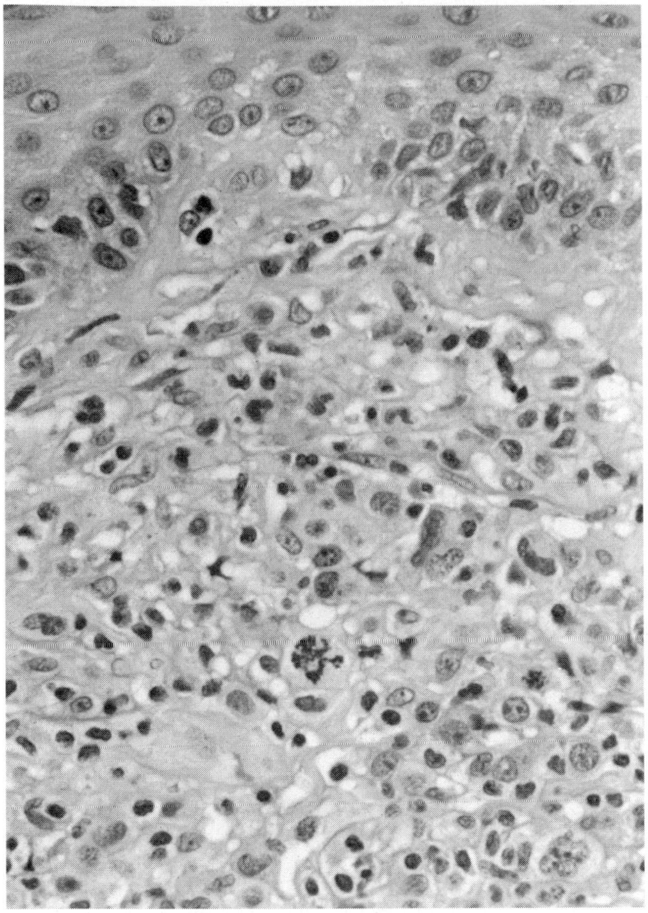

FIG. 17.41. Although this cutaneous lesion contains a polymorphous dermal infiltrate including Reed-Sternberg–like cells, clinical and immunophenotypic studies indicated that the lesion was most likely lymphomatoid papulosis. Primary cutaneous Hodgkin's disease is exceedingly rare (hematoxylin and eosin stain, original magnification: 480× magnification).

encountered over a 22-year period (232). All six were of the nodular sclerosis type. No case was considered to be primary in the breast; all were considered likely to have resulted from Hodgkin's disease in the intramammary or internal mammary lymph nodes or direct mediastinal extension into the chest wall and breast (232).

Historically, the gastrointestinal tract has been considered the most frequent extranodal site of Hodgkin's disease (219). Most of the earlier described cases of primary gastrointestinal Hodgkin's disease, however, likely were non-Hodgkin's lymphomas of the large cell or immunoblastic type (233). A morphologic diagnosis of gastrointestinal Hodgkin's disease requires immunologic confirmation (234) (Fig. 17.42). Most cases of intestinal Hodgkin's disease arise in a setting of inflammatory bowel or diverticular disease, have the characteristic immunophenotype of Hodgkin's disease, and are EBV-positive; such cases may be analogous to lymphomas arising in immunodeficent states (235–237). Waldeyer's ring is another uncommon site for Hodgkin's disease (13). Moreover, many cases purported to be Hodgkin's disease in

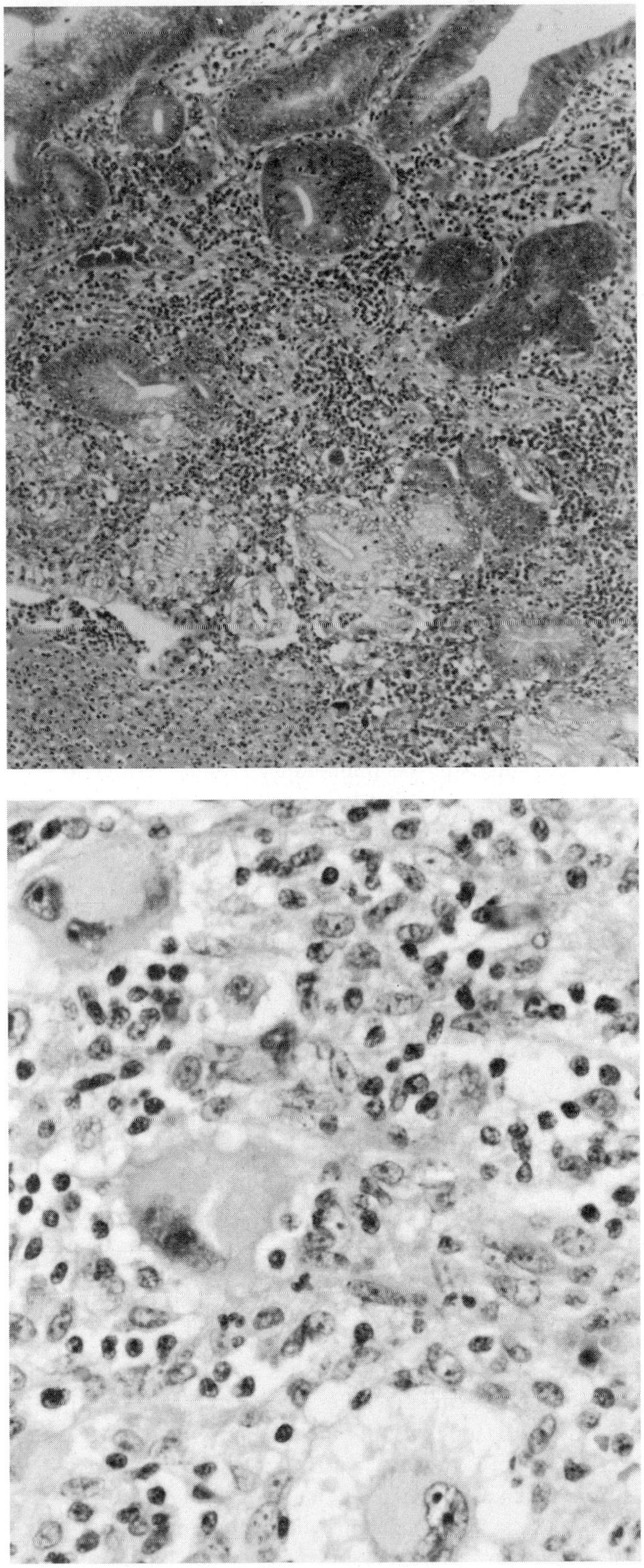

A

B

FIG. 17.42. **A:** A rare case of Hodgkin's disease in the stomach forms a large mass with a polymorphous infiltrate (hematoxylin and eosin stain, original magnification: 120× magnification). **B:** Detail of the infiltrate in the stomach wall including lacunar Reed-Sternberg cells. Gastrointestinal Hodgkin's disease requires immunologic verification (hematoxylin and eosin stain, original magnification: 480× magnification).

Waldeyer's ring likely represent non-Hodgkin's lymphomas of the Lennert type (185,238). There is one recent report of 16 cases of Waldeyer's ring Hodgkin's disease of predominantly mixed cellularity and nodular sclerosis types (239); immunohistochemical studies verified the diagnoses. EBV was detected in Reed-Sternberg cells in 67% of the cases studied; this high incidence was felt to reflect the fact that Waldeyer's ring is a reservoir for EBV (239). Most patients had stage I or II disease, and patients tended to respond to radiation or chemotherapy.

Hodgkin's disease also may present rarely as a primary solitary or multifocal bone tumor (240,241). In a recent review from the Mayo Clinic, 25 patients with osseous Hodgkin's disease were identified over a 70-year span (241); 17 patients initially presented with bone tumors, and the remainder had recurrent Hodgkin's disease involving bone. Bone pain was the main symptom, and most lesions were in the axial and proximal appendicular skeleton. Radiologic features included osteoblastic, osteolytic, and osteosclerotic patterns. Most patients subsequently were discovered to have nonosseous, particularly nodal Hodgkin's disease (240,241). In bone, Hodgkin's disease usually infiltrates between bony trabeculae and may be associated with reactive new bone formation. Although Reed-Sternberg cells were identifed in all cases, and there was immunophenotypic verification, necrosis also was seen that led to an occasional misdiagnosis of acute osteomyelitis (241). Most patients with primary Hodgkin's disease of bone do well with modern therapy (240,241).

PATHOLOGY OF RELAPSE

Notwithstanding the phenomenal success of modern therapy for Hodgkin's disease, slightly more than 30% of patients subsequently relapse, and 5% to 13% of them have late relapse 3 to 4 years after completion of therapy (242–244). The probability of relapse increases with the stage of disease, with the presence of systemic symptoms, and with bulky mediastinal disease (242,244). Patients with nodular sclerosis are more likely to have relapses than those with other histologies. Most patients experience relapse in sites of previously irradiated disease, particularly lymph nodes, but patients with stage I and II disease often have late relapses in unirradiated nodes (243). Late relapse also may occur in extranodal sites; for example, almost half of patients with Hodgkin's disease at autopsy are shown to have extranodal involvement, particularly in the liver and lung although any extranodal site may be involved (245,246).

Autopsy studies of patients with Hodgkin's disease reflect the effects of modern therapy and provide considerable data on relapse and persistent disease. Autopsy of patients who died of Hodgkin's disease before the current era of therapy often disclosed widespread Hodgkin's disease (13,16,247). Persistent Hodgkin's disease also was found in a small group of asymptomatic long-term survivors who died from apparently unrelated causes (245,247). Patients who die after treatment for Hodgkin's disease in the modern era often have a reduction in the extent of disease, and one third of patients has no evidence of residual Hodgkin's disease (245,246); the latter patients often die of complications of therapy. In fact, adults and children who are treated for Hodgkin's disease are at increased risk of dying of causes unrelated to progressive Hodgkin's disease compared with population-based statistics and despite successful therapy (248–250). The main causes of death include second malignancies, cardiac disease, and infections.

The histologic spectrum of Hodgkin's disease seen at autopsy is wide. Only a minority of patients (40% or less) have readily classifiable Hodgkin's disease or exhibit persistence of the original histologic type (245,246); in many patients, there is variation of pattern and histology either in the same site or among distant sites. For example, patients with nodular sclerosis frequently no longer demonstrate nodularity or sclerosis at autopsy (245). In most patients, there is histologic progression to a more aggressive histologic type, and there often is vascular invasion with dissemination to noncontiguous sites, including an increased incidence of extranodal Hodgkin's disease (66,246). Autopsy often discloses loss of lymphocytes and eosinophils and increased numbers of atypical, pleomorphic cells, including Reed-Sternberg cells. There may be associated necrosis and degeneration, including the presence of foamy macrophages in cases of nodular sclerosis and numerous regions of hyalinized scarring (143,245). The pleomorphic variants of Hodgkin's disease discovered at autopsy are almost impossible to classify accurately and are confused easily with diffuse large cell or immunoblastic non-Hodgkin's lymphomas. It remains unclear whether these changes in histology are a consequence of therapy or the result of intrinsically more aggressive malignant lymphoma (245).

The change in cell type of Hodgkin's disease at autopsy and at clinical relapse is well recognized and usually interpreted as histologic progression to a more aggressive form of Hodgkin's disease (16,32,114). Only cases of the nodular sclerosis type exhibit a high degree of persistence in sequential biopsies, although some studies indicate that nodular lymphocyte predominance also is characterized by histologic persistence (114,116). The immunophenotype of classic Reed-Sternberg cells also is relatively constant in sequential biopsy specimens of Hodgkin's disease. In one study, 82% of cases exhibited immunophenotypic stability, as opposed to a previous report of only 19% consistency in patients with Hodgkin's disease undergoing biopsies at different times (251,252). The latter study preceded the use of antigen-retrieval techniques in immunohistochemistry.

At relapse, the histologic appearance depends on whether relapse occurs in an untreated or previously treated site (Table 17.7) (253,254). The vast majority of patients (89%) maintain the histologic appearance in biopsy specimens from an untreated site experiencing a relapse (253). An increase in epithelioid cell granulomatous reactions is observed among those patients who have an interval before relapse greater

TABLE 17.7. *Hodgkin's disease at relapse*

Relapse	Patients, no. (%)
Untreated site	
Histologic Persistence	46/52 (89%)
Histologic Alteration	6/52 (11%)
NS to MC	
MC to NS	
NSCP to MS	
NSCP to LD	
Treated site	
Histologic Persistence	26/46 (54%)
Histologic Alteration	21/46 (46%)
Unclassifiable Cases	9/46 (20%)

NS, nodular sclerosis; MC, mixed cellularity; NSCP, nodular sclerosis cellular phase; LD, lymphocytic depletion. From Colby TV, Warnke RA. The histology of the initial relapse of Hodgkin's disease. *Cancer* 1980;45:289–292; and Dolginow D, Colby TV, Recurrent Hodgkin's disease in treated sites. *Cancer* 1981;48:1124–1126, with permission.

than 1 year. Histologic persistence is far less common in patients who develop relapse in treated sites. Almost half these patients exhibit some alteration from their original histology (Fig. 17.43), and 20% are unclassifiable because of an unusual appearance, with loss of lymphocytes and increased numbers of pleomorphic cells, including bizarre Reed-Sternberg cells (32,254) (Fig. 17.44). These findings are identical to those described at autopsy (245,246). Curiously, the histologic appearance or subclassification at relapse does not necessarily portend a poor prognosis (254).

It is important to stress that the development of a mass in a patient after treatment for Hodgkin's disease may not indicate recurrent disease. Large, bulky masses in the mediastinum or retroperitoneum may represent masses of fibrosis, with or without other degenerative changes, probably as a consequence of therapy (255,256). Patients with Hodgkin's disease also are susceptible to infections such as toxoplasmosis after therapy and can develop lymphadenopathy, which may simulate clinical recurrence. In order to document clinical relapse of Hodgkin's disease, rebiopsy is required, or a lymph node aspiration if lymphadenopathy or a mass develops at a site that otherwise may require a major surgical procedure for diagnosis (244,257).

Patients treated for Hodgkin's disease are prone to develop second malignancies including solid tumors, acute myeloid leukemias, and non-Hodgkin's lymphomas (82–85,248–250). The nonhematopoietic solid tumors appear to be late occurrences arising in patients clinically cured of Hodgkin's disease and include bone and soft-tissue sarcomas, malignant melanoma, and carcinomas of the head and neck, lung, and breast (82); the solid tumors largely are related to radiation. The development of acute myeloid leukemia or a myelodysplastic syndrome seems related to chemotherapy with alkylating agents but also is associated with splenectomy and an advanced stage of disease (82,84,85,249). The risk of therapy-related leukemia does not rise continuously over time and is present in the first 10 years after Hodgkin's disease. Patients who have Hodgkin's disease and later develop non-Hodgkin's lymphomas develop these secondary tumors late, usually after 6 years or more, with a cumulative risk of 4.1% at 20 years (82–85).

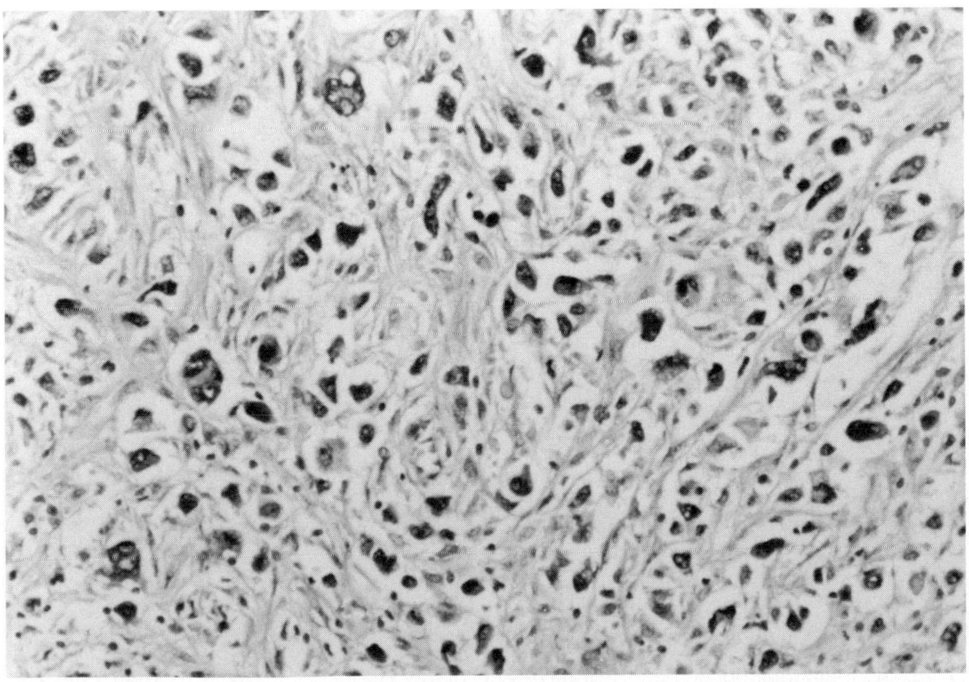

FIG. 17.43. Recurrent Hodgkin's disease in a treated site frequently exhibits histologic progression to a more aggressive type of Hodgkin's disease, such as lymphocytic depletion. This patient had an original diagnosis of nodular sclerosis (hematoxylin and eosin stain, original magnification: 240× magnification).

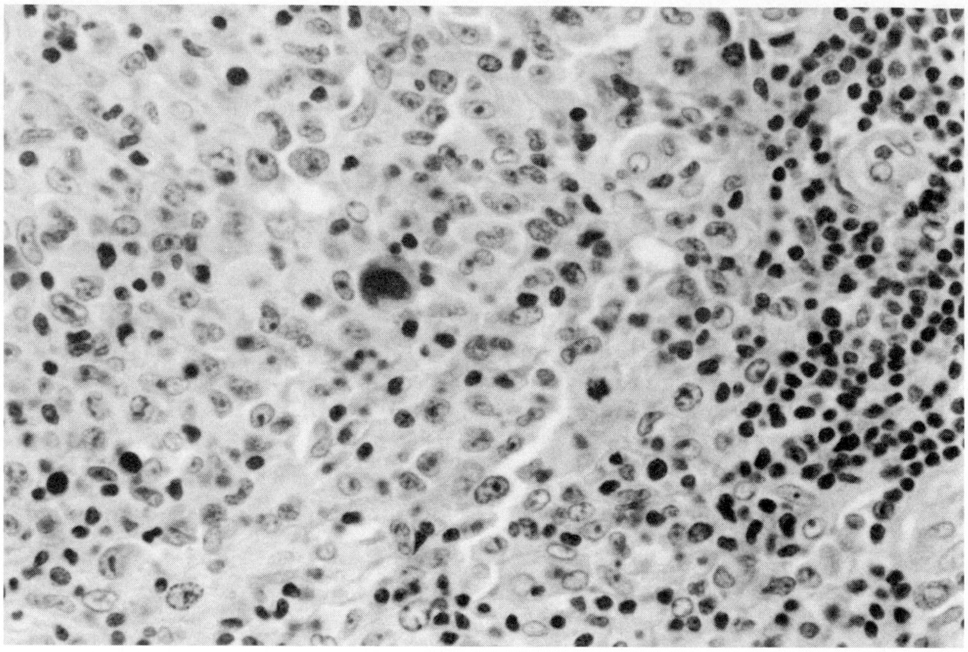

FIG. 17.44. Recurrent Hodgkin's disease in a treated site often is unclassifiable. This case resembles large cell lymphoma but was interpreted to be recurrent Hodgkin's disease based on morphologic and immunologic criteria. The original diagnosis was nodular sclerosis (hematoxylin and eosin stain, original magnification: 480× magnification).

A

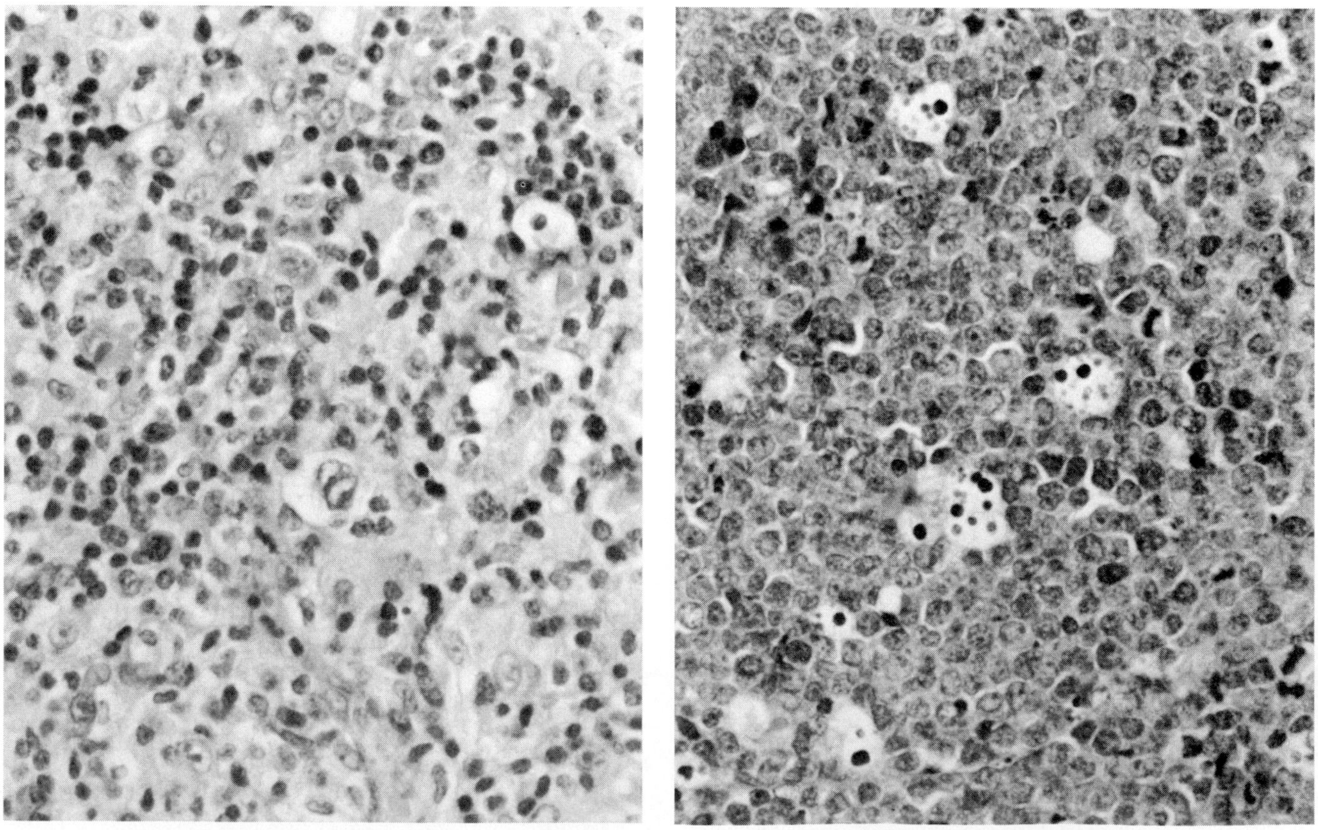

B

FIG. 17.45. A: Initial diagnostic biopsy of mixed cellularity Hodgkin's disease (hematoxylin and eosin stain, original magnification: 480× magnification). **B:** Burkitt's-like lymphoma of B-cell lineage presenting as an abdominal mass 6 years after the original diagnosis and combined-modality therapy (hematoxylin and eosin stain, original magnification: 480× magnification).

The risk of developing non-Hodgkin's lymphoma is greatest in patients receiving combined-modality therapy. Patients with lymphoma frequently have abdominal presentations, including involvement of the gastrointestinal tract, and mainly have B-cell lymphomas of the large cell or small noncleaved cell (Burkitt's-like and Burkitt's lymphoma) types (84,258,259) (Fig. 17.45). According to one case report, an aggressive B-cell non-Hodgkin's lymphoma was not related clonally to the preceding treated Hodgkin's disease (260). Rare cases of T-cell lymphoma have been reported after therapy for Hodgkin's disease (261). In a combined morphologic, immunophenotypic, and molecular genetic study of 12 patients who developed monomorphic lymphomas after therapy for Hodgkin's disease, seven lymphomas were B-cell malignancies (262). Two of the B-cell lymphomas arose in patients with lymphocyte predominance and likely were similar to other reported B-cell lymphomas developing in patients with this form of Hodgkin's disease (117–125). The remaining five cases of monomorphic lymphomas were $CD15^+$ and may have represented the pleomorphic, unclassifiable Hodgkin's disease described at autopsy and at relapse in treated sites, or the syncytial variant of nodular sclerosis (163,245,254,262). Two of the four $CD15^+$ patients expressed B-cell antigens, and in another patient the tumor cells expressed T-cell antigens, but all three patients showed some form of immunoglobulin gene rearrangement (262). These studies suggest that the causes of the aggressive lymphomas arising in patients with Hodgkin's disease are diverse. Some cases may represent morphologic transformation of Hodgkin's disease to a more pleomorphic variant; the B-cell lymphomas may be a consequence of either an immunosuppressive or a mutagenic effect of combined-modality therapy or develop secondary to Hodgkin's disease–associated defective immunity (258,259,263). Development of B-cell lymphoma after therapy does not appear to be related to EBV infection (263).

SUMMARY AND CONCLUSIONS

The advances in the understanding of Hodgkin's disease in the past 35 years have been multidisciplinary. Clinical progress sprang from the development of new diagnostic techniques including lymphangiography, staging laparotomy, computed tomography, and more recently magnetic resonance imaging, which led to the elucidation of the general orderly and contiguous pattern of dissemination of Hodgkin's disease. The employment of more accurate diagnostic methods also resulted in the worldwide acceptance of the Ann Arbor system for staging the extent of disease. The ability to stage Hodgkin's disease accurately culminated in the development of new therapeutic regimens with innovative modes of radiation therapy and the evolution of chemotherapy, combined-modality therapy, and bone marrow transplantation. Consequently, 80% or more of patients who develop Hodgkin's disease are cured at major centers in all parts of the world.

During this same era, the pathologic contributions to the understanding of Hodgkin's disease have been equally dynamic. The now historic clinicopathologic studies of Lukes and Butler resulted in a pathologic classification system, including the subsequent Rye modification, that has proven its relevance and reproducibility. Although the classification scheme of Lukes and Butler provides the base for the pathologic understanding of Hodgkin's disease, their concepts have undergone considerable redefinition and refinement and have been superseded by the modifications offered in the REAL and WHO classifications. In the lymphocyte predominance type of Hodgkin's disease, the nodular variant predominates and is a distinct entity, differing from other types of Hodgkin's disease in that the L&H variants of Reed-Sternberg cells, as well as most of the surrounding small lymphocytes, react with antibodies directed against CD45 and, significantly, express B cell lineage–restricted antigens but not the Hodgkin's disease–associated antigens CD15 and CD30. It has been proposed that the B-cell nature of nodular lymphocyte predominance Hodgkin's disease may be related histogenetically to PTGC, which has been reported to coexist with this type of Hodgkin's disease. Approximately 2% to 3% of patients with lymphocyte predominance evolve to a high-grade lymphoma of B-cell type but, like most patients with lymphocyte predominance, these patients also have localized clinical disease with a high rate of long-term survival.

Lymphocyte-rich classic Hodgkin's disease is the new category of Hodgkin's disease formalized in the REAL and WHO classifications. A small set of cases have a nodular or follicle-like architecture, and some cases of lymphocyte-rich classic Hodgkin's disease could be placed in either the cellular phase of nodular sclerosis or mixed-cell groups. Unlike lymphocyte predominance, the lymphocyte-rich form has identifiable classic Reed-Sternberg cells with a classic immunophenotypic profile ($CD15^+CD30^+CD20^-CD45^-$). The immunophenotype is significant, and an immunophenotypic panel is mandatory to differentiate lymphocyte-rich classic Hodgkin's disease absolutely from lymphocyte predominance and T cell– or histiocyte-rich B-cell lymphoma. Lymphocyte-rich classic Hodgkin's disease shares many clinical traits with lymphocyte predominance, most notably with respect to the manner of presentation; however, patients with lymphocyte-rich classic Hodgkin's disease behave more like patients with other types of classic Hodgkin's disease with respect to the patterns of relapse.

Classic nodular sclerosis is the most accurately diagnosed type of Hodgkin's disease, but there are histologic variants that may lead to a diagnostic conundrum. The two essential criteria for diagnosis of this type are sclerotic bands and clusters of the lacunar variants of Reed-Sternberg cells. There are cases, however, in which nodules of lacunar cells are found without fibrous septa; these cases raise the issue of the cellular phase of nodular sclerosis. The definition of the cellular phase is variable and its precise place remains controversial, although one important study suggested that these cases behave similar to cases of mixed cellularity. Other variants of nodular sclerosis include a fibroblastic type in which the fibroblasts almost mimic the appearance of malignant fibrous histiocytoma; this variant is associated with a shorter duration relapse-free survival. A third variant is a pleomorphic grade II type of Hodgkin's disease also referred to as the syncytial variant. These cases are mistaken easily for metastatic carcinoma or large cell lymphoma, and there is debate as to whether the syncytial variant or other cases of nodular sclerosis with anaplastic lacunar cells is associated with a worse rate of survival compared with the more common grade I type of nodular sclerosis.

Mixed-cell Hodgkin's disease has a highly variable morphologic appearance, because the classification essentially is a repository for cases that do not fit into the other types of Hodgkin's disease. Our understanding of the subtleties of the morphology of the mixed-cell type essentially derives from expansion of the differential diagnosis to refine the broad histologic criteria for this type of Hodgkin's disease. The differential diagnosis of mixed-cell Hodgkin's disease includes virus-induced florid reactive hyperplasias, AILD and AILD-like T-cell lymphoma, and other peripheral T-cell lymphomas of the mixed medium-sized and large cell type, as well as cases with epithelioid histiocytes (Lennert's lymphoma). Mixed-cell Hodgkin's disease also may be confused with B-cell lymphomas that are rich in reactive T cells. In all cases, morphologic criteria have been expounded, but an absolute diagnosis is dependent on verification by immunologic means. In addition, both the mixed-cell and nodular sclerosis types may affect only a portion of a lymph node; such cases have been designated as focal or interfollicular Hodgkin's disease.

Lymphocyte depletion is the least common type of Hodgkin's disease and, with the advances in both immunology and molecular genetics, the number of cases being filed in pathology archives under this type is being reduced further. Many historical cases identified as lymphocyte depletion were in fact the syncytial variant of nodular sclerosis, other types of Hodgkin's disease, and non-Hodgkin's lymphomas of large cell type, most notably anaplastic large cell lymphomas. Both morphologic reappraisal and immunophenotypic analysis are mandatory in the contemplation of any diagnosis of lymphocyte depletion.

The pathology of Hodgkin's disease at staging by laparotomy essentially has not changed, probably because of the almost universal abandonment of this diagnostic procedure. The pathologic criteria for involvement of spleen, abdominal lymph nodes, liver, and bone marrow at surgical staging remain those proposed at the Ann Arbor conference in 1971. The most significant proposal of the criteria for establishing Hodgkin's disease at staging is that a mononuclear cell with a single large nucleolus is acceptable for diagnosis in a small biopsy specimen from liver or bone marrow in patients with histologically established Hodgkin's disease. Extranodal Hodgkin's disease is rare, except in patients with AIDS, and should be regarded with initial skepticism. Genuine cases of extranodal Hodgkin's disease can arise in a variety of sites such as the lungs, gastrointestinal tract, and bone.

Studies of Hodgkin's disease at relapse indicate that almost all patients exhibit persistence of the original histologic appearance if relapse occurs in an untreated site. If relapse occurs in a treated site, the morphologic appearance becomes more pleomorphic and more difficult to classify, and the histology resembles that seen in Hodgkin's disease at autopsy. Curiously, there is no correlation of pleomorphism with prognosis. Patients who relapse also may develop an aggressive non-Hodgkin's lymphoma of B-cell type that seems related to combined-modality therapy. In other patients, relapse with an apparent non-Hodgkin's lymphoma actually may represent dedifferentiated Hodgkin's disease.

ACKNOWLEDGMENTS

The author thanks Diane Fletcher and Eric Gold for their assistance in the preparation of the manuscript.

REFERENCES

1. Hodgkin T. On some morbid appearances of the absorbent glands and spleen. *Med Chir Trans* 1832;17:68–114.
2. Wilks S. Cases of enlargement of the lymphatic glands and spleen (or, Hodgkin's disease), with remarks. *Guys Hosp Rep* 1865;11:56–67.
3. Rather LJ. Who discovered the pathognomonic giant cell of Hodgkin's disease? *Bull N Y Acad Med* 1972;48:943–950.
4. Sternberg C. Über eine eigenartige unter dem Bilde der Pseudoleukämie verlaufende Tuberculose des lymphatischen Apparates. *Ztschr Heilk* 1898;19:21–90.
5. Reed DM. On the pathological changes in Hodgkin's disease with especial reference to its relation to tuberculosis. *Johns Hopkins Hosp Rep* 1902;10:133–196.
6. Kaplan HS. Hodgkin's disease: unfolding concepts concerning its nature, management and prognosis. *Cancer* 1980;45:2439–2474.
7. Rosenberg SA. Hodgkin's disease: challenges for the future. *Cancer Res* 1989;49:767–769.
8. Urba WJ, Longo DL. Hodgkin's disease. *N Engl J Med* 1992;326: 678–687.
9. DeVita VT, Hubbard SM. Hodgkin's disease. *N Engl Med* 1993;328: 560–565.
10. Kanzler H, Küppers R, Hansmann M-L, et al. Hodgkin and Reed-Sternberg cells in Hodgkin's disease represent the outgrowth of a dominant tumor clone derived from (crippled) germinal center B cells. *J Exp Med* 1996;184:1495–1505.
11. Marafioti T, Hummel M, Anagnostopoulos I, et al. Origin of nodular lymphocyte-predominant Hodgkin's disease from a clonal expansion of highly mutated germinal-center B cells. *N Engl J Med* 1997;337: 453–458.
12. Ohno T, Stribley JA, Wu G, et al. Clonality in nodular lymphocyte-predominant Hodgkin's disease. *N Engl J Med* 1997;337:459–465.
13. Kaplan HS. *Hodgkin's disease,* 2nd ed. Cambridge, MA: Harvard University Press, 1980.
14. Rosenberg SA, Canellos GP. Hodgkin's disease. In: Canellos GP, Lister TA, Sklar JL, eds. *The lymphomas.* Philadelphia: WB Saunders, 1998:305–331.
15. Aisenberg AC. Problems in Hodgkin's disease management. *Blood* 1999;93:761–779.
16. Lukes RJ, Butler JJ. The pathology and nomenclature of Hodgkin's disease. *Cancer Res* 1966;26:1063–1081.
17. Lukes RJ, Butler JJ, Hicks EB. Natural history of Hodgkin's disease as related to its pathologic picture. *Cancer* 1966;19:317–344.
18. Jackson H Jr, Parker F Jr. *Hodgkin's disease and allied disorders.* New York: Oxford University Press, 1947.
19. Lukes RJ, Craver LF, Hall TC, et al. Report of the nomenclature committee. *Cancer Res* 1966;26:1311.

20. Harris NL, Jaffe ES, Stein H, et al. A revised European-American classification of lymphoid neoplasms: a proposal from the International Lymphoma Study Group. *Blood* 1994;84:1361–1392.
21. Stein H. Hodgkin's disease. *Am J Surg Pathol* 1997;21:119–120(abst).
22. Jaffe ES, Harris NL, Diebold J, et al. World Health Organization classification of lymphomas: a work in progress. *Ann Oncol* 1998; 9(Suppl 5):S25–S30.
23. Harris NL. Hodgkin's disease: classification and differential diagnosis. *Mod Pathol* 1999;12:159–176.
24. MacLennan KA, Bennett MH, Tu A, et al. Relationship of histopathologic features to survival and relapse in nodular sclerosing Hodgkin's disease: a study of 1659 patients. *Cancer* 1989;64:1686–1693.
25. Wijlhuizen TJ, Vrints LW, Jairam R, et al. Grades of nodular sclerosis (NSI-NSII) in Hodgkin's disease: are they of independent prognostic value? *Cancer* 1989;63:1150–1153.
26. Pittaluga S, Wlodarska I, Pulford K, et al. The monoclonal antibody ALK1 identifies a distinct morphological subtype of anaplastic large cell lymphoma associated with 2p23/ALK rearrangements. *Am J Pathol* 1997;151:343–351.
27. Pulford K, Lamant L, Morris SW, et al. Detection of anaplastic lymphoma kinase (ALK) and nucleolar protein nucleophosmin (NPM)-ALK proteins in normal and neoplastic cells with the monoclonal antibody ALK1. *Blood* 1997;89:1394–1404.
28. Benharroch D, Meguerian-Bedoyan Z, Lamant L, et al. ALK-positive lymphoma: a single disease with a broad spectrum of morphology. *Blood* 1998;91:2076–2084.
29. Falini B, Bigerna B, Fizzotti M, et al. ALK expression defines a distinct group of T/null lymphomas (''ALK lymphomas'') with a wide morphological spectrum. *Am J Pathol* 1998;153:875–886.
30. Lukes RJ. Criteria for involvement of lymph node, bone marrow, spleen, and liver in Hodgkin's disease. *Cancer Res* 1971;31:1755–1767.
31. Dorfman RF, Colby TV. The pathologist's role in management of patients with Hodgkin's disease. *Cancer Treat Rep* 1982;66:675–680.
32. Butler JJ, Pugh WC. Review of Hodgkin's disease. *Hematol Pathol* 1993;7:59–77.
33. Butler JJ. Relationship of histological findings to survival in Hodgkin's disease. *Cancer Res* 1971;31:1770–1775.
34. Berard CW, Thomas LB, Axtell LM, et al. The relationship of histopathological subtype to clinical stage of Hodgkin's disease at diagnosis. *Cancer Res* 1971;31:1776–1785.
35. Dorfman RF. Relationship of histology to site in Hodgkin's disease. *Cancer Res* 1971;31:1786–1793.
36. Tindle BH, Parker JW, Lukes RJ. ''Reed-Sternberg cells'' in infectious mononucleosis? *Am J Clin Pathol* 1972;58:607–617.
37. Strum SB, Park JK, Rappaport H. Observation of cells resembling Sternberg-Reed cells in conditions other than Hodgkin's disease. *Cancer* 1970;26:176–190.
38. Weiss LM, Crabtree GS, Rouse RV, et al. Morphologic and immunologic characterization of 50 peripheral T-cell lymphomas. *Am J Pathol* 1985;118:316–324.
39. Pinkus GS, O'Hara CJ, Said JW. Peripheral/post-thymic T-cell lymphomas: a spectrum of disease. Clinical, pathologic, and immunologic features of 78 cases. *Cancer* 1990;65:971–998.
40. Chittal SM, Brousset P, Voigt J-J, et al. Large B-cell lymphoma rich in T-cells and simulating Hodgkin's disease. *Histopathology* 1991; 19:211–220.
41. McBride JA, Rodriguez J, Luthra R, et al. T-cell-rich B large-cell lymphoma simulating lymphocyte-rich Hodgkin's disease. *Am J Surg Pathol* 1996;20:193–201.
42. Filippa DA, Ladanyi M, Wollner N, et al. CD30 (Ki-1)-positive malignant lymphomas: clinical, immunophenotypic, histologic, and genetic characteristics and differences with Hodgkin's disease. *Blood* 1996; 87:2905–2917.
43. Said JW. The immunohistochemistry of Hodgkin's disease. *Semin Diagn Pathol* 1992;9:265–271.
44. Carbone A, Gloghini A, Gattei V, et al. Expression of functional CD40 antigen on Reed-Sternberg cells and Hodgkin's disease cell lines. *Blood* 1995;85:780–789.
45. Pinkus GS, Pinkus JL, Langhoff E, et al. Fascin, a sensitive new marker for Reed-Sternberg cells of Hodgkin's disease. Evidence for a dendritic or B cell derivation? *Am J Pathol* 1997;150:543–562.
46. Kadin ME. The borderline between Hodgkin's lymphomas and anaplastic large cell lymphoma. *Am J Surg Pathol* 1998;22:133(abst).
47. Rüdiger T, Ott G, Ott MM, et al. Differential diagnosis between classic Hodgkin's lymphoma, T-cell-rich B-cell lymphoma, and paragranuloma by paraffin immunohistochemistry. *Am J Surg Pathol* 1998;22: 1184–1191.
48. Frizzera G, Wu CD, Inghirami G. The usefulness of immunophenoypic and genotypic studies in the diagnosis and classification of hematopoietic and lymphoid neoplasms: an update. *Am J Clin Pathol* 1999; 111(Suppl 1):S13–S39.
49. von Wasielewski R, Mengel M, Fischer R, et al. classic Hodgkin's disease: clinical impact of the immunophenotype. *Am J Pathol* 1997; 151:1123–1130.
50. MacMahon B. Epidemiology of Hodgkin's disease. *Cancer Res* 1966; 26:1189–1200.
51. Guinee VF, Giacco GG, Durand M, et al. The prognosis of Hodgkin's disease in older adults. *J Clin Oncol* 1991;9:947–953.
52. Glaser SL, Swartz WG. Time trends in Hodgkin's disease incidence: the role of diagnostic accuracy. *Cancer* 1990;66:2196–2204.
53. Medeiros LJ, Greiner TC. Hodgkin's disease. *Cancer* 1995;75: 357–369.
54. Kennedy BJ, Fremgen AM, Menck HR. The National Cancer Data Base report on Hodgkin's disease for 1985–1989 and 1990–1994. *Cancer* 1998;83:1041–1047.
55. Correa P, O'Conor GT. Epidemiologic patterns of Hodgkin's disease. *Int J Cancer* 1971;8:192–201.
56. Hu E, Hufford S, Lukes R, et al. Third-world Hodgkin's disease at Los Angeles County-University of Southern California Medical Center. *J Clin Oncol* 1988;6:1285–1292.
57. Zarate-Osorno A, Roman LN, Kingma DW, et al. Hodgkin's disease in Mexico: prevalence of Epstein-Barr virus sequences and correlations with histologic subtype. *Cancer* 1995;75:1360–1366.
58. Goedert JJ, Coté TR, Virgo P, et al. Spectrum of AIDS-associated malignant disorders. *Lancet* 1998;351:1833–1839.
59. Rubio R. Hodgkin's disease associated with human immunodeficiency virus infection: a clinical study of 46 cases. *Cancer* 1994;73: 2400–2407.
60. Herndier BG, Sanchez HC, Chang KL, et al. High prevalence of Epstein-Barr virus in the Reed-Sternberg cells of HIV-associated Hodgkin's disease. *Am J Pathol* 1993;142:1073–1079.
61. Bellas C, Santón A, Manzanal A, et al. Pathological, immunological, and molecular features of Hodgkin's disease associated with HIV infection: comparison with ordinary Hodgkin's disease. *Am J Surg Pathol* 1996;20:1520–1524.
62. Austin-Seymour MM, Hoppe RT, Cox RS, et al. Hodgkin's disease in patients over sixty years old. *Ann Intern Med* 1984;100:13–18.
63. Regula DP Jr, Hoppe RT, Weiss LM. Nodular and diffuse types of lymphocyte predominance Hodgkin's disease. *N Engl J Med* 1988; 318:214–219.
64. Neiman RS, Rosen PJ, Lukes RJ. Lymphocyte-depletion Hodgkin's disease: a clinicopathological entity. *N Engl J Med* 1973;288: 751–754.
65. Rosenberg SA, Kaplan HS. Evidence for an orderly progression in the spread of Hodgkin's disease. *Cancer Res* 1966;26:1225–1231.
66. Naeim F, Waisman J, Coulson WF. Hodgkin's disease: the significance of vascular invasion. *Cancer* 1974;34:655–662.
67. Strum SB, Hutchison GB, Park JK, et al. Further observations on the biologic significance of vascular invasion in Hodgkin's disease. *Cancer* 1971;27:1–6.
68. Strum SB, Allen LW, Rappaport H. Vascular invasion in Hodgkin's disease: its relationship to involvement of the spleen and other extranodal sites. *Cancer* 1971;28:1329–1334.
69. Lamoureux KB, Jaffe ES, Berard CW, et al. Lack of identifiable vascular invasion in patients with extranodal dissemination of Hodgkin's disease. *Cancer* 1973;31:824–825.
70. Glatstein E, Guernsey JM, Rosenberg SA, et al. The value of laparotomy and splenectomy in the staging of Hodgkin's disease. *Cancer* 1969;24:709–718.
71. Ferguson DJ, Allen LW, Griem ML, et al. Surgical experience with staging laparotomy in 125 patients with lymphoma. *Arch Intern Med* 1973;131:356–361.
72. Gamble JF, Fuller LM, Martin RG, et al. Influence of staging celiotomy in localized presentations of Hodgkin's disease. *Cancer* 1975; 35:817–825.

73. Ng A, Weeks JC, Mauch PM, et al. Laparotomy versus no laparotomy in the management of early-stage, favorable-prognosis Hodgkin's disease: a decision analysis. *J Clin Oncol* 1999;17:241–252.
74. Rosenberg SA. Laparotomy and splenectomy in Hodgkin's disease: a reappraisal after twenty years. *Scand J Haematol* 1985;34:289–292.
75. Connors JM. Evaluation and treatment of early-stage Hodgkin's disease. In: ASCO education book 1997. Philadelphia, PA: WB Saunders Co., 1997:240–243.
76. Rosenberg SA. Exploratory laparotomy and splenectomy for Hodgkin's disease: a commentary. *J Clin Oncol* 1988;6:574–575.
77. Diehl V, Sieber M, Rüffer U, et al. Treatment of early-stage Hodgkin's disease: considerations in the use of chemotherapy. In: ASCO education book 1998. Philadelphia, PA: WB Saunders Co., 1998:181–187.
78. Carbone PP, Kaplan HS, Musshoff K, et al. Report of the committee on Hodgkin's disease staging classification. *Cancer Res* 1971;31: 1860–1861.
79. Lister TA, Crowther D, Sutcliffe SB, et al. Report of a committee convened to discuss the evaluation and staging of patients with Hodgkin's disease: Cotswolds meeting. *J Clin Oncol* 1989;7:1630–1636.
80. Loeffler M, Brosteanu O, Hasenclever D, et al. Meta-analysis of chemotherapy versus combined modality treatment trials in Hodgkin's disease. *J Clin Oncol* 1998;16:818–829.
81. Horning SJ, Chao NJ, Negrin RS, et al. High-dose therapy and autologous hematopoietic progenitor cell transplantation for recurrent or refractory Hodgkin's disease: analysis of the Stanford University results and prognostic indices. *Blood* 1997;89:801–813.
82. Young RC, Bookman MA, Longo DL. Late complications of Hodgkin's disease management. *J Natl Cancer Inst Monograph* 1990;10: 55–60.
83. van Leeuwen FE, Klokman WJ, Hagenbeek A, et al. Second cancer risk following Hodgkin's disease: a 20-year follow-up study. *J Clin Oncol* 1994;12:312–325.
84. Mauch PM, Kalish LA, Marcus KC, et al. Second malignancies after treatment for laparotomy staged IA-IIIB Hodgkin's disease: long-term analysis of risk factors and outcome. *Blood* 1996;87:3625–3632.
85. Wolden SL, Lamborn KR, Cleary SF, et al. Second cancers following pediatric Hodgkin's disease. *J Clin Oncol* 1998;16:536–544.
86. Colby, TV, Hoppe RT, Warnke RA. Hodgkin's disease: a clinicopathologic study of 659 cases. *Cancer* 1982;49:1848–1858.
87. Poppema, S. Lymphocyte-predominance Hodgkin's disease. *Semin Diagn Pathol* 1992;9:257–264.
88. Mason DY, Banks PM, Chan J, et al. Nodular lymphocyte predominance Hodgkin's disease: a distinct clinicopathological entity. *Am J Surg Pathol* 1994;18:526–530.
89. Butler JJ. The histologic diagnosis of Hodgkin's disease. *Semin Diagn Pathol* 1992;9:252–256.
90. Hansmann M-L, Stein H, Dallenbach F, et al. Diffuse lymphocyte-predominant Hodgkin's disease (diffuse paragranuloma): a variant of the B-cell-derived nodular type. *Am J Pathol* 1991;138:29–36.
91. Delabie J, Vandenberghe Kennes C, et al. Histiocyte-rich B-cell lymphoma: a distinct clinicopathologic entity possibly related to lymphocyte predominant Hodgkin's disease, paragranuloma subtype. *Am J Surg Pathol* 1992;16:37–48.
92. Gascoyne RD, Delabie J, de Wolfe-Peeters C, et al. ''Paragranuloma-type'' T-cell rich B-cell lymphoma: a report of 50 cases. *Mod Pathol* 1999;137A(abst).
93. Wright DH. Lymphocyte predominance Hodgkin's disease [Letter]. *N Engl J Med* 1988;319:246.
94. Pinkus GS, Said JW. Hodgkin's disease, lymphocyte predominance type, nodular-further evidence for a B cell derivation: L&H variants of Reed-Sternberg cells express L26, a pan B cell marker. *Am J Pathol* 1988;133:211–217.
95. Stoler MH, Nichols GE, Symbula M, et al. Lymphocyte predominance Hodgkin's disease: evidence for a κ light chain-restricted monotypic B-cell neoplasm. *Am J Pathol* 1995;146:812–818.
96. von Wasielewski R, Wilkens L, Nolte M, et al. Light-chain mRNA in lymphocyte-predominant and mixed-cellularity Hodgkin's disease. *Mod Pathol* 1996;9:334–338.
97. Poppema S. The nature of the lymphocytes surrounding Reed-Sternberg cells in nodular lymphocyte predominance and in other types of Hodgkin's disease. *Am J Pathol* 1989;135:351–357.
98. Kamel OW, Gelb AB, Shibuya RB, et al. Leu 7 (CD57) reactivity distinguishes nodular lymphocyte predomince Hodgkin's disease from nodular sclerosing Hodgkin's disease, T-cell-rich B-cell lymphoma and follicular lymphoma. *Am J Pathol* 1993;142:541–546.
99. Poppema S, Kaiserling E, Lennert K. Hodgkin's disease with lymphocytic predominance, nodular type (nodular paragranuloma) and progressively transformed germinal centres-a cytohistological study. *Histopathology* 1979;3:295–308.
100. Hansmann M-L, Fellbaum C, Hui PK, et al. Progressive transformation of germinal centers with and without association to Hodgkin's disease. *Am J Clin Pathol* 1990;93:219–226.
101. Osborne BM, Butler JJ, Gresik MV. Progressive transformation of germinal centers: comparison of 23 pediatric patients to the adult population. *Mod Pathol* 1992;5:135–140.
102. Van den Oord JJ, de Wolf-Peeters C, Desmet VJ. Immunohistochemical analysis of progressively transformed follicular centers. *Am J Clin Pathol* 1985;83:560–564.
103. Osborne BM, Butler JJ. Clinical implications of progressive transformation of germinal centers. *Am J Surg Pathol* 1984;8:725–733.
104. Burns BF, Colby TV, Dorfman RF. Differential diagnostic features of nodular L&H Hodgkin's disease, including progressive transformation of germinal centers. *Am J Surg Pathol* 1984;8:253–261.
105. Ferry JA, Zukerberg LR, Harris NL. Florid progressive transformation of germinal centers: a syndrome affecting young men, without early progression to nodular lymphocyte predominance Hodgkins disease. *Am J Surg Pathol* 1992;16:252–258.
106. Hansmann M-L, Zwingers T, Boske A, et al. Clinical features of nodular paragranuloma (Hodgkin's disease, lymphocyte predominance type, nodular). *J Cancer Res Clin Oncol* 1984;108:321–330.
107. Trudel MA, Krikorian JG, Neiman RS. Lymphocyte predominance Hodgkin's disease: a clinicopathologic reassessment. *Cancer* 1987; 59:99–106.
108. Chang KL, Kamel OW, Arber DA, et al. Pathologic features of nodular lymphocyte predominance Hodgkin's disease in extranodal sites. *Am J Surg Pathol* 1995;19:1313–1324.
109. Siebert JD, Stuckey JH, Kurtin PJ, et al. Extranodal lymphocyte predominance Hodgkin's disease: clinical and pathologic features. *Am J Clin Pathol* 1995;103:485–491.
110. Bodis S, Kraus MD, Pinkus G, et al. Clinical presentation and outcome in lymphocyte-predominant Hodgkin's disease. *J Clin Oncol* 1997; 15:3060–3066.
111. Borg-Grech, Radford JA, Crowther D, et al. A comparative study of the nodular and diffuse variants of lymphocyte-predominant Hodgkin's disease. *J Clin Oncol* 1989;7:1303–1309.
112. Tefferi A, Zellers RA, Banks PM, et al. Clinical correlates of distinct immunophenotypic and histologic subcategories of lymphocyte-predominance Hodgkin's disease. *J Clin Oncol* 1990;8:1959–1965.
113. Diehl V, Sextro M, Franklin J, et al. Clinical presentation, course, and prognostic factors in lymphocyte-predominant Hodgkin's disease and lymphocyte-rich classic Hodgkin's disease: report from the European Task Force on Lymphoma project on lymphocyte-predominant Hodgkin's disease. *J Clin Oncol* 1999;17:776–783.
114. Strum SB, Rappaport H. Interrelations of the histologic types of Hodgkin's disease. *Arch Pathol* 1971;91:127–134.
115. Gelb AB, Dorfman RF, Warnke RA. Coexistence of nodular lymphocyte predominance Hodgkin's disease and Hodgkin's disease of the usual type. *Am J Surg Pathol* 1993;17:364–374.
116. Regula DP Jr, Weiss LM, Warnke RA, et al. Lymphocyte predominance Hodgkin's disease: a reappraisal based upon histological and immunophenotypical findings in relapsing cases. *Histopathology* 1987;11:1107–1120.
117. Miettinen M, Franssila KO, Saxen E. Hodgkin's disease, lymphocytic predominance nodular: increased risk for subsequent non-Hodgkin's lymphomas. *Cancer* 1983;51:2293–2300.
118. Sundeen JT, Cossman J, Jaffe ES. Lymphocyte predominant Hodgkin's disease nodular subtype with coexistent ''large cell lymphoma:'' histological progression or composite malignancy? *Am J Surg Pathol* 1988;12:599–606.
119. Hansmann M-L, Stein H, Fellbaum C, et al. Nodular paragranuloma can transform into high-grade malignant lymphoma of B type. *Hum Pathol* 1989;20:1169–1175.
120. Chittal SM, Alard C, Rossi J-F, et al. Further phenotypic evidence that nodular, lymphocyte-predominant Hodgkin's disease is a large B-cell lymphoma in evolution. *Am J Surg Pathol* 1990;14:1024–1035.
121. Grossman DM, Hanson CA, Schnitzer B. Simultaneous lymphocyte predominant Hodgkin's disease and large-cell lymphoma. *Am J Surg Pathol* 1991;15:668–676.
122. Greiner TC, Gascoyne RD, Anderson ME, et al. Nodular lymphocyte-

predominant Hodgkin's disease associated with large-cell lymphoma: analysis of Ig gene rearrangements byV-J polymerase chain reaction. *Blood* 1996;88:657–666.
123. Wickert RS, Weisenburger DD, Tierens A, et al. Clonal relationship between lymphocytic predominance Hodgkin's disease and concurrent or subsequent large-cell lymphoma of B lineage. *Blood* 1995;86: 2312–2320.
124. Pan LX, Diss TC, Peng HZ, et al. Nodular lymphocyte predominance Hodgkin's disease: a monoclonal or polyclonal B-cell disorder? *Blood* 1996; 87:2428–2434.
125. Hell K, Hansmann ML, Pringle JH, et al. Combination of Hodgkin's disease and diffuse large cell lymphoma: an in situ hybridization study for immunoglobulin light chain messenger RNA. *Histopathology* 1995;27:491–499.
126. Delabie J, Greiner TC, Chan WC, et al. Concurrent lymphocyte predominance Hodgkin's disease and T-cell lymphoma: a report of three cases. *Am J Surg Pathol* 1996;20:355–362.
127. Nguyen PL, Ferry JA, Harris NL. Progressive transformation of germinal centers and nodular lymphocyte predominance Hodgkin's disease; a comparative immunohistochemical study. *Am J Surg Pathol* 1999;23:27–33.
128. Ashton-Key M, Thorpe PA, Allen JP, et al. Follicular Hodgkin's disease. *Am J Surg Pathol* 1995;19:1294–1299.
129. von Wasielewski R, Werner M, Fischer R, et al. Lymphocyte-predominant Hodgkin's disease: an immunohistochemical analysis of 208 reviewed Hodgkin's disease cases from the German Hodgkin Study Group. *Am J Pathol* 1997;150:793–803.
130. von Wasielewski R, Seth S, Franklin J, et al. Prevalence, presentation and prognosis of lymphocyte-rich classic Hodgkin's disease. *Mod Pathol* 1999;12:147A(abst).
131. Schmidt U, Metz KA, Leder L-D. T-cell-rich B-cell lymphoma and lymphocyte-predominant Hodgkin's disease: two closely related entities? *Br J Haematol* 1995;90:398–403.
132. De Jong D, Van Gorp J, Sie-Go D, et al. T-cell rich B-cell non-Hodgkin's lymphoma: a progressed form of follicle centre cell lymphoma and lymphocyte predominance Hodgkin's disease. *Histopathology* 1996;28:15–24.
133. Patsouris E, Noel H, Lennert K. Lymphoplasmacytic/lymphoplasmacytoid immunocytoma with a high content of epithelioid cells: Histologic and immunohistochemical findings. *Am J Surg Pathol* 1990;14: 660–670.
134. Colby TV, Warnke RA, Burke JS, et al. Differentiation of chronic lymphocytic leukemia from Hodgkin's disease using immunologic marker studies. *Am J Surg Pathol* 1981;5:707–710.
135. Brecher M, Banks PM. Hodgkin's disease variant of Richter's syndrome: report of eight cases. *Am J Clin Pathol* 1990;93:333–339.
136. Williams J, Schned A, Cotelingam JD, et al. Chronic lymphocytic leukemia with coexistent Hodgkin's disease: implications for the origin of the Reed-Sternberg cell. *Am J Surg Pathol* 1991;15:33–42.
137. Weisenberg E, Anastasi J, Adeyanju M, et al. Hodgkin's disease associated with chronic lymphocytic leukemia: eight additional cases, including two of the nodular lymphocyte predominant type. *Am J Clin Pathol* 1995;103:479–484.
138. Hansmann ML, Fellbaum C, Hui PK, et al. Morphological and immunohistochemical investigation of non-Hodgkin's lymphoma combined with Hodgkin's disease. *Histopathology* 1989;15:35–48.
139. Momose H, Jaffe ES, Shin SS, et al. Chronic lymphocytic leukemia/ small lymphocytic lymphoma with Reed-Sternberg-like cells and possible transformation to Hodgkin's disease: mediation by Epstein-Barr virus. *Am J Surg Pathol* 1992;16:859–867.
140. Ohno T, Smir BN, Weisenburger DD, et al. Origin of the Hodgkin/ Reed-Sternberg cells in chronic lymphocytic leukemia with "Hodgkin's transformation." *Blood* 1998;91:1757–1761.
141. Shin SS, Ben-Ezra J, Burke JS, et al. Reed-Sternberg-like cells in low-grade lymphomas are transformed neoplastic cells of B-cell lineage. *Am J Clin Pathol* 1993;99:658–662.
142. Holman CDJ, Matz LR, Finlay-Jones LR, et al. Inter-observer variation in the histopathological reporting of Hodgkin's disease: an analysis of diagnostic subcomponents using kappa statistics. *Histopathology* 1983;7:399–407.
143. Variakojis D, Strum SB, Rappaport H. The foamy macrophages in Hodgkin's disease. *Arch Pathol* 1972;93:453–456.
144. Kadin ME, Glatstein E, Dorfman RF. Clinicopathologic studies of 117 untreated patients subjected to laparotomy for the staging of Hodgkin's disease. *Cancer* 1971;27:1277–1294.
145. Rappaport H, Berard CW, Butler JJ, et al. Report of the committee on histopathological criteria contributing to staging of Hodgkin's disease. *Cancer Res* 1971;31:1864–865.
146. Suster S. Transformation of Hodgkin's disease into malignant fibrous histiocytoma. *Cancer* 1986;57:264–268.
147. Strum SB, Rappaport H. Significance of focal involvement of lymph nodes for the diagnosis and staging of Hodgkin's disease. *Cancer* 1970;25:1314–1319.
148. Doggett RS, Colby TV, Dorfman RF. Interfollicular Hodgkin's disease. *Am J Surg Pathol* 1983;7:145–149.
149. Maheswaran PR, Ramsay AD, Norton AJ, et al. Hodgkin's disease presenting with the histological features of Castleman's disease. *Histopathology* 1991;18:249–253.
150. Mohrmann RL, Nathwani BN, Brynes RK, et al. Hodgkin's disease occurring in monocytoid B-cell clusters. *Am J Clin Pathol* 1991;95: 802–808.
151. Ohsawa M, Kanno H, Naka N, et al. Occurence of monocytoid B-lymphocytes in Hodgkin's disease. *Mod Pathol* 1994;7:540–543.
152. Keller AR, Kaplan HS, Lukes RJ, et al. Correlation of histopathology with other prognostic indicators in Hodgkin's disease. *Cancer* 1968; 22:487–499.
153. Coppleson LW, Rappaport H, Strum B, et al. Analysis of the Rye classification of Hodgkin's disease: the prognostic significance of cellular composition. *J Natl Cancer Inst* 1973;51:379–390.
154. Haybittle JL, Hayhoe FGJ, Easterling MJ, et al. Review of British National Lymphoma Investigation studies of Hodgkin's disease and development of prognostic index. *Lancet* 1985:967–972.
155. Ferry JA, Linggood RM, Convery KM, et al. Hodgkin's disease, nodular sclerosis type: implications of histologic subclassification. *Cancer* 1993;71:457–463.
156. Georgii A, von Wasielewski R, MacLennan KA, et al. Nodular sclerosing Hodgkin shows significant differences in clinical course when graded by histopathology. *Mod Pathol* 1998;11:129A(abst).
157. Masih AS, Weisenburger DD, Vose JM, et al. Histologic grade does not predict prognosis in optimally treated, advanced-stage nodular sclerosing Hodgkin's disease. *Cancer* 1992;69:228–232.
158. d'Amore ESG, Lee CKK, Aeppli DM, et al. Lack of prognostic value of histopathologic parameters in Hodgkin's disease, nodular sclerosis type: a study of 123 patients with limited stage disease who had undergone laparotomy and were treated with radiation therapy. *Arch Pathol Lab Med* 1992;116:856–861.
159. Hess JL, Bodis S, Pinkus G, et al. Histopathologic grading of nodular sclerosis Hodgkin's disease: lack of prognostic significance in 254 surgically staged patients. *Cancer* 1994;74:708–714.
160. Alavaikko MJ, Blanco G, Aine R, et al. Follicular dendritic cells have prognostic relevance in Hodgkin's disease. *Am J Clin Pathol* 1994; 101:761–767.
161. Baur AS, Meugé-Moraw C, Michel G, et al. Prognostic value of follicular dendritic cells in nodular sclerosing Hodgkin's disease. *Histopathology* 1998;32:512–520.
162. Butler JJ. The Lukes-Butler classification of Hodgkin's disease revisited. In: Bennett JM, ed. *Controversies in the management of lymphomas.* Boston: Martinus Nijhoff, 1983:1–18.
163. Strickler JG, Michie SA, Warnke RA, et al. The "syncytial variant" of nodular sclerosing Hodgkin's disease. *Am J Surg Pathol* 1986;10: 470–477.
164. Bacchi CE, Dorfman RF, Hoppe RT, et al. Metastatic carcinoma in lymph nodes simulating "syncytial variant" of nodular sclerosing Hodgkin's disease. *Am J Clin Pathol* 1991:96:589–593.
165. Zarate-Osorno A, Jaffe ES, Medeiros LJ. Metastatic nasopharyngeal carcinoma initially presenting as cervical lymphadenopathy: a report of two cases that resembled Hodgkin's disease. *Arch Pathol Lab Med* 1992;116:862–865.
166. Khalidi HS, Singleton TP, Weiss SW. Inflammatory malignant fibrous histiocytoma: distinction from Hodgkin's disease and non-Hodgkin's lymphoma by a panel of leukocyte markers. *Mod Pathol* 1997:10: 438–442.
167. Argani P, Facchetti F, Inghirami G, et al. Lymphocyte-rich well-differentiated liposarcoma: report of nine cases. *Am J Surg Pathol* 1997; 21:884–895.
168. Montgomery EA, Devaney KO, Giordano TJ, et al. Inflammatory myxohyaline tumor of distal extremities with virocyte or Reed-Stern-

berg-like cells: a distinctive lesion with features simulating inflammatory conditions, Hodgkin's disease, and various sarcomas. *Mod Pathol* 1998;11:384–391.

169. Perrone T, Frizzera G, Rosai J. Mediastinal diffuse large-cell lymphoma with sclerosis: a clinicopathologic study of 60 cases. *Am J Surg Pathol* 1986;10:176–191.
170. Cazals-Hatem D, Lepage E, Brice P, et al. Primary mediastinal large B-cell lymphoma: a clinicopathologic study of 141 cases compared wth 916 nonmediastinal large B-cell lymphomas, a GELA (''Groupe d'Etude des Lymphomes de l'Adulte'') study. *Am J Surg Pathol* 1996; 20:877–888.
171. Suster S, Moran CA. Pleomorphic large cell lymphomas of the mediastinum. *Am J Surg Pathol* 1996;20:224–232.
172. Higgins JP, Warnke RA. CD30 expression in mediastinal large B-cell lymphoma. *Mod Pathol* 1999;12:138A(abst).
173. Kim H, Hendrickson MR, Dorfman RF. Composite lymphoma. *Cancer* 1977;40:959–976.
174. Gonzalez CL, Medeiros LJ, Jaffe ES. Composite lymphoma: a clinicopathologic analysis of nine patients with Hodgkin's disease and B-cell non-Hodgkin's lymphoma. *Am J Clin Pathol* 1991;96:81–89.
175. Travis LB, Gonzalez CL, Hankey BF, et al. Hodgkin's disease following non-Hodgkin's lymphoma. *Cancer* 1992;69:2337–2342.
176. Zarate-Osorno A, Medeiros LJ, Kingma DW, et al. Hodgkin's disease following non-Hodgkin's lymphoma: a clinicopathologic and immunophenotypic study of nine cases. *Am J Surg Pathol* 1993;17: 123–132.
177. Ben-Ezra J, Sheibani K, Swartz W, et al. Relationship between eosinophil density and T-cell activation markers in lymph nodes of patients with Hodgkin's disease. *Hum Pathol* 1989;20:1181–1185.
178. Frizzera G, Moran EM, Rappaport H. Angio-immunoblastic lymphadenopathy: diagnosis and clinical course. *Am J Med* 1975;59:803–818.
179. Freter CE, Cossman J. Angioimmunoblastic lymphadenopathy with dysproteinemia. *Semin Oncol* 1993;20:627–635.
180. Nathwani BN, Rappaport H, Moran EM, et al. Malignant lymphoma arising in angio-immunoblastic lymphadenopathy. *Cancer* 1978;41: 578–606.
181. Weiss LM, Strickler JG, Dorfman RF, et al. Clonal T-cell populations in angioimmunoblastic lymphadenopathy and angioimmunoblastic lymphadenopathy-like lymphoma. *Am J Pathol* 1986;122:392–397.
182. Feller AC, Griesser H, Schilling CV, et al. Clonal gene rearrangement patterns correlate with immunophenotype and clinical parameters in patients with angioimmunoblastic lymphadenopathy. *Am J Pathol* 1988;133:549–556.
183. Schlegelberger B, Zhang Y, Weber-Matthiesen K, et al. Detection of aberrant clones in nearly all cases of angioimmunoblastic lymphadenopathy with dysproteinemia-type T-cell lymphoma by combined interphase and metaphase cytogenetics. *Blood* 1994;84:2640–2648.
184. Ree HJ, Kadin ME, Kikuchi M, et al. Angioimmunoblastic lymphoma (AILD-type T-cell lymphoma) with hyperplastic germinal centers. *Am J Surg Pathol* 1998;22:643–655.
185. Burke JS, Butler JJ. Malignant lymphoma with a high content of epithelioid histiocytes (Lennert's lymphoma). *Am J Clin Pathol* 1976; 66:1–9.
186. Kim H, Nathwani BN, Rappaport H. So-called ''Lennert's lymphoma: '' is it a clinicopathologic entity? *Cancer* 1980;45:1379–1399.
187. Patsouris E, Noel H, Lennert K. Histological and immunohistological findings in lymphoepithelioid cell lymphoma (Lennert's lymphoma). *Am J Surg Pathol* 1988;12:341–350.
188. Patsouris E, Noel H, Lennert K. Cytohistologic and immunohistochemical findings in Hodgkin's disease, mixed cellularity type, with a high content of epithelioid cells. *Am J Surg Pathol* 1989;13: 1014–1022.
189. Nguyen D, Nathwani BN, Ellison DJ, et al. Differential diagnosis between T-cell lymphoma and Hodgkin's disease: the value of mitotic counts and pericapsular infiltration. *Hematol Pathol* 1989;3:63–71.
190. Osborne BM, Uthman MO, Butler JJ, et al. Differentiation of T-cell Lymphoma from Hodgkin's disease: mitotic rate and S-phase analysis. *Am J Clin Pathol* 1990;93:227–232.
191. Banks PM. The distinction of Hodgkin's disease from T cell lymphoma. *Semin Diagn Pathol* 1992;9:279–283.
192. Medeiros LJ, Weiss LM, Warnke RA, et al. Utility of combining antigranulocyte with antileukocyte antibodies in differentiating Hodgkin's disease from non-Hodgkin's lymphoma. *Cancer* 1988;62: 2475–2481.
193. Wieczorek R, Burke JS, Knowles DM. Leu-M1 antigen expression in T-cell neoplasia. *Am J Pathol* 1985;121:374–380.
194. Sheibani K, Battifora H, Burke JS, et al. Leu-M1 antigen in human neoplasms: an immunohistologic study of 400 cases. *Am J Surg Pathol* 1986;10:227–236.
195. Meis JM, Osborne BM, Butler JJ. A comparative marker study of large cell lymphoma, Hodgkin's disease, and true histiocytic lymphoma in paraffin-embedded tissue. *Am J Clin Pathol* 1986;86:591–599.
196. Kinney MC, Kadin ME. The pathologic and clinical spectrum of anaplastic large cell lymphoma and correlation with ALK gene dysregulation. *Am J Clin Pathol* 1999;111(suppl 1):S56–S67.
197. Bearman RM, Pangalis GA, Rappaport H. Hodgkin's disease, lymphocyte depletion type: a clinicopathologic study of 39 patients. *Cancer* 1978;41:293–302.
198. Greer JP, Kinney MC, Cousar JB, et al. Lymphocyte-depleted Hodgkin's disease: clinicopathologic review of 25 patients. *Am J Med* 1986; 81:208–214.
199. Kant JA, Hubbard SM, Longo DL, et al. The pathologic and clinical heterogeneity of lymphocyte-depleted Hodgkin's disease. *J Clin Oncol* 1986;4:284–294.
200. Kinney MC, Greer JP, Collins RD. Assessment of lymphocyte depleted Hodgkin's disease, reticular variant (LDHD-R) by monoclonal antibodies reactive in paraffin sections. *Mod Pathol* 1991;4:75A(abst).
201. Leoncini L, Del Vecchio MT, Kraft R, et al. Hodgkin's disease and CD30-positive anaplastic large cell lymphomas: a continuous spectrum of malignant disorders. A quantitative morphometric and immunohistologic study. *Am J Pathol* 1990;137:1047–1057.
202. Frizzera G. The distinction of Hodgkin's disease from anaplastic large cell lymphoma. *Semin Diagn Pathol* 1992;9:291–296.
203. Pardmore RF, Finn WG, Singleton TP, et al. Fascin expression in immunophenotypic variants of classic Hodgkin's disease. *Mod Pathol* 1999;12:144A(abst).
204. Nakamura S, Nagahama M, Kagami Y, et al. Hodgkin's disease expressing follicular dendritic cell marker CD21 without any other B-cell marker. *Am J Surg Pathol* 1999;23:363–376.
205. R^{n}diger T, Jaffe ES, Delsol G, et al. Workshop report on Hodgkin's disease and related diseases (''grey zone'' lymphoma). *Ann Oncol* 1998;9(Suppl 5):S31–S38.
206. Zinzani PL, Martelli M, Magagnoli M, et al. Anaplastic large cell lymphoma Hodgkin's-like: a randomized trial of ABVD versus MACOP-B with and without radiation therapy. *Blood* 1998;92: 790–794.
207. Burke JS. Surgical pathology of the spleen: an approach to the differential diagnosis of splenic lymphomas and leukemias. Part I. Diseases of the white pulp. *Am J Surg Pathol* 1981;5:551–563.
208. Hoppe RT, Rosenberg SA, Kaplan HS, et al. Prognostic factors in pathological stage IIIA Hodgkin's disease. *Cancer* 1980;46: 1240–1246.
209. Kadin ME, Donaldson SS, Dorfman RF. Isolated granulomas in Hodgkin's disease. *N Engl J Med* 1970;283:859–861.
210. Sacks EL, Donaldson SS, Gordon J, et al. Epithelioid granulomas associated with Hodgkin's disease: clinical correlations in 55 previously untreated patients. *Cancer* 1978;41:562–567.
211. Burke JS, Osborne BM. Localized reactive lymphoid hyperplasia of the spleen simulating malignant lymphoma: a report of seven cases. *Am J Surg Pathol* 1983;7:373–380.
212. Thomas RM, Jaffe ES, Zarate-Osorno A, et al. Inflammatory pseudotumor of the spleen: a clinicopathologic and immunophenotypic study of eight cases. *Arch Pathol Lab Med* 1993;117:921–926.
213. Bagley CM Jr, Roth JA, Thomas LB, et al. Liver biopsy in Hodgkin's disease: clinicopathologic correlations in 127 patients. *Ann Intern Med* 1972;76:219–225.
214. Dich NH, Goodman ZD, Klein MA. Hepatic involvement in Hodgkin's disease: clues to histologic diagnosis. *Cancer* 1989;64: 2121–2126.
215. O'Carroll DI, McKenna RW, Brunning RD. Bone marrow manifestations of Hodgkin's disease. *Cancer* 1976;38:1717–1728.
216. Te Velde J, Den Ottolander GJ, Spaander PJ, et al. The bone marrow in Hodgkin's disease: the non-involved marrow. *Histopathology* 1978; 2:31–46.
217. Bartl R, Frisch B, Burkhardt R, et al. Assessment of bone marrow histology in Hodgkin's disease: correlation with clinical factors. *Br J Haematol* 1982;51:345–360.
218. Munker R, Hasenclever D, Brosteanu O, et al. Bone marrow involve-

ment in Hodgkin's disease: an analysis of 135 consecutive cases. *J Clin Oncol* 1995;13:403–409.

219. Wood NL, Coltman CA Jr. Localized primary extranodal Hodgkin's disease. *Ann Intern Med* 1973;78:113–118.
220. Radin AI. Primary pulmonary Hodgkin's disease. *Cancer* 1990;65:550–563.
221. Kern WH, Crepeau A, Jones JC. Primary Hodgkin's disease of the lung: report of four cases and review of the literature. *Cancer* 1961;14:1151–1165.
222. Yousem SA, Weiss LM, Colby TV. Primary pulmonary Hodgkin's disease: a clinicopathologic study of 15 cases. *Cancer* 1986;57:1217–1224.
223. Sapozink MD, Kaplan HS. Intracranial Hodgkin's disease: a report of 12 cases and review of the literature. *Cancer* 1983;52:1301–1307.
224. Ashby MA, Barber PC, Holmes AE, et al. Primary intracranial Hodgkin's disease: a case report and discussion. *Am J Surg Pathol* 1988;12:294–299.
225. Higgins SA, Peschel RE. Hodgkin's disease with spinal cord compression: a case report and review of the literature. *Cancer* 1995;75:94–98.
226. Smith JL Jr, Butler JJ. Skin involvement in Hodgkin's disease. *Cancer* 1980;45:354–361.
227. Sioutos N, Kerl H, Murphy SB, et al. Primary cutaneous Hodgkin's disease: unique clinical, morphologic, and immunophenotypic findings. *Am J Dermatopathol* 1994;16:2–8.
228. Kumar S, Kingma DW, Weiss WB, et al. Primary cutaneous Hodgkin's disease with evolution to systemic disease: association with the Epstein-Barr virus. *Am J Surg Pathol* 1996;20:754–759.
229. Willemze R, Beljaards RC. Spectrum of primary cutaneous CD30 (Ki-1)-positive lymphoproliferative disorders: a proposal for classification and guidelines for management and treatment. *Am Acad Dermatopathol* 1993;28:973–980.
230. Paulli M, Berti E, Rosso R, et al. CD30/Ki-1-positive lymphoproliferative disorders of the skin: clinicopathologic correlation and statistical analysis of 86 cases. A multicentric study from the European Organization for Research and Treatment of Cancer Cutaneous Lymphoma Project Group. *J Clin Oncol* 1995;13:1343–1354.
231. Willemze R, Kerl H, Sterry W, et al. EORTC classification for primary cutaneous lymphomas: a proposal from the Cutaneous Lymphoma Study Group of the European Organization for Research and Treatment of Cancer. *Blood* 1997;90:354–371.
232. Meis JM, Butler JJ, Osborne BM. Hodgkin's disease involving the breast and chest wall. *Cancer* 1986;57:1859–1865.
233. Soderstrom K-O, Joensuu H. Primary Hodgkin's disease of the stomach. *Am J Clin Pathol* 1988;89:806–809.
234. Devaney K, Jaffe ES. The surgical pathology of gastrointestinal Hodgkin's disease. *Am J Clin Pathol* 1991;95:794–801.
235. Vanbockrijck M, Cabooter M, Casselman J, et al. Primary Hodgkin's disease of the ileum complicating Crohn disease. *Cancer* 1993;72:1784–1789.
236. Thomas DB, Huston BM, Lamm KR, et al. Primary Hodgkin's disease of the sigmoid colon: a case report and review of the literature. *Arch Pathol Lab Med* 1997;121:528–532.
237. Kumar S, Kingma DW, Quintanilla-Martinez L, et al. EBV + primary gastrointestinal Hodgkin's disease: association with inflammatory bowel disease and immunosuppression. *Mod Pathol* 1999;12:141A(abst).
238. Todd GB, Michaels L. Hodgkin's disease involving Waldeyer's lymphoid ring. *Cancer* 1974;34:1769–1778.
239. Kapadia SB, Roman LN, Kingma DW, et al. Hodgkin's disease of Waldeyer's ring: clinical and histoimmunophenotypic findings and association with Epstein-Barr virus in 16 cases. *Am J Surg Pathol* 1995;19:1431–1439.
240. Ozdemirli M, Mankin HJ, Aisenberg AC, et al. Hodgkin's disease presenting as a solitary bone tumor: a report of four cases and review of the literature. *Cancer* 1996;77:79–88.
241. Ostrowski ML, Inwards CY, Strickler JG, et al. Osseous Hodgkin's disease. *Cancer* 1999;85:1166–1178.
242. Young RC, Canellos GP, Chabner BA, et al. Patterns of relapse in advanced Hodgkin's disease treated with combination chemotherapy. *Cancer* 1978;42:1001–1007.
243. Herman TS, Hoppe RT, Donaldson SS, et al. Late relapse among patients treated for Hodgkin's disease. *Ann Intern Med* 1985;102:292–297.
244. Brierley JD, Rathmell AJ, Gospodarowicz MK, et al. Late relapse after treatment for clinical stage I and II Hodgkin's disease. *Cancer* 1997;79:1422–1427.
245. Colby TW, Hoppe RT, Warnke RA. Hodgkin's disease at autopsy: 1972–1977. *Cancer* 1981;47:1852–1862.
246. Grogan TM, Berard CW, Steinhorn SC, et al. Changing patterns of Hodgkin's disease at autopsy: a 25-year experience at the National Cancer Institute, 1953–1978. *Cancer Treat Rep* 1982;66:653–665.
247. Strum SB, Rappaport H. The persistence of Hodgkin's disease in long term survivors. *Am J Med* 1971;51:222–240.
248. Van Rijswijk REN, Verbeek J, Haanen C, et al. Major complications and causes of death in patients treated for Hodgkin's disease. *J Clin Oncol* 1987;5:1624–1633.
249. Hancock SL, Hoppe RT. Long-term complications of treatment and causes of mortality after Hodgkin's disease. *Semin Radiat Oncol* 1996;6:225–242.
250. Hudson MM, Poquette CA, Lee J, et al. Increased mortality after successful treatment for Hodgkin's disease. *J Clin Oncol* 1998;16:3592–3600.
251. Vasef MA, Alsabeh R, Medeiros LJ, et al. Immunophenotype of Reed-Sternberg and Hodgkin's cells in sequential biopsy specimens of Hodgkin's disease: a paraffin-section immunohistochemical study using the heat-induced epitope retrieval method. *Am J Clin Pathol* 1997;108:54–59.
252. Chu W-S, Abbondanzo SL, Frizzera G. Inconsistency of the immunophenotype of Reed-Sternberg cells in simultaneous and consecutive specimens from the same patients: a paraffin section evaluation in 56 patients. *Am J Pathol* 1992;141:11–17.
253. Colby TV, Warnke RA. The histology of the initial relapse of Hodgkin's disease. *Cancer* 1980;45:289–292.
254. Dolginow D, Colby TV. Recurrent Hodgkin's disease in treated sites. *Cancer* 1981;48:1124–1126.
255. Chao N, Levine J, Horning SJ. Retroperitoneal fibrosis following treatment for Hodgkin's disease. *J Clin Oncol* 1987;5:231–232.
256. Chen JL, Osborne BM, Butler JJ. Residual fibrous masses in treated Hodgkin's disease. *Cancer* 1987;60:407–413.
257. Dmitrovsky E, Martin SE, Krudy AG, et al. Lymph node aspiration in the management of Hodgkin's disease. *J Clin Oncol* 1986;4:306–310.
258. Krikorian JG, Burke JS, Rosenberg SA, et al. Occurrence of non-Hodgkin's lymphoma after therapy for Hodgkin's disease. *N Engl J Med* 1979;300:452–458.
259. Zarate-Orsorno A, Medeiros LJ, Longo DL, et al. Non-Hodgkin's lymphomas arising in patients successfully treated for Hodgkin's disease: a clinical, histologic, and immunophenotypic study of 14 cases. *Am J Surg Pathol* 1992;16:885–895.
260. Ohno T, Trenn G, Wu G, et al. The clonal relationship between nodular sclerosis Hodgkin's disease with a clonal Reed-Sternberg cell population and a subsequent B-cell small noncleaved cell lymphoma. *Mod Pathol* 1998;11:485–490.
261. Gaulier A, Teillet F, Davi F, et al. Pleomorphic medium-sized T-cell lymphoma following Hodgkin's disease (nodular sclerosis type). *Arch Pathol Lab Med* 1997;121:411–416.
262. Casey TT, Cousar JB, Mangum M, et al. Monomorphic lymphomas arising in patients with Hodgkin's disease: correlation of morphologic, immunophenotypic, and molecular genetic findings in 12 cases. *Am J Pathol* 1990;136:81–94.
263. Kingma DW, Medeiros LJ, Barletta J, et al. Epstein-Barr virus is infrequently identified in non-Hodgkin's lymphomas associated with Hodgkin's disease. *Am J Surg Pathol* 1994;18:48–61.

CHAPTER 18

Hodgkin's Disease: Cell of Origin, Immunobiology, and Pathogenesis

Marshall E. Kadin

A conceptual understanding of Hodgkin's disease (HD) is based on the pivotal role of the Reed-Sternberg (RS) cell in the pathogenesis of HD. The RS cell has gained general acceptance as being the malignant cell in HD. In this chapter, new information regarding the nature of the RS cell is considered. Advances have been made in this regard because of the development of methods for analysis of genes in single cells using polymerase chain reaction (PCR) amplification. Most evidence points to the origin of the RS cell from a post–germinal center B lymphocyte that has undergone immunoglobulin gene hypermutations in classic HD and a germinal center B lymphocyte with ongoing mutations in nodular lymphocyte predominance (LP) HD. Derivation of the RS cell from a lymphocyte is supported by case reports and small patient series that show a clonal relationship between tumor cells in HD and in non-Hodgkin's lymphomas (NHLs). There are data to suggest that in a minority of HD cases, RS cells are derived from T lymphocytes, particularly those that contain cytotoxic molecules. A lymphoid origin for the RS cell is supported by the finding of nonrandom chromosome abnormalities associated with lymphoid neoplasms in HD tissues. Epstein-Barr virus (EBV) appears to play a role in the pathogenesis of HD through the interaction of latent membrane protein-1 (LMP-1) with signaling proteins of the tumor necrosis factor (TNF) receptor superfamily and the transcription factor, NF-κB. RS cells represent only a small proportion of the cellular constituents of HD, and the remaining cellular and fibrous tissue elements appear to be a consequence of cytokines or growth factors secreted by RS cells and the responding inflammatory cells in their microenvironment. Tumor-derived cytokines appear to be responsible for some important clinical manifestations of HD, including B symptoms and immunosuppression. Among these is a defect in the cytotoxic T-cell response to LMP-1 in the presence of EBV, probably mediated by transforming growth factor-β (TGF-β).

M. E. Kadin: Departments of Pathology, Beth Israel Deaconess Medical Center and Harvard Medical School, Boston, Massachusetts

NATURE OF THE REED-STERNBERG CELL

Evidence of Origin from a Germinal Center B Lymphocyte

Pioneering work on this subject was done by the group of Rajewsky in Cologne, Germany, who amplified immunoglobulin genes from single Hodgkin's–RS (HRS) cells and compared them with normal germinal center B cells (1–3). Sequence analysis of immunoglobulin heavy and light chain gene rearrangements amplified from isolated HRS cells in 13 cases of classic HD revealed that HRS cells harbored somatically mutated immunoglobulin variable region genes in 12 cases. "Crippling" mutations creating stop codons within in-frame potentially functional variable region genes were detected in 4 of these 12 cases. Rearrangements of variable region heavy or light chain genes were clonal, indicating a clonal derivation of HRS cells in these cases. The finding of somatic mutations within the rearranged immunoglobulin genes of HRS cells strongly suggests that they are derived from germinal center B cells or memory B cells in these cases. A scenario for the generation of HRS cells from germinal centers is depicted in Figure 18.1.

Not all groups initially found clonal immunoglobulin gene rearrangements in HRS cells (4,5). Some investigators failed to detect immunoglobulin gene rearrangements; others found only polyclonal or polyclonal and monoclonal immunoglobulin gene rearrangements in HD tissues. These different results could be explained by non–B cell precursors to

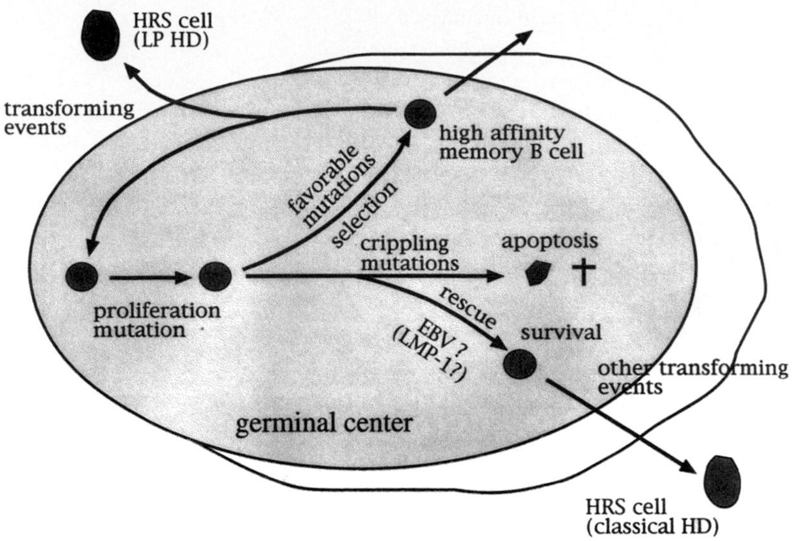

FIG. 18.1. Schema for development of Reed-Sternberg cells from germinal center B cells in lymphocyte predominance and classic Hodgkin's disease. (From Kuppers R, Rajewsky K. The origin of Hodgkin and Reed/Sternberg cells in Hodgkin's disease. *Ann Rev Immunol* 1998; 16:471–493.

HRS cells in a minority of patients with HD. Alternatively, the lack of clonal immunoglobulin gene rearrangements could result from technical artifacts in the amplification of immunoglobulin genes, resulting in the lack of detectable immunoglobulin gene rearrangements, or the amplification of immunoglobulin genes from surrounding non-malignant B lymphocytes in HD tissues, producing a pattern of polyclonal B lymphocytes in other cases (6). Further studies, including reinvestigation of some of the originally ''polyclonal'' cases, reached a consensus that most cases of classic HD contain HRS cells with clonal immunoglobulin gene rearrangements (7).

Lymphocyte Predominance HD Contains HRS Cells with Ongoing Immunoglobulin Mutations

As in classic HD, somatic mutations in immunoglobulin gene rearrangements have been detected in LPHD. There are differences in the mutation pattern between classic HD and LPHD. LPHD showed ongoing mutations within clonal immunoglobulin gene rearrangements with intraclonal diversity in 13 of 21 cases analyzed (8–10); somatic hypermutation of immunoglobulin genes appears to be ongoing in LPHD. The ongoing mutations identify mutating germinal center B cells as precursors of HRS cells in LPHD, whereas the lack of ongoing mutations indicate that the HRS cells in classic HD are derived from post-germinal center or memory B cells.

Derivation of HD from B Lymphocytes Is Supported by the Clonal Relationship between HD and B-cell Neoplasms

Further evidence to support a B-lymphocytic origin for most cases of HD comes from the demonstration of a common clonal immunoglobulin gene rearrangement in HD and B cell malignancies. Ohno and coworkers (11) found that IgH CDR3 sequences from HRS cells were identical to those from chronic lymphocytic leukemia B cells in two of three patients with Richter's syndrome in whom chronic lymphocytic leukemia had undergone transformation to a morphologic picture of HD. Wickert and coworkers (12) demonstrated a clonal relationship between LPHD and concurrent or subsequent large cell lymphoma of B lineage in two of nine cases analyzed. Kuppers and Rajewsky (13) found the same somatically mutated clonal immunoglobulin heavy and light chain gene rearrangements in a composite lymphoma of HD and follicular lymphoma occurring in the same lymph node. In this unusual case, several nucleotide differences between the tumor cells of the HD and follicular lymphoma indicated that they were derived from two distinct members of a germinal center B-cell clone. These studies demonstrate that in some cases of HD the HRS cells share a common clonal origin with tumor cells in B-cell leukemia or lymphoma, supporting the origin of HRS cells from a B lymphocyte in these cases.

Other evidence supporting a germinal center origin for HRS cells comes from their expression of BCL-6, a transcription factor expressed in germinal center B cells, and CD138, or syndecan-1 (SYN-1), a proteoglycan associated with post–germinal center terminal B-cell differentiation. Carbone and coworkers (14) found that tumor cells in LPHD consistently display a BCL-6–positive ($BCL\text{-}6^+$) SYN-1–negative ($SYN\text{-}1^-$) phenotype, consistent with derivation from germinal center B cells. In classic HD, the tumor cells have a more heterogeneous phenotype, because in a fraction of classic HD they are $BCL\text{-}6^-SYN\text{-}1^+$, characteristic of post germinal center B cells, whereas another fraction of classic HD consists of a mixture of tumor cells reflecting either a germinal center ($BCL\text{-}6^+SYN\text{-}1^-$) or a post-germinal center ($BCL\text{-}6^-SYN\text{-}1^+$) (14) phenotype.

Evidence for Origin of HRS cells from Dendritic Cells

Dendritic cells are potent antigen-presenting cells in germinal centers (follicular dendritic cells) and interfollicular areas (interdigitating dendritic cells) of lymph nodes. Similar to normal dendritic cells, HRS cells have been shown to be capable of antigen presentation (15) and to stimulate mixed leukocyte cultures (16). RS cells in HD also express the B7 costimulatory molecule present on antigen-presenting cells (17). Activated B and T lymphocytes, however, are also capable of antigen presentation and expression of costimulatory molecules (18,19).

Curran and Jones (20) were the first to propose that HRS cells might be derived from follicular dendritic cells, based on the similar silver impregnation staining patterns of HRS cells and follicular dendritic cells. Delsol and coworkers (21) further noted the intimate association of HRS cells with the follicular dendritic cell network and the similar expression of CD21 antigen by follicular dendritic cells and HRS cells. Moreover, they described the common expression of IgG Fc receptors and the presence of polyclonal IgG and IgE within the cytoplasm of follicular dendritic cells and HRS cells. Other evidence for a follicular dendritic cell origin for HRS cells comes from analysis of a series of 94 patients with HD by Nakamura and colleagues (22) in which they identified nine cases (9.6%) as positive for HRS cell expression of CD21 without any other B-cell marker. Of these nine patients, six had HRS cells with distinctive walnut-shaped or cerebriform nuclei and cytoplasmic processes and three had multinucleated RS cells with triangular nuclei, but without cytoplasmic processes. In none of these nine cases were rearrangements of immunoglobulin heavy chain or T-cell receptor (TCR) genes found. Kennedy and coworkers (23) described other similarities between the HRS cells and dendritic cells. Soderstrom and coworkers (24) detected an acid cysteine proteinase inhibitor characteristic of normal follicular dendritic cells in HRS cells of classic HD but not those of LPHD.

Hodgkin's–RS cells also share characteristics with interdigitating dendritic cells (25–27). HRS cells and interdigitating dendritic cells have highly irregular nuclei, are surrounded by T lymphocytes that indent their cytoplasmic projections, show minimal phagocytosis, and have similar cytochemical staining for acid nonspecific esterase and acid phosphatase (25,26). Pinkus and coworkers (27) demonstrated a similar staining profile for HRS and interdigitating dendritic cells for fascin, a 55-kd actin-bundling protein, in classic HD. Both HRS and interdigitating dendritic cells consistently show strong diffuse cytoplasmic staining for fascin, which reveals their dendritic outlines, particularly in nodular sclerosis (NS) (Fig. 18.2). Normal B and T lymphocytes are negative for fascin, and neoplasms of B and T

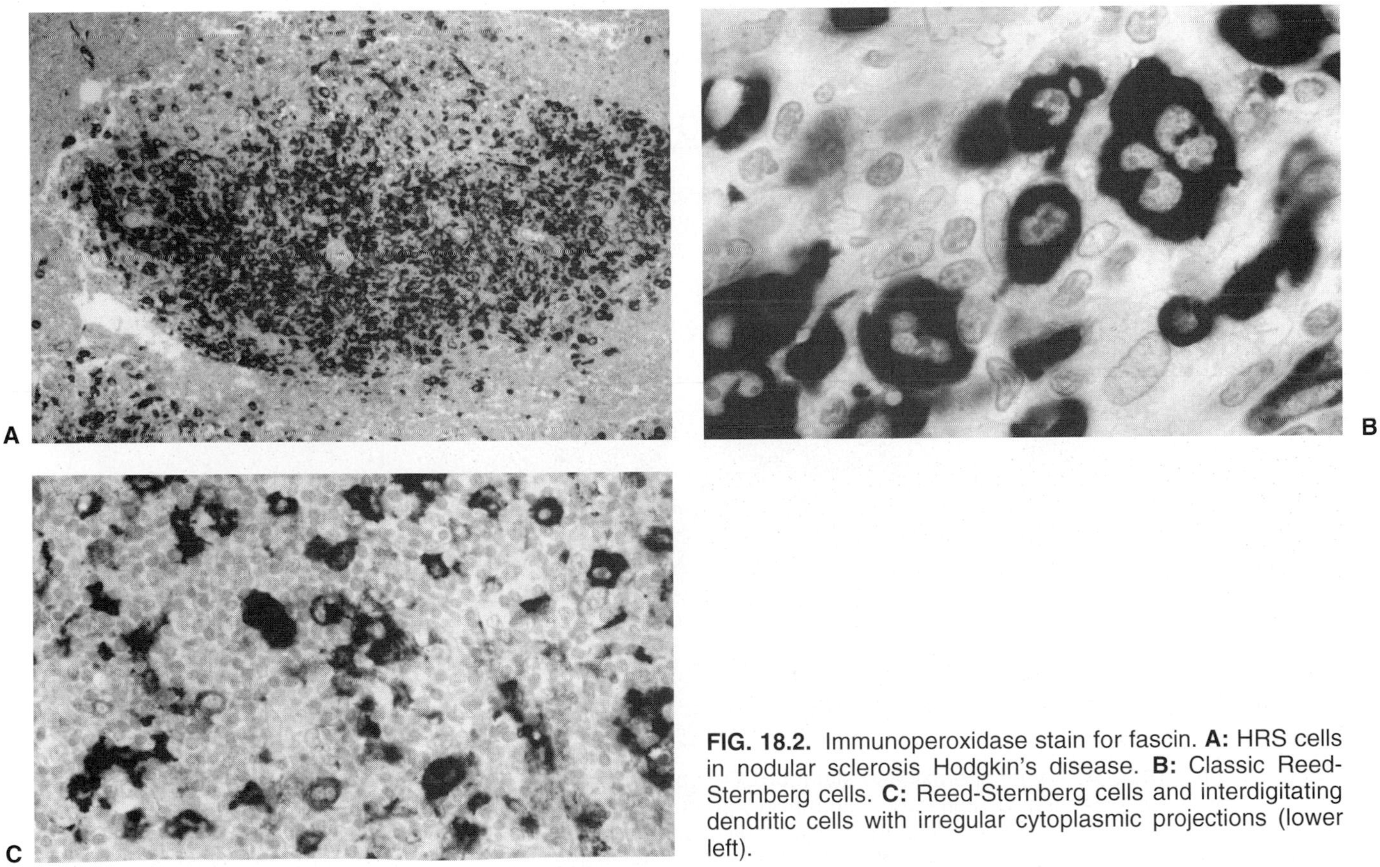

FIG. 18.2. Immunoperoxidase stain for fascin. **A:** HRS cells in nodular sclerosis Hodgkin's disease. **B:** Classic Reed-Sternberg cells. **C:** Reed-Sternberg cells and interdigitating dendritic cells with irregular cytoplasmic projections (lower left).

lymphocytes show infrequent and weak fascin staining. Tumor cells in anaplastic large cell lymphoma (ALCL) often are weakly reactive, in contrast to the strong fascin staining of HRS cells. Fascin expression can be induced in B cells after EBV infection. This observation would not provide an explanation for the discrepancy between fascin staining of HRS cells in all cases of classic HD and detection of EBV in only a fraction of HD cases, usually one third to one half (28).

Evidence of Origin of Hodgkin's–Reed-Sternberg Cells from T Lymphocytes

Several HD cell lines (L538, L540, CO, HDLM-1, HDLM-2, HDLM-3) have clonal TCR gene rearrangements and expression of T-cell antigens (reviewed by Drexler [29]). *In vivo* studies have noted the presence of T-cell antigens on the surface and often within the cytoplasm of HRS cells (30–34) (Fig. 18.3). There can be difficulty distinguishing true staining of HRS cells from that of surrounding T lymphocytes, and there is the possibility of absorption of T-cell antigens by HRS cells. Recently, several groups have noted the presence of cytotoxic molecules (granzyme B, perforin, and TIA-1) in HRS cells in 10% to 18% of patients with classic HD (35–38) (Fig. 18.4). Granzyme B, perforin, and TIA-1 normally are found in cytotoxic T lymphocytes and natural killer cells. Because HRS cells do not express other markers of natural killer cells but do express T-cell antigens in a similar percentage of cases, these studies sup-

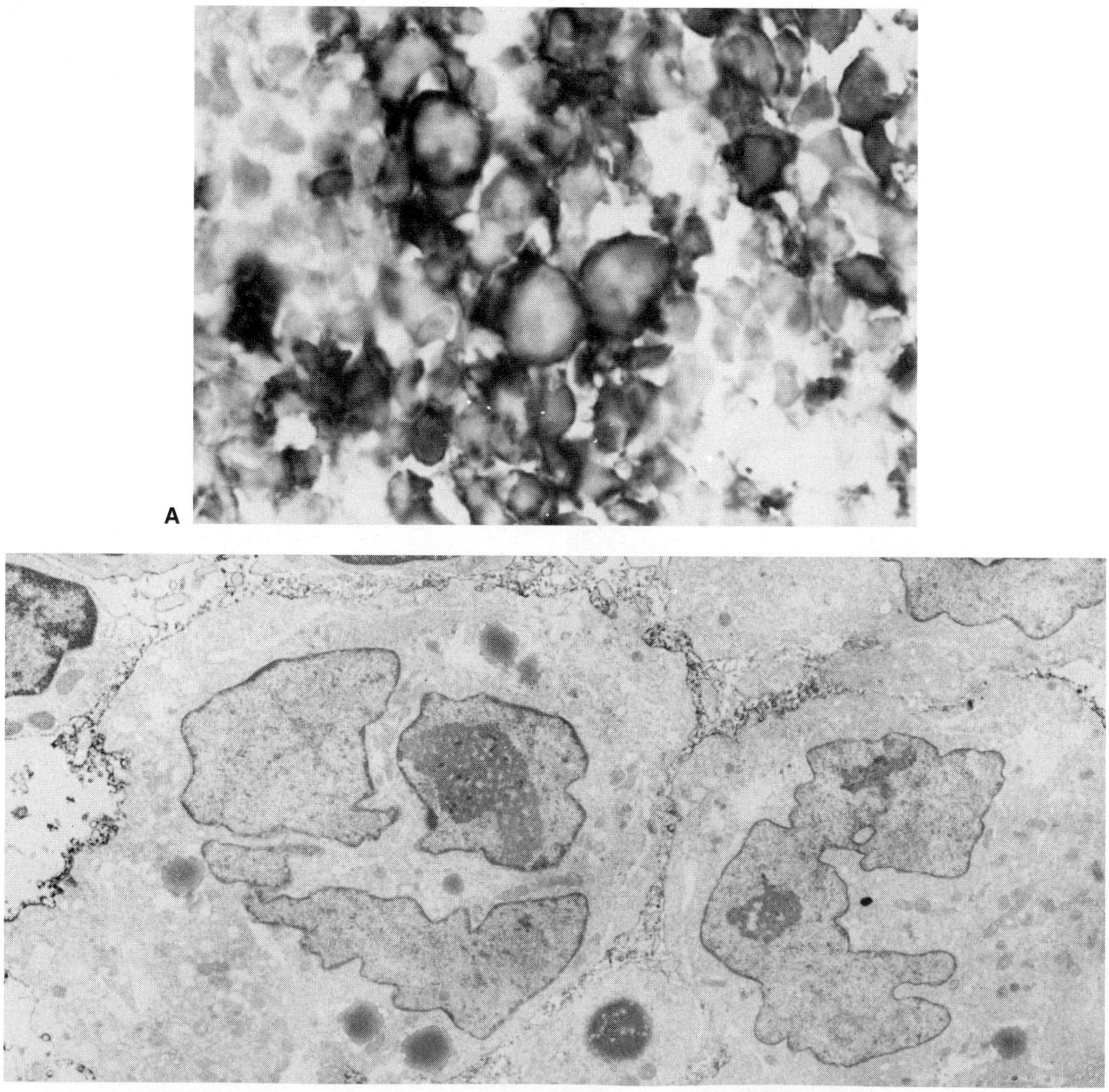

A

B

FIG. 18.3. A: Immunoperoxidase stain for CD4 antigen on Reed-Sternberg cells in mixed cellularity Hodgkin's disease. **B:** Immunoelectron micrograph shows surface staining for CD2 antigen on Reed-Sternberg cells in mixed cellularity Hodgkin's disease. (From Kadin ME, Muramoto L, Said J. Expression of T cell antigens by Reed-Sternberg cells in Hodgkin's disease. *Am J Pathol* 1988;130:345–353, with permission.)

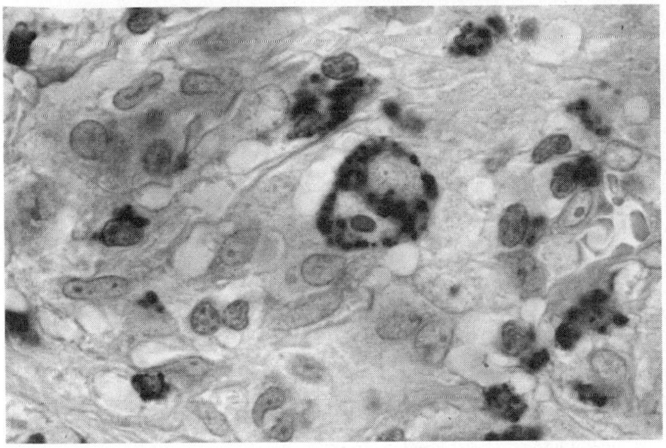

FIG. 18.4. Immunoperoxidase stain for cytotoxic protein TIA-1 shows cytoplasmic staining of Reed-Sternberg cell and surrounding lymphocytes.

port the origin of HRS cells from cytotoxic T lymphocytes in a minority of cases of classic HD.

Additional evidence for a T-cell origin of HRS cells in some cases of HD comes from the coexistence, and sometimes demonstrated clonal relationship, between HD and T-cell malignancies. HD has been associated with mycosis fungoides, lymphomatoid papulosis, and anaplastic or pleomorphic T-cell lymphomas in some patients (39–41). A clonal relationship among HD, mycosis fungoides, and lymphomatoid papulosis has been demonstrated in one patient (39). Cytotoxic molecules demonstrated in the HRS cells of this pateient suggest that the HRS cells are derived from cytotoxic T lymphocytes (M. E. Kadin, 1998, unpublished data). Absence of the ALK kinase gene of ALCL (42,43) supports the interpretation of HD. Three recent studies have shown that HRS cells in classic HD harbor clonal rearrangements of TCR genes in a small percentage of cases (1%–5%), whereas immunoglobulin heavy and light chain genes are in the germline configuration, (44,45). Using PCR amplification of antigen receptor genes from single HRS cells, Muschen and coworkers (44) found clonal TCR β chain VDJ rearrangement in one of three patients with HD in whom HRS cells expressed cytotoxic T-cell markers. Similarly, Hummel and colleagues (45) detected clonal TCR γ chain rearrangements in HRS cells in 2 of 13 patients with classic HD with T-cell marker–positive HRS cells. Finally, Willenbrock and collaborators (45a) detected identical clonal rearrangements of the TCR β chain gene in HRS cells of a cutaneous lymphoma and lymph node of mixed cellularity HD from a single patient. Thus, the derivation of HRS cells from T lymphocytes, particularly cytotoxic T lymphocytes, appears to occur in a small percentage of cases of classic HD.

Immunophenotype of the Reed-Sternberg Cell

Each type of HD is associated with a particular pattern of lymph node involvement, unique appearance, and immunophenotype of the RS cell. These features are summarized in Table 18.1.

Lymphocyte Predominance Hodgkin's Disease

The RS cell and its variants in nodular LPHD (NLPHD) have a B-cell phenotype (46). Lymphocytic and histiocytic (L&H) variants of RS cells express CD20, a pan–B cell marker detectable in both frozen and paraffin-fixed tissue sections (Fig. 18.5). Stein and colleagues (47) demonstrated the unique expression of J chain in RS cells in NLPHD. Since only B cells synthesize J chain, this finding provides further evidence that L&H variants are derived from B cells. The B-cell phenotype of L&H cells is consistent with their localization in altered germinal centers in NLPHD (48–50).

Poppema and colleagues (48,49) compared the histologic features of NLPHD with those of progressively transformed germinal centers, which are enlarged follicles showing a predominance of small lymphocytes and some residual ger-

TABLE 18.1. *Summary of morphology and phenotype of Reed-Sternberg cells in different histologic types of Hodgkin's disease*

Histologic type	Reed-Sternberg cell variant	Pattern	Phenotype	Appearance
Mixed cellularity	Classical	Interfollicular or diffuse	null>B>T; CD30$^+$, CD15$^+$, CD40$^+$, Fascin$^+$, CD45 –, CD74$^+$ CDW75$^-$, EMA$^-$, EBV$^\pm$	Binucleate/multinucleated with huge inclusion-like eosinophilic nucleoli
Nodular sclerosis	Lacunar cell	Inter- or intrafollicular	null>B>T; CD30$^+$, CD15$^+$, CD40$^+$, Fascin$^+$, CD45$^-$, CD74$^+$, CDW75$^-$, EMA$^-$, EBV$^\pm$	Pale retracted cytoplasm; one to many nuclei; small, sometimes basophilic nucleoli
Lymphocyte predominance	Lymphocytic and histiocytic or popcorn cell	Intrafollicular	B; CD30$^\pm$, CD15$^-$, CD40$^+$, Fascin$^-$, CD45$^+$, CD74$^+$, CDW75$^+$, EMA$^+$	Wrinkled, twisted nucleus, small nucleoli
Lymphocytic-depletion	Sarcomatous	Diffuse fibrosis	Unknown, CD30$^+$, CD15$^+$, CD40$^+$, Fascin$^+$, CD45$^-$, CD74$^+$, CDW75$^-$, EMA$^-$, EBV$^\pm$	Pleomorphic hyperchromatic nuclei, nucleoli often indistinct

EBV, Epstein-Barr virus; EMA, epithelial membrane antigen.

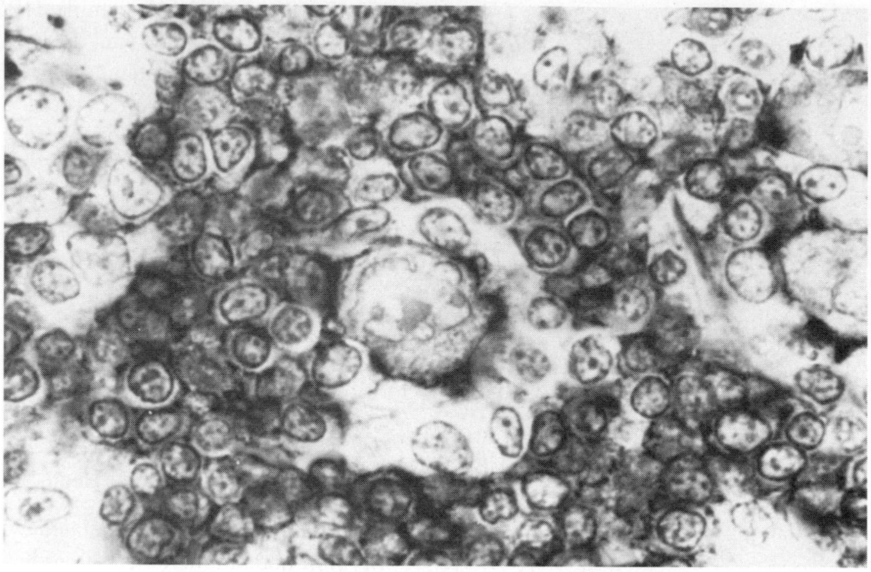

FIG. 18.5. Lymphocytic and histiocytic "popcorn" variant of Reed-Sternberg cell in nodular lymphocyte predominance Hodgkin's disease, stained for B-cell antigen L26 (CD20). Most surrounding lymphocytes also are stained.

minal center cells. Progressively transformed germinal centers sometimes are found in nonspecific lymphadenopathy (reactive hyperplasia) (49). The histologic similarity and coexistence or subsequent presence of both NLPHD and progressively transformed germinal centers in lymph nodes from the same patient suggest that NLPHD originates in progressively transformed germinal centers (48,49).

Timens and associates (50) provided further evidence that NLPHD is derived from germinal centers. They demonstrated that NLPHD is confined to follicles that contain predominantly small lymphocytes, usually more than 50% B cells, and large numbers of dendritic cells. The B lymphocytes are polyclonal. The T lymphocytes in these follicles are derived from a subpopulation of $CD4^+$ lymphocytes, which express the natural killer cell antigen CD57 and occur in normal germinal centers. These lymphocytes belong to a subpopulation of activated helper-inducer memory T cells ($CD4^+CD57^+CD45RO^+CD45RA^-$), which normally are confined to the light zone of germinal centers of secondary follicles (51). The function of $CD4^+CD57^+$ T cells in germinal centers in unknown, although their presence in late stages of germinal center reactions suggests a regulatory role in B-cell differentiation toward memory B cells. The exclusive presence of $CD4^+CD57^+$ T cells around RS cells establishes an additional immunohistochemical criterion for the diagnosis of NLPHD (51).

The B-cell phenotype of the RS cell in NLPHD may help to explain the progression of LPHD to large cell lymphoma of B-cell type in about 2% to 10% of patients (52–54). In a follow-up study of 537 patients with NLPHD, Hansmann and coworkers found the simultaneous presence of ($n = 11$) or subsequent transition to ($n = 3$) a large cell lymphoma in 14 cases. All patients studied showed a B-cell phenotype, with monotypic immunoglobulin demonstrated in five. Sundeen and coworkers (55) have described large clusters of B cells in lymph nodes of patients with NLPHD, which they have interpreted as early histologic progression to large cell lymphoma (Fig. 18.6). A longer duration of survival was found in patients with large cell lymphoma secondary to NLPHD than in patients with primary B-cell large cell lymphoma (54,55).

The diagnosis of LPHD may be difficult on the basis of morphology alone, as revealed by an immunohistochemical analysis of 208 cases of HD reviewed by the German Hodgkin's Disease Study Group (56). Immunohistochemistry disproved the morphologic diagnosis of LPHD of the expert panel in 25 of 104 cases, whereas 13 cases originally not confirmed by the panel as being LPHD showed an LPHD-like immunophenotype. Patients who were confirmed immunohistochemically as having LPHD had a significantly better likelihood of freedom from treatment failure ($P = 0.033$) than those with classic HD.

Reed-Sternberg Cells in Classic Hodgkin's Disease

Reed-Sternberg cells and their variants in classic HD commonly express activation antigens CD30 (Ki-1/Ber-H2), CD15 (Leu M1), CD25 (Tac), CD71 (transferrin receptor), and la (HLA-DR) (Fig. 18.7). The CD30 antigen was recognized first by monoclonal antibody Ki-1 raised against the HD cell line L428 (57). Expression of the CD30 antigen, together with the interleukin-2 (IL-2) receptor (CD25), can be induced on normal lymphoid cells of both T- and B-cell types by exposure to phytohemagglutinin, human T-cell leukemia viruses, EBV, or *Staphylococcus aureus* (58). The Ki-1 antibody reacts with RS cells and a subpopulation of

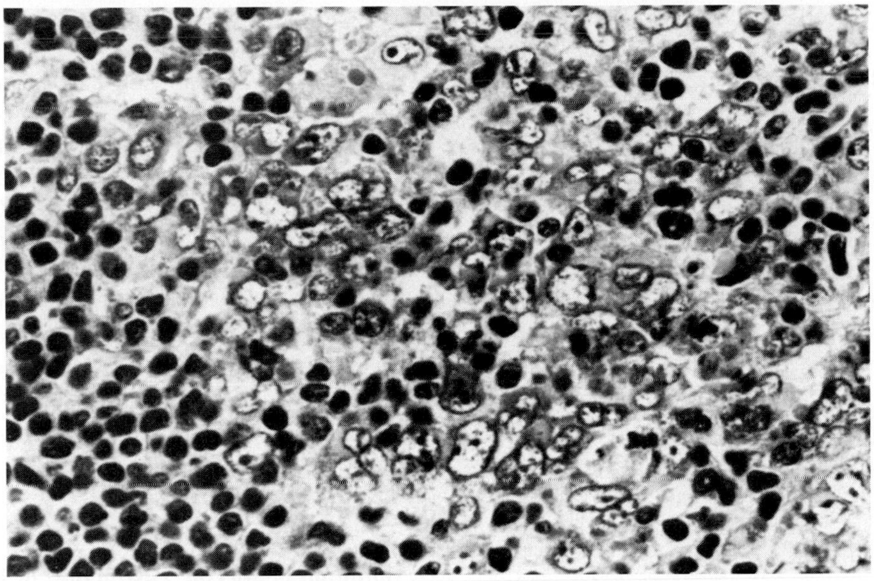

FIG. 18.6. Cluster of large cells in nodular lymphocyte predominance Hodgkin's disease. Such clusters have been interpreted as histologic evidence of an evolving large cell lymphoma.

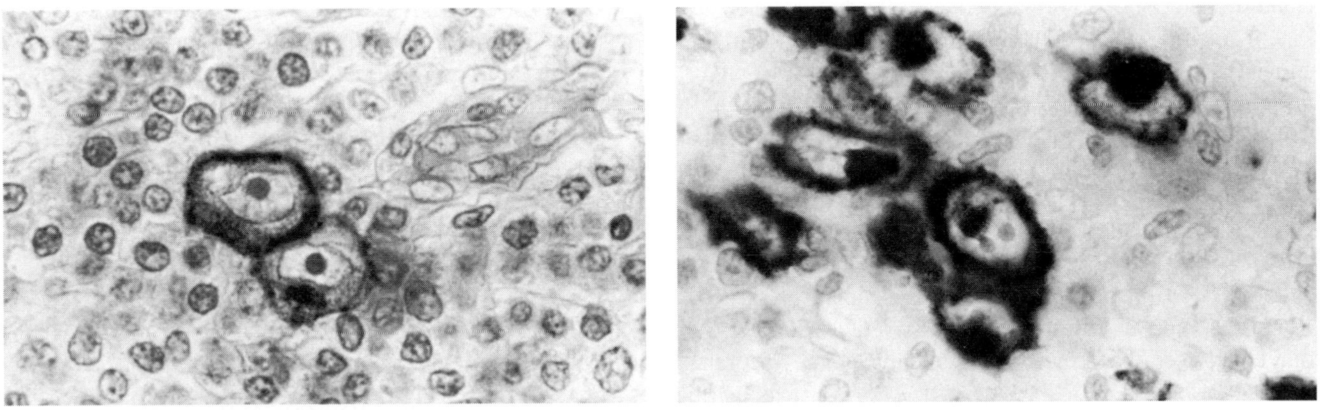

A B

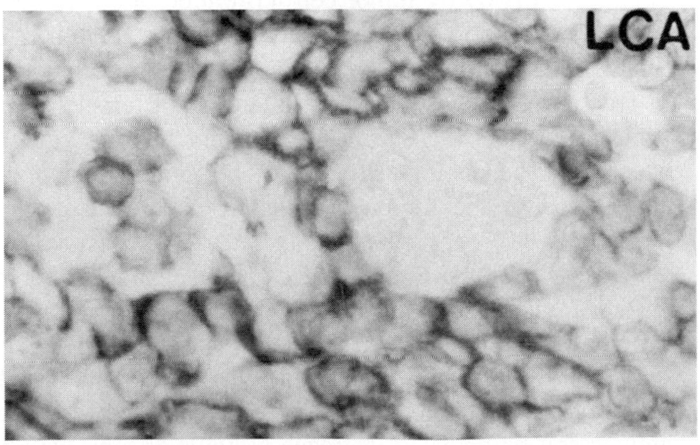

C

FIG. 18.7. Immunoperoxidase stain of Reed-Sternberg cells in paraffin sections. **A:** CD30 (Ber-H2); **B:** CD15 (Leu M1); **C:** CD45 (leukocyte common antigen). Note surface and cytoplasmic staining for CD30 and CD15; absence of staining for CD45.

nonmalignant lymphoid cells located between, around, and sometimes within B-cell follicles (57,58). Under some *in vitro* conditions, the CD30 antigen can be detected on activated monocytes as well (59,60). It has been argued that the binding of anti-CD30 antibodies to monocytes may be through a high-affinity Fcγ receptor that may be induced *in vitro* by interferon-γ (IFN-γ) (61).

The utility of the CD30 antigen for the diagnosis of HD has been expanded to paraffin-embedded tissues through the development of the Ber-H2 antibody, which detects a formalin-resistant epitope of the CD30 antigen (62). Unfortunately, the CD30 antigen is not reliably detected with the Ber-H2 antibody in B5-fixed tissues, which are used widely by American hematopathologists.

Expression of the CD30 antigen is not restricted to lymphoid neoplasms. Palleson and Hamilton-Dutoit (63) discovered expression of CD30 in a majority of embryonal carcinomas and some mixed germ cell tumors. Schwarting and associates (62) expanded the list of CD30$^+$ neoplasms to include pancreatic carcinomas, reactive in both frozen and paraffin tissues, and, infrequently, carcinomas of the breast, lung, urinary bladder, endometrium, and melanomas, weakly and diffusely positive in the cytoplasm of tumor cells in paraffin sections.

CD15, a granulocyte-related differentiation antigen, is detected by Leu M1, a highly effective antibody for the detection of diagnostic RS cells and their variants in paraffin-embedded tissues (64,65). Stein and colleagues (66) previously had described antigens specific to late cells of granulopoiesis in RS and mononuclear HD giant cells. Dorfman and colleagues (67) demonstrated that six monoclonal antigranulocyte antibodies reacted with RS cells in mixed cellularity HD and NSHD but not with RS and L&H variants in the NLPHD type. Agnarsson and Kadin (31) and Pinkus and coworkers (46) also found that CD15 is not expressed by RS cells in most cases of NLPHD. Hsu and associates (68) found, however, that after removal of sialic acid by neuraminidase, antibody Leu M1 reacts with L&H variants of RS cells in more than 50% of cases. Thus, L&H cells differ from RS cells in other types of HD in their ability to sialylate the 150-kd CD15 antigen. The CD15 antigen is also a late T-cell activation antigen (69). CD15 does not appear to be a reliable marker for the distinction of HD from T-cell malignancies in which neoplastic T cells express CD15 in 50% to 67% of cases (70,71).

Epithelial membrane antigen, which is also a lymphocyte-activation antigen (69,72), is expressed on L&H cells in most cases of NLPHD but not on RS cells in diffuse LPHD or in mixed cellularity HD and NSHD (73).

The CD25 (Tac) antigen corresponds to the p55 α chain of the IL-2 receptor. CD25 has been detected on the surface and in the cytoplasm of RS cells and their mononuclear variants in most patients with HD (31,74,75).

The transferrin receptor (CD71) is expressed on activated lymphocytes and can be detected on RS cells in virtually all patients with HD (31). RS cells commonly express several non–lineage restricted antigens normally expressed on activated lymphocytes.

The pattern of antigen expression on HRS cells may have clinical significance. A study of cases of classic HD by the German Hodgkin's Disease Study Group, using microwave epitope retrieval to optimize staining sensitivity, showed that 83% were CD15$^+$CD30$^+$CD20$^-$, 12% were CD15$^-$CD30$^-$CD20$^-$, and 5% showed other phenotypes (76). Clinical correlation showed significantly better probability of freedom from treatment failure (P = 0.0022) and overall survival (P = 0.0001) for patients with expression of CD15. Lack of CD15 expression was an independent prognostic factor for relapse (P = 0.022) and death (P = 0.0035) in a multivariate analysis, suggesting that immunophenotype is able to identify cases of classic HD with an unfavorable clinical outcome.

Immunophenotypic Distinction of Hodgkin's Disease from Non-Hodgkin's Lymphoma

There are several NHLs that resemble HD morphologically but appear to be biologically different from HD based on subtle differences in histology, tumor cell immunophenotype, principal sites of disease, and responses to therapy. Ree and associates (77) found that a panel of three markers including Ber-H2, Leu M1, and peanut agglutinin was most useful in detecting RS cells and distinguishing HD from NHL in paraffin sections (Fig. 18.7). Recently, fascin has been shown to be a useful marker for HRS cells that seldom is detected with similar strong staining of tumor cells in NHL (27). A comparison of HD with NHL resembling HD is presented in Table 18.2.

Anaplastic Large Cell Lymphoma

Anaplastic large cell lymphomas resemble HD in their focal involvement of lymph nodes and the presence of occasional RS cells (Fig. 18.8). ALCLs usually can be distinguished from HD by tumor cell infiltration of lymph node sinuses and monomorphous sheets of tumor cells in ALCL. Sinus infiltration of tumor cells, however, can occur rarely in HD, and sheets of tumor cells are characteristic of the syncytial variant of NSHD (78). In ambiguous cases ALCL usually can be distinguished from HD immunophenotypically, because the tumor cells in ALCL are most often CD15$^-$, CD40$^-$, epithelial membrane antigen–positive, and CD45$^+$, whereas RS cells have the opposite phenotype (79,80). This distinction can be more difficult if only paraffin-embedded tissues are available, because as many as one third of ALCLs may appear to be leukocyte common antigen–negative in paraffin sections (81). Leukocyte common antigen can be detected in frozen sections of most ALCLs (79). In the study of Delsol and coworkers (80), Leu M1 stained only 13 of 60 ALCLs, and staining was restricted to small granules in the cytoplasm in all but one case. T- and B-cell antigens usually are expressed on tumor cells with

TABLE 18.2. *Comparison of Hodgkin's disease with non-Hodgkin's lymphomas resembling Hodgkin's disease*

Disease	Histology	Principal sites of disease	Tumor cell immunophenotype
Hodgkin's disease	RS cells a constant feature; sinus infiltration usually absent, sheets of cells can surround areas of necrosis in syncytial variant	Peripheral LN, mediastinum, spleen, paraaortic LN	$CD30^+$, $CD40^+$, $Fascin^+$, $CD15^+$, $CD45^-$, $CD74^+$, EMA^-, $EBV^\pm$
Anaplastic large cell lymphoma	RS cells rare, sinus infiltration, usually sheets of cells with histiocyte-like appearance	Peripheral LN, extranodal sites (skin, gastrointestinal tract, bone)	$CD30^+$, $CD45^\pm$, $CD15^-$, Epithelial membrane antigen–positive, T>N>B, $CD40^-$, Fascin weakly positive
Postthymic or peripheral T-cell lymphoma	Some cases have numerous large cells which are similar to or indistinguishable from RS cells; A spectrum of medium and small atypical cells also is found	Generalized lymphadenopathy, spleen, skin	$CD30^-$, $CD45^+$, $CD15^\pm$, B^-, T^+, $CD40^-$, $Fascin^-$
Mediastinal large B-cell lymphoma with sclerosis	RS cells rare or absent-large immunoblast-like cells, no lacunar cells, bands of collagen surround individual and small groups of cells	Mediastinum (thymus), spread to kidneys, adrenal, liver	$CD30^{\pm a}$, $CD45^+$, $CD15^-$, B^+, T^-, $CD40^+$, $Fascin^-$.

[a] Weak CD30 expression with Ber-H2 on frozen sections or microwave-treated paraffin sections has been encountered by some investigators.
RS, Reed–Sternberg; LN, lymph node.

greater frequency in ALCL than in HD (58,79). Recent studies indicate that tumor cell expression of the NPM-ALK fusion protein and negative or weak staining for fascin favor a diagnosis of ALCL over HD (27,42,43). These immunophenotypic differences can be significant, because there are important clinical differences between ALCL and HD. ALCLs respond well to CHOP, COMP, or D-COMP chemotherapy for large cell NHL, whereas HD is treated with MOPP or ABVD. ALCLs more often present in extranodal sites, including the skin, gastrointestinal tract, bone, and soft tissues (82). Some ALCLs have long periods of remission after excision or only local therapy (83,84) (Chapter 25).

Postthymic or Peripheral T Cell Lymphoma

Postthymic T-cell lymphomas include angiocentric, lymphoepithelioid (Lennert's), angioimmunoblastic lymphadenopathy–like, and HD-like lymphomas (85). RS-like cells are often prominent and cause confusion with HD in the latter types. Most cases can be distinguished by the spec-

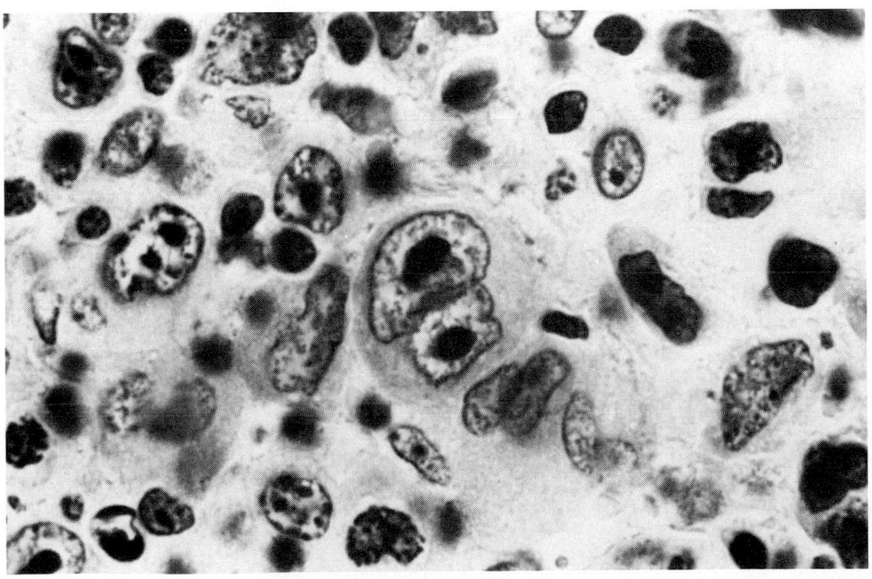

FIG. 18.8. Reed-Sternberg cell in anaplastic large cell lymphoma. Note surrounding atypical cells that help to distinguish this lesion from Hodgkin's disease.

trum of smaller atypical cells in T-cell NHL (86). Moreover, the atypical cells in peripheral T-cell lymphomas often have aberrant T-cell phenotypes (87), whereas the small T cells in HD are predominantly mature $CD4^+$ helper T cells (51,88). T-cell antigens CD2, CD4, and CD3 can be detected on HRS cells from patients with HD in frozen sections, but these cells generally do not react with monoclonal antibodies Leu-22, MT-1 (CD43), and UCHL-1 (CD45RO), which react with neoplastic cells in most peripheral T-cell lymphomas (73,89).

The RS-like cells in NHL are usually $CD30^-CD45^+$, although they may express CD15 in 50% to 67% of cases (70,71). TCR gene rearrangement results can help to distinguish between T-cell NHL and HD; relatively dense rearranged bands are expected in T-cell NHL and only faint bands or polyclonal patterns of T cells (absent 11-kb band in ECO RI digests) commonly are observed in HD (90) (Chapter 29).

Mediastinal Large B-Cell Lymphoma with Sclerosis

This is a B-cell lymphoma in which delicate sclerosis surrounds large noncleaved cells or immunoblasts. Patients are usually young females who present with mediastinal masses and local extension into thoracic structures. Addis and Isaacson (91) proposed that these tumors arise from B cells normally present in small numbers in the thymic medulla. RS-like cells may be found and cause confusion with HD, especially because there is sclerosis and a similarity to NSHD in the clinical presentation. Lacunar cells, characteristic of NSHD, are not found in mediastinal large cell lymphoma. Immunologic distinction can be made on the basis of CD15 staining, which is not found in mediastinal large cell lymphoma, and CD45- and B cell–specific antigens, which are detected more often in mediastinal large cell lymphoma than in HD. Monotypic immunoglobulin is detected in about one third of cases of mediastinal B-cell lymphoma (91); in contrast, the immunoglobulin associated with RS cells is not monotypic (92) (see Chapter 25).

Interleukins and Growth Factors in Hodgkin's Disease

A variety of cytokines and growth factors have been associated with the RS cell and appear to be responsible for many of the unique clinical and pathologic features of HD (58,93, 94) (Table 18.3). This working hypothesis first was proposed by Newcom and O'Rourke (95), resulting from their detection of a fibroblast-stimulating factor in supernatants of short-term cell cultures of lymph nodes from NSHD, and by Ford and colleagues (96), who described IL-1–like and fibroblast-stimulating activities in supernatants of involved spleen cultures from patients with HD. Further studies of fresh HD cell cultures and the L428 cell line derived from NSHD indicate that the fibroblast stimulating growth factor is not IL-1 but more likely TGF-β, a multifunctional growth factor that promotes the growth of fibroblasts and collagen synthesis, both *in vitro* and *in vivo* (97). TGF-β also recruits and activates histiocytes and macrophages (98) and thus may augment the collections of epithelioid histiocytes and granulomas often found in tissues affected by HD (99). TGF-β has been localized immunohistochemically to the surface of RS cells and lacunar variants in NSHD, where it is associated with newly formed collagen bands (100) (Fig. 18.9). Further studies suggest that TGF-β interacts with basic fibroblast

TABLE 18.3. *Interleukins/growth factors in Hodgkin's disease*

Interleukin/Growth Factor	Clinicopathologic Feature
Transforming growth factor-β	Nodular sclerosis, granulomas, immunosuppression
Interleukin-5	Eo-CSF, eosinophilia, IgA, IgM enhancement, enhanced interleukin of IgE
Granulocyte colony-stimulating factor	Myeloid hyperplasia
Interleukin-4	Autocrine growth factor for RS cell, B lymphocte proliferation, IgG1, IgE enhancement, macrophage activation, formation of polykaryons
Tumor necrosis factor-α, β (lymphotoxin)	T lymphocyte proliferation, recruitment of neutrophils and eosinophils, macrophage activation, fibroblast growth, endothelial/leukocyte interactions, prostaglandin synthesis
Interferon-γ	Fever, chills (B symptoms), lymphocyte/monocyte recruitment, formation of polykaryons
Interleukin-6	B symptoms
Interleukin-8	Neutrophil recruitment/activation
CD40L	Prevents apoptosis of HRS cells, stimulates interaction with T cells
Interleukin-13	Autocrine growth factor for HRS cells, induction of IgE and IgG4, differentiation of Th2 cells, stimulates fibroblasts
CD30L	Paracrine growth and activation factor for HRS cells

HRS, Hodgkin's Reed-Sternberg.

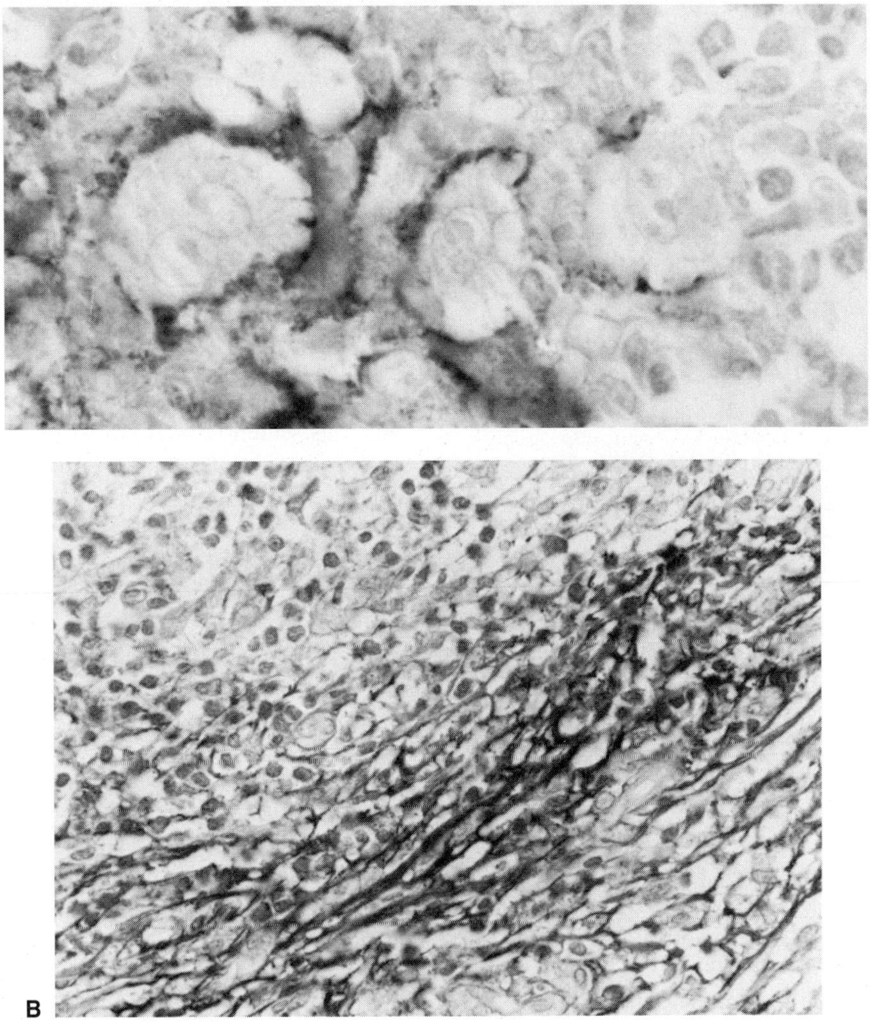

FIG. 18.9. Transforming growth factor-β localized immunohistochemically to the surface of Reed-Sternberg cells (**A**) and collagen fibers (**B**) in nodular sclerosis Hodgkin's disease. This is a multifunctional growth factor that promotes fibroblast growth and collagen synthesis. (**A:** From Kadin ME, Agnarsson BA, Ellingsworth LR, Newcom SR. Immunohistochemical evidence of a role for transforming growth factor beta in the pathogenesis of nodular sclerosing Hodgkin's disease. *Am J Pathol* 1990; 136:1209–1214, with permission.)

growth factor to cause fibrosis in HD. Simultaneous application of TGF-β and basic fibroblast growth factor causes persistent fibrosis in a murine model of cutaneous fibrosis (101). Ohshima and coworkers (102) demonstrated the presence of basic fibroblast growth factor using immunohistochemistry and *in situ* hybridization in RS cells, histiocytes, and stromal cells in NSHD.

Recently, Visser and Poppema (103) provided evidence that TGF-β is responsible for suppression of T-cell function in HD. They found that supernatants from the HD cell line L428 suppressed CD3- and CD28-induced T-cell activation. In the presence of L428 supernatants, T cells become $CD69^+$ but do not undergo blastic transformation, and they also have strongly reduced IL-2 and IFN-γ production and CD25 expression. Supernatants depleted of TGF-β have no effect, whereas TGF-β recovered from L428 supernatants produces suppression equal or superior to the complete supernatant. Depletion of IL-10 from supernatants has no effect. These results suggest that L428 cells inhibit T-cell activation through production of TGF-β, and that the lack of effective T-cell activation in patients may result from TGF-β production in their HD tumors.

Eosinophil chemotactic activity was discovered in supernatants from cultured HD lymph node cells (104). IL-5 messenger RNA (mRNA) has been detected in RS cells of HD with eosinophilia (105) (Fig. 18.10). Among the interleukins, IL-5 is involved most directly and specifically in eosinopoiesis (106). Recently, Feldstein and coworkers reported a strong correlation of tissue eosinophilia with expression of eotaxin-1 mRNA in HD tissues (107). Eotaxin-1 is an eosinophil-specific chemokine that has been identified in rodent models of asthma and allergic inflammation. Its

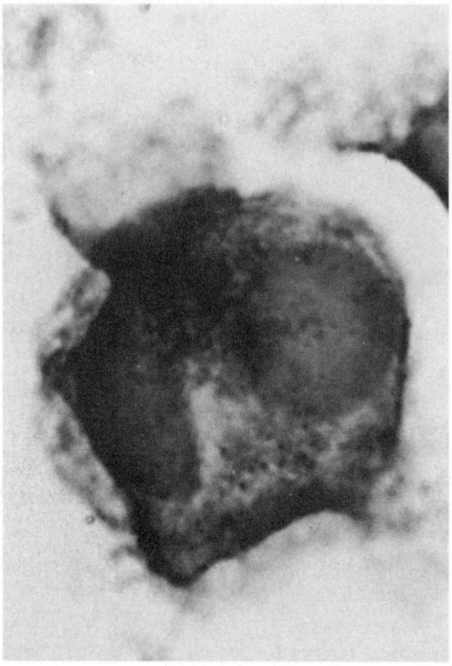

FIG. 18.10. Interleukin-5 messenger RNA in Reed-Sternberg cell of patient with Hodgkin's disease and eosinophilia. Cells from Hodgkin's disease were hybridized with a digoxigenin-labeled oligonucleotide probe directed to human interleukin-5. After development of the color reaction, there is abundant blue precipitate in the Reed-Sternberg cell, indicating transcriptional activation of the IL-5 gene and production of IL-5 messenger RNA. (Courtesy of Michael Samoszuk, M.D., University of California, Irvine, CA.)

expression is induced by IL-3. A high level expression of eotaxin-1 was found in NSHD compared with other histologic types. Supporting the hypothesis that the eosinophilia of HD is caused by a cytokine secreted by the malignant cells, instead of the reactive T cells, Ben-Ezra and colleagues (108) have shown an inverse relationship between tissue eosinophilia and the presence of $CD25^+$ T cells in HD lymph nodes.

Myeloid hyperplasia and granulocytosis are common features of HD. Burrichter and associates (109) have shown that conditioned medium from the HD cell line L428 induces myeloproliferation in semisolid media. The L428 cell line was established from a patient who developed a leukocytosis of 60,000 cells per microliter, with an eosinophilia of 92% shortly before death. However, predominantly neutrophil colonies were observed by Burrichter and associates in colonies stimulated by the L428 conditioned media. Eosinophil colony-stimulating factor was present in low concentrations. No evidence for macrophage growth factor was obtained. Further work is needed to define the nature and scope of bone marrow colony-stimulating factors produced and secreted by RS cells.

Newcom and colleagues (110) have provided evidence that IL-4 is the principal autocrine growth factor for the L428 RS cell line. IL-4 is a potent stimulator of B-cell growth and also enhances production of IgG1 and IgE (111), which may help to explain the B-cell hyperactivity characteristic of patients with HD. IL-4 also acts as a macrophage activation factor and stimulates the fusion of macrophages to form multinucleated giant cells, which could promote granulomas in HD (112).

A recent study has shown that IL-13 is secreted by and stimulates the growth of HRS cells (110a). IL-13 and IL-4 share a common α chain. *In situ* hybridization showed IL-13 mRNA transcripts in HRS cells in lymph nodes from patients with HD. An anti-IL-13 neutralizing antibody had an antiproliferative effect on HD cell line HDLM-2, but not on cell lines L428 or KIMH-2, possibly because of their vigorous secretion of IL-13.

It has been shown that inflammation or necrosis of tumors cannot explain the fever in most febrile patients with HD (113). The immunohistochemical demonstration of IL-1–bearing cells in HD does not correlate well with fever or other constitutional symptoms in HD (114). Ellis and coworkers (115) have shown that the HD cell line L428 produces IL-1–like accessory cell activity for CD3-driven T-cell proliferation and CD3-dependent IL-2 production; however, neither the genes for IL-1α nor IL-1β are transcribed by L428 cells.

Recent studies suggest that the IL-1–independent accessory cell activity of L428 HD cells may be cause by TNF-α. Kretschmer and associates demonstrated synthesis of both TNF-α and TNF-β (lymphotoxin) by HD cell lines L428 and L540 and TNF-α protein and mRNA directly in tissue biopsy specimens from patients with HD (116). Sappino and colleagues (117) demonstrated high levels of lymphotoxin mRNA in Northern blots of tissue extracts from LPHD. TNF-α and lymphotoxin have a broad range of biologic activities that include neutrophil and eosinophil recruitment (118), macrophage activation (119), stimulation of fibroblast growth (120), and endothelial cell–leukocyte interactions (121), each of which may contribute to the pathologic features of HD.

Interferon-γ mRNA and protein are produced by the cell line SUP-HD1, derived from the pleural effusion of a patient with NSHD (122). Injections of IFN-γ can cause the fever and chills that are frequent systemic symptoms of patients with HD. IFN-γ also causes lymphocyte proliferation, activation of mononuclear phagocytes, T-lymphocyte and monocyte recruitment, and formation of polykaryons and could contribute to the histologic manifestations of HD (123).

Presence of B symptoms in patients with HD has been found to correlate best with elevated serum IL-6 levels (124). Nine (60%) of 15 HD patients with B symptoms had detectable IL-6 levels, versus only 1 of 11 without B symptoms ($P < 0.01$). The median duration of survival of HD patients with IL-6 levels greater than 22 pg/mL was 10 months; the median survival of patients with lower serum IL-6 levels had not been reached at a median follow-up of 37.5 months ($P = 0.0012$).

Cytokines also affect the interaction of HRS cells with surrounding T lymphocytes, which adhere to HRS cells both *in vivo* and *in vitro*, imparting the appearance of a lymphocyte rosette around the giant cells (125,126). The T lymphocytes around HRS cells are polyclonal (127). The significance of these rosettes is poorly understood, but they suggest a functional interaction of HRS cells as antigen-presenting cells with T lymphocytes (15). HRS cells express B7/BB1 (CD80), which is present on the membrane of professional antigen-presenting cells and is the natural ligand of CD28, a membrane receptor of T lymphocytes (128). CD28 ligation on T cells augments their secretion of IL-2, lymphotoxin, TNF-α, IFN-γ, and granulocyte-macrophage colony-stimulating factor, potentially affecting further the histopathology and clinical features of HD (129).

CD40 is a 50-kd phosphoprotein expressed mainly on cells of B lineage, including most B-cell leukemias and lymphomas (130,131). CD40 acts as a receptor for a specific ligand (CD40L) that is a type II integral membrane glycoprotein and has homology to ligands for other receptors of the NGF-TNF receptor superfamily (132). CD40L is expressed primarily on activated CD4$^+$ helper T cells (133), including cells that form rosettes around HRS cells. Engagement of CD40 antigen by CD40L or monoclonal antibodies against CD40 prevents apoptosis of germinal center B cells (134,135) and may protect HRS cells from apoptosis. CD40 is expressed at high levels on primary and cultured HRS cells (136,137). Exposure of HD cell lines L428 and KM-H2 results in a dose-dependent enhancement of their clonagenic growth and increased colony formation in semisolid media (138). CD40L engagement also enhances cell line expression of the costimulatory molecule B7 (CD80) and intercellular adhesion molecule ICAM-1 (CD5) and induces release of cytokines IL-8, IL-6, TNF-α, and lymphotoxin-α (139).

CD30 is a late-activation antigen and marker for lymphoid cells, with normal expression being limited to antigen-stimulated and memory T cells (58,59,62,140). CD30 is expressed consistently by HRS cells in all types of HD, with the exception of NLPHD (56). CD30L is expressed on activated T cells, macrophages, and granulocytes (141). CD30L has pleiotropic effects on cell lines expressing CD30 (142). Recombinant CD30L and anti-CD30 antibodies were found to enhance proliferation of "T cell–like" HD-derived cell lines (HDLM-2 and L540) and adult T-cell leukemia cell lines in a time- and dose-dependent manner but did not enhance proliferation of "B cell–like" HD-derived cell lines (KM-H2 and L428). None of six HD-derived cell lines tested showed CD30L mRNA or protein expression constitutively or after stimulation with phorbol ester or a variety of cytokines (IL-1, IL-2, IL-4, IL-6, IL-9, TNF-α), indicating that these HD cell lines do not use CD30-CD30L interaction for autocrine growth stimulation. High levels of CD30L expression have been detected among T cells and granulocytes surrounding HRS cells in HD lesions (143). Native CD30L displayed on the cell surface was functionally active, as shown by the ability of fixed granulocytes to interact with CD30$^+$ cell lines.

The ability of multiple members of the TNF receptor superfamily, such as CD40 and CD30, to interact with various members of the TNF receptor–associated factor (TRAF) family of signal-transduction molecules and their coexpression in HRS cells likely results in a complex cascade of signaling events in HD. Although TRAF molecules have no intrinsic catalytic capability, their interaction with certain kinases appears to stimulate activity of those molecules. The NF-κB–inducing kinase is a mitogen-activated protein kinase (144). A substrate of the NF–κB-inducing kinase is the IκB complex, which consists of two subunits, I$\kappa\kappa\alpha$ and I$\kappa\kappa\beta$ (145,146). Available data suggest that the IκB complex is required for phosphorylation and inactivation of NF-κB inhibitor protein by IκB (145–149). IκB is found in the cytoplasm associated with NF-κB, maintaining the latter in an inactive state. On phosphorylation and degradation of IκB, NF-κB translocates into the nucleus in an activated state and can stimulate transcription of a variety of cellular genes (150). Constitutive activation of NF-κB-RelA appears to be required for proliferation and survival of HRS cells (151). As a consequence, Hodgkin's lymphoma cells depleted of constitutive NF-κB show impaired tumor growth in severe combined immunodeficiency mice (151).

Soluble Cellular Receptors in the Staging and Prognosis of Hodgkin's Disease

Soluble IL-2 receptors have been shown to be elevated in various lymphoproliferative disorders including adult T-cell leukemia, hairy cell leukemia, and undifferentiated lymphomas (152–154). Pizzolo and colleagues found that most patients with active HD have elevated levels of soluble IL-2 receptors (155). The level of these receptors correlates with the severity of HD, as suggested by the significantly higher levels seen in stage B compared with stage A (154).

These investigators also measured serum levels of soluble CD30 (sCD30) antigen in 58 patients with HD (156). sCD30 was detected only in patients with active HD and was not found in control sera or in patients in remission from HD. Among patients with active HD, the incidence of presence and mean level of sCD30 were higher in patients with progressive or relapsing disease then in those first presenting. Among patients presenting, detectable levels were observed more often in those with advanced-stage disease (stage III or IV) and with constitutional B symptoms than in early stages without B symptoms. Higher mean sCD30 levels were found in patients with stage III or IV disease and in patients with B symptoms than in those with stage I and II disease or without B symptoms, respectively. Interestingly, sCD30 appears to be a marker only for the neoplastic component and not for the reactive cells in HD. These results suggest a possible role for sCD30 as a tumor marker in HD.

Younes and coworkers (157) found that patients with high levels of serum sCD30 have low detectable levels of CD30L on their peripheral blood lymphocytes, compared with normal donors ($P = 0.0008$). Experimental introduction of exogenous sCD30 blocked membrane-bound CD30L-mediated apoptosis in a $CD30^+$ tumor cell line. These observations led the investigators to conclude that sCD30 decreases availability of CD30L on peripheral blood lymphocytes in patients with HD and other $CD30^+$ tumors, and that blocking of the apoptosis-inducing activity of CD30L by its soluble receptor could explain how $CD30^+$ tumors escape immune surveillance and the poor prognosis of patients who have elevated sCD30 levels.

Host and Environmental Factors in Hodgkin's Disease

Factors other than cytokines released by the RS cell likely contribute to the histopathology of HD. Unfavorable histologies of the mixed cellularity and lymphocytic depletion types are found more often in patients of advanced age and those from underdeveloped countries or lower socioeconomic groups in the United States who have poor nutrition, whereas the favorable histologies of LPHD and NSHD predominate in the first decade of life (158,159).

The immune status of patients also affects the type and stage of the HD they acquire. Mixed cellularity is the prevalent histology of HD in HIV-infected patients (160). HD lymph nodes of HIV-infected patients have relatively few $CD4^+$ T cells and a predominance of $CD8^+$ cells (161,162). In HIV-infected patients, stromal histiocytes appear abnormal, with indistinct borders, vesicular cytoplasm, and lack of a polygonal shape (163). The histology of HD in HIV-infected patients is influenced by the cytopathic effect of HIV on nonmalignant $CD4^+$ lymphocytes and histiocytes.

HIV-infected patients with HD commonly present in advanced stages, often involving extranodal sites (162,164). Most remarkable is the high frequency of HD in the skin and liver, the latter occasionally presenting without prior involvement of the spleen (164). These observations indicate that in HIV-infected patients HD often does not follow the orderly progression of spread characteristic of the disease in patients without HIV infection (165) (Chapter 28).

Nature of the Immunologic Derangement in Hodgkin's Disease

Most untreated patients with HD, including those with limited stage disease, exhibit a defect in cell-mediated immunity (166). Untreated patients have a decrease in $CD4^+$ cells that is associated with the extent of disease (167). A displacement of $CD4^+$ T lymphocytes from the blood to peripheral lymphoid organs has been demonstrated (168). Grimfors and colleagues (169) showed an increased clearance rate of isotope-labeled autologous $CD4^+$ cells in patients with active HD. There are frequent $CD4^+$ cells with cytolytic activity in spleens of patients with HD (170). These studies suggest that the observed T lymphocytopenia in HD may reflect a biologic response to the tumor (169).

In HD there are defects in T-lymphocyte function that include a depressed response to T-cell mitogens (166,171) and decreased capacity of T lymphocytes to respond in an autologous or syngeneic mixed lymphocyte response (172). Decreased *in vitro* synthesis of IL-2 and IFN-γ has been demonstrated in untreated patients with HD (173). A persistent functional immune defect of T cells has been demonstrated in long-term survivors of HD (174,175).

A lectin-binding site on the surface of cultured RS cells has been characterized (176). This site binds and stimulates T lymphocytes and is postulated to mutually activate and stimulate the growth and rosetting of RS cells and the $CD4^+$ T cells that surround them (177).

B-cell function appears to be normal in most patients with HD at the time of diagnosis. For example, pneumococcal vaccination results in normal antibody response, provided that no cytotoxic treatment is given for 10 to 14 days. Overwhelming bacterial sepsis with encapsulated organisms may occur, however, in patients with HD who have had surgical or therapeutic splenectomy (178). There is increased IgG synthesis by uninvolved or lightly involved spleens of patients with HD, similar to that by normal spleens after secondary antigenic stimulation (179). The IgG produced *in vitro* by HD splenic lymphocytes has antibody-dependent cellular cytotoxicity for a population of homologous lymphocytes (180). This antibody-dependent cytotoxicity could mediate the lymphopenia and anergy common to patients with HD.

The number of monocytes in the blood of untreated HD patients is usually normal. Monocytes in HD show a decreased chemotactic response (181); this may result from a chemotactic factor inhibitor in the serum (182). Monocytes of both untreated patients with HD and those whose disease is in long-term remission show decreased killing of candidal organisms and dysfunction in the generation of oxygen radicals associated with excessive production of prostaglandin E2 (183). Enhanced prostaglandin-mediated suppressor activity by monocytes from patients with HD has been described and is considered to be responsible for depressed lymphoproliferative responses (184,185) and reduced T cell colony formation (186).

It has been suggested that the immune derangement in HD may result from lymphocyte hyperactivity that can follow overstimulation of the immune system by an unknown antigen (187). Reactive follicular hyperplasia in lymph nodes surrounding HD, which accounts for negative biopsy results in many patients eventually found to have HD, has been interpreted as evidence of B-lymphocyte hyperactivity in HD (188). Polyclonal B-cell activation also has been demonstrated during the course of some infectious diseases, including infectious mononucleosis (189). Polyclonal B-cell activation may be responsible for dysfunction of T cells and enhanced monocyte suppressor function, as shown in some patients with sarcoidosis (190). Hyperactivity of B cells can in turn be stimulated by increased helper T-cell function of peripheral blood T cells, as seen in untreated patients with

HD (191). Considerable insight into the mechanism of altered immunity in HD may be gained if the antigens provoking B-cell hyperactivity are discovered.

Some of the immune derangements in HD result from the effects of cytokines produced and secreted directly by the RS cell. Among the cytokines described with potent immunomodulatory effects are TNF-α, lymphotoxin, and TGF-β. TNF-α and lymphotoxin are active in the cyclooxygenase pathway and can potentiate prostaglandin synthesis (192). TGF-β suppresses the growth and differentiation of T and B lymphocytes (193,194), the cytolytic activity and responsiveness to interferon of natural killer cells (195), and the proliferation and differentiation of precursors to natural killer cells (196). TGF-β2 first was isolated from a glioblastoma cell line and was characterized by its ability to suppress T-cell function (197). TGF-β2 from glioblastomas inhibits the generation of lymphokine-activated killer cells (198). The normal immune status of patients who have glioblastoma may be restored if their tumors are removed (199). Therefore, the successful treatment of HD, the elimination of RS cells, which secrete an active form of TGF-β (200), may help to restore normal immune function in patients who have HD.

PATHOGENESIS

Cytogenetics and Molecular Genetics

Seif and Spriggs (201) were the first to demonstrate evidence of a clone of malignant aneuploid cells with marker chromosomes in HD. Subsequent cytogenetic studies confirmed that HD giant cells are aneuploid and clonally related (202). Weber-Matthiesen and coworkers (203) verified numerical chromosome abnormalities within CD30$^+$ HRS cells in all types of HD by simultaneous fluoresecence immunophenotyping and interphase cytogenetic analysis. They found a high variability of copy numbers of certain chromosomes in different metaphases of individual cases. They demonstrated that this karyotype instability did not result from artifact but rather was an *in vivo* characteristic of HRS cells.

Recurrent nonrandom chromosome abnormalities have been found in fresh HD tissues and cell lines. The chromosome abnormalities identified by Cabanillas and colleagues (204) in fresh tissues from patients with HD are most consistent with a lymphoid origin for the malignant cell in HD. The most common abnormalities were at 11q23, 14q32, 6q11-21, and 8q22-24, sites of common breakpoints in B- and T-cell malignancies. Schouten and colleagues (205) found recurrent breakpoints at 4q32-q34, 6q24, 12q13, 12q23-q24, and 13p11-q13; three patients had two or more clones, and one had subclones. Tilly and coworkers (206) found that some chromosome regions altered in HD are also abnormal in NHL of either B-cell (e.g., 14q32, 8q24, 6q, and 11q21-q23) or T-cell (e.g., 4q28, 7q31-q35, 3q27) origin; significant differences occurred more often between HD and diffuse B-cell NHL than between HD and T-cell NHL. The recurrent 11q23 breakpoint is the site of the *ETS* oncogene. This breakpoint has been implicated in the pathogenesis of a unique type of childhood B-cell acute lymphoblastic leukemia characterized by simultaneous expression of myeloid and monocytic antigens (207); HRS cells also express myeloid and monocytic antigens, for example CD15 (66,208).

The t(14;18)(q32;q21) translocation that causes *BCL2* gene rearrangement and is characteristic of follicular lymphomas (209, 210) appears to be quite rare in HD. In a comparative study of cytogenetics and PCR amplification of t(14;18), Poppema and coworkers detected frequent involvement of the immunoglobulin heavy chain region at the 14q32 region but found translocations involving the region of *BCL2* at chromosome 18q21 in only one of 28 consecutive untreated patients (211). They concluded that *BCL2* gene rearrangements detected by PCR in 40% of these 28 cases were in small bystander B lymphocytes. *BCL2* gene rearrangements also have been detected in 30% of nonmalignant, hyperplastic tonsils (212). The 6q− abnormalities are in the region of the *MYB* oncogene, which frequently is involved in lymphoid malignancies (213, 214). The 8q24 breakpoint is at the site of the *MYC* oncogene (215). The *MYC* gene cooperates with *BCL2* to immortalize B cells (216) and was found to be activated in the evolution of a B-cell malignancy with a rearranged *BCL2* gene (217). These data suggest that *ETS*, *MYC-ETS*, *MYB*, *MYC*, and less frequently *BCL2* are involved in the pathogenesis of HD and other lymphoid malignancies.

Fonatsch and associates (218) studied the cytogenetics of HD cell lines and found nonrandom chromosomal abnormalities frequently associated with oncogenes and other genes. The most common abnormalities involved are 1p21-p22 associated with *RAS*, *LYM*, and *MYC*; 7q11.2-q36 associated with *MET* and TCR β chain genes; 11q21-23 associated with *ETS1*, *ETST3D*, and *ETSE* genes; 14q32 associated with IgH chain genes; 15p12 associated with the nucleolus organizing region; and 21q21-q22 associated with *ETS2*. These investigators also found increased chromosome instability in lymphocytes of several untreated patients with HD.

The DNA-binding phosphoprotein p53 is necessary for the regulation of the cell cycle and induction of apoptosis after DNA damage (219). Genetic alterations of p53 are the most frequent genetic abnormality observed in human tumors. Mutation of p53 generates a stable p53 protein with loss of sequence-specific DNA-binding activity and an abnormally long half-life, leading to overexpression detected by immunohistochemistry. Point mutations of p53 have been detected in cultured and primary HRS cells in all histologic types except for NLPHD (220,221). The identification of identical p53 gene mutations in multiple samples of HD from the same patient indicate a clonal relationship between the separate lesions, and furthermore that HD represents a clonal neoplasm (222).

Taken together these cytogenetic and molecular genetic data from both fresh tissues and cell lines indicate that HD is a clonal disorder of B- and T-lymphocyte origin; tumor suppressor genes, such as p53 and certain oncogenes such as *ETS*, *MYB*, *MYC*, and *BCL2*, are likely to be involved in the pathogenesis of HD; HRS cells have chromosome instability; and a prior defect in chromosome stability can lead to increased susceptibility to HD and a high incidence of secondary malignancies in patients treated for HD.

Epstein-Barr Virus

A role for EBV in the pathogenesis of HD long has been suspected. Lukes and Tindle (223) drew attention to the close morphologic resemblance between RS cells and immunoblasts in infectious mononucleosis. Epidemiologic and serologic studies have shown an increased risk for HD in patients with histories of infectious mononucleosis, elevated antibody titers, or an altered serologic pattern of antibody response to EBV, before or after the diagnosis of HD (224). Mueller and coworkers (224) demonstrated IgG and IgA antibodies against EBV in the serum of patients obtained more than 3 years before the diagnosis of HD, indicating that the development of HD in some patients is preceded by enhanced activation of EBV. About 5% of patients with HD studied by these investigators, however, had no evidence of EBV infection. A more recent study by Sleckman and colleagues (225) compared the detection of EBV in HD tissues with histology and history of infectious mononucleosis. Contrary to their original hypothesis, there was no association between a history of infectious mononucleosis and EBV positivity in HD tissues, with only 3 of 14 patients who once had infectious mononucleosis having EBV detected by *in situ* hybridization and immunohistochemistry in their HD tissues. Although these data suggest that EBV is not involved in the pathogenesis of some cases of HD, it remains possible that EBV infection is a step in the pathogenesis of HD but that in some instances all or most of the viral genome is lost in the setting of a vigorous cytotoxic T-cell response to viral latency antigens.

Epstein-Barr virus first was demonstrated by Poppema and colleagues (226) directly in HD tissues by immunoperoxidase staining of EBV nuclear antigen in RS cells in a single patient with chronic lymphadenopathy resembling mixed cellularity HD, after a chronic EBV infection. Since then EBV genomes have been detected by Weiss and others in RS cells in one third to one half of patients with HD (227–230). There is evidence that EBV is integrated clonally into RS cells, which indicates that the infection occurred prior to or at the time of malignant transformation and thereby implicates EBV directly in the pathogenesis of these cases of HD. Weiss and coworkers (227) showed that a subset of patients with HD has a clonal population of EBV-infected cells, and they localized EBV genomes to RS cells in most of these patients (Fig. 18.11). Similar results were obtained by Anagnostopoulos and coworkers (228), who showed by use of an EBV terminal region DNA probe that the EBV-infected cell population represents a clonal expansion of a progenitor cell infected by a single virion. The EBV genome is amplified 50-fold or more in EBV-positive HRS cells (229).

The frequency with which EBV is detected in HD varies considerably according to the methods used and the patient population studied. Using PCR, Herbst and colleagues (230)

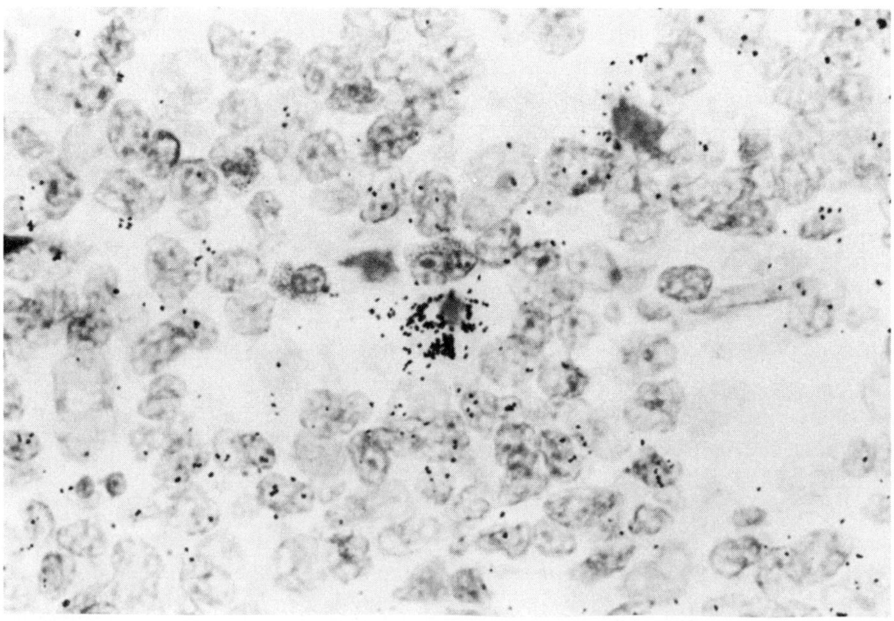

FIG. 18.11. *In situ* hybridization for Epstein-Barr virus nucleic acids in a splenic specimen from a patient with Hodgkin's disease. (Courtesy of Lawrence Weiss, MD, City of Hope National Medical Center, Duarte, CA.)

detected EBV-specific sequences in DNA extracts from frozen or paraffin-embedded tissues from 58% of 198 patients with HD. *In situ* hybridization revealed exclusive localization of viral DNA to HRS cells. Brousset and associates (231) demonstrated EBV mRNA in RS cells in 15 (27.3%) of 55 patients with HD. Because PCR detects EBV in bystander lymphocytes rather than in HRS cells in HD tissues, it has been recommended that *in situ* hybridization be used to determine the true frequency of EBV-associated HD. Correlation between EBV status and histology has shown that EBV is frequent in mixed cellularity disease, uncommon in NSHD, and very infrequent in NLPHD (232–234). EBV is most common in HD in children up to age 15 years and patients older than 50 years of age but is relatively uncommon in young adults (235,236). EBV-associated HD occurs at its highest frequency in patients from poor socioeconomic groups in underdeveloped countries. Gulley and coworkers (229) found that EBV was associated with Hispanic ethnicity in a series of cases from Mexico, Costa Rica, and the United States. Ambinder and colleagues (237) reported a 100% incidence of EBV in pediatric HD in Honduras. Chang and colleagues (238) detected EBV in 94% of patients with HD in an indigenous Indian population in Peru. The incidence of EBV in HD approaches 100% in HIV-infected patients (239). In cases in which multiple disease sites could be analyzed, EBV was detected in HRS cells at all anatomic sites (240). Recurrences of EBV-positive HD remain EBV-positive (241).

Epstein-Barr virus comprises two common strains, types A and B. Type A transforms lymphocytes more efficiently than type B. Most cases of HD are associated with type A EBV, although about 30% cases are associated with both type A and B viral sequences (242). Type B EBV is detectable in HD that develops in severely immunocompromised patients (243). The relative infrequency of type B EBV sequences in patients without prior HIV or immunosuppressive chemotherapy suggests that EBV-associated HD is not a result of a global deficiency of the immune system in the host (93).

Reed-Sternberg cells commonly express the EBV gene product LMP-1 (232), a transforming protein that can confer a growth advantage on HRS cells (244). Transcription of LMP-1 in HD is similar to that in nasopharyngeal carcinoma (245). Kaye and coworkers (246) found that the first 43 amino acids are critical for B-lymphocyte transformation by LMP-1. Partial deletions of the *LMP1* gene occur in approximately 10% of HD cases and are associated with necrosis, anaplasia, and numerous HRS cells (247). These deletions occur near the 3′ end of the *LMP1* gene; similar deletions in nasopharyngeal carcinoma have been associated with aggressive xenografts in nude mice (248). *LMP1* transfection appears to promote the formation of multinucleated cells in the EBV-negative HD cell line L428, and this effect is mediated by activation of NF-κB (249).

Latent membrane protein-1 is a homologue of the TNF receptor superfamily and engages signaling proteins of that superfamily (250–254). There are multiple signaling molecules that interact with domains of TNF receptors and other proteins that are involved directly in signal transduction. In most cases, these so-called adapter molecules have more than one family member, which function in slightly different manners and ultimately lead to different signals being transduced. The TRAF family of adapter molecules has at least six members, TRAF-1 through TRAF-6 (255–267). EBV LMP-1 interacts with TRAF family members to activate these pathways in EBV-positive cases of HD. The likelihood that LMP-1 can exert effects on HRS cell growth through the TRAF signaling pathway is supported by demonstrations of TRAF-mediated LMP-1 signaling *in vivo* in EBV-associated, AIDS-related NHLs and posttransplant lymphoproliferative disorders (250).

Latent membrane protein-1 may have additional effects on HRS cells in the development of HD. LMP-1 upregulates CD40, which prevents apoptosis of germinal center cells (134,135). There is controversy about whether LMP-1 also induces BCL-2 in HRS cells; BCL-2 protects germinal center B cells from apoptosis. Henderson and coworkers (268) showed that human B cells are protected from apoptosis by DNA transfection and expression of LMP-1, and that this effect results from upregulation of BCL-2. However, Jiwa and associates (269) found that expression of BCL-2 and MYC products in RS cells is independent of EBV infection and expression of LMP-1, and Khan and coworkers (270) found that coexpression of LMP-1 and BCL-2 occured in only 4% of patients with HD and BCL-2 was present in only a subset of LMP-1^{+} cells. EBV infection has been more closely associated with expression of BCL-x, a BCL-2–related protein in HD (271). Moreover, BAX, the product of a cell death–inducing gene, frequently is expressed in HRS cells, but usually in combination with BCL-2, BCL-x, or MCL-1, another antiapoptotic protein (272). It is possible that frequent expression of BAX in HRS cells may explain the relatively good responses of HD patients to therapy.

Latent membrane protein-1 normally is recognized by cytotoxic T cells; this could explain the better overall survival rate of patients with HD whose tumor cells express LMP1 (273,274). Surprisingly, increased numbers of cytotoxic T cells in HD tissues have been associated with an unfavorable clinical outcome of patients with HD (275), possibly reflecting impaired ability of cytotoxic T cells in HD to kill HRS cells. In support of this hypothesis, Frisan and coworkers (276) found an inverse correlation between the presence of EBV in HRS cells and EBV-specific cytotoxic lymphocytes in lymph nodes involved by HD. Although EBV-specific cytotoxic T cells were detected in three EBV-negative cases of HD, none of six EBV positive cases had detectable EBV-specific cytotoxic activity. One patient with EBV-positive HD from whom peripheral blood was available had circulating EBV-specific cytotoxic T cells. These observations suggest that local factors in the lymph node environment of HRS cells might suppress virus-specific cytotoxic T cells. T cells in patients with HD have a defect in cytolytic function associated with downregulation of the TCR ζ chain (277). Additionally, failure of HRS cells to express major histocompatibility complex class I antigens may permit them to escape immune surveillance by cytotoxic T cells (278). There is also evidence of a familial genetic defect in immunity (279); HD may in part result from the inability of affected individuals to control an EBV infection that in immunocompetent individuals would produce only a benign syndrome of infectious mononucleosis or would be clinically silent. The severe defect in T-cell immune surveillance is associated with a high frequency of advanced HD in patients with AIDS (164). Patients with HD may benefit from immunotherapy with bispecific monoclonal antibodies, which bridge human effector cells to HRS cells (280).

SUMMARY AND CONCLUSIONS

Recent studies, including PCR amplification of genes from single HRS cells, have provided evidence of somatic hypermutations within clonally rearranged immunoglobulin genes of HRS cells in classic HD, strongly suggesting that they are derived from post–germinal center B cells. HRS cells in LPHD have ongoing immunoglobulin variable region region mutations, indicating a germinal center origin for HRS variants in NLPHD. Studies of individual cases of HD and composite or prior B-cell malignancy have shown common clonal immunoglobulin gene rearrangements, providing additional evidence for a B-cell origin of HRS cells in these cases. A unique profile of HRS cells for expression of BCL-6, a transcription factor expressed by germinal center B cells, and CD138, or SYN-1, a proteoglycan associated with post–germinal center terminal B cell differentiation, supports the derivation of HRS cells from germinal center B cells in most cases.

An origin of HRS cells from follicular dendritic cells in some cases is suggested by their expression of CD21 without other B-cell antigens or clonal immunoglobulin gene rearrangements. An origin of HRS cells from T lymphocytes in 1% to 5% of cases is suggested by their expression of T-cell antigens, cytotoxic proteins (granzyme B, perforin, and TIA-1), and clonal TCR gene rearrangements. A possible origin of HRS cells from interdigitating dendritic cells is suggested by their similar unique morphology, close interaction with surrounding T cells, expression of fascin, and localized expression of non-specific esterase and acid phosphatase.

HRS cells have an immunophenotype consistent with an origin from activated lymphocytes ($CD30^+CD15^+CD25^+ CD71^+$ HLA-DR^+). Immunohistochemistry is useful in establishing the diagnosis of LPHD and determining the prognosis of classic HD. The differential diagnosis of HD from morphologically similar NHL is aided by use of a panel of antibodies reactive with CD30, CD15, CD45, epithelial membrane antigen, fascin, ALK-kinase, pan–T cell, and pan–B cell antigens. A diagnosis of NHL is favored over HD by the finding of strong nongermline bands in immunoglobulin or TCR gene rearrangement studies.

Hodgkin's disease is a tumor of cytokine-secreting HRS cells, which contribute to its unique histopathology and clinical features. Among the characteristics of HD attributed to cytokines are eosinophilia (IL-5 and eotaxin), myeloid hyperplasia (granulocyte-macrophage colony-stimulating factor), nodular sclerosis (TGF-β1 and basic fibroblast growth factor), immune suppression (TGF-β1), and systemic B symptoms (IL-6). Serum IL-2R and CD30 levels are markers of tumor burden in HD, and sCD30 may block apoptosis of $CD30^+$ tumor cells.

CD40 and CD30 are members of the TNF receptor superfamily expressed at high levels on HRS cells. Engagement of CD40 protects germinal center B cells and possibly HRS cells from apoptosis and induces adhesion of T lymphocytes which surround HRS cells. CD30L is expressed on activated T lymphocytes and granulocytes in HD tissues and likely affects growth or apoptosis of HRS cells. IL-4 and IL-13 are autocrine growth factors for the HD cell lines HDLM-2 and L428, respectively. A more complete understanding of the roles of cytokines and cytokine receptors in HD could lead to novel treatments for this disease.

Most untreated patients with HD, including those with limited stage disease, exhibit defects in cell-mediated immunity; B-cell function appears to be normal or even increased. Chemotaxis and killing by monocytes is impaired. Some of the immune derangements in HD appear to result from the effects of cytokines, such as TGF-β.

Cytogenetics has confirmed the clonality of HRS cells and detected recurrent chromosomal abnormalities in HRS cells that are common in other neoplasms of B- and T-lymphocyte origin. An abnormality at 11q23 is shared by a B-cell leukemia with simultaneous expression of myeloid antigens, similar to HRS cells. *BCL2* gene rearrangements detected by PCR often are not associated with t(14;18) in HD. Mutations affecting p53 expression detected in a minority of cases are identical in separate tissues and individual HRS cells, supporting their clonality. HRS cells have genetic instability that may be a preexisting condition in lymphocytes of patients who develop HD.

A likely role for EBV in the pathogenesis of HD is based on serologic, tissue hybridization, and immunohistochemical studies. EBV LMP-1, a transforming protein, has been detected in HRS cells in 30% to 50% of patients with HD. Expression of LMP-1 may aid "crippled" HRS cells in escaping apoptosis in germinal centers. LMP-1 engages signaling proteins of the TNF receptor superfamily through TRAF signaling molecules. These interactions are responsible for activation of NF-κB, which is required for survival and proliferation of HRS cells. Recognition of LMP-1 in patients with HD is impaired by an acquired T-cell defect, most likely resulting from secretion of activated TGF-β1 by HRS cells and eosinophils in the HD microenvironment.

REFERENCES

1. Kuppers R, Rajewsky K, Zhao M, et al. Hodgkin and Reed/Sternberg cells picked from histological setions show clonal immunoglobulin gene rearrangements and appear to be derived from B cells at various stages of development. *Proc Natl Acad Sci USA* 1994;91:962–966.
2. Kuppers R, Zhao M, Hansmann ML, et al. Tracing B cell development in human germinal centers by molecular analysis of single cells picked from histological sections. *EMBO J* 1993;12:4955–4967.
3. Kanzler H, Kuppers R, Hansmann ML, et al. Hodgkin and Reed/Sternberg cells in Hodgkin's disease represent the outgrowth of a domimant tumor clone derived from (crippled) germinal center B cells. *J Exp Med* 1996;184:1495–1505.
4. Hummel M, Ziemann K, Lammert H, et al. Hodgkin's disease with monoclonal and polyclonal populations of Reed-Sternberg cells. *N Engl J Med* 1995;333:901–906.
5. Delabie J, Tierens A, Gavril T, et al. Phenotype, genotype and clonality of Reed-Sternberg cells in nodular sclerosis Hodgkin's disease: results of single cell study. *Br J Haematol* 1996;94:198–205.
6. Kuppers R, Kanzler H, Hansmann ML, et al. immunoglobulin V genes in Reed-Sternberg cells [Letter]. *N Engl J Med* 1996;334:404.
7. Braeuninger A, Kuppers R, Strickler JG, et al. Hodgkin and Reed-Sternberg cells in lymphocyte predominance Hodgkin's disease represent clonal populations of germinal center-derived tumor cells. *Proc Natl Acad Sci USA* 1997;94:9337–9342.
8. Hummel M, Marafiotis T, Stein H. immunoglobulin V genes in Reed-Sternberg cells [Letter]. *N Engl J Med* 1996;334;405–406.
9. Marafioti TR, Hummel M, Anagnostopoulos I, et al. Origin of nodular lymphocyte-predominant Hodgkin's disease from a clonal expansion of highly mutated germinal-center B cells. *N Engl J Med* 1997;337: 453–458.
10. Ohno T, Stribley JA, Wu G, et al. Clonality in lymphocyte predominance Hodgkin's disease. *N Engl J Med* 1997;337:459–465.
11. Ohno T, Smir BN, Weisenburger DD, et al. Origin of the Hodgkin/Reed-Sternberg cells in chronic lymphocytic leukemia with "Hodgkin's transformation." *Blood* 1998;91:1757–1761.
12. Wickert RS, Weisenburger DD, Tierens A, et al. Clonal relationship between lymphocyte predominance Hodgkin's disease and concurrent or subsequent large cell lymphoma of B-lineage. *Blood* 1995;86: 2312–2320.
13. Kuppers R, Rajewsky K. The origin of Hodgkin and Reed/Sternberg cells in Hodgkin's disease. *Ann Rev Immunol* 1998;16:471–493.
14. Carbone A, Gloghini A, Gaidano G, et al. Expression status of bcl-6 and syndecan-1 identifies distinct histogenetic subtypes of Hodgkin's disease. *Blood* (*in press*).
15. Fisher RI, Cossman J, Diehl V, et al. Antigen presentation by Hodgkin's disease cells. *J Immunol* 1985;135:3568–3571.
16. Fisher RI, Bostick-Bruton F, Sauder DN, et al. Neoplastic cells obtained from Hodgkin's disease are potent stimulators of human primary mixed lymphocyte cultures. *J Immunol* 1983;130:2666–2670.
17. Munro JM, Freedman AS, Aster JC, et al. In vivo expression of the B7 costimulatory molecule by subsets of antigen-presenting cells and the malignant cells of Hodgkin's disease. *Blood* 1994;83:793–798.
18. Delabie J, Ceuppens JL, Vandenberghe P, et al. The B7/BB1 antigen is expressed by Reed-Sternberg cells of Hodgkin's disease and contributes to the stimulating capacity of Hodgkin's disease-derived cell lines. *Blood* 1993;82:2845–2852.
19. Azuma M, Yssel H, Phillips JH, et al. Functional expression of B7/BB1 and activated T lymphocytes. *J Exp Med* 1993;177:845–850.
20. Curran RC, Jones EL. Dendritic cells and B lymphocytes in Hodgklin's disease. *Lancet* 1977:349.
21. Delsol G, Meggetto F, Brousset P, et al. Relation of follicular dendritic reticulum cells to Reed-Sternberg cells of Hodgkin's disease with emphasis on the expression of CD21 antigen. *Am J Pathol* 1993;1729.
22. Nakamura S, Nagahama M, Kagami Y, et al. Hodgkin's disease expressing follicular dendritic cell marker CD21 without any other B-cell marker: a clinicopathologic study of nine cases. *Am J Surg Pathol* (*in press*).
23. Kennedy ICS, Hart DNJ, Colls BM, et al. Nodular sclerosing, mixed cellularity and lymphocyte-depleted variants of Hodgkin's disease are probable dendritic cell malignancies. *Clin Exp Immunol* 1989;76: 324–331.
24. Soderstrom K-O, Rinne R, Hopsu-Havu VK, et al. Hodgkin's disease: a malignancy of follicular dendritic cells? *Lancet* 1994;343:422–423.
25. Kadin ME. Possible origin of the Reed-Stenberg cell from an interdigitating reticulum cell. *Cancer Treat Rep* 1982;66:601–608.
26. Beckstead JH, Warnke R, Bainton DF. Histochemistry of Hodgkin's diasease. *Cancer Treat Rep* 1982;66:609–613.
27. Pinkus GS, Pinkus JL, Langhoff E, et al. Fascin, a sensitive new marker for Reed-Sternberg cells of Hodgkin's disease: evidence for a dendritic or B cell derivation? *Am J Pathol* 1997;150:543–562.
28. Weiss LM, Chang KL. Association of Epstein-Barr virus with hematolymphoid neoplasia. *Adv Anat Pathol* 1996.
29. Drexler HG. Recent results on the biology of Hodgkin and Reed-Sternberg cells: II. Continuous cell lines. *Leuk Lymphoma* 1993;9: 1–25.
30. Falini B, Stein H, Pileri S, et al. Expression of lymphoid-associated antigens on Hodgkin's and Reed-Sternberg cells of Hodgkin's disease: an immunocytochemical study on lymph node cytospins using monoclonal antibodies. *Histopathology* 1987;11:1229–1242.
31. Agnarsson BA, Kadin ME. The immunophenotype of Reed-Sternberg cells: a study of 50 cases of Hodgkin's disease using fixed frozen tissues. *Cancer* 1989;63:2083–2087.
32. Kadin ME, Muramoto L, Said J. Expression of T cell antigens by Reed-Sternberg cells in Hodgkin's disease. *Am J Pathol* 1988;130: 345–353.
33. Dallenbach FE, Stein H. Expression of T-cell receptor b-chain in Reed-Sternberg cells. *Lancet* 1989:828–830.
34. Casey TT, Olson SJ, Cousar JB, et al. Immunophenotypes of Reed-Sternberg cells: a study of 19 cases of Hodgkin's disease in plastic embedded sections. *Blood* 1989;74:2624–2628.
35. Oudejans JJ, Kummer JA, Jiwa M, et al. Granzyme B expression in Reed-Sternberg cells of Hodgkin's diasease. *Am J Pathol* 1996;148: 233–240.
36. Foss HD, Anagnostopoulos I, Araugo I, et al. Anaplastic large-cell lymphomas of T-cell and null-cell phenotype express cytotoxic molecules. *Blood* 1996;88:4005–4011.
37. Krenacs L, Wellmann A, Sorbara L, et al. Cytotoxic cell antigen experssion in anaplastic large cell lymphomas of T- and null-cell type and Hodgkin's disease: evidence for a distinct cellular origin. *Blood* 1997;89:980–989.
38. Felgar RE, Macon WR, Kinnney MC, et al. TIA-1 expression in lymphoid neoplasms. *Am J Pathol* 1997;150:1893–1900.
39. Davis TH, Morton CC, Miller-Cassman R, et al. Hodgkin's disease, lymphomatoid papulosis and cutaneous T-cell lymphoma derived from a common T-cell clone. *N Engl J Med* 1992;326:1115–1122.
40. Chan WC, Griem ML, Gozea PN, et al. Mycosis fungoides and Hodgkin's disease occurring in the same patient: report of three cases. *Cancer* 1979;44:1408–1413.
41. Hawkins KA, Schinella R, Schwartz M, et al. Simultaneous occurrence of mycosis fungoides and Hodgkin's disease: clinical and histologic correlations in three cases with ultrastructural studies in two. *Am J Hematol* 1983;14:355–362.
42. Morris SW, Kirstein MN, Valentine MB, et al. Fusion of a kinase gene, ALK, to a nucleolar protein gene, NPM, in non-Hodgkin's lymphoma. *Science* 1994;1281–1284.
43. Shiota M, Nakamura S, Ichinohasama R, et al. Anaplastic large cell lymphomas expressing the novel chimeric protein p80 NPM/ALK: a distinct clinicopathologic entity. *Blood* 1995;86:1954–1960.
44. Muschen M, Rajewsky K, Brauninger A, et al. Rare occurrence of classic Hodgkin's disease as a T cell lymphoma. *J Exp Med* 2000; 387–394.
45. Hummel SV, Hummel M, Marafioti T, et al. Detection of clonal T-cell receptor gamma-chain gene-rearrangements in Reed-Sternberg cells of classic Hodgkin's disease. *Blood* 2000 (*in press*).

45a. Willenbrock K, Ichinohasama R, Kadin ME, et al. Clonal rearrangement of the TCR-β chain gene in a cutaneous T cell lymphoma and classic Hodgkin's disease of the same patient. Manuscript in preparation.

46. Pinkus GS, Said JW. Hodgkin's disease, lymphocyte predominance type, nodular—further evidence for a B cell derivation: L & H variants of Reed-Sterberg cells express L26, a pan B cell marker. *Am J Pathol* 1988;133:211–217.
47. Stein H, Hansmann ML, Lennert K, et al. Reed-Sternberg and Hodgkin's cells in lymphocyte-predominant Hodgkin's disease of nodular subtype contain J chain. *Am J Clin Pathol* 1986;86:292–297.
48. Poppema S, Kaiserling E, Lennert K. Hodgkin's disease with lymphocyte predominance, nodular type (nodular paragranuloma) and pro-

gressively transformed germinal centers: a cytohistological study. *Histopathology* 1979;3:295–308.
49. Poppema S, Kaiserling E, Lennert K. Nodular paragranuloma and progressively transformed germinal centers: ultrastructural and immunohistologic findings. *Virchows Arch (Cell Pathol)* 1979;31:211–225.
50. Timens W, Visser L, Poppema S. Nodular lymphocyte predominance type of Hodgkin's disease is a germinal center lymphoma. *Lab Invest* 1986;54:457–461.
51. Poppema S. The nature of the lymphocytes surrounding Reed-Sternberg cells in nodular lymphocyte predominance and in other types of Hodgkin's disease. *Am J Pathol* 1989;135:351–357.
52. Miettinen M, Franssila KO, Saxen E. Hodgkin's disease, lymphocytic predominance nodular-increased risk for subsequent non-Hodgkin's lymphomas. *Cancer* 1983;54:2293–2300.
53. Lennert K, Hansmann ML. Progressive transformation of germinal centers: clinical significance and lymphocyte predominant Hodgkin's disease—the Kiel experience. *Am J Surg Pathol* 1987;11:149–150.
54. Hansmann ML, Stein H, Fellbaum C, et al. Nodular paragranuloma can transform into high-grade malignant lymphoma of B type. *Hum Pathol* 1989;20:1169–1175.
55. Sundeen JT, Cossman J, Jaffe ES. Lymphocyte predominant Hodgkin's disease nodular subtype with coexistent ''large cell lymphoma: '' histologic progression or composite malignancy? *Am J Surg Pathol* 1988;12:599–606.
56. von Wasielewski R, Werner M, Fischer R, et al. Lymphocyte-predominant Hodgkin's disease: an immunohistochemical analysis of 208 reviewed Hodgkin's disease cases from the German Hodgkin Study Group. *Am J Pathol* 1997;150:793–803.
57. Schwab U, Stein H, Gerdes J, et al. Production of a monoclonal antibody specific for Hodgkin and Sternberg-Reed cells of Hodgkin's disease and a subset of normal lymphoid cells. *Nature* 1982;299: 65–67.
58. Stein H, Mason DY, Gerdes J, et al. The expression of the Hodgkin's disease associated antigen Ki-1 in reactive and neoplastic lymphoid tissue: evidence that Reed-Sternberg cells and histiocytic malignancies are derived from activated lymphoid cells. *Blood* 1985;66: 848–858.
59. Andreesen R, Brugger W, Lohr GW, et al. Human macrophages can express the Hodgkin's cell-associated antigen Ki-1(CD30). *Am J Pathol* 1989;134:187–192.
60. Pfreundschuh M, Mommertz E, Meissner M, et al. Hodgkin and Reed-Sternberg cell associated monoclonal antibodies HRS-1 and HRS-2 react with activated cells of lymphoid and monocytoid origin. *Anticancer Res* 1988;8:217–224.
61. Stein H, Schwarting R, Dallenbach F, et al. Immunology of Hodgkin and Reed-Sternberg cells. In: Diehl V, Pfreundschuh M, Loeffler M, eds. *Recent results in cancer research.* Berlin: Springer-Verlag, 1990: 14–26.
62. Schwarting R, Gerdes J, Durkop H, et al. Ber-H2: a new anti-Ki-1 (CD30) monoclonal antibody directed at a formol-resistant epitope. *Blood* 1989;74:1678–1689.
63. Palleson G, Hamilton-Dutoit SJ. Ki-1(CD30) antigen is regularly expressed by tumor cells of embryonal carcinoma. *Am J Pathol* 1988; 133:446–450.
64. Pinkus GS, Thomas P, Said JW. Leu-M1—A marker for Reed-Sternberg cells in Hodgkin's disease: an immunoperoxidase study of paraffin-embedded tissues. *Am J Pathol* 1985;119:244–252.
65. Hsu SM, Jaffe ES. Leu-M1 and peanut agglutinin stain the neoplastic cells of Hodgkin's disease. *Am J Clin Pathol* 1984;82:29–32.
66. Stein H, Uchanska-Ziegler B, Gerdes J, et al. Hodgkin and Sternberg-Reed cells contain antigens specific to late cells of granulopoiesis. *Int J Cancer* 1982;29:283–290.
67. Dorfman RF, Gatter KC, Pulford KAF, et al. An evaluation of the utility of antigranulocyte and anti-leukocyte monoclonal antibodies in the diagnosis of Hodgkin's disease. *Am J Pathol* 1986;123:508–519.
68. Hsu SM, Ho Y-S, Li P-I, et al. L & H variants of Reed-Sternberg cells express sialylated Leu-M1 antigen. *Am J Pathol* 1986;122:199–203.
69. Chadburn A, Inghirami G, Knowles DM. T-cell activation antigen expression by neoplastic T-cells. *Lab Invest* 1990;60:17a(abst).
70. Wieczorek R, Burke JS, Knowles DM. Leu-M1 antigen expression in T-cell neoplasia. *Am J Pathol* 1985;121:374–380.
71. Sheibani K, Battifora H, Burke JS, et al. Leu-M1 antigen in human neoplasms: an immunohistologic study of 400 cases. *Am J Surg Pathol* 1986;10:227–236.
72. Delsol G, Gatter KC, Stein H, et al. Human lymphoid cells express epithelial membrane antigen: implications for the diagnosis of human neoplasms. *Lancet* 1984;2:1124–1128.
73. Chittal SM, Caveriviere P, Schwarting R, et al. Monoclonal antibodies in the diagnosis of Hodgkin's disease: the search for a rational panel. *Am J Surg Pathol* 1988;12:9–21.
74. Pizzolo G, Chilosi M, Semenzanto G, et al. Immunohistological analysis of Tac antigen expression in tissues involved by Hodgkin's disease. *Br J Cancer* 1984;50:415–417.
75. Sheibani K, Winberg CD, van de Velde S, et al. Distribution of lymphocytes with interleukin-2 receptors (TAC antigens) in reactive lymphoproliferative processes, Hodgkin's disease, and non-Hodgkin's lymphomas: an immunohistologic study of 300 cases. *Am J Pathol* 1987;127:27–37.
76. von Wasielewski R, Mengel M, Fischer R, et al. Classic Hodgkin's disease: clinical impact of the immunophenotype. *Am J Pathol* 1997; 151:1123–1130.
77. Ree HJ, Neiman RS, Martin AW, et al. Paraffin section markers for Reed-Sternberg cells: a comparative study of peanut agglutinin, Leu-M1, LN-2, and Ber-H2. *Cancer* 1989;63:2030–2036.
78. Strickler JG, Michie SA, Warnke RA, et al. The ''syncytial variant'' of nodular sclerosing Hodgkin's disease. *Am J Surg Pathol* 1986;10: 470–477.
79. Agnarsson BA, Kadin ME. Ki-1 positive large cell lymphoma: a morphologic and immunologic study of 19 cases. *Am J Surg Pathol* 1988; 12:264–274.
80. Delsol G, Al Saati T, Gatter KC, et al. Coexpression of epithelial membrane antigen (EMA), Ki-1, and interleukin-2 receptor by anaplastic large cell lymphomas: diagnostic value in so-called malignant histiocytosis. *Am J Pathol* 1988;130:59–70.
81. Falini B, Pileri S, Stein H, et al. Variable expression of leucocyte-common (CD45) antigen in CD30 (Ki-1) positive anaplastic large-cell lymphoma: implications for the differential diagnosis between lymphoid and nonlymphoid malignancies. *Hum Pathol* 1990;21: 624–629.
82. Kadin ME. Primary Ki-1-positive anaplastic large-cell lymphoma: a distinct clinicopathologic entity. *Ann Oncol* 1994;5(Suppl 1): S25–S30.
83. Salhany KE, Collins RD, Greer JP, et al. Longterm survivial in Ki-1 lymphoma: report of three cases. *Cancer* 1991;67:516–522.
84. Beljaards RC, Meijer CJLM, Scheffer E, et al. Prognostic significance of CD30 (Ki-1/Ber-H2) expression in primary cutaneous large-cell lymphomas of T-cell origin: a clinicopathologic and immunohistochemical study in 20 patients. *Am J Pathol* 1989;135:1169–1178.
85. Weis JW, Winter MW, Phyliky RL, et al. Peripheral T-cell lymphomas: histologic, immunohistologic and clinical characterization. *Mayo Clin Proc* 1986;61:411–426.
86. Waldron JA, Leech JH, Glick AD, et al. Malignant lymphoma of peripheral T-cell origin: immunologic, pathologic, and clinical features in six patients. *Cancer* 1977;40:1604–1617.
87. Weiss LM, Crabtree GS, Rouse RV, et al. Morphologic and immunologic characterization of 50 peripheral T-cell lymphomas. *Am J Pathol* 1985;118:316–324.
88. Knowles DM, Halper JP, Jakobiec FA. T-lymphocyte subpopulations in B-cell-derived non-Hodgkin's lymphomas and Hodgkin's disease. *Cancer* 1984;56:644–651.
89. Wieczorek R, Buck D, Bindl J, et al. Monoclonal antibody Leu-22 (L60) permits the demonstration of some neoplastic T cells in routinely fixed and paraffin-embedded tissue sections. *Hum Pathol* 1988; 19:1434–1443.
90. Knowles DM, Neri A, Pelicci PG, et al. immunoglobulin and T-cell receptor B-chain gene rearrangement analysis of Hodgkin's disease: implications for lineage determination and differential diagnosis. *Proc Natl Acad Sci USA* 1986;83:7942–7946.
91. Addis BJ, Isaacson PG. Large cell lymphoma of the mediastinum: a B-cell tumour of probable thymic origin. *Histopathology* 1986;10: 379–390.
92. Taylor CR. The nature of Reed-Sternberg cells and other malignant ''reticulum'' cells. *Lancet* 1974:802–806.
93. Gruss H-J, Kadin ME. Pathophysiology of Hodgkin's disease: functional and molecular aspects. In: Diehl V, ed. *Bailliere's clinical haematology: international practice and research*, vol 9. London: Bailliere Tindall, 1996:417–446.
94. Kadin ME, Leibowitz D. Cytokines and cytokine receptors in Hodg-

kin's disease. In: Mauch PM, Armitage JO, Diehl V, et al, eds. *Hodgkin's disease.* Philadelphia: Lippincott Williams & Wilkins, 1999: 139–158.
95. Newcom SR, O'Rourke L. Potentiation of fibroblast growth by nodular sclerosing Hodgkin's cell cultures. *Blood* 1982;60:228–237.
96. Ford RJ, Mehta S, Davis F, et al. Growth factors in Hodgkin's disease. *Cancer Treat Rep* 1982;66:633–638.
97. Roberts AB, Sporn MB, Assoian RK, et al. Transforming growth factor type beta: rapid induction of fibrosis and angiogenesis in vivo and stimulation of collagen formation in vitro. *Proc Natl Acad Sci USA* 1986;83:4167–4171.
98. Wahl SM, Hunt DA, Wakefield LM, et al. Transforming growth factor type B induces monocyte chemotaxis and growth factor production. *Proc Natl Acad Sci USA* 1987;84:5788–5792.
99. Kadin ME, Donaldson S, Dorfman RF. Isolated granulomas in Hodgkin's disease. *N Engl J Med* 1970;283:859–861.
100. Kadin ME, Agnarsson BA, Ellingsworth LR, et al. Immunohistochemical evidence of a role for transforming growth factor beta in the pathogenesis of nodular sclerosing Hodgkin's disease. *Am J Pathol* 1990;136:1209–1214.
101. Shinozaki M, Kawara HN, Kakinuma T, et al. Induction of subcutaneous tissue fibrosis in newborn mice by transforming growth factor–simultaneous application with basic fibroblast growth factor cause persistent fibrosis. *Biochem Biophys Res Commun* 1997;237:292–6.
102. Ohshima K, Sugihara M, Suzymiya H, et al. Basic fibroblast growth factor and fibrosis in Hodgkin's disease. *Am J Hematol (in press).*
103. Visser L, Poppema S. The absence of effective T-cell activation in Hodgkin's disease may be the result of TGFb production by Reed-Sternberg cells. *Leuk Lymphoma* 1998;29(Suppl 1):P38(abst).
104. Kay AB, Mc Vie JG, Stuart AE, et al. Eosinophil chemotaxis of supernatants from cultured Hodgkin's lymph node cells. *J Clin Pathol* 1975;28:502–505.
105. Samoszuk M, Nansen L. Detection of interleukin-5 messenger RNA in Reed-Sternberg cells of Hodgkin's disease with eosinophilia. *Blood* 1990;75:13–16.
106. Clutterbuck EJ, Hirst EMA, Sanderson CJ. Human interleukin-5 regulates the production of eosinophils in human bone marrow cultures: comparison and interaction with IL-1, IL-3, IL-6, and GMCSF. *Blood* 1989;73:1504–1512.
107. Teruya-Feldstein JT, Jaffe ES, Burd PR, et al. Differential chemokine expression in tissues involved by Hodgkin's disease: direct correlation of eotaxin-1 expression and tissue eosinophilia. *Blood* 1999;93:2463.
108. Ben-Ezra J, Sheibani K, Swartz W, et al. Relationship between eosinophil density and T-cell activation markers in lymph nodes of patients with Hodgkin's disease. *Hum Pathol* 1989;20:1181–1185.
109. Burrichter H, Heit W, Schaadt M, et al. Production of colony-stimulating factors by Hodgkin's cell lines. *Int J Cancer* 1984;31:269–274.
110. Newcom SR, Muth LH, Ansari A. Interleukin-4 is an autocrine growth factor secreted by the L428 Reed-Sternberg cell. *Blood* 1992;79: 191–197.
110a. Kapp U, Yeh WC, Patterson B, et al. Interleukin 13 is secreted by and stimulates the growth of Hodgkin and Reed-Sternberg cells. *J Exp Med* 1999;1939–1945.
111. Coffman RL, O Hara J, Bond MW, et al. B cell stimulatory factor-1 enhances the IgE response of lipopolysaccharide-activated B cells. *J Immunol* 1986;136:949–954.
112. McInnes A, Rennick DM. Interleukin-4 induces cultured monocytes/macrophages to form giant multinucleated cells. *J Exp Med* 1988; 167:598–611.
113. Ree HJ, Pezzullo JC. Inflammation and/or necrosis of tumors cannot account for fever in most febrile patients with Hodgkin's disease. *Cancer* 1987;60:1787–1789.
114. Ree HJ, Crowley JP, Dinarello CA. Anti-interleukin-1 reactive cells in Hodgkin's disease. *Cancer* 1987;59:1717–1720.
115. Ellis TM, McMannis JD, Chua AO, et al. Interleukin-1 independent activation of human T-lymphocytes stimulated by anti-CD3 and a Hodgkin's disease cell line with accessory cell activity. *Cell Immunol* 1988;116:352–366.
116. Kretschmer C, Jones DB, Morrison K, et al. Tumor necrosis factor alpha and lymphotoxin production in Hodgkin's disease. *Am J Pathol* 1990;137:341–351.
117. Sappino A-P, Seelentag W, Pelte M-F, et al. Tumor necrosis factor/cachectin and lymphotoxin gene expression in lymph nodes from lymphoma patients. *Blood* 1990;75:958–962.
118. Perussia B, Kobayashi M, Rossi ME, et al. Immune interferon enhances functional properties of human granulocytes: role of Fc receptor and effect of lymphotoxin tumor necrosis factor, and granulocyte-macrophage colony stimulating factor. *J Immunol* 1987;138:765–774.
119. Chang RJ, Lee SH. Effects of interferon-gamma and tumor necrosis factor-alpha on the expression of an la antigen on a murine macrophage cell line. *J Immunol* 1987;13:2853–2856.
120. Sugarman BJ, Aggarwal BB, Hass PE, et al. Recombinant human tumor necrosis factor-alpha: effects on proliferation of normal and transformed cells in vitro. *Science* 1985;230:943–945.
121. Pober JS, Lapierre LA, Stolpen AH, et al. Activation of cultured human endothelial cells by recombinant lymphotoxin: comparison with tumor necrosis factor and interleukin-1 species. *J Immunol* 1987; 138:3319–3324.
122. Naumovski L, Utz PJ, Bergstrom SK, et al. SUP-HD1: a new Hodgkin's disease-derived cell line with lymphoid features produces interferon-gamma. *Blood* 1989;74:2733–2742.
123. Murray HW. Interferon-gamma, the activated macrophage, and host defense against microbial challenge. *Ann Intern Med* 1988;108: 595–608.
124. Kurzrock R, Redman J, Cabanillas F, et al. serum interleukin 6 levels are elevated in lymphoma patients and correlate with survival in advanced Hodgkin's disease with B symptoms. *Cancer Res* 1993;53: 2118–22.
125. Kadin ME, Newcom SR, Gold SB, et al. Origin of Hodgin's cell. *Lancet* 1974,167.
126. Stuart AE, Williams AR, Habeshaw JA. Rosetting and oth er reactions of the Reed-Sternberg cell. J Pathol 1977;122:81.
127. Roers A, Montesinos-Rongen M, Hansmann ML, et al. T cells rosetting around Hodgkin and Reed-Sternberg cells in Hodgkin's disease are polyclonal. *Leuk Lymphoma* 1998;29(Suppl 1):P20.
128. Delabie J, Ceuppens JL, Vandenberghe P, et al. The B7/BB1 antigen is expressed by Reed-Sternberg cells of Hodgkin's disease and contributes to the stimulating capacity of Hodgkin's disease-derived cell lines. *Blood* 1993;82:2845–2852.
129. Thompson CB, Lindsten T, Ledbetter JA, et al. CD28 activation pathway regualtes the production of multiple T-cell-derived lymphokines/cytokines. *Proc Natl Acad Sci USA* 1989;86:1333–1337.
130. Stamenkovic I, Clark EA, Seed B. A B-lymphocyte activation molecule related to the nerve growth factor receptor and induced by cytokines in carcinomas. *EMBO J* 1989;8:1403–1410.
131. Law CL, Wormann B, LeBien TW. Analysis of expression and function of CD40 on normal and leukemic human B cell precursors. *Leukemia* 1990;4:732–738.
132. Smith CA, Farrah T, Goodwin RG. The TNF receptor superfamily of cellular and viral proteins: activation, costimulation, and death. *Cell* 1994;75:959–962.
133. Lane P, Traunecker A, Hubele S, et al. Activated human T cells express a ligand for the human B cell-associated antigen CD40 which participates in T cell-dependent activation of B lymphocytes. Eur *J Immunol* 1992;22:2573–2578.
134. Banchereau J, de Paoli P, Valle A, et al. Long-term human B cell lines dependent on interleukin-4 and antibody to CD40. *Science* 1991; 251:70–72.
135. Liu YJ, Mason DY, Johnson GD, et al. Germinal center cells express bcl-2 protein after activation by signals which prevent their entry into apoptosis. Eur *J Immunol* 1991;21:1905–1910.
136. O'Grady JT, Stewart S, Lowrey J, et al. CD40 expression in Hodgkin's disease [See comments]. *Am J Pathol* 1994;144:21–26.
137. Gruss HJ, Hirschstein D, Wright B, et al. Expression and function of CD40 on Hodgkin and Reed-Sternberg cells and the possible relevance for Hodgkin's disease. *Blood* 1994;84:2305–2314.
138. Carbone A, Gloghini A, Gattei V, et al. Expression of CD40 antigen on Reed-Sternberg cells and Hodgkin's disease cell lines. *Blood* 1995; 85:780–789.
139. Gruss HJ, Hirschstein D, Wright B, et al. Expression and function of CD40 on Hodgkin and Reed-Sternberg cells and the possible relevance for Hodgkin's disease. *Blood* 1994;84:2305–2314.
140. Ellis TM, Simms PE, Slivnick DJ, et al. CD30 is a signal-transducing molecule that defines a subset of human activated CD45RO + T cells. *J Immunol* 1993;151:2380–2389.
141. Smith CA, Gruss HJ, Davis T, et al. CD30 antigen, a marker for Hodgkin's lymphoma, is a receptor whose ligand defines an emerging family of cytokines with homology to TNF. *Cell* 1993;73:1349–1360.

142. Gruss HJ, Boinai N, Williams DE, et al. Pleiotropic effects of the CD30 ligand on CD30-expressing cells and lymphoma cell lines. *Blood* 1994;83:2045–2056.
143. Gruss HJ, Pinto A, Gloghini A, et al. CD30 ligand expression in nonmalignant and Hodgkin's disease-involved lymphoid tissues. *Am J Pathol* 1996;149:469–481.
144. Malinin NL, Boldin MP, Kovalenko AV, et al. MAP3K-related kinase involved in NF-kappaB induction by TNF, CD95 and IL-1. *Nature* 1997;385:540–544.
145. Regnier CH, Song HY, Gao X, et al. Identification and characterization of an IkappaB kinase. *Cell* 1997;90:373–383.
146. Woronicz JD, Gao X, Cao Z, et al. IkappaB kinase-beta: NF-kappaB activation and complex formation with IkappaB kinase-alpha and NIK [See comments]. *Science* 1997;278:866–869.
147. DiDonato JA, Hayakawa M, Rothwarf DM, et al. A cytokine-responsive IkappaB kinase that activates the transcription factor NF-kappaB [See comments]. *Nature* 1997;388:548–454.
148. Zandi E, Rothwarf DM, Delhase M, et al. The IkappaB kinase complex (IKK) contains two kinase subunits, IKKalpha and IKK beta, necessary for IkappaB phosphorylation and NF-kappaB activation. *Cell* 1997;91:243–252.
149. Mercurio F, Zhu H, Murray BW, et al. IKK-1 and IKK-2: cytokine-activated IkappaB kinases essential for NF-kappa B activation [See comments]. *Science* 1997;278:860–866.
150. Baldwin AS Jr. The NF-kappa B and I kappa B proteins: new discoveries and insights. *Annu Rev Immunol* 1996;14:649–683.
151. Bargou RC, Emmerich F, Krappmann D, et al. Constitutive nuclear factor-kB-RelA activation is required for proliferation and survival of Hodgkin's disease tumor cells. *J Clin Invest* 1997;100:2961–2969.
152. Yasuda N, Lai P, Ip SH, et al. Soluble interleukin 2 receptors in sera of Japanese patients with adult T cell leukemia mark activity of disease. *Blood* 1988;71:1021–1026.
153. Chilosi M, Semenzato G, Cetto GL, et al. Soluble interleukin-2 receptors in the sera of patients with hairy cell leukemia: relationship with the effect of recombinant alphainterferon therapy on clinical parameters and natural killer in vitro activity. *Blood* 1987;70:1530–1535.
154. Wagner D, Kiwanuka J, Edwards BK, et al. Soluble interleukin-2 receptor levels in patients with undifferentiated and lymphoblastic lymphomas: correlation with survival. *J Clin Oncol* 1987;5:1262–1274.
155. Pizzolo G, Chilosi M, Vinante F, et al. Soluble interleukin-2 receptors in the serum of patients with Hodgkin's disease. *Br J Cancer* 1987;55:427–428.
156. Pizzolo G, Vinante F, Chilosi M, et al. Serum levels of soluble CD30 molecule (Ki-1 antigen) in Hodgkin's disease: relationship with disease activity and clinical stage. *Br J Haematol* 1990;75:282–284.
157. Younes A, Consoli U, Snell V, et al. CD30 ligand in lymphoma patients with CD30 + tumors. *J Clin Oncol* 1997;15:3355–3362.
158. Burn C, Davies JNP, Dodge OG, et al. Hodgkin's disease in English and African children. *J Natl Cancer Inst* 1971;46:37–41.
159. Strum SB, Rappaport H. Hodgkin's disease in the first decade of life. *Pediatrics* 1970;46:748–759.
160. Ree HJ, Strauchen JA, Khan A, et al. Hodgkin's disease in HIV-infected patients: clinico-pathologic studies of 24 cases. Preponderance of mixed cellularity type. *Cancer* 1991;67:1614–1621.
161. Unger PD, Strauchen JA. Hodgkin's disease in AIDS complex patients: report of four cases and tissue immunologic marker studies. *Cancer* 1986;58:821–825.
162. Knowles DM, Chamulak GA, Subar M, et al. Lymphoid neoplasia associated with the acquired immunodeficiency syndrome (AIDS). *Ann Intern Med* 1988;108:744–753.
163. Ree HJ, Teplitz C, Khan AA, et al. HIV-associated Hodgkin's disease: abnormal histiocytes and extracellular changes detected by concanavalin A (Con-A) staining. *Lab Invest* 1991;64:83a(abst).
164. Schoeppel JL, Hoppe RT, Dorfman RF, et al. Hodgkin's disease in homosexual men with generalized lymphadenopathy. *Ann Intern Med* 1984;100:7–13.
165. Rosenberg SA, Kaplan HS. Evidence for an orderly progression in the spread of Hodgkin's disease. *Cancer Res* 1966;26:1225–1231.
166. Levy RA, Kaplan HS. Impaired lymphocyte function in untreated Hodgkin's disease. *N Engl J Med* 1974;290:181–186.
167. Bjorkholm M, Holm G, Mellstedt H. Immunocompetence in patients with Hodgkin's disease. In: Lacher MJ, Redman JR, eds. *Consequences of survival in Hodgkin's disease.* Philadelphia: Lea & Febiger, 1990:12.
168. Romagnani S, Del Prete GF, Maggi E, et al. Displacement of T lymphocytes with the ''helper/inducer'' phenotype from peripheral blood lymphoid organs in untreated patients with Hodgkin's disease. *Scand J Haematol* 1983;31:305–314.
169. Grimfors G, Holm G, Mellstedt H, et al. Increased blood clearance of indium-111 oxine-labeled autologous CD4 + Blood cells in untreated patients with Hodgkin's disease. *Blood* 1990;76:583–589.
170. Maggi E, Parronchi P, Del Prete G, et al. Frequent T4-positive cells with cytolytic activity in spleens of patients with Hodgkin's disease (a clonal analysis). *J Immunol* 1986;136:1516–1519.
171. Romagnani S, Amadori A, Biti G, et al. In vitro lymphocyte response to phytomitogens in untreated and treated patients with Hodgkin's disease. *Int Arch Allergy Appl Immunol* 1976;51:378–389.
172. Engleman EG, Benike CJ, Hoppe RT, et al. Autologous mixed lymphocyte reaction in patients with Hodgkin's disease: evidence for a T cell defect. *J Clin Invest* 1980;66:149–158.
173. Ford RJ, Tsao J, Kouttab NM, et al. Association of an interleukin abnormality with the T cell defect in Hodgkin's disease. *Blood* 1984;64:386–392.
174. Liberati AM, Ballatori E, Fizzoti M, et al. Immunologic profile in patients with Hodgkin's disease in complete remission. *Cancer* 1987;59:1906–1913.
175. Fisher RI, De Vita VT, Bostick F, et al. Persistent immunologic abnormalities in long-term survivors of advanced Hodgkin's disease. *Ann Intern Med* 1980;92:595–599.
176. Paietta E, Stockert RJ, Morell AG, et al. Unique antigen of cultured Hodgkin's cells: a putative sialyltransferase. *J Clin Invest* 1986;78:349–354.
177. Paietta E, Stockert RJ, McManus M, et al. Hodgkin's cell lectin, a lymphocyte adhesion molecule and mitogen. *J Immunol* 1989;143:2850–2857.
178. Hays D, Ternberg JL, Chen TT, et al. Complications related to 234 staging laparotomies performed in the Intergroup Hodgkin's Disease in Childhood Study. *Surgery* 1984;96:471–479.
179. Longmire RL, McMillan R, Yelenosky R, et al. In vitro splenic IgG synthesis in Hodgkin's disease. *N Engl J Med* 1973;289:763–767.
180. Longmire RL, Ryan S, McMillan R. Antibody-dependent lymphocytoxicity induced by immunoglobulin G from Hodgkin's disease splenic lymphocytes. *Science* 1978;199:71–72.
181. Leb L, Merrit JA. Decreased monocyte function in patients with Hodgkin's disease. *Cancer* 1978;41:1794–1803.
182. Petrini H, Polidori AR, Vatteroni ML, et al. Serum factors inhibiting leukocyte functions in Hodgkin's disease. *Clin Immunol Immunopathol* 1982;23:124–132.
183. Estevez ME, Ballart IJ, de Macedo MP, et al. Dysfunction of monocytes in Hodgkin's disease by excessive production of PGE-2 in long-term remission patients. *Cancer* 1988;62: 2128–2133.
184. Goodwin JS, Messner RP, Bankhurst AD, et al. Prostaglandin-producing suppressor cells in Hodgkin's disease. *N Engl J Med* 1977;297:963–968.
185. Schecter GS, Soehnlen F. Monocyte-mediated inhibition of lymphocyte blastogenesis in Hodgkin's disease. *Blood* 1978;52:261–271.
186. Bockman RS. Stage-dependent reduction in T-colony formation in Hodgkin's disease: coincidence with monocyte synthesis of prostaglandins. *J Clin Invest* 1980;66:523–531.
187. Romagnani S, Ferrine PLR, Ricci M. The immune derangement in Hodgkin's disease. *Semin Hematol* 1985;22:41–55.
188. Stuart AE. The pathogenesis of Hodgkin's disease. *J Pathol* 1978;126:239–254.
189. Johnsen HE, Madsen M, Kristensen T. Lymphocyte subpopulations in man: suppression of PWM-induced B cell proliferation by infectious mononucleosis T cells. *Scand J Immunol* 1979;10:251–255.
190. James DG, Williams WJ. Immunology of sarcoidosis. *Am J Med* 1982;72:5–8.
191. Romagnani S, Del Prete GF, Maggi E, et al. Abnormalities of in vitro immunoglobulin synthesis by peripheral blood lymphocytes from untreated patients with Hodgkin's disease. *J Clin Invest* 1983;71:1375–1382.
192. Bendtzen K. Interleukin-1, interleukin-6 and tumor necrosis factor in infection, inflammation and immunity. *Immunol Lett* 1988;19:183–192.

193. Kerhl JH, Wakefield LM, Roberts AB, et al. 1986; Production of transforming growth factor beta by human T lymphocytes and its potential role in the regulation of T cell growth. *J Exp Med* 1986; 163:1037–1050.
194. Kerhl JH, Roberts AB, Wakefield L, et al. Transforming growth factor beta is an important immunomodulation protein for human B lymphocytes. *J Immunol* 1986;137:3855–3860.
195. Rook AH, Kerhl JH, Wakefield SM, et al. Effects of transforming growth factor B on the functions of natural killer cells: depressed cytolytic activity and blunting of interferon responsiveness. *J Immunol* 1986;136:3916–3920.
196. Kasid A, Bell GI, Director EP: Effects of transforming growth factor-β on human lymphokine-activated killer cell precursors: autocrine inhibition of cellular proliferation and differentiation to killer cells. *J Immunol* 1988;141:690–697.
197. Wrann M, Bodmer S, de Martin R, et al. T cell suppressor factor from human glioblastoma cells is a 12.5 KD protein closely related to transforming growth factor-beta. *EMBO J* 1987;6:1633–1636.
198. Kuppner MC, Hamou M-F, Bodmer S, et al. The glioblastoma-derived T-cell suppressor/transforming growth factor beta2 inhibits the generation of lymphokine activated killer (LAK) cells. *Int J Cancer* 1988; 42:562–567.
199. Sporn MB, Roberts AB. Transforming growth factor-B. Multiple actions and potential clinical applications. JAMA 1989;262:938–941.
200. Newcom SR, Kadin ME, Ansari AA, et al. L428 nodular sclerosing Hodgkin's cell secretes a unique transforming growth factor-beta active at physiologic pH. *J Clin Invest* 1988;82:1915–1921.
201. Seif GSF, Spriggs AI. Chromosome changes in Hodgkin's disease. *J Natl Cancer Inst* 1967;39:557–570.
202. Boecker WR, Hossfeld DK, Gallmeier WM, et al. Clonal growth of Hodgkin's cells. *Nature* 1975;258:235–236.
203. Weber Matthiesen K, Deerberg J, Poetsch M, et al. Numerical chromosome aberrations are present within the CD30 + Hodgkin and Reed-Sternberg cells in 100% of analyzed cases of Hodgkin's disease. *Blood* 1995;86:1464–1168.
204. Cabanillas F, Pathak S, Trujillo J, et al: Cytogenetic features of Hodgkin's disease suggest possible origin from a lymphocyte. *Blood* 1988; 71:1615–1617.
205. Schouten HC, Sanger WG, Duggan M, et al: Chromosomal abnormalities in Hodgkin's disease. *Blood* 1989;73:2149–2154.
206. Tilly H, Bastard C, Delastre T, et al: Cytogenetic studies in untreated Hodgkin's disease. *Blood* 1991;77:1298–1304.
207. Strong RS, Korsmeyer SJ, Parkin JL, et al: Human acute leukemia cell line with the t(4:11) chromosomal rearrangement exhibits B lineage and monocytic characteristics. *Blood* 1985;65:21.
208. Hsu SM, Jaffe ES. Leu-M1 and peanut agglutinin stain the neoplastic cells of Hodgkin's disease. *Am J Clin Pathol* 1984;82:29–32.
209. Tsujimoto Y, Finger LR, Yunis JJ, et al. Cloning of the chromosome break-point of neoplastic B cells with the t(14;18) chromosome translocation. *Science* 1984;226:1098–1099.
210. Cleary ML, Sklar J. Nucleotide sequence of a t(14;18) chromosomal breakpoint in follicular lymphoma and demonstration of a breakpoint-cluster region near a transcriptionally active locus on chromosome 18. *Proc Natl Acad Sci USA* 1985;82:7439–7443.
211. Poppema S, Kaleta J, Hepperle B. Chromosomal abnormalities in patients with Hodgkin's disease: evidence for frequent involvement of the 14q chromosomal region but infrequent bcl-2 gene rearrangement in Reed-Sternberg cells. *J Natl Cancer Inst* 1992;84:1789–1793.
212. Limpens J, De Jong D, van Krieken JH, et al. Bcl-2/Jh rearrangements in benign lymphoid tissues with follicular hyperplasia. *Oncogene* 1991;6:2271–2276.
213. Oshimura M, Sandberg A. Chromosomal 6q-anomaly in acute lymphoblastic leukemia. *Lancet* 1977,1405.
214. Nowell PC, Finan JB, Vonderheid EC. Clonal characteristics of cutaneous T cell lymphomas: cytogenetic evidence from blood, lymph nodes, and skin. *J Invest Dermatol* 1982;78:69–75.
215. Pellici PG, Knowles DM, Magrath I, et al. Chromosomal breakpoints and structural alterations of the c-myc locus differ in endemic and spontaneous forms of Burkitt lymphoma. *Proc Natl Acad Sci USA* 1986;83:2984–2988.
216. Vaux DL, Cory S, Adams JM. Bcl-2 gene promotes hematopoietic cell survival and cooperates with c-myc to immortalize B cells. *Nature* 1988;335:440–424.
217. Gauwerky CE, Haluska FG, Tsujimoto Y, et al. Evolution of B-cell malignancy: pre-B-cell leukemia resulting from MYC activation in a B-cell neoplasm with a rearranged BCL-2 gene. *Proc Natl Acad Sci USA* 1988;85:8548–8552.
218. Fonatsch C, Gradt G, Rademacher JL. Genetics of Hodgkin's lymphoma. In: Diehl V, Pfreundschuh M, Loeffler M, eds. *Recent results in cancer research.* Berlin: Springer-Verlag, 1990:35–49.
219. Levine J, Momand J, Finaly CA. The p53 tumour suppressor gene. *Nature* 1991;351:453–456.
220. Gupta RK, Norton AJ, Thompson IW, et al. P53 expression in primary biopsy material and cell lines of Hodgkin's disease. *Proc Natl Acad Sci USA* 1993;90:2817–2821.
221. Trumper LH, Brady G, Bagg A, et al. Single-cell analysis of Hodgkin and Reed-Sternberg cells: molecular heterogeneity of gene expression and p53 mutations. *Blood* 1993;81:3097–3115.
222. Inghirmai G, Macri L, Rosati S, et al. The Reed-Sternberg cells of Hodgkin disease are clonal. *Proc Natl Acad Sci USA* 1994;91: 9842–9846.
223. Lukes RJ, Tindile BH, Parker JW. Reed-Sternberg-like cells in infectious mononucleosis. *Lancet* 1969,1003–1004.
224. Mueller N, Evans A, Harris NA, et al. Hodgkin's disease and Epstein-Barr virus: altered antibody pattern before diagnosis. *N Engl J Med* 1989;320:689–695.
225. Sleckman BG, Mauch PM, Ambinder RF, et al. EBV-associated Hodgkins disease, infectious mononucleosis and childhood risk factors. *Cancer Epidemiol Biomarkers Prev* 1998;7:117–121.
226. Poppema S, van Imhoff G, Torensma R, et al. Lymphadenopathy morphologically consistent with Hodgkin's disease associated with Epstein-Barr virus infection. *Am J Clin Pathol* 1985;84:385–390.
227. Weiss LM, Mohaved LA, Warnke RA, et al. Detection of Epstein-Barr viral genomes in Reed-Sternberg cells of Hodgkin's disease. *N Engl J Med* 1989;320:502–506.
228. Anagnostopoulos I, Herbst H, Niedobitek G, et al. Demonstration of monoclonal EBV genomes in Hodgkin's disease and Ki-1-positive large cell lymphoma by combined Southern blot and in situ hybridization. *Blood* 1989;74:810–816.
229. Gulley ML, Eagan PA, Quintanilla-Martinez L, et al. Epstein-Barr virus DNA is abundant and monoclonal in the Reed-Sternberg cells of Hodgkin's disease: association with mixed cellularity subtype and Hispanic American ethnicity. *Blood* 1994;83:1595–1602.
230. Herbst H, Niedobitek G, Kneba M, et al. High incidence of Epstein-Barr virus genomes in Hodgkin's disease. *Am J Pathol* 1990;137: 13–18.
231. Brousset P, Schlaifer D, Chittal S, et al. Detection of Epstein-Barr virus messenger RNA in Reed-Sternberg cells of Hodgkin's disease with in situ hybridization with biotinylated probes on specially processed modified acetone methyl benzoate xylene (ModAMeX) sections. *Blood* 1991;77:1781–1786.
232. Pallesen G, Hamilton-Dutoit MR, Young LS. Expression of Epstein-Barr virus latent gene products in tumor cells of Hodgkin's disease. *Lancet* 1991;337:320–322.
233. Herbst H, Pallesen G, Weiss LM, et al. Hodgkin's disease and Epstein-Barr virus. *Ann Oncol* 1992;suppl.3:S27.
234. Weiss LM, Chen Y-Y, Liu X-F, et al. Epstein-Barr virus and Hodgkin's disease: a correlative in situ hybridization and polymerase chain reaction study. *Am J Pathol* 1991;139:1259–1265.
235. Jarrett RF: Viral involvement in Hodgkin's disease. *Int J Cell Cloning* 1992;10:315–322.
236. Armstrong AA, Alexander FE, Paes RP, et al: Association of Epstein-Barr virus with pediatric Hodgkin's disease. *Am J Pathol* 1993;142: 1683.
237. Ambinder RF, Browning PJ, Lorenzana I, et al. Epstein-Barr virus in childhood Hodgkin's disease in Honduras and the United States. *Blood* 1993;81:462–467.
238. Chang KL, Albujar PF, Chen YY, et al. High prevalence of Epstein-Barr virus in the Reed-Sternberg cells of Hodgkin's disease occurring in Peru. *Blood* 1993;81:496–501.
239. Herndier BG, Sanchez HC, Chang KL, et al. High prevalence of Epstein-Barr virus in the Reed-Sternberg cells of HIV-associated Hodgkin's disease. *Am J Pathol* 1993;142:1073–1079.
240. Vasef MA, Kamel OW, Chen Y-Y, et al. Detection of Epstein-Barr virus in multiple sites involved by Hodgkin's disease. *Am J Pathol* 1995;147:1408–1415.
241. Coates PJ, Slavin G, d'Ardonne AJ. Persistence of Epstein-Barr virus

in Reed-Sternberg cells throughout the course of Hodgkin's disease. *J Pathol* 1991;77:1781–1786.
242. Lin J-C, Lin S-C, De BK, et al. Precision of genotyping of Epstein-Barr virus by polymerase chain reaction using three gene loci (EBNA-2, EBNA-3C and EBER): predominance of type A virus associated with Hodgkin's disease. *Blood* 1993;81:3372–3381.
243. Boyle MJ, Vasak E, Tschuchnigg M, et al. Subtypes of Epstein-Barr virus (EBV) in Hodgkin's disease: Association between B-type EBV and immunocompromise. *Blood* 1993;81:468–474.
244. Wang D, Liebowitz D, Kieff E: An EBV membrane protein expressed in immortalized lymphocytes transforms established rodent cells. *Cell* 1985;43:831–840.
245. Deacon EM, Pallesen G, Niedobitek G, et al. Epstein-Barr virus and Hodgkin's disease: transcriptional analysis of virus latency in the malignant cells. *J Exp Med* 1993;77:339–349.
246. Kaye KM, Izumi KM, Kieff E. Epstein-Barr virus latent membrane protein 1 is essential for B-lymphocyte growth transformation. *Proc Natl Acad Sci USA* 1993;90:9150–9154.
247. Knecht H, Bachmann E, Brousset P, et al. Deletions within the LMP1 oncogene of Epstein-Barr virus are clustered in Hodgkin's disease and identical to those observed in nasopharyngeal carcinoma. *Blood* 1993;82:2937–2942.
248. Chen ML, Tsai CN, Liang CL, et al. Cloning and characterization of the latent membrane protein (LMP) of a specific Epstein-Barr virus variant derived from the nasopharyngeal carcinoma in the Taiwanese population. *Oncogene* 1992;7:2131–2140.
249. Knecht H, McQuain C, Martin J, et al. Expression of the LMP1 oncoprotein in the EBV negative Hodgkin's disease cell line L428 is associated with Reed-Sternberg cell morphology. *Oncogene* 1996;13: 947–953.
250. Mosialos G, Birkenbach M, Yalamanchili R, et al. The Epstein-Barr virus transforming protein LMP1 engages signaling proteins for the tumor necrosis factor receptor family. *Cell* 1995;80:389–399.
251. Devergne O, Hatzivassiliou E, Izumi KM, et al. Association of TRAF1, TRAF2, and TRAF3 with an Epstein-Barr virus LMP1 domain important for B-lymphocyte transformation: role in NF-kappaB activation. *Mol Cell Biol* 1996;16:7098–7108.
252. Kaye KM, Devergne O, Harada JN, et al. Tumor necrosis factor receptor associated factor 2 is a mediator of NF-kappa B activation by latent infection membrane protein 1, the Epstein-Barr virus transforming protein. *Proc Natl Acad Sci USA* 1996;93:11085–11090.
253. Izumi KM, Kaye KM, Kieff ED. The Epstein-Barr virus LMP1 amino acid sequence that engages tumor necrosis factor receptor associated factors is critical for primary B lymphocyte growth transformation. *Proc Natl Acad Sci USA* 1997;94:1447–1452.
254. Liebowitz D. Asoociation of the Epstein-Barr virus latent membrane protein (LMP1) with a tumor necrosis factor receptor signaling pathway in post-transplant lymphoproliferative disease and AIDS-associated non-Hodgkin's lymphoma. *N Engl J Med* 1998;338:1413–1421.
255. Hu HM, K OR, Boguski MS, et al. A novel RING finger protein interacts with the cytoplasmic domain of CD40. *J Biol Chem* 1994; 269:30069–30072.
256. Rothe M, Wong SC, Henzel WJ, et al. A novel family of putative signal transducers associated with the cytoplasmic domain of the 75 kDa tumor necrosis factor receptor. *Cell* 1994;78:681–692.
257. Rothe M, Sarma V, Dixit VM, Goeddel DV. TRAF2-mediated activation of NF-kappa B by TNF receptor 2 and CD40. *Science* 1995;269: 1424–1427.
258. Cheng G, Cleary AM, Ye ZS, et al. Involvement of CRAF1, a relative of TRAF, in CD40 signaling. *Science* 1995;267:1494–1498.
259. Regnier CH, Tomasetto C, Moog Lutz C, et al. Presence of a new conserved domain in CART1, a novel member of the tumor necrosis factor receptor-associated protein family, which is expressed in breast carcinoma. *J Biol Chem* 1995;270:25715–25721.
260. Cao Z, Xiong J, Takeuchi M, et al. TRAF6 is a signal transducer for interleukin-1. *Nature* 1996;383:443–446.
261. Ishida T, Mizushima S, Azuma S, et al. Identification of TRAF6, a novel tumor necrosis factor receptor-associated factor protein that mediates signaling from an amino-terminal domain of the CD40 cytoplasmic region. *J Biol Chem* 1996;271:28745–28748.
262. Ishida TK, Tojo T, Aoki T, et al. TRAF5, a novel tumor necrosis factor receptor-associated factor family protein, mediates CD40 signaling. *Proc Natl Acad Sci USA* 1996;93:9437–9442.
263. Nakano H, Oshima H, Chung W, et al. TRAF5, an activator of NF-kappaB and putative signal transducer for the lymphotoxin-beta receptor. *J Biol Chem* 1996;271:14661–14664.
264. Takeuchi M, Rothe M, Goeddel DV. Anatomy of TRAF2: distinct domains for nuclear factor-kappa B activation and association with tumor necrosis factor signaling proteins. *J Biol Chem* 1996;271: 19935–19942.
265. Sato T, Irie S, Reed JC. A novel member of the TRAF family of putative signal transducing proteins binds to the cytosolic domain of CD40. *FEBS Lett* 1995;358:113–118.
266. Song HY, Donner DB. Association of a RING finger protein with the cytoplasmic domain of the human type-2 tumour necrosis factor receptor. *Biochem J* 1995;309:825–829.
267. Baker SJ, Reddy EP. Transducers of life and death: TNF receptor superfamily and associated proteins. *Oncogene* 1996;12:1–9.
268. Henderson S, Rowe D, Gregor C, et al. Induction of bcl-2 expression by Epstein-Barr virus latent membrane protein protects infected B cells from programmed cell death. *Cell* 1991;65:1107–1115.
269. Jiwa NH, van der Valk P, Walboomers JMM, et al. Expression of c-myc and bcl-2 oncogene products in Reed-Sternberg cells independent of presence of Epstein-Barr virus. *J Clin Pathol* 1993;46:211–217.
270. Khan G, Gupta RK, Coates PH, et al. Epstein-Barr virus infection and bcl-2 proto-oncogene expression: separate events in the pathogenesis of Hodgkin's disease? *Am J Pathol* 1993;143:1270–1274.
271. Shlaifer D, March M, Krajewski S, et al. High expression of bcl-x gene in Reed-Sternberg cells of Hodgkin's disease. *Blood* 1996;85: 2671–2674.
272. Brousset P, Benharroch D, Krajewski S, et al. Frequent expression of the cell death-inducing gene Bax in Reed-Sternberg cells of Hodgkin's disease. *Blood* 1996;87:2470–2475.
273. Murray RJ, Wang D, Young LS, et al. Epstein-Barr virus-specific cytotoxic T-cell recognition of transfectants expressing the virus-encoded latent membrane protein LMP. *J Virol* 1988;62:3747–3755.
274. Morente MM, Piris MA, Abraira V, et al. adverse clinical outcome in Hodgkin's disease is associated with loss of retinoblastoma protein experssion, high Ki67 proliferation index, and absence of Epstein-Barr virus-latent membrane protein. *Blood* 1997;90:2429–2436.
275. Oudejans JJ, Jiwa NM, Kummer GJ, et al. activated cytotoxic T cells as prognostic marker in Hodgkin's disease. *Blood* 1997;89: 1376–1382.
276. Frisan T, Sjoberg J, Dolcetti R, et al. Local suppression of Epstein-Barr virus (EBV)-specific cytotoxicity in biopsies of EBV-positive Hodgkin's disease. *Blood* 1995;86:1493–1501.
277. Renner C, Ohnesorge S, Held G, et al). T-cells from patients with Hodgkin's disease have a defective T-cell receptor zeta chain expression that is reversible by T-cell stimulation with CD3 and CD28. *Blood* 1996;88:236–241.
278. Poppema S, Visser L. Absence of HLA-class I expression by Reed-Sternberg cells. *Am J Pathol* 1994;145:37–41.
279. Merk K, Bjokholm M, Tullgren O, et al. Immune deficiency in family members of patients with Hodgkin's disease. *Cancer* 66:1938–1943.
280. Hartmann F, Tenner C, Jung W, et al. Treatment of refractory Hodgkin's disease with an anti-CD16/CD30 bispecific antibody. *Blood* 1997;89:2042–2047.

CHAPTER 19

Classification of Non-Hodgkin's Lymphomas

Nancy Lee Harris and Judith A. Ferry

HISTORY OF LYMPHOMA CLASSIFICATIONS

Controversy in lymphoma classification dates back to the first attempts to organize the variety of described neoplasms into a comprehensive scheme (1–15). This controversy stems from several factors, including the large variety of tumors that arise from cells of the lymphoid system, the relative insensitivity of the techniques of routine histopathology that are useful in other organ systems in recognizing defining features of lymphoid cells and their tumors, and the assumption of many authorities that there had to be a single guiding principle—a gold standard—for lymphoma classification. Many classifications were based purely on morphology (e.g., Gall and Mallory, Jackson and Parker, Rappaport, World Heath Organization); others utilized primarily clinical features (e.g., American Registry of Pathology, Working Formulation); and still others were based primarily on cell lineage and differentiation, in the belief that each neoplasm corresponded to a recognizable normal cell or differentiation stage (e.g., Robb-Smith, Kiel, Lukes and Collins). A review of the history of lymphoma classifications provides a useful perspective from which to view current attempts (16).

Early Lymphoma Classifications

The first century of lymphoma classification consisted of the sequential recognition by a variety of observers of different disease entities characterized by distinctive morphologies and clinical course (16) (Table 19.1). The earliest description of what later proved to be a lymphoma generally is attributed to Thomas Hodgkin (17), who in 1832 described six patients with ''disorders of the absorbent glands.'' Hodgkin believed that this disease was inflammatory, and later review of the original histologic material revealed that several of the cases were examples of tuberculosis (18). Other cases were examples of what in 1865 came to be called *Hodgkin's disease* (19); at least one case appears to be a non-Hodgkin's lymphoma. The first use of the term *lymphosarcoma* is attributed to Rudolf Virchow, who in 1863 distinguished it from leukemia, which he had described in 1845; the term *malignant lymphoma* was proposed by Theodore Billroth in 1871 (reviewed in ref. 16). The first clear description of the pathology of lymphosarcoma is attributed to Kundrat (20,21). In 1898 and 1902, Carl Sternberg (22) and Dorothy Reed (23) independently described the characteristic binucleate cell that came to be called the *Reed-Sternberg* (or Sternberg-Reed) *cell* and gave a more precise histologic definition of Hodgkin's disease. In 1908, Sternberg described an aggressive mediastinal tumor in young males (24); initially known as *Sternberg's sarcoma*, this was later recognized as *lymphoblastic lymphoma* (25). Jackson and Parker (21) credit Ewing with proposing in 1913 that tumors of lymphoid tissues could arise from reticulum cells (26). The term was adopted by Roulet (*retothelsarkom*) (27) and others (28). The term *reticulum cell* had been applied to a large cell found within the supporting fibrous reticulum of lymphoid tissues (it generally was not believed to produce the reticulum) (3, 21). Some observers considered it to be related to an endothelial cell; some believed it to be an immature lymphoid cell, some a pluripotential stem cell. Still others believed it was identical to the histiocyte or macrophage, also known as the ''clasmatocyte.'' The term *reticulum cell sarcoma* generally was applied to large cell neoplasms (3,29)—this uncertainty about the lineage of large cell neoplasms of lymphoid tissues persisted well into the latter half of the 20th century—and lymphosarcomas were considered to be composed of smaller cells recognized as lymphocytes. These terms were applied inconsistently, causing Gall and Mallory to comment that ''when such variation of opinion exists it seems probable that the individual authors . . . cannot be describing the same tumor'' (3). In 1925, Brill and colleagues (30) described an enlargement of lymph nodes

N. L. Harris and J. A. Ferry: Department of Pathology, Massachusetts General Hospital and Harvard Medical School, Boston, Massachusetts 02215.

TABLE 19.1. *Partial time line of lymphoma descriptions and classification*

Diseases defined
Hodgkin's disease: Hodgkin (1832), Wilkes (1865), Sternberg (1898), Reed (1902)
Leukemia: Virchow (1845)
Lymphosarcoma: Virchow (1863), Billroth (1871: malignant lymphoma), Kundrat (1893: distinction of lymphosarcoma from Hodgkin's disease)
Multiple myeloma: Bence Jones (1848), MacIntyre (1859), Wright (1933)
Reticulum cell sarcoma: Ewing (1913), Roulet (1930)
Follicular lymphoma: Brill (1925), Symmers (1927), Baehr (1932), Gall (1941)
Burkitt lymphoma: Burkitt (1958), O'Conor (1961)
Lymphoma classifications
American Registry of Pathology (1934)
Robb-Smith (1938)
Gall and Mallory (1942)
Jackson and Parker (1939, 1947)
Rappaport (1956, 1966)
Lennert (1967)
Lukes and Collins (1974)
Kiel (1974)
British National Lymphoma Investigation (1974)
Dorfman (1974)
World Health Organization (1976)

characterized by a proliferation of lymphoid follicles; additional cases were reported by Symmers (31). As with Hodgkin's disease, there was initial confusion about whether this represented a neoplasm or a progressive reactive process, and it is likely that initial reports contained, in addition to examples of what we would now call follicular lymphoma, cases of florid reactive follicular hyperplasia. By 1941, however, follicular lymphoma, or giant follicle lymphoma, was recognized and confirmed by Gall et al. (32) to be a distinctive form of lymphoid neoplasm, frequently disseminated and having a long natural history. In 1958, Burkitt (33) described a tumor in African children, which rapidly was recognized as a new and distinctive type of lymphoma (33–35) that also occurred in Western countries (36). Multiple myeloma first was described in 1846 by Bence Jones (37) and was recognized as a neoplasm of plasma cells by Wright in 1933 (38), with the application of the Wright's stain. Waldenstrom's macroglobulinemia, mycosis fungoides, and Sézary syndrome all were recognized as distinct entities by the mid-1940s.

Gall and Mallory, Jackson and Parker

In the first half of the 20th century, the existing terms—lymphoma, lymphosarcoma, giant follicle or follicular lymphoma, lymphocytoma, lymphoblastoma, reticulum cell sarcoma, and even Hodgkin's disease—were used heterogeneously by different pathologists and understood variably by clinicians. In the 1930s and 1940s, several attempts were made to develop a comprehensive list of the lymphomas that had been recognized, what might be called a classification, and these were published in both the United States and Europe . Although those nostalgic for what they believe to have been a simpler past are fond of suggesting that early classifications contained only three diseases—lymphosarcoma, reticulum cell sarcoma, and Hodgkin's disease—review of these early classifications actually reveals a far different picture. In fact, as early as 1948, Willis complained that "nowhere in pathology has a chaos of names so clouded clear concepts than in the subject of lymphoid tumors" (39). One of the earliest American attempts at a lymphoma classification came in 1934 from the American Registry of Pathology, the predecessor to the Armed Forces Institute of Pathology (1). This classification incorporated morphologic and clinical information into a scheme that included multiple categories for each morphologic type, depending on its clinical presentation and the extent of disease (Table 19.2). The paper in which the scheme was published illustrates the complexity that can come from attempts to categorize with insufficient data. In 1938, Robb-Smith (2) published a classification of benign and malignant disorders of lymph nodes, based on the concept of the reticuloendothelial system and the relationship of neoplasms to these normal counterparts, which escalated the complexity even further (Table 19.3). Several years later, Gall and Mallory (3), at Massachusetts General Hospital, reviewed their own extensive material—618 cases—and concluded that the American Registry of Pathology proposal was not a practical approach; they proposed a classification based predominantly on morphology but showed that the different categories described had distinctive clinical courses. In addition, the morphologic features of the different subtypes were described and illustrated carefully, so that pathologists could learn and use the classification. The classification included both of what have come to be known as non-Hodgkin's lymphomas and Hodgkin's disease; the classification of the non-Hodgkin's lymphomas appears to have been the first generally accepted classification of these

TABLE 19.2. *The American Registry of Pathology classification of lymphatic and reticular tumors (1934) (1)*

Lymphocytic
Leukemic lymphocytoma
Chronic
Acute
Aleukemic lymphocytoma
Diffuse
Nodular
Lymphosarcoma
Aleukemic
Leukemic
Reticulum cell
Leukemic reticulocytoma (monocytic leukemia)
Aleukemic reticulocytoma
Reticulum cell sarcoma

TABLE 19.3. *The Robb-Smith classification of reticulosis and reticulosarcoma (1938) (2)*

Reticuloses
Follicular reticuloses
Lymphoid (follicular lymphoblastoma of American writers)
Myeloid (experimental only)
Lymphoid and histiocytic (Flemming's centers: reactive hyperplasia)
Giant cell and fibrillary
Sinus reticuloses
Histiocytic (sinus catarrh)
Giant-cell histiocytic (Stengel-Wolbach sclerosis)
Histiosyncytial
Medullary reticuloses
Lymphoid (lymphoid leukosis)
Myeloid (myeloid leukosis)
Monocytic (monocytic leukosis)
Reticulum-celled (Letterer-Siwe syndrome)
Storage reticulum-celled (lipoidosis)
Histiocytic
Prohistiocytic–fibrillary
Fibromyeloid (Hodgkin's disease)
Reticulosarcoma
Undifferentiated reticulosarcoma (syncytial)
Diffuse
Trabecular (stroma reaction)
Differentiation to histioid cells
Dictyosyncytial (fibrillosyncytial) reticulosarcoma
Dictyocytic (fibrillary) reticulosarcoma
Differentiation to hemic cells
Lymphocytoma
Lymphoblastic sarcoma
Medullary
Follicular
Lymphosarcoma
Plasmocytoma
Monocytoma
Myeloblastoma
Erythroblastoma
Mixed type (polymorphic reticulosarcoma)
Differentiation to sinus lining cells
Undifferentiated cell type (reticuloendothelio-sarcoma)
Differentiated cell type (histiocytoma)

disorders in the United States (Table 19.4). In 1947, Jackson and Parker (21,29,40,41), at Boston University Hospital, also published a comprehensive lymphoma classification, with a primary focus on Hodgkin's disease. Their classification of Hodgkin's disease rapidly became the standard in the United States and was not challenged until 1966 (Table 19.5).

TABLE 19.4. *The Gall and Mallory classification (1942) (3)*

Reticulum cell sarcoma
Stem cell lymphoma
Clasmatocytic lymphoma
Lymphoblastic lymphoma
Lymphocytic lymphoma
Follicular lymphoma
Hodgkin's lymphoma
Hodgkin's sarcoma

TABLE 19.5. *The Jackson and Parker classification (1939, 1947) (21)*

Reticulum cell sarcoma
Lymphosarcoma
Giant follicle lymphoma
Lymphocytoma
Lymphoblastoma
Plasmocytoma
Hodgkin's disease
Paragranuloma
Granuloma
Sarcoma

Rappaport Classification

In the mid-1950s, Edward Gall and Henry Rappaport comoderated a workshop on lymphoma at the American Society of Clinical Pathology (42); out of this collaboration, Rappaport developed a new classification proposal, based on the principles of the Gall and Mallory classification (Table 19.6). The Rappaport classification, initially published in 1956 in a report primarily focused on follicular lymphoma (4) and fully developed in the Armed Forces Institute of Pathology fascicle of 1966 (5), took as its primary stratification the pattern of the lymphoma and assumed that all lymphomas—including Hodgkin's disease—could be either nodular or diffuse. Within each tumor type, those with a nodular pattern in general had a better prognosis than those with a diffuse pattern. In comparison with the Gall and Mallory classification, that of Rappaport provided some simplification—the unfortunate term "clasmatocytic" was dropped—and this classification also was characterized by clearly defined and well-illustrated categories, which made it accessible to pathologists. Unfortunately, the concept of nodularity represented a step backwards from the recognition of distinct biologic entities. The previously well-defined follicular lymphoma of Gall and Mallory became lost amid four categories of nodular lymphoma (well differentiated lymphocytic, poorly differentiated lymphocytic, mixed lymphocytic and histiocytic, and histiocytic), and its histologically obvious relationship to lymphoid follicles was de-

TABLE 19.6. *The Rappaport classification (1956, 1966) (4, 5)*

Nodular lymphomas	Diffuse lymphomas
Well differentiated lymphocytic	Well differentiated lymphocytic
Poorly differentiated lymphocytic	Poorly differentiated lymphocytic
Mixed lymphocytic and histiocytic	Mixed lymphocytic and histiocytic
Histiocytic	Histiocytic
Undifferentiated	Undifferentiated
Hodgkin's disease	Hodgkin's disease

nied. The nodular and diffuse variants of Hodgkin's disease also were listed with the other lymphomas, implying that there was no more difference between nodular Hodgkin's disease and nodular poorly differentiated lymphocytic lymphoma than between nodular the latter and the nodular mixed lymphocytic and histiocytic types. By 1966, when the classification was published in full, the phenomenon of lymphocyte transformation had been described, and it was known that large cells could be lymphoid in origin; despite this, the erroneous designation of "histiocytic" was retained for large cell neoplasms. Finally, the entity of lymphoblastic lymphoma was subsumed under diffuse poorly differentiated lymphocytic lymphoma, thus mingling the distinctive Sternberg sarcoma and nodal infiltrates of acute lymphoblastic leukemia with diffuse variants of follicle center lymphomas.

The Rappaport classification, despite its many attractive features, actually represented a step backwards in our understanding of the lymphomas. If it was biologically incorrect, one might wonder why it was so successful in predicting patient outcome? The reason lies in the frequency distribution of lymphomas in the United States and Western Europe. Follicular lymphoma, which accounts for the vast majority of lymphomas with a nodular pattern, comprises almost 40% of adult non-Hodgkin's lymphomas in the United States (14,43). Because the vast majority of these follow an indolent course, simple recognition of a nodular or follicular pattern identifies a large number of patients with an indolent disease. Diffuse large B-cell lymphoma (DLBCL), which comprises about 70% of diffuse lymphomas, is roughly equal in frequency to follicular lymphoma; because this is an aggressive disease, simple recognition of a diffuse pattern identifies an aggressive lymphoma in the majority of the cases. Because pattern recognition has been shown to be the only truly reproducible feature of these classifications, and because pattern alone identifies the two most common types of lymphoma, which have different clinical courses, this simple approach to classification proved to have "clinical relevance" even though it was biologically incorrect. It was not, however, useful for childhood lymphomas, because nodular variants are rare in children, and the category of lymphoblastic lymphoma was not recognized (44). It was also less useful in parts of the world in which follicular lymphoma is less common. In 1974, a large-scale study of patients from Stanford confirmed the clinical predictive value of the Rappaport classification for adult patients in the United States and ensured its adoption as the American standard (43,45).

Lukes and Butler Classification of Hodgkin's Disease

Although all previous classifications of lymphoma had addressed both Hodgkin's disease and other lymphomas, as well as lymphoid leukemias, Lukes and Butler published in 1966 a new proposal for the classification of Hodgkin's disease, based on material from the Armed Forces Institute of Pathology (46) (Table 19.5). Because at the time Hodgkin's disease accounted for almost half of all lymphomas in the United States, because it often affected young patients with long life expectancies, and because the work of Peters in Toronto (47) and Kaplan (48) at Stanford had shown that many cases could be cured with radiation therapy, the diagnosis and classification of Hodgkin's disease had taken on new importance. In fact, all other lymphomas were rapidly relegated to the category of *non-Hodgkin's lymphoma*.

The major contribution of the Lukes and Butler classification of Hodgkin's disease was to divide the Jackson and Parker category of *granuloma* into two subtypes: nodular sclerosis and mixed cellularity. Data from the Armed Forces Institute of Pathology clearly showed that these two types had different demographics, with a younger median age and increased mediastinal disease in nodular sclerosis Hodgkin's disease. In addition, the classification provided a clear description of nodular lymphocyte predominance Hodgkin's disease (paragranuloma in the Jackson and Parker classification) and its distinctive clinical behavior. The descriptions of the histologic subtypes were detailed, and criteria for the diagnosis were clear, enabling pathologists to apply the classification in practice. A clinical conference on Hodgkin's disease in Rye, New York, adopted a modified version of this classification, which rapidly became the world standard Rye classification of Hodgkin's disease (49).

Immunologic Advances of the 1960s and 1970s

In the 1960s, two discoveries revolutionized the understanding of the immune system and its neoplasms. These were the potential of lymphocytes—which had been thought to be end-stage, terminally differentiated cells—to transform into large, proliferating cells in response to mitogens or antigens (50); and the existence of several distinct lymphocyte lineages (T, B, and natural killer [NK]) that could not be predicted by morphology but had different functions and physiology (51). In the early 1970s, lymphoid cells were found to have surface antigens or receptors that could be exploited to identify the lineage of both normal and neoplastic cells (52). In response to the new information, pathologists quite appropriately began to try to apply it to the classification of lymphomas.

Kiel Classification

The first of these efforts was led by Karl Lennert, in Kiel, Germany, who first recognized that many lymphomas resembled germinal center cells and produced immunoglobulin, consistent with an origin from germinal center B cells (53). These studies led to the Kiel classification, published in final form in 1974 (9) and updated in 1988 (54). In this approach (Table 19.7), lymphomas were classified according to a hypothetical scheme of lymphocyte differentiation, and the nomenclature reflected the putative normal counterpart of the neoplastic cells. Although the majority of the neoplasms described were B-cell entities, several well-defined types of T-cell lymphomas were included. The neo-

TABLE 19.7. *The Kiel classification (1974, 1988) (9, 54)*

B-cell	T-cell
Low-grade malignancy	
Lymphocytic	Lymphocytic
CLL	CLL
Hairy cell leukemia	Small cerebriform cell
Lymphoplasmacytoid/cytic (immunocytoma)	Lymphoepithelioid (Lennert's)
Plasmacytic (plasmacytoma)	Angioimmunoblastic
Centroblastic/centrocytic	T-zone
Centrocytic	Pleomorphic, small cell (HTLV-$1^{\pm}$)
High-grade malignancy	
Centroblastic	Pleomorphic, medium and large cell (HTLV-$1^{\pm}$)
Immunoblastic	Immunoblastic (HTLV-$1^{\pm}$)
Lymphoblastic	Lymphoblastic
Burkitt lymphoma	
Anaplastic large cell (Ki-1^{+})	Anaplastic large cell (Ki-1^{+})

CLL, chronic lymphocytic leukemia; HTLV-1, human T-cell lymphotrophic virus type 1.

plasms were grouped according to histologic features into low-grade (predominance of small cells or ''-cytes'') and high-grade (predominance of ''-blasts'') malignancies. After its initial reporting in the form of a letter to *The Lancet*, a comprehensive description accompanied by many color illustrations was published by Lennert (13), and this classification became widely used in Europe. After the updated version of the Kiel classification was published in 1988 (54), revised definitions and illustrations were provided in 1992 (15).

The Kiel classification never achieved general acceptance in the United States. Possible reasons for this include the terminology, which included new names for most cell types and disease categories; the lack of inclusion of pattern as a major defining feature, and the lack of subclassification (grading) of nodular (follicular) lymphoma, which was perceived in the United States as having prognostic importance. Follicular lymphoma was reported at the time to be less common in Europe than in North America (13), a fact that probably influenced the attention paid by each of the classifications to this disease. These problems were more a matter of perception than reality. The terminology was not particularly difficult and reflected usage adopted by immunologists (such as the term *immunoblast*); newly described cell types had to be named, and the convention of hematologists was used: Small resting cells were named with the suffix *-cyte*, and large, transformed, or proliferating cells were named using *-blast*. Follicular lymphoma was recognized as an entity—given the cumbersome name *centroblastic/centrocytic* lymphoma—and subclassified as follicular, follicular and diffuse, or diffuse. It also was graded, in the sense that this category included only the low-grade categories of ''poorly differentiated lymphocytic'' and ''mixed lymphocytic and histiocytic'' in the Rappaport scheme; cases composed of predominantly large cells (Rappaport's ''nodular histiocytic'') were classified as follicular centroblastic—a category of high-grade lymphoma. Although cell type rather than pattern was the primary method of classification, the importance of pattern within this category was indeed recognized.

The Kiel classification represented the first major advance in classification since Gall and Mallory: it recognized and defined important disease entities and correctly predicted their relationship to normal cellular counterparts. The failure of American pathologists and oncologists to recognize the importance of this approach impeded progress in understanding the biology of lymphomas for the next 20 years.

Lukes and Collins Classification

In 1974, Lukes and Collins published an immunologically based classification of lymphomas (8) (Table 19.8). Although it was based on essentially the same observations and immunologic data as the Kiel classification, the approach to defining diseases was quite different. First, this scheme required primary division into T- and B-cell lineages, despite the fact that methods for doing this were not widely available at the time, and no data existed to indicate whether this was either possible or clinically important. Second, it did not recognize pattern at all, taking the extreme view that pattern was unimportant, and that cell type alone would predict clinical behavior—again, without data to support this contention. Third, one category, follicular center cell lymphoma, contained the vast majority of all neoplasms, from follicular lymphoma (small cleaved follicular center cell, large cleaved follicular center cell) to diffuse large-cell lymphoma (large cleaved follicular center cell, large noncleaved follicular center cell) to Burkitt's lymphoma (small noncleaved follicular center cell). The requirement for assigning lineage based on morphology, the lack of good illustrations, and the difficulty in relating the disease categories to the familiar categories of the Rappaport scheme resulted in resistance on the parts of both pathologists and oncologists to this classifica-

TABLE 19.8. *The Lukes and Collins classification (1974) (8)*

B-cell types
Small lymphocytic
Plasmacytoid lymphocytic
Follicular center cell lymphomas (follicular, follicular and diffuse, or diffuse)
Small cleaved
Large cleaved
Small noncleaved
Large noncleaved
Immunoblastic sarcoma of B cells
T-cell types
Convoluted lymphocytic
Immunoblastic sarcoma of T cells
Mycosis fungoides or Sezary's syndrome
Histiocytic (rare)
Undefined cell type

tion. A final problem was that neither in its original description nor in subsequent publications were clear criteria for diagnosis presented and illustrated; thus, it was difficult for pathologists to learn and apply the classification. It is unfortunate that, in some respects, the Lukes and Collins classification, because of its perceived impracticality, may have contributed to a degree of cynicism among American oncologists and pathologists about immunologic approaches to the classification of lymphomas.

Dorfman, British National Lymphoma Investigation, and World Health Organization Classifications

Shortly after the publication of the Kiel and the Lukes and Collins classifications, several other proposals appeared: the ''working classification'' of Dorfman (6), the proposal of Bennett and colleagues (7) that became the British National Lymphoma Investigation Classification, and the World Health Organization (WHO) Classification of Mathe and colleagues (11). To varying extents, these classifications attempted to apply terminology that reflected immunologic advances—that is, the recognition that large cell lymphomas were lymphoid, rather than histiocytic—to the basic framework of the Rappaport Classification (Tables 19.9–19.11). The British National Lymphoma Investigation classification was used for many years in Britain, but the other two never achieved widespread use.

International Working Formulation for Clinical Usage

By the mid-1970s, at least five new proposals for lymphoma classification had been made. This situation was the subject of much humor (10) but also a cause for consternation among oncologists, who were concerned that the results of clinical trials from different institutions would be impossible to interpret. Several meetings were organized by oncologists in both the United States and Europe in the mid-1970s, in an attempt to produce a consensus among the expert pathologists on a unified approach to lymphoma classification; unfortunately, this were unsuccessful.

In response to this unacceptable situation, the American National Cancer Institute, under the leadership of Vincent de Vita, undertook a large-scale project in which histologic slides and clinical data from patients enrolled in clinical trials at centers around the world would be reviewed, in an attempt to develop data that could be used to determine which of the classifications was most effective in predicting the clinical behavior of lymphomas. Proponents of each of the six classifications traveled to the different sites and reviewed histologic sections from 1,245 patients with non-Hodgkin's lymphomas, each classifying them according to his or her own scheme. In addition, six other pathologists reviewed all cases and attempted to classify each case according to all six schemes. Several endpoints were used as markers of the validity of each classification; the most important was the overall actuarial survival rate of patients whose slides were reviewed, but both inter- and intraobserver reproducibility also were evaluated.

TABLE 19.10. *The British National Lymphoma Investigation classification (1974) (7)*

Grade 1
Follicular lymphomas
Predominantly small follicular cell
Mixed small and large follicular cell
Predominantly large follicular cell
Diffuse lymphomas
Lymphocytic well differentiated (small round lymphocyte)
Lymphocytic intermediate differentiation (small follicular cell)
Grade 2
Lymphocytic poorly differentiated
Mixed small lymphoid and undifferentiated large cell
Undifferentiated large cell
Plasma cell
True histiocyte
Unclassified

TABLE 19.9. *Working classification of non-Hodgkin's lymphomas (6)*

Follicular lymphomas
Small lymphoid
Mixed small and large lymphoid
Large lymphoid
Diffuse lymphomas
Small lymphocytic
Atypical small lymphoid
Convoluted lymphocytic
Large lymphoid
Mixed small and large lymphoid
Histiocytic
Burkitt's lymphoma
Mycosis fungoides
Undefined

TABLE 19.11. *The World Health Organization classification of malignant lymphomas (1976) (11)*

Lymphosarcoma
Nodular lymphosarcoma
Prolymphocytic
Prolymphocytic, lymphoblastic
Diffuse lymphosarcoma
Lymphocytic
Lymphoplasmacytic
Prolymphocytic
Lymphoblastic
Immunoblastic
Burkitt's tumor
Mycosis fungoides
Plasmacytoma
Reticulosarcoma
Unclassified malignant lymphomas

TABLE 19.12. *The Working Formulation for clinical usage (1982) (14)*

Low-grade
Malignant lymphoma, small lymphocytic
Consistent with chronic lymphocytic leukemia
Plasmacytoid
Malignant lymphoma, follicular, predominantly small cleaved cell
Malignant lymphoma, follicular, mixed small cleaved and large cell
Intermediate-grade
Malignant lymphoma, follicular, predominantly large cell
Malignant lymphoma, diffuse, small cleaved cell
Malignant lymphoma, diffuse, mixed small and large cell
Malignant lymphoma, diffuse, large cell
Cleaved cell
Non-cleaved cell
High-grade
Malignant lymphoma, large cell, immunoblastic
Plasmacytoid
Clear cell
Polymorphous
Malignant lymphoma, lymphoblastic
Convoluted
Nonconvoluted
Malignant lymphoma, small non-cleaved cell
Burkitt's
Non-Burkitt's

After analysis of all the data, the survival curves showed that each of the classifications identified tumors with a broad spread of survival curves, and the statisticians were unable to identify any one classification as superior to the others in this respect. Intra- and interobserver reproducibility were relatively poor for all of the classifications. In the end, none of the classifications could be agreed upon as the standard, and the ''Working Formulation for Clinical Usage'' was developed to ''translate'' between the various classifications (14) (Table 19.12).

The Working Formulation (WF) essentially used the Rappaport categories of lymphomas but substituted terminology—primarily from the Lukes and Collins classification—that was believed to be biologically more correct, such as ''small lymphocytic'' instead of ''well differentiated lymphocytic,'' ''small cleaved cell'' instead of ''poorly differentiated lymphocytic,'' ''large cell'' instead of ''histiocytic,'' and ''follicular'' rather than ''nodular.'' It also recognized that not all lymphomas could have a truly follicular pattern. Unfortunately, in adapting the Lukes and Collins terminology, important modifying terms were left out, which led to a lack of specificity and clarity in the WF terminology. In the Lukes and Collins scheme, a ''small cleaved follicular center cell'' was a distinctive cell of the germinal center; this term did not apply to any cell with nuclear irregularity. Similarly, a ''small noncleaved follicular center cell'' was a distinctive blastic cell (corresponding to Burkitt's lymphoma cells), which was small only in comparison to ''large noncleaved follicular center cells.'' The term ''small noncleaved cell'' however, could be confusing, because a small lymphocyte is also small and ''noncleaved.''

The WF categories deliberately were defined broadly, so that all lymphomas could be classified, and all categories of all existing classifications could be accommodated, thus fulfilling its function as a sort of pathologic ''*lingua franca*'' or ''Esperanto.'' Thus, the category of ''diffuse mixed small and large cell'' included both diffuse follicular center lymphomas and peripheral T-cell lymphomas, and the category of ''large cell immunoblastic'' included both B- and T-cell cases. To further deemphasize the idea of disease entities, each category was given a letter designation (A through J), which could be used instead of the category name.

An important and novel feature of the WF was the separation of the lymphomas into clinical prognostic groups, or ''clinical grades,'' as they came to be called. These groupings differed from the ''histologic grades'' of the Kiel classification in that they were based on the actuarial survival curves of the patients in the international study, and not on morphologic features such as cell size, nuclear immaturity, or proliferative activity. The oncologists involved in the study believed that these groupings were necessary to help clinicians deal with the large number of morphologic categories, by combining them into groups that could be used to suggest appropriate treatment. ''Low-grade'' lymphomas could be treated palliatively, with an expectation of long survival unaffected by treatment; ''intermediate-grade'' lymphomas would be treated aggressively with an expectation of cure; and ''high-grade'' lymphomas would be treated intensively, often with central nervous system prophylaxis.

In the mid-1970s, clinical studies had begun to show that some aggressive lymphomas (diffuse histiocytic) could be cured with combination chemotherapy (55). At least one study appeared to show that histologic subclassification of these lymphomas could predict which cases could be cured with this treatment (56). There was considerable optimism that morphologic features could be used to predict the outcome of patients with large cell lymphomas. This hypothesis was tested in the National Cancer Institute study; unfortunately, the pathologists were unable to agree on subclassification of many of the cases. Nonetheless, in a subset of the cases that could be classified as immunoblastic, there was a small but statistically significant decrease in survival compared with the large cleaved and noncleaved types (14). The WF thus divided large cell lymphomas into two categories: large cell (cleaved or noncleaved) and immunoblastic. The immunoblastic category was placed in the high-grade clinical group, with Burkitt's and lymphoblastic lymphomas; the large cell category was considered intermediate-grade. Unfortunately, clear and reproducible criteria for separating large cell and large cell immunoblastic lymphomas were not given in the paper, and pathologists found this distinction difficult to make. Although the distinction theoretically could have led to important differences in treatment, it proved impossible for pathologists to make reliably (57).

Although much has been said about the clinical relevance

of the WF, it is clear that survival alone does not define a disease process, particularly if the patients in various different categories have not been treated uniformly. If different treatments for two entirely different diseases are equally effective, the survival curves for the two diseases may appear identical. Similarly, entirely different diseases may by chance have similar survival curves. Furthermore, patients with the same disease may have vastly different survival rates, depending on a variety of prognostic factors, such as age, stage, and performance status. Reflecting the fact that the prognostic groups defined by the WF do not really reflect the course of the tumors, many clinical trials of low-grade lymphoma include diffuse small cleaved cell lymphoma and follicular large cell lymphoma, although these are technically intermediate-grade in the WF (58), and trials of aggressive treatment for lymphoma usually include some but not all intermediate- (diffuse mixed and large cell but not diffuse small cleaved and follicular large cell) and some but not all high-grade (immunoblastic and sometimes small noncleaved cell, but not usually lymphoblastic) lymphomas (59,60). Some entities that were already recognized to have distinctive features, such as Burkitt's lymphoma, lymphoblastic lymphoma, hairy cell leukemia, and B-cell chronic lymphocytic leukemia (CLL), typically were treated according to disease-specific protocols.

As with the Rappaport classification, the WF seemed to ''work'' because the majority of non-Hodgkin's lymphomas seen in the United States were follicular lymphoma (40%) or DLBCL (30%) (14,61). This meant that over half of all lymphomas could be diagnosed and treated adequately according to the WF principles. Trials involving ''WF low-grade lymphoma'' are trials involving follicular lymphoma, contaminated by a small number of cases of mantle cell, small lymphocytic, and marginal zone lymphoma of mucosa-associated lymphoid tissue (MALT); trials involving ''WF intermediate- and high-grade lymphoma'' are trials involving DLBCL, contaminated by small numbers of peripheral T-cell lymphomas and other rare diseases. Lumping diverse entities into these broad prognostic groups tends to distort the data on common entities and to obscure the distinctive features of rare entities.

An additional result of the adoption of the WF, with its letter designations of categories and its clinical ''grades,'' was a growing disregard among oncologists for the pathologic classification of lymphomas. Thus, instead of ''follicular lymphoma,'' the designation ''WF B-D'' would be used, and rather than asking for a histologic diagnosis, many practicing oncologists simply wanted to know whether a tumor was low-, intermediate-, or high-grade in the WF. The ''crutch'' of the WF prognostic groups gave oncologists a sense of security, but it delayed recognition of and development of new therapies for diseases such as extranodal low-grade B-cell lymphoma of MALT, mantle cell lymphoma, and peripheral T-cell lymphomas.

Revised European–American Classification of Lymphoid Neoplasms from the International Lymphoma Study Group

Although the WF was not intended to be a freestanding classification, it rapidly replaced the Rappaport classification in the United States and became the standard American lymphoma classification. Both Lukes and Lennert, however, had published critical commentaries at its initial publication (14), and many American and European pathologists continued to use the Lukes and Collins and Kiel classifications, respectively. The lack of consensus on lymphoma classification and terminology persisted, with the WF being the standard in the United States and several other countries, and the Kiel classification being the standard in many European countries. This situation caused continued problems for both pathologists and clinicians and created difficulty in interpreting published studies. In the 1980s and 1990s, many new disease entities were described that were not included in either classification, leading to confusion among both pathologists and oncologists about which were ''real'' diseases that should be recognized in daily practice. Finally, the introduction of the new techniques of immunophenotyping and molecular genetic analysis led to confusion about what, if anything, should be the modern gold standard for defining disease entities.

Most experienced hematopathologists began in the late 1980s and early 1990s to modify both the WF and the Kiel classification to address these issues. This led to even more confusion, because not only were there differences between American and European classifications, but each institution was developing idiosyncratic internal classification schemes. Consideration was given to updating the WF or attempting to adopt the Kiel classification as the new international standard. Both classifications had limitations that made this impractical: The WF was not intended to be a freestanding classification, and its categories were intentionally broad and imprecise. In addition, the clinical data that were thought to give it validity were based on the original study patients; a similar large-scale clinical study theoretically would be required in order to provide an updated version with similar clinical relevance. The Kiel classification was intended for use on primary nodal lymphomas only; the issues of MALT lymphomas and their relationship to other lymphomas were not clarified, and other primary extranodal lymphomas other than mycosis fungoides were not addressed. In addition, the scheme for classifying peripheral T-cell lymphomas was based on morphologic criteria that were difficult to reproduce, and the histologic grades did not appear to correlate well with clinical behavior (62,63).

The International Lymphoma Study Group—an informal group of 19 hematopathologists from the United States, Europe, and Asia that had been meeting since 1991—adopted a new approach to lymphoma classification. In this approach, all available information—morphology, immunophenotype, genetic features, and clinical features—is used to define a disease entity. The relative importance of each of these features varies among diseases, and there is no one gold standard. Morphology is always important, and some diseases are defined primarily by morphology, such as follicular lymphoma, angioimmunoblastic T-cell lymphoma, and nodular sclerosis Hodgkin's disease, with immunophenotype as backup in difficult cases. Some diseases have a virtually specific immunophenotype—for example, mantle cell lymphoma, small lymphocytic lymphoma (SLL), and anaplastic large cell lymphoma (ALCL)—such that one would hesitate to make the diagnosis in the absence of the immunophenotype. In some lymphomas a specific genetic abnormality is an important defining criterion, such as the translocations t(11;14) in mantle cell lymphoma, t(8;14) in Burkitt's lymphoma, or t(14;18) in follicular lymphoma; others lack specific genetic abnormalities, such as MALT lymphoma and DLBCL. Still others require a knowledge of clinical features as well—for example, nodal versus extranodal presentation in marginal zone lymphoma and peripheral T-cell lymphomas, and mediastinal location in mediastinal large B-cell lymphoma. The inclusion of clinical criteria was one of the most novel aspects of the International Lymphoma Study Group approach. The emphasis on defining real disease entities, rather than focusing on subtleties of morphology or immunophenotype or primarily on patient survival, represented a new paradigm in lymphoma classification.

In 1993, the International Lymphoma Study Group undertook the development of a consensus list of diseases that its members recognized in daily practice and that appeared to be distinct clinical entities, using a combination of available morphologic, immunologic, and genetic information. This consensus approach represented the second major departure from previous classifications, most of which represented the work of one or a few individuals. The group recognized that the complexity of the field in the 1990s makes it impossible for a single person or small group to be completely authoritative, and also that broad agreement is necessary if the result is to be used by multiple pathologists, even if this requires compromise. The International Lymphoma Study Group consensus list of well-defined, real diseases was published in 1994 (64) (Table 19.13). Because it represented a revision of current and prior European and American lymphoma classifications (Table 19.14), it was called the Revised European–American Classification of Lymphoid Neoplasms (REAL). Although its initial publication incited considerable controversy, experience over the intervening years has shown that it can be used by most pathologists, and that the entities it describes have distinctive clinical features, making it a useful and practical classification, despite its apparent complexity (61,65–67).

World Health Organization Classification of Hematologic Malignancies

Since 1995, members of the European and American hematopathology societies have been collaborating on a new

TABLE 19.13. *The revised European–American classification of lymphoid neoplasms (REAL) (1994)(64)*

- B-cell neoplasms
  - Precursor B-cell neoplasm: B-lymphoblastic leukemia/lymphoma
  - Peripheral B-cell neoplasms
    - B-cell chronic lymphocytic leukemia/prolymphocytic leukemia/small lymphocytic lymphoma
    - Lymphoplasmacytoid lymphoma/Immunocytoma
    - Mantle cell lymphoma
    - Follicle center lymphoma, follicular
      - Provisional cytologic grades: 1 (small cell), II (mixed small and large cell), III (large cell)
      - Provisional subtype: diffuse, predominantly small cell type
    - Marginal zone B-cell lymphoma, extranodal mucosa-associated lymphoid tissue type ($\pm$ monocytoid B cells)
      - Provisional subtype: Nodal marginal zone lymphoma ($\pm$ monocytoid B cells)
      - Provisional entity: Splenic marginal zone lymphoma ($\pm$ villous lymphocytes)
    - Hairy cell leukemia
    - Plasmacytoma/plasma cell myeloma
    - Diffuse large B-cell lymphoma[a]
      - Subtype: Primary mediastinal (thymic) B-cell lymphoma
    - Burkitt's lymphoma
    - Provisional entity: High-grade B-cell lymphoma, Burkitt's-like[a]
- T-cell and putative natural killer-cell neoplasms
  - Precursor T-cell neoplasm: T-lymphoblastic lymphoma/leukemia
  - Peripheral T-cell and natural killer-cell neoplasms
    - T-cell chronic lymphocytic leukemia/prolymphocytic leukemia
    - Large granular lymphocyte leukemia
      - T-cell type
      - Natural killer-cell type
    - Mycosis fungoides/Sezary syndrome
    - Peripheral T-cell lymphomas, unspecified[a]
      - Provisional cytologic categories: medium-sized cell, mixed medium-sized and large cell, large cell, lymphoepithelioid cell
      - Provisional subtypes
        - Hepatosplenic $\gamma\delta$ T-cell lymphoma
        - Subcutaneous panniculitic T-cell lymphoma
    - Angioimmunoblastic T-cell lymphoma
    - Angiocentric lymphoma
    - Intestinal T-cell lymphoma ($\pm$ enteropathy-associated)
    - Adult T-cell lymphoma/leukemia
    - Anaplastic large cell lymphoma, $CD30^+$, T- and null cell types
    - Provisional entity: anaplastic large cell lymphoma, Hodgkin's-like
- Hodgkin's disease
  - Lymphocyte predominance
  - Classic Hodgkin's disease
  - Nodular sclerosis
  - Mixed cellularity
  - Lymphocyte depletion
  - Provisional entity: lymphocyte-rich classical Hodgkin's disease

[a] Likely to include more than one disease entity.

TABLE 19.14. *Comparison of the original REAL classification with the Kiel classification and the Working Formulation*

Kiel classification	REAL classification	Working Formulation
B-lymphoblastic	Precursor B-lymphoblastic lymphoma/leukemia	Lymphoblastic
B-lymphocytic, CLL B-lymphocytic, prolymphocytic leukemia Lymphoplasmacytoid immunocytoma	B-cell chronic lymphocytic leukemia/prolymphocytic leukemia/small lymphocytic lymphoma	**Small lymphocytic, consistent with CLL** Small lymphocytic, plasmacytoid
Lymphoplasmacytic immunocytoma	Lymphoplasmacytoid lymphoma	**Small lymphocytic, plasmacytoid** Diffuse, mixed small and large cell
Centrocytic Centroblastic, centrocytoid subtype	Mantle cell lymphoma	Small lymphocytic **Diffuse, small cleaved cell** Follicular, small cleaved cell Diffuse, mixed small and large cell Diffuse, large cleaved cell
	Follicular center lymphoma, follicular	
Centroblastic—centrocytic, follicular	Grade I	**Follicular, predominantly small cleaved cell**
	Grade II	**Follicular, mixed small and large cell**
Centroblastic, follicular	Grade III	Follicular, predominantly large cell
Centroblastic—centrocytic, diffuse	Follicular center lymphoma, diffuse, small cell (provisional)	**Diffuse, small cleaved cell** Diffuse, mixed small and large cell
—	Extranodal marginal zone B-cell lymphoma (low grade B-cell lymphoma of mucosa-associated lymphoid tissue type)	**Small lymphocytic** Diffuse, small cleaved cell Diffuse, mixed small and large cell
Monocytoid, including marginal zone Immunocytoma	Nodal marginal zone B-cell lymphoma (provisional)	**Small lymphocytic** Diffuse, small cleaved cell Diffuse, mixed small and large cell Unclassifiable
—	Splenic marginal zone B-cell lymphoma (provisional)	**Small lymphocytic** Diffuse small cleaved cell
Hairy cell leukemia	Hairy cell leukemia	—
Plasmacytic	Plasmacytoma/myeloma	Extramedullary plasmacytoma
Centroblastic (monomorphic, polymorphic and multilobated subtypes) **B-immunoblastic** B-Large cell anaplastic (Ki-1+)	Diffuse large B-cell lymphoma	**Diffuse, large cell** Large cell immunoblastic Diffuse, mixed small and large cell
—[a]	Primary mediastinal large B-cell lymphoma	**Diffuse, large cell** Large cell immunoblastic
Burkitt's lymphoma	Burkitt's lymphoma	Small noncleaved cell, Burkitt's
— some cases of centroblastic and immunoblastic?	High grade B-cell lymphoma, Burkitt's-like (provisional)	**Small noncleaved cell, non-Burkitt's** Diffuse, large cell Large cell immunoblastic
T-lymphoblastic	Precursor T-lymphoblastic lymphoma/leukemia	Lymphoblastic
T-lymphocytic, CLL type T-lymphocytic, prolymphocytic leukemia	T-cell chronic lymphocytic leukemia/prolymphocytic leukemia	**Small lymphocytic** Diffuse small cleaved cell
T-lymphocytic, CLL type	Large granular lymphocytic leukemia	**Small lymphocytic** Diffuse, small cleaved cell
—	T-cell type	
	Natural killer cell type	
Small cell cerebriform (mycosis fungoides, Sezary syndrome)	Mycosis fungoides/Sezary syndrome	Mycosis fungoides
T-zone Lymphoepithelioid Pleomorphic, small T-cell **Pleomorphic, medium-sized and large T-cell**	Peripheral T-cell lymphomas, unspecified (including provisional subtype: subcutaneous panniculitic T-cell lymphoma)	Diffuse, small cleaved cell **Diffuse, mixed small and large cell** Diffuse, large cell **Large cell immunoblastic**

(continued)

TABLE 19.14. *Continued.*

Kiel classification	REAL classification	Working Formulation
T-immunoblastic		
—	Hepatosplenic δ T-cell lymphoma (provisional)	—
Angioimmunoblastic (AILD, LgX)	Angioimmunoblastic T-cell lymphoma	**Diffuse, mixed small and large cell AILD** Diffuse, large cell **Large cell immunoblastic**
—[a]	Angiocentric lymphoma	Diffuse, small cleaved cell **Diffuse, mixed small and large cell** Diffuse, large cell **Large cell immunoblastic**
—	Intestinal T-cell lymphoma	Diffuse, small cleaved cell Diffuse, mixed small and large cell Diffuse, large cell **Large cell immunoblastic**
Pleomorphic small T-cell, HTLV-1$^+$ **Pleomorphic medium-sized and large T-cell, HTLV-1$^+$**	Adult T-cell lymphoma/leukemia	Diffuse, small cleaved cell Diffuse, mixed small and large cell Diffuse, large cell **Large cell immunoblastic**
T-large cell anaplastic (Ki-1$^+$)	Anaplastic large cell lymphoma, T- and null-cell types	Large cell immunoblastic

[a] Not listed in classification, but discussed as rare or ambiguous type.
HTLV-1, human T-cell lymphotrophic virus-type 1.

WHO classification of hematologic malignancies. It will use an updated version of the REAL classification for lymphomas and will expand the principles of the REAL classification to the classification of myeloid and histiocytic neoplasms (68,69) (Tables 19.15, 19.16). The WHO project includes over 50 pathologists from around the world, as well as a clinical advisory committee of more than 30 international expert hematologists and oncologists (70). Proponents of current classifications—WF, Kiel, REAL, and French–American–British—are in agreement that the final WHO consensus will replace existing classifications and represent the first true international consensus on the classification of hematologic malignancies.

Principles of the Revised European–American Classification of Lymphoid Neplasms and the World Health Organization Classification of Lymphoid Neoplasms

The REAL-WHO classification is a list of distinct disease entities, which are defined by a combination of morphology, immunophenotype, and genetic features, and which have distinct clinical features. It recognizes that all of these criteria are at best approximations, and that continued research and experience ARE needed to continue to improve the definition of these diseases. Morphology remains the first and most basic approach and is sufficient for both diagnosis and classification in many typical cases of lymphoma. Immunophenotyping and particularly molecular genetic studies are not needed in all cases; however, they are useful in difficult cases and improve interobserver reproducibility. It is the availability of these more objective methods that make possible now a consensus on lymphoma classification that was impossible in the 1970s, when classification was based purely on subjective morphologic features.

The classification includes all lymphoid neoplasms: Hodgkin's disease, non-Hodgkin's lymphomas, lymphoid leukemias, and plasma cell neoplasms. Both lymphomas and lymphoid leukemias are included, because both solid and circulating phases are present in many lymphoid neoplasms, and distinction between them is artificial. Thus, B-cell CLL and SLL are simply different manifestations of the same neoplasm, as are lymphoblastic lymphomas and acute lymphoblastic leukemias. In addition, Hodgkin's disease and plasma cell myeloma are recognized as lymphoid neoplasms of B-cell lineage and therefore belong in a compilation of lymphoid neoplasms. Immunodeficiency-associated lymphomas are classified according to the basic lymphoma classification; a separate classification of posttransplant lymphoid proliferations that do not fulfill criteria for lymphoma also is given (Table 19.16). Many of the neoplasms recognized in the classification have morphologic variants or clinical subtypes, which are shown in Tables 19.17 through 19.28.

Normal Counterparts of Neoplastic Cells

Attempting to understand the normal counterpart of the neoplastic cell is an important component of any tumor classification. At present, the normal counterpart—both in lineage and differentiation stage—of many hematologic malignancies can be postulated with reasonable certainty. Our understanding of the immune system is insufficient, however, to permit this to be done in all cases, and therefore

TABLE 19.15. *Proposed updated REAL/WHO classification of lymphoid neoplasms (major categories)*

B-cell neoplasms
- Precursor B-cell neoplasm: precursor B-lymphoblastic leukemia/lymphoma (precursor B-cell acute lymphoblastic leukemia)[a]
- Mature (peripheral) B-cell neoplasms[b]
  - B-cell chronic lymphocytic leukemia/small lymphocytic lymphoma[a]
  - B-cell prolymphocytic leukemia
  - Lymphoplasmacytic lymphoma
  - Splenic marginal zone B-cell lymphoma (± villous lymphocytes)
  - Hairy cell leukemia
  - Plasma cell myeloma[a]/plasmacytoma
  - Extranodal marginal zone B-cell lymphoma of mucosa-associated lymphoid tissue type[a]
  - Nodal marginal zone B-cell lymphoma (± monocytoid B cells)
  - Follicular lymphoma[a]
  - Mantle cell lymphoma[a]
  - Diffuse large B-cell lymphoma[a]
    - Mediastinal large B-cell lymphoma
    - Primary effusion lymphoma
  - Burkitt's lymphoma/Burkitt's cell leukemia[a]

T- and NK cell neoplasms
- Precursor T-cell neoplasm: Precursor T-lymphoblastic lymphoma/leukemia (precursor T-cell acute lymphoblastic leukemia)[a]
- Mature (peripheral) T-cell neoplasms[b]
  - T-cell prolymphocytic leukemia
  - T-cell granular lymphocytic leukemia
  - Aggressive NK-cell leukemia
  - Adult T-cell lymphoma/leukemia (HTLV1+)
  - Extranodal NK/T-cell lymphoma, nasal type
  - Enteropathy-type T-cell lymphoma
  - Hepatosplenic $\gamma\delta$ T-cell lymphoma
  - Subcutaneous panniculitis-like T-cell lymphoma
  - Mycosis fungoides[a]/Sezary syndrome
  - Anaplastic large cell lymphoma, T/null cell, primary cutaneous type
  - Peripheral T-cell lymphoma, not otherwise characterized[a]
  - Angioimmunoblastic T-cell lymphoma[a]
  - Anaplastic large cell lymphoma, T/null cell, primary systemic type[a]
- Hodgkin's lymphoma (Hodgkin's disease)[a]
  - Nodular lymphocyte predominance Hodgkin's lymphoma
  - Classical Hodgkin's lymphoma
    - Nodular sclerosis Hodgkin's lymphoma (Grades 1 and 2)[a]
    - Lymphocyte-rich classical Hodgkin's lymphoma
    - Mixed cellularity Hodgkin's lymphoma[a]
    - Lymphocyte depletion Hodgkin's lymphoma

[a] More common entities.
[b] B and T/NK cell neoplasms are grouped according to major clinical presentations (predominantly disseminated/leukemic, primary extranodal, predominantly nodal).
NK, natural killer.

TABLE 19.16. *Categories of posttransplant lymphoproliferative disorders*

Early lesions
- Reactive plasmacytic hyperplasia
- Infectious mononucleosis-like

Polymorphic
- Polyclonal (rare)
- Monoclonal

Monomorphic (classify according to lymphoma classification)
- B-cell lymphomas
  - Diffuse large B-cell lymphoma (immunoblastic, centroblastic, anaplastic)
  - Burkitt's/Burkitt's-like lymphoma
  - Plasma cell myeloma
- T-cell lymphomas
  - Peripheral T-cell lymphoma, not otherwise categorized
  - Other types (hepatosplenic, $\gamma\delta$, T natural killer)

Other types (rare)
- Hodgkin's disease-like lesions (associated with methotrexate therapy)
- Plasmacytoma-like lesions

TABLE 19.17. *Acute lymphoid leukemias in the WHO classification*

Precursor B-cell acute lymphoblastic leukemia (cytogenetic subgroups)
- t(9;22)(a34;q11) *BCR/ABL*
- t(v;11q23); *MLL* rearranged
- t(12;21)(p12;q22) *TEL/AML*1
- t(1;19)(q23;p13) *PBX/E2A*

Precursor T-cell acute lymphoblastic leukemia
Burkitt's cell leukemia

TABLE 19.18. *B-cell neoplasms, predominantly disseminated or leukemic types*

B-cell chronic lymphocytic leukemia/small lymphocytic lymphoma
- Variant: with monoclonal gammopathy/plasmacytoid differentiation

Hairy cell leukemia
- Variant: hairy cell leukemia variant

TABLE 19.19. *Follicular and mantle cell lymphomas: grading and variants*

- Follicular lymphoma
  - 1: 0–5 centroblasts/hpf
  - 2: 6–15 centroblasts/hpf
  - 3: >15 centroblasts/hpf
    - a: >15 centroblasts, but centrocytes are still present
    - b: Centroblasts form solid sheets with no residual centrocytes
  - Variants
    - Cutaneous follicle center lymphoma
    - Diffuse follicle center lymphoma
      - 1: 0–5 centroblasts/hpf
      - 2: 6–15 centroblasts/hpf
- Mantle cell lymphoma
  - Variant: blastoid

TABLE 19.20. *Diffuse large B-cell lymphoma*

- Morphologic variants
  - Centroblastic
  - Immunoblastic
  - T-cell or histiocyte-rich
  - Lymphomatoid granulomatosis type
  - Anaplastic large B-cell
  - Plasmablastic
- Subtypes
  - Mediastinal (thymic) large B-cell lymphoma
  - Primary effusion lymphoma
  - Intravascular large B-cell lymphoma

TABLE 19.21. *Burkitt's lymphoma*

- Morphologic variants
  - Burkitt's-like
  - With plasmacytoid differentiation (AIDS-associated)
- Subtypes (clinical and genetic)
  - Endemic
  - Sporadic
  - Immunodeficiency-associated

TABLE 19.22. *Plasma cell disorders*

- Monoclonal gammopathy of undetermined significance
- Plasma cell myeloma variants
  - Indolent myeloma
  - Smoldering myeloma
  - Osteosclerotic myeloma (POEMS syndrome)
  - Plasma cell leukemia
  - Nonsecretory myeloma
- Plasmacytoma variants
  - Solitary plasmacytoma of bone
  - Extramedullary plasmacytoma

TABLE 19.23. *Immunosecretory disorders (clinical manifestations of diverse lymphoid neoplasms)*

Clinical syndrome	Underlying neoplasm
Waldenstrom's macroglobulinemia	Lymphoplasmacytic lymphoma
Heavy chain diseases	
γ	Lymphoplasmacytic lymphoma
α	Extranodal marginal zone lymphoma (immunoproliferative small intestinal disorder)
μ	B-cell chronic lymphocytic leukemia
Immunoglobulin deposition diseases	
Systemic light chain disease	Plasma cell myeloma, monoclonal gammopathy
Primary amyloidosis	Plasma cell myeloma, monoclonal gammopathy

TABLE 19.24. *T-cell neoplasms, disseminated leukemic types*

- T-cell prolymphocytic leukemia, morphologic variants
  - Small cell
  - Cerebriform cell
- Adult T-cell leukemia/lymphoma (human T-cell lymphotrophic virus, type 1–positive), clinical variants
  - Acute
  - Lymphomatous
  - Chronic
  - Smoldering
  - Hodgkin's-like

TABLE 19.25. *Peripheral T-cell neoplasms, primary extranodal types*

- Mycosis fungoides variants
  - Pagetoid reticulosis
  - Follicular mucinosis
  - Granulomatous slack skin disease
- Primary cutaneous $CD30^{+}$ T-cell lymphoproliferative disorders
  - Lymphomatoid papulosis (type A and B)
  - Primary cutaneous anaplastic large cell lymphoma
  - Borderline lesions

TABLE 19.26. *Peripheral T-cell neoplasms, predominantly nodal types*

- Peripheral T-cell lymphoma (not otherwise categorized), variants
  - Lymphoepithelioid (Lennert's)
  - T-zone
- Anaplastic large cell lymphoma T/null cell type, variant:
  - Lymphohistiocytic
- Small cell

TABLE 19.27. *Differences between the original REAL and the updated REAL/WHO classifications*

WHO B-cell neoplasms: differences from REAL
Nomenclature
Follicular lymphoma
Lymphoplasmacytic lymphoma
Provisional entities now "real"
Nodal marginal zone lymphoma
Splenic marginal zone lymphoma
New, separated, or deleted entities
Separation of B-prolymphocytic leukemia from B-cell chronic lymphocytic leukemia
Immunodeficiency-associated lymphomas
Burkitt's-like type is a variant of Burkitt's lymphoma
WHO T-cell neoplasms: differences from REAL
Nomenclature
T-prolymphocytic leukemia (vs T-cell chronic lymphocytic leukemia)
Extranodal NK T-cell lymphoma, nasal-type (vs angiocentric)
Provisional entities now "real"
Hepatosplenic gamma/delta T-cell lymphoma
Subcutaneous panniculitis-like T-cell lymphoma
New, separated, or deleted entities
NK cell leukemia
Primary cutaneous ALCL
ALCL Hodgkin's-like is either HD or ALCL
WHO Hodgkin's lymphoma: differences from REAL
Nomenclature: Hodgkin's lymphoma?
Provisional entity now "real"
Classic Hodgkin's disease, lymphocyte-rich
Deleted entity
Anaplastic large cell lymphoma Hodgkin's-like is either Hodgkin's disease or anaplastic large cell lymphoma

TABLE 19.28. *Reproducibility of lymphoma diagnosis (61,67)*

Diagnosis	Contribution of immunophenotype, %
Reproducibility >85% (86%–96%)	
B-cell chronic or small lymphocytic leukemia	3
Mantle cell lymphoma	10
Follicular lymphoma	0
Marginal zone/mucosa-associated lymphoid tissue	2
Diffuse large B-cell lymphoma	15
T-lymphoblastic lymphoma	40
Anaplastic large cell lymphoma	39
Peripheral T-cell lymphoma, unspecified	41
Mycosis fungoides	
Reproducibility 80%	
Angioimmunoblastic T-cell lymphoma	
Extranodal natural killer or T-cell lymphoma	
Reproducibility <50%	
Burkitt's-like lymphoma	6
Lymphoplasmacytic lymphoma	

rigid adherence to classification by normal counterpart is not feasible at this time. Three major categories of lymphoid malignancies can be defined based on a combination of morphology and cell lineage: B-cell neoplasms, T- or NK cell neoplasms, and Hodgkin's disease or Hodgkin's lymphoma. Within the B- and T-cell categories, two major subcategories are recognized: precursor neoplasms, corresponding to the earliest lymphoblastic stages of differentiation (lymphoblastic lymphomas and acute lymphoblastic leukemias); and peripheral or mature neoplasms, corresponding to more differentiated B- and T-cell stages.

Grading and Prognostic Groups

The final classification includes over 20 distinct entities. These diseases are in most cases unrelated to one another—that is, we can no longer talk about lymphoma or non-Hodgkin's lymphoma as a single disease with a range of histologic grades and clinical aggressiveness. Now that lymphomas can be defined more precisely with the aid of immunophenotypes and genetic features, we find that many malignant lymphomas have—within the same disease entity—a spectrum of morphologic features and clinical aggressiveness. This has been known for years for follicular lymphoma, but it is also probably true for B-cell CLL, mantle cell lymphoma, and MALT lymphoma. Histologic grade is just one of many prognostic factors, which should be applied *within* a disease entity, not across the whole range of lymphoid neoplasms. Another corollary of defining distinct lymphoma entities is that it is neither possible nor helpful to sort them broadly according to histologic grade or clinical aggressiveness. For example, although it is true that many lymphomas composed of relatively small cells with a low proliferation fraction have generally indolent courses, at least one of them—mantle cell lymphoma—is rather aggressive. In addition, they each have a distinctive set of presenting features and, often, different treatments—hairy cell leukemia versus B-CLL versus extranodal marginal zone or MALT lymphoma. Thus, both the pathologist and the oncologist must "get to know" each disease entity, its spectrum of morphology and clinical course, and its peculiarities of occurrence and response to therapy. Although a group of oncologists recently published a suggested clinical grouping of the entities in the REAL classification (71), they since have recognized its impracticality, and the WHO clinical advisory committee agreed that clinical groupings of lymphoid neoplasms are of no practical value and may be misleading (70). In practice, treatment of a specific patient should be determined not by which broad prognostic group the patient's neoplasm falls into but by the specific type of neoplasm, with the addition of grade within the tumor type, if applicable, and clinical prognostic factors such as stage, age, performance status, and the International Prognostic Index (IPI) (72).

Because of the impracticality of arranging the list of B- and T-lymphoid neoplasms according to prognostic groups, the final WHO classification lists them first according to differentiation stage (precursor followed by mature or peripheral) and second according to predominant clinical presentation (predominantly disseminated or leukemic, primary extranodal, and predominantly nodal or systemic). This approach is intended for convenience and ease of learning; it places diseases that are likely to resemble one another both clinically and histologically in proximity in the list and in a text. It also has some biologic relevance, because there appear to be important biologic differences between primary nodal and primary extranodal lymphomas, particularly in the T- or NK cell diseases. Any principle of sorting these neoplasms is artificial, however, and the lists can be regrouped in different ways for different purposes.

Clinical Test of the Revised European–American Classification of Lymphoid Neoplasms

An initial criticism of the REAL Classification was that it had not been tested in a clinical study (73), although it only included diseases of which descriptions had been published and the clinical features were known (74). To address this issue, an international group of oncologists and pathologists devised a clinical study of the classification, in which five expert pathologists reviewed over 1,300 cases of non-Hodgkin's lymphoma at centers around the world (61,67). The aims of the study were to see whether the classification could be used in practice, to test its interobserver reproducibility, to determine the need for immunophenotyping in diagnosis, to determine whether the categories of disease identified in the classification were clinically distinctive either at presentation or in outcome, and to determine the relative frequency of these diseases in the populations studied.

This study convincingly demonstrated that the classification could be used by expert hematopathologists: More than 95% of the cases with adequate material could be classified into one of the categories. The interobserver reproducibility was substantially better than that for other classifications, higher than 85% for most diseases (Table 19.28). Immunophenotyping was helpful in some diseases, such as mantle cell lymphoma and DLBCL, in which it improved accuracy by 10% to 15%, and was essential for all types of T-cell lymphoma, improving reproducibility from around 50% to more than 90%. It was not required for many diseases, such as follicular lymphoma, B-cell SLL, and MALT lymphoma (61).

The relative frequency of the different B- and T- or NK cell lymphomas in the study population was similar to previous patterns reported in the literature (Table 19.29). The most common lymphoma was DLBCL, followed by follicular lymphoma; together, these comprised 50% of the lymphomas in the study. New entities not specifically recognized in the WF accounted for 27% of the cases: MALT 8%, mantle cell 7%, peripheral T-cell 6%, nodal marginal zone 2%, mediastinal large B-cell 2%, anaplastic large T- or null cell 2%. These results are reassuring, confirming that the majority of the cases that are encountered by oncologists and pathologists fall into only a few subtypes, with which they are already familiar. The results also underscore, however, the need for recognizing the more recently described entities, which although less common have important clinical differences. The study also found differences in geographic distribution of the lymphoma types, with follicular lymphoma being more common in North America and Western Europe, T-cell lymphomas more common in Hong Kong, and both mediastinal large B cell lymphoma and mantle cell lymphoma more common in Ticino (the Italian-speaking canton), Switzerland (75).

The different entities recognized by the classification had significantly different clinical presentations and survivals. For example, diffuse aggressive lymphomas, which would be lumped among intermediate- and high-grade entities in the WF, include DLBCL, mediastinal large B-cell lymphoma, peripheral T-cell lymphoma, and anaplastic large T-

TABLE 19.29. *Presenting features of common B- and T-cell neoplasms*

Neoplasm	Frequency, %	Age, y	Male, %	Stage, % I	Stage, % II	Stage, % III	Stage, % IV	B symptoms, %	Any extranodal site[a]	Bone marrow, %	Gastro-intestinal tract, %	International Prognostic Index Score, % 0/1	2/3	4/5
Large B-cell	31	64	55	25	29	13	33	33	71	16	18	35	46	9
Mediastinal	2	37	34	10	56	3	31	38	56	3	0	52	37	11
Follicular	22	59	42	18	15	16	51	28	64	42	4	45	48	7
Small or chronic lymphocytic leukemia	6	65	53	4	5	8	83	33	80	72	3	23	64	13
Mucosa-associated lymphoid tissue	8	60	48	39	28	2	31	19	98	14	50	44	48	8
Mantle cell	6	63	74	13	7	9	71	28	81	51	9	23	54	23
Peripheral T-cell	7	61	55	8	12	15	65	50	82	36	15	17	52	31
Anaplastic large cell lymphoma	2	34	69	19	32	10	39	53	59	13	9	61	18	21

[a] Include bone marrow.

or null cell lymphoma. The clinical features at presentation were strikingly different, with younger age groups for mediastinal large T-cell lymphoma and anaplastic large T- or null cell lymphoma, and striking differences in male : female ratios, suggesting that these are distinctive biologic entities (Table 19.29). Entities that would have been lumped together as low-grade or intermediate- and high-grade in the WF showed marked differences in overall survival rates, again confirming that they need to be recognized and treated as distinct entities (see Chapter 20).

A critical finding in this study was that classification is not the only predictor of clinical outcome. Patients with any of these diseases could be stratified into better and worse prognostic groups according to the IPI (72). For example, although patients with follicular lymphoma typically have IPI scores between 1 and 3, those patients with scores of 4 or 5 had a predicted median overall duration of survival of only 18 months. Thus, to plan treatment for an individual patient, the oncologist must know not only the diagnosis but also the clinical prognostic factors that influence that patient's course.

BIOLOGIC BASIS FOR CLASSIFICATION OF LYMPHOID NEOPLASMS

Although the normal counterpart of the neoplastic cell is not known for all types of lymphoid neoplasms, it can be postulated for many of them. Understanding the normal counterpart of neoplastic cells can provide a useful framework for understanding the morphology, immunophenotype, and to some extent the clinical behavior of the neoplasms (Figs. 19.1–19.3).

Anatomy and Morphology of Normal Lymphoid Tissues

Lymphoid tissues can be divided into two major categories: the central or primary lymphoid tissues, which harbor lymphoid precursor cells and provide for their maturation to a stage at which they are capable of performing their function in response to antigen; and the peripheral or secondary lymphoid tissue, in which antigen-specific reactions occur.

Primary (Central) Lymphoid Tissues

Bone Marrow (Bursa-equivalent)

Many of the early experiments that discovered the basic biology of the lymphoid system used chickens and other avian species as experimental animals; in avian species, an organ known as the bursa of Fabricius, located in the region of the cloaca, proved to be the source of cells capable of producing antibody. These cells were termed *B cells*, for *bursa-derived cells*. In mammals, the bursa does not exist, and experiments have shown that the precursors of antibody-producing cells come from the bone marrow. The bone marrow is also the source of other hematopoietic cells, including T cells (so named because their crucial maturation steps cannot occur in the absence of the thymus).

Thymus

The thymus, located in the anterior mediastinum, is the site at which immature T-cell precursors (prethymocytes)

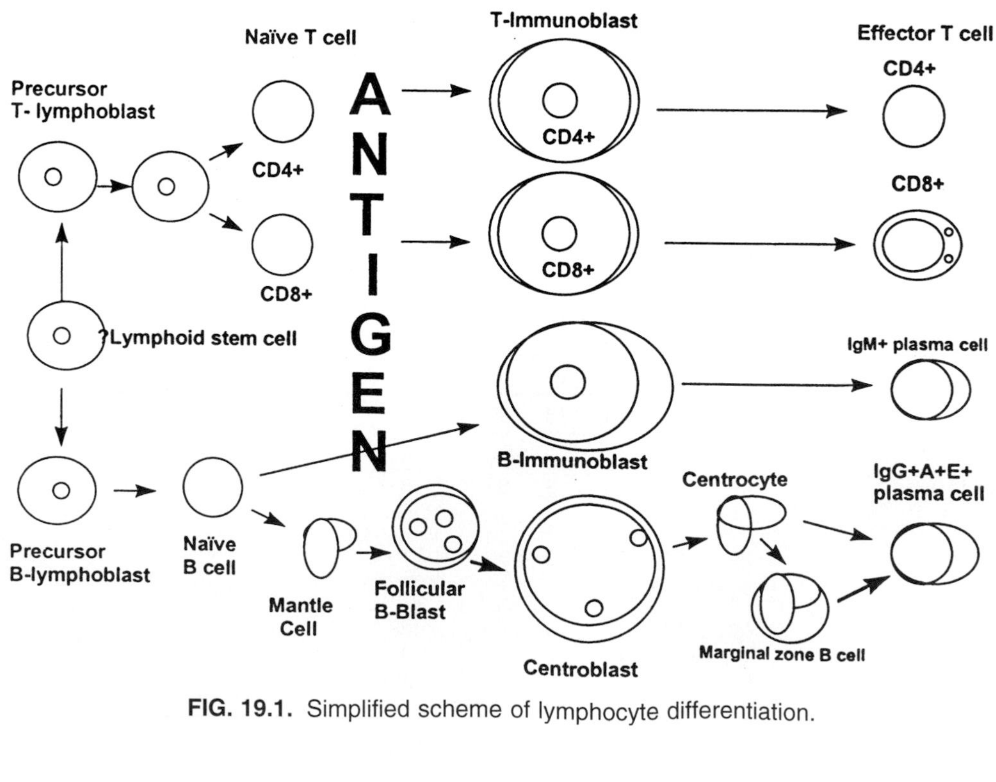

FIG. 19.1. Simplified scheme of lymphocyte differentiation.

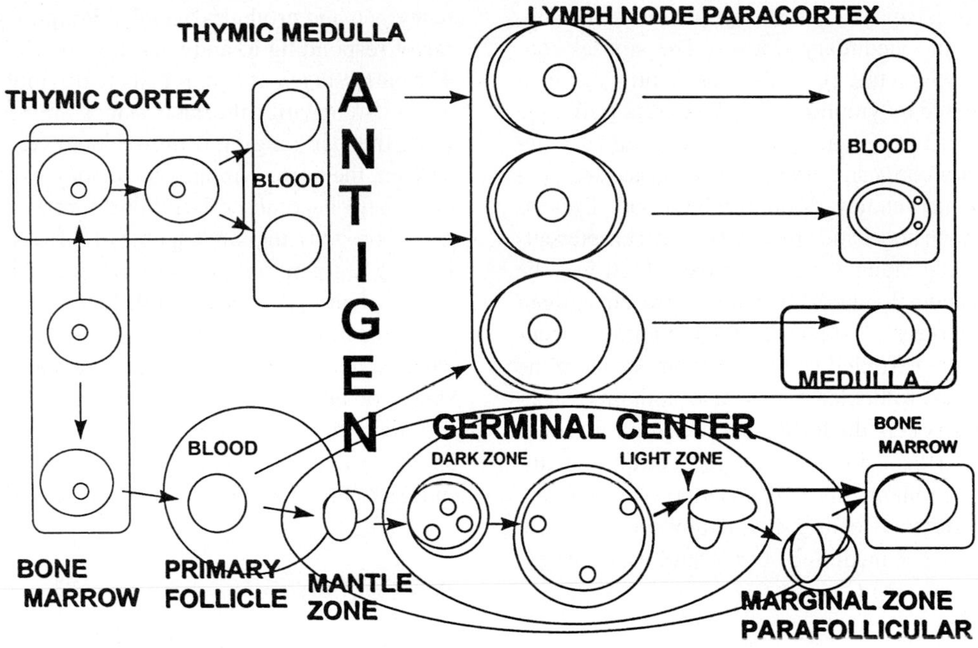

FIG. 19.2. Scheme of lymphocyte differentiation showing anatomic locations of various stages.

that migrate from the bone marrow undergo maturation and selection, to become mature, naive T cells that are capable of responding to antigen. The thymus is divided into a cortex and a medulla, each of which is characterized by specialized epithelium and accessory cells, which provide the milieu for T-cell maturation (see Chapter 6).

Secondary (Peripheral) Lymphoid Tissues

Lymph Nodes

Lymph nodes are located at sites throughout the body, strategically placed to process antigens present in lymph drained from most organs through the afferent lymphatics.

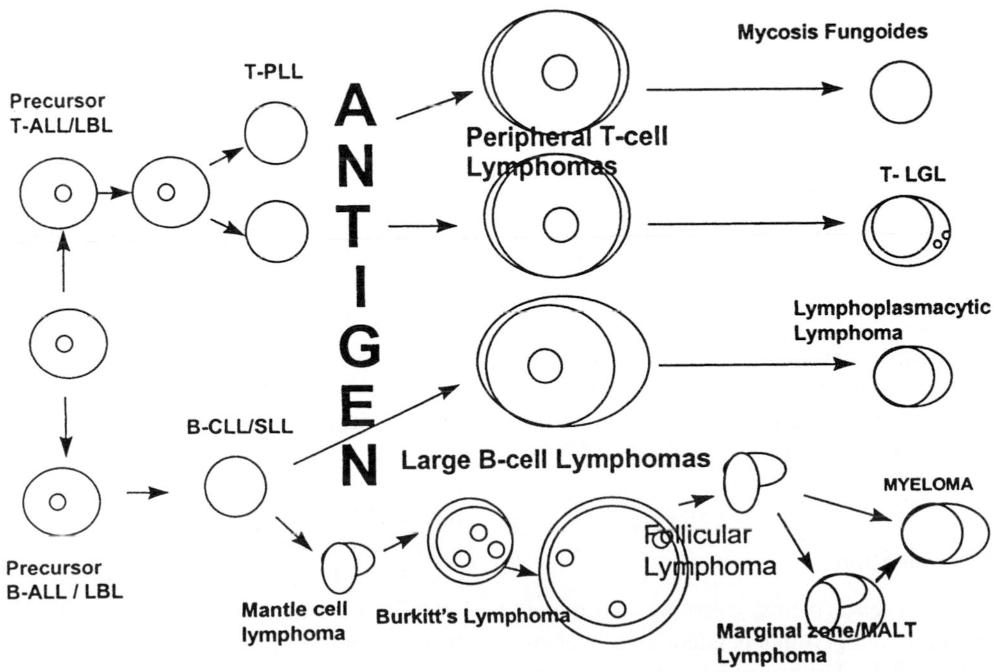

FIG. 19.3. Scheme of lymphocyte differentiation showing corresponding lymphoid neoplasms.

Lymph nodes have a capsule, a cortex, a medulla, and subcapsular, cortical, and medullary sinuses. The sinuses contain macrophages, which take up and process antigen, which then may be presented to lymphocytes. The cortex is divided into follicular and diffuse (paracortical) regions, and the medulla into medullary cords and sinuses. The paracortex contains high endothelial venules, through which both T and B lymphocytes enter the node, and specialized antigen-presenting cells, the interdigitating dendritic cells, which may be related to the cutaneous Langerhans cell and present antigen to T cells. T-cell and early B-cell reactions to antigen occur in the paracortex; the germinal center reaction occurs in the follicular cortex. The follicular cortex also contains a specific type of accessory cell, the follicular dendritic cell; adhesion to the follicular dendritic cell–antigen complex is important in the differentiation of B cells in response to antigen. Plasma cells and effector T cells generated by immune reactions accumulate in the medullary cords and exit through the medullary sinuses (see Chapter 6).

Spleen

The spleen, located in the left upper abdomen, has two major compartments: the red pulp, which functions as a filter for particulate antigens and for the formed elements of the blood, and the white pulp, which is virtually identical in its compartments to the lymphoid tissue of the lymph node. Follicles and germinal centers are found in the malpighian corpuscles; T cells and interdigitating dendritic cells are found in the adjacent periarteriolar lymphoid sheath. Plasma cells accumulate in the red pulp (see Chapters 6 and 53).

Mucosa-associated Lymphoid Tissue

Specialized lymphoid tissue is found in association with certain epithelia, in particular the naso- and oropharynx (Waldeyer's ring: adenoids, tonsils), the gastrointestinal tract (gut-associated lymphoid tissue: Peyer's patches of the distal ileum, mucosal lymphoid aggregates in the colon and rectum), and lung (bronchus-associated lymphoid tissue). Collectively, this is MALT. These tissues tend to have prominent B-cell follicles but also may have discrete T-cell zones, similar to the paracortex of lymph nodes. MALT is thought to function in responding to intraluminal antigens and the generation of mucosal immunity. Lymphoid cells that respond to antigen in the MALT acquire homing properties that enable them to return to these tissues (76,77) (see Chapters 33 and 35).

B- and T-cell Differentiation

In both the T- and B-cell systems, there are two major phases of differentiation: antigen-independent and antigen-dependent (Figs. 19.1, 19.2). Antigen-independent differentiation occurs in the primary lymphoid organs—bursa-equivalent (?bone marrow) and thymus—without exposure to antigen and produces a pool of lymphocytes that are capable of responding to antigen (naive or virgin T and B cells). The early stages are stem cells and lymphoid blasts, which are self-renewing; the later stages are resting cells with a finite lifespan ranging from weeks to years. On exposure to antigen, the naive lymphocyte undergoes ''blast transformation'' and becomes a large proliferating cell, which gives rise to progeny that are capable of direct activity against the inciting antigen: antigen-specific effector cells. The earlier stages of antigen-dependent differentiation are proliferating cells; the fully differentiated effector cells are less mitotically active. Neoplasms that correspond to proliferating stages of either antigen-independent or antigen-dependent differentiation are likely to be aggressive; those that correspond to naive or mature effector stages are likely to be indolent (Fig. 19.3) (see Chapters 2 and 3).

B-cell Differentiation

Antigen-independent B-cell Differentiation

Precursor B Cells. The earliest B cells have rearranged immunoglobulin heavy chain genes but lack surface immunoglobulin (sIg); the B cells at this stage are called precursor B cells, or pre–pre-B cells (78). At the next stage, pre-B cells make cytoplasmic μ heavy chain, but no light chain, and do not express sIg. Both types of cells are lymphoblasts, with dispersed chromatin and small nucleoli. They contain the intranuclear enzyme terminal deoxynucleotidyl transferase (TdT) and express CD34, a glycoprotein present on immature cells of both lymphoid and myeloid lineage, HLA-DR (class II major histocompatibility complex [MHC] antigens), and the common acute lymphoblastic leukemia antigen (CD10) (79–82). Expression of class II MHC antigens persists throughout the life of the B cell and is important in interactions with T cells. Pan–B-cell antigens are expressed sequentially on precursor B cells: CD19 and cytoplasmic CD22, followed by surface CD20. The leukocyte common antigen (CD45) does not appear until surface CD20; thus, staining for CD45 may not be useful in identifying early B-cell neoplams (83). Precursor B cells also express CD79a, a molecule that is associated with sIg, and is involved in transduction of signal after engagement of sIg with antigen (84,85), analogous to CD3 and the T-cell receptor (TCR) molecule.

Fetal early B-cell development occurs in the liver, bone marrow, and spleen; in adults, B-cell development is restricted to the bone marrow. Cells with the morphologic and immunologic features of precursor B cells can be found in normal and regenerating bone marrow, in which they correspond to the lymphocyte-like cells known as hematogones (86,87). Neoplasms of precursor B cells usually involve bone marrow and peripheral blood and are known as *common or precursor B acute lymphoblastic leukemia*; rarely, they present as solid tumors (*precursor B lymphoblastic lymphoma*).

Naive B Cells. The end stage of antigen-independent B-cell differentiation is the mature, naive (virgin) B cell, which expresses both complete sIgM and IgD, lacks TdT and common acute lymphoblastic leukemia antigen, and is capable of responding to antigen. Naive B cells have rearranged but unmutated immunoglobulin genes (88). Each individual B cell is committed to a single light chain, either κ or λ, and all of its progeny express the same light chain (89). In contrast to precursor B cells, naive B cells lack CD10 and CD34. In addition to sIg, naive B cells express pan–B-cell antigens (CD19, CD20, CD22, CD40, and CD79a), HLA class II molecules, complement receptors (CD21 and CD35), CD44, Leu-8 (L-selectin), CD23, and the pan–T cell antigen CD5 (90). Many of the surface antigens expressed by mature B cells are involved in "homing" or adhesion to vascular endothelium, interaction with antigen-presenting cells, and signal transduction. CD79a, CD19, CD20, and sIg appear to be involved in signal transduction (91); CD22 is involved in signaling (92); and CD40 is involved in interaction with T cells (93) and further differentiation of B cells. Resting B cells also produce the BCL-2 protein, which promotes survival in the resting state (94). CD5-positive ($CD5^+$) B cells produce immunoglobulin that often has broad specificity (cross-reactive idiotypes) and reactivity with self-antigens (autoantibodies) (90).

Naive B cells are small resting lymphocytes. In fetal tissues, they are the predominant lymphoid cell in the spleen; in adults, they circulate in the blood and also comprise a minor fraction of the B cells in primary lymphoid follicles and follicle mantle zones (so-called recirculating B cells) (90,95). Studies of single cells picked from the mantle zones of reactive follicles show that they are clonally diverse and contain unmutated immunoglobulin genes, consistent with naive B cells (96). Tumors of these cells are usually clinically indolent and histologically of low grade. In addition, they are often widespread and leukemic, consistent with the recirculating behavior of the normal naive B cell. Two neoplasms appear to correspond to $CD5^+$ B cells: B-cell CLL and mantle cell (centrocytic or intermediate) lymphoma (97–99).

Antigen-dependent B-cell Differentation

Immunoblastic or Plasma Cell Reaction. On encountering antigen, the naive B cell transforms into a proliferating cell, which ultimately matures into an antibody-secreting plasma cell. In T-cell–independent reactions, and in the early primary immune response, naive B cells transform into IgM^+ blast cells (B blasts or immunoblasts) in the T-cell zones, proliferate, and differentiate into IgM-secreting plasma cells, producing the IgM antibody of the primary immune response (89,100,101). These plasma cells have largely unmutated immunoglobulin genes. There is a loss of sIgD during blast transformation, as of some other antigens, such as CD21 and CD22. Other antigens associated with activation are upregulated. With maturation to plasma cells, most surface antigens are lost, including pan–B-cell antigens HLA-DR, and leukocyte common antigen, CD45 (102), and secretory cytoplasmic IgM accumulate. The corresponding neoplasm to the IgM-producing plasma cell may be lymphoplasmacytic lymphoma (immunocytoma), or Waldenstrom's macroglobulinemia.

Germinal Center Reaction. Later in the primary response (within 3–7 days of antigen challenge in experimental animals) and in secondary responses, the T cell–dependent germinal center reaction occurs. Each germinal center is formed from between 3 and 10 naive B cells and ultimately contains approximately 10,000 to 15,000 B cells; more than 10 generations are required to form a germinal center (96,101). Proliferating IgM^+ B blasts formed from naive B cells that have encountered antigen in the T-cell zone (paracortex) migrate into the center of the primary follicle and fill the follicular dendritic cell meshwork by about 3 days after antigen stimulation, forming a germinal center (101,103). These B blasts differentiate into immunoglobulin-negative centroblasts (large noncleaved follicular center cells), which appear at about 4 days and accumulate at one pole of the germinal center, forming the "dark zone." Centroblasts are large proliferating cells with vesicular nuclei, one to three prominent, peripheral nucleoli, and a narrow rim of basophilic cytoplasm. They lack sIg (101,104,105) and also switch off the gene that encodes the BCL-2 protein; thus, they and their progeny are susceptible to death through apoptosis (94). Germinal center cells express antigens associated with activation, most of which are involved with interaction with T cells, including CD23, CD71, CD40, and CD86 (93,106–110) as well as antigens associated with adhesion to follicular dendritic cells, including CD11a/18 and CD29/49d (111,112), and antigens that may promote apoptosis, such as CD95 (113). An important event in germinal center development is expression of BCL-6 protein, a nuclear zinc finger transcription factor that is expressed by both centroblasts and centrocytes but not by naive or memory B cells, mantle cells, or plasma cells (114,115). Interestingly, normal resting B cells express high levels of *BCL6* messenger RNA but lack the protein (116).

In centroblasts, a process of somatic mutation of the immunoglobulin gene variable (V) region begins, which alters the affinity for antigen of the antibody that will be produced by the cell (117,118). In addition, the cell may switch from IgM to IgG or IgA production (103,119); through these mechanisms, the germinal center reaction gives rise to the better-fitting IgG or IgA antibody of the late primary or secondary immune response (120). Studies on single centroblasts picked from the dark zone of germinal centers suggest that in the early stages, a germinal center may contain about 5 to 10 clones of centroblasts, which show only a moderate amount of immunoglobulin gene V-region mutation; later, the number of clones diminishes to as few as three, and the degree of somatic mutation increases (96).

Centroblasts mature to nonproliferating medium-sized cells with irregular nuclei, inconspicuous nucleoli, and scant cytoplasm, called *centrocytes* (small or large cleaved follicular center cells), which accumulate in the opposite pole of the germinal center, known as the "light zone," which also contains a high concentration of follicular dendritic cells. Centrocytes reexpress sIg, which has the same VDJ rearrangement as the parent naive B cell and the centroblast of the dark zone but which may have undergone heavy chain class switch, and which has an altered antibody combining site, because of the somatic mutations in the immunoglobulin V region (96). This process of somatic mutation thus results in marked intraclonal diversity of antibody-combining sites in a population of cells derived from only a few precursors. Also in the germinal center, the *BCL6* gene undergoes somatic mutation of the 5′ noncoding promoter region, at a lower frequency than is seen in the immunoglobulin genes (121–123). Thus, immunoglobulin gene mutation and *BCL6* mutation serve as markers of cells that have experienced the germinal center.

Centrocytes whose immunoglobulin gene mutations have resulted in decreased affinity for antigen rapidly die by apoptosis (programmed cell death); the prominent starry-sky pattern of phagocytic macrophages seen in germinal centers at this stage is a result of the apoptosis of centrocytes. In contrast, centrocytes whose immunoglobulin gene mutations have resulted in increased affinity are able to bind to native, unprocessed antigen trapped in antigen–antibody complexes by the complement receptors on the processes of follicular dendritic cells. The centrocytes are able to process the antigen and present it to T cells in the light zone of the germinal center. It is thought that this activation of T cells may induce them to express CD40 ligand (CD40L), which can engage CD40 on the B cell. Both ligation of the antigen receptor by antigen and ligation of CD40 on the surfaces of germinal center B cells can "rescue" them from apoptosis (89,103–105,124). Interaction with surface molecules expressed by follicular dendritic cells, such as CD23, appears to be important in directing differentiation of the centrocytes into plasma cells; interaction with the numerous T cells present in the light zone, through the CD40 molecule and its ligand on T cells, appears to be important in the generation of memory B cells (101,103). In addition, both antigen–receptor ligation and CD40 ligation switch off *BCL6* messenger RNA production and BCL-6 protein expression (116).

Follicular lymphomas are tumors of germinal center B cells, in which centrocytes fail to undergo apoptosis because they have a chromosomal rearrangement, t(14;18), that prevents the normal switching off of the antiapoptosis gene *BCL2* (94,125). Most large B-cell lymphomas are composed of cells that at least in part resemble centroblasts and have mutated immunoglobulin V-region genes and therefore are thought to derive from the germinal center stage of differentiation. Finally, it is possible that Burkitt's lymphoma corresponds to the early sIgM$^+$ B blast found in the early germinal center reaction in experimental animals (126).

Marginal Zone and Monocytoid (Parafollicular) B Cells. When the germinal center polarizes into a dark and a light zone, the mantle zone becomes better defined and eccentric, with the broader portion surrounding the light zone of the germinal center. Antigen-specific B cells generated in the germinal center reaction leave the follicle and reappear in the outer mantle zone, to form a "marginal zone"; these are particularly prominent in mesenteric lymph nodes, Peyer's patches, and the spleen (104,127–130). Marginal zone B cells have slightly irregular nuclei, resembling those of centrocytes, but with more abundant, pale cytoplasm. The term *centrocyte-like* has been applied to similar neoplastic cells (131). On rechallenge with antigen, splenic marginal zone B cells first migrate into the germinal center and then quickly appear in the T cell zone as immunoglobulin-positive blast cells, which give rise to antigen-specific plasma cells; thus, they are thought to be memory B cells (101). Memory B cells are also detectable in the peripheral blood, in which they may be IgM$^+$ and even CD5$^+$ (132,133). Studies on single marginal zone B cells from spleen and Peyer's patches show that they have mutated V-region genes, may be oligoclonal, and are not related clonally to the adjacent germinal center (134–136). Cells that resemble marginal zone B cells but with even more nuclear indentation and abundant cytoplasm, known as *monocytoid B lymphocytes*, are seen in clusters adjacent to subcapsular and cortical sinuses of some reactive lymph nodes (137), peripheral to and often continuous with the follicle marginal zone. In contrast to marginal zone B cells, the monocytoid B cells found in reactive lymph nodes appear either to have unmutated immunoglobulin V-region genes or to show only a small number of randomly distributed mutations that do not suggest selection by antigen (136). Nodal and splenic tumors resembling normal marginal zone and monocytoid B cells have been described (138–141). Analysis of immunoglobulin V-region genes suggest that most of these have mutations consistent with germinal center exposure and antigen selection (142,143).

Bone Marrow Plasma Cells. Immunoglobulin G–producing plasma cells accumulate in the lymph node medulla, but it appears that the immediate precursor of the bone marrow plasma cell leaves the node and migrates to the bone marrow. Plasma cells lose sIg, pan–B cell antigens, HLA-DR, CD40, and CD45, and cytoplasmic IgG or IgA accumulates. Plasma cells also express CD38. They have rearranged and mutated immunoglobulin genes but do not have the ongoing mutations seen in follicle center cells. Tumors of these marrow-homing plasma cells correspond to plasmacytoma and multiple myeloma.

Mucosa-associated Lymphoid Tissue. A subset of B cells, including all the differentiation stages listed previously, are programmed for gut-associated rather than nodal lymphoid tissue. In these tissues (Waldeyer's ring, Peyer's patches, and mesenteric nodes), similar responses occur to antigen, but both the intermediate and end-stage B cells that originate in the gut or mesenteric lymph nodes preferentially return there, rather than to peripheral lymph nodes or bone marrow. The plasma cells generated in gut-associated lymphoid tissue home preferentially to the lamina propria, rather than to the bone marrow (76,77). Many extranodal low-grade B-cell lymphomas are thought to arise from this MALT (131). Because most MALT lymphomas contain prominent marginal zone type B cells, in addition to small B lymphocytes and plasma cells, and similar lymphomas occur in non-MALT sites, the term *extranodal marginal zone lymphoma of MALT type* has been proposed for these tumors (64). MALT-type lymphomas have somatically mutated V-region genes, consistent with an antigen-selected post–germinal center B-cell stage (144).

T-cell Differentiation

Antigen-independent T-cell Differentiation

Cortical Thymocytes. As in the B-cell system, the earliest stages of T-cell differentiation involve characteristic rearrangement of the DNA encoding the antigen receptor molecule. The earliest antigen-independent stages of T-cell differentiation occur in the bone marrow; later stages occur in the thymic cortex. The exact site at which precursor cells become committed to the T lineage is not known, because the thymus contains cells that can differentiate into either T or NK cells but not B cells (reviewed in ref. 145). Cortical thymocytes are lymphoblasts, which contain the intranuclear enzyme TdT. The earliest committed T-cell precursors are $CD34^+CD45RA^+$, express the CD13 and CD33 antigens usually associated with myeloid cells, and are $CD3^-CD4^-CD8^-$ (''triple negative''); within the thymus they sequentially acquire CD1, CD2, CD5, and cytoplasmic CD3, and first the CD4 ''helper'' and then the CD8 ''suppressor'' antigens (''double positive''). In the thymus, rearrangement of the TCR genes is initiated, beginning with the γ and δ chains, followed by the β and then the α chain genes; these proteins are expressed on the cell surface. Surface CD3 expression appears at the same time as expression of the T-cell antigen receptor β chain, with which it is closely associated and participates in signal transduction. Cortical thymocytes express the CD45RO epitope of the leukocyte common antigen instead of CD45RA (146), and lack the antiapoptosis protein BCL-2 (94).

In addition to providing a pool of mature T cells through proliferation of precursor cells, the thymus plays a major role in the selection of T cells, so that the resulting pool of mature T cells does not react to self-antigens. Both positive and negative selection occur in the thymus at the double positive ($CD4^+CD8^+$) stage. Thymocytes that have anti-self specificity bind strongly through their $\alpha\beta$ TCR complex to self-antigens presented by the MHC on thymic dendritic cells, and they die by apoptosis. Those that lack anti-self reactivity undergo positive selection on thymic epithelial cells; they express increased levels of surface CD3, acquire CD27 and CD69, switch their CD45 isotype from RO back to RA, lose CD1, express BCL-2, and lose either CD4 or CD8 to become mature, naive T cells (145). The tumor that corresponds to the stages of T-cell differentiation in the thymic cortex is precursor T lymphoblastic lymphoma or leukemia; the variety of immunophenotypes and antigen receptor gene rearrangements found in precursor T-cell neoplasia correspond to the variety of stages of intrathymic T-cell differentiation.

Naive T Cells. Mature, naive (virgin) T cells have the morphologic appearance of small lymphocytes, have a low proliferation fraction, lack TdT and CD1, and express either (but not both) CD4 or CD8, as well as surface CD3 and CD5 (147), CD45RA, and BCL-2 (94,146). These cells leave the thymus and can be found in the circulation, in the paracortex of lymph nodes, and in the thymic medulla. Some cases of T-cell prolymphocytic leukemia and peripheral T-cell lymphoma may correspond to naive T cells.

Antigen-dependent T-cell Differentiation

A complex interaction of T-cell surface molecules with molecules on the surface of antigen-presenting cells is required for T-cell activation in response to antigen (reviewed in ref. 93). On the T cell, the CD4 or CD8 molecules bind to MHC class II or class I molecules, respectively, on the antigen-presenting cell. A complex of CD3 and the T-cell antigen receptor (which may be of either $\gamma\delta$ or $\alpha\beta$ type and has a combining site that ''fits'' the specific peptide antigen) binds to the antigen-MHC complex on the antigen-presenting cell. The adhesion molecule LFA-1 on the T cell binds to ICAM-1 on the antigen-presenting cell; the activation-associated molecule CD40L on the T cell binds to CD40; and CD28 and CTLA-4 on the T cell bind to B7-1 and B7-2 (CD86) on the antigen-presenting cell (109). The binding of CD40 and CD40L provides an activation stimulus for both the T cell and the antigen-presenting cell, and binding of CD28 or CTLA-4 to B7 provides a crucial second stimulus for the T cell, without which anergy develops (148). In addition, both the T cell and the antigen-presenting cell release stimulatory molecules, such as interferon-γ and interleukins, which provide further mutual activation stimuli (93).

T Immunoblasts. On encountering antigen, mature T cells transform into immunoblasts, which are large cells with prominent nucleoli and basophilic cytoplasm, that may be indistinguishable from B immunoblasts. T immunoblasts, in contrast to T lymphoblasts (thymocytes), are TdT-negative and $CD1^-$, strongly express pan–T-cell antigens, and continue to express either CD4 or CD8 but not both. Activated or proliferating T cells express HLA-DR, as well as CD25 (interleukin-2 receptor), and both CD71 and CD38. Antigen-dependent T-cell reactions occur in the paracortex of lymph nodes and the periarteriolar lymphoid sheath of the spleen, as well as at extranodal sites of immunologic reactions.

Effector T Cells. From the T-immunoblastic reaction come antigen-specific effector T cells of either CD4 or CD8 type, as well as memory T cells. Antigen-stimulated T cells switch their CD45 isotype from CD45RA to CD45RO. Effector T cells of the CD4 type typically act as helper cells, and those of the CD8 type as suppressor cells *in vitro*; however, both types can be cytotoxic (149). CD4 cells are cytotoxic to cells that display antigen complexed with MHC class II antigen; CD8 cells are cytotoxic to cells that display it complexed with MHC class I antigen. In addition to cytotoxicity, effector T cells produce a variety of cytokines that affect the function of B cells and antigen-presenting cells, which modulate the immune response. Fully differentiated T-effector cells are small lymphocytes, morphologically similar to other nonproliferating lymphocytes of either T or B type. In addition to differences in subset antigen (CD4 versus CD8 or double negative) expression, peripheral T cells may differ in their TCR expression ($\gamma\delta$ versus $\alpha\beta$). The majority of T cells in the circulation and in most lymphoid tissues are $\alpha\beta^+$; $\gamma\delta$ T cells are more numerous in mucosae and in the spleen (150).

Most cases of peripheral T-cell lymphoma are thought to correspond to stages of antigen-dependent T-cell differentation—for example, mycosis fungoides corresponds to a mature, effector CD4$^+$ cell, hepatosplenic $\gamma\delta$ T-cell lymphoma to a $\gamma\delta$ T cell, T-cell large granular lymphocyte leukemia to a mature effector CD8$^+$ cell; however, the relationship between neoplastic and normal T cells is not nearly as well understood as in the B-cell system. The systemic symptoms such as fever, skin rashes, and hemophagocytic syndromes associated with some peripheral T-cell lymphomas may be consequences of cytokine production by the neoplastic T cells.

Natural Killer Cells

A third line of lymphoid cells, called *natural killer* cells because they can kill certain targets without sensitization and without MHC restriction, appears to derive from a common progenitor with T cells (reviewed in ref. 145). NK cells recognize self–class I MHC molecules on the surfaces of cells and kill cells that lack these antigens. Immature NK cells have cytoplasmic CD3, but these cells do not rearrange their TCR genes or express TCRs or surface CD3. They are characterized by certain NK cell–associated antigens (CD16, CD56, and CD57), which also can be expressed on some T cells, and express some T cell–associated antigens (CD2, CD28, and CD8). NK cells appear in the peripheral blood as a small proportion of circulating lymphocytes; they are usually slightly larger than most normal T and B cells, with abundant pale cytoplasm containing azurophilic granules—so-called large granular lymphocytes (see Chapters 2 and 3). Angiocentric or nasal T- or NK cell lymphoma and some types of large granular lymphocyte leukemia appear to correspond to immature and mature NK cells, respectively.

Immunophenotyping of Lymphoid Cells

Individual B and T lymphoid cells as well as accessory cells of the mononuclear phagocyte system can be recognized in cell suspensions or tissue sections by the presence of surface or cytoplasmic molecules (antigens) that can be detected using antibodies labeled with either fluorescence or enzymatic (immunohistochemical) methods. Immunophenotyping with monoclonal antibodies can be done using viable cell suspensions, frozen tissue sections, or paraffin-embedded tissue sections. With monoclonal antibodies and acetone-fixed cryostat sections, many types of normal and neoplastic lymphoid cells have been classified (151,152). A series of international workshops have developed a standardized nomenclature for many of the antigens detected by more than one monoclonal antibody (153). For cells in body fluids, particularly the peripheral blood, flow cytometry with fluorescent-labeled antibodies is the method of choice; this method also can be applied to fine needle aspiration biopsy specimens and to cell suspensions prepared from fresh tissue specimens, but sampling problems occur because of selective loss of fragile neoplastic cells. Acetone-fixed frozen sections are the most reliable method for the pathologist to assess the phenotype of lymphoid cells in tissue sections. In recent years, however, the technology for detecting lymphocyte-associated antigens in paraffin-embedded tissue has improved greatly, so that most clinically necessary immunophenotyping can be accomplished using routinely processed tissue. It is still advisable to prepare fresh frozen tissue for all cases of suspected lymphoma, in case a diagnosis cannot be made with certainty through analysis of paraffin-embedded tissue, and also for possible molecular genetic analysis (see Chapters 3, 4, and 5).

Molecular Genetic Analysis of Lymphoid Cells

Lymphocyte differentiation involves rearrangement of the genes involved in antigen recognition. This process is required for development of a functional antigen receptor gene and serves to increase the diversity of these receptors beyond what can be ''hard-coded'' into the genome, so that lymphoid cells can develop a repertoire large enough to respond to the majority of antigens they may encounter. Analysis of these rearrangements has provided insights into normal T- and B-cell differentiation and also is useful in the diagnosis and classification of lymphoid neoplasms. In addition to these normal rearrangements, chromosome translocations frequently occur in lymphoid neoplasms, as they do in other tumors. In lymphomas, these translocations often involve ''hot spots'' in the antigen receptor genes; these translocations can be useful in the diagnosis and classification of lymphoid neoplasms (see Chapter 9).

Antigen Receptor Gene Rearrangement

Immunoglobulin Gene Rearrangement

Differentiation of B cells involves rearrangements of the genes involved in immunoglobulin production (78,154). The genes that encode the constant and variable regions of the immunoglobulin heavy and light chain molecules are located far apart on the chromosomes in germline cells. In order to produce RNA for an immunoglobulin protein, many thousands of base pairs of DNA must be deleted from the genome, to bring the different portions of the immunoglobulin gene together. These rearrangements change the position on the DNA of restriction sites: points at which restriction endonucleases cleave the DNA. Thus, fragments produced by digesting B-cell DNA with these enzymes are of a different size than those produced by digesting non–B cell (germline) DNA and migrate differently in an electrophoresis gel. If radiolabeled DNA probes (cloned segments of DNA produced by bacteria) that are complementary to specific portions of the immunoglobulin gene are applied to such a gel, they specifically mark the position of the immunoglobulin gene, which can be demonstrated on an autoradiograph. The exact size, and therefore position on the gel (Southern blot), of each immunoglobulin gene fragment is unique to an individual B cell; this technique provides not only a specific marker for B cells but also a true marker for monoclonality (see Chapter 7).

T-Cell Receptor Gene Rearrangement

A process of gene rearrangement analogous to that seen in B cells also occurs during T-cell differentiation (145). This process involves the DNA encoding a T cell–specific surface molecule that serves as the TCR for antigen, analogous to sIg on B cells. As in the B-cell system, the size of restriction fragments of the DNA encoding the TCR gene are specific for a single clone of T cells. TCR gene rearrangement is a specific marker for T cells, and also a true marker for monoclonality in T cells (see Chapter 7).

Oncogene Rearrangements

In addition to rearrangements of antigen receptor genes, hematologic malignancies frequently have specific chromosomal translocations (155). Cellular oncogenes (genes that can cause malignant transformation if transfected in activated or altered form into cultured normal cells) have been identified in association with some of the more common chromosome translocations that characterize lymphoid malignancies (156,157). These translocations can be detected using DNA probes that hybridize to the breakpoint regions on the chromosome carrying the oncogene. Using a technique for amplifying unique DNA segments (polymerase chain reaction), rare cells carrying a given translocation can be detected, using probes that span the breakpoint, or using a reverse transcriptase technique to detect RNA produced by the altered or fused gene (see Chapter 8). Numeric abnormalities of chromosomes are also common in lymphoid malignancies; these can be detected by fluorescence *in situ* hybridization, using probes to specific chromosomes (see Chapter 10).

To the extent to which specific histologic subtypes or prognostic groups of lymphomas are associated with specific gene rearrangements, detection of these rearrangements may prove useful in the characterization of lymphomas. In addition, this technique potentially could be used to detect disseminated or recurrent lymphoma on very small biopsy specimens, or in the blood. Finally, study of the function of the translocated oncogene is providing clues to the mechanisms of oncogenesis.

Use of Immunophenotyping and Genetic Studies in the Diagnosis of Lymphoid Neoplasms

Each of the lymphoid neoplasms has a characteristic morphology, which may be sufficient in a given case to permit diagnosis and classification on morphologic grounds alone, if well-prepared sections are available. There are many pitfalls in the histologic diagnosis of malignant lymphoma, however, and immunophenotyping or, less frequently, genetic studies can be useful in resolving major differential diagnostic problems (Table 19.30). Problems that can be

TABLE 19.30. *Immunohistologic and genetic features of common B-cell neoplasms*

Neoplasm	SIg; CIg	CD5	CD10	CD23	CD43[a]	CD103	Cyclin D1	Genetic abnormality	Immunoglobulin genes[b]
B-cell chronic or small lymphocytic lymphoma	+; −/+	+	−	+	+	−	−/+	Trisomy 12, 13q; t(9;14); del(6)(q23)	R,U
Lymphoplasmacytic lymphoma	+; +	−	−	−	−/+	−	−		R,M
Hairy cell leukemia	+; −	−	−	−	+	++	+/−	None known	R,M
Splenic marginal zone lymphoma	+; −/+	−	−	−	−	+	−	None known	R,M
Follicle center lymphoma	+; −	−	+/−	−/+	−	−	−	t(14;18); *BCL2*	R,M,O
Mantle cell lymphoma	+; −	+	−		+	−	+	t(11;14); *BCL1*	R,U
Mucosa-associated lymphoid tissue lymphoma	+; +/−	−	−	−/+	−/+	−	−	Trisomy 3; t(11;18)	R,M,O
Diffuse large B-cell lymphoma	+/−	−	−/+	NA	−/+	NA	−	t(14;18); t(8;14); 3q; *BCL2; MYC; BCL6*	R,M
Burkitt's	+	−	+	−	−	NA	−	t(8;14); t(2;8); *R,M* t(8;22); *MYC*; Epstein-Barr virus–positive	R,M

(continued)

TABLE 19.30. *Continued.*

Neoplasm	CD3; S,C	CD5	CD7	CD4	CD8	CD30	TCR	NK (16,56)	Cytotox granule[c]	EBV	Genetic abnormality	T receptor genes
T-PLL	+	−	+, +	+/−	−/+	−	$\alpha\beta$	−/+	−	−	inv(14), trisomy 8q	R
T-LGL	+	−	+, +	−	+	−	$\alpha\beta$	+, −	+	−	None known	R
NK LGL	−	−	+, −	−	+/−	−	−	−, +	+	+	None known	G
Extranodal NK/T-cell lymphoma	−; +	−	−/+	−	−	−	−	+	+	+ +	None known	G
Hepatospleninc $\gamma\delta$ T-cell lymphoma	+	−	+	−	−	−	$\gamma\delta$	+, −/+	+	−	iso(7q)	R
Enteropathy-type T-cell lymphoma	+	+	+	−	+/−	+/−	$\alpha\beta$	−	+	−	None known	R
Subcutaneous panniculitis-like T-cell	+	+	+	−	+	−/+	$\alpha\beta$	−	+	−	None known	R
PTCL-NOS	+/−	+/−	+/−	+/−	−/+	−/+	$\alpha\beta > \gamma\delta$	−/+	−/+	−/+	inv(14); complex	R
Angioimmunoblastic	+	+	+	+/−	−	−	$\alpha\beta$	−	NA	+/−	None known	R
ALCL												
Primary systemic	+/−	+/−	NA	−/+	−/+	+ +	$\alpha\beta$	−	+	−	t(2;5); NPM/ALK	R
Cutaneous	+/−	+/−	+/−	+/−	−	+ +	$\alpha\beta$	−	−/+	−	None known	R

[a] Positivity may vary depending on antibody used. R, rearranged; M, mutated; U, unmutated; O, ongoing mutations; + = > 90% positive; +/− = > 50% positive; +/− = < 50% positive; < 10% positive; NA, not applicable.
[b] Mutations in the immunoglobulin gene variable region indicate exposure to antigen
[c] TIA-1, perforin, or granzyme.

resolved by these techniques include reactive versus neoplastic lymphoid infiltrates, lymphoid versus nonlymphoid malignancies, and subclassification of lymphoma. If the morphology in a given case is typical of a given entity but the immunophenotypic or genetic features are unusual, the histologic sections should be reexamined; the case still might be an example of the entity suggested by morphologic features. If the morphology is atypical but the immunophenotype and genetic features are classic for a given entity, these features may override morphology in classification. If both the morphology and the immunophenotype are atypical, then the case is best regarded as unclassifiable or borderline.

LYMPHOID NEOPLASMS IN THE REVISED EUROPEAN–AMERICAN AND WORLD HEALTH ORGANIZATION CLASSIFICATION

The entities included in the REAL-WHO classification of lymphoid neoplasms are described briefly in the remainder of this chapter. For discussions of Hodgkin's disease and myeloid neoplasms, please refer to Chapters 17 and 18 and 47 through 49, respectively. Individual lymphoid neoplasms are described more completely in other chapters.

Any pathologist or oncologist involved in the diagnosis or treatment of hematologic malignancies must remember that any classification should be considered a work in progress. The diseases recognized and their definitions represent our current best approximation; the list will need to be updated periodically as long as there continues to be progress in our understanding of the biology of the immune system and of cancer in general. In the future, joint committees of the major hematopathology societies, together with clinical colleagues, will need to periodically review and update the classification of lymphoid and other hematologic neoplasms.

B-cell Neoplasms

Precursor B-lymphoblastic Leukemia/Lymphoma (Precursor B-cell Acute Lymphoblastic Leukemia/ Precursor B-lymphoblastic Lymphoma)

Definition

A neoplasm of lymphoblasts committed to the B-cell lineage, typically composed of small to medium-sized blast cells with scant cytoplasm, moderately condensed to dispersed chromatin and indistinct nucleoli, involving bone marrow and blood (acute lymphoblastic leukemia) and occasionally presenting with primary involvement of nodal or extranodal sites (lymphoblastic lymphoma).

Morphology

On smears, lymphoblasts vary from small cells with scant cytoplasm, condensed nuclear chromatin, and indistinct nucleoli to larger cells with a moderate amount of cytoplasm, dispersed chromatin, and multiple nucleoli. Azurophilic granules may be present. In tissue sections, the cells are small to medium-sized, with scant cytoplasm and round, oval, or convoluted nuclei with fine chromatin and indistinct or small nucleoli (Fig. 19.4). Occasional cases have larger cells. The pattern is infiltrative rather than destructive, with partial preservation of the subcapsular sinus and germinal

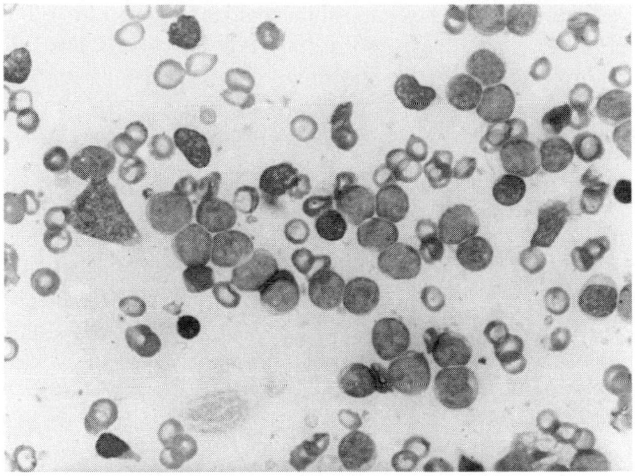

FIG. 19.4. Precursor B lymphoblastic lymphoma/leukemia. The lymphoblasts possess scanty cytoplasm and round to slightly irregular nuclei with dispersed chromatin and inconspicuous nucleoli (Wright-Giemsa).

centers. A starry-sky pattern may be present, but this is usually less prominent than in Burkitt's lymphoma.

Immunophenotype

The lymphoblasts are typically TdT^+ and variably express CD19, CD22, CD20, and CD79a, as well as CD45 and CD10. The constellation of antigens defines stages of differentiation, ranging from early precursor (membrane CD19 and CD79a and cytoplasmic CD22) to ''common'' ($CD10^+$) to late pre-B acyte lymphoblastic leukemia ($CD20^+$, cytoplasmic μ heavy chain). CD34 is expressed in 40%, and coexpression of myeloid antigens is seen in up to 30%, most commonly CD13 (14%) or CD33 (16%) (158,159). Expression of CD13 and CD33 is associated with rearrangement of *ETV6*—t(12;21)(p12;q22), *ETV6-CBFA2*, or *TEL-AML1*—and expression of CD68, CD15, and CD33 is seen in cases with 11q23/*MLL* abnormalities (159).

Genetic Features

Rearrangement of antigen receptor genes is variable in lymphoblastic neoplasms and may not be lineage-specific; thus, precursor B-cell neoplasms may have either or both immunoglobulin heavy chain and TCR γ or β chain gene rearrangements or may show no rearrangements (160–162).

Chromosomal abnormalties are common in precursor B-lymphoblastic neoplasms and are related to prognosis (Table 19.17). They are typically divided into hyperdiploidy with more than 50 chromosomes, hyperdiploidy with less than 50 chromosomes, and pseudodiploidy or translocations. The frequency of these abnormalities varies between children and adults, and some are associated with characteristic immunophenotypes or clinical behavior. Hyperdiploidy with 51 through 65 chromosomes (DNA index 1.16-1.6) is seen in up to 50% of cases of childhood precursor B acute lymphoblastic leukemia and is associated with a good prognosis; it is less common in adult acute lymphoblastic leukemia.

Translocations involving four recurrent sites are seen in precursor B acute lymphoblastic leukemia:

t(9;22)(a34;q11) *BCR/ABL*: poor prognosis, 25% of adults
t(v;11q23) *MLL* rearranged: poor prognosis, infants younger than 1 year of age and adults (163)
t(12;21)(p12;q22) *TEL/AML1*: good prognosis, children (164)
t(1;19)(q23;p13) *PBX/E2A*: poor prognosis, 25% of children

The t(9;22) and t(v;11q23) translocations often are associated with an early pre-B immunophenotype and a poor prognosis (158,163), although t(1;19) often is associated with a late pre-B immunophenotype (cytoplasmic μ-positive).

Postulated Normal Counterpart

Precursor B lymphoblast at varying stages of differentation.

Clinical Features

Precursor B acute lymphoblastic leukemia/lymphoma occurs most frequently in childhood, with a second peak in the elderly. The outcome is less favorable in infants younger than 1 year of age and in adults. In addition to cytogenetic features, risk groups are based on age, leukocyte count, sex, and response to therapy. In infants, many cases have translocations involving the *MLL* gene at 11q23, which is associated with a poor prognosis at any age (163); older children more often have hyperdiploidy or t(12;21), which confers a better prognosis (85%–90% long-term survival) (164). Adult precursor B acute lymphoblastic leukemia is associated more often with the poor prognosis of t(9;22) or t(v11q23), and the survival is much poorer than in childhood cases (158,165). Myeloid antigen expression does not seem to be an independent prognostic factor in acute lymphoblastic leukemia (159,166).

B-cell Chronic Lymphocytic Leukemia/Small Lymphocytic Lymphoma

Definition

A neoplasm of monomorphic, small round B lymphocytes in the peripheral blood and lymph nodes, admixed with prolymphocytes and paraimmunoblasts in lymph nodes, usually expressing CD5 and CD23. B-cell SLL is defined as a tissue infiltrate with the morphology and immunophenotype of B-cell CLL.

Morphology

The lymph node infiltrate of B-cell CLL/SLL is composed predominantly of small lymphocytes with condensed chro-

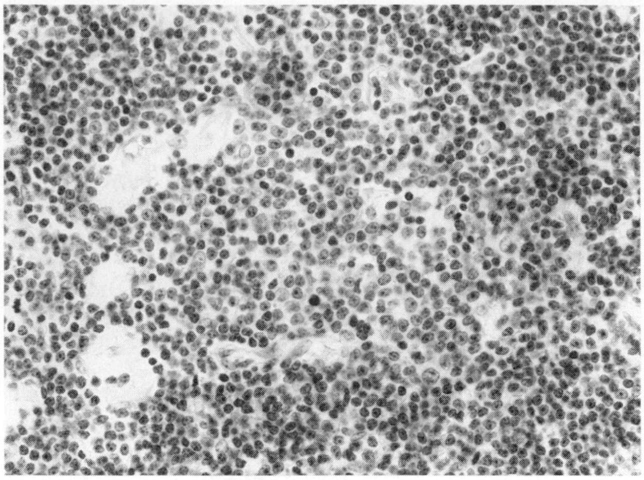

FIG. 19.5. B-cell small lymphocytic lymphoma/chronic lymphocytic leukemia. There is a diffuse infiltrate of lymphocytes, with a poorly defined pseudofollicle containing small lymphocytes, prolymphocytes, and paraimmunoblasts.

matin, round nuclei, and occasionally a small nucleolus (13,167). Larger lymphoid cells (prolymphocytes and paraimmunoblasts) with more prominent nucleoli and dispersed chromatin are always present, usually clustered in pseudofollicles (Fig. 19.5). In some cases, the cells show moderate nuclear irregularity, which can lead to a differential diagnosis of mantle cell lymphoma (168,169). Occasional cases show plasmacytoid differentiation (Table 19.18).

Immunophenotype

The tumor cells of B-CLL are faintly sIgM$^+$, and most coexpress IgD. The antigen specificity of the sIg in many cases has been shown to be against self-antigens, and these antibodies often have broad specificity—so-called cross-reactive idiotypes (170). Cytoplasmic immunoglobulin is detectable in about 5% of the cases. B cell–associated antigens (CD19, CD20, CD79a) are expressed, but CD20 may be very weak; tumor cells characteristically express both CD5 and CD23 (97). CD23 is particularly useful in distinguishing B-cell CLL/SLL from mantle cell lymphoma and should be evaluated in every case, if possible (97).

Genetic Features

Immunoglobulin heavy and light chain genes are rearranged. Most cases in early studies (75%) did not show somatic mutation of their V regions, suggesting that they corresponded to a cell that has not yet undergone antigen selection in the germinal center (171). Recent studies, however, have found that up to 40% of cases have V-region mutations, consistent with exposure to the germinal center. Cases with mutations are reported to express CD38 and to be associated with a better prognosis than cases without mutations or that are CD38$^-$ (172,173).

About 50% of cases have abnormal karyotypes (174). Trisomy 12 is reported in one third of the cases with cytogenetic abnormalities (175) and correlates with atypical histology and an aggressive clinical course (169,176). Abnormalities of 13q are reported in up to 25% of the cases and are associated with long survival. The t(11;14) transclocation and *BCL1* gene rearrangement have been reported (156,177), but many of these cases may be examples of leukemic mantle cell lymphoma. At least two clear-cut cases of B-cell CLL have been reported with *BCL1* gene rearrangement or cyclin D1 overexpression; in each the condition had an unusually aggressive clinical course (178,179). Abnormalities of 11q23 are found in a small subset of cases and are associated with lymphadenopathy and an aggressive course (180,181).

Postulated Normal Counterpart

Many cases of B-cell CLL are thought to correspond to the recirculating CD5$^+$CD23$^+$ naive B cells (90), which are found in the peripheral blood, primary follicle, and follicle mantle zone (89,95). It has been suggested that they are an anergic, self-reactive CD5$^+$ B-cell subset (182,183). Cases that show V-region mutations may correspond to a subset of peripheral blood CD5$^+$ and IgM$^+$ B cells that appear to be memory B cells (184).

Clinical Features

B-cell CLL comprises 90% of chronic lymphoid leukemias in the United States and Europe; nonleukemic B-cell SLL accounts for less than 5% of non-Hodgkin's lymphomas. In the International non-Hodgkin's Lymphoma Classification Project, 6.7% of 1,378 cases were diagnosed as B-cell CLL/SLL. The median age of patients affected was 65 years, and 83% had stage IV disease and 73% bone marrow involvement. Generalized lymphadenopathy, hepatosplenomegaly, and extranodal infiltrates may occur. Sixty-four percent of these patients had an IPI score of 2 or 3. The 5-year overall actuarial survival rate was 51%, with a failure-free survival rate of 25%. For those patients with an IPI score of 0 or 1 the overall actuarial survival rate was 76%; for those with a score of 4 or 5 it was only 38%. The extent of the disease at the time of the diagnosis is the best predictor of survival; however, chromosomal abnormalities and immunophenotype also may have prognostic importance (185). Occasional patients (<10%) present with aleukemic nodal involvement, but most ultimately are found to have or develop marrow and blood infiltration.

B-cell Prolymphocytic Leukemia

Definition

A rare B-cell neoplasm composed of prolymphocytes, with involvement of peripheral blood, bone marrow, and spleen.

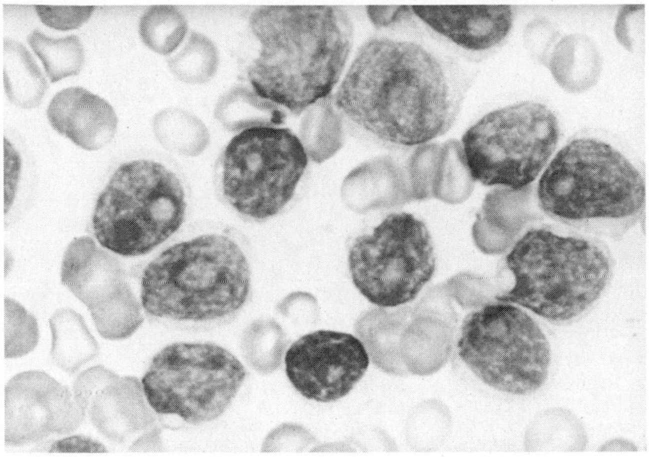

FIG. 19.6. B-cell prolymphocytic leukemia, peripheral smear, showing medium-sized cells with prominent central nucleoli. (Wright-Giemsa stain.)

Morphology

The peripheral blood prolymphocytes are medium-sized, approximately twice the size of a small lymphocyte, with moderately condensed chromatin and a single, prominent nucleolus; the nucleus is typically round, and the cytoplasm is usually scant and weakly basophilic (Fig. 19.6). These cells comprise by definition over 55% and typically over 90% of the neoplastic cells. The bone marrow is infiltrated in an interstitial pattern by similar cells. The spleen shows extensive white and red pulp infiltration by prolymphocytes. Involved lymph nodes may show vague nodularity, but pseudofollicles are absent (186–189).

Immunophenotype

The cells express bright sIgM and IgD and bright CD20 as well as other B-cell antigens (CD22, FMC7) and typically lack CD5 and CD23 (although up to one third of cases may express CD5).

Genetic Features

Translocations involving 14q32 are reported in two thirds of the cases; the most common of these is t(11;14)(q13;q32), which is characteristic of mantle cell lymphoma. It is possible that these cases are examples of leukemic mantle cell lymphoma. Trisomy 12 and complex karyotypes also are reported (190,191).

Clinical Features

This is an extremely rare disease, comprising less than 1% of cases of B-cell leukemia. If cases of mantle cell lymphoma, atypical CLL, and CLL or prolymphocytic leukemia are excluded, it may be vanishingly rare. The patients who have been reported typically present with very high white blood cell counts ($>100 \times 10^9$) and splenomegaly, with anemia cell and thrombocytopenia in 50%. The response to chemotherapy is poor. Responses have been reported to chemotherapy with cytoxan, adriamycin, vincristine, and prednisone; fludarabine; and 2-chlorodeoxyadenosine, and to splenic irradiation. Splenectomy may improve the patient's condition temporarily. Patients usually live less than 3 years.

Lymphoplasmacytic Lymphoma (with or without Waldenstrom's Macroglobulinemia)

Definition

A neoplasm of small B lymphocytes, plasmacytoid lymphocytes, and plasma cells involving bone marrow, lymph nodes, and spleen, lacking CD5, usually with a serum monoclonal protein with hyperviscosity or cryoglobulinemia. Plasmacytoid variants of other neoplasms are excluded. The term *lymphoplasmacytoid* (REAL) has been changed to *lymphoplasmacytic* (WHO).

Morphology

The tumor consists of a diffuse proliferation of small lymphocytes, plasmacytoid lymphocytes, and plasma cells, with variable numbers of immunoblasts (Fig. 19.7). In lymph nodes, sinuses are often open and may contain histiocytes reacting to secreted immunoglobulin seen with periodic acid–Schiff staining. In the spleen, both red and white pulp may be infiltrated. The pattern is usually diffuse, without a distinct marginal zone or nodularity in the red pulp. The bone marrow infiltrate may be either diffuse or nodular and often is interstitial and rather subtle; it is usually less massive than that of B-cell CLL and contains plasma cells and plasmacytoid cells in addition to small lymphocytes. Peripheral blood involvement is usually less prominent than in CLL, and the cells often have a plasmacytoid appearance.

Immunophenotype

The cells have surface and sometimes cytoplasmic immunoglobulin, usually IgM, usually lack IgD, and strongly express B cell–associated antigens (CD19, CD20, CD22, CD79a). The cells are $CD5^-$, $CD10^-$, $CD23^-$, $CD43^{\pm}$; CD25 or CD11c may be expressed faintly in some cases (97,151,192,193). Lack of CD5 and CD23, strong expression of sIg and CD20, and the presence of cytoplasmic immunoglobulin are useful in distinction from B-cell CLL.

Genetic Features

Immunoglobulin heavy and light chain genes are rearranged, and V-region genes show somatic mutations, suggesting that, in contrast to B-cell CLL, these cells arise from a population of B cells that have undergone antigen-driven selection (171,194–196). Translocation t(9;14)(p13;q32)

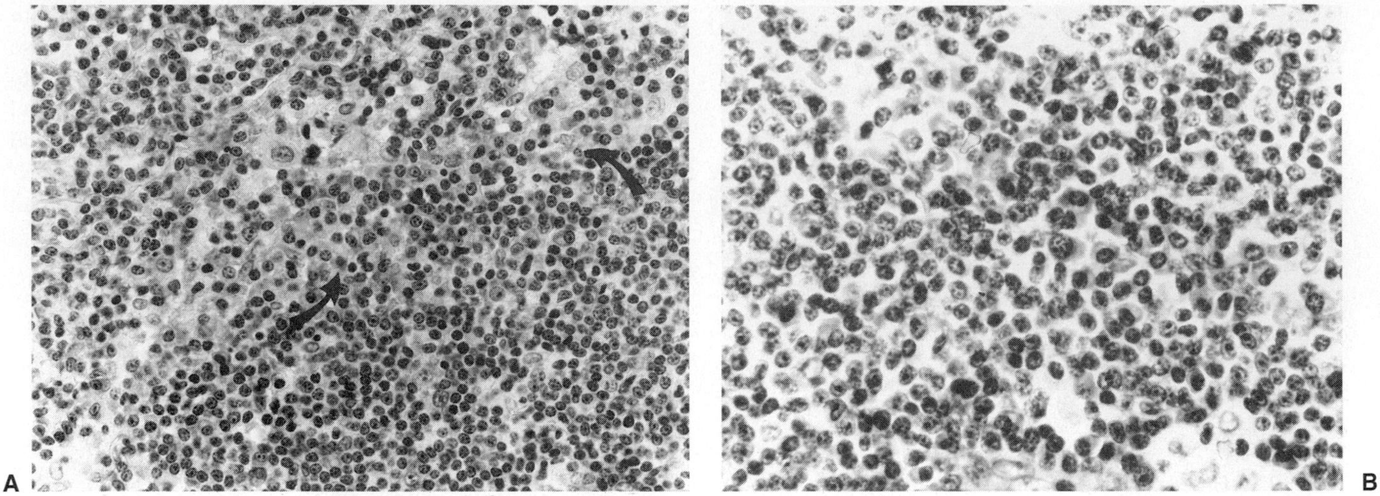

FIG. 19.7. Lymphoplasmacytic lymphoma. **A:** There is a diffuse infiltrate of lymphocytes with loose aggregates of plasma cells (*arrows*). **B:** Higher-power view showing lymphocytes and mature plasma cells.

and rearrangement of the *PAX5* gene is reported in up to 50% of cases. *PAX5* encodes a protein, B cell–specific activator protein (BSAP), that is important in early B-cell development. Expression of BSAP is restricted to B cells and appears to be independent of the translocation (197).

Postulated Normal Counterpart

Peripheral B lymphocyte stimulated to differentiate to a plasma cell, possibly corresponding to the primary immune response to antigen, or to a post–germinal center cell that has undergone somatic mutation but not heavy chain class switch.

Clinical Features

Lymphoplasmacytic lymphoma comprised only 1.2% (16/1378) of the cases in the REAL classification clinical study (61). Similar to B-cell CLL or SLL, the median age of patients affected was 63 years and 53% were male; most (73%) had bone marrow involvement. Sixty-nine percent had an IPI score of 2 or 3. Lymph node and splenic involvement are common. A monoclonal serum paraprotein of IgM type, with or without hyperviscosity syndrome (Waldenstrom's macroglobulinemia), is present in most patients (198); as with B-cell CLL, the paraprotein may have autoantibody or cryoglobulin activity.

Most cases of mixed cryoglobulinemia have been shown recently to be related to hepatitis C virus infection, even in patients who have demonstrable B-cell lymphoma in the bone marrow (199,200). Treatment of patients with hepatitis C virus infection and cryoglobulinemia with interferon to reduce viral load has been associated with regression of the lymphoma (201). Hepatitis C virus infection also has been documented in patients with B-cell lymphoma without cryoglobulinemia, most commonly in MALT-type or monocytoid B-cell lymphomas and in lymphomas of the salivary gland and liver (two sites of chronic viral infection) (202–205). Hepatitis C virus is an RNA virus that cannot integrate into the host genome, but it does infect lymphocytes, and viral proteins have been detected in lymphoid cells in these patients (206). It is not clear at this point whether the virus has transforming potential, or whether these neoplasms are antigen-driven, similar to MALT-type lymphomas.

The clinical course of lymphoplasmacytic lymphoma is indolent; in some European series it has been reported to be more aggressive than typical B-cell CLL (207, 208), but in the REAL clinical study, the 5-year overall actuarial (58%) and failure-free (25%) survival rates were identical to those of CLL or SLL (61).

Splenic Marginal Zone Lymphoma, with or without Villous Lymphocytes

Definition

A neoplasm of small B lymphocytes that surround and replace splenic white pulp germinal centers, merging with an outer marginal zone of larger cells with pale cytoplasm admixed with large transformed blasts. Both small and large cells infiltrate red pulp; often with villous lymphocytes in the peripheral blood (209).

Morphology

In the spleen, the neoplastic cells occupy both the mantle and marginal zone of the splenic white pulp, usually with a central residual germinal center, which may be either atrophic or hyperplastic (210–212) (Fig. 19.8). The mantle and marginal zones are expanded. The cells in the mantle zone are small, with slight nuclear irregularity and scant cyto-

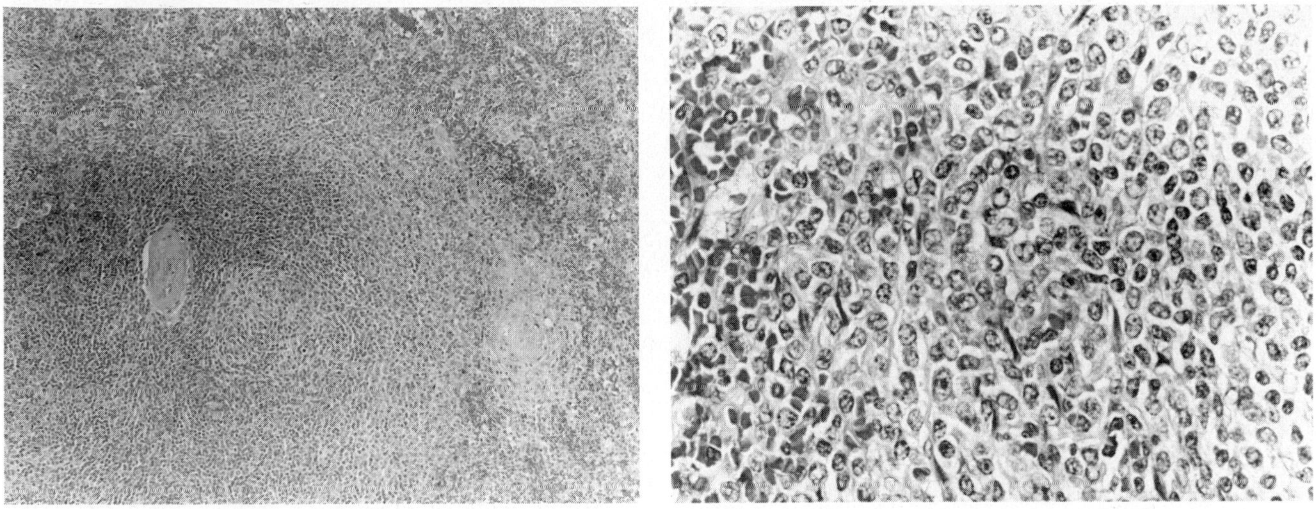

FIG. 19.8. Splenic marginal zone B-cell lymphoma. **A:** Low-power view shows replacement and expansion of the white pulp by an infiltrate of small lymphoid cells with scant cytoplasm, surrounded by a rim of small cells with slightly more abundant cytoplasm. The remnant of a reactive follicle is found in the center of the white pulp. **B:** High-power view shows small amount of red pulp (*left*), outer zone of white pulp containing small cells with clear cytoplasm and few large transformed cells, and inner zone of small cells with scant cytoplasm (*right*).

plasm; those in the marginal zone have more dispersed chromatin and abundant, pale cytoplasm, resembling marginal zone cells, and are admixed with centroblasts and immunoblasts. The red pulp is also involved, with diffuse and micronodular patterns and sinus infiltration. Epithelioid histiocytes may be present singly or in clusters and, particularly in the bone marrow, may give rise to the differential diagnosis of an infectious process. Splenic hilar lymph nodes often are involved; the neoplastic cells form vague nodules, often without a central germinal center, and a marginal zone pattern may or may not be present (213). Sinuses are often open. The marrow usually contains discrete lymphoid aggregates, without a marginal zone pattern, with or without diffuse lymphoid infiltration. If tumor cells are present in the peripheral blood they often have abundant cytoplasm with small surface ''villous'' projections or may appear plasmacytoid.

Immunophenotype

The tumor cells are IgM^+, IgD^+, and $CD5^-$ $CD10^-CD43^-CD23^-$, express B-cell antigens (CD19, CD20, CD22) and BCL-2, and lack CD11c and CD25 (211,214). In the majority of cases, lack of CD5 differentiates this disorder from B-cell CLL, and lack of CD103 and CD25 are useful in differentiating it from hairy cell leukemia. The cells are cyclin D1–negative with immunoperoxidase staining (215).

Genetic Features

Analysis of the immunoglobulin variable region genes indicates a high degree of somatic mutation, consistent with a post–germinal center stage of B-cell development (216). More recently, ongoing mutations of V-region genes, similar to germinal center cells, has been reported (142). BCL-2 is germline. Early reports that the translocation t(11;14)(q13;132), BCL-1 rearrangement, and cyclin D1 overexpresion were common probably reflected inclusion of cases of leukemic mantle cell lymphoma (217,218). Trisomy 3, found in nodal and extranodal marginal zone lymphoma, is detected in only a small number of cases (219,220).

Postulated Normal Counterpart

Post–germinal center memory B cell of splenic type.

Clinical Features

Splenic marginal zone lymphoma accounts for only 1% to 2% percent of cases of chronic lymphoid leukemia found on bone marrow examination, but up to 25% of low-grade B-cell neoplasms in splenectomy specimens (211,212,221,222). It may comprise the majority of chronic B-cell leukemias and low-grade splenic lymphomas that do not fit the defining criteria of B-cell CLL, lymphoplasmacytic lymphoma, mantle cell lymphoma, follicular lymphoma, or hairy cell leukemia. Patients typically present with splenomegaly, and lymphocytosis, usually without peripheral lymphadenopathy, and may have a small M-component (140). The course is extremely indolent, although the tumor may be surprisingly resistant to chemotherapy that would be effective for CLL. Splenectomy may be followed by prolonged remission.

Hairy Cell Leukemia

Definition

A neoplasm of small B lymphoid cells with oval nuclei and abundant cytoplasm with "hairy" projections in bone marrow and peripheral blood, diffusely infiltrating bone marrow and splenic red pulp and strongly expressing CD25, CD103, and CD11c.

Morphology

Hairy cells are small lymphoid cells with oval or bean-shaped nuclei, chromatin slightly less clumped than that of a normal lymphocyte, and abundant, pale cytoplasm with "hairy" projections on smear preparations. The bone marrow demonstrates a diffuse, interstitial infiltrate characterized by widely spaced, small nuclei, in contrast to the closely packed nuclei of most other low-grade lymphoid neoplasms involving the bone marrow. Lymphoid aggregates are not seen. Reticulin is increased, often resulting in a "dry tap." The diagnosis is best made through bone marrow biopsy. In the spleen, hairy cell leukemia involves the red pulp; the white pulp is usually atrophic (Fig. 19.9).

Immunophenotype

The tumor cells are sIg^+ ($M \pm D$, G, or A), and express B cell–associated antigens (CD19, CD20, CD22, CD79a). They are typically $CD5^-CD10^-CD23^-$ and express CD11c and CD25 strongly (85), FMC-7, and CD103 (223–226). Tartrate-resistant acid phosphatase is present in most cases but is neither necessary nor specific for the diagnosis. No one marker is specific for distinguishing hairy cell leukemia from other B-cell leukemias, because CD22, CD11c, CD25, FMC-7, and even TRAP can be present in disorders other than hairy cell leukemia. Strong expression of these markers in association with CD103, along with the characteristic morphologic features, is most useful. In tissue sections, the monoclonal antibody DBA.44 gives strong staining of hairy cells, but other lymphomas and normal B cells may express this antigen (227,228).

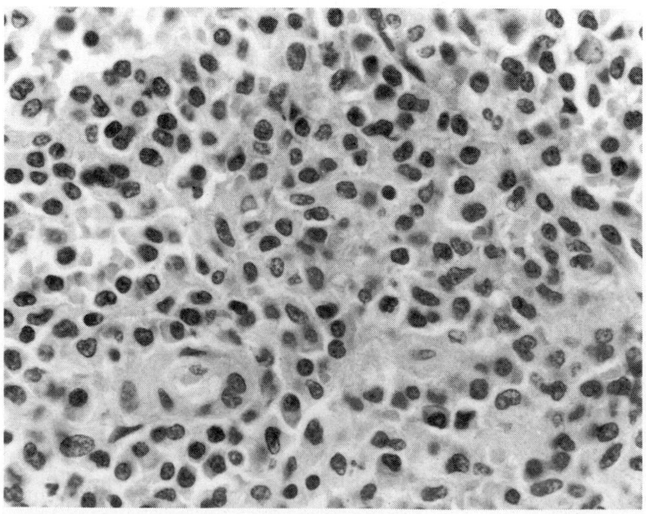

FIG. 19.9. Hairy cell leukemia. High-power view of a spleen involved by hairy cell leukemia shows medium-sized cells with oval or bean-shaped nuclei and abundant pale cytoplasm.

Genetic Features

Immunoglobulin heavy and light chain genes are rearranged (229). Immunoglobulin V-region genes are mutated, consistent with a post–germinal center cell (196). No specific cytogenetic abnormality has been described.

Postulated Normal Counterpart

Peripheral B cell of unknown post–germinal center stage.

Clinical Features

Patients are adults with splenomegaly and pancytopenia and may have few circulating neoplastic cells. Monocytopenia is usually present. Prolonged remission may follow splenectomy. There is increased susceptibility to opportunistic infections. Hairy cell leukemia does not respond well to conventional lymphoma chemotherapy, but interferon, deoxycoformycin, or 2-chlorodeoxyadenosine can induce long-term remission (230,231).

Plasma Cell Myeloma or Plasmacytoma

Definition

Plasma cell myeloma is a neoplasm of plasma cells with infiltration of bone marrow, skeletal destruction, and monoclonal immunoglobulin secretion. Plasmacytoma is a mass lesion composed of plasma cells that may be located within bone or in extramedullary sites.

Morphology

In plasma cell myeloma, the bone marrow contains more than 10% plasma cells (usually >30%), which are distributed in clusters and sheets in biopsy specimens, in contrast to the perivascular location of normal plasma cells (Fig. 19.10). In cases of plasmacytoma, there are sheets of neoplastic plasma cells forming a discrete tumor (Fig. 19.11). The neoplastic cells may resemble normal plasma cells or have more dispersed chromatin and nucleoli and decreased nuclear : cytoplasmic ratio, consistent with plasmablasts. Rare cases have multinucleated, polylobated, or pleomorphic cells (232). The 10% of patients with plasmablastic or other atypical morphologies have a worse prognosis.

Immunophenotype

The plasma cells contain monotypic IgG, IgA, or, less often, IgD or IgE type; 10% have light chains only. They

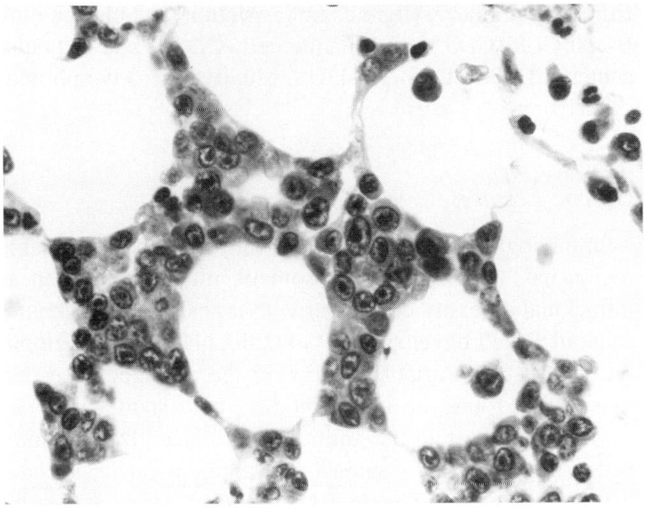

FIG. 19.10. Plasma cell myeloma. Normal hematopoietic elements have been replaced by an interstitial infiltrate of immature plasma cells with vesicular nuclei and prominent nucleoli.

typically lack CD20, variably express CD45, and express CD38 and CD138 (syndecan-1).

Genetic Features

Immunoglobulin heavy and light chain genes are rearranged and show variable region mutations consistent with post–germinal center cells (196). Cytogenetic abnormalities are common and are typically complex. The most common abnormalities involve the immunoglobulin heavy chain locus at 14q32 with a variety of partners. Some cases involve t(11;14) and cyclin D1 rearrangement and overexpression (233,234). Rare cases involve the translocation t(9;14) (p13q32) associated with lymphoplasmacytic lymphoma, involving rearrangement of the *PAX5* gene (235).

Extranodal Marginal Zone B-cell Lymphoma (Low-grade B-cell Lymphoma of Mucosa-associated Lymphoid Tissue)

Definition

An extranodal lymphoma comprised of heterogeneous small B cells, including marginal zone (centrocyte-like) cells, monocytoid cells, and small lymphocytes in varying proportions, and scattered immunoblast- and centroblast-like cells, with plasma cell differentiation in 40% of the cases. The infiltrate is in the marginal zone of reactive B-cell follicles and extends into the interfollicular region.

Morphology

Extranodal marginal zone B-cell (MALT) lymphoma reproduces the morphologic features of normal MALT (Fig. 19.12). It is characterized by a polymorphous infiltrate of small lymphocytes, marginal zone (centrocyte-like) B cells, monocytoid B cells, and plasma cells, as well as rare large basophilic blast cells (centroblast- or immunoblast-like). Reactive follicles are usually present, with the neoplastic marginal zone or monocytoid B cells occupying the marginal zone or the interfollicular region; occasionally follicles are "colonized" by marginal zone or monocytoid cells. In epithelial tissues, the marginal zone B cells typically infiltrate the epithelium, forming so-called lymphoepithelial lesions (131). Although blast cells are typically present, they are by definition in the minority. Clusters or sheets of blasts sufficiently large to warrant a diagnosis of large cell lymphoma are associated with a worse prognosis. In these cases, a separate diagnosis of DLBCL should be made. The term "high-grade MALT lymphoma" should be avoided for large B-cell lymphomas in MALT sites, because it may lead to inappropriate treatment with antibiotics instead of aggressive antilymphoma therapy (70,236–239).

A

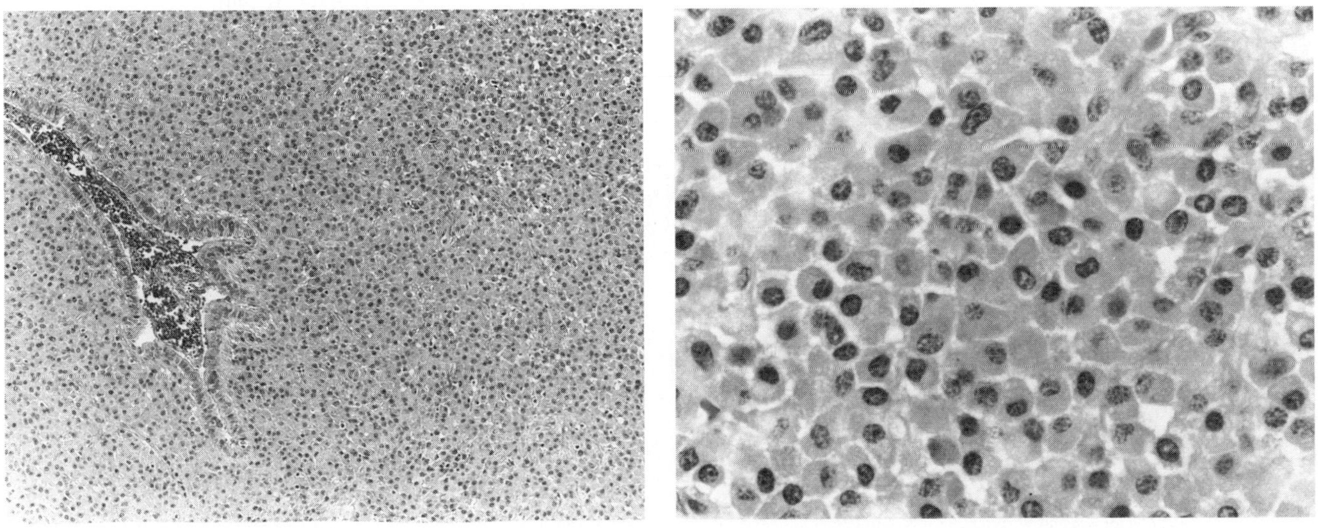

B

FIG. 19.11. Plasmacytoma. **A:** In this uncommon example of plasmacytoma of the lung, sheets of plasma cells surround a bronchiole. **B:** High-power view shows relatively mature plasma cells.

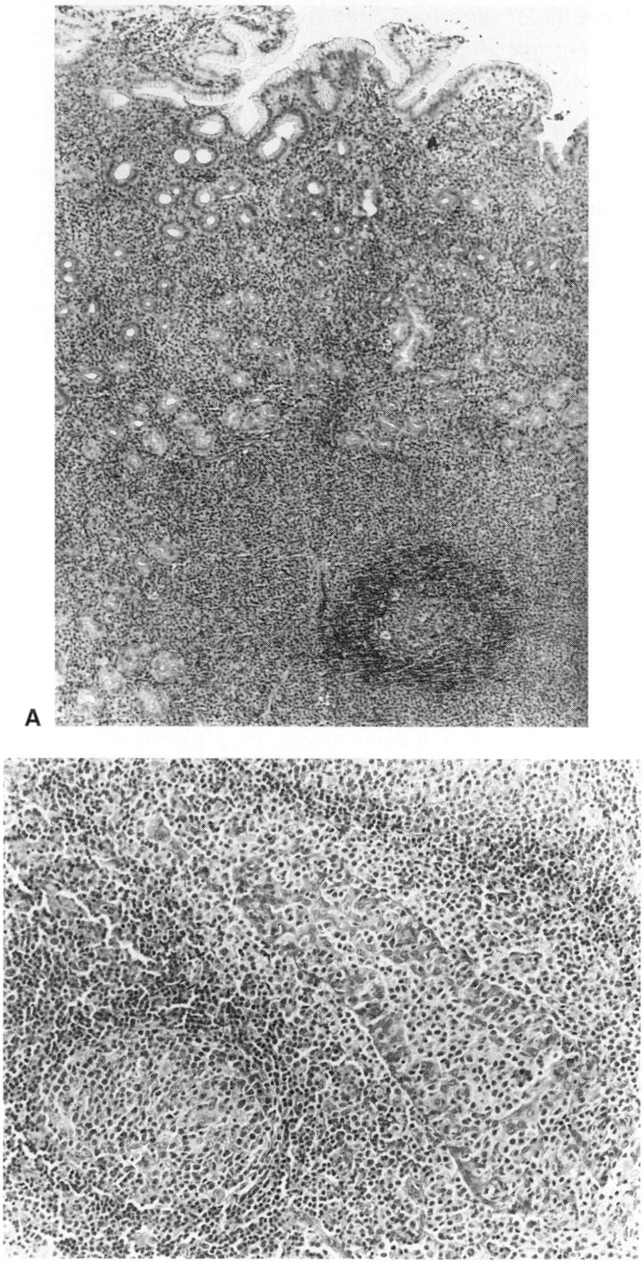

FIG. 19.12. Extranodal marginal zone lymphoma. A: Gastric lymphoma, showing infiltration of the lamina propria by small lymphocytes, marginal zone cells with epithelial infiltration, and plasma cells. B: Parotid lymphoma, with a reactive follicle adjacent to a lymphoepithelial lesion with a halo of monocytoid B cells.

Immunophenotype

The tumor cells express sIg (IgM more frequently than IgG, followed by IgA) and lack IgD, and 40% to 60% have monotypic cytoplasmic immunoglobulin, indicating plasmacytoid differentiation. They express B cell–associated antigens (CD19, CD20, CD22, CD79a) and are usually $CD5^-$ and $CD10^-$. Immunophenotyping studies are useful in confirming malignancy (light chain restriction) and in excluding B-cell CLL ($CD5^+$) and mantle cell ($CD5^+$) and follicular center ($CD10^+CD43^-CD11c^-$, usually CIg^-) lymphomas (97,210).

Genetic Features

Immunoglobulin genes are rearranged, and the variable region has a high degree of somatic mutation, as well as intraclonal diversity consistent with a post–germinal center stage of B-cell development (144,240,241). Immunoglobulin heavy chain variable regions in the analyzed cases are those often found in autoantibodies, consistent with prior studies showing that the antibodies produced by the tumor cells have specificity against self-antigens such as endothelial cells (144). The *BCL1* and *BCL2* genes are germline (242); trisomy 3 (60%) and t(11;18) (25%–40%) are the most common reported cytogenetic abnormalities (219,243,244). Interestingly, neither of these abnormalities is common in primary large cell lymphomas of the gastrointestinal tract (244,245). Recently, analysis of the t(11;18) breakpoint has shown fusion of the apoptosis-inhibiting gene *API2* to a novel gene at 18q21, named *MLT*, in two cases of MALT lymphoma (246). A gene involved in a breakpoint in MALT lymphomas with t(1;14) has recently been cloned; named *BCL10*, it is an apoptosis-promoting gene that in mutated form may cause cellular transformation (247).

Postulated Normal Counterpart

Post–germinal center memory B cell with the capacity to differentiate into marginal zone, monocytoid, and plasma cells.

Clinical Features

Extranodal marginal zone B-cell (MALT) lymphoma comprises the majority of low-grade gastric lymphomas and almost 50% of all gastric lymphomas (248); in other sites, such as the ocular adnexa, it comprises about 40% of the cases (249), and it comprises the majority of low-grade pulmonary lymphomas (250). Patients are usually older adults, although they may be in their twenties or thirties. A slight female predominance has been reported in some series (97). The majority of patients present with localized stage I or II extranodal disease, involving glandular epithelial tissues of various sites. The stomach is the most frequent site, but most low-grade lymphomas (and former pseudolymphomas) presenting in the lung, thyroid, salivary gland, or orbit are of this type; skin or soft tissues also may be the presenting site. Many patients have a history of autoimmune disease, such as Sjogren's syndrome or Hashimoto's thyroiditis, or of gastritis resulting from *Helicobacter pylori* in the case of gastric MALT lymphoma. "Acquired MALT" secondary to autoimmune disease or infection in these sites is thought to be the substrate for lymphoma development (251).

Proliferation of the cells of marginal zone lymphoma at certain sites depends on the presence of activated, antigen-driven T cells; in gastric tumors, it has been shown that the T-cells are driven by *H. pylori* antigens (252). Therapy directed at the antigen (*H. pylori* in gastric lymphoma) results in regression of most early lesions (253,254). The long-term prognosis of these patients is not known, however, and patients treated with antibiotic therapy require long and careful follow-up. The disease known as *Mediterranean abdominal lymphoma, alpha heavy chain disease*, or *immunoproliferative small intestinal disease*, which occurs in young adults in Eastern Mediterranean countries, is another example of a MALT-type lymphoma that may respond to antibiotic therapy in its early stages (251).

Localized MALT lymphomas of the stomach that do not respond to antibiotics, and those occurring in other sites, may be cured with local treatment, either surgery or radiation (250,255–257). Dissemination or recurrence may occur, often in other localized extranodal sites, with long disease-free intervals (258–260).

Nodal Marginal Zone B-cell Lymphoma

Definition

A primary nodal lymphoma with features identical to lymph nodes involved by MALT lymphoma, but without evidence of extranodal disease. Monocytoid B cells may be prominent. This diagnosis should not be made in patients with MALT lymphoma at other sites or Sjogren's syndrome, or if another low-grade B-cell lymphoma (follicular, mantle cell) is present in the same node.

Morphology

Tumors with morphologic features identical to those described for extranodal marginal zone (MALT-type) lymphoma occasionally have been reported with isolated or disseminated nodal involvement, in the absence of extranodal disease (138,261). Most reported cases of nodal monocytoid B-cell lymphoma have been in patients with Sjogren's syndrome and thus represent nodal involvement by a MALT-type lymphoma of the salivary gland (262,263) (Fig. 19.13). Others have been reported as "composite" lymphomas with other histologically low-grade lymphomas, chiefly follicular lymphoma. In these cases, however, this phenomenon represents focal differentiation to marginal zone or monocytoid B cells, and not a true composite lymphoma; these cases should be classified as follicular lymphoma (264). There are occasional cases that do not appear to be associated with other types of lymphoma. Two morphologic types have been described: cases that resemble MALT lymphoma, and cases that more closely resemble splenic marginal zone lymphoma (141). Those that resemble MALT lymphoma show aggregates of monocytoid B cells in a parafollicular, perivascular, and perisinusoidal distribution, with preserved germinal centers and mantle zones. Those that resemble splenic marginal zone lymphoma had infiltrates of marginal zone cells surrounding reactive follicles with germinal centers, but with attenuated mantle zones.

Immunophenotype and Genetic Features

The cases that resemble splenic marginal zone lymphoma are reported to express IgD and to lack CD5, CD23, and cyclin D1. Those that resemble MALT lymphoma are IgD$^-$

A

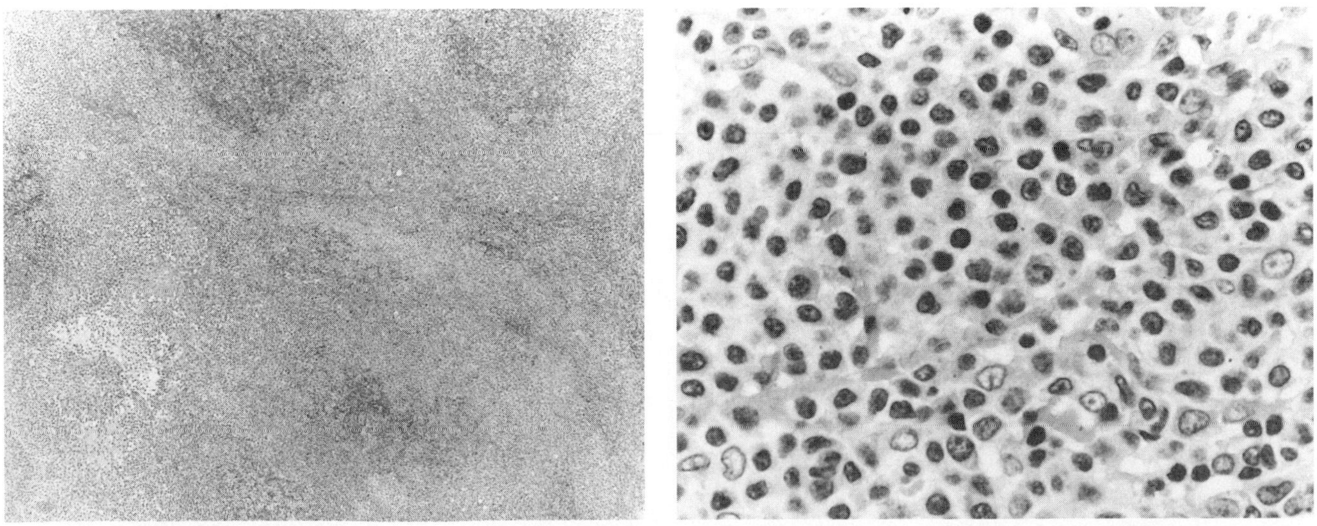

B

FIG. 19.13. Nodal marginal zone B-cell lymphoma with monocytoid B cells. **A:** The neoplastic monocytoid B cells occupy the parafollicular or perisinusoidal region, similarly to normal monocytoid B cells. **B:** High-power view of monocytoid B cells with abundant pale cytoplasm.

and have an immunophenotype identical to those of extranodal marginal zone B-cell lymphoma (MALT) (141).

Postulated Normal Counterpart

Nodal monocytoid or marginal zone B cell.

Clinical Features

This is a rare disorder, comprising 1% of the cases in the international study of the REAL classification (61). The patients presented with isolated or generalized nodal disease; bone marrow was involved in 30%; and rarely peripheral blood may be involved (67,265). Cases reported by Campo and associates (141) were predominantly localized at the time of the diagnosis. Of those that resembled MALT lymphoma, 44% on follow-up had an extranodal lymphoma; those resembling splenic marginal zone lymphoma did not. The overall and failure-free survival rates appear to be similar to those of follicular lymphoma or SLL (67).

Follicular Lymphoma

Definition

A lymphoma of follicle center B cells (centrocytes and centroblasts), which has at least a partially follicular pattern.

Morphology

The tumor is composed of follicle center cells, usually a mixture of centrocytes (cleaved follicular center cells) and centroblasts (large noncleaved follicular center cells) (Fig. 19.14). Centrocytes typically predominate; centroblasts are usually in the minority but by definition always are present. Rare lymphomas with a follicular growth pattern consist almost entirely of centroblasts. Occasional cases may show plasmacytoid differentiation or foci of marginal zone or monocytoid B cells (264). The proportion of centroblasts varies from patient to patient, and the clinical aggressiveness of the tumor increases with increasing numbers of centroblasts. Numerous criteria have been proposed for grading follicular lymphoma. The WHO classification (70) is adopting the cell-counting method of Mann and Berard (266) (Table 19.19). In addition to typical follicular lymphoma, two variants are recognized, whose relationship to follicular lymphoma remains controversial: cutaneous follicular center lymphoma and diffuse follicular center lymphoma.

Immunophenotype

The tumor cells of follicle center lymphoma are usually sIg^+; about 50% to 60% express IgM, about 40% express IgG, and rare cases express IgA. The tumor cells express pan–B cell associated antigens, about 60% are $CD10^+$, and they are $CD5^-$, $CD23^{\pm}$, $CD43^-$ in most cases, and $CD11c^-$. Tightly organized meshworks of follicular dendritic cells are present in follicular areas (151,267). Most cases are BCL-2^+, and nuclear BCL-6 is expressed by at least some of the neoplastic cells (115,268). The portion that is Ki-67^+ is smaller than in reactive follicles.

Genetic Features

Immunoglobulin heavy and light chain genes are rearranged, and analysis of the immunoglobulin V-region genes shows that most cases have extensive somatic mutations and a high frequency of intraclonal diversity, indicating ongoing mutations, similar to normal germinal center cells (269,270).

A

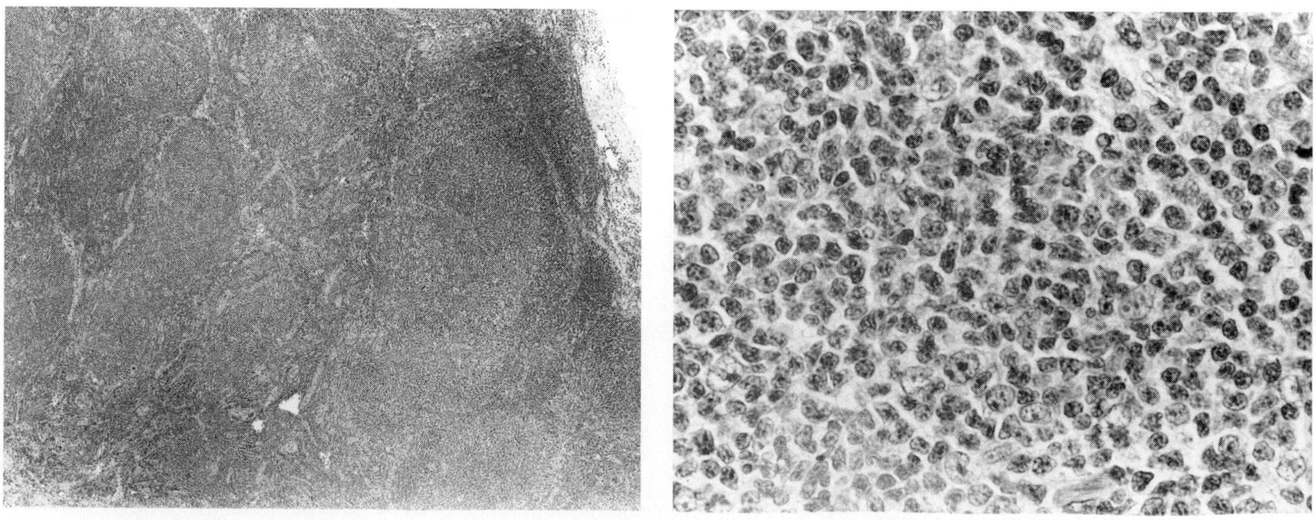

B

FIG. 19.14. Follicular lymphoma. **A:** Low-magnification view showing multiple poorly circumscribed, crowded follicles. **B:** High-magnification view showing cell types, with a majority of centrocytes (cleaved cells) and a minority of centroblasts (large noncleaved cells).

The translocation t(14;18) and *BCL2* gene rearrangement are present in the majority of the cases.

Postulated Normal Counterpart

Germinal center B cells, both centrocytes (small cleaved follicle center cells) and centroblasts (large noncleaved follicle center cells).

Clinical Features

Follicular lymphoma is the second most common lymphoma in the United States and western Europe, comprising 20% of all non-Hodgkin's lymphomas and up to 70% of low-grade lymphomas reported in American and European clinical trials (61,271). Thus, our understanding of the clinical features and response to treatment of low-grade lymphoma is essentially that of follicular lymphoma. Follicular lymphoma affects predominantly older adults, with a slight female predominance (14,61). Most patients have widespread disease at diagnosis, usually predominantly in the lymph nodes but also in the spleen, bone marrow, and occasionally peripheral blood or extranodal sites. Despite the advanced stage, the clinical course is generally indolent, with median duration of survival in excess of 8 years; however, the disease is not usually curable with available treatment. In the recent international study of the REAL classification, the few patients (7%) with IPI scores of 4 or 5 have a much worse prognosis, with a median duration of survival of only 1 year (61). In that study, cases with monocytoid B-cell differentiation had a worse prognosis than other cases (264).

Mantle Cell Lymphoma

Definition

A neoplasm of monomorphous small to medium-sized B cells with irregular nuclei, which resemble the cleaved cells (centrocytes) of germinal centers and overexpress cyclin D1; neoplastic transformed cells (centroblasts or immunoblasts) are absent. Tumor cells are typically CD5$^+$CD23$^-$.

Morphology

The pattern of mantle cell lymphoma may be diffuse, nodular, mantle zone, or a combination of the three. Some reports indicate a better prognosis for patients with a mantle zone pattern (272). Most cases are composed exclusively of small to medium-sized lymphoid cells, with slightly irregular or "cleaved" nuclei; however, the morphology in various cases can range from lymphocyte-like to large cleaved or lymphoblast-like (13,97,273–275) (Fig. 19.15, Table 19.19). Despite the small size and bland appearance, there is often more mitotic activity than in other histologically low-grade lymphomas. Single epithelioid histiocytes may be present, but clusters and granulomas are not seen. Transformed cells with basophilic cytoplasm (centroblast- or immunoblast-like cells) are extremely rare or absent.

Immunophenotype

The tumor cells express sIgM and IgD strongly, often of the λ light chain type, strongly express B cell–associated antigens, coexpress CD5 similar to B-cell CLL/SLL, but are CD23$^-$. In rare patients they may be CD5$^-$ or CD23$^+$ (276–278). In contrast to follicle center lymphoma, mantle cell lymphomas are usually CD10$^-$ and CD43$^+$. A prominent, irregular meshwork of follicular dendritic cells is found even in diffuse cases (97,151,267). The product of the cyclin D1 gene can be detected in the nuclei of neoplastic mantle cells in paraffin-embedded tissue sections with the immunoperoxidase technique and is useful in differentiating mantle

A B

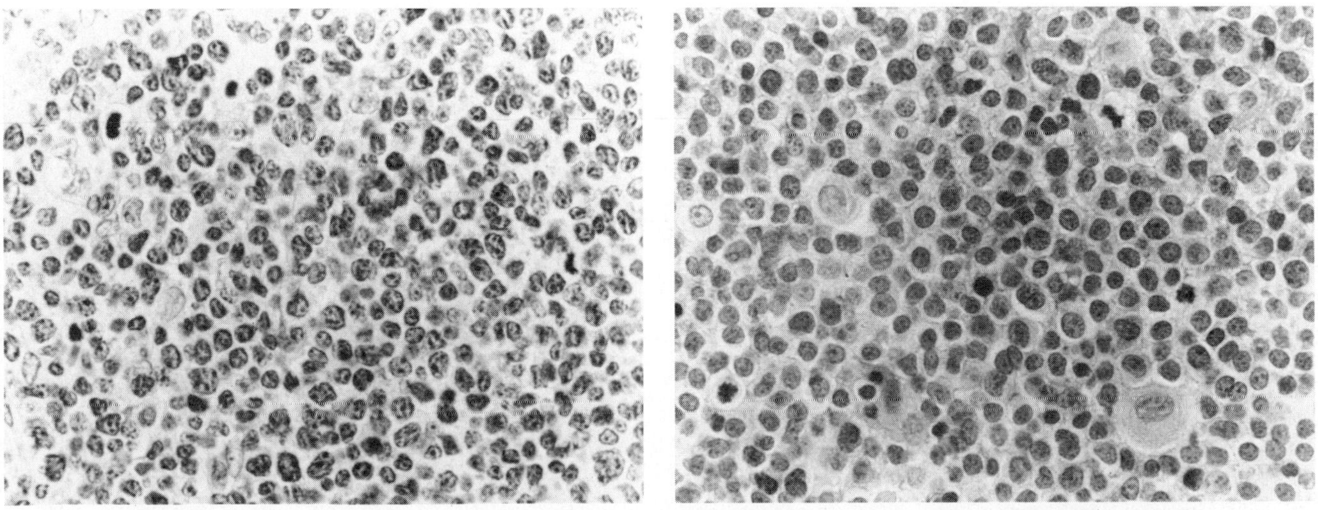

FIG. 19.15. Mantle cell lymphoma: **A:** There is a monomorphous population of cells with irregular nuclei. **B:** In this example of the blastic variant, the neoplastic cells are slightly larger, with more finely dispersed chromatin than in typical mantle cell lymphoma. Single epithelioid histiocytes are interspersed with neoplastic cells.

cell lymphomas from other low-grade B-cell lymphomas (178,233).

Genetic Features

Immunoglobulin heavy and light chain genes are rearranged. The immunoglobulin V-region genes lack somatic mutations, indicating a pre–germinal center stage of differentiation, consistent with an origin from the follicle mantle (99). A translocation t(11;14) in the majority of the cases results in overexpression of a gene known as *PRAD1* or cyclin D1, which encodes a cell-cycle associated protein that normally is not expressed in lymphoid cells (178,279,280). The protein is overexpressed even in patients lacking the translocation, suggesting that point mutations also may result in overexpression (281,282). Overexpression of this protein may explain the often high mitotic index and aggressive clinical course of this histologically low-grade lymphoma. Recent studies have shown abnormalities in expression of other genes associated with the cell cycle, including mutations of the CDK inhibitors p16 and p17 in blastoid variants and decreased expression of p27, another CDK inhibitor, in the majority of the cases (283). Cases of the blastoid variant have been reported to have high incidences of tetraploidy and p53 gene mutations (284–286). Acquisition of an *MYC* translocation has been reported in some fatal cases (287).

Postulated Normal Counterpart

A naive B cell of follicle mantle or germinal center origin that is distinct from both the recirculating B cell of B-cell CLL and SLL and the later centrocyte of follicle center lymphomas (95,151).

Clinical Features

Mantle cell lymphoma comprises about 7% of adult non-Hodgkin's lymphomas in the United States and Europe (13,61). In a recent review of 376 cases of disseminated low-grade lymphoma (WF categories A–E), mantle cell lymphoma comprised 10% of the cases (58). It is a tumor of older adults, with a male predominance (75%) (61). The majority (70%) of patients have stage IV disease at diagnosis; sites involved include lymph nodes, spleen, Waldeyer's ring, bone marrow (>60%), blood (up to 50%), and extranodal sites, especially the gastrointestinal tract (lymphomatous polyposis) (288). The course is moderately aggressive. The median overall duration of survival in most series is 3 years, with no plateau in the curve, and the duration of failure-free survival is around 1 year. The blastoid variant is reported in some studies to be more aggressive (58,61,277, 289–291). Therapy with anthracycline-containing regimens does not improve the outcome, and initial results with high-dose therapy and marrow transplantation have been disappointing (292–295). Fludarabine is reported to be less effective in mantle cell lymphoma than in CLL and follicular lymphoma (296).

Diffuse Large B-cell Lymphoma

Definition

A neoplasm of large, transformed B cells with prominent nucleoli and basophilic cytoplasm, with a diffuse growth pattern and a high proliferation fraction (>40%). The cells may resemble centroblasts, immunoblasts, multilobated cells, or anaplastic large cells. Rare cases involve only scattered large cells in a background of small T cells and epithelioid histiocytes (T cell– or histiocyte-rich large B-cell lymphoma).

Morphology

Diffuse large B-cell lymphomas are probably a heterogeneous group of neoplasms. They typically are composed of large cells that resemble centroblasts or immunoblasts, most often with a mixture of the two (Fig. 19.16). Several morphologic variants can be recognized, but their clinical significance is debated (Figs. 19.17–19.20, Table 19.20).

Centroblastic Variant. The monomorphic centroblastic (large noncleaved cell) type is composed of medium to large-sized lymphoid cells with oval to round vesicular nuclei with fine chromatin and two to four membrane-bound nucleoli. The cytoplasm generally is scanty and amphophilic to basophilic. The multilobated centroblastic type contains many large lymphoid cells with nuclei having more than three lobes. A polymorphic type shows a mixture of centroblasts and immunoblasts, and may contain up to 90% immunoblasts.

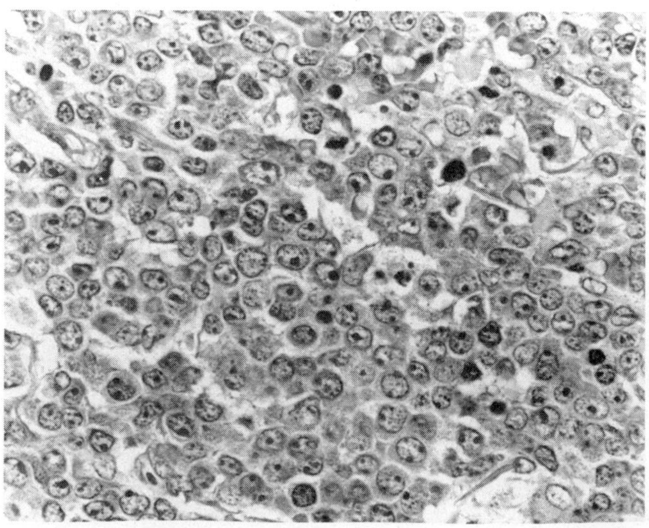

FIG. 19.16. Diffuse large B-cell lymphoma. The most common type shows a mixture of cells resembling centroblasts (one to three peripheral nucleoli) and cells resembling immunoblasts (single central nucleolus).

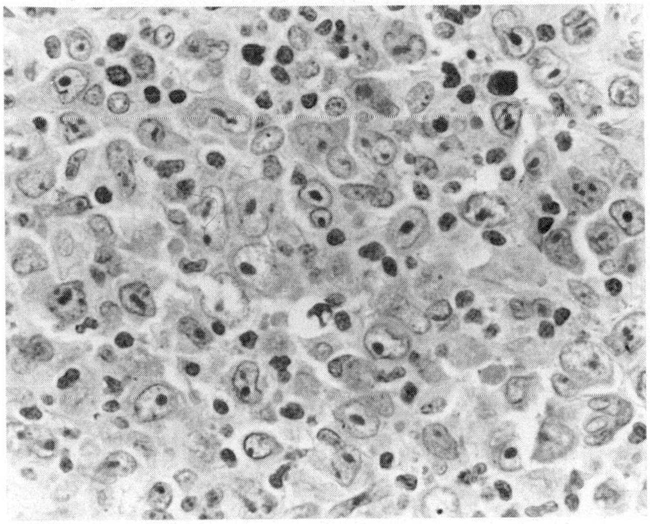

FIG. 19.17. Diffuse large B-cell lymphoma, immunoblastic. Neoplastic cells have large, vesicular nuclei and prominent central nucleoli.

Immunoblastic Variant. About 10% of the cases of DLBCL have over 90% immunoblasts with a prominent central nucleolus and abundant, basophilic cytoplasm. Plasmacytoid differentiation may be present. These cases are more common in immunosuppressed patients. In nonimmunosuppressed patients, they have been reported to have a worse prognosis (297) (Fig. 19.17).

Anaplastic Variant. In some cases of DLBCL, the cells are identical to those of large T- or null cell anaplastic lymphoma and strongly express CD30 (Ki-1) and T-cell antigens. Although these have been called B-cell ALCL, they do not have the same distinctive clinical or genetic features of T- or null cell ALCL and are considered a morphologic variant of large B-cell lymphoma in the REAL-WHO classification. The most significant differential diagnostic problem presented by such cases is with classical Hodgkin's disease expressing B-cell antigens (Chapters 17, 18, 25).

T cell– or Histiocyte-rich Large B-cell Lymphoma. Some cases of large B-cell lymphoma have a prominent background of reactive T cells and often histiocytes; this is the so-called T-cell– or histiocyte-rich large B-cell lymphoma. They may resemble Hodgkin's disease of either the lymphocyte predominance or mixed cellularity (298,299). In contrast to those with Hodgkin's disease, patients with T-cell or histiocyte-rich large B-cell lymphoma typically present with disseminated disease involving the liver and spleen and have a poor survival rate. The relationship of this disease to lymphocyte predominance or classic Hodgkin's disease remains to be discovered.

Large B-cell Lymphoma, Lymphomatoid Granulomatosis Type. The entity described as lymphomatoid granulomatosis, which had been thought to be related to nasal or angiocentric lymphoma, recently has been shown in most cases to be an Epstein-Barr virus (EBV)–positive large B-cell lymphoma with a T cell–rich background (300–303). The infiltrates show extensive necrosis, often with only a few atypical large B cells in a background of lymphocytes; the infiltrate may be both angiocentric and angioinvasive. Patients typically present with extranodal disease, most commonly involving the lung, brain, or kidneys. Evidence of past or present immunosuppression may be found. Although the infiltrates may resemble those of nasal or angiocentric lymphoma, there is no biologic and little clinical overlap, because the latter is an NK or T-cell neoplasm that involves the upper airway and midfacial region, the skin, sometimes

A

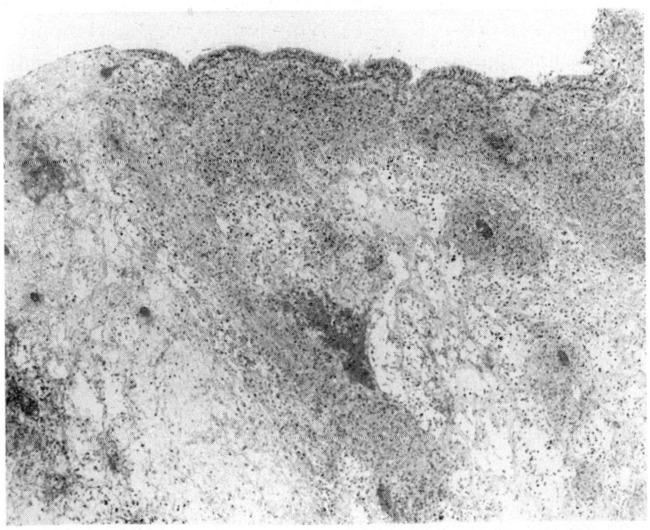

B

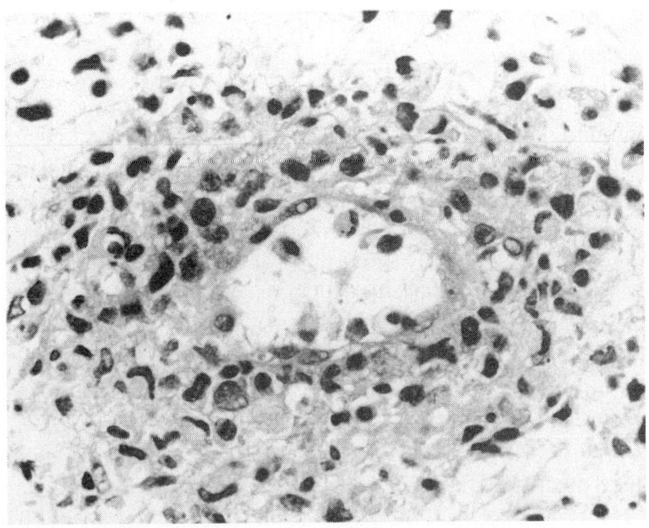

FIG. 19.18. Large B-cell lymphoma, lymphomatoid granulomatosis type. **A:** Low-power view shows edematous paranasal sinus mucosa with an atypical lymphoid infiltrate that is largely perivascular. **B:** High-power view shows medium-sized to large lymphoid cells with oval and irregular nuclei clustered around a blood vessel, with small lymphocytes scattered around the periphery.

A 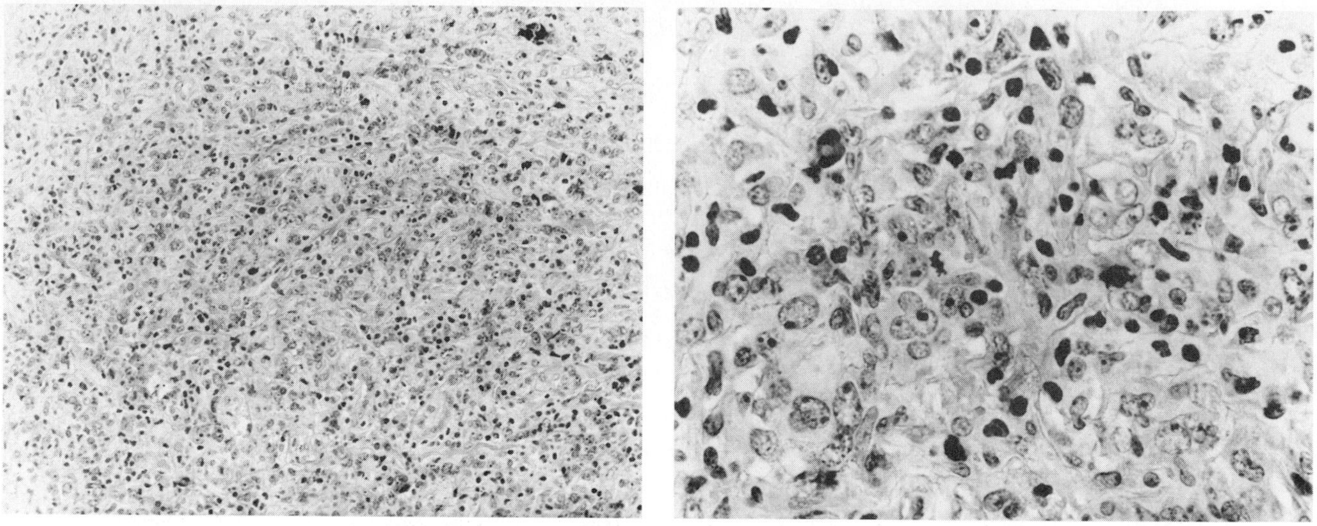 B

FIG. 19.19. Mediastinal (thymic) large B-cell lymphoma. **A:** Low-power view shows an infiltrate of atypical cells associated with packeting sclerosis. **B:** High-power view shows neoplastic cells with oval, irregular, and lobated nuclei and clear cytoplasm.

the gastrointestinal tract, and rarely the lung or central nervous system (Fig. 19.18).

Immunophenotype

Diffuse large B-cell lymphomas express one or more B cell–associated antigens (CD19, CD20, CD22, CD79a), as well as CD45, and often but not always sIg. They may coexpress CD5 or CD10 (151,304). In various studies 25% to 80% have been shown to express BCL-2 protein; this may be associated with a worse prognosis (305–309). Approximately 70% express BCL-6 protein, consistent with a germinal center origin (308,309); this expression is independent of *BCL6* gene rearrangement.

Genetic Features

Most patients with DLBCL have somatic mutations in the immunoglobulin V-region genes (133,310). The *BCL2* gene is rearranged in 15% to 30% of DLBCLs; this is associated with nodal and disseminated disease but not with a worse prognosis or BCL-2 expression (305). The *MYC* gene is rearranged in 5% to 15% of cases (155,311), and the *BCL6* gene is rearranged in 20% to 40% (311,312) of cases and shows mutations in the 5′ noncoding region in 70% (313,314). The 5′ noncoding mutations of the *BCL6* gene (121,123) and the immunoglobulin V-region gene mutations are found in normal germinal center cells (96); their presence in DLBCL is consistent with a germinal center or post–germinal center stage of differentiation.

Postulated Normal Counterpart

Proliferating peripheral B cells: centroblasts or immunoblasts in most cases.

Clinical Features

Diffuse large B-cell lymphoma was the most common lymphoma in the international study of the REAL classification, comprising 31% of the cases. Patients typically present with a rapidly enlarging, symptomatic mass, with B symptoms in one third of the cases (61,67). Localized (stage I or II) extranodal disease occurs in up to 30%; bone marrow involvement has been seen in only 16%. Up to 40% of DLBCL are extranodal; common sites include the gastrointestinal tract, bone, and central nervous system. The prognosis was highly associated with the IPI score (67), but not with histologic subclassification according to either the WF or the Kiel classification. Large B-cell lymphoma may occur as a high grade transformation of several low-grade B-cell lymphomas (B-cell CLL, lymphoplasmacytic lymphoma, follicular lymphoma, MALT lymphoma, splenic marginal zone lymphoma). DLBCL is usually treated with 6 months of combination chemotherapy including adriamycin (59); early-stage cases may be treated with shorter courses of chemotherapy followed by involved-field radiation therapy. DLBCL of certain extranodal sites, such as the central nervous system, may be clinically distinctive and may have specific treatment protocols. Distinctive subtypes of DLBCL are summarized in Table 19.20.

Primary Mediastinal (Thymic) Large B-cell Lymphoma

Morphology

Primary mediastinal large B-cell lymphoma usually involves the thymus at presentation (315,316). The tumor is composed of large cells with variable nuclear features, resembling centroblasts, large centrocytes, or multilobated cells, often with pale or "clear" cytoplasm. Less often, the tumor cells resemble immunoblasts. Reed-Sternberg–like cells may be present. Many cases have fine, compartmentalizing sclerosis (Fig. 19.19).

Immunophenotype

The tumor cells are often immunoglobulin-negative but express B cell–associated antigens (CD19, CD20, CD22, CD79a) and CD45 (316).

Genetic Features

Immunoglobulin heavy and light chain genes are rearranged; the *BCL2* gene is usually germline (316–318). *BCL6* gene rearrangements are uncommon (319). Amplification of the *REL* oncogene has been described in a minority of the cases (320).

Postulated Normal Counterpart

Putative thymic (medullary) B cell.

Clinical Features

Primary DLBCL of the mediastinum is a distinct clinicopathologic entity, requiring knowledge of both morphology, immunophenotype, and presenting site for the diagnosis (61). It comprised 7% of DLBCLs (2.4% of all non-Hodgkin's lymphoma) in the international REAL classification study (61,67). There is a female predominance and a median age in the fourth decade; patients present with a locally invasive anterior mediastinal mass originating in the thymus, with frequent airway compromise and superior vena cava syndrome (321). Relapses tend to be extranodal, with sites including the liver, gastrointestinal tract, kidneys, ovaries, and central nervous system. Although early studies suggested an unusually aggressive, incurable tumor, others have reported cure rates similar to those for other large cell lymphomas with aggressive therapy, usually combining chemotherapy with mediastinal irradiation (321,322).

Intravascular Large B-cell Lymphoma

Rare cases of large-cell lymphoma, usually of the B cell type, present with a disseminated intravascular proliferation of large lymphoid cells, involving small blood vessels, without an obvious extravascular tumor mass or leukemia (323). This tumor has been variously known as *intravascular lymphomatosis*, *angiotropic lymphoma*, and *malignant angioendotheliomatosis*. The neoplastic lymphoid cells are lodged mainly in the lumina of small vessels in many organs. The tumor cells are large, with vesicular nuclei, prominent nucleoli, and frequent mitotic figures (Fig. 19.20). Malignant cells rarely are seen in cerebrospinal fluid, blood, or bone marrow. The organs most commonly involved are the central nervous system, kidneys, lungs, and skin, but virtually any site may be involved. Patients present with a bewildering variety of symptoms related to organ dysfunction secondary to vascular occlusion, which may be transient. Because of this, the diagnosis is difficult, and many reported cases were diagnosed at autopsy. If a timely diagnosis is made and combination chemotherapy instituted, many patients achieve complete remission, and long-term survival appears to be possible (324).

Burkitt's Lymphoma

Definition

A B-cell lymphoma composed of monomorphic, medium-sized cells with basophilic cytoplasm and a high proliferation fraction, characterized by translocation and deregulation of

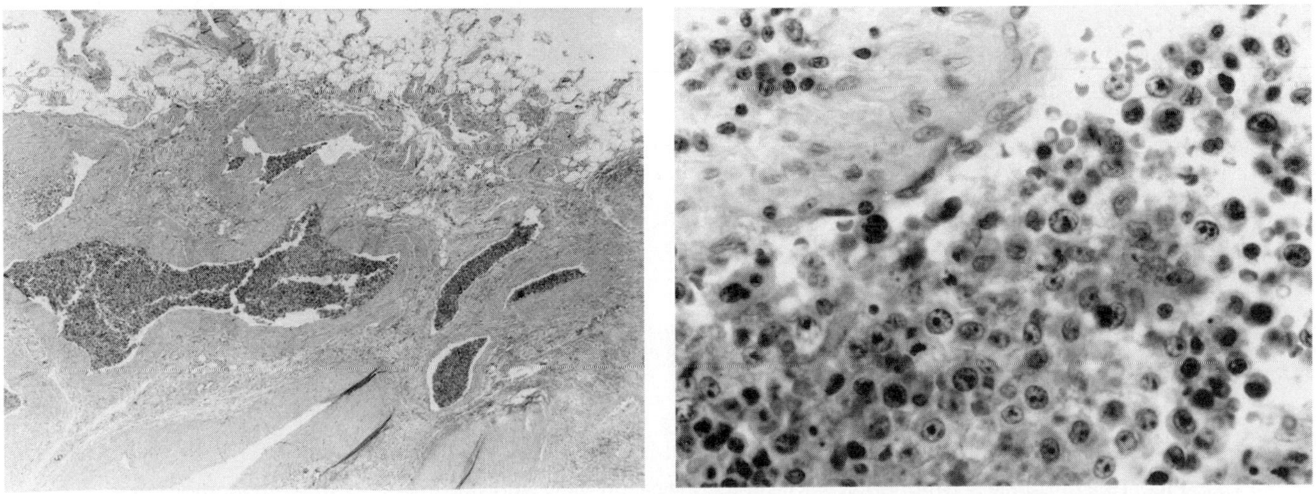

A B

FIG. 19.20. Intravascular large B-cell lymphoma. **A:** Multiple blood vessels are filled by atypical lymphoid cells. **B:** High-power view shows large lymphoid with the appearance of centroblasts and immunoblasts. (From Ferry JA, Harris NL, Young RH et al. *Am J Surg Pathol* 1994;18:376–390, with permission.)

the *MYC* gene on chromosome 8, which is often extranodal and occurs most often in children (endemic, sporadic) and immunocompromised hosts.

Morphology

Burkitt's tumor cells are monomorphic, medium-sized cells with round nuclei, multiple nucleoli, and basophilic cytoplasm (Fig. 19.21). Cytoplasmic lipid vacuoles are usually evident on imprints or smears. There is an extremely high rate of proliferation as well as a high rate of spontaneous cell death. A starry-sky pattern is usually present, imparted by numerous benign macrophages that have ingested apoptotic tumor cells. Although most patients present no problem in diagnosis, some may have larger cells or an admixture of immunoblast-like cells, and there is morphologic overlap with DLBCL. These borderline cases are often called ''non-Burkitt's'' (325) or ''Burkitt's-like'' (64) (Fig. 19.22). In children and HIV-positive patients these often have a *MYC* translocation and behave similarly to typical Burkitt's lymphoma; in adults, so-called ''Burkitt's-like'' lymphomas often have *BCL2* gene rearrangement and may represent an aggressive variant of DLBCL (326). In the international study of the REAL classification (61), Burkitt's-like lymphoma was a nonreproducible category, in which the pathologists agreed on the diagnosis only 50% of the time: Disagreements were equally split between large B-cell and Burkitt's lymphoma.

The most appropriate way to handle this confusion between Burkitt's lymphoma and DLBCL has been the subject of debate in the WHO classification project: Should DLBCL continue to be a separate, non-reproducible category, should it be a subtype of large B-cell lymphoma, or should it be a subtype of Burkitt's lymphoma? From a clinical standpoint, it is important to identify patients who should be treated as though they had Burkitt's lymphoma, because patients with Burkitt's lymphoma do not do well with treatment that would be effective for large-cell lymphoma. On the other hand, treatment for Burkitt's lymphoma is considerably more aggressive than that for large B-cell lymphoma, may cause significant treatment-related injury (327), and should not be used for usual large B-cell lymphomas. The question is how to draw the line between large-cell lymphoma and Burkitt's lymphoma so that morphologically borderline cases are assigned to the correct category.

The defining biologic feature of Burkitt's lymphoma is *MYC* deregulation, as a consequence of which the tumor cells remain constantly in cycle. It is this phenomenon that results in both its morphologic homogeneity and its clinical behavior. Unfortunately, detection of *MYC* translocation is not practical in all clinical specimens for technical reasons. In addition, some large B-cell lymphomas have t(8;14) and *MYC* deregulation, and it is not clear whether all such cases should be treated like Burkitt's lymphoma. The best practical surrogate for *MYC* deregulation is proliferation fraction: In a tumor with *MYC* deregulation, 100% of viable cells should be in cycle and express Ki-67. The WHO committees concluded that a *diagnosis of ''Burkitt's-like'' lymphoma should be made only in a tumor with morphologic features intermediate between Burkitt's lymphoma and DLBCL, in which the Ki-67 fraction of viable cells is at least 99%.* This tumor is considered a subtype of Burkitt's lymphoma in the WHO classification (70). Cases with morphologic features of large-cell lymphoma with a high proliferation fraction or t(8;14) and those that are morphologically borderline between Burkitt's lymphoma and large B-cell lymphoma with a lower proliferation fraction should be classified as DLBCL (Table 19.21).

A 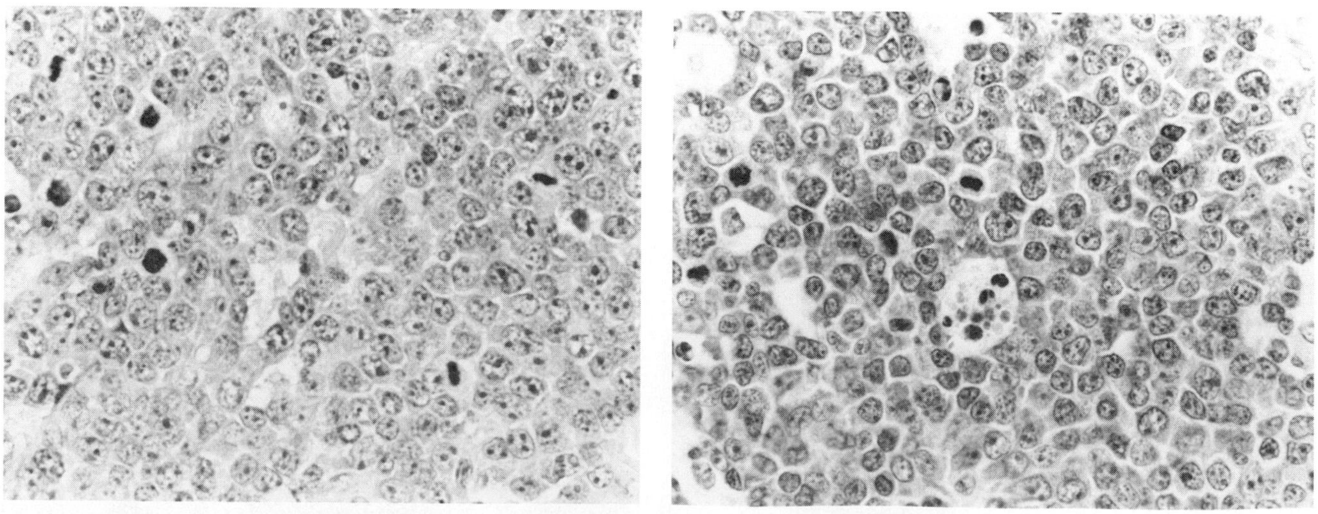 B

FIG. 19.21. Burkitt's lymphoma. **A:** High-magnification view showing medium-sized monomorphous cells with a high mitotic rate. **B:** In this example of African Burkitt's lymphoma, neoplastic cells are slightly more pleomorphic than those seen in **A**. Tingible body macrophages are also present.

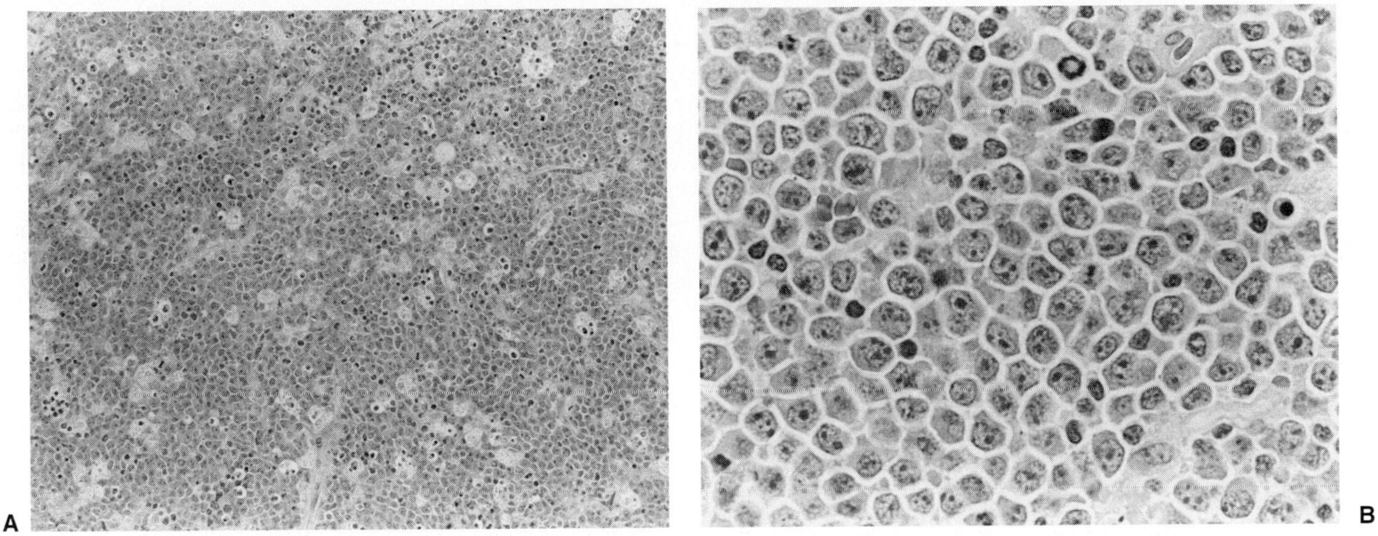

FIG. 19.22. Burkitt's-like lymphoma. **A:** Low-power view shows a diffuse infiltrate of atypical lymphoid cells with a prominent starry-sky pattern. **B:** High-power view shows cells that are, on average, medium-sized, although they are rather pleomorphic.

Immunophenotype

Burkitt's lymphoma cells express sIgM and B cell–associated antigens (CD19, CD20, CD22, CD79a), as well as CD10 and CD43; they lack CD5, BCL-2, and typically CD23 (328). They show nuclear staining for BCL-6 protein that is independent of *BCL6* gene rearrangement (329).

Genetic Features

Immunoglobulin heavy and light chain genes are rearranged. Studies of the immunoglobulin V-region genes show conflicting results: One study reported unmutated genes (330); others report somatic mutations and intraclonal heterogeneity, consistent with ongoing mutations (126,331,332). Most cases have a translocation of *MYC* from chromosome 8 to either the immunoglobulin heavy chain region on chromosome 14—t(8;14)—or light chain loci on 2—t(2;8)—or 22—t(8;22). In African (endemic) cases, the breakpoint on chromosome 14 involves the heavy chain joining region; in nonendemic cases, the translocation involves the heavy chain switch region (333,334). Mutations in the 5′ noncoding region of the *BCL6* gene, similar to those seen in large B-cell lymphoma, have been reported in 25% to 50% of cases (335). Most African cases contain EBV genomes, as do 25% to 40% of the cases associated with AIDS (336).

Postulated Normal Counterpart

Peripheral B cell of unknown stage, possibly a B blast of early germinal center reaction.

Clinical Features

Three distinct clinical forms of Burkitt's lymphoma can be recognized: endemic, sporadic, and immunodeficiency-associated (337) (Table 19.21). Although they are histologically identical and have similar clinical courses, there are differences in epidemiology, clinical presentation, and genetic features among the three forms. Endemic and sporadic Burkitt's lymphomas are both most common in children, but the median age is younger in endemic patients. Burkitt's lymphoma comprises 30% of nonendemic pediatric lymphomas but less than 1% of adult non-Hodgkin's lymphomas; in HIV-positive patients it typically affects those with a relatively high CD4 count and no opportunistic infections. In all groups, the majority of patients (3 : 1 or 4 : 1) are male. In endemic cases, the jaws and other facial bones often are involved, as well as the mesentery and gonads. The majority of sporadic cases present in the abdomen, most often involving distal ileum, cecum, or mesentery; ovaries, kidneys, or breasts may be involved (338). Immunodeficiency-related cases more often involve lymph nodes, and both these and sporadic cases may present as acute leukemia.

Patients typically present with rapidly growing tumor masses and often have very high serum lactate dehydrogenase levels. Burkitt's lymphoma is highly aggressive but potentially curable with very aggressive therapy (338).

T- and Natural Killer Cell Neoplasms

Precursor T-lymphoblastic Lymphoma/Leukemia (Precursor T-cell Acute Lymphoblastic Leukemia/ Precursor T-cell Lymphoblastic Lymphoma)

Definition

A neoplasm of lymphoblasts committed to the T-cell lineage, typically composed of small to medium-sized blast cells with scant cytoplasm, moderately condensed to dispersed chromatin and indistinct nucleoli, variably involving bone marrow and blood (precursor T-cell acute lymphoblastic leukemia) or thymus or lymph nodes (precursor T-cell lymphoblastic lymphoma).

Morphology

On smears, lymphoblasts vary from small cells with scant cytoplasm, condensed nuclear chromatin, and indistinct nucleoli to larger cells with a moderate amount of cytoplasm, dispersed chromatin, and multiple nucleoli. Azurophilic granules may be present. In tissue sections, the cells are small to medium-sized, with scant cytoplasm and round, oval, or convoluted nuclei, with fine chromatin and indistinct or small nucleoli (Fig. 19.23). Occasional patients have larger cells. The pattern is infiltrative rather than destructive, with partial preservation of the subcapsular sinus and germinal centers. A starry-sky pattern may be present but is usually less prominent than in Burkitt's lymphoma.

Immunophenotype

The lymphoblasts are typically TdT^+ and variably express CD2, CD7, CD3, CD5, CD1a, CD4, and CD8. Only CD3 is considered lineage-specific. The constellation of antigens defines stages of differentiation, ranging from early or pro-T (CD2, CD7 and cytoplasmic CD3) to ''common'' thymocyte (CD1a, sCD3, CD4 and CD8) to late thymocyte (CD4 or CD8). Although there is some correlation with presentation and differentiation stage—patients with bone marrow and blood presentation may show differentiation at an earlier stage than those with thymic presentation (339,340)—there is overlap (341).

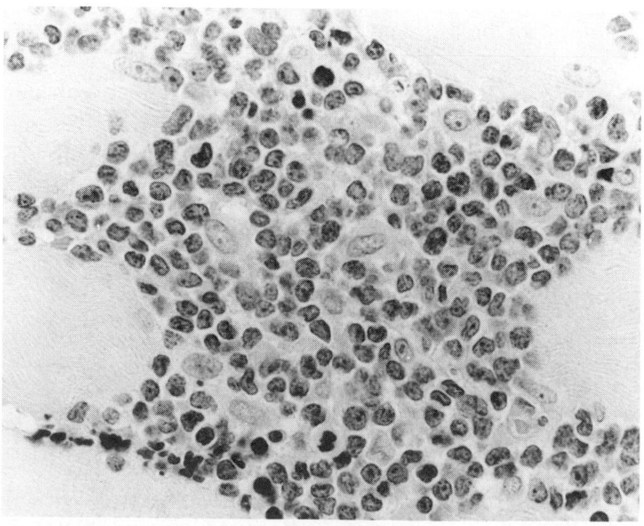

FIG. 19.23. T-cell precursor lymphoblastic lymphoma infiltrating skeletal muscle. In this case, most cells have irregular nuclei and nucleoli are inconspicuous. The appearance is similar to the B-cell precursor neoplasm.

Genetic Features

Rearrangement of antigen receptor genes is variable in lymphoblastic neoplasms and may not be lineage-specific; thus, precursor T-cell neoplasms may have either or both TCR β or γ chain gene rearrangements and immunoglobulin heavy chain gene rearrangements (342).

Chromosomal translocations involving the TCR alpha and delta loci at chromosome 14q11 and β and γ loci at 7q34 are present in about one third of patients (158,343); the partner genes are variable and include the transcription factors *MYC* (8q24), *TAL1/SCL* (1p32), *RBTN1* (11p35), *RBTN2* (11p13), and *HOX11* (10q24) and the gene expressing the cytoplasmic tyrosine kinase LCK (1p34). In an additional 25%, the *TAL1* locus at 1p32 has deletions in the 5′ regulatory region (344). Deletions of 9p involving deletion of the p16ink4a tumor suppressor gene (CDK4 inhibitor) is also seen in T-lymphoblastic neoplasms.

Postulated Normal Counterpart

Precursor T lymphoblast at varying stages of differentiation.

Clinical Features

Precursor T-cell neoplasms occur most frequently in late childhood, adolescence, and young adulthood, with a male predominance; they comprise 15% of childhood and 25% of adult acute lymphoblastic leukemias (165). The prognosis is typically worse than that for precursor B-cell neoplasms and is not affected by immunophenotype or genetic abnormalities. Patients typically present with a very high leukocyte count and often a mediastinal mass. Clinically, a case is defined as lymphoma if there is a mediastinal or other mass and less than 25% blasts in the bone marrow, and as leukemia if there are more than 25% bone marrow blasts, with or without a mass. In children, treatment is generally more aggressive than for precursor B acute lymphoblastic leukemia and typically the same as for lymphomatous and leukemic presentations (343).

T-cell Prolymphocytic Leukemia

Definition

An aggressive T-cell leukemia characterized by the proliferation of small to medium-sized prolymphocytes with a mature postthymic T-cell phenotype.

Morphology

The leukemic T cells usually are slightly larger than a normal lymphocyte and have prominent nucleoli, some nuclear irregularity, and moderately abundant nongranular cy-

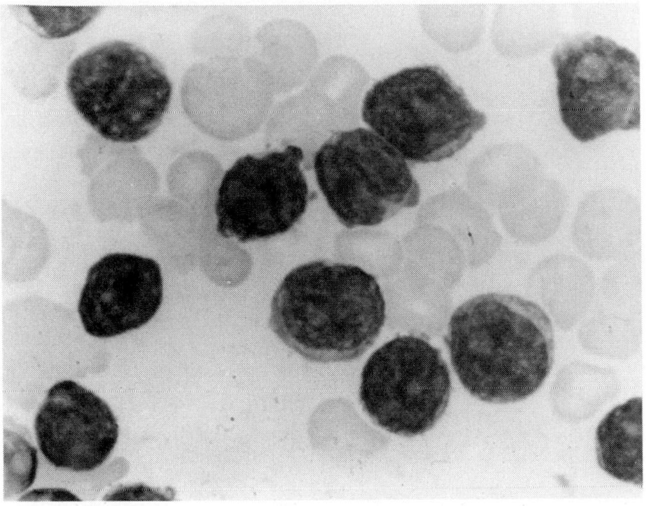

FIG. 19.24. T-cell prolymphocytic leukemia. Circulating cells have slight nuclear irregularity and prominent nucleoli. (Wright-Giemsa stain.)

toplasm, often with protrusions or blebs (Fig. 19.24). Some patients have smaller cells with inconspicuous nucleoli or cerebriform nuclei (345–347) (Table 19.24). Bone marrow involvement is diffuse. Lymph node involvement is often paracortical, with sparing of follicles, and pseudofollicles are absent. Prominent small vessels of the high endothelial venule type may be numerous and often contain atypical small lymphoid cells (348). Splenic red and white pulp are expanded and hepatic sinusoids may be infiltrated.

Immunophenotype

The tumor cells express CD2, CD3, CD5, and CD7 as well as the TCR $\alpha\beta$ chain and usually lack CD25; most cases are $CD4^+$ (65%), but some are $CD4^+CD8^+$ (21%), and rare cases are $CD4^-CD8^+$ (346,347,349).

Genetic Features

T-cell receptor genes are clonally rearranged; inv(14)(q11;q32) is found in 80%, and in 10% there is a reciprocal translocation t(14;14)(q11;q32). In 70% of cases there is also trisomy 8q, often as a consequence of iso(8q). Deletions or translocations of chromosome 11 are seen in 50% of cases.

Postulated Normal Counterpart

Circulating peripheral T cell.

Clinical Features

T-cell prolymphocytic leukemia comprises 1% of cases classified morphologically as CLL but up to 20% of prolymphocytic leukemias. Patients typically have a high white blood cell count (>100,000). Bone marrow, spleen, liver, and lymph nodes may be involved, as well as skin and mucosal sites. This leukemia is more aggressive than B-cell CLL and not usually curable with available therapy (347).

T-Cell Large Granular Lymphocyte Leukemia

Definition

A neoplasm of mature granular $CD8^+$ T lymphocytes with involvement of peripheral blood and bone marrow, typically associated with neutropenia.

Morphology

Peripheral blood cells have round or oval nuclei with moderately condensed chromatin and rare nucleoli, eccentrically placed in abundant pale blue cytoplasm with azurophilic granules. This disorder corresponds to cases described as T8 lymphocytosis with neutropenia, CD8 or Tγlymphoproliferative disease, and $CD8^+$ T-cell CLL (350). Bone marrow infiltration is usually sparse, with mild to moderate lymphocytosis and focal aggregates, sometimes resembling B-cell lymphoma. There may be a myeloid maturation arrest or erythroid hypoplasia.

The spleen is typically involved, with an infiltrate in the red pulp cords and sinuses (Fig. 19.25). Hepatic sinuses may be infiltrated (351). The cells appear small, sometimes with slight nuclear irregularity, and the cytoplasm appears less abundant that that of hairy cells.

Immunophenotype

T-cell large granular lymphocyte leukemia cells (350) express CD2, CD3, and usually CD8, as well as the NK

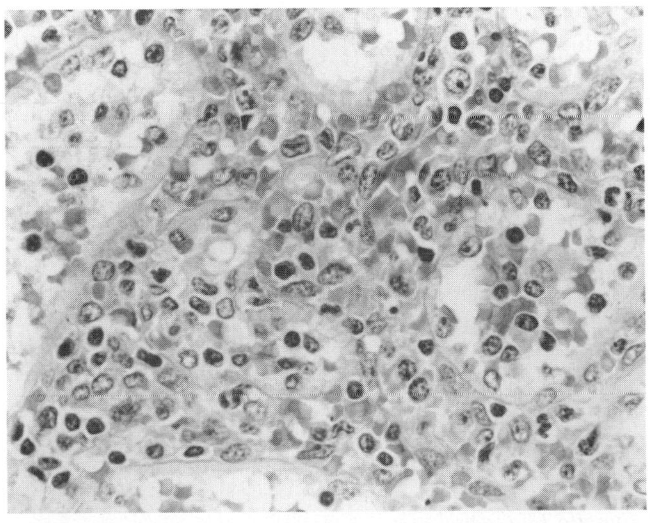

FIG. 19.25. T-cell large granular lymphocyte leukemia, showing splenic cords infiltrated and expanded by small to medium-sized cells with irregular nuclei.

cell–associated antigens CD16 and CD57 (Leu-7), but not CD56 and $\alpha\beta$ TCR.

Genetic Features

The TCR genes are clonally rearranged.

Postulated Normal Counterpart

Peripheral CD8$^+$ T lymphocyte with suppressor but no NK function.

Clinical Features

Most patients with T-cell large granular lymphocyte leukemia are adults with mild to moderate stable lymphocytosis (5,000–20,000 per cubic millimeter), often with neutropenia and anemia, and mild to moderate splenomegaly, without significant lymphadenopathy or hepatomegaly. The course is usually indolent, with injury related to cytopenias rather than tumor burden. Cyclosporine has been reported to ameliorate the neutropenia (352). Indolent cases may undergo histologic progression to a higher-grade neoplasm as a late event (350). Recently, aggressive T-cell large granular lymphocytes have been reported in immunosuppressed patients (353,354).

Aggressive Natural Killer Cell Leukemia

Definition

A neoplasm of immature NK cells with involvement of peripheral blood and an aggressive clinical course.

Morphology

Circulating leukemic cells in this condition are slightly larger than normal large granular lymphocytes and may have irregular, hyperchromatic nuclei and distinct nucleoli (Fig. 19.26). The cytoplasm is abundant and contains azurophilic granules. The marrow is often involved, with a diffuse interstitial pattern. Lymph nodes and the spleen show a diffuse infiltrate similar to that seen in acute leukemias. The cells often appear more primitive in tissue infiltrates than in the blood.

Immunophenotype

The cells are CD2$^+$CD56$^+$, do not express surface CD3, and may be CD11b$^+$. Expression of CD16 is variable, and CD57 usually is not expressed. Rare cases of CD3$^+$ aggressive large granular lymphocyte leukemia have been reported (355).

Genetic Features

The TCR genes are typically germline. Most contain EBV genomes, which are clonal.

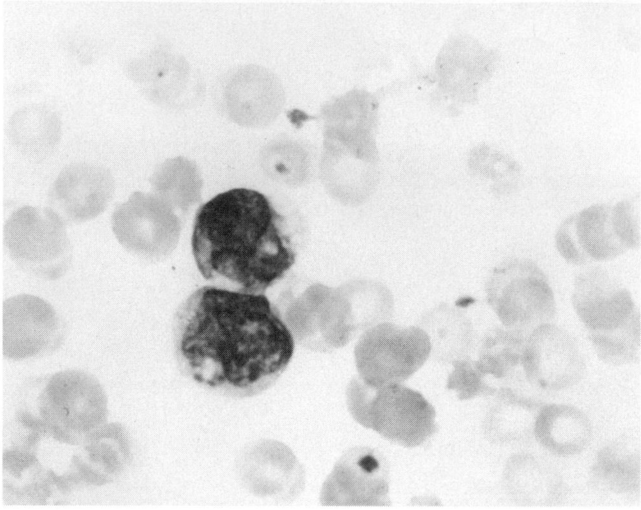

FIG. 19.26. NK cell large granular lymphocyte leukemia. Peripheral smear shows two large, highly atypical lymphoid cells with few cytoplasmic granules. Neoplastic cells were EBV-positive. (Wright stain.)

Normal Counterpart

Immature NK cell.

Clinical Features

Patients with aggressive NK cell leukemia are usually adolescents or young adults, more commonly Asian, who present with fever, hepatosplenomegaly, lymphadenopathy, and a leukemic blood picture (356,357). The disease is usually fatal in 1 to 2 years. Rare cases of nasal-type T- or NK cell lymphoma have progressed to aggressive NK large granular lymphocyte leukemia, and some investigators believe it may be a leukemic manifestation of this disorder (358).

Adult T-cell Lymphoma/Leukemia

Definition

A peripheral T-cell neoplasm caused by human T-cell lymphotrophic virus type 1.

Morphology

Cells with hyperlobated nuclei (flower cells) are common in the peripheral blood in leukemic cases. In addition, there is a small proportion of blast-like cells with a deep basophilic cytoplasm. Bone marrow infiltrates are usually patchy, ranging from sparse to moderate. In lymph nodes, the infiltrates are diffuse with architectural effacement (Fig. 19.27). Neoplastic cells are usually medium-sized to large, with nuclear pleomorphism; the cytoplasm is amphophilic, basophilic, or pale. Mitotic activity is variable. Reed-Sternberg–like cells and giant cells with convoluted or cerebriform nuclei may be present. Rare cases are composed of small atypical lym-

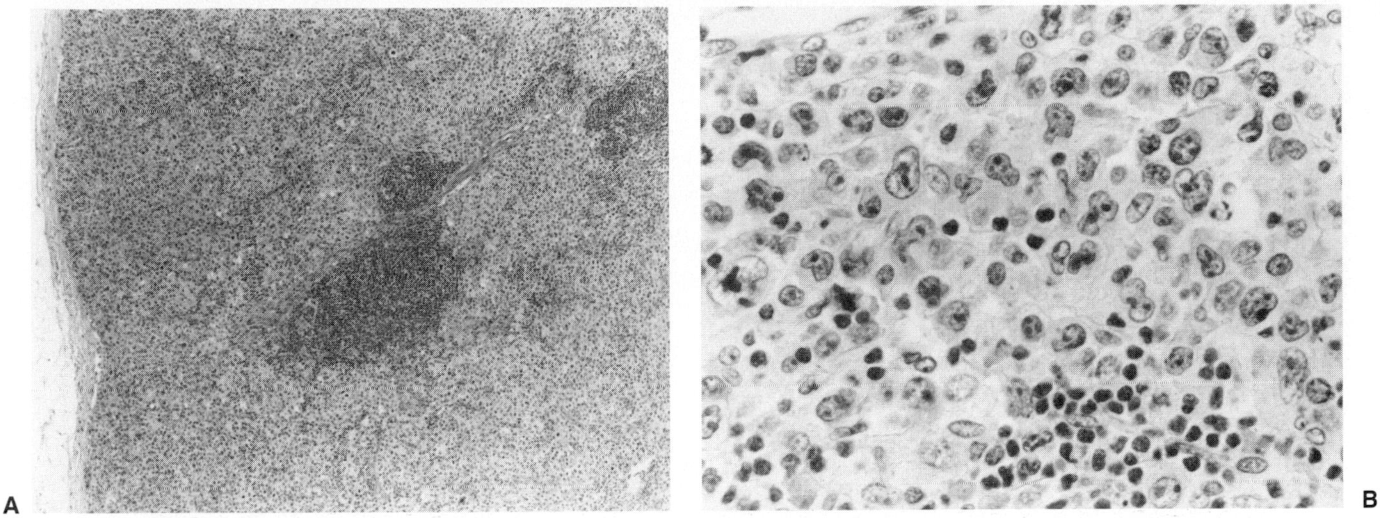

FIG. 19.27. Adult T-cell lymphoma/leukemia, in a patient with human T-cell lymphotrophic virus type 1. **A:** The lymph node is nearly replaced by an infiltrate of atypical lymphoid cells. A few primary follicles are spared. **B:** High-power view shows a mixture of pleomorphic small, medium-sized, and large cells, some with highly irregular nuclei.

phocytes with nuclear pleomorphism or resemble ALCL. In the background there is a mild to moderate proliferation of high endothelial venules.

Immunophenotype

Tumor cells express T cell–associated antigens (CD2, CD3, CD5), but usually lack CD7. Most cases are $CD4^+CD8^-$. Rare cases are $CD4^-CD8^+$ or $CD8^+CD4^+$. CD25 is expressed in a majority of the cases. Anaplastic large cell types express CD30 but not ALK (p80).

Genetics

Clonally integrated HTLV1 genes are found in all patients with this condition. The TCR genes are clonally rearranged.

Possible Normal Counterpart

Peripheral $CD4^+$ T cells in various stages of transformation.

Clinical Features

Patients are adults with antibodies to human T-cell lymphotrophic virus type 1. Most cases occur in Japan or in the Caribbean. Sporadic cases are found elsewhere in the world. Acute, lymphomatous, chronic, and smoldering variants have been described, depending on the clinical features (Table 19.24). The acute type, the most common, presents with neoplastic cells in the blood, skin rashes, generalized lymphadenopathy, hepatosplenomegaly, and hypercalcemia. The lymphomatous type is characterized by prominent lymphadenopathy but no blood involvement. The chronic type involves skin lesions and an increased white blood cell count with absolute lymphocytosis, but no hypercalcemia. In the smoldering type there are normal blood lymphocyte counts, with no more than 5% circulating neoplastic cells. Patients frequently have skin or pulmonary lesions, but hypercalcemia is not present. Progression from chronic and smoldering to acute types eventually occurs in up to 25% of patients.

Mycosis Fungoides

Definition

An epidermotropic cutaneous T-cell lymphoma consisting of small or medium-sized cells with cerebriform nuclei. The designation is reserved for cases with classic clinical features in which there is a progression from patches to plaques or tumors.

Morphology

Skin lesions show epidermotropic infiltrates consisting of small or medium-sized cells with irregular (cerebriform) nuclei (Fig. 19.28A). A minority of larger cells with similar nuclei may be present but are never prominent. So-called Pautrier microabcesses, consisting of groups of cerebriform cells in the epidermis, are highly characteristic but not seen in all cases. Epidermal involvement with single-cell exocytosis is more common. The dermal infiltrates may be patchy, band-like, or diffuse, depending on the stage of the disease. Involved lymph nodes may have the appearance of dermatopathic lymphadenitis or may show paracortical infiltrates of atypical cells similar to those seen in the skin, with architectural effacement (Fig. 19.28B,C).

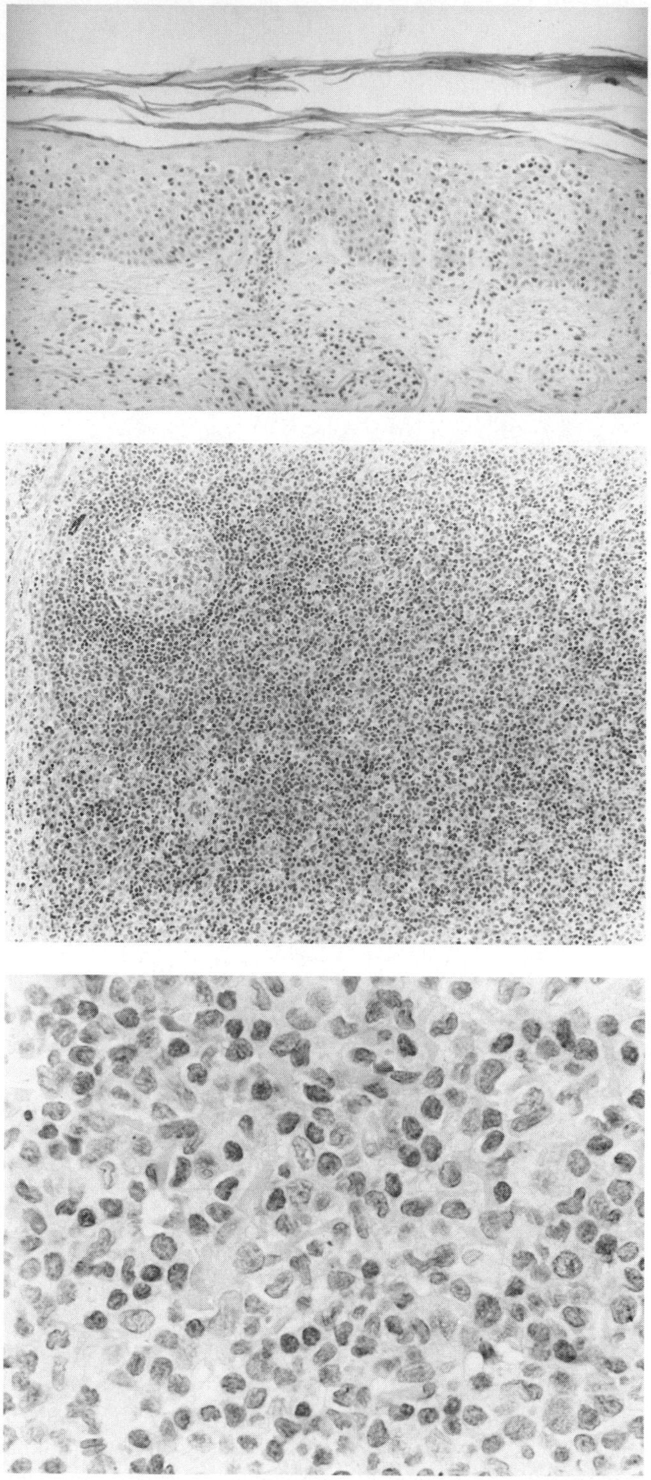

A
B
C

FIG. 19.28. Mycosis fungoides. **A:** This skin biopsy shows an infiltrate of atypical lymphoid cells in a band-like pattern in the papillary dermis and infiltrating the overlying epithelium. **B:** Low-power view of an involved lymph node shows paracortical expansion. **C:** High-power view of the lymph node shows atypical, medium-sized cells with irregular nuclei.

Immunophenotype

Tumor cells are $CD2^+CD3^+CD5^+CD7^\pm$ and express β TCR. Most cases are $CD4^+$. The expression of CD8 is less frequent. Aberrant T-cell phenotypes are frequent in tumor stages.

Genetics

The TCR genes are clonally rearranged. Consistent cytogenetic abnormalities have not been identified.

Possible Normal Counterpart

Peripheral, epidermotropic T cells.

Clinical Features

Patients are almost exclusively adults. The disease has an indolent course, with progression from patches to plaques and eventually tumors. Peripheral blood involvement is absent or subtle, and lymphadenopathy is a late occurrence. Long-term remissions can be obtained in the early stages. Prognosis in advanced stages is less favorable. As a terminal event, transformation to a large T-cell lymphoma or ALCL may occur.

Anaplastic Large-cell Lymphoma, Primary Cutaneous Type

Definition

Am ALCL presenting in the skin in patients with no preexisting lymphoproliferative disease and no evidence of extracutaneous disease at diagnosis.

Morphology

The cytologic features are similar to those in systemic ALCL, although cutaneous cases with less pronounced anaplastic features have been described (Fig. 19.29). Infiltrates are diffuse and involve both the upper and deep dermis and the subcutaneous tissue. Small, reactive lymphocytes may be present at the periphery of the lesions. Most cases are nonepidermotropic.

Immunophenotype

The neoplastic cells express T-cell antigens and are usually $CD4^+$. CD30 is expressed by a majority of the neoplastic cells. Unlike systemic ALCL, most cutaneous cases do not express ALK or epithelial membrane antigen (359,360). Half of the lesions are positive for the cutaneous lymphocyte antigen recognized by HECA-452 (361). Cytotoxic granule-associated proteins are probably expressed less frequently than in systemic cases.

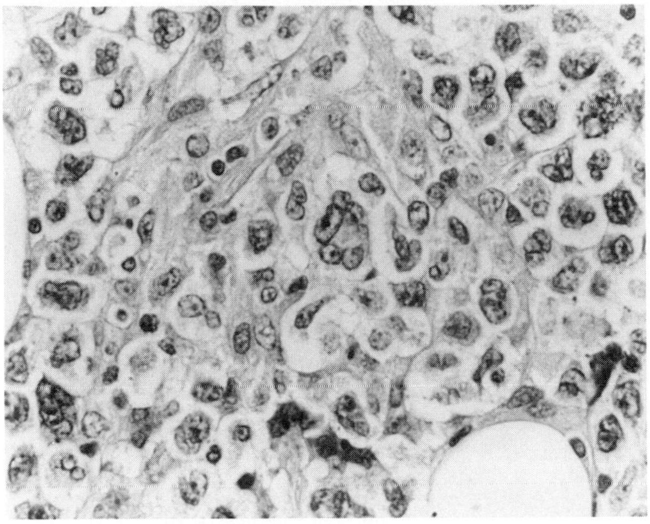

FIG. 19.29. Anaplastic large cell lymphoma, primary cutaneous type, with large, bizarre, sometimes multinucleated cells.

Genetic Features

The TCR genes are clonally rearranged. Although the translocation t(2;5) has been reported, it is rare, and its presence should raise the concern that the tumor is a cutaneous manifestation of systemic ALCL (362).

Clinical Features

Primary cutaneous ALCL affects predominantly older adults and is rare in children. Most cases show limited disease, with solitary or localized skin tumors or nodules. The prognosis is favorable, with long-term remissions or even spontaneous regressions. Systemic disease develops in approximately 25% of the patients. This disorder appears to represent one end of a biologic spectrum that includes lymphomatoid papulosis at the clinically benign end (361,363) (Table 19.25).

Extranodal Natural Killer or T-cell Lymphoma, Nasal Type (formerly Angiocentric Lymphoma)

Definition

An extranodal lymphoma, usually having an immature NK cell phenotype and expressing EBV, with a broad morphologic spectrum and frequent necrosis and angioinvasion, presenting most commonly in the midfacial region but also in other extranodal sites. It is designated as *NK or T-cell* because of uncertainty regarding lineage.

Morphology

Nasal NK or T-cell lymphoma typically is characterized by a polymorphous infiltrate composed of a mixture of normal-appearing small lymphocytes and atypical lymphoid cells of varying size (364,365), along with plasma cells and occasionally eosinophils and histiocytes (Fig. 19.30). Characteristic features are invasion of vascular walls and, usually but not always, occlusion of lumina by lymphoid cells with varying degrees of cytologic atypia. There is usually prominent ischemic necrosis of both tumor cells and normal tissue. The term *angiocentric lymphoma* has proven confusing, because angiocentricity is not evident in all cases. Because the most characteristic presentation is midfacial, and the cells have both T and NK features, the term extranodal *T- or NK cell lymphoma, nasal type* has been proposed (366).

Cases of pulmonary ''lymphomatoid granulomatosis'' were for a time considered to be part of the spectrum of angiocentric lymphoma. Recent studies suggest that most pulmonary cases are EBV-associated B-cell proliferations,

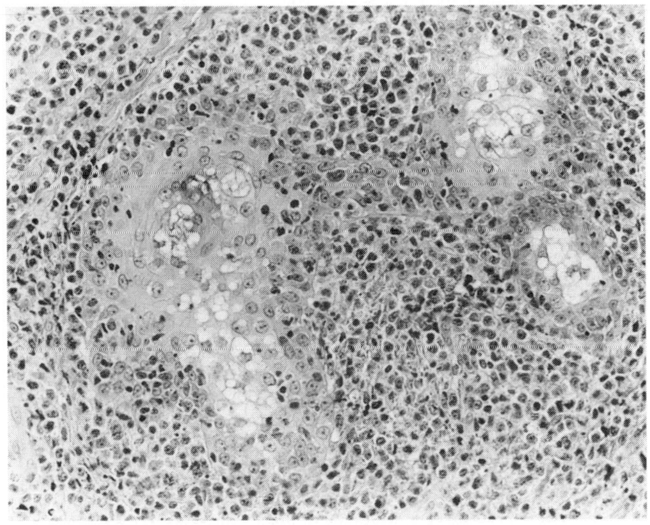

A

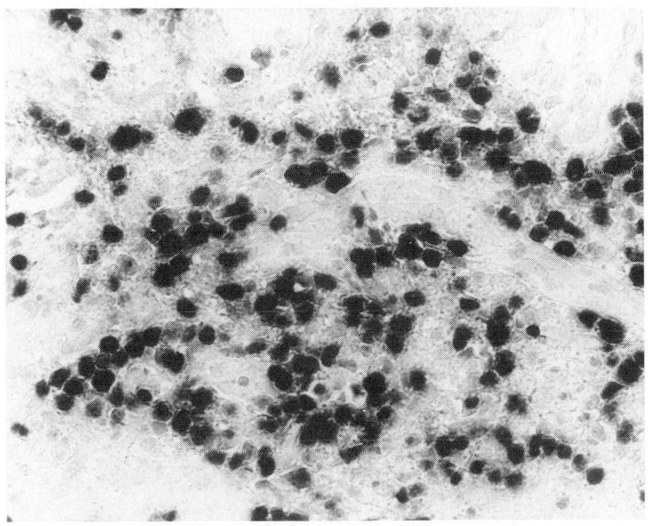

B

FIG. 19.30. Nasal NK or T-cell lymphoma. **A:** There is an infiltrate of medium-sized pleomorphic cells associated with squamous metaplasia of epithelial structures. **B:** *In situ* hybridization shows that neoplastic cells are uniformly positive for EBER.

and therefore a distinct disease category (300,303); however, some pulmonary lymphomas with histologic features of lymphomatoid granulomatosis lack $CD20^+$ cells and EBV and may be examples of peripheral T-cell lymphoma (303). Pulmonary lymphomas with angiocentric growth patterns and necrosis may be heterogeneous.

Immunophenotype

The atypical cells in most cases are $CD2^+CD56^+$ and express cytoplasmic but not surface CD3 (they do not express Leu 4 but are positive for the polyclonal anti-CD3, which detects the epsilon chain of CD3). They are typically $CD4^-CD8^-$ but may express CD4 or CD7 (365,367,368). Most cases express cytotoxic granule proteins such as granzyme B and TIA-1 (369).

Genetic Features

The TCR and immunoglobulin genes are usually germline; EBV genomes are usually present and are detectable in the majority of the cells in most cases by *in situ* hybridization for EBER-1 (368,370) (Fig. 19.30B).

Postulated Normal Counterpart

Immature NK cell.

Clinical Features

Nasal type T- or NK lymphoma is a rare disorder in the United States and Europe but is more common in Asia and in native populations in Peru. It may affect children or adults. Extranodal sites are invariably involved, including nose, palate, upper airway, gastrointestinal tract, and skin (364, 365,368,371,372). The clinical course is typically aggressive, with relapses in other extranodal sites (368,373,374). Hemophagocytic syndromes may occur. Some cases of the aggressive variant of NK cell leukemia or lymphoma may be related to this disorder (358).

Enteropathy-type T-cell Lymphoma

Definition

A tumor of intraepithelial T lymphocytes, usually associated with features of gluten-sensitive enteropathy, showing varying degrees of transformation but usually presenting as a high-grade (blastic) tumor.

Morphology

This disorder originally was termed *malignant histiocytosis of the intestine* but since has been shown conclusively to be a T-cell lymphoma (375). On gross examination, circumferentially oriented jejunal ulcers are present, often multiple, and often with perforation. A mass may or may not be present. The tumors contain a variable admixture of small, medium-sized, large, or anaplastic tumor cells, often with a high content of intraepithelial T cells in adjacent mucosa (Fig. 19.31). The adjacent mucosa may or may not show villous atrophy (376); this varies depending on the segment analyzed, because in sprue, villous atrophy is most prominent in the proximal small intestine and may be absent in distal jejunum or ileum. Early lesions may show mucosal ulceration with only scattered atypical cells and numerous reactive histiocytes, without formation of large masses (377); these lesions are nonetheless clonal. Intraepithelial lymphocytes in apparently nonneoplastic mucosa also may be clonal (378). Clonal TCR gene rearrangements have been found in cases of celiac disease unresponsive to a gluten-free diet, suggesting that these cases represent early T-cell

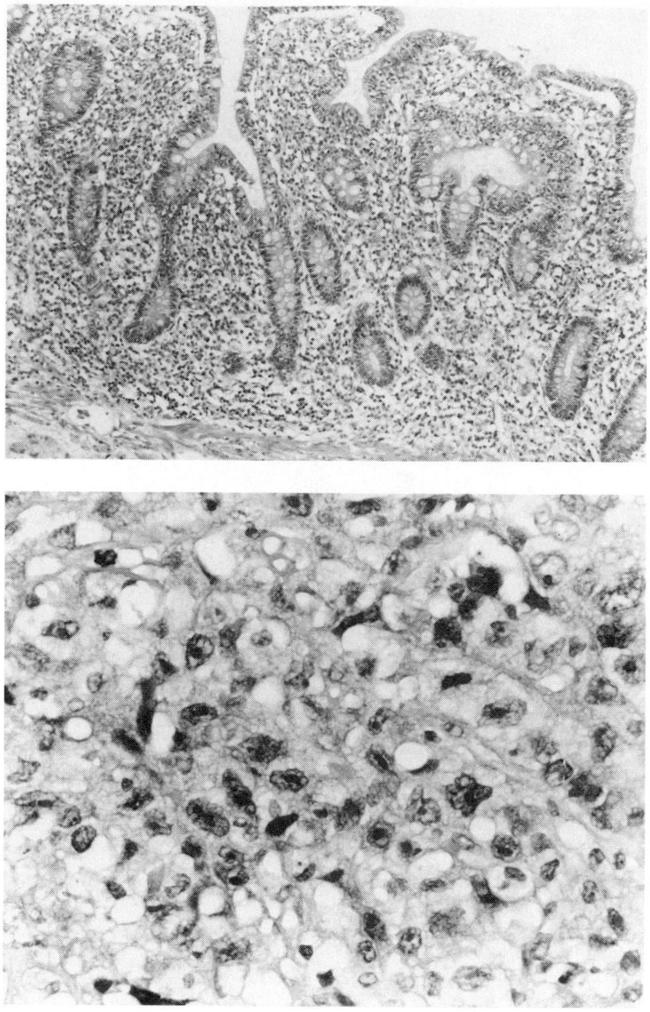

A

B

FIG. 19.31. Enteropathy-type T-cell lymphoma. **A:** Away from areas with obvious involvement by lymphoma, small intestinal villi are blunted, and crypts are hyperplastic. There are increased numbers of intraepithelial lymphocytes. **B:** In this case, the lymphoma is composed of large, highly atypical, pleomorphic lymphoid cells.

lymphomas (379) The tumor may involve liver, spleen, lymph nodes, and other viscera such as the gallbladder.

Immunophenotype

The tumor cells are T cells expressing pan–T cell antigens ($CD3^+CD7^+$), usually $CD8^+CD4^-$ and express the mucosal lymphoid antigen CD103 (380). CD30 may be expressed in some cells. Expression of cytotoxic T cell–associated proteins (granzyme B, TIA-1, perforin) is seen in many of the cases (381,382).

Genetic Features

The TCRβ gene is clonally rearranged (375); no specific cytogenetic abnormality has been described.

Postulated Normal Counterpart

Intestinal intraepithelial cytotoxic T cell in various stages of transformation.

Clinical Features

This disease occurs in adults, typically with a rather brief history of gluten-sensitive enteropathy, as the initial event in a patient found to have villous atrophy in the resected intestine or without evidence of enteropathy but with antigliadin antibodies, the typical HLA type (DQA1*0501, DQB1*0201) of patients with celiac disease, or both (383). It is uncommon in most areas of the United States and Europe but is being seen with increased frequency in areas in which gluten-sensitive enteropathy is common. Treatment of celiac disease with a gluten-free diet effectively prevents the development of lymphoma, so that patients diagnosed with celiac disease early in life usually do not develop lymphoma, and patients with lymphoma rarely have a long history of celiac disease (384,385). Patients present with abdominal pain, often associated with jejunal perforation; stomach or colon are affected less often (386), and other viscera, skin, or soft tissues may be involved (387,388). The course is aggressive, and death usually occurs from multifocal intestinal perforation, because of refractory malignant ulcers.

Hepatosplenic $\gamma\delta$ T-cell Lymphoma

Definition

A neoplasm of mature $\gamma\delta$ T cells with sinusoidal infiltration of spleen, liver, and bone marrow.

Morphology

Hepatosplenic $\gamma\delta$ T-cell lymphoma produces a sinusoidal infiltrate in liver and spleen, as well as bone marrow, of medium-sized lymphoid cells with round nuclei, moderately condensed chromatin, and moderately abundant, pale cytoplasm (389) (Fig. 19.32). The rate of mitotis generally is low (390). The white pulp is atrophic. Erythrophagocytosis may be prominent in splenic and bone marrow sinuses.

Immunophenotype

The tumor cells are $CD2^+CD3^+CD5^-CD4^-CD8^-$ $CD16^+CD56^{\pm}$ and lack the $\alpha\beta$ TCR protein, expressing instead the $\gamma\delta$ complex. Cytotoxic granule protein TIA-1 typically is expressed, but granzyme B and perforin are ab-

A 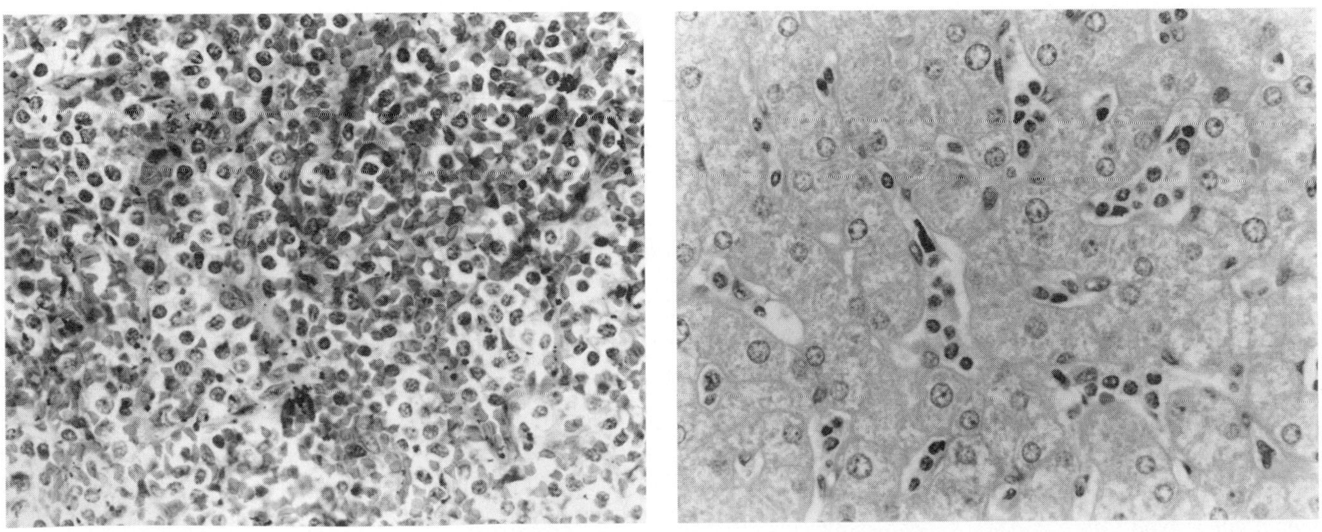 B

FIG. 19.32. Hepatosplenic T-cell lymphoma. **A:** The spleen contains a dense infiltrate of medium-sized, bland lymphoid cells with oval nuclei and clear cytoplasm. **B:** The hepatic sinusoids contain atypical lymphoid cells similar to those in the spleen.

sent, indicating a nonactivated cytotoxic T-cell phenotype (391–393).

Genetic Features

The TCR γ and δ genes are rearranged; the TCR β gene may be rearranged or germline. The tumor cells do not contain EBV. Isochromosome 7q and trisomy 8 have been reported in many cases (394–396).

Postulated Normal Counterpart

$\gamma\delta$ T cell of splenic type.

Clinical Features

This is a rare neoplasm, but because it only recently has been characterized, its frequency is not known; cases probably have been classified as T-cell CLL, prolymphocytic leukemia, or PTCL unspecified. Patients are predominantly adolescent and young adult males and present with marked hepatosplenomegaly; although circulating neoplastic cells are not usually prominent, subtle bone marrow involvement may be present (397,398). Interestingly, several cases have been reported in immunosuppressed recipients of solid-organ allografts (394,399). Despite the relatively bland appearance of the cells, this is an aggressive tumor; although there is often an initial response to chemotherapy, relapse and death are common (390). Neoplasms of $\gamma\delta$ T cells may occur in other sites, particularly mucosal or cutaneous tissues; these appear to behave similarly to primary extranodal $\alpha\beta$ T-cell or NK cell neoplasms of the same sites and do not disseminate to spleen and liver (400,401). The site of presentation appears to be an important defining criterion for this disease.

Subcutaneous Panniculitis-like T-cell Lymphoma

Definition

A T-cell lymphoma that preferentially infiltrates subcutaneous tissue, with atypical cells of varying size, showing prominent tumor necrosis and karyorrhexis.

Morphology

There is a variable mixture of small, medium, and large atypical cells, often containing irregular hyperchromatic nuclei and pale cytoplasm (Fig. 19.33). Reactive histiocytes with phagocytized nuclear debris or lipid are numerous. Granulomas may be present. Individual adipocytes are rimmed by neoplastic cells (402,403).

Immunophenotype

Most cases express pan–T cell antigens and usually CD8, although they may be $CD4^+$, and express cytotoxic granule proteins TIA-1 and perforin and, in most cases, the $\alpha\beta$ TCR (404). Occasional cases derive from $\gamma\delta$ T cells (403).

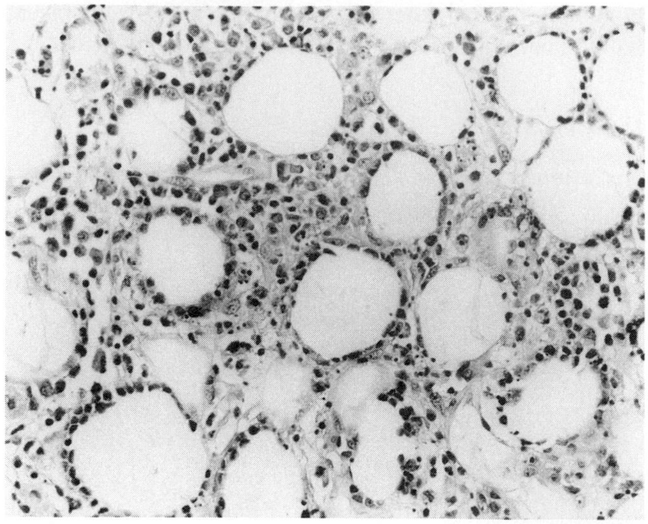

FIG. 19.33. Subcutaneous panniculitis-like T-cell lymphoma. The subcutaneous tissue contains a dense interstitial infiltrate of atypical lymphoid cells, with rimming of individual fat cells by the lymphoid cells.

Genetic Features

T-cell receptor γ genes are rearranged; usually β but occasionally δ chain genes are rearranged (403). No specific cytogenetic abnormalities have been described.

Postulated Normal Counterpart

Mature cytotoxic T cell.

Clinical Features

Patients present with one or more subcutaneous nodules and often are misdiagnosed as panniculitis. Hemophagocytic syndrome is common. The disease may present in an indolent fashion but typically becomes aggressive; patients may respond to aggressive therapy (402,403).

Peripheral T-cell Lymphoma Not Otherwise Categorized

Definition

A number of distinct entities have been defined, which correspond to recognizable subtypes of T-cell neoplasia. There remains a large group of predominantly nodal T-cell lymphomas, which are the most frequent T-cell neoplasms in Western countries. Although a variety of morphologic subtypes have been described, no consistent immunophenotypic, genetic, or clinical features have been associated with most of them. Therefore, for the time being, these presumably diverse cases are lumped under the heading of peripheral T-cell lymphoma not otherwise categorized, or unspecified. This category includes heterogeneous diseases that require further definition.

Morphology

Peripheral T-cell lymphomas typically contain a mixture of small and large atypical cells (348,405) and are classified as diffuse small cleaved, mixed, large cell, or immunoblastic in the WF (67,406) (Fig. 19.34). Admixed eosinophils or epithelioid histiocytes may be numerous (407); the term *lymphoepithelioid cell (Lennert's) lymphoma* has been used for cases rich in epithelioid cells (407) (Table 19.26). Because of their relative rarity and heterogeneity, it has been impossible to arrive at a generally useful classification (15,62,63,348,408). For the time being, these tumors are simply designated *peripheral T-cell lymphomas, unspecified.*

Immunophenotype

T cell–associated antigens are expressed variably ($CD3^{\pm}CD2^{+}CD5^{+}CD7^{\pm}$). CD4 is expressed more often than CD8, and tumors may be $CD4^{-}CD8^{-}$. B cell–associated antigens are lacking (405,409).

Genetic Features

The TCR genes are usually but not always rearranged; immunoglobulin genes are germline (410,411). No specific cytogenetic or oncogene abnormality has been reported, although complex karyotypes are common in cases with larger cells.

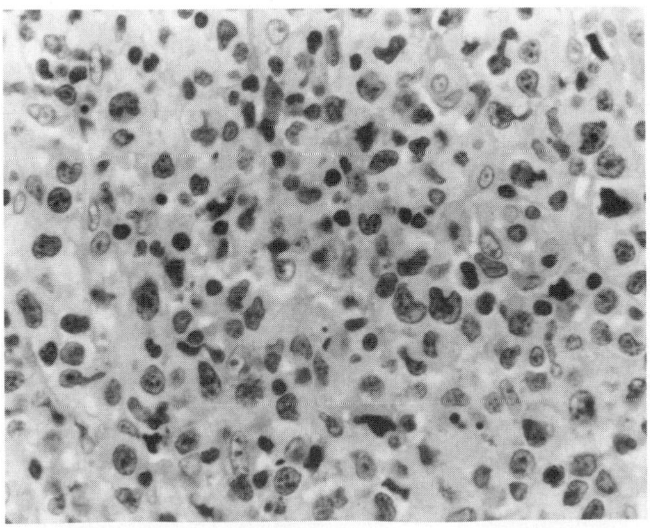

FIG. 19.34. Peripheral T-cell lymphoma not otherwise specified, composed predominantly of medium-sized and large cells with pleomorphic, irregular nuclei.

Postulated Normal Counterpart

Peripheral T cells in various stages of transformation.

Clinical Features

Peripheral T-cell lymphomas comprised only 6% of lymphomas in the international study of the REAL classification (61,67), reflecting their rarity in American and European populations. The median age was in the seventh decade, and 65% of the patients had stage IV disease. Blood eosinophilia, pruritis, and hemophagocytic syndromes may occur (412); lymph nodes, skin, liver, spleen, and other viscera may be involved (376,402). The clinical course is aggressive, and relapses are more common than in large B-cell lymphoma (61,408,413–415). In the international REAL classification study, this group had among the lowest overall and failure-free survival rates (61,67).

Angioimmunoblastic T-cell Lymphoma

Definition

A T-cell lymphoma characterized by systemic disease, a polymorphous infiltrate involving lymph nodes, with a prominent proliferation of high endothelial venules and follicular dendritic cells.

Morphology

The nodal architecture is effaced; peripheral sinuses are typically open and even dilated, but the abnormal infiltrate often extends beyond the capsule into the perinodal fat (Fig. 19.35). There are prominent arborizing high endothelial venules, many of which show thickened or hyalinized walls with periodic acid–Schiff staining. Clusters of epithelioid histiocytes and numerous eosinophils and plasma cells may be present. Expanded aggregates of follicular dendritic cells, visible on immunostained sections, surround the proliferating blood vessels and may have the appearance of ''burned-out'' germinal centers. The lymphoid cells are a mixture of small lymphocytes, immunoblasts, plasma cells, and medium-sized cells with round nuclei and clear cytoplasm. B immunoblasts may be numerous.

Immunophenotype

Tumor cells express T cell–associated antigens and usually CD4, but often many $CD8^{+}$ cells are present; expanded follicular dendritic cell clusters ($CD21^{+}$) are present around proliferated venules (416). The latter feature is useful in distinguishing this disorder from other T-cell lymphomas (15). Polyclonal plasma cells and B immunoblasts may be numerous.

Genetic Features

The TCR genes are rearranged in 75% of patients, and IgH in 10%, corresponding to expanded B-cell clones (416,417).

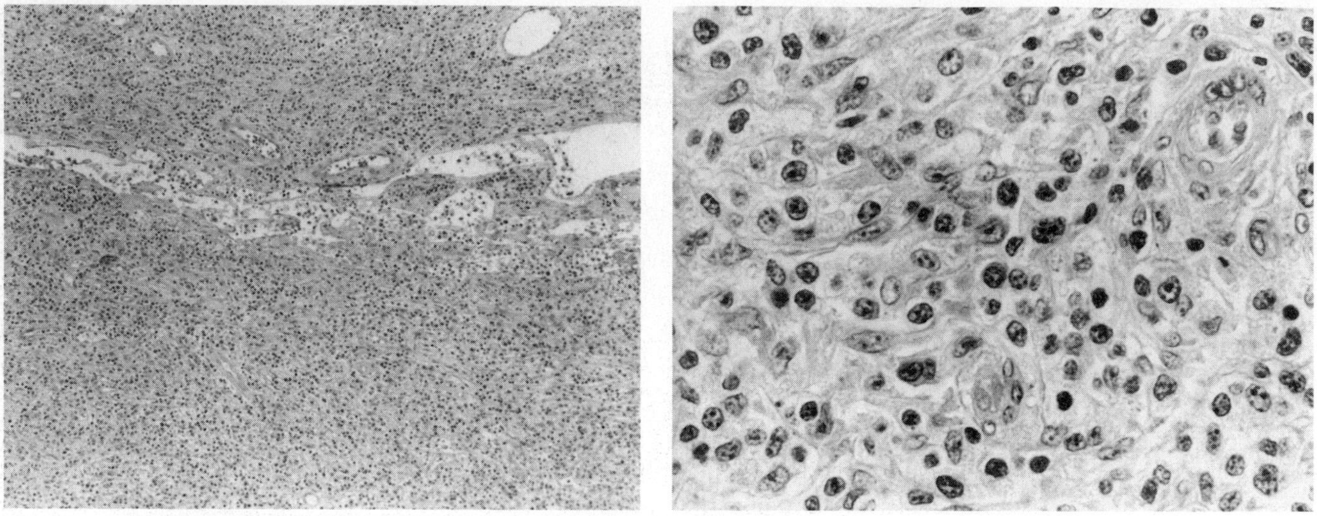

FIG. 19.35. Angioimmunoblastic T-cell lymphoma. **A:** Medium-power view showing diffuse architectural effacement with widely patent subcapsular sinus. **B:** The infiltrate contains medium-sized cells with clear cytoplasm and increased numbers of blood vessels.

EBV genomes are detected in many cases and may be present in either T or B cells (418,419); trisomy 3 or 5 may occur (420).

Postulated Normal Counterpart

Peripheral T cell of unknown subset in various stages of transformation.

Clinical Features

This is one of the more common peripheral T-cell lymphomas encountered in Western countries. In the Kiel registry, it accounted for 20% of all T-cell lymphomas, and about 4% of all lymphomas (15). Angioimmunoblastic T-cell lymphoma is clinically distinctive: patients typically have generalized lymphadenopathy, fever, weight loss, skin rash, and polyclonal hypergammaglobulinemia (421) and are susceptible to infections. The course is moderately aggressive, with occasional spontaneous remissions, and is not reliably predicted by the histologic appearance. About 30% of the patients may have initial remission on steroids alone, but most require some form of chemotherapy. Median duration of survival ranges from 15 ot 24 months, and the curability of this lymphoma has not been well established. Some patients develop a secondary EBV-positive large B-cell lymphoma.

Anaplastic Large T- or Null Cell Lymphoma, Primary Systemic Type

Definition

A neoplasm of large lymphoid cells with pleomorphic or multiple nuclei and abundant cytoplasm, a cohesive growth pattern, and sinusoidal spread in lymph nodes, expressing CD30 and either T-cell or no lineage-specific antigens, involving lymph nodes or extranodal sites not limited to the skin.

Morphology

The tumor usually is composed of large blastic cells with round or pleomorphic, often horseshoe-shaped or multiple nuclei with multiple or single prominent nucleoli and abundant cytoplasm, which gives the cells an epithelial or histiocyte-like appearance. The so-called hallmark cell has an eccentric nucleus and a prominent, eosinophilic golgi region (422) (Fig. 19.36). The tumor cells grow in a cohesive pattern and often involve the lymph node sinuses or paracortex

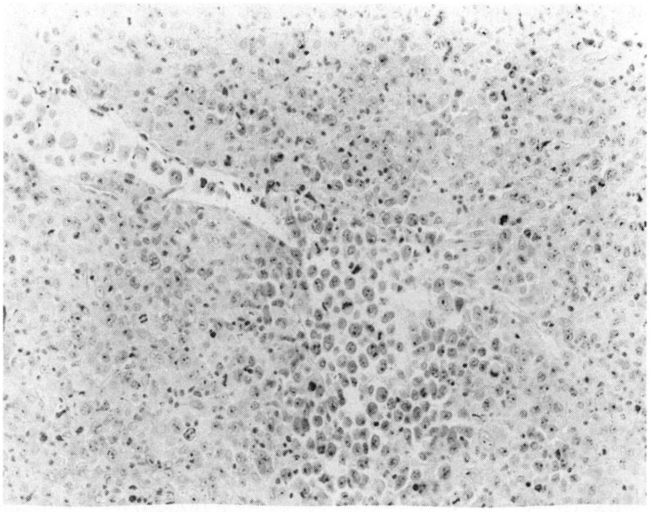

FIG. 19.36. Anaplastic large cell lymphoma, primary systemic type, in a lymph node, with invasion of sinuses.

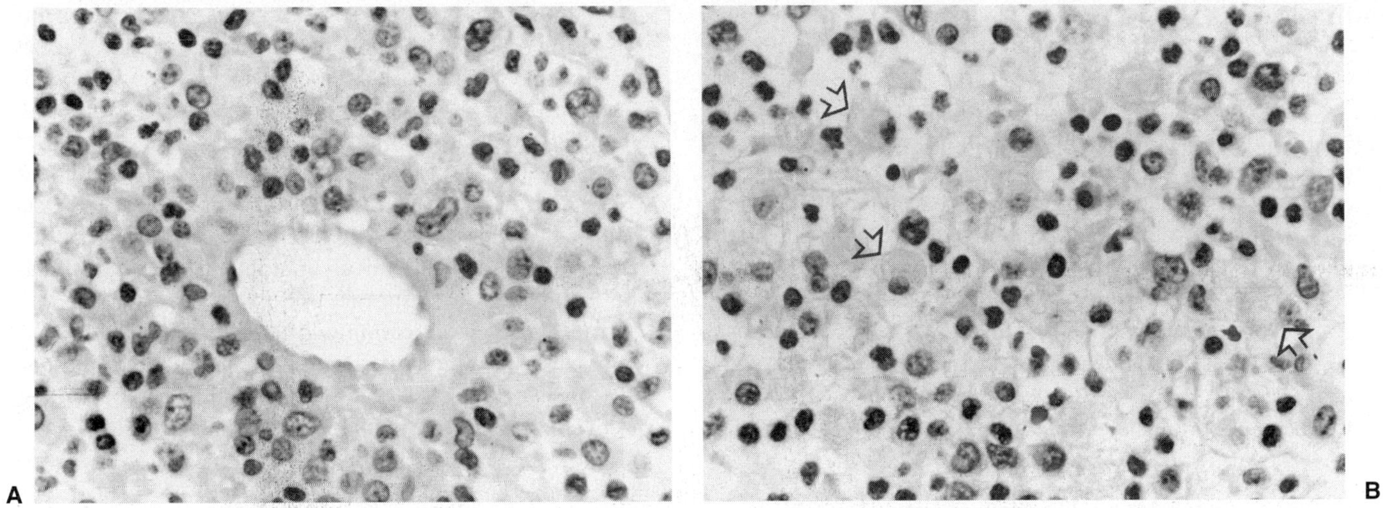

FIG. 19.37. Anaplastic large cell lymphoma, lymphohistiocytic variant. **A:** There is a mixture of lymphocytes, histiocytes and large atypical cells. The large cells show a tendency for perivascular localization. **B:** In areas, "plasmacytoid" histiocytes are seen (*arrows*).

preferentially (423). In some patients, the tumor cells have a more monomorphous appearance, with round to oval nuclei and no Reed-Sternberg–like cells; these cases have in common with the more anaplastic cases a low nuclear : cytoplasmic ratio, with dense, abundant cytoplasm and a cohesive, often sinusoidal growth pattern (424). Lymphohistiocytic and small cell variants have been described, again more commonly in children (425,426) (Fig. 19.37, Table 19.26). Study of cytogenetic and molecular genetic abnormalities as well as clinical features suggest that these cases belong to the same disease entity as the more anaplastic cases (422,427).

A variant of ALCL resembling Hodgkin's disease of nodular sclerosis type has been described (428,429), originally called *ALCL Hodgkin's-related* and included as a provisional entity under the name *ALCL Hodgkin's-like* (ALCL-HL) in the REAL classification (64). This subtype is defined as having architectural features of Hodgkin's disease (nodularity and sclerosis) but cytologic features of ALCL (sheets of neoplastic cells and sinusoidal infiltration). Many patients are young adults with mediastinal masses, and the outcome was said to be intermediate between that of typical ALCL and nodular sclerosis Hodgkin's disease. Several recent studies suggest that these are not true borderline cases. First, most cases of ALCL-HL lack the translocation t(2;5) or the ALK protein (360,430). Second, most cases of Hodgkin's disease are now thought to be B cell–derived, based on single-cell studies showing immunoglobulin gene rearrangement (431–435); ALCL is predominantly a T-cell disease, and there should be no true biologic borderline. Finally, a recent randomized study showed that patients with ALCL-HL responded equally well to the ABVD regimen for Hodgkin's disease as to a MACOP-B regimen for aggressive non-Hodgkin's lymphoma (436), suggesting a closer relationship to Hodgkin's disease than to typical ALCL. The current consensus is that the majority of these cases can be resolved as either Hodgkin's disease ($CD15^+CD30^+$, T-cell antigen–negative, ALK^-) or ALCL ($CD15^-CD30^+$, variable expression of T-cell antigen and ALK) by a combination of morphology and immunophenotype. This category will be eliminated from the WHO classification (70).

Immunophenotype

The tumor cells are $CD30^+$ and usually express CD25 and epithelial membrane antigen; they are typically $CD45^+CD15^-$; about 60% express one or more T cell–associated antigens (CD3, CD43, or CD45RO). Recent studies have shown cytotoxic granule proteins in many of the cases (437,438). The ALK protein can be detected in 40% to 60% of patients using the ALK-1 monoclonal antibody, showing both nuclear and cytoplasmic staining in cases with the translocation t(2;5), because nucleophosmin is a nuclear protein. ALK^+ patients are more commonly children and have a better prognosis than ALK^- patients (360,430,439).

Genetic Features

The majority of the cases have TCR genes rearranged; 20% to 30% have no rearrangement of TCR or immunoglobulin genes. Between 20% and 50% of primary systemic ALCL have a translocation t(2;5) (440,441), which results in a fusion of the nucleophosmin gene (*NPM*) on chromosome 5 to a novel tyrosine kinase gene on chromosome 2, *ALK* (anaplastic lymphoma kinase). The specificity of this translocation for ALCL has been debated, in part because of differing criteria for the diagnosis of ALCL. Using the reverse transcriptase polymerase chain reaction, or an antibody to the fusion protein, the fusion gene product can be detected in about 50% of patients with ALCL of T- and null cell types; however, it also is detected in some T-cell lymphomas without obvious anaplastic morphology (439,441,442). Based on published illustrations, the so-called nonanaplastic cases appear to represent examples of the monomorphic, small cell or histiocyte-rich variants (441). Rare cases of B-cell lymphoma with the translocation t(2;5) have been reported (439,443). Finally, variant translocations have been described, which also result in overexpression of ALK protein but without the nuclear localization (444).

Based on current information, the translocation t(2;5) and ALK expression are not defining features of ALCL, because negative cases exist; however, the positive cases appear clinically relatively homogeneous: young patients with a relatively good prognosis.

Clinical Features

Anaplastic large cell lymphoma represents about 2% of all lymphomas, but about 10% of childhood lymphomas and 50% of pediatric large cell lymphomas (15,61,65,67,445, 446).

Primary systemic ALCL may involve lymph nodes or extranodal sites, including the skin, but is not localized to the skin. Tumors that present with systemic disease (with or without skin involvement) have a bimodal age distribution in children and adults, and are associated with the translocation t(2;5), particularly in children, in 20% to 40% of patients. Patients may present with isolated lymphadenopathy or as extranodal disease in any site, including the gastrointestinal tract and bone (445). ALCL in children is characterized by frequent presentation in an advanced stage of disease but good response to therapy with overall excellent survival (441,445,446). In adults the tumor is aggressive but potentially curable, similar to other aggressive lymphomas (447). Cases with the translocation t(2;5) have a significantly better prognosis than those without t(2;5) (439).

SUMMARY AND CONCLUSIONS

Lymphoid neoplasms are a diverse group of tumors arising from cells of the immune system and, to various degrees, recapitulating stages of normal lymphocyte differentiation. A combination of morphologic, immunophenotypic, genetic, and clinical features defines each disease entity. The relative importance of these features varies from one entity to another, and there is no one "gold standard" at present. Although more than 30 distinct diseases can be recognized with current techniques, only about 10 of them are encountered in daily practice by most oncologists and pathologists. The less common entities must be recognized, however, and progress will be facilitated by defining homogeneous disease categories for clinical and basic research.

If pathologists are to contribute both to the care of patients with tumors and to research on these diseases, it is essential that agreed-on classifications, with agreed-on criteria for each entity, be used. Consensus is essential, even if it involves compromise: The only thing worse than an imperfect classification is multiple classifications. Reproducibility between observers is improved by having uniform criteria; in lymphoid neoplasms, immunophenotyping and—to a lesser extent—genetic studies are useful in some diseases but not essential in all cases if morphology is typical. Pathologists should take primary responsibility for the pathologic classification of diseases, but clinical input into any new classification is important to ensure its usefulness in practice.

Any disease classification will need to be updated for as long as there is progress in the field. In lymphoid neoplasms, new diseases will be defined, new defining criteria will be discovered, more information will become available about normal counterparts, and possibly some categories will prove not to be distinct diseases and will be deleted. It is essential that some mechanism be developed to do this that ensures periodic impartial review of new data by experts in the field, as well as a process for deciding when and how the classification should be updated.

For those who are daunted by the complexity of lymphomas, we observe that the immune system is complex, and that to understand its diseases a tolerance for diversity is essential. We do not hear astronomers complaining if a new celestial body is discovered: This is an opportunity to learn more about the universe. We do not hear infectious disease physicians complaining if a new microbe is discovered: This is an opportunity to develop new treatments and improve the human condition. The recent and ongoing explosion of information about lymphoid neoplasms and the immune system presents a tremendous opportunity to understand the pathogenesis and biology of these diseases, and to develop more specific diagnostic techniques, treatments, and—one hopes—preventive interventions. We agree with William of Ockham that "entities should not be multiplied unnecessarily" (448), but also with Albert Einstein that "things should be made as simple as possible, but not simpler" (449).

REFERENCES

1. Callendar GR. Tumors and tumor-like conditions of the lymphocyte, the myelocyte, the erythrocyte, and the reticulum cell. *Am J Pathol* 1934;10:443–465.
2. Robb-Smith AHT. Reticulosis and reticulosarcoma: a histological classification. *J Path Bact* 1938;47:457–480.
3. Gall EA, Mallory TB. Malignant lymphoma: a clinicopathologic survey of 618 cases. *Am J Pathol* 1942;18:381–395.
4. Rappaport H, Winter W, Hicks E. Follicular lymphoma: a re-evaluation of its position in the scheme of malignant lymphoma, based on a survey of 253 cases. *Cancer* 1956;9:792–821.
5. Rappaport H. Tumors of the hematopoietic system. In: *Atlas of tumor pathology*, section III. Washington, DC: Armed Forces Institute of Pathology, 1966.
6. Dorfman R. Classification of non-Hodgkin's lymphomas [Letter]. *Lancet* 1974;2:961–962.
7. Bennett M, Farrar-Brown G, Henry K, Jelliffe A. Classification of non-Hodgkin's lymphomas [Letter]. *Lancet* 1974;2.
8. Lukes R, Collins R. Immunologic characterization of human malignant lymphomas. *Cancer* 1974;34:1488–1503.

9. Gerard-Marchant R, Hamlin I, Lennert K, et al. Classification of non-Hodgkin's lymphomas. *Lancet* 1974;ii:406–408.
10. Kay HEM. Classification of non-Hodgkin's lymphomas [Letter]. *Lancet* 1974;ii:586.
11. Mathe G. Histological and cytological typing of neoplastic diseases of hematopoietic and lymphoid tissues. In: Rappaport H, O'Conor GT, Torlani H (eds). *WHO International Histological Classification of Tumors*, vol. 14, 1976.
12. Lennert K, Mohri N, Stein H, Kaiserling E. The histopathology of malignant lymphoma. *Br J Haematol* 1975;31[Suppl]:193–203.
13. Lennert K. *Malignant lymphomas other than Hodgkin's disease.* New York: Springer-Verlag, 1978.
14. Non-Hodgkin's lymphoma pathologic classification project. National Cancer Institute sponsored study of classifications of non-Hodgkin's lymphomas: summary and description of a Working Formulation for clinical usage. *Cancer* 1982;49:2112–2135.
15. Lennert K, Feller A. *Histopathology of non-Hodgkin's lymphomas.* New York: Springer-Verlag, 1992.
16. Dorfman RF. Hematopathology: a crescendo of scholarly activity. *Mod Pathol* 1994;7:226–241.
17. Hodgkin T. On some morbid appearances of the absorbent glands. *Med-Chir Trans* 1832;17:69–97.
18. Symmers WS. Museum piece. *Pathol Annu* 1984;19:375.
19. Wilks S. Cases of enlargement of the elymphatic glands and spleen (or, Hodgkin's disease), with remarks. *Guy's Hosp Rep* 1865;11: 56–67.
20. Kundrat H. Uber lymphosarkomatosis. *Wien klin Wochnschr* 1893;6: 211–213, 224–239.
21. Jackson H Jr, Parker F Jr. *Hodgkin's disease and allied disorders.* New York: Oxford University Press, 1947.
22. Sternberg C. Uber ene eigenartige unter dem bilde der pseudoleukamie verlaufend tuberkulose des lymphatischen apparates. *Ztschr Heilk* 1898;19:21–90.
23. Reed D. On the pathological changes in Hodgkin's disease, with especial reference to its relation to tuberculosis. *Johns Hopkins Hosp Rep* 1902;10:133–196.
24. Sternberg C. Uber leukosarcomatose. *Wien Klin Wochenschr* 1908; 21:475–480.
25. Barcos M, Lukes RJ. Malignant lymphoma of convoluted lymphocytes: a new entity of possible T-cell type. In: Sinks L, Godden J, eds. *Conflicts in childhood cancer: an evaluation of current management,* vol. 4. New York: Liss, 1975:147–178.
26. Ewing J. *Neoplastic diseases.* Philadelphia: WB Saunders, 1928.
27. Roulet F. Das primare retothelsarkom der lymphknoten. *Virchows Arch A* 1930;277:15–47.
28. Parker F, Jackson H. Primary reticulum cell sarcoma of bone. *Surg Gynec Obst* 1939;68:45–53.
29. Jackson H, Jr., Parker F, Jr. Hodgkin's disease and allied disorders. *N Engl J Med* 1939;220:26–30.
30. Brill N, Baehr G, Rosenthal N. Generalized giant lymph follicle hyperplasia of the lymph nodes and spleen: a hiterto undescribed type. *JAMA* 1925;84:668–671.
31. Symmers D. Follicular lymphadenopathy with splenomegaly: a newly recognized idsease of the lymphatic system. *Arch Pathol* 1927;3: 816–820.
32. Gall EA, Morrison HR, Scott AT. The follicular type of malignant lymphoma: a survey of 63 cases. *Ann Int Med* 1941;14:2073–2090.
33. Burkitt DP. A sarcoma involving the jaws in African children. *Br J Surg* 1958/59;46:218–223.
34. Burkitt DP, O'Conor GT. Malignant lymphoma in African children: I. A clinical syndrome. *Cancer* 1961;14:258–269.
35. O'Conor GT. Malignant lymphoma in African children: II. A pathological entity. *Cancer* 1961;14:270–283.
36. O'Conor GT, Rappaport H, Smith EB. Childhood lymphoma resembling "Burkitt tumor" in the United States. *Cancer* 1965;18:411–417.
37. Bence Jones H. On a new substance occurring in th eurine of a patient with millities and fragilitas ossium. *Philos Trans R Soc Lond* 1848; 55:673.
38. Wright JH. A case of multiple myeloma. *Bull Johns Hopkins Hosp* 1933;52:156.
39. Willis R. Pathology of lymphoid tissue tumors. In: *Pathology of Tumors.* St Louis: Mosby, 1948:760.
40. Jackson H Jr, Parker F Jr. Hodgkin's disease I: general considerations. *N Engl J Med* 1944;230:1–8.
41. Jackson H Jr, Parker F Jr. Hodgkin's disease II: pathology. *N Engl J Med* 1944;231:35–44.
42. Gall EA, Rappaport H. In: McDonald JR, ed. *Proceedings of Seminar on Diseases of Lymph Node and Spleen.* Chicago: ASCP Press, 1958.
43. Jones S, Fuks Z, Bull M, et al. Non-Hodgkin's lymphomas IV: clinicopathologic correlation in 405 cases. *Cancer* 1973;31:806–823.
44. Murphy S. Management of childhood non-Hodgkin's lymphoma. *Cancer Treat Rep* 1977;61:1161–1173.
45. Ezdinli E, Costello W, Wasser L, et al. Eastern Cooperative Oncology Group experience with the Rappaport classification of non-Hodgkin's lymphomas. *Cancer* 1979;43:544–550.
46. Lukes R, Butler J, Hicks E. Natural history of Hodgkin's disease as related to its patholgical picture. *Cancer* 1966;19:317–344.
47. Peters MV. A study of survivals in Hodgkin's disease treated radiologically. *Am J Roentgenol* 1950;63:299–311.
48. Kaplan H. *Hodgkin's disease.* Cambridge, MA: Harvard University Press, 1978.
49. Lukes R, Craver L, Hall T, et al. Report of the nomenclature committee. *Cancer Res* 1966;26:1311.
50. Nowell PC. Phytohemagglutinin: an initiator of mitosis in cultures of normal human leukocytes. *Cancer Res* 1960;20:462–466.
51. Cooper MD, Peterson RDA, Good RA. Delineation of the thymic and bursal lymphoid systems in the chicken. *Nature* 1965;205:143–146.
52. Wilson JD, Nossal GJV. Identification of human T and B lymphocytes in normal peripheral blood and in chronic lymphocytic leukemia. *Lancet* 1971;II:788–791.
53. Lennert K. Germinal centers and germinal center neoplasia. *Acta Haematol Jap* 1969;32:495–500.
54. Stansfeld A, Diebold J, Kapanci Y, et al. Updated Kiel classification for lymphomas. *Lancet* 1988;i:292–293.
55. Schein PS, Chabner BA, Canellos GP, et al. Potential for prolonged disease-free survival following combination chemotherapy of non-Hodgkin's lymphoma. *Blood* 1974;43:181–189.
56. Strauchen J, Young R, De Vita V, et al. Clinical relevance of the histopathological subclassification of diffuse "histiocyitc" lymphoma. *N Engl J Med* 1978;299:1382–1387.
57. Classification of non-Hodgkin's lymphomas: reproducibility of major classification systems. *Cancer* 1985;55:91–95.
58. Fisher RI, Dahlberg S, Nathwani BN, et al. A clinical analysis of two indolent lymphoma entities: mantle cell lymphoma and marginal zone lymphoma (including the mucosa-associated lymphoid tissue and monocytoid B-cell subcategories): a Southwest Oncology Group study. *Blood* 1995;85:1075–1082.
59. Fisher R, Gaynor E, Dahlberg S, et al. A phase III comparison of CHOP vs ProMACE-cytaBOM vs MACOP-B in patients with intermediate or high grade non-Hodgkin's lymphoma: results of SWOG-8576 (inter group 0067), the national high priority lymphoma study. *Ann Oncol* 1994;5(suppl2):91–95.
60. Longo DL, DeVita VT, Jaffe ES, et al. Lymphocytic Lymphomas. In: De Vita VT, Hellman S, Rosenberg S, eds. *Principles and practice of oncology.* Philadelphia: JB Lipincott Co, 1993:1859–1927.
61. A clinical evaluation of the International Lymphoma Study Group classification of non-Hodgkin's lymphoma. *Blood* 1997;89: 3909–3918.
62. Hastrup N, Hamilton-Dutoit S, et al. Peripheral T-cell lymphomas: an evaluation of reproducibility of the updated Kiel classification. *Histopathology* 1991;18:99–105.
63. Chott A, Augustin I, Wra F, et al. Peripheral T-cell lymphomas: a clinicopathologic study of 75 cases. *Hum Pathol* 1990;21:1117–1125.
64. Harris NL, Jaffe ES, Stein H, et al. A revised European-American classification of lymphoid neoplasms: a proposal from the International Lymphoma Study Group. *Blood* 1994;84:1361–1392.
65. Weisenburger D. The International Lymphoma Study Group (ILSG) classification of non-Hodgkin's lymphoma (NHL): pathology findings from a large multi center study. *Mod Pathol* 1997;10:136A.
66. Weisenburger D. The International Lymphoma Study Group (ILSG) classification of non-Hodgkin's lymphoma (NHL): clinical findings from a large multi-center study. *Mod Pathol* 1997;10:136A.
67. Armitage JO, Weisenburger DD. New approach to classifying non-Hodgkin's lymphomas: clinical features of the major histologic subtypes. *J Clin Oncol* 1998;16:2780–2795.
68. Jaffe ES, Harris NL, Chan JKC, et al. Proposed World Health Organization classification of neoplastic diseases of hematopoietic and lymphoid tissues. *Am J Surg Pathol* 1997;21:114–121.

69. Jaffe ES, Harris NL, Diebold J, et al. World Health Organization Classification of lymphomas: a work in progress. *Ann Oncol* 1998; 9[Suppl 5]:S25–30.
70. Harris NL, Jaffe ES, Diebold J, et al. The World Health Organization Classification of Hematological Malignancies: report of the Clinical Advisory Committee Meeting. *J Clin Oncol* 1999;17:3835–3849.
71. Hiddemann W, Longo DL, Coiffier B, et al. Lymphoma classification—the gap between biology and clinical management is closing. *Blood* 1996;88:4085–4089.
72. A predictive model for aggressive non-Hodgkin's lymphoma: the International non-Hodgkin's Lymphoma Project. *N Engl J Med* 1993; 329:987–994.
73. Rosenberg SA. Classification of lymphoid neoplasms. *Blood* 1994; 84:1359–1360.
74. Harris NL, Jaffe ES, Stein H, et al. Lymphoma classification proposal: clarification. *Blood* 1995;85.
75. Anderson JR, Armitage JO, Weisenburger DD. Epidemiology of the non-Hodgkin's lymphomas: distributions of the major subtypes differ by geographic locations. Non-Hodgkin's Lymphoma Classification Project. *Ann Oncol* 1998;9:717–720.
76. Gowans J, Knight E. The route of recirculation of lymphocytes in the rat. *Proc R Soc Lond B Biol Sci* 1964;159:257.
77. Butcher E. Cellular and molecular mechanisms that direct leukocyte traffic. *Am J Pathol* 1990;136:3–12.
78. Korsmeyer S, Hieter P, Ravetch J, et al. Developmental hierarchy of immunoglobulin gene rearrangements in leukemic pre-B cells. *Proc Natl Acad Sci USA* 1981;78:7096–7100.
79. Pesando J, Ritz J, Lazarus H, et al. Leukemia-associated antigens in ALL. *Blood* 1979;54:1240–1248.
80. Janossy G, Bollum F, Bradstock K, et al. Cellular phenotypes of normal and leukemic hematopoietic cells determined by selected antibody combinations. *Blood* 1980;56:430–441.
81. Shipp M, Richardson N, Sayre P, et al. Molecular cloning of the common acute lymphoblastic leukemia antigen (CALLA) identifies a type II integral membrane protein. *Proc Natl Acad Sci USA* 1988; 85:4819–1988.
82. Shipp M, Vuayaraghavan J, Schmidt E, et al. Common acute lymphoblastic leukemia antigen (CALLA) is active neutral endopeptidase 24.11 (''enkephalinase''): direct evidence by cDNA transfection analysis. *Proc Natl Acad Sci USA* 1989;86:297–301.
83. Quintanilla-Martinez L, Zukerberg L, Ferry J, et al. Extramedullary tumors of lymphoid or myeloid blasts: the role of immunohistology in diagnosis and classification. *Am J Clin Pathol* 1995;104:431–443.
84. Pleiman CM. The B-cell antigen receptor complex: structure and signal transduction. *Immunology Today* 1994;15:393–398.
85. Mason D, Cordell J, Tse A, et al. The IgM-associated protein mb-1 as a marker of normal and neoplastic B-cells. *J Immunol* 1991;147: 2474–2482.
86. Longacre T, Foucar K, Crago S, et al. Hematogones: a multiparameter analysis of bone marrow precursor cells. *Blood* 1989;73:543–552.
87. Loken M, Shah V, Dattilio K, et al. Flow cytometric analysis of human bone marrow: II. Normal B lymphocyte development. *Blood* 1987; 70:1317–1324.
88. Klein U, Kuppers R, Rejewsky K. Human IgM + IgD + B cells, the major B cell subset in the peripheral blood, express Vh genes with no or little somatic mutation throughout life. *Eur J Immunol* 1993; 23:3272.
89. MacLennan I, Liu Y, Oldfield S, Ahang J, Lane P. The evolution of B-cell clones. *Curr Top Microbiol Immunol* 1990;159:37–63.
90. Kipps T. The CD5 B cell. *Adv Immunol* 1989;47:117–185.
91. Tedder T, Penta A, Levine H, et al. Expression of the human leukocyte adhesion/homing molecule, LAM-1: identity with the TQ1 and Leu-8 differentiation antigens. *J Immunol* 1990;144:532–540.
92. Law C, Sidorenko S, Clark E. Regulation of lymphocyte activation by the cell-surface molecule CD22. *Immunol Today* 1994;15:442–449.
93. Durie FH, Foy TM, Masters SR, et al. The role of CD40 in the regulation of humoral and cell-mediated immunity. *Immunology Today* 1994;15:406–410.
94. Hockenbery D, Zutter M, Hickey W, et al. BCL2 protein is topographically restricted in tissues characterized by apoptotic cell death. *Proc Natl Acad Sci USA* 1991;88:6961–6965.
95. Inghirami G, Foitl D, Sabichi A, et al. Autoantibody-associated cross-reactive idiotype-bearing human B lymphocytes: distribution and characterization, including IgVH gene and CD5 antigen expression. *Blood* 1991;78:1503–1515.
96. Kuppers R, Zhao M, Hansmann M-L, et al. Tracing B cell development in human germinal centres by molecular analysis of single cells picked from histological sections. *EMBO J* 1993;12:4955.
97. Zukerberg L, Medeiros L, Ferry J, et al. Diffuse low-grade B-cell lymphomas: four clinically distinct subtypes defined by a combination of morphologic and immunophenotypic features. *Am J Clin Pathol* 1993;100:373–385.
98. Kuppers R, Ganse A, Rajewsky K. B cells of chronic lymphatic leukemia express V genes in unmutated form. *Leuk Res* 1991;15:487.
99. Hummel M, Tamaru J, Kalvelage B, et al. Mantle cell (previously centrocytic) lymphomas express Vh genes with no or very little somatic mutations like the physiologic cells of the follicle mantle. *Blood* 1994;84:403–407.
100. Veldman J, Keuning F, Molenaar I. Site of initiation of the plasma cell reaction in the rabbit lymph node. *Virchows Arch B* 1978;8:187–202.
101. Liu Y-J, Zhang J, Lane PJL, et al. Sites of specific B cell activation in primary and secondary responses to T cell-dependent and T cell-independent antigens. *Eur J Immunol* 1991;21:2951–2962.
102. Halper J, Fu S, Wang C, Winchester R, et al. Patterns of expression of IA-like antigens during the terminal stages of B cell development. *J Immunol* 1978;120:1480–1484.
103. MacLennan I. Germinal centers. *Annu Rev Immunol* 1994;12: 117–139.
104. Liu Y-J, Oldfield S, MacLennan I. Memory B cells in T-cell dependent antibody responses colonise the splenic marginal zones. *Eur J Immunol* 1988;18:355–362.
105. Liu Y-J, Johnson G, Gordon J, et al. Germinal centres in T-cell-dependent antibody responses. *Immunol Today* 1992;13:1–39.
106. Splawski JB. Immunoregulatory role of CD40 in human B cell differentiation. *J Immunol* 1993;150.
107. Freeman G, Freedman A, Segil J, et al. A new member of the Ig superfamily with unique expression on activated and neoplastic B cells. *J Immunol* 1989;143:2714–2722.
108. Freeman GJ, Gribben JG, Boussiotis VA, et al. Cloning of B7-2: a CTLA-4 counter-receptor that costimulates human T cell proliferation. *Science* 1993;262:909–911.
109. Engel P, Gribben J, Freeman G, et al. The B7-2 (B70) costimulatory molecule expressed by monocytes and activated B lymphocytes is the CD86 differentiation antigen. *Blood* 1994;84:1402–1407.
110. Munro J, Freedman A, Aster J, et al. In vivo expression of the B7 costimulatory molecule by subsets of antigen-presenting cells and the malignant cells of Hodgkin's disease. *Blood* 1994;83:793–798.
111. Freedman A, Munro M, Rice G, et al. Adhesion of human B cells to germinal centers in vitro involves VLA-4 and INCAM-110. *Science* 1990;249:1030–1033.
112. Freedman A. Expression of adhesion receptors on normal B cells and B-cell non-Hodgkin's lymphomas. *Semin Hematol* 1993;30:318–328.
113. Nguyen P, Harrisn N, Ritz J. Expression of CD95 in reactive lymphoid tissues and lymphomas. *Lab Invest* 1995;653(abst).
114. Cattoretti G, Chang CC, Cechova K, et al. BCL-6 protein is expressed in germinal-center B cells. *Blood* 1995;86:45–53.
115. Flenghi L, Bigerna B, Fizzotti M, et al. Monoclonal antibodies PG-B6a and PG-B6p recognize, respectively, a highly conserved and a formol-resistant epitope on the human BCL-6 protein amino-terminal region. *Am J Pathol* 1996;148:1543–1555.
116. Allman D, Jain A, Dent A, et al. BCL-6 expression during B-cell activation. *Blood* 1996;87:5257–5268.
117. French DL, Laskov R, Scharff MD. The role of somatic hypermutation in the generation of antibody diversity. *Science* 1989;244:1152.
118. Jacob J, Kelsoe G, Rajewsky K, et al. Intraclonal generation of antibody mutants in germinal centres. *Nature* 1991;354:389.
119. Wabl M, Forni L, Loor F. Switch in immunoglobulin production observed in single clones of committed lymphocytes. *Science* 1978;199: 1078–1079.
120. Berek C. The development of B cells and the B-cell repertoire in the microenvironment of the germinal centre. *Immunol Rev* 1992;126:5.
121. Peng HZ, Du MQ, Koulis A, et al. Nonimmunoglobulin gene hypermutation in germinal center B cells. *Blood* 1999;93:2167–2172.
122. Pasqualucci L, Migliazza A, Fracchiolla N, et al. BCL-6 mutations in normal germinal center B cells: evidence of somatic hypermutation acting outside Ig loci. *Proc Natl Acad Sci USA* 1998;95:11816–11821.
123. Shen HM, Peters A, Baron B, et al. Mutation of BCL-6 gene in normal

B cells by the process of somatic hypermutation of Ig genes. *Science* 1998;280:1750–1752.
124. Liu Y-J, Joshua DE, Williams GT, et al. Mechanism of antigen-driven selection in germinal centres. *Nature* 1989;342:929–931.
125. Pezzella F, Tse A, Cordell J, et al. Expression of the Bcl-2 oncogene protein is not specific for the 14-18 chromosomal translocation. *Am J Pathol* 1990;137:225–232.
126. Klein U, Klein G, Ehlin-Henriksson B, et al. Burkitt's lymphoma is a malignancy of mature B cells expressing somatically mutated V region genes. *Mol Med* 1995;1:495–505.
127. Van den Oord J, De Wolf-Peeters C, De Vos R, et al. Immature sinus histiocytosis: light- and electron-microscopic features, immunologic phenotype, and relationship with marginal zone lymphocytes. *Am J Pathol* 1985;1985:266–277.
128. van Krieken J, von Schilling C, Kluin P, et al. Splenic marginal zone lymphocytes and related cells in the lymph node: a morphologic and immunohistochemical study. *Hum Pathol* 1989;20:320–325.
129. Smith-Ravin J, Spencer J, Beverley P, et al. Characterization of two monoclonal antibodies (UCL4D12 and UCL3D3) that discriminate between human mantle zone and marginal zone B cells. *Clin Exp Immunol* 1990;82:181–187.
130. Spencer J, Finn T, Pulford K, et al. The human gut contains a novel population of B lymphocytes which resemble marginal zone cells. *Clin Exp Immunol* 1985;62:607–612.
131. Isaacson P, Spencer J. Malignant lymphoma of mucosa-associated lymphoid tissue. *Histopathology* 1987;11:445–462.
132. Klein U, Kuppers R, Rajewsky K. Evidence for a large compartment of IgM-expressing memory B cells in humans. *Blood* 1997;89: 1288–1298.
133. Klein U, Goossens T, Fischer M, et al. Somatic hypermutation in normal and transformed human B cells. *Immunol Rev* 1998;162: 261–280.
134. Dunn-Walters DK, Isaacson PG, Spencer J. Analysis of mutations in immunoglobulin heavy chain variable region genes of microdissected marginal zone (MGZ) B cells suggests that the MGZ of human spleen is a reservoir of memory B cells. *J Exp Med* 1995;182:559–566.
135. Dunn-Walters DK, Isaacson PG, Spencer J. Sequence analysis of rearranged IgVH genes from microdissected human Peyer's patch marginal zone B cells. *Immunology* 1996;88:618–624.
136. Tierens A, Delabie J, Michiels L, et al. Marginal-zone B cells in the human lymph node and spleen show somatic hypermutations and display clonal expansion. *Blood* 1999;93:226–234.
137. Cardoso de Almeida P, Harris N, Bhan A. Characterization of immature sinus histiocytes (monocytoid cells) in reactive lymph nodes by use of monoclonal antibodies. *Hum Pathol* 1984;15:330–335.
138. Nizze H, Cogliatti S, von Schilling C, et al. Monocytoid B-cell lymphoma: morphological variants and relationship to low-grade B-cell lymphoma of the mucosa-associated lymphoid tissue. *Histopathology* 1991;18:403–414.
139. Piris M, Rivas C, Morente M, et al. Monocytoid B-cell lymphoma, a tumour related to the marginal zone. *Histopathology* 1988;12: 383–392.
140. Melo J, Hegde U, Parreira A, et al. Splenic B cell lymphoma with circulating villous lymphocytes: differential diagnosis of B cell leukaemias with large spleens. *J Clin Pathol* 1987;40:642–651.
141. Campo E, Miquel R, Krenacs L, et al. Primary nodal marginal zone lymphomas of splenic and MALT type. *Am J Surg Pathol* 1999;23: 59–68.
142. Dunn-Walters DK, Boursier L, Spencer J, et al. Analysis of immunoglobulin genes in splenic marginal zone lymphoma suggests ongoing mutation. *Hum Pathol* 1998;29:585–593.
143. Kuppers R, Hajadi M, Plank L, et al. Molecular Ig gene analysis reveals that monocytoid B cell lymphoma is a malignancy of mature B cells carrying somatically mutated V region genes and suggests that rearrangement of the kappa-deleting element (resulting in deletion of the Ig kappa enhancers) abolishes somatic hypermutation in the human. *Eur J Immunol* 1996;26:1794–1800.
144. Du M, Diss T, Xu C, et al. Somatic mutations and intraclonal variations in MALT lymphoma immunoglobulin genes. *Blood* 1995; 86[Suppl]:181a.
145. Spits H, Lanier L, Phillips J. Development of human T and natural killer cells. *Blood* 1995;85:2654–2670.
146. Thomas M. The leukocyte common antigen family. *Ann Rev Immunol* 1989;7:339–369.
147. Bhan A, Reinherz E, Poppema S, et al. Location of T cell and major histocompatibility antigens in the human thymus. *J Exp Med* 1980; 152:771–682.
148. Gimmi C, Freeman J, Sugita K, et al. B7 provides a costimulatory signal which induces T cells to proliferate and secrete interleukin 2. *Proc Natl Acad Sci USA* 1991;88:6575–6579.
149. Meurer S, Schlossman S, Reinherz E. Clonal analysis of human cytotoxic T lymphocytes: T4 and T8 effector T cells recognize products of different major histocompatibility regions. *Proc Natl Acad Sci USA* 1982;79:4395–4399.
150. Inghirami G, Zhu B, Chess L, et al. Flow cytometric and immunohistochemical characterization of the γ/δ T-lymphocyte population in normal human lymphoid tissue and peripheral blood. *Am J Pathol* 1990; 136:357–367.
151. Stein H, Lennert K, Feller A, et al. Immunohistological analysis of human lymphoma: correlation of histological and immunological categories. *Adv Cancer Res* 1984;42:67–147.
152. Picker L, Weiss L, Medeiros L, et al. Immunophenotypic criteria for the diagnosis of non-Hodgkin's lymphma. *Am J Pathol* 1987;128: 181–201.
153. Knapp W, Dorken B, Rieber P, et al. *Leukocyte typing IV*. Oxford: Oxford University Press, 1989.
154. Arnold A, Cossman J, Bakhshi A, et al. Immunoglobulin gene rearrangements as unique clonal markers in human lymphoid neoplasms. *N Engl J Med* 1983;309:1594–1599.
155. Yunis J, Mayer M, Arnesen M, et al. Bcl-2 and other genomic alterations in the prognosis of large-cell lymphoma. *N Engl J Med* 1989; 320:1047–1054.
156. Tsujimoto Y, Yunis J, Onorato-Showe L, et al. Molecular cloning of the chromosomal breakpoint of B-cell lymphomas and leukemias with the t(11;14) chromosome translation. *Science* 1984;224:1403–1406.
157. Tsujimoto T, Cossman J, Jaffe E, et al. Involvement of the bcl-2 gene in human follicular lymphoma. *Science* 1985;288:1440–1443.
158. Khalidi HS, Chang KL, Medeiros LJ, et al. Acute lymphoblastic leukemia: survey of immunophenotype, French-American-British classification, frequency of myeloid antigen expression, and karyotypic abnormalities in 210 pediatric and adult cases. *Am J Clin Pathol* 1999; 111:467–476.
159. Pui CH, Rubnitz JE, Hancock ML, et al. Reappraisal of the clinical and biologic significance of myeloid-associated antigen expression in childhood acute lymphoblastic leukemia. *J Clin Oncol* 1998;16: 3768–3773.
160. Kitchingman G, Robigatti U, Mauer A, et al. Rearrangement of immunoglobulin heavy chain genes in T cell acute lymphoblastic leukemia. *Blood* 1985;65:725–729.
161. Tawa A, Hozumi N, Minden M, et al. Rearrangements of the T-cell receptor β chain gene in non-T-cell, non-B-cell acute lymphoblastic leukemia in childhood. *N Engl J Med* 1985;313:1033–1037.
162. Felix CA, Poplack DG, Reaman GH, et al. Characterization of immunoglobulin and T-cell receptor gene patterns in B-cell precursor acute lymphoblastic leukemia of childhood. *J Clin Oncol* 1990;8:431–442.
163. Pui CH, Behm FG, Downing JR, et al. 11q23/MLL rearrangement confers a poor prognosis in infants with acute lymphoblastic leukemia. *J Clin Oncol* 1994;12:909–915.
164. Rubnitz JE, Pui CH, Downing JR. The role of TEL fusion genes in pediatric leukemias. *Leukemia* 1999;13:6–13.
165. Boucheix C, David B, Sebban C, et al. Immunophenotype of adult acute lymphoblastic leukemia, clinical parameters, and outcome: an analysis of a prospective trial including 562 tested patients (LALA87). French Group on Therapy for Adult Acute Lymphoblastic Leukemia. *Blood* 1994;84:1603–1612.
166. Uckun FM, Sather HN, Gaynon PS, et al. Clinical features and treatment outcome of children with myeloid antigen positive acute lymphoblastic leukemia: a report from the Children's Cancer Group. *Blood* 1997;90:28–35.
167. Ben-Ezra J, Burke J, Swartz W, et al. Small lymphocytic lymphoma: a clinicopathologic analysis of 268 cases. *Blood* 1989;73:579–587.
168. Perry D, Bast M, Armitage J, et al. Diffuse intermediate lymphocytic lymphoma: a clinicopathologic study and comparison with small lymphocytic lymphoma and diffuse small cleaved cell lymphoma. *Cancer* 1990;66:1995–2000.
169. Bonato M, Pittaluga S, Tierens A, et al. Lymph node histology in typical and atypical chronic lymphocytic leukemia. *Am J Surg Pathol* 1998;22:49–56.

170. Kipps TJ, Carson DA. Autoantibodies in chronic lymphocytic leukemia and related systemic autoimmune diseases. *Blood* 1993;81:2475.
171. Aoki H, Takishita M, Kosaka M, et al. Frequent somatic mutations in D and/or Jh segments of Ig gene in Waldenstrom's macroglobulinemia and chronic lymphocytic leukemia (CLL) with Richter's syndrome but not in common CLL. *Blood* 1995;85:1913–1919.
172. Oscier DG, Thompsett A, Zhu D, et al. Differential rates of somatic hypermutation in V(H) genes among subsets of chronic lymphocytic leukemia defined by chromosomal abnormalities. *Blood* 1997;89:4153–4160.
173. Damle RN, Wasil T, Fais F, et al. Ig V gene mutation status and CD38 expression as novel prognostic indicators in chronic lymphocytic leukemia [See comments]. *Blood* 1999;94:1840–1847.
174. Juliusson G, Oscier D, Fitchett M, et al. Prognostic subgroups in B-cell chronic lymphocytic leukemia defined by specific chromosomal abnormalities. *N Engl J Med* 1990;323:720–724.
175. Knuutila S, Elonen E, Teerenhovi L, et al. Trisomy 12 in B cells of patients with B-cell chronic lymphocytic leukemia. *N Engl J Med* 1986;314:865–869.
176. Juliusson G, Merup M. Cytogenetics in chronic lymphocytic leukemia. *Semin Oncol* 1998;25:19–26.
177. Croce C, Tsujimoto Y, Erikson J, et al. Chromosome translocations and B cell neoplasia. *Lab Invest* 1984;51:258–267.
178. Yang WI, Zukerberg LR, Mokotura I, et al. BCL-1 (Cyclin D1) protein expression in low grade B-cell lymphomas and reactive hyperplasia. *Am J Pathol* 1994;145:86–96.
179. Bosch F, Jares P, Campo E, et al. PRAD-1/Cyclin D1 gene overexpression in chronic lymphoproliferative disorders: a highly specific marker of mantle cell lymphoma. *Blood* 1994;84:2726–2732.
180. Zhu Y, Monni O, El-Rifai W, et al. Discontinuous deletions at 11q23 in B cell chronic lymphocytic leukemia. *Leukemia* 1999;13:708–712.
181. Sembries S, Pahl H, Stilgenbauer S, et al. Reduced expression of adhesion molecules and cell signaling receptors by chronic lymphocytic leukemia cells with 11q deletion. *Blood* 1999;93:624–631.
182. Caligaris-Cappio F. B-chronic lymphocytic leukemia: a malignancy of anti-self B cells. *Blood* 1996;87:2615–2620.
183. Caligaris-Cappio F, Hamblin T. B-cell chronic lymphocytic leukemia: a bird of a different feather. *J Clin Oncol* 1999;17:399–408.
184. Klein U, Rajewsky K, Kuppers R. Human immunoglobulin (Ig)-M + IgD + peripheral blood B cells expressing the CD27 cell surface antigen carry somatically mutated variable region genes: CD27 as a general marker for somatically mutated (memory) B cells. *J Exp Med* 1998;188:1679–1689.
185. O'Brien A, del Giglio A, Keating M. Advances in the biology and treatment of B-cell chronic lymphocytic leukemia. *Blood* 1995;85:307–318.
186. Bearman RM, Pangalis GA, Rappaport H. Prolymphocytic leukemia. Clinical, histopathological and cytochemical observations. *Cancer* 1978;42:2360–2372.
187. Galton D, Goldman J, Wiltshaw E, et al. Prolymphocytic leukaemia. *Br J Haematol* 1974;27:7–23.
188. Lampert I, Catovsky D, Marsh G, et al. The histopathology of prolymphocytic leukaemia with particular reference to the spleen: a comparison with chronic lymphocytic leukemia. *Histopathology* 1980;4:3–19.
189. Melo J, Catovsky D, Galton D. The relationship between chronic lymphocytic leukaemia and prolymphocytic leukaemia: I. Clinical and laboratory features of 300 patients and characterization of an intermediate group. *Br J Haematol* 1985;63:377–387.
190. Lens D, Coignet LJ, Brito-Babapulle V, et al. B cell prolymphocytic leukaemia (B-PLL) with complex karyotype and concurrent abnormalities of the p53 and c-MYC gene. *Leukemia* 1999;13:873–876.
191. Sole F, Woessner S, Espinet B, et al. Cytogenetic abnormalities in three patients with B-cell prolymphocytic leukemia. *Cancer Genet Cytogenet* 1998;103:43–45.
192. Harris N, Bhan A. B-cell neoplasms of the lymphocytic, lymphoplasmacytoid, and plasma cell types: immunohistologic analysis and clinical correlation. *Hum Pathol* 1985;16:829–837.
193. Lennert K, Tamm I, Wacker H-H. Histopathology and immunocytochemistry of lymph node biopsies in chronic lymphocytic leukemia and immunocytoma. *Leuk Lymphoma* 1991;5[Suppl]:157–160.
194. Crouzier R, Martin T, Pasquali JL. Monoclonal IgM rheumatoid factor secreted by CD5-negative B cells during mixed cryoglobulinemia. Evidence for somatic mutations and intraclonal diversity of the expressed VH region gene. *J Immunol* 1995;154:413–421.
195. Sahota SS, Garand R, Bataille R, et al. VH gene analysis of clonally related IgM and IgG from human lymphoplasmacytoid B-cell tumors with chronic lymphocytic leukemia features and high serum monoclonal IgG. *Blood* 1998;91:238–243.
196. Wagner SD, Martinelli V, Luzzatto L. Similar patterns of Vk gene usage but different degrees of somatic mutation in hairy cell leukemia, prolymphocytic leukemia, Waldenstrom's macroglobulinemia, and myeloma. *Blood* 1994;83:3647–3653.
197. Krenacs L, Himmelmann AW, Quintanilla-Martinez L, et al. Transcription factor B-cell-specific activator protein (BSAP) is differentially expressed in B cells and in subsets of B-cell lymphomas. *Blood* 1998;92:1308–1316.
198. Dimopoulos MA, Alexanian R. Waldenstrom's macroglobulinemia. *Blood* 1994;83:1452–1459.
199. Agnello V, Chung RT, Kaplan LM. A role for hepatitis C virus infection in type II cryoglobulinemia [See comments]. *N Engl J Med* 1992;327:1490–1495.
200. Pozzato G, Mazzaro C, Crovatto M, et al. Low-grade malignant lymphoma, hepatitis C virus infection, and mixed cryoglobulinemia. *Blood* 1994;84:3047–3053.
201. Mazzaro C, Franzin F, Tulissi P, et al. Regression of monoclonal B-cell expansion in patients affected by mixed cryoglobulinemia responsive to alpha-interferon therapy. *Cancer* 1996;77:2604–2613.
202. Jorgensen C, Legouffe MC, Perney P, et al. Sicca syndrome associated with hepatitis C virus infection. *Arthritis Rheum* 1996;39:1166–1171.
203. Ascoli V, Lo Coco F, Artini M, et al. Extranodal lymphomas associated with hepatitis C virus infection [See comments]. *Am J Clin Pathol* 1998;109:600–609.
204. Zuckerman E, Zuckerman T, Levine AM, et al. Hepatitis C virus infection in patients with B-cell non-Hodgkin lymphoma [See comments]. *Ann Intern Med* 1997;127:423–428.
205. De Vita S, Sacco C, Sansonno D, et al. Characterization of overt B-cell lymphomas in patients with hepatitis C virus infection. *Blood* 1997;90:776–782.
206. Sansonno D, De Vita S, Cornacchiulo V, et al. Detection and distribution of hepatitis C virus-related proteins in lymph nodes of patients with type II mixed cryoglobulinemia and neoplastic or non-neoplastic lymphoproliferation. *Blood* 1996;88:4638–4645.
207. Brittinger G, Bartels H, Common H, et al. Clinical and prognostic relevance of the Kiel classification of non-Hodgkin lymphomas: results of a prospective multicenter study by the Kiel lymphoma study group. *Hematol Oncol* 1984;2:269–306.
208. Engelhard M, Brittinger G, Heinz R, et al. Chronic lymphocytic leukemia (B-CLL) and immunocytoma (LP-IC): clinical and prognostic relevance of this distinction. *Leukemia Lymphoma* 1991[Suppl]:161–173.
209. Pathology of the spleen: report on the workshop of the VIIIth meeting of the European Association for Haematopathology, Paris, 1996. *Histopathology* 1998;32:172–179.
210. Schmid C, Kirkham N, Diss T, Isaacson P. Splenic marginal zone cell lymphoma. *Am J Surg Pathol* 1992;16:455–466.
211. Isaacson PG, Matutes E, Burke M, et al. The histopathology of splenic lymphoma with villous lymphocytes. *Blood* 1995;85.
212. Mollejo M, Menarguez J, Lloret E. Splenic marginal zone lymphoma: a distinctive type of low-grade B-cell lymphoma: a clinicopathologic study of 13 cases. *Am J Surg Pathol* 1995;19:1146–1157.
213. Mollejo M, Lloret E, Menárguez J, et al. Lymph node involvement by splenic marginal zone lymphoma: morphological and immunohistochemical features. *Am J Surg Pathol* 1997;21:772–780.
214. Matutes E, Morilla R, Owusu-Ankomah K, et al. The immunophenotype of splenic lymphoma with villous lymphocytes and its relevance to the differential diagnosis with other B-cell disorders. *Blood* 1994;83:1558–1562.
215. Savilo E, Campo E, Mollejo M, et al. Absence of cyclin D1 protein expression in splenic marginal zone lymphoma. *Mod Pathol* 1998;11:601–606.
216. Zhu D, Oscier DG, Stevenson FK. Splenic lymphoma with villous lymphocytes involves B cells with extensively mutated Ig heavy chain variable region genes. *Blood* 1995;85:1603–1607.
217. Oscier DG, Matutes E, Gardiner A, et al. Cytogenetic studies in splenic lymphoma with villous lymphocytes. *Br J Hematol* 1993;85:487–491.
218. Jadayel D, Matutes E, Dyer MJS, et al. Splenic lymphoma with villous

lymphocytes: analysis of bcl-1 rearrangements and expression of cyclin D1 gene. *Blood* 1994;83:3664–3671.
219. Finn T, Isaacson P, Wotherspoon A. Numerical abnormality of chromosomes 3, 7, 12, and 18 in low grade lymphomas of MALT-type and splenic marginal zone lymphomas detected by interphase cytogenetics on paraffin embedded tissue. *J Pathol* 1993;170:335A.
220. Brynes RK, Almaguer R, Leathery K, et al. Numerical cytogenetic abnormalities of chromosomes 3, 7, and 12 in marginal zone B-cell lymphomas. *Mod Pathol* 1996;9:995–1000.
221. Pittaluga S, Verhoef G, Criel A, et al. ''Small'' B-cell non-Hodgkin's lymphomas with splenomegaly at presentation are either mantle cell lymphoma or marginal zone cell lymphoma: a study based on histology, cytology, immunohistochemistry, and cytogenetic analysis. *Am J Surg Pathol* 1996;20:211–223.
222. Arber DA, Rappaport H, Weiss LM. Non-Hodgkin's lymphoproliferative disorders involving the spleen. *Mod Pathol* 1997;10:18–32.
223. Moller P, Mielke B, Moldenhauer G. Monoclonal antibody HML-1, a marker for intraepithelial T cells and lymphomas derived thereof, also recognizes hairy cell leukemia and some B-cell lymphomas. *Am J Pathol* 1990;136:509–512.
224. Visser L, Shaw A, Slupsky J, et al. Monoclonal antibodies reactive with hairy cell leukemia. *Blood* 1989;74:320–325.
225. Moldenhauer G, Mielke B, Dorken B, et al. Identity of HML-1 antigen on intestinal intraepithelial T cells and of B-ly7 antigen on hairy cell leukaemia. *Scand J Immunol* 1990;32:77–82.
226. Flenghi L, Spinozzi F, Stein H, et al. LF61: a new monoclonal antibody directed against a trimeric molecule (150kD, 125kD, 105kD) associated with hairy cell leukaemia. *Br J Haematol* 1990;76: 451–459.
227. Falini B, Pileri S, Flenghi L, et al. Selection of a panel of monoclonal antibodies for monitoring residual disease in peripheral blood and bone marrow of interferon-treated hairy cell leukemia patients. *Br J Haematol* 1990;76:460–468.
228. Hounieu H, Shashikant C, Saati T, et al. Hairy cell leukemia: diagnosis of bone marrow involvement in paraffin-embedded sections with monoclonal antibody DBA.44. *Am J Clin Pathol* 1992;28:26–33.
229. Korsmeyer S, Greene W, Cossman J. Rearrangement and expression of immunoglobulin genes and expression of Tac antigen in hairy cell leukemia. *Proc Natl Acad Sci USA* 1983;80:4522–4528.
230. Spiers A, Moore D, Cassileth P, et al. Remissions in hairy-cell leukemia with pentostatin (2′-deoxycoformycin). *N Engl J Med* 1987;316: 825–830.
231. Piro L, Carrera C, Carson D, et al. Lasting remissions in hairy cell leukemia induced by a single infusion of 2′-chlorodeoxyadenosine. *Cancer* 1990;332:1117–1121.
232. Zukerberg L, Ferry J, Conlon M, et al. Plasma cell myeloma with cleaved, multilobated, and monocytoid nuclei. *Am J Clin Pathol* 1990; 93:657–661.
233. Zukerberg LR, Yang W-I, Arnold A, et al. Cyclin D1 expression in non-Hodgkin's lymphomas: detection by immunohistochemistry. *Am J Clin Pathol* 1995;102.
234. Vasef MA, Medeiros LJ, Yospur LS, et al. Cyclin D1 protein in multiple myeloma and plasmacytoma: an immunohistochemical study using fixed, paraffin-embedded tissue sections. *Mod Pathol* 1997;10: 927–932.
235. Sawyer J, Lukacs J, Munshi N, et al. Identification of new nonrandom translocation in multiple myeloma with multicolor spectral karyotyping. *Blood* 1998;92:4269–4278.
236. Harris NL, Jaffe ES, Diebold J, et al. The World Health Organization Classification of Hematological Malignancies: report of the Clinical Advisory Committee Meeting. *Ann Oncol* 1999;10:1419–1432.
237. Harris NL, Jaffe ES, Diebold J, et al. The World Health Organization classification of hematological malignancies: report of the Clinical Advisory Committee meeting. *Hematology Journal* 2000;1:53–66.
238. Harris NL, Jaffe ES, Diebold J, et al. The World Health Organization classification of hematological malignancies: report of the Clinical Advisory Committee meeting. *Mod Pathol* 2000;13:193–207.
239. Harris NL, Jaffe ES, Diebold J, et al. The World Health Organization classification of hematological malignancies: report of the Clinical Advisory Committee meeting. *Histopathology* 2000;36:69–87.
240. Qin Y, Greiner A, Trunk MJF, et al. Somatic hypermutation in low-grade mucosa-associated lymphoid tissue-type B-cell lymphoma. *Blood* 1995;86:3528–3534.
241. Miklos J, Swerdlow S, Bahler D. Analysis of immunoglobulin VH genes used by low grade salivary gland lymphomas of the mucosa-associated lymphoid tissue (MALT) type. *Blood* 1995;86[Suppl]: 182a.
242. Pan L, Diss T, Cunningham D, et al. The bcl-2 gene in primary B-cell lymphomas of mucosa associated lymphoid tissue (MALT). *Am J Pathol* 1989;135:7–11.
243. Auer IA, Gascoyne RD, Connors JM, et al. t(11;18)(q21;q21) is the most common translocation in Malt lymphomas. *Ann Oncol* 1997;8: 979–985.
244. Ott G, Katzenberger T, Greiner A, et al. The t(11;18)(q21;q21) chromosome translocation is a frequent and specific aberration in low-grade but not high-grade malignant non-Hodgkin's lymphomas of the mucosa-associated lympoid tisssue (MALT) type. *Cancer Res* 1997; 57:3944–3948.
245. Barth TF, Dohner H, Werner CA, et al. Characteristic pattern of chromosomal gains and losses in primary large B-cell lymphomas of the gastrointestinal tract. *Blood* 1998;91:4321–4330.
246. Dierlamm J, Baens M, Wlodarska I, et al. The apoptosis inhibitor gene API2 and a novel 18q gene, MLT, are recurrently rearranged in the t(11;18)(q21;q21) associated with mucosa-associated lymphoid tissue lymphomas. *Blood* 1999;93:3601–3609.
247. Willis TG, Jadayel DM, Du MQ, et al. Bcl10 is involved in t(1; 14)(p22;q32) of MALT B cell lymphoma and mutated in multiple tumor types [See comments]. *Cell* 1999;96:35–45.
248. Radaszkiewicz T, Dragosics B, Bauer P. Gastrointestinal malignant lymphomas of the mucosa-associated lymphoid tissue: factors relevant to prognosis. *Gastroenterology* 1992;102:1628–1638.
249. Ferry J, White W, Grove A, et al. Malignant lymphoma of ocular adnexa: a spectrum of B-cell neoplasia including low grade B-cell lymphoma of MALT type. *Lab Invest* 1992;66:77A.
250. Cogliatti S, Schmid U, Schumacher U, et al. Primary B-cell gastric lymphoma: a clinicopathological study of 145 patients. *Gastroenterology* 1991;101:1159–1170.
251. Isaacson PG. Gastrointestinal lymphoma. *Hum Pathol* 1994;25: 1020–1029.
252. Hussell T, Isaacson P, Crabtree J, et al. The response of cells from low-grade B-cell gastric lymphomas of mucosa-associated lymphoid tissue to Helicobacter pylori. *Lancet* 1993;342:571–574.
253. Wotherspoon A, Doglioni C, Diss T, et al. Regression of primary low-grade B-cell gastric lymphoma of mucosa-associated lymphoid tissue type after eradication of Helicobacter pylori. *Lancet* 1993;342: 575–577.
254. Pinotti G, Roggero E, Zucca E, et al. Primary low-grade gastric MALT lymphoma. *Proceedings of ASCO* 1995;14:393(abst).
255. Li G, Hansmann M, Zwingers T, et al. Primary lymphomas of the lung: morphological, immunohistochemical and clinical features. *Histopathology* 1990;16:519–531.
256. Fung CY, Grossbard ML, Linggood RM, et al. Mucosa-associated lymphoid tissue lymphoma of the stomach: long term outcome after local treatment. *Cancer* 1999;85:9–17.
257. Fung C, Ferry J, Linggood R, et al. Extranodal marginal zone (MALT type) lymphoma of the ocular adnexae: a localized tumor with favorable outcome after radiation therapy. Proceedings of ASTRO 37th Annual Meeting. *Int J Radiat Oncol Phys* 1996;36:199.
258. Mattia A, Ferry J, Harris N. Breast lymphoma: a B-cell spectrum including the low grade B-cell lymphoma of mucosa associated lymphoid tissue. *Am J Surg Pathol* 1993;17:574–387.
259. Bailey EM, Ferry JA, Harris NL, et al. Marginal zone lymphoma (low-grade B-cell lymphoma of mucosa-associated lymphoid tissue type) of skin and subcutaneous tissue: a study of 15 patients [See comments]. *Am J Surg Pathol* 1996;20:1011–1023.
260. Zinzani PL, Magagnoli M, Ascani S, et al. Nongastrointestinal mucosa-associated lymphoid tissue (MALT) lymphomas: clinical and therapeutic features of 24 localized patients. *Ann Oncol* 1997;8: 883–886.
261. Sheibani K, Burke J, Swartz W, et al. Monocytoid B cell lymphoma: clinicopathologic study of 21 cases of a unique type of low grade lymphoma. *Cancer* 1988;62:1531–1538.
262. Ngan B-Y, Warnke R, Wilson M, et al. Monocytoid B-cell lymphoma: a study of 36 cases. *Hum Pathol* 1991;22:409–421.
263. Shin S, Sheibani K, Fishleder A, et al. Monocytoid B-cell lymphoma in patients with Sjogren's syndrome: a clinicopathologic study of 13 patients. *Hum Pathol* 1991;22:422–430.
264. Nathwani BN, Anderson JR, Armitage JO, et al. Clinical significance

of follicular lymphoma with monocytoid B cells: Non-Hodgkin's Lymphoma Classification Project. *Hum Pathol* 1999;30:263–268.

265. Carbone A, Gloghini A, Pinto A, et al. Monocytoid B-cell lymphoma with bone marrow and peripheral blood involvement at presentation. *Am J Clin Pathol* 1989;92:228–236.
266. Mann R, Berard C. Criteria for the cytologic subclassification of follicular lymphomas: a proposed alternative method. *Hematol Oncol* 1982; 1:187–192.
267. Harris N, Nadler L, Bhan A. Immunohistologic characterization of two malignant lymphomas of germinal center type (centroblastic/centrocytic andf centrocytic) with monoclonal antibodies: follicular and diffuse lymphomas of small cleaved cell types are related but distinct entities. *Am J Pathol* 1984;117:262–272.
268. Pittaluga S, Ayoubi TA, Wlodarska I, et al. BCL-6 expression in reactive lymphoid tissue and in B-cell non-Hodgkin's lymphomas. *J Pathol* 1996;179:145–150.
269. Cleary M, Mecker T, Levy S, et al. Clustering of extensive somatic mutations in the variable region of an immunoglobulin heavy chain gene from a human B cell lymphoma. *Cell* 1986;44:97–106.
270. Bahler D, Campbell M, Hart s, et al. Ig V(H) gene expression among human follicular lymphomas. *Blood* 1991;78:1561.
271. Glass A, Karnell L, Menck H. The National Cancer Data Base report on non-Hodgkin's lymphoma. *Cancer* 1997;80:2311–2320.
272. Majlis A, Pugh WC, Rodriguez MA, et al. Mantle cell lymphoma: correlation of clinical outcome and biologic features with three histologic variants. *J Clin Oncol* 1997;15:1664–1671.
273. Lardelli P, Bookman M, Sundeen J, et al. Lymphocytic lymphoma of intermediate differentiation: morphologic and immunophenotypic spectrum and clinical correlations. *Am J Surg Pathol* 1990;14: 752–763.
274. Ott M, Ott G, Kuse R, et al. The anaplastic variant of centrocytic lymphoma is marked by frequent rearrangements of the Bcl-1 gene and high proliferation indices. *Histopathology* 1994;24:329–334.
275. Banks P, Chan J, Cleary M, et al. Mantle cell lymphoma: a proposal for unification of morphologic, immunologic, and molecular data. *Am J Surg Pathol* 1992;16:637–640.
276. Dorfman DM, Pinkus GS. Distinction between small lymphocytic and mantle cell lymphoma by immunoreactivity for CD23. *Mod Pathol* 1994;7:326–331.
277. Bosch F, Lopez-Guillermo A, Campo E, et al. Mantle cell lymphoma: presenting features, response to therapy, and prognostic factors. *Cancer* 1998;82:567–575.
278. Kaptain S. CD5-negative mantle cell lymphoma. *Mod Pathol* 1998.
279. Vandenberghe E, De Wolf-Peeters C, Van den Oord J, et al. Translocation (11;14): a cytogenetic anomaly associated with B-cell lymphomas of non-follicle centre cell lineage. *J Pathol* 1991;163:13–18.
280. Rosenberg C, Wong E, Petty E, et al. Overexpression of PRAD1, a candidate BCL1 breakpoint region oncogene, in centrocytic lymphomas. *Proc Natl Acad Sci USA* 1991;88:9638–9642.
281. Swerdlow SH, Yang WI, Zukerberg LR, et al. Expression of cyclin D1 protein in centrocytic/mantle cell lymphomas with and without rearrangement of the BCL1/cyclin D1 gene. *Hum Pathol* 1995;26: 999–1004.
282. de Boer CJ, Vaandrager JW, van Krieken JH, et al. Visualization of mono-allelic chromosomal aberrations 3′and 5′of the cyclin D1 gene in mantle cell lymphoma using DNA fiber fluorescence in situ hybridization. *Oncogene* 1997;15:1599–1603.
283. Quintanilla-Martinez L, Thieblemont C, Fend F, et al. Mantle cell lymphomas lack expresion of p27kip1, a cyclin-dependend kinase inhibitor. *Am J Pathol* 1998;153:175–182.
284. Greiner TC, Moynihan MJ, Chan WC, et al. p53 mutations in mantle cell lymphoma are associated with variant cytology and predict a poor prognosis. *Blood* 1996;87:4302–4310.
285. Ott G, Kalla J, Ott MM, et al. Blastoid variants of mantle cell lymphoma: frequent bcl-1 rearrangements at the major translocation cluster region and tetraploid chromosome clones. *Blood* 1997;89: 1421–1429.
286. Dreyling MH, Bullinger L, Ott G, et al. Alterations of the cyclin D1/ p16-pRB pathway in mantle cell lymphoma. *Cancer Res* 1997;57: 4608–4614.
287. Tirier C, Zhang Y, Plendl H, et al. Simultaneous presence of t(11; 14) and a variant Burkitt's translocation in the terminal phase of a mantle cell lymphoma. *Leukemia* 1996;10:346–350.
288. Isaacson P, MacLennan K, Subbuswamy S. Multiple lymphomatous polyposis of the gastrointestinal tract. *Histopathology* 1984;8: 641–656.
289. Meusers P, Engelhard M, Bartels H, et al. Multicentre randomized therapeutic trial for advanced centrocytic lymphoma: anthracycline does not improve the prognosis. *Hematol Oncol* 1989;7:365–380.
290. Berger F, Felman P, Sonet A, et al. Nonfollicular small B-cell lymphomas: a heterogeneous group of patients with distinct clinical features and outcome. *Blood* 1994;83:2829–2835.
291. Zukerberg L, Medeiros L, Ferry J, et al. Diffuse low grade B-cell lymphomas: identification of four major immunophenotypic subtypes. *Lab Invest* 1991;62:87(abst).
292. Stewart DA, Vose JM, Weisenburger DD, et al. The role of high-dose therapy and autologous hematopoietic stem cell transplantation for mantle cell lymphoma. *Ann Oncol* 1995;6:263–266.
293. Ketterer N, Salles G, Espinouse D, et al. Intensive therapy with peripheral stem cell transplantation in 16 patients with mantle cell lymphoma. *Ann Oncol* 1997;8:701–704.
294. Andersen NS, Donovan JW, Borus JS, et al. Failure of immunologic purging in mantle cell lymphoma assessed by polymerase chain reaction detection of minimal residual disease. *Blood* 1997;90:4212–4221.
295. Freedman AS, Neuberg D, Gribben JG, et al. High-dose chemoradiotherapy and anti-B-cell monoclonal antibody-purged autologous bone marrow transplantation in mantle-cell lymphoma: no evidence for long-term remission [See comments]. *J Clin Oncol* 1998;16:13–18.
296. Decaudin D, Bosq J, Tertian G, et al. Phase II trial of fludarabine monophosphate in patients with mantle-cell lymphomas. *J Clin Oncol* 1998;16:579–583.
297. Engelhard M, Brittinger G, Huhn D, et al. Subclassification of diffuse large B-cell lymphomas according to the Kiel Classification: distinction of centroblastic and immunoblastic lymphomas is a significant prognostic risk factor. *Blood* 1997;89:2291–2297.
298. Delabie J, Vandenberghe E, Kennes C, et al. Histiocyte-rich B-cell lymphoma: a distinct clinicopathologic entity possibly related to lymphocyte predominant Hodgkin's disease, paragranuloma subtype. *Am J Surg Pathol* 1992;16:37–48.
299. McBride JA, Rodriguez J, Luthra R, et al. T-cell-rich B large-cell lymphoma simulating lymphocyte-rich Hodgkin's disease [See comments]. *Am J Surg Pathol* 1996;20:193–201.
300. Guinee D, Kingma D, Fishback N, et al. Pulmonary lymphomatoid granulomatosis: evidence for a proliferation of Epstein-Barr virus infected B lymphocytes with a prominent T-cell component and vasculitis. *Am J Surg Pathol* 1994;18:753–764.
301. Haque AK, Myers JL, Hudnall SD, et al. Pulmonary lymphomatoid granulomatosis in acquired immunodeficiency syndrome: lesions with Epstein-Barr virus infection. *Mod Pathol* 1998;11:347–356.
302. Katzenstein A-L, Peiper S. Detection Epstein-Barr genomes in lymphomatoid granulomatosis: analysis of 29 cases by the polymerase chain reaction. *Mod Pathol* 1990;3:435.
303. Myers JL, Kurtin P, Katzenstein A, et al. Lymphomatoid granulomatosis: evidence of immunophenotypic diversity and relationship to Epstein-Barr virus infection. *Am J Surg Pathol* 1995;19:1300–1312.
304. Doggett R, Wood G, Horning S, et al. The immunologic characterization of 95 nodal and extranodal diffuse large cell lymphomas in 89 patients. *Am J Pathol* 1984;115:245–252.
305. Gascoyne RD, Adomat SA, Krajewski S, et al. Prognostic significance of Bcl-2 protein expression and Bcl-2 gene rearrangement in diffuse aggressive non-Hodgkin's lymphoma. *Blood* 1997;90:244–251.
306. Kramer MH, Hermans J, Parker J, et al. Clinical significance of bcl2 and p53 protein expression in diffuse large B-cell lymphoma: a population-based study. *J Clin Oncol* 1996;14:2131–2138.
307. Sanchez E, Chacon I, Plaza MM, et al. Clinical outcome in diffuse large B-cell lymphoma is dependent on the relationship between different cell-cycle regulator proteins. *J Clin Oncol* 1998;16:1931–1939.
308. Skinnider B, Horsman D, Dupuis B, et al. Bcl-6 and Bcl-2 protein expression in diffuse large B-cell lymphoma and follicular lymphoma: correlation with 3q27 and 18q21 chromosomal abnormalities. *Hum Pathol* 1999;30:803–808.
309. De Leval L, Shipp M, Neuberger D, et al. Diffuse large B-cell lymphomas are tumors of germinal center origin. *Blood* 1999 (*in press*).
310. Kuppers R, Rajewski K, Hansmann ML. Diffuse large cell lymphomas are derived from mature B cells carrying V region genes with a high load of somatic mutation and evidence of selection for antibody expression. *Eur J Immunol* 1997;27:1398–1405.
311. Kramer M, Hermans J, Wijburg E, et al. Clinical relevance of BCL2,

BCL6 and MYC rearrangements in diffuse large B-cell lymphoma. *Blood* 1998;92:3152–3162.
312. Bastard C, Deweindt C, Kerckaert JP, et al. LAZ3 rearrangements in non-Hodgkin's lymphoma: correlation with histology, immunophenotype, karyotype, and clinical outcome in 217 patients. *Blood* 1994; 83:2423–2427.
313. Migliazza A, Martinotti S, Chen W, et al. Frequent somatic hypermutation of the 5′noncoding region of the BCL6 gene in B cell lymphoma. *Proc Natl Acad Sci USA* 1995;91:12520–12524.
314. Vitolo U, Gaidano G, Botto B, et al. Rearrangements of bcl-6, bcl-2, c-myc and 6q deletion in B-diffuse large-cell lymphoma: clinical relevance in 71 patients. *Ann Oncol* 1998;9:55–61.
315. Addis B, Isaacson P. Large cell lymphoma of the mediastinum: a B-cell tumor of probable thymic origin. *Histopathology* 1986;10: 379–390.
316. Lamarre L, Jacobson JO, Aisenberg AC, et al. Primary large cell lymphoma of the mediastinum: a histologic and immunophenotypic study of 29 cases. *Am J Surg Pathol* 1989;13:730–739.
317. Moller P, Moldenhauer G, Momburg F, et al. Mediastinal lymphoma of clear cell type is a tumor corresponding too terminal steps of B cell differentiation. *Blood* 1987;69:1087–1095.
318. Scarpa A, Bonetti F, Menestrina F. Mediastinal large cell lymphoma with sclerosis: genotypic analysis establishes its B nature. *Virchows Arch A* 1987;412:17–21.
319. Tsang P, Cesarman E, Chadburn A, et al. Molecular characterization of primary mediastinal B cell lymphoma. *Am J Pathol* 1996;148: 2017–2025.
320. Joos S, Otano-Joos MI, Ziegler S, et al. Primary mediastinal (thymic) B-cell lymphoma is characterized by gains of chromosomal material including 9p and amplification of the REL gene. *Blood* 1996;87: 1571–1578.
321. Jacobson J, Aisenberg A, Lamarre L, et al. Mediastinal large cell lymphoma: an uncommon subset of adult lymphoma curable with combined modality therapy. *Cancer* 1988;62:1893–1898.
322. Lazzarino M, Orlandi E, Paulli M, et al. Treatment outcome and prognostic factors for primary mediastinal (thymic) B-cell lymphoma: a multicenter study of 106 patients. *J Clin Oncol* 1997;15:1646–1653.
323. Ferry J, Harris N, Picker L, et al. Intravascular lymphomatosis (malignant angioendotheliomatosis): a B-cell neoplasm expressing surface homing receptors. *Mod Pathol* 1988;1:444–452.
324. DiGiuseppe J, Nelson W, Seifter E, et al. Intravascular lymphomatosis: a clinicopathologic study of 10 cases and assessment of response ot chemotherapy. *J Clin Oncol* 1994;12:2573–2579.
325. Grogan T, Warnke R, Kaplan H. A comparative study of Burkitt's and non-Burkitt's "undifferentiated" malignant lymphoma: immunologic, cytochemical, ultrastructural, cytologic, histopathologic, clinical and cell culture features. *Cancer* 1982;49:1817–1828.
326. Yano T, van Krieken J, Magrath I, et al. Histogenetic correlations between subcategories of small noncleaved cell lymphomas. *Blood* 1992;79:1282–1290.
327. Sweetenham JW, Pearce R, Taghipour G, et al. Adult Burkitt's and Burkitt-like non-Hodgkin's lymphoma: Outcome for patients treated with high-dose therapy and autologous stem-cell transplantation in first remission or at relapse. Results from the European Group for Blood and Marrow Transplantation. *J Clin Oncol* 1996;14: 2465–2472.
328. Garcia C, Weiss L, Warnke R. Small noncleaved cell lymphoma: an immunophenotypic study of 18 cases and comparison with large cell lymphoma. *Hum Pathol* 1986;17:454–461.
329. Falini B, Fizzotti M, Pileri S, et al. Bcl-6 protein expression in normal and neoplastic lymphoid tissues. *Ann Oncol* 1997;8[Suppl 2]: 101–104.
330. Carroll WL, Yu M, Link MP, et al. Absence of Ig V region gene somatic hypermutation in advanced Burkitt's lymphoma. *J Immunol* 1989;143:692.
331. Chapman C, Mockridge C, Rowe M, et al. Analysis of VH genes used by neoplastic B cells in endemic Burkitt's lymphoma shows somatic hypermutation and intraclonal heterogeneity. *Blood* 1995;85: 2176–2181.
332. Chapman CJ, Zhou JX, Gregory C, et al. VH and VL gene analysis in sporadic Burkitt's lymphoma shows somatic hypermutation, intraclonal heterogeneity, and a role for antigen selection. *Blood* 1996; 88:3562–3568.
333. Neri A, Barriga F, Knowles D, et al. Different regions of the immunoglobulin heavy-chain locus are involved in chromosomal translocations in distinct pathogenetic forms of Burkitt lymphoma. *Proc Natl Acad Sci USA* 1988;85:2748–2752.
334. Pelicci P, Knowles D, Magrath I, et al. Chromosomal breakpoints and structural alterations of the c-myc locus differ in endemic and sporadic forms of Burkitt lymphoma. *Proc Natl Acad Sci USA* 1986;83: 2984–2988.
335. Capello D, Carbone A, Pastore C, et al. Point mutations of the BCL-6 gene in Burkitt's lymphoma. *Br J Haematol* 1997;99:168–170.
336. Hamilton-Dutoit S, Pallesen G, Franzmann M, et al. AIDS-related lymphoma: histopathology, immunophenotype, and association with Epstein-Barr virus as demonstrated by in situ nucleic acid hybridization. *Am J Pathol* 1991;138:149–163.
337. Wright DH. What is Burkitt's lymphoma [Editorial]? *J Pathol* 1997; 182:125–127.
338. Magrath I, Shiramizu B. Biology and treatment of small non-cleaved cell lymphoma. *Oncology* 1989;3:41–53.
339. Bernard A, Boumsell L, Reinherz L, et al. Cell surface characterization of malignant T cells from lymphoblastic lymphoma using monoclonal antibodies: evidence for phenotypic differences between malignant T cells from patients with acute lymphoblastic leukemia and lymphoblastic lymphoma. *Blood* 1981;57:1105–1110.
340. Gouttefangeas C, Bensussan A, Boumsell L. Study of the CD3-associated T-cell receptors reveals further differences between T-cell acute lymphoblastic lymphoma and leukemia. *Blood* 1990;74:931–934.
341. Quintanilla L, Zukerberg LR, Harris NL. Pre-thymic adult lymphoblastic lymphoma. *Am J Surg Pathol* 1992;16:1075–1084.
342. Szczepanski T, Pongers-Willemse MJ, Langerak AW, et al. Ig heavy chain gene rearrangements in T-cell acute lymphoblastic leukemia exhibit predominant DH6-19 and DH7-27 gene usage, can result in complete V-D-J rearrangements, and are rare in T-cell receptor alpha beta lineage. *Blood* 1999;93:4079–4085.
343. Uckun FM, Sensel MG, Sun L, et al. Biology and treatment of childhood T-lineage acute lymphoblastic leukemia. *Blood* 1998;91: 735–746.
344. Begley CG, Green AR. The SCL gene: from case report to critical hematopoietic regulator. *Blood* 1999;93:2760–2770.
345. Brouet J, Sasportes M, Flandrin G, et al. Chronic lymphocytic leukemia of T cell origin. *Lancet* 1975;ii:890–893.
346. Bennett J, Catovsky D, Daniel M-T, et al. Proposals for the classification of chronic (mature) B and T lymphoid leukemias. *J Clin Pathol* 1989;42:567–584.
347. Matutes E, Brito-Babapulle V, Swansbury J, et al. Clinical and laboratory features of 78 cases of T-prolymphocytic leukemia. *Blood* 1991; 78:3269–3274.
348. Suchi T, Lennert K, Tu L-Y. Histopathology and immunohistochemistry of peripheral T-cell lymphomas: a proposal for their classification. *J Clin Pathol* 1987;40:995–1015.
349. Knowles D. The human T-cell leukemias: clinical, cytomorphologic, immunophenotypic, and genotypic characteristics. *Hum Pathol* 1986; 17:14–33.
350. Loughran T. Clonal diseases of large granular lymphocytes. *Blood* 1993;82:1–14.
351. Agnarsson B, Loughran T, Starkebaum G, et al. The pathology of large granular lymphocyte leukemia. *Hum Pathol* 1989;20:643–651.
352. Sood R, Stewart CC, Aplan PD, et al. Neutropenia associated with T-cell large granular lymphocyte leukemia: long-term response to cyclosporine therapy despite persistence of abnormal cells. *Blood* 1998; 91:3372–3378.
353. Gentile TC, Hadlock KG, Uner AH, et al. Large granular lymphocyte leukaemia occurring after renal transplantation. *Br J Haematol* 1998; 101:507–512.
354. Gelb AB, van de Rijn M, Regula DP Jr, et al. Epstein-Barr virus-associated natural killer-large granular lymphocyte leukemia. *Hum Pathol* 1994;25:953–960.
355. Gentile T, Uner A, Hutchison R, et al. CD3+, CD56+ aggressive variant of large granular lymphocyte leukemia. *Blood* 1994;84:2315.
356. Imamura N, Kusunoki Y, Kawa-Ha K, et al. Aggressive natural killer cell leukaemia/lymphoma: report of four cases and review of the literature. Possible existence of a new clinical entity originating from the third lineage of lymphoid cells. *Br J Haematol* 1990:49.
357. Kwong Y, Chan A, Liang R. Natural killer cell lymphoma/leukemia: pathology and treatment. *Hematol Oncol* 1997;15:71–79.
358. Soler J, Bordes R, Ortuni F, et al. Aggressive natural killer cell leukae-

mia/lymphoma in two patients with lethal midline granuloma. *Br J Haematol* 1994;86:659–662.
359. Pittaluga S, Wiodarska I, Pulford K, et al. The monoclonal antibody ALK1 identifies a distinct morphological subtype of anaplastic large cell lymphoma associated with 2p23/ALK rearrangements. *Am J Pathol* 1997;151:343–351.
360. Pulford K, Lamant L, Morris S, et al. Detection of anplastic lymphoma kinase (ALK) and nucleolar protein nucleophosmin (NPM)-ALD proteins in normal and neoplastic cells with the monoclonal antibody ALK1. *Blood* 1997;89:1394–1404.
361. de Bruin P, Beljaards R, van Heerde P, et al. Differences in clinical behaviour and immunophenotype between primary cutaneous and primary nodal anaplastic large cell lymphoma of T-cell or null cell phenotype. *Histopathology* 1993;23:127–135.
362. Ott G, Katzenberger T, Siebert R, et al. Chromosomal abnormalities in nodal and extranodal CD30 + anaplastic large cell lymphomas: infrequent detection of the t(2;5) in extranodal lymphomas. *Genes Chromosomes Cancer* 1998;22:114–121.
363. Kaudewitz P, Stein H, Dallenbach F, et al. Primary and secondary cutaneous Ki-1 + (CD30 +) anaplastic large cell lymphomas: morphologic, immunohistologic, and clinical characteristics. *Am J Pathol* 1989;135:359–367.
364. Chan JKC, Sin VC, Wong KF, et al. Nonnasal lymphoma expressing the natural killer cell marker CD56: a clinicopathologic study of 49 cases of an uncommon aggressive neoplasm. *Blood* 1997;89: 4501–4513.
365. Chan J, Ng C, Lau W, et al. Most nasal/nasopharyngeal lymphomas are peripheral T cell neoplasms. *Am J Surg Pathol* 1987;11:418–429.
366. Jaffe E, Chan J, Su I, et al. Report of the workshop on nasal and related extranodal angiocentric T/NK cell lymphomas: definitions, differential diagnosis, and epidemiology. *Am J Surg Pathol* 1996;20: 103–111.
367. Ho F, Choy D, Loke S, et al. Polymorphic reticulosis and conventional lymphomas of the nose and upper aerodigestive tract: a clinicopathologic study of 70 cases, and immunophenotypic studies of 16 cases. *Hum Pathol* 1990;21:1041–1050.
368. Ferry J, Sklar J, Zukerberg L, et al. Nasal lymphoma: a clinicopathologic study with immunophenotypic and genotypic analysis. *Am J Surg Pathol* 1991;15:268–279.
369. Elenitoba-Johnson KS, Zarate-Osorno A, Meneses A, et al. Cytotoxic granular protein expression, Epstein-Barr virus strain type, and latent membrane protein-1 oncogene deletions in nasal T-lymphocyte/natural killer cell lymphomas from Mexico. *Modern Pathology* 1998;11: 754–761.
370. Chan JK, Yip TT, Tsang WY, et al. Detection of Epstein-Barr viral RNA in malignant lymphomas of the upper aerodigestive tract [published erratum appears in *Am J Surg Pathol* 1994;18:1274]. *Am J Surg Pathol* 1994;18:938–946.
371. Ho F, Srivastava G, Loke S, et al. Presence of Epstein-barr virus DNA in nasal lymphomas of B and T cell type. *Hematol Oncol* 1990;8: 271–281.
372. Lipford E, Margolich J, Longo D, et al. Angiocentric immunoproliferative lesions: a clinicopathologic spectrum of post-thymic T cell proliferations. *Blood* 1988;5:1674–1681.
373. Cuadra-Garcia I, Harris N, Proulx G, et al. Sinonasal lymphoma: an analysis of 57 cases. *Mod Pathol* 1999;12.
374. Cuadra-Garcia I, Proulx G, Wu C, et al. Sinonasal lymphoma: a clinicopathologic analysis of 58 cases. *Am J Surg Pathol* 1999;23: 1356–1369.
375. Isaacson P, Spencer J, Connolly C, et al. Malignant histiocytosis of the intestine: a T-cell lymphoma. *Lancet* 1985;ii:688–691.
376. Chott A, Dragosics B, Radaszkiewicz T. Peripheral T-cell lymphomas of the intestine. *Am J Pathol* 1992;141:1361–1371.
377. Ashton-Key M, Diss TC, Pan L, et al. Molecular analysis of T-cell clonality in ulcerative jejunitis and enteropathy-associated T-cell lymphoma. *Am J Pathol*1997;151:493–498.
378. Murray A, Cuevas EC, Jones DB, et al. Study of the immunohistochemistry and T cell clonality of enteropathy-associated T cell lymphoma. *Am J Pathol* 1995;146:509–519.
379. Carbonnel F, Grollet-Bioul L, Brouet JC, et al. Are complicated forms of celiac disease cryptic T-cell lymphomas? *Blood* 1998;92: 3879–3886.
380. Spencer J, Cerf-Bensussan N, Jarry A, et al. Enteropathy-associated T-cell lymphoma is recognized by a monoclonal antibody (HML-1) that defines a membrane molecule on human mucosal lymphocytes. *Am J Pathol* 1988;132:1–5.
381. Daum S, Foss HD, Anagnostopoulos I, et al. Expression of cytotoxic molecules in intestinal T-cell lymphomas: the German Study Group on Intestinal Non-Hodgkin Lymphoma. *J Pathol* 1997;182:311–317.
382. de Bruin PC, Connolly CE, Oudejans JJ, et al. Enteropathy-associated T-cell lymphomas have a cytotoxic T-cell phenotype [published erratum appears in *Histopathology* 1997;31:578]. *Histopathology* 1997; 31:313–317.
383. Howell WM, Leung ST, Jones DB, et al. HLA-DRB, -DQA, and -DQB polymorphism in celiac disease and enteropathy-associated T-cell lymphoma: common features and additional risk factors for malignancy. *Hum Immunol* 1995;43:29–37.
384. Collin P, Reunala T, Pukkala E, et al. Coeliac disease—associated disorders and survival [See comments]. *Gut* 1994;35:1215–1218.
385. Egan LJ, Stevens FM, McCarthy CF. Celiac disease and T-cell lymphoma [Letter, comment]. *N Engl J Med* 1996;335:1611–1612.
386. Case records of the Massachusetts General Hospital. Weekly clinicopathological exercises: Case 15-1996. A 79-year-old woman with anorexia, weight loss, and diarrhea after treatment for celiac disease [clinical conference; see comments]. *N Engl J Med* 1996;334: 1316–1322.
387. Mantovani G, Esu S, Astara G, et al. Primary T cell CD30-positive anaplastic large-cell lymphoma associated with adult-onset celiac disease and presenting with skin lesions. *Acta Haematol* 1995;94:48–51.
388. Shiboski CH, Greenspan D, Dodd CL, et al. Oral T-cell lymphoma associated with celiac sprue: a case report. *Oral Surg Oral Med Oral Pathol* 1993;76:54–58.
389. Gaulard P, Bourquelot P, Kanavaaros P. Expression of the $\alpha\beta$ and $\gamma\delta$T cell receptors in 57 cases of peripheral Tcell lymphomas: identification of a subset of $\gamma\delta$ T cell lymphomas. *Am J Pathol* 1990;137: 617–628.
390. Farcet J, Gaulard P, Marolleau J, et al. Hepatosplenic T-cell lymphoma: sinusal/sinusoidal localization af malignant cells expressing the T-cell receptor $\gamma\delta$. *Blood* 1990;75:2213–2219.
391. Boulland ML, Kanavaros P, Wechsler J, et al. Cytotoxic protein expression in natural killer cell lymphomas and in alpha beta and gamma delta peripheral T-cell lymphomas. *J Pathol* 1997;183: 432–439.
392. Salhany KE, Feldman M, Kahn MJ, et al. Hepatosplenic gammadelta T-cell lymphoma: ultrastructural, immunophenotypic, and functional evidence for cytotoxic T lymphocyte differentiation. *Hum Pathol* 1997;28:674–685.
393. Cooke CB, Krenacs L, Stetler-Stevenson M, et al. Hepatosplenic T-cell lymphoma: a distinct clinicopathologic entity of cytotoxic gamma delta T-cell origin [See comments]. *Blood* 1996;88:4265–4274.
394. François A, Lesesve J-F, Stamatoullas A, et al. Hepatosplenic gamma/delta T-cell lymphoma: a report of two cases in immunocompromised patients, associated with isochromosome 7q. *Am J Surg Pathol* 1997; 21:781–790.
395. Wang CC, Tien HF, Lin MT, et al. Consistent presence of isochromosome 7q in hepatosplenic T gamma/delta lymphoma: a new cytogenetic-clinicopathologic entity. *Genes Chromosomes Cancer* 1995;12: 161–164.
396. Jonveaux P, Daniel MT, Martel V, et al. Isochromosome 7q and trisomy 8 are consistent primary, non-random chromosomal abnormalities associated with hepatosplenic T gamma/delta lymphoma. *Leukemia* 1996;10:1453–1455.
397. Wong KF, Chan JKC, Matutes E. Hepatosplenic $\gamma\delta$T cell lymphoma: a distinctive aggressive lymphoma type. *Am J Surg Pathol* 1995;19: 718–726.
398. Cooke C, Greiner T, Raffeld M, et al. $\gamma\delta$T-cell lymphoma: a distinct clinicopathologic entity. *Mod Pathol* 1994;7:106A.
399. Ross CW, Schnitzer B, Scheldon S, et al. $\gamma\delta$T cell postransplantiation lymphoproliferative disorder primarily in the spleen. *Am J Clin Pathol* 1994;102:310–315.
400. Arnulf B, Copie-Bergman C, Delfau-Larue MH, et al. Nonhepatosplenic gamma delta T-cell lymphoma: a subset of cytotoxic lymphomas with mucosal or skin localization. *Blood* 1998;91:1723–1731.
401. Takimoto Y, Imanaka F, Sasaki N, et al. Gamma/delta T cell lymphoma presenting in the subcutaneous tissue and small intestine in a patient with capillary leak syndrome. *Int J Hematol* 1998;68:183–191.
402. Gonzalez C, Medeiros L, Braziel R, et al. T-cell lymphoma involving

subcutaneous tissue: a clinicopathologic entity commonly associated with hemophagocytic syndrome. *Am J Surg Pathol* 1991;15:17–27.
403. Salhany KE, Macon WR, Choi JK, et al. Subcutaneous panniculitis-like T-cell lymphoma: clinicopathologic, immunophenotypic, and genotypic analysis of alpha/beta and gamma/delta subtypes. *Am J Surg Pathol* 1998;22:881–893.
404. Kumar S, Krenacs L, Medeiros J, et al. Subcutaneous panniculitic T-cell lymphoma is a tumor of cytotoxic T lymphocytes. *Hum Pathol* 1998;29:397–403.
405. Weiss L, Crabtree G, Rouse R, et al. Morphologic and immunologic characterization of 50 peripheral T-cell lymphomas. *Am J Pathol* 1985;118:316–324.
406. Medeiros L, Lardelli P, Stetler-Stevenson M, et al. Genotypic analysis of diffuse, mixed cell lymphomas: comparison with morphologic and immunophenotypic findings. *Am J Clin Pathol* 1991;95:547.
407. Patsouris E, Noel H, Lennert K. Histological and immunohistological findings in lymphoepithelioid cell lymphoma (Lennert's lymphoma). *Am J Surg Pathol* 1988;12:341–350.
408. Weisenburger D, Linder J, Armitage J. Peripheral T cell lymphoma: a clinicopathologic study of 42 cases. *Hematol Oncol* 1987;5:175–187.
409. Borowitz M, Reichert T, Brynes R, et al. The phenotypic diversity of peripheral T-cell lymphomas: the Southeastern Cancer Study Group experience. *Hum Pathol* 1986;17:567.
410. Weiss L, Trela M, Cleary M, et al. Frequent immunoglobulin and T cell receptor gene rearrangement in "histiocytic" neoplasms. *Am J Pathol* 1985;121:369–373.
411. Weiss L, Picker L, Grogan T, et al. Absence of clonal beta and gamma T-cell receptor gene rearrangements in a subset of peripheral T-cell lymphomas. *Am J Pathol* 1988;130:436–443.
412. Falini B, Pileri S, De Solas I, et al. Peripheral T-cell lymphoma associated with hemophagocytic syndrome. *Blood* 1990;75:434–444.
413. Armitage J, Greer J, Levine A, et al. Peripheral T-cell lymphoma. *Cancer* 1989;63:158–163.
414. Lippman S, Miller T, Spier C, et al. The prognostic significance of the immunotype in diffuse large-cell lymphoma: a comparative study of the T-cell and B-cell phenotype. *Blood* 1988;72:436–441.
415. Coiffier B, Brousse N, Peuchmaur M, et al. Peripheral T-cell lymphomas have a worse prognosis than B-cell lymphomas: a prospective study of 361 immunophenotyped patients treated with the LNH-84 regimen. *Ann Oncol* 1990;1:45–50.
416. Feller A, Griesser H, Schilling C, et al. Clonal gene rearrangement patterns correlate with immunophenotype and clinical parameters in patients with angioimmunoblastic lymphadenopathy. *Am J Pathol* 1988;133:549–556.
417. Weiss L, Strickler J, Dorfman R, et al. Clonal T-cell populations in angioimmunoblastic lymphadenopathy and angioimmunoblastic lymphadenopathy-like lymphoma. *Am J Pathol* 1986;122:392–397.
418. Anagnostopoulos I, Hummel M, Finn T, et al. Heterogeneous Epstein-Barr virus infection patterns in peripheral T-cell lymphoma of angioimmunoblastic lymphadenopathy type. *Blood* 1992;80:1804–1812.
419. Weiss L, Jaffe E, Liu X, et al. Detection and localization of Epstein-Barr viral genomes in angioimmunoblastic lymphadenopathy and antioimmunoblastic lymphadenopathy-like lymphomas. *Blood* 1992; 79:1789.
420. Schlegelberger B, Feller A, Godde W, et al. Stepwise development of chromosomal abnormalities in angioimmunoblastic lymphadenopathy. *Cancer Genet Cytogenet* 1990;50:15.
421. Frizzera G, Moran E, Rappaport H. Angio-immunoblastic lymphadenopathy with dysproteinemia. *Lancet* 1974;i:1070–1073.
422. Benharroch D, Meguerian-Bedoyan Z, Lamant L, et al. ALK-positive lymphoma: a single disease with a broad spectrum of morphology. *Blood* 1998;91:2076–2084.
423. Stein H, Mason D, Gerdes J, et al. The expression of the Hodgkin's disease associated antigen Ki-1 in reactive and neoplastic lymphoid tissue: evidence that Reed-Sternberg cells and histiocytic malignancies are derived from activated lymphoid cells. *Blood* 1985;66: 848–858.
424. Chan J, NG C, Hui P, et al. Anaplastic large cell Ki-1 lymphoma: delineation of two morphological types. *Histopathology* 1989;15: 11–34.
425. Pileri S, Falini B, Delsol G, et al. Lymphohistiocytic T-cell lymphoma (anaplastic large cell lymphoma CD30+/Ki1+) with a high content of reactive histiocytes. *Histopathology* 1990;16:383–391.
426. Kinney M, Collins R, Greer J, et al. A small-cell-predominant variant of primary Ki-1 (CD30)+ T-cell lymphoma. *Am J Surg Pathol* 1993; 17:859–868.
427. Falini B, Bigerna B, Fizzotti M, et al. ALK expression defines a distinct group of T/null lymphomas ("ALK lymphomas") with a wide morphological spectrum. *Am J Pathol* 1998;153:875–886.
428. Pileri S, Bocchia M, Baroni C, et al. Anaplastic large cell lymphoma (CD30+/Ki-1+): results of a prospective clinicopathologic study of 69 cases. *Br J Haematol* 1994;86:513–523.
429. Zinzani P, Bendandi M, Martelli M, et al. Anaplastic large cell lymphoma (Ki-1/CD30+): clinical and prognostic evaluation of 90 adult patients. *J Clin Oncol* 1996;14:955.
430. Pittaluga S, Pulford K, Wlodarska I, et al. ALK-1 antibody staining pattern in anaplastic large cell lymphoma (ALCL) and ALCL-Hodgkin's like. *Mod Pathol* 1997;10:132A.
431. Kanzler H, Hansmann ML, Kapp U, et al. Hodgkin and Reed Sternberg cells in Hodgkin's disease represent the outgrowth of a dominant tumor clone derived from (crippled) germinal center B cells. *J Exp Med* 1996;184:1495–1505.
432. Kuppers R, Rajewsky K, Zhao M, et al. Hodgkin's disease: Hodgkin and Reed Sternberg cells picked from histological sections show clonal immunoglobulin gene rearrangements and appear to be derived from B cells at various stages of development. *Proc Natl Acad Sci USA* 1994;91:1092–1096.
433. Hummel M, Ziemann K, Lammert H, et al. Hodgkin's disease with monoclonal and polyclonal populations of Reed-Sternberg cells. *N Engl J Med* 1995;333:901–906.
434. Sundeen J, Lipford E, Uppenkamp J, et al. Rearranged antigen receptor genes in Hodgkin's disease. *Blood* 1987;70:96–103.
435. Weiss L, Strickler J, Hu E, et al. Immunoglobulin gene rearrangements in tissues involved by Hodgkin's disease. *Hum Pathol* 1986;17: 1006–1014.
436. Zinzani P, Martelli M, Magagnoli M, et al. Anaplastic large cell lymphoma, Hodgkin's-like: a randomized trial of ABVD versus MACOP-B with and without radiation therapy. *Blood* 1998;92:790–794.
437. Foss H, Anagnostopoulos I, Aranjo I, et al. Anaplastic large-cell lymphomas of T-cell and null-cell phenotype express cytotoxic molecules. *Blood* 1996;88:4005–4011.
438. Krenacs L, Wellman A, Sorbara L, et al. Cytoxic cell antigen expression in anaplastic large cell lymphomas of T- and null-cell type and Hodgkin's disease: evidence for distinct cellular origin. *Blood* 1997; 89:980–999.
439. Shiota M, Nakamura S, Ichinohasama R, et al. Anaplastic large cell lymphomas expressing the novel chimeric protein p80NPM/ALK: a distinct clinicopathologic entity. *Blood* 1995;86:1954–1960.
440. Mason D, Bastard C, Rimokh R, et al. CD30-positive large cell lymphomas ("Ki-1 lymphoma") are associated with a chromosomal translocation involving 5q35. *Br J Haematol* 1990;74:161–168.
441. Weisenburger D, Gordon B, Vose J, et al. Occurrence of the t(2; 5)(p23;q35) in non-Hodgkin's lymphoma. *Blood* 1996;87: 3860–3868.
442. Downing J, Shurtleff S, Zielenska M, et al. Molecular detection of the (2;5) translocation of non-Hodgkin's lymphoma by reverse transcriptase-polymerase chain reaction. *Blood* 1995;85:3416–3422.
443. Sandlund J, Pui C-H, Roberts W, et al. Clinicopathologic features and treatment outcome of children with large-cell lymphoma and the t(2; 5)(p23;q35). *Blood* 1994;84:2467–2471.
444. Wlodarska I, De Wolf-Peeters C, Falini B, et al. The cryptic inv(2)(p23q35) defines a new molecular genetic subtype of ALK-positive anaplastic large-cell lymphoma. *Blood* 1998;92:2688–2695.
445. Reiter A, Schrappe M, Tiemann M, et al. Successful treatment strategy for Ki-1 anaplastic large-cell lymphoma of childhood: a prospective analysis of 62 patients enrolled in three consecutive Berlin-Frankfurt-Munster group studies. *J Clin Oncol* 1994;12:899–908.
446. Sandlund J, Pui C-H, Santana V, et al. Clinical features and treatment outcome for children with CD30+ large-cell non-Hodgkin's lymphoma. *J Clin Oncol* 1994;12:895–898.
447. Greer J, Kinney M, Collins R, et al. Clinical features of 31 patients with Ki-1 anaplastic large-cell lymphoma. *J Clin Oncol* 1991;9: 539–547.
448. William of Okham. Quodlibeta. Miner M, Rawson H, editors. *The new international dictionary of quotations*. 2nd edition. NY: Penguin. 1997, p. 373.
449. Einstein A. Miner M, Rawson H, editors. *The new international dictionary of quotations.* 2nd edition. NY: Penguin. 1997, p. 394.

CHAPTER 20

Clinical Relevance of the Revised European–American Classification of Non-Hodgkin's Lymphomas

James O. Armitage

The ability of clinicians to care for patients with non-Hodgkin's lymphomas is tremendously influenced by the ability of pathologists to identify clinically relevant subgroups of patients. Throughout this century, our ability to group patients in clinically relevant categories has improved steadily. The distinction between Hodgkin's disease and non-Hodgkin's lymphoma was an important step. Improvements in the subclassification of non-Hodgkin's lymphomas, however, have been slow and, at times, agonizingly difficult.

Early methods for subclassifying non-Hodgkin's lymphomas focused almost exclusively on morphology, with some modifications based on immunologic typing. Non-Hodgkin's lymphomas were grouped based on cell size, shape, and growth pattern (1,2). The lymphomas, in some classifications, were divided into those of T cell or B cell origin (3–5). These systems had clinical relevance in that they identified subgroups with differing responses to therapy and survival. They would have been more helpful to clinicians, however, if they could have been applied accurately. Unfortunately, tests of the reproducibility of systems based primarily on morphology showed that they could divide non-Hodgkin's lymphomas into subtypes accurately only 50% to 60% of the time (6–8). Although not widely discussed, this problem slowed clinical research and made it difficult to identify specific subgroups of lymphoma in which unique therapies might be utilized.

New biologic insights in the 1980s and 1990s gave hope that it might be possible to improve our ability to identify specific subgroups of non-Hodgkin's lymphomas that represent "real" diseases. The recognition that certain groups of patients displayed unique genetic abnormalities was an important step in this regard. The existence of the translocation t(11;14) and the associated *BCL1* oncogene made it possible to recognize mantle cell lymphoma as a specific entity (9–18). In addition to the discovery of the CD30 antigen, discovery of t(2;5) led to recognition of anaplastic large T- or null cell lymphoma as a unique clinical entity (19–28). The discovery of the association of infection by *Helicobacter pylori* with a CD5-negative ($CD5^-$)small round cell lymphoma of the stomach was key in the development of the concept of mucosa-associated lymphoid tissue (MALT) lymphomas (29–34).

When these and other observations brought together a group of hematopathologists who called themselves the International Lymphoma Study Group in the early 1990s, an important step was taken toward revising our thinking about subdividing non-Hodgkin's lymphomas. The Revised European–American Classification of Lymphoid Neoplasms (REAL) brought together entities recognized through the knowledge accumulated to that point (35). Its most important contribution, however, was to change the emphasis on morphologic entities and instead try to identify clinical and pathologic entities that represented "real" diseases.

The REAL classification represented an important step forward in changing the way we think about non-Hodgkin's lymphomas. Many of the same ideas were being incorporated into the Working Formulation and the Kiel classification at the same time (36–38). The REAL classification, however, attempted to "wipe the slate clean" and change the way clinicians and pathologists think about non-Hodgkin's lymphomas. The proposal was important but needed to be tested to determine its ability to be applied clinically.

J. O. Armitage: College of Medicine, University of Nebraska Medical Center, Omaha, Nebraska 68198

INTERNATIONAL NON-HODGKIN'S LYMPHOMA CLASSIFICATION STUDY

Following the publication of the REAL classification, a group of experienced clinicians, pathologists, and biostatisticians joined together to test the application of this new approach (39). Specific goals of the study were to evaluate the ability of hematopathologists to apply the REAL classification to cases selected at sites around the world, to determine the role of immunophenotyping and knowledge of clinical data in diagnosis, to determine the clinical importance of immunophenotyping, to determine the intraobserver and interobserver reproducibility of diagnosis, to determine the clinical characteristics of the various entities, and to determine whether certain subgroups could be grouped together for prognostic or therapeutic purposes. The clinicians, pathologists, and biostatisticians who participated in the study are listed in Table 20.1. An attempt was made in choosing institutions to select those that as much as possible saw patients characteristic for the region.

Methods

Nine institutions in eight countries were chosen to provide up to 200 consecutive cases of previously untreated non-Hodgkin's lymphoma that were representative of the geographic region during the time between January 1, 1988, and December 31, 1990. The first 200 cases at each site that fulfilled the criteria were selected for the study. In all cases, tissue biopsy samples that were adequate for diagnosis and classification were required, and all diagnostic pathology materials obtained before initial therapy, including positive bone marrow specimens, were included in the pathology review. Immunologic characterization as to B- or T-cell origin, by whatever means in use at the institution, also was required in all cases. Leukemias were excluded from the study unless a biopsy of tissue other than bone marrow was performed before therapy. Clinical characteristics, treatment data, and some follow-up information also were required in all cases. The nine study sites, which provided a total of 1,403 cases, are shown in Table 20.2.

TABLE 20.2. *Number of cases by study site*

Site	Cases
Omaha, Nebraska	200
Vancouver, Canada	202
Cape Town, South Africa	196
London, UK	120
Locarno, Switzerland	80
Lyon, France	195
Wurzburg/Gottingen, Germany	210
Hong Kong	200

The clinical information for each case was abstracted from the medical record by a clinician or data manager and recorded on a standardized form for direct computerized data entry. These data included coded patient and site identifiers; patient gender, ethnic origin, and date of birth; the date and site of the diagnostic biopsy; and a tabulation of nodal and extranodal sites of involvement and Ann Arbor stage at the time of initial diagnosis. Laboratory data were recorded, in-

TABLE 20.1. *Participants in planning and carrying out the clinical evaluation of the REAL classification*

Category	Name	Institution
Site pathologists	Wing C. Chan	University of Nebraska
	Randy Gascoyne	Vancouver, Canada
	Pauline Close	Cape Town, South Africa
	Andrew Norton	London, UK
	Ennio Pedrinis	Lugano, Switzerland
	Francoise Berger	Lyon, France
	Faith Ho	Hong Kong, China
	German Ott	Wurzburg, Germany
	Alfred Schauer	Gottingen, Germany
Visiting pathologists	Jacques Diebold	Paris, France
	Kenneth A. MacLennan	Leeds, UK
	H. Konrad Muller-Hermelink	Wurzburg, Germany
	Bharat Nathwani	Los Angeles, California
	Dennis D. Weisenburger	Omaha, Nebraska
Consulting pathologist	Nancy L. Harris	Boston, Massachusetts
Clinicians	James O. Armitage	Omaha, Nebraska
	Joseph Connors	Vancouver, Canada
	Peter Jacobs	Cape Town, South Africa
	T. Andrew Lister	London, UK
	Franco Cavalli	Lugano, Switzerland
	Bertrand Coiffier	Lyon, France
	Raymond Ling	Hong Kong, China
	Wolfgang Hiddeman	Gottingen, Germany
Consulting clinician	Saul Rosenburg	Palo Alto, California
Biostatisticians	James R. Anderson	Omaha, Nebraska
	Pascal Roy	Lyon, France

cluding the serum lactate dehydrogenase level, absolute lymphocyte count, presence of circulating lymphoma cells, presence of monoclonal serum immunoglobulins, and a history of immunodeficiency and viral (human T-cell lymphotrophic virus type 1, [HTLV-1], human immunodeficiency virus [HIV]) status. Also recorded were the performance status and maximum diameter of the largest tumor mass. The initial therapy and therapeutic response, details of remission, progression, or relapse, and subsequent therapies and follow-up were tabulated in each case. For this report, all cases with clinical data were included regardless of the specific therapies given. For 73 patients, sufficient data were not available for the clinical and survival analyses.

At each institution, the pathology slides and reports for each patient were reviewed carefully by a designated site pathologist. The original stained slides and immunostains were organized for review, and additional sections, immunostains, and other studies were performed if deemed necessary by the site pathologist. The results of the immunologic studies for each case, as well as any available cytogenetic or molecular genetic data, were recorded on a standardized form for direct computerized data entry. Five expert hematopathologists then traveled as a group to each of the nine sites to review and classify each case in each of the three major classifications. The site visits occurred over a period of 8 months beginning in June 1995. All expert pathologists used a standard Labophot-2 microscope (Nikon, Melville, NY), including a 10× plan achromat objective lens (high-power field, 0.159 mm^2). The diagnostic categories in each of the three classifications were used according to published criteria. More specific criteria were developed for some of the entities, with Dr. Nancy L. Harris providing consultation regarding the International Lymphoma Study Group classification. The criteria of Mann and Berard (40) were used to grade follicular lymphoma in the International Lymphoma Study Group classification.

At each site, the diagnostic slides were reviewed and classified independently by each expert hematopathologist. The initial classification was based on examination of the hematoxylin and eosin– or Giemsa-stained slides with only the following clinical information from the time of initial diagnosis: patient age and sex, site of the biopsy, and the major site of disease (i.e., diagnosis 1). After recording a diagnosis in each classification, the expert was presented with the immunophenotypic profile, along with any available cytogenetic and molecular genetic data, and the immunostains or flow cytometry report. After review, a second diagnosis was rendered in each classification (i.e., diagnosis 2). The expert then was presented with all of the pretreatment clinical information, and a third diagnosis was made in each classification (i.e., diagnosis 3). No previous diagnosis could be changed based on information subsequently revealed. If a case was considered unclassifiable in any of the classifications, the expert was required to give a reason, such as inadequate material, poor slide preparation, additional phenotyping needed, or additional information needed. The expert was allowed to change the phenotype of a case if he or she interpreted the immunostains or phenotype data differently than the site pathologist. For some diagnostic categories, a research protocol also was completed by the expert pathologist. All information was recorded on standardized forms for direct computerized data entry. Approximately 40 to 50 cases were reviewed by each pathologist each day.

In addition to the independent diagnoses rendered by each of the expert pathologists, a consensus diagnosis also was reached in each case. A consensus was considered to have been reached if at least four of the five expert pathologists agreed on the third diagnosis (diagnosis 3) in the International Lymphoma Study Group classification. Diagnoses of follicular lymphoma of any grade were considered in agreement, and diagnoses of peripheral T-cell lymphoma of any type also were considered in agreement. In these two categories, agreement by three of the five expert pathologists with regard to the specific type was considered the consensus diagnosis; if there was no agreement with regard to the type, the case was arbitrated by Dr. Dennis Weisenburger based on the individual diagnoses and the research protocol. All other cases without a consensus diagnosis were reviewed jointly on a multiheaded microscope and discussed by the five expert pathologists and the site pathologist in a consensus conference at the end of each day, and an attempt was made to reach a consensus of at least four expert pathologists in each case. If additional sections, immunostains, molecular studies, or other information were required, a diagnostic algorithm was developed by the group and the additional materials were obtained, if possible, and reviewed at a subsequent consensus conference at the site. If the additional materials could not be obtained during the site visit, the required materials and information were sent to Dr. Weisenburger, who arbitrated the case based on the algorithm.

At the end of each site visit, after all cases had been reviewed, each expert pathologist rereviewed 20% of the cases. The cases for rereview were selected randomly by the statisticians. These cases were classified a second time by each expert, without knowledge of his or her initial interpretation, using all available pathology materials and pretreatment clinical information. Cases in which a consensus diagnosis had not yet been reached were excluded from the rereview.

Completed clinical and pathology forms were rereviewed and edited to detect any inconsistencies, and additional information or clarification was obtained if needed. After completion of the editing, the clinical and pathology data forms were entered into a computer for data analysis. The International Prognostic Index (41) was used to stratify patients within the various disease entities. Treatment outcome was measured using failure-free survival and overall survival. Duration of failure-free survival was defined as the time from diagnosis to the first occurrence of progression, relapse after response, or death from any cause. Follow-up of patients not experiencing one of these events was censored at their dates of last contact. Overall duration of survival was measured from diagnosis to death from any cause, with surviving patient

TABLE 20.3. *Distribution of non-Hodgkin's lymphoma cases by the consensus diagnosis*

Consensus diagnosis	No. of cases	% of total cases
Diffuse large B-cell	422	30.6
Follicular	304	22.1
Grade 1	131	9.5
Grade 2	85	6.2
Grade 3	88	6.4
Marginal zone B-cell, MALT	105	7.6
Peripheral T-cell	96	7.0
Medium-sized, mixed, and large	51	3.7
Angiocentric, nasal	19	1.4
Angioimmunoblastic	17	1.2
Intestinal	5	<1.0
Lymphoepithelioid	2	<1.0
Hepatosplenic	1	<1.0
Adult T-cell leukemia/ lymphoma	1	<1.0
Small B-lymphocytic (chronic lymphocytic leukemia)	93	6.7
Mantle cell	83	6.0
Primary mediastinal large B-cell	33	2.4
Anaplastic large T/null-cell	33	2.4
High grade B-cell, Burkitt-like	29	2.1
Marginal zone B-cell, nodal	25	1.8
Precursor T-lymphoblastic	23	1.7
Lymphoplasmacytoid	16	1.2
Marginal zone B-cell, splenic	11	<1.0
Mycosis fungoides	11	<1.0
Burkitt's	10	<1.0
All other types	84	6.1

MALT, mucosa-associated lymphoid tissue.

follow-up censored at the last contact date. Estimates of failure-free survival and overall survival distribution were calculated using the method of Kaplan and Meier (42). Time-to-event distributions were compared using the log-rank test (43).

Study Results

Of the 1,403 patients, 25 (1.8%) were found to have a diagnosis other than non-Hodgkin's lymphoma and were excluded from further analysis. The types of non-Hodgkin's lymphoma found in the remaining 1,378 cases are presented in Table 20.3. Approximately 31% of the patients had forms of diffuse large B-cell lymphoma, and approximately 22% of the cases had types of follicular lymphoma. All types of T-cell processes, including natural killer cell disorders, made up only 12% of the cases. Small lymphocytic lymphoma was observed in 6.7% of the cases, a higher percentage than sometimes is seen. The major newly recognized types of lymphoma that occurred most frequently were marginal zone B-cell lymphoma of MALT type (7.6%), mantle cell lymphoma (6.0%), primary mediastinal large B-cell lymphoma (2.4%), and anaplastic large T- or null cell lymphoma (2.4%). Only 2.8% of the 1,378 cases of non-Hodgkin's lymphoma could not be classified specifically using this system, usually because of technical factors.

Three diagnoses were made by each expert pathologist in each case: one based on only histology, the second on histology and immunophenotype data, and the third on a combination of histology, immunophenotype, and clinical data. In Table 20.4, the percentage of the review diagnoses that agreed with the consensus diagnosis is given for each major histologic type. For most of the histologic types, the percentage of third review diagnoses (using all available data) that

TABLE 20.4. *Expert pathologist agreement with the consensus diagnosis*

Consensus diagnosis	Diagnosis 1,[a] %	Change from 1 to 2, %	Diagnosis 2,[b] %	Change from 2 to 3, %	Diagnosis 3,[c] %
Follicular, any grade	93	1	94	0	94
Grade 1	72	1	73	0	73
Grade 2	61	0	61	0	61
Grade 3	60	1	61	0	61
Marginal zone B-cell, MALT	84	2	86	0	86
Small lymphocytic (chronic lymphocytic leukemia)	84	3	87	0	87
Lymphoplasmacytoid	53	3	56	0	56
High grade B-cell, Burkitt's-like	47	6	53	0	53
Primary mediastinal large B-cell	51	7	58	37	85
Marginal zone B-cell, nodal	55	8	63	0	63
Mantle cell	77	10	87	0	87
Diffuse large B-cell	73	14	87	0	87
Precursor T-lymphoblastic	52	35	87	2	89
Anaplastic large T/null-cell	46	39	85	0	85
Peripheral T-cell, all types	41	45	86	0	86

[a] Diagnosis 1 based only on histology.
[b] Diagnosis 2 based on histology and immunophenotype.
[c] Diagnosis 3 based on histology, immunophenotype, and clinical data.
MALT, mucosa-associated lymphoid tissue.

TABLE 20.5. *Pathologist agreement on re-review of 20% of the cases*

	Diagnosis 3/ consensus,[a] %	Near-miss,[b] %	None, %
Overall agreement	85	94	6
Expert pathologist			
A	89	97	3
B	87	96	4
C	85	93	7
D	82	93	7
E	82	92	8

[a] Agreement with either diagnosis 3 or the consensus diagnosis.
[b] Agreement including near-miss diagnosis.

agreed with the consensus diagnosis equaled or exceeded 85%. The agreement was only 53% for high-grade B-cell Burkitt's-like tumors, in which distinctions between Burkitt's lymphoma and diffuse large B-cell lymphoma often proved difficult. The agreement also was below 85% for lymphoplasmacytoid lymphoma and nodal marginal zone B-cell lymphoma, also at least in part because of the imprecise definitions of these entities. Whereas the accuracy of diagnosis of follicular lymphoma was 94%, the agreement for the various grades of the follicular lymphoma was only 61% to 73%. The agreement in follicular lymphoma, grade 3, increased to 74% if diagnoses of the condition with a diffuse component also were considered to be in agreement.

The usefulness of immunophenotyping in making the correct diagnosis depended on the specific disease (Table 20.4). For some lymphomas, such as follicular lymphoma, marginal zone B-cell lymphoma of MALT type, and the small lymphocytic and lymphoplasmacytoid lymphomas, information on the immunophenotype did not increase the diagnostic accuracy significantly. For the mantle cell, diffuse large B-cell, and T-cell lymphomas, however, immunophenotyping was helpful in many cases in reaching the correct diagnosis and improved the diagnostic accuracy by some 10% to 45%. In many such patients, the initial diagnosis based on histology only was unclassifiable malignant lymphoma. Immunophenotyping allowed the classification of such cases into specific categories. Detailed clinical data was helpful only in distinguishing primary mediastinal large B-cell lymphoma from the other diffuse large B-cell lymphomas, because there were no characteristic histologic or immunologic differences between these two categories.

The expert pathologists' rereview of 20% of the cases at each site showed that they reproducibly could make a diagnosis of non-Hodgkin's lymphoma (Table 20.5). Overall, the rereview diagnosis agreed exactly with the pathologist's initial diagnosis 3 or the consensus diagnosis (including the grading of follicular lymphoma) in 85% of the cases (range, 82%–89%). Because the consensus diagnosis for all of these cases was reached before the time of the rereview, the consensus process may have influenced the assessment of some cases at rereview. Therefore, the pathologists were allowed to agree with either their original diagnosis 3 or the consensus diagnosis at the time of rereview. For an additional 9% of the cases, the rereview diagnosis was nearly the same as the original diagnosis (i.e., follicular, grade 1, vs. follicular, grade 2; or follicular, grade 3, vs. follicular, grade 3, plus diffuse large B-cell). For 94% of the cases rereviewed (range, 92%–97%), the expert pathologists made a diagnosis consistent with either their original diagnosis 3 or the consensus diagnosis. In only 6% of the cases (range, 3% 8%), the pathologist's rereview diagnosis likely would have led to a different approach to therapy than the original diagnosis.

The clinical characteristics of the more common types of lymphoma are presented in Table 20.6. It is important to recognize that, although the average results vary between the various types, there was considerable overlap between

TABLE 20.6. *Patient characteristics by histologic type*

Consensus diagnosis	Male, %	Median age, yr	Stage 1 or 2, %	Marrow-positive, %	International Prognostic Index score, % 0/1	International Prognostic Index score, % 4/5	5-yr overall survival, %	5-yr failure-free survival, %
Follicular, all grades	42	59	33	42	39	6	72	40
Mantle cell	74	63	19	63	19	19	27	11
Marginal zone, B-cell, MALT	45	61	66	14	38	5	74	60
Marginal zone, B-cell, nodal	41	58	18	41	36	9	57	29
Small lymphocytic (chronic lymphocytic leukemia)	53	65	6	73	17	10	51	25
Lymphoplasmacytoid	53	63	20	73	20	13	59	25
Diffuse large B-cell	55	64	51	17	31	16	46	41
Primary mediastinal large B-cell	34	37	66	3	44	9	50	48
Burkitt's	89	31	56	33	44	22	44	44
High-grade B-cell, Burkitt's-like	59	55	50	21	25	18	47	43
Precursor T-lymphoblastic	74	25	13	43	35	22	26	24
Peripheral T-cell, all types	56	61	18	37	14	27	25	18
Anaplastic large T/null-cell	69	33	50	12	50	19	77	58

MALT, mucosa-associated lymphoid tissue.

TABLE 20.7. *Survival by histologic type and International Prognostic Index score*

Consensus diagnosis	5-yr overall survival, %		5-yr failure-free survival	
	Index score 0/1	Index score 4/5	Index score 0/1	Index score 4/5
Follicular, all grades	84	17	55	6
Mantle cell	57	0	27	0
Marginal zone B-cell, MALT	89	40	83	0
Marginal zone B-cell, nodal	76	50	30	0
Small lymphocytic (chronic lymphocytic leukemia)	76	38	35	13
Diffuse large B-cell	73	22	63	19
Primary mediastinal large B-cell	77	0	69	0
High grade B-cell, Burkitt's-like	71	0	71	0
Precursor T-lymphoblastic	29	40	29	40
Peripheral T-cell, all types	36	15	27	10
Anaplastic large T/null-cell	81	83	49	83

MALT, mucosa-associated lymphoid tissue.

the types for any particular characteristic. The newly recognized types of lymphoma appear to be distinctive. Marginal zone B-cell lymphoma of MALT type was characterized by a high frequency of localized extranodal disease and a prolonged duration of survival, whereas patients with nodal marginal zone (monocytoid) B-cell lymphoma more often presented with advanced-stage disease and had a shorter duration of survival. Mantle cell lymphoma had a striking male predominance, a high frequency of advanced-stage disease with marrow involvement, and the lowest 5-year survival rate of any type of lymphoma. Primary mediastinal large B-cell lymphoma occurred more frequently in young females and was often of a low stage, but the survival rate was no different from that of other diffuse large B-cell lymphomas. Anaplastic large T- or null cell lymphoma occurred mainly in young patients and had a surprisingly high 5-year survival rate compared with other lymphomas with large cell histology or a T-cell phenotype. This was not a result of the inclusion of a high proportion of patients with only skin involvement; such patients represented just 6% of the total.

The average overall survival rate allowed for division of the non-Hodgkin's lymphomas into four broad groupings by histologic type. Those with a 5-year overall survival of greater than 70% included follicular lymphoma, marginal zone B-cell lymphoma of MALT type, and anaplastic large T- or null cell lymphoma. Lymphomas with a 50% to 70% 5-year overall survival rate included the small lymphocytic, lymphoplasmacytoid, and nodal marginal zone B-cell lymphomas. Lymphomas with a 30% to 49% 5-year overall survival rate included diffuse large B-cell lymphomas, primary mediastinal large B-cell lymphoma, and the high-grade B-cell Burkitt's-like and Burkitt's lymphomas. Lymphomas with less than a 30% 5-year overall survival rate included peripheral T-cell lymphoma, precursor T-lymphoblastic lymphoma, and mantle cell lymphoma.

The histologic diagnosis of a specific type of lymphoma provided clinically important information; equally important prognostic information was obtained from the clinical characteristics of the individual patients. We found considerable variation within any particular histologic type for both overall survival and failure-free survival rates based on patient clinical characteristics using the International Prognostic Index (Table 20.7). For example, patients with follicular lymphoma had significantly different outcomes depending on their clinical prognostic characteristics (Fig. 20.1). Moreover, patients with follicular lymphoma with high (unfavorable) prognostic indexes had far worse overall and failure-free survival rates (17% and 6%, respectively) than patients with diffuse large B-cell lymphoma and low (favorable) prognostic indexes (73% and 63%).

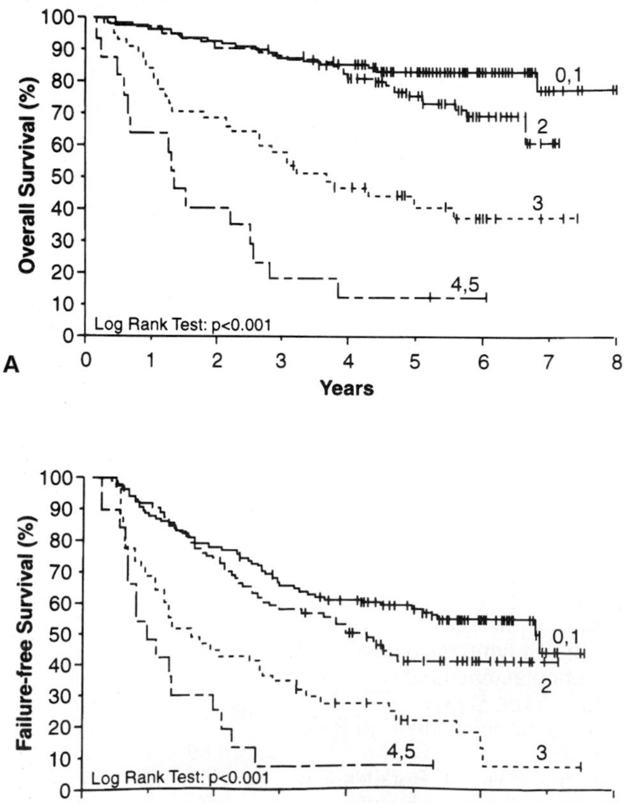

FIG. 20.1. Overall survival (**A**) and failure-free survival (**B**) for patients with follicular lymphoma stratified by International Prognostic Index scores.

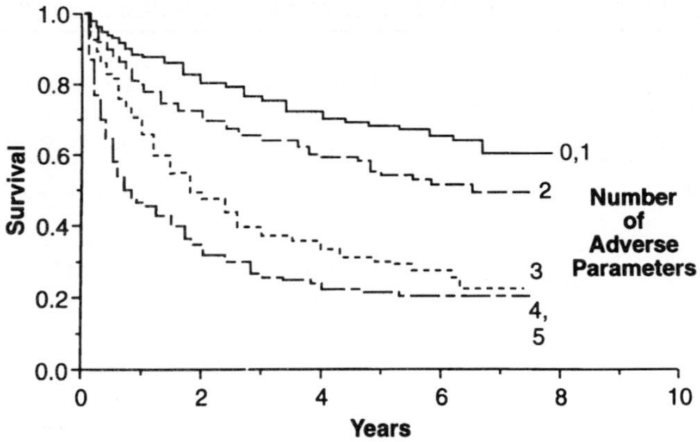

FIG. 20.2. Overall survival of 1,254 patients with all subtypes of non-Hodgkin's lymphoma grouped according to International Prognostic Index score.

WHAT DOES THE REVISED EUROPEAN–AMERICAN CLASSIFICATION OF LYMPHOID NEOPLASMS MEAN FOR CLINICIANS?

The REAL classification codifies a new way of thinking about non-Hodgkin's lymphomas. The development of this approach is seen in modifications of the Working Formulation and the Kiel classification, and it served as the basis for the REAL classification. The concept is that lymphomas should be thought of as clinical pathologic entities—that is, specific diseases—rather than morphologic subgroups. The study described previously showed that this approach can lead to a diagnostic accuracy that is superior to what was previously achieved, and that the clinical entities so defined are distinctive.

An equally important part of the study was the recognition that the correct diagnosis alone is insufficient information on which to base clinical decisions. Clinical parameters as evaluated in the International Prognostic Index (41) provide equally important information about patient outcome. In fact, clinical parameters alone could serve as a basis of a classification of lymphomas. Figure 20.2 plots the survival rates of approximately 1,400 patients with lymphoma included in the study based entirely upon their International Prognostic Index scores. The different therapies appropriate for different subtypes of lymphomas make this approach unreasonably simplistic; a similar comment might be made about the diagnostic subgroup alone without an accurate clinical evaluation.

The wide spectrum of clinical outcomes that can be seen in any particular subtype of lymphoma, based on the clinical characteristics, raises a new question about what should be thought of as an aggressive non-Hodgkin's lymphoma. For example, a patient with diffuse large B-cell lymphoma who has no adverse risk factors in the International Prognostic Index has a much longer anticipated duration of survival than a similar patient who has multiple adverse risk factors but has follicular lymphoma (Fig. 20.3).

Finally, neither the REAL classification nor the International Prognostic Index take into account certain unique characteristics about special subgroups of lymphomas that require special clinical care. For example, Burkitt's lymphoma, lymphoblastic lymphoma, and any subtype of lymphoma that involves the paranasal sinuses, epidural space, and probably testes require prophylactic therapy to the central nervous system to prevent an unacceptably high incidence of meningeal relapse. Patients who present with non-Hodgkin's lymphoma involving Waldeyer's ring need careful evaluation of the distal gastrointestinal tract because of a high incidence of concordant involvement. Patients with involvement of the distal gastrointestinal tract should have Waldeyer's ring evaluated for the same reason. These and many other examples must be known to clinicians caring for patients with these disorders in order for the patients to receive optimal care.

MAJOR LYMPHOMA SUBTYPES

The clinical and laboratory characteristics of the major subtypes of non-Hodgkin's lymphoma and their overall sur-

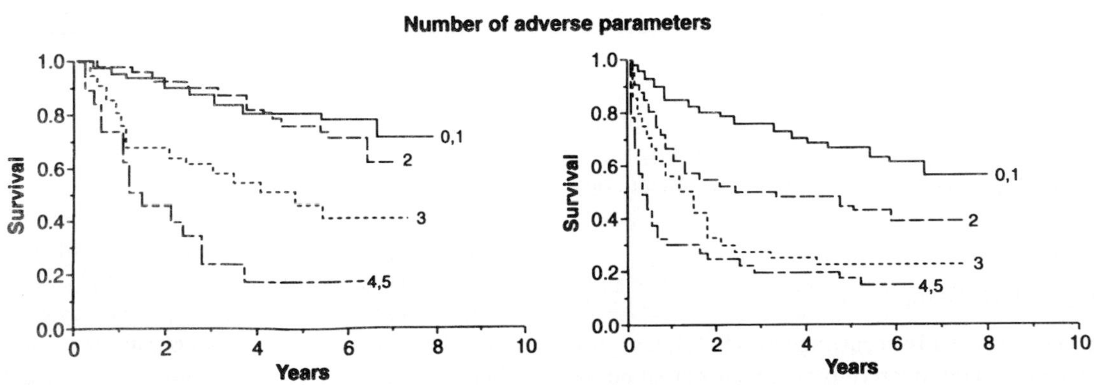

FIG. 20.3. Overall survival for 275 patients with follicular lymphoma (left) and 388 patients with diffuse large B-cell lymphoma (right) stratified by International Prognostic Index score.

TABLE 20.8. *Clinical characteristics of the*

Characteristics	Diffuse large B-cell lymphoma	Follicular lymphoma	Small lymphocytic lymphoma	Mantle cell lymphoma	Peripheral T-cell lymphoma	Marginal zone B-cell lymphoma, MALT type
Frequency, % (no.)	31 (422)	22 (306)	6 (88)	6 (83)	6 (76)	5 (72)
Age, yr						
Median	64	59	65	63	61	60
Range	14–98	23–90	21–91	37–82	17–90	19–91
Male, %	55	42	53	74	55	48
Stage						
I	12	16	4	10	1	0
IE	13	2	0	3	7	39
II	13	11	2	6	6	0
IIE	16	4	3	1	6	28
III	13	16	8	9	15	2
IV	33	51	83	71	65	31
B symptoms	33	28	33	28	50	19
Elevated LDH	53	30	41	40	64	27
Karnofsky score ≤70	24	9	11	21	32	15
Tumor bulk, %						
≥5 cm	76	61	59	69	65	68
≥10 cm	30	28	13	25	12	8
Any extranodal site, %	71	64	80	81	82	98
>1 extranodal site, %	29	23	29	51	45	31
Bone marrow involved, %	16	42	72	64	36	14
Gastrointestinal tract involved	18	4	3	9	15	50
International Prognostic Index score, %						
0/1	35	45	23	23	17	44
2/3	46	48	64	54	52	48
4/5	19	7	13	23	31	8
Typical immunophenotype	$CD20^+$, $CD3^-$	$CD20^+$, $CD3^-$ $CD10^+$, $CD5^-$	$CD20^+$, $CD3^-$ $CD10^-$, $CD5^+$ $CD23^+$	$CD20^+$, $CD3^-$ $CD10^-$, $CD5^+$ $CD23^-$, $PRAD1^+$	$CD20^-$, $CD3^+$	$CD20^+$, $CD3^-$ $CD10^-$, $CD5^-$ $CD23^-$
Characteristic cytogenetics	t(14;18) (q32; q21) t(8;14) (q24; q32) t(3;14) (q27; q32)	t(14;18) q(32; q21)	del(13q), $^+12$	t(11;14) (q13; q32)	Variable	t(11;18) (q21; q21) $^+3$,$^+18$
Oncogenes frequently involved	BCL-2 C-MYC BCL-6	BCL-2	Unknown	BCL-1 (PRAD1)	Unknown	Unknown

vival and failure-free survival rates, along with survival and failure-free survival rates based on International Prognostic Index Score, are presented here. The clinical characteristics of each subtype are listed in Table 20.8.

Diffuse Large B-Cell Lymphoma

This is the most frequently occurring non-Hodgkin's lymphoma. It contains predominantly lymphomas classified as diffuse large cell, diffuse mixed cell, or immunoblastic in the Working Formulation and lymphomas classified as diffuse centroblastic, diffuse centroblastic or centrocytic, or immunoblastic in the Kiel classification. In the Non-Hodgkin's Lymphoma Classification Project, using histology, immunophenotyping, and clinical information, diffuse large B-cell lymphoma was diagnosed accurately 87% of the time. Immunophenotyping improved the accuracy of diagnosis by 14%. Diffuse large B-cell lymphoma is curable by chemotherapy. Chance for cure is predicted by the International Prognostic Index score. There are a number of regimens major subgroups of non-Hodgkin's lymphomas

Primary mediastinal large B-cell lymphoma	Anaplastic large T-/null cell lymphoma	Lymphoblastic lymphoma (T/B)	Burkitt's-like lymphoma	Marginal zone B-cell lymphoma, nodal type	Lymphoplasmacytic lymphoma	Burkitt's lymphoma
2 (33)	2 (33)	2 (26)	2 (29)	1 (20)	1 (15)	<1 (10)
37	34	28	57	58	63	31
21–84	10–100	4–65	20–92	27–90	37–81	2–60
34	69	64	59	42	53	89
10	16	0	19	13	7	25
0	3	0	7	0	0	12
34	22	11	4	13	0	13
22	10	0	22	0	13	12
3	10	14	7	34	7	0
31	39	75	41	40	73	38
38	53	21	39	37	13	22
81	45	70	61	40	15	75
22	26	29	27	7	27	44
90	76	86	92	36	50	56
52	17	32	42	0	25	22
56	59	82	79	47	100	78
19	28	43	43	16	40	56
3	13	50	21	32	73	33
0	9	4	29	5	7	11
52	61	33	30	60	16	57
37	18	41	48	27	69	29
11	21	26	22	13	15	14
$CD20^+$, $CD3^-$	CD20, $CD3^+$ $CD30^+$, $CD15^-$ EMA^+, ALK^+	$CD20^-$, $CD3^+$ Tdt^+	$CD20^+$, $CD3^-$ $CD10^-$, $CD5^-$ Tdt^-	$CD20^+$, $CD3^-$ $CD10^-$, $CD5^-$ $CD23^-$	$CD20^+$, $CD3^-$ $CD10^-$, $CD5^-$ $CD23^-$, cyto Ig^+	$CD20^+$, $CD3^-$ $CD10^+$, $CD5^-$ Tdt^-
Variable	t(2;5) (p23;q35)	Variable	t(14;18) (q32; q21) t(8;14) (q24; q32)	$^+3$,$^+18$	t(9;14) (p13;q32) del 6(q23)	t(8;14) (q24; q32) t(2;8) (p12; q24) t(8;22) (q24; q11)
Unknown	ALK	TCL1–3	BCL-2, C-MYC	Unknown	Unknown	C-MYC

effective in diffuse large B-cell lymphoma, but all contain an anthracycline. Studies to date have failed to identify one superior regimen. See Insert 1.

Follicular Lymphoma

The combined group of follicular lymphomas makes up the second most frequent type of non-Hodgkin's lymphoma. These lymphomas are classified as follicular small cleaved cell, follicular mixed cell, and follicular large cell lymphoma in the Working Formulation and predominantly as follicular centroblastic or centrocytic or follicular centroblastic lymphoma in the Kiel classification. In the non-Hodgkin's Lymphoma Classification Project, follicular lymphoma was diagnosed accurately 94% of the time. Subtyping of follicular lymphomas was less accurate. Immunophenotyping improved the accuracy of diagnosis by only 1%. Although there was an overall 5-year survival rate of approximately 72%, patients with a high International Prognostic Index score had a poor survival rate. The optimal treatment for patients with

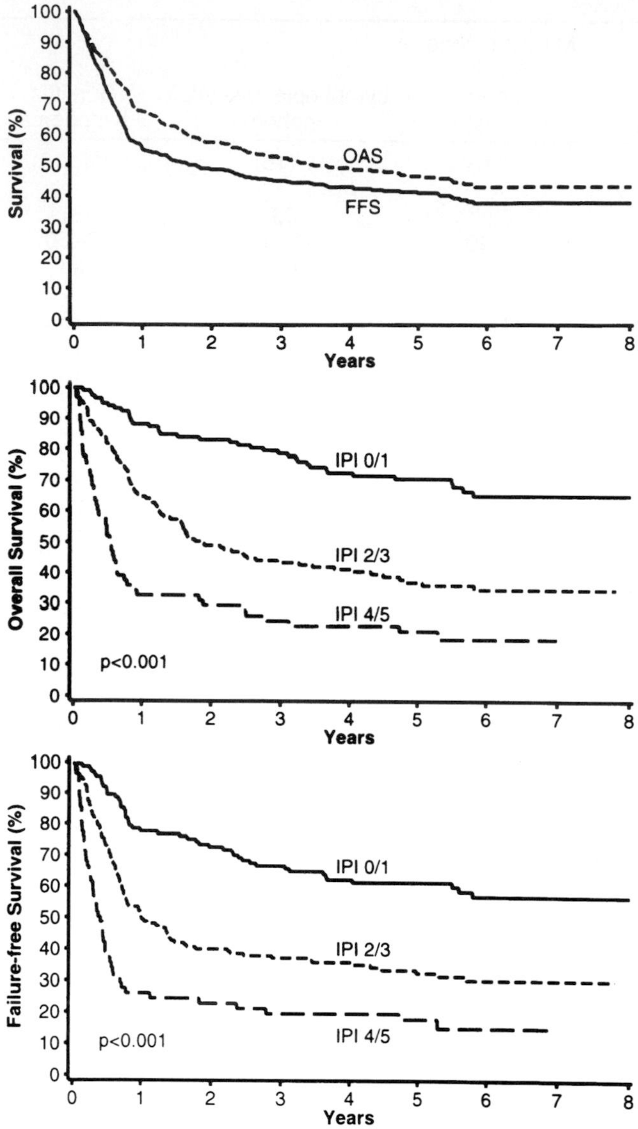

INSERT 1. Survival Curves for Diffuse Large B-Cell Lymphoma.

follicular lymphoma remains controversial. Some clinicians suggest no initial therapy for an asymptomatic patient; others suggest treatment aimed at achieving an initial complete remission. In some patients, the initial complete remissions can be extremely long. Until the question of which patients of follicular lymphoma can be cured with available therapies is resolved, controversy will persist. See Insert 2.

Small Lymphocytic Lymphoma

Small lymphocytic lymphoma makes up 6% of all non-Hodgkin's lymphomas. Because this often is the tissue manifestation of chronic lymphocytic leukemia, if patients who present with leukemia and predominantly blood and bone marrow involvement were included, the actual incidence would be higher. It contains predominantly lymphomas classified as small lymphocytic in the Working Formulation but is called *chronic lymphocytic leukemia* in the Kiel classification. In the non-Hodgkin's Lymphoma Classification Project, small lymphocytic lymphoma was diagnosed accurately 87% of the time. Immunophenotyping added only 3% to the diagnostic accuracy. The optimal treatment for patients with small lymphocytic lymphoma remains controversial. Few patients have localized disease and can benefit from local therapy. The use of chlorambucil, fludarabine, or combination chemotherapy for patients with disseminated disease frequently produces a response, but such disease rarely if ever is curable. See Insert 3.

Mantle Cell Lymphoma

Mantle cell lymphoma is among the most frequent of the newly recognized subtypes of non-Hodgkin's lymphoma. In

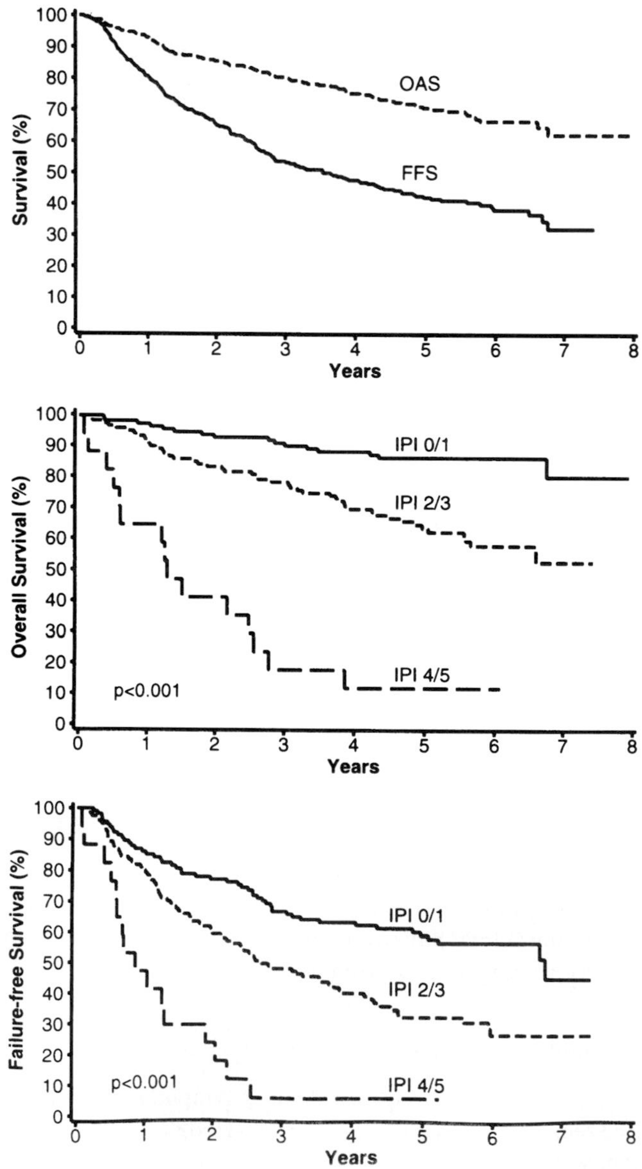

INSERT 2. Survival Curves for Follicular Lymphoma.

the Working Formulation, mantle cell lymphoma is classified as diffuse small cleaved cell lymphoma most frequently, but also as follicular small cleaved cell lymphoma, small lymphocytic lymphoma, diffuse large cell lymphoma, and lymphoblastic lymphoma. In the Kiel classification, this lymphoma most frequently is classified as centrocytic lymphoma or centrocytoid centroblastic lymphoma. In the non-Hodgkin's Lymphoma Classification Project, mantle cell lymphoma was diagnosed accurately 87% of the time. Immunophenotyping added 10% to the accuracy of diagnosis. Patients with mantle cell lymphoma are mostly male, usually have advanced disease, and have poor overall and failure-free survival rates, which belies the good chance of survival usually anticipated with small cell lymphomas. The optimal treatment for mantle cell lymphoma is unknown. Because of the extremely poor prognosis, many clinicians recommend a

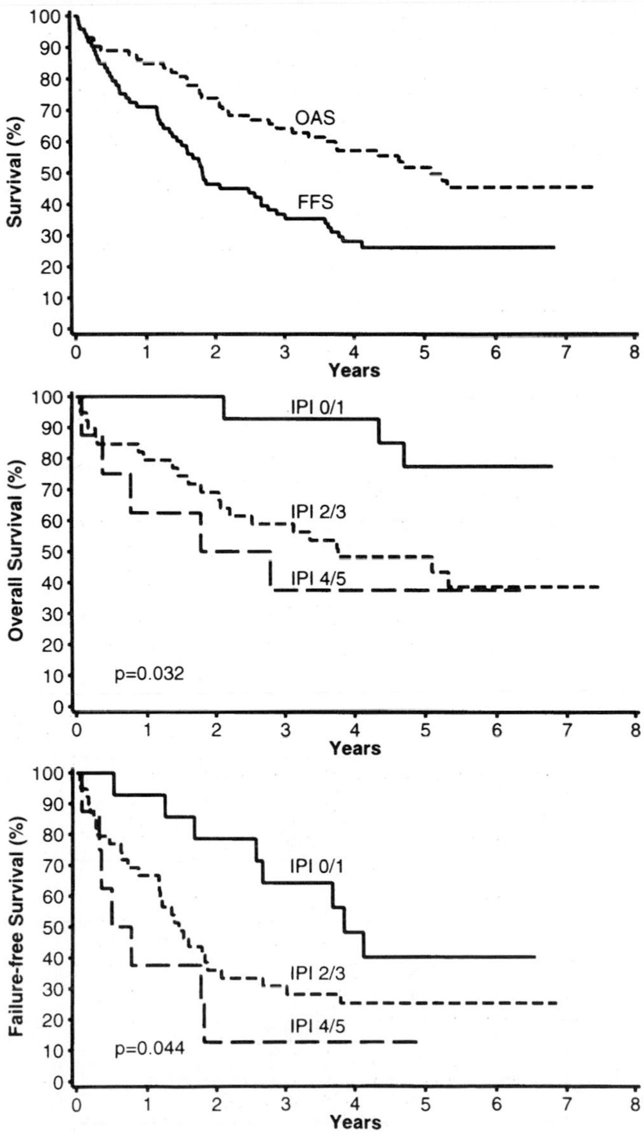

INSERT 3. Survival Curves for Small Lymphocytic Lymphoma.

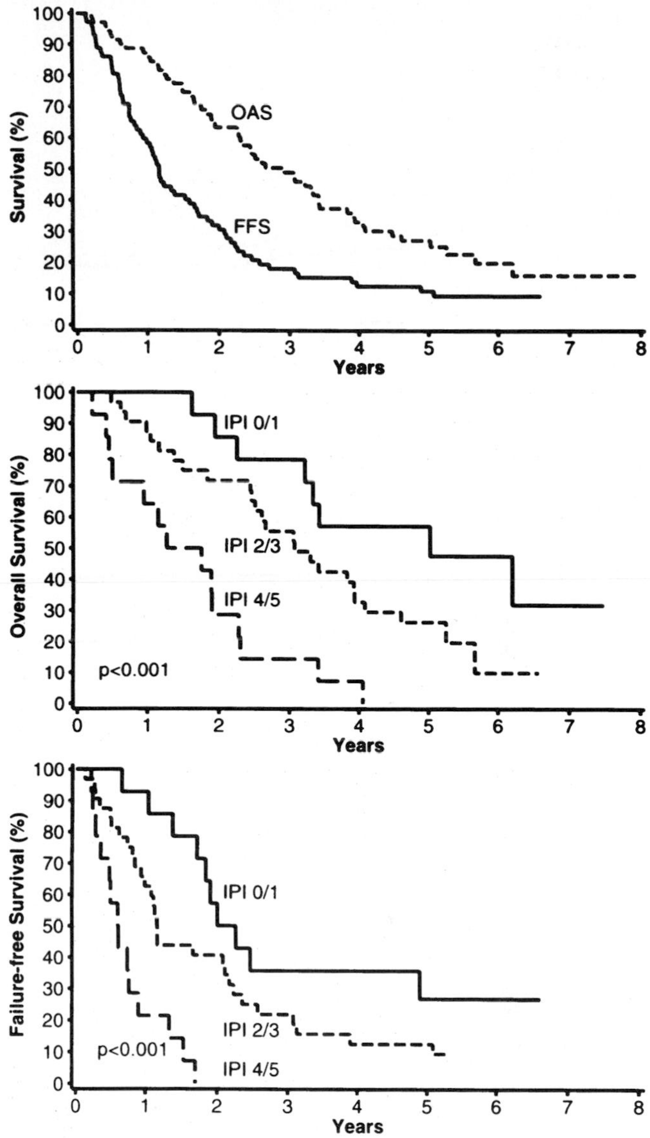

INSERT 4. Survival Curves for Mantle Cell Lymphoma.

bone marrow transplant as part of the primary treatment. See Insert 4.

Peripheral T-Cell Lymphoma

The subgroup of peripheral T-cell lymphoma not otherwise specified represents the largest group of T-cell lymphomas in the REAL classification. For this report, angiocentric nasal lymphomas and human T-lymphotropic virus type 1–associated lymphomas were excluded, which makes the results typical for those seen in most Western countries. Peripheral T-cell lymphoma includes lymphomas with a wide variety of histologic appearances. Tumors in this subgroup were classified as diffuse small cleaved cell, diffuse mixed cell, diffuse large cell, and immunoblastic in the Working Formulation. In the non-Hodgkin's Lymphoma Classification Project, peripheral T-cell lymphoma was diag-

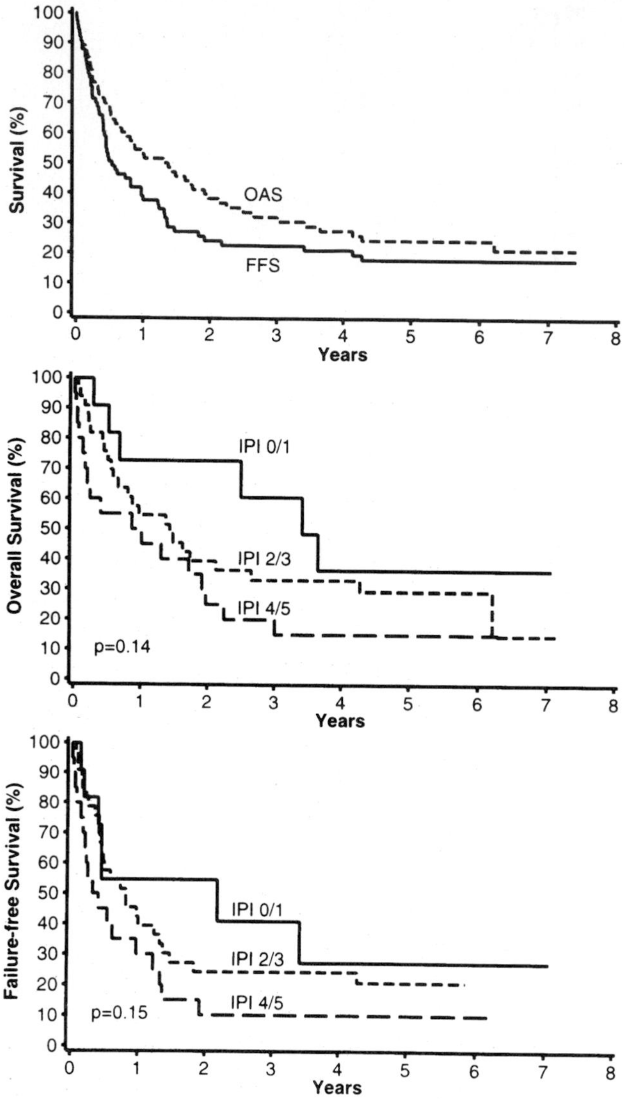

INSERT 5. Survival Curves for Peripheral T-Cell Lymphoma.

nosed accurately 86% of the time, if immunophenotyping was available. Immunophenotyping improved the accuracy of diagnosis by 45%. Peripheral T-cell lymphomas have one of the lowest overall and failure-free survival rates. The optimal treatment for peripheral T-cell lymphoma remains unknown. Patients with localized disease should receive combination chemotherapy and local radiotherapy. Patients with disseminated disease are treated in a manner similar to patients with diffuse large B-cell lymphoma but have a worse outcome. See Insert 5.

Marginal Zone B-Cell Lymphoma, MALT Type

This is among the most frequent of the newly recognized subtypes of non-Hodgkin's lymphoma. In this report, only low-grade MALT lymphomas are included. In the Working Formulation, MALT lymphomas were diagnosed most commonly as small lymphocytic lymphoma or small lymphocytic lymphoma with plasmacytoid characteristics, although some were called diffuse small cleaved cell lymphoma. In the non-Hodgkin's Lymphoma Classification Project, marginal zone lymphoma of the MALT type was diagnosed accurately 86% of the time. Immunophenotyping added only 2% to the accuracy of the diagnosis. MALT lymphomas have one of the highest survival rates of any subtype, and even patients with a high International Prognostic Index score have a 5-year overall survival rate of 40%. MALT lymphomas appear to be sometimes curable with local therapy. Patients with gastric MALT lymphoma who are infected with *Helicobacter pylori* often benefit from antibiotic therapy and by eradicating the bacteria. See Insert 6.

Primary Mediastinal Large B-Cell Lymphoma

Primary mediastinal large B-cell lymphoma is a diffuse lymphoma that cannot be distinguished histologically but presents as a clinical syndrome because of the presence of

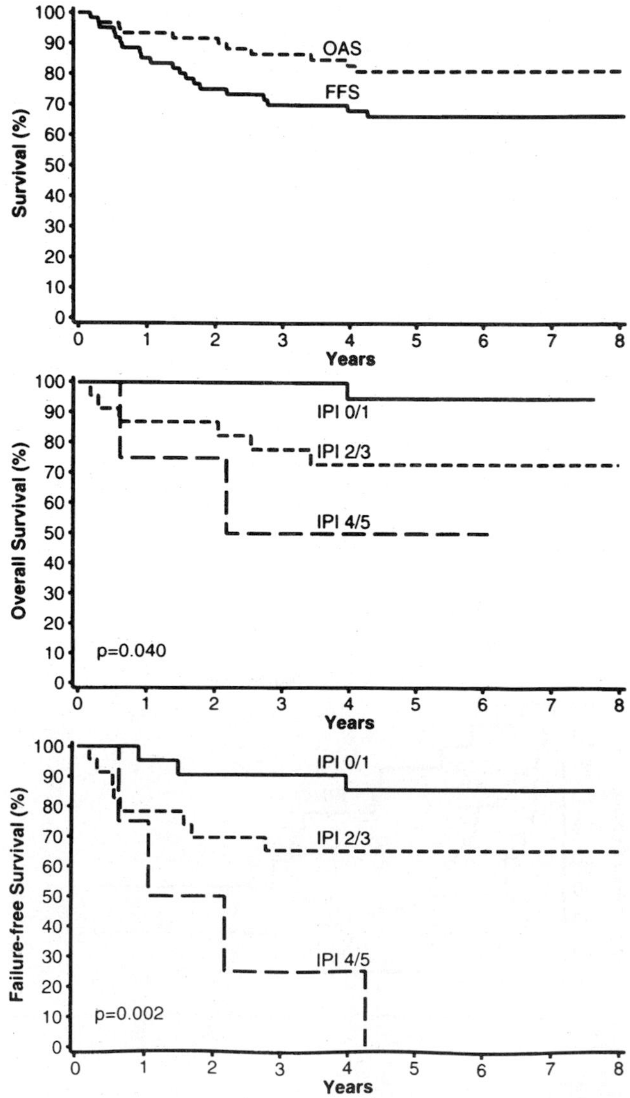

INSERT 6. Survival Curves for Marginal Zone B-Cell Lymphoma, MALT Type.

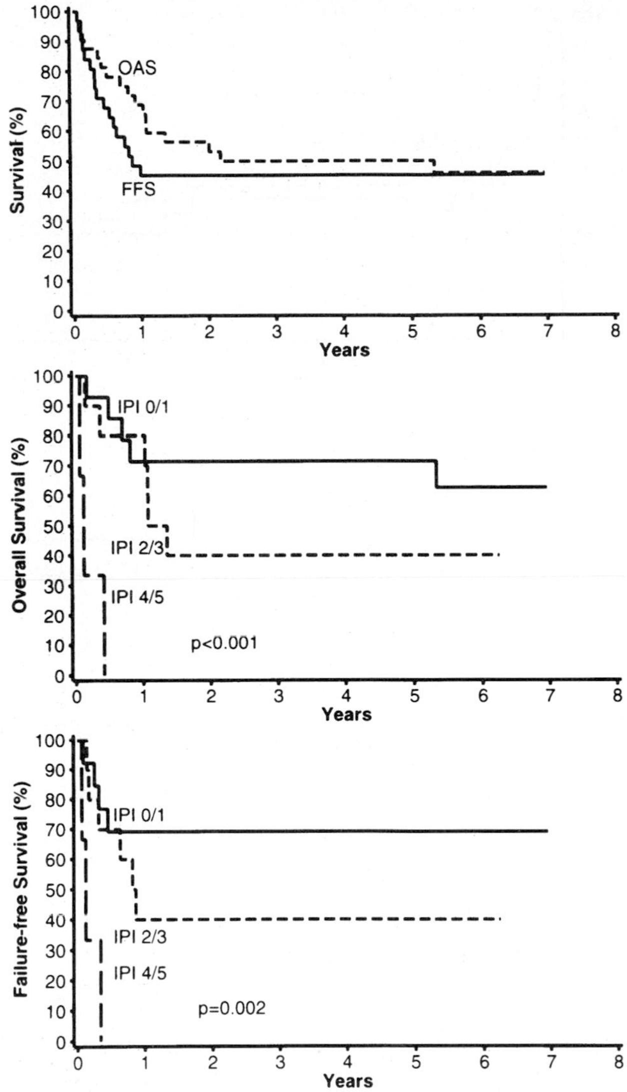

INSERT 7. Survival Curves for Primary Mediastinal Large B-Cell Lymphoma.

a large mediastinal mass. This syndrome is clinically distinctive because it occurs predominantly in younger patients and has a female predominance. In the International non-Hodgkin's Lymphoma Classification Project, mediastinal large B-cell lymphoma was diagnosed accurately 85% of the time. Immunophenotyping added 7% to the accuracy of diagnosis. The clinical course of these patients differed little from that of other patients with diffuse large B-cell lymphoma, although mediastinal radiotherapy may play an important role in their treatment. The optimal combination chemotherapy regimen would involve an anthracycline and is no different from other types of diffuse large B-cell lymphoma. See Insert 7.

Anaplastic Large T- or Null Cell Lymphoma

Anaplastic large T- or null cell lymphoma represents the second most common T-cell lymphoma in the REAL classification. Patients with anaplastic large T- or null cell lymphoma often were classified as having anaplastic carcinoma or an undifferentiated malignant neoplasm before staining for the CD30 antigen and discovery of the characteristic chromosomal translocation between chromosomes 2 and 5 led to its recognition as a distinctive non-Hodgkin's lymphoma. In the REAL classification, only anaplastic large-cell lymphomas with T or null immunophenotype are included in this category. In the non-Hodgkin's Lymphoma Classification Project, anaplastic large T- or null cell lymphoma was diagnosed accurately 85% of the time. Immunophenotyping contributed 39% to the accuracy of diagnosis. Patients with this subtype of lymphoma have a young median age and a male predominance and have the best overall and failure-free survival rates of any large cell lymphoma. The optimal treatment for this lymphoma is unknown. For patients with disseminated disease, an anthracycline containing combination chemotherapy regimen should be the initial treatment in almost all patients. See Insert 8.

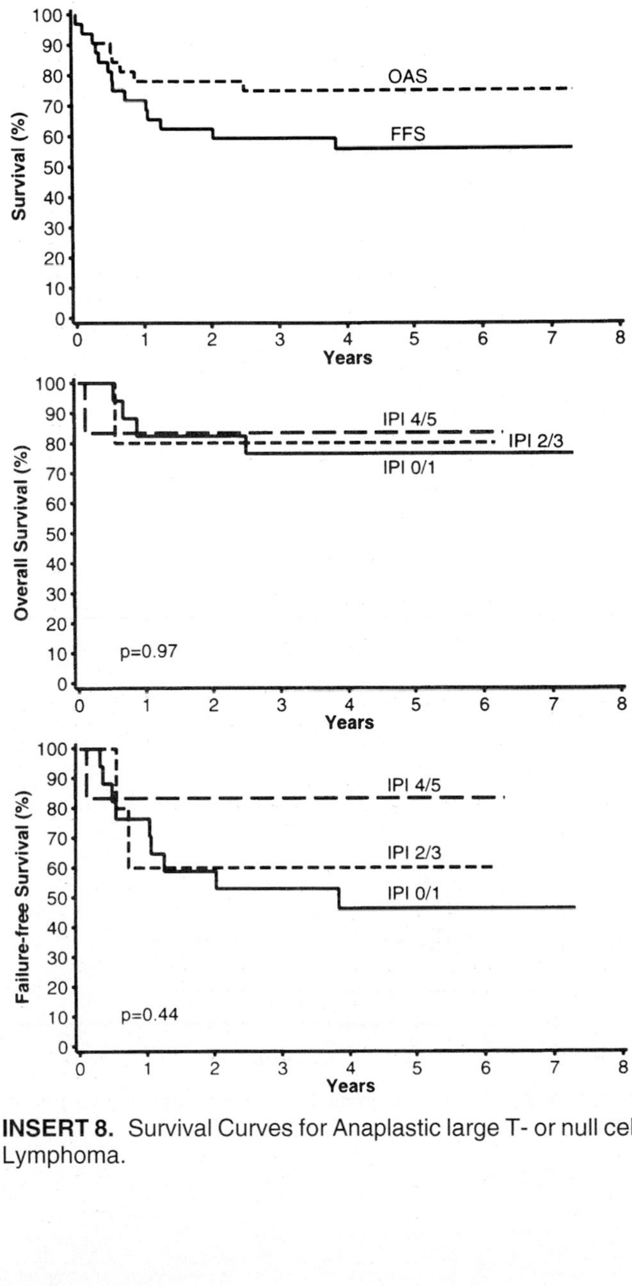

INSERT 8. Survival Curves for Anaplastic large T- or null cell Lymphoma.

Lymphoblastic Lymphoma

The lymphoblastic lymphomas make up a small proportion of all non-Hodgkin's lymphomas and are associated with a low median age, male predominance, and advanced stage. In the non-Hodgkin's Lymphoma Classification Project, lymphoblastic lymphomas were diagnosed accurately 89% of the time. Immunophenotyping contributed 35% to the accuracy of diagnosis. This is an aggressive lymphoma with low overall and failure-free survival rates.

This tumor is largely a pediatric disease. The most popular treatment regimens are protocols similar to those used for the treatment for acute leukemia. See Insert 9.

Burkitt's-Like Lymphoma

Burkitt's-like lymphomas could not be diagnosed accurately in the non-Hodgkin's Lymphoma Classification

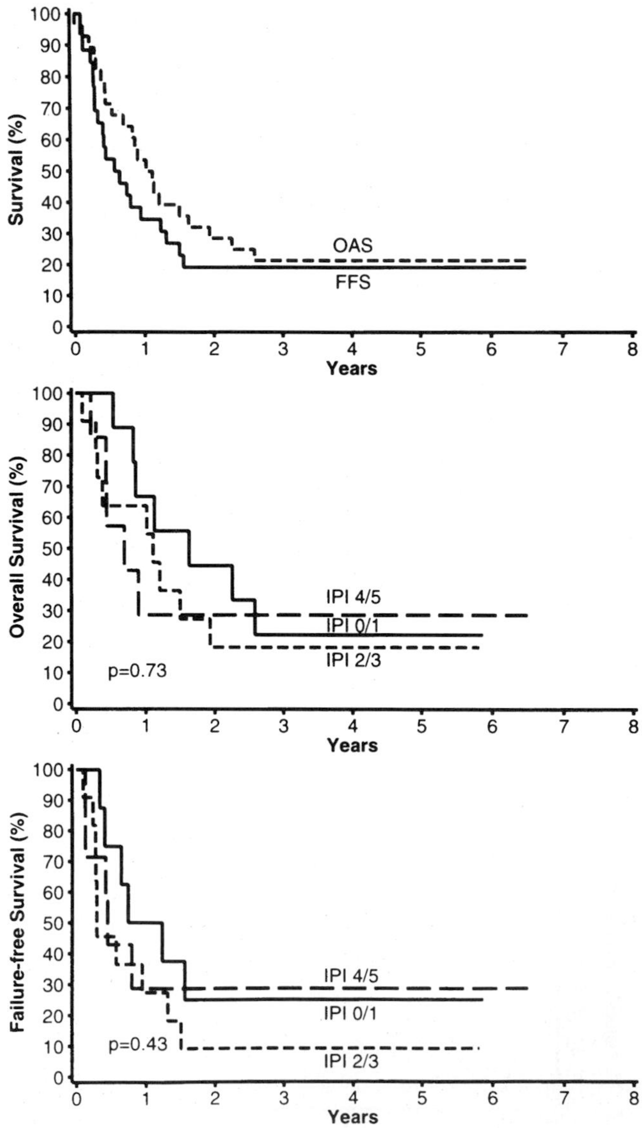

INSERT 9. Survival Curves for Lymphoblastic Lymphoma (T/B).

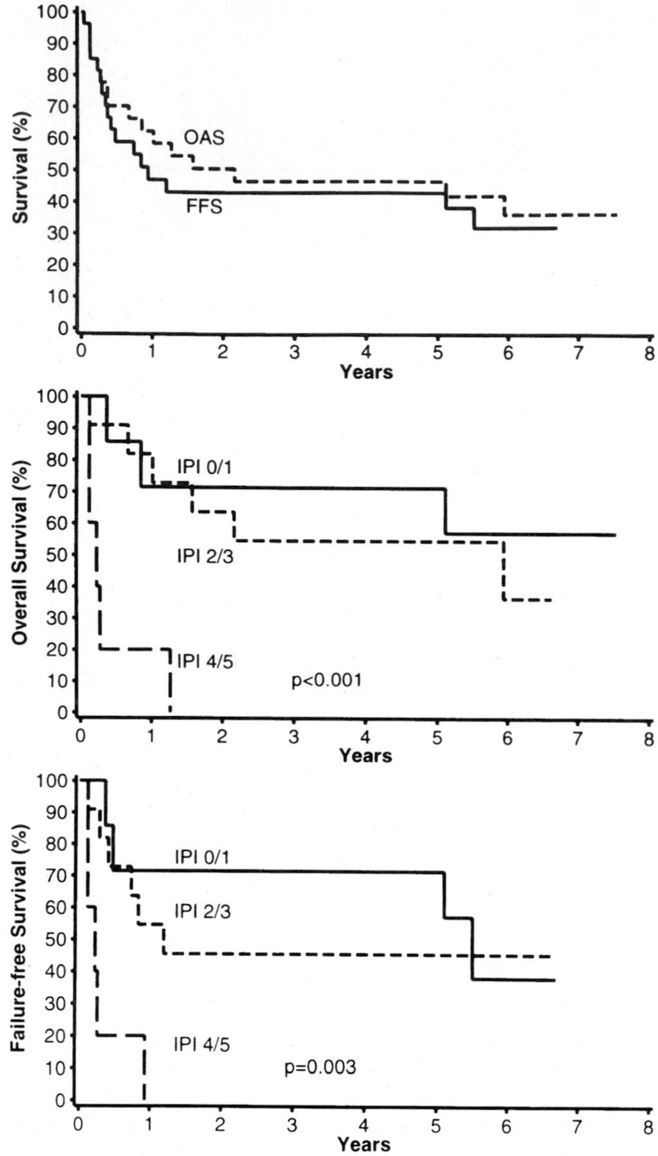

INSERT 10. Survival Curves for Burkitt's-Like Lymphoma.

Project. Based on histology, immunophenotyping, and clinical information, the diagnostic accuracy was only 53%. There was a lack of precise definitions separating this group from the diffuse large B-cell category or true Burkitt's lymphoma. The median age and clinical characteristics of this subgroup were intermediate between those of patients with diffuse large B-cell lymphoma and those with Burkitt's lymphoma but more closely approximated the former. See Insert 10.

Marginal Zone B-Cell Lymphoma, Nodal Type

Marginal zone B-cell lymphoma of the nodal type is one of the new forms of non-Hodgkin's lymphoma not recognized in the Working Formulation. In the Working Formulation, these lymphomas most commonly were placed in the small lymphocytic subcategory but also sometimes were diagnosed as diffuse small cleaved cell lymphoma, small lymphocytic lymphoma with plasmacytoid characteristics, or diffuse mixed cell lymphoma. In the non-Hodgkin's Lymphoma Classification Project using histology, immunophenotype, and clinical information, marginal zone B-cell lymphoma of the nodal type was diagnosed accurately 63% of the time. Immunophenotyping added 8% to the accuracy of diagnosis. These patients had overall and failure-free survival rates similar to those seen with small lymphocytic lymphoma. These lymphomas often are diagnosed as monocytoid B-cell lymphoma. The recent recognition of this subtype of lymphoma, and the difficulty in its diagnosis, makes comments about optimal therapy difficult. See Insert 11.

Lymphoplasmacytic Lymphoma

Lymphoplasmacytic lymphoma is an uncommon diagnosis in the REAL classification and includes patients who also

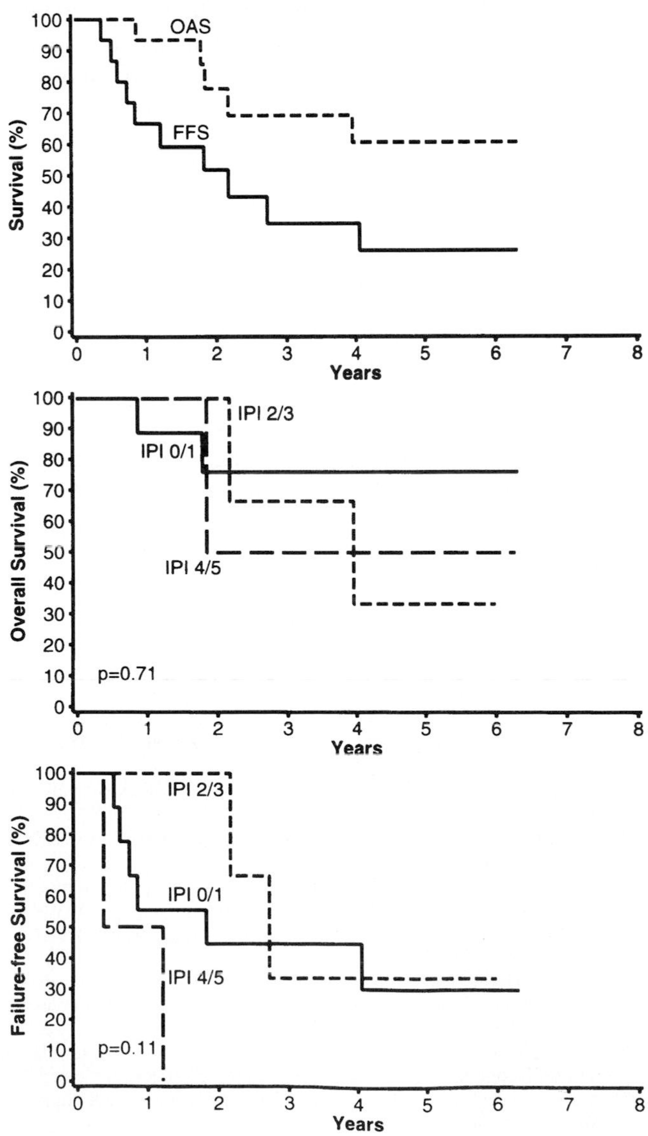

INSERT 11. Survival Curves for Marginal Zone B-Cell Lymphoma, Nodal Type.

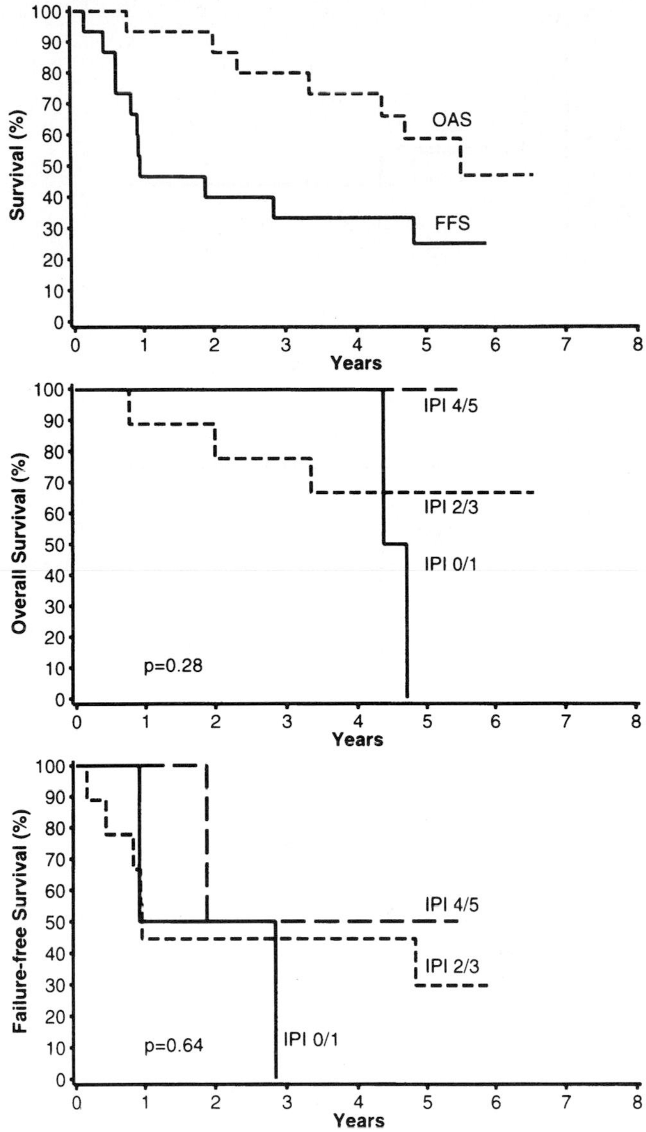

INSERT 12. Survival Curves for Lymphoplasmacytic Lymphoma.

might be diagnosed with Waldenstrom's macroglobulinemia. In the non-Hodgkin's Lymphoma Classification Project using histology, immunophenotyping, and clinical information, lymphoplasmacytic lymphoma was diagnosed accurately 56% of the time. Immunophenotyping contributed 3% to the diagnostic accuracy. The clinical characteristics of this lymphoma were similar to those of small lymphocytic lymphoma. See Insert 12.

Burkitt's Lymphoma

This is a rare lymphoma in a clinical series that includes predominantly adults. Although this is a highly aggressive and clinically distinctive lymphoma requiring unique treatment approaches, the overall and failure-free survival rates are similar to diffuse large B-cell lymphoma. This tumor

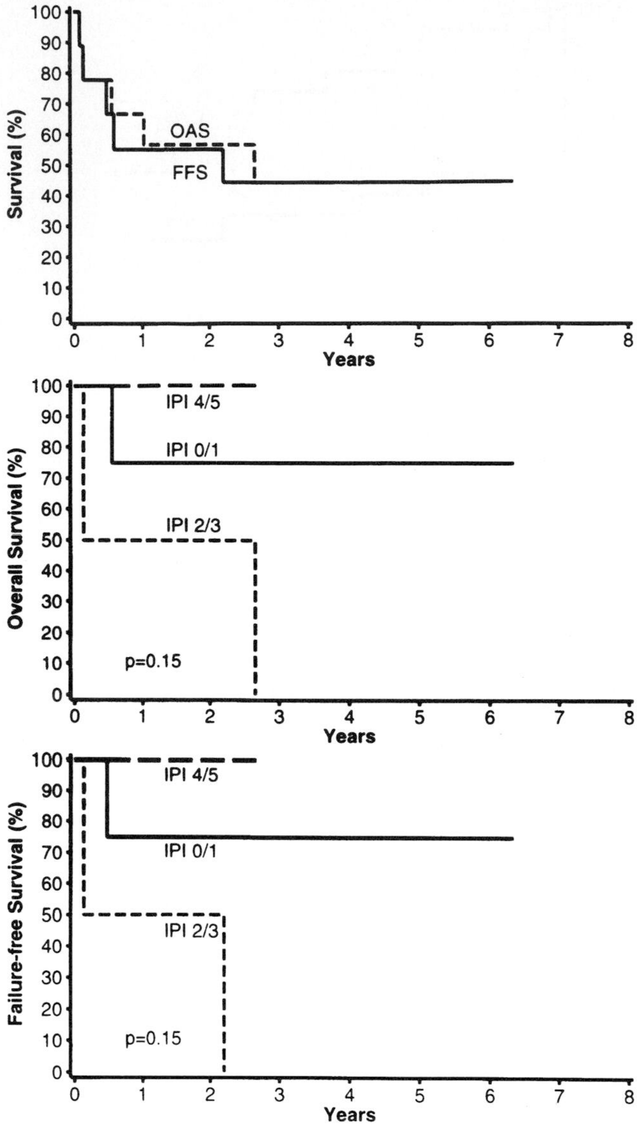

INSERT 13. Survival Curves for Burkitt's Lymphoma.

occurs predominantly in pediatric age groups. Short-course, very intensive chemotherapy regimens can achieve a high cure rate. See Insert 13.

THE FUTURE

It is important to understand that the classification of non-Hodgkin's lymphoma will continue to change. As long as pathologists and scientists continue to make new observations about the biology of the immune system, these observations will alter our knowledge of the malignancies that affect the immune system. From time to time, these insights will allow us to recognize new types of non-Hodgkin's lymphoma that we were not able to "see" previously.

The most likely immediate changes to come in our understanding of non-Hodgkin's lymphomas relate to genetic observations. Diffuse large B-cell lymphoma almost certainly represents a number of clinical entities. Patterns of gene activation might make it possible to subdivide these lymphomas in the next few years. Hopefully, this will allow better therapeutic decisions and improve survival for our patients.

SUMMARY AND CONCLUSIONS

Our understanding of non-Hodgkin's lymphoma continues to evolve. We are moving from a classification based on purely morphologic characteristics to a new system that identifies specific clinical and pathologic entities. This approach has been tested and can be applied more accurately than previous systems.

The two most common non-Hodgkin's lymphomas are diffuse large B-cell lymphoma and follicular lymphoma. They make up approximately 31% and 22% of lymphomas, respectively. Diffuse large B-cell lymphoma can be cured in a significant portion of patients but follows an aggressive course, with a short duration of survival, in patients who are not cured. Follicular lymphoma has a pattern of continuous relapse, but a long median survival. No other non-Hodgkin's lymphoma represents as many as 10% of the total cases. The most common other lymphomas include MALT lymphomas, small lymphocytic lymphoma or chronic lymphocytic leukemia, mantle cell lymphoma, and peripheral T-cell lymphoma. Despite being a small cell lymphoma, mantle cell lymphoma is associated with a poor clinical outcome. An unusual lymphoma, anaplastic large T- or null cell lymphoma, is associated with an excellent clinical outcome despite an unfavorable histologic appearance.

This new approach to classifying lymphomas improves treatment outcome. It is important that all clinicians who treat patients with lymphoma be able to use it.

REFERENCES

1. Gall EA, Mallory TB. Malignant lymphoma: a clinicopathologic survey of 618 cases. *Am J Pathol* 1942;18:381.
2. Rappaport H, Winter WI, Hicks EB. Follicular lymphoma: a re-evaluation of its position in the scheme of malignant lymphoma, based on a survey of 253 cases. *Cancer* 1954;9:792.
3. Lukes RF, Collins RD. Immunologic characterization of human malignant lymphomas. *Cancer* 1974;34:1488.
4. Lennert K, Mohri N, Stein H, et al. The histopathology of malignant lymphoma. *Br J Haematol* 1975;31[Suppl]:193.
5. Lennert K. *Malignant lymphomas other than Hodgkin's disease.* New York: Springer-Verlag, 1978.
6. Whitcomb CC, Crissman JD, Flint A, et al. Reproducibility of morphologic classification of non-Hodgkin's lymphomas using the Lukes-Collins system: the Southeastern Cancer Study Group experience. *Am J Clin Pathol* 1973;82:383.
7. NCI non-Hodgkin's Classification Project Writing Committee. Classification of non-Hodgkin's lymphoma: reproducibility of major classification systems. *Cancer* 1985;55:91.
8. Dick F, VanLier S, Banks P, et al. Use of the Working Formulation for non-Hodgkin's lymphoma in epidemiologic studies: agreement between reported diagnosis and a panel of experienced pathologists. *J Natl Cancer Inst* 1987;78:1137.
9. Lardelli P, Bookman MA, Sundeen J, et al. Lymphocytic lymphoma of intermediate differentiation: morphologic and immunophenotypic spectrum and clinical correlations. *Am J Surg Pathol* 1990;14:752.

10. Norton AJ, Mathews J, Pappa V, et al. Mantle cell lymphoma: natural history defined in a serially biopsied population over a 20 year period. *Ann Oncol* 1995;6:249.
11. Segal GH, Masih AS, Fox Ac, et al. CD5-expressing B-cell non-Hodgkin's lymphomas with bcl-1 gene rearrangement have a relatively homogeneous immunophenotype and are associated with an overall poor prognosis. *Blood* 1995;85:1570.
12. Zuckerbert LR, Medeiros JL, Ferry JA, et al. Diffuse low-grade B-cell lymphomas: four clinically distinct subtypes defined by a combination of morphologic and immunophenotypic features. *Am J Clin Pathol* 1993;100:373.
13. Weisenburger DD, Sanger WG, Armitage JO, et al. Intermediate lymphocytic lymphoma: immunophenotypic and cytogenetic findings. *Blood* 1987;69:1617.
14. Leroux D, Le Marc' hadour F, Gressin R, et al. non-Hodgkin's lymphomas with t(11;14)(q13;q32): a subset of mantle zone/intermediate lymphocytic lymphomas? *Br J Haematol* 1991;77:346.
15. Rimokh R, Berger F, Cornillet P, et al. Break in the bcl-1 locus is closely associated with intermediate lymphocytic lymphoma subtype. *Genes Chrom Cancer* 1990;2:223.
16. Rosenberg CL, Wong E, Petty EM, et al. Prad 1, a candidate BCL1 oncogene: mapping and expression in centrocytic lymphoma. *Proc Natl Acad Sci USA* 1991;88:9636.
17. Withers DA, Harvey RC, Faust JB, et al. Characterization of a candidate bel-1 gene. *Mol Cell Biol* 1991;11:4846.
18. Banks PM, Chan J, Cleary M, et al. Mantle cell lymphoma: a proposal for unification of morphologic, immunologic, and molecular data. *Ann J Surg Pathol* 1992;16:637.
19. Stein H, Mason DY, Gerdes J, et al. The expression of Hodgkin's disease associated antigen Ki-1 in reactive and neoplastic lymphoid tissue: evidence that Reed-Stenberg cells and histiocytic malignancies are derived from activated lymphoid cells. *Blood* 1985;66:848.
20. Agnarsson B, Kadin M. Ki-1 positive large cell lymphoma: a morphologic and immunologic study of 19 cases. *Am J Surg Pathol* 1988;12:264.
21. Kaudewitz P, Stein H, Dallenbach F, et al. Primary and secondary cutaneous Ki-1+ (CD30+) anaplastic large cell lymphomas. *Am J Pathol* 1989;135.359.
22. Mason D, Bastard C, Rimokh R, et al. CD30-positive large cell lymphomas (''Ki-1 lymphoma'') are associated with a chromosomal translocation involving 5q35. *Br J Haematol* 1990;74:161.
23. Greer J, Kinney M, Collins R, et al. Clinical features of 31 patients with Ki-1 anaplastic large-cell lymphoma. *J Clin Oncol* 1991;9:539.
24. De Bruin PC, Beljaards RC, van Heerde P, et al. Differences in clinical behavior and immunophenotype between primary cutaneous and primary nodal anaplastic large cell lymphoma of T-cell or null cell phenotype. *Histopathology* 1993;23:127.
25. Shulman LN, Frisard B, Antin JH, et al. Primary Ki-1 anaplastic large cell lymphoma in adults: clinical characteristics and therapeutic outcome. *J Clin Oncol* 1993;11:937.
26. Pileri S, Bocchia M, Baroni C, et al. Anaplastic large cell lymphoma (CD30+/Ki-1+): results of a prospective clinicopathologic study of 69 cases. *Br J Haematol* 1994;86:513.
27. Romaguera J, Garcia-Foncillas J, Cabanillas F. 16-year experience at MD Anderson Cancer Center with primary Ki-1 (CD30) antigen expression and anaplastic morphology in adult patients with diffuse large cell lymphoma. *Leuk Lymphoma* 1995;20:97.
28. Weisenburger DD, Gordon BG, Vose JM, et al. Occurrence of the t(2;5) (p23;q35) in non-Hodgkin's lymphoma. *Blood* 1996;87:3860.
29. Isaacson P, Wright D. Malignant lymphoma of mucosa-associated lymphoid tissue: a distinctive B-cell lymphoma. *Cancer* 1983;52:1410.
30. Isaacson P, Spencer J. Malignant lymphoma of mucosa-associated lymphoid tissue. *Histopathology* 1987;11:445.
31. Cogliatti S, Schmid U, Schumacher U, et al. Primary B-cell gastric lymphoma: a clinicopathologic study of 145 patients. *Gastroenterology* 1991;101:1159.
32. Radaszkiewicz T, Dragosics B, Bauer P. Gastrointestinal malignant lymphomas of the mucosa-associated lymphoid tissue: factors relevant to prognosis. *Gastroenterology* 1992;102:1628.
33. Wotherspoon A, Doglioni C, Diss T, et al. Regression of primary low-grade B-cell gastric lymphoma of mucosa-associated lymphoid tissue type after eradication of Helicobacter pylori. *Lancet* 1993;342:575.
34. Roggero E, Zucca E, Pinotti G, et al. Eradication of Helicobacter pylori infection in primary low-grade gastric lymphoma of mucosa-associated lymphoid tissue. *Ann Intern Med* 1995;122:767.
35. Harris NJ, Jaffe ES, Stein H, et al. A revised European-American classification of lymphoid neoplasms: a proposal from the International Lymphoma Study Group. *Blood* 1994;84:1361.
36. Stansfeld A, Diebold J, Kapanci Y, et al. Updated Kiel classification of lymphomas. *Lancet* 1988;i:292.
37. The non-Hodgkin's Lymphoma Classification Project. National Cancer Institute sponsored study of classifications of non-Hodgkin's lymphomas: summary and description of a working formulation for clinical usage. *Cancer* 1982;49:2112.
38. Nathwani B, Russell K, Brynes, et al. Classifications of non-Hodgkin's lymphomas. In: Knoules DM (ed). *Neoplastic Hematopathology*. Baltimore: Williams & Wilkins, 1992;555–601.
39. The non-Hodgkin's Lymphoma Classification Project. A clinical evaluation of the International Lymphoma Study Group Classification of non-Hodgkin's Lymphoma. *Blood* 1997;89:3909.
40. Mann RB, Berard CW. Criteria for the cytologic subclassification of follicular lymphoma: a proposed alternative method. *Hematol Oncol* 1982;1:187.
41. The International non-Hodgkin's Lymphoma Prognostic Factors Project. A predictive model for aggressive non-Hodgkin's lymphoma. *N Engl J Med* 1993;329:987.
42. Kaplan EL, Meier P. Nonparametric estimation from incomplete observations. *J Am Stat Assoc* 1958;53:457.
43. Cox DR. Regression models and life-tables. *J R Stat Soc* 1972;34:187.

CHAPTER 21

Small Lymphocytic Lymphoma

Jonathan Ben-Ezra

Small lymphocytic lymphoma (SLL) is a low-grade malignant lymphoma characterized morphologically by a proliferation of small, mature-appearing lymphocytes (1). It is classified as B-cell chronic lymphocytic leukemia in the Revised European–American Classification of Lymphoid Neoplasms (REAL) (2). In the Rappaport classification system (3), SLL is called *well-differentiated lymphocytic lymphoma*. It is classified as malignant lymphoma, lymphocytic, and SLL in the Kiel (4) and Lukes and Collins (5) systems, respectively. In all geographic areas, SLL comprises 3% to 10% of all non-Hodgkin's lymphomas (1,6–11). A similar percentage is seen among canine non-Hodgkin's lymphomas (12).

RELATIONSHIP TO OTHER LYMPHOPROLIFERATIVE DISORDERS

Small lymphocytic lymphoma biologically is related very closely to two other lymphoproliferative disorders: chronic lymphocytic leukemia (CLL) and lymphoplasmacytic lymphoma or immunocytoma (Waldenström's macroglobulinemia) (13–15). This is evidenced by the fact that the REAL classification has eliminated the category of SLL and has subsumed it under the category of B-cell CLL (see Chapter 19). There is much overlap between these clinicopathologic entities, and in some cases it may be impossible to distinguish them morphologically and clinically one from another. In many patients, the lymph node morphology in CLL is indistinguishable from that seen in SLL (16). Many patients with SLL present with an absolute lymphocytosis or bone marrow involvement (13,14,17–20), thus simulating CLL. Even in those patients with SLL who do not have overt involvement of the peripheral blood, circulating neoplastic cells can be detected by sensitive methods, such as polymerase chain reaction. Moreover, between 14% and 35% of patients with "pure" SLL, that is, nodal involvement by SLL without lymphocytosis at presentation, eventually develop a clinical picture simulating CLL, with an absolute peripheral lymphocytosis, during the course of their disease. A monoclonal gammopathy is present in 10% to 20% of patients with the lymph node histology of SLL; some of these patients also have an absolute lymphocytosis (13,14). In addition, 2% to 5% of patients with SLL have both an absolute lymphocytosis and a monoclonal gammopathy (13,14). In the past, it was thought that if the process was primarily nodal the diagnosis was SLL, and if the process primarily involved the peripheral blood and bone marrow it was CLL. This is no longer the case. The disease is a unified B-cell CLL: Only a small minority of patients have disease entirely limited to lymph nodes (2).

If a monoclonal gammopathy is detectable in the presence of plasmacytoid cells the process should be classified as lymphoplasmacytic lymphoma or immunocytoma (Waldenström's macroglobulinemia).

PATHOLOGIC FEATURES

The lymph node involved by SLL may be of normal size, but most often it is enlarged. The node is firm, with a white "fish-flesh" appearance. The tumor may extend into the surrounding soft tissues. SLL has a similar appearance if it involves extranodal tissues, such as orbit, stomach, or lung.

The neoplastic cell in SLL is a small, mature-appearing lymphocyte (Fig. 21.1). The cell is approximately 6 to 12 μm in size and is morphologically indistinguishable from a benign normal, nontransformed lymphocyte. In the usual form of SLL, the cytoplasm is scant; more cytoplasm is seen in the plasmacytoid variant. The cellular proliferation is usually monotonous, although some patients may have a heterogeneous population of malignant lymphoid cells. The nuclei are round, with only slight irregularity of the nuclear membrane contour; a diagnosis of mantle cell lymphoma

J. Ben-Ezra: Department of Pathology, Medical College of Virginia, Campus of Virginia Commonwealth University, Richmond, Virginia 23298-0250

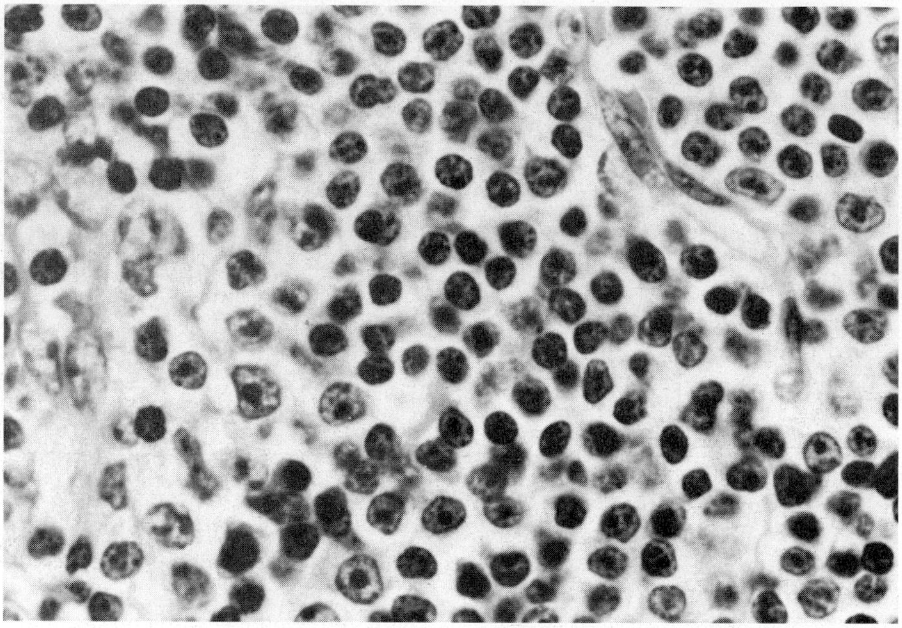

FIG. 21.1. Photomicrograph of small lymphocytic lymphoma, showing the small, mature-appearing lymphoid cells with clumped chromatin. Note the larger, paler cells in the right side of the photograph, which are part of a pseudofollicular proliferation center (hematoxylin and eosin stain, original magnification: 1,000× magnification).

(MCL) should be entertained if the nuclei have moderate irregularity. The lymphoid irregularity may be part of the SLL process, or it may be a technical artifact because of fixation or processing (14,21). In keeping with its mature appearance, the nuclear chromatin is condensed. Several small nucleoli may be observed. Electron microscopy reveals round, fairly large mitochondria concentrated near one pole of the cell (22).

In fine needle aspiration specimens and touch imprints (Fig. 21.2), the neoplastic cells appear morphologically similar to small, nontransformed lymphocytes (13,23). The cells have a scant or barely perceptible amount of cytoplasm, which is pale to basophilic. As in the tissue sections, the nuclei have several indistinct nucleoli and a clumped chromatin pattern. A variable number of prolymphocytes and large transformed cells (immunoblasts) also may be present, depending on the abundance of pseudofollicular proliferation centers. These cells have more cytoplasm than the typical cells of SLL. The large transformed cells have one to several prominent nucleoli but lack intense cytoplasmic basophilia (see Chapter 13).

Only a limited number of morphometric studies have been performed to analyze the nuclei in SLL (21,24). These studies have shown that the cells in SLL are different from the neoplastic cells of follicle center cell lymphomas. The cells in SLL show heterogeneity, both within a single case and between cases. No differences are found between the nuclei in "typical" SLL and those in the subgroup with plasmacytic differentiation; the morphologic differences between the variants result from cytoplasmic, not nuclear, parameters.

In up to 75% of patients, the lymph node architecture is completely effaced by the malignant process (17,25). In the remaining patients, residual lymph node structures may be present. These residual structures include germinal centers, present in 10% to 15% of cases (14,17), and patent sinuses

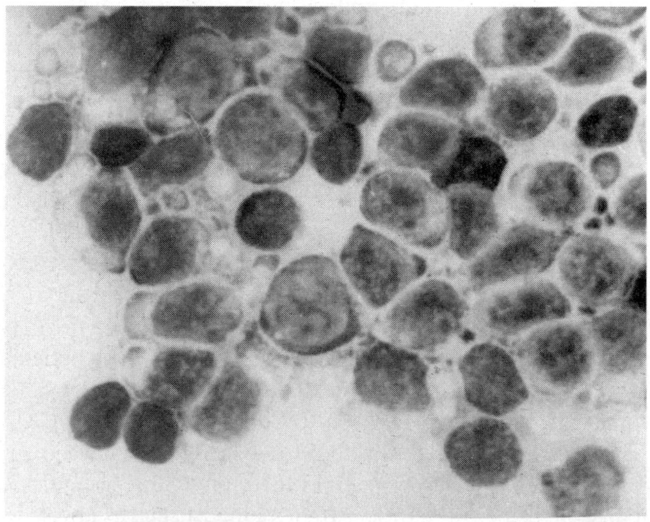

FIG. 21.2. Fine needle aspiration specimen from a patient with small lymphocytic lymphoma, showing small mature lymphoid cells and the larger cells of a pseudofollicular proliferation center (DiffQuik stain, original magnification: 1,000× magnification).

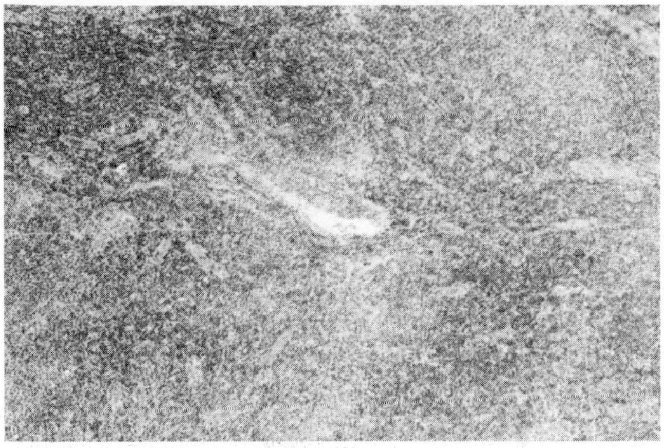

FIG. 21.3. A diffuse proliferation of small lymphoid cells is apparent, with preservation of a sinus (in center of figure) (hematoxylin and eosin stain, original magnification: 100× magnification).

(Fig. 21.3), present in 19% of cases (17). The patent sinuses may be empty, or they may contain lymphocytes or histiocytes. If germinal centers are present, the SLL usually encroaches directly on the secondary follicle, with resultant obliteration of the mantle zone. Capsular invasion is present in most cases (Fig. 21.4), and is massive in 13% to 36% of cases of SLL (14,17).

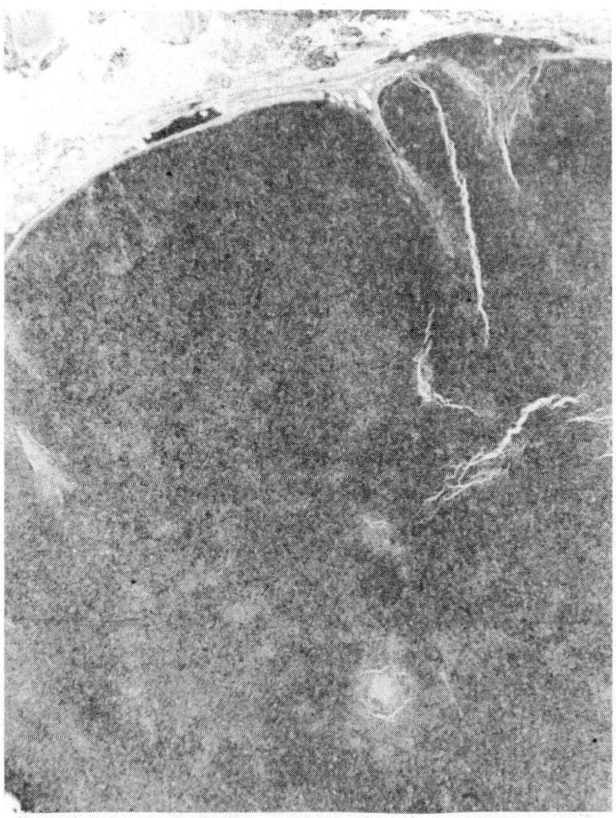

FIG. 21.4. Although the capsule of the lymph node is attenuated, some focal infiltration is noted. The lighter staining areas represent pseudofollicles (hematoxylin and eosin stain, original magnification: 20× magnification).

In the vast majority of cases, the overall pattern is one of a diffuse lymphoma. A rare case of nodular SLL may be observed (3,26). This pattern must be very extraordinary, however, because none of the 268 cases described by Ben-Ezra and colleagues (17) or the 84 described by Evans and coworkers (14) had a true nodular pattern. If a true nodular pattern is present, the lymphoid cells should be examined closely for the presence of irregularity of their nuclear contours, which would indicate that one is dealing with an MCL or a follicle center cell lymphoma (26) that may or may not have been colonized by marginal zone B cells.

In almost all cases of SLL, paler staining areas, referred to as *pseudofollicular proliferation centers* or *pseudofollicles*, are seen (13–17) (Figs. 21.4, 21.5). These areas tend to be round and faint with indistinct margins but may vary slightly in shape (27). These proliferation centers comprise prolymphocytes, larger lymphoid cells (immunoblasts), and small cleaved cells; the percentage of each of these cell types varies from case to case (13,14,17,27). Pseudofollicles may be seen in cases with and without residual germinal centers (27).

Cells other than neoplastic lymphocytes, those of the pseudofollicular proliferation centers, or those of the residual lymph node may be seen in lymph nodes involved by SLL. These include epithelioid histiocytes (25) or cells morphologically indistinguishable from Reed-Sternberg cells (16,28,29) (Fig. 21.6); if Reed-Sternberg–like cells are seen in a patient with SLL, the possibility of coexisting Hodgkin's disease or transformation to Hodgkin's disease should be considered (30). Mitotic figures are rare in lymph node sections, although occasional patients may have a brisk mitotic rate (14,17).

The bone marrow often is involved by SLL at diagnosis. The pattern of bone marrow involvement is almost always nodular (31,32), in contrast to CLL, in which the pattern of bone marrow involvement may be nodular, interstitial, diffuse, or mixed (32). The nodules are not preferentially paratrabecular in location but rather may be found throughout the marrow space. The cells in the nodules may be small, mature-appearing lymphoid cells, although a variable number of cells with a slightly cleaved nuclear contour may be present. The precise reason for this difference in histology between the nodal lesion and bone marrow involvement is not known, although it is probably related to fixation and tissue processing; touch imprint preparations or aspirate smears from bone marrows involved by SLL show the lymphocytes to be small and mature-appearing, morphologically similar to the neoplastic cells present in lymph nodes.

Without immunohistochemical studies, it may be difficult, if not impossible, to distinguish benign bone marrow lymphoid nodules from nodular involvement of the bone marrow by SLL. Clues to the malignant nature of the infiltrate, however, may be apparent. The more massive the involvement of the bone marrow, the more likely it is that the lymphoid nodules are malignant. Benign lymphoid nodules tend to be small and compact; malignant lymphoid nodules

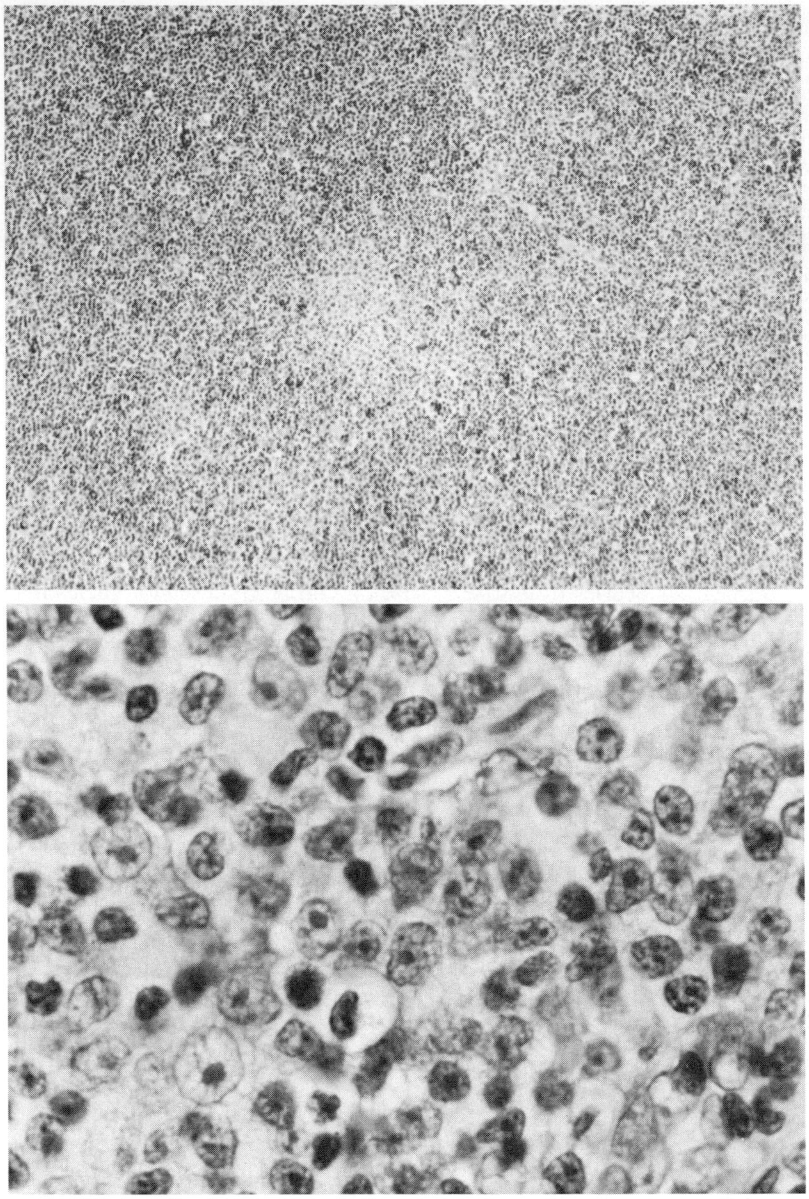

A

B

FIG. 21.5. A: Diffuse proliferation of small lymphoid cells in SLL, with a paler staining pseudofollicular proliferation center in the middle of the photomicrograph (hematoxylin and eosin stain, original magnification: 100× magnification). **B:** Higher power of a pseudofollicle which shows the large cells containing nuclei with a vesicular chromatin pattern and prominent nucleoli (hematoxylin and eosin stain, original magnification: 1,000× magnification).

may be large. Finally, benign lymphoid nodules in the bone marrow tend to be circumscribed, whereas the nodules of SLL may have cells at the periphery that ''leak'' out into the surrounding bone marrow parenchyma and surround residual hematopoietic elements (33). The lymphocytes in a malignant lymphoid nodule in the bone marrow express CD20 and BCL-2, but not CD3 (33).

Occasionally, SLL may be seen in the bone marrow of a patient with a higher grade lymphoma. Such a morphologic occurrence is termed *discordant histology*. These patients have the same prognosis as patients with large cell lymphoma who do not have bone marrow involvement, which is markedly better than those patients whose bone marrow is involved by the higher grade lymphoma (34,35).

The spleen involved by SLL is almost always enlarged, sometimes massively (36–38). Splenic weights in excess of 4 kg may be seen (38). SLL accounts for approximately 20% of the spleens that are involved by non-Hodgkin's lymphoma (39). The lymphoma predominantly involves the white pulp, with many small white nodules seen throughout the splenic parenchyma, simulating a miliary pattern. These small nodules sometimes coalesce, forming larger nodules or a diffuse pattern of involvement. Involvement of the red pulp, including the splenic cords and sinuses, also may be seen. Although splenic involvement most often is present in patients with known SLL, it may be the only site of involvement (39) (see Chapter 53).

Although SLL is primarily nodal in its tissue manifestation, it may involve other extranodal tissues and organs besides the spleen (see Chapter 31). These are primarily the orbit (40) and lung (41,42), although other organs and tissues, such as the skin and stomach, may be involved. In

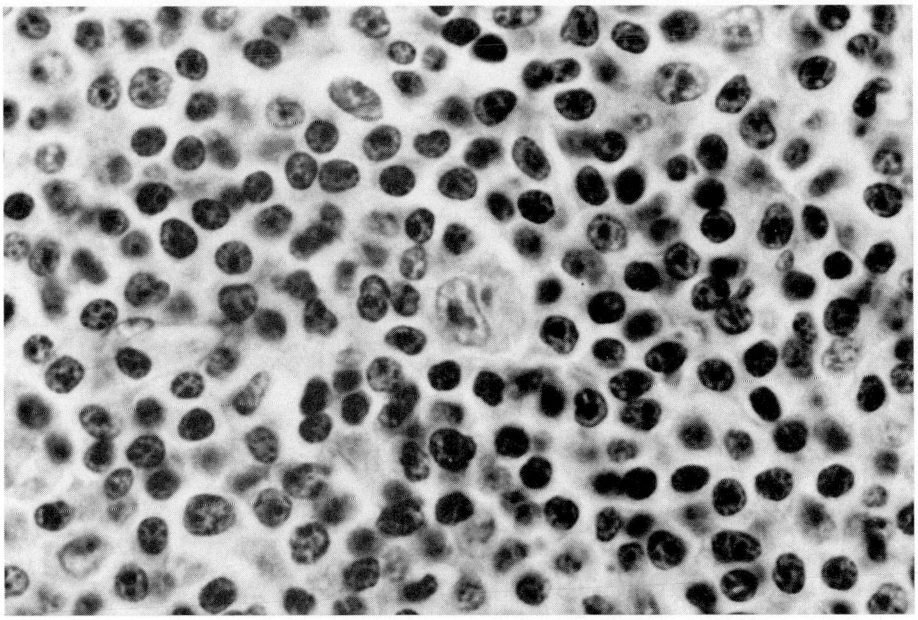

FIG. 21.6. A case of small lymphocytic lymphoma in which cells indistinguishable from Reed-Sternberg cells are present. In a different setting, one might consider the diagnosis of lymphocyte-rich Hodgkin's disease (hematoxylin and eosin stain, original magnification: 1,000× magnification).

these extranodal sites, the differentiation of SLL from other small B-cell lymphomas, such as MCL and marginal zone lymphoma, must be made; this distinction usually can be made based upon nuclear features, the lack of epithelial infiltration, and immunohistochemistry. The differentiation of SLL from reactive proliferations (''pseudolymphoma'') may be difficult. Morphologic clues to the malignant nature of the small lymphocytic infiltrate (in SLL) are the lack of reactive germinal centers, a monomorphous infiltrate, and massive infiltration with tissue destruction. The only definitive method of distinguishing SLL from pseudolymphoma, however, is the demonstration of monoclonality of the lymphocytic infiltrate.

IMMUNOLOGIC FEATURES

Small lymphocytic lymphoma is almost invariably of B-cell derivation (43–45). Of 298 cases of SLL analyzed at the City of Hope National Medical Center, 295 were of B-cell derivation, and only three were derived from T cells (J. Ben-Ezra, unpublished observations). Only approximately 1% of SLLs are comprised of neoplastic T cells. Conversely, only 2% of T-cell lymphomas are morphologically proven to be SLL (46).

The B-cell SLLs express a characteristic immunophenotype; they are HLA-DR—positive (HLA-DR$^+$), CD19$^+$, CD20$^+$, CD5$^+$, CD23$^+$, CD43$^+$, CD10-negative (CD10$^-$), CD22$^-$, CD11c$^\pm$, and CD25$^\pm$ (47) (Fig. 21.7). Similar to CLL, surface immunoglobulin expression by the neoplastic cells is weak; this is because of a surface immunoglobulin density approximately 10% of that of normal B lymphocytes (approximately 9,000 molecules of surface immunoglobulin per cell) (48). In more than 80% of cases, the cells also express CD5, a pan-T cell antigen (24,43–45). The expression of CD20 is weaker than that of normal B cells (49). The cells most commonly express surface IgM or IgM and IgD heavy chains (24,43–45). In keeping with the immunoglobulin light chain frequency of normal B cells, more than half of SLLs express κ, as opposed to λ, immunoglobulin light chains (15,24,43,45). Although determination of monoclonality is best done either on fresh cells in suspension or on fresh snap-frozen tissue, monoclonality occasionally may be determined on paraffin-embedded material, especially if the cells have plasmacytoid features (15), in which case intracytoplasmic immunoglobulin is detected. Approximately 60% to 75% of cases of SLL express CD21 (the C3d receptor) (24,43–45). The neoplastic cells also may express other antigens, including CD11c, CD25 (Tac antigen), and CD14 (50,51). Immunologically, the only known difference between the cells of SLL and of CLL is the expression of lymphocyte function-associated antigen (LFA-1), an adherence molecule, on the cells of SLL as opposed to those of CLL (52), and the higher mean percentage of mouse rosette-forming cells in the peripheral blood of CLL compared with the lymph nodes of SLL (53).

The exact benign immunologic counterpart in normal human blood and lymph nodes of the malignant lymphoid cells of SLL and CLL is not known. There is preferential usage of the *VH5*, *VH6*, and *VKIII* immunoglobulin variable gene families (54); gene families that are relatively small. The cell of origin in SLL is presumed to be a B cell of intermediate differentiation, based on the presence of CD19,

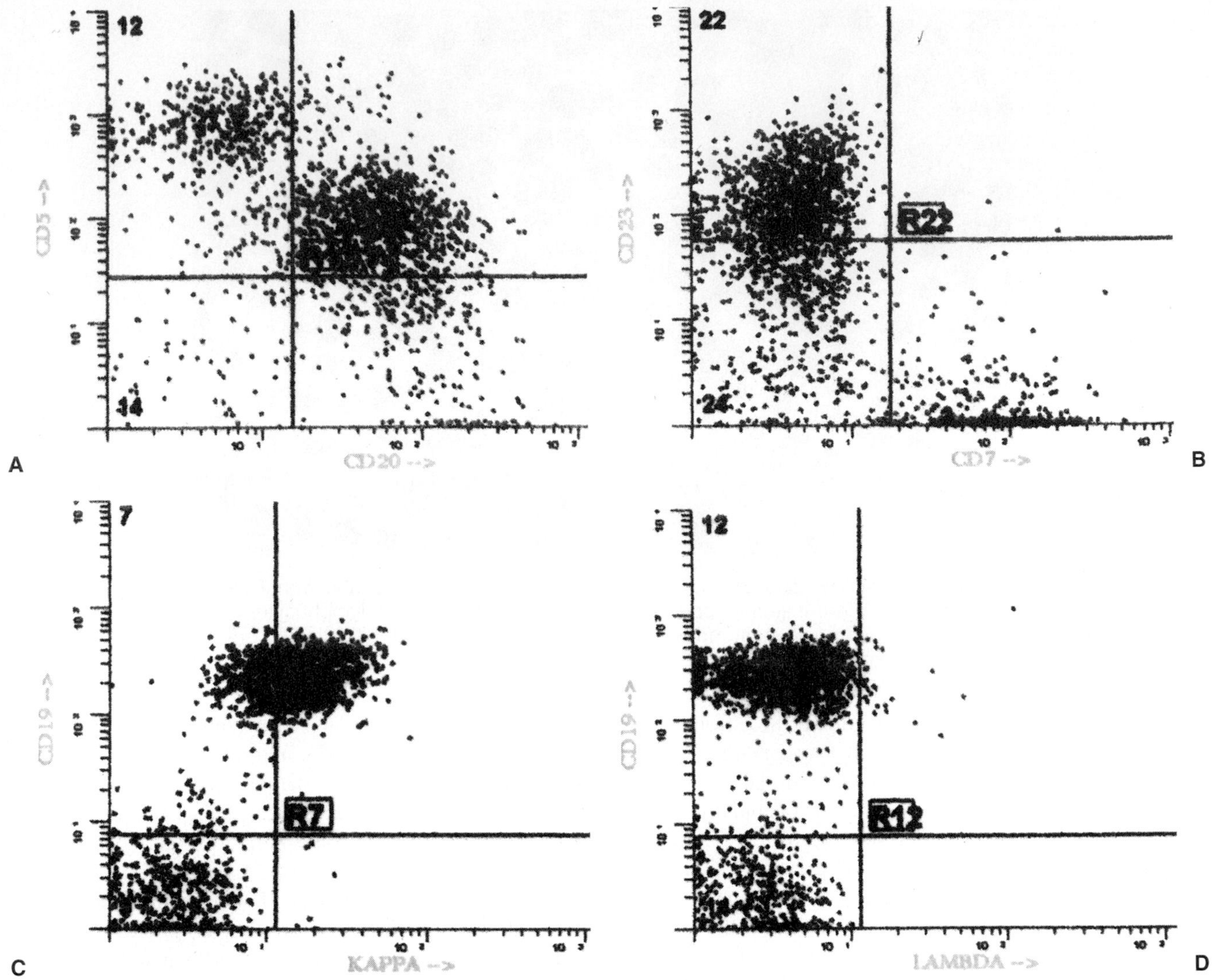

FIG. 21.7. Flow cytometric evaluation of a fine needle aspiration specimen from a small lymphocytic lymphoma (SLL) (same patient as in Fig. 21.2). **A:** Coexpression of CD20 and CD5 by the cells of SLL. Notice the slightly weaker intensity of CD5 on the neoplastic cells compared with the normal $CD5^+CD20^-$ T cells. **B:** The cells of SLL express CD23. **C,D:** Expression of κ (**C**) and λ (**D**) light chains on the B cells. Notice the weak intensity of the κ light chain staining, representing the low density of immunoglobulin on the cell surface.

CD20, CD5, and low levels of surface immunoglobulin on the surface of these cells (48). This most likely is a pre–germinal center B cell, based on the lack of somatic hypermutation of its immunoglobulin variable region genes (55).

Most cases of SLL coexpress CD5 and CD43 (56), which are considered to be T cell–associated antigens. Although these markers usually are expressed together, occasionally there is dyssynchronous expression of CD5 and CD43 (57). Although not easily identifiable, the $CD5^+$ B cell is a cell normally present in low numbers in the body, because variable numbers of $CD5^+$ B cells, ranging from 20% to 40% of the circulating B cells, may be found in the peripheral blood of normal individuals (50,51). In addition, $CD5^+$ B cells may be seen in the germinal centers of lymph nodes and tonsils (58) (Chapters 2,3).

Several attempts have been made to correlate the immunologic profiles of SLLs with their histologic and clinical characteristics (24,44,45). The results, in general, have been contradictory and unrewarding. It appears that patients with SLL with peripheral blood lymphocytosis more often express IgD heavy chains and CD5 than those who do not have an elevated white blood cell count. Plasmacytoid differentiation has been associated with CD25 and CD71 expression and with CD5 negativity (59). The association of CD21 expression with nodal versus extranodal location, and of CD5 negativity with extranodal location and plasmacytoid features, has not been uncontested in the literature (44,45,59,60). It appears that many cases that were considered to be extranodal $CD5^-$ SLLs may in fact have been examples of B-cell marginal zone lymphomas (59).

The immunoarchitecture of the pseudofollicles deserves special mention. In addition to bearing monotypic surface immunoglobulin (45), the cells within the proliferation centers also may strongly express antigens associated with dendritic reticulum cells, either CD21 (CRII) or DRC-1 (43,45,61,62). These antibodies only react with a minority of cases of SLL. In these cases, the DRC frameworks are diminished in size and number, compared with reactive germinal centers and the nodules of follicular lymphomas (61); this may indicate that pseudofollicular proliferation centers originate from atrophic germinal centers (43,61). The pseudofollicular proliferation centers have a higher concentration of Ki-67$^+$ cells than do the surrounding tissue (45,62). The cells in the pseudofollicular proliferation centers, compared with the diffuse portion of the SLL, may be 41H$^+$ and CD71$^+$ (45). In addition, in cases in which the diffuse portion of the tumor fails to express either CD38 or CD25, the pseudofollicular proliferation centers may express these antigens. On paraffin sections, the cells within the pseudofollicular proliferation centers may express S-100 (62), CD74, or CD75 (27).

CYTOGENETIC AND MOLECULAR FEATURES

As is characteristic of B-cell lymphomas, those SLLs that are derived from B cells exhibit clonal immunoglobulin gene rearrangements (63,64). Because SLL is derived from relatively mature B cells, both the immunoglobulin heavy chain and light chain genes are rearranged in most cases. Approximately 8% of patients with SLL also possess rearrangements of the T-cell receptor β-chain gene locus (63). SLL and CLL preferentially rearrange certain immunoglobulin heavy and light chain genes as opposed to others, including a highly conserved $V_K III$ gene, *HUMKV325* (55,65,66). In contrast to higher-grade B-cell non-Hodgkin's lymphomas, somatic hypermutation is not seen in cases of SLL and CLL, but instead the gene rearrangements appear to be stable (55,67); this is consistent with the pre–germinal center cell of origin of SLL.

As is characteristic of those with other non-Hodgkin's lymphomas, most patients with SLL possess chromosomal abnormalities (68–70). Although few, if any, are unique to SLL, some of these abnormalities are recurring. Abnormalities of chromosome 14 may be seen in 53%, and of chromosome 12 in 32%, of cases of SLL. Trisomy 12, which commonly is seen in B-cell CLL, may be seen in approximately 20% of cases of SLL (68,70,71). In approximately half of the cases of SLL with trisomy 12, this is the only cytogenetic abnormality present (68,70). Although not pathognomonic for SLL, abnormalities of 14q22 occur more frequently in SLL than in other non-Hodgkin's lymphomas (68,72). One of the most common cytogenetic abnormalities present may be a deletion of 13q, either 13q12 or 13q14.3, that encompasses the *BRACA2* oncongene (73–77); this change may be seen in up to 80% of cases. Other cytogenetic abnormalities that may be observed in SLL include trisomy 3, trisomy or monosomy 18, dic(4;7)(p11;p11), del(6)(q21q23), t(11;18)(q21;q21), abnormalities of 10q23-25, t(14;18), and t(13;17)(q12-14;p12-13) (68–70, 78–84). Those patients with monosomy 18 often have peripheral blood and bone marrow involvement (78), and those with trisomy 18 may have a shortened survival (83). Although patients with SLL with a cytogenetic abnormality have only one abnormal clone, up to 33% of cases may have an additional clone present at presentation (68,70). Those cases of SLL that in the past were described as having a t(11;14) translocation most likely represent cases of MCL.

Oncogene and tumor suppressor gene overexpression is variable in SLLs. Two thirds of SLLs have increased levels of *MYC* and one third have increased levels of *RAS* (85); although the quantity of the oncogene protein may be elevated, the increase is probably not due to mutations of these oncogenes (86,87). Levels of *ABL* are increased in 29% of cases of SLL and in 46% of cases of immunocytoma (SLL, plasmacytoid) (88); an increased level of *ABL* is associated with a more aggressive clinical course (88). Overexpression of *P53* is seen in approximately 20% of cases of SLL (89), and this overexpression results from mutation of the *P53* gene (87,90). The activity of the *SRC* protooncogene is low in SLL (91). The cytogenetic abnormality at 13q12.3 may be related to inactivation of the *BRCA2* gene (73,77).

Only a rare case of SLL is found to have a t(14;18) translocation on cytogenetic evaluation (68,69). Many cases of SLL have increases in the amount of the BCL-2 protein expressed by the lymphoma (33,92–94). Although in the past it was thought that abnormalities of *BCL1*, with a t(11;14) translocation, may be seen in cases of SLL (95,96), it currently is believed that those cases probably are examples of MCL. SLL lacks rearrangement of the *BCL1* oncogene or overexpression of its cyclin D1–PRAD-1 protein (71,97–101). Similarly, SLL lacks deletion or rearrangement of the cyclin-dependent kinase inhibitors p18 and p19, and overexpression of cyclin D3, although cyclin D2 may be overexpressed (71,102). Although the small lymphocytes in SLL do not express the retinoblastoma protein, it is expressed by the cells in the pseudofollicles (101).

Epstein-Barr virus (EBV) transcripts are not found in the small neoplastic cells of SLL (30), although the virus may be involved in the transformation of SLL to Hodgkin's disease or a higher-grade lymphoma (11,30,87,103,104).

In most cases of SLL, less than 5% of the cells are in S phase (71,105,106), and only a small fraction of cells express the MIB-1 proliferation protein (89); expression of MIB-1 is seen more frequently in the pseudofollicular proliferation centers than in the small neoplastic lymphoid cells of SLL. Approximately 90% of cases of SLL, with and without plasmacytoid features, are diploid (106).

DIFFERENTIAL DIAGNOSIS

Several other entities should be considered in the differential diagnosis of the lymph node thought to be involved by

SLL: lymphoid hyperplasia, Hodgkin's disease, MCL, marginal zone lymphoma, and diffuse small cleaved cell lymphoma. Diffuse interstitial hyperplasia may be confused with SLL, because both entities consist of a diffuse proliferation of small, mature-appearing lymphocytes. Some cases of SLL, particularly the interfollicular variety (27), have reactive follicles, patent sinuses, a lack of capsular infiltration, and expansion of the interfollicular areas, features present in a reactive lymph node. Pseudofollicular proliferation centers, however, are not present in reactive lymph nodes, whereas they are present in nearly all cases of SLL. Immunoblasts also are likely to be present in a reactive process; they are absent in SLL. If any doubt remains, immunologic studies should be performed. In a reactive process, the small mature interfollicular lymphocytes are T cells; in SLL they are almost invariably B cells.

The differential diagnosis between SLL and Hodgkin's disease, either nodular lymphocyte predominance or lymphocyte-rich, also may be difficult (28). In lymphocyte predominance and lymphocyte-rich Hodgkin's disease, diagnostic Reed-Sternberg cells are rare and may not be detected, particularly if the overall architecture of the lymph node does not suggest the diagnosis. In addition, occasional cases of SLL contain cells that are indistinguishable from Reed-Sternberg cells (Fig. 21.6). Helpful features in distinguishing the two entities are the presence of large nodules (which are distinguished easily from the pseudofollicles of SLL) and the possible presence of progressive transformation of germinal centers in the nodular lymphocyte predominance type (Chapter 17), and the presence of pseudofollicles in SLL. In an occasional specimen, it is not possible to distinguish between SLL and lymphocyte-rich Hodgkin's disease morphologically (28); one must resort to immunologic methods. The small lymphocytes of lymphocyte predominance Hodgkin's disease are T cells; those in SLL are monoclonal B cells.

Close attention to cellular detail in well-prepared sections is necessary to distinguish SLL from MCL (Chapter 22) or from diffuse, small cleaved cell lymphoma. It is important to make this distinction, because the clinical course and treatment of SLL are different from those of these other non-Hodgkin's lymphomas. In SLL, the neoplastic lymphocytes have round and regular nuclear membranes; those in MCL have slight to moderate nuclear irregularity (Fig. 21.8); and those in diffuse, small cleaved cell lymphoma have marked nuclear irregularity. Lymph nodes involved by SLL usually have pseudofollicles; those involved by diffuse, small cleaved cell lymphoma do not. In contrast to SLL, the cellular proliferation in MCL is very monotonous, with occasional histiocytic cells in the background. Although some cases of presumed MCL may contain pseudofollicles, the clinical course of these patients is similar to that of SLL (107), and these cases should be considered low-grade lymphomas similar, if not identical, to SLL. The nuclear chromatin in MCL is usually more dispersed than that seen in SLL, and the nucleus may contain inconspicuous nucleoli. In both SLL and MCL the mitotoic rate is usually low. In most patients it is prudent to perform immunologic studies to help distinguish these two entities. In SLL, the neoplastic cells are $CD20^+CD5^+CD23^+$ but negative for cyclin D1; those of MCL are $CD20^+CD5^+CD23^-$ and do not express cyclin D1 (97–100).

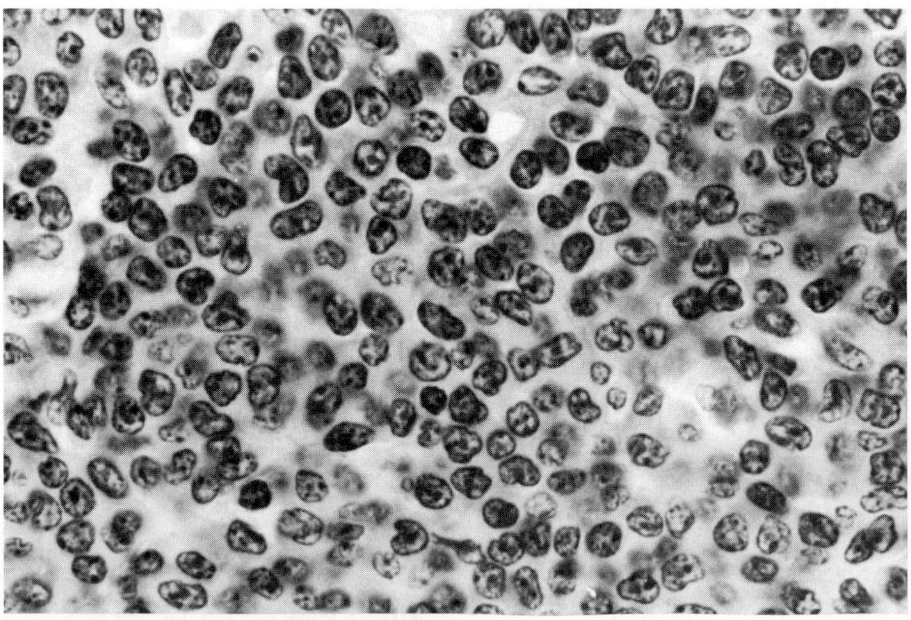

FIG. 21.8. A case of mantle cell lymphoma. Note the cleaved and angulated nuclei and compare them with the more regularly shaped nuclei in Figures 21.1, 21.7, and 21.9 (hematoxylin and eosin stain, original magnification: 1,000× magnification).

In addition, SLL must be distinguished from marginal zone lymphoma. In marginal zone lymphoma, the neoplastic cells are small, but they have curved nuclear contours and abundant clear cytoplasm. In contrast to the cells of SLL, the cells of marginal zone lymphoma lack CD5 and CD23.

Although the differential diagnosis involves many entities, the correct diagnosis can be made in the vast majority of cases, especially if a good clinical history is obtained and appropriate immunohistochemical studies are performed (10).

CLINICAL FEATURES

Small lymphocytic lymphoma is predominantly a disease of middle age and of the elderly, with a median age at diagnosis of 55 to 61 years (1,9,13,14,17–20,108). In the elderly, SLL comprises a greater percentage of non-Hodgkin's lymphomas than it does in younger age groups (109,110), and very few patients are younger than 40 years of age (1,17,18). The male-to-female ratio is approximately 2 : 1 (1,10,14, 17–19,108).

At presentation, most patients have advanced disease; stage IV disease is present in 61% to 90% of patients presenting with SLL (1,10,17–20,108). Between 69% and 82% of these patients have bone marrow involvement at diagnosis (1,10,13,14,17,18,20). Nodal involvement is present in 85% of patients initially, and approximately 30% of patients have extranodal involvement at the time of presentation (1). B symptoms (anemia, weight loss, or night sweats) are present in 15% to 43% of SLL patients (17,19,20,108). Only rare patients are found to be physically incapacitated at the time of initial diagnosis (18).

Almost all patients with SLL have generalized lymphadenopathy at presentation (13,14,17). Hepatic and splenic enlargement is seen in more than 50% of patients at presentation (13,14,17,20). Splenomegaly may be the presenting clinical finding in some patients with SLL; 19% to 55% of all primary splenic lymphomas are SLLs (36–39). A leukocytosis or an absolute lymphocytosis (4,000/mm^3) is seen initially in 33% to 66% of patients (13,14,17,18,20). In addition, 12% to 33% of patients have anemia (<11 g hemoglobin/dL) and 6% to 42% of patients have thrombocytopenia (< 150,000 platelets per cubic millimeter) (13,14,17–19).

MORPHOLOGIC TRANSFORMATION AND CLINICAL PROGRESSION

In approximately 3% to 20% of patients with CLL, the disease does not remain stable but instead progresses to a large cell lymphoma or undergoes prolymphocytic or blastic transformation, or the patient develops Hodgkin's disease. CLL progressing to large cell lymphoma is termed *Richter's syndrome* (see Chapter 40) (111). These changes are a poor prognostic sign, with the transformation usually heralding significantly shortened patient survival. Although the same processes theoretically should occur in SLL, such progressions to large cell lymphoma or a prolymphocytic transformation are only occasionally reported (20,105,111–114). In the solid tissue counterpart of classic Richter's syndrome, the large cell lymphoma may be derived from the same clone as (87,113,114) or a different clone than (87,113,115) the original small lymphocytic neoplasm. Although the large cell lymphoma may bear a different immunoglobulin heavy or light chain than the original SLL or CLL, this does not necessarily imply that the large cell lymphoma is derived from a different clone (113,114). This transformation to a large cell lymphoma may be related to mutations in the *P53* gene (87). The only way to definitively determine the clonal origin of the large cell lymphoma is to compare the clonal immunoglobulin heavy and light chain gene rearrangements of both the original and the subsequent tumors (87, 115–117).

Tissue manifestations of prolymphocytic transformation of SLL have been reported only rarely (105), although cases reported under other terms, such as the paraimmunoblastic variant of SLL (118,119), the tumor-forming subtype of B-cell CLL (120), or MCL (14), may represent such a transformation (105). The lymph nodes contain an admixture of small mature-appearing lymphocytes, characteristic of SLL, and other larger cells (Fig. 21.9). Most of these other cells are of intermediate size and have vesicular nuclei containing prominent, centrally placed nucleoli (105,118); similar cells are present in the pseudofollicular proliferation centers of typical SLL (17). Immunoblasts may be present. The cells have an increased S-phase fraction compared with SLL, although not as much so as in large cell transformation (105). These patients have accelerated clinical courses (118). Prolymphocytic transformation of SLL has a clinical course intermediate between that of SLL and large cell transformation of SLL.

Another transformation of SLL that deserves mention is that of transformation to Hodgkin's disease (30,121,122). In this variant, Hodgkin's disease develops after the diagnosis of SLL has been established; occasionally the Hodgkin's disease may be seen in the same lymph node as the SLL. This transformation occurs in approximately 0.5% of patients with SLL, with a median time to development of 45 months (122). It presents with an advanced stage of Hodgkin's disease and is relatively resistant to treatment. This process should be distinguished from those cases of SLL that involve Reed-Sternberg–like cells (29,30). In the latter situation, the lymph node does not contain the background of Hodgkin's disease but rather that of SLL, with the Reed-Sternberg–like cells present in a sea of the small lymphoid cells characteristic of SLL. If doubt exists about the correct diagnosis, immunohistochemical studies can be performed. In SLL with Reed-Sternberg–like cells, the large binucleated cells are $CD45^+CD15^-CD30^-$ B cells (29,30); in transformation to Hodgkin's disease, the cells have the classic immunophenotype of Reed-Sternberg cells ($CD15^+CD30^+$ $CD45^-$) (30,121).

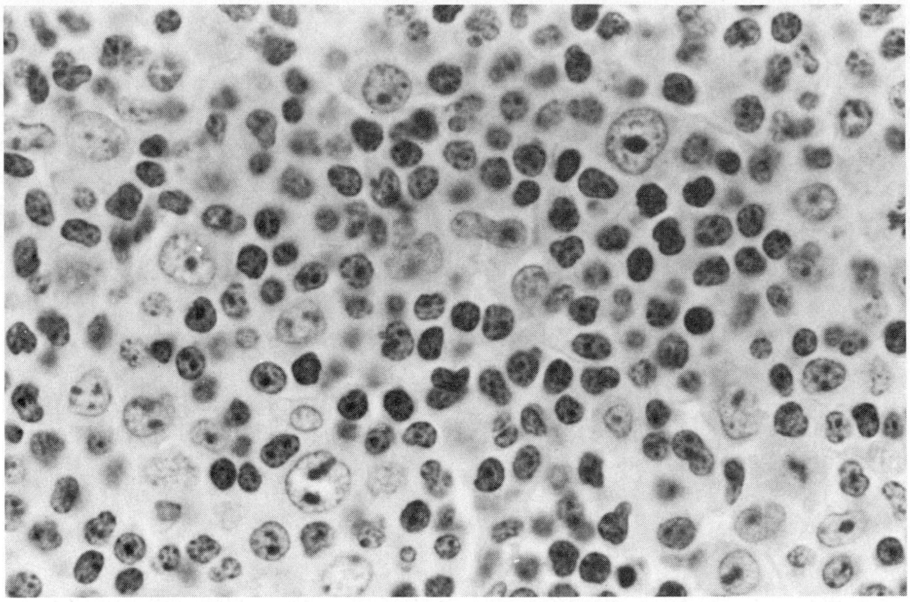

FIG. 21.9. A case of small lymphocytic lymphoma undergoing prolymphocytic transformation. Intermixed with the small, mature-appearing lymphoid cells are larger cells with abundant cytoplasm and a nucleus with a vesicular chromatin pattern and prominent nucleoli. These larger cells are similar to those seen in pseudofollicular transformation centers (hematoxylin and eosin stain, original magnification: 1,000× magnification).

SMALL LYMPHOCYTIC LYMPHOMA, PLASMACYTOID

All of the major classification schemes of non-Hodgkin's lymphomas recognize a subcategory of SLL in which the neoplastic cells exhibit plasmacytoid features (Fig. 21.10). In the Lennert classification system, three such categories of lymphomas with cytoplasmic plasmacytoid features exist: lymphoplasmacytic immunocytoma, lymphoplasmacytoid immunocytoma, and polymorphic immunocytoma (4,25, 120). The first two have been classified as subcategories of SLL, with differentiation between them depending on

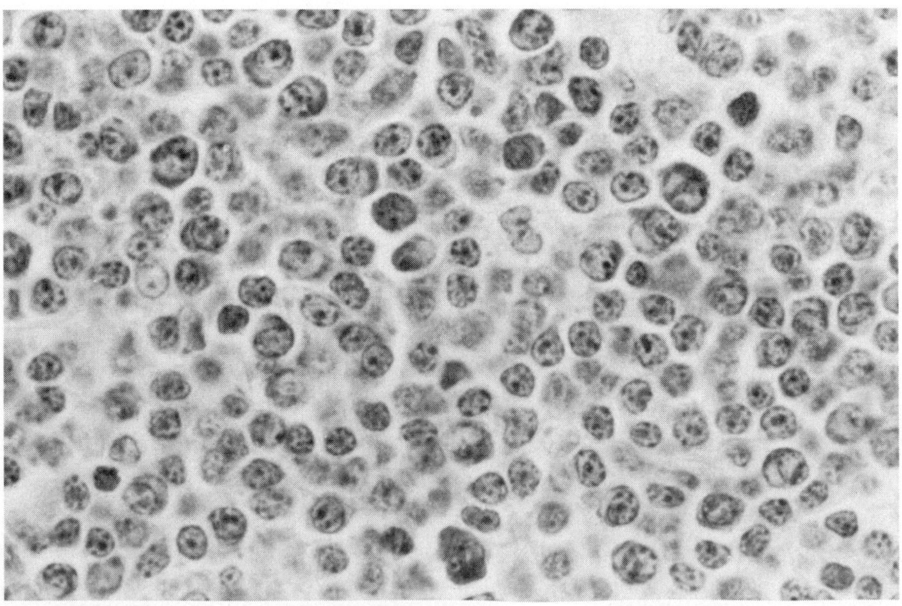

FIG. 21.10. Photomicrograph of the cells in the plasmacytoid variant of small lymphocytic lymphom. Note the presence of mature plasma cells and lymphoid cells with plasmacytoid features. The cells have eccentrically placed nuclei and abundant cytoplasm (hematoxylin and eosin stain, original magnification: 1,000× magnification).

whether there is an admixture of small malignant lymphocytes with mature plasma cells (lymphoplasmacytic immunocytoma) or with small lymphocytic cells with cytoplasmic plasma cell features (lymphoplasmacytoid immunocytoma). Polymorphic immunocytoma with small lymphoid cells, plasmacytoid cells, and larger lymphoid cells usually is classified under malignant lymphoma, diffuse mixed small and large cell, in the Working Formulation (1). In the REAL classification (2), the category of lymphoplasmacytoid lymphoma–immunocytoma is reserved for Lennert's lymphoplasmacytic type and comprises 1% of all non-Hodgkin's lymphomas (10).

Clinically, many of these patients have a serum monoclonal gammopathy, in which case they have Waldenström's macroglobulinemia (13,120,123). The age at presentation, as well as the percentage with advanced clinical stage, is similar to that seen in SLL without plasmacytoid differentiation (10,108,123). Some of the patients may have an associated autoimmune disorder, such as Sjögren's syndrome (25,44); in these patients, sheets of monocytoid B cells also may be present (25).

The overall architectural features of the lymph nodes are similar to those seen in SLL. Although the architecture is usually diffusely effaced, some cases have residual germinal centers (25). Globular periodic acid–Schiff stain–positive inclusions may be seen frequently in the cytoplasm of the plasmacytoid cells and occasionally form intranuclear inclusions called *Dutcher bodies* (13,15,25,120). In the lymphoplasmacytoid variant (Lennert's), the plasmacytoid cells are intermingled with the small lymphocytic cells; in the lymphoplasmacytic variant there are often sheets of small lymphocytes adjacent to sheets of plasma cells, with little blending of the two components (13,44). The nuclei of the small lymphocytes are identical to the nuclei of the plasmacytoid cells; the only difference between the two cellular subgroups is the amount and character of the cytoplasm (24). Immunoblasts, plasmablasts, eosinophils, neutrophils, mast cells, or epithelioid histiocytes also may be seen in these lymph nodes (25,120).

Similar to SLL but without plasmacytoid features, these tumors are derived from B cells (44). Monoclonal expression of immunoglobulin may be found on immunologic staining of the paraffin sections in these cases, because the immunohistochemical staining detects the abundant periodic acid–Schiff stain–positive immunoglobulin that is present in the cytoplasm of the plasma cells and plasmacytoid cells (15). The monoclonal immunoglobulin detected in and on these cells is of the same type as that seen in the serum in those patients with a monoclonal gammopathy (15).

The clinical and immunologic data support making lymphoplasmacytic immunocytoma its own category and subsuming the lymphoplasmacytoid variant under B-cell CLL (SLL). The cells of the lymphoplasmacytoid variant are $CD5^+$, similar to those of classic SLL; the cells of the lymphoplasmacytic variant are usually $CD5^-$ (120). Moreover, similar to SLL, patients with the lymphoplasmacytoid variant have more peripheral blood involvement, and a lower incidence of paraproteinemia, than patients with the lymphoplasmacytic type of immunocytoma (120).

These tumors generally are considered to be low-grade neoplasms (2,10,123) and have a median duration of survival of 49 to 59 months (10,123). Some studies have found no difference in survival duration between those tumors with and those without plasmacytoid features (10,13,14,17,19, 124). Other authors, however, have described poorer survival for those patients whose SLLs have plasmacytic or plasmacytoid features compared with those without these features (108,123). On multivariate analysis, Karnofsky index, age, and Binet stage have been found to be significant independent prognostic factors. Similar to typical SLL, cases may transform to a more aggressive non-Hodgkin's lymphoma (25).

PROGNOSTIC FACTORS

Several investigators have attempted to correlate histologic and clinical characteristics of SLL at presentation with the eventual clinical outcome (13,14,17–20,59,89, 123–125). The data, unfortunately, often have been conflicting. Althought bone marrow status (17,19) appears to have no influence on survival, and a positive response to treatment portends prolonged survival (17,18), the prognostic utility of other factors is subject to debate, both within and between studies. Although many studies conclude that the type of small lymphocytic proliferation (SLL vs. CLL vs. Waldenström's macroglobulinemia) (13,14,124), stage at presentation (14,17,19,124), number of large lymphocytes present in the cellular infiltrate (14,17), sex (17,124), and the presence of plasmacytoid features (17,19,124) have no influence on prognosis, the large study by Englehard and colleagues (123) found that advanced stage, increased numbers of large lymphocytes, male gender, and the presence of plasmacytoid features are poor prognostic factors. In this study, even bone marrow status in immunocytoma was determined to be prognostically significant. More than one study has found a correlation between age (14,17,123) or hemoglobin level (14,17,125) and survival, but others have not. The presence of complete lymph node effacement may affect prognosis adversely (14,17), but no study has shown a clearcut influence on survival. Some studies have shown prognostic significance in the presence of a high mitotic rate (14) or pseudofollicles (19,123); others have failed to show these factors to be important predictors of survival.

The influence of peripheral lymphocytosis on survival is the subject of much controversy and in some ways relates to the precise relationship between SLL and CLL. There appears to be no difference in survival rate between those patients who present predominantly with lymphadenopathy (SLL) or with lymphocytosis (13,14,124). Moreover, several investigators have found no difference in survival rate between those patients with SLL presenting with or without an absolute lymphocytosis (14,18,123,124). Ben-Ezra and coworkers (17), however, found a difference in survival rate between those patients with SLL who did or did not have a leukocytosis; if the two groups (white blood cell count greater than or less than 10,000 per cubic millimeter) were analyzed separately, differences in prognostic factors were observed between the two groups. Nonetheless, if the combined data were analyzed by multivariate analysis, white blood cell count was not found to be an independent prognostic variable. In addition, those patients with SLL who eventually develop CLL have a survival rate similar to that of patients who do not develop CLL (19). Lymphocytosis *per se* does not predict poorer survival independently in SLL (17,123).

Medeiros and coworkers (124) looked at immunologic markers, in addition to clinical and histologic parameters, that were associated with survival. Although the clinical and pathologic variables did not correlate with survival, some of the immunologic ones did. Greater than 25% Ki-67$^+$ cells, less than 25% CD3$^+$ cells, or less than 15% CD4$^+$ cells correlated with decreased survival. No significant correlation was seen with other B-cell, T-cell, or other markers. The prognostic significance of the proliferative index (Ki-67) is similar to the finding by others (14,89) that patients with actively dividing tumors do poorly. The correlation of survival rate with the number of CD3$^+$ and CD4$^+$ cells most likely results from a manifestation of host response to the tumor. Other clinical markers, such as serum β_2-microglobulin (20,125) and thymidine kinase (125) levels, indicate a poor prognosis, as does *MYC* gene amplification in the tumor cells (89).

TREATMENT AND SURVIVAL

Small lymphocytic lymphoma is a low-grade lymphoma and has a "favorable" prognosis. The 2-year survival rate is 67% to 76% (18,24), the 5-year rate between 47% and 76% (1,10,14,17,19), and the 10-year rate between 7% and 49% (14,17,19). The median duration of survival is between 4.3 and 5.8 years (1,14,17,18,123), although some other studies show a longer median survival (20,126). The survival curve does not show a plateau but rather shows a steady decline with time (1,14,17,123).

Most patients with SLL present with advanced (stage III or IV) disease; only approximately 10% of patients with SLL have limited (stage I or II) disease. In this subgroup of patients with localized disease, local irradiation is the treatment of choice, with excellent control of the disease. In the much larger group of patients with advanced disease, the choice of treatment modality, and even whether to treat, is much more difficult. Those patients who are treated have an approximately 50% complete response rate (1,18,20), and those that initially respond may be disease-free for over 5 years (1), although the failure-free 5-year survival is only 25% (10). In several studies, there did not appear to be any difference in survival rate between those patients who were treated initially with high-dosage chemotherapy and radiation and those patients who were followed without treatment and only received treatment if they become symptomatic (127–129). In these studies, patients in the "wait and watch" groups had a median of 3 years before they became symptomatic enough that treatment was warranted. For symptomatic patients with advanced disease, alkylating agents such as chlorambucil may decrease lymph node enlargement. In all studies, there is a steady decline in the number of survivors with the passage of time, without reaching a plateau.

SUMMARY AND CONCLUSIONS

Small lymphocytic lymphoma is a low-grade non-Hodgkin's lymphoma that is comprised predominantly of small, mature-appearing lymphoid cells. SLL is very closely related to CLL and Waldenström's macroglobulinemia, and there is much overlap of clinical and pathologic features among the three groups. Almost all of the tumors are derived from B cells, and almost all of the patients have advanced (stage III or IV) disease at presentation. Although SLL is a low-grade lymphoma, the survival curve shows an inexorable and steady decline, with the life line eventually descending below the relative plateau seen in high-grade non-Hodgkin's lymphomas.

ACKNOWLEDGMENTS

The author thanks Dr. Michael Kornstein and the editor of this book, Dr. Daniel Knowles, for reviewing the manuscript and for their helpful and thoughtful comments.

REFERENCES

1. Non-Hodgkin's Lymphoma Pathologic Classification Project. National Cancer Institute sponsored study of the non-Hodgkin's lymphomas: summary and description of a working formulation for clinical usage. *Cancer* 1982;49:2112–2135.
2. Harris NL, Jaffe ES, Stein H, et al. A revised European-American classification of lymphoid neoplasms: a proposal from the international lymphoma study group. *Blood* 1994;84:1361–1392.
3. Rappaport H. *Tumors of the hematopoietic system.* Washington D.C.: Armed Forces Institute of Pathology, 1966.
4. Lennert K, Mohri N, Stein H, et al. The histopathology of malignant lymphoma. *Br J Haematol* 1975;31[Suppl]:193–203.
5. Lukes RJ, Collins RD. New approaches to the classification of the lymphomata. *Br J Cancer* 1975;31:1–28.
6. Schultz HB, Ersboll J, Nissen NI, et al. A simplified working formulation of non-Hodgkin's lymphomas based on quantifiable histologic criteria. *Cancer* 1989;64:2532–2540.
7. Garg A, Dawar R, Agarwal V, et al. Non-Hodgkin's lymphoma in Northern India: a retrospective analysis of 238 cases. *Cancer* 1985; 56:972–977.
8. Salem P, Anaissie E, Allam C, et al. Non-Hodgkin's lymphomas in the Middle East: a study of 417 patients with emphasis on special features. *Cancer* 1986;58:1162–1166.
9. Newell GR, Cabanillas FG, Hagemeister FJ, et al. Incidence of lymphoma in the US classified by the working formulation. *Cancer* 1987; 59:857–861.
10. The Non-Hodgkin's Lymphoma Classification Project. A clinical evaluation of the international lymphoma study group classification of non-Hodgkin's lymphoma. *Blood* 1997;89:3909–3918.
11. Cool CD, Bitter MA. The malignant lymphomas of Kenya: morphol-

ogy, immunophenotype, and frequency of Epstein-Barr virus in 73 cases. *Hum Pathol* 1997;28:1026–1033.
12. Greenlee PG, Filippa DA, Quimby FW, et al. Lymphomas in dogs: A morphologic, immunologic, and clinical study. *Cancer* 1990;66: 480–490.
13. Pangalis GA, Nathwani BN, Rappaport H. Malignant lymphoma, well differentiated type: its relationship with chronic lymphocytic leukemia and macroglobulinemia of Waldenström. *Cancer* 1977;39:999–1010.
14. Evans HL, Butler JJ, Youness EL. Malignant lymphoma, small lymphocytic type: a clinicopathologic study of 84 cases with suggested criteria for intermediate lymphocytic lymphoma. *Cancer* 1978; 41:1440–1455.
15. Pangalis GA, Nathwani BN, Rappaport H. Detection of cytoplasmic immunoglobulin in well-differentiated lymphoproliferative diseases by the immunoperoxidase method. *Cancer* 1980;45:1334–1339.
16. Dick FR, Maca RD. The lymph node in chronic lymphocytic leukemia. *Cancer* 1978;41:283–292.
17. Ben-Ezra J, Burke JS, Swartz WG, et al. Small lymphocytic lymphoma: a clinicopathologic analysis of 268 cases. *Blood* 1989;73: 579–587.
18. Icli F, Ezdinili EZ, Costello W, et al. Diffuse well-differentiated lymphocytic lymphoma (DLWD): response and survival. *Cancer* 1978;42:1936–1942.
19. Morrison WH, Hoppe RT, Weiss LM, et al. Small lymphocytic lymphoma. *J Clin Oncol* 1989;7:598–606.
20. Berger F, Felman P, Sonet A, et al. Nonfollicular small B-cell lymphomas: a heterogeneous group of patients with distinct clinical features. *Blood* 1994;83:2829–2835.
21. Dardick I, Caldwell DR, Silver SS, et al. Lymphocyte nuclear morphology in diffuse well-differentiated lymphocytic lymphoma: comparative morphometry of normal lymphoid tissues, non-Hodgkin's lymphoma, and Hodgkin's disease. *Arch Pathol Lab Med* 1987;111: 130–138.
22. Mori Y, Lennert K. *Electron microscopy atlas of lymph node cytology and pathology*. Berlin, Germany: Springer-Verlag, 1969.
23. Koo CH, Rappaport H, Sheibani K, et al. Imprint cytology of non-Hodgkin's lymphomas based on a study of 212 immunologically characterized cases: correlation of touch imprints with tissue sections. *Hum Pathol* 1989;20[Suppl 1]:1–138.
24. Tosi P, Leoncini L, Del Vecchio MT, et al. Heterogeneous subgroups among malignant diffuse small B cell lymphomas: a combined nucleometric and immunocytologic study. *Lab Invest* 1990;62: 202–212.
25. Patsouris E, Noël H, Lennert K. Lymphoplasmacytic/lymphoplasmacytoid immunocytoma with a high content of epitheliod cells: Histologic and immunohistochemical findings. *Am J Surg Pathol* 1990;14: 660–670.
26. Chang KL, Arber DA, Shibata D, et al. Follicular small lymphocytic lymphoma. *Am J Surg Pathol* 1994;18:999–1009.
27. Ellison DJ, Nathwani BN, Cho SY, et al. Interfollicular small lymphocytic lymphoma: the diagnostic significance of pseudofollicles. *Hum Pathol* 1989;20:1108–1118.
28. Colby TV, Warnke RA, Burke JS, et al. Differentiation of chronic lymphocytic leukemia from Hodgkin's disease using immunologic marker studies. *Am J Surg Pathol* 1981;5:707–710.
29. Shin S, Ben-Ezra J, Burke JS, et al. Reed-Sternberg-like cells in low grade lymphomas are transformed neoplastic cells of B-cell lineage. *Am J Clin Pathol* 1993;99:658–662.
30. Momose H, Jaffe ES, Shin SS, et al. Chronic lymphocytic leukemia/small lymphocytic lymphoma with Reed-Sternberg-like cells and possible transformation to Hodgkin's diseases: mediation by Epstein-Barr Virus. *Am J Surg Pathol* 1992;16:859–867.
31. Pangalis GA, Roussou PA, Kittas C, et al. Clinical significance of patterns of bone marrow involvement in chronic lymphocytic leukemia and small lymphocytic (well-differentiated) non Hodgkin's lymphoma. *Bibltheca Haemat* 1984;50:87–97.
32. Pangalis GA, Roussou PA, Kittas C, et al. Patterns of bone marrow involvement in chronic lymphocytic leukemia and small lymphocytic (well differentiated) non-Hodgkin's lymphoma: its clinical significance in relation to their differential diagnosis and prognosis. *Cancer* 1984;54:702–708.
33. Ben-Ezra JM, King BE, Harris AC, et al. Staining for bcl-2 protein helps to distinguish benign from malignant lymphoid aggregates in bone marrow biopsies. *Mod Pathol* 1994;7:560–564.
34. Fisher DE, Jacobson JO, Ault KA, et al. Diffuse large cell lymphoma with discordant bone marrow histology: clinical features and biologic implications. *Cancer* 1989;64:1879–1887.
35. Conlan MG, Bast M, Armitage JO, et al. Bone marrow involvement by non-Hodgkin's lymphoma: the clinical significance of morphologic discordance between the lymph node and bone marrow. *J Clin Oncol* 1990;8:1163–1172.
36. Spier CM, Kjeldsberg CR, Eyre HJ, et al. Malignant lymphoma with primary presentation in the spleen: a study of 20 patients. *Arch Pathol Lab Med* 1985;109:1076–1080.
37. Kraemer BB, Osborne BM, Butler JJ. Primary splenic presentation of malignant lymphoma and related disorders: a study of 49 cases. *Cancer* 1984;54:1606–1619.
38. Narang S, Wolf BC, Neiman RS. Malignant lymphoma presenting with prominent splenomegaly: a clinicopathologic study with special reference to intermediate cell lymphoma. *Cancer* 1985;55: 1948–1957.
39. Arber DA, Rappaport H, Weiss LW. Non-Hodgkin's lymphoproliferative disease involving the spleen. *Mod Pathol* 1997;10:18–32.
40. Knowles DM, Jakobiec FA, McNally L, et al. Lymphoid hyperplasia and malignant lymphoma occurring in the ocular adnexa (orbit, conjunctiva, and eyelids): a prospective multiparametric analysis of 108 cases during 1977 to 1987. *Hum Pathol* 1990;21:959–973.
41. Kennedy JL, Nathwani BN, Burke JS, et al. Pulmonary lymphomas and other pulmonary lymphoid lesions: a clinicopathologic and immunologic study of 64 patients. *Cancer* 1985;56:539–552.
42. Ben-Ezra J, Winberg CD, Wu A, et al. Concurrent presence of two clonal populations in small lymphocytic lymphoma of the lung. *Hum Pathol* 1987;18:399–402.
43. Spier CM, Grogan TM, Fielder K, et al. Immunophenotypes in "well-differentiated" lymphoproliferative disorders, with emphasis on small lymphocytic lymphoma. *Hum Pathol* 1986;17:1126–1136.
44. Harris NL, Bhan AK. B-cell neoplasms of the lymphocytic, lymphoplasmacytoid, and plasma cell types: immunohistologic analysis and clinical correlation. *Hum Pathol* 1985;16:829–837.
45. Medeiros LJ, Strickler JG, Picker LJ, et al. "Well-differentiated" lymphocytic neoplasms: immunologic findings correlated with clinical presentation and morphologic features. *Am J Pathol* 1987;129: 523–535.
46. Jaffe ES. Post-thymic lymphoid neoplasia. In Jaffe ES, ed. *Surgical pathology of the lymph nodes and related organs.* Philadelphia: WB Saunders, 1985:218–248.
47. Jennings CD, Foon KA. Recent advances in flow cytometry: application to the diagnosis of hematologic malignancy. *Blood* 1997;90: 2863–2892.
48. Foon KA, Todd RF III. Immunologic classification of leukemia and lymphoma. *Blood* 1986;68:1–31.
49. Almasri NM, Duque RE, Iturraspe J, et al. Reduced expression of CD20 antigen as a characteristic marker for chronic lymphocytic leukemia. *Am J Hematol* 1992;40:259–263.
50. Wormsley SB, Baird SM, Gadol N, et al. Characteristics of CD11c + CD5 + chronic B-cell leukemias and the identification of novel peripheral blood B-cell subsets with chronic lymphoid leukemia immunophenotypes. *Blood* 1990;76:123–130.
51. Kipps TJ, Vaughan JH. Genetic influence on the levels of circulating CD5 B lymphocytes. *J Immunol* 1987;139:1060–1064.
52. Inghirami G, Wieczorek R, Zhu BY, et al. Differential expression of LFA-1 molecules in non-Hodgkin's lymphomas and lymphoid leukemia. *Blood* 1988;72:1431–1434.
53. Batata A, Shen B. Immunophenotyping of subtypes of B-chronic (mature) lymphoid leukemia. *Cancer* 1992;70:2436–2443.
54. Mayer R, Stone K, Han A, et al. Malignant CD5 B cells—biased immunoglobulin variable gene usage and autoantibody production. *Int Rev Immunol* 1991;7:189–203.
55. Pratt LF, Rassenti L, Larrick J, et al. Ig V region gene expression in small lymphocytic lymphoma with little or no somatic hypermutation. *J Immunol* 1989;143:699–705.
56. Contos MJ, Kornstein MJ, Innes DJ, et al. The utility of CD20 and CD43 in subclassification of low-grade B-cell lymphoma on paraffin sections. *Mod Pathol* 1992;5:631–633.
57. Lynch EF, Jones PA, Swerdlow SH. CD43 and CD5 antibodies define four normal and neoplastic B-cell subsets: a three color cytometric study. *Cytometry* 1995;22:223–231.
58. Caligaris-Cappio F, Gobbi M, Bofill M, et al. Infrequent normal B

lymphocytes express features of B-chronic lymphocytic leukemia. *J Exp Med* 1982;155:623–628.
59. Sundeen JT, Longo DL, Jaffe ES. CD5 expression in B-cell small lymphocytic malignancies: correlations with clinical presentation and sites of disease. *Am J Surg Pathol* 1992;16:130–137.
60. Martinsson U, Sundström C, Glimelius B. Immunophenotype analysis of B-CLL lymphoma and immunocytoma. *APMIS* 1989;97:1025–1032.
61. Ratech H, Sheibani K, Nathwani BN, et al. Immunoarchitecture of the "pseudofollicles" of well differentiated (small) lymphocytic lymphoma: a comparison with true follicles. *Hum Pathol* 1988;19:89–94.
62. Mori N, Oka K, Kojima M. DRC expression in B-cell lymphomas. *Am J Clin Pathol* 1988;89:488–492.
63. Kneba M, Bergholz M, Bolz I, et al. Heterogeneity of immunoglobulin gene rearrangements in B-cell lymphomas. *Int J Cancer* 1990;45:609–613.
64. Kamat D, Laszewski MJ, Kemp JD, et al. The diagnostic utility of immunophenotyping and immunogenotyping in the pathologic evaluation of lymphoid proliferations. *Mod Pathol* 1990;3:105–112.
65. Kipps TJ, Robbins BA, Tefferi A, et al. CD-5 B-cell malignancies frequently express cross-reactive idiotypes associated with IgM autoantibodies. *Am J Pathol* 1990;136:809–816.
66. Mayer R, Logtenberg T, Strauchen J, et al. CD5 and immunoglobulin V gene expression in B-cell lymphomas and chronic lymphocytic leukemia. *Blood* 1990;75:1518–1524.
67. de Jong D, Voetdijk BMH, van Ommen GJB, et al. Alterations in immunoglobulin genes reveal the origin and evolution of monotypic and bitypic B cell lymphomas. *Am J Pathol* 1989;134:1233–1242.
68. Levine EG, Arthur DC, Frizzera G, et al. There are differences in cytogenetic abnormalities among the histologic subtypes of the non-Hodgkin's lymphomas. *Blood* 1985;66:1414–1422.
69. Koduru PRK, Filippa DA, Richardson ME, et al. Cytogenetic and histologic correlations in malignant lymphomas. *Blood* 1987;69:97–102.
70. Fifth International Workshop on Chromosomes in Leukemia-Lymphoma. Correlation of chromosome abnormalities with histologic and immunologic characteristics in non-Hodgkin's lymphoma and adult T cell leukemia-lymphoma. *Blood* 1987;70:1554–1564.
71. Delmer A, Ajchenbaum-Cymbalista F, Tang R, et al. Overexpression of cyclin D2 in chronic B-cell malignancies. *Blood* 1995;85:2870–2876.
72. Tilly H, Bastard C, Halkin E, et al. Del (14)(q22) in diffuse B-cell lymphocytic lymphoma. *Am J Clin Pathol* 1988;89:109–113.
73. Garcia-Marco JA, Navarro B, Caldas C. Confirmation of frequent somatic deletion of the 13q12.3 locus encompassing BRCA2 in chronic lymphocytic leukaemia. *Br J Haematol* 1997;99:708–709.
74. Foroni L, Panayiotidis P, Hoffbrand AV. Lack of clonal BCRA2 gene deletion on chromosome 13 in chronic lymphocytic leukaemia: an update of recent scientific reports. *Br J Haematol* 1998;100:800.
75. Panayiotidis P, Ganeshaguru K, Rowntree C, et al. Lack of clonal BCRA2 gene deletion on chromosome 13 in chronic lymphocytic leukaemia. *Br J Haematol* 1997;97:844–847.
76. Panayiotidis P, Ganeshaguru K, Hoffbrand AV, et al. Deletion of 13q14.3 and not 13q12 is the most common genetic abnormality detected in chronic lymphocytic leukemia cells. *Blood* 1997;89:734–735.
77. Garcia-Marco JA, Caldas C, Price CM, et al. Frequent somatic deletion of the 13q12.3 locus encompassing BRCA2 in chronic lymphocytic leukemia. *Blood* 1996;88:1568–1575.
78. Younes A, Jendiroba D, Engel H, et al. High incidence of monosomy 18 in lymphoid malignancies that have bone marrow and peripheral blood involvement. *Cancer Genet Cytogenet* 1994;77:39–44.
79. Offit K, Louie DC, Parsa NZ, et al. Clinical and morphologic features of B-cell small lymphocytic lymphoma with del(6)(q21q23). *Blood* 1994;83:2611–2618.
80. Callet-Bauchu E, Rimokh R, Tigaud I, et al. dic(4;7)(p11;p11): a new recurrent chromosomal abnormality in chronic B-lymphoid disorders. *Genes Chromosomes Cancer* 1996;17:185–190.
81. Speaks SL, Sanger WG, Masih AS, et al. Recurrent abnormalities of chromosome bands 10q23-25 in non-Hodgkin's lymphoma. *Genes Chromosomes Cancer* 1992;5:239–243.
82. Griffin CA, Zehnbauer BA, Beschorner WE, et al. t(11;18)(q21;q21) is a recurrent chromosome abnormality in small lymphocytic lymphoma. *Genes Chromosomes Cancer* 1992;4:153–157.
83. Schouten HC, Sanger WG, Weisenburger DD, et al. Chromosomal abnormalities in untreated patients with non-Hodgkin's lymphoma: associations with histology, clinical characteristics, and treatment outcome. *Blood* 1990;75:1841–1847.
84. Leroux D, Sotto JJ, Jacob MC, et al. Translocation t(13;17)(q12-14; p12-13) in two patients with lymphocytic lymphoma. *Cancer Genet Cytogenet* 1989;43:243–247.
85. Mitani S, Sugawara I, Shiku H, et al. Expression of c-myc oncogene product and ras family oncogene products in various human malignant lymphomas defined by immunohistochemical techniques. *Cancer* 1988;62:2085–2093.
86. Neri A, Knowles DM, Greco A, et al. Analysis of RAS oncogene mutations in human lymphoid malignancies. *Proc Natl Acad Sci USA* 1988;85:9268–9272.
87. Matolcsy A, Inghirami G, Knowles DM. Molecular genetic demonstration of the diverse evolution of Richter's syndrome (chronic lymphocytic leukemia and subsequent large cell lymphoma). *Blood* 1994;83:1363–1372.
88. Greil R, Gattringer C, Fasching B, et al. Abl oncogene expression in non-Hodgkin lymphomas: correlation to histological differentiation and clinical status. *Int J Cancer* 1988;42:529–538.
89. Palestro G, Ponti R, Chiusa L, et al. Cell proliferation, bcl-2, c-myc, p53 and apoptosis as indicators of different aggressiveness in small lymphocytic lymphoma (SLL). *Eur J Haematol* 1997;59:148–154.
90. Gaidano G, Ballerini P, Gong JZ, et al. p53 mutations in human lymphoid malignancies: association with Burkitt lymphoma and chronic lymphocytic leukemia. *Proc Natl Acad Sci USA* 1991;88:5413–5417.
91. Lynch SA, Brugge JS, Fromowitz F, et al. Increased expression of the src proto-oncogene in hairy cell leukemia and a subgroup of B-cell lymphomas. *Leukemia* 1993;7:1416–1422.
92. Pezzella F, Tse AGD, Cordell JL, et al. Expression of the bcl-2 oncogene protein is not specific for the 14;18 chromosomal translocation. *Am J Pathol* 1990;137:225–232.
93. Nguyen PL, Harris NL, Ritz J, et al. Expression of CD95 antigen and Bcl-2 protein in non-Hodgkin's lymphomas and Hodgkin's disease. *Am J Pathol* 1996;148:847–853.
94. Zutter M, Hockenbery D, Silverman GA, et al. Immunolocalization of the bcl-2 protein within hematopoietic neoplasms. *Blood* 1991;78:1062–1068.
95. Meeker TC, Grimaldi JC, O'Rourke R, et al. An additional breakpoint region in the BCL-1 locus associated with the t(11;14)(q13;q32) translocation of B-lymphocytic malignancy. *Blood* 1989;74:1801–1806.
96. Ince C, Blick M, Lee M, et al. Bcl-1 gene rearrangements in B cell lymphoma. *Leukemia* 1988;2:343–346.
97. Swerdlow SH, Yang WI, Zukerberg LR, et al. Expression of cyclin D1 protein in centrocytic/mantle cell lymphomas with and without rearrangement of the BCL1/cyclin D1 gene. *Hum Pathol* 1995;26:999–1004.
98. Yang WI, Zukerberg LR, Motokura T, et al. Cyclin D1 (Bcl-1,PRAD1) protein expression in low grade B-cell lymphomas and reactive hyperplasia. *Am J Pathol* 1994;145:86–96.
99. Oka K, Ohno T, Kita K, et al. PRAD1 gene over-expression in mantle-cell lymphoma but not in other low-grade B-cell lymphomas, including extranodal lymphoma. *Br J Haematol* 1994;86:786–791.
100. Vasef MA, Medeiros LJ, Koo C, et al. Cyclin D1 immunohistochemical staining is useful in distinguishing mantle cell lymphoma from other low-grade B-cell neoplasms in bone marrow. *Am J Clin Pathol* 1997;108:302–307.
101. Zukerberg LR, Benedict WF, Arnold A, et al. Expression of the retinoblastoma protein in low-grade B-cell lymphoma: relationship to cylin D1. *Blood* 1996;88:268–276.
102. Williams ME, Whitefield M, Swerdlow SH. Analysis of cyclin-dependent kinase inhibitors p18 and p19 in mantle-cell lymphoma and chronic lymphocytic leukemia. *Ann Oncol* 1997;8:71–73.
103. Shimakage M, Nakamine H, Tamura S, et al. Detection of Epstein-Barr virus transcripts in anaplastic large cell lymphomas by mRNA in situ hybridization. *Hum Pathol* 1997;28:1415–1419.
104. Petrella T, Yaziji N, Collin F, et al. Implication of the Epstein-Barr virus in the progression of chronic lymphocytic leukaemia/small lymphocytic lymphoma to Hodgkin-like lymphomas. *Anticancer Res* 1997;17:3907–3913.
105. Traweek ST, Esteban JM, Rappaport H. Prolymphocytic transforma-

tion of small lymphocytic lymphoma: Cell cycle and ploidy analysis. *Lab Invest* 1990;62:101A(abst).
106. Lehtinen T, Aine R, Lehtinen M, et al. Flow cytometric DNA analysis of 199 histologically favourable or unfavourable non-Hodgkin lymphomas. *J Pathol* 1989;157:27–36.
107. Perry DA, Bast MA, Armitage JO, et al. Diffuse intermediate lymphocytic lymphoma: a clinicopathologic study and comparison with small lymphocytic lymphoma and diffuse small cleaved cell lymphoma. *Cancer* 1990;66:1995–2000.
108. Richards MA, Hall PA, Gregory WM, et al. Lymphoplasmacytoid and small cell centrocytic non-Hodgkin's lymphoma: a retrospective analysis from St. Bartholomew's Hospital 1972–1986. *Hematol Oncol* 1989;7:19–35.
109. Carbone A, Tirelli U, Volpe R, et al. Non-Hodgkin's lymphoma in the elderly: a retrospective clinicopathologic study of 50 patients. *Cancer* 1986;57:2185–2189.
110. Alkan S, Karcher DS. Low grade lymphomas in the elderly. *Ann Clin Lab Sci* 1995;25:218–227.
111. Harousseau JL, Flandrin G, Tricot G, et al. Malignant lymphoma supervening in chronic lymphocytic leukemia and related disorders: Richter's syndrome. A study of 25 cases. *Cancer* 1981;48:1302–1308.
112. Acker B, Hoppe RT, Colby TV, et al. Histologic conversion in the non-Hodgkin's lymphomas. *J Clin Oncol* 1983;1:11–16.
113. Chan WC, Dekmezian R. Phenotypic changes in large cell transformation of small cell lymphoid malignancies. *Cancer* 1986;57:1971–1978.
114. Sheibani K, Nathwani BN, Winberg CD, et al. Small lymphocytic lymphoma: morphologic and immunologic progression. *Am J Clin Pathol* 1985;84:237–243.
115. Matolcsy A, Casali P, Knowles DM. Different clonal origin of B-cell populations of chronic lymphocytic leukemia and large-cell lymphoma in Richter's syndrome. *Ann N Y Acad Sci* 1995;764:496–503.
116. van Dongen JJM, Hooijkaas H, Michiels JJ, et al. Richter's syndrome with different immunoglobulin light chains and different heavy chain gene rearrangements. *Blood* 1984;64:571–575.
117. Sun T, Susin M, Desner M, et al. The clonal origin of two cell populations in Richter's syndrome. *Hum Pathol* 1990;21:722–728.
118. Pugh WC, Manning JT, Butler JJ. Paraimmunoblastic variant of small lymphocytic lymphoma/leukemia. *Am J Surg Pathol* 1988;12:907–917.
119. Grosso LE, Kelley PD. bcl-1 translocations are frequent in the paraimmunoblastic variant of small lymphocytic lymphoma. *Mod Pathol* 1998;11:6–10.
120. Lennert K, Tamm I, Wacker H-H. Histopathology and immunocytochemistry of lymph node biopsies in chronic lymphocytic leukemia and immunocytoma. *Leuk Lymphoma* 1991;5[Suppl]:157–160.
121. Brecher M, Banks PM. Hodgkin's disease variant of Richter's syndrome: Report of eight cases. *Am J Clin Pathol* 1990;93:333–339.
122. Fayad L, Robertson LE, O'Brien S, et al. Hodgkin's disease variant of Richter's syndrome: experience at a single institution. *Leuk Lymphoma* 1996;23:333–337.
123. Engelhard M, Brittinger G, Heinz R, et al. Chronic lymphocytic leukemia (B-CLL) and immunocytoma (LP-IC): Clinical and prognostic relevance of this distinction. *Leuk Lymphoma* 1991;5[Suppl]:161–173.
124. Medeiros LJ, Picker LJ, Gelb AB, et al. Numbers of host ''helper'' T cells and proliferating cells predict survival in diffuse small-cell lymphomas. *J Clin Oncol* 1989;7:1009–1017.
125. Hallek M, Wanders L, Ostwald M, et al. Serum beta(2)-microglobulin and serum thymidine kinase are independent predictors of progression-free survival in chronic lymphocytic leukemia and immunocytoma. *Leuk Lymphoma* 1996;22:439–447.
126. Kamihira S, Hirakata Y, Atogami S, et al. CD5-expressing B-cell lymphomas/leukemias: relatively high frequency of CD5 + B-cell lymphomas with an overall poor prognosis in Nagasaki Japan. *Leuk Lymphoma* 1996;22:137–142.
127. Horning SA, Rosenberg SA. The natural history of initially untreated low-grade non-Hodgkin's lymphomas. *N Engl J Med* 1984;311:1471–1475.
128. Young RC, Longo DL, Glatstein E, et al. The treatment of indolent lymphomas: watchful waiting V aggressive combined modality treatment. *Semin Hematol* 1988;25[Suppl 2]:11–16.
129. Rosenberg SA. The low-grade non-Hodgkin's lymphomas: challenges and opportunities. *J Clin Oncol* 1985;3:299–310.

CHAPTER 22

Mantle Cell Lymphoma

Dennis D. Weisenburger

In the mid-1970s, Berard and colleagues (1–4) coined the term *lymphocytic lymphoma of intermediate differentiation* to describe a group of non-Hodgkin's lymphomas that were not readily classifiable as either well differentiated (small lymphocytic) or poorly differentiated (small cleaved cell) lymphoma. In lymph node sections, the tumors usually had a diffuse pattern of growth and were composed of a mixture of small lymphoid cells, some with round nuclei like those of small lymphocytic lymphoma and others with indented and cleaved nuclei like those of small cleaved cell lymphoma. The term *intermediate* was used to describe the intermediate morphologic appearance of the tumors. About the same time, Lennert and coworkers (5–7) described a lymphoma with a similar appearance, termed *centrocytic*, which was characterized by a predominance of irregular and cleaved lymphoid cells. Early immunologic studies of these tumors revealed a B-cell phenotype, with the neoplastic cells showing moderate to intense staining for monoclonal surface immunoglobulin (3,4,7). Cytochemical stains for surface alkaline phosphatase suggested to Berard and colleagues (3,4) that intermediate lymphocytic lymphoma corresponded to the cells of primary lymphoid follicles and the mantle zones of secondary follicles; Lennert and coworkers (5–7) believed that centrocytic lymphoma was a germinal center cell lymphoma. In the early 1980s, Weisenburger and associates (8) and Palutke and colleagues (9) described a distinctive type of follicular lymphoma that was characterized by the proliferation of atypical small lymphoid cells in wide mantles around benign germinal centers. Weisenburger and associates (8,10) coined the term *mantle zone lymphoma* for this entity and suggested that it represented the follicular counterpart of diffuse intermediate lymphocytic lymphoma.

More recent studies, which are detailed in this chapter, have further characterized all of these various lymphomas clinically, immunologically, and at the molecular level and have led to the conclusion that they represent a closely related spectrum of tumors that corresponds to a subset of normal lymphocytes in the primary lymphoid follicles and mantle zones of secondary follicles. *Mantle cell lymphoma* (MCL) is now accepted as the name for this group of lymphomas (11,12).

D. D. Weisenburger: Department of Pathology and Microbiology, University of Nebraska Medical Center, Omaha, Nebraska 68198

PATHOLOGIC FEATURES

The pathologic features of MCL have been refined and the histologic spectrum of the disease has been expanded in recent years through the use of immunologic, cytogenetic, and molecular techniques. A number of large, well-studied series with detailed descriptions of the pathology of the MCL have been published (13–23).

Lymph Nodes

The non-Hodgkin's lymphomas of mantle cell type usually consist of atypical small lymphoid cells and have either a nodular or diffuse pattern of growth or a combination of the two patterns. Nodularity is present, at least focally, in approximately 40% of patients with MCL at the time of initial diagnosis. Early in the course of disease, nodular MCL may have a distinctly nodular or a vaguely nodular growth pattern at low magnification, and the nodal architecture may show only partial effacement. In nodular MCL, some or many of the nodules may consist of follicles with reactive germinal centers surrounded by broad mantles of small lymphoid cells (Fig. 22.1), the so-called mantle zone pattern (8,20). In such cases, however, some neoplastic nodules without germinal centers, which mimic primary follicles, are also present. In other cases, these latter nodules may predominate or be present exclusively (Fig. 22.2), and the process may be confused with a follicle center cell lymphoma of the small cleaved cell type. Later in the course of the disease, invasion and obliteration of the reactive germinal centers and interfollicular areas by neoplastic cells result in a diffuse pattern of growth and effacement of the

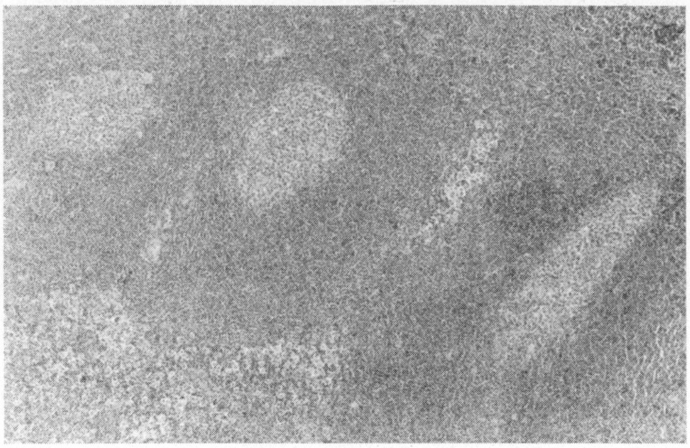

FIG. 22.1. Mantle cell lymphoma composed of nodules with reactive germinal centers surrounded by wide mantles of neoplastic small lymphoid cells (hematoxylin and eosin stain, original magnification: 40× magnification).

nodal architecture. Residual vague nodularity may be seen in such cases, and naked germinal centers lacking a normal lymphocyte cuff are found within the diffuse areas in approximately one quarter of patients (Fig. 22.3).

Cytologically, MCL usually consists of a monotonous population of atypical small lymphoid cells with irregular and indented nuclei, moderately coarse chromatin, inconspicuous nucleoli, and scant cytoplasm (typical ''intermediate'' cytology). Small round lymphocytes, some of which are T cells, are admixed in variable numbers, and neoplastic cells with cleaved nuclei are often present. Cases of MCL with predominantly round nuclei or only slight nuclear irregularity and cases with angulated and cleaved nuclei (''centrocytic'' cytology) or even cerebriform nuclei do occur. Although the neoplastic lymphoid cells show a spectrum of nuclear irregularity from case to case, ranging from slight to marked, the cells usually show little variation within an

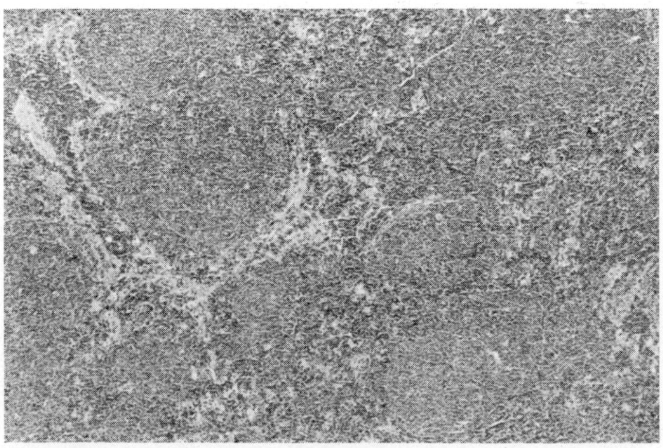

FIG. 22.2. Mantle cell lymphoma composed of nodules of neoplastic small lymphoid cells without reactive germinal centers (hematoxylin and eosin stain, original magnification: 40× magnification).

individual neoplasm (Fig. 22.4). In some cases, the cells in focal areas may have more abundant pale cytoplasm and resemble marginal zone or monocytoid B cells (21). In such cases, more typical areas are usually present, and it is unclear whether this finding is real or a result of problems with fixation or processing.

In about 20% of patients with MCL, the neoplastic cells are larger than usual and have more finely dispersed nuclear chromatin and small nucleoli. These high-grade variants have been referred to as *large cell* (''anaplastic centrocytic'') or *blastic* forms of MCL (6,15–17,22,23). Sometimes a mixture of atypical small cells and larger cells is present, imparting a more pleomorphic cytologic picture. In other patients, the blastic cells are quite monotonous, ranging from medium to large in size, with very fine chromatin and multiple small nucleoli (''blastoid'' or ''centrocytoid centroblastic'' cytology). These high-grade variants of MCL may occur *de novo* or as a transformation during the course of more typical disease (Fig 22.5). The diversity of morphologies seen in different cases of MCL is broad, ranging from small cells with round or slightly irregular nuclei at one end of the spectrum to large transformed cells with distinct nucleoli at the other end.

In general, large transformed lymphoid cells with vesicular nuclei and multiple prominent nucleoli (large noncleaved cells or centroblasts) are not seen in the lymphocytic forms of MCL, except in residual benign germinal centers. Plasma cells are usually absent or present in only small numbers in MCL and are polyclonal in nature. The rate of mitosis is generally low (<20 mitoses per 10 high-power fields) in the lymphocytic forms of MCL, but an increased rate usually is seen in the high-grade variants and often is accompanied by admixed benign histiocytes (10,14,15,20,23). These rather distinctive histiocytes have abundant pink cytoplasm and may contain phagocytized cellular debris (Fig. 22.6).

Histologic progression from a nodular pattern to a diffuse pattern of growth may be evident in a subsequent biopsy, and transformation from lymphocytic to high-grade cytology with a high rate of mitosis is not uncommon. Norton and colleagues (17) noted histologic transformation to high-grade cytology on rebiopsy in 17% of their patients with MCL and found evidence of transformation in 70% of their cases at autopsy. Transformation of MCL to the more common forms of diffuse large B-cell lymphoma, however, is an uncommon event.

Cytology, Peripheral Blood, and Bone Marrow

In lymph node touch preparations and other cytologic specimens, the neoplastic cells are small to medium-sized, with irregular, indented, and cleaved nuclear contours, moderately clumped (smudged) to more finely dispersed chromatin, one or more conspicuous nucleoli, and small to moderate amounts of cytoplasm (Fig. 22.7). Larger cells with round nuclei, fine chromatin, prominent nucleoli, and moderate amounts of basophilic cytoplasm are seen in the high-grade variants of MCL. Smears of involved bone marrow and pe-

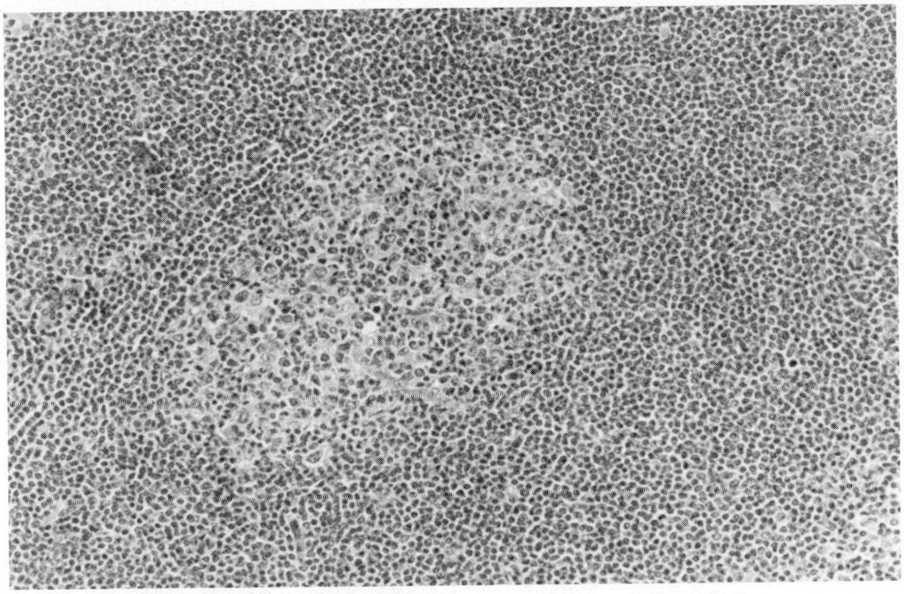

FIG. 22.3. Diffuse mantle cell lymphoma with a naked germinal center lacking a normal lymphocyte cuff (hematoxylin and eosin stain, original magnification: 100× magnification).

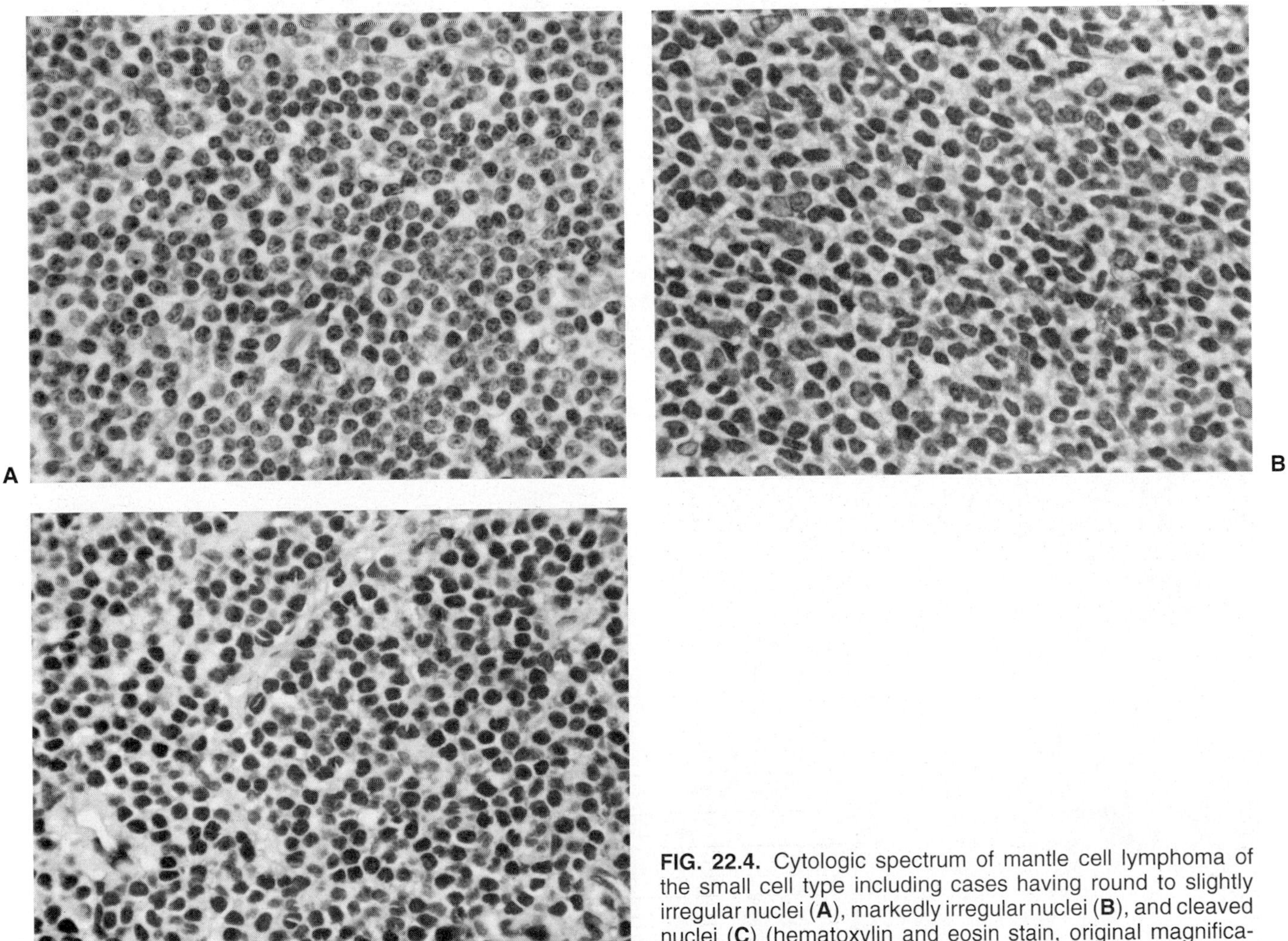

FIG. 22.4. Cytologic spectrum of mantle cell lymphoma of the small cell type including cases having round to slightly irregular nuclei (**A**), markedly irregular nuclei (**B**), and cleaved nuclei (**C**) (hematoxylin and eosin stain, original magnification: 200× magnification).

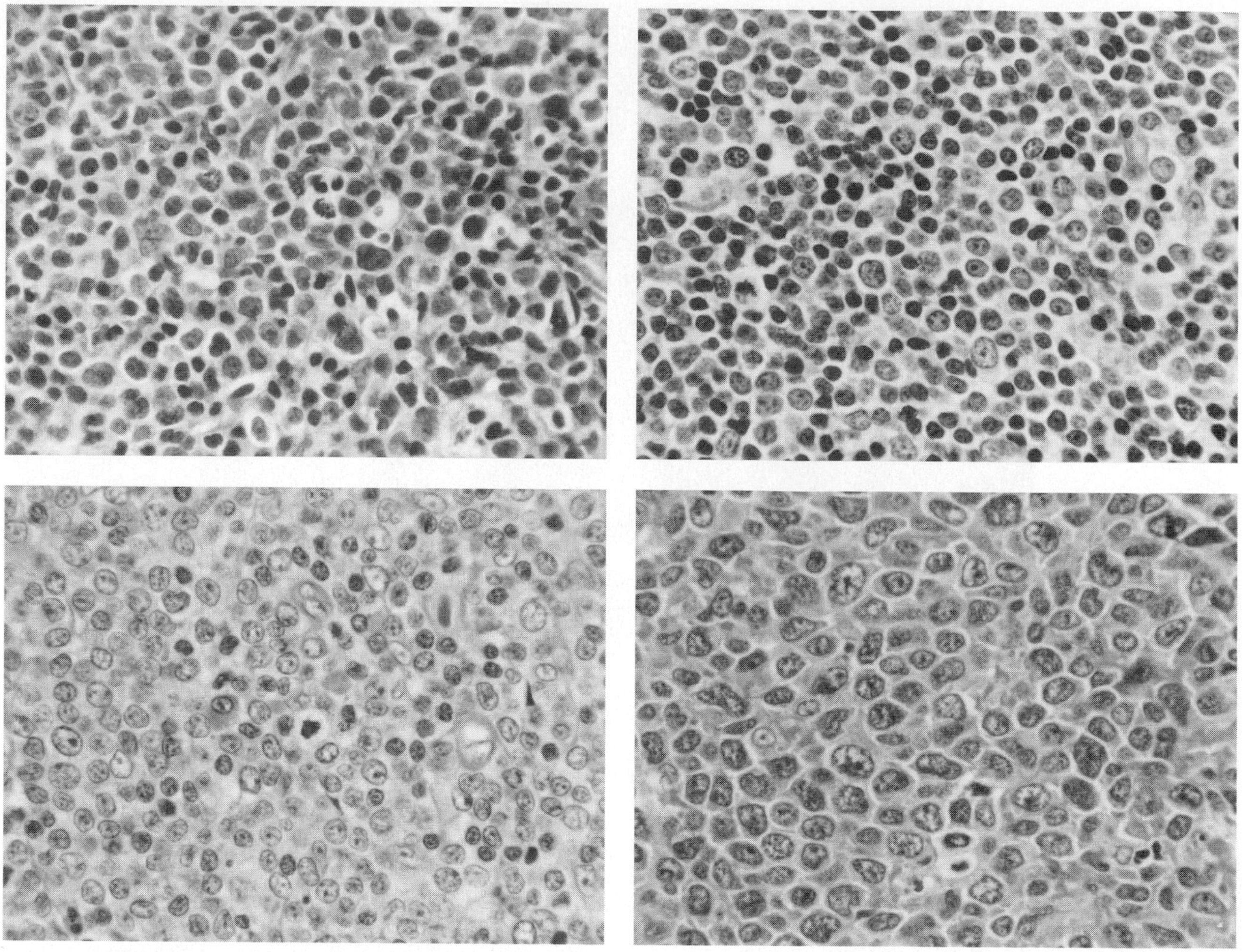

FIG. 22.5. Cytologic spectrum of high-grade mantle cell lymphoma including cases having pleomorphic cytology with larger "anaplastic" cells (**A**), pleomorphic cytology with medium-sized blastic cells (**B**), monotonous medium-sized blastic cells (**C**), and large transformed cells (**D**) (hematoxylin and eosin stain, original magnification: 200× magnification).

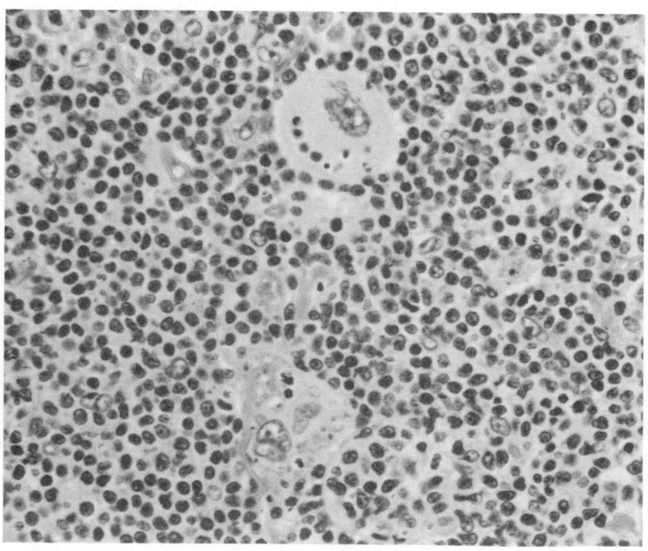

FIG. 22.6. Mantle cell lymphoma with admixed benign histiocytes that contain phagocytized cellular debris (hematoxylin and eosin stain, original magnification: 150× magnification).

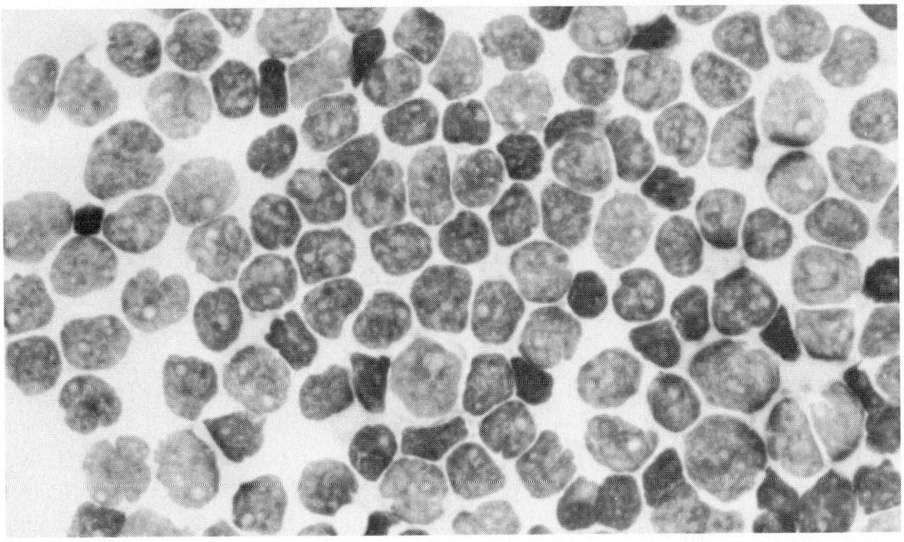

FIG. 22.7. Touch preparation of mantle cell lymphoma showing medium-sized lymphoid cells with irregular nuclear contours, moderately clumped (smudged) chromatin, small nucleoli, and scant cytoplasm (Wright-Giemsa stain, original magnification: 400× magnification).

ripheral blood generally reflect the lymphoid population present in the lymph nodes (10,24,25). The neoplastic cells in the blood and bone marrow of a given patient may be quite heterogeneous in appearance (Fig. 22.8). In bone marrow sections, the neoplastic cells may infiltrate in either a focal, often paratrabecular, pattern or a diffuse pattern (10,23,26, 27). One should not make a diagnosis of MCL based on the examination of peripheral blood or bone marrow alone, because of the lack of precise criteria for such a diagnosis. Immunologic analysis by flow cytometry (see Immunologic Features) may be very useful in the diagnosis of such specimens (24,25).

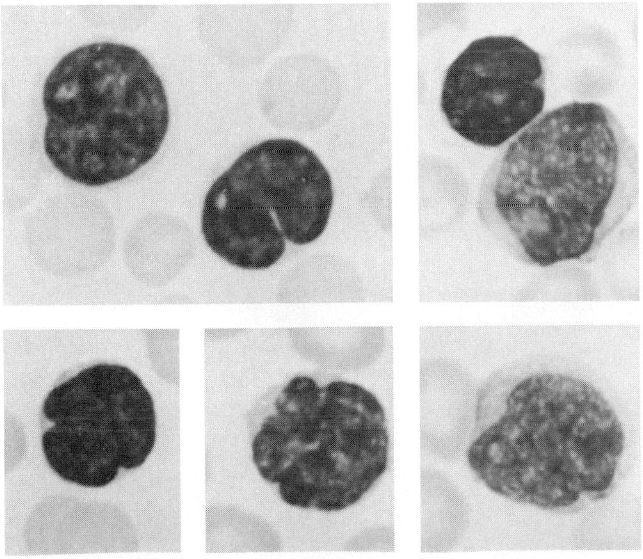

FIG. 22.8. Peripheral blood smear of mantle cell lymphoma showing a spectrum of lymphoma cells (Wright-Giemsa stain, original magnification: 1,000× magnification).

Spleen

The spleen often is enlarged in patients with MCL, and particularly in those with the nodular (mantle zone) type (8,20). Spleen weights range from 600 to 3700 g (8,13,28). Macroscopically, the cut surface often reveals numerous lymphoid nodules measuring 1 to 3 mm in diameter. Microscopically, the white pulp areas appear expanded by a proliferation of atypical lymphoid cells similar to those found in the lymph nodes. Residual benign germinal centers may be present in the white pulp areas, but the marginal zones are usually obliterated (Fig. 22.9). In small white pulp nodules, thin residual marginal zones may be present, but careful study often reveals infiltration of the marginal zones by

FIG. 22.9. Spleen in mantle cell lymphoma showing an expanded white pulp area without a marginal zone. Note the red pulp involvement (indicated in upper right area of the figure) (hematoxylin and eosin stain, original magnification: 40× magnification).

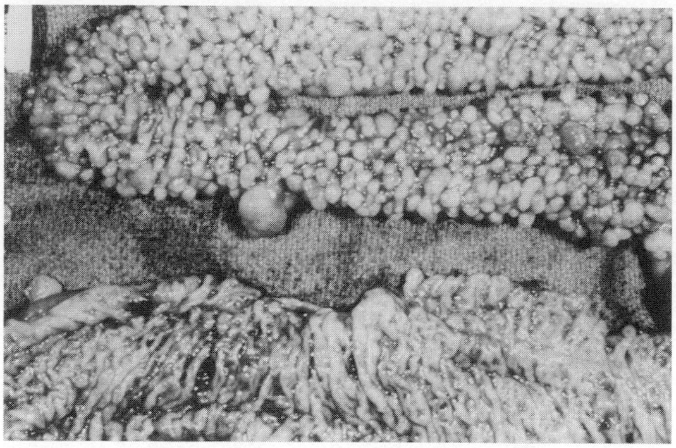

FIG. 22.10. Multiple lymphomatous polyposis of the intestine with a myriad of confluent polyps within the ileum (top) and scattered, more sessile polyps within the colon (bottom). (From Moynihan MJ, Bast MA, Chan WC, et al. Lymphomatous polyposis: a neoplasm of either follicular mantle or germinal center cell origin. *Am J Surg Pathol* 1996;20:442–452, with permission.)

tumor cells. Nodular infiltration of the red pulp is usually also present, albeit in varying degrees.

Other Organs

Involvement of other organs by MCL is not uncommon, because patients usually have disseminated disease at the time of diagnosis. Liver involvement is common and is characterized by atypical portal lymphoid infiltrates. Sinusoidal infiltration also is seen in those with blood involvement. Extranodal sites that are most likely to be involved primarily or as part of a disseminated process include the gastrointestinal tract and Waldeyer's ring (20%–30% of cases). Gastrointestinal involvement as multiple lymphomatous polyposis (Fig. 22.10), often accompanied by a large localized mass, is characteristic of MCL (29–31) but is not entirely specific for MCL (32).

IMMUNOLOGIC FEATURES

The immunohistologic features of MCL reveal a characteristic phenotype (13–15,19,33–36). In frozen sections, the cells have a monoclonal B-cell phenotype, almost always bearing surface IgM (sIgM) and often sIgD. Surface IgG is expressed along with sIgM in about 20% of cases. The $\kappa : \lambda$ light ratio is reversed in MCL, with about 60% of cases expressing monoclonal λ light chains, and the residual germinal centers are polyclonal. The neoplastic cells also stain for a variety of pan–B cell antigens (CD19, CD2, CD22, and CD24) and HLA-DR antigen. The cells are usually negative for CD23 antigen. The cells typically have the pan–T cell antigen CD5 on the surface (Fig. 22.11) and are negative for CD10 (CALLA) antigen. The neoplastic cells may also bear the T cell–associated antigens CD43 and Leu-8, but fail to stain for other pan–T-cell antigens. Aberrant expression of CD8 antigen has been reported in some cases (37). Antibodies to follicular dendritic cells reveal large aggregates of these cells in cases with a nodular or mantle zone pattern, whereas a more sparse and irregular meshwork of dendritic cells usually is found in diffuse areas. Patients with high-grade MCL are less likely to express sIgD, CD5, or CD43 and may express CD10 antigen. The phenotype of MCL is remarkably similar to that of small lymphocytic lymphoma and chronic lymphocytic leukemia, except for

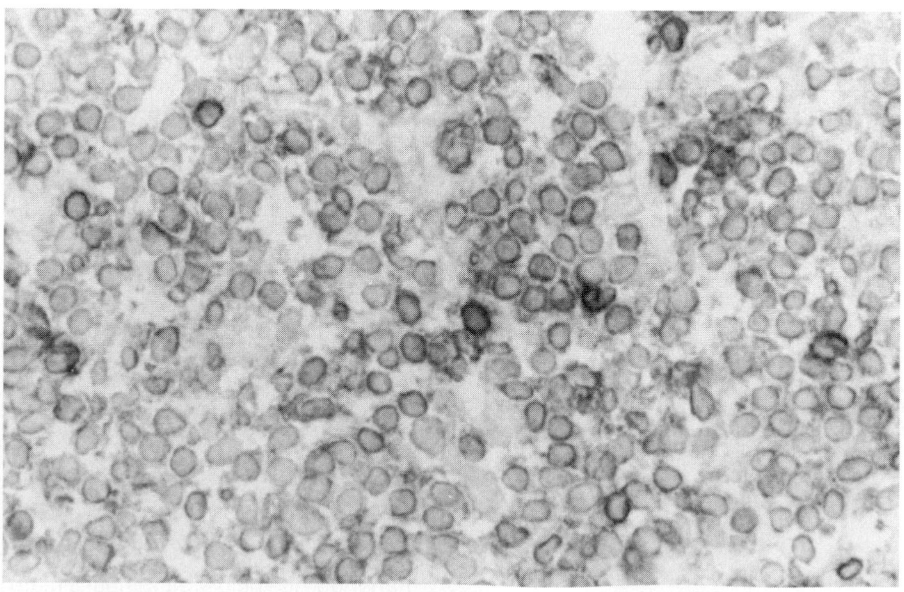

FIG. 22.11. Mantle cell lymphoma stained with CD5 antibody. Note that the tumor cells do not stain as intensely as the few admixed T cells (immunoperoxidase stain, original magnification: 200× magnification).

more intense sIg and CD20 staining, and lack of CD23 expression in MCL. Studies of cellular proliferation in MCL generally have found low rates in the lymphocytic forms and high rates in the high-grade variants, but with considerable overlap (15,19,38).

CYTOGENETIC AND MOLECULAR GENETIC FEATURES

The characteristic cytogenetic abnormality in MCL is the translocation t(11;14)(q13;q32), which is seen in the majority of cases (39–42). Variant translocations involving the 11q13 breakpoint also have been reported (42–44). Secondary abnormalities that appear to be nonrandom in MCL include the loss of chromosomes 13 and Y, deletions of chromosomes 6q, 11q22, and 13q14, a gain at chromosome 3q26-27, and various abnormalities of chromosome 6q15 (45–47). The presence of a complex karyotype with hyperdiploidy has been associated with high-grade cytology and suggests an aggressive clinical course in MCL (38,48). Similarly, secondary abnormalities involving the *MYC* oncogene on chromosome 8q24 are associated with a short duration of survival (49). Because the translocation t(11;14)(q13;q32) also occurs, albeit quite infrequently, in other types of non-Hodgkin's lymphoma, lymphocytic leukemia, and multiple myeloma, positive cytogenetic findings need to be correlated carefully with the pathologic and immunologic features to confirm a diagnosis of MCL.

The molecular counterpart of the translocation t(11;14) involves an error in Variable-Diversity-Joining (V-D-J) during immunoglobulin heavy chain gene rearrangement, resulting in the movement of a putative cellular oncogene adjacent to the *BCL1* (11q13) breakpoint into proximity of the enhancer region of the immunoglobulin heavy chain gene (14q32). Breaks in the latter region are thought to occur during early B-cell development and to be mediated by the recombinase system; 11q13 appears to be a common fragile site (50). The breakpoints in the *BCL1* locus are not tightly clustered, although about 30% to 40% of patients with MCL have breaks in the major translocation cluster region (51–54) (Fig. 22.12). Using multiple probes, including those for a number of minor breakpoint regions, a variety of investigators have detected clonal rearrangements in 50% to 70% of patients with MCL (51–54). A polymerase chain reaction assay detects most of the breaks in the major translocation cluster region and also may be used on DNA extracted from paraffin-embedded tissues (55–57). Fluorescence *in situ* hybridization has been used to detect the translocation t(11; 14) in interphase cells or in DNA from intact cells in nearly all cases tested, demonstrating the importance of this translocation in the pathogenesis of MCL (58–60). Both polymerase chain reaction and fluorescence *in situ* hybridization techniques are useful to detect minimal residual disease in MCL.

The putative oncogene deregulated by the translocation t(11;14) is located approximately 120 kilobases telomeric from the major translocation cluster breakpoint (Fig. 22.12)

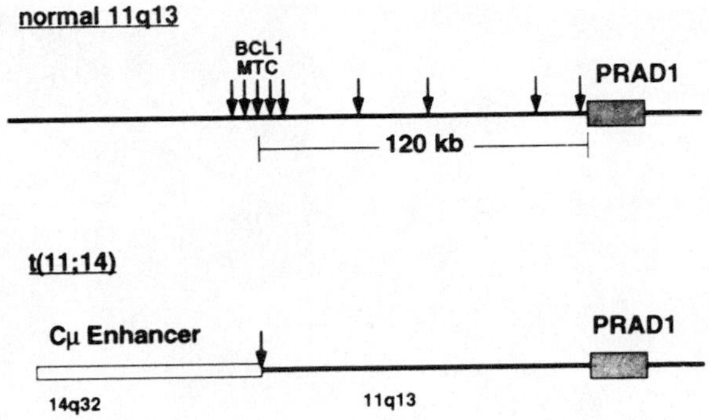

FIG. 22.12. Diagram of the translocation t(11;14) in mantle cell lymphoma. An 11q13 breakpoint at the *BCL1* major translocation cluster is shown; other described breakpoints (arrows in upper panel) exist as close as 1 kilobase to the first exon of the *PRAD1* gene. (From Arnold A. The cyclin D1/PRAD1 oncogene in human neoplasia. *J Invest Med* 1995; 43:543–549, with permission.)

(61,62). The gene was named *PRAD1* because of its original recognition in parathyroid adenoma (63) but officially has been named *CCND1*. The gene encodes for cyclin D1 and is overexpressed in MCL; it only rarely is expressed in other forms of hematopoietic cancer (52,54,61–65). Because overexpression of this gene has been found in nearly all cases of MCL, including those without detectable *BCL1* rearrangements, additional minor breakpoint sites outside of those detected by the available probes are likely to be involved in the translocation of chromosome 11q13. All of the known breakpoints leave the *CCND1* coding region structurally intact and result in increased protein expression. In about 10% of patients, loss of 3′ end regulatory sequences also may increase the half-life of cyclin D1 (44,66). Antibodies to cyclin D1 that stain paraffin-embedded material have been shown to be highly sensitive and specific markers for MCL and are very useful to confirm the diagnosis or elucidate the nature of diagnostically difficult cases (67–72). Nuclear staining is specific for cyclin D1, but only a subpopulation of the tumor cells may stain in MCL (Fig. 22.13). Although normal lymphoid tissues generally do not express detectable cyclin D1, one report described a few positive cells in the mantle zones of reactive follicles and the residual mantle zones of follicular lymphoma (65). Because cyclin D1 is quite labile and may be affected by poor fixation or harsh processing, positive staining of scattered internal control cells, such as stromal or endothelial cells, should be observed before interpreting a case as not expressing cyclin D1. A positive stain is not absolutely pathognomic of MCL, because other types of lymphocytic lymphoma or leukemia occasionally stain, and careful correlation with the pathologic and immunologic features is necessary to confirm a diagnosis of MCL.

The mechanism by which cyclin D1 overexpression facilitates lymphomagenesis is not yet well understood, but its key role in cell cycle regulation and the progression of cells

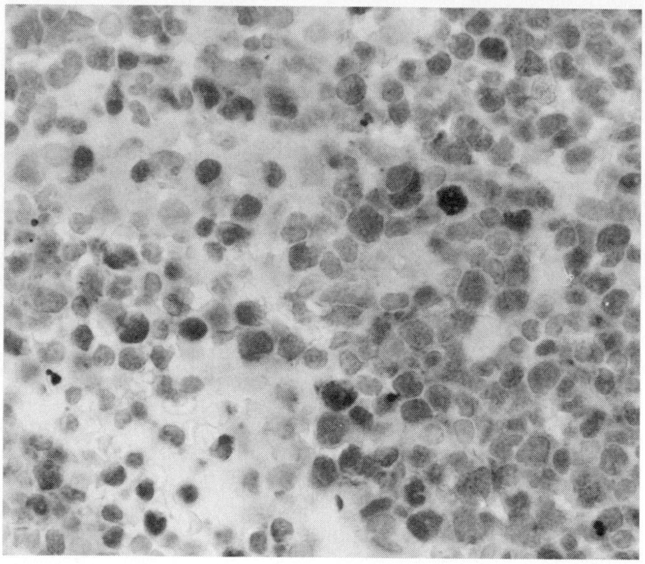

FIG. 22.13. Mantle cell lymphoma stained with a polyclonal antibody to cyclin D1. Note the nuclear positivity of variable intensity in a majority of the cells (immunoperoxidase stain, original magnification: 200× magnification).

through the main commitment checkpoint in G1 to S phase is certainly important (73–75). Overexpression of cyclin D1 results in a shortened G1 phase, probably through its physical interaction with the tumor suppressor retinoblastoma protein (76). Cyclin D1 binds to and activates important enzymes called *cyclin-dependent kinases* (CDKs)—mainly CDK4 and CDK6—whose activity is needed to propel cells through the G1 checkpoint. Cyclin D1–CDK complexes bind to and hyperphosphorylate retinoblastoma, which in turn prevents retinoblastoma from binding important transcription factors such as E2F. The growth-restraint effect of retinoblastoma through its binding of transcription factors is removed, and the cells are propelled into S phase (Fig. 22.14). Overexpression of cyclin D1 also can have complex effects on the expression of other genes that control cell cycle progression (77), such as the downregulation of cyclin D3 in MCL (78). High levels of retinoblastoma are found in MCL (79,80). The retinoblastoma appears to be unmutated and underphosphorylated and therefore should be in its active form. These findings suggest that cyclin D1 may inactivate retinoblastoma by a mechanism other than phosphorylation in MCL (80).

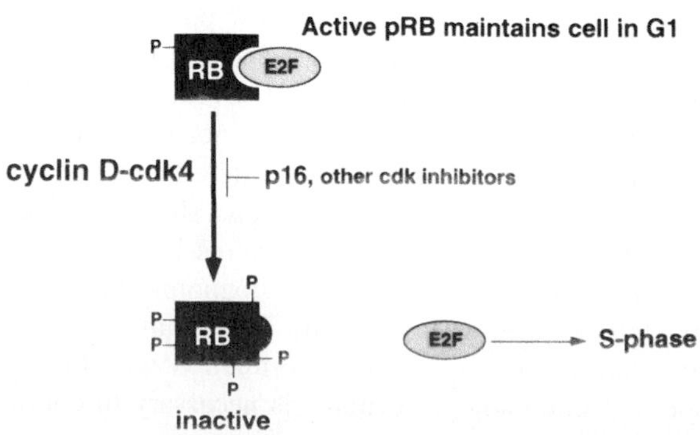

FIG. 22.14. Schematic diagram showing the functional interrelationships of cyclin D1. (From Arnold A. The cyclin D1/PRAD1 oncogene in human neoplasia. *J Invest Med* 1995; 43:543–549, with permission.)

A number of CDK inhibitor proteins bind to cyclin-CDK complexes and inhibit their function (75,81). These include the INK-4 family (p15, p16, p18, and p19) and the p21/p27 family of CDK inhibitors (Fig. 22.14). Deletions, mutations, and loss of expression of these genes has been reported in MCL, usually associated with high-grade cytology, and may enhance the effects of cyclin D1 overexpression (82–86). Mutations and deletions of the tumor suppressor *P53* gene also have been reported in high-grade variants of MCL (22,87–89). This gene regulates the expression of p21 protein, which is an important universal inhibitor of cyclin-CDK complexes. Loss or mutation of the *P53* gene, with resultant loss of this inhibition, could enhance the effects of overexpressed cyclin D1 further. The normal *P53* gene acts as a molecular monitor of the genome (90). If DNA is damaged, p21 protein accumulates and switches off replication to allow extra time for DNA repair. If the repair fails, *P53* may trigger cell suicide by apoptosis. Tumor cells in which *P53* is deleted or inactivated by mutation, however, cannot carry out this arrest and are genetically unstable. Such cells accumulate additional mutations and chromosomal abnormalities at an increased rate, thus leading to the rapid selection of highly malignant clones. *P53* and the CDK inhibitor genes play critical roles at the G1 checkpoint and alterations of these genes are important in the progression of MCL.

Evidence has accumulated that *CCND1* can function as an oncogene by causing abnormalities of cellular growth control, cell cycle progression, and gene expression, as well as malignant transformation (73,91–94). Studies using transgenic mice have shown that *CCND1* cooperates with the *MYC* genes in the generation of B-cell lymphomas, although *CCND1* is not oncogenic by itself (95,96). These studies demonstrated subtle alterations in cell cycle progression and the number of bone marrow B cells resulting from *CCND1* overexpression (95,96). Activation of cyclin D genes by proviral insertions in murine lymphomas has also been reported (97,98). Overexpression of cyclin D1 also was shown to induce mammary hyperplasia and carcinoma in a different transgenic model (99). It appears that *CCND1* is a bona fide oncogene whose activity appears to depend on the specific cell type and specific cooperating partner genes in order to induce tumors.

NORMAL CELLULAR COUNTERPART

Currently, the various types of B cell neoplasia are thought to represent cells arrested at various stages in the normal differentiation scheme (100). The histologic and immunologic features of MCL suggest that the neoplastic cells correspond to normal, naive B lymphocytes that home to and reside in primary lymphoid follicles and the mantle zones of secondary follicles. These cells seem to correspond phenotypically to a major population of fetal B cells that leave the bone marrow and form the primary lymphoid follicles in the lymph nodes and spleen (101–103). At birth, 68% of cord blood B cells and approximately half of peripheral blood B cells are CD5-positive ($CD5^+$) (104,105), and these cells are morphologically similar to the cells of MCL (106). In the adult, $CD5^+$ B cells circulate in small numbers (107–109) and are found in the inner area of the mantle zones of lymphoid follicles (107,110). Normal mantle cells have been shown to express a diverse repertoire of unmutated immunoglobulin heavy chain variable region genes, as one would expect of naive pre–germinal center B cells (111). Identical findings have been reported in MCL (112). Furthermore, $CD5^+$ B cells can be induced to differentiate to CD5-negative ($CD5^-$) cells with the immunologic features of germinal center cells (113). The cells of MCL appear to correspond to precursor cells of the normal germinal center reaction (100,114).

DIFFERENTIAL DIAGNOSIS

A diagnosis of MCL with a mantle zone pattern may be difficult to make if incomplete obliteration of the normal lymph node architecture and numerous benign-appearing germinal centers are present. The presence of wide follicular mantles in MCL, however, is distinctly different from the thin mantles found in most cases of reactive follicular hyperplasia. In the spleen, involvement of the red pulp by lymphoma is also a helpful diagnostic feature. In lymph nodes, mantle zone hyperplasia and angiofollicular lymphoid hyperplasia of the hyaline vascular type (Castleman's disease) are two uncommon reactive processes that may be difficult to distinguish from mantle zone lymphoma. Mantle zone hyperplasia usually occurs as an isolated, small node in the neck of a young individual. In mantle zone hyperplasia, the follicles are usually localized predominantly to the cortex of the node, and the architectural effacement and diffuse areas of involvement characteristic of lymphoma are lacking. Angiofollicular lymphoid hyperplasia also usually presents in young individuals, but as a large and localized mass, and is characterized by typical hyaline vascular germinal centers without diffuse areas of involvement. Immunohistochemical stains may be very helpful in distinguishing MCL with a mantle zone pattern from these reactive processes. The monoclonality and CD5, CD43, and cyclin D1 positivity of the neoplastic cells clearly separate MCL from the follicular center, mantle zone, and angiofollicular hyperplasias. These features are also useful for separating diffuse MCL from diffuse reactive lymphoid proliferations of B-cell type.

A variety of non-Hodgkin's lymphomas also may be confused with the lymphomas of mantle cell origin. Immunohistochemical studies are very useful in differentiating the various entities (Table 22.1). The nodular (primary follicular) form of MCL may be difficult to differentiate from follicular small cleaved cell lymphoma. The cells of MCL, however, are usually not as angulated and cleaved as those of follicle center cell lymphoma. Also, large transformed cells (large noncleaved cells or centroblasts) are usually absent in MCL, although residual large cells of invaded benign germinal centers may occasionally confuse the issue. Harris and Bhan (115) have described a rare form of follicle center cell lymphoma in which small cleaved cells exit the neoplastic germinal centers and accumulate in the adjacent mantle zones. Such cases should not be considered MCL, because they arise from germinal center cells. In difficult cases, immunohistochemical stains can be used to separate follicle center cell lymphoma from MCL by the fact that the former has monoclonal, $CD10^+$ germinal centers and thin, polyclonal, $CD5^-$ mantle zones, whereas polyclonal, $CD10^-$ germinal centers and large, monoclonal, $CD5^+$ mantle zones and nodules are seen in nodular MCL. Immunologic studies are also helpful in separating diffuse MCL from diffuse small cleaved follicle center cell lymphoma, which is $CD5^-$ negative and often $CD10^+$ and frequently exhibits immunoglobulin heavy chain switching to a more mature phenotype (116). Transformed large cells and small cells with the elongated and twisted nuclei of follicle center cell lymphoma are generally absent in diffuse MCL. Also, the former is always cyclin–D1 negative, whereas the latter is positive.

TABLE 22.1. *Phenotypes of the various B-lymphocytic lymphomas*

Subtype	sIg	cIg	CD5	CD10	CD23	CD43	DRC	Cyclin D1
Mantle cell lymphoma	M ± D	−	+	−	−	+	+	+
Follicle center cell lymphoma	G ± M	−	−	+/−	+/−	−	+	−
Small lymphocytic lymphoma/CLL	M ± D	−/+	+	−	+	+	−	−
Monocytoid B-cell lymphoma	M	−/+	−	−	−/+	−	−	−
Mucosa-associated lymphoma	M	−/+	−	−	−	−/+	−	−
Lymphoplasmacytic lymphoma	M	+	−	−	−	−	−	−
Splenic "marginal zone" lymphoma	M ± D	−/+	−	−	−	−	−	−

sIg, surface immunoglobulin; cIg, cytoplasmic immunoglobulin; DRC, dendritic reticulum cell network; CLL, chronic lymphocytic leukemia; +, >80% positive; +/−, >50% positive; −/+, <50% positive; −, <20% positive.

Adapted from Weisenburger DD, Armitage JO. Mantle cell lymphoma: an entity comes of age. *Blood* 1996;87:4483–4494, with permission.

Interfollicular small lymphocytic lymphoma may encroach on and invade reactive follicles and produce a pseudo–mantle zone pattern (117). This pattern is characterized by reactive germinal centers with thin, residual mantle zones that are surrounded by the neoplastic infiltrate. The predominance of small lymphocytes with uniformly round nuclei, however, and the presence of pseudofollicular proliferation centers, prolymphocytes, and paraimmunoblasts in small lymphocytic lymphoma are useful differential features, because they do not occur in MCL. Perry and associates (118) have shown that lymphocytic lymphomas, composed of cells with irregular nuclei but having pseudofollicular proliferation centers, should be classified as small lymphocytic lymphoma for clinical purposes. The immunophenotypes of MCL and small lymphocytic lymphoma are similar, but cyclin D1 expression and the presence of numerous follicular dendritic cells, as well as the absence of CD23 antigen in MCL, are useful diagnostic features.

A pseudo–mantle zone pattern also may be seen in nodal monocytoid B-cell lymphoma, small (centrocyte-like) B-cell lymphoma occurring in mucosa-associated lymphoid tissues, lymphoplasmacytic lymphoma, and peripheral T-cell lymphoma composed of atypical small lymphoid cells. These lymphomas arise in the parafollicular or interfollicular regions and may invade reactive lymphoid follicles secondarily. Each of these lymphomas has distinctive histologic and immunologic features that are useful in the differential diagnosis (Table 22.1). The presence of lymphoepithelial lesions is not useful in differentiating MCL from the small B-cell lymphoma of mucosa-associated lymphoid tissue, because they also have been described in MCL (30–32).

In the spleen, MCL also must be distinguished from so-called splenic marginal zone lymphoma (28,119,120). In MCL, the splenic marginal zones usually are obliterated by a monotonous lymphoid infiltrate, although thin residual marginal zones may be present focally in small white pulp nodules. In splenic marginal zone lymphoma, there is a prominent expansion of the marginal zones (119) or, more commonly, a biphasic pattern with involvement of the mantle and marginal zones (120). The cytology of splenic marginal zone lymphoma is characterized by small lymphoid cells with round nuclei in the mantle areas and cells with monocytoid and plasmacytoid features, along with large transformed cells, in the expanded marginal zones. The different phenotypes are also helpful diagnostically (Table 22.1). Although splenic marginal zone lymphoma is usually negative for cyclin D1 (120,121), a few positive cases have been reported (21,122). The pathologic features of any such case must be carefully integrated to arrive at the correct diagnosis.

The blastic variants of MCL sometimes are confused with precursor B-cell lymphoblastic lymphoma (123,124) or granulocytic sarcoma, although the chromatin pattern is usually somewhat more coarse in blastic MCL. Immunologic studies are usually helpful in this regard, because blastic MCL is surface immunoglobulin-positive, $CD5^+$, and terminal deoxynucleotide transferase–negative, and precursor B-cell lymphoblastic lymphoma is $CD5^-$, usually sIg^-, and terminal deoxynucleotide transferase–positive. The presence of CD10 is not helpful, because it may be expressed in either entity. In addition to these features, a number of myeloid markers including myeloperoxidase, lysozyme, and specific esterase usually delineate granulocytic sarcoma from MCL. Of these entities, only blastic MCL is cyclin D1–positive.

Although MCL may be diagnosed in extranodal sites, such as the gastrointestinal tract, one should hesitate to make a primary diagnosis of MCL in extranodal sites such as the bone marrow, liver, or soft tissue, because of the nuclear irregularities that may occur as a result of the surrounding fibrous tissue reaction. Such cases are better diagnosed as lymphocytic lymphoma, not further classified, if corroborating evidence for MCL cannot be obtained. Similarly, one should not make a diagnosis of MCL based on bone marrow or peripheral blood smears alone, because criteria for such a diagnosis are not well defined. A lymph node biopsy with immunologic studies is often necessary to categorize such cases precisely, although flow cytometric and molecular studies of blood and bone marrow may be very useful.

CLINICAL FEATURES

Mantle cell lymphoma comprises approximately 7% of all non-Hodgkin's lymphomas in North America, whereas higher rates are found in some parts of Europe and lower rates are found in Hong Kong (125). A number of detailed studies have defined the clinical features of MCL (10,13–15,17–20,31,126–139) (Table 22.2). Patients with MCL have a median age of approximately 60 years, and males predominate. Patients generally present with advanced (stage III/IV) disease, usually with generalized lymphadenopathy and bone marrow and liver involvement, but fewer

TABLE 22.2. *Clinical features of mantle cell lymphoma at initial presentation*

Median age	60 years
Male to female ratio	4:1
Generalized lymphadenopathy	90%
Splenomegaly	60%
Hepatomegaly	30%
Peripheral blood lymphocytosis	30%
Bone marrow infiltration	80%
Gastrointestinal involvement	20%
Waldeyer's ring involvement	10%
Ann Arbor stage III/IV	90%
B symptoms	40%
Bulky disease	30%
Poor performance status	20%
Elevated serum lactate dehydrogenase	40%
Elevated $\beta 2$ microglobulin	55%

From Weisenburger DD, Armitage JO. Mantle cell lymphoma: an entity comes of age. *Blood* 1996;87:4483–4494, with permission.

than one half of the patients have systemic (B) symptoms. Splenomegaly is present at initial diagnosis in approximately 60% of the patients. Other extranodal sites also are involved frequently, particularly the gastrointestinal tract and Waldeyer's ring (20%–30% of cases). A particularly striking extranodal presentation is multiple lymphomatous polyposis of the intestine, which should suggest a diagnosis of MCL (29–32). Central nervous system involvement is rare at the time of presentation but occurs during the course of disease in 10% of the patients (137). Mild anemia is not uncommon at presentation; thrombocytopenia occurs in fewer than 15% of the patients. A peripheral blood lymphocytosis of greater than 4,000 lymphocytes/mm^3 occurs in 20% to 40% of patients, but absolute counts higher than 20,000/mm^3 are uncommon. A positive Coombs' test, marked hypogammaglobulinemia, and a significant monoclonal gammopathy are also uncommon. Small amounts of monoclonal serum protein have been found in about 25% of patients with MCL (140). The significance of such a monoclonal serum protein is unclear, because it may not be produced by the neoplastic cells (137,140).

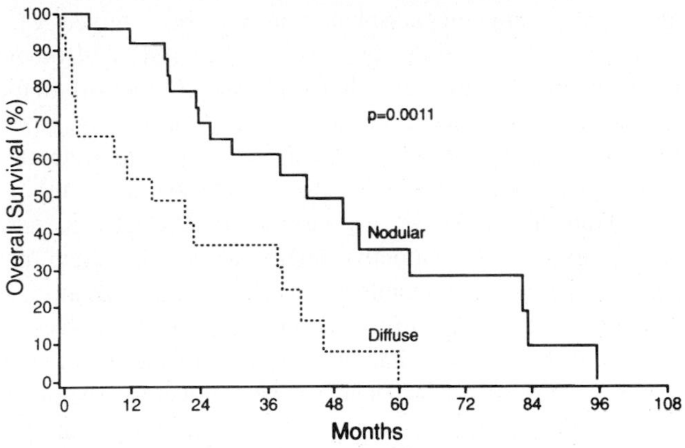

FIG. 22.16. Overall survival rates of patients with mantle cell lymphoma of the small cell type having a nodular growth pattern compared with those with a diffuse pattern. (From Weisenburger DD, Vose JM, Lynch JC, et al. Mantle cell lymphoma: a clinicopathologic study of 68 cases from the Nebraska Lymphoma Study Group. *Am J Hematol* (in press), with permission.

TREATMENT AND SURVIVAL

Mantle cell lymphoma is a vexing and increasingly frequent problem for oncologists. The disease brings together the worst characteristics of high-grade and low-grade lymphomas: The course is not indolent, and the disease is rarely curable. The median duration of survival of patients with MCL has ranged between 3 and 4 years in most series (10, 13–15, 17–20, 23, 31, 126, 127, 129–131, 133, 137–139) (Fig. 22.15). This is significantly shorter than the survival of patients with other forms of lymphocytic lymphoma (129,130,132,133,137,138). In a number of studies, patients with a nodular or mantle zone pattern of growth had a significantly longer median duration of survival compared with those with diffuse MCL (14,15,19,130,134,139,141) (Fig. 22.16); those with high-grade cytology are thought to have a very aggressive clinical course regardless of the growth pattern (15,17,22,23,130,136,137).

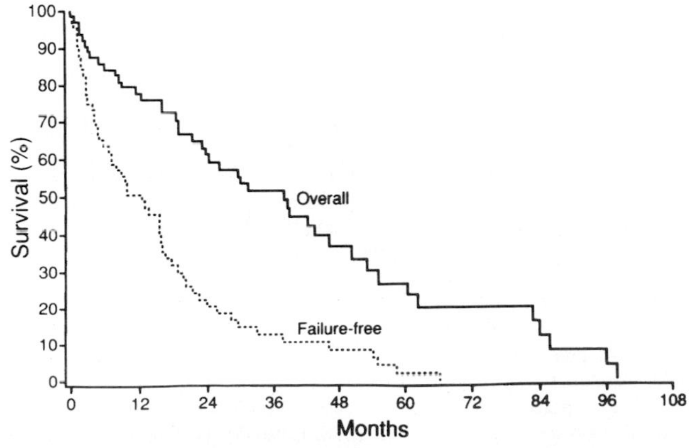

FIG. 22.15. Overall and failure-free survival rates of patients with mantle cell lymphoma. (From Weisenburger DD, Vose JM, Lynch JC, et al. Mantle cell lymphoma: a clinicopathologic study of 68 cases from the Nebraska Lymphoma Study Group. *Am J Hematol* (in press), with permission.

With the use of noncurative, pre–first generation combination chemotherapy, which usually did not contain doxorubicin, various investigators obtained complete remission rates of 20% to 40% (126–128,132,135,138). Meusers and colleagues (127) reported a complete remission rate of 58% using a combination of cyclophosphamide, doxorubicin, vincristine, and prednisone (CHOP), but few long-term remissions or cures have been reported in any series because of disease recurrence and progression. Zucca and associates (131) have reported a benefit from aggressive chemotherapy in a subset of patients with good prognostic indicators. Teodorovic and colleagues (132) have reported a complete remission rate of 52% for patients treated with aggressive chemotherapy and suggested that improved survival may be achieved if complete remission is obtained after CHOP-like chemotherapy. In elderly patients, less aggressive therapy such as cyclophosphamide, vincristine, and prednisone may be justified. Therapeutic experience with the purine analogues, fludarabine and 2-CDA, and interferon has been disappointing (12,132,142). Although a small proportion of patients may benefit from observation only (128,135), complete remission could not be obtained if such patients were treated later for progressive symptomatic disease. Most studies have shown, however, that patients who achieve an initial complete remission have a longer duration of survival than those who do not achieve a complete remission, but few patients are cured.

Because the long-term prognosis of patients receiving conventional therapy for MCL is rather poor (Fig. 22.15), aggressive combination chemotherapy with stem cell transplantation has been tried in younger patients. The results of autologous stem cell transplantation have been mixed, with some centers reporting poor results (143,144) and others reporting good results with short follow-up (145,146). In the largest reported series, Freedman and colleagues (147) used high-dose chemoradiotherapy and antibody-purged autologous marrow to treat patients in first or later partial remission but found no plateau in disease-free survival at a median follow-up time of 24 months. These authors suggested that cures may not be achievable using this approach because, at least in part, of its inability to adequately purge the harvested marrow (148) and the inherent resistance of the tumor cells to available therapy (147). Clearly, new and better therapeutic strategies are needed, including the exploration of allogeneic transplantation (148,149), immunotherapy with monoclonal antibodies (150,151), and innovative approaches that target the cell cycle (152–156).

A number of clinical and pathologic features are predictive of survival in MCL. The clinical features predicting a poor prognosis are generally the same as those for other lymphoma subtypes and include advanced age and stage, B symptoms, poor performance status, peripheral blood involvement, elevated lactate dehydrogenase or β2-microglobulin levels, intermediate or high risk with the International Prognostic Index, and failure to achieve a good clinical response to therapy (13,14,17,23,26,31,126,127,129,131, 133,135–139). The pathologic features that predict a poor prognosis are a diffuse growth pattern, a high rate of mitosis (>20 per 10 high-power fields) or high proliferative fraction, high-grade cytology, a complex karyotype with hyperdiploidy, and *P53* mutation or deletion (13–15,17,19,20,22,23, 38,48,54,87–89,126,130,133,134,136,137,139,141).

SUMMARY AND CONCLUSIONS

Numerous studies have confirmed that MCL is a distinct clinicopathologic entity. The neoplastic cells of MCL appear to correspond to naive B cells that normally home to and reside in primary lymphoid follicles and the mantle zones of secondary follicles. As such, they correspond to a subset of normal follicle B cells that are thought to transform into germinal center cells in response to antigen. The relationship between the nodular (mantle zone) and diffuse lymphocytic forms of MCL is biologically analogous to the germinal center cell lymphomas of follicular and diffuse types, respectively; the high-grade variants of MCL are analogous to the transformed lymphomas arising in other low-grade lymphomas. New and better therapies are needed for this group of lymphomas. Until such progress is made, MCL will continue to be one of the worst forms of non-Hodgkin's lymphoma, a clinically aggressive disease with little hope of a cure.

REFERENCES

1. Berard CW, Dorfman RF. Histopathology of malignant lymphomas. *Clin Haematol* 1974;3:39–76.
2. Berard CW. Reticuloendothelial system: an overview of neoplasia. In: Rebuck JW, Berard CW, Abell MR, eds. *The reticuloendothelial system.* International Academy of Pathology Monograph no. 16. Baltimore: Williams & Wilkins, 1975:301–317.
3. Jaffe ES, Braylan RC, Namba K, et al. Functional markers: a new perspective on malignant lymphomas. *Cancer Treat Rep* 1977;61: 1953–1962.
4. Namba K, Jaffe ES, Braylan RC, et al. Alkaline phosphatase-positive malignant lymphoma: subtype of B-cell lymphomas. *Am J Clin Pathol* 1977;68:535–542.
5. Lennert K, Stein H, Kaiserling E. Cytological and functional criteria for the classification of malignant lymphomata. *Br J Cancer* 1975; 31(Suppl II):29–43.
6. Lennert K. *Malignant lymphomas other than Hodgkin's disease.* Berlin: Springer-Verlag, 1978:284–302.
7. Tolksdorf G, Stein H, Lennert K. Morphological and immunological definition of a malignant lymphoma derived from germinal-center cells with cleaved nuclei (centrocytes). *Br J Cancer* 1980;41: 168–182.
8. Weisenburger DD, Kim H, Rappaport H. Mantle-zone lymphoma: a follicular variant of intermediate lymphocytic lymphoma. *Cancer* 1982;49:1429–1438.
9. Palutke M, Eisenberg L, Mirchandani I, et al. Malignant lymphoma of small cleaved lymphocytes of the follicular mantle zone. *Blood* 1982;59:317–322.
10. Weisenburger DD, Nathwani BN, Diamond LW, et al. Malignant lymphoma, intermediate lymphocytic type: a clinicopathologic study of 42 cases. *Cancer* 1981;48:1415–1425.
11. Banks PM, Chan J, Cleary ML, et al. Mantle cell lymphoma: a proposal for unification of morphologic, immunologic, and molecular data. *Am J Surg Pathol* 1992;16:637–640.
12. Zucca E, Stein H, Coffier B. European Lymphoma Task Force (ELTF): Report of the workshop on mantle cell lymphoma (MCL). *Ann Oncol* 1994;5:507–511.
13. Swerdlow SH, Habeshaw JA, Murray LJ, et al. Centrocytic lymphoma: a distinct clinicopathologic and immunologic entity. A multiparameter study of 18 cases at diagnosis and relapse. *Am J Pathol* 1983;113:181–197.
14. Weisenburger DD, Duggan MJ, Perry DA, et al. Non-Hodgkin's lymphomas of mantle-zone origin. In: Rosen PP, Fechner RE, eds. *Pathology annual.* East Norwalk, CT: Appleton & Lange, 1990:139–158.
15. Lardelli P, Bookman MA, Sundeen J, et al. Lymphocytic lymphoma of intermediate differentiation: morphologic and immunophenotypic spectrum and clinical correlations. *Am J Surg Pathol* 1990;14: 752–763.
16. Lennert K, Feller AC. *Histopathology of non-Hodgkin's lymphomas.* Berlin: Springer-Verlag, 1992:93–102.
17. Norton AJ, Mathews J, Pappa V, et al. Mantle cell lymphoma: natural history defined in a serially biopsied population over a 20-year period. *Ann Oncol* 1995;6:249–256.
18. Pittaluga S, Wlodarska I, Stul MS, et al. Mantle cell lymphoma: a clinicopathologic study of 55 cases. *Histopathology* 1995;26:17–24.
19. Segal GH, Masih AS, Fox AC, et al. CD5-expressing B-cell non-Hodgkin's lymphomas with bcl-1 gene rearrangement have a relatively homogeneous immunophenotype and are associated with an overall poor prognosis. *Blood* 1995:85;1570–1579.
20. Duggan MJ, Weisenburger DD, Ye YL, et al. Mantle zone lymphoma: a clinicopathologic study of 22 cases. *Cancer* 1990;66:522–529.
21. Swerdlow SH, Zukerberg LR, Yang WI, et al. The morphologic spectrum of non-Hodgkin's lymphomas with BCL1/Cyclin D1 gene rearrangements. *Am J Surg Pathol* 1996;20:627–640.
22. Zoldan MC, Inghirami G, Masuda Y, et al. Large cell variants of mantle cell lymphoma: cytologic characteristics and p53 anomalies may predict poor outcome. *Br J Haematol* 1996;93:475–486.
23. Agatoff LH, Connors JM, Klasa RJ, et al. Mantle cell lymphoma: a clinicopathologic study of 80 cases. *Blood* 1997;89:2067–2078.
24. Pombo de Oliveira MS, Jaffe ES, Catovsky D. Leukemic phase of mantle zone (intermediate) lymphoma: its characterization in 11 cases. *J Clin Pathol* 1989;42:962–972.
25. Criel A, Billiet J, Vandenberghe E, et al. Leukemia intermediate lymphocytic lymphomas: analysis of twelve cases diagnosed by morphology. *Leuk Lymphoma* 1992;8:381–387.
26. Pittaluga S, Verhoef G, Criel A, et al. Prognostic significance of bone

marrow trephine and peripheral blood smears in 55 patients with mantle cell lymphoma. *Leuk Lymphoma* 1996;21:115–125.
27. Wasman J, Rosenthal NS, Fahri D. Mantle cell lymphoma. Morphologic findings in bone marrow involvement. *Am J Clin Pathol* 1996; 106:196–200.
28. Pittaluga S, Verhoef G, Criel A, et al. "Small" B-cell non-Hodgkin's lymphomas with splenomegaly at presentation are either mantle cell lymphoma or marginal zone cell lymphoma: a study based on histology, cytology, immunohistochemistry, and cytogenetic analysis. *Am J Surg Pathol* 1996;20:211–223.
29. O'Briain DS, Kennedy MJ, Daley PA, et al. Multiple lymphomatous polyposis of the gastrointestinal tract: a clinicopathologically distinctive form of non-Hodgkin's lymphoma of B-cell centrocytic type. *Am J Surg Pathol* 1989;13:691–699.
30. Lavergne A, Brouland J, Launay E, et al. Multiple lymphomatous polyposis of the gastrointestinal tract: an extensive histopathologic and immunohistochemical study of 12 cases. *Cancer* 1994;74: 3042–3050.
31. Ruskone-Formestraux A, Delmer A, Lavergne A, et al. Multiple lymphomatous polyposis of the gastrointestinal tract: a prospective clinicopathologic study of 31 cases. *Gastroenterology* 1997;112:7–16.
32. Moynihan MJ, Bast MA, Chan WC, et al. Lymphomatous polyposis: a neoplasm of either follicular mantle or germinal center cell origin. *Am J Surg Pathol* 1996;20:442–452.
33. Zuckerberg LR, Medeiros JL, Ferry JA, Harris NL. Diffuse low-grade B-cell lymphomas: four clinically distinct subtypes defined by a combination of morphologic and immunophenotypic features. *Am J Clin Pathol* 1993;100:373–385.
34. Molot RJ, Meeker TC, Wittwar CT, et al. Antigen expression and polymerase chain reaction amplification in mantle cell lymphomas. *Blood* 1994;83:1626–1631.
35. Kilo MN, Dorfman DM. The utility of flow cytometric immunophenotypic analysis in the distinction of small lymphocytic lymphoma/chronic lymphocytic leukemia from mantle cell lymphoma. *Am J Clin Pathol* 1996;105:451–457.
36. Kumar S, Green GA, Teruya-Feldstein J, et al. Use of CD23 (BU38) on paraffin sections in the diagnosis of small lymphocytic lymphoma and mantle cell lymphoma. *Mod Pathol* 1996;9:925–929.
37. Hoffmann DG, Tucker SJ, Emmanoulides C, et al. CD8-positive mantle cell lymphoma: a report of two cases. *Am J Clin Pathol* 1998;109: 689–694.
38. Ott G, Kalla J, Ott M, et al. Blastoid variants of mantle cell lymphoma: frequent bcl-1 rearrangements at the major translocation cluster region and tetraploid chromosome clones. *Blood* 1997;89:1421–1429.
39. Weisenburger DD, Sanger WG, Armitage JO, et al. Intermediate lymphocytic lymphoma: immunophenotypic and cytogenetic findings. *Blood* 1987;69:1617–1621.
40. Rimokh R, Berger F, Cornillet P, et al. Break in the bcl-1 locus is closely associated with intermediate lymphocytic lymphoma subtype. *Genes Chromosomes Cancer* 1990;2:223–226.
41. Leroux D, Le Marc'hadour F, Gressin R, et al. Non-Hodgkin's lymphomas with t(11;14)(q13;q32): a subset of mantle zone/intermediate lymphocytic lymphomas. *Br J Haematol* 1991;77:346–353.
42. Vandenberghe E, de Wolfe-Peeters C, Wlodarska I, et al. Chromosome 11q rearrangements in B non-Hodgkin's lymphoma. *Br J Haematol* 1992;81:212–217.
43. Komatsu H, Iida S, Yamamoto K, et al. A variant chromosome translocation at 11q13 identifying PRAD1/Cyclin D1 as the bcl-1 gene. *Blood* 1994;84:1226–1231.
44. Rimokh R, Berger F, Bastard C, et al. Rearrangement of CCND1 (BCL1/PRAD1) 3′ untranslated region in mantle-cell lymphomas and the t(11q13)-associated leukemias. *Blood* 1994;10:3689–3696.
45. Johansson B, Mertens F, Mitelman F. Cytogenetic evolution patterns in non-Hodgkin's lymphoma. *Blood* 1995;86:3905–3914.
46. Stilgenbauer S, Nickolenko J, Wilhelm J, et al. Expressed sequences as candidates for a novel tumor suppressor gene at band 13q14 in B-cell chronic lymphocytic leukemia and mantle cell lymphoma. *Oncogene* 1998;16:1891–1897.
47. Monni O, Oinonen R, Elonen E, et al. Gain of 3q and deletion of 11q22 are frequent aberrations in mantle cell lymphoma. *Genes Chromosom Cancer* 1998;21:298–307.
48. Daniel MT, Tagaud I, Flexor MA, et al. Leukemic non-Hodgkin's lymphomas with hyperdiploid cells and t(11;14)(q13;q32): a subtype of mantle cell lymphoma? *Br J Haematol* 1995;90:77–84.
49. Tirier C, Zhang Y, Plendl H, et al. Simultaneous presence of t(11; 14) and a variant Burkitt's translocation in the terminal phase of a mantle cell lymphoma. *Leukemia* 1996;10:346–350.
50. Chary-Reddy S, Prasad VS, Ahuja YR. Expression of common fragile sites in untreated non-Hodgkin's lymphoma with aphidicolin and folate deficiency. *Cancer Lett* 1994;86:111–117.
51. Williams ME, Swerdlow SH, Rosenberg CL, et al. Chromosome 11 translocation breakpoint at the PRAD1/Cyclin D1 gene locus in centrocytic lymphoma. *Leukemia* 1993;7:241–245.
52. Rimokh R, Berger F, Delsol G, et al. Rearrangement and overexpression of the bcl-1/PRAD-1 gene in intermediate lymphocytic lymphomas and in t(11q13)-bearing leukemias. *Blood* 1993;81: 3063–3067.
53. de Boer CJ, Loyson S, Kluin PM, et al. Multiple breakpoints within the Bcl-1 locus in B-cell lymphoma: rearrangements of the cyclin D1 gene. *Cancer Res* 1993;53:4148–4152.
54. Bosch F, Jares P, Campo E, et al. PRAD1/Cyclin D1 gene overexpression in chronic lymphoproliferative disorders: a highly specific marker of mantle cell lymphoma. *Blood* 1994;84:2726–2732.
55. Rimokh R, Berger F, Delsol G, et al. Detection of the chromosomal translocation in t(11;14) by polymerase chain reaction in mantle cell lymphomas. *Blood* 1994;83:1871–1875.
56. Luthra R, Hai S, Pugh WC. Polymerase chain reaction detection of the t(11;14) translocation involving the bcl-1 major translocation cluster in mantle cell lymphoma. *Diagn Mol Pathol* 1995;4:4–7.
57. Pinyol M, Campo E, Nadal A, et al. Detection of the bcl-1 rearrangement at the major translocation cluster in frozen and paraffin embedded tissues of mantle cell lymphomas by polymerase chain reaction. *Am J Clin Pathol* 1996;105:532–537.
58. Monteil M, Callanan M, Dascalescu C, et al. Molecular diagnosis of t(11;14) in mantle cell lymphoma using two-color interphase fluorescence in situ hybridization. *Br J Haematol* 1996;93:656–660.
59. Vaandrager JW, Schuuring E, Zwikstra E, et al. Direct visualization of dispersed 11q13 chromosomal translocations in mantle cell lymphoma by multicolor DNA fiber fluorescence in situ hybridization. *Blood* 1996;88:1177–1182.
60. Siebert R, Matthiesen P, Harder S, et al. Application of interphase cytogenetics for the detection of t(11;14)(q13;q32) in mantle cell lymphomas. *Ann Oncol* 1998;9:519–526.
61. Rosenberg CL, Wong E, Petty EM, et al. PRAD 1, a candidate BCL1 oncogene: mapping and expression in centrocytic lymphoma. *Proc Natl Acad Sci USA* 1991;88:9636–9642.
62. Withers DA, Harvey RC, Faust JB, et al. Characterization of a candidate bcl-1 gene. *Mol Cell Biol* 1991;11:4846–4853.
63. Motokura T, Bloom T, Kim HG, et al. A novel cyclin encoded by a bcl 1-linked candidate oncogene. *Nature* 1991;350:512–515.
64. Oka K, Ohno T, Kita K, et al. PRAD1 gene overexpression in mantle-cell lymphoma but not in other low-grade B-cell lymphomas, including extranodal lymphoma. *Br J Haematol* 1994;86:786–791.
65. de Boer CJ, van Krieken JHJM, Kluin-Nelemans HC, et al. Cyclin D1 messenger RNA overexpression as a marker for mantle cell lymphoma. *Oncogene* 1995;10:1833–1840.
66. de Boer CJ, Vaandrager JW, van Krieken JHJM, et al. Visualization of mono-allelic chromosomal aberrations 3′ and 5′ of the cyclin D1 gene in mantle cell lymphoma using DNA fiber fluorescence in situ hybridization. *Oncogene* 1997;15:1599–1603.
67. Yang WI, Zukerberg LR, Motokura T, et al. Cyclin D1 (bcl-1, PRAD1) protein expression in low-grade B-cell lymphomas and reactive hyperplasia. *Am J Pathol* 1994;145:86–96.
68. Zuckerberg LR, Yang WI, Arnold A, et al. Cyclin D1 expression in non-Hodgkin's lymphomas: detection by immunohistochemistry. *Am J Clin Pathol* 1995;103:756–760.
69. Swerdlow SH, Yang WI, Zuckerberg LR, et al. Expression of cyclin D1 protein in centrocytic/mantle cell lymphomas with and without rearrangement of the BCL1/cyclin D1 gene. *Hum Pathol* 1995;26: 999–1004.
70. deBoer CJ, Schuuring E, Dreef E, et al. Cyclin D1 protein analysis in the diagnosis of mantle cell lymphoma. *Blood* 1995;86:2715–2723.
71. Oka K, Ohno T, Yamaguchi M, et al. PRAD1/cyclin D1 gene overexpression in mantle cell lymphoma. *Leuk Lymphoma* 1996;21:37–42.
72. Yatabe Y, Nakamura S, Seto M, et al. Clinicopathologic study of PRAD1/cyclin D1 overexpression with special reference to mantle cell lymphoma. *Am J Surg Pathol* 1996;20:1110–1122.
73. Lukas J, Jadayel D, Bartikova J, et al. BCL-1/cyclin D1 oncoprotein

oscillates and subverts the G1 phase control in B-cell neoplasms carrying the t(11;14) translocation. *Oncogene* 1994;9:2159–2167.
74. Arnold A. The cyclin D1/PRAD1 oncogene in human neoplasia. *J Invest Med* 1995;43:543–549.
75. Sherr CJ. Cancer cell cycles. *Science* 1996;274:1672–1677.
76. Daudy SF, Hinds PW, Louie K, et al. Physical interactions of the retinoblastoma protein with human D cyclins. *Cell* 1993;73:499–511.
77. Imoto M, Doki T, Jiang W, et al. Effects of cyclin D1 overexpression on G1 progression-related events. *Exp Cell Res* 1997;236:173–180.
78. Ott MM, Bartikova J, Bartek J, et al. Cyclin D1 expression in mantle cell lymphoma is accompanied by downregulation of cyclin D3 and is not related to proliferative activity. *Blood* 1997;90:3154–3159.
79. Jares P, Campo, E Pinyol M, et al. Expression of retinoblastoma gene product (pRB) in mantle cell lymphomas. Correlation with cyclin D1 (PRAD1/CCND1) mRNA levels and proliferative activity. *Am J Pathol* 1996;148:1591–1600.
80. Zuckerberg LR, Benedict WF, Arnold A, et al. Expression of the retinoblastoma protein in low-grade B-cell lymphoma: relationship to cyclin D1. *Blood* 1996;88:268–276.
81. Hirama T, Koeffler HP. Role of the cyclin dependent kinase inhibitors in the development of cancer. *Blood* 1995;86:841–854.
82. Koduru PRK, Zariwala M, Soni M, et al. Deletion of cyclin-dependent kinase 4 inhibitor genes p15 and p16 in non-Hodgkin's lymphoma. *Blood* 1995;86:2900–2905.
83. Pinyol M, Hernandez L, Carzola M, et al. Deletions and loss of expression of P16 INK4 and P21Waf1 genes are associated with aggressive variants of mantle cell lymphomas. *Blood* 1997;86:272–280.
84. Dreyling WH, Bullinger L, Ott G, et al. Alterations of the cyclin D1/p16-pRB pathway in mantle cell lymphoma. *Cancer Res* 1997;57:4608–4616.
85. Williams ME, Whitefield M, Swerdlow SH. Analysis of the cyclin-dependent kinase inhibitors p18 and p19 in mantle cell lymphoma and chronic lymphocytic leukemia. *Ann Oncol* 1997;8(Suppl 2):571–573.
86. Quintanilla-Martinez L, Thieblemont C, Fend F, et al. Mantle cell lymphomas lack expression of p27kip1, a cyclin-dependent kinase inhibitor. *Am J Pathol* 1998;153:175–182.
87. Louie DC, Offit K, Jaslow R, et al. p53 overexpression as a marker of poor prognosis in mantle cell lymphomas with the t(11;14)(q13;q32). *Blood* 1995;86:2892–2899.
88. Greiner TC, Moynihan MJ, Chan WC, et al. p53 mutations in mantle cell lymphoma are associated with variant cytology and predict a poor prognosis. *Blood* 1996;87:4302–4310.
89. Hernandez L, Fest T, Carzorla M, et al. p53 gene mutations and protein overexpression are associated with aggressive variants of mantle cell lymphomas. *Blood* 1996;87:3351–3359.
90. Lane DP. p53, guardian of the genome. *Nature* 1992;358:15–16.
91. Jiang W, Kahn SM, Zhou P, et al. Overexpression of cyclin-D1 in rat fibroblasts causes abnormalities in growth control, cell cycle progression and gene expression. *Oncogene* 1993;8:3447–3457.
92. Hinds PW, Daudy SF, Eaton EN, et al. Function of a human cyclin gene as an oncogene. *Proc Natl Acad Sci USA* 1994;91:709–713.
93. Lovec H, Sewing A, Lucibello FC, et al. Oncogenic activity of cyclin D1 revealed through cooperation with Ha-ras: link between cell cycle control and malignant transformation. *Oncogene* 1994;9:323–326.
94. Uchimaru K, Endo K, Fujinuma H, et al. Oncogenic collaboration of the cyclin D1 (PRAD1, bcl-1) gene with a mutated p53 and an activated ras oncogene in neoplastic transformation. *Jpn J Cancer Res* 1996;87:459–465.
95. Bodrug SE, Warner BJ, Bath ML, et al. Cyclin D1 transgene impedes lymphocyte maturation and collaborates in lymphomagenesis with the myc gene. *EMBO J* 1994;13:2124–2130.
96. Lovec H, Grzeschiezek A, Kowalski MB, et al. Cyclin D1/bcl-1 cooperates with myc genes in the generation of B-cell lymphoma in transgenic mice. *EMBO J* 1994;13:3487–3495.
97. Lammie GA, Smith R, Silver J, et al. Proviral insertions near cyclin D1 in mouse lymphomas: a parallel for BCL1 translocations in human B-cell neoplasms. *Oncogene* 1992;7:2381–2387.
98. Hanna Z, Jankowski M, Tremblay P, et al. The vin-1 gene, identified by proviral insertional mutagenesis, is the cyclin D2. *Oncogene* 1993;8:1661–1666.
99. Wang TC, Cardiff RD, Zukerberg L, et al. Mammary hyperplasia and carcinoma in MMTV-cyclin D1 transgenic mice. *Nature* 1994;369:669–671.
100. Weisenburger DD, Harrington DS, Armitage JO. B-cell neoplasia: a conceptual understanding based on the normal humoral immune response. In: Rosen PP, Fechner RE, eds. *Pathology annual.* East Norwalk, CT: Appleton and Lange, 1990;99–115.
101. Bofill M, Janossy G, Janossa M, et al. Human B cell development: II. Subpopulations in the human fetus. *J Immunol* 1985;134:1531–1538.
102. Antin JH, Emerson SG, Martin P, et al. Leu-1 + (CD5 +) B cells: a major lymphoid subpopulation in human fetal spleen: phenotypic and functional studies. *J Immunol* 1986;136:505–510.
103. Asano S, Akaike Y, Muramatsu T, et al. Immunohistologic detection of the primary follicle (PF) in human fetal and newborn lymph node anlages. *Pathol Res Prac* 1993;189:921–927.
104. Rabian-Herzog C, Lesage S, Gluckman E. Characterization of lymphocyte subpopulations in cord blood. *Bone Marrow Transplant* 1992;9(Suppl 1):64–67.
105. Durandy A, Thuillier L, Forvielle M, et al. Phenotypic and functional characteristics of human newborns' B lymphocytes. *J Immunol* 1990;144:60–65.
106. Hamburg A, Brynes RK, Reese C, et al. Human cord blood lymphocytes: ultrastructural and immunologic surface marker characteristics; a comparison with B- and T-cell lymphomas. *Lab Invest* 1976;34:207–215.
107. Gobbi M, Caligaris-Cappio F, Janossy G. Normal equivalent cells of B cell malignancies: analysis with monoclonal antibodies. *Br J Haematol* 1983;54:393–403.
108. Gadol N, Ault KA. Phenotypic and functional characterization of Leu-1 (CD5) B cells. *Immunol Rev* 1986;93:23–34.
109. Freedman AS, Boyd AW, Bieber FR, et al. Normal cellular counterparts of B cell chronic lymphocytic leukemia. *Blood* 1987;70:418–427.
110. Abe M, Tominga K, Wakesa H. Phenotypic characterization of human B-lymphocyte subpopulations, particularly human CD5 + B-lymphocyte subpopulation within the mantle zones of secondary follicles. *Leukemia* 1994;8:1039–1044.
111. Küppers R, Zhoa M, Hansmann ML, et al. Tracing B cell development in human germinal centers by molecular analysis of single cells picked from histological sections. *EMBO J* 1993;12:4955–4967.
112. Hummel M, Tamaru J, Kalvelage B, et al. Mantle cell (previously centrocytic) lymphomas express VH genes with no or very little somatic mutations like the physiologic cells of the follicle mantle. *Blood* 1994;84:403–407.
113. Caligaris-Cappio F, Riva M, Tesio L, et al. Human normal CD5 + B lymphocytes can be induced to differentiate to CD5-B lymphocytes with germinal center features. *Blood* 1989;73:1259–1263.
114. Holder MJ, Abbot SD, Milner AE, et al. Il-2 expands and maintains IgM plasmablasts from a CD5 + subset contained within the germinal centre cell-enriched (surface IgD-/CD39-buoyant) fraction of human tonsil. *Int Immunol* 1993;5:1059–1066.
115. Harris NL, Bahn AK. Mantle-zone lymphoma: a pattern produced by lymphomas of more than one cell type. *Am J Surg Pathol* 1985;9:872–882.
116. Weisenburger DD, Linder J, Daley DT, et al. Intermediate lymphocytic lymphoma: an immunohistologic study with comparison to other lymphocytic lymphomas. *Hum Pathol* 1987;18:781–790.
117. Ellison DJ, Nathwani BN, Cho SY, et al. Interfollicular small lymphocytic lymphomas: the diagnostic significance of pseudofollicles. *Hum Pathol* 1989;20:1108–1118.
118. Perry DA, Bast MA, Armitage JO, et al. Diffuse intermediate lymphocytic lymphoma: a clinicopathologic study with comparison to small lymphocytic lymphoma and diffuse small cleaved cell lymphoma. *Cancer* 1990;66:1995–2000.
119. Hammer RD, Glick AD, Greer JP, et al. Splenic marginal zone lymphoma: a distinct B-cell lymphoma. *Am J Surg Pathol* 1996;20:613–626.
120. Mollejo M, Manarquez J, Lloret E, et al. Splenic marginal zone lymphoma: a distinctive type of low-grade B-cell lymphoma. A clinicopathologic study of 13 cases. *Am J Surg Pathol* 1995;19:1146–1157.
121. Savilo E, Campo E, Mollejo M, et al. Absence of cyclin D1 protein expression in splenic marginal zone lymphoma. *Mod Pathol* 1998;11:601–606.
122. Troussard X, Mauvieux L, Radford-Weiss I, et al. Genetic analysis of splenic lymphomas with villous lymphocytes. *Br J Haematol* 1998;101:712–721.
123. Cheng AL, Su IJ, Tien HF, et al. Characteristic clinicopathologic features of adult B-cell lymphoblastic lymphoma with special empha-

sis on differential diagnosis with an atypical form probably of blastic lymphocytic lymphoma of intermediate differentiation origin. *Cancer* 1994;73:706–710.

124. Soslow RA, Zuckerberg LR, Harris NL, et al. BCL-1 (PRAD1/cyclin D1) overexpression distinguishes the blastoid variant of mantle cell lymphoma from B-lineage lymphoblastic lymphoma. *Mod Pathol* 1997;10:810–817.
125. Anderson JR, Armitage JO, Weisenburger DD, for the Non-Hodgkin's Lymphoma Classification Project. Epidemiology of the non-Hodgkin's lymphomas: distributions of the major subtypes differ by geographic locations. *Ann Oncol* 1998;9:717–720.
126. Brittinger G, Bartels H, Common H, et al. (Kiel Lymphoma Study Group). Clinical and prognostic relevance of the Kiel classification of non-Hodgkin's lymphomas: results of a prospective multicenter study by the Kiel Lymphoma Study Group. *Hematol Oncol* 1984;2: 269–306.
127. Meusers P, Engelhard M, Bartels H, et al. Multicentre randomized therapeutic trial for advanced centrocytic lymphoma. Anthracycline does not improve prognosis. *Hematol Oncol* 1989;7:365–380.
128. Bookman MA, Lardelli P, Jaffe ES, et al. Lymphocytic lymphoma of intermediate differentiation: morphologic, immunophenotypic, and prognostic factors. *J Natl Cancer Inst* 1990;82:742–748.
129. Berger F, Felman P, Sonet A, et al. Nonfollicular small B-cell lymphomas: a heterogeneous group of patients with distinct clinical features and outcome. *Blood* 1994;83:2829–2835.
130. Fisher RI, Dahlberg S, Nathwani BN, et al. A clinical analysis of two indolent lymphoma entities: mantle cell lymphoma and marginal zone lymphoma (including mucosa-associated lymphoid tissue and monocytoid B cell categories). A Southwest Oncology Group study. *Blood* 1995;85:1075–1082.
131. Zucca E, Roggero E, Pinotti G, et al. Patterns of survival in mantle cell lymphoma. *Ann Oncol* 1995;6:259–262.
132. Teodorovic I, Pittaluga S, Kluin-Nelemans JC, et al. Efficacy of four different regimens in 64 mantle-cell lymphoma cases: clinicopathologic comparison with 498 other non-Hodgkin's lymphoma subtypes. *J Clin Oncol* 1995;13:2819–2826.
133. Velders GA, Kluin-Nelemans JC, de Boer CJ, et al. Mantle-cell lymphoma: a population-based clinical study. *J Clin Oncol* 1996;14: 1269–1274.
134. Majlis A, Pugh WC, Rodriguez MA, et al. Mantle cell lymphoma: correlation of clinical outcome and biologic features with three histologic variants. *J Clin Oncol* 1997;15:1664–1667.
135. Vandenberghe E, de Wolf-Peeters C, Vaughn Hudson G, et al. The clinical outcome of 65 cases of mantle cell lymphoma initially treated with non-intensive therapy by the British National Lymphoma Investigation Group. *Br J Haematol* 1997;99:842–847.
136. Decaudin D, Bosq J, Munck JN, et al. Mantle cell lymphomas: characteristics, natural history and prognostic factors of 45 cases. *Leuk Lymphoma* 1997;26:539–550.
137. Bosch F, Lopez-Guillermo A, Campo E, et al. Mantle cell lymphoma: presenting features, response to therapy, and prognostic factors. *Cancer* 1998;82:567–575.
138. Hiddemann W, Unterhalt M, Herrmann R, et al. Mantle cell lymphomas have more widespread disease and slower response to chemotherapy compared with follicle-center lymphomas: results of a prospective comparative analysis of the German Low-grade Lymphoma Study Group. *J Clin Oncol* 1998;16:1922–1930.
139. Weisenburger DD, Vose JM, Lynch JC, et al. Mantle cell lymphoma: a clinicopathologic study of 68 cases from the Nebraska Lymphoma Study Group. *Am J Hematol* (in press).
140. Preud'homme JL, Gombert J, Brizard A, et al. Serum Ig abnormalities in mantle cell lymphoma. *Blood* 1997;90:894–896.
141. Plank L, Lennert K. Centrocytic lymphoma. *Am J Surg Pathol* 1993; 17:638–639.
142. Decaudin D, Bosq J, Tertian G, et al. Phase II trial of fludarabine monophosphate in patients with mantle cell lymphomas. *J Clin Oncol* 1998;16:579–583.
143. Stewart DA, Vose JM, Weisenburger DD, et al. The role of high-dose therapy and autologous hematopoietic stem cell transplantation for mantle cell lymphoma. *Ann Oncol* 1995;6:263–266.
144. Ketterer N, Salles G, Espinouse D, et al. Intensive therapy with peripheral stem cell transplantation in 16 patients with mantle cell lymphoma. *Ann Oncol* 1997;8:701–704.
145. Blay JY, Sebban C, Surbiquet C, et al. High-dose chemotherapy with hematopoietic stem cell transplantation in patients with mantle cell or diffuse centrocytic non-Hodgkin's lymphomas: a single center experience in 18 patients. *Bone Marrow Transplant* 1998;21:51–54.
146. Kröger N, Hoffknecht M, Dreger P, et al. Long-term disease-free survival of patients with advanced mantle-cell lymphoma following high-dose chemotherapy. *Bone Marrow Transplant* 1998;21:55–57.
147. Freedman AS, Neuberg D, Gribben JG, et al. High-dose chemoradiotherapy and anti-B-cell monoclonal antibody-purged autologous bone marrow transplantation in mantle cell lymphoma: no evidence for long term remission. *J Clin Oncol* 1998;16:13–18.
148. Anderson NS, Donovan JW, Borus JS, et al. Failure of immunologic purging in mantle cell lymphoma assessed by polymerase chain reaction detection of minimal residual disease. *Blood* 1997;90:4212–4221.
149. Corradini P, Ladetto M, Astolfi M, et al. Clinical and molecular remission after allogeneic blood cell transplantation in a patient with mantle cell lymphoma. *Br J Haematol* 1996;94:376–378.
150. Kaminski MS, Zasadny KR, Francis IR, et al. Radioimmunotherapy of B-cell lymphoma with [131I] anti-B1 (anti-CD20) antibody. *N Engl J Med* 1993;329:459–465.
151. McLaughlin P, Grillo-López AJ, Link BK, et al. Rituximab chimeric anti-CD20 monoclonal antibody therapy for relapsed indolent lymphoma: half of patients respond to a four-dose treatment program. *J Clin Oncol* 1998;16:2825–2833.
152. Zhau P, Jiang W, Zhang Y, et al. Antisense to cyclin D1 inhibits growth and reverts the transformed phenotype of human esophageal cancer cells. *Oncogene* 1995;11:571–580.
153. Ball KL, Lain S, Fahraeus E, et al. Cell-cycle arrest and inhibition of cdk4 activity by small peptides based on the carboxy-terminal domain of p21WAF1. *Curr Biol* 1996;7:71–80.
154. Kim HG, Miller DM. A novel triplex-forming oligonucleotide targeted to human cyclin D1 (bcl-1 proto-oncogene) promoter inhibits transcription in HeLa cells. *Biochemistry* 1998;37:2666–2672.
155. König A, Schwartz GK, Mohammed RM, et al. The novel cyclin-dependent kinase inhibitor flavopiridol downregulates bcl-2 and induces growth arrest and apoptosis in chronic B-cell leukemia lines. *Blood* 1997;90:4307–4312.
156. Arguello F, Alexander M, Sterry JA, et al. Flavopiridol induces apoptosis of normal lymphoid cells, causes immunosuppression, and has potent antitumor activity in vivo against human leukemia and lymphoma xenografts. *Blood* 1988;91:2482–2490.

CHAPTER 23

Nodal Marginal Zone B-Cell Lymphomas

Elias Campo and Elaine S. Jaffe

HISTORICAL BACKGROUND

Nodal marginal zone B-cell lymphomas (MZLs) were initially recognized by Sheibani and colleagues and Cousar and associates as monocytoid B-cell lymphomas and parafollicular lymphomas, respectively (1,2). These tumors were characterized by perisinusoidal, perivascular, and parafollicular infiltration by neoplastic lymphocytes resembling the monocytoid B cells observed in certain reactive lymphoid hyperplasias such as acquired toxoplasmosis (3) and human immunodeficiency virus (HIV)–associated lymphadenopathy (4). The initial descriptions and the terms used to designate these neoplasms emphasized the most frequent architectural (parafollicular) or cytologic (monocytoid) features of the tumors. Subsequent studies by different groups recognized considerable overlap in the clinical and pathologic characteristics of these lymphomas and lymphomas of mucosa-associated lymphoid tissue (MALT) (5–7). The similar morphologic, immunophenotypic, and genetic characteristics of these lymphomas and the fact that lymph node involvement by MALT lymphomas was similar to apparently primary monocytoid B-cell lymphomas led to the idea that nodal monocytoid B-cell lymphomas were the equivalent of primary extranodal MALT lymphomas (7–13). The frequent association of nodal and extranodal components in the same patients, even after a long time, raised speculation that a significant number, and perhaps all, of nodal monocytoid B-cell lymphomas could represent dissemination of primary extranodal MALT lymphomas (7,10,13,14). However, patients with nodal MZLs in which no extranodal involvement is detected after thorough clinical evaluation and follow-up have been described, indicating that primary nodal MZLs may also exist (15).

The relationship between the MALT lymphomas and the lymphocytes of the marginal zone of the Peyer's patches (8,16–18) suggested that these lymphomas may be derived from a post–germinal center memory cell localized in the marginal zone with the potential to differentiate into plasma cells and monocytoid B cells. Based on the similarities between monocytoid B-cell lymphomas and MALT lymphomas and their possible common histogenesis in a marginal zone B cell, the terms nodal and extranodal MZLs have been proposed to designate these neoplasms, respectively (19).

Splenic marginal zone lymphoma (SMZL) is a distinct entity characterized by marked splenomegaly, a relatively indolent clinical course, and frequent bone marrow and peripheral blood involvement (20–23). The tumor frequently involves splenic hilar lymph nodes and more rarely may spread to other lymph node groups. SMZL shows preferential expansion of the marginal zone, raising speculation that it too may be of marginal zone derivation. However, other data, such as the expression of IgD by the neoplastic cells, have raised questions regarding the precise histogenesis of SMZL. Moreover, it appears distinct from nodal and extranodal marginal zone (MALT) lymphomas of the usual type (21,24–27). We identified a primary nodal lymphoma with morphologic and immunophenotypic characteristics similar to SMZL that we designated marginal zone B-cell lymphoma of the splenic type (28). This type of MZL is contrasted with the more classic form of MZL, called MALT-type MZL (Table 23.1).

This chapter reviews the pathologic and clinical characteristics of nodal MZLs, their relationship to extranodal counterparts, and the differential diagnosis with other lymphomas, which may occasionally adopt a marginal zone pattern. The analysis of the literature on this subject is difficult because most of the studies have included extranodal MALT-type lymphomas along with apparently primary nodal tumors (6,29–31). Some series have also included other well-defined entities, such as follicular lymphoma, mantle cell lymphoma (MCL), or chronic lymphocytic leu-

E. Campo: Hematopathology Section, Laboratory of Pathology, Hospital Clinic, University of Barcelona, Barcelona, Spain

E. S. Jaffe: Hematopathology Section, Laboratory of Pathology, National Cancer Institute, National Institutes of Health, Bethesda, Maryland 20892

TABLE 23.1. *Differential diagnosis of nodal marginal zone lymphomas*

Feature	MALT type	Splenic type
Residual germinal centers	Prominent	Indistinct, regressed
Mantle zones	Prominent	Generally absent
Cytoplasmic membranes	Usually prominent	Indistinct
Monocytoid B cells	Often prominent	Absent
Admixed neutrophils	Common	Absent
Blast cells	May be present	May be present
Plasmacytoid features	May be present	May be present
IgD	Negative	Weakly positive
BCL-2 protein	Positive	Positive
Intrafollicular T cells	Not increased	Increased

kemia/small lymphocytic lymphoma (CLL/SLL) but with monocytoid B-cell differentiation (6,12,30,32). Some studies could have included tumors that, retrospectively, might have been SMZLs (33,34). The controversies regarding the relationship between nodal and extranodal MZL and the so-called composite lymphomas with a monocytoid B-cell component are discussed.

MONOCYTOID B LYMPHOCYTES AND FOLLICULAR MARGINAL ZONE

Monocytoid B cells were first identified by Lennert as a particular sinusoidal cell population in reactive lymphadenopathies and were interpreted as immature sinus histiocytes (35). The morphologic similarities with peripheral blood monocytes and the subsequent demonstration of a B-cell phenotype led to the designation of these cells as monocytoid B lymphocytes (3,36,37) (Fig. 23.1). The term *parafollicular B cells* was also proposed to reflect the predilection of these cells to proliferate in the parafollicular compartment of the lymph node (2). Monocytoid B cells are commonly seen in reactive lymphadenopathies with florid follicular hyperplasia, particularly toxoplasmic lymphadenitis and acquired immunodeficiency syndrome (AIDS)–associated lymphadenopathy, but they may also be seen in infectious mononucleosis, cytomegalovirus lymphadenitis, nonspecific lymphoid hyperplasias, granulomatous lymphadenitis, and purulent lymphadenopathies, among other reactive processes (38,39) (see Chapters 15 and 28). Clusters of reactive monocytoid B cells may be also present in Hodgkin's disease (40) and peripheral T-cell lymphomas (41).

Morphologically, the medium-sized lymphocytes have clear cytoplasm and a central rounded or slightly irregular nucleus with moderately clumped chromatin and inconspicuous nucleoli. Large cells are absent or occasional, although rare cases with predominant large cells have been recognized (38). Monocytoid B cells are distributed in focal aggregates in sinusoids and parasinusoidal areas, in surrounding reactive follicles, and in perivascular spaces. Usually, these aggregates are multifocal but not confluent. A certain concordance between the extent of the monocytoid B-cell hyperplasia and follicular hyperplasia has been noticed (30,37,38). Small clusters of neutrophils and eosinophils can be seen intermingled with the monocytoid cells. Phenotypically, they are B lymphocytes expressing IgM or IgG and polyclonal immunoglobulin light chains. T-cell–associated antigens, including CD5 and CD43, are absent (3,36,37,42). BCL-2 is usually absent in reactive monocytoid B cells but is present in a variable number of MZLs (32,43,44). The histiocytic marker Ki-M1p may show a fine granular immunoreactivity. CD30 and other activation-associated antigens are absent, but expression can be seen in isolated larger cells (38,45).

The biologic significance of this particular subpopulation of B lymphocytes is not well understood. The close association of these cells with reactive follicular hyperplasia suggests they may represent a transient B-cell differentiation stage related to follicular activation (3,36,37). A relationship between these cells and lymphocytes of the marginal zone has been suggested based on the topologic distribution and similar morphologic and phenotypic characteristics (3).

The follicular marginal zone is the most external area of the follicle outside the mantle cell corona. This area is well developed and easily identifiable morphologically in reactive spleen, Peyer's patches, and mesenteric lymph nodes, but it is less evident in other lymph node sites (46,47). In rodents, the splenic marginal zone is clearly separated from the mantle corona by a marginal sinus, but in humans, the transition between the mantle layer and the marginal zone is less well defined (47).

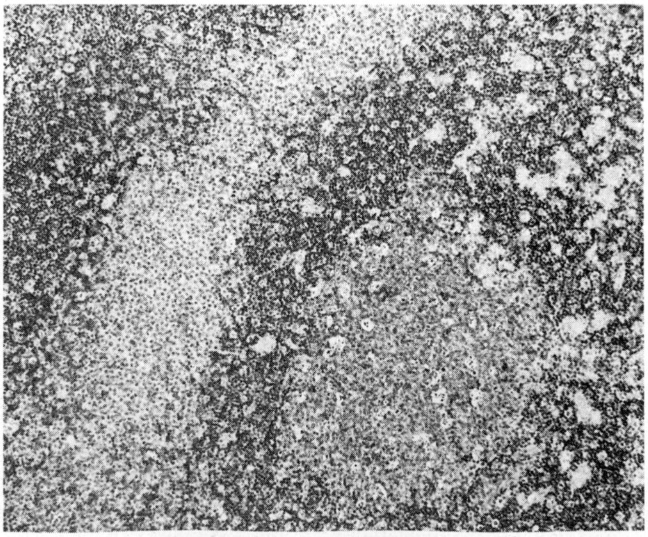

FIG. 23.1. Toxoplasmic lymphadenitis contains a prominent reaction of monocytoid B cells with a perivascular and perisinusoidal distribution (hematoxylin and eosin stain, original magnification: 100× magnification).

The cell composition is heterogeneous, with a main population of B cells, some T cells, and macrophages that may act as antigen presenting cells. The marginal zone lymphocytes have abundant, pale cytoplasm with slightly irregular nuclei. Phenotypically, they represent a characteristic subset of resting, nonactivated B cells expressing IgM; IgD is absent or weakly expressed. CD21 is present, but CD23 and CD10 are not present in these cells (48).

The functional activity of marginal zone lymphocytes is not clear. Some evidence indicates that the lymphoid population of the marginal zone is heterogeneous, with different types of memory B lymphocytes and cells involved in a T-cell–independent immunoresponse to poorly immunogenic antigens such as polysaccharides (TI-2 antigens) (49). After antigen stimulation, marginal zone B lymphocytes may undergo cycles of reentering the germinal center and become late memory cells that return to the marginal zone or evolve to plasma cells. Marginal zone lymphocytes may also participate in the transport of antigens to follicular dendritic cells. Analysis of immunoglobulin genes has shown that human marginal zone lymphocytes have somatic mutations, indicating that these cells have been through the germinal center and have become memory cells (50).

Nodal monocytoid B cells may have a heterogeneous origin. Molecular studies of reactive monocytoid cells have confirmed the constant expression of IgG and lack of IgM/IgD at the mRNA and protein levels. Mutational analysis of V_H genes has shown that 74% of these cells are naive, unmutated B cells and that only about 26% carry a low number of somatic mutations, indicating nonantigen-selected, post–germinal center B cells (51). Immunophenotypically and genetically, normal marginal zone B cells and parasinusoidal monocytoid B cells appear distinct.

NODAL MARGINAL ZONE LYMPHOMA

Nodal MZLs are characterized by a heterogeneous proliferation of atypical lymphocytes that includes medium-sized lymphocytes with clear cytoplasm (monocytoid B cells), small to medium-sized lymphocytes with irregular nuclei and scant cytoplasm (centrocyte-like cells), and a variable number of larger lymphocytes and plasma cells. The tumor cells adopt predominantly a sinusoidal, perivascular, and parafollicular pattern of infiltration but may evolve to a diffuse obliteration of the nodal architecture (Fig. 23.2). The tumor cells express B-cell markers with IgM expressed more frequently than IgG. They usually do not express IgD, CD5, CD23, CD10, and cyclin D1. Some cases may coexpress CD43. Genetic and molecular alterations are not well defined.

Morphologic Features

Architectural Patterns

The lymph nodes in MZL may show different patterns of involvement. In most cases, the nodal architecture is preserved or only partially effaced (1,2,7,29,52). In early lesions, the tumor cells are usually found in a sinusoidal and perisinusoidal distribution following the subcapsular and paratrabecular sinuses. Medullary sinuses may also be involved. In these cases, the nodal architecture is relatively preserved, with intact follicles and residual paracortical T-cell areas. The tumor cells may also be seen in a focal perivascular distribution surrounding small intranodal vessels. An increased number of epithelioid venules may be seen in the tumor infiltrates of some cases without associated T cells (7).

The most common infiltration is the parafollicular and interfollicular pattern in which the tumor cells grow around reactive follicles. This pattern is also called the *marginal zone pattern* because the tumor cells expand the external area of the follicle beyond the mantle cell cuff. In some cases, the parafollicular tumor cells tend to merge more extensively, producing a marked expansion of the interfollicular regions. In most of the cases, the parafollicular and interfollicular patterns coexist with the sinusoidal and perivascular infiltration of the tumor cells.

In a small number of cases, the tumor cells may widely efface the nodal architecture in a diffuse pattern of infiltration (7,52). Residual follicles may be scarce, poorly preserved, or absent. Immunohistochemical studies of follicular dendritic cells or IgD to detect residual mantle cells may help to identify remnants of follicles in these cases.

The lymphoid follicles usually show reactive features with a mixed population of centrocytes, centroblasts, and tingible body macrophages in the germinal centers and a relatively preserved mantle area. The size of the follicles may vary from large and hyperplastic to small and atrophic. The mantle cell cuff may be expanded, relatively normal, or attenuated, but it usually separates the tumor growth from the germinal center. In some cases, however, the boundaries between neoplastic lymphocytes and reactive germinal centers may be poorly defined (7,53). Similar to extranodal MZL of the MALT type, tumor cells of nodal MZL may colonize preexisting reactive germinal centers (7,13). In this situation, the mantle cuff may be preserved. Follicular colonization is usually more clearly identified when the tumor cells express monotypic cytoplasmic immunoglobulin.

The capsule of the lymph node is usually infiltrated by tumor cells and in up to 20% of the cases is associated with marked capsular sclerosis (7) (Fig. 23.3). The T-cell areas are relatively preserved or partially replaced by tumor cells in most of the cases but may be completely effaced in more advanced tumors. Hyperplasia of the T-cell areas can also be seen in occasional cases (7).

Cytologic Characteristics

Nodal MZLs are cytologically heterogeneous. The most characteristic cells are the monocytoid B lymphocytes resembling the monocytoid cells observed in reactive lym-

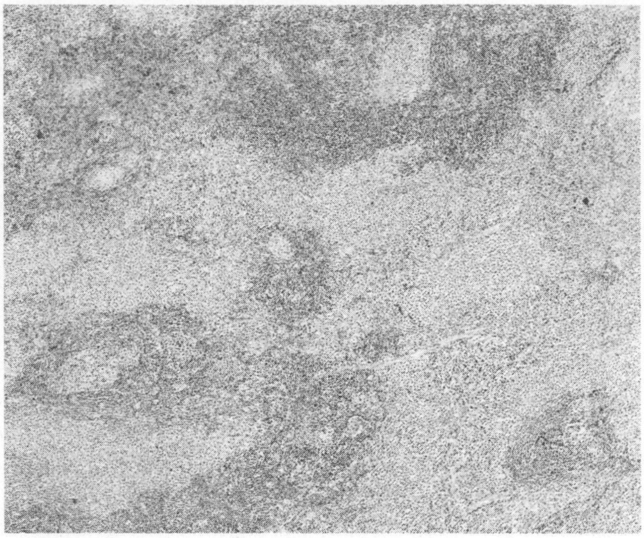
A

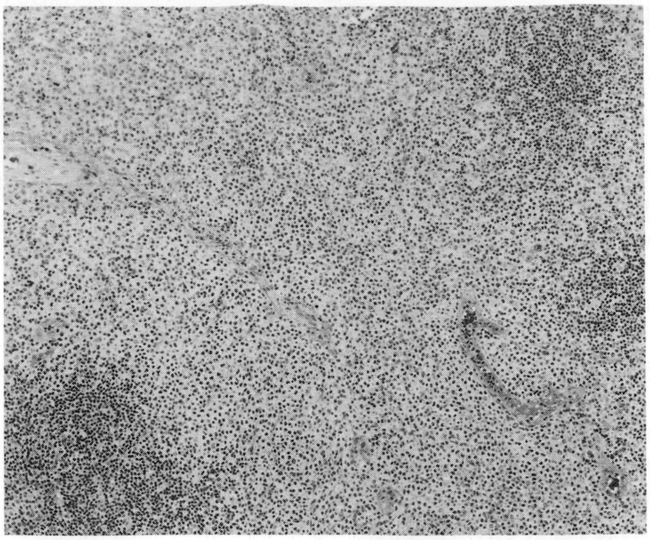
B

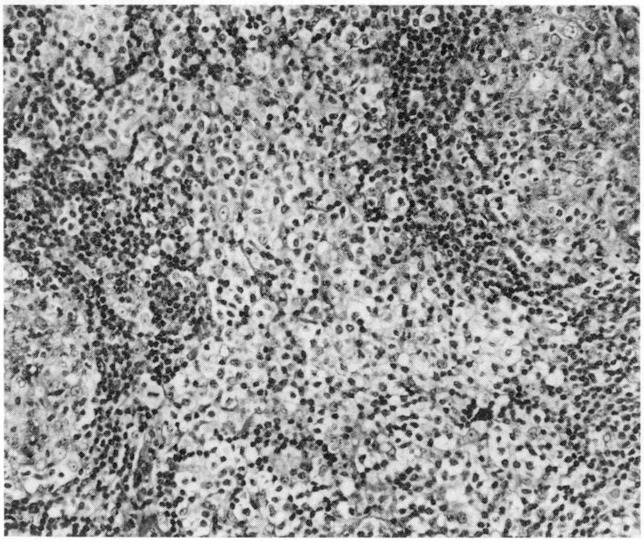
C

FIG. 23.2. Nodal marginal zone lymphoma. An extensive infiltrate of cells with pale cytoplasm involves the interfollicular region. **A:** Reactive follicles with intact mantle zones are evident (hematoxylin and eosin stain, original magnification: 50× magnification). **B:** The neoplastic cells are prominent surrounding blood vessels (hematoxylin and eosin stain, original magnification: 100× magnification). **C:** At higher power, the cells in the interfollicular region contain abundant pale cytoplasm (hematoxylin and eosin stain, original magnification: 200× magnification).

phadenopathies (Fig. 23.4). These cells show abundant clear cytoplasm with a well demarcated membrane, round or slightly irregular nuclei with coarse chromatin, and small or inconspicuous nucleoli. They may resemble hairy cell leukemia infiltrating tissues, but the cytochemical and immunophenotypic characteristics are different. In addition to the monocytoid B cells, smaller lymphocytes with irregular indented nuclei and scarce cytoplasm (i.e., centrocyte-like cells) may also be identified and in certain cases may predominate over the monocytoid cells (7). The tumor cells may include a variable proportion of larger blasts with oval or rounded nuclei and prominent nucleoli (Fig. 23.5). These larger cells are usually sparse but in some cases may be more abundant. The mitotic index in MZL is usually low but may increase in cases with a higher number of blasts or cases showing transformation to a large B-cell lymphoma.

Plasmacytoid differentiation is relatively common in these tumors, and in 30% of the cases, monotypic plasma cell proliferation may be the predominant feature (13,53) (Fig. 23.6). Russell and Dutcher bodies are recognized frequently in these cases. In some tumors, monotypic plasma cells are found within reactive germinal centers, indicating colonization by tumor cells (13,53). The presence of plasma cell differentiation has been associated with some degree of blastic transformation. A sharp separation between neoplastic monocytoid B cells and plasma cells in some tumors suggests displacement of tumor cells to different topologic compartments when they undergo plasmacytoid differentiation (13).

A relatively common finding is the presence of isolated or small clusters of polymorphonuclear leukocytes intermingled with the neoplastic monocytoid B cells. This feature recapitulates the association of neutrophils with reactive monocytoid B cells. In some cases, eosinophils may also be found, although marked eosinophilia is rare (7). Epithelioid histiocytes may be occasional or focal, and in certain cases,

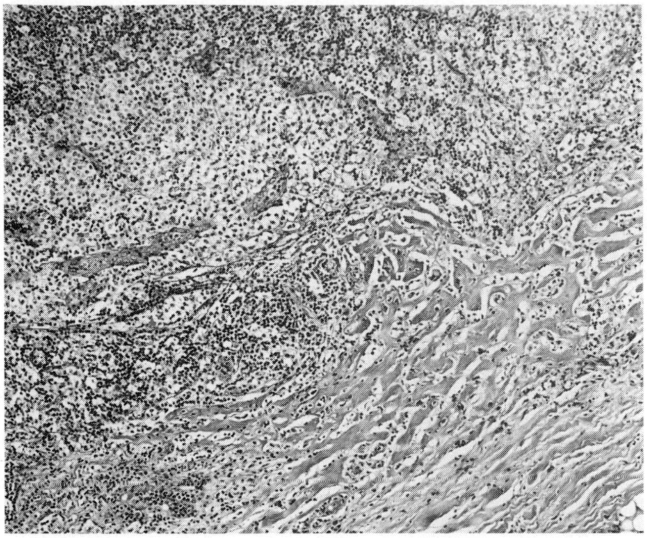

FIG. 23.3. Capsular fibrosis may be prominent in many cases of nodal marginal zone lymphoma (hematoxylin and eosin stain, original magnification: 100× magnification).

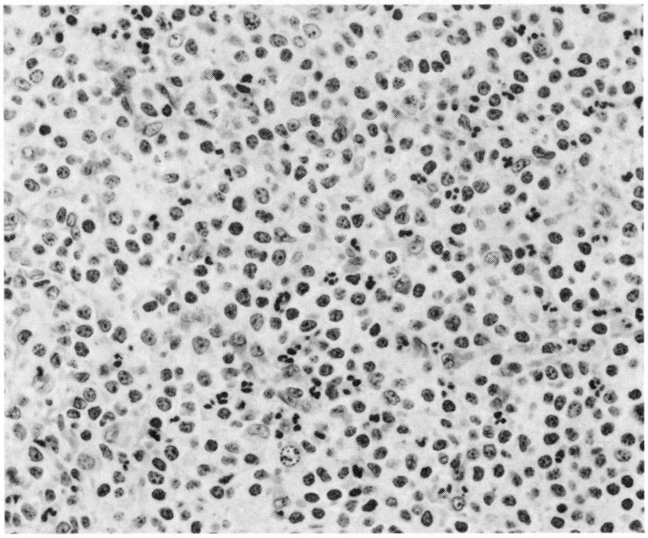

FIG. 23.4. Cytologic features of nodal marginal zone lymphoma. The neoplastic cells resemble monocytoid B cells with abundant clear cytoplasm. They are often associated with neutrophils, a feature that is seen in reactive monocytoid B-cell proliferations (hematoxylin and eosin stain, original magnification: 400× magnification).

A

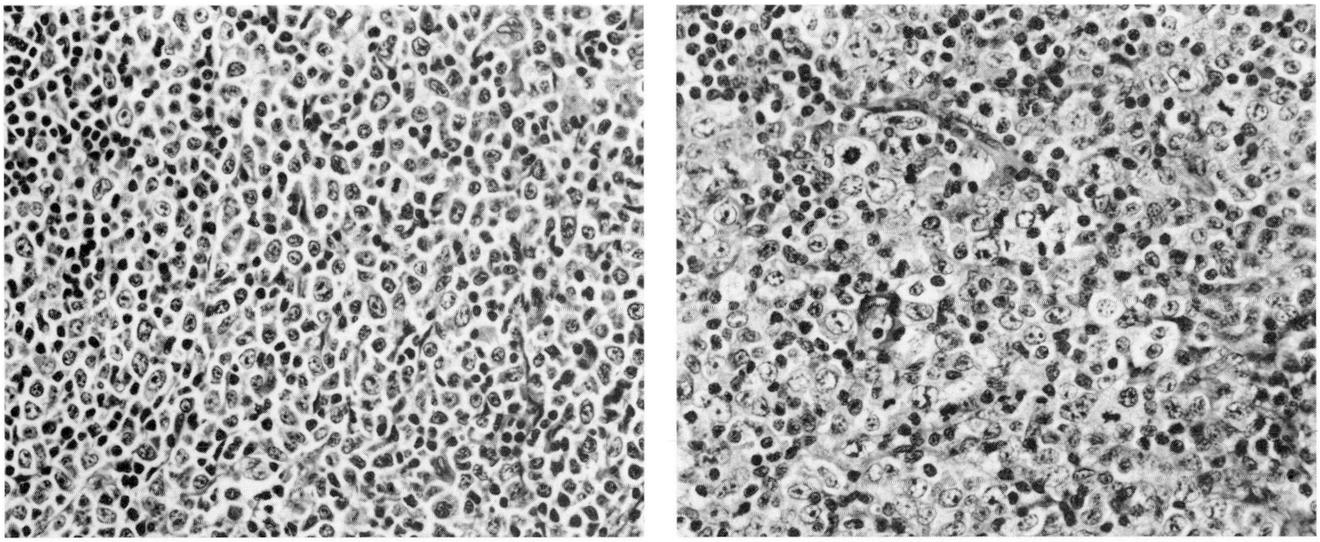

B

FIG. 23.5. Cytologic spectrum in nodal marginal zone lymphoma. **A:** Monocytoid B cells are inconspicuous, and interspersed blasts with vesicular nuclei and distinct basophilic nucleoli are seen (hematoxylin and eosin stain, original magnification: 400× magnification). **B:** Blast cells are more numerous, and mitoses are more readily seen. Cases with increased blasts may pursue a more aggressive clinical course (hematoxylin and eosin stain, original magnification: 400× magnification).

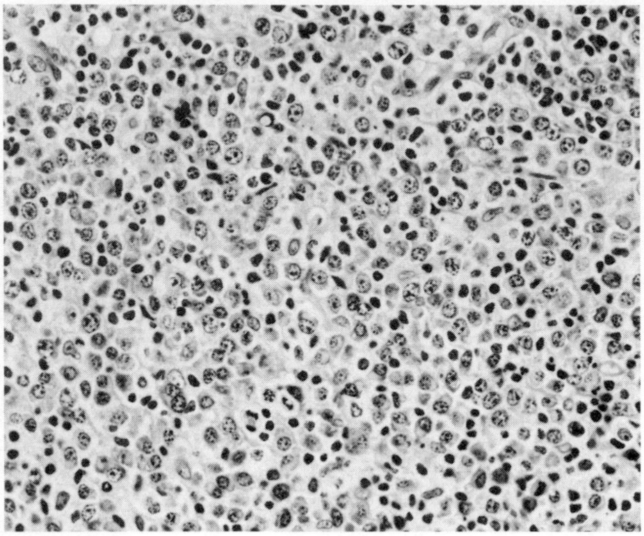

FIG. 23.6. Plasmacytoid differentiation may be conspicuous in some nodal marginal zone lymphomas. Cells with Dutcher bodies can be identified (hematoxylin and eosin stain, original magnification: 400× magnification).

they may extensively infiltrate the tumor cells (7,13,30). Massive deposition of crystalloid immunoglobulins in associated histiocytes has been described in MALT lymphomas with plasmacytic differentiation, but they may be also seen in the involved lymph nodes (54).

Ultrastructural Features

Electron microscopy studies have shown similarities between tumor cells in MZL and reactive monocytoid B lymphocytes (2,17,29). The tumor cells usually have an irregular shape with interdigitating processes and have abundant cytoplasm with glycogen, polyribosomes, inactive Golgi regions, polarized organelles, large mitochondria, and marked rough endoplasmic reticulum with occasional cisterns parallel to the cell surface. The nuclei are round, slightly irregular, or lobulated with a moderate quantity of marginated chromatin and evident nucleolus. No ribosomal-lamellar complexes have been observed. Cases with plasmacytic differentiation contain dilated cisternae of endoplasmic reticulum filled with proteinaceous material. Intermediate forms between monocytoid and plasma cells have been identified (53).

Pathology of Specific Organs

Bone marrow involvement has been considered uncommon in MZL, but it has been observed in 42% of cases in a series of 19 nodal and 6 extranodal MZLs (31). Similarly, a study by the Non-Hodgkin's Lymphoma Classification Project, in which nodal and extranodal MZLs have been analyzed separately, identified bone marrow involvement at presentation in 32% of nodal lymphomas but in only 16% of extranodal MZLs (55). Bone marrow biopsy seems to be more effective than smears to evaluate involvement in these tumors (31). The pattern of infiltration is usually focal with small, intertrabecular aggregates or interstitial infiltrates, although paratrabecular nodules have also been described (29). Liver biopsies have been reported in rare patients and have shown sinusoidal infiltration by tumor cells (29).

Transformation to Large B-Cell Lymphoma

Occasional blast cells with large nuclei and prominent nucleoli are a relatively common finding in MZL, but they usually represent less than 10% of the tumor (7,13). The presence of these isolated cells in low-grade MZL is probably of little clinical significance, and in some studies, they have been associated with plasmacytoid cell differentiation (13).

Aggressive transformation of a low-grade MZL to a diffuse large B-cell lymphoma has been described in several series (6,7,13,14,29,53). This phenomenon occurred 10 to 76 months after the original diagnosis of a low-grade tumor (13,14,53). However, focal transformation to a large cell lymphoma may also be recognized at diagnosis (30). The progressed lymphoma is usually found in a nodal recurrence, but it may also be seen at an extranodal site after a primary diagnosis of nodal MZL (14). The clinical course of these transformed tumors is aggressive with poor response to therapy and short survival (6 to 15 months after transformation) (13,53). Morphologically, the high-grade lymphomas are difficult to recognize as marginal zone neoplasms, and the tumor cells resemble other large cell lymphomas with centroblasts, immunoblasts, large cells with plasma cell differentiation, or large pleomorphic lymphocytes (7,13,30). Transformation is associated with an increase in the mitotic index and Ki-67 labeling of tumor cells (6). Focal necrosis and clusters of epithelioid histiocytes also may be associated with transformed cells (30). If transformation is observed, the term *diffuse large B-cell lymphoma*, rather than high-grade MZL, is preferred. Criteria for the grading of MZL without overt transformation have not been agreed on, and this remains a subject for future study.

Immunophenotype

Nodal MZLs are mature B-cell neoplasms expressing B-cell antigens CD19, CD20, and CD22 (6,7,13,29) (Table 23.2). Other B-cell antigens, such as CD45RA, CD74 (LN2), and CD75 (LN1), have been detected in a variable number of cases (56). Surface immunoglobulin is usually of the IgM class, and IgD usually is absent (Fig. 23.7). Some cases may express IgG or IgA. The κ light chain is more frequently detected than the λ light chain (6,7,13,29). Monotypic cytoplasmic immunoglobulins may be observed mainly in the perinuclear space of tumor cells. Larger blasts and cells with plasmacytoid differentiation show stronger and more diffuse cytoplasmic positivity. Progressed large B-cell lymphomas maintain the same immunoglobulin class as the low-grade

TABLE 23.2. *Immunophenotype in the differential diagnosis of marginal zone lymphomas*

Antigen	MZL, MALT type	MZL, splenic type	CLL/SLL	MCL	Follicular lymphoma	Hairy cell leukemia
CD20, CD19	+	+	+	+	+	+
CD10	−	−	−	−	+	−
CD5	−	−	+	+	−	−
CD23	−	−	+	−	−	−
CD43	±	±	+	+	−	−
CD21	−	−	−		+	−
CD25	−	−	±	−	−	+
IgM	+	+	+	+	±	−
IgD	−	+	+	+	−	−
BCL-2 protein	+	+	+	+	+ +	+
Cyclin D1	−	−	−	+	−	−

CLL/SLL, chronic lymphocytic leukemia/small lymphocytic lymphoma; MALT, mucosa-associated lymphoid tissue; MCL, mantle cell lymphoma; MZL, marginal zone lymphoma.

component, suggesting a clonal evolution of the tumor (53). Staining for cytoplasmic monotypic immunoglobulins may be useful to recognize follicular colonization by tumor cells. Polyclonal plasma cells may also be identified in some cases. Tumors with marked plasmacytic differentiation may be CD20$^-$ (28) and may express other plasma cell-related antigens such as EMA and PCA-1 (28,29,56). Other B-cell associated antigens, including CD10, CD23, CD21, and CD35, are usually absent (6,7,13,17,28,29).

T-cell specific antigens CD3, CD2, and CD7 are absent. However, the less restricted antigen CD43 may be coexpressed in 10% to 50% of these tumors (6,28,57,58). Variability in CD43 staining may be caused by differential reactivity of different clones, because negative results have been

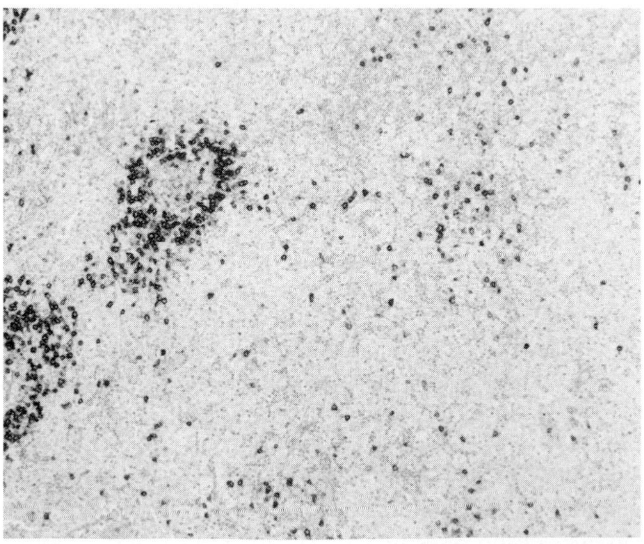

FIG. 23.7. Nodal marginal zone lymphomas are typically IgD$^-$, a feature seen in extranodal mucosa-associated lymphoid tissue (MALT) lymphomas. The IgD stain highlights residual mantle zones surrounding reactive germinal centers (immunoperoxidase stain, original magnification: 100× magnification).

reported using clone MT-1 (56). Contrary to B-cell CLL/SLL and MCL, CD43 expression in MZL is usually not associated with CD5 reactivity (28,58). Occasional CD5$^+$ extranodal MZLs have been described, and some controversy exits about whether these cases may have a more aggressive behavior (59,60). Some previously described CD5$^+$ MZLs may correspond to MCL or peculiar variants of CLL/SLL (12,34,61–63). One tumor diagnosed as a CD5$^+$ monocytoid B-cell lymphoma with leukemic involvement was shown to have unmutated rearranged V region genes similar to MCL or CLL/SLL. This finding contrasts with studies of monocytoid B-cell lymphoma that showed somatic mutations, suggesting that this case was a CLL/SLL or MCL with monocytoid differentiation (12). CD45RO is usually not expressed in MZL, but it has been observed in rare cases with plasmacytoid differentiation (28). Although mainly expressed in T-cell lymphomas, a switch between CD45RA and CD45RO may appear at a pre–plasma cell stage of B-cell differentiation (64,65).

Variable expression of some other antigens has been described in MZL. BCL-2 immunostaining may be observed in 50% to 80% of cases (14,28,43,44). Some studies have indicated that reactive monocytoid B cells are negative for BCL-2, whereas malignant monocytoid B cells are positive (32,43,44). This difference could help in the differential diagnosis between florid monocytoid B-cell hyperplasia and early involvement by MZL. BCL-6 usually is not expressed in low-grade MZL (66), but focal aggregates of positive cells have been described in high-grade gastric lymphomas (67).

DBA.44 is a monoclonal antibody that recognizes a subpopulation of B lymphocytes and is strongly positive in hairy cell leukemia. DBA.44 immunoreactivity has been observed in occasional cases of MZL (14,68,69). Ki-B3, which recognizes a B-cell–associated antigen, is reactive in monocytoid cells but not in the small centrocyte-like tumor cells (7). Early studies had detected CD11c expression in a high proportion of MZLs (6), but this finding has not been confirmed in other series (7,17,29). Ki-M1p, a histiocytic marker, has been detected in a variable number of tumor cells with a finely granular pattern that contrasts with the strong cytoplasmic reactivity of histiocytes (7,14). The activation marker CD25 has been expressed in some cases (17) but is not detected in other studies (7,29). Muscle-specific actin and vimentin immunoreactivity have been described in 50% and 30% of MZLs, respectively (56).

Cytogenetics

Cytogenetic studies performed in MZL show relatively similar alterations in nodal and extranodal tumors, supporting a common histogenetic origin. However, some controversy still exists concerning the relationship between the genetic anomalies of these tumors and those of SMZL. Trisomy 3 has been found in 50% to 62% of nodal MZLs using classic cytogenetic and fluorescence *in situ* hybridization techniques (11,24,70). This incidence is similar to that observed in extranodal MZL of the MALT type (56% to 85%) (11,24,70,71). However, a study using a sensitive double fluorescence *in situ* hybridization assay has detected trisomy 3 in only 20% of extranodal MALT lymphomas (72). Trisomy 3 has been detected in approximately 50% of cases of SMZL in some studies (11,24) but with a much lower incidence in other series (70,73,74). Different observations indicate that the relevant region in this alteration may be localized in the long arm of chromosome 3 (24,75). Usually, trisomy 3 is associated with other genetic alterations in MZL, suggesting that it may develop as a secondary change in the evolution of the tumors (71).

Trisomies 18, 7, 12, and structural alterations at 1q21 and 1p34 have also been described in nodal MZL with an incidence similar to extranodal MZL (24,70,76). Trisomy 13 and structural alterations in 13q14 have been occasionally reported (77,78). The relevance of these alterations in the pathogenesis of MZL is still unknown.

The t(11;18)(q21;q21) translocation appears to be the most common translocation in extranodal low-grade MZL, and it is usually present as a single clonal alteration (71). This translocation fuses the gene *IAP2,* which codes for an inhibitor of apoptosis, on chromosome 11 with a novel gene on chromosome 18 *(MLT1),* creating the chimeric gene *API2-MLT.* This gene may participate in the pathogenesis of these lymphomas by interfering with apoptotic pathways of the cell (79,80). Although this translocation can be detected in 27% of low-grade extranodal MALT lymphomas, it seems to be absent in nodal MZL, suggesting that these lymphomas may have a different pathogenetic origin (81).

Early cytogenetic studies of nodal MZL had detected trisomy 12, t(11;14)(q13;q32), and t(14;18)(q32;q21) in some cases (78). These alterations were usually found in so-called composite lymphomas in which the monocytoid B-cell lymphoma was associated with components of CLL/SLL, MCL, or follicular lymphoma. These chromosomal aberrations have not been found in pure MZL.

Molecular Biology

Molecular studies have demonstrated clonal rearrangements of the immunoglobulin heavy and light-chain genes, whereas the T-cell receptor gene is in the germline configuration (1,82). Analysis of the mutational status of the immunoglobulin genes in nodal MZL has shown the presence of somatic mutations similar to those in extranodal MZL, suggesting that these tumors are derived from a post–germinal center memory B cell (12,83).

No *BCL1, BCL2, BCL3,* or *MYC* gene rearrangements have been found in pure MZLs (6,24). However, *BCL1* and *BCL2* rearrangements may be detected in mantle cell and follicular lymphomas with monocytoid B-cell differentiation (14,32,84). *BCL6* gene rearrangements are usually negative but they have been described in occasional cases of extranodal MALT lymphoma (85). Molecular studies have not identified Epstein-Barr virus, human T-cell lymphotrophic virus type 1, human herpesvirus-8, and hepatitis C virus in MZL (77,86,87).

Differential Diagnosis

Typical cases of nodal MZL are not difficult to recognize. However, certain features in particular cases may raise the differential diagnosis with reactive processes, other lymphoproliferative disorders, or even leukemic infiltration of the lymph node. Monocytoid-like differentiation and a marginal zone growth pattern are not specific features of MZL and may occur in other lymphomas, such as follicular lymphoma, MCL, CLL/SLL, and SMZLs, involving lymph nodes and leading to possible confusion in the diagnosis of these disorders as MZL. Extensive plasma cell differentiation in MZL may suggest the diagnosis of lymphoplasmacytoid lymphoma or plasmacytoma. A problem in the differential diagnosis with other disorders such as hairy cell leukemia or mastocytosis, although possible, is uncommon.

Benign Versus Malignant Monocytoid B-Cell Proliferations

The differential diagnosis between florid reactive monocytoid B-cell proliferations and early involvement of a lymph node by MZL may be difficult (29). Morphologically, confluent areas of monocytoid cells, presence of cytologic atypia, transformed cells, and mitotic activity suggest lymphoma rather than a reactive process (30). BCL-2 expression has been reported as negative in reactive monocytoid B cells, whereas MZLs are positive (32,43,44). However, BCL-2 reactivity in these tumors may be irregular or weak, and up to 50% of the cases may be negative (28,32,43). Immunoglobulin light-chain restriction detected by immunohistochemistry or monoclonality by molecular techniques may be useful in the differential diagnosis (45).

Extensive monocytoid B-cell proliferations have been observed in cytomegalovirus (CMV) lymphadenitis. In these cases, cells infected by CMV are found intermingled with the monocytoid cells and may suggest malignant cells. However, the large size of the cells, the nuclear inclusion bodies, and the expression of CD15 by CMV infected cells may suggest Hodgkin's disease rather than monocytoid B-cell lymphoma. Immunohistochemical detection of CMV is helpful in the differential diagnosis (39).

Marginal Zone Pattern in Malignant Lymphomas Other Than Marginal Zone Lymphomas

Several types of B-cell lymphoma may occasionally display a monocytoid appearance, with abundant clear cytoplasm and/or a marginal zone growth pattern surrounding germinal centers that may lead to misdiagnosis as MZL. Some of these cases have been called composite lymphomas, and they include a combination of monocytoid B-cell lymphoma with CLL/SLL, immunocytoma, MCL, or follicular lymphoma. In these cases, it is usually possible to see a transition between the atypical monocytoid cells and the other tumor cells. The monocytoid B cells share an identical light-chain restriction and clonal immunoglobulin gene rearrangement with the other lymphomatous component. These findings indicate that both components are the same tumor and are clonally related (14,32,88,89). Genetic and molecular studies have demonstrated the presence of trisomy 12, t(11;14)/*BCL1* rearrangement, or t(14;18)/*BCL2* rearrangement in these composite lymphomas but not in pure monocytoid B-cell lymphomas (14,32,84), supporting the idea that the marginal zone differentiation in these tumors is a morphologic variant of the underlying lymphoma and not a different entity. Although the clinical information in these cases is limited, the biologic behavior seems to be concordant with that of the nonmonocytoid component. MCLs with monocytoid-like differentiation have followed a very aggressive clinical course rather than the indolent course of the typical MZL (84), and follicular lymphomas with monocytoid cells have had disseminated disease and bone marrow involvement at diagnosis, a finding less common in pure MZL (14,88).

Small Lymphocytic Lymphoma

Typical SLL/CLLs have a diffuse pattern, with pale proliferation centers containing prolymphocytes and paraimmunoblasts. However, some cases may have reactive germinal centers, with the tumor cells expanding in the interfollicular areas (90) (Fig. 23.8). Occasionally, the tumor cells surrounding the germinal centers may have more abundant pale cytoplasm, mimicking marginal zone differentiation (90,91). In these cases, the tumor cells are usually more monotonous than in MZL, with round nuclei and central nucleoli resembling prolymphocytes and paraimmunoblasts. Immunohistochemical studies should demonstrate CD5 and CD23 positivity, assisting in the diagnosis (see Chapter 21).

Follicular Lymphoma

MZLs occasionally resemble follicular lymphomas. Particularly when MZL cells massively colonize follicular centers, they may be interpreted morphologically as follicular lymphomas (32,88). Immunohistochemical demonstration of CD10 and BCL-6 may help in the differential diagnosis,

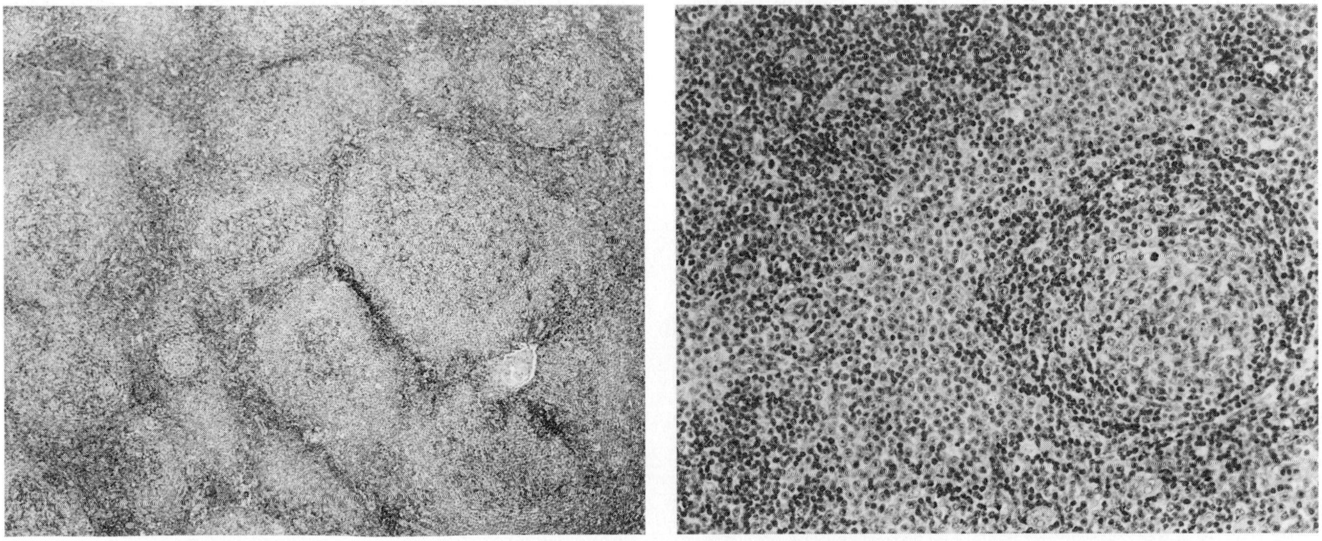

A B

FIG. 23.8. Chronic lymphocytic leukemia/small lymphocytic lymphoma (CLL/SLL) with a marginal zone pattern. **A:** At low power, the infiltrate of tumor cells with pale cytoplasm surrounds residual germinal centers (hematoxylin and eosin stain, original magnification: 100× magnification). **B:** The cytologic appearance is typical of CLL/SLL with admixed prolymphocytes and paraimmunoblasts. The neoplastic cells expressed CD5 and CD23 (hematoxylin and eosin stain, original magnification: 200× magnification).

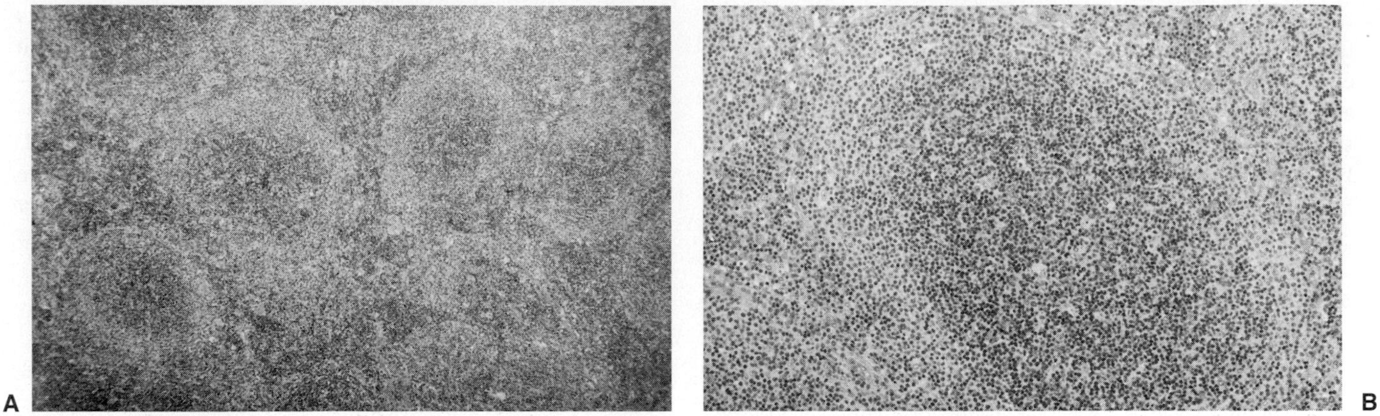

FIG. 23.9. Follicular lymphoma with a marginal zone pattern. **A:** An inverse follicular pattern is seen, with a dark center and a pale rim (hematoxylin and eosin stain, original magnification: 100× magnification). **B:** Neoplastic cells at the periphery of the follicle contain more abundant cytoplasm. The transition in cytologic appearance is gradual (hematoxylin and eosin stain, original magnification: 200× magnification).

because MZL has been reported to be negative for these markers. Molecular detection of *BCL2* gene rearrangement also is negative in these cases.

Follicular lymphomas may exhibit monocytoid differentiation. In these cases, neoplastic follicles are surrounded by a rim of large, transformed cells with pale cytoplasm, producing an ''inverse follicular pattern'' with the clear areas at the periphery and the dark areas in the center of the follicle (Fig. 23.9). Immunohistochemical studies for CD10 and BCL-6 and for *BCL2* gene rearrangement can help in the diagnosis. Although initially interpreted as composite lymphomas, it seems reasonable to consider these cases as follicular lymphomas with peculiar monocytoid B-cell differentiation. One study suggested that follicular lymphoma with monocytoid cells may behave more aggressively than conventional follicular lymphoma (92).

Mantle Cell Lymphoma

Some cases of MCL may have tumor cells with relatively abundant, pale cytoplasm that coupled with the presence of residual reactive germinal centers may suggest the diagnosis of MZL (84) (Fig. 23.10). Morphologically, the identification of areas of typical MCL and the absence of a mantle

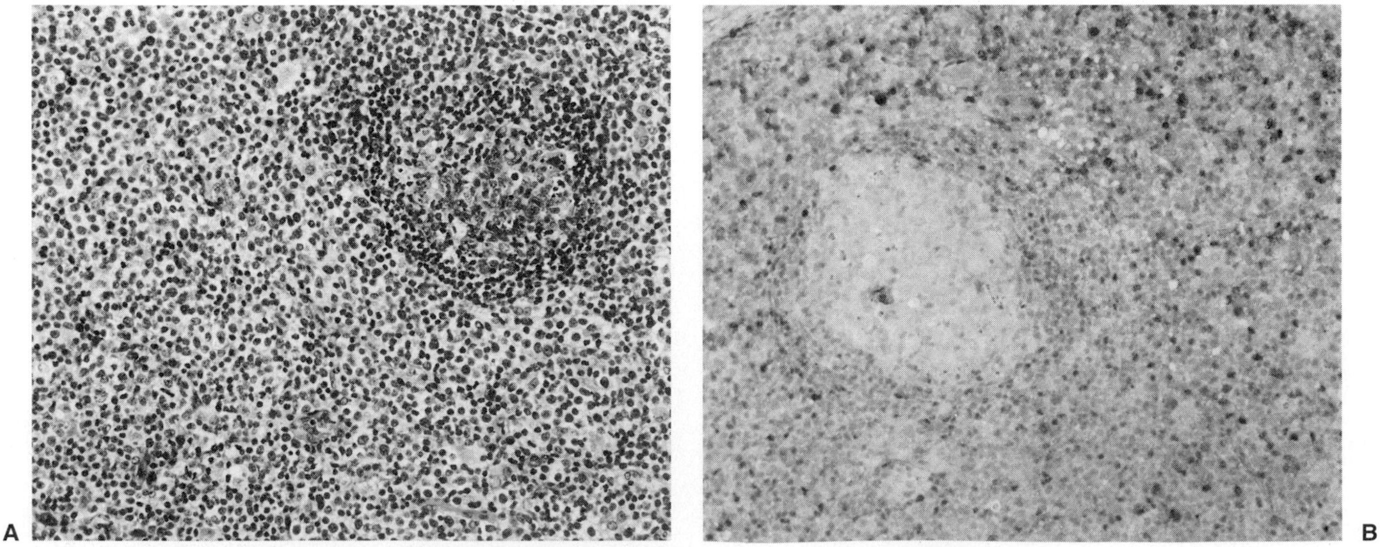

FIG. 23.10. Mantle cell lymphoma with a marginal zone pattern. **A:** At low power, the infiltrate simulates marginal zone lymphoma. An intact mantle zone appears to surround a residual germinal center (hematoxylin and eosin stain, original magnification: 200× magnification). **B:** A cyclin D1 stain is positive in the smaller "mantle cells" and in the interfollicular cells with more abundant cytoplasm. Both cellular components are neoplastic. The residual germinal center is IgD^- (immunoperoxidase stain, original magnification: 200× magnification).

cell corona in the reactive germinal centers (i.e., ''naked germinal centers'') may suggest the diagnosis of MCL. The immunophenotype and molecular characteristics of these tumors with CD5 and cyclin D1 expression and *BCL1* rearrangement can confirm the diagnosis. It is important to recognize these tumors as MCL, because the clinical behavior is aggressive, with extensive dissemination and a rapid clinical course. Some previously described cases of aggressive MZL with expression of CD5 may correspond to these variants of MCL (34,93) (see Chapter 22).

Lymphoplasmacytic Lymphoma

Early descriptions of composite lymphoma between monocytoid B-cell lymphoma and other components also included cases of lymphoplasmacytoid/lymphoplasmacytic lymphoma (6), and some cases of monocytoid B-cell lymphoma were initially diagnosed as nodal plasmacytomas (7). This differential diagnosis is complicated by the presence of extensive plasma cell differentiation in MZL (53). A polymorphic infiltrate associated with the atypical plasmacytoid cells and associated with reactive follicles, perhaps colonized by tumor cells, should suggest the diagnosis of MZL.

The differential diagnosis of lymphoplasmacytic lymphoma with MZL is difficult, and precise criteria to define the boundaries of MZL and lymphoplasmacytic lymphoma are lacking. Numerous Dutcher bodies, marked plasmacytic differentiation, and an absence of monocytoid B cells favor lymphoplasmacytic lymphoma. Clinical criteria, such as the presence of a monoclonal IgM spike indicative of Waldenström's macroglobulinemia, also may be of value.

Other Lymphoproliferative Disorders

Nodal infiltration by hairy cell leukemia may mimic MZL. However, the clinical presentation and the phenotype distinguish these entities (see Chapter 41). Mastocytosis involving tissues occasionally simulates MZL, particularly when the cells are round with clear cytoplasm. Mastocytosis is usually associated with perivascular fibrosis and tissue eosinophilia. Mast cells are $CD20^-$ but stain for tryptase and chloroacetate esterase (see Chapter 52). Monocytoid B-cell proliferations have been identified in Hodgkin's disease (40) and peripheral T-cell lymphomas (41).

Clinical Features and Natural History

Clinical Presentation and Laboratory Findings

Nodal MZL is a tumor mainly occurring in elderly females. The mean age at diagnosis is 60 to 65 years, with a range of 29 to 87 years (10,13,28–30,53), but the tumor may also be found in children and young patients (28,77). The male to female ratio has ranged from 1 to 1.5 men per 5 women in different series (13,28–30,53), although a similar number of males and females has been occasionally observed (10). In 50% to 65% of patients, the tumor manifests as localized stage I or II disease (10,29). However, in a study comparing pure nodal with extranodal MZL, patients with nodal tumors presented in an advanced stage more frequently (71%) than those with extranodal MZL (34%) (55).

The lymph node regions predominantly involved are head and neck, followed by inguinal and retroperitoneal areas. Lymphadenopathy is usually asymptomatic and may have been present for a few months to 2 years before the biopsy. The tumor grows slowly and in some cases may undergo spontaneous regression (10). Fever, B symptoms, or weight loss are uncommon but in some patients have been associated with tumor progression (6,82). Bone marrow involvement has been observed in 15% to 42% of cases in series in which nodal and extranodal cases were included (10,31,94) and in 32% of patients in a study of nodal MZL (55).

Laboratory findings are usually negative, although some patients may have an increased erythrocyte sedimentation rate and anemia. Monoclonal gammopathy has been reported in some cases (6,10).

Relationship to Extranodal Lymphoma

In 30% to 50% of cases diagnosed as nodal MZL, the tumor may represent dissemination of an extranodal MZL (6,7,10,13,14,28,29). In these patients, the extranodal lymphoma may be diagnosed simultaneously during staging maneuvers or may be detected before the diagnosis of the nodal tumor. Dissemination of extranodal MZL may occur many years after the original diagnosis. The extranodal sites more frequently involved are the gastrointestinal tract, salivary glands, and thyroid, but tumors in soft tissues, breast, lung, and other extranodal localizations have also been reported. In some patients, extranodal involvement may be detected during the progression of the disease, and aggressive transformation to a large cell lymphoma may occur at extranodal sites in patients originally diagnosed in a lymph node biopsy (14). Staging is important for patients who present with apparently primary nodal MZL to exclude the presence of extranodal disease. Nodal involvement may represent dissemination of an extranodal MALT lymphoma and may have a more aggressive evolution (31,95).

In some cases presenting as nodal MZL, it is not possible to detect extranodal involvement after extensive staging explorations. No extranodal lymphoma has been detected in some patients with a long follow-up up to 15 years in which only nodal recurrences occurred (28). These observations and the detection of nodal MZL in children (28,77), in whom extranodal MALT lymphomas are extremely rare, suggest that primary nodal MZL may occur. The finding of the t(11;18)(q21;q21) in extranodal low-grade MALT lymphomas but not in nodal MZLs confirms that at least a subset of these tumors do not represent the dissemination of an undetected extranodal lymphoma (81). However, given the relatively frequent association between nodal and extranodal lymphomas and the different biologic significance of these cases, extensive explorations are warranted in patients presenting with nodal disease before the diagnosis of primary nodal MZL is established.

Marginal Zone Lymphoma and Immunologic Disorders

MZLs are frequently associated with autoimmune disorders. In particular, Sjögren's syndrome has been reported in 15% to 30% of patients with MZL (94). Conversely, virtually all lymphomas in patients with Sjögren's syndrome seem to be low-grade MZLs or high-grade lymphomas probably derived from MZL (87). In most of these patients, the lymphoma is localized in the salivary glands or in salivary glands and lymph nodes. However, some cases of nodal MZL without apparent salivary gland involvement have been reported (87). MZLs may also occur in patients with rheumatoid arthritis, systemic lupus erythematosus, Raynaud's syndrome, polyclonal gammopathy, and cryoglobulinemia (6,13). MZLs also have been reported in patients with Hodgkin's disease (6) or other solid tumors (13,30)

MZLs may occur in patients with AIDS, particularly in the pediatric age group and young adults (96–98). Most of these lymphomas occur in extranodal sites, and contrary to the aggressive behavior of the usual high-grade lymphomas in AIDS patients, these tumors follow an indolent course and are Epstein-Barr virus negative. Nodal MZLs also have been reported in this patient population (99,100). The relationship between MZL and immunologic disorders suggest that dysregulation of the immune system may be an important factor in the development of these tumors. The pathogenesis of MZL in AIDS appears distinct from the high-grade B-cell lymphomas more commonly seen in immunodeficiency states.

Leukemic Phase: Does It Really Exist?

Peripheral blood involvement is not a common manifestation in MZL. However, a leukemic phase was detected at diagnosis or during the evolution of the disease in several cases (34,59,61,101,102). Retrospective interpretation of most of these cases suggests that they could be other types of lymphomas such as SMZL, MCL, or CLL/SLL. Some patients had massive splenomegaly (33,34,61,102), no or minimal peripheral lymphadenopathy, bone marrow involvement, and atypical lymphocytes in the peripheral blood with cytoplasmic hairy-like projections (61,93,102). These features suggest SMZL. Other cases were $CD5^+$, and the cells were described as having indented nuclei and expressing IgM/IgD. In these patients, the disease followed a very aggressive course, with a short survival period of 14 to 20 months. These characteristics are more concordant with MCL than with classic MZL (34,61). Nevertheless, some reported cases with peripheral blood involvement had clinicopathologic features of MZL, indicating that leukemic phase may occur in patients with these tumors (59,101). This complication is rare, and other entities must be considered before a definitive diagnosis of leukemic MZL is established.

Treatment and Survival

Patients in early stages have been treated with surgical excision, local radiotherapy, multiagent chemotherapy, or different combinations of these strategies, whereas diverse chemotherapy regimens have been used in patients with advanced stages of disease (10,29,31,95). Purine analogues have been suggested as a possible treatment alternative in MZL (103).

The clinical evolution is usually indolent, similar to other low-grade lymphomas. However, important differences may exist according to the stage of the tumor. Patients with early disease have a long survival, even after being treated only with local therapeutic regimens, although late relapses may occur (10). Patients in advanced stages have a worse prognosis with a higher risk of early recurrences and short survival (10). However, some contradictory results have been reported. One European study of patients presenting with nodal MZL showed a median survival of 4.1 years and early recurrences. This survival was worse than for patients with follicular lymphoma (31). In contrast, primary nodal MZL in stages III and IV have been reported to have a relatively long survival, with more than 50% of patients being alive at 10 years. Survival of patients with nodal MZL was longer than in advanced primary extranodal MALT, but this series is difficult to evaluate because cases of follicular lymphoma with marginal zone differentiation also were included in the group of primary nodal MZL (95).

SPLENIC MARGINAL ZONE LYMPHOMA

SMZL has been recognized as a distinct entity characterized by a clinical presentation with marked splenomegaly, absence or uncommon lymphadenopathy, and frequent bone marrow and peripheral blood involvement, occasionally with ''villous'' lymphocytes (20–23). Morphologically, the spleen exhibits a nodular expansion of the white pulp, with medium-sized lymphocytes surrounding and eventually replacing reactive follicle centers. In these nodules, larger lymphocytes with more abundant cytoplasm and higher proliferative activity tend to localize at the periphery, whereas smaller cells concentrate in the inner part of the follicle. This distribution of cells resembles a marginal zone pattern. However, a clear mantle cell corona is not recognized in these tumors. Phenotypically, SMZLs express B-cell antigens, are positive for IgM and IgD, and are negative for CD23, CD10, CD5, CD43, and cyclin D1. Although initially these tumors were interpreted as derived from the marginal zone and therefore were similar to MALT lymphomas, the relationship between these entities and the putative cell of origin of SMZL is not clear (21,24–27).

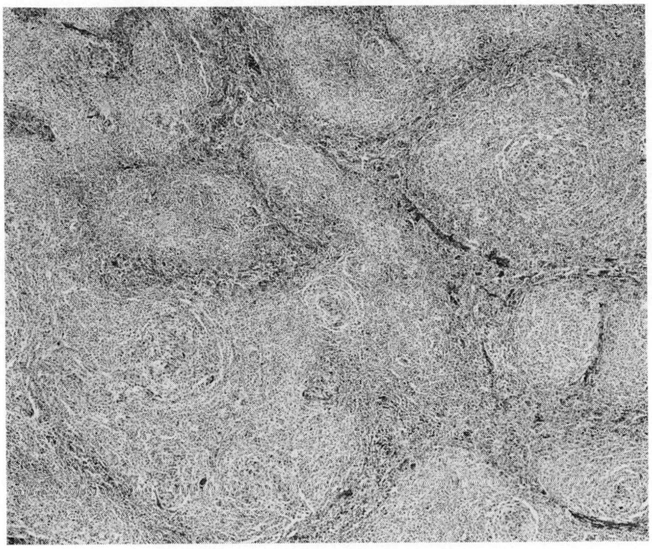

A

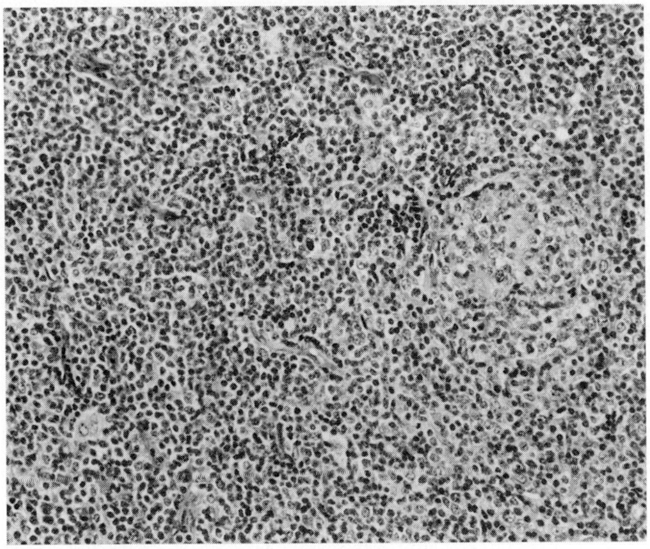

B

FIG. 23.11. Splenic type of nodal marginal zone lymphoma. **A:** Residual germinal centers are surrounded by an indistinct expansion of neoplastic cells, imparting a nodular appearance (hematoxylin and eosin stain, original magnification: 100× magnification). **B:** In this case, the germinal center remnant is nearly overrun by neoplastic cells (hematoxylin and eosin stain, original magnification: 200× magnification).

Splenic hilar and, less frequently, peripheral lymph nodes may be secondarily involved by SMZL (104). The morphologic features are reminiscent of the splenic pattern, with small, irregular lymphocytes surrounding and replacing preexisting follicles without evidence of a preserved mantle cuff. In some cases, a residual germinal center could only be identified after immunostaining for follicular dendritic cells. BCL-2 staining also may help to detect a residual negative germinal center that contrasts with the positivity of the tumor cells. Peripheral lymph nodes show a more effaced architecture than splenic hilar lymph nodes in which open sinusoids are usually seen.

We identified a group of primary nodal lymphomas with morphologic and immunophenotypic features resembling SMZL (28). Most of these patients had stage I or II disease without evidence of splenomegaly, peripheral blood, or bone marrow involvement. Three patients were alive with no evidence of disease 18 to 40 months after diagnosis, and one had recurrent disease after 24 months. The only patient presenting in stage III died of progressive disease.

The tumors showed a nodular or vaguely nodular pattern with a lymphoid proliferation surrounding residual germinal centers (Fig. 23.11). A mantle corona was absent or attenuated, and the limits of the germinal centers were usually poorly defined. Cytologically, the tumors were composed of small to medium-sized lymphocytes with pale cytoplasm, irregular nuclei, and inconspicuous nucleoli (Fig. 23.12). Occasional larger cells had a tendency to be localized at the periphery of the nodules. These tumors expressed B-cell antigens and IgD. CD23, CD5, and cyclin D1 were not detected. IgD expression was weaker than in residual mantle cells (Fig. 23.13). In cases with a nodular pattern, IgD staining highlighted an attenuated layer of mantle cells at the periphery of the nodules, suggesting a displacement of the mantle corona by the expansion of the tumor cells growing between a residual germinal center and the mantle cuff. This pattern may suggest an origin in follicular germinal center cells. However, CD10 staining was positive in the residual germinal center but negative in the tumor cells (Fig. 23.14). In contrast, the germinal center did not express BCL-2,

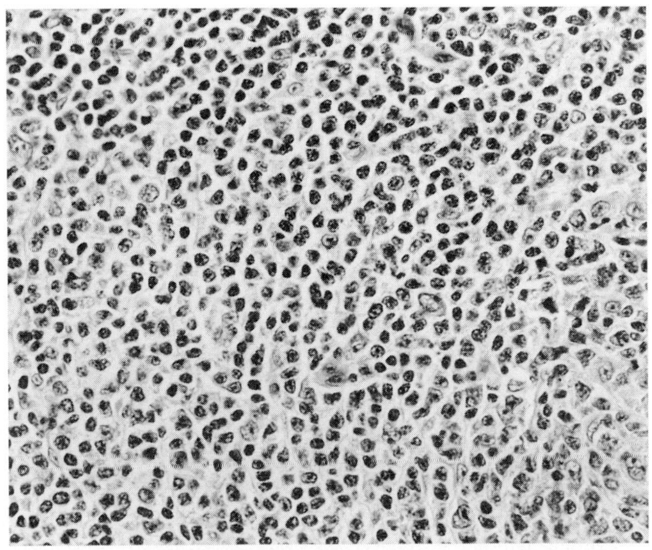

FIG. 23.12. Splenic type of nodal marginal zone lymphoma. The germinal center remnant is seen at lower right. The neoplastic cells are round to slightly irregular, with a rim of pale, indistinct cytoplasm (hematoxylin and eosin stain, original magnification: 400× magnification).

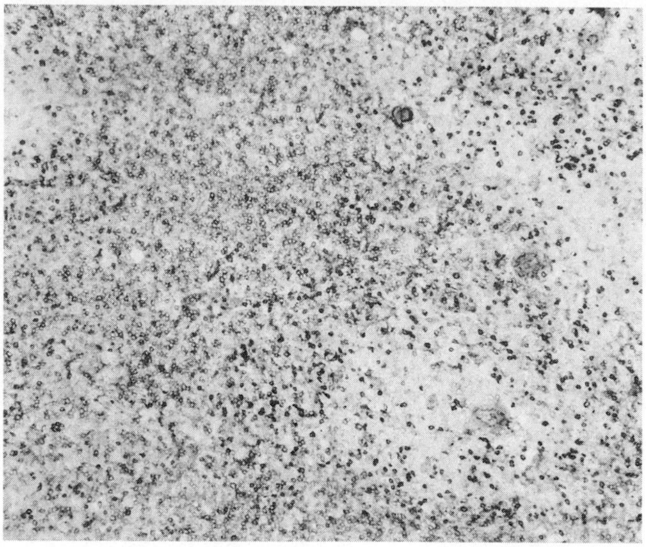

FIG. 23.13. IgD staining of a case of nodal marginal zone lymphoma of the splenic type. The tumor cells are weakly IgD$^+$, residual normal mantle cells are strongly IgD$^+$, but the residual germinal center cells are IgD$^-$ (immunoperoxidase stain, original magnification: 200× magnification).

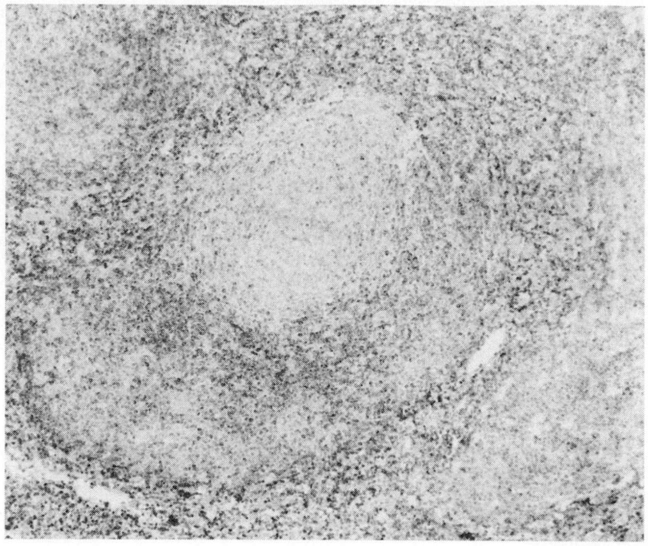

FIG. 23.15. BCL-2 staining of a case of nodal marginal zone lymphoma of the splenic type. Although the low-power appearance may suggest follicular lymphoma, germinal center remnants are BCL-2$^-$, in contrast to the neoplastic cells (immunoperoxidase stain, original magnification: 200× magnification).

whereas the tumor cells were positive (Fig. 23.15). *BCL2* gene rearrangement was not detected by polymerase chain reaction methods. T cells were numerous and in some cases showed a prominent nodular pattern because of a massive infiltration of the germinal centers (Fig. 23.16).

The growth pattern of these tumors, with tumor cells surrounding a reactive germinal center and a tendency of the larger cells to localize at the periphery of the nodules, is reminiscent of a marginal zone pattern. However, contrary to MZL of the MALT type, they are IgD$^+$ and do not have a preserved mantle corona between the tumor cells and the germinal center. Although the nodular pattern may suggest a follicle center cell origin, the residual germinal center has the appearance of being reactive with negativity for BCL-2. Moreover, the tumor cells are CD10$^-$, and *BCL2* gene rearrangement is not detected. The heterogeneous cytologic

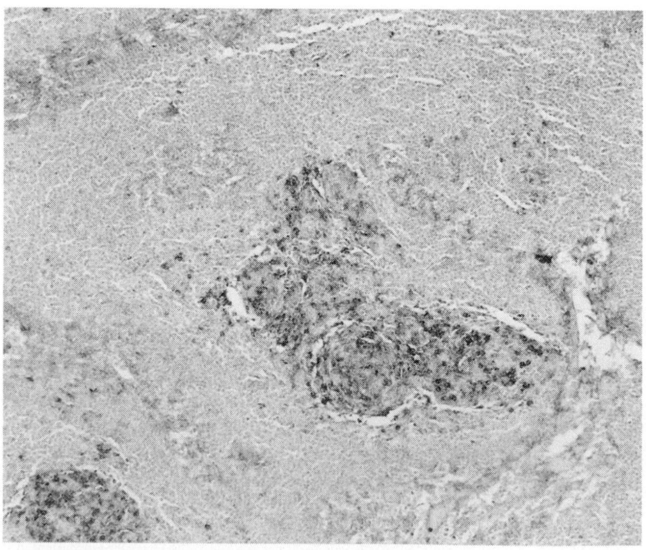

FIG. 23.14. CD10 staining in a case of nodal marginal zone lymphoma of the splenic type. The neoplastic cells are negative for staining, whereas the residual germinal center is positive (immunoperoxidase stain, original magnification: 100× magnification).

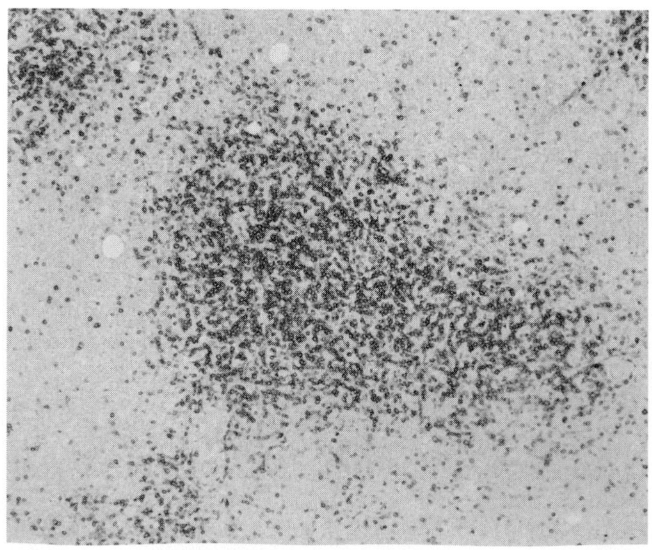

FIG. 23.16. CD3 staining in a case of nodal marginal zone lymphoma of the splenic type. T cells may be abundant in the residual germinal centers (immunoperoxidase stain, original magnification: 200× magnification).

appearance and the immunophenotype are not consistent with MCL or CLL/SLL. The most similar neoplasm to these nodal lymphomas seems to be SMZL, and therefore the term MZL of the splenic type was proposed (28). However, more studies are needed to determine the relationship of these neoplasms to other tumors with a marginal zone pattern.

SUMMARY AND CONCLUSIONS

Nodal MZL is an indolent lymphoma characterized by perisinusoidal, parafollicular, and perivascular infiltration of the lymph nodes by a heterogeneous proliferation of monocytoid B cells, small irregular lymphocytes, and a variable number of large blasts and plasma cells. These tumors are B-cell neoplasms that mainly express IgM but not IgD and that do not express CD5, CD10, CD23, and cyclin D1. The morphologic and immunophenotypic characteristics of the tumor cells and the presence of somatic mutations in the rearranged immunoglobulin genes suggest that they derive from a post–germinal center memory cell similar to the lymphocytes of the marginal zone. Nodal MZLs are similar to extranodal MZL of MALT type, and a relatively high number of these cases may represent a nodal dissemination of an extranodal MZL. However, detection of nodal tumors in children and young patients in whom MALT lymphomas are rare and the absence of extranodal involvement in some cases after extensive staging exploration and a relatively long follow-up suggest that primary nodal MZL may also exist. Nodal MZLs must be distinguished from other non-Hodgkin's lymphomas such as follicular lymphoma, MCL, or CLL/SLL, which occasionally may adopt a marginal zone distribution. The biologic behavior of these tumors seems more concordant with the underlying lymphoma than with the natural history of MZL.

Nodal MZLs with MALT-type features must be distinguished from lymph node involvement by SMZL. SMZL was originally described in the spleen, but secondary involvement of hilar and peripheral lymph nodes may occur. A primary nodal lymphoma with morphologic and immunophenotypic characteristics similar to SMZL also seems to exit. The relationships between the SMZL and the primary nodal tumors with similar characteristics and the potential normal counterpart of these lymphomas are unknown.

REFERENCES

1. Sheibani K, Sohn CC, Burke JS, et al. Monocytoid B-cell lymphoma: a novel B-cell neoplasm. *Am J Pathol* 1986;124:310–318.
2. Cousar JB, McGinn DL, Glick AD, et al. Report of an unusual lymphoma arising from parafollicular B-lymphocytes (PBLs) or so-called "monocytoid" lymphocytes. *Am J Clin Pathol* 1987;87:121–128.
3. van den Oord JJ, de Wolf-Peeters CH, de Vos R, et al. Immature sinus histiocytosis: light and electron microscopic features, immunologic phenotype, and relationship with marginal zone lymphocytes. *Am J Pathol* 1985;118:266–277.
4. Shon CC, Sheibani D, Winberg CD, et al. Monocytoid B-lymphocytes: their relation to the patterns of the acquired immunodeficiency syndrome (AIDS) and AIDS-related lymphadenopathy. *Hum Pathol* 1985;16:979–985.
5. Isaacson PG. Parafollicular B lymphocytes. *Am J Clin Pathol* 1987; 88:393–394.
6. Ngan B-Y, Warnke RA, Wilson M, et al. Monocytoid B-cell lymphoma: A study of 36 cases. *Hum Pathol* 1991;22:409–421.
7. Nizze H, Cogliatti SB, Von Schilling C, et al. Monocytoid B-cell lymphoma: morphological variants and relationship to low-grade B-cell lymphoma of the mucosa associated lymphoid tissue. *Histopathology* 1991;18:403–414.
8. Harris NL. Low-grade B-cell lymphoma of mucosa-associated lymphoid tissue and monocytoid B-cell lymphoma. *Arch Pathol Lab Med* 1993;117:771–775.
9. Isaacson PG, Spencer J. Malignant lymphoma of mucosa associated lymphoid tissue. *Histopathology* 1987;11:445–462.
10. Cogliatti SB, Lennert K, Hansmann M-L, et al. Monocytoid B-cell lymphoma: clinical and prognostic features of 21 patients. *J Clin Pathol* 1990;43:619–625.
11. Dierlamm J, Michaux L, Wlodarska I, et al. Trisomy 3 in marginal zone B-cell lymphoma: a study based on cytogenetic analysis and fluorescence in situ hybridization. *Br J Haematol* 1996;93:242–249.
12. Kuppers R, Hajadi M, Plank L, et al. Molecular Ig gene analysis reveals that monocytoid B cell lymphoma is a malignancy of mature B cells carrying somatically mutated V region genes and suggests that rearrangement of the kappa-deleting element (resulting in deletion of the Ig kappa enhancers) abolishes somatic hypermutation in the human. *Eur J Immunol* 1996;26:1794–1800.
13. Ortiz-Hidalgo C, Wright DH. The morphological spectrum of monocytoid B-cell lymphoma and its relationship to lymphomas of mucosa-associated lymphoid tissue. *Histopathology* 1992;21:555–561.
14. Mollejo M, Menarguez J, Cristobal E, et al. Monocytoid B cells: a comparative clinical pathological study of their distribution in different types of low-grade lymphomas. *Am J Surg Pathol* 1994;18: 1131–1139.
15. Schmitt-Graff A. Immunological and molecular classification of mucosa-associated lymphoid tissue lymphoma. *Recent Results Cancer Res* 1996;142:121–136.
16. Spencer J, Finn T, Pulford K, et al. The human gut contains a novel population of B lymphocytes which resemble marginal zone cells. *Clin Exp Immunol* 1985;62:607–612.
17. Piris MA, Rivas C, Morente M, et al. Monocytid B-cell lymphoma, a tumour related to the marginal zone. *Histopathology* 1988;12: 383–392.
18. Spencer J, Diss T, Isaacson P. A study of the properties of a low-grade mucosal B-cell lymphoma using a monoclonal antibody specific for the tumor immunoglobulin. *J Pathol* 1990;160:231–238.
19. Harris NL, Jaffe ES, Stein H, et al. A revised European-American classification of lymphoid neoplasms: a proposal from the International Lymphoma Study Group. *Blood* 1994;84:1361–1392.
20. Isaacson PG, Matutes E, Burke M, et al. The histopathology of splenic lymphoma with villous lymphocytes. *Blood* 1994;84:3828–3834.
21. Mollejo M, Menarguez J, Lloret E, et al. Splenic marginal zone lymphoma: a distinctive type of low-grade B-cell lymphoma. A clinicopathological study of 13 cases. *Am J Surg Pathol* 1995;19:1146–1157.
22. Schmid C, Kirkham N, Diss T, et al. Splenic marginal zone cell lymphoma. *Am J Surg Pathol* 1992;16:455–456.
23. Wu CD, Jackson CL, Medeiros LJ. Splenic marginal zone cell lymphoma: an immunophenotypic and molecular study of five cases. *Am J Clin Pathol* 1996;105:277–285.
24. Dierlamm J, Pittaluga S, Wlodarska I, et al. Marginal zone B-cell lymphomas of different sites share similar cytogenetic and morphologic features. *Blood* 1996;87:299–307.
25. Isaacson PG. Malignant lymphomas with a follicular growth pattern. *Histopathology* 1996;28:487–495.
26. Isaacson PG. Splenic marginal zone lymphoma. *Blood* 1996;88: 751–752.
27. Pittaluga S, Verhoef G, Criel A, et al. "Small" B-cell non-Hodgkin's lymphomas with splenomegaly at presentation are either mantle cell lymphoma or marginal zone cell lymphoma: a study based on histology, cytology, immunohistochemistry, and cytogenetic analysis. *Am J Surg Pathol* 1996;20:211–223.
28. Campo E, Miquel R, Krenacs L, et al. Primary nodal marginal zone lymphomas of splenic and MALT types. *Am J Surg Pathol* 1999;23: 59–68.
29. Sheibani K, Burke JS, Swartz WG, et al. Monocytoid B-cell lym-

phoma: clinicopathologic study of 21 cases of a unique type of low-grade lymphoma. *Cancer* 1988;62:1531–1538.

30. Nathwani BN, Mohrmann RL, Brynes RK, et al. Monocytoid B-cell lymphoma: an assessment of diagnostic criteria and a perspective on histogenesis. *Hum Pathol* 1992;23:1061–1071.
31. Pittaluga S, Bijnens L, Teodorovic I, et al. Clinical analysis of 670 cases in two trials of the European Organization for the Research and Treatment of Cancer Lymphoma Cooperative Group subtyped according to the Revised European-American classification of lymphoid neoplasms: a comparison with the Working Formulation. *Blood* 1996;87:4358–4367.
32. Hernandez AM, Nathwani BN, Nguyen D, et al. Nodal benign and malignant monocytoid B cells with and without follicular lymphomas: a comparative study of follicular colonization, light chain restriction, bcl-2, and t(14;18) in 39 cases. *Hum Pathol* 1995;26:625–632.
33. Fend F, Kraus-Huonder B, Müller-Hermelink H-K, et al. Monocytoid B-cell lymphoma: its relationship to and possible origin from marginal zone cells. *Hum Pathol* 1993;24:336–339.
34. Traweek ST, Sheibani K. Monocytoid B-cell lymphoma: the biologic and clinical implications of peripheral blood involvement. *Am J Clin Pathol* 1992;97:591–598.
35. Lennert K. Diagnose und atiologie der piringerschen lymphadenitis. *Verh Dtsch Ges Pathol* 1959;42:203–209.
36. De Almeida PC, Harris NL, Bhan AD. Characterization of immature sinus histiocytes (monocytoid cells) and reactive lymph nodes by use of monoclonal antibodies. *Hum Pathol* 1984;15:330–335.
37. Sheibani K, Fritz RM, Winberg CD, et al. ''Monocytoid'' cells in reactive follicular hyperplasia with and without multifocal histiocytic reactions: an immunohistochemical study of 21 cases including suspected cases of toxoplasmic lymphadenitis. *Am J Clin Pathol* 1984; 81:453–458.
38. Plank L, Hansmann HL, Fischer R. The cytologic spectrum of the monocytoid B-cell reaction: recognition of its large cell type. *Histopathology* 1993;23:425–431.
39. Rushin JM, Riordan GP, Heaton RB, et al. Cytomegalovirus-infected cells express Leu-M1 antigen: a potential source of diagnostic error. *Am J Pathol* 1990;136:989–995.
40. Mohrmann RL, Nathwani BN, Brynes RK, et al. Hodgkin's disease occurring in monocytoid B-cell clusters. *Am J Clin Pathol* 1991;95: 802–808.
41. Plank L, Hansmann ML, Fischer R. Monocytoid B-cell reaction associated with peripheral T-cell lymphomas. *Pathol Res Pract* 1995; 1152–1158.
42. Piris MA, Rivas C, Morente M, et al. Immature sinus histiocytosis a monocytoid B-lymphoid reaction. *J Pathol* 1986;148:159–167.
43. Wang T, Lasota J, Hanau CA, et al. Bcl-2 oncoprotein is widespread in lymphoid tissue and lymphomas but its differential expression in benign versus malignant follicles and monocytoid B-cell proliferations is of diagnostic value. *APMIS* 1995;103:655–662.
44. Lai R, Arber DA, Chang KL, et al. Frequency of bcl-2 expression in non-Hodgkin's lymphoma: a study of 778 cases with comparison of marginal zone lymphoma and monocytoid B-cell hyperplasia. *Mod Pathol* 1998;11:864–869.
45. Plank L, Hell K, Hansmann ML, et al. Reactive versus neoplastic monocytoid B-cell proliferations: in situ hybridization study of immunoglobulin light chain mRNA. *Am J Clin Pathol* 1995;103:330–337.
46. van den Oord JJ, Wolf-Peeters CH, Desmet VJ. The marginal zone in the human reactive lymph node. *Am J Clin Pathol* 1986;86:475–479.
47. van Krieken JHJM, von Schilling C, Kluin PHM, et al. Splenic marginal zone lymphocytes and related cells in the lymph node: a morphologic and immunohistochemical study. *Hum Pathol* 1989;20: 320–325.
48. Timens W, Boes A, Poppema S. Human marginal zone B cells are not an activated B cell subset: strong expression of CD21 as a putative mediator for rapid B cell activation. *Eur J Immunol* 1989;19: 2163–2166.
49. MacLennan ICM, Liu J-L. Marginal zone B cells respond both to polysaccharide antigens and protein antigens. *Res Immunol* 1991;142: 346–351.
50. Dunn-Walters DK, Isaacson PG, Spencer J. Analysis of mutations in immunoglobulin heavy chain variable region genes of microdissected marginal zone (MGZ) B cells suggests that the MGZ of human spleen is a reservoir of memory B cells. *J Exp Med* 1995;182:559–566.
51. Stein K, Hummel M, Korbjuhn P, et al. Monocytoid B cells are distinct from splenic marginal zone cells and commonly derive from unmutated naive B cells and less frequently from postgerminal center B cells by polyclonal transformation. *Blood* 1999;94:2800–2808.
52. Ng CS, Chan JKC. Monocytoid B-cell lymphoma. *Hum Pathol* 1987; 18:1069–1071.
53. Davis GC, York JC, Glick AD, et al. Plasmacytic differentiation in parafollicular (monocytoid) B-cell lymphoma: a study of 12 cases. *Am J Surg Pathol* 1992;16:1066–1074.
54. Llobet M, Castro P, Barcelo C, et al. Massive crystal-storing histiocytosis associated with low-grade malignant B-cell lymphoma of MALT-type of the parotid gland. *Diagn Cytopathol* 1997;17: 148–152.
55. Nathwani BN, Anderson JR, Armitage JO, et al. Marginal zone B-cell lymphoma: A clinical comparison of nodal and mucosa-associated lymphoid tissue types. *J Clin Oncol* 1999;17:2486–2492.
56. Stroup R, Sheibani K. Antigenic phenotypes of hairy cell leukemia and monocytoid B-cell lymphoma: an immunohistochemical evaluation of 66 cases. *Hum Pathol* 1992;23:172–177.
57. Contos MJ, Kornstein MJ, Innes DJ, et al. The utility of CD20 and CD43 in subclassification of low-grade B-cell lymphoma on paraffin sections. *Mod Pathol* 1992;5:631–633.
58. Zukerberg LR, Medeiros LJL, Ferry JA, et al. Diffuse low-grade B-cell lymphomas: four clinically distinct subtypes defined by a combination of morphologic and immunophenotypic features. *Am J Clin Pathol* 1993;100:373–385.
59. Ferry JA, Yang WI, Zukerberg LR, et al. $CD5^+$ extranodal marginal zone B-cell (MALT) lymphoma: a low grade neoplasm with a propensity for bone marrow involvement and relapse [see comments]. *Am J Clin Pathol* 1996;105:31–37.
60. Ballesteros E, Osborne BM, Matsushima AY. $CD5^+$ low grade marginal zone B-cell lymphomas with localized presentation. *Am J Surg Pathol* 1998;22:201–207.
61. Adami F, Semenzato G, Menestrina F, et al. $CD5^+$ leukemic monocytoid B-cell lymphoma and lymphocytic lymphomas. *Am J Clin Pathol* 1993;100:187–188.
62. Adami F, Chilosi M, Lestan M , et al. A $CD5^+$ leukemic lymphoma with monocytoid features: an unusual B-cell lymphoma mimicking hairy-cell leukemia. *Acta Haematol* 1993;89:94–99.
63. Leith CP, Mangalik A, Foucar K. A B-cell ''chameleon'': striking clinical, morphological, and immunophenotypic diversity of a single low-grade B cell clone. *Hum Pathol* 1997;28:104–108.
64. Jensen GS, Poppema S, Mant MJ, et al. Transition in CD45 isoform expression during differentiation of normal and abnormal B cells. *Int Immunol* 1989;1:229–236.
65. Marty LM, Caldwell CW, Feldbush TL. Expression of CD45 isoforms by Epstein-Barr virus-transformed human B lymphocytes. *Clin Immunol Immunopathol* 1992;62:8–15.
66. Flenghi L, Bigerna B, Fizzotti M, et al. Monoclonal antibodies PG-B6a and PG-B6p recognize, respectively, a highly conserved and formol-resistant epitope on the human bcl-6 protein amino-terminal region. *Am J Pathol* 1996;148:1543–1555.
67. Ree HJ, Kikuchi M, Kadin ME, et al. Up-regulation of bcl-6 protein expression is associated with high grade transformation of gastric MALT lymphomas. *Mod Pathol* 1998;11:139A(abst).
68. Ohsawa M, Kanno H, Machii T, et al. Immunoreactivity of neoplastic and non-neoplastic monocytoid B lymphocytes for DBA.44 and other antibodies [published erratum appears in *J Clin Pathol* 1994;47:1058]. *J Clin Pathol* 1994;47:928–932.
69. Hounieu H, Chittal SM, Al Saati T, et al. Hairy cell leukemia. Diagnosis of bone marrow involvement in paraffin embedded sections with monoclonal antibody DBA.44. *Am J Clin Pathol* 1992;98:26–33.
70. Brynes RK, Almaguer PD, Leathery KE, et al. Numerical cytogenetic abnormalities of chromosomes 3, 7, and 12 in marginal zone B-cell lymphomas. *Mod Pathol* 1996;9:995–1000.
71. Auer IA, Gascoyne RD, Connors JM, et al. t(11;18)(q21;q21) is the most common translocation in MALT lymphomas. *Ann Oncol* 1997; 8:979–985.
72. Ott G, Kalla J, Steinhoff A, et al. Trisomy 3 is not a common feature in malignant lymphomas of mucosa-associated lymphoid tissue type. *Am J Pathol* 1998;153:689–694.
73. Sole F, Woessner S, Florensa L, et al. Frequent involvement of chromosomes 1, 3, 7, and 8 in splenic marginal zone B-cell lymphoma. *Br J Haematol* 1997;98:446–449.
74. Wotherspoon AC, Finn TM, Isaacson PG. Trisomy 3 in low-grade

B-cell lymphomas of mucosa-associated lymphoid tissue. *Blood* 1995; 85:2000–2004.

75. Dierlamm J, Rosenberg C, Stul M, et al. Characteristic pattern of chromosomal gains and losses in marginal zone B cell lymphoma detected by comparative genomic hybridization. *Leukemia* 1997;11: 747–758.
76. Banerje SS, Harris M, Eyden BP, et al. Monocytoid B-cell lymphoma. *J Clin Pathol* 1991;44:39–44.
77. Elenitoba-Johnson KS, Kumar S, Lim MS, et al. Marginal zone B-cell lymphoma with monocytoid B-cell lymphocytes in pediatric patients without immunodeficiency: a report of two cases. *Am J Clin Pathol* 1997;107:92–98.
78. Slovak ML, Weiss LM, Nathwani BN, et al. Cytogenetic studies of composite lymphomas: monocytoid B-cell lymphomas and other B-cell non-Hodgkin's lymphomas. *Hum Pathol* 1993;24:1086–1094.
79. Akagi T, Motegi M, Tamura A, et al. A novel gene, MALT1 at 18q21, is involved in t(11;18)(q21;q21) found in low-grade B-cell lymphomas of mucosa-associated lymphoid tissue. *Oncogene* 1999;18: 5785–5794.
80. Dierlamm J, Baens M, Wlodarska I, et al. The apoptosis inhibitor gene AP12 and a novel 18q gene, MLT, are recurrently rearranged in the t(11;18)(q21;q21) associated with mucosa-associated lymphoid tissue lymphomas. *Blood* 1999;93:3601–3609.
81. Rosenwald A, Ott G, Stilgenbauer S, et al. Exclusive detection of the t(11;18)(q21;q21) in extranodal marginal zone B-cell lymphomas (MZBL) of MALT type in contrast to other MZBL and extranodal large B-cell lymphomas. *Am J Pathol* 1999;155:1817–1821.
82. Shin SS, Sheibani K, Fishleder A, et al. Monocytoid B-cell lymphoma in patients with Sjögren's syndrome: a clinicopathologic study of 13 patients. *Hum Pathol* 1991;22:422–430.
83. Tierens A, Delabie J, Pittaluga S, et al. Mutation analysis of the rearranged immunoglobulin heavy chain genes of marginal zone cell lymphomas indicates an origin from different marginal zone B lymphocytes subsets. *Blood* 1998;91:2381–2386.
84. Swerdlow SH, Zukerberg LR, Yang WI, et al. The morphologic spectrum of non-Hodgkin's lymphomas with BCL1/cyclin D1 gene rearrangements. *Am J Surg Pathol* 1996;20:627–640.
85. Dierlamm J, Pittaluga S, Stul M, et al. Bcl-6 gene rearrangements also occur in marginal zone B-cell lymphomas. *Br J Haematol* 1997; 98:719–725.
86. Chang KL, Chen Y-Y, Weiss LM. Lack of evidence of Epstein-Barr virus in Hairy cell leukemia and monocytoid B-cell lymphoma. *Hum Pathol* 1993;24:58–61.
87. Royer B, Cazals-Hatem D, Sibila J, et al. Lymphomas in patients with Sjögren's syndrome are marginal zone B-cell neoplasms, arise in diverse extranodal and nodal sites, and are not associated with viruses. *Blood* 1997;90:766–775.
88. Schmid U, Cogliatti SB, Diss TC, et al. Monocytoid/marginal zone B-cell differentiation in follicle centre cell lymphoma. *Histopathology* 1996;29:201–208.
89. Abou-Elella AA, Nathwani BN, Gascoyne R, et al. The relationship between monocytoid B-cell (MBC) lymphoma and coexisting follicular lymphoma. *Mod Pathol* 1998;11: 124A.
90. Ellison DJ, Nathwani BN, Cho SY, et al. Interfollicular small lymphocytic lymphoma: the diagnostic significance of pseudofollicles. *Hum Pathol* 1989;20:1108–1118.
91. Nguyen DT, Diamond LW, Schwonzen M, et al. Chronic lymphocytic leukemia with an interfollicular architecture: avoiding diagnostic confusion with monocytoid B-cell lymphoma. *Leuk Lymphoma* 1995;18: 179–184.
92. Nathwani BN, Anderson JR, Armitage JO, et al. Clinical significance of follicular lymphoma with monocytoid B cells. *Hum Pathol* 1999; 30:263–268.
93. Traweek ST, Sheibani K, Winberg CD, et al. Monocytoid B-cell lymphoma: its evolution and relationship to other low-grade B-cell neoplasms. *Blood* 1989;73:573–578.
94. Shin SS, Sheibani K. Monocytoid B-cell lymphoma. *Am J Clin Pathol* 1993;99:421–425.
95. Fisher RI, Dahlberg S, Nathwani BN, et al. A clinical analysis of two indolent lymphoma entities: mantle cell lymphoma and marginal zone lymphoma (including the mucosa-associated lymphoid tissue and monocytoid B-cell subcategories): a Southwest Oncology Group study. *Blood* 1995;85:1075–1082.
96. Teruya-Feldstein J, Temeck BK, Sloas MM, et al. Pulmonary malignant lymphoma of mucosa associated lymphoid tissue (MALT) arising in a pediatric HIV-positive patient. *Am J Surg Pathol* 1995;19: 357–363.
97. Wotherspoon AC, Diss TC, Pan L, et al. Low grade gastric B-cell lymphoma of mucosa associated lymphoid tissue in immunocompromised patients. *Histopathology* 1996;28:129–134.
98. Doshi VV, Gagnon GA, Chadwick EG, et al. The spectrum of mucosa-associated lymphoid tissue lesions in pediatric patients infected with HIV: a clinicopathologic study of six cases. *Am J Clin Pathol* 1997; 107:592–600.
99. Sheibani K, Ben-Ezra J, Swartz WG, et al. Monocytoid B-cell lymphoma in a patient with human immunodeficiency virus infection: demonstration of human immunodeficiency virus sequences in paraffin-embedded lymph node sections by polymerase chain reaction amplification. *Arch Pathol Lab Med* 1990;114:1264–1267.
100. Charton-Bain MC, Le Tourneau A, Weiss L, et al. Rare non-Hodgkin's lymphoma in the course of infection with human immunodeficiency virus: two cases with bone marrow invasion. *Ann Pathol* 1997; 17:38–40.
101. Carbone A, Gloghini A, Pinto A, et al. Monocytoid B-cell lymphoma with bone marrow and peripheral blood involvement at presentation. *Am J Clin Pathol* 1989;92:228–236.
102. Vasef M, Katzin WE. Monocytoid B-cell lymphoma with a distinctive clinical presentation. *Hum Pathol* 1993;24:558–561.
103. Horning SJ. Purine analogs in marginal-zone lymphomas. *Ann Oncol* 1996;7[Suppl 6]:S21–S26.
104. Mollejo M, Lloret E, Menarguez J, et al. Lymph node involvement by splenic marginal zone lymphoma: morphologic and immunohistochemical features. *Am J Surg Pathol* 1997;21:772–780.

CHAPTER 24

Follicular Lymphoma

Nancy Lee Harris and Judith A. Ferry

HISTORY OF FOLLICULAR LYMPHOMA CLASSIFICATION

The tumor now known as follicular lymphoma was first recognized as a distinct disorder by Brill, Baehr and Rosenthal (1), and Symmers (2) and was sometimes referred to as *Brill-Symmers disease.* The process was considered to represent an abnormal proliferation of lymphoid follicles, and there was some early confusion about whether it was reactive or neoplastic. Brill used the term *giant follicular hyperplasia* and Symmers the term *follicular lymphadenopathy*, but both eventually came to believe it was a form of lymphoma (3,4). Other terms used for this disorder included *giant follicle lymphoma* and *follicular lymphoblastoma.* Into the 1930s there continued a debate about the neoplastic nature of this disorder and its relationship to other lymphomas, including Hodgkin's disease (4,5).

Gall and colleagues at Massachusetts General Hospital, in 1941, provided the first clear description of the morphology and clinical features, advocating use of the term *follicular lymphoma* (6). In a report of 63 cases, they described its architectural and cytologic variability and proposed a grading scheme based on the architecture and the number of large cells (Table 24.1). In comparison to 500 cases of other lymphoma types, they demonstrated its clinical distinctiveness, including the equal incidence in females and males (which contrasted with other lymphomas), the older age group, infrequency of extranodal involvement, frequency of abdominal and retroperitoneal disease, responsiveness to treatment, and the long survival compared with other lymphomas (Table 24.2). These findings were expanded into a proposal for the classification of all types of lymphoma in a later study by Gall and Mallory (7). Follicular lymphoma accounted for only 7% of the 618 lymphomas in this later series, which included cases collected from 1917 through 1936.

In 1956, Rappaport published the largest series to that date—253 cases from the Armed Forces Institute of Pathology (AFIP)—and emphasized histologic features useful in distinction from follicular hyperplasia (8). This study included all lymphomas with a follicular pattern, including Hodgkin's disease. The investigators proposed four subtypes, based on cellular composition (Table 24.1). Rappaport was concerned by the frequency with which reactive hyperplasia and follicular lymphoma were confused in material submitted to the AFIP, and was at pains to refute the suggestion that follicular lymphoma was related to or could arise from follicular hyperplasia. Although Rappaport rejected the idea that neoplastic follicles arose from reactive germinal centers, he stated it was "conceivable that formation of follicle-like nodules may represent an attempted imitation of normal pattern, in other words, an attempt at differentiation such as we find in other malignant tumors. Such a concept not only would be consistent with the clinical behavior of these tumors, but also would make it unnecessary to postulate a change from one type of malignant lymphoma into another every time sequential tissue examinations reveal loss of follicular pattern." This concept is very close to our current understanding of the nature of neoplastic follicles. However, to emphasize the neoplastic nature of these so-called follicles or nodules of follicular lymphoma, he suggested changing the terminology from *follicular* to *nodular,* unfortunately eliminating the verbal connection of the tumor to its normal counterpart. In addition to introducing the term *nodular,* Rappaport changed the terminology of the cells comprising the tumors. Gall and associates, as did other pathologists at the time, considered slightly enlarged lymphoid cells within follicles to be lymphoblasts, and the largest cells to be reticulum cells (divided by Gall into *stem cells* (large lymphoid cells) or *clasmatocytes* (phagocytic cells)). Rappaport acknowledged the resemblance of the medium-sized cells to lymphoblasts but correctly doubted that they were related to the cells of acute lymphoblastic leukemia, and suggested that they were poorly differentiated lymphocytes. He further proposed in 1966 changing the name of the large cells in these lymphomas from reticulum cells to histiocytes, follow-

N. L. Harris and J. A. Ferry: Department of Pathology, Harvard Medical School and Massachusetts General Hospital, Boston, Massachusetts 02114

TABLE 24.1. *Comparison of Gall, Rappaport, and REAL/WHO classifications of follicular lymphoma*

Gall[a]	Rappaport, 1956	Rappaport, 1966	Working formulation	REAL/WHO
Follicular lymphoma, type I	Nodular lymphoma, lymphocytic type, well differentiated	Nodular well differentiated lymphocytic lymphoma	Follicular, predominantly small cleaved cell	Follicular lymphoma, grade 1
	Nodular lymphoma, lymphocytic type, poorly differentiated	Nodular poorly differentiated lymphocytic lymphoma		
Follicular lymphoma, type II	Nodular lymphoma, mixed type (lymphocytic and reticulum cell)	Nodular mixed lymphocytic and histiocytic lymphoma	Follicular, mixed small cleaved and large cell	Follicular lymphoma, grade 2
Follicular lymphoma, type III	Nodular lymphoma, reticulum cell type	Nodular histiocytic lymphoma	Follicular, predominantly large cell	Follicular lymphoma, grade 3
Follicular lymphoma, type IV	Nodular lymphoma, Hodgkin's type			

[a] Categories in corresponding rows are not necessarily equivalent in the different classifications.

ing then-current terminology for phagocytic cells. In contrast to Gall, who left open the possibility that the large cells of these lymphomas were also lymphoid, Rappaport introduced the idea that a single tumor could differentiate toward lymphoid cells and histiocytic cells.

Rappaport was also struck by the resemblance of the neoplastic cells of follicular lymphomas to those of diffuse lymphomas, and concluded that ''on the basis of our observation we do not regard follicular lymphoma as a separate and distinct disease entity but as a variant of diffuse lymphoma of corresponding cellular composition.'' He proposed eliminating the category of follicular lymphoma, and simply recognizing diffuse and nodular patterns in any of the recognized lymphoma subtypes (Table 24.1). This terminology and concept were further promulgated in the AFIP fascicle on hematologic malignancies in 1966 (9), and by the early 1970's, it had been generally accepted in the United States. This was a somewhat unfortunate development, in that it to some extent reversed what had been a generally correct understanding of follicular lymphoma by Gall and Mallory.

By the late 1960s, Karl Lennert, working at the University of Kiel, Germany, had recognized that the neoplastic cells of follicular lymphomas were morphologically identical to those found in the normal germinal center, which he called first *germinocytes* and *germinoblasts* and later modified to *centrocytes* and *centroblasts* (10,11). The term *cyte* referred to a nonproliferating cell, and the term *blast* referred to a proliferating cell. Lennert and colleagues proposed the term *centroblastic/centrocytic lymphoma* for neoplasms composed of both these cell types, which typically had at least a partially follicular pattern (12) (Table 24.3).

Lukes and Collins, using similar morphologic observations, concluded that most B-cell lymphomas were of follicle center cell origin, and could be categorized according to the predominant cell type. The Lukes-Collins classification recognized four categories of follicular center cell lymphoma: small cleaved follicular center cell, large cleaved follicular center cell, small noncleaved follicular center cell, and large noncleaved follicular center cell (13) (Table 24.1). Similar to Lennert, Lukes and Collins did not use pattern as a major criterion in classification, believing that cell type, rather than pattern, would be the major determinant of the behavior of the neoplasm.

These morphologic observations and subsequent immunologic studies (14–17) confirmed that the cells of follicular lymphoma are B cells, and that the follicular pattern of follicular lymphoma does reflect formation of neoplastic follicles by cells whose normal counterparts have this capacity, analogous to the formation of neoplastic glands by the cells of an adenocarcinoma. Although there is general agreement with Rappaport's contention that neoplastic follicles do not derive from reactive ones, it is now felt that they do represent true follicles. The term *follicular* has replaced *nodular* in current lymphoma classification schemes (12,13,18–20).

TABLE 24.2. *Clinical features of follicular lymphoma compared with other lymphomas (including Hodgkin's disease)*

Clinical features	Follicular lymphoma (n = 63)	Other lymphomas (n = 507)
Age at onset	50 years	42 years
Onset <20 yr	3.5%	14%
Onset >40 yr	72%	54%
Mean disease duration	6 years	3 years
Death <2 yr	21%	56%
5-yr survival	47%	19%
Male : female	1.2 : 1	2.4 : 1
Fever	16%	42%
Retroperitoneal lymph nodes	63%	48%
Mediastinal lymph nodes	29%	46%
Extranodal involvement		
Gastrointestinal	2%	14%
Genitourinary	5%	10%
Pulmonary	2%	9%
Cutaneous	5%	21%
Bone	9%	14%
Peripheral blood involvement	9%	29%

From Gall EA, Morrison HR, Scott AT. The follicular type of malignant lymphoma: a survey of 63 cases. *Ann Intern Med* 1941;14:2073–2090, with permission.

TABLE 24.3. *Nomenclature of normal and neoplastic B cells in different classifications*

Rappaport	Luke-Collins	Working formulation	Kiel classification	REAL/WHO
Well-differentiated lymphocyte	Small lymphocyte	Small lymphocyte	Lymphocyte	Small lymphocyte
Poorly differentiated lymphocyte	Small cleaved FCC	Small cleaved cell	Centrocyte (small)	Centrocyte
Histiocyte	Large noncleaved FCC	Large noncleaved cell	Centroblast	Centroblast
	Large cleaved FCC	Large cleaved cell	Centrocyte (large)	Centrocyte
	Immunoblast	Immunoblast	Immunoblast	Immunoblast
Undifferentiated cell	Small noncleaved FCC	Small noncleaved cell	? Centroblast (small) ? Burkitt's lymphoma cell	Burkitt lymphoma cell (follicular B-blast)

FCC, follicular center cell.

Despite general agreement on the term, *follicular,* and on the relationship of this lymphoma to lymphoid follicles, the definition of follicular lymphoma and its recognition as a distinct entity has differed in various classification schemes. Rappaport's concept that there were multiple types of lymphoma that could have a follicular pattern persisted in the categories of the Working Formulation, which defined three distinct categories of lymphoma with a follicular pattern (Table 24.1), but the Working Formulation recognized that not all lymphomas could have a true follicular pattern (18). The Kiel classification supported earlier concepts that follicular lymphoma was a distinct entity but defined it by cellular composition rather than pattern, such as a lymphoma containing centrocytes and centroblasts (21). Cases of centroblastic or centrocytic lymphoma are typically follicular but can be entirely diffuse, whereas lymphomas with a follicular pattern but with confluent sheets of centroblasts are called centroblastic, and are categorized together with diffuse centroblastic lymphoma as a high-grade malignancy. The Lukes-Collins classification took an extreme approach, contending that pattern was of no consequence biologically or clinically; although most cases of "small cleaved follicular center cell" lymphoma had a follicular pattern, they predicted that pattern would have no bearing on clinical behavior (13).

An important difference between the Kiel classification and the three American classifications (Rappaport, Lukes-Collins, and Working Formulation) was the recognition by Lennert that there were two distinct neoplasms of small lymphoid cells with irregular or "cleaved" nuclei. Centroblastic/centrocytic lymphoma was composed of centrocytes and centroblasts and typically had a follicular pattern; centrocytic lymphoma was composed entirely of centrocytes and typically had a predominantly diffuse pattern (21). The major reason that diffuse lymphomas of small irregular lymphoid cells (i.e., poorly differentiated lymphocytes) in the other classifications had a worse prognosis than follicular ones was not simply that they had a diffuse pattern; it was because they were different diseases. Rappaport included lymphoblastic lymphoma in his category of "diffuse poorly differentiated lymphocytic" lymphoma (PDL), and neither the Rappaport classification, the Lukes-Collins classification, nor the Working Formulation recognized that most cases of nonlymphoblastic diffuse PDL or small cleaved cell lymphomas corresponded to centrocytic lymphoma in the Kiel classification—the tumor we now know as mantle cell lymphoma. Lymphoblastic lymphoma and mantle cell lymphoma are aggressive diseases, which have no relationship to follicular lymphoma and are not "diffuse counterparts" of this disease (22–24). A purely diffuse variant of what we now know as follicular lymphoma is so rare that its existence is still debated (19,25).

Based on this accumulated experience, the Revised European-American classification of Lymphoid Neoplasms (REAL) proposed the term *follicle center lymphoma, follicular,* for a distinct entity composed of centrocytes and centroblasts, with at least a partially follicular pattern and a spectrum of histologic grade and clinical aggressiveness determined by the proportion of centroblasts (19). A category of *follicle center lymphoma, diffuse,* was considered provisional, to be used for rare purely diffuse cases in which the predominant cell is a centrocyte, with a minor component of centroblasts. In the new World Health Organization (WHO) classification (Table 24.4), the definition of the REAL classi-

TABLE 24.4. *Follicular lymphoma: grading and variants of the WHO classification*

Grading	Definition
Grade 1	0–5 centroblasts per hpf[a]
Grade 2	6–15 centroblasts per hpf[a]
Grade 3	>15 centroblasts per hpf[a]
3a	Centrocytes present
3b	Solid sheets of centroblasts
Reporting of pattern	*Proportion follicular*
Follicular	>75%
Follicular and diffuse	25–75%[b]
Focally follicular	<25%[b]
Follicular lymphoma: variants	
Diffuse follicle center lymphoma	
Grade 1	0–5 centroblasts/hpf[a]
Grade 2	6–15 centroblasts/hpf[a]
Cutaneous follicle center lymphoma	

[a] High-power field (hpf) of 0.159 mm^2 (40× objective, 10× 18mm ocular; count 10 hpf and divide by 10). If using a 10× 20-mm ocular, count 10 hpf and divide by 12; if using a 10× 22-mm ocular, count 10 hpf and divide by 15 to get the number of centroblasts/0.159 mm^2 hpf.

[b] Give approximate percentage in report.

fication is used, but the name is changed back to follicular lymphoma—we have returned to the original concept of Edward Gall, of 1941 (25–27) (see Chapter 19).

NORMAL B-CELL FOLLICLE

Because follicular lymphoma is a neoplasm of the germinal center, an understanding of normal germinal center B-cell development is useful as a background for understanding the lymphoma.

Germinal Center Reaction

The T-cell–dependent germinal center reaction occurs late in the primary immune response (within 3 to 7 days of antigen challenge in experimental animals) and in secondary

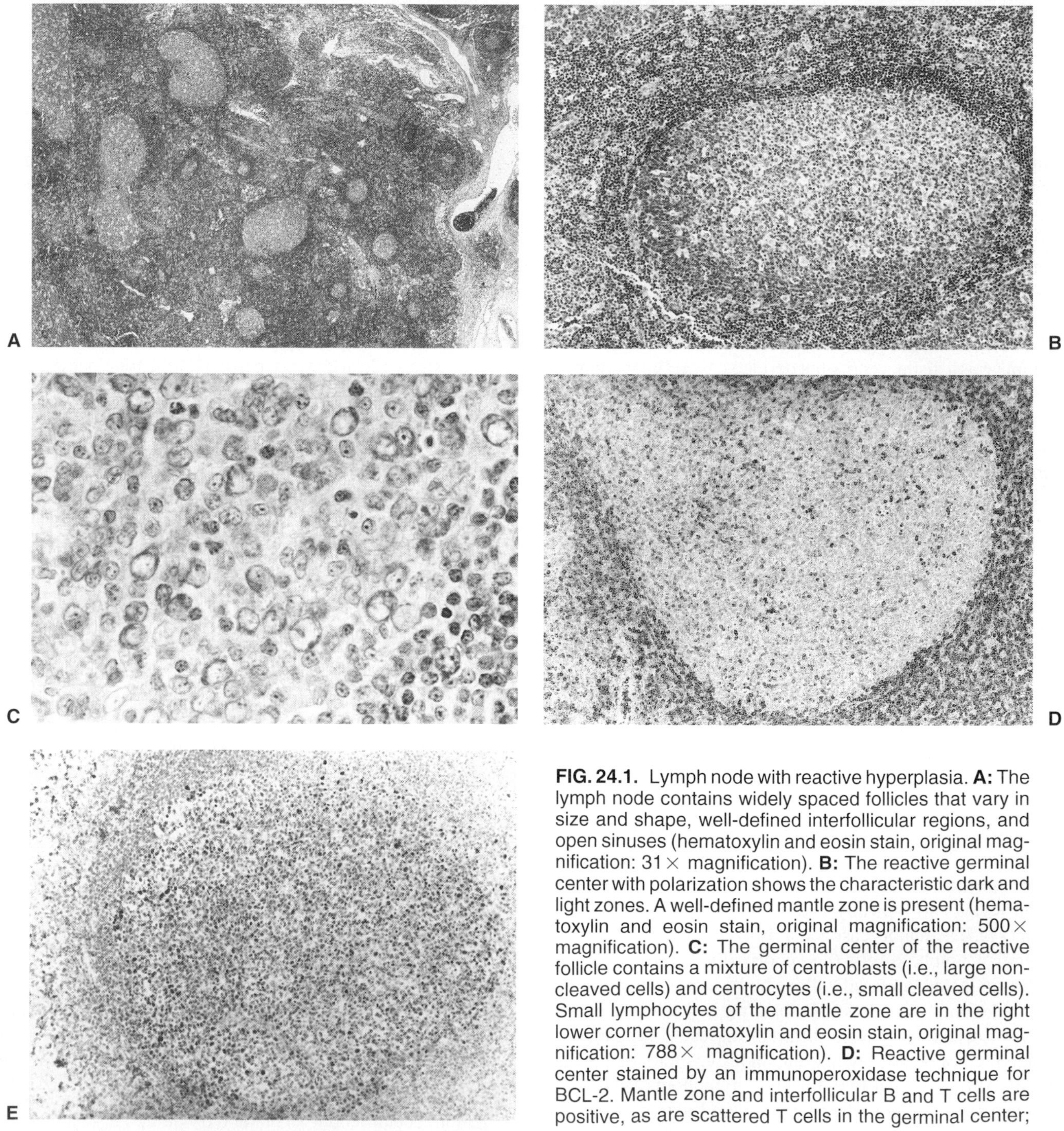

FIG. 24.1. Lymph node with reactive hyperplasia. **A:** The lymph node contains widely spaced follicles that vary in size and shape, well-defined interfollicular regions, and open sinuses (hematoxylin and eosin stain, original magnification: 31× magnification). **B:** The reactive germinal center with polarization shows the characteristic dark and light zones. A well-defined mantle zone is present (hematoxylin and eosin stain, original magnification: 500× magnification). **C:** The germinal center of the reactive follicle contains a mixture of centroblasts (i.e., large noncleaved cells) and centrocytes (i.e., small cleaved cells). Small lymphocytes of the mantle zone are in the right lower corner (hematoxylin and eosin stain, original magnification: 788× magnification). **D:** Reactive germinal center stained by an immunoperoxidase technique for BCL-2. Mantle zone and interfollicular B and T cells are positive, as are scattered T cells in the germinal center; germinal center B cells are negative (original magnification: 125× magnification). **E:** Germinal center stained for BCL-6 protein; the nuclei of most cells are positive (original magnification: 125× magnification). *(continued)*

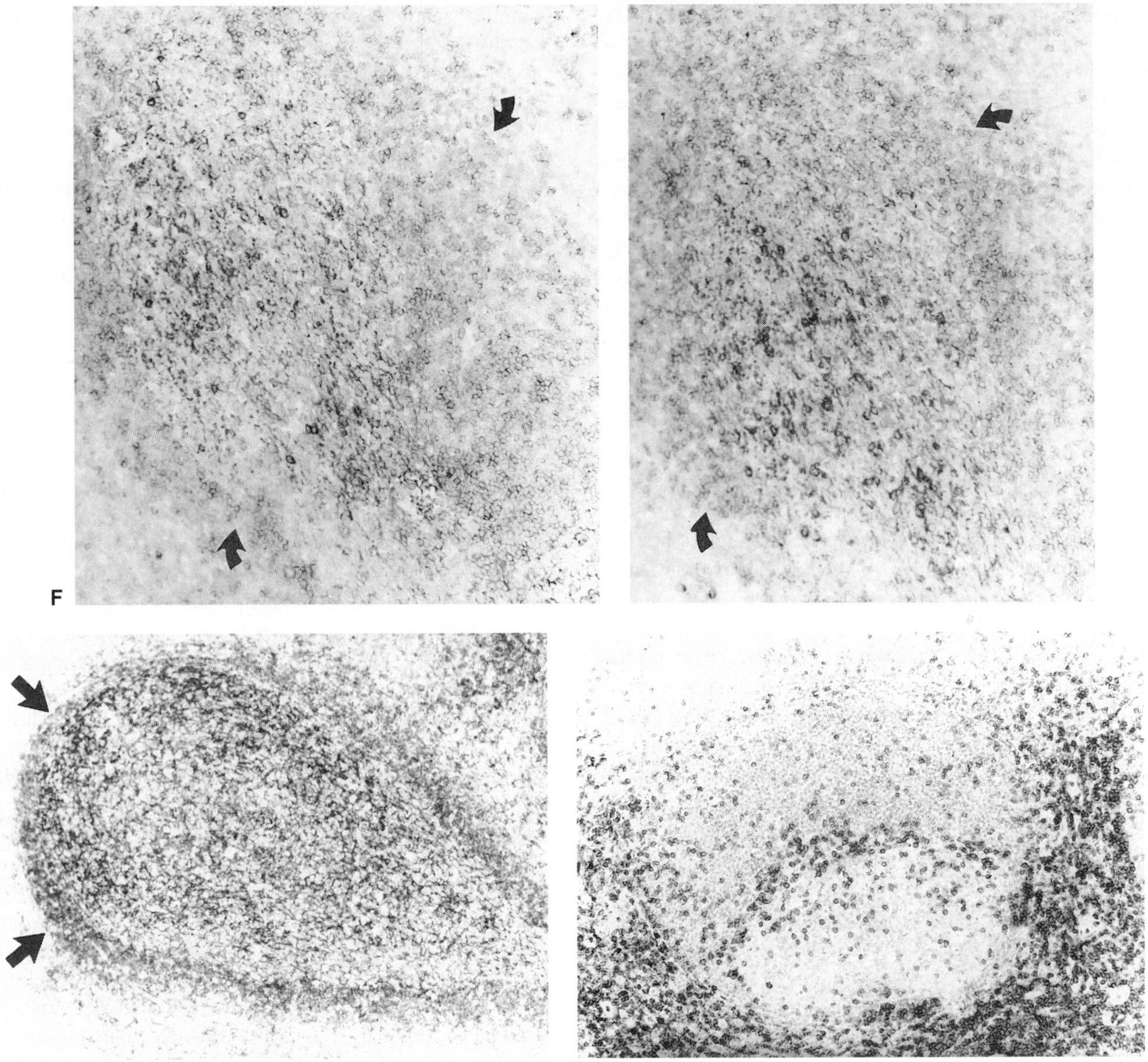

F G H

FIG. 24.1. *Continued.* **F:** Germinal center stained for κ *(left)* and λ *(right)* light chains (original magnification: 100× magnification). Notice also the mantle zones of the follicle *(arrows)*. **G:** Germinal center stained for CD21 shows follicular dendritic cell meshworks, which are more prominent in the light zone *(arrow)* (original magnification: 80× magnification). **H:** Germinal center stained for CD3 (pan-T) antigen. Numerous T cells are in the light zone (original magnification: 80× magnification). **D–H:** immunoperoxidase technique was used on frozen (**F**) or paraffin (**D, E, G, H**) sections.

responses to antigen. Each germinal center is formed by 3 to 10 naive B cells and ultimately contains approximately 10,000 to 15,000 B cells; more than 10 generations are required to form a germinal center (28,29). Proliferating IgM-positive (IgM^+) B blasts formed from naive B cells that have encountered antigen in the T-cell zone (paracortex) migrate into the center of the primary follicle and fill the follicular dendritic cell (FDC) meshwork by about 3 days after antigen stimulation, forming a germinal center (28,30) (Fig. 24.1A). These B-blasts differentiate into Ig^- centroblasts (large noncleaved follicular center cells), which appear at about 4 days, and accumulate at one pole of the germinal center, forming the ''dark zone'' (Fig. 24.1B). Centroblasts are large proliferating cells with vesicular nuclei; one to three prominent, peripheral nucleoli; and a narrow rim of basophilic cytoplasm (Fig. 24.1C). They lack surface immunoglobulin (sIg) (28,31,32) and switch off the gene that encodes the BCL-2 protein (Fig. 24.1D); they and their progeny are susceptible to death through apoptosis (33). Germinal center cells express antigens associated with activation, most of which are involved with interaction with T cells, including CD23, CD71, CD40, and CD86 (34–39), and antigens associated with adhesion to follicular dendritic cells (FDC), including CD11a/18 and CD29/49d (40,41), and antigens that may promote apoptosis, such as CD95 (42). An important event in germinal center development is expression of BCL-6 protein, a nuclear zinc-finger transcription factor that is expressed by centroblasts and centrocytes but not by naive or memory B cells, mantle cells, or plasma cells (43,44) (Fig. 24.1E). Normal resting B cells express high levels of BCL-6 messenger RNA (mRNA), while lacking the protein (45).

In centroblasts, a process of somatic mutation of the Ig gene variable (V) region begins, which alters the affinity for antigen of the antibody that will be produced by the cell (46,47). The cell may also switch from IgM to IgG or IgA production (30,48); through these mechanisms, the germinal center reaction gives rise to the better-fitting IgG or IgA antibody of the late primary or secondary immune response (49). Studies on single centroblasts picked from the dark zone of germinal centers suggest that in the early stages, a germinal center may contain about five to 10 clones of centroblasts, which show only a moderate amount of Ig gene V region mutation; later, the number of clones diminishes to as few as three, and the degree of somatic mutation increases (29).

Centroblasts divide and their progeny mature to nonproliferating medium-sized cells with irregular nuclei, inconspicuous nucleoli, and scant cytoplasm, called *centrocytes* (small or large cleaved follicular center cells), which accumulate at one pole of the germinal center. This area is known as the ''light zone'' and is typically toward the subcapsular sinus in lymph nodes or the epithelium in tonsillar tissue (Fig. 24.1B). It also contains a high concentration of FDCs. Centrocytes reexpress sIg, which has the same variable-diversity-joining (VDJ) gene rearrangement as the parent naive B-cell and the centroblast of the dark zone, but which has an altered antibody combining site, because of the somatic mutations in the Ig V region, and may have undergone heavy-chain class switch (29). The process of somatic mutation results in marked intraclonal diversity of antibody combining sites in a population of cells derived from only a few precursors. In the germinal center, the *BCL6* gene undergoes somatic mutation of the 5′ noncoding promoter region at a lower frequency than is seen in the Ig genes (50–52). The Ig gene mutation and *BCL6* mutation serve as markers of cells that have experienced the germinal center.

Centrocytes whose Ig gene mutations have resulted in decreased affinity for antigen rapidly die by apoptosis (programmed cell death); the prominent starry-sky pattern of phagocytic macrophages seen in germinal centers at this stage is a result of the apoptosis of centrocytes. In contrast, centrocytes whose Ig gene mutations have resulted in increased affinity are able to bind to native, unprocessed antigen trapped in antigen-antibody complexes by the complement receptors on the processes of FDCs (Fig. 24.1F, G). The centrocytes are able to present the antigen to T cells in the light zone of the GC (Fig. 24.1H). It is thought that this activation of T cells may induce them to express CD40 ligand (CD40L), which can engage CD40 on the B cell. Ligation of the antigen receptor by antigen and ligation of CD40 on the surfaces of GC B cells can ''rescue'' them from apoptosis (30–32,53,54). Interaction with surface molecules expressed by FDCs, such as CD23, appears to be important in inducing heavy-chain class switch and directing differentiation of the centrocytes into plasma cells, while interaction with the numerous T cells present in the light zone, through the CD40 molecule and its ligand on T cells, appears to be important in the generation of memory B cells (28,30). Antigen-receptor ligation and CD40 ligation switch off BCL-6 mRNA production and BCL-6 protein expression (45).

Marginal Zone and Monocytoid (Parafollicular) B Cells

When the germinal center polarizes into a dark and a light zone, the mantle zone becomes better defined and eccentric, with the broader portion surrounding the light zone of the germinal center. Antigen-specific B cells generated in the germinal center reaction leave the follicle and reappear in the outer mantle zone, to form a *marginal zone*; these are particularly prominent in mesenteric lymph nodes, Peyer's patches, and the spleen (31,55–58). Marginal zone B cells have slightly irregular nuclei, resembling those of centrocytes, but with more abundant, pale cytoplasm. The term *centrocyte-like* has been applied to similar neoplastic cells (59). On rechallenge with antigen, splenic marginal zone B cells migrate first into the germinal center, and then quickly appear in the T-cell zone as Ig^+ blast cells, which give rise to antigen-specific plasma cells; they are thought to be memory B cells (28). In the spleen, they are typically IgM^+ and IgD^-. Memory B cells are also detectable in the peripheral blood, where they may be IgM^+ and even $CD5^+$ (60,61). Studies on single marginal zone B cells from spleen and Peyer's patches show that they have mutated V region genes, may be oligoclonal, and are not clonally related to the adjacent germinal center (62–64).

Cells that resemble marginal zone B cells, but with even more nuclear indentation and abundant cytoplasm, known as *monocytoid B lymphocytes*, are seen in clusters adjacent to subcapsular and cortical sinuses of some reactive lymph nodes (65), peripheral to and often continuous with the follicle marginal zone. Monocytoid B cells express IgM or IgG without IgD and are positive for BCL-2 protein. In contrast to splenic marginal zone B cells, the monocytoid B cells found in reactive lymph nodes appear to have unmutated Ig V-region genes or to show only a small number of randomly distributed mutations that do not suggest selection by antigen (64,66). Tierens and colleagues also found a significant number of monocytoid B cells to be in cell cycle. The nature of these cells and their relationship to follicle center and marginal zone cells remains to be determined.

DEFINITION OF FOLLICULAR LYMPHOMA

Follicular lymphoma is defined in the updated REAL/WHO classification as a *lymphoma of follicle center B cells (centrocytes and centroblasts), which has at least a partially follicular pattern.* It is a tumor of germinal center B cells, in which centrocytes fail to undergo apoptosis because they have a chromosomal rearrangement, t(14;18), that prevents the normal switching off of the antiapoptosis gene, *BCL2* (33,67).

The term *follicle center lymphoma, follicular,* was proposed in the REAL classification to encompass most tumors classified as follicular lymphomas in the Working Formulation, most tumors with a follicular pattern classified as follicular center cell lymphoma in the Lukes-Collins classification, all cases in the Kiel classification category of centroblastic/centrocytic lymphoma with any follicular pattern, and centroblastic lymphoma with a purely follicular pattern. Although the term, *follicle center lymphoma, follicular,* was selected as the most precise term, it is somewhat cumbersome. The WHO classification returns to the old term, *follicular lymphoma,* but this term has been redefined more precisely to apply only to a lymphoma of follicle center cells with a follicular pattern, and not to other lymphomas with a nodular or follicular growth pattern. The existence and clinical significance of a purely diffuse lymphoma composed of centroblasts and centrocytes is controversial. A separate category of *follicle center lymphoma, diffuse,* is included in the WHO classification as a variant of follicular lymphoma.

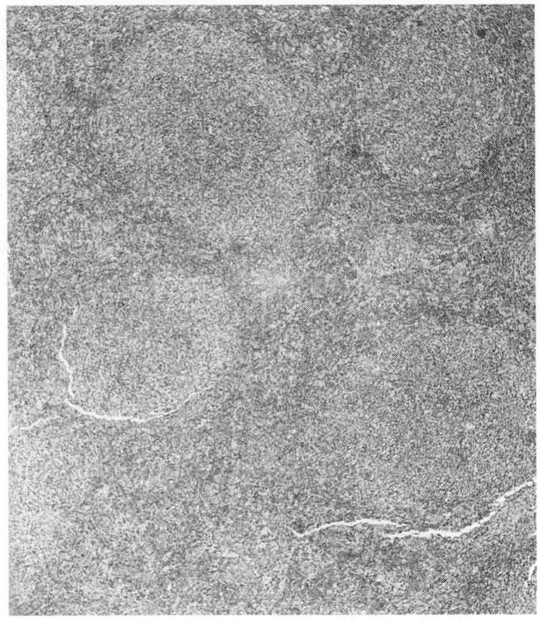

FIG. 24.2. Follicular lymphoma with relatively uniform follicles that are slightly larger than most reactive follicles (hematoxylin and eosin stain, original magnification: 50× magnification).

MORPHOLOGIC FEATURES OF FOLLICULAR LYMPHOMA

Pattern

General Features

More than 90% of lymphomas composed of centroblasts and centrocytes have a follicular pattern, at least in part. In the typical case of follicular lymphoma, the follicles are approximately the same size as a mature germinal center, uniform in size, closely packed, lacking a mantle zone, and evenly distributed throughout the lymph node, obliterating sinuses and extending outside the capsule (Fig. 24.2). However, at least five variables in pattern can be recognized: characteristics (size, shape, distribution) of the follicles, presence or absence and characteristics of a mantle zone, interfollicular involvement, presence of diffuse areas, and sclerosis.

Follicles

Neoplastic follicles may range in size from no larger than a primary follicle to much larger than the average reactive follicle; although usually round (Fig. 24.2), they may be irregular and serpiginous (Fig. 24.3), mimicking floridly reactive hyperplastic follicles. Within a given tumor, the follicles are likely to be relatively uniform and monotonous, but this is not absolute, and in some cases marked variation in size can be seen from one follicle to another. In most cases, the follicles appear paler at low magnification than the interfollicular region, because the follicles contain larger, paler cells than the small lymphocytes of the interfollicular region. In occasional cases, the "reverse" pattern appears, with darker follicles against a light background (68). In still other cases, the follicles may appear irregularly mottled, resembling progressively transformed germinal centers; this usually occurs in cases with increased large cells and has been called the *floral variant* of follicular lymphoma (69,70) (Fig. 24.3B).

Mantle Zone

In most cases, neoplastic follicles are not sharply delimited from the interfollicular region, and lack the typical mantle of small lymphocytes seen around reactive germinal centers. In a substantial minority, however, partial or complete mantle zones may be present around all or some of the follicles (16) (Fig. 24.3A). When present, these usually contain predominantly small round B lymphocytes, which are polyclonal IgM^+IgD^+ cells similar to those of the normal follicle mantle. These polyclonal mantle zone B cells are presumably attracted to neoplastic follicles by a mechanism analogous to that which results in the presence of FDCs and nonneoplastic T cells in these follicles.

Marginal Zone

In some follicular lymphomas, the outer cells of the follicles may resemble marginal zone or monocytoid B cells,

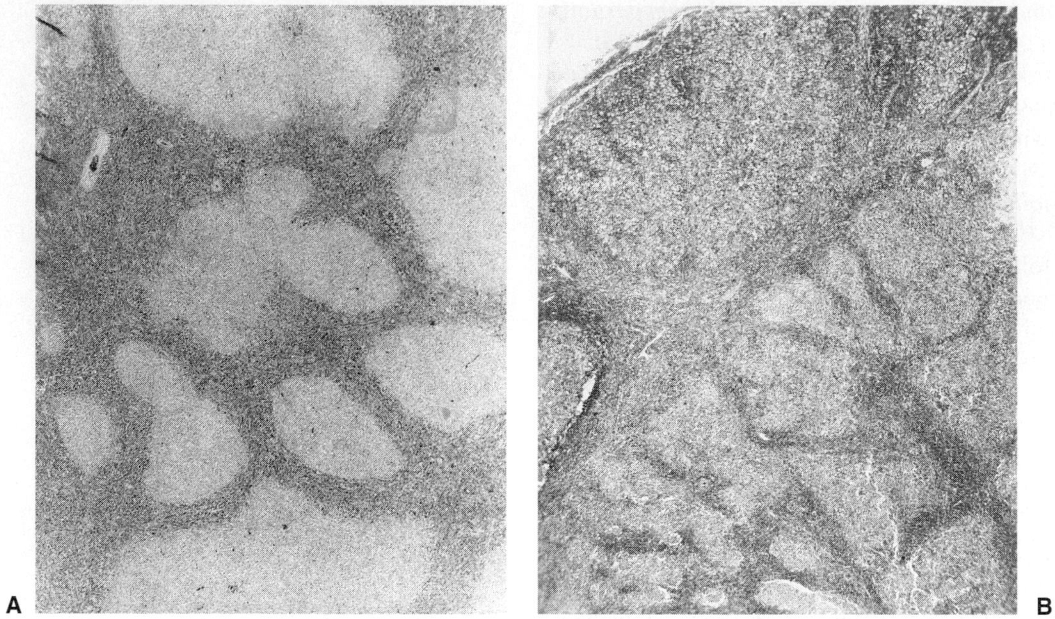

FIG. 24.3. **A:** Follicular lymphoma is composed of irregularly shaped follicle zones (hematoxylin and eosin stain, original magnification: 50× magnification). **B:** Floral variant of follicular lymphoma demonstrates broken up follicles within a mantle zone of small lymphocytes, resembling progressively transformed germinal centers or lymphocyte predominance Hodgkin's disease (hematoxylin and eosin stain, original magnification: 63× magnification).

with nuclei similar to centrocytes, but with more abundant, pale cytoplasm. These cells may form partial or complete ''marginal zones'' around some or most of the follicles in a given case, and may also have an interfollicular and perisinusoidal distribution (Fig. 24.4), resembling nodal involvement by extranodal marginal zone lymphoma of mucosa-associated lymphoid tissue (MALT) type, or nodal marginal zone lymphoma. This phenomenon has been regarded as ''composite lymphoma'' with follicular and monocytoid B-cell lymphoma by some investigators (71,72), but others consider it evidence of intratumoral differentiation, similar to plasmacytoid differentiation, in a follicular lymphoma (73). In the cases studied, a clonal relationship between the follicular and monocytoid B-cell components has been suggested, by virtue of common Ig isotype expression. Nathwani (74) has suggested that follicular lymphoma with marginal zone or monocytoid B cells represents a neoplasm of a memory B-cell ''capable of trafficking through the germinal center and differentiating into multiple cell types.'' In one study, the presence of significant marginal zone/monocytoid B-cell areas in follicular lymphomas was associated with a significantly worse prognosis compared with cases lacking this feature (75).

Capsular Invasion

Characteristically, subcapsular and medullary sinuses are largely obliterated by the infiltrate in follicular lymphoma, but sinuses may be partially or completely preserved. Extracapsular extension is also common but not universal; when it occurs, the capsule may be visible as a band of fibrous tissue within the tumor. Successive levels of extracapsular extension may appear as concentric parallel bands of fibrosis in the extranodal tissue (Fig. 24.5).

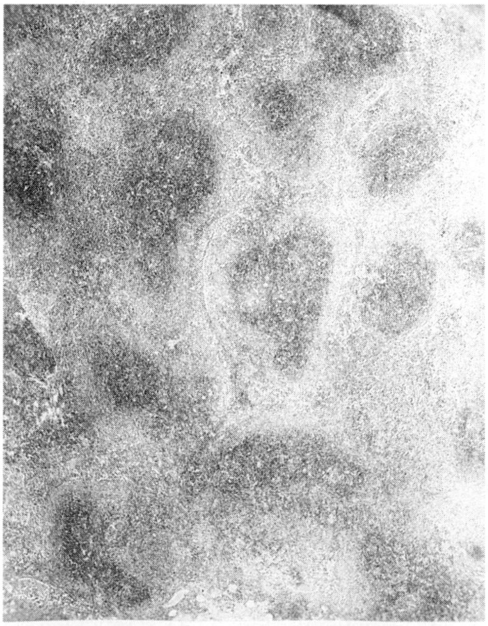

FIG. 24.4. Follicular lymphoma with marginal zone differentiation. Low magnification shows areas of pale cells surrounding dark follicle centers (hematoxylin and eosin stain, original magnification: 31× magnification). Compare with Figure 24.14.

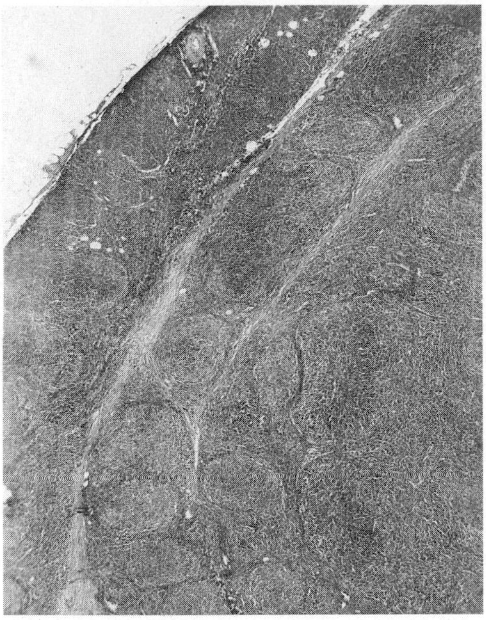

FIG. 24.5. Follicular lymphoma with concentric bands of fibrosis is associated with the infiltration of small, closely packed follicles beyond the nodal capsule (hematoxylin and eosin stain, original magnification: 31× magnification).

Interfollicular Region

In most cases of follicular lymphoma, the follicles are closely packed, with only a small amount of interfollicular tissue, and absence of the normal T zones. The interfollicular region may contain numerous small blood vessels of the high endothelial venule (HEV) type, but is poor in transformed lymphocytes and plasma cells, and usually contains neoplastic centrocytes (16,76). Two exceptions to this general rule occur. In some cases, the follicles may appear widely spaced, and the interfollicular region is expanded by large numbers of cells identical to those within the follicles (Fig. 24.6). In others, the widely spaced follicles may be surrounded by a relatively normal appearing interfollicular region, without evidence of extrafollicular neoplastic cells. The latter pattern is extremely difficult to distinguish from follicular hyperplasia, and immunohistologic studies are usually required for the diagnosis (68). This pattern may reflect early nodal involvement by follicular lymphoma (77).

Sclerosis

Neoplastic follicles are usually poor in reticulin fibers, similar to normal follicles. The interfollicular area may contain numerous fibers, which appear to be compressed by the expanded follicles, similar to the pattern that can be seen in reactive nodes. The interfollicular region may show an increase in collagen that is recognizable on routine stains, resulting in a nodular sclerosis pattern (78). Sclerosis appears to be more common in central lymph nodes (mediastinal, retroperitoneal), as opposed to peripheral lymph nodes. It may cause problems in diagnosis, because it tends to be more pronounced at the periphery of involved nodes or nodal masses, and may obscure the neoplastic cells in biopsies from the edges of nodal masses. In general, sclerosis is more marked in areas in which the infiltrate is becoming diffuse, and can be a useful differential diagnostic feature in distinguishing follicular lymphoma from follicular or diffuse lymphoid hyperplasia.

A

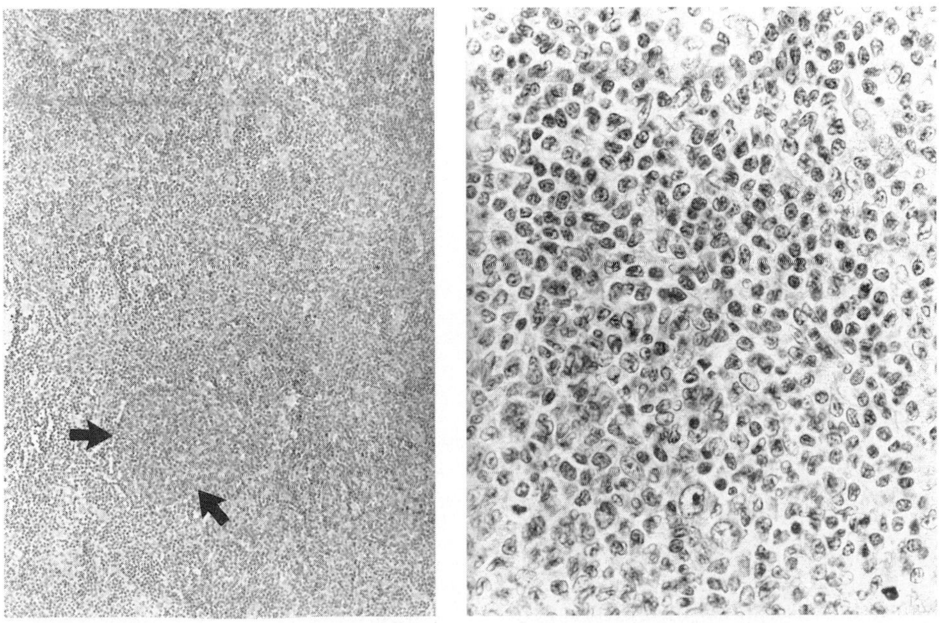

B

FIG. 24.6. A: Follicular lymphoma with prominent involvement of the interfollicular region and diffuse areas. Small, poorly circumscribed follicles are present. **B:** High magnification shows small, irregular lymphoid cells (hematoxylin and eosin stain, original magnification: 500× magnification).

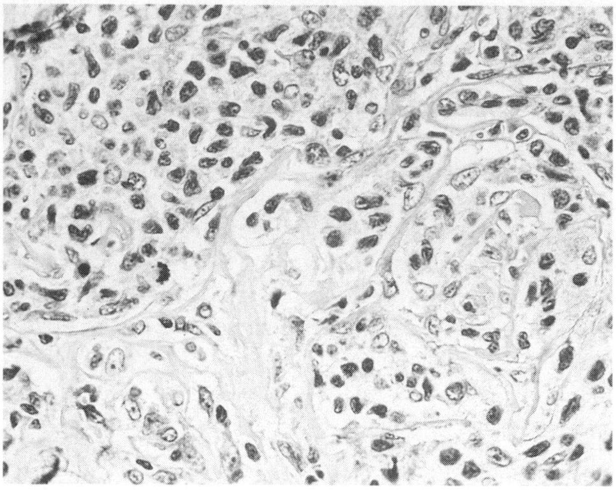

FIG. 24.7. Follicular lymphoma has a diffuse area showing numerous centrocytes with distorted, elongated nuclei and prominent sclerosis (hematoxylin and eosin stain, original magnification: 500× magnification).

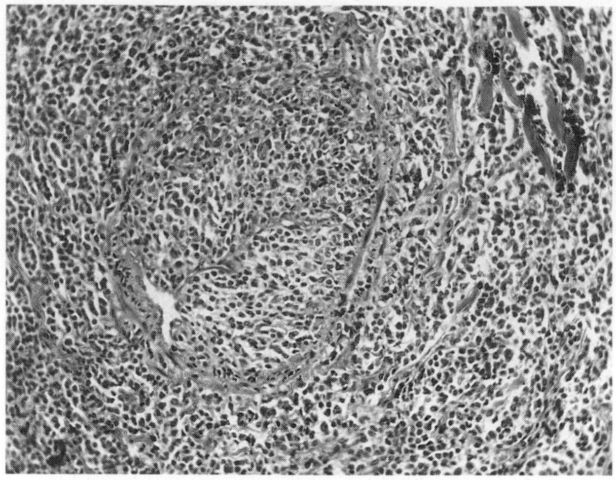

FIG. 24.8. Follicular lymphoma with vascular invasion. Neoplastic lymphoid cells infiltrate the wall of a small blood vessel, with compression of the lumen (hematoxylin and eosin stain, original magnification: 200× magnification).

In diffuse areas with sclerosis, the neoplastic centrocytes frequently assume an elongated shape, and may resemble the nuclei of fibroblasts (Fig. 24.7). This appearance may give rise to a differential diagnosis of sarcoma; with Giemsa stain, however, the lymphoid morphology of the centrocytes is more apparent, and centroblasts can always be recognized by their basophilic cytoplasm. Centrocytes are often more numerous in sclerotic areas than in diffuse areas lacking sclerosis, and the admixture of nonneoplastic lymphocytes is less apparent; in difficult cases, careful examination of the cells in areas of sclerosis is useful in establishing the diagnosis.

Vascular Invasion

Vascular invasion is a surprisingly common feature in follicular lymphomas within involved lymph nodes and in pericapsular veins (21). Neoplastic follicles themselves are not seen within veins, but centrocytes are commonly seen infiltrating through the walls of small and even larger veins, accumulating within the intimal layer (Fig. 24.8). In cases with large numbers of reactive T cells, the areas of vascular invasion, similar to the areas of sclerosis, often contain fewer reactive cells, permitting recognition of the neoplastic centrocytes. Vascular invasion may be seen within the lymph node or in surrounding soft tissue, and is a useful feature in the differential diagnosis with hyperplasia.

Infarction and Necrosis

Small foci of necrosis are uncommon in follicular lymphoma, compared with higher-grade lymphomas or Hodgkin's disease, but total infarction of the lymph node may be seen and appears to be more common in follicular lymphoma than in other lymphomas (21). This phenomenon may be related to the tendency toward invasion of extranodal vessels. The diagnosis may be confirmed in totally infarcted nodes by careful evaluation of the cells preserved in the extranodal tissue and by reticulin stains, which demonstrate the follicular pattern throughout the infarcted area. Molecular genetic analysis can occasionally successfully demonstrate immunoglobulin gene rearrangement in infarcted tissue, and immunohistochemistry can also be successfully used to document that the cells are $CD45^+$ and $CD20^+$ (79–81).

Diffuse Areas

A diffuse area in a follicular lymphoma is defined as an area that lacks any evidence of neoplastic follicles and contains a mixture of cells similar to that seen within the neoplastic follicles. Involvement of the interfollicular region by neoplastic cells is not considered evidence of a diffuse pattern in follicular lymphoma. An increase in reticulin fibers and often frank sclerosis are frequently seen in diffuse areas (21) (Fig. 24.7). The diffuse areas often resemble the interfollicular regions of follicular areas, with prominent high endothelial venules (HEV) and large numbers of admixed benign T lymphocytes.

Although the prognostic importance of diffuse areas is debated, the WHO Clinical Advisory Committee recommended that they be quantified. The WHO classification therefore recommends three categories of grade 1 and 2 follicular lymphoma that should recognize the most clinically important subgroups: follicular (>75% follicular), follicular and diffuse (25% to 75% follicular) and predominantly diffuse (<25% follicular) (Table 24.4). Diffuse areas in a grade 3 follicular lymphoma are diagnosed as diffuse large B-cell lymphoma.

Diffuse Follicle Center Lymphoma

Rare lymphomas composed of centrocytes and centroblasts have a purely diffuse pattern, equivalent to diffuse centroblastic/centrocytic lymphoma in the Kiel classification. In some of these cases it is likely that focal follicular areas are present, and that a sampling problem results in a purely diffuse pattern. The frequency of these cases is difficult to determine, because they are lumped with a variety of other lymphomas in the diffuse "mixed" categories of the Rappaport classification and the Working Formulation. Two studies analyzing the morphologic, immunophenotypic, and molecular genetic features of "diffuse mixed" lymphomas found that approximately 40% had morphologic, immunophenotypic, or genetic (*BCL2* rearrangement) evidence of follicle center derivation (82,83). Lennert reported that only 4% of CB/CC lymphomas in the Kiel registry were entirely diffuse, and commented that these were often follicular in other lymph nodes (21). Studies using the Kiel classification (23) suggest that purely diffuse cases of centroblastic/centrocytic lymphoma have a significantly worse prognosis that cases with a follicular or follicular and diffuse pattern. In the WHO classification, *diffuse follicle center lymphoma* is defined as a diffuse lymphoma composed of centrocytes and centroblasts, in which centrocytes predominate. It is proposed that these cases be graded as for follicular lymphoma into grade 1 and grade 2 (Table 24.4). A diffuse lymphoma with a predominance of large follicle center cells should be classified as diffuse large B-cell lymphoma.

Cellular Composition of Follicular Lymphoma

General Features

The centrocytes and centroblasts of most cases of follicular lymphoma are identical to those of normal germinal centers (Fig. 24.9). The centrocytes, although usually less than twice the size of small lymphocytes, have a spectrum of size and may be almost as large as centroblasts. The nuclei appear irregular or angulated in tissue sections; although the term

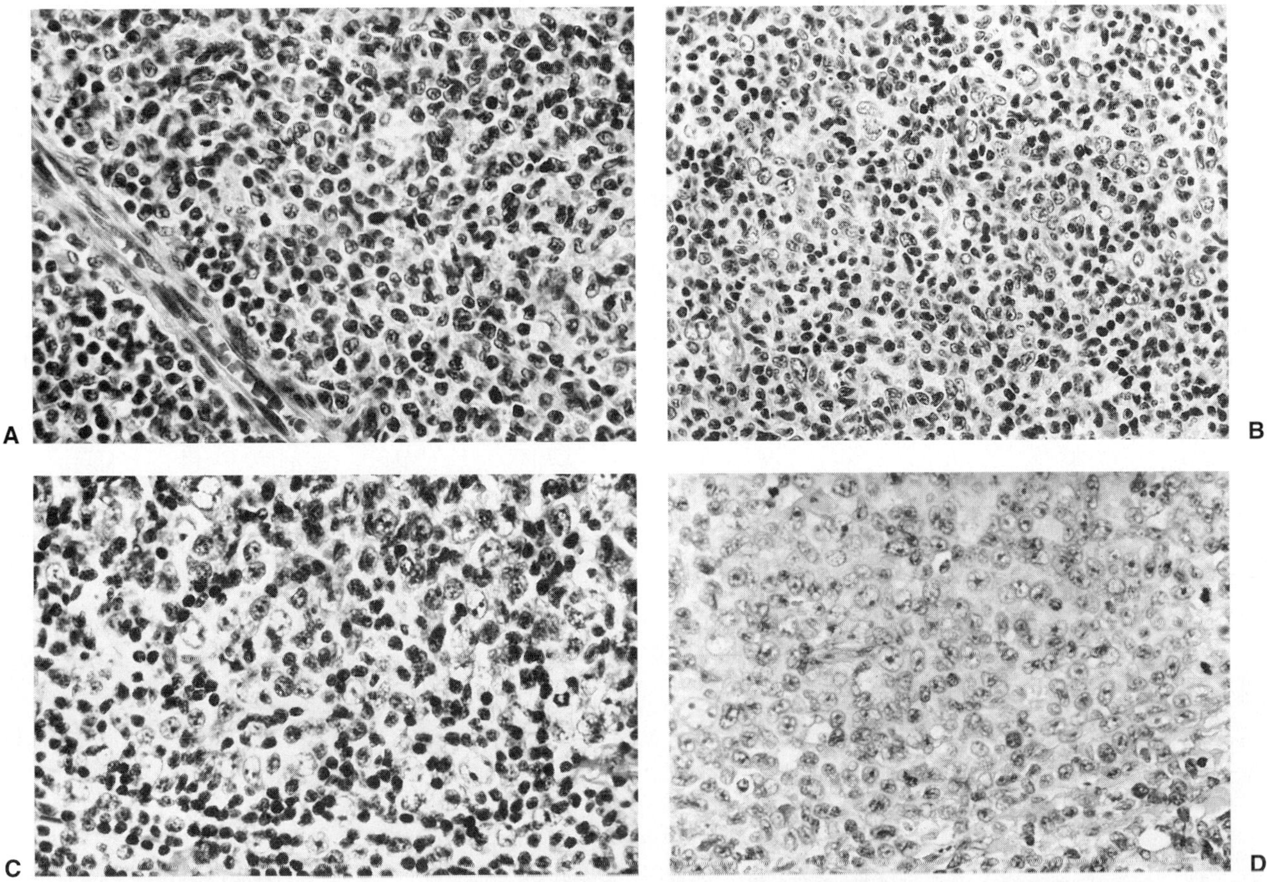

FIG. 24.9. Grading follicular lymphoma. **A:** Grade 1 follicular lymphoma has a predominance of centrocytes with rare centroblasts (hematoxylin and eosin stain, original magnification: 500× magnification). **B:** Grade 2 follicular lymphoma has a mixture of centrocytes with irregular, twisted, angular nuclei and many scattered centroblasts (hematoxylin and eosin stain, original magnification: 500× magnification). **C:** Grade 3a follicular lymphoma has large lymphoid cells predominating within the neoplastic follicle, but centrocytes are still present (hematoxylin and eosin stain, original magnification: 500× magnification). **D:** Grade 3b follicular lymphoma has solid sheets of centroblasts (hematoxylin and eosin stain, original magnification: 500× magnification).

cleaved is used, a distinct nuclear cleft is seldom seen. The chromatin is paler than that of small lymphocytes and is evenly dispersed, giving the nucleus a gray-blue appearance. Single or multiple small nucleoli may be present. The cytoplasm is scant and pale, and is not usually visible on hematoxylin and eosin– or Giemsa-stained sections. In most cases, the centrocytes appear more monomorphous than those of normal follicles, with most being of approximately the same size. Centroblasts are usually three to four times the size of small lymphocytes; the nuclei are round or oval, but they may be irregular, indented, or even have a cleft. The nucleus is vesicular, with a clear center and some peripheral condensation of chromatin; there are one to three basophilic nucleoli, usually apposed to the nuclear membrane. Centroblasts have a narrow rim of cytoplasm, which is intensely basophilic on Giemsa staining. In most cases, the centrocytes are relatively small, and the few centroblasts stand out sharply against the monotonous background of centrocytes. In some cases, however, the centrocytes are larger and may be almost as large as centroblasts. In these cases, the centrocytes may appear more pleomorphic, with more deeply indented or multilobated appearing nuclei, and the centroblasts also appear atypical, with variable nuclear size and shape, increased heterochromatin, and binucleate or multinucleated forms. In most cases, mitotic activity is low, and a starry-sky pattern with phagocytic histiocytes is absent. However, in cases with increased numbers of centroblasts, mitoses are more numerous, and phagocytosis of nuclear debris is rarely seen. Polarization, as seen in reactive follicles, is rare in follicular lymphomas, although in some cases with increased numbers of centroblasts, these cells may be more dense in one area of the follicle than another, creating an impression of polarization.

In addition to neoplastic cells, neoplastic follicles also contain FDCs; these have nuclei similar in size to centroblast nuclei, but have delicate nuclear membranes and central, small, eosinophilic nucleoli. Follicular dendritic cells are often binucleate, and the two nuclei are typically apposed to one another, with flattening of the adjacent nuclear membranes (Fig. 24.10). In contrast to centroblasts, their cytoplasm does not stain blue with the Giemsa stain. Small T cells may also be found in neoplastic follicles; these are usually less numerous than in reactive germinal centers, but occasionally they may be numerous.

Grading Follicular Lymphoma

Follicular lymphoma cannot be sharply divided into distinct subtypes, but rather shows a continuous gradation in the number of centroblasts (84). It has been repeatedly shown that an individual pathologist can effectively predict outcome in follicular lymphoma by grading according to proportion of large cells, but this is difficult to reproduce among groups of pathologists (85,86). Several studies suggest that the ''cell counting'' method of Mann and Berard is more reproducible and better in predicting prognosis than other methods of grading follicular lymphoma (85–87). In this method, the centroblasts (large nucleolated cells) per 40X high power microscopic field (hpf) are counted (10 to 20 hpf in different follicles). A case with up to 5 centroblasts per hpf is grade 1, one with 6 to 15 centroblasts is grade 2, and one with more than 15 centroblasts is grade 3 (84). Approximately 80% of follicular lymphomas are grade 1 (40% to 60%) or grade 2 (25% to 35%) (Fig. 24.9A–D).

This method has a technical drawback. It counts large cells per high-power microscopic field rather than as a percent of all cells, and variation in ocular diameter from one microscope to another can significantly affect the field size and potentially the grade of the tumor. The international study of the REAL classification used microscopes with a hpf of 0.159 mm^2; this is achieved with a 10× 18-mm diameter

A
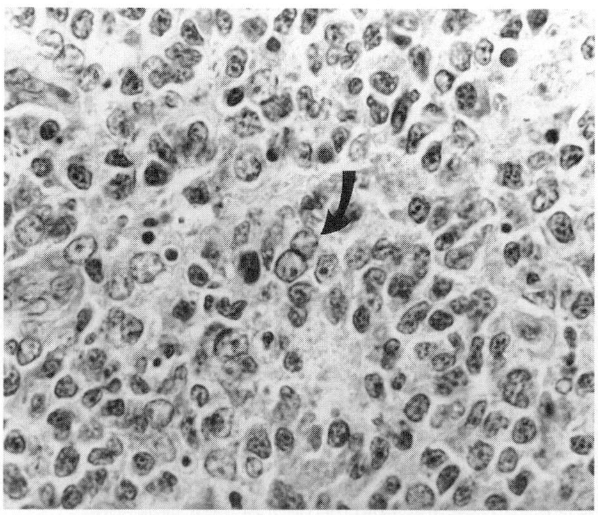
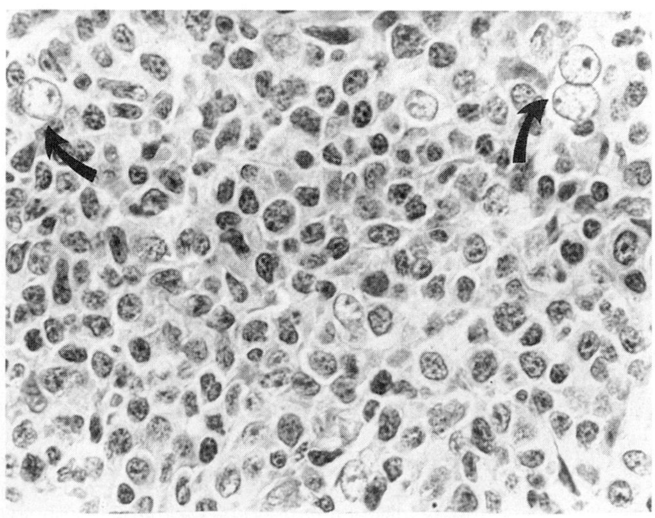
B

FIG. 24.10. Follicular dendritic cells in a reactive follicle **(A)** and follicular lymphoma **(B)**. The nuclei are similar in size to centroblast nuclei but have single, small nucleoli and are often binucleate *(arrows)* (hematoxylin and eosin stain, original magnification: 630× magnification).

ocular and a 40× objective (Table 24.4), and should be considered the standard hpf for the purpose of grading follicular lymphoma (88). A 10× 20-mm diameter ocular gives a hpf of 0.196 mm^2, and a 10× 22-mm diameter (wide field) ocular a field of 0.237 mm^2. Because 10 hpf at 0.159 mm^2 is a total area of 1.59 mm^2, counting 8 hpf using a 10× 20-mm ocular or 7 hpf using a 10× 22-mm ocular is roughly equivalent to counting 10 hpf with a 10× 18-mm ocular. The result is divided by 10 to get the number of large cells in a 0.159 mm^2 hpf. Using the standard 0.159 mm^2 hpf, the international study of the REAL classification found that a cutoff of 15 large cells/hpf (150 large cells/1.59 mm^2) had significant prognostic value for overall and disease-free survival in follicular lymphoma (89).

An additional problem is that, using the numeric cutoffs of Mann and Berard, the spectrum of follicular large cell lymphoma may be very broad, ranging from cases with 16 large cells per high-power field to cases in which most of the cells in the follicle are centroblasts (90) (Fig. 24.9D). Some investigators have suggested modifying the Mann and Berard method so that cases are not called *large cell* unless at least 50% of the cells are centroblasts or large centrocytes (91). There is some evidence that cases with solid sheets of centroblasts are biologically distinct from those with a mixture of centrocytes and centroblasts. For this reason, the WHO classification provides optional subtypes of grade 3 follicular lymphoma. Grade 3a is defined as more than 15 centroblasts/hpf, but centrocytes are still present, and grade 3b is defined by solid sheets of centroblasts.

Another criterion that could be evaluated in grading follicular lymphoma is proliferation rate, particularly using immunohistochemical staining for Ki-67. One would hope that more objective methods such as counting Ki-67^+ cells using an automated image analyzer would provide more uniformity; however, a study suggested that this method was less useful in predicting outcome than the Mann and Berard counting method (91). Additional studies of the utility of proliferation fraction in predicting outcome in follicular lymphoma are needed.

Although in most cases of follicular lymphoma the cytologic composition is relatively uniform throughout the involved tissue, it is not unusual for the relative proportion of centrocytes and centroblasts to vary from one follicle to another. Multiple sections should be examined, and estimation of the proportion of large cells should be done on a representative sample of follicles. Rarely, individual follicles or parts of the node may show an abrupt transition from a predominance of small centrocytes to a predominance of centroblasts. Areas of diffuse large cell lymphoma may also be found in lymph nodes showing follicular lymphoma; although this has been called a composite lymphoma, it actually represents transformation of the same tumor to a higher-grade lymphoma. Distinct areas of follicular grade 3 lymphoma or diffuse large B-cell lymphoma in a predominantly grade 1 or 2 follicular lymphoma should be specifically noted in the report, with a separate diagnosis. Occasional patients with follicular lymphoma have divergent histologic features in lymph nodes taken simultaneously from different sites, showing variation in grade or progression to diffuse large B-cell lymphoma (92).

Histologic Transformation and Progression in Follicular lymphoma

Patients with follicular lymphoma may develop a diffuse large cell lymphoma at some time during their course. The magnitude of this risk is difficult to assess, because not all patients undergo rebiopsy before repeat therapy. The early studies of Gall and Rappaport focused on the consistency of cellular composition of follicular lymphoma. Gall found that 6 of 8 autopsied cases showed some degree of progression from lower to higher grade, although only one case progressed to a diffuse high-grade lymphoma (6). Rappaport and associates reported analysis of sequential biopsies or autopsies in 104 of their cases of follicular lymphoma. Thirty-seven percent showed no change in cytology or pattern, 30% showed progression to a diffuse pattern without change in cytology, and 44% showed an increase in large cells with or without a diffuse pattern. The frequency of progression was highest in the mixed category, with 49% progressing to large cell type, most with a diffuse pattern. Eighty-six percent of the cases of nodular reticulum cell type progressed to a diffuse pattern (8). Later studies showed an actuarial risk of transformation of approximately 20% at 8 years (93–95).

Transformation of follicular lymphoma is usually to diffuse large B-cell lymphoma (Fig. 24.11), most commonly with cells resembling centroblasts but occasionally resembling anaplastic large cells, with CD30 expression (96) (Fig. 24.11). Cases of transformation to Burkitt's or Burkitt's-like lymphoma have been reported (97,98). Rare patients with follicular lymphoma have developed precursor B-cell lymphoblastic lymphoma or acute lymphoid leukemia (99–102). In several of these cases the leukemic cells, in addition to the t(14;18), acquired a t(8;14) translocation, similar to that seen in Burkitt's lymphoma, with rearrangement of the *MYC* gene (99–101). In one report, the lymphoblastic lymphoma and the follicular lymphoma had identical heavy- and light-chain gene rearrangements, and sequence analysis showed additional somatic mutations in the lymphoblastic lymphoma (102).

Transformation of follicular lymphoma in most cases represents evolution of the original neoplastic clone to a more rapidly proliferating cell type. Several studies have confirmed a common origin for the low- and high-grade components, showing identical clonal immunoglobulin heavy and light-chain gene rearrangements as well as *BCL2* rearrangements in both tumors (103–105).

This evolution can be understood as follows. the centroblast is assumed to be the precursor cell of the centrocyte; the centroblast is the proliferating cell, whose progeny retain the ability to mature into centrocytes. Centrocytes have a predilection to form (or home to) follicular structures. In early stages of the disease, most centroblasts mature to cen-

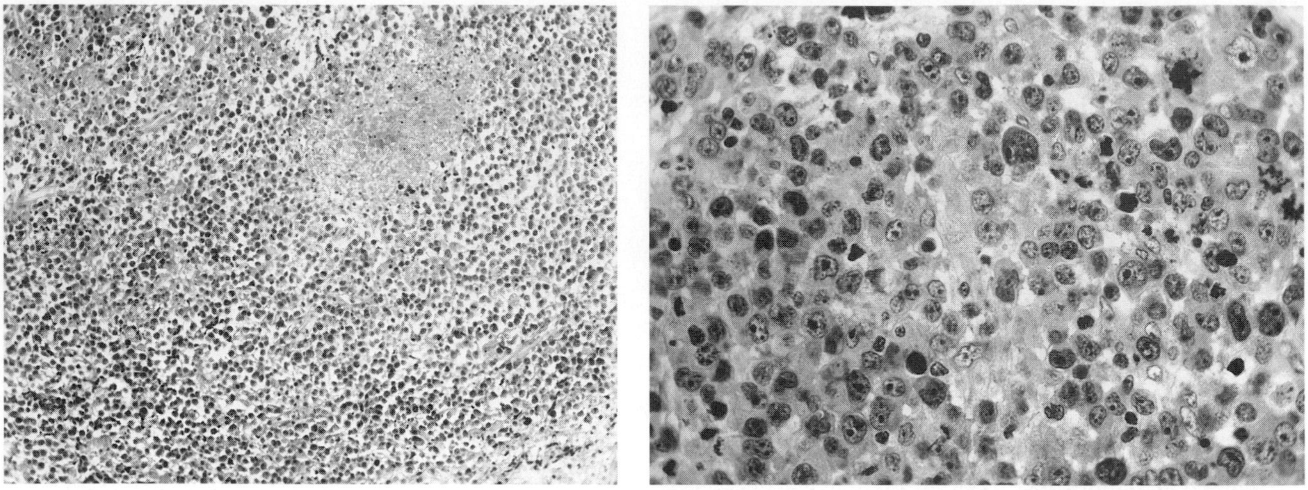

A B

FIG. 24.11. Follicular lymphoma with transformation to large B-cell lymphoma, anaplastic large cell variant. **A:** Twelve years after the diagnosis of follicular lymphoma, this patient developed a malignant lymphoma with a diffuse pattern and areas of necrosis (hematoxylin and eosin stain, original magnification: 125× magnification). **B:** Large, bizarre, pleomorphic lymphoid cells with prominent nucleoli and a high mitotic rate. The tumor cells were positive for B-cell antigen, CD20, and CD30 (hematoxylin and eosin stain, original magnification: 500× magnification).

trocytes, and the tumor has the appearance of a follicular low-grade lymphoma, with a relatively slow growth and indolent clinical course. With time, probably associated with additional genetic events, a subclone of centroblasts loses its ability to mature into centrocytes; these rapidly proliferating cells soon dominate the picture. Being less ''differentiated,'' they lack the ability to form or home to follicles. The histologic picture is that of a diffuse large cell lymphoma, and the clinical picture is that of a high-grade malignancy. *TP53* mutations and *MYC* gene rearrangement have been reported to be associated with transformation in follicular lymphoma (97,98,106,107).

Plasmacytoid Differentiation

Theoretically, because the end result of B-cell differentiation is the formation of plasma cells, any B-cell lymphoma could contain plasma cells, but plasmacytoid differentiation is common in some tumors and rare in others. Follicular lymphomas rarely contain appreciable numbers of plasma cells, a fact that can be useful in their differentiation from reactive hyperplasia. In some cases, evidence of plasmacytoid differentiation can be found; this can take two forms, both equally rare.

Follicular Lymphoma with Plasma Cells

Infrequent reported cases of follicular lymphoma contain neoplastic plasma cells (108–112). The neoplastic plasma cells are found in the follicles and in the interfollicular region, and monotypic immunoglobulin can be demonstrated in the plasma cells with the immunoperoxidase technique on paraffin-embedded tissue sections. The reported cases are heterogeneous; 8 of the 21 cases in the cited studies were extranodal, and one was confined to the spleen. It is likely that many of these cases would now be considered to be examples of marginal zone lymphomas of mucosa-associated lymphoid tissue (MALT), nodal, or splenic types (59,113–115).

Follicular Lymphoma with Signet Ring Cells

Several cases of follicular lymphoma have been reported in which the neoplastic centrocytes have large cytoplasmic vacuoles, which were clear or eosinophilic, giving them the appearance of signet ring cells (116–122) (Fig. 24.12).

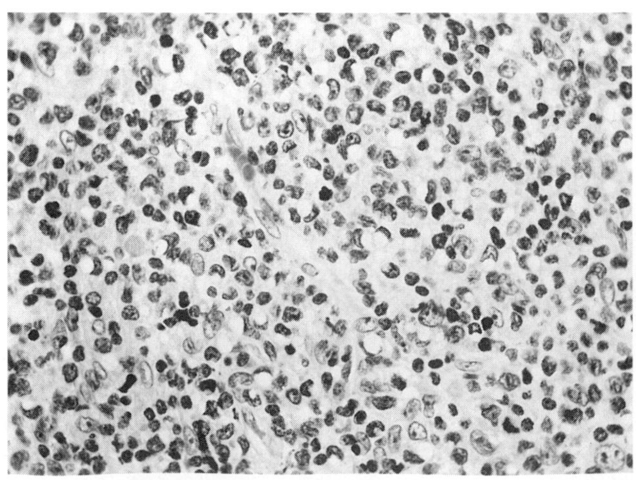

FIG. 24.12. Follicular lymphoma with signet ring cells. Many of the atypical lymphoid cells contain a large, clear cytoplasmic vacuole, simulating carcinoma cells of the signet ring cell type (hematoxylin and eosin stain, original magnification: 500× magnification).

These cases differ from those with plasma cells, because the immunoglobulin expression occurs in centrocytes rather than plasma cells. In most of these cases, cytoplasmic immunoglobulin can be demonstrated in the signet ring cells. Cases with clear cytoplasm typically express cytoplasmic IgG, with a predominance of λ light chain, whereas those with periodic acid–Schiff–positive (PAS^+) eosinophilic globules in the cytoplasm or nucleus more commonly express IgM (116,123). On ultrastructural examination, the clear inclusions are large, membrane-bound vacuoles containing multiple tiny coated vesicles, while the eosinophilic inclusions consist of dilated rough endoplasmic reticulum, filled with electron dense material, presumably immunoglobulin. The nature of the vacuoles in the clear cell cases is not well understood, but a relationship to multivesicular bodies has been suggested (124).

Clinically, follicular lymphomas with signet ring cell morphology do not appear to differ from typical follicular lymphomas. The patients are older adults; the reported clear cell cases have a striking female predominance, while those with eosinophilic inclusions are equally common in males and females, like typical follicular lymphoma. Virtually all reported cases are nodal, in contrast to cases with plasmacytoid differentiation; patients usually have disseminated disease and long survivals. Most are classified as grade 1 or grade 2. The factors that induce these cases, in contrast to most other follicular lymphomas, to express cytoplasmic immunoglobulin are not known.

Follicular Lymphoma with Amorphous Extracellular Material

Occasional cases of follicular lymphoma may have amorphous, eosinophilic, extracellular, often PAS^+ material deposited in an irregular fashion within the follicle centers (125,126). The nature of this material is not clear; Chittal and colleagues found that by ultrastructure, it contained membrane fragments, and by immunohistochemistry, contained many antigens found in and on the neoplastic cells (CD45, CD22, immunoglobulin). Others (125) have speculated that it represents deposition of antigen-antibody complexes on the processes of FDCs analogous to the deposits often seen in reactive follicles. Because follicular lymphomas rarely secrete immunoglobulin, this phenomenon is less common in neoplastic than in reactive follicles. However, in reactive follicles extracellular immunoglobulin deposition is rarely massive enough to be conspicuous by light microscopy, while in the few lymphomas that show this phenomenon, it may be impressive. Although uncommon and by no means diagnostic, massive extracellular deposition of amorphous material within follicles should raise the question of lymphoma.

Follicular Lymphoma with Other Types of Lymphoma

Follicular Lymphoma with Other Small B-Cell Lymphomas

Follicular lymphomas may show focal differentiation toward marginal zone B cells or plasma cells. Although this phenomenon has been called *composite lymphoma,* most observers believe it represents intratumoral differentiation rather than the occurrence of two distinct lymphomas. With advanced techniques, two case reports illustrated the range of possible biologic relationships between two apparent different histologic subtypes of small B-cell lymphoma (i.e., composite lymphoma) occurring in the same tissues.

In one report, Isaacson and colleagues (77) described a 44-year-old woman with Sjögren's syndrome, who sequentially developed a MALT lymphoma of the salivary gland and a follicular lymphoma involving mesenteric and inguinal lymph nodes and spleen and liver. The two components shared identical *BCL2* and immunoglobulin gene rearrangements, indicating a common clonal origin, although they differed with regard to CD10 expression. The investigators hypothesized that a B-cell containing a t(14;18) underwent malignant transformation into a MALT lymphoma in the salivary gland, and that during follicular colonization, in the microenvironment of the germinal center, the tumor cells subsequently acquired the characteristics of follicular lymphoma.

A second case was reported in which a follicular lymphoma at relapse contained broad mantle zones of atypical, small cleaved cells; flow cytometry showed two populations with a single light chain: one $CD5^+CD10^-$ and one $CD5^-CD10^+$. Molecular genetic analysis showed *BCL1* and *BCL2* gene rearrangements, but only one clonal IgH rearrangement with identical sequences in microdissected tissue from the follicular and mantle cell areas, suggesting a single tumor with features of mantle cell and follicular lymphoma (127).

Follicular Lymphoma and Hodgkin's Disease

Follicular lymphoma and diffuse large B-cell lymphoma are the most common lymphomas to occur in patients with Hodgkin's lymphoma. Follicular lymphoma may precede, follow, or occur simultaneously with Hodgkin's lymphoma (128–132). This may simply reflect the fact that follicular lymphoma and Hodgkin's disease are both relatively common, or it may reflect a relationship between them. The occurrence of Hodgkin's disease and follicular lymphoma in the same tissue is relatively rare, but many cases have been reported over the years (128) (Fig. 24.13). In two studies, single cell analysis of neoplastic cells from the Hodgkin's disease component and the follicular lymphoma component of composite or sequential lymphomas demonstrated identical immunoglobulin heavy-chain gene rearrangements in the two tumors, both showing somatic mutations, consistent with derivation from a common germinal center cell precursor (133,134). In both cases, divergent patterns of somatic mutation indicated that the two tumors originated from a common precursor, but diverged at the germinal center centroblast stage, with the follicular lymphoma continuing to acquire new somatic mutations. Cases of ''composite'' Hodgkin's disease and follicular lymphoma, like other com-

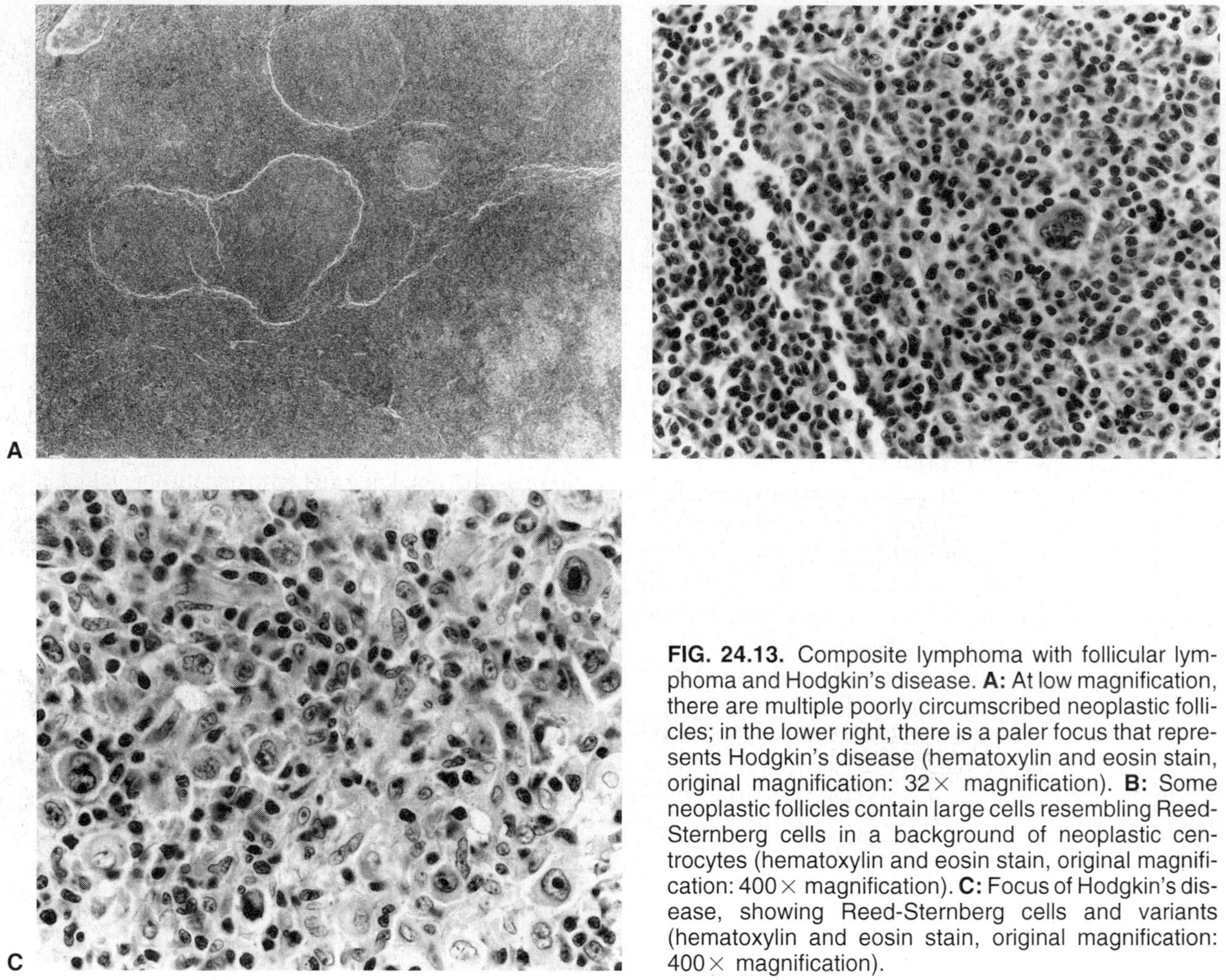

FIG. 24.13. Composite lymphoma with follicular lymphoma and Hodgkin's disease. **A:** At low magnification, there are multiple poorly circumscribed neoplastic follicles; in the lower right, there is a paler focus that represents Hodgkin's disease (hematoxylin and eosin stain, original magnification: 32× magnification). **B:** Some neoplastic follicles contain large cells resembling Reed-Sternberg cells in a background of neoplastic centrocytes (hematoxylin and eosin stain, original magnification: 400× magnification). **C:** Focus of Hodgkin's disease, showing Reed-Sternberg cells and variants (hematoxylin and eosin stain, original magnification: 400× magnification).

posite lymphomas, probably represent two morphologic manifestations of the same tumor clone.

Follicular Lymphoma in Extranodal Sites

Follicular lymphoma is predominantly a tumor of lymph nodes. Extranodal lymphoid tissue, such as the spleen and Waldeyer's ring, are often involved, as are the bone marrow and liver, common sites of stage IV involvement in other lymphomas (92). Follicular lymphoma may occasionally be truly extranodal, that is, involve areas that are not normally considered to contain lymphoid tissue, such as the skin and subcutis, ocular adnexa, gastrointestinal tract, and female genital tract. The relationship of these truly extranodal cases to nodal follicular lymphoma is debated; in particular, many primary cutaneous lymphomas believed to be of follicle center origin lack BCL2 and the t(14;18) (135–138).

Spleen

The appearance of follicular lymphomas at staging laparotomy was described in detail by Kim and Dorfman (92). In the spleen, there is typically a uniform pattern of white pulp involvement, resembling reactive hyperplasia on gross examination and at low magnification. This phenomenon has been postulated to reflect the ability of the neoplastic cells to ''home'' to normal B-cell regions. Kim and Dorfman observed that the gross pattern in follicular lymphomas was that of uniform, rounded nodules (Fig. 24.14A), compared with diffuse ''poorly differentiated lymphocytic'' lymphoma (corresponding to what we now know as mantle cell lymphoma), which produced irregularly shaped, variably sized nodules. The white pulp follicles in follicular lymphoma are increased in number and in size, and they show a monomorphous infiltrate of centrocytes and centroblasts similar to that in lymph nodes. The marginal zone may be preserved, or the lymphoma may show marginal zone differentiation, creating difficulty in differential diagnosis with splenic marginal zone lymphoma (Fig. 24.14B). The red pulp typically contains numerous small follicles, but diffuse red pulp involvement is not common in follicular lymphoma (see Chapter 53).

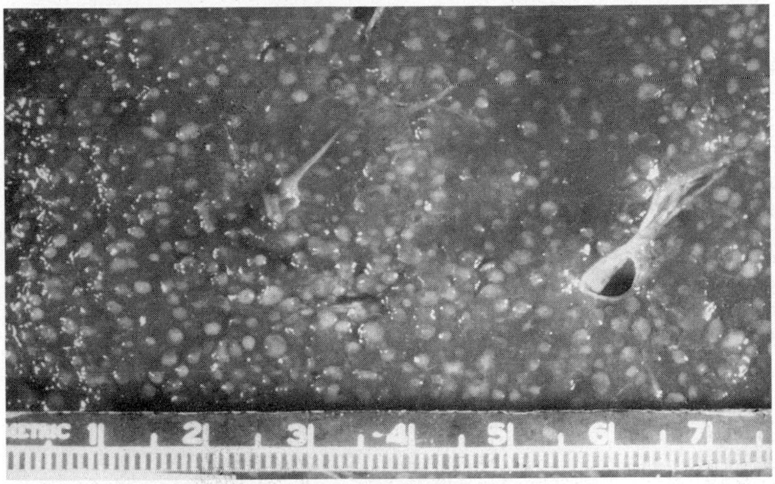

A

FIG. 24.14. Splenic involvement by follicular lymphoma. **A:** Photograph of a spleen involved by follicular lymphoma. The white pulp follicles are increased in size and number, and most are relatively round. **B:** Low magnification of follicular lymphoma involving the spleen shows marginal zones around the neoplastic follicles, creating a resemblance to splenic marginal zone lymphoma (hematoxylin and eosin stain, original magnification: 80× magnification). **C:** Higher magnification shows neoplastic centrocytes with irregular nuclei and scant cytoplasm *(right)* and marginal zone–type cells with irregular nuclei and more abundant, pale cytoplasm *(left)* (hematoxylin and eosin stain, original magnification: 500× magnification).

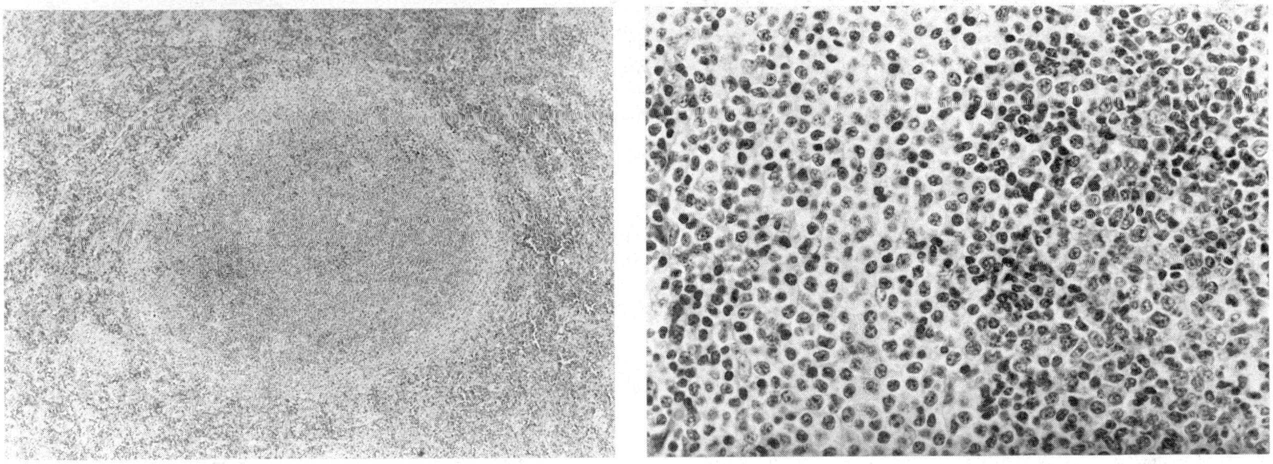

B C

Bone Marrow

Bone marrow involvement by follicular lymphoma is typically seen as circumscribed nodules, which often are situated adjacent to bony trabeculae (92) (Fig. 24.15). This feature is useful in distinguishing nodules of lymphoma from benign lymphoid aggregates, which are usually central within marrow spaces rather than paratrabecular. This criterion is not absolute, however, because occasional paratrabecular lymphoid aggregates can be seen in apparently healthy individuals (92). Infiltrates that appear to hug or wrap around bony trabeculae are highly suspicious for follicular lymphoma, in contrast to those that simply touch the trabeculae. Marrow aggregates of follicular lymphoma are typically composed predominantly of small centrocytes, with only rare centroblasts; the cellular composition may not reflect that of the lymph node, which may contain larger centrocytes and more centroblasts. Marrow involvement by identical cells can be seen in cases of diffuse large cell lymphoma—the so-called *discordant* bone marrow histology (139). Lymphomas cannot be accurately subclassified based on their appearance in the bone marrow, because this may not reflect the appearance of nodal tumor (see Chapter 39).

Peripheral Blood

Approximately 10% of patients with follicular lymphoma have an elevated lymphocyte count. The circulating cells are centrocytes, which are usually slightly larger than small lymphocytes and have a nuclear cleft (140). The term *chronic lymphosarcoma cell leukemia* was initially used to describe these cases and to distinguish them from typical chronic lymphocytic leukemia; however, this term encompasses cases of leukemic mantle cell lymphoma as well and should be replaced by the term *lymphoma (specific type) in leukemic phase* (141). The morphology of the circulating cells is similar in follicular and mantle cell lymphoma, and some cleaved cells may be seen in occasional patients with B-cell chronic lymphocytic leukemia (CLL). Immunophenotyping and often lymph node biopsy are usually necessary for correct subclassification.

A much greater number of patients with follicular lymphoma have occasional neoplastic cells in the blood, without an elevated lymphocyte count. These cells can be detected by flow cytometry or molecular genetic analysis to detect the t(14;18) in most patients with follicular lymphoma (142–144). The small centrocyte appears to circulate in vir-

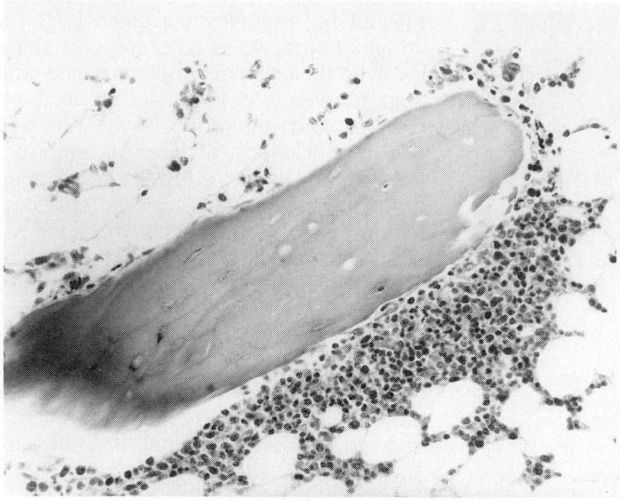
A

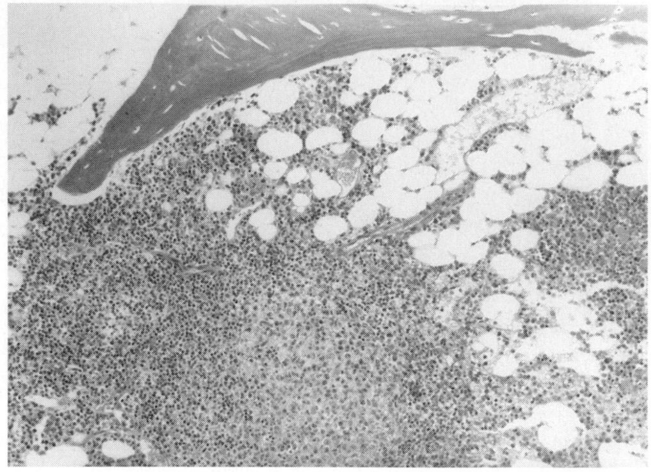
C

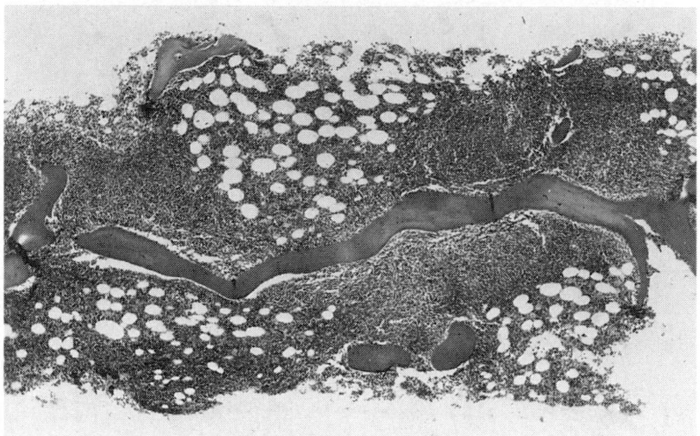
B

FIG. 24.15. Follicular lymphoma involving bone marrow. **A:** Bone marrow biopsy from a patient with follicular lymphoma shows a small paratrabecular lymphoid aggregate (hematoxylin and eosin stain, original magnification: 250× magnification). **B:** With more advanced involvement, a broad cuff of neoplastic lymphoid cells surrounds bony trabeculae. Residual normal hematopoietic marrow is present away from the bone and is recognizable as areas with normal distribution of fat (hematoxylin and eosin stain, original magnification: 50× magnification). **C:** Occasionally, recognizable neoplastic follicles *(lower center)* can be found in the bone marrow (hematoxylin and eosin stain, original magnification: 125× magnification).

tually all cases, which probably explains why so few patients have truly localized disease.

True Extranodal Sites

Cutaneous Follicle Center Lymphoma

Skin and soft tissue involvement may be seen in patients with advanced nodal follicular lymphoma, and follicular lymphoma can also present in the skin (145). A lymphoma composed of centrocyte and centroblast-like cells, often with a partially follicular but predominantly diffuse pattern, is reported to be the most common form of primary cutaneous B-cell lymphoma; the term, cutaneous follicle center lymphoma has been applied to this tumor by the European Organization for Research and Treatment of Cancer (EORTC) (146,147). The definition and normal counterpart of cutaneous follicle center lymphoma is still somewhat controversial. According to the definition of the EORTC, this is a neoplasm composed of follicle center cells, including cases with centrocytes and centroblasts and cases with a predominance of centroblasts and with a follicular or diffuse pattern. Some cases would be classified as follicular lymphoma in the REAL/WHO classification, but others would be called diffuse large B-cell lymphoma. However, most cases illustrated in the EORTC reports appear to be composed of both centrocytes and centroblasts and to have at least a partially follicular pattern.

The immunophenotype and genetic features of cutaneous follicle center lymphoma are reported to differ from those of nodal follicular lymphoma, in that most cases are reported to lack the BCL-2 protein and evidence of the t(14;18) or *BCL2* gene rearrangement. In contrast, follicular lymphoma secondarily involving the skin is more likely to show the typical immunophenotype and to have *BCL2* rearrangement (136,138,148,149). However, two studies showed BCL-2 staining in 60% to 75% of primary cutaneous follicular lymphoma and 5(14;18) by PCR in 25% (150,151).

The clinical features of primary cutaneous follicle center lymphoma are distinctive and make it important to distinguish from systemic cases of follicular lymphoma or diffuse large B-cell lymphoma (152–155). The tumors typically present as raised reddish nodules without ulceration, on the head (face or scalp) or trunk; they may be solitary or multiple, and may reach large size. They respond to radiation therapy, which is the treatment of choice for solitary lesions; multiple lesions can also be treated successfully with radiation to multiple sites, or with chemotherapy (154). Virtually none of these patients develop systemic lymphoma, and they only rarely die of their disease. This is in marked contrast to diffuse large B-cell lymphomas presenting on the lower extremities, which are typically multifocal, ulcerated lesions composed of centroblasts or immunoblasts, and usually develop systemic spread (154).

Follicular Lymphoma of the Gastrointestinal Tract

Most cases previously reported as follicular lymphoma in the gastrointestinal tract are now believed to be examples of marginal zone/MALT lymphoma or mantle cell lymphoma (156). However, follicular lymphoma may occasionally present with gastrointestinal involvement, typically of the small bowel, and usually associated with mesenteric lymph node involvement. Many of these cases appear to represent retrograde or secondary involvement from primary nodal lymphoma of the mesentery and retroperitoneum. Rare cases of follicular lymphoma presenting as lymphomatous polyposis of the intestinal tract have been reported (157) (see Chapter 33).

IMMUNOPHENOTYPE OF FOLLICULAR LYMPHOMA

Neoplastic follicles contain all elements of normal, reactive germinal centers, including follicular center B cells, mantle zone B cells, T cells, macrophages, and follicular dendritic cells.

Follicular lymphoma B cells express pan-B-cell antigens (CD19, CD20, CD22) and surface immunoglobulin (sIg) with light-chain restriction (Fig. 24.16A, Table 24.5). In more than 50% of the cases, the sIg is of μ heavy-chain

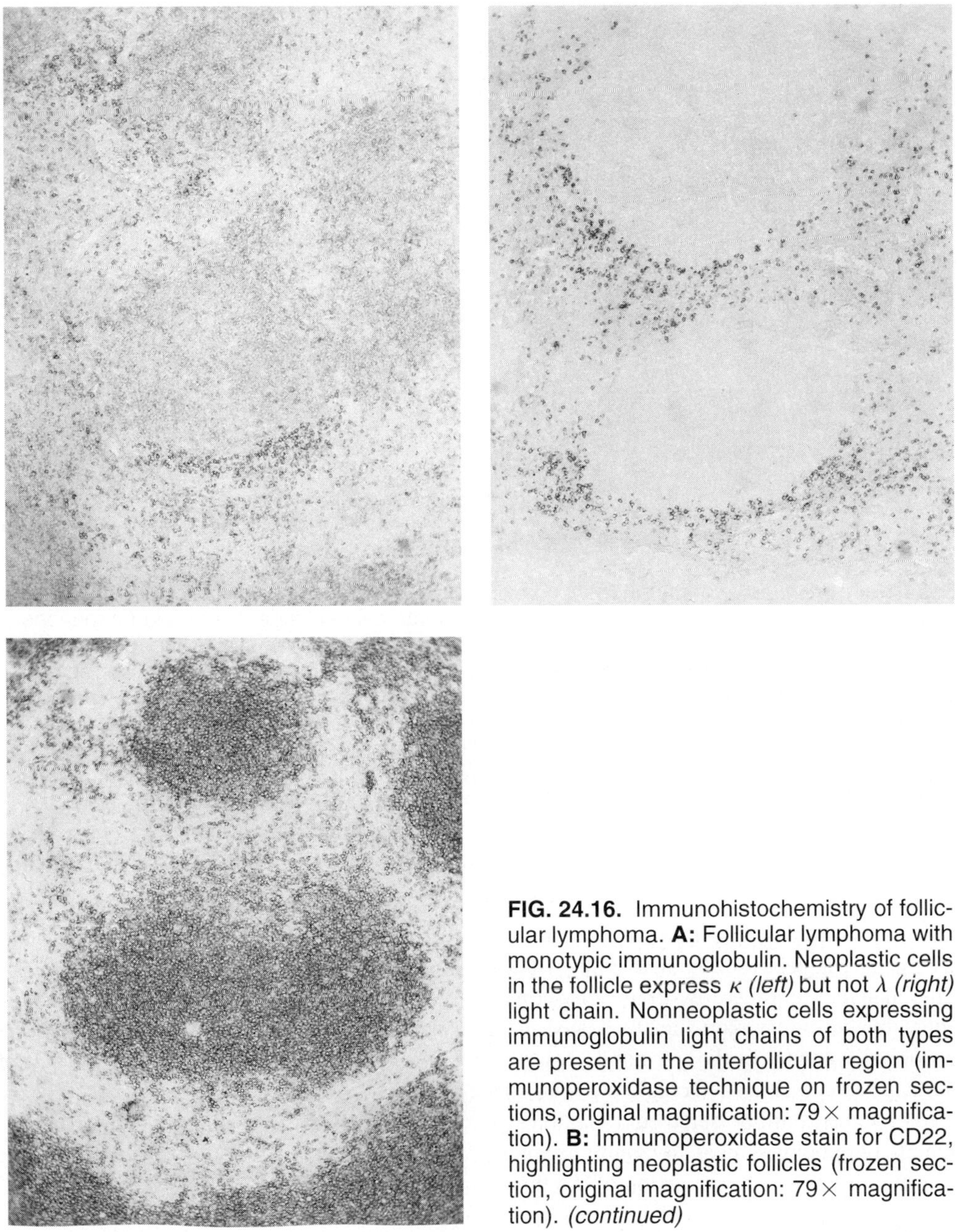

A

B

FIG. 24.16. Immunohistochemistry of follicular lymphoma. **A:** Follicular lymphoma with monotypic immunoglobulin. Neoplastic cells in the follicle express κ *(left)* but not λ *(right)* light chain. Nonneoplastic cells expressing immunoglobulin light chains of both types are present in the interfollicular region (immunoperoxidase technique on frozen sections, original magnification: 79× magnification). **B:** Immunoperoxidase stain for CD22, highlighting neoplastic follicles (frozen section, original magnification: 79× magnification). *(continued)*

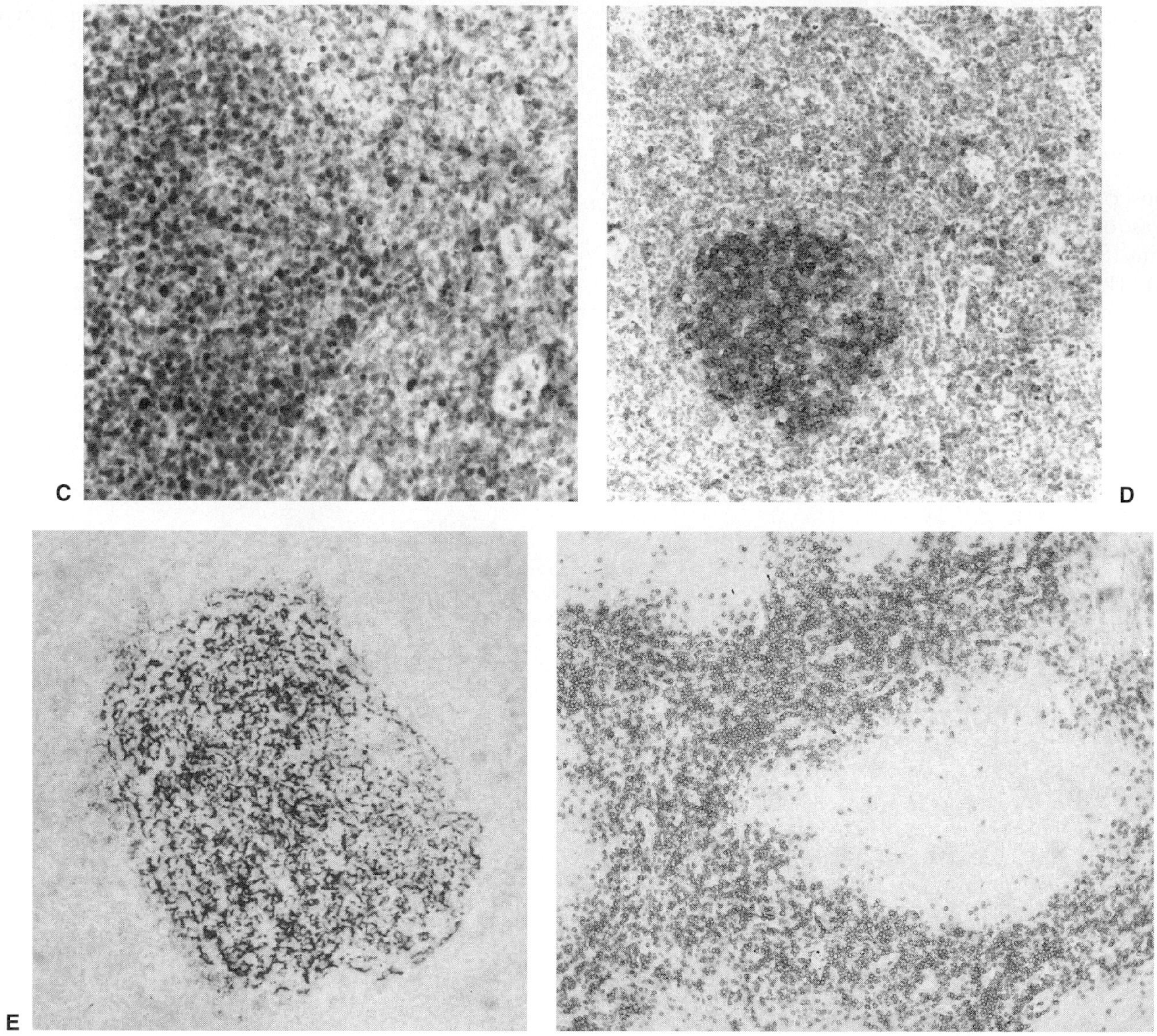

FIG. 24.16. *Continued.* **C:** Immunoperoxidase stain for BCL-6 protein in a follicular lymphoma provides nuclear staining of most cells in the follicle and scattered cells outside the follicle (immunoperoxidase stain on paraffin section, original magnification: 200× magnification). **D:** Immunoperoxidase stain for CD10 shows positive staining of follicles and scattered positive cells in the interfollicular region (immunoperoxidase stains, paraffin section, original magnification: 125× magnification). **E:** Neoplastic follicle with prominent staining for CD21 in a dendritic pattern (immunoperoxidase technique on frozen section, original magnification: 125× magnification). **F:** Follicular lymphoma stained for CD3. Neoplastic follicles contain few T cells, but numerous T cells are present in the interfollicular region (immunoperoxidase technique on frozen section, original magnification: 79× magnification).

class, with a minority also expressing δ; however, a large minority express γ heavy chains, and rare cases express α heavy chain (24). This frequency of Ig heavy-chain class switching is higher than that for other low-grade lymphomas and is consistent with the observation that Ig heavy-chain class switching normally occurs in the germinal center. In a minority of the cases, there is no detectable sIg, but pan-B-cell antigen expression can still be detected (24,158) (Fig. 24.16B). Follicular lymphomas also invariably express BCL-6 nuclear protein in at least a proportion of the tumor cells (159) (Fig. 24.16C). In approximately 60% of the cases, CD10 (CALLA) can be detected on the neoplastic follicle center cells (Fig. 24.16D); CD10 expression is often stronger in the follicles than in interfollicular neoplastic cells (24,76,160). Most cases express the BCL-2 protein (67); the frequency is highest in grade 1 and 2 cases, and as low as 50% in grade 3 cases (Fig. 24.16C) (161). Follicular lymphoma is $CD5^-$ and typically $CD43^-$ (162–164). Most $CD43^+$ cases are grade 3 with diffuse areas (164). Follicular lymphoma cells typically express the CD95/FAS protein

TABLE 24.5. *Small B-cell neoplasms: immunophenotypic and genetic features*

Neoplasm	sIg; cIg (F/P)	CD5 (F)	CD10 (F)	CD23 (F/P)	CD43 (F/P)	Cyclin D1 (P)	BCL-6 protein	Genetic abnormality	Ig V-region genes
Follicular lymphoma	+; −	−	+/−	−/+	−	−	+	t(14;18); *BCL*-2R	Mutated, ongoing
Mantle cell lymphoma	+; −	+	−	−	+	+	−	t(11;14); *BCL*-1R	Unmutated
Extranodal and nodal marginal zone lymphoma	+; +/−	−	−	−/+	−/+	−	−	Trisomy 3; t(11;18) (extranodal)	Mutated, ongoing (?)
B-CLL/SLL	+; −/+	+	−	+	+	−/+	−	Trisomy 12 (15%); 13q deletions	60% unmutated; 40% mutated
Lymphoplasmacytic lymphoma	+; +	−	−	−	−/+	−	−	t(9;14); *PAX*-5R	Mutated
Splenic marginal zone lymphoma	+; −/+	−	−	−	−	−/+	−	NA	Mutated

(165). CD21 expression by neoplastic germinal center B cells is difficult to assess, because of the prominent dendritic cell staining (Fig. 24.16E). In somewhat less than 50% of the cases, there appears to be some CD21 expression by the neoplastic cells. CD23 expression is similarly variable. Follicular lymphomas also express costimulatory molecules CD80 and CD86 (B7-1a and B7-2) and CD40 (76,166). Expression of these antigens is weak compared with that of normal germinal center B cells (166).

Follicular dendritic cells are readily demonstrated by use of monoclonal antibodies against the CD21 antigen; nodular aggregates of FDCs are virtually always present in follicular lymphomas, outlining the neoplastic follicles (Fig. 24.16E). In diffuse areas of follicular lymphomas, FDCs are typically absent; this fact may be useful in distinguishing diffuse follicle center lymphoma from mantle cell and marginal zone lymphomas, in which large, irregular aggregates of FDCs are seen even in areas that appear diffuse on routine staining (24).

T cells are usually less numerous in neoplastic than reactive follicles, and seldom show the crescentic arrangement at the junction with the mantle zone, that may be seen in reactive follicles (167,168). $CD4^+$ cells predominate, as in reactive follicles. The interfollicular region also contains numerous T cells of both subsets (Fig. 24.16F). In cell suspension studies, it is not unusual for the T cells to outnumber the neoplastic follicular center cells, although on average, they comprise about 25% of the cells. There is no consistent association of T-cell number or distribution with histologic subtype of follicular lymphoma or with stage or prognosis.

GENETIC FEATURES OF FOLLICULAR LYMPHOMA

Immunoglobulin Genes

Like other B-cell lymphomas, follicular lymphoma has rearranged immunoglobulin heavy- and light-chain genes, demonstrable as clonal bands on Southern blot analysis or polymerase chain reaction (PCR) (Table 24.5) (see Chapters 7 and 9). Like normal germinal center B cells, the cells of follicular lymphoma have somatic mutations in the variable regions of their immunoglobulin genes (105,169–171). In most cases studied, there is intraclonal variation in the somatic mutations, indicating that the mutation process is ongoing in these cells, similar to normal germinal center B cells (47,172). Studies of the frequency of replacement (R) to silent (S) mutations in the framework (FWR) and complementarity-determining (CDR) regions have been interpreted to indicate a role for antigen selection in these cases (105). As expected from normal germinal center cells, Ig heavy-chain class switching occurs in approximately 40% of the cases (173).

Detailed analysis of the Ig genes in cases of follicular lymphoma has revealed some unexpected findings. Using the technique of DNA fiber fluorescence *in situ* hybridization (FISH), the group at Leiden (173) have shown that IgG-expressing follicular lymphomas showed normal class switching on the functional allele and on the nonfunctional allele involved in the *BCL2* translocation. In contrast, in 85% of IgM-expressing follicular lymphomas, the translocated allele had undergone class switching, while the nontranslocated, functional allele showed a functional $C\mu$-$C\delta$ region with a complex pattern of downstream heavy-chain constant region (C_H) rearrangements. In cases showing this change, the rearranged $C\mu$ band on Southern blot was 1 to 2 kb smaller than the germline band, consistent with deletion of part of the μ switch ($S\mu$) region. The investigators suggested that deletion of the switch region and additional rearrangements might be seen in cells driven by selective pressure to express IgM, but in which the class switching mechanism remained operative.

Analysis of Ig genes in multiple samples from the same patient has also yielded interesting information. In patients with follicular lymphoma who relapse without transformation to large cell lymphoma, the Ig genes show identical VDJ rearrangements and the pattern of V region mutations continues to show intraclonal heterogeneity (105,174). In contrast, transformation to high grade lymphoma or leukemia has been reported to involve a single clone, without intraclonal diversity (104,175), suggesting that the hypermutation mechanism is switched off with high grade transformation.

Cytogenetic Abnormalities and Oncogenes

In most series, virtually 100% of follicular lymphomas have cytogenetic abnormalities (176) (Table 24.6). The proportion of abnormal metaphases, probably reflecting an increased proliferation fraction of the neoplastic cells, is inversely correlated with patient outcome (177). Follicular lymphomas have translocations involving the long arms of chromosomes 14 and 18—t(14;18)(q32;q21)—in 75% to 90% of the cases (178,179). The t(14;18) is not associated with a better or worse prognosis. Rare cases have a t(2;18)(p12;q21), which places the *BCL2* gene with the light-chain gene on chromosome 2. In cases with t(14;18), it is the sole abnormality in only 10%; the remainder have additional breaks (median of 6 in one study), most commonly involving chromosomes 1, 2, 4, 5, 13, and 17 or additions of X, 7, 12, or 18 (176). This study found that the presence of more than 6 chromosomal breaks was associated with a poor outcome; breaks at 6q23-26 or 17p conferred a worse prognosis and a shorter time to transformation (176,177). The 17p abnormalities may reflect alterations in the *TP53* gene at 7p13, which are associated with transformation in follicular lymphoma (107). Abnormalities at 6q23-36 are found in 10% to 40% of B-cell lymphomas of all types, and are the most common second abnormality in cases with the t(14;18). Three distinct deletions have been described at 6q21, 6q23, and 6q25-27, suggesting the presence of three distinct tumor suppressor genes (180). Deletions and other alterations of chromosome 9p, involving the p15 and p16 gene loci, have been reported in cases of follicular lymphoma that transform to diffuse large B-cell lymphoma (181,182) (see Chapter 10).

TABLE 24.6. *Follicular lymphoma: genetic abnormalities*

Abnormalities	Percent positive (approximate)
Cytogenetic	100
+7	20
+18	20
t(14;18)(q32;q21)	80
3q27–28	15
6q23–26[a]	15
17p[a]	15
Oncogene	
BCL2 rearranged	80
BCL6 rearranged	15
BCL6 5′ mutations	40

[a] Associated with a worse prognosis (176).

BCL2

Analysis of the t(14;18) breakpoint revealed a segment of DNA that was clonally rearranged in most follicular lymphomas and comigrated with the rearranged immunoglobulin gene in Southern blots of tumor DNA (183,184). The gene encoded by this segment was given the name *BCL2* (see Chapter 8). The BCL-2 protein is expressed by resting B and T cells, but not by normal germinal center cells, cortical thymocytes (33), or monocytoid B cells (185). Transgenic mice expressing the *BCL2* gene develop massive follicular lymphoid hyperplasia, with persistence of a mature B-cell population (186). Overexpression of BCL-2 protein confers a survival advantage on B cells *in vitro,* by preventing apoptosis under conditions of growth factor deprivation (187). Follicular lymphomas are tumors of germinal center B cells, in which centrocytes fail to undergo apoptosis because they have a chromosomal rearrangement, t(14;18), that prevents the normal switching off of the antiapoptosis gene, *BCL2* (67). This finding correlates with the morphologic appearance and biologic behavior of follicular lymphomas, consistent with tumors of resting rather than rapidly proliferating cells.

BCL2 gene rearrangement can be detected in 75% of follicular lymphomas by Southern blot; in one series the sensitivity of Southern blot was slightly lower than that of classic cytogenetics, but higher than that for PCR analysis of the breakpoint, which detected it in 65% of the cases (179).

BCL6

The *BCL6* gene was cloned from the breakpoint of the 3q27 translocation found in a subset of diffuse large B-cell lymphomas (188). This gene is a zinc finger transcriptional repressor (189) that is normally expressed in germinal center B cells (43,45) and in rare intrafollicular and interfollicular $CD4^+$ T cells; its presence is required for germinal center formation (190). The translocation, which involves a variety of other chromosomes, always involves the 5′ noncoding region of the *BCL6* gene, which is replaced by the promotor of the partner gene. It is presumed that these translocations prevent downregulation of *BCL6* and in some way prevent the cell from progressing past the germinal center stage, facilitating neoplastic transformation (43). The *BCL6* gene undergoes mutations in the 5′ noncoding region in normal germinal center B cells (50–52); an association of this process with immunoglobulin gene mutation has been suggested but not proven. One study found *BCL6* mutations in approximately 50% of cases of B-cell chronic lymphocytic leukemia, and these did not correlate with the presence of immunoglobulin gene mutations (191). Abnormalities of 3q27 and *BCL6* rearrangement are found in about 15% of follicular lymphomas, and 5′ mutations of the *BCL6* gene are found in approximately 40% (50) (see Chapter 8).

DIFFERENTIAL DIAGNOSIS OF FOLLICULAR LYMPHOMA

Follicular Hyperplasia

Reactive follicular hyperplasia is the major differential diagnosis in cases of follicular lymphoma. In most cases, typical architectural and cytologic features readily permit the diagnosis of follicular lymphoma based on histologic criteria alone (8,68). In difficult cases, immunophenotyping and, less often, molecular genetic studies can be helpful in establishing a diagnosis.

Morphologic Criteria

Pattern

Effacement of the normal architecture by closely packed, relatively uniform follicles that lack a mantle zone and extend outside the nodal capsule is the diagnostic appearance of follicular lymphoma (Table 24.7). However, one or more of these features may be lacking in many cases. Follicles may be widely spaced, vary in size and shape, have a mantle zone, or be confined within the capsule with preservation of some sinuses. Foci of uninvolved lymph node may be present, with some reactive follicles. In such cases, close attention must be paid to the other diagnostic features that are present. Several architectural criteria are useful in difficult cases. First, close packing of follicles, even focally, particularly if the follicles in this area are small and uniform, is very suggestive of lymphoma. Second, if the follicles are widely spaced, the interfollicular region should be examined at high magnification for the presence of centrocytes (small cleaved cells). Transformed cells (immunoblasts and occasionally centroblasts) can be seen in the interfollicular regions of reactive nodes, but centrocytes are virtually never found outside germinal centers in nonneoplastic lymph nodes (Fig. 24.6). A third helpful feature is extension of follicles outside the capsule in association with concentric bands of sclerosis (Fig. 24.5). In lymphadenitis, capsular fibrosis often occurs, with small lymphocytes and plasma cells present in perinodal fat, but germinal centers are rarely seen outside the capsule. Sclerosis within the lymph node, particularly in diffuse areas, is a fourth feature that is very suggestive of lymphoma; areas of sclerosis should be scrutinized at high magnification for the presence of centrocytes (Fig. 24.7). Transmural invasion of the walls of small or medium-sized veins by centrocytes, within the node or in perinodal tissue, is often seen and is highly suggestive of lymphoma (Fig. 24.8).

TABLE 24.7. *Histologic features useful in the differential diagnosis of follicular lymphoma and follicular hyperplasia*

Feature	Utility	Frequency
Predominance of centrocytes in follicles	Diagnostic	High
Interfollicular centrocytes	Diagnostic	High
Transmural vascular invasion	Diagnostic	High
Close packing of follicles	Highly suggestive	High
Diffuse areas/sclerosis	Highly suggestive	High
Extranodal extension (follicles)	Highly suggestive	High
Absence of mantle zone	Suggestive	High
Absence of "starry sky" cells	Suggestive	High
Presence of mantle zone	Not helpful	Low
Presence of some reactive follicles	Not helpful	Low
Size/shape/uniformity of follicles	Not helpful	—
"Cracking" artifact/reticulin	Not helpful	—

Cytology

The neoplastic follicles in most follicular lymphomas contain a monotonous population of centrocytes, which readily distinguishes them from germinal centers, in which centroblasts are more numerous. The cases that cause problems in diagnosis are typically of grade 2 or 3 (mixed or large cell type), in which the admixture of centroblasts more closely approximates that of the normal germinal center. In these cases, the absence of phagocytic "tingible body" macrophages, a low mitotic rate, lack of polarization, crowding of follicles, and lack of a mantle zone are all helpful features. In some cases, the centroblasts or large centrocytes may have a cytologically atypical appearance, with hyperchromatic or abnormally shaped nuclei. The cytology of the interfollicular, extranodal, and diffuse areas in these cases can be essential in establishing the diagnosis.

Immunophenotyping

Immunohistologic studies are not necessary for the diagnosis in most cases of follicular lymphoma, but can be very helpful in difficult cases. In the distinction of benign from malignant lymphoid infiltrates, the most reliable criterion is immunoglobulin light-chain restriction, which is best evaluated by immunohistochemistry on frozen tissue sections or in cell suspensions by flow cytometry. Evidence of light-chain restriction (κ or λ) within the follicles is diagnostic of lymphoma. Normal germinal centers contain a characteristic pattern of extracellular deposition of immunoglobulin on follicular dendritic cell processes; this pattern is almost always absent in neoplastic follicles (Fig. 24.1F and 24.16A). Rare cases of follicular lymphoma are Ig^-. Total absence of immunoglobulin staining is an abnormal finding, and is strongly suggestive of neoplastic follicles.

Immunohistochemical staining for BCL-2 protein is the most useful technique for distinguishing follicular lymphoma from follicular hyperplasia on paraffin tissue sections. Sections must be examined together with sections stained for CD20 and CD3, because numerous $BCL\text{-}2^+$ T cells may be present in reactive and neoplastic follicles;

staining of these cells should not be misinterpreted as BCL-2 expression by neoplastic cells. In many cases, the neoplastic follicle center cells express BCL-2 more strongly than surrounding mantle zone or interfollicular cells, but in some cases, staining of follicular lymphoma cells may be faint, and may be restricted to a subset of the cells, usually centrocytes. Unfortunately, BCL-2 positivity is less common in grade 3 follicular lymphomas, which cause the greatest problems in differential diagnosis with reactive hyperplasia (161).

Expression of CD10 (CALLA) is more easily detectable in neoplastic than in reactive follicles, but cannot be considered a criterion for malignancy, because CD10 is also expressed by normal germinal center cells (24). Detection of $CD10^+$ cells in the interfollicular region is suggestive of follicular lymphoma; however, interfollicular neoplastic cells may lack CD10 or express it more weakly than those within the follicles (24,76). Assessment of proliferation fraction using Ki-67 may be of some help, because in reactive follicles, most of the cells are in cycle, whereas even in grade 3 follicular lymphomas, the proliferation fraction is rarely more than 50%.

Molecular Genetic Analysis

Southern blot or PCR analysis for immunoglobulin or *BCL2* rearrangements can be more sensitive for detecting small clonal populations than conventional immunophenotyping, and may also prove clonality in Ig^- tumors. Southern blot analysis requires fresh tissue and can detect immunoglobulin gene rearrangements in most follicular lymphomas (179). PCR analysis is less sensitive, with only about 65% of follicular lymphomas showing clonal rearrangements; this lack of sensitivity has been attributed to the failure of consensus primers to bind because of extensive somatic mutations in the immunoglobulin genes in follicular lymphoma. In one study, 89% of follicular lymphoma cases had the t(14;18) by cytogenetic analysis, 75% had *BCL2* rearrangement by Southern blot and 65% had *BCL2* rearrangement detectable by PCR (179). PCR analysis has a significant false-negative rate for detection of immunoglobulin and *BCL2* rearrangement. Because *BCL2* rearrangement can be detected in some normal tonsils and lymph nodes, detection of a small clonal population by this technique is not diagnostic of malignancy (192).

Other Lymphomas

A true follicular pattern is virtually diagnostic of follicular lymphoma. However, other lymphomas with a vaguely nodular pattern may resemble follicular lymphoma; these include mantle cell lymphoma, marginal zone lymphoma, occasionally small lymphocytic lymphoma, and rarely Hodgkin's disease.

Small B-Cell Lymphomas: Mantle Cell, Marginal Zone, and Small Lymphocytic Lymphoma

Morphologic Features

The morphologic features of small B-cell lymphomas are summarized in Table 24.8. Cases of mantle cell lymphoma may have a vaguely nodular or, rarely, a truly follicular pattern. In most cases, the follicular pattern is only focal, with large diffuse areas. In contrast to follicular lymphoma, which always contains a mixture of neoplastic centroblasts and centrocytes, mantle cell lymphoma contains a monotonous population of small cells that resemble centrocytes, with virtually no blast cells. Occasional centroblasts can be seen in areas of partially overrun follicles. In many cases, foci of preserved germinal centers surrounded by a mantle zone of atypical cells can be found; this appearance would be unusual in follicular lymphoma. In many cases of mantle cell lymphoma, there is a characteristic infiltrate of single epithelioid histiocytes, which are nonphagocytic. Mantle cell lymphoma often has a higher mitotic rate than follicular lymphoma. The character of the blood vessels may also provide a clue as to the diagnosis. In mantle cell lymphoma, the small vessels that proliferate are not usually of the high endothelial venule type; they have flat endothelial cells and often have eosinophilic sclerosis of their walls. In diffuse areas of follicular lymphoma, the proliferating small vessels are usually of the HEV type and do not show prominent sclerosis. Compartmentalizing fibrosis, which is commonly seen at least focally in diffuse follicle center lymphoma, is rare in mantle

TABLE 24.8. *Small B-cell neoplasms: histological features*

Neoplasm	Pattern	Small cells	Transformed cells
Follicular lymphoma	Follicular +/− diffuse areas, rarely diffuse	Cleaved	Centroblasts
Mantle cell lymphoma	Diffuse, vaguely nodular, mantle zone, rarely follicular	Cleaved (rarely round or oval)	None
Marginal zone B-cell lymphoma	Diffuse, interfollicular, marginal zone, follicular colonization	Heterogeneous: round (small lymphocytes), cleaved (marginal zone/monocytoid B cells), plasma cells	Centroblast-like, immunoblast-like
B-CLL/SLL	Diffuse with pseudofollicles	Round (occasionally cleaved)	Prolymphocytes, paraimmunoblasts
Lymphoplasmacytic lymphoma	Diffuse; no pseudofollicles	Round (may be cleaved) Plasma cells	Centroblasts, immunoblasts

cell lymphoma. Diffuse areas of follicular lymphomas frequently contain large numbers of small, reactive T lymphocytes, while mantle cell lymphoma contains many fewer reactive cells.

Marginal zone lymphomas may have a partially follicular pattern, which results from the presence of follicles that have been "colonized" by neoplastic marginal zone cells. Typically, these follicles are widely spaced in a background of interfollicular marginal zone cells, but occasionally they can be numerous, and mimic follicular lymphoma. Marginal zone lymphoma also enters the differential diagnosis of diffuse follicle center lymphoma, because both contain a mixture of small cells with irregular nuclei and large centroblasts or immunoblasts. Problems can also arise when biopsy specimens are small, and a mixed population of centrocyte-like cells and centroblast-like cells is present without an obvious pattern.

Small lymphocytic lymphoma/chronic lymphocytic leukemia (SLL/CLL)typically has a pseudofollicular pattern in lymph nodes; this can be mistaken for a true follicular pattern and result in confusion with follicular lymphoma. In general, pseudofollicles are uniform in size and shape and evenly spaced throughout the node, like bacterial colonies on a culture dish, giving what some have called a "cloudy sky" pattern. They are poorly demarcated from the surrounding infiltrate, so that they seem to "disappear" at progressively higher magnifications. They contain cells with predominantly round nuclei, and show a subtle gradation from small lymphocytes to prolymphocytes to paraimmunoblasts, in contrast to the sharp dichotomy between centrocytes and centroblasts in follicular lymphoma. Sclerosis and extranodal extension are uncommon in SLL/CLL.

Immunophenotype

The immunophenotypic and genetic features of small B-cell lymphomas are summarized in Table 24.5. Mantle cell lymphoma and SLL/CLL characteristically express IgM, IgD, CD5, and CD43, and most cases are negative for CD10. In contrast, follicular lymphoma is usually IgD^-, IgG^+ or IgM^+, $CD5^-$, and 50% to 80% are $CD10^+$ (162). With antibodies to FDCs, follicular areas in follicular lymphoma are highlighted by concentric aggregates of FDCs, while diffuse areas show few if any FDCs. In contrast, mantle cell lymphomas and many marginal zone lymphomas show large, irregular FDC aggregates throughout the tumors (24,150). Staining for BCL-2 may highlight residual reactive follicles in mantle cell lymphoma and marginal zone lymphoma, whereas follicle centers are positive in follicular lymphoma. BCL-2 staining of the extrafollicular neoplastic cells is not helpful in the differential diagnosis of small B-cell lymphomas, because all are positive. Staining for cyclin D1 shows nuclear staining in virtually all mantle cell lymphomas, but follicular lymphoma is negative (193). This is particularly useful in the rare cases of $CD5^-$ mantle cell lymphoma (194).

Immunophenotyping is least useful in the differential diagnosis between follicular lymphoma and marginal zone lymphoma with follicular colonization. Reactive and neoplastic follicle center cells can be $CD10^+$, and marginal zone B cells within colonized follicles may be BCL-2^- (195). Expression of CD10 by extrafollicular B cells is potentially useful in this differential diagnosis, tending to confirm follicle center lymphoma (150,159), although extrafollicular neoplastic cells in follicular lymphoma may lack or weakly express CD10 (24,76). Similarly, the expression of BCL-6 by extrafollicular cells is seen in follicular lymphoma but not in marginal zone lymphoma (150,159).

Molecular Genetic Analysis

The *BCL2* gene rearrangement characteristic of follicular lymphoma is not found in mantle cell, small lymphocytic or marginal zone lymphoma, while *BCL1/PRAD1* gene rearrangement is detectable by PCR in about 40% of mantle cell lymphomas and not in follicular lymphoma (Table 24.5).

Hodgkin's Disease

Rarely, cases of follicular lymphoma with interfollicular sclerosis may resemble Hodgkin's disease, nodular sclerosis type (NSHD). This confusion occurs in cases with very atypical large centrocytes and centroblasts, in which the atypical cells may resemble mononuclear or diagnostic Reed-Sternberg cells. In these cases, the binucleate centroblasts do not have the abundant cytoplasm and multilobated nuclei of typical lacunar cells, and the background cells are centrocytes, rather than the lymphocytes, eosinophils, and plasma cells of NSHD. Nonetheless, in some cases, immunohistologic studies may be required to distinguish the two (HD: $CD15^+$, $CD30^+$, $CD45^{-/+}$, and $CD20^{-/+}$; follicular: $CD15^-$, $CD30^-$, $CD45^+$, $CD20^+$, and Ig^+).

Occasionally, follicular lymphoma and nodular lymphocyte predominance Hodgkin's disease (NLPHD) may resemble one another. This problem is most common in the so-called floral variant of follicular lymphoma. In this morphologic variant of follicular lymphoma, grade 3 (large cell), numerous small, polyclonal B cells are present around and within the nodules of large, neoplastic follicle center B cells (Fig. 24.3B). On morphologic examination, the size and shape of the follicles is useful, because those of follicular lymphoma tend to be more uniform and smaller than the very large, variably sized nodules of NLPHD. Centrocytes are much more numerous in the nodules of follicular lymphoma than in those of NLPHD. Immunohistologic criteria must be used with caution, because the atypical cells and the background lymphocytes of NLPHD share many antigens with normal germinal center cells and with follicular lymphoma. Demonstration of monotypic Ig is diagnostic of follicular lymphoma. BCL-2 positivity of the large cells is helpful, because the neoplastic cells of LPHD typically lack BCL-2. Demonstration of monotypic Ig by Southern blot or

PCR or demonstration of *BCL2* rearrangement would strongly favor a diagnosis of follicular lymphoma in this setting.

CLINICAL FEATURES OF FOLLICULAR LYMPHOMA

Demographic Features

Follicular lymphoma is a disease of adults, with a median age of 55 (6,8) (Table 24.2). In contrast to most other hematologic malignancies, in which males predominate, follicular lymphoma occurs with approximately equal frequency in men and women (6,8) (Table 24.2). Follicular lymphoma is more common in the United States and western Europe than in other parts of the world (88). In most American series, follicular lymphoma constitutes on average 40% of adult non-Hodgkin's lymphoma. It is uncommon in Japan, where T-cell lymphomas predominate, and is seen relatively infrequently in underdeveloped countries.

Follicular lymphoma occasionally occurs in individuals under age 20 years; patients are predominantly males with disease localized to the head and neck (often tonsils) and approximately 50% are of large cell (grade 3) type (196–201). The prognosis of these patients appears to be good, with most reported cases disease free at the time of last follow-up.

Stage and Sites of Involvement

Most patients with follicular lymphoma have widespread disease at the time of the diagnosis, even though they may feel relatively well (18,88). In most studies, the majority of patients are in stage III or IV. Most patients present with nodal involvement, and purely extranodal presentations are uncommon. The most common sites of stage IV disease are bone marrow and liver. Nonnodal presentations usually involve the spleen, Waldeyer's ring or the gastrointestinal tract; skin and soft tissue presentations occur less often, and primary lymphoma of bone or central nervous system is virtually never of follicular type (see Chapters 31 through 36). Most of the patients probably have circulating neoplastic cells, and 10% are frankly leukemic. In contrast to leukemic involvement in high-grade non-Hodgkin's lymphoma, this finding does not confer a worse prognosis in patients with follicular lymphoma (141).

Prognosis

Clinical Factors

Follicular lymphoma is an indolent lymphoma, and like most other indolent hematologic malignancies, most cases are not curable with available therapy (18,88). Most patients respond well to chemotherapy of almost any type and to local radiation therapy (202). Patients with advanced clinical stage and adverse clinical prognostic factors according to the International Prognostic Index (IPI) (high LDH, bulky disease, poor performance status) may have much shorter survival than the more typical patients without these factors (88). Cases of early stage (I and II) follicular lymphoma may have very long disease-free survival with local therapy (202). Some studies report very long disease-free survivals in patients treated with aggressive combination chemotherapy (203). However, the curability of follicular lymphoma is still debated. Initial therapy in advanced cases is directed at relief of symptoms, and care is taken not to compromise the ability of the patient to tolerate more aggressive therapy later, when the disease becomes more aggressive.

Histologic Grade

The prognostic value of grading follicular lymphomas clearly depends on the method used, and of course also on how the patients are treated in a given study. In studies using the "estimation of predominant cell" method, no clear difference was established between the small cleaved cell and mixed cell categories, in a number of studies (204), although cases classified as predominantly large cell had a more aggressive clinical course in most studies. Several early reports using the cell counting method showed a difference in response to treatment and survival for the mixed small and large cell type, compared with the small cleaved cell type (203,205). A subsequent study from a cooperative group (206) failed to show a potential for cure, but confirmed a significant difference in survival between the small cleaved and mixed cell types. The curability of grade 2 follicular lymphoma remains a subject of debate. Most published studies show a significantly more aggressive clinical course for grade 3 cases (90,91,205,207). These cases are typically treated with combination chemotherapy as for diffuse large B-cell lymphoma; their prognosis appears to be slightly better than that for diffuse large B-cell lymphoma, but with an increased likelihood of relapse (87,90,208–210). In a study of the REAL classification, grade 3 follicular lymphoma had a significantly worse overall survival when treated with non–Aadriamycin-containing regimens; the survival in the group treated with Adriamycin was identical to that of grade 1 and grade 2 cases (89).

Diffuse Areas

Many studies (8,18,21,211) have indicated that the presence of even very large diffuse areas in a follicular lymphoma of grade 1 or 2 (small cleaved or mixed small and large cell) does not significantly alter the prognosis; therefore, if any definite follicular areas are seen in a lymphoma of follicle center type, the tumor is classified as follicular lymphoma. However, some studies have suggested that the degree of nodularity does have an impact on survival (212,213). A study from Stanford University (213) suggested that patients with mixed small and large cell lymphomas showing less than 25% follicular pattern had a significantly worse survival than those whose tumors were more than 50% follicular; patients with tumors that were more than 50% follicular did not differ in outcome from those whose tumors were 100% follicular. A review of patients with follicular grade 1 and 2 (i.e., small cleaved and mixed small and large cell) lymphomas treated by a large cooperative group (212) revealed that cases with a predominantly (>75%) follicular pattern had a significantly longer median survival than patients with a follicular and diffuse (>25% diffuse) pattern (39.6 versus 68.2 months, $p < 0.003$). In grade 3 follicular lymphoma (follicular large cell), the presence of diffuse areas is more common than in grade 1 and grade 2 cases, and most observers believe that this finding is clinically significant. A Stanford study (211) showed that grade 3 follicular lymphomas with diffuse areas up to 50% had a prognosis intermediate between that of purely follicular cases and purely diffuse large cell lymphomas; a later study of follicular grade 3 lymphoma from the same institution confirmed pattern as an independent prognostic feature (90). However, studies from Nebraska suggest that pattern is not a significant prognostic factor in grade 3 follicular lymphoma (87,214).

Histologic Transformation

In 25% to 35% of patients with follicular lymphoma, transformation or "progression" to a large cell lymphoma, usually diffuse, occurs (94,95). This occurrence is usually associated with a rapidly progressive clinical course and death from tumor that is refractory to treatment (95,215).

Less commonly, patients with follicular lymphoma develop acute leukemia. This may take one of two forms. Patients who have received multiple or prolonged courses of alkylating agent therapy are at increased risk of developing acute nonlymphoid leukemia, similar to patients with other tumors such as ovarian cancer, myeloma, and Hodgkin's disease (216). The leukemias in these patients are believed to result from a direct oncogenic effect of the alkylating agents on bone marrow myeloid stem cells. Rare patients develop acute lymphoid leukemia, which in most cases appears to represent blast transformation of the original B-cell tumor (99).

SUMMARY AND CONCLUSIONS

Follicular lymphoma is a distinctive tumor that reproduces most of the morphologic, immunophenotypic, and genetic features of the lymphoid germinal center. The biologic behavior of the tumor is ordained by a chromosomal translocation resulting in activation of a gene, *BCL2,* that confers a survival advantage on nonproliferating neoplastic cells, averting the rapid cell death that is thought to be the fate of most normal germinal center cells. The diagnosis in most cases is relatively straightforward, relying on morphologic evidence of uncontrolled accumulation of centrocytes, accompanied by rare self-renewing centroblasts. The neoplastic germinal center cells appear to follow the migration routes of their normal counterparts, resulting in a tumor that shows widespread involvement of lymphoid tissues, with homing to normal follicular regions, and which is rarely truly extralymphatic in its presentation. Clinically, follicular lymphoma is an indolent malignancy, with a long median survival that is unaffected by treatment in most cases; the pace of the disease is predictable to some extent by the number of centroblasts in the neoplastic follicles. Transformation to an aggressive lymphoma may occur when additional chromosomal translocations or mutations result in activation of oncogenes or inactivation of suppressor genes, resulting in increased cell proliferation.

REFERENCES

1. Brill N, Baehr G, Rosenthal N. Generalized giant lymph follicle hyperplasia of the lymph nodes and spleen: a hitherto undescribed type. *JAMA* 1925;84:668–671.
2. Symmers D. Follicular lymphadenopathy with splenomegaly: a newly recognized disease of the lymphatic system. *Arch Pathol* 1927;3:816–820.
3. Baehr G. The clinical and pathological picture of follicular lymphoblastoma. *Trans Assoc Am Physicians* 1932;47:330–338.
4. Symmers D. Giant follicular lymphadenopathy with or without splenomegaly. *Arch Pathol* 1938;26:603–647.
5. Jackson H Jr, Parker F Jr. Hodgkin's disease and allied disorders. *N Engl J Med* 1939;220:26–30.
6. Gall EA, Morrison HR, Scott AT. The follicular type of malignant lymphoma: a survey of 63 cases. *Ann Intern Med* 1941;14:2073–2090.
7. Gall EA, Mallory TB. Malignant lymphoma: a clinicopathologic survey of 618 cases. *Am J Pathol* 1942;18:381–395.
8. Rappaport H, Winter W, Hicks E. Follicular lymphoma: a reevaluation of its position in the scheme of malignant lymphoma, based on a survey of 253 cases. *Cancer* 1956;9:792–821.
9. Rappaport H. Tumors of the hematopoietic system. In *Atlas of tumor pathology,* Vol 1, Section III. Washington, DC: Armed Forces Institute of Pathology, 1966.
10. Lennert K. Germinal centers and germinal center neoplasia. *Acta Haematol Jpn* 1969;32:495–500.
11. Lennert K, Mohri N, Stein H, et al. The histopathology of malignant lymphoma. *Br J Haematol* 1975;31[Suppl]:193–203.
12. Gerard-Marchant R, Hamlin I, Lennert K, et al. Classification of non-Hodgkin's lymphomas. *Lancet* 1974;2:406–408.
13. Lukes R, Collins R. Immunologic characterization of human malignant lymphomas. *Cancer* 1974;34:1488–1503.
14. Jaffe E, Shevach E, Frank M, et al. Nodular lymphoma: evidence for origin from follicular B lymphocytes. *N Engl J Med* 1974;290:813–819.
15. Warnke R, Levy R. Follicular lymphoma: a model of B lymphocyte homing. *N Engl J Med* 1974;298:481.
16. Harris N, Data R. The distribution of neoplastic and normal B-lymphoid cells in nodular lymphomas: use of an immunoperoxidase technique on frozen sections. *Hum Pathol* 1982;13:610–617.
17. Stein H, Gerdes J, Mason D. The normal and malignant germinal centre. *Clin Haematol* 1982;11:531–559.
18. Non-Hodgkin's lymphoma pathologic classification project. National Cancer Institute sponsored study of classifications of non-Hodgkin's lymphomas: summary and description of a Working Formulation for clinical usage. *Cancer* 1982;49:2112–2135.
19. Harris NL, Jaffe ES, Stein H, et al. A revised European-American classification of lymphoid neoplasms: a proposal from the International Lymphoma Study Group. *Blood* 1994;84:1361–1392.
20. Harris NL, Jaffe ES, Diebold J, et al. The World Health Organization classification of hematological malignancies. Report of the Clinical Advisory Committee Meeting. *Ann Oncol* 1999 (in press).
21. Lennert K. *Malignant lymphomas other than Hodgkin's disease.* New York: Springer-Verlag, 1978.

22. Nathwani BN, Diamond LW, Winberg CD, et al. Lymphoblastic lymphoma: a clinicopathologic study of 95 patients. *Cancer* 1981;48: 2347–2357.
23. Brittinger G, Bartels H, Common H, et al. Clinical and prognostic relevance of the Kiel classification of non-Hodgkin lymphomas: results of a prospective multicenter study by the Kiel lymphoma study group. *Hematol Oncol* 1984;2:269–306.
24. Harris N, Nadler L, Bhan A. Immunohistologic characterization of two malignant lymphomas of germinal center type (centroblastic/centrocytic and centrocytic) with monoclonal antibodies: follicular and diffuse lymphomas of small cleaved cell types are related but distinct entities. *Am J Pathol* 1984;117:262–272.
25. Harris NL, Jaffe ES, Diebold J, et al. The World Health Organization classification of hematological malignancies. Report of the Clinical Advisory Committee Meeting. *J Clin Oncol* 1999;17:3835–3849.
26. Harris NL, Jaffe ES, Diebold J, et al. The World Health Organization classification of hematological Malignancies. Report of the Clinical Advisory Committee Meeting. *Mod Pathol* 2000;13:193–207.
27. Jaffe ES, Harris NL, Diebold J, et al. World Health Organization classification of neoplastic diseases of the hematopoietic and lymphoid tissues: a progress report. *Am J Clin Pathol* 1999;111: S8–12.
28. Liu Y-J, Zhang J, Lane PJL, et al. Sites of specific B cell activation in primary and secondary responses to T cell-dependent and T cell-independent antigens. *Eur J Immunol* 1991;21:2951–2962.
29. Kuppers R, Zhao M, Hansmann M-L, et al. Tracing B cell development in human germinal centres by molecular analysis of single cells picked from histological sections. *EMBO J* 1993;12:49–55.
30. MacLennan I. Germinal centers. *Annu Rev Immunol* 1994;12: 117–139.
31. Liu Y-J, Oldfield S, MacLennan I. Memory B cells in T-cell dependent antibody responses colonise the splenic marginal zones. *Eur J Immunol* 1988;18:355–362.
32. Liu Y-J, Johnson G, Gordon J, et al. Germinal centres in T-cell–dependent antibody responses. *Immunol Today* 1992;13:1–39.
33. Hockenbery D, Zutter M, Hickey W, et al. BCL2 protein is topographically restricted in tissues characterized by apoptotic cell death. *Proc Natl Acad Sci USA* 1991;88:6961–6965.
34. Durie FH, Foy TM, Masters SR, et al. The role of CD40 in the regulation of humoral and cell-mediated immunity. *Immunol Today* 1994; 15:406–410.
35. Splawski JB. Immunoregulatory role of CD40 in human B cell differentiation. *J Immunol* 1993;150.
36. Freeman G, Freedman A, Segil J, et al. A new member of the Ig superfamily with unique expression on activated and neoplastic B cells. *J Immunol* 1989;143:2714–2722.
37. Freeman GJ, Gribben JG, Boussiotis VA, et al. Cloning of B7-2: a CTLA-4 counter-receptor that costimulates human T cell proliferation. *Science* 1993;262:909–911.
38. Engel P, Gribben J, Freeman G, et al. The B7-2 (B70) costimulatory molecule expressed by monocytes and activated B lymphocytes is the CD86 differentiation antigen. *Blood* 1994;84:1402–1407.
39. Munro J, Freedman A, Aster J, et al. In vivo expression of the B7 costimulatory molecule by subsets of antigen-presenting cells and the malignant cells of Hodgkin's disease. *Blood* 1994;83:793–798.
40. Freedman A, Munro M, Rice G, et al. Adhesion of human B cells to germinal centers in vitro involves VLA-4 and INCAM-110. *Science* 1990;249:1030–1033.
41. Freedman A. Expression of adhesion receptors on normal B cells and B-cell non-Hodgkin's lymphomas. *Semin Hematol* 1993;30:318–328.
42. Nguyen P, Harrisn N, Ritz J. Expression of CD95 in reactive lymphoid tissues and lymphomas. *Lab Invest* 1995;72:653 (abst).
43. Cattoretti G, Chang CC, Cechova K, et al. BCL-6 protein is expressed in germinal-center B cells. *Blood* 1995;86:45–53.
44. Flenghi L, Bigerna B, Fizzotti M, et al. Monoclonal antibodies PG-B6a and PG-B6p recognize, respectively, a highly conserved and a formol-resistant epitope on the human BCL-6 protein amino-terminal region. *Am J Pathol* 1996;148:1543–1555.
45. Allman D, Jain A, Dent A, et al. BCL-6 expression during B-cell activation. *Blood* 1996;87:5257–5268.
46. French DL, Laskov R, Scharff MD. The role of somatic hypermutation in the generation of antibody diversity. *Science* 1989;244:1152.
47. Jacob J, Kelsoe G, Rajewsky K, et al. Intraclonal generation of antibody mutants in germinal centres. *Nature* 1991;354:389.
48. Wabl M, Forni L, Loor F. Switch in immunoglobulin production observed in single clones of committed lymphocytes. *Science* 1978;199: 1078–1079.
49. Berek C. The development of B cells and the B-cell repertoire in the microenvironment of the germinal centre. *Immunol Rev* 1992;126:5.
50. Peng HZ, Du MQ, Koulis A, et al. Nonimmunoglobulin gene hypermutation in germinal center B cells. *Blood* 1999;93:2167–2172.
51. Pasqualucci L, Migliazza A, Fracchiolla N, et al. BCL-6 mutations in normal germinal center B cells: evidence of somatic hypermutation acting outside Ig loci. *Proc Natl Acad Sci USA* 1998;95:11816–11821.
52. Shen HM, Peters A, Baron B, et al. Mutation of BCL-6 gene in normal B cells by the process of somatic hypermutation of Ig genes. *Science* 1998;280:1750–1752.
53. Liu Y-J, Joshua DE, Williams GT, et al. Mechanism of antigen-driven selection in germinal centres. *Nature* 1989;342:929–931.
54. MacLennan I, Liu Y, Oldfield S, et al. The evolution of B-cell clones. *Current Topics in Microbiology and Immunology* 1990;159:37–63.
55. Van den Oord J, De Wolf-Peeters C, De Vos R, et al. Immature sinus histiocytosis. Light- and electron-microscopic features, immunologic phenotype, and relationship with marginal zone lymphocytes. *Am J Pathol* 1985;1985:266–277.
56. van Krieken J, von Schilling C, Kluin P, et al. Splenic marginal zone lymphocytes and related cells in the lymph node: A morphologic and immunohistochemical study. *Hum Pathol* 1989;20:320–325.
57. Smith-Ravin J, Spencer J, Beverley P, et al. Characterization of two monoclonal antibodies (UCL4D12 and UCL3D3) that discriminate between human mantle zone and marginal zone B cells. *Clin Exp Immunol* 1990;82:181–187.
58. Spencer J, Finn T, Pulford K, et al. The human gut contains a novel population of B lymphocytes which resemble marginal zone cells. *Clin Exp Immunol* 1985;62:607–612.
59. Isaacson P, Spencer J. Malignant lymphoma of mucosa-associated lymphoid tissue. *Histopathology* 1987;11:445–462.
60. Klein U, Kuppers R, Rajewsky K. Evidence for a large compartment of IgM-expressing memory B cells in humans. *Blood* 1997;89: 1288–1298.
61. Klein U, Goossens T, Fischer M, et al. Somatic hypermutation in normal and transformed human B cells. *Immunol Rev* 1998;162: 261–280.
62. Dunn-Walters DK, Isaacson PG, Spencer J. Analysis of mutations in immunoglobulin heavy chain variable region genes of microdissected marginal zone (MGZ) B cells suggests that the MGZ of human spleen is a reservoir of memory B cells. *J Exp Med* 1995;182:559–566.
63. Dunn-Walters DK, Isaacson PG, Spencer J. Sequence analysis of rearranged IgV_H genes from microdissected human Peyer's patch marginal zone B cells. *Immunology* 1996;88:618–624.
64. Tierens A, Delabie J, Michiels L, et al. Marginal-zone B cells in the human lymph node and spleen show somatic hypermutations and display clonal expansion. *Blood* 1999;93:226–234.
65. Cardoso de Almeida P, Harris N, Bhan A. Characterization of immature sinus histiocytes (monocytoid cells) in reactive lymph nodes by use of monoclonal antibodies. *Hum Pathol* 1984;15:330–335.
66. Stein K, Hummel M, Korbjuhn P, et al. Monocytoid B cells are distinct from splenic marginal zone cells and commonly derive from unmutated naive B cells and less frequently from postgerminal center B cells by polyclonal transformation. *Blood* 1999;94:2800–2808.
67. Pezzella F, Tse A, Cordell J, et al. Expression of the Bcl-2 oncogene protein is not specific for the 14-18 chromosomal translocation. *Am J Pathol* 1990;137:225–232.
68. Nathwani BN, Winberg CD, Diamond LW, et al. Morphologic criteria for the differentiation of follicular lymphoma from florid reactive follicular hyperplasia: a study of 80 cases. *Cancer* 1981;48: 1794–1806.
69. Osborne BM, Butler JJ. Follicular lymphoma mimicking progressive transformation of germinal centers. *Am J Clin Pathol* 1987;88: 264–269.
70. Goates JJ, Kamel OW, LeBrun DP, et al. Floral variant of follicular lymphoma. Immunological and molecular studies support a neoplastic process. *Am J Surg Pathol* 1994;18:37–47.
71. Ngan B-Y, Warnke R, Wilson M, et al. Monocytoid B-cell lymphoma: a study of 36 cases. *Hum Pathol* 1991;22:409–421.
72. Fisher RI, Dahlberg S, Nathwani BN, et al. A clinical analysis of two indolent lymphoma entities: mantle cell lymphoma and marginal zone lymphoma (including the mucosa-associated lymphoid tissue and

monocytoid B-cell subcategories): a Southwest Oncology Group study. *Blood* 1995;85:1075–1082.

73. Schmid U, Cogliatti SB, Diss TC, et al. Monocytoid/marginal zone B-cell differentiation in follicle centre cell lymphoma. *Histopathology* 1996;29:201–208.
74. Nathwani B, Mohrmann R, Brynes R, et al. Monocytoid B-cell lymphomas: an assessment of diagnostic criteria and a perspective on histogenesis. *Hum Pathol* 1992;23:1061–1071.
75. Nathwani BN, Anderson JR, Armitage JO, et al. Clinical significance of follicular lymphoma with monocytoid B cells. Non-Hodgkin's lymphoma classification project. *Hum Pathol* 1999;30:263–268.
76. Dogan A, Du MQ, Aiello A, et al. Follicular lymphomas contain a clonally linked but phenotypically distinct neoplastic B-cell population in the interfollicular zone. *Blood* 1998;91:4708–4714.
77. Aiello A, Du MQ, Diss TC, et al. Simultaneous phenotypically distinct but clonally identical mucosa-associated lymphoid tissue and follicular lymphoma in a patient with Sjögren's syndrome. *Blood* 1999;94: 2247–2251.
78. Bennett M, Millett Y. Nodular sclerotic lymphosarcoma: a possible new clinico-pathological entity. *Clin Radiol* 1969;20:339–343.
79. Maurer R, Schmid U, Davies JD, et al. Lymph-node infarction and malignant lymphoma: a multicentre survey of European, English and American cases. *Histopathology* 1986;10:571–588.
80. Norton AJ, Ramsay AD, Isaacson PG. Antigen preservation in infarcted lymphoid tissue: a novel approach to the infarcted lymph node using monoclonal antibodies effective in routinely processed tissues. *Am J Surg Pathol* 1988;12:759–767.
81. Laszewski MJ, Belding PJ, Feddersen RM, et al. Clonal immunoglobulin gene rearrangement in the infarcted lymph node syndrome. *Am J Clin Pathol* 1991;96:116–120.
82. Foucar K, Armitage J, Dick F. Malignant lymphomas, diffuse mixed small and large cell: a clinicopathologic study of 47 cases. *Cancer* 1983;51:2090–2099.
83. Medeiros L, Lardelli P, Stetler-Stevenson M, et al. Genotypic analysis of diffuse, mixed cell lymphomas: comparison with morphologic and immunophenotypic findings. *Am J Clin Pathol* 1991;95:547.
84. Mann R, Berard C. Criteria for the cytologic subclassification of follicular lymphomas: a proposed alternative method. *Hematol Oncol* 1982; 1:187–192.
85. Metter G, Nathwani B, Burke J, et al. Morphological subclassification of follicular lymphoma: variability of diagnosis among hematopathologists, a collaborative study between the Repository Center and Pathology Panel for Lymphoma Clinical Studies. *J Clin Oncol* 1985;3: 25–38.
86. Nathwani B, Metter G, Miller T, et al. What should be the morphologic criteria for the subdivision of follicular lymphomas? *Blood* 1986;68: 837–845.
87. Anderson JR, Vose JM, Bierman PJ, et al. Clinical features and prognosis of follicular large-cell lymphoma: a report from the Nebraska Lymphoma Study Group. *J Clin Oncol* 1993;11:218–224.
88. A clinical evaluation of the International Lymphoma Study Group classification of non-Hodgkin's lymphoma. *Blood* 1997;89: 3909–3918.
89. Weisenburger D, Anderson J, Armitage J, et al. Grading of follicular lymphoma: diagnostic accuracy, reproducibility, and clinical relevance. *Mod Pathol* 1998;11:142A.
90. Bartlett NL, Rizeq M, Dorfman RF, et al. Follicular large-cell lymphoma: intermediate or low grade? *J Clin Oncol* 1994;12:1349–1357.
91. Martin AR, Weisenburger DD, Chan WC, et al. Prognostic value of cellular proliferation and histologic grade in follicular lymphoma. *Blood* 1995;85:3671–3678.
92. Kim H, Dorfman R. Morphological studies of 84 untreated patients subjected to laparotomy for the staging of non-Hodgkin's lymphomas. *Cancer* 1974;33:657–674.
93. Acker B, Hoppe RT, Colby TV, et al. Histologic conversion in the non-Hodgkin's lymphomas. *J Clin Oncol* 1983;1:11–16.
94. Horning SJ, Rosenberg SA. The natural history of initially untreated low-grade non-Hodgkin's lymphomas. *N Engl J Med* 1984;311: 1471–1475.
95. Gallagher CJ, Gregory WM, Jones AE, et al. Follicular lymphoma: prognostic factors for response and survival. *J Clin Oncol* 1986;4: 1470–1480.
96. Alsabeh R, Medeiros LJ, Glackin C, et al. Transformation of follicular lymphoma into CD30–large cell lymphoma with anaplastic cytologic features. *Am J Surg Pathol* 1997;21:528–536.
97. Lee JT, Innes DJ Jr, Williams ME. Sequential bcl-2 and c-myc oncogene rearrangements associated with the clinical transformation of non-Hodgkin's lymphoma. *J Clin Invest* 1989;84:1454–1459.
98. Yano T, Jaffe ES, Longo DL, et al. MYC rearrangements in histologically progressed follicular lymphomas. *Blood* 1992;80:758–767.
99. de Jong D, Voetdujk B, Baverstock G, et al. Activation of the c-myc oncogene in a precursor B-cell blast crisis of follicular lymphoma, presenting as composite lymphoma. *N Engl J Med* 1988;318:1373.
100. Gauwerky C, Hoxie J, Nowell P. Pre-B-cell leukemia with a t(8; 14) and a t(14;18) translocation is preceded by follicular lymphoma. *Oncogene* 1988;2:431–435.
101. Fiedler W, Weh H, Zeller W. Translocation (14;18) and (8;22) in three patients with acute leukemia/lymphoma following centrocytic/ centroblastic non-Hodgkin's lymphoma. *Ann Hematol* 1991;63: 282–287.
102. Kroft S, Domiati-Saad R, Finn W, et al. Precursor B-lymphoblastic transformation of grade 1 follicle center lymphoma. *Am J Clin Pathol* 2000;113:411–418.
103. Raffeld M, Wright JJ, Lipford E, et al. Clonal evolution of t(14;18) follicular lymphomas demonstrated by immunoglobulin genes and the 18q21 major breakpoint region. *Cancer Res* 1987;47:2537–2542.
104. Zelenetz AD, Chen TT, Levy R. Histologic transformation of follicular lymphoma to diffuse lymphoma represents tumor progression by a single malignant B cell. *J Exp Med* 1991;173:197–207.
105. Ottensmeier CH, Thompsett AR, Zhu D, et al. Analysis of V_H genes in follicular and diffuse lymphoma shows ongoing somatic mutation and multiple isotype transcripts in early disease with changes during disease progression. *Blood* 1998;91:4292–4299.
106. Lo Coco F, Gaidano G, Louie DC, et al. P53 mutations are associated with histologic transformation of follicular lymphoma. *Blood* 1993; 82:2289–2295.
107. Sander CA, Yano T, Clark HM, et al. P53 mutation is associated with progression in follicular lymphomas. *Blood* 1993;82:1994–2004.
108. Frizzera G, Anaya J, Banks P. Neoplastic plasma cells in follicular lymphomas. Clinical and pathological findings in six cases. *Virchows Arch Pathol Anat* 1986;409:149–162.
109. Schmid U, Karow J, Lennert K. Follicular malignant non-Hodgkin's lymphoma with pronounced plasmacytic differentiation: a plasmacytoma-like lymphoma. *Virchows Arch A Pathol Anat Histopathol* 1985; 405:473–481.
110. Keith TA, Cousar JB, Glick AD, et al. Plasmacytic differentiation in follicular center cell (FCC) lymphomas. *Am J Clin Pathol* 1985;84: 283–290.
111. Vago JF, Hurtubise PE, Redden-Borowski MM, et al. Follicular center-cell lymphoma with plasmacytic differentiation, monoclonal paraprotein, and peripheral blood involvement: recapitulation of normal B-cell development. *Am J Surg Pathol* 1985;9:764–770.
112. Alberti V, Neiman R. Lymphoplasmacytic lymphoma. A clinicopathologic study of a previously unrecognized variant. *Cancer* 1984;53: 1103–1108.
113. Campo E, Miquel R, Krenacs L, et al. Primary nodal marginal zone lymphomas of splenic and MALT type. *Am J Surg Pathol* 1999;23: 59–68.
114. Mollejo M, Menarguez J, Lloret E. Splenic marginal zone lymphoma: a distinctive type of low-grade B-cell lymphoma: a clinicopathologic study of 13 cases. *Am J Surg Pathol* 1995;19:1146–1157.
115. Mollejo M, Lloret E, Menérguez J, et al. Lymph node involvement by splenic marginal zone lymphoma: morphological and immunohistochemical features. *Am J Surg Pathol* 1997;21:772–780.
116. Kim H, Dorfman RF, Rappaport H. Signet ring cell lymphoma: a rare morphologic and functional expression of nodular (follicular) lymphoma. *Am J Surg Pathol* 1978;2:119–132.
117. Vernon S, Voet RL, Naeim F, et al. Nodular lymphoma with intracellular immunoglobulin. *Cancer* 1979;44:1273–1279.
118. Silberman S, Fresco R, Steinecker PH. Signet ring cell lymphoma: a report of a case and review of the literature. *Am J Clin Pathol* 1984; 81:358–363.
119. Navas-Palacios JJ, Valdes MD, Lahuerta-Palacios JJ. Signet-ring cell lymphoma: ultrastructural and immunohistochemical features of three varieties. *Cancer* 1983;52:1613–1623.
120. Harris M, Eyden B, Read G. Signet ring cell lymphoma: a rare variant of follicular lymphoma. *J Clin Pathol* 1981;34:884–891.

121. Moir DH. Signet ring cell lymphoma: a case report. *Pathology* 1980; 12:119–122.
122. van den Tweel JG, Taylor CR, Parker JW, et al. Immunoglobulin inclusions in non-Hodgkin's lymphomas. *Am J Clin Pathol* 1978;69: 306–313.
123. Spagnolo D, Papadimitriou J, Matz L, et al. Nodular lymphomas with intracellular immunoglobulin inclusions: report of three cases and a review. *Pathology* 1982;14:415–427.
124. Eyden B, Cross P, Harris M. The ultrastructure of signet-ring cell non-Hodgkin's lymphoma. *Virchows Arch A Pathol Anat* 1990;417: 395–404.
125. Rosas-Uribe A, Variakojis D, Rappaport H. Proteinaceous precipitate in nodular (follicular) lymphomas. *Cancer* 1973;534–542.
126. Chittal SM, Caveriviere P, Voigt JJ, et al. Follicular lymphoma with abundant PAS-positive extracellular material. Immunohistochemical and ultrastructural observations. *Am J Surg Pathol* 1987;11:618–624.
127. Tsang P, Pan L, Cesarman E, et al. A distinctive composite lymphoma consisting of clonally related mantle cell lymphoma and follicle center cell lymphoma. *Hum Pathol* 1999;30:988–992.
128. Gonzalez C, Medeiros L, Jaffe E. Composite lymphoma: a clinicopathologic analysis of nine patients with Hodgkin's disease and B-cell non-Hodgkin's lymphoma. *Am J Clin Pathol* 1991;96:81–89.
129. Bennett M, MacLennan K, Hudson G, et al. Non-Hodgkin's lymphoma arising in patients treated for Hodgkin's disease in the BNLI: a 20-year experience. *Ann Oncol* 1991;2[Suppl 2]:83–92.
130. Travis LB, Gonzalez CL, Hankey BF, et al. Hodgkin's disease following non-Hodgkin's lymphoma. *Cancer* 1992;69:2337–2342.
131. Jaffe E, Zarate-Osorno A, Medeiros L. The interrelationship of Hodgkin's Disease and non-Hodgkin's lymphomas—lessons learned from composite and sequential malignancies. *Semin Diagn Pathol* 1992;9: 297–303.
132. Harris N. The relationship between Hodgkin's disease and non-Hodgkin's lymphoma. *Semin Diagn Pathol* 1992;9:304–310.
133. Brauninger A, Hansmann ML, Strickler JG, et al. Identification of common germinal-center B-cell precursors in two patients with both Hodgkin's disease and non-Hodgkin's lymphoma [see comments]. *N Engl J Med* 1999;340:1239–1247.
134. Marafioti T, Hummel M, Anagnostopoulos I, et al. Classical Hodgkin's disease and follicular lymphoma originating from the same germinal center B cell. *J Clin Oncol* 1999;17:3804–3809.
135. Neri A, Fracchiolla NS, Roscetti E, et al. Molecular analysis of cutaneous B- and T-cell lymphomas. *Blood* 1995;86:3160–3172.
136. Cerroni L, Volkenandt M, Rieger E, et al. Bcl-2 protein expression and correlation with the interchromosomal 14;18 translocation in cutaneous lymphomas and pseudolymphomas. *J Invest Dermatol* 1994; 102:231–235.
137. Delia D, Borrello MG, Berti E, et al. Clonal immunoglobulin gene rearrangements and normal T-cell receptor, bcl-2, and c-myc genes in primary cutaneous B-cell lymphomas. *Cancer Res* 1989;49: 4901–4905.
138. Geelen FA, Vermeer MH, Meijer CJ, et al. Bcl-2 protein expression in primary cutaneous large B-cell lymphoma is site-related. *J Clin Oncol* 1998;16:2080–2085.
139. Fisher D, Jacobson J, Ault K, et al. Diffuse large cell lymphoma with discordant bone marrow histology: clinical features and biological implications. *Cancer* 1989;64:1879–1887.
140. Spiro S, Galton D, Wiltshaw E, et al. Follicular lymphoma: a survey of 75 cases with special reference to the syndrome resembling chronic lymphocytic leukaemia. *Br J Haematol* 1975;31[Suppl II]:60–88.
141. Come S, Jaffe E, Andersen J, et al. Non-Hodgkin's lymphomas in leukemic phase: clinicopathologic correlations. *Am J Med* 1980;69: 667–674.
142. Ault K. Detection of small numbers of monoclonal B lymphocytes in the blood of patients with lymphoma. *N Engl J Med* 1979;300: 1401.
143. Berliner N, Ault K, Martin P, et al. Detection of clonal excess in lymphoproliferative disease by kappa/gamma analysis: correlation with immunoglobulin gene DNA rearrangement. *Blood* 1986;67: 80–85.
144. Gribben J, Freedman A, Woo S, et al. All advanced stage non-Hodgkin's lymphomas with a polymerase chain reaction amplifiable breakpoint of bcl-2 have residual cells containing the bcl-2 rearrangement at evaluation and after treatment. *Blood* 1991;78:3275.
145. Garcia CF, Weiss LM, Warnke RA, et al. Cutaneous follicular lymphoma. *Am J Surg Pathol* 1986;10:454–463.
146. Willemze R, Beljaards R, Meijer C, et al. Classification of primary cutaneous lymphomas. *Dermatology* 1994;189[Suppl 2]:8–15.
147. Willemze R, Sterry HKW, Berti E, et al. EORTC classification for primary cutaneous lymphomas: a proposal from the cutaneous lymphoma study group of the European organization for research and treatment of cancer. *Blood* 1997;90:354–371.
148. Vermeer MH, Geelen FA, van Haselen CW, et al. Primary cutaneous large B-cell lymphomas of the legs: a distinct type of cutaneous B-cell lymphoma with an intermediate prognosis. Dutch Cutaneous Lymphoma Working Group [see comments]. *Arch Dermatol* 1996; 132:1304–1308.
149. Chimenti S, Cerroni L, Zenahlik P, et al. The role of MT2 and anti-bcl-2 protein antibodies in the differentiation of benign from malignant cutaneous infiltrates of B-lymphocytes with germinal center formation. *J Cutan Pathol* 1996;23:319–322.
150. de Leval L, Harris NL, Longtine J, et al. Bcl-6, CD10, and CD21 expression in cutaneous B-cell lymphomas. *Mod Pathol* 2000;13:62A.
151. Aguilera N, Tomaszewski M, Moad J, et al. Cutaneous follicle center lymphoma (FCL): a study of 24 cases. *Mod Pathol* 2000;13:59A.
152. Santucci M, Pimpinelli N, Arganini L. Primary cutaneous B-cell lymphoma: a unique type of low-grade lymphoma. Clinicopathologic and immunologic study of 83 cases. *Cancer* 1991;67:2311–2326.
153. Gilliam AC, Wood GS. Primary cutaneous lymphomas other than mycosis fungoides. *Semin Oncol* 1999;26:290–306.
154. Bekkenk MW, Vermeer MH, Geerts ML, et al. Treatment of multifocal primary cutaneous B-cell lymphoma: a clinical follow-up study of 29 patients. *J Clin Oncol* 1999;17:2471–2478.
155. Kirova YM, Piedbois Y, Le Bourgeois JP. Radiotherapy in the management of cutaneous B-cell lymphoma: our experience in 25 cases. *Radiother Oncol* 1999;52:15–18.
156. Isaacson PG. Gastrointestinal lymphoma. *Hum Pathol* 1994;25: 1020–1029.
157. Hashimoto Y, Nakamura N, Kuze T, et al. Multiple lymphomatous polyposis of the gastrointestinal tract is a heterogeneous group that includes mantle cell lymphoma and follicular lymphoma: analysis of somatic mutation of immunoglobulin heavy chain gene variable region. *Hum Pathol* 1999;30:581–587.
158. Ngan B, Warnke A, Cleary ML. Variability of immunoglobulin expression in follicular lymphoma: an immunohistologic and molecular genetic study. *Am J Pathol* 1989;135:1139–1144.
159. Raible MD, Hsi ED, Alkan S. Bcl-6 protein expression by follicle center lymphomas: a marker for differentiating follicle center lymphomas from other low-grade lymphoproliferative disorders. *Am J Clin Pathol* 1999;112:101–107.
160. Hollema H, Poppema S. Immunophenotypes of malignant lymphoma centroblastic-centrocytic and malignant lymphoma centrocytic: an immunohistologic study indicating a derivation from different stages of B cell differentiation. *Hum Pathol* 1988;19:1053–1059.
161. Nguyen PL, Zukerberg LR, Benedict WF, et al. Immunohistochemical detection of p53, bcl-2, and retinoblastoma proteins in follicular lymphoma. *Am J Clin Pathol* 1996;105:538–543.
162. Zukerberg L, Medeiros L, Ferry J, et al. Diffuse low-grade B-cell lymphomas: four clinically distinct subtypes defined by a combination of morphologic and immunophenotypic features. *Am J Clin Pathol* 1993;100:373–385.
163. de Leon ED, Alkan S, Huang JC, et al. Usefulness of an immunohistochemical panel in paraffin-embedded tissues for the differentiation of B-cell non-Hodgkin's lymphomas of small lymphocytes. *Mod Pathol* 1998;11:1046–1051.
164. Lai R, Weiss LM, Chang KL, et al. Frequency of CD43 expression in non-Hodgkin lymphoma: a survey of 742 cases and further characterization of rare $CD43^+$ follicular lymphomas. *Am J Clin Pathol* 1999;111:488–494.
165. Nguyen PL, Harris NL, Ritz J, et al. Expression of CD95 antigen and Bcl-2 protein in non-Hodgkin's lymphomas and Hodgkin's disease [published erratum appears in *Am J Pathol* 1996;149:346]. *Am J Pathol* 1996;148:847–853.
166. Dorfman DM, Schultze JL, Shahsafaei A, et al. In vivo expression of B7-1 and B7-2 by follicular lymphoma cells can prevent induction of T-cell anergy but is insufficient to induce significant T-cell proliferation. *Blood* 1997;90:4297–4306.

167. Poppema S, Bhan A, Reinherz E, et al. Distribution of T cell subsets in human lymph nodes. *J Exp Med* 1981;153:30–41.
168. Harris N, Bhan A. Distribution of T cell subsets in follicular and diffuse lymphomas of B cell type. *Am J Pathol* 1983;113:172–180.
169. Cleary M, Mecker T, Levy S, et al. Clustering of extensive somatic mutations in the variable region of an immunoglobulin heavy chain gene from a human B cell lymphoma. *Cell* 1986;44:97–106.
170. Levy S, Mendel E, Kon S, et al. Mutational hot spots in Ig V region genes of human follicular lymphomas. *J Exp Med* 1988;168:475.
171. Zelenetz AD, Chen TT, Levy R. Clonal expansion in follicular lymphoma occurs subsequent to antigenic selection. *J Exp Med* 1992; 176:1137.
172. Bahler D, Campbell M, Hart S, et al. Ig V(H) gene expression among human follicular lymphomas. *Blood* 1991;78:1561.
173. Vaandrager JW, Schuuring E, Kluin-Nelemans HC, et al. DNA fiber fluorescence in situ hybridization analysis of immunoglobulin class switching in B-cell neoplasia: aberrant CH gene rearrangements in follicle center-cell lymphoma. *Blood* 1998;92:2871–2878.
174. Bahler DW, Levy R. Clonal evolution of a follicular lymphoma: evidence for antigen selection. *Proc Natl Acad Sci USA* 1992;89: 6770–6774.
175. Zhu D, Hawkins RE, Hamblin TJ, et al. Clonal history of a human follicular lymphoma as revealed in the immunoglobulin variable region genes. *Br J Haematol* 1994;86:505–512.
176. Tilly H, Rossi A, Stamatoullas A, et al. Prognostic value of chromosomal abnormalities in follicular lymphoma. *Blood* 1994;84: 1043–1049.
177. Levine EG, Arthur DC, Frizzera G, et al. Cytogenetic abnormalities predict clinical outcome in non-Hodgkin lymphoma. *Ann Intern Med* 1988;108:14–20.
178. Rowley J. Chromosome studies in the non-Hodgkin's lymphomas: the role of the 14;18 translocation. *J Clin Oncol* 1988;6:919–925.
179. Horsman DE, Gascoyne RD, Coupland RW, et al. Comparison of cytogenetic analysis, southern analysis, and polymerase chain reaction for the detection of t(14;18) in follicular lymphoma. *Am J Clin Pathol* 1995;103:472–478.
180. Offit K, Parsa NZ, Gaidano G, et al. 6q Deletions define distinct clinico-pathologic subsets of non-Hodgkin's lymphoma. *Blood* 1993; 82:2157–2162.
181. Pinyol M, Cobo F, Bea S, et al. P16(Ink4a) gene inactivation by deletions, mutations, and hypermethylation is associated with transformed and aggressive variants of non-Hodgkin's lymphomas. *Blood* 1998;91:2977–2984.
182. Elenitoba-Johnson KS, Gascoyne RD, Lim MS, et al. Homozygous deletions at chromosome 9p21 involving p16 and p15 are associated with histologic progression in follicle center lymphoma. *Blood* 1998; 91:4677–4685.
183. Tsujimoto T, Cossman J, Jaffe E, et al. Involvement of the bcl-2 gene in human follicular lymphoma. *Science* 1985;288:1440–1443.
184. Yunis J, Mayer M, Arnesen M, et al. Bcl-2 and other genomic alterations in the prognosis of large-cell lymphoma. *N Engl J Med* 1989; 320:1047–1054.
185. Lai R, Arber DA, Chang KL, et al. Frequency of bcl-2 expression in non-Hodgkin's lymphoma: a study of 778 cases with comparison of marginal zone lymphoma and monocytoid B-cell hyperplasia. *Mod Pathol* 1998;11:864–869.
186. McDonnell T, Deane N, Platt F, et al. Bcl-2–immunoglobulin transgenic mice demonstrate extended B cell survival and follicular lymphoproliferation. *Cell* 1989;57:79–88.
187. Nunez G, London L, Hockenbery D, et al. Deregulated bcl-2 gene expression selectively prolongs survival of growth factor–deprived hemopoietic cell lines. *J Immunol* 1990;144:3602–3610.
188. Ye BH, Lista F, Lo Coco F, et al. Alterations of a zinc finger-encoding gene, BCL-6, in diffuse large-cell lymphoma. *Science* 1993;262: 747–750.
189. Chang CC, Ye BH, Chaganti RS, et al. BCL-6, a POZ/zinc-finger protein, is a sequence-specific transcriptional repressor. *Proc Natl Acad Sci USA* 1996;93:6947–6952.
190. Ye BH, Cattoretti G, Shen Q, et al. The BCL-6 proto-oncogene controls germinal-centre formation and Th2-type inflammation. *Nat Genet* 1997;16:161–170.
191. Sahota S, Davis Z, Hamblin T, et al. Discordant somatic mutation of immunoglobulin variable region genes and BCL-6 genes in chronic lymphocytic leukemia. *Blood* 2000;95:3534–3540.
192. Limpens J, de Jong D, van Krieken J, et al. Bcl-2 in benign lymphoid tissue with follicular hyperplasia. *Oncogene* 1991;6:2271–2276.
193. Zukerberg LR, Yang W-I, Arnold A, et al. Cyclin D1 expression in non-Hodgkin's lymphomas: detection by immunohistochemistry. *Am J Clin Pathol* 1995;103:756–760.
194. Kaptain S, Zuckerberg LR, Ferry JA, et al. BCL-1 cyclin D1-positive CD5-negative mantle cell lymphoma. *Mod Pathol* 1998;11:133A.
195. Ashton-Key M, Biddolph S, Stein H, et al. Heterogeneity of bcl-2 expression in MALT lymphoma. *Histopathology* 1995;26:75–78.
196. Wright DH, Isaacson P. Follicular center cell lymphoma of childhood: a report of three cases and a discussion of its relationship to Burkitt's lymphoma. *Cancer* 1981;47:915–925.
197. Winberg CD, Nathwani BN, Bearman RM, et al. Follicular (nodular) lymphoma during the first two decades of life: a clinicopathologic study of 12 patients. *Cancer* 1981;48:2223–2235.
198. Frizzera G, Murphy SB. Follicular (nodular) lymphoma in childhood: a rare clinical-pathological entity. Report of eight cases from four cancer centers. *Cancer* 1979;44:2218–2235.
199. Finn LS, Viswanatha DS, Belasco JB, et al. Primary follicular lymphoma of the testis in childhood. *Cancer* 1999;85:1626–1635.
200. Pinto A, Hutchison R, Grant L, et al. Follicular lymphomas in pediatric patients. *Mod Pathol* 1990;3:308–313.
201. Dong H, Kozakewich H, Longtine J, et al. Pediatric follicle center lymphoma: a rare entity with distinctive features. *Mod Pathol* 2000; 13:147A.
202. Paryani SB, Hoppe RT, Cox RS, et al. The role of radiation therapy in the management of stage III follicular lymphomas. *J Clin Oncol* 1984;2:841–848.
203. Longo DL, Young RC, Hubbard SM, et al. Prolonged initial remission in patients with nodular mixed lymphoma. *Ann Intern Med* 1984;100: 651–656.
204. Jones S, Fuks Z, Bull M, et al. Non-Hodgkin's lymphomas IV. Clinicopathologic correlation in 405 cases. *Cancer* 1973;31:806–823.
205. Anderson T, Bender R, Fisher R, et al. Combination chemotherapy in non-Hodgkin's lymphoma: results of long-term follow-up. *Cancer Treat Rep* 1977;61:1057–1066.
206. Glick JH, Barnes JM, Ezdinli EZ, et al. Nodular mixed lymphoma: results of a randomized trial failing to confirm prolonged disease-free survival with COPP chemotherapy. *Blood* 1981;58:920–925.
207. McLaughlin P, Fuller LM, Velasquez WS, et al. Stage III follicular lymphoma: durable remissions with a combined chemotherapy-radiotherapy regimen. *J Clin Oncol* 1987;5:867–874.
208. Wendum D, Sebban C, Gaulard P, et al. Follicular large-cell lymphoma treated with intensive chemotherapy: an analysis of 89 cases included in the LNH87 trial and comparison with the outcome of diffuse large B-cell lymphoma. Groupe d'Etude des Lymphomes de l'Adulte. *J Clin Oncol* 1997;15:1654–1663.
209. Kantarjian HM, McLaughlin P, Fuller LM, et al. Follicular large cell lymphoma: analysis and prognostic factors in 62 patients. *J Clin Oncol* 1984;2:811–819.
210. Glick JH, McFadden E, Costello W, et al. Nodular histiocytic lymphoma: factors influencing prognosis and implications for aggressive chemotherapy. *Cancer* 1982;49:840–845.
211. Warnke R, Kim H, Fuks Z, et al. The co-existence of nodular and diffuse patterns in nodular non-Hodgkin's lymphomas. *Cancer* 1977; 40:1229–1233.
212. Ezdinli E, Costello W, Kucuk O, et al. Effect of the degree of nodularity on the survival of patients with nodular lymphomas. *J Clin Oncol* 1987;5:413–418.
213. Hu E, Weiss L, Hoppe R, et al. Follicular and diffuse mixed small cleaved and large cell lymphoma—a clinicopathologic study. *J Clin Oncol* 1985;3:1183–1187.
214. Vose JM, Bierman PJ, Lynch JC, et al. Effect of follicularity on autologous transplantation for large-cell non-Hodgkin's lymphoma. *J Clin Oncol* 1998;16:844–849.
215. Armitage JO, Dick FR, Corder MP. Diffuse histiocytic lymphoma after histologic conversion: a poor prognostic variant. *Cancer Treat Rep* 1981;65:413–418.
216. Collins A, Bloomfield C, Peterson B, et al. Acute nonlymphocytic leukemia in patients with nodular lymphoma. *Cancer* 1977;40: 1748–1754.
217. Harris NL. Hodgkin's disease: classification and differential diagnosis. *Mod Pathol* 1999;12:159–175.

CHAPTER 25

Diffuse Large Cell Lymphomas

Ioannis Anagnostopoulos, Friederike Dallenbach, and Harald Stein

By definition, diffuse large cell non-Hodgkin lymphomas (NHLs) are composed of large transformed lymphoid cells with nuclei at least twice the size of two small lymphocytes or larger than the size of a normal histiocyte. The nuclei can show a marked variation in their contour, have generally vesicular chromatin and prominent nucleoli. The amount of cytoplasm and its characteristics may vary. These lymphomas exhibit a moderate to high proliferation fraction. This lymphoma group is also heterogeneous regarding other features, including antigen profile, molecular genetic features, clinical features, and clinical behavior.

CONCEPTS INFLUENCING CLASSIFICATION AND SUBTYPING OF DIFFUSE LARGE CELL LYMPHOMAS

A given classification of lymphomas should accomplish a dual task. It must allow the definition of distinct lymphoma entities and form a sound basis for proper and reproducible diagnoses. At the same time, it must be clinically useful and enable clinicians to estimate the prognostic relevance of the entities diagnosed and to guide therapeutic decisions accordingly. The definition of lymphoma entities requires not only the consideration of morphologic criteria but also immunophenotypic, genetic, and clinical findings. The determination of the cell of origin is helpful but not essential for the definition of clinicopathologic disease entities.

We begin this chapter with a brief review of the historical cornerstones that significantly influenced the classification of diffuse large cell lymphomas, because the knowledge of the steps leading to the recognition of lymphoma entities is very helpful for its understanding (Table 25.1). This historical account also shows that the steps of progress in lymphoma classification closely correlate with the advent of new diagnostic techniques.

I. Anagnostopoulos, F. Dallenbach, and H. Stein: Institut of Pathology, Klinikum Benjamin Franklin, Free University of Berlin, Berlin, Germany

As this historical overview shows, large cell lymphomas consist of two main groups: one is of B-cell origin, and the other is of T-cell origin and displays ''anaplastic'' morphology. This concept serves as the basis for this chapter.

DIFFUSE LARGE B-CELL LYMPHOMAS

Diffuse large B-cell lymphomas (DLBCLs) represent the group of NHLs that is under continuous discussion about the existence of true subentities and their differentiation from variants occurring in this lymphoma group. The DLBCL group is one of the more common subtypes, representing up to 40% of all NHL cases. An aggressive natural history is usually documented, as well as a good response to chemotherapy. The complete remission rate is 75% to 80% with long-term disease-free survival approaching 50% or more in most series (1–5). DLBCLs may occur in lymph nodes or in extranodal sites at presentation. The most frequently involved extranodal sites include bone, skin, thyroid, gastrointestinal tract and lung. DLBCLs are heterogeneous in morphology. Part of this heterogeneity may reflect different cellular origins or different pathogenesis or development from the transformation of another less aggressive lymphoma (designated as secondary DLBCL).

Classification

Unfortunately, the subtyping of these lymphomas is still unsatisfactory in the various classifications. Most of these classifications (i.e., Lukes and Collins, Rappaport, Working Formulation, and the Kiel classification) are mainly based on morphology. It has been repeatedly demonstrated, however, that the reproducibility rate of subtyping of these lymphomas according to these classifications is low. The Revised European–American Lymphoma (REAL) classification proposed to subsume all aggressive B-cell lymphomas other than lymphoblastic and Burkitt's lymphoma under the generic term of *diffuse large B cell lymphoma* (DLBCL) (6). The initiators of the REAL classification

TABLE 25.1. *Some essential historical data related to the identification and subtyping of large cell lymphomas*

Year	Author	Method	Result
1832	Hodgkin	Gross pathology	Identification of peculiar lymph node tumors occurring in the cervical region, called Hodgkin's disease in 1865 by Wilks.
1858/63	Virchow	Histology	The terms *lymphoma* and *lymphosarcoma* were coined.
1892/93	Dreschfeld Kundrat	Histology	Hodgkin's disease and lymphosarcoma became recognized as separate lymphoma groups.
1930	Roulet	Histology	Lymphomas of larger cell size were separated from lymphosarcomas and related to reticular cells or sinus lining cells and called *reticulum cell sarcomas.*
1958 1960	Burkitt O'Connor and Davies	Gross pathology, histology	Burkitt described a unique tumor of the jaws and the abdomen that became recognized as a new lymphoma category.
1966	Rappaport	Histology	Lymphomas of larger cell size were called *histiocytic* in the belief that they were derived from histiocytes or phagocytic cells and not from reticular cells. Undifferentiated lymphomas became separated from histiocytic lymphomas. Latter ones are of intermediate size, with no evidence of a lymphoid or a histiocytic origin.
1972	Stein et al.	Histology, immunohistology	Identification that "reticulum cell sarcomas" of Roulet and "histiocytic lymphomas" of Rappaport were most commonly derived from transformed B cells
1974/75	Lennert and coworkers	Histology, immunology, immunohistology	Establishment of the Kiel classification. The terms lymphoblastic, centroblastic and immunoblastic were introduce to describe different forms of aggressive lymphomas. The lymphoblastic and centroblastic group included most of Rappaport's undifferentiated lymphomas. The centroblastic group also included together with the immunoblastic category most of Rappaport's histiocytic lymphomas.
1974	Lukes and Collins	Histology, immunohistology	The terms *large cleaved* and *large noncleaved* were coined for the distinction of different types of large cell lymphomas.
1976–1979	Vogler et al. Greaves et al. Brouet et al.	Immunology, immunocytochemistry	Lymphoblastic lymphomas were demonstrated to be derived from precursor B or T cells and were thus separated from other aggressive (i.e., centroblastic and immunoblastic) non-Hodgkin lymphomas (NHLs).
1982	National Cancer Institute	Histology, clinical data	The Working Formulation was established as a terminology compromise between earlier classifications (e.g., Lukes and Collins, Rappaport, Dorfman). The term *large cell lymphoma* was introduced as a generic form for an aggressive NHL of nonlymphoblastic and non-Burkitt type. In addition, the terms *cleaved, noncleaved,* and *immunoblastic* were adopted.
1985	Weiss et al.	Antigen receptor gene rearrangement analysis	Many cases of Rappaport's malignant histiocytosis were found to have a T-cell genotype.
1985	Stein et al.	Immunohistology	The Ki-1 (CD30)–positive anaplastic large cell lymphomas (ALCLs) were recognized as a distinct lymphoma group. They had been previously mistaken as malignant histiocytosis or as undifferentiated carcinoma or malignant melanoma or others. ALCLs were found to be mostly related to transformed T or B cells.
1985/88	Isaacson et al.	Histology, immunohistology, antigen receptor gene rearrangement analysis	Celiac disease-associated malignant histiocytosis of the intestine became recognized as being derived from intraepithelial T cells of the gut.
1982–1990	Wright, Isaacson et al.	Histology Immunohistology	Establishment of the concept that many low-grade extranodal lymphomas are derived from mucosa-associated lymphoid tissue (MALT).
1972–1986	van Heerden et al., Addis and Issacson, Benjamin et al., Menestrina et al., Möller et al.	Morphology, immunohistology, clinical data	Primary mediastinal large B-cell lymphoma was recognized as a distinct clinicopathological entity.

TABLE 25.1. *Continued.*

Year	Author	Method	Result
1989	Kaudewitz et al.	Clinical data, immunohistology	Separation of primary cutaneous ALCL from primary extracutaneous (systemic) ALCL.
1994	International Lymphoma Study Group	Morphology, immunohistology, molecular genetic techniques, clinical data	Establishment of the Revised European-American Classification of lymphoid neoplasms. All lymphomas consisting of large B cells were subsumed under the term *large B-cell lymphoma;* among them, primary mediastinal large B-cell lymphomas were recognized as a distinct disease entity. ALCL of T and null phenotypes were separated as a distinct entity.
1994–1999	Mason et al., Morris et al., Falini et al.	Immunohistology Molecular genetic techniques Clinical data	Identification of an ALCL group with constant presence of the t(2;5) translocation or a variant genetic alteration leading to the expression of an ALK fusion protein, most commonly NPM-ALK, that can be detected by immunohistology. ALK protein–positive lymphomas are in the process of being accepted as a distinct clinicopathologic entity different from ALK-negative tumors.
1996	Foss et al.	Immunohistology Molecular genetic techniques	Cytotoxic T cells were identified as the cell of origin of most ALCLs.

stated that the lymphomas subsumed under DLBCL are likely to include more than one disease entity, but that there are no presently described morphologic, immunologic and molecular parameters able to clearly define clinically relevant subentities and differentiate them from variants. There is one exception—that of the primary mediastinal large B-cell lymphoma. All other morphologic and immunophenotypic variations are regarded to reflect variants. The new World Health Organization (WHO) classification has adopted the REAL concept, with the only difference being that two additional subentities are distinguished: intravascular large B-cell lymphoma and primary effusion lymphoma. This section follows the WHO proposal and is accordingly divided into a part that describes the DLBCLs, their variants and a part that describes the subentities. Before starting with the description of the morphologic variants, an overview of the most important genetic and phenotypic structures is given because they help in understanding the pathogenesis and classification of these lymphomas.

Molecular Genetic and Immunophenotypic Markers

Immunoglobulin Genes

The clarification of the structure of the immunoglobulin (Ig) gene locus led to the discovery that in B cells, in contrast to other somatic cells, the Ig genes are rearranged (7). It could be further shown that this gene rearrangement takes place during the development of B cells. In the bone marrow, B-cell precursors assemble variable (V), heavy (H), and light (L) chain genes by the process of gene segment recombination. The enormous diversity among the V regions is generated by combinatorial permutation of different V, D, and J gene segments and by a random incorporation of nucleotides (known as N segments) at the VD and DJ joints. The result is that each single nonmalignant B cell contains distinct IgH and IgL chain gene rearrangements that are—like a fingerprint for a given human being—specific for an individual B cell. This specificity is predominantly located within the complementarity determining region (CDR) 3. In contrast to reactive B cells, neoplastic cells from B-cell lymphomas have identically rearranged Ig genes and therefore identical CDR3 sequences. This finding confirms that each B-cell lymphoma is derived from a single transformed B cell and represents a monoclonal B-cell population (see Chapter 7).

If the B cells within the bone marrow succeed in generating a functional, nonautoreactive receptor, they are released into the peripheral B-cell pool as naive B cells. On antigen encounter, the antibody expressed by a B cell may be modified by somatic hypermutation and class switch recombination. The process of somatic hypermutation appears to be restricted to B cells proliferating within the microenvironment of a germinal center (GC). Although this process has an element of randomness, selection toward an antigen tends to result in conservation of the Ig framework regions (FRs) and in clustering of replacement mutations within the CDRs. The presence of somatically mutated V region genes is a hallmark of GC B cells and their descendants (i.e., memory B cells and long-lived plasma cells). Examination of the rearranged V region genes of B-cell lymphomas by sequence analysis is useful to trace the developmental stage at which neoplastic transformation has occurred and assign the neoplastic cells to their normal counterparts. Moreover, V gene analysis may reveal pathogenic aspects in B-cell lymphomas, including possible bias in V_H gene usage. For instance, preferential V_H gene usage might implicate a possible role for B-cell superantigens in driving B-cell proliferation, because it is evident that certain antigens can bind to IgM antibodies through unmutated FRs.

Several groups have analyzed the clonally rearranged Ig gene variable regions in small cohorts of patients with

DLBCL. Regarding biased V_H gene usage the results of these groups are inconsistent. A biased V_H gene usage with overrepresentation of the V_H4 gene family and particularly of the V_H4-34 gene was reported in three studies (8–10), while three other studies found an unbiased V_H gene usage in DLBCL cases (11–13). The common finding of all studies, however, was the detection of a high number of somatic mutations in all rearranged V_H (up to 11%) and V_L genes. These values are higher than those determined for nonmalignant human B cells (average mutation frequency for memory B cells 4%, for IgM^+IgD^- peripheral blood memory cells, 2%). The finding of somatically mutated V region genes identified the GC B cells or their descendants as the precursors of the malignant cell clones in DLBCL. The observed high load of somatic mutations suggests that the precursors of the malignant cell clones have remained under the influence of the GC mutational machinery for a long time period. No clear evidence of ongoing mutations in DLBCLs has been reported.

To verify whether the cells with somatically mutated, rearranged V_H genes have been selected for the production of a high affinity antibody, the mutation patterns were analyzed. Because the framework regions (FRs) are important for the integrity of the variable domain, replacement mutations should be counterselected in the FRs (i.e., one should find lower replacement/silent (R/S) values than expected assuming random mutagenesis), whereas the antigen binding CDRs should be selected for affinity-increasing R mutations (i.e., high R/S values). The analysis of the pattern of somatic mutations within the rearranged V_H region genes revealed that the mutated B-cell clones of DLBCLs were selected for expression of a high affinity antigen receptor. In conclusion, the overview of the published data implies that DLBCLs are derived from antigen-experienced B cells that have participated in a GC reaction.

The BCL6 *Gene and its Alterations*

Chromosomal Translocations Involving 3q27

Structural aberrations of the distal part of the long arm of chromosome 3 had been observed in sporadic cases of NHLs during the 1970s, but these abnormalities did not attract much attention until 1983 when Kaneko and coworkers found an association between 3q abnormalities and diffuse large cell histology (14). In their series of 30 karyotypically abnormal lymphomas, 7 displayed 3q27-29 rearrangements, including a t(3;6)(q29;p15) and six translocations of an unidentified segment into the terminal region of 3q. Six of the patients with 3q27-29 rearrangements had a DLBCL. In the following years, there were only sporadic reports of cases harboring a translocation involving chromosomal band 3q27. The first report on the association of this translocation with the IgL genes was published in 1989 (15). This study identified the presence of a t(3;22)(q27;q11) in 8 (4.3%) of the 187 NHLs analyzed, recognizing it as the third most common recurring translocation in diffuse large cell lymphoma after t(14;18) and t(8;14). Since that study, several other investigators have agreed that the 3q27 translocation is one of the most common recurring translocations in B-cell NHLs (16,17). The most frequent translocation is the (3;14) (q27;q32) involving the IgH gene. In contrast to other translocations observed in B-cell neoplasms, 3q27 translocations are unique in that they can involve the IgH and IgL gene loci and involve numerous, as yet uncharacterized chromosomal loci as partners. More than 20 chromosomal sites, including the three Ig loci, have been reported to be translocation partners of 3q27. Some of the translocations have been described by two or more independent laboratories, indicating that they are recurrent chromosomal translocations and that they may play important roles in the development of B-cell NHL. However, it remains to be determined whether each partner locus affects the clinicopathologic profile of a B-cell NHL carrying a particular 3q27 translocation. The 3q27 abnormality is not a marker for a specific subtype of B-cell NHL (16,18). Regarding DLBCL, the overall incidence of 3q27 abnormalities has been estimated to be 23.1% (19). This incidence is likely to be underestimated because this terminal chromosomal alteration is sometimes difficult to detect cytogenetically.

It is of further interest that dual translocations may occur with concurrent 3q27 abnormality and a t(14;18) or t(8;14) translocation (18,20) in a small number of cases.

Cloning the BCL6 *Gene*

By analogy with other well-characterized translocations in B-cell neoplasms, cytogenetic observations of translocations involving 3q27 and one of the three Ig gene loci suggested that a potential oncogene was localized on this chromosome region. Four independent groups cloned junctional areas of these translocations using molecular probes for the IgH and IgL genes, and isolated the same genomic region from 3q27. By comparison with their data of junctional areas, the breakpoints were apparently clustered within a limited region. Genomic probes detected a transcriptional unit of about 3.8 kb, resulting in the cloning of cDNA of a novel gene from this region. This gene was differently designated by each study group (i.e., *BCL5* [21], *LAZ3* [22], *BLY3* [23], and *BCL6* [24]), and the name *BCL6* has been officially adopted (see Chapter 8).

The *BCL6* gene spans 26 kb and contains 10 exons (25). At least two types of mRNA are produced by alternative splicing, which do or do not contain exon 2. The BCL-6 protein contains two identical functional domains. The C-terminal region comprises six Cys^2-His^2 zinc finger motifs, each separated by a conserved stretch of seven amino acids, by which BCL-6 was classified as belonging to the Krüp-PEL-like subfamily of zinc finger proteins. The N-terminal region contains a conserved protein-protein interaction motif, the POZ (poxvirus and zinc finger) domain. The POZ domain plays a role in homodimerization and heterodimerization, raising the possibility that BCL-6 may act in conjunction with another POZ domain factor. The BCL-6 protein has structural features of DNA-binding transcriptional regulators, and a consensus binding sequence of the protein has been determined (26,27).

The transcriptional level of the *BCL6* gene has been studied in many types of hematologic tumor cell lines. The expression was limited to those of mature B-cell immunophenotype except for EBV-immortalized lymphoblastoid cell lines (28,29). High levels of expression were found in Burkitt's lymphoma and follicular lymphoma cell lines (30).

The role of BCL-6 in physiologic immune responses has been investigated by animal models in which the gene has been biallelically disrupted. Although these bcl-6$^{-/-}$ mice display normal B- and T-cell counts, they consistently fail to form germinal centers after injection of T-cell–dependent antigens. This failure is associated with a high incidence of infectious diseases and inflammatory processes leading to premature death (31). BCL-6 is required for germinal center formation and a normal antigen-dependent antigen response.

Genomic Structure of 3q27 Translocations and Mechanism of BCL6 *Deregulation*

Rearrangements of the *BCL6* gene result from chromosomal translocations that have been found to be clustered within a 4kb region spanning the noncoding exon 1 (major translocation cluster). In most cases, breakpoints are located immediately 3′ of exon 1. Although 3q27 translocations can coexist with other B-cell neoplasm–specific translocations or their molecular equivalents, the possibility that this translocation can be a primary genetic defect is strongly supported by the presence of cases in which it represents the sole chromosome abnormality (18,32,33). Detailed translocation analysis suggests that their critical molecular consequence is the replacement of 5′ regulatory elements of the *BCL6* gene by many types of regulatory sequences on partner chromosomes. The patterns of regulation of each regulatory sequence, however, have not yet been fully characterized. Several studies show that the coding region of the *BCL6* gene itself is not affected by the translocations (34). The translocated allele obviously encodes the wild-type BCL-6 protein.

In a later study, the regulation of expression of the promoters of the heterologous genes that fuse to the *BCL6* gene during B-cell differentiation has been analyzed to provide some insights into the functional consequences of the 3q27 translocation (35). This analysis showed that in contrast to *BCL6,* whose expression is restricted to mature B cells with a GC phenotype, all of the fusion partners studied displayed a different pattern of regulation, including persistence of expression to the plasmacytoid stage. This data suggest that, driven by the heterologous promoter, BCL6 expression is inappropriately continued and may block B-cell differentiation, inhibit apoptosis and maintain proliferation. This blockade of normal downregulation of *BCL6* may also expose the cells to genetic alterations ultimately leading to lymphoma development.

Analysis of BCL6 *Gene Rearrangements in Diffuse Large B-Cell Lymphomas*

Because all rearrangements reported are clustered within the major translocation cluster region of *BCL6,* they can be identified by Southern blot analysis using probes of this region. A significant number of cases, however, with a cytogenetically defined 3q27 translocation have been shown to lack rearrangements on Southern analysis, suggesting that breakpoints occur outside the area that can be covered by available probes. The occasional biallellic deletion of sequences in the major translocation cluster region may be the cause of negative Southern analysis (36), and cases with *BCL6* rearrangements have been found without visible chromosome breaks on 3q27 on conventional cytogenetic analysis. This lack of strict correlation between the two methods reflects their different sensitivities and approaches. A promising technique enabling rapid detection of 3q27 translocations is FISH, which can be successful even when cytogenetic analysis is noninformative (37,38).

Although the initial study on *BCL6* gene rearrangement indicated a specific association with DLBCL (24), later studies of NHL case panels invariably showed that a significant number of follicular lymphomas also carried such rearrangements (17,28,30,32,39). The published data report an incidence of *BCL6* rearrangements in DLBCL in Western countries as high as 28.6% to 35.5%. Considering that chromosomal defects can involve sequences outside the major breakpoint cluster, the real incidence of *BCL6* rearrangements may be even higher. This implies that abnormalities involving the *BCL6* gene are one of the most common genetic defects associated with DLBCL (see Chapters 8 and 9).

Prognostic Implications of BCL6 *Rearrangement*

Considerable interest was generated by reports of Offit and coworkers that DLBCLs with rearranged *BCL6* genes had a remarkably favorable outcome, in terms of overall survival and survival without disease progression, as compared with patients lacking rearrangement (19). The presence of *BCL6* rearrangement had independent prognostic value according to multivariate analysis. The same group has also found that cases of DLBCL with *BCL6* rearrangement have a reduced incidence of cytogenetic indices of disease progression and poor prognosis (40). Other studies have not confirmed the favorable prognosis of *BCL6* rearranged cases and demonstrated that clinical outcome varied from an indolent course to highly clinical aggressivity (32,41,42).

BCL6 *Gene Hypermutations*

Multiple, often biallelic mutations were initially reported to occur clustered within the 3.5-kb regulatory sequences encompassing exon 1 of *BCL6* (43). According to that study, the *BCL6* 5′ regulatory sequences were mutated in up to 73% of DLBCLs. Mutations were somatic in origin and were present with or without *BCL6* rerarrangements/3q27 translocations. The investigators attributed these mutations to the possible ectopic influence of the immunoglobulin variable region hypermutation process. Similar analysis of 123 carcinomas and glioblastomas did not reveal any *BCL6* gene mutations.

Later studies showed that *BCL6* gene mutations are not only present in B-NHLs but are also found in normal GC and memory B cells (44,45). This implies that the *BCL6* gene is apparently a real target for the somatic hypermutation process in normal B lymphocytes. It is therefore highly likely that the mutations seen in lymphomas were already present in their B-cell precursors before malignant transformation.

The BCL-6 Protein

Monoclonal and polyclonal antibodies have been generated against the BCL-6 protein facilitating its subcellular localization by appropriate immunostains. As expected from its structure containing the zinc-finger domain typical of transcriptional factors, the BCL-6 protein is strictly confined to the nucleus. There is a diffuse microgranular pattern sparing the nucleoli. Screening of lymphoid tissues established an intense labeling of GC B cells (centroblasts and centrocytes) (46–48), but the naive B cells of the follicle mantle lack BCL-6. No BCL-6 protein expression is found in immunoblasts, plasma cells, macrophages or follicular dendritic cells within the germinal centers. Most marginal zone B cells and a small percentage of $CD4^+$ T cells within follicles and in the interfollicular zones may show BCL-6 expression (48).

The highly restrictive expression of BCL-6 protein in GC B cells suggests that the *BCL6* gene product is involved in subtle processes of B-cell differentiation, including antigen-dependent proliferation, isotype class switching, somatic mutation in V genes of IgH and apoptosis. However, BCL-6 protein exhibits potent transcriptional repressive activity when bound to its consensus binding sequence (49,50).

BCL-6 Protein Expression Patterns in Diffuse Large B-Cell Lymphoma

In the various published series 55% to 97% of the DLBCL cases investigated showed BCL-6 expression (48,51–53). The reason for this variation is the variability of the antigen demasking techniques and the various hybridoma clones used. The application of newly generated monoclonal antibodies against formalin-resistant epitopes of BCL-6 protein (52) has been shown to be more sensitive than earlier antibodies leading to a significant increase of positivity (53). Within the DLBCL group, it was found that cases of the immunoblastic variant had a lower frequency of BCL-6 expression compared with cases with centroblastic morphology (27% versus 82%) (53). This finding correlates with the expression pattern of BCL-6 in normal lymphoid tissues. There was no expression difference found between nodal and extranodal DLBCL. In contrast to DLBCL, mantle cell lymphoma and low-grade marginal zone lymphoma were negative for expression. High-grade marginal zone lymphomas with a coexistent low-grade component were found also to express BCL-6 protein (54). This observation questions the generally accepted hypothesis that BCL-6 protein expression is always predictive of a GC cell origin of the given lymphoma. Combined studies of BCL-6 immunostains have shown that the level of BCL-6 expression does not correlate with the presence or absence of *BCL6* gene alterations (51,53). The prognostic significance of BCL-6 protein expression in DLBCL has not been analyzed.

The* BCL2 *Gene and its Alterations

Translocation (14;18) and the BCL2 *Protooncogene*

The *BCL2* gene located on chromosome 18 at q21 has been identified by virtue of its involvement in the t(14;18)(q32;q21) translocation frequently found in follicular lymphomas (55–57). This translocation places the *BCL2* gene into juxtaposition with the joining segment of the IgH gene. Despite the mature phenotype of t(14;18)-bearing lymphomas, the translocation appears to occur at a pre-B-cell stage (58). In most cases (about 70%), the breakpoints on chromosome 18 are clustered in the 3′ end of the last *BCL2* exon (major breakpoint region [MBR]), the remaining within the 3′ untranslated region of the gene (59) (minor cluster region [MCR]), which occurs 20 kb distal to MBR, leaving the open reading frame intact. The location of the breakpoints does not show any correlation with a specific lymphoma morphology (60). The precise mechanisms responsible for the localized DNA breaks in *BCL2* and its recombination with the Ig locus remain uncertain.

The cloning of the t(14;18) interchromosomal breakpoint revealed a new gene, *BCL2*. The t(14;18) translocation leads to overexpression of the BCL-2 protein by posing the *BCL2* gene under the constitutive activation of the IgH promoter. The BCL-2 protein is located in the mitochondrial inner membrane and functions as an antiapoptotic protein inhibiting cells from programmed cell death (61). In normal lymphoid cells, BCL-2 protein is expressed at pre GC-B-cell stages, but the expression usually decreases when the B cells migrate in GC.

The contribution of the t(14;18) to neoplasia was directly assessed by generating transgenic mice bearing a *BCL2*-Ig minigene that recapitulated the molecular consequences of the human translocation (62,63). These mice uniformly developed a polyclonal follicular lymphoid proliferation that selectively expanded small resting B cells. These recirculating B cells accumulated due to extended survival rather than increased proliferation. These mice showed a slow progression from indolent follicular hyperplasia to diffuse large cell lymphoma usually of immunoblastic morphology (64). Several of these diffuse large cell lymphomas harbored as a secondary genetic change *MYC* gene rearrangement. These observations indicate that prolonged cell survival is oncogenic (see Chapter 8).

Translocation (14;18) in Diffuse Large B-Cell Lymphoma

In addition to follicular lymphomas, t(14;18) has also been observed in 20% to 30% of DLBCLs (65,66). It has been suggested that the presence of t(14;18) in DLBCL can be explained by the previous history of follicular lymphoma (67). Analysis of *de novo* DLBCLs without history and histologic features of follicular lymphoma revealed the existence of *BCL2* rearrangements in 20% of the cases. These *de novo* DLBCLs with *BCL2* rearrangements had distinctive clinical features, including presenting with extranodal tumors of early stage, without association with mucosa, and were more often HLA-DR$^-$ than cases without *BCL2* rearrangement (66). The finding that DLBCL cases with *BCL2* rearrangement are frequently extranodal has also been reported in an earlier study (68) (see Chapter 9).

BCL2 *Amplification in Diffuse Large B-Cell Lymphoma*

BCL-2 protein overexpression has been reported to occur in 22% to 80% of DLBCLs, a much higher frequency than could be expected by the presence of t(14;18) alone (69–73). The t(14;18) alone does not explain the observed increased BCL-2 expression in these lymphomas. In several tumors, gene amplification has been shown to occur in response to a selection pressure for increased gene expression. In hematologic malignancies, hallmarks of gene amplification in G-banding analysis such as double minute chromosomes and homogeneously staining regions are fairly uncommon compared with solid tumors. This fact led many researchers to conclude that gene amplification might not play a very important role in the genesis of lymphomas. Comparative genomic hybridization (CGH) however has changed this view, because it allowed the study of amplified genes in NHLs. By using CGH, up to 32 DLBCLs of centroblastic variant have been analyzed by one group (74) leading to the detection of high level amplification of 18q21-23 in 21% of the patients with DNA copy number changes. By Southern blot hybridization this region was verified to include the *BCL2* gene in all cases with 18q21-23 overrepresentation in CGH analysis. FISH analysis disclosed that the extra material was present in marker (18q) chromosomes, and one case exhibited two complex translocations involving three or four chromosomes. Western blot analysis and immunohistology could then show that *BCL2* amplification had caused an increased BCL-2 protein expression. The cases were further studied for the presence of t(14;18) using a combination of various methods, including Southern blot analysis for *BCL2* rearrangement, PCR, and FISH. It could be demonstrated that *BCL2* rearrangement was never observed in cases with *BCL2* amplification (75). It seems that *BCL2* amplification is another mechanism, in addition to t(14;18), for BCL-2 protein overexpression. A later study of 96 DLBCLs revealed the presence of a 4- to 10-fold amplification of *BCL2* in 11% of the cases (76). These results support the hypothesis that gene amplification might play a role in the deregulation of *BCL2* gene in lymphomas.

Clinical Correlations of BCL2 *Gene Rearrangements*

Interpretations of the prognostic significance of *BCL2* rearrangement are controversial even though most studies have found no significant correlation with overall survival or disease-free survival (73,77–80). Yunis and colleagues reported that the presence of *BCL2* rearrangements in DLBCL indicated poor response to therapy and short survival (81). This was supported by another study observing an association between t(14;18) and worse disease-free survival in DLBCL patients (82). In contrast, Levine and associates found no differences in prognosis between patients with and without this translocation (77). Offit and coworkers later reported that DLBCL cases with t(14;18) at relapse have better survival than cases lacking this translocation (83). The drawbacks of most of the studies are that the number of cases investigated is often small, the follow-up period was fairly short and the included cases inhomogeneous as cases with previous history of follicular lymphoma are listed.

BCL2 *Gene Mutations*

Somatic mutations of the open reading frame of the translocated *BCL2* gene have been detected in the SU-DHL6 cell line and in some lymphomas carrying the t(14;18) translocation (84,85). The biologic significance of these mutations is highly debated. There are reports of follicular lymphoma carrying somatic mutations of the ORF leading to an alteration of the BCL-2 protein structure (85). These mutations may contribute to deregulation of BCL-2 protein by affecting its interactions with other *BCL2* family members or other oncogenes and tumor suppressor genes. Matolcsy and colleagues have also found that somatic mutations of the translocated *BCL2* gene are associated with morphologic transformation of follicular lymphoma to DLBCL. They consequently suggested that DLBCL cells might represent transformants of a preexisting follicular lymphoma clone, or may emerge from an unrelated B-cell clone containing a novel *BCL2* rearrangement. They also suggested that somatic mutations of the ORF of the *BCL2* are associated with higher-grade NHL (86). Studies on DLBCL cases for the presence of *BCL2* gene mutations have not been performed.

BCL-2 Protein Expression in Diffuse Large B-Cell Lymphoma

BCL-2 protein overexpression has been reported to occur in 22% to 80% of DLBCLs. Nodal tumors had a higher rate of BCL-2 reactivity compared with extranodal tumors (53). Although in the normal reactive secondary lymphoid follicle expression of BCL-2 and BCL-6 proteins show an inverse relationship, the situation in DLBCLs is different, because lymphomas with cytogenetically detected t(14;18) had usually a BCL-2^+/BCL-6^+ phenotype, while in those without this translocation the pattern is more variable without obvious relationship.

Not much is known about the impact of BCL-2 overexpression on survival in DLBCL. Although some studies have shown little evidence on the correlation of BCL-2 expression and poor clinical outcome (72,87), other groups report a clear correlation (73,80,88).

The antiapoptotic function of BCL-2 is thought to be modulated in part by its ability to heterodimerize with another member of the BCL-2 family named BAX, which promotes apoptosis countering the death repressor activity of BCL-2. It is the ratio of BCL-2 to BAX that determines survival or death after an apoptotic stimulus. Studies have suggested that in DLBCL the expression of BAX and BCL-2 are associated with poorer prognosis than high BCL-2 expression alone. However, BAX expression alone did not seem to have any association with prognosis, but tumors with low BAX expression and high BCL-2 expression had an improved 8-year disease-free survival (89). These results suggest that interactions between BCL-2 and BAX proteins may be crucial for tumor cells in deciding whether to survive or die and may provide novel insights into their functional and clinical significance.

The MYC *Gene and its Alterations*

The presence of the t(8;14)(q24;q32) translocation implies that the *MYC* oncogene located at chromosome 8 band q24 translocates into the IgH locus at 14q32 (90–92). In a minority of cases, the translocation is between chromosomes 2 and 8 or between 8 and 22, bringing *MYC* into the proximity of the IgL κ or λ region, respectively (93). This defect was initially reported in greater than 90% of Burkitt's lymphomas. It was recognized that all proliferating tissues express at least one member of the *MYC* family, usually *MYC*, that is downregulated when cells reach terminal differentiation or, in the case of lymphocytes, become long-lived memory cells resting in G_0 (94). Transfection experiments have shown that constitutive expression of *MYC* can prevent inducible differentiation, whereas repression of *MYC* by transfection with *MYC* antisense constructs can induce cell differentiation. *MYC* expression seems closely related to the decision between further proliferation and differentiation of the lymphoid tissue (see Chapter 8).

Several reports had described a certain rate of *MYC* rearrangements among DLBCLs (95). These rearrangements appeared to be structurally similar to those of sporadic Burkitt's lymphoma. However, subsequent studies unequivocally showed that *MYC* activation among primary DLBCLs is rare (96) and preferentially associates with very small numbers of extranodal DLBCLs or DLBCLs transformed from a previous follicular lymphoma (97). In a subsequent study of 156 cases of *de novo* DLBCLs, *MYC* rearrangements were found in 16% of primary extranodal lymphomas, compared with 2% of primary nodal cases. In particular, it became evident that *MYC* rearrangements occurred most frequently in primary gastrointestinal lymphomas (28% of the cases) (98). The distinct biologic behavior of these extranodal lymphomas was reflected by a high complete remission rate: 7 of 10 patients with *MYC* rearrangement attained complete remission, and 5 responders remained alive for more than 4 years.

*Nuclear Factor-κB/*REL *Gene Alterations*

Two members of the NF-κB/*REL* family of transcription factors appear to be involved in the pathogenesis of a fraction of DLBCLs, including NF-κB2 and REL. The *NF-κB2* gene maps to 10q24 and occasionally has been found to undergo rearrangement in DLBCL. These rearrangements are structurally similar to those more frequently found in T-cell NHL and cause the production of altered proteins that are unable to repress transcription and behave as constitutional transactivators (99–101). Genetic alterations of *REL* and more particular gene amplifications, appear to be a more frequent event, because they occur in 20% of DLBCLs, preferentially in cases with extranodal involvement (76,102).

The 6q Chromosomal Deletions

Nonrandom chromosomal deletions reflect the loss of genetic material and suggest the presence of tumor suppressor genes that are inactivated during the process of malignant transformation. Chromosomal deletions on the long arm of chromosome 6 (6q) have been found in a variety of human malignancies, including malignant melanoma (103), renal cell carcinoma (104), salivary gland adenocarcinoma (105), ovarian carcinoma (106), and hematologic malignancies. Among hematologic malignancies, 6q deletions occur most frequently in lymphoblastic leukemia and nodal NHLs of various types, including chronic lymphocytic leukemia, follicular lymphoma, and DLBCL (107). Regarding NHLs, cytogenetic studies have shown deletions in up to 15% (83) of the cases while studies on loss of heterozygosity have shown such alterations in 22% of NHLs (108). In nodal NHL, three regions (6q21, 6q23, and 6q25-27) were determined to show frequent deletions by cytogenetic analysis. However, an exclusive association of a specific 6q deletion with a distinct morphology and grade of NHL could not be confirmed (109–112). It is a matter of debate whether the presence of 6q deletions is of prognostic significance. Whereas one group concluded that breaks at 6q21-25 predicted a decreased probability of achieving remission (113), other studies failed to do so (42,111).

Epstein-Barr Virus

An additional molecular mechanism that may play a role in the development of DLBCL is infection of the tumor clone by oncogenic viruses. Epstein-Barr virus (EBV) represents the prototype of an oncogenic virus implicated in lymphomagenesis. Historically, EBV was initially identified in cases of endemic Burkitt's lymphoma of African children (114). Upon infection of a B cell, the EBV genome is transported into the nucleus where it is predominantly present as an extrachromosomal circular molecule (episome).

The pathogenetic relevance of EBV in lymphomagenesis is substantiated by the following data. EBV is able to significantly alter the growth of B cells *in vitro* and *in vivo* (115,116). EBV-infected cells can express the EBV-encoded proteins LMP-1 and more rarely EBNA-2, which are well-known transforming agents for B cells (117).

Despite these facts, several observations make the pathogenetic role of EBV in DLBCL difficult to understand. *In situ* hybridization for detection of EBV-encoded small nuclear RNA transcripts (EBER-1 and EBER 2) has shown that EBV infection of neoplastic cells is detectable only in a low percentage of cases. Only 15% of the 102 DLBCL cases analyzed (118) harbored the virus within the neoplastic cell population. Among the morphologic variants, the plasmablastic exhibited the highest association with EBV followed by the anaplastic, immunoblastic and centroblastic variants. Quantification of the infected neoplastic cells, however, complicated the picture as it revealed two different patterns among the EBV-associated DLBCLs: presence of the virus in all or nearly all neoplastic cells (about 50% of the EBV^+ cases) and presence of the virus in only a proportion (1% to 80%) of the neoplastic cells (about 50% of the EBV^+ cases). Although a role for the virus in the pathogenesis of the cases with infection of the total tumor cell population is conceivable, its role in the cases with partial infection is uncertain. It may be that EBV episomes get lost during progression of the tumor clones, an observation reported in longtime cultures of EBV-infected tumor cell lines (119,120). The latter hypothesis implies that EBV might have played a role at the time of tumor development.

CD10

CD10 is a proteolytic enzyme expressed on the surface of GCB cells and on a variety of other cells, including lymphoid precursor cells and some epithelial cells. *In vitro* and *in vivo* studies of B cells suggest a function of CD10 in the regulation of B-cell development (121). Expression of CD10 is a characteristic finding in lymphoblastic, Burkitt's and in follicular lymphoma. The precise frequency of CD10 expression in follicular lymphoma has not yet been established. Studies on a large number of DLBCL cases regarding CD10 expression in paraffin-embedded tissue specimens also have not been published. In a report analyzing cell suspensions by fluorescence-activated cell sorter for CD10 positivity, it was shown that 56% of DLBCL cases expressed this antigen (122) (see Chapter 3).

Syndecan-1/CD138

The syndecans are a family of cell surface proteoglycans (123). All four known members of the syndecan family (i.e., syndecan-1, -2, -3, and -4) are type I transmembrane proteins capable of mediating a broad range of functions, including cell-cell and cell–extracellular matrix adhesions, as well as acting as co-receptors in growth factor binding. Syndecan-1/CD138, the most extensively studied member of this family, is expressed predominantly on epithelial cells but also on hematopoietic B lineage cells. During normal murine B-cell differentiation, syndecan-1/CD138 is expressed on pre-B cells, lost on circulating B cells and is reexpressed on mature plasma cells (124). The expression of syndecan-1/CD138 correlates with stages of B-cell development in which the cells are sessile. Expression of syndecan-1/CD138 has been reported in lymphomas with terminally differentiated B cells, such as plasmacytomas (125) (see Chapter 3).

CD5

CD5 is expressed by the major subpopulation of B cells, the B-1 cells. The $CD5^+$ B cells show differences with the $CD5^-$ B cells in their anatomic localization, immunophenotype, gene usage and function (126–131). The number of $CD5^+$ B cells exhibits a variation throughout life: 40% to 60% in the fetus, 20% in the peripheral blood and spleen of adults, and 30% in adult lymph nodes and tonsils. In B-cell neoplasms, CD5 has been found to be a characteristic antigen of most cases of chronic lymphocytic leukemia/small lymphocytic lymphoma and mantle cell lymphoma, but only 5% to 10% of DLBCLs are known to express the CD5 antigen (132–134). It is unclear how many of these cases represent a transformed B-cell chronic lymphocytic leukemia (see Chapter 3).

CD30

The research team of Stein, while searching for viral antigens in the Hodgkin's disease cell line L428, generated among others the monoclonal antibody Ki-1 (135). In 1987, the Ki-1 molecule was clustered as a new B- and T-cell activation antigen, called CD30. By molecular cloning, the CD30 antigen was identified as a cytokine receptor of the tumor necrosis factor receptor family (136). Gene disruption and functional studies revealed that CD30 is involved in the negative selection of thymocytes and in the regulation of apoptosis and proliferation of activated lymphoid cells (137–139). The CD30 antigen proved to be an ideal marker for the Hodgkin and Reed-Sternberg cells of classic Hodgkin's disease. Screening of a large number of NHLs led to the identification of a group of lymphomas, the anaplastic large cell lymphomas, in which the CD30 molecule is expressed on all tumor cells (140). The detection of CD30 on some large perifollicular and intrafollicular blasts in normal lymphoid tissue and the finding that expression of this molecule can be induced on normal peripheral blood B and T cells by mitogens and viruses, indicate that CD30 represents a differentiation antigen whose expression is associated with activation of lymphoid cells (141) (see Chapter 3).

MUM1/IRF4 Protein

Chromosomal translocations affecting band 14q32 and unidentified partner chromosomes are common in multiple myeloma, suggesting that they may cause activation of novel oncogenes (142). The translocation t(6;14)(p25;q32) causes a juxtaposition of the IgH locus to the multiple myeloma oncogene 1 (*MUM1)/IRF4* gene (143,144). It has been suggested that as a consequence of this translocation, the *MUM1)/IRF4* gene is overexpressed, an event that may contribute to tumorigenesis.

The product of this gene, the MUM1/IRF4 protein (i.e., PIP, LSIRF, or ICSAT) (145–147) is a member of the interferon regulatory factor (IRF) family of transcription factors, known to play an important role in the regulation of gene expression in response to signalling by interferons and by other cytokines. By Northern blot analysis, strong expression of *MUM1)/IRF4* mRNA has been detected in mature B-cell derived lymphoma and myeloma cell lines (144) and in human T-cell lymphotropic virus type 1–infected T cells (147). The *MUM1)/IRF4*–deficient mice were unable to form GCs, lacked plasma cells in the spleen and lamina propria, and exhibited a profound reduction of serum immunoglobulin levels and an inability to mount detectable antibody responses or to generate cytotoxic T lymphocyte or antitumor responses (146). These findings provide evidence that the *MUM1)/IRF4* gene is essential for the function of mature B cells and cytotoxic lymphocytes. At the molecular level MUM1/IRF4 acts by forming a cooperative ternary complex with the transcription factor PU.1 at immunoglobulin enhancer elements (148–151).

A new monoclonal antibody generated against MUM1/IRF4 was used to study its expression patterns in a variety of tissues. MUM1 was found to be expressed in the nuclei of plasma cells and a small percentage of GC B light zone cells displaying some degree of plasmacellular differentiation. The phenotype of the latter cells was MUM1$^+$/BCL-6$^-$/Ki-67$^-$, different from that of most GC B cells (MUM1$^-$/BCL-6$^+$/Ki-67$^+$) and mantle zone B cells (MUM1$^-$/BCL-6$^-$/Ki-67$^-$). MUM1 expression was identified in 75% of the DLBCL cases analyzed. Unlike normal GC B cells, in which expression of MUM1 and BCL-6 were mutually exclusive, tumor cells of approximately 50% of the MUM1$^+$ DLBCLs also expressed BCL-6, suggesting that expression of these proteins is deregulated in these lymphomas (152).

The **TP53** *Gene and its Alterations*

The p53 transcription regulatory protein monitors the integrity of the genome by arresting cells at G_1 or programming them to cell death when DNA replication is defective or when DNA is damaged. Mutations of the *TP53* gene lead to a loss of function by a recessive or dominant negative process. Inactivation of *TP53* is reported to be virtually absent in DLBCLs arising *de novo,* but it frequently is associated with cases resulting from the histologic transformation from follicular lymphoma to DLBCL (153,154). It is likely that disruption of normal p53 functions may contribute to tumor progression directly by providing follicular lymphoma cells with a high proliferative rate or indirectly by following the accumulation of additional genetic lesions (see Chapter 8).

P27/KIP1

The p27 cyclin-dependent kinase (CDK) inhibitor downregulation is essential for the transition to the S phase of the cell cycle (155,156). Proliferating cells in reactive lymphoid tissue show no detectable p27 expression (157). Although most lymphomas analyzed exhibit a weak or no p27 expression (158) anomalous high p27 expression has been shown to exist in a group of aggressive lymphomas of Burkitt's and DLBCL type characterized by a high proliferation index and an adverse clinical outcome (159). This suggests that in these cases the abnormally accumulated p27 protein has been rendered functionally inactive. Analysis of the causes of the anomalous p27 presence revealed a statistically significant association between p27 and cyclin D3 expression. Cases with stronger cyclin D3 expression showed a higher p27 expression (160). These data support the hypothesis that there are cyclin D3/p27 complexes in a subset of aggressive lymphomas, including DLBCL, in which p27 lacks the inhibitory activity found when it is bound to cyclin E/CDK2 complexes. The cause of this anomalous p27 and cyclin D3 expression in these cases has not yet been identified.

MORPHOLOGIC VARIANTS OF DIFFUSE LARGE B-CELL LYMPHOMAS

Centroblastic Variant

Definition

This morphologic variant includes tumors with a cellular component exhibiting the morphologic features of centroblasts found in reactive GCs. These are medium to large-sized cells (10 to 14 μm) with relatively large round or oval vesicular nuclei, fine chromatin, two to four membrane-bound nucleoli and scanty basophilic cytoplasm (Fig. 25.1). The lymphomas of this variant encompass tumors containing cells that resemble immunoblasts. Because the percentage of the immunoblast-like cells within this entity ranges from

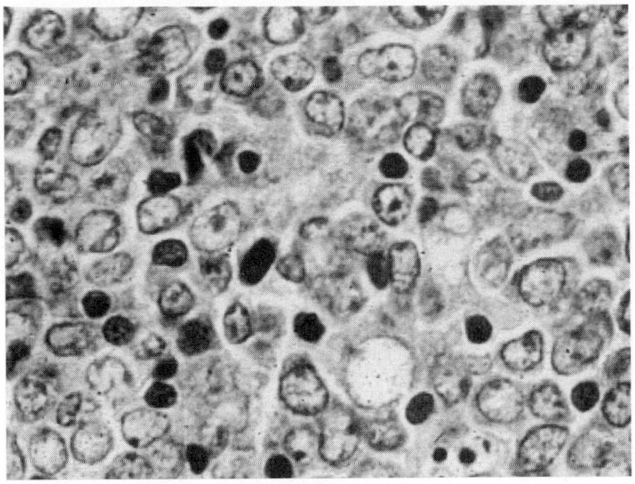

FIG. 25.1. Centroblastic variant of diffuse large B-cell lymphoma. The monomorphous infiltrate of cells resembles typical centroblasts (Giemsa-stained paraffin section).

0% to 90% of the entire population, it is evident that the border between the centroblastic and immunoblastic variant is not clear-cut. This indicates that the distinction between these two variants is problematic and arbitrary in daily routine diagnosis, reducing diagnostic reproducibility and that the centroblastic variant is the largest and most important group among the DLBCLs. According to the WHO concept, the pathologist has the possibility to further specify the given centroblastic lymphoma according to its cellular features in monomorphic, multilobated, and polymorphic subvariants.

In the monomorphic subvariant, most neoplastic cells resemble typical centroblasts, resulting in a monotonous-looking appearance. In the multilobated subvariant, the tumors contain many medium-sized to large cells with nuclei exhibiting more than three lobes. The chromatin is very fine, and it is often difficult to recognize the nucleoli. In the polymorphic subvariant, the tumors clearly consist of a mixture of centroblast-like cells, immunoblast-like cells and cells with overlapping features. The immunoblast-like cells may be present in variable numbers and can comprise up to 90% of the neoplastic cell population. In most cases they catch the eye because of their size and morphology (large central nucleoli; abundant basophilic cytoplasm).

Immunohistologic Findings

These lymphomas express various pan-B-cell markers such as CD19, CD20, CD22, and CD79a. Surface immunoglobulin can be demonstrated in most cases (IgM > IgG). CD5 is detectable in approximately 10% of the cases. The CD10 antigen can be found in a variable proportion of the cases (precise data are not available). A variable but usually very small proportion of the neoplastic cells may also show weak CD30 expression. The proliferative fraction as detected by Ki-67 staining is usually high (>40%).

Genetic Findings

Analysis of the IgH and IgL genes of 10 cases of the centroblastic variant revealed the presence of somatic mutations within the rearranged genes, indicating that the cells of origin are derived from GC or post-GC B cells (161). According to the experience of the investigators' laboratory, polymerase chain reaction (PCR) analysis of the IgH genes may led to negative results in 30% to 50% of the cases. This is most probably due to the high number of somatic mutations inhibiting primer annealing.

A cytogenetic study of 68 cases classified as centroblastic lymphoma according to the Kiel classification criteria showed that the most frequent numerical aberrations were gains of chromosomes X, 3, 5, 7, 12, and 18 and losses of chromosomes Y, 6, 13, 15, and 17 (162). Regarding the presence of chromosomal translocations, the t(14;18) translocation was the most frequent, because it was detected in 20 (29.4%) of 68 cases. This finding supports data of an earlier study (163). The t(3;14) was detected in 9 (12.3%) of 63 cases, and the typical Burkitt's lymphoma translocation t(8;14) was present in two cases of this variant (2.9%). No variant *MYC* translocations were seen (162).

Latent EBV infection of the neoplastic cells has been identified only in a minority of cases (8%) (164). In all positive cases, the virus was detectable only in a proportion of the neoplastic cell population, questioning the importance of EBV in the pathogenesis of these cases.

Immunoblastic Variant

Definition

By definition more than 90% of the cells of this variant show a single, centrally located nucleolus and have an appreciable amount of basophilic cytoplasm (Fig. 25.2). Plasma-

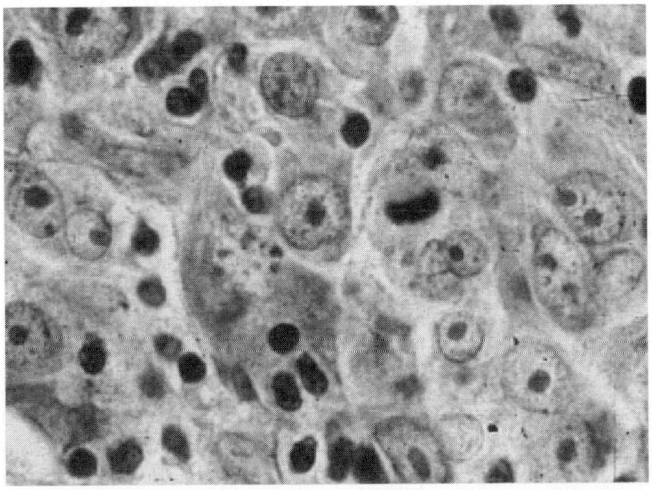

FIG. 25.2. Immunoblastic variant of diffuse large B-cell lymphoma. Notice the centrally located, prominent nucleoli (Giemsa-stained paraffin section).

cellular differentiation may or may not be seen and is evidenced by admixed plasma cells and plasmablasts.

According to the defining histologic criteria, this variant makes up only a very low percentage of DLBCLs. As calculated in the last version of the Kiel classification (165) only 4% of all NHLs would be included in the immunoblastic variant. The lumping of this variant in the DLBCL group by the REAL classification has ignited massive protest from the Kiel group. They were able to show in prospective, randomized, multicenter trials that the distinction between centroblastic and immunoblastic lymphomas according to the Kiel classification is a significant prognostic risk factor. Overall survival was significantly shorter in immunoblastic lymphoma than in centroblastic lymphoma; relapse-free survival also proved to be worse in cases of immunoblastic compared with centroblastic lymphomas, even when the patient collective analyzed was inhomogeneous regarding treatment (162,166). The study of Engelhard and associates has a significant drawback in its design, because all histopathologic diagnoses were made after reprocessing the specimens and embedding in resin and were at the end established by a single person. It remains to be seen whether studies at other centers will be able to identify the immunoblastic variant as the most aggressive group of DLBCLs.

Immunohistologic Findings

The immunophenotype is largely identical to that of the centroblastic variant. In addition to surface immunoglobulin (IgM > IgG > IgA), cases with plasmacellular differentiation also show the same immunoglobulin light chain within immunoblasts, plasmablasts, and proplasma cells.

Genetic Findings

The few cases analyzed harbored somatic mutations within the rearranged IgH and IgL genes, indicating a derivation from mature B cells that have participated in a GC reaction.

The study of the Kiel-Wien Lymphoma Study Group, showed that the most frequent numerical aberrations of this variant were gains of chromosomes 3,7,12, and 18 and losses of chromosomes Y, 8, 10, 14, and 21. When chromosomal abnormalities were compared for their frequency, losses of the whole chromosome 10, deletions in 8q and 14q, and structural abnormalities of 4p were significantly more frequent in the immunoblastic than in the centroblastic variant. Several differences in chromosomal translocations became clear. The typical Burkitt's translocation t(8;14) was not detectable within the 26 cases of immunoblastic variant. The t(14;18) was significantly rarer in 1 (3.6%) of 26 cases than in the centroblastic variant, whereas the t(3;14) translocation was observed as frequently as in the centroblastic variant in 5 (17.9%) of 21 cases (162). It seems that so far no characteristic chromosomal abnormalities of the immunoblastic DLBCL variant have been identified. Schouten and coworkers assumed that patients with an abnormal chromosome 6 had an increased frequency to suffer from immunoblastic lymphoma (167). This could not be verified by the Kiel-Wien Lymphoma Study Group where no significant difference in 6q deletions between centroblastic and immunoblastic lymphomas were found (162).

Latent EBV infection has been identified within the neoplastic cells of 14% of the cases (164), a higher incidence than observed in the centroblastic variant. However, EBV was never found to infect the entire neoplastic cell population, but only a proportion of it. The significance of EBV as an important factor in the pathogenesis of this variant seems therefore to be low.

Anaplastic Variant

Definition

Anaplastic large cell lymphoma is characterized by a proliferation of large neoplastic cells with bizarre, anaplastic morphology (Fig. 25.3A). As the neoplastic cells show immunoreactivity with antibodies against CD30 in almost all cases, this lymphoma has also been designated Ki-1 or $CD30^+$ lymphoma. In the past, anaplastic large cell lymphoma was often erroneously diagnosed as immunoblastic lymphoma, histiocytic malignancy, or metastatic carcinoma. Immunohistologic analysis led to the establishment of this lymphoma as a distinct entity in the updated Kiel classification. The wealth of data accumulated within the past years has completely changed the concepts of this lymphoma category. As extensively analyzed in the anaplastic large cell lymphoma (ALCL) section of this chapter, the non–B-ALCLs have been recognized to include distinct entities with specific clinicopathologic and molecular features. This fact and the observation that B-cell ALCLs do not show significant differences from the other DLBCL variants in the clinical course (168) have been taken into account by the REAL classification that has recognized ALCLs of T/null cell phenotype as an entity, while those with a B-cell phenotype have been grouped within the DLBCL category.

Unfortunately, the anaplastic DLBCL variant has not yet been sufficiently analyzed. This is mostly due to the fact that such cases constitute only a small percentage (less than 20%) of the anaplastic large cell lymphoma group (140,169). The morphologic distinction of these cases from other variants of DLBCL (i.e., centroblastic and immunoblastic) is not straightforward (168). These facts have hampered the collection of representative data regarding phenotype, molecular biologic features, and prognosis.

Histologic Findings

For a more extensive description of morphology the reader may refer to the ALCL section of this chapter. The tumor cells are large with abundant cytoplasm. Giant cells can be observed, whereas the so-called hallmark cells of ALCL are not frequently encountered.

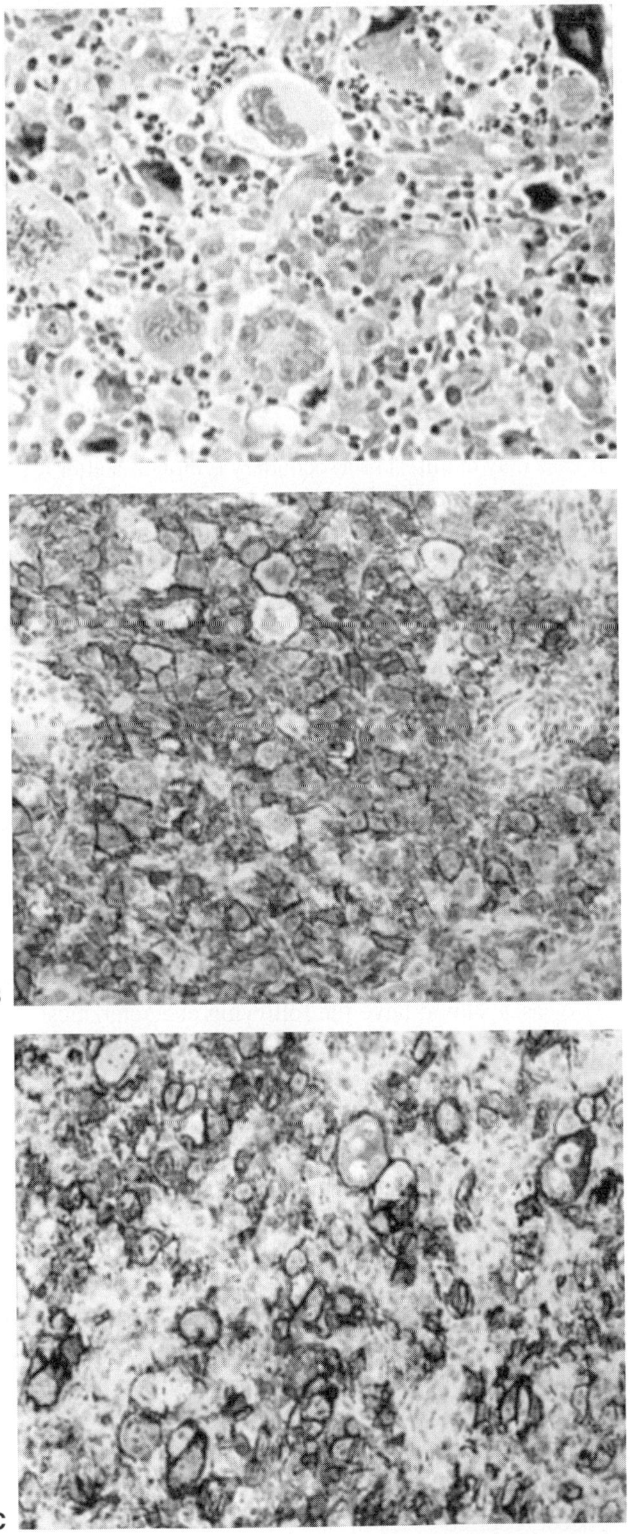

A

B

C

FIG. 25.3. Anaplastic variant of diffuse large B-cell lymphoma. **A:** The infiltrate is composed of large, bizarre, often multinucleated neoplastic cells (Giemsa-stained paraffin section). **B:** Expression of CD20 by the bizarre neoplastic cells (paraffin section, alkaline phosphatase and anti-alkaline phosphatase [APAAP] technique using monoclonal antibody L26). **C:** The neoplastic cells show membranous CD30 expression (paraffin section, APAAP technique with monoclonal antibody Ber-H2).

Immunohistologic Findings

By definition, the neoplastic cells show expression of B-cell associated antigens (CD19, CD20, CD22) combined with CD30 expression (Fig. 25.3B). The CD30 immunostaining is highly variable; it ranges from strong membrane-bound or dotlike to weakly diffuse cytoplasmic in contrast to the consistently strong cell membrane expression observed in the T/null cell ALCL (Fig 25.3C). In addition to CD30, further activation-related antigens have been found, including CD23, CD21, CD38, CD71, and CD25. CD45 is also detected on the neoplastic cells, but CD15 is usually absent (170,171).

Genetic Findings

Clonal rearrangements of the IgH genes have been reported in 3 of 5 cases studied by the Southern blot hybridization method (171). Using appropriate PCR methods, rearranged IgH genes have been found in 59% of the B-cell ALCL cases analyzed (172). Most cases (90%) harbored a high load of somatic mutations within the rearranged V_H region genes. The average mutation frequency was 13%, similar to that observed in other DLBCLs and in follicular lymphomas and classic Hodgkin's disease. The finding of the presence of somatic mutations suggests that the tumor cells of B-ALCL are derived from GC or post-GC B cells. The replacement to silent ratio of somatic mutations within the V_H genes was further analyzed to verify a possible selection for high-affinity antigen binding. The R/S value of the cases with in-frame rearrangement indicated that the mutations were selected for increased antibody affinity (173).

The presence of infection by EBV has been analyzed in some cases with variable results. In an early study using the Southern blot technique none of the ALCL cases with a B cell phenotype was found to harbor the EBV genome (174). However, later studies from a Japanese research group have shown a high association of these cases with EBV infection (6 [35%] of 17 cases) (170). In that study, EBV was detectable by Southern blot and PCR methods, including the demonstration of monoclonal EBV episomes in most of the cases. In the EBV-associated cases, *in situ hybridization* for EBER detection revealed labeling of the neoplastic cells. In all cases an additional expression of the latent membrane protein (LMP-1) of EBV was observed, as well as the additional presence of EBNA-2 expression in two cases. Similar findings have also been reported in three cases of an earlier study of the EBV association of ALCL (175). This data has to be interpreted with caution as such an EBV protein expression pattern (LMP-1$^+$, EBNA-2$^+$) is found mostly in lymphomas and lymphoid proliferations associated with various causes of immunodeficiency. As the published data imply that these EBV$^+$ cases have been induced by the viral infection, they should be considered separately. In another study encompassing 16 cases of the anaplastic variant, EBER$^+$ neoplastic cells were identified in 19% of the cases

(118). In these cases EBV protein expression restricted to LMP-1 was identified.

T-Cell–Rich/Histiocyte-Rich Variant

Concepts Influencing the Definition

This morphoimmunophenotypic variant of DLBCL was originally described in 1984 in abstract form by Jaffe and coworkers as pseudoperipheral T-cell lymphoma (176). All six cases were preceded by follicular lymphomas. The definition given by these investigators included a diffuse mixed or large cell morphology and a mixture of large neoplastic B cells with a predominant component of up to 75% reactive T cells. The latter cell component was thought to represent a "beneficial host response," given the indolent course of these patients' disease despite conversion to a large cell lymphoma. Mirchandani and coworkers also described seven B-cell lymphomas with a morphologic resemblance to T-cell lymphoma (177). Cell suspension studies revealed that 80% of the cellular population consisted of E-rosetting T lymphocytes. The tumor cells were found to be of B-cell origin, as demonstrated by the detection of a single class of surface or cytoplasmic immunoglobulin (178). Ramsay and coworkers coined the term *T-cell–rich B-cell lymphoma* in their study of five cases in which the small T cells exceeded 90% of the entire nodal population, and the B cells were found to be clonal as demonstrated by light-chain restriction in Ig expression (179). In this study, the tumors appeared to arise *de novo,* and the clinical course was aggressive. The observations of Ramsay and coworkers were soon confirmed by Ng and associates, who analyzed an additional 21 cases with T cells making up 50% to 90% of the cell population (180). Large B cells were present in all cases, and most were centroblast-like or immunoblast-like cells. Reed-Sternberg–like cells were also observed in eight cases. In fourteen cases monotypic light-chain restriction was identified.

A substantial number of further reports on lymphoid neoplasms fitting into the category of T-cell–rich large B-cell lymphoma have been added in the years that followed (181–187). A further part of the spectrum of this lymphoma variant was described by Delabie and coworkers showing numerous nonepithelioid histiocytes, a marked male predominance, advanced disease stage at presentation and an aggressive disease course. They coined the term *histiocyte-rich B-cell lymphoma* and argued that it shares a common origin with lymphocyte predominance Hodgkin's disease (188).

If one summarizes the features of the cases published as T-cell–rich large B-cell lymphoma, it is evident that the cases reported are heterogeneous with regard to the proportion of T cells, the relative number and morphology of the large cells, and the histologic pattern. This is easy to understand because strict criteria have not been used, leading to the unhappy situation of a broad spectrum of lymphomas lumped together in one category. This broad spectrum of lymphomas is underlined by the descriptive terms used (i.e., *poorly differentiated lymphocytic lymphoma, Lennert's lymphoma, mixed lymphocytic-histiocytic lymphoma, poorly histiocytic lymphoma, T-zone lymphoma, peripheral T-cell lymphoma Waldron's type,* and *Hodgkin's-like lymphoma* [189]). The lack of homogeneity of published cases is also reflected in the reported variable biology of the disease; some investigators described these tumors as following an indolent course, others found a highly variable outcome, and still others reported the cases to behave aggressively. According to the literature there seem to be manifold relationships between T-cell–rich large B-cell lymphoma and other lymphoma types. This can be deduced from the fact that this lymphoma does not always arise *de novo,* but may develop from, accompany, or transform into other lymphomas. The disease may manifest as a secondary lymphoma after follicular lymphoma or DLBCL or even lymphocyte predominance Hodgkin's disease. It has also transformed into follicular or DLBCL. Coexistence with follicular lymphoma has also been observed (189). These facts have led to the concept that T-cell–rich B-cell lymphoma does not represent an entity but comprises a heterogeneous group of B-cell lymphomas rich in reactive T cells or histiocytes, by which they mimic peripheral T-cell lymphoma or Hodgkin's disease. This concept has been adopted by the REAL classification, which has not separated T-cell–rich large B-cell lymphoma as an entity, but incorporated it as a variant in the DLBCL group.

Definition

Although there is not complete agreement on the criteria for diagnosis of the T-cell-/histiocyte-rich variant, the prototypic cases should have the following characteristics:

A diffuse growth pattern is seen throughout the entire specimen on hematoxylin and eosin stain.
Scattered large neoplastic B cells with a highly variable morphology make up less than 10% of the total cell population; they may show a nodular grouping in some instances.
The other cells present are mostly T cells and histiocytes.
Clonality of the neoplastic B cells can be demonstrated by immunohistologic and molecular techniques.
Despite sharing features with lymphocyte predominance Hodgkin's disease, it is usually associated with advanced clinical stage at presentation and aggressive behavior.

Clinical Presentation

Most reported cases of this DLBCL variant are nodal tumors, with rare examples occurring in a variety of extranodal sites such as skull, brain, nasopharynx, parotid, tongue, mediastinum, lung, common bile duct, spleen, skin, and soft tissues. The disease is usually at an advanced stage at presentation; more than 60% of the patients present with stage III or IV disease, frequently showing spleen and bone marrow involvement (190). There is a slight male predominance and most patients are in their fifth or sixth decade.

Histologic Findings

The infiltrate is diffuse and is composed of a mixture of lymphoid cells while the large cell population can be inconspicuous (Fig. 25.4A). The small lymphoid cells (which usually belong to the T lineage) have dark round, irregular and convoluted nuclei. Medium-sized lymphocytes (usually of T-cell lineage) with round or folded nuclei can be recognized. Interspersed, there are large lymphoid cells distributed diffusely or accumulated in groups. In some cases, they resemble immunoblasts or centroblasts, in other cases they mimic the lymphohistiocytic (L&H) cells found in lymphocyte predominance Hodgkin's disease. Multinucleated forms resembling Reed-Sternberg cells may be present.

High endothelial venules may or may not be prominent, but can be so striking that the lesion is reminiscent of an angioimmunoblastic T-cell lymphoma. Variable numbers of histiocytes, which may have an epithelioid appearance, are often intermingled, and a pattern mimicking lymphoepithelioid (i.e., Lennert's lymphoma) T-cell lymphoma can occur. Plasma cells and eosinophils may be prominent in some cases.

Bone marrow infiltrates can exhibit a paratrabecular or a diffuse growth pattern. The cellular composition is similar to that found in primary diagnostic biopsy specimens.

A

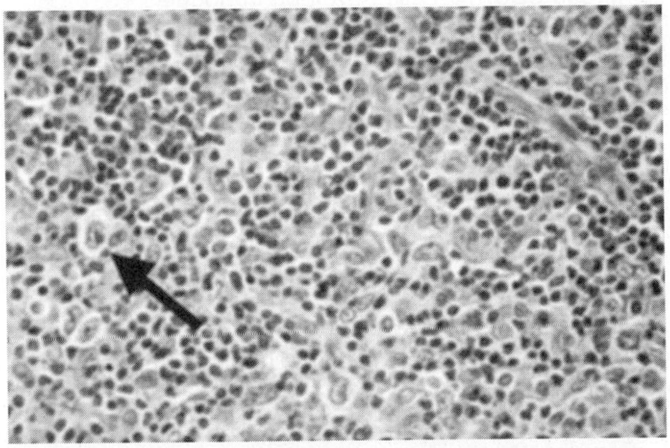

B

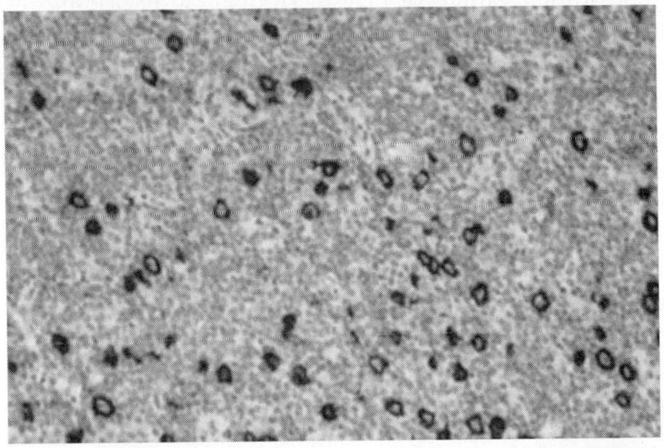

C

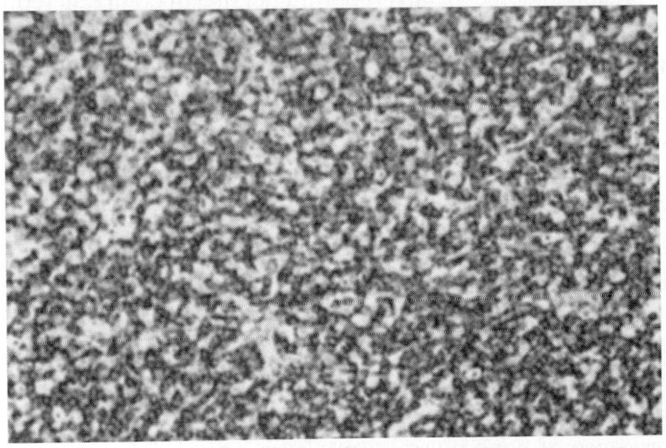

FIG. 25.4. T-cell–rich and histiocyte-rich variant of diffuse large B-cell lymphoma. **A:** By conventional histology, the scarce neoplastic cells *(arrow)* are not easily identifiable within the lymphocyte and histiocyte-rich background infiltrate (hematoxylin and eosin–stained paraffin section). **B:** Immunostaining for CD20 highlights the neoplastic cells (paraffin section immunostained with monoclonal antibody L26, alkaline phosphatase and anti-alkaline phosphatase [APAAP] technique). **C:** Immunostaining for CD3 reveals the T-cell–rich background infiltrate (paraffin section immunostained with anti-CD3 polyclonal antibody, APAAP technique).

Immunohistologic Findings

Immunohistologic analysis reveals a predominant T-cell population corresponding to more than 90% of the infiltrate (Fig. 25.4C) and scattered large cells with a B cell phenotype (Fig. 25.4B). The T cells are immunophenotypically normal, with $CD4^+$ cells usually predominating over CD8-expressing cells (179,183). Practically all the large atypical cells stain for various B-cell markers such as L26 (CD20), 4KB5 (CD45RA), and mb-1 (CD79a). In many cases monotypic surface or cytoplasmic immunoglobulin can be demonstrated on frozen and paraffin sections, respectively (179,180,183). Problems in interpretation of immunohistologic detection of immunoglobulin expression caused by the passive uptake of interstitial immunoglobulin can often be circumvented by the use of *in situ* hybridization for immunoglobulin mRNA (184). Expression of J-chain has been investigated only in the minority of the cases published. In one study, a percentage of 19% positivity was given (191). With few exceptions (183,185,187), the atypical large cells do not show any expression of the CD30 antigen. Expression of the epithelial membrane antigen (EMA) was reported to be common in one study (184), but other groups could not make similar observations.

Molecular Genetic Findings

Genotypic analysis by the Southern blot hybridization technique (182,183,186) or PCR (185) has demonstrated rearrangements of the IgH and IgL genes, but not the T-cell receptor (TCR) genes. Because of the low number of neoplastic cells it is possible that the tumor cell clone may escape detection (179).

The neoplastic atypical B-blasts have been isolated directly from specimens of six cases of the T-cell–rich DLBCL variant by means of a hydraulic micromanipulator (192). The DNA obtained from such single cells was analyzed for the presence of rearrangements in the variable region of the IgH and IgL chain genes. In all cases clonal Ig gene rearrangements were identified in the isolated large cells expressing B-cell antigen CD20. This data confirms that the large atypical blasts in this variant represent neoplastic cells. In all cases the rearranged Ig genes carried somatic mutations. These findings are similar to those reported for the other DLBCL variants and imply that the tumor cells are derived from mature B cells that have participated in a GC reaction (i.e., GC or post-GC B cells). Analysis of R/S mutations within the FRs revealed signs of selection toward an antigen. The sole molecular difference in the other DLBCLs was the finding of frequent intraclonal diversity of the somatic mutations. Because the process of somatic hypermutation appears to be restricted to GC B cells, the finding of intraclonal diversity points out that the precursors of the tumor clone in the T-cell–/histiocyte-rich variant are GC B cells. It is, however, unclear whether the somatic hypermutation machinery was still active in the tumor cells at the time of biopsy. It is therefore possible that the intraclonal diversity of the neoplastic cells resulted from ongoing mutations that occurred at a very early stage of the clonal expansion with subsequent outgrowth of the subclones.

BCL2 gene rearrangement is identified in some cases, suggesting that these cases may be related to follicular lymphoma (185–187). Viral DNA has been detected in a small proportion of cases (183).

Differential Diagnosis

Differentiation of the T-cell–/histiocyte-rich variant of DLBCL from Hodgkin's disease is of therapeutic and prognostic importance. Patients that had been initially misdiagnosed as having Hodgkin's disease showed only a partial response and an early relapse (193,194). These observations stress the importance of not confusing DLBCL of the T-cell–/histiocyte-rich variant with Hodgkin's disease.

Lymphocyte predominance Hodgkin's disease (LPHD) can be difficult to distinguish from the T-cell-/histiocyte-rich variant, particularly in specimens showing a largely diffuse growth pattern, because the cellular composition of both entities may be quite similar. However, immunohistologic studies for CD20, CD21, CD3, and CD57 can highlight the presence of nodular growth in a LPHD specimen by demonstrating even small nodular accumulations of B lymphocytes (i.e., small B cells), a concomitant meshwork of follicular dendritic cells and the presence of rosettes from CD3 or CD57$^+$ NK/T cells surrounding the large neoplastic blasts (Table 25.2).

Application of these criteria to a multinational study of a large collection of cases submitted as LPHD revealed that even cases of LPHD that show a diffuse growth pattern on hematoxylin and eosin stains usually contain small areas of

TABLE 25.2. *Immunophenotypic criteria for identifying the extent of nodularity in lymphocyte predominance Hodgkin's disease*

Nodular or vaguely nodular clusters of small B cells
Neoplastic B blasts within the small B-cell nodules
Nodular aggregates of CD21$^+$ follicular dendritic cells
Numerous CD57$^+$ T cells arranged in nodules

nodularity, while LPHD cases devoid of signs of nodularity are rare (Anagnostopoulos and coworkers, unpublished data). This raises the question as to whether completely diffuse LPHD cases really exist, or whether such cases represent DLBCLs of T-cell-/histiocyte-rich variant. Criteria that may help in the differentiation between this DLBCL variant and LPHD are listed in Table 25.3.

The differential diagnosis with Hodgkin's disease is difficult only when classic Hodgkin's disease cases are rich in lymphocytes and show a diffuse growth pattern. This lymphocyte-rich variant of classic Hodgkin's disease has also been found to have a background rich in CD3$^+$ T lymphocytes. The immunophenotype of the neoplastic cells can solve the diagnostic problem as these exhibit a classic Hodgkin's disease immunophenotype (CD30$^+$, usually CD15$^+$), entirely different from that of the T-cell–rich/histiocyte-rich variant. B-cell antigens may be expressed by the neoplastic cells in classic Hodgkin's disease but this expression is usually limited to a proportion of the neoplastic cell population and the intensity of expression varies greatly.

Prognosis

Whereas some groups reported persistent complete remissions with combination chemotherapy in 62% and 84% of the patients, respectively (185,194), others observed poor results in patients with liver involvement (195). In the series of Greer and colleagues, excellent results were achieved only in limited-stage patients, and patients with poor prognostic factors seemed to benefit from high-dose chemotherapy with marrow transplantation (196). Skinnider and colleagues reported a complete response in 60% of the patients, even with bone marrow infiltration, when the correct diagnosis was established at presentation (190). That study did not identify any differences in survival between patients with T-cell/histiocyte-rich and those with "common" DLBCL, even in the presence of bone marrow involvement.

Lymphomatoid Granulomatosis Variant

Concepts Influencing the Definition

Lymphomatoid granulomatosis (LYG) was first described as a distinct clinicopathologic entity by Liebow and coworkers in 1972. It was defined as an angiocentric and angiodestructive lymphoproliferative process (197). It typically involves the lung but has also been described as presenting at

TABLE 25.3. *Morphologic and immunohistologic features for differentiating between lymphocyte predominance Hodgkin's disease and T-cell/histiocyte–rich variant of diffuse large B-cell lymphoma*

Feature	LPHD	DLBCL T-cell-/histiocyte–rich variant
Morphology of the neoplastic cells		
L&H (popcorn)	Predominant	Minor proportion
Reed-Sternberg cells	Variable number	Rare
Centroblast-like	−	+
Immunoblast-like	−	+
Phenotype of neoplastic cells		
CD45	+	+
CD20	+ (appx. 100%)	+
CD79a	+ (80–100%)	+
J-chain	+ (92%)	−/+ (19%)
CD30	−	− (few exceptions)
CD15	−	−
EMA	54%	Up to 100%
Latent EBV infection of neoplastic cells		
EBER	−	?
LMP-1	−	9.5%
Composition of the cellular background		
$CD20^+$ small B cells	Many in nodular areas, few in diffuse	Few cells
$CD57^+$ T cells	Many within the nodules, occasionally forming rosettes, low number in diffuse areas	Few cells
TIA^- (T-cell–associated antigen) − 1^+ cells	Few cells	Large number of cells

several other sites (i.e., skin, kidney, liver, and central nervous system). As originally described, the diagnosis is based on recognition of a characteristic histologic triad: polymorphic lymphoid infiltrate composed of small lymphocytes, plasma cells, and a variable number of large immunoblasts; angiitis characterized by transmural infiltration of the walls of arteries and veins by mononuclear cells; and granulomatosis, a term used to describe necrosis occurring within lymphoid nodules rather than true granuloma formation.

Subsequent reports stated that many cases were malignant from the outset or went on to develop frank lymphomas (198–200). Subsequent immunohistologic studies on frozen sections identified most cells, including those infiltrating the blood vessels, as T cells, leading to the belief that LYG is a T-cell process. The term *angiocentric immunoproliferative lesion* was introduced by Jaffe to include lymphomatoid granulomatosis and polymorphic reticulosis (i.e., lethal midline granuloma) (201). A grading system was also proposed for these lesions (Table 25.4).

When T-cell receptor gene rearrangements were sought in LYG, little was found to support the hypothesis that LYG and polymorphic reticulosis represent different aspects of one entity: no TCR β chain or γ chain gene rearrangement could be found, and only one case with δ chain gene rearrangement was seen, this in a grade 3 lesion (202). A further interesting observation was made by Katzenstein and Peiper who identified EBV by PCR in most cases of LYG, implicating a viral infection in the pathogenesis of this disorder (203). In the REAL classification lymphomatoid granulomatosis/angiocentric immunoproliferative lesions have been classed together as angiocentric T-cell lymphomas, although cases with a B-cell phenotype were observed.

In the years that followed, the situation changed, because it could be repeatedly demonstrated that the atypical lymphoid cells harboring EBV-encoded EBER transcripts express a B-cell phenotype (204,205). These findings have supported the view that most cases of LYG, in particular grade 3, represent a T-cell–rich, EBV-associated B-cell lymphoproliferative disorder. This interpretation was underlined by the finding of oligoclonal or monoclonal immunoglobulin gene rearrangements in many cases by PCR or light-chain restriction by immunohistology (206). The findings that in LYG T cells, histiocytes and $CD57^+$ cells do not proliferate and that the average proliferation index of B cells

TABLE 25.4. *Criteria for histopathologic grading of angiocentric immunoproliferative lesions*

Grade 1	
	Polymorphous infiltrate (lymphoid cells, plasma cells, histiocytes, +/− eosinophils)
	Large lymphoid cells/immunoblasts are infrequent and lack cytologic atypia.
Grade 2	
	Polymorphous infiltrate (as grade 1)
	Cytologic atypia in small lymphoid cells
	Occasional large lymphoid cells/immunoblasts that lack marked cytologic atypia
Grade 3	
	Malignant lymphoma on cytologic grounds
	Monomorphic infiltrate with marked cytologic atypia in small and large lymphoid cells

in grade 3 LYG is similar to that observed in DLBCLs have led to the conclusion that grade 3 LYG is a morphologic variant of DLBCL and should be treated accordingly (207). It became evident that the previously mentioned features of LYG could accurately separate it from the EBV-associated angiocentric NK/T-cell lymphomas.

Definition

The LYG variant of DLBCL represents an angiocentric/angiodestructive T-cell–rich, EBV-associated B-cell lymphoma.

Histologic Features

There is a nodular growth of an angiocentric or angiodestructive lymphoid infiltrate in the involved organ. Necrosis is present in all cases. The infiltrate consists of small- to medium-sized lymphocytes with angulated nuclei and an interspersed population of medium to large-sized atypical cells making up to 40% of the total lymphoid population. Most of these large atypical cells exhibit vesicular nuclei containing coarsely clumped chromatin and prominent nucleoli, occasionally resembling Reed-Sternberg cells. In all cases there are also numerous histiocytes with scattered karyorrhectic debris. Mitotic figures can be frequent.

Immunohistologic Findings

Most of the background lymphocytes of small to medium-size stain positively with antibodies to CD3. These cells are also those that usually participate in the vascular lesions. The medium-sized to large atypical cells stain positively with antibodies to B-cell antigens and show a large growth fraction. These cells usually predominate adjacent to necrotic zones. In the cases tested these cells did not show CD30 or CD15 expression. Monoclonal immunoglobulin light-chain restriction can be observed in occasional cases.

Genetic Findings

Clonal rearrangements of the IgH genes can be demonstrated by PCR.

The number of infected cells as detected by EBER-ISH is high and ranges up to 40% of the total cell number. The labeled cells correspond to the medium to large-sized atypical B-blasts.

Clinical Features

In most series the median age of the patients is approximately 57 years (range, 24 to 76 years). There is always a clear-cut male over female predominance. Symptoms at presentation are usually cough, hemoptysis, dyspnea and chest pain. There is usually lung involvement at presentation, which can be unilateral or bilateral and is usually described as forming multiple nodules or consolidation or lobar collapse. Other organs that can be involved at presentation are the skin, the liver, central nervous system or kidney.

Differential Diagnosis

Pulmonary LYG shares histologic and clinical similarities with EBV-associated lymphoproliferative disorders (EBV-LPD) occurring in immunosuppressed patients. Both processes consist of a polymorphous infiltrate containing areas of necrosis and various numbers of large atypical cells, and they both can lead to overt lymphoma. The B cells in both processes have been found to harbor EBV and EBV-LPDs can show prominent vascular involvement. Clinically, there are multiple reports of LYG occurring in the setting of immunodeficiency, such as after organ transplantation or in AIDS. Both processes commonly affect multiple organs, including the lungs, kidneys, and central nervous system, among others. The pattern of lung involvement is also similar in both conditions.

Despite their similarities, the two processes differ in the following aspects. Unlike LYG, EBV-associated LPD consists predominantly of B cells without a prominent T-cell reaction. Clinically, LYG usually presents in the lung, while EBV^+ LPD mostly manifests in the gastrointestinal tract and head and neck. Cutaneous involvement is also common in LYG, but uncommon in EBV-associated LPD. These disorders have similarities but are not identical.

Plasmablastic Variant

Definition

This particular variant of DLBCL was recognized and described in the first edition of this textbook by the investigators. It was found that its morphology resembled immunoblastic lymphoma, while the antigen profile was similar to that of plasmacytoma. Because the tumor cells are apparently in the differentiation stage between a B-immunoblast and a plasma cell, they have been designated as plasmablastic. The first published collection of such cases drawn from the files of the Lymphoma Reference Center in Berlin has shown that the patients are usually human immunodeficiency virus positive (HIV^+) and that the lymphomas are located in the oral cavity (208). This type of lymphoma has not been included in any classification proposal but will be included in the forthcoming WHO classification as a DLBCL variant. The few published data point out that this DLBCL variant can be defined as extranodal large B-cell lymphomas usually associated with HIV infection exhibiting the morphologic features of immunoblasts and an immunophenotype of plasma cells.

We think this DLBCL variant does not only occur in the setting of HIV infection because we have identified examples occurring in immunocompetent patients. In all these cases, the predilection of this lymphoma to manifest in extranodal sites has remained constant. In the following section, only the well-established characteristics of the AIDS-related cases are presented, because data on the cases unassociated with HIV are incomplete.

Incidence

The real incidence of this DLBCL variant is still unknown. In the investigators' series, they make up to 4% of the DLBCLs diagnosed in the Reference Center in Berlin. In another study of 191 AIDS-related NHLs observed at one institution, the plasmablastic DLBCL variant accounted for 2.6% of cases (209).

Clinical Features

In most of the reported cases a predilection for the oral cavity mucosa, frequently with involvement of the gingiva, has been observed. In several instances, the bulk of the tumor infiltrated the adjacent bone, as assessed by radiographic analysis. In most patients the lymphoma was limited to the oral cavity at the time of diagnosis, but the extension of the tumor to distant sites (abdomen, retroperitoneum) and other organs (bones and ovary) was identified shortly after diagnosis. None of the patients exhibited a monoclonal immunoglobulin gradient in their serum.

Histologic Features

The neoplastic cells diffusely infiltrate the mucosal stroma (Fig. 25.5A). Extension to the submucosal compartment and to the mucosal surfaces with ulcerations also occurs. The histologic appearance of the infiltrate is relatively monomorphic. There is usually a cohesive growth pattern with large neoplastic cells exhibiting a squared-off appearance with interspersed tingible body macrophages. The neoplastic cells have a centrally or eccentrically placed nucleus with a single prominent nucleolus or several nucleoli (Fig.25.5B). Russell bodies and Dutcher bodies are not present. The cytoplasm is abundant and appears deeply basophilic after Giemsa staining. Apoptotic figures are numerous, and there are often single cell necrosis and numerous mitotic figures. The infiltrate is devoid of discernible proplasma cells and mature plasma cells. Only a few small reactive lymphocytes are found to be admixed with the neoplastic cell population.

Immunohistologic Features

The AIDS-related plasmablastic DLBCL variant is characterized by an absent or very faint expression of the most common lymphoid antigens such as CD45 (Fig. 25.5C) and CD20 (Fig. 25.5D). In more than half of the cases monotypic cytoplasmic expression of IgG (Fig. 25.5F) is found, and IgL chains are demonstrated in only one third of the cases. The plasmablastic variant cases usually display strong labeling with monoclonal antibody VS38C that reacts with plasma cells (Fig. 25.5E). The CD138 antigen also may be expressed. The phenotype of the plasmablastic DLBCL variant with negativity or weak positivity for CD45 and CD20, strong expression of CD79a in 50% of the cases and constant positivity for VS38C is consistent with a marked plasma cellular differentiation of the tumor (210,211). Expression of the BCL-2 protein has been found to be heterogeneous among the cases analyzed. BCL-6 proved to be expressed in a given case only in a proportion of the cells.

Genetic Characteristics

In all three tested cases, a monoclonal Ig gene rearrangement was demonstrated, confirming the B-cell origin of this lymphoma variant. In the three cases analyzed, no evidence for a gene rearrangement around the major breakpoint region of the *BCL2* gene could be identified.

EBV-infected neoplastic cells could be identified by means of *in situ* hybridization for EBV-encoded RNAs (EBERs) in 60% of the cases. In one half of the EBV^+ cases single neoplastic cells also showed expression of the EBV-encoded latent membrane protein-1, whereas EBNA-2 expression was not demonstrable in any of the cases. As evidence of a transition from a latent to a lytic virus cycle, most of the cases contained single neoplastic cells expressing the ZEBRA protein of the EBV. No sequences of the Kaposi's sarcoma–associated herpesvirus DNA could be detected in the three plasmablastic cases analyzed.

Differential Diagnosis

Awareness of the morphologic and immunohistologic features can greatly contribute to the diagnostic differentiation between the plasmablastic DLBCL variant and nonlymphoid malignancies. The observation of an undifferentiated large cell tumor lacking CD45 expression in HIV-infected individuals should therefore not erroneously lead to the exclusion of lymphoma from differential diagnosis. In this case, Giemsa staining and application of antibodies against VS38C, CD138, and CD79a and the search for immunoglobulin expression allow the diagnosis of plasmablastic DLBCL variant and avoid confusion with undifferentiated carcinomas and sarcomas.

HIV-related DLBCL can be differentiated from the plasmablastic variant as the cells of common DLBCL usually show strong expression of CD45 and CD20 and no or little expression of VS38C.

It would be interesting to determine whether the cases described in the literature as being intermediate between Burkitt's lymphoma and immunoblastic lymphoma with plasmacytoid differentiation in HIV^+ patients and Burkitt's lymphoma with intracytoplasmic Ig are more closely related to the plasmablastic DLBCL variant than to Burkitt's lymphoma and other NHL types.

The plasmablastic DLBCL variant can be differentiated from plasmacytoma with the help of analysis of the morpho-

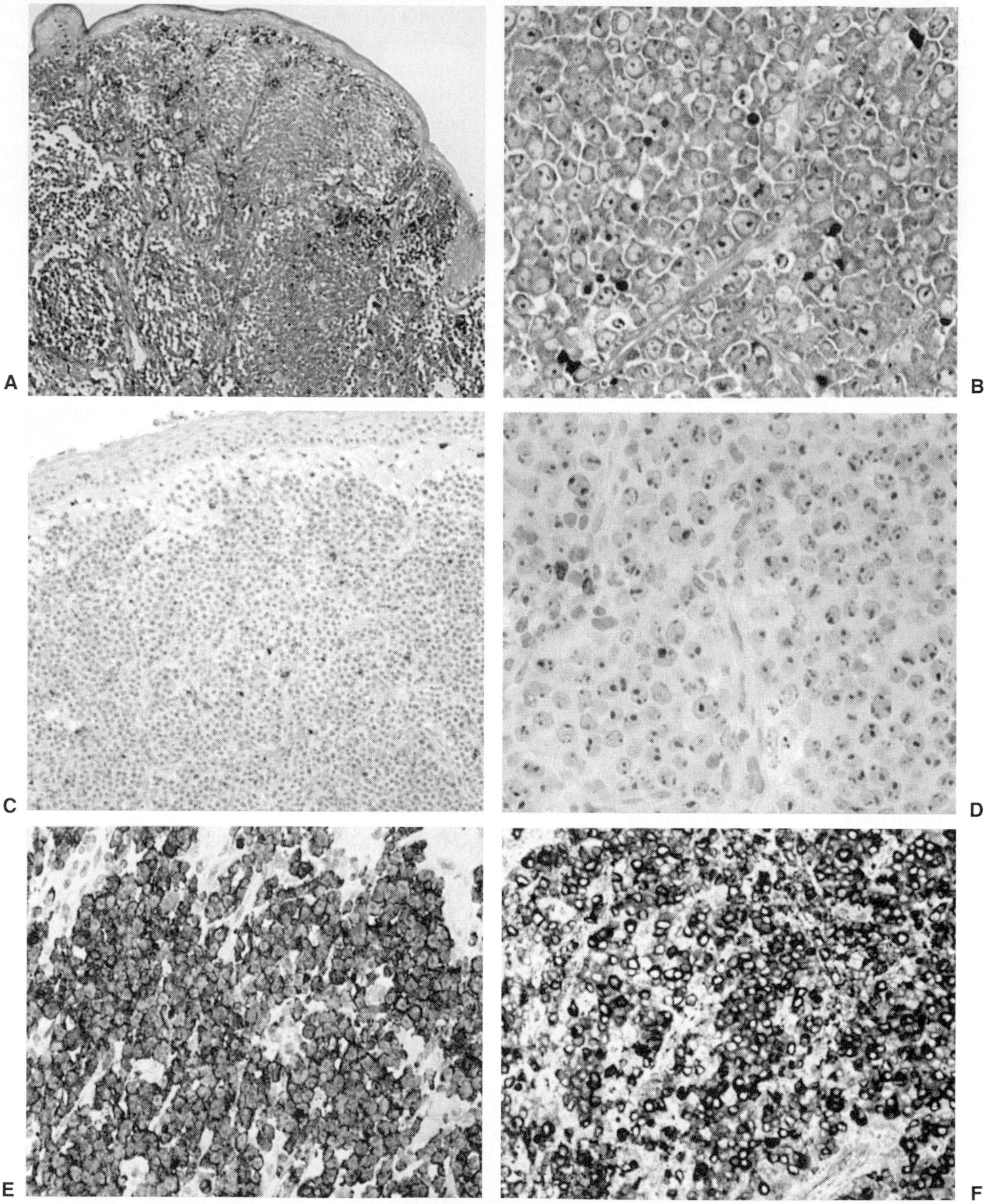

FIG. 25.5. Morphology and immunophenotype of the plasmablastic variant of diffuse large B-cell lymphoma. **A:** Diffuse infiltration of the mucosal stroma by neoplastic cells (Giemsa-stained paraffin section). **B:** The tumor cells resemble immunoblasts in terms of their central prominent nucleoli and plasma cells in terms of their strong basophilic, often abundant cytoplasm. **C:** Staining for CD45 shows absence of labeling from the neoplastic cells with only few labeled bystander lymphocytes (paraffin section, monoclonal antibody 2B11, alkaline phosphatase and anti-alkaline phosphatase [APAAP] technique). **D:** The tumor cells do not express CD20; only one bystander B cell is labeled (paraffin section, immunostaining using monoclonal antibody L26, APAAP technique). **E:** Strong immunoreactivity of the neoplastic cells for VS38C (paraffin section, APAAP technique). **F:** Expression of IgG by the neoplastic cells (paraffin section, peroxidase technique).

TABLE 25.5. *Differential diagnostic criteria for AIDS-related plasmablastic DLBCL variant, common DLBCL, and plasmacytoma*

Feature	Common DLBCL	Plasmablastic DLBCL variant	Plasmacytoma
Cytology	Centroblastic and/or immunoblastic	Immunoblastic	Plasma cell and proplasma cell
Size of the tumor cells	Large	Large	Intermediate
CD20	+	−[a]	−
CD79a	+	+ or −	+ (50%)
CD45	+	−[a]	−
VS38C	−	+	+
CD138	−	+	+
Ki-67	>40%	Prolif. index >90%	PI: 50%–60%
Ig heavy chain	M, G	G	G,A,M,D
EBV	12%+	60%+	6.7%+

[a] In some cases, weak (usually cytoplasmic) positivity in some cells.

logic details. Plasmablastic DLBCLs are entirely composed of blastic-appearing cells and do not contain the proplasma cells and mature plasma cells consistently present in plasmacytomas. Major difficulties may occur when a solitary plasmacytoma has acquired anaplastic features with a predominance of blastoid-appearing cells. Such cases usually contain various numbers of proplasma cells and plasma cells that are virtually absent from plasmablastic lymphoma. Table 25.5 lists features that are helpful in the differential diagnosis of plasmablastic from common DLBCL and from plasmacytoma. In particular, the extremely high proliferation index and the numerous mitotic figures are unusual for a plasmacytoma. Plasmablastic lymphomas show a high association with EBV infection, whereas the EBV genome has been found only in a minority of plasmacytomas.

Prognosis

All AIDS-related plasmablastic DLBCLs proved to be very aggressive, and the prognosis was poor (survival 1 to 6 months) despite chemotherapy with or without combined radiotherapy. Only the few patients with tumors limited to the oral cavity responded well to radiotherapy alone.

Burkitt's-like Lymphoma Variant: a Short-Lived Provisional Entity

In the REAL classification proposal a provisional entity called Burkitt's-like lymphoma had been included within the high-grade B-cell lymphomas (6). The separate mentioning of this group of tumors had been proposed to highlight the cases exhibiting morphologic features intermediate between Burkitt's lymphoma and the immunoblastic/centroblastic variants of DLBCL. These cases were described as showing a less monotonous cytologic appearance than Burkitt's lymphoma, including cells with immunoblastic features (i.e., medium-sized cells with a prominent central nucleolus). A starry sky pattern could be observed in a proportion of cases. The immunophenotype of this variant had been described as pan B-cell antigen positive, surface Ig^+ or Ig^-, cytoplasmic Ig^-, $CD5^-$, and $CD10^-$ or $CD10^+$. A finding similar to Burkitt's lymphoma was the extremely large growth fraction indicating that all viable cells are in cycle (Ki-67 index of 100%). The genotypic features reported were an infrequent occurrence of *MYC* rearrangements, whereas rearrangements of *BCL2* were present in 30% of the cases, implying a relationship with follicular lymphoma.

As in the REAL classification, the diagnosis of this variant was and is problematic. Clinical evaluation of the REAL classification found the least degree of consensus among pathologists in making the diagnosis of Burkitt's-like lymphoma (53%) with difficulty distinguishing it from Burkitt's or DLBCL (212). A similar low reproducibility of the diagnosis was also reported from the Children's Cancer Group (213).

The clinical and molecular studies performed on lymphomas with the diagnosis of Burkitt's-like could not establish an uniform picture. Some investigators have proposed that Burkitt's-like lymphoma could be distinguished from Burkitt's lymphoma in immunocompetent patients by the older patients' age, a frequent nodal presentation, a lower complete remission rate and shorter survival (214–216). However, other studies have not found any difference between the two groups (217,218). A study of 11 Burkitt's-like lymphomas that occurred in HIV^- patients showed that these tumors lacked the Burkitt's lymphoma characteristic *MYC* rearrangement (219). In contrast, three of them had a *BCL2* rearrangement, a rare finding in Burkitt's lymphoma. In a subsequent study of a large series of HIV^+ NHLs, 19 Burkitt's-like lymphomas were identified and molecularly analyzed. This revealed that most of the cases (68%) had a molecular profile identical to that of Burkitt's lymphoma (i.e., they harbored *MYC* rearrangements in the absence of *BCL2* rearrangements). The only difference between Burkitt's-like lymphoma and Burkitt's lymphoma was found to be the higher rate of EBV infection in the Burkitt's-like lymphomas (220). Another study of 10 cases of AIDS-related Burkitt's-like lymphoma also found *MYC* rearrangement but only in two cases (221). In a report including 39 cases of Burkitt's-like lymphoma studied with cytogenetic methods detecting also variant *MYC* rearrangements, three groups of cases were identified: cases with a *MYC* translocation (11 patients), cases with dual translocations of *MYC* and *BCL2* (13 cases), and cases with other cytogenetic abnormalities (13 cases) (222).

In the Airlie House meeting of the WHO committees, there was a consensus among the oncologists that it would be a mistake to consider Burkitt's-like lymphoma as a subtype of DLBCL. The oncologists felt that a Burkitt's-like lymphoma diagnosis in the pediatric age group would lead to an undertreatment of lymphomas behaving like Burkitt's lymphoma. It was emphasized that Burkitt's-like lymphoma is more related to Burkitt's lymphoma than to DLBCL, because a high incidence of *MYC* translocations has been observed. It was concluded that the Burkitt's-like lymphoma category should be eliminated from the classification and that Burkitt's-like cases should be classified as a variant of Burkitt's lymphoma (223).

LARGE B-CELL LYMPHOMA VARIANTS WITH DISTINCTIVE CLINICOPATHOLOGIC FEATURES

Primary Mediastinal (Thymic) Large B-Cell Lymphoma

Concepts Influencing the Definition

The history of primary B-cell lymphoma of the mediastinum is relatively short. The first descriptions appeared in the early 1980s. Miller and colleagues (224) described a diffuse histiocytic lymphoma with sclerosis as a clinicopathologic entity frequently causing superior vena cava obstruction. In this study the pathologic hallmarks of this lymphoma type were also given, including the large cell size and the occurrence of sclerosis. One year later, Trump and associates (225) outlined the peculiar mediastinal presentation of a similar series of cases, that were histologically classified as diffuse large cell and undifferentiated lymphoma. In 1984, Waldron summarized the cytologic and clinical features of this entity, introducing the definition of *primary large cell lymphoma of the mediastinum* (226). In the mid-1980s the B-cell lineage of the lymphoma cells was established by immunohistologic and genotypic studies (227–229). Addis and Isaacson were the first to suggest a possible thymic origin of the neoplastic cells and therefore designated it as *large cell lymphoma of the thymus* (230). As published in most papers, the clinical features of primary mediastinal large B-cell lymphoma (PMLBCL) seem to be unique; it occurs predominantly in young females, causing symptoms of a rapidly enlarging mass of the upper anterior mediastinum. The tumor is usually bulky, but extrathoracic manifestations have been reported to be uncommon at presentation.

The literature on this lymphoma is often confusing and contradictory because in several studies the definition of primary mediastinal and the exclusion of coexistent systemic lymphoma with secondary spread to the mediastinum is not always clearly stated (231–234). A stricter definition is therefore mandatory. The criteria proposed in a study from the Nebraska Lymphoma Study Group seems to be more appropriate as they define PMLBCL as a mediastinal mass of at least 5.0 cm in its maximal dimension, with no extramediastinal mass larger than that in the mediastinum (235). Another fact complicating the matters regards the identification of "thymic" PMLBCLs. After the original studies on mediastinal large cell lymphomas and the subsequent recognition of those of B-cell origin, it became apparent that some of these latter lymphomas might originate from a subset of thymic B cells. Although these primary "thymic" PMLBCs have peculiar immunophenotypic and genetic characteristics different from those presumably arising in mediastinal lymph nodes, most studies equate "mediastinal" and "thymic" lymphomas (233,234,236–238). Unfortunately the real thymic PMLBCL can be verified only by using a combination of extensive immunophenotypic and genotypic studies that can reveal their peculiar features (Table 25.6). This fact also implies that in the absence of extensive investigations, which would also require analysis of frozen tissue specimens, there cannot be any assurance that a given study on mediastinal LBCL evaluates lymphomas of thymic or nodal origin or of both. If the uncertainty on the criteria of patient selection persists, it is of no surprise that patient data, clinical characteristics, response to treatment and prognosis are and will remain variable from study to study.

Although the major features of PMLBCL had been recognized by numerous investigators, this lymphoma had difficulties in finding its place within the existing classifications. Within the Working Formulation, PMLBCL is classified heterogeneously, whereas the two earlier versions of the Kiel classification (239,240), by having exclusively focused on primary nodal lymphomas, did not mention PMLBCL. Only in its 1990 update has the Kiel classification tried to fill

TABLE 25.6. *Diagnostic criteria of primary mediastinal (thymic) large B-cell lymphoma*

Clinical features
Primary mediastinal localization
Predominantly young adults
Histologic features
Hydropic change of tumor cell cytoplasm
Moderate to marked interstitial sclerosis
Immunophenotypic features
B-cell phenotype (CD19, CD20, CD22, CD79a positive) with frequent absence of surface immunoglobulins
Expression of MAL protein in most studied cases
Abnormal major histocompatibility complex molecule expression
CD21 and CD10 negative
Characteristic adhesion receptor profile
Genetic features
BCL2 gene rearrangements: rare
BCL6 gene rearrangements: rare
MYC gene: infrequent rearrangements or mutations
TP53 gene: rare mutations
Occasional gains of chromosomes 2p, 9p, 12q, Xq with reported *REL* gene amplification

this gap by including this lymphoma among the "rare and ambiguous entities" with the definition of *large sclerosing lymphoma of mediastinum* (165). The International Lymphoma Study Group was the first to consider PMLBCL as a clinicopathologic subentity distinct from ordinary DLBCLs, a concept that has been followed by the new WHO classification.

Definition

The primary mediastinal (thymic) large B-cell lymphoma is a distinct, relatively common clinicopathologic subentity of DLBCLs that occurs predominantly in young adults.

Clinical Presentation

Most patients seek care because of symptoms related to a large mediastinal mass, such as chest pain, cough, superior vena cava syndrome, pleural and pericardial effusions. Elevated serum lactase dehydrogenase levels are usually present (241–243).

Regarding the sex of the patients there is a large number of studies indicating only a slight insignificant female predominance (230,244–251), others showing a clear-cut female predominance (242,252–257), and even a few reporting a male predominance (258–260). Although a predominance of one sex cannot be clearly established, all studies highlight the fact that patients with PMLBCL are significantly younger than those of the other DLBCLs.

As shown in several studies, PMLBCL can present in advanced stage like other DLBCLs (244,249,254,255,261). Bone marrow involvement has been reported to occur in up to 10% of the cases at presentation, a finding quite similar to that observed in other DLBCLs (244).

It is a popular notion stated in various reports that PMLBCL may commonly present or relapse at unusual anatomic sites. Lazzarino and colleagues (245) and two other groups (243,251) stated that PMLBCL exerts renal tropism, especially at relapse. The frequency of kidney involvement at presentation was 7% in one study (245), whereas the kidney involvement at relapse varied from 7% to 50% (243,245,251). Other studies could not identify significant differences in the involvement of extranodal sites at presentation or relapse of these lymphomas when compared with other DLBCLs (244,249,261).

Histologic Findings

PMLBCL is remarkably heterogeneous in morphology. Whereas the spectrum of the neoplastic cells within one individual lesion seems to be limited, this is not true for the PMLBCL entity itself. As summarized in a study of 109 cases the predominant tumor cells are large-sized centroblast-like with irregular round or oval nuclei (262) (Fig. 25.6A). In a minority of cases the neoplastic cells can be medium-sized or even very large, sometimes enormous, with cellular volumes at approximately 15 to 20 times that of a normal lymphocyte. Hodgkin-like and multinucleated Reed-Sternberg–like cells are only rarely identified, usually associated with a population of large-sized tumor cells.

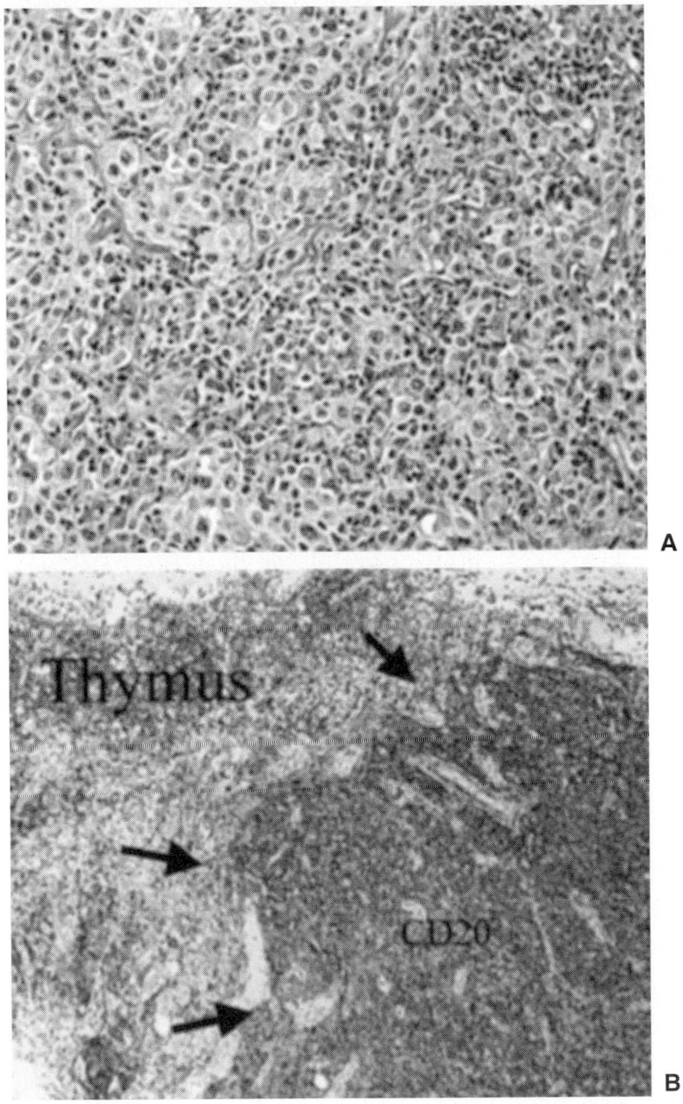

FIG. 25.6. Primary mediastinal large B-cell lymphoma. **A:** Large centroblast-like tumor cells with irregular nuclei and hydropic swelling of cytoplasm accompanied by sclerosis (hematoxylin and eosin–stained paraffin section). **B:** Infiltration of thymic tissue by $CD20^+$ neoplastic cells *(arrow)* (Paraffin section immunostained with monoclonal antibody L26, alkaline phosphatase and anti-alkaline phosphatase technique)

Hydropic change of the cytoplasm is a major cytologic characteristic in PMLBCL. This cytoplasmic alteration has been found not to be an artifact, because it can be also observed in frozen tissue sections. This hydropic swelling causes the "clear cell" morphology of PMLBCL (228). This feature can be observed at best in formalin-fixed material, while it might become less obvious in the cases of other types of fixation (263).

TABLE 25.7. *Histologic features of primary mediastinal large B-cell lymphoma in the various sites of involvement*

Feature	Thymus	Lymph node	Lung	Soft tissue
Growth pattern	Expansive	Expansive	Destructive angioinvasion	More infiltrative than destructive
Desmoplastic reaction	No	Eventual fibrosis of capsule	Frequent mild to extensive sclerosis	Frequent mild to extensive sclerosis
Necrosis	No	No	Often	Relatively rare

As summarized in Table 25.7, the histologic features of PMLBCL can vary depending on the involved tissue (262). In routine stains, involvement of thymic structures is usually not obvious as a component of the PMLBCL tumor mass. Thymic cells and structures can become highlighted by the immunohistologic detection of cytokeratin antigens in up to 40% of the cases. The thymic epithelial network is preserved in its original structure although it appears expanded due to the lymphoma infiltration. The PMLBCL colonizes the medullary and the cortical areas of the thymus. As a rule, there is no intrathymic sclerosis and no necrosis. Involvement of mediastinal and more rarely of supraclavicular or cervical lymph nodes occurs through continuous growth. The lymphoma invades the marginal sinuses in a carcinoma-like pattern and subsequently colonizes the perifollicular areas. Involvement of the lung occurs through continuous spread. The neoplastic cells lead characteristically to mucosal defects in small bronchi and terminal bronchioli. Ultimately, endobronchial growth can take place causing bronchial stenosis or obstruction. Invasion of the walls of larger vessels can be observed. Typically, infiltration of the lung induces stromal changes starting with interstitial fibrosis. This sclerosing reaction is thought to be an early event because it is found at the invasion frontiers. The full-blown picture of sclerosis, which is regarded as a classic histologic characteristic of PMLBCL, is found in most lung specimens infiltrated by this lymphoma. Correlation of the various histomorphologic features of PMLBCL with the disease course of the patients (disease-free and overall survival) revealed that routine histology failed to deliver any criteria with potential prognostic impact (262).

Immunohistologic Findings

All cases exhibit a B-cell phenotype (Fig 25.6B). This has been proven by the demonstration in frozen and paraffin-embedded tissues of CD19, CD20, CD22, and the immunoglobulin-associated molecule CD79a, whereas T-cell–associated antigens such as CD3 were absent from all cases studied (232,264,265). The leukocyte common antigen is reported to be positive in most cases (266,267).

PMLBCLs have severe defects regarding the expression of immunoglobulin heavy and light chains and frequently lack major histocompatibility complex (MHC) antigen molecules of the class I or II (227,228,264,268,269). Decreased MHC class I molecule expression has been suggested as an escape mechanism from immune tumor surveillance by cytotoxic T cells and as a possible explanation of the aggressive behavior of this lymphoma. The β_2-microglobulin, the light chain of MHC class I antigen, is expressed in low levels in PMLBCL patients in contrast to other aggressive NHLs (270,271). This low level of β_2-microglobulin may be caused by the reduced/absent expression of MHC class I by the tumor cells. CD10, CD21, and CD25 are not expressed (246,247,272).

Expression of the activation-associated antigen CD70 has been reported in the frozen tissue studies (232). Data regarding expression of the activation-antigen CD30 are quite variable in the literature. Although there are studies of frozen tissue samples with entirely negative results (247,272), Falini reported several cases expressing CD30 rather weakly and in a variable proportion of the neoplastic cells. Regarding CD30 expression in paraffin-embedded tissues, there are variable data, depending on the method of epitope unmasking used by the different investigators, with the most recent study of Higgins and Warnke reporting strong CD30 expression in 68% of the cases using high temperature antigen retrieval and trypsin predigestion as antigen unmasking procedures (266). According to their experience, CD30 is only weakly expressed by a low number of neoplastic cells even after high pressure cooking for antigen retrieval. CD15 has been reported to be not expressed in most cases.

Analysis of the very late antigen (VLA-*syn* β_1-integrin) family molecules binding to matrix molecules (fibronectin, laminin, epiligrin) has shown consistent absence of VLA-α_1, -α_2, -α_3, -α_5, and -α_6. Most PMLBCLs were found to be also devoid of CD11a expression, while the intercellular adhesion molecule (ICAM)-1 (CD54) was found to be expressed in almost all PMLBCLs. The adhesion receptor profile of PMLBCL is reminiscent of the pattern of normal thymic medullary B cells in some aspects (273).

Expression of BCL-2 protein has been analyzed in 141 PMLBCLs disclosing labeling of tumor cells in 30% of the cases (267). Promising data regarding the identification of PMLBCL by immunohistology have been published; in their study of mRNAs expressed in PMLBCLs and in peripheral DLBCLs, investigators identified the presence of an mRNA specifically expressed in PMLBCLs. Sequence analysis showed that this mRNA is encoded by the *MAL* gene, the expression of which was shown to be restricted to the T-cell lineage during hematopoiesis (274–276). *MAL* gene expression could be demonstrated by Northern blot and reverse transcription PCR in 8 of 12 PMLBCLs, but the peripheral DLBCLs showed only little or no *MAL* gene expression. Immunohistologic analysis revealed expression of MAL protein in the neoplastic B cells only of the PMLBCL type (277). Although the number of cases investigated is low, the results are promising for establishing MAL protein detection as a major criterion in the diagnosis of PMLBCL.

Postulated Cell of Origin

Initially, based on the lack of Ig, CD10, and CD21 expression, it was suggested that PMLBCL derives from terminally differentiated B cells or preplasma cells (264). However, this Ig^- and $CD21^-$ phenotype bears similarity to the noncirculating B cells of the thymus. It has been postulated that PMLBCLs arise from a noncirculating population of intramedullary thymic B lymphocytes (247). This is further supported by the frequent finding, or residual thymic tissue around the tumor (Fig. 25.6B) and a lack of additional nodal involvement.

Genetic Findings

The 22 cases of PMLBCL investigated by Southern blot analysis of extracted DNA showed clonal IgH and IgL chain gene rearrangements (229,278). The T-cell receptor β chain gene was found to be rearranged only in one case. These data confirm the B-cell origin of PMLBCL as concluded from the immunophenotypic analysis of this entity. Analysis of the rearranged IgH and IgL variable genes in five cases revealed the presence of somatic mutations comparable to those observed in the DLBCLs (12).

Analysis of 16 PMLBCLs revealed rearrangement of the *BCL6* gene only in one case. This finding suggests that *BCL6* gene alteration is not a significant pathogenetic event in these tumors (278). None of the cases studied revealed any evidence of *BCL2* gene rearrangement (278).

Investigations of PMLBCL by Southern blot analysis revealed that *MYC* gene rearrangements occur only rarely (279). Noncoding mutations near the 3′ end of exon 1 were detected by PCR-SSCP in up to 19% of the cases (278). Mutations in this region have been associated with deregulation of transcriptional control and have been consistently found in Burkitt's lymphoma.

Point mutations involving codons 12, 13, and 61 of the *HRAS, KRAS,* and *NRAS* genes could not be detected (278) in any of the PMLBCL cases studied. These data fail therefore to support an origin of PMLBCL from terminally differentiated B cells carrying mutations in these codons in up to one third of the cases (280).

Missense point mutations of the *TP53* gene in exon 5, 6, or 7, resulting in an amino acid substitution in the protein, were found in 3 (19%) of 16 of the cases (278). No rearrangements of the *MAL* gene have been reported in the cases analyzed (281).

CGH studies showed a characteristic pattern of chromosomal imbalances in PMLBCL, including gains of chromosomal material involving chromosomes 9, 12, and X (282). Chromosome 9 was overrepresented in 50% of the cases analyzed. This high incidence of chromosome 9 (in subregion 9p) overrepresentation has been characteristic for PMLBCL compared with other DLBCLs (282,283). Chromosome band 12q24 was overrepresented in 31% of the studied cases. Gain of chromosomal material was also found at two different sites of chromosome 2, 2p24-p25 and 2p13-p16, in 2 of 26 cases. Southern blot analysis of the latter two cases revealed an amplification of the protooncogene *REL.* This finding has been observed also in 2 cases of follicular lymphoma (284) and in a study of DLBCL showing that *REL* amplification was frequently observed in extranodal lymphomas (102). Overrepresentation of chromosome X was found in about one third of the analyzed PMLBCLs, a percentage similar to that found in other B-NHLs analyzed (109).

In situ hybridization data for detection of EBERs indicate a low presence of latent EBV infection in PMLBCL. Whereas in two studies no $EBER^+$ cells could be identified in each of the 18 patients studied (232,278), another larger study of 41 cases reported EBER-specific signals, albeit in a proportion of the neoplastic cells, in two cases (267).

Differential Diagnosis

PMLBCL can in some cases be difficult to diagnose because of limited amounts of diagnostic tissue supplied by fine-needle biopsy; crush artifacts produced during operative sampling; or inadequate material obtained from areas with prominent necrosis or sclerosis. Cytologic preparations are totally unsuitable for establishing the diagnosis.

In daily diagnostic practice, expression of CD30 by PMLBCL may lead to misdiagnosis of this lymphoma as classic Hodgkin's disease. Classic Hodgkin's disease differs from PMLBCL morphologically and immunohistologically. In classic Hodgkin's disease, there is the typical admixture of Reed-Sternberg cells and reactive elements associated with frequent nodularity and band-forming or diffuse sclerosis, which is usually more pronounced than that observed in PMLBCL. The neoplastic cells of classic Hodgkin's disease express the CD30 antigen definitely more strongly than PMLBCL and coexpress CD15 in most cases (285). Moreover, expression of B-cell antigens is not as constant and frequent as in PMLBCL, and when present these antigens are usually not detectable in the entire neoplastic cell population (286,287). Problems can arise with small specimens if needle biopsies are used for the diagnosis of mediastinal tumors. In these cases, immunophenotypic analysis with a limited panel of antibodies can assist in establishing the correct diagnosis (Table 25.8)

When compared with PMLBCL, the anaplastic variant of DLBCL shows larger cells and more bizarre cells with somewhat more abundant cytoplasm. The cells of the anaplastic variant exhibit strong CD30 expression in all neoplastic cells (288), quite different from the pattern observed in PMLBCL.

For malignant thymoma, carcinoma of the thymus, tera-

TABLE 25.8. *Immunophenotypic criteria useful in differential diagnosis of primary mediastinal large B-cell lymphoma and classic Hodgkin's disease*

Feature	PMLBCL	CHD
CD20	+	−/+[c]
CD79a	+	−/+[c]
Light chain restriction	+[a]	−
CD30	−/+[b]	+
CD15	−	+/−
EBV (EBER, LMP-1)	0%–5%	45%

[a] Detectable only in a minority of cases.
[b] Usually weak.
[c] The proportion of positive neoplastic cells and the level of expression is usually low.

toma, or neuroendocrine carcinoma of the mediastinum, the distinction is easy to make with the appropriate immunohistologic analysis because these tumors contain large numbers of epithelial cells expressing cytokeratins.

Mediastinal seminoma is best recognized by immunohistology because the neoplastic cells express placental alkaline phosphatase in the absence of epithelial and leukocyte markers.

Prognosis

Two studies encompassing a large number of cases (a total of 184 cases) did not identify any statistical differences in survival between PMLBCL and a similar control group of DLBCLs (235,267). Rodriguez and colleagues reviewed the literature on PMLBCL and stated that, although some studies report a poor prognosis for PMLBCL, most studies have found that the prognosis does probably not differ from that of other DLBCLs when patients are given curative chemotherapeutic regimens (236). Two reports described high-dose therapy and autologous hematopoietic stem cell transplantation as an effective salvage treatment for patients with persistent and relapsed PMLBCL (233,234).

Intravascular Large B-Cell Lymphoma

Concepts Influencing the Definition

Intravascular large B-cell lymphoma (IVLBCL) was first described by Pfleger and Tappeneimer in 1959 as angioendotheliomatosis proliferans systemisata (289). This name reflected their opinion that IVLBCL arose from endothelial cells. In the following years, the concept prevailed that this disease was a primary endothelial disorder (290–292). With the advent of immunohistologic studies, the lymphoid origin of the neoplastic cells in IVLBCL was established (293–298). This conclusion has been further supported by antigen receptor gene rearrangement studies (299–302). These findings, in conjunction with the characteristic clinical picture resulting from occlusion of small vessels by the disseminated intravascular proliferation of the tumor cells, have led the WHO committee to regard IVLBCL as a specific subtype of DLBCL.

Definition

Intravascular large B-cell lymphoma is a rare, aggressive variant of DLBCL in which the neoplastic cells have a predilection to remain confined within vascular lumina.

Clinical Presentation

Most patients are middle-aged or elderly, but a congenital case has also been reported (303). The symptoms result from occlusion of small blood vessels by tumor cells and fibrin. Patients most commonly present with symptoms attributable to involvement of the skin or central nervous system. Skin involvement usually manifests as erythematous or violaceous nodular subcutaneous masses or plaques that may ulcerate, often recurring in the trunk and extremities. Central nervous system (CNS) involvement usually manifests as confusing, bizarre and nonspecific neurologic symptoms attributable to multiple infarcts and resulting in progressive dementia, nonlocalizing neurologic deficits, and focal neurologic signs. Any organ or system can be involved, and a variety of clinical syndromes have been described (304–306). These include nephrotic syndrome, pyrexia and hypertension, breathlessness and hematologic involvement (autoimmune hemolytic anemia, leukopenia and disseminated intravascular coagulation).

Most studies reported on the absence of circulating neoplastic cells in the peripheral blood and rare involvement of the bone marrow (297,307). A later study showed that bone marrow could be the site of the initial manifestation of IVLBCL (308). This observation implies that subtle bone marrow manifestations may have escaped detection from earlier studies before the advent of immunohistology. Involvement of the cerebrospinal fluid is reported to be rare.

Histologic Findings

The principal feature of IVLCL is the disseminated intravascular proliferation of tumor cells. The neoplastic lymphoid cells are lodged in the lumina of small and medium-sized vessels in the various involved sites (Fig. 25.7A). These cells are large and usually exhibit round nuclei, vesicular chromatin, multiple prominent nucleoli, and a moderate rim of amphophilic cytoplasm.

The tumor cells may be palisaded along the luminal side of the blood vessels, giving the impression that they represent endothelial cells, or they may proliferate in the subendothelial layer. There is a tendency for these intravascular tumor cells to be enmeshed in fibrin or platelet thrombi. The involved blood vessels can also become tortuous or thrombosed with or without signs of recanalization. The resulting vascular occlusion can then lead to multiple infarcts in the

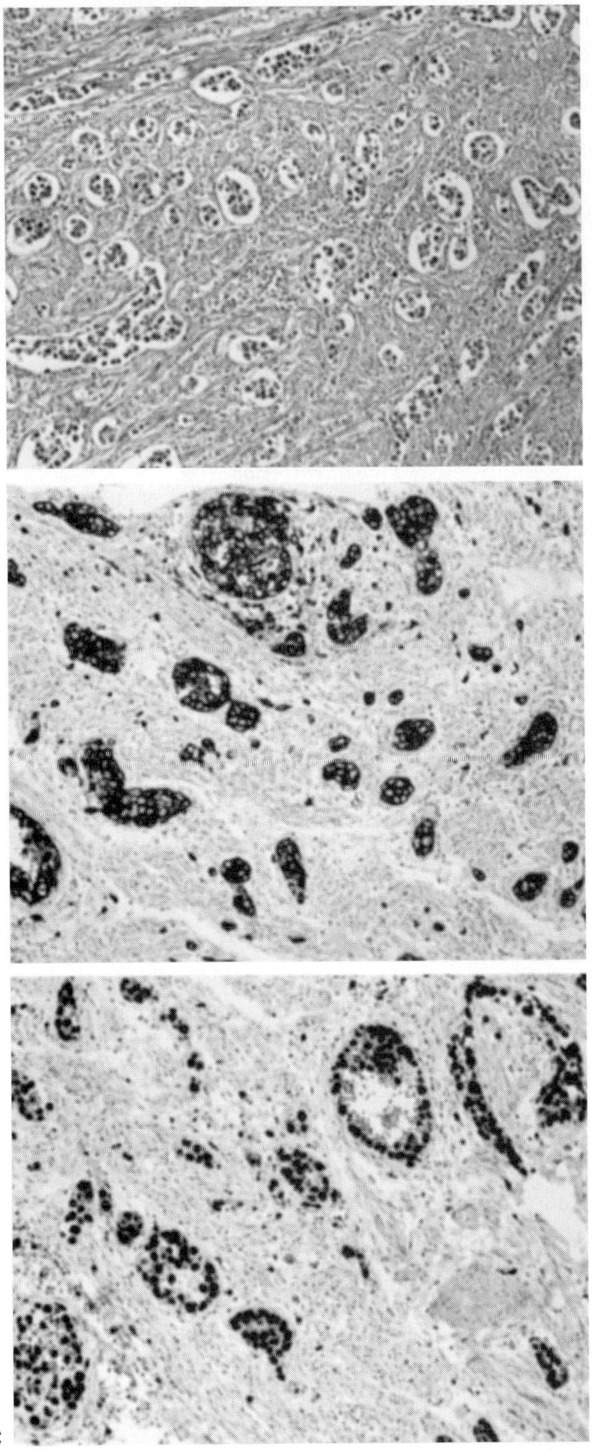

FIG. 25.7. Intravascular large B-cell lymphoma. **A:** Dissemination of neoplastic cells within the blood vessels of myometrium (hematoxylin and eosin–stained paraffin section). **B:** The B-cell nature of the intravascular cells is highlighted after immunostaining for CD79a (monoclonal antibody JCB117, alkaline phosphatase and anti-alkaline phosphatase [APAAP] technique). **C:** Demonstration of the large growth fraction of the neoplastic cells (immunostain for Ki-67 using monoclonal antibody MIB1, APAAP technique).

involved organs. In some cases IVLCL may eventually disseminate outside vascular spaces.

Immunohistologic Findings

The lymphoid nature of the neoplastic cells can be unequivocally confirmed by the demonstration of lymphoid antigens. More than 90% of IVLCLs has been of B-cell lineage, with expression of CD19, CD20, CD22, and CD79a (Fig. 25.7B). Expression of T-cell antigens has been reported in a small number of cases (up to 9%). However, the incidence of T-cell IVLCL cases in the literature is likely to represent an overestimation, because unusual examples of this entity are more likely to be reported and cases in which CD43 or CD45RO expression are taken as the sole evidence of T-cell lineage are not necessarily of T-cell origin as the aforementioned antigens are expressed in 20% to 40% of B-cell lymphomas (296,302,303,309). There are also single cases reported of presumed true histiocytic origin (310). Some investigators have suggested that B-cell IVLCL is a heterogeneous entity, because perhaps three different immunophenotypic categories were reported (311).

The first category expressing B-cell–associated antigens and being $CD10^+$ and $CD5^-$ may be related to GC B cells. There is also one case report of an IVLBCL that occurred in a patient with a history of follicular lymphoma, lending further support to this hypothesis (312).

The second category is characterized by the expression of CD5 by the neoplastic cells. The clinical significance of CD5 expression in IVLBCL is uncertain. It is unlikely that these cases represent Richter transformation of chronic lymphocytic leukemia, or the blastic variant of mantle cell lymphoma, because such cases have been reported to be $CD23^-$ and cyclin $D1^-$.

The third potential category of cases is $CD5^-$ and $CD10^-$.

Genetic Findings

A number of cases with B-cell phenotype have been shown to contain clonal Ig gene rearrangements. In one of the rare cases with a T-cell phenotype, clonally rearranged T-cell receptor genes were detectable, confirming its derivation from T cells (302). No consistent cytogenetic alterations have been reported up to now.

Postulated Normal Counterpart

The postulated normal counterpart is the proliferating peripheral B-cell in most of the cases. The predilection of IVLBCL for confinement within vascular channels has remained enigmatic. The homing receptor for high endothelial venules, as detected by the Hermes-3 antibody, is expressed by the lymphoma cells, and therefore this lymphocyte homing system appears to be intact (313). However, the lymphoma cells lack the leukocyte adhesion molecule CD11a/

CD18, which may contribute to their inability to extravasate to perivascular spaces (314). The significance of the latter finding remains unclear, because 36% of NHLs have also been found to be CD11a/CD18 negative. The molecular basis for the distinctive intravascular growth pattern seen in IVLBCL remains elusive.

Differential Diagnosis

Disseminated carcinoma or melanoma may mimic IVLBCL by conventional histology. The lymphoid nature of the neoplastic cells can be suspected by the noncohesive growth pattern and the presence of amphophilic to basophilic cytoplasm. Additional immunostains for lymphoid cell–specific antigens in conjunction with antibodies against epithelial and melanocytic antigens can lead to the appropriate diagnosis.

IVLBCL must also be distinguished from reactive angioendotheliomatosis, a rare reactive vasoproliferative lesion. The latter is associated with infective endocarditis, hypersensitivity reaction or other unknown causes. It is confined to the skin, the cellular proliferation is intravascular and composed of an admixture of plump spindled endothelial cells and pericytes. This can be made visible by immunohistologic demonstration of CD31, CD34, and factor VIII or of smooth muscle specific actin, respectively.

Prognosis

In general, the prognosis for IVLBCL is poor. In a literature review of 86 patients, almost half were diagnosed at postmortem examination. Of those patients diagnosed ante mortem, the median survival was only 5 months (300). Because of the rarity of this disease, a control study of response to various therapies has not been possible, and treatment recommendations are largely based on anecdotal experience. A review of cases treated in a single institution revealed that aggressive combination chemotherapy may induce a lasting complete remission (307).

Primary Effusion Lymphoma

Definition

Primary effusion lymphoma (PEL), otherwise known as body cavity based lymphoma, is a rare large B-cell lymphoma entity presenting as a lymphomatous effusion in the absence of a contiguous tumor mass. PEL usually occurs in immunodeficient patients and is consistently infected with the human herpesvirus (HHV)-8, also called Kaposi's sarcoma–associated herpesvirus (315) (see Chapter 28).

Clinical Features

PEL presents initially as lymphomatous effusions in the serous body cavities in the absence of contiguous solid tumor masses. These lymphomas remain restricted to the body cavity of origin and only rarely spread to local lymph nodes or distant sites. They usually occur in patients with an already established diagnosis of AIDS showing severe immunodeficiency. The median age of presentation in HIV-seropositive patients is 42.5 years, and HIV-seronegative patients show a higher median age at presentation (81.5 years) (315).

Cytomorphologic Features

The neoplastic cells exhibit cytologic features that seem to bridge the anaplastic and the immunoblastic variants: they possess moderately abundant basophilic cytoplasm, frequently with a perinuclear hof, but the nuclei display variable polymorphism, varying from large and round to irregular, multilobated, and pleomorphic with one or more large nucleoli.

Immunocytologic Features

The neoplastic cells usually do not express surface immunoglobulin and lack the B-cell associated antigens CD19, CD20, and CD22 but express CD45 and antigens related to the late stages of B-cell differentiation, such as CD30, CD38, CD71, CD138, and the epithelial membrane antigen (315–317). No expression of BCL-6 protein has been found (318).

Genetic Features

In all cases analyzed by Southern blot hybridization analysis or by PCR, clonal Ig gene rearrangements have been detected (315,316,319,320). Analysis of the V genes of the rearranged IgH and IgL genes revealed the presence of a high number of somatic mutations. No intraclonal heterogeneity of the expressed V_H and V_L sequences was found in almost all of the PEL cases analyzed. The pattern of somatic mutation and the immunophenotype suggest a post-GC cell and possibly a plasma cell origin for most PEL cases. Only one case displayed signs of ongoing somatic mutation in the V_H sequences. This finding suggests that PEL can be related to GC cells in rare instances (319). The distribution of replacement/silent mutations within the CDR and FRs regions of the rearranged V_H genes shows features of a selection toward an antigen.

PELs lack genetic alterations characterizing the other DLBCLs. They lack *BCL6*, *BCL2*, and *MYC* rearrangements and do not exhibit *RAS* and *TP53* gene mutations (315). Mutations in the 5′ noncoding regions of the *BCL6* gene have been found in most cases analyzed (321).

Infection by HHV-8 is the genetic hallmark of PEL and a conditio sine qua non for diagnosis of this lymphoma entity when compared with the whole spectrum of lymphomatous effusions (315,322,323). The infection is characterized by a high viral load, approximating 60 to 100 copies of the HHV-8 genome per neoplastic cell. The virus also displays a marked restriction of viral gene expression, consistent with a pattern of latent infection in most cells (324).

The precise pathogenetic contribution of HHV-8 to PEL is still under investigation. The formal proof that HHV-8 is tumorigenic is still lacking. However, HHV-8 is consistently associated with PEL when compared with other lymphoid neoplasms suggesting that it has an important role in the pathogenesis of this lymphoma. HHV-8 harbors genes with structural and functional homologies to those for *BCL-2*, interleukin-6, cyclin D, and interleukin-8 receptor (325). These HHV-8 genes are expressed by PEL cells constitutively or on adequate stimuli inducing viral activation and lytic viral phase (326–329). These data imply that deregulation of HHV-8 genes may be critical for AIDS-PEL development.

Because nonneoplastic B cells with HHV-8 infection are also detectable among HIV-infected individuals without AIDS-PEL (330), it is likely that infection by HHV-8 alone is not sufficient for lymphoma development and that other genetic alterations are required. One such alteration may be represented by EBV as such an infection has been detected in the majority, although not the totality, of PELs (315). Analysis of EBV latent gene expression revealed a latency type I with detectable EBNA-1 mRNA and EBERs, or a latency type II with additional LMP-1 and LMP2A mRNA detection. The levels of LMP-1 protein were low leading to its absence from EBV-infected PELs. In most cases a productive viral infection in a very small proportion of the neoplastic cells was identified (331).

Presumed Cell Of Origin

Collectively, the data suggest that AIDS-PEL derive from antigen-experienced B cells. The heterogeneous mutation profile of the rearranged V_H genes suggests that malignant transformation is apparently not restricted to specific stages of B cell development. Based on this hypothesis and the HHV-8 data, it is possible that B cells may carry HHV-8 in all stages of B cell maturation while the events leading to neoplastic transformation appear to be independent of the B-cell stage of development.

LARGE B-CELL LYMPHOMA TYPES NOT YET ESTABLISHED AS DISEASE ENTITIES

Primary Central Nervous System Large B-Cell Lymphoma

Definition

Primary central nervous system DLBCLs are NHLs strictly confined to the cerebrospinal axis without extracerebral manifestation or metastasis to other organs, including the lymphatic system.

Epidemiology

Immunocompromised Patients

Patients with acquired and congenital immunodeficiencies are at risk for the development of primary central nervous system lymphomas (PCNSLs). The two congenital immunodeficiency states most commonly associated with these lymphomas are severe combined immunodeficiency and the Wiskott-Aldrich syndrome. Iatrogenic immunodeficiency, commonly in the setting of solid organ transplantation, predisposes to the development of these lymphomas. The most frequent cause of PCNSL is however AIDS (see Chapter 28).

Primary CNS lymphoma has been established as a major cause of morbidity and mortality among HIV-infected individuals. The absolute incidence rate of brain lymphoma among persons with AIDS is 3600-fold higher than that of the general population (332). This type of lymphoma accounts for approximately 20% of the AIDS-related non Hodgkin lymphomas. Because the PCNSLs become apparent only at necropsy, the real incidence may be higher, even approximating 40% of the AIDS-related non-Hodgkin lymphomas in some series. Because this type of PCNSL is the most investigated and most common one, the AIDS-related lymphomas are discussed in the following text as representative of the tumors evolving in immunodeficient patients.

Immunocompetent Patients

A substantial increase of primary central nervous system lymphomas has been also observed among persons without AIDS (0.04 cases per 100,000 in 1982 to 0.28 cases per 100,000 persons in 1989). The reason for this increase in incidence is unknown (332).

Clinical Features

The median age at diagnosis is 55 years for immunocompetent patients and 31 years for AIDS patients. A male to female ratio of 3 : 2 is seen in the immunocompetent group, whereas most AIDS patients are male. AIDS-related primary central nervous system lymphomas are associated with advanced stages of HIV infection with profoundly disrupted immune function and very low levels of peripheral $CD4^+$ cells. In most reported cases, the patients present with multiple other systemic or cerebral AIDS-associated diseases, including the presence of a variety of infections (e.g., cytomegalovirus, *Pneumocystis carinii,* toxoplasmosis, HIV encephalitis), Kaposi's sarcoma, and progressive multifocal leukoencephalopathy. In immunocompetent and immunodeficient patients, these lymphomas are frequently located supratentorially, whereas multifocal manifestations appear to be more common in AIDS patients.

Histologic Findings

The tumors consist in the central areas of densely packed, large neoplastic cells, usually with features of centroblasts and immunoblasts, while the periphery exhibits a characteristic angiocentric infiltration with pericellular arrangement of reticulin fibers displaying multiple perivascular concentrically arranged hoops.

Immunohistologic Findings

All cases exhibit a B-cell phenotype with expression of CD20 and absence of T-cell specific antigens, while there are some differences in certain protein expression patterns between the AIDS-related– and non-AIDS–related groups.

Because all AIDS-related cases harbor an EBV infection, activation-associated antigens like CD23, CD30, CD38, CD39, and CD70 can be identified. An increased expression of the adhesion molecules CD18 (LFA1 complex), CD54 (ICAM-1), and CD58 (LFA3) can be detected (333). It has also been demonstrated that in cases expressing EBV-encoded LMP-1, a strong expression of BCL-2 is found, while BCL-6 protein is almost undetectable. In contrast, the AIDS-related cases without LMP-1 expression were characterized by BCL-6^+ neoplastic cells (334). These findings are consistent with data derived from *in vitro* models suggesting that LMP-1 is able to downregulate BCL-6, whereas LMP-1 upregulates BCL-2 expression. In contrast, all the AIDS-unrelated cases were found to express BCL-6 protein, but BCL-2 expression was rare (334).

Genetic Findings

All studies using the Southern blot hybridization technique or PCR have demonstrated clonal Ig gene rearrangements in the cases analyzed. Sequence analysis of the rearranged V_H genes has found different results for AIDS-related and -unrelated cases, although the number of the cases studied is very small.

In AIDS-related cases no preferential usage of one particular V_H family or one peculiar segment of gene was found. All cases contained somatic mutations in the rearranged IgV_H genes. However, no intraclonal variability of the somatic mutations was identified, suggesting that the hypermutation mechanism is no longer efficient in these malignant B cells. Probability analysis of the observed somatic mutations showed evidence for selection toward a specific antigen in a proportion of cases (335).

In AIDS-unrelated EBV^- cases two groups reported V_H gene usage restricted to the V4-34 gene (336,337). This finding supports the hypothesis that intracerebral stimuli direct the Ig repertoire and have an important influence on the development and biology of these lymphomas. Whether this biased usage of the V4-34 gene reflects a superantigen drive or the presence of intracerebral antigens stimulating expansion and intracerebral persistence of B cells, remains to be elucidated. In both studies, a significantly high number of somatic mutations was detected (13.2% to 18.4%). Whereas one group (336) found a very high frequency of mutations (18.4% ± 3.7%), higher than in all the other B-cell malignancies reported (131), the other group reported a 13.2% mutation rate. Intraclonal diversity of the rearranged gene sequences was observed in most cases. This pattern of somatic mutation and intraclonal variation suggests that these lymphomas are derived from GC B cells.

Because the patient series investigated are too small, it is imperative that more cases be analyzed to draw final conclusions on the cell of origin and on the open question whether AIDS-related and AIDS-unrelated primary CNS lymphomas represent distinct disease entities with a different pathogenesis.

Another intriguing phenomenon is the occurrence of multiple CNS lesions in AIDS-related tumors. Analysis of one case with two lesions occurring in widely separated areas of the brain has shown that both tumor sites contained the identical B-cell clone (338). This finding might imply that at least in the case of AIDS-related lymphomas the tumors begin as a monoclonal B-cell process within the systemic circulation and secondarily disseminate within the CNS. Of course such models can only become established after investigation of a representative number of cases.

Mutations of the 5′ noncoding regions of *BCL6* were found in 42.3% of the AIDS-related and 59.1% of the AIDS-unrelated cases. No gross rearrangements of the *BCL6* gene could be identified in the AIDS-related or unrelated cases (334). In all cases of AIDS-related lymphoma analyzed, no rearrangement of the *BCL2* gene within the major breakpoint region or the minor cluster region could be identified (333). All cases of AIDS-related and AIDS-unrelated lymphomas analyzed were devoid of molecular alterations of *MYC,* including rearrangements and mutations of the regulatory regions (334).

Virtually all AIDS-related cases harbor latent EBV infection, while EBV is absent from lymphomas of immunocompetent patients. EBV genome has been found with probing of Southern blots or by PCR analysis of DNA extracts (339), and *in situ* hybridization for EBERs confirmed the presence of the virus within the neoplastic cell population (340–342). EBV infection is associated with expression of the EBV-transforming LMP-1 in approximately 50% of the cases, suggesting a direct oncogenic role for the virus in the pathogenesis of these lymphomas. LMP-1 expression apparently induces sustained levels of BCL-2 protein, leading to the constant detection of this protein in the LMP-1 expressing cases (343). In addition to LMP-1, several cases show expression of EBNA-2, which transactivates viral and cellular genes (333). These facts imply that the AIDS-PCNSLs actually represent EBV-driven lymphoid proliferations arising in the setting of profound immunodeficiency in the protected environment of the CNS. This type of lymphoma may be also classified as an opportunistic infection. A further consequence of the EBV infection is the finding of the upregulated expression of a variety of cellular adhesion molecules that have also been found in lymphoblastoid cell lines.

In addition to latent EBV infection, there are also findings implying a transition toward a lytic viral cycle in some

AIDS-PCNSLs; within some cases expression of the replication activator ZEBRA-protein was found, while expression of viral capsid antigen and of membrane antigen was a rare phenomenon (333).

Data regarding the presence of human herpesvirus-8 within AIDS-PCNSL are quite variable. One study reported the identification of HHV-8 sequences by PCR in a significant proportion of such cases (344), but other studies have shown a complete absence of HHV-8 infection (345). Because all these studies have used DNA extracts, a sensitive *in situ* hybridization study or immunohistochemical demonstration of HHV-8 proteins is necessary to clarify the real association of this virus with AIDS-related PCNSL.

The overview of the presented data indicate that mutations of the 5′ noncoding regions of the *BCL6* gene represent the most frequent protooncogene lesion detectable among primary central nervous system large B-cell lymphomas. Because these mutations are regarded as a genetic marker specifically acquired by B cells at the time of transition through the germinal center, they support the Ig gene rearrangement data suggesting that a substantial fraction of these tumors may derive from B cells related to the GC subsequently localized in the CNS. The frequency of these mutations and their location in the proximity of *BCL6* promoter further suggest that they have been selected during tumorigenesis based on their potential ability to deregulate BCL-6 expression. It is, however, a curious finding that, despite the frequency of *BCL6* mutations, the primary CNS lymphomas appear to be devoid of *BCL6* gene rearrangements. The reason for that remains unexplained. It may be possible that a combination of *BCL6* mutations and EBV infection may be sufficient for development of these lymphomas in the context of AIDS, whereas an additional, presently unknown genetic alteration may substitute for EBV in the AIDS-unrelated cases.

Primary Cutaneous Large B-Cell Lymphoma

Primary cutaneous B-cell lymphomas account for approximately 20% to 25% of all primary cutaneous lymphomas. Most of these B-NHLs correspond according to their morphology to DLBCLs. The precise classification of this lymphoma group is under discussion. In particular, clinical findings have led to the concept that there exist two large subgroups.

Most primary cutaneous DLBCLs present with nodules or tumors on a restricted skin area on the head or trunk. In most reports, including the European Organization for Research and Treatment of Cancer (EORTC) classification for primary cutaneous lymphomas, these cases are included in the group of *primary cutaneous follicle center–cell lymphomas*. Studies have revealed that lymphomas of this subgroup are highly responsive to radiotherapy or chemotherapy, rarely disseminate to extracutaneous sites, and have an excellent prognosis, with a disease-related 5-year survival greater than 95% (344–348).

The other subgroup has been designated *primary cutaneous DLBCLs of the leg*. These lymphomas particularly affect elderly patients and have a higher relapse rate and a more unfavorable prognosis (disease-related 5-year survival rate of 58%) compared with those on the head or trunk (350,351).

The mechanisms that underline the different clinical behavior in these two subgroups are unknown. An intriguing difference in the BCL-2 protein expression pattern between these two subgroups has been described. Whereas all DLBCLs of the leg expressed this protein, all similar tumors of the head or trunk were constantly BCL-2 negative (352). In both groups, the t(14;18) translocation was not detectable. Although this finding supports the assumption that the two subgroups of primary cutaneous DLBCL are distinct disease entities, the studied series are two small and only a few parameters have been studied up to to now justify this separation. The clinical differences may be highly influenced by the patients' age as patients with DLBCL of the leg are significantly older than those with DLBCL of the head or trunk.

Although this classification proposal that is favored by the EORTC cutaneous lymphoma study group is of clinical importance, it cannot easily be followed by pathologists. The major problem is that the group of so-called cutaneous follicle center cell lymphomas is not homogeneous as it includes not only DLBCL cases but also those with features of follicular lymphoma. The reported immunophenotype is not entirely typical for follicle center cells as the CD10 antigen is stated to be not expressed in these cases (349). There is a need for additional studies on a large number of cases to verify whether it is justified to put these lymphomas in direct relationship to follicle center B cells or whether they represent a mixture of different lymphoma types (see Chapter 32).

Gastric Large B-Cell Lymphomas

Primary gastric lymphoma is the most common extranodal NHL, accounting for nearly 20% of the cases. Studies of these lymphomas have suggested that their clinicopathologic features are closely related to the structure and function of mucosa-associated lymphoid tissue (MALT), ultimately leading to the establishment of the disease entity called *marginal zone lymphoma of the MALT type*. Although initially restricted to low-grade lymphoma, the existence of a gastric high-grade lymphoma with features of DLBCL is well established. The low-grade lymphoma usually presents as an indolent disease, frequently showing a characteristic chromosomal translocation t(11;18)(q21;q21). In contrast, the situation regarding the molecular and cytogenetic alterations in the aggressive, high-grade large B-cell lymphomas originating in the stomach is less clear-cut. Deletions and mutations of the *TP53* gene have been observed in low- and high-grade extranodal, primarily gastrointestinal tract, lymphomas and it has been suggested that partial inactivation of the *TP53* gene might play an important role in the development of low-grade lymphomas, whereas complete inactivation might be associated with high-grade transformation (353). Some gastric high-grade DLBCLs overexpress the BCL-6 protein (54) or demonstrate *BCL6* rearrangements (354). Homozygous deletions of the p16 gene was reported in 14% of the patients with gastric high-grade DLBCL (355). One of the most frequent cytogenetic alterations in gastric high-grade DLBCLs is a loss of heterozygosity (LOH) on the long arm of chromosome 6q, because it has been demonstrated that up to 42% of these cases have a deletion of a part or the whole long arm of chromosome 6. Because cytogenetic studies of low-grade MALT lymphomas failed to identify such deletions, the 6q LOH appears to be a characteristic feature of high-grade gastric lymphoma implying that certain important gatekeeper genes should be situated on this chromosome playing a role in the transition from a low to a high-grade disease (356). Partial or whole gains of chromosomes 1, 3, 7, 11, 12, 18, and 21 have been detected in cytogenetic and CGH studies (356–362). The reported incidence of the latter alterations is often discrepant between the various reports. Various factors can contribute to such discrepancies (i.e., differences in case selection, methodology, technical approaches, and interpretations). Most of these chromosomal gains are apparently also present in the low-grade MALT lymphomas, albeit usually with a lower frequency.

There is also some debate as to whether gastric large B-cell lymphomas should be separated into primary and secondary subtypes. The secondary tumors, which are often designated as high-grade MALT lymphoma, have a history of or morphologically recognizable residual foci of low-grade MALT lymphoma in the same specimen. Additional findings implying an evolution from low-grade MALT lymphoma are the demonstration of identical clonal Ig gene rearrangements in the low- and high-grade component in the same patient (363), as well as the finding of similar genetic abnormalities such as trisomy (362).

It is unlikely that all diffuse large B-cell gastric NHLs represent transformed low-grade MALT lymphomas but most possibly primary tumors. Several facts support this assumption. Features of a low-grade component are only found in 30% of the cases (364); characteristic translocation t(11;18) of low-grade MALT lymphoma has not been detected in DLBCLs of the gastrointestinal tract; *BCL6* gene rearrangements and BCL-6 protein expression have been found in a proportion of extranodal DLBCLs, including those in the gut but not in low-grade MALT lymphomas; homozygous deletion of the p16 gene was found only in some high-grade gastric B-cell lymphomas but not in low-grade MALT lymphomas; and the finding that primary gastric DLBCLs appeared to contain fewer chromosomal alterations than secondary high-grade MALT lymphoma might also indicate that the two types of aggressive lymphomas have distinct oncogenic pathways (362). Although the distinction between primary and secondary gastric DLBCLs may be interesting, this separation is not favored by all investigators. Such a separation is also impossible to make in cases without any concomitant low-grade component and it remains uncertain whether such a distinction is of biologic or clinical significance (365).

In the REAL classification there is no separation between primary and secondary large B-cell lymphomas of the stomach and all such tumors are classified as DLBCLs. At the Airlie House Meeting of the WHO Clinical Advisory Committee, it was suggested that the term *high-grade MALT lymphoma* used by pathologists to denote a transformation from a low-grade MALT lymphoma or any DLBCL in an extranodal site should be avoided. Such a term can be misleading for clinicians used to accepting MALT lymphomas only as a low-grade disease entity synonymous with a lesion that may respond to antibiotic therapy for eradication of *Helicobacter pylori.* Because there are data showing differences in cytogenetic abnormalities between low-grade MALT lymphomas and primary DLBCLs of the stomach placing the relationship of these lymphomas into question, the following terminology was suggested. MALT lymphoma would be used only for the low-grade lymphoma originally described as low-grade B-cell lymphoma of MALT. Areas of large B-cell lymphoma, if present, should be separately diagnosed as DLBCL. Primary DLBCLs of the MALT sites should be diagnosed as DLBCLs and not as high-grade MALT lymphoma (223).

ALK-Positive Large B-Cell Lymphoma

As described in the ALCL section, many cases of this lymphoma are associated with a characteristic reciprocal chromosomal translocation, t(2;5)(p23;q35), juxtaposing the gene at 5q35 encoding nucleophosmin (NPM), a nucleolar-associated glycoprotein, with the gene of a receptor tyrosine kinase, the anaplastic lymphoma kinase (ALK), at 2p37. The resultant hybrid gene encodes a chimeric 80-kd protein in which part of the N-terminal portion of NPM is fused to the complete intracytoplasmic portion of ALK (366).

For the detection of ALK protein in tissues a variety of monoclonal and polyclonal antibodies has been produced. These antibodies have been raised against the intracellular portion of the ALK protein and react with the NPM-ALK fusion protein and the full-length ALK. Because it could be demonstrated that normal lymphoid cells do not express ALK, immunostaining with anti-ALK antibodies has been used as the method of choice for detecting ALCLs carrying the t(2;5) translocation. During screening of a large number of lymphomas with anti-ALK antibodies, Delsol and coworkers discovered that specific immunostaining could be achieved also in occasional cases without the t(2;5) translocation. Seven of these cases were collected and subsequently published (367). These cases represent a previously unreported type of DLBCL that can be defined as large B-cell lymphomas superficially resembling ALCL morphologically but lacking CD30 and expressing the full-length ALK receptor kinase.

Clinical Features

All but one of these patients were male, the median age being 51 years. Patients tended to present with advanced disease (mostly stage III or IV). Although lymphadenopathy at multiple sites was common, splenomegaly was only rarely observed. Most patients with advanced stage disease had a short survival. Only one boy treated with chemotherapy with stage I disease at presentation is in complete remission 13 years after diagnosis.

Histologic Findings

The lymph node architecture was obliterated in all cases with the exception of some preserved sinuses. A common feature was the prominent sinusoidal infiltration by the neoplastic cells, especially in small lymph nodes without massive tumor infiltration. By conventional histology alone, this sinusoidal pattern can even lead to the erroneous diagnosis of metastatic carcinoma or malignant melanoma.

The neoplastic cells had a monomorphic immunoblastic-like appearance (Fig. 25.8A). The nuclei were round and contained large single central nucleoli. The cytoplasm was basophilic and a paranuclear hof was sometimes seen, suggesting plasmablastic differentiation. Binucleate cells re-

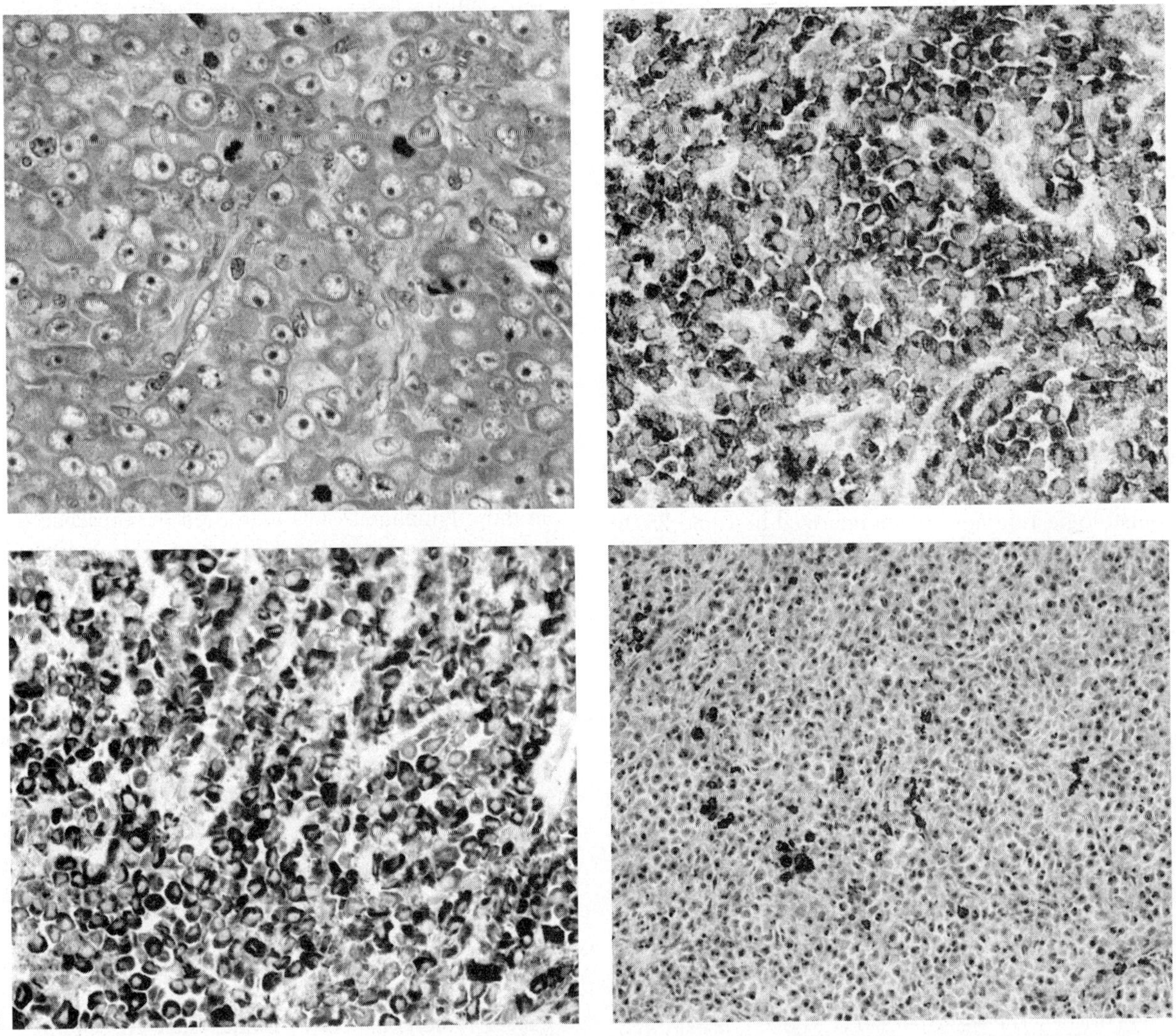

A B C D

FIG. 25.8. Anaplastic lymphoma kinase–positive (ALK^{+}) large B-cell lymphoma, a case from the Lymph Node Registry, Berlin. **A:** The neoplastic cells resemble plasmablasts morphologically (Giemsa-stained paraffin section). **B:** Immunostaining for ALK protein reveals exclusive labeling of the cytoplasm sparing the nucleus (paraffin section, alkaline phosphatase and anti-alkaline phosphatase [APAAP] technique using ALK1 monoclonal antibody). **C:** Monotypic expression of immunoglobulin light chain κ by the neoplastic cells (paraffin section, peroxidase technique using polyclonal primary antibody). **D:** Absence of CD20 expression by the neoplastic cells. Only a few bystander B cells are labelled (paraffin section, APAAP technique using L26 monoclonal antibody).

sembling Reed-Sternberg cells were seen in all cases, but giant cells were rare. In three cases, plasma cells were numerous while cells with morphology intermediate between mature plasma cells and large malignant cells were absent. Histiocytes and granulocytes were mainly found in the vicinity of necrotic areas.

Immunohistologic Findings

The hallmark of these lymphomas is strong EMA expression. This staining is usually present on the cell membrane, sometimes accompanied by dotlike staining of the Golgi area. Cytokeratin is not detectable. All cases express CD45. The staining is usually of weak to moderate intensity and often present in only a proportion of the malignant cells. Some cells also show cytoplasmic staining. In frozen sections all cases investigated clearly expressed the CD4 antigen, but the staining was weaker than that of the surrounding nonneoplastic T lymphocytes. Malignant cells are negative for other T-cell antigens (CD2, CD3, CD5,CD7, CD8, CD43, and CD45RO). Most of the B-cell associated antigens are not expressed (CD19, CD20, CD21, CD22, CD75, and CD79a) (Fig. 25.8D). Immunostains for macrophage-associated antigens CD14 and CD68 are negative. Most malignant cells in all cases are labeled by antibody VS38C, which reacts with an endoplasmic reticulum–associated molecule abundantly present in plasma cells. A proportion of the neoplastic cells in some cases are also labeled for CD57/natural killer–associated antigen, but the intensity varies from cell to cell. Most of the cases show cytoplasmic expression of the IgA molecule. Most cases studied demonstrate clonal expression of the immunoglobulin light chains (Fig. 25.8C). Immunohistologic findings are summarized in Table 25.9.

In all but one of the cases analyzed virtually all the malignant cells were strongly positive in immunostains with the antibody ALK-1. The staining was restricted to the cytoplasm of the malignant cells and appeared as scattered granules, usually associated with a clump of staining in the Golgi area (Fig. 25.8B). Nuclear or nucleolar ALK-1 staining was never observed.

The polyclonal ALK-AE antibody reacting with the extracellular portion of the ALK receptor gave clear membrane

TABLE 25.9. *Summary of immunohistologic findings in ALK-positive large B-cell lymphomas*

CD45	+
B-cell antigens (CD19, CD20, CD21, CD22, CD79a)	−
Plasma-cell antigens (VS38C, IgA, Ig-light chains)	+
T-cell antigens (CD2, CD3, CD7, CD8, CD43, CD45RO)	−
CD4 (in frozen sections)	(+)
CD57	+/−
CD30	−
ALK-1	+ (cytoplasmic)

staining of a proportion of the malignant cells. In contrast, cells harboring the t(2;5) were constantly negative.

Genetic Findings

One of the three cases investigated showed clonal IgH rearrangement by Southern blot analysis. The single case analyzed showed a trisomy 12 associated with a reciprocal translocation involving two of the three chromosomes.

No NPM-ALK transcripts were found in the cases tested by RT-PCR. All cases tested for ALK mRNA yielded the expected bands of the intracellular and extracellular ALK portions. Southern blot analysis of one case also did not reveal evidence of an *ALK* gene rearrangement. Western blot studies of that case demonstrated the presence of the full-length ALK protein in the tumor cells. This data in conjunction with the immunohistologic findings indicate that these lymphomas express the full-length ALK receptor and not a chimeric molecule. This type of ALK receptor expression is unique within lymphoid neoplasms. Although it implies that an *ALK* gene rearrangement should have caused its transcriptional activation, such an altered *ALK* gene configuration could not be identified under the conditions of Southern blot hybridization analysis used.

Novel Data Changing the Approach of DLBCL Classification: a Promising Outlook

All attempts to define subgroups on the basis of morphology within the DLBCLs have failed due to diagnostic discrepancies arising from interobserver and intraobserver reproducibility. Molecular analysis of the rearranged Ig genes in these lymphomas has identified the presence of somatic mutations characteristic of somatic hypermutation, a mechanism normally seen only within the GC, of secondary lymphoid organs. This evidence suggests that DLBCLs arise from germinal center B cells or from B cells at a later stage of differentiation.

A new approach is the analysis of genomic scale gene expression profiling (368). For this purpose, the DNA microarray technique that allows the quantification of the expression of thousands of genes in parallel using complementary DNA microarrays was used. This method has already been used to observe gene expression variation in a variety of human tumors. The investigators designed a specialized microarray by selecting genes preferentially expressed in lymphoid cells and genes with known and suspected roles in processes important in immunology and cancer. Among the cDNA clones selected, several were from a germinal center (GC) B-cell library, and others from genes that are induced or repressed during B- and T-cell activation by mitogens or cytokines. Analysis of *de novo,* previously untreated DLBCLs using these ''lymphochips'' revealed two large groups of cases: the *GC B-like DLBCLs* and the *activated B-like DLBCLs.* The GC B-like group expressed, to various degrees, all of the genes that define a GC B-cell signature. In contrast, the activated B-like group expressed such genes at low or undetectable levels for the most part. The gene expression signature of the activated B-like DLBCLs is reminiscent of the signature of activated peripheral blood B cells. Correlation with histology revealed that the gene expression subgroups defined with this approach did not show any relationship to the histologic subtypes of DLBCL. The investigators also tested a possible correlation of the gene expression patterns with the clinical characteristics of the patients. It became evident that GC B-like and activated B-like DLBCLs were associated with statistically significant differences in overall survival and event-free survival; 76% of the GC B-like DLBCL patients were still alive after 5 years, although this was the case for only 16% of the activated B-like DLBCL patients. The molecular differences between the two kinds of DLBCL were accompanied by a remarkable divergence in clinical behavior, suggesting that these molecularly defined lymphoma groups could be regarded as distinct entities.

This study has shown that a genomic view of gene expression can bring clarity to the DLBCL group. The two DLBCL subgroups identified are distinguished from each other by the differential expression of hundreds of different genes, and these genes relate each subgroup to a separate stage of B-cell differentiation and activation. It is unclear which of the genes that distinguish GC B-like from activated B-like DLBCL are the most important; they represent the marker genes of each group. An additional problem with this approach is that some of the genes identified in this study as being highly expressed in DLBCLs are T-cell specific. This is presumably caused by the reactive T cells present within the malignant B-cell infiltrate in various percentages (a few up to 90% of the infiltrate, as in the T-cell–rich DLBCL variant). It remains to be seen whether additional studies of more patients will reproduce these observations and whether the obtained data will ultimately lead to a novel DLBCL classification that will be prognostically relevant and allow the development of novel therapeutic approaches specifically directed against the genes contributing to the malignant behavior.

ANAPLASTIC LARGE CELL LYMPHOMA

Identification as a Distinct Lymphoma Entity

In 1982, the search for Hodgkin's and Reed-Sternberg–specific antigens led to the discovery of a new antigen initially called Ki-1 (369,370) and subsequently clustered as CD30 (371). Reactivity for the CD30 antigen was investigated in a large number of Hodgkin's and NHLs, as well as in lymph nodes and tissues infiltrated by poorly classified malignant lesions. This led in 1985 to the identification of a group of diffuse large cell neoplasms in which the CD30 molecule is expressed on all the tumor cells. The frequent presence of lymphoid markers and the constant absence of molecules associated with histiocytic or other cell lineages indicated a lymphocytic origin for this new tumor category. Because of the constant Ki-1/CD30 expression and the frequent anaplastic features, this tumor form was called *Ki-1$^+$ anaplastic large cell lymphoma* (ALCL) (372). These tumors had not been previously identified as a separate lymphoma entity but had been classified as true histiocytic lymphoma or malignant histiocytosis, or regressing atypical histiocytosis (RAH). A smaller number of cases had been also assigned to the categories of nodular sclerosis Hodgkin's disease, primary Hodgkin's sarcoma or sinusoidal large cell (histiocytic) lymphoma. Because of the sinusoidal infiltration in cases with partially involved lymph nodes, several tumors of this group had been mistaken for anaplastic (metastatic) carcinoma, malignant melanoma, seminoma or even for malignant fibrous histiocytoma (MFH). The lymphoid nature of this new entity was further confirmed by the demonstration of clonal rearrangements in antigen receptor genes (373,374). After the initial description of ALCL, lymphomas with the same morphology and identical antigen profile were described by several investigators (375–377) using the terms *lymphoma large cell anaplastic (LCA) CD30$^+$*, *Ki-1 lymphoma*, or *Ki-1$^+$ large cell lymphoma.* The Kiel classification was the first to incorporate Ki-1$^+$ ALCL as a separate entity with a T- and a B-cell immunophenotype (240). In the following years, the terms using Ki-1/CD30 positivity for the designation of this lymphoma have been found to be inadequate because CD30 is also expressed in some unrelated neoplasms such as Hodgkin's disease (372) or embryonal carcinoma (378). The designation that has been adopted by the REAL (379) and the new WHO classification is *anaplastic large cell lymphoma* (ALCL) (380).

Evolving Concepts of Classification

CD30$^+$ anaplastic large cell lymphoma (ALCL) is characterized by a frequent cohesive proliferation of large pleomorphic blasts and a constant expression of the CD30 molecule on all neoplastic cells. Despite these common features, heterogeneity in the cytology and in the antigen profile of the tumor cells and in the clinical features of patients affected by this condition was noticed in the original and later publications. This led to the distinction of several morphologic, immunophenotypic and clinical subforms of ALCL (376,381–384). A morphologic and immunophenotypic overlap with classic Hodgkin's disease was also recognized (372,385). In the late 1980s, several investigators could convincingly show that primary cutaneous ALCLs significantly differed from primary extracutaneous (systemic) ALCLs not only regarding phenotype but also in clinical features (386,387). This led to the concept that primary cutaneous and primary systemic ALCLs represent distinct disease entities. This concept has been considered in the REAL classification and in the new WHO classification. In 1989 and 1990, a translocation between chromosomes 2 and 5 was assigned to a proportion of systemic ALCL cases having a T/null cell immunophenotype (388–391). In 1994, the genes participating in this translocation (nucleophosmin *(NPM)* and anaplastic lymphoma kinase *(ALK)* were identified (392). It was subsequently shown that the *ALK* gene was normally not expressed in any human tissue, with the exception of a few brain cells (393), and that its expression is usually associated with fusion with another gene (in most instances *NPM*) causing *ALK* gene deregulation. Antibodies generated against ALK protein allowed studies on its expression patterns in a large number of ALCLs. Within the group of systemic ALCL a new distinct clinicopathologic entity has emerged, accounting for 50% to 60% of the cases (394). It is defined by the expression of an ALK fusion protein, an affection of young male patients and a more favorable clinical course. These data ultimately led to the recognition of three distinct ALCL disease entities:

Primary systemic ALK$^+$ ALCL
Primary systemic ALK$^-$ ALCL
Primary cutaneous ALCL

Since the initial description of ALCL, there has been discussion about whether there exists a distinct entity of primary systemic ALCL of B-cell type. In the Kiel classification this was included as its own disease entity (240), whereas in the REAL classification (379) and the new WHO classification (380), it is regarded as a variant of DLBCL (see the DLBCL section). Similar debates exist regarding HIV-related ALCL. Most HIV-related ALCLs have been proved to be DLBCLs with anaplastic morphology and EBV infection (395).

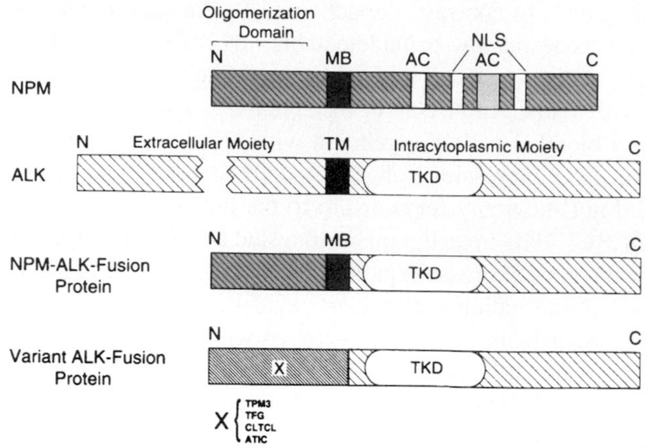

FIG. 25.9. Molecular structure of nucleophosmin (NPM), anaplastic lymphoma kinase (ALK), and ALK fusion proteins. The NPM protein consists of an an oligomerization domain (residues 1 through 83), a metal-binding domain (MB) (residues 104 through 115), two acidic amino acid clusters (AC) (residues 120 through 132 and 161 through 188) that function as acceptor regions for nucleolar targeting signals, and two nuclear localization signals (NLS). The ALK protein is a transmembrane tyrosine kinase receptor containing a transmembrane domain (TM) and a tyrosine kinase domain (TKD) in the N-terminal part of the intracytoplasmic tail. In the NPM-ALK fusion protein, the extracellular and transmembrane domains of ALK are replaced by the oligomerization domain of NPM (in approximately 75%) or of other proteins *(X)*. The fused part of NPM contains, in addition to the oligomerization domain, the metal-binding region. The fusion point is at codon 117. N, amino terminus; C, carboxyl terminus.

Genetic and Immunophenotypic Markers for Anaplastic Large Cell Lymphoma Classification

CD30

In 1982, Stein's group discovered a new molecule that was initially called Ki-1 and subsequently designated CD30. CD30 is strongly expressed on Hodgkin and Reed-Sternberg cells of classic Hodgkin's disease, but is absent from the cells of all normal tissues except scattered activated large lymphoid blasts preferentially located around B-cell follicles (372). Biochemical studies and molecular cloning have revealed that CD30 is a 120-kd transmembrane cytokine receptor of the TNF receptor family (396), for which the ligand (CD30L) (397) was identified. A soluble 85-kd form of CD30 was found to be released from the membrane bound molecule by proteolytic cleavage (398), and it is possible to detect it in the sera of patients with CD30$^+$ reactive and neoplastic lesions (399,400) (see Chapter 3).

NPM-ALK *Gene*

In the late 1980s it was found that a proportion of ALCLs are associated with a t(2;5) chromosomal translocation (389–391). As demonstrated by Morris and colleagues in 1994, the t(2;5) translocation causes the *NPM* gene located at 5q35 to fuse with a gene at 2p23 encoding the receptor tyrosine kinase alk (392). The properties of wild-type NPM and ALK, as well as their chimerized genes and proteins, are summarized in Figure 25.9. Wild-type NPM was first identified in the late 1970s and early 1980s as an ubiquitous acidic 37-kd phosphoprotein associated with nucleoli (401,402). NPM shuttles continuously between the cytoplasm and the nucleolus and functions as a carrier of newly synthesized proteins into the nucleolus (403). The NPM molecule exercises this function through an oligomerization motif at the N-terminal region (404), and two nuclear localizing signals at the C-terminal domain (Fig. 25.9) (405). The wild-type ALK protein is a 200-kd transmembrane receptor that is most closely related to leukocyte tyrosine kinase (LTK) and whose postnatal expression is restricted physiologically to a few scattered cells in the nervous system (some glia cells, a few endothelial cells, and some pericytes) (406–408). The intracellular tail of the ALK molecule carries the tyrosine kinase catalytic domain (Fig. 25.9), which becomes physiologically activated as a result of homodimerization after ligand binding (409).

The t(2;5) translocation juxtaposes the portion of the *NPM* gene encoding the N-terminal domain of NPM (amino acids 1 through 117) (Fig. 25.9) to the part of the *ALK* gene, which codes for the entire cytoplasmic region of the ALK protein (392,410). As a consequence, the *ALK* gene comes under

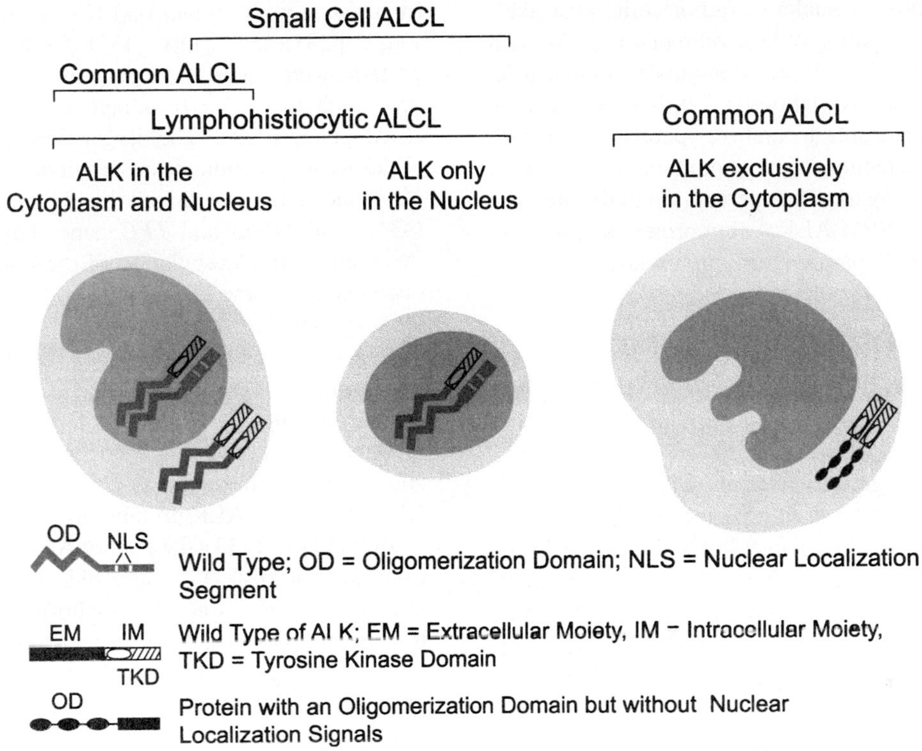

FIG. 25.10. Patterns of oligomerization and cellular distribution of NPM-ALK fusion and variant ALK fusion proteins in the various subforms of ALK^+ systemic anaplastic large cell lymphomas.

the control of the NPM promoter that induces a permanent transcription of the *NPM-ALK* hybrid gene, resulting in the production of a 80-kd chimeric protein called NPM-ALK (392) or p80 (411). This NPM-ALK protein contains the NPM oligomerization domain and the intracytoplasmic region of ALK. The C-terminal NPM domain carrying the nuclear localization signals and the extracellular and transmembrane region of the ALK are absent (392,410). The NPM-ALK protein can form homodimers (by crosslinking with other NPM-ALK molecules) or heterodimers (by crosslinking with wild-type NPM) (Fig. 25.10). The formation of homodimers results in the constitutive activation of the catalytic ALK domain contained in the NPM-ALK fusion protein (409,410). The activated ALK domain has been shown to bind GRB2, and to the SH2 domains of phospholipase C-γ, interactions that have been demonstrated to induce mitogenic activity and are likely to be involved in the neoplastic transformation (409,411,412). Transfection of murine hematopoietic cells with the *NPM-ALK* fusion gene induces transplantable lymphoid tumors further supporting the oncogenic property of the fusion protein (413).

Demonstration and Subcellular Distribution of the NPM-ALK Fusion Protein

The presence of the *NPM-ALK* gene was initially demonstrated in tissue samples by Southern blot analysis (414), reverse transcriptase–polymerase chain reaction (RT-PCR) (415–419), and *in situ* hybridization (420). The application of these techniques has confirmed the association of ALCL with the t(2;5) translocation. The Southern blot and RT-PCR techniques have, however, produced discrepant results over the frequency of the *NPM-ALK* fusion gene in ALCL, and the occurrence of this anomaly in large B-cell lymphoma, Hodgkin's disease and even in normal cells (421–423). Because RT-PCR is prone to artifact, the generation and application of polyclonal (424,425) and monoclonal antibodies specific for formol-fixative–resistant epitopes on the cytoplasmic tail of the ALK protein (393,394) and on the N-terminal domain of NPM (426) represented a significant advance in the detection of the NPM-ALK anomaly. Because ALK protein is absent in all normal tissues, with the exception of scattered cells in the brain, positive immunohistochemical staining in tissues (other than brain) indicates anomalous ALK expression, usually in the form of the t(2;5) associated NPM-ALK fusion protein (393,394,424,425). Thanks to the generation of a monoclonal antibody against the N terminus of NPM, the molecular association of the detected ALK with NPM can also be immunohistologically demonstrated because, in the presence of NPM-ALK, this antibody stains the cytoplasm and the nucleus (426), whereas in tissues devoid of NPM-ALK labeling is restricted to the nucleus (426,427). The putative mechanism that may account for the different subcellular distributions of NPM-ALK is presented in Fig. 25.10. The lack of nuclear localization signals in the chimeric NPM-ALK protein suggests that its transportation into the nuclei of tumor cells most likely occurs through the formation of heterodimers of NPM-ALK with wild-type NPM (428), which contains two nuclear localization signals. The availability of anti-ALK and anti-NPM antibodies applicable to archival paraffin-embedded tissues allowed the screening of large numbers of neoplasms to be performed, leading to a clear perception of the presence and frequency of the NPM-ALK fusion protein and the possibility of variant ALK proteins in lymphomas.

ALK Proteins Other Than NPM-ALK

Within the large series of ALCL investigated, 15% to 28% of chimeric ALK$^+$ lymphomas were found to be negative for the t(2;5) translocation (as detected by immunohistochemistry) and it was suggested that they may represent cases in which the *ALK* gene fuses to a partner other than *NPM* to produce variant X-ALK proteins (393,394,427,428). Such X-ALK$^+$ lymphomas are characterized by a cytoplasm-restricted expression of the ALK protein (Fig. 25.10) and a nucleus-restricted expression of wild-type NPM. Additional evidence to support the presence of chimeric ALK proteins other than NPM-ALK has been obtained from reports of genetic abnormalities affecting the *ALK* gene in ALK$^+$ ALCL. These include the inversion (2)(p23;q35) and the (1;2)(q21;p23) and (2;3)(p23;q21) translocations, suggesting the existence of genes other than *NPM* that can deregulate the *ALK* gene (429–431). The existence of variant ALK proteins has been confirmed by immunobiochemical studies using monoclonal antibodies to ALK and NPM (N-terminal domain) (432). Western blotting studies have demonstrated the presence of variant ALK proteins of 85, 97, 104, and 113 kd. These new ALK fusion partners have now been identified by 5′ RACE studies (Fig. 25.11). Lamant and coworkers disclosed the 104 kd ALK protein as being TPM3 (nonmuscle tropomyosin)-ALK in a tumor exhibiting the (1;2)(q21;p23) translocation (433). The 85- and the 97-kd ALK proteins were found to be generated by a fusion of the *ALK* gene with the *TFG* (tropomyosin receptor kinase (TRK)-fused gene) (434). The larger TFG-ALK fusion protein (TFG-ALK$_{long}$) contains an additional 165 bp TFG sequence (434) and is associated with the (2;3)(p23;q21) translocation (431). The *TPM3* and *TFG* genes have been found to be involved in the deregulation of the kinase domain of other oncogenic tyrosine kinases present in carcinomas (435). In common with NPM, TFG and TPM3 proteins contain dimerization regions. The possibility exists that the formation of homodimers of TPM3-ALK or TFG-ALK (to mimic ligand binding) results in the constitutive activation of the ALK kinase domain conferring oncogenic activity on these variant ALK proteins. In support of this is the finding that TFG-ALK and TPM3-ALK proteins are capable of autophosphorylation *in vitro* (433). Two other ALK fusion partners ATIC (5-aminoimidazole-4-carboxamide-1-β-D-ribonucleotide transformylase/inosine monophosphate cyclohydrolase), possibly caused by the inversion (2)(p23;q35), and CLTCL (clathrin heavy polypeptide-like gene), occurring as a result of the t(2;22)(p23;q11) translocation (436,437) (Fig. 25.11). These studies also documented the frequency with which the newly found ALK fusion variants occur. It is of pathogenic significance that all chimeric ALK variants contain the same functional kinase domain of ALK as that present in the NPM-ALK protein (Fig. 25.11). The lack of nuclear localization signals in all fusion proteins other than NPM-ALK accounts for the absence of these fusion proteins from the nucleus and their cytoplasm only distribution (Fig. 25.10).

ALK Expression Outside Lymphoid Tumors

Evidence is accumulating that ALK proteins may also be expressed in tumors other than lymphoid neoplasms. Falini

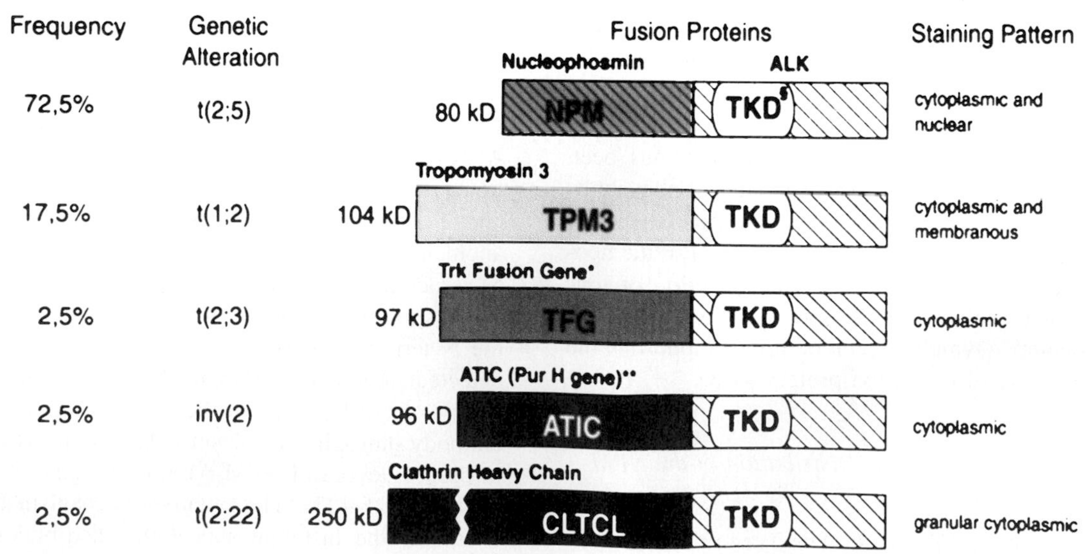

FIG. 25.11. Features of the various ALK fusion proteins occurring in ALK$^+$ systemic anaplastic large cell lymphomas.

and associates reported the presence of full-length ALK protein in a rhabdomyosarcoma (394). This is in keeping with the earlier observation by Morris and colleagues that the rhabdomyosarcoma cell line RH30 expresses the 200-kd wild-type ALK protein (392). Expression of ALK proteins has been observed in inflammatory myofibroblastic tumors (438) and in neuroblastomas (439). In the former tumor lesion ALK expression appears to be due to a rearrangement of the 2p23 region where the *ALK* gene is located.

Specificity of ALK *Gene Expression and Correlation with Lymphoma Immunophenotype and Morphology*

Using the highly specific monoclonal anti-ALK antibodies, ALK-1 and ALKc, expression of the chimeric ALK protein was found to be confined to ALCL of T/null cell type with a frequency ranging from 53% to 89% (393,394,428). The only other group of lymphoid neoplasms to express ALK proteins are the rare large B-cell lymphomas reported by Delsol and associates (440) and those by Gascoyne and coworkers (423). The ALK molecule could not be detected in any other lymphoma types, including most cases of $CD30^+$ primary cutaneous lymphoproliferative disorders (primary cutaneous ALCL and lymphomatoid papulosis), Hodgkin's disease, and most cases (>85%) of ALCL with Hodgkin-like appearance.

Cytotoxic Molecules

Among the wealth of cytotoxic molecules, perforin and granzyme B are two well-characterized proteins involved in one major pathway leading to apoptosis (441–443). Perforin allows the entry of granzyme molecules into the target cells, which then activate the apoptotic protease CPP32 (444). The genes for perforin and granzyme B have been cloned (442,445) and antibodies directed against these molecules have been generated (446). T-cell restricted intracellular antigen (TIA)-1, another molecule found in cytotoxic cells, is recognized by the antibody 2G9 (447). The precise function of TIA-1 has not been elucidated. Because it induces DNA fragmentation in digitonin-permeabilized thymocytes (448), it may be implicated in the killing induced by cytotoxic lymphocytes. The antibody 2G9 has been demonstrated to react also with another protein, called GMP-17 (granule membrane protein of 17 kd), which is found in the membrane of the granules of neutrophils and cytotoxic cells (449). With the exception of neutrophils, which are morphologically distinguishable from lymphoid cells, the expression of all the previously mentioned molecules appears to be largely restricted to cytotoxic cells.

Established Clinicopathologic Disease Entities

ALCL has been subdivided clinically into a primary (*de novo*) and a secondary (anaplastic transformation from another lymphoma) form. Among the primary ALCLs, a systemic and cutaneous category have been recognized in immunocompetent and HIV^+ (rare) patients.

Primary systemic ALCL is the most frequent subform, accounting for 2% to 8 % of NHLs in adults (379) and approximately 30% of large cell lymphomas in children (450,451). Wright and associates reported that the clinical features and the outcome of systemic ALCL are somewhat discrepant, probably due to the different diagnostic criteria employed, different age distribution of patients and inclusion in clinical trials of provisional categories such as ALCL HD-like and ALCL of B cell phenotype, as well as of primary cutaneous forms (452). An additional bias appears to be that in previous studies ALK expression was not investigated and therefore the two emerging entities of systemic ALCL (ALK^+ and ALK^-) were not distinguishable. Because the clinical features and outcome of systemic ALCL differ significantly in cases harboring and cases lacking a dysregulated *ALK* gene, ALK^+ and ALK^- ALCL cases deserve separate discussion.

Alk-Positive Systemic Anaplastic Large Cell Lymphoma

Definition

Lymphoma with expression of an ALK fusion protein; predominantly large anaplastic, sometimes also small neoplastic cells; constant expression of CD30 by the large neoplastic cells; and absence of B-cell antigens. The features of ALK^+ systemic ALCL are summarized in Table 25.10.

Clinical Features

It mostly occurs in children and young adults with male predominance that is particularly striking in the second and third decades of life (male to female ratio of 6.5) (423,428,453). This lymphoma frequently presents as ag-

TABLE 25.10. *ALK-positive anaplastic large cell lymphoma*

Histologic findings
Broad histologic spectrum (e.g., common type, small cell variant, lymphohistiocytic variant)
Immunohistologic findings
ALK^+, $CD30^+$, EMA^+, cytotoxic molecules$^+$, $CD3^{+/-}$, CD4>CD8
Genetic findings
T-cell receptor chain (β/γ) genes clonally rearranged
t(2;5) translocation in 75% of the cases; variant translocations or inversions in 25% of the cases, with constant participation of the *ALK* gene on chromosome 2p23
Clinical findings
Mean age at presentation 22–30 years
Male>female
Lymph node swelling (>90%), fever
Extranodal manifestations (60%) predominantly in soft tissue, bones, lungs, and bone marrow
Prognosis
Favorable; 10-year survival rates of 71% to 90%

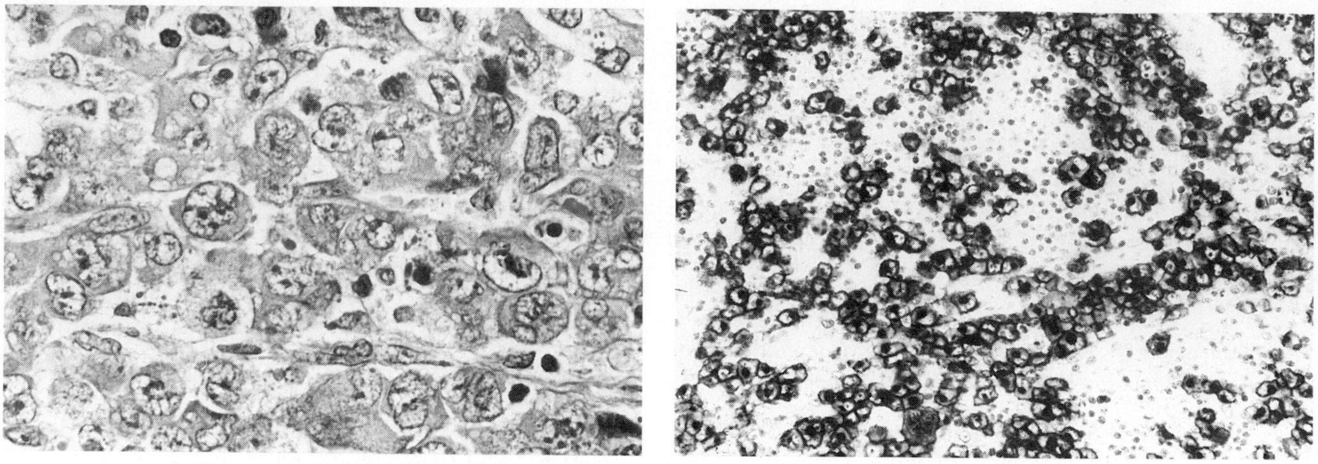

FIG. 25.12. Growth patterns of systemic anaplastic large cell lymphoma. **A:** Sinusoidal dissemination of neoplastic cells (paraffin section immunostained for CD30 with monoclonal antibody Ber-H2, alkaline phosphatase and anti-alkaline phosphatase technique). **B:** Perifollicular homing of the CD30$^+$ neoplastic cells (paraffin section processed).

gressive stage III or IV disease, usually associated with systemic symptoms (75%), especially high fever that possibly reflects the release of cytokines by tumor cells or accompanying inflammatory cells. A noncontiguous, often tender, multiple peripheral lymphadenopathy is observed in a high percentage of patients. Extranodal involvement is common (60%), with approximately 40% of patients showing two or more extranodal sites of disease. In a large study, the frequency of extranodal sites of lymphoma involvement was as follows: skin, 21%; bone (solitary or multiple lesions), 17%; soft tissues, 17%; lung, 11%; and liver, 8%, with involvement of the gut and CNS being a rare event (453). The incidence of bone marrow involvement is approximately 11% when analyzed with hematoxylin and eosin stains and approximately 30% when checked with immunohistochemistry because scattered ALCL cells are detectable in bone marrow trephines only when they are specifically labeled (454).

Histologic Findings

ALK$^+$ ALCL encompasses a broad spectrum of morphologic variants that are relevant for the diagnosis of ALCL but apparently not for the prognosis. All morphologic variants have in common a diffuse and often sinusoidal growth pattern (Fig. 25.12A), and in cases with partial involvement of lymph node, a preferential perifollicular spread (Fig. 25.12B) of the neoplastic cells. In all variants, there are large atypical neoplastic blasts and various proportions of smaller neoplastic cells. The large tumor cells usually exhibit a horseshoe- or kidney-shaped nucleus with multiple medium-sized nucleoli. The cytoplasm is broad, slightly basophilic and contains vacuoles (latter being visible only in imprint preparations). Cells with these cytologic features have been called hallmark cells because they are encountered in all ALCL variants (428). The smaller neoplastic cells show irregular nuclei and clear cytoplasm. These cells are only

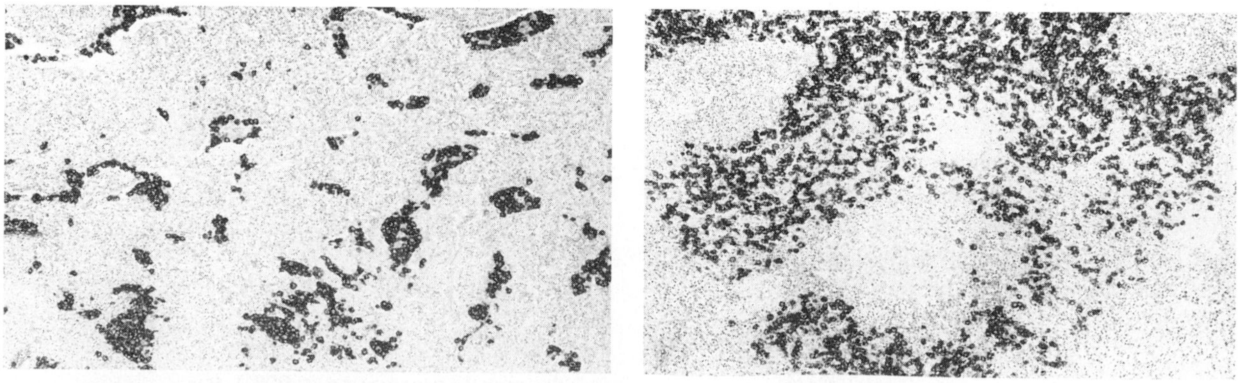

FIG. 25.13. Anaplastic large cell lymphoma of the common type. **A:** The tumor cells are large and have irregularly shaped nuclei, multiple prominent nucleoli, and a moderately abundant, grayish, basophilic cytoplasm (Giemsa-stained paraffin section). **B:** Immunoreactivity for CD30 shows strong staining of the cell membrane and of the Golgi area in all neoplastic cells (paraffin section, monoclonal antibody Ber-H2, alkaline phosphatase and anti-alkaline phosphatase technique).

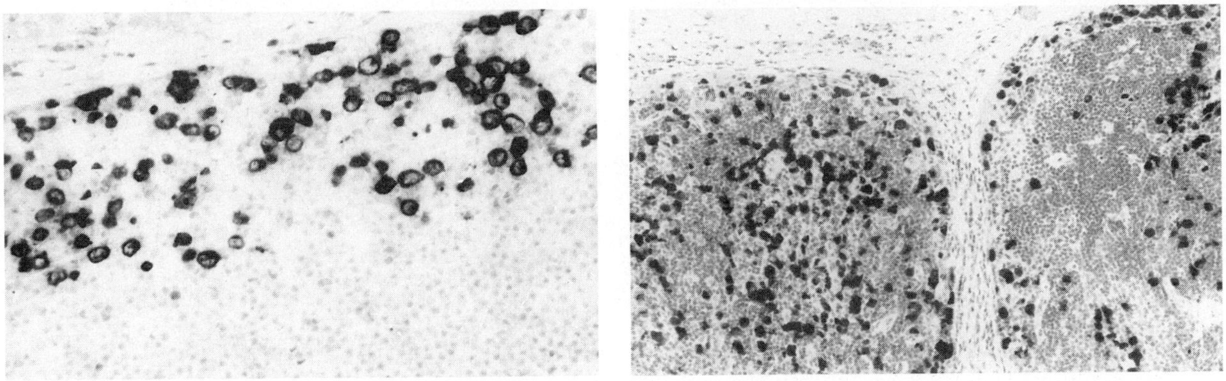

A B

FIG. 25.14. Immunophenotype of anaplastic lymphoma kinase–positive (ALK^+) systemic anaplastic large cell lymphoma. **A:** Immunoreactivity for the cytotoxic molecule perforin highlights the intrasinusoidal neoplastic cells (paraffin section immunostained with monoclonal antibody P1-8, alkaline phosphatase and anti-alkaline phosphatase [APAAP] technique). **B:** Immunoreactivity for ALK. The cells are strongly labeled in the cytoplasm and nucleus. This immunostain allows easy and selective detection of the neoplastic cells (paraffin section immunostained with the monoclonal ALK1 antibody, APAAP technique).

slightly larger than normal lymphocytes. The various morphologic variants of ALCL are recognized according to the histologic spectrum of the tumor cell population and the admixture of reactive cells:

The *common type* (372,455) is characterized by sheets of large lymphoid cells with chromatin-poor horseshoe-shaped nuclei containing multiple nucleoli (Fig. 25.13A). Multinucleated cells with a Reed-Sternberg–like appearance may also occur. The tumor cells have abundant cytoplasm that in imprint preparations frequently shows numerous vacuoles (Fig. 25.13B). The monomorphic subform probably represents a variant of the common type (377). Because of the cytologic resemblance of the latter to immunoblastic lymphoma, it can easily be confused with nonanaplastic large cell lymphomas when immunohistology is not applied (Fig. 25.14).

The *small cell variant* (381) is characterized by a mixture of small, medium-sized, and large lymphoid cells (Fig. 25.15A). The nuclei of the small and medium-sized cell population are often irregular. Large cells surrounding small vessels are a frequent and characteristic finding. In the past, the small cell variant was usually diagnosed as peripheral T-cell lymphoma, and some investigators still prefer this interpretation. The small cell variant may, however, contain areas with the morphology of ALCL common type (i.e., sheets of blasts) and can transform into the common type and vice versa (428,456). These observations strongly suggest that the small cell variant is part of the histologic spectrum of ALCL.

The dominant feature of the *lymphohistiocytic variant* is the large number of histiocytes that may mask the anaplastic tumor cell population (382) (Fig. 25.16A). Occasionally, the

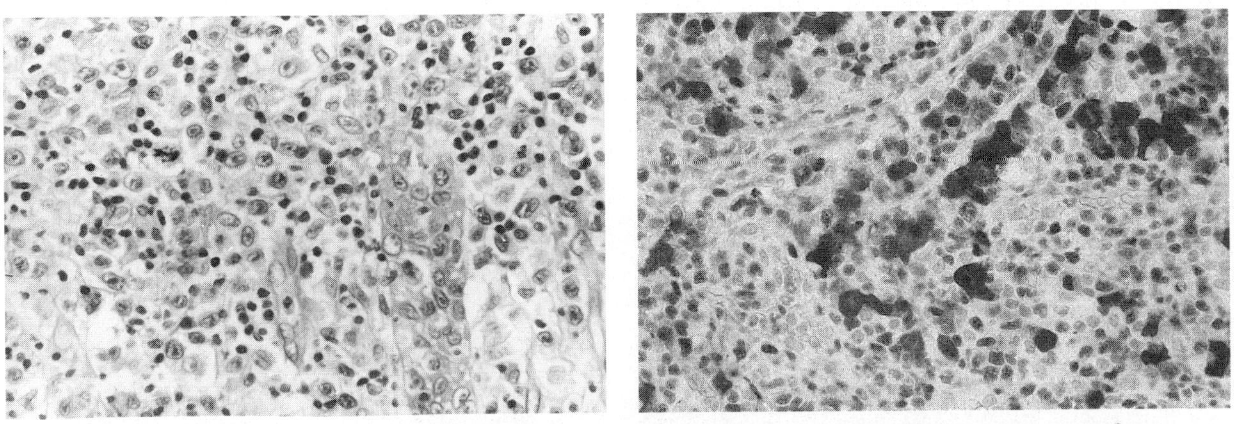

A B

FIG. 25.15. Morphology and immunophenotype of the small cell variant of ALK^+ systemic anaplastic large cell lymphoma. **A:** Most of the cells exhibit a small, irregular nucleus and light cytoplasm; larger cells tend to be located close to small vessels (Giemsa-stained paraffin section). **B:** Immunoreactivity for ALK protein shows that the larger cells located in the vicinity of small vessels are positive for ALK in the cytoplasm and nucleus, whereas in the smaller cells, the labeling is mainly restricted to the nucleus (paraffin section immunostained with the ALK1 monoclonal antibody, alkaline phosphatase and anti-alkaline phosphatase technique).

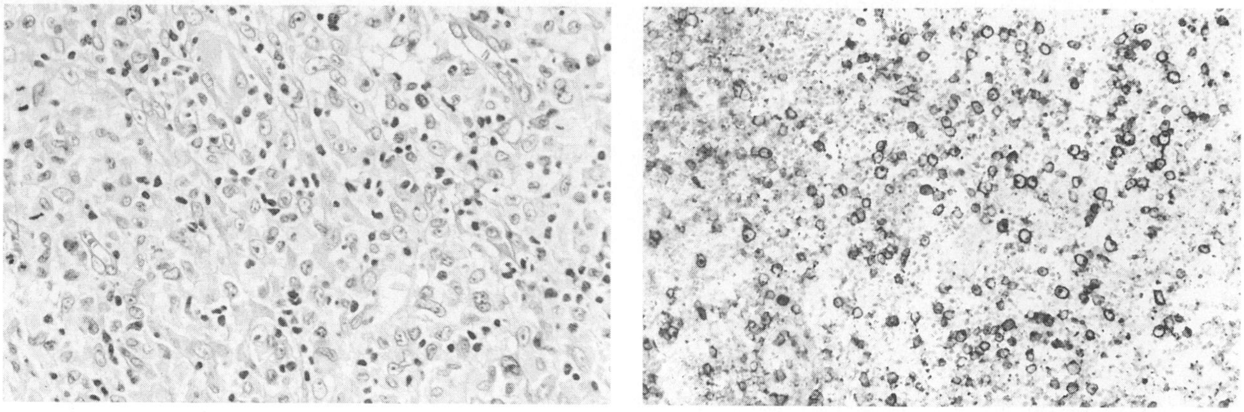

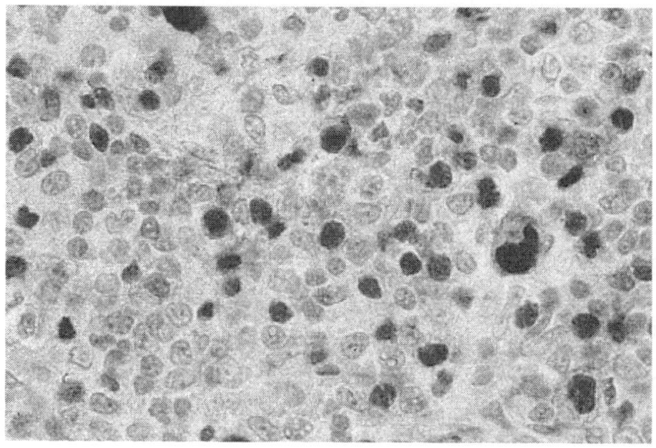

FIG. 25.16. Morphology and immunophenotype of the lymphohistiocytic variant of ALK$^+$ systemic anaplastic large cell lymphoma. **A:** Most cells correspond to histiocytes, but the neoplastic cells are not easily discernible in routine histologic sections (Giemsa-stained paraffin section). **B:** Immunostaining for CD30 highlights the scarce neoplastic cells (paraffin section immunostained with the Ber-H2 monoclonal antibody, alkaline phosphatase and anti-alkaline phosphatase [APAAP] technique). **C:** Immunostaining for ALK protein reveals variation in the size of the labeled cells, with a predominance of smaller cells. The smaller the cells, the more the labeling is restricted to the nucleus. The ALK$^-$ cells are bystander macrophages (paraffin section, monoclonal antibody ALK1, APAAP technique).

histiocytes show signs of erythrophagocytosis and often display a monomorphic appearance with eccentric nuclei, a feature that in the past often led to the misdiagnosis of malignant histiocytosis. The neoplastic cells of this variant are usually smaller than in the common ALCL type and therefore this subtype may be related to the small cell variant. Because of the small-sized tumor cell component, the lymphohistiocytic subform was not regarded as a variant of ALCL in the Kiel classification but erroneously categorized as a peripheral T-cell lymphoma.

In the *giant cell–rich variant* (455) a large number of the tumor cells contain more than one nucleus. The tumor cells are often very large and bizarre (Fig. 25.17A).

The *sarcomatoid variant* of ALCL (457) mimics soft tissue tumors, especially of malignant fibrous histiocytoma (MFH) type. The neoplastic cells of this rare variant are

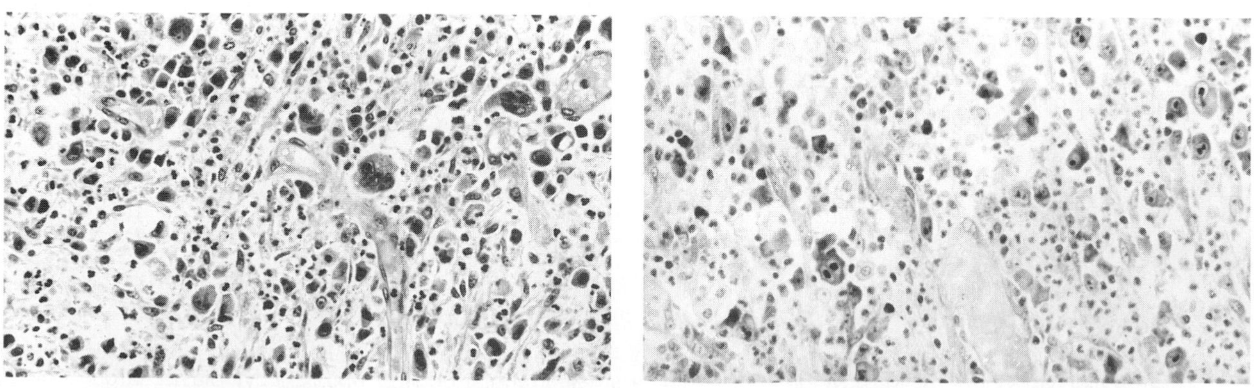

FIG. 25.17. Morphologic variants of systemic anaplastic large cell lymphoma. **A:** Giant cell–rich variant of anaplastic large cell lymphoma shows many multinucleated tumor cells (Giemsa-stained paraffin section). **B:** Anaplastic large cell lymphoma (Hodgkin's-like) contains various numbers of Hodgkin's- and Reed-Sternberg–like tumor cells embedded in a background with inflammatory cells (Giemsa-stained paraffin section).

large, bizarre, and often spindle shaped. Multinucleated forms are present in various numbers.

There are also some rare morphologic variants of ALCL characterized by an abundant admixture of eosinophils or neutrophils (383,458). Such cases may easily be mistaken for Hodgkin's disease, true histiocytic malignancies or even an acute inflammatory process. This is especially true for the *neutrophil-rich variant*, because it may mimic an acute inflammation and when located in the skin, a pustular lesion (459). An ALCL *variant with signet ring* appearance of the neoplastic cells has also been described (384,460).

Immunohistologic Findings

Essential for diagnosis is the immunohistologic demonstration of CD30 (Figs. 25.12A, 25.13) and ALK proteins (Fig. 25.14B) and the absence of B-cell specific antigens. CD30 is strongly expressed on the cell membrane and in the Golgi region (Fig. 25.13A), so that membrane-associated CD30 expression was included in the definition of ALCL (372). Immunostaining for CD30 highlights mostly the large anaplastic cells, whereas heterogeneous CD30 expression is seen in the small cell population with many small cells being $CD30^-$ (Fig.25.16B) (more commonly) or weakly $CD30^+$. The analysis of conventional T-cell markers reveals that the T-cell type is the most frequent (372,376,461). The most constantly expressed T-cell antigen is the ϵ-chain of the TCR/CD3 complex; a minority of cases express CD4 or CD8 with a predominance of CD4 (462). The frequency of the null cell type depends on the number of T-cell antigens investigated in a given study. Most, if not all, of the null cell cases have been found to belong to the T-cell type. This becomes evident when a large number of T-cell antigens or the configuration of the T-cell receptor genes are investigated and the immunohistologic studies are extended to detection of cytotoxic molecules. Most T/null ALCLs proved to express the cytotoxic molecules perforin, granzyme B, and TIA-1 (Fig. 25.14A), regardless of the expression of CD4 or CD8 (462–464). Because cytotoxic molecules are not only expressed by cytotoxic T cells but also by natural killer (NK) cells (442,465) and activated NK cells may express CD30 (466), there is the possibility that a minority of the T/null ALCLs are derived from NK cells rather than cytotoxic T cells. In support of this possibility is the expression of the NK cell–associated marker CD56 in some cases of ALCL (464) and the finding that approximately 10% of ALCLs lack detectable TCR gene rearrangements (463). Further studies are required to unequivocally clarify the relationship of some ALCL cases to NK cells. A nonspecific marker for cellular origin is epithelial membrane antigen (EMA), which can be demonstrated in most cases (386,467).

Immunohistologic demonstration of ALK protein expression has revealed the wide morphologic spectrum of the ALK^+ ALCLs, which ranges from the small cell to the giant cell variant of ALCL, with most cases falling into the category of ALCL common type (394,428,468). It became evident that, in addition to the large anaplastic cells, a variable proportion of small-sized elements (sometimes regarded as nonneoplastic on morphologic grounds and by the absence of CD30) express the ALK protein (394). There is a correlation between the size of ALK^+ tumor cells and the subcellular distribution of the ALK protein, the large anaplastic tumor cells being usually positive in the cytoplasm and the nucleus (less commonly only in the cytoplasm) while the small tumor cells exhibit nuclear-restricted ALK protein expression (394) (Figs. 25.15B, 25.16C). The large ALK^+ tumor cells make up the dominant population in the common and giant cell variants while the ALK^+ small cell elements are the dominant population in the small cell and lymphohistiocytic variants (394).

The fact that the ALK protein is detectable in the small and large tumor cells indicates that the genetic lesion leading to anomalous ALK expression is present in both cell populations, and the large and small cells therefore belong to the same neoplastic clone. For this reason, the hypothesis that the large cells observed in the small cell variant of ALCL represent a subclone that has arisen in a t(2;5) translocation-negative low-grade (small cell) lymphoma by acquiring the t(2;5) translocation, can be dismissed. According to one study, the transformation of the ALK^+ small cell ALCL variant into the ALCL common type may be linked, at least in some cases, to the acquisition of additional chromosomal abnormalities (e.g., those involving the sex chromosome and chromosomes 6, 7, 9, and 15) (456).

From the available data, it can be concluded that the wide morphologic spectrum observed in chimeric ALK^+ lymphomas results from the different ratios between the large and the small tumor elements (variable from case to case and within a given case at presentation and relapse), which appears to depend on whether the NPM-ALK protein is dimerized with wild-type NPM (Fig. 25.6); the different tissue distribution of neoplastic cells (e.g., perivascular pattern versus diffuse); the occasional occurrence of nodular sclerosis (producing a Hodgkin's-like appearance); and the presence of different reactive cells (e.g., histiocytes in the lymphohistiocytic variant).

Genetic Findings

Initial studies on the configuration of the antigen receptor genes in ALCL that were performed using the Southern blot technique demonstrated that one or more T-cell receptor genes were clonally rearranged in most cases (374,469). At that time, a divergence between a T-cell genotype and an immunophenotype with absent characteristic T-cell markers was noticed (374). Later investigations using PCR in conjunction with family specific primers demonstrated an almost complete concordance between the T-cell antigen profile and the presence of clonally rearranged TCR genes (463) (Table 25.2). The demonstration of clonally rearranged TCR β and γ genes in 90% cases of T and null type ALCL indicates that most or all null ALCLs are immunophenotypic variants of T-type ALCL (463) and ALCLs originating from NK cells seem to be extremely rare, despite the reported, although somewhat controversial, expression of CD56 in approximately one third of ALCLs.

The constant feature of t(2;5) cases is the presence of this translocation leading to expression of ALK fusion proteins. Infection with EBV is practically absent (470,471).

Differential Diagnosis

The prerequisite for the diagnosis of an ALK$^+$ ALCL is the immunohistologic detection of the ALK protein or the molecular detection of the corresponding translocation. The differential diagnosis encompasses other ALK$^+$ neoplasms. Expression of this protein has been reported only in soft tissue tumors (rhabdomyosarcoma, inflammatory myofibroblastic tumors (394,438,439) and in a rare form of DLBCL (440). In addition to morphologic differences, immunohistologic studies are of assistance for the correct diagnosis as rhabdomyosarcomas almost always express desmin and muscle-specific transcription factors (i.e., Myf4), and they are always CD30$^-$. The inflammatory myofibroblastic tumors express smooth muscle actin while they are CD30$^-$. The rare ALK$^+$ large B-cell lymphoma also does not show CD30 expression. These lymphomas frequently express IgA and J-chain and more rarely IgL chains.

The lymphohistiocytic ALCL variant may be confused with malignant histiocytosis (382). The neoplastic cells can be easily recognized within the dominant histiocytic populations after CD30 and ALK immunostains. The histiocytes hardly proliferate, as revealed by their negativity for the nuclear proliferation marker Ki-67, and therefore are reactive. In contrast, the tumor cells show a high Ki-67 index.

The distinction of the sarcomatoid variant from malignant fibrous histiocytoma is easily accomplished by immunohistology because this and other soft tissue tumors consistently lack CD30 and other lymphoid markers.

Prognosis

Patients with ALK$^+$ ALCL appear to benefit from chemotherapy more than those with ALK$^-$ forms of systemic ALCL. In a retrospective study of 53 patients suffering from systemic ALK$^+$ ALCL treated with antracyclin-containing regimens, the 5-year overall survival proved to be far better for this lymphoma than for ALK$^-$ ALCL (71 [15%] versus 15 [11%]) (453) (Fig. 25.18). Similar differences between ALK$^+$ and ALK$^-$ ALCL were reported by Shiota and colleagues (472) and confirmed by other investigators (423). Other studies have also reported an excellent outcome for systemic ALCL occurring in pediatric (473–475) and young adult patients (453,476,477). Although ALK expression was not investigated in those studies, the young age suggests that these series of patients contained a relatively large proportion of chimeric ALK$^+$ ALCL cases. In two patients, transformation of the ALK$^+$ small variant to common type ALCL

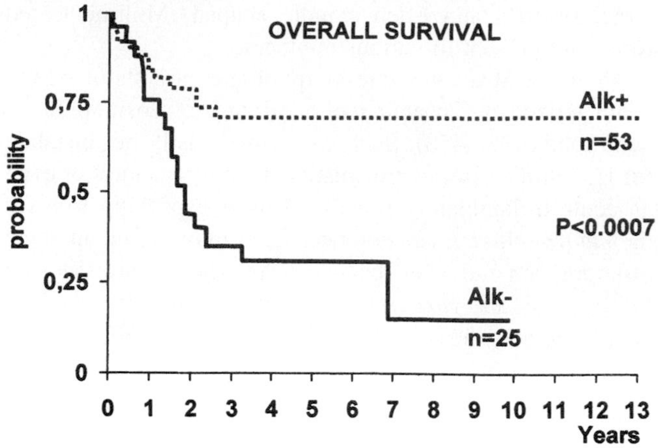

C

FIG. 25.18. The difference in the overall survival between ALK$^+$ systemic anaplastic large cell lymphoma and ALK$^-$ systemic anaplastic large cell lymphoma. (Data from Mora J, Filippa DA, Thaler HT, et al. Large cell non-Hodgkin lymphoma of childhood: analysis of 78 consecutive patients enrolled in two consecutive protocols at the Memorial Sloan-Kettering Cancer Center. *Cancer* 2000;88:186–197.)

was found to be predictive of a rapid clinical course (456), but this finding needs to be confirmed by study of a larger number of patients. There are no differences in the clinical features and outcome between the ALK$^+$ lymphomas bearing the common *NPM-ALK* fusion gene and those carrying variants(s) of the ALK fusion protein (427).

Falini and colleagues demonstrated that, within the good prognostic group of chimeric ALK$^+$ cases, the 5-year survival was 94% ± 5% for the low- and intermediate-risk group (age-adjusted International Prognostic Index = 0 to 1) and 41% ± 12% for the high- and intermediate-risk group (age-adjusted International Prognostic Index ≥2) (453). Similar findings were observed by Gascoyne and associates (423). These findings contrast with those of another report by the Non-Hodgkin's Lymphoma Classification Project in which no significant difference was observed between ALCL patients with a low or a high International Prognostic Index (478). However, this result was obtained in a less well defined group of ALCL patients that were not characterized with anti-ALK antibodies.

ALK-Negative Systemic Anaplastic Large Cell Lymphoma

Definition

Lymphoma composed of anaplastic large-sized blasts showing strong CD30 expression in the absence of B-cell antigens and of the ALK protein. The features of ALK$^-$ systemic ALCL are summarized in Table 25.11.

Clinical Features

The reported clinical features of ALK$^-$ systemic ALCLs are not consistent. According to one study, these lymphomas

TABLE 25.11. *ALK-negative anaplastic large cell lymphoma*

Histologic findings	
	Usually common type, rarely giant cell variant, or lymphohistiocytic or Hodgkin's–like variant
Immunohistologic findings	
	ALK^- $CD30^+$, $EMA^{-/+}$, cytotoxic molecules$^{+/-}$, $CD3^{+/-}$, CD4>CD8
Genetic findings	
	T-cell receptor (β/γ) chain genes clonally rearranged
Clinical findings	
	Mean age at presentation 46–61 years
	Male = female
	Lymph node swellings, extranodal tumors
Prognosis	
	Unfavorable; 10-year survival rates of 15% to 37%

occur in older individuals and are associated with a lower male to female ratio (0.9) and with a lower incidence of stage III or IV disease and extranodal involvement than ALK^+ ALCLs (427), whereas another study did not find such differences (423).

Histologic Findings

All morphologic variants described in the section of ALK^+ ALCL can be observed in the ALK^- ALCL group with one main exception: the small cell variant, which is a salient feature of the ALK^+ group of cases (394). The lymphohistiocytic and the giant cell variants are more rarely observed among the ALK^- than the ALK^+ cases.

Immunohistologic Findings

The immunophenotype is entirely similar to that of the ALK^+ ALCL with the exception of ALK expression. The differences between the entities are unknown. Only a few ALK^- cases have been investigated because most studies concentrate on ALK^+ cases.

Genetic Findings

For T-cell receptor genes, most cases, regardless of a T-cell or null cell immunophenotype, show a clonal rearrangement of the T-cell receptor genes (463).

Differential Diagnosis

ALK^- ALCL has to be differentiated from ALK^+ ALCL, classic Hodgkin's disease, and a variety of undifferentiated nonlymphoid neoplasms, including embryonal carcinoma of the testis and metastatic malignant melanoma. In most cases, immunohistologic analysis (Table 25.12) greatly facilitates establishment of the correct diagnosis. Only the differentiation from classic Hodgkin's disease may be problematic. In 1994 at the European Association of Hematopathology Workshop in Toledo, it became evident that markers such as CD15, BNH.9, and EMA—despite initial optimism—did not help in this distinction (479). This proved to be valid also for cytotoxic molecules because these may also be expressed by the Reed-Sternberg cells of Hodgkin's disease and by the tumor cells in ALCL. The *PAX5* gene encoded B-cell–specific activation transcription factor (BSAP) has been found to be expressed by Reed-Sternberg cells but not by cells of T-cell or null cell type ALCL (480,481). A preliminary study has demonstrated the usefulness of this antigen in the differential diagnosis of ALCL and Hodgkin's disease. Another entity that may cause differential diagnostic problems is that of the peripheral T-cell lymphomas of the gastrointestinal tract as they can exhibit anaplastic cytomorphologic features combined with strong CD30 expression. Clinical data of a history of celiac disease and histologic features indicative of a tumor cell tropism for gastrointestinal mucosa (infiltration of crypt and surface epithelia) allow correct classification as an intestinal T-cell lymphoma in most cases (482). In Japanese patients, ALK^- ALCL has to be differentiated from the human T lymphotropic virus type 1 (HTLV-1)–positive anaplastic variant of adult T-cell leukemia.

Prognosis

In all studies ALK^- ALCLs showed a poorer prognosis than ALK^+ ALCLs, with a 10-year overall survival of about 15% to 37% (423,453) (Fig. 25.18).

Primary Cutaneous Anaplastic Large Cell Lymphoma

Concepts Influencing the Definition

The classification of $CD30^+$ cutaneous T-cell lymphomas has changed in the last few years. Initially, only primary cutaneous lymphomas exhibiting anaplastic large-sized neoplastic cells with CD30 expression by 100% of the neoplastic cell population were classified as primary cutaneous ALCL. Meanwhile, it could be demonstrated that cutaneous T-cell lymphomas showing CD30 positivity in more than 75% of the neoplastic cells are characterized by a significantly better prognosis than the $CD30^-$ cases (with the exception of mycosis fungoides) (483). CD30 expression became more important for classification than tumor cell morphology. Real $CD30^+$ primary cutaneous ALCLs can be differentiated from the spontaneous disappearing lymphomatoid papulosis only after clinical observation. In the classification of cutaneous lymphomas proposed by the EORTC group it has been recommended that all T-cell lymphomas with CD30 expression by more than 75% of the tumor cells and a solitary cutaneous manifestation of at least 6 months should be clas-

TABLE 25.12. *Immunohistologic features for differentiating between classic Hodgkin's disease and systemic anaplastic large cell lymphoma*

Feature	Classic Hodgkin's disease	ALK-positive systemic ALCL	ALK-negative systemic ALCL
ALK protein	–	+	–
LMP-1 (EBV)	ca. 40–50% +	–	–
BSAP	80–90% +	–	–
CD20	ca. 20–30% +	–	–
CD15	ca. 90% +	<5% +	<50% +
CD3	ca. 20% +	frequently +	frequently +
CD4	ca. 5–10% +	frequently +	frequently +
Granzyme B/perforin	10–20% +	ca. 80–100% +	ca. 60–80% +
CD43	–	frequently +	frequently +

sified as primary cutaneous $CD30^+$ T-cell lymphoid proliferation (484). The final classification as primary cutaneous ALCL or lymphomatoid papulosis should be performed according to the clinical course. This EORTC concept will most likely be adopted by the new WHO classification. The features of primary cutaneous ALCL are summarized on Table 25.13.

Clinical Presentation

Primary cutaneous ALCL arises *de novo* in the skin and affects older patients with a median age of approximately 60 years. It accounts for approximately 9% of cutaneous lymphomas (484). The lesion usually presents as a solitary asymptomatic cutaneous or subcutaneous reddish violet tumor, which can be superficially ulcerated (485). Less commonly, the disease is characterized by multiple tumor nodules aggregated in a circumscribed area or as multicentric tumors at multiple sites.

TABLE 25.13. *Primary cutaneous anaplastic large cell lymphoma*

Histologic findings
- Large cell anaplastic or immunoblastic ("cutaneous ALCL")
- Large blasts with dense reactive infiltrate ("lymphomatoid papulosis")

Immunohistologic findings
- $CD30^+$ >75% of the neoplastic cells, $CD3^+$, $CD4^{+/-}$, cytotoxic molecules in about 70%
- ALK+<5%, Heca452+/−, EMA negative, Epstein-Barr virus proteins negative

Genetic findings
- T-cell receptor (β/γ) chain genes clonally rearranged

Clinical findings
- Mean age at presentation: 60 years
- At point of diagnosis, exclusively cutaneous manifestations

Clinical classification
- Progressive tumorous growth produces cutaneous ALCL
- Spontaneous regression produces lymphomatoid papulosis

Histologic Findings

Most cases show a more or less dense infiltrate of large immunoblast-like to anaplastic tumor cells, sometimes with admixed multinucleated giant cells in the upper dermis, often with ulceration of the epidermis (484). A varying amount of background infiltrate composed of reactive lymphocytes, histiocytes, neutrophils and eosinophils may complicate the diagnosis and lead to the erroneous interpretation of an inflammatory process.

Immunohistologic Findings

The diagnosis of primary cutaneous ALCL requires a proportion of tumor cells (>75%) to express CD30 antigen. T-cell antigens and particularly CD3 are more commonly detected than in systemic ALCLs. Expression of the cytotoxic molecules TIA-1/GMP17, perforin, and granzyme B is observed in about 70% of the cases. Primary cutaneous ALCL is usually negative for EMA and for the ALK protein (486–488). Moreover, nearly one half of the cases arising in the skin are positive for the cutaneous lymphocyte antigen recognized by monoclonal antibody HECA 452 (386).

Differential Diagnosis

Despite some differences, primary cutaneous ALCL and *lymphomatoid papulosis* overlap in histologic, immunophenotypic and clinical features. The major clinical difference is that lymphomatoid papulosis, despite relapses, runs a benign clinical course with spontaneous disappearance of individual skin lesions in most instances (484). Because a histologic and immunohistochemical distinction between primary cutaneous ALCL and lymphomatoid papulosis is often not possible because of the overlapping features, clinical criteria should be applied to determine whether the patient has a locally progressive disease that requires treatment (ALCL) or a relapsing condition that needs no treatment (i.e., lymphomatoid papulosis) (489).

Prognosis

Primary cutaneous ALCL has a more favorable prognosis than systemic ALCL (which may secondarily involve the skin). Approximately 25% of patients with primary cutaneous ALCL show partial or complete spontaneous regression, accounting for the previous designation of regressing atypical histiocytosis (RAH). Treatment of localized lesions is usually excision with or without radiation and is associated with long term survival (386,483–485). However, patients with disseminated skin disease appear to be at greater risk of developing extracutaneous involvement and may benefit from systemic polychemotherapy (485).

Hodgkin-like Anaplastic Large Cell Lymphoma: Is It a Distinct Entity?

Although there is accumulating evidence that ALCL and classic Hodgkin's disease are biologically distinct, the morphologic and immunophenotypic border between these two disease categories is not sharp in all instances (479). This applies especially to classic Hodgkin's disease cases rich in tumor cells, with lymphocytic depletion, nodular sclerosis grade II or syncytial growth pattern. To keep both entities, classic Hodgkin's disease and ALCL "clean," in the late 1980s, a category (basket) under the term *ALCL-HD–related* was created (490). The borderline cases, or gray zone cases, could then be collected in this basket for further studies. Under the designation ALCL-Hodgkin's-like, this type was adopted by the REAL classification as a preliminary category (379). The tumors falling into this category show features of ALCL and Hodgkin's disease. These ambiguous cases contain relatively dense nodules or sheets of tumor cells with features of classic Hodgkin and Reed-Sternberg cells (Fig. 25.17B). Tumor cells are usually present within sinuses and, due to capsule thickening and nodular or diffuse fibrosis, the sinusoidal dissemination is on occasion recognizable only by immunolabeling for CD30. The proportion of admixed reactive inflammatory cells is lower than that found in typical cases of Hodgkin's disease. The change from the term *ALCL-HD–related* to *ALCL-HD–like* reflects the early 1990s tendency to believe that most of these gray zone lymphomas represented ALCLs mimicking Hodgkin's disease. ALCL, Hodgkin's like has been reported to occur in young patients (like ALK^+ ALCL) but shows clinical features different from those observed in ALK^+ ALCL; there is a high frequency of mediastinal involvement (bulky disease in about 60% of cases), frequent stage II presentation, and lack of skin and bone involvement (491). These clinical findings, together with the absence of ALK protein and expression of the B-cell–specific activation protein (*PAX-5* gene product) in most cases, further support the view that that most cases of ALCL-HD-like represent a tumor cell–rich variant of classic Hodgkin's disease and not a true ALCL because the expression pattern is characteristic for Hodgkin's disease (480). Accordingly, the new WHO classification has abandoned the ALCL-HD-like subform and subsumes these cases under classic Hodgkin's Disease (492).

Other Forms of Anaplastic Large Cell Lymphoma Not Representing Disease Entities

Human Immunodeficiency Virus–Related Anaplastic Large Cell Lymphoma

True ALCL, especially the form bearing chimeric ALK proteins, is rare in HIV-infected patients (Falini B. and colleagues, personal communication, 1999). Most ALCLs reported to occur in HIV-associated patients are different from true ALCL and appear to be related to the anaplastic variant of DLBCL because they are of B cell origin and infected by EBV in most instances (395). Their prognosis usually relates to the immune status of the patient.

Secondary Anaplastic Large Cell Lymphoma

These neoplasms may arise in the progression of other lymphomas, most commonly during the course of mycosis fungoides, peripheral T-cell lymphomas, Hodgkin's disease or lymphomatoid papulosis. Such tumors mainly occur in older adults (493), are usually ALK^- and have a poor prognosis, indicating that appearance of CD30 expression in a previously $CD30^-$ lymphoma (most frequently being primary cutaneous T-cell lymphomas) is an unfavorable prognostic sign.

Clinical Value of Soluble CD30 in Anaplastic Large Cell Lymphoma

Increased levels of the soluble form of the CD30 molecule (higher than those in Hodgkin's disease) have been detected in virtually all patients with ALCL at diagnosis (399). The soluble CD30 level returns to the normal range on achievement of complete response but increases again after relapse (400). Moreover, a relationship between a risk of lower survival and increased pretreatment levels of sCD30 has been reported (400). However, it is not clear whether the determination of soluble CD30 can serve as an independent prognostic and disease monitoring indicator.

Reproducibility of the Diagnosis of Anaplastic Large Cell Lymphoma

The availability of monoclonal antibodies directed against CD30 and ALK protein was an enormous achievement in the recognition and diagnosis of ALCL. The detection of CD30 (in conjunction with other lymphoid and nonlymphoid markers) is also very important, not only in the differential diagnosis between ALCL and nonlymphoid anaplastic large cell tumors, but also in the distinction between ALCL and other types of lymphomas. The reproducibility of the diagnosis of ALCL on morphologic grounds is 46% but can be increased to 85% by immunostaining for CD30 (478). Application of EMA may further improve the reproducibility because its expression is mainly restricted to ALK$^+$ ALCL. The detection of ALK protein adds to our potential to distinguish ALCL of small cell and lymphohistiocytic types (whose small tumor cell components often lacks CD30) from peripheral T-cell lymphomas and even reactive conditions (393,394,428) and can greatly increase the diagnostic reproducibility of the ALK$^+$ ALCL to practically 100%. Given the absence of ALK protein in all normal tissues but the brain, ALK antibodies can be used to detect single tumor cells at the time of initial staging procedures or after therapy (minimal residual disease, as in the bone marrow).

Open Questions

Although the findings reviewed in this section indicate an enormous progress in the characterization of ALCL and its subforms since the first description of this lymphoma category 15 years ago, several questions still need to be answered. Is the ALK$^-$ primary systemic ALCL of T/null cell type one disease or a mixture of different diseases? Are all anaplastic large B-cell lymphomas variants of DLBCL or do all or a proportion of them represent a distinct disease entity? What is the mechanism by which the ALK fusion proteins cause malignant growth? Will it be possible to exploit the CD30 expression or an interference with chimeric ALK$^+$ activity for new more specific therapeutic strategies? Can all interface or gray zone cases between Hodgkin's disease and ALCL be assigned to one of these categories when more and more specific antigenic and genetic markers have been identified? What are the transforming events in ALK$^-$ systemic and primary cutaneous ALCL? Providing answers to these questions will increase our understanding of the tumorigenesis and the diagnostic reproducibility of the AKL$^-$ ALCL subforms, as well as improve the therapeutic management of patients who have ALCL.

REFERENCES

1. Miller TP, Jones SE. Initial chemotherapy for clinically localized lymphomas of unfavorable histology. *Blood* 1983;62:413–418.
2. Connors JM, Klimo P, Fairey RN, et al. Brief chemotherapy and involved field radiation therapy for limited-stage, histologically aggressive lymphoma. *Ann Intern Med* 1987;107:25–30.
3. Tondini C, Zanini M, Lombardi F, et al. Combined modality treatment with primary CHOP chemotherapy followed by locoregional irradiation in stage I or II histologically aggressive non-Hodgkin's lymphomas. *J Clin Oncol* 1993;11:720–725.
4. Dana BW, Dahlberg S, Miller TP, et al. m-BACOD treatment for intermediate- and high-grade malignant lymphomas: a Southwest Oncology Group phase II trial. *J Clin Oncol* 1990;8:1155–1162.
5. O'Reilly SE, Hoskins P, Klimo P, et al. MACOP-B and VACOP-B in diffuse large cell lymphomas and MOPP/ABVD in Hodgkin's disease. *Ann Oncol* 1991;2[Suppl 1]:17–23.
6. Harris NL, Jaffe ES, Stein H, et al. A revised European-American classification of lymphoid neoplasms: a proposal from the International Lymphoma Study Group [see comments]. *Blood* 1994;84:1361–1392.
7. Rajewsky K. Clonal selection and learning in the antibody system. *Nature* 1996;381:751–758.
8. Hsu FJ, Levy R: Preferential use of the V_H4 Ig gene family by diffuse large-cell lymphoma. *Blood* 1995;86:3072–3082.
9. Stevenson FK, Spellerberg MB, Treasure J, et al. Differential usage of an Ig heavy chain variable region gene by human B-cell tumors. *Blood* 1993;82:224–230.
10. Funkhouser WK, Warnke RA. Preferential IgH V4-34 gene segment usage in particular subtypes of B-cell lymphoma detected by antibody 9G4. *Hum Pathol* 1998;29:1317–1321.
11. Daley MD, Berinstein NL, Siminovitch KA. Immunoglobulin heavy chain variable gene utilization in human large cell and Burkitt's lymphoma cell lines. *Clin Invest Med* 1994;17:522–530.
12. Kuppers R, Rajewsky K, Hansmann ML. Diffuse large cell lymphomas are derived from mature B cells carrying V region genes with a high load of somatic mutation and evidence of selection for antibody expression. *Eur J Immunol* 1997;27:1398–1405.
13. Rosenquist R, Lindstrom A, Holmberg D, et al. V(H) gene family utilization in different B-cell lymphoma subgroups. *Eur J Haematol* 1999;62:123–128.
14. Kaneko Y, Rowley JD, Variakojis D, et al. Prognostic implications of karyotype and morphology in patients with non-Hodgkin's lymphoma. *Int J Cancer* 1983;32:683–692.
15. Offit K, Jhanwar S, Ebrahim SA, et al. T(3;22)(q27;q11): a novel translocation associated with diffuse non-Hodgkin's lymphoma [see comments]. *Blood* 1989;74:1876–1879.
16. Bastard C, Tilly H, Lenormand B, et al. Translocations involving band 3q27 and Ig gene regions in non-Hodgkin's lymphoma [see comments]. *Blood* 1992;79:2527–2531.
17. Ueda Y, Matsuda F, Misawa S, et al. Tumor-specific rearrangements of the immunoglobulin heavy-chain gene in B-cell non-Hodgkin's lymphoma detected by in situ hybridization. *Blood* 1996;87:292–298.
18. Michaud GY, Gascoyne RD, McNeil BK, et al. Bcl-6 and lymphoproliferative disorders. *Leuk Lymphoma* 1997;26:515–525.
19. Offit K, Lo CF, Louie DC, et al. Rearrangement of the bcl-6 gene as a prognostic marker in diffuse large-cell lymphoma [see comments]. *N Engl J Med* 1994;331:74–80.
20. Horsman DE, McNeil BK, Anderson M, et al. Frequent association of t(3;14) or variant with other lymphoma-specific translocations. *Br J Haematol* 1995;89:569–575.
21. Miki T, Kawamata N, Hirosawa S, et al. Gene involved in the 3q27 translocation associated with B-cell lymphoma, BCL5, encodes a Kruppel-like zinc-finger protein. *Blood* 1994;83:26–32.
22. Kerckaert JP, Deweindt C, Tilly H, et al. LAZ3, a novel zinc-finger encoding gene, is disrupted by recurring chromosome 3q27 translocations in human lymphomas. *Nat Genet* 1993;5:66–70.
23. Baron BW, Nucifora G, McCabe N, et al. Identification of the gene associated with the recurring chromosomal translocations t(3;14)(q27;q32) and t(3;22)(q27;q11) in B-cell lymphomas. *Proc Natl Acad Sci USA* 1993;90:5262–5266.
24. Ye BH, Lista F, Lo CF, et al. Alterations of a zinc finger-encoding gene, BCL-6, in diffuse large-cell lymphoma. *Science* 1993;262:747–750.
25. Kawamata N, Miki T, Fukuda T, et al. The organization of the BCL6 gene. *Leukemia* 1994;8:1327–1330.
26. Kawamata N, Miki T, Ohashi K, et al. Recognition DNA sequence of a novel putative transcription factor, BCL6. *Biochem Biophys Res Commun* 1994;204:366–374.
27. Baron BW, Stanger RR, Hume E, et al. BCL6 encodes a sequence-specific DNA-binding protein. *Genes Chromosomes Cancer* 1995;13:221–224.
28. Otsuki T, Yano T, Clark HM, et al. Analysis of LAZ3 (BCL-6) status in B-cell non-Hodgkin's lymphomas: results of rearrangement and gene expression studies and a mutational analysis of coding region sequences. *Blood* 1995;85:2877–2884.
29. Allman D, Jain A, Dent A, et al. BCL-6 expression during B-cell activation. *Blood* 1996;87:5257–5268.
30. Muramatsu M, Akasaka T, Kadowaki N, et al. Rearrangement of the BCL6 gene in B-cell lymphoid neoplasms: comparison with lymphomas associated with BCL2 rearrangement. *Br J Haematol* 1996;93:911–920.
31. Ye BH, Cattoretti G, Shen Q, et al. The BCL-6 proto-oncogene con-

trols germinal-centre formation and Th2-type inflammation. *Nat Genet* 1997;16:161–170.
32. Bastard C, Deweindt C, Kerckaert JP, et al. LAZ3 rearrangements in non-Hodgkin's lymphoma: correlation with histology, immunophenotype, karyotype, and clinical outcome in 217 patients. *Blood* 1994; 83:2423–2427.
33. Ohno H, Kerckaert JP, Bastard C, et al. Heterogeneity in B-cell neoplasms associated with rearrangement of the LAZ3 gene on chromosome band 3q27. *Jpn J Cancer Res* 1994;85:592–600.
34. Ye BH, Chaganti S, Chang CC, et al. Chromosomal translocations cause deregulated BCL6 expression by promoter substitution in B cell lymphoma. *EMBO J* 1995;14:6209–6217.
35. Chen W, Iida S, Louie DC, et al. Heterologous promoters fused to BCL6 by chromosomal translocations affecting band 3q27 cause its deregulated expression during B-cell differentiation. *Blood* 1998;91: 603–607.
36. Nakamura Y, Miki T, Kawamata N, et al. Biallelic DNA rearrangements and deletions within the BCL-6 gene in B-cell non-Hodgkin's lymphoma. *Br J Haematol* 1995;90:404–408.
37. Hebert J, Romana SP, Hillion J, et al. Translocation t(3;22)(q27;q11) in non-Hodgkin's malignant lymphoma: chromosome painting and molecular studies. *Leukemia* 1993;7:1971–1974.
38. Ueda Y, Nishida K, Miki T, et al. Interphase detection of BCL6/IgH fusion gene in non-Hodgkin lymphoma by fluorescence in situ hybridization. *Cancer Genet Cytogenet* 1997;99:102–107.
39. Lo CF, Ye BH, Lista F, et al. Rearrangements of the BCL6 gene in diffuse large cell non-Hodgkin's lymphoma. *Blood* 1994;83: 1757–1759.
40. Offit K, Louie DC, Parsa NZ, et al. BCL6 gene rearrangement and other cytogenetic abnormalities in diffuse large cell lymphoma. *Leuk Lymphoma* 1995;20:85–89.
41. Pescarmona E, De Sanctis V, Pistilli A, et al. Pathogenetic and clinical implications of Bcl-6 and Bcl-2 gene configuration in nodal diffuse large B-cell lymphomas. *J Pathol* 1997;183:281–286.
42. Vitolo U, Gaidano G, Botto B, et al. Rearrangements of bcl-6, bcl-2, c-myc and 6q deletion in B-diffuse large-cell lymphoma: clinical relevance in 71 patients. *Ann Oncol* 1998;9:55–61.
43. Migliazza A, Martinotti S, Chen W, et al. Frequent somatic hypermutation of the 5′ noncoding region of the BCL6 gene in B-cell lymphoma. *Proc Natl Acad Sci USA* 1995;92:12520–12524.
44. Shen HM, Peters A, Baron B, et al. Mutation of BCL-6 gene in normal B cells by the process of somatic hypermutation of Ig genes. *Science* 1998;280:1750–1752.
45. Pasqualucci L, Migliazza A, Fracchiolla N, et al. BCL-6 mutations in normal germinal center B cells: evidence of somatic hypermutation acting outside Ig loci. *Proc Natl Acad Sci USA* 1998;95:11816–11821.
46. Cattoretti G, Chang CC, Cechova K, et al. BCL-6 protein is expressed in germinal-center B cells. *Blood* 1995;86:45–53.
47. Flenghi L, Ye BH, Fizzotti M, et al. A specific monoclonal antibody (PG-B6) detects expression of the BCL-6 protein in germinal center B cells. *Am J Pathol* 1995;147:405–411.
48. Onizuka T, Moriyama M, Yamochi T, et al. BCL-6 gene product, a 92- to 98-kD nuclear phosphoprotein, is highly expressed in germinal center B cells and their neoplastic counterparts. *Blood* 1995;86:28–37.
49. Deweindt C, Albagli O, Bernardin F, et al. The LAZ3/BCL6 oncogene encodes a sequence-specific transcriptional inhibitor: a novel function for the BTB/POZ domain as an autonomous repressing domain. *Cell Growth Differ* 1995;6:1495–1503.
50. Seyfert VL, Allman D, He Y, et al. Transcriptional repression by the proto-oncogene BCL-6. *Oncogene* 1996;12:2331–2342.
51. Pittaluga S, Ayoubi TA, Wlodarska I, et al. BCL-6 expression in reactive lymphoid tissue and in B-cell non-Hodgkin's lymphomas. *J Pathol* 1996;179:145–150.
52. Flenghi L, Bigerna B, Fizzotti M, et al. Monoclonal antibodies PG-B6a and PG-B6p recognize, respectively, a highly conserved and a formol-resistant epitope on the human BCL-6 protein amino-terminal region. *Am J Pathol* 1996;148:1543–1555.
53. Skinnider BF, Horsman DE, Dupuis B, et al. Bcl-6 and Bcl-2 protein expression in diffuse large B-cell lymphoma and follicular lymphoma: correlation with 3q27 and 18q21 chromosomal abnormalities. *Hum Pathol* 1999;30:803–808.
54. Omonishi K, Yoshino T, Sakuma I, et al. bcl-6 protein is identified in high-grade but not low-grade mucosa-associated lymphoid tissue lymphomas of the stomach. *Mod Pathol* 1998;11:181–185.
55. Tsujimoto Y, Louie E, Bashir MM, et al. The reciprocal partners of both the t(14;18) and the t(11;14) translocations involved in B-cell neoplasms are rearranged by the same mechanism. *Oncogene* 1988; 2:347–351.
56. Bakhshi A, Jensen JP, Goldman P, et al. Cloning the chromosomal breakpoint of t(14;18) human lymphomas: clustering around J_H on chromosome 14 and near a transcriptional unit on 18. *Cell* 1985;41: 899–906.
57. Cleary ML, Sklar J. Nucleotide sequence of a t(14;18) chromosomal breakpoint in follicular lymphoma and demonstration of a breakpoint-cluster region near a transcriptionally active locus on chromosome 18. *Proc Natl Acad Sci USA* 1985;82:7439–7443.
58. Tsujimoto Y, Gorham J, Cossman J, et al. The t(14;18) chromosome translocations involved in B-cell neoplasms result from mistakes in VDJ joining. *Science* 1985;229:1390–1393.
59. Ngan BY, Nourse J, Cleary ML. Detection of chromosomal translocation t(14;18) within the minor cluster region of bcl-2 by polymerase chain reaction and direct genomic sequencing of the enzymatically amplified DNA in follicular lymphomas. *Blood* 1989;73:1759–1762.
60. Klefstrom J, Franssila K, Peltomaki P, et al. Major and minor breakpoint sites of chromosomal translocation t(14;18) in subtypes of non-Hodgkin's lymphomas. *Leuk Res* 1994;18:245–250.
61. Hockenbery D, Nunez G, Milliman C, et al. Bcl-2 is an inner mitochondrial membrane protein that blocks programmed cell death. *Nature* 1990;348:334–336.
62. McDonnell TJ, Nunez G, Platt FM, et al. Deregulated Bcl-2–immunoglobulin transgene expands a resting but responsive immunoglobulin M and D-expressing B-cell population. *Mol Cell Biol* 1990;10: 1901–1907.
63. McDonnell TJ, Deane N, Platt FM, et al. bcl-2–immunoglobulin transgenic mice demonstrate extended B cell survival and follicular lymphoproliferation. *Cell* 1989;57:79–88.
64. McDonnell TJ, Korsmeyer SJ. Progression from lymphoid hyperplasia to high-grade malignant lymphoma in mice transgenic for the t(14; 18). *Nature* 1991;349:254–256.
65. Weiss LM, Warnke RA, Sklar J, et al. Molecular analysis of the t(14; 18) chromosomal translocation in malignant lymphomas. *N Engl J Med* 1987;317:1185–1189.
66. Jacobson JO, Wilkes BM, Kwaiatkowski DJ, et al. Bcl-2 rearrangements in de novo diffuse large cell lymphoma. Association with distinctive clinical features. *Cancer* 1993;72:231–236.
67. Dalla-Favera R, Ye BH, Lo CF, et al. Identification of genetic lesions associated with diffuse large-cell lymphoma. *Ann Oncol* 1994;5[Suppl 1]:55–60.
68. Lee MS, Blick MB, Pathak S, et al. The gene located at chromosome 18 band q21 is rearranged in uncultured diffuse lymphomas as well as follicular lymphomas. *Blood* 1987;70:90–95.
69. Pezzella F, Tse AG, Cordell JL, et al. Expression of the bcl-2 oncogene protein is not specific for the 14;18 chromosomal translocation. *Am J Pathol* 1990;137:225–232.
70. Zutter M, Hockenbery D, Silverman GA, et al. Immunolocalization of the Bcl-2 protein within hematopoietic neoplasms. *Blood* 1991;78: 1062–1068.
71. Kondo E, Nakamura S, Onoue H, et al. Detection of bcl-2 protein and bcl-2 messenger RNA in normal and neoplastic lymphoid tissues by immunohistochemistry and in situ hybridization. *Blood* 1992;80: 2044–2051.
72. Tang SC, Visser L, Hepperle B, et al. Clinical significance of bcl-2–MBR gene rearrangement and protein expression in diffuse large-cell non-Hodgkin's lymphoma: an analysis of 83 cases. *J Clin Oncol* 1994;12:149–154.
73. Hill ME, MacLennan KA, Cunningham DC, et al. Prognostic significance of BCL-2 expression and bcl-2 major breakpoint region rearrangement in diffuse large cell non-Hodgkin's lymphoma: a British National Lymphoma Investigation Study. *Blood* 1996;88:1046–1051.
74. Monni O, Joensuu H, Franssila K, et al. DNA copy number changes in diffuse large B-cell lymphoma—comparative genomic hybridization study. *Blood* 1996;87:5269–5278.
75. Monni O, Joensuu H, Franssila K, et al. BCL2 overexpression associated with chromosomal amplification in diffuse large B-cell lymphoma. *Blood* 1997;90:1168–1174.
76. Rao PH, Houldsworth J, Dyomina K, et al. Chromosomal and gene amplification in diffuse large B-cell lymphoma. *Blood* 1998;92: 234–240.

77. Levine EG, Arthur DC, Frizzera G, et al. Cytogenetic abnormalities predict clinical outcome in non-Hodgkin lymphoma. *Ann Intern Med* 1988;108:14–20.
78. Pezzella F, Jones M, Ralfkiaer E, et al. Evaluation of bcl-2 protein expression and 14;18 translocation as prognostic markers in follicular lymphoma. *Br J Cancer* 1992;65:87–89.
79. Romaguera JE, Pugh W, Luthra R, et al. The clinical relevance of t(14;18)/BCL-2 rearrangement and DEL 6q in diffuse large cell lymphoma and immunoblastic lymphoma. *Ann Oncol* 1993;4:51–54.
80. Gascoyne RD, Adomat SA, Krajewski S, et al. Prognostic significance of Bcl-2 protein expression and Bcl-2 gene rearrangement in diffuse aggressive non-Hodgkin's lymphoma. *Blood* 1997;90:244–251.
81. Yunis JJ, Mayer MG, Arnesen MA, et al. bcl-2 and other genomic alterations in the prognosis of large-cell lymphoma [see comments]. *N Engl J Med* 1989;320:1047–1054.
82. Offit K, Koduru PR, Hollis R, et al. 18q21 Rearrangement in diffuse large cell lymphoma: incidence and clinical significance. *Br J Haematol* 1989;72:178–183.
83. Offit K, Jhanwar SC, Ladanyi M, et al. Cytogenetic analysis of 434 consecutively ascertained specimens of non-Hodgkin's lymphoma: correlations between recurrent aberrations, histology, and exposure to cytotoxic treatment. *Genes Chromosomes Cancer* 1991;3:189–201.
84. Seto M, Jaeger U, Hockett RD, et al. Alternative promoters and exons, somatic mutation and deregulation of the Bcl-2–Ig fusion gene in lymphoma. *EMBO J* 1988;7:123–131.
85. Reed JC, Tanaka S. Somatic point mutations in the translocated bcl-2 genes of non-Hodgkin's lymphomas and lymphocytic leukemias: implications for mechanisms of tumor progression. *Leuk Lymphoma* 1993;10:157–163.
86. Matolcsy A, Casali P, Warnke RA, et al. Morphologic transformation of follicular lymphoma is associated with somatic mutation of the translocated Bcl-2 gene. *Blood* 1996;88:3937–3944.
87. Piris MA, Pezzella F, Martinez-Montero JC, et al. P53 and bcl-2 expression in high-grade B-cell lymphomas: correlation with survival time [published erratum appears in *Br J Cancer* 1994;69:978]. *Br J Cancer* 1994;69:337–341.
88. Hermine O, Haioun C, Lepage E, et al. Prognostic significance of bcl-2 protein expression in aggressive non-Hodgkin's lymphoma. Groupe d'Etude des Lymphomes de l'Adulte (GELA). *Blood* 1996;87:265–272.
89. Gascoyne RD, Krajewska M, Krajewski S, et al. Prognostic significance of Bax protein expression in diffuse aggressive non-Hodgkin's lymphoma. *Blood* 1997;90:3173–3178.
90. Dalla-Favera R, Bregni M, Erikson J, et al. Human c-myc oncogene is located on the region of chromosome 8 that is translocated in Burkitt lymphoma cells. *Proc Natl Acad Sci USA* 1982;79:7824–7827.
91. Dalla-Favera R, Martinotti S, Gallo RC, et al. Translocation and rearrangements of the c-myc oncogene locus in human undifferentiated B-cell lymphomas. *Science* 1983;219:963–967.
92. Taub R, Kirsch I, Morton C, et al. Translocation of the c-myc gene into the immunoglobulin heavy chain locus in human Burkitt lymphoma and murine plasmacytoma cells. *Proc Natl Acad Sci USA* 1982;79:7837–7841.
93. Hollis GF, Mitchell KF, Battey J, et al. A variant translocation places the lambda immunoglobulin genes 3′ to the c-myc oncogene in Burkitt's lymphoma. *Nature* 1984;307:752–755.
94. Henriksson M, Luscher B. Proteins of the Myc network: essential regulators of cell growth and differentiation. *Adv Cancer Res* 1996;68:109–182.
95. Ladanyi M, Offit K, Jhanwar SC, et al. MYC rearrangement and translocations involving band 8q24 in diffuse large cell lymphomas. *Blood* 1991;77:1057–1063.
96. Volpe G, Vitolo U, Carbone A, et al. Molecular heterogeneity of B-lineage diffuse large cell lymphoma. *Genes Chromosomes Cancer* 1996;16:21–30.
97. Yano T, Jaffe ES, Longo DL, et al. MYC rearrangements in histologically progressed follicular lymphomas. *Blood* 1992;80:758–767.
98. Kramer MH, Hermans J, Wijburg E, et al. Clinical relevance of BCL2, BCL6, and MYC rearrangements in diffuse large B-cell lymphoma. *Blood* 1998;92:3152–3162.
99. Neri A, Fracchiolla NS, Migliazza A, et al. The involvement of the candidate proto-oncogene NFKB2/lyt-10 in lymphoid malignancies. *Leuk Lymphoma* 1996;23:43–48.
100. Neri A, Fracchiolla NS, Roscetti E, et al. Molecular analysis of cutaneous B- and T-cell lymphomas. *Blood* 1995;86:3160–3172.
101. Neri A, Chang CC, Lombardi L, et al. B cell lymphoma-associated chromosomal translocation involves candidate oncogene lyt-10, homologous to NF-kappa B p50. *Cell* 1991;67:1075–1087.
102. Houldsworth J, Mathew S, Rao PH, et al. REL proto-oncogene is frequently amplified in extranodal diffuse large cell lymphoma. *Blood* 1996;87:25–29.
103. Trent JM, Rosenfeld SB, Meyskens FL. Chromosome 6q involvement in human malignant melanoma. *Cancer Genet Cytogenet* 1983;9:177–180.
104. Morita R, Saito S, Ishikawa J, et al. Common regions of deletion on chromosomes 5q, 6q, and 10q in renal cell carcinoma. *Cancer Res* 1991;51:5817–5820.
105. Stenman G, Sandros J, Mark J, et al. Partial 6q deletion in a human salivary gland adenocarcinoma. *Cancer Genet Cytogenet* 1989;39:153–156.
106. Orphanos V, McGown G, Hey Y, et al. Allelic imbalance of chromosome 6q in ovarian tumours. *Br J Cancer* 1995;71:666–669.
107. Merup M, Moreno TC, Heyman M, et al. 6q deletions in acute lymphoblastic leukemia and non-Hodgkin's lymphomas. *Blood* 1998;91:3397–3400.
108. Gaidano G, Hauptschein RS, Parsa NZ, et al. Deletions involving two distinct regions of 6q in B-cell non-Hodgkin lymphoma. *Blood* 1992;80:1781–1787.
109. Hammond DW, Goepel JR, Aitken M, et al. Cytogenetic analysis of a United Kingdom series of non-Hodgkin's lymphomas. *Cancer Genet Cytogenet* 1992;61:31–38.
110. Schouten HC, Sanger WG, Weisenburger DD, et al. Chromosomal abnormalities in untreated patients with non-Hodgkin's lymphoma: associations with histology, clinical characteristics, and treatment outcome. The Nebraska Lymphoma Study Group. *Blood* 1990;75:1841–1847.
111. Whang-Peng J, Knutsen T, Jaffe ES, et al. Sequential analysis of 43 patients with non-Hodgkin's lymphoma: clinical correlations with cytogenetic, histologic, immunophenotyping, and molecular studies. *Blood* 1995;85:203–216.
112. Zhang Y, Weber-Matthiesen K, Siebert R, et al. Frequent deletions of 6q23-24 in B-cell non-Hodgkin's lymphomas detected by fluorescence in situ hybridization. *Genes Chromosomes Cancer* 1997;18:310–313.
113. Offit K, Wong G, Filippa DA, et al. Cytogenetic analysis of 434 consecutively ascertained specimens of non-Hodgkin's lymphoma: clinical correlations. *Blood* 1991;77:1508–1515.
114. Epstein MA, Achong BG, Barr YM. Virus particles in cultured lymphoblasts from Burkitt's lymphoma. *Lancet* 1964;1:702–703.
115. Henle W, Diehl V, Kohn G, et al. Herpes-type virus and chromosome marker in normal leukocytes after growth with irradiated Burkitt cells. *Science* 1967;157:1064–1065.
116. Henle G, Henle W, Diehl V. Relation of Burkitt's tumor-associated herpes-type virus to infectious mononucleosis. *Proc Natl Acad Sci USA* 1968;59:94–101.
117. Rowe M, Evans HS, Young LS, et al. Monoclonal antibodies to the latent membrane protein of Epstein-Barr virus reveal heterogeneity of the protein and inducible expression in virus-transformed cells. *J Gen Virol* 1987;68(Pt 6):1575–1586.
118. Hummel M, Anagnostopoulos I, Korbjuhn P, et al. Epstein-Barr virus in B-cell non-Hodgkin's lymphomas: unexpected infection patterns and different infection incidence in low- and high-grade types. *J Pathol* 1995;175:263–271.
119. Shimizu N, Tanabe-Tochikura A, Kuroiwa Y, et al. Isolation of Epstein-Barr virus (EBV)–negative cell clones from the EBV-positive Burkitt's lymphoma (BL) line Akata: malignant phenotypes of BL cells are dependent on EBV. *J Virol* 1994;68:6069–6073.
120. Trivedi P, Zhang QJ, Chen F, et al. Parallel existence of Epstein-Barr virus (EBV) positive and negative cells in a sporadic case of Burkitt lymphoma. *Oncogene* 1995;11:505–510.
121. Salles G, Chen CY, Reinherz EL, et al. CD10/NEP is expressed on Thy-1^{low} $B220^{+}$ murine B-cell progenitors and functions to regulate stromal cell-dependent lymphopoiesis. *Blood* 1992;80:2021–2029.
122. Almasri NM, Iturraspe JA, Braylan RC. CD10 expression in follicular lymphoma and large cell lymphoma is different from that of reactive lymph node follicles. *Arch Pathol Lab Med* 1998;122:539–544.

123. Carey DJ. Syndecans: multifunctional cell-surface co-receptors. *Biochem J* 1997;327(Pt 1):1–16.
124. Sanderson RD, Lalor P, Bernfield M. B lymphocytes express and lose syndecan at specific stages of differentiation. *Cell Regul* 1989; 1:27–35.
125. Sebestyen A, Berczi L, Mihalik R, et al. Syndecan-1 (CD138) expression in human non-Hodgkin lymphomas. *Br J Haematol* 1999;104: 412–419.
126. Hardy RR, Hayakawa K. Development and physiology of Ly-1 B and its human homolog, Leu-1 B. *Immunol Rev* 1986;93:53–79.
127. Hayakawa K, Hardy RR, Herzenberg LA, et al. Progenitors for Ly-1 B cells are distinct from progenitors for other B cells. *J Exp Med* 1985;161:1554–1568.
128. Kipps TJ. The CD5 B cell. *Adv Immunol* 1989;47:117–185.
129. Stall AM, Wells SM, Lam KP. B-1 cells: unique origins and functions. *Semin Immunol* 1996;8:45–59.
130. Muller-Hermelink HK, Greiner A. Molecular analysis of human immunoglobulin heavy chain variable genes (IgV_H) in normal and malignant B cells [comment]. *Am J Pathol* 1998;153:1341–1346.
131. Klein U, Goossens T, Fischer M, et al. Somatic hypermutation in normal and transformed human B cells. *Immunol Rev* 1998;162: 261–280.
132. Burns BF, Warnke RA, Doggett RS, et al. Expression of a T-cell antigen (Leu-1) by B-cell lymphomas. *Am J Pathol* 1983;113: 165–171.
133. Knowles DM, Halper JP, Azzo W, et al. Reactivity of monoclonal antibodies Leu 1 and OKT1 with malignant human lymphoid cells. Correlation with conventional cell markers. *Cancer* 1983;52: 1369–1377.
134. Matolcsy A, Chadburn A, Knowles DM. *De novo* CD5-positive and Richter's syndrome-associated diffuse large B cell lymphomas are genotypically distinct. *Am J Pathol* 1995;147:207–216.
135. Schwab U, Stein H, Gerdes J, et al. Production of a monoclonal antibody specific for Hodgkin and Sternberg-Reed cells of Hodgkin's disease and a subset of normal lymphoid cells. *Nature* 1982;299: 65–67.
136. Durkop H, Latza U, Hummel M, et al. Molecular cloning and expression of a new member of the nerve growth factor receptor family that is characteristic for Hodgkin's disease. *Cell* 1992;68:421–427.
137. Amakawa R, Hakem A, Kundig TM, et al. Impaired negative selection of T cells in Hodgkin's disease antigen CD30-deficient mice. *Cell* 1996;84:551–562.
138. Smith CA, Gruss HJ, Davis T, et al. CD30 antigen, a marker for Hodgkin's lymphoma, is a receptor whose ligand defines an emerging family of cytokines with homology to TNF. *Cell* 1993;73:1349–1360.
139. Shanebeck KD, Maliszewski CR, Kennedy MK, et al. Regulation of murine B cell growth and differentiation by CD30 ligand. *Eur J Immunol* 1995;25:2147–2153.
140. Stein H, Mason DY, Gerdes J, et al. The expression of the Hodgkin's disease associated antigen Ki-1 in reactive and neoplastic lymphoid tissue: evidence that Reed-Sternberg cells and histiocytic malignancies are derived from activated lymphoid cells. *Blood* 1985;66: 848–858.
141. Stein H, Mason DY, Gerdes J, et al. The expression of the Hodgkin's disease associated antigen Ki-1 in reactive and neoplastic lymphoid tissue: evidence that Reed-Sternberg cells and histiocytic malignancies are derived from activated lymphoid cells. *Blood* 1985;66: 848–858.
142. Hallek M, Bergsagel PL, Anderson KC. Multiple myeloma: increasing evidence for a multistep transformation process. *Blood* 1998;91:3–21.
143. Grossman A, Mittrucker HW, Nicholl J, et al. Cloning of human lymphocyte-specific interferon regulatory factor (hLSIRF/hIRF4) and mapping of the gene to 6p23-p25. *Genomics* 1996;37:229–233.
144. Iida S, Rao PH, Butler M, et al. Deregulation of MUM1/IRF4 by chromosomal translocation in multiple myeloma. *Nat Genet* 1997;17: 226–230.
145. Eisenbeis CF, Singh H, Storb U. Pip, a novel IRF family member, is a lymphoid-specific, PU.1-dependent transcriptional activator. *Genes Dev* 1995;9:1377–1387.
146. Mittrucker HW, Matsuyama T, Grossman A, et al. Requirement for the transcription factor LSIRF/IRF4 for mature B and T lymphocyte function. *Science* 1997;275:540–543.
147. Yamagata T, Nishida J, Tanaka S, et al. A novel interferon regulatory factor family transcription factor, ICSAT/Pip/LSIRF, that negatively regulates the activity of interferon-regulated genes. *Mol Cell Biol* 1996;16:1283–1294.
148. Brass AL, Kehrli E, Eisenbeis CF, et al. Pip, a lymphoid-restricted IRF, contains a regulatory domain that is important for autoinhibition and ternary complex formation with the Ets factor PU.1. *Genes Dev* 1996;10:2335–2347.
149. Yee AA, Yin P, Siderovski DP, et al. Cooperative interaction between the DNA-binding domains of PU.1 and IRF4. *J Mol Biol* 1998;279: 1075–1083.
150. Perkel JM, Atchison ML. A two-step mechanism for recruitment of Pip by PU.1. *J Immunol* 1998;160:241–252.
151. Glimcher LH, Singh H. Transcription factors in lymphocyte development—T and B cells get together. *Cell* 1999;96:13–23.
152. Falini B, Fizzotti M, Pucciarini A, et al. A monoclonal antibody (MUM1p) detects expression of the MUM1/IRF4 protein in a subset of germinal center B cells, plasma cells, and activated T cells. *Blood* 2000;95:2084–2092.
153. Lo CF, Gaidano G, Louie DC, et al. P53 mutations are associated with histologic transformation of follicular lymphoma. *Blood* 1993; 82:2289–2295.
154. Sander CA, Yano T, Clark HM, et al. P53 mutation is associated with progression in follicular lymphomas. *Blood* 1993;82:1994–2004.
155. Polyak K, Lee MH, Erdjument-Bromage H, et al. Cloning of p27Kip1, a cyclin-dependent kinase inhibitor and a potential mediator of extracellular antimitogenic signals. *Cell* 1994;78:59–66.
156. Reynisdottir I, Polyak K, Iavarone A, et al. Kip/Cip and Ink4 Cdk inhibitors cooperate to induce cell cycle arrest in response to TGF-beta. *Genes Dev* 1995;9:1831–1845.
157. Sanchez-Beato M, Saez AI, Martinez-Montero JC, et al. Cyclin-dependent kinase inhibitor p27KIP1 in lymphoid tissue: p27KIP1 expression is inversely proportional to the proliferative index. *Am J Pathol* 1997;151:151–160.
158. Quintanilla-Martinez L, Thieblemont C, Fend F, et al. Mantle cell lymphomas lack expression of p27Kip1, a cyclin-dependent kinase inhibitor. *Am J Pathol* 1998;153:175–182.
159. Saez A, Sanchez E, Sanchez-Beato M, et al. P27KIP1 is abnormally expressed in diffuse large B-cell lymphomas and is associated with an adverse clinical outcome. *Br J Cancer* 1999;80:1427–1434.
160. Sanchez-Beato M, Camacho FI, Martinez-Montero JC, et al. Anomalous high p27/KIP1 expression in a subset of aggressive B-cell lymphomas is associated with cyclin D3 overexpression. p27/KIP1-cyclin D3 colocalization in tumor cells. *Blood* 1999;94:765–772.
161. Kuppers R, Rajewsky K, Hansmann ML. Diffuse large cell lymphomas are derived from mature B cells carrying V region genes with a high load of somatic mutation and evidence of selection for antibody expression. *Eur J Immunol* 1997;27:1398–1405.
162. Schlegelberger B, Zwingers T, Harder L, et al. Clinicopathogenetic significance of chromosomal abnormalities in patients with blastic peripheral B-cell lymphoma. Kiel-Wien-Lymphoma Study Group. *Blood* 1999;94:3114–3120.
163. Nowotny H, Karlic H, Gruner H, et al. Cytogenetic findings in 175 patients indicate that items of the Kiel classification should not be disregarded in the REAL classification of lymphoid neoplasms. *Ann Hematol* 1996;72:291–301.
164. Hummel M, Anagnostopoulos I, Korbjuhn P, Stein H. Epstein-Barr virus in B-cell non-Hodgkin's lymphomas: unexpected infection patterns and different infection incidence in low- and high-grade types. *J Pathol* 1995;175:263–271.
165. Lennert K, Feller A. *Histopathology of non-Hodgkin's lymphomas (based on the updated Kiel classification)*, 2nd ed. New York: Springer-Verlag, 1990.
166. Engelhard M, Brittinger G, Huhn D, et al. Subclassification of diffuse large B-cell lymphomas according to the Kiel classification: distinction of centroblastic and immunoblastic lymphomas is a significant prognostic risk factor. *Blood* 1997;89:2291–2297.
167. Schouten HC, Sanger WG, Weisenburger DD, et al. Chromosomal abnormalities in untreated patients with non-Hodgkin's lymphoma: associations with histology, clinical characteristics, and treatment outcome. The Nebraska Lymphoma Study Group. *Blood* 1990;75: 1841–1847.
168. Noorduyn LA, de Bruin PC, Van Heerde P, et al. Relation of CD30 expression to survival and morphology in large cell B cell lymphomas. *J Clin Pathol* 1994;47:33–37.
169. Chan JK, Ng CS, Hui PK, et al. Anaplastic large cell Ki-1 lymphoma.

Delineation of two morphological types [see comments]. *Histopathology* 1989;15:11–34.
170. Kuze T, Nakamura N, Hashimoto Y, et al. Clinicopathological, immunological and genetic studies of CD30$^+$ anaplastic large cell lymphoma of B-cell type; association with Epstein-Barr virus in a Japanese population. *J Pathol* 1996;180:236–242.
171. Herbst H, Tippelmann G, Anagnostopoulos I, et al. Immunoglobulin and T-cell receptor gene rearrangements in Hodgkin's disease and Ki-1–positive anaplastic large cell lymphoma: dissociation between phenotype and genotype. *Leuk Res* 1989;13:103–116.
172. Kuze T, Nakamura N, Hashimoto Y, et al. Most of CD30$^+$ anaplastic large cell lymphoma of B cell type show a somatic mutation in the IgH V region genes. *Leukemia* 1998;12:753–757.
173. Kuze T, Nakamura N, Hashimoto Y, et al. Most of CD30$^+$ anaplastic large cell lymphoma of B cell type show a somatic mutation in the IgH V region genes. *Leukemia* 1998;12:753–757.
174. Anagnostopoulos I, Herbst H, Niedobitek G, et al. Demonstration of monoclonal EBV genomes in Hodgkin's disease and Ki-1–positive anaplastic large cell lymphoma by combined Southern blot and in situ hybridization [see comments]. *Blood* 1989;74:810–816.
175. Herbst H, Dallenbach F, Hummel M, et al. Epstein-Barr virus DNA and latent gene products in Ki-1 (CD30)-positive anaplastic large cell lymphomas. *Blood* 1991;78:2666–2673.
176. Jaffe ES, Longo DL, Cossman J, et al. Diffuse B-cell lymphomas with T-cell predominance in patients with follicular lymphoma or "pseudo T-cell lymphoma." *Lab Invest* 1984;50:27A-28A(abst).
177. Mirchandani I, Palutke M, Tabaczka P, et al. B-cell lymphomas morphologically resembling T-cell lymphomas [published erratum appears in *Cancer* 1986;57:1004]. *Cancer* 1985;56:1578–1583.
178. Mirchandani I, Palutke M, Tabaczka P, et al. B-cell lymphomas morphologically resembling T-cell lymphomas [published erratum appears in *Cancer* 1986;57:1004]. *Cancer* 1985;56:1578–1583.
179. Ramsay AD, Smith WJ, Isaacson PG. T-cell–rich B-cell lymphoma. *Am J Surg Pathol* 1988;12:433–443.
180. Ng CS, Chan JK, Hui PK, et al. Large B-cell lymphomas with a high content of reactive T cells. *Hum Pathol* 1989;20:1145–1154.
181. Scarpa A, Bonetti F, Zamboni G, et al. T-cell–rich B-cell lymphoma. *Am J Surg Pathol* 1989;13:335–337.
182. Osborne BM, Butler JJ, Pugh WC. The value of immunophenotyping on paraffin sections in the identification of T-cell rich B-cell large-cell lymphomas: lineage confirmed by J_H rearrangement [see comments]. *Am J Surg Pathol* 1990;14:933–938.
183. Baddoura FK, Chan WC, Masih AS, et al. T-cell–rich B-cell lymphoma: a clinicopathologic study of eight cases [see comments]. *Am J Clin Pathol* 1995;103:65–75.
184. Chittal SM, Brousset P, Voigt JJ, et al. Large B-cell lymphoma rich in T-cells and simulating Hodgkin's disease. *Histopathology* 1991; 19:211–220.
185. Krishnan J, Wallberg K, Frizzera G. T-cell–rich large B-cell lymphoma: a study of 30 cases, supporting its histologic heterogeneity and lack of clinical distinctiveness [see comments]. *Am J Surg Pathol* 1994;18:455–465.
186. Macon WR, Williams ME, Greer JP, et al. T-cell–rich B-cell lymphomas. A clinicopathologic study of 19 cases [see comments]. *Am J Surg Pathol* 1992;16:351–363.
187. De Jong D, Van Gorp J, Sie-Go D, et al. T-cell rich b-cell non-hodgkin's lymphoma: a progressed form of follicle centre cell lymphoma and lymphocyte predominance Hodgkin's disease [see comments]. *Histopathology* 1996;28:15–24.
188. Delabie J, Vandenberghe E, Kennes C, et al. Histiocyte-rich B-cell lymphoma. A distinct clinicopathologic entity possibly related to lymphocyte predominant Hodgkin's disease, paragranuloma subtype. *Am J Surg Pathol* 1992;16:37–48.
189. Schmidt U, Leder LD. T-cell–rich B-cell lymphoma—a distinct clinicopathologic entity? *Leuk Lymphoma* 1996;23:17–24.
190. Skinnider BF, Connors JM, Gascoyne RD. Bone marrow involvement in T-cell–rich B-cell lymphoma [see comments]. *Am J Clin Pathol* 1997;108:570–578.
191. Rudiger T, Ott G, Ott MM, et al. Differential diagnosis between classic Hodgkin's lymphoma, T-cell–rich B-cell lymphoma, and paragranuloma by paraffin immunohistochemistry. *Am J Surg Pathol* 1998;22: 1184–1191.
192. Brauninger A, Kuppers R, Spieker T, et al. Molecular analysis of single B cells from T-cell–rich B-cell lymphoma shows the derivation of the tumor cells from mutating germinal center B cells and exemplifies means by which immunoglobulin genes are modified in germinal center B cells. *Blood* 1999;93:2679–2687.
193. McBride JA, Rodriguez J, Luthra R, et al. T-cell–rich B large-cell lymphoma simulating lymphocyte-rich Hodgkin's disease [see comments]. *Am J Surg Pathol* 1996;20:193–201.
194. Rodriguez J, Pugh WC, Cabanillas F. T-cell–rich B-cell lymphoma. *Blood* 1993;82:1586–1589.
195. Khan SM, Cottrell BJ, Millward-Sadler GH, et al. T-cell–rich B-cell lymphoma presenting as liver disease. *Histopathology* 1993;23: 217–224.
196. Greer JP, Macon WR, Lamar RE, et al. T-cell–rich B-cell lymphomas: diagnosis and response to therapy of 44 patients. *J Clin Oncol* 1995; 13:1742–1750.
197. Liebow AA, Carrington CR, Friedman PJ. Lymphomatoid granulomatosis. *Hum Pathol* 1972;3:457–558.
198. Katzenstein AL, Carrington CB, Liebow AA. Lymphomatoid granulomatosis: a clinicopathologic study of 152 cases. *Cancer* 1979;43: 360–373.
199. Colby TV, Carrington CB. Pulmonary lymphomas simulating lymphomatoid granulomatosis. *Am J Surg Pathol* 1982;6:19–32.
200. Pisani RJ, DeRemee RA. Clinical implications of the histopathologic diagnosis of pulmonary lymphomatoid granulomatosis [see comments]. *Mayo Clin Proc* 1990;65:151–163.
201. Lipford EH Jr, Margolick JB, Longo DL, et al. Angiocentric immunoproliferative lesions: a clinicopathologic spectrum of post-thymic T-cell proliferations. *Blood* 1988;72:1674–1681.
202. Medeiros LJ, Peiper SC, Elwood L, et al. Angiocentric immunoproliferative lesions: a molecular analysis of eight cases. *Hum Pathol* 1991; 22:1150–1157.
203. Katzenstein AL, Peiper SC. Detection of Epstein-Barr virus genomes in lymphomatoid granulomatosis: analysis of 29 cases by the polymerase chain reaction technique. *Mod Pathol* 1990;3:435–441.
204. Guinee D Jr, Jaffe E, Kingma D, et al. Pulmonary lymphomatoid granulomatosis: Evidence for a proliferation of Epstein-Barr virus infected B-lymphocytes with a prominent T-cell component and vasculitis. *Am J Surg Pathol* 1994;18:753–764.
205. Wilson WH, Kingma DW, Raffeld M, et al. Association of lymphomatoid granulomatosis with Epstein-Barr viral infection of B lymphocytes and response to interferon-alpha 2b. *Blood* 1996;87:4531–4537.
206. Nicholson AG, Wotherspoon AC, Diss TC, et al. Lymphomatoid granulomatosis: evidence that some cases represent Epstein-Barr virus–associated B-cell lymphoma. *Histopathology* 1996;29:317–324.
207. Guinee DG Jr, Perkins SL, Travis WD, et al. Proliferation and cellular phenotype in lymphomatoid granulomatosis: implications of a higher proliferation index in B cells [see comments]. *Am J Surg Pathol* 1998; 22:1093–1100.
208. Delecluse HJ, Anagnostopoulos I, Dallenbach F, et al. Plasmablastic lymphomas of the oral cavity: a new entity associated with the human immunodeficiency virus infection. *Blood* 1997;89:1413–1420.
209. Carbone A, Gloghini A, Canzonieri V, et al. AIDS-related extranodal non-Hodgkin's lymphomas with plasma cell differentiation [Letter]. *Blood* 1997;90:1337–1338.
210. Delecluse HJ, Anagnostopoulos I, Dallenbach F, et al. Plasmablastic lymphomas of the oral cavity: a new entity associated with the human immunodeficiency virus infection. *Blood* 1997;89:1413–1420.
211. Carbone A, Gaidano G, Gloghini A, et al. AIDS-related plasmablastic lymphomas of the oral cavity and jaws: a diagnostic dilemma. *Ann Otol Rhinol Laryngol* 1999;108:95–99.
212. A clinical evaluation of the International Lymphoma Study Group classification of non-Hodgkin's lymphoma. The Non-Hodgkin's Lymphoma Classification Project. *Blood* 1997;89:3909–3918.
213. Lones MA, Auperin A, Raphael M, et al. Mature B-cell lymphoma/leukemia in children and adolescents: intergroup pathologist consensus with the revised European-American Lymphoma Classification. *Ann Oncol* 2000;11:47–51.
214. Miliauskas JR, Berard CW, Young RC, et al. Undifferentiated non-Hodgkin's lymphomas (Burkitt's and non-Burkitt's types): the relevance of making this histologic distinction. *Cancer* 1982;50: 2115–2121.
215. Payne CM, Grogan TM, Cromey DW, et al. An ultrastructural morphometric and immunophenotypic evaluation of Burkitt's and Burkitt's-like lymphomas. *Lab Invest* 1987;57:200–218.
216. Pavlova Z, Parker JW, Taylor CR, et al. Small noncleaved follicular

center cell lymphoma: Burkitt's and non-Burkitt's variants in the US. II. Pathologic and immunologic features. *Cancer* 1987;59: 1892–1902.
217. Kelly DR, Nathwani BN, Griffith RC, et al. A morphologic study of childhood lymphoma of the undifferentiated type. The Pediatric Oncology Group experience. *Cancer* 1987;59:1132–1137.
218. Hutchison RE, Murphy SB, Fairclough DL, et al. Diffuse small noncleaved cell lymphoma in children, Burkitt's versus non-Burkitt's types. Results from the Pediatric Oncology Group and St. Jude Children's Research Hospital. *Cancer* 1989;64:23–28.
219. Yano T, Van Krieken JH, Magrath IT, et al. Histogenetic correlations between subcategories of small noncleaved cell lymphomas. *Blood* 1992;79:1282–1290.
220. Davi F, Delecluse HJ, Guiet P, et al. Burkitt-like lymphomas in AIDS patients: characterization within a series of 103 human immunodeficiency virus-associated non-Hodgkin's lymphomas. Burkitt's Lymphoma Study Group. *J Clin Oncol* 1998;16:3788–3795.
221. Gaidano G, Pastore C, Gloghini A, et al. Genetic heterogeneity of AIDS-related small non-cleaved cell lymphoma. *Br J Haematol* 1997; 98:726–732.
222. Macpherson N, Lesack D, Klasa R, et al. Small noncleaved, non-Burkitt's (Burkitt-like) lymphoma: cytogenetics predict outcome and reflect clinical presentation. *J Clin Oncol* 1999;17:1558–1567.
223. Harris NL, Jaffe ES, Diebold J, et al. The World Health Organization classification of neoplastic diseases of the haematopoietic and lymphoid tissues: report of the Clinical Advisory Committee Meeting, Airlie House, Virginia, November 1997. *Histopathology* 2000;36: 69–86.
224. Miller JB, Variakojis D, Bitran JDU, et al. Diffuse histiocytic lymphoma with sclerosis: a clinicopathologic entity frequently causing superior venacaval obstruction. *Cancer* 1981;47:748–756.
225. Trump DL, Mann RB. Diffuse large cell and undifferentiated lymphomas with prominent mediastinal involvement. *Cancer* 1982;50: 277–282.
226. Waldron JA, Farber LL, Cadman E. Primary large cell lymphomas of the mediastinum: an analysis of 18 cases. *Lab Invest* 1984;50: 60A(abst).
227. Menestrina F, Chilosi M, Bonetti F, et al. Mediastinal large-cell lymphoma of B-type, with sclerosis: histopathological and immunohistochemical study of eight cases. *Histopathology* 1986;10:589–600.
228. Moller P, Lammler B, Eberlein-Gonska M, et al. Primary mediastinal clear cell lymphoma of B-cell type. *Virchows Arch A Pathol Anat Histopathol* 1986;409:79–92.
229. Scarpa A, Bonetti F, Menestrina F, et al. Mediastinal large-cell lymphoma with sclerosis: genotypic analysis establishes its B nature. *Virchows Arch A Pathol Anat Histopathol* 1987;412:17–21.
230. Addis BJ, Isaacson PG. Large cell lymphoma of the mediastinum: a B-cell tumour of probable thymic origin. *Histopathology* 1986;10: 379–390.
231. Kirn D, Mauch P, Shaffer K, et al. Large-cell and immunoblastic lymphoma of the mediastinum: prognostic features and treatment outcome in 57 patients. *J Clin Oncol* 1993;11:1336–1343.
232. Falini B, Venturi S, Martelli M, et al. Mediastinal large B-cell lymphoma: clinical and immunohistological findings in 18 patients treated with different third-generation regimens. *Br J Haematol* 1995;89: 780–789.
233. Popat U, Przepiork D, Champlin R, et al. High-dose chemotherapy for relapsed and refractory diffuse large B-cell lymphoma: mediastinal localization predicts for a favorable outcome. *J Clin Oncol* 1998;16: 63–69.
234. Sehn LH, Antin JH, Shulman LN, et al. Primary diffuse large B-cell lymphoma of the mediastinum: outcome following high-dose chemotherapy and autologous hematopoietic cell transplantation. *Blood* 1998;91:717–723.
235. Abou-Elella AA, Weisenburger DD, Vose JM, et al. Primary mediastinal large B-cell lymphoma: a clinicopathologic study of 43 patients from the Nebraska Lymphoma Study Group. *J Clin Oncol* 1999;17: 784–790.
236. Rodriguez J, Pugh WC, Romaguera JE, et al. Primary mediastinal large cell lymphoma. *Hematol Oncol* 1994;12:175–184.
237. Davis RE, Dorfman RF, Warnke RA. Primary large-cell lymphoma of the thymus: a diffuse B-cell neoplasm presenting as primary mediastinal lymphoma. *Hum Pathol* 1990;21:1262–1268.
238. Lazzarino M, Orlandi E, Paulli M, et al. Treatment outcome and prognostic factors for primary mediastinal (thymic) B-cell lymphoma: a multicenter study of 106 patients. *J Clin Oncol* 1997;15:1646–1653.
239. Lennert K, Mohri N, Stein H, et al. Malignant lymphomas other than Hodgkin's disease: histology, cytology, ultrastructure, immunology. Berlin: Springer, 1978.
240. Stansfeld AG, Diebold J, Noel H, et al. Updated Kiel classification for lymphomas [Letter] [published erratum appears in *Lancet* 1988; 1:372]. *Lancet* 1988;1:292–293.
241. Addis BJ, Isaacson PG. Large cell lymphoma of the mediastinum: a B-cell tumour of probable thymic origin. *Histopathology* 1986;10: 379–390.
242. Moller P, Lammler B, Eberlein-Gonska M, et al. Primary mediastinal clear cell lymphoma of B-cell type. *Virchows Arch A Pathol Anat Histopathol* 1986;409:79–92.
243. Perrone T, Frizzera G, Rosai J. Mediastinal diffuse large-cell lymphoma with sclerosis: a clinicopathologic study of 60 cases. *Am J Surg Pathol* 1986;10:176–191.
244. Abou-Elella AA, Weisenburger DD, Vose JM, et al. Primary mediastinal large B-cell lymphoma: a clinicopathologic study of 43 patients from the Nebraska Lymphoma Study Group. *J Clin Oncol* 1999;17: 784–790.
245. Lazzarino M, Orlandi E, Paulli M, et al. Primary mediastinal B-cell lymphoma with sclerosis: an aggressive tumor with distinctive clinical and pathologic features [see comments]. *J Clin Oncol* 1993;11: 2306–2313.
246. Yousem SA, Weiss LM, Warnke RA. Primary mediastinal non-Hodgkin's lymphomas: a morphologic and immunologic study of 19 cases. *Am J Clin Pathol* 1985;83:676–680.
247. al Sharabati M, Chittal S, Duga-Neulat I, et al. Primary anterior mediastinal B-cell lymphoma: a clinicopathologic and immunohistochemical study of 16 cases. *Cancer* 1991;67:2579–2587.
248. Lavabre-Bertrand T, Donadio D, Fegueux N, et al. A study of 15 cases of primary mediastinal lymphoma of B-cell type. *Cancer* 1992; 69:2561–2566.
249. Rohatiner AZ, Whelan JS, Ganjoo RK, et al. Mediastinal large-cell lymphoma with sclerosis (MLCLS). *Br J Cancer* 1994;69:601–604.
250. Chim CS, Liang R, Chan AC, et al. Primary B cell lymphoma of the mediastinum. *Hematol Oncol* 1996;14:173–179.
251. Menestrina F, Chilosi M, Bonetti F, et al. Mediastinal large-cell lymphoma of B-type, with sclerosis: histopathological and immunohistochemical study of eight cases. *Histopathology* 1986;10:589–600.
252. Jacobson JO, Aisenberg AC, Lamarre L, et al. Mediastinal large cell lymphoma: an uncommon subset of adult lymphoma curable with combined modality therapy. *Cancer* 1988;62:1893–1898.
253. Lamarre L, Jacobson JO, Aisenberg AC, et al. Primary large cell lymphoma of the mediastinum. A histologic and immunophenotypic study of 29 cases. *Am J Surg Pathol* 1989;13:730–739.
254. Cazals-Hatem D, Lepage E, Brice P, et al. Primary mediastinal large B-cell lymphoma: a clinicopathologic study of 141 cases compared with 916 nonmediastinal large B-cell lymphomas, a GELA ("Groupe d'Etude des Lymphomes de l'Adulte") study. *Am J Surg Pathol* 1996; 20:877–888.
255. Todeschini G, Ambrosetti A, Meneghini V, et al. Mediastinal large B-cell lymphoma with sclerosis: a clinical study of 21 patients. *J Clin Oncol* 1990;8:804–808.
256. Zinzani PL, Bendandi M, Frezza G, et al. Primary Mediastinal B-cell lymphoma with sclerosis: clinical and therapeutic evaluation of 22 patients. *Leuk Lymphoma* 1996;21:311–316.
257. Falini B, Venturi S, Martelli M, et al. Mediastinal large B-cell lymphoma: clinical and immunohistological findings in 18 patients treated with different third-generation regimens. *Br J Haematol* 1995;89: 780–789.
258. al Sharabati M, Chittal S, Duga-Neulat I, et al. Primary anterior mediastinal B-cell lymphoma: a clinicopathologic and immunohistochemical study of 16 cases. *Cancer* 1991;67:2579–2587.
259. Joos S, Otano-Joos MI, Ziegler S, et al. Primary mediastinal (thymic) B-cell lymphoma is characterized by gains of chromosomal material including 9p and amplification of the REL gene. *Blood* 1996;87: 1571–1578.
260. Kirn D, Mauch P, Shaffer K, et al. Large-cell and immunoblastic lymphoma of the mediastinum: prognostic features and treatment outcome in 57 patients. *J Clin Oncol* 1993;11:1336–1343.
261. Lazzarino M, Orlandi E, Paulli M, et al. Treatment outcome and prog-

nostic factors for primary mediastinal (thymic) B-cell lymphoma: a multicenter study of 106 patients. *J Clin Oncol* 1997;15:1646–1653.
262. Paulli M, Strater J, Gianelli U, et al. Mediastinal B-cell lymphoma: a study of its histomorphologic spectrum based on 109 cases. *Hum Pathol* 1999;30:178–187.
263. Perrone T, Frizzera G, Rosai J. Mediastinal diffuse large-cell lymphoma with sclerosis: a clinicopathologic study of 60 cases. *Am J Surg Pathol* 1986;10:176–191.
264. Moller P, Moldenhauer G, Momburg F, et al. Mediastinal lymphoma of clear cell type is a tumor corresponding to terminal steps of B cell differentiation. *Blood* 1987;69:1087–1095.
265. Kanavaros P, Gaulard P, Charlotte F, et al. Discordant expression of immunoglobulin and its associated molecule mb-1/CD79a is frequently found in mediastinal large B cell lymphomas. *Am J Pathol* 1995;146:735–741.
266. Higgins JP, Warnke RA. CD30 expression is common in mediastinal large B-cell lymphoma [see comments]. *Am J Clin Pathol* 1999;112: 241–247.
267. Cazals-Hatem D, Lepage E, Brice P, et al. Primary mediastinal large B-cell lymphoma: a clinicopathologic study of 141 cases compared with 916 nonmediastinal large B-cell lymphomas, a GELA (''Groupe d'Etude des Lymphomes de l'Adulte'') study. *Am J Surg Pathol* 1996; 20:877–888.
268. Momburg F, Herrmann B, Moldenhauer G, et al. B-cell lymphomas of high-grade malignancy frequently lack HLA-DR, -DP and -DQ antigens and associated invariant chain. *Int J Cancer* 1987;40: 598–603.
269. Moller P, Herrmann B, Moldenhauer G, et al. Defective expression of MHC class I antigens is frequent in B-cell lymphomas of high-grade malignancy. *Int J Cancer* 1987;40:32–39.
270. Rodriguez J, Pugh WC, Romaguera JE, et al. Primary mediastinal large cell lymphoma is characterized by an inverted pattern of large tumoral mass and low beta 2 microglobulin levels in serum and frequently elevated levels of serum lactate dehydrogenase. *Ann Oncol* 1994;5:847–849.
271. Lazzarino M, Orlandi E, Astori C, et al. A low serum beta 2-microglobulin level despite bulky tumor is a characteristic feature of primary mediastinal (thymic) large B-cell lymphoma: implications for serologic staging [Letter]. *Eur J Haematol* 1996;57:331–333.
272. Moller P, Matthaei-Maurer DU, Hofmann WJ, et al. Immunophenotypic similarities of mediastinal clear-cell lymphoma and sinusoidal (monocytoid) B cells. *Int J Cancer* 1989;43:10–16.
273. Eichelmann A, Koretz K, Mechtersheimer G, et al. Adhesion receptor profile of thymic B-cell lymphoma. *Am J Pathol* 1992;141:729–741.
274. Alonso MA, Barton DE, Francke U. Assignment of the T-cell differentiation gene MAL to human chromosome 2, region cen-q13. *Immunogenetics* 1988;27:91–95.
275. Alonso MA, Weissman SM. cDNA cloning and sequence of MAL, a hydrophobic protein associated with human T-cell differentiation. *Proc Natl Acad Sci USA* 1987;84:1997–2001.
276. Rancano C, Rubio T, Correas I, et al. Genomic structure and subcellular localization of MAL, a human T-cell–specific proteolipid protein. *J Biol Chem* 1994;269:8159–8164.
277. Copie-Bergman C, Gaulard P, Maouche-Chretien L, et al. The MAL gene is expressed in primary mediastinal large B-cell lymphoma. *Blood* 1999;94:3567–3575.
278. Tsang P, Cesarman E, Chadburn A, et al. Molecular characterization of primary mediastinal B cell lymphoma. *Am J Pathol* 1996;148: 2017–2025.
279. Scarpa A, Borgato L, Chilosi M, et al. Evidence of c-myc gene abnormalities in mediastinal large B-cell lymphoma of young adult age [see comments]. *Blood* 1991;78:780–788.
280. Portier M, Moles JP, Mazars GR, et al. *P53* and *RAS* gene mutations in multiple myeloma. *Oncogene* 1992;7:2539–2543.
281. Copie-Bergman C, Gaulard P, Maouche-Chretien L, et al. The MAL gene is expressed in primary mediastinal large B-cell lymphoma. *Blood* 1999;94:3567–3575.
282. Joos S, Otano-Joos MI, Ziegler S, et al. Primary mediastinal (thymic) B-cell lymphoma is characterized by gains of chromosomal material including 9p and amplification of the REL gene. *Blood* 1996;87: 1571–1578.
283. Offit K, Richardson ME, Ceng QQ, et al. Nonrandom chromosomal aberrations are associated with sites of tissue involvement in non-Hodgkin's lymphoma. *Cancer Genet Cytogenet* 1989;37:85–93.
284. Lu D, Thompson JD, Gorski GK, et al. Alterations at the rel locus in human lymphoma. *Oncogene* 1991;6:1235–1241.
285. von Wasielewski R, Mengel M, Fischer R, et al. Classical Hodgkin's disease: clinical impact of the immunophenotype. *Am J Pathol* 1997; 151:1123–1130.
286. Schmid C, Pan L, Diss T, et al. Expression of B-cell antigens by Hodgkin's and Reed-Sternberg cells. *Am J Pathol* 1991;139:701–707.
287. Korkolopoulou P, Cordell J, Jones M, et al. The expression of the B-cell marker mb-1 (CD79a) in Hodgkin's disease. *Histopathology* 1994;24:511–515.
288. Schwarting R, Gerdes J, Durkop H, et al. BER-H2: a new anti-Ki-1 (CD30) monoclonal antibody directed at a formol-resistant epitope. *Blood* 1989;74:1678–1689.
289. Pfleger L, Tappeiner J. Zur Kenntnis der systemisierten Endotheliomatose der kutanen Blutgefässe (Reticuloendotheliose). *Hautarzt* 1959;10:359–363.
290. Wick MR, Banks PM, McDonald TJ. Angioendotheliomatosis of the nose with fatal systemic dissemination. *Cancer* 1981;48:2510–2517.
291. Fulling KH, Gersell DJ. Neoplastic angioendotheliomatosis. Histologic, immunohistochemical, and ultrastructural findings in two cases. *Cancer* 1983;51:1107–1118.
292. Kitagawa M, Matsubara O, Song SY, et al. Neoplastic angioendotheliosis. Immunohistochemical and electron microscopic findings in three cases. *Cancer* 1985;56:1134–1143.
293. Ansell J, Bhawan J, Cohen S, et al. Histiocytic lymphoma and malignant angioendotheliomatosis: one disease or two? *Cancer* 1982;50: 1506–1512.
294. Bhawan J, Wolff SM, Ucci AA, et al. Malignant lymphoma and malignant angioendotheliomatosis: one disease. *Cancer* 1985;55:570–576.
295. Wrotnowski U, Mills SE, Cooper PH. Malignant angioendotheliomatosis: an angiotropic lymphoma? *Am J Clin Pathol* 1985;83: 244–248.
296. Sheibani K, Battifora H, Winberg CD, et al. Further evidence that ''malignant angioendotheliomatosis'' is an angiotropic large-cell lymphoma. *N Engl J Med* 1986;314:943–948.
297. Wick MR, Mills SE, Scheithauer BW, et al. Reassessment of malignant ''angioendotheliomatosis.'' Evidence in favor of its reclassification as ''intravascular lymphomatosis.'' *Am J Surg Pathol* 1986;10: 112–123.
298. Carroll TJ Jr, Schelper RL, Goeken JA, et al. Neoplastic angioendotheliomatosis: immunopathologic and morphologic evidence for intravascular malignant lymphomatosis. *Am J Clin Pathol* 1986;85: 169–175.
299. Otrakji CL, Voigt W, Amador A, et al. Malignant angioendotheliomatosis—a true lymphoma: a case of intravascular malignant lymphomatosis studied by Southern blot hybridization analysis. *Hum Pathol* 1988;19:475–478.
300. Domizio P, Hall PA, Cotter F, et al. Angiotropic large cell lymphoma (ALCL): morphological, immunohistochemical and genotypic studies with analysis of previous reports. *Hematol Oncol* 1989;7:195–206.
301. Petroff N, Koger OW, Fleming MG, et al. Malignant angioendotheliomatosis: an angiotropic lymphoma. *J Am Acad Dermatol* 1989;21: 727–733.
302. Sepp N, Schuler G, Romani N, et al. ''Intravascular lymphomatosis'' (angioendotheliomatosis): evidence for a T-cell origin in two cases. *Hum Pathol* 1990;21:1051–1058.
303. Tateyama H, Eimoto T, Tada T, et al. Congenital angiotropic lymphoma (intravascular lymphomatosis) of the T-cell type. *Cancer* 1991; 67:2131–2136.
304. Axelsen RA, Laird PP, Horn M. Intravascular large cell lymphoma: diagnosis on renal biopsy. *Pathology* 1991;23:241–243.
305. Banerjee SS, Harris M. Angiotropic lymphoma presenting in the prostate. *Histopathology* 1988;12:667–670.
306. D'Agati V, Sablay LB, Knowles DM, et al. Angiotropic large cell lymphoma (intravascular malignant lymphomatosis) of the kidney: presentation as minimal change disease. *Hum Pathol* 1989;20: 263–268.
307. DiGiuseppe JA, Nelson WG, Seifter EJ, et al. Intravascular lymphomatosis: a clinicopathologic study of 10 cases and assessment of response to chemotherapy. *J Clin Oncol* 1994;12:2573–2579.
308. Estalilla OC, Koo CH, Brynes RK, et al. Intravascular large B-cell lymphoma: a report of five cases initially diagnosed by bone marrow biopsy. *Am J Clin Pathol* 1999;112:248–255.
309. Shimokawa I, Higami Y, Sakai H, et al. Intravascular malignant lym-

phomatosis: a case of T-cell lymphoma probably associated with human T-cell lymphotropic virus. *Hum Pathol* 1991;22:200–202.
310. Snowden JA, Angel CA, Winfield DA, et al. Angiotropic lymphoma: report of a case with histiocytic features. *J Clin Pathol* 1997;50:67–70.
311. Khalidi HS, Brynes RK, Browne P, et al. Intravascular large B-cell lymphoma: the CD5 antigen is expressed by a subset of cases. *Mod Pathol* 1998;11:983–988.
312. Carter DK, Batts KP, de Groen PC, et al. Angiotropic large cell lymphoma (intravascular lymphomatosis) occurring after follicular small cleaved cell lymphoma. *Mayo Clin Proc* 1996;71:869–873.
313. Ferry JA, Harris NL, Picker LJ, et al. Intravascular lymphomatosis (malignant angioendotheliomatosis): a B-cell neoplasm expressing surface homing receptors. *Mod Pathol* 1988;1:444–452.
314. Jalkanen S, Aho R, Kallajoki M, et al. Lymphocyte homing receptors and adhesion molecules in intravascular malignant lymphomatosis. *Int J Cancer* 1989;44:777–782.
315. Nador RG, Cesarman E, Chadburn A, et al. Primary effusion lymphoma: a distinct clinicopathologic entity associated with the Kaposi's sarcoma-associated herpesvirus. *Blood* 1996;88:645–656.
316. Ansari MQ, Dawson DB, Nador R, et al. Primary body cavity-based AIDS-related lymphomas [see comments]. *Am J Clin Pathol* 1996; 105:221–229.
317. Gaidano G, Gloghini A, Gattei V, et al. Association of Kaposi's sarcoma-associated herpesvirus-positive primary effusion lymphoma with expression of the CD138/syndecan-1 antigen. *Blood* 1997;90: 4894–4900.
318. Gaidano G, Carbone A, Dalla-Favera R. Pathogenesis of AIDS-related lymphomas: molecular and histogenetic heterogeneity. *Am J Pathol* 1998;152:623–630.
319. Matolcsy A, Nador RG, Cesarman E, et al. Immunoglobulin V_H gene mutational analysis suggests that primary effusion lymphomas derive from different stages of B cell maturation [see comments]. *Am J Pathol* 1998;153:1609–1614.
320. Fais F, Gaidano G, Capello D, et al. Immunoglobulin V region gene use and structure suggest antigen selection in AIDS-related primary effusion lymphomas. *Leukemia* 1999;13:1093–1099.
321. Gaidano G, Capello D, Cilia AM, et al. Genetic characterization of HHV-8/KSHV-positive primary effusion lymphoma reveals frequent mutations of BCL6: implications for disease pathogenesis and histogenesis. *Genes Chromosomes Cancer* 1999;24:16–23.
322. Cesarman E, Nador RG, Aozasa K, et al. Kaposi's sarcoma-associated herpesvirus in non-AIDS related lymphomas occurring in body cavities. *Am J Pathol* 1996;149:53–57.
323. Cesarman E, Chang Y, Moore PS, et al. Kaposi's sarcoma-associated herpesvirus-like DNA sequences in AIDS-related body-cavity-based lymphomas [see comments]. *N Engl J Med* 1995;332:1186–1191.
324. Cesarman E, Knowles DM. Kaposi's sarcoma-associated herpesvirus: a lymphotropic human herpesvirus associated with Kaposi's sarcoma, primary effusion lymphoma, and multicentric Castleman's disease [published erratum appears in *Semin Diagn Pathol* 1997;14:161–2]. *Semin Diagn Pathol* 1997;14:54–66.
325. Russo JJ, Bohenzky RA, Chien MC, et al. Nucleotide sequence of the Kaposi sarcoma-associated herpesvirus (HHV8). *Proc Natl Acad Sci USA* 1996;93:14862–14867.
326. Chang Y, Moore PS, Talbot SJ, et al. Cyclin encoded by KS herpesvirus [Letter]. *Nature* 1996;382:410.
327. Moore PS, Boshoff C, Weiss RA, et al. Molecular mimicry of human cytokine and cytokine response pathway genes by KSHV. *Science* 1996;274:1739–1744.
328. Renne R, Zhong W, Herndier B, et al. Lytic growth of Kaposi's sarcoma-associated herpesvirus (human herpesvirus 8) in culture. *Nat Med* 1996;2:342–346.
329. Arvanitakis L, Geras-Raaka E, Varma A, et al. Human herpesvirus KSHV encodes a constitutively active G-protein-coupled receptor linked to cell proliferation [see comments]. *Nature* 1997;385: 347–350.
330. Moore PS, Kingsley LA, Holmberg SD, et al. Kaposi's sarcoma-associated herpesvirus infection prior to onset of Kaposi's sarcoma. *AIDS* 1996;10:175–180.
331. Horenstein MG, Nador RG, Chadburn A, et al. Epstein-Barr virus latent gene expression in primary effusion lymphomas containing Kaposi's sarcoma-associated herpesvirus/human herpesvirus-8. *Blood* 1997;90:1186–1191.
332. Cote TR, Manns A, Hardy CR, et al. Epidemiology of brain lymphoma among people with or without acquired immunodeficiency syndrome. AIDS/Cancer Study Group. *J Natl Cancer Inst* 1996;88:675–679.
333. Camilleri-Broet S, Davi F, Feuillard J, et al. AIDS-related primary brain lymphomas: histopathologic and immunohistochemical study of 51 cases. The French Study Group for HIV-Associated Tumors. *Hum Pathol* 1997;28:367–374.
334. Larocca LM, Capello D, Rinelli A, et al. The molecular and phenotypic profile of primary central nervous system lymphoma identifies distinct categories of the disease and is consistent with histogenetic derivation from germinal center-related B cells. *Blood* 1998;92: 1011–1019.
335. Julien S, Radosavljevic M, Labouret N, et al. AIDS primary central nervous system lymphoma: molecular analysis of the expressed V_H genes and possible implications for lymphomagenesis. *J Immunol* 1999;162:1551–1558.
336. Thompsett AR, Ellison DW, Stevenson FK, et al. V(H) gene sequences from primary central nervous system lymphomas indicate derivation from highly mutated germinal center B cells with ongoing mutational activity. *Blood* 1999;94:1738–1746.
337. Montesinos-Rongen M, Kuppers R, Schluter D, et al. Primary central nervous system lymphomas are derived from germinal-center B cells and show a preferential usage of the V4-34 gene segment. *Am J Pathol* 1999;155:2077–2086.
338. Ng VL, McGrath MS. The immunology of AIDS-associated lymphomas. *Immunol Rev* 1998;162:293–298.
339. Morgello S. Epstein-Barr and human immunodeficiency viruses in acquired immunodeficiency syndrome-related primary central nervous system lymphoma. *Am J Pathol* 1992;141:441–450.
340. MacMahon EM, Glass JD, Hayward SD, et al. Epstein-Barr virus in AIDS-related primary central nervous system lymphoma. *Lancet* 1991;338:969–973.
341. Hamilton-Dutoit SJ, Raphael M, Audouin J, et al. In situ demonstration of Epstein-Barr virus small RNAs (EBER-1) in acquired immunodeficiency syndrome-related lymphomas: correlation with tumor morphology and primary site. *Blood* 1993;82:619–624.
342. Bashir RM, Harris NL, Hochberg FH, et al. Detection of Epstein-Barr virus in CNS lymphomas by in-situ hybridization. *Neurology* 1989;39:813–817.
343. Camilleri-Broet S, Davi F, Feuillard J, et al. High expression of latent membrane protein 1 of Epstein-Barr virus and BCL-2 oncoprotein in acquired immunodeficiency syndrome-related primary brain lymphomas. *Blood* 1995;86:432–435.
344. Corboy JR, Garl PJ, Kleinschmidt-DeMasters BK. Human herpesvirus 8 DNA in CNS lymphomas from patients with and without AIDS [see comments]. *Neurology* 1998;50:335–340.
345. Morgello S, Tagliati M, Ewart MR. HHV-8 and AIDS-related CNS lymphoma. *Neurology* 1997;48:1333–1335.
346. Willemze R, Meijer CJ, Sentis HJ, et al. Primary cutaneous large cell lymphomas of follicular center cell origin. A clinical follow-up study of nineteen patients. *J Am Acad Dermatol* 1987;16:518–526.
347. Berti E, Alessi E, Caputo R, et al. Reticulohistiocytoma of the dorsum. *J Am Acad Dermatol* 1988;19:259–272.
348. Rijlaarsdam JU, Toonstra J, Meijer OW, et al. Treatment of primary cutaneous B-cell lymphomas of follicle center cell origin: a clinical follow-up study of 55 patients treated with radiotherapy or polychemotherapy. *J Clin Oncol* 1996;14:549–555.
349. Santucci M, Pimpinelli N, Arganini L. Primary cutaneous B-cell lymphoma: a unique type of low-grade lymphoma: clinicopathologic and immunologic study of 83 cases. *Cancer* 1991;67:2311–2326.
350. Willemze R, Kerl H, Sterry W, et al. EORTC classification for primary cutaneous lymphomas: a proposal from the Cutaneous Lymphoma Study Group of the European Organization for Research and Treatment of Cancer. *Blood* 1997;90:354–371.
351. Vermeer MH, Geelen FA, van Haselen CW, et al. Primary cutaneous large B-cell lymphomas of the legs: a distinct type of cutaneous B-cell lymphoma with an intermediate prognosis. Dutch Cutaneous Lymphoma Working Group [see comments]. *Arch Dermatol* 1996; 132:1304–1308.
352. Geelen FA, Vermeer MH, Meijer CJ, et al. Bcl-2 protein expression in primary cutaneous large B-cell lymphoma is site-related. *J Clin Oncol* 1998;16:2080–2085.
353. Du M, Peng H, Singh N, et al. The accumulation of p53 abnormalities is associated with progression of mucosa-associated lymphoid tissue lymphoma. *Blood* 1995;86:4587–4593.

354. Gaidano G, Volpe G, Pastore C, et al. Detection of BCL-6 rearrangements and p53 mutations in Malt-lymphomas. *Am J Hematol* 1997; 56:206–213.
355. Neumeister P, Hoefler G, Beham-Schmid C, et al. Deletion analysis of the p16 tumor suppressor gene in gastrointestinal mucosa-associated lymphoid tissue lymphomas. *Gastroenterology* 1997;112:1871–1875.
356. Starostik P, Greiner A, Schultz A, et al. Genetic aberrations common in gastric high-grade large B-cell lymphoma. *Blood* 2000;95: 1180–1187.
357. Chan WY, Wong N, Chan AB, et al. Consistent copy number gain in chromosome 12 in primary diffuse large cell lymphomas of the stomach. *Am J Pathol* 1998;152:11–16.
358. Ott G, Kalla J, Steinhoff A, et al. Trisomy 3 is not a common feature in malignant lymphomas of mucosa-associated lymphoid tissue type. *Am J Pathol* 1998;153:689–694.
359. Dierlamm J, Rosenberg C, Stul M, et al. Characteristic pattern of chromosomal gains and losses in marginal zone B cell lymphoma detected by comparative genomic hybridization. *Leukemia* 1997;11: 747–758.
360. Zhang Y, Cheung AN, Chan AC, et al. Detection of trisomy 3 in primary gastric B-cell lymphoma by using chromosome in situ hybridization on paraffin sections. *Am J Clin Pathol* 1998;110:347–353.
361. Barth TF, Dohner H, Werner CA, et al. Characteristic pattern of chromosomal gains and losses in primary large B-cell lymphomas of the gastrointestinal tract. *Blood* 1998;91:4321–4330.
362. Hoeve MA, Gisbertz IA, Schouten HC, et al. Gastric low-grade MALT lymphoma, high-grade MALT lymphoma and diffuse large B cell lymphoma show different frequencies of trisomy. *Leukemia* 1999;13: 799–807.
363. Peng H, Du M, Diss TC, et al. Genetic evidence for a clonal link between low and high-grade components in gastric MALT B-cell lymphoma. *Histopathology* 1997;30:425–429.
364. Chan JK, Ng CS, Isaacson PG. Relationship between high-grade lymphoma and low-grade B-cell mucosa-associated lymphoid tissue lymphoma (MALToma) of the stomach. *Am J Pathol* 1990;136: 1153–1164.
365. Isaacson PG. Mucosa-associated lymphoid tissue lymphoma. *Semin Hematol* 1999;36:139–147.
366. Morris SW, Kirstein MN, Valentine MB, et al. Fusion of a kinase gene, *ALK,* to a nucleolar protein gene, *NPM,* in non-Hodgkin's lymphoma [published erratum appears in *Science* 1995;267:316–317]. *Science* 1994;263:1281–1284.
367. Delsol G, Lamant L, Mariame B, et al. A new subtype of large B-cell lymphoma expressing the ALK kinase and lacking the 2;5 translocation. *Blood* 1997;89:1483–1490.
368. Alizadeh AA, Eisen MB, Davis RE, et al. Distinct types of diffuse large B-cell lymphoma identified by gene expression profiling [see comments]. *Nature* 2000;403:503–511.
369. Schwab U, Stein H, Gerdes J, et al. Production of a monoclonal antibody specific for Hodgkin and Sternberg-Reed cells of Hodgkin's disease and a subset of normal lymphoid cells. *Nature* 1982;299: 65–67.
370. Stein H, Gerdes J, Schwab U, et al. Identification of Hodgkin and Sternberg-Reed cells as a unique cell type derived from a newly-detected small-cell population. *Int J Cancer* 1982;30:445–459.
371. Beverley PCL. Activation antigens: new and previously defined clusters. In: McMichael AJ, ed. *Leucocyte typing,* III. Oxford: Oxford University Press, 1987:516–524.
372. Stein H, Mason DY, Gerdes J, et al. The expression of the Hodgkin's disease associated antigen Ki-1 in reactive and neoplastic lymphoid tissue: evidence that Reed-Sternberg cells and histiocytic malignancies are derived from activated lymphoid cells. *Blood* 1985;66: 848–858.
373. O'Connor NT, Stein H, Gatter KC, et al. Genotypic analysis of large cell lymphomas which express the Ki-1 antigen. *Histopathology* 1987; 11:733–740.
374. Herbst H, Tippelmann G, Anagnostopoulos I, et al. Immunoglobulin and T-cell receptor gene rearrangements in Hodgkin's disease and Ki-1–positive anaplastic large cell lymphoma: dissociation between phenotype and genotype. *Leuk Res* 1989;13:103–116.
375. Agnarsson BA, Kadin ME. Ki-1 positive large cell lymphoma. A morphologic and immunologic study of 19 cases. *Am J Surg Pathol* 1988;12:264–274.
376. Chan JK, Ng CS, Hui PK, et al. Anaplastic large cell Ki-1 lymphoma: delineation of two morphological types [see comments]. *Histopathology* 1989;15:11–34.
377. Chott A, Kaserer K, Augustin I, et al. Ki-1–positive large cell lymphoma. A clinicopathologic study of 41 cases [see comments]. *Am J Surg Pathol* 1990;14:439–448.
378. Pallesen G, Hamilton-Dutoit SJ. Ki-1 (CD30) antigen is regularly expressed by tumor cells of embryonal carcinoma. *Am J Pathol* 1988; 133:446–450.
379. Harris NL, Jaffe ES, Stein H, et al. A revised European-American classification of lymphoid neoplasms: a proposal from the International Lymphoma Study Group [see comments]. *Blood* 1994;84: 1361–1392.
380. Jaffe ES, Harris NL, Diebold J, et al. World Health Organization classification of lymphomas: a work in progress. *Ann Oncol* 1998; 9[Suppl 5]:S25–S30.
381. Kinney MC, Collins RD, Greer JP, et al. A small-cell-predominant variant of primary Ki-1 $(CD30)^+$ T-cell lymphoma. *Am J Surg Pathol* 1993;17:859–868.
382. Pileri S, Falini B, Delsol G, et al. Lymphohistiocytic T-cell lymphoma (anaplastic large cell lymphoma $CD30^+$/Ki-1^+ with a high content of reactive histiocytes). *Histopathology* 1990;16:383–391.
383. Mann KP, Hall B, Kamino H, et al. Neutrophil-rich, Ki-1–positive anaplastic large-cell malignant lymphoma. *Am J Surg Pathol* 1995; 19:407–416.
384. Falini B, Liso A, Pasqualucci L, et al. $CD30^+$ anaplastic large-cell lymphoma, null type, with signet-ring appearance. *Histopathology* 1997;30:90–92.
385. Chittal SM, Delsol G. The interface of Hodgkin's disease and anaplastic large cell lymphoma. *Cancer Surv* 1997;30:87–105.
386. de Bruin PC, Beljaards RC, Van Heerde P, et al. Differences in clinical behaviour and immunophenotype between primary cutaneous and primary nodal anaplastic large cell lymphoma of T-cell or null cell phenotype. *Histopathology* 1993;23:127–135.
387. Kaudewitz P, Stein H, Dallenbach F, et al. Primary and secondary cutaneous Ki-1^+ ($CD30^+$) anaplastic large cell lymphomas. Morphologic, immunohistologic, and clinical-characteristics. *Am J Pathol* 1989;135:359–367.
388. Rimokh R, Magaud JP, Berger F, et al. A translocation involving a specific breakpoint (q35) on chromosome 5 is characteristic of anaplastic large cell lymphoma (''Ki-1 lymphoma''). *Br J Haematol* 1989;71:31–36.
389. Mason DY, Bastard C, Rimokh R, et al. CD30-positive large cell lymphomas (''Ki-1 lymphoma'') are associated with a chromosomal translocation involving 5q35 [see comments]. *Br J Haematol* 1990; 74:161–168.
390. Bitter MA, Franklin WA, Larson RA, et al. Morphology in Ki-1 (CD30)–positive non-Hodgkin's lymphoma is correlated with clinical features and the presence of a unique chromosomal abnormality, t(2; 5)(p23;q35). *Am J Surg Pathol* 1990;14:305–316.
391. Kaneko Y, Frizzera G, Edamura S, et al. A novel translocation, t(2; 5)(p23;q35), in childhood phagocytic large T-cell lymphoma mimicking malignant histiocytosis. *Blood* 1989;73:806–813.
392. Morris SW, Kirstein MN, Valentine MB, et al. Fusion of a kinase gene, *ALK,* to a nucleolar protein gene, *NPM,* in non-Hodgkin's lymphoma [published erratum appears in *Science* 1995;267:316–317]. *Science* 1994;263:1281–1284.
393. Pulford K, Lamant L, Morris SW, et al. Detection of anaplastic lymphoma kinase (ALK) and nucleolar protein nucleophosmin (NPM)-ALK proteins in normal and neoplastic cells with the monoclonal antibody ALK1. *Blood* 1997;89:1394–1404.
394. Falini B, Bigerna B, Fizzotti M, et al. ALK expression defines a distinct group of T/null lymphomas (''ALK lymphomas'') with a wide morphological spectrum. *Am J Pathol* 1998;153:875–886.
395. Tirelli U, Vaccher E, Zagonel V, et al. CD30 (Ki-1)–positive anaplastic large-cell lymphomas in 13 patients with and 27 patients without human immunodeficiency virus infection: the first comparative clinicopathologic study from a single institution that also includes 80 patients with other human immunodeficiency virus-related systemic lymphomas. *J Clin Oncol* 1995;13:373–380.
396. Durkop H, Latza U, Hummel M, et al. Molecular cloning and expression of a new member of the nerve growth factor receptor family that is characteristic for Hodgkin's disease. *Cell* 1992;68:421–427.
397. Smith CA, Gruss HJ, Davis T, et al. CD30 antigen, a marker for

Hodgkin's lymphoma, is a receptor whose ligand defines an emerging family of cytokines with homology to TNF. *Cell* 1993;73:1349–1360.
398. Hansen HP, Kisseleva T, Kobarg J, et al. A zinc metalloproteinase is responsible for the release of CD30 on human tumor cell lines. *Int J Cancer* 1995;63:750–756.
399. Nadali G, Vinante F, Stein H, et al. Serum levels of the soluble form of CD30 molecule as a tumor marker in CD30$^+$ anaplastic large-cell lymphoma. *J Clin Oncol* 1995;13:1355–1360.
400. Zinzani PL, Pileri S, Bendandi M, et al. Clinical implications of serum levels of soluble CD30 in 70 adult anaplastic large-cell lymphoma patients. *J Clin Oncol* 1998;16:1532–1537.
401. Lischwe MA, Smetana K, Olson MO, et al. Proteins C23 and B23 are the major nucleolar silver staining proteins. *Life Sci* 1979;25:701–708.
402. Michalik J, Yeoman LC, Busch H. Nucleolar localization of protein B23 (37/5.1) by immunocytochemical techniques. *Life Sci* 1981;28: 1371–1379.
403. Borer RA, Lehner CF, Eppenberger HM, et al. Major nucleolar proteins shuttle between nucleus and cytoplasm. *Cell* 1989;56:379–390.
404. Kutzner H, Englert W, Hellenbroich D, et al. [Systemic proliferative angioendotheliomatosis: a cutaneous manifestation of malignant B-cell lymphomas. Histologic and immunohistologic studies of two cases]. *Hautarzt* 1991;42:384–390.
405. Adachi Y, Copeland TD, Hatanaka M, et al. Nucleolar targeting signal of Rex protein of human T-cell leukemia virus type I specifically binds to nucleolar shuttle protein B-23. *J Biol Chem* 1993;268: 13930–13934.
406. Iwahara T, Fujimoto J, Wen D, et al. Molecular characterization of ALK, a receptor tyrosine kinase expressed specifically in the nervous system. *Oncogene* 1997;14:439–449.
407. Morris SW, Naeve C, Mathew P, et al. ALK, the chromosome 2 gene locus altered by the t(2;5) in non-Hodgkin's lymphoma, encodes a novel neural receptor tyrosine kinase that is highly related to leukocyte tyrosine kinase (LTK) [published erratum appears in *Oncogene* 1997; 15:2883]. *Oncogene* 1997;14:2175–2188.
408. Shiota M, Fujimoto J, Semba T, et al. Hyperphosphorylation of a novel 80 kDa protein-tyrosine kinase similar to Ltk in a human Ki-1 lymphoma cell line, AMS3. *Oncogene* 1994;9:1567–1574.
409. Bischof D, Pulford K, Mason DY, et al. Role of the nucleophosmin (NPM) portion of the non-Hodgkin's lymphoma-associated NPM-anaplastic lymphoma kinase fusion protein in oncogenesis. *Mol Cell Biol* 1997;17:2312–2325.
410. Ladanyi M. The NPM/ALK gene fusion in the pathogenesis of anaplastic large cell lymphoma. *Cancer Surv* 1997;30:59–75.
411. Fujimoto J, Shiota M, Iwahara T, et al. Characterization of the transforming activity of p80, a hyperphosphorylated protein in a Ki-1 lymphoma cell line with chromosomal translocation t(2;5). *Proc Natl Acad Sci USA* 1996;93:4181–4186.
412. Bai RY, Dieter P, Peschel C, et al. Nucleophosmin-anaplastic lymphoma kinase of large-cell anaplastic lymphoma is a constitutively active tyrosine kinase that utilizes phospholipase C-γ to mediate its mitogenicity. *Mol Cell Biol* 1998;18:6951–6961.
413. Kuefer MU, Look AT, Pulford K, et al. Retrovirus-mediated gene transfer of NPM-ALK causes lymphoid malignancy in mice. *Blood* 1997;90:2901–2910.
414. Bullrich F, Morris SW, Hummel M, et al. Nucleophosmin (NPM) gene rearrangements in Ki-1–positive lymphomas. *Cancer Res* 1994; 54:2873–2877.
415. DeCoteau JF, Butmarc JR, Kinney MC, et al. The t(2;5) chromosomal translocation is not a common feature of primary cutaneous CD30$^+$ lymphoproliferative disorders: comparison with anaplastic large-cell lymphoma of nodal origin [see comments]. *Blood* 1996;87: 3437–3441.
416. Wellmann A, Otsuki T, Vogelbruch M, et al. Analysis of the t(2; 5)(p23;q35) translocation by reverse transcription–polymerase chain reaction in CD30$^+$ anaplastic large-cell lymphomas, in other non-Hodgkin's lymphomas of T-cell phenotype, and in Hodgkin's disease. *Blood* 1995;86:2321–2328.
417. Lopategui JR, Sun LH, Chan JK, et al. Low frequency association of the t(2;5)(p23;q35) chromosomal translocation with CD30$^+$ lymphomas from American and Asian patients: a reverse transcriptase-polymerase chain reaction study. *Am J Pathol* 1995;146:323–328.
418. Elmberger PG, Lozano MD, Weisenburger DD, et al. Transcripts of the npm-alk fusion gene in anaplastic large cell lymphoma, Hodgkin's disease, and reactive lymphoid lesions. *Blood* 1995;86:3517–3521.
419. Downing JR, Shurtleff SA, Zielenska M, et al. Molecular detection of the (2;5) translocation of non-Hodgkin's lymphoma by reverse transcriptase-polymerase chain reaction. *Blood* 1995;85:3416–3422.
420. Herbst H, Anagnostopoulos J, Heinze B, et al. ALK gene products in anaplastic large cell lymphomas and Hodgkin's disease. *Blood* 1995;86:1694–1700.
421. Orscheschek K, Merz H, Hell J, et al. Large-cell anaplastic lymphoma-specific translocation (t[2;5] [p23;q35]) in Hodgkin's disease: indication of a common pathogenesis? [see comments]. *Lancet* 1995;345: 87–90.
422. Trumper L, Pfreundschuh M, Bonin FV, et al. Detection of the t(2; 5)-associated NPM/ALK fusion cDNA in peripheral blood cells of healthy individuals. *Br J Haematol* 1998;103:1138–1144.
423. Gascoyne RD, Aoun P, Wu D, et al. Prognostic significance of anaplastic lymphoma kinase (ALK) protein expression in adults with anaplastic large cell lymphoma. *Blood* 1999;93:3913–3921.
424. Shiota M, Fujimoto J, Takenaga M, et al. Diagnosis of t(2;5)(p23; q35)-associated Ki-1 lymphoma with immunohistochemistry. *Blood* 1994;84:3648–3652.
425. Lamant L, Meggetto F, al Saati T, et al. High incidence of the t(2; 5)(p23;q35) translocation in anaplastic large cell lymphoma and its lack of detection in Hodgkin's disease: comparison of cytogenetic analysis, reverse transcriptase–polymerase chain reaction, and P-80 immunostaining. *Blood* 1996;87:284–291.
426. Cordell JL, Pulford KAF, Bigerna B, et al. Detection of normal and chimeric nucleophosmin in human cells. *Blood* 1999;93:632–642.
427. Falini B, Pulford K, Pucciarini A, et al. Lymphomas expressing ALK fusion protein(s) other than NPM-ALK. *Blood* 1999;94:3509–3515.
428. Benharroch D, Meguerian-Bedoyan Z, Lamant L, et al. ALK-positive lymphoma: a single disease with a broad spectrum of morphology. *Blood* 1998;91:2076–2084.
429. Pittaluga S, Wiodarska I, Pulford K, et al. The monoclonal antibody ALK1 identifies a distinct morphological subtype of anaplastic large cell lymphoma associated with 2p23/ALK rearrangements. *Am J Pathol* 1997;151:343–351.
430. Wlodarska I, De Wolf-Peeters C, Falini B, et al. The cryptic inv(2)(p23q35) defines a new molecular genetic subtype of ALK-positive anaplastic large-cell lymphoma. *Blood* 1998;92:2688–2695.
431. Rosenwald A, Ott G, Pulford K, Katzenberger T, et al. T(1;2)(q21; p23) and t(2;3)(p23;q21): two novel variant translocations of the t(2; 5)(p23;q35) in anaplastic large cell lymphoma. *Blood* 1999;94: 362–364.
432. Pulford K, Falini B, Cordell J, et al. Biochemical detection of novel anaplastic lymphoma kinase proteins in tissue sections of anaplastic large cell lymphoma. *Am J Pathol* 1999;154:1657–1663.
433. Lamant L, Dastugue N, Pulford K, et al. A new fusion gene TPM3-ALK in anaplastic large cell lymphoma created by a (1;2)(q25;p23) translocation. *Blood* 1999;93:3088–3095.
434. Hernandez L, Pinyol M, Hernandez S, et al. TRK-fused gene (TFG) is a new partner of ALK in anaplastic large cell lymphoma producing two structurally different TFG-ALK translocations. *Blood* 1999;94: 3265–3268.
435. Butti MG, Bongarzone I, Ferraresi G, et al. A sequence analysis of the genomic regions involved in the rearrangements between TPM3 and NTRK1 genes producing TRK oncogenes in papillary thyroid carcinomas. *Genomics* 1995;28:15–24.
436. Trinei M, Lanfrancone L, Campo E, et al. A new variant anaplastic lymphoma kinase (ALK)-fusion protein (ATIC-ALK) in a case of ALK-positive anaplastic large cell lymphoma. *Cancer Res* 2000;60: 793–798.
437. Touriol C, Greenland C, Lamant L, et al. Further demonstration of the diversity of chromosomal changes involving 2p23 in ALK-positive lymphoma: 2 cases expressing ALK kinase fused to CLTCL (clathrin chain polypeptide-like). *Blood* 2000;95:3204–3207.
438. Griffin CA, Hawkins AL, Dvorak C, et al. Recurrent involvement of 2p23 in inflammatory myofibroblastic tumors. *Cancer Res* 1999;59: 2776–2780.
439. Lamant L, Pulford K, Bischof D, et al. Expression of the ALK tyrosine kinase gene in neuroblastoma. *Am J Pathol* 2000;156:1711–1721.
440. Delsol G, Lamant L, Mariame B, et al. A new subtype of large B-cell lymphoma expressing the ALK kinase and lacking the 2;5 translocation. *Blood* 1997;89:1483–1490.
441. Liu CC, Walsh CM, Young JD. Perforin: structure and function. *Immunol Today* 1995;16:194–201.

442. Smyth MJ, Trapani JA. Granzymes: exogenous proteinases that induce target cell apoptosis. *Immunol Today* 1995;16:202–206.
443. Shresta S, MacIvor DM, Heusel JW, et al. Natural killer and lymphokine-activated killer cells require granzyme B for the rapid induction of apoptosis in susceptible target cells. *Proc Natl Acad Sci USA* 1995; 92:5679–5683.
444. Darmon AJ, Nicholson DW, Bleackley RC. Activation of the apoptotic protease CPP32 by cytotoxic T-cell–derived granzyme B. *Nature* 1995;377:446–448.
445. Lichtenheld MG, Podack ER. Structure and function of the murine perforin promoter and upstream region: reciprocal gene activation or silencing in perforin positive and negative cells. *J Immunol* 1992;149: 2619–2626.
446. Kummer JA, Kamp AM, van Katwijk M, et al. Production and characterization of monoclonal antibodies raised against recombinant human granzymes A and B and showing cross reactions with the natural proteins. *J Immunol Methods* 1993;163:77–83.
447. Anderson P, Nagler-Anderson C, O'Brien C, et al. A monoclonal antibody reactive with a 15-kDa cytoplasmic granule-associated protein defines a subpopulation of CD8$^+$ T lymphocytes. *J Immunol* 1990;144:574–582.
448. Tian Q, Streuli M, Saito H, et al. A polyadenylate binding protein localized to the granules of cytolytic lymphocytes induces DNA fragmentation in target cells. *Cell* 1991;67:629–639.
449. Medley QG, Kedersha N, O'Brien S, et al. Characterization of GMP-17, a granule membrane protein that moves to the plasma membrane of natural killer cells following target cell recognition. *Proc Natl Acad Sci USA* 1996;93:685–689.
450. Kadin ME, Sako D, Berliner N, et al. Childhood Ki-1 lymphoma presenting with skin lesions and peripheral lymphadenopathy. *Blood* 1986;68:1042–1049.
451. Mora J, Filippa DA, Thaler HT, et al. Large cell non-Hodgkin lymphoma of childhood: analysis of 78 consecutive patients enrolled in two consecutive protocols at the Memorial Sloan-Kettering Cancer Center. *Cancer* 2000;88:186–197.
452. Wright D, McKeever P, Carter R. Childhood non-Hodgkin lymphomas in the United Kingdom: findings from the UK Children's Cancer Study Group [see comments]. *J Clin Pathol* 1997;50:128–134.
453. Falini B, Pileri S, Zinzani PL, et al. ALK$^+$ lymphoma: clinicopathological findings and outcome. *Blood* 1999;93:2697–2706.
454. Fraga M, Brousset P, Schlaifer D, et al. Bone marrow involvement in anaplastic large cell lymphoma: immunohistochemical detection of minimal disease and its prognostic significance. *Am J Clin Pathol* 1995;103:82–89.
455. Kadin ME. Anaplastic large cell lymphoma and its morphological variants. *Cancer Surv* 1997;30:77–86.
456. Hodges KB, Collins RD, Greer JP, et al. Transformation of the small cell variant Ki-1$^+$ lymphoma to anaplastic large cell lymphoma: pathologic and clinical features. *Am J Surg Pathol* 1999;23:49–58.
457. Chan JK, Buchanan R, Fletcher CD. Sarcomatoid variant of anaplastic large-cell Ki-1 lymphoma [see comments]. *Am J Surg Pathol* 1990; 14:983–988.
458. McCluggage WG, Walsh MY, Bharucha H. Anaplastic large cell malignant lymphoma with extensive eosinophilic or neutrophilic infiltration. *Histopathology* 1998;32:110–115.
459. Camisa C, Helm TN, Sexton C, et al. Ki-1–positive anaplastic large-cell lymphoma can mimic benign dermatoses. *J Am Acad Dermatol* 1993;29:696–700.
460. Bellas C, Molina A, Montalban C, et al. Signet-ring cell lymphoma of T-cell type with CD30 expression. *Histopathology* 1993;22:188–189.
461. Penny RJ, Blaustein JC, Longtine JA, et al. Ki-1–positive large cell lymphomas, a heterogenous group of neoplasms. Morphologic, immunophenotypic, genotypic, and clinical features of 24 cases. *Cancer* 1991;68:362–373.
462. Krenacs L, Wellmann A, Sorbara L, et al. Cytotoxic cell antigen expression in anaplastic large cell lymphomas of T- and null-cell type and Hodgkin's disease: evidence for distinct cellular origin. *Blood* 1997;89:980–989.
463. Foss HD, Anagnostopoulos I, Araujo I, et al. Anaplastic large-cell lymphomas of T-cell and null-cell phenotype express cytotoxic molecules. *Blood* 1996;88:4005–4011.
464. Felgar RE, Salhany KE, Macon WR, et al. The expression of TIA-1$^+$ cytolytic-type granules and other cytolytic lymphocyte-associated markers in CD30$^+$ anaplastic large cell lymphomas (ALCL): correlation with morphology, immunophenotype, ultrastructure, and clinical features. *Hum Pathol* 1999;30:228–236.
465. Garcia-Sanz JA, MacDonald HR, Jenne DE, et al. Cell specificity of granzyme gene expression. *J Immunol* 1990;145:3111–3118.
466. Cambiaggi A, Cantoni C, Marciano S, et al. Cultured human NK cells express the Ki-1/CD30 antigen. *Br J Haematol* 1993;85:270–276.
467. Delsol G, al Saati T, Gatter KC, et al. Coexpression of epithelial membrane antigen (EMA), Ki-1, and interleukin-2 receptor by anaplastic large cell lymphomas. Diagnostic value in so-called malignant histiocytosis. *Am J Pathol* 1988;130:59–70.
468. Pileri SA, Pulford K, Mori S, et al. Frequent expression of the NPM-ALK chimeric fusion protein in anaplastic large-cell lymphoma, lympho-histiocytic type. *Am J Pathol* 1997;150:1207–1211.
469. Weiss LM, Picker LJ, Copenhaver CM, et al. Large-cell hematolymphoid neoplasms of uncertain lineage. *Hum Pathol* 1988;19:967–973.
470. Nakagawa A, Nakamura S, Ito M, et al. CD30-positive anaplastic large cell lymphoma in childhood: expression of p80npm/alk and absence of Epstein-Barr virus. *Mod Pathol* 1997;10:210–215.
471. Kasai K, Kon S, Kikuchi K, et al. Expression of carbohydrate antigens, p80NPM/ALK, cytotoxic cell–associated antigens, and Epstein-Barr virus gene products in anaplastic large cell lymphomas. *Pathol Int* 1998;48:171–178.
472. Shiota M, Nakamura S, Ichinohasama R, et al. Anaplastic large cell lymphomas expressing the novel chimeric protein p80NPM/ALK: a distinct clinicopathologic entity. *Blood* 1995;86:1954–1960.
473. Reiter A, Schrappe M, Tiemann M, et al. Successful treatment strategy for Ki-1 anaplastic large-cell lymphoma of childhood: a prospective analysis of 62 patients enrolled in three consecutive Berlin-Frankfurt-Munster group studies. *J Clin Oncol* 1994;12:899–908.
474. Vecchi V, Burnelli R, Pileri S, et al. Anaplastic large cell lymphoma (Ki-1$^+$/CD30$^+$) in childhood. *Med Pediatr Oncol* 1993;21:402–410.
475. Murphy SB. Pediatric lymphomas: recent advances and commentary on Ki-1–positive anaplastic large-cell lymphomas of childhood. *Ann Oncol* 1994;5[Suppl 1]:31–33.
476. Zinzani PL, Bendandi M, Martelli M, et al. Anaplastic large-cell lymphoma: clinical and prognostic evaluation of 90 adult patients [see comments]. *J Clin Oncol* 1996;14:955–962.
477. Tilly H, Gaulard P, Lepage E, et al. Primary anaplastic large-cell lymphoma in adults: clinical presentation, immunophenotype, and outcome. *Blood* 1997;90:3727–3734.
478. A clinical evaluation of the International Lymphoma Study Group classification of non-Hodgkin's lymphoma. The Non-Hodgkin's Lymphoma Classification Project. *Blood* 1997;89:3909–3918.
479. Stein H. Diagnosis of Hodgkin's disease, Hodgkin's like anaplastic large cell lymphoma, and T cell/histiocyte-rich B cell lymphoma. In: Mason DY, Harris NL, eds. *Human lymphoma: clinical implications of the REAL classification.* Berlin: Springer-Verlag, 1999.
480. Foss HD, Reusch R, Demel G, et al. Frequent expression of the B-cell–specific activator protein in Reed-Sternberg cells of classical Hodgkin's disease provides further evidence for its B-cell origin. *Blood* 1999;94:3108–3113.
481. Krenacs L, Himmelmann AW, Quintanilla-Martinez L, et al. Transcription factor B-cell–specific activator protein (BSAP) is differentially expressed in B cells and in subsets of B-cell lymphomas. *Blood* 1998;92:1308–1316.
482. Isaacson PG. Gastrointestinal lymphoma. *Hum Pathol* 1994;25: 1020–1029.
483. Beljaards RC, Meijer CJ, Scheffer E, et al. Prognostic significance of CD30 (Ki-1/Ber-H2) expression in primary cutaneous large-cell lymphomas of T-cell origin: a clinicopathologic and immunohistochemical study in 20 patients. *Am J Pathol* 1989;135:1169–1178.
484. Willemze R, Kerl H, Sterry W, et al. EORTC classification for primary cutaneous lymphomas: a proposal from the Cutaneous Lymphoma Study Group of the European Organization for Research and Treatment of Cancer. *Blood* 1997;90:354–371.
485. Paulli M, Berti E, Rosso R, et al. CD30/Ki-1–positive lymphoproliferative disorders of the skin—clinicopathologic correlation and statistical analysis of 86 cases: a multicentric study from the European Organization for Research and Treatment of Cancer Cutaneous Lymphoma Project Group. *J Clin Oncol* 1995;13:1343–1354.
486. Su LD, Schnitzer B, Ross CW, et al. The t(2;5)-associated p80 NPM/ALK fusion protein in nodal and cutaneous CD30$^+$ lymphoproliferative disorders. *J Cutan Pathol* 1997;24:597–603.
487. Beylot-Barry M, Lamant L, Vergier B, et al. Detection of t(2;5)(p23;

q35) translocation by reverse transcriptase polymerase chain reaction and in situ hybridization in CD30-positive primary cutaneous lymphoma and lymphomatoid papulosis. *Am J Pathol* 1996;149:483–492.

488. Vergier B, Beylot-Barry M, Pulford K, et al. Statistical evaluation of diagnostic and prognostic features of $CD30^+$ cutaneous lymphoproliferative disorders: a clinicopathologic study of 65 cases. *Am J Surg Pathol* 1998;22:1192–1202.
489. Harris NL, Jaffe ES, Diebold J, et al. The World Health Organization classification of neoplastic diseases of the haematopoietic and lymphoid tissues: report of the Clinical Advisory Committee Meeting, Airlie House, Virginia, November 1997. *Histopathology* 2000;36:69–86.
490. Stein H, Herbst H, Anagnostopoulos I, et al. The nature of Hodgkin and Reed-Sternberg cells, their association with EBV, and their relationship to anaplastic large-cell lymphoma. *Ann Oncol* 1991;2[Suppl 2]:33–38.
491. Pileri S, Bocchia M, Baroni CD, et al. Anaplastic large cell lymphoma ($CD30^+$/Ki-1^+): results of a prospective clinicopathological study of 69 cases. *Br J Haematol* 1994;86:513–523.
492. Harris NL, Jaffe ES, Diebold J, et al. The World Health Organization classification of neoplastic diseases of the hematopoietic and lymphoid tissues: report of the Clinical Advisory Committee meeting, Airlie House, Virginia, November, 1997. *Ann Oncol* 1999;10:1419–1432.
493. Salhany KE, Cousar JB, Greer JP, et al. Transformation of cutaneous T-cell lymphoma to large cell lymphoma: a clinicopathologic and immunologic study. *Am J Pathol* 1988;132:265–277.

CHAPTER 26

Lymphoblastic Lymphoma

Daniel M. Knowles

Lymphoblastic lymphoma (LBL) apparently first was recognized in 1916 by Sternberg (1), who described a mediastinal lymphoma that terminated in acute leukemia—hence the designation *Sternberg sarcoma*. In 1932, Cooke (2) critically reviewed the world literature to assemble a collection of 74 cases of Sternberg sarcoma. In addition, he described nine new patients, all young boys who had mediastinal masses and leukemia, either at presentation or shortly thereafter, and who died within 6 months of presentation. Cooke pointed out the distinctive age and sex distribution and natural history of this clinical entity, correctly hypothesized its thymic derivation, and suggested that it was considerably more common than previously believed. Subsequently, a series of clinicopathologic studies (3–8) led to widespread recognition (9) that a significant proportion of children who had non-Hodgkin's lymphoma exhibited the distinctive clinical features now associated with LBL.

At that time, the diffuse non-Hodgkin's lymphomas were classified into two broad categories: reticulum cell sarcoma and lymphosarcoma (10). Some pathologists subclassified lymphosarcoma as *lymphocytic*, predominantly composed of small round lymphocytes, or *lymphoblastic*, predominantly composed of immature or atypical lymphoid cells (10). Unfortunately, criteria for this subclassification were not well defined, so non-Hodgkin's lymphomas were classified variably by pathologists (10). Nonetheless, the term *lymphoblastic lymphosarcoma* already had been applied aptly at that time to designate the clinically distinctive childhood non-Hodgkin's lymphomas composed of neoplastic cells that bear a striking resemblance to those of *acute lymphoblastic leukemia* (ALL) (8).

The Rappaport classification for non-Hodgkin's lymphoma (11) was adopted widely throughout the United States during the 1960s. The terms *lymphosarcoma* and *reticulum cell sarcoma* were eliminated. The terms *lymphocytic* and *lymphoblastic lymphosarcoma* were replaced by *well differentiated* and *poorly differentiated lymphocytic lymphoma*, respectively. A new category, *undifferentiated*, also was introduced. Each category in the Rappaport classification and the criteria established to distinguish among the categories were well defined (11). As a result, many important clinicopathologic correlations previously obscured by the older, imprecise terminology were discovered. Rappaport's poorly differentiated lymphocytic category, however, consisted of a clinically, histopathologically, and immunologically diverse group of predominantly adult lymphomas that differ substantially from the childhood LBLs included within the same category. As the term *lymphoblastic* was abandoned in favor of *poorly differentiated lymphocytic*, the special clinical features of childhood LBL became increasingly blurred (10). To compound the problem, LBL sometimes was reclassified erroneously as undifferentiated (12), resulting in confusion with the newly described Burkitt's and Burkitt's-like lymphomas (13,14). As the distinctive clinical and morphologic features of LBL became obscured, pathologists and other physicians appeared to forget about its existence (10).

Lymphoblastic lymphoma was rediscovered as a clinicopathologic entity because of the application of B- and T-cell marker analysis and careful morphologic observation. In 1973, Smith and associates (15) showed that the neoplastic cells isolated from a case of Sternberg sarcoma were T cells and suggested that these mediastinal lymphomas are thymic in origin. One year later, Kaplan and colleagues (16) demonstrated the T-cell origin of four childhood LBLs. Several investigators demonstrated that approximately 20% of ALLs have T-cell origins and share many clinical characteristics, including a high frequency of mediastinal involvement, with T-cell LBL (17–19). McCaffrey and colleagues (20,21) and Kung and associates (22) suggested that both T-cell LBL and T-cell ALL are thymic in origin because they consistently express terminal deoxynucleotidyl transferase

D. M. Knowles: Department of Pathology, Weill Medical College of Cornell University, New York, New York 10021

(TdT), a marker of immature (thymic) T cells (23). In contrast, the undifferentiated Burkitt's and Burkitt's-like lymphomas and the majority of adult poorly differentiated lymphocytic lymphomas were shown to be of B-cell origin (24–26).

In 1975, Barcos and Lukes (27) described 27 cases of mediastinal lymphoma composed of immature-appearing lymphoid cells containing irregular, complex nuclei. These investigators pointed out the occurrence of these lymphomas in older children and adolescents, the male predominance, a high incidence of mediastinal involvement, and their frequent termination in acute leukemia. They designated these cases *convoluted lymphocytic lymphoma* and suggested that they represent a distinct clinical and morphologic entity, probably of T-cell origin.

Nathwani and colleagues (28) quickly and correctly pointed out that Barcos and Lukes had not described a new entity but instead had rediscovered LBL. Nathwani and colleagues (28) showed that convoluted nuclei are not a necessary feature of this distinct morphologic subtype of diffuse poorly differentiated lymphocytic lymphoma. They proposed that the term *lymphoblastic*, abandoned as imprecise 20 years earlier, be resurrected to designate specifically these lymphomas, and that it be used instead of the term *convoluted lymphocytic*. Their rationale was not all LBLs have convoluted nuclei (28,29), many ALLs have convoluted nuclei (30), and LBLs with and without convoluted nuclei exhibit similar clinical behavior and bear a striking clinical and morphologic resemblance to ALL (28,29).

RELATIONSHIP BETWEEN LYMPHOBLASTIC LYMPHOMA AND ACUTE LYMPHOBLASTIC LEUKEMIA

Acute lymphoblastic leukemia occurs most frequently in children and represents the most common malignancy of childhood (31). Approximately 80% of ALLs are derived from precursor B cells; the remaining 20% are derived from precursor (thymic) T cells. Children who possess precursor B- and T-cell ALL display different clinical features. Those who have precursor T-cell ALL are generally older, are more often male than female, and usually present with more advanced disease than those who have precursor B-cell ALL. Children who have precursor T-cell ALL often present with hyperleukocytosis (>100,000 leukocytes per cubic millimeter), an anterior mediastinal mass, massive peripheral lymphadenopathy, and organomegaly. Overall, they have a worse prognosis than those who have precursor B-cell ALL (32) (see Chapter 46).

Approximately 80% or more of LBLs are derived from precursor T cells, and the remainder are derived from precursor B cells (33–36). Precursor T- and B-cell LBL share overlapping clinical, pathologic, immunologic, cytogenetic, and molecular features with ALL of corresponding cellular derivation. For this reason, some investigators have suggested that LBL and ALL simply represent different manifestations of the same disease and lump them together as a single entity (37–40). This concept inspired the International Lymphoma Study Group to designate these diseases precursor B- and T-cell lymphoblastic lymphoma/leukemia in the Revised European–American Classification of Lymphoid Neoplasms (REAL) (41).

Lymphoblastic lymphoma and ALL do appear to be related biologically, perhaps analogous to the relationship between B-cell small lymphocytic lymphoma and chronic lymphocytic leukemia. Despite identical morphologic and other overlapping features, however, the majority of LBLs and ALLs of corresponding cellular derivation differ with respect to clinical presentation and immunophenotype. For example, patients who have precursor T-cell LBL usually have no or only minimal peripheral blood or bone marrow involvement, normal or only minimally decreased hemoglobin and hematocrit levels and white blood cell and platelet counts, and lack splenomegaly at presentation (28,29,39). Patients who have precursor T-cell ALL nearly always have massive peripheral blood or bone marrow involvement, anemia, and thrombocytopenia and often have splenomegaly at presentation (29,30,39). The majority of precursor T-cell LBLs express immunophenotypic profiles consistent with a more mature level of intrathymic T-cell differentiation than most precursor T-cell ALLs (33–35,42–46).

Despite these differences, the distinction between LBL and ALL is unclear sometimes, and these entities must be differentiated arbitrarily. The criterion that the presence of 25% or more lymphoblasts in the bone marrow signifies ALL (43) commonly is used to distinguish these two entities (31,35,39,47). A true discrimination cannot always be made, for example, between a leukemic conversion of LBL and *de novo* ALL (29). At least some cases diagnosed as ALL probably represent the leukemic conversion of LBL that occurs before a patient seeks medical attention. It has been suggested that the identification of convoluted lymphoblasts in peripheral blood smears is a useful marker for the leukemic conversion of LBL (48). Convoluted nuclei, however, can be identified in more than one half of patients with ALL, including those with and without a mediastinal mass (30). The presence of convoluted nuclei is not useful in distinguishing the leukemic phase of LBL from *de novo* ALL (30). An attempt should be made to separate cases of LBL and ALL clinically, to permit identification and prevent masking of subtle but significant clinical and biologic differences that may exist.

HISTOPATHOLOGY

Lymphoblastic lymphoma and ALL are morphologically indistinguishable in tissue sections and in bone marrow aspirate smears, both light microscopically and ultrastructurally (29,30,40,41). Lymphoblastic lymphoma exhibits a diffuse, aggressive pattern of infiltration. In the majority of instances, the neoplastic cells completely obliterate the lymph node

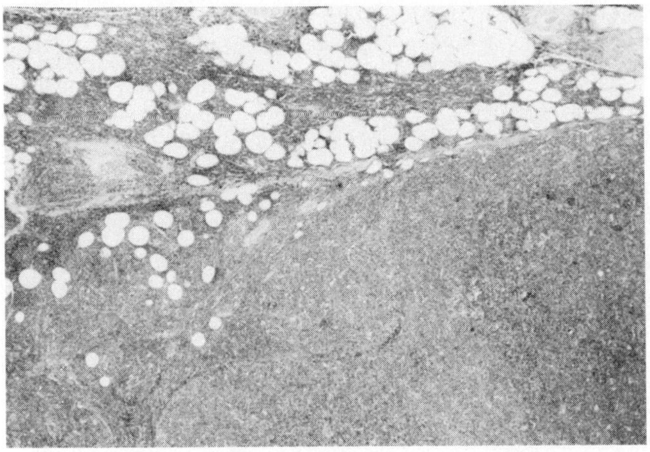

FIG. 26.1. Lymphoblastic lymphoma characteristically displays a diffuse and aggressive pattern of infiltration. The malignant lymphoblasts obliterate the lymph node architecture, infiltrate the lymph node capsule, and invade the surrounding perinodal fibroadipose tissue (hematoxylin and eosin stain, original magnification: 40× magnification).

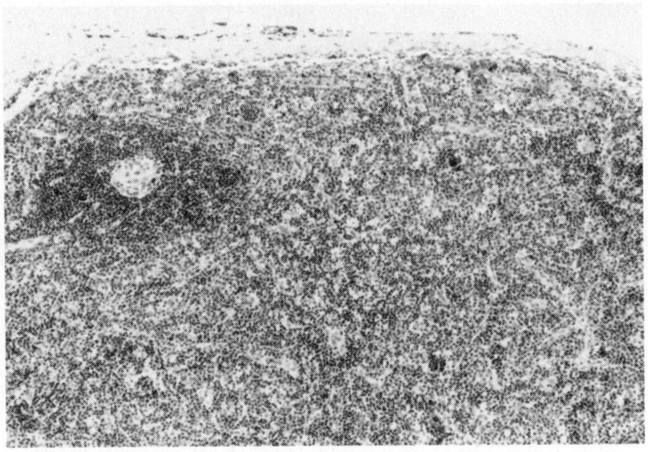

FIG. 26.3. In approximately one third of cases, the malignant T lymphoblasts preferentially infiltrate the interfollicular and paracortical (T-cell) areas, leaving small islands of residual normal lymphoid tissue that often contain germinal centers (B-cell areas) intact (hematoxylin and eosin stain, original magnification: 100× magnification).

architecture and invade the capsule and pericapsular tissue (Fig. 26.1). The neoplastic cells often characteristically split the pericapsular collagen fibers and infiltrate between them in a single-file arrangement (Fig. 26.2). Invasion and destruction of the walls of variably sized vessels located inside and outside the lymph node, accompanied by entrance of the neoplastic cells into the lumina, commonly is seen. In about one third of cases, the neoplastic cells selectively involve the interfollicular and paracortical (T-cell) zones, leaving small islands of residual normal lymphoid tissue that often contain intact germinal centers (Fig. 26.3). The peripheral or medullary sinuses sometimes remain partially patent as well. A starry-sky pattern caused by the presence of interspersed macrophages may be present focally but is only infrequently as diffuse and prominent as in Burkitt's lymphoma (Fig. 26.4). These macrophages often display phagocytosis. A crush artifact of variable but sometimes extensive numbers of neoplastic cells within the lymph node

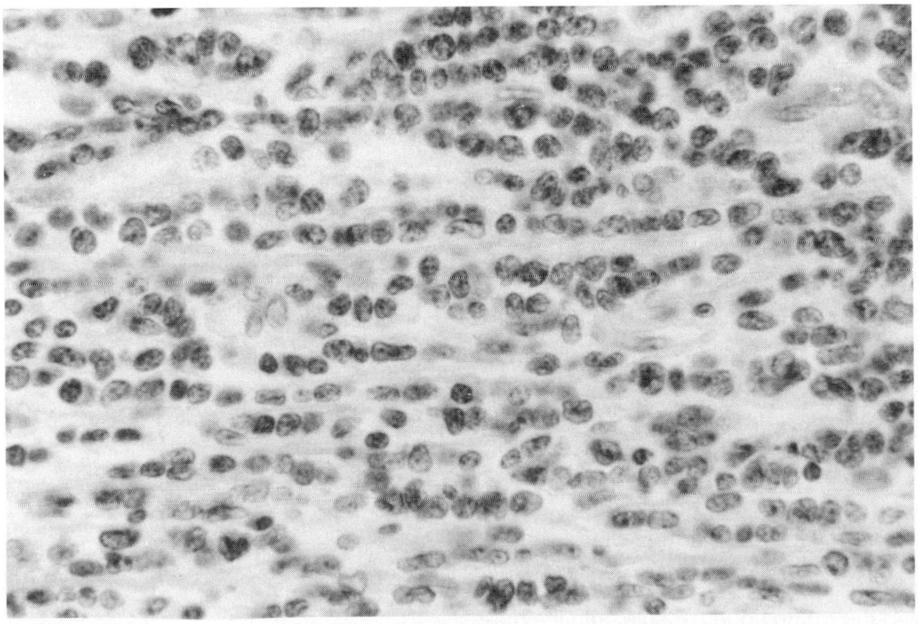

FIG. 26.2. The infiltrating malignant lymphoblasts characteristically split the pericapsular collagen fibers and infiltrate between them in Indian file (single-cell) fashion (hematoxylin and eosin stain, original magnification: 400× magnification).

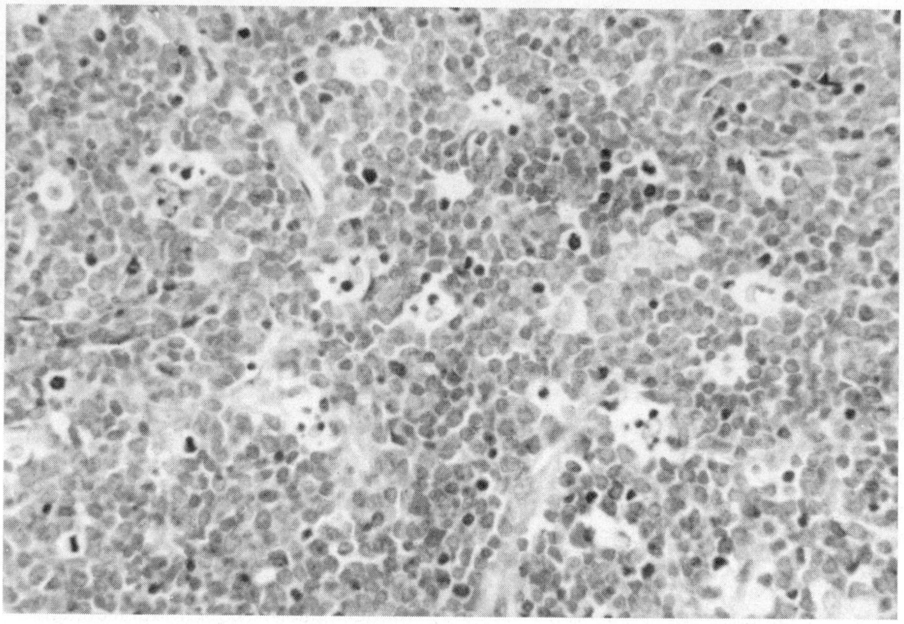

FIG. 26.4. A starry-sky pattern caused by the presence of tingible body macrophages may be present focally in lymphoblastic lymphoma (hematoxylin and eosin stain, original magnification: 250× magnification).

(as well as those infiltrating the pericapsular tissues) is observed in approximately 85% of cases, a feature characteristic of LBL (Figs. 26.5, 26.6). Mitotic figures are usually numerous; they average about 10 but can range up to more than 40 per high power field (400× magnification) (28,29) (Table 26.1).

Lymphoblastic lymphomas have been subclassified into convoluted and nonconvoluted morphologic subtypes according to the nuclear configuration of the neoplastic cells (28). The presence of only occasional convoluted nuclei qualifies an LBL as the convoluted subtype (28). Approximately 85% of LBLs can be classified as convoluted based on this criterion (29,49). Convoluted LBLs may contain anywhere from fewer than 10% to more than 90% convoluted nuclei.

The neoplastic cells of convoluted and nonconvoluted LBL share characteristic cytomorphologic features. These include scanty cytoplasm, poorly defined cell borders as

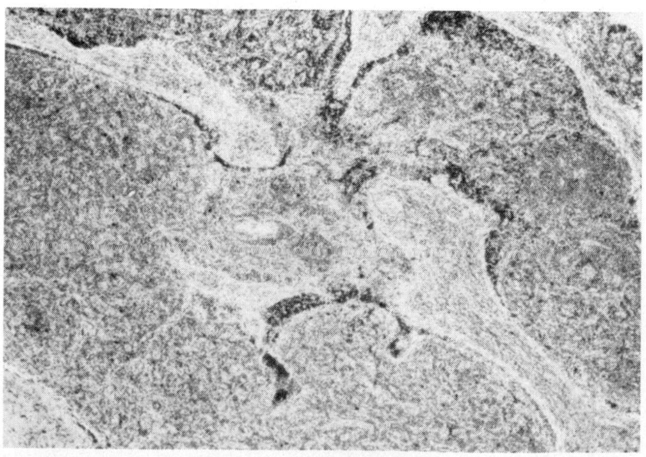

FIG. 26.5. Low-power examination of this lymph node involved by lymphoblastic lymphoma illustrates two of the features observed in approximately 85% of lymphoblastic lymphomas: The malignant lymphoblasts diffusely infiltrate beyond the confines of the lymph node capsule, and the malignant lymphoblasts positioned along the lymph node capsule show extensive crush artifact (hematoxylin and eosin stain, original magnification: 63× magnification).

TABLE 26.1. *Histopathologic features observed in 95 patients with lymphoblastic lymphoma*

Microscopic finding	Percentage of patients
Starry-sky pattern	
Prominent	10
Focal	15
Some sinuses open	16
Residual follicles or lymphoid islands	31
Invasion of pericapsular tissue	87
Single-file arrangement	46
Invasion of vessel walls	41
Crush artifact	85
Convoluted	84
Nonconvoluted	16
Moderate to marked variations in nuclear size	66
Small, inconspicuous nucleoli	28
Plasma cells	15
Eosinophils	16

Modified from Nathwani BN, Diamond LW, Winberg CD, et al. Lymphoblastic lymphoma: A clinicopathologic study of 95 patients. *Cancer* 1981;48:2347–2357, with permission.

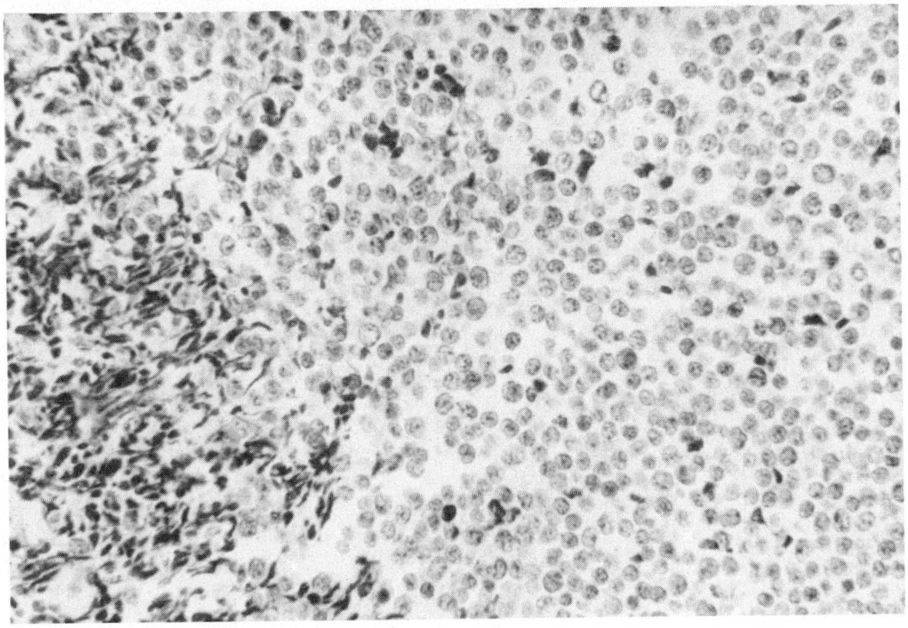

FIG. 26.6. Crush artifact of the malignant lymphoblasts is seen in approximately 85% of cases (hematoxylin and eosin stain, original magnification: 250× magnification).

viewed in tissue sections, thin but distinct nuclear membranes, finely dispersed and evenly distributed dust-like chromatin, and inconspicuous nucleoli. If nucleoli are present, they usually are single, small, and centrally located (Fig. 26.7). These small nucleoli are sometimes difficult to distinguish from condensation of nuclear chromatin, especially in poorly fixed preparations (28,29).

Nuclei are classified as convoluted if they possess one or more deep clefts or infoldings, resulting in a lobulated appearance (48) initially likened to a ''chicken footprint'' (27) or ''baseball catcher's mitt'' (50). Convoluted nuclei display great variability in shape and moderate variability in size. The majority measure 12 ± 2 μm (28). This is smaller than the nuclei of reactive histiocytes but larger than the cells of chronic lymphocytic leukemia or small lymphocytic lymphoma (51). The convolutions usually are most conspicuous in the larger cells, in which deep irregular clefts may be seen (28). Convoluted nuclei are most easily identified in cytocentrifuge preparations or in thin, well-prepared histologic sections, in which they are best appreciated by

A

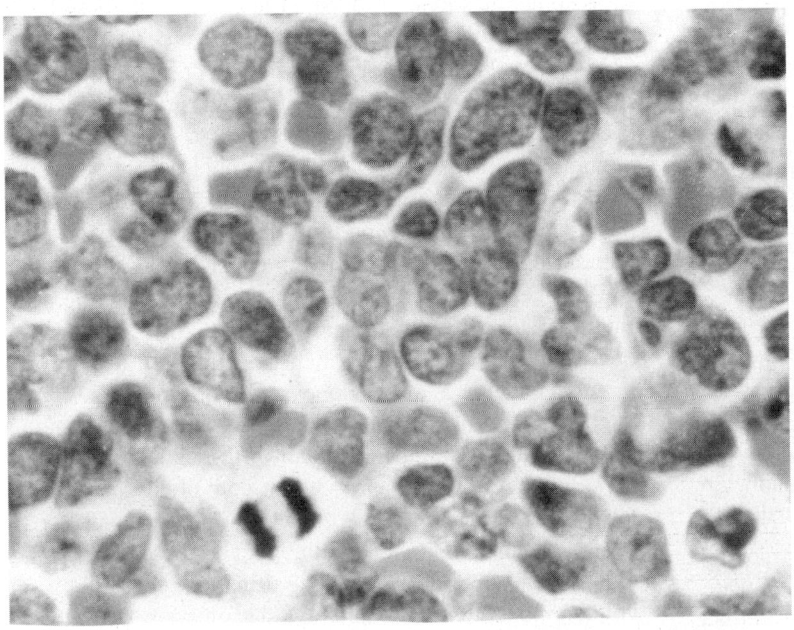

FIG. 26.7. Characteristic cytomorphology of lymphoblastic lymphoma as viewed in a histopathologic section (**A**). *(continued)*

B 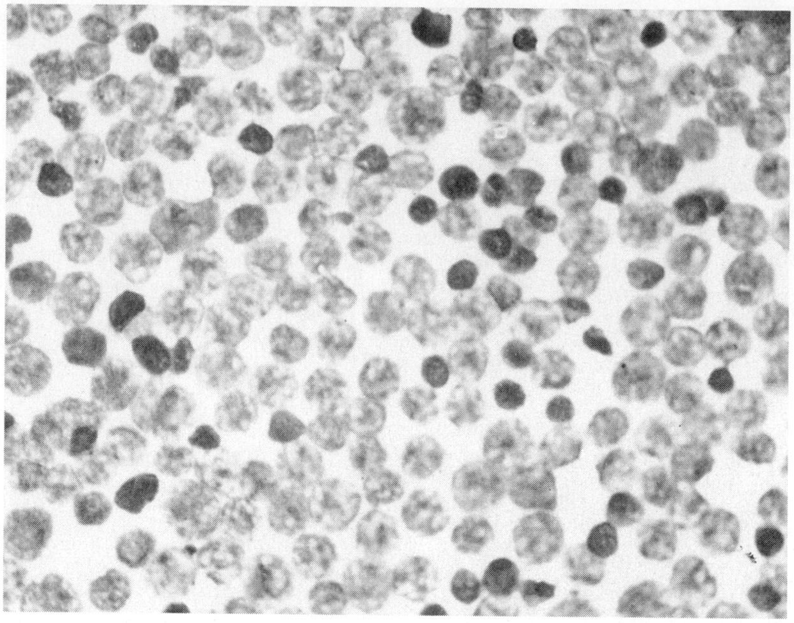

FIG. 26.7. *Continued.* A touch preparation (**B**) of a lymph node diffusely replaced by lymphoblastic lymphoma. The malignant lymphoblasts characteristically contain scant cytoplasm and have thin but distinct nuclear membranes, and their nuclei contain finely dispersed and evenly distributed dust-like chromatin with inconspicuous nucleoli. (**A:** Hematoxylin and eosin, original magnification: 1,000× magnification; **B:** Wright-Giemsa stain, original magnification: 630× magnification.)

constant manipulation of the fine focusing adjustment of the microscope (28,38). They are most striking if viewed ultrastructurally (52). Nuclear convolutions also can be identified readily in well-prepared Wright-stained peripheral blood and bone marrow smears and tissue imprints (30) (Fig. 26.8). Nonconvoluted nuclei are monotonous, round to ovoid, with little variation in size or shape; they measure about 14 ± 2 μm (28). In Romanowsky-stained imprints, the majority of the lymphoblasts correspond to the L1 ALL category (51) of the French–American–British (FAB) classification (53,54).

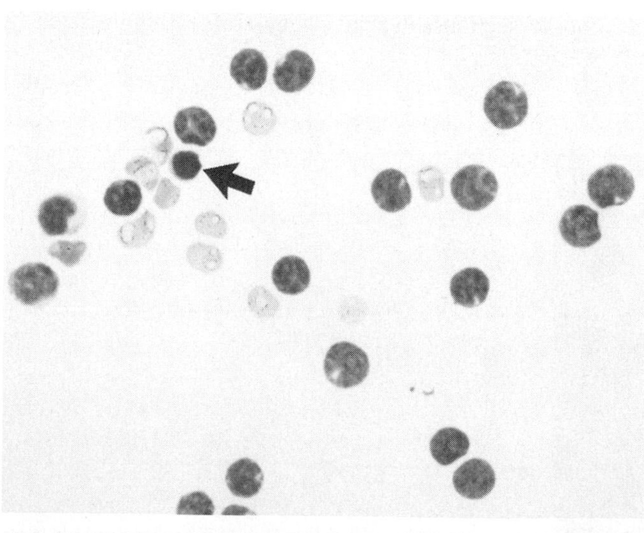

FIG. 26.8. The cells, predominantly malignant lymphoblasts, present within a sample of aspirated bone marrow, were harvested by ficoll-hypaque density gradient centrifugation. An aliquot of cells then was placed onto a glass slide by cytocentrifugation, and Wright-Giemsa staining was performed. Many of the malignant lymphoblasts have convoluted nuclei, as evidenced by nuclear notching and indentation. A benign lymphocyte (*arrow*) is present for comparison (Wright-Giemsa stain, original magnification: 630× magnification).

A third distinctive morphologic subtype of LBL, variously called the *atypical*, *large cell*, *pleomorphic*, or *L2* variant, also has been described (49,51). This subtype is said to comprise about 10% of all cases of LBL (49). The lymphoblasts of this variant generally are larger in size and possess more abundant cytoplasm and frequently have convoluted nuclei that contain one or two relatively prominent nucleoli (49,51) (Fig. 26.9). Morphologically, these lymphoblasts resemble more closely the L2 ALL category of the FAB classification in imprint preparations (51). These cytomorphologic features sometimes make it difficult to distinguish these LBLs from some Burkitt's-like and diffuse large cell lymphomas. The best and only absolute criterion for separating these LBLs from other intermediate- and high-grade lymphomas is recognition of the finely dispersed, dust-like chromatin structure characteristic of all lymphoblasts. Other nuclear or cytoplasmic features, the mitotic index, and histologic patterns of proliferation and infiltration are not consistently helpful in making this distinction (49).

The age and sex distribution, clinical presentation and findings, laboratory parameters, natural history, incidence of leukemic conversion, response to therapy, and median duration of survival do not appear to differ among the convoluted, nonconvoluted, and atypical morphologic subtypes (29,49). These parameters do not differ significantly in patients with ALL, with and without convoluted nuclei (30). Furthermore, none of these histologic subtypes of LBL appears to express unique immunophenotypic characteristics (33,43). The morphologic subclassification of LBL into convoluted, nonconvoluted, and atypical subtypes does not appear to have any obvious clinical value.

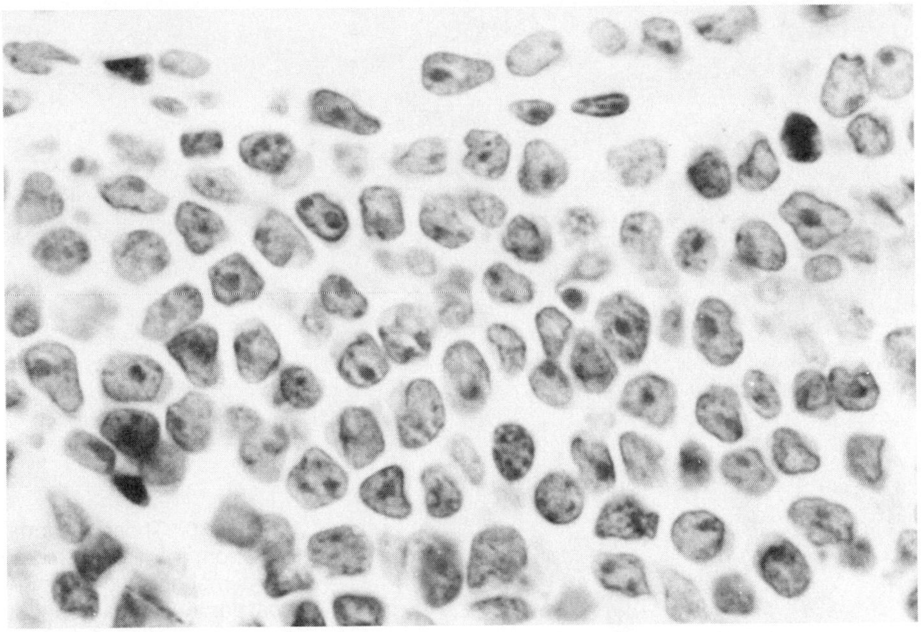

FIG. 26.9. The malignant lymphoblasts in this case frequently contain one nucleolus and sometimes two relatively prominent nucleoli but otherwise have the finely dispersed and evenly distributed chromatin characteristic of lymphoblastic lymphoma. This morphologic subtype has been called the "L2" variant because of its resemblance to the L2 acute lymphoblastic leukemia category of the French–American–British classification (hematoxylin and eosin stain, original magnification: 1000× magnification).

IMMUNOPHENOTYPIC CHARACTERISTICS

Recognition of the T-cell origin of mediastinal LBL initially was based on the observation that the malignant lymphoblasts form sheep erythrocyte rosettes (15–17), a property of normal human T cells (55), or react with various anti-human T cell heteroantisera (56–58). Recognition of the immature (thymic) nature of the T-cell lymphoblasts initially was based on the fact that they form heat-stable sheep erythrocyte rosettes (59) and express TdT (20–22,37,60), markers of thymocytes (21,37,59). Those LBLs that did not form sheep erythrocyte rosettes, failed to react with anti-human T cell heteroantisera, and lacked the mature B-cell marker surface immunoglobulin were designated *null* or *non-B, non-T cell* (18,19).

Jaffe and associates (61) and Stein and coworkers (62) further demonstrated the phenotypic heterogeneity of LBL by showing that both sheep erythrocyte rosette–positive and sheep erythrocyte rosette–negative LBLs variably express complement receptors. The dual expression of sheep erythrocyte rosette and complement receptors is a feature of many fetal thymocytes (63). In addition, Catovsky and colleagues (64,65), Stein and coworkers (62), and others (66) demonstrated that sheep erythrocyte rosette–positive ALL and LBL express strong focal paranuclear acid phosphatase activity, another feature of fetal thymocytes (62,63). A positive acid phosphatase reaction was believed to be so highly associated with T-cell ALL and LBL that the term *acid phosphatase–positive ALL or LBL* was proposed to designate this clinical entity (62,66) (Fig. 26.10). Some T-cell LBLs are acid phosphatase–negative, however, and some non–T cell LBLs and mature postthymic T-cell leukemias and lymphomas are acid phosphatase–positive (47,67,68). Therefore, use of the term *acid phosphatase–positive ALL or LBL* to indicate a distinct clinical entity was discouraged (65,67), and this term fell into disuse.

Our contemporary understanding of the lineage and stage of differentiation of LBLs is based on extensive immunophenotypic studies of normal and neoplastic T and B cells using large panels of monoclonal antibodies in conjunction with cytofluorometric and immunohistochemical techniques (69–73). These studies have led to the development of hypothetical schema of normal T and B cell differentiation. In these schema, discrete developmental stages are defined according to reactivity with a panel of monoclonal antibodies that detects differentiation and subset-associated antigens (Figs. 26.11, 26.12) (see Chapter 3). The central thesis in these immunophenotyping studies is that lymphoid neoplasms represent clonal proliferations of neoplastic cells frozen or blocked at a particular stage in T- or B-cell ontogeny. This thesis may not be entirely correct. Furthermore, differentiation is a continuous and not a discrete process. These schema are overly simplified and probably are not entirely accurate. Neoplastic cell immunophenotypes that do not reflect these differentiation schema have been encountered. Whether this is because the models of normal B- and T-cell differentiation are incorrect, because the normal counterparts of some malignant lymphoid cells are uncommonly identified, or because they aberrantly express B- and T-cell differentiation–associated antigens has not yet been determined.

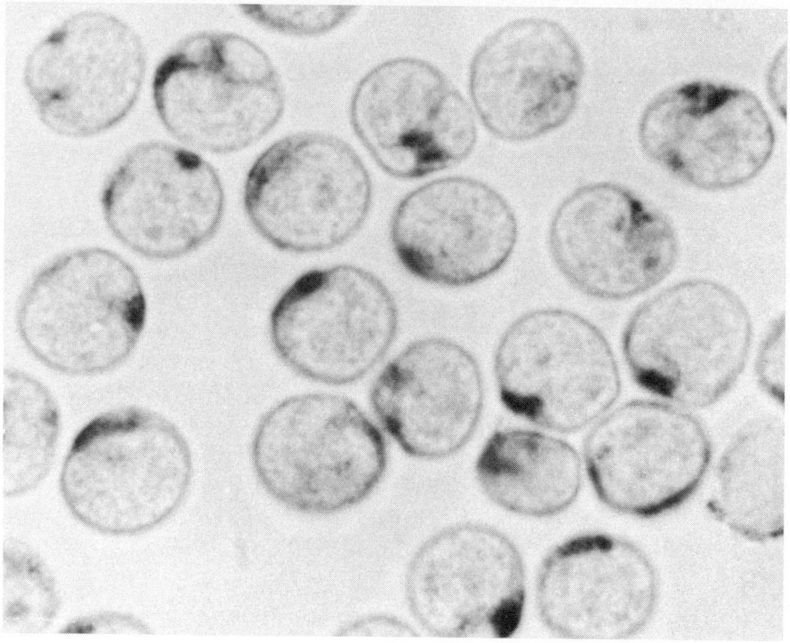

FIG. 26.10. These malignant lymphoblasts isolated from a patient with mediastinal precursor T-cell lymphoblastic lymphoma express strong focal paranuclear acid phosphatase activity (original magnification: 1,100× magnification).

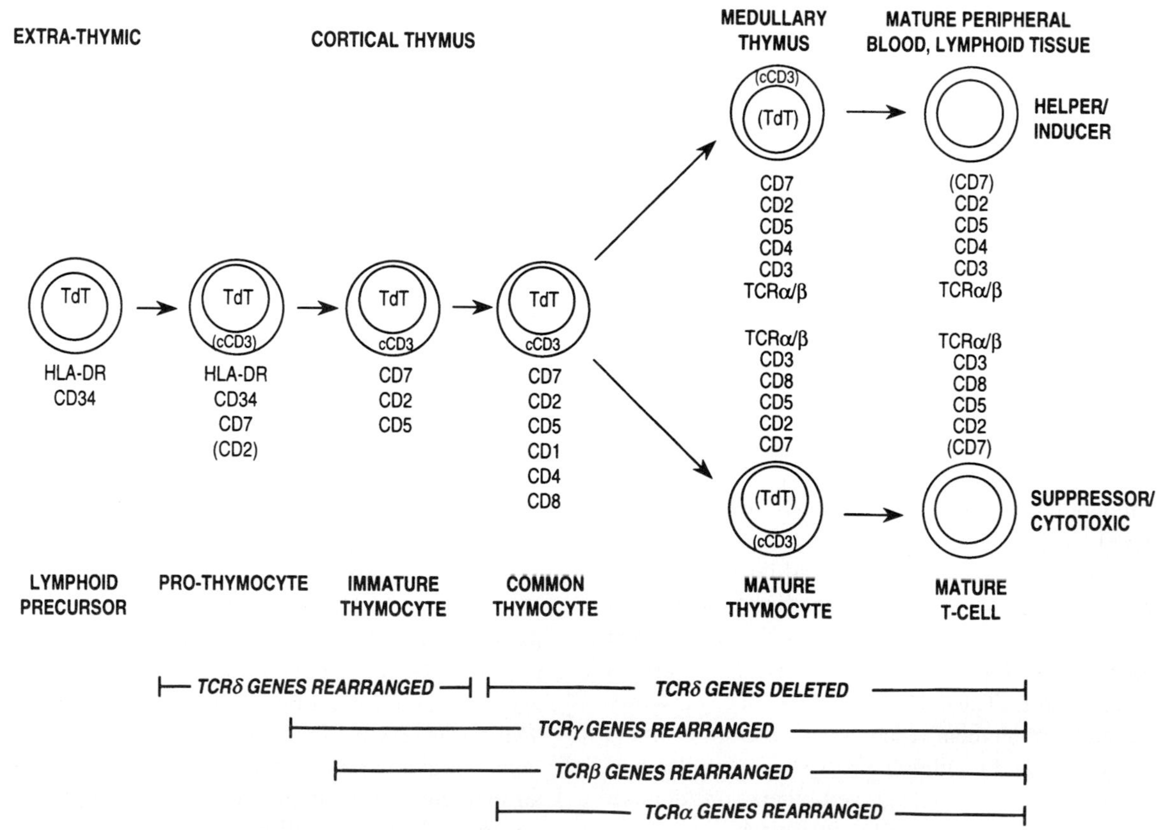

FIG. 26.11. Hypothetical schema of T-cell differentiation.

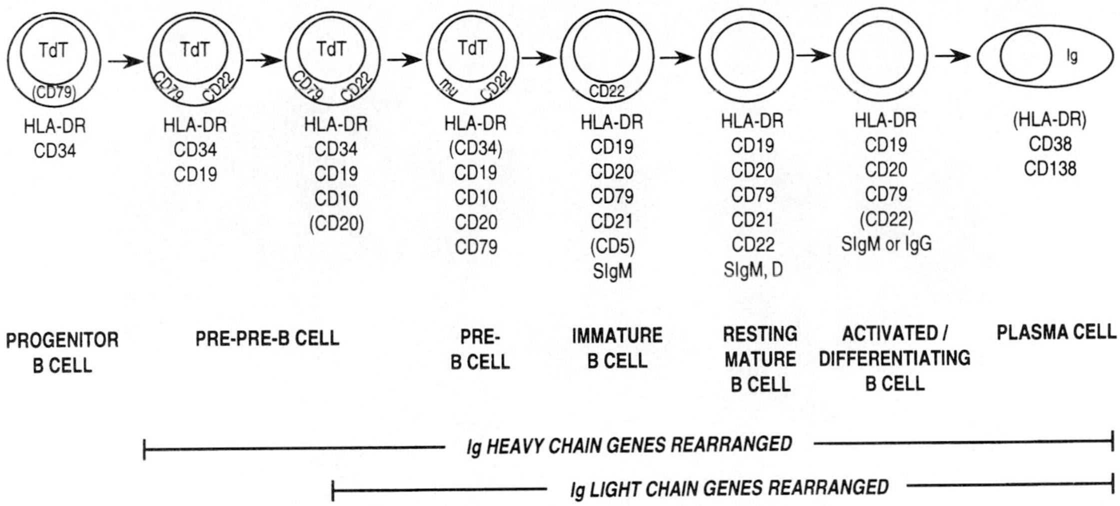

FIG. 26.12. Hypothetical schema of B-cell differentiation.

Nonetheless, these schemas are helpful in understanding precursor T- and B-cell LBL immunophenotypes and their relationship to normal T- and B-cell differentiation.

Terminal deoxynucleotidyl transferase is a unique nuclear DNA polymerase that catalyzes the polymerization of deoxyribonucleotides in the absence of a template (23). It apparently is responsible for the addition of non–germline-encoded nucleotides called *N regions* during the process of antigen receptor gene rearrangement (74) (see Chapter 3). TdT is expressed by precursor B and T cells at the earliest recognizable stages of lymphoid cell ontogeny (75). Under normal conditions, TdT-positive cells are confined to the thymus and bone marrow in which these precursor cells reside; TdT-positive cells are not observed normally in the peripheral blood or peripheral lymphoid tissue (21,23,37, 76). The presence of TdT-positive cells in such circumstances is considered diagnostic of precursor LBL or ALL (76).

The usefulness of TdT as a marker of immature hematopoietic cells was recognized early and has been exploited widely in the diagnosis and characterization of non-Hodgkin's lymphomas and acute leukemias (23). Essentially all malignant lymphoblasts comprising virtually all cases of precursor B- or T-cell LBL or ALL and cases of chronic myelogenous leukemia in lymphoid blast crisis express TdT (10,20–23,34,37,76–79). Functional biochemical assays can be used to detect TdT activity in leukolysates of bone marrow or tissue extracts (77). For purposes of routine immunophenotypic analysis, immunocytochemical and immunohistochemical assays offer the advantages of technical simplicity, applicability to smears and tissue sections, and the ability to evaluate cell morphology (76). Dual marker evaluation by immunoenzymatic techniques is also possible (76). Therefore, TdT routinely is detected by immunofluorescent (21,67), immunoperoxidase (80,81), or immunoalkaline phosphatase (82) staining of cytocentrifuge slide preparations (Fig. 26.13), cytofluorometric analysis of isolated viable lymphoblasts in suspension (83), or immunoperoxidase staining of frozen (84) or paraffin tissue (85) sections (Fig. 26.14). The application of antigen-retrieval techniques (86) has simplified the immunohistochemical demonstration of TdT and significantly increased the sensitivity of its detection in paraffin tissue sections (87). This has facilitated reliable and reproducible TdT detection by automated instrumentation (Knowles, unpublished observations).

According to current concepts, T-cell ontogeny—that is, the differentiation of lymphoid precursor cells in the bone marrow into mature, peripheral immunocompetent T cells—can be divided operationally into several discrete stages according to the expression of T-cell lineage–restricted and –associated cytoplasmic and surface membrane antigens. These stages can be referred to as *prothymocyte*, *immature thymocyte*, *common thymocyte*, *mature thymocyte*, and *mature peripheral T cell* (32,42,71–73,88–92) (Fig. 26.11). The majority of bone marrow pleuripotential lymphoid precursor cells express intranuclear TdT, HLA-DR, and CD34 antigens. Prothymocytes are the earliest identifiable T-cell precursors to appear in the bone marrow. In addition to TdT, HLA-DR, and CD34, prothymocytes express CD7, generally believed to be the first T-cell lineage–restricted antigen to appear during T-cell ontogeny (92–94). $CD7^+CD3^-CD4^-CD8^-$ precursor T cells, referred to as "triple negative," can be identified in 7-week fetal tissues prior to the development of the thymus (92). CD3 gene transcription apparently begins during the prothymocyte stage, prior to entrance into the thymus, and cytoplasmic CD3ϵ (cCD3ϵ) appears after CD7 but before CD2 (90,91). Thus, these prothymocytes also appear to variably express cCD3 and CD2. $CD7^+cCD3^+$ and $CD7^+cCD3^-$ prothymocytes then migrate to and colonize the epithelial thymic rudiment. These T-cell precursors undergo all further maturation under the influence of the thymic epithelium

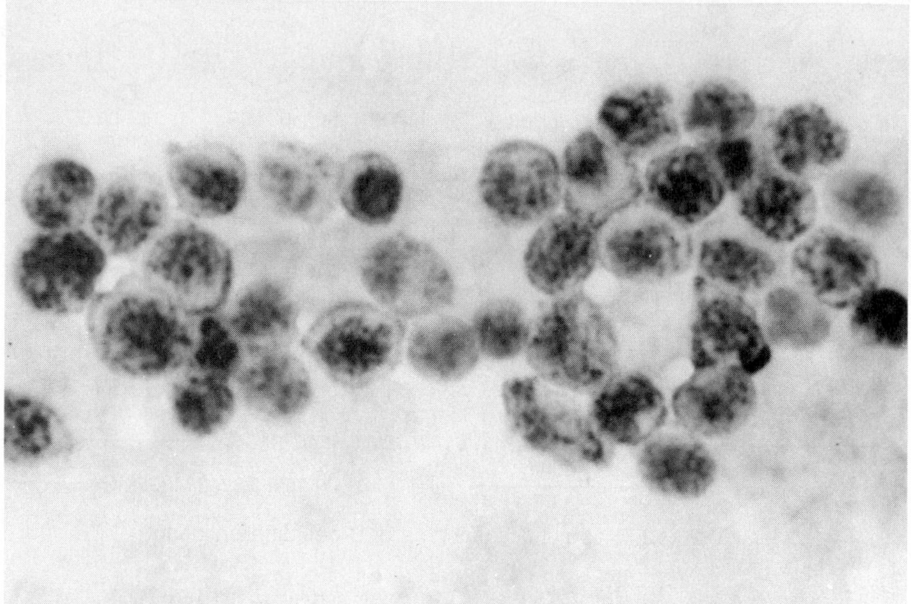

FIG. 26.13. The malignant lymphoblasts were isolated from this lymphoblastic lymphoma and placed into cell suspension. The cells then were placed onto a glass slide by cytocentrifugation, and the cytospin preparation was stained for the presence of intranuclear terminal deoxynucleotidyl transferase by immunoperoxidase. Essentially all the malignant lymphoblasts express strong intranuclear terminal deoxynucleotidyl tranferase positivity (immunoperoxidase stain, original magnification: 1,000× magnification).

(95,96). T-cell development in the thymus is characterized by distinct and sequential patterns of surface antigen expression and loss, accompanied by the progressive and orderly rearrangements of the genes encoding the T-cell receptor (TCR) (95,96). The prothymocytes lose HLA-DR and CD34, and continue to acquire cCD3 and CD2, as well as CD5,

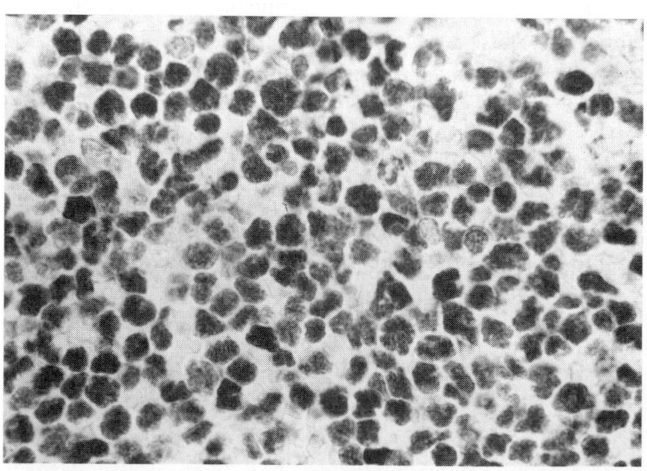

FIG. 26.14. The malignant lymphoblasts that constitute this mediastinal precursor T-cell lymphoblastic lymphoma were stained for intranuclear terminal deoxynucleotidyl transferase by immunoperoxidase staining of formalin-fixed, paraffin-embedded tissue sections. The majority of the malignant lymphoblasts express strong terminal deoxynucleotidyl transferase positivity (immunoperoxidase stain, original magnification: 630× magnification).

to become the immature thymocyte population. Immature thymocytes retain cCD3, CD7, CD2 and CD5 and acquire CD1, CD4 and CD8 to become common thymocytes, which comprise approximately 70% of all thymocytes. Those thymocytes that coexpress CD4 and CD8 are referred to as "double positive." The prothymocyte, immature thymocyte, and common thymocyte populations reside in the cortex. Common thymocytes lose CD1 and acquire the completely assembled TCR-CD3 surface membrane complex and differentiate along one of two pathways, either retaining CD4 and losing CD8 or retaining CD8 and losing CD4, to become mature (medullary) thymocytes. These cells variably express cCD3 and TdT. The mature thymocytes subsequently peripheralize, losing cCD3 and TdT entirely, and become the mature $CD4^+CD8^-$ (helper-inducer) and $CD4^-CD8^+$ (suppressor-cytotoxic) T-cell subsets, respectively. In addition to the T-cell differentiation–associated antigens discussed here and illustrated in Figure 26.11, thymocytes variably express a wide range of other molecules, including CD38, CD71 (the transferrin receptor), and various integrins and other receptors (97) (see Chapters 2, 3, and 6).

Investigators initially believed that CD3 was expressed by only about 10% to 15% of normal thymocytes (42) and was not commonly expressed by precursor T-cell LBLs (33,42–44). These findings were based on the cell suspension analysis of isolated thymocytes and lymphoblasts, which used cytofluorometric and immunofluorescent techniques to detect surface membrane but not cytoplasmic antigens. Immunohistochemical analysis performed on frozen tissue sections detects cytoplasmic and surface membrane antigens. Immunohistochemical studies have demonstrated that cytoplasmic CD3 is expressed before surface membrane CD3 in thymocytes (98), that more than 80% of thymocytes express surface membrane or cytoplasmic CD3 (98,99), and that CD3 frequently is expressed in the cytoplasm but not on the surface of malignant T lymphoblasts (34,90,98,100). This fact probably accounts for the discrepancies in the reported frequency of CD3 antigen expression by precursor T-cell LBLs described by investigators who have used cell suspension (33,42–44), compared with frozen tissue section (34,35,99,100), techniques.

Mammalian B cells are generated in the bone marrow and undergo differentiation (B-cell ontogeny) by direct interaction with cellular components and soluble factors within the bone marrow microenvironment (101). According to current concepts, B-cell ontogeny can be divided into several discrete stages according to the expression of B cell–restricted and associated cytoplasmic and surface membrane antigens. These stages can be referred to as *progenitor B cell, pre-pre-B cell, pre-B cell, immature B cell,* and *resting mature (naive) B cell* (69–72,76,102–105) (Fig. 26.12). The earliest identifiable B cells—progenitor B cells, express intranuclear TdT, HLA-DR, CD34, and CD79. Progenitor B cells acquire B-cell lineage–associated antigens CD19 and cCD22 to become pre-pre-B cells. Next, they acquire CD10 followed by B cell–associated antigen CD20. They begin to lose CD34 and continue to acquire CD20 and express surface membrane CD79 and cytoplasmic μ heavy chains unaccompanied by light chains as they enter the pre-B cell stage. Pre-B cells lose TdT, CD34, cytoplasmic μ heavy chains, and CD10; retain CD19, cCD22, CD20 and CD79; and acquire CD21 and surface IgM (sIgM) to become immature B cells. CD5 is expressed by a subset of immature B cells. As normal development proceeds, CD22 is exported to the cell surface, the average amount of sIgM decreases, an increasing amount of sIgD appears, and the cells become resting mature (naive) B cells. The naive B cell is a small lymphocyte that expresses HLA-DR, CD19, CD20, CD79, CD22, CD21, sIgM, and sIgD; is in the G_0 stage of the cell cycle; and has not yet undergone the events associated with activation. The naive B cell is the first B cell to exit the bone marrow and circulate in the peripheral blood, from which it can enter the lymph nodes, spleen, and mucosa-associated lymphoid tissues. Further differentiation into activated or differentiating B cells and secretory B cells (plasma cells) is antigen-dependent and occurs in the peripheral lymphoid tissues. The molecular events and other immunophenotypic changes that occur during antigen-independent and -dependent B-cell differentiation are discussed in Chapters 2, 6, and 7.

Based on monoclonal antibody studies, we now know that about 80% of LBLs are derived from precursor (thymic) T cells (33–36). We also have learned that approximately 20% of precursor T-cell LBLs lack sheep erythrocyte rosette receptors or are incapable of forming sheep erythrocyte rosettes (36,43,44). Reactivity with anti-T cell heteroantisera was helpful in identifying the T-cell origin of some sheep erythrocyte rosette–negative LBLs (57). Most heteroantisera suffer from impurities, low titer, or limited availability, however, making their specificity, sensitivity, and general application suboptimal. Reactivity with monoclonal antibodies that detect T-cell differentiation–associated antigens has proved to be the best indicator of the T-cell origin of an LBL. Many of the LBLs reported in the literature before the mid-1980s as ''null'' or ''non-B, non-T'' LBL (44,52,56) are actually of T-cell origin.

Precursor T-cell LBLs display a wide array of immunophenotypic profiles comparable to those expressed by developing T cells during the prethymic and intrathymic stages of normal T-cell differentiation (33,71–73,99). The non–T cell LBLs are derived from precursor B cells (33–35). These neoplasms display the pre-pre-B cell and pre-B cell immunophenotypes expressed by developing B cells during normal B cell differentiation (70,72). Very rarely, cases of LBL are derived from mature B cells and express monoclonal surface immunoglobulin (35). Both precursor T- and B-cell LBLs may be partially or wholly composed of neoplastic cells displaying convoluted or nonconvoluted nuclei. The nuclear configurations of the malignant lymphoblasts do not correlate with, nor can they be used to predict accurately, the lineage or the immunophenotypic profile of an LBL (29,33,35,43).

More than two thirds of precursor T-cell LBLs express immunophenotypic profiles consistent with the common and medullary thymocyte stages of T-cell differentiation (33–35,43–45,99,100). Virtually every precursor T-cell LBL is $CD7^+$; the vast majority express CD5, CD2, or CD3 (surface or cytoplasmic); and many express CD1, CD4, or CD8 as well. Fewer than one third of precursor T-cell LBLs express prothymocyte or immature thymocyte phenotypes, that is, express only CD5, CD2, or CD7 and lack CD3, CD1, CD4, and CD8 (33–35,43–45,94,99,100). Many precursor T-cell LBLs express CD71 and CD38 as well (34,35,43,44). Some investigators have claimed that many precursor T-cell LBLs express HLA-DR antigens (35). The majority of investigators, however, have found that only occasional precursor T-cell LBLs displaying prothymocyte and immature thymocyte immunophenotypes express HLA-DR antigens (33,94,99), paralleling normal T-cell differentiation (71–73). Precursor T-cell LBLs only very rarely express T-cell activation–associated antigen CD25 (interleukin-2 receptor) and CD15 and virtually never express CD30 (34,35,106–108). The expression of specific T cell–associated antigens and various immunophenotypic profiles by precursor T-cell LBLs does not appear to explain variabilities in clinical behavior among these patients or have prognostic significance (35,43–47). An exception may be the rare cases of adult prethymic ($CD7^+CD2^-$) LBLs associated with relatively indolent lymph node disease and, inexplicably, Langerhans' cell histiocytosis (109). This may represent a point of distinction with T-cell ALL, in which CD2 antigen expression has been found to be a powerful predictor of event-free survival (110).

Precursor T-cell LBLs often display considerable intratumor as well as intertumor immunophenotypic heterogeneity (33,34,43,111). Individual cases of precursor T-cell LBL often contain lymphoblasts that variably express multiple T-cell differentiation–associated antigens. In one instance, two immunophenotypically discrete neoplastic cell populations were demonstrated within the same neoplasm (112). These findings suggest that most precursor T-cell LBLs contain multiple neoplastic subpopulations that reflect a spectrum of T-cell developmental stages rather than one neoplastic cell population frozen at a single point in T-cell differentiation. Many precursor T-cell LBLs express immunophenotypes that do not parallel precisely the discrete stages defined in the hypothetical model of T-cell differentiation presented in Fig 26.11 and cannot be assigned precisely to one of the four major stages of thymic differentiation (35,43,44). This is probably because this scheme does not take into account the likely existence of additional transitional stages of T-cell maturation or the variable loss of T-cell differentiation–associated antigens that probably occurs during malignant transformation.

The TCR, the antigen recognition molecule on T cells, is a heterodimer composed of covalently linked α and β or, alternatively, γ and δ polypeptide chains (113) (see Chapters 3 and 7). Monoclonal antibodies WT31 (114) and βF1 (115) detect the $\alpha\beta$ TCR heterodimer, which is expressed by more than 90% of thymocytes and mature peripheral blood and lymphoid tissue T cells (114–117). Approximately 60% of precursor T-cell LBLs express $\alpha\beta$ TCR (116–118), making $\alpha\beta$ TCR the pan–T cell antigen least commonly expressed by precursor T-cell LBLs (116). The $\alpha\beta$ TCR–negative tumors tend to display a less mature phenotype (116,118), because the majority of surface $CD3^+$ precursor T-cell LBLs express $\alpha\beta$ TCR (119); this correlation is not absolute, however (116,118). $\alpha\beta$ TCR negative precursor T-cell LBLs tend to lack other pan–T cell antigens as well (116), raising the possibility that this anomalous immunophenotypic expression may be related to aberrant gene expression by the malignant lymphoblasts (116). Antibodies recognizing the δ chain detect the $\gamma\delta$ TCR heterodimer (120), which is expressed by less than 5% of benign normal T cells (121). Only approximately 10% to 20% of $CD3^+$ $\alpha\beta$ TCR–negative precursor T-cell LBLs express the $\alpha\beta$ TCR heterodimer, and these tumors are often $CD4^-CD8^-$ (122), the phenotype associated with normal $\alpha\beta$ TCR cells (121). In contrast, about two thirds of $CD3^+$ $\alpha\beta$ TCR–negative precursor T-cell ALLs express the $\gamma\delta$ TCR heterodimer (119). These findings support the contention that certain fundamental biologic differences exist between precursor T-cell LBL and precursor T-cell ALL.

Expression of the common ALL antigen CD10 initially was believed to be restricted to, and therefore was used as a specific immunodiagnostic marker for, common precursor B-cell ALL (123); however, CD10 is actually expressed by a wide range of B and T cell–derived hematopoietic neoplasms (70,124), including 20% or more of precursor T-cell LBLs (33–35,43,62,94,99,107,124). Therefore, the CD10 antigen is not useful in distinguishing between precursor B- and T-cell LBL. Moreover, $CD10^+$ and $CD10^-$ precursor T-cell LBLs do not appear to exhibit any obvious clinical differences, and CD10 antigen expression by precursor T-cell LBLs does not appear to carry prognostic significance (35). In contrast, both children and adults who have $CD10^+$ precursor T-cell ALL are significantly more likely to achieve a complete remission and have an increased duration of event-free survival than those who have $CD10^-$ precursor T-cell ALL (125,126).

A small number of precursor T-cell LBLs express natural killer cell–associated antigens CD16, CD56, or CD57 (35,127–131). These neoplasms are morphologically identical to other LBLs (35,127,128) except for the occasional ultrastructural identification of cytoplasmic membrane-bound, electron-dense granules (129–131). Parallel tubular arrays are absent (129–131). They similarly express TdT, cCD3, and immunophenotypic profiles comparable to those of precursor T-cell LBLs lacking natural killer cell–associated antigens, except perhaps for the frequent expression of HLA-DR antigens (127–131). Also, these LBLs often exhibit the germline configuration of the T-cell receptor and immunoglobulin genes (129–131). Human fetal thymus appears to contain a T- or natural killer cell bipolar progenitor cell population possessing the ability to differentiate into T cells and natural killer cells through separate precursors (132). It has been suggested that these natural killer cell antigen–positive LBLs are derived from this cell population (130). Also, it has been suggested that these patients differ clinically in that they are predominantly female and nonwhite, usually respond only briefly or not at all to aggressive combination chemotherapy and radiation therapy, and often die shortly after diagnosis (35,127,128). These natural killer cell antigen–positive precursor T-cell LBLs may represent a clinically and biologically distinct subgroup of LBLs, although more information is needed to support that conclusion.

The majority of precursor B-cell LBLs express pre-pre-B cell or pre-B cell immunophenotypes (34,35), similar or identical to those expressed by common type and pre-B cell ALL (47) (see Chapter 46). In addition, virtually all precursor B-cell LBLs express HLA-DR antigens and B cell–associated antigens CD19, CD79, or CD22 (surface or cytoplasmic) (34,35,47,70–72,104,133–137), and the majority variably express B cell–associated antigens CD20, CD24, and CD9 (35,70–72,135), the C3d receptor CD21 (34,70), the transferrin receptor CD71 (34,35), the activation antigen CD38 (33,34), and the hematopoietic progenitor cell-associated antigen CD34 (135,138). Exceptionally rare cases of LBL simultaneously express TdT and surface immunoglobulin (Knowles, unpublished observations) or apparently lack TdT but express surface immunoglobulin (35,139). These LBLs may represent the neoplastic counterpart of a pre-B cell in transition to a mature B cell. Leukemic counterparts coexpressing TdT and sIgM have been described and referred to as *transitional pre-B-cell ALL* (140). The expression of certain antigens, for example, CD10, CD13, CD15, CD24, CD33, and CD34, and particular immunophenotypic profiles by precursor B-cell ALLs carries clinical and prognostic significance (135,138,141–148). These clinical immunophenotypic correlations also may hold true for the precursor B-cell LBLs, but this has not been determined conclusively, most likely because insufficient numbers of cases have been analyzed. (These correlations are discussed in Chapter 46.)

The results of immunophenotypic analysis of precursor B- and T-cell LBLs or ALLs reported in the literature generally have been based on newly diagnosed and untreated patients. The malignant lymphoblasts appearing in relapsing patients usually, but not always, express the identical pretreatment immunophenotypic profile. The most common immunophenotypic alteration in precursor B-cell LBL or ALL appears to be a change in CD10 expression, most often diminution or loss and less commonly gain of the antigen at relapse (149–152). HLA-DR antigens may be lost or gained (150–152). Pui and colleagues (152) reported loss of TdT in 25% of cases. Both Bernard and coworkers (153) and Roper and associates (44) have reported losses, gains, and changes in density of various T cell–associated antigens among precursor T-cell LBLs at relapse, suggesting a shift in the differentiation status of the malignant cell population. A systematic investigation of a large cohort of newly diagnosed and relapsed patients who have lymphoblastic malignancies using extensive antibody panels has not been performed. The true incidence and complete nature of immunophenotypic alterations among these tumors at relapse is therefore unknown.

MOLECULAR GENETIC AND CYTOGENETIC FEATURES

Extensive molecular genetic and cytogenetic studies of precursor B- and T-cell ALL have been performed during the past decade. Substantially fewer comparable studies of precursor B- and T-cell LBL have been performed during the same period. This is because of the greater availability of leukemic specimens and the fact that these analyses are generally less difficult to perform on leukemia than on lymphoma specimens. ALL and LBL of corresponding cellular derivation, however, share overlapping clinicopathologic and immunophenotypic features: they sometimes are distinguished merely on the basis of arbitrary clinical criteria (31,35,39,43,47). Many investigators have suggested that ALL and LBL are related biologically and represent different manifestations of the same disease (37–40). At least some and perhaps many literature reports describing molecular genetic and cytogenetic analyses of ALL actually include cases of LBL. It remains difficult to summarize accurately the molecular genetic and cytogenetic characteristics of LBL *per se*. The following discussion is based on our current knowledge and understanding of the molecular genetic and cytogenetic characteristics of precursor B- and T-cell LBL and ALL. These features are discussed in more detail in Chapters 9, 10, and 46.

Immunoglobulin and TCR molecules represent the antigen-recognition molecules of B and T cells, respectively (154,155). The human genome contains three sets of immunoglobulin genes: the heavy chain locus (IgH) and the κ (IgL_κ) and λ light chain (IgL_λ) loci. A functional immunoglobulin protein molecule consists of the product of the rearranged IgH gene and either the rearranged IgL_κ or the IgL_λ gene (156). Four TCR loci have been identified: TCR_α, TCR_β, TCR_γ, and TCR_δ. The products of these genes are expressed in mutually exclusive pairs, $\alpha\beta$ and $\gamma\delta$ TCR (113). The structures of all these antigen receptor gene loci are similar: a series of discontinuously arranged coding regions designated constant (C), variable (V), joining (J), and diversity (D, only present in the IgH, TCR_β, and TCR_δ loci. Immunologic diversity is generated if individual elements of these regions within a gene are combined, allowing for transcription of an RNA message that can be translated to a unique immunoglobulin or TCR protein (73,157,158). Recombination (rearrangement) of the immunoglobulin and TCR genes occurs very early in B- and T-cell differentiation, respectively, and is generally but not entirely restricted to the B- and T-cell lineages (73,157,158). Rearrangement also occurs in a specific sequence, correlating with discrete stages of B- and T-cell differentiation (157). Consequently, clonal immunoglobulin and TCR gene rearrangements have been used widely as markers of B- and T-cell lineage, clonality, and differentiation (32,73,156–163) (see Chapters 7 and 9).

Until about 15 years ago, the majority of ALLs and a significant proportion of LBLs were designated *non-B, non-T* because their precise lineage was not demonstrable by immunophenotypic analysis (18,19,68). The discovery and mapping of the immunoglobulin and TCR gene loci, the cloning of numerous probes for these genes, and the widespread application of immunogenotypic analysis has permitted the lineage assignment of the lymphoblastic malignancies (156–158,164). Approximately 80% of LBLs and 20% of ALLs are of precursor T-cell origin, and the remaining 20% of LBLs and 80% of ALLs are of precursor B-cell origin (32–36).

A small subset (5%) of precursor B-cell LBLs and ALLs, predominantly those occurring in infants, express HLA-DR antigens and B-cell lineage–restricted antigen CD19 but do not exhibit clonal IgH or IgL gene rearrangements and customarily lack clonal TCR_γ and TCR_β gene rearrangements as well (165,166). Approximately 95% of precursor B-cell LBLs and ALLs, however, including virtually all of those occurring in children and young adults, exhibit clonal immunoglobulin gene rearrangements (156,164,167,168). Approximately two thirds of these cases exhibit IgH gene rearrangements, consistent with their immature stage of B-cell differentiation, and the remaining one third of cases exhibit both IgH and IgL gene rearrangements (156,157,164,167).

Correlative phenotypic and genotypic studies have demonstrated that those patients exhibiting IgH and IgL gene rearrangements express a more mature B-cell phenotype than those cases only exhibiting IgH gene rearrangement (167).

Precursor T-cell LBLs or ALLs expressing the prothymocyte phenotype (TdT-positive, $CD7^+$) may not rearrange any TCR genes or may rearrange only the TCR_δ gene (94,166,169–174). In some precursor T-cell LBLs and ALLs that express immature thymic phenotypes, the TCR_γ or TCR_δ gene may be rearranged, with the TCR_β gene in the germline configuration (166,169,172–174). Rarely, the opposite occurs (166). The TCR_α gene usually remains in the germline configuration in those precursor T-cell LBLs and ALLs expressing prothymocyte and immature thymocyte phenotypes and rearranges in those expressing more mature thymic phenotypes (175,176). The majority of precursor T-cell LBLs express mature thymic phenotypes, however, and exhibit rearrangement or deletion of the TCR_δ, TCR_γ, TCR_β, and TCR_α genes (73,94,166,168,169,171–173,175–180).

Immunoglobulin and TCR gene rearrangements are not entirely lineage-specific. Immunoglobulin genes rearrange in some T-cell malignancies, and TCR genes rearrange in some B-cell malignancies (181). This phenomenon has been referred to as *lineage promiscuity* (182); it occurs most commonly among precursor B- and T-cell neoplasms, that is, the lymphoblastic malignancies (168,177,179–186) (Fig. 26.15). This probably reflects the presence of common recombinase enzymes capable of recognizing similar recombination signals in the two types of loci (187).

The TCR genes rearrange more commonly among precursor B-cell LBL or ALL than do the immunoglobulin genes among precursor T-cell LBL or ALL (166–168,175,177, 184,188). The approximate incidence of TCR gene rearrangements in precursor B-cell LBL or ALL is 60% to 80% for TCR_δ, 40% to 80% for TCR_γ, 40% to 60% for TCR_α, and 20% to 40% for TCR_β (166,168,172,174,175,177,179–181, 183–186,188–191). The incidence of TCR gene rearrangements among precursor B-cell LBLs and ALLs correlates with the age of the patient and the stage of differentiation of the leukemic cell population (165,192). Common precursor B-cell ALLs occurring in children older than 2 years of age are more likely to exhibit TCR gene rearrangements than are pre-B cell or mature immunoglobulin-positive B-cell ALLs occurring in children younger than 2 years of age (165,192).

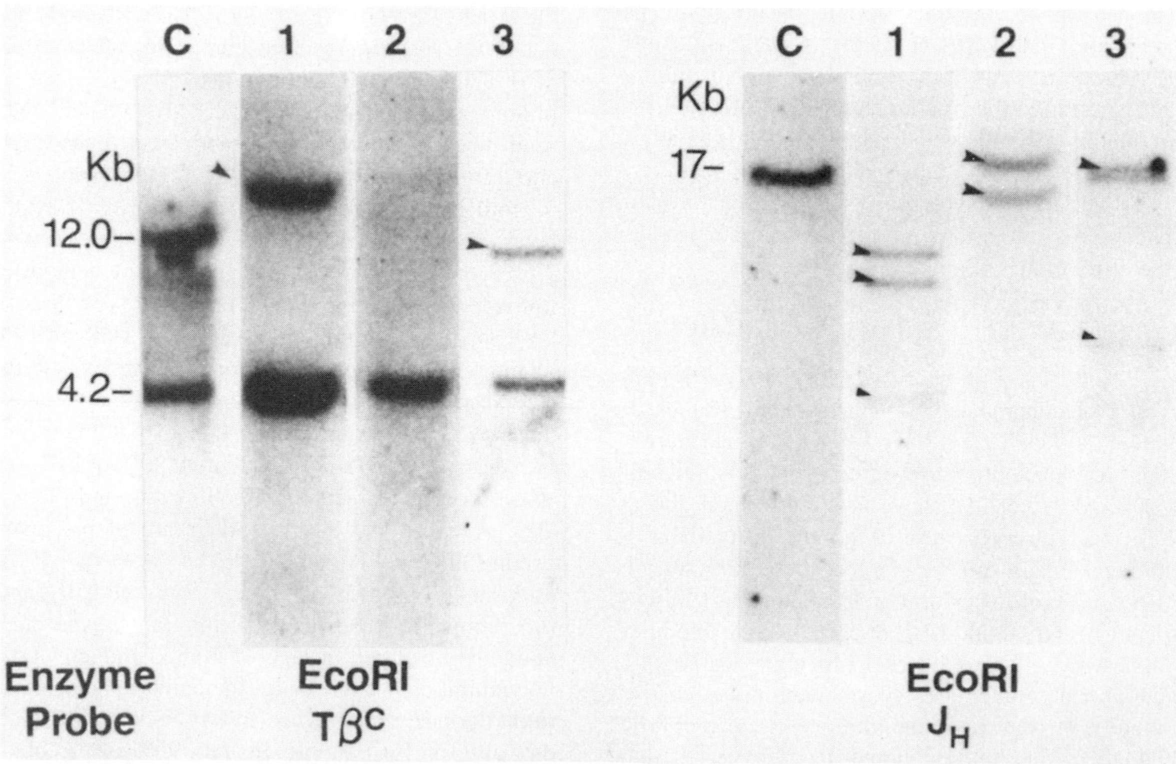

FIG. 26.15. Antigen receptor gene rearrangement analysis of three bigenotypic lymphoid neoplasms. Aliquots of DNA extracted from the three cases (lanes 1 through 3) and from normal human placenta were digested with EcoRI and hybridized to immunoglobulin heavy chain joining region and T-cell receptor β chain DNA probes. The control lane (*C*) shows the germline configuration. *Arrows* indicate rearrangement bands. Each neoplasm displays both immunoglobulin and T-cell receptor gene rearrangements or deletions. Despite this bigenotypism, each neoplasm expressed a B- or T-cell lineage–restricted immunophenotype. (From Pelicci PG, Knowles DM, Dalla-Favera R. Lymphoid tumors displaying rearrangements of both immunoglobulin and T cell receptor genes. *J Exp Med* 1985;162:1015–1024, with permission.)

Clonal IgH gene rearrangements occur in about 10% to 25% of precursor T-cell LBLs and ALLs (166,167,181,191, 193,194). In contrast, IgL gene rearrangements traditionally have been considered to be restricted to B cell–lineage neoplasms (159,160,166,167); however, IgL gene rearrangements have been reported, albeit rarely, in T-cell malignancies, including precursor T-cell LBL or ALL (195–197). IgL gene rearrangement is a reasonably specific but not a restricted molecular genetic marker for the B-cell lineage.

The interpretation of the results of immunogenotypic analysis of the lymphoblastic malignancies may be complicated by their complex genetic heterogeneity and lineage promiscuity. Most B cell–lineage neoplasms rearrange both IgH gene alleles (167,179), however, and most T cell–lineage neoplasms rearrange both TCR_β gene alleles (161,162,166, 168,180). B cell–lineage neoplasms that rearrange both TCR_β gene alleles and T cell–lineage neoplasms that rearrange both IgH gene alleles are uncommon (168,180,193, 198). Furthermore, T cell–lineage neoplasms only rarely rearrange the IgL genes (195–197) and precursor B- and T-cell LBL and ALL differ substantially with respect to the choice of joining and constant regions used for TCR_γ gene rearrangement (166,177,179,180,183). Nevertheless, the heterogeneous patterns of immunoglobulin and TCR gene rearrangement among the lymphoblastic malignancies underscore the necessity to exercise caution in assigning lineage based on the results of these assays alone. The results of immunogenotypic analysis, especially that of precursor B- and T-cell LBL or ALL, always should be interpreted in conjunction with morphologic examination and the results of immunophenotypic analysis.

As in the case of immunophenotypic analysis of precursor B- and T-cell LBL or ALL, the results of immunogenotypic analysis reported in the literature generally have been based on newly diagnosed and untreated patients. The malignant lymphoblasts in relapsing patients appear to represent reemergence of the original clone in about 80%, based on antigen receptor gene rearrangement patterns identical to those at diagnosis (199). In the remaining patients, changes in the antigen receptor gene rearrangement patterns at relapse suggest either clonal evolution or the development of an entirely new neoplasm (199). A significant proportion of the latter represent secondary acute myeloid leukemias (AML) exhibiting translocations involving 11q23 (199).

The overall frequency of chromosomal abnormalities in ALL or LBL ranges from 50% to 90% (200). These can be divided broadly into abnormalities of chromosome number and chromosome structure. The most common abnormalities that occur nonrandomly are hyperdiploidy (more than 50 chromosomes), t(1;19)(q23;p13), t(4;11)(q21;q23), del(6q), del(9p)t(9p), and del(12p)t(12p). Many of these recurring karyotypic abnormalities define clinicopathologically and immunologically distinct subgroups of patients, and some also appear to have prognostic relevance (200).

Approximately 30% to 40% of children (201–204) and 20% of adults (205–207) who have precursor B-cell ALL possess hyperdiploid blasts, that is, contain more than 46 chromosomes. A distinct clinicopathologic subgroup of children have FAB L1 or L2 lymphoblasts containing 51 to 65 chromosomes. These patients often have a simple gain of many chromosomes containing few structural abnormalities (204–207). They invariably have precursor B-cell ALL and usually are $CD10^+$. These patients usually also have other ''good prognosis'' factors, including age between 3 and 7 years and low white blood cell count (201,203,208); however, hyperdiploidy is an important, highly favorable independent prognostic factor (201,208,209). Combined trisomy of chromosomes 4 and 10 appears to account for the beneficial effect of hyperdiploidy (210). These patients enjoy the longest duration of disease-free survival of any cytogenetically defined ALL patient subgroup (200). These cases can be identified easily by DNA cytofluorometric analysis; they correspond to samples with a DNA index of about 1.16 to 1.60 (211) (see Chapter 5).

Other abnormalities in chromosome number are considerably less common and do not appear to constitute distinct syndromes (203,204). Hyperdiploid patients having 47 to 50 chromosomes should be distinguished from those having 51 to 65 chromosomes because they do not share the same favorable prognosis (204,212). Near tetraploidy occurs in about 1% of patients with ALL and appears to be preferentially associated with precursor T-cell ALL (213).

Abnormalities of chromosome structure involve translocations or other breaks at particular bands of a given chromosome. Some of these abnormalities have been defined at the molecular level and shown to involve activation of a cellular oncogene (see Chapter 8). Certain recurring translocations assist in defining distinct clinicopathologic entities. Two of the most widely studied translocations are the Philadelphia chromosome, t(9;22)(q34;q11), in which the *ABL* oncogene is translocated from chromosome 9 into the *BCR* gene on chromosome 22 (214,215), and the t(8;14)(q24;q32) and its variant translocations t(2;8)(p12;q24), t(8;22)(q24;q11), in which there is a reciprocal translocation between the *MYC* oncogene on chromosome 8 and the immunoglobulin gene loci on chromosome 14, 2, or 22 (216,217). The t(9;22) translocation results in the formation of one of two variants of the chimeric fusion gene *BCR/ABL*, a 190-kd product in t(9;22) childhood ALL or a 210-kd product in one third of patients with t(9;22) adult ALL (218). The t(9;22) translocation is associated commonly with precursor B-cell LBL or ALL (219) and only very rarely with precursor T-cell LBL or ALL (220). The t(9;22) imparts a particularly unfavorable prognosis in ALL (205,218,221,222). The t(8;14) is associated closely with Burkitt's lymphoma and FAB L3 immunoglobulin-positive B-cell ALL (223,224) and not LBL. (These translocations are discussed in more detail in Chapters 8, 10, and 46.)

Williams and associates (225) recognized and described the association of the t(1;19)(q23;p13) reciprocal translocation with the pre-B cell immunophenotype, that is, cytoplasmic μ chain–positive, in 1984. This translocation creates a molecular abnormality involving site-specific fusion of the *E2A* gene and the *PBX1* homeobox gene (226,227). The E2A-PBX-1 fusion protein likely acts as a transcriptional regulator (226,227). The translocation t(1;19)(q23;p13) occurs in about 20% to 30% of precursor B-cell ALLs displaying the pre-B cell immunophenotype, and only rarely in cases displaying other immunophenotypes (224,225, 227–229). Patients who have t(1;19)(q23;p13) characteristically present with low white blood cell counts, and their neoplastic cells express the CD10 antigen (230). Patients who have pre-B cell ALL with t(1;19)(q23;p13) have a less favorable outcome than those patients who lack this karyotypic abnormality and who express other precursor B-cell immunophenotypes if treated with antimetabolite-based therapy (230). Detection of the fusion gene product by polymerase chain reaction methods is useful in identifying t(1; 19) and detecting minimal residual disease (227).

Translocations involving chromosome band 11q23 and a variety of reciprocal breakpoint regions occur frequently in hematologic malignancies, including approximately 8% of ALLs, in which the translocation t(4;11) predominates (204–206,221,231,232). The t(4;11) results in the fusion of the *MLL* (mixed lineage leukemia) gene on 11q23 with the *AF4* gene on 4q21 (233). Among the ALL patients whose lymphoblasts exhibit t(4;11), approximately one half are adults and the other half are children, predominantly infants younger than 1 year of age (231,234–238). In most cases, the blasts are classifiable as FAB L1 or L2 lymphoblasts (239,240). Occasionally, blasts appear monocytoid and not lymphoid, and monocytoid blasts may coexist within the same case (241). The leukemic cells express a distinctive immunophenotype. They are TdT-positive and usually express HLA-DR and B cell–associated antigens CD19 and CD9 but not CD24 or CD10 (231,240–242). They often express CD15 (231,236,240,241), and a variable proportion of the cells may be myeloperoxidase, Sudan Black B, and nonspecific esterase stain–positive (241,242). They lack surface and cytoplasmic immunoglobulin- and T cell–associated antigens. This immunophenotype has caused many of these precursor B-cell ALLs to be referred to as *mixed lineage leukemias* (243). However, the neoplastic cells usually exhibit clonal IgH, and in some instances clonal IgL, gene rearrangements (239,242). Consequently, they probably are best regarded as a clinically and biologically distinct subset of precursor B-cell ALL (244,245). The patients usually present with hyperleukocytosis, often more than 200×10^9 leukocytes per liter, and hepatosplenomegaly, possess other aggresive clinical features, and have poor outcomes (231,234,236–238,246).

A variety of 12p12 rearrangements, including partial deletions and translocations, have been reported as nonrandom abnormalities in approximately 10% of childhood precursor B-cell ALLs (225,247). The translocation t(12;21)(p12;q22) was discovered in a fluorescent *in situ* hybridization analysis of ALLs with del(12)(p12) (248). The t(12;21) translocation results in fusion between the helix–loop–helix domain of the *TEL* gene on 12p (249) and the DNA-binding and transactivation domains of the *AML1* gene on 21q (250,251). The t(12;21) only rarely is identified by conventional cytogenetic banding techniques (252,253). With the use of fluorescent *in situ* hybridization, Southern blotting, and reverse transcriptase–polymerase chain reaction assays, *TEL* is found to be rearranged in about 25% of ALLs, with more than 90% of patients expressing a TEL-AML-1 chimeric gene product (253,254). The t(12;21) has become recognized as the most frequent molecular genetic abnormality in pediatric precursor B-cell ALL (253). It occurs much less frequently among patients with adult precursor B-cell ALLs (255). Furthermore, *TEL* gene rearrangement identifies a relatively homogeneous patient subgroup characterized by age between 1 and 10 years, lymphoblasts exhibiting a precursor B-cell ALL phenotype and nonhyperdiploid DNA content, and an exceptionally good outcome independent of other risk-stratifying factors, such as age and initial leukocyte count (253–256). The t(12;21) translocation is the first genetic abnormality to be associated with a favorable prognosis in childhood ALL.

Abnormalities of the short arm of chromosome 9, particularly those leading to the loss of material in the p21-22 region, are observed in about 10% of ALLs (204,257–260). Multiple tumor suppressor genes 1 and 2, encoding two previously identified inhibitors (p16 and p15) of the cyclin D–cyclin-dependent protein kinase 4 complex (261), are located within 9p21 (262). Abnormalities of 9p typically result in homozygous deletions (but not point mutations) of *MST1* and *MST2* gene sequences (263–268), which have been reported in as many as 95% of precursor T-cell LBLs and ALLs and in some precursor B-cell LBLs and ALLs using molecular techniques (263,267,268). *MST1* and *MST2* gene deletions and mutations have not been identified in other lymphoid malignancies (267). These data suggest that *MST1* or *MST2* gene inactivation may play a role in the pathogenesis of precursor T-cell LBL and ALL. Chilcote and coworkers (257) reported that 9p21 abnormalities are associated with lymphomatous features, namely, mediastinal enlargement, massive lymphadenopathy, splenomegaly, and T-cell phenotype at presentation. Murphy and colleagues (258) reported a statistically significant association between 9p abnormalities and high-risk factors at diagnosis, including older age, massive splenomegaly, high white blood cell count, and T-cell phenotype. However, 9p abnormalities and these same clinical features also may be seen in precursor B-cell ALL (269).

Hypereosinophilia has been described in association with precursor B- and T-cell LBL or ALL (270–274). The hypereosinophilia may be discovered prior to, concurrent with, or subsequent to the diagnosis of lymphoblastic malignancy (274). The translocation t(5;14)(q31;q32) has been described in several of these cases (272–274). The region 5q23-q33 includes the genes for the only known eosinophil growth factors (interleukin-3, interleukin-5, and granulocyte-macrophage colony-stimulating factor) (275). In at least two cases, the chromosomal translocation was cloned and found to involve the joining of the immunoglobulin heavy chain gene enhancer region to the promoter region for interleukin-3 (273,276). Thus, this translocation may activate the interleukin-3 gene, resulting in abnormal expansion of the eosinophil population (273).

Deletions of 6q occur in about 10% of ALLs as well (204–207,260). These cases lack a characteristic immunophenotype, and their prognostic significance is unclear. Not all of the structural chromosomal changes commonly observed in LBL and ALL appear to be associated with particular clinical features.

The first recurring karyotypic abnormality to be defined in precursor T-cell ALL was t(8;14)(q24;q11) (225). Subsequently, a distinct pattern of nonrandom karyotypic abnormalities began to emerge in precursor T-cell ALL; the same abnormalities also have been observed in precursor T-cell LBLs (277,278). Raimondi and colleagues (279) and Berger and associates (260) discovered abnormal karyotypes in 72% of pediatric T-cell ALLs and 75% of pediatric and adult T-cell ALLs, respectively. Kaneko and colleagues (278) discovered abnormal karyotypes in 73% and 94% of precursor T-cell ALLs and LBLs, respectively. Between 30% and 50% of the abnormal karyotypes included a breakpoint at 14q11, 7q34-36, or 7p15 (260,278,279).

The TCR_α and TCR_δ genes have been mapped to band q11 on chromosome 14 (280,281), and the TCR_β and TCR_γ genes have been mapped to bands q34-36 and p15 on chromosome 7, respectively (282,283). Molecular analysis of the translocation t(11;14)(p13;q11) in T-cell ALL provided evidence that the breakpoint on chromosome 14 occurs within the TCR_δ gene (284,285). Analysis of eight other recurring abnormalities in T-cell neoplasms involving breakpoints in 14q11, 7q35-36, and 7p15 have revealed that the break also occurs within the corresponding TCR gene in each instance (286). Analogous to B-cell neoplasms in which translocations frequently involve the chromosomal bands containing the IgH and IgL gene loci (158), the TCR gene loci frequently are involved in translocations specific for T-cell neoplasms, especially precursor T-cell LBLs and ALLs (260,287). These recurring translocations involving the TCR gene loci are of significant biological interest. Unlike those involving the immunoglobulin gene loci, however, they do not appear to carry prognostic significance (40).

Translocations involving band 14q11, the site of the TCR_α gene (280,286,288), occur in 20% or more of cases of precursor T-cell ALL and appear to be specific for the disease (260,279). The most common partner for the translocation is band 11p13 or 11p15 (260,279,286,288,289), the site of the putative oncogene, *TCL2*. A t(10;14)(q24;q11) translocation involving the *TCL3* oncogene occurs in 5% to 10% of cases of precursor T-cell LBL or ALL (290,291). A less common translocation, t(1;14)(p32;q11), has been shown to involve the *TAL1* gene on chromosome 1, which codes for a helix–loop–helix transcription factor (292). Chromosome 7 appears to be involved in several recurring abnormalities that occur preferentially in precursor T-cell ALL and LBL. These include t(7;7)(q32;q36), t(7;7)(p15;q11), t(7;14)(p15;q11), t(7;14)(q34-36;q11), t(7;9)(q34-36;q34), t(7;9)(q34-36;q32), and t(7;19)(q34-36;p13), among others (260, 277,293). In addition, Berger and colleagues (260) described deletions or translocations involving 11q14-q21 in several patients with T-cell ALL, and Kaneko and associates (294) described a novel translocation, t(9;17)(q24;q23), in three children who had clinically aggressive precursor T-cell LBL.

DIFFERENTIAL DIAGNOSIS

Under normal conditions, TdT-positive precursor B and T cells are confined to the thymus and bone marrow; they are not normally observed in the peripheral blood or in peripheral lymphoid tissue (21,23,37,76). TdT-positive cells, many of which also express CD10 (295,296), represent about 2% to 7% of bone marrow cells in neonates and children up to 5 years of age, and 1% to 2% of those in adults (297,298). Under certain physiologic conditions, such as regenerating bone marrow following chemotherapy and bone marrow transplantation, TdT-positive cells may account for up to 20% of the bone marrow cellularity (296–301). Malignant lymphoblasts must be distinguished from these benign TdT-positive progenitor cells or "hematogones" (295). If this phenomenon occurs in patients who have a history of precursor LBL or ALL, distinguishing these nonneoplastic hematogones from residual or recurrent malignant lymphoblasts can be problematic, because they resemble FAB L1 lymphoblasts morphologically (302). They may be distinguished by their relatively more compact nuclear chromatin and lack of discernable cytoplasm (295). Also, they nearly always can be distinguished from malignant lymphoblasts by further immunophenotypic characterization, expecially using multiparameter flow cytometry (295,302). This is because they are more heterogeneous in their expression of B lineage–associated antigens than are malignant lymphoblasts (295,303). Finally, they are not monoclonal and can be distinguished from malignant lymphoblasts at the molecular level, if necessary (301).

Lymphoblastic lymphoma may be confused histologically with several categories of non-Hodgkin's lymphoma and several other hematopoietic and nonhematopoietic neoplasms (see Chapter 30). In children, the principal differential diagnosis of LBL includes Burkitt's and diffuse large cell lymphoma (31,304). Depending on the location of disease, the differential diagnosis of LBL also may include Ewing's sarcoma, neuroblastoma, primitive neuroectodermal tumor, and embryonal rhabdomyosarcoma (305–307). In adults, the differential diagnosis of LBL must be extended to include small lymphocytic lymphoma, mantle cell lymphoma (especially the lymphoblastic variant), and follicular and diffuse follicle center cell lymphoma, neuroendocrine neoplasms, such as oat cell carcinoma and cutaneous Merkel cell carcinoma, and thymoma (308–312). These entities are not usually included in the differential diagnosis of pediatric LBL because they occur either very rarely or not at all in children (31,37,304,309,311,312). It is important that the pathologist be capable of identifying LBL correctly and distinguishing it from these other entities because the therapy, management, and prognosis of LBL differ substantially from those of these other neoplasms (49,304,309,311).

Knowledge of the clinical presentation and principal site of disease is very helpful in the differential diagnosis of pediatric LBL. Among children, the distribution of LBL is nearly always supradiaphragmatic, especially mediastinal, and only rarely abdominal, whereas the distribution of Burkitt's lymphoma is nearly always abdominal and almost never mediastinal (31,51,313,314). The primary site of childhood diffuse large cell lymphoma is highly variable and includes nodal and extranodal locations, with the general exception of the mediastinum (31,51). Those apparently arising in the mediastinum resemble the primary mediastinal large B-cell lymphomas of adults and account for nearly all the rare mediastinal nonlymphoblastic lymphomas of childhood (314). Each of these categories of non-Hodgkin's lymphoma displays distinctive morphologic and cytochemical features that serve as useful criteria in their differential diagnosis (51,304,314) (Fig. 26.16, Table 26.2) (see Chapters 25 and 27).

In adults, LBL may be misinterpreted as small lymphocytic lymphoma, mantle cell lymphoma, or diffuse follicle center cell lymphoma. In addition, LBL rarely may exhibit a pseudofollicular growth pattern, because of the tendency of malignant lymphoblasts to be compartmentalized by con-

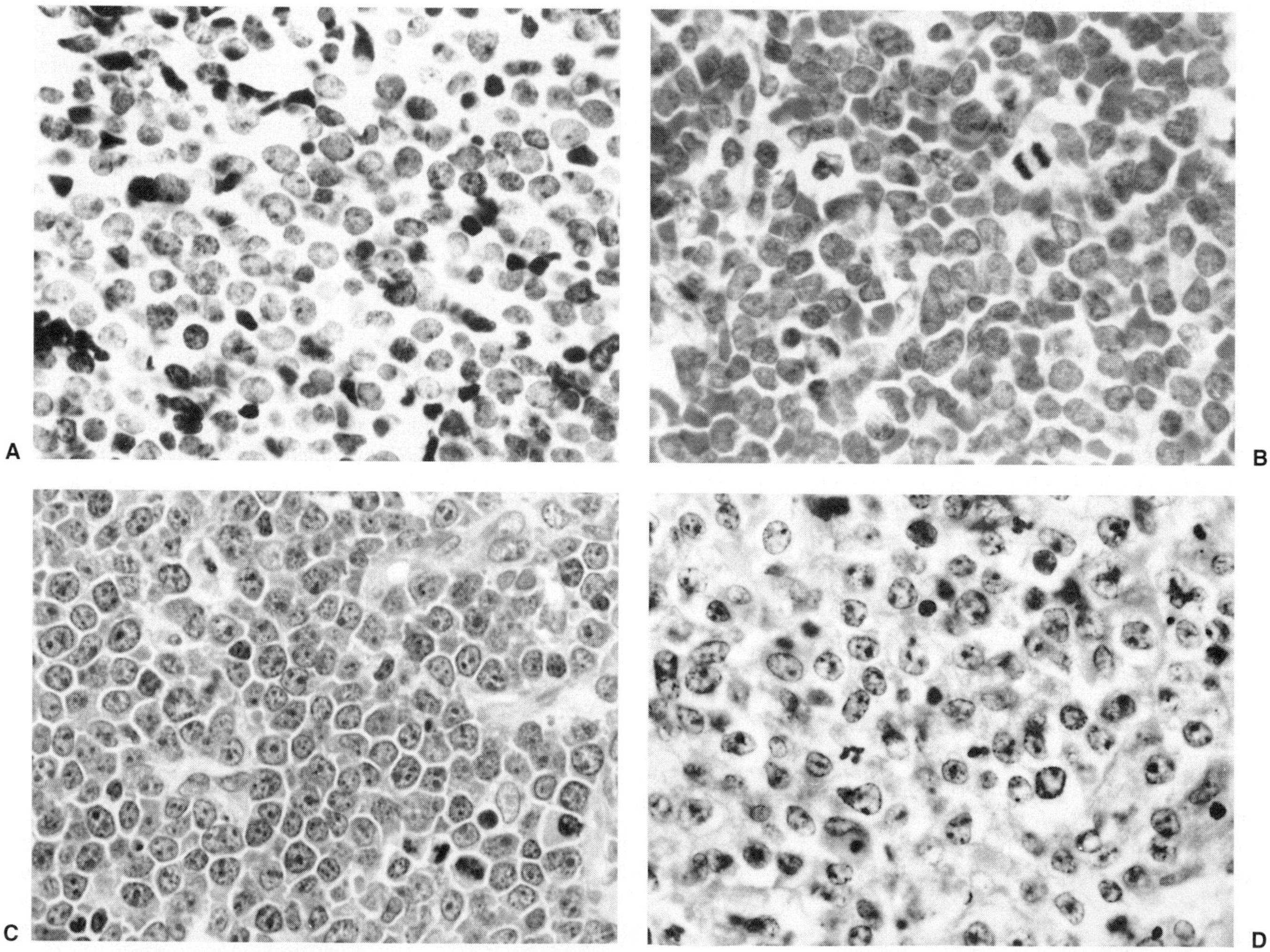

FIG. 26.16. Comparison of the histopathologic features of lymphoblastic lymphoma (**A,B**), Burkitt's lymphoma (**C**), and large B-cell lymphoma (**D**). The neoplastic cells of lymphoblastic lymphoma characteristically contain scant cytoplasm and have either round monotonous nuclei or variably irregular nuclei with convolutions. They also have finely dispersed and evenly distributed nuclear chromatin and small and inconspicuous nucleoli. The malignant cells of Burkitt's lymphoma contain a moderate amount of cytoplasm, have round and monotonous nuclei, and have clumped chromatin with two to five nucleoli. The malignant cells of large B-cell lymphoma contain moderately abundant cytoplasm, have large round to slightly irregular nuclei, and usually contain one prominent nucleolus adjacent to the nuclear membrane (hematoxylin and eosin stain, original magnification: 630× magnification).

TABLE 26.2. *Comparison of the morphologic and cytochemical features of lymphoblastic, Burkitt's, and large cell lymphoma*

	Lymphoblastic	Burkitt's	Burkitt's-like	Large cell
Imprint cytology Wright stain	FAB L1; occasional FAB L2 blasts	FAB L3 blasts	FAB L3 blasts	Variable large transformed lymphocytes, immunoblasts
Nuclear size	Smaller than macrophage nucleus	Approximates macrophage nucleus	Approximates macrophage nucleus but variable	Larger than macrophage nucleus
Nuclear shape	Round and monotonous or variably irregular with convolutions	Round and monotonous	Variably round to ovoid	Variable
Nuclear chromatin	Fine, dust-like	Diffusely clumped	Diffusely clumped	Variably vesicular
Nucleoli	Small, inconspicuous	2–5, often prominent	1–3, occasionally single, central and prominent	Variable, from inconspicuous to central and prominent
Mitotic index	High	High	High	Moderate to high
Cytoplasm	Scant	Moderate	Moderate	Moderate to abundant
Cytoplasmic vacuoles	Inconspicuous	Prominent oil red O positive	Prominent oil red O positive	Inconspicuous
Periodic acid–Schiff stain	Occasionally positive	Negative	Negative	Occasionally positive
Methyl green pyronin stain	Usually negative or focal positive	Strongly positive	Strongly positive	Usually positive

FAB, French–American–British classification.

Modified from Wilson JF, Jenkin RDT, Anderson JR, et al. Studies on the pathology of non-Hodgkin's lymphoma of childhood I: the roles of routine histopathology as a prognostic factor. A report from the Children's Cancer Study Group. *Cancer* 1984;53:1695–1704, with permission.

nective tissue planes. This may result in the formation of variably sized and shaped nodules of lymphoblasts separated by collagen strands and small aggregates of residual, non-neoplastic lymphocytes that may mimic a cytologic grade I follicle center cell (follicular, predominantly small cleaved cell) lymphoma (315,316). Small lymphocytic lymphoma is composed predominantly of monomorphic small lymphocytes containing round, regular nuclei with peripheral clumped chromatin. Follicle center cell lymphoma, cytologic grade I, is composed predominantly of small lymphocytes containing angulated, indented, and cleaved nuclei with clumped chromatin and variable numbers of large ''transformed'' lymphocytes with vesicular nuclei containing one or more distinct nucleoli. These large transformed lymphocytes form pseudofollicular proliferation centers in small lymphocytic lymphoma. Mantle cell lymphoma represents a diffuse or vaguely nodular mantle zone proliferation of small lymphocytes possessing slightly irregular nuclei containing evenly distributed, condensed chromatin and inconspicuous nucleoli. Rarely, nuclear irregularities may be marked, approaching a convoluted appearance. Epithelioid histiocytes are usually present, interspersed among the lymphoma cells (312). These lymphomas generally exhibit a low proliferation index (308) (see Chapters 21, 22, and 24). In contrast, LBL represents a diffuse monomorphic proliferation of lymphoblasts possessing round to ovoid or convoluted nuclei containing evenly distributed, finely dispersed, dust-like chromatin and inconspicuous nucleoli and exhibiting a very high proliferation index. The lymphoblastic variant of mantle cell lymphoma may represent the most difficult morphologic differential diagnosis, because the neoplastic cells resemble lymphoblasts and display a large amount of mitotic activity, although epithelioid histiocytes are usually abundant, in contrast with LBL, in which the latter cells are absent and tingible body macrophages may be present (28,29,51,304,312) (Figs. 26.7, 26.16). Careful attention to the monomorphism, cytomorphology, and mitotic activity of the neoplastic proliferation usually permits the recognition of LBL and its distinction from these other entities. These same morphologic features can be used to recognize LBL in fine needle aspiration biopsy specimens (317,318) (Fig. 26.17) (see Chapter 13).

Immunophenotypic analysis, particularly the demonstration of TdT positivity, is a useful adjunct to the morphologic diagnosis of LBL and is often very helpful in distinguishing LBL from the other categories of non-Hodgkin's lymphoma and from other hematopoietic neoplasms with which it may be confused morphologically. Virtually all malignant lymphoblasts comprising essentially all precursor B- and T-cell LBLs are TdT-positive (10,20–23,34,37,77–79). In contrast, none of the malignant lymphoid cells comprising essentially any cases of nonlymphoblastic non-Hodgkin's lymphoma express TdT (10,73,78,297,319). AMLs occasionally are confused with LBL, especially if they present in lymph nodes, the skin, or in the mediastinum (320,321). The majority of AMLs are also TdT-negative (22,23,79,322,323), but

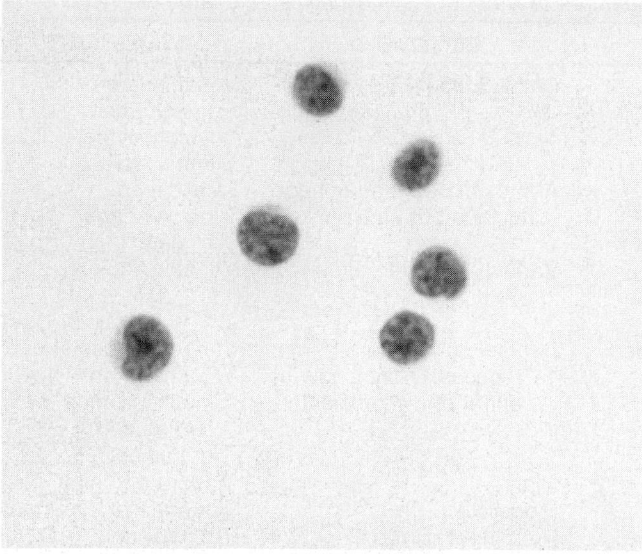

FIG. 26.17. Fine needle aspiration biopsy specimen from a lymph node that contains lymphoblastic lymphoma. The malignant cells display the characteristic cytomorphologic features of malignant lymphoblasts (papanicolaou stain, original magnification: 1,000× magnification).

as many as 20% of AMLs apparently contain TdT-positive malignant cells (324). In these cases, the proportion of TdT-positive blasts coexpressing myeloid-associated antigens is variable and often represents only a small subset of the total malignant cell population. In most series, TdT-positive AML is diagnosed if as few as 5% to 10% TdT-positive malignant cells are identified (324). The determination of TdT expression remains valid and useful in the differential diagnosis of LBL and AML but should be employed in the context of a thorough immunophenotypic analysis (76).

Because precursor T- and B-cell LBLs are morphologically identical and TdT-positive, additional immunophenotypic analyses are necessary to differentiate between them. Such studies are also useful in distinguishing LBLs from other non-Hodgkin's lymphomas and from AMLs. The most sensitive, although not the most specific, marker for precursor T-cell LBL is CD7. More than 95% of precursor T-cell LBLs, even those exhibiting the most immature phenotypes and lacking clonal T cell receptor gene rearrangements, express CD7 (34,35,45,47,73,76,325,326). CD7 expression does not necessarily imply a T cell lineage derivation, however. Approximately 5% to 20% of *de novo* AMLs, primarily those belonging to the FAB M0 and M1 categories, express CD7 as well (327–333). The most specific marker for precursor T-cell LBL is cytoplasmic CD3 (cCD3), which is expressed by nearly all patients (34,98,334,335) and is uniformly absent from precursor B-cell LBLs and AMLs (71–73,334,336–338). In addition, the majority of T-cell LBLs express surface membrane CD5, CD2, CD4, or CD8 (32,34,35,42–47,71–73,98–100,338). Virtually no precursor T-cell LBLs express CD19, CD20, CD22, or CD24 (34,35,44,47,71,94,133,134,338). In contrast, approximately 95% or more precursor B-cell LBLs express C19, CD79, and surface or cytoplasmic CD22 (34,45,47,69–71,104,133, 134,136,137,338–340), about 50% express CD20 (34,71,337,341–343) and none express CD7, CD3, CD5, CD2, CD4, or CD8 (34,35,47,69,71–73,325,326,338). In addition, nearly all precursor B-cell LBLs, but only a small number of precursor T-cell LBLs, express HLA-DR (45,135); approximately 90% of precursor B-cell LBLs but only 25% of precursor T-cell LBLs express CD10 (34,125,144,344–347), and 75% of precursor B-cell LBLs but only 5% of precursor T-cell LBLs express CD34 (348–351). A varied but generally small proportion of AMLs express CD7 (182,322,327–333), CD2 (333, 352–354), a cytoplasmic protein that cross-reacts with CD22 (133,134), CD4 (333), and CD79 (355), and only rare AMLs express CD19 (134,338) and CD20 (331). The majority of AMLs, even those that are TdT-positive or myeloperoxidase-negative, express myeloid-associated antigen CD13 or CD33 (322,323), which are expressed much less commonly by precursor T- and B-cell LBLs (47,135). Finally, virtually all non-Hodgkin's lymphomas of nonlymphoblastic type express either mature B cell (often accompanied by monotypic surface immunoglobulin) or mature, postthymic T-cell immunophenotypes (47,71–73,338). A judiciously planned cytofluorometric analysis of viable cells in suspension or immunohistochemical analysis of frozen or even paraffin tissue sections usually can distinguish precursor B- and T-cell LBL from each other and from all other hematopoietic neoplasms with which they may be confused morphologically.

In adults, LBL presenting as an anteriosuperior mediastinal mass must be distinguished from thymoma, a neoplasm derived from thymic epithelium (309). The neoplastic thymic epithelial cells possess poorly defined cytoplasmic borders and large round to slightly irregular nuclei that sometimes contain a single small nucleolus; they are differentiated easily from the lymphoblasts of LBL (309) (Fig. 26.18). The majority of thymomas, however, also contain variable numbers of benign thymocytes. These may be numerous enough to obscure the epithelial component and thereby simulate malignant lymphoma, especially LBL (309,356). This diagnostic dilemma most commonly occurs in small mediastinoscopic biopsy specimens, in which the other morphologic features of thymoma, such as "perivascular lakes," may be absent. This differential diagnosis often is morphologically resolvable because, in contrast to malignant lymphoblasts, benign thymocytes generally contain clumped chromatin and are mitotically inactive (309) (Fig. 26.18). Immunophenotypic analysis is not usually helpful, because benign thymocytes and malignant T lymphoblasts express similar immunophenotypic profiles including TdT positivity (47,357–359). Electron microscopy is usually helpful, because it readily demonstrates the presence of thymic epithelial cells and their numerous long cytoplasmic processes containing dense bundles of tonofilaments and desmosomes (309,356). The simplest and most practical diagnostic adjunct is immunohistochemical staining of frozen or paraffin

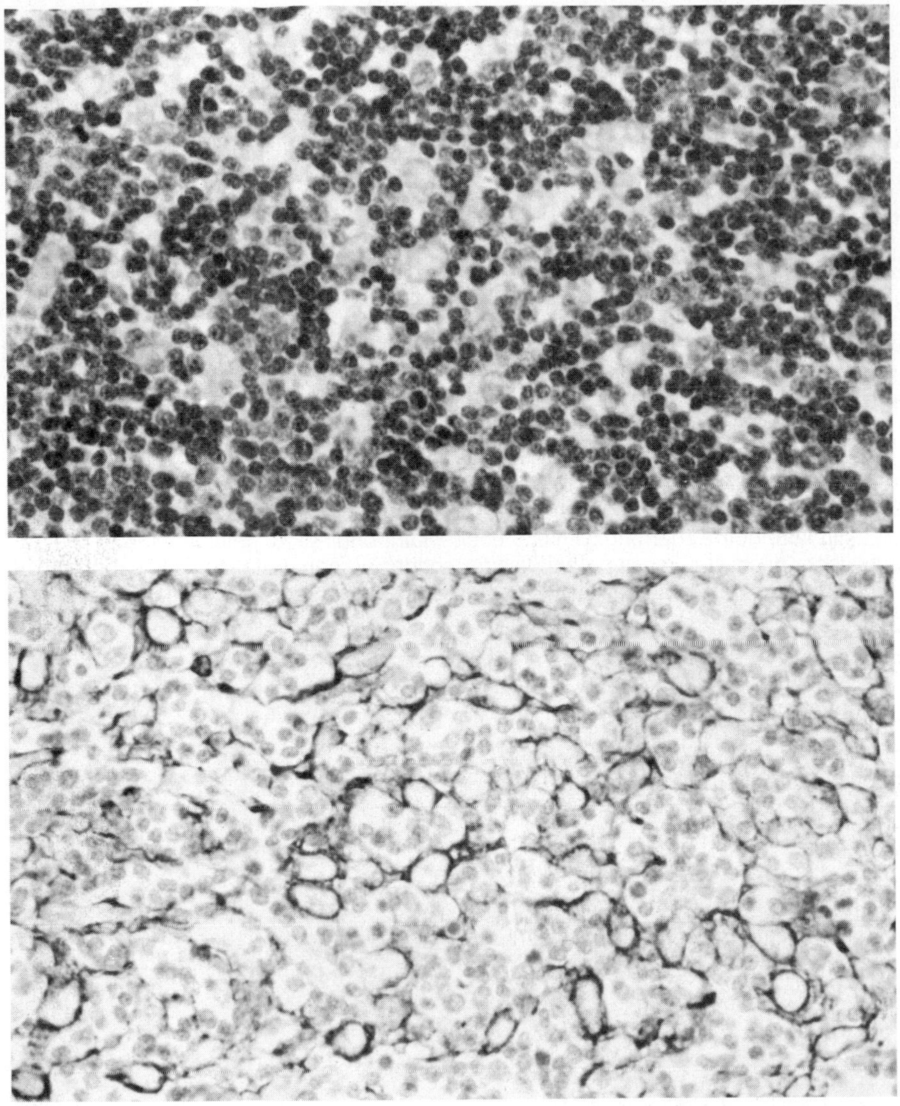

FIG. 26.18. **A:** Histopathologic section of a thymoma containing large numbers of monotonous small round lymphoid cells that simulate a lymphoblastic lymphoma. A starry-sky pattern of tingible body macrophages and mitotic figures indicative of rapid lymphoid proliferation are absent, however, and epithelial cells containing large, round to slightly irregular nuclei, sometimes with a small nucleolus, punctuate the lesion (hematoxylin and eosin stain, original magnification: 630× magnification). **B:** Immunohistochemical staining of paraffin tissue sections reveals the presence of numerous cytokeratin positive epithelial cells and a dendritic pattern of cytokeratin positive processes throughout the neoplasm, confirming the diagnosis of thymoma (immunoperoxidase stain, original magnification: 630× magnification).

tissue sections for cytokeratin, however (356,360) (Fig. 26.18). Thymic epithelial cells and their long cytoplasmic processes contain cytokeratin and, therefore, form a conspicuous fluorescent or peroxidase-positive network throughout all thymomas that permits their differentiation from LBL and all other malignant lymphomas that virtually always lack cytokeratin (356,360). If all these approaches fail, antigen receptor gene rearrangement analysis usually provides a definitive diagnosis. The vast majority of LBLs exhibit clonal rearrangements of the antigen receptor genes (157,158,161); these genes remain in the germline configuration in thymomas (358,361).

An LBL sometimes may be misinterpreted as a nonhematopoietic neoplasm, including, for example, Ewing's sarcoma, neuroblastoma, primitive neuroectodermal tumor, embryonal rhabdomyosarcoma, oat cell carcinoma, or Merkel cell carcinoma (305–307,309–311) (Fig. 26.19). This usually happens if LBL manifests clinically as a solitary neoplasm involving bone, skin, or another extranodal site. Each of these entities displays distinctive histopathologic features that usually permit their differential diagnosis (307,309,310,362–365). In those instances in which an unequivocal morphologic diagnosis cannot be made and fresh tissue is not available for immunophenotypic analysis, im-

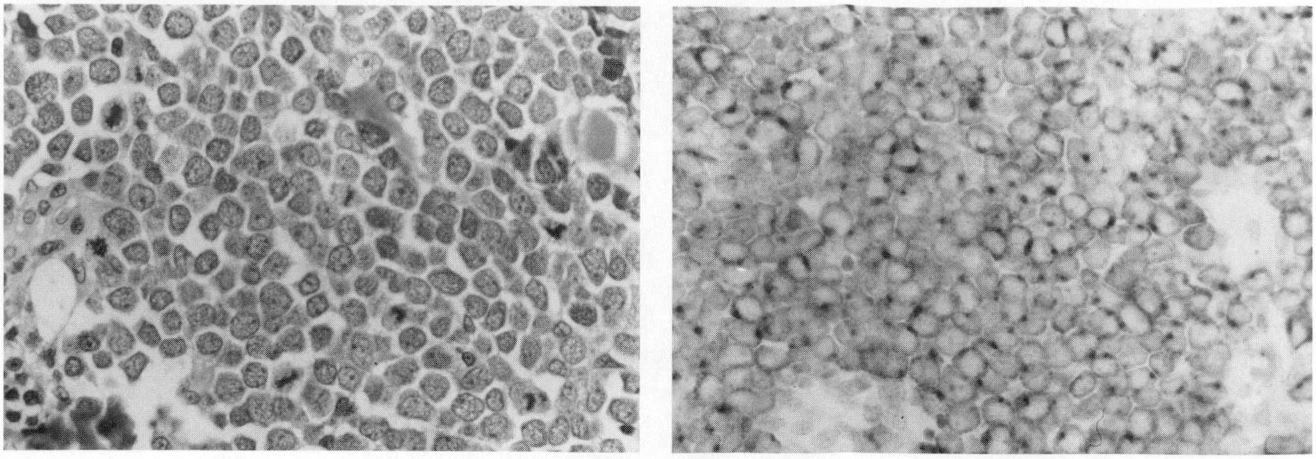

FIG. 26.19. Cutaneous Merkel cell carcinoma that simulates cutaneous presentation of lymphoblastic lymphoma. **A:** Clusters of neoplastic cells that exhibit cytomorphologic features closely resembling those of lymphoblastic lymphoma (hematoxylin and eosin stain, original magnification: 630× magnification). **B:** Immunohistochemical staining of paraffin tissue sections demonstrates that the neoplastic cells exhibit characteristic dot-like cytokeratin positivity (immunoperoxidase stain, original magnification: 400× magnification).

munohistochemical staining of paraffin tissue sections usually results in a definitive diagnosis. LBLs virtually always lack the markers expressed by nonhematopoietic neoplasms, namely, cytokeratin, epithelial membrane antigen, neuron-specific enolase, chromagranin, synaptophysin, muscle-specific actin, myoglobin, and desmin. One should not rely solely on the determination of CD45 (leukocyte common antigen) expression to distinguish betweeen LBL and epithelial and mesenchymal neoplasms. As many as 20% of LBLs lack CD45, and among those LBLs that do express CD45 the intensity varies greatly (135,341,366–373) (Fig. 26.20) (see Chapter 30).

CLINICAL CHARACTERISTICS AND NATURAL HISTORY

Lymphoblastic lymphoma constitutes approximately one third to one half of all pediatric non-Hodgkin's lymphomas

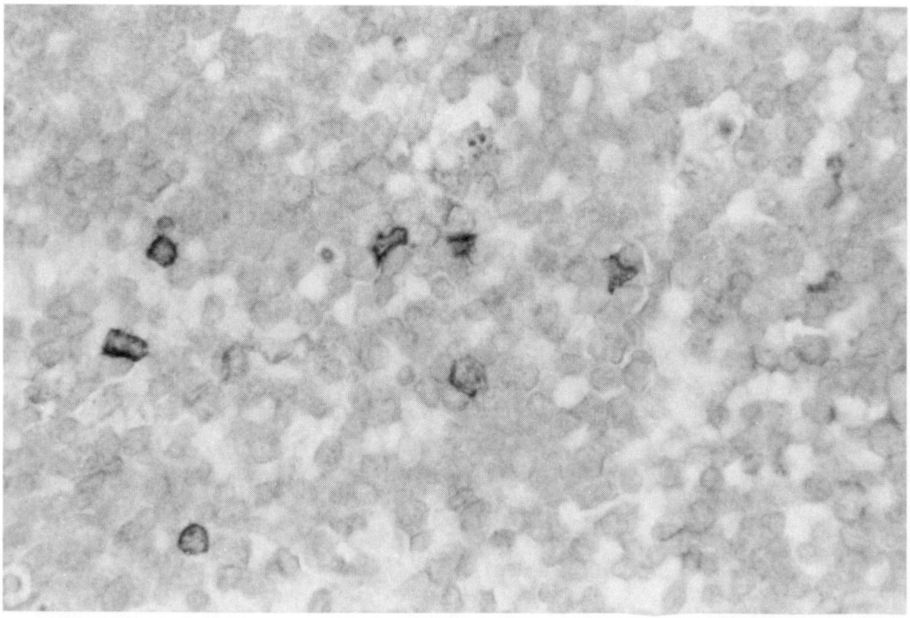

FIG. 26.20. Mediastinal precursor T-cell lymphoblastic lymphoma immunostained for CD45 (leukocyte common antigen) in formalin-fixed, paraffin-embedded tissue sections. A small number of cells, probably benign thymocytes, are strongly CD45-positive. The majority of malignant lymphoblasts, however, express CD45 in very low density (immunoperoxidase stain, original magnification: 400× magnification).

(31,49,51). In contrast, LBL occurs much less frequently among adults, accounting for only 3% to 5% of all adult non-Hodgkin's lymphomas (52,374). About 50% of children who have LBL are 10 years of age or older (51), and the majority of adults who have LBL are younger than 30 years of age (28,36,375). The peak incidence of LBL occurs in the second and third decades. Nathwani and coworkers (29), however, identified a bimodal age distribution among adults, with a second peak incidence in the seventh decade. Men appear to exhibit this bimodal age distribution; in women LBL appears to be evenly distributed over all decades (29). Men predominate in all age groups; male-to-female ratios between 2 : 1 and 10 : 1 have been reported (27–29,35,36, 49,51,375). There is a strong predilection for LBL to occur in older children, adolescents, and young adults, predominantly males (27–29,36,49,52,375), although LBL has been reported to occur in males and females of all ages, from the first year (376) through the tenth decade of life (374). LBL does not exhibit any obvious racial predilections (28,29).

The majority of children and adults have advanced disease, Murphy stages 3 and 4 (31,377) and Ann Arbor stages III and IV (378), respectively, at presentation (29,36,39,45, 49,52,375,379). Among 106 children who had LBL accessioned by the Pediatric Oncology Group, 64% presented with a mediastinal mass and 74% presented with peripheral lymphadenopathy, which was distributed as follows: 46% with mediastinal mass and peripheral lymphadenopathy, 28% with peripheral lymphadenopathy without a mediastinal mass, and 18% with a mediastinal mass without peripheral lymphadenopathy (49). The distribution of disease among adults appears to be comparable (29,36,52,374,375,379). Nathwani and colleagues (29) found that adult men and women who have mediastinal masses are significantly younger than those who do not, with medians of 23.5 versus 45 and 25 versus 54 years of age, respectively. They also found that a mediastinal mass is more common in males than in females (29).

Mediastinal involvement is often massive in patients who have LBL; the diameter of the tumor frequently reaches between 10 and 17 cm (374,379). This commonly results in progressive airway obstruction leading to dyspnea (27,39,52, 374,375,380), bilateral pleural effusions, pericardial effusion, and sometimes esophageal compression leading to dysphagia (52,379–381). Most patients who have mediastinal masses present with 2- to 4-week histories of upper respiratory tract infections with malaise and cough, progressive dyspnea, or chest pain (27,31). Some patients present with the superior vena cava syndrome (9,36,374,380). Occasionally, patients experience an acute onset of symptoms that may be life-threatening, precipitating a medical emergency (27,52,380).

Most patients who lack symptomatology attributable to a mediastinal mass present with peripheral lymphadenopathy. This is nearly always supradiaphragmatic in distribution and predominantly cervical, supraclavicular, or axillary (27,36,374). Asymptomatic mediastinal involvement sometimes is discovered during the evaluation of peripheral lymphadenopathy (51). Occasionally, patients also complain of single or multiple subcutaneous nodules that may grow rapidly (27,51,375,382). Fewer than 5% of patients present with predominantly abdominal disease (49,51). Hepatosplenomegaly because of disease involvement is uncommon at presentation (28,374,375). Approximately one third to one half of patients complain of B symptoms, that is, fevers, night sweats, and weight loss (29,36,374,375,379). In rare instances, myasthenia gravis accompanies mediastinal precursor T-cell LBL and resolves spontaneously following therapeutically induced clinical remission of the LBL (383–386).

Lymphoblastic lymphoma has the highest incidence of secondary involvement of the central nervous system (CNS) of any category of non-Hodgkin's lymphoma (387,388). Lymphoblastic histology has been identified as an independent predictive factor for CNS involvement by multivariate analysis (389). The CNS is involved at presentation in approximately 20% of patients (374,375,388,390,391) and is often the initial site of relapse (36,51,374). Progressive CNS involvement commonly occurs among these patients; as many as one half have CNS disease at some point during their clinical course (28,52,374,375,387,388,390,391). CNS involvement consists of leptomeningeal infiltration and frequently is accompanied by malignant cells in the cerebrospinal fluid (51,374,387,388). This may manifest clinically as lethargy, headaches, visual disturbances, extremity weakness, or cranial nerve disorders (374,387,388). Symptoms referable to the spinal cord may be produced by meningeal infiltration, extradural compression, or ischemia (51,388).

The testes and ovaries may be involved at presentation (36), may serve as initial sites of relapse (51), or may be involved during the course of the disease (27,374). Gonadal involvement usually manifests clinically as an asymptomatic or painful enlarging mass. More than 20% of patients are discovered to have gonadal involvement at autopsy (27,28,390).

Variable numbers of lymphoblasts can be identified in the peripheral blood or bone marrow in about one third of patients at presentation (27–29,36,52,374,375,379). Because bone marrow infiltration is not usually massive, however, the majority of patients have normal or near normal hemoglobin and hematocrit levels as well as white blood cell and platelet counts at presentation (27–29,36,375,379). About 10% to 15% of patients have a leukemic blood picture indistinguishable from ALL at presentation (29,36,375); these patients are believed to have the leukemic phase of LBL and not ALL based on other clinical parameters. It is these patients who largely account for the fewer than 10% of LBL patients who have anemia or thrombocytopenia at presentation (27). Patients who have LBL virtually never have monoclonal gammopathies (29).

Sixty percent or more of patients undergo leukemic conversion or develop massive bone marrow replacement during their clinical course (27–29,391). The incidence of leukemic conversion has been reported to approach 90% among children who have mediastinal LBL (9,392). At this point, LBL usually becomes indistinguishable from ALL. The incidence of leukemic conversion appears to be roughly equivalent in males and females. The incidence of leukemic conversion is significantly higher, however, among males younger than 30 than among those older than 30 years of age (29). Following leukemic conversion, LBL usually disseminates rapidly and widely in a noncontiguous fashion (31). Postmortem examination of patients who die from LBL often reveals widespread disease, including involvement of the mediastinum, lungs, pleura, lymph nodes, bone marrow, peripheral blood, leptomeninges, gonads, liver, spleen, and viscera (27–29).

Although precursor T- and B-cell LBLs are morphologically indistinguishable, cell lineage correlates with clinical presentation. Those patients who have precursor T-cell LBL tend to exhibit the classical clinical features of LBL described previously. In particular, virtually all LBLs involving the mediastinum express a precursor T-cell phenotype (33–36,393). In contrast, precursor B-cell LBLs may involve a variety of anatomic sites above and below the diaphragm, but mediastinal involvement is exceptionally rare (394).

For example, some patients who have precursor B-cell LBL present with involvement of noncutaneous, extranodal sites as the initial or the only manifestation of LBL. Most commonly, this is a solitary lytic bone lesion, which may be associated with bone pain. The most frequent osseous sites are the femur (306,395,396) and the tibia (33,396,397). Other osseous sites include the ribs (395,396), vertebrae (398,399), scapula (400), pelvis (306), and bones of the feet (306). Rarely, patients present with multiple osteolytic lesions in the absence of other organ involvement (401). Other extranodal sites reported include the paraspinal area (402), tonsil (403), nasopharynx (34,393), parotid gland (393,395), submaxillary gland (398), gastrointestinal tract (403,404) and the heart (405). Also, we have documented LBL initially localized to the kidney and CNS (Knowles, unpublished observations). These patients include both children and adults, and males and females are affected equally. In virtually all of these patients, the malignant lymphoblasts express precursor B-cell immunophenotypes (33,395,397,398,400–402). Precursor T-cell LBL exhibiting isolated involvement of noncutaneous extranodal sites, such as the kidneys and gastrointestinal tract, is extremely uncommon (406–408). Precursor T-cell LBL, however, has been reported to occur in immunosuppressed individuals, including those who have undergone organ transplantation (Chapter 16). Rarely, precursor T-cell LBL occurs in association with thymoma (409,410).

A small number of patients presents with cutaneous involvement as the initial or only manifestation of LBL, suggesting origination in the skin (376,382,393,395,411–414). The neoplastic cells in these patients are morphologically identical to those comprising mediastinal and lymph node LBL; they may have convoluted or nonconvoluted nuclei

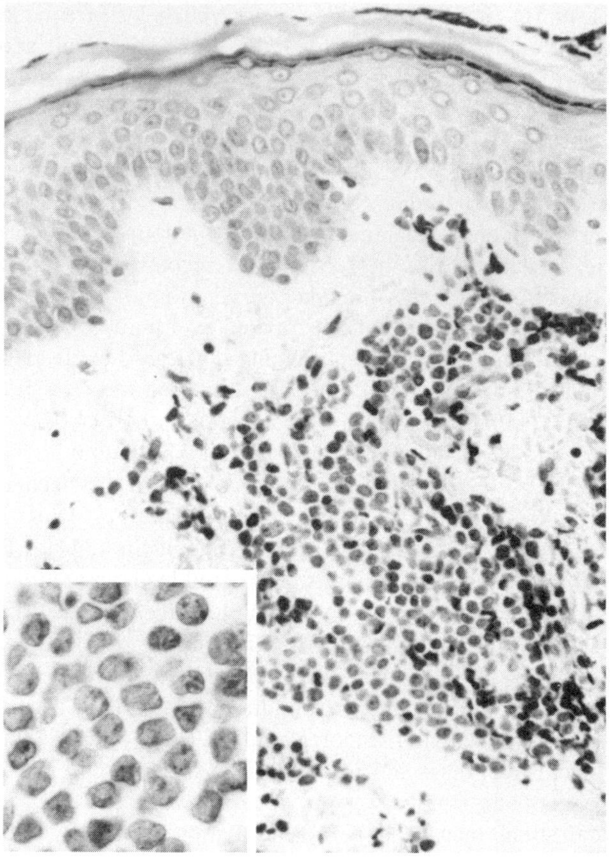

FIG. 26.21. Cutaneous precursor B-cell lymphoblastic lymphoma. The patient is a 6-year-old girl who presented with a cutaneous nodule on the back of the neck. The nodule contains a dermal infiltrate of malignant lymphoblasts with the cytomorphologic features of lymphoblastic lymphoma. Immunophenotypic studies performed on frozen tissue sections demonstrated the precursor B-cell nature of these malignant lymphoblasts (hematoxylin and eosin stain, original magnification: 250× magnification; **Inset:** original magnification: 630× magnification).

(Fig. 26.21). Patients who have primary cutaneous LBL appear to exhibit a unique constellation of clinical and immunologic features. Frequently, they are very young children, ranging from about 5 months to 6 years in age (376,382,393, 395,411–415); occasionally, they are adolescents or adults (35,374,382,416). Males and females are affected equally. They present with solitary, several, or multiple cutaneous lesions, most commonly on the scalp, forehead, face, and neck but sometimes elsewhere. The lesions are usually firm, nodular, plaque-like, erythematous, and nontender. They may wax and wane for several months, or they may grow rapidly. These patients almost never have a mediastinal mass. Occasionally, regional lymph node or focal bone marrow involvement may be present. The cutaneous lesions usually regress in response to chemotherapy, and most patients achieve a complete remission. Like most patients who have LBL, however, they may relapse in the bone marrow, CNS, and gonads or undergo leukemic conversion. Overall, those patients appear to have the same prognosis as those who have extracutaneous LBL (382,416). These primary cutaneous LBLs characteristically express precursor B-cell phenotypes, most commonly the pre-B cell phenotype—TdT, HLA-DR, CD19, CD10, and cytoplasmic μ heavy chains (35,376,382,393,395,411–416)—similar or identical to that of most childhood ALLs (19,20). In summary, patients who have primary cutaneous LBL differ from the vast majority of LBL patients by their younger age, lack of male predominance, primarily cutaneous disease, absent mediastinal mass, and precursor B-cell immunophenotype. This unique constellation of findings suggests that primary cutaneous LBL represents a distinct clinical entity in children (413).

Approximately 5% of children who have ALL, predominantly those who have T-cell ALL, develop secondary AML within 6 years of initial hematologic remission following antileukemic therapy (417). Some patients who present initially with precursor T-cell LBL also develop secondary AML following therapy (418–420). Many of these secondary AMLs exhibit monocytic differentiation and possess translocations involving the *MLL* gene locus at 11q23 (417). In the majority of these instances, the original karyotype is replaced completely when the secondary AML develops, suggesting induction of a second, independent malignancy (417). In addition, some patients who have precursor T-cell ALL have exhibited progressive conversion to AML, with cytogenetic evidence of the same clone or clonal evolution shortly after beginning therapy with deoxycoformycin (421,422). This phenomenon has been referred to as *lineage switch* by some investigators (423). A case of biphenotypic LBL exhibiting simultaneous evidence of thymic T-cell and myeloid differentiation also has been described (424). In some instances, molecular genetic studies have provided evidence for the same clonal origin of the initial LBL and the terminal AML (425), suggesting that this phenomenon represents phenotypic conversion of a single malignant cell population derived from a pleuripotential leukemic cell. The clinical outcome of patients who develop secondary AML is extremely poor (417).

Finally, numerous literature reports over the past 20 years have described patients who have LBL or ALL and who have developed a variety of benign and malignant, presumably histiocytic, proliferations following therapy (426). Most of these reports were published prior to the application of immunohistochemical and immunogenotypic techniques, to the recognition of hemophagocytic syndromes associated with viral infection (427) and the definition of new categories of non-Hodgkin's lymphomas, such as anaplastic large cell lymphoma (428) and histiocyte-rich B-cell lymphoma (429). Consequently, the true cell lineage and the reactive or malignant nature of most of these so-called histiocytic proliferations is unclear. Recently, however, Soslow and colleagues (426) documented the occurrence of clinically aggressive neoplasms possessing the morphologic and immunophenotypic features of true histiocytic lymphoma in three patients following therapy for LBL or ALL. Whether these tumors represent transformation of the original lymphoblastic malignancy or arose secondarily as a consequence of therapy or the posttreatment immunosuppressed state is unclear, as is the true incidence of this phenomenon.

THERAPY AND SURVIVAL

Lymphoblastic lymphoma is a histologic high-grade, clinically aggressive lymphoma (308). The principal clinicopathologic studies that established LBL as a distinct clinical entity reported median durations of survival of 8 to 17 months among children and adults, with very few long-term survivors (27–29,52,375,391). The neoplasms of the patients included in those studies, however, initially had been classified variably and, consequently, had been treated variably. Furthermore, the therapeutic protocols employed were generally inadequate to treat this particularly aggressive non-Hodgkin's lymphoma, with its propensity for leukemic conversion and CNS spread. Although LBL often responded dramatically to therapy initially, complete remissions were generally infrequent and of short duration (29,52,375). They frequently were interrupted by bone marrow, CNS, and gonadal relapses and leukemic conversion, usually resulting in rapid death. These experiences demonstrated that LBL is a chemotherapeutically responsive neoplasm in which long-term survival is sometimes possible, but that the protocols used to treat other non-Hodgkin's lymphomas are inadequate to treat LBL. In particular, LBL requires systemic therapy including CNS prophylaxis, regardless of stage. These principles have remained true, even as new therapeutic regimens have been employed (430).

The poor results obtained by treating LBL with conventional antilymphoma therapy and the obvious overlap between LBL and ALL led some investigators to treat childhood LBL with intensive, multidrug, ALL-like protocols that included CNS prophylaxis, which yielded encouraging results (431). Experience with a regimen including doxorubicin, vincristine, and prednisone plus radiation therapy resulted in a marked improvement in the prognosis of childhood mediastinal LBL (432,433). The first really successful therapeutic regimen for childhood LBL, however, was a modified 10-drug protocol (LSA_2-L_2), including cyclophosphamide, vincristine, methotrexate, daunomycin, prednisone, cytarabine, thioguanine, asparaginase, hydroxyurea, and carmustine, devised by Wollner and colleagues (434,435). The efficacy of LSA_2-L_2 in treating childhood LBL, including its superiority to a regimen (CHOP) including cyclophosphamide, vincristine, methotrexate, and prednisone, in treating disseminated disease was demonstrated by the Children's Cancer Study Group (436), the Pediatric Oncology Group (437), and others (438,439). The Children's Cancer Study Group confirmed these findings in a long-term follow-up of pediatric LBL patients treated with these protocols (440). They found 5-year disease-free survival rates of 84% for children who had localized LBL treated with either protocol but 64% and 35% for children who had disseminated LBL treated with LSA_2-L_2 and

COMP, respectively. The 3-year disease-free survival rate was 58%, and the 3-year actuarial survival rate was 72% in another study of pediatric LBL treated with LSA_2-L_2 (441). The incidence of CNS relapse was only 7% using cranial radiation with intrathecal chemotherapy or intrathecal chemotherapy alone (LSA_2-L_2) as CNS prophylaxis (441). Only 3 of 11 children with Murphy stage 4 disease in that study remained disease-free, however (441). Eden and colleagues (442) reported more encouraging results in 95 consecutively diagnosed children with stage III and IV precursor T-cell LBL treated between 1985 and 1990 with the United Kingdom Children's Cancer Study Group protocol 8503. This is an intensive, multidrug leukemia-type regimen that includes cranial irradiation, CNS prophylaxis, and continuing chemotherapy for 2 years following remission. They reported a 4-year event-free survival rate of 65% and an overall survival rate of 78%, with no significant difference between those with stage III and IV disease. The fact that some children relapsed widely suggests that this protocol is still not intensive enough or sustained sufficiently long enough to achieve lasting remission in 10% to 15% of children who have advanced stage LBL.

The results obtained treating adult LBL with conventional antilymphoma therapy were similarly dismal (29,52,375, 443), prompting several investigators to treat adult LBL with intensive, multidrug ALL-like protocols that included CNS prophylaxis. Coleman and associates (443) achieved a 100% complete response rate and a 3-year actuarial disease-free survival rate of 56% in 14 patients. Using a modified LSA_2-L_2 protocol, Levine and colleagues (444) achieved a 73% complete response rate, a 3-year actuarial disease-free survival rate of 50% among those who responded completely, an actuarial survival rate of 40% at 5 years, and a median duration of survival of 28 months in 15 patients. CNS relapse remained a problem in both clinical trials (443,444). Coleman and coworkers (445) reduced the incidence of CNS relapse to 3% by initiating CNS prophylaxis earlier and combining cranial radiation and intrathecal methotrexate, although this modified protocol did not affect the overall survival rate. The high rate of control of CNS disease using this protocol has not been confirmed by some others, however (446). Using a series of five different intensive chemotherapy protocols for ALL, Slater and colleagues (447) achieved an 80% complete response rate, with the 5-year disease-free survival rate projected at 45%. Other investigators (379) have reported results comparable to those of Slater and coworkers (447) and Levine and associates (444). Following these studies, investigators began to focus on adding chemotherapeutic agents with non–cross-resistant activity and nonoverlapping toxicity (448–450). The impact of these additional drugs in the treatment of LBL remains to be determined. Aggressive, multidrug, ALL-like protocols that include CNS prophylaxis appear to be capable of inducing complete remission in 80% or more of adult LBL patients, yielding results comparable to those obtained in childhood LBL (379). The prognosis for patients who failed to respond to first-line therapy in these series was very poor; they achieved a median duration of survival of only about 9 months, and less than 10% survived for a long term.

Both allogeneic and autologous bone marrow transplantation have been used effectively to prolong disease-free survival in some LBL patients who have relapsed (451,452). These results have stimulated interest in using transplantation to treat LBL patients in their first clinical remission. Groups employing this approach have reported 4- to 5-year actuarial survival rates of approximately 60% to 75% in adult patients who have LBL, achieving equivalent results with allogeneic and autologous transplants (453–455). This has led to the suggestion that high-dose chemotherapy (LSA_2-L_2 type protocol) to induce complete remission followed by autologous bone marrow transplantation may improve long-term, disease-free survival rates in advanced-stage adult LBL (453,455). The European Group for Bone Marrow Transplantation reported an overall actuarial survival rate of 42% at 6 years in 214 adult precursor B- and T-cell LBL patients from 36 United States and European centers treated with high-dose chemotherapy and autologous bone marrow transplantation. The 6-year actuarial survival rate was 63% for patients transplanted in first clinical remission, compared with 24% for those in partial, second, or subsequent remission and 15% for those with chemorefractory disease at transplantation. Transplantation in second complete remission resulted in a 31% actuarial survival rate at 6 years; these results are superior to those for conventional dose salvage regimens (456). These findings suggest that autologous bone marrow transplantation may be an effective therapeutic approach for adult LBL in a number of clinical situations. The precise role of allogeneic and autologous bone marrow transplantation in the treatment of childhood and adult LBL remains to be determined (457).

These clinical studies have contributed to our understanding of the prognostic variables in LBL. In a series of 80 adult LBL patients, Morel and coworkers (379) found that a higher complete remission rate was associated with age less than 40 years, lactate dehydrogenase level less than two times the upper limit of normal, and no or only one extranodal site of disease. Short duration of survival was associated with a failure to achieve complete remission, age older than 40 years, B symptoms, a lactate dehydrogenase level more than two times the upper limit of normal, and a hemoglobin level less than 100 g/L (379). Age younger than 30 years (381,447), the extent of disease defined by Ann Arbor stage (294,360), a white blood cell count greater than 50,000 per cubic millimeter (445), and elevated lactate dehydrogenase levels (381) have been identified as significant prognostic factors in other series. A short time (4 to 6 weeks) to complete response also has been correlated with long-term survival (445,447). In the Stanford series, serum lactate dehydrogenase combined with Ann Arbor stage distinguished two patient subgroups: a low-risk group with a five-year actual rate of freedom from relapse of greater than 90%, and a high-risk group with projected rate of freedom from relapse of only approximately 20% over a similar time (445). In contrast, Slater and colleagues did not find serum lactate dehydrogenase to be a significant prognostic indicator (447). Neither the presence nor the size of a mediastinal mass has been found to be prognostically significant (379,381,445, 447). Shepard and coworkers (458) reported, however, that the 5-year event-free and overall survival of children with Murphy stage 3 mediastinal LBL is statistically significantly better in those whose chest radiographs were normal within 60 days of commencing treatment; early resolution of a mediastinal mass probably reflects tumor chemosensitivity. Neither the presence nor the extent of bone marrow involvement have been found to be prognostically significant (379,440,445), and leukemic presentation has been found not to have prognostic value in some series (379,447). The development of an accurate prognostic index should prove helpful in identifying those patients who are at greatest risk of relapse and might benefit from more intensive therapy earlier or from bone marrow transplantation. The optimal prognostic staging system remains unclear (379,457).

DETECTION OF MINIMAL RESIDUAL DISEASE

Clinically silent, diffuse infiltration by malignant lymphoblasts can occur in ''privileged sites'' such as the CNS and testes, as well as the bone marrow and peripheral blood (76). Recent studies suggest that the detection of minimal residual disease and the ability to predict relapse may be important prognostic factors in lymphoblastic malignancy (459,460). Consequently, the pathologist frequently is asked to evaluate a patient's therapeutic response by detecting evidence of persistent or recurrent minimal residual disease in these and other sites. The histopathologic evaluation of bone marrow aspirates and biopsy core specimens following chemotherapy is difficult and fraught with pitfalls (Chapter 50). Clear distinction between malignant lymphoblasts and benign lymphocytes in small surgical biopsy specimens from the testes or other solid organs also may be difficult. Fine needle aspiration biopsy has been advocated as a less traumatic technique that offers more representative sampling than surgical biopsy, and one with which this diagnostic distinction often can be made morphologically (317, 318,461). In all these instances, however, immunophenotypic analysis represents a useful tool for monitoring minimal residual disease following chemotherapy and for detecting the reemergence of malignant lymphoblasts during clinically apparent complete remission of precursor B- and T-cell LBL or ALL (462–466). The immunophenotypic demonstration of TdT-positive cells is an extremely useful adjunct to morphology in documenting the presence of malignant lymphoblasts (318). The immunocytochemical demonstration of TdT-positive cells in cerebrospinal fluid samples is diagnostic of precursor LBL or ALL, because TdT-positive cells are never found there under normal conditions (467). The immunohistochemical demonstration of TdT-positive cells in the testis is similarly diagnostic (468), as is the cytofluorometric or immunocytochemical demonstration of TdT-positive cells in the peripheral blood (76). This is not true in the case of the bone marrow, in which the known increase in TdT-positive cells, that is, hematogones, in regenerating bone marrow following chemotherapy (295–298) may hamper the immunophenotypic detection of persistent or recurrent lymphoblastic malignancy in some clinical situations.

For these reasons, many investigators have utilized Southern blot hybridization and polymerase chain reaction analysis for clonal antigen receptor gene rearrangements (469–471) to detect minimal persistent or recurrent lymphoblastic malignancy. Other molecular approaches to detect minimal residual disease that have been employed in patients who have lymphoblastic malignancy include reverse transcriptase–polymerase chain reaction assays to detect leukemia-specific fusion transcripts in cases harboring t(1;19), t(4;11), and t(9;22) translocations (472–474). Another application of polymerase chain reaction in the detection of minimal residual disease has been the generation of probes specific for the rearranged immunoglobulin heavy chain of the leukemic clone (459,475,476). Using a variation of this approach, Brisco and colleagues (477) demonstrated a significant correlation between detection of minimal residual disease and probability of relapse. The exquisite sensitivity of these molecular biologic techniques has led to the frequent demonstration of residual disease during complete remission as defined traditionally. Whether early therapeutic intervention based on the detection of relapse in advance of overt clinical manifestations alters the course of the disease is still unclear, however. The evaluation of postchemotherapy bone marrow specimens and the detection of minimal lymphoblastic malignancy are discussed in Chapters 7, 9, 45, 46, and 50.

SUMMARY AND CONCLUSIONS

Lymphoblastic lymphoma is recognized universally as a clinicopathologic entity that exhibits a distinctive age and sex distribution; clinical, morphologic, and immunophenotypic characteristics; and natural history. LBL occurs most commonly in older children, adolescents, and young adults, predominantly males, and typically presents with supradiaphragmatic disease, usually consisting of a mediastinal mass or cervical, supraclavicular, and axillary lymphadenopathy. It is composed of neoplastic lymphoid cells that are morphologically indistinguishable from those of ALL and similarly express precursor T- and B-cell immunophenotypes. LBL has a high incidence of bone marrow, CNS, and gonadal involvement and frequently terminates in acute leukemia with widespread organ infiltration. LBLs of precursor T- and B-cell origin share many features with ALLs of corresponding cellular derivation. The distinction between LBL and ALL sometimes is unclear, and these entities must be differentiated arbitrarily, customarily on the basis of the presence or absence of significant bone marrow involvement. The treatment of LBL with intensive, multidrug, ALL-like protocols that include CNS prophylaxis has resulted in a marked improvement in the prognosis of both children and adults who have LBL. Recent advances in the application of sensitive molecular genetic approaches to detect minimal disease should aid considerably in monitoring patients who have malignant lymphoblastic disease and improve clinical outcome even further.

ACKNOWLEDGMENTS

The author thanks Al Lamme for preparing the excellent photomicrographs.

REFERENCES

1. Sternberg G. Leukosarkomatose und myeloblastenleukamie. *Beitr z Path Anat uz allg Path* 1916;61:75–100.
2. Cooke JV. Mediastinal tumor in acute leukemia: a clinical and roentgenologic study. *Am J Dis Child* 1932;44:1153–1177.
3. Rosenberg SA, Diamond HD, Dargeon HW, et al. Lymphosarcoma in children. *N Engl J Med* 1958;259:505–512.
4. Webster R. Lymphosarcoma of the thymus: its relation to acute lymphatic leukemia. *Med J Aust* 1961;48:582–586.
5. Bailey RJ, Burgert EO, Dahlin DC. Malignant lymphoma in children. *Pediatrics* 1961;28:985–992.
6. Sullivan MP. Leukemic transformation in lymphosarcoma of childhood. *Pediatrics* 1962;29:589–599.
7. Davis LA, McCreadie SR. The enlarged thymus gland in leukemia in childhood. *Am J Roentgenol* 1962;88:924–927.
8. Jones B, Klingberg WG. Lymphosarcoma in children: a review of 43 cases and review of the recent literature. *J Pediatr* 1963;63:11–20.
9. Jenkin RDT, Sonley MJ. The management of malignant lymphoma in childhood. In: *Neoplasia in childhood.* Chicago: Year Book Medical Publishers, 1969:305–319.
10. Jaffe ES, Berard CW. Lymphoblastic lymphoma, a term rekindled with new precision. *Ann Intern Med* 1978;89:415–417.
11. Rappaport H. Tumors of the hematopoietic system. In: *Atlas of tumor pathology*, section 3, fascicle 8. Washington, DC: US Armed Forces Institute of Pathology, 1966.
12. Pinkel D, Johnson W, Aur RJA. Non-Hodgkin's lymphoma in children. *Br J Cancer* 1975;31[Suppl II]:298–323.
13. Berard C, O'Conor GT, Thomas LB, et al. Histopathologic definition of Burkitt's tumor. *Bull World Health Organ* 1969;40:601–607.
14. Carbone PP, Berard CW, Bennett JM, et al. NIH clinical staff conference: Burkitt's tumor. *Ann Intern Med* 1969;70:817–832.
15. Smith JL, Barker CR, Clein GP, et al. Characterization of malignant mediastinal lymphoid neoplasm (Sternberg sarcoma) as thymic in origin. *Lancet* 1973;i:74–77.
16. Kaplan J, Mastrangelo R, Peterson WD. Childhood lymphoblastic lymphoma, a cancer of thymus-derived lymphocytes. *Cancer Res* 1974;34:521–525.
17. Borella L, Sen L. T cell surface markers on lymphoblasts from acute lymphocytic leukemia. *J Immunol* 1973;111:1257–1260.
18. Sen L, Borella L. Clinical importance of lymphoblasts with T markers in childhood acute leukemia. *N Engl J Med* 1975;292:828–832.
19. Tsukimoto I, Wong KY, Lampkin BC. Surface markers and prognostic factors in acute lymphoblastic leukemia. *N Engl J Med* 1976;294:245–248.
20. McCaffrey R, Smoler DF, Baltimore D. Terminal deoxynucleotidyl transferase in a case of childhood acute lymphoblastic leukemia. *Proc Natl Acad Sci USA* 1973;70:521–525.
21. McCaffrey R, Harrison TA, Parkman P, et al. Terminal deoxynucleotidyl transferase activity in human leukemic cells and in normal human thymocytes. *N Engl J Med* 1975;292:775–780.
22. Kung PC, Long JC, McCaffrey RP, et al. Terminal deoxynucleotidyl transferase in the diagnosis of leukemia and malignant lymphoma. *Am J Med* 1978;64:788–794.
23. Bollum FJ. Terminal deoxynucleotidyl transferase as a hematopoietic cell marker. *Blood* 1979;54:1203–1215.
24. Jaffe ES, Shevack EM, Frank MM, et al. Nodular lymphomas. Evidence for origin from follicular B lymphocytes. *N Engl J Med* 1974;290:813–819.
25. Lukes RJ, Collins RD. Immunologic characterization of human malignant lymphomas. *Cancer* 1974;34:1488–1503.
26. Jaffe ES, Shevack EM, Sussman EH, et al. Membrane receptor sites for the identification of lymphoreticular cells in benign and malignant conditions. *Br J Cancer* 1975;31[Suppl 2]:107–120.
27. Barcos MP, Lukes RJ. Malignant lymphoma of convoluted lymphocytes: a new entity of possible T-cell type. In: Sinks LF, Godden JO, eds. *Conflicts in childhood cancer: an evaluation of current management*, vol 4. New York: Alan R. Liss, 1975:147–178.
28. Nathwani BN, Kim H, Rappaport H. Malignant lymphoma, lymphoblastic. *Cancer* 1976;38:964–983.
29. Nathwani BN, Diamond LW, Winberg CD, et al. Lymphoblastic lymphoma: a clinicopathologic study of 95 patients. *Cancer* 1981;48:2347–2357.
30. Pangalis GA, Nathwani B, Rappaport H, et al. Acute lymphoblastic leukemia: the significance of nuclear convolutions. *Cancer* 1979;43:551–557.
31. Murphy SB. Classification, staging and end results of treatment of childhood non-Hodgkin's lymphomas: dissimilarities from lymphomas in adults. *Semin Oncol* 1980;7:332–339.
32. Knowles DM. The human T-cell leukemias: clinical, cytomorphologic, immunophenotypic, and genotypic characteristics. *Hum Pathol* 1986;17:14–33.
33. Cossman J, Chused TM, Fisher RI, et al. Diversity of immunologic phenotypes of lymphoblastic lymphoma. *Cancer Res* 1983;43:4486–4490.
34. Weiss L, Bindl JM, Picozzi VJ, et al. Lymphoblastic lymphoma: an immunophenotype study of 26 cases with comparison to T cell acute lymphoblastic leukemia. *Blood* 1986;67:474–478.
35. Sheibani K, Nathwani BN, Winberg CD, et al. Antigenically defined subgroups of lymphoblastic lymphoma: relationship to clinical presentation and biological behavior. *Cancer* 1987;60:183–190.
36. Salloum E, Henry-Amar M, Caillou B, et al. Lymphoblastic lymphoma in adults: a clinicopathological study of 34 cases treated at the Institut Gustave-Roussy. *Cancer Clin Oncol* 1988;24:1609–1616.
37. McCaffrey RP. Case records of the Massachusetts General Hospital: weekly clinicopathological exercises. *N Engl J Med* 1978;299:296–303.
38. Williams AH, Taylor CR, Higgins GR, et al. Childhood lymphoma-leukemia: I. Correlation of morphology and immunological studies. *Cancer* 1978;42:171–181.
39. Mitchell CD, Gordon I, Chessells JM. Clinical, haematological, and radiological features in T-cell lymphoblastic malignancy in childhood. *Clin Radiol* 1986;37:257–261.
40. Head DR, Behm FG. Acute lymphoblastic leukemia and the lymphoblastic lymphomas of childhood. *Semin Diagn Pathol* 1995;12:325–334.
41. Harris NL, Jaffe ES, Stein H, et al. A revised European-American classification of lymphoid neoplasms: a proposal from the International Lymphoma Study Group. *Blood* 1994;84:1361–1392.
42. Reinherz EL, Kung PC, Goldstein G, et al. Discrete stages of human intrathymic differentiation: analysis of normal thymocytes and leukemic lymphoblasts of T-cell lineage. *Proc Natl Acad Sci USA* 1980;77:1588–1592.
43. Bernard A, Boumsell L, Reinherz EL, et al. Cell surface characterization of malignant T cells from lymphoblastic lymphoma using monoclonal antibodies: evidence for phenotypic differences between malignant T cells from patients with acute lymphoblastic leukemia and lymphoblastic lymphoma. *Blood* 1981;57:1105–1110.
44. Roper M, Crist WM, Metzgar R, et al. Monoclonal antibody characterization of surface antigens in childhood T-cell lymphoid malignancies. *Blood* 1983;61:830–837.
45. MaGrath IT. Malignant non-Hodgkin's lymphomas in children. *Hematol Oncol Clin North Am* 1987;1:577–602.
46. Crist WM, Shuster JJ, Falletta J, et al. Clinical features and outcome in childhood T-cell leukemia-lymphoma according to stage of thymocyte differentiation: a Pediatric Oncology Study Group study. *Blood* 1988;72:1891–1897.

47. Borowitz MJ, Falleta JM. Leukemias and lymphomas of thymic differentiation. *Clin Lab Med* 1988;8:119–134.
48. Lukes RJ, Parker JW, Taylor CR, et al. Immunologic approach to non-Hodgkin's lymphomas and related leukemias: analysis of the results of multiparameter studies of 425 cases. *Semin Hematol* 1978;15: 322–356.
49. Griffith RC, Kelly DR, Nathwani BN, et al. A morphologic study of childhood lymphoma of the lymphoblastic type: the pediatric oncology group experience. *Cancer* 1987;59:1126–1131.
50. Greenberg BR, Peter CR, Glassy F, et al. A case of T-cell lymphoma with convoluted lymphocytes. *Cancer* 1976;38:1602–1607.
51. Kjeldsberg CR, Wilson JF, Berard CW. Non-Hodgkin's lymphoma in children. *Hum Pathol* 1983;14:612–627.
52. Rosen PJ, Feinstein DI, Pattengale PK, et al. Convoluted lymphocytic lymphoma in adults: a clinicopathologic entity. *Ann Intern Med* 1978; 89:319–324.
53. Bennett JM, Catovsky D, Daniel MT, et al. Proposals for the classification of the acute leukaemias. *Br J Haematol* 1976;33:451–458.
54. Bennett JM, Catovsky D, Daniel MT, et al. The morphologic classification of acute lymphoblastic leukaemia: concordance among observers and clinical correlations. *Br J Haematol* 1981;47:553–561.
55. Jondal M, Holm G, Wigzell H. Surface markers on human T and B lymphocytes: I. A large population of lymphocytes forming nonimmune rosettes with sheep red blood cells. *J Exp Med* 1972;136: 207–215.
56. Kersey J, Nesbit M, Hallgren H, et al. Evidence for origin of certain childhood acute lymphoblastic leukemias and lymphomas in thymus-derived lymphocytes. *Cancer* 1975;36:1348–1352.
57. Bernard A, Boumsell L, Bayle C, et al. Subsets of malignant lymphoma in children related to the cell phenotype. *Blood* 1979;54: 1058–1068.
58. Melvin S. Comparison of techniques for detecting T cell acute lymphocytic leukemia. *Blood* 1979;54:210–215.
59. Borella L, Sen L. E receptors on blasts from untreated acute lymphocytic leukemia (ALL): comparison of temperature dependence of E rosettes formed by normal and leukemic lymphoid cells. *J Immunol* 1975;114:187–190.
60. Donlon JA, Jaffe ES, Braylan RC. Terminal deoxynucleotidyl transferase activity in malignant lymphomas. *N Engl J Med* 1977;297: 461–464.
61. Jaffe ES, Braylan RC, Frank MM, et al. Heterogeneity of immunologic markers and surface morphology in childhood lymphoblastic lymphoma. *Blood* 1976;48:213–222.
62. Stein H, Petersen N, Gaedicke G, et al. Lymphoblastic lymphoma of convoluted or acid phosphatase type: a tumor of T precursor cells. *Int J Cancer* 1976;17:292–295.
63. Stein H, Muller-Hermelink HK. Simultaneous presence of receptors for complement and sheep red blood cells in human fetal thymocytes. *Br J Haematol* 1977;96:225–230.
64. Catovsky D, Galette J, Okos A, et al. Cytochemical profile of B and T leukemic lymphocytes with special reference to acute lymphoblastic leukemia. *J Clin Pathol* 1974;27:767–771.
65. Catovsky D. T-cell origin of acid phosphatase positive lymphoblasts. *Lancet* 1975;ii:327–328.
66. Ritter J, Gaedicke G, Winkler K, et al. Possible T cell origin of lymphoblasts in acid phosphatase positive acute lymphatic leukemia. *Lancet* 1975;ii:75.
67. Knowles DM. Non-Hodgkin's lymphomas: I. Immunologic and enzymatic markers useful in their evaluation. *Prog Surg Pathol* 1980;2: 71–105.
68. Knowles DM. Non-Hodgkin's lymphomas: II. Current immunologic concepts. *Prog Surg Pathol* 1980;2:107–143.
69. Nadler LM, Korsmeyer SJ, Anderson KC, et al. B cell origin of non-T cell acute lymphoblastic leukemia a model for discrete stages of neoplastic and normal pre-B cell differentiation. *J Clin Invest* 1984; 74:332–340.
70. Anderson KC, Bates MP, Slaughenhoupt BL, et al. Expression of human B cell-associated antigens on leukemias and lymphomas: a model of human B cell differentiation. *Blood* 1984;63:1424–1433.
71. Knowles DM. Lymphoid cell markers: their distribution and usefulness in the immunophenotypic analyses of lymphoid neoplasms. *Am J Surg Pathol* 1985;9[Suppl]:85–108.
72. Foon KA, Todd RF. Immunologic classification of leukemia and lymphoma. *Blood* 1986;68:1–31.
73. Knowles DM. Immunophenotypic and antigen receptor gene rearrangement analysis in T cell neoplasia. *Am J Pathol* 1989;134: 761–785.
74. Alt FW, Oltz EM, Young F, et al. VDJ recombination. *Immunol Today* 1992;13:306–314.
75. Silverstone AE, Cantor H, Goldstein G, et al. Terminal deoxynucleotidyl transferase is found in prothymocytes. *J Exp Med* 1976;144: 543–548.
76. Chilosi M, Pizzolo G. Review of terminal deoxynucleotidyl transferase: biological aspects, methods of detection, and selected diagnostic applications. *Appl Immunohistochem* 1995;3:209–221.
77. Mertelsmann R, Mertelsmann I, Koziner B, et al. Improved biochemical assay for terminal deoxynucleotidyl transferase in human blood cells: results in 89 adult patients with lymphoid leukemias and malignant lymphomas in leukemic phase. *Leuk Res* 1978;2:57–69.
78. Murphy S, Jaffe ES. Terminal transferase activity and lymphoblastic neoplasms. *N Engl J Med* 1984;311:1373–1374.
79. Marks SM, Baltimore D, McCaffrey R. Terminal transferase as a predictor of initial responsiveness to vincristine and prednisone in blastic crisis chronic myelogenous leukemia. *N Engl J Med* 1978; 298:812–814.
80. Stass SA, Dean L, Peiper SC, et al. Determination of terminal deoxynucleotidyl transferase on bone marrow smears by immunoperoxidase. *Am J Clin Pathol* 1982;77:174–176.
81. Fetterhoff TJ, McCarthy RC. Avidin-biotin amplification procedures for the detection of human terminal deoxynucleotidyl transferase in cell smears. *Am J Clin Pathol* 1985;83:565–570.
82. Erber WN, Mason DY: Immunoalkaline phosphatase labeling of terminal transferase in hematologic samples. *Am J Clin Pathol* 1987;88: 43–50.
83. Bardales RH, Carrato A, Fleischer M, et al. Detection of terminal deoxynucleotidyl transferase (TdT) by flow cytometry in leukemic disorders. *J Histochem Cytochem* 1989;37:509–513.
84. Racklin B, Bearman R, Sheibani K, et al. The demonstration of terminal deoxynucleotidyl transferase on frozen tissue sections and smears by the avidin-biotin complex (ABC) method. *Leuk Res* 1983;7: 431–437.
85. Said JW, Shintaku IP, Pinkus GS. Immunohistochemical staining for terminal deoxynucleotidyl transferase (TdT): an enhanced method in routinely processed formalin-fixed tissue sections. *Am J Clin Pathol* 1988;89:649–652.
86. Gown AM, de Wever N, Battifora H. Microwave-based antigenic unmasking. A revolutionary new technique for routine immunohistochemistry. *Appl Immunohistochem* 1993;1:256–266.
87. Orazi A, Cattoretti G, John K, Neiman RS: Terminal deoxynucleotidyl transferase staining of malignant lymphomas in paraffin sections. *Mod Pathol* 1994;7:582–586.
88. Reinherz EL, Schlossman SF. The differentiation and function of human T lymphocytes. *Cell* 1980;19:821–827.
89. Reinherz EL, Schlossman SF. Regulation of the immune response-inducer and suppressor T lymphocyte subsets in human beings. *N Engl J Med* 1980;303:370–373.
90. van Dongen JJM, Quertermous T, Bartram CR, et al. T cell receptor-CD3 complex during early T cell differentiation: analysis of immature T cell acute lymphoblastic leukemias (T-cell ALL) at DNA, RNA, and cell membrane level. *J Immunol* 1987;138:1260–1269.
91. Campana D, Janossy G, Coustan-Smith E, et al. The expression of T cell receptor-associated proteins during T cell ontogeny in man. *J Immunol* 1989;142:57–66.
92. Haynes BF, Denning SM, Singer KH, et al. Ontogeny of T-cell precursors: a model for the initial stages of human T-cell development. *Immunol Today* 1989;10:87–91.
93. Van Dongen JJM, Hooijkaas H, Comans-Bitter M, et al. Human bone marrow cells positive for terminal deoxynucleotidyl transferase (TdT), HLA-DR, and a T cell marker may represent prothymocytes. *J Immunol* 1985; 135:3144–3150.
94. Pittaluga S, Raffeld M, Lipford EH, et al. 3A1 (CD7) expression precedes Tβ gene rearrangements in precursor T (lymphoblastic) neoplasms. *Blood* 1986;68:134–139.
95. van Ewijk W. T-cell differentiation is influenced by thymic microenvironments. *Annu Rev Immunol* 1991;9:591–615.
96. Anderson G, Moore NC, Owen JJ, Jenkinson EJ. Cellular interactions in thymocyte development. *Annu Rev Immunol* 1996;14:73–99.

97. von Boehmer H. The developmental biology of T lymphocytes. *Annu Rev Immunol* 1988;6:309–326.
98. Link MP, Stewart SJ, Warnke RA, et al. Discordance between surface and cytoplasmic expression of the Leu-4 (T3) antigen in thymocytes and in blast cells from childhood T lymphoblastic malignancies. *J Clin Invest* 1985;76:248–253.
99. Feller AC, Parwaresch MR, Stein H, et al. Immunophenotyping of T-lymphoblastic lymphoma/leukemia: correlation with normal T-cell maturation. *Leuk Res* 1986;10:1025–1031.
100. Mori N, Oka K, Yoda Y, et al. Leu-4 (CD3) antigen expression in the neoplastic cells from T-cell ALL and T-lymphoblastic lymphoma. *Am J Clin Pathol* 1988;90:244–249.
101. Rosenberg N, Kincade PW. B-lineage differentation in normal and transformed cells and the microenvironment that supports it. *Curr Opin Immunol* 1994;6:203–211.
102. Nadler LM, Anderson KC, Marti G, et al. B4, a human B lymphocyte associated antigen expressed on normal, mitogen activated, and malignant B lymphocytes. *J Immunol* 1983;131:244–250.
103. Strauss LC, Rowley SD, La Russa VF, et al. Antigenic analysis of hematopoiesis: V. Characterization of My-10 antigen expression by normal lymphohematopoietic progenitor cells. *Exp Hematol* 1986;14: 878–886.
104. Dörken B, Pezzutto M, Kohler M, et al. Expression of cytoplasmic CD22 in B-cell ontogeny. In: McMichael AJ, Beverley PCL, Cobbold S, et al, eds. *Leukocyte typing III: white cell differentiation antigens.* Oxford: Oxford University Press, 1987L:474–476.
105. Mason DY, van Noesel CJM, Cordell JL, et al. The B29 and mb-1 polypeptides are differentially expressed during human B cell differentiation. *Eur J Immunol* 1992;22:2753–2756.
106. Wieczorek R, Buck D, Bindl J, et al. Monoclonal antibody Leu-22 (L60) permits the demonstration of some neoplastic T cells in routinely fixed and paraffin-embedded tissue sections. *Hum Pathol* 1988; 19:1434–1443.
107. Hollema H, Poppema S. T-lymphoblastic and peripheral T-cell lymphomas in the Northern part of the Netherlands: an immunologic study of 29 cases. *Cancer* 1989;64:1620–1628.
108. Chadburn A, Inghirami G, Knowles DM. T cell activation associated antigen expression by neoplastic T cells. *Hematol Pathol* 1992;6: 131–141.
109. Quintanilla-Martinez L, Zuckerberg LR, Harris NL. Prethymic adult lymphoblastic lymphoma: a clinicopathologic and immunohistochemical analysis. *Am J Surg Pathol* 1992;16:1075–1084.
110. Uckun FM, Steinherz PG, Sather H, et al. CD2 antigen expression on leukemic cells as a predictor of event-free survival after chemotherapy forT-lineage acute lymphoblastic leukemia: a Children's Cancer Study Group study. *Blood* 1996;88:4288–4295.
111. Knowles DM, Halper JP. Human T cell malignancies: correlative clinical, histopathologic, immunologic and cytochemical analysis of 23 cases. *Am J Pathol* 1982;106:187–203.
112. Ruco LP, Vitolo PR, Paliotta D, et al. Evidence for neoplastic cell differentiation in mediastinal T lymphoblastic lymphoma. *Virchows Arch A* 1987;410:443–447.
113. Marrack P, Kappler J. The T-cell receptor. *Science* 1987;238: 1073–1079.
114. Spits H, Borst J, Tax W, et al. Characteristics of a monoclonal antibody (WT31) that recognizes a common epitope on the human T cell receptor for antigen. *J Immunol* 1985;135:1922–1928.
115. Brenner MB, McLean J, Scheft H, et al. Characterization and expression of the human $\alpha\beta$T cell receptor using a framework monoclonal antibody. *J Immunol* 1987;138:1502–1509.
116. Picker LJ, Brenner MB, Weiss LM, et al. Discordant expression of CD3 and T-cell receptor beta-chain antigens in T lineage lymphomas. *Am J Pathol* 1987;129:434–440.
117. Chan WC, Borowitz MJ, Hammami A, et al. T cell receptor antibodies in the immunohistochemical studies of normal and malignant lymphoid cells. *Cancer* 1988;62:2118–2124.
118. Ng CS, Chan JKC, Hui PK, et al. Application of a T cell receptor antibody βF1 for immunophenotypic analysis of malignant lymphomas. *Am J Pathol* 1988;132:365–371.
119. Gouttenfangeas C, Bensussan A, Boumsell L. Study of the CD3 associated T cell receptors reveals further differences between T cell acute lymphoblastic lymphoma and leukemia. *Blood* 1990;75:931–934.
120. Band H, Hochstenbach F, McLean J, et al. Immunochemical proof that a novel rearranging gene encodes the T cell receptor δ subunit. *Science* 1987;238:682–684.
121. Inghirami G, Zhu BY, Chess L, et al. Flow cytometric and immunohistochemical characterization of the γ/δ T lymphocyte population in normal human lymphoid tissue and peripheral blood. *Am J Pathol* 1990;136:357–367.
122. Picker LJ, Brenner MB, Michie S, et al. Expression of T cell receptor delta chains in benign and malignant T lineage lymphoproliferations. *Am J Pathol* 1988;132:401–405.
123. Greaves MF, Brown G, Rapson NT, et al. Antisera to acute lymphoblastic leukemia cells. *Clin Immunol Immunopathol* 1975;4:67–84.
124. Ritz J, Nadler LM, Ghan AK, et al. Expression of common acute lymphoblastic leukemia antigen (cALLa) by lymphomas of B-cell and T-cell lineage. *Blood* 1981;8:648–652.
125. Dowell BL, Borowitz MJ, Boyett JM, et al. Immunologic and clinicopathological features of common acute lymphoblastic leukemia antigen-positive childhood T-cell leukemia: a Pediatric Oncology Group study. *Cancer* 1987;59:2020–2026.
126. Boucheix C, David B, Sebban C, et al. Immunophenotype of adult acute lymphoblastic leukemia, clinical parameters, and outcome: an analysis of a prospective trial including 562 tested patients. (LALA87). *Blood* 1994;84:1603–1612.
127. Swerdlow SH, Habeshaw JA, Richards MA, et al. T lymphoblastic lymphoma with Leu-7 positive phenotype and unusual clinical course: a multiparameter study. *Leuk Res* 1985;9:167–173.
128. Sheibani K, Winberg CD, Burke JS, et al. Lymphoblastic lymphoma expressing natural killer cell-associated antigens: a clinicopathologic study of six cases. *Leuk Res* 1987;11:371–377.
129. Kawano S, Tatsumi E, Yoneda N, et al. Novel leukemic lymphoma with probable derivation from immature stage of natural killer (NK) lineage in an aged patient. *Hematol Oncol* 1995;13:1–11.
130. Ichinohasama R, Endoh K, Ishizawa K, et al. Thymic lymphoblastic lymphoma of committed natural killer cell precursor origin: a case report. *Cancer* 1996;77:2592–2603.
131. Koita H, Suzumiya J, Ohshima K, et al. Lymphoblastic lymphoma expressing natural killer cell phenotype with involvement of the mediastinum and nasal cavity. *Am J Surg Pathol* 1997;21:242–248.
132. Sanchez MJ, Muench MO, Roncarolo MG, et al. Identification of a common T/natural killer cell progenitor in human fetal thymus. *J Exp Med* 1994;180:569–576.
133. Mason DY, Stein H, Gerdes J, et al. Value of monoclonal anti-CD22 (p135) antibodies for the detection of normal and neoplastic B lymphoid cells. *Blood* 1987;69:836–840.
134. Boue DR, Le Bien TW. Expression and structure of CD22 in acute leukemia. *Blood* 1988;71:1480–1486.
135. Borowitz MJ. Immunologic markers in childhood acute lymphoblastic leukemia. *Hematol Oncol Clin N Am* 1990;4:743–765.
136. Buccheri V, Mihaljevic B, Matutes E, et al. mb-1: A new marker for B-lineage lymphoblastic leukemia. *Blood* 1993;82:853–857.
137. Mason DY, Cordell JL, Brown MH, et al. CD79a: a novel marker for B-cell neoplasms in routinely processed tissue samples. *Blood* 1995;86:1453–1459.
138. Borowitz MJ, Shuster JJ, Civin CI, et al. Prognostic significance of CD34 expression in childhood B-precursor acute lymphocytic leukemia: a Pediatric Oncology Group study. *J Clin Oncol* 1990;8: 1389–1398.
139. Stroup R, Sheibani K, Misset JL, et al. Surface immunoglobulin positive lymphoblastic lymphoma: a report of three cases. *Cancer* 1990; 65:2559–2563.
140. Koehler M, Behm FG, Shuster J, et al. Transitional pre-B-cell acute lymphoblastic leukemia of childhood is associated with favorable prognostic clinical features and an excellent outcome: a Pediatric Oncology Group study. *Leukemia* 1993;7:2064–2068.
141. Kersey J, Goldman A, Abramson C, et al. Clinical usefulness of monoclonal antibody phenotyping in childhood acute lymphoblastic leukemia. *Lancet* 1982;ii:1419–1423.
142. Hoelzer D, Thiel E, Loffler H, et al. Intensified therapy in acute lymphoblastic and acute undifferentiated leukemia in adults. *Blood* 1984; 64:38–47.
143. Crist WM, Boyett J, Roper M, et al. Pre-B cell leukemia responds poorly to treatment: a Pediatric Oncology Group study. *Blood* 1984; 63:407–414.
144. Hurwitz CA, Loken MR, Graham ML, et al. Asynchronous antigen

expression in B lineage acute lymphoblastic leukemia. *Blood* 1988; 72:299–307.
145. Vannier JP, Bene MC, Faure GC, et al. Investigation of the CD10 (cALLa) negative acute lymphoblastic leukaemia: further description of a group with poor prognosis. *Br J Haematol* 1989;72:156–160.
146. Sobol RE, Mick R, Royston I, et al. Clinical importance of myeloid antigen expression in adult acute lymphoblastic leukemia. *N Engl J Med* 1989;316:1111–1117.
147. Crist W, Boyett J, Jackson J, et al. Prognostic importance of the pre-B cell immunophenotype and other presenting features in B lineage childhood acute lymphoblastic leukemia. *Blood* 1989;74:1256–1259.
148. Boldt DH, Kopecky KJ, Head D, et al. Expression of myeloid antigens by blast cells in acute lymphoblastic leukemia of adults: the Southwest Oncology Group experience. *Leukemia* 1994;8:2118–2126.
149. Greaves MF, Paxton A, Janossy G, et al. Acute lymphoblastic leukemia associated antigen: III. Alterations in expression during treatment and relapse. *Leuk Res* 1980;4:1–14.
150. Lauer S, Piaskowaski V, Camitta B, et al. Bone marrow and extramedullary variations of cell membrane antigen expression in childhood lymphoid neoplasias at relapse. *Leuk Res* 1982;6:769–774.
151. Pullen DJ, Boyett JM, Crist WM, et al. Pediatric Oncology Group utilization of immunologic markers in the designation of acute lymphocytic leukemia: subgroups influence on treatment response. *Ann NY Acad Sci* 1984;428:226–248.
152. Pui CH, Raimondi SC, Behm FG, et al. Shifts in blast cell phenotype and karyotype at relapse of childhood lymphoblastic leukemia. *Blood* 1986;68:1306–1310.
153. Bernard A, Raynal B, Lemerle J, et al. Changes in surface antigens on malignant T cells from lymphoblastic lymphomas at relapse: an appraisal with monoclonal antibodies and microfluorometry. *Blood* 1982;59:809–815.
154. Tonegawa S. Somatic generation of antibody diversity. *Nature* 1983; 301:575–581.
155. Hood L, Kronenberg M, Hunkapiller T. T-cell antigen receptors and the immunoglobulin supergene family. *Cell* 1985;40:225–229.
156. Korsmeyer SJ, Waldmann TA. Immunoglobulin genes: rearrangement and translocation in human lymphoid malignancy. *J Clin Immunol* 1984;4:1–11.
157. Waldmann TA. The arrangement of immunoglobulin and T-cell receptor genes in human lymphoproliferative disorders. *Adv Immunol* 1987;40:247–321.
158. Dalla-Favera R, Neri A, Knowles DM. Molecular genetic markers in the diagnosis and classification of non-Hodgkin's Lymphomas. In: Magrath IT, ed. *The non-Hodgkin's lymphomas.* London: Edward Arnold, 1990: 109–121.
159. Arnold A, Cossman J, Bakhaski A, et al. Immunoglobulin gene rearrangements as unique clonal markers in human lymphoid neoplasms. *N Engl J Med* 1983;309:1593–1599.
160. Cleary ML, Chao J, Warnke R, et al. Immunoglobulin gene rearrangement as a diagnostic criterion of B-cell lymphoma. *Proc Natl Acad Sci USA* 1984;81:593–597.
161. Flug F, Pelicci PG, Bonetti F, et al. T cell receptor gene rearrangements as markers of lineage and clonality in T cell neoplasms. *Proc Natl Acad Sci USA* 1985;82:3460–3464.
162. Waldmann TA, Davis MM, Bongiovanni KF, et al. Rearrangements of gene for the antigen receptor on T cells as markers of lineage and clonality in human lymphoid neoplasms. *N Engl J Med* 1985;313: 776–783.
163. Knowles DM, Neri A, Pelicci PG, et al. Immunoglobulin and T cell receptor beta chain gene rearrangement analysis of Hodgkin's disease: implications for lineage determination and differential diagnosis. *Proc Natl Acad Sci USA* 1986;83:7942–7946.
164. Korsmeyer SJ, Hieter PA, Ravetch JV, et al. Developmental hierarchy of immunoglobulin gene rearrangements in human leukemic pre-B-cells. *Proc Natl Acad Sci USA* 1981;78:7096–7100.
165. Felix CA, Reaman GH, Korsmeyer SJ, et al. Immunoglobulin and T-cell receptor gene configuration in acute lymphoblastic leukemia in infancy. *Blood* 1987;70:536–541.
166. Felix CA, Wright JJ, Poplack DG, et al. T cell receptor α, β, and γ genes in T cell and pre-B cell acute lymphoblastic leukemia. *J Clin Invest* 1987;80:545–556.
167. Korsmeyer SJ, Arnold A, Bakhshi A, et al. Immunoglobulin gene rearrangement and cell surface antigen expression in acute lymphocytic leukemias of T cell and B cell precursor origins. *J Clin Invest* 1983;71:301–313.
168. Tawa A, Hozumi N, Minden M, et al. Rearrangement of the T-cell receptor beta-chain gene in non-T, non-B acute lymphoblastic leukemia of childhood. *N Engl J Med* 1986;313:1033–1037.
169. Davey MP, Bongiovanni KF, Kaulfersch W, et al. Immunoglobulin and T-cell receptor gene rearrangement and expression in human lymphoid leukemia cells at different stages of maturation. *Proc Natl Acad Sci USA* 1986;83:8759–8763.
170. Greenberg JM, Kersey JH. Terminal deoxynucleotidyl transferase expression can precede T cell receptor β chain and γ chain rearrangement in T cell acute lymphoblastic leukemia. *Blood* 1987;69:356–360.
171. Pittaluga S, Uppenkamp M, Cossman J. Development of T3/T cell receptor gene expression in human pre-T neoplasms. *Blood* 1987;69: 1062–1067.
172. Hara J, Benedict SH, Champagne E, et al. T cell receptor δ gene rearrangements in acute lymphoblastic leukemia. *J Clin Invest* 1988; 82:1974–1982.
173. de Villartay J-P, Pullman A, Andrade R, et al. Gamma/delta lineage relationship within a consecutive series of human precursor T-cell neoplasms. *Blood* 1989;74:2508–2518.
174. Kimura N, Takihara Y, Akiyoshi T, et al. Rearrangement of T-cell receptor δ chain gene as a marker of lineage and clonality in T-cell lymphoproliferative disorders. *Cancer Res* 1989;49:4488–4492.
175. Hara J, Benedict SJ, Mak TW, et al. T-cell receptor alpha-chain rearrangements in B-precursor leukemia are in contrast to the findings in T cell acute lymphoblastic leukemia. *J Clin Invest* 1987;80: 1770–1777.
176. Hara J, Benedict SH, Champagne E, et al. Comparison of T-cell receptor α, β and γ gene rearrangement and expression in T cell acute lymphoblastic leukemia. *J Clin Invest* 1988;81:989–996.
177. Greenberg JM, Quertermous T, Seidman JG, et al. Human T-cell γ-chain gene rearrangement in acute lymphoid and non-lymphoid leukemia: comparison with the T cell receptor β-chain gene. *J Immunol* 1986;137:2043–2049.
178. Knowles DM, Pelicci PG, Dalla-Favera R. T-cell receptor beta chain gene rearrangements: genetic markers of T cell lineage and clonality. *Hum Pathol* 1986;17:546–551.
179. Chen Z, Le Paslier D, Dausset J, et al. Human T cell γ genes are frequently rearranged in B-lineage acute lymphoblastic leukemias but not in chronic B cell proliferations. *J Exp Med* 1987;165:1000–1015.
180. Tawa A, Benedict SH, Hara J, et al. Rearrangement of the T cell receptor γ-chain gene in childhood acute lymphoblastic leukemia. *Blood* 1987;70:1933–1939.
181. Pelicci PG, Knowles DM, Dalla-Favera R. Lymphoid tumors displaying rearrangements of both immunoglobulin and T cell receptor genes. *J Exp Med* 1985;162: 1015–1024.
182. Greaves MF, Chan LC, Furley AJW, et al. Lineage promiscuity in hematopoietic differentiation and leukemia. *Blood* 1986;67:1–11.
183. Subar M, Pelicci PG, Neri A, et al. Patterns of T cell receptor gamma gene rearrangement and expression in B and T lymphoid malignancies. *Leukemia* 1988;2:19–26.
184. Dyer MJS. T-cell receptor δ/α rearrangements in lymphoid neoplasms. *Blood* 1989;74:1073–1083.
185. Griesinger F, Greenberg JM, Kersey JH. T-cell receptor gamma and delta rearrangements in hematologic malignancies. *J Clin Invest* 1989; 84:506–516.
186. Felix CA, Poplack DG, Reaman GH, et al. Characterization of immunoglobulin and T-cell receptor gene patterns in B-cell precursor acute lymphoblastic leukemia of childhood. *J Clin Oncol* 1990;8:431–442.
187. Yancopoulous GD, Blackwell KT, Suh H, et al. Introduced T-cell receptor variable region gene segments recombine in pre-B cells: evidence that B and T cells use a common recombinase. *Cell* 1986;44: 251–259.
188. Goorha R, Bunin M, Mirro J Jr, et al. Provocative pattern of rearrangements of the genes for the gamma and beta-chains of the T-cell receptor in human leukemias. *Proc Natl Acad Sci USA* 1987;84:4547–4551.
189. Minden MD, Mak TW. The structure of the T cell antigen receptor genes in normal and malignant T cells. *Blood* 1986;68:327–339.
190. Hara J, Benedict SH, Champagne E, et al. Relationship between rearrangement and transcription of the T-cell receptor α, β and γ genes in B-precursor acute lymphoblastic leukemia. *Blood* 1989; 73:500–508.
191. Kitchingman GR, Mirro J Jr, Stass A. The molecular biology of mixed

lineage leukemia. In: Cossman J, ed. *Molecular genetics in cancer diagnosis*. New York: Elsevier, 1990:223–248.
192. Nuss R, Kitchingman G, Cross A, et al. T cell receptor gene rearrangements in B-precursor acute lymphoblastic leukemia correlate with age and the stage of B cell differentiation. *Leukemia* 1988;2:722–727.
193. Kitchingman GR, Rovigatti U, Mauer AM, et al. Rearrangement of immunoglobulin heavy chain genes in T cell acute lymphoblastic leukemia. *Blood* 1985;65:725–729.
194. Pugh WC, Stass SA. Immunoglobulin gene rearrangement and its implications for the study of B cell neoplasia. *Clin Lab Med* 1988;8:45–64.
195. Ha-Kawa K, Hara J, Keiko Y, et al. Kappa-chain gene rearrangement in an apparent T-lineage lymphoma. *J Clin Invest* 1986;78:1439–1442.
196. Sheibani K, Wu A, Ben-Ezra J, et al. Rearrangement of β-chain and T-cell receptor β-chain genes in malignant lymphomas of "T-cell" phenotype. *Am J Pathol* 1987;129:201–207.
197. Hanson CA, Thamilarasan M, Ross CW, et al. Kappa light chain gene rearrangement in T-cell acute lymphoblastic leukemia. *Am J Clin Pathol* 1990;93:563–568.
198. Aisenberg AC, Wilkes BM. The genotype and phenotype of T cell and non-T, non-B acute lymphoblastic leukemia. *Blood* 1985;66:1215–1218.
199. Bunin NJ, Raimondi SC, Mirro J, et al. Alterations in immunoglobulin or T cell receptor gene rearrangement at relapse: involvement of 11q23 and changes in immunophenotype. *Leukemia* 1990;4:727–731.
200. Third International Workshop on Chromosomes in Leukemia. *Cancer Genet Cytogenet* 1981;4:95–142.
201. Williams DL, Tsiatis A, Brodeur GMG, et al. Prognostic importance of chromosome number in 136 untreated children with acute lymphoblastic leukemia. *Blood* 1982;60:864–871.
202. Look AT. The cytogenetics of childhood leukemia: clinical and biologic implications. *Pediatr Clin N Am* 1988;35:723–741.
203. Secker-Walker LM, Chessells JM, Stewart EL, et al. Chromosomes and other prognostic factors in acute lymphoblastic leukemia: a long-term follow-up. *Br J Haematol* 1989;72:336–342.
204. Raimondi SC. Current status of cytogenetic research in childhood acute lymphoblastic leukemia. *Blood* 1993;81:2237–2251.
205. Bloomfield CD, Secker-Walker LM, Goldman AI, et al. Six-year follow-up of the clinical significance of karyotype in acute lymphoblastic leukemia. *Cancer Genet Cytogenet* 1989;40:171–185.
206. Secker-Walker LM, Prentice HG, Durrant J, et al. Cytogenetics adds independent prognostic information in adults with acute lymphoblastic leukemia on MRC trial UKALL XA. *Br J Haematol* 1997;96:601–610.
207. Faderl S, Kantarjian WM, Talpaz M, et al. Clinical significance of cytogenetic abnormalities in adult lymphoblastic leukemia. *Blood* 1998;91:3995–4019.
208. Look AT, Roberson PK, Williams DL, et al. Prognostic importance of blast cell DNA content in childhood acute lymphoblastic leukemia. *Blood* 1985;65:1079–1085.
209. Kalwinsky DK, Roberson P, Dahl G, et al. Clinical relevance of lymphoblast biological features in children with acute lymphoblastic leukemia. *J Clin Oncol* 1985;3:477–484.
210. Harris MB, Shuster JJ, Carroll A, et al. Trisomy of leukemic cell chromosomes 4 and 10 identifies children with B-progenitor cell acute lymphoblastic leukemia with a very low risk of treatment failure: a Pediatric Oncology Group study. *Blood* 1992;79:3316–3324.
211. Land VJ, Shuster JJ, Carroll AJ, et al. A DNA index greater than 1.16 in B-precursor childhood acute lymphoblastic leukemia predicts a 95% 3-year event-free survival. *Blood* 1990;76:292a.
212. Pui C-H. Childhood leukemia. *N Engl J Med* 1995;332:1618–1630.
213. Pui C-H, Carroll AJ, Head D, et al. Near-triploidy or near-tetraploidy acute lymphoblastic leukemia of childhood. *Blood* 1990;76:590–596.
214. Rowley JD. A new consistent chromosomal abnormality in chronic myelogenous leukemia identified by quinacrine flourescence and Giemsa staining. *Nature* 1973;243:290–292.
215. Groffen J, Stephenson JR, Heisterkamp N, et al. Philadelphia chromosomal breakpoints are clustered with a limited region, bcr, on chromosome 22. *Cell* 1984;36:93–99.
216. Dalla-Favera R, Bregni M, Erikson J, et al. Human c-myc onc gene is located on the region of chromosome 8 that is translocated in Burkitt lymphoma cells. *Proc Natl Acad Sci USA* 1982;79:7824–7827.
217. Taub R, Kirsch I, Morton C, et al. Translocation of the c-myc gene into the immunoglobulin heavy chain locus in human Burkitt lymphoma and murine plasmacytoma cells. *Proc Natl Acad Sci USA* 1982;79:7837–7841.
218. Suryanarayan K, Hunger SP, Kohler S, et al. Consistent involvement of the BCR gene by 9;22 breakpoints in pediatric acute leukemias. *Blood* 1991;77:324–330.
219. Ribeiro R, Abromowitch M, Raimondi SC, et al. Clinical and biological hallmarks of the Philadelphia chromosome in childhood acute lymphoblastic leukemia. *Blood* 1987;70:948–953.
220. Gramatzki M, Bartram CR, Muller D, et al. Early T cell differentiated chronic myeloid leukemia blast crisis with rearrangement of the breakpoint cluster region but not of the T cell receptor β chain genes. *Blood* 1987;69:1082–1086.
221. The Groupe Francais de Cytogenetique Hematologique. Cytogenetic abnormalities in adult acute lymphoblastic leukemia: correlations with hematologic findings and outcome. A collaborative study of the Groupe Francais de Cytogenetique Hematologique. *Blood* 1996;87:3135–3142.
222. Schlieben S, Borkhardt A, Reinsch I, et al. Incidence and clinical outcome of children with BCR/ABL-positive acute lymphoblastic leukemia (ALL): a prospective RT-PCR study based on 673 patients enrolled in the German pediatric multicenter therapy trials ALL-BFM-90 and CoALL-05-92. *Leukemia* 1996;10:957–963.
223. Croce CM, Nowell PC. Molecular basis of human B cell neoplasia. *Blood* 1985;65:1–7.
224. Berger R, Bernheim A, Brouet JC, et al. t(8;14) translocation in a Burkitt's type of lymphoblastic leukaemia (L3). *Br J Haematol* 1979;43:87–90.
225. Williams DL, Look AT, Melvin SL, et al. New chromosomal translocations correlate with specific immunophenotypes of childhood acute lymphoblastic leukemia. *Cell* 1984;36:101–109.
226. Mellentin JD, Murre C, Donlon TA, et al. The gene for enhancer binding proteins E12/E47 lies at t(1;19)breakpoint in acute leukemias. *Science* 1989;246:379–382.
227. Hunger SP, Galili N, Carroll AJ, et al. The t(1;19)(q23;p13) results in consistent fusion of E2A and PBX1 coding sequences in acute lymphoblastic leukemias. *Blood* 1991;77;687–693.
228. Michael PM, Levin MD, Garson OM. Translocation 1;19: a new cytogenetic abnormality in acute lymphocytic leukemia. *Cancer Genet Cytogenet* 1984;12:333–341.
229. Carroll AJ, Crist WM, Parmley MT, et al. Pre-B cell leukemia associated with chromosome translocation 1;19. *Blood* 1984;63:721–724.
230. Crist WM, Carroll AJ, Shuster JJ, et al. Poor prognosis of children with pre-B acute lymphoblastic leukemia is associated with the t(1;19)(q23;p13): a Pediatric Oncology Group study. *Blood* 1990;76:117–122.
231. Pui C-H, Frankel LS, Carroll AJ, et al. Clinical characteristics and treatment outcome of childhood acute lymphoblastic leukemia with the t(4;11)(q21;q23): a collaborative study of 40 cases. *Blood* 1991;77:440–447.
232. Johansson B, Moorman AV, Haas OA, et al. Hematologic malignancies with t(4;11)(q21;q23): a cytogenetic, morphologic, immunophenotypic and clinical study of 183 cases. *Leukemia* 1998;12:779–787.
233. Gu Y, Nakamura T, Alder H, et al. The t(4;11) chromosomal translocation of human acute leukemias fuses the ALL-1 gene, related to drosophila trithorax to the AF-4 gene. *Cell* 1992;71:701–708
234. Stark B, Umiel T, Mammon Z, et al. Leukemia of early infancy: early B-cell lineage associated with t(4;11). *Cancer* 1986;58:1265–1271.
235. Lampert F, Harbott J, Ludwig WD, et al. Acute leukemia with chromosome translocation (4;11): 7 new patients and analysis of 71 cases. *Blut* 1987;54:325–335.
236. Chen C-S, Sorenson PHB, Domer PH, et al. Molecular rearrangements on chromosome 11q23 predominate in infant acute lymphoblastic leukemia and are associated with specific biologic variables and poor outcome. *Blood* 1993;81:2386–2393.
237. Rubnitz JE, Link MP, Shuster JJ, et al. Frequency and prognostic significance of HRX rearrangements in infant acute lymphoblastic leukemia: a Pediatric Oncology Group study. *Blood* 1994;84:570–573.
238. Cimino G, Rapanotti MC, Rivolta A, et al. Prognostic relevance of ALL-1 gene rearrangement in infant acute leukemias. *Leukemia* 1995;9:391–395.
239. Stong RC, Korsmeyer SJ, Parkin JL, et al. Human acute leukemia

cell line with the t(4;11) chromosomal rearrangement exhibits B lineage and monocytic characteristics. *Blood* 1985;65:21–31.
240. Arthur DC, Bloomfield CD, Lindquist LL, et al. Translocation 4;11 in acute lymphoblastic leukemia: clinical characteristics and prognostic significance. *Blood* 1982;59:96–99.
241. Parkin JL, Arthur DC, Abramson CS, et al. Acute leukemia associated with the t(4;11) chromosome rearrangement: ultrastructural and immunologic characteristics. *Blood* 1982;60:1321–1331.
242. Mirro J, Kitchingman G, Williams D, et al. Clinical and laboratory characteristics of acute leukemia with the 4;11 translocation. *Blood* 1986;67:689–697.
243. Childs CC, HirschGinsberg C, Gulbert SJ, et al. Lineage heterogeneity in acute leukemia with the t(4;11) abnormality: implications of acute mixed lineage leukemia. *Hematol Pathol* 1988;2:145–148.
244. Pui C-H, Behm FG, Crist WM. Clinical and biologic relevance of immunologic marker studies in childhood acute lymphoblastic leukemia. *Blood* 1993;82:343–362.
245. Copelan EA, McGuire EA. The biology and treatment of acute lymphoblastic leukemia in adults. *Blood* 1995;85:1151–1168.
246. Bloomfield CD, Goldman AI, Alimena G, et al. Chromosomal abnormalities identify high-risk and low-risk patients with acute lymphoblastic leukemia. *Blood* 1986;67:415–420.
247. Raimondi SC, Williams DL, Callihan T, et al. Non random involvement of the 12p12 breakpoint in chromosome abnormalities of childhood acute lymphoblastic leukemia. *Blood* 1984;68:69–75.
248. Romana SP, Le Coniat M, Berger R. t(12;21): A new recurrent translocation in acute lymphoblastic leukemia. *Genes Chromosomes Cancer* 1994;9:186–191.
249. Golub TR, Barker GF, Lovett M, et al. Fusion of PDGF receptor beta to a novel ets-like gene, tel, in chronic myelomonocytic leukemia with t(5;21) chromosomal translocation. *Cell* 1994;77:307–316.
250. Golub TR, Barker GF, Bohlander SK, et al. Fusion of the TEL gene on 12p13 to the AML1 gene on 21q22 in acute lymphoblastic leukemia. *Proc Natl Acad Sci USA* 1995;92:4917–4921.
251. Romana SP, Machauffe M, Le Coniat M, et al. The t(12;21) of acute lymphoblastic leukemia results in a TEL-AML1 gene fusion. *Blood* 1995;85:3662–3670.
252. Romana SP, Poirel H, LeConiat M, et al. High frequency of t(12;21) in childhood B-lineage acute lymphoblastic leukemia. *Blood* 1995; 86:4263–4269.
253. Shurtleff SA, Buijs A, Behm FG, et al. TEL/AML1 fusion resulting from a cryptic t(12;21) is the most common genetic lesion in pediatric ALL and defines a subgroup of patients with an excellent prognosis. *Leukemia* 1995;9:1985–1989.
254. Rubnitz JE, Downing JR, Pui C-H, et al. TEL gene rearrangement in acute lymphoblastic leukemia: a new genetic marker with prognostic significance. *J Clin Oncol* 1997;15:1150–1157.
255. McLean TW, Ringold S, Neuberg D, et al. TEL/AML-1 dimerizes and is associated with a favorable outcome in childhood acute lymphoblastic leukemia. *Blood* 1996;88:4252–4258.
256. Borkhardt A, Cazzaniga G, Viehmann S, et al. Incidence and clinical relevance of TEL/AML-1 fusion genes in children with acute lymphoblastic leukemia enrolled in the German and Italian multicenter therapy trials. *Blood* 1997;90:571–577.
257. Chilcote RR, Brown E, Rowley JD. Lymphoblastic leukemia with lymphomatous features associated with abnormalities of the short arm of chromosome 9. *N Engl J Med* 1985;313:286–291.
258. Murphy SB, Raimondi SC, Rivera GK, et al. Non-random abnormalities of chromosome 9p in childhood acute lymphoblastic leukemia: association with high-risk clinical features. *Blood* 1989;74:409–415.
259. Diaz MO, Rubin CM, Harden A, et al. Deletions of interferon genes in acute lymphoblastic leukemia. *N Engl J Med* 1990;322:77–82.
260. Berger R, Le Coniat M, Vecchione D, et al. Cytogenetic studies of 44 T-cell acute lymphoblastic leukemias. *Cancer Genet Cytogenet* 1990;44:69–75.
261. Serrano M, Hannon GJ, Beach D. A new regulatory motif in cell cycle control causing specific inhibition of cyclin D/CDK4. *Nature* 1993;366:704–707.
262. Kamb A, Gruis NA, Weaver-Feldhaus J, et al. A cell cycle regulator potentially involved in genesis of many tumor types. *Science* 1994; 264:436–440.
263. Herbert J, Cayuela JM, Berkely J, et al. Candidate tumor suppressor genes MTS1 (p16INK4A) and MST2 (p15INK4B) display frequent homozygous deletions in primary cells from T but not from B cell lineage acute lymphoblastic leukemias. *Blood* 1994;84:4038–4044.
264. Quesnel B, Preudhomme C, Philippe N, et al. p16 gene homozygous deletions in acute lymphoblastic leukemia. *Blood* 1995;85:657–663.
265. Takeuchi S, Bartram CR, Seriu T, et al. Analysis of family of cyclin dependent kinase inhibitors: p15/MTS2/INK4B, p16/MTS/INK4A and p18 genes in acute lymphoblastic leukemia of childhood. *Blood* 1995;86:755–760.
266. Okuda T, Shurtleff SA, Valentine MB, et al. Frequent deletion of p16INK4A/MTS1 and p15INK4B/MTS2 in pediatric acute lymphoblastic leukemia. *Blood* 1995;85:2321–2330.
267. Otsuki T, Clark HM, Wellman A, et al. Involvement of CDKN2 (p16INK4A)/MST1) and p15INK4B/MST2) in human leukemias and lymphomas. *Cancer Res* 1995;55:1436–1440.
268. Iolscon A, Faienza MF, Coppola B, et al. Homozygous deletions of cyclin-dependent kinase inhibitor genes, p16 INK4A and p18, in childhood T cell lineage acute lymphoblastic leukemias. *Leukemia* 1996;10:255–260.
269. Carroll AJ, Castleberry RP, Crist WM. Lack of association between abnormalities of the chromosome 9 short arm and either ''lymphomatous'' features or T-cell phenotype in childhood acute lymphocytic leukemia. *Blood* 1987;69:735–738.
270. Spitzer G, Garson DM. Lymphoblastic leukemia with marked eosinophilia: A report of two cases. *Blood* 1973;42:377–384.
271. Catovsky D, Bernasconi C, Verdonck PJ, et al. The association of eosinophilia with lymphoblastic leukemia or lymphoma: A study of seven patients. *Br J Haematol* 1980;45:523–534.
272. Hogan TF, Koss W, Murgo AJ, et al. Acute lymphoblastic leukemia with chromosomal 5;14 translocation and hypereosinophilia: case report and literature review. *J Clin Oncol* 1987;5:382–390.
273. Meeker TC, Hardy D, William C, et al. Activation of the interluekin-3 gene by chromosome translocation in acute lymphocytic leukemia with eosinophilia. *Blood* 1990;76:285–289.
274. Fishel RS, Farmer JP, Hanson CA, et al. Acute lymphoblastic leukemia with eosinophilia. *Medicine* 1990;69:232–243.
275. Wasmuth J, Ferrell R. Report of the committee on the genetic constitution of chromosome 5, Interim Human Gene Mapping Workshop 9.5. *Cytogenet Cell Genet* 1988;49:55–57.
276. Grimaldi JC, Meeker TC. The t(5;14) chromosomal translation in a case of acute lymphocytic leukemia joins the interleukin-3 gene to the immunoglobulin heavy chain gene. *Blood* 1989;73:2081–2085.
277. Trent JM, Kaneko Y, Mitelman F. Report of the committee on structural chromosome changes in neoplasia: human gene mapping 10 (1989). *Cytogenet Cell Genet* 1989;51:533–562.
278. Kaneko Y, Frizzera G, Shikano T, et al. Chromosomal and immunophenotypic patterns in T cell acute lymphoblastic leukemia (T-cell ALL) and lymphoblastic lymphoma (LBL). *Leukemia* 1989;3: 886–892.
279. Raimondi SC, Behm FG, Roberson PK, et al. Cytogenetics of childhood T-cell leukemia. *Blood* 1988;72:1560–1566.
280. Croce CM, Isobe M, Palumbo A, et al. Gene for α-chain of human T-cell receptor: location on chromosome 14 region involved in T cell neoplasms. *Science* 1985;227:1044–1047.
281. Coccia N, Bruns GAP, Kirsch IR, et al. T cell receptor α-chain genes are located on chromosome 14 at 14q 11-14q 12 in humans. *J Exp Med* 1985;161:1255–1260.
282. Le Beau MM, Diaz MO, Rowley JD, et al. Chromosomal localization of the human T cell receptor beta chain genes. *Cell* 1985;41:335.
283. Murre C, Waldmann RA, Morton CC, et al. Human γ-chain genes are rearranged in leukemic T cells and map to the short arm of chromosome 7. *Nature* 1985;316:549–552.
284. Erikson J, Williams DL, Finan J, et al Locus of the alpha-chain of the T-cell receptor is split by chromosome translocations in T-cell leukemia. *Science* 1985;229:784–786.
285. Lewis WA, Michalopoulos EE, Williams DL, et al. Breakpoints in the human T-cell antigen receptor α-chain locus in two T-cell leukemia patients with chromosomal translocations. *Nature* 1985;317:544–546.
286. LeBeau MM, McKeighan TW, Shima EA, et al. T-cell receptor α-chain gene is split in a human T-cell leukemia cell line with a t(11; 14)(p15;q11). *Proc Natl Acad Sci USA* 1986;83:9744–9748.
287. Berger R, Baranger L, Berheimm A, et al. Cytogenetics of T-cell malignant lymphoma: report of 17 cases and review of the chromosomal breakpoints. *Cancer Genet Cytogenet* 1988;36:123–130.
288. Champagne E, Takihara Y, Sagman U, et al. The T-cell receptor delta

chain locus is disrupted in the T-cell ALL associated t(11;14)(p13; q11) translocation. *Blood* 1989;73:1672–1676.
289. Lampert F, Harbott J, Ritterbach J, et al. T-cell acute childhood lymphoblastic leukemia with chromosome 14q11 anomaly: a morphologic, immunologic, and cytogenetic analysis of 10 patients. *Blut* 1988;56: 117–123.
290. Dube ID, Raimondi SC, Pi D, et al. A new translocation, t(10:14) (q24;q11), in T cell neoplasia. *Blood* 1986;67:1181–1184.
291. Zutter M, Hockett RD, Roberts CWM, et al. The t(10;14)(q24;q11) of T-cell acute lymphoblastic leukemia juxtaposes the δT cell receptor with TCL3, a conserved and activated locus at 10q24. *Proc Natl Acad Sci USA* 1990; 87:3161–3165.
292. Chen Q, Cheng J-T, Tsai LT, et al. The tal gene undergoes chromosome translocation in T cell leukemia and potentially encodes a helix-loop-helix protein. *EMBO J* 1990; 9:415–424.
293. Smith SD, Morgan R, Gemmell R, et al. Clinical and biologic characterization of T-cell neoplasias with rearrangements of chromosome 7 band q34. *Blood* 1988;71:395–402.
294. Kaneko Y, Frizzera G, Maseki N, et al. A novel translocation, t(9; 17)(q34;q23), in aggressive childhood lymphoblastic lymphoma. *Leukemia* 1988;2:745–748.
295. Longacre TA, Foucar K, Crago S, et al. Hematogones: a multiparameter analysis of bone marrow precursor cells. *Blood* 1989;73:543–552.
296. Gore SD, Kastan MB, Civin CI. Normal human bone marrow precursors that express terminal deoxynucleotidyl transferase include T-cell precursors and possible lymphoid stem cells. *Blood* 1991;77: 1681–1690.
297. Bearman RM, Winberg CD, Maslow WC, et al. Terminal deoxynucleotidyl transferase activity in neoplastic and non-neoplastic hematopoietic cells. *Am J Clin Pathol* 1981;75:794–802.
298. Muehleck SD, McKenna RW, Gale PF, et al. Terminal deoxynucleotidyl transferase (TdT)-positive cells in bone marrow in the absence of hematologic malignancy. *Am J Clin Pathol* 1983;79:277–284.
299. Caldwell CW, Patterson WP. Relationship between T200 antigen expression and stages of B cell differentiation in resurgent hyperplasia of bone marrow. *Blood* 1989;70:1165–1172.
300. Kobayashi SD, Seki K, Suwa N, et al. The transient appearance of small blastoid cells in the marrow after bone marrow transplantation. *Am J Clin Pathol* 1991;96: 191–195.
301. Sandhaus LM, Chen TL, Ettinger LJ, et al. Significance of increased proportions of CD10-positive cells in nonmalignant bone marrow of children. *Am J Pediatr Hematol Oncol* 1993;15:65–70.
302. Arber DA, Weiss LM. CD10: a review. *Appl Immunohistochem* 1997; 5:125–140.
303. Loken MR, Shah VO, Dattilio KL, et al. Flow cytometric analysis of human bone marrow: II. Normal B lymphocyte development. *Blood* 1987;70:1316–1324.
304. Wilson JF, Jenkin RDT, Anderson JR, et al. Studies on the pathology of non-Hodgkin's lymphoma of childhood: I. The role of routine histopathology as a prognostic factor, a report from the Children's Cancer Study Group. *Cancer* 1984;53:1695–1704.
305. Kant JA, Hicks DG. Interpretation of non-lymphoid elements in lymph node biopsy specimens. In: Jaffe E, ed. *Surgical pathology of the lymph nodes and related organs*, 2nd edition. Philadelphia: WB Saunders, 1995;594–623.
306. Furman WL, Fitch S, Hustu O, et al. Primary lymphoma of bone in children. *J Clin Oncol* 1989;7:1275–1280.
307. Yunis EJ. Ewing's sarcoma and related small round cell neoplasms in children. *Am J Surg Pathol* 1986;10(Suppl):54–62.
308. The Non-Hodgkin's Lymphoma Pathologic Classification Project. National Cancer Institute sponsored study of classification of non-Hodgkin's lymphomas: summary and description of a working formulation for clinical usage. *Cancer* 1982;49:2112–2135.
309. Rosai J, Levine GD. Tumors of the thymus. In: *Atlas of tumor pathology*, series 2, fascicle 13. Washington, DC: Armed Forces Institute of Pathology, 1976.
310. Battifora H, Silva EG. The use of antikeratin antibodies in the immunohistochemical distinction between neuroendocrine (Merkel cell) carcinoma of the skin, lymphoma, and oat cell carcinoma. *Cancer* 1986;58:1040–1046.
311. Visscher D, Cooper PH, Zarbo RJ, et al. Cutaneous neuroendocrine (Merkel cell) carcinoma: an immunophenotypic, clinicopathologic, and flow cytometric study. *Mod Pathol* 1989;2:331–338.
312. Lardelli P, Bookman MA, Sundeen J, et al. Lymphocytic lymphoma of intermediate differentiation: morphologic and immunophenotypic spectrum and clinical correlations. *Am J Surg Pathol* 1990;14: 752–763.
313. Mazza P, Bertini M, Macchi S, et al. Lymphoblastic lymphoma in adolescents and adults: clinical, pathological and prognostic evaluation. *Eur J Cancer Clin Oncol* 1986;22:1503– 1510.
314. Piira T, Perkins SL, Anderson JR, et al: Primary large B cell lymphoma in children: a report from the Children's Cancer Group. *Pediatr Pathol Lab Med* 1995:15:561–570.
315. Ioachim HL, Finkbeiner JA. Pseudonodular pattern of T-cell lymphoma. *Cancer* 1980;45:1370–1378.
316. Schwartz JE, Grogan TM, Hicks MJ, et al. Pseudonodular T cell lymphoblastic lymphoma. *Am J Med* 1984;77:947–949.
317. Kardos TF, Sprague RI, Wakely PE, et al. Fine-needle aspiration biopsy of lymphoblastic lymphoma and leukemia: a clinical, cytologic and immunologic study. *Cancer* 1987;60:2448–2453.
318. Jacobs JC, Katz RL, Shaff N, et al. Fine needle aspiration of lymphoblastic lymphoma: a multiparameter diagnostic approach. *Acta Cytol* 1992;36:887–894.
319. Braziel RM, Keneklis T, Donlon JA, et al. Terminal deoxynucleotidyl transferase in non-Hodgkin's lymphoma. *Am J Clin Pathol* 1983;80: 655–659.
320. Neiman RS, Barcos M, Berard C, et al. Granulocytic sarcoma: a clinicopathologic study of 61 biopsied cases. *Cancer* 1981;48:1426–1437.
321. Garaventa A, Dallorso S, Savioli C, et al. Granulocytic sarcoma presenting as an isolated mediastinal mass: a difficult diagnostic problem. *Acta Paediatr Scand* 1989;78:473–475.
322. Seremetis SV, Pelicci PG, Tabilio A, et al. High frequency of clonal immunoglobulin or T cell receptor gene rearrangements in acute myelogenous leukemia expressing terminal deoxyribonucleotidyl transferase. *J Exp Med* 1987;165:1703–1712.
323. Stark AN, MacKarill ID, Limbert HJ, et al. TdT expression in acute myeloid leukemia. *Blut* 1988;56:33–38.
324. Drexler HG, Sperling C, Wolf-Dieter L. Terminal deoxynucleotidyl transferase (TdT) expression in acute myeloid leukemia: review. *Leukemia* 1993;7:1142–1150.
325. Link M, Warnke R, Finlay J, et al. A single monoclonal antibody identifies T cell lineage of childhood lymphoid malignancies. *Blood* 1983;62:722–728.
326. Vodenelich L, Tax W, Bai Y, et al. A monoclonal antibody (WT1) for detecting leukemias of T-cell precursors (T-cell ALL). *Blood* 1983; 62:1108–1113.
327. Osada H, Emi N, Ueda R, et al. Genuine CD7 expression in acute leukemia and lymphoblastic lymphoma. *Leuk Res* 1990;14:869–877.
328. Eto T, Akashi K, Harada M, et al. Biological characteristics of CD7 positive acute myelogenous leukaemia. *Br J Haematol* 1992;82: 508–514.
329. Kondo S, Okamura S, Harada N, et al. CD7-positive acute myeloid leukemia: further evidence of cellular immaturity. *J Cancer Res Clin Oncol* 1992;118:386–388.
330. Buccheri V, Matutes E, Dyer MJS, et al. Lineage commitment in biphenotypic acute leukemia. 1993;9:919–927.
331. Drexler H, Thiel E, Ludwig W-D. Acute myeloid leukemias expressing lymphoid-associated antigens: diagnostic incidence and prognostic significance. *Leukemia* 1993;7:489–498.
332. Traweek ST. Immunophenotypic analysis of acute leukemia. *Am J Clin Pathol* 1993;99:504–512.
333. Venditti A, Del Poeta G, Buccisano F, et al. Minimally differentiated acute myeloid leukemia (AML-M0): comparison of 25 cases with other French-American-British subtypes. *Blood* 1997;89:621–629.
334. Campana D, Thompson JS, Amlot P, et al. The cytoplasmic expression of CD3 antigens in normal and malignant cells of the T lymphoid lineage. *J Immunol* 1987;138:648–655.
335. van Dongen JJM, Krissansen GW, Wolvers-Tettero ILM, et al. Cytoplasmic expression of the CD3 antigen as a diagnostic marker for immature T cell malignancies. *Blood* 1988;71:603–612.
336. Davey FR, Gatter KC, Ralfkiaer E, et al. Immunophenotyping of non-Hodgkin's lymphomas using a panel of antibodies on paraffin-embedded tissues. *Am J Pathol* 1987;129:54–63.
337. Kurec AS, Cruz VE, Barrett D, et al. Immunophenotyping of acute leukemias using paraffin-embedded tissue sections. *Am J Clin Pathol* 1990;93;502–509.
338. Jennings CD, Foon KA. Recent advances in flow cytometry: applica-

tion to the diagnosis of hematologic malignancy. *Blood* 1997;90: 2863–2892.
339. Mason DY, Cordell JL, Tse AG, et al. The IgM-associated protein mb-1 as a marker of normal and neoplastic B cells. *J Immunol* 1991; 147:2474–2482.
340. Janossy G, Coustan-Smith E, Campana D. The reliability of cytoplasmic CD3 and CD22 antigen expression in the immunodiagnosis of acute leukemia: a study of 500 cases. *Leukemia* 1989;3:170–181.
341. Hall PA, d'Ardenne AJ, Stansfeld AG. Paraffin section immunohistochemistry: I. Non-Hodgkin's lymphoma. *Histopathology* 1988;13: 149–160.
342. Linder J, Ye Y, Armitage JO, et al. Monoclonal antibodies marking B-cell non-Hodgkin's lymphoma in paraffin-embedded tissue. *Mod Pathol* 1988;1:29–34.
343. Norton J, Isaacson PG. Lymphoma phenotyping in formalin-fixed and paraffin wax-embedded tissues: II. Profiles of reactivity in the various tumour types. *Histopathology* 1989;14:557–579.
344. Kaplan SS, Penchansky L, Stoic V, et al. Immunophenotyping in the classification of acute leukemia in adults. Interpretation of multiple lineage reactivity. *Cancer* 1989;63:1520–1527.
345. Kurec AS, Belair P, Stefanu C, et al. Significance of aberrant immunophenotypes in childhood acute lymphoid leukemia. *Cancer* 1991;67: 3081–3086.
346. Rosanda C, Cant-Rajnoldi A, Ivernizzi R, et al. B-cell acute lymphoblastic leukemia (B-cell ALL): a report of 17 pediatric cases. *Haematologica* 1992;77:151–155.
347. Pui C, Rivera GK, Hancock ML, et al. Clinical significance of CD10 expression in childhood acute lymphoblastic leukemia. *Leukemia* 1993;7:35–40.
348. Civin CI, Trischman TM, Fackler MJ, et al. Report on the CD34 cluster workshop. In: Knapp W, Dörken B, Gilks WR, et al, eds. *Leukocyte typing IV: white cell differentiation antigens.* New York: Oxford University Press, 1989:818–825.
349. Borowitz MJ, Shuster JJ, Civin CI, et al. Prognostic significance of CD34 expression in childhood B-precursor acute lymphocytic leukemia: a Pediatric Oncology Group study. *J Clin Oncol* 1990;8: 1389–1398.
350. Pui CH, Hancock ML, Head DR, et al. Clinical significance of CD34 expression in childhood acute lymphoblastic leukemia. *Blood* 1993; 82:889–894.
351. Greaves MF, Titley I, Colman SM, et al. CD34 cluster workshop report. In: Schlossman SF, Boumsell L, Gilks WR, et al, eds. *Leukocyte typing V: white cell differentiation antigens.* New York: Oxford University Press, 1995;840–846.
352. Mirro J, Antouin GR, Zipf TF, et al. The E-rosette associated antigen of T cells can be identified on blasts from patients with acute myeloblastic leukemia. *Blood* 1985;65:363–367.
353. Adriaansen HJ, te Boekhorst PAW, Hagemeijer AM, et al. Acute myeloid leukemia M4 with bone marrow eosinophilia (M4Eo) and inv(16) (p13q22) exhibits a specific immunophenotype with CD2 expression. *Blood* 1993;81:3043–3051.
354. Paietta E, Wiernik PH, Andersen J, et al. Acute myeloid leukemia M4 with inv(16) (p13q22) exhibits a specific immunophenotype with CD2 expression, correspondence. *Blood* 1993;82:2595.
355. Arber DA, Jenkins KA, Slovak ML. CD79α expression in acute myeloid leukemia: high frequency of expression in acute promyelocytic leukemia. *Am J Pathol* 1996;149:1105–1110.
356. Battifora H, Sun TT, Bahu RM, et al. The use of antikeratin antiserum as a diagnostic tool: thymoma versus lymphoma. *Hum Pathol* 1980; 11:635–642.
357. Mokhtar N, Hsu SM, Lad RP, et al. Thymoma: lymphoid and epithelial components mirror the phenotype of normal thymus. *Hum Pathol* 1984;15:978–984.
358. Inghirami G, Chilosi M, Knowles DM. Western thymomas lack Epstein-Barr virus by Southern blotting and by polymerase chain reaction. *Am J Pathol* 1990;136:1429–1436.
359. Ichikawa Y, Shimizu H, Yoshida M, et al. Two-color flow cytometric analysis of thymic lymphocytes from patients with myasthenia gravis and/or thymoma. *Clin Immunol Immunopathol* 1992;62:91–96.
360. Azumi N, Battifora H. The distribution of vimentin and keratin in epithelial and nonepithelial neoplasms. A comprehensive immunohistochemical study on formalin and alcohol fixed tumors. *Am J Clin Pathol* 1987;88:286–296.
361. Katzin WE, Fishleder AJ, Linden MD, et al. Immunoglobulin and T-cell receptor genes in thymomas: genotypic evidence supporting the non-neoplastic nature of the lymphocytic component. *Hum Pathol* 1988;19:323–328.
362. Carter D, Eggleston JC. Tumors of the lower respiratory tract. In: *Atlas of tumor pathology*, series 2, fascicle 17. Washington, DC: Armed Forces Institute of Pathology, 1980.
363. Leong AS-Y, Phillips GE, Pieterse AS, et al. Criteria for the diagnosis of primary endocrine carcinoma of the skin (Merkel cell carcinoma): a histological, immunohistochemical and ultrastructural study of 13 cases. *Pathology* 1987;18:393–399.
364. Enzinger FM, Weiss SW. *Soft tissue tumors*, 2nd edition. St. Louis: CV Mosby, 1988.
365. Triche TJ. Neuroblastoma and other childhood neural tumors: a review. *Pediatr Pathol* 1990;10:175–193.
366. Kurtin PJ, Pinkus GS. Leukocyte common antigen-a diagnostic discriminant between hematopoietic and nonhematopoietic neoplasms in paraffin sections using monoclonal antibodies: correlation with immunologic studies and ultrastructural localization. *Hum Pathol* 1985;16: 353–365.
367. Salter DM, Krajewski AS, Dewar AE. Immunohistochemical staining of non-Hodgkin's lymphoma with monoclonal antibodies specific for the leucocyte common antigen. *J Pathol* 1985;146:345–353.
368. Norton AJ, Isaacson PG. An immunocytochemical study of T-cell lymphomas using monoclonal and polyclonal antibodies effective in routinely fixed wax embedded tissues. *Histopathology* 1986;10: 1243–1260.
369. Michels S, Swanson PE, Frizzera G, et al. Immunostaining for leukocyte common antigen using an amplified avidin-biotin-peroxidase complex method and paraffin sections. *Arch Pathol Lab Med* 1987; 111:1035–1039.
370. Strickler JG, Weiss LM, Copenhaver CM, et al. Monoclonal antibodies reactive in routinely processed tissue sections of malignant lymphoma, with emphasis on T-cell lymphomas. *Hum Pathol* 1987;18: 808–814.
371. Wieczorek R, Buck D, Bindl J, et al. Monoclonal antibody Leu-22 (L60) permits the demonstration of some neoplastic T cells in routinely fixed and paraffin-embedded tissue sections. *Hum Pathol* 1988; 19:1434–1443.
372. Elghetany MT, Kurec AS, Schuehler K, et al. Immunophenotyping of non-Hodgkin's lymphomas in paraffin-embedded tissue sections: a comparison with genotypic analysis. *Am J Clin Pathol* 1991;95: 517–525.
373. Behm FG, Raimondi SC, Schell MJ, et al. Lack of CD45 antigen on blast cells in childhood acute lymphoblastic leukemia is associated with chromosomal hyperdiploidy and other favorable prognostic features. *Blood* 1992;79:1011–1016.
374. Baldit C, Trojani M, Eghbali H, et al. Lymphoblastic lymphoma with convoluted nuclei: a report of 19 cases. *Oncology* 1984;41:252–256.
375. Streuli RA, Kaneko Y, Variakojis D, et al. Lymphoblastic lymphoma in adults. *Cancer* 1981;47:2510–2516.
376. Meyers L, Hakami N. Pre-B cell cutaneous lymphoma in infancy: a unique clinical entity. *Med Pediatr Oncol* 1984;12:252–254.
377. Murphy SB: Childhood non-Hodgkin's lymphoma. *N Engl J Med* 1978;299:1446–1448.
378. Carbone PP, Kaplan HS, Musshoff K, et al. Report of the committee on Hodgkin's disease staging classification. *Cancer Res* 1971;31: 1860–1861.
379. Morel P, Lepage E, Brice P, et al. Prognosis and treatment of lymphoblastic lymphoma in adults: a report on 80 patients. *J Clin Oncol* 1992; 10:1078–1085.
380. Lichtenstein AK, Levine A, Taylor CR, et al. Primary mediastinal lymphoma in adults. *Am J Med* 1980;68:509–514.
381. Zinzani PL, Bendandi M, Visani, G, et al. Adult lymphoblastic lymphoma: clinical features and prognostic factors in 53 patients. *Leuk Lymphoma* 1996;23:577–582.
382. Sander CA, Medeiros LJ, Abruzzo LV, et al. Lymphoblastic lymphoma presenting in cutaneous sites: a clinicopathologic analysis of six cases. *J Am Acad Dermatol* 1991;25:1023–1031.
383. Hansen BA, Sorensen PS, Lauritzen MI, et al. A case of malignant lymphoma and myasthenia gravis. *Scand J Hematol* 1983;31: 155–160.
384. Bowen JD, Kidd P. Myasthenia gravis associated with T helper cell lymphoma. *Neurology* 1987;37:1405–1408.
385. Mortimer JE, Kidd P. Myasthenia gravis and lymphoblastic lym-

phoma antiacetylcholine receptor antibody as a tumor marker: a case report. *Cancer Invest* 1989;7:327–331.

386. Liu KL, Herbrecht R, Tranchant C, et al. Malignant thymic lymphoblastic lymphoma and myasthenia gravis: an exceptional association. *Nouv Rev Fr Hematol* 1992;34:221–223.
387. Herman TS, Hammond N, Jones SE, et al. Involvement of the central nervous system by non-Hodgkin's lymphoma: the Southwest Oncology Group experience. *Cancer* 1979;943:390–397.
388. Ersbell HB, Schultz JB, Thomsen BLR, et al. Meningeal involvement in non-Hodgkin's lymphoma: symptoms, incidence, risk factors and treatment. *Scand J Haematol* 1985;35:487–496.
389. Keldsen N, Michalski W, Bentzen SM, et al. Risk factors for central nervous system involvement in non-Hodgkin's lymphoma. *Acta Oncologica* 1996;35:703–708.
390. Hausner RJ, Rosas-Uribe A, Wickstrum DA, et al. Non-Hodgkin's lymphoma in the first two decades of life: a pathological study of 30 cases. *Cancer* 1977;40:1533–1546.
391. Kaneko Y, Variakojis D, Kluskens L, et al. Lymphoblastic lymphoma: cytogenetic, pathologic and immunologic studies. *Int J Cancer* 1982; 30:273–279.
392. Jaffe N, Buell D, Cassady JR, et al. Role of staging in childhood non-Hodgkin's lymphoma. *Cancer Treat Rep* 1977;61:1001–1007.
393. Bernard A, Murphy SB, Melvin S, et al. Non-T, non-B lymphomas are rare in childhood and associated with cutaneous tumor. *Blood* 1982;59:549–554.
394. Sander CA, Jaffe ES, Gebhardt FC, et al. Mediastinal lymphoblastic lymphoma with an immature B-cell immunophenotype. *Am J Surg Pathol* 1992;16:300–305.
395. Knowles DM, Dodson L, Burke JS, et al. sIg-E-("null-cell") non-Hodgkin's lymphomas: multiparametric determination of their B- or T-cell lineage. *Am J Pathol* 1985;120:356–370.
396. Loeffler JS, Tarbell NJ, Kozakewich H, et al. Primary lymphoma of bone in children: analysis of treatment results with adriamycin, prednisone, oncovin (APO), and local radiation therapy. *J Clin Oncol* 1986;4:496–501.
397. Kamps WA, Poppema S. Pre-B-cell non-Hodgkin's lymphoma in childhood. *Am J Clin Pathol* 1988;90:103–107.
398. Schwob VS, Weiner L, Hudes G, et al. Extranodal non-T-cell lymphoblastic lymphoma in adults: a report of two cases. *Am J Clin Pathol* 1988;90:602–605.
399. Nieman TH, Thomas PA. Primary lymphoma of bone: diagnosis by fine-needle aspiration biopsy in a pediatric patient. *Diagn Cytopathol* 1995;12:165–167.
400. Castella A, Neuberg RW, Kurec AS, et al. Non-Hodgkin's lymphoma with immunologic phenotype similar to non-T, non-B acute lymphocytic leukemia. *Hum Pathol* 1982;13:777–779.
401. Lands R, Karnad A. Non-T cell lymphoblastic lymphoma with extensive osteolytic lesions and hypercalcemia. *South Med J* 1991;84: 1405–1406.
402. Smith RG. Parosteal lymphoblastic lymphoma: a human counterpart of Abelson virus-induced lymphosarcoma of mice. *Cancer* 1984;54: 471–476.
403. Papadimitriou CS, Papacharalampous NX, Kittas C. Primary gastrointestinal malignant lymphomas: a morphologic and immunohistochemical study. *Cancer* 1985;55:870–879.
404. Grody WW, Weiss LM, Warnke RA, et al. Gastrointestinal lymphomas: Immunohistochemical studies on the cell of origin. *Am J Surg Pathol* 1985;9:328–337.
405. Kuo TT, Yang CP, Lin CH, et al. Lymphoblastic lymphoma presenting as a huge intracavitary cardiac tumor causing heart failure. *Pediatr Pathol* 1987;7:341–349.
406. Camitta BM, Casper JT, Kun LE, et al. Isolated bilateral T-cell renal lymphoblastic lymphoma. *Am J Ped Heme/Oncol* 1986;8:8–12.
407. Cunningham D, Gilchrist NL, Lee FD, et al. T cell lymphoblastic lymphoma of the uterus complicated by Chlamydia trachomatis pneumonia. *Postgrad Med J* 1986;62:55–57.
408. Chiu EKW, Loke SL, Chan ACL, et al. T-lymphoblastic lymphoma arising in the small intestine. *Pathology* 1991;23:356–359.
409. Macon WR, Rynalski TH, Swerdlow SH, et al. T cell lymphoblastic leukemia/lymphoma presenting in a recurrent thymoma. *Mod Pathol* 1991;4:524–528.
410. Friedman HD, Inman DA, Hutchinson RE, et al. Concurrent invasive thymoma and T cell lymphoblastic leukemia and lymphoma: a case report with necropsy findings and literature review of thymoma and associated hematologic neoplasm. *Am J Clin Pathol* 1994;101: 432–437.
411. Vogler LB, Crist WM, Bockman DE, et al. Pre-B cell leukemia. A new phenotype of childhood lymphoblastic leukemia. *N Engl J Med* 1978;298:872–878.
412. Kukreja S, Zarkowsky H. Cutaneous lymphoma in an infant: case report. *Med Pediatr Oncol* 1979;7:17–18.
413. Link MP, Roper M, Dorfman RF, et al. Cutaneous lymphoblastic lymphoma with pre-B markers. *Blood* 1983;61:838–841.
414. Borowitz MJ, Croker BP, Metzgar RS. Lymphoblastic lymphoma with the phenotype of common acute lymphoblastic leukemia. *Am J Clin Pathol* 1983;79:387–391.
415. Grumayer ER, Ladenstein RL, Slave I, et al. B cell differentiation pattern of cutaneous lymphomas in infancy and childhood. *Cancer* 1988;61:303–308.
416. Vaillant L, Lorette G, Colombat P, et al. Primary cutaneous lymphoblastic lymphoma of non-B, non-T phenotype. *Arch Dermatol* 1990; 126:400–401.
417. Pui C-H, Behm FG, Raimondi SC, et al. Secondary acute myeloid leukemia in children treated for acute lymphoid leukemia. *N Engl J Med* 1989;321:136–142.
418. Kjeldsberg CR, Nathwani BN, Rappaport H. Acute myeloblastic leukemia developing in patients with mediastinal lymphoblastic lymphoma. *Cancer* 1979;44:2316–2323.
419. Hermann R, Han T, Barcos MP, et al. Malignant lymphoma of pre-T cell type terminating in acute myelocytic leukemia: a case report with enzymic and immunologic marker studies. *Cancer* 1980;46: 1383–1388.
420. Posner MR, Said J, Pinkus GS, et al. T-cell lymphoblastic lymphoma with subsequent acute non-lymphocytic leukemia: a case report. *Cancer* 1982;50:118–124.
421. Murphy SB, Stass S, Kalwinsky D, et al. Phenotypic conversion of acute leukaemia from T lymphoblastic to myeloblastic induced by therapy with 2′-deoxycoformycin. *Br J Haematol* 1983;55:285–293.
422. Herschfield MS, Kurtzberg J, Harden E, et al. Conversion of a stem cell leukemia from a T lymphoid to a myeloid phenotype induced by the adenosine deaminase inhibitor 2′-deoxycoformycin. *Proc Natl Acad Sci USA* 1984;81:253–257.
423. Stass S, Mirro J, Melvin S, et al. Lineage switch in acute leukemia. *Blood* 1984;64:701–706.
424. Childs CC, Chrystal GS, Strauchen JA. Biphenotypic lymphoblastic lymphoma: an unusual tumor with lymphocytic and granulocytic differentiation. *Cancer* 1986;57:1019–1023.
425. Nosaka T, Ohno H, Doi S, et al. Phenotypic conversion of T lymphoblastic lymphoma to acute biphenotypic leukemia composed of lymphoblasts and myeloblasts: molecular genetic evidence of the same clonal origin. *J Clin Invest* 1988;81:1824–1828.
426. Soslow RA, Davis RE, Warnke RA, et al. True histiocytic lymphoma following therapy for lymphoblastic neoplasms. *Blood* 1996;87: 5207–5212.
427. Risdall RJ, McKenna RW, Nesbit ME: Virus-associated hemophagocytic syndrome: a benign histiocytic proliferation distinct from malignant histiocytosis. *Cancer* 1979;44:993–1002.
428. Kinney MC, Greer JP, Glick AD, et al. Anaplastic large-cell Ki-1 malignant lymphomas. Recognition, biological and clinical implications. *Pathol Annu* 1991;26:1–24.
429. Delabie J, Vandenberghe E, Kennes C, et al. Histiocyte-rich B-cell lymphoma: a distinct clinicopathologic entity possibly related to lymphocyte predominant Hodgkin's disease, paragranuloma subtype. *Am J Surg Pathol* 1992;16:37–48.
430. Liang R, Todd D, Chan TK, et al. Intensive therapy for adult lymphoblastic lymphoma. *Cancer Chemother Pharmacol* 1991;29:80–82.
431. Aur RJA, Hustu HO, Simone JV, et al. Therapy of localized and regional lymphosarcoma of childhood. *Cancer* 1971;27:1328–1331.
432. Weinstein HJ, Vance ZB, Jaffe N, et al. Improved prognosis for patients with mediastinal lymphoblastic lymphoma. *Blood* 1979;53: 687–694.
433. Camitta BM, Lauer SJ, Casper JT, et al. Effectiveness of a six-drug regimen (APO) without local irradiation for treatment of mediastinal lymphoblastic lymphoma in children. *Cancer* 1985;56:738–741.
434. Wollner N, Burchenal JH, Lieberman PH, et al. Non-Hodgkin's lymphoma in children: a comparative study of two modalities of therapy. *Cancer* 1976;37:123–134.
435. Wollner N, Exelby PR, Lieberman PH. Non-Hodgkin's lymphoma in

children: a progress report on the original patients treated with the LSA2-L2 protocol. *Cancer* 1979;44:1990–1999.
436. Anderson JR, Wilson JF, Jenkin DT, et al. Childhood non-Hodgkin's lymphoma: the results of a randomized therapeutic trial comparing a 4-drug regimen (COMP) with a 10-drug regimen (LSA2-L2). *N Engl J Med* 1983;308:559–565.
437. Sullivan MP, Boyett J, Pullen J, et al. Pediatric Oncology Group experience with modified LSA2-L2 therapy in 107 children with non-Hodgkin's lymphoma (Burkitt's lymphoma excluded). *Cancer* 1985; 55:323–336.
438. Pichler E, Jurgenssen OA, Radaszkiewicz T, et al. Results of LSA2-L2 therapy in 26 children with non-Hodgkin's lymphoma. *Cancer* 1982;50:2740–2746.
439. Zintl F, Herman J, Katenkamp D, et al. Results of LSA2-L2 therapy in children with high-risk acute lymphoblastic leukaemia and non-Hodgkin's lymphoma. *Haematol Blood Trans* 1983;28:62–66.
440. Anderson JR, Jenkin RDT, Wilson JF, et al. Long-term follow-up of patients treated with COMP or LSA2 L2 therapy for childhood non-Hodgkin's lymphoma: a report of CCG-551 from the Children's Cancer Group. *J Clin Oncol* 1993;11:1024–1032.
441. Hvizdala EV, Berard C, Callihan BT, et al. Lymphoblastic lymphoma in children: a randomized trial comparing LSA2-L2 with the A-COP + therapeutic regimen. A Pediatric Oncology Group study. *J Clin Oncol* 1988;6:26–33.
442. Eden OB, Hann I, Imeson J, et al. Treatment of advanced stage T cell lymphoblastic lymphoma: results of the United Kingdom Children's Cancer Study Group (UKCCSG) protocol 8503. *Br J Hematol* 1992, 82:310–316.
443. Coleman CN, Cohen JR, Burke JS, et al. Lymphoblastic lymphoma in adults: results of a pilot protocol. *Blood* 1981;57:679–684.
444. Levine AM, Forman SJ, Meyer PR, et al. Successful therapy of convoluted T-lymphoblastic lymphoma in the adult. *Blood* 1983;61:92–98.
445. Coleman CN, Picozzi VJ, Cox RS, et al. Treatment of lymphoblastic lymphoma in adults. *J Clin Oncol* 1986;4:1628–1637.
446. Sweetenham JW, Mead GM, Whitehouse JMA. Adult lymphoblastic lymphoma: High incidence of central nervous system relapse in patients treated with the Stanford University protocol. *Ann Oncol* 1992; 3:839–841.
447. Slater DE, Mertelsman R, Koziner B, et al. Lymphoblastic lymphoma in adults. *J Clin Oncol* 1986;4:57–67.
448. Colgon J, Anderson J, Glick J, et al. Treatment of lymphoblastic lymphoma in adults. *Proc Am Soc Clin Oncol* 1987;6:194.
449. Picozzi VJ, Coleman CN. Lymphoblastic lymphoma. *Semin Oncol* 1990;17:96–103.
450. Kersey J, Krailo M, Meadows A, et al. Childhood lymphoblastic lymphoma: a randomized trial comparing LSA-2 to ADCOMP. *Proc Am Soc Clin Oncol* 1991;10:289.
451. Appelbaum FR, Sullivan KM, Buckmer CD, et al. Treatment of malignant lymphoma in 100 patients with chemotherapy, total body irradiation, and marrow transplantation. *J Clin Oncol* 1987;5:1344–1347.
452. Philip T, Armitage JO, Spitzer G, et al. High dose therapy and autologous bone marrow transplantation after failure of conventional chemotherapy in adults with intermediate or high grade non-Hodgkin's lymphoma. *N Engl J Med* 1987;316:1493–1498.
453. Santini G, Coser P, Chisesi T, et al. Autologous bone marrow transplantation for advanced stage adult lymphoblastic lymphoma in first complete remission: a pilot study of the non-Hodgkin's Lymphoma Co-operative Study Group (NHLCSG). *Bone Marrow Transplant* 1989;4:399–404.
454. Milpied N, Ifrah N, Kuentz M, et al. Bone marrow transplantation for adult poor prognosis lymphoblastic lymphoma in first complete remission. *Br J Haematol* 1989;73:82–87.
455. Santini G, Congiu AM, Coser P, et al. Autologous bone marrow transplantation for adult advanced stage lymphoblastic lymphoma in first CR. A study of the NHLCSG. *Leukemia* 1991;5[Suppl 1]:42–45.
456. Sweetenham JW, Liberti G, Pearce R, et al. High-dose therapy and autologous bone marrow transplantation for adult patients with lymphoblastic lymphoma: results of the European Group for Bone Marrow Transplantation. *J Clin Oncol* 1994;12:1358–1365.
457. Picozzi VJ. Lymphoblastic lymphoma. In: Dana B, Ed. *Malignant lymphoma including Hodgkin's disease: diagnosis, management, and special problems.* Boston: Kluwer Academic Publishers, 1993:81–94.
458. Shepard SF, Hern RP, Pinkerton CR, on behalf of the United Kingdom Children's Cancer Study Group (UKCCSG). Childhood T cell lymphoblastic lymphoma: does early resolution of mediastinal mass predict for final outcome? *Br J Cancer* 1995;72:752–756.
459. Cave H, ten Bosch JVDW, Suciu S, et al. Clinical significance of minimal residual disease in childhood acute lymphoblastic leukemia. *N Engl J Med* 1998;339:591–598.
460. Coustan-Smith E, Behm FG, Sanchez J, et al. Immunological detection of minimal residual disease in children with acute lymphoblastic leukaemia. *Lancet* 1998;351:550–554.
461. Katz RL, Caraway NP. FNA lymphoproliferative diseases: myths and legends. *Diagn Cytopathol* 1995;12:99–100.
462. Bradstock KF, Janossy G, Tidman N, et al. Immunological monitoring of residual disease in treated thymic acute lymphoblastic leukaemia. *Leuk Res* 1981;5:301–309.
463. Van Dongen JJM, Hooijkaas H, Adriaansen HJ, et al. Detection of minimal residual acute lymphoblastic leukemia by immunological marker analysis: possibilities and limitations. In: Hagenbeek A, Lowenberg B, eds. *Minimal residual disease in acute leukemia.* Dordecht: M. Nijhoff, 1986:113–121.
464. Campana D, Coustan-Smith E, Janossy G. The immunological detection of minimal residual disease in acute leukemia. *Blood* 1990;76: 163–171.
465. Campana D, Coustan-Smith E, Behm FG. The definition of remission in acute leukemia with immunologic techniques. *Bone Marrow Transplant* 1991;8:429–437.
466. Drach J, Drach D, Glassl H, et al. Flow cytometric determination of atypical antigen expression in acute leukemia for the study of minimal residual disease. *Cytometry* 1992;13:893–901.
467. Hooijkaas H, Hahlen K, Adriaansen HJ, et al. Terminal deoxynucleotidyl transferase (TdT)-positive cells in cerebrospinal fluid and development of overt CNS leukemia: a 5-year follow-up study in 113 children with a TdT-positive leukemia or non-Hodgkin's lymphoma. *Blood* 1989;74:416–422.
468. Thomas JA, Janossy G, Eden OB, et al. Nuclear terminal deoxynucleotidyl transferase in leukaemic infiltrates of testicular tissue. *Br J Cancer* 1982;45:709–717.
469. Katz F, Ball L, Gibbons B, et al. The use of DNA probes to monitor minimal residual disease in childhood acute lymphoblastic leukemia. *Br J Haematol* 1989;73:173–180.
470. D'Auriol L, MacIntyre E, Galibert F, et al. In vitro amplification of T-cell γ-gene rearrangements: a new tool for the assessment of minimal residual disease in acute lymphoid blastic leukemias. *Leukemia* 1989; 3:155–158.
471. Hansen-Hagge TE, Yokota S, Bartram CR. Detection of minimal residual disease in acute lymphoblastic leukemia by in vitro amplification of rearranged T-cell receptor δ chain sequences. *Blood* 1989;74: 1762–1767.
472. Devaraj PE, Foroni L, Kitra-Roussos V, et al. Detection of BCR-ABL and E2A-PBX1 fusion genes by RT-PCR in acute lymphoblastic leukemia with failed or normal cytogenetics. *Br J Haematol* 1996; 89:349–355.
473. Devaraj PE, Foroni L, Janossy G, et al. Expression of the E2A-PBX fusion transcripts in t(1;19)(q23;p13) and der(19)t(1;19) at diagnosis and in remission of acute lymphoblastic leukemia with different B lineage immunophenotypes. *Leukemia* 1995;9:821–825.
474. Cimino G, Elia L, Rivolta A, et al. Clinical relevance of residual disease monitoring by polymerase chain reaction in patients with ALL-1/AF-4 positive-acute lymphoblastic leukemia. *Br J Haematol* 1996;92:659–664.
475. Yamada M, Hudson S, Tournay O, et al. Detection of minimal disease in hematopoietic malignancies of the B-cell lineage by using third-complementarity-determining region (CDR-III)-specific probes. *Proc Natl Acad Sci USA* 1989;86:5123–5127.
476. Yamada M, Wasserman R, Lange B, et al. Minimal residual disease in childhood B-lineage lymphoblastic leukemia. Persistence of leukemic cells during the first 18 months of treatment. *N Engl J Med* 1990; 323:448–455.
477. Brisco MJ, Condon J, Hughes E, et al. Outcome prediction in childhood acute lymphoblastic leukemia by molecular quantification of residual disease at the end of induction. *Lancet* 1994;343:196–200.

CHAPTER 27

Burkitt's Lymphoma

Ian Magrath, Elaine S. Jaffe, and Kishor Bhatia

NOMENCLATURE

The term *Burkitt's lymphoma* (BL) first was used to describe a common tumor in children in equatorial Africa, the characteristic clinical features of which were described by Burkitt (1) at approximately the same time as O'Conor (2) reported that 50% of the childhood malignant tumors in their series in Uganda were diffuse lymphomas, the majority of which were histologically identical. Of Ugandan patients with this rapidly progressive tumor, 60% to 70% presented with jaw tumors and 50% had abdominal masses. Because of its high frequency, apparently restricted geographic distribution (subsequently shown to be caused by climatic limitations of the distribution of the tumor in equatorial Africa), and quite well defined histologic and clinical features, it seems likely that the equatorial African form of the disease, sometimes referred to as *endemic* BL, is a single pathologic entity. The histologic category of *small noncleaved cell lymphoma*, however, as defined in the Working Formulation for Clinical Usage (3), which was divided into BL and non-BL subtypes, encompassed entities that differed with respect to immunopathology as well as cytogenetics and molecular genetics. The term was used because of the morphologic resemblance of the tumor cells to a population of normal cells in the germinal centers of lymph nodes, and it is important to recognize that the classification was based on tumors from the United States and Europe, not Africa (4). In the recent Revised European–American Classification of Lymphoid Neoplasms (REAL), *small noncleaved cell lymphoma* was replaced by the terms *BL* and *BL-like lymphoma* (BLL), with the important distinction that such lymphomas were exclusively of B-cell origin (5). Burkitt's-like lymphoma fell into the histologic no-man's land between BL and the REAL classification's large B-cell lymphoma (LBCL), which are entities on a continuous histologic spectrum (6). There is no doubt that BLL is heterogeneous, because it encompasses not only tumors that have the same nonrandom chromosomal translocations first described in African BL—t(8;14) or variant translocations such as t(2;8) or t(8;22)—but others that bear the cytogenetic hallmark of the majority of follicular lymphomas, t(14;18), a translocation that also occurs in some 25% of LBCLs (7), as well as, occasionally, cytogenetic abnormalities that also occur in LBCL. Some BLLs contain both t(8;14) or a variant translocation and t(14;18). A small proportion (5–10% overall) of instances of LBCL, particularly extranodal tumors, apparently contain the same translocations that occur in BL (although there could be differences at the molecular level) (8).

Histology and cytogenetics are not consonant with respect to these three categories of B-cell lymphomas (BL, BLL, and LBCL). Although the histologic borders of BL are not highly reproducible among histopathologists, using a strict histologic definition the vast majority of BLs examined by highly experienced lymphoma pathologists have been shown to contain t(8;14) or variant chromosomal translocations, and not t(14;18). This is an easier task in children, in whom the proportion of LBCLs is much lower than in adults, as is the proportion of BLLs (Fig. 27.1). There can be little doubt that BL is also a true entity outside equatorial Africa, but the border dividing it from other B-cell lymphomas is not sharp, because of the continuous histologic spectrum on which BL, BLL, and LBCL lie. Because most BLLs behave clinically like BLs, that is, in a very aggressive manner, and appear to require similar treatment approaches (9,10), those that are not true BLs, defined at molecular and immunophenotypic levels, but closely resemble BL histologically could be considered a separate subset of B-cell lymphomas. Whether these tumors fall within the heterogeneous mixture of tumors known as LBCL or should be classified separately is something of a moot point. The gradual histologic transition between BLL and LBCL and the occasional presence in BLL of chromosomal translocations, such as t(14;18), that

I. Magrath: Department of Pediatrics, University of the Uniformed Services in the Health Sciences, Bethesda, Maryland

E. S. Jaffe and K. Bhatia: Lymphoma Biology Section, National Cancer Institute, Bethesda, Maryland 20892

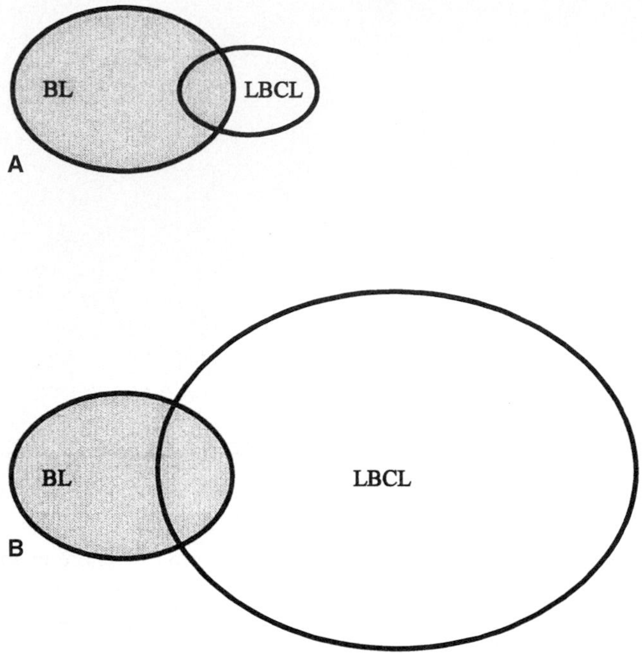

FIG. 27.1. The overlap between diseases defined on the basis of histology and cytogenetics in children (**A**) and adults (**B**). The difference in the proportions of Burkitt's lymphoma and large B-cell lymphomas is shown, and at the overlap point the differences in the proportions of Burkitt's-like lymphoma (BLL) are indicated (not drawn to scale). In adults, a higher proportion of tumors are BLL than in children, which corresponds to the higher proportion of large B-cell lymphomas. Some 5% to 10% of histologically typical large B-cell lymphomas contain t(8;14) or variant translocations (not shown). The likelihood that BLL differs with respect to the relative proportions of true Burkitt's lymphoma and cytogenetically or molecularly different tumors in adults versus children can be seen.

are encountered with high frequency (approximately 20%) in LBCL supports their inclusion among the LBCLs, but this issue is unlikely to be resolved until the issue of heterogeneity in LBCLs also has been resolved—presumably by adopting a classification based on their molecular features. The very aggressive clinical behavior of BLL suggests that it represents at least a specific subset of LBCL. One possibility worthy of consideration is that BLL, if indeed this represents a separate entity, contains a deregulated *MYC* gene like BL (hence its aggressive behavior and high growth fraction) but deregulation, unlike BL, does not always occur as a consequence of t(8;14) or a variant translocation.

Evolution from Follicular Lymphoma

Some BLLs appear to originate as subclinical indolent lymphomas, because not only has transformation from overt follicular lymphoma to BLL, based both on histology and the presence of a t(8;14) or a variant translocation been well described (11–14), but the occurrence of follicular lymphoma after presentation with BLL also is well known. This explains the occasional occurrence of lymphomas bearing both t(14;18) as well as t(8;14) or variant translocations, a situation that has a parallel in mice transgenic for *Bcl2* (the gene that is deregulated in lymphomas that bear the translocation t[14;18]), in which progression to aggressive diffuse lymphoma associated with rearrangement of the *MYC* gene also has been observed (15). The expression of *BCL2*, and the consequent prevention by this antiapoptotic gene of programmed cell death, may provide one of several functional requirements for the major molecular abnormality of BL, namely *MYC* deregulation, to lead to neoplasia (16), although the prevention of apoptosis is not brought about by *BCL2* in BL. Apparently in some tumors (e.g., BLL) it can be. Of course, the possibility that tumors bearing the translocation t(14;18) but histologically resembling BL also may occur *de novo*, that is, in the absence of a preexisting indolent lymphoma, cannot be excluded. Indolent lymphomas are rare in most developing countries, suggesting that those forms of BL or BLL that arise from a preexisting indolent lymphoma, subclinical or not, also would be rare in Africa, but there is presently no available information about this. Indolent lymphomas are also rare, however, in children, and BLL, whether arising from a preexisting indolent lymphoma or not, is correspondingly uncommon in children. As is shown in Figure 27.1, LBCL also is relatively uncommon in children compared with adults, so that the composition and frequency of BLL are likely to differ between adults and children. BLL appears to be a heterogeneous mixture of true BL, in which the histology is not as classic as usual, and one or more tumors more closely related to LBCL that, like BL, have high growth fractions and aggressive clinical behavior. Whether the occasional case of histologically classic LBCL with a translocation t(8;14) belongs properly in the BLL category is a debatable point at present. More information regarding the growth fractions of these tumors and their clinical behavior and response to therapy is required in order to provide a more satisfactory answer to this question.

World Health Organization Classification

Whatever the origins of lymphomas that resemble BL but have a more pleomorphic appearance, and may differ at a molecular level, the available evidence suggests that such lymphomas ought to be treated in the same way as BL, because they respond in an essentially identical fashion to the same therapy. In developing the new World Health Organization classification scheme, which is derived from the REAL classification, pathologists proposed initially that BLL should be defined as a subtype of large B-cell lymphoma. There was a consensus among oncologists, however, that this probably would lead to patients with such lymphomas receiving less than adequate therapy—that is, the same therapy that is given for LBCL (17). In an attempt to identify particularly aggressive tumors requiring the same therapy as BL, the pathologists suggested the term *atypical* BL for such tumors, but because this designation implies that the tumors are closely related to BL, which may not always be the case at a molecular level, it was decided to retain the term BLL, albeit with a more narrow definition than the REAL category of BLL, so that tumors felt to be LBCLs with high growth fractions would be excluded. Although more research is required to clarify the origins of BLL, because essentially 100% of cells in BL are "cycling"—that is, their growth fraction is 100% (a possible reason for their high curability)—only tumors in which more than 99% of cells are stained by Ki-67 or MIB-1, indicators of proliferating cells, are considered, in the World Health Organization classification, to fall within the category of BL or BLL. In addition, three subcategories were proposed—*endemic*, *nonendemic*, and *imunodeficiency-associated*—on the grounds that these are the major subtypes of the disease. Unfortunately, the first two categories beg a number of questions, and because they represent geographic rather than histologic variants, it is not clear how helpful this categorization is. In addition, how much the World Health Organization category of BLL differs from the REAL category of BLL with respect to the spectrum of lymphomas encompassed is unknown, and because this category was not reproducible among pathologists (there was only 50% agreement), it is likely to remain relatively poorly defined, although the addition of the need to demonstrate a proliferation fraction greater than 99% should result in an improvement in reproducibility. The lack of histological correlation with cytogenetics is demonstrated even more clearly in patients with HIV-associated non-Hodgkin's lymphomas, in whom a relatively high fraction (compared with non–HIV associated lymphomas) of tumors histologically classified as BLL or LBCL have molecular abnormalities typical of BL (18,19) (see Chapter 28). Of possible relevance to this and to the issue of variable histology in molecularly defined BL is the finding that cell lines derived from BL can be induced to alter their histologic appearances by treatment with phorbol esters (20). This suggests that the precise histologic appearance may reflect the totality of molecular changes in the tumor cell, a suggestion that is supported by some experimental data. The possibility that the microenvironment also may influence the histology of the tumor, however, cannot be discounted.

Burkitt's Leukemia

Another nomenclatural issue involves acute B-cell leukemia. It long has been recognized that a small fraction (2–4%) of patients who present with a clinical syndrome consistent with acute lymphoblastic leukemia actually have neoplasms of mature B-cell phenotype; that is, they express surface immunoglobulin, have morphology similar to BL (referred to in the French–American–British classification of acute lymphoblastic leukemia as *L3* acute lymphoblastic leukemia [21]), and often bear the same chromosomal translocations as BL (22–26). In other cases, either t(14;18) or both t(8;14) or a variant translocation and a translocation t(14;18) are present (27,28). Clearly, these leukemias, or at least those with a t(8;14) or both t(8;14) and t(14;18) translocations, which closely parallel the lymphomas (with or without bone marrow involvement) with respect to their immunophenotypic and molecular abnormalities, should be considered to be simply BL or BLL in leukemic phase. Even the rare cases in which a translocation t(14;18) but no t(8;14) is present are likely to be the equivalent of transformed follicular lymphoma and are the leukemic equivalent of at least one subset of BL or BLL. The presence in bone marrow or peripheral blood is thus a prognostic factor or staging issue, as recognized in the World Health Organization classification, rather than signifying a separate entity. Not all leukemias with L3 morphology are Burkitt's leukemia. Some lack the characteristic translocations of BL, and some have been reported to possess T-cell characteristics (29–31). Also, not all patients present with a leukemic syndrome. Many present with solid masses and then are shown to have bone marrow involvement, so that there is no clear dividing line between BL and Burkitt's leukemia, or between BLL and its leukemic counterpart. In pediatric oncology, the term *acute B-cell leukemia* has been used widely if BL involves the bone marrow to the extent that 25% or more of the nucleated cells are BL cells. In adult oncology, a dividing line between leukemia and lymphoma has not been accepted universally, although many use a figure of 30% or more blasts in the bone marrow to signify leukemia. Because many lymphoid neoplasms of B-cell origin involve the bone marrow, the acute B-cell leukemia probably encompasses a rather heterogeneous group of diseases, although most should be distinguishable clearly from BL or BLL. Cases that clearly meet the criteria for a diagnosis of BL or a BLL should be considered Burkitt's leukemia rather than acute B-cell leukemia. In children, because BL is much more common than BLL, it seems likely that Burkitt's leukemia is a more homogeneous disease than in adults.

Burkitt's Leukemia with an Immature Immunophenotype

Rare cases reported as acute lymphoblastic leukemia of L3 type contain a t(8;14) translocation but express cytoplasmic μchains without surface immunoglobulin and may express terminal deoxyribonucleotidyl transferase (TdT), indicating a more immature phenotype than that of BL (32–35): Not only is the expression of cytoplasmic μ chains a hallmark of pre-B cells, but TdT is expressed during immunoglobulin gene rearrangement. This is consistent with the hypothesis that the chromosomal translocations occur early in B-cell differentiation, but these cases are sufficiently rare that not all pathologists are convinced of their existence. Some leukemias with BL or BLL morphology may not express immunoglobulin at all, although they do not have an immature immunophenotype. In some cases this may be because of the involvement of both 14 chromosomes by a translocation: t(14;18) on one and t(8;14) on the other (27,36,37). In others, however, either a translocation t(14;18) or t(8;14) is present, without an explanation for the lack of immunoglobulin synthesis (unless the leukemia has an immature phenotype, as described previously) (38,39).

In addition to acute B-cell leukemias with L3 (BL) morphology, occasional cases of acute lymphoblastic leukemia express surface immunoglobulin but morphologically conform to the L1 or L2 French–American–British types. Such leukemias also may express TdT (as do the majority of L1 and L2 leukemias) but do not have a translocation t(8;14) (40). Some of these have t(14;18) with or without translocations other than t(8;14) (41–43). In interpreting atypical findings of these kinds, one should be aware that the reproducibility of French–American–British subtype classification is not 100% accurate even in the most expert hands; however, it would appear that neither a morphologic diagnosis of L3 leukemia nor the detection of surface immunoglobulin provides sufficient grounds for concluding that the neoplasm is the pathologic equivalent of BL or BLL. Definitive diagnosis requires immunophenotyping *and* cytogenetics or molecular characterization.

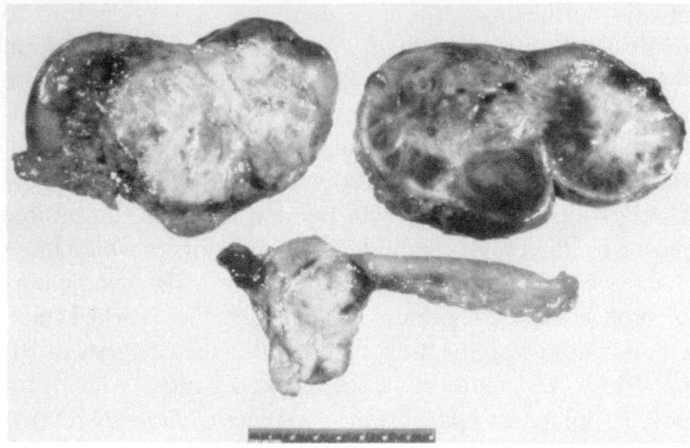

FIG. 27.2. Gross pathologic appearance of bilateral ovarian tumors removed from a 25-year-old North American woman who had Burkitt's lymphoma. The tumor has a creamy appearance and the consistency of ripe brie cheese and is relatively avascular. No other tumor was present in this patient, and she achieved long-term survival after chemotherapy.

Definitions of BL and BLL

Given the problems of definition and the rarity of BL, it is not surprising that it has been difficult to establish the true incidence of this disease in many parts of the world, even in the United States. Accuracy of diagnosis would be increased if a combination of histology, immunophenotype, cytogenetics, and, wherever possible, molecular genetics, were used routinely. Incongruency among these diagnostic modalities, however, remains a problem for the taxonomist; the clinical significance of discordance also remains to be determined. Molecular genetics ultimately may prove to be the most definitive diagnostic tool, but studies must be performed to determine the clinical significance of genetically defined subtypes. Meanwhile, BL may be defined best as a B-cell lymphoma with characteristic histology, a high growth fraction (expression of Ki-67 in more than 99% of the cells), and a chromosomal translocation that results in the juxtaposition of the *MYC* gene to immunoglobulin sequences, with resultant *MYC* deregulation. The definition of BLL is more difficult, but requirements should include at least B-cell characteristics, consistent histology, and a high growth fraction. It is likely that this will remain a heterogeneous group of lymphomas with respect to cytogenetics and molecular genetic characteristics but if the behavior and response to therapy are sufficiently similar to BL, retention of this diagnostic category is appropriate. In the meantime, correlation of clinical findings and response to therapy should be made with cytogenetic or molecular genetic studies to the extent that this is possible, so that ultimately the value (or lack thereof) of subdividing the BLL group becomes apparent.

GROSS PATHOLOGIC APPEARANCE

Burkitt's lymphoma and BLL may grow as large solid masses or diffusely infiltrate organs or tissues. In the abdomen, which is involved in 80% of cases, there may be thickening (usually patchy) of the peritoneum omentum, bowel mesentery, or bowel wall, with frequent development into masses that continue to grow, displacing normal organs. The ovaries (Fig. 27.2), testes, kidneys, liver, adrenals (Fig. 27.3), and spleen (which is involved more often in BLL, rarely in endemic BL) may be enlarged, sometimes massively, as a result of tumor infiltration, which may be manifested as either discrete, frequently multiple masses or diffuse infiltration (44). If the tumor is extensive it may be impossible to determine the organ or tissue from which it originally arose, and extensive involvement of the peritoneum may give rise to ascites. Similar involvement of the pleura or pericardium results in pleural or pericardial effusions, the former being considerably more common. Mesenteric lymph nodes, particularly those in the catchment region

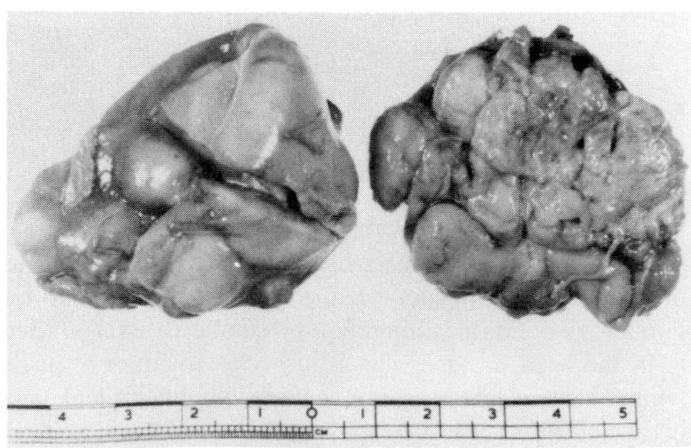

FIG. 27.3. Gross pathologic appearance of bilateral adrenal tumors removed at autopsy in an African child who had Burkitt's lymphoma. The glands are grossly expanded and replaced by lobulated tumor.

of a bowel mass, often are enlarged and are involved by tumor inconsistently. Jaw tumors in African children are expansile and may push out the deciduous teeth. They may ulcerate inside the mouth (and infrequently through the skin surface), leading to superficial necrosis. Such ulceration is rare in subcutaneous or breast tumors but can occur in the latter if they reach massive size. Tumor may grow within the orbit (quite commonly in African children, rarely in the United States or Europe) and nasal sinuses, frequently occluding the latter completely, or pharynx; occasionally, isolated tonsillar or lymph node swelling is observed as a result of tumor infiltration. At autopsy, the cut surface of marrow-containing bones may be yellowish-white in involved regions, which often are patchy in distribution. Cranial nerves may be thickened because of direct tumor infiltration (44,45). Occasionally, myocardial involvement may be revealed by creamy white regions of infiltrating tumor; the lungs and thymus almost never are involved at a macroscopic level, although if tumor is widespread, microscopic involvement may be detectable in the lungs. The frequencies of involvement of various organs in a series of autopsies of Ugandan patients with BL is provided in Table 27.1.

The cut surface of solid masses of BL is yellowish-white in color and homogeneous in appearance. These tumors have the consistency of thick cream or brie cheese and sometimes are semiliquid. Scattered areas of hemorrhage may be seen, but often the entire surface appears to be uniformly avascular.

TABLE 27.1. *Percentage involvement of various organs at autopsy in African patients with Burkitt's lymphoma*

	Children (n = 65)	Adults (n = 23)	Total (n = 88)
Skeleton			
Jaw	57	30	48
Skull vault	9	26	14
Other bones	12	30	17
Central nervous system			
Brain	18	13	17
Spinal cord (paraplegia)	9	17	11
Thoracic cavity			
Pericardium	3	4	5
Heart	32	22	30
Pleura	9	13	10
Lung	17	9	15
Digestive system			
Salivary glands	9	13	10
Peritoneum	12	9	11
Stomach	26	13	23
Small intestine	28	26	27
Large intestine	14	13	14
Liver	37	43	39
Gall bladder	5	9	6
Pancreas	43	39	42
Lymphoreticular system			
Lymph nodes	69	70	68
Spleen	31	35	32
Genitourinary system			
Kidney	77	70	73
Bladder	3	9	5
Prostate[a]	2	1	
Testes[a]	12	5	10
Ovaries[b]	82	75	81
Breast	2	13	3
Endocrine system			
Pituitary	12	13	12
Thyroid	37	35	34
Adrenals	58	48	56

[a] Percentages based on the number of men in the series.
[b] Percentages based on the number of women in the series.
From Wright D. Gross distribution and hematology. In: Burkitt D, Wright D, eds. *Burkitt's lymphoma.* London: E & S Livingstone, 1970:64–81, with permission.

HISTOLOGIC AND CYTOLOGIC APPEARANCE

Burkitt's lymphoma is a diffuse lymphoma, once characterized as having an ''undifferentiated'' appearance—that is, it did not resemble mature lymphocytes or histiocytes and had instead a blastic appearance. The cells are of medium size, not as large as those of large cell lymphomas or centroblasts nor as small as those of small cell lymphomas or mature lymphocytes. The previous designation of *small noncleaved cell lymphoma* was used by Lukes and Collins (4) because they thought that BL cells were morphologically similar to the smaller of two types of noncleaved cells in germinal centers; it was not meant to indicate that the tumor cells are small in a more specific sense. Both histologically and cytologically, BL has a similar appearance throughout the world, and endemic and sporadic forms of the disease do not differ with respect to cytomorphology (46). In histologic sections (Figs. 27.4, 27.5), the tumor cells are seen to be closely approximated to each other, with little or no stroma, and rather few infiltrating normal cells other than the prominent macrophages that give rise to the so-called starry-sky appearance (referring to the pale cytoplasm of the interspersed macrophages contrasting with the overwhelming blue in hematoxylin and eosin–stained sections) of the surrounding tumor cell nuclei, with minimal cytoplasm in evidence. The presence of these ''tingible body macrophages'' (nuclear debris is readily discernible in their cytoplasm) almost certainly is related to the high apoptotic rate of the tumor cells, and the cytoplasmic debris is the remains of ingested apoptotic nuclei. The starry-sky pattern is not pathognomonic and may be seen in any rapidly proliferating lymphoma with a high cell turnover. It is rarely observed in carcinomas, however, and its appearance is helpful in making this distinction. Perhaps because of the high proliferative rate, infiltrated tissue appears to include normal areas interspersed with clumps or streams of tumor cells. Little damage appears to be done to the adjacent normal cells, as attested to by complete recovery of normal organ or nerve function (unless compressive neuropathy or ischemia has resulted in neuronal death) in successfully treated patients. In partially

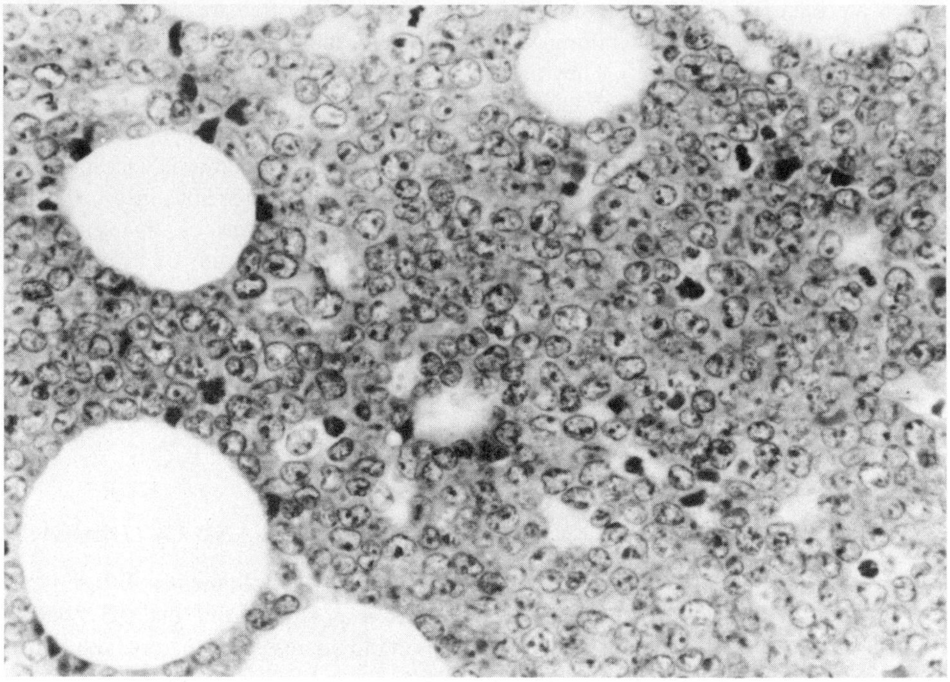

A

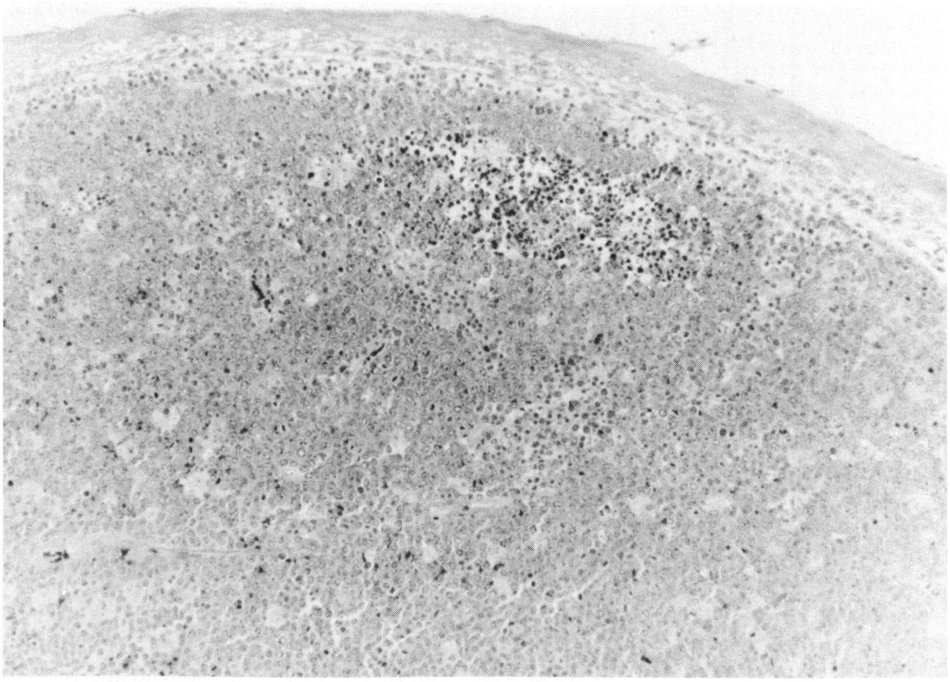

B

FIG. 27.4. A: Histologic appearance at low power of Burkitt's lymphoma in a normal individual. The cells diffusely infiltrate omental fat (hematoxylin and eosin stain, original magnification: 132× magnification). **B:** Burkitt's lymphoma in an HIV-positive patient. The tumor diffusely infiltrates tonsil. A starry-sky pattern with interspersed macrophages is seen (hematoxylin and eosin stain, original magnification: 33× magnification).

involved lymph nodes or tonsils, normal lymphoid tissue is sometimes apparent immediately adjacent to tumor, but the overall impression is one of rapid expansion of tumor cell colonies rather than cohabitation of normal and tumor cells in the lymph node environment, and in most involved nodes there is complete effacement of the normal nodal architecture. Occasionally, selective involvement of germinal centers is observed in mesenteric lymph nodes in the drainage area of a bowel mass, a phenomenon first noted by Mann and coworkers in 1976 (47) and more recently observed in lymphomas of mucosa-associated lymphoid tissue.

The tumor cells have a round or oval nucleus that is

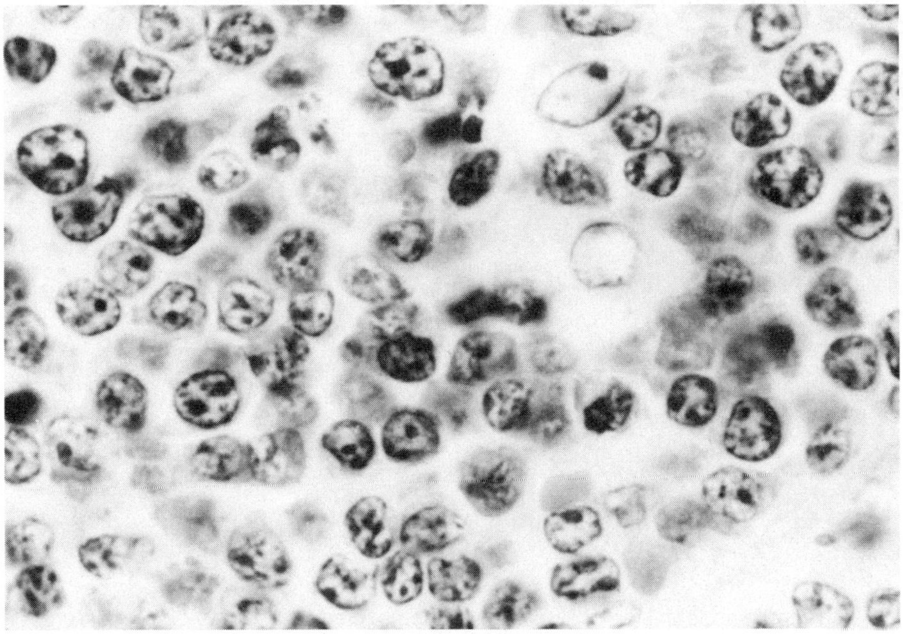

A

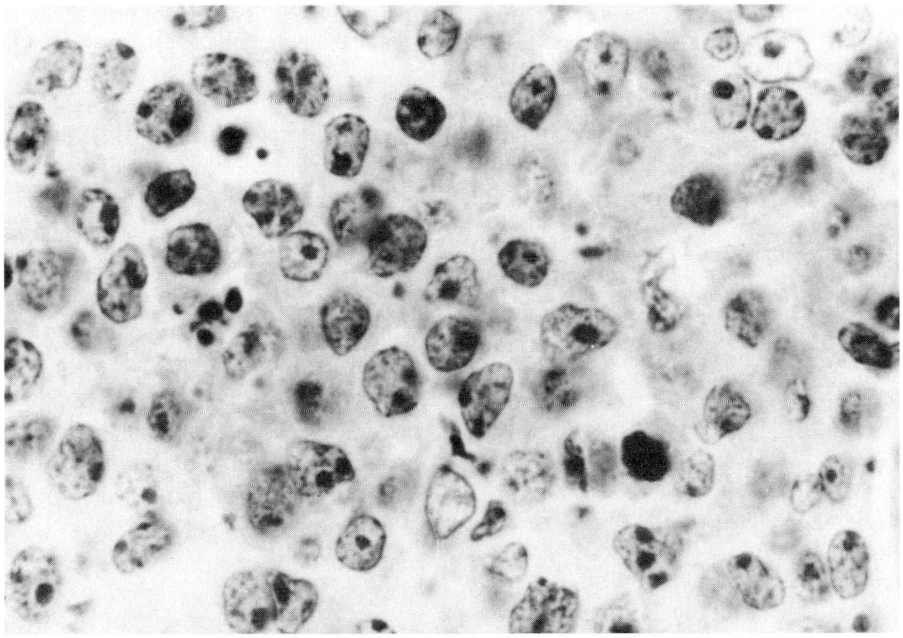

B

FIG. 27.5. A: Histologic appearance at high power of Burkitt's lymphoma. Cells are uniform in size and shape and contain multiple basophilic nucleoli (hematoxylin and eosin stain, original magnification: 330× magnification). **B:** Burkitt's-like lymphoma. Cell size and shape are more variable and many cells have prominent nucleoli (hematoxylin and eosin stain, original magnification: 330× magnification).

slightly smaller than or similar in size to a macrophage nucleus, except in BLL, in which the nuclei, which are more pleomorphic, range in size from those of the typical BL cell to those of the typical LBCL cell (i.e., larger than a macrophage nucleus), many being intermediate in size. The chromatin is noticably clumped in well-fixed material, with a clear parachromatin. This creates the appearance of fenestrations in the nucleus, a feature that contrasts with the fine stippled chromatin of lymphoblastic lymphoma cells. The majority of cells contain multiple (usually two to five), readily discernible nucleoli, although occasional cells with single central nucleoli are present. If such cells are frequent, most pathologists diagnose BLL. The rim of cytoplasm is very basophilic (staining intensely with methyl green pyronine) because of the high RNA content, and it usually contains numerous lipid vacuoles (which can be stained with lipid stains such as oil red O).

Cytologic preparations (Fig. 27.6) stained with a Romanowsky stain are simple to prepare and often provide additional information. Sources of cells for cytology include fine

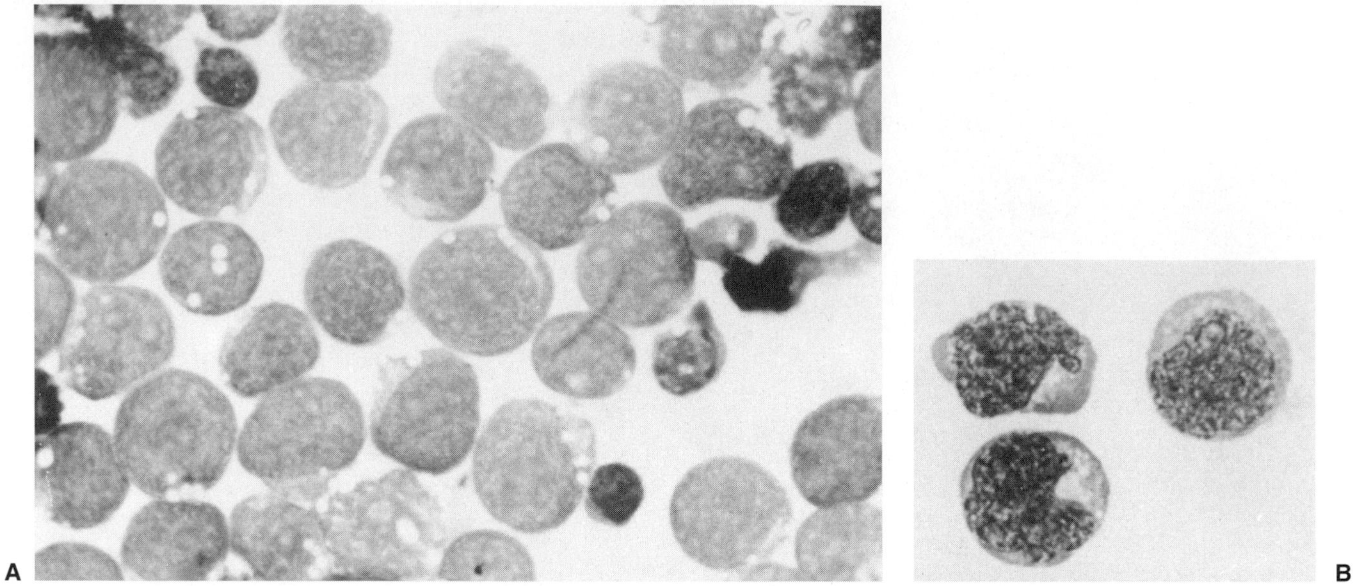

FIG. 27.6. A: Cytologic appearance of Burkitt's lymphoma. Needle aspirate obtained from a jaw tumor of a Ugandan child. **B:** Smears of ascitic fluid prepared from a child in the United States who had an abdominal mass and ascites. The cytoplasm in both cases has a deep basophilic appearance and numerous cytoplasmic vacuoles are visible (Wright's stain, original magnification: 330× magnification).

needle aspirates, fresh tumor imprints, smears or cytocentrifuge preparations of cells from serous effusions or cerebrospinal fluid, and bone marrow smears. In an appropriate setting such preparations may be sufficient to establish a diagnosis (e.g., in equatorial Africa or in patients who have AIDS) (48), particularly if immunophenotyping is performed. In general, tumor cells are more pleomorphic in cytologic preparations, and the distinction between typical BL and BLL is made less readily.

IMMUNOPHENOTYPE

Burkitt's lymphoma is a neoplasm of B lymphoid cells and has the phenotype of a germinal center cell. Thus, both pan–B cell markers and proteins expressed on a broad range of B cells such as CD19, CD20, and CD22 are expressed, as well as proteins expressed on germinal center B cells, such as CD10, CD38, and CD40. CD5, which is expressed by a subset of B cells and their derivative neoplasms—those that give rise to chronic lymphocytic leukemia and mantle cell lymphoma—is not expressed in BL. In essentially all cases of BL, and most cases of BLL, surface immunoglobulin (in most cases IgM, rarely IgG or IgA) is present. This is nearly always associated with either κ or λ light chain expression, as well as the immunoglobulin-associated proteins, including Igα (Mb-1 or CD79a), Igβ, and Igγ. BL, particularly sporadic BL, also may secrete immunoglobulin (49), although usually in such small amounts that special techniques are required to detect it in serum (50).

Additional evidence that BL is the neoplastic counterpart of a germinal center cell is provided by the presence of hypervariable region mutations in its immunoglobulin genes (51,52). Although these are typical of other hypervariable mutations, they are not as numerous as in other B-cell neoplasms, such as follicular lymphoma and large cell lymphoma (53). T-cell markers are not expressed by BL cells, and markers of natural killer cells (CD56, CD57) are not detectable. BL does not express TdT, which, being involved in the generation of antigen receptor diversity by the insertion of additional nontemplated nucleotides at VD and DJ junctions (54), is a marker of lymphoid precursor cells. This provides an objective means of excluding the diagnosis of lymphoblastic lymphoma, which is nearly always TdT-positive, whether it is of precursor B- or T-cell origin (55). Rare pre-B cell phenotypes of TdT-positive leukemias that contain t(8;14) or a variant translocation, however, have been described.

Burkitt's lymphoma, particularly the subset associated with Epstein-Barr virus (EBV), also expresses a protein, CD21 (CR2), that can bind both a complement subcomponent (C3d) and EBV (56–58), these separate sites in the molecule being detected respectively by the monoclonal antibodies B2 or OKB7 and by HB5 (59,60). The human leukocyte A, B, C, and D antigens also are invariably present (61), although class I molecules may be expressed in low amounts compared with, for example, B cells transformed by EBV. This fact, as well as decreased expression of leukocyte adhesion molecules such as LFA-1, ICAM-1, and LFA-3, appears to explain in part the decreased sensitivity of BL cell lines to killing by cytotoxic T cells. It has been reported that *MYC* expression causes a downregulation of LFA-1 and major histocompatibility complex molecules, and it is probable that the low levels of these molecules result from t(8;14) or variant chromosomal translocations associated with BL, which cause deregulation of *MYC* (62).

CYTOGENETICS AND MOLECULAR BIOLOGY

Burkitt's lymphoma and some BLLs contain characteristic, nonrandom, reciprocal chromosomal translocations, either t(8;14), which occurs in some 80% of tumors (63), or one of the variant translocations—t(8;22) or t(2;8) (64) (Fig. 27.7). The recognition of these translocations led to critically important insights into the pathogenesis of this disease, because the breakpoint on chromosome 8 coincides with the location of the protooncogene transcription factor, *MYC*, on band q24 (65,66), and the breakpoint on the partner chromosome is in an immunoglobulin chain locus—either that of the heavy chains (chromosome 14, band q32) or that of one of the light chains (chromosome 22, band q11, or chromosome 2, band p11/p12, the loci of λ and κ genes, respectively) (67). In translocation t(8;14), the *MYC* gene is translocated from chromosome 8 to the heavy chain locus on chromosome 14 (7,65–68), whereas in the variant translocations that involve immunoglobulin light chains, a part of the light chain constant region is translocated to chromosome 8, distal to the *MYC* gene (67). The common feature of all three translocations is the juxtaposition of the *MYC* gene with immunoglobulin-constant region sequences, whether of heavy or light chain origin. This leads, in turn, to the subordination of the regulation of *MYC*, whose own regulatory regions invariably are damaged (by point mutation or deletion) as a consequence of the chromosomal translocation, to the immunoglobulin gene regulatory sequences that now lie adjacent to it on the same chromosome (i.e., in cis configuration) (67–69) (Figs. 27.8, 27.9). The *MYC* gene is regulated as if it were an immunoglobulin gene and, because immunoglobulin genes are expressed constantly in B cells, the *MYC* gene remains switched on, even if it should not be expressed. This paradigm—the deregulation of one gene (frequently, but not always, a transcription factor) by juxtaposition to immunoglobulin sequences, first identified in BL in the three types of *MYC*-immunoglobulin translocation—has proved to be a recurring theme in B-cell neoplasia and extends to T-cell neoplasia, in which juxtaposition of protooncogenes, again predominantly transcription factors (including *MYC*), to the T-cell antigen receptor is a frequent consequence of nonrandom chromosomal translocations. The same mechanism results in deregulation of the *BCL2* gene in the neoplasms associated with translocation t(14;18). including a fraction of BLLs.

In BL, the normal *MYC* allele, present on the untranslocated chromosome 8, is usually silent (70). This suggests that the normal counterpart cell of BL does not express *MYC*. The alternative possibility—that the untranslocated allele is silenced because of overexpression of the translocated allele and operation of the normal feedback regulatory control mechanism—is unlikely for two reasons. First, this mechanism is inactivated in tumors that overexpress *MYC* (71), and

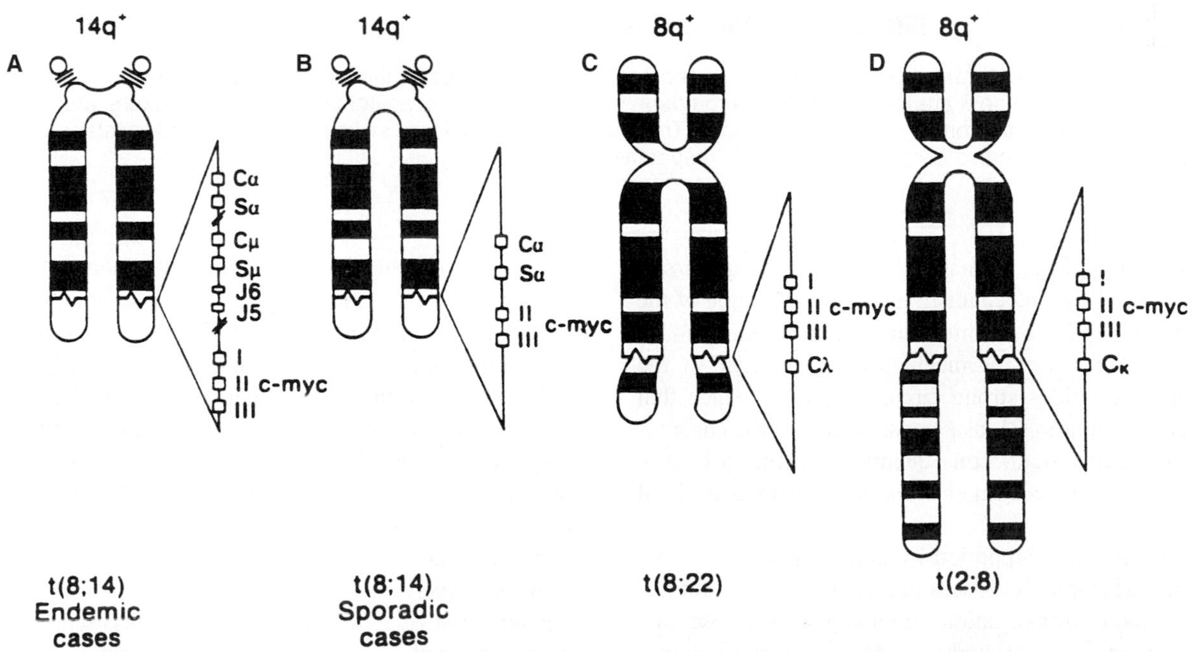

FIG. 27.7. Diagrammatic depiction of the cytogenetic abnormalities observed in the small, noncleaved cell lymphomas. **A,B:** The 14q + chromosome is shown for typical endemic and sporadic cases. **C,D:** The 8q + chromosomes that result from the variant translocations are shown. In each case the configuration of the *MYC*-immunoglobulin genes are illustrated. (From Haluska FG, Tsujimoto Y, Croce CM: The molecular genetics of non-Hodgkin's lymphomas. In Magrath IT, ed. *The non-Hodgkin's lymphomas.* London: Edward Arnold, 1990:96–108, with permission.)

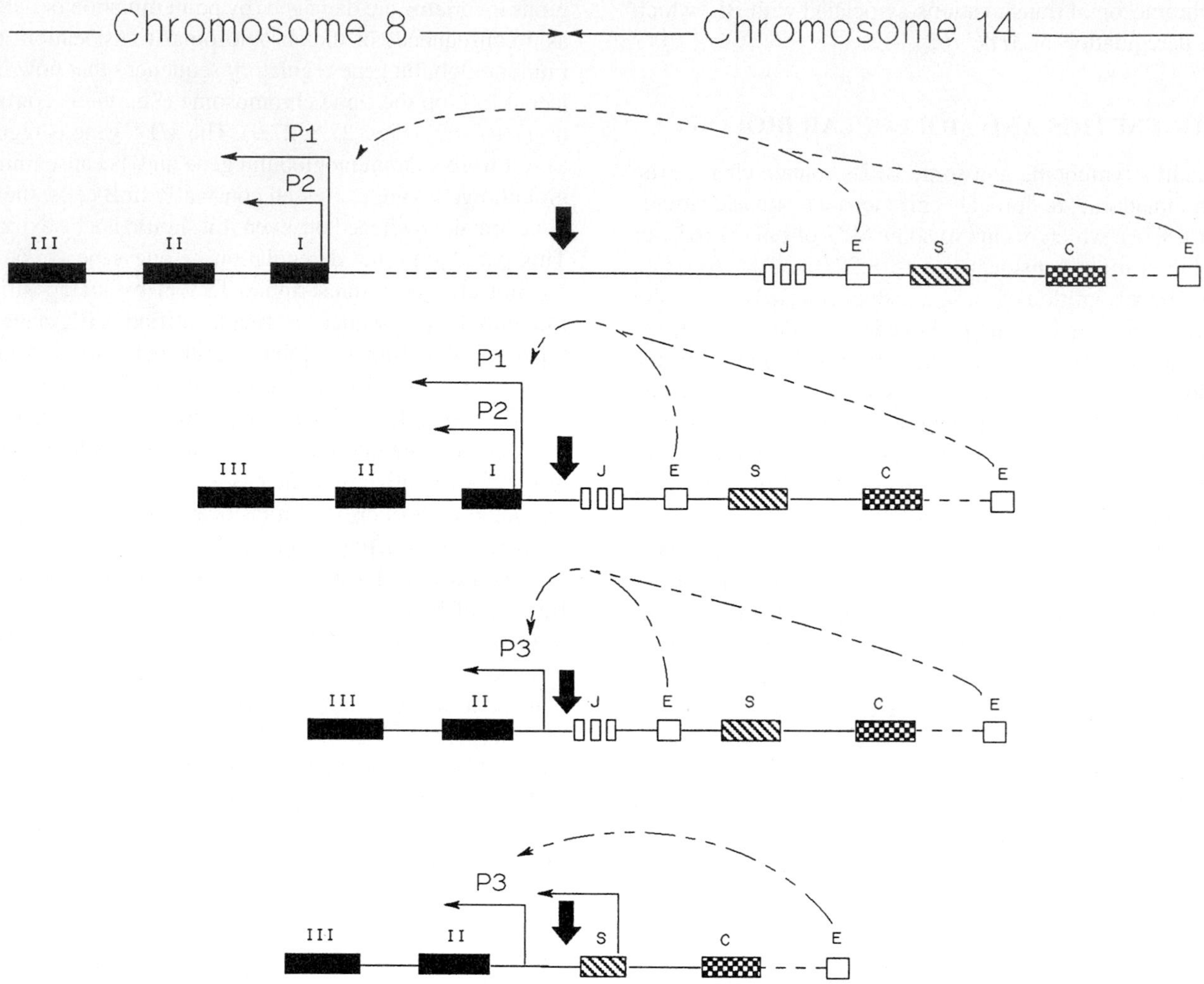

FIG. 27.8. Diagrammatic depiction of the molecular consequences of the translocation t(8;14). Parts of chromosome 8 are translocated to chromosome 14 in a head-to-head configuration; *MYC* exons are indicated by the roman numerals I, II, and III. The immunoglobulin joining, switch, enhancer, and constant regions are indicated as J, S, E, and C, respectively.

second, silencing of the normal *MYC* allele in BL appears to be accomplished by a mechanism involving alteration of the protein structure of the chromosome region in which *MYC* resides (72). Whatever the mechanism, the silence of the normal allele provides strong circumstantial evidence that *MYC* is deregulated in BL as a consequence of the chromosomal translocation and, consequently, that this a central element, perhaps *the* central element, in the pathogenesis of BL.

This conclusion is supported by animal models. In both mouse plasmacytomas and rat immunocytomas, *Myc*-immunoglobulin locus translocations homologous to those that occur in human BL are found (73). Moreover, plasmacytomas that do not contain translocations can be induced if deregulated *Myc* expression is provided by infection with a *Myc*-containing retrovirus (74). Evidence of deregulation of *Myc* has been provided by a classic series of experiments conducted by Cory and Adams and colleagues. These investigators introduced a *Myc* transgene to the mouse B-cell compartment (by coupling the gene to the μ immunoglobulin enhancer, E) and demonstrated that such transgenic mice have a high incidence of B-cell and pre-B cell lymphomas (75,76). Prior to the development of tumors, the bone marrows of the mice are grossly infiltrated by rapidly dividing polyclonal pre-B cells. The B-cell neoplasms that subsequently develop are monoclonal, indicating that abnormal *Myc* expression creates hyperplasia but not neoplasia, and that neoplastic transformation requires additional genetic lesions. Complementation experiments, such as those involving infection of E-μ-*Myc* transgenic mice with nononcogenic Moloney retroviruses, which cause expression of genes near their insertion sites into the cellular genome (insertional mutagenesis), have demonstrated that a number of inappropriately expressed genes may hasten the development of overt, monoclonal tumors (77,78). These early experiments have been supplemented by crossing E-μ-*Myc*

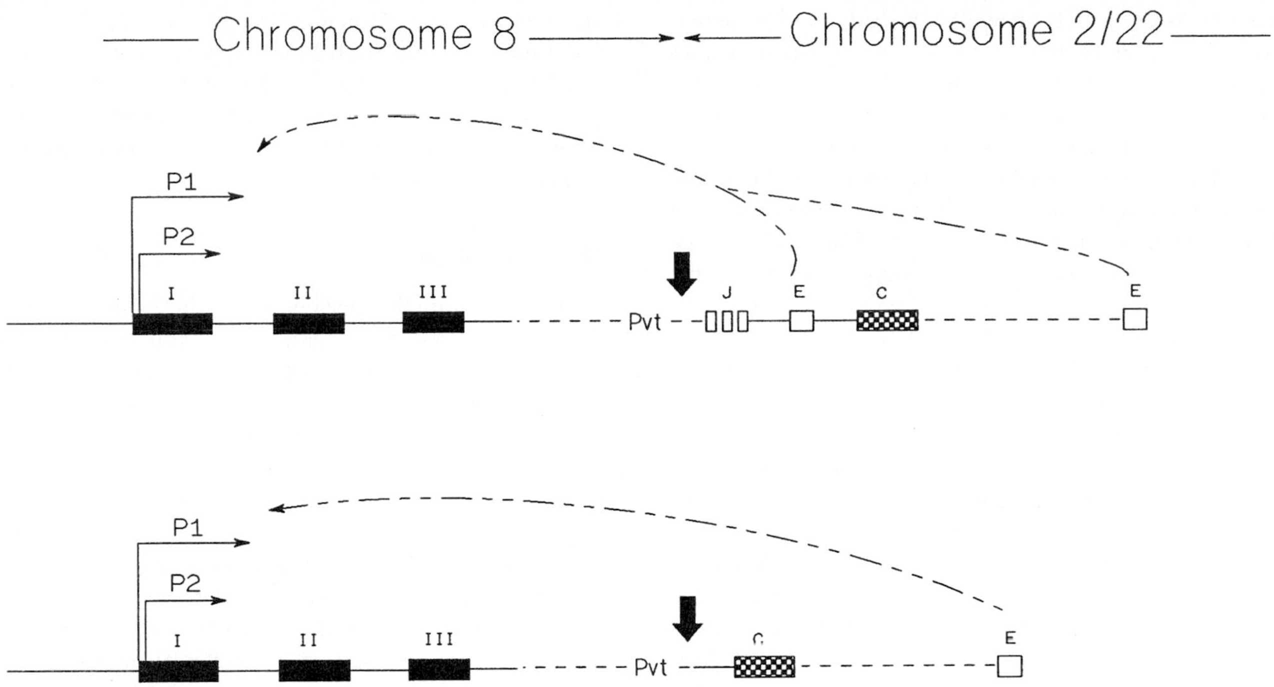

FIG. 27.9. Diagrammatic depiction of the consequences of the translocations t(2;8) and t(8;22). A part of the light chain locus is translocated to chromosome 8 and comes to lie distal to *MYC* in a head-to-tail configuration; *MYC* exons are indicated by the roman numerals *I*, *II*, and *III*. The immunoglobulin joining, enhancer, and constant regions are indicated as J, E, and C, respectively. *Pvt* indicates the presumptive "plasmacytoma variant translocation" locus.

transgenic mice with mice made transgenic for other genes such as *Bcl2*, *Pim1*, and *Bmi1*. The doubly transgenic mice have a greatly enhanced rate of tumor development (79). There is decreased development to mature lymphocytes in E-μ-*Myc* mice (80), and although this may be a result in part of a differentiation failure, it is likely that cells that fail to differentiate undergo apoptosis. This is consistent with the observation that inappropriate expression of the MYC protein leads to apoptosis (81) and suggests that at least some of the additional genetic lesions result in the inhibition of apoptosis, because otherwise, the presence of a *MYC*-deregulating chromosomal translocation would lead to cell death rather than tumorigenesis. The possibility that EBV can provide the equivalent of one or more of these complementary genetic lesions is discussed subsequently.

Further discussion of the pathogenesis of BL focuses on the genetic lesions that have been recognized in this neoplasm to date. A detailed discussion of the possible pathogenetic mechanisms that apply to BLL in which t(14;18) chromosomal translocations are present is not provided, because this topic is covered in Chapters 8 and 10.

Functions of *MYC* and the Potential Consequences of its Deregulation

First identified as the transforming element of the myelocytomatosis retrovirus, *MYC* is known to be important to the proliferation of most cell types, including lymphoid cells (82–86), providing an immediate explanation of its potential as an important oncogene. Expression of the protein product of *MYC* is curtailed in quiescent cells, but if induced to proliferate, MYC levels increase during the first 4 hours after stimulation and the gene continues to be expressed throughout the cell cycle. Similarly, the induction of MYC expression is sufficient to drive quiescent cells to proliferate, and the inhibition of MYC expression by highly specific antisense molecules results in the inhibition of cell proliferation (87,88). *MYC*, like a number of other crucial genes involved in cellular proliferation, is linked to apoptotic pathways; clear evidence for this first was provided by Evan and colleagues in 1992 (89), who showed that *Myc* overexpression is sufficient to cause apoptosis in primary rodent embryo fibroblasts or established rat fibroblasts (*Rat1*) deprived of growth factors. MYC plays a central role in the regulation of critical cellular functions associated with cellular proliferation and survival, a conclusion that is confirmed by the observations that targeted homozygous deletion of *Myc* in mice causes these mice (so-called double knockouts) to die early in embryonic development (90), and homozygous deletion in rat fibroblasts causes a marked prolongation in cell doubling time (91).

As is perhaps not surprising for a gene with such broad and essential attributes, *MYC* is a transcription factor located in the nucleus (92,93), and there is little doubt that its actions are mediated largely through its ability to regulate (either to transactivate or to repress) the expression of other genes. Its structure has been investigated extensively, and numerous proteins have been shown to bind to it and modify its actions in various ways. The precise consequences, however, in the context of normal cell physiology, of its binding to many of these genes, the target genes with which it interacts *in vivo*, of which more than 30 candidates have been identified, and the precise pathways through which it mediates its major functions remain enigmatic (81,91,92). The available evidence suggests that there are not specific domains within *MYC* that are associated with its different effects on cells. Rather, the protean effects of the MYC protein all appear to be mediated through its ultimate function as a transcription factor, that is, its ability to bind DNA and to transactivate adjacent promoters.

The MYC protein consists of two major domains: the amino-terminal region, in which resides the transactivating domain, and the carboxy-terminal region, which bears several structural motifs common to a family of DNA-binding proteins known to regulate transcription, basic helix–loop–helix (HLH) zipper proteins. The HLH structure (i.e., a region that consists of two amphipathic α helices on either side of a looped-out segment) is contained within residues 368 through 410, immediately upstream of which is a highly basic region (B) extending from amino acid 355 through 368. The leucine zipper is encoded in amino acid residues 411 through 439 (Fig. 27.10). It is so named because of the projection of leucine residues from every other turn of an α helix (every seventh amino acid is a leucine). The zipper is able to mediate dimerization by interdigitating with leucine residues that jut from a similar leucine zipper lying adjacent in parallel orientation. Dimerization of B HLH/LZ, proteins (a process in which both zipper and HLH regions participate) is believed to result in a surface that can bind specifically to DNA through the basic region upstream of the HLH motif. All the MYC family proteins—c-MYC, N-MYC, L-MYC, S-MYC and B-MYC—are B HLH/LZ proteins, and there is no doubt that the carboxy-terminal motifs are essential, through dimerization and DNA binding, to the ability of MYC to transactivate target genes, and hence to all of its functions. Mutational analysis of *Myc* has shown, for example, that the B-HLH and zipper regions are essential to its ability to cooperate with *Ras* in the transformation of primary rat embryo fibroblasts, for it to negatively regulate itself, and for it to inhibit the differentiation of Friend erythroleukemia cells (94,95).

MAX and MAD

Such data initially appeared to conflict with the observation that purified MYC protein was found to bind only weakly to DNA, a puzzle that was solved by the identification of several proteins that bind to MYC through its carboxy-terminal region motif and that function as regulators of its ability to bind to DNA. The first of these proteins to be identified was MAX (96). MAX also belongs to the B HLH zipper group of proteins (Fig. 27.10), and by binding to MYC through the carboxy-terminal motifs confers on the dimeric complex the ability to bind strongly to a DNA sequence, CACGTG, identified by using synthetic oligonucleotides. This canonic sequence, known as an "E box," is present in the promoter regions of several growth-promoting genes. By itself, MYC binds weakly to E boxes, and MAX is unable to bind at all. MAX is a smaller protein than MYC, because it lacks the transactivational domain of the latter, demonstrating that it is purely a regulatory protein. MAX is expressed in a wide range of cells and binds readily to all members of the MYC family of proteins, but not to other proteins that bear HLH zipper motifs. It appears that heterodimerization with MAX is essential to their function. Moreover, MAX homodimers cannot bind to DNA, and so MAX does not appear to be able to function as a transcriptional repressor, although MYC/MAX dimers are themselves capable of suppressing the expression of some genes: those involved with inhibition of the cell cycle, such as *GADD45* and *GADD34* (97,98). These genes cause growth arrest in the presence of DNA damage (hence their names) as well as during nutritional deprivation and cell differentiation. The importance of *GADD45* as an MYC target gene is empha-

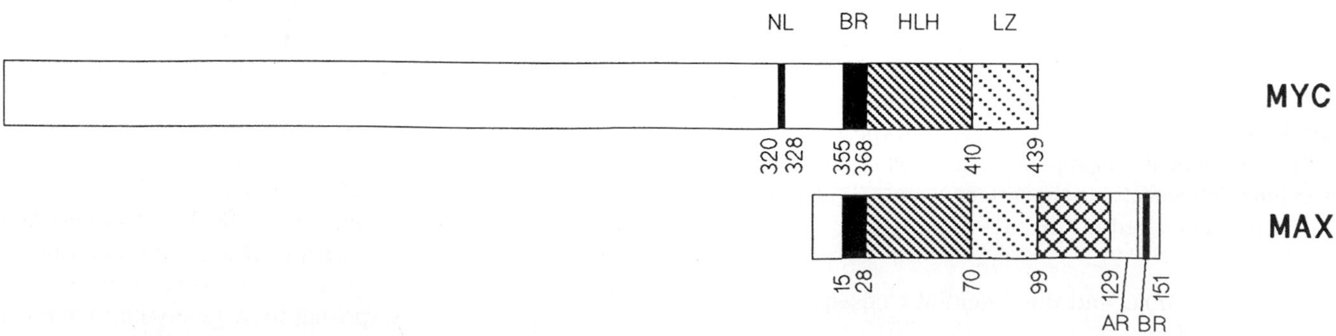

FIG. 27.10. Diagrammatic depiction of the structure of the MYC and MAX proteins. Heterodimer formation occurs between MYC and MAX, a protein that confers specificity for a particular DNA sequence on Myc. *AR*, acidic region; *BR*, basic region; *NL*, nuclear localization signal; *HLH*, helix–loop–helix region; *LZ*, leucine zipper region. Numbers indicate amino acid residues encompassing each region.

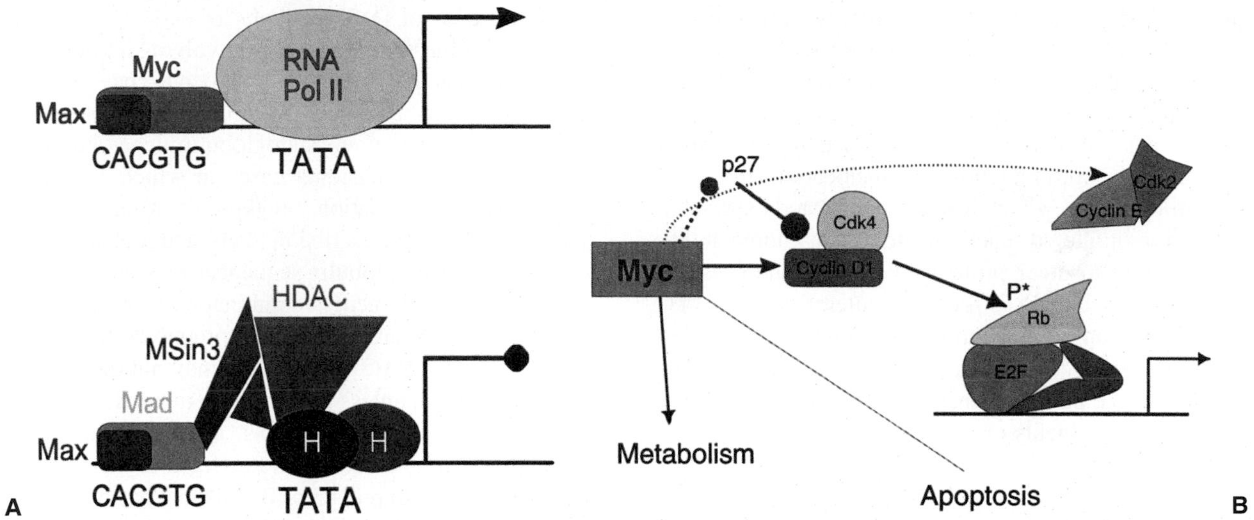

FIG. 27.11. Diagrammatic depiction of MYC-MAX and MYC-MAD dimerization at the cannonical CACGTG binding sites (**A**) and interaction of the MYC protein with cell cycle proteins and other relevant pathways (**B**). *HDAC*, histone deacetylases.

sized by the observation that it is one of only two genes whose expression is altered consistently in *MYC* null cells (99). This, coupled with the evidence that MYC directly activates cyclin D2, with consequent phosphorylation of the retinoblastoma protein and progression through the G_1 checkpoint, and at the same time causes sequestration of the cyclin inhibitor p27 (100), strongly suggests that MYC/MAX dimers activate genes involved in progression through the cell cycle and suppress genes that inhibit such progression, resulting in cell proliferation. Both functions may be critical to its ability to transform cells (Fig. 27.11).

The reversal of the ability of MYC to induce proliferation is brought about by another family of proteins able to bind to MAX, namely the MAD proteins, four of which have been identified so far (101). MAD/MAX heterodimers bind to the same E boxes as MYC/MAX dimers but result in repression of the relevant target genes. Repression domains have been demonstrated in MAD proteins (102). MAD is expressed if cells differentiate and appears to be an antagonist of MYC, permitting cells to exit from the cell cycle and undergo differentiation (101,103,104). MAD appears to exert its effect by binding the mammalian homolog of the yeast protein SIN-3, a corepressor protein (105,106), which in turn recruits other proteins into the complex, including histone deacetylases (Fig. 27.11). The suppression of transcription appears to result from an alteration in chromatin structure (107).

The amino terminus of MYC is structurally similar to the transcriptional activation domains of other proteins and contains clusters of proline and glutamine residues as well as several stretches of highly conserved amino acids, which are known as *MYC box motifs* (81). The two MYC box motifs MB1 and MB11, contained between residues 45 and 63 and 129 and 143, respectively, have been shown to be necessary for transactivation and for the transforming ability of *MYC*. The amino terminus also contains several phosphorylation sites, mutations of which affect transcription and transformation functions (108,109).

This picture is complicated further by the ability of MYC to bind to a large number of other proteins, including amino terminus–binding proteins such as a-tubulin and a number of adaptor proteins including BIN-1, MM-1, PAP, TRRAP, p107, and AMY-1; the carboxy-terminal domain binds others including YY-1, AP-2, BRCA-1, TF-2, and MIZ-1. These proteins are linked to the transcription machinery, the cell cycle, chromatin modeling, and apoptosis and appear to represent an additional level of MYC regulation (110). The functional effects of MYC are likely to differ according to the levels of these various MYC-binding proteins in different cell types, or in the same cell exposed to various concentrations of external (cytokine) regulators of growth and viability (including genes capable of downregulating MYC such as transforming growth factor-β and interferons); the pattern of gene expression for the range of MYC target genes also is governed by the structure of the target gene promoters themselves, including the number and accessibility (at least in part dependent on chromatin structure) of E boxes and probably the presence or absence of adjacent sites to which other regulatory proteins may bind. Potential MYC target genes are involved in a broad range of cellular processes, including the cell cycle (*GADD45*, *CDC25A*, cyclins A and E, *P27*, *P19*), apoptosis (*P19*^{ARF} and *P53*), DNA metabolism (*DFR*, *CAD*, *TK*), DNA dynamics (telomerase), energy metabolism (*LDHA*, H-ferritin), and macromolecular synthesis (*ECA39*, *ELF2A*, *ELF4E*) to name but a few (93,111). MYC influences a variety of pathways relevant to cell proliferation, and its role in cell transformation is complex and likely involves different pathways in different cell types. A common feature appears to be that it is relatively overexpressed in neoplastic cells. It may be overexpressed relative to expression in a normal counterpart cell, either because genetic changes in other genes drive its expression inappropriately, because of amplification, or because of structural changes resulting from mutation or translocation (the situation pertaining in BL), which lead to deregulated expression or degradation or altered function, such as an altered ability of MYC to bind to other proteins. Whatever the cause of the augmentation of MYC function, alterations in MYC expression alone are unlikely to be sufficient to induce neoplasia. Multiple defects, involving both the regulation of its expression and the pathways influenced by its target genes, are necessary components of cell transformation (112,113).

Occurrence and Anatomy of *MYC*-Immunoglobulin Translocations

Although there is no doubt that the deregulation of *MYC*, brought about by the nonrandom chromosomal translocations associated with BL, represents the central pathogenetic feature of this disease, a full understanding of the pathogenesis of BL requires not only a complete description of all the associated genetic lesions but also a detailed description of the mechanism or mechanisms that create the translocation as well as the environmental and inherited factors that predispose to the development of the genetic lesions. Understanding at this level has not been achieved, although recent developments in the ability to examine the expression of thousands of genes at the level of mRNA as well as of protein have made knowledge of the sum total of functional aberrations in the BL cell a realizable goal. The extensive analysis of single nucleotide polymorphisms in a wide range of genes in patients with BL may represent the beginning of an understanding of genetic predisposition to BL. More rapid progress in this area may be possible through the detailed study of familial BL, which has been described in Tanzania (114). Genetic predisposition is likely to be closely linked to environmental factors; for example, genetic factors influence the immunologic response to infectious agents, such as malaria and EBV, both of which are relevant to the pathogenesis of BL. Many other factors are likely to influence the incidence of a relevant chromosomal translocation or of the development of complementary genetic changes. Little information is available with respect to any of these factors. The cell type in which the *MYC*-immunoglobulin translocations occur has yet to be identified clearly. It is likely that the chromosomal translocation occurs in a proliferating cell, because DNA replication is almost certainly a prerequisite for the development of any translocation. In this context, it is tempting to associate the occurrence of translocations involving immunoglobulin genes to immature B cells, either during or close to the time of immunoglobulin gene rearrangement, that is, VDJ recombination, because of the need for a change in the chromatin pattern at this time that permits enzyme-mediated rearrangement of DNA and the generation of "free" ends of DNA is likely to render the cell particularly susceptible to translocations involving immunoglobulin genes. Consistent evidence for the occurrence of translocation break points at or close to signal sequences pertinent to the rearrangement of immunoglobulin genes has not been found (although occasional cases in which the sequences adjacent to translocation breakpoints resemble such sequences have been described [114]), and it appears unlikely that *MYC*-immunoglobulin sequences represent "mistakes" of immunoglobulin gene recombination in which the wrong strands of DNA are religated. Immunoglobulin recombinases, known as *RAG* genes (115), may not be mediators of the translocation, unless they are able to mediate recombinational events, on rare occasions, at sites other than those presently recognized as substrates for these enzymes.

An alternative to precursor B cells that has been proposed as the anatomic site at which chromosomal translocations occur is the germinal center of lymphoid tissue. Translocation could occur, at least theoretically, during or around the time of switch immunoglobulin recombination (although only about one third of BLs have rearrangements in a switch region), which occurs primarily in germinal centers. Recent evidence that remodeling of immunoglobulin gene rearrangement with respect to the VDJ region, involving *RAG* gene expression, occurs in germinal centers also makes it possible that the cell may be susceptible to translocations in and around the regions of immunoglobulin genes involved in such recombinational events during passage through a germinal center. Knowledge regarding this issue is limited, although the presence of breakpoints in or around the J or switch regions of immunoglobulin genes suggests that physiologic recombinational events in immunoglobulin genes predispose, even if only because of alterations in chromatin structure, to the occurrence of translocations involving these loci. The demonstration that pro-B cells, derived by EBV transformation of immature cells present in fetal liver, are highly susceptible to translocations involving immunoglobulin switch regions (116) supports the possibility that translocation may occur in precursor B cells and also indicates that the involvement of switch regions in translocations does not imply that the translocation occurred in a germinal center.

Additional evidence for the occurrence of the translocation in immature cells--prior to VDJ rearrangement—has been provided by Southern blot analysis of the immunoglobulin region from the translocated allele (117). Such analysis demonstrates that a significant fraction of BLs carry an unrearranged J region. Because essentially all BLs synthesize immunoglobulin, at least one of the immunoglobulin genes must be rearranged functionally. Not surprisingly, in the majority of BLs, immunoglobulin is transcribed from the immunoglobulin locus not involved in the translocation (67). These observations suggest that the translocation involves an immunoglobulin locus that has not rearranged its J segment. The J segment is, however, one of the first segments to be recombined (with D) during the process of VDJ joining.

It is believed that DJ joining occurs simultaneously on both the alleles of chromosome 14. A probable explanation of this finding is that the translocation occurred prior to the initiation of the immunoglobulin gene rearrangement, that is, in a pro-B cell. Another possibility is that the translocation preferentially targets rare cells that have rearranged only one immunoglobulin allele. Such cells are not observed within the peripheral blood, although they occasionally are encountered in the bone marrow. It is not at all apparent why the translocation would favor such cells, and their rarity would argue against them as a requirement for the translocation to occur, but there are no additional data on this issue. The presence of precursor B-cell neoplasms bearing *MYC*-immunoglobulin translocations suggests that the translocation, at least on some occasions, may occur in immature B cells.

The study of the integrity of the J region in BL (117) revealed that a large proportion of breakpoints on chromosome 14 do not occur within the chromosomal region involved in VDJ joining. Some of the breakpoints are in regions upstream of J sequences or between the J and switch-μ sequences. These findings also argue against the possibility that most *MYC*-immunoglobulin translocations result from simple mistakes in VDJ joining.

Expression of a Functional Immunoglobulin Molecule in BL

If the translocations associated with BL occur around the same time as VDJ joining, it might be expected, in view of the high frequency of production of nonfunctional immunoglobulin genes during this process, that at least some BLs fail to express a functional immunoglobulin molecule. This is rarely the case, although occasional BLLs in which both 14 chromosomes are involved, including those with both t(8; 14) and t(14;18), fail to express Ig. This suggests either that functional rearrangement of an immunoglobulin gene invariably occurs before the translocation, which takes place on the allele that has failed to produce a functional antibody molecule, or that cells that bear a translocation have an absolute requirement for a functional immunoglobulin molecule, with those that fail to produce one succumbing to apoptosis. Genetic changes disabling the physiologic process leading to the elimination, through apoptosis, of differentiating B cells that fail to express a functional Ig molecule theoretically could obviate the need for this; it would seem, however, on a statistical basis alone that the avoidance of apoptosis in a translocation bearing cell is much more likely to be accomplished through the physiologic process already in place, which permits programmed cell death to be avoided in differentiating B cells, than through the random generation of relevant genetic changes.

Geographic Variability in Chromosomal Breakpoint Location

An interesting observation that may provide clues to the nature of genetic and environmental factors that predispose to the generation of *MYC*-immunoglobulin translocations is that in BL, the breakpoint location on chromosome 8 varies with the geographic origin of the tumor (Fig. 27.12). Unlike

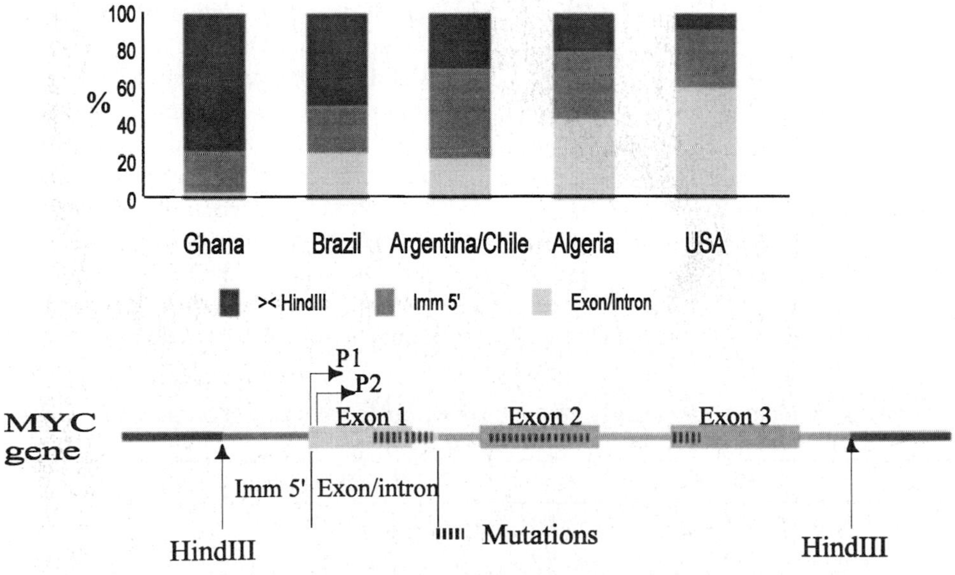

FIG. 27.12. Differences in the breakpoint regions on chromosome 8 in tumors from various world regions. The breakpoint regions are classified into three main regions: outside the HINDIII fragment encompassing *MYC*, in the immediate 5′ region of *MYC*, and within the first exon or intron of *MYC*. These regions are shown as differently shaded areas in both the histogram, which shows the breakpoint patterns (i.e., relative proportions of each of these three breakpoint regions) in countries from which tumors have been studied, and in the drawing, which depicts the three main breakpoint regions in and around the *MYC* gene on chromosome 8 as well as the regions of *MYC* known to bear point mutations in Burkitt's lymphoma.

several other translocations, in which breakpoints are confined to one or more relatively small regions of each of the involved genes, in the chromosomal translocations associated with BL breakpoints may be spread over a wide region of chromosome 8 and its partner chromosomes. With respect to chromosome 8, three major breakpoint regions can be defined: outside the *MYC* gene—that is, either upstream, in t(8;14), or downstream, in variant translocations of the the *HINDIII* fragment containing the *MYC* gene; in the immediate 5′ flanking region of the gene—that is, within the *HINDIII* fragment but upstream of the P1 promoter; and within the gene. Breakpoints within the gene are invariably in the first exon or the first one third of the first intron of *MYC*, so that major disruptions in the MYC protein, which is encoded by the second exon and most of the third, do not occur, although a minor, slightly larger protein species, which contains 14 amino acids derived from exon 1, is not expressed if the gene is truncated. The ratio of these two protein species may have importance to some aspects of MYC function, but there is limited information presently available on this.

Based on a study that eventually included 120 BLs from North and South America and equatorial and North Africa, clear patterns in the breakpoint locations on chromosomes 8 and 14 emerge (67,118–122) (Table 27.2). In endemic (equatorial African) lymphomas, represented by those found in Ghana, the breakpoint is usually (in 74% of tumors) outside the *MYC* gene, and often a considerable distance—hundreds of kilobases—upstream or downstream of *MYC*. In this circumstance, in which the transcriptional unit of *MYC* is not grossly disrupted, mutations are found in elements of the 5′ region of the gene that regulate *MYC* transcription—particularly in the 3′ end of the first exon (a region that is involved in regulating transcript elongation) and an intronic region known to bind several proteins referred to as *MYC intronic factors* (123). Such mutations almost certainly contribute to the transcriptional deregulation of *MYC*. Chromosomal breakpoints in the immediate flanking region of *MYC* or within the first exon or intron of the gene occur in only 26% of Ghanaian patients with BLs. Similarly, relatively few (22%) of the breakpoints on chromosome 14 are in the switch-μ region of the heavy chain locus on chromosome 14 (118–122). Such breakpoints result in the major μ-enhancer being moved from chromosome 14 to chromosome 8, so that only enhancer elements lying downstream of the switch-μ (124) are available to regulate the *MYC* gene.

In sporadic North American BLs, breakpoints far outside *MYC* occur in less than 10% of tumors, and the breakpoint is usually within the gene (60%) or in its immediate upstream flanking sequences (31%)—that is, in regions important to the regulation of *MYC* expression (67,125). Such translocations result in the deletion of a variable stretch of *MYC* regulatory elements, sometimes including the major promoters P1 and P2, and can cause mutations in those elements that remain immediately downstream of the translocation breakpoint. These gross structural changes in *MYC* are clearly critical elements in the deregulation of the gene. Almost one third of the breakpoints on chromosome 14 in tumors from North America are in switch-μ.

Although the patterns of chromosomal breakpoint locations differ markedly between equatorial Africa and North America, those in South American BL appear to be, in some senses, intermediate. Breakpoints in temperate South American BL, represented by tumors in Argentinean and Chilean patients, are, like those in North Americans, usually within the *HINDIII* fragment encompassing *MYC*, but unlike North American BL the majority (48%) are in the immediate 5′ region of the *MYC* gene. In Brazilian BL, the breakpoint pattern appears to be intermediate between those in equatorial African and temperate South American tumors, with a higher fraction (50%) having breakpoints distant from the *MYC* gene (121,122). Switch-μ breakpoints appear to be approximately twice as common in temperate South American BL than in Brazilian BL.

Only a small number of BLs from North Africa (e.g., Algeria) have been examined for chromosomal breakpoint location, but even the small numbers involved leave little doubt that the pattern is different from that of BL in equatorial Africa, because a high fraction of North African tumors have breakpoints within the *MYC* gene itself. In this small group of Algerian tumors, rearrangements within the switch-μ region appear to be uncommon.

In all of the countries examined, chromosomal breakpoints in the switch-μ region of chromosome 14 almost al-

TABLE 27.2. *Percentage of tumors from various countries/geographic regions with breakpoints in designated regions of chromosomes 8 and 14*

Chromosome breakpoints	Ghana	Brazil	Argentina/Chile	Algeria	United States
Hind III[a]	74	50	30	21	9
Immediate 5′[b]	22	25	48	36	31
Exon/intron[c]	4	25	22	43	60
Sμ[d]	22	20	38	7	31
non-Sμ[e]	78	80	62	93	69

[a] Breakpoint location outside the HINDIII fragment that encompasses *MYC*.
[b] Breakpoint location in the immediately 5′ region of *MYC* (HINDIII-SmaI).
[c] Breakpoint location in the first exon or in the first intron of c-myc (SmaI-PstI).
[d] μ: Breakpoint within the switch-μ region of the IgH gene (HINDIII-EcoRI fragment).
[e] Any breakpoint outside the switch-μ region.

TABLE 27.3. *Chromosome 8 and 14 breakpoint combinations in various geographic regions*

Geographic region (no. of tumors)	R/Sμ %	R/non-Sμ, %	U/Sμ, %	U/non-Sμ, %
Ghana (23)	3 (13)	3 (13)	2 (9)	15 (65)
Brazil (24)	5 (20)	7 (30)	0	12 (50)
Argentina/Chile (25)	9 (35)	9 (35)	1 (3)	7 (27)
Algeria (12)	1 (7)	9 (75)	0	2 (17)
USA (32)	9 (28)	20 (63)	1 (3)	2 (6)
Epstein-Barr Virus association	55%	58%	50%	76%

R, rearranged *MYC-BKP* within the HindIII fragment; U, unrearranged *MYC*; Sμ, breakpoint within the switch-μ region (HindIII-EcoRI fragment) of the IgH gene; non-Sμ, any breakpoint outside the Sμ region.

ways are associated with chromosome 8 breakpoints that are either in the immediate 5′ region of *MYC* or in the first intron or first exon of *MYC*—that is, those breakpoints that result in a rearrangement, seen on a Southern blot, of the *MYC* gene (Table 27.3). Chromosomal breakpoints outside the *HINDIII* fragment, which do not result in a rearrangement of *MYC*, rarely are associated with switch-μ breakpoints in any region of the world (122). A possible explanation for this observation is that the μ-enhancer, which is upstream of switch-μ, and therefore not "in cis" with *MYC* when the chromosome 14 breakpoint is in switch-μ (Fig 27.8), is required to be on the same chromosome as *MYC* if the latter remains unrearranged. In this circumstance, *MYC* is usually a considerable distance from the immunoglobulin locus with which it is juxtaposed. Rare cases in which the breakpoint is just outside the *HINDIII* fragment occur, however, and examination of their likelihood of association with a switch-μ breakpoint could be revealing. Locations outside the switch-μ region, which usually result in juxtaposition of the μ-enhancer with the translocated *MYC* gene, are the predominant breakpoint locations on chromosome 14 in all of the regions studied, accounting for between 62% and 93% of the breakpoints in this series (Table 27.2).

The reasons for geographic differences in the chromosomal breakpoint location patterns remain unknown, but the possibility that the chromosomal location may be influenced by environmental factors must be considered. Differences in environmental factors, such as prevalent infections, could alter the proportions of cells at various stages of B-cell differentiation, each of which may be more or less susceptible to different breakpoint locations. Differences in environmental factors that predispose to potentially complementary genetic changes may favor the survival of neoplastic cells with particular types of *MYC* deregulation. Further study of the breakpoint location patterns within large countries with differing environments (tropical and temperate), such as Brazil, and in other regions of the world clearly is justified, and detailed epidemiologic studies coupled with analyses of breakpoint locations may shed more light on this issue, although they are difficult to accomplish. Whether the molecular differences are associated with differences in clinical behavior or response to therapy remains unknown.

Mutations in the MYC Protein

In addition to mutations in the first exon and intron, in a high proportion (approximately 60%) of BLs mutations are found in the protein-coding region of the gene, predominantly in exon 2 (126,127). These mutations do not involve the dimerization and DNA-binding domains in the carboxy-terminal region of the protein, as might be anticipated, because these domains are essential to the functional activities of MYC. The pattern of mutations appears to be different in endemic versus sporadic BL; in the former, the distance over which the mutations are spread is more restricted—many more cluster around the phosphorylation sites at residues threonine 58 and serine 62. The functional significance of these mutations remains unclear, and most of the effort in identifying their effect on MYC function has been put into the mutations in and around the 58 and 62 and other nearby phosphorylation sites. Two hypotheses have been put forward on the basis of experimental evidence: that the mutations interfere with the ability of p107, a protein belonging to the retinoblastoma family of proteins, to inhibit the ability of MYC to transactivate its target genes (although not with the ability of p107 to bind to MYC [128]), and that the mutations prolong the life span of the MYC protein by inhibiting ubiquitin-mediated proteosomal degradation (or possibly other degradation mechanisms) of the protein (129,130). Information required for MYC degradation is known to be contained in the two highly conserved MYC boxes in the amino-terminal domain, the first of which, between residues 45 and 63, encompasses the phosphorylation sites at residues 58 and 62 (129). Whichever of these possibilities applies (and the possibility that they are not mutually exclusive must be considered), the net consequence would be further deregulation of MYC function, and such mutations, therefore, are likely to be relevant to the pathogenesis of BL.

The mutations present in the terminal region of exon 1 may interfere with the normal inhibition of mRNA chain elongation of *MYC* transcribed from the P1 promoter, leading to a shift in the relative proportions of mRNA derived from P1 versus P2 (the latter predominates in normal cells, the former in BL, in which P1 and P2 are both present) and to an increased level of mRNA production (131). It is easy to see how this transcriptional deregulation would be complemented by functional deregulation, whether mediated through prolongation of the half-life of the *MYC* message, for which there is independent evidence in BL (132), by stabilization of the MYC protein, or by decoupling of a mechanism designed to limit, perhaps at specific time points during the cell cycle, the ability of the MYC protein to transactivate its target genes. The latter possibility is supported by evidence that phosphorylation of MYC at codons 58 and 62 is dependent on cyclin A (133).

Lesions in Apoptotic Pathways

The ability of MYC to cause apoptosis if overexpressed in cells that have been deprived of growth factors has been described. This is unlikely to be a simple mechanism, because MYC has connections with multiple apoptotic pathways (81). Moreover, the ability of MYC to induce apoptosis appears to be linked absolutely to its functional properties as a transcription factor, requires binding to MAX, and is prevented by mutations in the dimerization and DNA-binding regions. The conclusion must be drawn that MYC primes the cell for apoptosis—that is, activates apoptotic pathways—and drives proliferation. For proliferation to occur in normal cells, presumably, antiapoptotic proteins are required to inhibit apoptosis, and genetic events that cause the overexpression of antiapoptotic proteins or the inhibition of proapoptotic proteins are likely to contribute to the pathogenesis of BL. Although BCL-2, the first antiapoptotic protein to be identified, is not overexpressed in BL, there is little doubt that its overexpression can contribute to tumorigenesis in the presence of MYC deregulation, because crosses between mice transgenic for *Myc* with mice transgenic for *bcl2* greatly enhance the development of tumors in the resultant doubly transgenic mice (79). Particularly aggressive lymphomas and leukemias in which both t(8;14) and t(14;18) have been identified are well known.

Although MYC may ''prime'' apoptotic pathways, it remains unknown whether apoptosis requires a specific initiating signal for apoptosis to occur (for example, the binding of a tumor necrosis factor family protein to its cognate receptor), or whether in the absence of inhibitors of apoptosis, MYC expression is sufficient to trigger apoptosis. These are not mutually exclusive possibilities and may depend on the cell lineage as well as the cellular microenvironment. At least in some systems, overexpression of MYC in growth-arrested cells does not result in apoptosis, suggesting that a second, triggering signal is required (81,134), and in *Rat1* fibroblasts transfected with *MYC*, apoptosis but not proliferation is prevented by inhibition of CD95-FAS signaling (81,135). MYC expression appears to sensitize cells to apoptosis induced by tumor necrosis factor family receptors, including CD95-FAS (81). It is perhaps not surprising that inhibition of the CD95-FAS–triggered apoptotic pathway can be demonstrated in BL. Studies by Gutierrez and colleagues (136) have shown that BL cell lines fall into three categories in this respect: those in which the pathway appears to be intact, those in which it is inhibited but the inhibition can be released by treatment with cycloheximide, and those in which inibition is not released by cycloheximide. A high proportion of the latter cell lines have frame-shift mutations in the proapoptotic BAX protein that result in its truncation and inactivation. Absence of a full-length BAX protein has been demonstrated in approximately one third of BL biopsy specimens by immunohistochemistry. Further elucidation of the relevant pathways is required, but CD95-FAS–triggered apoptosis is known to occur through one of two different pathways, one of which is dependent on and one of which is independent of mitochondria (Fig 27.13). One of these pathways is favored in type I versus type II cells. In type I cells, binding of caspase 8 to the CD95-FAS receptor through the adaptor protein FADD leads to direct activation of caspase 3 and apoptosis. In type II cells, activation of caspase 8 is weaker and delayed. Eventually, the BCL-2 family protein BID is cleaved and activated by caspase 8, resulting in cytochrome C release from mitochondria and activation of caspase 9 through APAF-1. This stimulates caspase 3 activity and apoptosis. It is the permeability of the mitochondrial membrane to cytochrome C that is influenced by BCL-2 family proteins, so that a role for BAX in MYC-induced apoptosis seems likely. BCL-2 family proteins form heterodimers that inhibit cytochrome C release (e.g., BCL-2-BAX heterodimers) or promote its release (e.g., BAX homodimers). BID probably acts by displacing antiapoptotic proteins from their proapoptotic partners, and recently described BCL-2 family members may act directly on APAF-1. Whether the BAX mutations described in BL simply prevent type II CD95-FAS–induced apoptosis in BL cells, or whether there is another role for BAX in CD95-FAS pathways in BL, remains to be seen, but these data leave little room for doubt that lesions on apoptotic pathways are an essential component of the pathogenesis of BL.

Mutations in another protein capable of inducing apoptosis, p53, also have been described in approximately 40% to 50% of patients with BL (137,138). If DNA is damaged p53 is induced and causes either cell cycle arrest—during which DNA repair can be induced—or apoptosis. It seems less likely that mutations in *P53* are relevant to pathogenesis, because in many BLs, *P53* mutations are found in only a fraction of the tumor cells; a role for *P53* mutations in tumor progression seems more likely. This is supported by evidence that p53 influences the tumorigenicity of BL cell lines in nude mice (139). Whether such mutations influence the response to chemotherapy—which sometimes causes cell death through the p53 apoptotic pathway because of the ability of cytotoxic drugs to cause DNA damage—is likely to depend on the chemotherapy regimen used, but evidence that *P53* mutations impair the ability of BL cells to undergo apoptosis if exposed to radiation or specific chemotherapeutic drugs, as well as some clinical data, suggests that at least in some circumstances, *P53* mutations may be associated with poor response to treatment (140–142). Whether or not MYC is involved in apoptotic pathways in-

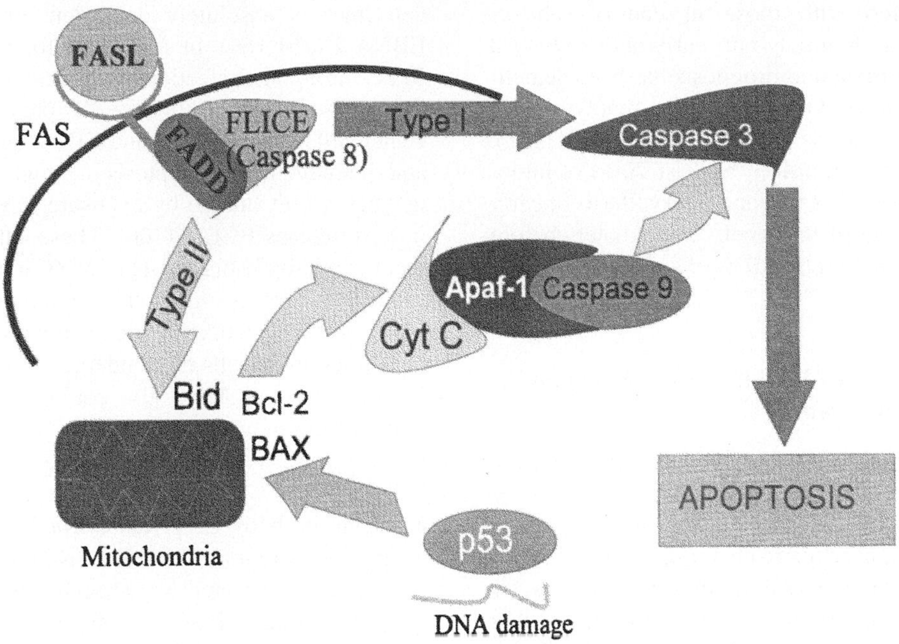

FIG. 27.13. Diagrammatic depiction of apoptotic pathways involved in CD95-FAS receptor–induced apoptosis (types I and II) and following DNA damage through induction of p53. Both pathways may be coupled to MYC.

volving p53 in BL is unknown, but there is evidence that in at least some circumstances MYC expression may be required for p53-induced apoptosis to occur. One potential connecting link is the cell cycle inhibitory protein, INK-4, which encodes both p16 and $p19^{ARF}$. The latter is involved in the regulation of p53-MDM-2 complexes and is a potential MYC target gene. The introduction of MYC into wild-type mouse embryo fibroblasts elevates $p19^{ARF}$ and p53 with resultant apoptosis, but MYC is unable to induce either p53 or apoptosis in $p19^{ARF}$ null fibroblasts (81). There are no data available on the expression or functional integrity of $p19^{ARF}$ in BL, but further exploration of this connection in the context of the p53 pathway may be revealing.

ASSOCIATION WITH EPSTEIN-BARR VIRUS

Epstein-Barr virus was discovered in 1964 in cell lines derived from BL biopsies sent to Epstein's laboratory from Uganda (143). Since then, EBV DNA has been demonstrated to be present in 95% of endemic BL, in some 20% of sporadic tumors, and in 30% to 40% of HIV-related BLs (and approximately 80% of LBCLs, including all central nervous system [CNS] lymphomas) (67,120,122,144,145). In BL in North Africa and South America, and in a number of developing countries in which EBV association has been determined, intermediate frequencies of association (60–88%) are observed (120–122,146–151). The possible role of EBV in the pathogenesis of BL long has been the subject of debate, but although the International Agency for Research in Cancer has determined that there is enough evidence to conclude that EBV is of pathogenetic significance in BL, an absolutely definitive conclusion would require a detailed understanding of the pathways through which EBV proteins interact with cellular proteins in predisposing or contributing to the pathogenesis of BL.

The EBV genome is complex and encodes three major groups of proteins, classified according to their expression in relation to viral replication. Latent genes are expressed if the virus is in a nonreplicative state; their expression consists of six Epstein-Barr nuclear antigens (EBNAs) and three latent membrane proteins, LMP-1, LMP-2A, and LMP-2B (sometimes referred to as *terminal proteins*, or TP-1 and TP-2). Only this set of genes can be relevant to cell transformation, because viral replication is associated with cell lysis. Antigens expressed if viral production (the ''lytic cycle'') has been initiated include the immediate early protein zebra, which is necessary and sufficient to initiate viral replication, and various other proteins required for and expressed prior to DNA synthesis, such as the early antigens themselves, or after viral DNA synthesis, such as the late antigens (structural proteins such as the virus capsid antigen). Because viral replication is associated with cell lysis, virion synthesis occurs, at most, in only a small minority of neoplastic cells, and virus particles as well as early and late EBV antigens are difficult to find in fresh biopsy specimens from patients with EBV-associated BL, although good evidence that both zebra expression and viral replication occurs in a fraction of the cells in some tumors has been published (152,153). In patients with African BL, however, the serum levels of antibodies to both early antigens and the virus capsid antigen are elevated compared with those in control subjects (151,154). An association among anti-early antigen titer at presentation, tumor burden, and prognosis has been demonstrated (155), consistent with the observation that lytic virus replication occurs in a small percentage of tumor cells (153). It is known that a high proportion (at least 70%) of tumor cell progeny do not survive (156), and the synthesis of early antigens in at least some of these cells immediately before their death could account for elevations of anti-early antigens in BL.

Latent Gene Expression in Burkitt's Lymphoma and Relevance to Lymphomagenesis

Although there is little doubt that EBV is of pathogenetic significance to EBV-associated BL, there is also no doubt that the mechanisms of transformation and the maintenance of the transformed state differ from those responsible for EBV-induced transformation of normal B lymphocytes—a phenomenon observed *in vitro* many years ago, and one that at the time (which was prior to the discovery of EBV latent genes) was felt to provide evidence for a pathogenetic role for EBV in BL. It since has become clear, however, that the pattern of expression of EBV latent genes differs in normal B cells transformed by EBV and BL. EBV-containing BLs and BL cell lines immediately after explantation express EBNA-1 in the absence of other EBNAs and LMPs, although occasional cells in biopsy samples can be seen to express LMP-1 or EBNA-2 (157–159). In contrast, B lymphocytes transformed *in vitro* by EBV express the full set of latent proteins, that is, the six EBNAs and three membrane proteins. These patterns of latent gene expression are known respectively as *type I* and *type III* (159). It has been shown that EBNA-2 and LMP-1 are critical to the transformation of normal B cells (151,160), and it must be concluded that either these proteins are not required during the pathogenesis of BL or they are downregulated once the cell has developed a *MYC*-immunoglobulin chromosomal translocation. Either of these possibilities is consistent with the observation that MYC can replace the need for EBNA-2 and LMP-1 in the proliferation of EBV-transformed lymphoblastoid cell lines (161). In this study, cells driven by MYC rather than EBNA-2 and LMP-1 had the morphology and immunophenotype of BL cells rather than of lymphoblastoid cell lines. MYC overexpression, however does not lead simply to a lack of a requirement for the major EBV-transforming proteins, EBNA-2 and LMP-1, because the forced expression of either of these genes in BL cell lines causes downregulation of both MYC and immunoglobulin expression (the latter finding is consistent with the decreased expression of immunoglobulin in cells with a type III latent gene expression pattern compared with type I cells) as well as growth suppression (162–164). In contrast, in EBV-transformed lymphoblastoid cell lines, EBNA-2 induces the expression of both MYC and LMP-1, although it still downregulates immunoglobulin gene expression (165). The continued proliferation of these cell lines is absolutely dependent on the expression of EBNA-2 (161,164). In such cells, forced overexpression of MYC through transfection also leads to conversion to a BL-like phenotype, with increased expression of the germinal center cell markers CD10 and CD38, vacuolated cytoplasm, and the induction of apoptosis in a high fraction of cells, the last being preventable by exposure to CD40 ligand, which in turn induces BCL-2 (166). These data, together, suggest that the relatively high level of MYC expression is responsible for conferring on BL the immunophenotype and morphology of germinal center cells (as well as, probably, for the high fraction of cells that undergo apoptosis in this tumor). It is possible that MYC also could drive the hypervariable mutation of immunoglobulin genes without the need for antigen exposure—antigen, after all, also induces, directly or indirectly, MYC expression. These data also indicate that, although in both EBV-transformed cells and BL MYC expression is required to drive proliferation, this is accomplished quite differently: through EBNA-2 expression in lymphoblastoid cell lines, and through a *MYC*-immunoglobulin translocation in BL. It is because of the translocation that the ability of EBNA-2 and LMP-1 to downregulate immunoglobulin genes also results in down regulation of *MYC* in BL. Not only do BL cells not require EBNA-2 and LMP-1, but their expression could inhibit rather than stimulate proliferation. In one *in vivo* situation this is certainly true, although its relevance to the pathogenesis of BL is not entirely clear: Just as lymphoblastoid cell lines generally undergo spontaneous regression in nude mice, BL cells expressing LMP-1, either transfected or introduced by somatic cell hybridization, undergo spontaneous regression in nude mice, whereas the same cell lines proliferate indefinitely in nude mice in the absence of LMP-1 expression (167,168).

The expression of EBNA-2 and LMP-1 (or of other latent genes) would be deleterious to BL for other reasons. The epitopes present in these proteins are expressed as processed peptides at the cell surface in the context of major histocompatibility complex class I antigens, so that they are able to excite an EBV-specific cytotoxic T-cell response (169). This is the basis for the ability of EBV to persist in normal humans without inducing a lymphoproliferative process (beyond, that is, the self-limited lymphoproliferation associated with the acute stages of infectious mononucleosis prior to the development of a T cell–mediated immune response). If these antigens were expressed in BL cells, it is likely that the tumor would be destroyed by T cells.

These observations regarding the deleterious effect of EBNA-1 and LMP-1 in BL cells provoke a teleologic argument with respect to the role of EBV in the pathogenesis of BL. Given that relatively few B cells contain EBV in the normal host (approximately 1–10 per million circulating B cells), it would appear highly unlikely that BLs, containing as they do a deregulated *MYC* gene, would be associated with EBV at all unless EBV is capable, in the absence of the proteins primarily responsible for the transformation of normal B cells, of playing a crucial role in pathogenesis.

Even if EBV played a passive role, that is, could be considered a ''passenger virus'' (unlikely in view of the deleterious effect of some of its genes), the chance that it would be present in BL, even based solely on the frequency of EBV infected cells in the body, would seem to be small. Yet the viral genomes in BL not only are present in every cell but are clonal (170). This indicates that all EBV genomes arose from a single virus particle infecting a single original cell—that is, EBV must have been present at the time of transformation of the tumor cell clone. This observation does not speak to the issue of the sequence of transformational events, whether EBV infects a cell already containing a *MYC*-immunoglobulin chromosomal translocation and represents a late, if not final, transformational event, or whether the translocation occurs in an EBV-infected cell, which otherwise would have remained benign. A topic for discussion some years ago, when little was known of the functions of latent EBV proteins, this issue now seems of less importance than an understanding of the mechanisms through which EBV contributes to pathogenesis, which is likely to lead, in any event, to an answer to this question.

Potential Pathogenetic Mechanisms

Although EBV can integrate into the cellular genome, this appears to be an uncommon occurrence, and EBV persists in most cells as circular plasmid molecules that are replicated once per cell cycle (171). A mechanism based on an integration site (such as promoter insertion) is highly unlikely. If EBV is an important factor in the pathogenesis of BL, the relevant molecular pathways presumably involve one or more of the two viral proteins and two nontranslated small RNA molecules that are known to be regularly expressed in EBV-associated BL. These are EBNA-1, a transcription factor involved in maintenance of EBV latent genomes in infected cells (171,172); the recently described protein BARF-0 (173), of unknown function; and the small untranslated proteins EBER-1 and EBER-2 (159), also of unknown function. A recent study of fresh biopsy specimens from patients with BL from equatorial Africa also identified the presence of BAMHI-A rightward transcripts (BART) in 7 of 7 tumors and LMP-2A transcripts in 5 of 7 tumors with well-preserved RNA (174). In this study, transcripts for the other EBNAs and for LMP-1 were not detected in any tumor. The lack of expression of these genes in BL (except in rare cells), coupled with their deleterious effects on BL cells, strongly suggests that they are unimportant to pathogenesis, but a role in the early steps of the multistep process of pathogenesis cannot be excluded. If the *MYC*-immunoglobulin translocation occurs in an EBV-containing cell, these genes at least are involved in the infection of the cell in the first place, although this hardly can be considered a pathogenetic role.

Among the products of the EBV genes that are expressed in BL, and therefore are strong candidates for a pathogenetic role, there is no information on BARF-0 and BART or LMP-2A, whose functions in the normal life cycle remain unknown. EBER-1 and EBER-2, however, are potential candidates for a role in lymphomagenesis in view of the recent observation that the oncogenicity of EBV-negative subclones of the EBV-positive BL cell line Akarta is restored by transfection of *EBER* genes (175). *EBNA1* is also a potential candidate, in view of its reported ability to induce lymphomas if introduced as a transgene into mouse lymphocytes (176), although alone it cannot restore oncogenicity to EBV-negative subclones of Akarta (177). Whatever the functional role of EBER-1 and EBER-2, which remains to be examined in models that go beyond the exceptional situation of a cell line, Akarta, from which EBV-negative clones can be produced, EBNA-1 is still, presumably, essential to any pathogenetic process subserved by EBV, because it is responsible for maintenance of EBV genomes in the cell. A single report of fragments of EBV genomes in EBV-negative BL (178), suggesting that in some circumstances EBV may be relevant during the initiation of tranformation but is not required for maintenance, leaves open the possibility of a ''hit-and-run'' mechanism that could apply to a subset of apparently EBV-negative tumors, but further investigation of such a possibility would be difficult. Identification of mechanisms is explored most logically in EBV-positive tumors, which account for the majority of BLs worldwide.

Whatever role EBV genes may have in pathogenesis, they ultimately must act through cellular genes relevant to the control of proliferation and to cell viability (or, conversely, apoptosis). Although similar or identical effects could be produced by a series of genetic changes in cellular genes, the requirement for multiple changes would mean that EBV-negative tumors would be expected to be much less common than EBV-positive tumors. Although this proves to be true on a global scale—the incidence of EBV-positive BL in children in equatorial Africa is some 25-fold or more greater than the incidence of EBV-negative BL in, for example, children in the United States (155)—it begs some questions in the study of specific world regions. For example, the incidence of EBV-positive BL in North American children is even lower than that of EBV-negative BL, a fact that must be taken into account in considering epidemiologic aspects of the role of EBV in BL.

Potential Role for EBNA-1 in the Pathogenesis of Burkitt's Lymphoma

EBNA-1 is present in all neoplasms known to be associated with EBV (151), at least in part because of its role in maintaining the presence of EBV genomes in the cell. It is known that in the type I latency pattern, which occurs in peripheral lymphocytes and BL, EBNA-1 is transcribed from a promoter in the Q *BAMH1* fragment of EBV: Qp (179,180). This differs greatly from the situation in lymphoblastoid cells with type III latency, in which EBNA-1 is transcribed from promoters in the W (immediately after infection) or C (from 48-72 hours after infection) *BAMH1* fragments as part of a large, polycistronic transcript that contains all six EBNAs (181,182). The latency type I pattern appears to be relevant to the maintenance of the viral reservoir in B lymphocytes. Because such cells are not in cycle (although they may enter the cell cycle if stimulated appropriately), and because there is, in general, no requirement for virus multiplication in circulating lymphocytes (infection of other hosts appears to be through release of EBV in saliva, possibly after amplification in epithelial cells overlying the nasopharyngeal lymphoid tissue), the expression of other genes is not required. It can be argued that the expression of EBNA-1 is not required either, and it is possible that some EBV-containing cells do not express any EBV proteins for much of their lifespan. The restricted pattern of EBNA-1 expression, that in which it is transcribed from Qp, can be detected, however, in normal resting B lymphocytes in EBV-positive individuals (183), although the level of EBNA-1 mRNA is lower than that present in cycling cells. This is probably a consequence of the regulation of Qp through cell cycle genes, because this promoter region contains E2F binding sites and can be regulated, through E2F, by retinoblastoma (184,185).

In addition to its role in viral genome persistence, EBNA-1 has other unique properties that may be important in its potential role in tumorigenesis. Unlike the other latent proteins, and related to the fact that it is the only EBV gene expressed in the B-cell reservoir, EBNA-1 is not processed in proteasomes and presented at the cell surface in the context of major histocompatibility complex class I antigens, which would lead to recognition and elimination of EBV-carrying B lymphocytes by T cells. This property, which also may account for the very long half-life of EBNA-1, is conferred on the protein by its internal alanine–glycine repeat region (186). The lack of immunogenicity, at least with respect to cytotoxic T cells, of EBNA-1, along with the lack of expression of the immunogenic latent proteins, is relevant to the escape of BL cells from immunosurveillance mediated by cytotoxic T cells directed against EBV proteins; this neat story, however, may need to be modified if other proteins capable of mediating an immune response against EBV-containing cells, such as BARF-0 and LMP-2A, prove to be regularly expressed in BL. The ability of EBNA-1, because of its alanine-glycine repeat region, to escape antigen processing could be irrelevant in the context of BL; in BL cells, all antigen processing and expression in the context of class I major histocompatibility complex proteins is impaired because of downregulation of the transporter proteins, TAP-1 and TAP-2, associated with this process (187,188). Some human leukocyte antigen class I molecules and adhesion molecules are poorly expressed at the cell surface (189–192). The net consequence of these changes is that BL presents a poor target to cytotoxic T cells (193). If LMP-1 is transfected into BL cells, upregulation of TAP proteins and human leukocyte antigens with restoration of antigen processing occurs (187,194), providing yet another reason why latent gene expression in BL is restricted.

Consistent with the recognition that LMP-1 uses signal-transduction pathways also utilized by CD40, so that LMP-1, at least in part, is able to substitute for CD40 antigen ligation, treatment of BL cell lines with soluble CD40 ligand also has been shown to upregulate peptide transporter expression and restore endogenous antigen processing in BL cells, although without full restoration of the immunogenicity of viral proteins (195). The defective antigen processing pathways in BL and impaired immunogenicity probably would be largely abrogated if type II or III latency were the rule. Perhaps more interesting than this, however, is the fact that some of the latent genes appear to simulate the effects of molecules that would be expected to interact with normal B cells passing through a germinal follicle: antigen in the case of EBNA-2 (which induces MYC expression), and CD40 in the case of LMP-1. Not only are these effects of the latent EBV proteins not required by BL, but they could lead to the extinction of any budding BL cell.

The focus naturally returns to the restricted EBV latency manifested in BL, and how this might be relevant to pathogenesis. There are two possibilities worthy of consideration: that these cells are predisposed to the development of a *MYC*-immunoglobulin translocation (or perhaps any translocation involving immunoglobulin genes), and that the type I latency pattern is able to inhibit at least some of the apoptotic pathways (those likely to be engaged in BL cells). The first possibility might be related to the capacity of EBNA-1 to upregulate the immunoglobulin recombinases, RAG-1 and RAG-2 (196). Although the enzymes mediating chromosomal translocation in BL remain poorly defined, it is possible that EBNA-1 could increase the likelihood that *MYC*-immunoglobulin translocations will arise in B cells, as a consequence of preparation of the cells to undergo immunoglobulin gene recombination. The *RAG* genes are expressed in immature B cells and in some germinal center B cells (197–199), each of which is a location at which chromosomal translocations may occur. In this respect it is of interest that EBV can infect very immature B cells (116), and also that there is evidence to support the possibility that circulating B cells that contain EBV, in both normal individuals and patients with acute malaria, are derived from virgin B cells recently released from the bone marrow, which have a life span measured in months in the absence of antigen stimulation. This suggests that the EBV reservoir may be maintained in immature B cells (200), which is consistent with the observation that BL cells frequently have unrearranged J regions, supporting the possibility that the translocations arise in immature B cells (117). It is possible that the translocations occur in germinal centers during further recombination of the VDJ region, however, presumably in cells that do not bind strongly to antigen and are given a second chance to create a high-affinity binding region. Although under normal circumstances antigen binding has been shown to limit further VDJ recombination in germinal center cells (201), the occurrence of a *MYC*-immunoglobulin translocation may have the same inhibitory effect at this anatomic location. In immature cells, the opposite is the case:

The presence of a translocation does not prevent rearrangement of the other immunoglobulin allele. Whether BL cells have been exposed to antigen or seem to have been exposed (e.g., with respect to hypervariable region mutations) because of activation of the same pathways (and ultimately MYC) must remain an unanswered question for now; despite the phenotype of a germinal center cell (also likely to be induced by MYC), however, it is intriguing that the cells maintain a latent gene expression pattern consistent with that found in peripheral lymphocytes. These findings leave open the hypothesis that BL cells would be virgin B cells if it were not for the effect of the deregulated *MYC* gene (67).

A role for the restricted latent gene pattern in BL in the inhibition of apoptosis at first seems unlikely. Many EBV genes influence apoptosis, either directly, like the lytic cycle gene, *BHRF1*, or indirectly, through upregulation of cellular BCL-2, as has been shown for the latent genes *LMP1* and *EBNA2* (202–204). BL cell lines with restricted latency patterns appear to be quite susceptible to apoptosis, and the conversion of type I latency to type III reduces this susceptibility, at least *in vitro* (203). Such effects are unlikely to be important to the pathogenesis of BL, except possibly in an early step. The evidence from these systems, transfected EBV-negative cell lines, and the Akata model suggests that EBNA-1 has little effect on inhibiting apoptosis; although such *in vitro* experiments do not exclude an antiapoptotic role for EBNA-1 in specific microenvironments, there is no evidence to support such a role. In the Akata model, restoration of EBV to EBV-negative subclones increased resistance to apoptosis even if *LMP1*– and *EBNA2*–defective viruses were used, but EBNA-1 alone was not able to accomplish this, although restoration to a full type 1 latency pattern was (177,205). The suggestion that other latent genes also may influence apoptosis has been proved by the demonstration that oncogenicity and resistance to apoptosis is mediated solely by the *EBER* genes (175). The simplest model with respect to the role of EBV latent genes in the pathogenesis of BL is that *EBNA1* maintains the EBV genome and may cause the cell to be predisposed to the development of an *MYC*-immunoglobulin translocation, and the *EBER* genes protect against apoptosis. This model probably is oversimplified, and more evidence than is presently available is required, with respect to both the potential of *RAG* gene expression to predispose to translocations involving immunoglobulin genes and the possible role of *EBER* genes as inhibitors of apoptosis, before it can be evaluated critically. A role not previously conceived for EBNA-1, through either the transactivation of cellular genes (206) or the binding of cellular proteins, cannot be excluded; several proteins able to bind to EBNA-1 recently have been identified (207–209). The development of lymphomas in mice transgenic for *EBNA1* cannot be overlooked, although confirmation of this observation is required (176). Support of a different kind comes from recent evidence suggesting that *EBNA1* sequence variants may segregate differently in EBV-associated neoplasias than in normal lymphocytes (210,211). Although the latter finding provides no hint of a potential pathogenetic mechanism, and a geographic element to the distribution of *EBNA1* subtypes may exist, there is evidence that the *EBNA* subtypes arise *in vivo*, and that the subtype found most commonly in peripheral lymphocytes is found uncommonly in BL. In BL, two subtypes, one of which is not readily detected in normal peripheral blood lymphocytes, predominate (211,212), but more information is necessary about BL (as well as *EBNA1* subtypes in peripheral lymphocytes) in different world regions to determine whether these observations are correct. These data are consistent with the possibility that mutation is required in *EBNA1* for it to play a role in neoplasia. This novel notion raises the possibility that experiments with *EBNA1* which have, in general, failed to show an effect of *EBNA1* on oncogenicity or resistance to apoptosis, may have been performed with nononcogenic *EBNA1* variants.

Although further studies are required to elucidate the mechanisms through which EBV contributes to pathogenesis in BL, the sum total of evidence strongly favors a causal role, as recently was concluded by the International Agency for Research in Cancer (151). One final issue must be addressed: the rarity of EBV-associated BL in Europe and the United States compared with equatorial Africa and most other developing countries. The most likely explanation is that early infection (perinatal or infancy) with EBV predisposes to EBV-associated BL (213), perhaps in association with simultaneous exposure to other chronic infectious diseases, such as malaria. Why this should be remains a subject for speculation.

MALARIA AS A COFACTOR IN THE PATHOGENESIS OF BURKITT'S LYMPHOMA

The possibility that malaria is a cofactor in the pathogenesis of Burkitt's lymphoma evolved from Burkitt's observation that the high incidence area in sub-Saharan Africa could be demarcated on the basis of environmental factors (151,214,215), and the recognition by Davies that the distribution of BL in Africa was similar to that of mosquito-vectored diseases such as yellow fever (plotted by Haddow), suggesting that the disease might be caused by an agent transmitted by an arthropod (151,216). Given the recent demonstration of the viral causation of certain mouse leukemias, the most likely candidate seemed to be a mosquito-vectored virus. It was this theory that led directly to the discovery of EBV in 1964 (143). Subsequently, given the strong epidemiologic evidence linking EBV with BL, the absence of data supporting the possibility that EBV is vectored by arthropods, and the recognized occurrence of BL outside Africa, the notion that holoendemic malaria, which has a distribution similar to that of endemic BL, might be a cofactor for the development of BL was accepted increasingly as being the most likely explanation for the climatic determinants of the distribution of BL in tropical regions. This hypothesis, originally proposed by Dalldorf and colleagues (217), has been supported over the years by much indirect evidence, such as the demonstration that mice infected with *Plasmodium berghei* more readily develop "aleukemic leukemia" or lymphomas inducible by Maloney virus (218), the observation that the percentage of EBV-positive B cells is higher in the peripheral blood (219–221) and lymph nodes (222) of individuals with acute malaria, and evidence that the intensity of exposure to malaria measured by malaria parasitemia rates, which is higher in rural than urban regions, influences the incidence of BL (223). A possible mechanism is suggested by the finding that mouse malaria causes hyperplasia of precursor B cells (224). B-cell hyperplasia induced by malaria could increase the likelihood of the development of BL, by increasing the population of target cells susceptible to the development of genetic changes leading to BL, permitting the survival of a greater number of EBV-containing B cells in the body, or both. BL in equatorial Africa is almost invariably EBV-associated, and although occasional EBV-negative cases occur (approximately 5%), the incidence of such cases may be similar to that found elsewhere. The alteration of T-cell immunity to EBV brought about by malaria may be more important than the B-cell hyperplasia it induces. In this context, it is possible that a further requirement is infection at an early age by malaria—that is, at around the time at which EBV infection occurs, which could explain why a relationship between the distributions of malaria and BL has not been established outside the holoendemic malarial regions. These regions are also predominantly regions in which *Plasmodium falciparum* predominates, but whether the type of malaria is a relevant factor remains unknown.

In order to study the possibility that malaria is a cofactor for the development of BL directly, a controlled trial of malaria prophylaxis (with chloroquine) was carried out in the Mara Masai area of Tanzania. Although the incidence of BL was significantly reduced during the period of the trial (225), there was some evidence that this reduction was already in progress immediately prior to the commencement of the trial, and these results have not been considered as proving conclusively that malaria can predispose to BL. There remains, however, no better explanation for the climatic determinants of the distribution of BL in tropical regions such as equatorial Africa and New Guinea.

The likelihood that BL, and particularly EBV-associated BL, is related to malaria, and perhaps particularly malaria acquired perinatally or early in infancy, as occurs in holoendemic regions, raises the possibility that other chronic infections, particularly those that are associated with a TH2 type of immune response, that is, with reduced cell-mediated immunity, also may predispose to BL in other world regions. Potential candidates include other parasitic diseases, and suggestive evidence that this could be the case for schistomiasis has been reported from Brazil, where, once again, most BL is EBV-associated (226).

The possibility that B-cell hyperplasia—if sufficiently marked and prolonged--predisposes to the development of translocations involving immunoglobulin genes also is supported by another situation in which BL is more common than in normal populations: the presence of immunosuppression, whether inherited or acquired.

ASSOCIATION OF BURKITT'S LYMPHOMA WITH IMMUNODEFICIENCY STATES

Because lymphomas arise from the constituent cells of the immune system, it is not surprising that disorders associated with abnormal regulation of lymphocytes, that is, inherited, acquired, or iatrogenic immunosuppression, are associated with an increased incidence of non-Hodgkin's lymphomas (227,228). This is probably a consequence of alterations in the size and self-renewal potential of selected lymphoid subpopulations. EBV also appears to be important in the pathogenesis of lymphomas in immunodeficiency states, because a majority of these lymphomas and lymphoproliferative syndromes contain EBV genomes (145,151,227,228). As in malaria, it appears that defective T-cell regulation permits the expansion of EBV-infected clones of B cells, so that these are present in increased numbers in both peripheral lymphocytes (229) and lymph nodes (230). Not all of the B-cell lymphomas in these diseases, however, bear the characteristic *MYC*-immunoglobulin chromosomal abnormalities, and many have large B-cell (often referred to in the past as immunoblastic lymphoma) morphology (Chapter 16). In HIV-associated lymphomas, BL is less often associated with EBV (30–40%) than is LBCL and also is more likely to occur early in the illness, before marked immunosuppression has developed; the reverse applies to LBCL. LBCL appears to be more likely than BL to arise from neoplastic progression occurring in EBV-transformed B lymphocytes, permitted to increase in number by the defective immune response. Why AIDS (and sometimes other immunodeficiency syndromes) predisposes patients to both EBV-positive and EBV-negative BL is unknown, but B-cell hyperplasia is likely one factor; the age at which EBV infection occurs may influence the likelihood of EBV association. Many other factors in patients with immunodeficiency syndromes probably influence the likelihood of the development of BL, including the association of some inherited immunodeficiency syndromes associated with chromosomal replication abnormalities (such as ataxia telangiectasia, Bloom syndrome, and xeroderma pigmentosum) with defects in DNA repair. There is no doubt that HIV itself has no direct role in pathogenesis, because it cannot be found in the lymphoma cells themselves.

In general, the molecular characteristics of BL in immunodeficiency syndromes, best studied in HIV-associated BL, are similar to those observed in BL occurring in the absence of an underlying immunodeficiency (231,232), although the border between BL and LBCL may be even less well defined (18,231–234). Tumors that have the molecular characteristics of BL and are associated with EBV but have a much more differentiated phenotype, including plasmacytoid features, have been described in HIV-associated lymphomas

(19). The significance of this is unknown, but it is possible that histologic borders are even less distinct in HIV-associated lymphomas than in those in individuals not infected by HIV (Chapter 28).

CLINICAL CHARACTERISTICS

Burkitt's lymphoma is a rare tumor that occurs predominantly in the first two decades of life but has been observed at all ages between 2 and 80 years. The male : female ratio is 2 : 1 or 3 : 1, and the incidence ranges from 1 to 3 per million in the United States to 50 to 100 per million in Equatorial Africa.

The disease is primarily extranodal, and most patients within the United States and Europe present with abdominal pain or swelling or changes in bowel habits, because involvement of intraabdominal organs and tissues, particularly the terminal ileum, appendix, ascending colon, and peritoneum (often resulting in ascites), is the most frequent manifestation of the disease, present in some 90% of patients in the United States (235) (Fig. 27.14). Organs less commonly involved at presentation include the bone marrow, pleura, CNS, breast (Fig. 27.15), kidneys, testes, and ovary. Involvement of the jaw (frequently of both the maxilla and mandible) and orbital tumors are seen more commonly in African patients, occurring in some 60% at presentation (155). This may present as loose teeth or early loss of deciduous teeth, or there may be one or more large intraoral masses with necrotic areas, giving the patient's breath a characteristic fetid odor. The maxillary antrum may be filled with tumor, and penetration through the floor of the orbit is not uncommon. These tumors grow sufficiently quickly that the skin of the face becomes taught and shiny, but rarely does the tumor penetrate the skin. Orbital tumors may protrude around the eye or, as is usually the case, push the eye forward. There is often gross chemosis of the conjunctiva. Involvement of the cranial nerves or paraspinal epidural space is also more common in African patients, but bone marrow involvement is seen much less frequently (236). A comparison of the frequency of involvement of various anatomic sites at presentation is shown in Table 27.4. More detailed comparisons of the clinical features of African and American patients have been provided elsewhere (151,155,235,237).

Jaw involvement probably occurs with intermediate frequency in some parts of the world, such as Turkey, but appears to occur at high frequency only in children in equatorial Africa (147,238). Although jaw tumors are uncommon in Brazilian children, those that do occur often have the features of the African jaw tumors: They are prominent tu-

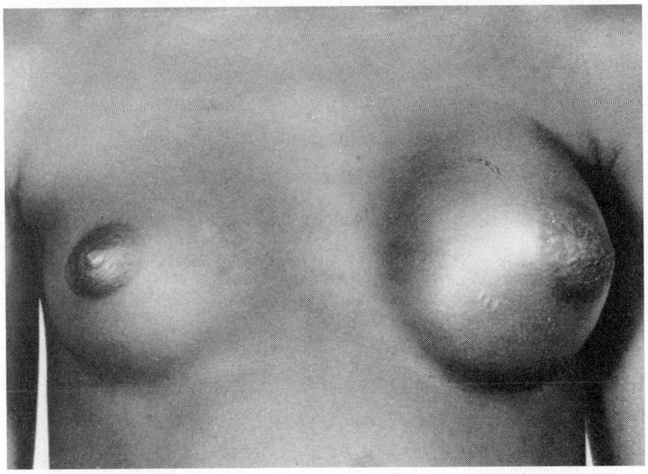

FIG. 27.15. Bilateral breast involvement in an adolescent African girl with Burkitt's lymphoma. The tumor presented as rapid enlargement of the breast buds. The consistency of the breasts was very firm, and the skin of the distended left breast can be seen to be taut and shiny, with flattening of the nipple.

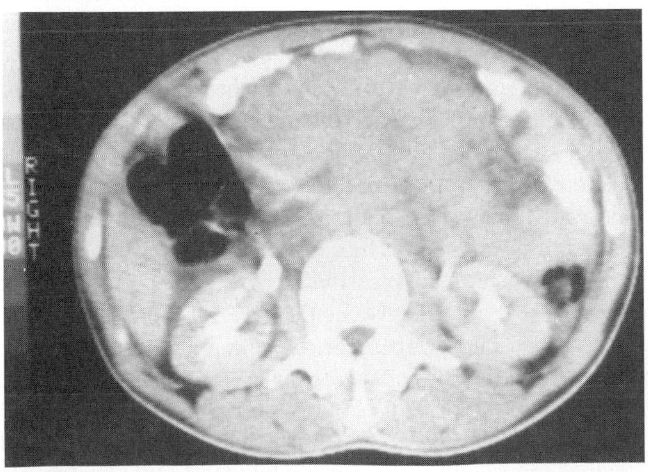

FIG. 27.14. Computerized tomogram of the abdomen in a male patient aged 18 years showing a large abdominal mass that displaces contrast filled loops of bowel. (From Levine AS, ed. *Cancer in the young.* New York: Academic Press, 1991, with permission.)

TABLE 27.4. *Percentages of patients with involvement at designated disease sites at presentation in Burkitt's lymphoma*

	Endemic	Sporadic
Abdomen (all)	58	91
Pleural effusion	3	19
Bone marrow	7	20
Peripheral nodes	9	13
Bone	8	9
Cerebrospinal fluid–central nervous system	19	14
Paraspinal	17	2
Testis	2	6
Pharynx	0	10
Jaw	58	7
Mediastinum	1	3
Orbit	11	1
Miscellaneous[a]	17	15

Note. Many patients had multiple sites of disease.
[a] Includes thyroid, breast, skin, shoulder, and thigh.

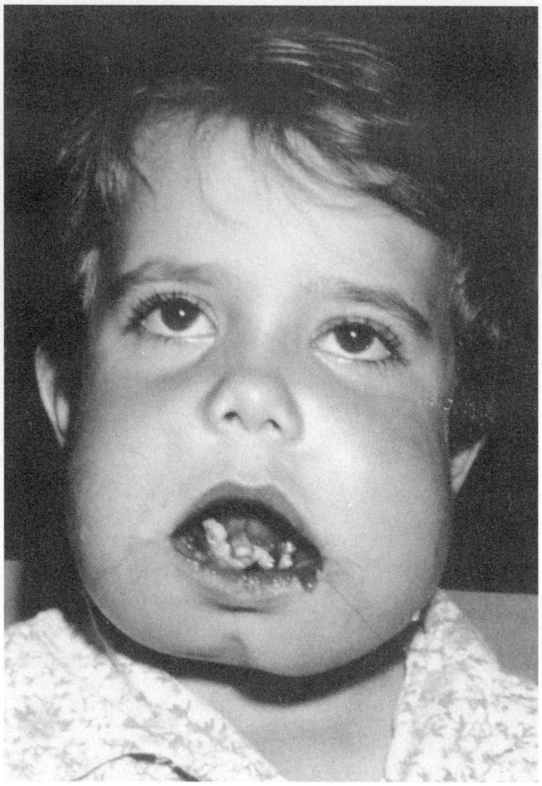

FIG. 27.16. Brazilian child with bilateral maxillary and mandibular Burkitt's lymphoma. (Courtesy of Dr. Sidnei Epelman, Carmago Hospital, Sao Paulo.)

mors usually originating around the molar tooth buds, occurring in young children, and frequently involving multiple jaw quadrants (Fig. 27.16). In North America, there is no association between age and the likelihood of jaw tumors, and if jaw involvement does occur, it frequently is accompanied by involvement of other bony sites of disease and the bone marrow (235).

Many patients have weight loss before presentation, but few develop fevers unless there is superimposed infection, for example because of neutropenia from bone marrow involvement. Infrequently involved sites include lymph nodes, the pharynx, the liver, the spleen, the heart and pericardium, bones, salivary glands, adrenals, the brain, and the skin.

Serious complications can result from tumor deposits in some organs (235). Gastrointestinal bleeding or perforation, ureteric obstruction, intraabdominal venous obstruction (rarely with consequent pulmonary embolus), and obstructive jaundice may result from abdominal involvement, and paraplegia can occur from epidural tumor. Mediastinal tumor, although uncommon (thymic involvement almost never is seen), may lead to pericardial effusion and cardiac tamponade. Uric acid nephropathy may arise from the high cell turnover (and hence increased pool of oxypurines) in patients who have a large tumor burden. Such patients are at high risk to develop renal failure after the commencement of chemotherapy, at which time hyperkalemia and hyperphosphatemia may be life-threatening (235,239).

POTENTIAL ROLE OF GROWTH FACTORS IN DETERMINING ANATOMIC DISTRIBUTION OF TUMOR

Some evidence supports the likelihood that the microenvironment of tumor cells is an important factor in determining tumor distribution. In most patients overt tumor is confined to certain organs, although the tumor cells almost certainly circulate in the blood stream. Jaw tumors and orbital tumors in Africa have a much higher frequency in young children. In the case of jaw tumors, there is a close association with the developing molar teeth, tumor spreading into the pulp and through the laminar dura into the marrow of the jaw (although without dissemination throughout the bone marrow). This is likely related to the presence of a microenvironment conducive to tumor cell growth and viability, although whether this relates to growth factors for the molar teeth or to the presence of lymphoid tissue in this region is unknown. The latter could relate to the presence of infection in African children, similar to the inducement of lymphoid tissue in the stomach by *Helicobacter pylori*. This parallel is not at all inappropriate, because although it usually is not designated as such, BL is in essence an aggressive tumor of mucosa-associated lymphoid tissue. Its distribution is quite similar to that of extranodal marginal zone lymphoma, that is, mucosa-associated lymphoid tissue lymphomas: A very high fraction of patients has involvement of the gastrointestinal tract and, in African children at least, involvement of the thyroid and salivary glands is not uncommon. If the breasts are involved, patients are usually pubertal girls or lactating women (241–243). In the latter, this may relate to the influx of mucosa-associated lymphoid tissue lymphoblasts that occurs in the early stages of lactation.

Burkitt's lymphoma cells express receptors for many growth factors, including low levels of interleukin-2 receptors (244), which may influence growth-regulating pathways. The MYC promoter contains a response element for tranforming growth factor-β, which causes downregulation of MYC (245). Direct effects of growth factor receptors on MYC expression clearly depend on the presence of appropriate regulatory elements in the *MYC* promoter, which in turn differs in tumors with different chromosomal breakpoint locations. It is possible that differences in the clinical presentation of BL between equatorial Africa and other world regions could be accounted for by a mechanism of this kind. Factors that influence the expression of EBV genes relevant to the pathogenesis of BL also could have relevance to the anatomic distribution of tumor, by influencing the growth or viability of the BL cells. Potentially important in this regard is the observation that the Q promoter of EBNA-1 is positively regulated by STATS, proteins that are important to signal transduction of many cytokines (246). Factors that influence the expression of latent genes not normally expressed in BL also could have a negative influence on the growth of BL cells and could excite an immune response against BL cells or even induce lytic cycle genes, as does

EBNA2 in Akata cells (247). The expression of lytic cycle genes, of course, results in cell lysis. Factors of this kind also could influence the response of BL to chemotherapy, which probably occurs through the induction of apoptosis. In one recently published study, prognosis of African children with BL was shown to differ according to the expression of lytic cycle genes, the latter being associated with a better response (152). This finding appears to be contrary to the much earlier recognition that the serum titer of antibodies to early antigens correlated with prognosis (248–250). Such an association could result either from actual differences in the expression of these antigens in tumors, or, if a small fraction of cells in any tumor expresses them, from differences in tumor burden. A correlation between the serum antibody titer and tumor burden has been demonstrated (250). The expression of protein zebra in tumor cells, however, does not necessarily correlate with the titer of antibodies to early antigens.

NATURAL HISTORY

Burkitt's lymphoma is a rapidly progressive tumor with a short doubling time (156). Tumors can increase in size with remarkable and frightening speed. The serum lactate dehydrogenase (250) and interleukin-2 receptor (235) levels correlate well with tumor burden and progressively rise in the face of tumor cell proliferation. Ultimately, with large tumors, hyperuricemia and lactic acidemia ensue. These progressively worsen as the tumor burden increases; such worsening may be confounded by renal failure caused by ureteric compression or diffuse renal involvement. If untreated, patients usually die from fluid, electrolyte, or metabolic disturbances associated with any combination of renal failure, bone marrow failure, intestinal obstruction, serous effusions, airway or major venous obstruction, and CNS spread. In the presence of marrow involvement, bleeding and infection may occur consequent to thrombocytopenia and granulocytopenia. The prognosis depends on the extent of tumor at the time of commencement of chemotherapy and, of course, on the efficacy of therapy. Involvement of the bone marrow and the CNS (stage IV disease) carries a worse prognosis, although with modern, intensive treatment regimens, the difference in survival rates of such patients from others with less extensive disease is not marked, and the previous assumption that CNS disease was a major obstacle to cure has not been borne out (251).

TREATMENT AND SURVIVAL

Prompt staging (determination of the extent of disease) and treatment are essential in BL because of the very short doubling time of the tumor. Surgery may be needed initially to make a histologic diagnosis and to treat urgent complications such as gastrointestinal bleeding or perforation of the bowel, both of which are uncommon (patients who undergo ill-advised attempts to resect extensive abdominal disease may be predisposed to the latter). Patients in whom all abdominal tumor can be resected (stage II in the St. Jude staging system) have an excellent prognosis if chemotherapy is administered within a few days of surgery (252), but although it is possible that surgery provides a significant advantage if low-intensity chemotherapy regimens are used, this is probably not the case with the high-intensity regimens used more recently in the United States and Europe (253,254). It is likely that the good prognosis in such patients is a consequence more of the small size of the tumor, which makes it readily resectable, than of the fact that the tumor was resected (253). Radiation has no primary role in the treatment of BL, which is considered to be disseminated widely from the outset, even in patients with localized disease (255). The major treatment modality is chemotherapy.

Effective combination chemotherapy regimens consist of high doses of alkylating agents (cyclophosphamide or ifosfamide) in various combinations with methotrexate, vincristine, etoposide, doxorubicin, cytarabine, and usually a corticosteroid (235). The most recent and effective regimens in use in Europe and in the United States for patients who have extensive tumor include high-dose methotrexate and often high-dose cytosine arabinoside as well (256–259). These drugs are effective against systemic and CNS disease, although they are supplemented by intrathecal drugs (methotrexate and cytosine arabinoside) to prevent CNS spread, which otherwise would occur in perhaps 50% of patients who have extensive disease. These and other regimens currently used are intensive: Repeated doses of chemotherapeutic agents are administered as rapidly as possible, at least for patients with disseminated disease, for short durations (the total duration of therapy can be as short as 3 months, even for patients with the most extensive disease). Vigorous hydration and close monitoring are needed during initial therapy to prevent the metabolic complications that could arise from the rapid lysis of the tumor by cytotoxic agents (235,239). The most serious of these complications is hyperkalemia, which originally brought the rapid tumor lysis syndrome to attention, because of the occurrence of fatal cardiac arrest (260). Hyperkalemia may occur within hours of initial therapy but, like acute renal failure in this situation, is not seen if a high urine flow can be maintained.

Almost all patients with limited BL can be cured with currently available treatment, and the outlook for patients who have advanced disease has improved steadily as regimens have increased in intensity and additional effective drugs have been incorporated into the regimens. The most recently reported results from Germany, France, and the United States suggest that 85% to 90% of patients with extensive disease can be cured, and it is difficult to define a poor prognostic group (256–259). Preliminary evidence suggests that adults with BL or BLL treated with similar regimens are likely to enjoy similar survival rates, although this may not apply to elderly patients, who may be less well able to tolerate the intensive therapy required (257,261). Fortunately, if relapse occurs in BL, it does so within 1 year, and few relapses occur after 8 months from initial chemotherapy. Patients who survive free of disease for at least 1 year after diagnosis can be considered cured.

Potential New Therapeutic Approaches

Although the results of intensive combination chemotherapy regimens have been excellent, these treatment protocols have a high toxic cost, both in inconvenience to the patient and in the incidence of potentially serious infectious complications of chemotherapy-induced granulocytopenia. Deaths caused by toxicity occur, although fortunately usually in less than 5% of patients once oncologists have become familiar with the protocols. Nevertheless, therapy more specific for the tumor cells would provide major benefits to patients. In this respect, approaches directed towards altering the fine balance between survival and apoptosis of tumor cells, for example by modifying pathways through which MYC induces apoptosis, and using EBV as a potential target for therapy, or even a therapeutic tool, are the most promising. The former is premature at this point, because the apoptotic pathways used by MYC still are defined imprecisely. With respect to EBV, a number of possible approaches can be envisioned. These include forcing the expression of latent genes not normally expressed in BL, for example by using agents such as 5-azacytidine that inhibit methylation, one of the mechanisms believed to be relevant to the restricted latent gene expression in BL (262,263), or by treatment with CD40 ligand (195). Approaches of this kind, at least theoretically, could lead to the development of a host immune response against the tumor. The use of gene therapy, in which vectors driven by EBNA-1 include ori-P in the gene construct to limit their activation to EBV-containing cells, is worthy of consideration, although such an approach has significant logistic problems related to the identification of appropriate vectors. Nonetheless, destruction of tumor cells *in vitro* has been accomplished using suicide genes such as a prodrug-activating enzyme, to enhance the concentration of drug in tumor cells, or the zebra gene, to induce the EBV lytic cycle (264,265). Such *in vitro* studies demonstrate proof of principle and are likely to be more important as stimuli for the development of tumor-specific therapies based on an understanding of pathogenesis of BL than to be realistic therapeutic alternatives at the present time. Of particular interest for the near future is the capacity to design low molecular weight drugs capable of specifically affecting pathways known to be relevant to pathogenesis and maintenance of the transformed phenotype. Before such ''designer'' therapies can be embarked on, however, a much greater understanding of the cellular pathways that are affected by the genetic abnormalities in BL and by the presence of EBV is needed. Given the progress that has been made in the 40 years since the discovery of BL, it seems likely that such therapies will be available before the middle of this century.

Prevention

Vaccination against EBV is an appealing approach to the prevention of BL in equatorial Africa, but whether this would be effective and cost-effective remains speculative and a matter of some controversy. Coupled to a clinical trial, the outcomes seen with such a vaccination also would provide direct evidence for or against the involvement of EBV in the pathogenesis of BL. Avoidance of exposure to the medicinal plant *Euphorbia tiruncalli*, which has been implicated as a cause of BL through its reputed induction of translocations and the ability of EBV to transform cells (266), perhaps should be mentioned as another potential approach; however, the absence of strong epidemiologic support for this plant as a factor in the cause of BL, as well as the logistic difficulties of clinical studies and implementing such a policy in Africa, where this plant is found and used, are likely to dampen enthusiasm for the approach. A more feasible approach to prevention in Africa is to develop a vaccine against malaria—in which case the potential for the prevention of BL would be a side benefit of much less value than the prevention of malaria itself. This is a difficult task, but one that is being explored (267,268). The chemoprevention of malaria is difficult, for reasons including resistance of the parasite to available drugs and the need for repeated administration. Malarial prevention, if it could be achieved effectively and an appropriate control group could be found for studies, like EBV prevention would provide direct evidence for a pathogenetic role for malaria in BL.

REFERENCES

1. Burkitt D. A sarcoma involving the jaws in African Children. *Br J Surg* 1958;46:218–223.
2. O'Conor G. Malignant lymphoma in African children: II. A pathological entity. *Cancer* 1961;14:270–283.
3. National Cancer Institute sponsored study of the classifications of non-Hodgkin's lymphomas: summary and description of a working formulation for clinical usage. *Cancer* 1982;49:2112–2135.
4. Lukes RJ, Collins RD. New approaches to the classification of the lymphomata. *Br J Cancer* 1975;31[Suppl II]:1–28.
5. Harris N, Jaffe ES, Stein H, et al. A revised European-American classification of lymphoid neoplasms: a proposal from the International Lymphoma Study Group. *Blood* 1994;84:1361–1392.
6. Sigaux F, Berger R, Bernheim A, et al. Malignant lymphomas with band 8q24 chromosome abnormality: a morphologic continuum extending from Burkitt's to immunoblastic lymphoma. *Br J Haematol* 1984;57:393–405.
7. Yano T, Van Krieken JHJM, Magrath IT, et al. Histogenetic correlations between subcategories of small non-cleaved cell lymphomas. *Blood* 1992;79:1282–1290.
8. Kramer MH, Hermans J, Wijburg E. Clinical relevance of BCL2, BCL6, and MYC rearrangements in diffuse large B-cell lymphoma. *Blood* 1998;92:3152–3162.
9. Magrath I, Adde M, Shad A, et al. Adults and children with small non-cleaved cell lymphoma have a similar excellent outcome when treated with the same chemotherapy regimen. *J Clin Oncol* 1996;13:925–935.
10. Adde M, Shad A, Venzon D, et al. Additional chemotherapy agents improve treatment outcome for children and adults with advanced B-cell lymphomas. *Semin Oncol* 1998;2[Suppl 4]:33–39.
11. Garvin AJ, Simon RM, Osborne CK, et al. An autopsy study of histologic progression in non-Hodgkin's lymphomas: 192 cases from the National Cancer Institute. *Cancer* 1983;52:393–398.

12. Mintzer DM, Andreeff M, Filippa DA, et al. Progression of nodular poorly differentiated lymphocytic lymphoma to Burkitt's-like lymphoma. *Blood* 1984;64:415–421.
13. Gauwerky CE, Haluska FG, Tsujimoto Y, et al. Evolution of B-cell malignancy: pre-B-cell leukemia resulting from MYC activation in a B-cell neoplasm with a rearranged BCL2 gene. *Proc Natl Acad Sci USA* 1988;85:8548–8552.
14. Gauwerky CE, Hoxie J, Nowell PC, et al. Pre-B-cell leukemia with a t(8;14) and a t(14;18) translocation is preceded by follicular lymphoma. *Oncogene* 1988;2:431–435.
15. McDonnell TJ, Korsmeyer SJ. Progression from lymphoid hyperplasia to high-grade malignant lymphoma in mice transgenic for the t(14; 18). *Nature* 1991;349:254–256.
16. Cory S, Vaux DL, Strasser A, et al. Insights from Bcl-2 and Myc: malignancy involves abrogation of apoptosis as well as sustained proliferation. *Cancer Res* 1999;59[Suppl 7]:1685–1692.
17. Harris NL, Jaffe ES, Diebold J, et al. The World Health Organization Classification of Hematological Malignancies: report of the Clinical Advisory Committee Meeting, Airlie House, Virginia, November 1997. *J Clin Oncol* 1999;17:3835–3849.
18. Gaidano G, Pastore C, Gloghini A, et al. AIDS-related non-Hodgkin's lymphomas: molecular genetics, viral infection and cytokine deregulation. *Acta Haematol* 1996;95:193–198.
19. Davi F, Delecluse HJ, Guiet P, et al. Burkitt-like lymphomas in AIDS patients: characterization within a series of 103 human immunodeficiency virus-associated non-Hodgkin's lymphomas. Burkitt's Lymphoma Study Group. *J Clin Oncol* 1998;16:3788–3795.
20. Benjamin D, Magrath IT, Triche T, et al. Induction of plasmacytoid differentiation by phorbol ester in B cell lymphoma cell lines bearing 8;14 translocations. *Proc Natl Acad Sci USA* 1984;81:3547–3551.
21. Bennett JM, Catovsky D, Daniel MT, et al. Proposals for the classification of the acute leukaemias: French-American-British (FAB) cooperative group. *Br J Haematol* 1976;33:451–458.
22. Flandrin G, Brouet JC, Daniel MT, et al. Acute leukemia with Burkitt's tumor cells: a study of six cases with special reference to lymphocyte surface markers. *Blood* 1975;45:183–188.
23. Magrath IT, Ziegler JL. Bone marrow involvement in Burkitt's lymphoma and its relationship to acute B-cell leukemia. *Leuk Res* 1980; 4:33–59.
24. Roos G, Nordenson I, Osterman B, et al. Patient with acute B-cell leukemia of Burkitt's type (L3) and marker chromosomes including an (8;14) translocation. *Leuk Res* 1982;8:27–31.
25. Mitelman F, Andersson-Anvret M, Brandt L, et al. Reciprocal 8:14 translocation in EBV-negative B-cell acute lymphocytic leukemia with Burkitt-type cells. *Int J Cancer* 1979;24:27–33.
26. Berger R, Bernheim A, Brouet JC, et al. t(8;14) translocation in a Burkitt's type of lymphoblastic leukemia (L3). *Br J Haematol* 1979; 43:87–90.
27. Gluck WL, Bigner SH, Borowitz MJ, et al. Acute lymphoblastic leukemia of Burkitt's type (L3 ALL) with 8;22 and 14;18 translocations and absent surface immunoglobulins. *Am J Clin Pathol* 1986;85: 636–640.
28. Geisler C, Philip P, Plesner T, et al. Simultaneous presence of translocations t(14;18) and t(2;8) in a case of chronic lymphocytic leukemia. *Cancer Genet Cytogenet* 1986;22:35–44.
29. Mangan KF, Rauch AE, Bishop M, et al. Acute lymphoblastic leukemia of Burkitt's type (L-3 ALL) lacking surface immunoglobulin and the 8;14 translocation. *Am J Clin Pathol* 1985;83:121–126.
30. Aso T, Hirota Y, Matsumoto I, et al. Acute lymphoblastic leukemia of Burkitt's type (L3-ALL) without chromosome abnormality and lacking surface and cytoplasmic immunoglobulins. *Jpn J Med* 1989; 28:632–635.
31. Azza KM, Assem MM, Jaffe ES, et al. Immunological phenotypic pattern of acute lymphoblastic leukemia in Egypt. *Leuk Res* 1989;13: 519–525.
32. Secker-Walker L, Stewart E, Norton E, et al. Multiple chromosome abnormalities in a drug resistant TdT positive B cell leukemia. *Leuk Res* 1987;11(2):155–161.
33. Drexler HG, Messmore HL, Menon M, et al. A case of TdT positive B-cell acute lymphoblastic leukemia. *Am J Clin Pathol* 1986;85: 735–738.
34. Ganick DL, Finlay JL. Acute lymphoblastic leukemia with Burkitt cell morphology and cytoplasmic immunoglobulin. *Blood* 1980;56: 311–314.
35. Navid F, Mosijczuk AD, Head DR, et al. Acute lymphoblastic leukemia with the (8;14)(q24;q32) translocation and FAB L3 morphology associated with a B-precursor immunophenotype: the Pediatric Oncology Group experience. *Leukemia* 1999;13:135–141.
36. Smith SR, Bown N, Wallis JP, et al. Acute lymphoblastic leukemia of Burkitt type (L3) with a (14;18) and an atypical (8;22) translocation. *Cancer Genet Cytogenet* 1992;62:197–199.
37. Gladstone B, Kadam PR, Balsara BR, et al. Cytogenetic studies on patients of acute lymphoblastic leukemia Burkitt's type with (8;14) & (14;18) translocations. *Indian J Med Res* 1994 99:264–266.
38. Kramer MH, Raghoebier S, Beverstock GC, et al. De novo acute B-cell leukemia with translocation t(14;18): an entity with a poor prognosis. *Leukemia* 1991;5:473–478.
39. Borrego S, Antinolo G, Parody R, et al. Translocation (14;18) in a patient with common acute lymphoblastic leukemia. *Cancer Genet Cytogenet* 1993;65:177–178.
40. Michiels JJ, Adriaansen HJ, Hagemeijer A, et al. TdT positive B-cell acute lymphoblastic leukemia (B-ALL) without Burkitt characteristics. *Br J Haematol* 1988;68:423–426.
41. Collett JM, Begley CG, Sammann ME, et al. Two cases of de novo precursor B-cell acute lymphoblastic leukemia with t(14;18), but without cytogenetic evidence of an associated Burkitt's or Burkitt's variant translocation. *Am J Clin Pathol* 1994;101:587–589.
42. Kouides PA, Phatak PD, Wang N, et al. B-cell acute lymphoblastic leukemia with L1 morphology and coexistence of t(1;19) and t(14; 18) chromosome translocations. *Cancer Genet Cytogenet* 1994;78: 23–27.
43. Rowe D, Devaraj PE, Irving JA, et al. A case of mature B-cell ALL with coexistence of t(1;19) and t(14;18) and expression of the E2A/PBX1 fusion gene. *Br J Haematol* 1996;94:133–135.
44. Wright D. Gross distribution and hematology. In: Burkitt D, Wright D, eds. *Burkitt's lymphoma.* London: E & S Livingstone, 1970:64–81.
45. Magrath IT, Mugerwa J, Bailey I, et al. Intracerebral Burkitt's lymphoma: pathology, clinical features, and treatment. *Quart J Med* 1974; 43:489–508.
46. Berard CW, O'Conor G, Thomas LB, et al. Histopathological definition of Burkitt's tumor. *Bull World Health Organ* 1969;40:601–607.
47. Mann RB, Jaffe ES, Braylan RC, et al. Non-endemic Burkitt's lymphoma: a B cell tumor related to germinal centers. *N Engl J Med* 1976;295:685–691.
48. Wright DH. Microscopic features, histochemistry, histogenesis and diagnosis. In: Burkitt D, Wright D, eds. *Burkitt's lymphoma.* London: E & S Livingstone, 1970:82–102.
49. Benjamin D, Magrath IT, Maguire R, et al. Immunoglobulin secretion by cell lines derived from African and American undifferentiated lymphomas of Burkitt's and non-Burkitt's type. *J Immunol* 1982;129: 1336–1342.
50. Magrath I, Benjamin D, Papadopoulos N. Serum monoclonal immunoglobulin bands in undifferentiated lymphomas of Burkitt and non-Burkitt types. *Blood* 1983;61:726–731.
51. Klein U, Klein G, Ehlin-Hendridsson B, et al, Burkitt's lymphoma is a malignancy of mature B cells expresssing somatically mutated V region genes. *Mol Med* 1995;1:495–505.
52. Chapman CJ, Mockridge CI, Rowe M, et al. Analysis of VH genes used by neoplastic B cells in endemic Buritt's lymphoma shows somatic hypermutation and intraclonal heterogeneity. *Blood* 1995;85: 2176–2181.
53. Kuppers R, Rajewsky K, Hansmann ML. Diffuse large cell lymphomas are derived from mature B cells carrying V region genes with a high load of somatic mutation and evidence of selection for antibody expression. *Eur J Immunol* 1997;27:1398–1405.
54. Desiderio SV, Yancopoulos GD, Paskind M, et al. Insertion of N regions into heavy-chain genes is correlated with expression of terminal deoxytransferase in B cells. *Nature* 1984;311:752–755.
55. Braziel RM, Keneklis T, Donlon JA, et al. Terminal deoxynucleotidyl transferase in non-Hodgkin's lymphoma. *Am J Clin Pathol* 1983;80: 655–659.
56. Magrath IT, Freeman CB, Pizzo P, et al. Characterization of lymphoma derived cell lines: comparison of cell lines positive and negative for Epstein-Barr virus nuclear antigen. II. Surface markers. *J Natl Cancer Inst* 1980;64:477–483.
57. Fingeroth JD, Weis JJ, Tedder TF, et al. Epstein-Barr virus receptor of human B lymphocytes is the C3d receptor CR2. *Proc Natl Acad Sci USA* 1984;81:4510–4514.

58. Magrath I, Freeman C, Santaella M, et al. Induction of complement receptor expression in cell lines derived from human undifferentiated lymphomas: II. Characterization of the induced complement receptors and demonstration of the simultaneous induction of EBV receptor. *J Immunol* 1981;127:1039–1043.
59. Carel JC, Myones BL, Frazier B, et al. Structural requirements for C3d,g/Epstein-Barr virus receptor (CR2/CD21) ligand binding, internalization, and viral infection. *J Biol Chem* 1990;265:12293–12299.
60. Petzer AL, Schulz TF, Stauder R, et al. Structural and functional analysis of CR2/EBV receptor by means of monoclonal antibodies and limited tryptic digestion. *Immunology* 1988;63:47–53.
61. Avila CJ, Torsteinsdottir S, Ehlin HB, et al. Paired Epstein-Barr virus (EBV)-negative and EBV-converted Burkitt lymphoma lines: stimulatory capacity in allogeneic mixed lymphocyte cultures. *Int J Cancer* 1987;40:691–697.
62. Inghirami G, Grignani F, Sternas L, et al. Down-regulation of LFA-1 adhesion receptors by C-myc oncogene in human B lymphoblastoid cells. *Science* 1990;250:682–686.
63. Zech L, Haglund U, Nilsson K, et al. Characteristic chromosomal abnormalities in biopsies and lymphoid-cell lines from patients with Burkitt and non-Burkitt lymphomas. *Int J Cancer* 1976;17:47–56.
64. Bernheim A, Berger R, Lenoir G. Cytogenetic studies on African Burkitt's lymphoma cell lines: t(8;14), t(2;8) and t(8;22) translocations. *Cancer Genet Cytogenet* 1981;3:307–345.
65. Taub R, Kirsch I, Morton C, et al. Translocation of the c-myc gene into the immunoglobulin heavy chain locus in human Burkitt lymphoma and murine plasmacytoma cells. *Proc Natl Acad Sci USA* 1982; 79:7837–7841.
66. Dalla-Favera R, Bregni M, Erikson J, et al. Human c-myc onc gene is located on the region of chromosome 8 that is translocated in Burkitt lymphoma cells. *Proc Natl Acad Sci USA* 1982;79:7824–7827.
67. Magrath IT. The pathogenesis of Burkitt's lymphoma. In: Vande Woude GF, Klein G, eds. *Advances of Cancer Research.* New York: Academic Press, 1990;55:133–270.
68. Adams JM, Cory S. Myc oncogene activation in B and T lymphoid tumours. *Proc R Soc Lond B Biol Sci* 1985;226:59–72.
69. Krolewski JJ, Dalla Favera R. Molecular genetic approaches in the diagnosis and classification of lymphoid malignancies. *Hematol Pathol* 1989;3:45–61.
70. Ar-Rushdi A, Nishikura K, Erikson J, et al. Differential expression of the translocated and the untranslocated c-myc oncogene in Burkitt lymphoma. *Science* 1983;222:390–393
71. Grignani F, Lombardi L, Inghirami G, et al. Negative autoregulation of c-myc gene expression is inactivated in transformed cells. *EMBO J* 1990;9:3913–3922.
72. Nishikura K, Murray JM. The mechanism of inactivation of the normal c-myc gene locus in human Burkitt lymphoma cells. *Oncogene* 1988; 2:493–498.
73. Klein G. Immunological aspects of B-cell derived tumos in humans and rodents. *Princess Takamatsu Symp* 1988;19:3–13.
74. Potter M, Mushinski JF, Mushinski EB, et al. Avian v-myc replaces chromosomal translocation in murine plasmacytomagenesis. *Science* 1987;235:787–789.
75. Adams JM, Harris AW, Pinkert CA, et al. The c-myc oncogene driven by immunoglobulin enhancers induces lymphoid malignancy in transgenic mice. *Nature* 1985;318:533–538.
76. Cory S, Adams JM. Transgenic mice and oncogenesis. *Annu Rev Immunol* 1986;6:25–48.
77. Van Lohuizenm M, Verbeek S, Scheijen B, et al. Identification of cooperating oncogenes in E-μ-myc transgenic mice by provirus tagging. *Cell* 1991;65:737–752.
78. Haupt Y, Alexander W, Barri G, et al. Novel zinc finger gene implicated as myc collaborator by retrovirally accelerated lymphomagenesis in E-μ-myc transgenic mice. *Cell* 1991;65:753–763.
79. Adams JM, Harris AW, Strasser, et al. Transgenic models of lymphoid neoplasia and development of a pan-hematopoietic vector. *Oncogene* 1999:18:5268–5277.
80. Langdon WY, Harris AW, Cory S, et al. The c-myc oncogene perturbs B lymphocyte development in E-μ-myc transgenic mice. *Cell* 1986; 47:11–18.
81. Prendergast GC. Mechanisms of apoptosis by c-Myc. *Oncogene* 1999; 18:2967–2987.
82. Armelin HA, Armelin MC, Kelly K, et al. Functional role for c-myc in mitogenic response to platelet-derived growth factor. *Nature* 1984; 310:655–660.
83. Kelly K, Siebenlist U. Mitogenic activation of normal T cells leads to increased initiation of transcription in the c-myc locus. *J Biol Chem* 1988;263:4828–4831.
84. Kelly K, Underwood B. Cell growth associated regulation of c-myc and c-fos in normal human T cells. *Adv Exp Med Biol* 1987;213: 241–247.
85. Kelly K, Siebenlist U. The regulation and expression of c-myc in normal and malignant cells. *Annu Rev Immunol* 1986;4:317–338.
86. Kelly K, Siebenlist U. The role of c-myc in the proliferation of normal and neoplastic cells. *J Clin Immunol* 1985;5:65–77.
87. Heikkila R, Schwab G, Wickstrom E, et al. A c-myc antisense oligodeoxynucleotide inhibits entry into S phase but not progress from G0 to G1. *Nature* 1987;328:445–449.
88. McManaway ME, Neckers LM, Loke SL, et al. Specific inhibition of proliferation of a subset of Burkitt's lymphoma cell lines by a c-myc intron antisense oligodeoxynucleotide. *Lancet* 1990;335: 807–811.
89. Evan GI, Wyllie AH, Gilbert CS, et al. Induction of apoptosis in fibroblasts by c-myc protein. *Cell* 1992;69:119–128.
90. Davis AC, Wims M, Spotts GD, et al. A null c-myc mutation causes lethality before 10.5 days of gestation in homozygotes and reduced fertility in heterozygous female mice *Genes Dev* 1993;7:671–682.
91. Mateyak MK, Obaya AJ, Adachi S, et al. Phenotypes of c-Myc deficient rat fibroblasts isolated by targeted homologous recombination. *Cell Growth Differ* 1997;8:1039–1048.
92. Henriksson M, Luscher B. Proteins of the Myc network: essential regulators of cell growth and differentiation. *Adv Cancer Res* 1996; 68:109–182.
93. Dang CV. C-Myc target genes involved in cell growth, apoptosis, and metabolism. *Mol Cell Biol* 1999;19:1–11.
94. Stone J, de Lange T, Ramsay G, et al. Definition of regions in human c-myc that are involved in transformation and nuclear localization. *Mol Cell Biol* 1987;7:1697–1709.
95. Smith MJ, Charron-Prochownik DC, Prochownik EV. The leucine zipper of c-myc is required for full inhibition of erythroleukemia differentiation. *Mol Cell Biol* 1990;10:5333–5339.
96. Blackwood EM, Eisenman RN. Max: a helix-loop-helix zipper protein that forms a sequence-specific DNA binding complex with myc. *Science* 1991;251:1211–1217.
97. Marhin WW, Chen S, Facchini LM et al. Myc represses the growth arrest gene gadd45. *Oncogene* 1997;14:2825–2834.
98. Amundson SA, Zhan Q, Penn LZ, et al. Myc suppresses induction of the growth arrest genes gadd34, gadd45, and gadd 153 by DNA-damaging agents. *Oncogene* 1998;17:2149–2154.
99. Bush A, Mateyak M, Dugan K, et al. c-myc null cells misregulate cad and gadd45 but not other proposed c-Myc targets *Genes Dev* 1998;12:3797–3802.
100. Bouchard C, Thieke K, Maier A, et al. Direct induction of cyclin D2 by Myc contributes to cell cycle progression and sequestration of p27. *EMBO J* 1999;18:5321–5333.
101. Queva C, Hurlin PJ, Foley KP, et al. Sequential expression of the MAD family of transcriptional repressors during differentiation and development. *Oncogene* 1998;16:967–977.
102. Ayer DE, Laherty CD, Lawrence QA, et al. Mad proteins contain a dominant transcription repression domain. *Mol Cell Biol* 1996;16: 5772–5781.
103. Foley KP, Eisenman RN. Two MAD tails: what the recent knockouts of Mad1 and Mxi1 tell us about the MYC/MAX/MAD network. *Biochim Biophys Acta* 1999;1423:M37–47.
104. Foley KP, McArthur GA, Queva C, et al. Targeted disruption of the MYC antagonist MAD1 inhibits cell cycle exit during granulocyte differentiation. *EMBO J* 1998;17:774–785.
105. Ayer DE, Lawrence QA, Eisenman RN. Mad-Max transcriptional repression is mediated by ternary complex formation with mammalian homologs of yeast repressor Sin3. *Cell* 1995;80:767–776.
106. Koskinen PJ, Ayer DE, Eisenman RN. Repression of Myc-Ras cotransformation by Mad is mediated by multiple protein-protein interactions. *Cell Growth Differ* 1995;6:623–629.
107. Heinzel T, Levinsky RM, Mullen TM, et al. A complex containing N-Cor, mSin3 and histone deacetylase mediates transcriptional repression. *Nature* 1997;387:43–48.
108. Beijersbergen RL, Hijmans EM, Zhu L, et al. Interaction of c-Myc

with the pRb-related protein p107 results in inhibition of c-Myc-mediated transactivation. *EMBO J* 1994;13:4080–4086.
109. Gu WM, Bhaia K, Magrath IT, et al. Binding and suppression of the Myc transcriptional activation domain by p107. *Science* 1994;264: 251–254.
110. Sakamuro D, Prendergast GC. New Myc-interacting proteins: a second Myc network emerges. *Oncogene* 1999;18:2942–2954.
111. Wu KJ, Polack A, Dalla-Favera R. Coordinated regulation of iron-controlling genes, H-ferritin and IRP2, by c-MYC. *Science* 1999;283: 676–679.
112. Cole MD, McMahon SB. The Myc oncoprotein: a critical evaluation of transactivation and target gene regulation. *Oncogene* 1999;18: 2916–2924.
113. Brubaker G, Levin AG, Steel CM, et al. Multiple cases of Burkitt's lymphoma and other neoplasms in families in the North Mara district of Tanzania. *Int J Cancer* 1980;26:165–170.
114. Haluska FG, Finver S, Tsujimoto Y, et al. The t(8;14) translocation occurring in B-cell malignancies results from mistakes in V-D-J joining. *Nature* 1986;324:158–161.
115. Oettinger MA, Schatz DG, Gorka C, et al. RAG-1 and RAG-2, adjacent genes that synergistically activate V(D)J recombination. *Science* 1990;248:1517–1523.
116. Altiok E, Klein G, Zech L, et al. Epstein-Barr virus-transformed pro-B cells are prone to illegitimate recombination between the switch region of the mu chain gene and other chromosomes. *Proc Natl Acad Sci USA* 1989;86:6333–6337.
117. Bhatia K, Gutierrez MI, Magrath IT. Burkitt's lymphoma cells frequently carry monoallelic DJ rearrangements. *Curr Top Microbiol Immunol* 1992;182:319–324.
118. Pelicci PG, Knowles DM, Magrath I, et al. Chromosomal breakpoints and structural alterations of the c-myc locus differ in endemic and sporadic forms of Burkitt lymphoma. *Proc Natl Acad Sci USA* 1986; 83:2984–2988.
119. Neri A, Barriga F, Knowles DM, et al. Different regions of the immunoglobulin heavy-chain locus are involved in chromosomal translocations in distinct pathogenetic forms of Burkitt lymphoma. *Proc Natl Acad Sci USA* 1988;85:2748–2752.
120. Shiramizu B, Barriga F, Neequaye J, et al. Patterns of chromosomal breakpoint locations in Burkitt's lymphoma: relevance to geography and EBV association. *Blood* 1991;77:1516–1526.
121. Gutierrez M, Bhatia K, Barriga R, et al. Molecular epidemiology of Burkitt's lymphoma from South America: differences in breakpoint locations and EBV association from tumors in other world regions. *Blood* 1992;79:3261–3266.
122. Gutierrez MI, Hamdy N, Bhatia K, et al. Geographic variation in t (8;14) chromosomal breakpoint locations and EBV association in Burkitt's lymphoma. *Int J Pediatr Hematol Oncol* 1999;6:161–168.
123. Zajac-Kaye M, Yu B, Ben-Baruch N. Downstream regulatory elements in the c-myc gene. *Curr Top Microbiol Immunol* 1990;166: 279–284.
124. Madisen L, Groudine M. Identification of a locus control region in the immunoglobulin heavy-chain locus that deregulates c-myc expression in plasmacytoma and Burkitt's lymphoma cells. *Genes Dev* 1994; 8:2212–2226.
125. Snyder RC, Miller DM. Regulation of c-myc transcription initiation and elongation. *Crit Rev Oncog* 1992;3:283–291.
126. Bhatia K, Huppi, K, Spangler G, et al. Point mutations in the c-Myc transactivation domain are common in Burkitt's lymphoma and mouse plasmacytoma. *Nat Genet* 1993;5:56–61.
127. Yano T, Sander CA, Clark HM, et al. Clustered mutations in the second exon of the MYC gene in sporadic Burkitt's lymphoma. *Oncogene* 1993;8:2741–2748.
128. Gu W, Bhatia K, Magrath IT, et al. Binding and suppression of the Myc transcriptional activation domain by p107. *Science* 1994;264: 251–260.
129. Flinn EM, Busch CM, Wright AP, et al. Myc boxes, which are conserved in myc family proteins, are signals for protein degradation via the proteasome. *Mol Cell Biol* 1998;18:5961–5969.
130. Gavine PR, Neil JC, Crouch DH, et al. Protein stabilization: a common consequence of mutations in independently derived v-Myc alleles. *Oncogene* 1999;18:7552–7558.
131. Krumm A, Meulia T, Brunvand M, et al. The block to transcriptional elongation within the human c-myc gene is determined in the promoter-proximal region *Genes Dev* 1992;6:2201–2213.
132. Eick D, Piechaczyk M, Henglein B, et al. Aberrant c-myc RNAs of Burkitt's lymphoma cells have longer half-lives. *EMBO J* 1985;4: 3717–3725.
133. Hoang AT, Lutterbach B, Lewis BC, et al. A link between increased transforming activity of lymphoma-derived MYC mutant alleles, their defective regulation by p107, and altered phosphorylation of the c-Myc transactivation domain. *Mol Cell Biol* 1995;15:4031–4042.
134. Ryan KM, Birnie GD. Cell-cycle progression is not essential for c-Myc to block differentiation. *Oncogene* 1997;14:2835–2843.
135. Hueber AO, Zornig M, Lyon D, et al. Requirement for the CD95 receptor-ligand pathway in c-Myc-induced apoptosis. *Science* 1997; 278:1305–1309.
136. Gutierrez MI, Cherney B, Hussain A, et al. Bax is frequently compromised in Burkitt's lymphomas with irreversible resistance to Fas-induced apoptosis. *Cancer Res* 1999;59:696–703.
137. Gaidano G, Ballerine P, Gong JZ, et al. P53 mutations in human lymphoid malignancies: association with Burkitt's lymphoma and chronic lymphocytic leukemia. *Proc Natl Acad Sci USA* 1991;88: 5413–5417.
138. Bhatia K, Gutierrez MI, Huppi K, et al. The pattern of p53 mutations in Burkitt's lymphoma differs from that of solid tumors. *Cancer Res* 1992;52:1–4.
139. Cherney BW, Bhatia KG, Sgadari C, et al. Role of the p53 tumor suppressor gene in the tumorigenicity of Burkitt's lymphoma cells. *Cancer Res* 1997;57:2508–2515.
140. O'Connor PM, Jackman J, Jondle D, et al. Role of the p53 tumor suppressor gene in cell cycle arrest and radio-sensitivity of Burkitt's lymphoma cell lines. *Cancer Res* 1993;53:4776–4780.
141. Fan S, el-Deiry W S, Bae I, et al. p53 gene mutations are associated with decreased sensitivity of human lymphoma cells to DNA damaging agents. *Cancer Res* 1994;54:5824–5830.
142. Gutierrez MI, Bhatia K, Diez B, et al. Prognostic significance of p53 mutations in small noncleaved cell lymphomas. *Int J Oncol* 1994;4: 567–571.
143. Epstein MA, Achong BG, Barr YM. Virus particles in cultured lymphoblasts from Burkitt's lymphoma. *Lancet* 1964;i:702–703.
144. Subar M, Neri A, Inghirami G, et al. Frequent c-myc oncogene activation and infrequent presence of Epstein-Barr virus genome in AIDS-associated lymphoma. *Blood* 1988;72:667–671.
145. Ernberg I. Epstein-Barr virus and acquired immunodeficiency syndrome. *Adv Viral Oncol* 1989;8:203–217.
146. Anwar N, Kingma D, Block AR, et al. The investigation of Epstein-Barr viral sequences in 41 cases of Burkitt's lymphoma from Egypt: epidemiological correlations. *Am J Pathol Cancer* 1995;76: 1245–1252.
147. Cavdar AO, Yavuz G, Babacan E, et al. Burkitt's lymphoma in Turkish children: clinical, viral [EBV] and molecular studies. *Leuk Lymphoma* 1994;14:323–330.
148. Meziane F, Aguercif M, Chevallier A, et al. Burkitt's lymphoma-Epstein-Barr virus association in western Algeria: clinical, cytological and serological aspects apropos of 34 pediatric cases. *Pediatrie* 1985; 40:87–98.
149. Ladjadj Y, Philip T, Lenoir GM, et al. Abdominal Bur-kitt-type lymphomas in Algeria. *Br J Cancer* 1984;49:503–512.
150. Bacchi MM, Bacchi CE, Alvarenga M, et al. Burkitt's lymphoma in Brazil: strong association with Epstein-Barr virus. *Mod Pathol* 1996; 9:63–67.
151. Epstein-Barr virus. *IARC Monogr Eval Carcinog Risks Hum* 1997; 70:47–373.
152. Labrecque LG, Xue SA, Kazembe P, et al. Expression of Epstein-Barr virus lytically related genes in African Burkitt's lymphoma: correlation with patient response to therapy. *Int J Cancer* 1999;81:6–11.
153. Gutierrez MI, Bhatia K, Magrath I. Replicative viral DNA in Epstein-Barr virus associated Burkitt's lymphoma biopsies. *Leuk Res* 1993; 17:285–289.
154. Henle W, Henle G. Seroepidemiology of the virus. In: Epstein MA, Achong BG, eds. *The Epstein-Barr virus*. New York: Springer, 1979: 61–78.
155. Magrath IT. African Burkitt's lymphoma: history, biology, clinical features, and treatment. *Am J Pediatr Hemat Oncol* 1991;13:222–246.
156. Iverson U, Iverson OH, Ziegler JL, et al. Cell kinetics of African cases of Burkitt's lymphoma: a preliminary report. *Eur J Cancer* 1972;8:305–310.
157. Rowe DT, Rowe M, Evan GI, et al. Restricted expression of EBV

latent genes and T-lymphocyte-detected membrane antigen in Burkitt's lymphoma cells. *EMBO J* 1986;5:2599–2607.
158. Rowe M, Rowe DT, Gregory CD, et al. Differences in B cell growth phenotype reflect novel patterns of Epstein-Barr virus latent gene expression in Burkitt's lymphoma cells. *EMBO J* 1987;6:2743–2751.
159. Niedobitek G, Agathanggelou A, Rowe M, et al. Heterogeneous expression of Epstein-Barr virus latent proteins in endemic Burkitt's lymphoma. *Blood* 1995;86:659–665.
160. Manet E, Bourillot PY, Waltzer L, et al. EBV genes and B cell proliferation. *Crit Rev Oncol Hematol* 1998;28:129–137.
161. Polack A, Hortnagel K, Pajic A, et al. c-myc activation renders proliferation of Epstein-Barr virus (EBV)-transformed cells independent of EBV nuclear antigen 2 and latent membrane protein 1. *Proc Natl Acad Sci USA* 1996;93:10411–10416.
162. Jochner N, Eick D, Zimber-Strobl U, et al. Epstein-Barr virus nuclear antigen 2 is a transcriptional suppressor of the immunoglobulin mu gene: implications for the expression of the translocated c-myc gene in Burkitt's lymphoma cells. *EMBO J* 1996;15:375–382.
163. Floettmann JE, Ward K, Rickinson AB, et al. Cytostatic effect of Epstein-Barr virus latent membrane protein-1 analyzed using tetracycline-regulated expression in B cell lines. *Virology* 1996;223:29–40.
164. Zimber-Strobl U, Strobl L, Hofelmayr H, et al. EBNA2 and c-myc in B cell immortalization by Epstein-Barr virus and in the pathogenesis of Burkitt's lymphoma. *Curr Top Microbiol Immunol* 1999;246: 315–320
165. Kaiser C, Laux G, Eick D, et al. The proto-oncogene c-myc is a direct target gene of Epstein-Barr virus nuclear antigen 2. *J Virol* 1999;73: 4481–4484.
166. Cutrona G, Ulivi M, Fais F, et al. Transfection of the c-myc oncogene into normal Epstein-Barr virus-harboring B cells results in new phenotypic and functional features resembling those of Burkittlymphoma cells and normal centroblasts. *Cell* 1991;65:1107–1115.
167. Wolf J, Klevenz B, Pawlita M, et al. Regressing nude mouse grafts of Burkitt's lymphoma x lymphoblastoid cell hybrids show deregulation of the c-myc gene and expression of the EBV latent membrane protein. *Int J Cancer* 1991;47:99–104.
168. Cherney BW, Sgadari C, Kanegane C, et al. Expression of the Epstein-Barr virus protein LMP1 mediates tumor regression in vivo. *Blood* 1998;91:2491–2500.
169. Masucci MG, Gavioli R, de Campos-Lima PO, et al. Transformation-associated Epstein-Barr virus antigens as targets for immune attack. *Ann NY Acad Sci* 1993;690:86–100.
170. Neri A, Barriga F, Inghirami G, et al. Epstein-Barr virus infection precedes clonal expansion in Burkitt's and acquired immunodeficiency syndrome-associated lymphoma. *Blood* 1991;77:1092–1095.
171. Kirchmaier AL, Sugden B. Plasmid maintenance of derivatives of oriP of Epstein-Barr virus. *J Virol* 1995;69:1280–1283.
172. Lee MA, Diamond ME, Yates JL. Genetic evidence that EBNA-1 is needed for efficient, stable latent infection by Epstein-Barr virus. *J Virol* 1999;73:2974–2982.
173. Kienzle N, Buck M, Greco S, et al. Epstein-Barr virus-encoded RK-BARF0 protein expression. *J Virol* 1999;73:8902–8906.
174. Tao Q, Robertson KD, Manns A, et al. Epstein-Barr virus (EBV) in endemic Burkitt's lymphoma: molecular analysis of primary tumor tissue. *Blood* 1998;91:1373–1381.
175. Komano J, Maruo S, Kurozumi K, et al. Oncogenic role of Epstein-Barr virus-encoded RNAs in Burkitt's lymphoma cell line Akata. *J Virol* 1999;73:9827–9831.
176. Wilson JB, Bell JL, Levine AJ. Expression of Epstein-Barr virus nuclear antigen-1 induces B cell neoplasia in transgenic mice. *EMBO J* 1996;15:3117–3126.
177. Ruf IK, Rhyne PW, Yang H, et al. Epstein-barr virus regulates c-MYC, apoptosis, and tumorigenicity in Burkitt lymphoma. *Mol Cell Biol* 1999;19:1651–1660.
178. Razzouk BI, Srinivas S, Sample CE, et al. Epstein-Barr Virus DNA recombination and loss in sporadic Burkitt's lymphoma. *J Infect Dis* 1996;173:529–535.
179. Schaefer BC, Strominger JL, Speck SH. Redefining the Epstein-Barr virus-encoded nuclear antigen EBNA-1 gene promoter and transcription initiation site in group I Burkitt lymphoma cell lines. *Proc Natl Acad Sci USA* 1995;92:10565–10569.
180. Tsai CN, Liu ST, Chang YS. Identification of a novel promoter located within the Bam HI Q region of the Epstein-Barr virus genome for the EBNA 1 gene. *DNA Cell Biol* 1995;14:767–776.
181. Szeles A, Falk KI, Imreh S, et al. Visualization of alternative Epstein-Barr virus expression programs by fluorescent in situ hybridization at the cell level. *J Virol* 1999;73:5064–5069.
182. Yoo LI, Mooney M, Puglielli MT, et al. B-cell lines immortalized with an Epstein-Barr virus mutant lacking the Cp EBNA2 enhancer are biased toward utilization of the oriP-proximal EBNA gene promoter Wp1. *J Virol* 1997;71:9134–9142.
183. Chen F, Zou JZ, di Renzo L, et al. A subpopulation of normal B cells latently infected with Epstein-Barr virus resembles Burkitt lymphoma cells in expressing EBNA-1 but not EBNA-2 or LMP1. *J Virol* 1995; 69:3752–3758.
184. Ruf IK, Sample J. Repression of Epstein-Barr virus EBNA-1 gene transcription by pRb during restricted latency. *J Virol* 1999;73: 7943–7951.
185. Davenport MG, Pagano JS. Expression of EBNA-1 mRNA is regulated by cell cycle during Epstein-Barr virus type I latency. *J Virol* 1999;73:3154–3161.
186. Levitskaya J, Coram M, Levitsky V, et al. Inhibition of antigen processing by the internal repeat region of the Epstein-Barr virus nuclear antigen-1. *Nature* 1995;375:685–688.
187. Rowe M, Khanna R, Jacob CA, et al. Restoration of endogenous antigen processing in Burkitt's lymphoma cells by Epstein-Barr virus latent membrane protein-1: coordinate up-regulation of peptide transporters and HLA-class I antigen expression. *Eur J Immunol* 1995; 25:1374–1384.
188. Frisan T, Zhang QJ, Levitskaya J, et al. Defective presentation of MHC class I-restricted cytotoxic T-cell epitopes in Burkitt's lymphoma cells. *Int J Cancer* 1996;68:251–258.
189. Gavioli R, De Campos-Lima PO, Kurilla MG, et al. Recognition of the Epstein-Barr virus-encoded nuclear antigens EBNA-4 and EBNA-6 by HLA-A11-restricted cytotoxic T lymphocytes: implications for down-regulation of HLA-A11 in Burkitt lymphoma. *Proc Natl Acad Sci USA* 1992:89:5862–5866.
190. Imreh MP, Zhang QJ, de Campos-Lima PO. Mechanims of allele selective down regulation of HLA class I in Burkitt's lymphoma. *Int J Cancer* 1995;62:90–96.
191. Gregory CD, Murray RJ, Edwards CF, et al. Downregulation of cell adhesion molecules LFA-3 and ICAM-1 in Epstein-Barr virus-positive Burkitt's lymphoma underlies tumor cell escape from virus-specific T cell surveillance. *J Exp Med* 1988;167:1811–1824.
192. Billaud M, Rousset F, Calender A, et al. Low expression of lymphocyte function-associated antigen (LFA)-1 and LFA-3 adhesion molecules is a common trait in Burkitt's lymphoma associated with and not associated with Epstein-Barr virus. *Blood* 1990;75:1827–1833.
193. Rickinson AB, Murray RJ, Brooks J, et al. T cell recognition of Epstein-Barr virus associated lymphomas. *Cancer Surv* 1992;13:53–80.
194. de Campos-Lima PO, Torsteinsdottir S, Cuomo L et al. Antigen processing and presentation by EBV-carrying cell lines: cell-phenotype dependence and influence of the EBV-encoded LMP1. *Int J Cancer* 1993;53:856–862.
195. Khanna R, Cooper L, Kienzle N, et al. Engagement of CD40 antigen with soluble CD40 ligand up-regulates peptide transporter expression and restores endogenous processing function in Burkitt's lymphoma cells. *J Immunol* 1997;159:5782–5785.
196. Srinivas SK, Sixbey JW. Epstein-Barr virus induction of recombinase-activating genes RAG1 and RAG2. *J Virol* 1995;69:8155–8158.
197. Papavasiliou F, Casellas R, Suh H, et al. V(D)J recombination in mature B cells: a mechanism for altering antibody responses. *Science* 1997;278:298–301.
198. Han S, Dillon SR, Zheng B, et al. V(D)J recombinase activity in a subset of germinal center B lymphocytes. *Science* 1997;278:301–305.
199. Giachino C, Padovan E, Lanzavecchia A, et al. Re-expression of RAG-1 and RAG-2 genes and evidence for secondary rearrangements in human germinal center B lymphocytes. *Eur J Immunol* 1998;28: 3506–3513.
200. Lam KM, Whittle H, Grzywacz M, et al. Epstein-Barr virus-carrying B cells are large, surface IgM, IgD-bearing cells in normal individuals and acute malaria patients. *Immunology* 1994;82:383–388.
201. Meffre E, Papavasiliou F, Cohen P, et al. Antigen receptor engagement turns off the V(D)J recombination machinery in human tonsil B cells. *J Exp Med* 1998;188:765–772.
202. Henderson S, Rowe M, Gregory G, et al. Induction of bcl-2 expression by Epstein-Barr virus latent membrane protein 1 protects infected B cells from programmed cell death. *Cell* 1991;65:1–20.

203. Gregory CD, Dive C, Henderson S, et al. Activation of Epstein-Barr virus latent genes protects human B cells from death by apoptosis. *Nature* 1991;349:612–614
204. Finke J, Fritzen R, Ternes P, et al. Expression of bcl-2 in Burkitt's lymphoma cell lines: induction by latent Epstein-Barr virus genes. *Blood* 1992;80:459–469.
205. Komano J, Sugiura M, Takada K. Epstein-Barr virus contributes to the malignant phenotype and to apoptosis resistance in Burkitt's lymphoma cell line Akata. *J Virol* 1998;72:9150–9156.
206. Horner D, Lewis M, Farrell PJ. Novel hypotheses for the roles of EBNA-1 and BHRF1 in EBV-related cancers. *Intervirology* 1995; 38(3-4):195–205.
207. Wang Y, Finan JE, Middeldorp JM, et al. P32/TAP, a cellular protein that interacts with EBNA-1 of Epstein-Barr virus. *Virology* 1997;236: 18–29.
208. Chen MR, Yang JF, Wu CW, et al. Physical association between the EBV protein EBNA-1 and P32/TAP/hyaluronectin. *J Biomed Sci* 1998;5:173–179.
209. Ito S, Ikeda M, Kato N, et al. Epstein-Barr virus nuclear antigen-1 binds to nuclear transporter karyopherin alpha1/NPI-1 in addition to karyopherin alpha2/Rch1. *Virology* 2000;266:110–119.
210. Bhatia, K, Raj MI, Guierrez MI, et al. Variation in the sequence of Epstein Barr virus nuclear antigen-1 in normal peripheral blood lymphocytes and in Burkitt's lymphomas. *Oncogene* 1996;13:177–181.
211. Guttiérez M, Raj A, Spangler G, et al. Sequence variations in EBNA-1 may dictate restriction of tissue distribution of Epstein-Barr virus in normal and tumor cells. *J Gen Virol* 1997;78:1663–1670.
212. Gutierrez MI, Spangler G, Kingma D, et al. Epstein-Barr virus in nasal lymphomas contains multiple ongoing mutations in the EBNA-1 gene. *Blood* 1998;92:600–606.
213. de Thé. Is Burkitt's lymphoma related to perinatal infection by Epstein-Barr virus. *Lancet* 1977;i:335–337.
214. Burkitt D. Determining the climatic limitations of a children's cancer common in Africa. *Br Med J* 1962;2:1019–1026.
215. Burkitt D. A children's cancer dependent on climatic factors. *Nature* 1962;194:232–234.
216. Haddow AJ. An improved map for the study of Burkitt's lymphoma syndrome in Africa. *East Afr Med J* 1963;40:429–432.
217. Dalldorf G, Linsell CA, Marnhart FE, et al. An epidemiological approach to the lymphomas of African children and Burkitt's sarcoma of the jaws. *Perspect Biol Med* 1964;7:435–449.
218. Wedderburn N. Effect of concurrent malarial infection on development of virus-induced lymphoma in Balb-c mice. *Lancet* 1970;ii: 1114–1116.
219. Whittle HC, Brown J, Marsh K, et al. T-cell control of Epstein-Barr virus infected B-cells is lost during P. falciparum malaria. *Nature* 1984;312:449–450.
220. Gunapala DE, Facer CA, Davidson R, et al. In vitro analysis of Epstein-Barr virus: host balance in patients with acute Plasmodium falciparum malaria. *Parasitol Res* 1990;76:531–535.
221. Lam KM, Syed N, Whittle H, et al. Circulating Epstein-Barr virus-carrying B cells in acute malaria. *Lancet* 1991;13;337:876–878.
222. Facer C, Khan G. Detection of EBV RNA (EBER-1 and EBER-2) in malaria lymph nodes by in situ hybridization. *Microbiol Immunol* 1997;41:891–894.
223. Biggar RJ, Nkrumah FK. Burkitt's lymphoma in Ghana: urban-rural distribution, time-space clustering and seasonality. *Int J Cancer* 1979; 23:330–336.
224. Osmond DG, Priddle S, Rico-Vargas S. Proliferation of B cell precur sors in bone marrow of pristane-conditioned and malaria-infected mice. Implications for B cell oncogenesis. *Curr Top Microbiol Immunol* 1990;166:149–157.
225. Geser A, de Thé G, Lenoir G, et al. Final case reporting from the Ugandan prospective study of the relationship between EBV and Burkitt's lymphoma. *Int J Cancer* 1982;29:397–400.
226. Araujo I, Foss HD, Bittencourt A, et al. Expression of Epstein-Barr virus-gene products in Burkitt's lymphoma in Northeast Brazil. *Blood* 1996;87:5279–5286.
227. Seibel N, Cossman J, Magrath IT. Lymphoproliferative Disorders. In: Pizzo PA, Poplack DG, eds. *Principles and practice of pediatric oncology*, 3rd ed. Philadelphia: JB Lippincott Co., 1997:589–615.
228. Magrath IT, Shad AT, Sandlund JT. Lymphoproliferative disorders in immunocompromised individuals. In: Magrath IT, ed. *The non-Hodgkin's lymphomas*, 2nd ed. London, Edward Arnold, 1997: 955–974.
229. Birx DL, Redfield RR, Tosato G. Defective regulation of Epstein-Barr virus infection in patients with acquired immunodeficiency syndrome (AIDS). *N Engl J Med* 1986;314:874–879.
230. Dolcetti R, Gloghini A, De Vita S. Characteristics of EBV-infected cells in HIV-related lymphadenopathy: implications for the pathogenesis of EBV-associated and EBV-unrelated lymphomas of HIV-seropositive individuals. *Int J Cancer* 1995;63:652–659.
231. Whang-Peng J, Lee EC, Sieverts H, et al. Burkitt's lymphoma in AIDS; a cytogenetic study. *Blood* 1984;63:818–822.
232. Chaganti RSK, Jhanwar S, Kozinar B, et al. Specific translocations characterize Burkitt's like lymphoma of homosexual men with the acquired immunodeficiency syndrome. *Blood* 1983;61:1269–1272.
233. Gaidano G, Pastore C, Gloghini A, et al. Genetic heterogeneity of AIDS-related small non-cleaved cell lymphoma. *Br J Haematol* 1997; 98:726–732.
234. Kersten MJ, Van Gorp J, Pals ST, et al. Expression of Epstein-Barr virus latent genes and adhesion molecules in AIDS-related non-Hodgkin's lymphomas: correlation with histology and CD4-cell number. *Leuk Lymphoma* 1998;30:515–524.
235. Magrath IT. Therapy of the small non-cleaved cell lymphomas. In: Magrath IT, ed. *The non-Hodgkin's lymphomas*, 2nd ed. London, Edward Arnold, 1997:779–881.
236. Magrath IT, Ziegler J. Bone marrow involvement in Burkitt's lymphoma and its relationship to acute B cell leukemia. *Leuk Res* 1980; 4:33–59.
237. Magrath IT. Non-Hodgkin's lymphomas in children. In: Peckham M, Pineda H, Veronesi U (eds). Oxford textbook of oncology, 2nd ed. New York: Oxford University press (*in press*).
238. Ertem U, Duru F, Pamir A, et al. Burkitt's lymphoma in 63 Turkish children diagnosed over a 10 year period. *Pediatr Hematol Oncol* 1996;13:123–134.
239. Cohen LF, Balow JE, Magrath IT. Acute tumor lysis syndrome: a review of 37 patients with Burkitt's lymphoma. *Am J Med* 1980;68: 486–491.
240. Adatia AK. Significance of jaw lesions in Burkitt's lymphoma. *Br Dent J* 1978;145:263–266.
241. Plantaz D, Bachelot C, Dyon JF, et al. Massive breast involvement in Burkitt's lymphoma. *Arch Pediatr* 1987;44:199–200.
242. Armitage JO, Feagler JR, Skoog DP. Burkitt lymphoma during pregnancy with bilateral breast involvement. *JAMA* 1977;237:151.
243. Durodola JI. Burkitt's lymphoma presenting during lactation. *Int J Gynaecol Obstet* 1976;14:225–231.
244. Wagner D, Kiwanuka J, Edwards B, et al. Soluble interleukin II receptor levels in patients with undifferentiated and lymphoblastic lymphomas. *J Clin Oncol* 1987;5:1262–1274.
245. Moses HL, Yang EY, Pietenpol JA. TGF-beta stimulation and inhibition of cell proliferation: new mechanistic insights. *Cell* 1990;63: 245–247.
246. Chen H, Lee JM, Wang Y, et al. The Epstein-Barr virus latency BamHI-Q promoter is positively regulated by STATs and Zta interference with JAK/STAT activation leads to loss of BamHI-Q promoter activity. *Proc Natl Acad Sci USA* 1999;96:9339–9344.
247. Epstein-barr virus (EBV) nuclear protein 2-induced disruption of EBV latency in the Burkitt's lymphoma cell line Akata: analysis by tetracycline-regulated expression. *J Virol* 1999;73:5214–5219.
248. Henle W, Henle G, Gunvén P, et al. Patterns of antibodies to Epstein-Barr virus-induced early antigens in Burkitt's lymphoma: comparison of dying patients with long-term survivors. *J Natl Cancer Inst* 1973; 50:1163–1173.
249. Nkrumah F, Henle W, Henle G, et al. Burkitt's lymphoma: its clincal course in relation to immunologic reactivities to Epstein-Barr virus and tumor related antigens. *J Natl Cancer Inst* 1976;57:1051–1056.
250. Magrath IT, Lee YJ, Anderson T, et al. Prognostic factors in Burkitt's lymphoma: importance of total tumor burden. *Cancer* 1980;45: 1507–1515.
251. Haddy TB, Adde MA, Magrath IT. Central nervous system involvement in small non-cleaved cell lymphoma: is CNS disease per se a poor prognostic sign? *J Clin Oncol* 1991;9:1973–1982.
252. Magrath IT, Lwanga S, Carswell W, et al. Surgical reduction of tumour bulk in management of abdominal Burkitt's lymphoma. *Br Med J* 1974;2:308–312.
253. LaQuaglia MP, Stolar CHJ, Krailo M, et al. The role of surery in

abdominal non-Hodgkin's lymphoma: experience from the Children's Cancer Study Group. *J Pediatr Surg* 1992;27:230–235.
254. Reiter A, Zimmermann W, Zimmermann M, et al. The role of initial laparotomy and second-look surgery in the treatment of abdominal B-cell non-Hodgkin's lymphoma of childhood: a report of the BFM Group. *Eur J Pediatr Surg* 1994;4:74–81.
255. Link MP, Shuster JJ, Donaldson SS, et al. Treatment of children and young adults with early-stage non-Hodgkin's lymphoma. *N Engl J Med* 1997;337:1259–1266.
256. Reiter A, Schrappe M, Parwaresch R, et al. Non-Hodgkin's lymphomas of childhood and adolescence: results of a treatment stratified for biologic subtypes and stage. A report of the Berlin-Frankfurt-Munster Group. *J Clin Oncol* 1995;13:359–372.
257. Magrath I, Adde M, Shad A, et al. Adults and children with small non-cleaved cell lymphoma have a similar excellent outcome when treated with the same chemotherapy regimen. *J Clin Oncol* 1996;13: 925–935.
258. Patte C. Non-Hodgkin's lymphoma. *Eur J Cancer* 1998;34:359–363.
259. Adde M, Shad A, Venzon D, et al. Additional chemotherapy agents improve treatment outcome for children and adults with advanced B-cell lymphomas. *Semin Oncol* 1998;2[Suppl 4]:33–39.
260. Arseneau JC, Bagley CM, Anderson T, et al. Hyperkalemia, a sequel to chemotherapy of Burkitt's lymphoma. *Lancet* 1973;i:10–14.
261. Soussain C, Patte C, Ostronoff M, et al. Small noncleaved cell lymphoma and leukemia in adults: a retrospective study of 65 adults treated with the LMB pediatric protocols. *Blood* 1995;85:664–674.
262. Masucci MG, Contreras-Salazar B, Ragnar E, et al. 5-Azacytidine up regulates the expression of Epstein-Barr virus nuclear antigen 2 (EBNA-2) through EBNA-6 and latent membrane protein in the Burkitt's lymphoma line rael. *J Virol* 1989;63:3135–3141.
263. Robertson KD, Barletta J, Samid D, et al. Pharmacologic activation of expression of immunodominant viral antigens: a new strategy for the treatment of Epstein-Barr-virus-associated malignancies. *Curr Top Microbiol Immunol* 1995;194:145–154.
264. Judde JG, Spangler G, Magrath I, et al. The use of EBV virus associated genes as determinants in targeting molecular therapy of EBV associated neoplasia. *Hum Gene Ther* 1996;7:646–653.
265. Gutierrez MI, Judde JG, Magrath IT, et al. Switching viral latency to viral lysis: a novel therapeutic approach for Epstein-Barr virus-associated neoplasia. *Cancer Res* 1996;56:969–972.
266. Aya T, Kinoshita T, Imai S, et al. Chromosome translocation and c-MYC activation by Epstein-Barr virus and Euphorbia tirucalli in B lymphocytes. *Lancet* 1991;337:1190.
267. O'Donnell RA, Saul A, Cowman AF, et al. Functional conservation of the malaria vaccine antigen MSP-119 across distantly related Plasmodium species. *Nat Med* 2000;6:91–95.
268. Gardner MJ. The genome of the malaria parasite. *Curr Opin Genet Dev* 1999;9:704–708.

CHAPTER 28

Lymphadenopathy and the Lymphoid Neoplasms Associated with the Acquired Immune Deficiency Syndrome

Daniel M. Knowles and Amy Chadburn

The medical community was alerted to the existence of the acquired immunodeficiency syndrome (AIDS) by the Centers for Disease Control (CDC) in the summer of 1981 (1,2). This was based on reports from New York and California of previously healthy young homosexual men who developed severe, life-threatening opportunistic infections such as *Pneumocystis carinii* pneumonia and clinically aggressive, extracutaneous Kaposi's sarcoma similar to the lymphadenopathic form of the disease observed in Africa (3,4). By the end of 1996, 581,429 persons (84% men, 15% women, and 1% children younger than 13 years old) diagnosed with AIDS in the United States had been reported to the CDC (5,6). Over 60% of these individuals already have died, after a median time period of approximately 14 months (5–7). Since 1994, AIDS has emerged as the leading cause of death among persons aged 25 to 44 years in the United States; it accounts for 19% of deaths from all causes in this age group (6). The number of persons who are living with AIDS continues to increase (5). It has been estimated that approximately 223,000 adults and adolescents in the United States were living with AIDS by mid-1996 (5).

ETIOLOGY AND EPIDEMIOLOGY

Human immunodeficiency virus (HIV) type 1 has been identified as the primary agent responsible for AIDS (8,9), although HIV-2 has been shown to be associated with the development of AIDS in a small number of patients (10). Infection by these retroviruses most frequently is spread by sexual contact, by inoculation or infusion of infected blood and blood products, or perinatally from mother to child (11,12). The epidemiologic patterns of the AIDS epidemic are diverse and vary according to geographic location. In the United States, the major groups at risk for AIDS are men who have sex with men (MSM) and injecting drug users (IDUs) (6). These groups account for 44% and 26%, respectively, and heterosexual transmission for 12% of the prevalent AIDS cases reported to the CDC through 1996 (6). Heterosexual transmission has been responsible for the largest proportionate increase (19%) in AIDS prevalence recently, however, primarily reflecting transmission from the large population of HIV-infected IDUs, predominantly men, to their heterosexual partners, primarily women (6). In the United States, regardless of the mode of transmission, blacks and Hispanics have been disproportionately affected by the epidemic (6). The prevalence of HIV infection in western Europe similarly is highest in MSM and IDUs. The relative proportion of HIV-positive individuals accounted for by homosexual or bisexual transmission decreased from 50% to 25%, however, and the proportion accounted for by injecting drug use increased from 31% to 42% in western Europe over the 10-year period between 1984 and 1993 (13). More than 90% of these IDU cases were concentrated in southwestern Europe, especially in Spain, and to a somewhat lesser extent in Italy, Portugal, and France (14). The proportion of cases of HIV infection accounted for by heterosexual transmission increased from 7% to 18% in western Europe over the same time period (13), once again a reflection of the spread of HIV infection from male IDUs to their female non-IDU partners (14). Percentage increases in AIDS incidence in this community have been projected to be 26% for injecting drug use and 50% for heterosexual transmission (13). As of the end of 1996, more than 7,600 children in the United States

D. M. Knowles and A. Chadburn: Department Of Pathology, Weill Medical College of Cornell University, New York, New York 10021.

with AIDS had been reported to the CDC (5). Approximately 90% of these children acquired HIV infection by perinatal exposure (vertical transmission) from their HIV-infected mothers, who largely had acquired infection by injecting drug use or by heterosexual transmission from a male IDU partner (5,14,15).

The epidemiology of the AIDS epidemic is strikingly different in developing countries. In Africa, the principal population at risk for AIDS is sexually active heterosexuals (16). It has been estimated that more than 7.5 million people in sub-Saharan Africa, about one half of whom are women of childbearing age, were HIV-infected by the end of 1993 (16). More than 700,000 African children were HIV-infected by 1993 as well, primarily as a result of mother-to-child transmission (16). In Africa, the probability of infants acquiring HIV infection from their mother is about 30% (16); approximately 80% of these infants progress to AIDS within 5 years after infection. The AIDS epidemic has spread by variable combinations of heterosexual, homosexual, bisexual, and injecting drug use behaviors in Latin America and the Caribbean, which has progressively shifted the epidemic to the female population (16). South and Southeast Asia have experienced an explosion in HIV infection related to injecting drug use and heterosexual transmission by female prostitutes to their partners (16).

By the end of 1996, nearly 84,000 HIV-positive individuals without AIDS had been reported to the CDC (5). It is estimated that more than 1.2 million people in the United States and approximately 24 million people worldwide are HIV-infected. The World Health Organization projected a cumulative total of 30 to 40 million HIV-positive individuals by the year 2000, 90% of whom reside in developing countries and nearly half of whom are women (17). This is exerting great social and economic strains on many countries, particularly those in the developing world, where AIDS will serve as a formidable obstacle to further development.

PATHOGENESIS

The pathogenesis of HIV infection has not been delineated fully, although extensive investigative studies performed during the past 15 years have increased our knowledge of the pathophysiology of HIV infection greatly (18). HIV consists of several strains and subtypes, making it extremely heterogeneous, and possesses the ability to infect a wide variety of cells—thus it is also polytropic (18). It is HIV infection of certain cells of the immune system and the central nervous system (CNS), however, resulting in immunosuppression and neuropsychologic deficits, respectively, that has the most devastating consequences for the host. The main receptor for HIV on human cells is the CD4 molecule (19,20), which is expressed primarily by helper or inducer T lymphocytes and monocytes or macrophages (see Chapter 3), to which HIV binds through envelope gp120 (21). Although the precise mechanism of viral entry is not known, it now is believed that the CD4-gp120 interaction is neither sufficient for nor the sole method of viral binding, because HIV-infected CD4-negative ($CD4^-$) T lymphocytes have been identified (18). In addition, at least two chemokine receptors, CXCR-4 and CCR-5, are thought to function as coreceptors for HIV entry into the cell. These chemokine receptors appear to be used by different HIV strains, however. The CXCR-4 chemokine has been shown to act as a coreceptor for strains that have a syncytial-inducing phenotype and are T-lymphocyte tropic; the CCR-5 chemokine is associated with those strains that have a non–syncytial-inducing phenotype and preferentially infect monocytes or macrophages (18).

CD4-positive ($CD4^+$) helper or inducer T lymphocytes are involved either directly or indirectly in most of the body's immunologic functions (see Chapter 2). The HIV-related destruction of this cell population and the consequent loss of these functions results in progressive impairment of the immune response and ultimately in the marked immunodeficiency characteristic of AIDS (18,22,23). A variety of mechanisms is thought to be involved in the destruction of CD4 T lymphocytes. These include direct cytopathic effects (syncytium formation with both HIV-infected and HIV-uninfected cells, cytoplasmic accumulation of viral cDNA, alteration of cell membrane permeability), induction of apoptosis (including increasing the sensitivity of the cells to FAS), and induction of anti-CD4 (both normal and HIV-infected) cytotoxic activity mediated primarily by $CD8^+$ T lymphocytes (18). The progressive depletion of the CD4 T lymphocyte population is reflected in the histologic appearance and immunophenotype of the cells that populate the lymph nodes of HIV-positive individuals at the different clinical stages of their disease.

Numerous studies have demonstrated a strong association between the absolute number or percentage of peripheral blood CD4 T cells and the development of life-threatening opportunistic illnesses (24–32). Most AIDS-defining conditions, especially opportunistic infections, occur if the number of CD4 T cells in HIV-infected patients falls below 200 per microliter (32–36). For this reason, measurements of CD4 T cells are used to guide the clinical and therapeutic management of HIV-infected persons in the United States (31). The use of zidovudine monotherapy and prophylaxis specific to some AIDS-defining opportunistic infections has reduced the number of certain infections, such as *P. carinii* pneumonia and those resulting from toxoplasmosis and herpes simplex virus, in these individuals (37–41). Recently, new therapeutic strategies involving combinations of antiretroviral compounds, including nucleoside reverse transcriptase inhibitors and protease inhibitors (42–44), have made it possible to suppress viral replication markedly in HIV-infected individuals (45). Increases in CD4 T-cell counts, which are transient during zidovudine monotherapy, now persist for extended periods (46). The incidence of nearly all AIDS-defining events occurring in HIV-infected persons treated with these potent antiretroviral combination regimens has declined (46,47). These novel therapeutic approaches have altered the profile and time course of AIDS-defining conditions significantly, prolonged the time interval between HIV infection and the development of AIDS, and improved survival rates (6,7,44,46,48).

The steady improvement in survival rates among persons with AIDS is thought to reflect these improvements in management and therapy as well as improved access to healthcare (7). Because of better recognition and greater knowledge of HIV disease and more accurate statistical models, it now is believed that the HIV-AIDS incubation period is 12.8 years (49), with only a 60% probability of progressing to AIDS and 48% probability of death within 10 years of seroconversion (48). The increase in the number of HIV-infected individuals and their longer duration of survival suggests that HIV-related pathology is likely to continue to increase in amount and perhaps also in scope.

DEFINITION AND CLASSIFICATION OF HIV-RELATED DISEASE

Adults and Adolescents 13 Years of Age or Older

Various systems designed to classify the clinical stages of HIV infection have been proposed and periodically revised throughout the AIDS epidemic, in response to our increasing understanding of the pathophysiology of HIV infection, enhanced knowledge of the natural history of HIV disease, recognition of new HIV-related illnesses, improved laboratory and other diagnostic methods, and improved clinical management (50–57). The AIDS surveillance case definition originally published by the CDC in 1982 (58) has been revised several times. In 1982, the CDC surveillance definition of AIDS was ''a disease, at least moderately predictive of a defect in cell-mediated immunity, occurring in a person with no known cause for diminished resistance to that disease'' (58). Diseases that qualified a person for the diagnosis of AIDS included Kaposi's sarcoma; *P. carinii* pneumonia; pneumonia, meningitis, or encephalitis caused by various organisms, such as those of *Cryptococcus*, *Toxoplasma*, *Aspergillus*, *Candida*, and *Strongyloides* species, atypical mycobacteria, and cytomegalovirus; esophagitis caused by candidal organisms, cytomegalovirus, or herpes simplex; progressive multifocal leukoencephalopathy; chronic enterocolitis caused by organisms of *Cryptospiridium* species; and unusual and extensive mucocutaneous herpes simplex virus (HSV) (58,59). The CDC expanded the AIDS surveillance case definition in 1985 (60) and again in 1987 (61), to include, for example, primary CNS lymphoma and high- and intermediate-grade B-cell and phenotypically indeterminate lymphomas as qualifying diseases (60,61). The definition also was expanded to include laboratory test results for HIV infection (60,61). Finally, the 1993 Revised Classification System for HIV Infection and Expanded Surveillance Case Definition for AIDS among Adolescents and Adults (62) was proposed by the CDC to replace the 1987 case definition (61), which had been developed prior to the widespread use of CD4 T-lymphocyte testing.

The 1993 AIDS Expanded Surveillance Case Definition was instituted to simplify the classification of HIV infection, to categorize HIV-related morbidity more reliably, to emphasize the clinical importance of the CD4 T-lymphocyte count, and to reflect the current standard of care of HIV-positive individuals (62). It has been employed in the United States since January 1, 1993. The system categorizes persons on the basis of three ranges of CD4 T-lymphocyte counts and three clinical categories and is represented by a matrix of nine mutually exclusive categories (62) (Table 28.1). In contrast to previous CDC classifications, all HIV-infected persons who have CD4 T-cell counts of less than 200 per microliter or CD4 T-cell percentages (of total lymphocytes) less than 14% are included in the 1993 AIDS Expanded Surveillance Case Definition in recognition of the high correlation between the number of CD4 T cells and the development and severity of HIV-related illnesses (62). The intent was to enable the AIDS surveillance data to represent more accurately those individuals who are recognized as being immunosuppressed, have the greatest need for close medical follow-up, and are at the greatest risk for developing the full spectrum of HIV-related morbidity (62). In addition, the 1993 system adds three clinical conditions (pulmonary tuberculosis, recurrent pneumonia, and invasive cervical

TABLE 28.1. *1993 Revised classification system for HIV infection and expanded AIDS surveillance case definition for adolescents and adults (62)*

CD4-positive T-cell categories	A. Asymptomatic, acute (primary) HIV or PGL[a]	B. Symptomatic, not A or C conditions[b]	C. AIDS indicator conditions[c]
1. $\geq$500/μl	A1	B1	C1
2. 200–499/μl	A2	B2	C2
3. <200/μl AIDS indicator T-cell count	A3	B3	C3

Note. Categories A3, B3, and C represent the expanded AIDS surveillance case definition. Persons with category C AIDS indicator conditions as well as those with $CD4^+$ T-lymphocyte counts <200/μl (categories A3 or B3) are reportable as AIDS cases in the United States and territories, effective January 1, 1993.

[a] Clinical Category A includes acute (primary) HIV infection (63, 64).

[b] See text for discussion.

[c] See Table 28.3.

PGL, persistent generalized lymphadenopathy.

cancer) to the previous list of 23 AIDS-defining illnesses to reflect their importance in the AIDS epidemic (62).

The three CD4 T-lymphocyte categories are defined as follows:

Category 1: at least 500 cells/μl
Category 2: 200 to 499 cells/μl
Category 3: less than 200 cells/μl

The lowest accurate, and not necessarily the most recent, CD4 T-lymphocyte count is used for classification purposes. The percentage of CD4 T cells may be substituted for the absolute CD4 T-cell count. The corresponding percentages of CD4 T cells for the categories are at least 29%, 14% to 28%, and less than 14%, respectively (62).

The clinical categories of HIV infection are defined as follows: *Category A* consists of one or more of the conditions listed here in an adult or adolescent at least 13 years of age with documented HIV infection. Conditions listed in categories B and C must not be present.

Asymptomatic HIV infection
Persistent generalized lymphadenopathy
Acute (primary) HIV infection with accompanying illness or history of acute HIV infection (63,64)

Category B consists of symptomatic conditions in an HIV-infected adult or adolescent at least 13 years of age that are not included among the conditions listed in clinical category C and that are attributed to HIV infection, are indicative of a defect in cell-mediated immunity, or are considered by physicians to have a clinical course or require management that is complicated by HIV infection. Category B conditions (Table 28.2) take precedence over category A conditions for classification purposes. For example, someone previously treated for oropharyngeal candidiasis who is now asymptomatic and who has not developed a category C disease is classified in clinical category B.

TABLE 28.2. *Conditions included in category B of the Centers for Disease Control 1993 revised classification system for HIV infection and expanded surveillance case definition for AIDS among adolescents and adults (62)*

Bacillary angiomatosis
Candidiasis, oropharyngeal (thrush)
Candidiasis vulvovaginal; persistent, frequent, or poorly responsive to therapy
Cervical dysplasia (moderate to severe) or cervical carcinoma *in situ*
Constitutional symptoms such as fever (≥38.5°C) or diarrhea lasting >1 month
Hairy leukoplakia, oral
Herpes zoster (shingles), involving at least two distinct episodes or more than one dermatome
Idiopathic thrombocytopenia purpura
Listeriosis
Pelvic inflammatory disease, particularly if complicated by tuboovarian abscess
Peripheral neuropathy

TABLE 28.3. *Conditions included in category C of the Centers for Disease Control 1993 revised classification system for HIV infection and expanded surveillance case definition for AIDS among adolescents and adults (62)*

Candidiasis of bronchi, trachea, or lungs
Candidiasis, esophageal
Cervical cancer, invasive
Coccidioidomycosis, disseminated or extrapulmonary
Cryptococcosis, extrapulmonary
Crytosporidiosis, chronic intestinal (>1 month's duration)
Cytomegalovirus disease (other than liver, spleen, or nodes)
Cytomegalovirus retinitis (with loss of vision)
Encephalopathy, HIV-related
Herpes simplex: chronic ulcers (>1 month's duration); or bronchitis, pneumonitis, or esophagitis
Histoplasmosis, disseminated or extrapulmonary
Isosporiasis, chronic intestinal (>1 month's duration)
Kaposi's sarcoma
Lymphoma, Burkitt's (or equivalent term)
Lymphoma, immunoblastic (or equivalent term)
Lymphoma, primary, of brain
Mycobacterium avium complex or *M. kansasii,* disseminated or extrapulmonary
M. tuberculosis, any site (pulmonary[a] or extrapulmonary)
Mycobacterium spp, other species, or unidentified species, disseminated or extrapulmonary
Pneumocystis carinii pneumonia
Pneumonia, recurrent[a]
Progressive multifocal leukoencephalopathy
Salmonella septicemia, recurrent
Toxoplasmosis of brain
Wasting syndrome caused by HIV

[a] Added in the 1993 expansion of the AIDS surveillance case definition.

Category C includes the clinical conditions listed in the AIDS surveillance case definition (Table 28.3). For classification purposes an individual remains in category C once a category C condition has occurred (62).

Based on these criteria, individuals are classified into one of nine mutually exclusive categories (Table 28.1) based on clinical characteristics (categories A–C) and CD4 T-lymphocyte count (categories 1–3). HIV-positive individuals classified in the subcategories A3, B3, and C3 meet the immunologic criteria of the AIDS Expanded Surveillance Case Definition; those in categories C1, C2, and C3 meet the clinical criteria for surveillance purposes (62).

The adoption of the AIDS Expanded Surveillance Case Definition in 1993 had a substantial impact on the number of reported cases of AIDS. The number of AIDS cases reported to the CDC in 1993 was double the number reported in 1992 (6), largely because of the addition of immunosuppression to the definition (62). This increase was followed by a yearly decline in the number of AIDS cases reported to the CDC in 1994 through 1996 (6), but the 68,473 AIDS cases reported in 1996 remained almost 50% higher than the number reported in 1992 (6).

The CDC 1993 AIDS Expanded Surveillance Case Definition met with opposition in Europe, where some but not all of the revisions were adopted, with variation across the

TABLE 28.4. *Pediatric HIV classification (70)*

	Clinical categories			
Immunologic categories	N. No signs/ symptoms	A. Mild signs/ symptoms	B. Moderate signs/ symptoms[a]	C. Severe signs/symptoms
1. No evidence of suppression	N1	A1	B1	C1
2. Evidence of moderate suppression	N2	A2	B2	C2
3. Severe suppression	N3	A3	B3	C3

Note. Children whose HIV infection status is not confirmed are classified by using the above grid with a letter E (for perinatally exposed) placed before the appropriate classification code (e.g., EN2).

[a] Both Category C and lymphoid interstitial pneumonitis in Category B are reportable to state and local health departments as acquired immunodeficiency syndrome.

continent. The European Centre for the Epidemiological Monitoring of AIDS agreed that monitoring CD4 T-cell counts is essential for staging HIV infection and clinical care (65). Nonetheless, they elected to add the three indicator diseases (pulmonary tuberculosis, recurrent pneumonia, and invasive cervical cancer) but not individuals who have CD4 T-cell counts below 200 per microliter (65,66). The reasons cited for the decision included the lack of availability and standardization of CD4 T-cell quantitation in Europe, the possible lack of completeness of AIDS surveillance based on HIV testing and CD4 T-cell enumeration among AIDS risk groups, and the consequent misinterpretations of trends because of selection biases, as well as the detrimental psychological and social consequences for asymptomatic individuals labeled as having AIDS only on the basis of CD4 T-cell counts (65,66). The revised AIDS surveillance case definition for Europe resulted in only a 6.8% overall increase in reported AIDS cases during its first year of use (67).

Children

It has been evident for many years that the clinical characteristics of AIDS in children differ from those in adults (68). In 1987, the CDC published a system for classifying the clinical manifestations of HIV infection in children based on the limited information available early in the AIDS epidemic (69). The knowledge gained in the ensuing years concerning the progression of HIV disease in children prompted the CDC to propose the 1994 Revised Classification System for HIV Infection in Children less than 13 years of Age (70). In this system, children are classified into mutually exclusive categories according to three parameters: infection status, clinical status, and immunologic status (70) (Table 28.4). Once classified, an HIV-infected child cannot be reclassified in a less severe category even if the child's clinical or immunologic status improves (70). This revised classification reflects the stage of the child's disease and provides greater medical accuracy (70).

Virtually all children born to HIV-infected women are HIV antibody–positive at birth, because maternal anti-HIV IgG antibodies cross the placenta. Only 15% to 30% of these children, however, actually acquire HIV infection (70). The HIV-uninfected children can remain HIV antibody–positive up to 18 months of age (71). Standard anti-HIV IgG antibody tests cannot be relied on to determine a child's HIV status until after this age. Consequently, it is difficult to diagnose HIV infection in children born to HIV-infected women (70,71). Strict criteria have been established for the diagnosis of pediatric HIV infection (Table 28.5). Polymerase chain reaction (PCR) and viral culture are probably the most sensitive and specific assays for detecting HIV infection in children born to HIV-infected mothers (72–74). These assays identify approximately 30% to 50% of infected infants at birth and almost 100% of infected infants by 3 to 6 months

TABLE 28.5. *Diagnosis of HIV infection in children (70)*

HIV infected
- A child <18 months of age who is known to be HIV seropositive or born to an HIV-infected mother and:
  - Has positive results on two separate determinations (excluding cord blood) from one or more of the following HIV detection tests:
    - HIV culture
    - HIV polymerase chain reaction
    - HIV antigen (p24) or
  - Meets criteria for AIDS diagnosis based on the 1987 AIDS surveillance case definition (61)
- A child ≥18 months of age born to an HIV-infected mother or any child infected by blood, blood products, or other known modes of transmission (e.g., sexual contact) who;
  - Is HIV-antibody positive by repeatedly reactive EIA and confirmatory test (e.g., Western blot or IFA) or
  - Meets any of the criteria for children <18 months

Perinatally exposed (prefix E)
- A child who does not meet the criteria above who:
  - Is HIV seropositive by EIA and confirmatory test (e.g., Western blot or IFA) and is <18 months of age at the time of test or
  - Has unknown antibody status, but was born to a mother known to be infected with HIV

Seroreverter (SR)
- A child who is born to an HIV-infected mother and who:
  - Has been documented as HIV-antibody negative (i.e., two or more negative EIA tests performed at 6–18 months of age or one negative EIA test after 18 months of age) and
  - Has had no other laboratory evidence of infection (has not had two positive viral detection tests, if performed) and
  - Has not had an AIDS-defining condition

TABLE 28.6. *Immunologic categories based on age-specific CD4-positive T-lymphocyte counts and percentage of total lymphocytes (70)*

Immunologic categories	Age of child		
	<12 months, μl (%)	1–5 years, μl (%)	6–12 years, μl (%)
No evidence of suppression	≥1,500(≥25)	≥1,000(≥25)	≥500(≥25)
Evidence of moderate suppression	750–1,499(15–24)	500–999(15–24)	200–499(15–24)
Severe suppression	<750(<15)	<500(<15)	<200(<15)

of age (75). The standard p24 antigen assay is less sensitive than PCR or viral culture (76), and other laboratory tests are used infrequently (70). Some children develop severe HIV-related illnesses before their HIV infection status has been established sufficiently. A child meeting the 1987 case definition criteria for AIDS (61) is considered HIV-infected even in the absence of definitive laboratory tests. Children born to HIV-infected mothers are designated *seroreverters* and considered uninfected if they become HIV antibody–negative after 6 months of age, lack other laboratory evidence of HIV infection, and do not meet the AIDS surveillance case definition criteria (70).

The three immunologic categories (Table 28.6) were established to classify children according to the severity of immunosuppression attributable to HIV infection. The guidelines established for employing CD4 T cell counts to assess HIV-induced immunosuppression in adults and adolescents, however, are complicated by certain special circumstances if applied to children (70). For example, normal CD4 T-cell counts are higher in infants and young children than in adults and decline during the first 5 years of life (77–81). Also, children appear to develop opportunistic infections at higher CD4 T-cell counts than do adults (82–84). Low age-specific CD4 T-cell counts, however, appear to correlate with conditions associated with immunosuppression in children (77,82,85,86), and classification based on age-specific CD4 T-cell counts appears to be useful in describing the immune status of HIV-infected children (70). The immunologic category classification is based on either the absolute CD4 T-cell count or the percentage of CD4 T cells. If the CD4 T-cell count and the percentage of CD4 T cells indicate different categories, the child is classified in the more severe category (70). A child is not reclassified in a less severe category regardless of subsequent CD4 T-cell counts (70).

Children who are HIV-infected or exposed to HIV perinatally may be classified into one of four mutually exclusive clinical categories based on signs, symptoms, or diagnoses related to HIV infection (Table 28.7). Like the immunologic categories, the clinical categories were defined to provide a staging system (70). The prefix *E* is attached for children who are at risk for HIV but whose HIV infection status has not been firmly established (Table 28.5). Category N, "not symptomatic," includes children with no signs or symptoms considered to be the result of HIV infection or with only one of the conditions listed in category A. Category B,

TABLE 28.7. *Clinical categories for children with HIV infection (70)*

Category N: Not symptomatic
- Children who have no signs or symptoms considered to be the result of HIV infection or who have only one of the conditions listed in category A

Category A: Mildly symptomatic
- Children with two or more of the conditions listed below but none of the conditions listed in Categories B and C
  - Lymphadenopathy (≥0.5 cm at more than two sites; bilateral = one site)
  - Hepatomegaly
  - Splenomegaly
  - Dermatitis
  - Parotitis
  - Recurrent or persistent upper respiratory infection, sinusitis, or otitis media

Category B: Moderately symptomatic
- Children who have symptomatic conditions other than those listed for category A or C that are attributed to HIV infection. Examples of conditions in clinical category B include but are not limited to:
  - Anemia (<8 g/dL), neutropenia (<1,000/mm^3), or thrombocytopenia (<100,000/mm^3) persisting ≥30 days
  - Bacterial meningitis, pneumonia, or sepsis (single episode)
  - Candidiasis, oropharyngeal (thrush), persisting (>2 months) in children >6 months of age
  - Cardiomyopathy
  - Cytomegalovirus infection, with onset before 1 month of age
  - Diarrhea, recurrent or chronic
  - Hepatitis
  - HSV stomatitis, recurrent (more than two episodes within 1 year)
  - HSV bronchitis, pneumonitis, or esophagitis with onset before 1 month of age
  - Herpes zoster (shingles) involving at least two distinct episodes or more than one dermatome
  - Leiomyosarcoma
  - LIP or pulmonary lymphoid hyperplasia complex
  - Nephropathy
  - Nocardiosis
  - Persistent fever (lasting >1 month)
  - Toxoplasmosis, onset before 1 month of age
  - Varicella, disseminated (complicated chickenpox)

Category C: Severely symptomatic
- Children who have any condition listed in the 1987 surveillance case definition for acquired immunodeficiency syndrome (61), with the exception of LIP (Table 28.8).

HSV, herpes simplex virus; LI, lymphoid interstitial pneumonia.

TABLE 28.8. *Conditions included in clinical category C (severely symptomatic) for children infected with HIV (70)*

Serious bacterial infections, multiple or recurrent (i.e., any combination of at least two culture-confirmed infections within a 2-year period), of the following types: septicemia, pneumonia, meningitis, bone or joint infection, or abscess of an internal organ or body cavity (excluding otitis media, superficial skin or mucosal abscesses, and indwelling catheter-related infections)
Candidiasis, esophageal or pulmonary (bronchi, trachea, lungs)
Coccidioidomycosis, disseminated (at site other than or in addition to lungs or cervical or hilar lymph nodes)
Cryptococcosis, extrapulmonary
Cryptosporidiosis or isosporiasis with diarrhea persisting >1 month
Cytomegalovirus disease with onset of symptoms at age >1 month (at a site other than liver, spleen, or lymph nodes)
Encephalopathy (at least one of the following progressive findings present for at least 2 months in the absence of a concurrent illness other than HIV infection that could explain the findings): a failure to attain or loss of developmental milestones or loss of intellectual ability, verified by standard developmental scale or neuropsychological tests; impaired brain growth or acquired microcephaly demonstrated by head circumference measurements or brain atrophy demonstrated by computerized tomography or magnetic resonance imaging (serial imaging is required for children <2 years of age); acquired symmetric motor deficit manifested by two or more of paresis, pathologic reflexes, ataxia, and gait disturbance
Herpes simplex virus infection causing a mucocutaneous ulcer that persists for >1 month, or bronchitis, pneumonitis, or esophagitis for any duration affecting a child >1 month of age
Histoplasmosis, disseminated (at a site other than or in addition to lungs or cervical or hilar lymph nodes)
Kaposi's sarcoma
Lymphoma, primary, in brain
Lymphoma, small, noncleaved cell (Burkitt's), or immunoblastic or large cell lymphoma of B-cell or unknown immunologic phenotype
Mycobacterium tuberculosis, disseminated or extrapulmonary
Mycobacterium spp, other species, or unidentified species, disseminated (at a site other than or in addition to lungs, skin, or cervical or hilar lymph nodes)
Mycobacterium avium complex or *M. kansasii,* disseminated (at site other than or in addition to lungs, skin or cervical or hilar lymph nodes)
Pneumocystis carinii pneumonia
Progressive multifocal leukoencephalopathy
Salmonella (nontyphoid) septicemia, recurrent
Tomoplasmosis of the brain with onset at >1 month of age
Wasting syndrome in the absence of a concurrent illness other than HIV infection that could explain the following findings: persistent weight loss >10% of baseline; downward crossing of at least two of the following percentile lines on the weight-for-age chart (e.g., 95th, 75th, 50th, 25th, 5th) in child ≥1 year of age; or <5th percentile on weight-for-height chart on two consecutive measurements, ≥30 days apart; *plus* chronic diarrhea (i.e., at least two loose stools per day for ≥30 days) or documented fever (for ≥30 days, intermittent or constant)

Note. See the 1987 AIDS surveillance case definition (61) for diagnosis criteria.

"moderately symptomatic," includes all children with signs and symptoms thought to be caused by HIV infection but not specifically listed in categories A or C. The conditions listed in Table 28.7 are only examples; any HIV-related condition not included in categories A or C should be included in category B. Category C includes all children who have AIDS-defining conditions except lymphoid interstitital pneumonitis (70) (Table 28.8). Lymphoid interstitial pneumonitis has been separated from the other AIDS-defining conditions in category C and placed in category B, because several reports suggest that the prognosis for children who have lymphoid interstitial pneumonitis is significantly better than that for children who have other AIDS-defining conditions (85,87,88). According to the 1994 Revised Classification System for HIV Infection in Children less than 13 Years of Age, all children classified in clinical category C, that is, as C1, C2, or C3, or in clinical category B because of lymphoid interstitial pneumonitis are reportable as having AIDS (70).

HIV-RELATED BENIGN LYMPHADENOPATHY

General Comments

In 1982, unexplained, persistent diffuse lymphadenopathy not attributable to previously known causes was reported in homosexual men in major metropolitan areas of the United States, especially New York and San Francisco, in which cases of Kaposi's sarcoma and opportunistic infections previously had been described (89). This was designated *persistent generalized lymphadenopathy syndrome* and was defined as lymphadenopathy of at least 3 months' duration involving two or more noncontiguous, extrainguinal sites in the absence of any illness or drug use known to cause lymphadenopathy and displaying hyperplastic histopathology on lymph node biopsy (89). Most patients were aware of the lymphadenopathy for 10 to 18 months before presentation (89–93). In some individuals, persistent generalized lymphadenopathy was accompanied by fever, night sweats, malaise, weight loss, diarrhea, cutaneous anergy, hypergammaglobulinemia, diminished CD4 T-cell counts, and other phenomena associated with HIV infection; this was referred to as the *AIDS-related complex* (59,94). Although any lymph node or lymph node group might be enlarged, the lymphadenopathy often involved unusual sites, such as epitrochlear and submandibular lymph nodes (95). The enlarged lymph nodes usually were tender, and they sometimes fluctuated in size with illness or stress (95).

Biopsy examination of such lymph nodes frequently was performed in the early years of the AIDS epidemic to exclude AIDS-defining conditions such as Kaposi's sarcoma, opportunistic infections, or non-Hodgkin's lymphoma (NHL), as the cause of the enlargement. Consequently, many benign, reactive lymph nodes obtained from HIV-seropositive individuals who had varying levels of immunosuppression were examined. The various histopathologic patterns

TABLE 28.9. *Histopathologic classifications of HIV-related benign lymphadenopathy*

Current	Biberfield et al. (104)	Chadburn et al. (107)	Ewing et al. (102)	Iaochim et al. (108)	Pallesen et al. (105)	Pileri et al. (106)
Florid follicular hyperplasia	Follicular hyperplasia; follicular involution with fragmentation	Explosive follicular hyperplasia	Type I	Type A	Stage I	Follicular hyperplasia
Mixed follicular hyperplasia and follicular involution		Mixed follicular hyperplasia/ follicular involution		Type B	Stage II	Mixed follicular and interfollicular hyperplasia
Follicular involution	Follicular involution with atrophy	Follicular involution	Type II	Type C	Stage III	Lymphocytic depletion
Lymphocyte depletion	Follicular depletion	Lymphocyte depletion	Type III			

of reactive hyperplasia observed in these lymph nodes were described (91,94,96–104), although the cause of the lymphadenopathy was unknown. Several classification schemes were proposed (102,104–108) (Table 28.9), based primarily on the morphologic features of the common lymph node patterns, often without regard for their clinical relevance or prognostic value. Some investigators noticed, however, that certain histopathologic patterns appeared to correlate with peripheral blood CD4:CD8 ratios and the clinical stage of HIV infection (104,106,107,109–112). Patients who had certain lymph node histologies, such as florid follicular hyperplasia, had a relatively stable clinical course, sometimes lasting for several years; those who had other histologies, such as follicular involution and lymphocyte depletion, rapidly developed some of the stigmata of AIDS (102,104,107–109). For example, approximately 90% of the reactive lymph nodes examined in biopsies in individuals who had persistent generalized lymphadenopathy displayed florid follicular hyperplasia or mixed follicular hyperplasia and follicular involution, and the remaining 10% displayed follicular involution (90–93,97,102–104,107,108,111). In contrast, approximately one third of the reactive lymph nodes undergoing biopsy in individuals who had AIDS-related complex displayed florid follicular hyperplasia or mixed follicular hyperplasia and follicular involution; the remaining two thirds exhibited follicular involution (90,104,106,107,111). By examining sequential lymph node biopsies from HIV-infected persons, it has become known that lymph node histology transforms in a consistent pattern throughout the course of HIV infection (107). Although recent studies have shed light on the events underlying these morphologic changes, the mechanisms involved in the progressive destruction of the lymph node, and of the immune system in general, have not been elucidated completely. Nonetheless, it is clear that the temporal progression of lymph node histopathology, observed in routine histologic sections, correlates with other features of HIV disease progression, such as peripheral blood CD4 T-cell counts, viremia, and the development of opportunistic infections, and has prognostic implications for the HIV-infected patient (107).

Histopathology

Florid Follicular Hyperplasia

Grossly, most lymph nodes are soft and moderately enlarged (2–4 cm) and do not show evidence of necrosis or hemorrhage (91,104). Histologically, they are composed of large, hyperplastic follicles, sometimes with serrated borders. The follicles may coalesce, become very large, and form "dumbbell" and other irregular shapes—hence the term *geographic follicles* (91,94,96,102,104,107) (Fig. 28.1). These hyperplastic follicles may be present in the medulla (96,97) as well as the cortex and may extend outside the lymph node capsule (95). In some instances, the follicles occupy more than two thirds of the cross-sectional area of the lymph node (106). The reactive follicles contain various lymphoid cells; however, large cleaved, large noncleaved, and small noncleaved cells predominate (96,104,107). In addition, numerous tingible body macrophages and abundant mitotic figures are usually present within the reactive follicles, giving them a prominent starry-sky appearance

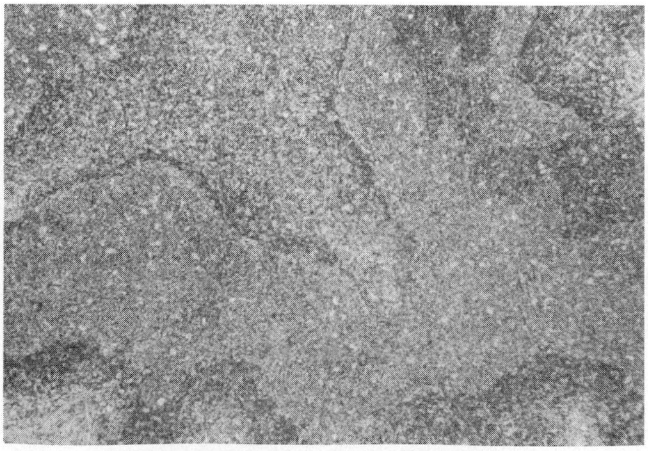

FIG. 28.1. HIV-related florid follicular hyperplasia. The hyperplastic follicles often coalesce to form extremely large and irregularly shaped follicles referred to as *geographic follicles* (hematoxylin and eosin stain, original magnification: 40× magnification).

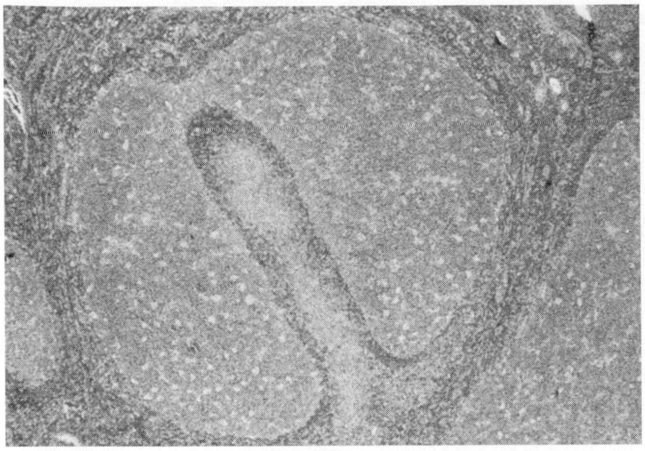

FIG. 28.2. HIV-related florid follicular hyperplasia. The large hyperplastic follicles have a prominent starry-sky appearance caused by the presence of numerous tingible body macrophages and abundant mitotic figures, indicative of a high rate of proliferation. Adjacent to this hyperplastic follicle is a zone of monocytoid B cells (hematoxylin and eosin stain, original magnification: 40× magnification).

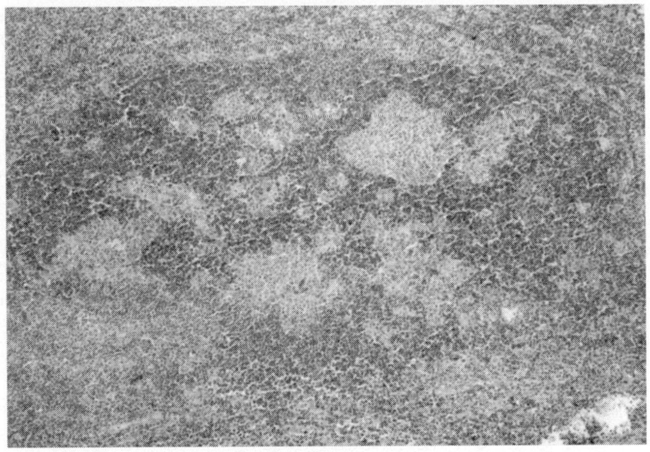

FIG. 28.4. HIV-related florid follicular hyperplasia. This hyperplastic follicle has undergone follicle lysis characterized by the infiltration of small lymphocytes into the germinal center, accompanied by hemorrhage, resulting in the formation of irregularly shaped clusters of follicle center cells (hematoxylin and eosin stain, original magnification: 63× magnification).

(91,96,100,104,107) (Fig. 28.2). The surrounding mantle zones often exhibit focal disruption, extensive attenuation, or even total effacement (91,96,101,104,106,107), so that the germinal centers are poorly defined and appear to merge with the surrounding interfollicular area. In some instances the mantle zones are entirely absent, and only ''naked'' germinal centers are present (98) (Fig. 28.3).

Follicle lysis, also known as *follicular fragmentation*, is characterized by germinal centers transected by invaginating small lymphocytes, with or without erythrocytes (91,95,99, 105–107,113). Follicle lysis is identified in a minority of follicles in approximately 50% of lymph nodes that exhibit florid follicular hyperplasia (99,113). The infiltrating small lymphocytes, which sometimes appear to track along small blood vessels (94,100), eventually break the follicle up into separate clusters of follicle center B cells (99) (Fig. 28.4). The combination of follicle lysis and mantle zone effacement obscures normal lymph node architecture and can cause con-

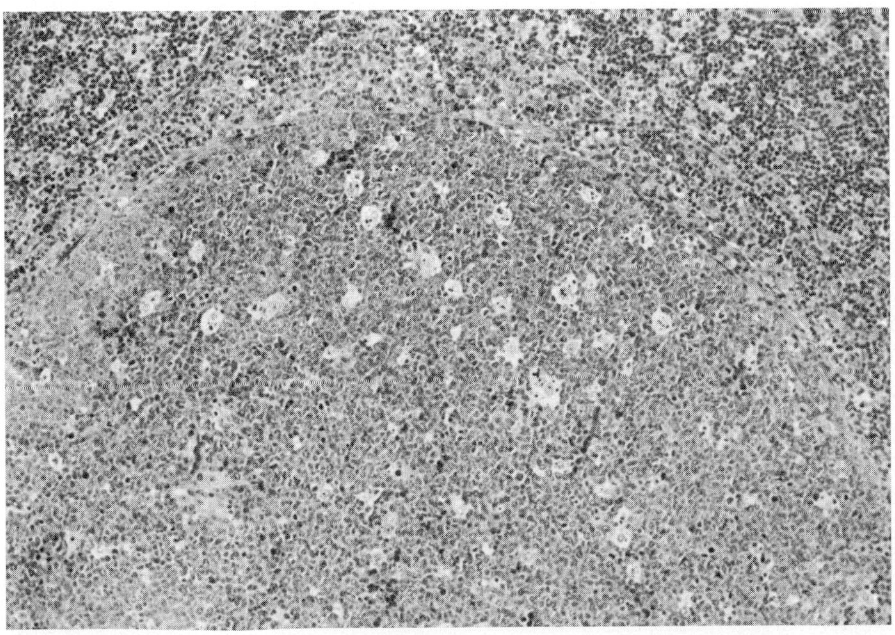

FIG. 28.3. HIV-related florid follicular hyperplasia. The large hyperplastic follicles sometimes lack a mantle zone and appear to merge with the surrounding interfollicular lymphoid cells (hematoxylin and eosin stain, original magnification: 100× magnification).

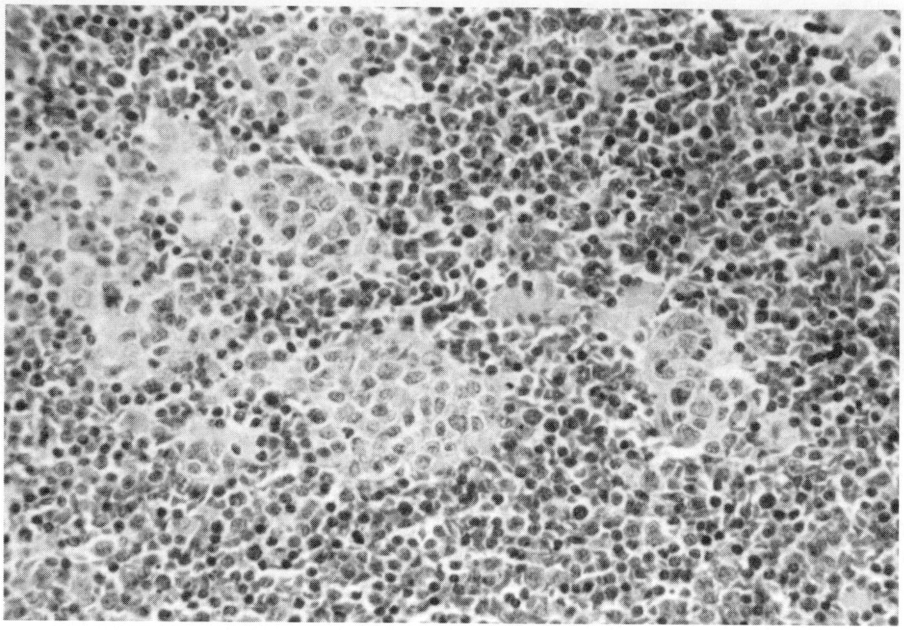

FIG. 28.5. HIV-related florid follicular hyperplasia. The irregularly shaped clusters of large transformed follicle center B cells may be confused with malignant lymphoma by the inexperienced observer (hematoxylin and eosin stain, original magnification: 250× magnification).

fusion with malignant lymphoma for the inexperienced observer (95) (Fig. 28.5).

Collections of monocyte-like cells often are seen surrounding trabecular vessels in the sinusoids between the floridly hyperplastic germinal centers (91,96,99,102,106,114, 115) (Figs. 28.2, 28.6). These monocytoid cells possess bland, oval, slightly indented nuclei containing inconspicuous nucleoli and relatively abundant pale to clear cytoplasm. Immunophenotypic studies have shown that these cells are polyclonal B lymphocytes (114). In HIV-related florid follicular hyperplasia, monocytoid B cells usually are seen in sinusoids associated with neutrophils (91,95,96,114,115); occasionally, monocytoid B cells also are seen partially encircling a reactive follicle (91,114).

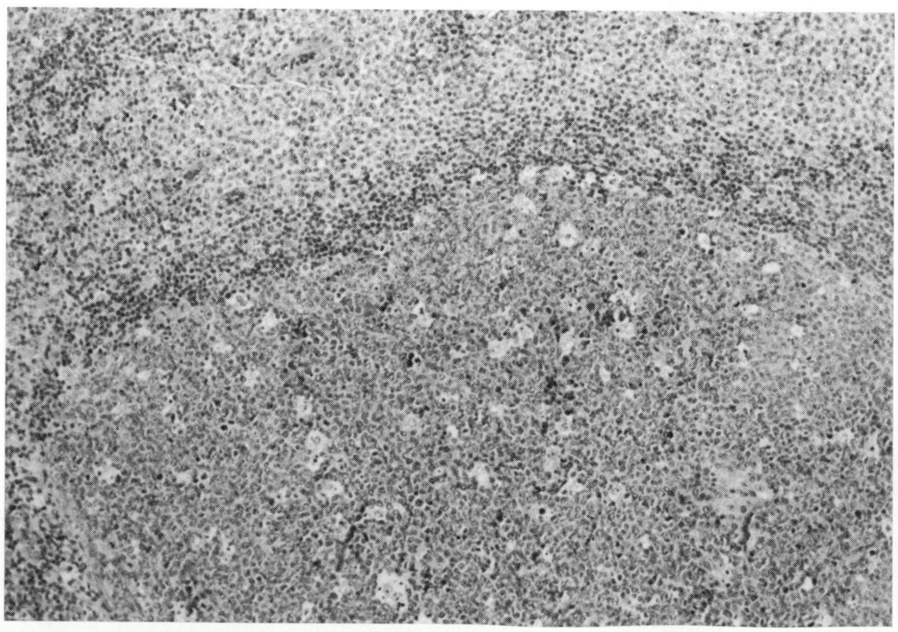

FIG. 28.6. HIV-related florid follicular hyperplasia. A zone of monocytoid B cells lies adjacent to a large hyperplastic follicle lined by an attenuated mantle zone (hematoxylin and eosin stain, original magnification: 100× magnification).

The interfollicular areas of lymph nodes exhibiting florid follicular hyperplasia contain numerous small blood vessels with prominent endothelium and a mixed population of small lymphocytes, immunoblasts, plasma cells, histiocytes, and sometimes eosinophils (95,97,102,104). Increased numbers of neutrophils also may be seen (106). The subcapsular sinuses are usually patent and contain histiocytes admixed with scattered neutrophils, lymphocytes, and erythrocytes (102,106). Multinucleated giant cells of the Warthin-Finkeldy type, which are identified in 9% to 25% of lymph nodes exhibiting florid follicular hyperplasia, are seen in the follicular or interfollicular areas (94,99,102,104,105,116). Hemophagocytosis also has been identified in lymph nodes displaying florid follicular hyperplasia (102). Rarely, foci of necrosis or noncaseating granulomas, with no organisms identified by special stains, have been identified (92). Some lymph nodes display the classic triad of toxoplasmic lymphadenitis comprising follicular hyperplasia, sinusoidal monocytoid B cells, and epithelioid histiocytes that encroach on the follicles (99). Focal dermatopathic change, with or without melanin pigment, has been seen in lymph nodes exhibiting florid follicular hyperplasia, even in patients without skin lesions (99). Lymph nodes displaying florid follicular hyperplasia also may have foci of Kaposi's sarcoma. These can be focal, present only in the subcapsular sinuses or along the perivascular septae, or partially replace the lymph node parenchyma (91,94,107).

Several of the histologic features of lymph nodes exhibiting florid follicular hyperplasia have been thought to be diagnostic or at least highly characteristic of HIV-related lymphadenopathy (115,117,118). The most important among these features include the large and irregularly shaped (geographic) hyperplastic follicles, disrupted and attenuated mantle zones, Warthin-Finkeldy–type multinucleated giant cells, and sinusoidal monocytoid B cells, especially if associated with small numbers of neutrophils (115,117,118). Comparison of lymph nodes from patients at risk for AIDS with those from patients without AIDS risk factors has shown that few, if any, of these morphologic findings are specific for HIV-related lymphadenopathy (115,117,118). Polykaryocytes, large and irregularly shaped hyperplastic follicles, sinusoidal monocytoid B cells, and effaced mantle zones all have been reported to occur statistically significantly more often in patients who have AIDS risk factors (117,118). Studies also have found, however, that multinucleated cells in lymph nodes from HIV-infected persons are present too infrequently to be of much diagnostic significance (118). Although mantle zone effacement, sinusoidal monocytoid B cells, and large, irregularly shaped hyperplastic follicles occur more frequently in patients who have persistent generalized lymphadenopathy, these features are also seen in a significant number of lymph nodes from patients who have no AIDS risk factors. Monocytoid B cells, for example, represent one of the three diagnostic features of toxoplasmic lymphadenitis (119). Furthermore, follicle lysis, which first was described in patients at risk for AIDS (99), is said to occur with equal or greater frequency in follicular hyperplasia not associated with HIV (118). Nonetheless, these histopathologic features, if present in the correct clinical and epidemiologic setting, for example identified in the lymph node of a 35-year-old never married white man living in New York city, can be considered highly suggestive of HIV-related lymphadenopathy (115,117).

Mixed Follicular Hyperplasia and Follicular Involution

Mixed follicular hyperplasia and follicular involution is histologically transitional between florid follicular hyperplasia and follicular involution (94,107,108). Grossly, the lymph nodes usually are enlarged (104). A combination of histopathologic features that encompasses those characteristic of florid follicular hyperplasia and follicular involution are observed (97,103,105,107,108). The lymph nodes contain distinct areas of florid follicular hyperplasia, with large, irregularly shaped germinal centers that account for less than two thirds of the cross-sectional area of the lymph node (106) and areas of follicular involution, with small, hyalinized follicles (97,103,105,107,108) (Fig. 28.7). The mantle zones surrounding the large follicles are effaced, as in florid follicular hyperplasia; those surrounding the involuted follicles may be thick, thin, or absent (103). In most patients, the percentage of involuted follicles does not exceed 50% of the total number of germinal centers (103). The interfollicular area appears expanded, compared with florid follicular hyperplasia, and widely separates the follicles (103,105,106). Vascular proliferation (which is most prominent around the germinal centers), lymphocytes, plasma cells, immunoblasts, and histiocytes are evident in the interfollicular area (105,106,108). In some patients, however, lymphocytes are relatively depleted throughout the lymph node, especially compared with patients with florid follicular hyperplasia (97,108). Foci of sinusoidal monocytoid B cells are seen in over 80% of cases (106). Warthin-Finkeldy–type giant cells also are seen occasionally (105).

Follicular Involution

In contrast to florid follicular hyperplasia, the germinal centers in lymph nodes exhibiting follicular involution are small, atrophic, and hypocellular (94,102–104,107,108,111) (Figs. 28.8, 28.9). The involuted germinal centers are hyalinized or epithelialized and consist primarily of concentric layers of follicular dendritic cells and occasional follicle center cells (95,97,99,103,107,108) (Fig. 28.10). Sometimes, only a fibrous scar remains of what once was a follicle (102,105) (Fig. 28.9B). Small, hyalinized blood vessels penetrate the atrophic germinal centers, often at right angles, leading to a "lollipop" appearance similar to that seen in Castleman's disease (103,104,108) (Figs. 28.9A, 28.10). Some of the follicles have a rim of small mantle zone lymphocytes; others do not; the latter consist only of "naked" germinal centers

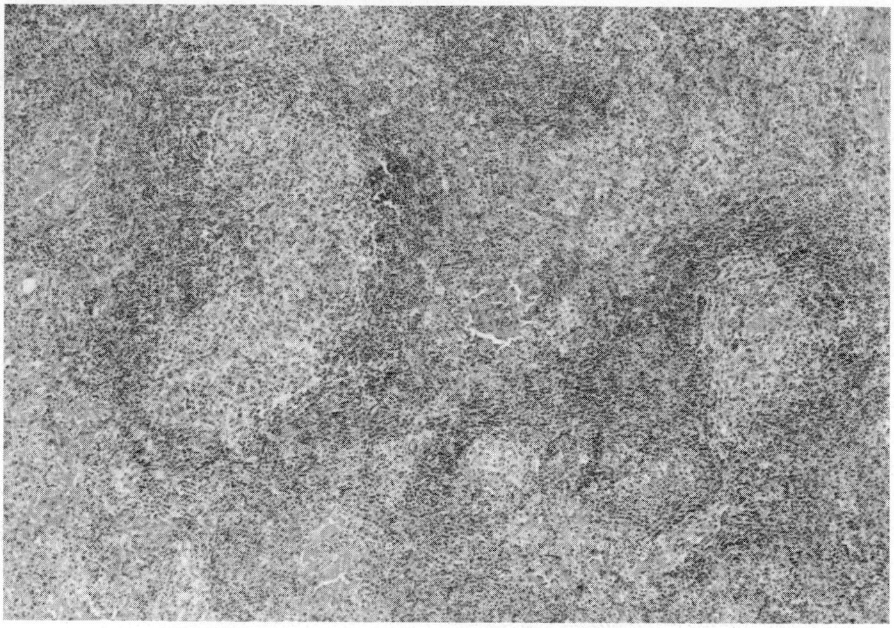

FIG. 28.7. HIV-related mixed follicular hyperplasia and follicular involution. A large hyperplastic follicle is present on the left, and smaller, atrophic follicles representative of follicular involution are present on the right (hematoxylin and eosin stain, original magnification: 63× magnification).

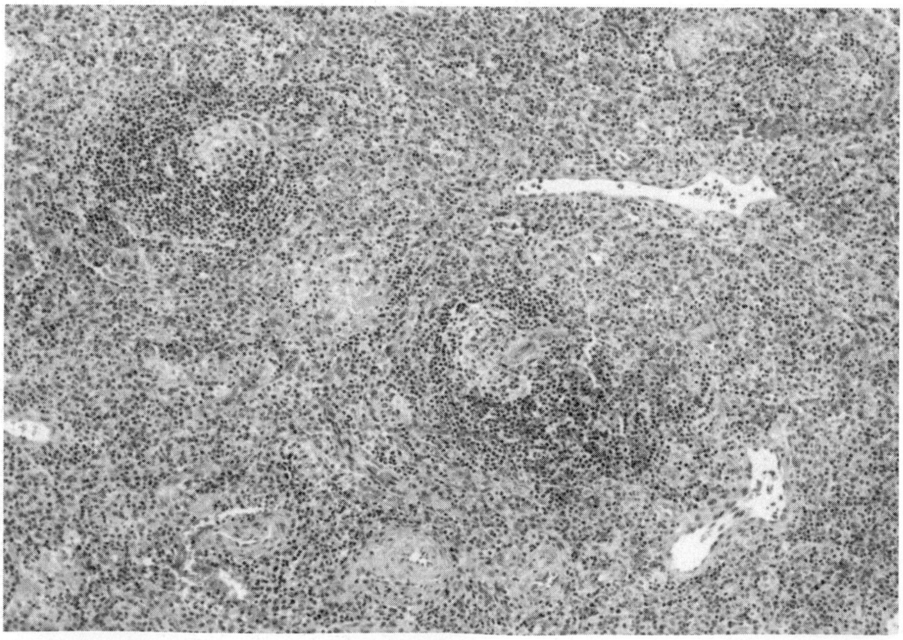

FIG. 28.8. HIV-related follicular involution. The germinal centers are small, atrophic, and hypocellular (hematoxylin and eosin stain, original magnification: 100× magnification).

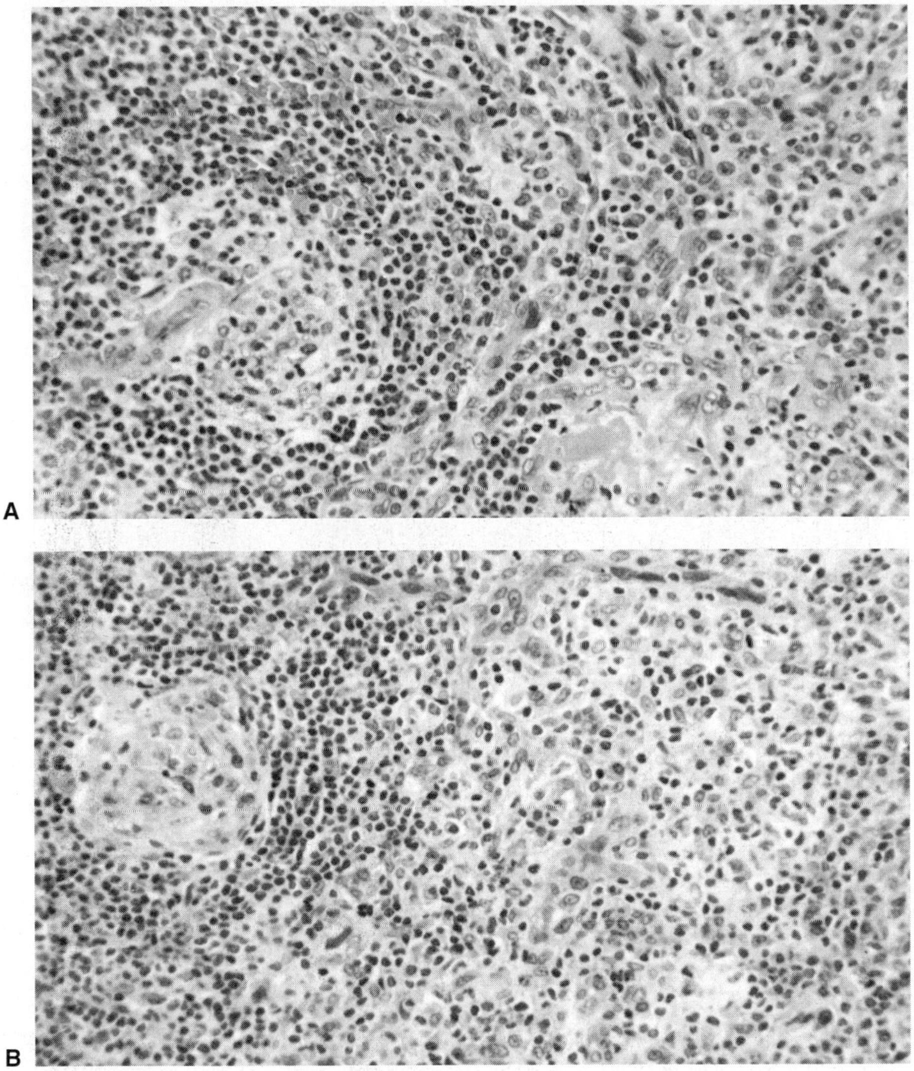

FIG. 28.9. HIV-related follicular involution. **A:** This small atrophic germinal center contains a penetrating hyalinized blood vessel and is surrounded by a thin mantle zone. **B:** This small fibrous scar surrounded by a thin mantle zone is all that remains of this germinal center. Both the atrophic germinal center and the germinal center scar lie adjacent to an expanded interfollicular area containing prominent vascular proliferation and a polymorphous cell population composed of small lymphocytes, plasma cells, and histiocytes (hematoxylin and eosin stain, original magnification: 250× magnification).

(104). Extracellular hyalinized eosinophilic material that stains with the periodic acid–Schiff stain sometimes is associated with the atrophic follicles (94,104,108,111).

The interfollicular area is expanded widely and yet lymphoid-depleted (99,107,108,111,113) (Fig. 28.11). Although small lymphocytes remain the major cell type in the paracortical area, they are decreased in number and are associated with an increased number of histiocytes and plasma cells (94,96,107,108,111). Occasionally, Russell bodies are seen (102). Normal numbers of immunoblasts as well as mast cells, eosinophils, and scattered mitotic figures also are identified in the interfollicular areas (102,105,111). Warthin-Finkeldy–like polykaryocytes are identified in 50% to 70% of lymph nodes exhibiting HIV-related follicular involution (91,102,105). Vascular proliferation with endothelial cell hyperplasia and fibrous thickening of the vessel walls are prominent (96,102,105,108,111). Many of these vessels are the size of postcapillary venules, and the number of lymphocytes that traverses them is increased (96,102). Sinus histiocytosis may or may not be prominent (96,102,105,111); however, neutrophils as well as histiocytes can be identified within the sinuses (102,111). In some lymph nodes, increased amounts of background eosinophilic material, which may represent necrotic debris (95), are present, and there may be fibrosis of the medullary region (102). Fibrosis of the lymph node capsule is often present (96,102,105), and this occasionally extends down into and obliterates the subcapsular sinuses (91,96). Erythrophagocytosis has been identified in 13% of patients with follicular involution (102).

The histologic picture of HIV-related follicular involution

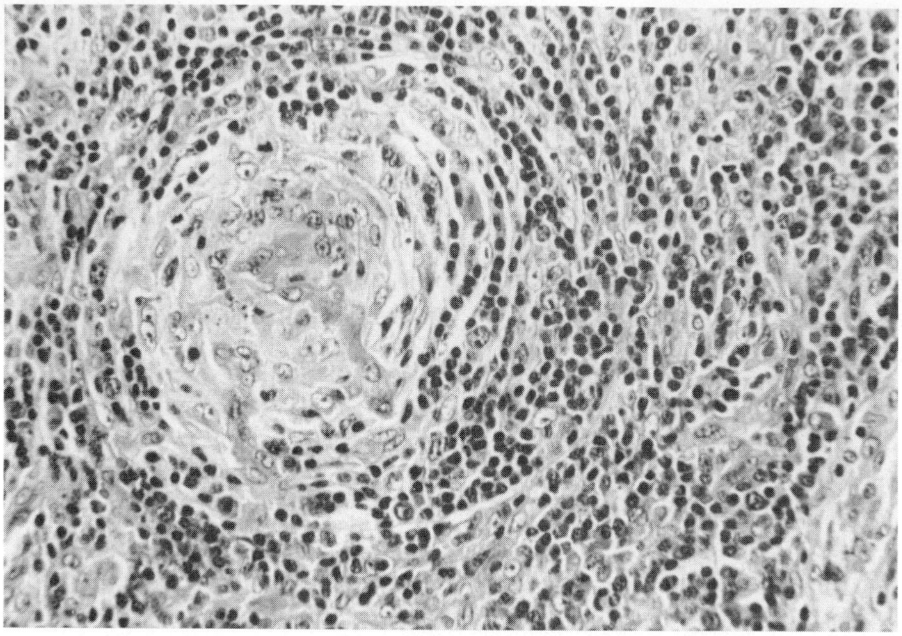

FIG. 28.10. HIV-related follicular involution. The involuted germinal centers consist primarily of concentric layers of follicular dendritic cells, often contain penetrating hyalinized blood vessels, and are surrounded by concentric layers of small lymphocytes that mimic the appearance of the germinal centers frequently seen in Castleman's disease (hematoxylin and eosin stain, original magnification: 250× magnification).

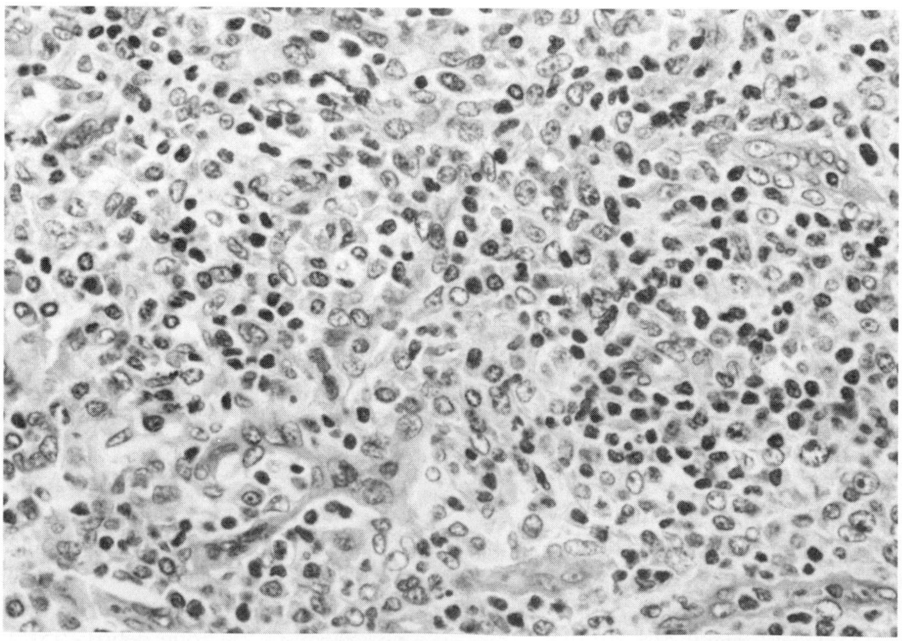

FIG. 28.11. HIV-related follicular involution. The interfollicular area is widely expanded and displays prominent vascular proliferation and a polymorphous cell population composed of small lymphocytes, plasma cells, and histiocytes (hematoxylin and eosin stain, original magnification: 400× magnification).

may be confused with the hyaline vascular form of Castleman's disease and angioimmunoblastic lymphadenopathy, because many of the morphologic features, such as hyalinized atrophic follicles, expanded interfollicular areas, and prominent vascular proliferation, are shared by all these entities (see Chapter 16). Furthermore, HIV-infected individuals who have the follicular involution phase of HIV-related lymphadenopathy and HIV-uninfected individuals who have Castleman's disease or angioimmunoblastic lymphadenopathy share many clinical features (107,103,120–124) (see Chapter 16). For these reasons, it is not surprising that there have been several reports describing the occurrence of Castleman's disease and angioimmunoblastic lymphadenopathy in young HIV-seropositive homosexual men, many of whom also have Kaposi's sarcoma (125–130). Most of these cases were reported early in the AIDS epidemic, prior to widespread awareness of the follicular involution pattern of HIV-related lymphadenopathy. In all probability, most of these cases represent HIV-related follicular involution and not Castleman's disease or angioimmunoblastic lymphadenopathy.

Several subtle morphologic differences and certain clinical features may be useful in distinguishing between these entities. For example, the interfollicular cell population tends to be more polymorphous in HIV-related follicular involution than in Castleman's disease (107). Also, the relatively small number of immunoblasts, as well as the presence of residual follicles and sinusoids, in HIV-related follicular involution makes the diagnosis of angioimmunoblastic lymphadenopathy unlikely (97,102,105). In addition, immunohistochemical studies have shown that more CD4 T cells than CD8 T cells are present in the interfollicular areas of lymph nodes that exhibit Castleman's disease (131,132); the opposite is true for lymph nodes that exhibit HIV-related follicular involution (98,133,134). The clinical settings of Castleman's disease, angioimmunoblastic lymphadenopathy, and HIV-related follicular involution differ. Individuals who have Castleman's disease and angioimmunoblastic lymphadenopathy are usually between 55 and 80 years old and are HIV-seronegative (120–123); those who have HIV-related follicular involution are usually in their thirties or early forties and are HIV-seropositive (126–130). Although patients who have Castleman's disease may have a decreased peripheral blood CD4:CD8 ratio, it is usually not as severe as that seen in HIV-related follicular involution, and it is usually the result of an increase in CD8 T cells and not a decrease in CD4 T cells (135). In fact, most individuals who have HIV-related follicular involution have CD4 T-cell counts of less than 200 per microliter (108).

Several recent studies have identified a strong association between the Kaposi's sarcoma–associated herpesvirus (KSHV) and multicentric Castleman's disease in both HIV-infected and HIV-uninfected individuals, including those with and those without Kaposi's sarcoma (136–138). Although the histologic features of HIV-related follicular involution and KSHV-associated multicentric Castleman's disease in HIV-seropositive individuals are very similar, some investigators believe that subtle morphologic differences between the two entities exist (139). It has been suggested that the lack of concentric layers of mantle cells surrounding atrophic germinal centers and marked lymphoid depletion are more suggestive of HIV-related follicular involution, and increases in hyalinized blood vessels and plasma cells are more suggestive of KSHV-associated multicentric Castleman's disease in an HIV-infected individual (139). Many HIV-seropositive individuals who have benign lymphadenopathy exhibiting the follicular involution pattern are not infected with KSHV (140). These findings suggest that multicentric Castleman's disease is a separate entity, even if it occurs in HIV-seropositive individuals, and is distinct from the follicular involution and other histologic patterns of HIV-related lymphadenopathy. HIV-seropositive individuals in all stages of HIV disease may be KSHV-infected, and it is possible to identify KSHV-infected individuals who have HIV-related lymphadenopathy exhibiting any of the four histopathologic patterns (i.e., florid follicular hyperplasia, mixed follicular hyperplasia and involution, follicular involution, or lymphocyte depletion) (140).

Both Castleman's disease and angioimmunoblastic lymphadenopathy exhibit relatively constant histopathologic patterns in separate lymph node biopsies obtained several months apart from the same patient (120–123). In contrast, HIV-related lymphadenopathy is in dynamic evolution: Progressive changes in lymph node histopathology correlate with a constantly changing clinical picture that parallels the patient's deteriorating immune status. HIV-related follicular involution is only one of several histopathologic patterns seen in the dynamic continuum of HIV-related lymphadenopathy (103,107,108).

Lymphocyte Depletion

The lymph nodes in HIV seropositive persons who exhibit lymphocyte depletion usually are obtained at autopsy (94,102,107,111,141). Grossly, the lymph nodes are small, usually measuring less than 1.0 cm in diameter (94,97). Histologically, the lymph nodes are characterized by severe lymphoid depletion and a complete loss of germinal centers (94,97,102,107,141); they are composed primarily of medullary cords and sinusoids (102,107,141). Subcapsular and sinusoidal fibrosis is present, with focal hyaline deposits in sites of degenerated follicles (94,107,141) (Fig. 28.12). The lymph nodes are populated primarily by histiocytes, plasma cells, and scattered immunoblasts (94,102,107,141). Some of the plasma cells are large and atypical; they may contain multiple nuclei and display bizzare shapes (102). Russell bodies also sometimes are seen (102,141). Sinus histiocytosis can be extensive (111). Phagocytosis of blood cells, including erythrocytes, neutrophils, and lymphocytes by sinus histiocytes can be seen in up to 90% of lymphocyte-depleted lymph nodes (102). The venules are usually thin-walled and contain few, if any, transversing lymphocytes

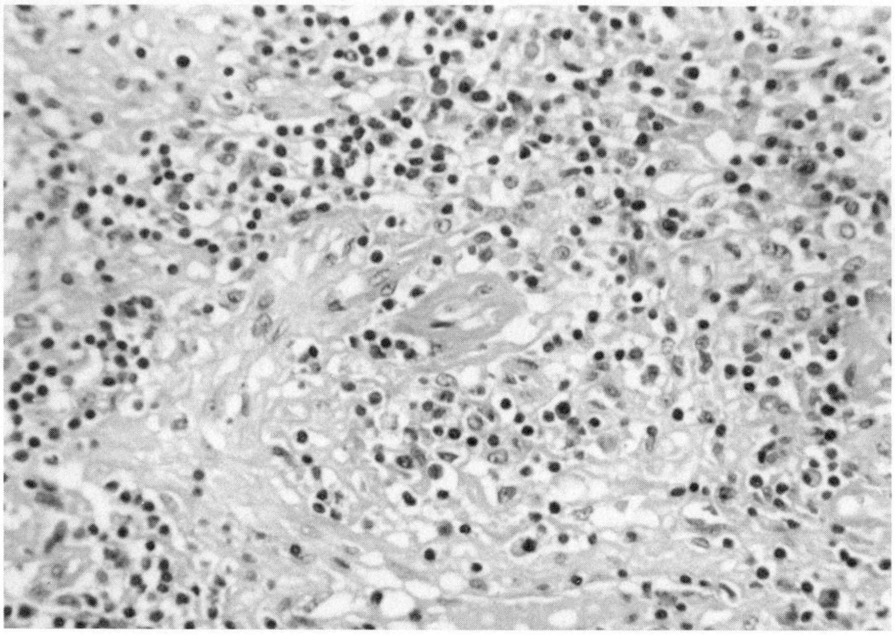

FIG. 28.12. HIV-related lymphocyte depletion. The lymph node displays severe lymphoid depletion, a total loss of germinal centers, and focal hyaline deposits in sites of degenerated follicles. The cell population is composed largely of histiocytes and plasma cells, with scattered immunoblasts (hematoxylin and eosin stain, original magnification: 250× magnification).

(102). Small lymphocytes, lying either singly or in small clusters, can be identified scattered diffusely throughout lymphocyte-depleted lymph nodes (102,111). In addition, some investigators believe that lymph nodes that are totally replaced by infectious organisms, such as *Mycobacterium avium intracellulare*, should be classified as lymphocyte-depleted lymph nodes (97,111).

Ultrastructure

The human immunodeficiency virions have been characterized ultrastructurally as 80- to 120-nm particles containing a central core composed of the viral p24 gag capsid protein. The majority of virions contain one cone-shaped core measuring 60 nm at the broad end (which contains the viral RNA) and 20 nm at the narrow end (9,18,142). A small percentage of virions contain a single tubular-shaped core approximately 40 nm in diameter. Two to several cores, however, cone-shaped, tubular-shaped, or both, may be present in one virion (142). Irregularly shaped electron-dense masses, known as the *lateral bodies*, are situated parallel to the long axis of the core and appear to be continuous with the membrane-associated matrix protein (MA) shell. This p17 MA, which is about 7 nm thick, is tightly bound to the inner layer of the viral envelope. This intimate attachment, which is mediated by myristoylation of an amino-terminal glycine, is necessary for viral budding (142). The HIV viral envelope is studded with 72 nine- to ten-nanometer long envelope glycoprotein projections, known as *knobs*, which are arranged symmetrically on the viral surface. The knobs are comprised of oligomers (probably trimers) composed of the surface envelope glycoprotein, gp120, and the transmembrane protein, gp41 (18,142–144). Progressive loss of these knobs, which are shed from the viral surface at a rate dependent on strain, virion age, and temperature, is associated with a gradual decrease in infectivity. It is thought that a minimal number of knobs is necessary for a virion to be infectious (142,145). The mechanism by which HIV actually enters the cell is still unclear. Thin-section electron microscopic studies have demonstrated both direct fusion and receptor-mediated uptake of the virus into the cell (18,142,144). In addition, HIV can be transmitted either by syncytium formation or by cell-to-cell contact without cell membrane fusion (18).

Systemic dissemination occurs during the acute phase of HIV infection, which covers a period of approximately 3 to 6 weeks after initial infection (146). Virus has been found in lymphoid organs within 1 week of infection and prior to seroconversion in animal models of simian immunodeficiency virus infection (146). Human immunodeficiency virus has been identified in a variety of lymphoid organs, including lymph nodes, tonsils, spleen, and thymus, as early as 2 weeks after seroconversion (147,148). During the early and clinically latent stages of the disease, viral particles have been found primarily in the germinal centers of lymph nodes, in which they have been identified most commonly along the cellular processes of the follicular dendritic cells (18,146,148–155). During the latent stage the viral load associated with the follicular dendritic cells is thought to be 100- to 10,000-fold greater than in the peripheral blood (18). Most studies examining lymph nodes obtained from HIV-infected individuals have identified virions in the extracellular spaces between the dendritic cells, usually complexed with antibody and complement. Some studies have reported viral budding from follicular dendritic cells; others have found immune complexed viral proteins or complete virus within these cells (148–158). Recently, a second population of dendritic cells, more akin to circulating peripheral blood dendritic cells, has been identified in germinal centers. These germinal center dendritic cells are potent antigen-presenting cells that regulate the activation of naive T cells. They are $CD4^+$ and are potential targets for HIV infection (159,160). The HIV-infected dendritic cells present within germinal centers may not be follicular dendritic cells but rather these recently described $CD4^+$ germinal center dendritic cells.

Whether the follicular dendritic cells are infected by HIV directly or only trap the virus, it is clear that the destruction of these cells, as demonstrated by ultrastructural studies, is an important factor in the pathobiology and clinical behavior of HIV disease. Early in HIV infection the follicular dendritic cells may resemble those seen in the hyperplastic follicles of lymph nodes obtained from HIV-uninfected individuals. In most lymph nodes morphologically classified as representing florid follicular hyperplasia, however, the labyrinthine structure is expanded and may be composed of hyperplastic follicular dendritic cells. The follicular dendritic cell cytoplasmic extensions are more voluminous and extensive than those found in most reactive lymph nodes in HIV-uninfected individuals. In addition, the dendritic meshwork often contains relatively large groups of blast cells between the cellular extensions (150,153,161,162). Within the cells the rough endoplasmic reticulum cisterns are often swollen, and increased numbers of lysosomes are present (161). Numerous viral particles are seen in association with the dendritic processes (150,155,163) (Fig. 28.13). At this stage there is little or no evidence of cytolysis of the follicular dendritic cells (164). Ultrastructural characterization, however, shows that although some follicles, presumably earlier in the disease process, exhibit the same spectrum of follicular dendritic cell subtypes as those found in HIV-uninfected individuals, other follicles have follicular dendritic cells that are more frequently of the less differentiated subtypes (4 and 5) and the more regressive subtypes (6 and 7), indicating

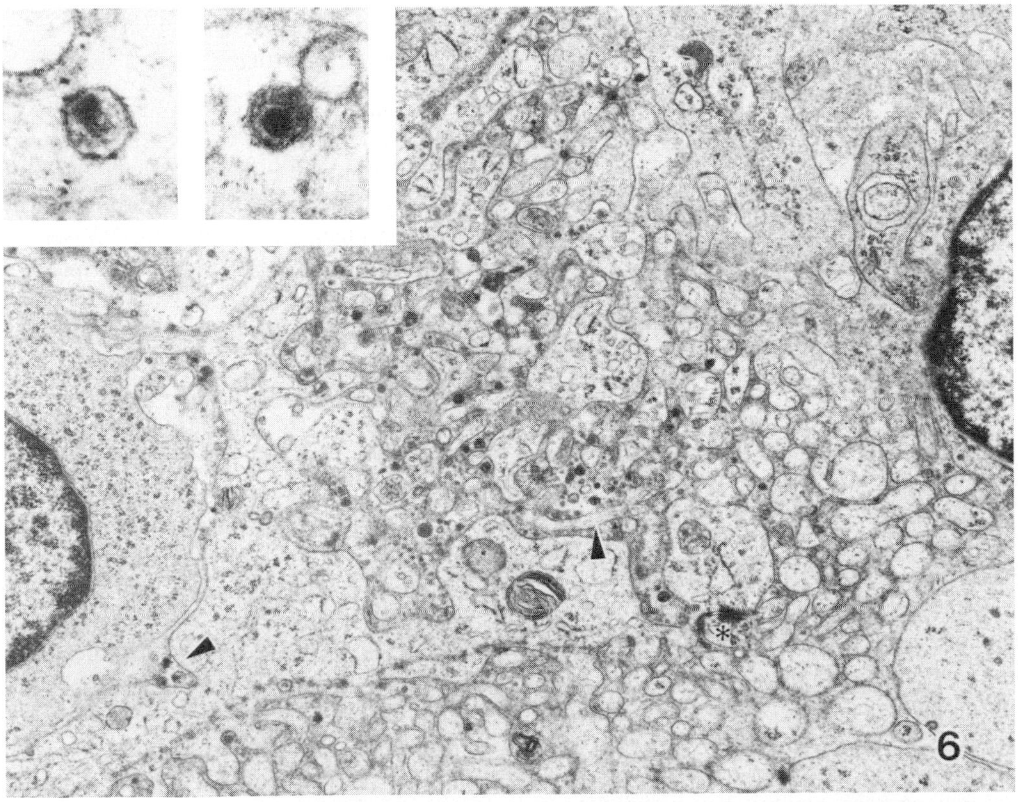

FIG. 28.13. Follicular dendritic cell containing viral particles. An electron micrograph of a germinal center in a lymph node obtained from a homosexual man who had persistent generalized lymphadenopathy demonstrates hyperplastic labyrinthine processes from a follicular dendritic cell identified by the presence of desmosome-like junctions (*asterisks*). Numerous round viral particles are present in spaces between the processes (*arrowheads*). High-magnification electron micrographs (**top**) illustrate the fine structure of the viral particles. Note the peripheral capsule and central nucleus (**top right**) or rectangular eccentric nucleus with tapering apex (**top left**) (uranyl acetate, lead citrate stain, original magnifications: 12,000× magnification; **Inset:** 75,000× magnification). (From Said JW. AIDS-related lymphadenopathies. *Semin Diagn Pathol* 1988;5:365–375, with permission.)

altered cellular physiology (161,162,165). As HIV disease progresses, fragmentation, degeneration, and lysis of the follicular dendritic cells occur (151,154,157). The cause of follicular dendritic cell destruction is unclear. Several hypotheses have been suggested, including HIV-mediated mitochondrial damage, abnormal cytokine production, viral or viral product toxicity, and cytotoxic T-cell destruction (18,148,155,158,166–168). The ultrastructural destruction of the follicular dendritic cells, however, is associated with disease progression, follicle involution, and loss of virus-trapping capability (146,154,157). The stage of lymphocyte depletion is associated with virtual loss of follicular dendritic cells (154).

Although the majority of HIV has been identified ultrastructurally within germinal centers associated with follicular dendritic cells, HIV has been identified in other cell types within lymph nodes, primarily by *in situ* hybridization or immunohistochemistry (146,147,157,169). Prior to the destruction of the follicular dendritic cells, HIV is only rarely, if ever, identified ultrastructurally outside of the germinal center (153,154). Once the dendritic meshwork has been destroyed, however, HIV particles often are observed scattered throughout the lymph node, where they are found most frequently in macrophages (170). Viral particles also have been seen rarely within endothelial cells and mononuclear cells, often associated with the endoplasmic reticulum (8,168).

Tubuloreticular structures and test tube– and ring-shaped forms, also known as *cylindric conformational cisternae* (171), have been identified frequently in cells populating the lymph nodes of HIV-infected individuals (100,150,153,171, 172). The percentage of cells containing these structures and forms appears to increase with HIV disease progression (172). The tuboreticular structures seen in HIV-infected patients are intracellular structures composed of anastomosing tubules, measuring 24 nm in diameter, and are located within the cisternae of the endoplasmic reticulum (172) (Fig. 28.14). These structures also have been associated with other viral infections and autoimmune diseases (171–174). The test tube– and ring-shaped forms are observed less commonly than tuboreticular structures (172). They are tubal in appearance on longitudinal section and ring-shaped on cross-section and are composed of two or more cisternae of endoplasmic reticulum, one inside the other, separated by a 24-nm layer of electron-dense material (172). The tuboreticular structures and test tube– and ring-shaped forms are found most frequently in lymphocytes, monocytes, and endothelial cells, but they also have been identified in macrophages, plasma cells, interdigitating dendritic cells, and follicular dendritic cells (153,172). Initially they were thought to represent viral constituents and to possess diagnostic significance (172); it is now believed that they arise from the rough endoplasmic reticulum membrane in the setting of elevated interferon-α levels (175,176). They are mentioned here primarily for historical interest.

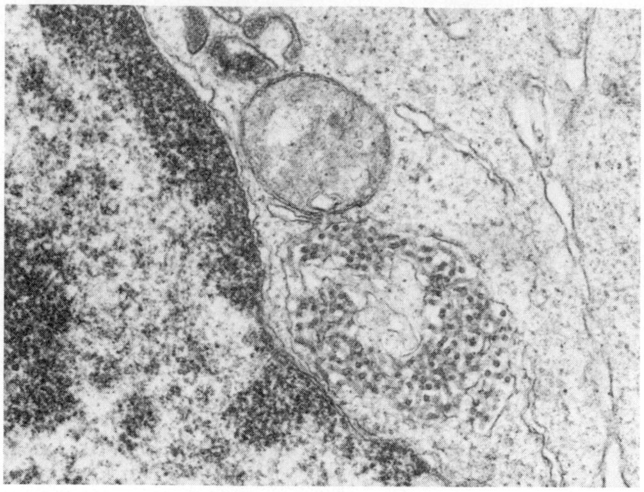

FIG. 28.14. Tubuloreticular structures. Electron micrograph showing tubuloreticular structure consisting of anastomosing tubules measuring 24 nm in diameter. These are frequently identified in lymph nodes of HIV-infected patients but also are found in other viral infections and autoimmune diseases (uranyl acetate, lead citrate, original magnification: 35,000× magnification). (From Said JW. AIDS-related lymphadenopathies. *Semin Diagn Pathol* 1988;5:365–375, with permission.)

Immunoarchitecture

The immunoarchitecture of lymph nodes exhibiting florid follicular hyperplasia in HIV-infected persons in some ways is similar to, and in other ways is distinctly different from, that of lymph nodes exhibiting follicular hyperplasia attributable to other causes. In both HIV-seropositive and HIV-uninfected individuals the transformed germinal center B cells present in such lymph nodes are polyclonal (94,113,177). In HIV-seropositive individuals, however, the germinal centers of such lymph nodes contain increased numbers of T cells, in contrast to those in HIV-negative persons (100,110,178–180). These T cells, nearly all of which are $CD8^+$, are present in small clusters around small penetrating blood vessels or are scattered diffusely throughout the follicles (105,116,179–183). The CD8 T cells present within the germinal centers almost exclusively represent $CD45RO^+$ memory T cells (184). Conflicting reports, however, have described these cells as either suppressor or cytotoxic CD8 T cells. Early reports suggested that these cells are suppressor T cells, based on their lack of CD28 expression (178). Recent studies, however, have demonstrated increased levels of cytotoxic T cell–associated enzymes and proteins such as TIA-1, serine esterase B, granzyme B, and perforin in the follicles of HIV-positive individuals compared with HIV-uninfected persons, indicating that they most likely are cytotoxic CD8 T cells (167,179–181,184). The lack of CD28 expression by intrafollicular cytotoxic CD8 T cells may be explained at least partially by the progressive downregulation and eventual loss of surface CD28 antigen expression by both CD4 and CD8 T cells during the course of HIV infection (185,186). The increase in CD8

T cells results in a marked decrease in the intrafollicular CD4:CD8 T-cell ratio from the normal range of greater than 10:1 to not more than 2.5:1 (101,106,116,178,183,187). The number of CD4 T cells present within the germinal centers has been reported to be approximately the same, slightly increased, or decreased compared with non–HIV-related follicular hyperplasia (94,100,101,178,183, 187–189). Approximately 30% to 50% of these CD4 T cells express CD57 (187,190). These $CD4^+CD57^+$ T cells appear to be the most abundant productively HIV-infected cells within the germinal centers of lymph nodes exhibiting florid follicular hyperplasia (190).

The destruction of the follicular dendritic cell meshwork is a consistent immunoarchitectural feature of HIV-related lymphadenopathy. As seen with immunostaining using a variety of monoclonal antibodies such as anti-DRC-1, anti-CD21, and anti-CD35, the usual interwoven concentric pattern of the follicular dendritic cell meshwork is lost (94,104,105,113,156,157,165, 180,182,188,191). In HIV-related florid follicular hyperplasia this meshwork is disrupted extensively with focal areas of negative staining that correspond to areas infiltrated by small lymphocytes as seen in routine histologic sections (94,104,111,113,155,165,169, 182,188,192). In other germinal centers, the follicular dendritic cell meshwork is destroyed completely, leaving behind only residual small clusters of cells exhibiting loss of their cytoplasmic dendritic extensions (105,189).

It is not completely clear why or how the follicular dendritic cell meshwork is destroyed during the course of HIV infection (179,180). Both a direct cytolytic effect of the virus, either by lytic infection of the follicular dendritic cells or by the lytic action of entrapped viral antigens, and lysis by cytotoxic T cells have been suggested as mechanisms of follicular dendritic cell destruction (104,156,167,179–181, 184,187). Some investigators have suggested that HIV, through a complex and incompletely understood mechanism, is directly responsible for the death of the follicular dendritic cells and dissolution of the meshwork (104–106,148,177, 188,189). Within weeks of seroconversion, scattered viral particles are seen within germinal centers (148), and immunostaining for HIV p17 and p24 proteins and follicular dendritic cell-associated antigens has shown identical staining patterns within the germinal centers (169,181,182,187,189, 192–194), indicating an intimate relationship between the virus and the follicular dendritic cells. Although follicular dendritic cells generally are CD4-negative (195), they occasionally express CD4 (113,177,196) and can be infected by HIV *in vitro* (197,198). Along with the identification of budding viral particles by electron microscopy and the localization of viral DNA and mRNA by *in situ* hybridization within the cells, this suggests that follicular dendritic cells can be infected productively by HIV (148,150,151,155,156,179, 199). In time this may lead to direct cell lysis. Furthermore, the association of free cytoplasmic virus and the presence of cellular degenerative changes, particularly involving the mitochondria, suggests that HIV directly damages follicular dendritic cells (155,168). In most instances, HIV is found in the intrafollicular dendritic cell spaces and not within the follicular dendritic cells themselves (94,153,157,164,188, 193). In addition, recent studies have identified a second, much smaller population of dendritic cells within lymph node germinal centers that expresses CD4 and is thought to be derived from peripheral blood dendritic cells (159,160). These may be the productively HIV-infected dendritic cells identified rarely by some investigators (151,155,156). It is unlikely that a direct cytopathic effect of HIV significantly contributes to the destruction of follicular dendritic cells in most instances.

In HIV infection, there is a significant increase in the number of intrafollicular CD8 T cells, which frequently are found in clusters in the areas of negative immunostaining within the follicular dendritic cell meshwork, suggesting that the follicular dendritic cells are destroyed by these cells (94,148,187). The follicular dendritic cells most likely are destroyed as innocent bystanders. The intrafollicular CD8 T cells, the majority of which are cytotoxic T cells based on the expression of TIA-1, perforin, serine esterase B, and granzyme (166,167,180,181,184), are thought to be recruited to the germinal center by a chemotactic effect of HIV or specific HIV components (200). These clusters of cytotoxic T cells often contain HIV p24 antigen–positive cells (187). The cytotoxic CD8 T cells may exert lysis through class I restricted lysis after antigen recognition (200). Alternatively, because there is a high degree of similarity between HIV gp41 and gp120 and human class II major histocompatibility complex $\beta1$ domain and β chain, resulting in a large number of pseudo–class II determinants, the CD8 T cells may destroy HIV-containing immune complexes attached to the follicular dendritic cells by antibody-dependent cell-mediated cytotoxicity or lysis (200–202). In this instance, follicular dendritic cells theoretically are damaged and eventually destroyed in a retrograde manner resulting in dissolution of the meshwork (200).

The presence of HIV in the follicular dendritic cell meshwork and its subsequent destruction is a critical component in the pathogenesis of HIV disease. The follicular dendritic cells trap HIV in the form of immune complexes on the surface of the cell membrane (149,157,160,165,187,194, 199). This trapped virus is highly infectious and readily can infect CD4 T cells (158,160). In addition, follicular dendritic cells can transform neutralized HIV into an infectious form, even in the setting of a vast excess of neutralizing antibody (158), further propagating the infection. Once the follicular dendritic cell meshwork is destroyed, the germinal center no longer has the capability to trap HIV, resulting in a marked increase in the number of circulating virions and the onset of more severe symptoms (146,157). Furthermore, electron microscopic studies have shown that in the majority of lymph nodes displaying florid follicular hyperplasia, the follicular dendritic cells exhibit undifferentiated and regressive morphology that is associated with an inversion in the ratio of germinal center B-cell blasts (centroblasts) to centrocytes

(161). The destruction of the follicular dendritic cell meshwork and associated imbalance of the microenvironment in the germinal center may contribute to the B-cell dysregulation and functional abnormalities seen in HIV-infected individuals (148,189,203).

B cells represent the most common cell within the germinal centers of lymph nodes exhibiting florid follicular hyperplasia. These B cells express CD19, CD20, CD22, and IgM or IgG but not IgD (93,104,182,192) and are polyclonal with respect to immunoglobulin light chain determinants (94,113,116,204). These cells also express class II major histocompatibility comples antigens, CD10, CD21, CD38 (weakly), and CD71 (weakly) (113,177,182,192,204). The germinal center B cells are highly proliferative, with more than 90% in the G_1 or G_2 phases of the cell cycle, as measured by Ki-67 expression (187,188). As the follicular dendritic cell meshwork is destroyed, the number of total B cells and proliferating B cells within the germinal center is reduced (189,191,192,204). In addition, a significant number of cytoplasmic immunoglobulin-containing follicular center cells (centroblasts) and plasma cells is found within the germinal centers (155,192).

In HIV-related florid follicular hyperplasia, as in other types of follicular hyperplasia, the mantle zone lymphocytes surrounding the germinal centers are polyclonal B cells that express both IgM and IgD (94,95,113,177,204). These mantle zone B cells also express HLA-DR and CD62L and lack CD38 and CD71 (113,177). Mirroring the architectural features of the mantle zones observed on routine histologic sections, immunohistochemical staining shows that these IgM^+ and IgD^+ B-cell mantle zones are usually disrupted, attenuated, or even focally absent in cases of HIV-related florid follicular hyperplasia (95,101,104,105,177). Small lymphocytes invaginate into the germinal centers, often along small penetrating blood vessels, into areas of negative staining with anti-DRC-1, anti-CD21, or anti-CD35 antibodies (104,113,155,165,182,187). These invaginating lymphocytes are thought by some investigators to be mantle zone B cells associated with a variable number of CD4 or CD8 T cells (105,111,113,182). Other investigators have suggested that most, if not all, of the cells that infiltrate into areas devoid of follicular dendritic cells are T cells (94,104,148, 155,182,192). There are decreased numbers of CD4 helper T cells and increased numbers of CD8 suppressor T cells in the mantle cell zone (95,178, 187).

Immunophenotypic analysis of the paracortical regions of lymph nodes exhibiting HIV-related florid follicular hyperplasia may show a decrease in the overall number of T cells (178) as a result of the decrease in the number of CD4 helper T cells (178). Although there may be a decrease in the number of $CD8^+CD28^+$ cytotoxic T cells, there is usually a significant increase in $CD8^+CD28^-$ suppressor T cells, resulting in an overall increase in the number of CD8 T cells in the paracortex (95,101,106,110,178,180,183,191,205). Increased numbers of serine esterase B–positive and $TIA\text{-}1^+$ cells also are found in the paracortex in comparison with HIV-negative control subjects (181,184), again suggesting that at least some of the CD8 T cells are cytotoxic in nature. It may be that these $CD8^+CD28^-$ T cells, similar to those in the follicle, are actually cytotoxic cells that have downregulated and lost surface CD28 antigen expression secondary to HIV infection (185,186). Only a relatively small increase in the number of granzyme B–positive cells, however, is seen in the paracortical area of lymph nodes exhibiting florid follicular hyperplasia (180).

Early in HIV disease the CD4:CD8 T-cell ratio in lymph nodes may be relatively normal (105). In most cases, the CD4:CD8 T-cell ratio in the paracortex is decreased or inverted compared with that in HIV-negative control subjects (94,106,116,178,182,183,188,191). The CD4:CD8 T-cell ratio in the lymph nodes is usually not as low as that in the peripheral blood (104,110,111,165,187). In addition, the number of paracortical CD62L positive cells is reduced (178). The CD62L antigen is expressed by a wide variety of cell types, including some CD4 and CD8 T cells, natural killer cells, monocytes, and granulocytes (178). It is the expression of CD62L by the CD4 T cells, however, that separates the helper T-cell population into two main functional groups: $CD4^+CD62L^-$ T cells that help B cells to differentiate, and $CD4^+CD62L^+$ T cells that are involved in other types of inducer functions (178,205). This relative loss of one of the CD4 T-cell subsets (inducer) and the relative excess of the other subset (helper) may account at least partially for the florid follicular hyperplasia and hypergammaglobulinemia that occurs in HIV-infected individuals (90,92,178,206).

The sinusoidal monocytoid B cells are polyclonal B cells (114). Interdigitating dendritic cells, as identified by immunostaining with antibodies to CD1 and S-100 protein, are increased in the paracortical regions of lymph nodes from HIV-infected patients (94,105,110,165,182,187, 191). These cells may be seen in clusters (104,105) or associated with cytoplasmic IgG-containing $CD38^+$ lymphocytes, immunoblasts, and plasma cells (182,191). This increase may be caused by an influx of interdigitating dendritic cells that present antigen to CD4 T cells (111,165,194). It is thought by some to indicate the continuous exposure of antigen to T cells that have lost the capacity of adequate responsiveness (165). This increase may not be caused by HIV infection itself but may be secondary to dermatopathic lymphadenopathy attributable to other HIV-related diseases such as dermatopathic Kaposi's sarcoma or HIV-related dermatitis (99,177,205). In addition, the number of natural killer cells and histiocytes usually are increased in the interfollicular areas of lymph nodes that exhibit HIV-related florid follicular hyperplasia (177,178,191). There is also an increase in the numbers of polyclonal plasma cells in the paracortex (191) and arborizing HLA-DR–, factor VIII–, and ulex-positive blood vessels (182,191).

Immunohistochemistry, *in situ* hybridization, and *in situ* hybridization PCR studies have helped localize HIV to specific areas and cells within lymph nodes exhibiting florid follicular hyperplasia. Immunohistochemical staining for the HIV p24 core protein shows a pattern of positive staining in the germinal center that parallels that of immunostaining for follicular dendritic cells using the anti-DRC-1 antibody (155,156,169,181,182,187,192,194,199,207). A similar pattern and intensity of reactivity in the germinal center can be seen using antibodies to HIV-related core and envelope antigens p15, p17, p18, and gp120 (156,165,187,192,194, 199). Immunostaining for gp41 in the germinal center, however, is somewhat less extensive and less intense (156,165,194). Immunostaining for HIV-related antigens outside of the germinal center shows scattered positive cells in the paracortical area, which occasionally are seen in a perivascular location (169). Furthermore, a few $p24^+$ and $gp41^+$ endothelial cells have been observed (165,169,182, 194). *In situ* hybridization studies for viral RNA, identifying cells that are infected productively, have demonstrated two patterns of reactivity in lymph nodes displaying HIV-related florid follicular hyperplasia: a diffuse or reticular pattern in the germinal centers (107,149,157,164,181,199,208), which is thought to correlate with the HIV particles present in the extracellular space between the follicular dendritic cells (107, 149,164, 208), and an intense, dot-like labeling of scattered individual cells in both the follicular and paracortical areas (107,157,164,165,181,194,199,208). In the majority of studies, the individual positive germinal center cells, which represent the actively replicating HIV-infected cells, have been found to be not follicular dendritic cells (149,164,208) but rather $CD4^+CD45RO^+CD57^+$ T cells (149,190,208). The scattered individual viral RNA–positive cells in the paracortical area appear to be CD4 T cells, S-100 protein–positive interdigitating dendritic cells, or rarely macrophages (149,208). In tonsils and benign lymphoepithelial cysts of the parotid salivary gland, the number of productively infected dendritic cells and macrophages, located primarily in and beneath the epithelium, is increased (208,209), and rare positive marginal sinus cells also have been identified using *in situ* hybridization (187). Although the number of productively infected cells appears to be relatively small as determined using *in situ* hybridization PCR, which identifies viral DNA, and limiting dilution assays, the number of latently infected cells is much higher (149,210). The latently infected CD4 T cells appear to be present most frequently in and around germinal centers and paracortical regions and around blood vessels (149). In addition, scattered latently infected monocytes and macrophages are also present (149).

Immunohistochemical staining of lymph nodes exhibiting mixed follicular hyperplasia and involution demonstrates a decrease in the number of and area covered by follicles, as seen by staining for follicular dendritic cells and B cells (105,191,204). In addition, there is often a decrease in the number and percentage of CD4 T cells and an increase in the number and percentage of CD8 T cells in the germinal centers, mantle zones, and interfollicular areas, compared with these same areas in lymph nodes exhibiting florid follicular hyperplasia attributable to HIV or other causes (105,191,204). Overall, the percentage of CD3 T cells is increased in the mixed follicular hyperplasia and involution pattern of HIV-related lymphadenopathy, compared with florid follicular hyperplasia (204).

In HIV-related lymph nodes exhibiting follicular involution, immunohistochemical studies show that the follicular remnants consist of only a small number of follicular dendritic cells present in small shrunken nests, associated with few, if any, IgM^+ B cells (94,104,105,133,191,192). The number of proliferating cells in the germinal center is low (105,187,192). The number of such lymph nodes containing plasma cells in the germinal centers is increased compared with HIV-related lymph nodes exhibiting florid follicular hyperplasia (192,207). In comparison with lymph nodes from both HIV-negative and HIV-positive individuals who exhibit follicular hyperplasia, the number of CD4 T cells is decreased and the number of CD8 T cells is increased within the germinal centers (187,191,192). $CD68^+$ macrophages also have been identified within the atrophic germinal centers (191). Furthermore, the expanded interfollicular region contains decreased numbers of T cells based on CD3 expression compared with HIV-negative individuals who have follicular hyperplasia (133). In addition, there is a relative depletion of CD4 T cells with increased or normal numbers of CD8 T cells (104,111,191) in the interfollicular area, leading to an inverted CD4:CD8 T-cell ratio that varies between 0.6 and 1.1 (133,183). Numerous $CD1^+$ or S-100 protein–positive interdigitating dendritic cells usually are identified, often in the subcapsular area of the paracortex (94,105,111). Histiocytes are present in increased number in the interfollicular area (133). Cytoplasmic immunoglobulin positive plasma cells are seen in aggregates and diffusely scattered throughout the lymph nodes but are most prominent in the medullary area; these cells usually contain polyclonal IgG and only rarely IgM (111,192). The number of $CD57^+$ natural killer cells is not increased over that in control subjects (133), but the number of $TIA\text{-}1^+$ $CD8^+$ cells in the interfollicular area is greater than that seen in lymph nodes from HIV-negative individuals (184).

Overall, the percentage of B cells, based on immunostaining for pan–B cell antigens or surface immunoglobulin, present in cases of follicular involution is approximately the same as in both the florid follicular hyperplasia and mixed follicular hyperplasia and involution patterns of HIV-related lymphadenopathy (106,192,211). Furthermore, based on morphometric studies, the total B-cell area does not decrease in follicular involution, because the B cells are often present in small clusters or scattered diffusely throughout the lymph nodes (192). In comparison with florid follicular hyperplasia, however, in which the B cells (follicle center cells) usually express CD10, the B cells present in follicular involution express only pan–B cell antigens or surface immunoglobulin (192). The overall percentage of T cells, based on CD3 expression, is somewhat increased; the overall percentage of $CD4^+$ cells is decreased or approximately the same (207,210,211) compared with that seen in florid follicular hyperplasia and mixed follicular hyperplasia and involution (192,211).

Viral proteins, as determined by immunohistochemical staining for the p17 and p24 gag proteins, have been identified in at least 80% of lymph nodes exhibiting follicular involution (194); however, the density of these viral proteins is less than in florid follicular hyperplasia (194). *In situ* hybridization for viral RNA shows that the majority of the cells with a positive signal are present in the interfollicular areas of the lymph node (157,194). The number of positive cells in the interfollicular areas is increased compared with that in patients showing florid follicular hyperplasia (157). Furthermore, in contrast with the predominently diffuse extracellular pattern of reactivity seen in the germinal centers of florid follicular hyperplasia and mixed follicular hyperplasia and involution, only scattered individual positive cells are identified by *in situ* hybridization in the atrophic follicles of follicular involution (212). There is an overall decrease in the number of productively infected cells per area compared with lymph nodes exhibiting florid follicular hyperplasia (170).

Immunohistochemical studies of lymph nodes exhibiting lymphocyte depletion reveal their lymphocyte-depleted state. Variable numbers of T cells are present, either scattered singly or in small groups (111). Most of them are CD8 T cells; CD4 T cells are virtually absent (104,111,210). Collections of B cells expressing pan–B cell markers or immunoglobulin are also present (104,111,194) and may be the predominant cell population (210). In some cases there are numerous polyclonal IgG^+ plasma cells, including those cells with Russell bodies (213). In others, the lymph nodes are characterized by fibrosis (213). Immunostaining with anti-DRC-1 demonstrates that virtually no follicular dendritic cells are present (111,156,212). Immunostaining for p17, p24, and gp41 HIV proteins identifies scattered positive cells in the interfollicular area (194); however, they are present in smaller numbers than in lymph nodes displaying florid follicular hyperplasia (194). *In situ* hybridization and *in situ* hybridization PCR studies show that lymphocyte depletion lymph nodes generally contain fewer HIV-positive cells than do lymph nodes that exhibit the other three patterns of HIV-related lymphadenopathy (170,214). The positive cells are dispersed throughout the lymph node but tend to be more concentrated near the subcapsular sinuses (214). Serial section immunostaining, *in situ* hybridization, and *in situ* hybridization PCR indicate that virutally all of the $CD4^+$ cells in lymphocyte depletion lymph nodes are infected productively with HIV (214), reflecting the CD4 T-cell and follicular dendritic cell loss characteristic of this stage.

Clinical Correlations

Relatively early in the AIDS epidemic it was realized that the incubation period between initial HIV infection and seroconversion and the development of AIDS can be quite long (215,216). The institution of antiretroviral therapy and the use of prophylactic medications for a variety of opportunistic infections has been changing the natural history of HIV-related disease (217). Because of these therapeutic advances, the time from seroconversion to the development of opportunistic infections and other HIV-related illnesses has and will continue to become even longer (217).

Between 40% and 90% of individuals who are acutely infected with HIV become clinically ill within days to weeks of their initial exposure (146,218). The most common symptoms are fever, fatigue, a maculopapular rash, myalgias, and, in up to 70% of patients, lymphadenopathy (218,219). Following infection, there is a rapid increase in plasma viremia, which results in dissemination of the virus to the lymphoid tissues (146,218). Dendritic cells are thought to be the initial cellular target of HIV, and lymphoid tissues such as tonsils and adenoids, which are rich in these cells, are thought to facilitate the transmission of the virus to the CD4 T cells (209,218). The virus is cleared from the blood relatively rapidly by cytotoxic T cells and by follicular dendritic cells that trap viral particles (146,218,219). After the acute infection stage, lymphoid tissue serves as the primary reservoir for HIV and as one of the principal sites for the progressive infection and death of CD4 T cells (149,157,158,210).

Following the initial acute illness, HIV-infected individuals are usually asymptomatic. Over time they develop a variety of symptoms such as fever, weight loss, diarrhea, and oral thrush (24,220) and deteriorate clinically, in parallel with a declining absolute CD4 T-cell count, a dropping CD4:CD8 T-cell ratio, and an increasing viral load in the peripheral blood (26, 32,219,221–224). Likewise, lymph node histology in HIV-related lymphadenopathy is progressive over the course of HIV-related disease (103,107,108, 157,204,225). As the lymph node histology progresses from florid follicular hyperplasia to mixed follicular hyperplasia and follicular involution, to follicular involution, and finally to lymphocyte depletion, there is a progressive loss of follicles and lymphocytes, which can be observed histologically and immunohistochemically. In addition, accompanying the progressive destruction of the follicles, there is a loss of viral trapping by the follicular dendritic cells, resulting in higher levels of circulating virus (146,157) and the redistribution of HIV outside of the lymphoid system (226). It appears that the baseline for this temporal progression is determined early in HIV infection by the level of viremia and CD4 T-cell count after the acute HIV infection stage (224). Specifically, patients who have higher plasma levels of virus and lower CD4 T-cell counts progress more rapidly to AIDS (218,224,227–229). It is believed that the natural course of the disease can be altered by lowering the viral load and raising the peripheral blood CD4 T-cell count with antiretroviral therapy (37,218,230).

That the histopathologic patterns in the lymph nodes of HIV-seropositive individuals are progressive and predictive of their clinical status was suggested by several studies (94,95,102,104,109,112,191,231). Only by examining multiple, sequential lymph node biopsy specimens obtained

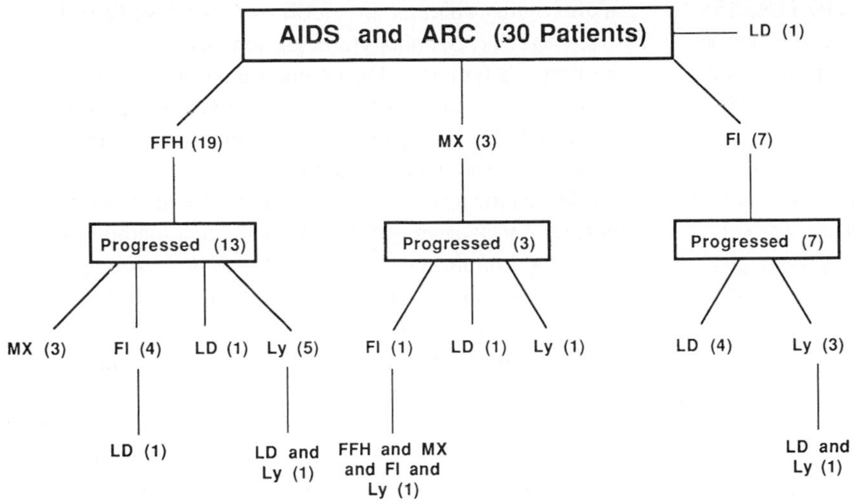

FIG. 28.15. Progression of lymph node histology in 30 patients who had AIDS and AIDS-related complex. (From Chadburn A, Metroka C, Mouradian J. Progressive lymph node histology and its prognostic value in patients with acquired immunodeficiency syndrome and AIDS-related complex. *Hum Pathol* 1989;20:579–587, with permission.)

from patients at risk for HIV infection, however, has it been shown definitively that, with only rare exceptions, lymph node histology changes over time in a consistent pattern, from florid follicular hyperplasia to mixed follicular hyperplasia and follicular involution, to follicular involution, to lymphocyte depletion (103,107,204,225) (Fig 28.15). The clinical course of the patients parallels this dynamic morphologic transformation, indicative of the prognostic significance of lymph node histopathology (107,108,191,204) (Table 28.10). Persons whose lymph nodes display florid follicular hyperplasia or mixed follicular hyperplasia and follicular involution appear to have the best prognosis (107,108,191); they do not appear to develop opportunistic infections or die as long as their lymph nodes display these early histologies. It appears that HIV-infected patients only develop many of the complications of AIDS after their lymph node histology has progressed to either follicular involution or lymphocyte depletion (107,191,231). No matter how long the lymph node pattern of florid follicular hyperplasia persists in an HIV-infected person, however, at some point the lymph node pattern changes, signaling progression of the disease (107,112). In the era before highly active antiretroviral therapy (HAART), for all patients who had persistent generalized lymphadenopathy, the incidence of AIDS increased after 3 years of lymphadenopathy, leading to a cumulative incidence progression to AIDS within 5 years of approximately 30% (232,233). For those patients who had no other symptoms except persistent generalized lymphadenopathy and who had CD4 T-cell counts greater than 400 per cubic millimeter, the 5-year incidence of developing AIDS was 19%, with none developing AIDS until the fourth year after the onset of lymphadenopathy (233). The lymph nodes of HIV-infected individuals diagnosed with AIDS usually show follicular involution or lymphocyte depletion, especially in those who have opportunistic infections. The impact of HAART on this time course of disease progression has yet to be determined.

It is often years before HIV-infected individuals whose lymph nodes display florid follicular hyperplasia progress histologically and clinically to AIDS. None of 57 HIV-infected persons who had florid follicular hyperplasia or mixed follicular hyperplasia and follicular involution histologies

TABLE 28.10. *Clinical correlations of progressive HIV-related lymphadenopathy*

	Number of patients	Persistent histology, n (%)	Progressive histology, n (%)	Developing opportunistic infections, % (mo)	Developing Ks, % (mo)	Developing lymphoma, % (mo)	Developing AIDS, % (mo)	Dead, % (mo)
ARC								
FFH	15	6 (40)	9 (60)	33 (69)	13 (5)	40 (67)	47 (24)	47 (34)
MX	5	1 (20)	4 (80)	40 (27)	0	40 (30)	80 (23)	80 (30)
FI	8	1 (13)	7 (83)	63 (5)	63 (4)	38 (34)	87 (3)	87 (7)
LD	7	NA	NA	86 (NA)	57 (NA)	29 (NA)	100 (NA)	100 (NA)
AIDS								
FFH	4	0 (0)	4 (100)	50 (20)	100 (NA)	25 (26)	NA	100 (22)
MX	1	1 (100)	0 (NA)	100 (19)	100 (NA)	0 (11)	NA	100 (30)
FI	4	1 (25)	3 (75)	75 (<6)	50 (NA)	50 (9)	NA	100 (11)
LD	3	NA	NA	100 (NA)	67 (NA)	0 (11)	NA	100 (<2)

ARC, AIDS-related Complex; FFH, florid follicular hyperplasia; FI, follicular involution; LD, lymphocyte depletion; MX, mixed follicular hyperplasia and follicular involution; NA, not applicable.

followed for 1 to 53 months developed AIDS (107,108,225). With longer clinical follow-up (up to 7.2 years after lymph node biopsy), however, 40% to 50% of those whose lymph nodes displayed florid follicular hyperplasia and 65% to 80% of those whose lymph nodes displayed mixed follicular hyperplasia and follicular involution progressed to AIDS (107,108). In addition, the patients whose lymph node histology indicated florid follicular hyperplasia had a median duration of survivial that varied from 30 to 54 months after lymph node biopsy, whereas the median survival was 30 to 35 months for those who had mixed follicular hyperplasia and follicular involution histology (107,108). The mixed follicular hyperplasia and follicular involution pattern most likely represents a transition from the immunosuppressed florid follicular hyperplasia stage to the immunodeficient follicular involution stage (94,97,107,234). Although most patients are not ill with full-blown AIDS, HIV-infected patients whose lymph nodes display florid follicular hyperplasia and mixed follicular hyperplasia and follicular involution histologies have decreased CD4:CD8 T-cell ratios in both the peripheral blood (0.2–1.0) and lymph nodes (0.4–3.7) (108,110–112,141,183,210,225). In patients with florid follicular hyperplasia, plasma viremia is at levels that are low or undetectable using coculture techniques (228). A significant amount of virus, however, is detected in the plasma by reverse transcriptase–PCR, although in general the viral load is less than in patients with follicular involution (210).

Histologic progression to follicular involution signals a marked change not only in histology, as evidenced by the loss of hyperplastic germinal centers that have become hyalinzed atrophic follicles, but also in the immunologic and clinical status of the HIV-infected person (107,108,112,210, 225). A significantly higher percentage of patients who are symptomatic (AIDS-related complex) have follicular involution rather than florid follicular hyperplasia or mixed follicular hyperplasia and follicular involution (104,107,112); the majority of the remaining patients with follicular involution, including 20% to 40% with opportunistic infections, has AIDS at the time of lymph node biopsy (102,104,107,112, 210,231,234). Immunologic studies indicate marked immunodeficiency with peripheral blood CD4:CD8 T-cell ratios lower than 0.5 (98,104,108,111,112,210,225) and absolute CD4 T-cell counts that average less than 400 per cubic millimeter and are frequently less than 200 per cubic millimeter (98,108,210,225). There is an increase in viral load in the peripheral blood during this stage (157). This plasma viremia is thought to be secondary to the loss of follicular dendritic cells, which trap HIV particles within germinal centers and thereby effectively remove virus from the circulation (146,157). It is also during this stage of histologic progression of HIV-related lymphadenopathy that HIV-infected individuals develop opportunistic infections, with 65% to 95% of patients developing an opportunistic infection a median of less than 1 year after a lymph node biopsy exhibiting follicular involution. The median duration of survival for patients with follicular involution is also less than 1 year (107,108). The lymphocyte depletion pattern is seen most commonly in lymph nodes obtained at autopsy but occasionally is seen in *ante mortem* lymph node biopsies as well (94,102,107,108,111,213). This pattern appears to reflect the near complete destruction of the immune system.

Although the development of opportunistic infections and length of survival are predicted by the histopathologic pattern of the lymph nodes, the development of Kaposi's sarcoma and malignant lymphoma are not (107). HIV-infected patients who develop Kaposi's sarcoma can exhibit any one of the four histologic patterns of HIV-related lymphadenopathy (94,98,107). Malignant lymphoma also has been identified in association with all four histologic patterns of HIV-related lymphadenopathy (103,107). Although HIV-seropositive patients who have Kaposi's sarcoma and florid follicular hyperplasia do not usually live as long as HIV-seropositive patients who have only florid follicular hyperplasia, they live nearly twice as long as those patients diagnosed with AIDS on the basis of an opportunistic infection (107). The immunologic status of AIDS patients who have florid follicular hyperplasia and Kaposi's sarcoma is more like that of HIV-infected individuals who have only florid follicular hyperplasia, as reflected by peripheral blood CD4:CD8 T-cell ratios of 0.7 and 0.5, respectively (98,101,116,210, 225). AIDS patients who have opportunistic infections and, therefore, usually follicular involution often have a CD4:CD8 T-cell ratio of less than 0.2 (210,235). Lymph node histology may be a more important prognostic indicator than the diagnosis of AIDS. The institution of HAART in the later stages of HIV disease, however, also can increase CD4 T-cell counts significantly and lower the viral load in both the peripheral blood and lymphoid tissues, resulting in at least partial reconstitution of the immune system (146,236–240) and potentially influencing the temporal progression of the disease and the histologic features of the lymph nodes.

OTHER HIV-ASSOCIATED LESIONS THAT MAY INVOLVE LYMPH NODES

Benign Lymphoepithelial Lesion

The benign lymphoepithelial lesion (BLEL) is a nodular or diffuse salivary gland enlargement characterized histologically by atrophy of salivary gland parenchyma, replacement of ducts by collections of epithelial and myoepithelial cells, and lymphocytic infiltration (241). It occurs most frequently in patients who have autoimmune diseases such as Sjögren's syndrome or as an isolated salivary gland lesion caused by periductal sialadenitis, localized autoimmune sialadenitis, or reactive lymphoid proliferation of intraglandular or periglandular lymph nodes (241) (see Chapter 30).

Salivary gland enlargement as a result of apparent BLEL first was recognized in HIV-infected individuals by Ryan and colleagues in 1985 (242). We now know that this lesion, designated *BLEL* by Smith and coworkers in 1988 (241), occurs in a small percentage of HIV-infected patients; its significance is unknown. Initially, it was hypothesized that HIV-associated BLELs are related to Sjögren's syndrome (243); however, HIV-infected patients who have this lesion lack the signs, symptoms and laboratory abnormalities of Sjögren's syndrome, including antinuclear SS-A and SS-B antibodies as well as rheumatoid factor (244–246). The BLELs occurring in association with HIV infection are bilateral, multiple, and cystic far more frequently than those occurring in Sjögren's syndrome (247); HIV-associated BLEL appears to represent a distinctive clinicopathologic subtype of BLEL related to HIV infection. Most investigators believe that HIV-associated BLELs actually arise in incompletely encapsulated intraglandular lymph nodes that contain salivary ducts or acinar inclusions. It is believed that the progressive lymphoid hyperplasia causes obstruction, squamous metaplasia, and cystification of the intranodal ductal structures, eventually resulting in the BLEL (241,245,248–250). According to this hypothesis, HIV-associated BLELs are a localized manifestation of persistent generalized lymphadenopathy. The presence of *EBER1* expression, indicative of latent Epstein-Barr virus (EBV) infection, in the lymphocyte nuclei of HIV-associated BLELs but not of Sjögren's syndrome–related or other BLELs has been cited in support of this hypothesis (251). Some authors have referred to HIV-associated BLELs as *cystic BLELs* (252,253) or prefer the term *benign lymphoepithelial cyst* (244,250,254) because of the prominent cyst formation in these cases and their distinction from the BLELs occurring in Sjögren's syndrome.

The gross specimens of HIV-associated BLELs are usually 2 to 5 cm in diameter and consist of one or multiple tan, fleshy, or rubbery nodules surrounded by varying amounts of salivary gland tissue. Multiple cysts ranging from a few millimeters to 3 centimeters and containing clear yellow to turbid, watery to gelatinous material are present within the nodules in many of the specimens (241,243,244,249) (Fig. 28.16). Stensen's duct is normal, without evidence of sialolithiasis or periductal fibrosis in most, if not all, patients (242,249).

Histologically, the nodules are partially to completely delimited by fibrous capsules, beneath which a peripheral sinus may be present focally (241,244). The nodules are comprised of masses of lymphoid tissue containing epithelial structures of presumed ductal origin embedded within them (241–243,249,252) (Fig. 28.17). The ducts often are dilated cystically and lined by cuboidal, columnar, or variably keratinized stratified squamous epithelium (241,242,244). The cysts contain pale, eosinophilic homogeneous material (244). Epimyoepithelial islands are present in the majority of patients (241,243–245,249,252). The lymphoid tissue usually exhibits the histologic features of HIV-related florid follicular hyperplasia: large, irregularly shaped hyperplastic follicles, mantle zone effacement, follicle lysis, interfollicular monocytoid B cells, and Warthin-Finkeldey cells (241,243,245,248,252) (Fig. 28.16). In occasional patients, the lymphoid tissue displays the small shrunken follicles and other histologic features of HIV-related follicular involution (241,242,244). Immunohistochemical studies demonstrate an increase in CD8 T cells, including their presence within germinal centers, and a decrease in CD4 T cells (245,252,255), similar to HIV-related benign lymphadenop-

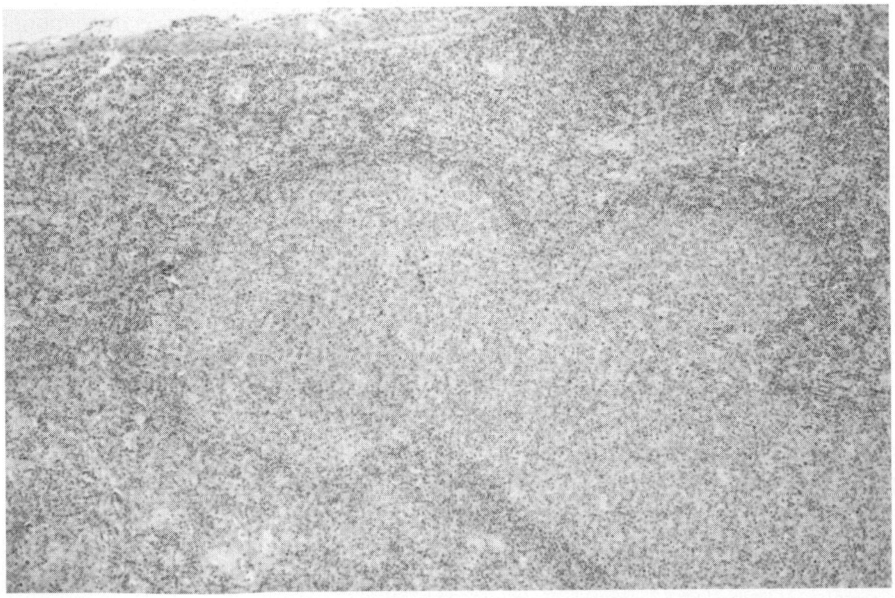

FIG. 28.16. HIV-related benign lymphoepithelial lesion. This lesion contained a grossly visible cyst. The squamous epithelial lining of this cyst is evident in the upper lefthand corner. The lymphoid tissue within this lesion exhibits the histopathologic changes seen in HIV-related florid follicular hyperplasia. A large hyperplastic follicle is present (hematoxylin and eosin stain, original magnification: 63× magnification).

A

B

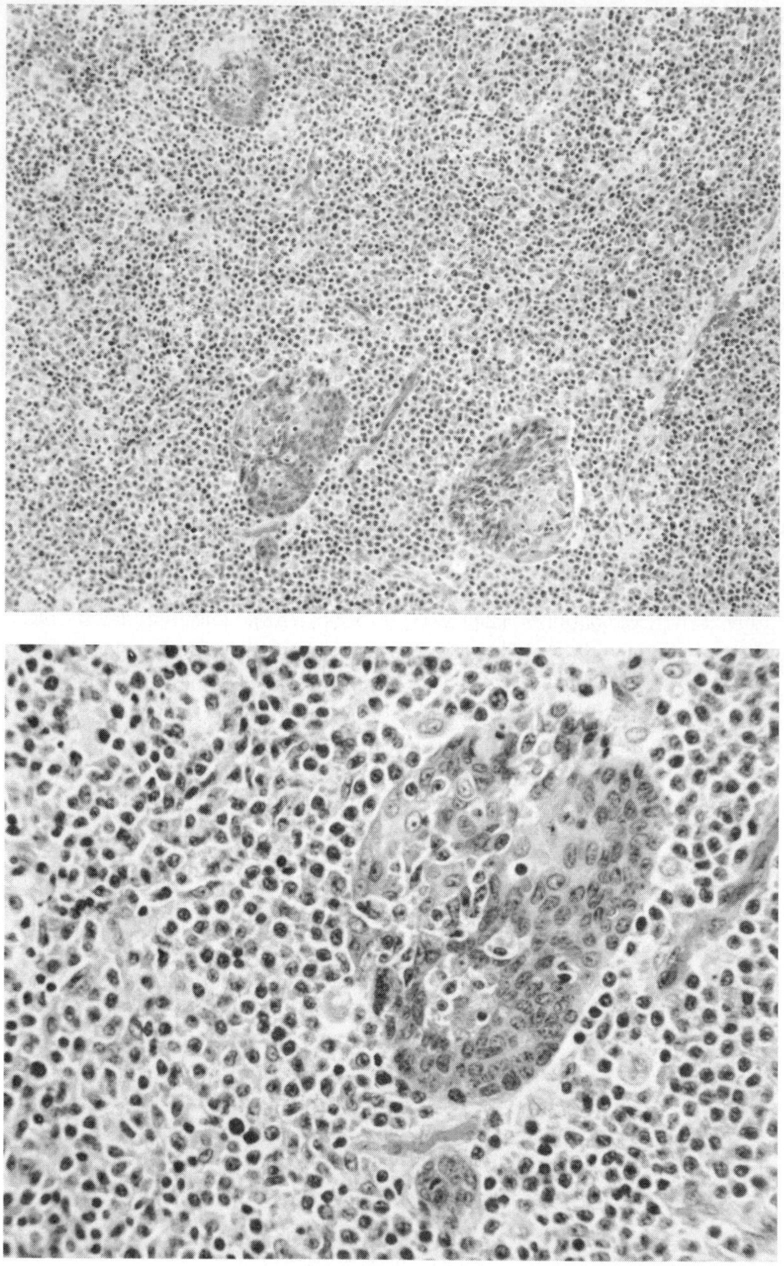

FIG. 28.17. HIV-related benign lymphoepithelial lesion. **A:** Numerous epithelial structures are present within the lymphoid tissue (hematoxylin and eosin stain, original magnification: 100× magnification). **B:** Higher magnification shows this ductular inclusion, which has undergone squamous metaplasia and is infiltrated by small lymphocytes (hematoxylin and eosin stain, original magnification: 250× magnification).

athy (94,110,116,178,191). In addition, CD8 T cells predominate within the epimyoepithelial islands (245). This is in contrast with Sjögren's syndrome, in which CD4 T cells predominate (256). The adjacent salivary gland tissue is usually unremarkable, except for interstitial and periductal lymphoid infiltration that appears to represent expansion of the lymphoid cell population and extension through capsular defects (241,245). The intraglandular and periglandular lymph nodes in BLELs exhibit histologic features identical to those of the lymphoid tissue comprising the BLEL nodules (241).

Virtually all the patients who develop HIV-related BLELs are adults, predominantly men and mostly IDUs, with an average age in the late thirties (241,244,246,247,249,257). Members of all AIDS risk groups (241,247,249,257,258), however, apparently even children born to HIV-infected women (259), may develop BLELs. The patients are usually in the early stages of HIV infection, possess CD4 T-cell counts greater than 200 per microliter, and only rarely have received a prior diagnosis of AIDS (241,247,249,257). BLELs often are the initial manifestation of HIV infection in these individuals (241,249). The patients are usually asymptomatic except for dull aching pain and mild tenderness in the affected area (244,246,247,257). The HIV-infected individuals described as having persistent generalized lymphadenopathy, salivary gland lymphocytic infiltration, and the sicca complex (260,261) likely have the CD8 lymphocytosis syndrome described by Itescu and colleagues

(262,263), and not HIV-associated BLELs. Patients usually complain of unilateral or sometimes bilateral parotid salivary gland enlargement (241,244,249,264,265). Computed tomographic and magnetic resonance imaging demonstrate multiple intraparotid cystic lesions bilaterally, accompanied in the majority of patients by bilateral cervical lymphadenopathy (264,265). The submandibular and submaxillary glands also may be involved (241–243,249,252). Salivary gland enlargement usually evolves slowly, often over 1 to 4 years (241,249). The majority of the patients have the persistent generalized lymphadenopathy syndrome as well (241,243,245,249), and BLELs develop and persist concurrently with persistent generalized lymphadenopathy in most of them.

A uniform set of recommendations concerning the management of HIV-associated BLELs has not been accepted universally. Superficial parotidectomy (246) or local excision of the lesions (257), which predominantly are located in the tail of the parotid gland (244,257), has been recommended to exclude malignant lymphoma unequivocally and to provide cosmetic improvement and pain relief to the patient. These patients appear to have an indolent clinical course, however. In the largest series with long-term follow-up, almost 50% of patients developed AIDS, at a median interval of 4 years following the diagnosis of HIV-associated BLELs (247). Very few patients develop AIDS-defining conditions within the first 2 years following diagnosis of BLELs (241,242,244,246,247,249). For this reason, observation and periodic fine needle aspiration biopsy has been advocated in the diagnosis and management of asymptomatic lesions that are cosmetically acceptable (247,249). Zidovudine therapy may be helpful in some instances (247). Even if surgically excised, these lesions may recur on the same or on the opposite side (247,248). Malignant lymphoma, and rarely even Kaposi's sarcoma, may originate or present within an HIV-associated BLEL (244,248; Knowles, unpublished observations).

Kaposi's Sarcoma

Between the time of its discovery by Moritz Kaposi in 1872 (266), and the recognition of its epidemic spread among homosexual men in the early 1980s heralding the AIDS epidemic (2,4,267), Kaposi's sarcoma largely was considered an enigmatic dermatologic curiosity whose incidence and natural history varied geographically (268,269). Four clinicoepidemiologic forms of Kaposi's sarcoma are now recognized. These are classic Mediterranean Kaposi's sarcoma, which occurs rarely in elderly individuals, predominantly men, of Mediterranean and Eastern Europe descent, in whom it usually exhibits benign, indolent clinical behavior; endemic African Kaposi's sarcoma, which occurs frequently in HIV-uninfected patients in equatorial Africa, in whom it often exhibits aggressive clinical behavior; iatrogenic Kaposi's sarcoma, which occurs relatively frequently in solid organ transplant recipients, in whom it often undergoes spontaneous regression following the withdrawal of immunosuppressive therapy (268,269); and AIDS epidemic Kaposi's sarcoma, which is a defining condition for the diagnosis of AIDS (61,62) and the most common neoplasm occurring in HIV-infected individuals (270), in whom it often behaves aggressively (270,271). The many special clinical, epidemiologic, and pathologic peculiarities of Kaposi's sarcoma have led to significant debate concerning its cell of origin, its hyperplastic versus neoplastic nature, and its cause, infectious or otherwise (268,269,272–275).

Patients in all AIDS risk groups possess an extraordinary risk of developing Kaposi's sarcoma. One to three percent of HIV-infected transfusion recipients and IDUs present with Kaposi's sarcoma, and female and heterosexual males who have AIDS have a 10,000-fold increase in the incidence of Kaposi's sarcoma relative to the general population. The risk of developing Kaposi's sarcoma in HIV-infected MSM is astronomic. The incidence of Kaposi's sarcoma in MSM who have an initial AIDS diagnosis other than Kaposi's sarcoma is increased 73,000-fold compared with the general population (270). In recent years, 15% to 20% of MSM who develop AIDS have presented with Kaposi's sarcoma (276). The significantly higher Kaposi's sarcoma risk in MSM initially was thought to be related to environmental or genetic factors (269). It is more likely, however, that the higher Kaposi's sarcoma risk in this population is because of the preferential or enhanced transmission of an infectious agent, such as KSHV, among this AIDS risk group because of certain sexual practices, especially those involving orofecal contact.

AIDS epidemic Kaposi's sarcoma exhibits a variable clinical course, ranging from minimal disease presenting as an incidental finding and exhibiting slow progression over many years to the explosive onset of widespread, rapidly progressive disease resulting in significant injury and mortality rate (271). During the past decade, AIDS epidemic Kaposi's sarcoma has shifted progressively from being an index diagnosis for AIDS to being an opportunistic neoplasm occurring later in the course of the disease and resulting in enhanced morbidity and mortality rates (271). Both corticosteroid therapy and opportunistic infections have been associated with the *de novo* appearance of Kaposi's sarcoma and with the exacerbation of preexisting Kaposi's sarcoma in HIV-infected persons (271,277). The most frequent site of involvement is the skin (267,271); although lesions can occur anywhere, they are concentrated on the face, genitalia, and lower extremities in many patients (271). Extracutaneous spread of AIDS epidemic Kaposi's sarcoma, however, is very common (274,278). The oral cavity, especially the palate and gingiva, frequently is involved (271,279). Pulmonary and gastrointestinal tract involvement are also quite common; the latter is highly associated with oral Kaposi's sarcoma and is detectable in 40% of patients who have Kaposi's sarcoma at initial diagnosis and in as many as 80% at autopsy (271). Both may occur in the absence of mucocutaneous disease (271). No organ has been spared from involvement by AIDS epidemic Kaposi's sarcoma. Investigators have described invasion by Kaposi's sarcoma into solid organs such as the heart, liver, pancreas, testis, and bone marrow (274), and metastasis to the brain (280). Extracutaneous involvement by AIDS epidemic Kaposi's sarcoma ranges from a solitary small nodule to multiple, variably sized nodules, to a large confluent hemorrhagic tumor mass of 10 cm or even greater in size (274).

Lymph node involvement by AIDS epidemic Kaposi's sarcoma is also common and may occur in the absence of mucocutaneous disease (271). AIDS epidemic Kaposi's sarcoma may occur in benign lymph nodes exhibiting any of the histopathologic patterns: florid follicular hyperplasia, mixed follicular hyperplasia and involution, follicular involution, or lymphocyte depletion (91,94,98,107,125–130,281,282), as well as in lymph nodes containing malignant lymphoma (283). Early in the clinical course, lymph nodes involved by AIDS epidemic Kaposi's sarcoma are usually between 1 and 2 cm in diameter and are discrete, mobile, firm or fleshy, and nontender (284). On cross-section, foci of purple or red-brown discoloration as well as firm, white to tan areas sometimes are grossly discernible (125,129). Early lesions as well as small foci of involvement usually are seen in or adjacent to the capsule, in the hilum, or occasionally in the perinodal adipose tissue (91,94,99,125,129,282) (Fig. 28.18). Diagnosis of these early lesions and small foci of Kaposi's sarcoma can be difficult, especially if they involve only the pericapsular tissue. They can be overlooked easily or may be dismissed as areas of fibrosis (94). Late in the clinical course, lymph nodes involved by AIDS epidemic Kaposi's sarcoma may appear grossly as hemorrhagic tumors measuring several centimeters in diameter (274).

AIDS epidemic Kaposi's sarcoma generally is histopathologically indistinguishable from the other clinicoepidemiologic forms of the disease (285). Kaposi's sarcoma is comprised of a variable mixture of ectatic, irregularly shaped, round capillary and slit-like endothelial-lined vascular spaces and spindle-shaped cells accompanied by a variable mixed mononuclear inflammatory cell infiltrate. The endothelial cells may be thin and spindle-shaped or oval to round. They generally lack cytologic atypia and mitotic activity. Erythrocytes and hemosiderin pigment are frequently present, often extravasated between the spindle cells. Small refractile, eosinophilic, hyaline globules that stain with the periodic acid–Schiff stain, representing the breakdown products of phagocytosed erythrocytes, may be present extracellularly or within macrophages (Fig. 28.19). The earliest patch and plaque stage lesions sometimes may be difficult to distinguish from granulation tissue. The spindle cells increasingly become the predominant cell population, forming fascicles that compress the vascular slits, and the lesions may progress to form nodules and tumors. The latter consist primarily of interwoven fascicles of spindle cells displaying prominent cytologic atypia, numerous mitotic figures, and often striking pleomorphism (94,99,125,285,286). The histogenesis of the spindle cell component of Kaposi's sarcoma, believed to be the ''tumor cell,'' has been controversial (269). Most investigators now favor a vascular endothelial cell origin for the spindle cells as well as the vascular lining cells of Kaposi's sarcoma (287–289).

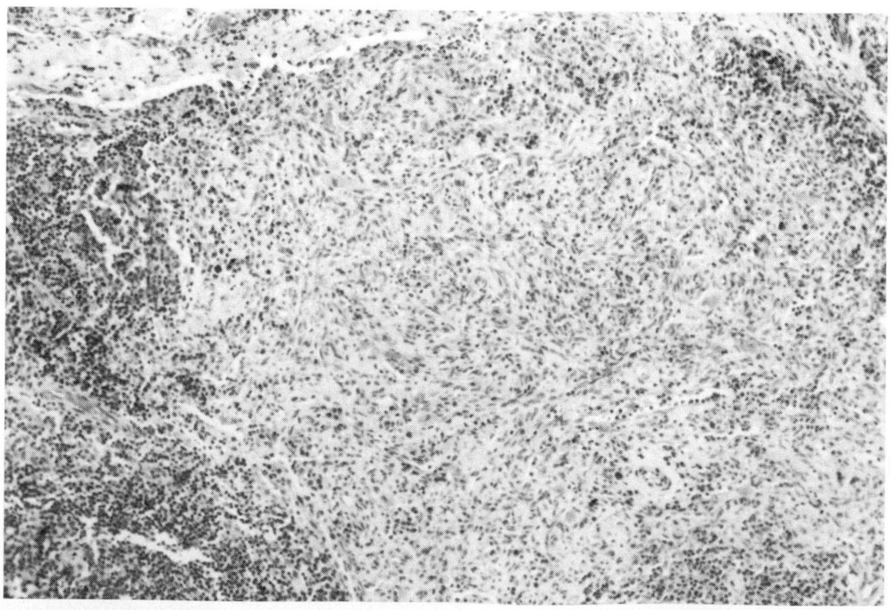

FIG. 28.18. Lymphadenopathic Kaposi's sarcoma. The peripheral subcapsular area of this lymph node is replaced by Kaposi's sarcoma (hematoxylin and eosin stain, original magnification: 100× magnification). (From Knowles DM, Chadburn A. The neoplasms associated with AIDS. In: Joshi VV, ed. *Pathology of AIDS and other manifestations of HIV infection.* New York: Igaku-Shoin, 1990:83–120, with permission.)

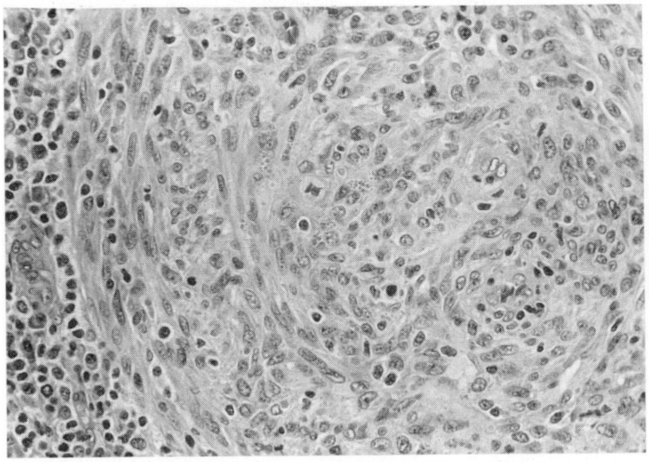

FIG. 28.19. Lymphadenopathic Kaposi's sarcoma. The lesion is comprised of a variable mixture of ectatic, irregularly shaped, round capillary and slit-like endothelial-lined vascular spaces and spindle-shaped cells accompanied by a variable mixed mononuclear inflammatory cell infiltrate. The endothelial cells may be thin and spindle-shaped or oval to round. They generally lack cytologic atypia and mitotic activity. Erythrocytes and hemosiderin pigment are frequently present, often extravasated between the spindle cells. Small refractile, eosinophilic, hyaline globules that stain with the periodic acid–Schiff stain, representing the breakdown products of phagocytosed erythrocytes, may be present extracellularly or with macrophases (hematoxylin and eosin stain, original magnification: 250× magnification).

Extracutaneous Kaposi's sarcoma may differ slightly histologically from and may exhibit a different developmental chronology than cutaneous Kaposi's sarcoma (285). The earliest histopathologic changes in lymph nodes involved by Kaposi's sarcoma are those that have been referred to as *hypervascular follicular hyperplasia* (290). Vascular channels within the lymph node are prominent, increased in number, and associated with increased numbers of plasma cells (291). Over time, these areas may develop the classical histopathologic features of Kaposi's sarcoma, including interwoven fascicles of spindle cells, vascular slits and extravasated erythrocytes (285,291). Kaposi's sarcoma involving lymph nodes extends along the sinusoids, infiltrates the interfollicular areas (125,282), and eventually may replace the entire lymph node (91,94).

A considerable body of clinical observations and epidemiologic data suggests that Kaposi's sarcoma has an infectious cause and is spread most frequently by sexual transmission of this infectious agent to an immunocompromised host (268,269,292,293). Herpes-type virus particles were identified electron microscopically in cultured cells derived from Kaposi's sarcoma lesions in African patients as early as 1972 (294). No known organism, however, including all those previously suspected of being the causal agent of Kaposi's sarcoma, had been shown to be associated causally with Kaposi's sarcoma (268,269). In search of the elusive cause of Kaposi's sarcoma, Chang and collaborators (295) utilized representational difference analysis to identify unique nonhuman, herpesvirus-like DNA sequences in a Kaposi's sarcoma lesion obtained from a homosexual man who had died from AIDS (296). They showed that these sequences belong to a novel, previously unidentified herpesvirus exhibiting homology with herpesvirus saimiri and EBV (296–299). They named the virus descriptively *Kaposi's sarcoma–associated herpesvirus* (296); this agent also has been designated *human herpesvirus-8* (297). We now know that KSHV is a transmissable, B-cell lymphotropic herpesvirus belonging to the $\gamma 2$ sublineage (genus *Rhadinovirus*) of the *Gammaherpesvirinae* subfamily (297–300), organisms of which are characterized by their ability to replicate in lymphoblastoid cells (301) (Fig. 28.20). This virus exhibits extensive sequence and positional homology and colinearity with herpesvirus saimiri (298), which appears to represent its closest relative. KSHV is detectable by PCR in virtually all Kaposi's sarcoma lesions occurring in more than 90% of individuals who have any of the four clinicoepidemiologic forms of the disease (297) (Fig. 28.21). The DNA sequence of KSHV appears to be highly conserved among these samples, suggesting that similar KSHV strains are present in Kaposi's sarcoma lesions worldwide. KSHV can be visualized in the nuclei of the spindle cells and the flat vascular lining cells of Kaposi's sarcoma lesions by *in situ* techniques (302,303). Furthermore, KSHV is absent, according to most studies, from the wide array of vascular tumors and inflammatory conditions that resemble Kaposi's sarcoma in their cellular composition (296,297,304). Further support for a causal relationship between KSHV and Kaposi's sarcoma comes from studies showing that the presence of KSHV DNA sequences

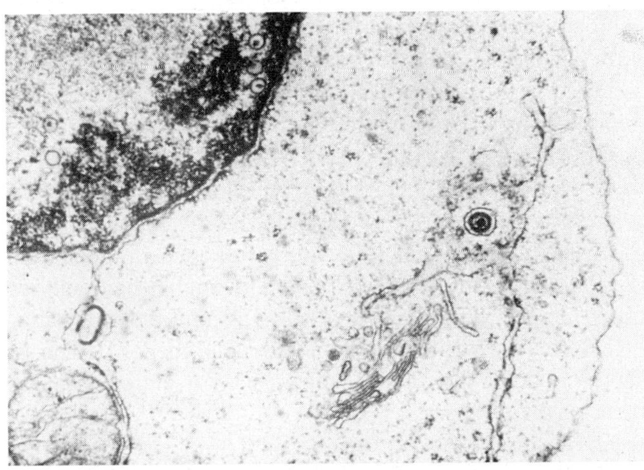

FIG. 28.20. Kaposi's sarcoma–associated herpesvirus (human herpesvirus-8). A primary effusion lymphoma cell containing nuclear capsids and a cytoplasmic virion within the dilated endoplasmic reticulum (uranyl acetate, lead acetate stain, original magnification: 44,000× magnification). (From Said JW, Chien K, Takeuchi S, et al. Kaposi's sarcoma-associated herpesvirus (KSHV or HHV-8) in primary effusion lymphoma: ultrastructural demonstration of herpesvirus in lymphoma cells. *Blood* 1996;87:4937–4943.)

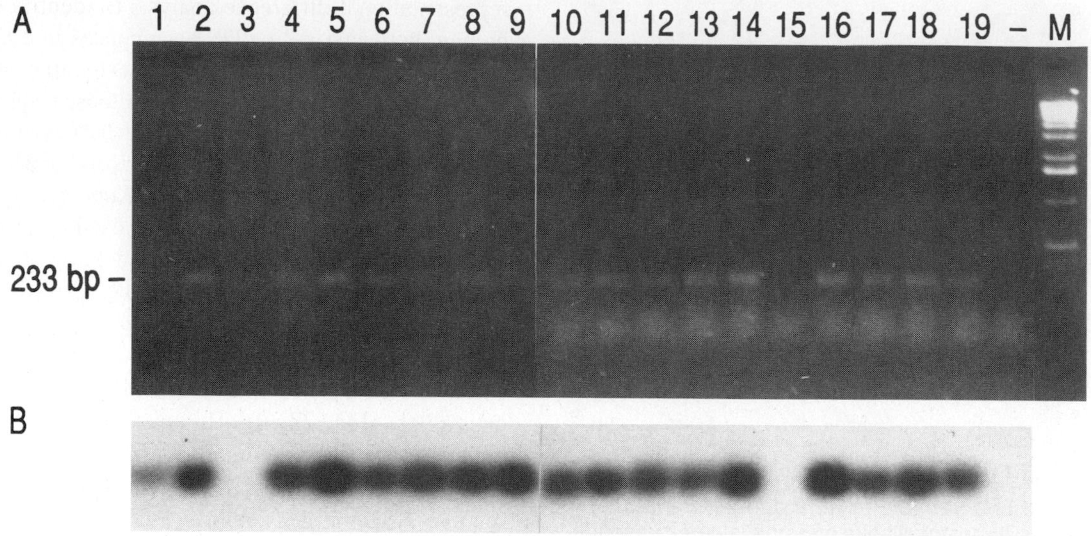

FIG. 28.21. Detection of Kaposi's sarcoma–associated herpesvirus (human herpesvirus-8) in Kaposi's sarcoma by polymerase chain reaction. The numbers above each lane indicate the number of the case. Lane 20 is a negative control, and *M* refers to a molecular size marker. **A:** Agarose gel of the amplification products from 19 Kaposi's sarcoma samples (lanes 1–19). **B:** Hybridization of the polymerase chain reaction products to a 32p end-labeled 25–base pair internal oligonucleotide after transfer of the gel to a nitrocellulose filter. All samples were positive for Kaposi's sarcoma–associated herpesvirus (human herpesvirus-8) except for cases 3 and 15, which lacked microscopically detectable Kaposi's sarcoma. (From Chang Y, Cesarman E, Pessin MS, et al. Identification of herpesvirus-like DNA sequences in AIDS-associated Kaposi's sarcoma. *Science* 1994;266:1865–1869, with permission.)

in the peripheral blood often antedates, and may predict, the subsequent development of Kaposi's sarcoma (305,306). Seroconversion to positivity for antibodies against KSHV-related nuclear antigens has been found to occur before the clinical appearance of Kaposi's sarcoma in a significant proportion of patients who have AIDS-related Kaposi's sarcoma (307). Finally, KSHV cyclin D and G protein–coupled receptor cellular gene homologues, which appear to represent viral oncogenes, are expressed at the RNA level in Kaposi's sarcoma lesions (299). KSHV, which appears to be oncogenic, almost definitely represents the elusive, long-sought agent causing Kaposi's sarcoma and very likely plays a role in its pathogenesis. The development of Kaposi's sarcoma is probably a multistep process that involves the interplay of KSHV with impaired immune surveillance, immune stimulation, and multiple genetic, environmental, behavioral, and other factors. The discovery of KSHV and the elucidation of its precise role in the complex development of Kaposi's sarcoma should facilitate the diagnosis, prevention and treatment of the disease.

KSHV also is consistently present in a specific type of NHL designated *primary effusion lymphoma*, which occurs principally, but not exclusively, in patients who have AIDS (297), as well as in a significant proportion of cases of AIDS-related and non–AIDS-related multicentric Castleman's disease (136,138,297).

Opportunistic Infections

Various opportunistic infectious agents have been identified within the lymph nodes of HIV-infected patients (94,141,278,281,282). Among the most common infectious agents are *M. avium complex*, *Cryptococcus neoformans*, *Histoplasmosis capsulatum*, and cytomegalovirus. Many other organisms may be seen (94,99,141,278,281,282). Opportunistic infections are identified in approximately 5% of lymph nodes from HIV-infected persons who have persistent generalized lymphadenopathy and who undergo lymph node biopsy (308). If tissue biopsy and cytology specimens from all sites are evaluated, approximately 42% of HIV-seropositive patients are diagnosed with opportunistic infections prior to death (281). Autopsy studies indicate that up to 95% of the AIDS population has at least one opportunistic infection at death (280,309). The development of opportunistic infections occurs relatively late in the course of HIV infection, when the patients usually have CD4 T-cell counts lower than 400 per microliter and CD4:CD8 T-cell ratios lower than 0.5 (98,104,111,112,235). In addition, there frequently is clinical regression of the lymphadenopathy 6 to 11 months before the diagnosis of an opportunistic infection (90). Histologically, the lymph nodes in the areas not replaced by organisms usually exhibit either the follicular involution or lymphocyte depletion pattern (91,102,107,112). Prior to the HAART era, patients who developed an opportunistic infection, whether in a lymph node or elsewhere in the body, had a median duration of survival of approximately 1 year (97,101).

Grossly, the lymph nodes may be enlarged (94,102) and may be necrotic (94). Histologically, lymph nodes involved by acid-fast bacilli or fungus usually contain poorly formed granulomas consisting of poorly defined collections of histiocytes possessing relatively abundant eosinophilic cytoplasm that, in heavy infections, may replace the entire lymph node (99,309). Granulomas with multinucleated giant cells, palisading histiocytes, caseous necrosis, and other characteristic tissue responses to mycobacteria or fungi occasionally are seen but usually are absent (104,309). Fungal organisms often can be identified on routine tissue sections, with or without a granulomatous response. Special stains, such as gomori-methanimine-silver, periodic acid–Schiff, and mucicarmine, highlight their presence. Cytomegalovirus inclusions also can be identified within lymph nodes, often within endothelial cells (104,141,309).

It appears that the natural history of at least some opportunistic infections, including their clinical presentation and possibly the histopathologic appearance of the involved lymph nodes, is impacted substantially by HAART (217). It was found recently that within a few weeks of initiation of HAART some patients who have extremely low CD4 T-cell counts develop fever and lymphadenopathy in the setting of a substantial increase in the CD4 T-cell count and a decrease in the viral load (240,310,311). Lymph node biopsies in these patients, many of whom have no prior history of *M. avium complex*, show the presence of granulomatous inflammation consisting primarily of histiocytes accompanied by a variable number of acute and chronic inflammatory cells (240,310,311). Some of these lymph nodes contain many acid-fast bacilli; others do not. This onset of symptomatic *M. avium complex* infection in patients with improved CD4 T-cell counts is thought to be a result of HAART-induced immunorestoration, which results in an inflammatory response to a previously clinically silent infectious organism (217,240,311). A similar phenomenon has been described in cytomegalovirus-related retinitis (217,238). How HAART impacts other opportunistic infections, particularly with respect to the presentation and histopathology of opportunistic infection-related lymphadenopathy, has not yet been delineated.

Bacillary Angiomatosis

Bacillary angiomatosis is an uncommon pseudoneoplastic vasoproliferative disorder with an infectious cause. It first was recognized in 1983 by Stoler and colleagues (312), who observed in an HIV-seropositive man bacteria within subcutaneous lesions that mimicked Kaposi's sarcoma. Four years later, unaware of Stoler's report, Cockerell and coworkers (313) described the same lesions but failed to recognize their infectious nature, designating them "epithelioid angiomatosis," emphasizing their distinction from Kaposi's sarcoma. LeBoit and colleagues (314) identified the relationship between these lesions and a cat-scratch disease bacillus–like organism in 1988. One year later they defined the entity histopathologically and coined the term *bacillary angiomatosis* to reflect the infectious and proliferative nature of the lesions (315). This term has been accepted generally as the preferred designation.

Bacillary angiomatosis occurs primarily in HIV-infected individuals (312–317) but has been described in other immunocompromised individuals, including organ transplant recipients (318–320) and individuals who have an underlying malignancy (321–323), and rarely in some apparently healthy immunocompetent hosts (324–327). Bacillary angiomatosis results from infection by *Bartonella henselae* and *B. quintana* (318,328,329), small gram-negative bacilli previously classified among the genus *Rochalimaea* (330). These and other organisms belonging to this genus have been associated with an array of diseases besides bacillary angiomatosis, including bacillary peliosis of the liver and spleen, a bacteremic syndrome, cat-scratch disease, and trench fever (331). Bacillary peliosis hepatis and splenis are now believed to represent visceral manifestations of bacillary angiomatosis (332). The domestic cat is a reservoir for *B. henselae* (333,334); as many as 40% of cats have been documented to be bacteremic with this organism (334). Exposure to cats and a history of a cat scratch or bite is associated with a significant proportion, although not all, of the cases of bacillary angiomatosis (331,335).

Cutaneous disease is the most frequent clinical manifestation of bacillary angiomatosis (312–315,323,324,327,331, 335). Patients usually have multiple and sometimes large numbers, greater than 1,000, of variably sized, superficial, cutaneous red to purple or flesh-colored papules that may mimic pyogenic granulomas and dermal and subcutaneous nodules that may be misinterpreted as Kaposi's sarcoma (312–315,331). Indurated hyperpigmented plaque-like lesions also have been described (336). An occasional patient, especially one who is immunocompetent, may have a solitary or only a few skin lesions (324,327,337,338). The lesions may occur anywhere on the skin surface including on the scalp (338), the palmar and plantar surfaces (334) and the penis (339). They range from 1 mm to several centimeters in diameter. The lesions may be tender or even painful and tend to bleed (331,336). Usually, they increase rapidly in size and number (313,331,336); rarely, they may undergo spontaneous regression (313). Patients often have associated constitutional signs and symptoms, such as fever, chills, malaise, headache, and anorexia, sometimes accompanied by weight loss (317,331,336).

Cutaneous bacillary angiomatosis may be accompanied by mucosal and visceral involvement. Conversely, extracutaneous bacillary angiomatosis often is accompanied by multiple cutaneous lesions, although it may occur in the absence of skin involvement (331). For example, approximately 20% of patients present with lymphadenopathy alone (340). The gastrointestinal and respiratory mucosal surfaces (313,317, 341–345) and most organ systems have been reported to be involved by bacillary angiomatosis. These include the heart (346), liver and spleen (317–319,325,347,348), bone marrow and lymph nodes (317–320,349–352), bones (316), muscles and soft tissues (317,351), female genital tract (353), and even CNS (317,354). Patients with extracutaneous disease usually have constitutional symptoms, including fever, anorexia, nausea, vomiting, and weight loss (316,331,340,352). They usually suffer from marked immu-

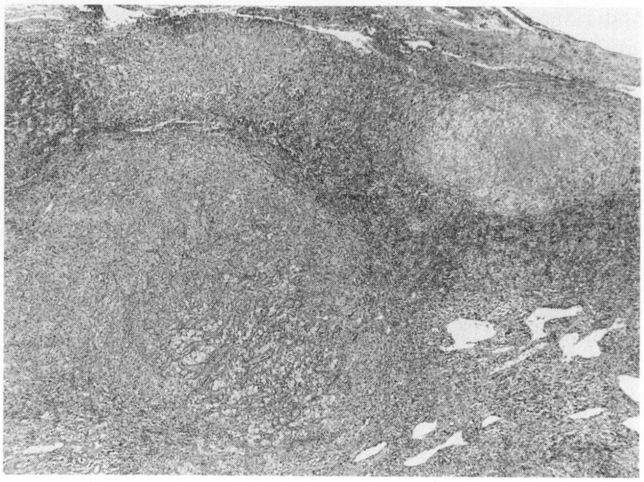

FIG. 28.22. Bacillary angiomatosis. Lymph node containing the variably sized nodular proliferations of small blood vessels typical of bacillary angiomatosis (hematoxylin and eosin stain, original magnification: 100× magnification). (Courtesy of Dr. John Chan, Queen Elizabeth Hospital, Hong Kong.)

nodeficiency, manifested by severely depressed CD4 T-cell counts (340); some patients have concomitant AIDS-associated opportunistic infections (316,331,340,343,348,353). These findings suggest that bacillary angiomatosis occurs late in the course of HIV infection, and consequently it has been suggested that bacillary angiomatosis should be considered an AIDS-defining opportunistic infection (340). There does not appear to be a predominant AIDS risk factor among individuals who have bacillary angiomatosis (313,340).

The peripheral, mediastinal, and abdominal lymph nodes are the ones most commonly involved by bacillary angiomatosis (317,352). The involved lymph nodes usually are enlarged, firm in consistency, and pale brown to red brown in color (320). Bacillary angiomatosis involves lymph nodes as discrete variably sized nodules, some of which may coalesce to form large masses. The underlying lymph node architecture may survive intact (320) (Fig. 28.22). Cutaneous and extracutaneous bacillary angiomatosis are essentially identical histopathologically. Bacillary angiomatosis characteristically is comprised of variably sized, circumscribed lobules of small blood vessels, some well formed, some barely canalized, and some ectatic, that are situated in an alternately mucinous and fibrotic stroma. The vessels are lined by protuberant, plump, polygonal endothelial cells that contain abundant pale cytoplasm, and ovoid nuclei containing one to several small nucleoli. They sometimes exhibit mild nuclear pleomorphism and mitotic figures. Occasional polygonal cells exhibiting similar cytologic features, and probably also of endothelial origin, lie between the vesssels. Aggregates of granular acidophilic to amphophilic material, which represent clumps and tangled masses of the causative bacteria, lie in the interstitium separating the vessels. Numerous neutrophils, accompanied by leukocytoclastic debris (''nuclear dust''), usually are scattered throughout the lesions and frequently aggregate around the bacterial clumps (312,313,315, 320,323,331,342,351,353) (Fig. 28.23).

The bacteria can be visualized with the Warthin-Starry stain (Fig. 28.24) but not with Gram's, methenamine silver, periodic acid–Schiff, or Ziehl-Neelsen stains (312,314,315, 320). Electron microscopy can be used to identify the bacteria, which are located extracellularly and exhibit an electron dense core surrounded by a trilaminar cell wall (312,314,320,351), characteristic of gram-negative bacilli. *B. henselae* and *B. quintana* are fastidious organisms. They

A

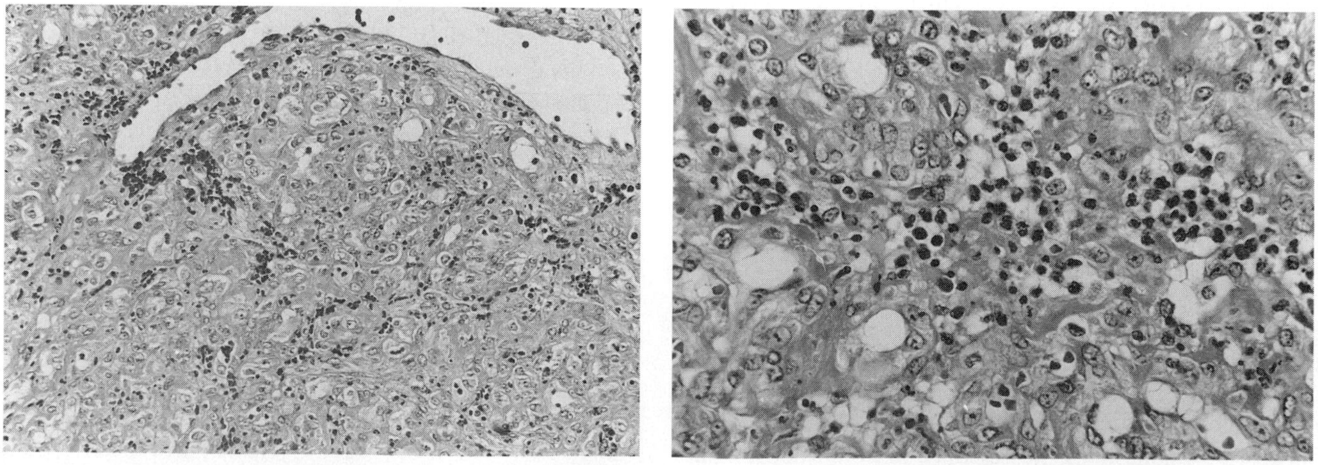

B

FIG. 28.23. Bacillary angiomatosis. **A:** Bacillary angiomatosis characteristically is comprised of variably sized, circumscribed lobules of small blood vessels, some well formed, some barely canalized, and some ectatic chemotoxylin and eosin stain, original magnification: 250× magnification. **B:** The vessels are lined by protuberant, plump, polygonal endothelial cells with abundant pale cytoplasm and ovoid nuclei containing one to several small nucleoli. Numerous neutrophils usually are scattered throughout the lesion, frequently aggregated around clumps of the causative bacteria (hematoxylin and eosin stain, original magnification: 400× magnification). (Courtesy of Dr. John Chan, Queen Elizabeth Hospital, Hong Kong.)

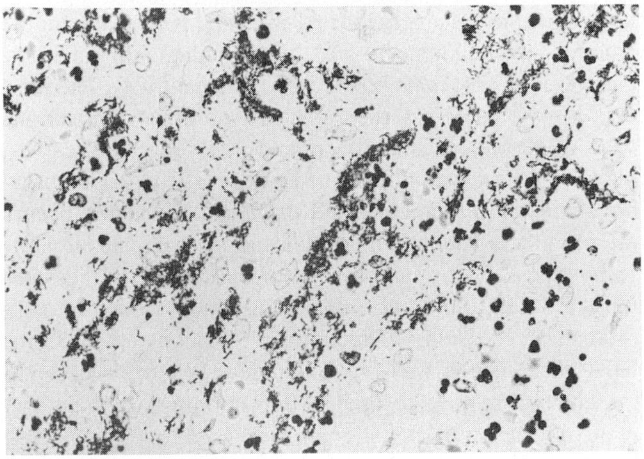

FIG. 28.24. Bacillary angiomatosis. The Warthin-Starry stain allows visualization of the clumps and tangled masses of the causative bacteria (original magnification: 100× magnification). (Courtesy of Dr. John Chan, Queen Elizabeth Hospital, Hong Kong.)

can be cultured from tissue lesions or from the peripheral blood, but this is often technically difficult and time-consuming (324,329,346); this approach is utilized infrequently for clinical diagnosis. Definitive identification of these organisms also can be made by PCR amplification of characteristic genetic sequences (318,329).

The principal differential diagnosis of bacillary angiomatosis involving a lymph node includes Kaposi's sarcoma (320,331), with which it can occur simultaneously in the same patient (316,342,348,354), epithelioid hemangioma, and angiosarcoma (320). Careful assessment of the clinical features of the patient and of the gross appearance and histopathology of the lesions, however, should lead to suspicion of bacillary angiomatosis (331), which can be confirmed readily by Warthin-Starry stain or electron microscopic demonstration of the bacteria (312,314,315,320,331,351). The accurate recognition of bacillary angiomatosis is important because appropriate antibiotic therapy, erythromycin or deoxycycline, leads to regression of both the cutaneous and extracutaneous lesions and resolution of the disease in virtually all patients (331). If bacillary angiomatosis remains undiagnosed or untreated, death may result from local complications, such as laryngeal obstruction (313), or overwhelming disseminated infection (313,317,343).

AIDS-RELATED NON-HODGKIN'S LYMPHOMA

Background

A relationship between immune deficiency and neoplasia has been recognized for more than 30 years (355–358). The incidence of cancer is 100 times greater than expected in individuals who have congential immune deficiency states such as ataxia-telangiectasia and the Wiscott-Aldrich syndrome; malignant lymphomas comprise the majority of these malignancies (358–360). A spectrum of lymphoproliferative disorders, including high-grade malignant lymphomas, also occurs with greatly increased incidence in solid organ transplant recipients, in the setting of iatrogenic immunosuppression and chronic antigenic stimulation (361–363). Malignant lymphomas occur with increased frequency among individuals with acquired autoimmune disorders such as collagen vascular diseases, Sjögren's syndrome, and Hashimoto's thyroiditis (355,364,365). Recurrent themes among these immunodeficiency-associated malignant lymphomas include origination in or involvement of extranodal and unusual anatomic sites, high-grade histopathology, aggressive clinical behavior, B-cell lineage derivation, and a frequent association with EBV infection (359,361,363). Persons suffering from HIV-induced immunosuppression are also at greatly increased risk for developing malignant lymphomas that exhibit some of these same clinical and biologic features.

Epidemiology

In May 1982, approximately 1 year after the initial cases of AIDS were described (1–3), Doll and List (366) reported an immunocompromised young homosexual man who had Burkitt's lymphoma. A few months later, Ziegler and colleagues (367–369) reported four additional cases of advanced Burkitt's-like lymphoma occurring in immunocompromised homosexual men. At that time, the relationship between malignant lymphoma and AIDS was uncertain. The CDC, however, included the occurrence of primary CNS NHL in persons younger than 60 years of age without a known cause of immunosuppression as an additional criterion for the diagnosis of AIDS in 1982 (58). The CDC excluded NHLs occurring in other sites from the criteria at that time, because malignant lymphoma is known to cause immunosuppression (58). The incidence of clinically aggressive, high-grade NHL in persons at risk for AIDS, however, increased in parallel with the AIDS epidemic. This led the CDC to revise their criteria for the diagnosis of AIDS in 1985 to include HIV-seropositive persons who had diffuse, undifferentiated (Burkitt's and Burkitt's-like) lymphoma occurring in all anatomic sites (60). A multiinstitutional study of 90 MSM who had malignant lymphoma (369), several large clinical series of AIDS-related malignant lymphoma reported from the endemic areas of Los Angeles (370,371), Houston (372), and New York City (373–375), and numerous additional reports of smaller numbers of cases of AIDS-related NHL (283,376–385) led to widespread recognition of this new AIDS-defining malignancy. These reports prompted the CDC to expand its criteria for the diagnosis of AIDS again in 1987 to include all HIV-seropositive persons who had intermediate or high grade NHLs of B-cell or indeterminate phenotype (61). AIDS-related NHLs displaying comparable clinical, pathologic, and immunologic characteristics were observed with similarly increasing frequency worldwide (386–390). NHL now is recognized widely as the second most common neoplasm occurring among HIV-infected individuals and the most common neoplasm occurring among HIV-infected IDUs and hemophiliacs (385,391).

Unfortunately, an accurate assessment of the incidence of NHL among HIV-infected individuals, and consequently the true scope of the epidemic of AIDS-related malignancies, cannot be ascertained. This is largely because of the problems associated with selective reporting, retrospective analysis, and short-term follow-up. The CDC has calculated the risk of NHL among individuals in the United States to be 60 times greater among those who have AIDS than among those in the general population, and the incidence of NHL in AIDS to be 2.9% (391). This is based on reports of 2,824 NHLs occurring among 97,258 patients with AIDS in the United States reported to the CDC between 1981 and mid-1989 (391). A similar percentage has been reported from Europe (392). Although primary CNS lymphoma and Burkitt's lymphoma, however, have been reportable conditions since 1981, immunoblastic lymphoma has been a reportable condition only since 1985 (61). Immunoblastic lymphoma frequently occurs as a secondary manifestation of AIDS late in the course of HIV infection (393). Once an individual has been diagnosed with the initial AIDS-defining illness, notification regarding subsequent AIDS-defining illnesses is not required by the CDC (391). For this reason, the subsequent development of malignant lymphoma following the initial notification of an AIDS case frequently is not reported to the CDC (391). The magnitude of this underreporting is unclear. Within a cohort of 60 patients reported by Levine and colleagues (394), for example, 75% of the patients with primary CNS lymphoma and 37% of the patients with systemic lymphoma had been diagnosed with AIDS prior to the development of lymphoma. None of these cases would have been reported to the CDC. In one large teaching hospital in the United Kingdom, malignant lymphoma has accounted for 12% to 16% of all AIDS-related deaths (395), suggesting that the true incidence is higher than 3%. The overall incidence may be further underestimated because the spectrum of AIDS-related illnesses may reduce the likelihood that the diagnosis of malignant lymphoma will be pursued. In several autopsy series of AIDS patients, relatively high rates of previously undiagnosed NHLs, especially primary CNS lymphoma, were identified (396–398). Presumably, many other AIDS-related NHLs go unrecognized because of the failure to perform *post mortem* examinations. Data collected from cohort studies and cancer registries may be more informative regarding the true incidence and risk factors for AIDS-related NHL (399). For these and other reasons, it is clear that the true incidence of AIDS-related NHL has been substantially underestimated. The incidence is more likely to be about 200-fold in excess of expected rates (400), and estimates placing the overall incidence of NHL in AIDS between 4% and 10% probably are more accurate (390,401–403).

Malignant lymphoma appears to be a relatively late manifestation of HIV infection. Epidemiologic studies have demonstrated that the increased incidence of NHL actually lagged behind the emergence of epidemic Kaposi's sarcoma among the young homosexual male population in San Francisco at high risk for AIDS by 1 to 2 years (404). The incidences of Kaposi's sarcoma and opportunistic infections were increased statistically as early as 1981; a true lymphoma epidemic was not defined until 1985 (405). Comparable studies have demonstrated that NHL frequently occurs after Kaposi's sarcoma in immunosuppressed renal allograft recipients. Kaposi's sarcoma and NHL develop in these patients at 16 and 30 months after transplantation, respectively (406,407). The delay in recognizing NHL as an AIDS-related phenomenon was probably secondary to its delay in presentation relative to other AIDS-defining illnesses. The relatively late onset of malignant lymphoma in HIV-infected individuals was confirmed by Pluda and colleagues (408,409) in their analysis of 55 patients with symptomatic HIV disease who had been enrolled in various antiretroviral trials between 1985 and 1987. They found that the probability of developing malignant lymphoma after the initiation of zidovudine antiretroviral therapy was 12% at two years (409), and the observed risk was 29% at 3 years (408). The probability of developing malignant lymphoma was 19% at 36 months in a group of 116 patients with symptomatic HIV infection receiving either zidovudine or dideoxyinosine (408). Among a cohort of 1,065 HIV-infected patients with hemophilia, the incidence of NHL increased exponentially as the duration of HIV infection increased, with the risk doubling every 2.4 years (410). These observations support the contention that the incidence of NHL in AIDS has risen steadily as other AIDS-related illnesses have become better controlled and the length of survival following HIV seroconversion has increased (411). Currently, about 10% of all NHLs occurring in the United States are thought to be AIDS-related (402). It has been suggested that eventually up to 25% of malignant lymphomas in the United States will be HIV-related (412).

In the United States, approximately 3% of patients with AIDS present with malignant lymphoma (402,405,413). In addition to MSM and IDUs, AIDS-related NHLs may develop in individuals of all ages who have been transfused with HIV-infected blood and blood products (368,375, 378,391), children born to HIV-infected mothers (391), and the heterosexual partners of HIV-infected persons (270,391,414). The risk of developing NHLs is relatively consistent among all population groups at risk for AIDS (270,414), without regard for geography (391,402), although it is highest in hemophiliacs (391). In the United States, approximately 80% of persons who develop AIDS-related NHLs are MSM, and the majority of the remainder are IDUs, once again predominantly men (375,415). In western Europe, approximately two thirds of persons who develop AIDS-related NHLs are IDUs (389,416). This is because MSM and IDUs represent the principal populations at risk for AIDS. The differences between their representation in the United States and Europe reflect the epidemiologic variations in the spread of the AIDS epidemic in these different regions. Similar to the distribution of conventional NHLs occurring in the HIV-uninfected general population, the incidence of AIDS-related NHL appears to be higher in men than in women (391,402), and in whites than in blacks (391). The incidence of AIDS-related NHL appears to increase with age among MSM and hemophiliacs, although not in IDUs (402). The clinicopathologic features of AIDS-related NHLs occurring in the various AIDS risk groups appear to be similar, based on data collected on MSM, IDUs, hemophiliacs, and transfusion recipients from the United States and Europe (369,370,375,391,410,417–420). One possible exception is that primary oral and anorectal NHLs appear to occur preferentially in MSM (368,370,391,410,416–418,420).

The AIDS status of patients at the time of diagnosis of AIDS-related NHL has changed over the course of the AIDS epidemic. In the multiinstitutional study published by Ziegler and coworkers in 1984 (369), 47% of the patients with NHL carried a prior diagnosis of AIDS, based on the presence of severe opportunistic infections, Kaposi's sarcoma, or both. In contrast, in results from a series in San Francisco published in 1989 (417) and a Washington-area study published in 1990 (421), only 27% and 25% of patients, respectively, had received a prior diagnosis of AIDS. These changes may be because of earlier recognition of HIV infection status, changes in risk factors, or the impact of antiretroviral therapy on the natural history of the disease (413,421).

Site of Origin

AIDS-related NHLs are divisible into three broad categories according to their anatomic sites of origin: those arising systemically (nodally or extranodally), those arising in the CNS, and those arising in the body cavities (422,423).

Systemic

The systemic lymphomas comprise approximately 80% of all AIDS-related NHLs. The majority of patients who have AIDS-related systemic NHL already have widely disseminated disease, including a high frequency of extranodal involvement, at initial presentation; only a small proportion present with localized lymph node–based disease (369,371,375,389,415,416,419). Approximately 65% of these individuals have clinical stage III or IV disease, and another almost 20% of them have clinical stage IE disease initially (375,389,416,419). Even the patients with clinical stage IE disease often have large bulky tumors, however (375). All together, about 85% of the patients have extranodal involvement at presentation (369,371,372,374, 375, 389,403,416,417). The CNS, the gastrointestinal tract, the bone marrow, and the liver are the most common sites of extranodal disease at presentation (369,371,375,389,415, 417,419,424). Furthermore, certain extranodal locations that uncommonly serve as primary sites of conventional lymphoma in the HIV-uninfected general population, such as the CNS, the anorectal region, and the heart, among others, have become recognized as frequent sites of origin for AIDS-related NHL (369,375,425–430). An extranodal biopsy is used to make the initial diagnosis of malignant lymphoma in approximately two thirds of patients (375). Not infrequently, the diagnosis is based on the biopsy of a particularly unusual extranodal site, such as the gingiva, anorectal region, mandible, or orbit, or the cytologic examination of an abdominal or pleural effusion (375).

The CNS is the most common extranodal site of involvement by AIDS-related NHLs (403,423). Approximately 20% to 40% of patients who have AIDS-related systemic lymphoma, especially those who have bone marrow infiltration, have CNS infiltration at presentation (369,371,372,375,415, 422), and two thirds of them are found to have CNS infiltation at *post mortem* examination (396). The majority of patients who have systemic NHL accompanied by secondary CNS involvement have leptomeningeal infiltration (Fig. 28.25) and not solid parenchymal masses (396). These patients usually present with lymphomatous meningitis and commonly have nuccal rigidity, headaches, cranial neuropathies, or numbness of the chin (390), although they may be asymptomatic (426). Cerebrospinal fluid samples obtained from these patients may contain neoplastic cells. Therefore, cytologic examination of the cerebrospinal fluid should be performed as part of the initial staging evaluation of all patients with AIDS-related systemic lymphoma, in order to rule out CNS involvement (425,431).

The second most common extranodal site of involvement by AIDS-related NHL is the gastrointestinal tract (403,423,431) (Fig. 28.26). Of the patients who had AIDS-related NHL reported from the Los Angeles County–University of Southern California (LAC-USC) (425) and New York University (375) Medical Centers, 27% and 28%, respectively, had gastrointestinal tract involvement initially. In addition, 10% and 16% of the patients, respectively, had liver involvement initially (375,425) (Fig. 28.27). The majority of patients who have AIDS-related systemic NHL are discovered to have gastrointestinal tract and liver involvement at the time of autopsy examination (396).

The gastrointestinal tract is also a common primary extranodal site of AIDS-related NHL (375,425,431). The most frequent sites of origin within the gastrointestinal tract are the stomach and the small intestine (425); however, any region from the oropharynx to the rectum and anus, including the liver (432,433), may serve as the primary site of NHL. Alternatively, patients may have extensive lymphomatous involvement of the entire gastrointestinal tract (425).

The signs and symptoms may be related to primary gastrointestinal tract involvement or result from extension into abdominal lymph nodes. Patients initially may complain of gingival swelling and bleeding, dysphagia, abdominal pain, symptoms related to ulceration, obstipation, bowel obstruction, abdominal swelling because of ascites or a palpable mass, jaundice or perirectal abscess, and ulceration (375,431). Organomegaly with or without ascites, abdominal

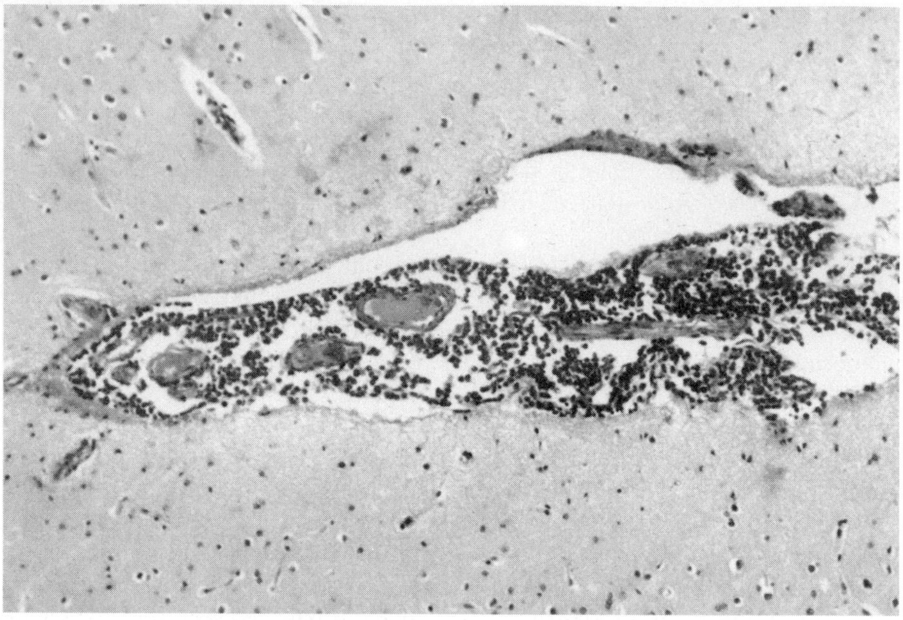

FIG. 28.25. An HIV-positive heterosexual woman presented with massive bone marrow replacement and peripheral blood involvement by B-cell acute lymphoblastic leukemia (Fig. 28.60), accompanied by meningeal signs. Malignant lymphoid cells were identified in a cerebrospinal fluid sample. Examination at autopsy revealed extensive infiltration of the leptomeninges by neoplastic lymphoid cells but no solid parenchymal masses, consistent with secondary involvement of the central nervous system (hematoxylin and eosin stain, original magnification: 100× magnification).

masses, retroperitoneal lymphadenopathy, and nonhealing perirectal ulcers or abscesses should prompt a tissue biopsy to rule out malignant lymphoma (431).

Non-Hodgkin's lymphoma arising or presenting in the anus or rectum of homosexual men is recognized as a frequent manifestation of AIDS (425,428–430). Primary anorectal lymphoma occurs infrequently in the general population. Malignant lymphomas of all histologic types comprise only 0.1 to 1.3% of all malignant tumors of the rectum (428,434), and rectal lymphomas represent only approximately 5% of all gastrointestinal tract lymphomas (434–436). Burkes and colleagues (428) and Ioachim and associates (430) reported series of four patients who had primary anorectal lymphoma diagnosed within brief time spans at the Los Angeles County–University of Southern California Medical Center and Lenox Hill Hospital in New York City, respectively. The patients usually are young MSM between 22 and 45 years of age (median 35) who have a history of practicing passive rectal intercourse with multiple anonymous sexual partners. They usually complain of rectal bleeding, pain on defecation, or a mucoid rectal discharge and B symptoms and have a palpable rectal mass on examination. The lymphomas tend to occur in the lower rectum and anal canal and display intermediate- and high-

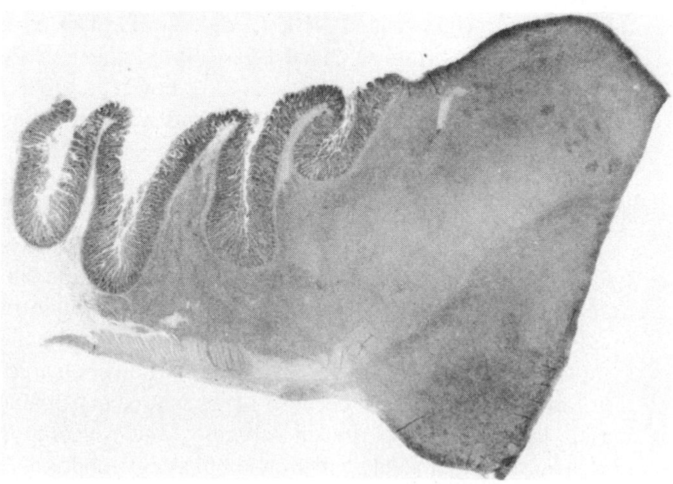

FIG. 28.26. AIDS-related non-Hodgkin's lymphoma occurring in the small bowel, in which it forms a large, bulky tumor mass. The gastrointestinal tract is the second most common extranodal site of origin for AIDS-related non-Hodgkin's lymphoma. (From Knowles DM, Chamulak GA, Subar M, et al. Clinicopathologic, immunophenotypic, and molecular genetic analysis of AIDS-associated lymphoid neoplasia. In: Rosen PP, Fechner RE, eds. *Pathology annual 1988, part 2.* East Norwalk, CT: Appleton and Lange, 1988:33–67, with permission.)

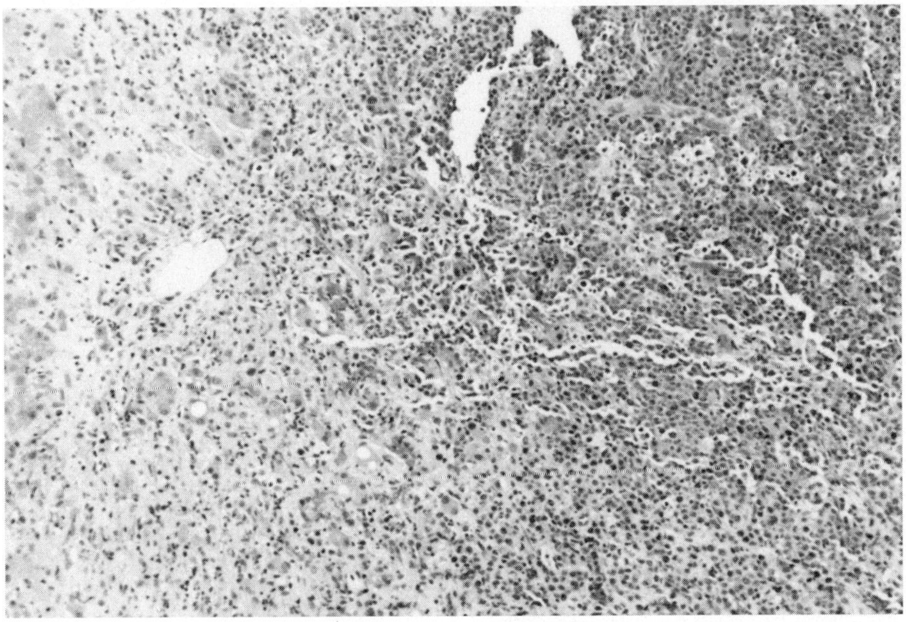

FIG. 28.27. AIDS-related Burkitt's lymphoma initially diagnosed by percutaneous liver needle biopsy. Note the extensive replacement of the liver parenchyma by malignant lymphoma displaying a prominent starry-sky pattern (*right*) and a small area of residual liver parenchyma (*left*). (Hematoxylin and eosin stain, original magnification: 100× magnification).

grade histologies. Although most patients present with clinical stage IE disease, nearly all of them develop disseminated lymphoma shortly thereafter. The median duration of survival has been approximately 7 months, with only rare patients sustaining a complete remission (428–430). In contrast, primary anorectal lymphomas occurring in the HIV-uninfected general population affect men and women equally, usually occur in the sixth and seventh decades of life, generally develop higher up in the rectum, and often exhibit low-grade histology (430,434). The significance of the development of anorectal lymphoma in MSM in association with AIDS at a specific site of sexual activity is unknown. Anal intercourse has been shown to be a risk factor, however, for the development of anal carcinoma (437,438) and, by analogy, may play a contributory role in the development of anorectal lymphoma as well.

AIDS-related systemic NHLs may originate or present in virtually any extranodal site, regardless of how isolated or obscure. They have been reported, for example, in the orbit (374,375,439), oropharynx (369,375,440), mandible (374,375,380), heart (441,442), lungs (374,375,440), skin (374,375,443), salivary glands (248,375), common bile duct (444), muscles (440), bones (369,440), kidneys (369,389), gonads (375,419,440), and adrenal glands (375) and even in the placenta and products of conception (445) (Figs. 28.28–28.31). Neoplastic cells even may circulate in the peripheral blood (375). In many instances, involvement of these extranodal sites is the result of extensive, widely disseminated disease; however, the malignant lymphoma often appears to have originated in the extranodal site. For example, Constantino and coworkers (441) described a malignant lymphoma arising in, and remaining limited to, the heart of a 34-year-old IDU (Fig. 28.32); we have observed similar cases (Knowles, unpublished observations). Levecq and colleagues (446) described a histologic high-grade B-cell lymphoma arising in an ileostomy stoma in a 73-year-old heterosexual man who apparently acquired HIV infection following transfusion. Kaplan and associates (444) described a Burkitt's lymphoma originating in the common bile duct that subsequently spread to the bone marrow and CNS. Malignant lymphoma should be considered if an individual at risk for AIDS presents with a tumor, regardless of the mode of presentation. The atypical presentation of a diffuse aggressive NHL involving an unusual extranodal site should raise suspicion of HIV infection. The factors that influence the development of malignant lymphoma in a particular location are unclear but may include site-specific chronic antigenic stimulation (447) and trauma (448).

Central Nervous System

In addition to the high frequency of secondary lymphomatous involvement of the CNS, approximately 20% of all AIDS-related NHLs are primary CNS lymphomas, that is, present as intracranial parenchymal mass lesions limited to the CNS (369,374,385,396,415,416,439). Before the emergence of AIDS, primary CNS lymphomas occurred rarely, constituting less than 1.5% of all primary brain tumors (449). In a study of 12,000 patients who had malignant lymphoma, involvement was limited to the brain in only 0.2% of the patients (450), and this usually occurred in the elderly (449) and among patients who had collagen vascular disorders

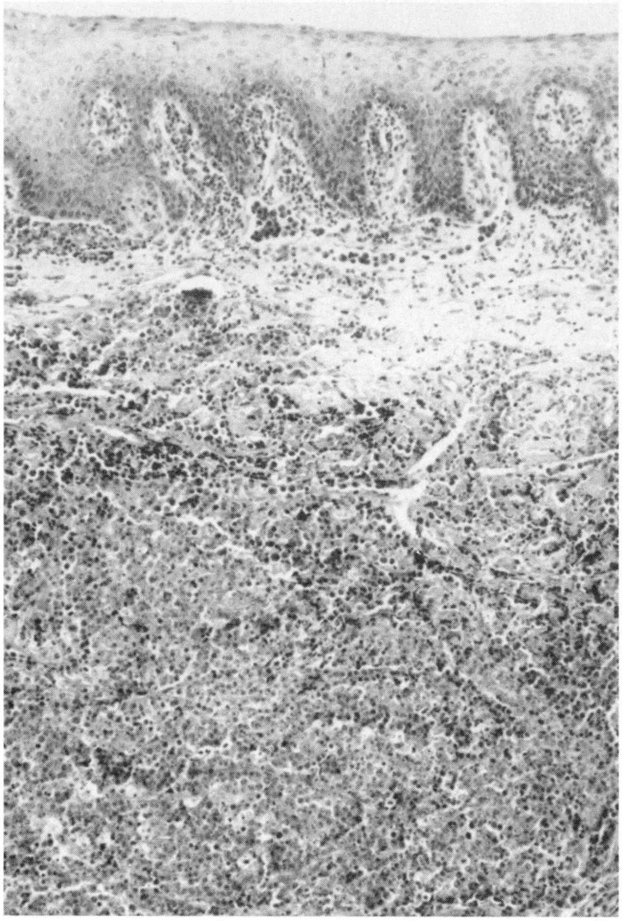

FIG. 28.28. AIDS-related immunoblastic lymphoma presenting as a gingival mass in a 36-year-old homosexual man. Note the presence of numerous tumor cells in the submucosal lymphatics (hematoxylin and eosin stain, original magnification: 100× magnification). (From Knowles DM, Chadburn A. The neoplasms associated with AIDS. In: Joshi VV, ed. *Pathology of AIDS and other manifestations of HIV infection.* New York: Igaku-Shoin, 1990:83–120, with permission.)

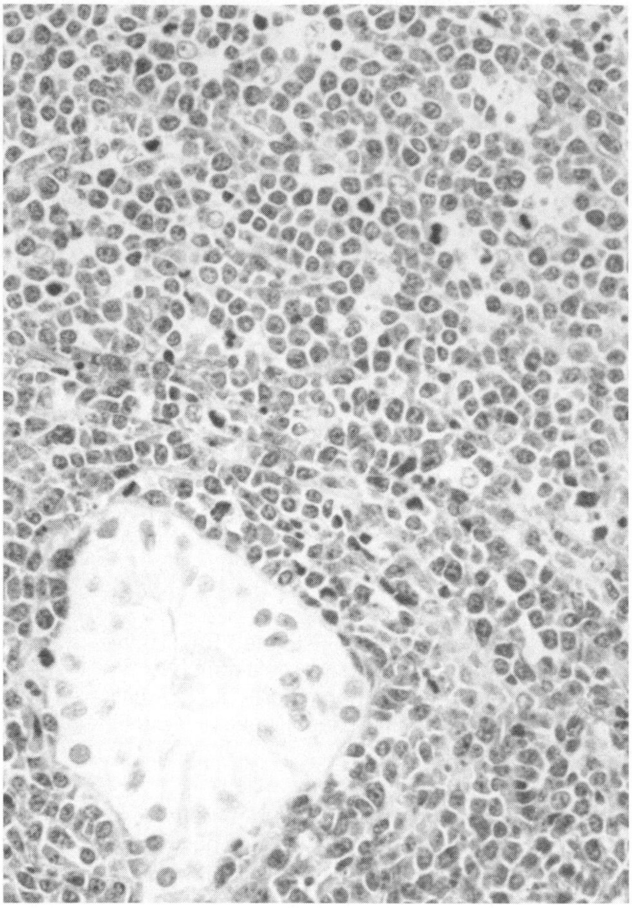

FIG. 28.29. AIDS-related Burkitt's-like lymphoma presenting as a testicular mass in a 43-year-old homosexual man. On further evaluation, this patient was discovered to have pulmonary, bone marrow, and central nervous system involvement by malignant lymphoma as well (hematoxylin and eosin stain, original magnification: 320× magnification). (From Knowles DM, Chadburn A. The neoplasms associated with AIDS. In Joshi VV, ed. *Pathology of AIDS and other manifestations of HIV infection.* New York: Igaku-Shoin, 1990:83–120).

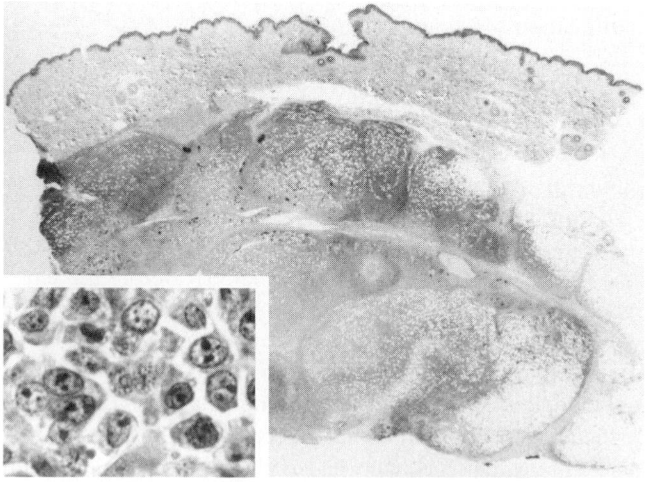

FIG. 28.30. AIDS-related immunoblastic lymphoma presenting as a subcutaneous mass in a 40-year-old homosexual man. The subcutaneous fat is infiltrated extensively by neoplastic lymphoid cells containing large, eccentrically placed nuclei and abundant amphophilic cytoplasm, sometimes with a paranuclear hof. The patient was considered to have clinical stage IE disease and achieved a complete remission with radiation therapy. He developed central nervous system lymphoma, however, and died 1 month later (hematoxylin and eosin stain, original magnifications: 4× magnification; **Inset:** 630× magnification).

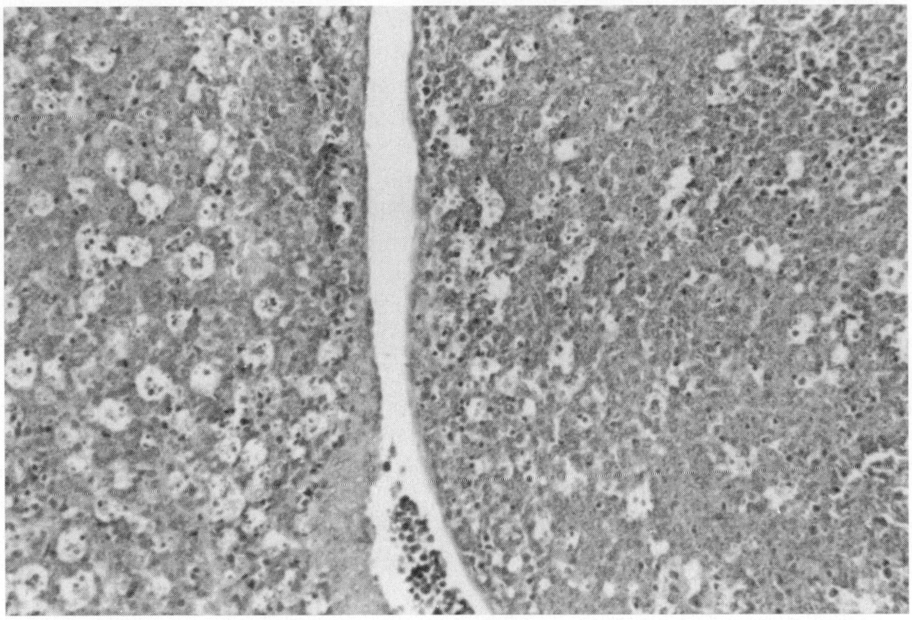

FIG. 28.31. AIDS-related Durkitt's lymphoma occurring in a benign lymphoepithelial cyst. Note the residual layer of focally attenuated stratified squamous epithelium overlying the malignant lymphoma, which exhibits a prominent starry sky pattern (hematoxylin and eosin stain, original magnification: 250× magnification).

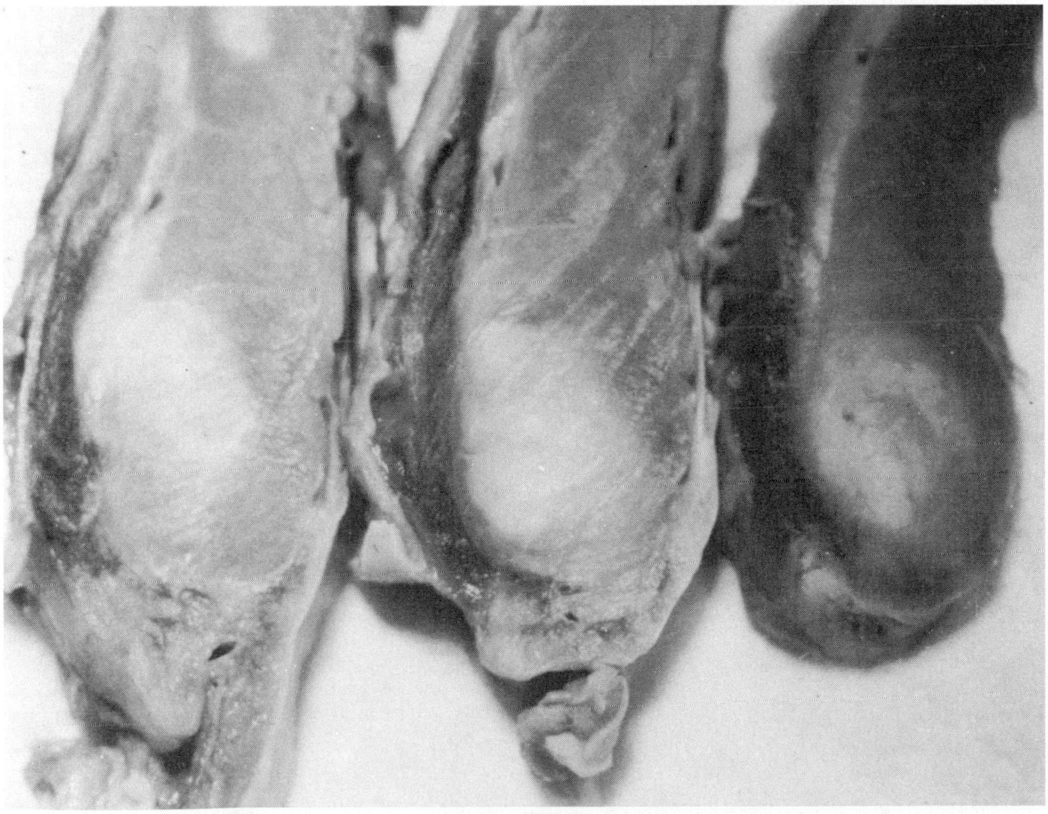

FIG. 28.32. Primary cardiac non-Hodgkin's lymphoma occurring in an HIV-positive 34-year-old injecting drug user. Autopsy examination failed to demonstrate any evidence of lymphoma beyond the heart. (From Constantino A, West TE, Gupta M, et al. Primary cardiac lymphoma in a patient with acquired immune deficiency syndrome. *Cancer* 1987;60:2801–2805, with permission.)

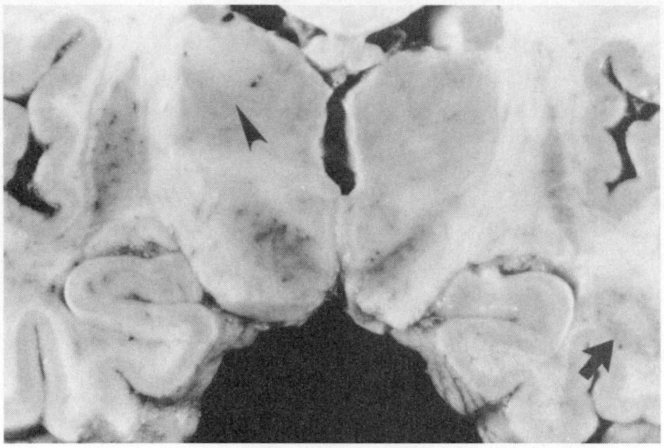

FIG. 28.33. AIDS-related central nervous system lymphoma. The infiltrative nature of this lymphoma is manifested on the left by the uniform enlargement of the thalamus and subthalamic area; its tendency to be multifocal is illustrated by more localized tumor foci in the dorsolateral thalamus (*arrowhead*) and contralateral temporal white matter (*arrow*). (Courtesy of Dr. James Powers, University of Rochester, Rochester, NY.)

(451) and various congenital and acquired immune deficiencies, including renal transplant recipients (356,407,447). Data collected by the CDC suggest that primary CNS lymphomas occur about 1,000 times more frequently in AIDS patients than in the general population (391). AIDS now represents the most common risk factor, by far, for the development of primary CNS lymphoma.

AIDS-related primary CNS lymphomas are intracranial parenchymal tumors. They are often large, sometimes larger than 3 cm, and frequently are multifocal (427,452,453). Grossly, they are characterized by indistinct borders and a granular surface (427) (Fig. 28.33). At autopsy, they nearly always are discovered to be multicentric, especially on microscopic examination (396,427). They occur most commonly in the cerebrum but also occur frequently in the cerebellum, basal ganglia, and brain stem (427,452–454). The lymphoma cells tend to be distributed along vascular channels as perivascular cuffs (427,453,454) (Fig. 28.34). Because the lesions are primarily intracranial, cerebrospinal fluid samples often do not contain diagnostic malignant cells (427); however, concurrent leptomeningeal involvement accompanied by malignant cells within the cerebrospinal fluid sometimes is observed (426,427). The lymphomas are of B-cell origin and display large cell and immunoblastic histologies (375,396,426,427,439,440,453,454).

The majority of patients who have AIDS-related primary CNS NHL are profoundly immunocompromised young homosexual men with very advanced HIV disease who have CD4 T-cell counts below 50 per microliter (396,415,426, 427,439). Approximately two thirds or more of them have AIDS-defining conditions, often severe opportunistic infections or Kaposi's sarcoma, before the development of primary CNS lymphoma (369,394,415,427,439,453,455). Approximately one half of patients experience focal seizures and a subacute progression of focal neurologic symptoms over days or weeks (427). Occasionally, clinical progression may be strikingly rapid, causing difficulty in distinguishing neoplastic, vascular, and infectious causes (427). Headaches, confusion, lethargy, and memory loss are other common symptoms, and subtle changes in behavior and personality

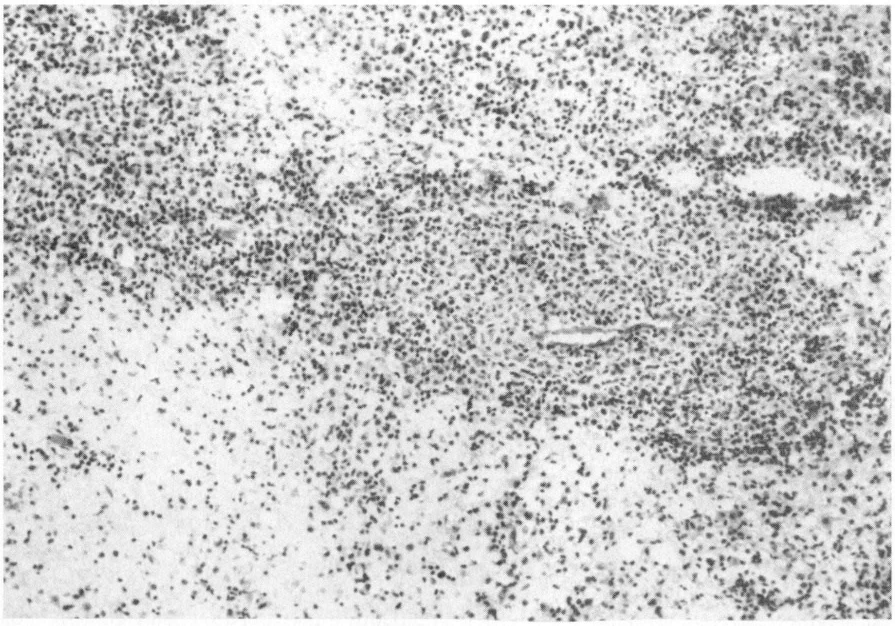

FIG. 28.34. AIDS-related primary central nervous system lymphoma. Note that the tumor cells tend to cluster around and along vascular channels (hematoxylin and eosin stain, original magnification: 100× magnification).

may be seen (425–427,439,453,455). Many patients eventually show signs suggesting an intracranial mass lesion; however, because many of them are seriously ill from their underlying systemic illness, these relatively nonspecific symptoms may not raise suspicion of such a lesion, and primary CNS lymphoma may not be diagnosed until after death (375,396,415,419,427). Only 11 of 20 patients who had AIDS-related primary CNS lymphoma at the University of California at San Francisco were diagnosed correctly after death; the remaining nine patients were correctly diagnosed only at autopsy (427).

The majority of persons who have AIDS-related primary CNS lymphoma exhibit abnormalities on computed tomographic scans consistent with an intracranial mass lesion (427,456). Solitary discrete and multiple discrete lesions are seen in equal proportions (427) (Figs. 28.35, 28.36). Computed tomographic scans have been used widely to distinguish between intracranial lymphoma and toxoplasmosis, based on the belief that malignant lymphoma exhibits a homogeneous, isodense, or hyperdense pattern, and toxoplasmosis displays a ring-enhancing pattern (426,457) This is generally true of conventional primary CNS lymphomas occurring in the general population, because these lymphomas usually consist of tightly packed tumor cells without necrosis (456). AIDS-related primary CNS lymphomas, however, frequently contain extensive necrosis and show some degree of enhancement, although the pattern is variable. This often makes it difficult or impossible to distinguish between AIDS-related primary CNS lymphoma and toxoplasmosis by computed tomographic scan (427,456). Brain biopsy is essential for accurate diagnosis in these patients (376,427,453,456,458–461) (Figs. 28.37, 28.38).

Body Cavities

Several years ago Knowles and colleagues (462) reported an uncommonly occurring subset of AIDS-related NHLs that grow almost exclusively in the pleural, pericardial, or peritoneal cavities as lymphomatous effusions, usually in the absence of a contiguous tumor mass. They also described several of the special properties of these malignant lymphomas, including their immunoblastic cytomorphology, indetermi-

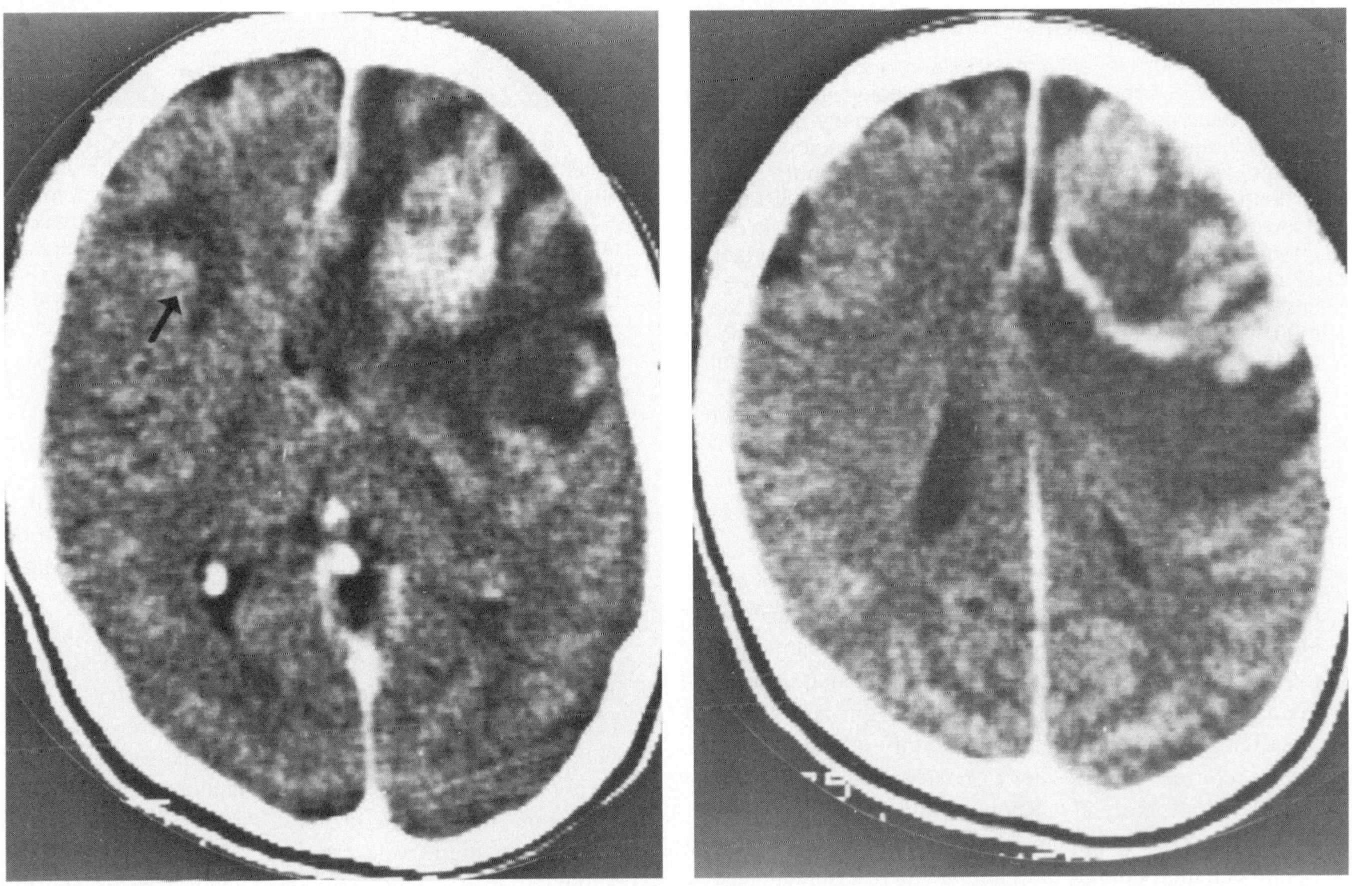

A B

FIG. 28.35. A,B: Left frontal irregular, rim-enhancing lesion with partial solid nodular mass in a 35-year-old man who had AIDS. This pathologically proven necrotic non-Hodgkin's lymphoma cannot be distinguished from glioblastoma multiforme. An additional small, solid-enhancing lesion is seen in the right frontal corticomedullary junction (*arrow*). (From Lee YY, Bruner JM, Van Tassel P, et al. Primary central nervous system lymphoma: CT and pathologic correlation. *Am J Neuroradiol* 1986;7:599–604, with permission.)

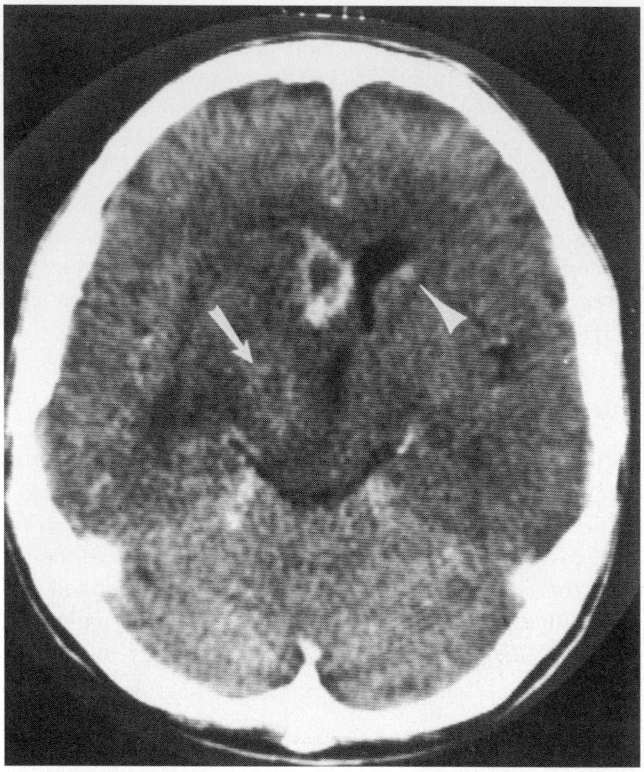

FIG. 28.36. Multiple, enhancing lesions in a 32-year-old man who had AIDS. Irregular rim-enhancing lesion is seen in head of right caudate nucleus, in addition to a poorly defined rim-enhancing lesion in the right thalamus and posterior limb of internal capsule (*arrow*) and a solid nodular-enhancing lesion in head of the left caudate nucleus (*arrowhead*). Needle biopsy of the right caudate lesion revealed non-Hodgkin's lymphoma. The patient received whole brain irradiation. Autopsy 42 months after the initial diagnosis revealed extensive necrotic lymphoma in both basal ganglia and in the right thalamus. There was no evidence of intracranial infection and no evidence of dissemination of lymphoma beyond the central nervous system. (From Lee YY, Bruner JM, Van Tassel P, et al. Primary central nervous system lymphoma: CT and pathologic correlation. *Am J Neuroradiol* 1986;7:599–604, with permission.)

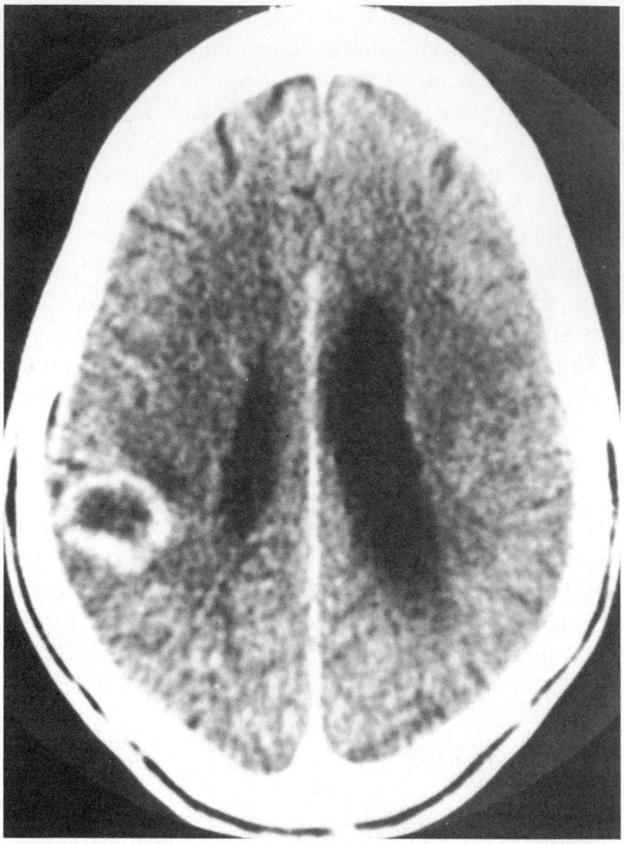

FIG. 28.37. Well-defined right parietal, thick, ring-enhancing lesion in a 24-year-old man who had AIDS. Open biopsy demonstrated that this lesion was a non-Hodgkin's lymphoma with extensive necrosis (Fig. 28.38). Autopsy examination 2 months later confirmed the diagnosis of primary central nervous system lymphoma without intracranial infection. (From Lee YY, Bruner JM, Van Tassel P, et al. Primary central nervous system lymphoma: CT and pathologic correlation. *Am J Neuroradiol* 1986;7:599–604, with permission.)

nate immunophenotype, B-cell genotype, presence of clonal EBV genome, and absence of *MYC* gene rearrangements. Other investigators subsequently described similar cases (463–465). Because these malignant lymphomas usually remain localized to the body cavity of origin and spread to local lymph nodes or to distant sites only infrequently, they were referred to as *body cavity–based lymphomas* (422,423,464). Recently, Knowles and colleagues demonstrated that these lymphomas exhibit a unique constellation of clinical, morphologic, immunophenotypic, and molecular characteristics, including the consistent presence of the recently described KSHV (466), and represent a distinct clinicopathologic entity. They have designated them *primary effusion lymphomas* (467). These lymphomas are described in more detail subsequently.

Histopathology

The histopathologic distribution of NHLs occurring in HIV-infected persons differs from that of conventional NHLs occurring in the HIV-uninfected general population, and also somewhat from those of NHLs occurring in other immune deficiency states.

In a study of all 89 AIDS-related NHLs investigated at the New York University Medical Center during the first 6 years of the AIDS epidemic (375), 40% were classified as Burkitt's lymphoma, and the remaining cases were divided evenly between immunoblastic lymphoma and large cell lymphoma; thus, approximately 70% of AIDS-related NHLs belong to a high-grade category, and the remaining 30% belong to an intermediate-grade category (375). The morphologic heterogeneity of diffuse, aggressive AIDS-related NHLs renders the precise classification of some patients into one of these three categories difficult (403,440,468). Patients exhibiting transitional histopathologic features also have been described. The French Study Group, however, reported

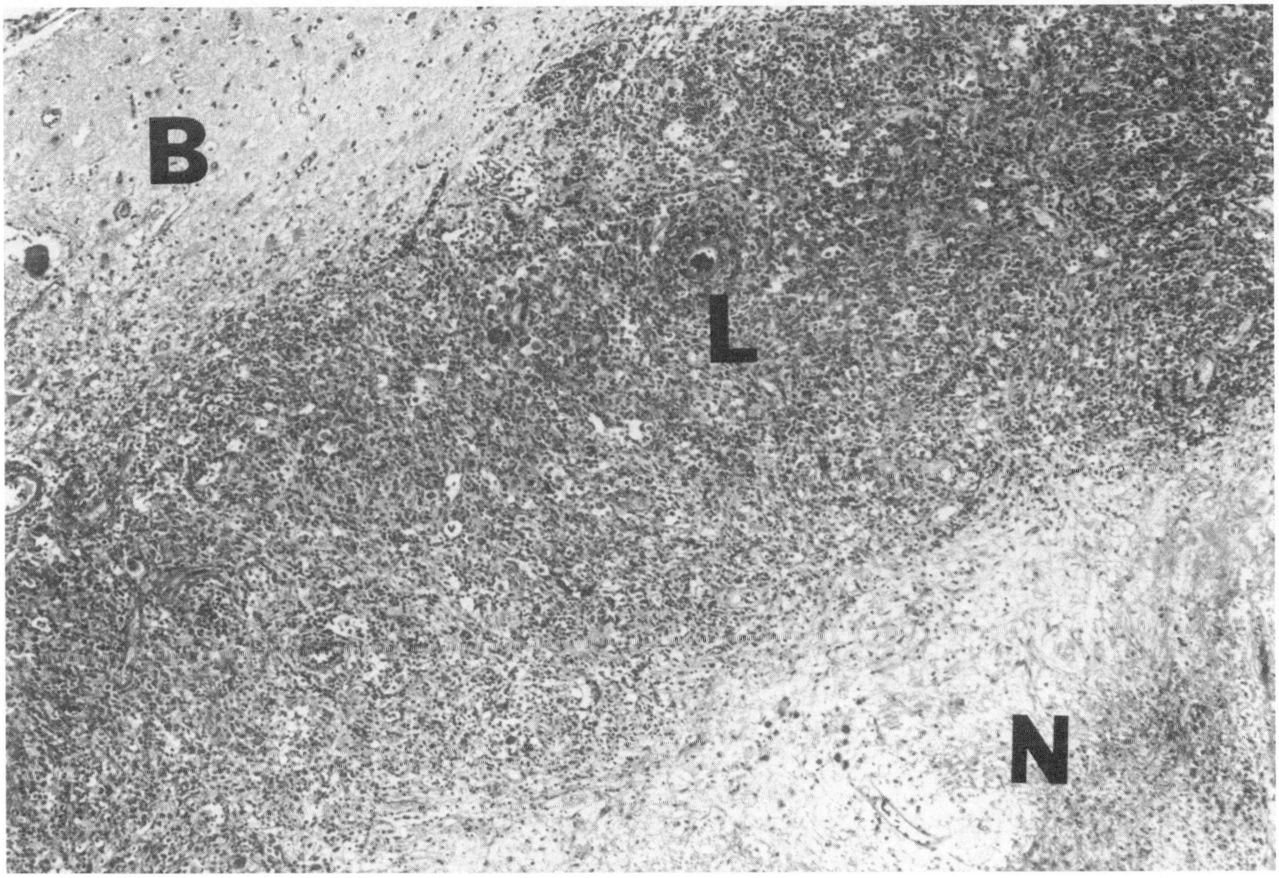

FIG. 28.38. Histopathologic section of the brain taken during autopsy examination of the patient illustrated in Figure 28.37. Extensive central necrosis (*N*) is surrounded by a rim of viable non-Hodgkin's lymphoma (*L*). Normal brain (*B*) is identified outside the lymphoma (hematoxylin and eosin stain, original magnification: 200× magnification). (From Lee YY, Bruner JM, Van Tassel P, et al. Primary central nervous system lymphoma: CT and pathologic correlation. *Am J Neuroradiol* 1986;7:599–604, with permission.)

virtually identical histopathologic distributions among 113 AIDS-related NHLs (440), and other large series have produced similar findings (369,375,389,417,418). In contrast, Burkitt's lymphoma and immunoblastic lymphoma comprise only approximately 10% of all conventional NHLs occurring in the HIV-uninfected general population in the United States (469). Based on cases reported to the CDC between 1981 and 1989, Burkitt's lymphoma appears to be 1,000 times more frequent in individuals who have AIDS than in the general population (391). The histopathologic distribution of AIDS-related NHLs also contrasts with that of other immunodeficiency states, in which the vast majority of NHLs exhibit large cell or immunoblastic morphology, and only a small minority exhibit Burkitt's lymphoma morphology (363,391).

Unlike most investigators, Carbone and colleagues (416,471) have reported that almost 15% of all AIDS-related systemic NHLs studied in Italy are $CD30^+$ anaplastic large cell lymphomas. These cases, however, exclusively expressed B-cell or non-B, non-T cell indeterminate immunophenotypes (470), and the majority of them demonstrated EBV (471). Anaplastic large cell lymphoma represents a distinct clinicopathologic entity characterized by T-cell derivation and the lack of association with EBV (472). B cell–derived NHLs exhibiting anaplastic large cell morphology are included among the morphologic variants of diffuse large B-cell lymphoma in the Revised European-American Classification of Lymphoid Neoplasms proposed by the International Lymphoma Study Group (472). Most of the cases designated *anaplastic large cell lymphoma* by Carbone and colleagues (416,471) probably have been included among the large cell and immunoblastic morphologic categories by other investigators. For example, the French Study Group identified only one case that they designated anaplastic large cell lymphoma among 113 AIDS-related NHLs that they examined (440). This may explain why Carbone and colleagues have failed to detect any clinical differences, including risk group, stage of HIV disease, performance status, CD4 T-cell counts, clinical presentation, clinical stage, disease distribution, eventual outcome, or cause of death, between cases that they have classified as non–T cell anaplastic large cell lymphoma and other AIDS-related systemic B-

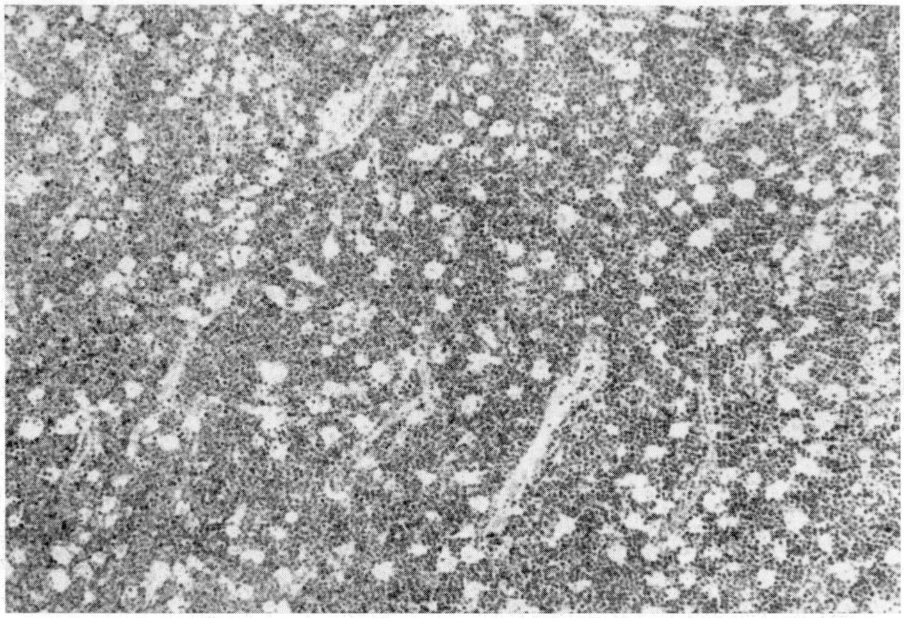

FIG. 28.39. AIDS-related Burkitt's lymphoma. Note the prominent starry-sky pattern, which is distributed evenly throughout the entire tumor (hematoxylin and eosin stain, original magnification: 100× magnification).

cell NHLs (470). Legitimate cases of anaplastic large cell lymphoma of T cell origin have been reported rarely in HIV-infected individuals (473).

AIDS-related NHLs exhibit morphologic features similar to those exhibited by conventional NHLs belonging to the same histopathologic categories. In general, AIDS-related NHLs appear to exhibit a higher frequency of mitotic figures, increased cellular debris, and a greater tendency to necrosis than conventional NHLs, suggesting a higher proliferation index and a more rapid rate of growth, which is consistent with their natural history (422,423).

AIDS-related Burkitt's lymphomas include those lymphomas displaying the histopathology of classical endemic (African) Burkitt's lymphoma as defined by the World

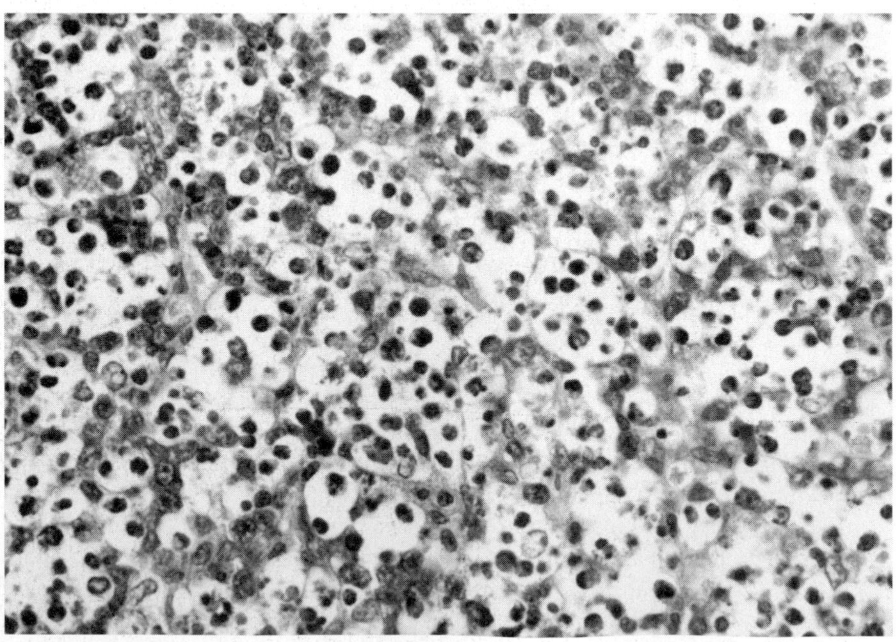

FIG. 28.40. AIDS-related Burkitt's lymphoma. This tumor possessed focal areas containing such large numbers of pyknotic nuclei, nuclear debris, and tingible body macrophages that the neoplastic cells are difficult to identify (hematoxylin and eosin stain, original magnification: 400× magnification).

Health Organization (474) and the so-called Burkitt's-like lymphomas. The latter lymphomas are those originally classified by Rappaport (475) as diffuse undifferentiated, non-Burkitt's type. They have been referred to as *Burkitt's lymphoma with plasmablastic differentiation* by Hui and coworkers (476). Burkitt's lymphomas characteristically contain numerous, evenly distributed tingible body macrophages possessing abundant clear cytoplasm that impart a prominent starry-sky pattern (Figs. 28.39, 28.40). These macrophages contain phagocytosed remnants of neoplastic cell debris, indicative of the high proliferation index of the lymphoma. Mitotic figures are extremely numerous, scattered nuclear debris is abundant, and there is a tendency for these lymphomas to undergo necrosis. Burkitt's lymphomas are characterized by a diffuse, monotonous proliferation of small to intermediate-sized neoplastic lymphoid cells containing moderately abundant basophilic cytoplasm and round, regular nuclei possessing two to five distinct nucleoli (Fig. 28.41). Numerous, well-defined cytoplasmic vacuoles staining with oil red O stain can be seen in air-dried Romanowsky-stained imprints (Fig. 28.42). Burkitt's-like lymphomas are morphologically similar to Burkitt's lymphomas, with the exception that the neoplastic cells are more variable in size and shape, some nuclei may be located more eccentrically, and some nuclei contain only one prominent, centrally placed nucleolus (422,423) (Fig. 28.41).

Immunoblastic lymphomas also often exhibit a starry-sky pattern, although it is usually less prominent than in Burkitt's

A

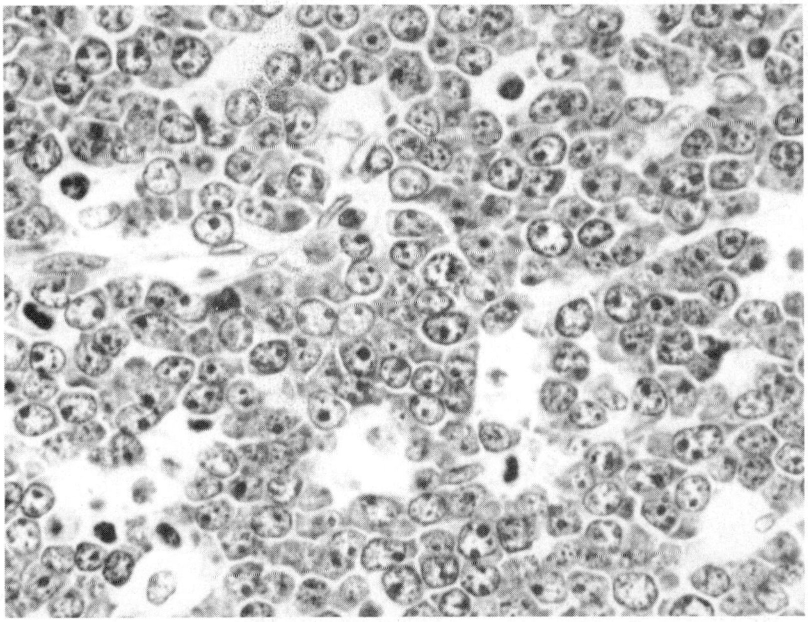

B

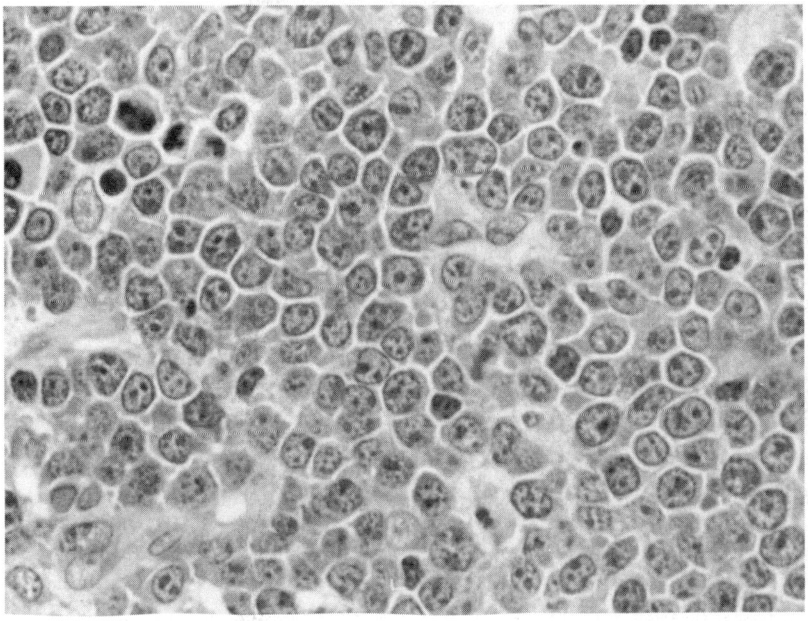

FIG. 28.41. AIDS-related Burkitt's and Burkitt's-like lymphomas. **A:** Burkitt's lymphoma. A monotonous proliferation of uniformly sized neoplastic cells containing round regular nuclei and generally two to four nucleoli. The nuclei are surrounded by a small rim of cytoplasm. Numerous tingible body macrophages impart a starry-sky pattern. **B:** Burkitt's-like lymphoma. The neoplastic cells as well as the nuclei show slightly more variability in size and shape. Many nuclei contain only one nucleolus. Nonetheless, the cells display the characteristic squared-off or "bathroom tile" appearance associated with Burkitt's lymphoma (hematoxylin and eosin stain, original magnification: 630× magnification).

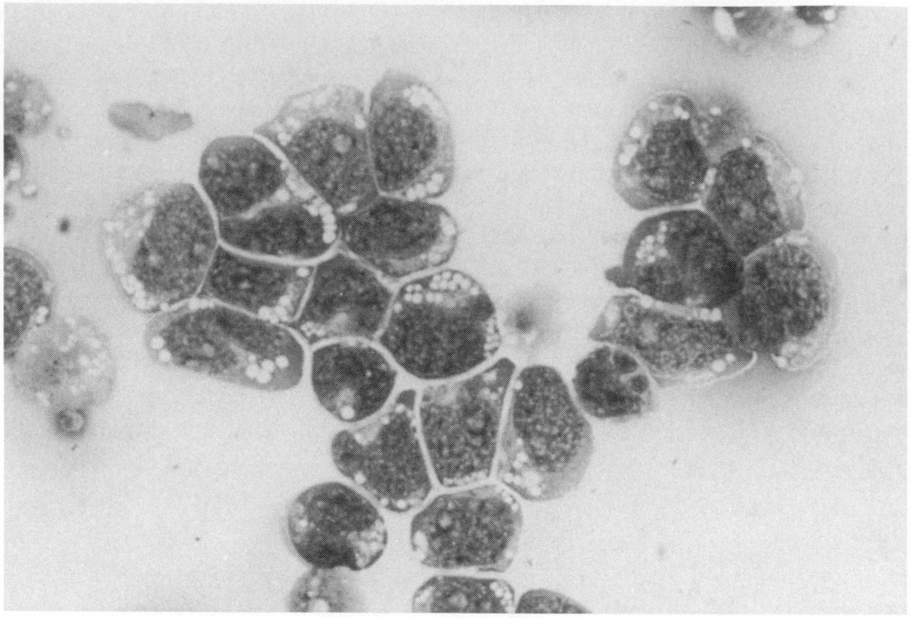

FIG. 28.42. Cytospin preparation of an AIDS-related Burkitt's lymphoma that presented as a massive abdominal effusion. The neoplastic cells possess abundant cytoplasm containing numerous small, round vacuoles. The nuclei contain one or more nucleoli (Wright stain, original magnification: 630× magnification).

lymphomas. Mitotic figures are extremely numerous, scattered nuclear debris is abundant, and these lymphomas also have a tendency to undergo necrosis. The neoplastic cells are larger than those comprising Burkitt's or large cell lymphomas. They are round, ovoid, or polygonal and often contain abundant, deeply basophilic cytoplasm, sometimes with a paranuclear hof indicative of their plasmacytoid differentiation. The nuclei are round to ovoid and often contain a solitary prominent, centrally placed nucleolus (Fig. 28.43). Binucleate and even multinucleate cells often are present

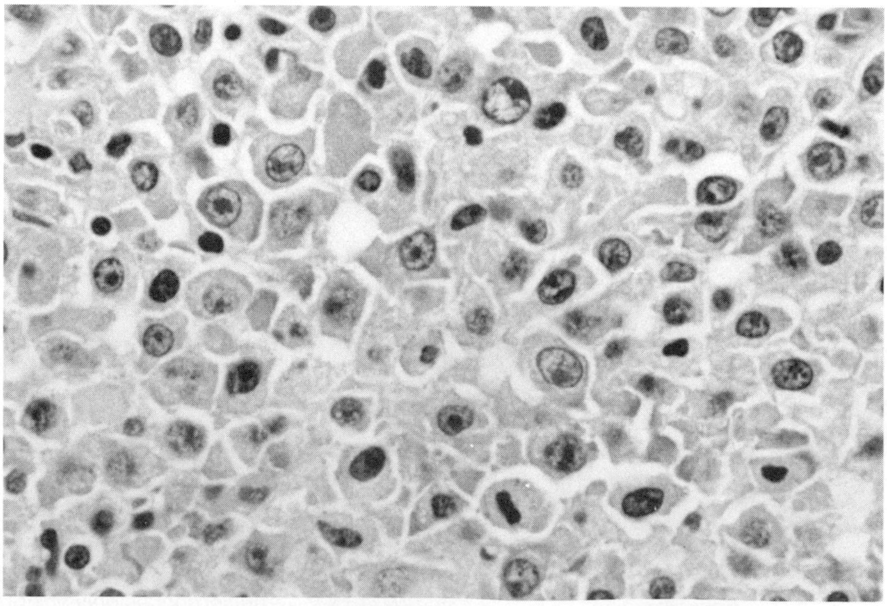

FIG. 28.43. AIDS-related immunoblastic lymphoma. The neoplastic cells are larger and show more variability in size and shape than those of Burkitt's and large cell lymphomas. The nuclei sometimes are placed eccentrically and are surrounded by abundant amphophilic cytoplasm with a paranuclear hof that imparts a plasmacytoid appearance to the neoplastic cells (hematoxylin and eosin stain, original magnification: 630× magnification).

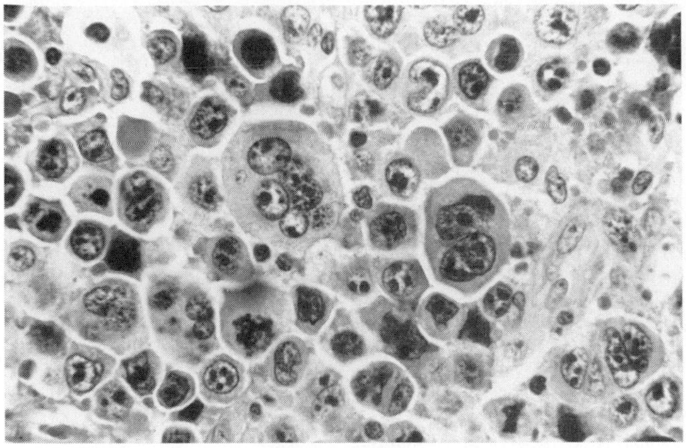

FIG. 28.44. AIDS-related immunoblastic lymphoma. This neoplasm is composed of large, pleomorphic tumor cells, many of which are binucleated and even multinucleated. Some resemble the pleomorphic Reed-Sternberg cells of Hodgkin's disease. The tumor cells expressed CD45 and a variety of activation-associated antigens but lacked B-cell lineage–restricted antigens. They displayed clonal immunoglobulin heavy and light chain gene rearrangements, consistent with a B-cell derivation, and contained Epstein-Barr virus (hematoxylin and eosin stain, original magnification: 630× magnification). (From Knowles DM, Dalla-Favera R. AIDS-associated malignant lymphoma. In: Broder S, Merigan TC, Bolognesi D, editors. *Textbook of AIDS medicine.* Baltimore: Williams & Wilkins, 1994:431–464, with permission.)

(422,423). Occasional immunoblastic lymphomas exhibit marked cellular pleomorphism (462). These cases are composed of large, pleomorphic tumor cells that contain abundant acidophilic to amphophilic cytoplasm and large, round, and regular to highly irregular and hyperconvoluted nuclei containing one or more prominent nucleoli, sometimes reminiscent of Reed-Sternberg cells (375,462) (Fig. 28.44).

The large cell lymphomas usually lack a prominent starry-sky pattern, because of the presence of fewer tingible body macrophages. Mitotic figures are less numerous, scattered nuclear debris is less abundant, and necrosis occurs less frequently than in the Burkitt's and immunoblastic lymphomas. The neoplastic cells are intermediate in size between those of Burkitt's and immunoblastic lymphoma and usually are round to slightly ovoid. They generally have scant to moderately abundant acidophilic cytoplasm, without a paranuclear hof or other evidence of plasmacytoid differentiation. The nuclei tend to be round and regular and have one to several small, but distinct, nucleoli adjacent to the nuclear membrane (322,323) (Fig. 28.45). Some large cell lymphomas contain variable proportions or even are composed entirely of neoplastic cells containing cleaved or multilobated nuclei (440) (Fig. 28.46).

Lineage and Clonality

Many investigators have demonstrated that the more than 90% of AIDS-related systemic and primary CNS lymphomas that display Burkitt's, immunoblastic, and large cell morphology are of B-cell derivation. This conclusion is based on their expression of monotypic surface immunoglobulin or B-cell lineage–associated antigens CD19, CD20,

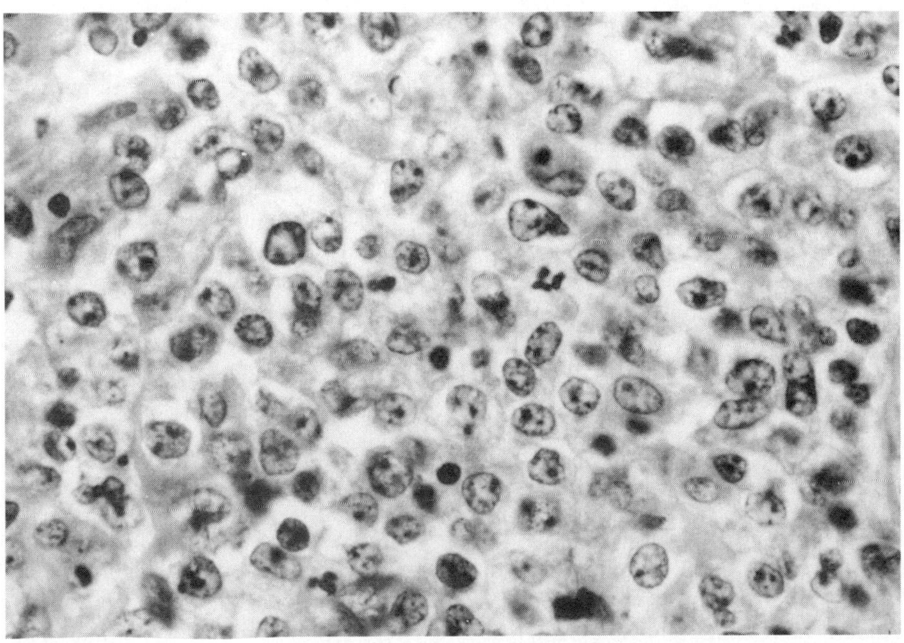

FIG. 28.45. AIDS-related large cell lymphoma (hematoxylin and eosin stain, original magnification: 500× magnification).

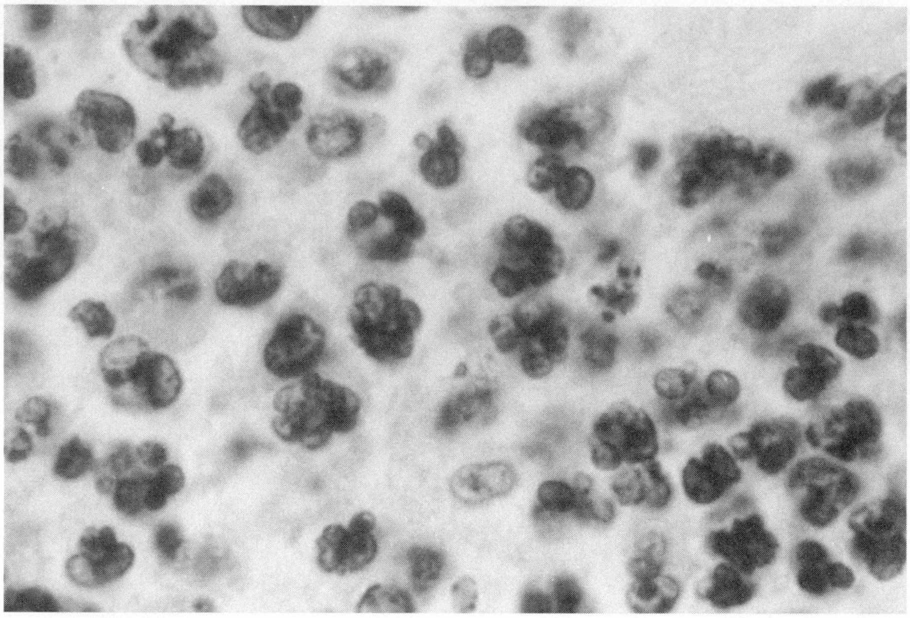

FIG. 28.46. AIDS-related large cell lymphoma comprised of tumor cells containing multilobated nuclei. The tumor cells were shown to be of B-cell origin by immunophenotypic analysis (hematoxylin and eosin stain, original magnification: 630× magnification).

and CD22, in the absence of T-cell lineage–associated antigens (369–371,375,401,418,424,440,468,477,478). Most of the remaining small proportion, approximately 3%, of AIDS-related NHLs represent body cavity–based (primary effusion) lymphomas. These tumors often express indeterminate phenotypes, that is, lack surface immunoglobulin and B cell– and T cell–associated antigens, and express non–lineage-specific antigens associated with activation (462–466). Occasional T-cell lineage–derived NHLs and lymphoid leukemias have been reported in HIV-infected individuals, but their relationship to HIV infection and the AIDS epidemic remains unclear (403,422,423). AIDS lymphomagenesis can be regarded as a B-cell phenomenon. Nearly all AIDS-related Burkitt's lymphomas express surface immunoglobulin, most commonly IgMκ, and approximately 75% express CD10. They express CD21 (the C3d-EBV receptor) uncommonly. Only about 50% of large cell and immunoblastic lymphomas express monotypic surface immunoglobulin, and the isotype is variable. The large cell and immunoblastic lymphomas express CD10 and CD21 heterogeneously (375,422,423). AIDS-related B-cell NHLs appear to express immunophenotypes that are similar to those expressed by conventional B-cell NHLs of comparable morphology occurring in the immunocompetent, HIV-uninfected general population (375,422,423,468).

Numerous investigators have demonstrated that most AIDS-related NHLs, including the body cavity–based lymphomas expressing indeterminate immunophenotypes, display clonal immunoglobulin heavy and light gene chain rearrangements in the absence of clonal T-cell receptor gene rearrangements, thus confirming their B-cell derivation (375,466,468,477,479–481). These malignant lymphomas appear to contain one dominant clonal B-cell population, based on the presence of one or two nongermline hybridizing bands of high intensity on Southern blotting. This dominant clonal B-cell population, representing the malignant lymphoma, sometimes is accompanied by additional minor B-cell clones that are detectable as additional faint bands following prolonged exposure on Southern blotting (477) (Fig. 28.47). Minor B-cell clones lacking evidence of malignant transformation have been identified in about 20% of hyperplastic lymph nodes obtained from HIV-infected patients (477). Possibly these clones persist in some lymph nodes that become replaced by malignant lymphoma, thus accounting for the additional faint rearranged bands observed in these cases.

A conspicuous exception to these findings are the studies published by McGrath, Herndier, and colleagues (482–485). These investigators have reported that approximately one third of all AIDS-related lymphomas from the San Francisco Bay area that they have studied are polyclonal. This conclusion was based on their inability to detect clonal immunoglobulin heavy chain gene rearrangements in biopsy specimens by Southern blotting or in some instances by reverse transcriptase–PCR (482–484). These lymphoid proliferations were described as exhibiting large cell morphology and expressing a spectrum of mixed immunophenotypes based on the presence of variable numbers of B cells, T cells, and macrophages (482–484). These ''polyclonal lymphomas'' were reported to lack EBV and *MYC* gene rearrangements and to have a more favorable clinical outcome than other AIDS-related NHLs (485). It was suggested by these investi-

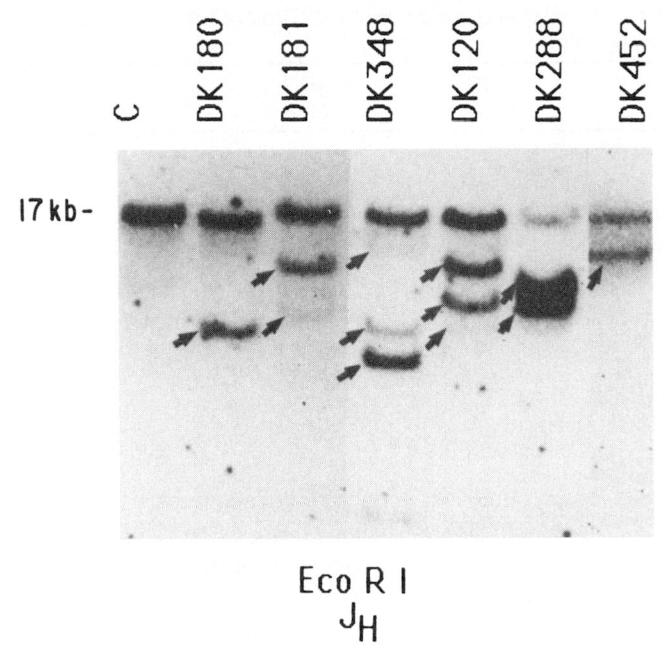

FIG. 28.47. Immunoglobulin gene rearrangement analysis of AIDS-related non-Hodgkin's lymphomas. The DNA extracted from the indicated cases and from normal human placenta (control, *C*) were digested with Eco RI and hybridized to an immunoglobulin heavy chain joining region probe. *Arrows* indicate rearrangement bands. The control lane shows the germline configuration. All AIDS-related non-Hodgkin's lymphomas exhibiting B-cell immunophenotypes display clonal immunoglobulin heavy chain gene rearrangements, consistent with a clonal B-cell derivation. Some of the tumors display more than two rearrangement bands, often of varying intensity, in addition to the germline band. These may represent minor B-cell clones in addition to the dominant malignant B-cell clone. In addition, histopathologically and immunophenotypically identical neoplasms taken from separate anatomic sites in the same patient (*DK180, DK181*) sometimes display distinct clonal immunoglobulin heavy chain gene rearrangement patterns, suggesting that each tumor may represent a distinct clonal proliferation. (From Pelicci PG, Knowles DM, Arlin Z, et al. Multiple monoclonal B-cell expansions and c-myc oncogene rearrangements in AIDS-related lymphoproliferative disorders: implications for lymphomagenesis. *J Exp Med* 1986;164:2049–2076, with permission from the Rockefeller University Press by copyright.)

gators that these polyclonal lymphomas represent a new category of AIDS-related lymphoma. These findings are unusual in that they are at odds with the vast literature concerning AIDS-related NHL, as well as with the widely held concept of monoclonality in lymphomagenesis.

The explanation for these discordant findings is unclear. McGrath and coworkers may have identified a novel subset of AIDS-related NHLs. Alternatively, tissue sampling or other technical factors may explain their findings. For example, these investigators often failed to analyze their cases for immunoglobulin light chain gene rearrangements (482–484). Furthermore, the absence of clonal immunoglobulin gene rearrangements by Southern blotting does not necessarily indicate polyclonality. Other scientific explanations can be offered to account for such findings (486).

In order to resolve the controversy surrounding the clonal nature of AIDS-related NHLs, we performed a comprehensive correlative molecular genetic and morphologic analysis of 74 AIDS-related systemic NHLs originating from the east and west coasts (37 cases each) of the United States (487) (Table 28.11). We were able to detect a solitary, dominant monoclonal B-cell population in 66 (89%) of the 74 patients by Southern blot immunoglobulin heavy chain gene rearrangement analysis, using two probes specific to different segments of the immunoglobulin heavy chain gene joining region. We were able to determine the monoclonal B-cell nature of 71 (96%) of the 74 cases if immunoglobulin heavy chain gene, immunoglobulin κ and λ light chain genes, and EBV terminal repeat analyses were used in conjunction. The occasional AIDS-related NHLs that apparently lack clonal immunoglobulin heavy chain gene rearrangements usually exhibit clonal immunoglobulin light chain gene rearrangements. Furthermore, many of those AIDS-related NHLs that apparently lack clonal immunoglobulin heavy and light chain gene rearrangements contain evidence of clonal EBV infection (Fig. 28.48). We failed to determine a clonal nature in only 1 (3%) of 37 east coast cases and 2 (6%) of 37 west coast cases, employing multiple approaches (487). None of these three cases resembled morphologically the so-called polyclonal lymphomas reported by McGrath and colleagues (482–485).

Our findings confirm that AIDS-related systemic NHLs exhibiting a germline immunoglobulin gene configuration exist but clearly demonstrate that such cases are quite uncommon. The results of Raphael and colleagues (468), who reported only rare cases of AIDS-related NHLs exhibiting a germline immunoglobulin gene configuration on Southern blot hybridization, are consistent with our findings. Whether these germline cases are truly polyclonal or clonality is not detectable with the methods employed remains to be determined.

Finally, studies concerning structural alterations of protooncogenes and tumor suppressor genes have provided considerable additional evidence in support of the widely held belief that most AIDS-related NHLs are monoclonal neoplasms. For example, the fact that only one rearranged *MYC* allele is detectable in each AIDS-related NHL (477,480,481) also supports the concept that each malignant lymphoma contains one vastly predominant clone, that is, is monoclonal. This conclusion is further supported by the presence of a solitary *P53* gene mutation, a solitary *BCL6* gene rearrangement, and so on in AIDS-related NHLs (481,488). Additional studies are necessary to confirm the authenticity of so-called polyclonal AIDS-related NHLs, as well as the significance of the observation that some AIDS-related NHLs apparently lack evidence of clonal immunoglobulin gene rearrangements. We have failed to find evidence to support the contention that true polyclonal lymphomas, those in

TABLE 28.11. *Immunoglobulin gene rearrangement patterns in 74 east and west coast AIDS-related non-Hodgkin's lymphomas* lymphomol

Region	Cases, n	IgHR IgLR	IgHR IgLG	IgHG IgLR	IgHG IgLG	T cell receptor β
East coast	37	30	4	2	1	0
West coast	37	24	8	1	4[a]	0

[a] Two cases clonal Epstein-Barr virus.
IgH, immunoglobulin heavy chain; IgL, immunoglobulin light chain; R, rearranged; G, germline.

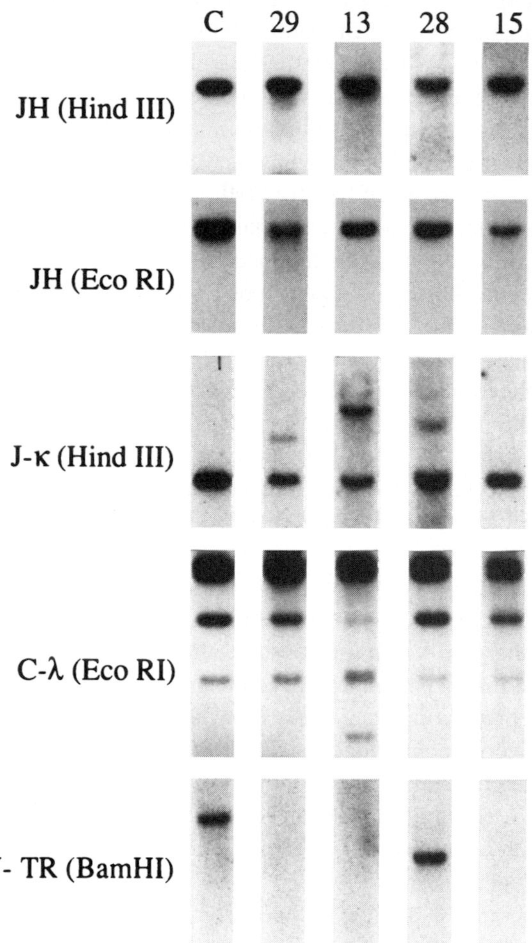

FIG. 28.48. Molecular genetic analysis of AIDS-related non-Hodgkin's lymphomas exhibiting a germline immunoglobulin heavy chain gene configuration on Southern blot hybridization. The number above each lane indicates the case number. *C* indicates a control lane (HL60 cell line), except in the case of EBV-TR, in which an EBV-containing Burkitt's lymphoma cell line (Daudi) was used. Each of these four cases exhibited a germline immunoglobulin heavy chain gene configuration. However, cases 29, 13, and 28 exhibit clonal κ light chain gene rearrangement, and case 13 also exhibits clonal λ light chain gene rearrangement. Case 28 contains evidence of clonal EBV infection. Case 15 apparently lacks clonal immunoglobulin heavy and light chain gene rearrangements, as well as evidence of clonal EBV infection. (From Knowles DM. Etiology and pathogenesis of AIDS-related non-Hodgkin's lymphoma: hematologic and oncologic aspects of HIV infection. *Hematol Oncol Clin North Am* 1996;10:1081–1109, with permission.)

which the neoplastic cell population is derived from multiple clones, exist.

Molecular Genetics

Several dominantly acting protooncogenes, *MYC*, *BCL1*, *BCL2*, and *BCL6*, are believed to play roles in lymphomagenesis in the immunocompetent host through chromosomal translocation or point mutation. The structural alterations involving these oncogenes occur nonrandomly in association with specific histopathologic categories of conventional NHL. It also is believed that inactivation of the *P53* and the retinoblastoma tumor suppressor genes is involved in lymphomagenesis (see Chapter 8). Structural alterations in some of these genes, and also in the *RAS* gene family, variably occur among AIDS-related NHLs as well.

Reciprocal chromosomal translocations occurring between the *MYC* oncogene on chromosome 8 and the immunoglobulin heavy chain, κ light chain, or λ light chain gene on chromosomes 14, 2, and 22, respectively, are associated highly with endemic (African) and sporadic (Western) Burkitt's lymphoma (489–491). These translocations are observed infrequently in other categories of conventional NHL occurring in the HIV-uninfected general population (491). The initial cytogenetic studies performed in the early years of the AIDS epidemic revealed the frequent occurrence of chromosomal translocations involving band 8q24, the site of the *MYC* gene, in AIDS-related NHLs, suggesting their molecular similarity to Burkitt's lymphoma occurring in immunocompetent hosts (377,380,381). These findings were confirmed and expanded by molecular analysis of the *MYC* locus in AIDS-related NHLs. Pelicci and colleagues (477) and Subar and coworkers (480) identified *MYC* gene rearrangements in approximately 75% of AIDS-related NHLs. These included most patients exhibiting Burkitt's morphology and, surprisingly, some exhibiting large cell and immunoblastic morphology. In addition, conventional Burkitt's lymphomas carrying the t(2;8) translocation usually express kappa light chains, and those carrying the t(8;22) translocation usually express λ light chains (492). A lack of correlation between the type of translocation and light chain expression has been described in AIDS-related Burkitt's lymphoma (493,494).

With respect to those AIDS-related large cell and immunoblastic lymphomas carrying *MYC* gene rearrangements, Delecluse and coworkers (495) have proposed that they actually represent a subset of AIDS-related Burkitt's lymphomas that have adopted large cell or immunoblastic morphology in the context of impaired immune surveillance. These investigators have suggested that severe perturbation of the immune system acts as a permissive factor for the morphologic switch of Burkitt's to large cell or immunoblastic histology and maintains the genetic distinction of Burkitt's lymphoma, namely, *MYC* gene activation (495). Supporting this hypothesis, AIDS-related NHLs displaying cytomorphologic features intermediate between those of Burkitt's lymphoma and large cell or immunoblastic lymphoma have been observed (468,496,497). Conventional Burkitt's lymphoma cells, especially if infected by EBV, often undergo immunoblastic transformation during serial passages in culture *in vitro*. This may be accompanied by immunophenotypic variations and by a change in the pattern of EBV latent gene expression (498–500). It has been suggested that AIDS-related large cell lymphomas exhibiting *MYC* gene activation display hybrid clinical features, namely, the host immunosuppression typical of AIDS-related large cell lymphoma and the preferential association with preexistent persistent generalized lymphadenopathy often seen in AIDS-related Burkitt's lymphoma (485). Another hypothesis that has been suggested is that the *MYC* gene activation observed in these cases may reflect simply the pathogenetic heterogeneity of AIDS lymphomagenesis (501).

Several differences exist between endemic and sporadic Burkitt's lymphoma. In nearly all patients with endemic Burkitt's lymphoma, the tumor cells contain the EBV genome, express Fc receptors and CD21 (the EBV receptor), lack CD10, and do not secrete IgM. Only a small proportion of sporadic Burkitt's lymphomas contain the EBV genome, and the tumor cells usually lack Fc receptors and CD21, express CD10, and secrete IgM (502). Dalla-Favera (503) has demonstrated that the translocations involving chromosome 8 lead to *MYC* gene deregulation by molecular mechanisms that vary according to the geographic origin of the Burkitt's lymphoma (503–505). The *MYC* gene is activated by point mutations or small rearrangements occurring within regulatory regions spanning its first exon–first intron border in the translocation t(8;14) associated with endemic Burkitt's lymphoma and the variant translocations t(2;8) and t(8;22) associated with both endemic and sporadic Burkitt's lymphoma. In contrast, the *MYC* gene is activated by truncations occurring within its first exon, first intron, or 5′ flanking sequences in the translocation t(8;14) associated with sporadic Burkitt's lymphoma (504–507). The pattern of chromosome 14 involvement in t(8;14) is also heterogeneous. *MYC* recombines preferentially with the joining region of the immunoglobulin heavy chain gene in all Burkitt's lymphomas, but more often with the switch region of the immunoglobulin heavy chain gene in sporadic Burkitt's lymphoma than in endemic Burkitt's lymphoma (504–507). The pathogeneses of endemic and sporadic Burkitt's lymphoma appear to differ, probably as a consequence of differences in the differentiation state of the target cells in which the translocational events occur (505) (see Chapter 27).

Most AIDS-related systemic Burkitt's lymphomas exhibit *MYC* gene rearrangement, but many of them do not contain EBV, and the tumor cells lack Fc and EBV receptors (CD21) but express CD10 (375,422,423,477,480), analogous to sporadic Burkitt's lymphoma (502). In additon, the molecular mechanisms leading to *MYC* gene activation in these lymphomas are similar to those operational in sporadic Burkitt's lymphoma (480,481,503,506). The bulk of the accumulated immunologic and molecular genetic data suggests that most AIDS-related systemic Burkitt's lymphomas resemble sporadic rather than endemic Burkitt's lymphoma.

The *BCL6* gene is located on 3q27 (508), the site of frequent chromosomal breaks in conventional and some AIDS-related NHLs (509–511). The *BCL6* gene encodes a zinc finger protein that shares homologies with several transcription factors (512–514). The BCL-6 protein normally is expressed at high levels by mature germinal center B cells (515) and is believed to control germinal center formation (516). Chromosomal translocations between 3q27 and a heterogeneous chromosomal partner cause the truncation of the *BCL6* gene within its 5′ noncoding regulatory sequences (512) in about 40% of diffuse large B-cell lymphomas occurring in immunocompetent hosts (517). *BCL6* gene rearrangements generally are not found in other categories of NHL, except for a small proportion of follicular center cell lymphomas (517). Rearrangements of the *BCL6* gene are detectable in approximately 20% of AIDS-related systemic NHLs, including both EBV-positive and EBV-negative cases (488). As in the case of conventional NHLs, however, they are associated overwhelmingly with those AIDS-related NHLs exhibiting large cell and immunoblastic morphology and are absent from those exhibiting classic Burkitt's morphology (488). *BCL6* and *MYC* gene rearrangements do not occur in the same tumor, suggesting that these genetic lesions represent mutually exclusive molecular pathways in lymphomagenesis. It has been suggested that *BCL6* gene rearrangement occurs preferentially among extranodal large cell lymphomas and is a favorable prognostic indicator for these lymphomas (518). Whether this holds true for *BCL6* gene rearrangement in AIDS-related NHLs has not been determined.

Activation of the *RAS* family of genes by single nucleotide substitutions at codons 12, 13, and 61 has been associated with a variety of human malignancies (519). Mutations involving *NRAS* gene codons 12 or 13 are detectable in almost 20% of precursor B-cell acute lymphoblastic leukemias (ALLs), and mutations involving *NRAS* gene condon 61 are detectable in approximately one third of cases of multiple myeloma or plasmacytoma (520–522). *RAS* gene mutations are not detectable in conventional NHLs occurring in the HIV-uninfected general population, however, including those exhibiting Burkitt's, large cell, or immunoblastic morphology (520,521). In contrast, activating point mutations involving *NRAS* or, less commonly, *KRAS*, are detectable in about 15% of AIDS-related systemic lymphomas (481). *RAS* gene mutations are more likely to be distinctive features in AIDS-related NHLs than in conventional NHLs of comparable morphology arising in immunocompetent persons. The biologic significance of this association is unknown. It is likely, however, that the mutated *RAS* genes contribute to the pathogenesis of those AIDS-related lymphomas in which they are present, because their role in the tumorigenic conversion of EBV-infected B cells *in vitro* is established (523).

Rearrangements of the *BCL1* gene, associated with translocation t(11;14), are associated preferentially with mantle cell lymphoma and occur in about 50% of these lymphomas (524). Rearrangements of the *BCL2* gene, associated with t(14:18), are associated highly with malignant lymphomas of follicular center cell origin. They occur in more than 80% of such cases displaying a follicular growth pattern and in the 20% of diffuse large B-cell lymphomas preceded by a follicular phase (525,526). AIDS-related NHLs consistently lack *BCL1* and *BCL2* gene rearrangements (462,480,527). These findings strongly suggest that AIDS-related NHLs are not derived from mantle or follicular center B cells and that they originate *de novo* and are not preceded by a follicular phase, as is a subset of conventional diffuse large B-cell lymphomas (526).

Certain tumor suppressor genes, including the *P53* gene, the retinoblastoma gene, and putative genes on chromosome 6q, are believed to play an important role in the development and progression of human neoplasia if deletions or mutations in these loci relieve cells from normal negative regulatory signals (528–531). The *P53* gene, mapping to 17p13, encodes a nuclear phosphoprotein that is believed to play an essential role in cell cycle control (529,530). Inactivation of the *P53* gene is usually the result of point mutations in the coding sequence of exons 5 through 8 in one allele, with or without loss of the corresponding allele (529,530). Mutations of the *P53* gene occur relatively frequently in many categories of human malignancy (532,533). Among lymphoid neoplasms, *P53* gene mutations are highly associated with Burkitt's lymphoma, large cell transformation of B-cell chronic lymphocytic leukemia (Richter's syndrome) and adult T-cell lymphoma or leukemia (534,535). *P53* gene mutations occur uncommonly among other categories of conventional NHL (534). Mutations involving the *P53* gene occur in about 37% of AIDS-related systemic NHLs (481) but are associated preferentially with Burkitt's morphology (481). This includes both EBV-positive and EBV-negative tumors (481). The frequent association between *P53* gene mutation and *MYC* gene deregulation in both AIDS-related and non–AIDS-related Burkitt's lymphomas suggests a pathogenetic relationship between these two genetic lesions that may have a synergistic effect on the development of these tumors (536). This hypothesis is supported by the finding that the MYC protein may be involved in the regulation of *P53* gene expression (537). The mutations similarly occur in exons 5 though 8 in AIDS-related NHLs. The most frequently encountered mutations are transitions at CpG dinucleotides (481), as is the case for conventional NHLs and some other tumors (529,530). This type of mutation is believed to occur as a DNA replication error, with no direct causal relationship with any known carcinogen (529). In some instances, *P53* gene mutations are accompanied by loss of the corresponding allele (481). The molecular mechanisms of *P53* gene inactivation in AIDS-related systemic NHLs are similar to those occurring in other human tumors (530), and the mutational spectrum is comparable to that of conventional NHLs occurring in immunocompetent hosts (534).

Deletions of the long arm of chromosome 6 long have been recognized as one of the predominant genetic lesions, as well as an indicator of poor prognosis, among B-cell lymphomas (531). Deletions of 6q are present in approximately 25% of AIDS-related NHLs and may play a role in their pathogenesis (536). The 6q deletions cluster in two discrete regions along the long arm of chromosome 6 mapping to 6q27 (region of minimal deletion-1 [*RMD1*]) and 6q21-23 (*RMD2*) (538). These two regions represent the sites of two putative tumor suppressor genes, which appear to be relevant to lymphomagenesis, leukemiagenesis, and tumorigenesis (538–541). *RMD1* and *RMD2* exhibit preferential association with low- and high-grade B-cell lymphomas, respectively (542). It is thought that *RMD2* lesions participate in AIDS lymphomagenesis, although the precise mechanism is unclear.

The retinoblastoma gene, located on chromosome 13q14 (543), encodes 110- to 114-kd phosphorylated proteins that are normally present in all human tissues and are believed to inhibit cell growth (544). Mutational inactivation of the retinoblastoma gene has been documented in a large variety of malignant tumors, suggesting that functional loss of this gene is involved in the initiation or progression of many human malignancies (545). Point mutations, encountered in 80% of lesions, represent the most frequent mechanism of retinoblastoma gene inactivation; gross rearrangements or large intragenic deletions occur much less commonly (546). A small proportion of diffuse aggressive conventional NHLs occurring in the HIV-uninfected general population exhibit retinoblastoma gene mutations or deletions (547). Investigators have failed to find evidence of retinoblastoma gene inactivation in AIDS-related NHLs (481,548), suggesting that this gene does not play a role in AIDS lymphomagenesis.

These molecular genetic alterations do not appear to occur entirely randomly among the AIDS-related NHLs, however. Previous molecular genetic analyses have suggested that distinct molecular differences exist among AIDS-related NHLs according to their histopathologic categories and anatomic sites of origin, that is, systemic versus primary CNS (418,419,454,480,481,488). These studies have suggested that virtually 100% of patients with Burkitt's lymphoma exhibit *MYC* gene rearrangements, two thirds display *P53* gene mutations, one third have EBV, and essentially none exhibit *BCL6* gene rearrangements. In the case of immunoblastic lymphoma, these studies have suggested that nearly 100% of

TABLE 28.12. *Molecular characteristics of 64 AIDS-related systemic non-Hodgkin's lymphomas*

Lesion	Burkitt's lymphoma (n = 6)	Burkitt's-like lymphoma (n = 20)	Large cell lymphoma (n = 12)	Immunoblastic lymphoma (n = 26)	Total (n = 64)
EBV	83%	40%	9%	50%	43%
KSHV	0%	0%	0%	15%	6%
C-MYC	84%	45%	50%	31%	44%
BCL6	0%	15%	25%	15%	16%
RAS	0%	5%	0%	8%	5%
P53	50%	30%	17%	31%	30%

patients have EBV, 25% display *MYC* gene rearrangements, 20% display *BCL6* gene rearrangements, and very few exhibit *P53* gene mutations. *RAS* gene mutations occur in a comparable proportion, about 20%, of patients with Burkitt's and immunoblastic lymphomas. These studies also have suggested, in the case of large cell lymphoma, that about 25% contain EBV, 50% exhibit *MYC* gene rearrangements, 25% exhibit *BCL6* gene rearrangements, and none contain *P53* or *RAS* gene mutations (481,488). Most of these studies, however, have involved only a small number of patients, often seen at a single institution where some but not all of the parameters were investigated.

We performed a comprehensive analysis of the viral content and the oncogene and tumor suppressor gene status of a cohort of 64 AIDS-related systemic NHLs originating on the east and west coasts of the United States and correlated the findings with the histopathology of the lesions (487) (Table 28.12). The incidence, type, and clonal pattern of EBV infection and the type and frequency of molecular genetic lesions were similar among the east and west coast cases, suggesting no evidence of geographic distinctions. We detected clonal EBV infection in 41% of the AIDS-related systemic NHLs by Southern blot hybridization analysis of the EBV terminal repeat region, consistent with previous studies (480,481). Type A EBV was found in two thirds of the patients, and type B in the remaining one third. We identified *MYC* gene rearrangements, *P53* gene mutations or deletions, *BCL6* gene rearrangements, and *RAS* gene mutations in 44%, 30%, 17%, and 6% of patients with these AIDS-related systemic NHLs, respectively. We failed to detect *BCL1* or *BCL2* gene rearrangements or retinoblastoma gene mutations or deletions among these patients. We found that more than 80% of the patients with Burkitt's lymphomas have EBV and *MYC* gene rearrangements, and approximately one half have *P53* gene mutations in the absence of *BCL6* gene rearrangements and *RAS* gene mutations. We found that the Burkitt's-like lymphomas exhibit a comparable constellation of genetic alterations, except that a smaller proportion of patients have EBV infection, *MYC* gene rearrangements, and *P53* gene mutations, and that *BCL6* gene rearrangements occur in a small percentage of patients. Among the large cell lymphomas, we found that only very few patients have EBV, approximately one half have *MYC* gene rearrangements, a small percentage have *P53* gene mutations, and approximately 25% exhibit *BCL6* gene rearrangements. We found that the immunoblastic lymphomas exhibit a constellation of molecular genetic alterations that closely resemble those of the Burkitt's-like lymphomas (487).

Comprehensive molecular genetic analysis of AIDS-related primary CNS lymphomas has not been performed. We know that they uniformly contain the EBV genome and lack *MYC* gene rearrangements, in contrast with AIDS-related systemic NHLs (454,549). The body cavity-based (primary effusion) lymphomas nearly always contain EBV and lack *MYC* gene rearrangements, and they also usually lack *BCL6* gene rearrangements, *RAS* gene mutations, and *P53* gene deletions or mutations (297,466,467).

These findings indicate that AIDS-related lymphomas are characterized by the accumulation of multiple distinct genetic lesions, involving viruses, protooncogenes, and tumor suppressor genes. These genetic lesions apparently accrue rather quickly, during the brief 4- to 6-year period between HIV infection and the development of malignant lymphoma (391,403). This contrasts sharply with the widely held belief that multistep tumorigenesis occurs over a long period of time, perhaps as long as 30 years (550,551). These findings also support the contentions that multiple alternative molecular pathways operate in AIDS lymphomagenesis, and that some of these pathways may be associated preferentially with specific histopathologic categories or anatomic sites of origin (552). Although EBV infection and certain molecular genetic alterations are associated with distinct histopathologic categories, however, the correlations do not appear to be as specific as previously suggested. AIDS-related NHLs appear to represent a morphologic and molecular genetic spectrum of high grade lymphoid neoplasia (487). Future clinical studies, including therapeutic trials, should include a comprehensive correlative morphologic and molecular genetic analysis of the lymphomas in order to verify and extend these findings. Such studies eventually may yield a classification, based at least partially on genetic features, that is clinically and prognostically more relevant than the current classification of AIDS-related lymphomas, which is based largely on histopathologic evaluation alone.

Clinical Characteristics Including Correlations with Anatomic Site of Origin and Histopathology

Approximately 95% of AIDS-related NHLs occur in adult men (369–375,385,391,393,403). This is largely because adult men predominate among the principal AIDS risk groups, that is, MEM and IDUs. The median age of patients is between 37 and 38 years in the largest clinical series reported from the United States (371,375,415) and 27 and 29 years in the largest western European series (389,416); however, AIDS-related NHLs occasionally occur in the very young or in the elderly who have other AIDS risk factors. The age distribution for patients with AIDS-related NHL conforms closely to that of AIDS in general (369). Approximately 50% of patients develop one or more severe opportunistic infections, and as many as 25% of patients (primarily MSM) have been reported to develop Kaposi's sarcoma before, concurrent with, or after the onset of NHL (369,372,375,415). The majority of patients exhibit the alterations in cellular immunity commonly associated with HIV infection, including cytopenias, cutaneous anergy, polyclonal hypergammaglobulinemia, and greatly decreased numbers of peripheral blood CD4 T cells, resulting in markedly reduced CD4:CD8 T-cell ratios (369,371,372,375). The majority of patients also have serologic evidence of preceeding or active cytomegalovirus or EBV infection (371,372,415,419).

Approximately 75% or more of patients who have AIDS-related NHLs complain of B symptoms as defined by the Ann Arbor staging system (553): unexplained fever, night sweats, or weight loss in excess of 10% of usual body weight (371,394,403,419,425). The B symptoms are secondary to malignant lymphoma in the majority of patients (425). Aside from B symptoms, patient complaints at initial presentation are variable because of the diverse and multiple organ systems involved by malignant lymphoma. The complaints may be local or systemic and usually depend on the principal location of lymphomatous disease (431).

AIDS-related NHLs belonging to all histopathologic categories were lumped together initially in most clinical studies for purposes of management, therapy, and clinicopathologic analysis. Knowles and colleagues (375), however, demonstrated that each histopathologic category of AIDS-related NHL actually exhibits distinctive clinical characteristics, including specific associations with clinical stage, preferential involvement of certain extranodal sites, and perhaps even statistically significant differences in median survival. For example, approximately two thirds of patients who have Burkitt's lymphoma, but only approximately 40% of patients who have immunoblastic or large cell lymphoma, present with clinical stage IV disease. This is partially because AIDS-related NHLs differ in their propensity to involve the bone marrow according to their histopathology. In a series of 89 patients with AIDS-related NHLs, 39% of those who had Burkitt's lymphoma, only 16% of those who had immunoblastic lymphoma, and none of 25 patients who had large cell lymphoma had bone marrow involvement at initial presentation (375). AIDS-related NHLs differ in their propensity to involve the gastrointestinal tract according to their histopathology. In that same series, 48% of immunoblastic, 36% of large cell, but only 8% of Burkitt's lymphomas involved the gastrointestinal tract initially (375). The French Study Group, based on an analysis of 113 AIDS-related NHLs, confirmed and extended these findings (440). They demonstrated that Burkitt's lymphoma more frequently involves lymph nodes, the bone marrow, and skeletal muscles; that immunoblastic lymphoma and large cell lymphoma more frequently involve the oral cavity, the gastrointestinal tract, and the CNS; and that these associations are statistically significant (440). The vast majority of primary CNS lymphomas express immunoblastic or large cell morphology (393,394,419,440,454). It appears that AIDS-related Burkitt's lymphomas usually originate in lymph nodes and then rapidly disseminate to involve distant lymph node groups, the bone marrow, and obscure extranodal sites; AIDS-related immunoblastic and large cell lymphomas more often originate in extranodal sites such as the gastrointestinal tract, grow to a large size at the primary site of origin, spread to regional lymph nodes, and subsequently disseminate to other lymph node groups and extranodal sites (375).

In addition to these findings, a number of observations suggest that other significant clinical distinctions exist among AIDS-related NHLs according to their histopathologic category and anatomic site of origin. For example, those individuals who develop AIDS-related Burkitt's lymphoma tend to be younger, usually do not have a prior diagnosis of AIDS, and tend to have higher mean CD4 T-cell counts at the time of diagnosis. In contrast, those individuals who develop AIDS-related immunoblastic lymphoma tend to be older, frequently have a prior diagnosis of AIDS, and tend to have lower mean CD4 T-cell counts at diagnosis (391,393,419). Burkitt's lymphoma tends to be an earlier manifestation of HIV infection than does immunoblastic lymphoma, which represented a secondary AIDS diagnosis in 87% of patients in one study (393). Immunodeficiency appears to be more severe and the HIV-associated illnesses appear to be more extensive in HIV-infected individuals who develop primary CNS lymphoma than in those who develop systemic lymphoma. In one study, the median CD4 T-cell count in patients with primary CNS lymphoma was only 30 cells per microliter; it was 189 cells per microliter in those patients who developed systemic lymphoma (394). In that same study, more than 70% of the patients who developed primary CNS lymphoma had a prior diagnosis of AIDS; only 37% of those who developed systemic lymphoma had documented AIDS (394).

The primary effusion lymphomas more closely resemble immunoblastic lymphoma than Burkitt's lymphoma and primary CNS lymphomas than systemic lymphomas, with respect to these various clinical characteristics. The primary effusion lymphomas tend to occur in slightly older HIV-infected individuals (median age 42 years), who are usually severely immune-deficient (median CD4 T-cell count 84 cells per microliter) and two thirds of whom have prior diagnoses of AIDS (467).

We have suggested that the therapeutic response and eventual outcome appear to differ according to the histopathologic category of NHL (375). In a clinicopathologic study of 89 patients who had AIDS-related NHL, Knowles and colleagues (375) found that 52% of patients who had large cell, 26% of patients who had Burkitt's, and 21% of patients who had immunoblastic lymphoma achieved complete responses. The patients who had large cell, Burkitt's, and immunoblastic lymphoma had median durations of survival of 7.5, 5.5, and 2.0 months, respectively (375). These survival rates are significantly shorter than those of HIV-uninfected patients in the general population who have histologically identical conventional NHLs (469). These findings strongly suggest that patients who have AIDS-related immunoblastic lymphoma fare the worst. These conclusions were based on a retrospective series of patients who had been treated with a variety of chemotherapeutic regimens and who were not stratified in terms of prognostic factors, however. Further studies are necessary to confirm these findings.

It is likely that the significance of these clinical observations will be solidified, and other distinctions having etiologic, therapeutic, and prognostic significance will become evident as more data are accumulated.

Prognostic Factors

Several factors are associated with shorter durations of survival among HIV-uninfected individuals who have conventional intermediate and high-grade NHL. These include older age, the presence of systemic B symptoms, increased tumor burden, and lower patient performance status (554,555). These factors, however, have not been uniformly applicable to patients who have AIDS-related NHL, among whom prognostic factors related to HIV infection and associated illnesses appear to be more important than those related to malignant lymphoma *per se*. For example, no correlation was found between clinical stage or histologic grade and complete response in the first large multiinstitutional series (369). In a multivariate analysis of 49 patients with AIDS-related systemic NHL from a single institution, Levine and colleagues (394) found that a prior history of AIDS, a Karnofsky performance status less than 70%, and bone marrow involvement each predicted for shorter survival. Lower CD4 T-cell counts also appeared to imply shorter duration of survival (394). Systemic B symptoms, tumor size, histopathologic category, elevated lactic dehydrogenase levels, and leptomeningeal disease did not predict shorter survival (394).

A series of 84 patients with AIDS-related NHL reported from San Francisco (417) confirmed the dominance of prognostic factors related to HIV infection and AIDS. In that series, the total number of CD4 T cells was the most important predictor of survival. Patients who had a total CD4 T-cell count greater than 100 cells per microliter had a median duration of survival of 24 months; for those whose CD4 T-cell count was less than 100 cells per microliter, the duration of survival of only 4.1 months. If CD4 T-cell counts were available, no other factors contributed prognostic information. In the absence of CD4 T cell counts, however, the best predictor of survival was a prior diagnosis of AIDS. The median survival of those patients without a prior AIDS diagnosis was 8.3 months, versus 2.2 months for those patients with a prior AIDS diagnosis. Less important prognostic factors were the Karnofsky performance status and the presence of extranodal disease. A Karnofsky performance status greater than 70% was associated with a median duration of survival of 6.8 months; one less than 70% was associated with a median duration of survival of 3.8 months. The median survival of those patients with extranodal disease was only 3.4 months, versus 12.2 months for those patients who had lymphadenopathy alone. Survival was not influenced by the specific extranodal site or the total number of extranodal sites. In this series, the use of more intensive chemotherapy regimens also correlated with decreased duration of survival (417). The survival of patients who have AIDS-related NHL appears to be most dependent on their level of immunodeficiency. The prognostic significance of the histopathologic category of AIDS related NHL within the context of this immunodeficiency remains unclear and requires expert pathologic review of the NHLs occurring in a large cohort of homogeneously treated patients for clarification.

Clinical Evaluation, Treatment, and Survival

The staging procedures routinely employed in the evaluation of patients who have AIDS-related NHLs are the same as those for HIV-uninfected patients who have conventional NHLs. They include a complete blood count; serum biochemistry studies including liver function tests and creatinine and lactic acid dehydrogenase measurements; chest radiograph and bone marrow aspiration and biopsy; and computed tomography of the chest, abdomen, and pelvis, with oral and intravenous contrast administration. In addition, a diagnostic lumbar puncture should be performed and the cerebrospinal fluid checked for cytology, cell count, and protein and glucose levels. Other workup depends on whether or not there are other unusual extranodal sites of involvement. It is desirable to check on the status of the HIV infection with CD4 T-cell counts and measurements of HIV load with plasma RNA levels (556).

The diagnosis of primary CNS lymphoma usually is established firmly by brain biopsy performed at craniostomy or with a computed tomography–guided stereotactic procedure. Some clinicians are reluctant to perform these diagnostic procedures, however, because of the associated risks and the poor therapeutic outcome (557). For this reason, noninvasive diagnostic procedures that may obviate the need for brain biopsy in some patients are being investigated. For example, one universal and potentially diagnostic feature of AIDS-related primary CNS lymphoma is the presence of the EBV genome (454). Cinque and colleagues (558) investigated as a possible diagnostic test a PCR assay of EBV in the cerebrospinal fluid of patients with AIDS-related primary CNS lymphoma. They reported that EBV DNA is consistently present in the cerebrospinal fluid of patients who have AIDS-related primary CNS lymphoma before the lesions can be visualized by computed tomographic scan or by magnetic resonance imaging, and that it is consistently absent from the cerebrospinal fluid of HIV-infected patients who die with other neurologic disorders, including toxoplasmosis and other infections. DeLuca and colleagues (559) have reported similar findings.

Sometimes the diagnosis of AIDS-related NHL is made first at autopsy, especially in the case of primary CNS lymphoma (369,374,375,419,427). In other instances, malignant lymphoma is so widespread at initial presentation and the patient is so ill that death occurs almost immediately following diagnosis, before therapy can be initiated (369,375,415, 419). In approximately 85% of patients, however, a tissue diagnosis of AIDS-related NHL is established *antemortem*, and the patient is treated. The treatment of AIDS-related systemic NHL is complicated by the fact that most patients have high- or intermediate-grade NHL and present with clinical stage III or IV disease, and many patients have secondary lymphomatous involvement of the bone marrow or the CNS. With these factors in mind, early treatment strategies employed dosage-intensive chemotherapeutic regimens comparable to those used to treat HIV-uninfected patients in the general population who have high- or intermediate-grade NHL (375,415). These approaches generally achieved dismal results, however. In one study, those patients who were treated more intensively actually experienced a significantly shorter duration of survival than those who were treated less intensively (417). HIV-infected patients often tolerate systemic chemotherapy poorly because of the severe underlying immune deficiency, recurring opportunistic infections, and leukopenia (431,560).

Complete response rates to the various, often dosage-intensive, chemotherapy regimens utilized in these early treatment strategies ranged between 20% and 67% (375,389,415, 419,560–562). Complete remission occurred primarily in those patients who presented with clinical stage I or II disease, without bone marrow or CNS involvement, and who had not experienced AIDS-related symptomatology (415). Even those responses were usually of short duration, and second-line chemotherapeutic regimens were rarely effective in inducing a second remission (375). CNS relapses were particularly problematic, and the use of prophylactic intrathecal chemotherapy did not prevent this phenomenon consistently (375,415,425,561). The median duration of survival usually was brief, ranging from 5 to 11 months (371,375,385,415,560–562).

Based on this information, the AIDS Clinical Trials Group initiated a prospective multiinstitutional trial using a low-dosage modification of the M-BACOD regimen (563), accompanied by early CNS prophylaxis with intrathecal cytosine arabinoside, and zidovudine at the completion of chemotherapy (564). A complete remission rate of approximately 50%, including long-term lymphoma-free survival in 75% of complete responders, was achieved among all patients, including those with poor prognostic indicators. Intrathecal CNS prophylaxis was effective: No patient experienced isolated CNS relapse. The median duration of survival was 6.5 months for all patients and 15 months for complete responders (565). Shortly thereafter, the availability of hematopoietic growth factors permitted the AIDS Clinical Trials Group (566) and Kaplan and colleagues (567), among others, to abrogate leukopenia and administer full doses of chemotherapy.

These and other therapeutic trials have led to some progress in achieving longer survival among patients who have AIDS-related systemic NHL (403). For example, it is now known that very low dosage multiagent chemotherapy may be effective in achieving long-term, lymphoma-free survival (564); CNS prophylaxis is necessary and intrathecal chemotherapy is effective in this regard (564,568); and hematopoietic growth factors may ameliorate the hematologic toxicity of chemotherapy in these patients (566,567). Individuals who have AIDS-related systemic NHL should receive antilymphoma therapy, because relatively longlasting remissions may be obtained even in those who have poor prognostic indicators (564). Successful salvage therapy, however, has not been achieved in patients who fail initial therapy or who experience relapse after initial remission, even among those who have undergone bone marrow transplantation (403). Only occasional patients are long-term survivors (372,375,415). The patients usually die from progressive lymphoma, opportunistic infections, or a combination of the two (369,374,375,389,415,419). Stratification of patients into good and poor risk categories should be part of the design and evaluation of future therapeutic trials (394,417).

Because the majority of patients who develop AIDS-related NHLs do poorly, investigators have been exploring new therapeutic strategies. These do not include bone marrow transplantation, however, for which there has been little enthusiasm because of its toxicity (556). Several groups have investigated or are now investigating concomitant antiretroviral and antilymphoma therapy in the treatment of individuals who have AIDS-related NHL. The toxicity of the first generation antiretroviral agents, however, including myelosuppression with zidovudine and the neurologic toxicity of zalcitabine, has limited their use in conjunction with antilymphoma chemotherapy. Other groups are evaluating intravenous interleukin-2 (IL-2) infusion, anti-IL-6 monoclonal antibody therapy, and the use of immunotoxins and radioimmunotherapy (556). Finally, the potential benefit of the temporary lowering of HIV load on overall clinical outcome has not been established. Investigation in these areas is likely to continue (556).

Patients who have AIDS-related primary CNS lymphoma usually are treated with intracranial irradiation, sometimes in combination with intrathecal chemotherapy (427,439). This approach often leads to regression of the lesions (426,439). These patients generally have very severe immune deficiency, however, as manifested by CD4 T-cell counts below 50 cells per microliter and multiple prior or concurrent opportunistic infections (394,420). They often die as a result of severe opportunistic infections (439,455). Some patients have a fulminant course and die within weeks following diagnosis (427). The mean duration of survival of patients following the onset of CNS symptoms was shorter than 2 months for those diagnosed and cared for at both the Los Angeles County–University of Southern California and University of California at San Francisco Medical Centers (426,427). In the largest clinical series of such patients reported to date, the median duration of survival was about 1 month for those patients who received no treatment and 4 months for those patients who received radiation therapy (455). Only rare patients survive for longer than 1 year (439,569,570), and these are usually the ones who have CD4 T-cell counts greater than 200 cells per microliter (569). This is substantially worse than the prognosis for conventional primary CNS lymphoma occurring in the HIV-uninfected general population (571). It has been suggested that the use of systemic chemotherapy in addition to intracranial radiation may be helpful in patients who have AIDS-related primary CNS lymphoma (570). The severe immune deficiency in these individuals, however, usually renders them unable to tolerate the additional immune suppression caused by systemic chemotherapy. The optimal therapeutic approach for these patients remains undefined.

The underlying HIV-induced immune deficiency, coexistent systemic and neuropathic opportunistic infections, and other illnesses associated with AIDS account for the overall poor prognosis in patients who have AIDS-related NHLs. Effective treatment for the underlying HIV infection and reconstitution of the immune system, in addition to antilymphoma therapy, may be necessary to significantly improve the survival rate of these patients. This certainly appears to be the case for individuals who have AIDS-related primary CNS lymphoma. One patient who had Burkitt's lymphoma, was treated successfully, and enjoyed a 3-year disease-free survival developed a second, clonally distinct Burkitt's lymphoma (479). This case emphasizes the greatly increased risk for HIV-infected persons to develop malignant lymphoma, as well as the guarded long-term outlook for these patients, even among those whose lymphomas seemingly are cured.

Uncommon Clinicopathologic Categories

Primary Effusion Lymphoma

After the discovery of KSHV (296), Cesarman and colleagues (466) examined DNA extracted from a clinically and pathologically diverse panel of 42 patients with AIDS-related NHLs and 151 with conventional lymphoid neoplasms occurring in HIV-uninfected individuals for the presence of KSHV by Southern blotting, PCR, or both. They discovered KSHV sequences in only eight patients with AIDS-related NHLs. All eight, and only these eight, cases had been classified as body cavity-based lymphomas (Fig. 28.49). These eight cases included ones that had been reported previously by Knowles and colleagues (462), Chadburn and coworkers (473), and Walts and colleagues (463). None of the remaining 185 DNA samples from patients with

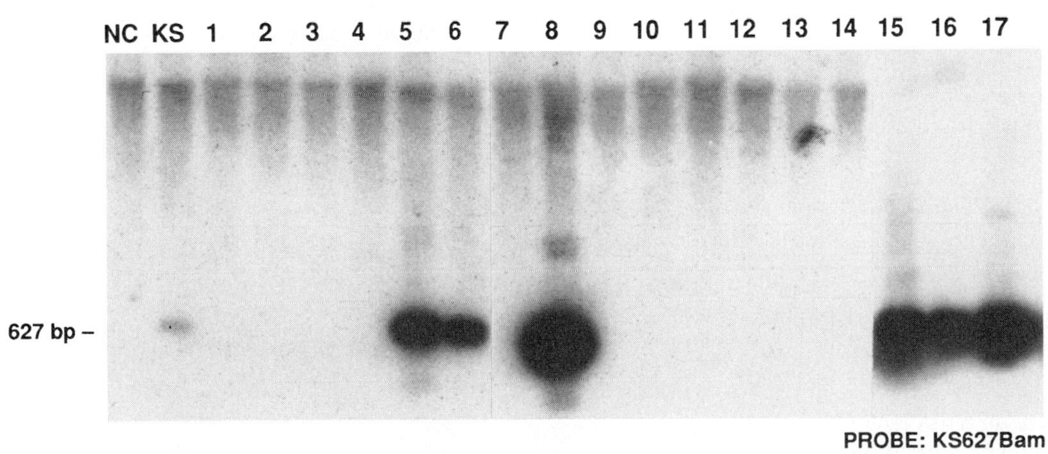

FIG. 28.49. Southern blot hybridization analysis of AIDS-related non-Hodgkin's lymphomas for Kaposi's sarcoma–associated herpesvirus (KSHV). The numbers above each lane indicate the number of the case. *NC* refers to a negative control (HL60 cell line). The Kaposi's sarcoma–positive control exhibits a weak but definite signal indicative of the presence of KSHV within this AIDS-related Kaposi's sarcoma lesion. Lanes 5, 6, 8, 15, 16, and 17 exhibit very strong hybridization signals on hybridization to the KS627Bam probe, indicative of the presence of KSHV in these six samples. All six positive samples represent cases of AIDS-related primary effusion lymphoma. The negative samples represent examples of AIDS-related and non-AIDS-related NHLs. (From Cesarman E, Chang Y, Moore PS, et al. Kaposi's sarcoma-associated herpesvirus-like DNA sequences are present in AIDS-related body cavity based lymphomas. *N Engl J Med* 322: 1186–1191, 1995, copyright 1995, Massachusetts Medical Society, with permission.)

AIDS-related and non–AIDS-related NHL, Hodgkin's disease (HD), or lymphoid leukemia contained KSHV. Between 40 and 80 copies of KSHV were present per lymphoma cell, in comparison with an average of one copy of KSHV per cell in Kaposi's sarcoma tissue (466). Other investigators from the United States and Europe later confirmed the unique association between KSHV and those AIDS-related NHLs arising as lymphomatous effusions (572–575). Rarely, it has been claimed that KSHV is present in other malignant lymphomas (576), but the authenticity and biologic significance of these anecdotal reports remains to be determined. Some investigators have claimed that KSHV is frequently present in AIDS-related and non–AIDS-related primary CNS lymphomas (577–579). Other investigators have failed to confirm these findings (580). Gaidano and colleagues (581) have shown clearly that, if present, the KSHV load in such lymphomas is extremely low and merely reflects the presence of bystander KSHV-infected nonneoplastic B cells. The KSHV load is 2×10^6 times greater in primary effusion lymphomas than in those primary CNS lymphomas in which KSHV is detected (581). Taken together, these findings underscore the unique nature of these so-called body cavity–based lymphomas and strongly suggest that this novel herpesvirus plays a role in their pathogenesis. These KSHV-positive lymphomas appear to account for about 3% of all AIDS-related NHLs (574). They also rarely occur in the HIV-uninfected general population, in which they comprise far less than 1% of all conventional NHLs.

Another infrequently occurring subset of NHLs also arises in the pleural cavity and can be considered body cavity–based lymphomas. These are the pyothorax-associated lymphomas, which have been reported largely from Japan (582,583). The pyothorax-associated lymphomas arise in the pleural cavity following a multiyear history of pyothorax resulting from artificially induced pneumothorax for the treatment of pulmonary tuberculosis or tuberculous pleuritis (582,583). Although they exhibit immunoblastic morphology, are of B-cell origin, and contain EBV, they grow as solid tumor masses instead of as lymphomatous effusions (582–584). Cesarman and colleagues (585) have shown that the pyothorax-associated lymphomas do not contain KSHV; thus the KSHV-containing body cavity–based lymphomas and the pyothorax-associated lymphomas are distinct clinicopathologic entities. Cesarman and coworkers proposed replacing the term *body cavity-based lymphoma* with the term *primary effusion lymphoma*, because the latter term describes these KSHV-containing lymphomas more accurately and avoids their confusion with other lymphomas that arise in the body cavities, including the pyothorax-associated lymphomas (585).

Kaposi's sarcoma–associated herpesvirus appears to be absent from lymphomatous effusions that develop secondary to a contiguous tumor mass or that are associated with disseminated disease (466,573–575). Not all lymphomatous effusions occurring in the absence of a tumor mass necessarily contain KSHV and represent primary effusion lymphomas (586). In our experience, those cases presenting as lymphomatous effusions that exhibit Burkitt's morphology and contain *MYC* gene rearrangements lack KSHV and probably represent an unusual presentation of Burkitt's lymphoma (467).

Since our initial studies, we have had the opportunity to investigate many AIDS-related and non–AIDS-related lymphoid malignancies for the presence of KSHV and to evaluate the clinical, morphologic, immunologic, and molecular features of those lymphoid neoplasms that contain KSHV (466,467,587–590). These studies have confirmed that the primary effusion lymphomas exhibit a unique and unusual constellation of characteristics that distinguish them from all other categories of malignant lymphoma, establishing them as a distinct clinicopathologic and biologic entity (Table 28.13). These characteristics include an epidemiology similar to Kaposi's sarcoma, that is, a younger median

TABLE 28.13. *Clinicopathologic, immunologic, and molecular characteristics of KSHV-positive lymphomas*

Parameter	n	Total no.	Percentage
Epidemiology similar to Kaposi's sarcoma			
HIV-positive 42 years of age, HIV-negative 73 years			
Male predominance	29	32	91
HIV seropositive	28	32	88
Homosexuality as a risk factor	28	28	100
Initial presentation as an effusion	24	32	75
Disease remains restricted to the body cavity	21	24	88
Initially solid, subsequently develop an effusion	4	8	50
Presence of Kaposi's sarcoma	9	27	33
Median survival 5 months			
CD45 expression	29	31	94
Absence of B cell–associated antigens	27	30	90
Lack of immunoglobulin expression	19	22	86
Clonal immunoglobulin gene rearrangements	27	27	100
Epstein-Barr virus genome	27	32	84
Absence of *MYC* gene rearrangements	23	24	96
Absence of other genetic alterations	18	20	90

age at presentation in HIV-infected than in HIV-uninfected individuals (42 versus 73 years) and a vast predominance in men. Nearly all of the men are HIV-seropositive, and homosexuality is the risk factor in the vast majority of them, except in southern Europe, where injecting drug use often is also a risk factor. HIV-seropositive MSM are the AIDS group at highest risk for the development of Kaposi's sarcoma (268–270), in which KSHV is also consistently present (297). We have identified KSHV-containing primary effusion lymphomas in two elderly HIV-seronegative men without AIDS risk factors (467,588). Among the HIV-seropositive individuals, the median CD4 T-cell count is 84 cells per microliter. Approximately one third of individuals who have primary effusion lymphomas also have Kaposi's sarcoma. Most patients present initially with a malignant lymphomatous effusion in the peritoneal, pleural, or abdominal cavity, usually in the absence of a contiguous tumor mass and without associated lymphadenopathy or organomegaly. In most patients, the lymphoma remains restricted to the body cavity of origin. The median survival is only about 5 months, comparable to other HIV-infected individuals who have severe immune deficiency and develop systemic lymphoma (466,467,587–590).

A KSHV-containing primary effusion lymphoma has been described in an HIV-infected woman whose AIDS risk factors are unknown (465). We have identified two HIV-uninfected women who developed KSHV-containing primary effusion lymphomas (589). One was an 85-year-old Russian immigrant who had classic Mediterranean Kaposi's sarcoma involving both lower extremities prior to the onset of primary effusion lymphoma in the pleural cavity. The other was a 46-year-old woman who had bilateral breast implants for 5 years. A primary effusion lymphoma developed in an artificial cavity between the breast implant and its capsule in the absence of a mass. In each case the malignant lymphoma was localized to the body cavity of origin and displayed the morphologic and immunophenotypic features characteristic of primary effusion lymphoma, except that it was EBV-negative (589).

We have identified two HIV-infected MSM who presented initially with KSHV-containing solid primary bowel lymphomas and who subsequently developed lymphomatous effusions (590). One patient had coexistent Kaposi's sarcoma. These cases otherwise resemble the primary effusion lymphomas clinically, as well as morphologically, immunophenotypically, and molecularly, including the presence of EBV (590). For these reasons, we believe that the spectrum of primary effusion lymphoma should be extended to include such patients.

In Wright-Giemsa–stained air-dried cytocentrifuge preparations, the malignant cells display cytomorphologic features that appear to bridge those of immunoblastic and anaplastic large cell lymphoma. The majority of the malignant cells are large, sometimes extremely large, and are round or ovoid to polygonal. They contain moderate to abundant amphophilic to deeply basophilic cytoplasm and nuclei ranging from large, round, and regular to highly irregular and pleomorphic. The nuclei possess coarsely reticular chromatin and one to four large prominent nucleoli. Most cells display plasmacytoid or immunoblastic features. Some of the cells are binucleated or multinucleated and resemble Reed-Sternberg cells. Mitotic figures, sometimes atypical, are numerous. The lymphoma cells appear somewhat more uniform in size and shape in cell block sections and in hematoxylin and eosin–stained tissue sections. They possess moderate to abundant lightly eosinophilic cytoplasm and round to slightly irregular nuclei that contain one or more prominent nucleoli. Occasional large pleomorphic cells are present. Some of these resemble Reed-Sternberg cells, and others have wreath-like nuclei, reminiscent of anaplastic large cell lymphoma (467,587) (Fig. 28.50).

In nearly all patients, the lymphoma cells express CD45 and a variety of activation-associated antigens, most commonly HLA-DR, CD30, CD38, CD71, and epithelial membrane antigen. In most but not all patients, the lymphoma cells lack surface immunoglobulin and B-cell lineage associated antigens, as well as T-cell, myeloid, and monocyte- or macrophage-associated antigens (466,467,587–590). Some investigators have detected monotypic cytoplasmic immunoglobulin in some patients (574,575). All patients exhibit clonal immunoglobulin heavy chain rearrangements, and most also exhibit κ light chain gene rearrangements, indicating a B-cell derivation (467). Rare patients also display clonal T-cell receptor gene rearrangements and are bigenotypic (575,587); there is a report of one such patient who was biphenotypic (575). The primary effusion lymphomas uniformly contain KSHV and nearly always contain clonal EBV (type A or type B) (Fig. 28.51). They consistently lack *MYC* gene rearrangements and mutations and usually also lack *RAS* and *P53* gene mutations and *BCL1*, *BCL2*, and *BCL6* gene rearrangements (467,591) (Table 28.13). In contrast, approximately 60% of all primary effusion lymphomas, irrespective of EBV content and occurring in both HIV-infected and HIV-uninfected individuals, exhibit mutations involving the 5′ noncoding region of the *BCL6* gene (591). They display a hyperdiploid karyotype with numerous chromosomal abnormalities (587,591). Partial or complete trisomy 12, complete trisomy 7, and abnormalities of 1q21-25 are observed frequently (591).

The consistent presence of clonal immunoglobulin heavy chain and κ light chain gene rearrangements in conjunction with the expression of cell surface antigens associated with the late stages of B-cell differentiation or activation, in the absence of antigens associated with the early and middle stages of B-cell differentiation, strongly suggest that the primary effusion lymphomas represent the malignant counterpart of a mature stage of B-cell ontogeny. Because the lymphoma cells usually also lack surface immunoglobulin but sometimes express cytoplasmic immunoglobulin, this would appear to be a stage following antigenic stimulation and lying somewhere between a mature B cell and a plasma cell.

Analysis of the nucleotide sequences of immunoglobulin

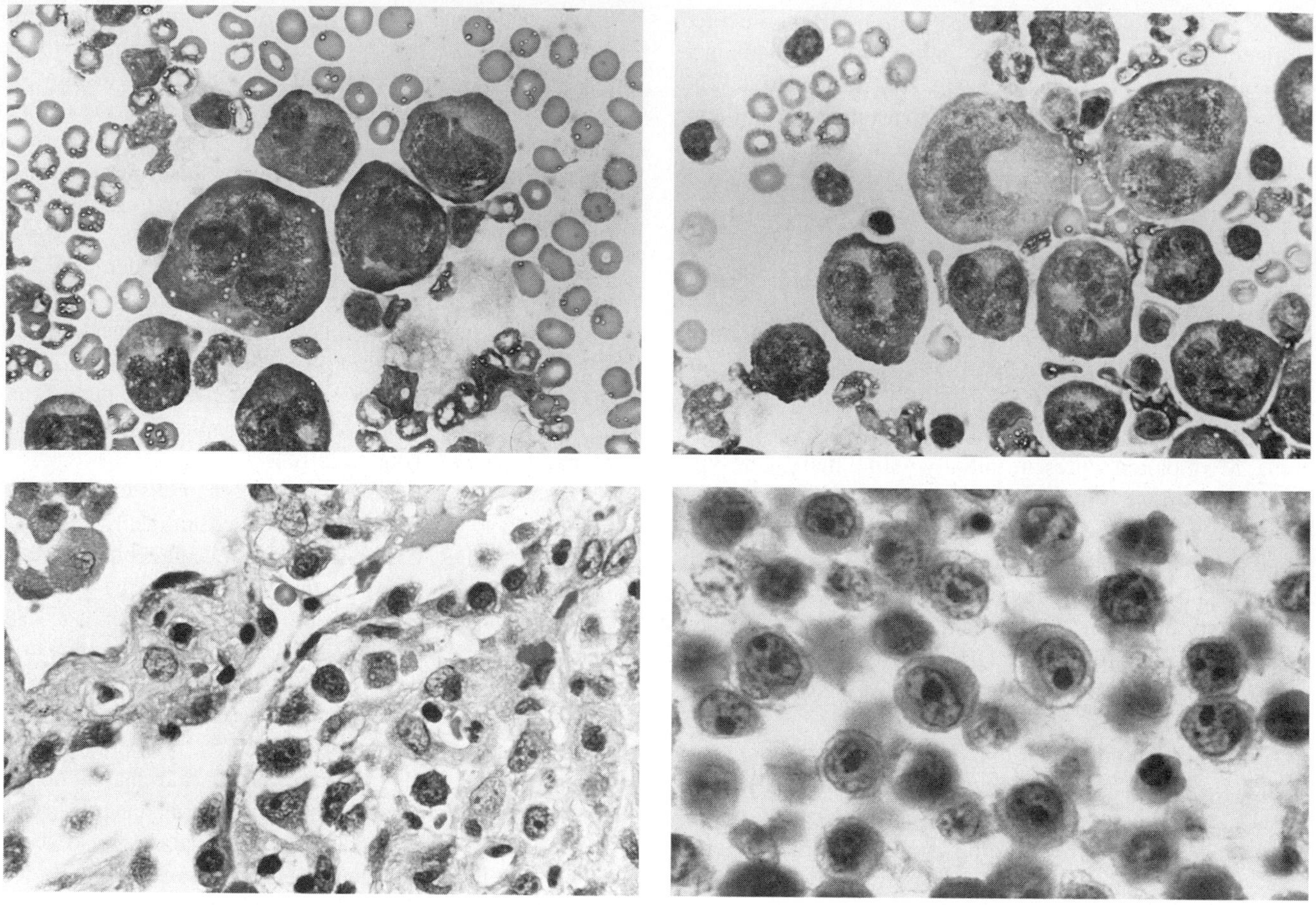

A B C D

FIG. 28.50. A,B: Air-dried cytocentrifuge preparation of a primary effusion lymphoma containing Kaposi's sarcoma–associated herpesvirus. The cells are considerably larger than normal benign lymphocytes and red blood cells and exhibit cytomorphologic features that bridge immunoblastic large cell lymphoma and anaplastic large cell lymphoma. The cells display variable polymorphism and generally possess moderately abundant amphophilic to deeply basophilic cytoplasm. A prominent clear perinuclear Golgi zone is frequently present. Small cytoplasmic vacuoles are occasionally present. The nuclei vary from large and round to highly irregular, multilobated and pleomorphic and often contain one or more large prominent nucleoli (Wright stain, original magnification: 630× magnification). (From Nador RG, Cesarman E, Chadburn A, et al. Primary effusion lymphoma: a distinct clinicopathologic entity associated with the Kaposi's sarcoma-associated herpes virus. *Blood* 1996;88:645–656). **C:** Section of a primary effusion lymphoma involving the pulmonary lymphatics (hematoxylin and eosin stain, original magnification: 630× magnification). (From Nador RG, Cesarman E, Chadburn A, et al. Primary effusion lymphoma: a distinct clinicopathologic entity associated with the Kaposi's sarcoma-associated herpes virus. *Blood* 1996;88:645–656, with permission.) **D:** Pleural fluid cell block section of a primary effusion lymphoma containing Kaposi's sarcoma–associated herpesvirus. The neoplastic cells are large, but appear more uniform in size and shape and less polymorphic in these histologic sections than in cytospin preparations. They contain moderately abundant, lightly eosinophilic cytoplasm, sometimes with a perinuclear hof, and generally large round to ovoid nuclei containing prominent nucleoli (hematoxylin and eosin stain, original magnification: 1,000× magnification). (From Ansari MQ, Dawson DB, Nador R, et al. Primary body cavity-based AIDS-related lymphomas. *Am J Clin Pathol* 1996;105:221–229, with permission.)

heavy chain variable region (IgHV) genes can provide insight into the stage of B-cell development at which clonal expansion occurs in B-cell tumors. Pre–germinal center B cells contain IgHV genes with a germline sequence; post–germinal center B cells contain mutated IgHV genes. Antigen-selected post–germinal center B cells display somatic mutations clustered in the complementary determining region sequences. Germinal center B cells are characterized by ongoing mutation, which is absent in post–germinal center B cells (592,593). We analyzed the nucleotide sequences of the IgHV region genes expressed by several primary effusion lymphomas, in order to determine the stage of B-cell development at which clonal expansion of these lymphoma cells occur (594). We found that all the EBV-positive primary effusion lymphomas obtained from HIV-infected individuals contained IgHV genes exhibiting numerous point

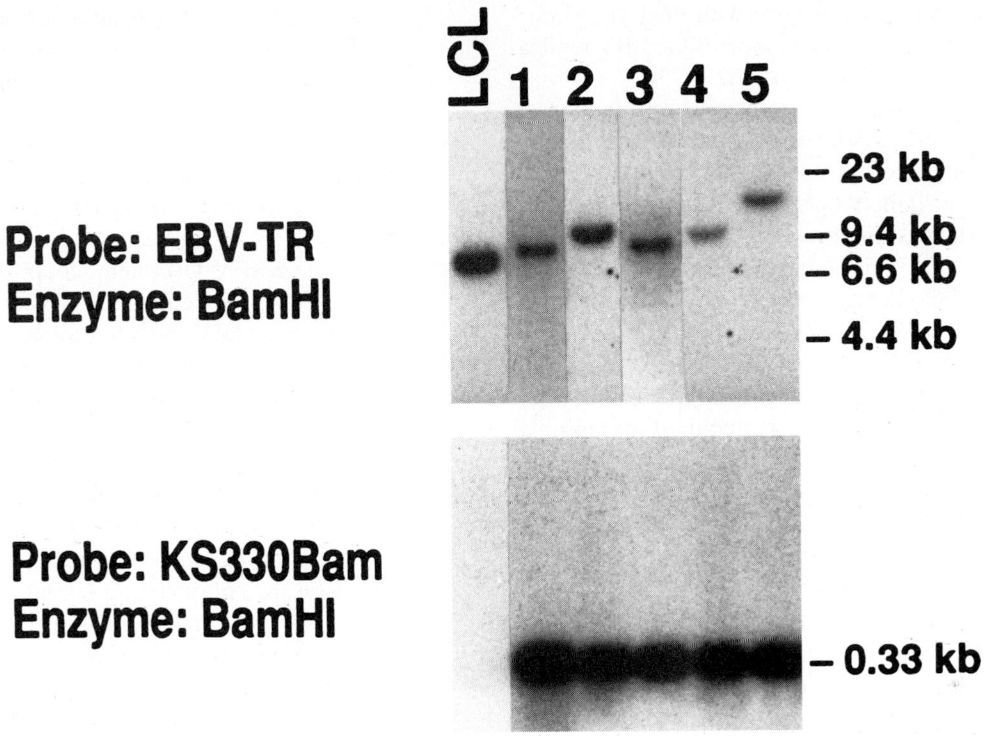

FIG. 28.51. Southern blot hybridization analysis of five primary effusion lymphomas (PELs) for Epstein-Barr virus (EBV) terminal repeat and Kaposi's sarcoma–associated herpesvirus (KSHV). DNA samples were digested with the BamHI restriction enzyme and hybridized to the BamHI NJ-het probe (**top**) and to the KS330BAM probe (**bottom**). UH1, an established lymphoblastoid cell line, was used as a positive control for EBV and as a negative control for KSHV. The number above each lane corresponds to the PEL case. All five PELs contained KSHV and EBV. (From Horenstein MG, Nador RG, Chadburn A, et al. Epstein Barr virus latent gene expression in primary effusion lymphomas containing Kaposi's sarcoma-associated herpesvirus/human herpesvirus 8. *Blood* 1997;90:1186–1191, with permission.)

mutations relative to the putative germline VH gene sequences. In all but one instance, the expressed IgHV gene sequences did not show intraclonal heterogeneity, suggesting that the final tumorigenic event occurred at a post–germinal center stage, at which the cells no longer are influenced by the somatic hypermutation mechanism. The significant clustering of replacement mutations in the complementary determining regions in these cases indicates that the tumor cells have been selected by antigen, or in other words have undergone affinity maturation. In one patient, considerable intraclonal heterogeneity was detected, analogous to the situation with follicular center cell lymphomas (595,596). This indicates that the tumor cells are still under the influence of the somatic hypermutation mechanism, subsequent to malignant transformation, suggesting a germinal center origin for this particular primary effusion lymphoma. In contrast, the IgHV gene segment of an EBV-negative primary effusion lymphoma occurring in an HIV-uninfected individual displayed complete nucleotide sequence identity with its putative germline precursor, suggesting a naive pre–germinal center B-cell origin for this particular lymphoma. In most cases of primary effusion lymphoma, the cell of origin is a germinal center or post–germinal center B cell. The development of primary effusion lymphoma, however, may not be restricted to one specific stage of B-cell differentiation; they may represent transformants of B cells at different stages of B-cell ontogeny (594).

EBV-infected normal B cells display IgHV genes with somatic hypermutation and evidence of intraclonal heterogeneity (597). EBV-infected malignant B cells, including those of endemic Burkitt's lymphoma (598) and lymphoproliferative disorders after transplantation (599) as well as the Reed-Sternberg cells of HD (600), express mutated IgHV genes. These findings suggest that EBV infection plays a role in preneoplastic events by driving B-cell proliferation, activation, and immunoglobulin gene mutation. EBV may make a comparable contribution to the pathogenesis of the primary effusion lymphomas.

It is rather remarkable in this regard that most primary effusion lymphomas contain clonal EBV genome in addition to KSHV (466,467,587) (Fig. 28.51). This is the only example of a consistent dual herpesviral infection in a human neoplasm. A critical question is the relative contribution of each virus to the pathogenesis of these lymphomas. It is well known, for example, that EBV is capable of immortalizing B cells *in vitro* but alone may be insufficient for tumorigenesis, as exemplified by the complementation of EBV and an activated *MYC* gene in Burkitt's lymphoma (601). Genetic complementation can occur *in vitro* with dual viral infections, an example of which is activation of the EBV replicative cycle by human herpesvirus-6 (602).

In order to better appreciate the respective contributions of KSHV and EBV to the pathogenesis of the primary effusion lymphomas, we analyzed the pattern of EBV latent gene expression in these lymphomas (603). Understanding the pattern of EBV latent gene expression is important for evaluating the role of EBV in these lymphomas, because the degree of activity of the latent virus correlates with its transforming properties. EBV infection of B cells gives rise to three patterns based on the selective expression of nine latent genes (604). In its most restricted pattern (latency I), EBV principally expresses *EBNA1*, a gene required for episomal replication that allows for maintenance of its genome. Latency I is characteristic of Burkitt's lymphoma (605) and circulating mononuclear cells of healthy EBV-infected individuals (606). In its most unrestricted pattern (latency III), EBV expresses nine genes, including the transforming *EBNA2* and *LMP1* genes, and may represent the principal driving force for cell proliferation. Latency III is found in lymphoblastoid cell lines (607) and in the lymphoproliferative disorders that occur after transplantation (608). An intermediate pattern (latency II) is found in cases of EBV-positive HD (609). We discovered that Qp-initiated mRNA, encoding only *EBNA1* and characteristic of latencies I and II, is positive, and Wp- and Cp-initiated mRNAs, encoding all EBNAs and characteristic of latency III, are negative in cases of primary effusion lymphoma. In addition, *LMP1* mRNA, which is expressed in latencies II and III, is only present at very low levels and is undetectable at the protein level by immunohistochemistry in primary effusion lymphomas (603). The primary effusion lymphomas exhibit a restricted pattern of EBV latent gene expression, suggesting that EBV is not solely responsible for their malignant transformation. It is highly likely that KSHV plays the major role in the pathogenesis of the primary effusion lymphomas. This conclusion is supported by a considerable body of evidence, including the existance of primary effusion lymphomas that contain KSHV but lack EBV (467,588,589).

The presence of KSHV in the primary effusion lymphomas and its conspicuous absence from all other categories of lymphoid neoplasia strongly suggest that this virus plays an important role in the pathogenesis of the primary effusion lymphomas. The accumulated evidence suggests that KSHV is an oncogenic herpesvirus that is important in malignant lymphoid transformation in these lymphomas: First, KSHV belongs to the *Gammaherpesvirinae* subfamily of herpesvirus, which is characterized by the ability to replicate in lymphoblastoid cells (301). Herpesvirus saimiri and EBV, the two herpesviruses having the most structural homology to KSHV, possess the ability to induce latent infection of peripheral lymphocytes of their natural host, immortalize lymphocytes *in vitro*, and lead to the development of malignant lymphomas (301,610,611). Herpesvirus saimiri, a squirrel monkey virus, can be isolated from the peripheral blood mononuclear cells of healthy animals but causes fulminant T-cell lymphomas in New World primates that are not its natural host (610). Herpesvirus saimiri also is capable of transforming human T cells to grow continuously *in vitro* (611).

Second, Cesarman and colleagues (299) have demonstrated that KSHV possesses homologues to known viral and cellular genes, including G protein–coupled receptors and cyclin D. The KSHV G protein–coupled receptor is most homologous with the cellular IL-8 receptors and also has homology with the HIV chemokine coreceptor, CCR-5. The KSHV cyclin gene is related closely to the cellular type D cyclins (299). Both genes are expressed at the RNA level in Kaposi's sarcoma and in primary effusion lymphomas (299). This is important because both genes encode functional proteins (612,613) and likely represent viral oncogenes. Cellular homologues of these genes have been shown to be involved in malignant transformation (614–621). Finally, because the entire coding region of KSHV has been sequenced, we know that KSHV encodes homologues to multiple cellular genes that are involved in inflammation and cellular proliferation (622). The expression of these KSHV genes in the primary effusion lymphomas lends additional strong support to the notion that this viral agent plays an active role in the pathogenesis and pathobiology of these lymphomas (Fig. 28.52).

The fact that benign $CD19^+$ B cells in HIV-infected individuals may be KSHV-infected in the absence of malignant lymphoma or Kaposi's sarcoma (300) suggests that latent infection by KSHV precedes malignant transformation. It is possible that B cells at multiple maturational stages carry KSHV, and that the events leading to malignant transformation occur independent of the stage of B-cell development. This hypothesis is consistent with the heterogeneous profile of IgHV gene mutations found in these lymphomas (594). Nonetheless, it is likely that additional molecular events are necessary to initiate malignant transformation of KSHV-infected B cells. Mutations of the 5′ noncoding region of the *BCL6* gene represent the most frequent consistent genetic alteration occurring in these lymphomas (591). Because *BCL6* gene mutations are regarded as a genetic marker of B-cell transition through the germinal center (623), this is consistent with other data suggesting that many, if not most, primary effusion lymphomas are derived from germinal center or post–germinal center B cells. Alterations involving the principle genes associated with lymphomagenesis—*BCL1*, *BCL2*, *MYC*, *RAS*, and *P53*—occur uncommonly or not at all in the primary effusion lymphomas (467,591). The molecular genetic mechanisms involved in their pathogenesis are incompletely understood.

Polymorphic Lymphoproliferative Disorder

The clinically and histopathologically heterogeneous group of EBV-driven lymphoid proliferations that arise following solid organ transplantation are referred to collec-

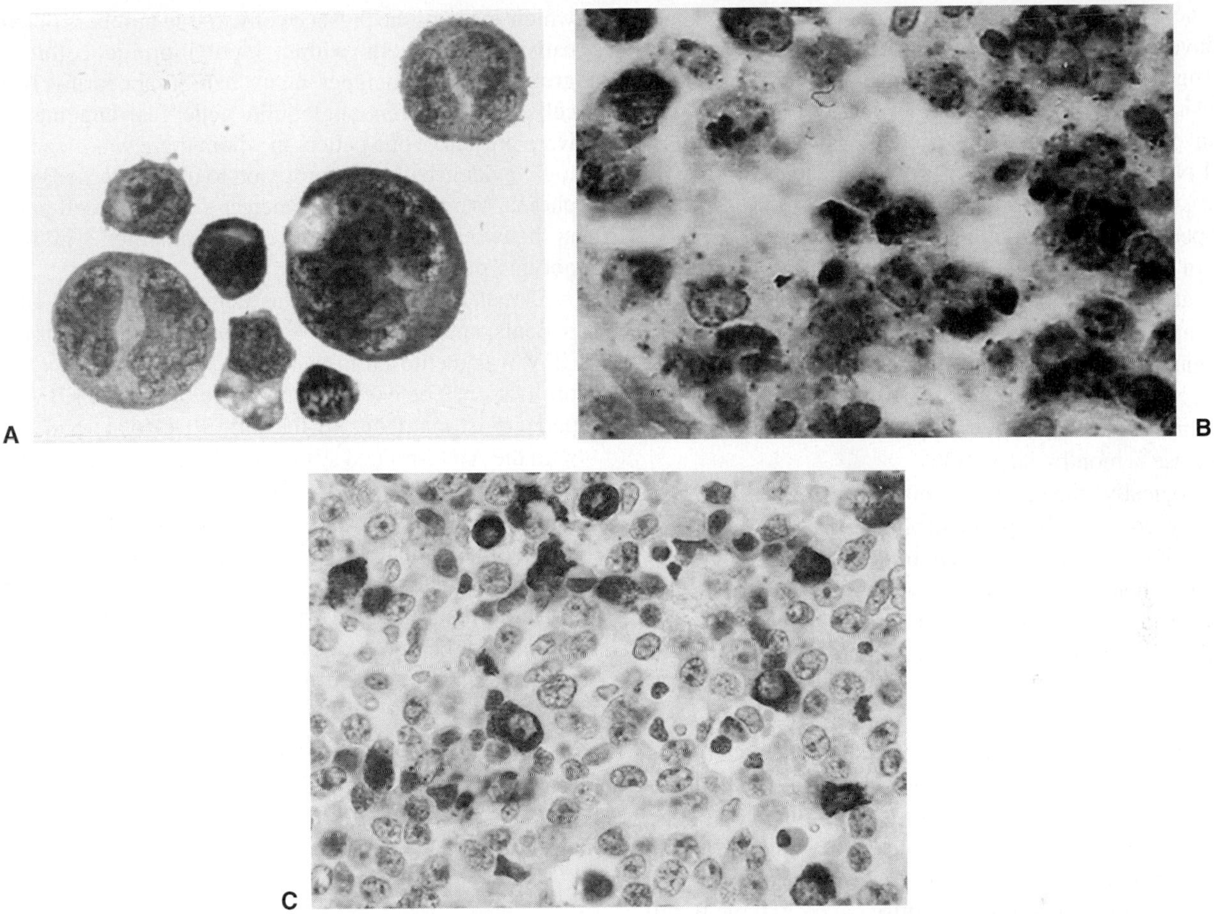

FIG. 28.52. Kaposi's sarcoma–associated herpesvirus (KSHV) in primary effusion lymphomas. **A:** Air-dried cytocentrifuge preparation of a KSHV-positive primary effusion lymphoma. The cells are considerably larger than normal benign lymphocytes and exhibit cytomorphologic features that appear to bridge immunoblastic lymphoma and anaplastic large cell lymphoma. The cells display significant polymorphism and possess moderately abundant amphophilic to deeply basophilic cytoplasm. A prominent clear perinuclear Golgi zone is frequently present. The nuclei vary from large and round to highly irregular, multilobated, and pleomorphic and often contain one or more prominent nucleoli (Wright-Giemsa stain, original magnification: 1,000× magnification). **B:** *In situ* hybridization for KSHV using a viral cyclin probe. A case of primary effusion lymphoma with solid tissue involvement shows cytoplasmic and nuclear hybridization signals in nearly all lymphoma cells. A spindle-shaped cell that is negative for KSHV hybridization signals is seen in the lower left corner of this panel (original magnification: 630× magnification). **C:** Abundant viral interleukin-6 protein expression is seen in numerous lymphoma cells using immunohistochemistry with a rabbit polyclonal antiserum raised against a virus interleukin-6–specific peptide (immunoperoxidase stain, original magnification: 400× magnification). (From Cesarman E, Knowles DM. The role of Kaposi's sarcoma-associated herpesvirus (KSHV/HHV-8) in lymphoproliferative diseases. *Semin Cancer Biol* 1999;9:165–174, with permission.)

tively as *posttransplantation lymphoproliferative disorders* (PT-LPD) (624). Many PT-LPDs comprise polymorphous cell populations of varying clonal composition (361,624–627). These features often make it difficult to determine their benign or malignant nature, classify those thought to be malignant by the standard lymphoma classifications, or reliably predict their clinical behavior (624,625,628,629). This is in marked contrast with the vast majority of AIDS-related NHLs, which are monomorphic, high-grade, monoclonal B-cell tumors; are easily recognized as malignant; and are usually readily classifiable, and whose aggressive clinical behavior is predictable. Furthermore, unlike AIDS-related NHLs, the polymorphic PT-LPDs consistently lack *MYC* gene rearrangements, *P53* gene mutations, *BCL6* gene rearrangements, and *RAS* gene mutations (363) (see Chapter 16). These clinical, morphologic, and molecular differences between the PT-LPDs and the AIDS-related NHLs suggest that distinct mechanisms are operational in their pathogenesis.

Reviewing a large collection of cases previously classified as AIDS-related NHL, however, we identified a subset displaying morphologic features resembling the polymorphic PT-LPDs in 10 HIV-infected individuals (630). We designated these cases *polymorphic lymphoproliferative disor-*

ders. These lesions appear to arise in both men and women who have acquired HIV infection through various routes, including homosexual and heterosexual contact and blood transfusion. Patients range in age from 28 to 55 years, with a mean of 38 years, similar to patients who have AIDS-related NHLs. None of the 10 individuals had a history of Kaposi's sarcoma or opportunistic infections. The lesions developed in lymph nodes as well as in extranodal sites. Seven of the 10 individuals had only clinical stage I or IE disease at presentation; two patients presented with generalized lymph node involvement (clinical stage III). Information regarding therapy and outcome was limited. Four patients received chemotherapy, one of whom died disease-free 28 months later and one of whom was alive with recurrent disease 7 months later (630).

Histologically, the lesions exhibit a diffuse growth pattern. They consist of a polymorphic cell population comprised of lymphocytes, plasmacytoid lymphocytes, plasma cells, immunoblasts, and histiocytes. The lesions display variable degrees of plasmacytoid differentiation and cytologic atypia and variable numbers of atypical immunoblasts (630) (Fig. 28.53).

Immunophenotypic analysis demonstrated a monotypic B-cell population in six of the eight patients in whom immunoglobulin expression was evaluated. A clonal B-cell population was detected in 7 of 10 patients by immunoglobulin heavy and light chain gene rearrangement analysis, and in one additional patient by EBV terminal repeat analysis. This included all six patients having significant monotypic B-cell populations, and the two in whom immunoglobulin expression was not assessed but who had large numbers of B cells. The nongermline hybridizing bands were usually faint, indicating that the clonal B-cell population represented only a subset of the total cells in each lesion. This finding is consistent with the histopathologic appearance of the lesions, which suggests the presence of variable numbers of cytologically atypical cells within a polymorphic cellular background, which includes many benign-appearing lymphoid cells. Strong immunoglobulin gene rearrangement bands were present in one patient in whom there was clear morphologic evidence of transformation to diffuse large B-cell lymphoma. We were unable to detect a clonal B-cell population in the two patients who expressed a polyclonal immunophenotypic profile (630).

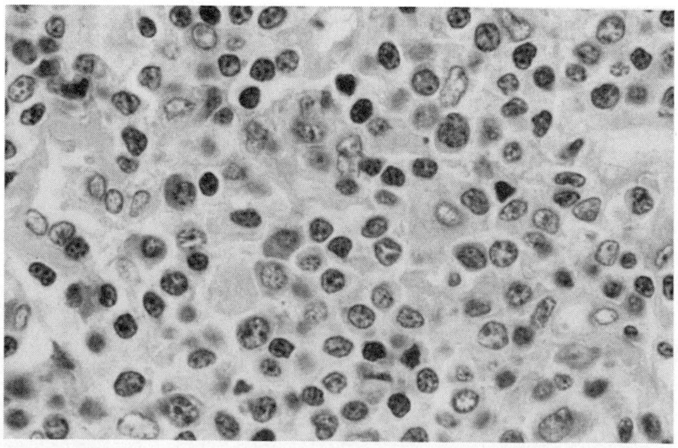

FIG. 28.53. AIDS-related polymorphic lymphoproliferative disorder. This lesion consists of a polymorphic cell population comprised of variable numbers of lymphocytes, plasmacytoid lymphocytes, plasma cells, immunoblasts and histiocytes (hematoxylin and eosin stain, original magnification: 630× magnification).

Clonal EBV infection was demonstrable in 4 of the 10 patients, and type A EBV was identified in all four of those. EBV was identified in two additional lesions by *in situ* hybridization. The exclusive presence of type A EBV in these patients is analogous to the PT-LPDs (631) and contrasts with the AIDS-related systemic NHLs, in which type B EBV is often present (632). KSHV, which is highly associated with the primary effusion lymphomas and not with solid lymphomas (466,467) or HIV-associated lymphadenopathy (140), was detectable in two cases by PCR but not by Southern blotting. *In situ* hybridization demonstrated KSHV in some of the benign, reactive cells and in some of the cytologically malignant-appearing cells in both lesions. The two cases containing KSHV occurred in MSM (630). Conceivably, herpesviruses may play a role in the development of these polymorphic lymphoproliferative disorders.

The one patient with polymorphic lymphoproliferative disorder who had focal areas of morphologic transformation to diffuse large B-cell lymphoma exhibited mutations involving the *MYC*, *BCL6*, and *P53* genes. One additional patient also displayed *P53* gene mutation. The remaining eight patients lacked structural alterations of the *MYC*, *BCL6*, *RAS*, or *P53* genes (630). Once again, these molecular features resemble those of the polymorphic PT-LPDs more closely than those of most AIDS-related systemic NHLs.

The malignant nature of the polymorphic PT-LPDs is controversial. Their morphologic appearance is atypical for a conventional malignant lymphoma, and a significant proportion of the lesions regress following a reduction in immunosuppressive therapy (624,633). One possible explanation for the development of these lesions is strong antigenic stimulation attributable to EBV infection, resulting in sequential polyclonal and oligoclonal lymphoid proliferations, which sometimes eventuate into monoclonal B cell lymphomas (624). The lack of oncogene and tumor suppressor gene alterations in these lesions, however, suggests that the clonal, cytologically atypical B cells in these lesions are not fully transformed (363,624).

Somatic mutations involving the 5′ noncoding region of the *BCL6* gene occur independent of translocation of the *BCL6* gene (623). They are present in about 70% of diffuse large B-cell lymphomas (623) and 60% of AIDS-related NHLs (591). They have been identified in that subset of polymorphic PT-LPDs exhibiting unresponsiveness to immune reconstitution. In our experience, none of the PT-LPDs that regress following reduction of immune suppression exhibit *BCL6* gene mutation, whereas all of the PT-LPDs that fail to regress exhibit *BCL6* gene mutation (634). Mutational analysis of the *BCL6* gene appears to be a reliable predictor of the biologic behavior of polymorphic PT-LPDs (634). The fact that *BCL6* gene mutation was identified only in the one patient with AIDS-related polymorphic lymphoproliferative disorder in transformation to diffuse large B-cell lymphoma, and not in other patients (630), supports the hypothesis that structural alteration of this gene may represent one of the earliest indicators of full malignant transformation and progression identified thus far. Like the polymorphic PT-LPDs, AIDS-related polymorphic lymphoproliferative disorders display a histologic spectrum ranging from polymorphic hyperplasia to malignant lymphoma, and the distinction between the two may be difficult at the morphologic level (630). The presence or absence of *BCL6* gene mutations in these lesions may serve to subdivide them into distinct biologic categories, analogous to the polymorphic PT-LPDs. This hypothesis is supported by the fact that the one patient whose lesion contained a *BCL6* gene mutation developed recurrent and disseminated disease, but many of the other patients exhibited only localized disease (630). The lack of *BCL6* gene mutation may represent a favorable prognostic indicator for these AIDS-related polymorphic lymphoproliferative disorders. More detailed clinical information concerning additional cases of AIDS-related polymorphic lymphoproliferative disorders clearly is needed, however, to substantiate this hypothesis.

These polymorphic lymphoproliferative disorders appear to represent a small but distinct subset of HIV-related lymphoid proliferations that are distinguishable from the traditional pathologic categories of AIDS-related NHL based on their morphologic and molecular characteristics and probably their clinical features as well. The polymorphic histopathology, the low "clonal strength," the general lack of oncogene and tumor suppressor gene alterations, the ability to transform to a high-grade malignant lymphoma, and the apparently lower disease load and better outcome suggest that these lymphoid proliferations resemble the polymorphic PT-LPDs more closely than they resemble the common categories of AIDS-related NHL. As in the case of the polymorphic PT-LPDs, the malignant nature and biologic significance of these lesions and their relationship to monomorphic B-cell lymphomas remains to be determined.

Plasmablastic Lymphoma

In 1997, Delecluse and colleagues (635) described a subset of NHLs that displays blastoid morphology and plasma cell–like immunophenotypic features and preferentially occurs in the oral cavity of HIV-infected individuals. They designated these cases *plasmablastic lymphomas* (635). Among 16 cases, 15 occurred in HIV-infected individuals, comprised of 12 MSM, one male IDU, one female IDU, and one male whose risk factors were unknown. The sole HIV-uninfected individual was an elderly woman. The median age of the patients was 39 years. About one third of the patients had B symptoms. None had a monoclonal gammopathy. The tumors were localized in the mucosa of the oral cavity, usually in the gingiva but sometimes in the floor of the mouth or the palate. Jaw bone infiltration occurred in one patient. At the time of diagnosis 11 patients had stage IE disease, and the remaining five patients had stage IV disease. The lymphoma sometimes extended to involve the abdomen, retroperitoneum, soft tissues of the extremities, and bone marrow. Occasional patients who had lymphoma limited to the oral cavity responded well to radiation therapy, but despite multi-drug chemotherapy most patients died in 7 months on average, often of unrelated or multiple causes (635).

The plasmablastic lymphomas grow diffusely. They often have a starry-sky appearance because of the presence of scattered interspersed tingible body macrophages. The lymphoma cells are large and possess abundant, deeply basophilic cytoplasm, eccentrically placed nuclei, and a paranuclear hof. The nuclei are round to ovoid and possess little chromatin and either a single prominent, centrally placed nucleolus or several peripherally located nucleoli. The proliferation index is very high, as evidenced by numerous apoptotic figures, single cell necrosis, and mitotic figures and greater than 90% positivity with MAb MIB-1 (635).

The plasmablastic lymphomas exhibit a distinctive immunophenotype characterized by diminished or absent CD45 or CD20 expression and strong immunoreactivity with the monoclonal anti-plasma cell antibody, VS38c. Approximately one half of patients display complete absence of CD45 and B-cell lineage–associated antigen CD20. In the remaining one half of patients, variable proportions of the lymphoma cells weakly express cytoplasmic CD45 or CD20, sometimes accompaned by weak surface membrane expression in a small number of cells. A variable proportion, 5% to 90%, of the lymphoma cells express CD79a. Intracytoplasmic IgG, but not other heavy chain isotypes, is detectable in about one half of patients. Sometimes this is accompaned by monotypic light chain expression. In all patients, the lymphoma cells exhibit strong immunoreactivity with VS38c. Occasional patients express BCL-6 protein (635). In summary, the plasmablastic lymphomas express the immunophenotypic features of plasma cells.

The small number of patients studied exhibited clonal immunoglobulin heavy gene rearrangements and lacked *BCL2* gene rearrangements and evidence of KSHV. About 60% of these patients exhibit EBV-encoded nuclear RNA transcripts (EBER), but in the absence of EBNA-2 expression, and only extremely small numbers of cells express LMP-1 or BZLF-1 (635). The plasmablastic lymphomas appear to be unrelated to follicular center cell lymphomas and those large cell lymphomas of follicular center cell origin.

The plasmablastic lymphomas appear to exhibit a unique constellation of clinical, morphologic, and immunophenotypic characteristics and represent a distinct clinicopathologic and biologic category of NHLs that is preferentially associated with AIDS. The blastoid morphology and immunophenotype of these lymphomas suggest that they most closely resemble plasmablasts, cells that still retain the blastoid feature of immunoblasts but already have acquired the antigen profile of plasma cells—hence the designation *plasmablastic lymphoma* (635). These lymphomas may be mistaken for diffuse large B-cell lymphomas with plasmacytoid differentiation or plasmacytomas, but careful attention to their distinctive clinical, morphologic, and immunophenotypic features should result in an accurate diagnosis. Factors that contribute especially to the pathogenesis of these lymphomas are unclear. Not all cases involve EBV, and those that do exhibit an EBV latent gene pattern of expression that is inconsistent with EBV-driven lymphoproliferative disorders. The plasmablastic lymphomas also lack KSHV (635). Molecular genetic analyses of these lymphomas, which have been limited thus far, should contribute to our understanding of their pathogenesis and relationship to other categories of NHL.

Pathogenesis

HIV

Initially, it was thought that HIV might be directly responsible for the B-cell NHLs that develop in HIV-infected patients, because HIV can infect EBV-transformed cells (636) and is endemic in regions of Africa in which Burkitt's lymphoma is common (637). Laurence and Astrin (638) provided some experimental support for this hypothesis when they were able to infect peripheral blood B cells obtained from HIV-seronegative, EBV-seropositive donors with HIV and derive continuously proliferating cell lines. If inoculated into severe combined immune deficiency (SCID) or nude mice, the HIV-transformed B cells gave rise to lymphoid proliferations resembling malignant lymphomas (638). These findings led these investigators to conclude that HIV may play a direct role in AIDS lymphomagenesis. We and numerous other investigators, however, consistently have failed to find evidence of HIV DNA by Southern blot hybridization analysis in the genomes of freshly isolated AIDS-related lymphomas and lymphoma cell lines established *in vitro* (369,462,477,480,493,548,639). PCR analysis of AIDS-related lymphoma tissues has demonstrated HIV levels consistent with the presence of infiltrating benign T cells within the tissues and inconsistent with HIV infection of the malignant lymphoma B cells (640). It is generally accepted that HIV is not involved directly in the *in vivo* malignant transformation of B cells or, consequently, in the direct induction of AIDS-related B-cell lymphomas. High-grade B-cell lymphomas develop in a similar setting in a primate model 5 to 15 months after infection by simian immunodeficiency virus and coincidentally with the onset of severe immune deficiency (641). These simian immunodeficiency virus–associated lymphomas are devoid of simian immunodeficiency virus genomes (641), consistent with the absence of HIV genome from AIDS-related lymphomas. It is more likely that the NHLs arising in HIV-infected individuals are the consequence of the immunosuppression and lack of immunosurveillance that develops in these individuals. HIV may play an indirect role in AIDS lymphomagenesis by inducing cytokine deregulation of the microenvironment (642) or by chronic antigen stimulation by HIV antigens (643–645).

Impaired Immune Surveillance

Diffuse aggressive B-cell NHLs, many of which share clinical and morphologic characteristics with AIDS-related NHLs, occur with an increased incidence in individuals who have congenital or acquired immune defects (359,407,447). HIV infection is associated with a variety of immunologic observations, including quantitative changes and functional defects in the CD4 T-cell population (22,646). Several investigators have demonstrated that the greatest risk for the development of AIDS-related NHLs occurs if CD4 T-cell counts are less than 50 per microliter (394,647,648), as is often the case in patients who have AIDS-related systemic immunoblastic lymphomas and primary CNS lymphomas (391,393,394). Prolonged exposure to immunosuppression appears to be another critical factor. Pluda and colleagues (648) estimated that the risk of individuals who have less than 50 CD4 T-cells per microliter for 24 months developing an AIDS-related NHL is more than double that of individuals with AIDS who are not selected for their CD4 T-cell counts. HIV-infected individuals suffer from selective impairment of immune surveillance against EBV-infected B cells, which are present in increased numbers in the peripheral blood and lymphoid tissues and may be responsible for minor clonal B-cell expansions that precede malignant transformation (649). Some investigators have suggested that these clonal expansions represent the precursors of AIDS-related NHLs (536).

AIDS lymphomagenesis likely also is affected by a failed local T-cell response *in situ*. The magnitude of the local response by tumor-infiltrating T cells has been suggested as an independent predictor of clinical outcome (650). Fewer tumor-infiltrating T cells are present in biopsy specimens from large cell lymphomas occurring in patients who have AIDS than in those from immunocompetent hosts (651). This is consistent with the description of profound functional defects of CD8 T cells in HIV-infected persons (642).

Cytokines and Growth Factors

Although it is unlikely that HIV participates in AIDS lymphomagenesis directly, it may participate indirectly by inducing the release of cytokines. Numerous cytokines and growth factors, including for example IL-1, IL-2, IL-4, IL-6, IL-7, IL-10, interferon-γ, tumor necrosis factor, lymphotoxin, and B-cell growth factors of 25 kD and 50 kD, are responsible for B-cell differentiation and proliferation (652–658). The ongoing activation of various cytokine networks and the release of these stimuli contributes to the state of chronic B-cell proliferation that characterizes HIV-induced immunosuppression (403). Experimental evidence suggests that at least some of these factors may play roles in the development and growth of malignant lymphoma.

Deregulation of the normal cytokine networks is a key feature of HIV infection (642). This may contribute to AIDS lymphomagenesis in two ways: First, cytokine deregulation may assist in maintaining HIV infection, or even making it more severe, in turn worsening immune function and facilitating the development of AIDS-related NHL (536). For example, in persons who have AIDS, the intense antigenic exposure of B cells *in vivo* directly activates IL-6 and tumor necrosis factor-α production. In turn, IL-6 and tumor necrosis factor-α induce HIV expression, maintaining viral infection (642). Second, deregulation by HIV of the numerous cytokines that normally control B-cell differentiation and proliferation may induce or sustain the growth of B-cell malignancies (536). For example, B cells from HIV-infected individuals who have hypergammaglobulinemia constitutively secrete high levels of tumor necrosis factor-α and IL-6 *in vitro* in the absence of exogenous stimuli (642).

There is considerable experimental evidence to support a role for IL-6 and IL-10 in AIDS lymphomagenesis. It is known that IL-6 potentiates the tumorigenicity of EBV-infected B cells (659,660) and plays a role in the development of B-cell lymphomas in immunocompetent hosts (661–664). IL-6 functions as an autocrine growth factor in tumor cell lines derived from non–AIDS-related, EBV-negative NHLs (665) and in multiple myeloma (661). Constitutive expression of the *IL6* gene has been demonstrated in chronic lymphocytic leukemia (666). With respect to AIDS lymphomagenesis, HIV directly stimulates IL-6 production by monocytes and macrophages (667), which in turn promotes the chronic proliferation of activated B cells, thereby driving immunoglobulin synthesis and causing the nonspecific hypergammaglobulinemia commonly seen in early HIV infection (668–670). IL-6 also is produced by activated B cells, which further contributes to the relatively high IL-6 serum levels observed in HIV-infected persons (671). Once a malignant lymphoma is established firmly, its continuous growth and expansion may be driven by IL-6 through paracrine loops (672). Macrophages and endothelial cells intermingled with the tumor cells release IL-6, which acts on IL-6 receptors expressed at high levels on the tumor cells (672). Consistent with this hypothesis, high levels of IL-6 have been demonstrated in both AIDS-related and non–AIDS-related immunoblastic and large cell lymphomas, independent of their EBV status (672). The number of IL-6 expressing cells has been found to be substantially higher in large cell lymphomas containing a high proportion of immunoblasts than in Burkitt's lymphomas, in which immunoblasts are absent (672), consistent with the purported role of IL-6 in the terminal stages of B-cell differentiation. Finally, clinical support for the role of IL-6 in the development of AIDS-related NHL comes from Pluda and colleagues (408,648) who discovered that elevated IL-6 serum levels may predict the future development of malignant lymphoma among individuals with symptomatic HIV infection.

Interleukin-10 is a pleiotropic cytokine with striking homology to BCRF-1, an EBV protein, and is a potent EBV stimulator (673). IL-10 production is absent from endemic and sporadic Burkitt's lymphoma occurring in non–HIV-infected individuals (674). Benjamin and colleagues (674), however, demonstrated that B-cell lines derived from AIDS-related Burkitt's lymphoma constitutively express IL-10 in large amounts, suggesting that IL-10 production is especially associated with AIDS lymphomagenesis. These findings were confirmed by Masood and coworkers (675), who also showed that IL-10 acts as an autocrine growth factor in these cell lines. It has been suggested that IL-10 contributes to AIDS lymphomagenesis by impairing immune surveillance against EBV-infected B cells through inhibition of T-cell production of IL-2 and interferon-α (676,677), by inhibiting B-cell apoptosis (678), or through its B cell–differentiating activity (679).

Epstein-Barr Virus

Epstein-Barr virus initially was implicated as a cause of endemic Burkitt's lymphoma. It was theorized that a compromised immune system permits EBV infection, resulting in polyclonal B-cell activation in the context of aberrant B-cell regulation, and that the inherent genetic instability of the EBV-immortalized B cells eventually leads to *MYC* gene rearrangement and the development of malignant lymphoma (680,681). Support for this hypothesis includes the facts that EBV infection occurs prior to the development of endemic Burkitt's lymphoma (682) and that the EBV genome is found consistently in endemic Burkitt's lymphoma cells (683). Subsequently, EBV has been implicated in the pathogenesis of an array of lymphoproliferative disorders occurring in individuals who have congenital, acquired, and iatrogenic immunodeficiency. For example, boys who have the X-linked lymphoproliferative disorder develop malignant lymphoma after primary EBV infection (684,685). The majority of lymphoproliferative disorders occurring in solid organ and bone marrow transplant recipients, in the setting of iatrogenic immunosuppression, contain the EBV genome (363,631) (see Chapter 16).

More than 90% of HIV-infected individuals are EBV-infected, and reactivation of EBV infection is a common occurrence in AIDS (686). HIV-infected individuals often suffer from a profound defect in T-cell immunity to EBV and possess abnormally high numbers of circulating EBV-infected B cells (649). EBV-infected B cells are long-lived and are capable of replicating *in vivo* and *in vitro,* where they can be established readily as long-term cell lines (687). It has been suggested frequently that EBV plays a role in AIDS lymphomagenesis; however, the precise nature of that role remains unclear.

Many investigators, including us, have identified EBV DNA or nuclear antigen in AIDS-related lymphomas (383,390,418,419,462,468,479–481,493). Within an individual EBV-positive AIDS-related NHL, essentially all the tumor cells carry the EBV genome and express viral genes (688). Neri and colleagues (689) have demonstrated that each EBV-containing AIDS-related NHL is infected by a single form of EBV, suggesting that EBV infection occurred prior to clonal expansion, and that the malignant lymphoma represents the clonally expanded progeny of a single EBV-infected cell. This concept has been corroborated by Shibata and coworkers (690), who detected a single identical form of EBV in multiple sites of involvement by a disseminated AIDS-related NHL. This is strong evidence in support of an important role for EBV in AIDS lymphomagenesis.

Based on these observations and findings, Pelicci and co-workers (477) and others (377,383) have suggested that AIDS lymphomagenesis is a multistep process that shares pathogenetic mechanisms with endemic Burkitt's lymphoma and other immunodeficiency-associated lymphomas. The hypothesis that has been advanced is that the immunosuppression induced by HIV infection permits frequent, continuous, and massive EBV infections, leading to polyclonal B-cell activation and the development of EBV-infected and immortalized B-cell clones. Such clones would be unstable and susceptible to genetic alterations, that is, the reciprocal chromosomal translocations associated with *MYC* gene rearrangement, resulting in the emergence of a fully transformed monoclonal B-cell population that contains EBV sequences in its genome and the development of a clinically overt B-cell NHL. This hypothesis is supported by studies showing that the introduction of an activated *MYC* gene into EBV-infected lymphoblasts obtained from AIDS patients leads to their malignant conversion (601).

The existence of two distinct EBV strains has been established on the basis of differences in the *EBNA* coding regions (631,691). Type A EBV can be identified in the oropharynx and peripheral blood B cells of immunocompetent individuals worldwide and is associated with efficient B-cell immortalization. Type B EBV initially was identified in individuals from central Africa, is present only rarely in peripheral blood B cells, and is associated with poor B-cell immortalization (624). An increased incidence of peripheral blood B cells infected with EBV type B has been identified in immunosuppressed individuals, especially in those who are HIV-infected or who have undergone solid organ transplantation (692). Many AIDS-related NHLs contain type B EBV (632). These findings suggest that type B EBV may play a role in the pathogenesis of lymphoproliferative disorders associated with immune suppression.

Nonetheless, a significant proportion of AIDS-related NHLs lack EBV. We have been able to detect EBV DNA sequences in only about 40% of AIDS-related systemic NHLs by Southern blot hybridization analysis (480,481,487). Utilizing the more sensitive technique of *in situ* hybridization, Hamilton-Dutoit and co-workers (390) demonstrated EBV in about 50% of patients. Many of the AIDS-related lymphoma cell lines established *in vitro* also lack EBV (548,639). Even if the model that has been proposed to explain the role of EBV in EBV-containing AIDS-related systemic NHLs is valid, alternative models must be formulated to explain those lymphomas lacking EBV. Ganser and coworkers (639) have speculated that these lymphomas occur through a different although comparable mechanism from that proposed by Pelicci and associates (477). They suggested that nonspecific B-cell activation caused by chronic antigenic stimulation by bacterial, fungal, or viral agents, which occurs in persons who have AIDS-induced immune alterations (22,477), results in monoclonal B-cell expansions (477), increasing the risk of a chromosomal translocation and rearrangement of *MYC* and immunoglobulin loci at the time of immunoglobulin gene rearrangement.

In contrast with the presence of EBV in only about 50% of AIDS-related systemic lymphomas, virtually all AIDS-related primary CNS lymphomas contain EBV. MacMahon and colleagues (454) detected EBV early region (EBER-1) transcripts, indicative of latent EBV infection, by *in situ* hybridization in 100% of the 21 AIDS-related primary CNS lymphomas that they studied. They found EBER-1 in only 43% of AIDS-related systemic lymphomas (as expected) and in only 7% of non-AIDS-related primary CNS lymphomas. In addition, they found that 45% of the AIDS-related, but none of the non–AIDS-related, primary CNS lymphomas expressed EBV LMP-1 (454), which is known to have transforming and oncogenic properties (693). It is possible that the pathogeneses of AIDS-related systemic and primary CNS lymphomas differ. Evidence has accumulated to suggest that AIDS-related NHLs exhibit distinct clinical and biologic differences according to their anatomic sites of origin and histopathologic categories. Most AIDS-related primary CNS lymphomas, including those analyzed by MacMahon and coworkers (454), exhibit large cell or immunoblastic morphology (393,394,419,440), and EBV is preferentially associated with these histopathologic categories (481). Whether the difference in EBV content between AIDS-related systemic and primary CNS lymphomas is a function of the anatomic site or the histopathologic category has been debated.

The role of EBV in AIDS lymphomagenesis and its preferential association with certain anatomic sites or histopathologic categories actually may be determined by the level of host immune surveillance (536). The highest frequency of EBV infection among AIDS-related NHLs occurs in the primary CNS lymphomas (454), which are associated with the lowest CD4 T-cell counts (394) and the lowest level of host immune function. Among AIDS-related systemic lymphomas, EBV occurs more frequently in immunoblastic than Burkitt's lymphomas (481,688). The former are associated with significantly lower CD4 T-cell counts than the latter (391). In addition, Pedersen and colleagues (419) have shown that among all AIDS-related systemic NHLs, the EBV-infected instances are associated with significantly lower CD4 T-cell counts and lower CD8 T-cell counts as well. Expression of the highly immunogenic EBV transforming antigens EBNA-2 and LMP-1 is restricted to AIDS-related lymphomas arising in the context of severely impaired immunity (496,688). The accumulated data strongly suggest that the involvement of EBV in AIDS lymphomagenesis is dependent on the level of immunity against EBV and requires highly permissive immunologic conditions (536).

Other Viruses

In addition to EBV, a number of viruses, including human T-cell lymphotrophic virus type 1 (HTLV-1), HTLV-2, human herpesvirus-6, and cytomegalovirus, have been claimed to be associated with AIDS-related NHLs (694–697). Aside from KSHV, however, which is highly associated with the primary effusion lymphomas (467), there is no definitive evidence for the presence of these viruses within the actual lymphoma cells and, hence, their involvement in AIDS lymphomagenesis.

Chronic B-Cell Stimulation and Proliferation

HIV infection also is characterized by a state of chronic stimulation of B cells by various environmental antigens and self-antigens (642), mitogens, and viruses, including EBV (649,685) and HIV itself (643). This leads to polyclonal hypergammaglobulinemia (642,643) and florid follicular (B-cell) hyperplasia (646) within enlarged, reactive lymph nodes, which is referred to as the *persistent generalized lymphadenopathy syndrome* (90,92). That HIV is one direct cause of polyclonal B-cell activation is evidenced by the frequent oligoclonal bands displaying anti-HIV reactivity that accompany the hypergammaglobulinemia (698,699).

The crucial role of antigens in normal B-cell development is well documented (700). A role for antigen stimulation in B-cell expansion and selection associated with the development of malignant lymphoma in immunocompetent hosts has been established (595,596). The studies performed by Riboldi and colleagues (701) provide evidence that chronic antigenic stimulation is involved in AIDS lymphomagenesis as well. These investigators discovered that some AIDS-related Burkitt's lymphomas produce autoantibodies. Furthermore, they demonstrated somatic hypermutation of the immunoglobulin gene hypervariable regions utilized by these lymphoma cells. An antigen-driven process of clonal selection may play a role in the emergence or expansion of a neoplastic B-cell clone in AIDS lymphomagenesis.

The persistent generalized lymphadenopathy syndrome precedes the development of AIDS-related NHL in as many as one third of individuals (369,375,440). This is of particular interest in view of the previously mentioned model of AIDS lymphomagenesis and the long-held belief that chronic antigenic stimulation is associated with the development of B-cell lymphoma (447). One report suggested that malignant lymphoma develops 850 times more frequently than expected in individuals who have persistent generalized lymphadenopathy (702). These observations suggest that a pathogenetic relationship may exist between B-cell hyperplasia and the development of B-cell lymphoma in HIV-infected individuals.

Pelicci and coworkers (477) investigated that relationship by performing a correlative immunophenotypic and molecular genetic analysis of hyperplastic lymph nodes obtained from HIV-infected individuals. They discovered that about 20% of the lymph nodes exhibiting polyclonal florid follicular hyperplasia contained one or more discrete immunoglobulin heavy chain gene rearrangements as determined by Southern blot hybridization, indicating the presence of one or more clonal B-cell expansions. The new rearranged bands often were of low intensity and sometimes were accompanied by a hybridization smear, suggesting the presence of additional oligoclonal B-cell populations (Fig. 28.54). These results suggest that the hyperplastic lymph nodes of HIV-infected patients often contain occult clonal B-cell populations that are not identifiable by morphologic examination or by immunophenotypic analysis. Comparable analysis of hyperplastic lymph nodes obtained from HIV-uninfected individuals generally fails to demonstrate the presence of clonal B-cell expansions, suggesting that the presence of oligoclonal B-cell expansions is preferentially associated with the immunosuppressed state of AIDS. Pelicci and associates (477) demonstrated that these B-cell clones do not carry *MYC* gene rearrangements, suggesting that they are immortalized but not yet fully transformed (Fig. 28.55). They hypothesized that these oligoclonal B-cell populations represent the EBV-infected and immortalized B-cell clones in their proposed multistep process of AIDS lymphomagenesis. The investigators theorized that the oligoclonal B-cell expansions occurring in these hyperplastic lymph nodes may represent a premalignant condition for the future development of AIDS-related B-cell lymphoma.

Unfortunately, Pelicci and coworkers (477) were unable to obtain subsequent tissue biopsy samples from these patients. Therefore, they were unable to ascertain whether those patients whose hyperplastic lymph nodes contained clonal B-cell populations actually later developed malignant lymphoma. Longitudinal studies of serial biopsy specimens obtained from individuals who present with persistent generalized lymphadenopathy and florid follicular (B-cell) hyperplasia and who subsequently develop malignant lymphoma are necessary to determine if a direct clonal relationship exists between HIV-associated hyperplastic lymphadenopathy and AIDS-related lymphomas.

Some experimental evidence is available to support this hypothesis. Shibata and colleagues (703) identified EBV DNA in 37% of reactive lymph nodes obtained from HIV-infected individuals. They demonstrated a statistically significant positive correlation between the presence of detectable amounts of EBV DNA in these reactive lymph nodes and the concurrent occurrence or subsequent development of EBV-containing malignant lymphoma (703). Chromosomal abnormalities have been identified in hyperplastic lymph nodes obtained from HIV-infected individuals who later developed malignant lymphoma (704).

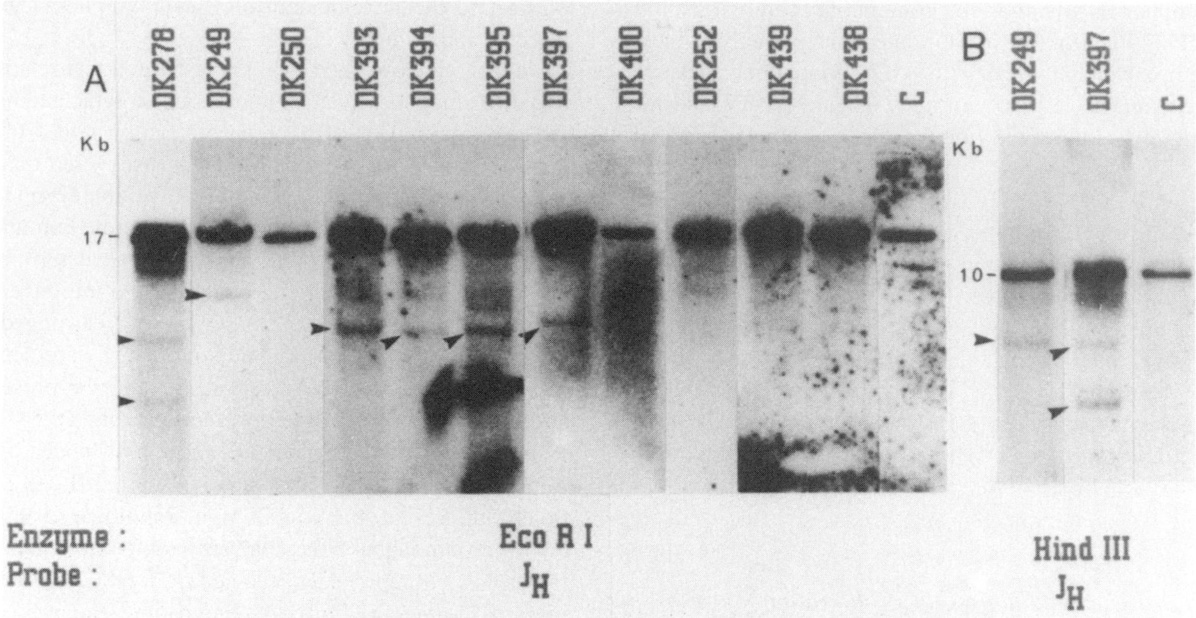

FIG. 28.54. Immunoglobulin gene rearrangement analysis of histopathologically benign and immunophenotypically polyclonal lymph nodes obtained from patients who had AIDS and AIDS-related complex. The DNA extracted from the indicated cases and from normal human placenta (control, *C*) were digested with Eco RI or HIND-III and hybridized to an immunoglobulin heavy chain joining region probe. Arrows indicate rearrangement bands. The control lane shows the germline configuration. Many of these hyperplastic lymph nodes display one or more rearrangement bands, often of low intensity, indicating the presence of one or more small clonal B-cell expansions. The rearrangement bands sometimes are accompanied by a hybridization smear, suggesting the presence of additional oligoclonal B-cell populations. These results suggest that the hyperplastic lymph nodes of HIV-infected persons often contain occult clonal B-cell populations not identifiable by morphologic examination or by immunophenotypic analysis. (From Pelicci PG, Knowles DM, Arlin Z, et al. Multiple monoclonal B-cell expansions and c-myc oncogene rearrangements in AIDS-related lymphoproliferative disorders: implications for lymphomagenesis. *J Exp Med* 1986;164:2049–2076, with permission from the Rockefeller University Press by copyright.)

Hyperplastic lymphadenopathy precedes the development of AIDS-related lymphoma in only approximately one third of individuals (369,375). Only about 5% to 10% of patients who have persistent generalized lymphadenopathy actually develop malignant lymphoma (90,705). It has been reported that HIV-infected individuals who previously have had persistent generalized lymphadenopathy have NHL restricted to lymph nodes significantly more frequently (440). Nevertheless, a high proportion of those lymphomas originate outside of lymph nodes, often in obscure extranodal sites (375). Once again, only about 50% of AIDS-related systemic NHLs contain EBV (390,418,480,481). AIDS-related NHL clearly occurs in a large number of individuals at risk for AIDS who do not have a prior history of persistent generalized lymphadenopathy and who develop AIDS-related systemic lymphomas that do not contain EBV. For all these reasons, the precise relationship among EBV infection, the persistent generalized lymphadenopathy syndrome, and the eventual development of AIDS-related malignant lymphoma remains unclear.

Role of Protooncogenes and Tumor Suppressor Genes

Several investigators have suggested that the hyperstimulated clonal B-cell populations undergoing physiologic immunoglobulin gene rearrangement in the milieu of the HIV-induced immunodeficiency state are inherently genetically unstable. Hence, they have a propensity to undergo specific chromosomal translocations involving the immunoglobulin heavy and light chain genes, for example, t(8;14), t(8;22), and t(2;8). Such translocations permit deregulation of the *MYC* gene on chromosome 8, either by *MYC* gene rearrangement as in sporadic Burkitt's lymphoma or by point mutations as in endemic Burkitt's lymphoma (504,505), ultimately resulting in the development of malignant lymphoma. Pelicci and coworkers (477) and Subar and coworkers (480) demonstrated *MYC* gene rearrangements in about 75% to 80% of AIDS-related systemic lymphomas, respectively, which is consistent with this hypothesis. It is likely that *MYC* gene deregulation contributes to AIDS lymphomagenesis. This may occur through disruption of the normal control of *MYC* gene expression by mechanisms analogous to those in

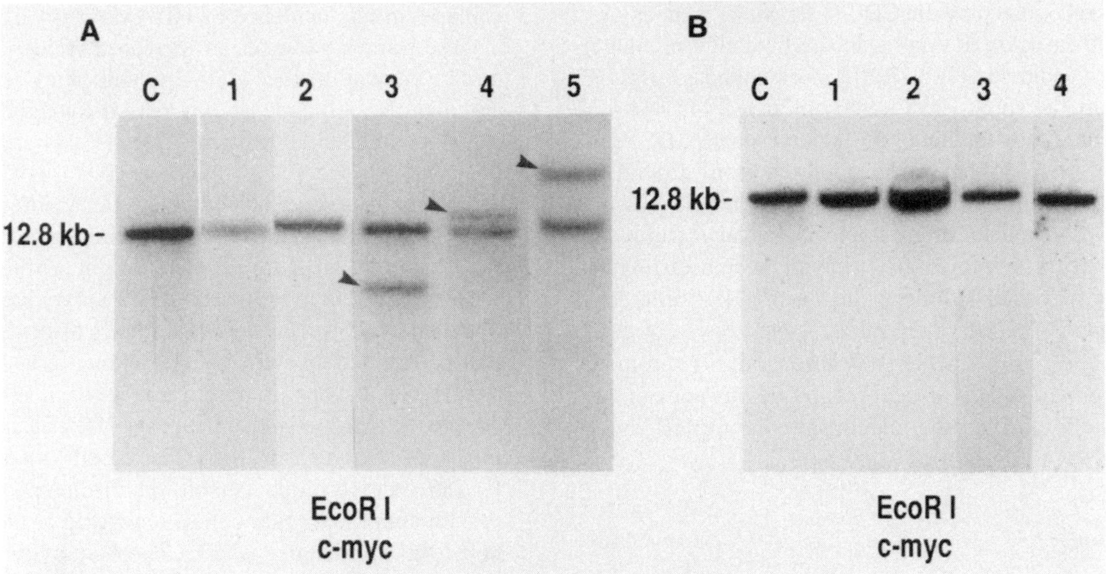

FIG. 28.55. Southern blot hybridization analysis for *MYC* gene rearrangements in AIDS-related non-Hodgkin's lymphomas (**A**) and hyperplastic lymph nodes (**B**). The DNA extracted from the indicated cases and from normal human placenta (control, *C*) were digested with Eco RI and hybridized to probe MC413RC, representative of the third exon of the human *MYC* gene. Rearrangement bands that indicate *MYC* gene rearrangement are indicated with arrowheads. The control lane shows the germline configuration. The majority of AIDS-related non-Hodgkin's lymphomas exhibit *MYC* gene rearrangement; the hyperplastic lymph nodes, despite the fact that they may contain small clonal B-cell expansions, consistently lack *MYC* gene rearrangements. (From Pelicci PG, Knowles DM, Arlin Z, et al. Multiple monoclonal B-cell expansions and c-myc oncogene rearrangements in AIDS-related lymphoproliferative disorders: implications for lymphomagenesis. *J Exp Med* 1986;164:2049–2076, with permission from the Rockefeller University Press by copyright.)

conventional Burkitt's lymphoma occurring in the immunocompetent host (536). Also, cells in which translocations involving the immunoglobulin and *MYC* genes have occurred may acquire specific properties that render them especially well suited to expand and progress to malignancy in the context of HIV-induced immunodeficiency (536). Once such alteration may be downregulation of the integrin receptor lymphocyte function antigen-1 (LFA-1), which is controlled by *MYC* in B cells (706) and is involved in many biologic functions, including cell conjugate formation between B cells and cytotoxic T cells, natural killer cells, and vascular endothelia (536). Burkitt's lymphoma cells lack LFA-1, which is involved in immunorecognition by T cells and are unable to elicit either autologous or allogeneic responses *in vitro* (707,708). The occurrence of a *MYC* gene rearrangement in a B cell that already carries EBV increases growth and confers full tumorigenic potential and, in addition, downregulates the surface LFA antigens, allowing the tumor cells to escape immune surveillance (536). The effects of such alterations would be amplified greatly in the immunodeficient environment associated with HIV infection.

AIDS lymphomagenesis involves multiple factors, including the state of HIV-induced immunosuppression, impaired immune surveillance, cytokine and growth factor release and deregulation, chronic B-cell stimulation, differentiation, and proliferation, and EBV infection. This milieu appears to be conducive to the occurrence of genetic alterations in critical oncogenes or tumor suppressor genes, leading for example to *MYC* gene activation and *P53* gene inactivation, subsequent clonal selection, and the development of monoclonal B-cell lymphoma. Because the risk of developing malignant lymphoma is similar in all AIDS risk groups, environmental cofactors may not be very important in the etiology of HIV-related NHL (411). The same factors may cause certain lymphomas regardless of whether they are associated with HIV infection or not. This process may be heterogeneous, however, and distinct pathogenetic mechanisms may account for different anatomic sites or histopathologic categories of AIDS-related lymphoma. Although multiple immunologic and molecular steps in this process have been elucidated, considerably more work is required to acquire a complete understanding of AIDS lymphomagenesis.

HODGKIN'S DISEASE

Background

The initial cases of HD occurring in individuals at risk for AIDS were reported from the United States in 1984 and 1985 (373,709–712), as early as 3 years after the AIDS epidemic was recognized by the CDC (1,2). Since then, approximately 400 cases of HIV-associated HD, including numerous isolated incidents (713–728), many collected as small series from a single institution (375,385,415,416,424, 729–737), and most gathered through national AIDS registries (389,738–746), have been reported from around the world. These reports have served to characterize HIV-associated HD, including its often atypical clinical features and frequently aggressive biologic behavior, which distinguish it from conventional HD occurring in the HIV-uninfected general population. These reports, however, have not determined unequivocally whether HIV infection truly promotes the development of HD or merely modifies its course; they have not fully clarified the relationship among HIV infection, AIDS, and HD.

Epidemiology

Many investigators have suggested that the atypical manifestations peculiar to HD occurring in HIV-infected individuals justifies its recognition as an AIDS-related neoplasm and therefore as an AIDS-defining condition (715,716,731, 732,747). HD occurring in individuals who have primary immunodeficiency and in solid organ transplant recipients, however, similarly displays a preponderance of unfavorable histopathologic subtypes and aggressive clinical behavior (359,748), although its incidence is not increased in these patient populations (749,750). Alternatively, the atypical clinical features and aggressive biologic behavior of HIV-associated HD may represent simply an epiphenomenon of the underlying immunodeficiency state induced by HIV infection. AIDS-related neoplasms have been defined as those occurring in statistically increased numbers in HIV-infected persons compared with the general population (270). Currently, these include Kaposi's sarcoma, diffuse aggressive B-cell NHL, and invasive cervical carcinoma, each of which has been accepted by the CDC as an AIDS-defining condition (62). Although innumerable cases of HD occurring in patients at risk for AIDS have been reported, the relationship between HD and HIV infection has been difficult to evaluate because of the relatively high incidence of HD in the age group at greatest risk for HIV infection. The initial population-based studies of AIDS-associated neoplasms conducted in the 1980s failed to detect a statistically significant increase in the incidence of HD among young, never married men in San Francisco, New York, and Los Angeles, the epicenters of the then-emerging AIDS epidemic (404,414,751,752). For this reason, it was concluded that the relationship between HD and HIV infection is merely coincidental (401,751). Consequently, the CDC has never accepted HD as an AIDS-defining malignancy. Two critical issues require consideration in this regard, however.

First, the decision to investigate young, never married men as a surrogate population for homosexual men at risk for AIDS rather than HIV-infected individuals in these studies may have limited the ability of these studies to detect subtle increases in the incidence of HD. Alternatively, the failure of these studies to detect an increased incidence of HD in the first 5 years of the AIDS epidemic may reflect the requirement for a longer latency period for the development of HIV-associated HD. In any case, Hessol and colleagues (753) reported an excess risk of HD of 19.3 cases per 100,000 person years attributable to HIV infection among 6,704 homosexual men residing in the San Francisco area from 1978 through 1989. By linking the California Tumor Registry and the San Francisco AIDS Surveillance Registry, Reynolds and coworkers (754) similarly discovered a significantly increased incidence of HD among HIV-positive men with AIDS in the San Francisco area between 1980 and 1987. More recently, Lyter and colleagues (755) detected a statistically significant, nearly 20-fold increased risk of developing HD (85 cases/100,000 person years) among the HIV-infected homosexual male cohort registered at the Pittsburgh site of the Multicenter AIDS Cohort Study between 1984 and 1993. Despite the fact that the actual number of cases of HD identified in these epidemiologic studies was small, these findings suggest that the incidence of HD has increased among HIV-infected persons in the United States.

Second, determination of the incidence of HD in HIV-infected individuals has been based largely on epidemiologic data gathered from the United States, which is based primarily on homosexual men and not on IDUs. Although Ahmed and coworkers (385) failed to detect a significant increase in the overall incidence of HD among HIV-infected New York City prisoners from 1981 through 1984, they found that the incidence was 3 to 10 times higher among prisoners who were IDUs than among those who were not. Since then, National Registry surveys from Italy (389,746), France (739,742,744), and Spain (745) and several other studies (732,753) have shown that the ratio of NHL to HD is significantly lower in HIV-infected IDUs than in HIV-infected homosexual men, suggesting that HIV-associated HD occurs significantly more frequently among HIV-infected IDUs than among HIV-infected homosexual men. Despite these findings, HIV-associated HD does not appear to have a restricted distribution among AIDS-risk groups. HIV-associated HD has been described in HIV-infected hemophiliacs (410,718,735,745) and in women who have apparently acquired HIV infection through heterosexual contact with IDUs (731,740,744,745), in addition to MSM (424,730,733, 740), although the incidence does not appear to be increased in these latter groups (410). More data is probably necessary to determine unequivocally whether or not HD should be considered an AIDS-related neoplasm and an AIDS-defining condition. This requires additional larger, carefully designed epidemiologic studies that consider both the route of HIV transmission and the geographic location of the populations at risk for AIDS.

Pathology

The pathologic spectrum of conventional HD varies in different parts of the world and in different socioeconomic groups within the United States. Large referral centers in the United States and western Europe have reported the following approximate histopathologic distribution of types of conventional HD: nodular sclerosis, 52% to 62%; mixed cellularity, 24% to 27%; lymphocytic depletion, 3% to 6%; and lymphocyte predominance, the remaining 7% to 11% (756–758). In contrast, mixed cellularity and lymphocytic depletion are the most common histologic subtypes in underdeveloped countries (759,760). Similar increases in mixed cellularity and lymphocytic depletion HD have been observed in minority populations of lower socioeconomic status within the United States (761).

The pathologic spectrum of HIV-associated HD is similar to that of underdeveloped countries and patients of lower socioeconomic status within the United States. The approximate histopathologic distribution is mixed cellularity, 50%; nodular sclerosis, 28%; lymphocytic depletion, 14%, and unclassified, 5% (373,375,389,415,709–711,713,715,716, 729–732,734–746). Only rare cases of lymphocyte predominance HD have been reported (732,745,746). The mixed cellularity and lymphocytic depletion subtypes of HD occur significantly more frequently among HIV-infected than among HIV-uninfected individuals. Increases in the incidences of unfavorable histopathologic subtypes and a corresponding decrease in the prevalence of the more favorable nodular sclerosis subtype similarly is found in HD occurring in patients who have primary immunodeficiency (359, 748,762).

Cases of HIV-associated HD exhibit morphologic features comparable to those of conventional HD of corresponding histopathologic subtype (Fig. 28.56). Frequently, however, cases of HIV-associated HD display a distinct decrease in the number of benign lymphocytes making up the background host response cell population (735). This imparts a relative lymphocyte-depleted appearance compared with cases of conventional HD. The relative lymphocytic depletion probably reflects the decrease in CD4 T cells associated with HIV infection (375,729,735). Reed-Sternberg cells and variants sometimes are particularly numerous and may appear even more so against a relatively lymphocyte-depleted background. Histiocytes are often abundant, as is multifocal necrosis (735). These slightly atypical features sometimes render the histopathologic diagnosis of HD problematic in the setting of HIV infection. For example, these features may cause some cases of HIV-associated HD to be misinterpreted as diffuse large B-cell lymphoma or peripheral T-cell lymphoma. This diagnostic problem may be compounded by the presence of the HD lesion in the bone marrow or in another, often unusual, extranodal site. Bone marrow involvement by HIV-associated HD often is confluent, but it may be focal and patchy (424,735,736). In the latter cases, diagnostic Reed-Sternberg cells may be sparse and difficult to identify. In these instances, the bone marrow lesions of HIV-associated HD may be overlooked as benign lymphohistiocytic aggregates or thought to have an infectious cause (736). This is especially true in the absence of documented

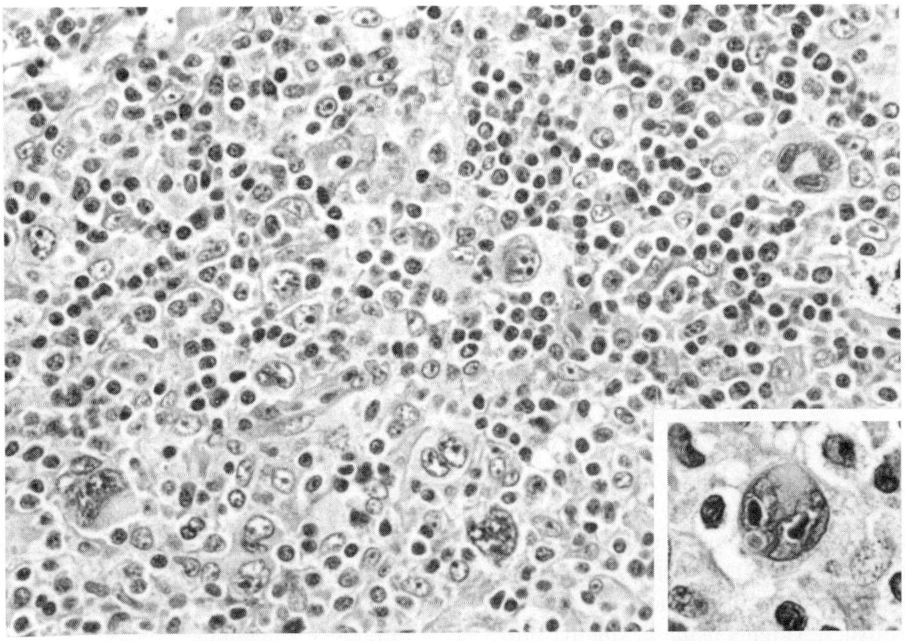

FIG. 28.56. HIV-associated mixed cellularity Hodgkin's disease that exhibits the same polymorphic cellular composition, including the presence of classic Reed-Sternberg cells, as mixed-cell Hodgkin's disease occurring in the general population unassociated with AIDS (hematoxylin and eosin stain, original magnifications: 320× magnification; **Inset:** 630× magnification). (From Knowles DM, Chadburn A. The neoplasms associated with AIDS. In: Joshi VV, ed. *Pathology of AIDS and other manifestations of HIV infection.* New York: Igaku-Shoin, 1990:83–120, with permission.)

lymph node involvement and clinical suspicion of HD. Recognition of these histopathologic features of HIV-associated HD and the appropriate use of immunohistochemical studies as adjuncts to morphologic interpretation should prevent misdiagnosis in these cases.

Immunophenotypic and Immunogenotypic Characteristics

HIV-associated and non–HIV-associated HD share similar immunophenotypic and immunogenotypic characteristics. In each instance, the lesions contain a variable mixture of CD4 and CD8 T cells, polyclonal B cells, histiocytes, Reed-Sternberg cells, and Reed-Sternberg cell variants (375,735). The Reed-Sternberg cells in HIV-associated HD similarly lack CD45 and usually express CD30 and CD15 when immunostained in paraffin tissue sections (375,735). The benign host response T-cell populations present within the HD lesions usually differ, however. The majority of T cells in most cases of non-HIV associated HD belong to the $CD4^{+}CD8^{-}$ subset (763). In contrast, fewer than usual numbers of T cells, reduced numbers of CD4 T cells, and increased numbers of CD8 T cells are often present in the lesions of HIV-associated HD (375,729,735). These differences are probably a consequence of the progressive depletion of the CD4 T-cell subset in HIV-infected patients caused by the cytopathic effect of HIV on CD4 T cells (18,22,23). It has been suggested that the presence of an inappropriate T-cell population and altered immunity in the HD lesions contributes to their biologic aggressiveness and the poor prognosis of patients who have HIV-associated HD (729,735).

We and others have demonstrated that most cases of conventional HD unassociated with HIV infection lack clonal immunoglobulin heavy and light chain and T-cell receptor gene rearrangements by Southern blot hybridization analysis (764,765). The lesions of HIV-associated HD also lack clonal antigen receptor gene rearrangements, as demonstrated if they are studied in a similar fashion (375,746), and thus are immunogenotypically identical to conventional HD. These characteristics are sometimes useful in distinguishing among HIV-associated HD and AIDS-related B- and T-cell NHLs; the latter nearly always exhibit clonal immunoglobulin or T-cell receptor gene rearrangements (375,462,477, 480).

Epstein-Barr Virus

It has been suggested that EBV may be involved in the pathogenesis of conventional HD, because early EBV RNAs, LMP-1, or both are detectable in the Reed-Sternberg cells of almost 50% of such patients using *in situ* hybridization and immunohistochemical techniques (766,767). EBV is preferentially associated with the mixed cellularity and lymphocytic depletion subtypes (766–769) and the peripheral form of the disease (769) and is found far less commonly in the nodular sclerosis subtype and the central form of the disease (766–769). EBV is frequently present in the Reed-Sternberg cells of HD occurring in developing countries (770), where these histopathologic subtypes and peripheral HD are more prevalant (771). It is not altogether surprising that in a significantly higher percentage (approximately 80–100%) of patients with HIV-associated HD than of those with conventional HD, the Reed-Sternberg cells contain EBER or LMP-1 (746,772,773). This finding partially reflects the significantly higher frequency of these unfavorable histopathologic subtypes and the peripheral form of the disease in HIV-infected individuals (731,732,743–747). Even in cases of HIV-associated nodular sclerosis HD, however, the Reed-Sternberg cells consistently contain the EBV genome (772,773). The presence of clonal EBV genomes in a very high proportion of cases of HIV-associated HD, in comparison with conventional HD (746), and the same EBV genome in multiple metachronous HD lesions in some HIV-seropositive individuals (746) further suggests an etiologic role for EBV in the pathogenesis of HIV-associated HD. These findings suggest that in at least a subset of cases of HD, the Reed-Sternberg cells represent a clonal expansion of a single EBV-infected cell, which continues to express EBV latent gene products. In contrast with EBV-containing, non–HIV-associated HD, in which type B EBV is present uncommonly (746,767), type A and type B EBV have approximately equal distributions in EBV-containing, HIV-associated HD (746,774). This finding suggests that type B EBV may be involved in the pathogenesis of HD in the setting of HIV infection, analogous to AIDS-related NHL (775). Further studies are needed to clarify the relationship between EBV and HD, including its precise role in the development of HD in HIV-infected individuals.

Clinical Features

Individuals who develop HIV-associated HD display a distinct constellation of clinical features that is remarkably consistent among all AIDS risk groups, regardless of geographic location (375,389,415,424,730,731,733,735,740, 743–746). These features contrast sharply with those of conventional HD occurring in the HIV-uninfected general population. In the United States, only approximately 30% of newly diagnosed patients with conventional HD, or 60% in the case of those of low socioeconomic status, complain of B symptoms (757,761), only 30% lack mediastinal disease, and only 40% have stage III or IV disease at presentation (756,757). Extranodal involvement is uncommon; bone marrow infiltration occurs in less than 5% of patients overall (756) and only approaches 30% even in those patients who have the mixed cellularity or lymphocytic depletion subtypes (775). Comparable findings have been reported in western European patients who have conventional HD (732,746,776).

Approximately 90% or more of the patients who have HIV-associated HD are adult men (415,416,424,729–733, 735,740,743–746). In the United States, the majority are MSM (375,415,729,730,733,735,740), but in western Europe most are male IDUs (389,731,732,741,743–746). Initially, this difference was believed to reflect the epidemiologic patterns of the AIDS epidemic, because the majority of patients with AIDS in the United States are MSM, but in Europe they are IDUs (732,741,744,745). Many investigators, however, now believe that this difference reflects a genuine predilection for HIV-associated HD to occur in IDUs. The median ages of patients who have HIV-associated HD are about 35 years in the United States (375,424,733, 740) and about 28 years in western Europe (389,732,741, 743–746), comparable to the median ages of patients in these regions who have AIDS-related NHL (375,389).

HIV-associated HD usually occurs prior to an AIDS-defining illness and thus usually is the first manifestation of HIV infection in these individuals (389,415,745). Among 114 patients with HIV-associated HD studied by the Italian Cooperative Group on AIDS and Tumors, 33% were asymptomatic, 28% had persistent generalized lymphadenopathy, 22% had AIDS-related complex, and only 17% had a diagnosis of AIDS (746). Only 11% of patients with HIV-associated HD in the French Registry had been diagnosed previously with AIDS (744). As many as 60% to 70% of individuals, especially IDUs, who develop HIV-associated HD have histories of persistent generalized lymphadenopathy (389,741). The persistent generalized lymphadenopathy precedes the diagnosis of HD by between 1 month and more than 3 years, although the median is 8 months (741). The clinical presentations of HIV-associated HD and persistent generalized lymphadenopathy, that is, enlarged peripheral lymph nodes accompanied by malaise, fever, night sweats, weight loss, and splenomegaly, may overlap significantly. In a European series of IDUs with HIV-associated HD, the diagnosis of HD was made in lymph nodes already known to exhibit persistent generalized lymphadenopathy in almost 40% of cases (741). HD even may coexist with the florid follicular hyperplasia (710) or follicular involution (424,735) phase of HIV-associated lymphadenopathy in individual lymph nodes. Accurate diagnosis and distinction between persistent generalized lymphadenopathy and HD requires a tissue biopsy. An increase in the size of persistently enlarged lymph nodes or the development of B symptoms warrants biopsy evaluation, possibly of multiple sites.

Patients who have HIV-associated HD exhibit a variable spectrum of the laboratory findings associated with HIV infection, that is, cutaneous anergy, polyclonal hypergammaglobulinemia, cytopenias, and a reduction in the number of peripheral blood CD4 T cells (375,731–733,745). Approximately 30% have active opportunistic infections at the time of diagnosis of HD (743,746). Kaposi's sarcoma occurs infrequently in patients who have HIV-associated HD (744,745) and only rarely prior to the diagnosis of HD (744). This may relate partially to the lesser degree of immune suppression and higher CD4 T-cell counts in these individuals than in those who have AIDS-related NHL. Median CD4 T-cell counts of between 201 and 306 per microliter have been reported in multiple series of patients with HIV-associated HD (740,741,743,744,746). Like Burkitt's lymphoma, HIV-associated HD appears to occur relatively early in the clinical course of HIV infection, prior to the onset of severe immunodeficiency and the development of AIDS-related illnesses. This finding is consistent with the fact that, like Burkitt's lymphoma, HD occurs infrequently in other immunodeficiency states (749,750). Factors other than HIV-induced immunosuppression may be involved in the development of HIV-associated HD.

Approximately 80% to 90% of patients who have HIV-associated HD complain of B symptoms (fever, drenching night sweats, or weight loss in excess of 10% of normal body weight) at presentation (731,732,743–746). Other symptomatic complaints are variable, because of the diverse and multiple organ systems involved by HIV-associated HD, and usually depend on the principal location of disease. These individuals normally already possess widely disseminated disease at the time of initial presentation. Approximately 75% to 90% have clinical stage III or IV disease (375,389,415,709–711,713,715,716,729–735,740, 743–746) and about two thirds have extranodal involvement (375,389,731,732,740,745,746) at diagnosis. The most common extranodal site is the bone marrow, which is involved in up to 40% to 50% of cases in some series (731,732,740, 745) (Fig. 28.57). Not infrequently, this is the first indication of the presence of HD in these individuals (424,735,740). About one third of patients have involvement of other extranodal sites initially, most commonly the liver, spleen, and lungs (375,389,732,743,745). Lung involvement in the absence of mediastinal lymphadenopathy, which is observed regularly in North American MSM, appears to occur less commonly among European IDUs, however (741). HIV-associated HD often involves unusual extranodal sites (740,743), including even the CNS (726) (Fig. 28.58). HIV-associated HD has been reported to originate or present in the oropharynx (415,740), the anorectal region (719,728), and the skin (710,724) (Fig. 28.59). As in AIDS-related NHL, the diagnosis of HIV-associated HD often is established on the basis of a biopsy of an extranodal site (375,740).

HIV-associated HD often has an atypical presentation and spreads in a random, noncontiguous fashion. There is a conspicuous absence of the classic presentation of supradiaphragmatic peripheral as well as mediastinal and hilar lymph node disease (375,415,710,744,746). Patients often have involvement of multiple, noncontiguous lymph node groups, extensive liver or bone marrow disease in the absence of splenic involvement, widespread disease with sparing of the mediastinum and hilar lymph nodes, and involvement of unusual extranodal sites (375,415,710). Mediastinal lymph node involvement occurs infrequently in HIV-associated HD (732,744,746). Only 23% of the Italian cohort (746) and only 13% of the French cohort (744) with HIV-associated HD had mediastinal involvement, and these generally were individuals who had clinical stage IV disease. A very high frequency of the peripheral form of HD (absence of mediastinal involvement) is a specific feature of HIV-associated HD. Andrieu and colleagues (744) have pointed out

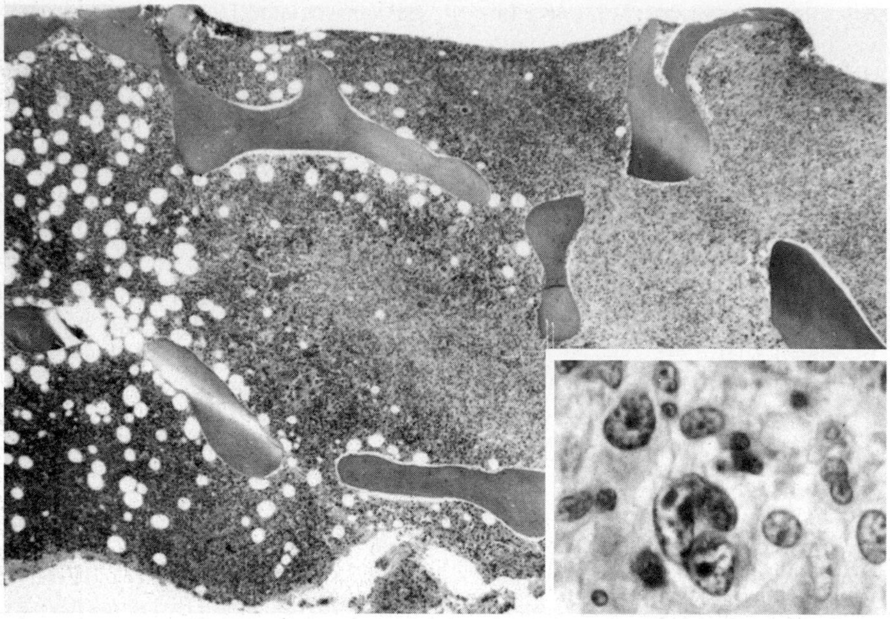

FIG. 28.57. Bone marrow biopsy core obtained at the time of initial presentation of the patient whose lymph node biopsy is illustrated in Figure 28.56. Large areas of the bone marrow are replaced by Hodgkin's disease, indicating stage IVB Hodgkin's disease. The areas of bone marrow involvement show delicate fibrosis and a sparsely cellular infiltrate composed of Reed-Sternberg cells, Reed-Sternberg cell variants, and histiocytes. Small lymphocytes, plasma cells, and eosinophils are reduced in number, consistent with lymphocytic depletion Hodgkin's disease (hematoxylin and eosin stain, original magnifications: 40× magnification; **Inset:** 630× magnification).

that the mixed cellularity subtype occurs in 37% of patients with conventional HD lacking mediastinal involvement, and in 48% of such patients if only men aged 23 to 50 years are considered. The mixed cellularity subtype is highly associated with peripheral HD in both HIV-infected and HIV-uninfected individuals. An increase in the incidence of the peripheral but not the central form of HD may account for the higher incidence of HD among HIV-infected individuals. HIV seropositivity should be suspected in patients with HD who exhibit atypical clinical manifestations or a hyperaggressive disease course. The identification of patients who have HIV-associated HD rather than conventional HD has significant therapeutic, managerial, and prognostic implications.

Treatment and Survival

A few patients who have HIV-associated HD are not treated because of poor performance status or short life expectancy or because the diagnosis is made after death (745,746). An additional few patients are treated with radiation therapy alone, primarily for palliation of local disease (745,746); radiation therapy may induce a complete response in patients who have stage IA HIV-associated HD (375,745). Most patients who have HIV-associated HD are treated with standard mechlorethamine, oncovin[vincristine], procarbazine, prednisone/adriamycin[doxorubicin], bleomycin, vinblastine, decarbizine protocols that are employed in treating patients with conventional HD (777). These protocols may be administered alone or followed by radiation therapy. These protocols achieve a complete remission in almost 90% of patients who have conventional HD (778) and render more than 70% of all patients who have conventional HD permanently disease-free (777,779). They are associated with complete remission in 70% to 80% of patients and with long-term disease-free survival in 60% to 70% of patients with stage III or IV conventional HD (777). Conventional HD is considered curable even in the presence of widely disseminated disease.

The prognosis of patients who have HIV-associated HD is significantly worse than that of those who have conventional HD, however. Complete remission rates of only about 40% to 70% (415,732,741,743,745,746) and median durations of survival of only 8 to 18 months (389,732,733,740,741,743,745,746) have been reported in virtually all large series of HIV-associated HD if these chemotherapeutic protocols have been employed. One problem is that these regimens often cause significant hematologic toxicity, including further cytopenias, disproportionate to the dosages employed if they are administered to HIV-infected patients, who often have extensive bone marrow disease and are already cytopenic (375,710,731,732,734,744–746). The increased hematologic toxicity and the propensity of these patients to develop multiple severe opportunistic infections often delays or necessitates dosage reductions of scheduled chemotherapy, compromising therapy and management (732,740,741,743). Errante and coworkers (780) discovered that the addi-

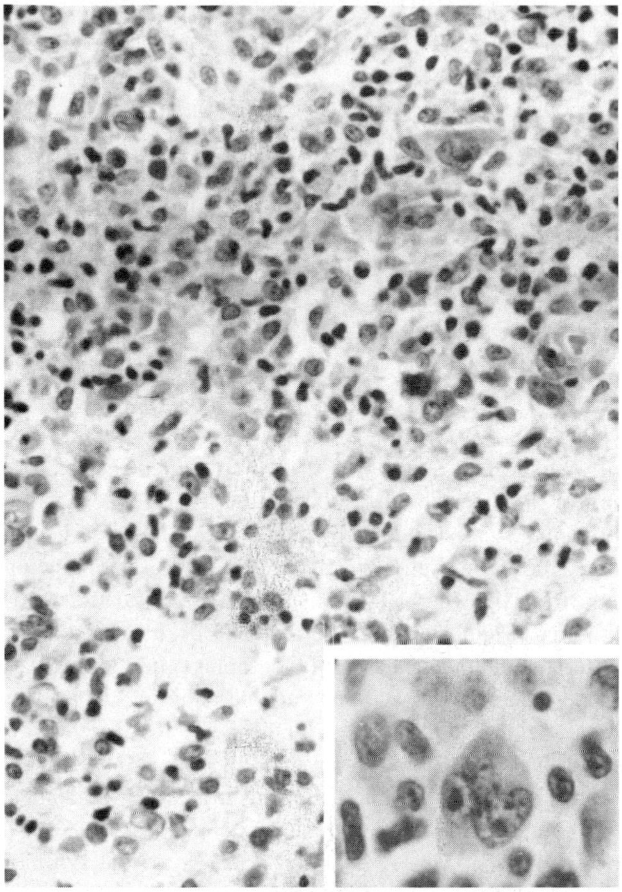

FIG. 28.58. HIV-associated mixed-cell Hodgkin's disease involving the central nervous system. This 35-year-old HIV-positive intravenous drug user with clinical stage IVB Hodgkin's disease developed central nervous system involvement on chemotherapy. Note the typical polymorphic cellular composition of mixed cellularity Hodgkin's disease (above) blending into the adjacent normal brain parenchyma (below). Characteristic Reed-Sternberg cells are readily identifiable (hematoxylin and eosin stain, original magnifications: 250× magnification; **Inset:** 630× magnification).

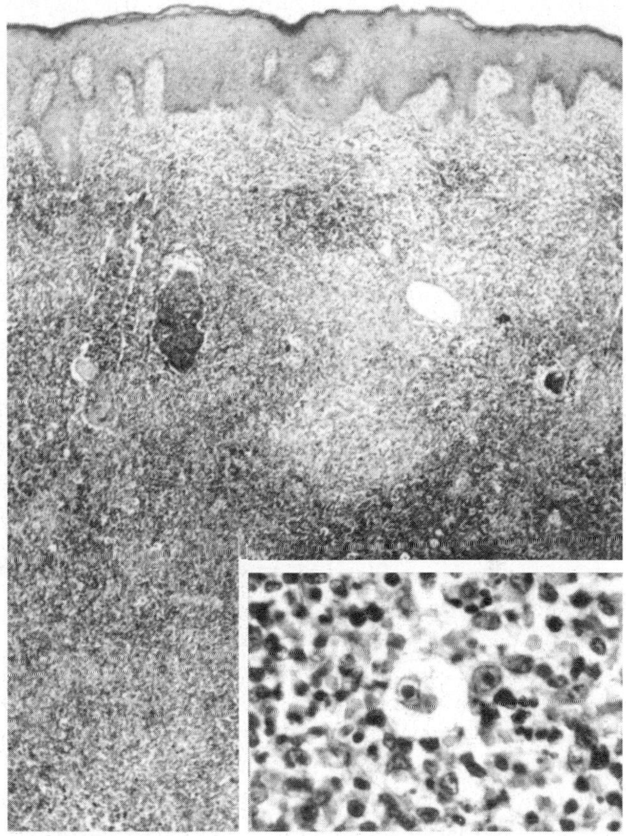

FIG. 28.59. Cutaneous involvement by HIV-associated nodular sclerosis Hodgkin's disease. A 25-year-old homosexual intravenous drug user with widely disseminated nodular sclerosis Hodgkin's disease developed cutaneous involvement. Reed-Sternberg cell lacunar variants are readily identifiable (hematoxylin and eosin stain, original magnifications: 40× magnification; **Inset:** 400× magnification). (Courtesy of Professor Ronald F. Dorfman, Stanford University, Palo Alto, CA.)

tion of antiretroviral therapy to standard antineoplastic chemotherapy regimens significantly decreased the occurrence of opportunistic infections both during and after chemotherapy, although it did not significantly increase the complete remission rate or the median survival. Newcom and colleagues (737), however, achieved a complete remission rate of 100% and a median duration of survival of 38 months in a small group of patients with HIV-associated HD by employing truncated standard chemotherapy regimens individualized to induce a clinical remission in conjunction with *P. carinii* pneumonia prophylaxis. The optimal therapeutic approach for treating HIV-associated HD is unclear. Prospective clinical trials are needed to define better therapeutic strategies for these patients. The inclusion of hematopoietic growth factors, which may permit the administration of higher-dosage chemotherapy, and the prolonged use of antiretroviral drugs should be considered in future therapeutic approaches (743,780).

Patients who have HIV-associated HD experience a high incidence of severe, life-threatening opportunistic infections during and after chemotherapy, often in the terminal phase in which HD relapses (731,732,741,743,744,746,781). These infections include *P. carinii* pneumonia, Legionella pneumonia, cerebral toxoplasmosis, cryptococcal meningitis, cryptosporidiosis, and disseminated cytomegalovirus, candidiasis, and *M. avium complex* infections (730,731,740,744, 745). These severe opportunistic infections occur only rarely in conventional HD, in which bacterial infections predominate (732,782,783). The predilection for individuals with HIV-associated HD to develop serious opportunistic infections is related to the underlying HIV-induced immunodeficiency. Patients who have HIV-associated HD occasionally develop Kaposi's sarcoma, either during or after therapy (375,713,714,734,744,745). Rarely, an HIV-seropositive individual develops HD prior to (727), concurrent with (723), or after development of an AIDS-related NHL (725). Approximately one third of patients who have HIV-associated HD die as a direct result of tumor progression. The majority of patients die as a result of opportunistic infections, either alone or in conjunction with tumor progression, and a minority die as a result of severe cytopenias (389,732,740,741, 743,744,746). Investigators must study the underlying HIV-induced immunodeficiency that permits the development of these opportunistic infections if significant improvements in long-term survival are to be attained among patients who have HIV-associated HD.

Little is known about prognostic factors for survival in HIV-associated HD. A prior diagnosis of AIDS, pretreatment cytopenias, failure to attain complete remission, and CD4 T-cell counts lower than 250 per microliter have been found to be associated with a significantly shorter duration of survival (732,743,746). AIDS risk group, stage of disease, histologic subtype, bone marrow involvement, therapeutic regimen, and presence of opportunistic infections have not proven to be significant prognostic factors (732,746), but multivariate analysis of large numbers of uniformly treated patients has not been performed (781).

The incidence of HD may be increased in HIV-infected individuals. HIV-associated HD occurs more frequently among IDUs than among other AIDS risk groups and displays atypical clinical manifestations and aggressive biologic behavior that is distinct from that of conventional HD. These features include significantly higher frequencies of B symptoms, advanced stage disease, and bone marrow and other extranodal involvement at initial presentation; random, noncontiguous spread; absence of mediastinal disease; unfavorable histopathologic (mixed cellularity and lymphocytic depletion) subtypes; poor response to and enhanced hematologic toxicity from chemotherapy; and shortened durations of survival; often because of the development of severe opportunistic infections associated with the underlying HIV-induced immunodeficiency.

OTHER HEMATOPOIETIC NEOPLASMS

A variety of other hematopoietic neoplasms occurring in HIV-infected persons, some of whom have AIDS, have been reported. These include B-cell ALLs (784–794), plasma cell tumors (283,795–809), histologic low grade B-cell leukemias and NHLs (369,371,373,415,810–813), an array of T-cell neoplasms (375,473,814–831), angiocentric immunoproliferative lesions (832–834), and a spectrum of myeloproliferative disorders, including various subtypes of acute myeloid leukemia (AML) (835–850). The true incidence of these neoplasms in individuals at risk for AIDS is uncertain and may be underestimated because these cases are not reported to the CDC. Nonetheless, these neoplasms only appear to occur sporadically in these individuals, and there is no definitive epidemiologic evidence to suggest that their incidence has increased in parallel with the AIDS epidemic. Because the relationship of these hematologic neoplasms to HIV infection and AIDS is generally unclear, these neoplasms are not recognized as meeting the criteria for the diagnosis of AIDS in HIV-infected individuals by the CDC at the present time.

A notable exception should be made for B-cell ALL, however. A minimum of 15 cases of B-cell ALL occurring in persons at risk for AIDS have been described in the literature (784–793), and we have studied three additional cases that have not been reported. AIDS risk factors have included homosexuality (11), injecting drug use (3), heterosexual contact with an HIV-seropositive person (2), being the infant child of an HIV-seropositive mother (1), and unknown (1). Two patients fulfilled the current CDC criteria for AIDS, and four had the persistent generalized lymphadenopathy syndrome. The remaining 12 patients were HIV-seropositive only. All patients presented with involvement of the bone marrow and peripheral blood, without evidence of lymphomatous masses. In 16 patients, the lymphoblasts displayed the cytomorphologic features of the L3 ALL category of the French–American–British (FAB) classification (851), which is virtually identical to that of Burkitt's lymphoma: moderately abundant basophilic cytoplasm containing variable numbers of well-defined vacuoles staining with oil red O stain, and a round nucleus with one to four nucleoli. In one instance, the lymphoblasts displayed abundant, nonvacuolated, deeply basophilic cytoplasm and large, round nuclei with solitary, centrally prominent nucleoli (Fig. 28.60). In another instance, the lymphoblasts displayed the cytomorphologic features of L3 ALL but cytochemical, immunophenotypic, and cytogenetic features of both L3 ALL and M4 AML, indicative of a unique hybrid acute leukemia (793). Further investigation of several of these B-cell ALLs has demonstrated surface immunoglobulin expression, usually IgMκ, absence of CD21 (C3d-EBV receptors), and the presence of the chromosomal translocation t(8;14) associated with *MYC* oncogene rearrangement. Most of the patients have had a rapidly fatal course despite aggressive systemic chemotherapy.

The only neoplasms recognized by the CDC as satisfying criteria for AIDS are Kaposi's sarcoma, intermediate- and high-grade NHLs of B-cell or indeterminate phenotype, and invasive cervical carcinoma occurring in HIV-seropositive patients (62). Therefore, 16 of these 18 cases of B-cell ALL do not meet the current CDC criteria for AIDS, despite the following facts:

B-cell ALL occurs rarely in adults (785).

B-cell ALL nearly always displays the morphologic, immunologic, and molecular genetic features of Burkitt's lymphoma: FAB L3 morphology, monotypic surface immunoglobulin, and t(8;14), t(8;22), or t(2;8) chromosomal translocations associated with *MYC* oncogene rearrangement (785,851,852).

Burkitt's lymphoma is the most common NHL type occurring in AIDS (375).

Most of these patients have the hyperaggressive clinical

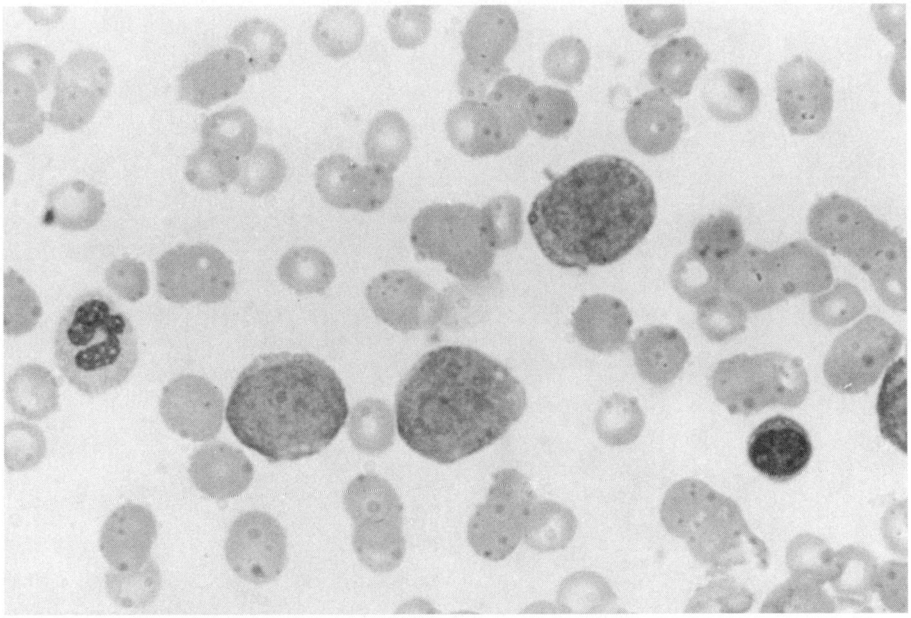

FIG. 28.60. Peripheral blood smear of AIDS-related B cell acute lymphoblastic leukemia. The patient presented in leukemic phase with extensive bone marrow replacement but without peripheral lymphadenopathy. The neoplastic cells are large, have a high nuclear:cytoplasmic ratio, and contain large, often centrally prominent nucleoli. Central nervous system involvement in this patient is illustrated in Fig. 28.25 (Wright stain, original magnification: 630× magnification).

course characteristically seen in AIDS-related lymphoid neoplasia.

For all intents and purposes, these patients have Burkitt's lymphoma in leukemic phase. For all these reasons, the development of B-cell ALL in these patients is most likely HIV-related and is not merely coincidental. We strongly believe that the current criteria for AIDS should be expanded to include the occurrence of B-cell ALL in an HIV-seropositive person.

A minimum of 21 cases of plasma cell neoplasia occurring in AIDS-risk persons have been described in the literature (283,795–809) (Fig. 28.61). All 21 patients were men who ranged in age from 22 to 65 years, with a median of 34 years. Most of them were severely immunosuppressed and had CD4:CD8 T-cell ratios of 1.0 or lower. AIDS risk factors were homosexuality (7), injecting drug use (6), transfused blood products (2), and unknown (6). All patients tested were HIV-seropositive. Only four patients fulfilled the CDC criteria for AIDS on the basis of severe opportunistic infections or Kaposi's sarcoma; the remaining patients had the AIDS-related complex, the persistent generalized lymphadenopathy syndrome, or otherwise asymptomatic HIV infection. The neoplasms included solitary and disseminated extramedullary plasmacytomas and secretory and nonsecretory myelomas associated with osteolytic bone disease and marrow plasmacytosis. Some extramedullary plasmacytomas arose in unusual anatomic sites including the skin (806), the oropharynx (800), and the penis (801). In two instances, myeloma involved the serous cavities and presented as massive peritoneal effusions (807), which is very rare in conventional multiple myeloma (853). Many of the patients exhibited elevated serum lactate dehydrogenase levels and, despite chemotherapy, experienced disease progression and died within a few months of presentation.

Unlike the case of B-cell ALL, it is difficult to prove that the occurrence of plasmacytomas and multiple myeloma in persons at risk for AIDS is related specifically to HIV infection and is not merely coincidental. Plasma cell malignancies, however, generally occur in the sixth decade and beyond; less than 2% of all patients who have conventional myeloma are younger than 40 years of age (854,855). The frequent development of multiple extramedullary plasmacytomas in individuals at risk for AIDS represents an unusual clinical course for conventional plasma cell neoplasia. HIV is capable of infecting B cells directly (856), and retroviral infection has been shown to promote the growth of murine plasmacytomas (857). Konrad and colleagues (805) reported an HIV-seropositive man with multiple myeloma whose IgGγ paraprotein specifically recognized the HIV p24 *gag* antigen. This plasma cell neoplasm may have developed at least in part because of an antigen-driven response to circulating p24 antigen, suggesting a direct pathogenetic role for HIV. Also, the EBV genome has been detected in several AIDS-associated myelomas (747,807,808), and clonal EBV populations have been demonstrable in some of these tumors (807), analogous to AIDS-related B-cell NHLs (477,480). These plasma cell neoplasms may have similar pathogeneses and fall within the spectrum of HIV-associated aggressive

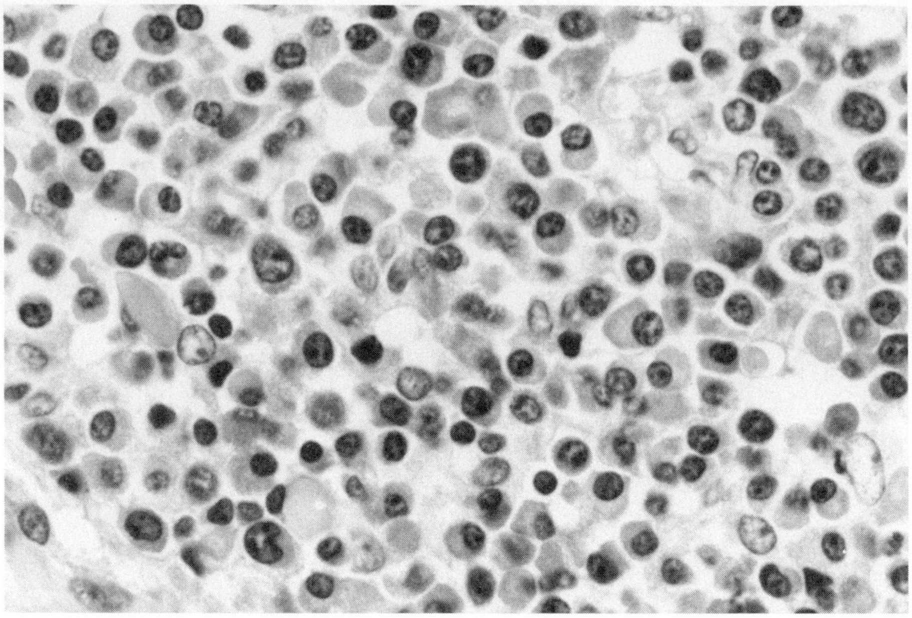

FIG. 28.61. AIDS-associated extramedullary plasmacytoma (hematoxylin and eosin stain, original magnification: 400× magnification).

B-cell neoplasia. The definition of AIDS eventually may be expanded to include plasma cell malignancies.

The sporadic occurrence of B-cell chronic lymphocytic leukemia and histologic low-grade B-cell NHLs, including small lymphocytic lymphoma, follicular center cell lymphoma, marginal zone (monocytoid B-cell) lymphoma, and mantle cell lymphoma, in MSM and IDUs has been reported (369–371,415,810–813). Some of these patients have been HIV-seronegative, and many of those who were HIV-infected lacked evidence of severe immune deficiency and AIDS-defining illnesses. Some of these patients even have enjoyed prolonged survival with no or minimal therapy, as would be expected in similar patients who are not HIV-infected (858). No evidence currently exists to suggest that these low-grade B-cell neoplasms are specifically associated with HIV infection or that their incidence has increased in parallel with the AIDS epidemic. It is likely that their occurrence in this patient population is merely coincidental, and that their pathogenesis is similar to that of comparable neoplasms occurring in the general population unassociated with HIV infection.

Several well-documented cases of precursor T-cell lymphoblastic lymphoma (815,819) and adult T-cell lymphoma/leukemia (816,820) and a minimum of 34 cases of cutaneous T-cell lymphoma (821–824,828,830,831) and peripheral T-cell lymphoma (817,818,823,827) occurring in HIV-infected persons have been described in the literature. Of the latter 34 cases, 21 were reported from a single institution, the University of California at San Francisco (831). Several cases of HIV-associated T cell–derived anaplastic large cell lymphoma have been reported (473,825,826,829). Other cases of purported HIV-associated T-cell lymphoma described in the literature (859–862) are poorly documented or unconvincing. Several cases of so-called lymphomatoid granulomatosis and lethal midline granuloma have been reported in persons at risk for AIDS (832–834). These cases appear to represent a heterogeneous group of neoplasms whose precise histopathologic classification and lineage derivation is unclear.

All 34 HIV-seropositive individuals who developed cutaneous or peripheral T-cell lymphoma were men. They ranged in age from 23 to 62 years. The mean age of the 20 University of California at San Francisco patients was 39 years and of the 13 literature cases was 42 years. AIDS risk factors were homosexuality (27), injecting drug use (2), and unknown or unstated (5) (817,818,821–824,827,828,830, 831). Kerschmann and colleagues (831) suggested that the individuals who have cutaneous presentations are divisible into two distinct clinical groups: those who have epidermatropic mycosis fungoides–like patches and plaques or Sezary syndrome–like exfoliative erythroderma, early HIV disease without AIDS, relative immunocompetence, and an indolent clinical course with a mean duration of survival longer than 3 years; and those who have nonepidermatropic large cell or immunoblastic lymphoma manifesting as papules or nodules, advanced HIV disease and often AIDS, significant immunosuppression, and a rapid clinical course, with a mean duration of survival of less than 7 months. The other literature reports generally support these findings. The epidermatropic mycosis fungoides—like cutaneous T-cell lymphomas are $CD30^-$ and lack EBV; a majority of the nonepidermatropic cutaneous T-cell lymphomas express CD30 and contain EBV. Many of the latter tumors might be considered anaplastic large cell lymphomas. Unlike in conventional cutaneous anaplastic large cell lymphoma (863), however, neither CD30 expression nor EBV content correlated with survival among these patients. Those HIV-infected individuals who have peripheral T-cell lymphoma generally possess advanced HIV disease, have severe immunosuppression and sometimes AIDS, often exhibit disseminated lymphoma at presentation, and experience a rapidly fatal course. The HIV-infected individuals who have anaplastic large cell lymphoma similarly have been severely immunosuppressed MSM or male IDUs in the third to fifth decades of life. They present with localized or extensive cutaneous disease, which sometimes is accompanied by disseminated lymph node and organ involvement. The clinical course has varied from sustained complete remission following chemotherapy to a rapidly fatal outcome because of disease progression or other AIDS-related illnesses (473,825, 826,829). T-cell subset antigen expression was not studied in the University of California at San Francisco cohort. Among six cutaneous T-cell lymphomas, six peripheral T-cell lymphomas, and two anaplastic large cell lymphomas analyzed, eight expressed the $CD4^+CD8^-$ (helper-inducer) phenotype, four expressed the $CD4^-CD8^+$ (suppressor-cytotoxic) phenotype, and two expressed the $CD4^-CD8^-$ phenotype (817,818,821–823,825,827–830). Some of these lesions exhibited clonal T-cell receptor β chain gene rearrangements.

Several cases of apparent T-cell chronic lymphocytic leukemia occurring in HIV-infected persons have been reported (283,375,814). In the three cases described by Knowles and associates (375), the lymphoid cells resembled small mature lymphocytes; expressed the mature peripheral suppressor-cytotoxic ($CD4^-CD8^+$) T-cell subset phenotype; lacked the azurophilic granule-rich basophilic cytoplasm characteristic of large granular lymphocytes and natural killer cells and their associated antigens CD16 and CD57, said to be characteristic of Tγ lymphoproliferative disease (864); and exhibited clonal T cell receptor β chain gene rearrangements (375). These findings are indicative of a clonal expansion of the mature $CD4^-CD8^+$ (suppressor-cytotoxic) T-cell subset. They detected a single specific HTLV-1 hybridizing band in one of these clonal T-cell proliferations (375), strongly suggesting clonal integration of the HTLV-1 genome. Harper and associates (814) also described an HIV-seropositive MSM who had AIDS-related complex and a comparable CD8 lymphocytosis possessing clonal integration of HTLV-1. The significance of a solitary report of $CD3^-$ Tγ lymphoproliferative disease occurring in an HIV-seropositive, HTLV-1 seronegative MSM following an acute viral illness (865) is not certain.

In addition to these T-cell malignancies, nonneoplastic CD8 lymphocytoses occurring in HIV-infected persons have been described (262,263,866,867). Itescu and colleagues have described "diffuse infiltrative CD8 lymphocytosis syndrome" associated with the HLA-DR5 haplotype (262,263). These patients are predominantly black men who characteristically have persistent peripheral blood CD8 lymphocytosis accompanied by clinically significant diffuse visceral CD8 infiltration, most commonly involving the salivary glands, lungs, and lymph nodes and sometimes the gastrointestinal tract, the nervous system, and other viscera. The most common clinical manifestations are bilateral salivary gland and lymph node enlargement, sicca symptoms, and lymphocytic interstitial pneumonitis leading to dyspnea (309). The patients have polyclonal hypergammaglobulinemia but usually lack the rheumatoid factors and anti-nuclear antibodies associated with Sjögren's syndrome. They generally have borderline normal or slightly subnormal CD4 T-cell counts, lack AIDS-defining illnesses, and do not appear to develop lymphoproliferative malignancies. A small number of African children displaying some or all of these clinical features has been reported as well (868).

Oksenhendler and colleagues (867) have described a clinical syndrome involving CD8 lymphocytosis associated with the HLA-DR3 haplotype. The patients are caucasian and have peripheral blood and bone marrow CD8 lymphocytosis, marked hypergammaglobulinemia, and massive pseudotumoral splenomegaly. The CD8 lymphocytes are activated suppressor T cells that exhibit the germline T-cell receptor gene configuration, consistent with the polyclonal expansion of a CD8 T-cell population aimed at suppressing viral replication. The association with specific haplotypes suggests that these clinical syndromes represent genetically determined distinct immune host responses to HIV. These systemic CD8 lymphocytoses should not be misinterpreted as T-cell malignancies.

Whether the occurrence of some or all of the various T-cell neoplasms reported in HIV-infected persons is directly related to HIV infection or is merely coincidental is unclear. Precursor T-cell lymphoblastic lymphomas and peripheral T-cell lymphomas, however, have been described in renal transplant recipients (869–873), another immunosuppressed patient population with an increased incidence of lymphoid neoplasia (407). It has been suggested that HIV itself may be a causal agent in the development of T-cell neoplasia, based on similarities between the transactivator genes in HIV, HTLV-1, and HTLV-2 (817). The transactivator gene product in HTLV-1 and HTLV-2 is believed to activate the expression of growth-promoting genes, which in turn may lead ultimately to the immortalization and malignant transformation of the infected cells (817). Southern blot hybridization studies have identified clonal integration of HIV provirus only in the neoplastic T cells of a single HIV-associated T-cell neoplasm (827), however; all the other T-cell neoplasms examined have been negative (375,815,817–819). HTLV-1, whose mode of transmission is similar to HIV, also has been suggested as a causal agent, and rare cases of adult T-cell lymphoma/leukemia occurring in individuals coinfected with HIV and HTLV-1 have been reported (816,820). We (375) and Harper and associates (814) described HIV-seropositive persons who had CD8 lymphocytosis with clonal integration of HTLV-1 in the CD8 T cells. HTLV-1 rarely may contribute to the development of clinically indolent, clonal $CD4^{-}CD8^{+}$ T-cell proliferations in HIV-infected patients depleted of CD4 T cells. These clonal CD8 proliferations could develop as a result of destruction of CD4 cells by HIV and the subsequent loss of control over a group of CD8 cells infected with HTLV-1 caused by the immunosuppression induced by HIV. Alternatively, prior infection with HTLV-1 and subsequent destruction of CD4 T cells may select for a CD8 T-cell population that is transformed more easily on subsequent exposure to HTLV-1 (814). Dual infection by HIV and HTLV-1 has been documented frequently in populations at risk for AIDS worldwide, especially in IDUs (874–877). None of the HIV-seropositive patients who developed T-cell lymphomas, however, has been discovered to have serum antibodies to HTLV-1, and Southern blot hybridization analyses have failed to find HTLV-1 in the majority of HIV-associated T-cell neoplasms (815,817–819,821–824,827,828,830,831). EBV has been suggested as a possible causative factor in HIV-associated T-cell neoplasia (823). Human T cells may be immortalized following transfection with EBV DNA (878). Furthermore, Harabuchi and associates (879) described five angiocentric immunoproliferative lesions containing EBV, and Jones and colleagues (880) described two peripheral T-cell lymphomas exhibiting clonal integration of EBV DNA. Some AIDS-associated T-cell lymphomas contain EBV (829,831), and EBV may contribute to the pathogenesis of T-cell neoplasms in HIV-infected individuals who are known to experience severe, massive, and continuous EBV infections. Additional studies, however, are needed to clarify the relationship between HIV infection and the development of T-cell neoplasia.

The occurrence of various myeloproliferative disorders in HIV-seropositive individuals also has been reported. AIDS risk factors for these individuals primarily have been homosexuality, injecting drug use, and transfusion of HIV-contaminated blood products. Only a few of these individuals meet the CDC criteria for AIDS. Myelodysplasia similar to that observed in the myelodysplastic or preleukemic syndromes has been described frequently in HIV-infected persons (881). AML arising in myelodysplastic syndrome (404), *de novo* AML (836,838–843,845–850), chronic myeloid leukemia (844), and agnogenic myeloid metaplasia (837) have been described. One individual developed NHL 4 months after chemotherapy-induced remission of AML (850). Among the 12 cases of AML reported in HIV-infected persons for which information is available, five were classified as FAB M2 (835,840–842,850), four as FAB M4 (acute myelomonocytic leukemia) (843,845,846), and three as FAB M5 (acute monocytic leukemia) (847–849).

The significance of the association between these myeloproliferative disorders and HIV infection is uncertain. Two patients who had transfusion-associated AIDS and AML were 58 and 62 years old (835). Nearly all the MSM and IDUs with myeloproliferative disorders, however, have been in the third and fourth decades of life. The incidence of myelodysplasia and AML in men younger than 45 years of age is low (882). It is possible that these disorders, rather than merely being coincidental, are a consequence of the severe T-cell immunodeficiency caused by HIV infection, either because of a failure of immune surveillance or because of defective T-cell control of hematopoiesis. The incidence of AML equals or exceeds that of ALL in at least two immunodeficiencies associated with chronic T-cell abnormalities, the Wiskott-Aldrich syndrome and severe combined immunodeficiency (883). HIV has been shown to infect the HL-60 promyelocytic cell line and other myelomonocytic cell lines expressing the CD4 antigen (884–886), bone marrow myeloid precursors in AIDS patients (887), and myeloid progenitor cells lacking CD4 (888). In one HIV-infected patient with AML, the circulating myelomonocytic leukemia cells were found to be infected productively by HIV (846). These observations suggest that HIV may play a direct, or at least an indirect, role in the malignant transformation of these cell populations. Additional studies, however, are necessary to explain the relationships among HIV infection, immunodeficiency, myelodysplasia, and leukemiagenesis.

SUMMARY AND CONCLUSIONS

Since AIDS was described initially in 1981, it has spread as a fatal epidemic among high-risk groups—MSM, IDUs, and recipients of HIV-infected blood products—and its incidence has increased steadily among the heterosexual contacts of HIV-infected persons and among children born to woman who have AIDS. The causal agent of AIDS is HIV-1. The main receptor for HIV on human cells is the CD4 molecule, which is expressed primarily by helper-inducer T cells and monocytes or macrophages. The HIV infection and subsequent cytopathic destruction of CD4 helper T cells results in their progressive depletion, progressively worsening immune deficiency, and eventually the collapse of the immune system. Most AIDS-defining conditions, especially opportunistic infections, occur if the level of CD4 T cells in an HIV-infected patient falls below 200 per microliter. For this reason, measurements of CD4 T cells have been used to guide the clinical and therapeutic management of HIV-infected persons in the United States. The progressive depletion of the CD4 T-cell population is reflected in the shifting cell populations and consequent changing histopathologic appearance of the lymph nodes of HIV-infected individuals in different clinical stages of the disease. Four distinct histopathologic patterns of HIV-related lymphadenopathy have been described; these are now commonly designated *florid follicular hyperplasia*, *mixed follicular hyperplasia and involution*, *follicular involution*, and *lymphocyte depletion*. The HIV-associated BLEL occurring in the salivary glands may be a localized manifestation of persistent generalized lymphadenopathy and usually exhibits florid follicular hyperplasia. HIV-related lymphadenopathy is in a state of dynamic evolution. Over time, the lymph nodes consistently and progressively transform histologically from florid follicular hyperplasia to mixed follicular hyperplasia and involution to follicular involution and, finally, to lymphocyte depletion. The temporal progression of HIV-related lymphadenopathy parallels the patient's deteriorating immune status and has clinical prognostic implications. In general, patients who have the histologic patterns of florid follicular hyperplasia or mixed follicular hyperplasia and involution appear to have the best prognosis because they do not seem to develop severe opportunistic infections or die from HIV-associated illnesses as long as they display these ''early'' histologies. HIV-infected patients develop the complications of AIDS only after the lymph node histology has progressed to either follicular involution or lymphocyte depletion. Although the development of severe opportunistic infections and length of survival are predicted by the histopathologic pattern of the lymph nodes, however, the development of Kaposi's sarcoma and malignant lymphoma are not. HIV-infected persons who have Kaposi's sarcoma or malignant lymphoma may exhibit any one of these four histopathologic patterns in their lymph nodes, including those lymph nodes actually involved by Kaposi's sarcoma or malignant lymphoma.

Various severe opportunistic infections, which represent AIDS-defining conditions, frequently are identified within the lymph nodes of HIV-infected patients who are severely immune-deficient. The most common infectious agents identified within the lymph nodes of these individuals are *M. avium complex*, *C. neoformans*, *H. capsulatum*, and cytomegalovirus. Opportunistic infections are identified in approximately 5% of lymph nodes from HIV-infected persons who have persistent generalized lymphadenopathy exhibiting florid follicular hyperplasia, but in up to 95% of AIDS patients at the time of autopsy. Bacillary angiomatosis is a rare pseudoneoplastic vasoproliferative disorder of infectious origin that occurs primarily in HIV-infected individuals. It is caused by *B. henselae* and *B. quintana*, cat-scratch disease bacillus-like organisms. Cutaneous disease is the most frequent clinical manifestation of bacillary angiomatosis, but this may be accompanied by mucosal, visceral, and lymph nodal involvement. Clumps and tangled masses of the causative organisms can be identified within the lesions with a Warthin-Starry stain. Bacillary angiomatosis must not be mistaken for Kaposi's sarcoma clinically or histopathologically. Appropriate antibiotic therapy leads to regression of the lesions and resolution of the disease.

Kaposi's sarcoma is the most common neoplasm occurring in association with HIV infection and is an AIDS-defining condition. Kaposi's sarcoma occurs most frequently in MSM and uncommonly in persons in other AIDS risk groups. AIDS-related Kaposi's sarcoma exhibits a variable clinical course ranging from an asymptomatic incidental finding to the explosive onset of widespread, rapidly progessive disease resulting in significant illness and even death. The lesions occur most commonly on the skin but can occur anywhere, particularly in the lungs and gastrointestinal tract. Lymph node involvement by AIDS-related Kaposi's sarcoma is also common and may occur in the absence of mucocutaneous disease. Kaposi's sarcoma often involves lymph nodes as small foci in or adjacent to the capsule, in the hilum, or occasionally in the perinodal adipose tissue. These lesions may be overlooked by an inexperienced observer. AIDS-related Kaposi's sarcoma is histopathologically indistinguishable from the other clinicoepidemiologic forms of the disease. The many special clinical, epidemiologic, and pathologic percularities of Kaposi's sarcoma have led to controversy concerning the cell of origin, nature, and cause of the disease. It is generally believed, however, that the spindle cells of Kaposi's sarcoma are of endothelial cell origin and that the disease has an infectious cause. A novel, transmissible B-cell lymphotropic herpesvirus designated *KSHV*, also known as human herpesvirus-8, is detectable in virtually all Kaposi's sarcoma lesions occurring in more than 90% of individuals who have any of the four clinicoepidemiologic forms of the disease. The development of Kaposi's sarcoma is probably a multistep process involving the interplay of the KSHV with impaired immune surveilance, immune stimulation, and multiple genetic environmental, behavioral, and other factors.

Malignant lymphoma is the second most common neoplasm occuring in association with HIV infection and AIDS. The CDC has adopted the occurrence of intermediate- or high-grade NHL of B-cell or indeterminate phenotype in an HIV-seropositive person as a criterion for the diagnosis of AIDS. NHLs occur in persons who belong to all AIDS risk groups worldwide, although the majority of the patients are MSM and male IDUs. The clinical and pathologic characteristics of the NHLs occurring in these various AIDS risk groups are similar, although primary oral and anorectal NHLs appear to preferentially occur in MSM. AIDS-related NHLs are divisible into three broad catagories according to their anatomic site of origin: those arising systemically (nodal or extranodal), those arising in the CNS, and those arising in the body cavities. Approximately 80% of all NHLs arise systemically. At initial presentation, approximately two thirds of patients who have systemic NHL already have widely disseminated disease, including a high frequency of extranodal involvement; the majority of the remaining patients have clinical stage IE disease but have large bulky tumor masses in these sites. The CNS and the gastrointestinal tract are the most common extranodal sites of primary and secondary involvement by NHL, respectively. AIDS-related NHLs, however, may arise or present at virtually any anatomic site, including, for example, the anorectal region and the heart. AIDS-related NHL should always be given diagnostic consideration in an individual at risk for AIDS who presents with a tumor mass, regardless of the site or mode of presentation, and the atypical presentation of diffuse, aggressive NHLs involving unusual extranodal sites should raise suspicion of HIV infection. Approximately 20% of all AIDS-related NHLs arise in the CNS; AIDS now represents the most common risk factor, by far, for the development of primary CNS lymphoma. The majority of these patients are profoundly immunocompromised young MSM with far-advanced HIV disease. Primary CNS lymphoma is often a secondary manifestation of AIDS in these patients. Less than 5% of all AIDS-related NHLs arise in the body cavities as lymphomatous effusions in the absence of a tumor mass. These so-called primary effusion lymphomas exhibit a unique constellation of clinical, morphologic, immunophenotypic, and molecular characteristics, including the presence of KSHV, and represent a distinct clinopathologic entity. Investigators also have described an apparently distinct subset of AIDS-related NHL designated *plasmablastic lymphoma* that preferentially occurs in the oral cavity, and a group of HIV-associated lymphoid proliferations of uncertain malignant potential referred to as *polymorphic lymphoproliferative disorders*.

The histopathologic distribution of NHLs occurring in HIV-infected persons differs from that of conventional NHLs occurring in the HIV-uninfected general population, and also from that of NHLs occurring in other immune-deficient states. Approximately 40% of AIDS-related NHLs are Burkitt's lymphomas, and the remainder are evenly divided between immunoblastic lymphomas and large cell lymphomas. Some patients exhibit transitional morphologic features. Each of these histopathologic categories of AIDS-related NHL exhibits distinctive clinical characteristics. The prognostic significance of the histopathologic category of AIDS-related NHL within the context of this immune deficiency remains unclear. The survival of patients who have AIDS-related NHLs appears to be most dependent on their levels of immune deficiency.

Generally speaking, the treatment of AIDS-related NHL is complicated by the fact that most patients have widely disseminated disease, including CNS and bone marrow involvement; have intermediate- and high-grade histologies; and have an underlying immune deficiency that causes them to tolerate chemotherapy poorly. Survival is frequently brief, and long-term remissions are uncommon. However, therapeutic trials employing low-dosage multiagent chemotherapy, in conjunction with antiretroviral therapy and hematopoietic growth factors, suggest that longer durations of survival may be achieved.

More than 95% of AIDS-related NHLs express B-cell immunophenotypes comparable to those expressed by B-cell NHLs of similar morphology occurring in the general population. Most of the remaining cases are primary effusion lymphomas, which characteristically often express indeterminate immunophenotypes. More than 95% of AIDS-related NHLs, including those displaying indeterminate immunophenotypes, exhibit clonal immunoglobulin gene rearrangements. Structural alterations involving several protooncogenes and tumor supressor genes occur nonrandomly in association with specific histopathologic categories of conventional NHL and are believed to play a role in their pathogenesis. Structural alterations of some of these genes—*MYC*, *BCL6*, *RAS*, and *P53*—as well as infection by EBV occur in AIDS-related NHLs as well. We detected *MYC* gene rearrangements, clonal EBV, *P53* gene mutations or deletions, *BCL6* gene rearrangements, and *RAS* gene mutations in 44%, 41%, 30%, 17%, and 6% of 64 AIDS-related systemic NHLs, respectively. These molecular genetic alterations do not appear to occur entirely randomly among the AIDS-related NHLs, however. They may vary among AIDS-related NHLs according to their histopathologic category and anatomic site of origin. We found that more than 80% of the Burkitt's lymphomas contain EBV and *MYC* gene rearrangements, and approximately one half contain *P53* gene mutations in the absence of *BCL6* gene rearrangements and *RAS* gene mutations. We found that the Burkitt's-like lymphomas exhibit a comparable constellation of genetic alterations, except that smaller proportions of patients have EBV infection, *CMYC* gene rearrangements, and *P53* gene mutations, and *BCL6* gene rearrangements occur in a small percentage of cases. Among the large cell lymphomas, we found that only very few patients have EBV, approximately one half have *MYC* gene rearrangements, a small percentage have *P53* gene mutations, and approximately 25% exhibit *BCL6* gene rearrangements. We found that the immunoblastic lymphomas exhibit a constellation of molecular genetic alterations that closely resemble those of the Burkitt's-like lymphomas. Although a comprehensive molecular genetic analysis of AIDS-related primary CNS lymphomas has not been performed, we know that they uniformly contain the EBV genome and lack *MYC* gene rearrangements, in contrast with AIDS-related systemic NHLs. The primary effusion lymphomas nearly always contain EBV and lack *MYC* gene rearrangements and also usually lack *BCL6* gene rearrangements, *RAS* gene mutations, and *P53* gene deletions or mutations.

AIDS-related NHLs are characterized by the accumulation of multiple distinct genetic lesions, which apparently accrue quickly. Diverse molecular genetic pathways may operate in AIDS lymphomagenesis.

More than 400 cases of HD occurring in HIV-infected persons, many collected through national AIDS registries, have been reported. These reports have not determined unequivocally whether HIV infection truly promotes the development of HD or merely modifies its course, and thus they have not fully clarified the relationship among HIV infection, AIDS, and HD. Although the incidence of HD apparently is not increased among MSM or individuals who have acquired HIV infection through heterosexual contact, it may be significantly increased among IDUs. Nonetheless, the occurrence of HD in an HIV-seropositve person has not been accepted by the CDC as an AIDS-defining condition. HD occurring in association with HIV infection displays distinctive clinical pathologic characteristics. The pathologic spectrum of HIV-associated HD, that is, a significant increase in the proportion of the unfavorable histologic subtypes (mixed cellularity and lymphocytic depletion), is similar to that of underdeveloped countries and patients of lower socioeconomic status in the United States. The lesions of HIV-associated and non–HIV-associated HD share similar immunophenotypic and genotypic characteristics, although the lesions of HIV-associated HD contain diminished numbers of CD4 T cells, and the Reed-Sternberg cells of HIV-associated HD of all histologic subtypes more frequently contain EBV. HIV-infected individuals belonging to any AIDS risk group who develop HD display a distinct constellation of clinical features that contrast sharply with those of conventional HD. These features include a significantly higher frequency of B symptoms, a higher propensity for advanced stage (III or IV) disease, and bone marrow and other extranodal involvement at initial presentation; random, noncontiguous spread of the diseae; a high incidence of the peripheral form of the disease (absent mediastinal disease); an atypical and particularly aggressive clinical course; poor response to and enhanced hematologic toxicity from chemotherapy; and shortened duration of survival, often because of the development of severe opportunistic infections associated with the underlying HIV-induced immune deficiency.

A variety of other neoplasms occurring in HIV-infected persons, some of whom have AIDS, have been reported. These include B-cell ALL, plasmacytomas and multiple myeloma, histologic low-grade NHLs and lymphoid leukemias, an array of T-cell neoplasms, and a spectrum of subtypes of AML. The cases of B-cell ALL essentially represent Burkitt's lymphoma in leukemic phase; their development is most likely HIV-related and not merely coincidental. The other neoplasms apparently only occur sporadically in HIV-seropositive individuals, and there is no epidemiologic evidence to suggest that their incidence has increased in parallel with the AIDS epidemic. It is likely, for example, that the occurrence of low-grade NHLs and lymphoid leukemias in this patient population is merely coincidental. The CDC does not recognize the occurrence of any of these neoplasms in HIV-seropositive individuals as an AIDS-defining condition. Their relationship to HIV infection and the development of AIDS remains to be determined.

The spread of HIV infection and the consequent increase in the number of patients with AIDS worldwide ensures an increase in the overall occurrence of AIDS-related pathology and the likelihood that pathologists, hematologists, oncologists, and other physicians will come into frequent contact with patients who have HIV-related illnesses.

ACKNOWLEDGMENTS

The authors thank Drs. Ethel Cesarman, Yuan Chang, Riccardo Dalla-Favera, Giorgio Inghirami, Patrick Moore, Roland Nador, Pier-Giuseppe Pelicci, Bruce Raphael, and Milayna Subar for their collaborative participation in portions of the studies summarized here, and Al Lamme and Scientific Photographic Services, Edgewater, New Jersey, for the excellent photomicrographs and figures.

REFERENCES

1. Centers for Disease Control. Pneumocystis pneumonia: Los Angeles. *MMWR* 1981;30:250–252.
2. Centers for Disease Control. Kaposi's sarcoma and Pneumocystis pneumonia among homosexual men: New York City and California. *MMWR* 1981;30:305–308.
3. Gottlieb MS, Schroff R, Schanker HM, et al. Pneumocystis carinii pneumonia and mucosal candidiasis in previously healthy homosexual men: Evidence of a new acquired cellular immunodeficiency. *N Engl J Med* 1981;305:1425–1431.
4. Centers for Disease Control Task Force on Kaposi's Sarcoma and Opportunistic Infections. Epidemiologic aspects of the current outbreak of Kaposi's sarcoma and opportunistic infections. *N Engl J Med* 1982;306:248–252.
5. Centers for Disease Control. *HIV AIDS surveillance report*. 1996;8: 1–39.
6. Centers for Disease Control. Update: trends in AIDS Incidence, Deaths, and Prevalence. United States, 1996. *MMWR* 1996;46: 166–172.
7. Blum S, Singh TP, Gibbons J, et al. Trends in survival among persons with acquired immunodeficiency syndrome in New York City: the experience of the first decade of the epidemic. *Am J Epidemiol* 1994; 139:351–361.
8. Barre-Sinoussi F, Chermann JC, Rey F, et al. Isolation of a T lymphotrophic retrovirus from a patient at risk for acquired immune deficiency syndrome (AIDS). *Science* 1983;220:868–871.
9. Gallo RC, Salahuddin SZ, Popovic M, et al. Frequent detection and isolation of cytopathic retroviruses (HTLV-III) from patients with AIDS and at risk for AIDS. *Science* 1984;224:500–503.
10. DeCock KM, Adjorlolo G, Ekpini E, et al. Epidemiology and transmission of HIV-2: why there is no HIV-2 pandemic. *JAMA* 1993; 270:2083–2086.
11. Friedland GH, Klein RS. Transmission of the human immunodeficiency virus. *N Engl J Med* 1987;317:1125–1135.
12. Curran JW, Jaffe HW, Hardy AM, et al. Epidemiology of HIV infection and AIDS in the United States. *Science* 1988;239:610–616.
13. Downs AM, Heisterkamp SH, Brunet JB, et al. Reconstruction and prediction of the HIV/AIDS epidemic among adults in the European Union and in the low prevalence countries of central and eastern Europe. *AIDS* 1997;11:649–662.
14. Hamers FF, Batter V, Downs AM, et al. The HIV epidemic associated with injecting drug use in Europe: geographic and time trends. *AIDS* 1997;11:1365–1374.
15. Rogers MF, Caldwell MB, Gwinn ML, et al. Epidemiology of pediatric human immunodeficiency virus infection in the United States. *Acta Paediatr Suppl* 1994;400:5–7.
16. Stoneburner RL, Sato P, Burton A, Mertens T. The global HIV pandemic. *Acta Paediatr Suppl* 1994;400:1–4.
17. Mertens E, Low-Beer D. HIV and AIDS: where is the epidemic going? *Bull World Health Organ* 1996;74:121–129.
18. Levy JA. *HIV and the pathogenesis of AIDS*, 2nd edition. Washington, DC: ASM Press, 1998.
19. Dalgleish AG, Beverley PCL, Clapham PR, et al. The CD4 (T4) antigen is an essential component of the receptor for the AIDS retrovirus. *Nature* 1984;312:763–767.
20. Klatzmann D, Champagne E, Chamaret S, et al. T-lymphocyte T4 molecule behaves as the receptor for human retrovirus LAV. *Nature* 1984;312:767–768.
21. Robey WG, Safai B, Oroszlan S, et al. Characterization of envelope and core structural gene products of HTLV-III with sera from AIDS patients. *Science* 1985;228:593–595.
22. Fauci AS. The human immunodeficiency virus: infectivity and mechanisms of pathogenesis. *Science* 1988;239:617–622.
23. Greene WC. The molecular biology of human immunodeficiency virus type 1 infection. *N Engl J Med* 1991;324:308–317.
24. Goedert JJ, Biggar RJ, Melbye M, et al. Effect of T4 count and cofactors on the incidence of AIDS in homosexual men infected with human immunodeficiency virus. *JAMA* 1987;257:331–334.
25. Nicholson JKA, Spira TJ, Aloisio CH, et al. Serial determinations of HIV-1 titers in HIV-infected homosexual men: association of rising titers with CD4 T cell depletion and progression to AIDS. *AIDS Res Hum Retroviruses* 1989;5:205–215.
26. Lang W, Perkins H, Anderson RE, et al. Patterns of T lymphocyte changes with human immunodeficiency virus infection: from seroconversion to the development of AIDS. *J Acquir Immune Defic Syndr* 1989;2:63–69.
27. Taylor JM, Fahey JL, Detels R, et al. CD4 percentage, CD4 numbers,

and CD4:CD8 ratio in HIV infection: which to choose and how to use. *J Acquir Immune Defic Syndr* 1989;2:114–124.
28. Masur H, Ognibene FP, Yarchoan R, et al. CD4 counts as predictors of opportunistic pneumonias in human virus (HIV) infection. *Ann Intern Med* 1989;111:223–231.
29. Fahey JL, Taylor JMG, Detels R, et al. The prognostic value of cellular and serologic markers in infection with human immunodeficiency virus type 1. *N Engl J Med* 1990;322:166–172.
30. Fernandez-Cruz E, Desco M, Garcia Montes M, et al. Immunological and serological markers predictive of progression to AIDS in a cohort of HIV-infected drug users. *AIDS* 1990;4:987–994.
31. National Institutes of Health. State-of-the-art conference on azidothymidine therapy for early HIV infection. *Am J Med* 1990;89:335–344.
32. Crowe S, Carlin JB, Steward KI, et al. Predictive value of CD4 lymphocyte numbers for the development of opportunistic infections and malignancies in HIV-infected persons. *J Acquir Immune Defic Syndr* 1991;4:770–776.
33. Pluda JM, Yarchoan R, Broder S. The occurrence of opportunistic non-Hodgkin's lymphomas in the setting of infection with the human immunodeficiency virus. *Ann Oncol* 1991;2[Suppl 2]: S191–S200.
34. Schwartlander B, Horsburgh Jr CR, Hamouda O, et al. Changes in the spectrum of AIDS-defining conditions and decrease in CD4 + lymphocyte counts at AIDS manifestation in Germany from 1986 to 1991. *AIDS* 1992;6:413–420.
35. Katz MH, Hessol NA, Buchbinder SP, et al. Temporal trends of opportunistic infections and malignancies in homosexual men with AIDS. *J Infect Dis* 1994;170:198–202.
36. Hoover DR, Rinaldo C, He Y, et al. Long-term survival without clinical AIDS after CD4+ cell counts fall below 200×10^6/l. *AIDS* 1995; 9:145–152.
37. Fischl MA, Richman DD, Grieco MH, et al. The efficacy of azidothymidine (AZT) in the treatment of patients with AIDS and AIDS-related complex: a double-blind, placebo-controlled trial. *N Engl J Med* 1987;317:185–191.
38. Graham NM, Zeger SL, Park LP, et al. Effect of zidovudine and Pneumocystis carinii pneumonia prophylaxis on progression of HIV-1 infection to AIDS: the Multicenter AIDS Cohort Study. *Lancet* 1991;338:265–269.
39. Moore RD, Keruly J, Richman DD, et al, the Zidovudine Epidemiology Study Group. Natural history of advanced HIV disease in patients treated with zidovudine. *AIDS* 1992;6:671–677.
40. Hoover DR. The effects of long term zidovudine therapy and Pneumocystis carinii prophylaxis on HIV disease: a review of the literature. *Drugs* 1995;49:20–36.
41. Jones JL, Hanson DL, Chu SY, et al. Toxoplasmic encephalitis in HIV-infected persons: risk factors and trends. *AIDS* 1996;10: 1393–1399.
42. Delta Coordinating Committee: Delta: a randomised double-blind controlled trial comparing combinations of zidovudine plus didanosine or zalcitabine with zidovudine alone in HIV-infected individuals. *Lancet* 1996;348:283–291.
43. Collier AC, Coombs RW, Schoenfeld DA, et al, for the AIDS Clinical Trials Group. Treatment of human immunodeficiency virus infection with saquinavir, zidovudine, and zalcitabine. *N Engl J Med* 1996;334: 1011–1017.
44. Hammer SM, Katzenstein DA, Hughes MD, et al, for the AIDS Clinical Trials Group Study 175 Study Team. A trial comparing nucleoside monotherapy with combination therapy in HIV-infected adults with CD4 cell counts from 200 to 500 per cubic millimeter. *N Engl J Med* 1996;335:1081–1090.
45. Gullick R, Mellors J, Havlir D, et al. Potent and sustained antiretroviral activity of indinavir (IDV) in combination with zidovudine (ZDV) and lamivudine (3TC). Abstract LB-7. Presented at the Third Conference on Retroviruses and Opportunistic Infections, Washington, DC, January 1996.
46. Brodt HR, Kamps BS, Gute P, et al. Changing incidence of AIDS-defining illnesses in the era of antiretroviral combination therapy. *AIDS* 1997;11:1731–1738.
47. Staszewski S, Hill AM, Bartlett J, et al. Reductions in HIV-1 disease progression for zidovudine/lamivudine relative to control treatments: a meta-analysis of controlled trials. *AIDS* 1997;11:477–483.
48. UK Register of HIV Seroconverters Steering Committee. The AIDS incubation period in the UK estimated from a national register of HIV seroconverters. *AIDS* 1998;12:659–667.
49. Bailey NTJ. A revised assessment of the HIV-AIDS incubation period, assuming a very short early period of high infectivity and using only San Francisco public health data on prevalence and incidence. *Stat Med* 1997;16:2447–2458.
50. Haverkos HW, Gotlieb MS, Killen JY, et al. Classification of HTLV-III/LAV-related diseases. *J Infect Dis* 1985;152:1095.
51. Kaplan MH, Pahwa SG, Popovic M, et al. A classification of HTLV-III infection based on 75 cases seen in a suburban community. *Cancer Res* 1985;45[Suppl]:4655S–4658S.
52. Redfield RR, Wright DC, Tramont EC. The Walter Reed staging classification for HTLV-III/LAV infection. *N Engl J Med* 1986;314: 131–132.
53. Centers for Disease Control. Classification system for human T-lymphotropic virus type III/lymphadenopathy-associated virus infections. *MMWR* 1986;35:334–339.
54. Zolla-Pazner S, DesJarlais DC, Friedman SR, et al. Nonrandom development of immunologic abnormalities after infection with human immunodeficiency virus: implications for immunologic classification of the disease. *Proc Natl Acad Sci USA* 1987;84:5404–5408.
55. Justice AC, Feinstein AR, Wells CK. A new prognostic staging system for the acquired immunodeficiency syndrome. *N Engl J Med* 1989; 320:1388–1393.
56. WHO. Interim proposal for a WHO staging system for HIV infection and diseases. *Weekly Epidemiol Record* 1990;65:221–224.
57. Royce RA, Luckmann RS, Fusaro RE, et al. The natural history of HIV-1 infection: staging classifications of disease. *AIDS* 1991;5: 355–364.
58. Centers for Disease Control. Update on acquired immune deficiency syndrome (AIDS): United States. *MMWR* 1982;31:507–508, 513–514.
59. Centers for Disease Control: Recommendations. *Eur J Cancer Clin Oncol* 1984;20:169–173.
60. Centers for Disease Control. Revision of the case definition of acquired immunodeficiency syndrome for national reporting: United States. *MMWR* 1985;34:373–375.
61. Centers for Disease Control. Revision of the CDC surveillance case definition for acquired immunodeficiency syndrome. *MMWR* 1987; 36[Suppl]:1S–15S.
62. Centers for Disease Control. 1993 revised classification system for HIV infection and expanded surveillance case definition for AIDS among adolescents and adults. *MMWR* 1992;41:1–19.
63. Ho DD, Sarngadharan MG, Resnick L, et al. Primary human T-lymphotropic virus type III infection. *Ann Intern Med* 1985;103:880–883.
64. Tindall B, Cooper DA. Primary HIV infection: host responses and intervention strategies. *AIDS* 1991;5:1–14.
65. Ancelle-Park RA. European AIDS definition. *Lancet* 1992;339:671.
66. Ancelle-Park RA. Expanded European AIDS case definition. *Lancet* 1993;341:441.
67. Ancelle-Park RA, Alix J, Downs AM, et al and National Coordinators for AIDS Surveillance in 38 European Countries. Impact of 1993 revision of adult/adolescent AIDS surveillance case-definition for Europe. *Lancet* 1995;345:789–790.
68. Centers for Disease Control. Unexplained immunodeficiency and opportunistic infection in infants: New York, New Jersey, California. *MMWR* 1982;31:665–667.
69. Centers for Disease Control. Classification system for human immunodeficiency virus (HIV) infection in children under 13 years of age. *MMWR* 1987;36:225–229, 235.
70. Centers for Disease Control. 1994 revised classification system for human immunodeficiency virus infection in children less than 13 years of age. *MMWR* 1994;43:1–10.
71. Simpson BJ, Andiman WA. Difficulties in assigning human immunodeficiency virus-1 infection and seroreversion status in a cohort of HIV-exposed children using serologic criteria established by the CDC and Prevention. *Pediatrics* 1994;93:840–842.
72. Rogers MF, Ou C-Y, Rayfield M, et al. Use of the polymerase chain reaction for early detection of the proviral sequences of human immunodeficiency virus in infants born to seropositive mothers. *N Engl J Med* 1989;320:1649–1654.
73. Krivine A, Firtion G, Cao L, et al. HIV replication during the first weeks of life. *Lancet* 1992;339:1187–1189.
74. Burgard M, Mayaux MJ, Blanche S, et al. The use of viral culture and p24 antigen testing to diagnose human immunodeficiency virus infection in neonates. *N Engl J Med* 1992;327:1192–1197.

75. Report of a consensus workshop, Siena, Italy, January 17–18, 1992: early diagnosis of HIV infection in infants. *J Acquir Immune Defic Syndr* 1992;5:1169–1178.
76. Rogers M, Ou C, Kilbourne B, et al. Advances and problems in the diagnosis of human immunodeficiency virus infection in infants. *Pediatr Infect Dis J* 1991;10:523–531.
77. Erkeller-Yuksel FM, Deneys V, Yukeel B, et al. Age-related changes in human blood lymphocyte sub-populations. *J Pediatr* 1992;120: 216–222.
78. Denny T, Yogev R, Gelman R, et al. Lymphocyte subsets in healthy children during the first 5 years of life. *JAMA* 1992;267:1484–1488.
79. McKinney RE, Wilfert CM. Lymphocyte subsets in children younger than 2 years old: normal values in a population at risk for human immunodeficiency virus infection and diagnostic and prognostic application to infected children. *Pediatr Infect Dis J* 1992;11:639–644.
80. The European Collaborative Study. Age-related standards for T-lymphocyte subsets based on uninfected children born to human immunodeficiency virus-1-infected women. *Pediatr Infect Dis J* 1992;11: 1018–1026.
81. Waecker NJ, Ascher DP, Robb ML, et al. Age adjusted CD4+ lymphocyte parameters in HIV at risk uninfected children. *Clin Infect Dis* 1993;17:123–126.
82. Leibovitz E, Rigaud M, Pollack H, et al. Pneumocystis carinii pneumonia in infants infected with the human immunodeficiency virus with more than 450 CD4 T lymphocytes per cubic millimeter. *N Engl J Med* 1990;323:531–533.
83. Connor E, Bagarazzi M, McSherry G, et al. Clinical and laboratory correlates of Pneumocystis carinii pneumonia in children infected with HIV. *JAMA* 1991;265:1693–1697.
84. Kovacs A, Frederick T, Church J, et al. CD4 T-lymphocyte counts and Pneumocystis carinii pneumonia in pediatric HIV infection. *JAMA* 1991;265:1698–1703.
85. de Martino M, Tovo PA, Galli L, et al. Prognostic significance of immunologic changes in 675 infants perinatally exposed to human immunodeficiency virus. *J Pediatr* 1991; 119:702–709.
86. Butler KM, Husson RN, Lewis LL, et al. CD4 status and p24 antigenemia: are they useful predictors of survival in HIV-infected children receiving antiretroviral therapy. *Am J Dis Child* 1992;146:932–936.
87. Blanche S, Tardieu M, Dullege AM, et al. Longitudinal study of 94 symptomatic infants with perinatally acquired human immunodeficiency virus infection. *Am J Dis Child* 1990;144:1210–1215.
88. Tovo PA, deMartino M, Gabiano C, et al. Prognostic factors and survival in children with perinatal HIV-1 infection. *Lancet* 1992;339: 1249–1253.
89. Centers for Disease Control. Persistent, generalized lymphadenopathy among homosexual males. *MMWR* 1982;31:249–251.
90. Metroka CE, Cunningham-Rundles S, Pollack MS, et al. Generalized lymphadenopathy in homosexual men. *Ann Intern Med* 1983;99: 585–591.
91. Ioachim HL, Lerner CW, Tapper M. Lympadenopathies in homosexual men: relationships with the acquired immune deficiency syndrome. *JAMA* 1983;250:1306–1309.
92. Mathur-Wagh U, Enlow RW, Spigland I, et al. Longitudinal study of persistent generalised lymphadenopathy in homosexual men: relation to acquired immunodeficiency syndrome. *Lancet* 1984;i:1033–1038.
93. Fishbein DB, Kaplan JE, Spira TJ, et al. Unexplained lymphadenopathy in homosexual men: a longitudinal study. *JAMA* 1985;254: 930–935.
94. Diebold J, Marche C, Audouin J, et al. Lymph node modification in patients with the acquired immunodeficiency syndrome (AIDS) or with AIDS related complex (ARC): a histological, immunohistopathological and ultrastructural study of 45 cases. *Pathol Res Pract* 1985; 180:590–611.
95. Said JW. AIDS-related lymphadenopathies. *Semin Diagn Pathol* 1988;5:365–375.
96. Brynes RK, Chan WC, Spira TJ, et al. Value of lymph node biopsy in unexplained lymphadenopathy in homosexual men. *JAMA* 1983; 250: 1313–1317.
97. Marche C, Neguesse Y, Bouton C, et al. Histopathologic studies of lymphadenopathy in AIDS: tentative classification. Preliminary report. *Antibiot Chemother* 1984;32:76–86.
98. Meyer PR, Yanagihara ET, Parker JW, et al. A distinctive follicular hyperplasia in the acquired immune deficiency syndrome (AIDS) and the AIDS related complex: a prelymphomatous state for B cell lymphomas? *Hematol Oncol* 1984;2:319–347.
99. Burns BF, Wood GS, Dorfman RF. The varied histopathology of lymphadenopathy in the homosexual male. *Am J Surg Pathol* 1985; 9:287–297.
100. Baroni CD, Pezzella F, Stoppacciaro A, et al. Systemic lymphadenopathy (LAS) in intravenous drug abusers: histology, immunohistochemistry and electron microscopy. Pathogenic correlations. *Histopathology* 1985;9:1275–1293.
101. Raphael M, Pouletty P, Cavaille-Coll M, et al. Lymphadenopathy in patients at risk for acquired immunodeficiency syndrome: histopathology and histochemistry. *Arch Pathol Lab Med* 1985;109:128–132.
102. Ewing EP, Chandler FW, Spira TJ, et al. Primary lymph node pathology in AIDS and AIDS-related lymphadenopathy. *Arch Pathol Lab Med* 1985;109:977–981.
103. Turner RR, Levine AM, Gill PS, et al. Progressive histopatholgic abnormalities in the persistent generalized lymphadenopathy syndrome. *Am J Surg Pathol* 1987;11:625–632.
104. Biberfeld P, Ost A, Porwit A, et al. Histopathology and immunohistology of HTLV-III/LAV related lymphadenopathy and AIDS. *Acta Pathol Microbiol Immunol Scand Sect A* 1987;95:47–65.
105. Pallesen G, Gerstoft J, Mathiesen L. Stages in LAV/HTLV-III lymphadenitis: I. Histological and immunohistological classification. *Scand J Immunol* 1987;25:83–91.
106. Pileri S, Rivano MT, Raise E, et al. The value of lymph node biopsy in patients with the acquired immunodeficiency syndrome (AIDS) and the AIDS-related complex (ARC): a morphological and immunohistochemical study of 90 cases. *Histopathology* 1986;10:1107–1129.
107. Chadburn A, Metroka C, Mouradian J. Progressive lymph node histology and its prognostic value in patients with acquired immunodeficiency syndrome and AIDS-related complex. *Hum Pathol* 1989;20: 579–587.
108. Ioachim HL, Cronin W, Roy M, et al. Persistent lymphadenopathies in people at high risk for HIV-infection: clinicopathologic correlations and long-term follow-up in 79 cases. *Am J Clin Pathol* 1990;93: 208–218.
109. Fernandez R, Mouradian J, Metroka C, et al. The prognostic value of histopathology in persistent generalized lymphadenopathy in homosexual men. *N Engl J Med* 1983;309:185–186.
110. Chan WC, Brynes RK, Spira TJ, et al. Lymphocyte subsets in lymph nodes of homosexual men with generalized unexplained lymphadenopathy: correlation with morphology and blood changes. *Arch Pathol Lab Med* 1985;109:133–137.
111. Schuurman HJ, Kluin PM, Meijling FHJG, et al. Lymphocyte status of lymph node and blood in acquired immunodeficiency syndrome (AIDS) and AIDS-related complex disease. *J Pathol* 1985;147: 269–280.
112. Gerstoft J, Pallesen G, Mathiesen L, et al. Stages in LAV/HTLV-III lymphadenitis: II. Correlation with clinical and immunological findings. *Scand J Immunol* 1987;25:93–99.
113. Wood GS, Garcia CF, Dorfman RF, et al. The immunohistology of follicle lysis in lymph node biopsies from homosexual men. *Blood* 1985;66:1092–1097.
114. Sohn CC, Sheibani K, Winberg CD, et al. Monocytoid B lymphocytes: their relation to the patterns of the acquired immunodeficiency syndrome (AIDS) and AIDS-related lymphadenopathy. *Hum Pathol* 1985;16:979–985.
115. Butler JJ, Osborne BM. Lymph node enlargement in patients with unsuspected human immunodeficiency virus infections. *Hum Pathol* 1988;19:849–854.
116. Carbone A, Manconi R, Poletti A. Lymph node immunohistology in intravenous drug abusers with persistent generalized lymphadenopathy. *Arch Pathol Lab Med* 1985;109:1007–1012.
117. Stanley MW, Frizzera G. Diagnostic specificity of histologic features in lymph node biopsy specimens from patients at risk for the acquired immunodeficiency syndrome. *Hum Pathol* 1986;17:1231–1239.
118. O'Murchadha MT, Wolf BC, Neiman RS. The histologic features of hyperplastic lymphadenopathy in AIDS-related complex are nonspecific. *Am J Surg Pathol* 1987;11:94–99.
119. Miettinen M. Histological differential diagnosis between lymph node toxoplasmosis and other benign lymph node hyperplasias. *Histopathology* 1981;5:205–216.
120. Frizzera G, Moran EM, Rappaport H. Angio-immunoblastic lymphadenopathy: diagnosis and clinical course. *Am J Med* 1975;59:803–818.

121. Frizzera G, Massarelli G, Banks PM, et al. A systemic lymphoproliferative disorder with morphologic features of Castleman's disease: pathologic findings in 15 patients. *Am J Surg Pathol* 1983;7:211–231.
122. Frizzera G, Peterson BA, Bayrd ED, Goldman A. A systemic lymphoproliferative disorder with morphologic features of Castleman's disease: clinical findings and clinicopathologic correlations in 15 patients. *J Clin Oncol* 1985;3:1202–1216.
123. Weisenburger DD, Nathwani BN, Winberg CD, et al. Multicentric angiofollicular lymph node hyperplasia: a clinicopathologic study of 16 cases. *Hum Pathol* 1985;16:162–172.
124. Tirelli U, Vaccher E, Carbone A, et al. Persistent generalized lymphadenopathy: clinical characteristics of a lymphadenopathy syndrome in intravenous drug abusers. *AIDS Res* 1986;2:227–230.
125. Finkbeiner WE, Egbert BM, Groundwater JR, et al. Kaposi's sarcoma in young homosexual men: a histopathologic study with particular reference to lymph node involvement. *Arch Pathol Lab Med* 1982; 106:261–264.
126. Perlow LS, Taff ML, Orsini JM, et al. Kaposi's sarcoma in a young homosexual man: association with angiofollicular lymphoid hyperplasia and a malignant lymphoproliferative disorder. *Arch Pathol Lab Med* 1983;107:510–513.
127. Blumenfeld W, Beckstead JH. Angioimmunoblastic lymphadenopathy with dysproteinemia in homosexual men with acquired immune deficiency syndrome. *Arch Pathol Lab Med* 1983;107:567–569.
128. Harris NL. Hypervascular follicular hyperplasia and Kaposi's sarcoma in patients at risk for AIDS. *N Engl J Med* 1984;310:462–463.
129. Lachant NA, Sun NCJ, Leong LA, et al. Multicentric angiofollicular lymph node hyperplasia (Castleman's disease) followed by Kaposi's sarcoma in two homosexual males with the acquired immunodeficiency syndrome (AIDS). *Am J Clin Pathol* 1985;83:27–33.
130. Lowenthal DA, Filippa DA, Richardson ME, et al. Generalized lymphadenopathy with morphologic features of Castleman's disease in an HIV-positive man. *Cancer* 1987;60:2454–2458.
131. van Den Oord JJ, de Wolf-Peeters C, Tricot G, et al. Distribution of lymphocyte subsets in a case of angiofollicular lymph node hyperplasia. *Am J Clin Pathol* 1984;82:491–495.
132. Carbone A, Manconi R, Volpe R, et al. Immunohistochemical, enzyme histochemical, and immunologic features of giant lymph node hyperplasia of the hyaline-vascular type. *Cancer* 1986;58:908–916.
133. Wood GS, Burns BF, Dorfman RF, et al. Fatal post-transfusion acquired immunodeficiency in a heterosexual man: quantitative lymph node immunopathology. *Hum Pathol* 1988;19:236–238.
134. Davis JM, Chadburn A, Mouradian JA. Lymph node biopsy in patients with human immunodeficiency virus infections. *Arch Surg* 1988;123: 1349–1352.
135. Dickson D, Ben-Ezra JM, Reed J, et al. Multicentric giant lymph node hyperplasia, Kaposi's sarcoma, and lymphoma. *Arch Pathol Lab Med* 1985;109:1013–1018.
136. Soulier J, Grollet L, Oksenhendler E, et al. Kaposi's sarcoma-associated herpesvirus-like DNA sequences in multicentric Castleman's disease. *Blood* 1995;86:1276–1280.
137. Gessain A, Sudaka A, Briere J. Kaposi's sarcoma-associated herpes-like virus (human herpesvirus type 8) DNA sequences in multicentric Castleman's disease: is there any relevant association in non-human immunodeficiency virus-infected patients? *Blood* 1996;87:414–416.
138. Chadburn A, Cesarman E, Nador RG, et al. Kaposi's sarcoma-associated herpesvirus sequences in benign lymphoid proliferations not associated with human immunodeficiency virus. *Cancer* 1997;80: 788–797.
139. Oksenhendler E, Duarte M, Soulier J, et al. Multicentric Castleman's disease in HIV infection: a clinical and pathological study of 20 patients. *AIDS* 1996;10:61–67.
140. Chadburn A, Nador R, Cesarman E, et al. Kaposi's sarcoma-associated herpesvirus (KSHV) infection in HIV-related lymphadenopathy (HIV-LAP). *Lab Invest* 1997;76[Suppl]:121A.
141. Ambros RA, Lee EY, Sharer LR, et al. The acquired immunodeficiency syndrome in intravenous drug abusers and patients with a sexual risk: clinical and postmortem comparisons. *Hum Pathol* 1987;18: 1109–1114.
142. Gelderblom HR. Assembly and morphology of HIV: potential effect of structure on viral function. *AIDS* 1991;5:617–638.
143. Gelderblom HR, Hausmann EHS, Özel M, et al. Fine structure of human immunodeficiency virus (HIV) and immunolocalization of structural proteins. *Virology* 1987;156:171–176.
144. Özel M, Pauli G, Gelderblom HR. The organization of the envelope projections on the surface of HIV. *Arch Virol* 1998;100:255–266.
145. McKeating JA, McKnight A, Moore JP. Differential loss of envelope glycoprotein gp120 from virions of human immunodeficiency virus type 1 isolates: effects on infectivity and neutralization. *J Virol* 1991; 65:852–860.
146. Panteleo G, Cohen OJ, Schwartzentruber DJ, et al. Pathogenic insights from studies of lymphoid tissue from HIV-infected individuals. *J Acquir Immune Defic Syndr Hum Retrovirol* 1995;10[Suppl 1]:S6–S14.
147. Pekovic DD, Gornitsky M, Ajdukovic D, et al. Pathogenicity of HIV in lymphatic organs of patients with AIDS. *J Pathol* 1987;152:31–35.
148. Tenner-Racz K. Human immunodeficiency virus-associated changes in germinal centers of lymph nodes and relevance to impaired B-cell function. *Lymphology* 1988;21:36–43.
149. Embretson J, Zupancic M, Ribas JL, et al. Massive covert infection of helper T lymphocytes and macrophages by HIV during the incubation period of AIDS. *Nature* 1993;362:359–362.
150. Armstrong JA, Horne R. Follicular dendritic cells and virus-like particles in AIDS-related lymphadenopathy. *Lancet* 1984;ii:370–372.
151. Armstrong JA, Dawkins RL, Horne R. Retroviral infection of accessory cells and the immunological paradox in AIDS. *Immunol Today* 1985;6:121–122.
152. Tenner-Racz K, Racz P, Dietrich M, et al Altered follicle dendritic cells and virus-like particles in AIDS and AIDS-related lymphadenopathy. *Lancet* 1985;i:105–106.
153. Le Tourneau A, Audouin J, Diebold J, et al. LAV-like viral particles in lymph node germinal centers in patients with the persistent lymphadenopathy syndrome and the acquired immunodeficiency syndrome-related complex: an ultrastructural study of 30 cases. *Hum Pathol* 1986;17:1047–1053.
154. Cameron PU, Dawkins RL, Armstrong JA, et al. Western blot profiles, lymph node ultrastructure and viral expression in HIV-infected patients: a correlative study. *Clin Exp Immunol* 1987;68:465–478.
155. Tacchetti C, Favre A, Moresco L, et al. HIV is trapped and masked in the cytoplasm of lymph node follicular dendritic cells. *Am J Pathol* 1997;150:533–542.
156. Parmentier HK, van Wichen D, Sie-Go DMD, et al. HIV-1 infection and virus production in follicular dendritic cells in lymph nodes. *Am J Pathol* 1990;137:247–251.
157. Panteleo G, Graziosi C, Demarest JF, et al. HIV infection is active and progressive in lymphoid tissue during the clinically latent stage of disease. *Nature* 1993;362:355–358.
158. Heath SL, Tew JG, Tew JG, Szakal AK, et al. Follicular dendritic cells and human immunodeficiency virus infectivity. *Nature* 1995; 377:740–744.
159. Grouard G, Durand I, Filgueira L, et al. Dendritic cells capable of stimulating T cells in germinal centres. *Nature* 1996;384:364–367.
160. Grouard G, Clark EA. Role of dendritic and follicular dendritic cells in HIV infection and pathogenesis. *Curr Opin Immunol* 1997;9: 563–567.
161. Rademakers LH, Schuurman HJ, de Frankrijker JF, et al. Cellular composition of germinal centers in lymph nodes after HIV-1 infection: evidence for an inadequate support of germinal center B lymphocytes by follicular dendritic cells. *Clin Immunol Immunopathol* 1992;62: 148–159.
162. Rademakers LH, Schuurman HJ, de Frankrijker JF. Ultrastructural analysis of human lymph node follicles after HIV-1 infection. *Adv Exp Med Biol* 1993;329:359–363.
163. Schmitz J, van Lunzen J, Tenner-Racz K, et al. Follicular dendritic cells (FDC) are not productively infected with HIV-1 in vivo. *Adv Exp Med Biol* 1994;355:165–168.
164. Schmitz J, van Lunzen J, Tenner-Racz K, et al. Follicular dendritic cells retain HIV-1 particles on their plasma membrane, but are not productively infected in asymptomatic patients with follicular hyperplasia. *J Immunol* 1994;153:1352–1359.
165. Schuurman HJ, Joling P, van Wichen DF, et al. Follicular dendritic cells and infection by human immunodeficiency virus type 1—a crucial target cell and virus reservoir. *Curr Top Microbiol Immunol* 1995; 201:161–188.
166. Laman JD, van den Eertwegh AJM. Cytotoxic potential of CD8 + T-cells in lymphoid follicles during HIV-1 infection. *AIDS* 1992;6: 333–334.
167. Sunila I, Vaccarezza M, Pantaleo G, et al. Activated cytotoxic lymphocytes in lymph nodes from human immunodeficiency virus (HIV) 1-

infected patients: a light and electronmicroscopic study. *Histopathology* 1997;30:31–40.
168. Carbonari M, Pesce AM, Cibati M, et al. Death of bystander cells by a novel pathway involving early mitochondrial damage in human immunodeficiency virus-related lymphadenopathy. *Blood* 1997;90: 209–216.
169. Baroni CD, Pezzella F, Pezzella M, et al. Expression of HIV in lymph node cells of LAS patients: immunohistology, in situ hybridization, and identification of target cells. *Am J Pathol* 1988;133:498–506.
170. Orenstein JM, Fox C, Wahl SM. Macrophages as a source of HIV during opportunistic infections. *Science* 1997;276:1857–1861.
171. Ewing EP, Spira TJ, Chandler FW, et al. Ultrastructure of AIDS lymph nodes: reply. *N Engl J Med* 1983;309:1190.
172. Sidhu GS, Stahl RE, El-Sadr W, et al. The acquired immunodeficiency syndrome: an ultrastructural study. *Hum Pathol* 1985;16:377–386.
173. Helder AW, Feltkamp-Vroom TM. Tubuloreticular structures and antinuclear antibodies in autoimmune and non-autoimmune disease. *J Pathol* 1976;119:49–56.
174. Jackson D, Tabor E, Gerety RJ. Acute non-A, non-B hepatitis: specific ultrastructural alterations in endoplasmic reticulum of infected hepatocytes. *Lancet* 1979;i:1249–1250.
175. Grimley PM, Davis GL, Kang YH, et al. Tubuloreticular inclusions in peripheral blood mononuclear cells related to systemic therapy with α-Interferon. *Lab Invest* 1985;52:638–649.
176. Luu J, Bockus D, Remington F, et al. Tubuloreticular structures and cylindrical confronting cisternae: a review. *Hum Pathol* 1989; 20: 617–627.
177. Wood GS, Burns BF, Dorfman RF, et al. The immunohistology of non-T cells in the acquired immunodeficiency syndrome. *Am J Pathol* 1985;120:371–379.
178. Wood GS, Burns BF, Dorfman RF, et al. In situ quantitation of lymph node helper, suppressor, and cytotoxic T cell subsets in AIDS. *Blood* 1986;67:596–603.
179. Parmentier HK, Van Wichen DF, Peters PJ, et al. No histological evidence for cytotoxic T cells in destruction of lymph-node follicle centres after HIV infection? *AIDS* 1991;5:778–780.
180. Koopman G, Wever PC, Ramkema MD, et al. Expression of granzyme B by cytotoxic T lymphocytes in the lymph nodes of HIV-infected patients. *AIDS Res Human Retroviruses* 1997;13:227–233.
181. Devergne O, Peuchmaur M, Crevon MC, et al. Activation of cytotoxic cells in hyperplastic lymph nodes from HIV-infected patients. *AIDS* 1991;5:1071–1079.
182. Baroni C, Vitolo D, Uccini S. Immunohistopathogenesis of persistent generalized lymphadenopathy in HIV-positive patients. *Res Clin Lab* 1990;20:1–10.
183. Said JW, Shintaku IP, Teitelbaum A, et al. Distribution of T-cell phenotypic subsets and surface immunoglobulin-bearing lymphocytes in lymph nodes from male homosexuals with persistent generalized adenopathy: an immunohistochemical and ultrastructural study. *Hum Pathol* 1984;15:785–790.
184. Tenner-Racz K, Racz P, Thomé C, et al. Cytotoxic effector cell granules recognized by the monoclonal antibody TIA-1 are present in CD8+ lymphocytes in lymph nodes of human immunodeficiency virus-1-infected patients. *Am J Pathol* 1993;142:1750–1758.
185. Choremi-Papadopoulou H, Viglis V, Gargalianos P, et al. Downregulation of CD28+ T lymphocytes during HIV-1 infection. *J Acquir Immune Defic Syndr* 1994;7:245–253.
186. Borthwick NJ, Bofill M, Gombert WM, et al. Lymphocyte activation in HIV-1 infection: II. Functional defects of CD28-T cells. *AIDS* 1994; 8:431–441.
187. Tenner-Racz K, Racz R. Follicular dendritic cells initiate and maintain infection of the germinal centers by human immunodeficiency virus. *Curr Top Microbiol Immunol* 1995;201:141–155.
188. Piris MA, Rivas C, Morente M, et al. Persistent and generalized lymphadenopathy: a lesion of follicular dendritic cells? *Am J Clin Pathol* 1987;87:716–724.
189. Mori S, Ezaki Y, Mori M, et al. Deterioration of B cell proliferation correlates with dendritic reticulum cell destruction in germinal centers of an AIDS patient: case study. *Acta Pathol Jpn* 1988;38:1205–1214.
190. Hufert FT, van Lunzen J, Janossy G, et al. Germinal centre CD4 + T cells are an important site of HIV replication in vivo. *AIDS* 1997; 11:849–857.
191. Muller H, Falk S, Schmidts HL, et al. In situ immunophenotyping of lymphocytes/macrophages: grading of lymphadenopathy, staging and pathophysiology of HIV infection. *Res Virol* 1990;141:171–184.
192. Porwit A, Böttiger B, Pallesen G, et al. Follicular involution in HIV lymphadenopathy. *APMIS* 1989;97:153–165.
193. Tenner-Racz K, Racz P, Bofill M. HTLV-III/LAV viral antigens in lymph nodes of homosexual men with persistent generalized lymphadenopathy and AIDS. *Am J Pathol* 1986;123:9–15.
194. Schuurman HJ, Krone WJA, Broekhuizen R, et al. Expression of RNA and antigens of human immunodeficiency virus type-1 (HIV-1) in lymph nodes from HIV-1 infected individuals. *Am J Pathol* 1988; 133:516–524.
195. Schriever F, Freedman AS, Freeman G, et al. Isolated human follicular dendritic cells display a unique antigenic phenotype. *J Exp Med* 1989; 169:2043–2058.
196. Wood GS, Turner RR, Shiurba RA, et al. Human dendritic cells and macrophages: in situ immunophenotypic definition of subsets that exhibit specific morphologic and microenvironmental characteristics. *Am J Pathol* 1985;119:73–82.
197. Parravinici CL, Vago L, Costanzi GC, et al. Follicle lysis in lymph nodes from homosexual men. *Blood* 1986;68:595–596.
198. Stahmer I, Zimmer JP, Ernst M, et al. Isolation of normal human follicular dendritic cells and CD4-independent in vitro infection by human immunodeficiency virus (HIV-1). *Eur J Immunol* 1991:21: 1873–1878.
199. Spiegel H, Herbst H, Niedobitek G, et al. Follicular dendritic cells are a major reservoir for human immunodeficiency virus type 1 in lymphoid tissues facilitating infection of CD4+ T-helper cells. *Am J Pathol* 1992;140:15–22.
200. Laman JD, Claassen E, Van Rooijen N, et al. Immune complexes on follicular dendritic cells as a target for cytolytic cells in AIDS. *AIDS* 1989;3:543–548.
201. Golding H, Robey FA, Gates FT, et al. Identification of homologous regions in human immunodeficiency virus I gp41 and human MHC class II β 1 domain. *J Exp Med* 1988;167:914–923.
202. Young JA. HIV and HLA similarity. *Nature* 1988;333:215.
203. Gerdes J, Flad HD. Follicular dendritic cells and their role in HIV infection. *Immunol Today* 1992;13:81–83.
204. Turner RR, Meyer PR, Taylor CR, et al. Immunohistology of persistent generalized lymphadenopathy: evidence for progressive lymph node abnormalities in some patients. *Am J Clin Pathol* 1987;88: 10–19.
205. Lash RH, Tubbs RR, Calabrese LH. Paracortical immunoregulatory subpopulations in lymph nodes from homosexual men with persistent generalized lymphadenopathy. *Hum Pathol* 1988;19:419–422.
206. Nicholson JKA, McDougal JS, Spira TJ, et al. Immunoregulatory subsets of the T helper and T suppressor cell populations in homosexual men with chronic unexplained lymphadenopathy. *J Clin Invest* 1984;73:191–201.
207. Burke AP, Anderson D, Mannan P, et al. Systemic lymphadenopathic histology in human immunodeficiency virus-1-seropositive drug addicts without apparent acquired immunodefiency syndrome. *Hum Pathol* 1994;25:248–256.
208. Tenner-Racz K, von Stemm AMR, Gühlk B, et al. Are follicular dendritic cells, macrophages and interdigitating cells of the lymphoid tissue productively infected by HIV? *Res Virol* 1994;145:177–182.
209. Frankel SS, Wenig BM, Burke AP, et al. Replication of HIV-1 in dendritic cell-derived syncytia at the mucosal surface of the adenoid. *Science* 1996;272:115–117.
210. Rosok B, Brinchmann JE, Voltersvik P, et al. Correlates of latent and productive HIV type-1 infection in tonsillar $CD4^+$ T cells. *Proc Natl Acad Sci USA* 1997;94:9332–9336.
211. Turner RR, Boone DC, Levine AM, et al. Flow cytometric lymphocyte immunophenotyping in homosexual men with the persistent generalized lymphadenopathy syndrome: a longitudinal study of lymph nodes and blood. *Diagn Clin Immunol* 1987;5:194–200.
212. Fox CH, Tenner-Rácz K, Rácz P, et al. Lymphoid germinal centers are reservoirs of human immunodeficiency virus type 1 RNA. *J Infect Dis* 1991;164:1051–1057.
213. Walewska-Zielecka B, Nowoslawki A. HIV lymphadenopathy: a histo-pathological and immunomorphological study of 65 cases. *Pol J Pathol* 1995;46:211–217.
214. Nuovo GJ, Becker J, Burk MW, et al. In situ detection of PCR-amplified HIV-1 nucleic acids in lymph nodes and peripheral blood in

patients with asymptomatic HIV-1 infection and advanced-stage AIDS. *J Acquir Immune Defic Syndr* 1994;7:916–923.
215. Anderson RM, May RM. Epidemiological parameters of HIV transmission. *Nature* 1988;333:514–519.
216. Giesecke J, Scalia-Tomba G, Hakansson C, et al. Incubation time of AIDS: progression of disease in a cohort of HIV-infected homo- and bisexual men with known dates of infection. *Scand J Infect Dis* 1990; 22:407–411.
217. Sepkowitz KA. Effect of HAART on natural history of AIDS-related opportunistic disorders. *Lancet* 1998;351:228–230.
218. Kahn JO, Walker BD. Acute human immunodeficiency virus type 1 infection. *N Engl J Med* 1998;339:33–39.
219. Saag MS. Evolving understanding of the immunopathogenesis of HIV. *AIDS Res Hum Retrovir* 1994;10:887–892.
220. Murray HW, Godblod JH, Jurica K, et al. Progression to AIDS in patients with lymphadenopathy or AIDS-related complex: reappraisal of risk and predictive factors. *Am J Med* 1989;86:533–538.
221. Krohn KJE, Antonen J, Valle SL, et al. Clinical and immunological findings in HTLV-III infection. *Cancer Res* 1985;45[Suppl]: 4612S–4615S.
222. Gritti FM, Raise E, Gualandi G, et al. A clinical-immunological evaluation of AIDS cases and related syndromes. *J Exp Pathol* 1987;3: 723–736.
223. Loveday C, Hill A. Prediction of progression to AIDS with serum HIV-1 RNA and CD4 count. *Lancet* 1995;345:790–791.
224. Mellors JW, Kingsley LA, Rinaldo CR, et al. Quantitation of HIV-1 RNA in plasma predicts outcome after seroconversion. *Ann Intern Med* 1995;122:573–579.
225. Turner RR, Boone DC, Levine AM, et al. Flow cytometric lymphocyte immunophenotyping in homosexual men with the persistent generalized lymphadenopathy syndrome: a longitudinal study of lymph nodes and blood. *Diagn Clin Immunol* 1987;5:194–200.
226. Donaldson YK, Bell JE, Ironside JW, et al. Redistribution of HIV outside the lymphoid system with onset of AIDS. *Lancet* 1994;343: 382–385.
227. Schechter MT, Craib KJP, Le TN, et al. Susceptibility to AIDS progression appears early in HIV infection. *AIDS* 1990;4:185–190.
228. Lafeuillade A, Tamalet C, Pellegrino P, et al. High viral burden in lymph nodes during early stages of HIV-1 infection. *AIDS* 1993;7: 1527–1528.
229. Mellors JW, Rinaldo CR, Gupta P, et al. Prognosis in HIV-1 infection predicted by the quantity of virus in plasma. *Science* 1996;272: 1167–1170.
230. Jacobson MA, Bacchetti P, Kolokathis A, et al. Surrogate markers for survival in patients with AIDS and AIDS related complex treated with zidovudine. *Br Med J* 1991;302:73–78.
231. Paiva DD, Morais JC, Pilotto J, et al. Spectrum of morphologic changes of lymph nodes in HIV infection. *Mem Inst Oswaldo Cruz* 1996;91:371–379.
232. Kaplan JE, Spira TJ, Fishbein DB, et al. Lymphadenopathy syndrome in homosexual men: evidence for continuing risk of developing the acquired immunodeficiency syndrome. *JAMA* 1987;257:335–337.
233. Kaplan JE, Spira TJ, Fishbein DB, et al. A six-year follow-up of HIV-infected homosexual men with lymphadenopathy: evidence for an increased risk for developing AIDS after the third year of lymphadenopathy. *JAMA* 1988;260:2694–2697.
234. Diebold J, Audouin J, Le Tourneau A. Lymphoid tissue changes in HIV-infected patients. *Lymphology* 1988;21:22–27.
235. Formenti SC, Turner RR, DeMartini RM, et al. Immunophenotypic analysis of peripheral blood leukocytes at different stages of HIV infection: an analysis of asymptomatic, ARC and AIDS populations. *Am J Clin Pathol* 1989;92:300–307.
236. Cavert W, Notermans DW, Staskus K, et al. Kinetics of response in lymphoid tissues to antiretroviral therapy of HIV-1 infection. *Science* 1997;276:960–964.
237. Lafeuillade A, Chouraqui M, Hittinger G, et al. Lymph node expansion of CD4 + lymphocytes during antiretroviral therapy. *J Infect Dis* 1997;176:1378–1382.
238. Jacobson MA, Zegans M, Pavan PR, et al. Cytomegalovirus retinitis after initiation of highly active antiretroviral therapy. *Lancet* 1997; 249:1443–1445.
239. Tenner-Racz K, Stellbrink HJ, van Lunzen J, et al. The unenlarged lymph nodes of HIV-1-infected, asymptomatic patients with high CD4 T cell counts are sites for virus replication and CD4 T cell proliferation: the impact of highly active antiretroviral therapy. *J Exp Med* 1998;187:949–959.
240. Race EM, Adelson-Mitty J, Kriegel GR, et al. Focal mycobacterial lymphadenitis following initiation of protease-inhibitor therapy in patients with advanced HIV-1 disease. *Lancet* 1998;351:252–255.
241. Smith FB, Rajdeo H, Panesar N, et al. Benign lymphoepithelial lesion of the parotid gland in intravenous drug users. *Arch Pathol Lab Med* 1988;112:742–745.
242. Ryan JR, Ioachim HL, Marmer J, et al. Acquired immune deficiency syndrome-related lymphadenopathies presenting in the salivary gland lymph nodes. *Arch Otolaryngol* 1985;111:554–556.
243. Ulirsch RC, Jaffe ES. Sjögren's syndrome-like illness associated with the acquired immunodeficiency syndrome-related complex. *Hum Pathol* 1987;18:1063–1068.
244. Finfer MD, Schinella RA, Rothstein SG, et al. Cystic parotid lesions in patients at risk for the acquired immunodeficiency syndrome. *Arch Otolaryngol Head Neck Surg* 1988;114:1290–1294.
245. Kornstein MJ, Parker GA, Mills AS. Immunohistology of the benign lymphoepithelial lesion in AIDS-related lymphadenopathy: a case report. *Hum Pathol* 1988;19:1359–1361.
246. Tunkel DE, Loury MC, Fox CH, et al. Bilateral parotid enlargement in HIV-seropositive patients. *Laryngoscope* 1989;99:590–595.
247. Terry JH, Loree TR, Thomas MD, et al. Major salivary gland lymphoepithelial lesions and the acquired immunodeficiency syndrome. *Am J Surg* 1991;162:324–329.
248. Ioachim HL, Ryan JR, Blaugrund SM. Salivary gland lymph nodes: the site of lymphadenopathies and lymphomas associated with human immunodeficiency virus infection. *Arch Pathol Lab Med* 1988;112: 1224–1228.
249. Sperling NM, Lin PT, Lucente FE. Cystic parotid masses in HIV infection. *Head Neck* 1990;12:337–341.
250. Som PM, Brandwein MS, Silvers A. Nodal inclusion cysts of the parotid gland and parapharyngeal space: a discussion of lymphoepithelial, AIDS-related parotid, and branchial cysts, cystic Warthin's tumors, and cysts in Sjögren's syndrome. *Laryngoscope* 1995;105: 1122–1128.
251. DiGiuseppe JA, Wu TC, Corio RL. Analysis of Epstein-Barr virus-encoded small RNA 1 expression in benign lymphoepithelial salivary gland lesions. *Mod Pathol* 1994;7:555–559.
252. d'Agay MF, de Roquancourt A, Peuchmaur M, et al. Cystic benign lymphoepithelial lesion of the salivary glands in HIV-positive patients. Virchows *Arch A Pathol Anat* 1990;417:353–356.
253. Labouyrie E, Merlio JPH, Beylot-Barry M, et al. Human immunodeficiency virus type 1 replications within cystic lymphoepithelial lesion of the salivary gland. *Am J Clin Pathol* 1993;100:41–46.
254. Cleary KR, Batsakis JG. Lymphoepithelial cysts of the parotid region: a "new face" on an old lesion. *Ann Otol Rhinol Laryngol* 1990;99: 162–164.
255. Poletti A, Manconi R, Volpe R, et al. Study of AIDS-related lymphadenopathy in the intraparotid and perisubmaxillary gland lymph nodes. *J Oral Pathol* 1988;17:164–167.
256. Fox RI, Howell FU, Bone RC, et al. Primary Sjögren's syndrome: clinical and immunopathologic features. *Semin Arthritis Rheum* 1988; 14:77–105.
257. Shaha AR, DiMaio T, Webber C, et al. Benign lymphoepithelial lesions of the parotid. *Am J Surg* 1993;166:403–406.
258. De Vries EJ, Kapadia SB, Johnson JT, et al. Salivary gland lymphoproliferative disease in acquired immune disease. *Otolaryngol Head Neck Surg* 1988;99:59–62.
259. Soberman N, Leonidas JC, Berdon WE, et al. Parotid enlargement in children seropositive for human immunodeficiency virus: imaging findings. *Am J Roentgenol* 1991;157:553–556.
260. Gordon JJ, Golbus J, Kurtides ES. Chronic lymphadenopathy and Sjögren's syndrome in a homosexual man. *N Engl J Med* 1984;311: 1441–1442.
261. Couderc LJ, D-Agay MF, Danon F, et al. Sicca complex and infection with human immunodeficiency virus. *Arch Intern Med* 1987;147: 898–901.
262. Itescu S, Brancato LJ, Winchester R. A sicca syndrome in HIV infection: association with HLA-DR5 and CD8 lymphocytosis. *Lancet* 1989;ii:466–468.
263. Itescu S, Brancato LJ, Buxbaum J, et al. A diffuse infiltrative CD8 lymphocytosis syndrome in human immunodeficiency virus (HIV)

infection: a host immune response associated with HLA-DR5. *Ann Intern Med* 1990;112:3–10.
264. Holliday RA, Cohen WA, Schinella RA, et al. Benign lymphoepithelial parotid cysts and hyperplastic cervical adenopathy in AIDS-risk patients: a new CT appearance. *Radiology* 1988;168:439–441.
265. Shugar JMA, Som PM, Jacobson AL, et al. Multicentric parotid cysts and cervical adenopathy in AIDS patients: a newly recognized entity: CT and MR manifestations. *Laryngoscope* 1988;98:772–775.
266. Kaposi M: Idiopatisches multiples pigmentsarkorn der haut. *Arch Dermatol Syphillis* 1872;4:265–273.
267. Friedman-Kien AE, Laubenstein LJ, Rubinstein P, et al. Disseminated Kaposi's sarcoma in homosexual men. *Ann Intern Med* 1982;96: 693–700.
268. Beral V: Epidemiology of Kaposi's sarcoma. In Beral V, Jaffe HW, Weiss RA, eds. *Cancer surveys: cancer, HIV and AIDS.* New York: Cold Spring Harbor Laboratory, 1991;10:5–22.
269. Peterman TA, Jaffe HW, Friedman-Kein AE, et al. The etiology of Kaposi's sarcoma. In Beral V, Jaffe HW, Weiss RA, eds. *Cancer surveys: cancer, HIV and AIDS.* New York: Cold Spring Harbor Laboratory, 1991;10:23–27.
270. Biggar RJ, Rabkin CS. The epidemiology of AIDS-related neoplasms. *Hematol Oncol Clin North Am* 1996;10:997–1010.
271. Dezube BJ. Clinical presentation and natural history of AIDS-related Kaposi's sarcoma. *Hematol Oncol Clin North Am* 1996;10: 1023–1029.
272. Costa J, Rabson AS. Generalised Kaposi's sarcoma is not a neoplasm. *Lancet* 1983;i:58.
273. Brooks JJ. Kaposi's sarcoma: a reversible hyperplasia. *Lancet* 1986; 2:1309–1310.
274. Ioachim HL, Adsay V, Giancotti FR, et al. Kaposi's sarcoma of internal organs: a multiparameter study of 86 cases. *Cancer* 1995;75: 1376–1385.
275. Rabkin CS, Bedi G, Musaba E, et al. AIDS-related Kaposi's sarcoma is a clonal neoplasm. *Clin Cancer Res* 1995;1:257–260.
276. Centers for Disease Control: First 500,000 AIDS cases: United States. *MMWR* 1995;41:1–19.
277. Gill PS, Loureiro C, Bernstein-Singer M, et al. Clinical effect of glucocorticoids on Kaposi's sarcoma related to the acquired immunodeficiency syndrome. *Ann Intern Med* 1989;110:937–940.
278. Niedt GW, Schinella RA. Acquired immunodeficiency syndrome: clinicopathologic study of 56 autopsies. *Arch Pathol Lab Med* 1985; 109:727–734.
279. Nichols CM, Flaitz CM, Hicks MJ. Treating Kaposi's lesions in the HIV-infected patient. *JADA* 1993;124:78–84.
280. Gorin FA, Bale JF, Halks-Miller M, et al. Kaposi's sarcoma metastatic to the CNS. *Arch Neurol* 1985;42:162–165.
281. Welch K, Finkbeiner W, Alpers CE, et al. Autopsy findings in the acquired immune deficiency syndrome. *JAMA* 1984;252:1152–1159.
282. Amberson JB, DiCarlo EF, Metroka CE, et al. Diagnostic pathology in the acquired immunodeficiency syndrome: surgical pathology and cytology experience with 67 patients. *Arch Pathol Lab Med* 1985; 109:345–351.
283. Kaplan MH, Susin M, Pahwa SG, et al. Neoplastic complications of HTLV-III infection: lymphomas and solid tumors. *Am J Med* 1987; 82:389–396.
284. Steis RG, Longo DL. Clinical, biologic, and therapeutic aspects of malignancies associated with the acquired immunodeficiency syndrome: Part I. *Ann Allergy* 1988;60:310–314.
285. Cockerell CJ: Histopathological features of Kaposi's sarcoma in HIV-infected individuals. In Beral V, Jaffe HW, Weiss RA, eds. *Cancer surveys: cancer, HIV and AIDS.* New York: Cold Spring Harbor Laboratory, 1991;10:73–90.
286. Santucci M, Pimpinelli N, Moretti S, et al. Classic and immunodeficiency-associated Kaposi's sarcoma: clinical, histologic, and immunologic correlations. *Arch Pathol Lab Med* 1988;112:1214–1220.
287. Rutgers JL, Wieczorek R, Bonetti F, et al. The expression of endothelial cell surface antigens by AIDS-associated Kaposi's sarcoma. *Am J Pathol* 1986;122:493–499.
288. Scully PA, Steinman HK, Kennedy C, et al. AIDS-related Kaposi's sarcoma displays differential expression of endothelial surface antigens. *Am J Pathol* 1988;130:244–251.
289. Kraffert C, Planus L, Penneys NS. Kaposi's sarcoma: further immunohistologic evidence of a vascular endothelial origin. *Arch Dermatol* 1991;127:1734–1735.
290. Lubin J, Rywlin AM. Lymphoma-like lymph node changes in Kaposi's sarcoma. *Arch Pathol* 1971;92:338–341.
291. Amazon K, Rywlin AM. Subtle clues to the diagnosis by conventional microscopy: lymph node involvement in Kaposi's sarcoma. *Am J Dermatopathol* 1979;1:173–176.
292. Beral V, Peterman TA, Berkelman RL, et al. Kaposi's sarcoma among persons with AIDS: a sexually transmitted infection? *Lancet* 1990; 335:123–128.
293. Beral V, Bull D, Darby S, et al. Risk of Kaposi's sarcoma and sexual practices associated with fecal contact in homosexual or bisexual men with AIDS. *Lancet* 1992;339:632–635.
294. Giraldo G, Beth E, Haguenau F. Herpes-type virus particles in tissue culture of Kaposi's sarcoma from different geographic regions. *J Natl Cancer Inst* 1972;49:1509–1526.
295. Lisitsyn N, Wigler M. Cloning the differences between two complex genomes. *Science* 1993;259:946–951.
296. Chang Y, Cesarman E, Pessin MS, et al. Identification of herpesvirus-like DNA sequences in AIDS-associated Kaposi's sarcoma. *Science* 1994;266:1865–1869.
297. Cesarman E, Knowles DM. Kaposi's sarcoma-associated herpes virus (KSHV/HHV -8): a lymphotropic human herpesvirus associated with Kaposi's sarcoma, primary effusion lymphoma and multicentric Castleman's disease. *Semin Diagn Pathol* 1997;14:54–66.
298. Moore PS, Gao S-J, Dominiguez G, et al. Primary characterization of a herpesvirus agent associated with Kaposi's sarcoma. *J Virol* 1996; 70:549–558.
299. Cesarman E, Nador RG, Bai F, et al. KSHV/HHV-8 contains G protein-coupled receptor and cyclin D homologues which are expressed in Kaposi's sarcoma and malignant lymphoma. *J Virol* 1996;70: 8218–8223.
300. Mesri EA, Cesarman E, Arvanitakis L, et al. Human herpesvirus-8/ Kaposi's sarcoma-associated herpesvirus is a new transmissible virus that infects B cells. *J Exp Med* 1996;183:2385–2390.
301. Roizman B: Herpesviridae: a brief introduction. In: Fields BN, ed. *Virology.* New York: Raven Press, 1990:1787–1793.
302. Boshoff C, Schulz TF, Kennedy MM, et al. Kaposi's sarcoma-associated herpesvirus infects endothelial and spindle cells. *Nature Med* 1995;1:1274–1278.
303. Reed JA, Nador RG, Spaulding D, et al. Demonstration of Kaposi's sarcoma-associated herpesvirus cyclin D homolog in cutaneous Kaposi's sarcoma by colorimetric in situ hybridization using a catalyzed signal amplification system. *Blood* 1998;91:3825–3832.
304. Knowles DM, Cesarman E. The Kaposi's sarcoma-associated herpesvirus (human herpesvirus-8) in Kaposi's sarcoma, malignant lymphoma, and other diseases. *Ann Oncol* 1997;8[Suppl 2]:5123–5129.
305. Whitby D, Howard MR, Tenant-Flowers M, et al. Detection of Kaposi's sarcoma associated herpesvirus in peripheral blood of HIV-infected individuals and progression to Kaposi's sarcoma. *Lancet* 1995;346:799–802.
306. Moore PS, Kingsley A, Holmberg SD, et al. Kaposi's sarcoma-associated herpesvirus infection prior to onset of Kaposi's sarcoma. *AIDS* 1996;10:175–180.
307. Gao SJ, Kingsley L, Hoover DR, et al. Seroconversion to antibodies against Kaposi's sarcoma-associated herpesvirus-related nuclear antigens before the development of Kaposi's sarcoma. *N Engl J Med* 1996;335:233–241.
308. Levine AM, Meyer PR, Gill PS, et al. Results of initial lymph node biopsy in homosexual men with generalized lymphadenopathy. *J Clin Oncol* 1986;4:165–169.
309. Guarda LA, Luna MA, Smith JL, et al. Acquired immune syndrome: postmortem findings. *Am J Clin Pathol* 1984;81:549–557.
310. Dworkin MS, Kaplan JE. Mycobacterium avium complex lymph node abscess after use of highly active antiretroviral therapy in a patient with AIDS. *Arch Intern Med* 1998;158:1828.
311. Ball SC, Chadburn A. HAART-associated lymphadenopathy. *AIDS Reader* 1999;9:11–12,17.
312. Stoler MH, Bonfiglio TA, Sheigbigel RT, et al. An atypical subcutaneous infection associated with acquired immune deficiency syndrome. *Am J Clin Pathol* 1983;80:714–718.
313. Cockerell CJ, Whitelow MA, Webster GF, et al. Epithelioid angiomatosis: a distinct vascular disorder in patients with the acquired immunodeficiency syndrome or AIDS-related complex. *Lancet* 1987; ii:654–656.
314. LeBoit PE, Egbert BM, Stoler MH, et al. Epithelioid haemangioma-

like vascular proliferation in AIDS: Manifestation of cat scratch disease bacillus infection? *Lancet* 1988;i:960–963.
315. LeBoit PE, Berger TG, Egbert BM, et al. Bacillary angiomatosis: the histopathology and differential diagnosis of a pseudoneoplastic infection in patients with human immunodeficiency virus disease. *Am J Surg Pathol* 1989;13:909–920.
316. Baron AL, Steinbach LS, LeBoit PE, et al. Osteolytic lesions and bacillary angiomatosis in HIV infection: radiologic differentiation from AIDS-related Kaposi sarcoma. *Radiology* 1990;177;77–81.
317. Moore EH, Russell LA, Klein JS, et al. Bacillary angiomatosis in patients with AIDS: multiorgan imaging findings. *Radiology* 1995; 197:67–72.
318. Relman DA, Loutit JS, Schmidt TM, et al. The agent of bacillary angiomatosis: an approach to the identification of uncultured pathogens. *N Engl J Med* 1990;323:1573–1580.
319. Kemper CA, Lombard CM, Deresinski SC, et al. Visceral bacillary epithelioid angiomatosis: possible manifestations of disseminated cat scratch disease in the immunocompromised host. A report of two cases. *Am J Med* 1990;89:216–222.
320. Chan J KC, Lewin KJ, Lombard CM, et al. Histopathology of bacillary angiomatosis of lymph node. *Am J Surg Pathol* 1991;15:430–437.
321. Meyers SA, Prose NS, Garcia JA, et al. Bacillary angiomatosis in a child undergoing chemotherapy. *J Pediatr* 1992;121:574–578.
322. Torok L, Viragh SZ, Borka I, et al. Bacillary angiomatosis in a patient with lymphocytic leukaemia. *Br J Dermatol* 1994;130:665–668.
323. Milde P, Brunner M, Borchard F, et al. Cutaneous bacillary angiomatosis in a patient with chronic lymphocytic leukemia. *Arch Dermatol* 1995;131:933–936.
324. Cockerell CJ, Bergstresser PR, Myrie-Williams C, et al. Bacillary epithelioid angiomatosis occurring in an immunocompetent individual. *Arch Dermatol* 1990;126:787–790.
325. Tappero JW, Koehler JE, Berger TG, et al. Bacillary angiomatosis and bacillary splenitis in immunocompetent adults. *Ann Intern Med* 1993;118:363–365.
326. Paul MA, Fleischer AB, Wiselthier JS, et al. Bacillary angiomatosis in an immunocompetent child: the first reported case. *Pediatr Dermatol* 1994;11:338–341.
327. Smith KJ, Skelton HG, Larson PL, et al. Bacillary angiomatosis in an immunocompetent child. *Am J Dermatol* 1996;18:597–600.
328. Welch DF, Pickett DA, Slater LN, et al. Rochalimaea henslelae, sp. nov., a cause of septicemia, bacillary angiomatosis, and parenchymal bacillary peliosis. *J Clin Microbiol* 1992;30:275–274.
329. Koehler JE, Quinn FD, Berger TG, et al. Isolation of Rochalimaea species from cutaneous and osseous lesions of bacillary angiomatosis. *N Engl J Med* 1992;327:1625–1631.
330. Brenner DJ, O'Connor SP, Winkler HH, et al. Proposals to unify the genera Bartonella and Rochalimaea with descriptions of Bartonella quintana comb. nov., Bartonella vinsonii comb. nov., Bartonella henselae comb. nov., and Bartonella elizabethae comb. nov., and to remove the family Bartonellaceae from the order Rickettsiales. *Int J Syst Bacteriol* 1993;43:777–786.
331. Adal KA, Cockerell CJ, Petri WA. Cat scratch disease, bacillary angiomatosis, and other infections due to Rochalimaea. *N Engl J Med* 1994;330:1509–1515.
332. Perkocha LA, Geaghan SM, Benedict Yen TS, et al. Clinical and pathological features of bacillary peliosis hepatis in association with human immunodeficiency virus infection. *N Engl J Med* 1990;323: 1581–1586.
333. Regnery R, Martin M, Olson J. Naturally occurring "Rochalimaea henselae" infection in domestic cat. *Lancet* 1992;340:557–558.
334. Koehler JE, Glaser CA, Tappero JW. Rochalimaea henselae infection: a new zoonosis with the domestic cat as reservoir. *JAMA* 1994;271: 531–535.
335. Tappero JW, Mohle-Boetani J, Koehler JE, et al. The epidemiology of bacillary angiomatosis and bacillary peliosis. *JAMA* 1993;269: 770–775.
336. Webster GF, Cockerell CJ, Friedman-Kien AF. The clinical spectrum of bacillary angiomatosis. *Br J Dermatol* 1992;126:535–541.
337. Bastug DF, Ness DT, DeSantis JG. Bacillary angiomatosis mimicking pyogenic granuloma in the hand: a case report. *J Hand Surg* 1994; 307–308.
338. Malane MS, Laude TA, Chen CK, et al. An HIV-1-positive child with fever and a scalp nodule. *Lancet* 1995;346:1466.
339. Eden CG, Marker A, Pryor JP. Human immunodeficiency virus-related bacillary angiomatosis of the penis. *Br J Urol* 1996;77:323–324.
340. Mohle-Boetani JC, Koehler JE, Berger TG, et al. Bacillary angiomatosis and bacillary peliosis in patients infected with human immunodeficiency virus: clinical characteristics in a case-control study. *Clin Infect Dis* 1996;22:794–800.
341. Szaniawski WK, Don PC, Bitterman SR, et al. Epithelioid angiomatosis in patients with AIDS: report of seven cases and review of the literature. *J Am Acad Dermatol* 1990;23:41–48.
342. Walford N, Van der Wouw PA, Das PK, et al. Epithelioid angiomatosis in the acquired immunodeficiency syndrome: morphology and differential diagnosis. *Histopathology* 1990;16:83–88.
343. Slater LN, Min KW. Polypoid endobronchial lesions. *Chest* 1992; 102:972–974.
344. Chang AD, Drachenberg CI, James SP. Bacillary angiomatosis associated with extensive esophageal polyposis: a new mucocutaneous manifestation of acquired immunodeficiency disease (AIDS). *Am J Gastroenterol* 1996;91:2220–2223.
345. Huh YB, Rose S, Schoen RE, et al. Colonic bacillary angiomatosis. *Ann Intern Med* 1996;124:735–737.
346. Spach DH, Callis KP, Paauw DS, et al. Endocarditis caused by Rochalimaea quintana in a patient infected with human immunodeficiency virus. *J Clin Microbiol* 1993;31:692–694.
347. Slater LN, Welch DF, Min KW. Rochalimaea henselae causes bacillary angiomatosis and peliosis hepatis. *Arch Intern Med* 1992;152: 602–606.
348. Steeper TA, Rosenstein H, Weiser J, et al. Bacillary epithelioid angiomatosis involving the liver, spleen, and skin in an AIDS patient with concurrent Kaposi's sarcoma. *Am J Clin Pathol* 1992;97:713–718.
349. Milam MW, Balerdi MJ, Toney JF, et al. Epithelioid angiomatosis secondary to disseminated cat scratch disease involving the bone marrow and skin in a patient with acquired immune deficiency syndrome: a case report. *Am J Med* 1990;88:180–183.
350. Krekorian TD, Radner AB, Alcorn JM, et al. Biliary obstruction caused by epithelioid angiomatosis in a patient with AIDS. *Am J Med* 1990;89:820–822.
351. Schinella RA, Greco MA. Bacillary angiomatosis presenting as a soft-tissue tumor without skin involvement. *Hum Pathol* 1990;21: 567–569.
352. Haught WH, Steinbach J, Zander DS, et al. Case report: bacillary angiomatosis with massive visceral lymphadenopathy. *Am J Med Sci* 1993;306:236–240.
353. Long SR, Whitfeld MJ, Eades C, et al. Bacillary angiomatosis of the cervix and vulva in a patient with AIDS. *Obstet Gynecol* 1996;88: 709–711.
354. Spach DH, Panther LA, Thorning DR, et al. Intracerebral bacillary angiomatosis in a patient infected with human immunodeficiency virus. *Ann Intern Med* 1992;116:740–742.
355. Miller DG. The association of immune disease and malignant lymphoma. *Ann Intern Med* 1967;66:507–521.
356. Penn I, Hammond A, Brett Scheider L, et al. Malignant lymphomas in transplantation patients. *Transplant Proc* 1969;1:106.
357. Gatti RA, Good RA. Occurrence of malignancy in immunodeficiency disease: a literature review. *Cancer* 1971;28:89–98.
358. Penn I. Occurrence of cancer in immune deficiencies. *Cancer* 1974; 34:858–866.
359. Frizzera G, Rosai J, Dehner LP, et al. Lymphoreticular disorders in primary immunodeficiencies: new findings based on an up-to-date histologic classification of 35 cases. *Cancer* 1980;46:692–699.
360. Morrell D, Cromartie E, Swift M. Mortality and cancer incidence in 263 patients with ataxia-telangiectasia. *J Natl Cancer Inst* 1986;77: 89–92.
361. Cleary ML, Warnke R, Sklar J. Monoclonality of lymphoproliferative lesions in cardiac transplant recipients: clonal analysis based on immunoglobulin gene rearrangements. *N Engl J Med* 1984;310:477–482.
362. Penn I. Cancers complicating organ transplantation. *N Engl J Med* 1990;323:1767–1769.
363. Knowles DM, Cesarman E, Chadburn A, et al. Correlative morphologic and molecular genetic analysis demonstrates three distinct categories of posttransplantation lymphoproliferative disorders. *Blood* 1995;85:552–565.
364. Burke JS, Butler JJ, Fuller LM. Malignant lymphomas of the thyroid: a clinical pathologic study of 35 patients including ultrastructural observations. *Cancer* 1977;39:1587–1602.

365. Zulman J, Jaffe R, Talal N. Evidence that the malignant lymphoma of Sjogren's syndrome is a monoclonal B cell neoplasm. *N Engl J Med* 1978;299:1215–1220.
366. Doll DC, List AF. Burkitt's lymphoma in a homosexual. *Lancet* 1982; i:1026–1027.
367. Centers for Disease Control. Diffuse, undifferentiated non-Hodgkin's lymphoma among homosexual males: United States. *MMWR* 1982; 31:277–279.
368. Ziegler JL, Miner RC, Rosenbaum E, et al. Outbreak of Burkitt's like-lymphoma in homosexual men. *Lancet* 1982;ii:631–633.
369. Ziegler JL, Beckstead JA, Volberding PA, et al. Non-Hodgkin's lymphoma in 90 homosexual men: relation to generalized lymphadenopathy and the acquired immunodeficiency syndrome (AIDS). *N Engl J Med* 1984;311:565–570.
370. Levine AM, Meyer PR, Begandy MK, et al. Development of B-cell lymphoma in homosexual men. *Ann Intern Med* 1984;100:7–13.
371. Levine AM, Gill PS, Meyer PR, et al. Retrovirus and malignant lymphomas in homosexual men. *JAMA* 1985;254:1921–1925.
372. Kalter SP, Riggs SA, Cabanillas F, et al. Aggressive non-Hodgkin's lymphomas in immunocompromised homosexual males. *Blood* 1985; 55:655–659.
373. Ioachim HL, Cooper MC, Hellman GC. Lymphomas in men at high risk for acquired immunodeficiency syndrome (AIDS): a study of 21 cases. *Cancer* 1985;56:2831–2842.
374. DiCarlo EF, Anderson JB, Metroka CE, et al. Malignant lymphomas and the acquired immunodeficiency syndrome. *Arch Pathol Lab Med* 1986;110:1012–1016.
375. Knowles, DM, Chamulak GA, Subar M, et al. Lymphoid neoplasia associated with the acquired immunodeficiency syndrome (AIDS): the New York University Medical Center experience with 105 patients (1981–1986). *Ann Intern Med* 1988;108:744–753.
376. Snider WD, Simpson DM, Aronyk KE, et al. Primary lymphoma of the nervous system associated with acquired immune-deficiency syndrome. *N Engl J Med* 1983;308:45.
377. Chaganti RSK, Jhanwar SC, Koziner B, et al. Specific translocations characterize Burkitt's-like lymphoma of homosexual men with the acquired immunodeficiency syndrome. *Blood* 1983;61:1265–1268.
378. Gordon EM, Berkowitz RJ, Strandjord SE, et al. Burkitt's lymphoma in a patient with classic hemophilia receiving Factor VIII concentrates. *J Pediatr* 1983;103:75–77.
379. Shibuya A, Saitoh A, Tsuneyoshi H, et al. Burkitt's lymphoma in a haemophiliac. *Lancet* 1983;ii:1432.
380. Whang-Peng J, Lee EC, Sieverts H, et al. Burkitt's lymphoma in AIDS: cytogenetic study. *Blood* 1984;63:818–822.
381. Petersen JM, Tubbs RR, Savage RA, et al. Small non-cleaved Burkitt-like lymphoma with chromosome t(8;14) translocation and Epstein-Barr virus nuclear-associated antigen in a homosexual man with acquired immune deficiency syndrome. *Am J Med* 1985;78:141–148.
382. Ragni MV, Lewis JH, Bontempo FA, et al. Lymphoma presenting as a traumatic hematoma in an HTLV-III antibody positive hemophiliac. *N Engl J Med* 1985;313:640.
383. Groopman J, Sullivan JL, Mulder C, et al. Pathogenesis of B-cell lymphoma in a patient with AIDS. *Blood* 1986;67:612–615.
384. Mernick MH, Malamud SC, Haubenstock A, et al. Non-Hodgkin's lymphoma in AIDS: report of 11 cases and literature review. *Mt Sinai J Med* 1986;53:664–667.
385. Ahmed T, Wormser GP, Stahl RE, et al. Malignant lymphomas in a population at risk for acquired immune deficiency syndrome. *Cancer* 1987;60:719–723.
386. Payan MJ, Gambarelli D, Routy JP, et al. Primary lymphoma of the brain associated with AIDS. *Acta Neuropathol (Berl)* 1984;64:78–80.
387. Casadei GP, Gambacorta M. A clinico-pathologic study of seven cases of primary high grade malignant non-Hodgkin's lymphoma of the central nervous system. *Tumori* 1985;71:501–507.
388. Raphael M, Tulliez M, Bellfqih S, et al. Les lymphomes et le SIDA. *Ann Pathol* 1986;278:281–286.
389. Monfardini S, Tirelli U, Vaccher E, et al. Malignant lymphomas in patients with or at risk for AIDS. *J Natl Cancer Inst* 1988;80:855–860.
390. Hamilton-Dutoit SJ, Pallesen G, Karkov J, et al. Identification of EBV-DNA in tumour cells of AIDS-related lymphomas by in-situ hybridization. *Lancet* 1989;i:554–555.
391. Beral V, Peterman T, Berkelman R, et al. AIDS-associated non-Hodgkin lymphoma. *Lancet* 1991;337:805–809.
392. Casabona J, Melbye M, Biggar R, and The AIDS Registry Contributors.Kaposi's sarcoma and non-Hodgkin's lymphoma in European AIDS cases. No excess risk of Kaposi's sarcoma in Mediterranean countries. *Int J Cancer* 1991;47:49–53.
393. Roithman R, Tourani JM, Andrieu JM. AIDS-associated non-Hodgkin's lymphoma. *Lancet* 1991;338:884–885.
394. Levine AM, Sullivan-Halley J, Pike MC, et al. HIV-related lymphoma: prognostic factors predictive of survival. *Cancer* 1991;68: 2466–2472.
395. Peters BS, Beck EJ, Coleman DG, et al. Changing disease patterns in patients with AIDS in referral center in the United Kingdom: the changing face of AIDS. *Br Med J* 1991;302:203–206.
396. Loureiro C, Gill PS, Meyer PR, et al. Autopsy findings in AIDS-related lymphoma. *Cancer* 1988;62:735–739.
397. Klatt, EC. Diagnostic findings in patients with acquired immune deficiency syndrome (AIDS). *J Acquir Immune Defic Syndr* 1988;1: 459–465.
398. Wilkes MS, Fortin AH, Felix JC, et al. Value of necropsy in acquired immunodeficiency syndrome. *Lancet* 1988;ii:85–88.
399. Rabkin CS. Epidemiology of AIDS-related malignancies. *Curr Opin Oncol* 1994;6:492–496.
400. Biggar RJ, Curtis RE, Cote TR, et al. Risk of other cancers following Kaposi's sarcoma: relation to acquired immunodeficiency syndrome. *Am J Epidemiol* 1994;139:362–368.
401. Levine AM. Non-Hodgkin's lymphomas and other malignancies in the acquired immunodeficiency syndrome. *Semin Oncol* 1987; 14[Suppl 3]:34–39.
402. Biggar RJ, Rabkin CS. The epidemiology of acquired immunodeficiency syndrome-related lymphomas. *Curr Opin Oncol* 1992;4: 883–893.
403. Levine AM. Acquired immunodeficiency syndrome-related lymphoma. *Blood* 1992;80:8–20.
404. Harnly ME, Swan SH, Holly EA, et al. Temporal trends in the incidence of non-Hodgkin's lymphoma and selected malignancies in a population with a high incidence of acquired immunodeficiency syndrome. *Am J Epidemiol* 1988;128:261–267.
405. Ross R, Dworsky R, Paganini-Hill A, et al. Non-Hodgkin's lymphomas in never married men in Los Angeles. *Br J Cancer* 1985;52: 785–787.
406. Penn I. Kaposi's sarcoma in immunosuppressed patients. *J Clin Lab Immunol* 1983;12:1–10.
407. Penn I. Lymphomas complicating organ transplantation. *Transplant Proc* 1983;15[Suppl]:2790–2797.
408. Pluda JM,Vanzon D, Tosato G, et al. Factors which predict for the development of non-Hodgkin's lymphoma in patients with HIV infection receiving antiretroviral therapy. *Blood* 1991;78:285a(abst).
409. Pluda JM, Yarchoan R, Jaffe ES, et al. Development of non-Hodgkin's lymphoma in a cohort of patients with severe human immunodeficiency virus (HIV) infection on long term antiretroviral therapy. *Ann Intern Med* 1990;113:276–282.
410. Rabkin CS, Hilgartner MW, Hedberg KW, et al. Incidence of lymphomas and other cancers in HIV-infected and HIV-uninfected patients with hemophilia. *JAMA* 1992; 267:1090–1094.
411. Bernstein L, Hamilton AS. The epidemiology of AIDS-related malignancies. *Curr Opin Oncol* 1993;5:822–830.
412. Gail MH, Pluda JM, Rabkin CS, et al. Projections of the incidence of AIDS-related non-Hodgkin's lymphoma. *J Natl Cancer Inst* 1991; 83:695–701.
413. Obrams GI, Grufferman S. Epidemiology of HIV associated non-Hodgkin lymphoma. In: Beral V, Jaffe HW, Weiss RA, eds. *Cancer surveys: cancer, HIV and AIDS*. New York: Cold Spring Harbor Laboratory, 1991:91–102.
414. Rabkin CS, Biggar RJ, Horm JW. Increasing incidence of cancers associated with the human immunodeficiency virus epidemic. *Int J Cancer* 1991;47:692–696.
415. Lowenthal DA, Straus DJ, Campbell SW, et al. AIDS-related lymphoid neoplasia: the Memorial Hospital experience. *Cancer* 1988; 61:2325–2337.
416. Carbone A, Tirelli U, Vaccher E, et al. A clinicopathologic study of lymphoid neoplasias associated with human immunodeficiency virus infection in Italy. *Cancer* 1991;68:842–852.
417. Kaplan LD, Abrams DI, Feigal E, et al. AIDS-associated non-Hodgkin's lymphoma in San Francisco. *JAMA* 1989;261:719–724.
418. Hamilton-Dutoit SJ, Pallesen G, Franzmann MB, et al. AIDS-related lymphoma: histopathology, immunophenotype, and association with

EBV as demonstrated by in situ nucleic acid hybridization. *Am J Pathol* 1991;138:149–163.

419. Pedersen C, Gerstoft J, Lundgren JD, et al. HIV-associated lymphoma: histopathology and association with Epstein-Barr virus genome related to clinical, immunological and prognostic features. *Eur J Cancer* 1991;27:1416–1423.
420. Monfardini S, Vaccher E, Foa R, et al. AIDS-associated non-Hodgkin's lymphoma in Italy: intravenous drug users versus homosexual men: the Italian Cooperative Group on AIDS-Related Tumors (GICAT). *Ann Oncol* 1990;1:203–211.
421. Freter CE. Acquired immunodeficiency syndrome-associated lymphomas. *J Natl Cancer Inst Monogr* 1990;10:45–54.
422. Knowles DM, Dalla-Favera R. AIDS-associated malignant lymphoma. In: Broder S, Merrigan TC, Bolognesi D, eds. *Textbook of AIDS medicine.* Baltimore: Williams & Wilkins, 1994:431–463.
423. Knowles DM. The pathology and the pathogenesis of non-Hodgkin's lymphomas associated with HIV infection. In: Magrath I, ed. *The non-Hodgkin's lymphomas.* London: Arnold, 1997:471–494.
424. Ioachim HL, Dorsett B, Cronin W, et al. Acquired munodeficiency syndrome associated lymphomas: clinical, pathological, immunologic and viral characteristics of 111 cases. *Hum Pathol* 1991;22:659–673.
425. Levine AM, Gill PS. AIDS-related malignant lymphoma: clinical presentation and treatment approaches. *Oncology* 1987;1:41–46.
426. Gill PS, Levine AM, Meyer PR, et al. Primary central nervous system lymphoma in homosexual men: clinical, immunologic, and pathologic features. *Am J Med* 1985;78:742–748.
427. So YT, Beckstead JH, Davis RL: Primary central nervous system lymphoma in acquired immune deficiency syndrome: a clinical and pathological study. *Ann Neurol* 1986;20:566–572.
428. Burkes RL, Meyer PR, Gill PS, et al. Rectal lymphoma in homosexual men. *Arch Intern Med* 1986;146:913–915.
429. Lee MH, Waxman M, Gillooley JF. Primary malignant lymphoma of the anorectum in homosexual men. *Dis Colon Rectum* 1986;29:413–416.
430. Ioachim HL, Weinstein MA, Robbins RD, et al. Primary anorectal lymphoma: a new manifestation of the acquired immune deficiency syndrome (AIDS). *Cancer* 1987;60:1449–1453.
431. Subar M, Chadburn A, Knowles DM. Gastrointestinal neoplasms in AIDS. In: Kotler DP, ed. *Gastrointestinal and nutritional manifestations of the acquired immunodeficiency syndrome.* New York: Raven Press, 1991:93–117.
432. Reichart CM, O'Leary TJ, Levens DL, et al. Autopsy pathology in the acquired immune deficiency syndrome. *Am J Pathol* 1983;112:357–382.
433. Caccamo D, Pervez NK, Marchevsky A. Primary lymphoma of the liver in the acquired immunodeficiency syndrome. *Arch Pathol Lab Med* 1986;110:553–555.
434. Vanden Heule B, Taylor CR, Terry R, et al. Presentation of malignant lymphoma in the rectum. *Cancer* 1982;49:2602–2607.
435. Loehr WJ, Mujahed Z, Zahn FD, et al. Primary lymphoma of the gastrointestinal tract: a review of 100 cases. *Ann Surg* 1969;170:232–238.
436. Dragosics B, Bauer P, Radaszkiewicz T. Primary gastrointestinal non-Hodgkin's lymphomas: a retrospective clinicopathologic study of 150 cases. *Cancer* 1985;55:1060–1073.
437. Daling JR, Weiss NS, Klopfenstein LL, et al. Correlates of homosexual behavior and the incidence of anal cancer. *JAMA* 1982;247:1988–1990.
438. Peters RK, Mack TM. Patterns of anal cancinoma by gender and marital status in Los Angeles County. *Br J Cancer* 1983;48:629–636.
439. Formenti SC, Gill PS, Lean E, et al. Primary central nervous system lymphoma in AIDS: results of radiation therapy. *Cancer* 1989;63:1101–1107.
440. Raphael J, Gentilhomme O, Tulliez M, et al. Histopathologic features of high grade non-Hodgkin's lymphomas in acquired immunodeficiency syndrome. *Arch Pathol Lab Med* 1991;115:15–20.
441. Constantino A, West TE, Gupta M, et al. Primary cardiac lymphoma in a patient with acquired immune deficiency syndrome. *Cancer* 1987;60:2801–2805.
442. Gill PS, Chandraratna AN, Meyer PR, et al. Malignant lymphoma: cardiac involvement at initial presentation. *J Clin Oncol* 1987;5:216–224.
443. Brooks HL, Downing J, McClure JA, et al. Orbital Burkitt's lymphoma in a homosexual man with acquired immune deficiency. *Arch Ophthalmol* 1984;102:1533–1537.
444. Kaplan LD, Kahn J, Jacobson M, et al. Primary bile duct lymphoma in the acquired immunodeficiency syndrome (AIDS). *Ann Intern Med* 1989;110:161–162.
445. Pollack RN, Sklarin NT, Rao S, et al. Metastatic placental lymphoma associated with maternal human immunodeficiency virus infection. *Obstet Gynecol* 1993;81:856–857.
446. Levecq H, Hautefeuille M, Hoang C, et al. Primary stomal lymphoma: an unusual complication of ileostomy in a patient with transfusion-related acquired immune deficiency syndrome. *Cancer* 1990;65:1028–1032.
447. Louie S, Daoust PR, Schwartz RS. Immunodeficiency and the pathogenesis of non-Hodgkin's lymphoma. *Semin Oncol* 1980;7:267–284.
448. Krivitzky A, Bentata-Pessayre M, et al. Lymphome malin initialement fessier: rôle possible des injections intra-musculaires repeteöes. *Ann Intern Med* 1984;135:205–207.
449. Henry JM, Heffner RR Jr, Dillard SH, et al. Primary malignant lymphomas of the central nervous system. *Cancer* 1974;34:1293–1302.
450. Freeman C, Berg JW, Cutler SJ. Occurrence and prognosis of extranodal lymphomas. *Cancer* 1972;29:252–260.
451. Good AE, Russo RH, Schnitzer B, et al. Intracranial histiocytic lymphoma with rheumatoid arthritis. *J Rheumatol* 1978;5:75–78.
452. Gill PS, Graham RA, Boswell W, et al. A comparison of imaging, clinical and pathologic aspects of space occupying lesions within the brain in patients with acquired immunodeficiency syndrome. *Am J Physiol Imaging* 1986;1:134–141.
453. Goldstein JD, Dickson DW, Moser FG, et al. Primary central nervous system lymphoma in acquired immunodeficiency syndrome: a clinical and pathologic study with results of treatment with radiation. *Cancer* 1991;67:2756–2765.
454. MacMahon EME, Glass JD, Hayward SD, et al. Epstein Barr virus in AIDS-related primary central nervous system lymphoma. *Lancet* 1991;338:969–973.
455. Baumgartner JE, Rachlin JR, Beckstead JH, et al. Primary central nervous system lymphomas: natural history and response to radiation therapy in 55 patients with acquired immunodeficiency syndrome. *J Neurosurg* 1990;73:206–211.
456. Lee YY, Bruner JM, Van Tassle P, et al. Primary central nervous system lymphoma: CT and pathologic correlation. *Am J Neurol Radiol* 1986;7:599–604.
457. Kelly WM, Brant-Zawadski M. Acquired immunodeficiency syndrome: neuroradiologic findings. *Radiology* 1983;49:485–491.
458. Edwards KR, Pendlebury WW. Central nervous system lymphoma versus toxoplasmosis in a patient with AIDS. *N Engl J Med* 1987;317:1540.
459. Levine AM. AIDS-related malignancies: the emerging epidemic. *J Natl Cancer Inst* 1993;85:1382–1397.
460. Bishburg E, Eng RHK, Slim J, et al. Brain lesions in patients with acquired immunodeficiency syndrome. *Arch Intern Med* 1989;149:941–943.
461. Ciricillo SF, Rosenblum ML. Use of CT and MR imaging to distinguish intracranial lesions and to define the need for biopsy in AIDS patients. *J Neurosurg* 1990;73:720–724.
462. Knowles DM, Inghirami G, Ubraico A, et al. Molecular genetic analysis of three AIDS-associated neoplasms of uncertain lineage demonstrates their B-cell derivation and the possible pathogenetic role of the Epstein-Barr virus. *Blood* 1989;73:792–799.
463. Walts AE, Shintaku IP, Said JW. Diagnosis of malignant lymphoma in effusions from patients with AIDS by gene rearrangement. *Am J Clin Pathol* 1990;94:170–175.
464. Karcher DS, Dawkins F, Garrett CT, et al. Body cavity-based non-Hodgkin's lymphoma (NHL) in HIV-infected patients: B-cell lymphoma with unusual clinical, immunophenotypic, and genotypic features. *Lab Invest* 1992;66[Suppl]:80A.
465. Green I, Espiritu E, Ladanyi M, et al. Primary lymphomatous effusions in AIDS: amorphological, immunophenotypic, and molecular study. *Mod Pathol* 1995;8:39–45.
466. Cesarman E, Chang Y, Moore PS, et al. Kaposi's sarcoma-associated herpesvirus-like DNA sequences are present in AIDS-related body cavity based lymphomas. *N Engl J Med* 1995;332:1186–1191.
467. Nador RG, Cesarman E, Chadburn A, et al. Primary effusion lymphoma: a distinct clinicopathologic entity associated with the Kaposi's sarcoma-associated herpesvirus. *Blood* 1996;88:645–656.

468. Raphael MM, Audouin J, Lamine M, et al. Immunophenotypic and genotypic analysis of acquired immunodeficiency syndrome-related non-Hodgkin's lymphoma: correlation with histologic features in 36 cases. *Am J Clin Pathol* 1994;101:773–782.
469. The Non-Hodgkin's Lymphoma Classification Project. National Cancer Institute sponsored study of classification of non-Hodgkin's lymphomas: summary and description of a working formulation for clinical usage. *Cancer* 1982;49:2112–2135.
470. Tirelli U, Vaccher E, Zagonel V, et al. CD30 (Ki-1)-positive anaplastic large-cell lymphomas in 13 patients with and 27 patients without human immunodeficiency virus infection: the first comparative clinicopathologic study from a single institution that also includes 80 patients with other human immunodeficiency virus-related systemic lymphomas. *J Clin Oncol* 1995;13:373–380.
471. Carbone A, Gloghini A, Volpe R, et al, and the Italian Cooperative Group on AIDS and Tumors. High frequency of Epstein-Barr virus latent membrane protein-1 expression in acquired immunodeficiency syndrome-related Ki-1 (CD30)-positive anaplastic large cell lymphomas. *Am J Clin Pathol* 1994;101:768–772.
472. Harris NL, Jaffe ES, Stein H, et al. A revised European-American classification of lymphoid neoplasms: a proposal from the International Lymphoma Study Group. *Blood* 1994;84:1361–1392.
473. Chadburn A, Cesarman E, Jagirdar J, et al. CD30 (Ki-1) positive anaplastic large cell lymphomas in individuals infected with the human immunodeficiency virus. *Cancer* 1993;72:3078–3090.
474. Berard C, O'Connor GT, Thomas LB, et al. Histopathological definition of Burkitt's tumor. *Bull World Health Organ* 1969;40:601–607.
475. Rappaport H. Tumors of the hematopoietic system. In: *Atlas of tumor pathology*, section 3, fascicle 8. Washington, DC: Armed Forces Institute of Pathology, 1966.
476. Hui PK, Feller AC, Lennert K. High-grade non-Hodgkin's lymphoma of B-cell type: I. histopathology. *Histopathology* 1988;12:127–143.
477. Pelicci PG, Knowles DM, Arlin Z, et al. Multiple monoclonal B-cell expansions and c-myc oncogene rearrangements in AIDS-related lymphoproliferative disorders: implications for lymphomagenesis. *J Exp Med* 1986;164:2049–2060.
478. Egerter DA, Beckstead JH. Malignant lymphomas in the acquired immunodeficiency syndrome: additional evidence for a B-cell origin. *Arch Pathol Lab Med* 1988;112:602–609.
479. Barriga F, Whang-Peng J, Lee E, et al. Development of a second clonally discrete Burkitt's lymphoma in a human immunodeficiency virus-positive homosexual patient. *Blood* 1988;72:792–795.
480. Subar M, Neri A, Inghirami G, et al. Frequent c-myc oncogene activation and infrequent presence of Epstein-Barr virus genome in AIDS-associated lymphoma. *Blood* 1988;72:667–671.
481. Ballerini P, Gaidano G, Gong JZ, et al. Multiple genetic lesions in AIDS-related non-Hodgkin lymphoma. *Blood* 1993;81:166–176.
482. McGrath MS, Shiramizu B, Meeker TC, et al. AIDS-associated polyclonal lymphoma: identification of a new HIV-associated disease process. *J Acquir Immune Defic Syndr* 1991;4:408–415.
483. Meeker TC, Shiramizu B, Kaplan L, et al. Evidence for molecular subtypes of HIV associated lymphoma: division into peripheral monoclonal, polyclonal and central nervous system lymphoma. *AIDS* 1991; 5:669–674.
484. Shiramizu B, Herndier B, Meeker T, et al. Molecular and immunophenotypic characterization of AIDS-associated, Epstein-Barr virus-negative polyclonal lymphoma. *J Clin Oncol* 1992;10:383–389.
485. Kaplan LD, Shiramizu B, Herndier B, et al. Influence of molecular characteristics on clinical outcome in human immunodeficiency virus-associated non Hodgkin's lymphoma: identification of a subgroup with favorable clinical outcome. *Blood* 1995;85:1727–1735.
486. Seiden M, Sklar J. AIDS and non-Hodgkin's lymphoma: a pre-B cell monoclonal lymphoma versus a novel mechanism of polyclonality. *J Clin Oncol* 1992;10:1650–1651.
487. Nador RG, Chadburn A, Cesarman E, et al. Correlative morphologic and molecular genetic analysis of 74 AIDS-related systemic non-Hodgkin lymphomas. (*submitted*).
488. Gaidano G, Lo Coco F, Ye BH, et al. Rearrangements of the BCL-6 gene in AIDS-associated non-Hodgkin's lymphoma: association with diffuse large cell subtype. *Blood* 1994;84:397–402.
489. Dalla-Favera R, Bregni M, Erikson J, et al. Human c-myc oncogene is located on the region of chromosome 8 that is translocated in Burkitt's lymphoma cells. *Proc Natl Acad Sci USA* 1982;79:7824–7827.
490. Dalla-Favera R, Martinotti S, Gallor RC, et al. Translocation and rearrangement of the c-myc oncogene locus in human undifferentiated B-cell lymphomas. *Science* 1983;219:963–967.
491. Croce CM, Nowell PC. Molecular genetics of human B cell neoplasia. *Adv Immunol* 1986;38:245–274.
492. Lenoir GM, Preud'homme JL, Bernheim A, et al. Correlation between immunoglobulin light chain expression and variant translocation in Burkitt's lymphoma. *Nature* 1982;298:474–476.
493. Rechavi G, Ben-Bassat I, Berkowicz M, et al. Molecular analysis of Burkitt's leukemia in two hemophilic brothers with AIDS. *Blood* 1987;70:1713–1717.
494. Magrath I, Erikson J, Whang-Peng J, et al. Synthesis of kappa light chains by cell lines containing an 8:22 chromosomal translocation derived from a male homosexual with Burkitt's lymphoma. *Science* 1983;222:1094–1098.
495. Delecluse HJ, Raphael M, Magaud JP, et al. Variable morphology of human immunodeficiency virus-associated lymphomas with c-myc rearrangements: the French Study Group of Pathology for Human Immunodeficiency Virus-Associated Tumors. *Blood* 1993;82: 552–563.
496. Carbone A, Tirelli U, Gloghini A, et al. Human immunodeficiency virus-associated systemic lymphomas may be subdivided into two main groups according to Epstein-Barr viral latent gene expression. *J Clin Oncol* 1993;11:1674–1681.
497. Carbone A, Gloghini A, Gaidano G, et al. AIDS-related Burkitt's lymphoma. *Am J Clin Pathol* 1995;103:561–567.
498. Rooney CM, Gregory CD, Rowe M, et al. Endemic Burkitt's lymphoma: phenotypic analysis of tumor biopsy cells and of derived tumor cell lines. *J Natl Cancer Inst* 1986;77:681–687.
499. Rowe DT, Rowe M, Evan GI, et al. Restricted expression of EBV latent genes and T-lymphocyte-detected membrane antigen in Burkitt's lymphoma cells. *EMBO J* 1986;5:2599–2607.
500. Rowe M, Rowe DT, Gregory CD, et al. Differences in B cell growth phenotype reflect novel patterns of Epstein-Barr virus latent gene expression in Burkitt's lymphoma cells. *EMBO J* 1987;6:2743–2751.
501. Gaidano G, Dalla-Favera R. Molecular pathogenesis of AIDS-related lymphomas. *Antibiot Chemother* 1994;46:117–124.
502. Magrath IT. Burkitt's lymphoma as a human tumor model: new concepts in etiology and pathogenesis. In: Pochedly C, ed. *Pediatric hem/oncology reviews.* New York: Praeger, 1985:1–57.
503. Dalla-Favera R. Chromosomal translocations involving the c-myc oncogene and their role in the pathogenesis of B-cell neoplasia. In Brugge J, Curran T, Harlow E, McCormick F (eds). *Origins of human cancer: a comprehensive review.* Cold Spring Harbor: Cold Spring Harbor Laboratory Press, 1991; 543–551.
504. Pelicci PG, Knowles DM, MaGrath I, et al. Chromosomal breakpoints and structural alterations of the c-myc locus differ in endemic and sporadic forms of Burkitt lymphoma. *Proc Natl Acad Sci USA* 1986; 83:2984–2988.
505. Shiramizu B, Barriga F, Neequaye J, et al. Patterns of chromosomal breakpoint locations in Burkitt's lymphoma: relevance to geography and Epstein-Barr virus association. *Blood* 1991;77:1516–1526.
506. Lanfrancone L, Pelicci PG, Dalla-Favera R. Structure and expression of translocated c-myc oncogenes: specific differences in endemic, sporadic and AIDS-associated forms of Burkitt lymphomas. *Curr Top Microbiol Immunol* 1986;132:257–265.
507. Neri A, Barriga F, Knowles DM, et al. Different regions of the immunoglobulin heavy-chain locus are involved in chromosomal translocations in distinct pathogenetic forms of Burkitt lymphoma. *Proc Natl Acad Sci USA* 1988;85:2748–2752.
508. Ye BH, Rao PH, Chaganti RSK, et al. Cloning of BCL-6, the locus involved in chromosome translocations affecting band 3q27 in B-cell lymphoma. *Cancer Res* 1993;53:2732–2735.
509. Offit K, Jhanwar S, Ebrahim S, et al. t(3;22)(q27;q11): a novel translocation associated with diffuse non-Hodgkin's lymphoma. *Blood* 1989; 74:1876–1879.
510. Bastard C, Tilly H, Lenormand B, et al. Translocations involving band 3q27 and Ig gene regions in non-Hodgkin's lymphoma. *Blood* 1992; 79:2527–2531.
511. Bastard C, Tilly H. Response to t(2;3)(p12;q27) in Hodgkin's disease of a human immunodeficiency virus-positive patient with hemophilia. *Blood* 1993;81:265.
512. Ye BH, Lista F, Lo Coco F, et al. Alterations of a zinc-finger encoding gene, BCL-6, in diffuse large cell-lymphoma. *Science* 1993;262: 747–750.

513. Kerckaert J-P, Deweindt C, Tilly H, et al. LAZ3, a novel zinc-finger encoding gene, is disrupted by recurring chromosome 3q27 translocations in human lymphoma. *Nat Genet* 1993;5:66–70.
514. Baron BW, Nucifora G, McCabe N, et al. Identification of the gene associated with the recurring chromosomal translocations t(3;14)(q27; q32) and t(3; 22) (q27; q11) in B-cell lymphomas. *Proc Natl Acad Sci USA* 1993;90:5262–5266.
515. Cattoretti G, Chang CC, Cechova K, et al. BCL-6 protein is expressed in germinal center B cells. *Blood* 1995;86:45–53.
516. Ye BH, Cattoretti G, Shen Q, et al. The BCL-6 proto-oncogene controls germinal center formation and Th2-type inflammation. *Nat Genet* 1997;16:161–170.
517. Lo Coco F, Ye BH, Lista F, et al. Rearrangements of the BCL6 gene in diffuse large cell non-Hodgkin's lymphoma. *Blood* 1994,83: 1757–1759.
518. Offit K, LoCoco F, Louie DC, et al. Rearrangement of the bcl-6 gene as a prognostic marker in diffuse large cell lymphoma. *N Engl J Med* 1994;331:74–80.
519. Bos JL. Ras oncogenes in human cancer: a review. *Cancer Res* 1989; 49:4682--4689.
520. Neri A, Baldini L, Ferrero D, et al. Frequency and type of ras oncogenes in lymphoid malignancies. In: *Molecular diagnostics of human cancer: cancer cells*, vol. 7. Cold Spring Harbor Laboratory, 1989; 101–105.
521. Neri A, Knowles DM, McCormick F, et al. Analysis of ras oncogene mutations in human lymphoid malignancies. *Proc Natl Acad Sci USA* 1988;85:9268–9272.
522. Neri A, Murphy J, Cro L, et al. Ras oncogene mutation in multiple myeloma. *J Exp Med* 1989;170:1715–1725.
523. Seremetis S, Inghirami G, Ferrero D, et al. Transformation and plasmacytoid differentiation of EBV-infected human B lymphoblasts by ras oncogenes. *Science* 1989;243:660–663.
524. Raffeld M, Jaffe ES. bcl-1, t(11;14), and mantle cell-derived lymphomas. *Blood* 1991;78:259–263.
525. Tsujimoto Y, Cossman J, Jaffe E, et al. Involvement of the bcl-2 gene in human follicular lymphoma. *Science* 1985;228:1440–1443.
526. Weiss LM, Warnke RA, Sklar J, et al. Molecular analysis of the t(14; 18) chromosomal translocation in malignant lymphomas. *N Engl J Med* 1987;317:1185–1189.
527. Athan E, Foitl DR, Knowles DM. bcl-1 gene rearrangement: frequency and clinical significance among B cell chronic lymphocytic leukemias and non-Hodgkin's lymphomas. *Am J Pathol* 1991;138: 591–599.
528. Goodrich DW, Lee WH. The molecular genetics of retinoblastoma. *Cancer Surv* 1990;9:529–554.
529. Hollstein M, Sidransky D, Vogelstein B, et al. p53 mutations in human cancers. *Science* 1991;253:49–53.
530. Levine AJ, Momand J, Finlay CA. The p53 tumor suppressor gene. *Nature* 1991; 351:453–456.
531. Offit K, Wong G, Filippa DA, et al. Cytogenetic analysis of 434 consecutively ascertained specimens of non-Hodgkin's lymphoma: clinical correlations. *Blood* 1991;77:1508–1515.
532. Baker SJ, Fearon ER, Nigro JM, et al. Chromosome 17 deletion and p53 gene mutations in colorectal carcinomas. *Science* 1989;244: 217–221.
533. Nigro JM, Baker SJ, Preisinger AC, et al. Mutations in the p53 gene occur in diverse human tumour types. *Nature* 1989;342:705–708.
534. Gaidano G, Ballerini P, Gong JZ, et al. p53 mutations in human lymphoid malignancies: association with Burkitt's lymphoma and chronic lymphocytic leukemia. *Proc Natl Acad Sci USA* 1991;88: 5413–5427.
535. Cesarman E, Chadburn A, Inghirami G, et al. Structural and functional analysis of oncogenes and tumor suppressor genes in adult T cell leukemia/lymphoma (ATLL) reveals frequent p53 mutations. *Blood* 1992;80:3205–3216.
536. Gaidano G, Dalla-Favera R. Molecular pathogenesis of AIDS-related lymphomas. *Adv Can Res* 1995;67:113–153.
537. Ronen D, Rotter V, Reisman D. Expression from the murine p53 promoter is mediated by factor binding to a downstream helix-loop-helix recognition motif. *Proc Natl Acad Sci USA* 1991;88:4128–4132.
538. Gaidano G, Dalla-Favera R. Molecular biology of lymphoid neoplasms. In: Mendelsohn J, Howley PM, Israel MA, eds. *The molecular basis of cancer*. Philadelphia: WB Saunders, 1995:251–272.
539. Hayashi Y, Raimondi SC, Look AT, et al. Abnormalities of the long arm of chromosome 6 in childhood acute lymphoblastic leukemia. *Blood* 1990;76:1626–1630.
540. Millikin D, Meese E, Vogelstein B, et al. Loss of heterozygocity for loci on the long arm of chromosome 6 in human malignant melanoma. *Cancer Res* 1991;51:5449–5453.
541. Morita S, Saito S, Ishikawa J, et al. Common regions of deletion on chromosomes 5q,6q, and 10q in renal cell carcinoma. *Cancer Res* 1991;51:5817–5820.
542. Offit K, Parsa NZ, Gaidano G, et al. 6q deletions define distinct clinico-pathologic subsets of non-Hodgkin's lymphoma. *Blood* 1993;82: 2157–2162.
543. Dryja TP, Rapaport JM, Joyce JM, et al. Molecular detection of deletions involving band q14 of chromosome 13 in retinoblastoma. *Proc Natl Acad Sci USA* 1986;83:7391–7394.
544. Ludlow JW, Shon J, Pipas JM, et al. The retinoblastoma susceptibility gene product undergoes cell cycle-dependent dephosphorylation and binding to and release from SV40 large T. *Cell* 1990;60:387–396.
545. Goodrich DW, Lee WH. The molecular genetics of retinoblastoma. *Cancer Surv* 1990;9:529–554.
546. Yandell DW, Campbell TA, Dayton SH, et al. Oncogenic point mutations in the human retinoblastoma gene: their application to genetic counseling. *N Engl J Med* 1989;321:1689–1695.
547. Haber MM, Inghirami G, Dalla-Favera R, et al. Retinoblastoma (Rb) gene product expression in B cell non-Hodgkin's lymphomas (NHLs) and lymphoid leukemias (LLs). *Lab Invest* 1991;64:73a.
548. Gaidano G, Parsa NZ, Tassi V, et al. In vitro establishment of AIDS-related lymphoma cell lines: phenotypic characterization, oncogene and tumor suppressor ene lesions, and heterogeneity in Epstein-Barr virus infection. *Leukemia* 1993;7:1621–1629.
549. Baumgartner J, Rachlin J, Rosenblum M, et al. Patterns of gene rearrangement in AIDS-associated primary central nervous system lymphoma (PCNSL). *Proc ASCO* 1989; 8:991.
550. Weinberg RA. Oncogenes, anti-oncogenes and the molecular bases of multistep carcinogenesis. *Cancer Res* 1989;49:3713–3721.
551. Fearon ER, Vogelstein B. A genetic model for colorectal tumorigenesis. *Cell* 1990;61:759–767.
552. Knowles DM. The molecular pathology of AIDS-related non-Hodgkin's lymphoma. *Semin Diagn Pathol* 1997;14:67–82.
553. Carbone PP, Kaplan HS, Musshoff K, et al. Report of the Committee on Hodgkin's Disease Staging Classification. *Cancer Res* 1971;31: 1860–1861.
554. Shipp MA, Harrington DP, Klatt MM, et al. Identification of major prognostic subgroups with large cell lymphoma treated with m-BACOD or M-BACOD. *Ann Intern Med* 1986;104:757–765.
555. Hoskins PJ, Ng V, Spinelli JJ, et al. Prognostic variables in patients with diffuse large cell lymphoma treated with MACOP-B. *J Clin Oncol* 1991;9:220–226.
556. Straus DJ. Human immunodeficiency virus-associated lymphomas. *Med Clin North Am* 1997;81:495–510.
557. Galetto G, Levine A. AIDS-associated primary central nervous system lymphoma. *JAMA* 1993;269:92–93.
558. Cinque P, Brytting M, Vago L, et al. Epstein-Barr virus DNA in cerebrospinal fluid from patients with AIDS-related primary lymphoma of the central nervous system. *Lancet* 1993;342:398–401.
559. DeLuca A, Antinori A, Cingolani A, et al. Evaluation of cerebrospinal fluid EBV-DNA and IL-10 as markers for in vivo diagnosis of AIDS-related primary central nervous system lymphoma. *Br J Haematol* 1995;90:844–849.
560. Raphael B, Knowles DM. AIDS-associated non-Hodgkin's lymphoma. *Semin Oncol* 1990;17:361–366.
561. Gill PS, Levine AM, Krailo M, et al. AIDS-related malignant lymphoma: results of prospective treatment trials. *J Clin Oncol* 1987;5: 1322–1328.
562. Bermudez MA, Grant KM, Rovien R, et al. Non-Hodgkin's lymphoma in a population with or at risk for AIDS: indications for intensive chemotherapy. *Am J Med* 1989;86:71–76.
563. Skarin AT, Canellos GP, Rosenthal DS, et al. Improved prognosis of diffuse histiocytic and undifferentiated lymphoma by use of high dose methotrexate alternating with standard agents (M-BACOD). *J Clin Oncol* 1983;1:91–98.
564. Levine AM, Wernz JC, Kaplan L, et al. Low-dose chemotherapy with central nervous system prophylaxis and azidothymidine maintenance in AIDS-related lymphoma: a prospective multi-institutional trial. *JAMA* 1991;266:84–88.

565. Levine AM, Wernz JC, Kaplan L, et al. Low dose chemotherapy with central nervous system prophylaxis and zidovudine maintenance in AIDS-related lymphoma: a prospective multi-institutional trial. *JAMA* 1991;266:84–88.
566. Walsh C, Wernz, J, Levine AM, et al. Phase I study of M-BACOD and GM-CSF in AIDS-associated non-Hodgkin's lymphoma. *J AIDS* 1993;6:265–271.
567. Kaplan LD, Kahn JO, Crowe S, et al. Clinical and virologic effects of recombinant human granulocyte-macrophage colony-stimulating factor in patients receiving chemotherapy for human immunodeficiency virus-associated non-Hodgkin's lymphoma: results of a randomized trial. *J Clin Oncol* 1991;9:929–940.
568. Haddy TB, Adde MA, Magrath IT. CNS involvement in small noncleaved cell lymphoma: is CNS disease per se a poor prognostic sign? *J Clin Oncol* 1991;9: 973–982.
569. Chamberlain MC. Long survival in patients with acquired immune deficiency syndrome-related primary central nervous system lymphoma. *Cancer* 1994;73:1728–1730.
570. Forsyth PA, Yahalom J, DeAngelis LM. Combined modality therapy in the treatment of primary central nervous system lymphoma in AIDS. *Neurology* 1994;44:1473–1479.
571. Woodman R, Shin K, Pineo G. Primary non-Hodgkin's lymphoma of the brain: a review. *Medicine* 1985;64:425–430.
572. Karcher DS, Alkan S. Herpes-like DNA sequences. AIDS-related tumors, and Castleman's disease. *N Engl J Med* 1995;333:797–798.
573. Pastore C, Gloghini A, Volpe G, et al. Distribution of Kaposi's sarcoma herpesvirus sequences among malignancies in Italy and Spain. *Br J Haematol* 1995;91:918–920.
574. Carbone A, Tirelli U, Gloghini A, et al. Herpesvirus-like DNA sequences selectively cluster with body cavity-based lymphomas throughout the spectrum of AIDS-related lymphomatous effusions. *Eur J Cancer* 1996;32A:555–556.
575. Otsuki T, Kumar S, Ensoli B, et al. Detection of HHV-8/KSHV DNA sequences in AIDS-associated extranodal lymphoid malignancies. *Leukemia* 1996;10:1358–1362.
576. Robert C, Agbalika F, Blanc F, et al. HIV-negative patient with HHV-8 DNA follicular B-cell lymphoma associated with Kaposi's sarcoma. *Lancet* 1996;347:1042–1043.
577. Luppi M, Barozzi P, Marasca R, et al. HHV-8-associated primary cerebral B-cell lymphoma in HIV-negative patient after long-term steroids. *Lancet* 1996;347:980.
578. Corboy JR, Garl PJ, Kleinschmidt-DeMasters BK. Human herpesvirus 8 DNA in CNS lymphomas from patients with and without AIDS. *Neurol* 1998;50:335–340.
579. Mikol DM, Deplanche M, Moulinier A, et al. Herpes virus-like DNA sequences in primary non-Hodgkin's lymphomas of the central nervous system. *J Neuropathol Exp Neurol* 1996;55:623.
580. Morgello S, Tagliati M, Ewart MR. HHV-8 and AIDS-related CNS lymphoma. *Neurology* 1997;48:1333–1335.
581. Gaidano G, Capello D, Pastore C, et al. Analysis of human herpesvirus type 8 infection in AIDS-related and AIDS-unrelated primary central nervous system lymphoma. *Am J Pathol* 1996;149:1193–1197.
582. Iuchi K, Ichimiya A, Akashi A, et al. Non-Hodgkin's lymphoma of the pleural cavity developing from long-standing pyothorax. *Cancer* 1987;60:1771–1775.
583. Iuchi K, Aozasa K, Yamamoto S, et al. Non-Hodgkin's lymphoma of the pleural cavity developing from long-standing pyothorax: summary of clinical and pathological findings in thirty-seven cases. *Jpn J Clin Oncol* 1989;19:249–257.
584. Fukayama M, Ibuka T, Hayashi Y, et al. Epstein-Barr virus in pyothorax-associated pleural lymphoma. *Am J Pathol* 1993;143:1044–1049.
585. Cesarman E, Nador RG, Aozasa K, et al. Kaposi's sarcoma-associated herpesvirus in non-AIDS-related lymphomas occurring in body cavities. *Am J Pathol* 1996;149:53–57.
586. Hermine O, Michel M, Buzyn-Veil A, et al. Body-cavity-based lymphoma in an HIV-seronegative patient without Kaposi's sarcoma-associated herpesvirus-like DNA sequences. *N Engl J Med* 1996;334: 272.
587. Ansari MQ, Dawson DB, Nador R, et al. Primary body cavity based AIDS-related lymphomas. *Am J Clin Pathol* 1996;105:221–229.
588. Nador RG, Cesarman E, Knowles DM, et al. Herpes-like DNA sequences in a body-cavity-based lymphoma in an HIV-negative patient. *N Engl J Med* 1995; 333:943.
589. Said JW, Tasaka T, Takeuchi S, et al. Primary effusion lymphoma in women: report of two cases of Kaposi's sarcoma herpes virus-associated effusion-based lymphoma in human immunodeficiency virus-negative women. *Blood* 1996;88:3124–3128.
590. de Pond W, Said JW, Tasaka T, et al. Kaposi's sarcoma associated herpesvirus/human herpesvirus 8 (KSHV/HHV8)-associated lymphoma of the bowel: report of two cases in HIV-positive men with secondary effusion lymphomas. *Am J Surg Pathol* 1997;21:719–724.
591. Gaidano G, Capello D, Cilia AM, et al. Genetic characterization of HHV-8/KSHV-positive primary effusion lymphoma reveals frequent mutations of BCL6: implications for disease pathogenesis and histogenesis. *Genes Chromosomes Cancer* 1999;24:16–23.
592. Küppers R, Zhao M, Hansmann ML, et al. Tracing B cell development in human germinal centres by molecular analysis of single cells picked from histological sections. *EMBO J* 1993;12:4955–4967.
593. Pascual V, Liu YJ, Magalski A, et al. Analysis of somatic mutation in five B cell subsets of human tonsil. *J Exp Med* 1994;180:329–339.
594. Matolcsy A, Nador RG, Cesarman E, et al. Immunoglobulin VH gene mutational analysis suggests that primary effusion lymphoma derive from different stages of B cell maturation. *Am J Pathol* 1998;153: 1609–1614.
595. Bahler DW, Levy R. Clonal evolution of a follicular lymphoma: evidence for antigen selection. *Proc Natl Acad Sci USA* 1992;89: 6770–6774.
596. Zelenetz AD, Chen TT, Levy R. Clonal expansion in follicular lymphoma occurs subsequent to antigenic selection. *J Exp Med* 1992; 176:1137–1148.
597. Chapman CJ, Spellerberg MB, Hamblin TJ, et al. Pattern of usage of the VH4-21 gene by B lymphocytes in a patient with EBV infection indicates ongoing mutation and class switching. *Mol Immunol* 1995; 32:347–353.
598. Chapman CJ, Mockridge CI, Rowe M, et al. Analysis of VH genes used by neoplastic B cell in endemic Burkitt's lymphoma shows somatic hypermutation and intraclonal heterogeneity. *Blood* 1995;85: 2176–2181.
599. Miklos JA, Locker J, Bahler DW. Evidence for antigen selection in post-transplant lymphoproliferative disorders. *Lab Invest* 1995; 72[Suppl]:116A.
600. Kanzler H, Küppers R, Hansmann ML, et al. Hodgkin and Reed-Sternberg cells in Hodgkin's disease represent the outgrowth of a dominant tumor clone derived from (crippled) germinal center B cells. *J Exp Med* 1996;184:1495–1505.
601. Lombardi L, Newcomb EW, Dalla-Favera R. Pathogenesis of Burkitt lymphoma: expression of an activated c-myc oncogene causes the tumorigenic conversion of EBV-infected human B lymphoblasts. *Cell* 1987;49:161–170.
602. Flamand L, Stefanescu I, Ablashi DV, et al. Activation of the Epstein-Barr virus replicative cycle by human herpesvirus 6. *J Virol* 1993; 67:6768–6777.
603. Horenstein MG, Nador RG, Chadburn A, et al. Epstein-Barr virus latent gene expression in primary effusion lymphomas containing Kaposi's sarcoma-associated herpesvirus/human herpesvirus-8. *Blood* 1997;90:1186–1191.
604. Rickinson AB, Kieff E. Epstein-Barr virus. In Fields BN, ed. *Virology*. Philadelphia: Lippincott-Raven, 1996:2397–2446.
605. Rowe M, Rowe D, Gregory C, et al. Differences in B cell growth phenotype reflect novel patterns of Epstein-Barr virus latent gene expression in Burkitt's lymphoma cells. *EMBO J* 1987;6:2743–2751.
606. Tierney R, Steven N, Young L, et al. Epstein-Barr virus latency in blood mononuclear cells: analysis of viral gene transcription during primary infection and in the carrier state. *J Virol* 1994;68:7374–7385.
607. Kieff E. Epstein-Barr virus and its replication. In Fields BN, ed. *Virology*. Philadelphia: Lippincott-Raven, 1996:2343–2396.
608. Young L, Alfieri C, Hennessy K, et al. Expression of Epstein-Barr virus transformation-associated genes in tissues of patients with EBV lymphoproliferative disease. *N Engl J Med* 1989;321:1080–1085.
609. Herbst H, Dallenbach F, Hummel M, et al. Epstein-Barr virus latent membrane protein expression in Hodgkin and Reed-Sternberg cells. *Proc Natl Acad Sci USA* 1991;88:4766–4770.
610. Fleckenstein B, Desrosiers RC. Herpesvirus saimiri and herpesvirus ateles. In: Roizman B, ed. *The herpesviruses*. New York: Plenum Press, 1982:253–332.
611. Biesinger B, Muller-Fleckenstein J, Simmer B, et al. Stable growth transformation of human T lymphocytes by herpesvirus saimiri. *Proc Natl Acad Sci USA* 1992;89:3116–3119.

612. Chang Y, Moore PS, Talbot SJ, et al. Cyclin encoded by Kaposi's sarcoma herpesvirus. *Nature* 1996;382:410.
613. Arvanitakis L, Geras-Raaka E, Gershengorn MC, et al. Kaposi's sarcoma herpesvirus encodes a constitutively active G protein-coupled receptor linked to cell proliferation. *Nature* 1997;385:347–350.
614. Tsujimoto Y, Finger LR, Yunis J, et al. Cloning of the chromosome breakpoint of neoplastic B cells with the t(14:18) chromosome translocation. *Science* 1984;226:1097–1099.
615. Young D, Waitches G, Birchmeier C, et al. Isolation and characterization of a new cellular oncogene encoding a protein with multiple potential transmembrane domains. *Cell* 1986;45:711–719.
616. Jackson TR, Blair LA, Marshall J, et al. The mas oncogene encodes an angiotensin receptor. *Nature* 1988;335:437–440.
617. Arnold A, Kim HG, Gaz RD, et al. Molecular cloning and chromosomal mapping of DNA rearranged with the parathyroid hormone gene in a parathyroid adenoma. *J Clin Invest* 1989;83:2034–2040.
618. Motokura T, Bloom T, Kim HG, et al. A novel cyclin encoded by a bell-linked candidate oncogene. *Nature* 1991;350:512–515.
619. Zhang YJ, Jiang W, Chen CJ, et al. Amplification and overexpression of cyclin D1 in human hepatocellular carcinoma. *Biochem Biophys Res Commun* 1993;196:1010–1016.
620. Parma J, Duprez L, Van Sande J, et al. Somatic mutations in the thyrotropin receptor gene cause hyperfunctioning thyroid adenomas. *Nature* 1993;365:649–651.
621. Russo D, Arturi F, Schlumberger M, et al. Activating mutations of the TSH receptor in differentiated thyroid carcinomas. *Oncogene* 1995;11:1907–1911.
622. Russo JJ, Bohenzky RA, Chien M-C, et al. Nucleotide sequence of the Kaposi's sarcoma-associated herpesvirus (HHV8). *Proc Natl Acad Sci USA* 1996;93: 14862–14867.
623. Migliazza A, Martinotti S, Chen W, et al. Frequent somatic hypermutation of the 5′ noncoding region of the BCL-6 gene in B-cell lymphoma. *Proc Natl Acad Sci USA* 1995;92:12520–12524.
624. Chadburn A, Cesarman E, Knowles DM. Molecular pathology of the post-transplantation lymphoproliferative disorders. *Semin Diagn Pathol* 1997;14:15–26.
625. Frizzera G, Hanto DW, Gajl-Peczalska KJ, et al. Polymorphic diffuse B-cell hyperplasias and lymphomas in renal transplant recipients. *Cancer Res* 1981;41:4262–4279.
626. Cleary ML, Sklar J. Lymphoproliferative disorders in cardiac transplant recipients are multiclonal lymphomas. *Lancet* 1984;ii:489–493.
627. Cleary ML, Nalesnik MA, Shearer WT, et al. Clonal analysis of transplant-associated lymphoproliferations based on the structure of the genomic termini of the Epstein-Barr virus. *Blood* 1988;72:349–352.
628. Nalesnik MA, Jaffe R, Starzl TE, et al. The pathology of posttransplant lymphoproliferative disorders occurring in the setting of cyclosporine A-prednisone immunosuppression. *Am J Pathol* 1988;133:173–192.
629. Locker J, Nalesnik M. Molecular genetic analysis of lymphoid tumors arising after organ transplantation. *Am J Pathol* 1989;135:977–987.
630. Nador, RG, Chadburn A, Gundappa G, et al. AIDS-related polymorphic lymphoproliferative disorders. (*Submitted*).
631. Frank D, Cesarman E, Liu YF, et al. Posttransplantation lymphoproliferative disorders frequently contain type A and not type B Epstein-Barr virus. *Blood* 1995;85:1396–1403.
632. Boyle MJ, Sewell WA, Sculley TB, et al. Subtypes of Epstein-Barr virus in human immunodeficiency virus-associated non-Hodgkin's lymphoma. *Blood* 1991; 78: 3004–3011.
633. Chadburn A, Chen JM, Hsu DT, et al. The morphologic and molecular genetic classification of post-transplantation lymphoproliferatie disorders (PT-LPDs) has clinical relevance. *Cancer* 1998;82:1978–1987.
634. Cesarman E, Chadburn A, Liu YF, et al. BCL-6 gene mutations in post-transplantation lymphoproliferative disorders (PT-LPDs) as predictors of response to therapy and clinical outcome. *Blood* 1998;92: 2294–2302.
635. Delecluse HJ, Anagnostopoulos F, Dallenbach F, et al. Plasmablastic lymphomas of the oral cavity: a new entity associated with the human immunodeficiency virus infection. *Blood* 1997;89:1413–1420.
636. Montagnier L, Gruest J, Chamaret S, et al. Adaptation of lymphadenopathy associated virus (LAV) to replication in EBV-transformed B lymphoblastoid cell lines. *Science* 1984;225:63–66.
637. Saxinger WC, Levine PH, Dean AG, et al. Evidence for exposure to HTLV-III in Uganda before 1973. *Science* 1985;227:1036–1038.
638. Laurence J, Astrin SM. Human immunodeficiency virus induction of malignant transformation in human B lymphocytes. *Proc Natl Acad Sci USA* 1991;88:7635–7639.
639. Ganser A, Carlo-Stella C, Bartram CR, et al. Establishment of two Epstein-Barr virus negative Burkitt cell lines from a patient with AIDS and B-cell lymphoma. *Blood* 1988;72:1255–1260.
640. Shibata D, Brynes RK, Nathwani B, et al. Human immunodeficiency viral DNA is readily found in lymph node biopsies from seropositive individuals. *Am J Pathol* 1989;135:697–702.
641. Feichtinger H, Rutkonen P, Parravicini C, et al. Malignant lymphomas in cynomolgus monkeys infected with simian immunodeficiency virus. *Am J Pathol* 1990;137:1311–1315.
642. Fauci AS, Schnittman SM, Poli G, et al. Immunopathogenic mechanisms in human immunodeficiency virus (HIV) infection. *Ann Intern Med* 1991;114:678–693.
643. Schnittman SM, Lane HC, Higgins SE, et al. Direct polyclonal activation of human B lymphocytes by the acquired immune deficiency syndrome virus. *Science* 1986;233:1084–1086.
644. Amariglio N, Vonsover A , Hakim I, et al. Immunoglobulin VH 3-positive AIDS-related Burkitt's lymphoma: a possible role for the HIV gp120 superantigen. *Acta Haematol* 1994;91:103–105.
645. Ng VL, Hurt MH, Fein CL, et al. IgMs produced by two acquired immune deficiency syndrome lymphoma cell lines: Ig binding specificity and VH-gene putative somatic mutation analysis. *Blood* 1994; 83:1067–1078.
646. Pantaleo G, Graziosi C, Fauci AS: Mechanisms of disease: the immuno-pathogenesis of human immunodeficiency virus infection. *N Engl J Med* 1993;328:327–335.
647. Moore RD, Kessler H, Richman DD, et al. Non-Hodgkin's lymphoma in patients with advanced HIV infection treated with zidovudine. *JAMA* 1991;265:2208–2211.
648. Pluda JM, Venzon DJ, Tosato G, et al. Parameters affecting the development of non-Hodgkin's lymphoma in patients with severe human immunodeficiency virus infection receiving antiretroviral therapy. *J Clin Oncol* 1993;11:1099–1107.
649. Birx DL, Redfield RR, Tosato G. Defective regulation of Epstein-Barr virus infection in patients with acquired immunodeficiency syndrome (AIDS) or AIDS-related disorders. *N Engl J Med* 1986;14:874–879.
650. Ramsay AD, Smith WJ, Isaacson PG. T-cell-rich B-cell lymphoma. *Am J Surg Pathol* 1988;12:433–443.
651. List AF, Spier CM, Miller TP, et al. Deficient tumor-infiltrating T-lymphocyte response in malignant lymphoma: relationship to HLA expression and host immunocompetence. *Leukemia* 1993;7:398–403.
652. Hirano T, Yasukawa K, Harada H, et al. Complementary DNA for a novel human interleukin (BSF-2) that induces B lymphocytes to produce immunoglobulin. *Nature* 1986;324:73–76.
653. Jelinek DF, Splawski JB, Lipsky PE. The roles of interleukin-2 and interferon-gamma in human B cell activation, growth and differentiation. *Eur J Immunol* 1986;16:925–932.
654. Jelinek DF, Lipsky PE. Enhancement of human B cell proliferation and differentiation by tumor necrosis factor-alpha and interleukin 1. *J Immunol* 1987;139:2970–2976.
655. Paul WE. Interleukin 4/B cell stimulatory factor 1: one lymphokine, many functions. *FASEB J* 1987;1:456–461.
656. Sharma S, Mehta S, Morgan J, et al. Molecular cloning and expression of a human B-cell growth factor gene in Escherichia coli. *Science* 1987;235:1489–1492.
657. Saeland S, Duvert V, Pandrau D, et al. Interleukin-7 induces the proliferation of normal human B cell precursors. *Blood* 1991;78: 2229–2238.
658. Zlotnik A, Morre KW. Interleukin 10. *Cytokine* 1991;3:366–371.
659. Scala G, Quinto I, Ruocco MR, et al. Expression of an exogenous interleukin 6 gene in human Epstein-Barr virus B cells confers growth advantage and in vivo tumorigenicity. *J Exp Med* 1990;172:61–68.
660. Tanner J, Tosato G. Impairment of natural killer functions by interleukin 6 increases lymphoblastoid cell tumorigenicity in athymic mice. *J Clin Invest* 1991;88:239–247.
661. Kawano M, Hirano T, Matsuda T, et al. Autocrine generation and requirement of BSF-2/IL-6 for human multiple myelomas. *Nature* 1988;332:83–85.
662. Kishimoto T. The biology of interleukin-6. *Blood* 1989;74:1–10.
663. Levy Y, Tsapis A, Brouet JC. Interleukin-6 antisense oligonucleotides inhibit the growth of human myeloma cell lines. *J Clin Invest* 1991; 88:696–699.
664. Schwab G, Siegall CB, Aarden LA, et al. Characterization of an in-

terleukin-6-mediated autocrine growth loop in the human multiple myeloma cell line, U266. *Blood* 1991;77:587–593.

665. Yee C, Biondi A, Wang XH, et al. A possible autocrine role of IL-6 in two lymphoma cell lines. *Blood* 1989;74:789–804.
666. Biondi A, Rossi V, Bassan R, et al. Constitutive expression of IL-6 gene in chronic lymphocytic leukemia. *Blood* 1989;73:1279–1284.
667. Nakajima K, Martinez-Maza O, Hirano T, et al. Induction of IL-6 (B cell stimulatory factor-2/IFN-beta-2) production by human immunodeficiency virus. *J Immunol* 1989;142:531–536.
668. Emilie D, Peuchmaur M, Maillot MC, et al. Production of interleukins in humanimmunodeficiency virus-1-replicating lymph nodes. *J Clin Invest* 1990;86:148–159.
669. Birx DL, Redfield RR, Tencer K, et al. Induction of interleukin-6 during human immunodeficiency virus infection. *Blood* 1990;76: 2303–2310.
670. Amadori A, Zamarchi R, Veronese ML, et al. B cell activation during HIV-1 infection: II. Cell-to-cell interactions and cytokine requirement. *J Immunol* 1991;146:57–62.
671. Breen EC, Rezai AR, Nakajima K, et al. Infection with HIV is associated with elevated IL-6 levels and production. *J Immunol* 1990;144: 480–484.
672. Emilie D, Coumbaras J, Raphael M, et al. Interleukin-6 production in high-grade B lymphomas: correlation with presence of malignant immunoblasts in acquired immunodeficiency syndrome and in human immunodeficiency virus seronegative patients. *Blood* 1992;80: 498–504.
673. Vieira P, deWaal-Malefyt R, Dang MN, et al. Isolation and expression of human cytokine synthesis inhibitory factor cDNA clones: homology to Epstein-Barr virus open reading frame BCRF1. *Proc Natl Acad Sci USA* 1991;88:1172–1176.
674. Benjamin D, Knobloch TJ, Abrams J, et al. Human B cell IL-10: B cell lines derived from patients with AIDS and Burkitt's lymphoma constitutively secrete large quantities of IL-10. *Blood* 1991;78:384a.
675. Masood R, Bond M, Scadden D, et al. Interleukin-10: autocrine B-cell growth factor for human B-cell lymphoma and the progenitors. *Blood* 1992;80:115a.
676. Fiorentino DF, Zlotnik A, Vieira P, et al. IL-10 acts on the antigen-presenting cell to inhibit cytokine production by Th1 cells. *J Immunol* 1991;146:3444–3451.
677. de Waal Malefyt R, Haanen J, Spits H, et al. Interleukin 10 (IL-10) and viral IL-10 strongly reduce antigen-specific human T cell proliferation by diminishing the antigen-presenting capacity of monocytes via downregulation of class II major histocompatibility complex expression. *J Exp Med* 1991;174:915–924.
678. Go BNF, Castle BE, Barrett R, et al. Interleukin 10, a novel B cell stimulatory factor: unresponsiveness of X chromosome-linked immunodeficiency B cells. *J Exp Med* 1990;172:1625–1631.
679. Rousset F, Garcia E, Defrance T, et al. Interleukin 10 is a potent growth and differentiation factor for activated human B lymphocytes. *Proc Natl Acad Sci USA* 1992;89:1890–1893.
680. de-The G, Geser A, Day NE, et al. Epidemiological evidence for casual relationship between Epstein-Barr virus and Burkitt's lymphoma from Ugandan prospective study. *Nature* 1978;274:756–761.
681. Klein G, Klein E. Evolution of tumors and the impact of molecular oncology. *Nature* 1985;315:190–195.
682. Geser A, de-The G, Lenoir G, et al. Final case reporting from the Uganda prospective study of the relationship between EBV and lymphoma. *Int J Cancer* 1982;29:397–400.
683. Lindahl T, Klein G, Reedman BM, et al. Relationship between Epstein-Barr virus (EBV) DNA and the EBV-determined nuclear antigen (EBNA) in Burkitt lymphoma biopsies and other lymphoproliferative malignancies. *Int J Cancer* 1974;13:764–772.
684. Purtilo DT. opportunistic non-Hodgkin's lymphoma in X-linked recessive immunodeficiency and lymphoproliferative syndrome. *Semin Oncol* 1977;4:335–343.
685. Purtilo DT, Klein G. Introduction to Epstein-Barr virus and lymphoproliferative diseases in immunodeficient individuals. *Cancer Res* 1981;41:4209.
686. Peiper SC, Myers JL, Broussard EE, et al. Detection of Epstein-Barr virus genomes in archival tissues by polymerase chain reaction. *Arch Pathol Lab Med* 1990;114:711–714.
687. Tosato G, Blaese RM. Epstein-Barr virus infection and immunoregulation in man. *Adv Immunol* 1985;37:99–149.
688. Hamilton-Dutoit SJ, Raphael M, Audouin J, et al. In situ demonstration of Epstein-Barr virus small RNAs (EBER 1) in acquired immunodeficiency syndrome-related lymphomas: correlation with tumor morphology and primary site. *Blood* 1993;82:619–624.
689. Neri A, Barriga F, Knowles DM, et al. Epstein-Barr virus infection precedes clonal expansion in Burkitt's and AIDS-associated lymphoma. *Blood* 1991;77:1092–1095.
690. Shibata D, Weiss LM, Hernandez AM, et al. Epstein-Barr virus-associated non-Hodgkin's lymphoma in patients infected with the human immunodeficiency virus. *Blood* 1993;81:2102–2109.
691. Sample J, Young L, Martin B, et al. Epstein-Barr virus types 1 and 2 differ in their EBNA-3A, EBNA-3B, and EBNA-3C genes. *J Virol* 1990;64:4084–4092.
692. Kyaw MT, Hurren L, Evans L, et al. Expression of B-type Epstein-Barr virus in HIV-infected patients and cardiac transplant recipients. *AIDS Res Hum Retroviruses* 1992;8:1869–1874.
693. Wang D, Liebowitz D, Kieff E. An EBV membrane protein expressed in immortalized lymphocytes transforms established rodent cells. *Cell* 1985;43:831–840.
694. Borisch B, Ellinger K, Neipel F, et al. Lymphadenitis and lymphoproliferative lesions associated with the human herpesvirus-6 (HHV-6). *Virchows Arch B Cell Pathol* 1991;61:179–187.
695. Karp JE, Broder S. Acquired immunodeficiency syndrome and non-Hodgkin's lymphomas. *Cancer Res* 1991; 51:4743–4756.
696. Torelli G, Marasca R, Luppi M, et al. Human herpesvirus-6 in human lymphomas: identification of specific sequences in Hodgkin's lymphomas by polymerase chain reaction. *Blood* 1991;77:2251–2258.
697. Paulus W, Jellinger K, Hallas C, et al. Human herpesvirus-6 and Epstein-Barr virus genome in primary cerebral lymphomas. *Neurology* 1993;43:1591–1593.
698. Ng VL, Hwang KM, Reyes GR, et al. High titer anti-HIV antibody reactivity associated with a paraprotein spike in a homosexual male with AIDS related complex. *Blood* 1988;71:1397–1401.
699. Ng VL, Chen KH, Kwang KM, et al. The clinical significance of human immunodeficiency virus type 1-associated paraproteins. *Blood* 1989;74:2471–2475.
700. Berek C, Milstein C. Mutation drift and repertoire shift in the maturation of the immune response. *Immunol Rev* 1987;96:23–41.
701. Riboldi P, Gaidano G, Schettino EW, et al. Two acquired immunodeficiency syndrome-associated Burkitt's lymphomas produce specific anti-i IgM cold agglutinins using somatically mutated VH4-21 segments. *Blood* 1994;83:2952–2961.
702. Levine AM, Gill PS, Krailo M, et al. Natural history of persistent generalized lymphadenopathy (PGL) in gay men: risk of lymphoma and factors associated with development of lymphoma. *Blood* 1986; 68:130a.
703. Shibata D, Weiss LM, Nathwani BN, et al. Epstein-Barr virus in benign lymph node biopsies from individuals infected with the human immunodeficiency virus is associated with concurrent or subsequent development of non-Hodgkin's lymphoma. *Blood* 1991;77: 1527–1533.
704. Alonso ML, Richardson ME, Metroka CE, et al. Chromosome abnormalities in AIDS-associated lymphadenopathy. *Blood* 1987;69: 855–858.
705. Mathur-Wagh U, Mildvan D, Senie RT. Follow-up at 4 1/2 years on homosexual men with generalized lymphadenopathy. *N Engl J Med* 1985;313:1542–1543.
706. Inghirami G, Grignani F, Sternas L, et al. Down-regulation of LFA-1 adhesion receptors by c-myc oncogene in human B lymphoblastoid cells. *Science* 1990;250:682–686.
707. Clayberger C, Wright A, Medeiros LJ, et al. Absence of cell surface LFA-1 as a mechanism of escape from immunosurveillance. *Lancet* 1987;2:533–536.
708. Inghirami G, Wieczorek R, Zhu BY, et al. Differential expression of LFA-1 molecules in non-Hodgkin's lymphoma and lymphoid leukemia. *Blood* 1988;72:1431–1434.
709. Robert NJ, Schneiderman H. Hodgkin's disease and the acquired immunodeficiency syndrome. *Ann Intern Med* 1984;101:142–143.
710. Schoeppel JL, Hoppe RT, Dorfman RF, et al. Hodgkin's disease in homosexual men with generalized lymphadenopathy. *Ann Intern Med* 1985;102:68–70.
711. Scheib RG, Siegel RS. Atypical Hodgkin's disease and the acquired immunodeficiency syndrome. *Ann Intern Med* 1985;102:554.
712. Moore GE, Cook DD. AIDS in association with malignant melanoma and Hodgkin's disease. *J Clin Oncol* 1985;3:1437.

713. Baer DM, Anderson ET, Wilkinson LS. Acquired immune deficiency syndrome in homosexual men with Hodgkin's disease. *Am J Med* 1986;80:738(740.
714. Mitsuyasu RT, Colman MF, Sun NCJ. Simultaneous occurrence of Hodgkin's disease and Kaposi's sarcoma in a patient with the acquired immune deficiency syndrome. *Am J Med* 1986;80:954–958.
715. Temple JJ, Andes WA. AIDS and Hodgkin's disease. *Lancet* 1986; 2:454–455.
716. Cid JA, Cid JL, Sanudo EF, et al. AIDS and Hodgkin's disease. *Lancet* 1986;ii:1104–1105.
717. Góngora-Biachi RA, González-Martínez P, Bastarrachea-Ortíz J. Hodgkin disease as the initial manifestation of acquired immunodeficiency syndrome. *Ann Intern Med* 1987;107:112.
718. Bello JL, Magallón M, Villar JM. Hodgkin disease in hemophilia. *Ann Intern Med* 1987;107:257.
719. Picard O, De Gramont A, Krulik M, et al. Rectal Hodgkin disease and the acquired immunodeficiency syndrome. *Ann Intern Med* 1987; 106:775.
720. Colbourn D, Staszewski H, Goldenberg S, et al. Fulminant lymphocyte depleted Hodgkin disease in a homosexual man with HIV infection. *NY State J Med* 1987;10:570–571.
721. Bassetti D, Luzzati R, Malena M, et al. Hodgkin's disease in AIDS patients. *AIDS* 1988;ii:138.
722. Keyserlingk H, Ludwig WD, Seibt H, et al. Atypical presentation of Hodgkin's disease in a patient at risk for the acquired immunodeficiency syndrome. *Cancer Detect Prev* 1988;12:243–248.
723. De Mascarel A, Merlio JP, Laborie V, et al. Hodgkin's disease and malignant lymphoma in acquired immunodeficiency syndrome. *Arch Pathol Lab Med* 1989;113:328.
724. Shaw MT, Jacobs SR. Cutaneous Hodgkin's disease in a patient with human immunodeficiency virus infection. *Cancer* 1989;64: 2585–2587.
725. Senaldi E, Lee MH, Toth I, et al. Hodgkin's disease after non-Hodgkin's malignant lymphoma in acquired immune deficiency syndrome. *Cancer* 1990;66:960–964.
726. Hair LS, Rogers JD, Chadburn A, et al. Intracerebral Hodgkin's disease in a human immunodeficiency virus-seropositive patient. *Cancer* 1991;67:2931–2934.
727. Lichtman SM, Brody J, Kaplan MH, et al. Hodgkin's disease and non-Hodgkin's lymphoma in an HIV positive patient. *Leuk Lymphoma* 1993;9:393–398.
728. Ranganathan V. Primary rectal Hodgkin's lymphoma: initial manifestation of HIV. *Am J Gastroenterol* 1996;91:180.
729. Unger PD, Strauchen JA. Hodgkin's disease in AIDS complex patients: report of four cases and tissue immunologic marker studies. *Cancer* 1986;58:821–825.
730. Prior E, Goldberg AF, Conjalka MS, et al. Hodgkin's disease in homosexual men: an AIDS-related phenomenon? *Am J Med* 1986;81: 1085–1088.
731. Alfonso PG, Sanudo EF, Carretero JM, et al. Hodgkin's disease in HIV-infected patients. *Biomed Pharmacother* 1988;42:321–325.
732. Serrano M, Bellas C, Campo E, et al. Hodgkin's disease in patients with antibodies to human immunodeficiency virus: a study of 22 patients. *Cancer* 1990;65:2248–2254.
733. Gold JE, Altarac D, Ree HJ, et al. HIV-associated Hodgkin disease: a clinical study of 18 cases and review of the literature. *Am J Hematol* 1991;36:93–99.
734. Ree HJ, Strauchen JA, Khan A, et al. HIV-associated Hodgkin's disease: clinicopathologic studies of 24 cases. Preponderance of mixed cellularity type characterized by the occurrence of fibro-histiocytoid stromal cells. *Cancer* 1991;67:1614–1621.
735. Pelstring RJ, Zellmer RB, Sulak LE, et al. Hodgkin's disease in association with human immunodeficiency virus infection. *Cancer* 1991; 67:1865–1873.
736. Karcher DS. Clinically unsuspected Hodgkin's disease presenting initially in the bone marrow of patients infected with the human immunodeficiency virus. *Cancer* 1993;71:1235–1238.
737. Newcom SR, Ward M, Napoli VM, et al. Treatment of human immunodeficiency virus-associated Hodgkin disease: is there a clue regarding the cause of Hodgkin's disease? *Cancer* 1993;71:3138–3145.
738. Tirelli U, Vaccher E, Rezza G, et al. Hodgkin's disease and infection with the human immunodeficiency virus (HIV) in Italy. *Ann Intern Med* 1988;108:309–310.
739. Roithmann S, Tourani JM, Andrieu JM. Hodgkin's disease in HIV-infected intravenous drug abusers. *N Engl J Med* 1990;323:275–276.
740. Ames ED, Conjalka MS, Goldberg AF, et al. Hodgkin's disease and AIDS. *Hematol Oncol Clin North Am* 1991;5:343–356.
741. Monfardini S, Tirelli U, Vaccher E, et al for the Gruppo Italian Cooperativo AIDS & Tumori (GICAT). Hodgkin's disease in 63 intravenous drug users infected with human immunodeficiency virus. *Ann Oncol* 1991;2[Suppl 2]:201–205.
742. Garnier G, Taillan B, Michiels JF. HIV-associated Hodgkin disease. *Ann Intern Med* 1991;115:233.
743. Tirelli U, Errante D, Vaccher E, et al. for the GICAT (Italian Cooperative Group on AIDS and Tumors). Hodgkin's disease in 92 patients with HIV infection: the Italian experience. *Ann Oncol* 1992;3[Suppl 4]: 69–72.
744. Andrieu JM, Roithmann S, Tourani JM, et al. Hodgkin's disease during HIV1 infection: the French Registry experience. *Ann Oncol* 1993; 4:635–641.
745. Rubio R. Hodgkin's disease associated with human immunodeficiency virus infection. *Cancer* 1994;73:2400–2407.
746. Tirelli U, Errante D, Dolcetti R, et al. Hodgkin's disease and human immunodeficiency virus infection: clinicopathologic and virologic features of 114 patients from the Italian Cooperative Group on AIDS and tumors. *J Clin Oncol* 1995;13:1758–1767.
747. Serraino D, Carbone A, Franceschi S, et al for the Italian Cooperative Group on AIDS and Tumours. Increased frequency of lymphocyte depletion and mixed cellularity subtypes of Hodgkin's disease in HIV-infected patients. *Eur J Cancer* 1993;29A:1948–1950.
748. Doyle TJ, Venkatachalam KK, Maeda K, et al. Hodgkin's disease in renal transplant recipients. *Cancer* 1983;51:245–247.
749. Elenitoba-Johnson Kaposi's sarcomaJ, Jaffe ES. Lymphoproliferative disorders associated with congential immunodeficiencies. *Semin Diagn Pathol* 1997;14:35–47.
750. Swerdlow SH. Classification of the posttransplant lymphoproliferative disorders: from the past to the present. *Semin Diagn Pathol* 1997; 14:2–7.
751. Biggar RF, Burnett W, Mikl J, et al. Cancer among New York men at risk of acquired immunodeficiency syndrome. *Int J Cancer* 1989; 43:979.
752. Bernstein L, Levin D, Mench H, et al. AIDS-related secular trends in cancer in Los Angeles county men: a comparison by marital status. *Cancer Res* 1989;49:466–470.
753. Hessol NA, Katz MH, Liu JY, et al. Increased incidence of Hodgkin disease in homosexual men with HIV infection. *Ann Intern Med* 1992; 117:309–311.
754. Reynolds P, Saunders LD, Layefsky ME, et al. The spectrum of acquired immunodeficiency syndrome (AIDS)-associated malignancies in San Francisco, 1980–1987. *Am J Epidemiol* 1993;137:19–30.
755. Lyter DW, Bryant J, Thackeray R, et al. Incidence of human immunodeficiency virus-related and nonrelated malignancies in a large cohort of homosexual men. *J Clin Oncol* 1995;13:2540–2546.
756. Colby TV, Hoppe RT, Warnke RA. Hodgkin's disease: a clinicopathologic study of 659 cases. *Cancer* 1982;49:1848–1858.
757. Davis S, Dahlberg S, Myers MH, et al. Hodgkin's disease in the United States: a comparison of patient characteristics and survival in the centralized cancer patient data system and the surveillance, epidemiology, and end results program. *J Natl Cancer Inst* 1987;78: 471–478.
758. Henry-Amar M. Workshop statistical report. In: Somers R, Henry-Amar M, Meerwaldt JK, et al, eds. *Treatment strategy in Hodgkin's disease.* Paris: Editions INSERM, 1990:169–190.
759. Correa P, O'Connor GT. Epidemiologic pattern of Hodgkin's disease. *Int J Cancer* 1972;8:192–201.
760. Riyat MS. Hodgkin's disease in Kenya. *Cancer* 1992;69:1047–1051.
761. Hu E, Hufford S, Lukes R, et al. Third world Hodgkin's disease at the Los Angeles County-University of Southern California Medical Center. *J Clin Oncol* 1988;6:1285–1292.
762. Robinson LL, Stoker V, Frizzera G, et al. Hodgkin's disease in pediatric patients with naturally occurring immunodeficiency. *Am J Pediatr Hematol Oncol* 1987;9:189–192.
763. Knowles DM, Halper JP, Jakobiec FA. T-lymphocyte subpopulations in B-cell derived non-Hodgkin's lymphomas and Hodgkin's disease. *Cancer* 1984;56:644–651.
764. Knowles DM, Neri A, Pelicci PG, et al. Immunoglobulin and T cell receptor beta chain gene rearrangement analysis of Hodgkin's disease: implications for lineage determination and differential diagnosis. *Proc Natl Acad Sci USA* 1986;83:7942–7946.

765. Linden MD, Fishleder AJ, Katzin WE, et al. Absence of B-cell or T-cell clonal expression in nodular, lymphocyte predominant Hodgkin's disease. *Hum Pathol* 1988;19:591–594.
766. Pallesen G, Hamilton-Dutoit SJ, Rowe M, et al. Expression of Epstein-Barr virus latent gene products in tumour cells of Hodgkin's disease. *Lancet* 1991;337:320–322.
767. Armstrong AA, Weiss LM, Gallagher A, et al. Criteria for the definition of Epstein-Barr virus association in Hodgkin's disease. *Leukemia* 1992;6:869–874.
768. Carbone A, Gloghini A, Zanette I, et al. Co-expression of Epstein-Barr virus latent membrane protein and vimentin in "aggressive" histological subtypes of Hodgkin's disease. *Virchows Arch A Pathol Anat Histopathol* 1993;422:39–45.
769. O'Grady J, Stewart S, Elton RA, et al. Epstein-Barr virus in Hodgkin's disease and site of origin of tumour. *Lancet* 1994;343:265–266.
770. Briere J, Beldjord K, Belkaid MI, et al. Epstein-Barr virus (EBV) markers in 46 Hodgkin's disease (HD) patients from France and Algeria. *Blood* 1992;80[Suppl 1]:465.
771. Glaser SL. Hodgkin's disease in a black population: a review of the epidemiologic literature. *Semin Oncol* 1990;17: 643–659.
772. Uccini S, Monardo F, Stoppacciaro A, et al. High frequency of Epstein-Barr virus genome detection in Hodgkin's disease of HIV-positive patients. *Int J Cancer* 1990;46:581–585.
773. Audouin J, Diebold J, Pallesen G. Frequent expression of Epstein-Barr virus latent membrane protein-1 in tumour cells of Hodgkin's disease in HIV-positive patients. *J Pathol* 1992;167:381–384.
774. De Re V, De Vita S, Dolcetti R, et al. Association between B-type Epstein-Barr virus and Hodgkin's disease in immunocompromised patients. *Blood* 1993;82:328–330.
775. O'Carroll DJH, McKenna RW, Brunning RD. Bone marrow manifestation of Hodgkin's disease. *Cancer* 1976;38:1717–1728.
776. Errante D, Zagonel V, Vaccher E, et al. Hodgkin's disease in patients with HIV infection and in the general population: comparison of clinicopathological features and survival. *Ann Oncol* 1994;5[Suppl 2]: 37–40.
777. Canellos GP, Anderson JR, Propert KJ, et al. Chemotherapy of advanced Hodgkin's disease with MOPP, ABVD, or MOPP alternating with ABVD. *N Engl J Med* 1992;327:1478–1484.
778. Bonadona G, Valagussa P, Santoro A. Alternating non-cross-resistant combination chemotherapy or MOPP in stage IV Hodgkin's disease: a report of 8-year results. *Ann Intern Med* 1986;104:739–746.
779. Urba WJ, Longo DL. Hodgkin's disease. *N Engl J Med* 1992;326: 678–687.
780. Errante D, Tirelli U, Gastaldi R, et al. for the Italian Cooperative Group on AIDS and Tumors (GICAT). Combined antineoplastic and antiretroviral therapy for patients with Hodgkin's disease and human immunodeficiency virus infection. *Cancer* 1994;73:437–444.
781. Levine AM. HIV-associated Hodgkin's disease. *Hematol Oncol Clin North Am* 1996;10:1135–1148.
782. Notter DT, Grossman PL, Rosenberg SA, et al. Infections in patients with Hodgkin's disease: a clinical study of 300 consecutive adult patients. *Rev Infect Dis* 1980;2:761–800.
783. Coker DD, Morris DM, Coleman JJ, et al. Infection among 210 patients with surgically staged Hodgkin's disease. *Am J Med* 1983;75: 97–109.
784. Berman M, Minowada J, Lewy LM, et al. Burkitt cell acute lymphoblastic leukemia with partial expression of T-cell markers and subclonal chromosome abnormalities in a man with acquired immunodeficiency syndrome. *Cancer Genet Cytogenet* 1985;16:341–347.
785. Gill PS, Meyer PR, Pavlova Z, et al. B cell acute lymphocytic leukemia in adults: clinical, morphologic, and immunologic findings. *J Clin Oncol* 1986;4:737–743.
786. Ernberg I, Bjorkholm M, Zech L, et al. An EBV genome carrying pre-B cell leukemia in a homosexual man with characteristic karyotype and impaired EBV-specific immunity. *J Clin Oncol* 1986;4: 1481–1488.
787. Rossi G, Gorla R, Cadeo GP, et al. Acute lymphoblastic leukemia of B cell origin in an anti-HIV positive intravenous drug abuser. *Br J Haematol* 1988;68:140–141.
788. Flanagan P, Chowdhury V, Costello C. HIV-associated B cell ALL. *Br J Haematol* 1988;69:287.
789. Milpied N, Bourhis JH, Garand R, et al. B cell ALL in an anti-HIV positive patient: achievement of a complete response with aggressive chemotherapy. *Br J Haematol* 1988;70:501–502.
790. Bernheim A, Berger R. Cytogenetic studies of Burkitt lymphoma-leukemia in patients with acquired immunodeficiency syndrome. *Cancer Genet Cytogenet* 1988;32:67–74.
791. Garavelli PL. Acute lymphoblastic leukemia, L3 type, in a HIV positive patient. *Hematologica* 1988;73:89.
792. Gold JE, Castella A, Zalusky R. B-cell acute lymphocytic leukemia in HIV antibody-positive patients. *Am J Hematol* 1989;32:200–204.
793. Gold JE, Babu A, Penchaszadeh V, et al. Hybrid acute leukemia in an HIV-antibody-positive patient. *Am J Hematol* 1989;30:240–247.
794. Arico M, Caselli D, D'Argenio P, et al. Malignancies in children with human immunodeficiency virus type 1 infection. *Cancer* 1991;68: 2473–2477.
795. Israel AM, Koziner B, Strauss DJ. Plasmacytoma and the acquired immunodeficiency syndrome. *Ann Intern Med* 1983;99:635–636.
796. Vandermolen LA, Fehir KM, Rice L. Multiple myeloma in a homosexual man with chronic lymphadenopathy. *Arch Intern Med* 1985; 145:745–746.
797. Gold JWM, Weikel CS, Godbold J, et al. Unexplained persistent lymphadenopathy in homosexual men and the acquired immune deficiency syndrome. *Medicine* 1985;64:203–213.
798. Thomas MAB, Ibels LS, Wells JV, et al. IgA kappa multiple myeloma and lymphadenopathy syndrome associated with AIDS virus infection. *Aust NZ J Med* 1986;16:402–404.
799. Karnad AB, Martin AW, Koh HK, et al. Non-secretory multiple myeloma in a 26-year-old man with acquired immunodeficiency syndrome, presenting with multiple extramedullary plasmacytomas and osteolytic bone disease. *Am J Hematol* 1989;32:305–310.
800. Voelkerding KV, Sandhaus LM, Kim HC, et al. Plasma cell malignancy in the acquired immune deficiency syndrome. *Am J Clin Pathol* 1989;92:222–228.
801. Gold JE, Schwam L, Castella A, et al. Malignant plasma cell tumors in HIV-infected patients. *Cancer* 1990;66:363–368.
802. von Keyserlingk H, Baur R, Stein H, et al. Multiple myeloma in a patient at risk for AIDS. *Cancer Detect Prev* 1990;14:403–404.
803. Nogues X, Supervia A, Knobel H, et al. Multiple myeloma and AIDS. *Am J Hematol* 1996;53:210–211.
804. Shokunbi WA, Okpala IE, Shokunbi MT, et al. Multiple myeloma co-existing with HIV-1 infection in a 65-year-old Nigerian man. *AIDS* 1991;5:115–116.
805. Konrad RJ, Kricka LJ, Goodman DBP, et al. Myeloma-associated paraprotein directed against the HIV-1 p24 antigen in an HIV-1 seropositive patient. *N Engl J Med* 1993;328:1817–1819.
806. Pizarro A, Gamallo C, Sanchez-Munoz JF, et al. Extramedullary plasmacytoma and AIDS-related Kaposi's sarcoma. *J Am Acad Dermatol* 1994;30:797–800.
807. Kumar S, Kumar D, Schnadig VJ, et al. Plasma cell myeloma in patients who are HIV-positive. *Am J Clin Pathol* 1994;102:633–639.
808. Ventura G, Lucia MB, Damiano F, et al. Multiple myeloma associated with Epstein-Barr virus in an AIDS patient: a case report. *Eur J Haematol* 1995;55:332–334.
809. Nosari AM, Landonio G, Cantoni S, et al. Multiple myeloma associated to HIV infection: report of two patients. *Eur J Haematol* 1996; 56:98–99.
810. Sewell HF, Walker F, Bennett B, et al. Chronic lymphocytic leukaemia contemporaneous with HIV infection. *Br Med J* 1987;294: 938–939.
811. Turner RR, Brynes RK, Nathwani BN, et al. Low grade B-cell lymphomas and leukemias in homosexual men. *Lab Invest* 1988;58:96A.
812. Sheibani K, Ben-Ezra J, Swartz WG, et al. Monocytoid B cell lymphoma in a patient with human immunodeficiency virus infection. *Arch Pathol Lab Med* 1990;114:1264–1267.
813. Bilgrami S, Shafi N, Pesanti EL, et al. Mantle cell lymphoma in a patient with human immunodeficiency viral infection. *Acta Haematol* 1995;93:101–104.
814. Harper ME, Kaplan MH, Marselle LM, et al. Concomitant infection with HTLV-1 and HTLV-III in a patient with T8 lymphoproliferative disease. *N Engl J Med* 1986;315:1073–1078.
815. Presant CA, Gala K, Wiseman C, et al. Human immunodeficiency virus-associated T-cell lymphoblastic lymphoma in AIDS. *Cancer* 1987;60:1459–1461.
816. Baurmann H, Miclea JM, Ferchal F, et al. Adult T cell leukemia associated with HTLV-1 and simultaneous infection by human immunodeficiency virus type 2 and human herpesvirus 6 in an African

woman: a clinical, virologic, and familial serologic study. *Am J Med* 1988;85:853–857.

817. Nasr SA, Brynes RK, Garrison CP, et al. Peripheral T-cell lymphoma in a patient with acquired immune deficiency syndrome. *Cancer* 1988; 61:947–951.
818. Lust JA, Banks PM, Hooper WC, et al. T cell non-Hodgkin lymphoma in human immunodeficiency virus-1-infected individuals. *Am J Hematol* 1989;31:181–187.
819. Ruff P, Bagg A, Papadopoulos K. Precursor T-cell lymphoma associated with HIV-1 infection: first reported case. *Cancer* 1989;64:39–42.
820. Shibata D, Brynes RK, Rabinowitz A, et al. Human T-cell lymphotropic virus type I (HTLV-I)-associated adult T-cell leukemia-lymphoma in a patient infected with human immunodeficiency virus type 1 (HIV-1). *Ann Intern Med* 1989;111:871–875.
821. Parker SC, Fenton DA, McGibbon DH. Homme rouge and the acquired immunodeficiency syndrome. *N Engl J Med* 1990;321: 906–907.
822. Goldstein J, Becker N, DelRowe J, et al. Cutaneous T cell lymphoma in a patient infected with human immunodeficiency virus type 1. *Cancer* 1990;66:1130–1132.
823. Crane GA, Variakojis D, Rosen ST, et al. Cutaneous T cell lymphoma in patients with human immunodeficiency virus infection. *Arch Dermatol* 1991;127:989–994.
824. Nahass GT, Kraffert CA, Penneys NS. Cutaneous T cell lymphoma associated with the acquired immunodeficiency syndrome. *Arch Dermatol* 1991;127:1020–1022.
825. González-Clemente JM, Ribera JM, Campo E, et al. Ki-1 + anaplastic large-cell lymphoma of T-cell origin in an HIV-infected patient. *AIDS* 1991;5:751–755.
826. Diekman MJM, Bresser P, Noorduyn LA, et al. Spontaneous regression of Ki-1 positive T-cell non-Hodgkin's lymphoma in a patient with HIV infection. *Br J Haematol* 1992;82:477–478.
827. Herndier BG, Shiramizu BT, Jewett NE, et al. Acquired immunodeficiency syndrome-associated T-cell lymphoma: evidence for human immunodeficiency virus type 1-associated T-cell transformation. *Blood* 1992;79:1768–1774.
828. Burns MK, Cooper KD. Cutaneous T cell lymphoma associated with HIV infection. *J Am Acad Dermatol* 1993;29:394–399.
829. Dreno B, Milpied-Homsi B, Moreau P, et al. Cutaneous anaplastic T-cell lymphoma in a patient with human immunodeficiency virus infection: detection of Epstein-Barr virus DNA. *Br J Dermatol* 1993; 129:77–81.
830. Berger TG, Kerschmann RL, Roth R, et al. Sezary's syndrome and human immunodeficiency virus infection. *Arch Dermatol* 1995;131: 739–740.
831. Kerschmann RL, Berger TG, Weiss LM, et al. Cutaneous presentations of lymphoma in human immunodeficiency virus disease: predominance of T cell lineage. *Arch Dermatol* 1995;131:1281–1288.
832. Montillo P, Dronda F, Moreno S, et al. Lymphomatoid granulomatosis and the acquired immunodeficiency syndrome. *Ann Intern Med* 1987; 106:166–167.
833. Anders KH, Latta H, Chang BS, et al. Lymphomatoid granulomatosis and malignant lymphomas of the central nervous system in the acquired immunodeficiency syndrome. *Hum Pathol* 1989;20:326–334.
834. Gold JE, Ghali V, Brown JC, et al. Angiocentric immunoproliferative lesions and the acquired immune deficiency syndrome: a case report and review of the literature. *Cancer* 1990;66:2407–2413.
835. Napoli VM, Stein SF, Spira TJ, et al. Myelodysplasia progressing to acute myeloblastic leukemia in an HTLV-III virus-positive homosexual man with AIDS-related complex. *Am J Clin Pathol* 1986;86: 788–791.
836. Darne C, Solal-Celigny P, Herrera A, et al. Acute myelofibrosis and infection with the lymphadenopathy-associated virus/human T-lymphotropic virus type III. *Ann Intern Med* 1986;104:130–131.
837. Solal-Celigny P, Leporrier M, Brousse N, et al. Splenomegalie myeloide et infection a virus LAV/HTLV-III. *Nouv Rev Fr Hematol* 1986; 28:163–169.
838. Willumsen L, Ellegaard J, Pedersen B. HIV infection in acute myeloblastic leukemia. *Am J Clin Pathol* 1987;88:536–537.
839. Diebold J, Audouin J. Lymphomes malins et autres proliferations malignes des organes hematopoietiques chez les sujets HIV positifs. *Arch Anat Cytol Path* 1988;36:5–11.
840. Garavelli PL, Azzini M. Leucosi in corso de infezione da HIV. *Minerva Med* 1988;79:105–107.
841. Monfardini S, Vaccher E, Pizzocaro G, et al. Unusual malignant tumours in 49 patients with HIV infection. *AIDS* 1989;3:449–452.
842. Wijermans PW, Ten Kate RW. Successful chemotherapy for acute myeloid leukemia in HIV-infected patients. *Eur J Haematol* 1990;41: 136–138.
843. Peters BS, Matthews J, Gompels M, et al. Acute myeloblastic leukaemia in AIDS. *AIDS* 1990;4:367–368.
844. Lorand-Metze I, Morais SL, Souza CA. Chronic myeloid leukemia in a homosexual HIV-seropositive man. *AIDS* 1990;4:923–933.
845. Puppo F, Scudeletti M, Murgia L, et al. Acute myelomonocytic leukaemia in an HIV-infected patient. *AIDS* 1991;6:136–137.
846. Murthy AR, Ho D, Goetz MB. Relationship between acute myelomonoblastic leukemia and infection due to human immunodeficiency virus. *Rev Infect Dis* 1991;13:254–256.
847. Mansberg R, Rowlings PA, Yip M-Y, et al. First and second complete remissions in a HIV positive patient following remission induction therapy for acute non-lymphoblastic leukaemia. *Aust NZ J Med* 1991; 21:55–57.
848. Rivers JK, Laubenstein LJ, Postel AH. Acute monocytic leukaemia in a HIV-seropositive man. *Clin Exp Dermatol* 1992;17:203–205.
849. De La Salmoniere P, Janier M, Gilquin J, et al. Chicken pox and acute monocytic leukaemia skin lesions in an HIV-seropositive man. *Clin Exp Dermatol* 1994;19:505–506.
850. Rabaud C, Dorvaux V, May T, et al. Acute myelogenous leukaemia followed by non-Hodgkin's lymphoma in a patient with AIDS. *J Infect* 1995;31:69–70.
851. Bennett JM, Catovsky D, Daniel M-T, et al. Proposals for the classification of acute leukemias: French-American-British (FAB) co-operative group. *Br J Haematol* 1976;33:451–458.
852. Minerbrook M, Schulman P, Budman DR, et al. Burkitt's leukemia: a re-evaluation. *Cancer* 1982;49:1444–1448.
853. Sasser RL, Yam LT, Li CY. Myeloma with involvement of the serous cavities. *Acta Cytol* 1990;34:479–485.
854. Kyle RA. Multiple myeloma: a review of 869 cases. Mayo Clin *Proc* 1975;50:29–40.
855. Meis JM, Butler JJ, Osborne BM, et al. Solitary plasmacytomas of bone and extramedullary plasmacytomas: a clinicopathologic and immunohistochemical study. *Cancer* 1987;59:1475–1485.
856. Salahuddin SZ, Albashi DV, Hunter EA, et al. HTLV-III infection of EBV-genome-positive B-lymphoid cells with or without detectable T4 antigens. *Int J Cancer* 1987;39:198–202.
857. Potter M, Mushinski JF, Mushinski E, et al. Avian V-myc replaces chromosomal translocation in murine plasmacytoma genesis. *Science* 1987;235:787–789.
858. Horning SJ, Rosenberg SA. The natural history of initially untreated low grade non-Hodgkin's lymphomas. *N Engl J Med* 1984;311:1471.
859. Ciobanu N, Andreeff M, Safai B, et al. Lymphoblastic neoplasia in homosexual patient with Kaposi's sarcoma. *Ann Intern Med* 1983; 98:151–155.
860. Kobayashi M, Yoshimoto S, Fujishita S, et al. HTLV-I positive T-cell lymphoma-leukemia in an AIDS patient. *Lancet* 1984;i:1361–1362.
861. Howard MR, McVerry BA. T-cell lymphoma in a haemophiliac positive for antibody to HIV. *Br J Haematol* 1987;67:115.
862. Sternlieb J, Mintzer D, Kwa D, Gluckman S. Peripheral T cell lymphoma in a patient with the acquired immunodeficiency syndrome. *Am J Med* 1988;85:445.
863. Beljaards RC, Kaudewitz P, Berti E, et al. Primary cutaneous CD30-positive large cell lymphoma: definition of a new type of cutaneous lymphoma with a favorable prognosis. A European Multicenter Study of 47 patients. *Cancer* 1993;71:2097–2104.
864. Reynold CW, Foon KA. Tγ-lymphoproliferative disease and related disorders in human and in experimental animals: a review of the clinical, cellular, and functional characteristics. *Blood* 1984;64: 1146–1158.
865. Ghali V, Castella A, Louis-Charles A, et al. Expansion of large granular lymphocytes (natural killer cells) and limited antigen expression (CD2 + , CD3-, CD4-, CD8-, CD16 + , NKH-1-) in an HIV-positive homosexual male. *Cancer* 1990;65:2243–2247.
866. Guillon JM, Fouret P, Mayaud C, et al. Extensive T8-positive lymphocytic visceral infiltration in a homosexual man. *Am J Med* 1987;82: 655–661.
867. Oksenhendler E, Autran B, Gorochov G, et al. CD8 lymphocytosis and pseudotumoral splenomegaly in HIV infection. *Lancet* 1992;340: 207–208.

868. Goddart D, Francois A, Ninane J, et al. Parotid gland abnormality found in children seropositive for the human immunodeficiency virus (HIV). *Pediatr Radiol* 1990;20:355–357.
869. Lippman SM, Grogan TM, Carry P, et al. Post-transplantation T cell lymphoblastic lymphoma. *Am J Med* 1987;82:814–816.
870. Garvin AJ, Self S, Sahovic EA, et al. The occurrence of a peripheral T-cell lymphoma in a chronically immunosuppressed renal transplant patient. *Am J Surg Pathol* 1988;12:64–70.
871. Ulrich W, Chott A, Watschinger B, et al. Primary peripheral T cell lymphoma in a kidney transplant under immunosuppression with cyclosporine A. *Hum Pathol* 1989;20:1027–1030.
872. Griffith RC, Saha BK, Janney CM, et al. Immunoblastic lymphoma of T-cell type in a chronically immunosuppressed renal transplant recipient. *Am J Clin Pathol* 1990;93:280–285.
873. Kemnitz J, Cremer J, Gebel M, et al. T-cell lymphoma after heart transplantation. *Am J Clin Pathol* 1990;94:95–101.
874. Robert-Guroff M, Weiss SH, Giron JA, et al. Prevalence of antibodies to HTLV-I, -II and -III in intravenous drug abusers from an AIDS endernic region. *JAMA* 1986;255:3133–3137.
875. De Rossi A, Gassa OD, del Mistro A, et al. HTLV-III and HTLV-I infection in populations at risk in the Veneto region of Italy. *Eur J Cancer Clin Oncol* 1986;22:411–418.
876. Bartholomew C, Saxinger CW, Clark JW, et al. Transmission of HTLV-1 and HIV among homosexual men in Trinidad. *JAMA* 1987; 257:2604–2608.
877. Cortes E, Detels R, Aboulafia D, et al. HIV-1, HIV-2, and HTLV-1 infection in high risk groups in Brazil. *N Eng J Med* 1989;320: 953–958.
878. Stevenson M, Volsky B, Hedenskog M, et al. Immortalization of human T lymphocytes after transfection of Epstein-Barr virus DNA. *Science* 1986;233:980–984.
879. Harabuchi Y, Yamanaka N, Kataura A, et al. Epstein-Barr virus in nasal T-cell lymphomas in patients with lethal midline granuloma. *Lancet* 1990;335:128–130.
880. Jones JF, Shurin S, Abramowsky C, et al. T-cell lymphoma containing Epstein-Barr viral DNA in patients with chronic Epstein-Barr virus infections. *N Engl J Med* 1988;318:733–741.
881. Schneider DR, Picker LJ. Myelodysplasia in the acquired immune deficiency syndrome. *Am J Clin Pathol* 1985;84:144–152.
882. Bennett JM, Catovsky D, Daniel MT, et al. Proposal for the classification of the myelodysplastic syndromes. *Br J Haematol* 1982;51: 189–199.
883. Spector BD, Perry GS III, et al. Genetically determined immunodeficiency disease and malignancy: report from the immunodeficiency-cancer registry. *Clin Immunol Immunopathol* 1978;11:12–29.
884. Levy JA, Shimabukuro J, McHugh T, et al. AIDS-associated retroviruses (ARV) can productively infect other cells besides human T helper cells. *Virology* 1985;147:441–448.
885. Cortes E, Koeffler HP, Gaynor R, et al. Infectivity and genetic regulation of human immunodeficiency virus (HIV) in myeloid leukemia cell lines. *Blood* 1986;68[Suppl 1]:123a.
886. Clapham PR, Weiss RA, Dalgleish AG, et al. Human immunodeficiency virus infection of monocytic and T lymphocytic cells: receptor modulation and differentiation induced by phorbol ester. *Virology* 1987;158:44–51.
887. Busch M, Beckstead J, Gantz D, et al. Detection of human immunodeficiency virus infection of myeloid precursors in bone marrow samples from AIDS patients. *Blood* 1986;68[Suppl 1]:122a(abst 367).
888. Folks TM, Kessler SW, Orenstein JM, et al. Infection and replication of HIV-I in purified progenitor cells of normal human bone marrow. *Science* 1988;242:919–922.

CHAPTER 29

Peripheral T-Cell Lymphomas

Geraldine S. Pinkus and Jonathan W. Said

T-cell malignancies represent a minor proportion of non-Hodgkin's lymphomas in the United States but are relatively more frequent in other geographic areas, particularly in Asia (1–22). In an international study (23), the combined group of peripheral T-cell and natural killer (NK) cell lymphomas constituted only 9.4% of non-Hodgkin's lymphomas. T-cell neoplasms correspond to proliferations derived from lymphoid cells at prethymic, intrathymic, or postthymic stages of T-cell differentiation. Stages of T-cell differentiation are associated with acquisition and loss of a variety of antigens and expression of terminal deoxynucleotidyl transferase (TdT) (24,25). The unifying feature for the diverse group of peripheral T-cell lymphomas is their derivation from mature T cells, such as T lymphocytes at a postthymic stage of T-cell differentiation. In contrast to precursor T-cell lymphoblastic leukemia/lymphoma, which derives from TdT^+ T cells at prethymic or intrathymic stages of differentiation, these lesions consistently lack TdT and CD1. Other phenotypic features of peripheral T-cell neoplasms include loss of pan-T-cell antigens and the occurrence of aberrant phenotypes. This chapter addresses neoplasms of mature T cells, NK-like T cells, and NK/T cells. Cutaneous T-cell lymphomas of mycosis fungoides type, precursor T-cell neoplasms, and leukemias other than adult T-cell leukemia/lymphoma are discussed elsewhere (see Chapters 26, 32, and 46).

Peripheral T-cell lymphomas are characterized by extreme morphologic diversity that has compromised the formulation of a reproducible classification for many years. The Kiel classification (26) recognized the immunologic derivation of these neoplasms and divided them into two groups based on cytologic composition (Table 29.1). However, these subdivisions do not necessarily reflect the biologic potential of these lesions and certain clinical entities are not recognized. In 1994, the Revised European-American Lymphoma (REAL) classification was proposed by the International Lymphoma Study Group, which grouped the T-cell and postulated NK cell lymphomas into clinical entities (27). The diverse histologic lesions that do not represent specific clinical entities were encompassed in the group of unspecified peripheral T-cell lymphomas. This classification was further refined, culminating in the World Health Organization (WHO) classification of peripheral T-cell and NK cell lymphomas (28) (Table 29.2). These disorders can be divided into three general groups (leukemic/disseminated, nodal, or extranodal) based on their clinical features (29) (Table 29.3). Characterization of entities included in this classification has integrated morphologic, clinical, phenotypic, genotypic, cytogenetic, and for some lesions, viral studies.

Phenotypic and genotypic studies have been extremely relevant in our recognition and understanding of these disorders that may be difficult to identify histologically. In contrast to B-cell lymphomas in which a normal nonneoplastic counterpart can be recognized, a normal morphologic counterpart is not well defined for most T-cell and NK cell lymphomas. Some T-cell lymphomas may be difficult to distinguish from reactive lesions. In contrast to B-cell lymphomas in which clonality may potentially be established by immunohistochemistry, a predominant T-cell population, even of a single subset, is insufficient to establish a diagnosis of a T-cell malignancy. Studies that may be helpful include identification of abnormal T-cell subsets (i.e., $CD4^+CD8^+$ or $CD4^-CD8^-$) or an anomalous T-cell phenotype characterized by deletion of pan-T-cell antigens or expression of markers not typically present (e.g., anaplastic lymphoma kinase, CD56). Additional studies for certain cytogenetic abnormalities, such as t(2;5) in anaplastic large cell lymphoma or isochromosome 7q in hepatosplenic T-cell lymphoma, or molecular biologic evaluation for T-cell receptor gene rearrangements

G. S. Pinkus: Department of Pathology, Brigham and Women's Hospital, Boston, Massachusetts 02115

J. W. Said: Division of Anatomic Pathology, University of California Los Angeles School of Medicine, Los Angeles, California 90095

TABLE 29.1. *Updated Kiel classification for T-cell malignancies*

Low grade
Lymphocytic (chronic lymphocytic and prolymphocytic leukemia)
Small cerebriform cell (mycosis fungoides, Sezary's syndrome)
Lymphoepithelioid (Lennert's lymphoma)
Angioimmunoblastic (AILD)
T zone
Pleomorphic small cell (HTLV-1 $\pm$)
High grade
Pleomorphic medium and large cell (HTLV-1 $\pm$)
Immunoblastic (HTLV-1 $\pm$)
Anaplastic large cell (Ki-1 +)
Lymphoblastic
Rare types

Adapted from Stansfeld AG, Diebold J, Kapanci Y, et al. Updated Kiel classification for lymphomas. *Lancet* 1988;1: 292–293.

TABLE 29.2. *Proposed World Health Organization (WHO) classification of T-cell and natural killer cell neoplasms*

Precursor T-cell neoplasm
Precursor T-lymphoblastic lymphoma/leukemia (precursor T-cell acute lymphoblastic leukemia)
Mature (peripheral) T-cell neoplasms
T-cell prolymphocytic leukemia
T-cell granular lymphocytic leukemia
Aggressive NK-cell leukemia
Adult T cell lymphoma/leukemia (HTLV-1^+)
Extranodal NK/T cell lymphoma, nasal type
Enteropathy-type T cell lymphoma
Subcutaneous panniculitis-like T-cell lymphoma
Mycosis fungoides/Sezary syndrome
Hepatosplenic $\gamma\delta$ T cell lymphoma
Anaplastic large cell lymphoma, T/null cell, primary cutaneous type
Anaplastic large cell lymphoma, T/null cell, primary systemic type
Peripheral T-cell lymphoma, not otherwise characterized
Angioimmunoblastic T-cell lymphoma

From Harris NL, Jaffe ES, Diebold J, et al. World Health Organization classification of neoplastic diseases of the hematopoietic and lymphoid tissues: report of the clinical advisory committee meeting, Arlie House, Virginia, November 1997. *J Clin Oncol* 1999;17:3835–3849, with permission.

TABLE 29.3. *Proposed World Health Organization (WHO) classification of peripheral T-cell and natural killer (NK) cell neoplasms according to clinical distribution of disease*

Predominantly nodal
Peripheral T-cell lymphoma, not otherwise characterized
Anaplastic large cell lymphoma, T/null cell, primary systemic type
Angioimmunoblastic T-cell lymphoma
Predominantly extranodal
Extranodal NK/T-cell lymphoma, nasal type
Subcutaneous panniculitis-like T-cell lymphoma
Enteropathy-type T-cell lymphoma
Hepatosplenic $\gamma\delta$ T cell lymphoma
Anaplastic large cell lymphoma, T/null cell, primary cutaneous type
Mycosis fungoides or Sezary syndrome
Predominantly leukemic/disseminated
Adult T-cell leukemia/lymphoma (HTLV-1^+)
Aggressive NK cell leukemia
T-cell granular lymphocytic leukemia
T-cell prolymphocytic leukemia

may be required for diagnosis. The consistent association of certain lymphomas with viral agents, such as Epstein-Barr virus (EBV) in NK/T-cell lymphomas of nasal type and HTLV-1 in adult T-cell leukemia/lymphoma, provides a further basis for accurate evaluation.

GENERAL CLINICAL FEATURES

Peripheral T-cell lymphomas generally affect older individuals (>50 years of age), with males affected more frequently than females (6,12–18,20–22,30). The only exception is anaplastic large cell type that tends to involve children and young adults, although a bimodal age distribution has been observed (i.e., second peak occurs in elderly patients [31–36]). Most patients present with lymphadenopathy. Mediastinal involvement is unusual (13,22,37,38). T-cell lymphomas may be stage III or IV at presentation. Extranodal disease may be observed in association with lymphadenopathy or as the mode of presentation. Extranodal sites of involvement include skin, soft tissue, gastrointestinal tract, lung, spleen, nasopharynx, bone, and nervous system. Placental involvement by a peripheral T-cell lymphoma has also been described (39). B symptoms are common. Hypercalcemia is rare, except in patients with adult T-cell leukemia/lymphoma (22,40,41). Approximately 15% of patients may have a prior history of an immune abnormality or a lymphoproliferative disorder (12,17,18,20–22,37,38,42). In a small number of cases, T-cell lymphomas may occur in patients with a prior history of a B-cell lymphoma, concurrent with a B-cell lymphoma, or may precede the development of a B-cell lymphoma (43). Immunosuppressed patients, including those with organ transplants or patients with congenital or acquired immune deficiency syndromes, may develop peripheral T-cell lymphomas (44–49), but most non-Hodg-

TABLE 29.4. *Comparison of survival in various non-Hodgkin's lymphomas*

Lymphoma type	Five-year survival (%)	Five-year disease-free survival (%)
Peripheral T-cell lymphoma[a]	25	18
Anaplastic large cell lymphoma (T/null cell type)	77	58
Diffuse large B-cell lymphoma	46	41
Marginal zone B-cell, MALT type	74	60

[a] Exclusive of anaplastic large cell type, T or null cell phenotype.

From The Non-Hodgkin's Lymphoma Classification Project. A clinical evaluation of the international lymphoma study group classification of non-Hodgkin's lymphoma. *Blood* 1997;89:3909–3918, with permission.

kin's lymphomas in these clinical settings are of B-cell phenotype (see Chapters 16 and 28). Controversy has existed as to whether the T-cell lymphomas are associated with a worse prognosis than their B-cell counterparts (13,18,21,22, 37,50). Although the clinical course may vary, peripheral T-cell lymphomas, exclusive of anaplastic large cell lymphoma, are regarded as an aggressive form of non-Hodgkin's lymphoma. Patients with T-cell lymphomas may achieve complete remission, but relapses frequently occur. In a study using the REAL classification, T-cell lymphomas, exclusive of anaplastic large cell lymphoma of T-cell or null cell type, had an extremely poor prognosis with an overall 5-year survival of only 25% and a 5-year disease-free survival of 18% (23). The International Prognostic Factor Index strongly predicts outcome for patients with peripheral T-cell lymphoma (51). Survival data for these tumors and several B-cell lymphomas are compared in Table 29.4. Clinical features are summarized in Table 29.5.

TABLE 29.5. *Clinical features of peripheral T-cell and NK/T-cell lymphomas*

Affect older adults (>50 years of age)
  Exception is anaplastic large cell type (bimodal age distribution)
Males > females
Lymphadenopathy most common presentation
Often stage III or IV at presentation
Extranodal presentation may occur involving upper respiratory tract, skin, soft tissue, lung, gastrointestinal tract, bone, spleen, nervous system
B symptoms common
Hypercalcemia rare, except in adult T-cell leukemia/lymphoma
History of immune/lymphoproliferative disorders (15%)
  Sjögren's syndrome
  Hashimoto's thyroiditis
  Angioimmunoblastic lymphadenopathy
  Immune thrombocytopenia purpura
  B-cell lymphoma
  Hodgkin's disease
  Gluten-sensitive enteropathy
  Polyclonal hypergammaglobulinemia
  After transplantation
  Immunodeficiency states

GENERAL HISTOLOGIC FEATURES

Histologically, these lesions demonstrate marked heterogeneity. Generally, a spectrum of lymphoid cells is evident, although a single cell size may predominate. In contrast to B-cell lymphomas, cytologic features are not predictive of biologic outcome. Sequential biopsies have provided evidence for cytologic progression or transformation in peripheral T-cell lymphomas. In occasional cases, such biopsies have also demonstrated a change from a cytologically high-grade tumor to a low-grade malignancy. Lymphoid cells exhibit various degrees of nuclear complexity and include multilobated, bizarre, anaplastic and Reed-Sternberg–like cells. In rare cases, tumor cells of signet ring (52,53) or multilobated type (8,54–57) may be observed. Cells of all sizes may reveal moderate to abundant pale/clear cytoplasm. Clear cells are particularly striking in angioimmunoblastic T-cell lymphomas. Histiocytes, eosinophils and plasma cells may be prominent. In some lymphomas, increased reticulin and compartmentalization are observed. Increased vascularity is frequently observed and is characterized by prominent arborizing high endothelial venules in angioimmunoblastic T-cell lymphomas. The latter lesions are also associated with prominent networks of dendritic cells ($CD21^+$, $CD35^+$, fascin$^+$) that occur outside follicles and frequently surround vascular structures, particularly high endothelial venules. Prominent dendritic networks are not a feature of peripheral T-cell lymphomas of other types. Extensive necrosis may be observed and is a striking feature in extranodal nasal-type NK/T lymphomas.

With nodal involvement, architecture may be completely obliterated or the process may exhibit a paracortical (T zone) or interfollicular pattern, with preservation of B-cell zones (Fig. 29.1). Subcapsular and sinusoidal involvement may be observed, as in anaplastic large cell lymphoma, a tumor that constitutes about 30% to 40% of pediatric large cell lymphomas. Sinusoidal involvement is also a feature of hepatosplenic T-cell lymphoma. Splenic involvement may exhibit a periarteriolar distribution, may occur as nodules produced by coalescence of contiguous areas of involved white pulp, or occasionally exhibit a red pulp distribution (58–62). Rare cases have been associated with spontaneous splenic rupture (63). Skin involvement usually assumes a dermal pattern of infiltration, without epidermotropism (Fig. 29.2), except in adult T-cell leukemia/lymphoma or mycosis fungoides (discussed elsewhere). In one subtype, a panniculitis-type infiltrate is observed. In occasional T-cell lymphomas, prominent erythrophagocytosis by benign histiocytes may involve bone marrow, spleen, or other sites, simulating malignant histiocytosis or virus-associated hemophagocytic syndrome

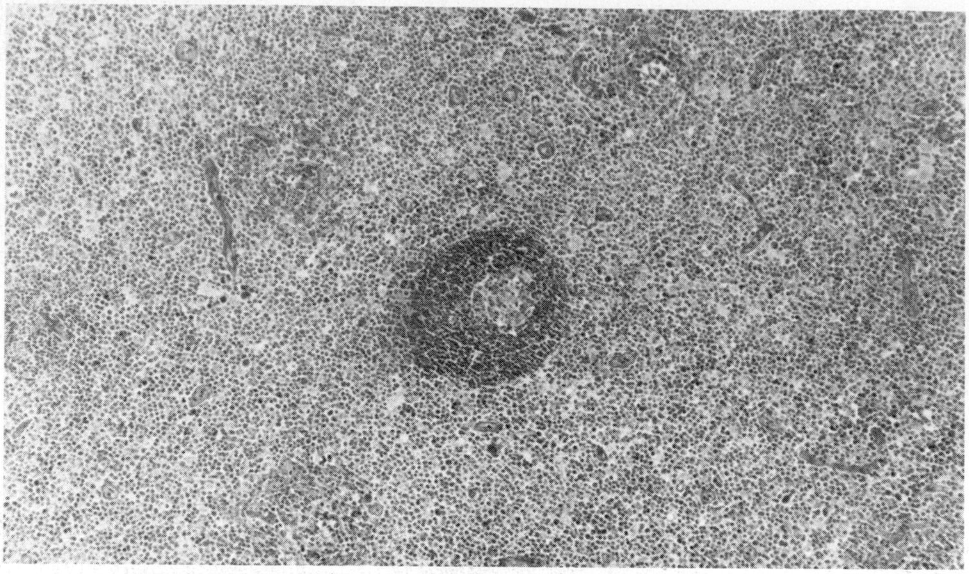

FIG. 29.1. In this node involved by a peripheral T-cell lymphoma not otherwise characterized, the infiltrate extensively involves the interfollicular region with preservation of a follicular B-cell area. Vascularity is mildly increased (periodic acid–Schiff stain, original magnification: 80× magnification).

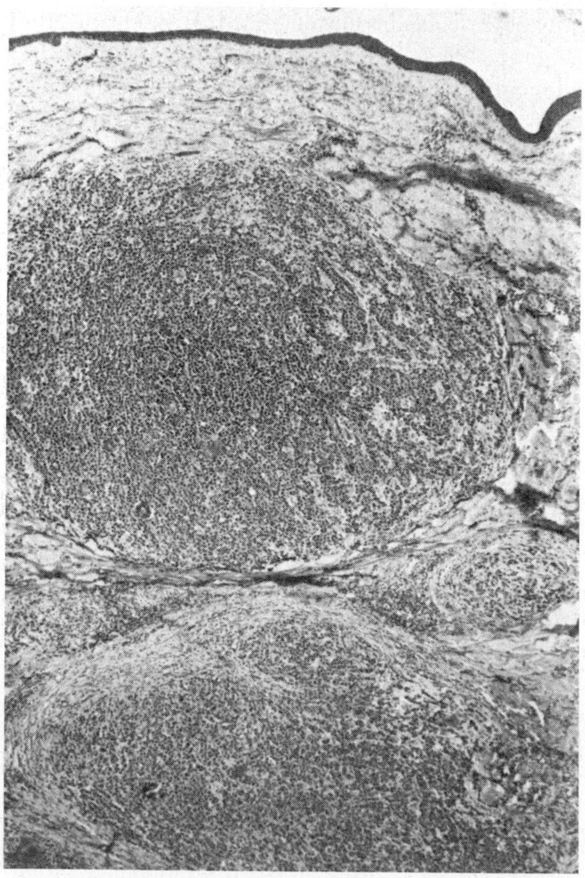

FIG. 29.2. Skin involvement in peripheral T-cell lymphomas is generally characterized by dermal infiltration without evidence of epidermotropism, as observed in this biopsy. Prominent nodular aggregates of neoplastic T cells are present in the dermis (hematoxylin and eosin stain, original magnification: 40× magnification).

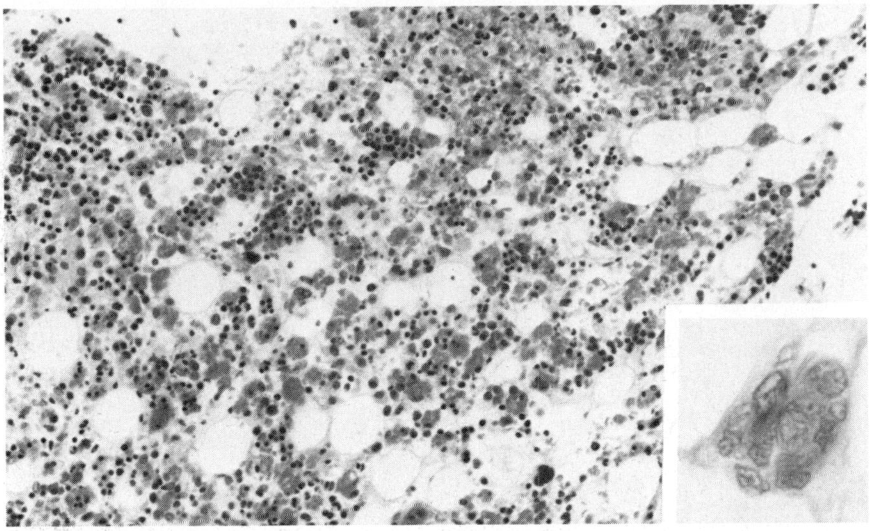

FIG. 29.3. Hemophagocytic syndrome characterized by exuberant phagocytosis of erythrocytes and other hematopoietic cells by benign histiocytes, as observed in this bone marrow biopsy, may be associated with a peripheral T-cell lymphoma, particularly subcutaneous panniculitis-like T-cell lymphoma and extranodal nasal-type natural killer/T-cell lymphoma (hematoxylin and eosin stain, original magnification: 180× magnification). **Inset:** Histiocyte with abundant phagocytosed erythrocytes (original magnification: 840× magnification). (From Pinkus GS, O'Hara CJ, Said JW. Peripheral/post-thymic T cell lymphomas: a spectrum of disease. *Cancer* 1990;65:971–998, with permission).

(Fig. 29.3). This finding may be related to lymphokine production by the neoplastic T cells. A recent article provides an excellent summary of the features of peripheral T-cell and NK cell neoplasms (29). The general morphologic features of these neoplasms are summarized in Table 29.6.

PERIPHERAL T-CELL LYMPHOMAS NOT OTHERWISE CHARACTERIZED

In the REAL (27) and WHO (28) classifications, peripheral T-cell lymphomas that do not correspond to clinicopathologic entities are placed in the category of *not otherwise characterized.* Because these tumors comprise a major proportion of peripheral T-cell lymphomas and are clinically aggressive, their recognition is highly relevant. The clinical and morphologic features of these lesions are highly variable. In the small group of tumors with a predominance of small cells, various degrees of nuclear irregularity are observed (Fig. 29.4), although relatively round nuclei may be observed in occasional cases (Fig. 29.5). Chromatin is heavily clumped and nucleoli are inconspicuous. Cytoplasm varies from scant to abundant and may appear pale or clear. Proliferation centers are not observed. Mitoses vary but may be frequent.

Peripheral T-cell lymphomas comprised of a spectrum of lymphoid cells or a predominant population of large cells represent most of the lesions in this category. The small- to intermediate-sized cells reveal moderate to marked nuclear irregularity and generally various quantities of pale cytoplasm. Larger lymphoid cells exhibit various degrees of nuclear complexity, with two or more distinct nucleoli, and pale to clear cytoplasm (Fig. 29.6). The large cell component may occur dispersed through the process or as clusters or

TABLE 29.6. *General morphologic features of peripheral T-cell lymphomas*

Extensive morphologic heterogeneity
Spectrum of lymphoid cells; single cell size may predominate
Various degrees of nuclear complexity
Abundant pale or clear cytoplasm
Presence of abundant pale/clear cytoplasm in full spectrum of cell sizes,[a] most striking in angioimmunoblastic type
Large transformed cells usually exhibit fine chromatin, single to several distinct nucleoli, and delicate nuclear membranes
Large bizarre or Reed-Sternberg–like cells may occur, particularly in cases with Hodgkin-like features or anaplastic large cell lymphomas
Increased vascularity, prominent in angioimmunoblastic T-cell lymphomas
Histiocytes increased; may be abundant
Eosinophils variable; conspicuous in lymphomas with Hodgkin-like features
Prominent necrosis in nasal and nasal-type lymphomas; infrequent in other types
Dendritic cell networks in angioimmunoblastic lymphomas
Sinusoidal growth patterns may occur, notably in anaplastic large cell type
T zone growth pattern may occur
Transformation in cell type may occur

[a] Quantity of cytoplasm may vary; appearance is contingent on fixative, with cytoplasmic clearing most marked with formalin fixation compared with pale eosinophilic cytoplasm with B5 fixative.

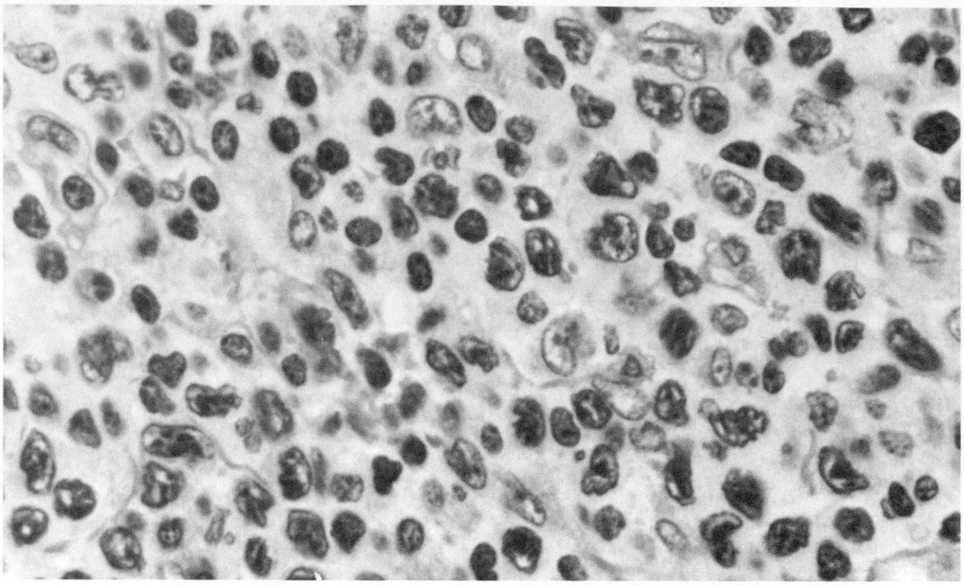

FIG. 29.4. In this peripheral T-cell lymphoma not otherwise characterized, the infiltrate consists mainly of small lymphoid cells with heavily clumped chromatin and moderate to marked nuclear irregularity (hematoxylin and eosin stain, original magnification: 850× magnification).

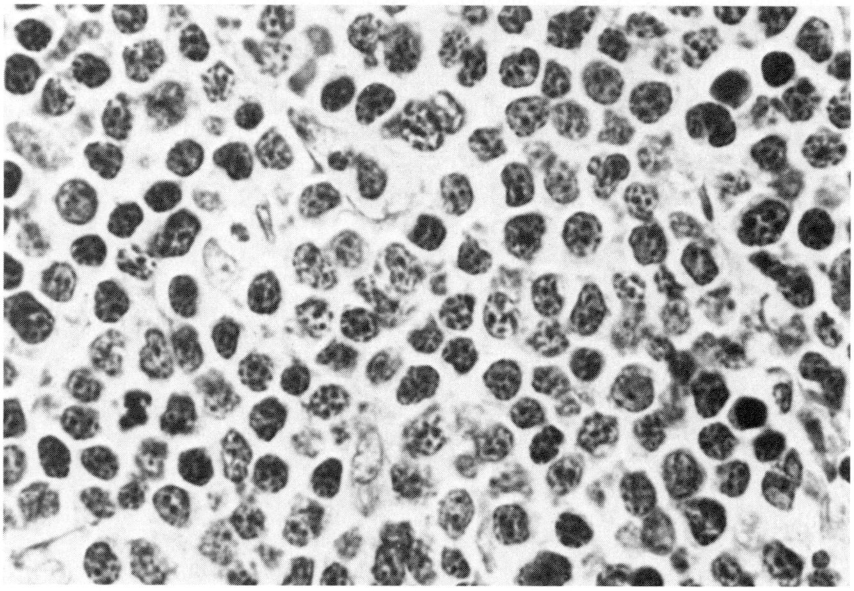

FIG. 29.5. In rare cases of peripheral T-cell lymphoma not otherwise characterized, small lymphoid cells with round nuclei and heavily clumped chromatin, resembling cells of small lymphocytic lymphoma of B-cell type, constitute the infiltrate. In contrast to the B-cell lesions, neoplastic T cells contain more abundant cytoplasm, proliferation centers are absent, and the mitotic rate is much greater. In this case, transformation to a lymphoma composed of large cells occurred with progressive disease and a survival time of only 27 months (periodic acid–Schiff stain, original magnification: 840× magnification).

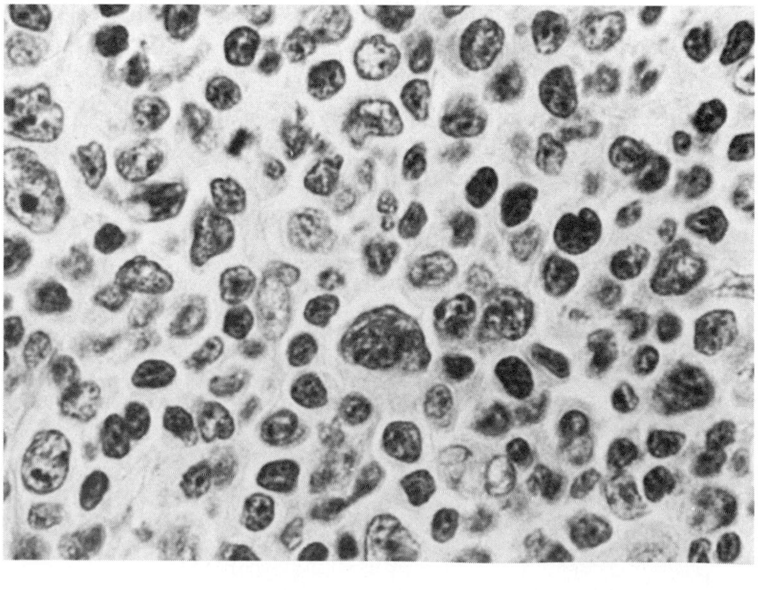

FIG. 29.6. The broad cytologic spectrum of peripheral T-cell lymphomas not otherwise characterized includes proliferations composed of a spectrum of lymphoid cells that exhibit various degrees of nuclear irregularity, which are most prominent in the large neoplastic cells in this case. Moderate quantities of pale cytoplasm are observed for cells of all sizes (hematoxylin and eosin stain, original magnification: 900× magnification). (From Pinkus GS, O'Hara CJ, Said JW. Peripheral/post-thymic T-cell lymphomas: a spectrum of disease. *Cancer* 1990; 65:971–998, with permission.)

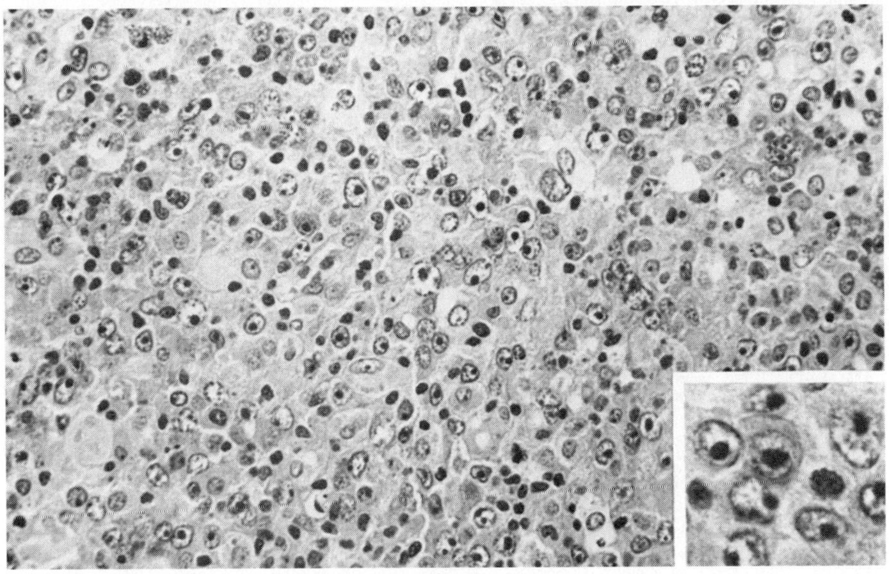

FIG. 29.7. Large neoplastic cells with immunoblastic features may dominate the proliferation of some peripheral T-cell lymphomas not otherwise characterized. Neoplastic T cells contain relatively regular nuclei, dispersed chromatin, one or more prominent nucleoli (some centrally placed), and moderate to abundant cytoplasm. Scattered histiocytes and small lymphocytes are also seen (hematoxylin and eosin stain, 400× magnification; **Inset**: original magnification: 900× magnification).

aggregates. T-cell lymphomas comprised mainly of large cells may arise *de novo* or represent transformation of other cytologic types of T-cell lymphoma. The morphologic features of the large cells may vary considerably. Some lesions consist of large cells with relatively regular nuclei with dispersed chromatin and several small to medium, distinct (occasionally inclusion-like) nucleoli, and moderate to abundant pale or clear to basophilic cytoplasm, corresponding to an immunoblastic type of cell (Fig. 29.7). In other proliferations, various degrees of nuclear irregularity occur, which may be extreme in some cases (Fig. 29.8). The infiltrate may include hyperlobated and polyploid forms or large highly pleomorphic cells, some of which may resemble Reed-Sternberg cells (Fig. 29.9). Histologic features may suggest a neo-

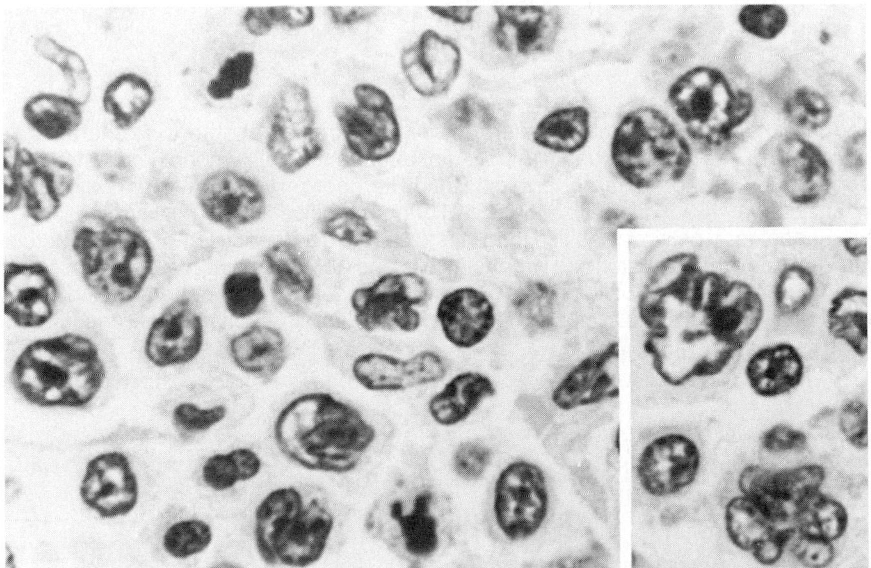

FIG. 29.8. Some peripheral T-cell lymphomas not otherwise characterized may be composed of an infiltrate of large neoplastic cells with striking degrees of nuclear irregularity, including occasional multilobated forms (**inset**). Chromatin is fine and nucleoli are small or inconspicuous (hematoxylin and eosin stain, original magnification: 1,000× magnification; **Inset**: original magnification: 1,200× magnification).

A
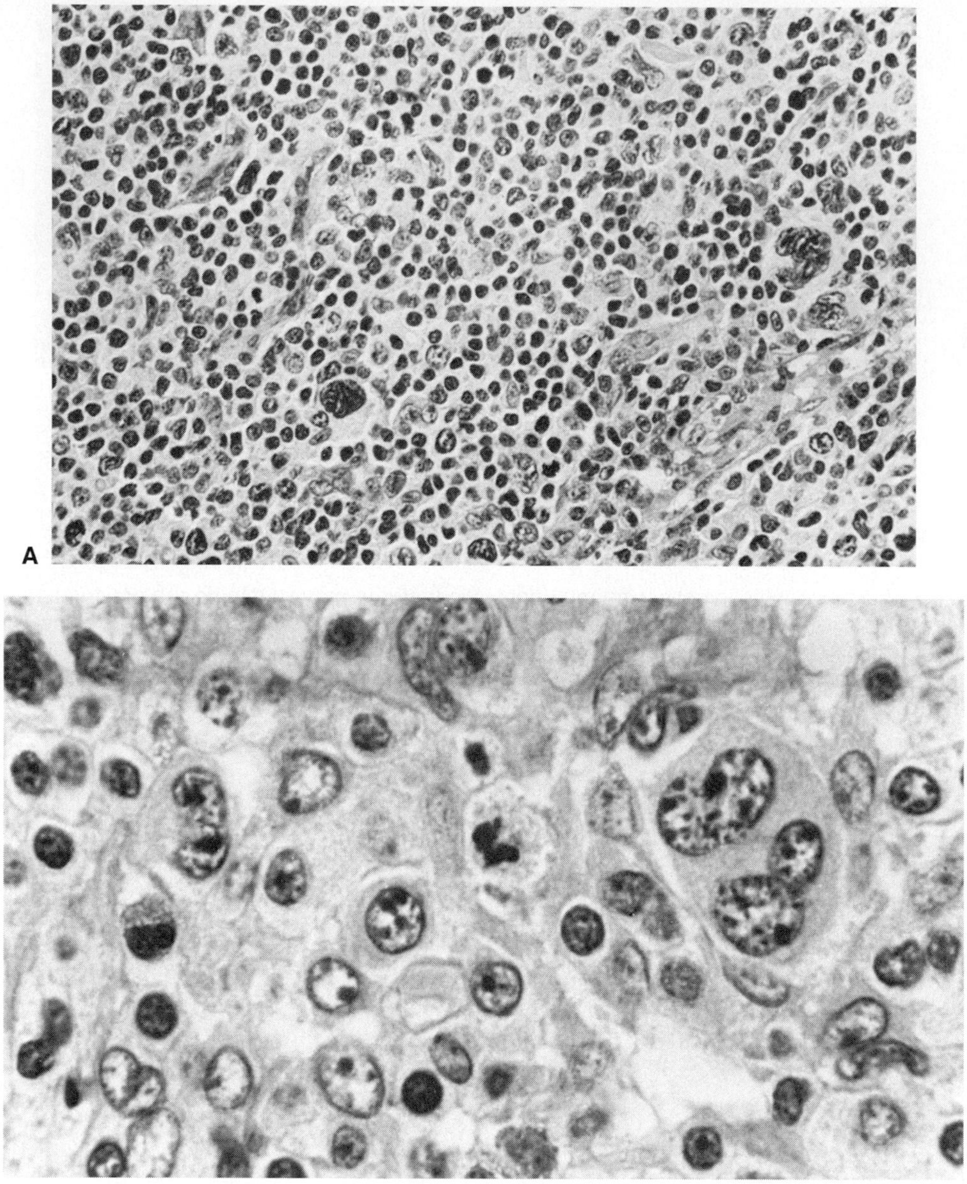
B

FIG. 29.9. A: The features of some peripheral T-cell lymphomas not otherwise characterized resemble Hodgkin's disease, with a background composed of abundant small lymphoid cells, frequent histiocytes and eosinophils, and scattered, large, atypical Reed-Sternberg–like cells (hematoxylin and eosin stain, original magnification: 400× magnification). **B:** Higher magnification shows that the large cells are not typical of the neoplastic cells of classic Hodgkin's disease. The spectrum of the background lymphoid cells, which includes large transformed lymphoid cells and abundant cytoplasm in most lymphoid forms, is inconsistent with a diagnosis of Hodgkin's disease. In difficult cases, phenotypic and genotypic studies may be required for accurate diagnosis (hematoxylin and eosin stain, original magnification: 1,000× magnification).

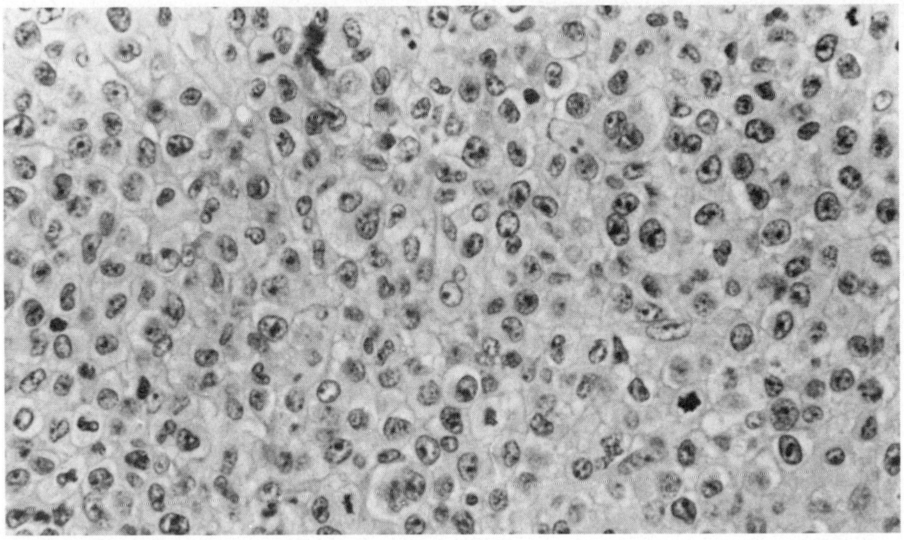

FIG. 29.10. This peripheral T-cell lymphoma is composed of large cells with various degrees of nuclear irregularity, dispersed chromatin, and one to several distinct nucleoli. A particularly striking feature in this B5-fixed section is the abundance of pale cytoplasm in the tumor cells associated with delicate cell borders (hematoxylin and eosin stain, original magnification: 600× magnification). (From Pinkus GS, O'Hara CJ, Said JW. Peripheral/post-thymic T-cell lymphomas: a spectrum of disease. *Cancer* 1990; 65:971–998, with permission).

plasm of true histiocytic type, such as malignant histiocytosis. Analysis of proliferations previously regarded as true histiocytic neoplasms have revealed markers compatible with T-cell lymphomas (33,64–66).

The cytoplasm of the large neoplastic T cells may vary from pale to clear (Fig. 29.10), or even appear amphophilic, a cytologic feature more suggestive of a B-cell neoplasm. A clear cell appearance appears contingent on the fixative employed, and is more apparent in formalin-fixed tissue as compared with B5 fixative. The presence of "clear cells" is highly suggestive of a T-cell neoplasm, but may also be observed in B-cell proliferations. The large cells in T-cell lymphomas may be accompanied by various numbers of smaller atypical lymphoid cells. In some cases, histiocytes may be conspicuous and eosinophils or plasma cells may be observed. Vascular proliferation is variable. In T-cell lymphomas containing large Reed-Sternberg–like cells and an infiltrate that includes histiocytes, eosinophils, and plasma cells, the process may closely resemble Hodgkin's disease and pose a difficult diagnostic problem. Cytologically, careful inspection of the lymphoid population may assist in this distinction. Peripheral T-cell lymphomas are characterized by a spectrum of lymphoid forms, frequently associated with marked nuclear irregularity. In Hodgkin's disease, the lymphoid cells exhibit little cytologic atypia, and cells at various stages of transformation, including large transformed lymphoid cells (immunoblasts), are not a feature of the disease. Cell marker studies may further assist in distinguishing these lesions. The large Reed-Sternberg–like cells of peripheral T-cell lymphomas (other than those of angioimmunoblastic type; discussed subsequently) typically express leukocyte common antigen (CD45) and T-cell antigens, and generally lack CD15 (Leu-M1; a granulocytic/histiocytic-associated antigen) and fascin, although some cases reportedly express these antigens (67,68). In classic Hodgkin's disease, Reed-Sternberg cells generally lack leukocyte common antigen and T-cell antigens, but express CD15, with a membranous/paranuclear/cytoplasmic staining pattern (69,70), and are strongly reactive for fascin (i.e., cytoplasmic reactivity [68]). In classic Hodgkin's disease and T-cell lymphomas, the background lymphoid cells are typically of T-cell type. In T-cell lymphomas, frequently an anomalous phenotype with deletion of T-cell antigens is observed for the lymphoid cells (71,72), in contrast with Hodgkin's disease, in which preservation of T-cell antigens is observed with a predominance of helper/inducer T cells. CD30 (Ki-1) antigen, a relatively consistent feature of Reed-Sternberg cells of Hodgkin's disease, may also be observed for large cells of some non-Hodgkin's lymphomas (33,35). In some cases, gene rearrangement studies may be required for the distinction between Hodgkin's disease and peripheral T-cell lymphoma. A distinct rearranged band for the T-cell receptor β chain gene strongly favors a T-cell lymphoma but cannot be regarded as an unequivocal marker. A comparison of features of T-cell lymphoma and Hodgkin's disease are presented in Table 29.7. In cases with equivocal immunophenotypic and genotypic studies, the lymphoma is best regarded as unclassifiable.

Another lesion that may pose a diagnostic problem is a B-cell lymphoma associated with a striking T-cell infiltrate,

TABLE 29.7. *Comparison of features of peripheral T-cell lymphomas and classic Hodgkin's disease*

Feature	T-Cell lymphoma	Hodgkin's Disease
Background	Spectrum of cells, with atypia	Small lymphocytes, little atypia
Predominant cell type	T cell	T cell
Reed-Sternberg–type cells	Atypical forms	Classic
LCA	+	−
CD15	−[a]	+
T-cell antigens	+	−[b]
Fascin	−[a]	+
B-cell antigens	−	Occasional +
TCR rearrangement	+	− to +/−

[a] Observed in some cases.
[b] Rarely seen in paraffin sections.

the *T cell–rich B-cell lymphoma* (73–76). These lesions may also contain abundant histiocytes. Although this lymphoma is actually a B-cell malignancy, the presence of abundant T cells and possibly also histiocytes, may obscure the minor population of neoplastic B cells, leading to an erroneous interpretation of a T-cell lymphoma. Careful analysis of these lesions should verify that the background T-cell proliferation is a reactive process, associated with a neoplastic component of B-cell derivation, generally of large cell type. In some cases it may be difficult to demonstrate unequivocal clonality for the B-cell population, particularly if only paraffin tissue sections are available. In such lesions, however, the use of pan-B-cell antibodies (CD20, CD79a) should permit identification and characterization of the true B-cell nature of the malignancy. In some instances, gene rearrangement studies may be required for definitive evaluation.

Several other unusual variants of T-cell lymphoma have been described and would be included in this category. The peripheral T-cell lymphoma that previously had been designated as *lymphoepithelioid cell lymphoma (Lennert's lymphoma)* would be included in this group (77–81). This lesion was first described by Lennert in 1968, who regarded the disorder as a mixed entity that included cases of Hodgkin's disease (77). Older individuals are generally affected. Splenomegaly and lymphadenopathy may be prominent features, with involvement by Waldeyer's ring also observed in European cases. The disease is generally disseminated, with involvement of liver and bone marrow. Histologically, an exuberant proliferation of epithelioid histiocytes is present in clusters and sheets, presumably occurring in response to lymphokines produced by neoplastic T cells. Eosinophils and plasma cells may be seen. The abnormal small lymphoid cells are of particular diagnostic importance and are oval to elongated with slightly irregular (''squiggly'') nuclear configurations; various numbers of medium- and large-sized cells may also occur (Fig. 29.11). Transformation to a lymphoma of large cell type may occur (82). In some cases, distinction from Hodgkin's disease or from a B-cell lymphoma with a high content of epithelioid histiocytes must be made by appropriate studies.

T zone lymphomas, although infrequent in this country, are often observed in other regions, such as China (30). These proliferations are characterized by an infiltrate that involves T-cell areas of the lymph node and are composed of small- to intermediate-sized lymphoid cells with limited pleomorphism, and generally abundant pale to clear cytoplasm. The number of high endothelial venules also is increased. Initially, follicular areas are preserved and may be hyperplastic. The infiltrate may include occasional large transformed cells and reactive cells (e.g., eosinophils, plasma cells, histiocytes). These lymphomas are considered low grade but may progress to high-grade neoplasms.

T-cell lymphomas with unusual nuclear features have also been described that may pose diagnostic problems in their morphologic distinction from other tumors. T-cell lymphomas of signet ring cell type have been observed and are associated with skin involvement and a relatively favorable prognosis (52,53). T-cell lymphomas of multilobated cell type are unusual neoplasms that frequently involve extranodal sites (8,54–57). Angiotropic (intravascular) T-cell lymphomas have been reported (83–87). Signet ring, multilobated, or angiotropic types of lymphoma may represent tumors of T- or B-cell type (88–90); marker studies are required for definitive assessment.

ANGIOIMMUNOBLASTIC T-CELL LYMPHOMA

Recognition of patterns of lymphoid proliferation in association with abnormal immune states can be traced to descriptions of entities called *lymphogranulomatosis-X* by Lennert (91), *immunoblastic lymphadenopathy (IBL)* by Lukes and Tindle (92), *and angioimmunoblastic lymphadenopathy with dysproteinemia (AILD)* by Frizzera, Moran, and Rappaport (93). These disorders appear to represent a spectrum of closely related, although not identical, diseases in which the boundary between benign and malignant may be problematic. Patients with these disorders are usually in their sixth or seventh decades, with a slight male predominance. Typically, these patients exhibit evidence of hyperimmunity, including polyclonal hypergammaglobulinemia, Coombs'-positive hemolytic anemia, fever, pruritis, rash, and generalized lymphadenopathy. Allergic reactions to an-

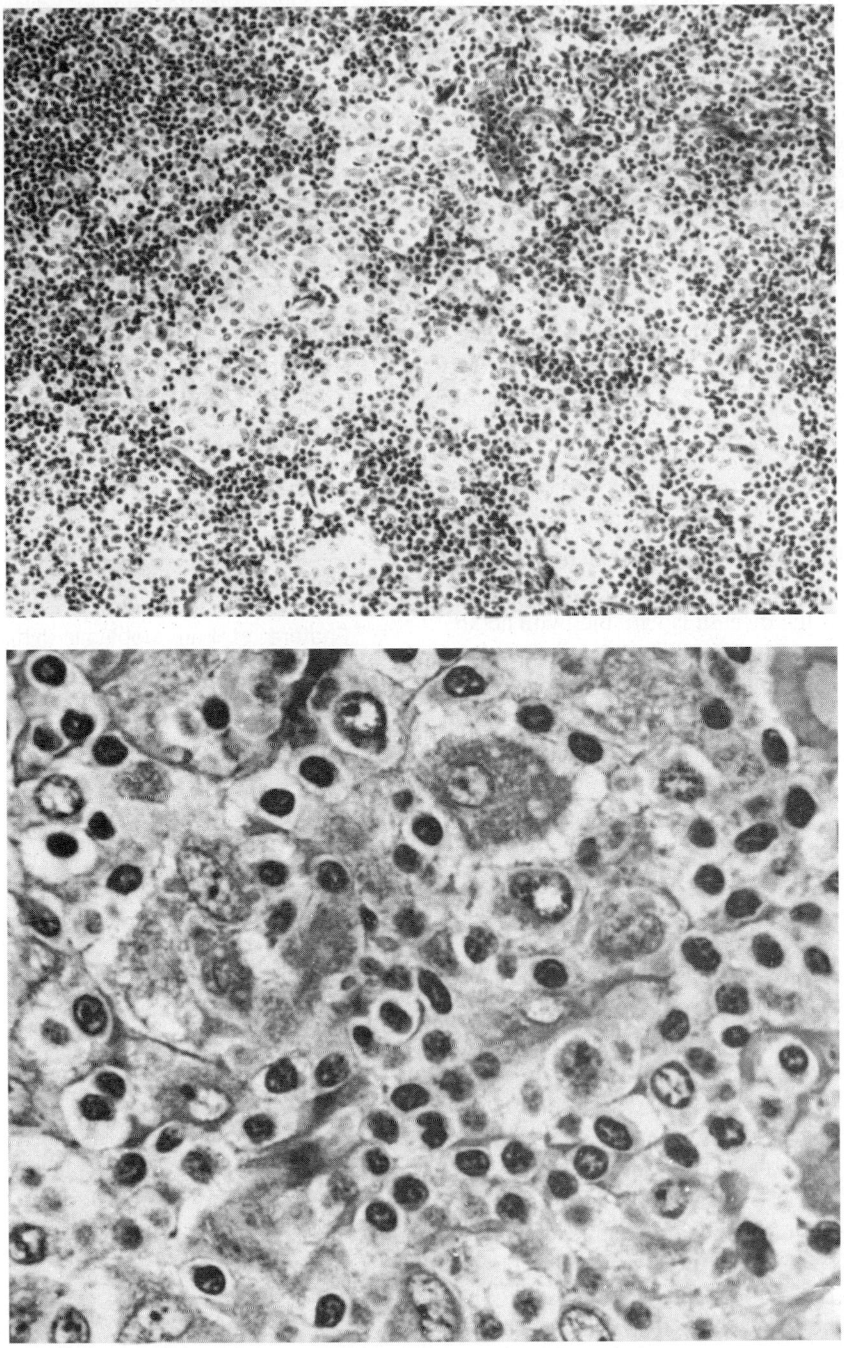
A
B

FIG. 29.11. **A:** This variant of peripheral T-cell lymphoma not otherwise characterized is associated with a prominent proliferation of epithelioid histiocytes admixed with small lymphoid cells and would be classified as a lymphoepithelioid lymphoma (Lennert's lymphoma) in the Kiel classification (hematoxylin and eosin stain, original magnification: 120× magnification). **B:** Higher magnification demonstrates small lymphoid cells with heavily clumped chromatin, minimal nuclear irregularity, and frequent, interspersed epithelioid histiocytes. A few medium to large lymphoid cells are also seen (hematoxylin and eosin stain, original magnification: 800× magnification). (From Pinkus GS, O'Hara CJ, Said JW. Peripheral/post-thymic T-cell lymphomas: a spectrum of disease. *Cancer* 1990;65:971–998, with permission.)

tibiotics commonly develop. Carcinomas occur as second malignancies in up to 11% of these patients (94).

Histologic features of IBL and AILD include complete loss of normal architecture and nodal effacement with overall lymphoid depletion. A characteristic feature is the presence of an anastomosing network of small blood vessels with prominent endothelial cells associated with a mixed B-cell and T-cell infiltrate composed of a spectrum of cells that includes small lymphocytes, plasma cells, histiocytes, eosinophils, and variable numbers of large transformed lymphoid cells or immunoblasts. The presence of interstitial deposits of periodic acid–Schiff–positive granular eosinophilic material in IBL has been emphasized by Lukes and Tindle (92). Ultrastructurally, this material can be shown to consist of debris from dying and degenerating cells (95). Unlike IBL, the presence of amorphous eosinophilic material is not essential for the diagnosis of AILD. Residual or ''burned-out'' germinal centers are described in AILD but not in IBL. Similar proliferations may be seen in tissues other than lymph nodes in IBL or AILD, including spleen, liver, bone marrow, and skin. The outcome of the disease is variable, with about half the patients dying relatively soon after diagnosis regardless of therapy. The remainder have a more prolonged course with exacerbations and remissions.

In one study of AILD, 36 of 84 patients revealed histologic features of a large cell malignant lymphoma, identified by clustering of monomorphous populations of immunoblasts (96). This relationship was first appreciated in Japan (96,97) in a series of adult patients with IBL-like T-cell lymphoma. These neoplasms were associated with polyclonal hypergammaglobulinemia and generalized lymphadenopathy. Most tumors that evolve in this setting are peripheral T-cell lymphomas, although B-cell neoplasms may develop in the setting of AILD or IBL (98–100). Evolution to lymphoma is generally characterized by greater cellularity, greater pleomorphism, and an increased population of large transformed lymphoid cells (Table 29.8). In addition to histologic similarities with IBL or AILD, including prominent arborizing blood vessels and effacement of architecture (Fig. 29.12A, B), the infiltrate is more cellular, with a more uniform population of small T lymphocytes with slightly irregular nuclei, small nucleoli and moderate to abundant cytoplasm. The background proliferation may contain reactive epithelioid histiocytes, plasma cells and eosinophils. A prominent population of large transformed T lymphoid cells with clear or amphophilic cytoplasm is essential to the diagnosis. In contrast to many T-cell lymphomas that exhibit marked nuclear irregularity, these cells tend to have relatively regular nuclear contours and may be scattered in the infiltrate or occur focally in clusters or sheets (Fig. 29.12C). ''Burned-out'' germinal centers may be seen but are less common than in cases of AILD (30). Meshworks of proliferating follicular dendritic cells that are associated with small blood vessels are present (Fig. 29.12D), a finding not typically observed for other peripheral T-cell lymphomas (101–103). Complete agreement is lacking as to whether this feature alone in a

TABLE 29.8. *Histologic comparison of angioimmunoblastic lymphadenopathy with dysproteinemia and angioimmunoblastic T-cell lymphoma*

AILD
Architectural effacement
Poorly cellular
Mixed-cell infiltrate with small cells and immunoblasts
Eosinophilic sludgy material[a]
Arborizing venules
Burnt-out germinal centers
Angioimmunoblastic T-cell lymphoma
Architectural effacement
Greater cellularity
Increased immunoblasts including clusters and sheets
Clear cells
Occasional Reed-Sternberg–type EBV$^+$ B cells in some cases
Arborizing venules
Absence of eosinophilic sludgy material
Burnt-out germinal centers variable
Proliferation of dendritic cells

AILD, angioimmunoblastic lymphadenopathy with dysproteinemia.

[a] Feature of immunoblastic lymphadenopathy, but not AILD.

peripheral T-cell neoplasm is sufficient to categorize the process as an angioimmunoblastic T-cell lymphoma. Occasional Reed-Sternberg–like B cells (discussed further subsequently) may be observed.

Phenotypic and cytogenetic studies may be helpful in categorizing angioimmunoblastic T-cell lymphomas and differentiating between AILD and lymphoma (Table 29.8). Immunoblastic lymphadenopathy and AILD are associated with a mixture of B and T lymphocytes (104). T cells include CD4$^+$ and CD8$^+$ lymphocytes, without loss of normal T-cell differentiation antigens. In most cases of angioimmunoblastic T-cell lymphoma, CD4$^+$ cells predominate, frequently associated with aberrant T-cell phenotype, with loss of CD5, CD7, or CD3. Although the first cases reported in Japan had a predominance of CD8$^+$ cells (96), later studies have revealed a CD4 helper/inducer phenotype for these lymphomas (105). DNA hybridization studies reveal clonal rearrangements of the T-cell receptor β chain gene in most angioimmunoblastic T-cell lymphomas, as well as in cases that exhibit the histologic features of AILD (99,106,107). Rearrangements of immunoglobulin heavy- and light-chain genes, as well as T-cell receptor genes, are also found in up to 30% of cases (107,108). In other types of T-cell lymphoma, immunoglobulin gene rearrangements are an unusual finding. In some cases, large lymphoid cells of B-cell phenotype that resemble classic Reed-Sternberg cells and variants may be identified in the background of the T-cell proliferation. These cells have the appearance and immunophenotype of Reed-Sternberg cells (CD15$^+$, CD30$^+$), are CD20$^+$, and harbor Epstein-Barr virus (EBER$^+$, LMP$^+$) (109). In a lesion associated with limited cytologic atypia of the T-cell

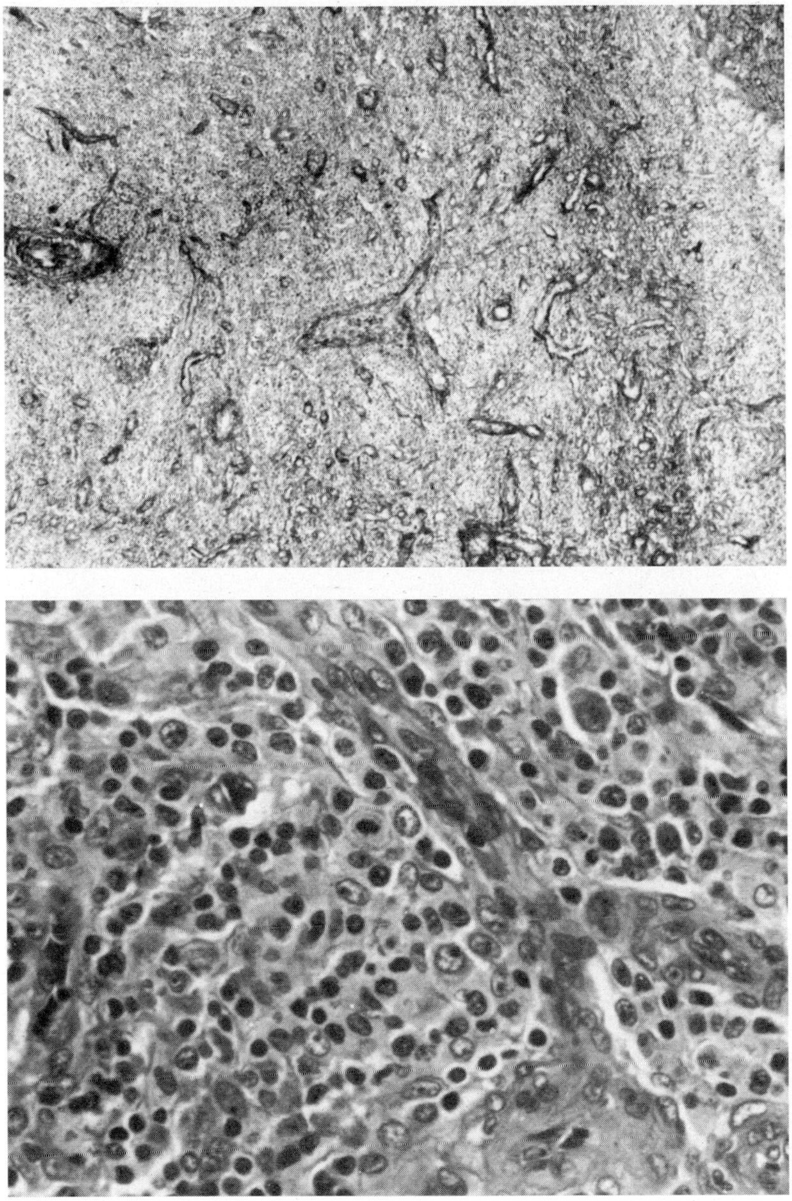

A

B

FIG. 29.12. Angioimmunoblastic T-cell lymphoma. **A:** This type of peripheral T-cell lymphoma is characterized by a prominent branching vascular proliferation that is delineated in this node by a reticulin stain (reticulin stain, original magnification: 120× magnification). **B:** At higher magnification, blood vessels with prominent endothelial cells are present in the proliferation, which is composed of small lymphoid cells with slightly irregular nuclei, histiocytes, and scattered, large lymphoid cells. Most lymphoid forms contain moderate to abundant cytoplasm (hematoxylin and eosin stain, original magnification: 350× magnification). *(continued)*

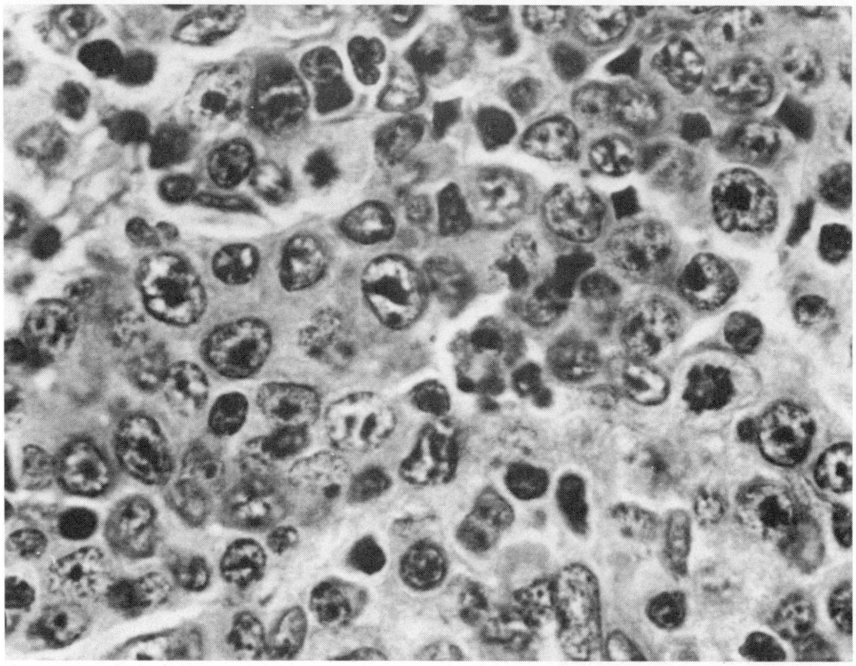

C

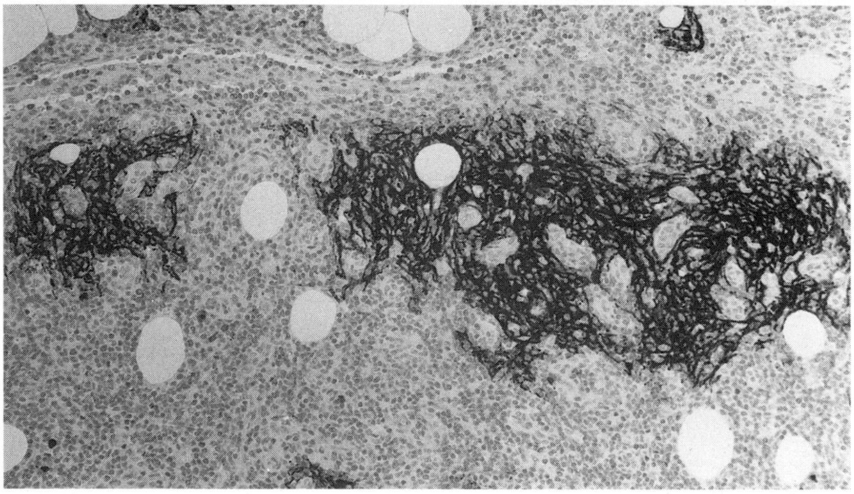

D

FIG. 29.12. *Continued.* **C:** Large, transformed lymphoid cells are present in clusters or aggregates, a feature helpful in the distinction of this lesion from angioimmunoblastic lymphadenopathy with dysproteinemia (hematoxylin and eosin stain, original magnification: 500× magnification). **D:** This immunohistochemical study for the dendritic cell marker CD21 demonstrates a feature observed in angioimmunoblastic T-cell lymphomas that is not typically observed in other T-cell neoplasms. Notice the meshworks of dendritic cells that are associated with small blood vessels consistent with high endothelial venules (immunoperoxidase study, hematoxylin counterstain, original magnification: 120× magnification).

population, distinction from classic Hodgkin's disease may be difficult. Polymerase chain reaction (PCR) analysis of microdissected Reed-Sternberg–type cells for immunoglobulin heavy-chain gene rearrangements have demonstrated an oligoclonal pattern. Clonal rearrangements of the T-cell receptor γ chain gene were observed in these cases. These patients do not appear to be at high risk for progression to Hodgkin's disease. The patients' underlying immune abnormalities may be the basis for the oligoclonal expansion of EBV-infected large B cells.

Characteristic chromosome patterns described in AILD and angioimmunoblastic lymphoma include the frequent presence of karyotypically unrelated abnormal clones, cells with nonclonal abnormalities, and a high incidence of trisomies of 3 and 5 (110,111). Interphase cytogenetic studies have demonstrated multiple unrelated aberrant clones in angioimmunoblastic T-cell lymphomas and in AILD. The significance of these findings is unclear, although they suggest that AILD may represent a prelymphomatous state and that, in some instances, clonal evolution to a T-cell lymphoma may occur at a genomic level, even before histologic evidence of lymphomatous transformation is apparent. The presence of clonal genomic populations in AILD has been used as evidence that these are neoplastic entities *de novo* but, as in other abnormal immune states, a monoclonal cell population cannot indubitably be equated with malignancy. Genotypic studies have demonstrated that clones can appear and disappear or new clones can emerge. Apparently, one or more events must supervene for the development of overt lymphoma. Many cases of AILD have an abrupt onset after

TABLE 29.9. *Phenotypic and genotypic findings in angioimmunoblastic lymphadenopathy and angioimmunoblastic T-cell lymphoma*

Angioimmunoblastic lymphadenopathy with dysproteinemia
Mixed T- and B-cell proliferation
Mixed population of $CD4^+$ and $CD8^+$ lymphocytes
No loss of T-cell antigens
$T\beta$, $T\gamma$, and J_H chain gene rearrangement variable
Angioimmunoblastic T-cell lymphoma
$CD4^+$ lymphocytes predominate
Aberrant T-cell phenotypes common
Loss of CD5, CD7, CD3
Occasional EBV^+ Reed-Sternberg type B cells[a]
$T\beta$ gene rearrangement common
J_H gene rearrangement variable
Nonrandom chromosomal abnormalities common

[a] $CD15^+$, $CD30^+$, $CD20^+$ (109).

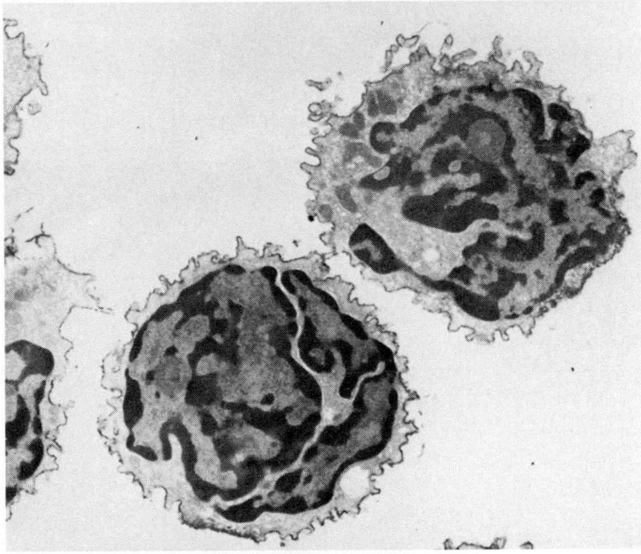

FIG. 29.13. Adult T-cell lymphoma/leukemia. Electron micrograph of neoplastic T cells from cerebrospinal fluid illustrates the highly irregular nuclear outlines with clumped heterochromatin and prominent nucleoli. Immunoperoxidase labeling with CD4 reveals a linear staining pattern *(black)* along the cell membrane. Phenotypically, the neoplastic T cells in this disorder are uniformly CD4 positive and express large amounts of interleukin-2 receptors (CD25, not shown) (uranyl acetate, lead citrate stain, original magnification: 20,000× magnification).

exposure to an allergic stimulus (e.g., drugs, virus) and a fluctuating clinical course, suggesting that they may represent the manifestation of an abnormal immune reaction. Phenotypic and genotypic studies for these lesions are summarized in Table 29.9.

ADULT T-CELL LEUKEMIA/LYMPHOMA

The term *adult T-cell lymphoma/leukemia* (ATLL) encompasses a morphologic spectrum of disorders associated with the human retrovirus HTLV-1 (112–117). HTLV-1 is endemic in southern Japan, but cases have been reported from the Caribbean, United Kingdom, and the United States. Characteristic clinical features include adult onset with widespread disease at presentation associated with generalized lymphadenopathy and early dissemination to liver, spleen, skin, peripheral blood and the central nervous system. The mediastinum is usually spared. Paraneoplastic syndromes, including hypercalcemia and susceptibility to opportunistic infections, contribute to the aggressive clinical course and poor survival (41). The disease is generally rapidly progressive despite aggressive chemotherapy (115). However, because ATLL may respond to interferon and antiviral therapy (e.g., zidovudine), recognition of this disorder is of clinical relevance. Chronic or smoldering forms of the disease are less common in the West but may be associated with pulmonary infiltrates and predisposition to infection.

Histologically, ATLL is most readily diagnosed by the appearance of characteristic pleomorphic lobated lymphoid cells in the peripheral blood or cerebrospinal fluid (Fig. 29.13). Similar cells may be observed in lymph nodes that, if incompletely involved, exhibit a leukemic pattern of infiltration by pleomorphic medium to large lymphoid forms (Fig. 29.14). Bizarre polyploid cells may occur. Small cell lymphomas with irregular nuclei may also be associated with HTLV-1 infection. Skin involvement may simulate mycosis fungoides, with epidermotropism, including the presence of Pautrier-type abscesses. Phenotypically, the neoplastic cells in ATLL are uniformly of mature helper/inducer T-cell type ($CD4^+$) and express large amounts of IL-2 receptor (TAC antigen, CD25). Neoplastic cells are $CD2^+$, $CD3^+$, and $CD5^+$ with variable expression of CD7. All cases reveal clonally integrated HTLV-1 genes. Features of this disorder are discussed elsewhere in more detail (see Chapter 44).

ANAPLASTIC LARGE CELL LYMPHOMA

Anaplastic large cell lymphoma (ALCL) represents an unusual variant of non-Hodgkin's lymphoma, accounting for less than 2% of these tumors in large series. This tumor typically exhibits anaplastic morphology and was initially identified on the basis of immunoreactivity of all or nearly all neoplastic cells for the activation antigen Ki-1 (CD30) (Fig. 29.15). The latter antigen was first recognized in 1982 during a search for Hodgkin's disease–related antigens and has been observed for Reed-Sternberg cells and variants, activated T and B lymphoid cells, EBV-infected B cells, and for some non-Hodgkin's lymphomas other than those with anaplastic large cell morphology (33,35,118,119). CD30 expression has also been detected in some epithelial tumors, particularly embryonal carcinoma, some pancreatic and salivary gland malignancies, and some mesenchymal neoplasms (120–122). In reactive lymphoid tissue, a few $CD30^+$ cells generally occur as scattered large cells surrounding germinal centers. Studies have established that the CD30 molecule is

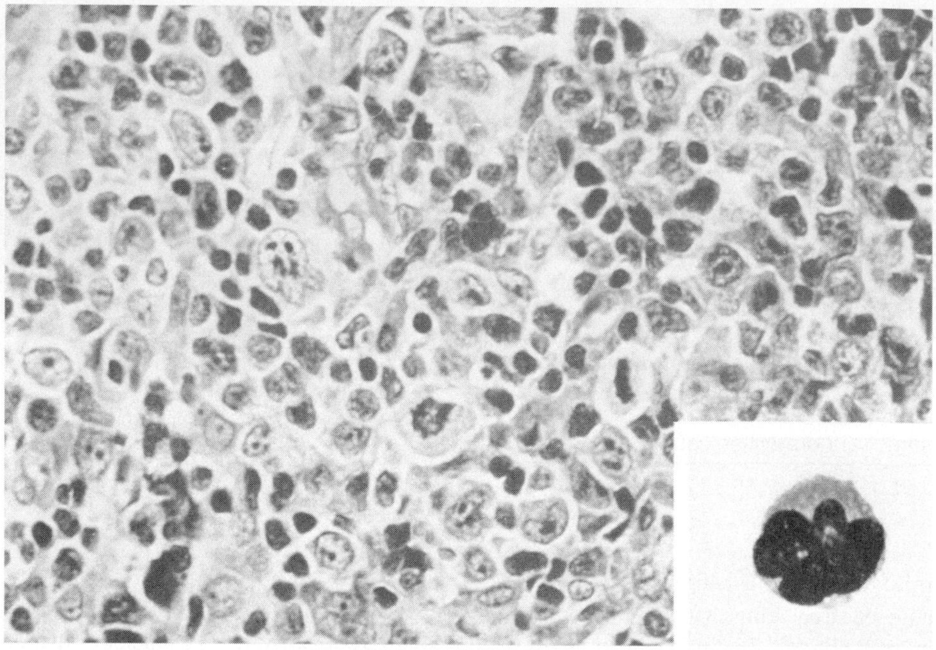

FIG. 29.14. Human T-cell lymphotrophic virus type 1–positive adult T-cell lymphoma/leukemia. The nodal infiltrate includes a spectrum of lymphoid cells, with a predominance of intermediate to large forms with prominent nucleoli. A cerebriform giant cell and frequent mitoses are apparent (hematoxylin and eosin stain, original magnification: 250× magnification). **Inset:** A typical lobated (flower-like) cell was present in the patient's cerebrospinal fluid (Wright's stain, original magnification: 800× magnification).

a member of the nerve growth factor/tumor necrosis factor receptor (TNFR) superfamily characterized by cysteine rich pseudorepeats (123). The CD30 gene is located on chromosome 1p36 near other TNFR family genes (124). The biologic role of CD30 still remains to be defined (see Chapter 3).

Recognition of ALCL is of particular importance in view of its anaplastic morphology, in combination with a sinusoidal or sheetlike growth pattern in lymph nodes, which simulates metastatic carcinoma or melanoma and malignant histiocytosis (Fig. 29.16). Many cases that had previously been regarded as malignant histiocytosis have been reclassified

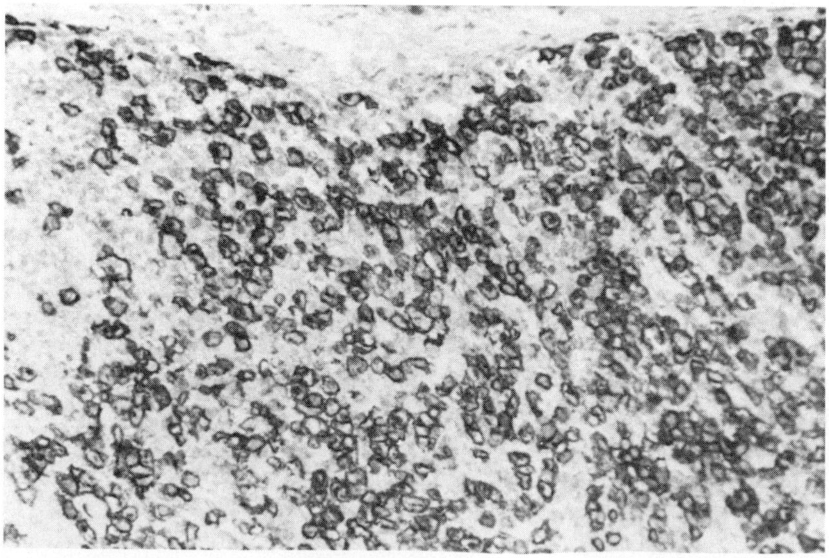

FIG. 29.15. Primary systemic type of anaplastic large cell lymphoma. In this cryostat section, essentially all the neoplastic cells in the nodal infiltrate strongly express CD30 (Ki-1 antigen), a characteristic feature of these neoplasms (immunoperoxidase technique, methyl green counterstain, original magnification: 150× magnification).

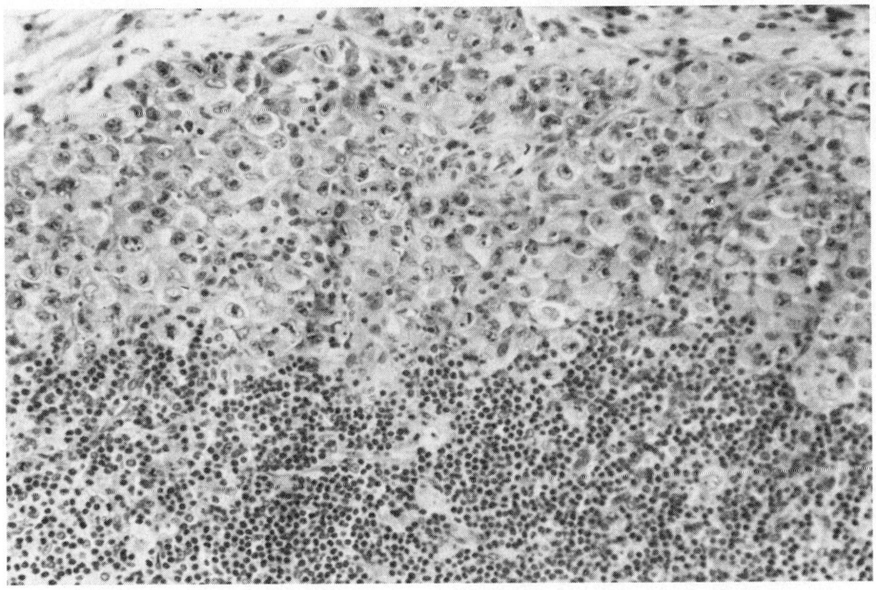

FIG. 29.16. Primary systemic type of anaplastic large cell lymphoma. The infiltrate involving the node exhibits a subcapsular or sinusoidal growth pattern that simulates metastatic carcinoma, a finding frequently observed in these neoplasms (hematoxylin and eosin stain, original magnification: 300× magnification).

as ALCL on the basis of current data (33,34). Accurate identification of ALCL is also relevant in regard to prognosis, because lesions of T-cell or null cell types are associated with a much better prognosis than the overall group of peripheral T-cell lymphomas (Table 29.4). These tumors may occur as primary lymphomas (more common) or as secondary lymphomas, associated with a variety of T-cell neoplasms (125). In prior studies, this category has included the less common B-cell neoplasms, including those of follicular center cell derivation, with anaplastic morphology (35,126). However, cases of large B-cell lymphoma with anaplastic morphology are not classified as anaplastic large cell lymphoma because this category is relegated to a specific clinicopathologic entity, with a T-cell or null cell phenotype (28).

ALCL, systemic type, displays a bimodal age distribution, with peaks in the second and seventh decades, and is most common in children and adolescents. ALCL represents the most common type of peripheral T-cell lymphoma in children. Peripheral lymphadenopathy is frequent. Mediastinal involvement is unusual. Skin represents the most common site of extranodal involvement. It is important to distinguish cases of systemic ALCL with cutaneous involvement from cases of localized cutaneous ALCL. Patients with systemic ALCL require aggressive chemotherapy, while those with localized cutaneous ALCL may be treated conservatively or with local therapy. The cutaneous type of ALCL generally is ALK protein negative and appears to represent part of a spectrum of cutaneous lymphoproliferative disorders that includes lymphomatoid papulosis, a clinically relapsing disorder that resolves spontaneously (discussed elsewhere). Other sites of involvement in systemic ALCL include Waldeyer's ring, gastrointestinal tract, spleen, bone and brain. Bone marrow involvement is unusual, except for the small cell variant of ALCL (36). A rare case of ALCL of maternal origin involving the placenta has also been reported (127).

Cytologically, in the common or classic type of ALCL, the neoplastic cells are large (10 to 50 μm) and contain round, oval, lobulated, wreathlike, horseshoe-shaped, Reed-Sternberg–like, and bizarre nuclei with one or more often prominent nucleoli, and abundant pale amphophilic to basophilic cytoplasm (Fig. 29.17). Frequent mitoses are observed. Neutrophils or histiocytes may be abundant (128). Other reactive cells are generally present in limited numbers. In one study, patients with proliferations composed of relatively monomorphic large cells, rather than pleomorphic anaplastic–appearing cells, including multinucleated and Reed-Sternberg–like cells, frequently presented with a more advanced stage of disease, often with bone marrow involvement, and had shorter survival times (119). In ALCL, the morphology may change after therapy. Lesions with highly anaplastic cells on initial biopsy may reveal monomorphous large lymphoid cells (lacking anaplastic features) or even assume the appearance of a T-cell lymphoma, small lymphocytic type, on rebiopsy after therapy.

In addition to the common type of ALCL, several variants have been described. In the small cell predominant variant (SCV), the infiltrate contains abundant small lymphoid cells with irregular nuclei (generally $CD30^-$) and a minor population of large cells occurring singly or in small clusters, often in a perivascular distribution or in sinuses, most readily delineated with studies for CD30 (36). Clinically, this variant is associated predominantly with skin and peripheral lymph node involvement at diagnosis. Lymph node involvement may be partial, with preservation of B-cell areas, causing

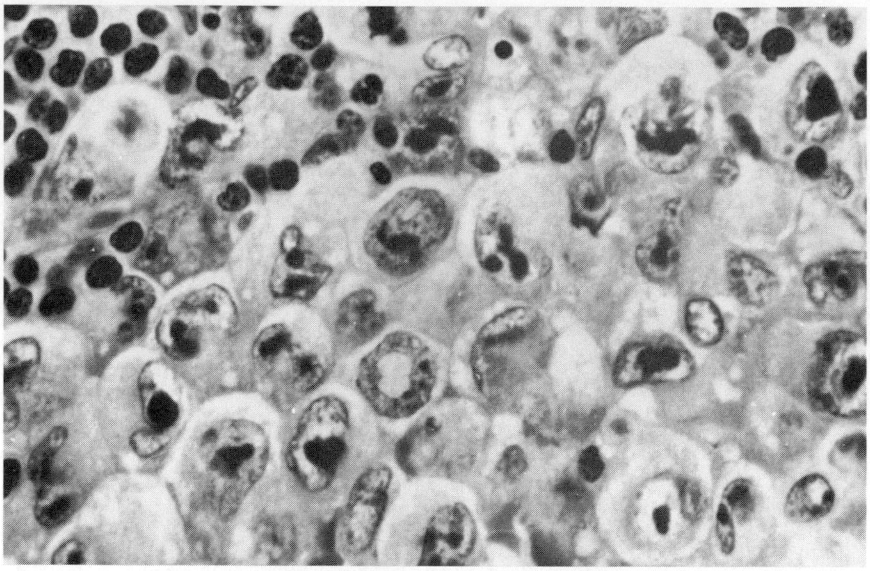

FIG. 29.17. Primary systemic type of anaplastic large cell lymphoma. The infiltrate involving this node is characteristic of that observed for the common or prototypic type of this lymphoma. Tumor cells are extremely large, contain wreathlike, horseshoe-shaped, lobated, and bizarre nuclei with prominent nucleoli and abundant pale to amphophilic or basophilic cytoplasm (hematoxylin and eosin stain, original magnification: 900× magnification).

confusion with a reactive process. Dissemination may occur in patients with SCV, with bone marrow and blood involvement apparent in about one third of cases. In patients with this ALCL variant, blood smears should be carefully reviewed for the presence of large (<20 μm) dysplastic vacuolated basophilic cells. Marrow involvement may be subtle and is optimally detected by immunohistochemical studies for CD30. Immunophenotypically, the SCV represents a homogeneous group of cases of T-cell phenotype, with most (80%) expressing epithelial membrane antigen (EMA). Cases evaluated cytogenetically have demonstrated a t(2;5). Sequential biopsies have demonstrated evolution to ALCL of large cell type in some patients.

A histiocyte-rich or lymphohistiocytic variant has also been reported, characterized by an exuberant histiocytic background with scattered large $CD30^+$ neoplastic cells (129–132) (Fig. 29.18). Clinically, superficial lymphadenopathy and systemic symptoms are observed. The latter variant and the SCV may pose diagnostic difficulties in their distinction from inflammatory or atypical reactive processes. Both variants predominantly affect young patients. Immunophenotypic studies for CD30 may be helpful for recognition of these disorders. Detection of the NPM-ALK chimeric fusion protein is highly valuable for accurate diagnosis (discussed subsequently). Other variants of ALCL include neutrophil-rich, sarcomatoid, and giant cell types.

A Hodgkin's-like variant of ALCL was initially proposed as a provisional category to encompass cases clinically associated with bulky disease that tend to involve the mediastinum of young adults, with histologic features that appear to overlap between Hodgkin's disease and anaplastic large cell lymphoma (27). Findings include a sheetlike proliferation of large cells, including forms with clear cytoplasm, the presence of fibrous bands, nodule formation, and possibly sinus involvement. At least some of these cases appear to represent a syncytial variant of nodular sclerosis Hodgkin's disease. The neoplastic cells are $CD30^+$, with variable expression for CD45, EMA and CD15. The cell of origin reported in these cases has been variable, with 50% T cell, 20% B cell, 30% null, and 1% to 2% hybrid B and T cell. Epstein-Barr virus has been detected in some cases (17%). In cases lacking typical morphologic or immunophenotypic features, the distinction between Hodgkin's disease and anaplastic large cell lymphoma may be extremely difficult. Features that would favor ALCL include cohesive groups of neoplastic cells with a sinus growth pattern, a high mitotic rate, expression of T-cell antigens or ALK protein, detection of T-cell receptor gene rearrangements, and absence of CD15. Cases with anaplastic cells with large inclusion-like nucleoli with few mitoses, an associated inflammatory infiltrate and expression of CD15 or B-cell antigens would be more in keeping with a diagnosis of Hodgkin's disease. Neoplastic cells of Hodgkin's disease are reportedly consistently nonreactive for ALK protein (133,134).

Cytogenetic studies have demonstrated the association of a nonrandom chromosomal translocation t(2;5)(p23;q35) for ALCL (135). In 1994 the t(2;5) was cloned and the gene involved in the translocation was identified (136). Nucleophosmin (NPM), a constitutively expressed nucleolar phosphoprotein located on 5q35, is involved in ribosomal shuttling between the nucleus and the cytoplasm. ALK (anaplastic lymphoma kinase), located on 2p23, represents a new tyrosine kinase. As a consequence of the translocation, ALK expression is controlled by the NPM promoter and is

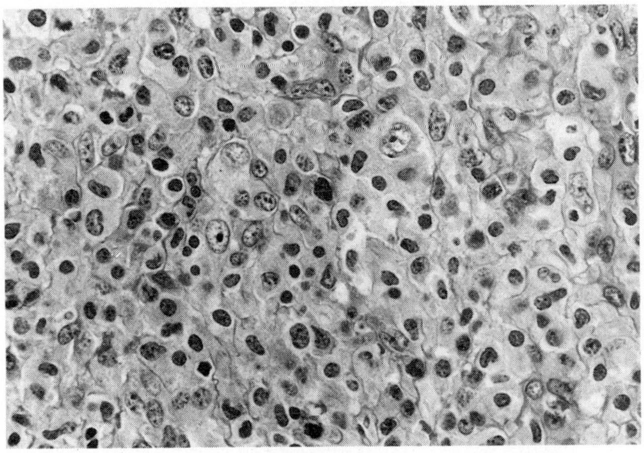

A

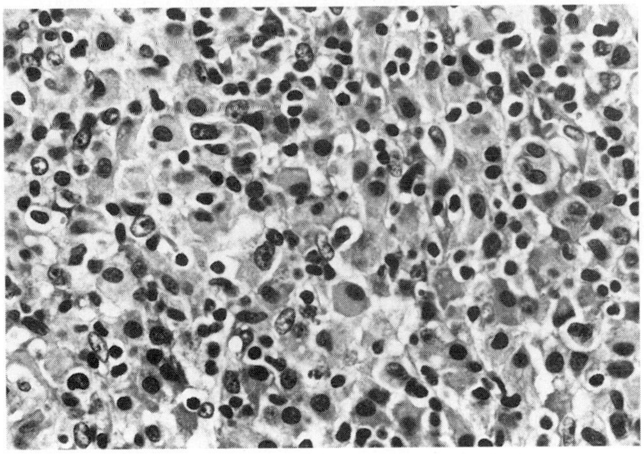

B

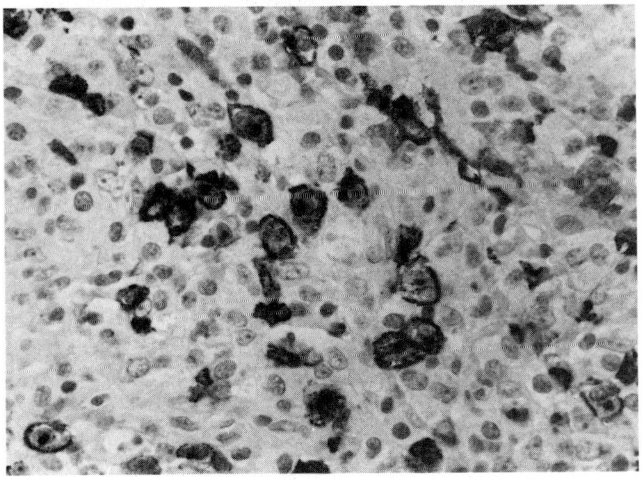

C

FIG. 29.18. Lymphohistiocytic variant of the primary systemic type of anaplastic large cell lymphoma (ALCL). **A:** The striking feature in this variant of ALCL is the presence of abundant histiocytes, which tend to obscure the neoplastic infiltrate. A few large, atypical cells can be recognized. In this variant, neoplastic cells may appear less anaplastic than those in the classic form of ALCL (hematoxylin and eosin stain, original magnification: 500× magnification). **B:** In some cases, some histiocytes may exhibit features suggesting plasma cells. A few large, atypical cells are observed (hematoxylin and eosin stain, original magnification: 500× magnification). **C:** An immunoperoxidase study for CD30 delineates the neoplastic cells, which are more abundant than apparent by routine histology (immunoperoxidase technique, hematoxylin counterstain, original magnification: 500× magnification).

increased. A novel hyperphosphorylated protein tyrosine kinase, p80, was found in a human $CD30^+$ lymphoma with a t(2;5). Cloning studies demonstrated that p80 represented the fusion protein of two different genes, the novel tyrosine kinase gene on chromosome 2p23 and the nucleophosmin gene on 5q35. A polyclonal antibody is available that detects the kinase domain of the *ALK* gene portion of the fusion protein p80 NPM/ALK (137,138). Monoclonal antibodies (designated ALK/ALKc-1) against the ALK protein have also become available (139,140). Because normal lymphoid cells do not express ALK, immunohistochemical studies permit detection of dysregulation of the *ALK* gene and are extremely valuable for diagnosis. ALK expression is highly correlated with t(2;5) and cases with this feature appear to define a patient group with a relatively good prognosis. However, absence of a t(2;5) or reactivity for ALK in cases with typical morphology does not exclude the diagnosis of ALCL. In a small proportion of cases, other cytogenetic abnormalities have been documented, including t(1;2), t(2;3), inv(2), and t(2;22) (141). In the latter cases, the staining pattern for ALK may be cytoplasmic, membranous, or granular (varies with abnormality), in comparison with the nuclear/nucleolar/cytoplasmic pattern observed in association with lymphomas with t(2;5) (Fig. 29.19).

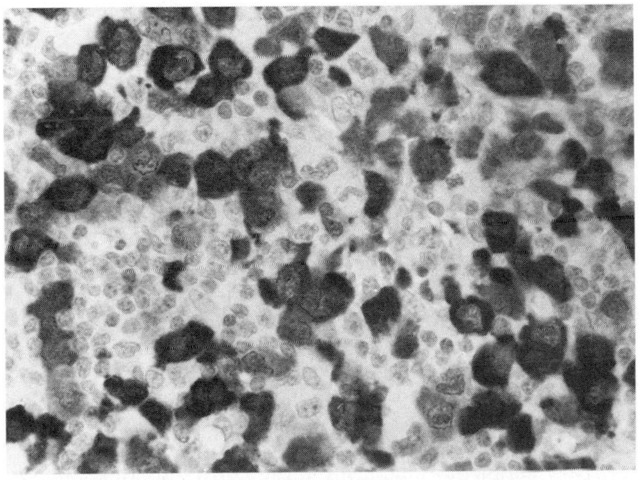

FIG. 29.19. Primary systemic type of anaplastic large cell lymphoma. Neoplastic cells display strong immunoreactivity for ALK protein and exhibit nuclear, nucleolar, and cytoplasmic staining, a finding observed in many cases with a t(2;5) cytogenetic abnormality (immunoperoxidase technique, methyl green counterstain, original magnification: 400× magnification). The staining pattern may vary in cases associated with other cytogenetic abnormalities (not shown).

Potentially, the most specific marker for ALCL is t(2;5)

as determined by cytogenetics, molecular genetics, or immunohistochemistry (p80 or ALK protein). Variability in detection of t(2;5) probably results from several factors, including analytical technique, heterogeneity in cases evaluated, and primary versus secondary tumors (usually lack translocation). Kinney and colleagues found p80 expression in 80 well-characterized cases of ALCL and found p80 expression in 58% of cases (142). Reactivity was observed for 80% of monomorphic, 76% of small cell variant, and 44% of the pleomorphic variant, suggesting a pathogenetic relationship for these cases. Most p80$^+$ cases were of T or null cell phenotype, and expressed EMA. Most primary cutaneous ALCLs are t(2;5) negative (143–145). This translocation also has been lacking in the limited number of cases of human immunodeficiency virus–associated ALCL and secondary ALCL that have been evaluated. In another study, Nakamura and colleagues (146) demonstrated p80 immunoreactivity in 43 (64%) of 67 cases of ALCL. This group of cases was characterized by uniformity of features, including younger patient age, more favorable clinical course, and an identical phenotype (p80$^+$, CD30$^+$, EMA$^+$, CD15$^-$, BCL-2$^-$, EBV$^-$, T- and null cell phenotype) and common type morphology (except for 3 cases of lymphohistiocytic/small cell types). No reactivity for p80 was observed for 63 cases of Hodgkin's disease. Studies using a new anti-ALK antibody, ALKc, demonstrated immunoreactivity in 60 of 100 cases of ALCL of various types (140). Reactivity for ALKc was observed in the cytoplasm and nucleus of large neoplastic cells, with nuclear restricted staining present in the small cells, suggesting that the *NPM-ALK* gene must be present in both cell types. Immunoreactivity for ALK appears to define a clinicopathologic entity of T/null cell phenotype that is characterized by a wide morphologic spectrum.

In paraffin tissue sections, one may have great difficulty detecting T-cell antigens or even leukocyte common antigen in cases of ALCL, because these lesions typically are associated with extensive T-cell antigen deletion. CD43 reactivity may be observed, and although supportive of a T-cell derivation, this marker is not specific for the T-cell lineage. Neoplastic cells of ALCL may also reveal cytotoxic proteins, a finding that is unusual in cases of Hodgkin's disease (10%) and is not observed in large B-cell lymphomas (147–149). CD30 expression and reactivity for ALK or p80 and for epithelial membrane antigen are more readily detected.

PRIMARY CUTANEOUS CD30$^+$ T-CELL LYMPHOPROLIFERATIVE DISORDERS

This group of disorders includes lymphomatoid papulosis, primary cutaneous anaplastic large cell lymphoma and borderline lesions, all of which tend to be associated with a favorable prognosis (150,151). In some cases, distinction between lymphomatoid papulosis (LyP) and primary cutaneous ALCL may be difficult or even impossible. Both lesions are associated with T-cell receptor gene rearrangement and deletion of pan-T-cell antigens, precluding these studies as a basis for definitive diagnosis. Patients present with chronic recurrent skin lesions that tend to regress spontaneously, although progression to lymphoma may occur in a minor proportion of cases. The unifying features of these lesions is the presence of CD30$^+$ large atypical cells. Variable reactivity for T-cell markers, EMA, and cutaneous lymphocyte antigen (HECA-452) is observed, expression of cytotoxic granules is common, and cytogenetic studies rarely reveal t(2;5) (143–145,152). These disorders appear to represent a morphologic and clinical spectrum of disease. LyP occurs over a wide age range (median, 41 years) and is usually associated with numerous small lesions (generally less than 2 cm), which tend to enlarge rapidly, centrally ulcerate and then regress over a 3- to 8-week period. This cycle may recur within several months and continue for a period of years (some reportedly for 40 years or more). Lymphadenopathy is not a feature. Histologically, LyP reveals a highly atypical infiltrate, usually with a prominent inflammatory background. Epidermotropism may be present. Cutaneous ALCL may evolve in a small proportion (10% to 20%) of these patients. In primary cutaneous ALCL, one or several tumor nodules may occur. The infiltrate is typically nonepidermotropic and consists of a relatively monomorphous population of large cells that may exhibit anaplastic or nonanaplastic features. Although neutrophils may occur, even in the absence of ulceration, the prominent inflammatory component typical of LyP is lacking. Other features that favor ALCL rather than LyP include size of tumor nodules (>2 cm) and extension of the infiltrate into the subcutaneous fat. Spontaneous regression may occur. Evidence of lymph node involvement is the most reliable criterion for malignancy. Progression to systemic disease occurs only in a small proportion of cases. Some patients with skin and nodal involvement who have achieved complete remission after chemotherapy have subsequently relapsed with skin involvement only, associated with clinical and histologic features compatible with lymphomatoid papulosis. Primary cutaneous ALCL differs from the systemic form of ALCL in that patients are generally older and t(2;5) is typically absent in these cases. Phenotypically, however, both types are similar, including expression of cytotoxic molecules, although epithelial membrane antigen expression is usually found only in the systemic form. Both types display clonal T-cell receptor gene rearrangements. These lesions are discussed in greater detail in Chapter 32.

For lesions restricted to the skin, it has been recommended that extreme caution be taken before a diagnosis of ALCL is rendered. Close monitoring of lesions for possible regression appears warranted before initiation of therapy. In cases with lymph node involvement, a diagnosis of malignancy and ALCL may be confidently established. Of clinical relevance is the fact that some ALCLs show a tendency to regress spontaneously, including cutaneous lymphomas, underscoring proposals for a conservative approach to management of the latter patients.

SUBCUTANEOUS PANNICULITIS-LIKE T-CELL LYMPHOMA

Subcutaneous panniculitis-like T-cell lymphoma represents an unusual and distinct disorder that may simulate erythema nodosum or chronic panniculitis and is characterized by multiple subcutaneous nodules generally involving the extremities, and occasionally the trunk (153–155). The disease is typically restricted to subcutaneous tissue, even at autopsy. Hemophagocytic syndrome frequently accompanies this disorder and may pursue a fulminant course. In those cases, benign histiocytes throughout the reticuloendothelial system exhibit exuberant phagocytosis of erythrocytes and other hematopoietic cells (Fig. 29.3). Clinical features associated with this complication include fever, hepatoplenomegaly, and pancytopenia. Histologically, in areas of lymphomatous involvement, atypical lymphoid cells infiltrate between fat cells of subcutaneous tissue in a lacelike pattern, with little or absent dermal involvement (Fig. 29.20A, B). This pattern of infiltration differs from that of other T-cell lymphomas involving skin and subcutaneous tissue that tend to exhibit a more sheetlike growth pattern. The lymphoid infiltrate varies in cell size and in degree of nuclear atypicality. In cases with limited cytologic atypia, the proliferation may be misdiagnosed as a reactive process. Although blood vessel invasion may occur, the lesion is not typically angiocentric or angiodestructive. Fat necrosis and prominent karyorrhexis may be observed. T-cell antigen deletion and clonal T-cell receptor gene rearrangements are usually observed, with most involving TCRβ. EBV has not been identified in these lesions. Studies reveal that the neoplastic cells are CD8^{+}, in contrast to most T-cell neoplasms, which are CD4^{+} and express cytotoxic granules (i.e., TIA-1, perforin, and granzyme B [156]). In tissue sections, the CD8^{+} neoplastic cells appear to outline or rim the clear space of the fat cells (Fig. 29.20C). This disease may pursue a chronic clinical course although a poor prognosis is often observed in cases associated with hemophagocytic syndrome.

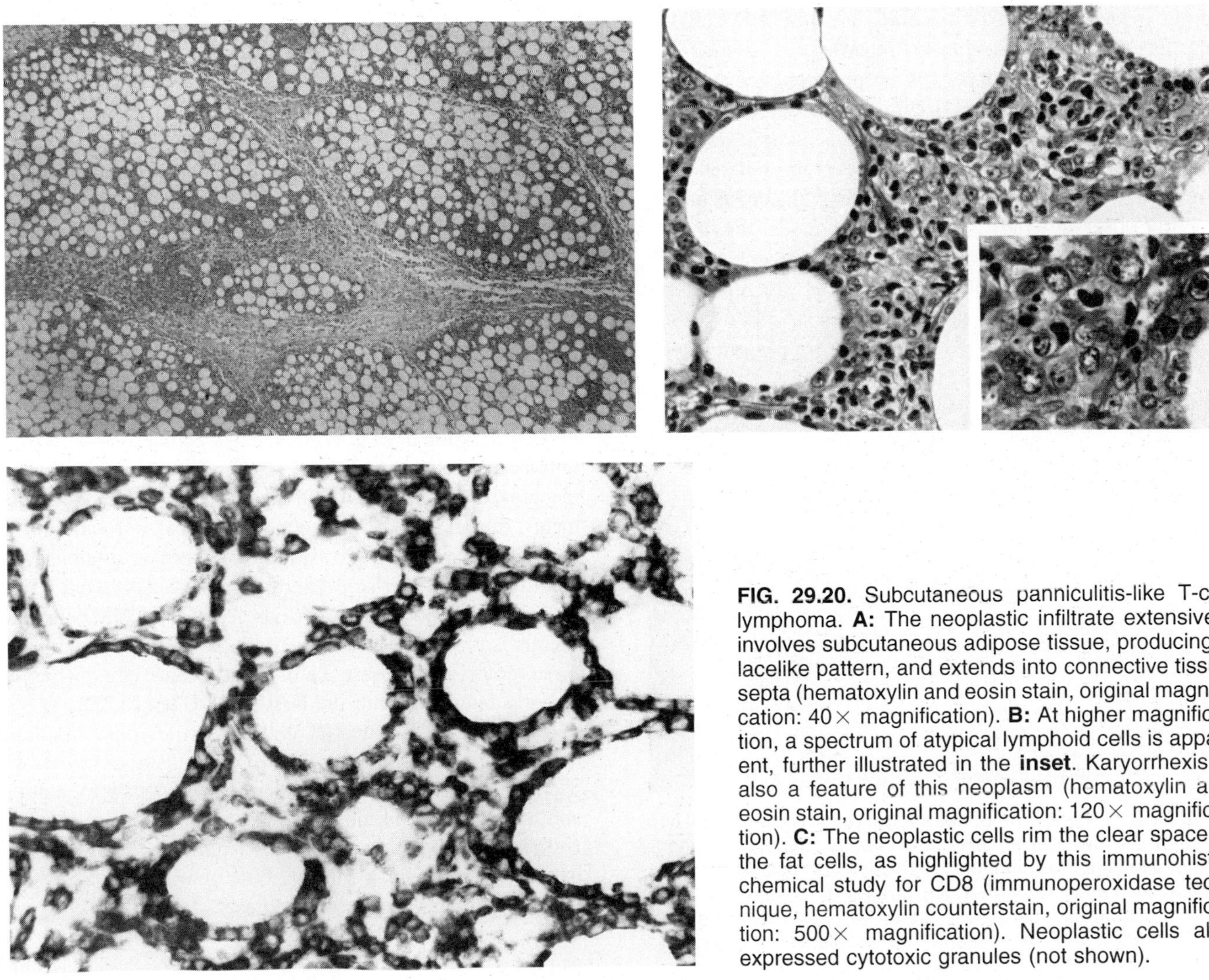

A B C

FIG. 29.20. Subcutaneous panniculitis-like T-cell lymphoma. **A:** The neoplastic infiltrate extensively involves subcutaneous adipose tissue, producing a lacelike pattern, and extends into connective tissue septa (hematoxylin and eosin stain, original magnification: 40× magnification). **B:** At higher magnification, a spectrum of atypical lymphoid cells is apparent, further illustrated in the **inset**. Karyorrhexis is also a feature of this neoplasm (hematoxylin and eosin stain, original magnification: 120× magnification). **C:** The neoplastic cells rim the clear space of the fat cells, as highlighted by this immunohistochemical study for CD8 (immunoperoxidase technique, hematoxylin counterstain, original magnification: 500× magnification). Neoplastic cells also expressed cytotoxic granules (not shown).

EXTRANODAL NATURAL KILLER/T-CELL LYMPHOMA, NASAL-TYPE

These lymphomas represent a group of distinct extranodal neoplasms that are more common in the Orient, Mexico and South and Central America as compared with the United States and encompass cases previously designated as *lethal midline granuloma, polymorphic reticulosis,* and some *angioimmunoproliferative lesions* and *angiocentric T-cell lymphomas.* Sites of involvement include the sinonasal area, upper and lower aerodigestive tract, skin, soft tissue and testis, generally in the absence of lymphadenopathy (17,19,20,157–167).

Patients with nasal natural killer or T-cell (NK/T-cell) lymphomas may present with a mass lesion associated with obstruction and bleeding or with facial destruction. This lymphoma tends to disseminate to other extranodal sites. These tumors are generally highly aggressive. Patients are also at increased risk for development of hemophagocytic syndrome. It has been proposed that these neoplasms be regarded as NK/T-cell lymphomas due to uncertainties associated with defining their precise lineage, although accumulating evidence suggests that most are true NK cell neoplasms. Although previously regarded as angiocentric lymphomas, this terminology is not preferred because some tumors may not exhibit angiocentric growth. Angiocentricity is not unique to this group of neoplasms and may be found in lymphomas of other lineages. However, prominent angioinvasion and angiodestruction or extensive necrosis are frequently observed (Fig. 29.21). In some cases, the necrosis or inflammatory infiltrate may obscure the neoplastic cells, making diagnosis difficult. These neoplasms reveal a broad cytologic spectrum with variable cytologic atypia. Cytologic preparations often demonstrate neoplastic cells with azurophilic granules.

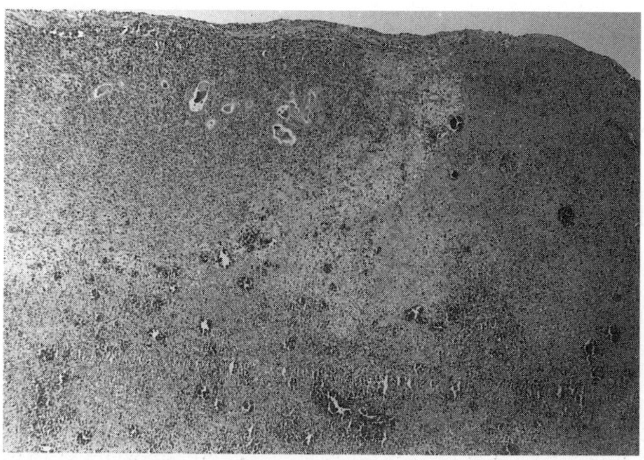

FIG. 29.21. Nasal type of extranodal natural killer/T-cell lymphoma. At low power, this nasal biopsy reveals commonly associated findings, including extensive necrosis *(right)*, reactive and inflammatory changes *(lower)*, and limited areas of preserved neoplastic tissue *(upper left)*. Extensive necrosis and inflammation may obscure the neoplastic process creating a difficult diagnostic problem (hematoxylin and eosin stain, original magnification: 50× magnification).

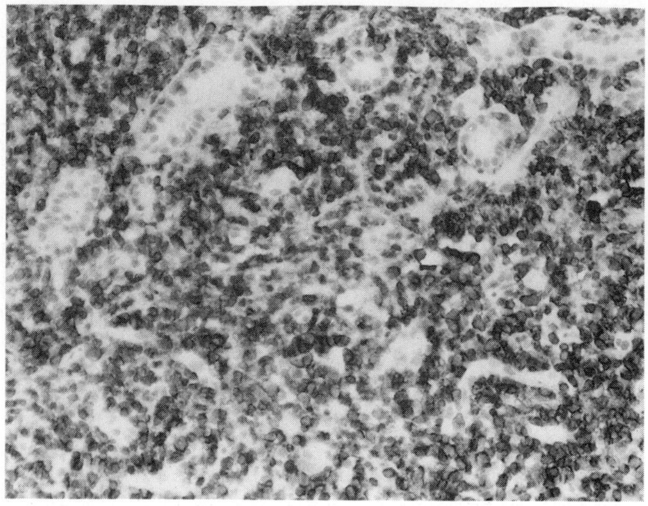

FIG. 29.22. Nasal-type of natural killer/T-cell lymphoma. Of particular importance is the demonstration of reactivity of the neoplastic cells for CD56, which can be detected in paraffin sections, as observed in this case. Essentially all cells comprising the dense infiltrate stain for CD56. Residual glands and ducts are nonreactive (immunoperoxidase technique, hematoxylin counterstain, original magnification: 300× magnification).

These tumors exhibit some T-cell surface antigens (usually $CD2^+$, surface $CD3^-$, $CD43^+$), and are reactive for CD56 (Fig. 29.22), the neural cell adhesion molecule (NCAM), but CD57 and CD16 are not typically expressed. Tumor cells lack surface CD3, but most cases are reactive for cytoplasmic CD3 in paraffin tissue sections using a polyclonal antibody that recognizes the ϵ chain of CD3 (Fig. 29.23). Because the latter portion of the CD3 molecule is present in T cells, fetal NK cells, and activated NK cells, its identification does not indicate a T-cell derivation. These tumors also consistently fail to demonstrate clonal T-cell receptor or immunoglobulin heavy-chain gene rearrangements, further supporting a putative NK cell derivation. The tumor cells are usually positive for cytotoxic granules, including TIA-1, perforin, and granzyme (148,168) (Fig. 29.24). A comparison of various features of NK cells and T cells is presented in Table 29.10. A consistent finding in these tumors is the presence of Epstein-Barr virus, which is clonally integrated into the host DNA (Fig. 29.25).

Rare cases of blastic NK cell leukemia/lymphoma have been described (165,169). This unusual disorder affects elderly patients and is associated with a cutaneous presentation and an aggressive clinical course with progression to overt leukemia. Nodal and marrow involvement is characterized by a monomorphous infiltrate of medium-sized cells resembling myeloblasts or lymphoblasts. In Wright-Giemsa–stained cytologic preparations, the cells have a blastic appearance (e.g., fine chromatin, many with nucleoli, variable quantities of cytoplasm), lack granules, or contain few azuro-

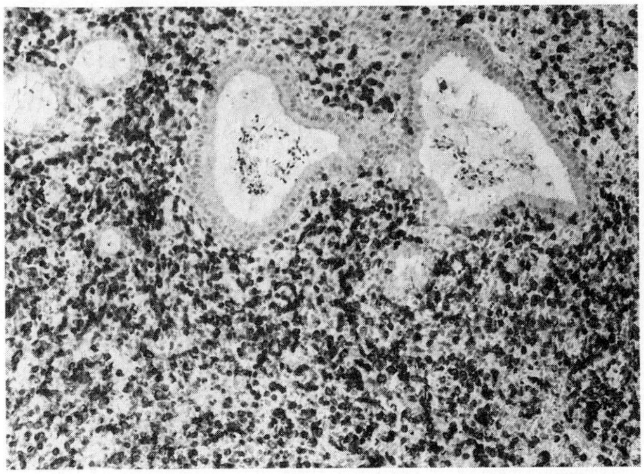

FIG. 29.23. Nasal type of natural killer/T-cell lymphoma. In these areas of viable tissue (paraffin section), the neoplastic cells are strongly immunoreactive for CD3, a pan-T-cell marker that also detects natural killer cells (immunoperoxidase technique, hematoxylin counterstain, original magnification: 140× magnification). Tumor cells in this type of lymphoma are nonreactive for surface CD3, as evaluated in cryostat sections or by flow cytometry (not shown).

TABLE 29.10. *Comparison of characteristics of T cells and natural killer cells*

Characteristic	T cell	NK cell
CD2	+	+
CD3 (surface)	+	−
CD3 (cytoplasmic)	+	+
CD4 or CD8	+	−
CD5	+	−
CD7	+	[a]
CD43	+	+
CD45RO	+	+ (usually)
CD56	(+)[b]	+
Toxic granules (TIA-1, granzyme, perforin)	+[b]	+
TCR[c]	+	−

[a] Occasional $CD7^+$ NK cells.
[b] Minor population.
[c] T-cell receptor $\alpha\beta$ or $\gamma\delta$ by immunohistochemistry.

philic granules. Phenotypically, the neoplastic cells are negative for CD2, CD4, CD56, and HLA-DR and are negative for CD3 (surface and cytoplasmic) and CD5. T-cell receptor gene rearrangements are not observed. The neoplastic cells are negative for EBV.

Another lesion that was previously regarded as part of the spectrum of angiocentric T-cell lymphomas is lymphomatoid granulomatosis, now recognized as an unusual B-cell lymphoma in most cases. This disorder involves extranodal sites, including the lungs, upper respiratory tract, central nervous system, skin and kidneys. Lymphomatoid granulomatosis of the lung was initially described by Liebow and Carrington (170,171) as an angiitis and granulomatosis, similar to the limited form of Wegener's granulomatosis. The process was considered to be benign, but capable of evolving to a malignant disorder. Later, Colby and Carrington revised this concept and recognized that almost all their cases represented primary lymphoma of the lungs (172,173). Katzenstein and colleagues (174) found that prognosis varied and was related to the degree of pleomorphism of the infiltrate. The Epstein-Barr virus (EBV) genome has been detected in tissue from most cases, supporting the hypothesis

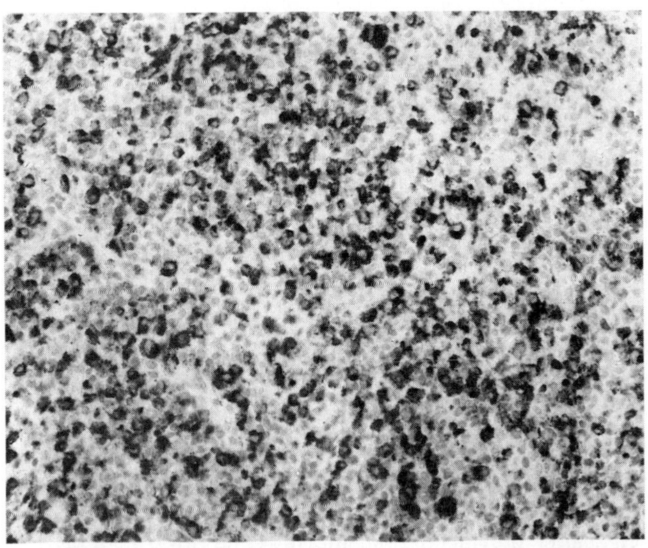

FIG. 29.24. Nasal-type natural killer/T-cell lymphomas are usually positive for cytotoxic granules as demonstrated in this immunohistochemical study for granzyme B. Nearly all the neoplastic cells reveal strong granular cytoplasmic reactivity (immunoperoxidase study, hematoxylin counterstain, original magnification: 200× magnification).

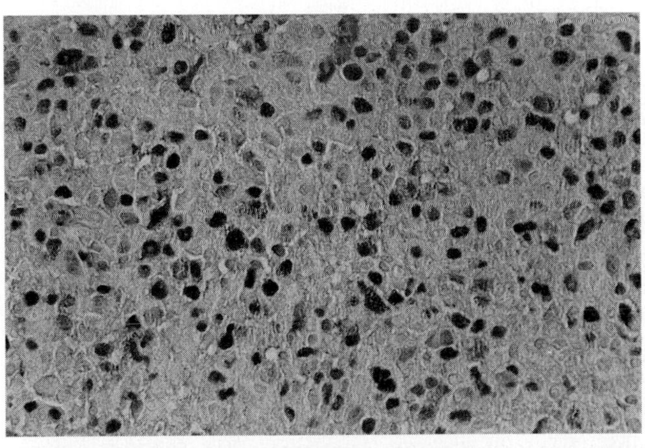

FIG. 29.25. A consistent feature in nasal-type natural killer/T-cell lymphomas is the presence of Epstein-Barr virus (EBV) as illustrated in this *in situ* hybridization study for EBV-encoded RNA (EBER) transcripts, which are localized in the nuclei *(black)* of infected cells. Variation in staining intensity probably reflects the state of preservation of the neoplastic cells in this lesion associated with prominent necrosis (*in situ* hybridization study, methyl green counterstain, original magnification: 500× magnification).

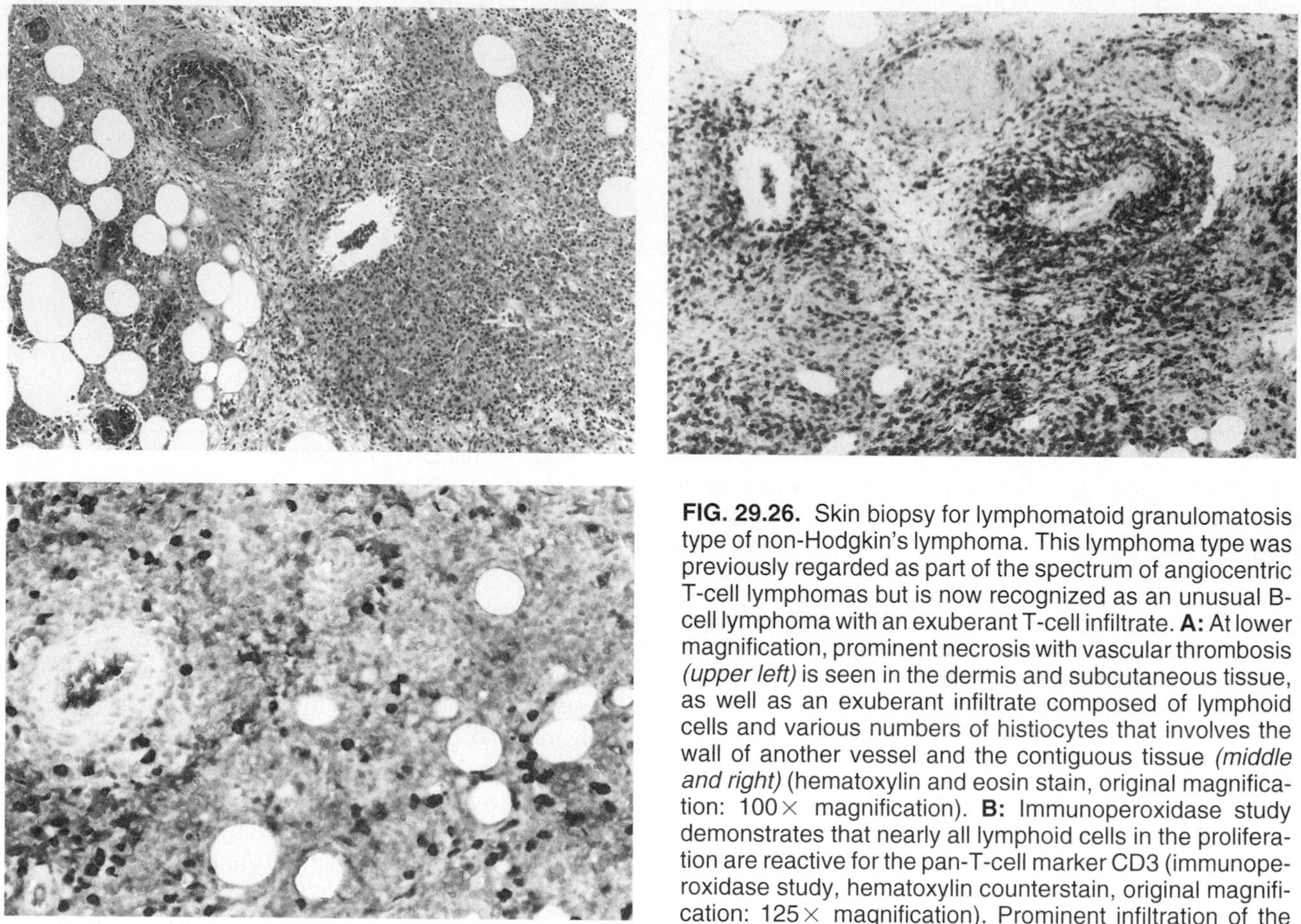

FIG. 29.26. Skin biopsy for lymphomatoid granulomatosis type of non-Hodgkin's lymphoma. This lymphoma type was previously regarded as part of the spectrum of angiocentric T-cell lymphomas but is now recognized as an unusual B-cell lymphoma with an exuberant T-cell infiltrate. **A:** At lower magnification, prominent necrosis with vascular thrombosis *(upper left)* is seen in the dermis and subcutaneous tissue, as well as an exuberant infiltrate composed of lymphoid cells and various numbers of histiocytes that involves the wall of another vessel and the contiguous tissue *(middle and right)* (hematoxylin and eosin stain, original magnification: 100× magnification). **B:** Immunoperoxidase study demonstrates that nearly all lymphoid cells in the proliferation are reactive for the pan-T-cell marker CD3 (immunoperoxidase study, hematoxylin counterstain, original magnification: 125× magnification). Prominent infiltration of the vessel wall has occurred. These lesions typically do not display T-cell receptor gene rearrangements (not shown). **C:** A minor component of large clonal B cells was present in the infiltrate, as illustrated by this study for λ light chains (immunoperoxidase study, hematoxylin counterstain, original magnification: 200× magnification). These cells were also reactive for CD20 and were positive for Epstein-Barr virus by *in situ* hybridization (not shown).

that lymphomatoid granulomatosis represents a unique form of B-cell lymphoma, possibly related to EBV infection (175), which is associated with an exuberant T-cell infiltrate that involves vessel walls (Fig. 29.26). Using double labeling techniques and PCR studies, most of these cases have been shown to represent EBV$^+$ B-cell lymphomas with clonal rearrangement of the immunoglobulin heavy-chain gene (i.e., a form of T-cell–rich B-cell lymphoma) (176–179). In nearly all cases, molecular studies for T-cell receptor genes have demonstrated a germline configuration. However, occasional cases of lymphomatoid granulomatosis of T-cell type have also been observed (177). Lymphomatoid granulomatosis appears to represent an EBV-driven lymphoproliferative disorder that occurs in patients with defects in cytotoxic T-cell function. This disorder is common in immunodeficiency states, including AIDS, Wiskott-Aldrich syndrome, and after transplantation (178). Although some cases may regress spontaneously, therapy is required in most cases.

Unusual true T-cell neoplasms occur that express the NK cell–associated antigen CD56 and have been designated as *NK-like T-cell lymphomas* (180,181). A separate designation for these tumors has not been assigned in the REAL or WHO classifications. These tumors are true T-cell neoplasms that express T-cell antigens, including surface CD3, express T-cell antigen receptor and reveal clonal T-cell receptor gene rearrangements. The neoplastic cells generally are CD2$^+$, CD3$^+$, variably express CD5, CD7, and CD8, express the T-cell antigen receptor $\alpha\beta$ or $\gamma\delta$, and express cytotoxic granule proteins TIA-1, perforin, and granzyme B. Clonal T-cell receptor gene rearrangements are observed. The group of $\gamma\delta$ hepatosplenic T-cell lymphomas (a distinct entity described subsequently) would fall into this category. In contrast to the group of nasal or nasal-type NK/T lymphomas, these cases are not typically associated with Epstein-Barr virus. Clinically, these lesions may affect any age group. Some cases have occurred in a background of immunosuppression (e.g., after transplantation, ulcerative colitis). Patients are generally extremely symptomatic, with fever, night sweats and weight loss, associated with hepatosplenomegaly, involvement of extranodal sites (e.g., skin, gastrointestinal tract, lung, kidney). Lymph node involvement is unusual. Bone marrow involvement is observed in cases associated with a leukemic phase. Because patients with a leukemic presentation by a disorder regarded as an aggressive variant of large granular cell leukemia also have prominent hepatosplenomegaly, perhaps NK-like T-cell lymphoma and aggressive variants of $CD3^+CD56^+$ leukemias of large granular lymphocytes represent different manifestations of the same disorder. The prognosis for NK-like T-cell lymphoma/leukemia is poor. Histologically, the infiltrate consists of medium- to large-sized cells with round to irregular nuclei, clumped chromatin and variably prominent nucleoli and pale/clear cytoplasm. The infiltrate tends to involve tissue sinusoids. In Wright-Giemsa–stained cytologic preparations, neoplastic cells include a spectrum of cell sizes, with variably irregular nuclei with prominent nucleoli, pale to deeply basophilic cytoplasm, and azurophilic granules. Erythrophagocytosis by the neoplastic cells is occasionally observed. Angiocentricity is not a feature of this disorder.

ENTEROPATHY-TYPE INTESTINAL T-CELL LYMPHOMA

Enteropathy-type intestinal T-cell lymphoma generally occurs in adults (median age, 60 years) with a short or prolonged history of celiac disease, although sporadic cases are also observed (182–185). Clinical presentation includes malabsorption associated with abdominal pain, weight loss or evidence of intestinal ulceration and stricture formation. Grossly, jejunal ulcers are present, are frequently multiple and are often associated with perforation. A tumor mass may also be seen. The neoplasm is usually multifocal and disseminated to other sites at initial diagnosis, including mesenteric lymph nodes, liver, spleen, bone marrow, lung and skin. Lymphoid cells comprising the infiltrate may vary considerably from relatively small cells to highly atypical bizarre tumor cells (Fig. 29.27). Frequent tumor cells may be present in the epithelium. A prominent inflammatory infiltrate may occur, obscuring the neoplastic cells. In early lesions (i.e., ''ulcerative jejunitis''), mucosal ulceration with scattered intraepithelial atypical cells and frequent histiocytes may occur. T-cell clonality with identical clones has been demonstrated in the ulcers of ulcerative jejunitis and enteropathy-type intestinal T-cell lymphoma, suggesting that ulcerative jejunitis complicating celiac disease is actually a manifestation of the lymphoma (186). These findings support the proposal that a low-grade intraepithelial T-cell lymphoma may precede the development of a higher-grade lesion. In uninvolved areas, villous atrophy and frequent intraepithelial lymphocytes may be observed. Involved lymph nodes may exhibit a sinusoidal or paracortical pattern of infiltration.

The neoplastic cells are usually $CD3^+$, $CD4^-$, and $CD8^-$, but they react with antibody HML-1 (CD103), which detects the normal intestinal intraepithelial T-cell population. The latter antigen is also observed in hairy cell leukemia but is rarely found in non-Hodgkin's lymphomas. In most

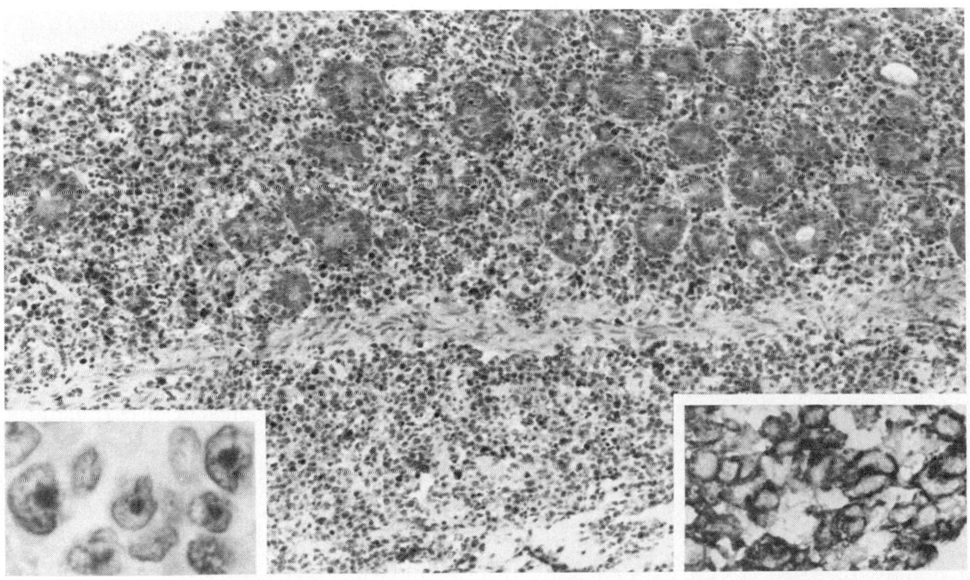

FIG. 29.27. Enteropathy-type T-cell lymphoma. This unusual T-cell lymphoma involved the small intestine of a patient with a history of malabsorption. The mucosa appears atrophic and contains a dense infiltrate of neoplastic cells in the lamina propria, mainly between glands, with extension to the submucosa. A few neoplastic cells are in the epithelium (hematoxylin and eosin stain, original magnification: 110× magnification). **Left inset:** At higher magnification, neoplastic cells reveal variable nuclear irregularity, finely dispersed chromatin, and distinct nucleoli (hematoxylin and eosin stain, original magnification: 850× magnification). **Right inset:** In cryostat section studies, neoplastic cells were reactive for pan-T-cell antigens, including CD3 (immunoperoxidase technique, methyl green counterstain, original magnification: 350× magnification).

cases, neoplastic cells exhibit a cytotoxic phenotype (148). In some cases, generally those composed of a monomorphic infiltrate of small- to medium-sized neoplastic cells, the infiltrate is $CD8^+$ and $CD56^+$ (185). Varying proportions of neoplastic cells are $CD30^+$. These tumors display clonal TCR β chain gene rearrangements that may also be observed for the contiguous areas of intestine that exhibit features of enteropathy. The $\gamma\delta$ intestinal T-cell lymphomas have also been described (187,188). EBV has been identified in neoplastic cells. The clinical course is generally aggressive.

HEPATOSPLENIC T-CELL LYMPHOMA

These lymphomas represent an unusual but distinctive disorder. In contrast to most T-cell lymphomas that derive from the $\alpha\beta$ subset of T cells, nearly all of these neoplasms originate from the minor subset of $\gamma\delta$ T cells (58,60,62). A small number of cases of $\alpha\beta$ T-cell derivation associated with clinicopathologic features of the more typical $\gamma\delta$ type of this disorder have also been described (189). Most patients with hepatosplenic T-cell lymphomas are young adult males who present with hepatosplenomegaly without associated lymphadenopathy. This lymphoma has been described in immunocompromised patients, including after transplantation (44,46,190) and in association with hepatitis B virus infection (191). The peripheral blood may be involved. Bone marrow involvement may occur, is typically subtle, and exhibits a sinusoidal pattern. In the spleen the infiltrate involves pulp cords and sinuses (Fig. 29.28), is monomorphous and composed of T cells of intermediate size with round to oval nuclei, condensed chromatin, inconspicuous nucleoli, and abundant pale to eosinophilic cytoplasm. Marked sinusoidal infiltration is typically observed in spleen and liver and is also apparent in other involved tissues, such as the bone marrow. The neoplastic cells are usually $CD3^+$, $CD4^-$, $CD8^-$, $CD2^+$, $CD7^+$, $CD5^-$, $CD56^+$, $CD16^+$, and $CD57^-$, and are immunoreactive for TCR $\gamma\delta$. Occasional cases are $CD8^+$. Neoplastic cells are generally positive for cytotoxic molecules and are EBV^-. Isochromosome 7q has been shown to be a characteristic feature of this disease (192–195). An associated trisomy 8 has been found in some cases. This lymphoma is associated with an aggressive clinical course (median survival, less than 2 years).

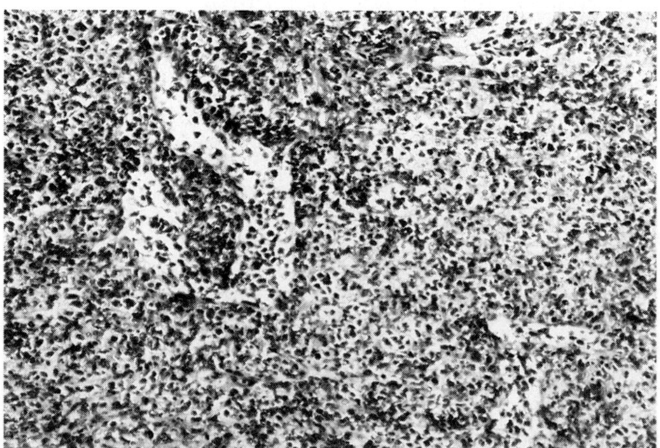

FIG. 29.28. Hepatosplenic $\gamma\delta$ T-cell lymphoma. Both splenic sinuses and pulp cords contain a prominent infiltrate of medium-sized, relatively monomorphic neoplastic cells that distort the splenic architecture (hematoxylin and eosin stain, original magnification: 200× magnification). In this disorder, a sinusoidal pattern of involvement also occurs in other involved tissues, such as the liver and bone marrow (not shown).

A nodal $\gamma\delta$ T-cell lymphoma associated with EBV has been described in Japan (196). This tumor initially occurred as a T zone lymphoma and, after complete remission, recurred with high-grade transformation. Neoplastic cells in this case were $CD56^-$. A small number of $\gamma\delta$ T-cell lymphomas involving skin or other extranodal sites, such as the nose, thyroid, and intestine, have also been described but do not represent distinct entities (197,198). Cutaneous lesions may involve subcutaneous tissue or exhibit epidermotropism.

STUDIES OF T-CELL LYMPHOMAS

Immunologic Studies

Initial recognition of T-cell lymphomas was based on the ability of the neoplastic cells to form spontaneous rosettes with sheep erythrocytes (Fig. 29.29). Examination of cytologic preparations permitted verification that the cells interpreted as the neoplastic components of these lymphomas were those forming E rosettes. Subsequent availability of monoclonal antibodies for pan-T-cell antigens and T-cell subset antigens, which could be used for evaluation of cell suspensions, cryostat, and paraffin tissue sections, provided greater refinement in the delineation of these tumors.

Phenotypically, the peripheral T-cell lymphomas correspond to neoplasms of postthymic lymphocytes. All cases lack CD1 and terminal deoxynucleotidyl transferase (TdT). Nonneoplastic mature T cells express the pan-T-cell antigens CD2, CD3, CD5, and CD7, and may be further subtyped as $CD4^+$ (helper/inducer) or $CD8^+$ (suppressor/cytotoxic). Neoplastic T cells present in peripheral T-cell lymphomas are phenotypically heterogeneous and frequently express abnormal phenotypes, with loss of one or more pan-T-cell antigens (13,15,17,19,20,22,50,71,72). CD5 and CD7 are most frequently lost, with deletion of CD3 and CD2 observed less often. Most cases evaluated for T-cell subsets (in this country) have demonstrated a helper/inducer ($CD4^+$) phenotype. A minor proportion demonstrate a suppressor/cytotoxic ($CD8^+$) phenotype, such as subcutaneous panniculitis-like T-cell lymphoma (Fig. 29.20C). A predominance of $CD4^+$ or $CD8^+$ cells cannot be equated with clonality, because reactive proliferations may exhibit subset predominance. Some T-cell lymphomas are $CD4^-$ and $CD8^-$ or express the anomalous $CD4^+CD8^+$ phenotype (71,72).

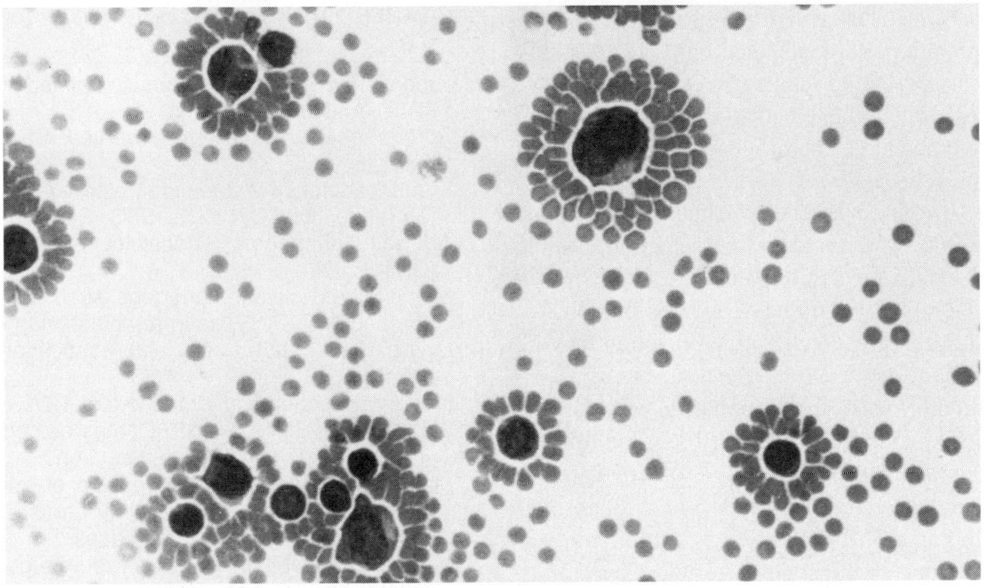

FIG. 29.29. Initial characterization of T cells and T-cell lymphomas was determined by the ability of the cells to form spontaneous rosettes with sheep erythrocytes. This cytocentrifuge preparation of a cell suspension of a lymph node involved by a T-cell lymphoma demonstrates a spectrum of T cells that form rosettes and correspond to lymphoid elements in the nodal infiltrate of histologic sections (Wright's stain, original magnification: 600× magnification).

Some tumors may exhibit a cytotoxic phenotype with reactivity for perforin, granzyme B (Fig. 29.24), or TIA-1. Tumor cells often express HLA-DR (Ia), and some cases are associated with expression of CD30 (Fig. 29.15), IL-2 receptor (CD25), or anomalous expression of epithelial membrane antigen (e.g., anaplastic large cell lymphomas, primary systemic type). Some tumors express NK cell–associated antigens CD56 (Fig. 29.22), CD57, CD16 (Leu-11b), or NKHI (199). Expression of CD15 is not generally observed in T-cell neoplasms, but if present, it is usually characterized by focal granular cytoplasmic staining (69,70). The membranous-paranuclear-cytoplasmic staining pattern that is observed for Reed-Sternberg cells of Hodgkin's disease is not typically observed for peripheral T-cell lymphomas, although it has occasionally been described for these tumors, such as for the tumor phase of mycosis fungoides (67,200). The large neoplastic T cells also differ in their phenotypic staining profile from Reed-Sternberg cells in that they are frequently leukocyte common antigen positive (201) and express T-cell antigens. Reed-Sternberg cells typically lack these antigens in routinely fixed, paraffin-embedded tissue sections.

A large number of T-cell antigens (e.g., CD1a, CD2, CD3, CD4, CD5, CD7, CD8, CD43, CD45RO) may be detected in routine paraffin sections mainly using monoclonal antibodies (202–209; personal observations). Antigen retrieval techniques are generally required for optimal immunoreactivity. CD3 represents a more specific pan-T-cell marker than CD43 (Fig. 29.30) or CD45RO, both of which may detect histiocytes or myeloid cells. Cytoplasmic reactivity for CD3 in paraffin sections may also be observed for NK cells because the polyclonal antibody detects the ϵ chain of CD3 (Fig. 29.23). CD43 is not detected in normal B cells, but it may be observed in some B-cell neoplasms and in myeloid leukemias (203,205,206). Evaluation of a panel that includes a highly effective pan-B-cell antibody for detection

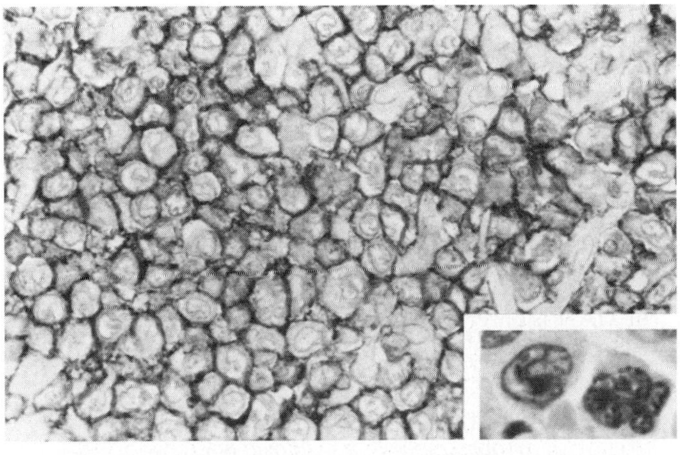

FIG. 29.30. This T-cell lymphoma was readily characterized in paraffin tissue sections using monoclonal antibodies and an immunoperoxidase technique. Antigen retrieval techniques may be required for optimal results. This section demonstrates immunoreactivity of neoplastic T cells for CD43 with strong membrane staining (immunoperoxidase technique, methyl green counterstain, original magnification: 650× magnification). Neoplastic cells were also reactive for other pan-T-cell markers (not shown). **Inset:** Prominent nuclear irregularity of the neoplastic cells (hematoxylin and eosin stain, original magnification: 1,000× magnification).

of CD20 (e.g., L26) or CD79a should assist in elimination of errors of interpretation. Particular caution is necessary for a proliferation that is reactive only for CD43. The type of fixative also plays a role in the effectiveness of immunophenotyping paraffin-embedded material, with B5-fixed tissues generally proving superior for some antigens (CD43, CD45RO) while, in our experience, formalin fixed tissue with antigen retrieval is preferred for the detection of most T-cell antigens. Certain precautions must be employed in the interpretation of paraffin tissue section immunohistochemical studies. Extensive T-cell antigen deletion may be present in anaplastic large cell lymphoma. In paraffin sections, demonstration of reactivity of neoplastic cells for leukocyte common antigen may be difficult for some tumors, such as ALCL. Detection of ALK (Fig. 29.19) or p80 protein may be helpful in defining this tumor type. Occasional small lymphocytic lymphomas of B-cell type may exhibit minimal reactivity for CD20 and strong staining for CD43, resulting in a possible erroneous interpretation of a T-cell lymphoma. A panel that includes CD3 and CD5 should prevent this type of error. Myeloblastomas (granulocytic sarcoma) may also pose problems in that these tumors are $CD43^+$. Tumors that are reactive only for CD43 should not be regarded as T-cell neoplasms without a more extensive immune phenotypic profile. Studies for myeloperoxidase or lysozyme should aid in accurate identification of infiltrates of acute myeloid leukemia. Antibodies to CD43 and CD45RO detect histiocytes and neoplasms derived from these cells, NK cells, and normal and neoplastic T cells (Table 29.10).

The assessment of T or NK cell lymphomas may reveal anomalous phenotypes with expression of markers not normally identified for T cells, such as anaplastic lymphoma kinase (ALK) (137–140). These tumors may express markers observed normally in only a minor population of T cells, such as CD56 (210), cytotoxic molecules (148,149,168), or TCR $\gamma\delta$. NK or NK/T-cell neoplasms may express CD2, CD45 and CD45RO. The NK cell marker CD56 can be readily detected in paraffin sections (210). NK cell and some peripheral T-cell neoplasms (Table 29.11) exhibit a cytotoxic phenotype that can be demonstrated using antibodies to TIA-1, granzyme B, and perforin (147–149). Expression of TIA-1 is observed for cytotoxic cells, regardless of activation status, whereas the presence of perforin and granzyme is highly increased in activated cytotoxic cells.

TABLE 29.11. *Peripheral T-cell and natural killer cell neoplasms with a cytotoxic phenotype*

Extranodal NK/T-cell lymphomas, nasal-type
Anaplastic large cell lymphoma, T/null cell, primary systemic type
Anaplastic large cell lymphoma, T/null cell, primary cutaneous type
Subcutaneous panniculitis-like T-cell lymphoma
Enteropathy-type T-cell lymphoma
Hepatosplenic $\gamma\delta$ T cell lymphoma
Aggressive NK cell leukemia
T-cell granular lymphocytic leukemia

TABLE 29.12. *Immunologic findings in peripheral T-cell lymphomas*

Predominant T-cell population as defined by one or more pan-T-cell antigens
Subset restriction may be observed, $CD4^+$ (most common) or $CD8^+$
Frequent deletion of one or more pan-T-cell antigens, in order of frequency: CD7, CD5, CD3, CD2
Aberrant phenotypes possible, such as $CD4^+CD8^+$ or $CD4^-CD8^-$
May express activation antigens, such as HLA-DR, CD30, IL-2 receptor (CD25), as in anaplastic large cell lymphomas
May express natural killer cell–associated antigens (CD56, CD16)
Immunohistochemical detection of CD2, CD3, CD4, CD5, CD7, CD8, CD43, CD45RO; may be helpful in characterizing proliferations in paraffin sections
May exhibit anomalous expression of epithelial membrane antigen and/or ALK protein/p80 protein
Cytotoxic phenotype in some cases
May lack all T-cell antigens and require gene rearrangement studies for characterization; some cases may lack gene rearrangements

In summary, for cell suspension, cryostat, or paraffin tissue section studies, a predominance of T cells with subset restriction is helpful in characterizing T-cell neoplasms, with aberrant expression of T-cell subset antigens and deletion of one or more pan-T-cell antigens providing more convincing evidence of a neoplastic process in histologically equivocal cases. The presence of unique markers also assists in diagnosis. An extensive profile is required to assess these neoplasms adequately due to overlapping characteristics of T cell, NK-like T cell, NK/T-cell neoplasms, and other proliferations (Table 29.12) (see Chapter 3).

Cytogenetic Studies

Certain cytogenetic abnormalities appear to be highly correlated with specific types of T-cell lymphoma (111). A cytogenetic abnormality of particular importance is t(2;5), which is observed in ALCL of T-cell type, except for the primary cutaneous lesions (135,136,141,143–145,211). In a few cases, a t(2;2) or other cytogenetic abnormalities have been described (141,212). The presence of the t(2;5) translocation in cases of anaplastic large cell lymphoma is reportedly associated with a much better prognosis compared with cases lacking this cytogenetic abnormality (146). A high incidence of trisomy 3 and 5 has been observed in angioimmunoblastic T-cell lymphoma (109,110). Isochromosome 7q is a characteristic feature of hepatosplenic $\gamma\delta$ T-cell lymphoma (192–194). Trisomy 8 has also been described in the latter disorder. The cytogenetic abnormalities in various T-cell neoplasms are summarized in Table 29.13.

TABLE 29.13. *Cytogenetic abnormalities in various T-cell neoplasms*

Tumor type	Cytogenetic abnormality
Anaplastic large cell lymphoma, T/null cell, primary systemic type	t(2;5), most common t(1;2), t(2;2), t(2;3), t(2;22), inv(2)
Hepatosplenic T-cell lymphoma	Isochromosome 7q; trisomy 8
Angioimmunoblastic T-cell lymphoma	Trisomy 3, trisomy 5, multiple unrelated clones
Peripheral T-cell lymphoma, not otherwise characterized	Trisomy 3, deletions in 6q, trisomy 7q, monosomy 13
T-cell prolymphocytic leukemia	Inversion (14), trisomy 8, deletion of 11q 22.3–23.1 segment

Viral Studies

Some of the T-cell or NK/T-cell neoplasms exhibit a strong association with specific viruses. Adult T-cell leukemia/lymphoma is associated with HTLV-1 infection and may respond to antiviral therapy (interferon and zidovudine). Nasal-type NK/T-cell lymphomas are strongly associated with Epstein-Barr virus. Only a small percentage of the overall group of peripheral T-cell lymphomas are associated with EBV. In angioimmunoblastic T-cell lymphoma, EBV transcripts may be found in some large transformed cells, particularly of B-cell type, which may exhibit features of Reed-Sternberg cells and variants. Occasional large EBV^+ B cells may also be detected in other types of T-cell lymphoma (213). These findings are summarized in Table 29.14. The presence of EBV is detected with a high level of sensitivity using *in situ* hybridization for EBV-encoded early RNA (EBER).

Role of Molecular Studies in the Diagnosis of T-Cell Proliferations

Because of the difficulties inherent in differentiating between reactive and neoplastic T-cell proliferations, as well as the importance of assigning a peripheral T or NK cell category to an individual neoplasm, it is imperative to adopt an integrated approach that takes into consideration the clinical features, morphologic findings, immunohistochemical profile, and molecular genetic data (29).

TABLE 29.14. *Viral association in peripheral T-cell and natural killer cell neoplasms*

Tumor type	Viral association
Adult T-cell leukemia/ lymphoma	Human T-cell lymphotropic virus, type 1 (HTLV-1)
Extranodal NK/T-cell lymphoma, nasal type	Epstein-Barr virus
Aggressive NK cell leukemia	Epstein-Barr virus
Angioimmunoblastic T-cell lymphoma	Epstein-Barr virus may be identified in large B cells[a]
Anaplastic large cell lymphoma	Epstein-Barr virus in minor population of t(2;5)–negative cases
Enteropathy-type T-cell lymphoma	Epstein-Barr virus in some cases

[a] Large Reed-Sternberg–like B cells

Clonality in B-cell neoplasms may be determined on the basis of surface immunoglobulin or cytoplasmic immunoglobulin studies. However, analogous immunophenotypic markers do not exist to define clonality in T-cell proliferations. Molecular biologic analysis of T-cell receptor (TCR) genes in these lesions represents an extremely sensitive method to define cell lineage, to distinguish between polyclonal and monoclonal proliferations, and possibly to classify the proliferation according to developmental stage (72,214–217). The basis for these studies is the knowledge that each human T-cell has an antigen receptor complex that activates the cell in response to a given antigen. To respond to a wide diversity of antigens, rearrangements of the TCR genes are required. During ontogeny, DNA segments rearrange to yield functional genes, in a process analogous to that of immunoglobulin gene rearrangements in B cells. The rearrangements occur in thymocytes early in T-cell differentiation, and follow a certain hierarchical order, with TCR-α and TCR-δ rearrangements (together with expression of CD7) occurring early, followed by TCR-β rearrangement (217). CD2 is detectable when TCR-β rearranges. TCR-α genes are fully transcribed in T cells with surface expression of CD3, CD4 and CD8 antigen (218). Most T cells (about 95%) recognize antigens with a receptor composed of an $\alpha\beta$ heterodimer, with about 5% of cells expressing an antigen receptor composed of $\gamma\delta$ chains. The rearrangements that occur in nonneoplastic T-cell proliferations generate many gene configurations of unique specificities. In a clonal or neoplastic T-cell process, the proliferating cells all reveal identically rearranged genes, providing the basis for detection using DNA probes to TCR genes. With these techniques, clonal populations comprising as little as 1% to 2% of the tissue DNA are detectable as nongermline bands in Southern blots.

Nearly all cases of peripheral T-cell lymphoma reveal clonally rearranged TCR-γ and TCR-β genes, and in some cases, also TCR-δ gene, without rearrangement of immunoglobulin genes (72,214–217,219). Limited knowledge exists regarding TCR-α gene rearrangements in T-cell neoplasms, because of technical difficulties inherent in detection with available probes, related to the extremely large physical nature of the gene (very large joining segment) (220). Rearrangement of the TCR-β chain gene appears to represent the most valuable genetic marker of clonality in analyzing these lesions (Fig 29.31). TCR-β gene rearrangement occurs early in T-cell differentiation and is a genetic marker of T-cell lineage; its presence, in combination with the absence of immunoglobulin gene rearrangement, is strong support for a T-cell derivation (221). TCR-γ rearrangements are less restrictive than TCR-β rearrangements as a genetic marker, because one third of immature B-cell neoplasms exhibit rear-

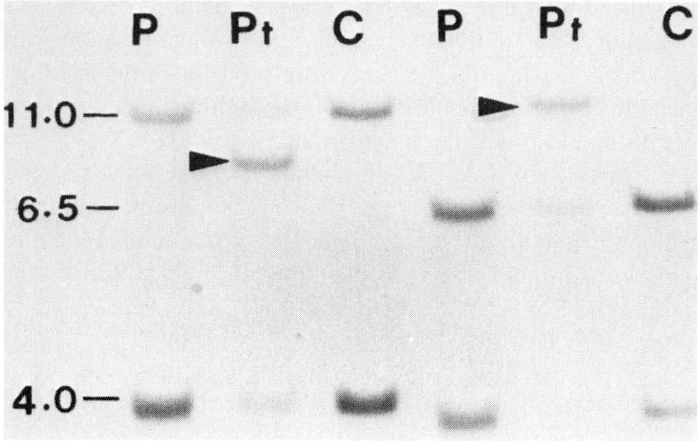

FIG. 29.31. Southern blot demonstrates T-cell receptor β chain gene rearrangements *(arrowhead)* in *Eco*R1 *(left three lanes)* and *Hin*dIII *(right three lanes)* digests from a patient with peripheral T-cell lymphoma (Pt). Germline bands are seen in control placental DNA (P) and DNA from a nonneoplastic lymph node (C). Dashes indicate molecular weights of the germline bands in kilobases.

rangement of the Tγ gene locus. In evaluating TCR-γ gene rearrangements, care must also be taken to exclude pseudoclonality. Because of the limited number of functionally rearranging V_γ genes (probably 7 or 8), benign polyclonal T cells, accounting for as little as 10% of the DNA, may produce nongermline bands, suggesting T-cell clones. Concurrent analysis of the TCR-β gene should serve to corroborate the clonality or pseudoclonality of such proliferations. TCR-δ rearrangement is a useful marker of clonality of immature T-cell tumors, which may reveal rearrangement of this gene alone. This finding is not specific for T-cell lineage, and TCR-δ deletion, rather than rearrangement, is more commonly observed in mature T-cell neoplasms (222). About 10% of T- and B-cell neoplasms, most with immature phenotypes, appear bigenotypic. However, immunophenotypic analysis of these lesions reveals expression of T- or B-cell lineage but not both (72). Occasional peripheral T-cell lymphomas may exhibit extensive deletion of pan-T-cell antigens and may also lack clonal rearrangements of the TCR-β or TCR-γ genes. These findings do not exclude the possibility of a T-cell malignancy (223). Morphologic, immunologic and genotypic data must be analyzed and correlated for accurate assessment of these proliferations.

Chromosomal mapping studies have localized the TCR-α gene to chromosome 14, band q11.2 (224). The TCR-β gene has been mapped to chromosome 7, near the bands 7q34q36 (225). Although extensive studies are not available, analysis of T-cell malignancies has demonstrated a high frequency of chromosomal abnormalities involving these genes. The TCR-α gene is especially prone to translocation (226).

Because frozen tissue is frequently unavailable for performing Southern blots to detect T-cell receptor gene rearrangements, increasing use is being made of the PCR to amplify DNA from formalin-fixed, paraffin embedded tissues. In cases where there is only a small amount of material (for example skin punch biopsies from patients with cutaneous T-cell lymphoma), PCR may be the only suitable technique for molecular analysis (227). Clonal gene rearrangements have been described in 50% to 83% of biopsies from patients with patch, patch/plaque, and erythrodermic stages, which often pose a diagnostic challenge (228). In our laboratory, sufficient DNA can usually be obtained by cutting 10 or more paraffin sections (depending on the size of the block) at 5 μm and collecting these in an uncontaminated 5 ml tube. A nonradioactive method to detect T-cell receptor γ (TCR-γ) gene rearrangements by PCR single-strand conformational polymorphism (PCR-SSCP) in paraffin-embedded tissue has been described (229). $V_\gamma1$–8, $V_\gamma9$, $V_\gamma10$, $V_\gamma11$, and $J_\gamma1/J_\gamma2$ consensus primers are suitable for TCR-γ gene rearrangement amplification, and PCR products can be analyzed by nonradioactive SSCP. Monoclonal controls from known T-cell lymphomas should yield a well-defined banded pattern, whereas polyclonal T-cell controls yield a smear pattern. Using these methods monoclonality may be demonstrated in up to 95% of T-cell lymphoma cases, and sensitivity has been reported as less than 5% (229).

SUMMARY AND CONCLUSIONS

Peripheral T-cell and NK/T-cell neoplasms are unusual lymphomas that vary geographically in their incidence and represent about 10% of non-Hodgkin's lymphomas. The marked morphologic and phenotypic heterogeneity of these tumors has compromised their classification for many years. The proposed WHO classification of these tumors, a scheme based on the REAL classification, recognizes distinct clinical entities and relegates the remaining neoplasms to a composite group (not further characterized). These tumors generally involve older adults, except for anaplastic large cell lymphoma (bimodal age distribution), who frequently present with lymphadenopathy, often with advanced stage disease. Some of the recognized clinical entities are associated with extranodal disease, including subcutaneous panniculitis-like T-cell lymphoma, nasal-type NK/T-cell lymphoma, enteropathy-type intestinal T-cell lymphoma, hepatosplenic T-cell lymphoma, and anaplastic large cell lymphoma. Although the overall group of peripheral T-cell lymphomas is associated with poor prognosis, a highly favorable prognosis is associated with anaplastic large cell lymphoma of T/null cell type, both systemic and cutaneous forms. Certain entities are highly associated with the presence of a specific virus, such as HTLV-1 in adult T-cell leukemia/lymphoma and Epstein-Barr virus in nasal type NK/T-cell lymphomas, with large EBV^+ cells observed in angioimmunoblastic T-cell lymphomas. Anaplastic large cell lymphoma, primary systemic type, is associated with a distinctive cytogenetic abnormality, t(2;5), and the presence of the chimeric protein ALK (anaplastic lymphoma kinase) as a consequence of this translocation. Other cytogenetic abnormalities may be present in these ALK⁺ neoplasms. This overall group of neoplasms is derived from mature T cells or putative NK cells (nasal-type), and are heterogenous in their expression of T-cell antigens and other markers, with frequent antigen deletion and anomalous phenotypes. Most tumors that express subset antigens are of CD4 (helper/inducer) type. Subcutaneous panniculitis-like T-cell lymphoma, however, is a $CD8^+$ neoplasm. These tumors frequently exhibit a cytotoxic phenotype, with the presence of cytotoxic granules as detected by antibodies to perforin, granzyme B, or TIA-1. Despite the ability to detect many T-cell antigens and other markers characteristic of these lesions in paraffin tissue sections, some tumors may require T-cell receptor gene rearrangements to define a T-cell derivation. Nasal type NK/T-cell lymphomas typically lack T-cell receptor gene rearrangements. Molecular studies can be performed on paraffin-embedded tissues using PCR techniques. Optimal analysis of this unusual group of tumors requires an integrated approach that incorporates clinical, histologic, immunophenotypic, viral, cytogenetic, and molecular features.

REFERENCES

1. Lukes RJ, Taylor CR, Parker JW, et al. A morphologic and immunologic surface marker study of 299 cases of non-Hodgkin's lymphomas and related leukemias. *Am J Pathol* 1978;90:461–586.
2. Kikuchi M, Mitsui T, Matsui N, et al. T cell malignancies in adults: histopathological studies of lymph nodes in 100 patients. *Jpn J Clin Oncol* 1979;9[Suppl]:407–422.
3. Watanabe S, Nakajima T, Shimosato Y, et al. T cell malignancies: subclassification and interrelationship. *Jpn J Clin Oncol* 1979; 9[Suppl]:423–442.
4. Kinoshita K, Kamihira S, Ikeda S, et al. Clinical, hematologic, and pathologic features of leukemic T cell lymphoma. *Cancer* 1982;50: 1554–1562.
5. Kadin ME, Berard CW, Nanba K, et al. Lymphoproliferative diseases in Japan and western countries. *Hum Pathol* 1983;14:745–772.
6. Waldron JA, Leech JH, Glick AD, et al. Malignant lymphoma of peripheral T lymphocyte origin: immunologic, pathologic and clinical features in six patients. *Cancer* 1977;40:1604–1617.
7. Pinkus GS, Said JW. Characterization of non-Hodgkin's lymphomas using multiple cell markers: immunologic, morphologic, and cytochemical studies of 72 cases. *Am J Pathol* 1978;94:349–380.
8. Pinkus GS, Said JW, Hargreaves H. Malignant lymphoma, T cell type: a distinct morphologic variant with large multilobated nuclei, with report of four cases. *Am J Clin Pathol* 1979;72:540–550.
9. Palutke M, Tabaczka P, Weise RW, et al. T cell lymphomas of large cell type—a variety of malignant lymphomas: "histiocytic" and mixed lymphocytic-"histiocytic." *Cancer* 1980;46:87–101.
10. Knowles DM, Halper JP. Human T cell malignancies: correlative clinical, histopathologic, immunologic and cytochemical analysis of 23 cases. *Am J Pathol* 1982;106:187–203.
11. Said JW, Shintaku IP, Chien K, et al. Peripheral T cell lymphoma (immunoblastic sarcoma of T cell type): an immuno-ultrastructural study. *Hum Pathol* 1984;15:324–329.
12. Greer JP, York JC, Cousar JB, et al. Peripheral T cell lymphoma: a clinicopathologic study of 42 cases. *J Clin Oncol* 1984;2:788–798.
13. Grogan TM, Fielder K, Rangel C, et al. Peripheral T cell lymphoma: aggressive disease with heterogenous phenotypes. *Am J Clin Pathol* 1985;83:279–288.
14. Weisenburger DD, Astorino RN, Glassy FJ, et al. Peripheral T cell lymphomas: a clinicopathologic study of a morphologically diverse entity. *Cancer* 1985;56:2061–2068.
15. Weiss LM, Crabtree GS, Rouse RV, et al. Morphologic and immunologic characterization of 50 peripheral T cell lymphomas. *Am J Pathol* 1985;118:316–324.
16. Schneider DR, Taylor CR, Parker JW, et al. Immunoblastic sarcoma of T and B cell types. *Hum Pathol* 1985;16:885–900.
17. Weis JW, Winter MW, Phyliky RL, et al. Peripheral T cell lymphomas: histologic, immunohistologic and clinical characterization. *Mayo Clin Proc* 1986;61:411–426.
18. Weisenburger DD, Linder J, Armitage JO. Peripheral T cell lymphoma: a clinicopathologic study of 42 cases. *Hematol Oncol* 1987; 5:175–187.
19. Jaffe ES. The morphologic spectrum of T cell lymphoma. *Am J Surg Pathol* 1988;12:158–159.
20. Jaffe ES. Post-thymic lymphoid neoplasia. In: Jaffe ES, ed. *Surgical pathology of the lymph nodes and related organs.* Philadelphia: WB Saunders, 1985:218–248.
21. Armitage JO, Greer JP, Levine AM, et al. Peripheral T cell lymphoma. *Cancer* 1989;63:158–163.
22. Pinkus GS, O'Hara CJ, Said JW. Peripheral/post-thymic T cell lymphomas: a spectrum of disease; clinical, pathologic and immunologic features of 78 cases. *Cancer* 1990;65:971–998.
23. The Non-Hodgkin's Lymphoma Classification Project. A clinical evaluation of the International lymphoma study group classification of non-Hodgkin's lymphoma. *Blood* 1997;89:3909–3918.
24. Reinherz EL, Schlossman SF. Regulation of the immune response-inducer and suppressor T lymphocyte subsets in human beings. *N Engl J Med* 1980;303:370–373.
25. Hsu S-M, Jaffe ES. Phenotypic expression of T lymphocytes in thymus and peripheral lymphoid tissues. *Am J Pathol* 1985;121:69–78.
26. Stansfeld AG, Diebold J, Kapanci Y, et al. Updated Kiel classification for lymphomas. *Lancet* 1988;1:292–293.
27. Harris NL, Jaffe ES, Stein H, et al. A revised European-American classification of lymphoid neoplasms proposed by the International Lymphoma Study Group. *Blood* 1994;84:1361–1392.
28. Harris NL, Jaffe ES, Diebold J, et al. World Health Organization classification of neoplastic diseases of the hematopoietic and lymphoid tissues: report of the clinical advisory committee meeting, Arlie House, Virginia, November 1997. *J Clin Oncol* 1999;17: 3835–3849.
29. Chan JKC. Peripheral T cell and NK-cell neoplasms: an integrated approach to diagnosis. *Mod Pathol* 1999;12:177–199.
30. Suchi T, Lennert K, Tu L-Y, et al. Histopathology and immunohistochemistry of peripheral T cell lymphomas: a proposal for their classification. *J Clin Pathol* 1987;40:995–1015.
31. Kadin ME, Sako D, Berliner N, et al. Childhood Ki-1 lymphoma presenting with skin lesions and peripheral adenopathy. *Blood* 1986; 68:1042–1049.
32. Agnarsson BA, Kadin ME. Ki-1 positive large cell lymphoma: a morphologic and immunologic study of 19 cases. *Am J Surg Pathol* 1988; 12:264–274.
33. Stein H, Mason DY, Gerdes J, et al. The expression of the Hodgkin's disease associated antigen Ki-1 in reactive and neoplastic lymphoid tissue: evidence that Reed-Sternberg cells and histiocytic malignancies are derived from activated lymphoid cells. *Blood* 1985;66: 848–858.
34. Chan JKC, Ng CS, Hui PK, et al. Anaplastic large cell Ki-1 lymphoma. Delineation of two morphological types. *Histopathology* 1989;15: 11–34.
35. Penny RJ, Blaustein JC, Longtine JA, et al. Ki-1 positive large cell lymphomas—a heterogenous group of neoplasms: morphologic, immunophenotypic, genotypic and clinical features in 24 cases. *Cancer* 1991;68:362–373.
36. Kinney MC, Collins, RD, Greer JP, et al. A small cell predominant variant of primary Ki-1 (CD30) and T cell lymphoma. *Am J Surg Pathol* 1993;17:859–868.
37. Levine AM, Taylor CR, Schneider DR, et al. Immunoblastic sarcoma of T cell versus B cell origin. I. Clinical features. *Blood* 1981;58: 52–61.
38. Borowitz MJ, Reichert TA, Brynes, et al. The phenotypic diversity of peripheral T-cell lymphomas: the Southeastern Cancer Study Group experience. *Hum Pathol* 1986;17:567–574.
39. Kurtin PJ, Gaffey TA, Habermann TM. Peripheral T cell lymphoma involving the placenta. *Cancer* 1992;70:2963–2968.
40. Blayney DW, Jaffe ES, Fisher RI, et al. The human T cell leukemia/lymphoma virus, lymphoma, lytic bone lesions, and hypercalcemia. *Ann Intern Med* 1983;98:144–151.
41. Grossman B, Schechter GP, Horton JE, et al. Hypercalcemia associ-

ated with T cell lymphoma-leukemia. *Am J Clin Pathol* 1981;75: 149–155.
42. Loughran TP, Kadin ME, Deeg HJ. T cell intestinal lymphoma associated with celiac sprue. *Ann Intern Med* 1986;104:44–47.
43. Abruzzo LV, Griffith LM, Nandedkar M, et al. Histologically discordant lymphomas with B-cell and T-cell components. *Am J Clin Pathol* 1997;108:316–323.
44. Ross CW, Schnitzer B, Sheldon S, et al. Gamma/delta T cell posttransplantation lymphoproliferative disorder primarily in the spleen. *Am J Clin Pathol* 1994;102:310–315.
45. Yasunaga C, Kasai T, Nishihara G, et al. Early development of Epstein-Barr virus-associated T cell lymphoma after a living-related renal transplantation. *Transplantation* 1998;65:1642–1644.
46. Kraus MD, Crawford DF, Kaleem Z, et al. T gamma/delta hepatosplenic lymphoma in a heart transplant patient after an Epstein-Barr virus positive lymphoproliferative disorder: a case report. *Cancer* 1998;82:983–992.
47. Garvin AJ, Self S, Sahovic EA, et al. The occurrence of a peripheral T cell lymphoma in a chronically immunosuppressed renal transplant patient. *Am J Surg Pathol* 1988;12:64–70.
48. Aydin F, Bartholomew PM, Vinson DG. Primary T cell lymphoma of the brain in a patient at advanced stage of acquired immunodeficiency syndrome. *Arch Pathol Lab Med* 1998;122:361–365.
49. Gottesman SR, Haas D, Ladanyi M, et al. Peripheral T cell lymphoma in a patient with common variable immunodeficiency disease: case report and literature review. *Leuk Lymphoma* 1999;32:589–595.
50. Lippman SM, Miller TP, Spier CM, et al. The prognostic significance of the immunophenotype in diffuse large cell lymphomas: a comparative study of the T-cell and B-cell phenotype. *Blood* 1988;72: 436–441.
51. Ansell SM, Habermann TM, Kurtin PJ, et al. Predictive capacity of the International Prognostic Factor Index in patients with peripheral T cell lymphoma. *J Clin Oncol* 1997;15:2296–3001.
52. Vaillant L, Monegier du Sorbier C, Arbeille B, et al. Cutaneous T cell lymphoma of signet ring cell type: a specific clinicopathologic entity. *Acta Derm Venereol* 1993;73:255–258.
53. Weiss LM, Wood GS, Dorfman RF. T cell signet ring lymphoma: a histologic, ultrastructural, and immunohistochemical study of two cases. *Am J Surg Pathol* 1985;9:273–280.
54. Pallesen G, Madsen M, Hastrup J. Large cell T lymphoma with hypersegmented nuclei. *Scand J Haematol* 1981;26:72–79.
55. Pileri S, Brandi G, Rivano MT, et al. Report of a case of non-Hodgkin's lymphoma of large multilobated cell type with B cell origin. *Tumors* 1982;68:543–548.
56. Van der Putte SCJ, Toonstra J, De Weger RA, et al. Cutaneous T cell lymphoma, multilobated type. *Histopathology* 1982;6:34–54.
57. Marzano AV, Alessi E, Berti E. CD30-positive multilobated peripheral T cell lymphoma primarily involving the subcutaneous tissue. *Am J Dermatopathol* 1997;19:284–288.
58. Farcet MF, Gaulard P, Marolleau J, et al. Hepatosplenic T cell lymphoma: sinusal/sinusoidal localization of malignant cells expressing the T cell receptor gamma-delta. *Blood* 1990;75:2213–2219.
59. Cooke C-B, Krenacs L, Stetler-Stevenson M, et al. Hepatosplenic T cell lymphoma: a distinct clinicopathologic entity of cytotoxic $\gamma\delta$-T cell origin. *Blood* 1996;88:4265–4274.
60. Kadin ME, Kamoun M, Lamberg J. Erythrophagocytic T gamma lymphoma—a clinicopathologic entity resembling malignant histiocytosis. *N Engl J Med* 1981;304:648–653.
61. Cuevas E, Ortiz-Hidalgo C, Oliva H, et al. Primary pleomorphic T cell lymphoma of the spleen. *Leuk Lymphoma* 1993;9:265–267.
62. Nosari A, Oreste PL, Biondi A, et al. Hepato-splenic gamma/delta T-cell lymphoma: a rare entity mimicking the hemophagocytic syndrome. *Am J Hematol* 1999;60:61–65.
63. Haj M, Zaina A, Wiess M, et al. Pathologic spontaneous rupture of the spleen as a presenting sign of splenic T-cell lymphoma—case report with review. *Hepatogastroenterology* 1999;46:193–195.
64. Isaacson PG, O'Connor NT, Spencer JO, et al. Malignant histiocytosis of the intestine: a T cell lymphoma. *Lancet* 1985;2:688–691.
65. Delsol G, Al Saati T, Gatter KC, et al. Coexpression of epithelial membrane antigen (EMA), Ki-1, and interleukin-2 receptor by anaplastic large cell lymphomas: diagnostic value in so-called malignant histiocytosis. *Am J Pathol* 1988;130:59–70.
66. Wilson MS, Weiss LM, Gatter KC, et al. Malignant histiocytosis—a reassessment of cases previously reported in 1975 based on paraffin section immunophenotyping studies. *Cancer* 1990;66:530–536.
67. Wieczorek R, Burke JS, Knowles DM. Leu-M1 antigen expression in T cell neoplasia. *Am J Pathol* 1985;121:374–380.
68. Pinkus GS, Pinkus JL, Langhoff E, et al. Fascin, a sensitive new marker for Reed-Sternberg cells of Hodgkin's disease: evidence for a dendritic B cell derivation? *Am J Pathol* 1997;150:543–562.
69. Hsu S-M, Jaffe ES. Leu-M1 and peanut agglutinin stain the neoplastic cells of Hodgkin's disease. *Am J Clin Pathol* 1984;82:29–32.
70. Pinkus GS, Thomas P, Said JW. Leu-M1—a marker for Reed-Sternberg cells in Hodgkin's disease. *Am J Pathol* 1985;119:244–252.
71. Picker LJ, Weiss LM, Medeiros LJ, et al. Immunophenotypic criteria for the diagnosis of non-Hodgkin's lymphoma. *Am J Pathol* 1987; 128:181–201.
72. Knowles DM. Immunophenotypic and antigen receptor gene rearrangement analysis in T cell neoplasia. *Am J Pathol* 1989;134: 761–785.
73. Ramsay AD, Smith WJ, Isaacson PG. T-cell rich B-cell lymphoma. *Am J Surg Pathol* 1988;12:433–443.
74. Ng CS, Chan JKC, Hui PK, et al. Large B cell lymphomas with a high content of reactive T cells. *Hum Pathol* 1989;20:1145–1154.
75. Macon WR, Williams ME, Greer JP, et al. T-cell rich B-cell lymphomas: a clinicopathologic study of 19 cases. *Am J Surg Pathol* 1992;16:351–363.
76. Rodriguez J, Pugh WC, Cabanillas F. T-cell rich B-cell lymphoma. *Blood* 1993;82:1586–1589.
77. Lennert K, Mestdagh J. Lymphogranulomatosen mit konstant hohem epithelioidzellgehalt. *Virchows Arch (Pathol Anat)* 1968;344:1–20.
78. Burke J, Butler JJ. Malignant lymphoma with a high content of epithelioid histiocytes (Lennert's lymphoma). *Am J Clin Pathol* 1976;66: 1–9.
79. Palutke M, Varadachari C, Weise RW, et al. Lennert's lymphoma: a T cell neoplasm. *Am J Clin Pathol* 1978;69:643–646.
80. Kim H, Nathwani BN, Rappaport H. So-called Lennert's lymphoma—is it a clinicopathologic entity? *Cancer* 1980;45:1379–1399.
81. Feller AC, Griesser GH, Mak TW, et al. Lymphoepithelioid lymphoma (Lennert's lymphoma) is a monoclonal proliferation of helper/inducer T cells. *Blood* 1986;68:663–667.
82. Klein MA, Jaffe R, Neiman RS. "Lennert's lymphoma" with transformation to malignant lymphoma, histiocytic type (immunoblastic sarcoma). *Am J Clin Pathol* 1977;68:601–605.
83. Sepp N, Schuler G, Romani N, et al. Intravascular lymphomatosis (angioendotheliomatosis): evidence for a T cell origin in two cases. *Hum Pathol* 1990;21:1051–1058.
84. Sheibani K, Battifora H, Winberg CD, et al. Further evidence that malignant angioendotheliomatosis is an angiotropic large cell lymphoma. *N Engl J Med* 1986;31:943–948.
85. Shimokawa I, Higami Y, Sakai H, et al. Intravascular malignant lymphoma: a case of T-cell lymphoma probably associated with human T cell lymphotropic virus. *Hum Pathol* 1991;22:200–202.
86. Stroup RM, Sheibani K, Moncada A, et al. Angiotropic (intravascular) large cell lymphoma: a clinicopathologic study of seven cases with unique clinical presentations. *Cancer* 1990;66:1781–1788.
87. Tateyama H, Eimoto T, Tada T, et al. Congenital angiotropic lymphoma (intravascular lymphomatosis) of the T cell type. *Cancer* 1991; 67:2131–2136.
88. O'Hara CJ, Said JW, Pinkus GS. Non-Hodgkin's lymphoma, multilobated B cell type: report of nine cases with immunohistochemical and immunoultrastructural evidence for a follicular center cell derivation. *Hum Pathol* 1986;17:593–599.
89. Von Baarlen J, Schuurman H-J, Van Unnik JAM. Multilobated non-Hodgkin's lymphoma—a clinicopathologic entity. *Cancer* 1988;61: 1371–1376.
90. Cerezo L. B cell multilobated lymphoma. *Cancer* 1983;52: 2277–2280.
91. Lennert K. Pathologisch-histologische Klassifizieurung der maligne lymphome. In: Stacher A, ed. *Leukamien und maligne lymphome.* Berlin: Urban and Schwarzenberg, 1973:181–194.
92. Lukes RJ, Tindle BH. Immunoblastic lymphadenopathy: a hyperimmune entity resembling Hodgkin's disease. *N Engl J Med* 1975;292: 1–8.
93. Frizzera G, Moran EM, Rappaport H. Angio-immunoblastic lymphadenopathy: diagnosis and clinical course. *Am J Med* 1975;59:803–818.
94. Patsouris E, Noel H, Lennert K. Angioimmunoblastic lymphadenopa-

thy-type of T cell lymphoma with a high content of epithelioid cells. *Am J Surg Pathol* 1989;13:262–275.
95. Neiman RS, Dervan P, Haudenschild C, et al. Angioimmunoblastic lymphadenopathy: an ultrastructural and immunologic study with review of the literature. *Cancer* 1978;41:507–518.
96. Shimoyama M, Minato K, Saito H, et al. Immunoblastic lymphadenopathy (IBL)–like T cell lymphoma. *Jpn J Clin Oncol* 1979; 9[Suppl]:347–356.
97. Watanabe S, Shimosato Y, Shimoyama M, et al. Adult T cell lymphoma with hypergammaglobulinemia. *Cancer* 1980;46:2473–2483.
98. Nathwani BN, Rappaport H, Moran EM, et al. Malignant lymphoma arising in angioimmunoblastic lymphadenopathy. *Cancer* 1978;41: 578–606.
99. Weiss LM, Strickler JG, Dorfman RF, et al. Clonal T-cell populations in angio-immunoblastic lymphadenopathy and angioimmunoblastic lymphadenopathy-like lymphoma. *Am J Pathol* 1986;122:392–397.
100. Abruzzo LV, Schmidt K, Weiss LM, et al. B cell lymphoma after angioimmunoblastic lymphadenopathy: a case with oligoclonal gene rearrangements associated with Epstein-Barr virus. *Blood* 1993;82: 241–246.
101. Chan JKC. Proliferative lesions of follicular dendritic cells: an overview, including a detailed account of follicular dendritic cell sarcoma, a neoplasm with many faces and uncommon etiologic associations. *Adv Anat Pathol* 1997;4:387–411.
102. Lennert K. Conceptual basis of the classification of malignant lymphomas. *Med J Kagoshima U* 1995;47[Suppl]:7–31.
103. Leung CY, Ho FCS, Srivastava G, et al. Usefulness of follicular dendritic cell pattern in classification of peripheral T cell lymphomas. *Histopathology* 1993;23:433–438.
104. Rudders RA, DeLellis R. Immunoblastic lymphadenopathy. A mixed proliferation of T and B lymphocytes. *Am J Clin Pathol* 1977;68: 518–521.
105. Doi S, Nasu K, Arita Y, et al. Immunohistochemical analysis of peripheral T cell lymphoma in Japanese patients. *Am J Clin Pathol* 1989; 91:152–158.
106. Tobinai K, Minato K, Ohtsu T, et al. Clinicopathologic, immunophenotypic, and immunogenotypic analyses of immunoblastic lymphadenopathy-like T cell lymphoma. *Blood* 1988;72:1000–1006.
107. Feller AC, Griesser H, Schilling CV, et al. Clonal gene rearrangement patterns correlated with immunophenotype and clinical parameters in patients with angioimmunoblastic lymphadenopathy. *Am J Pathol* 1988;133:549–556.
108. Griesser H, Feller A, Lennert K, et al. Rearrangement of the beta chain of the T cell antigen receptor and immunoglobulin genes in lymphoproliferative disorders. *J Clin Invest* 1986;78:1179–1184.
109. Quintanilla-Martinez L, Fend F, Moguel LR, et al. Peripheral T-cell lymphoma with Reed-Sternberg like cells of B-cell phenotype and genotype associated with Epstein-Barr virus infection. *Am J Surg Pathol* 1999;23:1233–1240.
110. Kaneko Y, Maseki N, Sakurai M, et al. Characteristic karyotypic pattern in T cell lymphoproliferative disorders with reactive "angioimmunoblastic lymphadenopathy with dysproteinemia-type" features. *Blood* 1988;72:413–421.
111. Schlegelberger B, Feller AC. Classification of peripheral T cell lymphomas: cytogenetic findings support the updated Kiel classification. *Leuk Lymphoma* 1996;20:411–416.
112. Uchiyama T, Yodoi J, Sagawa K, et al. Adult T cell leukemia: clinical and hematologic features of 16 cases. *Blood* 1977;50:481–492.
113. Catovsky D, Greaves MF, Rose M, et al. Adult T cell lymphoma-leukemia in blacks from the West Indies. *Lancet* 1982;1:639–643.
114. Blayney DW, Jaffe ES, Blattner WA, et al. The human T cell leukemia/lymphoma virus associated with American adult T cell leukemia/ lymphoma. *Blood* 1983;62:401–405.
115. Bunn PA, Schechter GP, Jaffe ES, et al. Clinical course of retrovirus-associated adult T cell lymphoma in the United states. *N Engl J Med* 1983;309:257–264.
116. Jaffe ES, Cossman J, Blattner WA, et al. The pathologic spectrum of adult T cell leukemia/lymphoma in the United States. *Am J Surg Pathol* 1984;8:263–275.
117. Swerdlow SH, Habeshaw JA, Rohatiner AZS, et al. Caribbean T cell lymphoma/leukemia. *Cancer* 1984;54:687–696.
118. Schwab U, Stein H, Gerdes J, et al. Production of a monoclonal antibody specific for Hodgkin's and Sternberg-Reed cells of Hodgkin's disease and a subset of normal lymphoid cells. *Nature* 1982;299: 65–67.
119. Chott A, Kaserer K, Augustin I, et al. Ki-1 positive large cell lymphoma: a clinicopathologic study of 41 cases. *Am J Surg Pathol* 1990; 14:439–448.
120. Pallesen G, Hamilton-Dutort H, et al. Ki-1 (CD30) antigen is regularly expressed by tumor cells of embryonal carcinoma. *Am J Pathol* 1988; 133:466–450.
121. Schwarting R, Gerdes J, Durkop H, et al. A new Ki-1 (CD30) monoclonal antibody directed at a formal resistant epitope. *Blood* 1989;74: 1678–1689.
122. Mechtersheimer G, Moller P. Expression of Ki-1 antigen (CD30) in mesenchymal tumors. *Cancer* 1990;66:1732–1737.
123. Falini B, Pileri S, Pizzolo G. CD30 (Ki-1) molecule: a new cytokine receptor of the tumor necrosis factor receptor superfamily as a tool for diagnosis and immunotherapy. *Blood* 1995;85:1–14.
124. Fonatsch C, Latza U, Durkop H, et al. Assignment of the human CD30 (Ki-1) gene to 1p36. *Genomics* 1992;14:825–826.
125. Lennert K, Feller AC. Large cell anaplastic lymphoma of T cell type (Ki-1^{+}). In: *Histopathology of non-Hodgkin's lymphomas.* New York: Springer-Verlag, 1992:229.
126. Alsabeth R, Medeiros LJ, Glackin C, et al. Transformation of follicular lymphoma into CD30-large cell lymphoma with anaplastic cytologic features. *Am J Surg Pathol* 1997;21:528–536.
127. Meguerian-Bedoyan Z, Lamant L, Hopfner C, et al. Anaplastic large cell lymphoma of maternal origin involving the placenta: case report and literature survey. *Am J Surg Pathol* 1997;21:1236–1241.
128. McCluggage WG, Walsh MY, Bharucha H. Anaplastic large cell malignant lymphoma with extensive eosinophilic or neutrophilic infiltration. *Histopathology* 1998;32:110–115.
129. Pileri S, Falini B, Delsol G, et al. Lymphohistiocytic T cell lymphoma (anaplastic large cell lymphoma). CD30^{+}/Ki-1^{+} with a high content of reactive histiocytes. *Histopathology* 1990;16:383–391.
130. Pileri S, Sabatini E, Poggi S, et al. Lymphohistiocytic T cell lymphoma. *Histopathology* 1994;25:191–193.
131. Pileri SA, Pulford K, Mori S, et al. Frequent expression of the NPM-ALK chimeric fusion protein in anaplastic large cell lymphoma, lympho-histiocytic type. *Am J Pathol* 1997;150:1207–1211.
132. Ott G, Bastian BC, Katzenberger T, et al. A lymphohistiocytic variant of anaplastic large cell lymphoma with demonstration of the t(2; 5)(p23;q35) chromosome translocation. *Br J Haematol* 1998;100: 187–190.
133. Herbst H, Anagnostopoulos J, Heinze B, et al. ALK gene products in anaplastic large cell lymphomas and Hodgkin's disease. *Blood* 1995;86:1694–1700.
134. Lamant L, Meggetto F, Saati T, et al. High incidence of the t(2;5)(p23; q35) translocation in anaplastic large cell lymphoma and its lack of detection in Hodgkin's disease. Comparison of cytogenetic analysis, reverse transcriptase-polymerase chain reaction, and P-80 immunostaining. *Blood* 1996;87:284–291.
135. Bitter MA, Franklin WA, Larson RA, et al. Morphology in Ki-1 (CD30)-positive non-Hodgkin's lymphoma is correlated with clinical features and the presence of a unique chromosomal abnormality, t(2; 5)(p23;q35). *Am J Surg Pathol* 1990;14:305–316.
136. Morris SW, Kirstein MN, Valentine MB, et al. Fusion of a kinase gene, ALK, to the nucleolar protein gene, NPM, in non-Hodgkin's lymphoma. *Science* 1994;263:1281–1284.
137. Shiota M, Fujimoto J, Takenaga M, et al. Diagnosis of t(2;5)(p23; q35)–associated Ki-1 lymphoma with immunohistochemistry. *Blood* 1994;84:3648–3652.
138. Shiota M, Nakamura S, Ichinohasama R, et al. Anaplastic large cell lymphomas expressing the novel chimeric protein p80 NPM/ALK a distinct clinicopathologic entity. *Blood* 1995;86:1954–1960.
139. Pulford K, Lamaut L, Morris SW, et al. Detection of anaplastic lymphoma kinase (ALK) and nuclear protein nucleophosmin (NPM)-ALK proteins in normal and neoplastic cells with the monoclonal antibody ALK-1. *Blood* 1997;89:1394–1404.
140. Pulford K, Falini B, Cordell J, et al. Biochemical detection of novel anaplastic lymphoma kinase proteins in tissue sections of anaplastic large cell lymphoma. *Am J Pathol* 1999;154:1657–1663.
141. Delsol G, Touriol C, Pulford K, et al. Diversity of chromosomal changes involving 2p23 in ALK-positive anaplastic large cell lymphoma. Proceedings of European Association for Haematopathology Meeting X. London, England, May 2000(abst).

142. Kinney MC, Greer JP, Kadin ME, et al. P80npm/alk expression in Ki-1+ lymphomas: histologic and immunophenotypic correlation. *Lab Invest* 1996;74:114A(abst).
143. DeCoteau JF, Butmarc JR, Kinney MC, et al. The t(2;5) chromosomal translocation is not a common feature of primary cutaneous CD30+ lymphoproliferative disorders: comparison with anaplastic large cell lymphoma of nodal origin. *Blood* 1996;87:3437–3441.
144. Beylot-Barry M, Lamant L, Vergier B, et al. Detection of the t(2;5)(p23;q35) translocation by reverse transcriptase polymerase chain reaction and in-situ hybridization in CD30-positive primary cutaneous lymphoma and lymphomatous papulosis. *Am J Pathol* 1996;149:483–492.
145. Wood GS, Hardman DL, Boni R, et al. Lack of the t(2;5) or other mutations resulting in expression of anaplastic lymphoma kinase catalytic domain in CD30+ primary cutaneous lymphoproliferative disorders and Hodgkin's disease. *Blood* 1996;88:1765–1770.
146. Nakamura S, Shiota M, Nakagawa A, et al. Anaplastic large cell lymphoma: a distinct molecular pathologic entity: a reappraisal with special reference to p80 (NPM/ALK) expression. *Am J Surg Pathol* 1997;21:1420–1432.
147. Krenaes L, Wellmann A, Sorbara L, et al. Cytotoxic cell antigen expression in anaplastic large cell lymphomas of T- and null-cell type and Hodgkin's disease: evidence for distinct cellular origin. *Blood* 1997;89:980–989.
148. Felgar RE, Macon WR, Kinney MC, et al. TIA-1 expression in lymphoid neoplasms: identification of subsets with cytotoxic T lymphocyte or natural killer cell differentiation. *Am J Pathol* 1997;150:1893–1900.
149. Foss HD, Anagnostopoulos I, Araujo I, et al. Anaplastic large cell lymphomas of T-cell and null-cell phenotype express cytotoxic molecules. *Blood* 1996;88:4005–4011.
150. Paulli M, Berti E, Rosso R, et al. CD30/Ki-1 positive lymphoproliferative disorders of the skin: clinicopathologic correlation and statistical analysis of 86 cases. A multicenter study from the European Organization for Cancer Research and Treatment of Cancer Cutaneous Lymphoma Project Group. *J Clin Oncol* 1995;13:1343–1354.
151. Willemze R, Kerl H, Sterry W, et al. EORTC classification for primary cutaneous lymphomas: a proposal from the Cutaneous Lymphoma Study Group of the 3 European Organization for Research and Treatment of Cancer. *Blood* 1997;90:354–71.
152. Noorduyn LA, Belijaards RC, Pals ST, et al. Differential expression of the HECA-452 antigen (cutaneous lymphocyte associated antigen; CLA) in cutaneous and noncutaneous T cell lymphomas. *Histopathology* 1992;21:59–64.
153. Gonzalez CL, Medeiros MJ, Braziel RM, et al. T cell lymphoma involving subcutaneous tissue: a clinicopathologic entity commonly associated with hemophagocytic syndrome. *Am J Surg Pathol* 1991;15:17–27.
154. Perniciaro C, Zalla MJ, White JW, et al. Subcutaneous T cell lymphoma. Report of two additional cases and further observations. *Arch Dermatol* 1993;129:1171–1176.
155. Mehregan DA, Su WPD, Kurtin PJ. Subcutaneous T-cell lymphoma: a clinical, histopathologic and immunohistochemical study of six cases. *J Cutan Pathol* 1994;21:110–117.
156. Kumar S, Krenacs L, Medeiros J, et al. Subcutaneous panniculitic T-cell lymphoma in a tumor of cytotoxic T lymphocytes. *Hum Pathol* 1998;29:397–403.
157. DeRemee RA, Weiland LH, McDonald TJ. Polymorphic reticulosis, lymphomatoid granulomatosis: two diseases or one? *Mayo Clin Proc* 1978;53:634–640.
158. Yamanaka N, Harabuchi Y, Sambe S, et al. Non-Hodgkin's lymphoma of Waldeyer's ring and nasal cavity: clinical and immunologic aspects. *Cancer* 1985;56:768–776.
159. Chott A, Rappersberger K, Schlossarek W, et al. Peripheral T cell lymphoma presenting primarily as lethal midline granuloma. *Hum Pathol* 1988;19:1093–1101.
160. Ng CS, Lo STH, Chan JKC, et al. CD56-positive putative natural killer cell lymphomas: production of cytolytic effectors and related proteins mediating tumor cell apoptosis? *Hum Pathol* 1997;28:1276–1282.
161. Jaffe ES, Chan JKC, Su IJ, et al. Report of the workshop in nasal and related extranodal angiocentric T/NK-cell lymphomas: definition, differential diagnosis and epidemiology. *Am J Surg Pathol* 1996;20:103–111.
162. Kern WF, Spier CM, Hanneman EH, et al. NCAM-positive peripheral T cell lymphoma: a rare variant with a propensity for unusual sites of involvement. *Blood* 1992;79:2432–2437.
163. Wong KF, Chan JKC, Ng CS, et al. CD56 (NKH1)-positive hematolymphoid malignancies: an aggressive neoplasm featuring frequent cutaneous/mucosal involvement, cytoplasmic azurophilic granules, and angiocentricity. *Hum Pathol* 1992;23:798–804.
164. Nakamura S, Suchi T, Koshikawa T, et al. Clinicopathologic study of CD56 (NCAM)-positive angiocentric lymphoma occurring in sites other than the upper and lower respiratory tract [see comments]. *Am J Surg Pathol* 1995;19:284–296.
165. Chan JKC, Sin VC, Wong KF, et al. Non-nasal lymphoma expressing the natural killer cell marker, CD56: a clinicopathologic study of 49 cases of an uncommon aggressive neoplasm. *Blood* 1997;89:4501–4513.
166. Ansai S, Maeda K, Yamakawa M, et al. CD56-positive (nasal-type T/NK cell) lymphoma arising on the skin: report of two cases and review of the literature. *J Cutan Pathol* 1997;24:468–476.
167. Kato N, Yasukawa K, Onozuka T, et al. Nasal and nasal-type T/NK cell lymphoma with cutaneous involvement. *J Am Acad Dermatol* 1999;40:850–856.
168. Jaffe ES, Krenacs L, Kumar S, et al. Extranodal peripheral T cell and NK-cell neoplasms. *Am J Clin Pathol* 1999;111[Suppl 1]:S46–55.
169. DiGiuseppe JA, Louie DC, Williams JE, et al. Blastic natural killer cell leukemia/lymphoma: a clinicopathologic study. *Am J Surg Pathol* 1997;21:1223–1230.
170. Liebow AA, Carrington CB, Friedman PJ. Lymphomatoid granulomatosis. *Hum Pathol* 1972;3:457–558.
171. Liebow AA, Carrington CB. Diffuse pulmonary lymphoreticular infiltrations associated with dysproteinemia. *Med Clin North Am* 1973;57:809–843.
172. Colby TV, Carrington CB. Pulmonary lymphomas simulating lymphomatoid granulomatosis. *Am J Surg Pathol* 1982;6:19–32.
173. Colby TV, Carrington CB. Pulmonary lymphomas: current concepts. *Hum Pathol* 1983;14:884–887.
174. Katzenstein AA, Carrington CB, Liebow AA. Lymphomatoid granulomatosis. A clinicopathologic study of 152 cases. *Cancer* 1979;43:360–373.
175. Katzenstein AA, Peiper SC. Detection of Epstein-Barr virus genome in lymphomatoid granulomatosis: analysis of 29 cases by the polymerase chain reaction technique. *Mod Pathol* 1990;3:435–442.
176. Guinee DJN, Jaffe E, Kingma D, et al. Pulmonary lymphomatoid granulomatosis. Evidence for a proliferation of Epstein-Barr virus infected B-lymphocytes with a prominent T-cell component and vasculitis. *Am J Surg Pathol* 1994;18:753–764.
177. Myers JL, Kurtin JP, Katzenstein AL, et al. Lymphomatoid granulomatosis. Evidence of immunophenotypic diversity and relationship to Epstein-Barr virus infection. *Am J Surg Pathol* 1995;19:1300–1312.
178. Jaffe ES, Wilson WH. Lymphomatoid granulomatosis: pathogenesis, pathology and clinical implications. *Cancer Surv* 1997;30:233–248.
179. Guinee DG, Perkins SL, Travis WD, et al. Proliferation and cellular phenotype in lymphomatoid granulomatosis. *Am J Surg Pathol* 1998;22:1093–1100.
180. Macon WR, Williams ME, Greer JP, et al. Natural killer-like T cell lymphomas: aggressive lymphomas of T large granular lymphocytes. *Blood* 1996;87:1474–1483.
181. Gentile TC, Uner AH, Hutchinson RE, et al. CD3+ CD56+ aggressive variant of large granular lymphocyte leukemia. *Blood* 1994;84:2315–2321.
182. Isaacson PG, Wright DH. Intestinal lymphoma associated with malabsorption. *Lancet* 1978;1:67–70.
183. Isaacson PG, O'Connor NT, Spencer J, et al. Malignant histiocytosis of the intestine: a T cell lymphoma. *Ann Intern Med* 1985;104:44–47.
184. Murray A, Cuevas EC, Jones DB, et al. Study of the immunohistochemistry and T cell clonality of enteropathy-associated T cell lymphoma. *Am J Pathol* 1995;146:509–519.
185. Isaacson PG. Gastrointestinal lymphomas of T- and B-cell types. *Mod Pathol* 1999;12:151–158.
186. Ashton-Key M, Diss TC, Pan L, et al. Molecular analysis of T cell clonality in ulcerative jejunitis and enteropathy-associated T cell lymphoma. *Am J Pathol* 1997;151:493–498.
187. Lavergne A, Brocheriou I, Delfau MH, et al. Primary intestinal gamma-delta T cell lymphoma with evidence of Epstein-Barr virus. *Histopathology* 1998;32:271–276.

188. Tsujikawa T, Itoh A, Bamba M, et al. Aggressive jejunal gamma delta T cell lymphoma derived from intraepithelial lymphocytes: an autopsy case report. *J Gastroenterol* 1998;33:280–284.
189. Macon WR, Levy NB, Casey TT, et al. Hepatosplenic $\alpha\beta$ T-cell lymphomas: a report of four cases with features similar to hepatosplenic $\gamma\delta$ T-cell lymphomas. *Mod Pathol* 1998;11:135A(abst).
190. Francois A, Lesesve JF, Stamatoullas A, et al. Hepatosplenic gamma/delta T cell lymphoma: a report of two cases in immunocompromised patients, associated with isochromosome 7q. *Am J Surg Pathol* 1997; 21:781–790.
191. Ozaki S, Ogasahara K, Kosaka M, et al. Hepatosplenic gamma delta T-cell lymphoma associated with hepatitis B virus infection. *J Med Invest* 1998;44:215–217.
192. Wang CC, Tien HF, Lin MT, et al. Consistent presence of isochromosome 7q in hepatosplenic T-$\gamma\delta$ lymphoma: a new cytogenetic-clinicopathologic entity. *Genes Chromosomes Cancer* 1995;12:161–164.
193. Jonveaux P, Daniel MT, Martel V, et al. Isochromosome 7q and trisomy 8 are consistent primary, nonrandom, chromosomal abnormalities associated with hepatosplenic T-$\gamma\delta$ lymphoma. *Leukemia* 1996; 10:1453–1455.
194. Alonsozana EL, Stamberg J, Kumar D, et al. Isochromosome 7q: the primary cytogenetic abnormality in hepatosplenic gamma-delta T cell lymphoma [Letter]. *Leukemia* 1997;11:1367–1372.
195. Salhany KE, Feldman M, Kahn, MJ, et al. Hepatosplenic gamma/delta T cell lymphoma: ultrastructural, immunophenotypic and functional evidence for cytotoxic T lymphocyte differentiation. *Hum Pathol* 1997;26:674–685.
196. Kagami Y, Nakamura S, Suzuki R, et al. A nodal gamma/delta T cell lymphoma with an association of Epstein-Barr virus. *Am J Surg Pathol* 1997;21:729–736.
197. Arnulf B, Copic-Bergman C, Delfau-Larue MH, et al. Nonhepatosplenic gamma-delta T cell lymphoma: a subset of cytotoxic lymphomas with mucosal or skin localization. *Blood* 1998;91:1723–1731.
198. Yamaguchi M, Ohno T, Nakamine H, et al. Gamma-Delta T cell lymphoma: a clinicopathologic study of 6 cases, including extrahepatosplenic type. *Int J Hematol* 1999;69:186–195.
199. Ng CS, Chan JKC, Lo STH. Expression of natural killer cell markers in non-Hodgkin's lymphomas. *Hum Pathol* 1987;18:1257–1262.
200. Wieczorek R, Suhrland M, Ramsay D, et al. Leu-M1 antigens in advanced (tumor) stage mycosis fungoides. *Am J Clin Pathol* 1986; 86:25–32.
201. Kurtin PJ, Pinkus GS. Leukocyte common antigen: a diagnostic discriminant between hematopoietic and nonhematopoietic neoplasms in paraffin sections using monoclonal antibodies. *Hum Pathol* 1985;16: 353–365.
202. Norton AJ, Ramsay AD, Smith SH. Monoclonal antibody (UCHL-1) that recognizes normal and neoplastic T cells in routinely fixed tissues. *J Clin Pathol* 1986;39:399–405.
203. Strickler JG, Weiss LM, Copenhaver CM, et al. Monoclonal antibodies reactive in routinely processed tissue sections of malignant lymphoma, with emphasis on T cell lymphomas. *Hum Pathol* 1987;18: 808–814.
204. Linder J, Ye Y, Harrington DS, et al. Monoclonal antibodies marking T lymphocytes in paraffin-embedded tissue. *Am J Pathol* 1987;127: 1–8.
205. Wieczorek R, Buck D, Bindl J, et al. Monoclonal antibody Leu-22 [L60] permits the demonstration of some neoplastic T cells in routinely fixed and paraffin-embedded tissue sections. *Hum Pathol* 1988; 19:1434–1443.
206. Said JW, Stoll PN, Shintaku P, et al. Leu-22: a preferential marker for T lymphocytes in paraffin sections. *Am J Clin Pathol* 1989;91: 542–549.
207. Chan JKC, Tsang WYW, Ng CS, et al. Discordant CD3 expression in lymphomas as studied in frozen and paraffin sections. *Hum Pathol* 1995;26:1139–1143.
208. Mason DY, Cordell J, Brown M, et al. Detection of T cells in paraffin wax-embedded tissue using antibodies against a peptide sequence from the CD3 antigen. *J Clin Pathol* 1989;42:1194–2000.
209. Chadburn A, Knowles DM. Paraffin-resistant antigens detectable by antibodies L26 and polyclonal CD3 predict the B- or T-cell lineage of 95% of diffuse, aggressive, non-Hodgkin's lymphomas. *Am J Clin Pathol* 1994;102:284–291.
210. Tsang WYW, Chan JKC, Ng CS, et al. Utility of a paraffin section-reactive CD56 antibody (123C3) for characterization and diagnosis of lymphomas. *Am J Surg Pathol* 1996;20:202–210.
211. Ott G, Katzenberger T, Siebert R, et al. Chromosomal abnormalities in nodal and extranodal $CD30^+$ anaplastic large cell lymphomas: infrequent detection of the t(2;5) in extranodal lymphomas. *Genes Chromosomes Cancer* 1998;22:114–121.
212. Mitev L, Christova S, Hadjiev E, et al. A new variant chromosomal translocation t(2;2)(p23;q23) in $CD30^+$/Ki-1^+ anaplastic large cell lymphoma. *Leuk Lymphoma* 1998;28:613–616.
213. Ho JW, Ho FC, Chan AC, et al. Frequent detection of Epstein-Barr virus-infected B cells in peripheral T cell lymphomas. *J Pathol* 1998; 185:79–85.
214. Knowles DM, Pelicci P-G, Dalla-Favera R. T cell receptor beta chain gene rearrangements: genetic markers of T cell lineage and clonality. *Hum Pathol* 1986;17:546–551.
215. Cossman J, Uppenkamp M, Sundeen J, et al. Molecular genetics and the diagnosis of lymphoma. *Arch Pathol Lab Med* 1988;112:117–127.
216. Korsmeyer SJ. Antigen receptor genes as molecular markers of lymphoid neoplasms. *J Clin Invest* 1987;79:1291–1295.
217. Griesser H, Tkachuk D, Reis MD, et al. Gene rearrangements and translocations in lymphoproliferative diseases. *Blood* 1989;73: 1402–1415.
218. Davey MP, Bongiovanni KF, Kaulfersch W, et al. Immunoglobulin and T cell receptor gene rearrangement and expression in human lymphoid leukemia cells at different stages of maturation. *Proc Natl Acad Sci USA* 1986;83:8759–8763.
219. Tkachuk D, Griesser H, Takihara Y, et al. Rearrangement of the T cell delta locus in lymphoproliferative disorders. *Blood* 1988;72:353–357.
220. Griesser H, Champagne E, Tkachuk D, et al. The human T cell receptor alpha-delta locus: a physical map of the variable, joining, and constant region genes. *Eur J Immunol* 1988;18:641–644.
221. Flug F, Pelicci PG, Bonetti F, et al. T cell receptor gene rearrangements as markers of lineage and clonality in T cell neoplasms. *Proc Natl Acad Sci USA* 1985;82:3460–3464.
222. Dyer MJS. T cell receptor delta-alpha rearrangements in lymphoid neoplasms. *Blood* 1989;74:1073–1083.
223. Weiss LM, Picker LJ, Grogan TM, et al. Absence of clonal beta and gamma T cell receptor gene rearrangements in a subset of peripheral T cell lymphomas. *Am J Pathol* 1988;130:436–442.
224. Jones C, Morse HG, Kao F-T, et al. Human T cell receptor alpha-chain genes: location on chromosome 14. *Science* 1985;228:83–85.
225. Isobe M, Erikson J, Emanuel BS, et al. Location of gene for beta subunit in human T cell receptor at band 7q35, a region prone to rearrangements in T cells. *Science* 1985;228:580–582.
226. Erikson J, Williams DL, Finan J, et al. Locus of the alpha-chain of the T cell receptor is split by chromosome translocation in T cell leukemia. *Science* 1985;229:784–786.
227. Hayashi Y, Fukayama M, Funata N, et al. Polymerase chain reaction screening of immunoglobulin heavy chain and T cell receptor gamma gene rearrangements: a practical approach to molecular DNA analysis of non-Hodgkin's lymphoma in a surgical pathology laboratory. *Pathol Int* 1999;49:110–117.
228. Bergman R. How useful are T cell receptor gene rearrangement studies as an adjunct to the histopathologic diagnosis of mycosis fungoides? *Am J Dermatopathol* 1999;21:498–502.
229. Signoretti S, Murphy M, Cangi MG, et al. Detection of clonal T cell receptor gamma gene rearrangements in paraffin embedded tissue by polymerase chain reaction and nonradioactive single-strand conformational polymorphism analysis. *Am J Pathol* 1999;154:67–75.

CHAPTER 30

Nonhematopoietic Elements in Lymph Nodes

Robert A. Soslow and Daniel M. Knowles

The pathologist is frequently asked to evaluate a lymph node biopsy specimen to determine the presence of any one of a wide spectrum of benign and malignant lymphoid proliferations that commonly involve lymph nodes. Various nonhematopoietic elements and nonlymphoid hematopoietic proliferations may be encountered in lymph nodes, and some of them may mimic benign or malignant lymphoid proliferations to an extraordinary degree.

Nonhematopoietic elements that occur in lymph nodes may be benign or malignant. The benign elements include a variety of congenital malformations and inclusions that may be misinterpreted as malignant neoplasms metastatic to lymph nodes. Rarely, a nonhematopoietic neoplasm may even originate from these ectopic elements, giving rise to a nonhematopoietic neoplasm primary in a lymph node. Malignant nonhematopoietic proliferations that involve lymph nodes include a large number of epithelial and mesenchymal proliferations that may mimic malignant lymphoma. Several nonlymphoid hematopoietic processes (e.g., granulocytic sarcoma, mast cell disease) may occur in lymph nodes and be mistaken for malignant lymphoma.

The recognition and correct interpretation of these nonhematopoietic elements and nonlymphoid hematopoietic proliferations often carry considerable clinical significance. The proper management, treatment, and prognosis of the patient may depend entirely on the pathologist's diagnosis. Fortunately, in recent years, the sometimes difficult pathologic differential diagnosis caused by these lesions has been aided by the application of frozen and paraffin tissue section immunohistochemistry that uses panels of polyclonal and monoclonal antibodies whose reactivity patterns characterize specific clinicopathologic entities.

In this chapter, we describe the morphologic features of the nonhematopoietic developmental ectopias and the benign and malignant nonhematopoietic and nonlymphoid hematopoietic proliferations that involve lymph nodes, and we discuss their differential diagnosis with lymphoid proliferations, including the contribution of immunohistochemistry (Table 30.1).

R. A. Soslow and D. M. Knowles: Department of Pathology, Weill Medical College of Cornell University, New York, New York 10021

APPROACH TO DIAGNOSIS

A variety of clinical and morphologic clues may enable the pathologist to distinguish benign and malignant nonhematolymphoid elements from hematolymphoid proliferations and to categorize further the nonhematolymphoid neoplasms. However, the histopathologic features of malignant lymphomas and nonlymphoid neoplasms occasionally overlap. When confronted with the difficult histopathologic differential diagnosis of a poorly differentiated malignant neoplasm of unknown origin compared with malignant lymphoma, multiple sections should be obtained to ensure that areas of specific cellular differentiation (i.e., squamous, glandular, and melanocytic) can be demonstrated. Histochemical stains can be performed for reticulin fibers, mucin, glycoprotein, glycogen, melanin, and endocrine granules (1). Even these approaches still leave many diagnostic dilemmas unresolved, however.

Electron Microscopy

In the past, ultrastructural studies were used frequently and widely to classify neoplasms that could not be identified by light microscopy. For example, the presence of desmosomal junctions and tonofilaments was taken to indicate a squamous epithelial origin, well-developed cell junctions and microvilli to indicate glandular derivation, melanosomes or premelanosomes to indicate a melanocytic proliferation, neurosecretory granules to indicate a neuroendocrine tumor such as neuroblastoma, and actin-myosin complexes to indicate rhabdomyosarcoma (1). Malignant lymphomas do not possess distinctive ultrastructural features (1). Moreover, many undifferentiated neoplasms cannot be classified on the

TABLE 30.1. *Nonhematopoietic elements in lymph nodes*

Congenital malformations and inclusions
Ectopic nevus cells
Ectopic mesothelial cells
Ectopic mullerian and celomic epithelium
Ectopic salivary gland
Ectopic thyroid gland
Ectopic breast and sweat gland tissue
Epithelial lesions primary in lymph nodes
Malignant melanoma
Lymphoepithelial lesion
Warthin's tumor
Acinic cell and mucoepidermoid carcinoma
Thyroid carcinoma
Breast carcinoma
Mesenchymal lesions primary in lymph nodes
Lipomatosis of lymph nodes
Fibrosis of lymph nodes
Vascular transformation
Nodal angiomatosis
Angiomyomatous hamartoma
Angiolipomatous hamartoma
Hemangioma
Vascular neoplasm of Castleman's disease
Lymphangioma
Lymphangiomyomatosis
Lymphangioleiomyomatosis
Epithelioid hemangioendothelioma
Kaposi's sarcoma
Angiomyolipoma
Bacillary angiomatosis
Inflammatory pseudotumor of lymph node
Palisaded myofibroblastoma
Mycobacterial spindle cell pseudotumor
Leiomyomatosis
Deciduosis
Other sarcomas
Metastatic neoplasms in lymph nodes
Poorly differentiated carcinomas
Undifferentiated nasopharyngeal carcinoma
Poorly differentiated neuroendocrine carcinoma
Mammary lobular carcinoma
Signet ring cell lesions
Other poorly differentiated carcinomas
Differentiated adenocarcinomas
Malignant melanoma
Germ cell tumors
Small round cell sarcomas
Ewing's sarcoma
Primitive neuroectodermal tumor
Rhabdomyosarcoma
Desmoplastic small round cell tumor
Synovial sarcoma and epithelioid sarcoma
Clear cell sarcoma
Metastatic sarcoma with glandular differentiation
Nonlymphoid hematopoietic disorders that mimic malignant lymphoma
Extramedullary myeloid tumor (granulocytic sarcoma)
Mast cell disease
Dendritic cell neoplasms

basis of electron microscopic examination (1). These factors, in addition to the requirement for costly facilities, specially trained personnel, and the large amount of time necessary to actually perform ultrastructural studies, render them neither practical nor cost effective in routine diagnosis. Such studies are now almost exclusively reserved for research.

Immunohistochemistry

Immunohistochemistry has become the principal method employed by pathologists to resolve difficult histopathologic dilemmas in the diagnosis and classification of neoplasms. Immunohistochemistry obviates all the disadvantages of electron microscopy. Extensive panels of well-characterized polyclonal and monoclonal antibodies that recognize a wide range of surface membrane and cytoplasmic structural proteins and cellular products are now available commercially. Nearly every major category of malignant neoplasia, including the most undifferentiated tumors, exhibits a constellation of immunohistochemical markers that permits diagnosis and classification (2,3) (Table 30.2). The malignant lymphomas express specific markers that readily permit their separation from the large variety of epithelial and other neoplasms that may simulate them (see Chapter 3). Moreover, this technology does not require costly or extensive facilities or specially trained and skilled laboratory personnel. The technical protocols must be followed carefully and the actual procedures must be performed meticulously. In general, however, the techniques are easy to teach to even inexperienced personnel. Most assays can be performed on routinely prepared paraffin tissue sections, are relatively inexpensive to perform, and can be completed within a few hours (4).

Whenever possible, the pathologic material subjected to immunostaining should be collected, stored, and processed under optimal conditions. Standard formalin fixation and paraffin embedding are the optimum methods of handling tissue to demonstrate most antigens in routine diagnostic pathology. However, certain antigens expressed by hematolymphoid neoplasms are still best detected in unfixed tissue (see Chapter 3). Fresh tissue can be used for ancillary cytogenetic and molecular diagnostic procedures. Ideally, in the case of all pathologic specimens of neoplasms but especially those that may require immunohistochemical examination, the specimens should be collected fresh and unfixed and some representative portions should be snap frozen and cryopreserved while other representative portions should be fixed and processed in the usual manner. This approach permits reliable immunohistochemical demonstration of the greatest range of antigenic markers.

A number of important factors must be considered in the performance and interpretation of immunohistochemical staining of human neoplasms in routine diagnosis. These are discussed in Chapter 4. Some of these factors, such as antigen retrieval, decalcification, and controls, deserve brief mention here. Antigen retrieval usually improves and, in some instances, may be necessary to demonstrate certain

TABLE 30.2. *Immunohistochemical staining profiles of neoplasms*

Stain	Non-Hodgkin's lymphoma	Carcinoma	Neuro-endocrine carcinoma	Malignant melanoma	Germ cell tumor	ES/PNET	Rhabdomyo-sarcoma	Sarcomas with epithelial differentiation
CD45	+	–	–	–	–	–	–	–
Cytokeratin	–	+	+	–	+/–	–	–	+
EMA	–/+	+	+	–	+/–	–	–	+
S-100	–	–/+	–	+	–	–/+	–	–/+
Chromogranin/ synaptophysin	–	–/+	+	–	–	+/–	–	–
CD99	–/+	–	–/+	–	–	+	–/+	–/+
HMB-45	–	–	+/–	–	–	–	–	–
AFP/PLAP	–	–	–	–	+/–	–	–	–
Desmin/(smooth muscle) actin	–	–	–	–	–	–	+	–
CD34	–/+	–	–	–	–	–	–	–/+

ES, Ewing's sarcoma; PNET, primitive neuroectodermal tumor.

antigens immunohistochemically in routinely prepared paraffin tissue sections. Because tissue fixation often results in rendering antigen domains (epitopes) inaccessible to antibody, antigen retrieval techniques can be useful in unmasking the antigen of interest. A variety of antigen retrieval techniques have been found to be helpful. These include heat, delivered by microwave, oven, or hot plate; heat and pressure, delivered by a pressure cooker; and partial proteolysis, using an enzyme such as trypsin (5,6). We hesitate to endorse any one system because optimal retrieval techniques depend on the specifics of fixation, antibody clones and dilution, and immunohistochemical protocols, all of which vary significantly from laboratory to laboratory. The antigen retrieval techniques must be monitored carefully, each antibody must be evaluated carefully to determine if pretreatment is beneficial or detrimental, and appropriate retrieval and nonretrieval controls must be used. Similarly, when dealing with neoplasms that have undergone decalcification, the potential loss of immunoreactivity should be kept in mind and appropriate controls that have been processed in an identical manner should be used. The specificity and sensitivity of all immunohistochemical studies must always be monitored carefully with the use of appropriate positive and negative controls.

The demonstration of a single antigenic marker should never be relied on to determine the histogenesis of a particular neoplasm or to make a definitive diagnosis. A carefully selected panel of antibody reagents that reflects positive and negative staining results of entities in the differential diagnosis should be used. This maximizes the specificity of the immunodiagnosis and minimizes the possibility of diagnostic error.

For example, one may arrive at a diagnosis of anaplastic large cell lymphoma after obtaining immunohistochemical reactivity with antibodies against epithelial membrane antigen and leukocyte common antigen, but not cytokeratin. Similarly, mesothelioma is characterized by the expression of cytokeratins and epithelial membrane antigen in the absence of monoclonal carcinoembryonic antigen (mCEA). Interpretation of immunophenotypic data should also include attention to the intensity and distribution of immune reactivity and the morphology of the immunoreactive cells. For example, mCEA positivity is commonly found in neutrophils (7), which does not have a bearing on the immunophenotype of the neoplasm in question. Paranuclear cytoplasmic ''dot'' positivity is characteristic of anti-cytokeratin antibodies in neuroendocrine tumors (8) (Fig. 30.1). Rare cytokeratin-positive cells may indicate epithelial differentiation in the appropriate setting, but only strong and diffuse nuclear

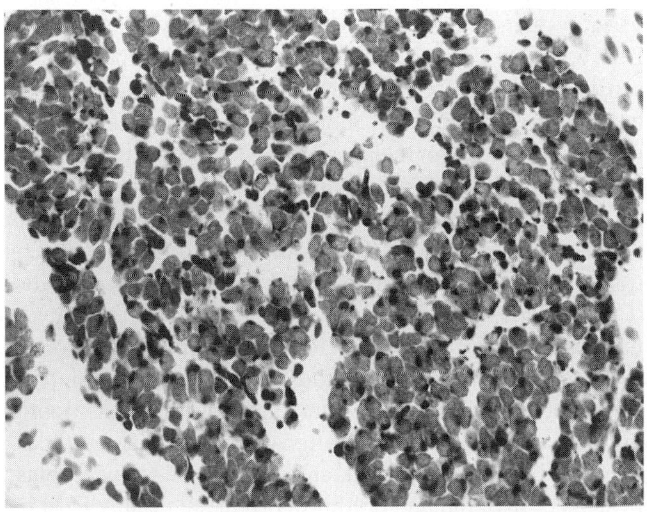

FIG. 30.1. Metastatic neuroendocrine carcinoma immunostained with the cell adhesion molecule (CAM) 5.2 monoclonal anti-cytokeratin antibody. Note the prominent perinuclear "dot" reactivity, a finding that is characteristic, but not necessarily indicative, of neuroendocrine neoplasms (immunoperoxidase stain, original magnification: 400× magnification). (Photomicrograph courtesy of Dr. Ronald DeLellis, Weill Medical College of Cornell University, New York, NY).

and cytoplasmic S-100 protein expression permits the identification of melanocytic differentiation (9). The results of immunohistochemical studies should be used as an adjunct to histopathologic diagnosis; all diagnostic conclusions should be based on correlation of the immunohistochemical findings with careful examination of the histopathologic sections.

For the initial evaluation of neoplasms that appear undifferentiated on routine hematoxylin and eosin sections we recommend an antibody panel capable of identifying the following antigens: leukocyte common antigen (CD45), cytokeratins (i.e., CAM 5.2, AE1/AE3, or both), and S-100 protein. In most cases, this antibody panel permits distinction among malignant lymphoma, carcinoma, and malignant melanoma (10). However, uniformly negative or unanticipated results should prompt the use of relevant ''backup'' antibodies, which is discussed in the context of the lesions discussed later in this chapter.

A brief discussion of the antigens recognized by the most commonly employed antibodies follows. These antigens represent an abbreviated list; Table 30.2 and the discussion of individual lesions provide a more comprehensive treatment of other important antigens and antibodies.

Leukocyte Common Antigen

Leukocyte common antigen (LCA, CD45) represents a family of surface membrane glycoproteins, ranging in size from 180 to 240 kd, that are found on all hematopoietic cells except erythrocytes and their precursors (11). Six to eight isoforms of LCA are expressed differentially on leukocyte subpopulations (11); B and T lymphocytes express LCA strongly whereas macrophages and histiocytes express LCA variably and neutrophils express LCA very weakly (11). Leukocyte common antigen is a remarkably specific and sensitive marker for hematopoietic neoplasms and should be used in evaluating all morphologically undifferentiated neoplasms to rule out the possibility of malignant lymphoma (12–16). The neoplastic cells that comprise most B- and T-cell non-Hodgkin's lymphomas and lymphoid leukemias express LCA (CD45) (12–16) (Fig. 30.2). Notable exceptions are immunoblastic lymphomas, CD30 positive ($CD30^+$) anaplastic large cell lymphomas, and plasmacytomas, which may be $CD45^-$ (17–19). All nonhematopoietic neoplasms, including those most commonly mistaken for hematopoietic neoplasms histopathologically, i.e., poorly differentiated carcinomas, malignant melanoma, neuroblastoma, and Ewing's sarcoma, are $CD45^-$ (12–16). Neoplastic cells of myeloid and erythroid origin are usually $CD45^-$ as well (11) (see Chapter 3).

Cytokeratins

Cytokeratins are the cytoskeletal intermediate filament proteins characteristic of almost all epithelial cells (20,21). There are at least 19 distinct keratin subsets that are divisible into two families: A (acidic) or B (basic), according to their molecular weights and isoelectric points (20). Low-molecular-weight keratins are typical of simple, nonstratified epithelia. High-molecular-weight keratins are found in stratified epithelia whose keratin composition is more complex (20,21). Malignant lymphomas almost never contain keratins (22). In contrast, virtually all carcinomas, except adrenal cortical carcinomas, regularly contain keratins (20). Biphasic tumors, such as synovial sarcomas and epithelioid sarcomas, also show immunoreactivity for keratins, but this is usually limited to the glandular elements, although the spindle cell component occasionally may express keratin (20,23). Fifty percent to 100% of leiomyosarcomas have been claimed to contain tumor cells that express cytokeratin as well (24–26). The exact nature of this finding is not well understood, but normal myometrium has been shown to contain keratin (27). Several other sarcomas (i.e., Ewing's sarcoma, rhabdomyosarcoma, and malignant fibrous histiocytoma) and malignant melanomas rarely have been reported to express cytokeratins (20,28,29). Although most adenocarcinomas do not demonstrate specific immunophenotypes, the use of antibodies against cytokeratins 7 and 20 permit separation into groups used to narrow the differential diagnosis (30).

Epithelial Membrane Antigen

Epithelial membrane antigen (EMA) is the name given to the incompletely characterized glycoprotein of apocrine cells. Epithelial membrane antigen is located in the milk fat globules, where it originally was identified with an antiserum (31,32), hence, it has been also called milk fat globule protein (31). For the most part, monoclonal antibodies are now used to demonstrate EMA, which is found on almost all benign and malignant epithelial cells (31,33,34); however, EMA is not specific for epithelial neoplasms, and it can be found in mesotheliomas (35), synovial sarcomas (36), leiomyosarcomas (26), perineural epithelium and their neoplasms (37), plasma cells and plasmacytoid neoplasms (38), meningiomas (36), and $CD30^+$ anaplastic large cell lymphomas (39) (Fig. 30.3). The frequent expression of EMA and lack of LCA by anaplastic large cell lymphomas probably accounts for their occasional misdiagnosis as poorly differentiated carcinomas or other nonhematopoietic neoplasms.

Vimentin

Vimentin is a cytoskeletal intermediate filament protein with a molecular mass of 57,000 daltons (40). Vimentin is present in mesenchymal cells, fibroblasts, endothelial cells, chondrocytes, histiocytes, lymphocytes, melanocytes, many glial cells, and some smooth muscle cells, especially vascular smooth muscle (20). It has been used as a general marker for sarcomas (20). Many poorly differentiated carcinomas, especially those of renal, thyroid, and endometrial origin,

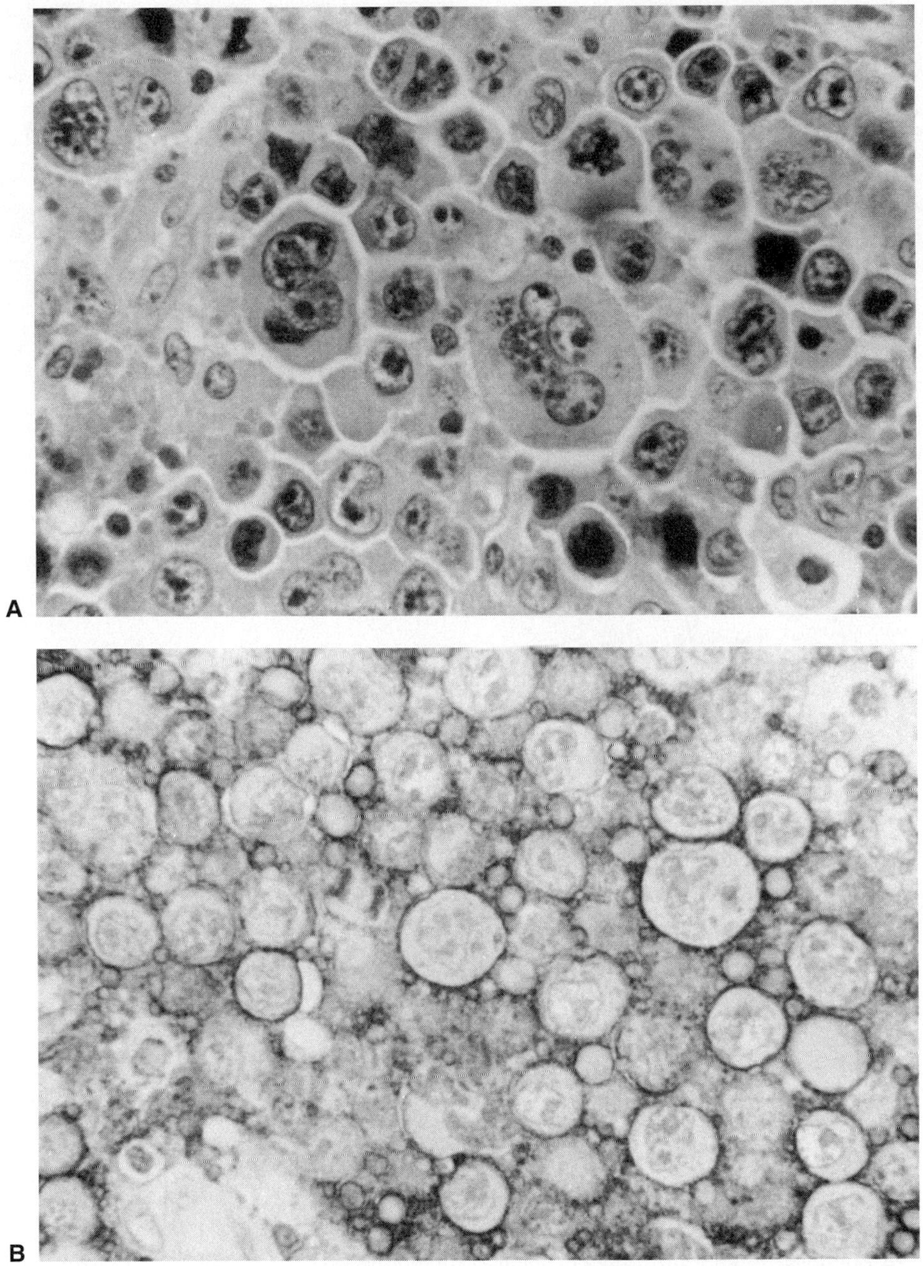

FIG. 30.2. Pleomorphic immunoblastic large cell non-Hodgkin's lymphoma. **A:** This pleomorphic tumor was considered possibly to represent an undifferentiated carcinoma or undifferentiated sarcoma on initial examination by the reviewing pathologist (hematoxylin and eosin, original magnification: 630× magnification). **B:** Immunostaining performed in paraffin tissue sections demonstrates that the pleomorphic tumor cells express CD45 (i.e., leukocyte common antigen), consistent with a hematopoietic neoplasm. Additional immunophenotypic and genotypic studies demonstrated that this tumor represents a B-cell non-Hodgkin's lymphoma (immunoperoxidase stain, original magnification: 400× magnification).

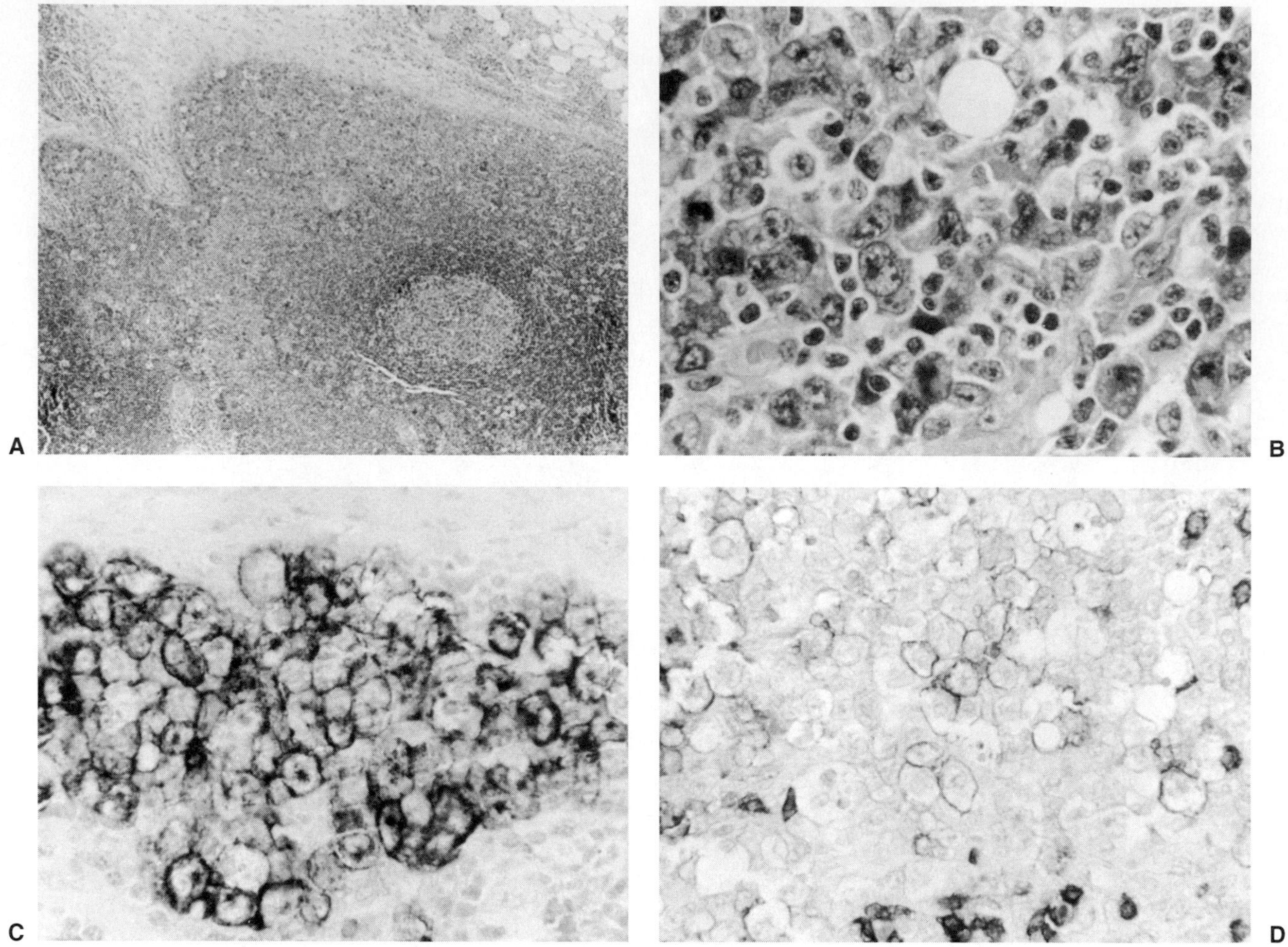

FIG. 30.3. CD30-positive anaplastic large cell lymphoma. This category of non-Hodgkin's lymphoma frequently exhibits the growth pattern and cellular characteristics of epithelial neoplasms. **A:** The neoplastic cells show a marked predilection for sinusoidal infiltration, hence mimicking metastatic carcinoma (hematoxylin and eosin, original magnification: 40× magnification). **B:** The neoplastic cells exhibit considerable pleomorphism and often contain large, bizarre nuclei surrounded by abundant cytoplasm. Binucleate and multinucleate cells are sometimes present. Mitotic figures are numerous. Once again, these cytologic features, in conjunction with the sinusoidal growth pattern, are often mistaken for metastatic carcinoma (hematoxylin and eosin, original magnification: 400× magnification). **C:** Immunoperoxidase staining of paraffin tissue sections demonstrates that these large neoplastic cells strongly express epithelial membrane antigen. Approximately 75% of CD30-positive anaplastic large cell lymphomas, however, are epithelial membrane antigen positive (immunoperoxidase stain, original magnification: 250× magnification). **D:** Additional immunostaining demonstrates that these neoplastic cells express T cell-associated antigen CD43 on immunostaining of paraffin tissue sections with monoclonal antibody Leu22 (immunoperoxidase stain, original magnification: 250× magnification).

and malignant melanomas and lymphomas also express vimentin (20,41). Its utility in the differential diagnosis of human neoplasms is very limited.

Desmin- and Muscle-Associated Antigens

Desmin is a muscle cell type of intermediate filament protein with a molecular mass of 53,000 daltons, which is believed to link myofilaments together (42). Desmin is almost always expressed by smooth muscle cells and skeletal and cardiac muscle cells and their neoplastic counterparts (43). Numerous other tumors also have been reported to be desmin positive, including liposarcomas, Schwann cell tumors, desmoplastic melanoma, fibromatosis, and malignant fibrous histiocytomas (43,44). Desmin positivity also has been described in squamous and small cell carcinomas and small cell carcinomas of the lung in frozen section material (43). Malignant lymphomas are desmin negative.

Actins that measure 6 nm in diameter are found in all cell types (45). α-Actins are present in muscle cells, β-actins are present in nonmuscle cells, and γ-actins are found in muscle and in some nonmuscle cells (45,46). The HHF-35 antibody to muscle actin selectively reacts with the α- and γ-actins of muscle cells and immunoreacts with all striated muscle cells as does desmin. It also reacts with all smooth muscle cells, including the desmin negative subsets of vascular smooth muscle cells (47,48). Pericytes and myoepithelial cells of salivary gland, skin, and breast are also HHF-35$^+$, although they do not contain desmin (48). In general, myofibroblasts are desmin negative but positive for HHF-35 (48). Muscle actins are typically found in leiomyosarcomas, rhabdomyosarcomas, and benign mixed tumors of salivary gland and skin adnexal origin (46,48).

Factor VIII– and Endothelial-Associated Antigens

Factor VIII–related antigen (factor VIIIRAg), also called von Willebrand's factor, is part of the factor VIII complex of the clotting system and is produced by vascular endothelial cells (49). Factor VIII–related antigen is a very specific marker for endothelial cells and vascular neoplasms of endothelial cell origin (50). It is helpful for distinguishing angiosarcoma and occasionally Kaposi's sarcoma (KS) from other pleomorphic and spindle cell tumors of nonendothelial cell origin, for example, fibrosarcomas, leiomyosarcomas, and malignant fibrous histiocytomas (51,52). Factor VIII–related antigen is consistently expressed by well differentiated angiosarcomas that possess vasoformative papillary patterns. Less well differentiated solid tumors are weakly or not at all immunoreactive for factor VIIIRAg (52); therefore, factor VIIIRAg is not a very sensitive marker for endothelial cells (50).

In contrast, CD31, also known as platelet/endothelial cell adhesion molecule-1 (PECAM-1), is a very useful marker because it is extremely sensitive for endothelial differentiation. It is expressed in the lateral borders between endothelial cells, on platelets, neutrophils, monocytes and subpopulations of T cells (53). Although it is not entirely specific for endothelial differentiation, it is only rarely expressed in neoplasms that resemble those with endothelial properties.

Antibodies against CD34, a transmembrane cell surface glycoprotein, are also useful in the identification of endothelial differentiation (54). However, the utility of this antibody is limited by its very broad range of reactivity. In addition to endothelial cells, anti-CD34 antibodies recognize hematopoietic stem cells, immature thymocytes, a subpopulation of blasts in acute lymphoblastic and myeloid leukemias, interstitial dendritic cells and numerous spindle cell proliferations and neoplasms (54,55) (see Chapter 3).

S-100 Protein

S-100 protein is a calcium-binding protein of unknown function that originally was described in bovine brain extract and is 100% soluble in neutral ammonium sulfate (56), hence, its name. The S-100 protein is present in glial cells, Schwann cells, melanocytes, epidermal Langerhans cells, interdigitating dendritic cells, chondrocytes, adipocytes, and myoepithelial cells (57). Schwann cell tumors, granular cell tumors, benign and malignant melanocytic proliferations, salivary gland myoepitheliomas, cartilaginous tumors, lipomatous tumors, and Langerhans cell histiocytosis (histiocytosis X) all are S-100 protein positive (57–62). Many carcinomas are also S-100$^+$ (63,64). The sustentacular or supportive cells in pheochromocytomas, ganglioneuroblastomas, and paragangliomas are S-100$^+$, but the predominant neural component of these tumors is S-100$^-$ (65). The text discusses the use of monoclonal antibodies HMB-45 and A103, which are more specific but less sensitive for melanocytic differentiation.

Neuron-Specific Enolase and Neuroendocrine/Neural-Associated Antigens

Neuron-specific enolase (NSE) designates the γ subunit of the dimeric enzyme enolase typical of neural cells (66) Initial studies suggested a high cell type specificity for NSE (66), hence the name. Later studies on a wide spectrum of tumors, however, revealed NSE positivity in numerous nonneural and nonneuroendocrine tumors (67), limiting its use in diagnostic pathology. In general, NSE should be used in conjunction with more specific neural/neuroendocrine markers such as chromogranin, synaptophysin, nerve growth factor receptor protein, and neurofilament proteins. Synaptophysin is a protein found in the membranes of neuronal cell vesicles (68). It is present in peripheral nerves, in central and peripheral nervous system neurons, and in neuroendocrine cells (68). Synaptophysin is consistently positive in neuroendocrine tumors, paragangliomas, and neuroblastomas (68). Nerve growth factor receptor is consistently positive in Schwann cell neoplasms, although some nonneural tumors have been reported to be positive; these include synovial sarcomas and hemangiopericytomas (69).

CONGENITAL MALFORMATIONS AND INCLUSIONS

Ectopic Nevus Cells

Not uncommonly, nevus cell aggregates occur in peripheral lymph nodes, most often those in the axillary region, and less frequently in the cervical and inguinal regions (70–73). The overall incidence of benign nevus cell aggregates has ranged from 0.33% to 6.2% in patients who have undergone axillary lymph node dissections for breast carcinoma or malignant melanoma (70,71). Benign nevus cell aggregates have been encountered in about 3% of patients who have malignant melanoma and who have had regional lymph node dissections (70).

In 1977, Azzopardi and colleagues (72) described the occurrence of blue nevi in lymph nodes. About 10 cases have been reported; they occur in both sexes and most commonly involve axillary lymph nodes (72,73). Intranodal blue nevi, in contrast to ectopic nevus cell aggregates, have not been identified in patients who have cutaneous malignant melanoma. Intranodal nevus cell aggregates and blue nevi morphologically resemble their dermal counterparts, intradermal nevi and common blue nevi, respectively. Both lesions are discovered incidentally in peripheral lymph nodes, where they occur in the capsular and pericapsular tissues (72,73) (Fig. 30.4). Ectopic nevus cells are only rarely encountered within the substance of a lymph node. The presence of cells thought to be benign nevus cells within a lymph node should lead to careful study of the cell population. Some malignant melanoma cells show only slight atypia and few mitotic figures. For a diagnosis of benign ectopia of nevus cells, the cells should not show any cytologic atypia, nuclear pleomorphism, or mitotic activity. Rarely, these cells may contain small amounts of melanin.

A

B

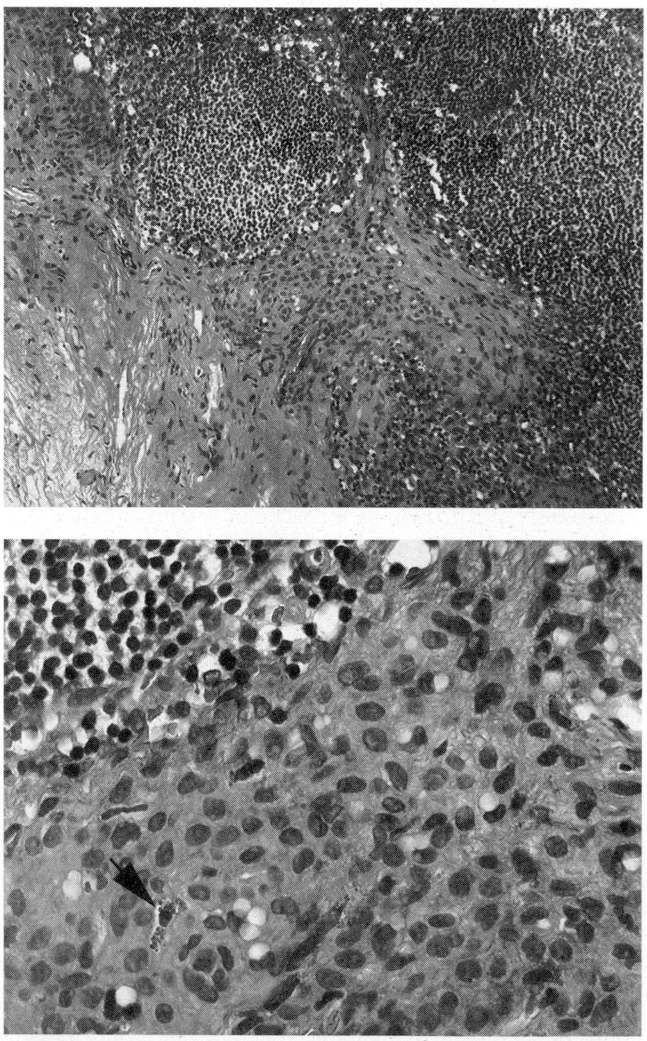

FIG. 30.4. Intranodal nevus cells. **A:** An aggregate of melanocytes is situated in the lymph node capsule (hematoxylin and eosin, original magnification: 200× magnification). **B:** High-power examination demonstrates bland nevus cells without significant cytologic atypia or mitotic activity. Note the melanin-containing melanophage *(arrow)* (hematoxylin and eosin, original magnification: 400× magnification).

Benign metastasis of cutaneous nevi and arrested migration of neural crest cells are the most appealing hypotheses advanced to explain the presence of nevus cell aggregates and blue nevi in lymph nodes. The occurrence of these benign nevus cells in lymph node capsules suggests that these cells migrate into the capsules of lymph nodes during embryonic migration of neural crest cells (74). The presence of benign nevus cells in the lymph node itself would suggest *benign metastasis* (74).

Ectopic Mesothelial Cells

The occurrence of mesothelial cell inclusions in lymph nodes is rare (75–77). Brooks and colleagues (76) described benign mesothelial cell aggregates in mediastinal lymph nodes that mimic metastatic carcinoma. Both patients had histories of pleuritis and pleural effusion with mediastinal widening. More recently, Argani and Rosai described benign mesothelial cell aggregates in cervical, hilar and mediastinal lymph nodes that mimic metastatic carcinoma (77). Recognition of this rare entity in the appropriate clinical setting may avoid the misdiagnosis of carcinoma of unknown origin.

The mesothelial cells, which were cytologically benign and mitotically inactive, occurred as individual cells and in small clusters and appeared only in the lymph node sinuses. On immunohistochemical examination, these cells were found to contain cytokeratin and lack epithelial membrane antigen, CD15, and carcinoembryonic antigen and, for the most part, were negative for B72.3 (76). The cells appeared to be mesothelial cells morphologically and immunohistochemically. Some inclusions that occur in pelvic and retroperitoneal lymph nodes also have been interpreted as mesothelial cell inclusions.

Ectopic Mullerian and Celomic Epithelium

Benign glandular inclusions that occur in pelvic and periaortic lymph nodes have been described almost exclusively in women (78–80). These inclusions have been referred to as *endometriosis, endometriosis-like inclusions, mullerian epithelial inclusions, endosalpingiosis,* and *mesothelial cell inclusions.* Endosalpingiosis refers to ectopic epithelium that resembles benign tubal epithelium (Fig. 30.5). In contrast to endometriosis, endosalpingiosis is usually found incidentally, especially in the setting of pelvic inflammatory disease and ovarian neoplasms. The most important differential diagnostic concern is to distinguish endosalpingiosis from a serous neoplasm, especially implants of serous borderline tumors (serous tumors of low malignant potential and atypically proliferating serous tumors). Endosalpingiosis lacks the tufting, stratification and arborizing architecture that

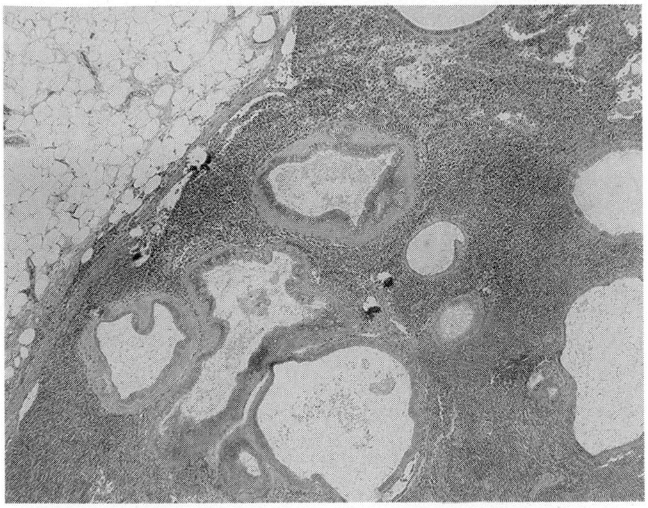

A

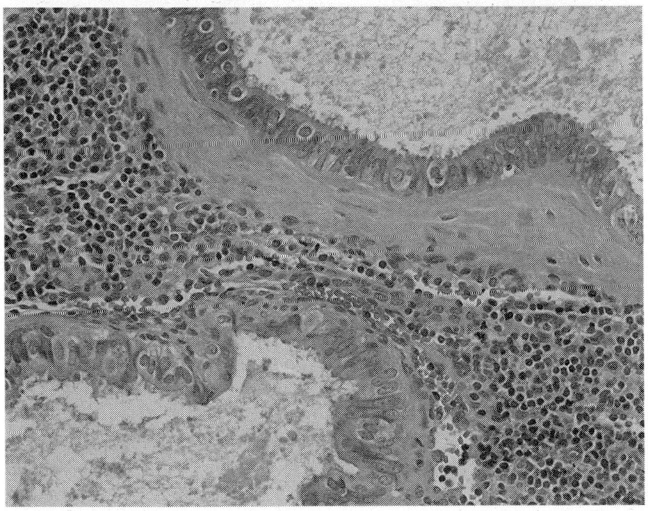

B

FIG. 30.5. Endosalpingiosis. **A:** Low-power examination depicts tubular and cystically dilated glands with psammoma bodies in a pelvic lymph node. This patient had a concurrent serous borderline tumor of the ovary (hematoxylin and eosin, original magnification: 100× magnification). **B:** High-power magnification shows the cytologic features of endosalpingiosis: a monolayer of bland ciliated columnar cells without apparent endometrial stroma, intracytoplasmic mucin, or squamous metaplasia. The presence of endosalpingiosis in a lymph node does not indicate tumor dissemination, nor does it have a bearing on prognosis (hematoxylin and eosin, original magnification: 400× magnification).

characterizes serous borderline tumors. Gynecologic pathologists recognize ''atypical endosalpingiosis,'' a lesion that shows histologic features that are intermediate between endosalpingiosis and serous borderline tumors; in the absence of clear-cut evidence for a serous borderline tumor, these lesions probably pursue a benign course.

Ectopic endometrium has been attributed to several mechanisms, including mullerian and wolffian duct rests (80). Such rests, however, are a less likely explanation than the theory of celomic metaplasia of mesothelial cell inclusions (79) or the regurgitation theory (81). In the metaplastic theory, these inclusions are believed to occur as the result of a metaplastic proliferation of peritoneal mesothelial implants within lymph nodes. Because peritoneal and mullerian epithelium derive from the embryonic celomic epithelium, it is not surprising that metaplastic mesothelium can resemble Mullerian epithelium. According to the regurgitation hypothesis, endometrial tissue is believed to be released through the fallopian tubes during menstruation and then implants on pelvic organs or travels through lymphatic or venous channels to distant organs and lymph nodes (82).

Intranodal endometrial gland inclusions have been found in 14% of women in surgical and autopsy series alike (83). Infrequent case reports have identified similar benign glandular inclusions in mediastinal and perinephric lymph nodes in men (84,85). These benign inclusions potentially could be misinterpreted as metastases to regional lymph nodes. On histologic examination, however, these inclusions are composed of small tubular structures lined by a single layer of cuboidal to columnar cells that contain round uniform nuclei. Occasionally, cilia may be found on their luminal surfaces, and endometrial-type stroma may accompany these glandular or tubular structures. The endometrial stroma may undergo a decidual reaction; this may be misinterpreted as a metastatic tumor, especially on a frozen section. The stromal cells become large but have abundant cytoplasm and uniform nuclei.

Ectopic Salivary Gland

Salivary gland elements frequently are found in intraparotid lymph nodes and, to a lesser degree, in nearby upper cervical lymph nodes (86–88). This tissue most often consists of striated ducts, intercalated ducts, and less commonly, acini (86). Parotid glandular tissue normally becomes incorporated into these lymph nodes during embryologic development. The parotid salivary gland develops from an outpouching of the primitive oral cavity while lymphoid tissue is condensing into parotid lymph nodes. Most of the intranodal glandular tissue fails to develop as the lymphoid tissue enlarges, but many of these lymph nodes retain small islands of the glandular tissue. All this is functioning salivary gland tissue connected to the adjacent parotid gland; occasionally, a fortuitous section or serial section shows the connection between the parotid gland and the intranodal glandular tissue. This ectopic tissue is subject to the same disease processes as the normal salivary gland. Salivary gland ductal inclusions can give rise to proliferative sialometaplasia (89) and lymphoepithelial cysts (90), a condition that has been frequently identified in human immunodeficiency virus (HIV)–infected patients (91,92) (see Chapter 28). Many lymphoepithelial cysts positioned in the high neck and in the parotid salivary gland are thought to arise from these intranodal glandular inclusions rather than from the branchial cleft apparatus, as previously believed. These inclusions occasionally also produce salivary gland tumors, both benign and malignant.

Ectopic Thyroid Gland

Small clusters of microscopically normal appearing thyroid follicles may be encountered rarely within cervical lymph nodes (93–97). These thyroid follicles probably become incorporated inside lymph nodes during the migration of thyroid tissue from the foramen cecum of the tongue to its final midline location and, perhaps, from the primitive intestinal tract in the area of the pharyngobranchial pouches. The occurrence of thyroid tissue in the lateral neck should not be automatically assumed to represent heterotopic or ''lateral aberrant thyroid'' tissue (98–100). Whereas midline thyroid rests seldom represent metastatic thyroid carcinoma, intranodal thyroid tissue in the lateral cervical chains should be considered to be metastatic carcinoma until proven otherwise. Unfortunately, the location of thyroid follicles within a lymph node, such as in the capsule, subcapsular sinus, or the medullary portion, does not help in distinguishing benign ectopic thyroid follicles from metastatic thyroid carcinoma. Even when intranodal thyroid follicles appear well formed, with cytologically benign cuboidal cells containing colloid, and having the appearance of normal thyroid follicles (94,95), the possibility of a malignancy cannot be entirely excluded (Fig. 30.6). The thyroid carcinomas that spread to regional lymph nodes include papillary carcinomas and their variants and mixed papillary and follicular carcinoma (96). These neoplastic follicles contain papillary structures, psammoma bodies, or cells with optically clear nuclei and nuclear grooves, and often do not contain colloid (96). Pure follicular carcinomas only rarely metastasize to cervical lymph nodes (97); in these cases, the cells have cytologically malignant nuclei. There are rare reports of primary intranodal papillary thyroid carcinoma (101–103). In the presence of a presumed intranodal thyroid inclusion, the patient should undergo a thorough thyroid evaluation, including a technetium thyroid scan and ultrasound examination, to search for a primary thyroid carcinoma. If no thyroid lesion is found and the intranodal lesion fulfills the morphologic criteria for ectopic thyroid tissue, then no further treatment is likely to be required.

Ectopic Breast and Sweat Gland Tissue

Ectopic ducts and acini that have the appearance of normal breast or sweat gland tissue rarely may be found in axillary lymph nodes (104,105) (Fig. 30.7). Because breast tissue represents a modified sweat gland, it may be difficult to distinguish between the two when they are present in axillary lymph nodes. The possible presence of these benign glandular inclusions should be kept in mind when evaluating axillary node dissections for the presence of metastatic carcinoma. Ectopic glandular tissue usually has a double cell layer, which is cytologically benign and does not resemble breast carcinoma. Immunohistochemical stains do not help in differentiating this ectopic tissue

A

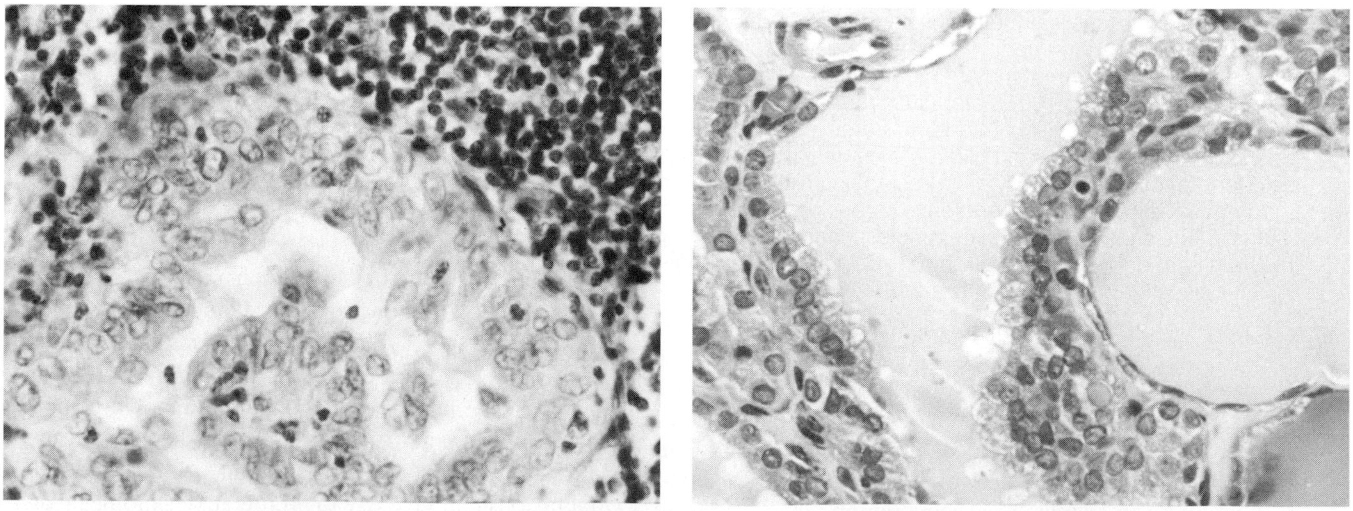

B

FIG. 30.6. Metastatic papillary and follicular thyroid carcinoma. **A:** This papillary thyroid carcinoma metastatic to a lymph node shows neoplastic follicles that lack colloid and contain a central papillary structure. The cells often contain optically clear and grooved nuclei (hematoxylin and eosin, original magnification: 400× magnification). **B:** The follicles that comprise this metastatic follicular thyroid carcinoma are irregular in size and shape and are lined by large atypical nuclei that occasionally contain prominent nucleoli (hematoxylin and eosin, original magnification: 400× magnification).

A
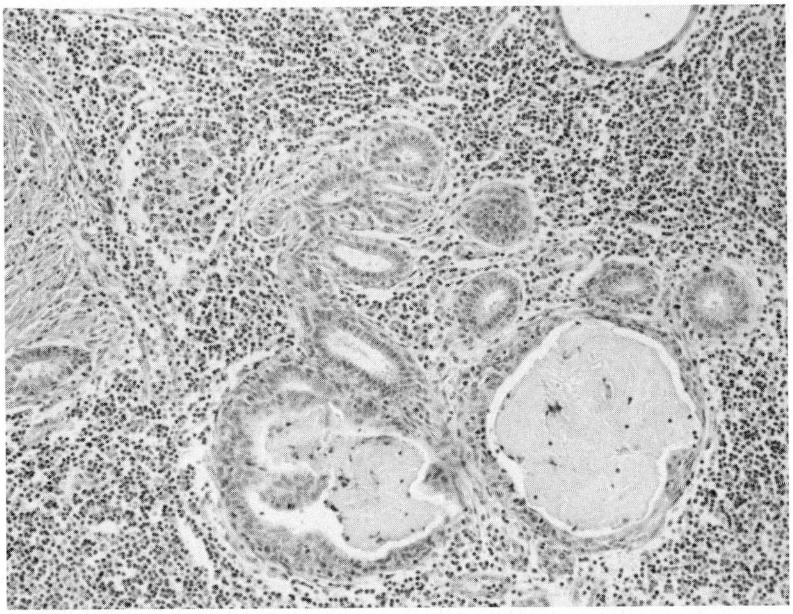

B
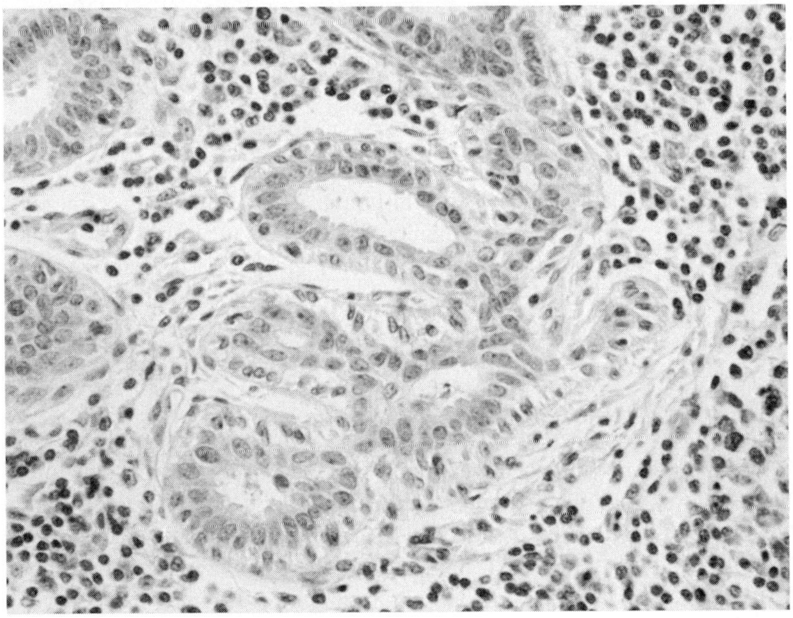

FIG. 30.7. Intranodal ectopic breast tissue. **A:** This microscopic focus of intranodal ectopic breast tissue was discovered as an incidental finding in a lymph node removed as part of an axillary dissection in the treatment of breast cancer. The patient had no evidence of carcinoma metastatic to lymph nodes and had no clinical evidence of metastatic disease (hematoxylin and eosin, original magnification: 100× magnification). **B:** Higher magnification demonstrates that the ducts are lined by a double cell layer and that the cells show bland cytologic features and possess apocrine snouts (hematoxylin and eosin, original magnification: 250× magnification).

from carcinoma but can support, however, their breast or sweat gland origin.

EPITHELIAL LESIONS PRIMARY IN LYMPH NODES

Malignant Melanoma

When malignant melanoma occurs in a lymph node, it is presumed to be a metastasis, and the primary cutaneous or mucosal process is discovered to be active, previously excised, spontaneously regressed, or occult (106–108). Intranodal nevus cell aggregates and blue nevi, as already described, are well-documented lesions that occur in lymph nodes. It has been hypothesized that these intranodal nevoid inclusions may serve as progenitors of primary intranodal malignant melanoma (109). A malignant melanoma that occurs in an axillary lymph node in conjunction with an intranodal blue nevus has been described; no other evidence of melanoma was found in this patient (109). As many as 4% of patients who show nodal involvement by malignant melanoma have no known primary lesion (110,111). The lymph nodes most often involved are axillary or cervical in men and inguinal in women (110). Spontaneous regression of a cutaneous primary malignant melanoma—always a possibility—can be demonstrated in some patients (106, 107,111). When a primary melanoma cannot be found elsewhere, however, the possibility exists that a malignant melanoma has developed primarily in ectopic intranodal nevus cells.

Lymphoepithelial Lesion

The lymphoepithelial lesion, once a rare entity referred to as *Mikulicz's disease* (112), is now encountered frequently. These lesions usually present as solitary nodules in the parotid salivary gland and occasionally in the periparotid tissue (90,113). They are intraparotid and periparotid lymph nodes in which the lymphoid tissue has undergone marked follicular hyperplasia. These lymph nodes often contain cysts of varying sizes lined by cuboidal to squamous epithelium. These cysts represent ectopic salivary gland ductal inclusions that have become cystically dilated. Ectopic salivary gland tissue that occurs in intraparotid and periparotid lymph nodes is functioning glandular tissue connected to the adjacent parotid salivary gland. The hyperplastic lymphoid tissue probably obstructs the ductal tissue, leading to the production of the cysts. Other islands of ectopic ductal tissue frequently demonstrate epimyoepithelial cell hyperplasia, in which small ducts are plugged by proliferating, cytologically benign epithelial and myoepithelial cells; this probably also represents a reactive hyperplasia. The lymphoepithelial lesion is now most commonly found in HIV-infected persons (91,92); the associated florid follicular hyperplasia most likely corresponds to the generalized lymphoid hyperplasia that is frequently observed in these patients (91) (see Chapter 28).

Warthin's Tumor

Warthin's tumor occurs most often in intraparotid lymph nodes but occasionally also may be seen in extraparotid cervical lymph nodes (90,114). These tumors are composed of cystic and papillary structures lined by oncocytic epithelial cells, histologically similar to striated duct cells. The lymphoid component represents the residual or hyperplastic lymphoid tissue of the lymph node in which the tumor arose, presumably from ectopic salivary gland tissue normally found in these lymph nodes (90). In resection specimens of the parotid salivary gland, other intraparotid lymph nodes may contain incidental microscopic Warthin's tumors. These are commonly found in patients who have clinically evident Warthin's tumors and, occasionally, in specimens resected for other lesions (90).

Warthin's tumor is seen most frequently in men older than 50 years of age and may be bilateral, occurring synchronously or metachronously (90). Primary non-Hodgkin's lymphomas and Hodgkin's disease have developed in Warthin's tumor (115–119); the presence of one lesion does not preclude the occurrence of a second lesion. Rarely, poorly differentiated carcinomas have developed in lymph nodes that contain Warthin's tumor (120,121). Whether these carcinomas arose in the Warthin's tumor cell population or in other ectopic salivary gland tissue cannot be determined conclusively.

Acinic Cell and Mucoepidermoid Carcinoma

Occasionally, other types of salivary gland tumors, including acinic cell carcinomas and mucoepidermoid carcinomas, may occur in ectopic salivary gland tissue in cervical nodes (122–125). These well-documented cases can only be accepted as primary tumors if thorough histologic evaluation of the salivary gland shows the tumor to be limited to lymph nodes. If neoplastic tissue is identified outside of lymph nodes, then the lesion may have developed in extranodal tissue and extended secondarily into lymph nodes.

Thyroid Carcinoma

Rare case reports have described intranodal papillary thyroid carcinoma with no apparent evidence of a primary carcinoma in a total thyroidectomy specimen (126). Of course, the possibility always remains that the thyroid tissue was examined or sampled incompletely, or that the primary carcinoma developed in ectopic thyroid tissue that occurred elsewhere, such as in the mediastinum (127) or as a component of a thyroglossal duct cyst (128). Apparently, benign thyroid elements can occur in lymph nodes. Presumably, these intranodal thyroid elements are subject to all the same neoplastic possibilities as nonectopic thyroid tissue and potentially could produce primary intranodal thyroid carcinoma.

Breast Carcinoma

A single case of breast carcinoma in an axillary lymph node has been reported (129). The tumor was a cystic, micropapillary carcinoma that also contained cytologically benign glandular inclusions. Although this must be an extraordinarily rare event, epithelial inclusions in lymph nodes should be examined carefully with the possibility of malignant transformation in mind. When a carcinoma with the histologic features of a breast carcinoma is discovered in an axillary lymph node, however, in almost all cases the tumor has arisen in the breast and secondarily involved the axillary lymph node. In some of these cases, the tumor can be shown to have developed in nearby breast tissue, such as in the axillary tail. In other cases, careful examination of a mastectomy specimen demonstrates the primary lesion in the breast.

MESENCHYMAL LESIONS PRIMARY IN LYMPH NODES

Lipomatosis of Lymph Nodes

Much of the normal architecture of a lymph node may be obscured by mature adipose tissue. Fatty replacement of nodal tissue has been called *lipomatosis, adipose metaplasia,* and "*lipo lymph node*." This is most frequently observed in the axillary lymph nodes that accompany breast resections for carcinoma. These lymph nodes can be recognized clinically and on gross examination as lymph nodes, but on histologic examination, only a rim of lymphoid tissue surrounds mature adipose tissue, which compresses the bulk of the lymph node. The fat probably extends into and compresses the lymph node from the hilar region. This fatty infiltration can be considered a normal finding associated with advancing age, obesity, and lymphoid depletion. This common finding should not mislead the pathologist into thinking that there may not be a lymphoma or metastatic neoplasm involving the lymph node as well, because fat does not appear to be a protective phenomenon.

Fibrosis of Lymph Nodes

Diffuse fibrosis of a lymph node usually involves the hilar region but may advance into the medullary and subcapsular sinuses, eventually separating the lymph node into regions or nodules. The observer should take special care not to misdiagnose such lesions as nodular sclerosis Hodgkin's disease. Fibrosis is found frequently in the inguinal and obturator lymph nodes and, most likely, represents the end-stage process of a nodal inflammatory lesion. Other processes that can commonly lead to areas of lymph node fibrosis include resolved granulomatous diseases, inflammatory pseudotumor of lymph nodes, and chronic lymphadenitis of any cause. Previous treatment of lymph nodes for malignant lymphoma or nonlymphoid malignancies may lead to fibrosis, especially if radiation has been used in the therapy.

Benign Vascular Lesions

Vascular Transformation

Vascular transformation of lymph nodes superficially resembles a hemangioma. This lesion is characterized, however, by congestion and striking reorganization of all subcapsular and medullary sinuses, the normal sinusoidal structure being replaced by an anastomosing network of small vascular channels lined by reactive endothelial cells (Fig. 30.8). The hilar and perinodal veins tend to be obliterated (130,131). This nonneoplastic lesion can easily be mistaken for Kaposi's sarcoma (KS). The absence of capsular involvement and the periodic acid–Schiff (PAS)–positive hyaline globules frequently observed in KS help in the differential diagnosis (132,133).

Nodal Angiomatosis

In nodal angiomatosis, the cortical and medullary sinuses are replaced by irregular cords of proliferating endothelial cells, but the underlying lymph node architecture remains intact. In pannodal hemangiomatoid lesions, vessels radially fan out around a central fibrovascular core and involve perinodal tissues; this architecture is the most prominent feature of this lesion (134). Like vascular transformation, nodal angiomatosis probably represents a reactive process rather than a true neoplasm (131).

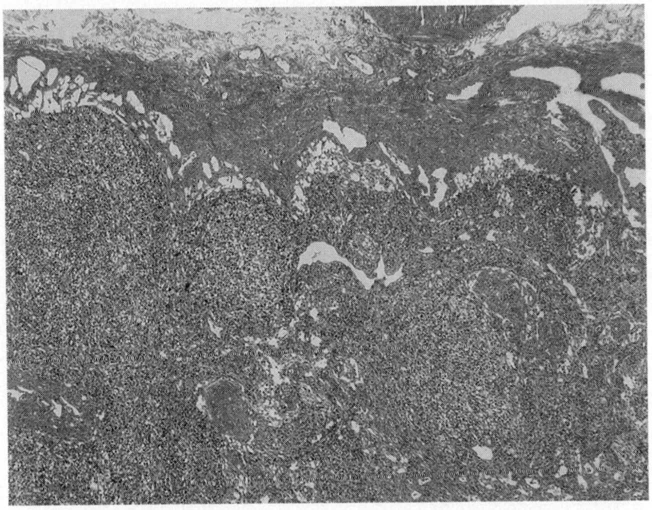

A

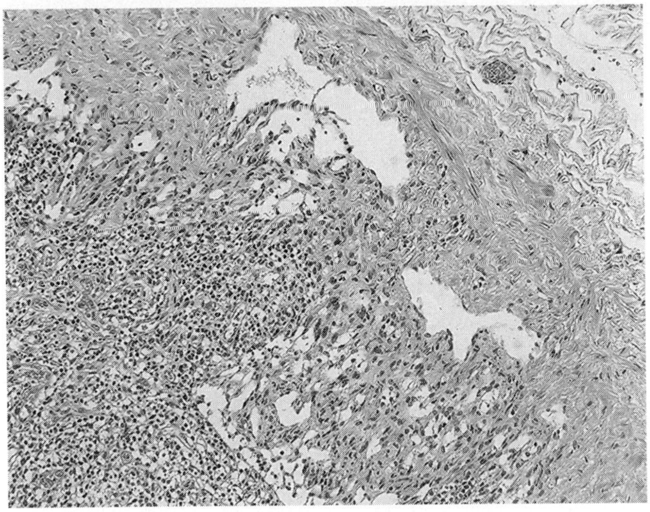

B

FIG. 30.8. Vascular transformation of a lymph node. **A:** The lymph node architecture is preserved, as is the integrity of the capsule, although endothelial cell proliferation is present in the subcapsular sinus (hematoxylin and eosin, original magnification: 100× magnification). **B:** Vascular transformation consists of a cytologically bland endothelial cell proliferation restricted to the subcapsular sinus without involvement of the capsule. The latter finding is helpful in excluding Kaposi's sarcoma (hematoxylin and eosin, original magnification: 200× magnification).

Angiomyomatous Hamartoma

This innocuous lesion is characterized by a proliferation of thick-walled blood vessels and bland smooth muscle cells centered on the lymph node hilum (135) (Fig. 30.9). It is believed to occur almost exclusively in inguinal lymph nodes (135).

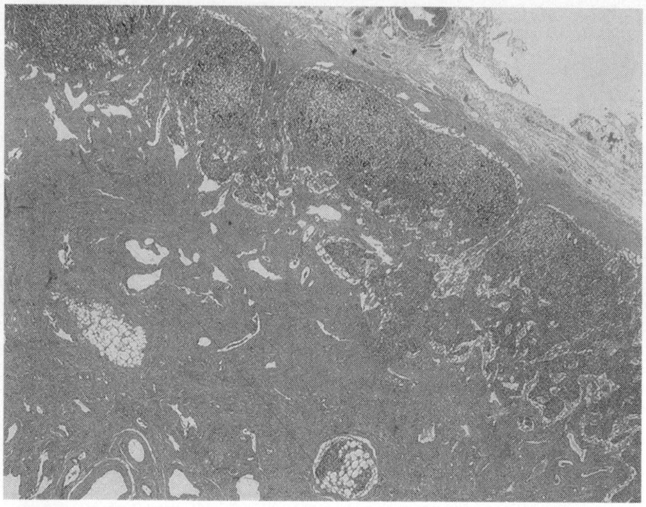

FIG. 30.9. Intranodal angiomyomatous hamartoma. The connective tissue framework of the lymph node is replaced by a proliferation of blood vessels and smooth muscle. The lymph node capsule, subcapsular sinus, and cortex are histologically unremarkable (hematoxylin and eosin, original magnification: 40× magnification).

Angiolipomatous Hamartoma

Angiolipomatous hamartoma is a rare lesion that may accompany lymph nodes involved by the hyaline-vascular form of Castleman's disease. Well-developed blood vessels are interspersed between mature adipocytes in extranodal soft tissue (136,137).

Hemangiomas

Hemangiomas occur in lymph nodes uncommonly, but several well-characterized intranodal hemangiomas have been reported (138–140). These lesions frequently demonstrate distinct feeder vessels, as seen in hemangiomas in other sites. The space-occupying effect, shown by the displacement of normal lymph nodal tissue to the periphery, supports the neoplastic nature of these lesions. Epithelioid hemangioma, also known as angiolymphoid hyperplasia with eosinophilia, is now considered a hemangioma variant instead of analogous to Kimura's disease (141). This proliferation shows well-formed vascular channels lined by epithelioid endothelium. The interstitium is frequently rich in chronic inflammatory cells, including lymphocytes and eosinophils.

Vascular Neoplasm of Castleman's Disease

The vascular neoplasm that arises in the setting of Castleman's disease is a proliferation of blood vessels, some of which resemble high endothelial venules and others that appear to be branching capillaries (142,143) (Fig. 30.10). Staghorn-shaped blood vessels may also be encountered. This vascular proliferation distorts and obscures the underlying lymph node architecture, and frequently, it may be difficult to identify the hyalinized follicles that are characteristic of hyaline-vascular Castleman's disease. The cytologic features range from bland to overtly malignant. This may have some bearing on the biologic behavior of the lesion because recurrence and metastasis have been reported (142,143).

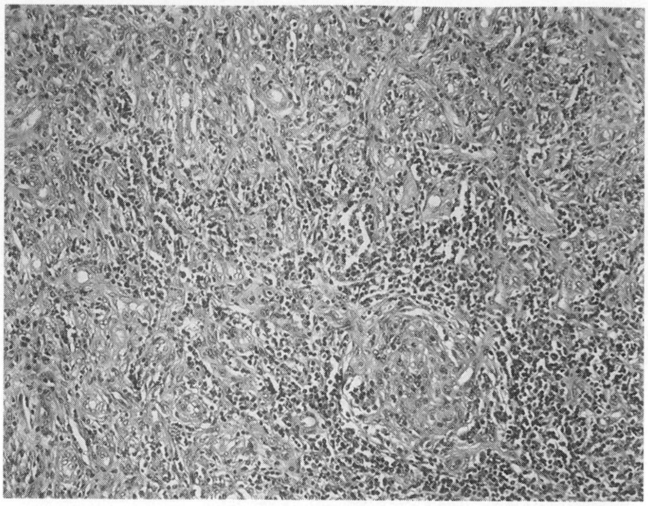

A

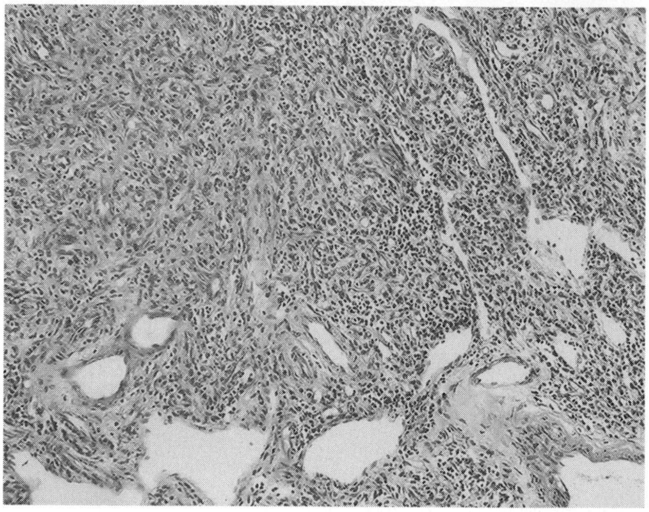

B

FIG. 30.10. Vascular neoplasm of Castleman's disease. **A:** The affected lymph node shows a prominent hyaline-vascular follicle, lymphoid depletion, and a prominent endothelial cell proliferation (hematoxylin and eosin, original magnification: 100× magnification). **B:** Higher-power magnification illustrates the pericytomatous "staghorn," branching, thin-walled blood vessels that can be seen in this lesion. Also shown are the compressed, slitlike, and focally storiformed small-caliber vessels lined by cytologically bland endothelium (hematoxylin and eosin, original magnification: 200× magnification).

Lymphangiomas

Intranodal lymphangiomas occur not infrequently and most commonly affect cervical and axillary lymph nodes.

They are histologically identical to their soft tissue counterparts and are composed of vascular channels lined by flattened endothelium, resembling normal lymphatics (144). Lymphangiomas are benign, well-delimited, space-occupying lesions. The lymphatic channels occasionally are cystically dilated; the cysts may be recognized grossly. Little or no smooth muscle is found in the walls of these lymphatic-like channels, which usually are filled with eosinophilic proteinaceous fluid, lymphocytes, and scattered red blood cells. Intranodal lymphangiomas displace the normal lymph node architecture as would a neoplasm, distinguishing them from the vascular transformative and reactive lesions of lymph nodes (144).

Lymphangioleiomyomatosis

Lymphangiomyomatosis, frequently associated with tuberous sclerosis, can involve lymph nodes as well. These lesions tend to dissect lymph nodes into compartments because they initially develop in the subcapsular and medullary sinuses. They do not usually represent a solitary lesion then but, rather, a multifocal process that eventually can obliterate the lymph node. Compared with lymphangiomas, the smooth muscle component of their vascular walls is prominent (145,146) (Fig. 30.11). Intranodal lymphangiomyomatosis that occurs in patients who have tuberculosis sclerosis is thought by some investigators to be a precursor of intranodal angiomyolipoma (147,148). In contrast to angiomyomatous hamartoma, lymphangioleiomyomatosis occurs exclusively in females, is not limited to inguinal lymph nodes, does not show significant sclerosis and expresses HMB-45 (149, 150).

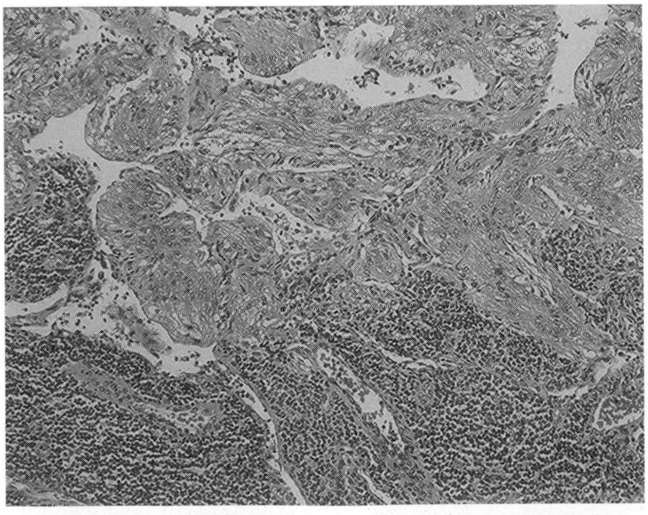

FIG. 30.11. Intranodal lymphangioleiomyomatosis. This entity is best known as a pulmonary and thoracic lesion but occasionally affects pelvic and abdominal retroperitoneal lymph nodes, causing clinical confusion with a primary gynecologic neoplasm and/or a retroperitoneal sarcoma. This lesion is composed of fascicles and small bundles of cytologically innocuous smooth muscle cells derived from lymphatic vessels (hematoxylin and eosin, original magnification: 40× magnification).

Epithelioid Hemangioendothelioma

Epithelioid hemangioendothelioma is a malignant endothelial-derived tumor that may originate in the lymph nodes or present as a metastasis from another site, including the skin, soft tissue and visceral organs (151,152). The spindled and epithelioid cells are arranged singly, in cords and trabeculae, and occasionally, in poorly formed nests. The stroma ranges from hyalinized to myxomatous. The identification of intracellular lumens that entrap blood cells and cellular aggregates around vascular channels are morphologic clues to the diagnosis. The nuclear features are usually bland to moderately atypical. Although the boundary between epithelioid hemangioendothelioma and epithelioid angiosarcoma is not strictly defined, severe atypia with brisk mitotic activity, in combination with a paucity of intracellular lumens, are more in keeping with a diagnosis of epithelioid angiosarcoma. Like epithelioid angiosarcoma, epithelioid hemangioendothelioma expresses the endothelial cell–associated markers CD31, CD34, and factor VIIIRAg (151). Because there are numerous reports of epithelioid vascular tumors that express cytokeratins, it is important to use an immunohistochemical panel that includes endothelial markers to make the correct diagnosis.

The polymorphous hemangioendothelioma is characterized by a low power variegated appearance: solid nests and primitive vascular structures lined by endothelial cells (135). There may be evidence of incomplete or primitive angiomatous differentiation in the form of cytoplasmic vacuoles, slit-like clefts, anastomosing vascular channels and papillary structures. The tumor cells are positive for *Ulex europaeus* but not factor VIIIRAg. This is an uncommon tumor about which little is known. The lesion is considered a low-grade malignancy and has the capability of metastasis (135).

Kaposi's Sarcoma

Between the time of its discovery in 1872 (153) and the recognition of its epidemic spread among homosexual men in the early 1980s heralding the AIDS epidemic (154–156), KS was largely considered an enigmatic dermatologic curiosity whose incidence and natural history varied geographically (157,158). Four clinical-epidemiologic forms of KS are now recognized; these are classic-Mediterranean, endemic-African, iatrogenic, and AIDS-epidemic KS (157,158). The classic-Mediterranean form of KS occurs in the United States uncommonly, having an incidence of only approximately 0.02% in the general population (159). This form of KS usually occurs as an indolent, nonprogressive neoplasm that primarily affects the skin of the lower extremities of the elderly, particularly those of Mediterranean descent (160). This form usually only involves lymph nodes secondarily and generally late in the course of the disease (160,161).

AIDS-epidemic KS is by far the most common clinical-epidemiologic form of the disease occurring in the United States at the present time (157,162). The presence of KS in an HIV-infected individual is an AIDS-defining condition (163,164); it remains the most common neoplasm overall in this patient population (162). However, while all AIDS-risk groups possess an extraordinary risk of developing KS, the risk among homosexual men is astronomical; therefore, these individuals represent the vast majority of patients who have AIDS-epidemic KS (162) (see Chapter 28).

The many special clinical, epidemiologic, and pathologic features of KS have led to significant debate concerning its cell of origin, its hyperplastic versus neoplastic nature, and its cause, infectious or otherwise (157,158,165–168). Most investigators now favor a vascular endothelial cell origin for the spindle cells as well as the vascular lining cells of KS (169–171). The hyperplastic versus neoplastic nature of KS continues to be debated, although at least some cutaneous nodular tumor masses of KS have been shown to be clonal (172). It has been hypothesized that the significantly higher incidence of KS among homosexual men is because of the preferential or enhanced transmissibility of an infectious agent related to the sexual practices of this group, especially those involving oral-fecal contact (173,174). A considerable body of clinical observations and epidemiologic data suggests that KS has an infectious cause and is spread most frequently by sexual transmission of this infectious agent to an immunocompromised host (157,158,173,174).

In 1994, Chang, Moore, Cesarman, Knowles, and collaborators identified a novel, previously unidentified herpesvirus exhibiting homology with herpesvirus saimiri and Epstein-Barr virus (EBV) (175–178), in a KS lesion obtained from a homosexual man who had died from AIDS (175). They named the virus descriptively Kaposi's sarcoma–associated herpesvirus (KSHV) (175); this agent has been also designated human herpesvirus-8 (176). We now know that KSHV is a transmissible, B-cell lymphotropic herpesvirus belonging to the γ-2 sublineage (genus Rhadinovirus) of the Gammaherpesvirinae subfamily (176–179), which are characterized by their ability to replicate in lymphoblastoid cells (180). This virus is detectable in virtually all KS lesions occurring in more than 90% of individuals who have any of the four clinical-epidemiologic forms of the disease (176). It can be visualized in the nuclei of the spindle cells and the flat vascular lining cells of KS lesions by *in situ* techniques (181,182). According to most studies, KSHV is absent from the wide array of vascular tumors and inflammatory conditions that resemble KS (175,176,183). KSHV, which appears to be oncogenic, almost definitely represents the elusive, long sought after etiologic agent of KS and probably plays a role in its pathogenesis. The development of KS is probably a multistep process that involves the interplay of KSHV with impaired immune surveillance, immune stimulation and multiple genetic, environmental, behavioral, and other factors.

In all forms of the disease, the skin is the most frequent site of involvement (156,157,184). Among individuals who have AIDS-epidemic KS, the lesions are often concentrated on the face, genitalia and lower extremities (184). However, extracutaneous spread is very common among individuals who have AIDS-epidemic KS (167,185); frequent sites of involvement include the oral cavity, the lungs and the gastrointestinal tract (184,186), all of which may be involved in the absence of mucocutaneous disease (184).

Lymph node involvement by AIDS-epidemic KS is also common and, similarly, may occur in the absence of mucocutaneous disease (184). AIDS-epidemic KS may occur in benign lymph nodes exhibiting florid follicular hyperplasia, follicular involution and lymphocyte depletion (187–191), as well as in lymph nodes containing malignant lymphoma (192). Early lesions as well as small foci of involvement are usually observed in or adjacent to the capsule, in the hilum, or, occasionally, in the perinodal adipose tissue (187,189, 193,194). Diagnosis of these early lesions and small foci of KS can be difficult, particularly when they only involve the pericapsular tissue. They can be easily overlooked or may be dismissed as an area of fibrosis (187). Late in the clinical course, lymph nodes involved by AIDS-epidemic KS may appear grossly as hemorrhagic tumors measuring several cm in diameter (167).

AIDS-epidemic KS generally is histopathologically indistinguishable from the other clinical-epidemiologic forms of the disease (195) (Fig. 30.12) (see Chapter 28). KS is composed of a variable mixture of ectatic, irregularly shaped, round capillary and slitlike endothelial-lined vascular spaces and spindle-shaped cells accompanied by a variable, mixed mononuclear cell infiltrate. The endothelial cells may be thin and spindle-shaped or oval to round; they generally lack cytologic atypia and mitotic activity. Erythrocytes and hemosiderin pigment are frequently present, often extravasated between the spindle cells. Small refractile, eosinophilic, PAS-positive hyaline globules, representing the breakdown products of phagocytosed erythrocytes, may be present extracellularly or within macrophages. The latter are highly associated with KS and assist in its differential diagnosis with angiosarcoma and other vascular proliferations (132). The spindle cells increasingly become the predominant cell population, forming fascicles that compress the vascular slits, and the lesions may progress to form nodules and tumors. The latter consist primarily of interwoven fascicles of spindle cells displaying prominent cytologic atypia, numerous mitotic figures and often striking pleomorphism (187, 189,195,196).

Extracutaneous KS may differ slightly histologically and may exhibit a different developmental chronology than cutaneous KS (195). The earliest histopathologic changes in lymph nodes involved by KS have been referred to as "hypervascular follicular hyperplasia" (197). Vascular channels within the lymph node are prominent, increased in number and are associated with increased numbers of plasma cells (198). Over time, these areas may develop the classic histopathologic features of KS, including interwoven fascicles of

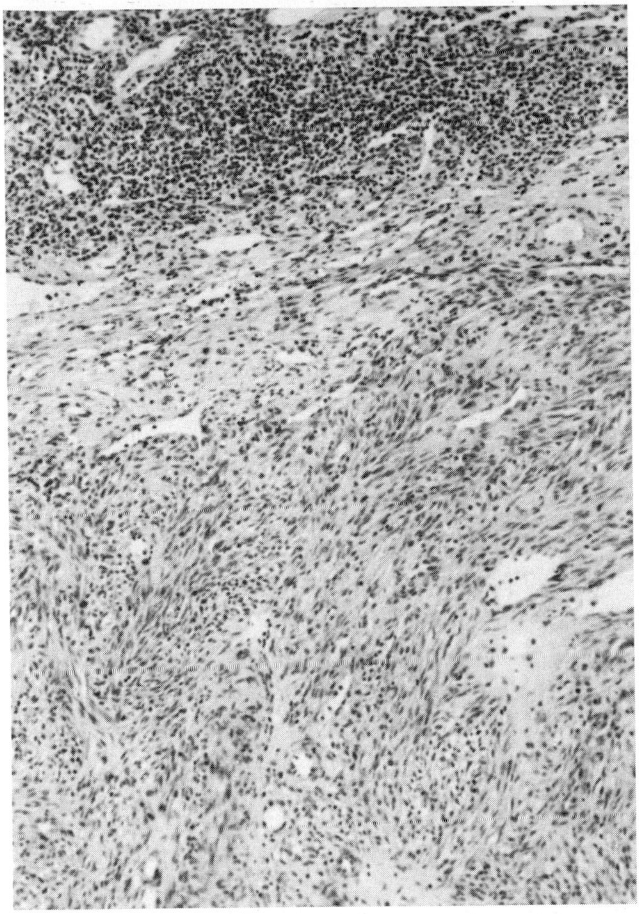

FIG. 30.12. Intranodal Kaposi's sarcoma. This lymph node is almost totally replaced by Kaposi's sarcoma. The lesion consists of interwoven bundles of closely packed spindle cells that extend in various directions and that sometimes produce cleft-like vascular channels. Red blood cells sometimes percolate through these vascular channels, and extravasated erythrocytes and hemosiderin are frequently present in the surrounding tissue (hematoxylin and eosin, original magnification: 100× magnification).

spindle cells, vascular slits and extravasated erythrocytes (195,198). KS involving lymph nodes extends along the sinusoids, infiltrates the interfollicular areas (189,194), and eventually may replace the entire lymph node (187,193).

Immunohistochemical studies demonstrate that the spindle cells and the vascular lining cells of KS express a variety of endothelial cell–associated antigens. These include factor VIII–related antigen, CD34, and CD31 (199–201). A variety of antibodies that are immunoreactive with normal vascular but not lymphatic endothelium (i.e., E92, B74, E431, OKM5, and HCL-1) are immunoreactive with the spindle cells and the vascular lining cells of KS (169,170). Ultrastructural studies demonstrate Weibel-Palade bodies in the cytoplasm of some KS cells (202,203).

In addition to angiosarcoma, KS must be distinguished from vascular transformation of the sinuses, nodal angiomatosis, intranodal hemangioma, bacillary angiomatosis, inflammatory pseudotumor of lymph node, and most muscle tumors. Some of these entities have already been discussed, and the remainder are discussed in later sections.

Angiomyolipoma

Renal angiomyolipomas that also involve lymph nodes are rare (204). The regional periaortic lymph nodes are the nodes typically involved (205). Histologically, this lesion is composed of a mixture of adipose tissue, smooth muscle arranged in fascicles, and thick-walled blood vessels. Focally, the smooth muscle cells may have mildly to moderately atypical nuclei; however, mitoses are found only infrequently (205). Nonetheless, because nodal involvement by a tumor implies malignancy, some investigators have raised the possibility of malignant transformation of this tumor (204). It is generally accepted, however, that nodal involvement by a renal angiomyolipoma most likely represents a multicentric growth pattern and not a true nodal metastasis (205). Follow-up studies in 12 cases show that the patients were well from 1 to 15 years (median, 3 years) after excision (204). This finding supports the interpretation that these lesions are benign. DNA analysis of nodal angiomyolipoma in three cases demonstrated a diploid DNA content (204), further supporting the benign nature of these lesions. The perivascular myoid cells in angiomyolipoma express HMB-45, a phenotype shared by lymphangioleiomyomatosis (150). A purely epithelioid angiomyolipoma that simulates the histologic appearance of an oncocytic neoplasm has been described (206); this tumor shows diffuse HMB-45 reactivity, which is consistent with the perivascular myoid cell derivation that is proposed.

Bacillary Angiomatosis

Bacillary angiomatosis is an uncommon pseudoneoplastic vasoproliferative disorder resulting from infection by *Bartonella henselae* and *Bartonella quintana* (207–209). The lesion was first described by Stoller and colleagues in 1983 (210). LeBoit and coworkers defined the entity histopathologically, identified the relationship between the lesions and the cat scratch bacillus-like organisms found within them and coined the term bacillary angiomatosis to reflect their infectious as well as their proliferative nature (211,212). The disease generally occurs in immunocompromised individuals, predominantly those who are HIV-infected and have AIDS (207,211–216) (see Chapter 28).

Cutaneous disease is the most frequent clinical manifestation of bacillary angiomatosis (210–213,217–219). The patients usually have multiple to very large numbers of variably sized, superficial cutaneous papules that may mimic pyogenic granuloma to dermal and subcutaneous nodules that may be misinterpreted as KS (210–213,217). Cutaneous disease may be accompanied by mucosal, visceral, or lymph node involvement (207,213,215,216,219–227). The peripheral, mediastinal and abdominal lymph nodes are the ones most commonly involved by bacillary angiomatosis (215,227).

Bacillary angiomatosis involves lymph nodes as discrete, variably sized nodules, some of which may coalesce to form large masses. The underlying lymph node architecture may survive intact. Bacillary angiomatosis is composed of variably sized, circumscribed lobules of small blood vessels (some well formed, some barely canalized, and some ectatic) that are situated in an alternately mucinous and fibrotic stroma. The vessels are lined by protuberant plump, polygonal endothelial cells containing abundant pale cytoplasm and ovoid nuclei that contain one to several small nucleoli. They sometimes exhibit mild nuclear pleomorphism and mitotic figures. Aggregates of granular acidophilic to amphophilic material, representing clumps of the causative bacteria, lie in the interstitium separating the vessels (220). The bacteria can be visualized with the Warthin-Starry stain (210–212,220). Numerous neutrophils accompanied by ''nuclear dust'' usually are scattered throughout the lesions and frequently aggregate around the bacterial clumps (210, 212,213,220,221) (see Chapter 28).

The principal differential diagnosis of bacillary angiomatosis involving a lymph node includes KS (217,220), with which it can occur simultaneously in the same patient (214,221,225); epithelioid hemangioma; and angiosarcoma (220). Careful assessment of the clinical features of the patient and of the gross appearance and histopathology of the lesions should lead to suspicion of bacillary angiomatosis (217), which can be readily confirmed by a Warthin-Starry stain (211,212,220,221). The accurate recognition of bacillary angiomatosis is important because appropriate antibiotic therapy leads to regression of the lesions and resolution of the disease in virtually all patients (217).

Inflammatory Pseudotumor of Lymph Node

The main histologic feature of this lesion is a spindle cell proliferation arranged in a storiform pattern, accompanied by proliferating small blood vessels and inflammatory cells (228,229) (Fig. 30.13). This proliferation predominantly involves the connective tissue framework of the lymph node that results in expansion of the hilum, trabeculae, and capsule. Frequently, this proliferation extends into the paracortical region and the perinodal soft tissues. As in nodular fasciitis that involves soft tissues, myxoid as well as fibrotic areas may be identified. The spindle cells appear to be a mixture of fibroblasts and myofibroblasts, as shown by their positivity for muscle actin. However, some investigators have reported inflammatory pseudotumors that exhibit the immunophenotypic features of follicular dendritic cells (230). The spindle cells and lymphocytes of inflammatory pseudotumors have been found to contain EBV genome in a significant number of cases (231). The proliferating vessels are usually straight, rarely ramifying. The vessels are lined by plump, reactive appearing endothelial cells and are surrounded by one or two layers of spindle cells. In the paracortical region, these vessels are mixed with postcapillary venules. Small benign lymphocytes, immunoblasts, histiocytes, and many plasma cells are present. Neutrophils may be seen infrequently, and some cases may have a prominent eosinophilic infiltrate. Multinucleated giant cells also can be found. Necrosis and a high mitotic rate are not usual features of inflammatory pseudotumors (229).

There is controversy surrounding the nomenclature of histologically similar lesions that have been reported to recur, metastasize and involve extranodal tissues. When these lesions extend into the perinodal soft tissue and irregularly entrap normal structures, they may be considered ''inflammatory myofibroblastic tumors'' that have recurring potential (232). Some investigators have reported histologically similar lesions in visceral organs and have used the term ''inflammatory fibrosarcoma'' to describe those with cytologic atypia and an aggressive clinical course (232,233).

Palisaded Myofibroblastoma

Palisaded myofibroblastoma is also known as *hemorrhagic spindle cell tumor with amainthoid fibers.* As the names imply, this rare tumor is composed of myofibroblasts with interstitial hemorrhage and amainthoid fibers (234,235). This benign lesion occurs predominantly in the inguinal lymph nodes, although presentation in other sites has also been reported. The constituent spindle cells appear bland and mitotically inactive. The so-called amainthoid fibers are ovoid and stellate regions of collagen deposition that may be calcified. The myofibroblast nuclei appear to palisade around the amainthoid fibers. The tumor cells express antigens shared with myofibroblasts in other lesions: vimentin, muscle-specific actin, but not desmin or S-100 protein. The morphologic and immunophenotypic features permit distinction from other lesions in the differential diagnosis, including KS, true dendritic cell sarcoma, and smooth muscle lesions such as metastatic leiomyosarcoma and leiomyomatosis.

Mycobacterial Spindle Cell Pseudotumor

This proliferation shows a significant degree of histologic overlap with inflammatory pseudotumor; one can observe short fascicles and storiform arrangements of spindle cells admixed with capillaries and chronic inflammatory cells, including plasma cells (236,237). Evaluation with a histochemical stain for acid-fast bacilli permits the correct diagnosis (236,237). The mycobacterial spindle cell tumor characteristically arises in the setting of Mycobacterium avium intracellulare infection in immunocompromised patients. The spindle cell population is thought to be histiocytic, however, immunoreactivity with anti-desmin antibodies has been reported (236).

Leiomyomatosis

Tumor-forming nodules of smooth muscle without the cytologic features of malignancy are occasionally encountered

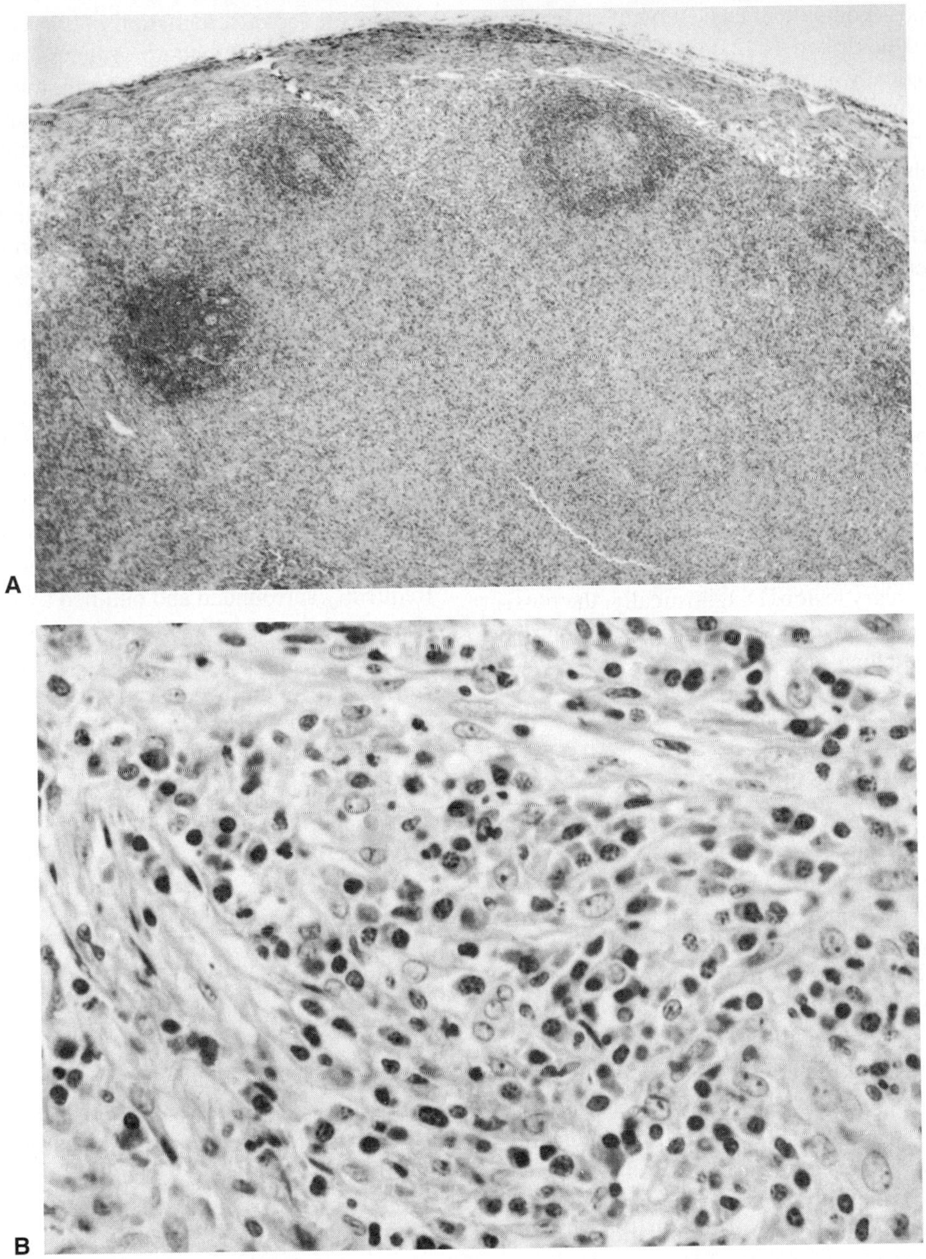

FIG. 30.13. Inflammatory pseudotumor of lymph node. **A:** Low-power examination of this lymph node demonstrates the presence of residual benign germinal centers, which are largely surrounded by an interfollicular spindle cell and inflammatory cell proliferation. This process extends focally into the paracortical region and into the perinodal tissue (hematoxylin and eosin, original magnification: 40× magnification). **B:** Higher magnification demonstrates that the proliferation consists of spindle cells, blood vessels, and a mixed inflammatory cell population. Cellular pleomorphism, necrosis, and frequent mitotic figures are absent (hematoxylin and eosin, original magnification: 400× magnification).

in lymph nodes (238–241). That is, these proliferations should not be considered metastatic leiomyosarcoma unless there is significant nuclear pleomorphism and necrosis. The distinction between an intranodal tumor and a primary soft tissue tumor is important because even small and cytologically bland smooth muscle tumors of the soft tissue can recur and metastasize. Nodal leiomyomatosis can result from deposits of benign metastasizing leiomyoma and leiomyomatosis peritonealis disseminata, or may represent a primary nodal lesion (238–241). The differential diagnosis is lengthy, and includes most of the spindle cell lesions discussed in this chapter. In contrast to the other spindle cell lesions, nodal leiomyomatosis is a homogeneous-appearing lesion that is indistinguishable from uterine leiomyoma (238–241).

Deciduosis

Intranodal, tumor-forming decidual cells can occur during pregnancy. They may be associated with endometriosis, although decidual deposits outside of the setting of endometriosis have been well described (242,243). The constituent cells are morphologically similar to decidual cells found within the endometrium. However, because of their intraabdominal or retroperitoneal distribution, there is often concern about the possibility of metastatic carcinoma, especially squamous cell carcinoma. The relatively bland cytologic appearance of the decidual cells and the absence of immunoreactivity for cytokeratins permit distinction from metastatic carcinoma.

Other Sarcomas

Rare cases have been reported in which an intranodal sarcoma, i.e., leiomyosarcoma, rhabdomyosarcoma, or malignant fibrous histiocytoma, has been found with no other evidence of disease elsewhere (244). The extreme rarity of such lesions, however, should always prompt a thorough clinical investigation for a primary lesion. Diagnostically, the possibility should always be left open of a primary lesion that has occurred in some other site.

METASTATIC NEOPLASMS IN LYMPH NODES THAT MIMIC MALIGNANT LYMPHOMA

Poorly Differentiated Carcinomas

Metastatic carcinomas that involve lymph nodes secondarily often recapitulate features of their primary lesion, displaying squamous, glandular, or transitional cell differentiation and therefore are readily recognizable. In cases in which it is unknown, the primary site sometimes can be inferred from the histologic features of the metastasis. In other instances, the clinical history, including the age and sex of the patient, can be used as well as the anatomic location of the involved lymph node to develop a likely differential diagnosis. Not infrequently, however, metastatic carcinomas may present a diagnostic problem in that they occasionally lack any obvious morphologic features of differentiation and thus mimic other malignant neoplasms. For example, they may simulate a malignant lymphoma if they are poorly differentiated and the cells lack cohesion; a sarcoma, if the cells undergo spindle cell metaplasia, and a melanoma, if the cells are characterized by solitary, prominent, centrally placed nucleoli. It is very important for the pathologist to make the correct histopathologic diagnosis in these instances because the therapeutic and prognostic implications of each diagnosis differ markedly.

The most common situation is one in which a poorly differentiated carcinoma replaces a lymph node in a diffuse sheetlike matter, mimicking a diffuse large cell lymphoma. The clinical history and a thorough clinical evaluation may distinguish between these two diagnostic possibilities and ascertain the primary site of metastatic carcinoma. Several histopathologic criteria may be helpful in distinguishing carcinoma from malignant lymphoma. In the absence of obvious cellular differentiation of the carcinoma cells, these criteria include the pattern of lymph node involvement, the cohesive nature and the cytomorphologic features of the neoplastic cells, and the pattern of necrosis, if it is present (1).

In malignant lymphomas, the interface between the neoplastic cells and the uninvolved lymph node tissue is often indiscrete, with lymphoma cells infiltrating freely into the adjacent benign lymph node parenchyma. In contrast, in carcinomas, prominent sinusoidal involvement results in large islands of neoplastic cells that often form a broad, clearly distinct border that appears to push against the benign residual lymphoid tissue (1).

Epithelial cells tend to be cohesive; epithelial neoplasms are frequently characterized by the formation of nests of cells. These cell nests may be well defined and readily apparent in routine histologic sections. Alternatively, they may be ill defined and only become apparent with a reticulin stain (1). In epithelial neoplasms, solid nests of tumor cells are frequently surrounded and outlined by reticulin fibers; these fibers are not present within the nests themselves. In contrast, malignant lymphomas often have a heavy reticulin fiber network, with reticulin fibers found near most tumor cells. In contrast to malignant lymphomas, poorly differentiated carcinomas are more likely to exhibit a greater degree of cellular anaplasia and pleomorphism, a higher frequency of multiple nuclei, and larger, more prominent nucleoli (1).

If necrosis is present, the pattern may serve as an additional feature to help establish a differential diagnosis. Carcinomas display areas of necrosis that are zonal and well demarcated from surrounding viable tumor. In contrast, individual cell necrosis is more common in malignant lymphomas. The single cell necrosis of lymphomas is associated with the presence of numerous phagocytic tingible body macrophages, resulting in a starry-sky pattern. Even in very aggressive carcinomas with extensive necrosis, broad areas of well-delimited necrosis are usually found and a starry-sky pattern is not seen. Because the pattern of necrosis in carcinomas is frequently related to the blood supply, viable tumor cells often are adjacent to intact blood vessels (1). The previously held belief that this pattern of perivascular starring of tumor is characteristic of carcinoma is no longer considered valid, however, because it also may be seen in certain aggressive lymphomas.

Carcinomas metastatic to lymph nodes may mimic malignant lymphoma if the tumor cells lack cohesiveness and grow diffusely. In cervical lymph nodes, metastatic carcinomas from the nasopharynx and occasionally from other areas of Waldeyer's ring are prime suspects in this differential diagnosis. Occasionally, only a few carcinoma cells may be present, and these may be obscured even more by a marked histiocytic and lymphocytic proliferation. An obvious nesting pattern is frequently absent. Such lesions may be diagnosed incorrectly as large cell lymphoma or mixed small and large cell lymphoma. Medullary and apocrine breast carcinomas may also resemble large cell lymphomas. Small cell carcinomas of the breast and lung may mimic small lymphocytic lymphoma, Burkitt's lymphoma and lymphoblastic lymphoma, depending on their particular cytologic features.

CD30^{+} anaplastic large cell lymphoma (ALCL) represents one category of malignant lymphoma that frequently has been misdiagnosed in the past because these lymphoid neoplasms often exhibit the growth pattern and cellular characteristics of epithelial neoplasms (245). The anaplastic large cell lymphomas exhibit a marked predilection for sinusoidal infiltration and, hence, often grow in an epithelial pattern (245) (Fig. 30.3). Moreover, the neoplastic cells of ALCL often exhibit marked pleomorphism and have one to many large, prominent nucleoli (246) (see Chapter 25).

In all these situations, immunohistochemical staining of routinely prepared paraffin tissue sections for CD45, cytokeratins, EMA, CD15, CD30, and B- and T-cell–associated antigens usually leads to the correct diagnosis.

The most common poorly differentiated carcinomas that may be confused with malignant lymphoma are undifferentiated nasopharyngeal carcinoma, pulmonary small cell undifferentiated carcinoma and mammary lobular carcinoma. Signet ring cell carcinomas also enter into the differential diagnosis, but less commonly.

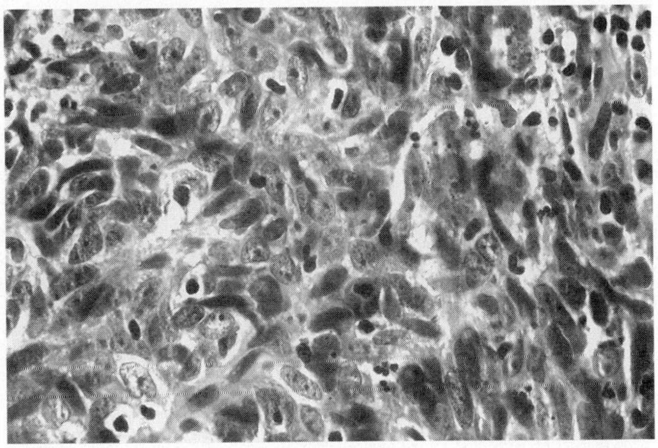

FIG. 30.14. Metastatic undifferentiated nasopharyngeal carcinoma. This lesion can easily be confused with a lymphoproliferative disorder because of the frequent presence of a heavy reactive lymphoid infiltrate that imparts the appearance of a lymphoepithelial lesion. This carcinoma can be recognized by its focal epithelial characteristics, which are usually manifested by nested growth and classic cytologic features including a vesicular nucleus and a centrally placed, prominent nucleolus (hematoxylin and eosin, original magnification: 400× magnification).

Undifferentiated Nasopharyngeal Carcinoma

Because of its peculiar epidemiology and usual site of presentation, the diagnosis of undifferentiated nasopharyngeal carcinoma (UNC) may be suspected before morphologic examination. Occurrence in young to middle-aged Southern Chinese is typical, as is dissemination to cervical and mediastinal lymph nodes. However, other presentations are not uncommon (247).

Morphologically, UNC is a tumor composed of single or aggregated large cells possessing scanty cytoplasm, and vesicular nuclei containing a single prominent eosinophilic nucleolus (Fig. 30.14). Because these lesional cells may be rare, one's low power impression is often that of a "blue" tumor, with a dense background of small, round lymphocytes. Despite a superficial resemblance to small lymphocytic lymphoma, T-cell–rich B-cell lymphoma and lymphocyte predominance Hodgkin's disease, UNC is an epithelial tumor that expresses cytokeratins and lacks CD45. One should be cautious about the interpretation of CD45 positivity in UNC, however. One may encounter the CD45^{-} UNC cells ringed by background CD45^{+} lymphocytes, which may confer on them the false appearance of CD45 expression. Determination of CD45 status in UNC should probably only be performed in clusters of cohesive UNC cells, thereby lessening the chance for misinterpretation.

Undifferentiated nasopharyngeal carcinoma is associated with EBV infection (248,249). Although detection of EBV genome and virus-associated proteins is straightforward in UNC, it is probably not contributory to its distinction from malignant lymphoma. A variety of malignant lymphomas are associated with EBV infection (250).

Poorly Differentiated Neuroendocrine Carcinoma

Poorly differentiated neuroendocrine carcinoma (PDNC) represents a spectrum of related tumors that encompasses small cell carcinoma, neuroendocrine carcinoma not-otherwise-specified, and large cell neuroendocrine carcinoma. The most common PDNC is the pulmonary small cell carcinoma, which in many cases may be correctly recognized in lymph nodes on the basis of the history of a pulmonary mass. When the history is not forthcoming or when a PDNC originates in an extrapulmonary organ, diagnosis can be difficult, however.

Small cell carcinoma may be easily mistaken for malignant lymphoma because the constituent cells possess inapparent cytoplasm and small, hyperchromatic nuclei (Fig. 30.15). Other carcinomas in this spectrum contain nuclei with finely stippled chromatin and small nucleoli. Cohesive, nestlike growth favors the diagnosis of carcinoma over lymphoma, but this finding is not specific. Smudged nuclear chromatin, including the well-recognized *Azzopardi effect* may be present, but this feature is shared in part by some lymphoid proliferations, including in the setting of systemic lupus erythematosus (251).

When PDNC is a possibility, immunohistochemical evaluation may aid in its distinction from malignant lymphoma and, perhaps, in tumor subtyping. Most PDNCs express cytokeratin and many demonstrate a characteristic paranuclear "dot" staining pattern for cytokeratin (252). Epithelial membrane antigen expression may be seen in the absence of cytokeratin expression and may be considered supportive of epithelial differentiation, especially when CD45 is absent and anaplastic large cell lymphoma is not a consideration

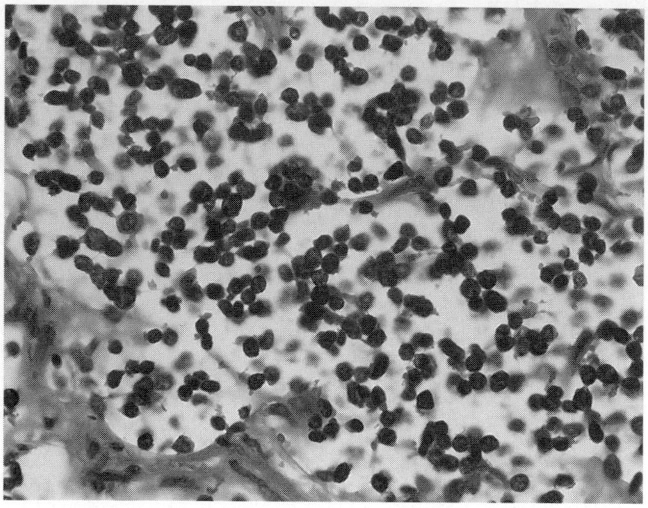

FIG. 30.15. Metastatic pulmonary small cell carcinoma. In this poorly preserved example of metastatic small cell carcinoma, the malignant cells have inapparent cytoplasm and small hyperchromatic nuclei resembling a lymphoproliferative disorder. Attention to morphologic detail in a well preserved specimen, a complete clinical history, and immunohistochemical evaluation all contribute to the distinction between metastatic small cell carcinoma and malignant lymphoma (hematoxylin and eosin, original magnification: 400× magnification).

(253). Many small cell carcinomas also express neuroendocrine-associated and neural markers (252–254). However, the distinction of a neuroendocrine carcinoma from a carcinoma that expresses neuroendocrine markers is unclear. The characteristic morphologic appearance of small cell carcinoma and carcinoid tumors permits distinction from other metastatic tumors. However, the criteria for separating non-small cell neuroendocrine carcinomas from other carcinomas is vague and appears arbitrary (255–257).

Nevertheless, chromogranin or synaptophysin reactivity is considered confirmatory of neuroendocrine differentiation. In some laboratories, NSE is used, but NSE is considered to be nonspecific by some investigators. Significant numbers of small cell carcinomas express CD57, and smaller numbers express CD99 (MIC-2 antigen) (258,259).

The use of antibodies to cytokeratins 7 and 20 (CK7 and CK20) may aid in the separation of cutaneous neuroendocrine carcinoma (i.e., Merkel cell carcinoma) from other PDNCs. In addition to the expression of pancytokeratins and neuroendocrine antigens, Merkel cell carcinoma is apparently unique among the PDNCs in the expression of CK20; many other PCNCs express only CK7 (30,260).

Mammary Lobular Carcinoma

Isolated axillary lymphadenopathy in a postpubertal woman should be considered likely to represent metastatic breast carcinoma until proven otherwise (261). In many cases a complete clinical history, including mammographic data, is helpful in diagnosing a diffuse round cell proliferation as metastatic breast carcinoma in the proper setting.

Although the distinction from malignant lymphoma is not always straightforward, infiltrating ductal carcinomas often form glands or large, cohesive tumor cell clusters in lymph nodes, which is typical of epithelial neoplasms. In contrast, however, metastatic lobular carcinoma of the breast is generally a small cell neoplasm that can infiltrate the lymph node parenchyma in single cells and form vague, confluent masses that mimic malignant lymphoma and sinus histiocytosis at low power (Fig. 30.16).

The first challenge confronted by the morphologist is determining that a lesion actually exists at all. Any low power abnormality that suggests a mass lesion or prominent sinuses should be examined at high magnification. Sinus histiocytosis should not form a mass lesion. Its high power morphology includes a moderate amount of vacuolated cytoplasm and small nuclei with reniform or oval shapes with nuclear grooves. This appearance is also shared, in part, by sinus histiocytosis with massive lymphadenopathy (Rosai-Dorfman disease) and Langerhans cell histiocytosis (see Chapter 51). In contrast, lobular carcinoma of the breast usually demonstrates monotonous, round nuclei of small to intermediate size, with small or inapparent nucleoli. The cytoplasm is generally scant; however, at low power, a mass of lobular carcinoma cells may impart the impression of a pink mass, generally because of the contrast between its epithelioid features and those of lymphocytes and histiocytes. Both these epithelioid characteristics and the fact that metastases are frequently focal may permit distinction from malignant lymphoma.

However, these features are neither specific nor exclusive;

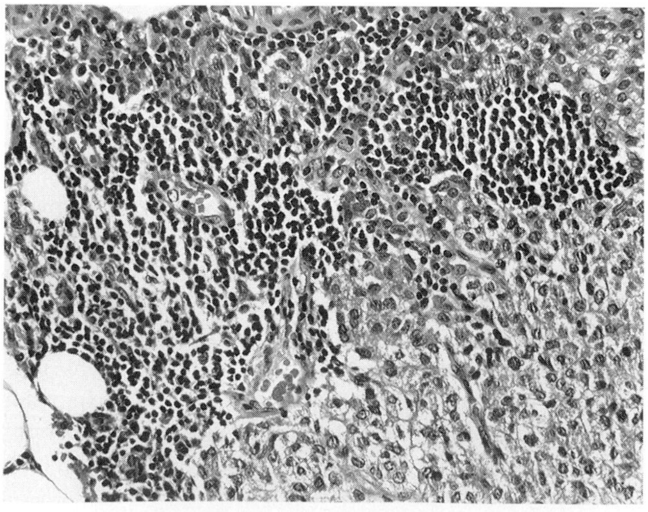

FIG. 30.16. Metastatic lobular carcinoma of breast. Metastatic lobular breast carcinoma can easily be overlooked because of its histologic similarity to sinus histiocytosis. The keys to diagnosis in this case are the nested pattern of growth, the relatively large nuclear size, and the absence of twisted, bean-shaped and reniform nuclei (hematoxylin and eosin, original magnification: 200× magnification).

immunohistochemical evaluation may be helpful. The screening panel (i.e., CD45, cytokeratin, and S-100) enables distinction from malignant lymphoma and a histiocytic proliferation. Lobular carcinoma expresses pancytokeratins, and as many as 50% of cases express the S-100 protein (262). Malignant lymphoma demonstrates the expected CD45$^+$, S-100, and cytokeratin-negative phenotype, and the histiocytes of sinus histiocytosis may express CD45 but are more likely to express CD68.

The morphologic appearance of lobular carcinoma may be heterogeneous. Lobular carcinoma variants include the alveolar, solid, pleomorphic and signet ring cell subtypes (263). Awareness of these lobular carcinoma variants may help in the distinction from malignant lymphoma and other metastatic neoplasms.

Once the correct diagnosis of metastatic carcinoma has been made, it may become necessary to determine the primary site of origin, especially when a complete physical examination and mammogram have not been performed. Using antibodies to estrogen and progesterone receptors, human cystic disease fluid protein (HCDFP/brst-2), mCEA, CK7, and CK20, it may be possible to distinguish a breast primary from an extramammary primary. Expression of estrogen, progesterone, or both receptors and brst-2 expression with negative or focally reactive mCEA are characteristic of breast carcinoma (264). The CK7$^+$CK20$^-$ phenotype is also supportive, although not entirely specific, of a mammary primary (30). Because the immunohistochemical results should not be considered diagnostic, but merely confirmatory of a type of differentiation, one should interpret the results in light of the clinical and light microscopic findings. For example, estrogen and progesterone receptors have been reported in numerous neoplasms (265) and the phenotype, as well as the morphology, of breast carcinoma may be indistinguishable from skin adnexal and salivary gland neoplasms (266).

Signet Ring Cell Lesions

The presence of vacuolated signet ring cells should not automatically lead to a diagnosis of adenocarcinoma. In some instances, the vacuoles may not represent intracellular mucin but instead may contain immunoglobulin. The tumor may be an uncommon variety of follicle center cell lymphoma, so-called signet ring cell lymphoma, in which lymphoma cells produce and retain immunoglobulin in large intracytoplasmic vacuoles (267) (see Chapter 24). Demonstration of intracellular mucin with an appropriate histochemical stain suggests epithelial differentiation, but is not specific for it. Evaluation with antibodies to cytokeratin, CD45, and immunoglobulin light chains may also be useful, especially when intracytoplasmic mucin is not readily identified. Rarely, liposarcomas, epithelioid hemangioendotheliomas, malignant melanomas, and rhabdoid carcinomas may contain cytoplasmic inclusions with eccentric, deformed nuclei (268). Nodal muciphages (269) and macrophages that contain mucicarmine-positive polyvinyl-pyrrolidone (PVP) (270) may also mimic metastatic poorly differentiated carcinoma. Attention to the clinical history and immunophenotype prevents misdiagnosis.

Other Poorly Differentiated Carcinomas

Adrenal cortical carcinoma can be difficult to diagnose because of its histologic overlap with renal clear cell carcinomas, hepatocellular carcinomas, pheochromocytomas and melanomas. Its very frequent lack of expression of cytokeratin and EMA (271) may even cause confusion with a mesenchymal neoplasm. Although vimentin expression could be useful, recent reports concerning monoclonal antibody A103 are very promising; this antibody recognizes Melan-A, an antigen associated with melanocytic differentiation in melanocytes (272).

Metastatic carcinosarcomas, also known as malignant mixed mullerian tumors when they occur in the female genital tract, are relatively uncommon tumors. They can sometimes be distinguished from metastatic carcinoma because they usually demonstrate malignant mesenchymal and malignant epithelial differentiation, at least focally. However, it is not uncommon for the metastases of carcinosarcoma to fail to show biphasic (mixed epithelial and mesenchymal) characteristics. That is, carcinosarcoma may be associated with metastatic deposits that appear carcinomatous or sarcomatous only (273).

It is well known that carcinomas and malignant melanomas can exhibit a spindle cell morphology. In these instances, in addition to a thorough clinical history, immunohistochemical evaluation can be very informative. Cytokeratin expression is usually supportive of epithelial differentiation. Although this usually indicates carcinoma, carcinosarcoma or sarcomatous carcinoma, one should not exclude primary soft tissue tumors that show epithelial differentiation, such as monophasic synovial sarcoma, based on the immunohistochemistry results alone. Most primary soft tissue spindle cell sarcomas also express cytokeratin (274). In these tumors, cytokeratin expression is generally not strong or diffuse or detectable with numerous cytokeratin antibodies. If a primary soft tissue spindle cell sarcoma is considered, one should be in the possession of a complete and supportive clinical history and should be aware of the fact that nodal metastasis of primary soft tissue spindle cell sarcomas is rare. S-100 protein expression supports the diagnosis of metastatic melanoma, although it does not exclude soft tissue spindle cell sarcoma, especially metastatic malignant peripheral nerve sheath tumor. Knowledge of the patient's clinical history is particularly important in such distinctions.

Differentiated Adenocarcinoma

The most common and most important obviously glandular lesion to recognize in lymph nodes is metastatic adenocarcinoma. Because of the presence of glands, this entity should not be confused with malignant lymphoma unless the lymphoma demonstrates numerous pseudorosettes, which may simulate glands (275,276). We include a discussion of these well and moderately differentiated adenocarcinomas in this chapter to outline effective ways of determining the primary site of origin. A complete clinical history is often contributory, of course. When the clinical history and the morphologic features of the lesion in question do not aid in determination of the primary site of origin, immunohistochemical analysis may be beneficial.

Some metastatic adenocarcinomas, such as prostatic and well differentiated thyroid carcinoma, exhibit very characteristic immunophenotypes that aid in their correct identification. More than 90% of prostatic adenocarcinomas express prostate-specific antigen (PSA), prostatic acid phosphatase (PSAP), or both (277–280). However, because very poorly differentiated prostatic carcinomas may not express these antigens, other antibodies should be included in the panel; strong expression of CK7 and CK20, mCEA, and CA 19-9 are unusual in prostate carcinoma (30,280,281). Hindgut carcinoids may express PSAP as well (282,283). If carcinoid tumor is in the differential diagnosis, the appropriate neuroendocrine markers should be included in the panel, but caution is advised because some aggressive prostate cancers express neuroendocrine markers (284).

Papillary and follicular carcinomas of the thyroid gland express thyroglobulin and many papillary carcinomas express S-100 and mCEA (285,286); thyroglobulin is very useful in identifying tumors with thyroid differentiation. Medullary carcinomas express calcitonin in addition to neuroendocrine markers (287). Anaplastic carcinomas may lack thyroglobulin and cytokeratin expression (288).

Although most of the other adenocarcinomas do not demonstrate specific immunophenotypes, the use of cytokeratins 7 and 20 permits separation into groups used to narrow the differential diagnosis (30) (Fig. 30.17). The $CK7^{+}CK20^{+}$ phenotype is characteristic of transitional cell carcinoma, pancreatic/biliary adenocarcinoma, and ovarian mucinous adenocarcinoma; these tumors often express mCEA and CA 19-9 as well (289,290). Antibodies against estrogen and progesterone receptors and CA 125 may permit separation of ovarian mucinous tumors from the others, although none of these markers is specific.

Pulmonary, breast, nonmucinous ovarian, and endometrial carcinomas, as well as mesotheliomas, demonstrate a $CK7^{+}CK20^{-}$ phenotype (30). Some subtypes of renal cell carcinomas also exhibit the $CK7^{+}CD20^{-}$ phenotype (291). Strong, diffuse, cytoplasmic mCEA reactivity often permits distinction of pulmonary adenocarcinoma from the other possibilities (292). The expression of villin appears to support the diagnosis of a pulmonary carcinoma in the $CK7^{+}CK20^{-}$ category (293). CD15 expression, in addition to mCEA, Ber-EP4, and B72.3 expression, helps separate pulmonary adenocarcinomas from mesothelioma, which lacks these antigenic markers (294–299). There are reports

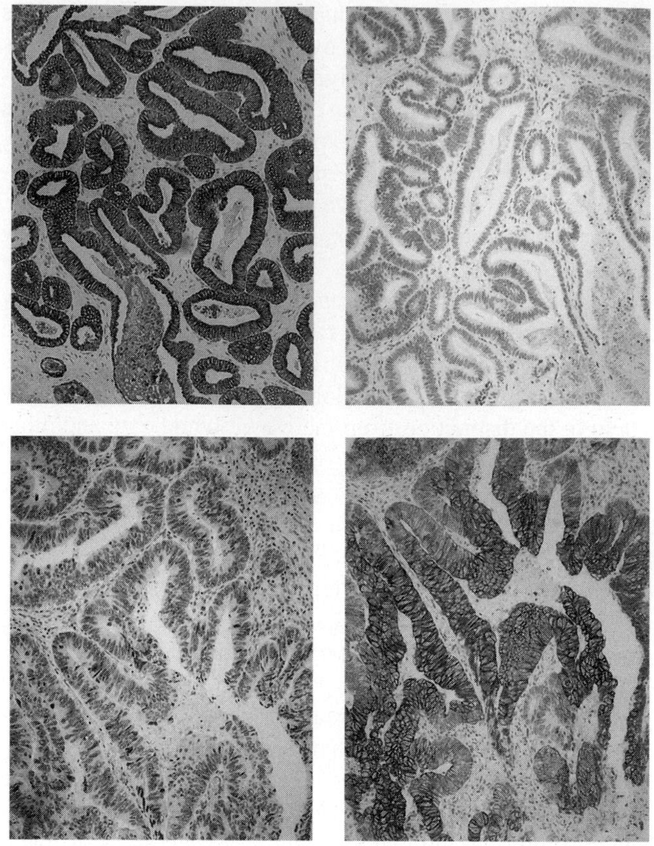

A,C

B,D

FIG. 30.17. Immunostaining with monoclonal anti-cytokeratin 7 and 20 antibodies. Immunostaining with antibodies recognizing cytokeratins 7 and 20 is useful in the distinction between gynecologic and lower gastrointestinal tract carcinomas. The left panels show a metastatic endometrioid adenocarcinoma from the ovary that expresses cytokeratin 7 (**A**) but not cytokeratin 20 (**B**). The right panels show a metastatic colonic adenocarcinoma that lacks cytokeratin 7 (**C**) but expresses cytokeratin 20 (**D**) (immunoperoxidase stain, original magnification: 40× magnification).

that calretinin and cytokeratins 5 and 6 are useful in the positive identification of mesothelioma (300–302). Breast, ovarian, and endometrial carcinomas frequently express estrogen, progesterone, or both receptors. At least 40% to 50% of breast carcinomas express brst-2 (303,304). More details on the immunophenotype of breast carcinoma was provided earlier in the discussion on mammary lobular carcinoma. Colorectal adenocarcinoma is predominantly $CK7^{-}CK20^{+}$. Other tumors that are less commonly $CK7^{-}CK20^{+}$ include gastric and, rarely, prostatic adenocarcinomas (30).

Hepatocellular and prostatic adenocarcinomas, as well as some renal cell carcinomas, are characteristically predominantly $CK7^{-}CK20^{-}$ (30). Because a significant minority of hepatocellular (HCC) and pancreaticobiliary carcinomas may express the $CK7^{+}CK20^{-}$ phenotype, additional antibodies may be useful. Less than 30% of HCCs express α-fetoprotein (305). Canalicular staining with polyclonal CEA is even more commonly encountered in HCC (306,307). Distinctive cytokeratin expression is commonly observed in HCC; low-molecular-weight cytokeratins (e.g., CAM 5.2) are expressed in HCC, whereas pancytokeratins (AE1/AE3) and high-molecular-weight cytokeratin expression is less common (308). Pancreaticobiliary carcinomas generally express both AE1/AE3 and CAM 5.2. They also express CA 19-9 and CU18, while expression of these antigens in HCC is rare (309,310).

Malignant Melanoma

Malignant melanomas often exhibit an intrasinusoidal distribution within lymph nodes. The cells tend to be less cohesive then those that comprise most other epithelial neoplasms. Moreover, melanoma cells often possess abundant eosinophilic cytoplasm and large vesicular nuclei that contain large prominent, centrally placed nucleoli (311) (Fig. 30.18). For these reasons, malignant melanomas may closely resemble malignant lymphomas in their growth pattern and cytomorphologically. They may be confused easily with immunoblastic and $CD30^+$ anaplastic large cell lymphomas and vice versa. Malignant melanoma is also well known for its propensity to recur and metastasize after a prolonged asymptomatic period. For all these reasons a complete clinical history may aid in the diagnosis of malignant melanoma that is metastatic to lymph nodes.

An epithelial pattern may be demonstrated with a reticulin stain, and melanin granules may be demonstrated with a silver stain or ultrastructurally. Identification of melanin pigment in a malignant neoplasm is generally considered confirmatory of malignant melanoma, although many melanomas are not pigmented, and other neoplasms, such as psammomatous melanotic schwannoma (312) and pheochromocytoma (313), may contain melanin. Benign melanocytic nevi of lymph nodes also may be pigmented (70–73). Attention to morphologic detail and clinical history is useful. The classic morphologic appearance of metastatic malignant melanoma is an epithelioid neoplasm comprising round to polygonal cells with large nucleoli that contain prominent nucleoli. However, melanoma may assume other appearances, including spindle cell and rhabdoid morphology (314). Rarely, melanomas may contain vacuolated cytoplasm similar to that seen in signet ring cells (268). Because of these features, the differential diagnosis of malignant melanoma is lengthy and includes poorly differentiated carcinoma, malignant lymphoma, and certain sarcomas.

When the clinical history is not forthcoming or it is confounding and the lesion in question is not obviously pigmented, immunohistochemical analysis may be useful and supersede these other ancillary approaches in supporting the diagnosis of malignant melanoma. Malignant melanoma is almost always negative for cytokeratins and CD45 (315,316). More than 90% of malignant melanomas express the S-100 protein (317). However, because S-100 protein expression is not specific for melanocytic differentiation, one must interpret S-100 expression in combination with the results of other immunohistochemical studies and the morphologic impression. Carcinomas (318–320), various

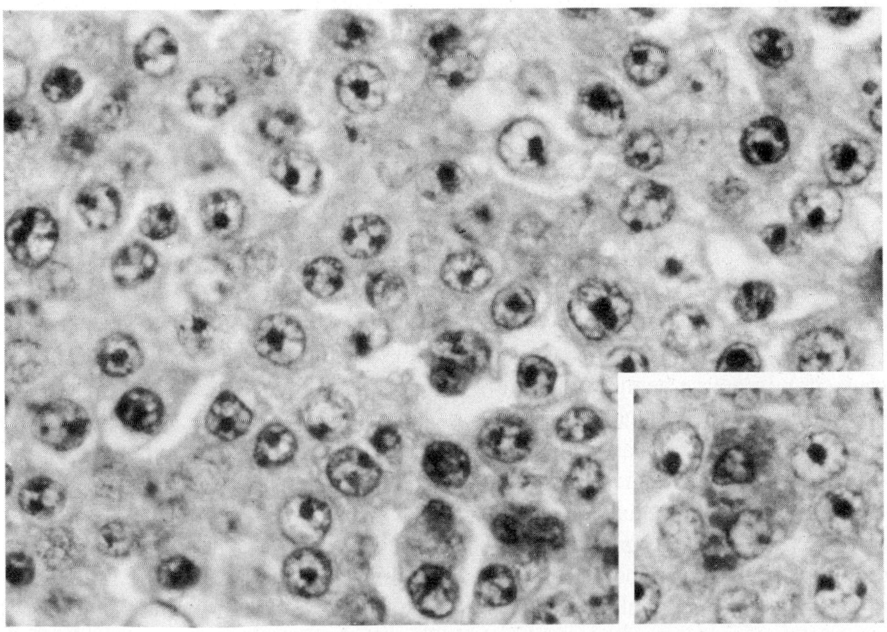

FIG. 30.18. Malignant melanoma metastatic to lymph node. The malignant melanoma cells grow in a diffuse sheet. They possess abundant cytoplasm and large round nuclei that contain prominent central nucleoli, simulating diffuse large cell lymphoma. In this case, melanophages that contain melanin pigment were found within the tumor, providing evidence of the melanocytic nature of this neoplasm (hematoxylin and eosin, original magnification: 630× magnification).

sarcomas (e.g., clear cell sarcoma, malignant peripheral nerve sheath sarcoma), and some hematolymphoid neoplasms, including histiocytic (321,322) and dendritic cell tumors (323), may express S-100 protein. HMB-45 is also expressed in more than 50% of melanomas and is more specific for melanocytic differentiation than S-100 (324,325). However, melanomas with spindle-shaped cells rarely express HMB-45 (326). HMB-45 may be expressed in angiomyolipoma and lymphangioleiomyomatosis, benign lesions that rarely involve lymph nodes (327,328). Expression of Melan-A, recognized by monoclonal antibody A103, may be more sensitive for melanocytic differentiation than HMB-45 (272). Rare melanomas with rhabdoid cytoplasm have been reported to express desmin (314). Malignant melanomas also have been reported to express CD10 and CD57 (329).

Germ Cell Tumors

Seminomas and other germ cell tumors may be mistaken for malignant lymphoma morphologically because the tumor cells possess abundant, often clear, cytoplasm and large vesicular nuclei containing prominent nucleoli; exhibit frequent mitotic figures; and grow diffusely (330). They are most commonly mistaken for immunoblastic lymphoma, anaplastic large cell lymphoma or even Hodgkin's disease. The distinction between seminoma and malignant lymphoma is often straightforward, however, given a complete clinical history and careful morphologic examination. For example, testicular seminoma characteristically affects men in the third and fourth decades, whereas testicular non-Hodgkin's lymphoma principally affects men in the seventh decade and beyond (331); the exception is testicular lymphoma occurring in HIV-infected men (332). It may be more difficult to distinguish between germ cell tumors, especially seminoma, and malignant lymphoma when disease is limited to the mediastinum. Evaluation for α-fetoprotein (AFP) and β-human chorionic gonadotrophin (β-HCG) may aid in the differential diagnosis between germ cell tumors and malignant lymphomas in some instances.

The malignant cells comprising seminoma in the male and dysgerminoma in the female may occur in variably sized nests that may be separated by aggregates of small lymphocytes and even by fibrous strands. These benign small lymphocyte aggregates are absent from immunoblastic lymphomas. The sinusoidal architecture of anaplastic large cell lymphoma is absent as are large malignant cells with wreathlike nuclei. Conceivably, some seminoma cells may be mistaken for mononuclear Reed-Sternberg cell variants, but classic Reed-Sternberg cells should be absent. Lacunae are distinctly uncommon as are well-developed fibrous septa. Occasionally, granulomatous inflammation can obscure the classic histopathologic features of seminoma, resulting in misdiagnosis (333) (Fig. 30.19).

Immunohistochemical studies may be of additional help in distinguishing between these entities. In general, seminoma

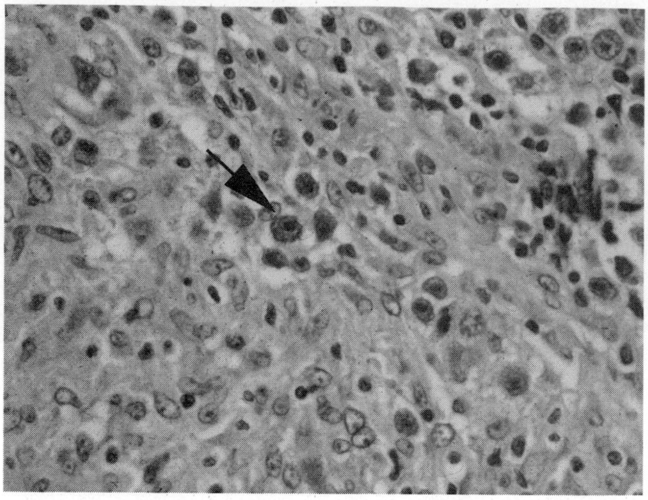

FIG. 30.19. Metastatic seminoma. The identification of metastatic seminoma is usually straightforward when the complete clinical history is known and the lesion demonstrates all of the classic histopathologic features. However, on occasion, the neoplastic cells of seminoma may be obscured by a prominent granulomatous response, as illustrated here. The arrow indicates an isolated seminoma cell surrounded by abundant epithelioid histiocytes. The neoplastic cells characteristically possess clear cytoplasm and round vesicular nuclei containing a prominent, centrally placed nucleolus (hematoxylin and eosin, original magnification: 400× magnification).

cells do not express CD45 (334) or other lymphoid cell antigens but do express placental alkaline phosphatase (PLAP) (335,336). Although PLAP was once thought to be specific for seminoma, trophoblasts, and the cells of intratubular germ cell neoplasms, it has become clear that PLAP expression alone is insufficient to support an unequivocal diagnosis of seminoma because it is expressed in carcinomas and other germ cell tumors (337,338). If metastatic carcinoma is a possibility, immunohistochemical staining for cytokeratin may be helpful. However, although seminoma was once considered to be a cytokeratin-negative neoplasm, there are numerous reports of cytokeratin expression in seminoma (339,340). Cytokeratin expression in seminoma is probably not common, however, and when it occurs, it is usually weak and patchy in distribution. Strong, diffuse cytokeratin expression in a lesion thought to be seminoma is unusual, and it should prompt the pathologist to consider metastatic carcinoma or another germ cell tumor. The syncytiotrophoblastic giant cells in seminoma express β-HCG; choriocarcinoma should not be diagnosed unless a biphasic proliferation of both cytotrophoblasts and syncytiotrophoblasts is identified. β-HCG is also expressed by a variety of poorly differentiated carcinomas (341). Identification of AFP in the serum or in sections from a lesion thought to be a pure seminoma should probably prompt a search for a yolk sac tumor.

Yolk sac tumors, choriocarcinoma, and embryonal carcinoma may share many features with other carcinomas, including cellular cohesion and growth in nests, tubules, trabeculae, and sheets. These features, in addition to expression of cytokeratins, aid in the distinction from malignant lymphoma. However, embryonal carcinoma and some lymphomas, including Hodgkin's disease, express CD30 (342). Expression of CD30 in nonhematopoietic tumors is unusual and, for the most part, limited to embryonal carcinoma. There are rare reports of CD30 expression in other carcinomas (342,343).

Sarcomas

Sarcomas arising in the soft tissues metastasize infrequently to lymph nodes (244,344). Recognition of metastatic sarcoma is usually relatively straightforward. As in the case of poorly differentiated carcinomas, malignant melanomas, and other neoplasms, sarcomas occasionally may be incorrectly diagnosed as malignant lymphoma and vice versa. Those sarcomas that resemble malignant lymphoma and therefore most commonly lead to difficulties in differential diagnosis are the small round cell sarcomas, such as Ewing's sarcoma, synovial sarcoma, and epithelioid sarcoma. In a background of diffuse fibrosis, some sarcomatous spindle cell proliferations may mimic lymphocyte depletion Hodgkin's disease. Cases of Hodgkin's disease that contain numerous neutrophils may mimic inflammatory fibrous histiocytoma. Focal cellular areas of malignant fibrous histiocytoma may simulate a large cell lymphoma, just like those sarcomas in which the malignant cells lack cohesion.

Small Round Cell Sarcomas

Ewing's sarcoma, primitive neuroectodermal tumor, embryonal and alveolar rhabdomyosarcoma, and desmoplastic small round cell tumor occur most commonly in children and young adults (345). They may mimic a small cell carcinoma, neuroblastoma, lymphoblastic lymphoma, or diffuse large cell lymphoma. Clinical features may help in the differential diagnosis. Morphologic features, such as the presence of rosette formation, rhabdomyoblasts, or desmoplastic stroma, for example, may be helpful; however, these tumors often have cells with scant cytoplasm and small- to moderate-sized nuclei with finely dispersed chromatin, features that may result in the mistaken diagnosis of lymphoblastic lymphoma. In these instances, the presence of glycogen in the cytoplasm may lead to a diagnosis of Ewing's sarcoma, although this is not, by any means, specific for Ewing's sarcoma. The identification of cytoplasmic cross-striations justifies the diagnosis of rhabdomyosarcoma; unfortunately, this finding is uncommon (345).

In most instances, immunohistochemical studies should be performed to provide a definitive answer. Ewing's sarcoma may be distinguished from all malignant lymphomas by its lack of CD45 and B- and T-cell–associated antigens. However, Ewing's sarcoma cells express CD99 (346,347), a product of the *MIC2* pseudoautosomal gene (348), and lymphoblastic lymphomas also express CD99 (349,350). Immunostains for terminal deoxynucleotidyl transferase (TdT) (positive in lymphoblastic lymphoma) (351) and desmin (positive in rhabdomyosarcoma) (43) should be performed in addition to CD99 when confronted with this differential diagnosis. Other markers (i.e., NSE and CD57) are occasionally expressed, and cytokeratins are rarely expressed in Ewing's sarcoma (352–354). Because there is controversy regarding the distinction of Ewing's sarcoma from primitive neuroectodermal tumor, some investigators accept chromogranin and synaptophysin in Ewing's sarcoma (355). Both tumors demonstrate the t(11;22) (356,357) and are treated identically.

Rhabdomyosarcomas are characteristically positive for desmin and muscle actin (HHF-35) (43). Desmin-positive tumor cells are also inconspicuous in less well differentiated rhabdomyosarcomas (358). Neuron-specific enolase and CD57 can be detected in myogenic tumors. MyoD1, an antigen recognized in frozen tissue, and myogenin have been identified in rhabdomyosarcoma and are thought to be specific for skeletal muscle differentiation (359). There are only rare reports of CD99 expression in rhabdomyosarcoma (346,347,350). Rhabdomyosarcomas consistently lack S-100 and HMB-45 and similarly lack CD45 and B- and T-cell–associated antigens. Because the prognosis and therapy for embryonal rhabdomyosarcomas and alveolar rhabdomyosarcomas differ significantly (360), attention to morphologic detail is essential; however, consistent immunohistochemical differences have not been described. The characteristic presence of t(2;13) and t(2;8) in alveolar rhabdomyosarcomas permits their distinction from embryonal rhabdomyosarcomas (361).

Desmoplastic small round cell tumor (DSRCT) shares the t(11;22) with Ewing's sarcoma and primitive neuroectodermal tumor, although the fusion protein differs (362). Desmoplastic small round cell tumor is also immunohistochemically distinct from these neoplasms; DSRCT expresses cytokeratins, desmin, and S-100 protein and lacks CD99 (363).

Neuroblastoma can mimic lymphoblastic lymphoma histologically. Both of these lesions are characterized by a sheetlike growth pattern of small- to medium-sized cells that possess scanty cytoplasm, nuclei containing finely stippled nuclear chromatin, and abundant mitotic figures. Rosettes are not always a conspicuous feature of neuroblastoma (364). Clinical correlation sometimes may be useful in distinguishing between these two entities; however, clinical correlation often does not provide a definitive answer, and immunohistochemical studies should then be used. Neuroblastoma cells frequently express NSE, synaptophysin, CD57, S-100 and neural filaments. They consistently lack CD45, TdT, and B- and T-cell–associated antigens (364,365), all immunophenotypic characteristics associated with lymphoblastic lymphoma. CD99 is not expressed, making the distinction from Ewing's sarcoma, primitive neuroectodermal tumor, and lymphoblastic lymphoma relatively straightforward (346,347,350) (see Chapter 26).

Synovial Sarcoma and Epithelioid Sarcoma

These sarcomatous lesions infrequently involve lymph nodes and therefore only occasionally present a diagnostic problem to the pathologist. If the epithelial component predominates or is the exclusive component in the lymph node metastasis, the possibility of confusing either of these with a carcinoma or malignant lymphoma becomes evident. The features previously attributed to undifferentiated carcinomas hold true for the epithelial components of both of these biphasic sarcomas. Immunohistochemically, they usually express cytokeratin and EMA, but they consistently lack CD45 and B- and T-cell–associated antigens (366). To help in the distinction from carcinoma, many epithelioid sarcomas express CD34 (367), and many synovial sarcomas express CD99 (368); both of these markers are only rarely expressed in carcinoma (369,370). Synovial sarcoma possesses a distinctive genotype: t(x;18) (371). Poorly differentiated variants of synovial sarcoma have been described recently (372,373); these tumors show considerable morphologic similarity to Ewing's sarcoma/primitive neuroectodermal tumor but can be distinguished from this group of neoplasms with immunohistochemistry and genotyping.

Clear Cell Sarcoma

Clear cell sarcoma is similarly a neoplasm of young adults and only rarely involves lymph nodes (374). It is characterized by aggregates of tumor cells that possess clear cytoplasm and prominent, centrally placed nucleoli (374). Clear cell sarcoma was previously known as malignant melanoma of soft parts (374). Reports confirm a unique genotype, t(12; 22), that has not been identified in malignant melanomas (375). In any case, it is worthwhile to remember its previous designation only to emphasize the similarity in immunophenotype to malignant melanoma; clear cell sarcomas almost uniformly express S-100 protein and HMB-45 (376).

Metastatic Sarcoma with Glandular Differentiation

Rarely, sarcomas demonstrating glandular differentiation can metastasize to lymph nodes. These sarcomas include synovial sarcoma, malignant peripheral nerve sheath tumor and endometrial stromal sarcoma.

NONLYMPHOID HEMATOPOIETIC DISORDERS THAT MIMIC MALIGNANT LYMPHOMA

Extramedullary Myeloid Tumor

Extramedullary myeloid tumor (i.e., granulocytic sarcoma) is a localized, tumor-like proliferation of immature cells that belongs to the myeloid lineage (377). Extramedullary myeloid tumor may occur as a localized tissue manifestation in patients who have acute myeloid leukemia, as a sign of impending blast crisis in chronic myelogenous leukemia or leukemic transformation in patients who have myelodysplastic disorders, or as a forerunner of acute myeloid leukemia in nonleukemic patients (377). Extramedullary myeloid tumors most frequently involve soft tissues, lymph nodes, and skin or occur as isolated lytic bone lesions (377).

Extramedullary myeloid tumors exhibit a spectrum of morphologic features (Fig. 30.20). Approximately 50% of cases contain occasional to numerous eosinophilic myelocytes indicative of myeloid differentiation. These cases are generally recognizable in routine histologic sections. The remaining 50% of cases are composed of cells that contain round, ovoid, or reniform immature blastlike nuclei with finely stippled chromatin and one or two small nucleoli. These neoplastic cells of myeloid derivation may be mistaken for those that constitute various intermediate and high-grade malignant lymphomas (377,378). Alternatively, especially in children, these lesions may be misinterpreted as rhabdomyosarcomas, neuroblastomas, or other nonhematopoietic neoplasms (378). A correct diagnosis usually can be made with the assistance of appropriate immunohistochemical studies capable of demonstrating myeloid-associated antigens, lysozyme, or naphthol-ASD-chloracetate esterase (i.e., Leder stain) in the neoplastic cells. However, several antigens, including CD45, CD43, and CD34 (377), are expressed by extramedullary myeloid tumors and by malignant lymphomas (see Chapter 47).

Mast Cell Disease

An uncontrolled proliferation of mast cells that occurs locally or systemically is usually referred to as mastocytosis or mast cell disease. Mast cell proliferations most commonly involve the dermis, where they form small, localized tumors (mastocytomas) or disseminate throughout the dermis, resulting in urticaria pigmentosa (379). Mast cell proliferations may involve multiple organs, however, including lymph nodes, whether accompanied by cutaneous manifestations or not. These are referred to as systemic mast cell disease (SMCD) (380).

Lymph nodes appear to be involved in about 25% or more of cases of SMCD (381). The mast cells preferentially infiltrate the cortical and paracortical areas where they surround and partially infiltrate the follicles and vessels. Most mast cells are round, have abundant clear cytoplasm, and contain only a few metachromatic granules; fusiform mast cells are usually infrequent. Even when present, however, spindle mast cells cannot be distinguished from connective tissue fibroblasts without special stains. These morphologic features, combined with the failure to consider SMCD in the differential diagnosis, frequently lead to the mistaken diagnosis of malignant lymphoma or sometimes hairy cell leukemia (380,381).

The clinical findings may be helpful in pointing the pathologist toward the correct diagnosis. Histologically, the dimorphic nature of the infiltrate, when present, is helpful, as is the frequent accompaniment of the mast cells by clusters of eosinophils. Wright-Giemsa–stained touch prepara-

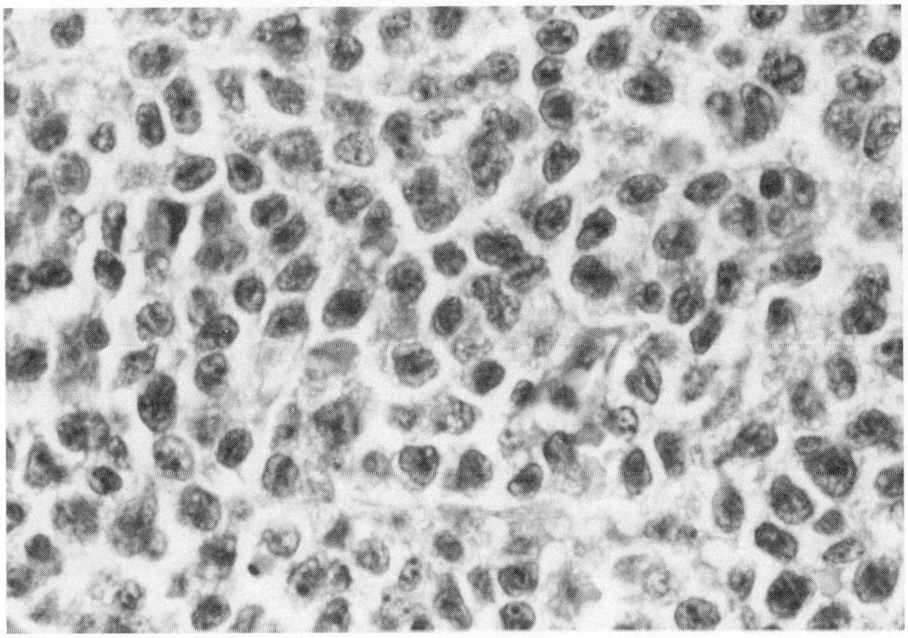

FIG. 30.20. Granulocytic sarcoma in lymph node. This 35-year-old man presented with cervical lymphadenopathy, and malignant lymphoma was suspected. The lymph node biopsy showed diffuse replacement by a monotonous population of neoplastic cells that contained moderately abundant cytoplasm and irregularly shaped, ovoid to reniform nuclei with stippled chromatin and one or two small nucleoli. These neoplastic cells contained lysozyme and chloroacetate esterase, consistent with a myeloid derivation and granulocytic sarcoma. Overt acute myeloid leukemia developed 4 months later (hematoxylin and eosin, original magnification: 630× magnification).

tions of the lymph node biopsy provide an excellent means of identifying the mast cells. Alternatively, toluidine blue stains of paraffin tissue sections are useful in highlighting the metachromatic granules (1). Immunophenotypic analysis of frozen and paraffin tissue sections sometimes may be helpful because mast cells exhibit immunophenotypic features distinct from those of B and T cells (see Chapter 52).

Dendritic Cell Neoplasms

It is extremely uncommon to encounter a neoplasm derived from follicular dendritic cells, interdigitating dendritic cells and fibroblastic reticular cells. These neoplasms all share storiform and interlacing fascicular growth. The constituent ovoid and spindle cells contain nuclei with smooth nuclear membranes and small central eosinophilic nucleoli. Cytologically atypical multinucleate cells with prominent nuclear pseudoinclusions have also been reported. Admixed lymphocytes and plasma cells are common. These tumors may also show hemorrhage and necrosis as well as significant mitotic indices (382–385) (Fig. 30.21).

The distinction among follicular dendritic cell, interdigitating dendritic cell, and fibroblastic reticular cell neoplasms depends primarily on the immunohistochemical profile and the ultrastructural features. Follicular dendritic cells express vimentin, CD21, CD68, and occasionally, CD35 and S-100 (386–388). The Epstein-Barr virus genome has been found in follicular dendritic cell tumors as well (230). Interdigitating dendritic cell tumors express vimentin, CD68 and S-100, but they lack CD21 and CD35 (386,389). The fibroblastic reticular cell tumor expresses vimentin, CD68, smooth muscle actin or desmin, and factor XIII (386, 390,391).

The prognosis of these tumors can be difficult to predict because of the variation in morphologic appearance from case to case and the paucity of large clinicopathologic studies with adequate follow-up data. The follicular dendritic cell tumor, often referred to as *follicular dendritic sarcoma,* is capable of recurrence and metastasis, resulting in death (382–384,392). Significant cytologic atypia, necrosis, and an elevated mitotic index are features that have been suggested to indicate the possibility of an aggressive clinical course. Follicular dendritic cell tumors may coexist with Castleman's disease of the hyaline-vascular, plasma cell, and mixed types (393). Interdigitating dendritic cell tumors are said to be more aggressive than follicular dendritic cell tumors (384,385,394). The two cases of fibroblastic reticular cell tumors with reported follow-up have pursued a benign clinical course (386) (see Chapter 51).

One must consider numerous entities in the differential diagnosis of dendritic cell neoplasms. If metastatic carcinoma, malignant melanoma, and other primary and metastatic sarcomas are excluded with attention to clinical history, morphologic detail, and immunophenotype, palisaded myofibroblastoma, true histiocytic lymphoma, and thymoma should also be considered. The distinction between reticu-

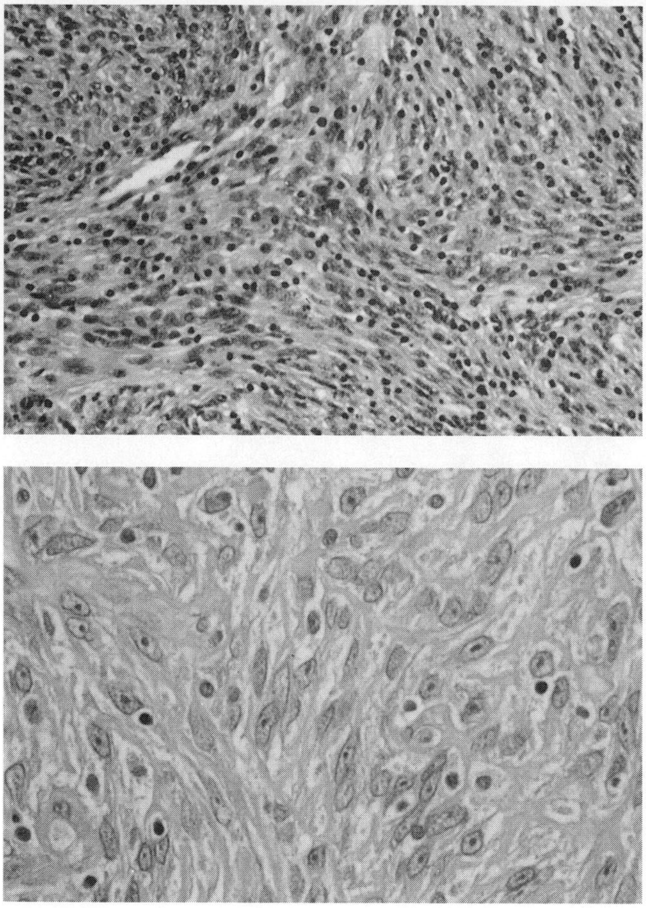

A

B

FIG. 30.21. Follicular dendritic cell tumor. The histologic appearance of the follicular dendritic cell tumor is reminiscent of other spindle cell proliferations such as neoplasms exhibiting fibroblastic, smooth muscle, neuroplastic, or metaplastic epithelial differentiation. **A:** Follicular dendritic cell tumor is composed of fascicles of spindle cells possessing pointed and elongated hyperchromatic nuclei. A reactive lymphoid infiltrate is present. The distinction of this lesion from other primary and metastatic lesions rests on clinical history and immunohistochemical findings. Follicular dendritic cell tumors express CD21, CD68, and, occasionally, CD35 and S-100 (hematoxylin and eosin, original magnification: 200× magnification). **B:** In this instance, the constituent cells possess elongate, vesicular nuclei containing prominent nucleoli (hematoxylin and eosin, original magnification: 400× magnification). (Photomicrographs courtesy of Dr. Glauco Frizzera, Weill Medical College of Cornell University, New York, NY.)

lum cell tumors and carcinomas can be difficult, especially given the report of cytokeratin-positive tumors with reticulum cell morphology (395).

SUMMARY AND CONCLUSIONS

A large and diverse variety of benign and malignant nonhematopoietic elements and proliferations may be encountered in lymph nodes. The benign elements include epithelial and mesenchymal congenital malformations, inclusions, and proliferations that must be distinguished from malignant neoplasms that secondarily involve lymph nodes. The malignant elements include a spectrum of primary and secondary epithelial and mesenchymal neoplasms that must be distinguished from a lymphoproliferative disorder, usually malignant lymphoma. Several nonlymphoid hematopoietic proliferations also may occur in lymph nodes and can be confused with malignant lymphoma. These pathologic processes usually can be recognized and interpreted correctly, based on careful evaluation of their histopathologic features in conjunction with the clinical findings. The judicious use of immunohistochemistry serves as a useful adjunct to diagnosis and may contribute significantly to the accurate diagnosis of poorly differentiated neoplasms difficult to classify by histopathologic criteria alone.

REFERENCES

1. Kant JA, Jaffe ES. The interpretation of non-lymphoid elements in lymph node biopsy specimens. In: Jaffe E, ed. *Surgical pathology of the lymph nodes and related organs.* Philadelphia: WB Saunders, 1985:412–437.
2. Ramaekers FC, Puts JJ, Moesker O, et al. Antibodies to intermediate filament proteins in the immunohistochemical identification of human tumours: an overview. *Histochem J* 1983;15:691–713.
3. Miettinen M. Immunohistochemistry of soft-tissue tumors: possibilities and limitations in surgical pathology. *Pathol Annu* 1990;25:1–36.
4. Sheibani K, Tubbs RR. Enzyme immunohistochemistry: technical aspects. *Semin Diag Pathol* 1984;1:235–250.
5. Miller RT, Estran C. Heat-induced epitope retrieval with a pressure cooker: suggestions for optimal use. *Appl Immunohistochem* 1995;3:190–193.
6. Fan Z, Clark V, Nagle RB. An evaluation of enzymatic and heat epitope retrieval methods for the immuhohistochemical staining of the intermediate filaments. *Appl Immunohistochem* 1997;5:49–58.
7. Kuroki M, Yamanaka T, Matsuo T, et al. Immunohistochemical analysis of carcinoembryonic antigen (CEA) related antigens differentially localized in intracellular granules of human neutrophils. *Immunol Invest* 1996;219:842–847.
8. Alvarez-Gago T, Bullon MM, Rivera F, et al. Intermediate filament aggregates in mitoses of primary cutaneous neuroendocrine (Merkel cell) carcinoma. *Histopathology* 1996;28:349–355.
9. Blessing K, Sanders DS, Grant JJ. Comparison of immunohistochemical staining of the novel antibody melan-A with S100 protein and HMB-45 in malignant melanoma and melanoma variants. *Histopathology* 1998;32:139–146.
10. Michie SA, Spagnolo DV, Dunn KA, et al. A panel approach to the evaluation of the sensitivity and specificity of antibodies for the diagnosis of routinely processed histologically undifferentiated human neoplasms. *Am J Clin Pathol* 1987;88:457–462.
11. Thomas ML, Lefrancois L. Differential expression of the leucocyte-common antigen family. *Immunol Today* 1988;9:320–326.
12. Pizzolo G, Sloane J, Beverley P, et al. Differential diagnosis of malignant lymphoma and nonlymphoid tumors using monoclonal anti-leukocyte antibody. *Cancer* 1980;46:2640–2647.
13. Battifora H, Trowbridge IS. A monoclonal antibody useful for the differential diagnosis between malignant lymphoma and non-hematopoietic neoplasms. *Cancer* 1983;51:816–821.
14. Warnke RA, Gatter KC, Falini B, et al. Diagnosis of human lymphoma with monoclonal antileukocyte antibodies. *N Engl J Med* 1983;309:1275–1281.
15. Kurtin PJ, Pinkus GS. Leukocyte common antigen, a diagnostic discriminant between hematopoietic and nonhematopoietic neoplasms in paraffin sections using monoclonal antibodies: correlation with immunologic studies and ultrastructural localization. *Hum Pathol* 1985;16:353–365.
16. Mason DY, Gatter KC. The role of immunohistochemistry in diagnostic pathology. *J Clin Pathol* 1987;40:1042–1054.

17. Harris NL, Bhan AK. Distribution of leukocyte common antigen (T-200) in B-cell neoplasia: T200 is lost in terminal B cell differentiation. *Lab Invest* 1985;52:28A.
18. Leoncini L, DelVecchio MT, Kraft R, et al. Hodgkin's disease and CD30 positive anaplastic large cell lymphomas, a continuous spectrum of malignant disorders: a quantitative morphometric and immunohistologic study. *Am J Pathol* 1990;137:1047–1057.
19. Strickler JG, Audeh MW, Copenhaver CM, et al. Immunophenotypic differences between plasmacytoma/multiple myeloma and immunoblastic lymphoma. *Cancer* 1988;61:1782–1786.
20. Azumi N, Battifora H. The distribution of vimentin and keratin in epithelial and nonepithelial neoplasms: a comprehensive immunohistochemical study on formalin- and alcohol-fixed tumors. *Am J Clin Pathol* 1987;88:286–296.
21. Thomas P, Battifora H. Keratins versus epithelial membrane antigen in tumor diagnosis: an immunohistochemical comparison of five monoclonal antibodies. *Hum Pathol* 1987;18:728–734.
22. Gustmann C, Altmannsberger M, Osborn M, et al. Cytokeratin expression and vimentin content in large cell anaplastic lymphomas and other non-Hodgkin's lymphomas. *Am J Pathol* 1991;138:1413–1422.
23. Miettinen M, Virtanen I, Damjanov I. Coexpression of keratin and vimentin in epithelioid sarcoma. *Am J Surg Pathol* 1985;9:460–463.
24. Brown DC, Theaker JM, Banks PM, et al. Cytokeratin expression in smooth muscle and smooth muscle tumors. *Histopathology* 1987;11: 477–486.
25. Norton AJ, Thomas JA, Isaacson PG. Cytokeratin-specific monoclonal antibodies are reactive with tumors of smooth muscle derivation: an immunocytochemical and biochemical study using antibodies to intermediate filament cytoskeletal proteins. *Histopathology* 1987; 11:487–499.
26. Miettinen M. Immunoreactivity for cytokeratin and epithelial membrane antigen in leiomyosarcoma. *Arch Pathol Lab Med* 1988;112: 637–640.
27. Huitfeldt HS, Brandtzaeg P. Various keratin antibodies produce immunohistochemical staining of human myocardium and myometrium. *Histochemistry* 1985;83:381–390.
28. Miettinen M, Fransila K. Immunohistochemical spectrum of malignant melanoma: the common presence of keratins. *Lab Invest* 1989; 61:623–628.
29. Zarbo RJ, Gown AM, Nagle RB, et al. Anomalous cytokeratin expression in malignant melanoma: one and two dimensional Western blot analysis and immunohistochemical survey of 100 melanomas. *Mod Pathol* 1990;3:494–501.
30. Wang NP, Zee S, Zarbo RJ, et al. Coordinate expression of cytokeratins 7 and 20 defines unique subsets of carcinomas. *Appl Immunohistochem* 1995;3:99–107.
31. Ceriani RL, Thompson K, Peterson JA, et al. Surface differentiation antigens of human mammary epithelial cells carried on the human milk fat globule. *Proc Natl Acad Sci USA* 1977;74:582–586.
32. Heyderman E, Steele K, Ormerod MG. A new antigen on the epithelial membrane: its immunoperoxidase localization in normal and neoplastic tissue. *J Clin Pathol* 1979;32:35–39.
33. Heyderman E, Strudley I, Powell G, et al. A new monoclonal antibody to epithelial membrane antigen (EMA)-E29: a comparison of its immunocytochemical reactivity with polyclonal anti-EMA antibodies and with another monoclonal antibody, HMFG-2. *Br J Cancer* 1985; 52:355–361.
34. Mattes MJ, Major PP, Goldenberg DM, et al. Patterns of antigen distribution in human carcinomas. *Cancer Res* 1990;50:880s–884s.
35. Strickler JG, Herndier BG, Rouse RV. Immunohistochemical staining in malignant mesotheliomas. *Am J Clin Pathol* 1987;88:610–614.
36. Pinkus GS, Kurtin PJ. Epithelial membrane antigen, a diagnostic discriminant in diagnostic pathology: immunohistochemical profile in epithelial, mesenchymal and hematopoietic neoplasms using paraffin sections and monoclonal antibodies. *Hum Pathol* 1985;19:929–940.
37. Ariza A, Bilbao JM, Rosai J. Immunohistochemical detection of epithelial membrane antigen in normal perineurial cells and perineurioma. *Am J Surg Pathol* 1988;12:678–683.
38. Delsol G, Gatter KC, Stein H, et al. Human lymphoid cells express epithelial membrane antigen: implications for diagnosis of human neoplasms. *Lancet* 1984;2:1124–1129.
39. Delsol G, Al-Saati TA, Gatter KC, et al. Coexpression of epithelial membrane antigen (EMA), Ki-1, and interleukin-2 receptor by anaplastic large cell lymphomas: diagnostic value in so-called malignant histiocytosis. *Am J Pathol* 1988;130:59–70.
40. Franke WW, Schmid E, Osborn M, et al. Different intermediate-sized filaments distinguished by immunofluorescence microscopy. *Proc Natl Acad Sci USA* 1978;75:5034–5038.
41. Dabbs DJ, Geisinger KR, Norris HT. Intermediate filaments in endometrial and endocervical carcinomas: the diagnostic utility of vimentin patterns. *Am J Surg Pathol* 1986;10:568–576.
42. Miettinen M, Lehto VP, Badley RA, et al. Alveolar rhabdomyosarcoma: demonstration of the muscle type of intermediate filament protein, desmin, as a diagnostic aid. *Am J Pathol* 1982;108:246–251.
43. Truong LD, Rangdaeng S, Cagle P, et al. The diagnostic utility of desmin: a study of 584 cases and review of the literature. *Am J Clin Pathol* 1990;93:305–314.
44. Seidal T, Kindblom LG, Angervall L. Myoglobin, desmin and vimentin in ultrastructurally proven rhabdomyomas and rhabdomyosarcomas: an immunohistochemical study utilizing a series of monoclonal and polyclonal antibodies. *Appl Pathol* 1987;5:201–219.
45. Miller F, Lazarides E, Elias J. Application of immunologic probes for contractile proteins to tissue sections. *Clin Immunol Immunopathol* 1976;5:416–428.
46. Miettinen M. Antibody specific to muscle actins in the diagnosis and classification of soft tissue tumors. *Am J Pathol* 1988;130:205–215.
47. Tsukada T, Tippens D, Gordon D, et al. HHF35, a muscle-actin-specific monoclonal antibody. I: Immunocytochemical and biochemical characterization. *Am J Pathol* 1987;126:51–60.
48. Tsukada T, McNutt MA, Ross R, et al. HHF35, a muscle-actin-specific monoclonal antibody. II: Reactivity in normal, reactive and neoplastic human tissues. *Am J Pathol* 1987;127:389–402.
49. Ozge-Anwar AH, Connell GE, Mustard JF. The activation of factor VIII by thrombin. *Blood* 1965;26:500–509.
50. McComb RD, Jones TR, Pizzo SV, et al. Specificity and sensitivity of immunohistochemical detection of factor VIII/von Willebrand factor antigen in formalin-fixed paraffin-embedded tissue. *J Histochem Cytochem* 1982;30:371–377.
51. Mukai K, Rosai J, Burgdorf WH. Localization of factor VIII-related antigen in vascular endothelial cells using an immunoperoxidase method. *Am J Surg Pathol* 1980;4:273–276.
52. Ordonez NG, Batsakis JG. Comparison of *Ulex europaeus* I lectin and factor VIII related antigen in vascular lesions. *Arch Pathol Lab Med* 1984;108:129–132.
53. Miettinen M, Lindenmayer AE, Chaubal A. Endothelial cell markers CD31, CD34, and BNH9 antibody to H- and Y-antigens: evaluation of their specificity and sensitivity in the diagnosis of vascular tumors and comparison with von Willebrand factor. *Mod Pathol* 1994;7: 82–90.
54. Traweek ST, Kandalaft PL, Mehta P, et al. The human hematopoietic progenitor cell antigen (CD34) in vascular neoplasia. *Am J Clin Pathol* 1991;96:25–31.
55. Ramani P, Bradley NJ, Fletcher CD. QBEND/10, a new monoclonal antibody to endothelium: assessment of its diagnostic utility in paraffin sections. *Histopathology* 1990;17:237–242.
56. Moore BW. A soluble protein characteristic of the nervous system. *Biochem Biophys Res Commun* 1965;19:739–744.
57. Nakajima T, Watanabe S, Sato Y, et al. An immunoperoxidase study of S-100 protein distribution in normal and neoplastic tissues. *Am J Surg Pathol* 1982;6:715–727.
58. Cocchia D, Lauriola L, Stolfi VM, et al. S-100 antigen labels neoplastic cells in liposarcoma and cartilaginous tumours. *Virchows Arch A Pathol Anat Histopathol* 1983;402:139–145.
59. Watanabe S, Nakajima T, Shimosato Y, et al. Malignant histiocytosis and Letterer-Siwe disease: neoplasms of T-zone histiocyte with S-100 protein. *Cancer* 1983;51:1412–1424.
60. Cochran AJ, Wen DR. S-100 protein as a marker for melanocytic and other tumours. *Pathology* 1985;17:340–345.
61. Kawahara E, Oda Y, Ooi A, et al. Expression of glial fibrillary acidic protein (GFAP) in peripheral nerve sheath tumors: a comparative study of immunoreactivity of GFAP, vimentin, S-100 protein, and neurofilament in 38 schwannomas and 18 neurofibromas. *Am J Surg Pathol* 1988;12:115–120.
62. Mazur MT, Shultz JJ, Myers JL. Granular cell tumor: immunohistochemical analyses of 21 benign tumors and one malignant tumor. *Arch Pathol Lab Med* 1990;114:692–696.
63. Drier JK, Swanson PE, Cherwitz DL, et al. S-100 protein immuno-

reactivity of poorly differentiated carcinomas: immunohistochemical comparison with malignant melanoma. *Arch Pathol Lab* Med 1987; 111:447–452.

64. Herrara GA, Turbat-Herrar EA, Lott RL. S-100 protein expression by primary and metastatic adenocarcinomas. *Am J Clin Pathol* 1988; 89:168–174.
65. Lloyd RV, Blaivas M, Wilson BS. Distribution of chromogranin and S-100 protein in normal and abnormal adrenal medullary tissues. *Arch Pathol Lab Med* 1985;109:633–635.
66. Marangos PJ, Polak JM, Pearse AGE. Neuron-specific enolase: a probe for neurons and neuroendocrine cells. *Trends Neurosci* 1982; 5:193–198.
67. Leader M, Collins M, Patel J, et al. Antineuron specific enolase staining reactions in sarcomas and carcinomas: its lack of neuroendocrine specificity. *J Clin Pathol* 1986;39:1186–1192.
68. Wiedenmann B, Franke WW. Identification and localization of synaptophysin, an integral membrane glycoprotein of MW 38,000 characteristic of presynaptic vesicles. *Cell* 1985;41:1017–1028.
69. Trojanowski JO. Immunohistochemistry of neural filament proteins and their diagnostic applications. In: DeLellis RA, ed. *Advances in immunohistochemistry*. New York: Raven Press, 1988:237–260.
70. Ridolfi RL, Rosen PP, Thaler H. Nevus cell aggregates associated with lymph nodes: estimated frequency and clinical significance. *Cancer* 1977;39:164–171.
71. Gadaleanu V, Muresan R. Inclusions of benign nevus cells in the capsule of axillary lymph nodes in three cases of breast cancer. *Morphol Embryol* 1984;30:137–139.
72. Azzopardi JG, Ross CM, Frizzera G. Blue naevi of lymph node capsule. *Histopathology* 1977;1:451–461.
73. Bansal RK, Bhaduri AS, Pancholi YJ, et al. Cellular blue nevus with nevus cells in regional lymph nodes: a lesion that mimics melanoma. *Indian J Cancer* 1989;26:149–150.
74. Johnson WT, Helwig EB. Benign nevus cells in the capsule of lymph nodes. *Cancer* 1969;23:747–753.
75. Hsu YK, Parmley TH, Rosenshein NB, et al. Neoplastic and non-neoplastic mesothelial proliferations in pelvic lymph nodes. *Obstet Gynecol* 1980;55:83–88.
76. Brooks JS, LiVolsi VA, Pietra GG. Mesothelial cell inclusions in mediastinal lymph nodes mimicking metastatic carcinoma. *Am J Clin Pathol* 1990;93:741–748.
77. Argani P, Rosai J. Hyperplastic mesothelial cells in lymph nodes: report of six cases of a benign process that can simulate metastatic involvement by mesothelioma or carcinoma. *Hum Pathol* 1988;29: 339–346.
78. Schnurr RC, Delgado G, Chun B. Benign glandular inclusions in para-aortic lymph nodes in women undergoing lymphadenectomies. *Am J Obstet Gynecol* 1978;130:813–816.
79. Mills SE. Decidua and squamous metaplasia in abdominopelvic lymph nodes. *Int J Gynecol Pathol* 1983;2:209–215.
80. Clement PB. Diseases of the peritoneum (including endometriosis) In: Kurman RJ, ed. *Blaustein's pathology of the female genital tract.* New York: Springer-Verlag, 1995:647–782.
81. Sampson JA. Peritoneal endometriosis due to menstrual dissemination of endometrial tissue into the peritoneal cavity. *Am J Obstet Gynecol* 1927;14:422–425.
82. Javert CT. Pathogenesis of endometriosis based upon endometrial homeoplasia, direct extension, exfoliation, and implantation: lymphocytic and hematogenous metastasis—including 5 case reports of endometrial tissue in pelvic lymph nodes. *Cancer* 1949;2:399–403.
83. Karp LA, Czernobilsky B. Glandular inclusions in pelvic and abdominal para-aortic lymph nodes: a study of autopsy and surgical material in males and females. *Am J Clin Pathol* 1969;52:212–218.
84. Huntrakoon M. Benign glandular inclusions in the abdominal lymph nodes of a man. *Hum Pathol* 1985;16:644–646.
85. Zanetti G. Epithelial inclusions and Tamm-Horsfall protein in para-nephric lymph nodes: a light microscopy and immunocytochemical study. *Virchow's Arch A Pathol Anat Histopathol* 1986;408:593–601.
86. Micheau C. Salivary ectopia: general review. *Arch Anat Pathol* 1969; 17:179–186.
87. Mair IW, Bjrang G, Kearney MS. Lateral cervical anomalies and salivary heterotopia. *Clin Otolaryngol* 1979;4:175–182.
88. Gricouroff G. Epithelial inclusions in the lymph nodes: diagnostic, histogenetic,and prognostic problems. *Diagn Gynecol Obstet* 1982;4: 285–293.
89. Goldman RL, Klein HZ. Proliferative sialometaplasia arising in an intraparotid lymph node. *Am J Clin Pathol* 1986;86:116–119.
90. Ellis GL, Auclair PL. Tumors of the salivary glands. Washington, DC: Armed Forces Institute of Pathology, 1996.
91. Ryan JR, Ioachim HL, Marmer J, et al. Acquired immune deficiency syndrome-related lymphadenopathies presenting in salivary gland lymph nodes. *Arch Otolaryngol* 1985;111:554–556.
92. Smith FB, Rajdeo H, Panesar N, et al. Benign lymphoepithelial lesions of the parotid gland in intravenous drug abusers. *Arch Pathol Lab Med* 1988;112:742–745.
93. Niwayama G. Inclusions of non-neoplastic thyroid tissue within cervical lymph nodes. *Tohoku J Exp Med* 1968;96:45–62.
94. Meyer JS, Steinberg LS. Microscopically benign thyroid follicles in cervical lymph nodes: serial section study of lymph node inclusions and entire thyroid gland in 5 cases. *Cancer* 1969;24:302–311.
95. Ibrahim NB, Milewski PJ, Gillett R, et al. Benign thyroid inclusions within cervical lymph nodes: an alarming incidental finding. *Aust N Z J Surg* 1981;51:188–189.
96. Russell WO, Ibanez ML, Clark RL, et al. Thyroid carcinoma: classification, intraglandular dissemination and clinicopathological study based upon whole organ sections of 80 thyroid glands. *Cancer* 1963; 16:1425–1460.
97. Franssila KO, Ackerman LV, Brown CL, et al. Follicular carcinoma. *Semin Diagn Pathol* 1985;2:101–122.
98. LiVolsi VA, Perzin KH, Savetsky L. Carcinoma arising in median ectopic thyroid (including thyroglossal duct tissue). *Cancer* 1974;34: 1303–1315.
99. Dalgaard JG, Wetteland P. Lateral cervical thyroid metastases: a follow-up study of 30 cases. *Acta Chir Scand* 1956;111:431–433.
100. Block MA, Wylie JH, Patton RB, et al. Does benign thyroid tissue occur in the lateral part of the neck? *Am J Surg* 1996;112:476–481.
101. Sampson RJ, Oka H, Key CR, et al. Metastases from occult thyroid carcinoma: an autopsy study from Hiroshima and Nagasaki, Japan. *Cancer* 1970;25:803–811.
102. Zapatero J, Baamonde C, Gonzalez F, et al. Ectopic goiters of the mediastinum: presentation of two cases and review of the literature. *Jpn J Surg* 1988;18:105–109.
103. LiVolsi VA, Perzin KH, Savetsky L. Carcinoma arising in median ectopic thyroid (including thyroglossal duct tissue). *Cancer* 1974;34: 1303–1315.
104. Walker AN, Fechner RE. Papillary carcinoma arising from ectopic breast tissue in an axillary lymph node. *Diagn Gynecol Obstet* 1982; 4:141–145.
105. Mesa-Tejada R, Palakodety RB, Leon JA, et al. Immunocytochemical distribution of a breast carcinoma associated glycoprotein identified by monoclonal antibodies. *Am J Pathol* 1988;130:305–314.
106. Das Gupta T, Bowden L, Berg JW. Malignant melanoma of unknown primary origin. *Surg Gynecol Obstet* 1963;117:341–345.
107. Baab GH, McBride CM. Malignant melanoma: the patient with an unknown site of primary origin. *Arch Surg* 1975;110:896–900.
108. Cochran AJ, Duan-Ren W, Morton DL. Occult tumor cells in the lymph nodes of patients with pathological stage I malignant melanoma. *Am J Surg Pathol* 1988;12:612–618.
109. Shenoy BV, Fort L, Benjamin SP. Malignant melanoma primary in lymph node: the case of the missing link. *Am J Surg Pathol* 1987; 11:140–146.
110. Sussman J, Rosai J. Lymph node metastasis as the initial manifestation of malignant mesothelioma: report of six cases. *Am J Surg Pathol* 1990;14:819–828.
111. Jonk A, Kroon BB, Rumke P, et al. Lymph node metastasis from melanoma with an unknown primary site. *Br J Surg* 1990;77:665–668.
112. Morgan WS, Castleman B. A clinicopathologic study of ''Mikulicz's disease.'' *Am J Pathol* 1953;29:471–495.
113. Hirota J, Maeda Y, Ueta E, et al. Immunohistochemical and histologic study of cervical lymphoepithelial cysts. *J Oral Pathol Med* 1989;18: 202–205.
114. Nishikawa H, Kirkham N, Hogkin BM. Synchronous extra-parotid Warthin's tumor. *J Laryngol Otol* 1989;103:792–793.
115. Miller R, Yanagihara ET, Dubrow AA, et al. Malignant lymphoma in the Warthin's tumor: report of a case. *Cancer* 1982;50:2948–2950.
116. Hall G, Tesluk H, Baron S. Lymphoma arising in adenolymphoma. *Hum Pathol* 1985;16:424–427.
117. Bunker ML, Locker J. Warthin's tumor with malignant lymphoma:

DNA analysis of paraffin-embedded tissue. *Am J Clin Pathol* 1989; 91:341–344.
118. Medeiros LJ, Rizzi R, Lardelli P, et al. Malignant lymphoma involving a Warthin's tumor: a case with immunophenotypic and gene rearrangement analysis. *Hum Pathol* 1990;21:974–977.
119. Melato M, Falconieri G, Fanin R, et al. Hodgkin's disease occurring in a Warthin's tumor: first case report. *Pathol Res Pract* 1986;181: 615–620.
120. Morrison GA, Shaw HJ. Squamous carcinoma arising within a Warthin's tumor of the parotid gland. *J Laryngol Otol* 1988;102: 1189–1191.
121. Onder T, Tiwari RM, van der Waal I, et al. Malignant adenolymphoma of the parotid gland: report of carcinomatous transformation. *J Laryngol Otol* 1990;104:656–661.
122. Healey WV, Perzin KH, Smith L. Mucoepidermoid carcinoma of salivary gland origin: classification, clinical-pathologic correlation and results of treatment. *Cancer* 1970;26:368–288.
123. Perzin KH, LiVolsi VA. Acinic cell carcinoma arising in ectopic salivary gland tissue. *Cancer* 1980;45:967–972.
124. Smith A, Winkler B, Perzin KH, et al. Muco-epidermoid carcinoma arising in an intraparotid lymph node. *Cancer* 1985;55;400–403.
125. Adkins GF, Hinckley DM. Primary muco-epidermoid carcinoma arising in a parotid lymph node. *Aust N Z J Surg* 1989;59:433–435.
126. Sampson RJ, Oka H, Key CR, et al. Metastases from occult thyroid carcinoma: an autopsy study from Hiroshima and Nagasaki, Japan. *Cancer* 1970;25:803–811.
127. Zapatero J, Baamonde C, Gonzalez F, et al. Ectopic goiters of the mediastinum: presentation of two cases and review of the literature. *Jpn J Surg* 1988;18:105–109.
128. LiVolsi VA, Perzin KH, Savetsky L. Carcinoma arising in median ectopic thyroid (including thyroglossal duct tissue). *Cancer* 1974;34: 1303–1315.
129. Walker AN, Fechner RE. Papillary carcinoma arising from ectopic breast tissue in an axillary lymph node. *Diagn Gynecol Obstet* 1982; 4:141–145.
130. Haferkamp O, Rosenau W, Lennert K. Vascular transformation of lymph node sinuses due to venous obstruction. *Arch Pathol* 1971;92: 81–83.
131. Bedrosian SA, Goldman RL. Nodal angiomatosis: relationship to vascular transformation of lymph nodes. *Arch Pathol Lab Med* 1984; 108:864–865.
132. Dorfman RF. Kaposi's sarcoma revisited. *Hum Pathol* 1984;15: 1013–1017.
133. Chan JK, Warnke RA, Dorfman RF. Vascular transformation of sinuses in lymph nodes: a study of its morphological spectrum and distinction from Kaposi's sarcoma. *Am J Surg Pathol* 1991;15: 732–743.
134. Fayemi AO, Toker C. Nodal angiomatosis. *Arch Pathol* 1975;99: 170–172.
135. Chan JK, Frizzera G, Fletcher CD, et al. Primary vascular tumors of lymph nodes other than Kaposi's sarcoma: analysis of 39 cases and delineation of two new entities. *Am J Surg Pathol* 1992;16:335–350.
136. Al-Jabi M, Tonai G, McCaughey WT. Angiofollicular lymphoid hyperplasia in an angiolipomatous mass. *Arch Pathol Lab Med* 1980; 104:313–315.
137. Madero S, Onate JM, Garzon A. Giant lymph node hyperplasia in an angiolipomatous mediastinal mass. *Arch Pathol Lab Med* 1986;110: 853–855.
138. Gupta IM. Hemangioma in a lymph node. *Indian J Pathol Bacteriol* 1964;71:110–114.
139. Almagro UO, Choi H, Rouse TM. Hemangioma in a lymph node. *Arch Pathol Lab Med* 1985;109:576–578.
140. Kasznica J, Sideli RV, Collins MH. Lymph node hemangioma. *Arch Pathol Lab Med* 1989;113:804–807.
141. Urabe A, Tsuneyoshi M, Enjoji M. Epithelioid hemangioma versus Kimura's disease: a comparative clinicopathologic study. *Am J Surg Pathol* 1987;11:758–766.
142. Gerald W, Kostianovsky W, Rosai J. Development of vascular neoplasia in Castleman's disease: report of seven cases. *Am J Surg Pathol* 1990;14:603–614.
143. Tsang WY, Chan JK, Dorfman RF, et al. Vasoproliferative lesions of lymph node. *Pathol Annu* 1994;29:63–133.
144. Williams HB. Hemangiomas and lymphangiomas. *Adv Surg* 1981;15: 317–349.
145. Wolff M. Lymphangiomyoma: clinicopathologic study and ultrastructural confirmation of its histogenesis. *Cancer* 1973;31:988–1007.
146. McIntosh GS, Dutoit SH, Chronos NV, et al. Multiple unilateral renal angiomyolipomas with regional lymphangioleiomyomatosis. *J Urol* 1989;142:1305–1307.
147. Monteforte WJ, Kohnen PW. Angiomyolipomas in a case of lymphangiomyomatosis syndrome: relationship to tuberous sclerosis. *Cancer* 1974;34:317–321.
148. Kaku T, Toyoshima S, Enjoji M. Tuberous sclerosis with pulmonary and lymph node involvement: relationship to lymphangiomyomatosis. *Acta Pathol Jpn* 1983;33:395–401.
149. Corrin B, Liebow AA, Friedman PJ. Pulmonary lymphangiomyomatosis. *Am J Pathol* 1975;79:348–382.
150. Chan JK, Tsang WY, Pau MY, et al. Lymphangiomyomatosis and angiomyolipoma: closely related entities characterized by hamartomatous proliferation of HMB-45 positive smooth muscle. *Histopathology* 1993;22:445–455.
151. van Haelst UJ, Pruszczynski M, ten Cate LN, et al. Ultrastructural and immunohistochemical study of epithelioid hemangioendothelioma of bone: coexpression of epithelial and endothelial markers. *Ultrastruct Pathol* 1990;14: 141–149.
152. Weiss SW, Enzinger FM. Epithelioid hemangioendothelioma: a vascular tumor often mistaken for a carcinoma. *Cancer* 1982;50: 970–981.
153. Kaposi M: Idiopatisches multiples Pigmentsarkorn der Haut. *Arch Dermatol Syphilis* 1872;4:265–273.
154. Centers for Disease Control. Kaposi's sarcoma and *Pneumocystis* pneumonia among homosexual men—New York City and California. *MMWR Morb Mortal Wkly Rep* 1981;30:305–308.
155. Centers for Disease Control Task Force on Kaposi's Sarcoma and Opportunistic Infections. Epidemiologic aspects of the current out break of Kaposi's sarcoma and opportunistic infections. *N Engl J Med* 1982;306:248–252.
156. Friedman-Kien AE, Laubenstein LJ, Rubinstein P, et al. Disseminated Kaposi's sarcoma in homosexual men. *Ann Intern Med* 1982;96: 693–700.
157. Beral V: Epidemiology of Kaposi's sarcoma. *Cancer Surv* 1991;10: 5–22.
158. Peterman TA, Jaffe HW, Friedman-Kein AE, et al. The etiology of Kaposi's sarcoma. *Cancer Surv* 1991;10:23–27.
159. Penn I. Lymphomas complicating organ transplantation. *Transplant Proc* 1983;15[Suppl]:2790–2797.
160. Safai B, Good RA. Kaposi's sarcoma: a review and recent developments. *Clin Bull* 1980;10:62–69.
161. Santucci M, Pimpinelli N, Moretti S. Classic and immunodeficiency-associated Kaposi's sarcoma: clinical, histologic, and immunologic correlations. *Arch Pathol Lab Med* 1988;112:1214–1220.
162. Biggar RJ, Rabkin CS. The epidemiology of AIDS-related neoplasms. *Hematol Oncol Clin North Am* 1996;10:997–1010.
163. Centers for Disease Control. Revision of the CDC surveillance case definition for acquired immunodeficiency syndrome. *MMWR Morb Mortal Wkly Rep* 1987;36[Suppl]:1S–15S.
164. Centers for Disease Control. 1993 Revised classification system for HIV infection and expanded surveillance case definition for AIDS among adolescents and adults. *MMWR Morb Mortal Wkly Rep* 1992; 41:1–19.
165. Costa J, Rabson AS. Generalised Kaposi's sarcoma is not a neoplasm. *Lancet* 1983;1:58.
166. Brooks JJ. Kaposi's sarcoma: a reversible hyperplasia. *Lancet* 1986; 2:1309–1310.
167. Ioachim HL, Adsay V, Giancotti FR, et al. Kaposi's sarcoma of internal organs: a multiparameter study of 86 cases. *Cancer* 1995;75: 1376–1385.
168. Rabkin CS, Bedi G, Musaba E, et al. AIDS-related Kaposi's sarcoma is a clonal neoplasm. *Clin Cancer Res* 1995;1:257–260.
169. Rutgers JL, Wieczorek R, Bonetti F, et al. The expression of endothelial cell surface antigens by AIDS-associated Kaposi's sarcoma. *Am J Pathol* 1986;122:493–499.
170. Scully PA, Steinman HK, Kennedy C, et al. AIDS-related Kaposi's sarcoma displays differential expression of endothelial surface antigens. *Am J Pathol* 1988;130:244–251.
171. Kraffert C, Planus L, Penneys NS. Kaposi's sarcoma: further immunohistologic evidence of a vascular endothelial origin. *Arch Dermatol* 1991;127:1734–1735.

172. Rabkin CS, Bedi G, Musba E, et al. AIDS-related Kaposi's sarcoma is a clonal neoplasm. *Clin Cancer Res* 1995;1:257–260.
173. Beral V, Peterman TA, Berkelman RL, et al. Kaposi's sarcoma among persons with AIDS: a sexually transmitted infection? *Lancet* 1990; 335:123–128.
174. Beral V, Bull D, Darby S, et al. Risk of Kaposi's sarcoma and sexual practices associated with fecal contact in homosexual or bisexual men with AIDS. *Lancet* 1992;339:632–635.
175. Chang Y, Cesarman E, Pessin MS, et al. Identification of herpesvirus-like DNA sequences in AIDS-associated Kaposi's sarcoma. *Science* 1994;266:1865–1869.
176. Cesarman E, Knowles DM. Kaposi's sarcoma-associated herpes virus (KSHV/HHV-8): a lymphotropic human herpesvirus associated with Kaposi's sarcoma, primary effusion lymphoma and multicentric Castleman's disease. *Semin Diagn Pathol* 1997;14:54–66.
177. Moore PS, Gao S-J, Dominiguez G, et al. Primary characterization of a herpesvirus agent associated with Kaposi's sarcoma. *J Virol* 1996; 70:549–558.
178. Cesarman E, Nador RG, Bai F, et al. KSHV/HHV-8 contains G protein-coupled receptor and cyclin D homologues which are expressed in Kaposi's sarcoma and malignant lymphoma. *J Virol* 1996;70: 8218–8223.
179. Mesri EA, Cesarman E, Arvanitakis L, et al. Human herpesvirus-8/ Kaposi's sarcoma-associated herpesvirus is a new transmissible virus that infects B cells. *J Exp Med* 1996;183:2385–2390.
180. Roizman B: Herpesviridae: a brief introduction. In: Fields BN, ed. *Virology*. New York: Raven Press, 1990:1787–1793.
181. Boshoff C, Schulz TF, Kennedy MM, et al. Kaposi's sarcoma-associated herpesvirus infects endothelial and spindle cells. *Nat Med* 1995; 1:1274–1278.
182. Reed JA, Nador RG, Spaulding D, et al. Demonstration of Kaposi's sarcoma by colorimetric in situ hybridization using a catalyzed signal amplification system. *Blood* 1998;91:3825–3832.
183. Knowles DM, Cesarman E. The Kaposi's sarcoma-associated herpesvirus (human herpesvirus-8) in Kaposi's sarcoma, malignant lymphoma, and other diseases. *Ann Oncol* 1997;8[Suppl 2]:5123–5129.
184. Dezube BJ. Clinical presentation and natural history of AIDS-related Kaposi's sarcoma. *Hematol Oncol Clin North Am* 1996;10: 1023–1029.
185. Niedt GW, Schinella RA. Acquired immunodeficiency syndrome: clinicopathologic study of 56 autopsies. *Arch Pathol Lab Med* 1985; 109:727–734.
186. Nichols CM, Flaitz CM, Hicks MJ. Treating Kaposi's lesions in the HIV-infected patient. *JADA* 1993;124:78–84.
187. Diebold J, Marche C, Audouin J, et al. Lymph node modification in patients with the acquired immunodeficiency syndrome (AIDS) or with AIDS related complex (ARC): a histological, immunohistopathological and ultrastructural study of 45 cases. *Pathol Res Pract* 1985; 180:590–611.
188. Chadburn A, Metroka C, Mouradian J. Progressive lymph node histology and its prognostic value in patients with acquired immunodeficiency syndrome and AIDS-related complex. *Hum Pathol* 1989;20: 579–587.
189. Finkbeiner WE, Egbert BM, Groundwater JR, et al. Kaposi's sarcoma in young homosexual men: a histopathologic study with particular reference to lymph node involvement. *Arch Pathol Lab Med* 1982; 106:261–264.
190. Perlow LS, Taff ML, Orsini JM, et al. Kaposi's sarcoma in a young homosexual man: association with angiofollicular lymphoid hyperplasia and a malignant lymphoproliferative disorder. *Arch Pathol Lab Med* 1983;107:510–513.
191. Harris NL. Hypervascular follicular hyperplasia and Kaposi's sarcoma in patients at risk for AIDS. *N Engl J Med* 1984;310:462–463.
192. Kaplan MH, Susin M, Pahwa SG, et al. Neoplastic complications of HTLV-III infection: lymphomas and solid tumors. *Am J Med* 1987; 82:389–396.
193. Ioachim HL, Lerner CW, Tapper M. Lymphadenopathies in homosexual men: relationships with the acquired immune deficiency syndrome. *JAMA* 1983;250:1306–1309.
194. Amberson JB, DiCarlo EF, Metroka CE, et al. Diagnostic pathology in the acquired immunodeficiency syndrome: surgical pathology and cytology experience with 67 patients. *Arch Pathol Lab Med* 1985; 109:345–351.
195. Cockerell CJ: Histopathological features of Kaposi's sarcoma in HIV-infected individuals. *Cancer Surv* 1991;10:73– 90.
196. Santucci M, Pimpinelli N, Moretti S, et al. Classic and immunodeficiency-associated Kaposi's sarcoma: clinical, histologic, and immunologic correlations. *Arch Pathol Lab Med* 1988;112:1214–1220.
197. Lubin J, Rywlin AM. Lymphoma-like lymph node changes in Kaposi's sarcoma. *Arch Pathol* 1971;92:338–341.
198. Amazon K, Rywlin AM. Subtle clues to the diagnosis by conventional microscopy: lymph node involvement in Kaposi's sarcoma. *Am J Dermatopathol* 1979;1:173–176.
199. Beckstead JH, Wood GS, Fletcher V. Evidence for the origin of Kaposi's sarcoma from lymphatic endothelium. *Am J Pathol* 1985; 119:294–300.
200. Schulze HJ, Rutten A, Mahrle G, et al. Initial lesions of HIV-related Kaposi's sarcoma a histological, immunohistochemical and ultrastructural study. *Arch Dermatol Res* 1987;279:499–503.
201. Russell Jones R, Orchard G, Zelger B, et al. Immunostaining for CD31 and CD34 in Kaposi sarcoma. *J Clin Pathol* 1995;48:1011–1016.
202. Dictor M, Carlen B, Bendsoe N, et al. Ultrastructural development of Kaposi's sarcoma in relation to the dermal microvasculature. *Virchows Arch A Pathol Anat Histopathol* 199;419:35–43.
203. Marquart KH. Weibel-Palade bodies in Kaposi's sarcoma cells. *J Clin Pathol* 1987;40:933.
204. Ro JY, Ayala AG, El-Naggar A, et al. Angiomyolipoma of kidney with lymph node involvement: DNA flow cytometric analysis. *Arch Pathol Lab Med* 1990;114:65–67.
205. McIntosh GS, Dutoit SH, Chronos NV, et al. Multiple unilateral renal angiomyolipomas with regional lymphangioleiomyomatosis. *J Urol* 1989; 142:1305–1307.
206. Martignoni G, Pea M, Bonetti F, et al. Carcinoma like monotypic epithelioid angiomyolipoma in patients without evidence of tuberous sclerosis: a clinicopathologic and genetic study. *Am J Surg Pathol* 1998;22:663–672.
207. Relman DA, Loutit JS, Schmidt TM, et al. The agent of bacillary angiomatosis: an approach to the identification of uncultured pathogens. *N Engl J Med* 1990;323:1573–1580.
208. Welch DF, Pickett DA, Slater LN, et al. *Rochalimaea henslelae*, sp. Nov., a cause of septicemia, bacillary angiomatosis, and parenchymal bacillary peliosis. *J Clin Microbiol* 1992;30:275–274.
209. Koehler JE, Quinn FD, Berger TG, et al. Isolation of *Rochalimaea* species from cutaneous and osseous lesions of bacillary angiomatosis. *N Engl J Med* 1992;327:1625–1631.
210. Stoler MH, Bonfiglio TA, Sheigbigel RT, et al. An atypical subcutaneous infection associated with acquired immune deficiency syndrome. *Am J Clin Pathol* 1983;80:714– 718.
211. LeBoit PE, Egbert BM, Stoler MH, et al. Epithelioid haemangioma-like vascular proliferation in AIDS: manifestation of cat scratch disease bacillus infection? *Lancet* 1988;1:960–963.
212. LeBoit PE, Berger TG, Egbert BM, et al. Bacillary angiomatosis: the histopathology and differential diagnosis of a pseudoneoplastic infection in patients with human immunodeficiency virus disease. *Am J Surg Pathol* 1989;13:909–920.
213. Cockerell CJ, Whitelow MA, Webster GF, et al. Epithelioid angiomatosis: a distinct vascular disorder in patients with the acquired immunodeficiency syndrome or AIDS-related complex. *Lancet* 1987; 2:654–656.
214. Baron AL, Steinbach LS, LeBoit PE, et al. Osteolytic lesions and bacillary angiomatosis in HIV infection: radiologic differentiation from AIDS-related Kaposi sarcoma. *Radiology* 1990;177;77–81.
215. Moore EH, Russell LA, Klein JS, et al. Bacillary angiomatosis in patients with AIDS: multiorgan imaging findings. *Radiology* 1995; 197:67–72.
216. Kemper CA, Lombard CM, Deresinski SC, et al. Visceral bacillary epithelioid angiomatosis: possible manifestations of disseminated cat scratch disease in the immunocompromised host. A report of two cases. *Am J Med* 1990;89:216–222.
217. Adal KA, Cockerell CJ, Petri WA. Cat scratch disease, bacillary giomatosis, and other infections due to *Rochalimaea*. *N Engl J Med* 1994; 330:1509–1515.
218. Tappero JW, Mohle-Boetani J, Koehler JE, et al. The epidemiology of bacillary angiomatosis and bacillary peliosis. *JAMA* 1993;269: 770–775.
219. Szaniawski WK, Don PC, Bitterman SR, et al. Epithelioid angi-

omatosis in patients with AIDS: report of seven cases and review of the literature. *J Am Acad Dermatol* 1990;23:41–48.
220. Chan JKC, Lewin KJ, Lombard CM, et al. Histopathology of bacillary angiomatosis of lymph node. *Am J Surg Pathol* 1991;15:430–437.
221. Walford N, Van der Wouw PA, Das PK, et al. Epithelioid angiomatosis in the acquired immunodeficiency syndrome: morphology and differential diagnosis. *Histopathology* 1990;16:83–88.
222. Chang AD, Drachenberg CI, James SP. Bacillary angiomatosis associated with extensive esophageal polyposis: a new mucocutaneous manifestation of acquired immunodeficiency disease (AIDS). *Am J Gastroenterol* 1996;91:2220–2223.
223. Huh YB, Rose S, Schoen RE, et al. Colonic bacillary angiomatosis. *Ann Intern Med* 1996;124:735–737.
224. Spach DH, Callis KP, Paauw DS, et al. Endocarditis caused by *Rochalimaea quintana* in a patient infected with human immunodeficiency virus. *J Clin Microbiol* 1993;31:692–694.
225. Steeper TA, Rosenstein H, Weiser J, et al. Bacillary epithelioid angiomatosis involving the liver, spleen, and skin in an AIDS patient with concurrent Kaposi's sarcoma. *Am J Clin Pathol* 1992;97:713–718.
226. Schinella RA, Greco MA. Bacillary angiomatosis presenting as a soft-tissue tumor without skin involvement. *Hum Pathol* 1990;21:567–569.
227. Haught WH, Steinbach J, Zander DS, et al. Case report: bacillary angiomatosis with massive visceral lymphadenopathy. *Am J Med Sci* 1993;306:236–240.
228. Perrone T, De Wolf Peeters C, Frizzera G. Inflammatory pseudotumor of lymph nodes: a distinctive pattern of nodal reaction. *Am J Surg Pathol* 1988;12:351–361.
229. Davis RE, Warnke RA, Dorfman RF. Inflammatory pseudotumor of lymph nodes: additional observations and evidence for an inflammatory etiology. *Am J Surg Pathol* 1991;15:744–756.
230. Selves J, Meggetto F, Brousset P, et al. Inflammatory pseudotumor of the liver: evidence for follicular dendritic reticulum cell proliferation associated with clonal Epstein-Barr virus. *Am J Surg Pathol* 1996; 20:747–753.
231. Arber DA, Kamel OW, van de Rijn M, et al. Frequent presence of the Epstein-Barr virus in inflammatory pseudotumor. *Hum Pathol* 1995;26:1093–1098.
232. Coffin CM, Watterson J, Priest JR, et al. Extrapulmonary inflammatory myofibroblastic tumor (inflammatory pseudotumor): a clinicopathologic and immunohistochemical study of 84 cases. *Am J Surg Pathol* 1995;19:859–872.
233. Meiss JM, Enzinger FM. Inflammatory fibrosarcoma of the mesentery and retroperitoneum: a tumor closely simulating inflammatory pseudotumor. *Am J Surg Pathol* 1991;15:1146–1156.
234. Weiss SW, Gnepp DR, Bratthauer GL. Palisaded myofibroblastoma: a benign mesenchymal tumor of lymph node. *Am J Surg Pathol* 1989; 13:341–346.
235. Suster S, Rosai J. Intranodal hemorrhagic spindle cell tumor with ''amianthoid'' fibers: report of six cases of a distinctive mesenchymal neoplasm of the inguinal region that simulates Kaposi's sarcoma. *Am J Surg Pathol* 1989;13:347–357.
236. Umlas J, Federman M, Crawford C, et al. Spindle cell pseudotumor due to *Mycobacterium avium-intracellulare* in patients with acquired immunodeficiency syndrome (AIDS): positive staining of mycobacteria for cytoskeleton filaments. *Am J Surg Pathol* 1991;15: 1181–1187.
237. Chen KT. Mycobacterial spindle cell pseudotumor of lymph nodes. *Am J Surg Pathol* 1992;16:276–281.
238. Abell MR, Littler ER. Benign metastasizing uterine leiomyoma, multiple lymph node metastasis. *Cancer* 1975;36:2206–2213.
239. Hsu YK, Rosenshein NB, Parmley TH, et al. Leiomyomatosis in pelvic lymph nodes. *Obstet Gynecol* 1981;57:91s–93s.
240. Mazzoleni G, Salerno A, Sntini D, et al. Leiomyomatosis of pelvic lymph nodes. *Histopathology* 1992;21:588–589.
241. Fujii S, Odamura H, Nakashima N, et al. Leiomyomatosis peritonealis disseminata. *Obstet Gynecol* 1980;55:79s–83s.
242. Mills SE. Decidua and squamous metaplasia in abdominopelvic lymph nodes. *Int J Gynecol Pathol* 1983;2:209–215.
243. Zaytsev P, Taxy JB. Pregnancy-associated ectopic decidua. *Am J Surg Pathol* 1987;11:526–530.
244. Mazeron JJ, Suit HD. Lymph nodes as sites of metastases from sarcomas of soft tissue. *Cancer* 1987;60:1800–1808.
245. Kinney MC, Greer JP, Glick AD, et al. Anaplastic large-cell Ki-1 malignant lymphomas: recognition, biological and clinical implications. *Pathol Annu* 1991;26:1–24.
246. Leoncini L, DelVecchio MT, Kraft R, et al. Hodgkin's disease and CD-30 positive anaplastic large cell lymphomas—a continuous spectrum of malignant disorders: a quantitative morphometric and immunohistologic study. *Am J Pathol* 1990;137:1047–1057.
247. Coffin CM, Rich SS, Dehner LP. Familial aggregation of nasopharyngeal carcinoma and other malignancies: a clinicopathologic description. *Cancer* 1991;68:1323–1328.
248. Ambinder RF, Mann RB. Detection and characterization of Epstein-Barr virus in clinical specimens. *Am J Pathol* 1994;145:239–252.
249. Raab-Traub N. Epstein-Barr virus and nasopharyngeal carcinoma. *Semin Cancer Biol* 1992;3:297–307.
250. Smith RD. Is Epstein-Barr virus a human oncogene or only an innocent bystander? [Editorial]. *Hum Pathol* 1997;28:1333–1335.
251. Medeiros LJ, Kaynor B, Harris NL. Lupus lymphadenitis: report of a case with immunohistologic studies on frozen sections. *Hum Pathol* 1989;20:295–299.
252. van Muijen GNP, Ruiter DJ, van Leeuwen C, et al. Cytokeratin and neurofilament in lung carcinomas. *Am J Pathol* 1984;116:363–369.
253. Guinee DG Jr, Fishback NF, Koss MN, et al. The spectrum of immunohistochemical staining of small-cell lung carcinoma in specimens from transbronchial and open-lung biopsies. *Am J Clin Pathol* 1994; 102:406–414.
254. Loy TS, Darkow GV, Quesenberry JT. Immunostaining in the diagnosis of pulmonary neuroendocrine carcinomas: an immunohistochemical study with ultrastructural correlations. *Am J Surg Pathol* 1995; 19:173–182.
255. Fushimi H, Kikui M, Morino H, et al. Detection of large cell component in small cell lung carcinoma by combined cytologic and histologic examinations and its clinical implication. *Cancer* 1992;70: 599–605.
256. Capella C, Heitz PU, Hofler H, et al. Revised classification of neuroendocrine tumours of the lung, pancreas and gut. *Virchows Arch A Pathol Anat Histopathol* 1995;425:547–560.
257. Jiang S, Kameya T, Shoji M, et al. Large cell neuroendocrine carcinoma of the lung: a histologic and immunohistochemical study of 22 cases. *Am J Surg Pathol* 1998;22:526–537.
258. Lumadue JA, Askin FB, Perlman EJ. MIC2 analysis of small cell carcinoma. *Am J Clin Pathol* 1994;102:692–694.
259. Michels S, Swanson PE, Robb JA, et al. Leu-7 in small cell neoplasms: an immunohistochemical study with ultrastructural correlations. *Cancer* 1987;60:2958–2964.
260. Moll I, Kuhn C, Moll R. Cytokeratin 20 is a general marker of cutaneous Merkel cells while certain neuronal proteins are absent. *J Invest Dermatol* 1995;104:910–915.
261. Rosen PP, Kimmel M. Occult breast carcinoma presenting with axillary lymph node metastases: a follow-up study of 48 patients. *Hum Pathol* 1990;21:518–523.
262. Matsushima S, Mori M, Adachi Y, et al. S100 protein positive human breast carcinomas: an immunohistochemical study. *J Surg Oncol* 1994;55:108–113.
263. Fechner RE. Histologic variants of infiltrating lobular carcinoma of the breast. *Hum Pathol* 1975;6:373–378.
264. Brown RW, Campagna LB, Dunn JK, et al. Immunohistochemical identification of tumor markers in metastatic adenocarcinoma: a diagnostic adjunct in the determination of primary site. *Am J Clin Pathol* 1997;107:12–19.
265. Su JM, Hsu HK, Chang H, et al. Expression of estrogen and progesterone receptors in non-small cell lung cancer: immunohistochemical study. *Anticancer Res* 1996;16:3803–3806.
266. Wallace ML, Longacre TA, Smoller BR. Estrogen and progesterone receptors and anti-gross cystic disease fluid protein 15 (BRST-2) fail to distinguish metastatic breast carcinoma from eccrine neoplasms. *Mod Pathol* 1995;8:897–901.
267. Kim H, Dorfman RF, Rappaport H. Signet ring cell lymphoma: a rare morphologic and functional expression of nodular (follicular) lymphoma. *Am J Surg Pathol* 1978;2:119–132.
268. LiVolsi VA, Brooks JJ, Soslow R, et al. Signet cell melanocytic lesions. *Mod Pathol* 1992;5:515–520.
269. De Petris G, Lev R, Siew S. Peritumoral and nodal muciphages. *Am J Surg Pathol* 1998;22:545–549.
270. Kuo T, Hsueh S. Mucicarminophilic histiocytosis: a polyvinylpyrroli-

done (PVP) storage disease simulating signet-ring cell carcinoma. *Am J Surg Pathol* 1984;8:419–428.
271. Sheahan K, O'Brien MJ, Burke B, et al. Differential reactivities of carcinoembryonic antigen (CEA) and CEA-related monoclonal and polyclonal antibodies in common epithelial malignancies. *Am J Clin Pathol* 1990;94:157–164.
272. Jungbluth AA, Busam KJ, Gerald WL, et al. A103: an anti-Melan-A monoclonal antibody for the detection of malignant melanoma in paraffin-embedded tissues. *Am J Surg Pathol* 1998;22:595–602.
273. Clement PB, Scully RE. Uterine tumors with mixed epithelial and mesenchymal elements. *Semin Diagn Pathol* 1988;5:199–222.
274. Swanson PE. Heffalumps, jaguars, and chesire cats: a commentary on cytokeratins and soft tissue sarcomas. *Am J Clin Pathol* 1991;96: 673–675.
275. Frizzera G, Gajl-Peczalska K, Sibley RK, et al. Rosette formation in malignant lymphoma. *Am J Pathol* 1985;119:351–356.
276. Tsang WY, Chan JK, Tang SK, et al. Large cell lymphoma with fibrillary matrix. *Histopathology* 1992;20:80–82.
277. Bates RJ, Chapman CM, Prout GJ, et al. Immunohistochemical identification of prostatic acid phosphatase: correlation of tumor grade with acid phosphatase distribution. *J Urol* 1982;127:574–580.
278. Jobsis AC, De Vries GP, Meijer EFH. The immunohistochemical detection of prostatic acid phosphatase: its possibilities and limitations in tumour histochemistry. *Histochemistry J* 1981;13:961–973.
279. Nadji M, Tabei SZ, Castro A, et al. Prostatic-specific antigen: an immunohistologic marker for prostatic neoplasms. *Cancer* 1981;48: 1229–1232.
280. Purnell DM, Heatfield BM, Trump BF. Immunocytochemical evaluation of human prostatic carcinomas for carcinoembryonic antigen, nonspecific cross-reacting antigen, beta-chorionic gonadotrophin, and prostate-specific antigen. *Cancer Res* 1984;44:285–292.
281. Loy TS, Sharp SC, Andershock CJ, et al. Distribution of CA 19-9 in adenocarcinomas and transitional cell carcinomas: an immunohistochemical study of 527 cases. *Am J Clin Pathol* 1993;99:726–728.
282. Azumi N, Traweek ST, Battifora H. Prostatic acid phosphatase in carcinoid tumors: immunohistochemical and immunoblot studies. *Am J Surg Pathol* 1991;15:785–790.
283. Federspiel BH, Burke AP, Sobin LH, et al. Rectal and colonic carcinoids: a clinicopathologic study of 84 cases. *Cancer* 1190;65: 135–140.
284. di Sant'Agnese PA, Cockett AT. Neuroendocrine differentiation in prostatic malignancy. *Cancer* 1996;78:357–361.
285. McLaren KM, Cossar DW. The immunohistochemical localization of S100 in the diagnosis of papillary carcinoma of the thyroid. *Hum Pathol* 1996;27;633–636.
286. Wilson NW, Pambakian H, Richardson TC, et al. Epithelial markers in thyroid carcinoma: an immunoperoxidase study. *Histopathology* 1986;10:815–829.
287. DeLellis RA, Wolfe H. Calcitonin immunohistochemistry. In: DeLellis RA, ed. *Diagnostic immunohistochemistry.* New York: Masson Publishing, 1981:61–74.
288. Carcangiu ML, Steeper T, Zampi G, et al. Anaplastic thyroid carcinoma: a study of 70 cases. *Am J Clin Pathol* 1985;83:135–158.
289. Jautzke G, Altenaehr E. Immunohistochemical demonstration of carcinoembryonic antigen (CEA) and its correlation with grading and staging on tissue sections of urinary bladder carcinomas. *Cancer* 1982; 50:2052–2056.
290. Soslow RA, Rouse RV, Hendrickson MR, et al. Transitional cell neoplasms of the ovary and urinary bladder: a comparative immunohistochemical analysis. *Int J Gynecol Pathol* 1996;15:257–265.
291. Pitz S, Moll R, Storkel S, et al. Expression of intermediate filament proteins in subtypes of renal cell carcinomas and in renal oncocytomas: distinction of two classes of renal cell tumors. *Lab Invest* 1987; 56:642–653.
292. Raab SS, Berg LC, Swanson PE, et al. Adenocarcinoma in the lung in patients with breast cancer: a prospective analysis of the discriminatory value of immunohistology. *Am J Clin Pathol* 1993;100:27–35.
293. Tan J, Sidhu G, Greco A, et al. Villin, cytokeratin 7, and cytokeratin 20 expression in pulmonary adenocarcinoma with ultrastructural evidence of microvilli with rootlets. *Hum Pathol* 1998;29:390–396.
294. Corson JM, Pinkus GS. Mesothelioma: profile of keratin proteins and carcinoembryonic antigen. An immunoperoxidase study of 20 cases and comparison with pulmonary adenocarcinomas. *Am J Pathol* 1982; 108:80–87.
295. Holden J, Churg A. Immunohistochemical staining for keratin and carcinoembryonic antigen in the diagnosis of malignant mesothelioma. *Am J Surg Pathol* 1984;8:277–279.
296. Sheibani K, Battifora H, Burke JS. Antigenic phenotype of malignant mesotheliomas and pulmonary adenocarcinomas: an immunohistologic analysis demonstrating the value of Leu MI antigen. *Am J Pathol* 1986;123:212–219.
297. Wang NS, Huang SN, Gold P. Absence of carcinoembryonic antigen-like material in mesothelioma: an immunohistochemical differentiation from other lung cancers. *Cancer* 1979;44:937–943.
298. Wick MR, Loy T, Mills SE, et al. Malignant epithelioid pleural mesothelioma versus peripheral pulmonary adenocarcinoma: a histochemical, ultrastructural and immunohistological study of 103 cases. *Hum Pathol* 1990;21:759–766.
299. Garcia-Prats MD, Ballestin C, Sotelo T, et al. A comparative evaluation of immunohistochemical markers for the differential diagnosis of malignant pleural tumours. *Histopathology* 1998;32:462–472.
300. Ordonez NG. Value of cytokeratin 5/6 immunostaining in distinguishing epithelial mesothelioma of the pleura from lung adenocarcinoma. *Am J Surg Pathol* 1998;22:1215–1221.
301. Clover J, Oates J, Edwards C. Anti-cytokeratin 5/6: a positive marker for epithelioid mesothelioma. *Histopathology* 1997;31:140–143.
302. Doglioni C, Tos AP, Laurino L, et al. Calretinin: a novel immunocytochemical marker for mesothelioma. *Am J Surg Pathol* 1996;20: 1037–1046.
303. Monteagudo C, Merino MF, LaPorte N, et al. Value of gross cystic disease fluid protein-15 in distinguishing metastatic breast carcinomas among poorly differentiated neoplasms involving the ovary. *Hum Pathol* 1991;22:368–372.
304. Wick MR, Lillemoe TJ, Copland GT, et al. Gross cystic disease fluid protein-15 as a marker for breast cancer: immunohistochemical analysis of 690 human neoplasms and comparison with alpha-lactalbumin. *Hum Pathol* 1989;20:281–287.
305. Palmer PE, Wolfe WJ. Immunocytochemical localization of oncodevelopmental proteins in human germ cell and hepatic tumors. *J Histochem Cytochem* 1978;26:523–531.
306. Ma CK, Zarbo RJ, Frierson HJ, et al. Comparative immunohistochemical study of primary and metastatic carcinomas of the liver. *Am J Clin Pathol* 1993;99:551–557.
307. Sheahan K, O'Brien MJ, Burke B, et al. Differential reactivities of carcinoembryonic antigen (CEA) and CEA-related monoclonal and polyclonal antibodies in common epithelial malignancies. *Am J Clin Pathol* 1990;94:157–164.
308. Johnson DE, Herndier BG, Medeiros LJ, et al. The diagnostic utility of the keratin profiles of hepatocellular carcinoma and cholangiocarcinoma. *Am J Surg Pathol* 1988;12:187–197.
309. Loy TS, Chapman RK, Diaz AA, et al. Distribution of BCA-225 in adenocarcinomas: an immunohistochemical study of 446 cases. *Am J Clin Pathol* 1991;96:326–329.
310. Loy TS, Sharp SC, Andershock CJ, et al. Distribution of CA 19-9 in adenocarcinomas and transitional cell carcinomas: an immunohistochemical study of 527 cases. *Am J Clin Pathol* 1993;99:726–728.
311. Murphy GF, Mihm MC Jr. Histological reporting of malignant melanoma. *Monogr Pathol* 1998;30:70–93.
312. Carney JA. Psammomatous melanotic schwannoma: a distinctive, heritable tumor with special associations, including cardiac myxoma and the Cushing syndrome. *Am J Surg Pathol* 1990;14:206–222.
313. Unger PD, Hoffman K, Thung SN, et al. HMB-45 reactivity in adrenal pheochromocytomas. *Arch Pathol Lab Med* 1992;16:151–153.
314. Chang ES, Wick MR, Swanson PE, et al. Metastatic malignant melanoma with "rhabdoid" features. *Am J Clin Pathol* 1994;102: 426–431.
315. Kurtin PJ, Pinkus GS. Leukocyte common antigen—a diagnostic discriminant between hematopoietic and nonhematopoietic neoplasms in paraffin sections using monoclonal antibodies: correlation with immunologic studies and ultrastructural localization. *Hum Pathol* 1985;16: 353–365.
316. Spagnolo DV, Michie SA, Crabree GS, et al. Monoclonal antikeratin (AE1) reactivity in routinely processed tissue from 166 human neoplasms. *Am J Clin Pathol* 1985;84:697–704.
317. Argenyi ZB, Cain C, Bromely C, et al. S-100 protein-negative malignant melanoma: fact or fiction? A light-microscopic and immunohistochemical study. *Am J Dermatopathol* 1994;16:233–240.
318. Drier JK, Swanson PE, Cherwitz DL, et al. S100 protein immunoreac-

tivity in poorly differentiated carcinomas: immunohistochemical comparison with malignant melanoma. *Arch Pathol Lab Med* 1987;111: 447–452.
319. Nakajima T, Watanabe S, Sato Y, et al. An immunoperoxidase study of S-100 protein distribution in normal and neoplastic tissues. *Am J Surg Pathol* 1982;6:715–727.
320. Schmitt FC, Bacchi CE. S-100 protein: is it useful as a tumour marker in diagnostic immunocytochemistry? *Histopathology* 1989;15: 281–288.
321. Soslow RA, Davis RE, Warnke RA, et al. True histiocytic lymphoma following therapy for lymphoblastic neoplasms. *Blood* 1996;87: 5207–5212.
322. Writing Group of the Histiocyte Society. Histiocytosis syndromes in children. *Lancet* 1987;1:208–209.
323. Pallesen G, Myhre-Jensen O. Immunophenotypic analysis of neoplastic cell in follicular dendritic cell sarcoma. *Leukemia* 1987;1:549–557.
324. Gown AM, Vogel AM, Hoak D, et al. Monoclonal antibodies specific for melanocytic tumors distinguish subpopulations of melanocytes. *Am J Pathol* 1986;123:195–203.
325. Fernando SS, Johnson S, Bate J. Immunohistochemical analysis of cutaneous malignant melanoma: comparison of S-100 protein, HMB-45 monoclonal antibody and NK1/C3 monoclonal antibody. *Pathology* 1994;26:16–19.
326. Anstey A, Cerio R, Ramnarain N, et al. Desmoplastic malignant melanoma: an immunocytochemical study of 25 cases. *Am J Dermatopathol* 1994;16:14–22.
327. Pea M, Bonetti F, Zamboni G, et al. Melanocyte-marker-HMB-45 is regularly expressed in angiomyolipoma of the kidney. *Pathology* 1991;23:185–188.
328. Bonetti F, Chiodera PL, Pea M, et al. Transbronchial biopsy in lymphangiomyomatosis of the lung: HMB-45 for diagnosis. *Am J Surg Pathol* 1993;17:1092–1102.
329. Duray PH, Ernstoff MS, Titus-Ernstoff L. Immunohistochemical phenotyping of malignant melanoma: a procedure whose time has come in pathology practice. *Pathol Annu* 1990;25:351–377.
330. Mostofi FK, Sesterhenn IA. Pathology of germ cell tumors of testes. *Prog Clin Biol Res* 1985;203:1–34.
331. Mostofi FK. Testicular tumors: epidemiologic, etiologic, and pathologic features. *Cancer* 1973;32:1186–1201.
332. Knowles DM, Chadburn AC. The neoplasms associated with AIDS. In: Joshi VV, ed. *Pathology of AIDS and other manifestations of HIV infection.* New York: Igaku-Shoin, 1990:83–120.
333. Richter HJ, Leder LD. Lymph node metastases with PAS-positive tumor cells and massive epithelioid granulomatous reaction as diagnostic clue to occult seminoma. *Cancer* 1979;44:245–249.
334. Mostofi FK, Sesterhenn IA, Davis CJ Jr. Immunopathology of germ cell tumors of the testis. *Semin Diagn Pathol* 1987;4:320–341.
335. Manivel JC, Jessurun J, Wick MR, et al. Placental alkaline phosphatase immunoreactivity in testicular germ cell neoplasms. *Am J Surg Pathol* 1987;11:21–29.
336. Ramaekers F, Feitz W, Moesker O, et al. Antibodies to cytokeratin and vimentin in testicular tumor diagnosis. *Virchows Arch A Pathol Anat Histopathol* 1985;408:127–142.
337. Riley D, Marks A, Stratis M, et al. Immunohistochemical staining of germ cell tumors and intratubular malignant germ cells of the testis using antibody to placental alkaline phosphatase and a monoclonal anti-seminoma antibody. *Mod Pathol* 1991;4:167–171.
338. Wick MR, Swanson PE, Manivel JC. Placental-like alkaline phosphatase reactivity in human tumors: an immunohistochemical study of 520 cases. *Hum Pathol* 1987;18:946–954.
339. Miettinen M, Virtanen I, Talerman A. Intermediate filament proteins in human testis and testicular germ cell tumors. *Am J Pathol* 1985; 120:402–410.
340. Suster S, Moran CA, Dominguez-Malagon H, et al. Germ cell tumors of the mediastinum and testis: a comparative immunohistochemical study of 120 cases. *Hum Pathol* 1998;29:737–742.
341. Kuida CA, Braunstein GD, Shintaku P, et al. Human chorionic gonadotropin expression in lung, breast and renal carcinoma. *Arch Pathol Lab Med* 1988;112:282–285.
342. Pallesen G, Hamilton-Dutoit SJ. Ki-1 (CD30) antigen is regularly expressed by tumor cells of embryonal carcinoma. *Am J Pathol* 1988,133:446–450.
343. Millward C, Weidner N. CD30 (Ber-H2) expression in nonhematopoietic tumors. *Appl Immunohistochem* 1998;6:164–168.
344. Haagensen CD. The spread of cancer in the lymphatic system. In: Haagensen CD, et al., eds. *Lymphatics in cancer.* Philadelphia: WB Saunders, 1972.
345. Enzinger FM, Weiss SW. *Soft tissue tumors,* 3rd ed. St. Louis: Mosby, 1995.
346. Ambros IM, Ambros PJ, Strehl S, et al. MIC2 is a specific marker for Ewing's sarcoma and peripheral primitive neuroectodermal tumors. *Cancer* 1991;67:1886–1893.
347. Fellinger EF, Garin-Chesa P, Triche TJ, et al. Immunohistochemical analysis of Ewing's sarcoma cell surface antigen p30/32 MIC2. *Am J Pathol* 1991;139:317–325.
348. Smith MJ, Goodfellow PJ, Goodfellow PN. The genomic organization of the human pseudoautosomal gene MIC2 and the detection of a related locus. *Hum Mol Genet* 1993;2:417–422.
349. Levy R, Dilley J, Fox RI, et al. A human thymus-leukemia antigen defined by hybridoma monoclonal antibodies. *Proc Natl Acad Sci USA* 1979;76:6552–6556.
350. Ramani P, Rampling D, Link M. Immunocytochemical study of 12E7 in small round-cell tumors of childhood: an assessment of its sensitivity and specificity. *Histopathology* 1993;23:557–561.
351. Soslow RA, Bhargava V, Warnke RA. MIC2, TdT, bcl-2, and CD34 expression in paraffin-embedded high-grade lymphoma/acute lymphoblastic leukemia distinguishes between distinct clinicopathologic entities. *Hum Pathol* 1997;28:1158–1165.
352. Carter RL, al-Sams SZ, Corbett RP, et al. A comparative study of immunohistochemical staining for neuron-specific enolase, protein gene product 9.5 and S-100 protein in neuroblastoma, Ewing's sarcoma and other round cell tumours in children. *Histopathology* 1990; 16:461–467.
353. Dierick AM, Roels H, Langlois M. The immunophenotype of Ewing's sarcoma: an immunohistochemical analysis. *Pathol Res Pract* 1993; 189:26–32.
354. Pinto A, Grant LH, Hayes FA, et al. Immunohistochemical expression of neuron-specific enolase and Leu 7 in Ewing's sarcoma of bone. *Cancer* 1989;64:1266–1273.
355. Parham DM, Hijazi Y, Steinberg SM, et al. Neuroectodermal differentiation in Ewing's sarcoma family of tumors does not predict tumor behavior. *Hum Pathol* 1999;30:911–918.
356. Dellatre O, Zucman J, Melot T, et al. The Ewing family of tumors: a subgroup of small-round-cell tumors defined by specific chimeric transcripts. *N Engl J Med* 1994;331:294–299.
357. Ladanyi M, Lewis R, Garin-Chesa P, et al. EWS rearrangements in Ewing's sarcoma and peripheral neuroectodermal tumor: molecular detection and correlation with cytogenetic analysis and MIC2 expression. *Diagn Mol Pathol* 1993;2:141–146.
358. Molenaar WM, Oosterhuis JW, Oosterhuis AM, et al. Mesenchymal and muscle-specific intermediate filaments (vimentin and desmin) in relation to differentiation in childhood rhabdomyosarcoma. *Hum Pathol* 1985;16:838–843.
359. Dias P, Parham DM, Shapiro DN, et al. Myogenic regulatory protein (MyoD1) expression in childhood solid tumors: diagnostic utility in rhabdomyosarcoma. *Am J Pathol* 1990;137:1283–1291.
360. Wijnaendts LC, van der Linden JC, van Unnik AJ, et al. Histopathological classification of childhood rhabdomyosarcomas: relationship with clinical parameters and prognosis. *Hum Pathol* 1994;25: 900–907.
361. Downing JR, Khandekar A, Shurtleff SA, et al. Multiple RT-PCR assay for the differential diagnosis of alveolar rhabdomyosarcoma and Ewing's sarcoma. *Am J Pathol* 1995;146:626–634.
362. Gerald WL, Rosai J, Ladanyi M. Characterization of the genomic breakpoint and chimeric transcripts in the EWS-WTI gene fusion of desmoplastic small round cell tumor. *Proc Natl Acad Sci USA* 1995; 92:1028–1032.
363. Gerald WL, Miller HK, Battifora H, et al. Intraabdominal desmoplastic small round-cell tumor: report of 19 cases of a distinctive type of high-grade polyphenotypic malignancy affecting young individuals. *Am J Surg Pathol* 1991;15:499–513.
364. Triche TJ, Askin FB. Neuroblastoma and the differential diagnosis of small-, round-, blue-cell tumors. *Hum Pathol* 1983;14:569–595.
365. Oppendale BR, Brandtzaeg P, Kemshead T. Immunohistochemical differentiation of neuroblastomas from other small round cell neoplasms of childhood using a panel of mono- and polyconal antibodies. *Histopathology* 1987;11:363–374.

366. du Boulay CE. Immunohistochemistry of soft tissue tumors: a review. *J Pathol* 1985;146:77–94.
367. Arber DA, Kandalaft PL, Mehta P, et al. Vimentin-negative epithelioid sarcoma: the value of immunohistochemical panel that includes CD34. *Am J Surg Pathol* 1994;17:302–307.
368. Dei Tos AP, Wadden C, Calonje E, et al. Immunohistochemical demonstration of glycoprotein p30/32MIC2 (CD99) in synovial sarcoma: a potential cause of diagnostic confusion. *Appl Immunohistochem* 1995;3:168–173.
369. Ramani P, Bradley NJ, Fletcher CD. QBEND/10, a new monoclonal antibody to endothelium: assessment of its diagnostic utility in paraffin sections. *Histopathology* 1990;17:237–242.
370. Weidner N, Tjoe J. Immunohistochemical profile of monoclonal antibody O13: antibody that recognizes glycoprotein p30/32MIC2 and is useful in diagnosing Ewing's sarcoma and peripheral neuroepithelioma. *Am J Surg Pathol* 1994;18:486–494.
371. Dal Cin P, Rao U, Jani-Sait S, et al. Chromosomes in the diagnosis of soft tissue tumors: I. Synovial sarcoma. *Mod Pathol* 1992;5:357–362.
372. Folpe AL, Schmidt RA, Chapman D, et al. Poorly differentiated synovial sarcoma: immunohistochemical distinction from primitive neuroendocrine tumors and high-grade malignant peripheral nerve sheath tumors. *Am J Surg Pathol* 1988;22:673–682.
373. van de Rijn M, Barr FG, Xiong QB, et al. Poorly differentiated synovial sarcoma: an analysis of clinical, pathologic, and molecular genetic features. *Am J Surg Pathol* 1999;23:106–112.
374. Chung EB, Enzinger FM. Malignant melanoma of soft parts: a reassessment of clear cell sarcoma. *Am J Surg Pathol* 1983;7:405–413.
375. Bridge JA, Borek DA, Neff JR, et al. Chromosomal abnormalities in clear cell sarcoma: implications for histogenesis. *Am J Clin Pathol* 1990; 93:26–31.
376. Swanson PE, Wick MR. Clear cell sarcoma: an immunohistochemical analysis of six cases and comparison with other epithelioid neoplasms of soft tissue. *Arch Pathol Lab Med* 1989;113:55–60.
377. Meis JM, Butler JJ, Osborne BM, et al. Granulocytic sarcoma in nonleukemic patients. *Cancer* 1986;58:2697–2709.
378. Zimmerman LE, Font RL. Ophthalmologic manifestations of granulocytic sarcoma (myeloid sarcoma or chloroma). *Am J Ophthalmol* 1975;80:975–990.
379. Klaus SN, Winkelmann RK. The clinical spectrum of urticaria pigmentosa. *Mayo Clin Proc* 1965;40:923–931.
380. Travis WD, Li C-Y, Bergstralh EJ, et al. Systemic mast cell disease: analysis of 58 cases and literature review. *Medicine (Baltimore)* 1988; 67:345–368.
381. Travis WD, Li C-Y. Pathology of the lymph node and spleen in systemic mast cell disease. *Mod Pathol* 1988;1:4–14.
382. Chan JKC, Fletcher CDM, Nayler SJ, et al. Follicular dendritic cell sarcoma: clinicopathologic analysis of 17 cases suggesting a malignant potential higher than currently recognized. *Cancer* 1997;79: 294–313.
383. Perez-Ordonez B, Erlandson RA, Rosai J. Follicular dendritic cell tumor: report of 13 additional cases of a distinctive entity. *Am J Surg Pathol* 1996;20:944–955.
384. Weiss LM, Berry GJ, Dorfman RF, et al. Spindle cell neoplasms of lymph nodes of probable reticulum cell lineage: true reticulum cell sarcoma. *Am J Pathol* 1990;14:405–414.
385. Chan WC, Zaatari G. Lymph node interdigitating reticulum cell sarcoma. *Am J Pathol* 1986;85:739–744.
386. Andriko JW, Kaldjian EP, Tsokos M, et al. Reticulum cell neoplasms of lymph nodes: a clinicopathologic study of 11 cases with recognition of a new subtype derived from fibroblastic reticular cells. *Am J Surg Pathol* 1998;22:1048–1058.
387. Pallesen G, Myhre-Jensen O. Immunophenotypic analysis of neoplastic cells in follicular dendritic cell sarcoma. *Leukemia* 1987;1: 549–557.
388. Parwaresch R, Radzun HJ, Hansmann M, et al. Monoclonal antibody Ki-M4 specifically recognizes human dendritic reticulum cells (follicular dendritic cells) and their precursors in blood. *Blood* 1983;62: 585–590.
389. Cline MJ. Histiocytes and histiocytosis. *Blood* 1994;84:2840–2853.
390. Toccanier-Pelte MF, Skalli O, Kapanci Y, et al. Characterization of stromal cells with myoid features in lymph nodes and spleen in normal and pathologic conditions. *Am J Pathol* 1987;129:109–118.
391. Pinkus GS, Warhol MJ, O'Connor EM, et al. Immunohistochemical localization of smooth muscle myosin in human spleen, lymph node, and other lymphoid tissues: unique staining patterns in splenic white pulp and sinuses, lymphoid follicles, and certain vasculature, with ultrastructural correlations. *Am J Pathol* 1986;123:440–453.
392. Hollowood K, Pease C, Mackay AM, et al. Sarcomatoid tumours of lymph nodes showing follicular dendritic cell differentiation. *J Pathol* 1991;163:205–216.
393. Chan JK, Tsang WY, Ng CS. Follicular dendritic tumor and vascular neoplasm complicating hyaline-vascular Castleman's disease. *Am J Surg Pathol* 1994;18:517–525.
394. Nakamura S, Hara K, Suchi T, et al. Interdigitating cell sarcoma: a morphologic, immunohistologic and enzyme histochemical study. *Cancer* 1988;61:562–568.
395. Chan ACL, Serrano-Olmo J, Erlandson RA, et al. Cytokeratin-positive malignant tumors with reticulum cell morphology: a subtype of fibroblastic reticulum cell neoplasm? *Am J Surg Pathol* 2000;24:107–116.

CHAPTER 31

Extranodal Lymphoid Proliferations: General Principles and Differential Diagnosis

Jerome S. Burke

Many pathologists and clinicians have the misconception that extranodal lymphomas are an uncommon and exotic category of malignant lymphomas. Only extranodal presentation of Hodgkin's disease is rare; among non-Hodgkin's lymphomas, extranodal presentations are relatively common. Depending on whether the definition of extranodal lymphoma includes cases that present in certain extranodal lymphoid tissue-bearing sites, such as Waldeyer's ring, up to 40% of non-Hodgkin's lymphomas present in extranodal locations (1–5), and the incidence is rising. Based on Surveillance, Epidemiology, and End Results data from the National Cancer Institute of the United States, extranodal lymphomas increased 4% between the periods from 1973 to 1977 and from 1983 to 1987 (4). Some histologic categories of malignant lymphoma, specifically Burkitt's lymphoma and large B-cell lymphomas, consistently present in extranodal locations (6). Extranodal lymphomas may present or originate in any site, but in virtually every study, the gastrointestinal tract, mainly the stomach, is the most common location (1–5). In the Surveillance, Epidemiology, and End Results data, the stomach is followed by the skin, oral cavity, small intestine, and central nervous system (4) (Table 31.1). In other studies, however, Waldeyer's ring follows the gastrointestinal tract in frequency (5). Between 1973 and 1987, the age-adjusted incidence rates for extranodal lymphomas increased 68%, and for some lymphomas, such as those of the skin, central nervous system, and colon or rectum, the incidence rates increased 100%; the rates for the gastrointestinal tract increased up to 50% (4). The increasing incidence of primary gastric lymphomas involves both men and women but largely is limited to those patients older than 60 years of age (7). This may be a true increase, because the study period precedes the general recognition of many extranodal lymphomas as low-grade marginal zone lymphomas of extranodal mucosa-associated lymphoid tissue (MALT) type (8). The increase in central nervous system lymphomas also appears genuine, with a greater number of cases in the general population as well as in the central nervous system secondary to AIDS (9). AIDS is the best known of the immunodeficiency states associated with the onset of extranodal lymphomas. Eighty percent of patients who have AIDS and who develop malignant lymphoma have extranodal presentations, and the extranodal sites are frequently unusual, such as the brain or heart (10,11) (see Chapter 28).

To be categorized as having an extranodal lymphoma, the patient must present with localized, clinical stage IE or IIE disease (5). An even stricter definition recently was proposed for primary extranodal cutaneous lymphomas. In a study from the European Organization for Research and Treatment of Cancer, the diagnosis of primary cutaneous lymphoma was restricted to patients who not only declared exclusively in the skin but who also had no evidence of extracutaneous lymphoma both at the time of diagnosis and within the first 6 months afterwards (12). Patients who have clinical stage IIIE or IV disease and who are diagnosed in an extranodal site are not included as cases of extranodal lymphoma, because the extranodal site is assumed to be a manifestation of disseminated and frequently occult lymphoma. Patients with known lymphoma who relapse in an extranodal site also are excluded.

The past two decades have witnessed an increasing interest in extranodal lymphomas, particularly since the advent of immunologic cell marker and molecular genetic techniques to analyze lymphomas (13,14). The most obvious source of an increasing awareness of extranodal lymphomas is the numerous publications about extranodal lymphomas and their relationship to MALT (15–18). The varying proposals, nomenclature, and merits of MALT and its association with extranodal lymphomas are not addressed in this

J. S. Burke: Department of Anatomic Pathology, Alta Bates Medical Center, Berkeley, California 94705

TABLE 31.1. *Extranodal lymphomas: age-adjusted incidence rate per 100,000*

	1973–1977	1983–1987
Stomach	0.4	0.6
Skin	0.3	0.6
Oral cavity or pharynx	0.3	0.4
Small intestine	0.2	0.3
Brain or central nervous system	0.1	0.2
Colon or rectum	0.1	0.2
Thyroid	0.1	0.1
Soft tissues	0.1	0.1
Lung or pleura	0.1	0.1
Orbit	0.0	0.1
All extranodal sites	1.9	3.2

Adapted from Greiner TC, Medeiros JL, Jaffe ES. Non-Hodgkin's lymphoma. *Cancer* 1995;75:370–380, with permission.

chapter. Isaacson, the main proponent of the concept of MALT-derived extranodal lymphomas, discusses these in Chapter 33. This chapter develops the general diagnostic principles employed in separating extranodal malignant lymphomas from extranodal lymphoid hyperplasias, or so-called pseudolymphomas. The histologic criteria that allow this distinction are emphasized here, and the role of immunophenotypic and genotypic studies in the refinement and alteration of these histologic criteria is examined.

TRADITIONAL DIAGNOSTIC CRITERIA

In establishing a histologic diagnosis of an extranodal lymphoma, pathologists are aware that various reactive lymphoid hyperplasias exist that mimic extranodal lymphomas clinically and pathologically. Examples of extranodal florid lymphoid hyperplasias that simulate extranodal lymphomas include lymphoid hyperplasia of the ileocecal region, myoepithelial sialadenitis or benign lymphoepithelial lesions (MESA-BLEL) of salivary glands, chronic lymphocytic thyroiditis, and the many types of cutaneous lymphoid hyperplasia. To complicate matters, malignant lymphomas may develop in association with some of these reactive and autoimmune conditions (8). Patients who have Sjögren's syndrome and chronic lymphocytic thyroiditis (Hashimoto's thyroiditis) have increased risk of developing malignant lymphoma (19,20). One explanation for the predisposition of patients who have Sjögren's syndrome and Hashimoto's thyroiditis to develop malignant lymphomas is the observation that many histologically benign lymphoid infiltrates in the salivary and thyroid glands represent occult monoclonal and oligoclonal B-cell proliferations (21–23).

The morphologic criteria for distinguishing extranodal lymphoma from extranodal lymphoid hyperplasia traditionally have been extrapolated from those used to distinguish malignant lymphoma from lymphoid hyperplasia in lymph nodes (24). The major criteria that allow this distinction include monomorphic lymphocytic infiltrates, cellular atypia, and disruption of the normal architecture. Identical criteria have been used as the histologic standards for the diagnosis of extranodal lymphomas (Table 31.2). Because 60% to 85% of all extranodal lymphomas are large B-cell lymphomas with associated monomorphism, cellular atypia, and architectural destruction of the extranodal site (for example, obliteration of glands or follicles), these traditional criteria generally have proven to be reliable and applicable (3,25). Reactive lymphoid conditions that are at the opposite end of the spectrum also do not pose diagnostic problems (26). Lymphocytic infiltrates that are polymorphous, that display a range of mature lymphocytes (including plasma cells and immunoblasts), that are associated with well-defined germinal centers, and that do not destroy completely the architectural landmarks of an extranodal site can be diagnosed confidently as benign and reactive.

The main difficulty in the separation of extranodal lymphomas from lymphoid hyperplasias concerns the low-grade MALT lymphomas, such as those in the ocular adnexa and lung, that are composed of small lymphocytes and frequently associated with germinal center formation (27–31). In such cases, the traditional histologic criteria are not fully applicable (32). Multiparameter studies have revealed that many histologically ambiguous extranodal small lymphocytic proliferations are monoclonal; they are presumed to be malignant lymphomas (13,23,33). The application of immunologic and molecular genetic analyses to extranodal small lymphocytic proliferations has altered the traditional histologic criteria and has revealed myriad inconsistencies in these criteria (Table 31.3). For example, in a recent review of 97 cases originally diagnosed as gastric pseudolymphoma between 1970 and 1985, 79% were reclassified as malignant lymphoma, with fully two thirds of the newly classified lymphomatous cases interpreted as lymphomas of MALT type (34). The remaining cases were regarded as examples of lymphoid hyperplasia or atypical lymphocytic infiltrates. Similarly, many cases previously interpreted as MESA-BLEL or as Hashimoto's thyroiditis also are low-grade lymphomas and commonly arise secondary to "acquired" MALT (35–37). Consequently, the term *pseudolymphoma*

TABLE 31.2. *Traditional histologic criteria for distinguishing extranodal lymphomas from lymphoid hyperplasias*

Extranodal lymphomas	Lymphoid hyperplasias
Infiltrate monomorphous	Infiltrate polymorphous (lymphocytes in stages of transformation)
Cytologic atypia	Cytologic maturity (lymphocytes, plasma cells, and immunoblasts)
Germinal centers uncommon	Germinal centers common (usually in center of infiltrate)
Massive infiltration with architectural destruction	Random infiltration with architectural retention

TABLE 31.3. *Modifications of the traditional histologic criteria for distinguishing extranodal lymphomas from lymphoid hyperplasia*

Extranodal lymphomas may be polymorphous (including peripheral T-cell lymphomas)
Extranodal lymphomas may be composed of cytologically mature-appearing lymphocytes (small lymphocytic and other low-grade lymphomas with or without plasma cell differentiation)
Germinal centers may be observed at the periphery of extranodal lymphomas and in the centers of many low-grade extranodal lymphomas, especially those of mucosa-associated lymphoid tissue type
Degree of infiltration, architectural and epithelial destruction highly variable in benign and malignant extranodal lymphocytic infiltrates

is regarded as imprecise and anachronistic and no longer is acceptable as a diagnostic category (38).

Cases in which extranodal lymphoma coexist with reactive lymphoid hyperplasia and technical artifacts, found mainly in small biopsy specimens, are other common factors that lead to diagnostic problems in the evaluation of extranodal lymphocytic infiltrates.

MODIFICATIONS OF THE TRADITIONAL HISTOLOGIC CRITERIA FOR THE DIAGNOSIS OF EXTRANODAL LYMPHOMAS

Polymorphous Extranodal Lymphomas

A polymorphous or mixed lymphoid proliferation in an extranodal site usually infers a benign reactive state. In extranodal lymphoid hyperplasia, the polymorphous cell population exhibits a spectrum of lymphocytic transformation, including small lymphocytes, intermediate-sized lymphocytes, plasma cells, and immunoblasts. This proliferation frequently is accompanied by germinal centers. If there are no germinal centers, it is the *range* of lymphocytic transformation and its orderliness that indicate that the lymphocytic population is hyperplasia and not lymphoma.

The morphologic interpretation of extranodal florid immunoblastic hyperplasia may be demanding, because florid hyperplasia often leads to obliteration of the normal histologic landmarks of that extranodal site (Fig. 31.1). In this setting, the immunoblasts may appear atypical, with the increased mitotic activity that results from an antigenic stimulus (32). Distinction from malignant lymphoma relies on recognizing that the lymphocytes have some symmetry in their proliferative activity, even if dominated by immunoblasts (Fig. 31.2). Unlike malignant lymphomas, the small lymphocytes in reactive lymphoid hyperplasias are round and appear mature. Malignant lymphoma, small lymphocytic lymphoma or chronic lymphocytic leukemia that contains admixed large cells or paraimmunoblasts, and marginal zone lymphoma of MALT type dominated by small lymphocytes that evolves to large cell lymphoma are exceptions; the small lymphocytes have no significant cytologic atypia

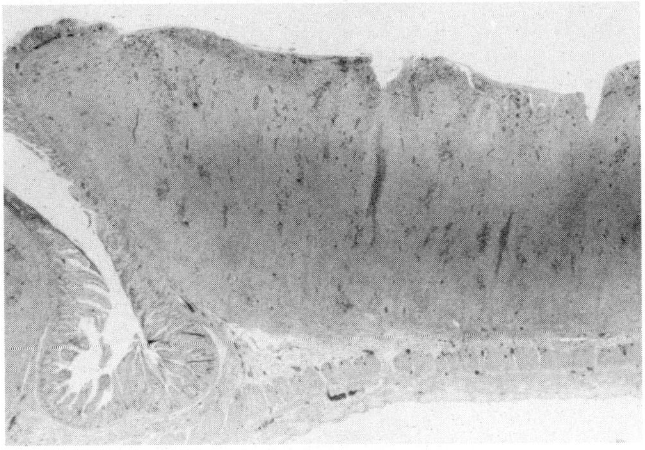

FIG. 31.1. Florid lymphoid hyperplasia of the terminal ileum results in a tumor mass that obliterates the mucosa and submucosa. Despite the massive size of the hyperplastic process, the proliferating lymphocytes do not invade the muscularis propria (hematoxylin and eosin stain, original magnification: 15× magnification).

(31,39). Such cases can be distinguished from reactive states because the cellular proliferation in the lymphomas usually is dense and destructive, and there often is an abrupt transition from the small lymphocytes to the large cells. In cases in which frank large cell lymphoma has developed, the large cells are monomorphous and form microscopic sheets or masses. In some extranodal sites, such as the stomach, however, the large malignant B cells are arcane and may form only small clusters or diffusely intermingle with the small lymphocytes of a low-grade MALT lymphoma. The observation of a diffuse large cell component in 1% to 10% with and without nonconfluent clusters of large cells predicts a significantly worse prognosis in an otherwise low-grade gastric MALT lymphoma (40). Hodgkin's disease is another malignant lymphoma with a polymorphous cell population and without atypia among the small lymphocytes; however, extranodal Hodgkin's disease is uncommon and usually presents in an extranodal site as a consequence of direct invasion from adjacent lymph nodes or by retrograde lymphatic spread (41).

Most extranodal polymorphous or mixed small to medium-sized and large cell lymphomas are characterized by nuclear membrane irregularities and atypia in the small lymphocytes (Fig. 31.3). This includes the peripheral T-cell and natural killer cell lymphomas of extranodal sites. Fortunately, noncutaneous extranodal natural killer cell and T-cell lymphomas are uncommon, except for those in the upper nasal air passages and those in the intestine associated with gluten sensitivity; the latter have been referred to as *enteropathy-type intestinal T-cell lymphomas* (42–44). In some cases the distinction of a polymorphous lymphoma from extranodal florid lymphoid hyperplasia may not be possible using only histologic criteria; immunologic and, at times, gene rearrangement studies are required for a definite diagnosis (8,13,14,33,45).

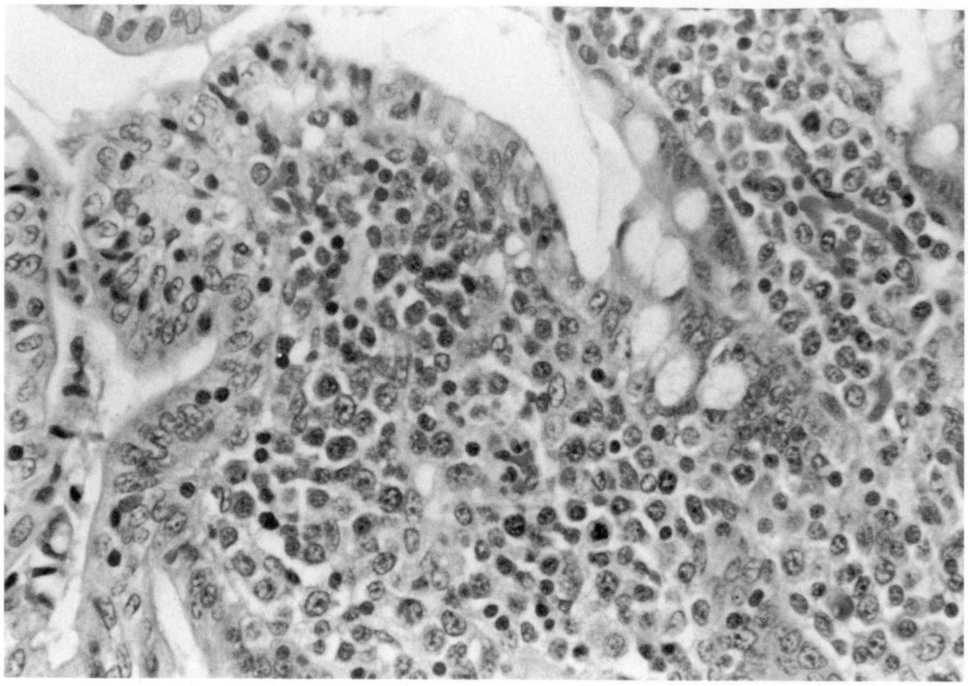

FIG. 31.2. Although numerous large immunoblasts appear in the lamina propria of the ileum, there is an orderly range of lymphocytic transformation indicative of florid reactive hyperplasia (hematoxylin and eosin stain, original magnification: 375× magnification).

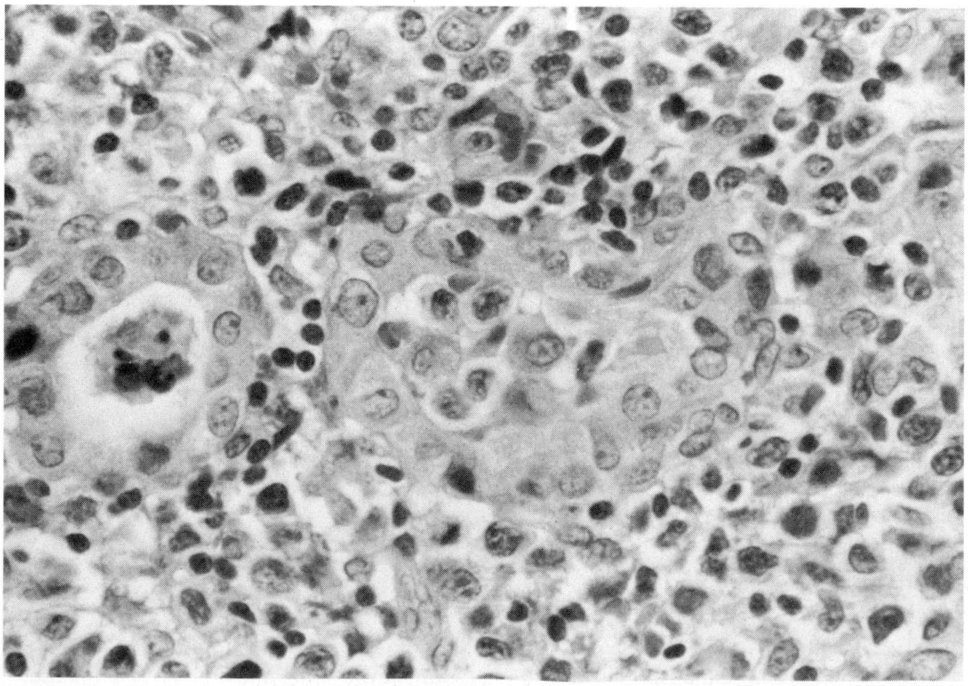

FIG. 31.3. Large cell or immunoblastic lymphoma, with a polymorphous cell population, displays nuclear membrane irregularities in small and large lymphocytes alike. Note the invasion of thyroid follicles (hematoxylin and eosin stain, original magnification: 600× magnification).

Cytologically Mature Extranodal Lymphomas

The conventional view is that extranodal lymphomas are characterized by nuclear membrane irregularities or atypia. Low-grade marginal zone lymphomas of MALT type, however, are cytologically mutable (31). Although MALT lymphomas typically are composed of centrocyte-like cells in the marginal zones, they also may have a monocytoid appearance, or they be composed of plasma cells or have no or only subtle nuclear membrane irregularities, similar to the cells of small lymphocytic lymphoma or chronic lymphocytic leukemia (16,17,31); the latter variant often is confused with extranodal lymphoid hyperplasia. With the widespread use of immunologic markers, it is recognized that many extranodal small lymphocytic proliferations, such as those in the ocular adnexa, lung, and gastrointestinal tract, are low-grade malignant lymphomas, mainly of MALT type (17,27–30,46).

Small biopsy specimens that contain a predominance of small lymphocytes represent the most difficult problem in the diagnosis of extranodal lymphocytic lesions (32). A small lymphocytic proliferation that appears mature is the histologic norm in cases of extranodal lymphoid hyperplasia, but cytologic maturity or minimal atypia also is the histologic hallmark of most low-grade malignant lymphomas. How can these two groups be distinguished in a small biopsy specimen? In many cases this is impossible if only histologic criteria are applied. This histologic dilemma prompted the use of the noncommittal term *extranodal small lymphocytic proliferation* to describe histologically ambiguous or indeterminate extranodal lymphocytic infiltrates (47). Morphologic criteria currently used to separate benign from malignant small lymphocytic infiltrates includes whether the infiltrate is monomorphous, is dense, or exhibits cytologic atypia or Dutcher bodies, and whether this results in destruction of glands, follicles, or other structures indigenous to that extranodal site (32,33,48) (Fig. 31.4). If these morphologic features are unequivocally present, then the lymphocytic infiltrate likely is malignant lymphoma. In the stomach, a histologic scoring system for MALT has been proposed in which invasion of epithelial structures (''lymphoepithelial lesions'' of MALT) are considered essential to the diagnosis (49). Employing the scoring system, a definite diagnosis of low-grade B-cell lymphoma of MALT is based on the presence of a dense diffuse infiltrate of centrocyte-like cells in the lamina propria, with prominent lymphoepithelial lesions. Cases regarded as suspicious lymphocytic infiltrates are those in which reactive follicles are surrounded by centrocyte-like cells that diffusely infiltrate into the lamina propria and into epithelium in small groups (49). There may be dense infiltrates, slight cytologic atypia, and lymphoepithelial-like lesions in cases of lymphoid hyperplasia in many extranodal sites, including the stomach (29,36,50,51). Morphologic interpretation also is obscured by the observation of germinal centers in most extranodal marginal zone lymphomas of MALT and in many mantle cell lymphomas (13,17,18,32,51,52). Frequently, in lymphomas such as the mantle cell lymphomas found in the gastrointestinal mucosa, including cases of multiple lymphomatous polyposis of the intestine, the germinal centers appear atrophic and are encircled by dense, monomorphous neoplastic lymphocytes (52,53) (Fig. 31.5).

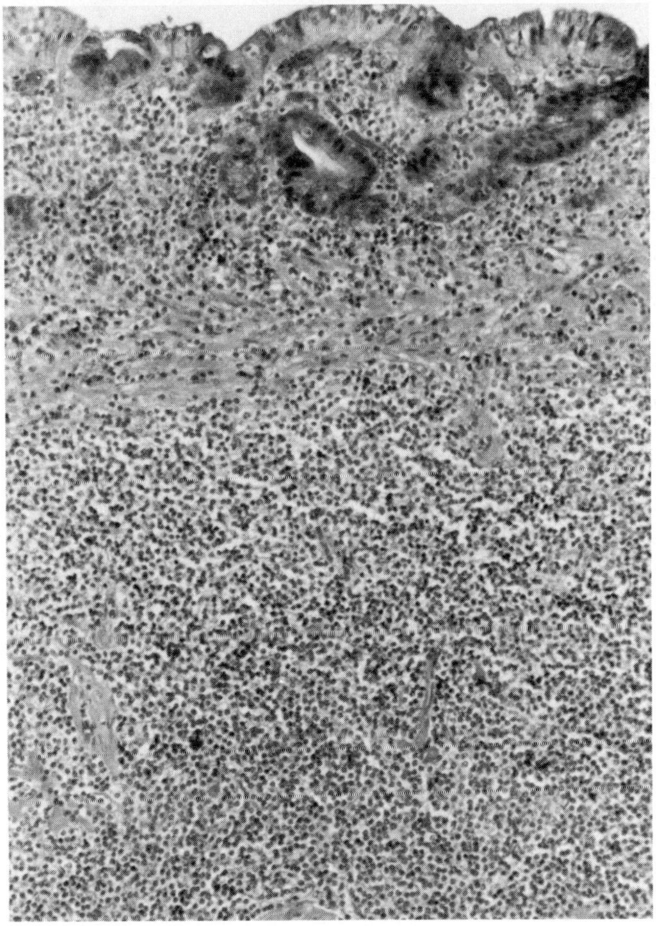

FIG. 31.4. A low-grade lymphoma composed of small lymphocytes in the stomach is characterized by a dense uniform infiltrate with destruction of normal gastric glands. Immunologic studies confirmed that the lymphocytes were B cells with λ light chain restriction (hematoxylin and eosin stain, original magnification: 150× magnification).

Our perspective of small extranodal lymphocytic proliferations that appear mature has been revised dramatically with the application of immunologic markers to analyze the clonality of these lesions (13,14,33). Immunologic studies have indicated that many extranodal small lymphocytic proliferations that fulfill the current histologic criteria are monoclonal B-cell proliferations; such cases usually are equated with low-grade MALT lymphomas (13,16,27,29,46). Correlative immunopathologic studies of monoclonal B-cell lymphoproliferative lesions, such as those in the ocular adnexa, have reduced the number of cases regarded as atypical or indeterminate (27,28,54). Naturally, there still are cases, especially small biopsy specimens, in which the histologic features or

A 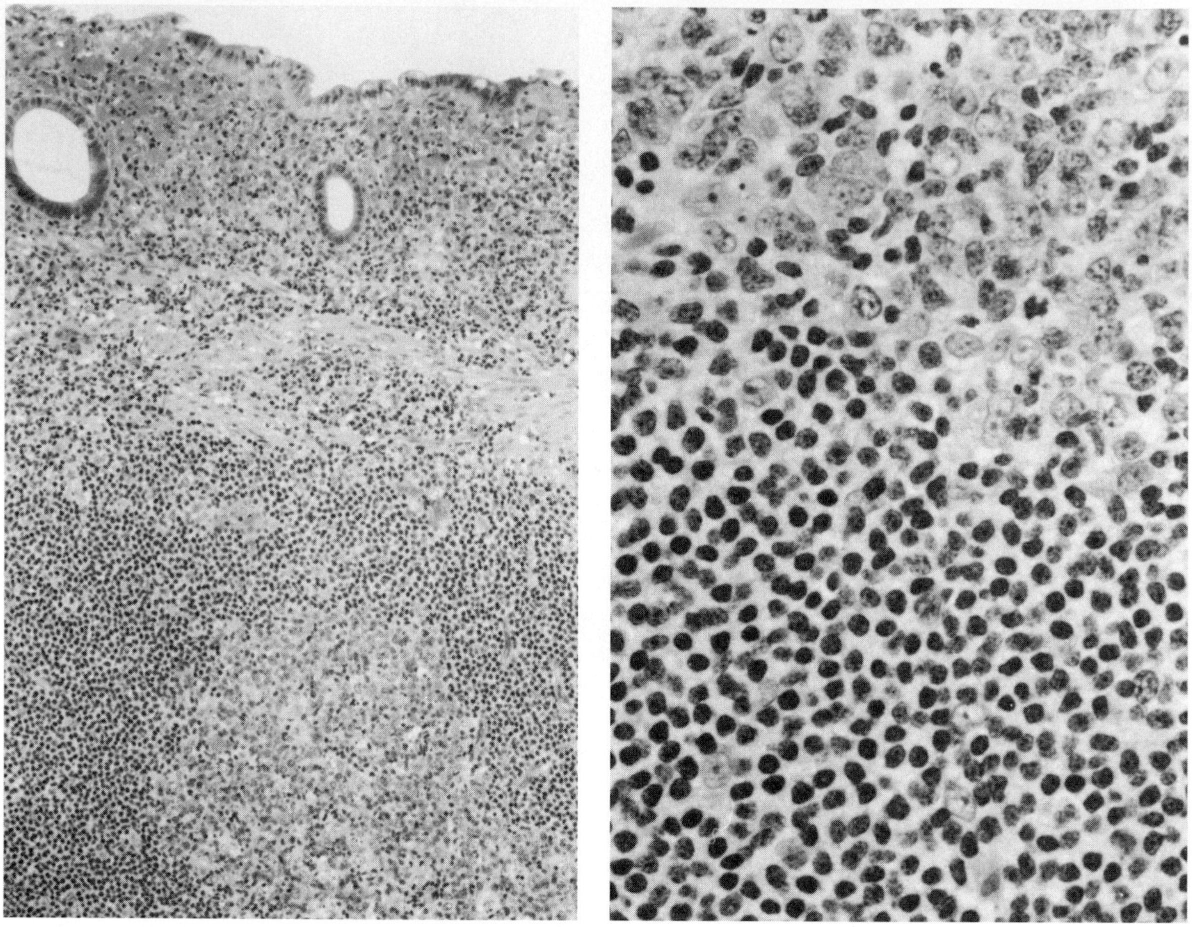 B

FIG. 31.5. A: Mantle cell lymphoma of the small intestine surrounds a germinal center in a case of multiple lymphomatous polyposis (hematoxylin and eosin stain, original magnification: 120× magnification). **B:** Detail of the atypical mantle zone lymphocytes that infiltrate into the margin of the germinal center; the lymphocytes expressed only κ light chains and IgM heavy chains (hematoxylin and eosin stain, original magnification: 480× magnification).

immunologic findings remain equivocal (Fig. 31.6); these cases should receive not only a descriptive diagnosis but also a request for a repeat biopsy with reservation of fresh tissue to determine clonality, by immunohistochemistry, flow cytometry, molecular techniques, or a combination thereof (17,31,55,56). If only fixed, paraffin-embedded tissues are available, a consistent determination of clonality in a biopsy specimen dominated by small lymphocytes usually is not possible in most laboratories. In some cases, immunologic studies of paraffin-embedded tissue can reveal an aberrant phenotype in the suspicious small lymphocytic population, such as the coexpression of B-cell antigen CD20 and T-cell antigen CD43 (57,58) (Fig. 31.7). Although caution is required in the interpretation of CD43-positive B-cell populations, in most instances the aberrant immunophenotype supports the diagnosis of an extranodal B-cell lymphoma (33). Prudence also is necessary in the evaluation of immunoglobulin gene rearrangement studies employing polymerase chain reaction techniques in fixed paraffin-embedded tissues (33,45); small monoclonal bands may occur in extranodal reactive lymphoid hyperplasias, as for example in chronic active gastritis associated with *Helicobacter pylori* (59).

Germinal Centers in Extranodal Lymphomas

The presence of germinal centers is a commonly accepted histologic attribute of extranodal lymphoid hyperplasias. Germinal centers, however, are regular constituents of many extranodal lymphomas. Germinal centers often are observed at the periphery of large cell lymphomas, such as those in the thyroid (36,60). In the thyroid, a histologic continuum frequently occurs between areas of chronic lymphocytic thyroiditis with germinal centers and areas of adjacent large cell lymphoma, usually devoid of germinal centers (36) (Fig. 31.8); this finding has suggested that thyroid lymphomas evolve from chronic lymphocytic thyroiditis (60).

There is increasing recognition that germinal centers also may be identified in the middle of an aggressive lymphoma, for example, mantle cell lymphomas of intestinal lymphom-

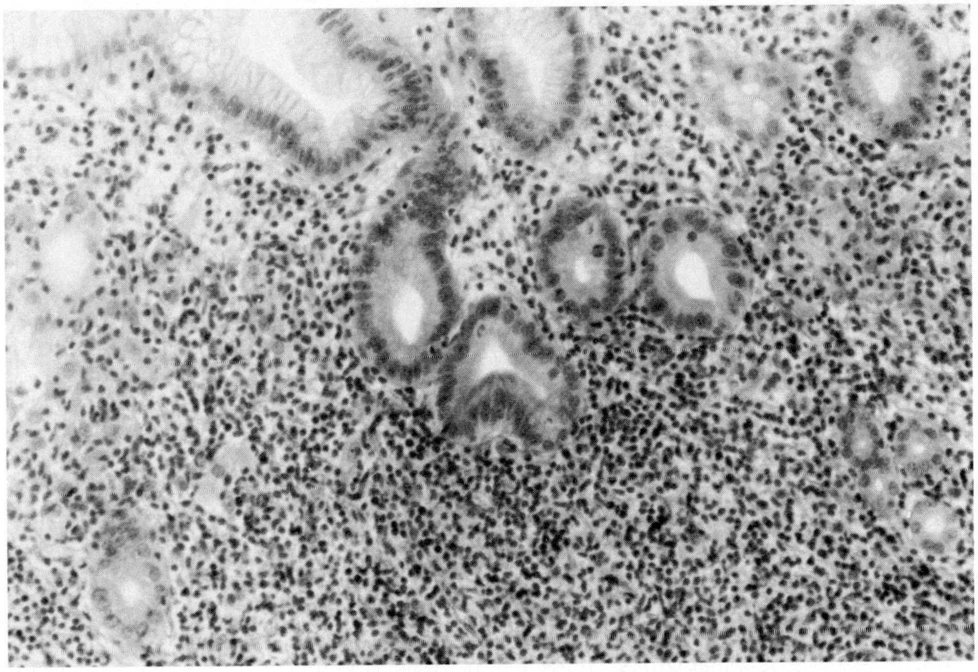

FIG. 31.6. This gastric biopsy specimen contains a variably dense lymphocytic infiltrate composed of small lymphocytes without cytologic atypia. The morphologic features were not regarded as completely diagnostic of malignant lymphoma, but a subsequent biopsy in which tissue was snap-frozen demonstrated a monoclonal B-cell population characterized as IgMκ (hematoxylin and eosin stain, original magnification: 240× magnification).

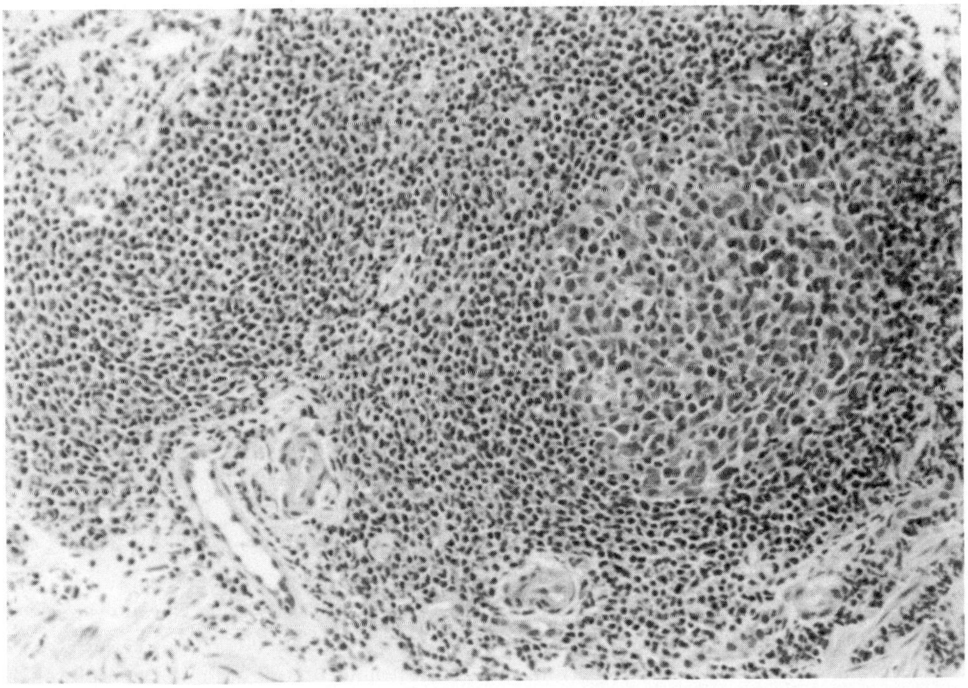

FIG. 31.7. A histologically equivocal small lymphocytic infiltrate in a stomach biopsy surrounds a germinal center. Both the germinal center and the surrounding lymphocytes expressed the B-cell antigen CD20 (L26), but the infiltrating small lymphocytes coexpressed the T-cell antigen CD43 (Leu 22), supporting the diagnosis of a MALT lymphoma (hematoxylin and eosin stain, original magnification: 240× magnification).

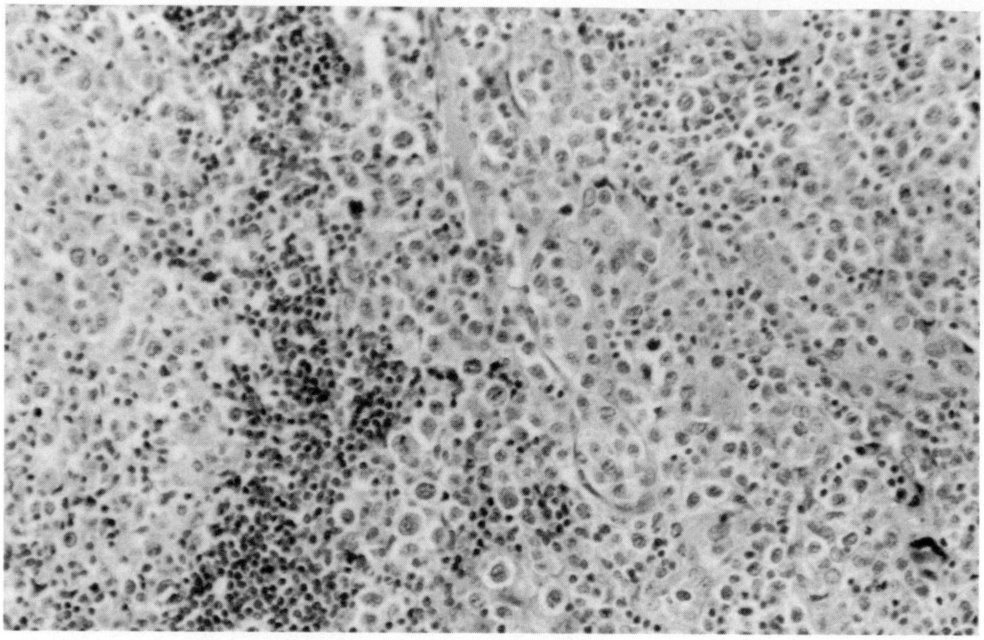

FIG. 31.8. A reactive germinal center on the left that reflects chronic lymphocytic thyroiditis merges with large cell lymphoma in the thyroid gland (hematoxylin and eosin stain, original magnification: 240× magnification).

atous polyposis and lymphoblastic lymphomas of the scalp (32,52,53). Germinal centers also are an integral component of the center of many low-grade lymphomas of MALT type. The essential morphologic characteristic of MALT lymphomas is their emulation of normal MALT, as typified by Peyer's patches found in the terminal ileum (17). The neoplastic B cells of MALT lymphomas are found in marginal-type zones surrounding reactive follicles, and frequently in attenuated rims of mantle zone lymphocytes. In MALT lymphomas of the lung, for example, germinal centers frequently are observed in the expanded alveolar walls surrounded by the proliferating neoplastic small lymphocytes (29,30) (Fig. 31.9). The germinal centers vary in appearance but commonly appear atrophic as a result of impingement by the surrounding small lymphocytes. In low-grade MALT lymphomas of the stomach associated with peptic ulceration, germinal centers occur at the base of the ulcer and in the adjacent mucosa, in which they seem encroached on and entrapped by the monotonous marginal zone lymphomatous population (46,51). In some cases, the neoplastic B cells in the marginal zone invade the germinal centers in a process referred to as *follicular colonization* (51,61). Follicular colonization may simulate follicular lymphoma in patients in whom there are numerous follicles. At times, the lymphomatous proliferation may be so extensive as to result in architectural obliteration with masking of any residual germinal centers; however, the presence of former germinal centers can be highlighted by the immunohistochemical demonstration of follicular dendritic cells employing an antibody against CD21 (31,51).

The finding of germinal centers in a small lymphocytic infiltrate in either the lung or stomach could be construed as examples of extranodal lymphoid hyperplasia; however, in both extranodal sites, replacement of the mantle zones is a histologic indication that the small lymphocytes likely are neoplastic. The mantle zones often are intact in MALT lymphomas dominated by monocytoid B cells that affect salivary glands, but in such patients the mantle zones and the germinal centers appear attenuated by the surrounding monocytoid B cells (35,62) (Fig. 31.10). The characteristic, well-developed lucent cytoplasm in the monocytoid B cells contrasts with the lack of visible cytoplasm in the residual mantle zone lymphocytes (Fig. 31.11).

Incomplete Architectural Effacement in Extranodal Lymphomas

Architectural effacement as a consequence of malignant lymphoma is a standard diagnostic tenet. Extranodal lymphomas usually obliterate and destroy normal epithelial structures and extend beyond the margins of that organ. For example, in the gastrointestinal tract, most aggressive lymphomas invade beyond the muscularis propria to the serosa and often into adjacent mesenteric fat. Gastrointestinal lymphoid hyperplasia generally is restricted to the mucosa or submucosa, with conservation of mucosal glands and crypts. Gastrointestinal lymphoid hyperplasias and malignant lymphomas deviate from these norms (51,63). Gastrointestinal lymphomas, particularly of MALT type, may be exceedingly subtle and confined to the mucosa and submucosa, without violation of the muscularis propria and with preservation of most mucosal glands (46,51) (Fig. 31.12). Alternatively, rare

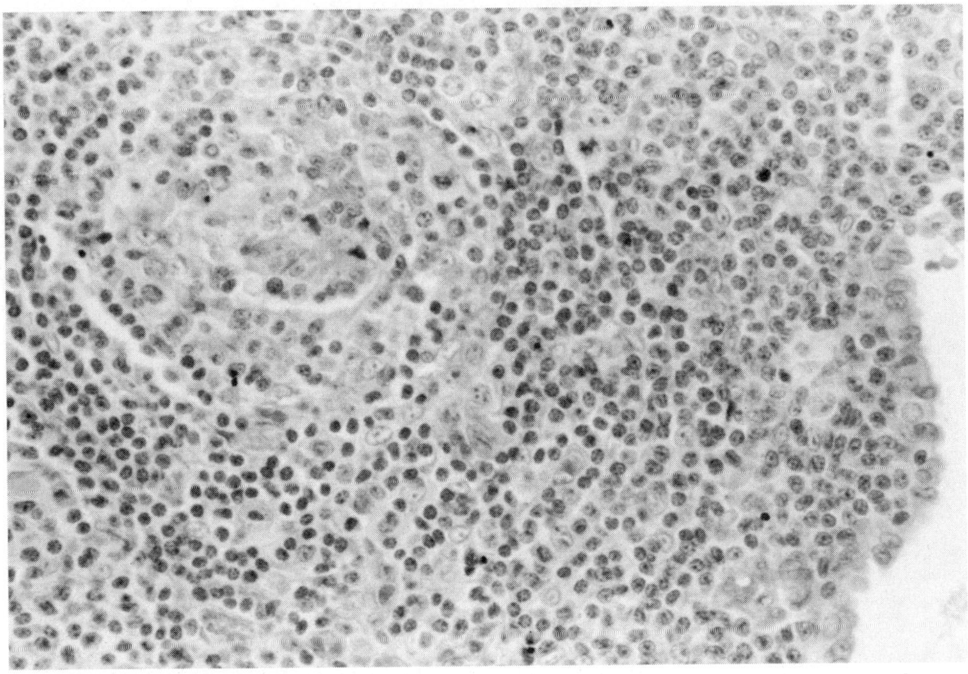

FIG. 31.9. In MALT lymphoma of the lung, a germinal center is entrapped and infiltrated by the neoplastic small lymphocytes with obliteration of the mantle zone. The small lymphocytes proved to be monoclonal B cells of IgMλ type (hematoxylin and eosin stain, original magnification: x375 magnification).

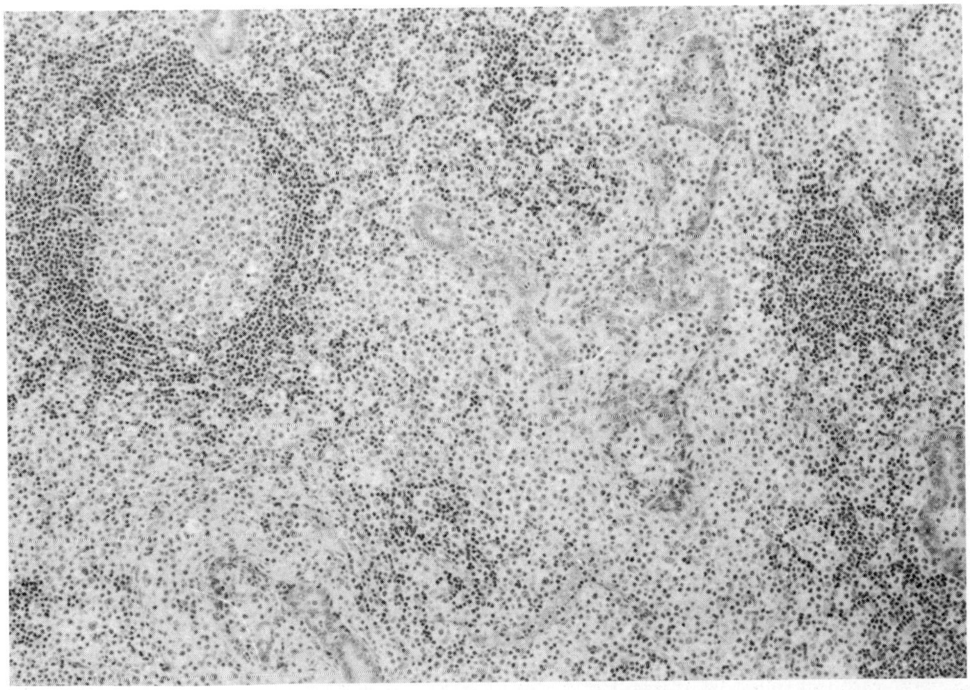

FIG. 31.10. MALT lymphoma, composed mainly of monocytoid B cells, that developed in a setting of myoepithelial sialadenitis. The monocytoid cells form wide interconnecting strands. A germinal center on the left with a variably intact mantle zone is distinct from the light staining cytoplasm of the monocytoid cells (hematoxylin and eosin stain, original magnification: 120$\times$ magnification).

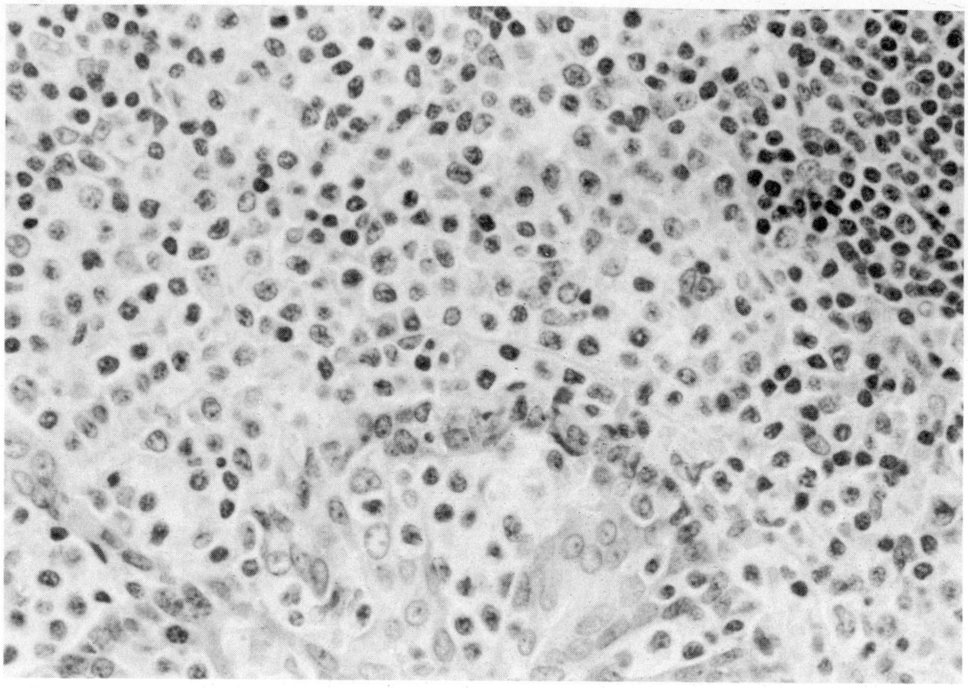

FIG. 31.11. The pale, almost lucent cytoplasm of the monocytoid cells contrasts with the mantle zone lymphocytes in the upper right. The neoplastic monocytoid B cells invade an epimyoepithelial island (hematoxylin and eosin stain, original magnification: 480× magnification).

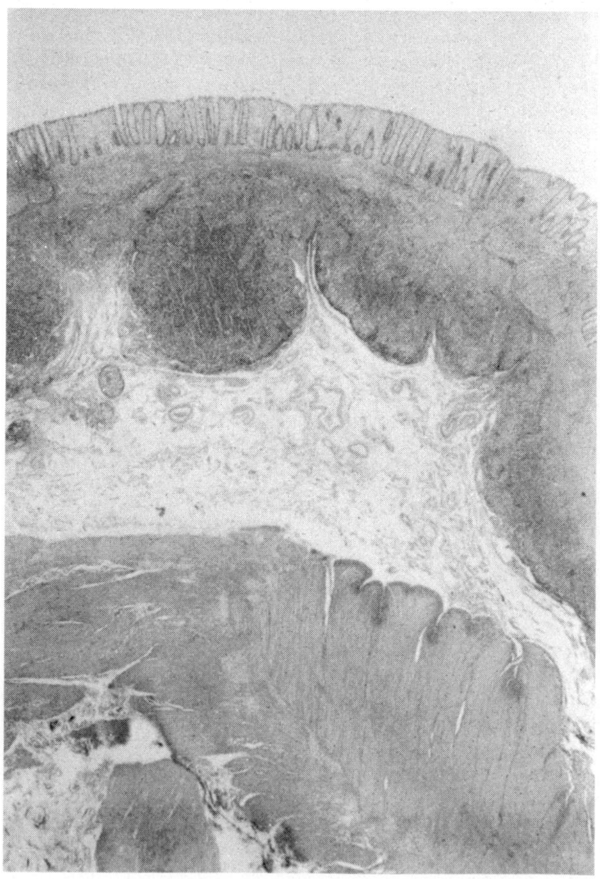

FIG. 31.12. A monoclonal B-cell lymphoma of low-grade type forms a localized polyp in the colon without destruction of the mucosa. The pattern mimics gastrointestinal lymphoid hyperplasia (hematoxylin and eosin stain, original magnification: 15× magnification).

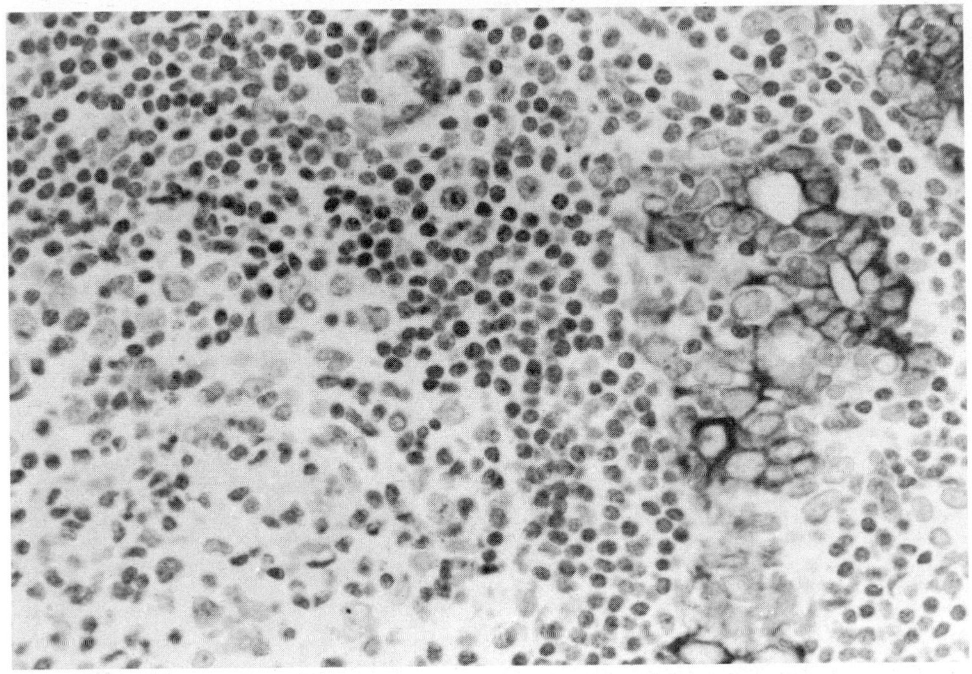

FIG. 31.13. In chronic lymphocytic thyroiditis, invasion of residual thyroid follicles may be observed; in this case it is highlighted with a stain for cytokeratin. Epithelial invasion or a lymphoepithelial-like lesion is not an absolute diagnostic criterion for extranodal lymphoma (immunoperoxidase stain, original magnification: 480× magnification).

cases of lymphoid hyperplasia may be florid and involve the entire depth of the gastrointestinal wall (63). In skin, malignant lymphomas may have a patchy, perivascular distribution in early lesions, may surround cutaneous adnexa, and even may be "top heavy," similar to cutaneous lymphoid hyperplasia (64–66). Conversely, cases of cutaneous lymphoid hyperplasia may invade cutaneous adnexa and be "bottom heavy," with infiltration into subcutaneous fat (67).

Invasion of epithelial structures, or "lymphoepithelial lesions" in the context of lymphomas of MALT, is an architectural feature purported to be significant in the diagnosis of extranodal lymphomas (15–18). Personal experience suggests that epithelial invasion by neoplastic lymphocytes actually may be difficult to identify, especially in the assessment of a small biopsy specimen if the differential diagnosis rests between a low-grade MALT lymphoma and lymphoid hyperplasia. In both conditions, epithelial structures are reduced by the lymphoid proliferation, but frank epithelial infiltration may not be prominent even with the use of keratin stains, which accentuate a lymphoepithelial lesion (36). Epithelial invasion virtually indistinguishable from a lymphoepithelial lesion may be found in various extranodal lymphoid hyperplasias, such as in the lung, salivary gland, thyroid, ileocecal region, and skin (29,35,36,50,67) (Fig. 31.13). Lymphoepithelial lesions are thought to be most significant as a diagnostic criterion of MALT lymphomas in the stomach, but even in this site lymphoid hyperplasia associated with *H. pylori* infection can exhibit infiltration of gastric epithelium and resemble a lymphomatous lymphoepithelial lesion (38,51). Vascular invasion is a more consistent morphologic feature of lymphomas than of extranodal lymphoid hyperplasias. In the rare cases of intravascular lymphomatosis, such as those in the skin and central nervous system, vascular involvement may be the only sign of extranodal lymphoma (68).

Although massive infiltration with architectural destruction is the general rule for most extranodal lymphomas, each case and each specific site must be assessed independently. Interpretation of architectural features in extranodal lymphocytic infiltrates depends on knowledge of the topography and histologic uniqueness of a specific site, in addition to a thorough evaluation of the cytologic composition of the lymphocytic infiltrate.

JUXTAPOSITION OF EXTRANODAL LYMPHOMA AND LYMPHOID HYPERPLASIA

One idiosyncracy that results in diagnostic problems in the pathologic evaluation of extranodal lymphoid proliferations is that lymphomas commonly are juxtaposed with areas of lymphoid hyperplasia (35,36,51,60,64). This problem is accentuated in small biopsy specimens, in which it may prove impossible to sort out the reactive from the neoplastic areas. Frequently, the sample is delusory and contains only the hyperplastic area. In the skin, for example, reactive T cells often proliferate in the superficial dermis, with lymphoma confined to the deeper portion of the dermis (66)

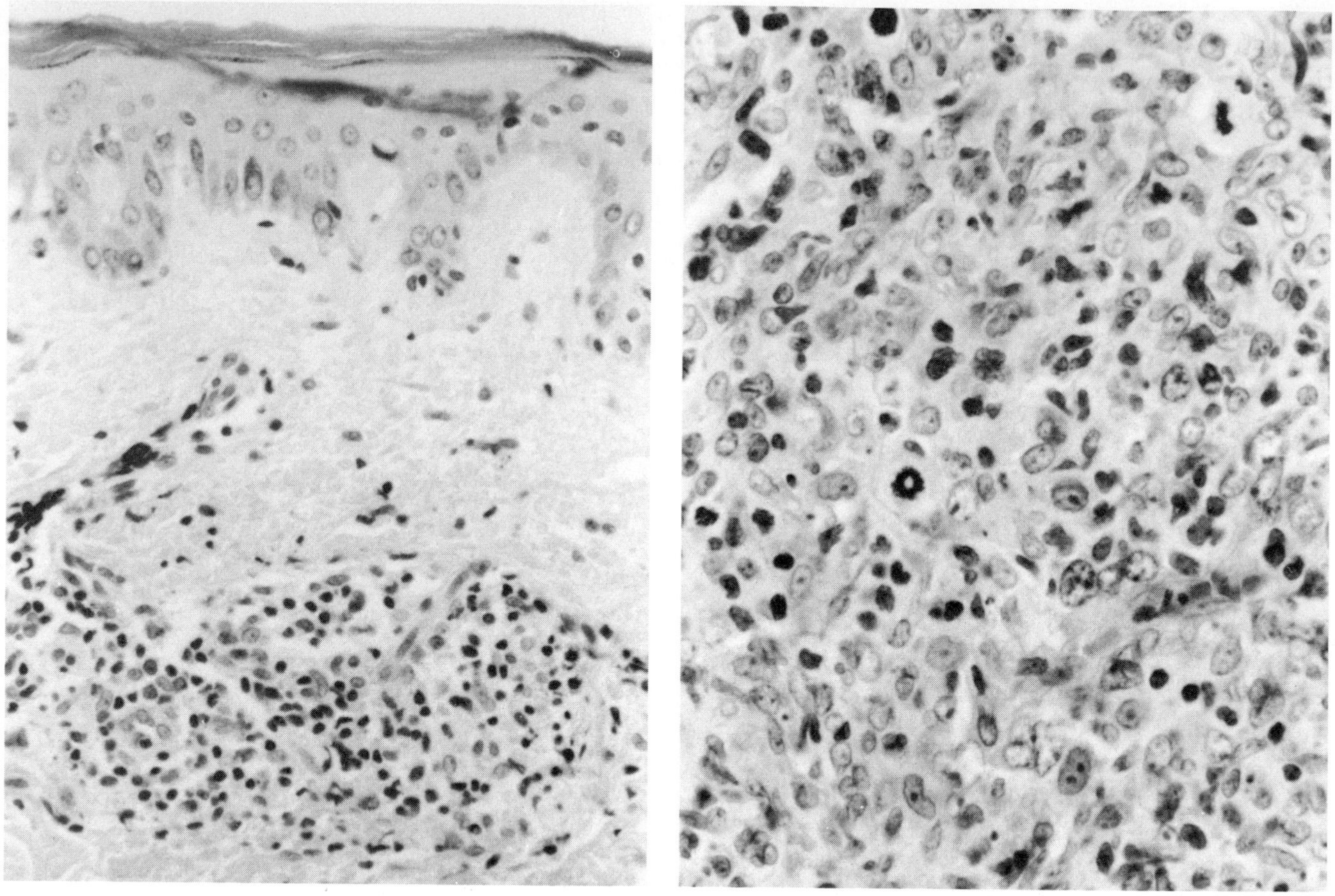

A B

FIG. 31.14. A: The superficial dermis in this skin biopsy specimen contains only a reactive T-cell population (hematoxylin and eosin stain, 375× magnification). **B:** The areas diagnostic of large cell lymphoma were present only in the deep dermis (hematoxylin and eosin stain, original magnification: 600× magnification).

(Fig. 31.14). In this setting, a shaved biopsy specimen is inadequate.

In large surgical resections of extranodal lymphoid lesions, there frequently is a continuous spectrum between areas of lymphoid hyperplasia and malignant lymphoma. This is especially true in the salivary and thyroid glands and correlates with the observation that patients who have Sjögren's syndrome and Hashimoto's disease have an increased risk of developing malignant lymphoma (19–22,35,36,60,62). The propensity for malignant lymphoma in the salivary and thyroid glands, as well as in other extranodal sites, probably is related to abnormal immune surveillance, decreased normal suppressor T-cell modulation, and development of a neoplastic clone that follows persistent antigenic B-cell stimulation and lymphoid hyperplasia with possible immunoglobulin gene hypermutation (69–73). In the salivary glands of patients with Sjögren's syndrome, for example, MESA-BLEL–associated clonal infiltrates derived from different patients bind the identical or similar antigens to suggest that MESA-BLEL clones begin as nonmalignant antigen-selected expansions (74). These investigations and hypotheses support molecular genetic studies that have detected clonal immunoglobulin gene rearrangements in patients who have clinical Sjögren's syndrome and Hashimoto's disease and who do not have histologic evidence of malignant lymphoma (21–23,75,76).

Although large cell lymphomas may be relatively straightforward to diagnose, even if found contiguous to lymphoid hyperplasia, lymphoma may be masked when it is focal and the hyperplasia prolific. An unequivocal diagnosis of malignant lymphoma in this setting rests on the conviction that a discrete homogeneous zone of lymphoid cells appears to be malignant. This zone must be more than the small cluster or aggregate of atypical lymphocytes that can be present in cases of lymphoid hyperplasia.

The most demanding diagnostic problem occurs when the malignant lymphoma that develops in the setting of lymphoid hyperplasia is not a high-grade but a low-grade lymphoma. This situation is best exemplified in patients who have Sjögren's syndrome and histologic MESA-BLEL in a salivary gland. In MESA-BLEL, there are multiple confluent lymphocytic aggregates that include germinal centers and

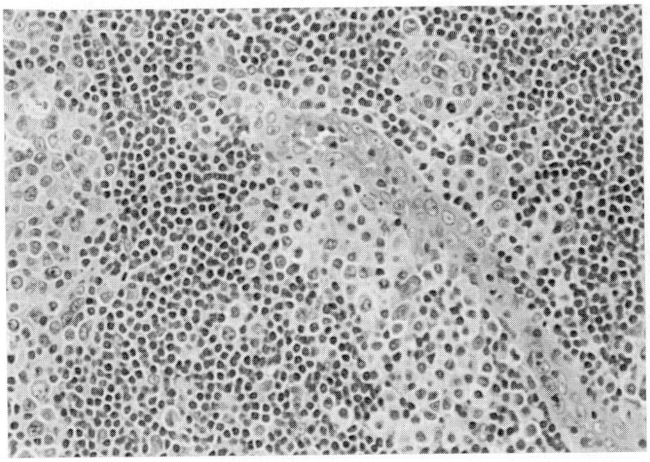

FIG. 31.15. A halo-like lesion composed of pale-staining monocytoid cells forms against a background of MESA-BLEL in a salivary gland. Many such halos prove to be monoclonal, but there is no consensus as to whether these cases should be interpreted as early MALT lymphomas (hematoxylin and eosin stain, original magnification: 300× magnification).

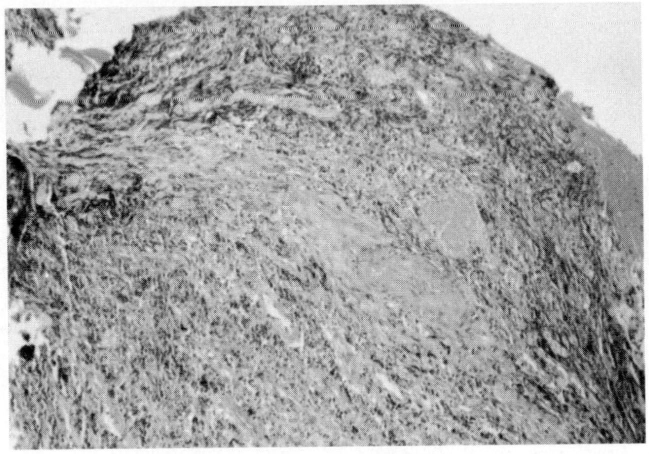

FIG. 31.16. An endoscopic biopsy specimen of the duodenum is not diagnostic, because of severe crush artifact (hematoxylin and eosin stain, original magnification: 120× magnification).

surrounding mantle zones (35). Epimyoepithelial islands are observed with partial destruction and obliteration of salivary gland ducts and acini. The malignant lymphomas that arise in this background frequently are subtle and histologically are lymphomas of MALT that usually are dominated by monocytoid B cells and often display some plasma cell differentiation (22,31,35,62). The recognition of concentrated monomorphous areas of monocytoid B cells sufficient to be morphologically diagnostic of malignant lymphoma is frequently problematic, and immunologic confirmation is important. If the histologic features are equivocal, such as the formation of nonconfluent monocytoid or clear cell ''halos'' (Fig. 31.15), a diagnosis of focal malignant lymphoma is controversial and may not be justifiable even if a monoclonal cell population can be demonstrated with the use of molecular methods, such as polymerase chain reaction (22,75,76). Moreover, clonality does not predict progression to the eventual development of clinically overt lymphoma (76).

TECHNICAL CONSIDERATIONS

In the assessment of extranodal lymphomas, technical considerations are a common and vexing problem (32). An accurate histologic diagnosis depends on the nature and quality of the tissue sample. Many initial biopsy specimens of extranodal lesions are small, such as shave and punch biopsies of skin, incisional biopsies of ocular lesions, and bronchoscopic, gastroscopic, and endoscopic specimens. These specimens often are subject to various alterations, including crush artifact and smudging, as well as the fact that a small sample may not be representative of the extranodal infiltrate (Fig. 31.16).

If the extranodal lesion is composed mainly of large cells, these may be insufficient in quantity, and the pattern may be developed insufficiently to exclude absolutely the possibility of another large cell malignant neoplasm, for example carcinoma. In small biopsy specimens that contain a malignant large cell neoplasm, immunoperoxidase stains for cytokeratin, leukocyte common antigen (CD45), pan–B cell and pan–T cell antigens such as CD20 and CD3, and possibly S-100 protein should be performed routinely (8,32) (Fig. 31.17). Should reactivity for these markers be negative, then appropriate stains with antimyeloid antibodies, such as myeloperoxidase, ought to follow, particularly for cases in which a malignant hematopoietic neoplasm is suspected (Fig. 31.18).

Some extranodal large cell infiltrates are not neoplastic and are mere clusters of reactive immunoblasts in patients with florid lymphoid hyperplasia (Fig. 31.19). Reactive immunoblasts may appear monomorphous and do not always show a range of lymphocytic transformation in a small biopsy specimen. Should a diagnosis of large cell lymphoma in this setting be at odds with the clinical setting, or if there is any suggestion of a reactive condition, it is sensible to offer a descriptive diagnosis, such as ''atypical,'' and to request a second biopsy with reservation of fresh tissues for immunologic studies. Similar discretion should be used for small biopsy specimens that contain only small lymphocytes, particularly if the infiltrate is focal or insufficiently dense or monomorphous, to be absolutely certain about whether the small lymphocytes are reactive or neoplastic. Both reactive and neoplastic small lymphocytes may mask an underlying, deeper high-grade lymphoma, such as in the stomach or skin (51,66); only the small lymphocytic, often reactive

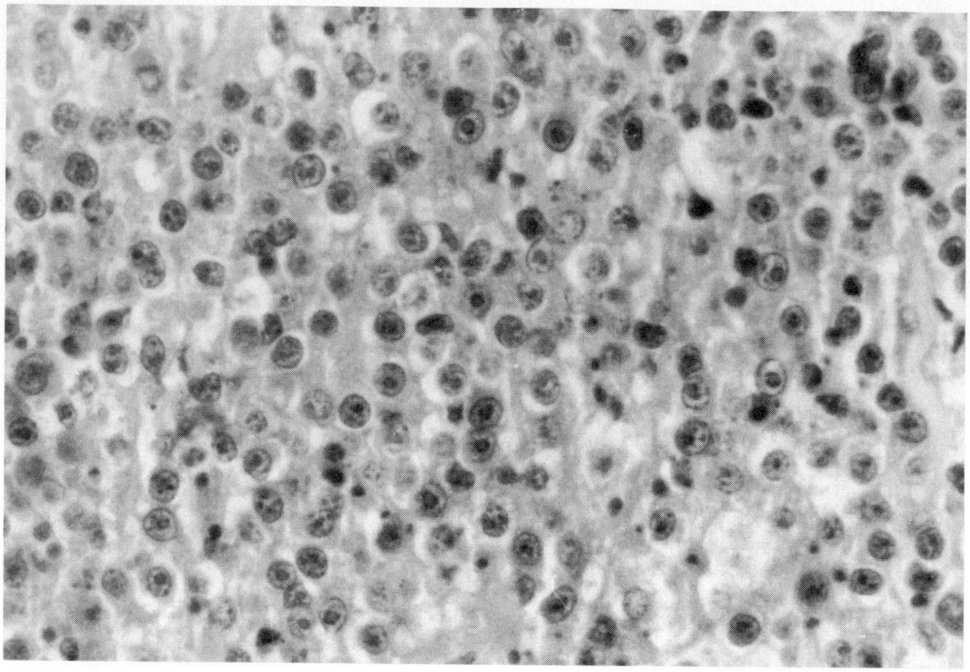

FIG. 31.17. Diffuse large cell lymphoma of plasmacytoid type was found in another small biopsy fragment from the duodenum (same patient as in Fig. 31.16). The diagnosis of lymphoma was verified by positive reactivity for the CD20 antigen and a negative stain for cytokeratin (hematoxylin and eosin stain, original magnification: 720× magnification).

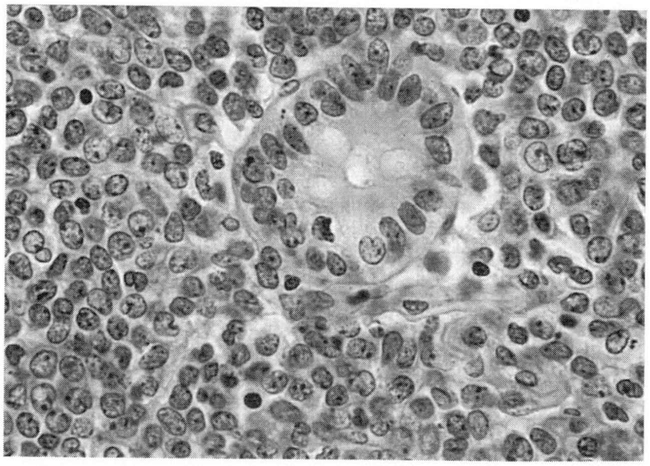

FIG. 31.18. A large cell malignant neoplasm in the small intestine did not express B- or T-cell lineage–specific antigens or cytokeratin; however, the neoplastic cells subsequently were shown to express myeloperoxidase to justify the diagnosis of an extramedullary myeloid tumor (granulocytic sarcoma) (hematoxylin and eosin stain, original magnification: 600× magnification).

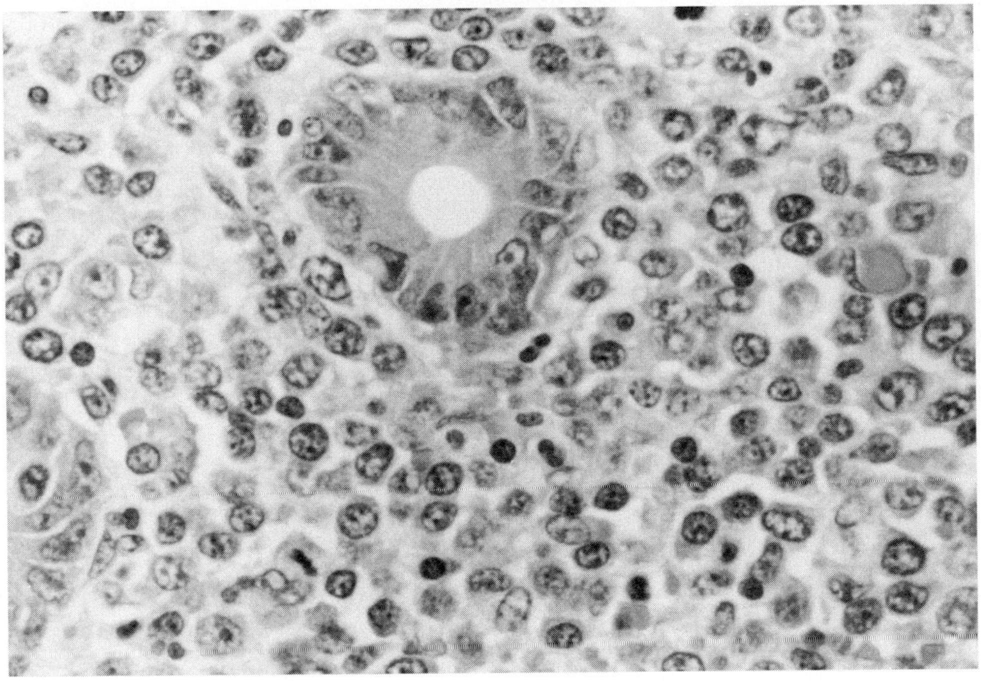

FIG. 31.19. Monomorphous-like groups of reactive immunoblasts are easily confused with malignant lymphoma in a small endoscopic biopsy specimen (hematoxylin and eosin stain, original magnification: 720× magnification).

component may be submitted for pathologic examination in a gastroscopic or superficial shave biopsy specimen.

IMPLICATIONS OF IMMUNOLOGIC CELL MARKER AND MOLECULAR GENETIC STUDIES ON EXTRANODAL LYMPHOID PROLIFERATIONS

The use of immunologic cell marker and molecular genetic studies has offered an entirely new perspective for the interpretation of lymphoid lesions, including those in extranodal sites (13,14,23,33,45). With simple immunoperoxidase techniques, an extranodal large cell neoplasm can be classified definitively as malignant lymphoma, as opposed to undifferentiated carcinoma, malignant melanoma, or an extramedullary myeloid tumor (granulocytic sarcoma) (8,32,77). In addition, the B- or T-cell lineage of a malignant lymphoma can be ascertained in both fresh and fixed tissues (22,27,29,35,36,46,52,53,62,66). Extranodal B-cell small lymphocytic lesions that formerly were regarded as histologically indeterminate can be phenotyped precisely as polyclonal, and therefore reactive, or monoclonal. The demonstration of monoclonality in an extranodal small lymphocytic proliferation generally has been equated with malignant lymphoma and has reduced the number of cases that are interpreted as extranodal pseudolymphomas (13,17,18,34). Molecular genetic analysis of extranodal lymphomas is contributing new information that points to the possibility of a unique pathogenesis for these neoplasms. For example, low-grade gastrointestinal MALT lymphomas generally do not exhibit *BCL1* or *BCL2* rearrangements, and both low- and high-grade MALT lymphomas may exhibit *MYC* gene mutations (78–80). The *MYC* gene rearrangements found in high-grade gastrointestinal lymphomas differ from their nodal counterparts (80,81). Partial inactivation of the *P53* gene also may be significant in the pathogenesis of low-grade MALT lymphomas, although others dispute this finding (82,83). Extranodal lymphomas, including those of MALT, likewise appear to have a higher frequency of somatic *FAS* mutations (84). Chronic antigenic stimulation resulting from infections is related pathogenetically to some extranodal lymphomas; these infections comprise *Helicobacter pylori* with gastric lymphomas, Epstein-Barr virus and sinonasal lymphomas of natural killer cell or T-cell type, and the association of hepatitis C virus with extranodal lymphomas of liver and major salivary glands (44,49,85).

A major concern is the appropriateness of classifying an extranodal small lymphocytic proliferation as a malignant lymphoma based largely on immunophenotypic or molecular criteria, particularly if the extranodal lesion is histologically equivocal and shows no clinical evidence of lymphoma. Some extranodal monoclonal B-cell proliferations may represent the tissue equivalent of a benign monoclonal gammopathy (13). This contention is supported by gene rearrangement studies of a variety of histologically benign and immunologically polyclonal extranodal lymphoid hyperplasias that demonstrated clonal immunoglobulin gene rearrangements without evidence of overt malignant lymphoma (21–23,59,76). The cases studied were in the salivary gland, ocular adnexa, breast, thyroid, and stomach. Knowles and associates concluded that most cases with occult monoclonal B-cell populations that appear benign are still reactive, although possibly at a prelymphomatous stage, and that there is a spectrum of clonal B-cell proliferations up to and including cases of malignant lymphoma (23). Other investigators echo these conclusions and stress that histologically benign clonal extranodal lymphocytic infiltrates are not synonymous with morphologically overt low-grade lymphomas, and that the demonstration of clonality does not predict inevitable progression to clinically obvious malignant lymphoma (22,76). Nonetheless, B-cell monoclonality may have clinical ramifications in some patients with extranodal lymphoid hyperplasia, and such lesions could be viewed as prelymphomatous or borderline; for example, clonality in *H. pylori*–associated chronic gastritis may precede the onset of gastric MALT lymphoma by 3 to 4 years (86,87). The discovery of occult clonal B-cell populations in clinical and histologic cases of extranodal lymphoid hyperplasia parallels the discovery of clonal T-cell populations in various clinically benign cutaneous lymphocytic infiltrates, such as lymphomatoid papulosis and *pityriasis lichenoides et varioliformis acuta* (Mucha-Habermann disease) (88,89).

The biologic significance of finding a clonal B- or T-cell population in the setting of a histologically reactive and clinically benign extranodal lymphocytic proliferation is uncertain. Because many extranodal clonal B-cell populations are antigen-driven, early clonal lesions may be reversible and even susceptible to antibiotic therapy, such as *H. pylori*–related clonal gastric lymphocytic infiltrates (49,69–74). An analogy has been drawn between this phase of a monoclonal small lymphocytic proliferation in the gastrointestinal tract and a colonic adenoma (90); both lesions often are clinically and histologically benign, with only a limited growth potential. At an undetermined point, the small lymphocytic lesion may become autonomous and transform into malignant lymphoma, probably with the onset of cytogenetic alterations, for instance trisomy 3 or a novel translocation t(11;18)(q21;q21) (23,90–92). The latter translocation is a crucial structural anomaly found in approximately 50% of cytogenetically abnormal low-grade MALT lymphomas. The *AP12* gene, an inhibitor of apoptosis, and a singular gene on 18q21 named *MLT* are rearranged in the translocation t(11;18)(q21;q21), and the *AP12-MLT* fusion likely is significant in the oncogenesis of MALT lymphomas (93).

From a clinical perspective, extranodal lymphoid proliferations with only occult clonal populations that appear to be histologically benign should continue to be designated as lymphoid hyperplasia and not as malignant lymphoma (8,22,23,59,76). It is appropriate to regard cases of extranodal small lymphocytic infiltrates that are immunophenotypically monoclonal and histologically monomorphous as low-grade lymphomas. Nonetheless, little evidence exists to suggest that even an unequivocal histologic and immunologic low-grade stage IE extranodal lymphoma pursues a malignant clinical course, unlike histologically similar low-grade lymphomas that present in lymph nodes. For example, among patients who have lymphoid proliferations in the ocular region, no differences in clinical prognosis exist between those with immunologically verified monoclonal B-cell lymphomas and those with polyclonal lymphoid hyperplasias; most patients who have clinical stage IE ocular lymphoid lesions have benign and indolent clinical courses (27). Survival statistics for low-grade MALT lymphomas in other sites, including skin, lung, salivary gland, thyroid, and stomach, are equally excellent and generally are not different from the statistics in normal age-matched control subjects (12,18,29–31,35,40,51). In the Non-Hodgkin's Lymphoma Classification Project, patients who had low-grade marginal zone lymphomas of MALT type manifested one of the highest survival rates of any lymphoma subtype (6); at 5 years, overall survival was 81% and failure-free survival 65%, which were significantly higher than in patients who had node-based marginal zone lymphomas (94). In another study of 75 patients who had nongastrointestinal low-grade MALT lymphomas, there was a response rate of 100% and an estimated 5-year survival rate of 95% (95). At the time of diagnosis, patients who have stage IE low-grade MALT lymphomas probably do not require any further management apart from local treatment or observation and continuous follow-up (23,31,95).

Despite the apparent excellent prognosis for patients who have stage IE monoclonal low-grade MALT lymphomas, the risk for the development of more clinically overt lymphoma and histologic progression remains unknown (8). Because there may be significant therapeutic repercussions from rendering a diagnosis of low-grade extranodal marginal zone lymphoma of MALT type, and because there are wide disparities (with a range from 1–85%) in published incidences of clonality in benign-appearing extranodal lymphocytic infiltrates, specifically in cases of *H. pylori*–associated lymphoid hyperplasia, it is proposed that many patients would be better served by the diagnosis of a neoplasm or a clonal disorder of "uncertain malignant potential" (45,46,59,96–98). Despite the indecisiveness that is inherent in this term, the diagnosis of extranodal low-grade lymphomas of MALT, or other lymphoma subtypes, depends not on the discovery of an occult clonal cell population but on strict histopathologic criteria augmented by immunophenotypic, molecular, and cytogenetic studies (8).

SUMMARY AND CONCLUSIONS

The pathologic interpretation of a lymphoid proliferation in an extranodal site is demanding, particularly with the many exceptions and pitfalls in the histologic criteria traditionally used to separate extranodal malignant lymphomas from lymphoid hyperplasias. Despite these exceptions, most extranodal lymphoid proliferations are readily diagnosable. The traditional histologic criteria generally are fully applicable but must be tempered by the newer concepts discovered as a result of immunopathologic correlations and viewed in the context of the clinical setting. The initiation of long-term clinical studies and the discovery of new genetic markers to precisely determine malignant transformation of extranodal lymphoid proliferations will define further their natural history and increase the accuracy of distinguishing between extranodal lymphoid hyperplasias and malignant lymphomas.

REFERENCES

1. Paryani S, Hoppe RT, Burke JS, et al. Extralymphatic involvement in diffuse non-Hodgkin's lymphoma. *J Clin Oncol* 1983;1:682–688.
2. Otter R, Gerrits WBJ, Sandt MMVD, et al. Primary extranodal and nodal non-Hodgkin's lymphomas: a survey of a population-based registry. *Eur J Cancer Clin Oncol* 1989;25:1203–1210.
3. D'Amore F, Christensen BE, Brincker H, et al. Clinicopathological features and prognostic factors in extranodal non-Hodgkin lymphomas. *Eur J Cancer* 1991;27:1201–1208.
4. Greiner TC, Medeiros JL, Jaffe ES. Non-Hodgkin's lymphoma. *Cancer* 1995;75:370–380.
5. Gospodarowicz MK, Sutcliffe SB. The extranodal lymphomas. *Semin Radiat Oncol* 1995;4:281–300.
6. Armitage JO, Weisenburger DD. New approach to classifying non-Hodgkin's lymphomas: clinical features of the major histologic subtypes. *J Clin Oncol* 1998;16:2780–2795.
7. Severson RK, Davis S. Increasing incidence of primary gastric lymphoma. *Cancer* 1990; 1283–1287.
8. Burke JS. Extranodal hematopoietic/lymphoid disorders: an introduction. *Am J Clin Pathol* 1999;111[Suppl 1]:S40–S45.
9. Corn BW, Marcus SM, Topham A, et al. Will primary central nervous system lymphoma be the most frequent brain tumor diagnosed in the year 2000? *Cancer* 1997;79:2409–2413.
10. Knowles DM, Chamulak GA, Subar M, et al. Lymphoid neoplasia associated with the acquired immunodeficiency syndrome (AIDS): the New York University Medical Center experience with 105 patients (1981-1986). *Ann Intern Med* 1988;108:744–753.
11. Gill PS, Chandraratna AN, Myer PR, et al. Malignant lymphoma: cardiac involvement at initial presentation. *J Clin Oncol* 1987;5:216–224.
12. Willemze R, Kerl H, Sterry W, et al. EORTC Classification for primary cutaneous lymphomas: a proposal from the Cutaneous Lymphoma Study Group of the European Organization for Research and Treatment of Cancer. *Blood* 1997;90:354–371.
13. Knowles DM, Jakobiec FA. Cell marker analysis of extranodal lymphoid infiltrates: to what extent does the determination of mono- or polyclonality resolve the diagnostic dilemma of malignant lymphoma v pseudolymphoma in an extranodal site? *Semin Diagn Pathol* 1985;2: 163–168.
14. Frizzera G, Wu CD, Inghirami G. The usefulness of immunophenotypic and genotypic studies in the diagnosis and classification of hematopoietic and lymphoid neoplasms: an update. *Am J Clin Pathol* 1999; 111[Suppl 1]:S13–S39.
15. Isaacson P, Wright DH. Extranodal malignant lymphoma arising from mucosa-associated lymphoid tissue. *Cancer* 1953:2515–2524.
16. Isaacson PG, Spencer J. Malignant lymphoma of mucosa-associated lymphoid tissue. *Histopathology* 1987;11:445–462.
17. Isaacson PG, Norton AJ. *Extranodal lymphomas*. Edinburgh: Churchill Livingstone, 1994:5–14.
18. Isaacson PG. Mucosa-associated lymphoid tissue lymphoma. *Semin Hematol* 1999;36:139–147.
19. Kassan SS, Thomas TL, Moutsopoulos HM, et al. Increased risk of lymphoma in sicca syndrome. *Ann Intern Med* 1978;89:888–892.
20. Holm L-E, Blomgren H, Lowhagen T. Cancer risks in patients with chronic lymphocytic thyroiditis. *N Engl J Med* 1985;312:601–604.
21. Fishleder A, Tubbs R, Hesse B, et al. Uniform detection of immunoglobulin-gene rearrangement in benign lymphoepithelial lesions. *N Engl J Med* 1987;316:1118–1121.
22. Quintana PG, Kapadia SB, Bahler DW, et al. Salivary gland lymphoid infiltrates associated with lymphoepithelial lesions: a clinicopathologic, immunophenotypic, and genotypic study. *Hum Pathol* 1997;28: 850–861.
23. Knowles DM, Athan E, Ubriaco A, et al. Extranodal noncutaneous lymphoid hyperplasias represent a continuous spectrum of B-cell neoplasia: demonstration by molecular genetic analysis. *Blood* 1989;73: 1635–1645.
24. Saltzstein SL. Extranodal malignant lymphomas and pseudolymphomas. *Pathol Annu* 1969;4:159–184.
25. Economopoulos T, Asprou N, Stathakis N, et al. Primary extranodal non-Hodgkin's lymphoma in adults: clinocopathologic and survival characteristics. *Leuk Lymphoma* 1996;21:131–136.
26. Knowles DM. The extranodal lymphoid infiltrate: a diagnostic dilemma. *Semin Diagn Pathol* 1985;2:147–151.
27. Knowles DM, Jakobiec FA, McNally L, et al. Lymphoid hyperplasia and malignant lymphoma occurring in the ocular adnexa (orbit, conjunctiva, and eyelids): a prospective multiparametric analysis of 108 cases during 1977 to 1987. *Hum Pathol* 1990;21:959–973.
28. Wotherspoon AC, Diss TC, Pan LX, et al. Primary low-grade B-cell lymphoma of the conjunctiva: a mucosa-associated lymphoid tissue type lymphoma. *Histopathology* 1993;23:417–424.
29. Li G, Hansmann M-L, Zwingers T, et al. Primary lymphomas of the lung: morphological, immunohistochemical and clinical features. *Histopathology* 1990;16:519–531.
30. Fiche M, Captron F, Berger F, et al. Primary pulmonary non-Hodgkin's lymphomas. *Histopathology* 1995;26:529–537.
31. Burke JS. Are there site-specific differences among the MALT lymphomas: morphologic, clinical? *Am J Clin Pathol* 1999;111[Suppl 1]:S133–S143.
32. Burke JS. Histologic criteria for distinguishing between benign and malignant extranodal lymphoid infiltrates. *Semin Diagn Pathol* 1985; 2:152–162.
33. Kurtin PJ. How do you distinguish benign from malignant extranodal small B-cell proliferations? *Am J Clin Pathol* 1999;111[Suppl 1]:S119–S126.
34. Abbondanzo SL, Sobin LH. Gastric "pseudolymphoma:" a retrospective morphologic and immunophenotypic study of 97 cases. *Cancer* 1997;79:1656–1663.
35. Hyjek E, Smith WJ, Isaacson PG. Primary B-cell lymphoma of salivary glands and its relationship to myoepithelial sialadenitis. *Hum Pathol* 1988;19:766–776.
36. Hyjek E, Isaacson PG. Primary B cell lymphoma of the thyroid and its relationship to Hashimoto's thyroiditis. *Hum Pathol* 1988;19: 1315–1326.
37. Isaacson PG, Spencer J. Malignant lymphoma and autoimmune disease. *Histopathology* 1993;22:509–510.
38. Isaacson PG. Lymphomas of mucosa-associated lymphoid tissue (MALT). *Histopathology* 1990;16:617–619.
39. Ben-Ezra J, Burke JS, Swartz WG, et al. Small lymphocytic lymphoma: a clinicopathologic analysis of 268 cases. *Blood* 1989;73:579–587.
40. De Jong D, Boot H, Van Heerde P, et al. Histological grading in gastric lymphoma: pretreatment criteria and clinical relevance. *Gastroenterology* 1997;112:1466–1474.
41. Smith JL, Butler JJ. Skin involvement in Hodgkin's disease. *Cancer* 1980;45:354–361.
42. Jaffe ES, Chan JKC, Su IH, et al. Report of the workshop on nasal and related extranodal angiocentric T/natural killer cell lymphomas: definitions, differential diagnosis, and epidemiology. *Am J Surg Pathol* 1996;20:103–111.
43. Chott A, Vesely M, Simonitsch I, et al. Classification of intestinal T-cell neoplasms and their differential diagnosis. *Am J Clin Pathol* 1999; 111[Suppl 1]:S68–S74.
44. Jaffe ES, Krenacs L, Kumar S, et al. Extranodal peripheral T-cell and NK-cell neoplasms. *Am J Clin Pathol* 1999;111[Suppl 1]:S46–S55.
45. Torlakovic E, Cherwitz DL, Jessurun J, et al. B-cell gene rearrangement in benign and malignant lymphoid proliferations of mucosa-associated lymphoid tissue and lymph nodes. *Hum Pathol* 1997;28:166–173.
46. Burke JS, Sheibani K, Nathwani BN, et al. Monoclonal small (well-differentiated) lymphocytic proliferations of the gastrointestinal tract resembling lymphoid hyperplasia: a neoplasm of uncertain malignant potential. *Hum Pathol* 1987;18:1238–1245.
47. Evans HL. Extranodal small lymphocytic proliferation: a clinicopathologic and immunocytochemical study. *Cancer* 1982;49:84–96.
48. Zukerberg LR, Ferry JA, Southern JF, et al. Lymphoid infiltrates of the stomach: evaluation of histologic criteria for the diagnosis of low-grade gastric lymphoma on endoscopic biopsy specimens. *Am J Surg Pathol* 1990;14:1087–1099.
49. Wotherspoon AC, Doglioni C, Diss TC, et al. Regression of primary low-grade B-cell gastric lymphoma of mucosa-associated lymphoid tissue type after eradication of Helicobacter pylori. *Lancet* 1993;342: 575–577.

50. Rubin A, Isaacson PG. Florid reactive lymphoid hyperplasia of the terminal ileum in adults: a condition bearing a close resemblance to low-grade malignant lymphoma. *Histopathology* 1990;17:19–26.
51. Isaacson PG. Gastrointestinal lymphomas of T- and B-cell types. *Mod Pathol* 1999;12:151–158.
52. Fraga M, Lloret E, Sanchez-Verde L, et al. Mucosal mantle cell (centrocytic) lymphomas. *Histopathology* 1995;26:413–422.
53. Moynihan MJ, Bast MA, Chan WC, et al. Lymphoid polyposis: a neoplasm of either follicular mantle or germinal center cell origin. *Am J Surg Pathol* 1996;20:442–452.
54. Medeiros LJ, Harris NL. Lymphoid infiltrates of the orbit and conjunctiva: a morphologic and immunophenotypic study of 99 cases. *Am J Surg Pathol* 1989;13:459–471.
55. Almasri NM, Zaer FS, Iturraspe JA, et al. Contribution of flow cytometry to the diagnosis of gastric lymphomas in endoscopic biopsy specimens. *Mod Pathol* 1997;10:650–656.
56. Osborne BM, Pugh WC. Practicality of molecular studies to evaluate small lymphocytic proliferations in endoscopic gastric biopsies. *Am J Surg Pathol* 1992;16:838–844.
57. Gelb AB, Rouse RV, Dorfman RF, et al. Detection of immunophenotypic abnormalities in paraffin-embedded B-lineage non-Hodgkin's lymphomas. *Am J Clin Pathol* 1994;102:825–834.
58. de Leon ED, Alkan S, Huang JC, et al. Usefulness of an immunohistochemical panel in paraffin-embedded tissues for the differentiation of B-cell non-Hodgkin's lymphomas of small lymphocytes. *Mod Pathol* 1998;11:1046–1051.
59. Hsi ED, Greenson JK, Singleton TP, et al. Detection of immunoglobulin heavy chain gene rearrangement by polymerase chain reaction in chronic active gastritis associated with Helicobacter pylori. *Hum Pathol* 1996;27:290–296.
60. Burke JS, Butler JJ, Fuller LM. Malignant lymphomas of the thyroid: a clinical pathologic study of 35 patients including ultrastructural observations. *Cancer* 1977;39:1587–1602.
61. Isaacson PG, Wotherspoon AC, Pan L. Follicular colonization in B-cell lymphoma of mucosa-associated lymphoid tissue. *Am J Surg Pathol* 1991;15:819–828.
62. Shin SS, Sheibani K, Fishleder A, et al. Monocytoid B-cell lymphoma in patients with Sjögren's syndrome: a clinicopathologic study of 13 patients. *Hum Pathol* 1991;22:422–430.
63. Ranchod M, Lewin KJ, Dorfman RF. Lymphoid hyperplasia of the gastrointestinal tract: a study of 26 cases and review of the literature. *Am J Surg Pathol* 1978;2:383–400.
64. Burke JS. Malignant lymphomas of the skin: their differentiation from lymphoid and nonlymphoid cutaneous infiltrates that simulate lymphoma. *Semin Diagn Pathol* 1985;2:169–182.
65. LeBoit PE, McNutt NS, Reed JA, et al. Primary cutaneous immunocytoma: a B-cell lymphoma that can easily be mistaken for cutaneous lymphoid hyperplasia. *Am J Surg Pathol* 1994;18:969–978.
66. Gilliam AC, Wood GS. Primary cutaneous lymphomas other than mycosis fungoides. *Semin Oncol* 1999;26:290–306.
67. Baldassano MF, Bailey EM, Ferry JA, et al. Cutaneous lymphoid hyperplasia and cutaneous marginal zone lymphoma: comparison of morphologic and immunophenotypic features. *Am J Surg Pathol* 1999;23:88–96.
68. DiGiuseppe JA, Nelson WG, Seifter EJ, et al. Intravascular lymphomatosis: a clinicopathologic study of 10 cases and assessment of response to chemotherapy. *J Clin Oncol* 1994;12:2573–2579.
69. Fox RI, Adamson TC, Fong S, et al. Lymphocyte phenotype and function in pseudolymphoma associated with Sjögren's syndrome. *J Clin Invest* 1983;72:52–62.
70. Matsubayashi S, Tamai H, Morita T, et al. Possible disorder of B-cell-related surveillance and malignant lymphoma of the thyroid. *Cancer* 1989;64:2259–2261.
71. Hussell T, Isaacson PG, Crabtree JE, et al. The response of cells from low-grade B-cell gastric lymphomas of mucosa-associated lymphoid tissue to Helicobacter pylori. *Lancet* 1993;342:571–574.
72. Du M, Diss TC, Xu C, et al. Ongoing mutation in MALT lymphoma immunoglobulin gene suggests that antigen stimulation plays a role in the clonal expansion. *Leukemia* 1996;10:1190–1197.
73. Bahler DW, Miklos JA, Swerdlow SH. Ongoing Ig gene hypermutation in salivary gland mucosa-associated lymphoid tissue-type lymphomas. *Blood* 1997;89:3335–3344.
74. Bahler DW, Swerdlow SH. Clonal salivary gland infiltrates associated with myoepithelial sialadenitis (Sjögren's syndrome) begin as nonmalignant antigen-selected expansions. *Blood* 1998;91:1864–1872.
75. Diss TC, Wotherspoon AC, Speight P, et al. B-cell monoclonality, Epstein Barr virus, and t(14;18) in myoepithelial sialadenitis and low-grade B-cell MALT lymphoma of the parotid gland. *Am J Surg Pathol* 1995;19:531–536.
76. Hsi ED, Siddiqui J, Schnitzer B, et al. Analysis of immunoglobulin heavy chain gene rearrangement in myoepithelial sialadenitis by polymerase chain reaction. *Am J Clin Pathol* 1996;106:498–503.
77. Menasce LP, Banerjee SS, Beckett E, et al. Extra-medullary myeloid tumor (granulocytic sarcoma) is often misdiagnosed: a study of 26 cases. *Histopathology* 1999;34:391–398.
78. Pan L, Diss TC, Cunningham D, et al. The bcl-2 gene in primary B cell lymphoma of mucosa-associated lymphoid tissue (MALT). *Am J Pathol* 1989;135:7–11.
79. Peng H, Diss T, Isaacson PG, et al. c-myc gene abnormalities in mucosa-associated lymphoid tissue (MALT) lymphomas. *J Pathol* 1997;181:381–386.
80. van Krieken JHJM, Raffeld M, Raghoebier S, et al. Molecular genetics of gastrointestinal non-Hodgkin's lymphomas: unusual prevalence and pattern of c-myc rearrangements in aggressive lymphomas. *Blood* 1990;76:797–800.
81. Raghoebier S, Kramer MHH, van Krieken JHJM, et al. Essential differences in oncogene involvement between primary nodal and extranodal large cell lymphoma. *Blood* 1991;78:2680–2685.
82. Du M, Peng H, Singh N, et al. The accumulation of p53 abnormalities is associated with progression of mucosa-associated lymphoid tissue lymphoma. *Blood* 1995;86:4587–4593.
83. Levy V, Miller C, Koeffler HP, et al. p53 in lymphomas of mucosal-associated lymphoid tissues. *Mod Pathol* 1996;9:245–248.
84. Grønbæk K, thor Straten P, Ralfkiaer E, et al. Somatic Fas mutations in non-Hodgkin's lymphoma: association with extranodal disease and autoimmunity. *Blood* 1998;92:3018–3024.
85. DeVita S, Sacco C, Sansonno D, et al. Characterization of overt B-cell lymphomas in patients with hepatitis C virus infection. *Blood* 1997;90:776–782.
86. Zucca E, Bertoni F, Roggero E, et al. Molecular analysis of the progression from Helicobacter pylori-associated chronic gastritis to mucosa-associated lymphoid-tissue lymphoma of the stomach. *N Engl J Med* 1998;338:804–810.
87. Nakamura S, Aoyagi K, Furuse M, et al. B-cell monoclonality precedes the development of gastric MALT lymphoma in Helicobacter pylori-associated chronic gastritis. *Am J Pathol* 1998;152:1271–1279.
88. Weiss LM, Wood GS, Trela M, et al. Clonal T-cell populations in lymphomatoid papulosis: evidence of a lymphoproliferative origin for a clinically benign disease. *N Engl J Med* 1986;315:475–479.
89. Weiss LM, Wood GS, Ellisen LW, et al. Clonal T-cell populations in pityriasis lichenoides et varioliformis acuta (Mucha-Habermann disease). *Am J Pathol* 1987;126:417–421.
90. Sigal SH, Saul SH, Auerbach HE, et al. Gastric small lymphocytic proliferation with immunoglobulin gene rearrangement in pseudolymphoma versus lymphoma. *Gastroenterology* 1989;97:195–201.
91. Blanco R, Lyda M, Davis B, et al. Trisomy 3 in gastric lymphomas of extranodal marginal zone B-cell (mucosa-associated lymphoid tissue) origin demonstrated by FISH in intact paraffin tissue sections. *Hum Pathol* 1999;30:706–711.
92. Auer IA, Gascoyne RD, Connors JM, et al. t(11;18)(q21;q21) is the most common translocation in MALT lymphomas. *Ann Oncol* 1997;8:979–985.
93. Dierlamm J, Baens M, Wlodarska I, et al. The apoptosis gene AP12 and a novel 18q gene, MLT, are recurrently rearranged in the t(11;18)(q21;q21) associated with mucosa-associated lymphoid tissue lymphomas. *Blood* 1999;93:3601–3609.
94. Nathwani BN, Drachenberg MR, Hernandez AM, et al. Nodal monocytoid B-cell lymphoma (nodal marginal-zone B-cell lymphoma). *Semin Hematol* 1999;36:128–138.
95. Zinzani PL, Magagnoli M, Galieni P, et al. Nongastrointestinal low-grade mucosa-associated lymphoid tissue lymphoma: analysis of 75 patients. *J Clin Oncol* 1999;17:1254–1258.
96. de Mascarel A, Dubus P, Belleannée G, et al. Low prevalence of monoclonal B cells in Helicobacter pylori gastritis patients with duodenal ulcer. *Hum Pathol* 1998;29:784–790.
97. Genta RM. Le lymphome imaginaire. *Hum Pathol* 1998;29:769–770.
98. Collins RD. Is clonality equivalent to malignancy: specifically, is immunoglobulin gene rearrangement diagnostic of malignant lymphoma? *Hum Pathol* 1997;28:757–759.

CHAPTER 32

Benign and Malignant Cutaneous Lymphoproliferative Disorders Including Mycosis Fungoides

Gary S. Wood

CLASSIFYING CUTANEOUS LYMPHOMAS

The two main classification systems used for cutaneous lymphomas are the Revised European-American Lymphoma (REAL) classification (1) (see Chapters 19 and 20) and the system created by the European Organization for Research and Treatment of Cancer (EORTC) (2). Both schema refine and extend older systems such as the Working Formulation (3) (see Chapter 19) because they are based on a combination of clinicopathologic, immunophenotypic, and molecular biologic characteristics. The REAL classification covers all lymphomas, whereas the EORTC classification pertains to primary cutaneous lymphomas. Mycosis fungoides (MF) and its leukemic variant, the Sezary syndrome (SS), are included as primary skin disorders, although SS and sometimes MF manifest as systemic lymphomas with concurrent cutaneous and extracutaneous involvement. Except possibly for solitary lesions, most primary cutaneous lymphomas are probably biologically systemic disorders in which tumor cells selectively home to or proliferate in the skin. They appear to represent proliferative disorders of lymphocytes belonging to the so-called skin-associated lymphoid tissue (SALT) (4), which includes lymphocytes and antigen-presenting cells that traffic between the skin and draining peripheral lymph nodes through the lymphatics and blood.

The REAL and EORTC classifications represent significant departures from prior schema, because they strive to define biologic entities rather than purely morphologic subtypes and because they recognize that the same biologic entity can have multiple morphologic variants or developmental phases. They avoid use of outdated, inaccurate terms such as *reticulum cell sarcoma* and *histiocytic lymphoma* to refer to lymphomas of B-cell or T-cell differentiation.The EORTC classification is shown in Table 32.1 along with the corresponding lymphomas in the REAL classification that can present with primary skin involvement. This chapter follows an alternative classification that covers all cutaneous lymphomas, including those that are systemic disorders. It is presented in Tables 32.2 and 32.3. This approach deals with MF/SS and variants as one group of diseases and non-MF/SS lymphomas as another.

Most patients presenting with cutaneous involvement have lesions of T-cell rather than B-cell differentiation (5). The most common primary cutaneous lymphoma is MF/SS and its variants, accounting for about 50% of cases. The remaining non-MF/SS cases are divided equally between T-cell and B-cell types (roughly 25% of the total for each). Viewed from an alternate perspective, 30% of total cases are non-MF/SS tumors composed of various large cell lymphomas, including $CD30^+$ and $CD30^-$ large T-cell types, follicle center large B-cell lymphomas, and so-called large B-cell lymphomas of the legs. The remaining 20% are composed of a wide variety of other T-cell and B-cell lymphomas that manifest in the skin more rarely (Table 32.3) (2). Concurrent and secondary cutaneous involvement by lymphomas also occurs. Systemic T-cell lymphomas frequently present or relapse in the skin (6). For example, the peripheral T-cell lymphoma (PTL)–unspecified group of the REAL classification shows skin involvement in 25% to 50% of cases. A large percentage of B-cell lymphomas presenting in the skin prove to be primary cutaneous tumors (6). The most common types presenting with skin involvement are follicle center cell lymphoma, marginal zone B-cell lymphoma, and diffuse large B-cell lymphoma. Approximately

G. S. Wood: Department of Dermatology, Louis Stokes VA Medical Center, Cleveland, Ohio 44106

TABLE 32.1. *Comparison of EORTC and REAL classifications of primary cutaneous lymphomas*

EORTC	REAL
Indolent T-cell lymphomas	
Mycosis fungoides (MF)	Mycosis fungoides
MF-associated follicular mucinosis	
Pagetoid reticulosis	
Lymphomatoid papulosis	
CD30$^+$ large T-cell lymphoma	Anaplastic large cell lymphoma
Aggressive T-cell lymphomas	
Sezary syndrome	Sezary syndrome
CD30$^-$ large T-cell lymphoma	Peripheral T-cell lymphoma
	Angiocentric lymphoma
Provisional T-cell lymphomas	
Granulomatous slack skin	
Pleomorphic small/medium-sized cell lymphoma	Peripheral T-cell lymphoma
Subcutaneous panniculitis-like T-cell lymphoma	Subcutaneous panniculitic T-cell lymphoma
Indolent B-cell lymphomas	
Follicle center cell lymphoma	Follicle center lymphoma
Marginal zone B-cell lymphoma	Extranodal marginal zone B-cell lymphoma
Intermediate B-cell lymphomas	
Large B-cell lymphoma of the legs	Diffuse large B-cell lymphoma
Provisional B-cell lymphomas	
Plasmacytoma	Plasmacytoma
Intravascular large B-cell lymphoma	

TABLE 32.2. *Mycosis fungoides, Sezary syndrome, and variants*

Primary cutaneous involvement
- MF (stages IA–IIIB)
- MF-associated follicular mucinosis
- Syringolymphoid hyperplasia
- Pagetoid reticulosis
- Granulomatous slack skin
- Juvnenile lymphogranulomatosis

Concurrent cutaneous/extracutaneous involvement
- MF (stage IV)
- Sezary syndrome

MF, mycosis fungoides; SS, Sezary syndrome.

TABLE 32.3. *Major non–mycosis fungoides/Sezary syndrome lymphomas with cutaneous involvement*

Primary cutaneous T-cell lymphomas (≈50% of primary tumors)[a]

Indolent type (5YS: 85–100%)
- CD30$^+$ large cell PTL (20% of PCTCLs)

Intermediate type (5YS: 50–60%)
- Pleomorphic, small/medium-sized PTL (5% of PCTCLs)

Aggressive (5YS: 10–20%)
- CD30$^-$ large cell PTL (15% of PCTCLs)
- Subcutaneous panniculitic PTL (<5% of PCTCLs)

Variable (survival depends on stage ± subtype)
- Other PCTCLs[b]

Primary cutaneous B-cell lymphomas (≈50% of primary tumors)[a]

Indolent type (5YS: 85–100%)
- Follicle center cell lymphoma (35% of PCBCLs)
- Marginal zone lymphoma (5% of PCBCLs)

Intermediate type (5YS: 50–60%)
- Large B-cell lymphoma of the legs (5% of PCBCLs)

Variable (survival depends on stage ± subtype)
- Other PCBCLs[c]

Systemic natural killer/T-cell lymphomas[d]

Precursor T-lymphoblastic leukemia/lymphoma
T-cell chronic lymphocytic leukemia/prolymphocytic leukemia
Adult T-cell leukemia/lymphoma
Angioimmunoblastic lymphoma
Systemic CD30$^+$ large cell PTL
Natural killer/T-cell angiocentric lymphoma
Aggressive natural killer cell leukemia
Intravascular large T-cell lymphoma
Other T-cell lymphomas[e]

Systemic B-cell lymphomas[d]

Precursor B-lymphoblastic leukemia/lymphoma
Small lymphocytic lymphoma/B-cell chronic lymphocytic leukemia
Follicle center cell lymphoma
Marginal zone lymphoma
Lymphomatoid granulomatosis
Mantle cell lymphoma
Diffuse large B-cell lymphoma
Other B-cell lymphomas[e]

5YS, 5-year disease-related survival; PCBCLs, primary cutaneous B-cell lymphomas; PCTCLs, primary cutaneous T-cell lymphomas; PTL, non–mycosis fungoides/Sezary syndrome peripheral T-cell lymphomas (includes cases with null phenotype).

[a] Any of the primary cutaneous lymphomas can also manifest with systemic involvement. The proportions of various lymphomas and 5-year disease-related survival are based on data from references 2, 7, 70, 71, and 241.

[b] Includes rare cases of primary cutaneous neoplasms such as angiocentric natural killer/T-cell lymphoma, intravascular T-cell lymphoma, and angioimmunoblastic lymphoma.

[c] Includes rare cases of primary cutaneous neoplasms such as plasmacytoma, intravascular B-cell lymphoma, pre-B lymphoblastic lymphoma, mantle cell lymphoma, small lymphocytic B-cell lymphoma, and lymphomatoid granulomatosis.

[d] Lymphomas with concurrent or secondary skin involvement.

[e] Includes rare cases of all other T-cell or B-cell lymphomas.

10% of systemic B-cell lymphomas involve the skin secondarily (7). This is usually a poor prognostic sign.

DIAGNOSING CUTANEOUS LYMPHOMAS

As with all extranodal lymphoid proliferations, the importance of adequate sampling of a suspected cutaneous lymphoma cannot be overemphasized (see Chapter 31). The pathologist should approach possible cutaneous lymphomas in a manner analogous to possible cutaneous squamous cell carcinomas and insist on a biopsy specimen that includes the deepest portion of the lesion. It is this region that may contain the only diagnostic area. The more superficial aspects of the biopsy specimen often contain only a nonspecific inflammatory infiltrate that probably represents a host response to the subjacent tumor (8,9).

In many cases, the histopathologic evaluation of suspected cutaneous lymphomas may be complemented by immunodiagnostic studies such as immunophenotyping (i.e., immunologic analysis of cellular antigen expression) and immunogenotyping (i.e., molecular biologic analysis of antigen receptor genes and chromosomal translocations) (5). The skin can be involved by several diseases, such as lymphomatoid papulosis, in which the demonstration of cytologic atypia, immunophenotypic abnormalities, or monoclonality does not necessarily correlate with the presence of clinically overt lymphoma (3,10) (Table 32.4). Because of this, clinicopathologic correlation is extremely important for the accurate interpretation of immunodiagnostic studies applied to cutaneous lymphoid infiltrates. Although epidermotropic cutaneous lymphomas usually are of T-cell lineage, exceptions exist (11). The lineage of nonepidermotropic cutaneous lymphomas usually cannot be predicted on the basis of histopathologic features alone (5,8,11). Special immunodiagnostic studies are required, but the relatively small size of most skin biopsies creates certain restrictions for these analyses. For example, immunophenotyping is best performed using immunohistologic rather than cell suspension techniques. Besides requiring a smaller cell sample, immunohistologic methods have the added advantages of retaining architectural detail and preserving fragile cells that may be lost during the preparation of cell suspensions.

Southern blot analysis of immunoglobulin (Ig) or T-cell receptor (TCR) gene rearrangements can generally detect a monoclonal T-cell or B-cell population down to a sensitivity limit of about 5% of the total lesional DNA (5). Although this is usually more than adequate for most node-based lymphomas, it may not be sensitive enough to consistently detect monoclonal populations in certain cutaneous lymphoproliferative disorders such as early MF. This is because the monoclonal cells may make up less than 5% of an otherwise adequately dense lymphoid infiltrate. Alternatively, the lymphoid infiltrate may itself contain a detectable percentage of monoclonal cells, but if the infiltrate is too sparse, the monoclonal DNA may become undetectable because of dilution by DNA from other constituent skin cells. In these situations, more sensitive techniques, such as gene amplification using the polymerase chain reaction (PCR), may be required to demonstrate the presence of a monoclonal lymphoid cell population. If the tumor clone gene rearrangement is known, PCR assays can be designed to be tumor specific and sensitive down to a limit of about 1 in 100,000 cells (12). More commonly, they involve consensus primers capable of amplifying a wide spectrum of potential TCR or Ig gene rearrangements. For cutaneous T-cell lymphomas, the most widely applied PCR assays involve amplification of the TCR-γ gene, which is rearranged although not expressed in most cases. A particularly useful method involves PCR amplification of TCR-γ gene rearrangements followed by their separation using denaturing gradient gel electrophoresis (PCR/DGGE method) (13). This method has a sensitivity threshold of about 1%. A variety of PCR assays involving PCR amplification of IgH gene rearrangements have also been described, but caution must be used when applying

TABLE 32.4. *Cutaneous pseudolymphomas*

Type	Lymphoid subset	Microenvironment	Associated findings
Cutaneous lymphoid hyperplasia	B or T	Reticular dermis	Sometimes associated with foreign antigens (e.g., drugs, infections, infestations)
Kimura's disease	B	Reticular dermis, subcutis	Lymphadenopathy, eosinophilia
Castleman's disease	B	Subcutis	Lymphadenopathy, POEMS syndrome, HHV-8 infection
Pseudo-MF/SS	T	Papillary dermis, epidermis	Drug
Follicular mucinosis	T	Hair follicle, perifollicular dermis	Alopecia
Lymphomatoid contact dermatitis	T	Papillary dermis, epidermis	Contact allergen
Actinic reticuloid	T	Dermis, epidermis	Photosensitivity, lymphadenopathy, circulating atypical lymphocytes
Lymphomatoid papulosis	T	Dermis, epidermis	Lymphoma
Lymphocytic infiltration of the skin	T	Perivascular and periadnexal dermis	—

HHV, human herpesvirus; MF, mycosis fungoides; POEMS, polyneuropathy, organomegaly, endocrinopathy, M protein, and skin changes; SS, Sezary syndrome.

these methods to skin lesions because my colleagues and I have seen examples of false-positive monoclonal or oligoclonal patterns arising from sparse reactive B cells within predominantly T-cell infiltrates or even normal skin. Some PCR methods have been adapted for analysis of paraffin-embedded skin samples, (14–16), but this technology is still evolving.

Immunophenotyping and immunogenotyping have additional limitations (see Chapters 3 through 9). Although abnormal patterns of antigen expression may suggest lymphoma by virtue of their uniformity within a suspect T-cell or B-cell population, they cannot be taken as direct evidence of clonality (5). Alternatively, clonal TCR gene rearrangements have been documented in lesions with independent evidence of B-cell differentiation, and rearrangements of certain Ig genes have been demonstrated in lesions with independent evidence of T-cell differentiation (5). These findings indicate that a combined immunophenotypic and genotypic approach is generally better than either alone. From a diagnostic perspective, the major value of immunogenotyping is to determine whether a clonal population is present within a lymphoid infiltrate. Its major application is in cases for which the diagnosis of lymphoma is suspected but not confirmed. The pattern of antigens expressed by a known lymphoma and detected by immunophenotyping is generally a better way of determining the B-cell or T-cell differentiation of the neoplasm.

Southern blot analysis of Ig/TCR gene rearrangements is also subject to additional interpretative errors (5,17). False-positive results may be caused by heritable differences in the location of restriction enzyme digestion sites resulting in restriction fragment length polymorphisms. False-positive results can also be obtained from incomplete digests. For example, an artifactual approximately 9-kb Cβ TCR gene band is sometimes seen in *Eco*RI restriction endonuclease digests. Multiple discrete TCR-γ gene rearrangements have been reported in polyclonal T-cell populations, presumably because the small number of V_γ and J_γ genes results in limited rearrangement options. False-negative results can arise from sampling error, a clonal percentage below the limits of detection, comigration of the clonal bands with the germline bands, or deletion of rearranged genes.

Even when bands are not artifactual, determining the number of clones responsible for them is not always straightforward. In monoclonal tumors, one or a pair of nongermline bands is present in genomic Southern blots if one or both alleles have been rearranged. Three or more rearranged bands may imply more than one clone of tumor cells (i.e., biclonal or multiclonal), as occurs in lymphomas in transplant recipients (18). Additional bands can sometimes arise from a monoclonal tumor as a result of divergent VDJ recombination in a transformed stem cell, V region substitution, hyperdiploidy, or somatic point mutations after prior rearrangements (19). In contrast, subsequent deletions of rearranged alleles may decrease the number of rearranged bands detectable by immunogenotyping (19).

STAGING CUTANEOUS LYMPHOMAS

Patients with cutaneous involvement by lymphoproliferative disorders can present with cutaneous disease alone, concurrent cutaneous and extracutaneous disease, or extracutaneous disease followed by subsequent development of secondary skin lesions (5,8). Although different cutaneous lymphomas can often be grouped into indolent or aggressive types, disease stage is still important for prognosis. The Ann Arbor staging system is used most commonly. In this system, most primary cutaneous lymphomas are staged as IEA (i.e., solitary or localized skin lesions, asymptomatic) or as IVEA (i.e., generalized skin lesions, asymptomatic). Localized lesions are seen more commonly with primary cutaneous B-cell lymphomas, and generalized skin lesions are more characteristic of primary cutaneous T-cell lymphomas (7). In general, the more localized the skin lesions, the better is the prognosis for any given lymphoma type. Involvement of lymph nodes is generally associated with a worse prognosis, but studies suggest that some localized cutaneous lymphomas with only regional nodal involvement may behave similarly to those without any nodal disease. This includes cutaneous B-cell lymphomas and CD30$^+$ anaplastic large T-cell lymphoma (2,20). As with other types of lymphomas, staging should be based on a thorough battery of appropriate tests and not merely physical examination and skin biopsy. Typically, this includes a complete blood count with differential and general blood chemistry panel; computed tomography (CT) scans of the chest, abdomen, and pelvis; and bone marrow sampling. Clinically abnormal lymph nodes and other extracutaneous masses should be biopsied to determine if they are involved by lymphoma. To qualify as a primary cutaneous lymphoma, some observers require the absence of extracutaneous lesions for at least 6 months after initial staging (7,21,22). This is particularly relevant for CD30$^+$ anaplastic large T-cell lymphoma and some of the cutaneous B-cell lymphomas that may present with skin lesions as part of a systemic lymphoma that soon manifests itself.

CUTANEOUS T-CELL LYMPHOPROLIFERATIVE DISORDERS

The term *cutaneous T-cell lymphoma* (CTCL) is used often to refer to MF and related entities. It has been useful as a unifying concept that has facilitated our understanding of these disorders, but because there are many clinicopathologically distinct T-cell lymphomas that involve the skin, it is preferable to refer to specific diseases by their individual names when considering diagnosis, prognosis, or management. Most CTCLs are postthymic T-cell lymphomas, which are lymphomas that lack thymic involvement and lymphoblastic cytologic features (5,8,23–28). Regardless of their histopathologic subtype, CTCLs often exhibit deficiencies of one or more antigens that are generally expressed by nonneo-

TABLE 32.5. *Deficient antigen expression in T-cell lymphoproliferative disorders affecting the skin*

Diagnosis[a]	Immunophenotype[b] CD2	CD3	CD5	CD7
MF—patch/plaque	+	+	+	−
MF—tumor	±	±	±	−
MF—nodal	±	±	±	−
SS—skin	±	+	±	−
SS—blood	+	+	+	−
ATL—skin, nodal	+	+	±	−
PTL—all sites	±	±	±	±
T-LBL—all sites	±	±	+	+
LYP—skin	±	±	−	−

ATL, adult T-cell leukemia/lymphoma; LYP, lymphomatoid papulosis; MF, mycosis fungoides; PTL, peripheral T-cell lymphoma; SS, Sezary syndrome; T-LBL, T-cell lymphoblastic lymphoma.

[a] Antigen deficiency was defined as <50% (minority) of tumor cells that were antigen positive.

[b] Immunophenotype was scored as follows: + (≤10% of cases antigen deficient), ± (11–49% of cases antigen deficient), − (≥50% of cases antigen deficient).

plastic T cells (Table 32.5) (5,8,23–30). In many cases, these deficiencies are present in a uniform manner throughout the infiltrate. Such immunophenotypic data can be helpful in establishing the T-cell lineage of the tumor, in distinguishing it from an inflammatory infiltrate, and in suggesting that it is monoclonal. Monoclonality can then be confirmed by demonstrating monoclonally rearranged TCR genes using molecular biologic methods. Most T-cell lymphomas involving the skin express TCR-$\alpha\beta$ rather than TCR-$\gamma\delta$ heterodimers. Antibodies directed against V_β gene families have also been used to detect tumor cells in MF/SS and other T-cell lymphomas (31,32). Because a limited number of genes encode the V region of the TCR-β gene, it has been possible to use monoclonal antibodies specific for a particular V_β gene product to identify monoclonal tumor cells. In a polyclonal T-cell population, no more than 3% to 5% of cells react with any one anti-Vβ monoclonal antibody, whereas in a T-cell lymphoma, all the neoplastic cells react with the particular anti-Vβ antibody specific for the V_β gene they express (31). Although one study found that most MF/SS cases express $V_\beta 8$ gene family products in their TCR-β chains (33), subsequent studies have not confirmed this type of restricted use of V_β gene families in MF/SS (34,35).

Molecular biologic analysis of TCR gene rearrangements has been performed on most T-cell lymphoproliferative disorders that can involve the skin (36–49). Among these are MF, SS, adult T-cell leukemia/lymphoma (ATL), other PTLs, and precursor T-cell lymphoblastic lymphomas. Monoclonal or oligoclonal rearrangement of the TCR-β gene has been demonstrated in each of these diseases and correlates with immunophenotypic evidence of T-cell antigen deficiencies (Table 32.5). This indicates that each of these diseases is a monoclonal or oligoclonal T-cell lymphoproliferative disorder. With rare exception, these types of clonal TCR-β gene rearrangements have not been observed in unequivocal inflammatory T-cell infiltrates or in normal tissues (13,32,50,51).

MYCOSIS FUNGOIDES OR SEZARY SYNDROME

Clinical Features

In its advanced cutaneous tumor phase, MF was first described by Alibert in 1806 (52). Later in the 19th century, additional cutaneous manifestations of MF were recognized (53–55), but it was not until 1938 that Sezary described peripheral blood involvement (56). MF is a type of peripheral T-cell lymphoma that classically manifests in the skin as flat patches that may evolve into raised, infiltrated plaques and tumor nodules with subsequent involvement of lymph nodes and ultimately viscera (57) (Fig. 32.1). Sometimes other types of cutaneous lesions may be present. Poikilodermatous lesions exhibit epidermal atrophy, telangiectasia, and mottled hypopigmentation and hyperpigmentation clinically. Lesions that contain follicular mucinosis manifest as boggy, infiltrated plaques with alopecia if they involve hairy areas. In the erythrodermatous variant of MF, usually the entire skin is erythematous and scaly. Patients who have SS classically exhibit erythroderma, lymphadenopathy, and leukemic involvement of the peripheral blood. It is not uncommon for other types of MF patients to have small numbers of circulating tumor cells at some point in their clinical course. Leukemic involvement usually is defined as circulating tumor cells exceeding 5% to 10% of the total leukocytes, 20% of total lymphocytes, or an absolute level of 1,000 cells/mm^3 of blood (57–60). In addition to the latter criterion, the EORTC group suggests two more criteria: monoclonality and a CD4 to CD8 ratio of less than 10 (2).

The peripheral lymph nodes are the most common site of extracutaneous involvement by MF. In various reports, 40% to 70% of MF/SS patients have had palpable lymphadenopathy, most often affecting the regional lymph node groups draining the sites of greatest cutaneous involvement (57,58,61–63). Using routine histopathologic examination, it is unusual to detect extracutaneous involvement of tissues other than lymph nodes during life. Liver biopsy has shown involvement by MF in fewer than 18% of patients (58,62,64). Bone marrow biopsy or aspiration has been positive in fewer than 7% of cases (58,61,62). However, revised criteria for bone marrow involvement have suggested prognostically significant levels of marrow infiltration in a larger proportion of cases (65).

Lymph nodes and viscera have each been involved in 70% to 75% of cases at autopsy (61,66). The most common sites of visceral involvement are spleen, lungs, and liver (approximately 50% of cases for each). Occasionally, MF has been found to involve almost any organ system. Transformation of MF to various types of large cell lymphoma has been observed at autopsy and during life (57,58,66–69).

Patients with MF/SS are commonly staged according to

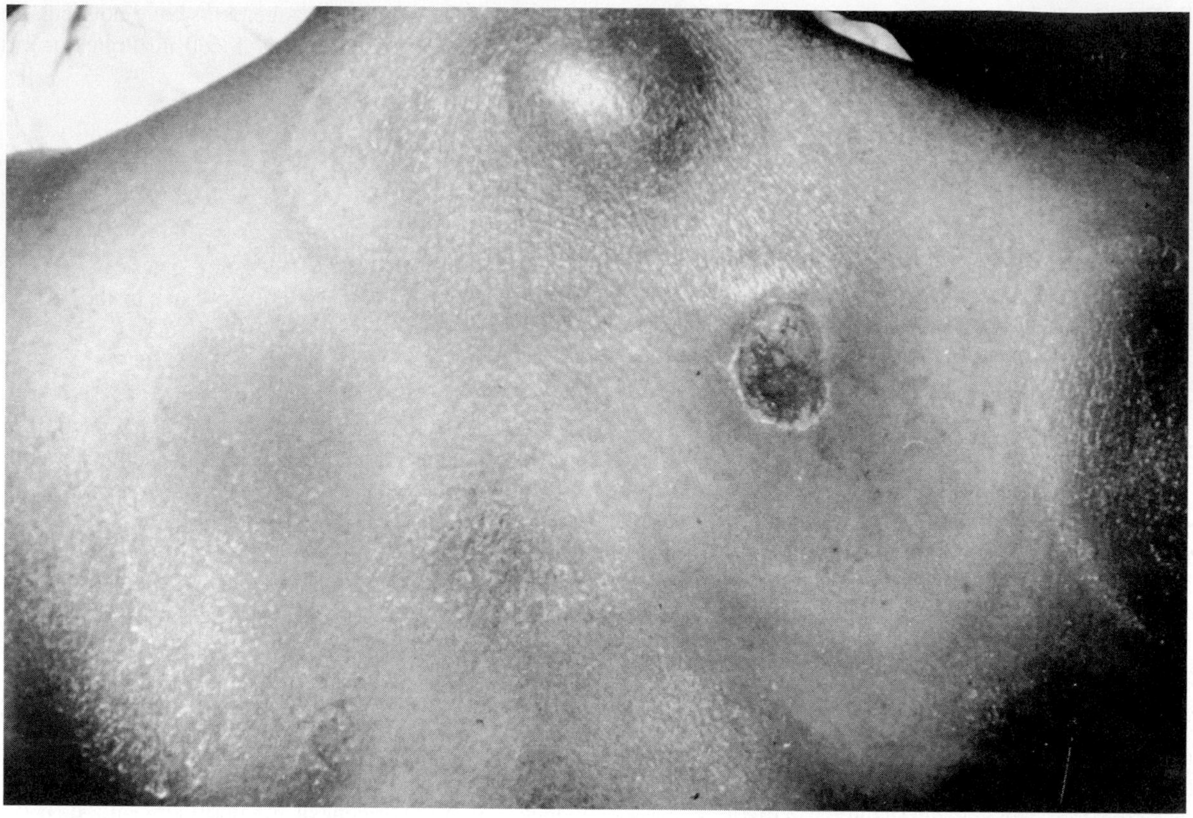

FIG. 32.1. Clinical features of mycosis fungoides. This patient's back demonstrates several different types of lesions, including flat, scaly patches; elevated plaques; and protuberant tumor nodules, one of which is ulcerated.

a tumor, lymph node, metastases (TNM) system (57,58,60) (Table 32.6). Using one form of this system in conjunction with evaluation of peripheral blood and a histopathologic grading of lymph node involvement, it has been possible to define three risk groups of MF/SS patients (58). The favorable-risk group has a median survival exceeding 12 years and includes patients with only T1 or T2 disease. The intermediate-risk group has a median survival of about 5 years and includes patients with T1 or T2 disease who also have lymph node or blood involvement and any patients with T3 or T4 disease. The poor-risk group has a median survival of only 2.5 years and includes all patients with visceral involvement or lymph node effacement by tumor. Studies indicate that the survival of patients with stage IA disease is similar to that of age-matched controls (70). Among erythrodermic (T4) patients, an unfavorable risk group can be identified based on the presence of at least two of the following three features: age 65 or older, peripheral blood involvement, and lymph node or visceral involvement (71). Patients lacking all of these features had the best prognosis, and those with only one had an intermediate outcome.

MF/SS is associated with other lymphoproliferative disorders. It may be preceded by large plaque parapsoriasis (72) or clonal dermatitis (73), or it may transform into a large cell lymphoma (57,58,66–69). Lymphomatoid papulosis or

TABLE 32.6. *TNM staging system for mycosis fungoides and Sezary syndrome*

Stage	T[a]	N[b]	M[c]
IA	1	0	0
IB	2	0	0
IIA	1–2	1	0
IIB	3	0–1	0
IIIA	4	0	0
IIIB	4	1	0
IVA	1–4	2–3	0
IVB	1–4	0–3	1

MF, mycosis fungoides.

[a] T1, cutaneous patches and/or plaques covering <10% of body surface; T2, cutaneous patches and/or plaques covering >10% of body surface; T3, one or more cutaneous tumor nodules; T4, erythroderma.

[b] N0, lymph nodes clinically normal and histologically negative for MF; N1, lymph nodes clinically enlarged but histologically negative for MF; N2, lymph nodes clinically normal but histologically positive for MF; N3, lymph nodes clinically enlarged and histologically positive for MF.

[c] M0, visceral involvement absent; M1, visceral involvement present.

Adapted from Bunn PA, Lamberg SI. Report of the committee on staging and classification of cutaneous T-cell lymphomas. *Cancer Treat Rep* 1979;63:725–728.

Hodgkin's disease may also precede, follow, or appear concurrently with MF/SS (74). Rarely, MF/SS has been associated with low-grade B-cell lymphoproliferative disorders (75).

Ultrastructure

The classic MF/SS tumor cell contains a convoluted or cerebriform nucleus, which has a serpiginous, folded configuration when examined ultrastructurally (76,77). Large and small variants have been described (76). Quantitative electron microscopic or light microscopic measurement of nuclear shape, area, chromatin dispersion, or nuclear to cytoplasmic ratio has been used to derive several values that have been used to discriminate between MF/SS and benign lesions with variable success (78–81). The main problem is a tradeoff between sensitivity and specificity. For example, the nuclear contour index (NCI) is one assessment of nuclear membrane irregularity (78–81). The presence of cells with an NCI exceeding 11.5 is highly specific for MF/SS, but a significant number of MF/SS patients do not have tumor cells with NCI values that are this high.

Cytogenetics

Cytogenetic studies have demonstrated some nonrandom chromosomal abnormalities in MF/SS cells, but none of these defects has been present consistently (62,82–85). This is characteristic of T-cell lymphomas and contrasts with the more consistent structural abnormalities present in certain types of B-cell lymphomas such as Burkitt's lymphoma [t(8; 14) translocation] and the follicular lymphomas [t(14;18) translocation] (86,87). Evidence has been presented to support the concept that MF/SS is derived from "genotraumatic" T cells (i.e., those with a predisposition to accumulate somatic mutations) (88).

DNA Cytophotometry

Flow cytometric and microscopic studies of DNA content have demonstrated aneuploidy or hypertetraploidy among MF/SS cells in many cases (89–91). As with NCI values, criteria have been established for the differential diagnosis of MF/SS from reactive cutaneous T-cell infiltrates, but some cases of MF/SS overlap with inflammatory T-cell infiltrates in terms of their DNA content profiles (i.e., they show only diploid and some tetraploid cells). Aneuploid and hypertetraploid DNA values can be seen in skin diseases other than overt lymphomas, including lymphomatoid papulosis and lymphomatoid contact dermatitis (80).

Immunophenotyping

The antigen expression of MF/SS tumor cells has been extensively characterized by immunophenotyping using monoclonal antibodies directed against a wide variety of lymphoid differentiation and activation antigens (see Chapter 3). In general, MF/SS expresses an immunophenotype consistent with a mature, memory, helper T-cell SALT lymphoma. In most cases, the tumor cells express a $CD4^+CD8^-$ (helper or inducer) T-cell phenotype (5,92–95). Rarely, the tumor cells may instead express a $CD4^-CD8^+$ (cytotoxic or suppressor) T-cell phenotype. Preliminary studies of these rare $CD8^+$ cases suggest that those that are $CD2^-CD7^+$ have a worse prognosis than those that are $CD2^+CD7^-$ (96). In contrast to precursor T-cell lymphoblastic lymphoma/leukemia, it is uncommon for MF/SS cells to be $CD1^+$, $CD4^-CD8^-$, or $CD4^+CD8^+$ (5). The cutaneous lymphocyte-associated antigen (CLA), which is the ligand for vascular E-selectin (ELAM-1) and a marker of SALT T cells, is expressed by MF/SS. In most cases, so is CD45RO, a marker of memory T cells (97). The latter feature suggests that the MF/SS tumor cell encountered its target antigen before malignant transformation. My colleagues and I have seen some cases of MF that express the cytolytic granule-associated marker TIA-1.

Unlike most other types of T-cell lymphoma, MF/SS generally retains expression of pan-T-cell antigens such as CD2, CD3, CD5, and TCR-β until the development of cutaneous tumors or lymph node involvement (5,92–96). In these advanced lesions, one or more pan-T-cell antigens are often absent and MF/SS becomes similar immunophenotypically to other types of peripheral T-cell lymphoma. This progression is sometimes accompanied by a transformation of MF/SS into a large cell lymphoma that may express CD30 (1,2,68,69).

In about 10% of cases, MF/SS skin lesions may exhibit deficiency of one or more pan-T-cell antigens exclusively among T cells infiltrating the epidermis (98,99). In most such cases, this is the only immunophenotypic abnormality identified. Such intraepidermal T-cell antigen deficiencies were not detected in more than 40 inflammatory skin lesions. This suggests that epidermal or dermal immunophenotypic discordance can be a useful differential diagnostic feature in some cases.

A characteristic feature of approximately two thirds of MF/SS cases is deficiency of Leu-8 (L-selectin), CD7 antigens, or both, with deficiency defined as expression of these antigens by less than 50% of lesional T cells (100,101). Leu-8 is a homing receptor antigen. Its deficiency is a nonspecific feature that is often observed in a variety of inflammatory and neoplastic cutaneous T-cell infiltrates. However, Leu-8 deficiency in reactive lymph nodes (excluding acquired immunodeficiency syndrome) is uncommon and suggests involvement by MF/SS or other T-cell lymphomas (30,101). Leu-8–deficient T cells have also been observed in some lymph nodes involved by Hodgkin's disease (30). The issue of CD7 deficiency as a differential diagnostic criterion for MF has been further investigated (102,103). CD7 deficiency is observed in about 10% to 20% of benign cutaneous T-cell infiltrates (30,100,104); therefore, isolated CD7 deficiency is suggestive but not conclusive proof of skin involvement by MF/SS or other T-cell lymphoma. The optimal CD7 percentage cut point appears to be around 33% (102,103). In reactive lymph nodes, however, CD7 deficiency is rare and strongly suggests neoplastic T-cell involvement (30,101). Among MF patients without microscopically detectable circulating tumor cells, there are normal numbers of Leu-8^{+} and CD7^{+} T cells in the peripheral blood (105).

In contrast to antigens that may be deficient in MF/SS, there are other antigens that tend to be preferentially expressed by T cells in MF/SS compared with inflammatory dermatoses. These antigens include CD38, CD71, BE1, and BE2, but there are insufficient data in the literature to determine if quantitation of these antigens is useful for differential diagnosis (5). CD25 (TAC) expression is generally more extensive in ATL than in MF/SS, but there is enough overlap to preclude CD25 expression as a useful distinguishing feature (5). There is also a wide range of CD25^{+} cells in inflammatory cutaneous T-cell infiltrates.

CD103 is expressed selectively on epidermotropic MF/SS cells, with loss of this antigen in the nonepidermotropic tumor phase of disease (106). This marker is absent on tumor cells clustered within Pautrier microabscesses. Epidermotropism has also been associated with expression of interferon-γ–inducible protein-10 (IP-10) by lesional keratinocytes and correlated with epidermotropism of CD4^{+} but not CD8^{+} T cells (107). Expression of very late activation (VLA) antigen-1 (VLA-1) through VLA-6 and CD44 splice variants have also been studied in MF/SS, and specific patterns appear to influence tumor cell trafficking behavior and correlate with disease stage (108–110). Most cell nuclei in typical MF/SS lesions are Ki-67^{-}, suggesting that tumor cells are not actively proliferating (111,112). One study of 14 cases suggested that the minority of Ki-67^{+} cells that are present in MF/SS skin lesions are preferentially localized within the epidermis (111), but a larger study of more than 50 cases suggested variability in the location of proliferating cells (113). A preliminary study of SS suggests that tumor cells increase in number because they have an inherent defect in expression of FAS (CD95) and activation-induced cell death; however, biochemical manipulations can overcome this defect and result in tumor cell apoptosis (114). These findings suggest that SS may be more of a ''lymphoaccumulative'' disorder than a lymphproliferative disorder.

Antibodies directed against specific TCR-Vβ families can be helpful in demonstrating T-cell monoclonality in MF/SS (31,32). The principal limiting factor is the unavailability of a comprehensive panel of such antibodies. Tumor clone–specific anti-TCR idiotype monoclonal antibodies have been used to detect MF/SS tumor cells immunohistologically and to monitor the tumor response to intravenous therapy with anti-idiotype antibody (115).

Although there is some controversy concerning the pattern of cytokines produced in early MF, advanced MF and SS appear to express a predominantly helper T cell type 2 (T_H2) cytokine profile (e.g., interleukin-4 [IL-4], IL-5, IL-10) rather than a T_H1 profile (e.g., IL-2, interferon-γ [IFN-γ]) (116,117).

In addition to plasma cells and eosinophils, certain other types of nonneoplastic cells are admixed with tumor cells in MF/SS skin lesions, each with its own characteristic immunophenotype. These include reactive T cells of the CD4^{+} and CD8^{+} subsets, CD1^{+} Langerhans cells or indeterminate cells, various types of macrophages, and occasionally with reactive polytypic B cells (5).

Immunogenotyping

The use of molecular biologic methods to determine T-cell clonality in MF has been reviewed (102). Southern blot analysis of TCR gene rearrangements in MF/SS cells infiltrating thick cutaneous plaques, tumors, blood, and lymph nodes has demonstrated that MF/SS is typically a monoclonal T-cell lymphoproliferative disorder. Although additional clones have been detected in a few cases (49), all sites of disease usually involve the same clone (5,10,36). Demonstration of a monoclonal population in the peripheral blood of erythrodermic patients has proven useful in distinguishing cases of SS from inflammatory skin diseases (118,119). Monoclonality does not always correlate with the presence of circulating Sezary cells and is probably a better indicator of blood involvement in MF/SS patients, despite the fact that dominant T-cell clones can sometimes be found in the blood of healthy elderly patients (120). Nevertheless, some studies have found a relatively high prevalence (about 50%) of dominant clonality in the blood of MF patients, including those with only stage I disease (121,122). The clinical significance of findings such as these may ultimately prove to depend more on quantitative than qualitative features. In patch and thin plaque lesions of MF/SS, monoclonal TCR gene rearrangements have not always been detected by Southern blotting (44–46), but these lesions contain fewer T cells than thick plaques and tumors. This creates the potential for false-negative results because of inadequate sampling. Sensitive molecular biologic techniques involving TCR-β or TCR-γ gene amplification using PCR have documented the monoclonality of most early MF/SS skin lesions, including some that were negative by conventional Southern blot analysis (13,32,102,121,123–131). Single-cell PCR analysis suggests enrichment of clonal tumor cells within the epidermis (132). Highly sensitive PCR methods employing RNase protection assays have detected the tumor clone in clinicopathologically uninvolved lymph nodes, blood, and bone marrow from MF patients, including those with only very early stage IA disease (133). This is consistent with the view that, rather than being a true primary skin lymphoma, MF is a neoplasm of the SALT T-cell type. Although MF cells may spend most of their time in the skin, they have the ability to traffic at low levels to extracutaneous lymphoid tissues through the blood and lymphatics (134). This behavior has been highlighted by studies showing that MF tumor cells can traffic into sites of allergic contact dermatitis induced in patients with MF (135) and by studies showing that low-level circulation of MF tumor cells is greater in the arterial than venous circulation because of clearance in the skin (136).

After a tumor clone has been identified in an MF/SS patient, Southern blot or PCR analysis of various tissues can be used to determine the distribution of the neoplastic clone throughout the body (i.e., immunogenotypic staging), to monitor the response to therapy, or to follow the patient for evidence of disease relapse. These studies have demonstrated that gene rearrangement analysis is more sensitive and specific than light microscopic examination or immunophenotyping for determining lymph node or blood involvement by MF/SS (3,137–141). For example, when lymph nodes from MF/SS patients were examined, six (75%) of eight nodes that were histopathologically negative for MF/SS were immunogenotypically positive, and three of eight were immunophenotypically positive (3). Occult lymph node involvement detectable by Southern blotting was associated with a poor prognosis among patients with LN2 grade biopsies (137). In this same set of cases, Southern blotting and PCR methods were equally sensitive in predicting poor outcome (142). Serial TCR gene rearrangement studies of blood lymphocytes from patients with leukemic MF/SS have been used to monitor changes in the circulating tumor cell burden in response to therapy (47,48). In one study, there was evidence for the emergence of new neoplastic clones or subclones over time (47). Mutations of *TP53* were found in tumor stage MF (without large cell transformation) but not in earlier patch-plaque lesions (143). Gene rearrangement analysis has shown that the skin can be a reservoir of minimal residual disease in MF/SS patients who are in complete clinical remission (144). Failure to detect dominant clonality in cases of early MF has been proposed as a favorable prognostic indicator, the theory being that this is a false-negative result implying a very low tumor clone density (145).

Histopathology

Skin

The histopathologic appearance of lesional skin biopsies depends on the clinical type of MF sampled (i.e., patch, plaque, tumor, or erythroderma) and whether associated changes are present such as poikiloderma, follicular mucinosis, or granulomatous inflammation. Well-developed plaques characteristically exhibit a dense bandlike infiltrate of atypical lymphoid cells with hyperchromatic, convoluted nuclei and scant cytoplasm within the upper dermis (Fig. 32.2). These atypical cells may vary considerably in size. The overlying epidermis contains similar cells singly and in clusters known as Pautrier microabscesses or microaggregates (Figs. 32.3, 32.4). The epidermis is often acanthotic but usually lacks significant intercellular edema (i.e., spongiosis). The dermal infiltrate often contains a variable number of histiocytes (i.e., macrophages and dendritic cells), eosinophils, and plasma cells. The deep dermis and subcutis are generally histologically normal in plaque lesions.

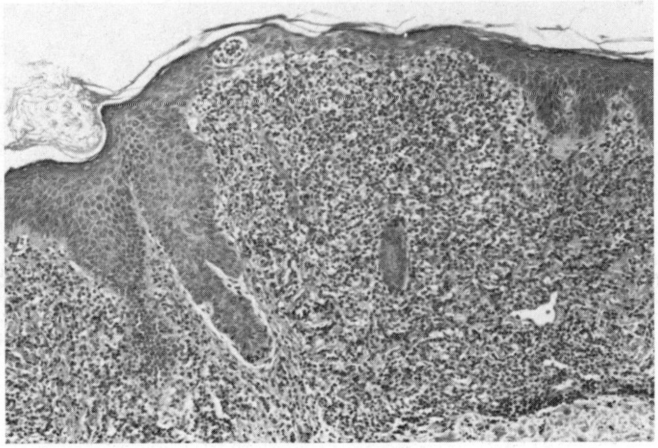

FIG. 32.2. Mycosis fungoides: well-developed plaque. A dense, bandlike upper dermal lymphoid infiltrate obscures the dermoepidermal junction centrally and extends into the epidermis, forming a Pautrier microaggregate (original magnification: 120× magnification).

Earlier patch lesions typically show a sparser upper dermal lymphoid infiltrate that may be patchy and perivascular rather than bandlike. Pautrier microaggregates may be rare or absent and cytologic atypia may be minimal. However, many lymphoid cells are still present within a nonspongiotic epidermis. Nevertheless, some patch and plaque lesions exhibit significant spongiosis in conjunction with a cytologically atypical lymphoid infiltrate. The spongiosis is sometimes caused by superimposed impetiginization or contact dermatitis, and it may resolve after appropriate therapy. Clinicopathologic correlation is required to rule out alternate diagnoses such as lymphomatoid contact dermatitis and MF-like drug eruptions.

Later tumor lesions contain a dense infiltrate of tumor cells within the upper and lower dermis that may extend into the subcutis. Tumor cells in these lesions appear to have lost their epidermotropism and often spare the epidermis and a thin superficial layer of papillary dermis known as the *Grenz zone*. From an architectural standpoint, tumor lesions of MF may resemble other forms of cutaneous lymphoma if they spare the epidermis and involve the full thickness of the dermis. From a cytologic standpoint, tumor lesions of MF often retain characteristic cytologic features (i.e., hyperchromatic, convoluted nuclei and scant cytoplasm) that generally allow them to be distinguished from other types of cutaneous lymphoma.

Erythrodermatous lesions of MF are similar to those seen in SS. In many cases, histopathologic features diagnostic of MF are present, but other cases exhibit only nonspecific spongiotic dermatitis (59,89). The diagnosis must then be based on microscopic examination of the peripheral blood or lymph node biopsies. Patches and thin plaques of MF that show poikiloderma clinically exhibit epidermal atrophy,

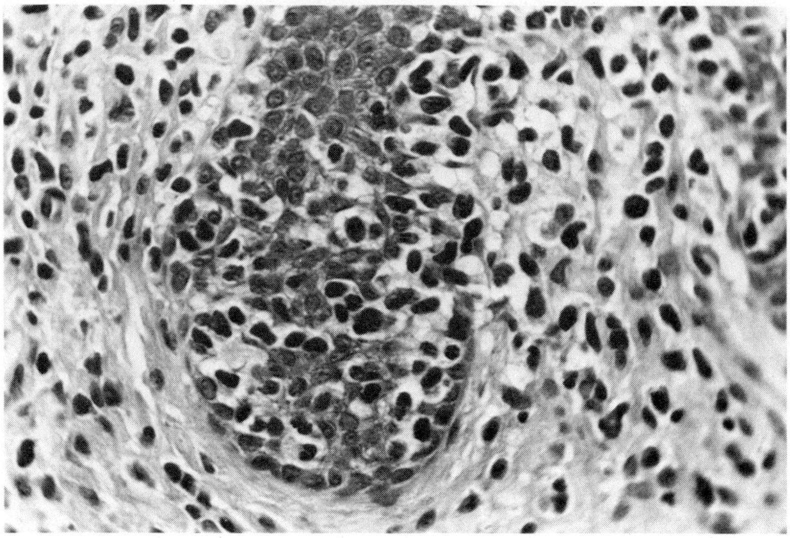

FIG. 32.3. Mycosis fungoides: epidermal involvement. Numerous atypical lymphocytes, characterized by hyperchromatic, irregularly shaped, variably sized nuclei, extend from the papillary dermis into the epidermis of the rete ridge in the center of the field (original magnification: 480× magnification).

vascular ectasia, and pigment incontinence histopathologically (72,146). Lesions of MF/SS associated with follicular mucinosis exhibit tumor cell infiltration of hair follicles and deposits of mucin in the intercellular spaces between the follicular epithelial cells (147). Sometimes there may be preferential follicular involvement by MF without mucinosis (148). Occasionally, the dermal infiltrate of MF/SS may contain a granulomatous component usually manifesting as small tuberculoid granulomas or individual histiocytic giant cells but in other cases resembling granuloma annulare (149).

Lymph Nodes

Enlarged lymph nodes obtained from MF patients are discrete, not matted, with a soft or rubbery consistency. Transected surfaces are homogeneous and tan with variable amounts of melanin pigmentation. In some cases, lymph nodes may exhibit only nonspecific histopathologic features such as reactive follicular hyperplasia, sinusoidal hyperplasia, or fibrosis. In other cases, there may be partial or complete effacement of lymph node architecture by a diffuse infiltrate of MF cells with or without transformation to large cell lymphoma (1,2,58,66–69,150–154). Transformation may be associated with the presence of cells resembling Reed-Sternberg cells. Plasma cells and eosinophils may be admixed. However, the most common histopathologic finding is dermatopathic lymphadenopathy, in which the paracortex is expanded by a mixture of interdigitating dendritic cells, macrophages containing melanin or lipid, lymphocytes, plasma cells, and sometimes eosinophils (155). Mitotic figures may be present. Reactive follicles and medullary cords are usually identifiable but may be compressed. Various numbers of atypical lymphoid cells with hyperchro-

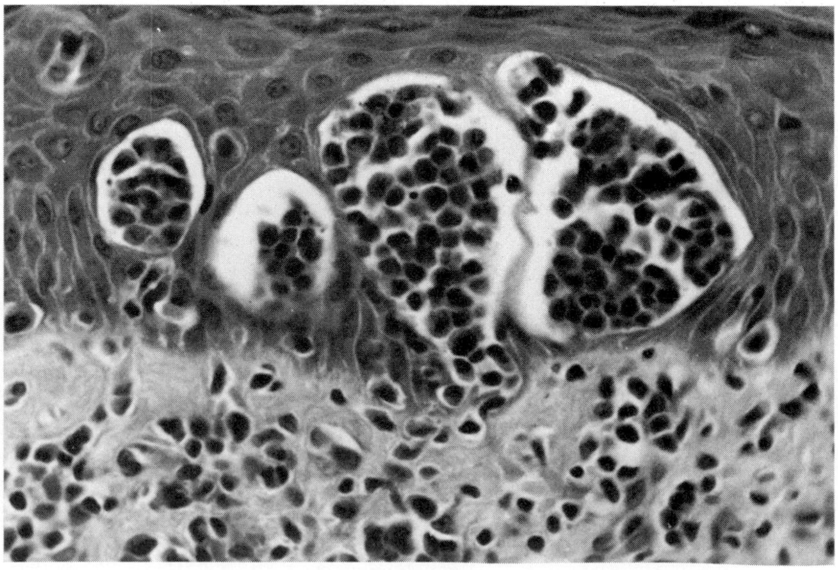

FIG. 32.4. Mycosis fungoides: Pautrier microaggregates. Atypical lymphocytes breach the epidermal basement membrane zone and collect within the epidermis in discrete nests. The epidermis surrounding these nests lacks intercellular edema (i.e., spongiosis), an important feature that helps to distinguish them from the spongiotic simulants of mycosis fungoides, occasional cases of spongiotic (eczematous) dermatitis that contain atypical lymphocytes (original magnification: 480× magnification).

TABLE 32.7. *Histopathologic scheme for grading dermatopathic and neoplastic changes in lymph nodes from patients with mycosis fungoides and Sezary syndrome*

Grade	Histopathologic features
LN-1	DL with occasional AL
LN-2	DL with AL singly or in small clusters (<6 cells)
LN-3	DL with numerous AL, singly or in large clusters (>15 cells)
LN-4	Partial or complete effacement by MF/SS ± DL.

AL, atypical lymphocytes; DL, dermatopathic lymphadenopathy; MF, mycosis fungoides; SS, Sezary syndrome.

matic, convoluted nuclei are often observed within this background of reactive changes (58,67–69,150–154).

A grading system has been created to divide such lymph nodes into four categories (LN1 through LN4) based on their content of atypical lymphoid cells (Table 32.7) (150). The major histopathologic features are illustrated in Figures 32.5 through 32.8. For staging purposes, only LN3 and LN4 lymph nodes have generally been considered to be involved by MF. The proportion of these cases varies, depending on the series reported, but molecular biologic studies suggest that some lymph nodes showing LN1 or LN2 features also may be involved by MF to a clinically significant degree (36,140). More than 80% of LN2 lymph nodes and all LN3 lymph nodes have shown cytogenetic or other evidence of MF involvement (61). These findings may help to explain reported discrepancies in the correlation between survival and the LN grade (153) and explain why even the largest studies show that, although lymph node grade can be a significant prognostic indicator, it is a dependent variable that parallels the extent of cutaneous and visceral involvement (58). The specificity of the LN3 grade for MF/SS has been brought into question by the demonstration of LN3 changes in dermatopathic lymph nodes from patients without evidence of lymphoma (154).

Viscera

Hepatic involvement by MF/SS usually consists of nodular aggregates of tumor cells in the portal zones or lobules. In patients with leukemic involvement, it is not unusual for tumor cells to be identified within the hepatic sinusoids, but this is not considered evidence of hepatic involvement (64). Bone marrow involvement by MF/SS is usually manifested as nodular aggregates of small atypical lymphoid cells (61). Criteria for involvement were defined in one study to include diffuse infiltration or lymphoid aggregates (i.e., paratrabecular or nonparatrabecular) containing atypical lymphoid cells with small convoluted or large transformed nuclei (65). Using these guidelines, 25 (28%) of 90 cases were considered to have clinically significant marrow involvement, including 4 in stages I through IIA, 4 in stages IIB through III, 5 in stage IVA, and 12 in stage IVB.

Potential Variants

Some additional cutaneous T-cell lymphoproliferative disorders are regarded as variants of MF by some observers. These diseases include MF-associated follicular mucinosis,

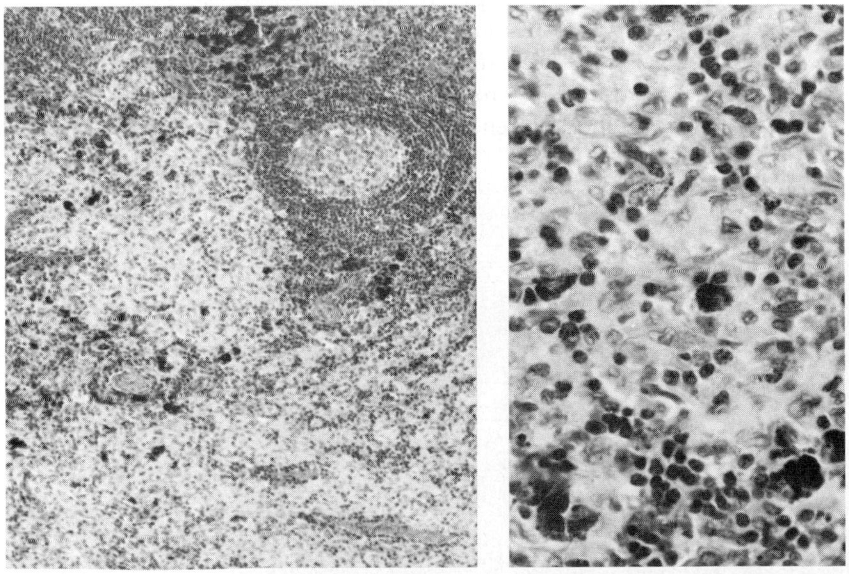

FIG. 32.5. Dermatopathic lymphadenopathy: LN1 category. **A:** The paracortical region has been expanded by numerous pale-staining interdigitating dendritic cells and macrophages. A residual secondary B-cell follicle is in the upper part of the field (original magnification: 120× magnification). **B:** Higher magnification shows the pale-staining interdigitating dendritic cells and macrophages admixed with a few normal lymphocytes (original magnification: 480× magnification). In both fields, the dense black structures are macrophages laden with melanin pigment.

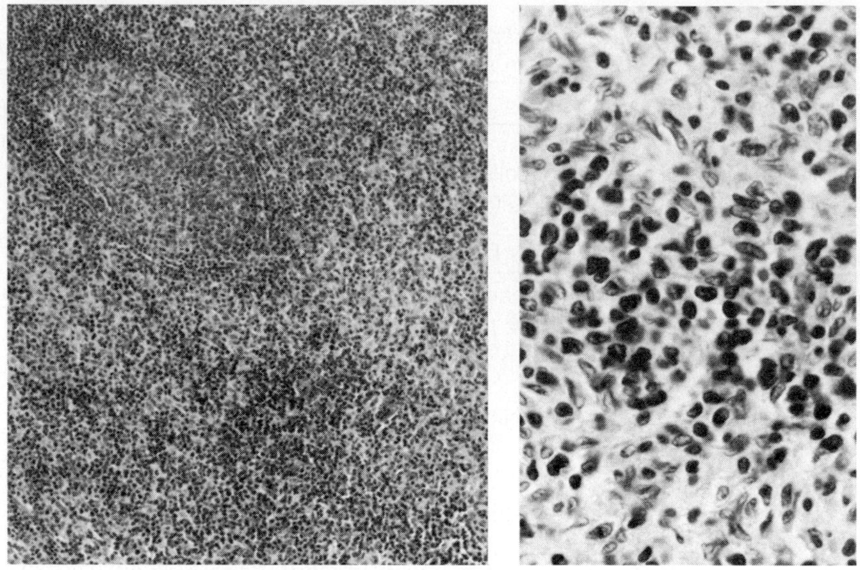

FIG. 32.6. Dermatopathic lymphadenopathy: LN3 category. **A:** The paracortex contains a large number of lymphoid cells as well as interdigitating dendritic cells and macrophages. One of the few remaining secondary B-cell follicles *(upper field)* is partially obscured (original magnification: 120× magnification). **B:** Higher magnification shows large clusters of atypical lymphocytes within a background of LN1-type changes (original magnification: 480× magnification).

syringolymphoid hyperplasia, pagetoid reticulosis, granulomatous slack skin, and juvenile lymphogranulomatosis.

Follicular Mucinosis

Also known as alopecia mucinosa (156), follicular mucinosis is a benign dermatosis when not arising from MF or other lymphomas. It is characterized clinically by boggy, sometimes pruritic, pink to yellow-white papules and plaques on the head and neck or occasionally elsewhere that are associated with alopecia when they involve hairy areas such as the scalp (147,156–158). Several clinical presentations have been reported: solitary or few lesions, usually on the head or neck of a child, that resolve spontaneously within a few years; widespread lesions in adults that may persist or recur indefinitely, sometimes arising in patients with chronic lymphocytic leukemia (CLL), Hodgkin's disease, or Kaposi's sarcoma (3,157,159,160); and secondary lesions within cutaneous lymphoid infiltrates of MF, SS, other cutaneous lymphomas, discoid lupus erythematosus, or angiolymphoid hyperplasia with eosinophilia (ALHE). Histopathologically, there is a lymphohistiocytic infiltrate within the dermis that surrounds and infiltrates hair follicles. The follicles contain pools of acid mucopolysaccharides associated

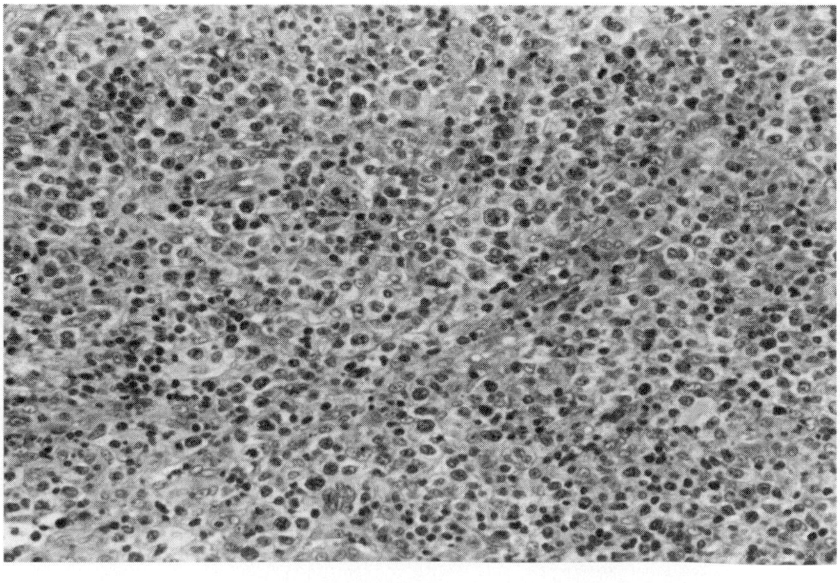

FIG. 32.7. Lymph node effacement by mycosis fungoides: LN4 category. The nodal architecture is diffusely effaced by a pleomorphic, atypical lymphoid infiltrate (original magnification: 240× magnification).

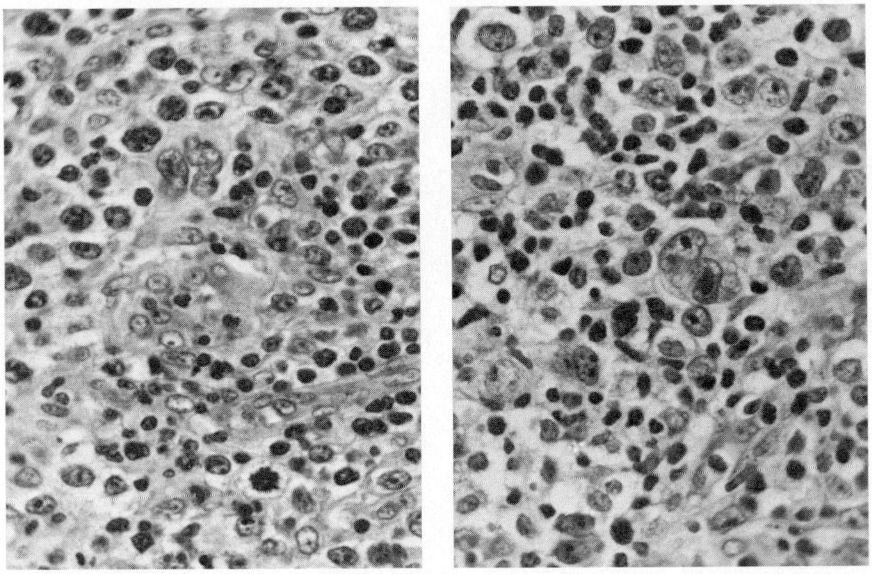

FIG. 32.8. Lymph node effacement by mycosis fungoides: transformed cells. Two fields showing higher magnification of the same case illustrated in Figure 32.7. Several tumor cells contain large nuclei with prominent nucleoli. Some cells are binucleate or contain bilobed nuclei resembling Reed-Sternberg cells. Infiltrates of mycosis fungoides–containing clusters of transformed cells or more than 25% transformed cells diffusely are said to exhibit transformation to large cell lymphoma (original magnification: 480× magnification).

with disruption of the follicular structure. This histopathologic alteration is also known as follicular mucinosis. Histiocytes and eosinophils may be admixed. In cases of MF/SS-associated follicular mucinosis, typical MF-type tumor cells can be identified in the follicular epithelium, the epidermis, or the dermis. Atypical lymphocytes are rare in other types of follicular mucinosis and reportedly do not form Pautrier-like microaggregates (147), but others have had difficulty distinguishing benign follicular mucinosis from the MF-associated variety on histopathologic grounds alone (160). Eosinophils have been observed in benign and MF-associated types (147,160). Gene rearrangement studies have documented dominant T-cell clonality in idiopathic and MF-associated follicular mucinosis, indicating that the primary type is also a lymphoproliferative disorder that cannot be differentiated from MF on the basis of dominant clonality alone (158,161,162).

Syringolymphoid Hyperplasia

This rare lymphoproliferative disorder presents with localized lesions exhibiting infiltration of eccrine units by small, cerebriform, monoclonal, $CD4^+$ lymphoid cells (7,163–165). There may also be involvement of hair follicles, without mucinosis, which can result in circumscribed alopecia.

Pagetoid Reticulosis

Also known as Woringer-Kolopp disease, pagetoid reticulosis consists of a clinically indolent, hyperkeratotic, or psoriasiform plaque localized to one body region, which contains an atypical lymphoid infiltrate of cerebriform or noncerebriform cells concentrated within the epidermis (166–168). Usually, there are only cytologically normal lymphocytes or no lymphocytes within the upper dermis (Fig. 32.9). Pagetoid reticulosis is a monoclonal T-cell lymphoproliferative disorder (167) and may contain predominantly $CD4^+$ or $CD8^+$ cells (166). CD30 may be expressed (169). Local treatment is usually curative, although disseminated relapse has occurred long after local therapy (170). It is considered by some to be a highly epidermotropic variant of MF that belongs to a continuum of unilesional, localized, and generalized presentations of this lymphoma (2,7,171,172), although others believe that its features are distinct enough to separate it from unilesional MF (168). A generalized dermatosis with lesions resembling pagetoid reticulosis was reported in the older literature as Ketron-Goodman syndrome, but these cases probably would be regarded now simply as MF with highly epidermotropic features. In support of this concept, transformation to $CD30^+$ anaplastic large T-cell lymphoma has been reported in a long-standing case with disseminated lesions (173). A $\gamma\delta$ T-cell phenotype has also been reported in a case with generalized lesions (174). Long-term survival is excellent, although some patients may develop local or distant recurrences, sometimes as typical MF (168).

Granulomatous Slack Skin

Granulomatous slack skin is a rare condition in which redundant skin folds develop in intertriginous areas such as the axillae and groin (7,175–177). Lesional skin contains a dense, diffuse dermal infiltrate of atypical lymphoid cells

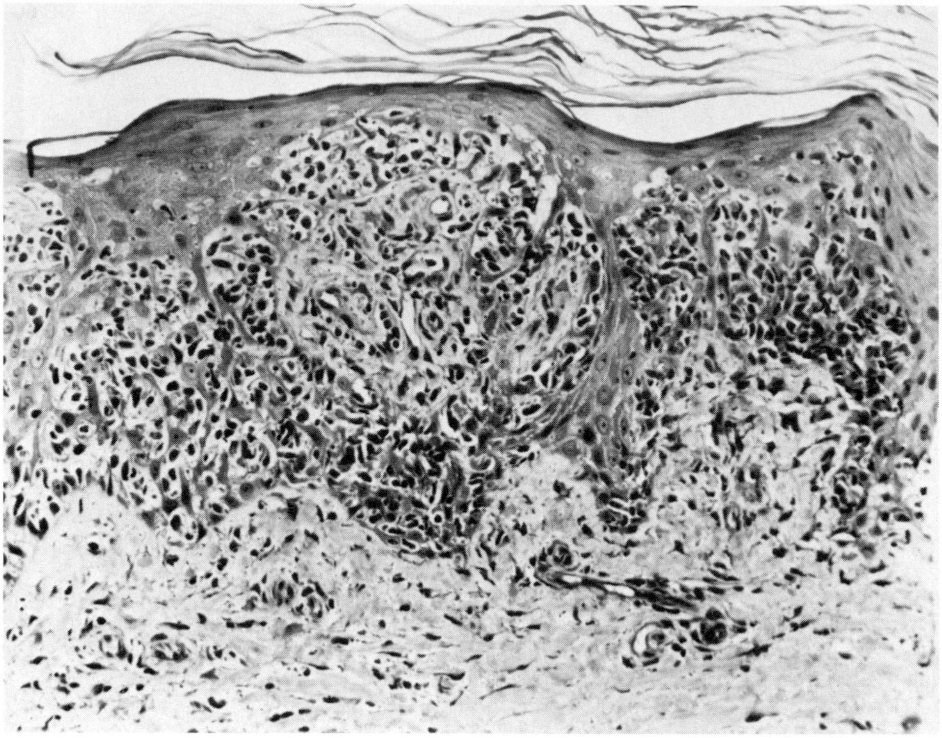

FIG. 32.9. Pagetoid reticulosis. The epidermis exhibits hyperkeratosis and irregular acanthosis. It is infiltrated by cytologically atypical mononuclear cells. The underlying dermis is largely uninvolved in this case. In others, it may contain a heavier mononuclear cell infiltrate, but these cells are usually not atypical (original magnification: 240× magnification).

similar to MF/SS cells. Atypical cells are also present singly and in small aggregates within the epidermis. Admixed with the dermal cells are scattered granulomatous tubercles, multinucleated giant cells, or both (Fig. 32.10). Elastic–van Gieson stains show nearly complete absence of elastic fibers within lesional dermis. Elastic fibers can be identified within the giant cells. Immunodiagnostic studies have demonstrated that granulomatous slack skin is a monoclonal T-cell lymphoproliferative disorder of $CD4^+$ cells (175,176). It is debatable whether granulomatous slack skin belongs within the spectrum of the rare granulomatous variants of MF/SS or represents a distinct cutaneous T-cell lymphoproliferative disorder (149), but as with MF/SS, there is an increased risk of Hodgkin's disease and non-Hodgkin's lymphomas (2,7,175,177). Granulomatous slack skin is readily distinguished from classic MF on clinical grounds. Histopathologically, the characteristic multinucleated giant cells facilitate the distinction of granulomatous slack skin from the diffuse dermal infiltrate seen in MF tumor nodules.

Juvenile Lymphogranulomatosis

Juvenile lymphogranulomatosis is a rare disorder. It manifests in children or young adults as poikilodermatous patches or nodules that may be localized or widespread (7). Histopathologically, there is a sarcoid granulomatous infiltrate composed of histiocytes, including epithelioid and sparse multinucleated forms, admixed with a minor component of small, mature, monoclonal T lymphocytes. Despite an initially indolent, slowly progressive clinical course that may last for years or decades, most patients die after developing nodal involvement by Hodgkin's disease or $CD30^+$ anaplastic large cell lymphoma. The differential diagnosis includes infectious and noninfectious granulomas and granulomatous lymphoproliferative disorders such as granulomatous slack skin and granulomatous MF. Juvenile lymphogranulomatosis lacks the pendulous skin folds and prominent multinucleated giant cells of granulomatous slack skin. It differs from typical cases of granulomatous MF in that the lymphocytic rather than the granulomatous component predominates in MF; nevertheless, this entity may ultimately prove to be an early-onset, granulomatous variant of MF.

Histopathologic Differential Diagnosis of Mycosis Fungoides or Sezary Syndrome

Early Mycosis Fungoides Versus Other Diseases

An important problem in the histopathologic recognition of MF is the lack of uniformly accepted minimal criteria for diagnosis. As a result, the threshold for the diagnosis of MF varies considerably among pathologists. Fortunately, in most cases, this problem can be overcome eventually by clinicopathologic correlation, repeated skin biopsies, biopsies of

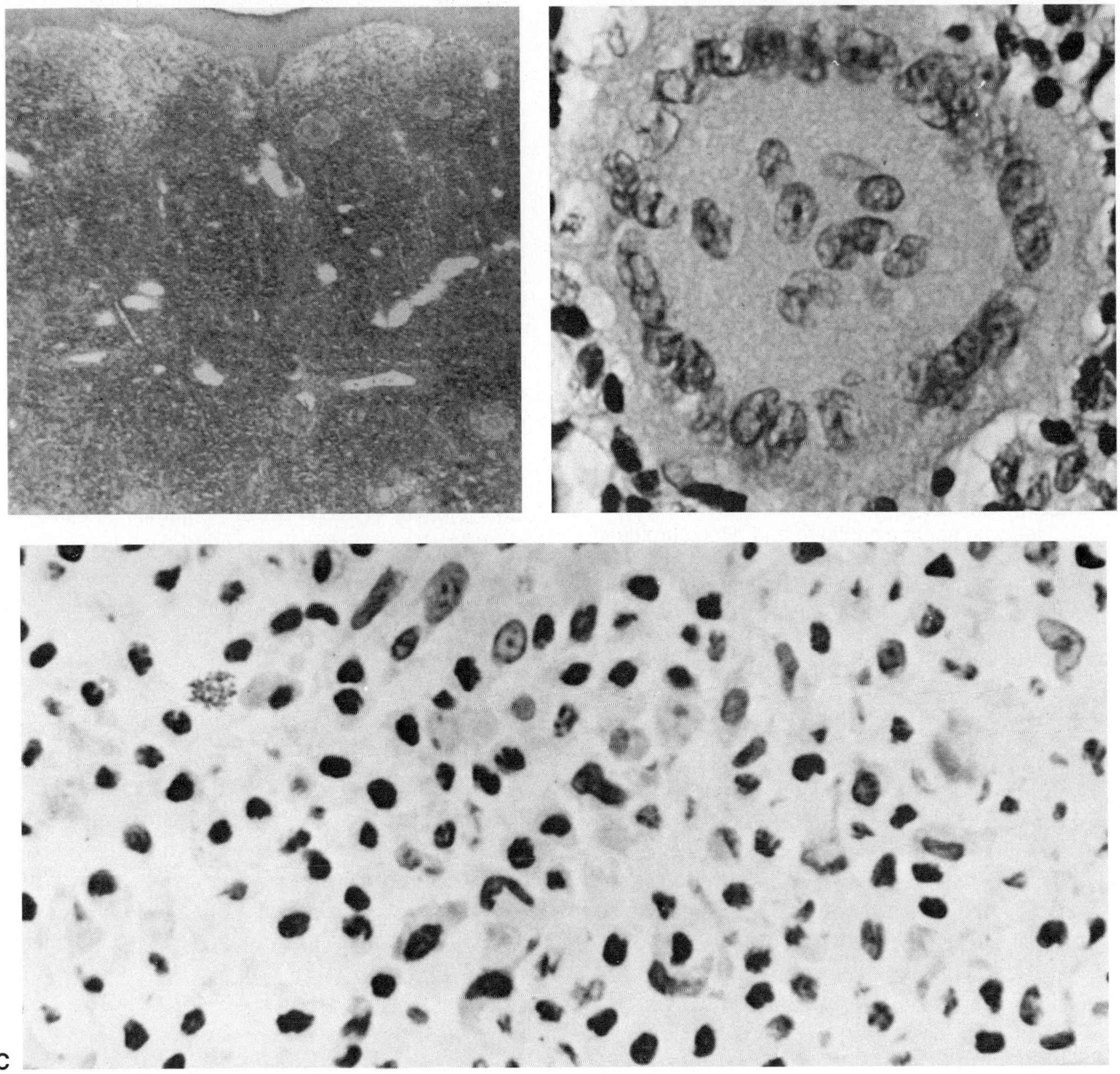

A

B

C

FIG. 32.10. Granulomatous slack skin. **A:** The dense, diffuse, superficial and deep dermal mononuclear cell infiltrate contains scattered multinucleated giant cells. The epidermis is typically involved at least to a minor degree (original magnification: 50× magnification). **B:** Higher magnification illustrates the cytologic features of the multinucleated giant cells and surrounding lymphoid cells (original magnification: 480× magnification). **C:** The dermal infiltrate is composed predominantly of small to medium lymphoid cells with hyperchromatic, irregular nuclei similar to those seen in mycosis fungoides (original magnification: 480× magnification).

other involved tissues, immunopathologic studies, and molecular biologic analysis. One set of histopathologic criteria that can be used to evaluate lesional skin biopsies from patients suspected clinically of having MF was developed at Stanford University and is listed in Table 32.8. These criteria allow skin biopsies to be classified into five categories based on histopathologic features alone. These include ''diagnostic of,'' ''consistent with,'' and ''suggestive of'' MF, as well as two other implicit categories: a mild, nonspecific spongiotic, psoriasiform, or interface dermatitis and a specific diagnosis other than MF. Patients with clinical features compatible with early MF whose skin biopsies are classified as ''diagnostic of'' MF (Figs. 32.2–32.4) or ''consistent with'' MF (Fig. 32.11) are diagnosed as having MF. Those whose skin biopsies are ''suggestive of'' MF (Fig. 32.12) or nonspecific are generally diagnosed as having ''large plaque parapsoriasis'' and periodically rebiopsied to monitor for the development of more overt MF. Other histologic criteria have also been developed to facilitate the differential diagnosis of MF (103,178–181), but no single set of criteria have gained widespread acceptance.

The most common challenge in the histopathologic diagnosis of MF is the distinction of early lesions (i.e., patches or thin plaques) from inflammatory dermatoses showing

TABLE 32.8. *Histopathologic criteria for the diagnosis of mycosis fungoides*

1. Multiple Pautrier microaggregates
2. Diffuse infiltration of many individual atypical lymphocytes[a] into the epidermis[b]
3. A few small intraepidermal clusters of a few atypical lymphocytes
4. A few individual intraepidermal atypical lymphocytes
5. Dense upper dermal bandlike interface infiltrate that includes atypical lymphocytes
6. Mild to moderate polymorphous upper dermal infiltrate that includes atypical lymphocytes and has a focal interface pattern
7. Extension of the infiltrate into the deep dermis

Categories diagnostic of MF: 1, 2, 3 + 4 + 5, 3 + 4 + 6 + 7

Categories consistent with MF: 3 + 5, 3 + 6, 4 + 5, 4 + 6 + 7

Categories suggestive of MF: 3, 4, 5, 6

MF, mycosis fungoides.

[a] Lymphocytes with scant cytoplasm and hyperchromatic, convoluted (cerebriform) nuclei. Cell size may vary.

[b] Epidermal involvement is characteristically not associated with prominent intercellular edema (spongiosis).

Based on the criteria of Alvin J. Cox, M.D., former Professor Emeritus of Dermatology and Pathology, Stanford University.

spongiotic, psoriasiform, or interface dermatitis histopathologically (Table 32.9). A variety of cutaneous lymphoid infiltrates can mimic early and more advanced forms of MF/SS. These include pseudo-T-cell lymphomas with bandlike infiltrates, lichenoid drug eruptions, poikilodermas, secondary syphilis, small and large plaque parapsoriasis, clonal dermatitis, lymphomatoid contact dermatitis, and actinic reticuloid.

Pseudo-T-Cell Lymphomas

Pseudolymphomas exhibiting a bandlike or MF/SS-like histopathologic appearance may occur *de novo* or in association with B-cell CLL, the eruption of lymphocyte recovery after iatrogenic bone marrow aplasia, or various drugs such as anticonvulsants and antihistamines (182–188). Typically, lesions manifest as one or a few cutaneous plaques, although a larger number of plaques or a Sezary-like syndrome occurs occasionally. The epidermis may be acanthotic and may contain an atypical lymphoid infiltrate. Compared with MF, epidermotropism is usually much less extensive, and Pautrier microabscess-like aggregates of lymphoid cells are uncommon. The upper dermis contains a bandlike interface infiltrate that obscures the dermoepidermal junction. There is no Grenz zone of subepidermal sparing. The lymphoid cells are small and medium sized, and their nuclei may exhibit clefted or cerebriform contours. Eosinophils and plasma cells are generally rare, although histiocytes may be seen in moderate numbers. One variant with a more prominent histiocytic component reminiscent of granuloma annulare has been called *interstitial granulomatous drug reaction* (188). These cases contain a diffuse dermal lymphohistiocytic, granulomatous infiltrate including histiocytic giant cells, fragmentation of collagen and elastic fibers, and variable mucin deposition. Most of these cases also exhibit a vacuolar interface dermatitis, sometimes with Sezary cell–like atypia and epidermotropism of lymphoid cells. The clinical and histopathologic differential diagnosis of all these pseudo-MF/SS reaction patterns from true MF/SS relies on the tendency toward a small number of lesions, minimal epidermotropism in most instances, and resolution after drug

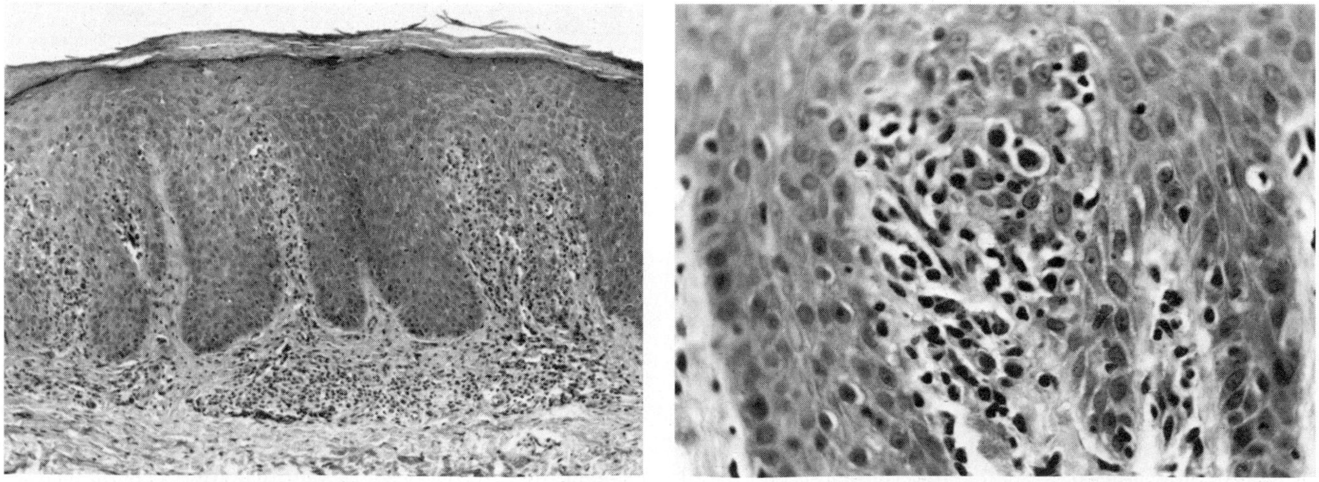

A B

FIG. 32.11. Differential diagnosis of mycosis fungoides (MF): features that are "consistent with MF." **A:** There is a moderate upper dermal mononuclear cell infiltrate with a focal interface pattern and epidermal involvement (original magnification: 120× magnification). **B:** The infiltrate is lymphocytic and contains several cells with hyperchromatic, irregular nuclei that form a few small groups within a nonspongiotic epidermis (original magnification: 480× magnification). This biopsy specimen was obtained from a patient with prior biopsies that were "diagnostic of MF." Compare with Figures 32.2, 32.3, 32.4, and 32.12.

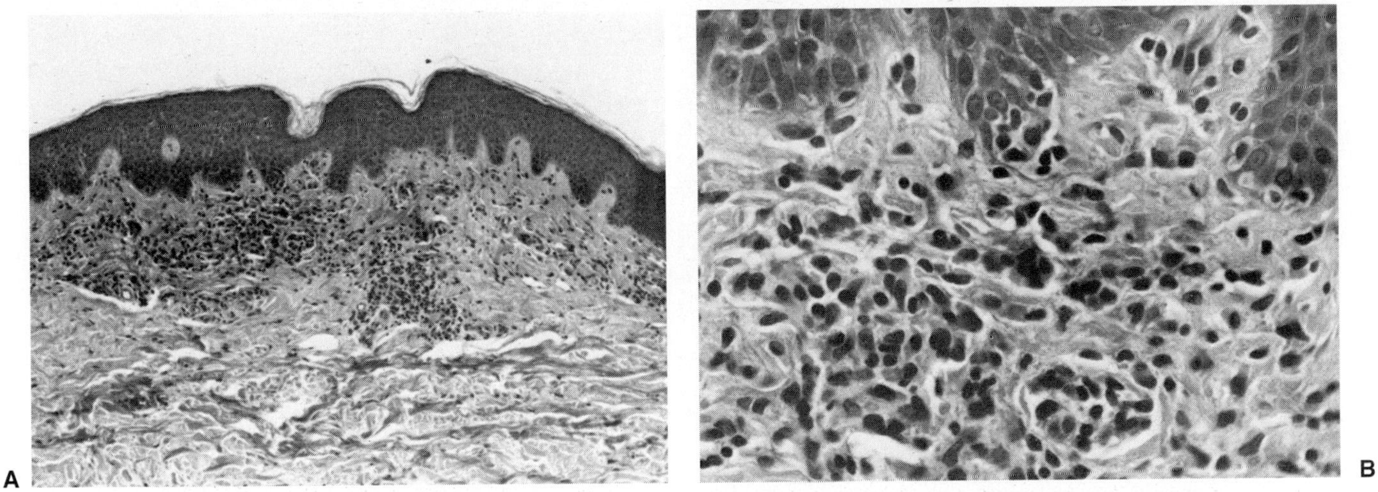

FIG. 32.12. Differential diagnosis of mycosis fungoides (MF): features that are "suggestive of MF." **A:** There is a mild to moderate upper dermal mononuclear cell infiltrate (original magnification: 120× magnification). **B:** The infiltrate is lymphocytic and contains some cells with hyperchromatic, irregular nuclei that very focally invade the basal region of a nonspongiotic epidermis (original magnification: 480× magnification). This biopsy specimen was obtained from a patient with prior biopsies that were "diagnostic of MF." Compare with Figures 32.2, 32.3, 32.4, and 32.11.

discontinuation or local treatment with topical corticosteroids or excision.

Classic Lichenoid Drug Eruptions

Classic lichenoid drug eruptions are reactions that can be produced by agents such as antimalarials, thiazides, and gold (Fig. 32.13). They can mimic atrophic forms of large plaque parapsoriasis or MF when they produce lesions with an atrophic epidermis overlying a bandlike lichenoid lymphoid infiltrate that may also contain eosinophils and plasma cells. In contrast to MF, these lesions have the clinical features of typical lichenoid drug rashes, lack cytologic atypia within their lymphoid infiltrates, and eventually resolve after the offending drug is stopped, although this may require several months.

TABLE 32.9. *Selected types of dermatitis sometimes considered in the histopathologic differential diagnosis of early mycosis fungoides and Sezary syndrome*

Spongiotic dermatitis
Large plaque parapsoriasis
Some drug eruptions
Allergic contact dermatitis
Gianotti-Crosti syndrome
Nummular dermatitis
Small plaque parapsoriasis
Pityriasis rosea
Psoriasiform dermatitis
Chronic spongiotic dermatitis
Lichen simplex chronicus
Psoriasis
Interface dermatitis
Large plaque parapsoriasis
Erythema dyschromicum perstans
Actinic reticuloid
Some drug eruptions
Collagen vascular poikiloderma
Secondary lues
Lichen planus
Lichen striatus
Lichenoid and granulomatous dermatitis of acquired immunodeficiency syndrome (AIDS)

Poikiloderma

The poikiloderma lesion is characterized clinically by cutaneous atrophy, telangiectasia, and mottled hyperpigmentation and hypopigmentation. The histopathologic correlates include epidermal thinning, dilated papillary dermal blood vessels, and pigment incontinence. In addition to MF and large plaque parapsoriasis, poikiloderma can be caused by collagen vascular diseases, certain genodermatoses and ionizing radiation. Poikiloderma related to collagen vascular diseases or genodermatoses differs from MF in its associated clinical and laboratory features, less intense lymphoid infiltration, and lack of lymphoid atypia. The collagen vascular disorders can exhibit dermal mucin, thickening of the epidermal basement membrane, immune deposits and characteristic epidermal alterations such as vacuolar degeneration, and follicular plugging. Chronic radiodermatitis may resemble MF clinically but exhibits many distinguishing features, including the relevant clinical history, sparsity of lymphoid infiltration, cytologic atypia of keratinocytes and fibroblasts, dermal fibrosis, and loss of adnexal structures.

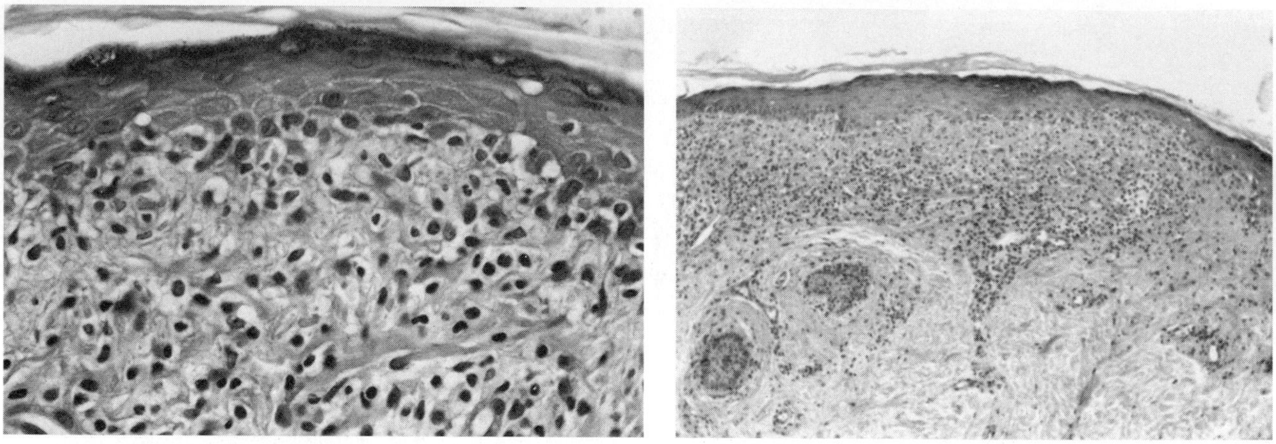

A B

FIG. 32.13. Differential diagnosis of mycosis fungoides (MF): lichenoid drug eruption. **A:** There is a bandlike upper dermal mononuclear cell infiltrate that obscures the dermoepidermal junction and invades the epidermis, which is focally atrophic. These features are also typical of atrophic MF and atrophic large plaque parapsoriasis (original magnification: 120× magnification). **B:** Higher magnification shows an interface infiltrate with vacuolar degeneration of the basal epidermis and epidermal atrophy. Although these features can be seen in MF, this infiltrate lacks the nuclear atypia characteristic of MF cells (original magnification: 480× magnification). Compare with Figure 32.3. These lesions showed the clinical features of a lichenoid drug eruption and occurred in a patient with rheumatoid arthritis after the institution of gold therapy.

Secondary Syphilis

Lues can mimic MF histopathologically when its lesions contain a dense, bandlike, interface lymphoid infiltrate that invades a nonspongiotic epidermis (Fig. 32.14). In contrast to MF, the infiltrate lacks atypia, has more plasma cells and fewer lymphocytes, and may contain epidermal neutrophils. Secondary syphilis typically exhibits perivascular infiltration of the deep dermis. This is uncommon in MF, except in the tumor phase. Clinically, the differential diagnosis is aided by the history, appearance of the lesions, positive serology, and response to antibiotic therapy.

Large Plaque Parapsoriasis

Patients with large plaque parapsoriasis (LPP) exhibit slightly scaly, variably erythematous patches, with or without poikiloderma, that clinically resemble patches of MF (72,146). The term *plaque* is somewhat misleading in this

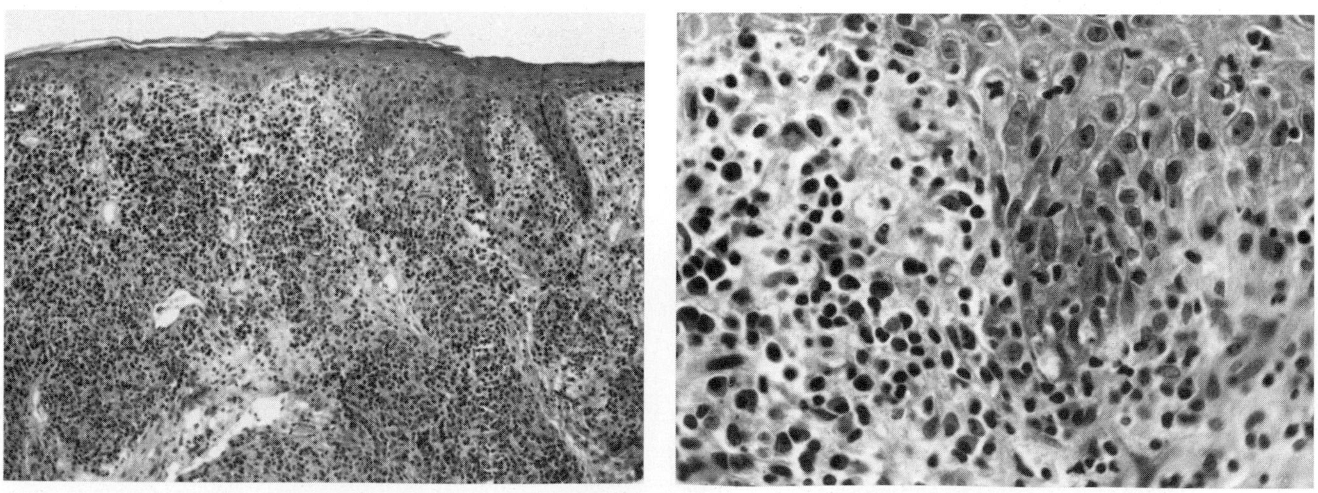

A B

FIG. 32.14. Differential diagnosis of mycosis fungoides (MF): secondary lues. **A:** There is a dense upper dermal mononuclear cell infiltrate that focally invades a nonspongiotic epidermis. This pattern mimics MF. The infiltrate also extensively involves the lower dermis in a perivascular pattern (not shown). This is unusual for MF except in tumor lesions (original magnification: 120× magnification). **B:** Higher magnification shows that the infiltrate contains more plasma cells than expected in MF and that the lymphocytes lack the nuclear atypia characteristic of MF cells (original magnification: 480× magnification). Compare with Figure 32.3. Serologic studies revealed a positive RPR titer of 1:512.

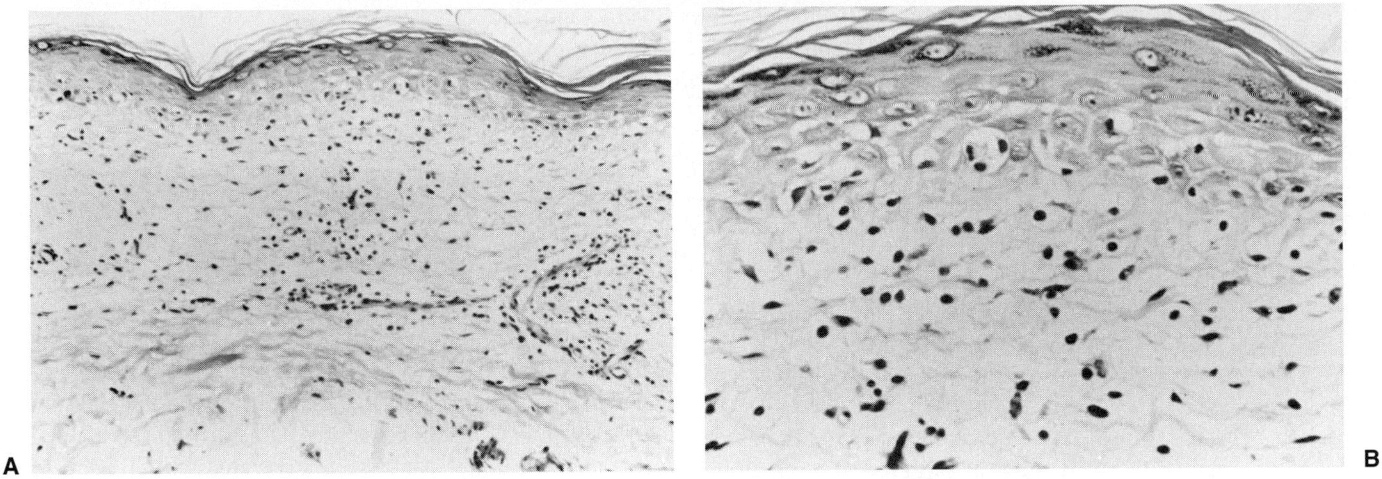

FIG. 32.15. Differential diagnosis of mycosis fungoides (MF): atrophic large plaque parapsoriasis. **A:** A mild upper dermal mononuclear cell infiltrate with an interface component invades the overlying, atrophic, nonspongiotic epidermis (original magnification: 100× magnification). **B:** Higher magnification shows that the infiltrate is lymphocytic and lacks the nuclear atypia characteristic of MF cells (original magnification: 400× magnification). Although the infiltrate in this biopsy is much less than that seen in the lichenoid drug eruption (Fig. 32.13), this patient eventually progressed from atrophic large plaque parapsoriasis to overt MF.

context because it is derived from the French terminology of Brocq in which plaque actually means ''patch'' in English (i.e., a flat rather than elevated or infiltrated lesion) (73). LPP is best regarded as an evolving or precursor form of early patch-phase MF (189) with the histopathologic features of a nonspecific mild spongiotic or interface dermatitis with a predominance of $CD4^+$ T cells (Fig. 32.15). Approximately 10% of LPP patients progress to overt MF over a 10-year period (72), and many lesions that satisfy the criteria for LPP have been shown to harbor dominant T-cell clones by PCR-based analysis of TCR gene rearrangements (13,73). Periodic reevaluation of LPP patients is indicated for the early detection of disease progression.

Small Plaque Parapsoriasis

Small plaque parapsoriasis (SPP) patients have small (<5 cm) patches that are slightly scaly and pink to yellowish (73). When they are arranged along the flanks in parallel arrays, they are known as *digitate dermatosis*. This variant has lesions that are narrow such as finger marks but often much longer than 5 cm. As with LPP, these lesions are flat patches rather than elevated or infiltrated plaques. Dominant T-cell clonality has been detected in most cases tested but often requires the enhanced sensitivity of PCR-based methods (190). Histopathologically, lesions show only mild, spongiotic dermatitis composed predominantly of $CD4^+$ T cells. Lesions may persist indefinitely or gradually resolve, spontaneously or in response to treatment. In contrast to LPP, SPP rarely progresses to MF. Although there are those who consider SPP to be an early form of MF, its nonspecific histology and lack of progression to overt lymphoma are distinguishing features. There are some clonal cutaneous T-cell lymphoproliferative disorders that characteristically fail to progress to recognizable lymphomas. The term *abortive lymphomas* has been used to refer to them, and SPP has been included in this group (7).

Clonal Dermatitis

The term *clonal dermatitis* was coined to refer to cases of clinically and histopathologically nonspecific cutaneous T-cell infiltrates that exhibit dominant T-cell clonality (13). Most of these are chronic, eczematous eruptions that respond poorly to treatment and have the histopathologic features of mild to moderately intense chronic spongiotic dermatitis. Some cases have progressed to overt MF within only a few months to years of observation (73,102,191). Those amenable to serial analysis have shown the same dominant clone in the clonal dermatitis and MF, indicating that clonal dermatitis can be a direct precursor to T-cell lymphoma of the skin. Clonal dermatitis has also been used to refer to that stage in the evolution of several skin disorders where a detectable, dominant T-cell clone has developed but the histologic features are not yet those of lymphoma. In this context, clonal dermatitis can be viewed as a transitional phase in the evolution of those cases of LPP, follicular mucinosis, and chronic eczema that are destined to develop into overt MF (73).

Lymphomatoid Contact Dermatitis

Lymphomatoid contact dermatitis presents clinically as generalized, pruritic, erythematous, scaly papules and plaques that may coalesce into erythroderma (192). It is essentially a persistent form of allergic contact dermatitis.

Patch tests for various common allergens (e.g., ethylenediamine dihydrochloride) may be positive. Histopathologically, lymphomatoid contact dermatitis can mimic MF/SS because lesions contain an epidermotropic, atypical lymphoid infiltrate composed of cells cytologically similar to small and medium-sized MF cells. Nevertheless, lymphomatoid contact dermatitis is a spongiotic simulant of MF (193); the intraepidermal atypical lymphoid cells are associated with significant intercellular edema between keratinocytes. There is frequently edema of the papillary dermis. These features argue against a diagnosis of MF that classically shows no edema, but the distinction may be challenging based on histologic grounds alone, because some cases of proven MF do exhibit a variable degree of superimposed spongiotic dermatitis. In lymphomatoid contact dermatitis, there is less tendency for the intraepidermal lymphoid cells to form cell aggregates than in MF. The clinical history, patch test results, and eventual resolution of lesions after avoidance of relevant allergens facilitate the differential diagnosis. Immunopathologic studies have shown lymphomatoid contact dermatitis to be a T-cell disorder. There have been rare cases in which lymphoma is said to have evolved from lymphomatoid contact dermatitis, but there is concern that these cases were lymphomas from the outset.

Actinic Reticuloid

The term *actinic reticuloid* refers to the severe end of the spectrum of chronic photosensitivity dermatitis that tends to affect older men; begins on sun-exposed skin as pruritic, lichenified papules and plaques that may be associated with a leonine facies and alopecia; may eventually generalize to erythroderma; and may bear a close clinicopathologic resemblance to MF/SS (157,194–197). Generalized lymphadenopathy is common. There is sensitivity to ultraviolet light and sometimes also to visible light, the minimal erythema dose level is reduced, and it may be possible to document photoallergic contact dermatitis to a variety of agents including compositae plants and fragrances. The histopathologic features are classically those of lichen simplex chronicus superimposed on chronic photoallergic contact dermatitis. Lesional skin exhibits an upper dermal lymphohistiocytic infiltrate that may be bandlike and contains plasma cells, eosinophils, mast cells, large stellate fibroblasts, and a variable number of atypical lymphoid cells (Fig. 32.16). There are often features of lichenification, including hyperkeratosis, focal hypergranulosis, acanthosis, and papillary dermal fibrosis. Parakeratosis may also be observed. The epidermis may be invaded by the subjacent cellular infiltrate, usually as single cells. In some cases, Pautrier-like microabscesses have been described resembling those seen in MF/SS. Sezary-like lymphocytes are also found in the peripheral blood of many patients, but in contrast to MF/SS cells that are generally $CD4^+$, there is a predominance of $CD8^+$ cells in the lesional skin and blood of most cases of actinic reticuloid (194,198,199).

Skin lesions have been reported to contain IgE^+ Langerhans cells in association with elevated serum IgE (194). Cytogenetic studies in a few patients have not shown evidence of clonality. Although a small percentage of metaphases exhibited karyotypic abnormalities, none was consistently present (194). Similarly, gene rearrangement analyses have shown actinic reticuloid to be a polyclonal T-cell disorder (200,201). The polyclonality, $CD8^+$ T-cell predominance and the photosensitivity help to distinguish actinic reticuloid from MF/SS. Actinic reticuloid may improve or persist indefinitely. Total avoidance of ultraviolet and sometimes visible light can be helpful but is difficult to maintain. Actinic reticuloid has not been associated with the development of overt lymphoma except in rare cases that may have been lymphomas from the beginning (157,196,202).

In addition to the diseases already mentioned, certain other entities pose special problems for the differential diagnosis of MF/SS. These disorders include tumor d'emblée MF and the transformation of MF into large cell lymphoma.

Tumor d'Emblée Mycosis Fungoides

Sometimes, it may be difficult to distinguish tumor lesions of MF from other cutaneous PTLs. In general, this is not a problem because MF tumor lesions are usually preceded or accompanied by typical patches and plaques, but cutaneous tumors are the initial skin lesions in some patients with CTCLs (55,57,60). Although this has been referred to as the tumor d'emblée form of MF in the past, this term should be abandoned. Cases not meeting all the criteria for MF are best regarded as non-MF cutaneous PTLs. They should be classified according to the REAL or EORTC terminology or other schemes designed specifically for T-cell lymphomas (1,2,203) (see Chapters 19 and 29). These cases are usually large T-cell lymphomas (with or without CD30), or pleomorphic small to medium-sized T-cell lymphomas.

Large Cell Transformation of Mycosis Fungoides

One factor that obscures the distinction between MF and other CTCLs is the transformation of typical MF into a cytologically distinct form of large cell lymphoma (57,58,66–69) (Fig. 32.8) (see Chapters 19 and 29). In general, lesions are defined as transformed if large cell lymphoma cells form microscopic nodules or exceed 25% of the total infiltrate. Roughly 50% of these tumors are $CD30^+$ large cell PTLs, and the remainder are $CD30^-$ large cell PTLs (1,2,68). Unlike the favorable clinical course of primary cutaneous $CD30^+$ anaplastic large T-cell lymphomas, transformation suggests a poor prognosis. Median survivals of only 1 to 2 years have been reported (68,69). In one series (68), patients with transformation confined to the skin had a slightly longer

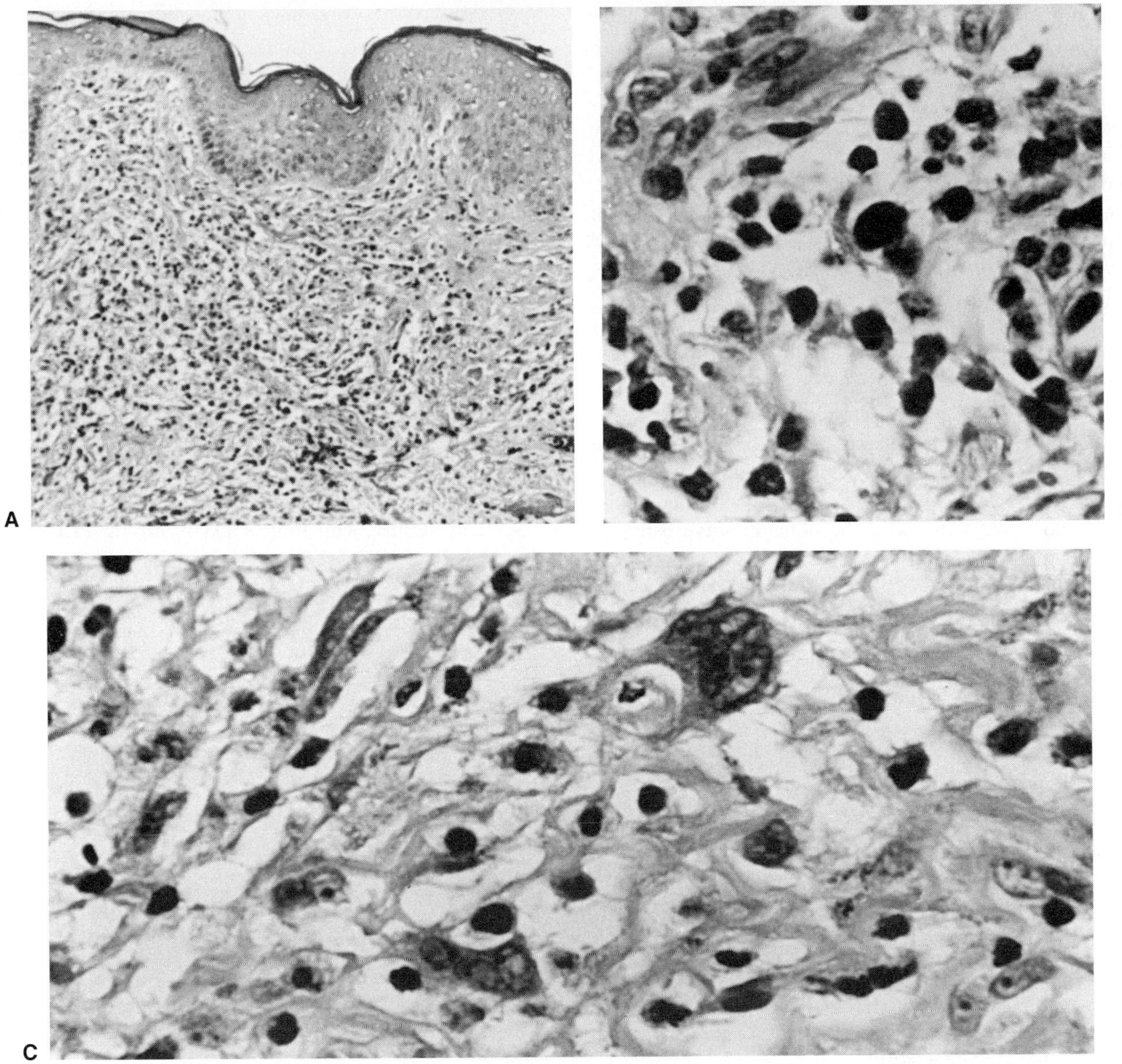

FIG. 32.16. Differential diagnosis of mycosis fungoides: actinic reticuloid. **A:** There is a band-like mononuclear cell infiltrate in the upper dermis. Although epidermal involvement is minimal in this field, it may be prominent (original magnification: 120× magnification). **B:** Higher magnification reveals a predominantly lymphoid infiltrate often containing some cells with atypical nuclei as shown here (original magnification: 480× magnification). **C:** There are also scattered large, multinucleated fibroblasts with irregular or stellate contours (original magnification: 480× magnification).

median survival than those with transformation in extracutaneous sites.

In most cases, the original MF appears to be clonally related to the transformed lymphoma. For example, in one patient, the same TCR-β gene rearrangement was detectable in plaques of MF and nodules of $CD30^+$ large cell lymphoma obtained 4 years apart (204). One retrospective study suggested that CD25 expression by MF/SS tumor cells may be associated with subsequent large cell transformation (205). Another study of serial biopsies showed p53 overexpression without *TP53* mutation in large cell transformation but not in preexisting MF/SS lesions from the same patients (206). Others have reported mutation of the *TP53* gene in several cases of tumor stage and transformed MF (143).

PRIMARY CUTANEOUS NON–MYCOSIS FUNGOIDES T-CELL LYMPHOPROLIFERATIVE DISORDERS

Pityriasis Lichenoides and Lymphomatoid Papulosis

The term *pityriasis lichenoides* encompasses two disorders: *pityriasis lichenoides chronica* (PLC) and *pityriasis lichenoides et varioliformis acuta* (PLEVA), also known as *Mucha-Habermann disease*. These conditions are generally regarded as two ends of a clinicopathologic spectrum of disease (157,207–209). This view is supported by two key clinical observations. First, some patients have lesions that are clinicopathologically intermediate between classic PLC and PLEVA. Second, some patients develop PLC and PLEVA lesions serially or concurrently. There is controversy about whether lymphomatoid papulosis (LYP) is a variant of PLEVA (208,209) or a separate disease (210,211); however, individual patients have been described who exhibit lesions of PLEVA and LYP concurrently or serially (209). This strongly suggests that LYP belongs within the PLC-PLEVA spectrum (157,212). There is also controversy about whether LYP should be regarded as a lymphoma outright or considered to be the clinically benign end of another continuum with primary cutaneous $CD30^+$ anaplastic large T-cell lymphoma at its extreme. Although these disorders share many features and intergrades exist, the nonaggressive behavior of most cases of LYP argues against its classification as an overt lymphoma.

Pityriasis Lichenoides

Patients with PLC exhibit slightly erythematous, scaly papules on the trunk and extremities. Individual lesions can persist indefinitely but usually resolve gradually, sometimes leaving hypopigmented macules. Unlike the indolent PLC, PLEVA presents with recurrent generalized crops of papules that become vesicles, pustules, or crusts, resolve within several weeks, and can leave residual varioliform scars (Fig. 32.17). The entire disorder can remit spontaneously or persist indefinitely. Neither PLC nor PLEVA is associated with CTCLs except in rare instances (213). PLC and PLEVA lesions contain a superficial perivascular and interface lymphocytic infiltrate that involves the epidermis (Fig. 32.18). The infiltrate is denser in PLEVA, where it extends deeper into the dermis, tapering to form a V-shaped pattern. Lymphocytic ''vasculitis'' has been noted in some studies, but true fibrinoid destruction of blood vessels is not usually prominent. The principal manifestation of vascular injury is erythrocyte extravasation. The epidermis is parakeratotic in PLC. In early PLEVA lesions, the epidermis may be normal, but as the lesions evolve, the epidermis becomes edematous or necrotic with eventual crust, vesicle, or pustule formation.

PLC and PLEVA lesions contain mixed $CD4^+$ and $CD8^+$ T-cell infiltrates, with more $CD8^+$ cells in PLEVA than in PLC (208,209,213,214). Molecular biologic studies have demonstrated T-cell monoclonality in three of three PLEVA cases (50). The more sparsely infiltrated lesions of PLC are more difficult to analyze, but PCR/DGGE has shown one of two cases to have detectable dominant clonality (215). PLC and PLEVA can usually be differentiated from MF/SS on the basis of clinical features, the circumscribed histopathologic configuration of the lesional infiltrate, and the presence of extravasated erythrocytes. PLEVA exhibits exten-

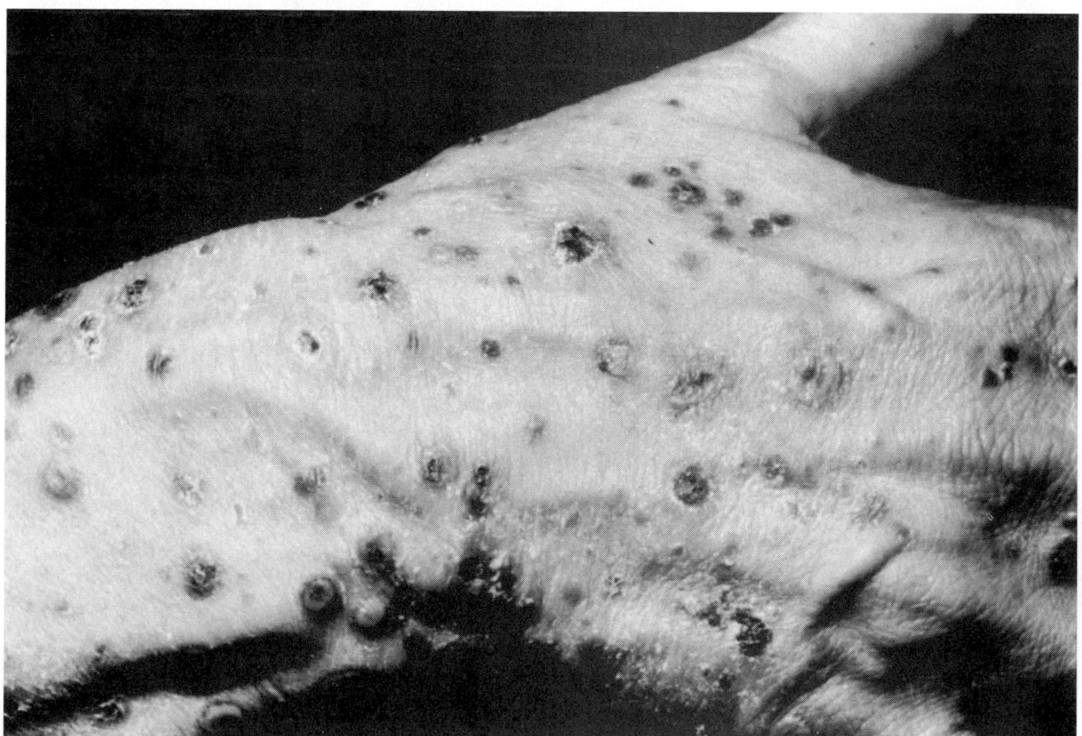

FIG. 32.17. Pityriasis lichenoides et varioliformis acuta. Lesions of different ages are characteristically present concurrently. They evolve from erythematous papules to vesicopustules to crusted papules and finally resolve with or without varioliform scars. Lymphomatoid papulosis may have a similar clinical appearance.

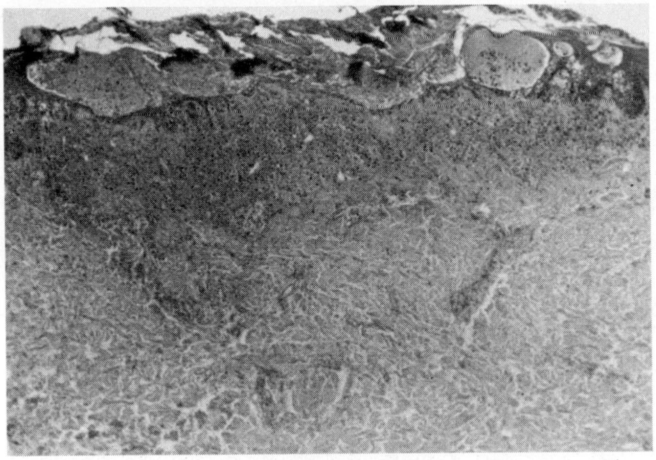

FIG. 32.18. Lymphomatoid papulosis. There is a wedge-shaped mononuclear cell infiltrate associated with invasion and destruction of the overlying epidermis. A similar architectural pattern is seen in pityriasis lichenoides et varioliformis acuta (original magnification: 70× magnification).

sive epidermal destruction. Cytologically atypical lymphocytes are absent in PLC. Some authorities allow a small percentage of such cells in PLEVA (207,209) while others consider these cases to be lymphomatoid papulosis (157).

Lymphomatoid Papulosis

LYP can mimic PLEVA clinically or can present with crops of papules that regress spontaneously without developing into vesicles, pustules, or crusts (29,157,207,209,216) (Fig. 32.17). The number of papules can vary from one to hundreds. Nodules or plaques can be admixed and occasionally predominant. The various stages of LYP lesions resemble those of PLEVA histopathologically (Fig. 32.18) except that LYP lesions contain a variable, often high percentage of large atypical lymphoid cells classified as type A or type B (217) (Figs. 32.19, 32.20). Type A cells resemble Reed-Sternberg cells and their mononuclear variants. Type B cells resemble the larger variants of MF/SS cells containing hyperchromatic, convoluted nuclei. Individual patients can have type A and type B cells in various lesions. A type C LYP lesion has been described in which there are sheets or clusters of type A cells, raising concern for $CD30^+$ anaplastic large T-cell lymphoma (2). There is a follicular variant of LYP in which mixed type A and B infiltrates surround the remnants of hair follicles (218).

Two distinctive immunopathologic features of LYP have been described. In the first, the type A large atypical cells are $CD30^+$ like the Reed-Sternberg cells of Hodgkin's disease. In the second, type A and B cells often show abnormal patterns of T-cell antigen expression analogous to T-cell lymphomas (29,219–224). Results for CD15 and epithelial membrane antigen (EMA) are usually negative. Type A LYP expresses a T_H2 cytokine pattern (i.e., IL-4, IL-5, and IL-10) (225). Molecular biologic studies have demonstrated monoclonal T-cell populations in most cases of LYP (216,226–229). The t(2;5)(p23;q35) translocation, which is present in about half of nodal $CD30^+$ anaplastic large T-cell lymphomas, is rarely found in LYP (2,230,231).

The clinical presentation of spontaneously resolving crops of papules, together with the mixed nature of the cellular

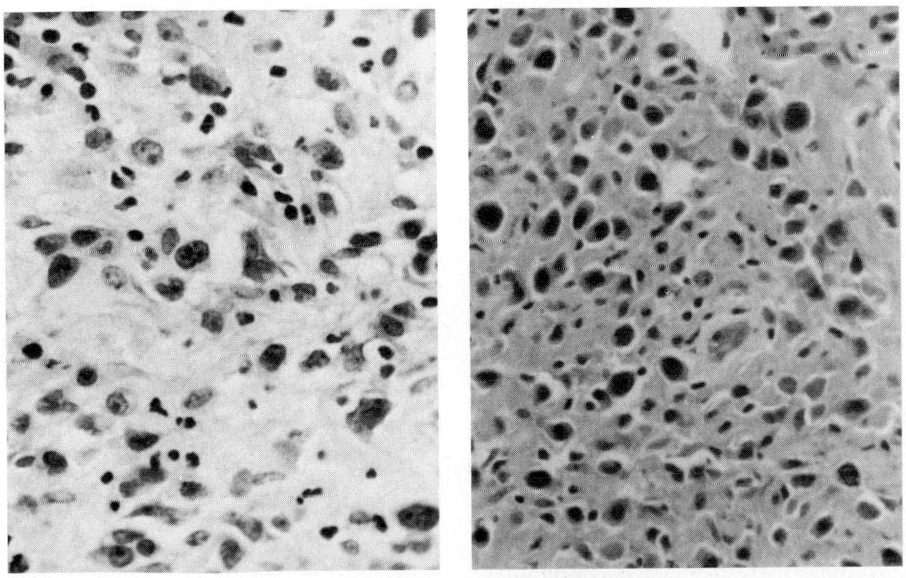

FIG. 32.19. Lymphomatoid papulosis. **A:** This polymorphous infiltrate contains several large atypical lymphoid cells with prominent nucleoli. These are the so-called type A cells. Similar cells can also be seen in Hodgkin's disease and pseudo-Hodgkin's disease (see Fig. 32.20) (original magnification: 480× magnification). **B:** This infiltrate contains several large atypical lymphoid cells with dense, irregular, hyperchromatic nuclei similar to those seen in mycosis fungoides. These are the so-called type B cells (original magnification: 480× magnification).

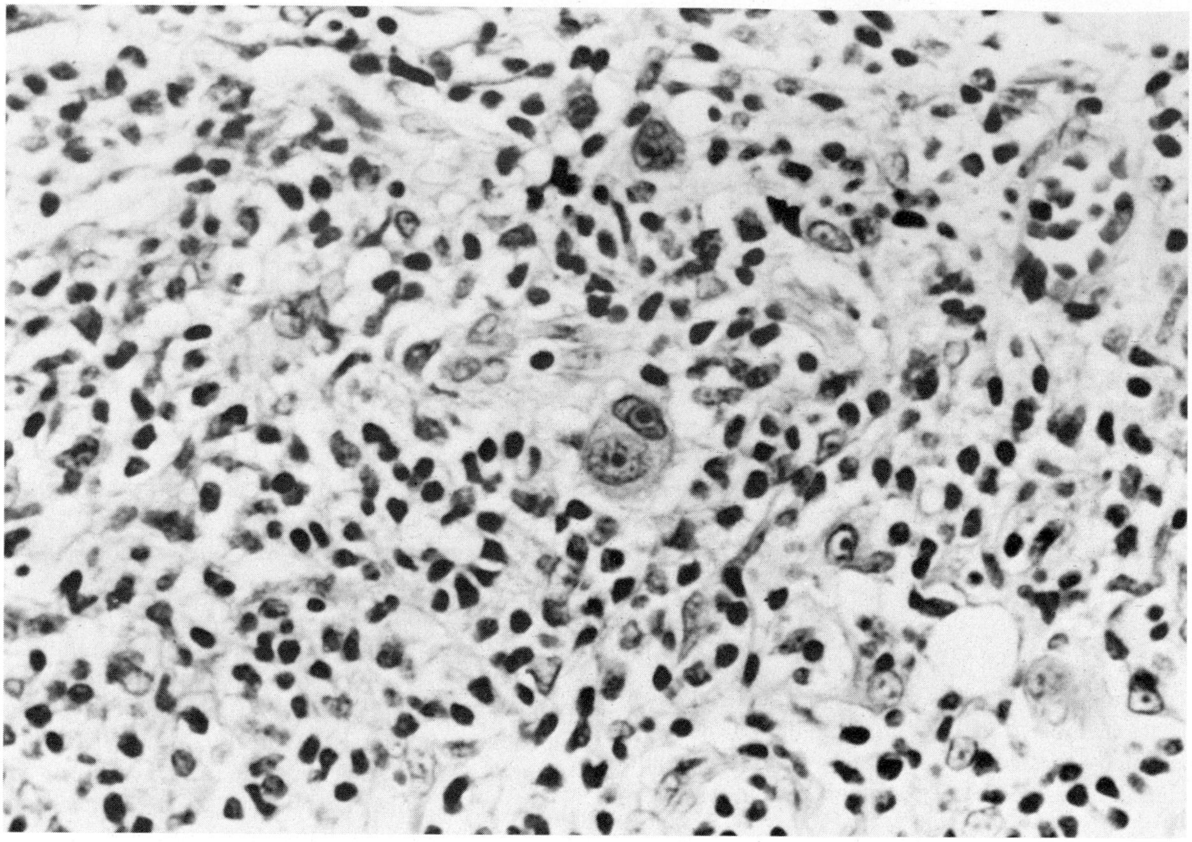

FIG. 32.20. Primary cutaneous Hodgkin's disease. This patient presented with a solitary nodule involving the arm. There was a dense dermal infiltrate composed predominantly of small lymphocytes. Shown here is a field containing scattered, large, atypical cells closely resembling Reed-Sternberg cells and their mononuclear variants. These cells also satisfy the cytologic criteria for the type A cells of lymphomatoid papulosis. The systemic workup for Hodgkin's disease was negative (original magnification: 480× magnification).

infiltrate, helps to distinguish type A LYP from primary cutaneous $CD30^+$ anaplastic large T-cell lymphoma. Nevertheless, intergrades exist with the clinical appearance of lymphoma (more persistent, nodular lesions) and the histology of LYP or *vice versa.* These are best regarded as cases in evolution along the LYP to $CD30^+$ lymphoma spectrum. The type B variant is the most difficult to distinguish from MF because the cytologic features and pattern of infiltration are similar. Nevertheless, all types of LYP can generally be recognized on the basis of clinical information, the circumscribed papular nature of the lesional infiltrate, extravasation of erythrocytes, and epidermal destruction. $CD30^+$ cells are present in type A and C LYP lesions but are absent or rare in typical MF/SS lesions.

Lymphoma, typically MF/SS, $CD30^+$ large T-cell lymphoma, or Hodgkin's disease, occurs in 10% to 20% of LYP patients (29,211,224,232). The lymphoma may precede, follow, or be concurrent with the LYP. Molecular biologic studies of patients with LYP and these associated lymphomas have generally shown identical dominant clonal TCR gene rearrangements in each type of lesion from individual cases (228,229,233). This evidence suggests that, in these individuals, the clinicopathologically distinct diseases arose as subclones of a common lymphoproliferative disorder. The underlying mechanism probably involves sequential somatic mutations of genes such as *TP53* and the type II TGF-β receptor that likely confer a survival or proliferative advantage to the newly mutated subclone (206,234,235).

The term *rhythmic paradoxical eruptions* has been proposed as an umbrella designation to include LYP and other spontaneously regressing yet histopathologically atypical cutaneous lymphoid infiltrates that lack the classic clinicopathologic features of LYP (236). Diseases satisfying these criteria include some that remain clinically benign and others that may progress to systemic involvement. The former group includes rare cases described as *lymphomatoid panniculitis* and possibly also those reported as *eosinophilic histiocytosis.* The latter group includes the early stages of some cutaneous large cell lymphomas (including so-called *regressing atypical histiocytosis*) and *primary cutaneous Hodgkin's disease.*

Lymphomatoid Panniculitis

Rarely, patients can present with tender, spontaneously regressing nodules centered in the subcutis that resemble

LYP or subcutaneous panniculitic T-cell lymphoma. The lesions may be few. My colleagues and I have seen a case associated with systemic lupus erythematosus, raising the possibility that this disorder may be an atypical presentation of lupus panniculitis. Lesions respond to low-dose prednisone and methotrexate. Unlike subcutaneous panniculitic T-cell lymphoma, they are clinically indolent. Progression to overt lymphoma or systemic involvement has not been observed within available follow-up of a few years (237).

Eosinophilic Histiocytosis

The term *eosinophilic histiocytosis* has been used to describe cases clinicopathologically similar to LYP except for an abundance of eosinophils and histiocytes (238). The histiocytes are S-100$^+$. The large atypical lymphoid cells have hyperchromatic nuclei and are CD45RO$^+$ but CD30$^-$ (239).

Regressing Atypical Histiocytosis

Regressing atypical histiocytosis manifests as a predominantly cutaneous proliferation of pleomorphic, large mononuclear cells (Fig. 32.21) that form skin nodules that may spontaneously regress, but the disease can eventually disseminate and prove fatal (240). Although initially suspected to exhibit ''histiocytic'' differentiation, this disorder is recognized to be the same as CD30$^+$ anaplastic large T-cell lymphoma on the basis of immunophenotyping and clonal rearrangement of TCR-β and TCR-γ genes (240) (see Chapter 51). This term should be used only for historical purposes.

Primary Cutaneous Hodgkin's Disease

Patients with this rare disorder develop one or a few clinically indolent cutaneous tumor nodules that may be ulcerated (179,210,241,242). Occasionally, the lesions may appear as plaques or papules. The overall potential of these lesions to regress spontaneously is unknown because they are often excised for diagnostic evaluation, but some cases have shown slow resolution, scarring, and recurrence. These lesions closely mimic Hodgkin's disease histopathologically (Fig. 32.20), but in contrast to the also rare secondary cutaneous involvement by nodal Hodgkin's disease, systemic workup is negative. Development of nodal involvement is possible, even years after therapy. This same condition has also been referred to as pseudo-Hodgkin's disease or as a variant of LYP.

CD30$^+$ Anaplastic Large T-Cell Lymphoma

This peripheral T-cell lymphoma is the most common form of non-MF primary CTCL. It exists on a continuum of CD30$^+$ cutaneous lymphoproliferative disorders with type A LYP at the clinically benign end. Clinical and histopathologic intergrades occur occasionally, making it impossible to definitively classify all cases. Because both disorders often respond well to treatment with low-dose oral methotrexate (243), this distinction becomes less important than correctly recognizing that a case belongs somewhere within this disease spectrum. Cases previously diagnosed as ''regressing atypical histiocytosis'' belong to this entity (Fig. 32.21). Patients typically present with localized or generalized tumor nodules that may exhibit some spontaneous regression, especially in early disease. It is important to distinguish primary cutaneous CD30$^+$ anaplastic large T-cell lymphoma from the morphologically similar systemic or primary nodal variety because of their different clinical behavior. Because the systemic variety may present with skin lesions soon followed by evidence of internal involvement, some observers require the absence of extracutaneous involvement for at least 6 months before the presumptive diagnosis of primary cutaneous CD30$^+$ anaplastic large T-cell lymphoma can be confirmed. Histopathologically, there is usually a dense, diffuse, nonepidermotropic dermal infiltrate of large lymphoid cells with round to bizarrely shaped pleo-

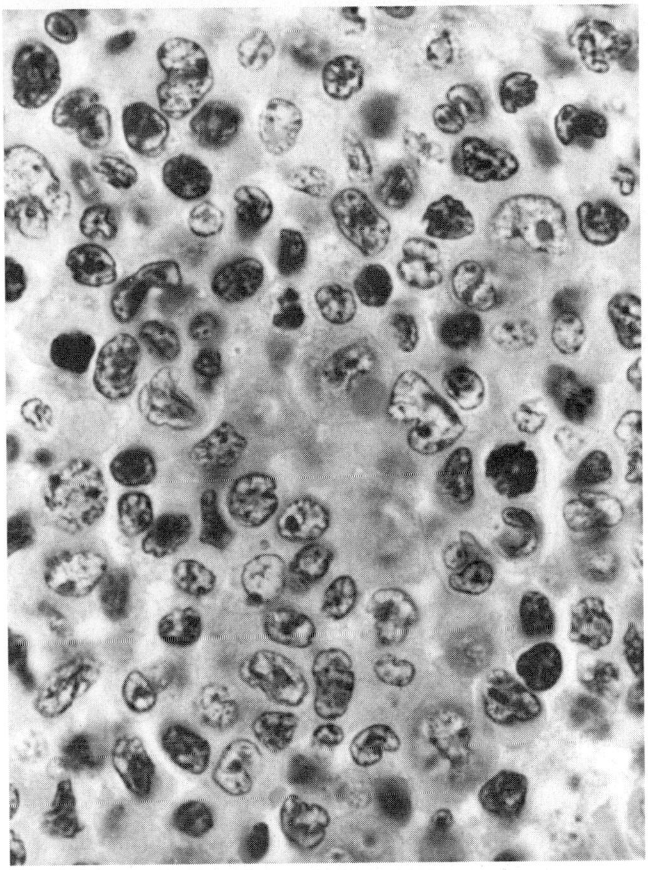

FIG. 32.21. Anaplastic large cell lymphoma (i.e., regressing atypical histiocytosis). There is a dense, diffuse infiltrate of large, pleomorphic mononuclear cells with variably prominent nucleoli and abundant cytoplasm. An erythrocyte is present within the cytoplasm of a cell in the center of the field (original magnification: 825× magnification). (From Headington JT, Roth MS, Ginsburg D, et al. T-cell receptor gene rearrangement in regressing atypical histiocytosis. *Arch Dermatol* 1987; 123:1183–1187, with permission.)

morphic nuclei, prominent nucleoli, and abundant cytoplasm that grow in a cohesive sheetlike array. Small lymphocytes, histiocytes, eosinophils and neutrophils may be admixed but the atypical large cells generally predominate. Some cases contain numerous inflammatory cells, imparting a LYP-type histologic appearance. Tumor cells usually express a CD4$^+$ T-cell phenotype but often lack one or more mature pan-T-cell antigens. Rare cases are CD8$^+$. A few have been shown to produce T_H2 cytokines (225). In addition to the requisite CD30 expression, tumor cells usually express CD25 and HLA-DR activation antigens. In contrast to the primary nodal form, the primary skin type is generally CD15$^-$ EMA$^-$CLA$^+$ (2). Clonal TCR gene rearrangements are present in most cases. The t(2;5)(p23;q35) is uncommon; however, I have seen two pediatric cases with a natural killer (NK) cell phenotype that had the t(2;5). Studies have shown that division of cases into morphologic subtypes (i.e., anaplastic, immunoblastic, pleomorphic, other) is not reproducible and has no prognostic relevance (244). Nevertheless, the term *anaplastic* is retained in the name of this lymphoma to maintain consistency with the terminology used to refer to its nodal counterpart. Expression or absence of p53 or BCL-2 is not prognostically relevant (243). Clinical course depends on stage of disease. Localized skin lesions are typically indolent, even if there is involvement of regional lymph nodes (2). Generalized skin lesions or extracutaneous dissemination are more worrisome, but 5-year survival is about 90% overall.

Differentiation of these lymphomas from nonepidermotropic tumor phase MF and CD30$^-$ large cell lymphomas is based on their distinctive cytology and CD30 expression. Lymphomas containing only a small proportion of CD30$^+$ tumor cells do not qualify as CD30$^+$ anaplastic large T-cell lymphomas. The distinction from LYP is usually straightforward. When intergrades are encountered, the clinical behavior of the lesions is the best guide to their correct classification as lymphoma or LYP. Differentiation from poorly differentiated melanomas and carcinomas sometimes requires an appropriate immunodiagnostic panel. To avoid misdiagnosing these lymphomas as nonlymphoid malignancies based on paraffin section immunohistology, it is important to recognize that a significant minority of cases are CD45$^-$.

CD30$^+$ Small Cell Variant

A small cell predominant variant of CD30$^+$ lymphoma has been described that can present in the subcutis, bears the t(2;5), and tends to transform into classic CD30$^+$ anaplastic large T-cell cytology (22). Some of these cases are CD8$^+$. A histiocyte-rich variant of CD30$^+$, anaplastic large T-cell lymphoma has also been reported but manifests typically in lymph nodes rather than skin and appears biologically similar to classic nodal forms of this disease (22).

CD30$^+$ Anaplastic Large T-Cell Lymphoma Secondary to Mycosis Fungoides

Roughly one half of all cases of "transformed MF" are CD30$^+$ anaplastic large T-cell lymphomas (68). In contrast to the truly primary cutaneous type, these second malignancies have a poor prognosis (1,2,7,68,69) and are discussed further in the section on transformation of MF.

Pleomorphic, Small or Medium-Sized T-Cell Lymphoma

These primary skin lymphomas present as solitary or multiple tumor nodules (2). The lesional infiltrates may or may not be epidermotropic, often extend into the subcutis, and are composed of small to medium-sized, atypical lymphoid cells with hyperchromatic, pleomorphic nuclei and a scant cytoplasmic rim. Despite the designation of small or medium sized, a small proportion of large pleomorphic cells may also be present, as well as some small lymphocytes and histiocytes. Some cases exhibit angiocentricity but usually not to the degree seen in primary extracutaneous angiocentric lymphomas. Most cases are CD4$^+$ with variable loss of mature T-cell antigens. Some cases are CD8$^+$. Most contain clonal TCR gene rearrangements. Overall, these tumors exhibit intermediate aggressiveness, with a 5-year survival of about 60%. A more favorable prognosis has been reported for patients with pleomorphic small cell type disease (246–248). Differentiation from MF can be difficult on histopathologic grounds alone. The clinical absence of preexisting patches and plaques argues strongly against MF. Pleomorphic large cell lymphoma is defined as containing more than about one third large cells. T-cell types of cutaneous lymphoid hyperplasia (pseudolymphoma) are generally distinguished by their polyclonality, normal immunophenotype, and greater heterogeneity of reactive cell types.

CD30$^-$ Large T-Cell Lymphoma

Like other non-MF PTLs, these cases usually present with cutaneous tumor nodules devoid of prior patches or plaques (2,7) (Fig. 32.22). Lesions may be single or multiple. The infiltrates are similar to those seen in pleomorphic small or medium-sized lymphomas, except that, by definition, more than one third large pleomorphic cells must be present (Fig. 32.23). Some cases may show angiocentricity but differ in several respects from classic angiocentric lymphomas as discussed in the section about that disorder. Differentiation from CD30$^+$ anaplastic large T-cell lymphoma is made on the basis of minimal or absent CD30 expression. A few CD30$^+$ cells are allowed in many types of lymphoma, whereas CD30$^+$ anaplastic large T-cell lymphomas express CD30 on most tumor cells. Cytologic features are less helpful because CD30$^+$ anaplastic large T-cell lymphomas may contain cells with anaplastic, pleomorphic, immunoblastic, or unclassified nuclear features. CD30$^-$ large T-cell lym-

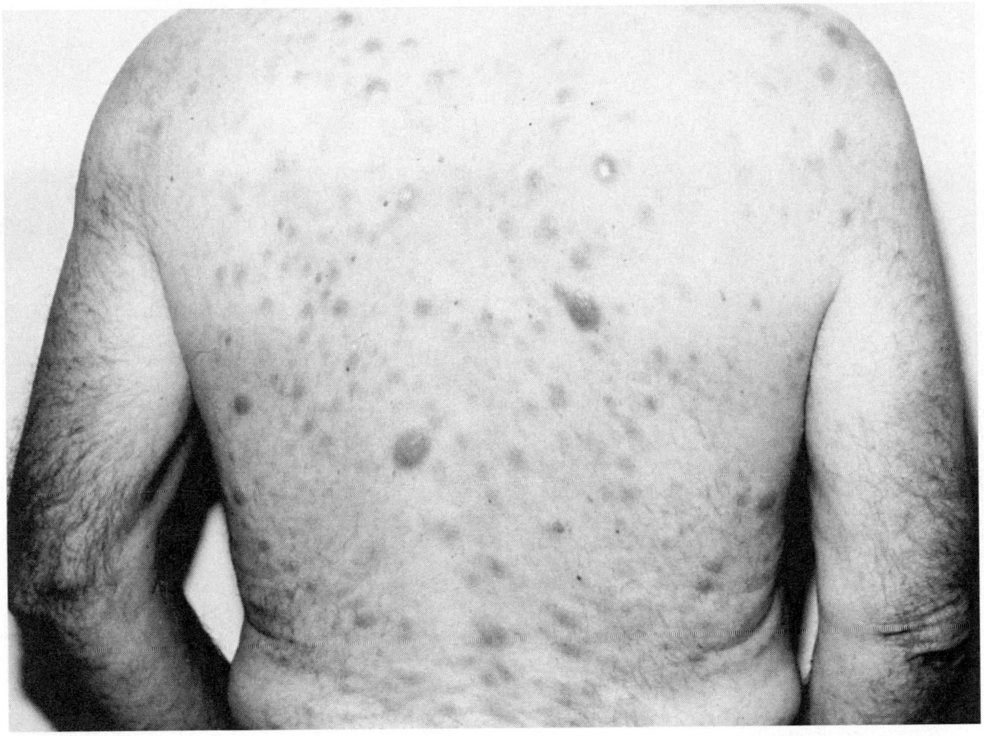

FIG. 32.22. Non–mycosis fungoides (MF) peripheral T-cell lymphoma: cutaneous lesions. In contrast to MF, which usually involves the skin initially as patches or plaques, these non-MF T-cell lymphomas usually involve the skin as discrete tumor nodules. This is also true of B-cell lymphomas.

phomas are aggressive, with an overall 5-year survival of only 10% to 20%. Decreased survival appears to parallel the proportion of large cells. Expression or absence of BCL-2 or p53 is not prognostically relevant (245). About one half of the cases of large cell transformation of MF are morphologically similar to primary cutaneous $CD30^-$ large T-cell lymphomas (7,68). The distinction is made on the basis of clinical history.

Subcutaneous Panniculitic T-Cell Lymphoma

Subcutaneous panniculitic T-cell lymphoma is an uncommon but distinctive form of cutaneous lymphoma. It manifests as deep-seated, subcutaneous tumor nodules that may spontaneously regress or persist (2,249–251). Relapses are characteristically confined to the subcutis, even at autopsy. Lesions are often accompanied by systemic abnormalities such as fever, weight loss, and cytopenia from a hemophagocytic syndrome. Many cases described previously as ''cytophagic histiocytic panniculitis'' probably belong to this category (252). The subcutaneous adipose tissue is replaced by a dense, diffuse infiltrate of pleomorphic lymphoid cells of different sizes mixed with histiocytes exhibiting erythrophagocytosis. There is often abundant necrosis and associated secondary alterations. Tumor cells express a T-cell phenotype of the $CD8^+$ or less commonly $CD4^+$ subset. Several cases express TIA-1. Occasional cases express CD30, CD56, or TCR-$\gamma\delta$ (253–256). Interferon-γ production has been documented in at least one case (253). Most cases contain clonally rearranged TCR genes. The clinical course is aggressive, with death from sepsis or other systemic complications rather than to widespread dissemination of tumor, which is uncommon. Median survival is less than 3 years (6). Differentiation from other types of cutaneous lymphoma is based primarily on the subcutaneous localization of lesions and the systemic manifestations. Immunophenotypic features are less helpful because some of these tumors may express markers such as CD30 that define a different type of lymphoma in other contexts.

Other Primary Cutaneous T-Cell Lymphomas

The peripheral T-cell lymphomas described previously constitute most primary CTCLs. Rarely, other types of T-cell lymphomas may manifest in the skin, but in aggregate, they probably account for less than 5% of cases. There are many ways to classify T-cell lymphomas, including cytologic features (e.g., large cell), immunophenotype (e.g., $CD30^+$), tissue localization (e.g., subcutaneous), and architectural pattern (i.e., angiocentric). Because lymphomas share these characteristics in an overlapping fashion, their classification according to only one parameter at a time would create a highly redundant and confusing array of categories. In contrast, the classification terminology presented in this chapter was selected to reflect fairly well-defined clinicopathologic entities with predictable outcomes and re-

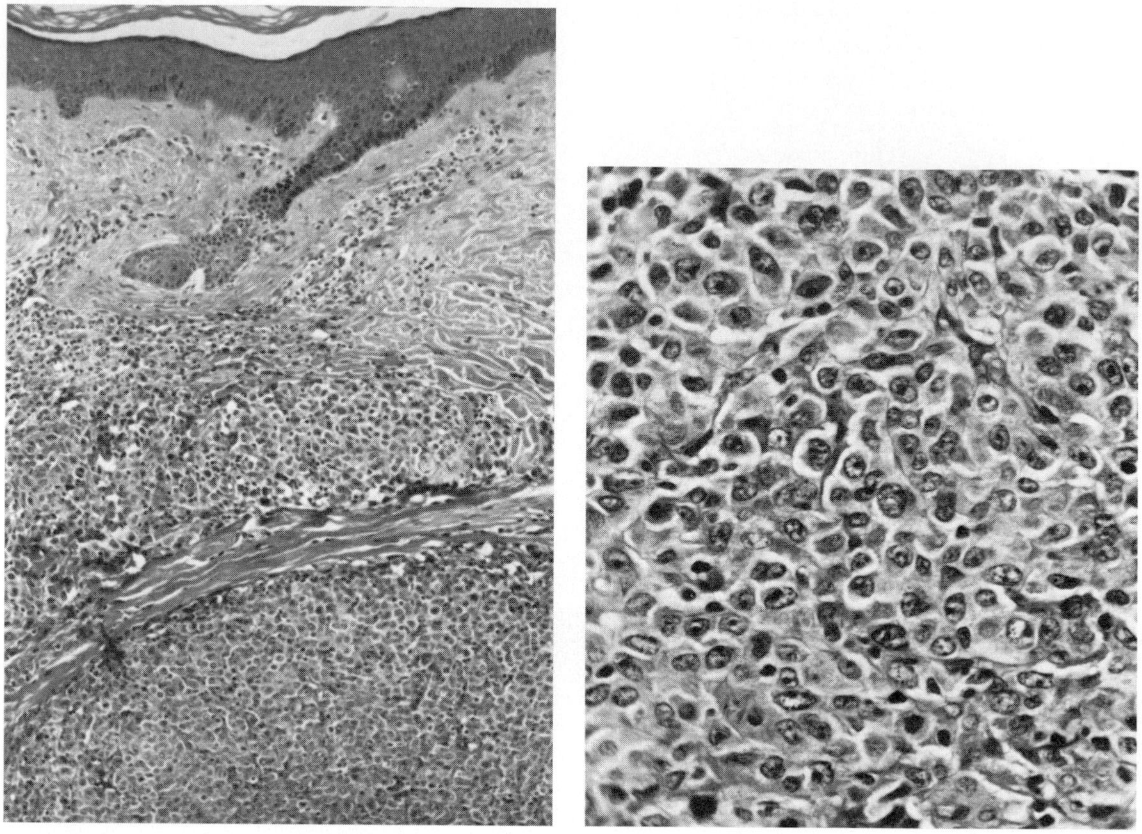

A B

FIG. 32.23. CD30$^-$ large T-cell lymphoma. **A:** There is a dense infiltrate of monomorphous mononuclear cells in the middle and deep dermis. The epidermis is uninvolved and separated from the infiltrate by a Grenz zone within the papillary dermis. This pattern of skin involvement is typical of most non–mycosis fungoides cutaneous lymphomas regardless of their T-cell or B-cell lineage. Notice the sparse perivascular infiltrate within the upper dermis. This common finding is a nonspecific host response composed of small, nonneoplastic lymphocytes. The diagnostic areas lie deeper in the dermis and illustrate the need for deep biopsies in the evaluation of possible skin lymphomas (original magnification: 120× magnification). **B:** Higher magnification of the deep dermal infiltrate shows the cytologic features of diffuse, large cell lymphoma. This tumor expressed a T-cell immunophenotype (original magnification: 480× magnification).

sponses to therapy. Among the primary skin lymphomas, there are certain rare subtypes defined by others that are not emphasized in this chapter's classification, because based on available data, they overlap with too many otherwise distinct disease entities. These include primary CTCLs with TCR-$\gamma\delta$, CD8$^+$, CD56$^+$, or angiocentric features (2,7,257, 258). Primary cutaneous TCR-$\gamma\delta$ lymphomas occur among cases with the features of MF, widespread pagetoid reticulosis or subcutaneous panniculitic lymphoma. Primary cutaneous CD8$^+$ lymphomas occur in two main subgroups as described subsequently. Primary cutaneous CD56$^+$ lymphomas occur among CD30$^+$ large cell lymphomas, subcutaneous panniculitic lymphomas and CD30$^-$ non-MF types. Primary cutaneous angiocentric lymphomas occur among the pleomorphic small or medium-sized and CD30$^-$ large cell varieties. There is incomplete overlap between CD56$^+$ and angiocentric lymphomas with cutaneous involvement. In one study, two of five CD56$^+$ lymphomas involving skin were angiocentric. In contrast, two of three angiocentric lymphomas involving skin were CD56$^+$ (259).

Although it has been reported that these lymphomas are often associated with more aggressive clinical behavior than comparable tumors lacking these features, it is not clear whether this behavior is independent of or secondary to more fundamental characteristics such as disease stage. In any event, numerous exceptions exist. For example, CD8$^+$ lymphomas that otherwise resemble typical cases of pagetoid reticulosis, MF or CD30$^+$ large T-cell lymphomas do not appear to have enhanced clinical aggressiveness. In contrast, those presenting as eruptive, ulcerating, epidermotropic lymphomas of the pleomorphic small or medium-sized or large cell type do appear to behave more aggressively than their CD4$^+$ counterparts (2). Two stage IEA primary cutaneous CD30$^+$ large cell lymphomas that also expressed CD56, other NK markers, and the t(2;5) behaved in an indolent fashion similar to typical stage IEA primary cutaneous CD30$^+$ anaplastic large T-cell lymphomas that do not share these other characteristics (231,258). A case of subcutaneous panniculitic T-cell lymphoma that also expressed TCR-$\gamma\delta$, CD1, CD30, and CD56 behaved like other subcutaneous panniculitic T-cell lymphomas lacking these additional features (i.e., death within a few years despite relapses confined to the subcutis) (253). A primary cutaneous T-cell or NK cell lymphoma that was $CD30^-$ and $CD56^+$ displayed an indolent clinical course rather than the aggressive clinical behavior typical of systemic $CD56^+$, angiocentric NK or T-cell lymphomas (260). When certain rare immunophenotypic or architectural features are exhibited by a cutaneous lymphoma, it would seem preferable at present to continue to use the lymphoma classification listed in Tables 32.2 and 32.3, with an added comment on the potential significance of the special features, rather than create a new lymphoma subtype based solely on these unusual characteristics. However, as more studies of these unusual cases are published, distinct new clinicopathologic entities may emerge.

CONCURRENT AND SECONDARY NON–MYCOSIS FUNGOIDES CUTANEOUS T-CELL LYMPHOMAS

Intravascular Large T-Cell Lymphoma

Intravascular large cell lymphomas are rare overall, and most are of B-cell lineage. However, occasional cases exhibit a T-cell phenotype (7). The clinicopathologic features of intravascular lymphomas are discussed in the section on the more common B-cell variety.

Adult T-Cell Leukemia/Lymphoma

ATL is a type of peripheral T-cell lymphoproliferative disorder associated with human T-cell lymphotrophic virus type 1 (HTLV-1) retrovirus infection (5,24,26,261–266) (see Chapter 44). ATL occurs in endemic foci of HTLV-1 infection throughout the world, such as Japan, Taiwan, the Caribbean basin, and central Africa, as well as scattered cases elsewhere. Most cases of ATL manifest as rapidly progressive lymphomas with cutaneous, lymphoid, visceral, and leukemic involvement. Serum calcium, lactate dehydrogenase, and bilirubin are often elevated and there may be lytic bone lesions. In addition to this fulminant form of disease, there are other variants of ATL and related conditions known as the asymptomatic carrier state, pre-ATL, lymphomatous ATL, smoldering ATL, and chronic ATL (Table 32.10). Overall, about two thirds of ATL cases involve the skin (6). Acute ATL and all its variants are characterized by seropositivity for antibodies against HTLV-1. Each of these conditions is also associated with integration of the intact HTLV-1 provirus into host T cells, eventually resulting in neoplastic transformation and ultimately monoclonal expansion. Histopathologically, these ATL cases are often classified as pleomorphic small, medium, or large cell lymphomas, but not all lymphomas of this type are associated with HTLV-1 infection. Involvement of skin, blood and lymph nodes can resemble MF/SS clinically and histopathologically, but the neoplastic cells in such cases have nuclei that are more lobated than cerebriform and have been referred to as ''flower'' cells. The characteristic geographic clustering, hypercalcemia, aggressive clinical behavior, and seropositivity for HTLV-1 facilitate the distinction of ATL from MF/SS. Although there has been some controversy about whether MF/SS is also associated with HTLV-1 proviral integration, most studies do not support this view (267,268). ATL characteristically expresses a $CD4^+CD8^-$ (helper or inducer) T-cell phenotype with variable deficiencies of pan-T-cell antigens (Table 32.5) and clonal TCR gene rearrangements (5,261–264). Like MF/SS, the most common deficiencies involve CD7 and CD5. CD25 expression was initially felt to distinguish ATL from MF/SS, but overlapping numbers of $CD25^+$ cells have been observed in these two disorders.

Systemic $CD30^+$ Anaplastic Large T-Cell Lymphoma

Systemic $CD30^+$ anaplastic large T-cell lymphomas are primary nodal lymphomas with morphologic features similar to their counterparts arising in the skin (1). They have a bimodal age distribution, occurring in children and adults. They may involve the skin as part of their systemic manifestations, but these tumors differ biologically from the primary cutaneous form in several ways. First, they are more aggressive clinically. Second, they are typically EMA^+, CLA^-, whereas the opposite is true of the primary cutaneous form. Third, they contain the t(2;5)(p23;q35) in about 40% of cases in contrast to the rarity of this translocation in the primary cutaneous type (see Chapter 25).

Angioimmunoblastic T-Cell Lymphoma

Previously regarded as an abnormal immune reaction called angioimmunoblastic lymphadenopathy with dyspro-

TABLE 32.10. *Adult T-cell leukemia/lymphoma variants*

Diagnosis	Skin lesions	Abnormal blood cells	Lymph node involvement	Visceral involvement
Asymptomatic carrier	Absent	Absent	Absent	Absent
Pre-ATL	Absent	Present	Absent	Absent
Lymphomatous ATL	Absent	Absent	Present	Absent
Smoldering ATL	Minimal	Minimal	Present	Absent
Chronic ATL	Minimal	Present	Present	Absent
Acute ATL	Variable	Prominent	Present	Present

ATL, adult T-cell leukemia/lymphoma.

teinemia or immunoblastic lymphadenopathy, this disorder is considered to be a moderately aggressive form of T-cell lymphoma (1). It is a systemic disease that usually presents in the elderly and can include generalized lymphadenopathy, hepatosplenomegaly, polyclonal hypergammaglobulinemia, Coombs' positive hemolytic anemia, and skin lesions in slightly less than one half of all cases (1,157,203,269–272) (see Chapter 16). The disease is chronic and can remit or progress to high-grade lymphoma, generally diffuse large cell immunoblastic T-cell or occasionally B-cell type. Clonal TCR gene rearrangements are present in most cases, although about 10% contain rearranged IgH genes (203,269,270,273–275). Some have proposed that angioimmunoblastic T-cell lymphoma exists as a clinicopathologic disease spectrum. Gene rearrangement and karyotypic studies suggest that progression along this continuum involves the outgrowth of a dominant lymphoid clone from a polyclonal or oligoclonal background (273,274). Clonal Epstein-Barr virus (EBV) genomes are present in several cases, suggesting an EBV-driven mechanism for lymphomagenesis (276–279). Some of these lymphomas have increased levels of various cytokines that may contribute to the immune dysfunction characteristic of this disease and foster growth of EBV-infected cells (280). Skin lesions are often the first clinical manifestation. They consist of a generalized, pruritic, maculopapular eruption, or less commonly, petechiae, plaques or nodules. The histopathologic features range from nonspecific perivascular dermatitis in the maculopapular lesions, to dense polymorphous lymphoid infiltrates with vascular proliferation or overt diffuse large cell (immunoblastic) lymphoma in the plaques and nodules. Lesions may contain plasma cells, small lymphocytes, and lymphocytic "vasculitis" with erythrocyte extravasation. The differential diagnosis of skin lesions can be difficult because of their frequently nonspecific features. Drug eruptions must be excluded by clinicopathologic correlation. Angioimmunoblastic T-cell lymphoma is distinguished from MF/SS by its systemic manifestations and the lack of epidermotropic, cerebriform lymphoid cells in lesional skin. The related high-grade lymphomas involving the skin are uncommon but similar to other lymphomas with the same morphology.

Natural Killer or T-Cell Angiocentric Lymphoma

NK or T-cell angiocentric lymphomas (see Chapter 29) usually arise in extranodal, extracutaneous sites such as the upper respiratory tract but may involve the skin secondarily (1,2,7,281,282). The most common primary site is nasal. *Polymorphic reticulosis, lethal midline granuloma*, and *angiocentric immunoproliferative lesion* (grades 2 and 3) are older terms that include cases of this disorder. Some prefer the terms *nasal* and *nasal-type NK or T-cell lymphoma* because not all cases are angioinvasive (6). Histopathologically, there is typically an angiocentric, angioinvasive infiltrate of small lymphocytes, atypical lymphoid cells of various sizes, immunoblasts, plasma cells and sometimes histiocytes and eosinophils. Vascular occlusion by atypical cells is characteristic and frequently associated with ischemic necrosis. The atypical lymphoid cells generally express a mixture of T-cell antigens ($CD2^+$, $CD5^{+/-}$, $CD7^{+/-}$) and NK cell antigens ($CD16^+$, $CD56^+$, $CD57^{+/-}$) but are often $CD3^-$. They may be $CD4^+$ or $CD8^+$. Clonal TCR and Ig gene rearrangements are typically absent but EBV is usually present. These tumors are generally aggressive and may result in central nervous system involvement. Clinical aggressiveness appears to parallel the proportion of large tumor cells. Primary cutaneous cases are uncommon, fall into the pleomorphic small, medium-sized, or large cell lymphoma categories, do not always express NK markers such as CD56 (259), less often contain EBV, and are less aggressive than classic angiocentric lymphomas of the upper aerodigestive tract (2,283). The differential diagnosis includes other lymphomas and leukemias with NK characteristics, including aggressive NK cell leukemia, the blastoid variant of NK cell leukemia/lymphoma (284), lymphoblastic lymphoma with NK features (285,286), myeloid or NK acute leukemia (287), and myeloid or NK acute precursor leukemia (288).

Aggressive Natural Killer Cell Leukemia

This disorder is included among the large granular lymphocyte leukemias and appears to be the leukemic counterpart of angiocentric NK or T-cell lymphoma. Like this latter neoplasm, it is more common in Asia than elsewhere, expresses a similar immunophenotype and immunogenotype, and often contains EBV (6,282,289,290). Patients develop disseminated disease that frequently includes the skin. Tumor cells are large with eccentric nuclei and abundant cytoplasm rich in azurophilic granules (7). The clinical presentation is relatively acute and the course is generally aggressive.

T-Cell Chronic Lymphocytic Leukemia or T-Prolymphocytic Leukemia

This disorder is generally regarded as a single entity and comprises about 1% CLL and 20% prolymphocytic leukemia (1). Skin and mucosal involvement are common and occur more frequently than in B-cell CLL (6,203,291). The clinical course is also more aggressive than B-cell CLL. Most cases exhibit prolymphocytic cytologic features and a high white blood cell count. Cutaneous infiltrates are usually nonepidermotropic but concentrated in the upper dermis. Cases generally express a mature T-cell phenotype; most are $CD4^+$, some are $CD4^+CD8^+$, and $CD8^+$ variants are rare. In contrast to other $CD4^+$ leukemias such as ATL and MF/SS, tumor cells are $CD7^+$. They are also; $CD25^-$. TCR genes are clonally rearranged, and inv14(q11;q32) is common as well as trisomy 8q.

Precursor T-Cell Lymphoblastic Lymphoma

Occasional CTCLs are of the precursor T-cell lymphoblastic subtype (5,6,292) (see Chapter 26). They can involve the thymus, blood, and marrow at some point in their course. They are usually immunophenotypically distinct from PTL because they are generally $CD7^+$ and many are also $CD1^+$ (Table 32.5). These tumors are typically $HLA\text{-}DR^-$, and MF/SS and PTL are variably $HLA\text{-}DR^-$. Compared with PTL, T-cell lymphoblastic lymphomas are also more heterogeneous in regard to expression of major T-cell subset markers. Usually, they are $CD4^+CD8^+$ or $CD4^-CD8^-$. They may also be $CD4^+CD8^-$ or $CD4^-CD8^+$. As with PTL, antigens such as CD2, CD3, and CD5 may be deficient. Some T lymphoblastic lymphomas may also exhibit NK features (285,286).

Other T-Cell Lymphomas

In addition to the types of T-cell lymphomas discussed previously, virtually all other types may involve the skin occasionally in a secondary fashion at some point in their clinical course.

CUTANEOUS B-CELL LYMPHOPROLIFERATIVE DISORDERS

Most cutaneous B-cell lymphomas have a diffuse rather than follicular pattern (2,5,8,9,21,293–298). These tumors may be Ig^+ or Ig^-. Ig^- cases are recognized by their expression of non-Ig B-cell surface antigens such as CD19, CD20, CD22, and CD79a. Occasionally, CD20 may be expressed by clonal cutaneous T cells (299). Some reports indicate that a higher percentage of cutaneous B-cell lymphomas are Ig^- than are nodal B-cell lymphomas (9). This may reflect a tendency for extranodal B-cell lymphomas as a group to be Ig^- more commonly. Ig^+ B-cell lymphomas are monotypic; all tumor cells express the same Ig light chain (κ or λ). In contrast, reactive polyclonal B-cell infiltrates are composed of a mixture of κ^+ and λ^+ cells, typically with κ predominance (104,300,301). The distinction between a reactive and a neoplastic B-cell infiltrate is often straightforward. Nevertheless, in some cases, a heavy inflammatory T-cell infiltrate may obscure a minority population of neoplastic B cells (5,9). These lesions have been called *pseudo-peripheral T-cell lymphomas* (302) or *T-cell–rich B-cell lymphomas* (7). Multiple biopsies and careful study of serial immunoperoxidase stained sections may be needed to make the correct diagnosis. Another complicating feature is the fact that some types of cutaneous B-cell lymphomas may contain residual reactive B-cell follicles similar to those seen in cutaneous lymphoid hyperplasia (2,7,303). Molecular biologic studies of Ig gene rearrangements are also often helpful because they are well suited for the detection of minor tumor cell populations. B-cell lymphomas of various histologic subtypes have been studied with immunogenotypic techniques (1,2,7,18,37,40,304). In most cases, immunogenotyping has indicated a monoclonal process, although evidence for multiclonality has been obtained for B-cell lymphomas in transplant recipients (18). Molecular biologic studies have also been used to monitor the emergence of new clones or subclones in cases of B-cell lymphoma undergoing histologic transformation (305) and in B-cell lymphoma patients receiving antiidiotype monoclonal antibody therapy whose tumors lose reactivity with the original antiidiotype antibody because of somatic point mutations in their Ig genes (19). Some of the key features distinguishing cutaneous B-cell lymphomas from cutaneous lymphoid hyperplasias are listed in Table 32.11.

PRIMARY CUTANEOUS B-CELL LYMPHOMAS

Follicle Center Cell Lymphomas

Primary cutaneous follicle center cell lymphomas usually manifest as solitary or localized thick plaques or nodules involving the head, neck, or trunk (2,7,9,21,294–298) (see Chapter 24). Included within this category is the so-called *reticulohistiocytoma of the dorsum* or *Crosti's lymphoma*

TABLE 32.11. *Differential diagnosis of primary cutaneous B-cell lymphoma and cutaneous lymphoid hyperplasia*

Feature	CBCL	CLH
Clinical appearance		
Size	Large nodules or plaques	Smaller lesions
Location	Localized or generalized	Usually solitary or localized
Histopathology		
Architecture	Usually diffuse, bottom heavy	Often follicular and diffuse, top-heavy
Cytology	Large cell lymphoma most common	Variety of cell types usually present in a single lesion
Reactive B-cell follicles	Usually absent except in some follicle center cell, marginal zone, and mantle cell lymphomas	Common
Immunopathology		
B cells	Monotypic or Ig^-	Polytypic
Follicular dendritic cells	Monotypic or Ig^- when surrounded by tumor cells	Polytypic
Gene rearrangements		
Ig genes	Monoclonal	Polyclonal except in a minority of cases (clonal CLH)
t(14;18)	Usually absent, even in follicle center cell CBCL	Absent

CBCL, cutaneous B-cell lymphoma; CLH, cutaneous lymphoid hyperplasia.

(7,297). Lesions contain dense, superficial and deep, dermal lymphoid infiltrates that spare the epidermis and are separated from it by a narrow Grenz zone of uninvolved papillary dermis. The infiltrates are often bottom heavy, and it is in these deeper foci where the most diagnostic fields frequently can be found. The subcutis may be involved. In most cases, these lymphomas exhibit a diffuse rather than follicular architecture. Sometimes, immunophenotyping may reveal a histologically inapparent follicular tumor architecture that had been obscured by dense interfollicular infiltrates of T cells and B cells (9). Cytologically, these lymphomas consist of a variable mixture of small cleaved and large noncleaved follicle center cells (Working Formulation), also known as centrocytes and centroblasts (Kiel classification). Early lesions are composed predominantly of smaller follicle center cells and may harbor residual reactive B-cell follicles, and more established lesions contain a greater proportion of large cells (Fig. 32.24). Overexpression of p53 may play a role in this process because progression has been associated with an increase in the proportion of $p53^+$ tumor cells (206). In contrast to their nodal counterparts, these predominantly diffuse large cell variants do not appear to behave in a more aggressive fashion (2). Available data suggest that they are biologically distinct from morphologically similar primary cutaneous tumors occurring on the legs (so-called large B-cell lymphoma of the leg) (2,306,307). Approximately one half of follicle center cell lymphomas are Ig^-. The remainder are Ig light-chain restricted (monotypic), although as with any Ig^+ B-cell lymphomas, one or more Ig heavy chains may be expressed. These patterns of Ig expression facilitate the distinction of follicle center cell lymphoma from cutaneous lymphoid hyperplasia (Table 32.11) (7,9,104,300,301).

Another feature helpful in this differential diagnosis of the rare follicular cases (Fig. 32.25) is their follicular dendritic cell network. Follicular dendritic cells are accessory cells that form a meshwork within reactive and neoplastic B-cell follicles (9,303). In reactive follicles, this network contains polytypic immune complexes bound to its surface. It stains for κ and λ Ig light chains. In contrast, Ig^- follicular lymphomas lack Ig staining of their follicular dendritic cell networks. In Ig^+ follicular lymphomas, this network is obscured by the monotypic staining of the tumor cells within the neoplastic follicles. It is important to recognize that B cells may also exist in the skin as scattered cells or in aggregates devoid of a follicular dendritic cell network. The major features of each type of cutaneous B-cell formation are listed in Table 32.12 (9,104).

Like their primary nodal counterparts, most primary cutaneous follicle center cell lymphomas exhibit monoclonal rearrangements of Ig heavy and light chain genes (297,308), but they differ from nodal primaries in that they usually lack the t(14;18) translocation and lack expression of BCL-2 and CD10 (298,303,309,310). Clinically, these lymphomas re-

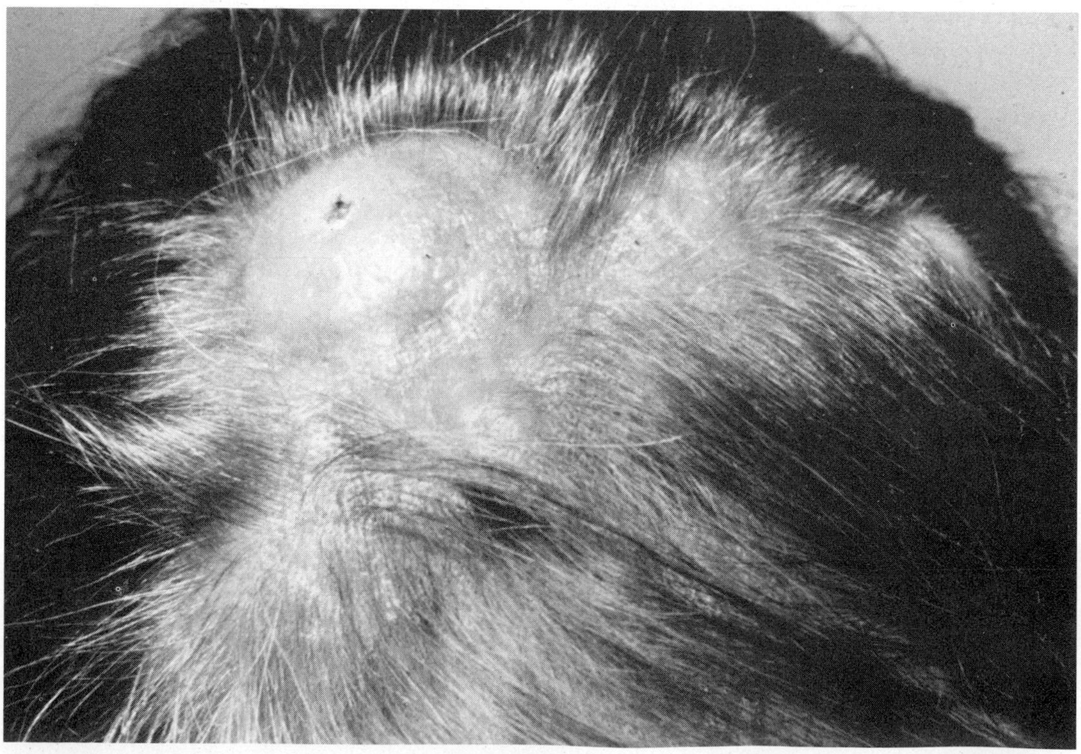

FIG. 32.24. Cutaneous follicle center B-cell lymphoma, diffuse pattern. This patient presented with a large scalp nodule surrounded by several smaller nodules. The lesions proved to be caused by a diffuse, large cell lymphoma of B-cell lineage that also involved lymph nodes concurrently. Localized, non–mycosis fungoides cutaneous T-cell lymphomas may exhibit an identical clinical appearance.

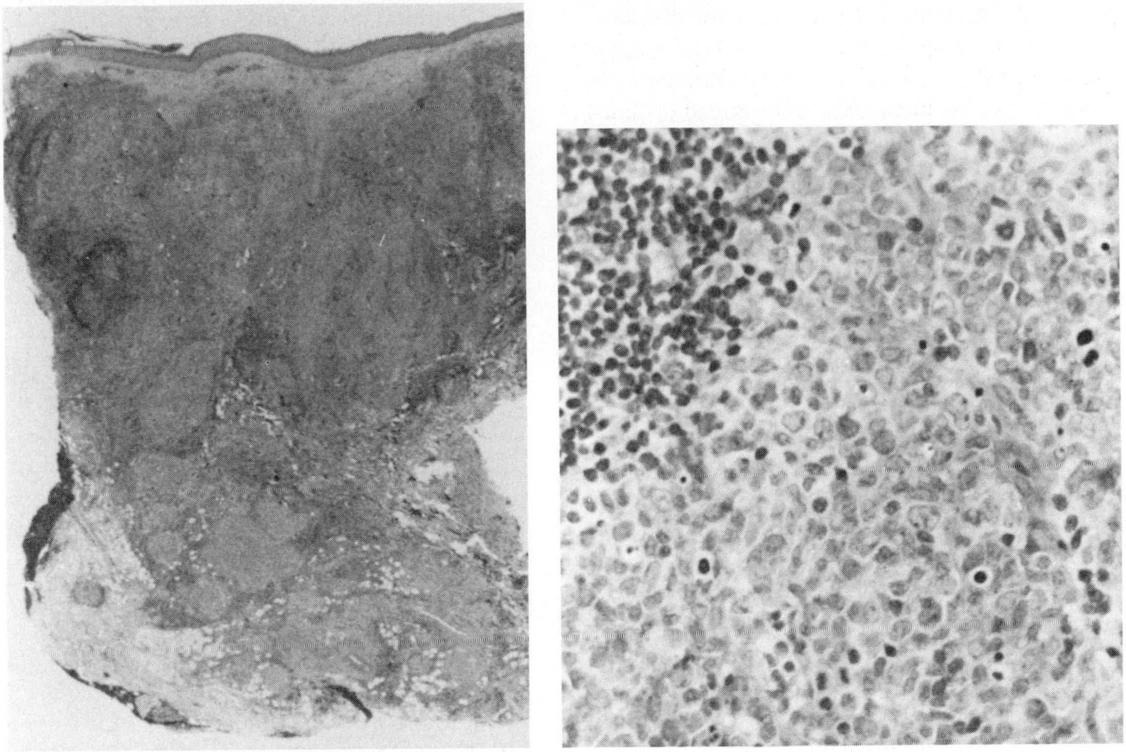

A B

FIG. 32.25. Cutaneous follicle center B-cell lymphoma, follicular pattern. **A:** There is a dense superficial and deep dermal infiltrate that extends into the subcutis and is separated from the overlying epidermis by an uninvolved Grenz zone. Even at scanning magnification, the paler staining follicular structures can be discerned (original magnification: 10× magnification). **B:** Higher magnification shows the follicles to be composed of relatively monomorphous large, noncleaved lymphoid cells. These cells were of Ig^- B-cell lineage. Small lymphocytes surround the neoplastic follicles and are seen in one corner of this field (original magnification: 480× magnification). Compare with Figure 32.27. (From Garcia CF, Weiss LM, Warnke RA, et al. Cutaneous follicular lymphoma. *Am J Surg Pathol* 1986;10:454–463, with permission.)

TABLE 32.12. *Differential diagnosis of cutaneous B-cell aggregates*

Type of B-cell aggregate	Zonation	FDC network	B-cell phenotype
B-cell cluster	Absent	Absent	Pan-B antigen positive, including 41H, polytypic Ig light-chain staining, variable Ig heavy-chain staining, Ki-67^+ <10%
Primary follicle	Absent	Present; FDC Ig staining obscured by surrounding Ig^+ B cells	Pan-B antigen positive, including 41H, polytypic Ig light-chain expression, μ/δ Ig heavy-chain expression, Ki-67^+ <10%
Secondary follicle	Mantle and germinal center are fully developed; germinal centers exhibit light (cleaved cell) and dark (noncleaved cell) zones.	Present; polytypic Ig light-chain staining apparent in germinal center	Mantle: similar to primary follicle. Germinal center: some pan-B antigens (CD22) only weakly expressed, $41H^-$; Ig expression polytypic but only trace positive, KI-67^+ >10%
Ig^- follicular lymphoma	Mantle may be present around tumor cells.	Present; no polytypic Ig light-chain staining	Mantle: similar to mantle of secondary follicle. Tumor cells: variable pan-B antigen expression, Ig^-, 41H may be positive, Ki-67^+ often >10%
Ig^+ follicular lymphoma	Mantle may be present around tumor cells.	Present; FDC Ig staining obscured by surrounding Ig^+ B cells	Mantle: similar to mantle of secondary follicles. Tumor cells: variable pan-B antigen expression, monotypic Ig light-chain expression, variable Ig heavy-chain expression, 41H may be positive, Ki-67^+ often >10%

FDC, follicular dendritic cell; Ig, immunoglobulin.

spond well to local treatment and have an indolent course with a 5-year survival of more than 95% (2). Data suggest that the prognosis remains favorable even when there is regional lymph node involvement (20). Widespread dissemination outside the skin is infrequent. Some cases are associated with *Borrelia burgdorferi* infection (264,311,312). Although it has been proposed that most B-cell lymphomas in this category are actually marginal zone lymphomas rather than follicle center cell lymphomas, the weight of current evidence favors their germinal center origin (308,309,313). Consistent with this view, follicle center cell lymphomas lack markers such as CD11c and CD43, which are expressed by many marginal zone neoplasms (1). They also show evidence of ongoing somatic mutations within their clonally rearranged Ig genes (314,315). This is consistent with arrest at the germinal center stage of B-cell differentiation.

Marginal Zone B-Cell Lymphoma

As currently defined, marginal zone B-cell lymphoma is an uncommon form of primary cutaneous lymphoma and has several synonyms, including mucosa-associated lymphoid tissue (MALT)–type lymphoma, monocytoid B-cell lymphoma, primary cutaneous immunocytoma, and low-grade B-cell lymphoma of SALT (1,2,6,7,21,308,311,316–323). Lesions appear as single or multiple papulonodules or tumors, with a predeliction for the extremities, but trunk and head may also be involved. There is a nonepidermotropic, dermal, or subcutaneous infiltrate composed of a heterogeneous mixture of small lymphocytes, marginal zone cells (centrocyte-like cells with a bit more cytoplasm), monocytoid B cells, lymphoplasmacytoid cells, and plasma cells, as well as occasional centroblasts and immunoblasts. Reactive B-cell follicles are usually present and surrounded by the neoplastic marginal zone or monocytoid cells. Because of their distinct rim of cytoplasm, these tumor cells sometimes create a "reverse germinal center" appearance with smaller reactive B cells surrounded by paler, slightly larger tumor cells. The extent of plasmacytoid differentiation varies, with more established lesions often showing the greatest degree and giving rise to the term *primary cutaneous immunocytoma.* Intranuclear inclusions (i.e., Dutcher bodies) may be present. This neoplasm is distinct from primary extracutaneous immunocytoma or lymphoplasmacytoid lymphoma of the REAL classification, which is frequently associated with monoclonal IgM serum paraprotein. Tumor cells express CD19, CD20, CD22, and CD79a, monotypic surface Ig and frequently cytoplasmic Ig. IgM is common. IgD is absent. Plasma cells may be monotypic or polytypic. Tumor cells are $CD5^-$, often $CD11c^+$, and sometimes $CD43^+$. These features help distinguish marginal zone lymphomas from B-cell CLL and mantle cell lymphomas ($CD5^+$) and follicle center cell lymphomas ($CD11c^-$, $CD43^-$, and cytoplasmic Ig^-). The observation of $\alpha_4\beta_7$ integrin on tumor cells and mucosal addressin cell adhesion molecule-1 (MAdCAM-1) on cutaneous endothelial cells (324) suggests that cutaneous and gastrointestinal forms of this lymphoma may be related neoplasms. Clonal Ig gene rearrangements are present (308). Although trisomy 3 and the t(11;18) translocation have been reported in some extranodal cases, they have not been observed in primary cutaneous cases (7). These lymphomas behave in an indolent fashion, with 100% 5-year survival (316). Although they may recur after treatment, they tend to relapse in the skin and other extranodal sites. Some cases are associated with *Borrelia burgdorferi* infection (312,316,317) or anetoderma (325).

Large B-Cell Lymphoma of the Leg

Large B-cell lymphoma of the leg is a variant of primary cutaneous B-cell lymphoma. It manifests most commonly in elderly females as nodules involving one or both legs (2,7,21,306,307). The dense, diffuse, nonepidermotropic infiltrate of large lymphoid cells with centroblastic or immunoblastic features may extend into the subcutis. Tumor cells express the usual mature B-cell antigens (CD19, CD20, CD22, CD79a) and monotypic Ig. Clonally rearranged Ig genes are detectable. Like primary cutaneous follicle center cell lymphomas, these tumors lack the t(14;18) translocation, but they differ in that they express BCL-2 strongly. This form of lymphoma displays intermediate aggressiveness with a 5-year survival of about 50% to 60% (2,7). My colleagues and I have seen one case that relapsed as intravascular large B-cell lymphoma, suggesting that, relative to primary cutaneous follicle center cell lymphomas of similar large cell cytology, poorer survival may be related to intravascular involvement in some cases (326).

As discussed in the section on follicle center cell lymphomas, primary cutaneous diffuse large B-cell lymphomas have been conceptualized in the EORTC classification as belonging to one of two groups: those arising on the head, neck, or trunk, which behave indolently and are considered to be a form of follicle center cell lymphoma, and those arising on the legs, which are more aggressive and conceptualized as a distinct type of cutaneous B-cell neoplasm (314). Nevertheless, single-cell PCR analysis and sequencing of clonal Ig gene rearrangements revealed similar features and suggested a germinal center cell origin for both types of lymphomas (314). Future studies may address the issue of whether variables such as patient age, clinical stage of disease or genetic alterations might account for this difference in prognosis between these two neoplasms. For example, localized cases appear to have a better prognosis than disseminated cases (327), and the t(8;14) translocation has been found in one case (328).

Other B-Cell Lymphomas

Most varieties of B-cell lymphoma not discussed previously can also manifest in the skin rarely. For example, occasional precursor B-cell lymphoblastic lymphomas manifest with skin lesions without extracutaneous tissue involvement or circulating tumor cells, although disseminated disease usually becomes apparent soon thereafter. They can exhibit a pre-B-cell immunophenotype (i.e., expression of cytoplasmic μ Ig heavy chain without light chain or surface Ig) (6,292,329) (see Chapter 26). These cases also express CD10, CD34, and TdT (7). Among miscellaneous types of primary cutaneous B-cell lymphoma are rare T-cell–rich B-cell lymphomas (a type of diffuse large cell lymphoma), CD30$^+$ anaplastic large B-cell lymphomas and EBV-associated lymphomas occurring in transplant recipients (6,7) (see Chapter 16).

CONCURRENT AND SECONDARY CUTANEOUS B-CELL LYMPHOMAS

Systemic B-Cell Lymphomas

Primary nodal or extracutaneous B-cell lymphomas may involve the skin concurrently or secondarily in about 10% of cases (7). These include follicle center cell, diffuse large cell, marginal zone, and precursor B-cell lymphoblastic lymphomas. Thorough staging is important for determining proper therapy and prognosis. I have seen patients with localized or generalized cutaneous B-cell lymphoma lesions, normal physical examinations and normal blood counts who were found to have disseminated internal disease after CT scans or bone marrow biopsies. Posttransplant lymphoproliferative disorders occasionally manifest in the skin and may be of B-cell (330) or T-cell (331) type (see Chapter 16). Additional types of B-cell lymphoma that typically involve the skin secondarily rather than primarily are discussed subsequently.

B-Cell Small Lymphocytic Lymphoma or Chronic Lymphocytic Leukemia

B-cell small lymphocytic lymphoma or CLL presents with skin lesions rarely, but B-cell CLL is the most common secondary cutaneous B-cell neoplasm (6,332). Peripheral blood evaluation is important in cases of small lymphocytic lymphoma to rule out CLL (see Chapter 40). The histopathologic pattern is variable but often shows nonepidermotropic, diffuse or superficial and deep perivascular dermal infiltrates. Differential diagnosis of the latter cases includes lupus erythematosus and Jessner's lymphocytic infiltrate, but these conditions are easily distinguished immunophenotypically because they are T-cell infiltrates. Only rare cases of small lymphocytic lymphoma or CLL possess a T-cell immunophenotype. Most express mature B-cell antigens (CD19, CD20, CD79a, but often not CD22), monotypic Ig, CD5, CD23, and CD43. This phenotype aids differentiation from marginal zone lymphoma (CD5$^-$) and mantle cell lymphoma (CD23$^-$).

Mantle Cell Lymphoma

Primary cutaneous mantle cell lymphoma is rare (333–335). Most cutaneous cases are secondary, this occurs in 17% of patients with stage IV disease (335,336). Lesions show a patchy infiltrate of monomorphous small to medium-sized atypical lymphoid cells with centrocyte-like features. Nonneoplastic cells such as eosinophils and plasma cells are rare. Follicular structures with follicular dendritic cells are absent (7). Mantle cell lymphomas express monotypic Ig (λ more often than κ), IgM, IgD, B-cell antigens (CD20, CD79a), CD5, and CD43, but not CD11c or CD23 (335). Most cases have a t(11;14) translocation that results in expression of cyclin D1 (BCL-1, PRAD-1) (337–339).

These tumors are aggressive, with an overall median survival of 3 to 5 years (1). Phenotypic features aid differentiation from marginal zone and follicle center cell lymphomas (CD5$^-$, cyclin D1$^-$), small lymphocytic lymphoma/B-cell CLL (CD23$^+$) and T-cell lymphomas.

Intravascular Large B-Cell Lymphoma

One uncommon type of diffuse large B-cell lymphoma that involves the skin is an intravascular variant known formerly as *malignant angioendotheliomatosis* or *neoplastic proliferating angioendotheliomatosis* (7,340–345) (see Chapter 34). Patients may present with sometimes indurated and painful patches, plaques, ulcerated tumors, and subcutaneous nodules in association with disseminated disease and an aggressive clinical course. My colleagues and I have seen one case of large B-cell lymphoma of the leg relapse as intravascular large B-cell lymphoma (326). Histopathologically, there is partial or complete occlusion of cutaneous vessels by large, pleomorphic mononuclear cells (Fig. 32.26) with similar intravascular and extravascular lesions manifest in multiple organs. The lymphomatous nature of this disease has been substantiated by demonstration of the expression of CD45 (leukocyte common antigen) and B-cell or occasionally T-cell antigens by the lesional cells. This lymphoma is often clinically aggressive, although variants that appear to be predominantly cutaneous may behave more favorably (2). The distinction of this disease from *reactive proliferating angioendotheliomatosis,* a self-limited endothelial cell disorder that produces clinically similar skin lesions, is made on the basis of cytologic atypia, lymphoid antigen expression, and rapidly fatal extracutaneous involvement.

Plasmacytoma

Primary cutaneous plasmacytoma is rare, accounting for less than 5% of extramedullary plasmacytomas (346–350). Most cases with skin involvement result from multiple myeloma, and these are uncommon as well (351). Lesions are solitary or multiple skin nodules that contain a dense, monomorphous dermal, and sometimes subcutaneous infiltrate of monotypic plasma cells that are CD38$^+$, variably CD79a$^+$, CD20$^-$, and CD45$^-$. Primary cutaneous cases show highly mature plasma cells, including multinucleated variants, and other cases contain variable degrees of maturation. Clonal Ig gene rearrangements are detectable (7). The clinical

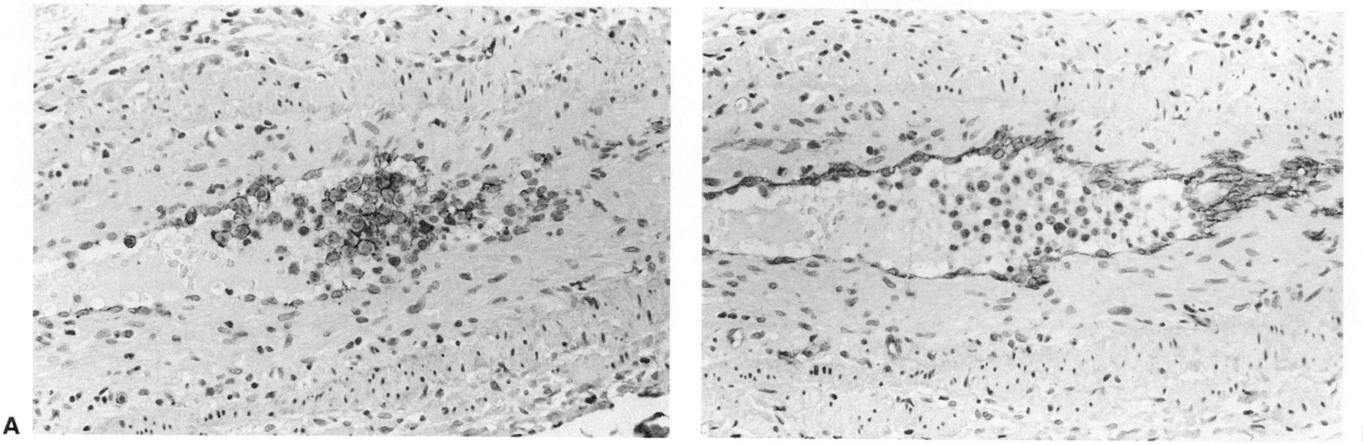

FIG. 32.26. Intravascular large B-cell lymphoma. **A:** Intravascular cluster of large, atypical, $CD20^+$ lymphoid cells. **B:** Serial section shows the $CD31^+$ vascular lining. (**A** and **B**, immunoperoxidase stain with hematoxylin counterstain, original magnification: 200× magnification).

course of primary cases is indolent without report of disease-specific deaths. In contrast, secondary involvement of the skin is a poor prognostic sign. Differential diagnosis includes reactive plasma cell infiltrates (which are polytypic) and cutaneous immunocytomas (which include monotypic lymphocytes with intranuclear periodic acid–Schiff-positive Dutcher bodies).

Lymphomatoid Granulomatosis

Lymphomatoid granulomatosis is a pulmonary lymphoproliferative disorder with systemic manifestations that had been considered previously to be part of a continuum of ''angiocentric immunoproliferative lesions'' with angiocentric lymphoma at its malignant extreme, but combined immunopathologic and gene rearrangement studies indicate that at least a subset of these cases are T-cell–rich, B-cell lymphomas characterized by EBV infection of tumor cells and an exuberant T-cell response (352,353) (see Chapter 34). Nevertheless, others appear to be T-cell lymphomas based on clonal TCR gene rearrangements and related evidence. This suggests that lymphomatoid granulomatosis is probably a heterogeneous mixture of B-cell and T-cell lymphomas with shared clinicopathologic features. Others have raised the suspicion that cases diagnosed as lymphomatoid granulomatosis in the past may also have included cases of Hodgkin's disease, angioimmunoblastic lymphadenopathy with dysproteinemia, and miscellaneous disorders (354). Lymphomatoid granulomatosis skin lesions precede pulmonary lesions in more than 10% of cases (355). Another 30% to 50% develop skin lesions after the onset of pulmonary involvement. Skin lesions include an erythematous or violaceous maculopapular eruption and nodules in the dermis or subcutis. Lesions are often symmetric and occasionally pruritic or tender. They may be localized or generalized, disappear spontaneously, persist, or develop into ulcers. Patients with cutaneous involvement by lymphomatoid granulomatosis exhibit a clinically aggressive course. They have a median survival time of only about 12 months. It is not uncommon for them to die of overt systemic lymphomas (356). Histopathologically, blood vessels in the lower dermis or subcutis are typically surrounded and invaded by a polymorphous infiltrate, including small lymphocytes, plasma cells, histiocytes, a variable number of immunoblasts, and small and large atypical lymphoid cells. Eosinophils may be present. The epidermis and adnexa are generally spared and Pautrier's microaggregates or microabscesses are absent. The subcutis and deep dermis are often more extensively involved than the upper dermis. Cases representing overt angiocentric lymphoma exhibit the histopathologic features of diffuse mixed or large cell lymphoma (Working Formulation) combined with angiocentricity, angioinvasion, and necrosis. Some cases have shown T-cell antigen deficiencies and clonal TCR gene rearrangements similar to other T-cell lymphomas (357), but others have shown evidence of B-cell lymphoma (353). Lymphomatoid granulomatosis can be distinguished histopathologically from MF/SS and LYP by its prominent angiocentricity and relative lack of epidermal and adnexal involvement. The crops of spontaneously resolving lesions that recur without extracutaneous involvement clinically differentiate LYP from lymphomatoid granulomatosis and MF.

CUTANEOUS PSEUDOLYMPHOMAS

The term *cutaneous pseudolymphoma* often causes confusion because it refers to a diverse group of disorders whose only common features are that they mimic true lymphomas and comprise the clinically benign end of a lymphoproliferative continuum having an overt cutaneous lymphoma at its malignant extreme. Often included under this umbrella category are predominantly B-cell disorders such as cutaneous lymphoid hyperplasia, Kimura's disease, angiolymphoid hyperplasia with eosinophilia, and Castleman's disease and T-cell disorders such as pseudo-MF/SS, follicular mucinosis, lymphomatoid contact dermatitis, actinic reticuloid, pityriasis lichenoides, lymphomatoid papulosis, and lymphocytic infiltration of the skin. Table 32.4 contains a classification of these disorders arranged according to the principal lymphoid subset involved, the main microenvironmental localization within the skin, and major associated clinical and laboratory findings. Several of these diseases have been discussed elsewhere in this chapter. The remainder are presented in the following sections.

Cutaneous Lymphoid Hyperplasia

Dense cutaneous lymphoid infiltrates can occur as idiopathic lesions or in response to arthropods (i.e., bites, stings, or infestations), trauma, cowpox vaccinations, herpes zoster, tattoos, antigen injections, or drugs such as phenytoin and antihistamines (104,184,212,358,359). Some cases associated with tick bites are caused by *Borrelia burgdorferi* (360). All of these lesions are referred to generally as *cutaneous lymphoid hyperplasia* (CLH) or *cutaneous lymphocytoma.* The former term is preferred because it is less likely to cause confusion with the term *cutaneous lymphoma.* Cutaneous lymphoid hyperplasia is usually a mixed B-cell and T-cell disorder (104,300,301,308,361), although some cases are composed almost exclusively of T cells (so-called T-cell CLH) (182,362,363).

Patients with CLH typically exhibit one or a few nodules or plaques involving the head or neck (104). Less often, CLH may involve localized areas on the trunk or extremities. Occasionally, it may manifest as generalized papules. *Nodular scabies* is a well-known form of persistent CLH that often has multiple lesions. Histopathologically, there is a dense, diffuse, or patchy lymphoid infiltrate in the dermis, sometimes extending into the subcutis but often diminishing in the deeper dermis. The infiltrate typically spares the epidermis, from which it is separated by a thin Grenz zone (Fig. 32.27). Although often regarded as morphologic evidence of lymphoma, features such as focal epidermal involvement, adnexal infiltration, vascular proliferation or invasion, infil-

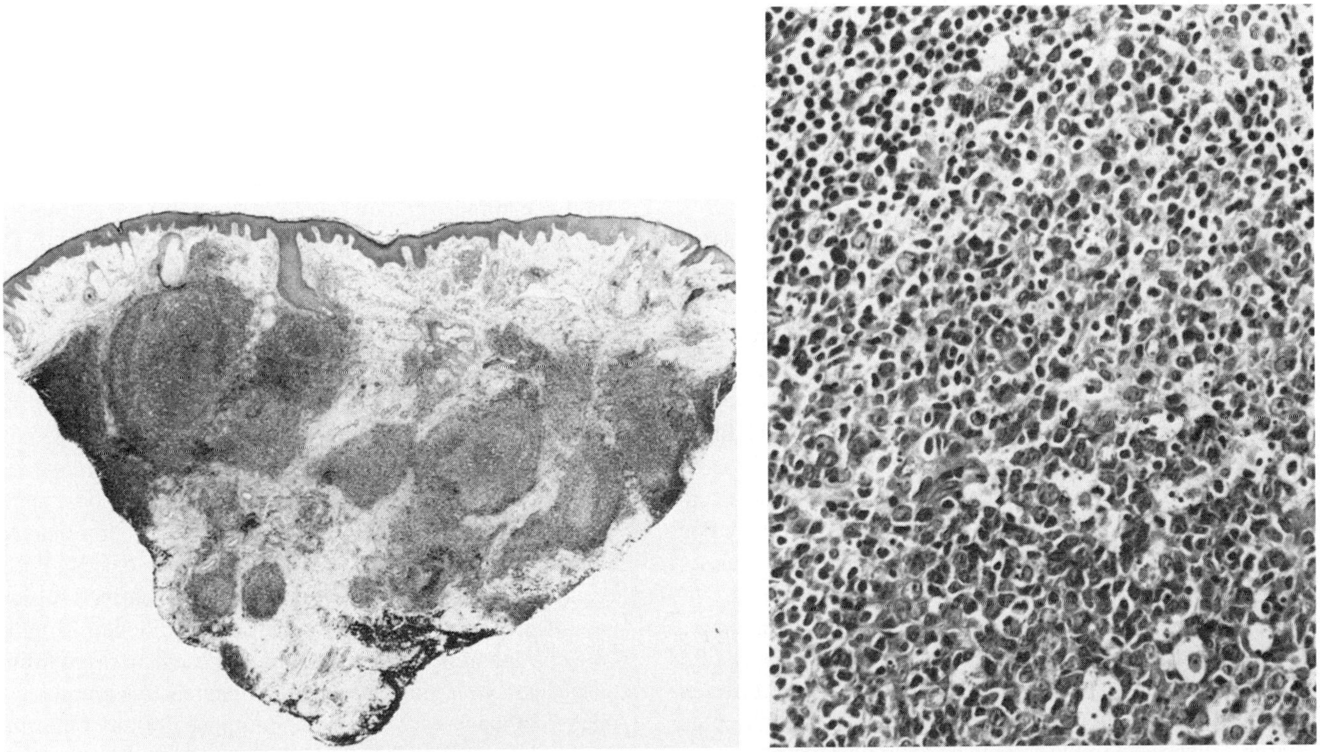

A B

FIG. 32.27. Cutaneous lymphoid hyperplasia. **A:** Scanning magnification reveals a patchy dermal infiltrate that diminishes in the deep dermis. It also spares the epidermis, from which it is separated by an uninvolved Grenz zone. Multiple follicular structures are evident. They contain peripheral mantle zones of small, dark cells. Their centers contain tingible body macrophages that impart a starry-sky pattern even at low magnification (original magnification: 10× magnification). **B:** Higher magnification of one reactive follicle shows its characteristic zonation. At the bottom of the field is the dark zone of the germinal center, which contains noncleaved follicular center cells and tingible body macrophages. In the middle of the field is the light zone of the germinal center, which contains cleaved follicular center cells. At the top of the field is the mantle zone, which contains small mature lymphocytes (original magnification: 400× magnification). Compare with Figure 32.25. (From Medeiros LJ, Picker LJ, Abel EA, et al. Cutaneous lymphoid hyperplasia: immunologic characteristics and assessment of criteria recently proposed as diagnostic of malignant lymphoma. *J Am Acad Dermatol* 1989;21:929–942, with permission.)

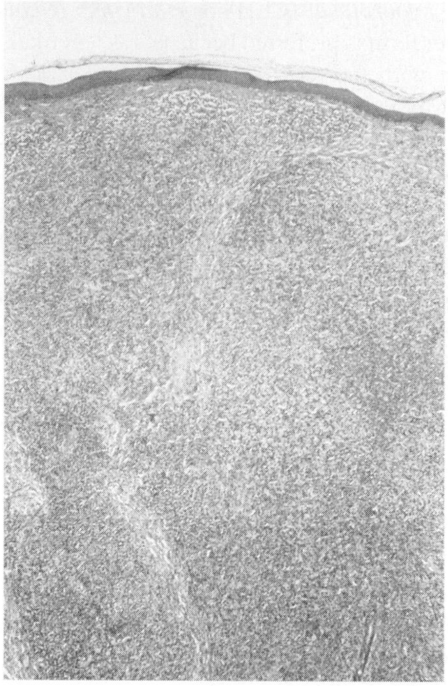

FIG. 32.28. Cutaneous lymphoid hyperplasia, diffuse pattern. This solitary nodule appeared on the neck. There is a narrow Grenz zone with overlying epidermal atrophy and a subjacent dense, diffuse dermal lymphoid infiltrate composed of phenotypically normal B cells, plasma cells, T cells, and histiocytes (original magnification: 40× magnification).

tration of surrounding dermal collagen, and preferential deep dermal involvement can be seen in CLH (104). Cytologically, the infiltrate is composed of mature lymphocytes, often with an admixture of large lymphoid cells and sometimes scattered plasma cells and eosinophils. The recognition of lymphoid follicles in routine sections of many cases has resulted in the subdivision of cases into follicular and diffuse types (Figs. 32.27, 32.28), but at least one half of the so-called diffuse cases also exhibit B-cell follicles when examined immunopathologically (104). This raises doubts concerning the value of making this distinction on the basis of routine histopathology alone. When identifiable, the lymphoid follicles often have well-developed zonation and numerous tingible body macrophages similar to reactive follicles in lymphoid tissues. This can facilitate their differential diagnosis from follicular lymphoma, as can the other features discussed in the section on follicular lymphoma and summarized in Table 32.11 (9,104). Like reactive lymphoid follicles in other tissues, those in CLH are negative for the t(14;18) translocation and associated BCL-2 expression (158,309,313).

The immunophenotypic features of CLH are similar to those of reactive lymphoid hyperplasia in other tissues. B cells are present in most cases, generally as secondary follicles but sometimes as primary follicles, B-cell clusters without a follicular dendritic cell network, or as scattered, individual B cells (Table 32.12). Even in cases with prominent secondary B-cell follicles, there are many T cells ($CD4^+$ more than $CD8^+$) with a normal pattern of pan-T-cell antigen expression. In some cases, CD7 antigen may be moderately deficient. A variable number of macrophages are also present.

In a minority of cases of CLH defined by clinicopathologic and immunophenotypic criteria, molecular biologic analysis of Ig or TCR gene rearrangements has shown evidence of occult lymphoid clones (182,308,361–364). These cases are known as clonal CLH. Some have shown progression to overt B-cell or T-cell lymphoma. These B-cell tumors can involve the same cutaneous site and show the same clonal Ig gene rearrangement as the prior CLH lesion (364) (Fig. 32.29). A study of 10 T-cell–rich CLH cases (five also containing some B cells) documented an occult T-cell clone in one case (362). This patient developed overt non-MF CTCL with subsequent lymph node involvement within 1 year. Another case of the transition from cutaneous T-cell–rich lymphoid hyperplasia to CTCL has also been reported (363). These findings indicate that cutaneous B-cell or T-cell lymphomas can sometimes evolve from preexisting CLH. From a pathogenetic standpoint, these findings support the view that at least some cases of CLH, clonal CLH, and cutaneous lymphomas exist as a lymphoproliferative continuum. Progression across this spectrum can occur, most likely through sequential somatic mutations in the emerging dominant lymphoid clone. CLH patients, especially those harboring occult B-cell or T-cell clones, require long-term follow-up evaluation.

The main differential diagnostic challenge involving CLH is its distinction from primary cutaneous lymphomas, usually of the B-cell type (Table 32.11). The lesions of CLH tend to be small with top-heavy lymphoid infiltrates. Lymphomas tend to form larger lesions that are bottom heavy. The most common types of primary cutaneous B-cell lymphomas are large cell lymphomas, including follicle center large B-cell lymphomas and large B-cell lymphoma of the leg (2). The latter are diffuse and monomorphous, and the former are usually diffuse and composed predominantly of large centrocytic or centroblastic lymphoid cells. Follicle center cell lymphomas that exhibit a well-defined follicular architecture are rare, although subtle follicular structures may be apparent on close scrutiny. These neoplastic follicles have less cytologic heterogeneity than reactive lymphoid follicles. In many cases, they are composed of monomorphous small or large B cells lacking the zonation typical of reactive follicles. Neoplastic B cells are Ig^- or Ig light-chain restricted. The t(14;18) translocation is not useful for differential diagnosis, because CLH and primary cutaneous B-cell lymphomas generally lack it, in contrast to nodal follicle center cell lymphomas. Despite the absence of the t(14;18), large B-cell lymphomas of the legs typically express BCL-2 protein strongly (2,7). Reactive lymphoid follicles can be present in some cutaneous B-cell lymphomas such as the marginal zone and mantle cell types. However, both of these tumors also contain monotypic neoplastic B cells with other

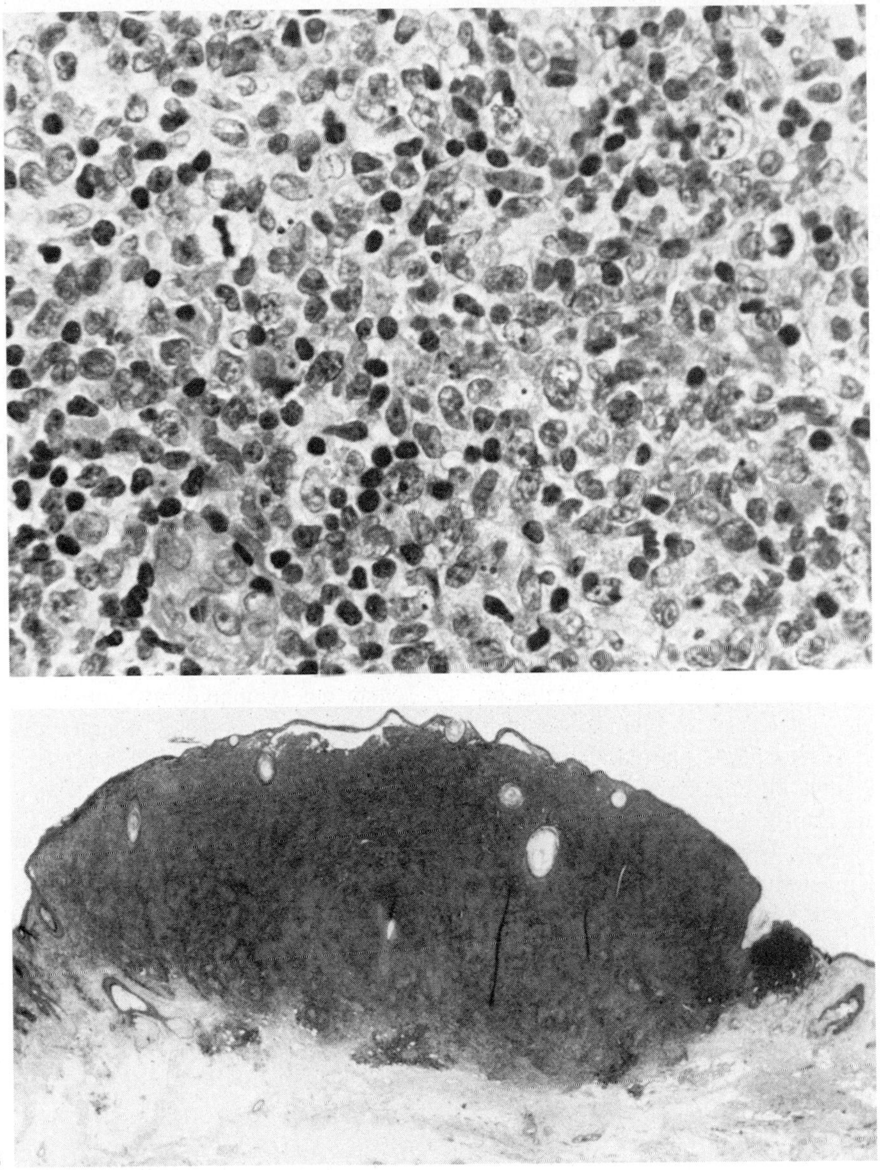

A

B

FIG. 32.29. Cutaneous follicle center B-cell lymphoma that arose from clonal cutaneous lymphoid hyperplasia. **A:** Scanning magnification shows a massive superficial and deep dermal infiltrate with extension into the superficial subcutis (original magnification: 5× magnification). **B:** Higher magnification shows a diffuse infiltrate of large, predominantly noncleaved lymphoid cells admixed with scattered small lymphocytes (original magnification: 480× magnification). This B-cell lymphoma evolved from a preexisting lesion of cutaneous lymphoid hyperplasia involving the same site. It contained a clonal immunoglobulin gene rearrangement identical to that present in an occult fashion within the earlier reactive lesion. (From Wood GS, Ngan B-Y, Tung R, et al. Clonal rearrangements of immunoglobulin genes and progression to B-cell lymphoma in cutaneous lymphoid hyperplasia. *Am J Pathol* 1989;135:13–19, with permission.)

characteristic features. For example, marginal zone lymphoma cells usually show a mix of monocytoid and plasmacytoid types combined with CD11c expression. They often surround smaller reactive lymphoid cells, imparting a ''reverse germinal center'' appearance to nodular aggregates within the lesions. Mantle cell lymphoma cells are usually CD5$^+$ and cyclin D1$^+$, bear the t(11;18) translocation, and almost always involve the skin secondary to known extracutaneous disease. Reactive lymphoid follicles can also be seen in Kimura's disease, angiolymphoid hyperplasia with eosinophilia, Castleman's disease, the inflammatory stage of morphea, inflammatory pseudotumor of the skin (i.e., solitary benign proliferation of myofibroblasts and inflammatory cells) (365), and within the host response to tumors such as basal cell carcinoma.

T-cell CLH must be distinguished from CTCLs. MF/SS exhibits marked epidermotropism and often Pautrier microabscesses, neither of which is typical of T-cell CLH, which may show mild focal epidermal infiltration but frequently has a Grenz zone such as usual CLH. It mainly requires differentiation from non-MF peripheral T-cell lymphomas, which are also nonepidermotropic. These tumors usually exhibit loss of one or more T-cell antigens, may express CD30, and are generally diffuse large cell lymphomas. Small cell or mixed small and medium-sized cell lymphomas are much less common. T-cell CLH may have an admixture of atypical cells (i.e., cerebriform cells and immunoblasts) and histiocytes, but small mature lymphocytes usually predominate.

It is also important to distinguish CLH from other lymphocytic infiltrates, including CLL, deep figurate erythemas, polymorphous light eruption, discoid lupus erythematosus, and Jessner's lymphocytic infiltration of the skin (LIS). These diseases all tend to produce perivascular and sometimes periadnexal lymphoid infiltrates that are much less dense than those typical of CLH. Many have associated clinical or laboratory abnormalities. With the exception of CLL, all are T-cell disorders. CLL is typically a monotypic, $CD5^+$ B-cell disorder with blood and marrow involvement. Cutaneous lymphoid hyperplasia lesions rich in plasma cells require differentiation from those of secondary syphilis, primary cutaneous plasmacytoma, and myeloma. Secondary syphilis lesions are typically richer in plasma cells and histiocytes than in small lymphoid cells, there is epidermal hyperplasia and an interface infiltrate without the Grenz zone typical of CLH, and serology is positive. The plasma cells in plasmacytoma and myeloma are monotypic and often atypical with mitotic figures, immaturity, and multinucleated forms. The broad differential diagnosis of CLH also includes histiocytoses (especially Rosai-Dorfman disease) and small round cell tumors such as Merkel cell carcinoma, oat cell carcinoma, neuroblastoma and Ewing's sarcoma.

Large Cell Lymphocytoma

Caution is warranted about making the diagnosis of CLH when lesions exhibit a diffuse dermal infiltrate of monomorphous small or large lymphoid cells or when lymphoid follicles are composed of monomorphous small or large lymphoid cells. In the first two instances, diffuse small lymphocytic lymphoma and diffuse large cell lymphoma, respectively, must be excluded. In the latter instances, follicular small cleaved cell or large cell lymphoma must be excluded. Diffuse mixed cell lymphomas and follicular mixed cell lymphomas can also present with primary skin involvement (5,8,9,293). Some of these cases in the literature might have been diagnosed *large cell lymphocytoma* (366,367). It has been argued that these cases do not represent true lymphomas because of continued survival throughout the reported follow-up period. However, most of these cases have not been well characterized using immunophenotypic or molecular biologic methods. Many of these patients have never undergone a complete lymphoma staging workup, the available follow-up intervals may be inadequate for low- or intermediate-grade lymphomas, some of these patients have progressed to more extensive skin involvement, and many of those in clinical remission have received definitive treatment such as radiation therapy for lesions that would have been classified as stage IEA if they had been diagnosed as lymphomas. Unequivocal primary cutaneous B-cell lymphomas may remain well localized and exhibit an indolent clinical course (9,293). For these reasons, use of the term *large cell lymphocytoma* is discouraged.

Hydantoin-Associated Pseudolymphoma Syndrome

In most cases of hydantoin-associated pseudolymphoma syndrome, which is caused by anticonvulsant drugs such as phenytoin, the skin is involved only by a generalized pruritic maculopapular eruption, with nonspecific histopathologic features reminiscent of typical hypersensitivity reactions to other drugs (157,158,368). The pseudolymphomatous nature of this syndrome is based more on its extracutaneous features, which include generalized lymphadenopathy, hepatosplenomegaly, fever, arthralgias, and peripheral eosinophilia. Only occasionally does phenytoin result in the dense cutaneous lymphoid infiltrates typical of CLH. The latter may contain aggregates of large cells mimicking lymphoma. Nevertheless, B cells and T cells are polyclonal (158).

Acral Pseudolymphomatous Angiokeratoma of Children

Acral pseudolymphomatous angiokeratoma of children is a rare disorder. It consists of unilateral angiomatous papules involving the extremities (369). These lesions are probably a variant of CLH resulting from arthropod bites. Biopsies show a dense lymphoid infiltrate associated with prominent thickened capillaries, histiocytes, and plasma cells.

Kimura's Disease and Angiolymphoid Hyperplasia with Eosinophilia

There is debate about whether Kimura's disease and ALHE are distinct disorders or part of one clinicopathologic entity, although the weight of evidence favors their distinction (157,370–373). Kimura's disease presents as one or more cutaneous or subcutaneous 1 to 10-cm nodules, usually on the head of a young or middle-aged adult. Peripheral blood eosinophilia and regional reactive lymphadenopathy are characteristic. In the subcutis or dermis, there is a proliferation of small vessels lined by prominent endothelial cells reminiscent of those in the high endothelial venules of lymphoid tissues. There is an associated, typically dense inflammatory infiltrate of lymphocytes, plasma cells, histiocytes, and eosinophils. The latter are usually prominent, but rarely, they may be absent. The cellular infiltrate usually contains multiple secondary lymphoid follicles with well-developed germinal centers, especially in subcutaneous lesions (Fig. 32.30). It is possible that Kimura's disease is essentially a florid, deep-seated variant of CLH.

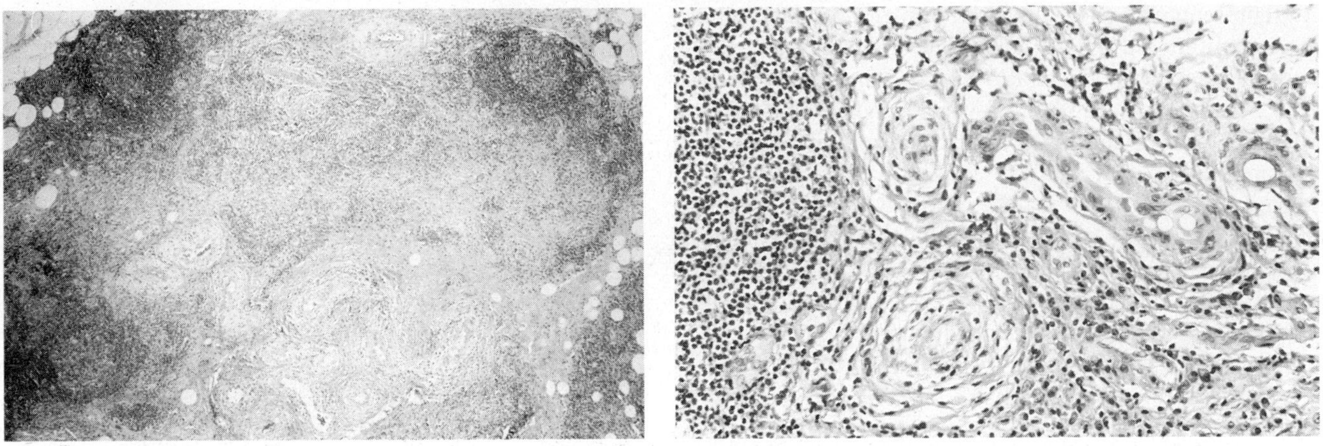

FIG. 32.30. Kimura's disease and angiolymphoid hyperplasia with eosinophilia. **A:** Low-power view shows replacement of subcutaneous adipose tissue by fibrous stroma containing increased blood vessels and several reactive lymphoid follicles (original magnification: 40× magnification). **B:** Higher power shows lymphoid aggregate adjacent to hyperplastic blood vessels lined by plump endothelial cells, some containing vacuolated cytoplasm. The surrounding inflammatory infiltrate is rich in lymphocytes, eosinophils, and plasma cells (original magnification: 200× magnification).

The terms *epithelioid hemangioma* and *pseudopyogenic granuloma* have been used as synonyms for ALHE. Those who favor a separation of ALHE from Kimura's disease regard the former as a malformation of blood vessels resulting from an underlying arteriovenous shunt with the CLH-like features developing as a secondary phenomenon. According to this view, ALHE lesions tend to be smaller, contain a more prominent vascular component manifested as a proliferation of small vessels lined by cells with abundant eosinophilic vacuolated cytoplasm and sometimes atypical nuclei, often show evidence of arteriovenous anastomoses, exhibit less lymphoid infiltration, and contain secondary lymphoid follicles only in a minority of cases.

Castleman's Disease

Also called giant lymph node hyperplasia and angiofollicular lymphoid hyperplasia, Castleman's disease is a lymphoproliferative disorder that usually presents with an isolated mediastinal mass or with multicentric involvement (374–377) (see Chapter 16). Presentation as a solitary tumor in the subcutaneous tissue or skin occurs rarely, and the clinical outcome is favorable. Castleman's disease is sometimes associated with the POEMS syndrome, which consists of polyneuropathy, organomegaly, endocrinopathy, M protein, and skin changes. Elevated levels of lesional and peripheral blood IL-1β and IL-6 have been documented in the multicentric form of the disease, raising speculation that cytokine imbalances may mediate the systemic manifestations of POEMS syndrome (378–380). Kaposi's sarcoma–associated herpesvirus (i.e., human herpesvirus type 8) has been detected in lesions of Castleman's disease arising in HIV-infected patients (381) and in some HIV-negative cases (see Chapter 28). Of the two histopathologic variants of Castleman's disease, the hyaline vascular variant occurs more commonly and consists of small, concentrically whorled lymphoid follicles surrounded by small lymphocytes arrayed in a concentric, onion skin pattern. The interfollicular areas contain a florid proliferation of capillaries. The plasma cell variant occurs more rarely and features large secondary lymphoid follicles separated by a highly vascular interfollicular zone rich in plasma cells. The differential diagnosis of subcutaneous and cutaneous Castleman's disease includes Kimura's disease, ALHE, CLH, follicular forms of cutaneous B-cell lymphoma, plasmacytoma and myeloma. However, these disorders lack the characteristic features of the reactive lymphoid follicles and interfollicular regions seen in the two histopathologic variants of Castleman's disease. Prominent vascular hyperplasia is absent from these diseases, except for Kimura's disease and ALHE, which have their own distinctive endothelial cell characteristics. Plasmacytoma and myeloma exhibit sheets of atypical, monotypic plasma cells and differ from Castleman's disease in their associated clinical findings. Cutaneous lymphoid hyperplasia is typically centered in the dermis, whereas Castleman's disease almost always involves the subcutis rather than the dermis when it occurs in these tissues. Most primary cutaneous B-cell lymphomas are architecturally diffuse rather than follicular. All are Ig^- or monotypic. Those with neoplastic follicles lack the zonation characteristic of the reactive lymphoid follicles seen in Castleman's disease.

Lymphocytic Infiltration of the Skin

LIS, also known as Jessner's lymphocytic infiltrate, presents typically as localized, chronic, asymptomatic papules and plaques, usually located on the face, neck, upper trunk, or arms (157,212,382,383). There is debate about whether

LIS represents a distinct entity or a nonspecific manifestation of other entities such as discoid lupus erythematosus, polymorphous light eruption, or as reported in one case, lymphocytic lymphoma (157,384). However, studies have shown that intradermal T cells in discoid lupus erythematosus usually are Leu-8$^-$, HLA-DR$^+$, and admixed with CD1a$^+$ Langerhans cells, whereas those in LIS are usually Leu-8$^+$, HLA-DR$^-$, and lack a Langerhans cell admixture (385,386). The lesional T cells in LIS are polyclonal (158). Histopathologically, there is a superficial and deep perivascular and periadnexal dermal infiltrate of mature T cells, often with a few macrophages and plasma cells admixed. The epidermis is uninvolved. Lymphoid follicles and eosinophils are not seen. Direct immunofluorescence is negative or nonspecific. The differential diagnosis of LIS includes skin lesions showing superficial and deep perivascular small cell lymphocytic infiltrates. LIS lacks the epidermal alterations and immune deposits typical of discoid lupus erythematosus. The tumid variant of lupus has abundant dermal mucin, which is not seen in LIS, although some mucin may be present. Polymorphous light eruption exhibits papillary dermal edema, whereas LIS does not. Patients with the former are also photosensitive, and observers disagree about whether LIS lesions can ever be photoexacerbated. CLL is a monoclonal B-cell disorder with circulating tumor cells in leukemic individuals. Erythema chronicum migrans is associated with active *Borrelia burgdorferi* infection. This is unusual in LIS. Reticulated erythematous mucinosis favors the trunk, has a reticulated clinical appearance, and contains bipolar fibroblasts. All of these are lacking in LIS. Cutaneous lymphoid hyperplasia contains much denser lymphoid infiltrates than LIS and is richer in B cells that often form reactive follicles. Drug eruptions often contain eosinophils that are absent in LIS. Female carriers of chronic granulomatous disease may develop skin lesions called *arcuate dermal erythema* that are clinicopathologically similar to LIS (387), but they have other distinctive clinical and laboratory features.

OTHER BONE MARROW–DERIVED PROLIFERATIVE DISORDERS INVOLVING THE SKIN

In addition to T-cell lymphomas, B-cell lymphomas, and lymphoid hyperplasias, the skin may be involved by other proliferative disorders of bone marrow–derived cells. These diseases include lymphoid and nonlymphoid leukemias (see Chapters 40, 41, 46, 47, and 49), histiocytosis X, benign non-X histiocytoses, and malignant histiocytosis (see Chapter 51).

Systemic Hodgkin's Disease

Although it is not unusual for patients with systemic Hodgkin's disease to develop various inflammatory skin diseases, specific cutaneous involvement by systemic Hodgkin's disease is an uncommon, often preterminal event found in less than 4% of cases (157,236,388) (see Chapter 17). The lesions appear as nodules, plaques, or large papules that tend to persist and may ulcerate. In rare cases, these cutaneous lesions exhibit a generalized distribution consistent with hematogenous dissemination, but they generally develop by retrograde lymphatic flow from involved regional lymph nodes or by direct spread of disease from an underlying extracutaneous lesion. As such, the skin lesions are often localized or regionalized, persistent, and associated with obvious extracutaneous disease. These features facilitate their clinical differentiation from LYP, which is typically a generalized, spontaneously waxing and waning papular eruption without extracutaneous involvement. Classic LYP can occasionally develop in patients who are in complete remission from Hodgkin's disease and should not be regarded as evidence of Hodgkin's disease relapse.

Histopathologically, cutaneous Hodgkin's disease exhibits a dense dermal or subcutaneous infiltrate including Reed-Sternberg cells or their mononuclear variants, small lymphocytes, plasma cells, eosinophils, macrophages, and sometimes neutrophils. Unlike classic LYP, the infiltrate tends to spare the epidermis. In some cases, it has been possible to subclassify lesions according to the Rye classification, but in many instances this is not possible (157,389). Immunophenotypically the Reed-Sternberg cells and variants are CD30$^+$ and often also CD15$^+$. The T cells are mixed CD4$^+$ and CD8$^+$. The plasma cells and B cells are polytypic and the latter may be organized into lymphoid follicles (389).

Disseminated Dermal Dendrocytoma

Disseminated dermal dendrocytoma is a rare disease that may belong to the broad category of bone marrow–derived proliferative disorders. Lesions manifest as multiple, generalized, firm cutaneous nodules and plaques without evidence of extracutaneous involvement (390). Histopathologically, there is an intradermal proliferation of spindled and nonspindled ''histiocytoid'' cells reminiscent of those seen in cutaneous fibrous histiocytomas (Fig. 32.31). Many of the cells express an antigen profile, including factor XIIIa, which is consistent with that of dermal dendrocytes. These cells are a constituent of normal skin that are believed to function as immune-associated accessory cells. They are increased in a number of cutaneous lesions including Kaposi's sarcoma, dermatofibroma, malignant fibrous histiocytoma, granuloma annulare, and early wound healing reactions. It is uncertain whether disseminated dermal dendrocytoma represents a primary proliferative disorder of dermal dendrocytes or a hyperplasia of these cells secondary to a fibroblastic proliferative disorder, as proposed for macrophages in malignant fibrous histocytomas (391). Other lesions that may be related to disseminated dermal dendrocytoma include giant dermal dendrocytoma of the face (392), dermal dendrocyte hamartoma with stubby white hair (393), and multiple clustered histiocytofibroma (394).

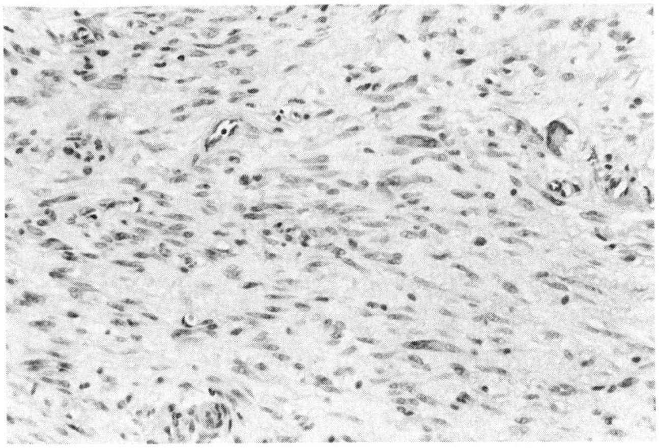

FIG. 32.31. Disseminated dermal dendrocytoma. Intradermal proliferation of spindled and nonspindled cells with a few giant cells set in a fibrous stroma. Approximately one half of the cells expressed factor XIIIa (original magnification: 200× magnification).

SUMMARY AND CONCLUSIONS

Cutaneous lymphoproliferative disorders constitute a diverse array of diseases that can manifest significant differential diagnostic challenges for pathologists and clinicians alike. There has been an explosion of information concerning the lineage and clonality of the lymphoid infiltrates comprising these disorders. This has resulted in an improved understanding of their relation to one another and to lymphoproliferative disorders presenting in extracutaneous sites. It has also resulted in new diagnostic tools. This chapter emphasizes the value of a multiparametric approach to diagnosis that incorporates clinical, microscopic, immunophenotypic, and immunogenotypic data when possible. In some instances, excessive reliance on any one of these without adequate consideration of the others can result in misdiagnosis. In the management of patients with cutaneous lymphoproliferative disorders, immunodiagnostic methods have proven valuable for more accurate diagnosis, staging, and detection of early relapse. As the types of primary cutaneous lymphomas have become better defined, it has become evident that they are often biologically distinct from their primary nodal counterparts and frequently require less aggressive treatment.

REFERENCES

1. Harris NL, Jaffe ES, Stein H, et al. A revised European-American classification of lymphoid neoplasms: a proposal from the International Lymphoma Study Group. *Blood* 1994;84:1361–1392.
2. Willemze R, Kerl H, Sterry W, et al. EORTC classification for primary cutaneous lymphomas: a proposal from the Cutaneous Lymphoma Study Group of the European Organization for Research and Treatment of Cancer. *Blood* 1997;90:354–371.
3. The Non-Hodgkin's Lymphoma Pathologic Classification Project. National Cancer Institute–sponsored study of classifications of non-Hodgkin's lymphomas: summary and description of working formulation for clinical usage. *Cancer* 1982;49:2112–2135.
4. Bos JD. *Skin immune system.* Boca Raton, FL: CRC Press, 1990.
5. Wood GS, Weiss LM, Warnke RA, et al. The immunopathology of cutaneous lymphomas: immunophenotypic and immunogenotypic characteristics. *Semin Dermatol* 1986;5:334–345.
6. Sander C, Kind P, Kaudewitz P, et al. The Revised European-American Classification of Lymphoid Neoplasms (REAL): a new perspective for the classification of cutaneous lymphomas. *J Cutan Pathol* 1997;24:329–341.
7. Burg G, Kempf W, Haeffner A, et al. Cutaneous lymphomas. *Dermatology* 1997;9:137–204.
8. Wood GS, Burke JS, Horning S, et al. The immunologic and clinicopathologic heterogeneity of cutaneous lymphomas other than mycosis fungoides. *Blood* 1983;62:464–472.
9. Garcia CF, Weiss LM, Warnke RA, et al. Cutaneous follicular lymphoma. *Am J Surg Pathol* 1986;10:454–463.
10. Wood GS. Recent advances in the molecular biology of cutaneous lymphomas and related disorders. *Semin Dermatol* 1991;10:172–177.
11. Burke JS. Malignant lymphomas of the skin: their differentiation from lymphoid and nonlymphoid cutaneous infiltrates that simulate lymphoma. *Semin Diagn Pathol* 1985;2:169–181.
12. Wood GS, Dummer R, Haeffner A, et al. Molecular biologic techniques for the diagnosis of CTCL. In: Burg G, Kerl H, Thiers B, eds. *Dermatologic clinics of North America: cutaneous lymphomas.* Philadelphia: WB Saunders, 1994:231–241.
13. Wood GS, Tung RM, Haeffner AC, et al. Detection of clonal T-cell receptor gamma gene rearrangements in early mycosis fungoides/Sezary syndrome by polymerase chain reaction and denaturing gradient gel electrophoresis (PCR/DGGE). *J Invest Dermatol* 1994;103:34–41.
14. Tok J, Mikkola D, Wood GS. A novel assay for analyzing the clonality of T-cell receptor (TCR)-γ gene rearrangements in paraffin embedded tissues. *J Invest Dermatol* 1998;110:577.
15. Sander CA, Kind P, Flaig M, et al. Genotypic analysis in cutaneous lymphoproliferative disease—a reliable test? *J Cutan Pathol* 1998;25:511.
16. Kohler H, Jones CD, Warnke RA, Zehnder JL. Heteroduplex analysis of T-cell receptor γ gene rearrangement on paraffin embedded skin biopsies. *J Cutan Pathol* 1998;25:501.
17. Cossman J, Uppenkamp M, Sundeen J, et al. Molecular genetics and the diagnosis of lymphoma. *Arch Pathol Lab Med* 1988;112:117–127.
18. Cleary ML, Sklar J. Lymphoproliferative disorders in cardiac transplant recipients are multiclonal lymphomas. *Lancet* 1984;2:489–493.
19. Bird J, Galili N, Link M, et al. Continuing rearrangement but absence of somatic hypermutation in immunoglobulin genes of human B-cell precursor leukemia. *J Exp Med* 1988;168:229–245.
20. Santucci M, Pimpinelli N. Cutaneous B-cell lymphoma: a SALT-related tumor? In: Lambert WC, Giannotti B, Van Vloten WA, eds. *Basic mechanisms of physiologic and aberrant lymphoproliferation in the skin.* New York: Plenum Press, 1994:301–315.
21. Kerl H, Cerroni L. Primary B-cell lymphomas of the skin. *Ann Oncol* 1997;2:29–32.
22. Krenacs L, Wellman A, Sorbara L, et al. Cytotoxic cell antigen expression in anaplastic large cell lymphomas of T- and null-cell type and Hodgkin's disease: evidence for distinct cellular origin. *Blood* 1997;89:980–989.
23. Weiss LM, Crabtree GS, Rouse RV, et al. Morphologic and immunologic characterization of 50 peripheral T-cell lymphomas. *Am J Pathol* 1985;188:316–324.
24. Nasu K, Said J, Vonderheid E, et al. Immunopathology of cutaneous T-cell lymphomas. *Am J Pathol* 1985;119:436–447.
25. Grogan TM, Fielder K, Rangel C, et al. Peripheral T-cell lymphoma: aggressive disease with heterogeneous immunotypes. *Am J Clin Pathol* 1985;83:279–288.
26. Lennert K, Kikuchi M, Sato E, et al. HLTV-positive and negative T-cell lymphomas: morphological and immunohistochemical differences between European and HTLV-positive Japanese T-cell lymphomas. *Int J Cancer* 1985;35:65–72.
27. Beljaards RC, Meijer CJ, Scheffer E, et al. Prognostic significance of CD30 (Ki-1/Ber-H2) expression in primary cutaneous large-cell lymphomas of T-cell origin: a clinicopathologic and immunohistochemical study in 20 patients. *Am J Pathol* 1989;135:1169–1178.
28. Smolle J, Ortner R, Ehall R, et al. Cutaneous large cell lymphomas—an immunohistological and morphometrical study. *J Cutan Pathol* 1986;13:463–463.
29. Wood GS, Strickler JG, Deneau DG, et al. Lymphomatoid papulosis

expresses immunophenotypes associated with T cell lymphoma but not inflammation. *J Am Acad Dermatol* 1986;15:444–458.
30. Picker LJ, Weiss LM, Medeiros LJ, et al. Immunophenotypic criteria for the diagnosis of non-Hodgkin's lymphoma. *Am J Pathol* 1987; 128:181–201.
31. Clark DM, Boylston AW, Hall PA, et al. Antibodies to T-cell antigen receptor beta chain families detect monoclonal T-cell proliferation. *Lancet* 1986;2:835–836.
32. Mielke V, Staib G, Boehncke WH, et al. Clonal disease in early cutaneous T-cell lymphoma. *Dermatol Clin* 1994;12:351–360.
33. Jack AS, Boylston AW, Carrel S, et al. Cutaneous T-cell lymphoma cells employ a restricted range of T-cell antigen receptor variable region genes. *Am J Pathol* 1990;136:17–21.
34. Kono DH, Baccala R, Balderas RS, et al. Application of a multiprobe RNase protection assay and junctional sequences to define Vβ gene diversity in Sezary syndrome. *Am J Pathol* 1992;140:823–830.
35. Bahler DW, Berry G, Oksenberg J, et al. Diversity of T-cell antigen receptor variable genes used by mycosis fungoides cells. *Am J Pathol* 1992;140:1–8.
36. Weiss LM, Hu E, Wood GS, et al. Clonal rearrangements of the T cell receptor gene in mycosis fungoides and dermatopathic lymphadenopathy. *N Engl J Med* 1985;313:539–544.
37. Cleary ML, Chao J, Warnke R, et al. Immunoglobulin gene rearrangements as a diagnostic criterion of B-cell lymphoma. *Proc Natl Acad Sci USA* 1984;81:593–597.
38. O'Connor NTJ, Weatherall DJ, Feller AC, et al. Rearrangement of the T-cell–receptor B-chain gene in the diagnosis of lymphoproliferative disorders. *Lancet* 1985;6:1295–1297.
39. Aisenberg AC, Wilkes BM. The genotype and phenotype of T-cell and non-T, non-B acute lymphoblastic leukemia. *Blood* 1985;66: 1215–1218.
40. Pelicci PG, Knowles DM, Favera RD. Lymphoid tumors displaying rearrangements of both immunoglobulin and T-cell receptor genes. *J Exp Med* 1985;162:1015–1024.
41. Minden MD, Mak TW. The structure of the T-cell antigen receptor genes in normal and malignant T-cells. *Blood* 1986;68:327–336.
42. Waldmann TA, Davis MM, Bongiovanni KF, et al. Rearrangements of genes for the antigen receptor on T-cells as markers of lineage and clonality in human lymphoid neoplasms. *N Engl J Med* 1985;313: 776–783.
43. Bertness V, Kirsch I, Hollis G, et al. T-cell receptor gene rearrangements as clinical markers of human T-cell lymphomas. *N Engl J Med* 1985;313:534–538.
44. Ralfkiaer E, O'Connor NTJ, Crick J, et al. Genotypic analysis of cutaneous T-cell lymphomas. *J Invest Dermatol* 1987;88:762–765.
45. Dosaka N, Tanaka T, Fujita M, et al. Southern blotting analysis of clonal rearrangements of T-cell receptor genes in plaque lesions of mycosis fungoides. *J Invest Dermatol* 1989;93:626–629.
46. Zelickson BD, Peters MS, Muller SA, et al. Study of T-cell receptor gene rearrangements in cutaneous T-cell lymphoma, parapsoriasis, benign dermatoses. *J Cutan Pathol* 1989;16:331.
47. Berger C, Lee M, Tien J, et al. Loss of initial clone and emergence of a novel genotype in cutaneous T-cell lymphoma treated with photochemotherapy. *J Invest Dermatol* 1990;94:506.
48. Zelickson B, Thibodeau SN, Peters M, et al. Serial T-cell receptor gene rearrangement analysis in Sezary syndrome. *J Invest Dermatol* 1990;94:594.
49. Bignon, Y-J, Souteyrand P, Roger H, et al. Clonotypic heterogeneity in cutaneous T-cell lymphomas. *Cancer Res* 1990;50:6620–6625.
50. Weiss LM, Wood GS, Ellisen LW, et al. Clonal T cell populations in pityriasis lichenoides et varioliformis acuta (Mucha-Habermann disease). *Am J Pathol* 1987;126:417–421.
51. Griffiths CEM, Nickoloff BJ. Keratinocyte intercellular adhesion molecule-1 (ICAM-1) expression precedes dermal T-lymphocytic infiltration in allergic contact dermatitis (Rhus dermatitis). *Am J Pathol* 1989; 135:1045–1053.
52. Alibert JL. *Description des maladies de la peau. Observees a l'hopital St. Louis et exposition des meilleures methodes suivries pour leur traitement.* Paris: Barrois L'Aine & Fils, 1806;167.
53. Bazin E. *Lecons sur le traitement des maladies chroniques en general affections de la peau en particular par l'emploi compare des eaux minerales de l'hydrotherapie et des moyins pharmaceutiques.* Paris: Adrien Delahaye, 1870;425.
54. Besnier E, Hallopeau H. On the erythroderma of mycosis fungoides. *J Cutan Genitourin Dis* 1892;10:453.
55. Vidal E, Brocq L. Etude sur le mycosis fungoides. *France Med* 1855; 2:946.
56. Sezary A, Bouvrain Y. Erythrodermie avec presence de cellules monstrueuses dans le derme et le sang circulant. *Bull Soc Fr Dermatol Syphil* 1938;45:254–260.
57. Hoppe RT, Wood GS, Abel EA. Mycosis fungoides and the Sezary syndrome: pathology, staging, and treatment. *Curr Probl Cancer* 1990;XIV:295–371.
58. Sausville EA, Eddy JL, Makuch RW, et al. Histopathologic staging at initial diagnosis of mycosis fungoides and the Sezary syndrome: definition of three distinctive prognostic groups. *Ann Intern Med* 1988;109:372–382.
59. Buechner SA, Winklemann RD. Sezary syndrome: a clinicopathologic study of 39 cases. *Arch Dermatol* 1983;119:979–986.
60. Bunn PA, Lamberg SI. Report of the committee on staging and classification of cutaneous T-cell lymphomas. *Cancer Treat Rep* 1979;63: 725–728.
61. Bunn PA, Huberman MS, Whang-Peng J, et al. Prospective evaluation of patients with cutaneous T-cell lymphomas: demonstration of a high frequency of extracutaneous dissemination. *Ann Intern Med* 1980;93: 223–230.
62. Hoppe RT, Cox RS, Fuks Z, et al. Electron-beam therapy for mycosis fungoides: the Stanford University experience. *Cancer Treat Rep* 1979;63:691–700.
63. Hoppe RT, Abel EA, Deneau DG, et al. Mycosis fungoides: management with topical nitrogen mustard. *J Clin Oncol* 1987;5:1796–1803.
64. Huberman M, Bunn PAJ, Matthews MJ, et al. Hepatic involvement in the cutaneous T-cell lymphomas: results of percutaneous biopsy and peritoneoscopy. *Cancer* 1980;45:1683–1688.
65. Graham S, Sharpe R, Steinberg SM, et al. Prognostic implications of a bone marrow histopathologic classification system in mycosis fungoides and the Sezary syndrome. *Cancer* 1993;72:726–734.
66. Rappaport H, Thomas LB. Mycosis fungoides: the pathology of extracutaneous involvement. *Cancer* 1974;34:1198–1229.
67. Dmitrovsky E, Matthews MJ, Bunn PA, et al. Cytologic transformation in cutaneous T-cell lymphoma: a clinicopathologic entity associated with poor prognosis. *J Clin Oncol* 1987;5:208–215.
68. Salhany KE, Cousar JB, Greer JP, et al. Transformation of cutaneous T-cell lymphoma to large cell lymphoma: a clinicopathologic and immunologic study. *Am J Pathol* 1988;132:265–277.
69. Cerroni L, Hodl S, Rieger E, et al. Transformation of mycosis fungoides to large cell lymphoma. *J Cutan Pathol* 1990;17:290.
70. Kim YH, Jensen RA, Watanabe GL, et al. Clinical stage IA (limited patch and plaque) mycosis and fungoides: a long-term outcome analysis. *Arch Dermatol* 1996;132:1309–1313.
71. Kim YH, Bishop K, Varghese A, et al. Prognostic factors in erythrodermic mycosis fungoides and the Sezary syndrome. *Arch Dermatol* 1995;131:1003–1008.
72. Lambert WC, Everett MA. The nosology of parapsoriasis. *J Am Acad Dermatol* 1981;5:373–395.
73. Wood GS, Hu CH. Parapsoriasis. In: Freedberg IM, Eisen AZ, Wolff K, et al, eds. *Dermatology in general medicine.* New York: McGraw-Hill, 1998.
74. Kadin ME. Common activated helper-T-cell origin for lymphomatoid papulosis, mycosis fungoides, and some types of Hodgkin's disease. *Lancet* 1985;2:864–865.
75. Liu YC, Tomashefski JF, Cleveland RP, et al. Composite cutaneous T-cell lymphoma and small B-cell lymphocytic lymphoma: morphologic, immunologic, and molecular genetic documentation of concurrent lymph node involvement. *Mod Pathol* 1994;7:641–646.
76. Lutzner MA, Emerit I, Durepaire R, et al. Cytogenetic, cytophotometric and ultrastructural study of large cerebriform cells of the Sezary syndrome and description of a small cell variant. *J Natl Cancer Inst* 1973;50:1145–1162.
77. Guccion JG, Fischmann AB, Bunn PA, et al. Ultrastructural appearance of cutaneous T-cell lymphomas in skin, lymph nodes and peripheral blood. *Cancer Treat Rep* 1979;63:565–570.
78. Meijer CJL, Van der Loo EM, Van Vloten WA, et al. Early diagnosis of mycosis fungoides and Sezary syndrome by morphometric analysis of lymphoid cells in the skin. *Cancer* 1981;45:2864–2871.
79. McNutt N, Crain WR. Quantitative electron microscopic comparison

of lymphocyte nuclear contour in mycosis fungoides and benign infiltrates in skin. *Cancer* 1981;47:698–709.
80. Willemze R, Cornelisse CJ, Hermans J, et al. Quantitative electron microscopy in the early diagnosis of cutaneous T-cell lymphomas: a long-term follow-up study of 77 patients. *Am J Pathol* 1986;123:166–173.
81. Fletcher V, Zackheim HS, Beckstead JH. Circulating Sezary cells: a new preparatory method for their identification and enumeration. *Arch Pathol Lab Med* 1984;108:954–958.
82. Erkman-Balis B, Rappaport H. Cytogenetic studies in mycosis fungoides. *Cancer* 1974;34:626–633.
83. Edelson RL, Berger CL, Raafat J, et al. Karyotype studies of cutaneous T-cell lymphoma: evidence for a clonal origin. *J Invest Dermatol* 1979;73:548–550.
84. Whang-Peng J, Bunn P, Knutson T, et al. Cytogenetic abnormalities in patients with cutaneous T-cell lymphomas. *Cancer Treat Rep* 1979;63:575–580.
85. Karenko L, Hyytinen E, Sarna S, et al. Chromosomal abnormalities in cutaneous T-cell lymphoma and in its premalignant conditions as detected by G-banding and interphase cytogenetic methods. *J Invest Dermatol* 1997;108:22–29.
86. Koduru PRK, Filippa DA, Richardson ME, et al. Genetic and histologic correlations in malignant lymphoma. *Blood* 1987;69:97–102.
87. Raimondi SC, Pui C, Behm FG, et al. Translocations in childhood T-cell leukemia: cytogenetic evidence for involvement of the T-cell receptor β-chain gene. *Blood* 1987;69:131–134.
88. Kaltoft K, Holm-Hansen B, Thestrup-Pedersen K. Cytogenetic findings in cell lines from cutaneous T-cell lymphoma. *Dermatol Clin* 1994;12:295–304.
89. Sentis HJ, Willemze R, Scheffer E. Histopathologic studies in Sezary syndrome and erythrodermic mycosis fungoides: a comparison with benign forms of erythroderma. *J Am Acad Dermatol* 1986;15:1217–1226.
90. Van Vloten WA, Schaberg A, Van der Ploeg M. Cytophotometric studies on mycosis fungoides and other cutaneous reticuloses. *Bull Cancer* 1977;64:249–258.
91. Van Vloten WA, Scheffer E, Meijer CJLM. DNA cytophotometry of lymph node imprints from patients with mycosis fungoides. *J Invest Dermatol* 1979;73:275–277.
92. Wood GS, Deneau D, Miller R, et al. Subtypes of cutaneous T cell lymphoma (CTCL) defined by expression of Leu-1 and Ia. *Blood* 1982;59:876–882.
93. Vonderheid EC, Tan E, Sobel EL, et al. Clinical implications of immunologic phenotyping in cutaneous T-cell lymphoma. *J Am Acad Dermatol* 1987;17:40–52.
94. Ralfkiaer E, Wantzin GL, Mason DY, et al. Phenotypic characterization of lymphocyte subsets in mycosis fungoides. *Am J Clin Pathol* 1985;84:610–619.
95. Van der Putte SCJ, Toonstra J, Van Wichen DF, et al. Aberrant immunophenotypes in mycosis fungoides. *Arch Dermatol* 1988;124:373–380.
96. Agnarsson BA, Vonderheid EC, Kadin ME. Cutaneous T-cell lymphoma with suppressor/cytotoxic (CD8) phenotype: identification of rapidly progressive and chronic subtypes. *J Am Acad Dermatol* 1990;22:569–577.
97. Heald P, Yan SL, Edelson RL, et al. Selective lymphocyte homing mechanisms in the pathogenesis of leukemia cutaneous T-cell lymphoma. *J Invest Dermatol* 1993;101:222–226.
98. Michie SA, Abel EA, Hoppe RT, et al. Expression of T-cell receptor antigens in mycosis fungoides and inflammatory skin lesions. *J Invest Dermatol* 1989;93:116–120.
99. Michie SA, Abel EA, Hoppe RT, et al. Discordant expression of antigens between intraepidermal and intradermal T-cells in mycosis fungoides. *Am J Pathol* 1990;137:1447–1451.
100. Wood GS, Abel EA, Hoppe RT, et al. Leu-8 and Leu-9 antigen phenotypes: immunologic criteria for the distinction of mycosis fungoides from cutaneous inflammation. *J Am Acad Dermatol* 1986;14:1006–1013.
101. Weiss LM, Wood GS, Warnke RA. Immunophenotypic differences between dermatopathic lymphadenopathy and lymph node involvement in mycosis fungoides. *Am J Pathol* 1985;120:179–180.
102. Bergman R, Faclieru D, Sahar D, et al. Immunophenotyping and T-cell receptor γ gene rearrangement analysis as a adjunct to the histopathologic diagnosis of mycosis fungoides. *J Am Acad Dermatol* 1998;39:554–559.
103. Smoller BR, Bishop K, Glusac E, et al. Reassessment of histologic parameters in the diagnosis of mycosis fungoides. *Am J Surg Pathol* 1995;19:1423–1430.
104. Medeiros LJ, Picker LJ, Abel EA, et al. Cutaneous lymphoid hyperplasia: Immunologic characteristics and assessment of criteria recently proposed as diagnostic of malignant lymphoma. *J Am Acad Dermatol* 1989;21:929–942.
105. Wood GS, Hong SR, Sasaki DT, et al. Leu8/Leu9 antigen expression by Leu4 T cells: comparative analysis of skin and blood in mycosis fungoides/Sezary syndrome relative to normal blood values. *J Am Acad Dermatol* 1990;22:602–607.
106. Dietz SB, Jensen PJ, Murphy GF, et al. The role of $\alpha_E\beta_7$ integrin (CD103) and E-cadherin in epidermotropism in cutaneous T-cell lymphoma (CTCL). *Abstracts* 1995;104:665.
107. Tensen CP, Vermeer MH, van der Stoop PM, et al. Epidermal interferon-γ inducible protein-10 (IP-10) and monokine induced by γ-interferon (MIG) but not IL-8 mRNA expression is associated with epidermotropism in cutaneous T cell lymphomas. *J Invest Dermatol* 1998;111:222–226.
108. Orteu CH, Li W, Allen MH, et al. CD44 variant expression in cutaneous T-cell lymphoma. *J Cutan Pathol* 1997;24:342–349.
109. Miyazawa M, Takahashi S, Kawaguchi H, et al. Low expression of adhesion molecules in a case of cutaneous T-cell lymphoma. *J Dermatol* 1995;22:659–664.
110. Sterry W, Mielke V, Konter U, et al. Role of beta 1-integrins in epidermotropism of malignant T cells. *Am J Pathol* 1992;141:855–860.
111. Nickoloff BJ, Griffiths CEM. Intraepidermal but not dermal T-lymphocytes are positive for a cell-cycle–associated antigen (Ki-67) in mycosis fungoides. *Am J Pathol* 1990;136:261–266.
112. Michie SA, Wood GS. Unpublished data, 1989.
113. Dummer R, Michie SA, Kell D, et al. Expression of BCL-2 protein and Ki-67 nuclear proliferation antigen in benign and malignant cutaneous T-cell infiltrates. *J Cutan Pathol* 1995;22:11–17.
114. Meech S, Ricketts K, Walsh P, et al. Failure of Fas mediated activation induced cell death in Sezary cells derived from a patient with Sezary syndrome. *J Invest Dermatol* 1999;112:626.
115. Maloney DG, Wood GS. Unpublished data, 1989.
116. Rook AH, Vowels BR, Jaworsky C, et al. The immunopathogenesis of cutaneous T-cell lymphoma: abnormal cytokine production by Sezary T cells. *Arch Dermatol* 1993;129:486–489.
117. Fivenson DP, Schaffer J, Saed G, et al. Absence of HTLV-I genomic determinants in canine mycosis fungoides. *Arch Dermatol* 1996;132:841–842.
118. Bakels V, van Oostveen JW, Gordijn RJL, et al. Diagnostic value of T-cell receptor β gene rearrangement analysis on peripheral blood lymphocytes of patients with erythroderma. *J Invest Dermatol* 1991;97:782.
119. Weinberg JM, Jaworsky C, Benoit BM, et al. The clonal nature of circulating Sezary cells. *Blood* 1995;86:4257–4262.
120. Moss P, Gillespie G, Frodsham P, et al. Clonal populations of $CD4^+$ and $CD8^+$ T cells in patients with multiple myeloma and paraproteinemia. *Blood* 1996;87:3297–3306.
121. Theodorou I, Delfau-Larue MH, Bigorgne C, et al. Cutaneous T-cell infiltrates: analysis of T-cell receptor-γ gene rearrangement by polymerase chain reaction and denaturing gradient gel electrophoresis. *Blood* 1995;86:305–310.
122. Muche JM, Lukowsky A, Asadullah K, et al. Demonstration of frequent occurrence of clonal T cells in the peripheral blood of patients with primary cutaneous T-cell lymphoma. *Blood* 1997;90:1636–1642.
123. Wood GS. Molecular biologic techniques for the diagnosis of cutaneous lymphomas. In: Barnhill R, ed. *Textbook of dermatopathology*. New York: McGraw-Hill, 1998;864–869.
124. Lessin SR, Rook AH, Rovera G. Molecular diagnosis of cutaneous T-cell lymphoma: polymerase chain reaction amplification of T-cell antigen receptor β-chain gene rearrangements. *J Invest Dermatol* 1991;96:299–302.
125. Bourguin A, Tung R, Galili N, et al. Rapid, non-radioactive detection of clonal T-cell receptor gene rearrangements in lymphoid neoplasms. *Proc Natl Acad Sci USA* 1990;87:8536–8540.
126. Volkenandt M, Soyer HP, Kerl H, et al. Development of a highly

specific and sensitive molecular probe for detection of cutaneous lymphoma. *J Invest Dermatol* 1991;97:137–140.
127. van Oostveen JW, Bakels V, Meijer CJLM, et al. Comparison of Southern blot and PCR/DGGE T-cell receptor gene rearrangement analysis in the diagnosis of cutaneous T-lymphoma. *J Invest Dermatol* 1993;100:448.
128. Staib G, Mielke V, Griesser H, et al. PCR analysis of T-cell-receptor (TCR)-γ genes to differentiate between malignant and reactive T-cell infiltrates of the skin. *J Invest Dermatol* 1993;100:458.
129. Bachelez H, Bioul L, Flageul B, et al. Detection of clonal T-cell receptor γ gene rearrangements with the use of the polymerase chain reaction in cutaneous lesions of mycosis fungoides and Sezary syndrome. *Arch Dermatol* 1995;131:1027–1031.
130. Tok J, Szabolcs MJ, Silvens DN, et al. Detection of clonal T-cell receptor γ gene rearrangement by polymerase chain reaction and dematuring gradient gel electrophoresis (PCR/DGGE) in archival specimens from patients with early cutaneous T-cell lymphoma: correlation of histologic findings with PCR/DGGE. *J Am Acad Dermatol* 1998; 38:453–460.
131. Ashton-Key M, Diss TC, Du MQ, et al. The value of the polymerase chain reaction in the diagnosis of cutaneous T-cell infiltrates. *Am J Surg Pathol* 1997;21:743–747.
132. Gellrich S, Lukowsky A, Rutz S, et al. Clonally expanded T lymphocytes in mycosis fungoides detected by micromanipulation and single-cell PCR. *J Invest Dermatol* 1999;112:631–631.
133. Veelken H, Wood GS, Sklar J. Molecular staging of cutaneous T cell lymphoma: evidence for systemic involvement in early disease. *J Invest Dermatol* 1995;104:889–894.
134. Wood GS. Lymphocyte activation in cutaneous T-cell Lymphoma. *J Invest Dermatol* 1995;105:105S-109S.
135. Veelken H, Sklar JL, Wood GS. Detection of low-level tumor cell trafficking to allergic contact dermatitis induced by mechlorethamine in patients with mycosis fungoides. *J Invest Dermatol* 1996;106: 685–688.
136. Li G, Rook AH, Lessin SR. The arteriolymphatic circulation of cutaneous T-cell lymphoma (CTCL). *J Invest Dermatol* 1997;108:636.
137. Kern DE, Kidd PG, Moe R, et al. T cell receptor gene rearrangement analysis from lymph nodes of patients with mycosis fungoides: prognostic implications. *Arch Dermatol* 1998;134:158–164.
138. Lynch JW, Linoilla I, Sausville EA, et al. Prognostic implications of evaluation for lymph node involvement by T-cell antigen gene rearrangement in mycosis fungoides. *Blood* 1992;79:3293–3299.
139. Bakels V, van Oostveen JW, Geerts ML, et al. Diagnostic and prognostic significance of clonal T-cell receptor beta gene rearragements in lymph nodes of patient with mycosis fungoides. *J Pathol* 1993; 170:249–255.
140. Wood GS. Using molecular biological analysis of T-cell receptor gene rearrangements to stage cutaneous T-cell lymphoma. *Arch Dermatol* 1998;134:221–223.
141. Wolfe JT, Chooback L, Finn DT, et al. Large cell transformation following detection of minimal residual disease in cutaneous T-cell lymphoma: molecular and in situ analysis of a single neoplastic T-cell clone expression the identical T-cell receptor. *J Clin Oncol* 1995; 13:1751–1757.
142. Haycox C, Juarez T, Sabath DE, et al. Analysis of t-cell receptor gene rearrangement for predicting clinical outcome inpatients with mycosis fungoides: a comparison of Southern blot and polymerase chain reaction methods. *J Invest Dermatol* 1999;112:617.
143. McGregor JM, Crook T, Fraser-Andrews EA, et al. Spectrum of p53 gene mutations suggests a possible role for ultraviolet radiation in the pathogenesis of advanced cutaneous lymphomas. *J Invest Dermatol* 1999;112:317.
144. Lessin SR, Benoit BM, Jaworsky C, et al. Skin as a reservoir of minimal residual disease in cutaneous T cell lymphoma after complete clinical response to biological response modifier therapy. *J Invest Dermatol* 1993;100:507.
145. Delfau-Larue MH, Dalac S, Lepage E, et al. Prognostic significance of a PCR-detectable dominant T-lymphocyte clone in cutaneous lesions of patients with mycosis fungoides. *Blood* 1998;92:3376–3380.
146. Lindae ML, Abel EA, Hoppe RT, et al. Poikilodermatous mycosis fungoides and atrophic large plaque parapsoriasis exhibit similar abnormalities of T-cell antigen expression. *Arch Dermatol* 1988;124: 366–372.
147. Nickoloff BJ, Wood C. Benign idiopathic versus mycosis-fungoides–associated follicular mucinosis. *Pediatr Dermatol* 1985;2: 201–226.
148. Flaig M, Kind P, Kaudewitz P, et al. Folliculocentric mycosis fungoides. *J Cutan Pathol* 1998;25:494.
149. LeBoit PE, Zackheim HS, White CRJ. Granulomatous variants of cutaneous T-cell lymphoma: the histopathology of granulomatous mycosis fungoides and granulomatous slack skin. *Am J Surg Pathol* 1988; 12:83–95.
150. Clendenning WE, Rappaport H. Report on the committee on pathology of cutaneous T-cell lymphomas. *Cancer Treat Rep* 1979;63: 719–724.
151. Scheffer E, Meijer CJL, van Vloten WA. Dermatopathic lymphadenopathy and lymph node involvement in mycosis fungoides. *Cancer* 1980;45:137–148.
152. Sausville EA, Worsham GF, Matthews MJ, et al. Histologic assessment of the lymph nodes in mycosis fungoides/Sezary syndrome (cutaneous T-cell lymphoma): clinical correlation and prognostic import of a new classification system. *Hum Pathol* 1985;16:1098–1109.
153. Colby TV, Burke JS, Hoppe RT. Lymph node biopsies in mycosis fungoides. *Cancer* 1981;47:351–359.
154. Burke JS, Colby TV. Dermatopathic lymphadenopathy: comparison of cases associated and unassociated with mycosis fungoides. *Am J Surg Pathol* 1981;5:343–352.
155. Cooper RA, Dawson PJ, Rambo ON. Dermatopathic lymphadenopathy: a clinicopathologic analysis of lymph node biopsies over a 15 year period. *Calif Med* 1967;106:170–175.
156. Pinkus H. Alopecia mucinosa. *Arch Dermatol* 1957;76:419.
157. Lever WF, Lever GS. *Histopathology of the skin*, 7th ed. Philadelphia: JB Lippincott, 1990.
158. Weinberg JM, Rook AH, Lessin SR. Molecular diagnosis of lymphocytic infiltrates of the skin. *Arch Dermatol* 1993;129:1491–1491.
159. Stewart M, Smoller BR. Follicular mucinosis (FM) in a patient with Hodgkin's disease (HD): a poor prognostic sign? *Cutan Pathol* 1990; 17:320.
160. Mehregan DA, Gibson LE, Muller SA. Follicular mucinosis: histopathologic review of 33 cases. *Mayo Clin Proc* 1991;66:387.
161. LeBoit PE, Abel EA, Cleary ML, et al. Clonal rearrangement of the T-cell receptor beta gene in the circulating lymphocytes of erythrodermic follicular mucinosis. *Blood* 1988;71:1329.
162. Zelickson B, Peters MS, Muller SA, et al. T-cell receptor gene rearrangement analysis: cutaneous T-cell lymphoma, peripheral T-cell lymphoma, and premalignant and benign cutaneous lymphoproliferative disorders. *J Am Acad Dermatol* 1991;25:787.
163. Vakilzadeh F, Brocker EB. Syringoloymphoid hyperplasia with alopecia. *Br J Dermatol* 1984;110:95–101.
164. Burg G, Schmoeckel C. Syringolymphoid hyperplasia with alopecia: a syringotropic cutaneous T-cell lymphoma? *Dermatology* 1992;184: 306–307.
165. Zelger B, Sepp N, Weyrer K, et al. Syringotropic cutaneous T-cell lymphoma: a variant of mycosis fungoides? *Br J Dermatol* 1994;130: 765–769.
166. Deneau DG, Wood GS, Beckstead JH, et al. Woringer-Kolopp disease (pagetoid reticulosis): four cases with histopathologic, ultrastructural, and immunohistologic observations. *Arch Dermatol* 1984;120: 1045–1051.
167. Wood GS, Weiss LM, Hu CH, et al. T-cell antigen deficiencies and clonal T-cell receptor gene rearrangements in pagetoid reticulosis (Woringer-Kolopp disease). *N Engl J Med* 1988;318:164–167.
168. Haghighi B, Smoller BR, LeBoit P, et al. Woringer-Kolopp disease: an immunophenotypic and clinicopathologic study with long term follow-up. *J Cutan Pathol* 1998. 25:497.
169. Burns MK, Chan LS, Cooper KD. Woringer-Kolopp disease (localized pagetoid reticulosis) or unilesional mycosis fungoides? *Arch Dermatol* 1995;131:325.
170. Yagi H, Hagiwara T, Shirahama S, et al. Disseminated pagetoid reticulosis: need for long-term follow-up. *J Am Acad Dermatol* 1994;30: 345–349.
171. Degreef H, Holvoet C, van Vloten WA, et al. Woringer-Kolopp disease: an epidermotropic variant of mycosis fungoides. *Cancer* 1976; 38:2154–2165.
172. Tan RS, MacLeod TI, Dean SG. Pagetoid reticulosis, epidermotropic mycosis fungoides and mycosis fungoides: a disease spectrum. *Br J Dermatol* 1987;116:67–77.

173. Ralfkiaer E, Thomsen K, Agdal N, et al. The development of a Ki-1–positive large cell non-Hodgkins's lymphoma in pagetoid reticulosis. *Acta Derm Venereol* 1989;69:206–211.
174. Berti E, Cerri A, Cavicchini S, et al. Primary cutaneous gamma/delta T-cell lymphoma presenting as disseminated pagetoid reticulosis. *J Invest Dermatol* 1991;96:718–723.
175. LeBoit PE, Beckstead JH, Bond B, et al. Granulomatous slack skin: clonal rearrangement of the T-cell receptor gene is evidence for the lymphoproliferative nature of a cutaneous elastolytic disorder. *J Invest Dermatol* 1987;89:183–186.
176. Helm KF, Cerio R, Winkelmann RK. Granulomatous slack skin: an immunohistochemical study of three cases. *J Cutan Pathol* 1990;12: 299.
177. LeBoit PE. Granulomatous slack of skin. *Dermatol Clin* 1994;12: 375–389.
178. Ackerman AB, Troy JL, Rosen LB, et al. *Differential diagnosis in dermatopathology II*. Philadelphia: Lea and Febiger, 1988;66–69.
179. Guitart J, Fretzin D. Skin as the primary site of Hodgkin's disease: a case report of primary cutaneous Hodgkin's disease and review of its relationships with non-Hodgkin's lymphoma. *Am J Dermatopathol* 1998;20:218–222.
180. Shapiro PE, Pinto FJ. The histologic spectrum of mycosis fungoides/ Sezary syndrome (cutaneous T-cell lymphoma). *Am J Surg Pathol* 1994;18:645–667.
181. Nickoloff BJ. Light-microscopic assessment of 100 patients with patch/plaque stage mycosis fungoides. *Am J Dermatopathol* 1988;10: 469–477.
182. Rijlaarsdam JU, Scheffer C, Meijer CJ, et al. Cutaneous pseudo-T-cell lymphomas: a clinicopathologic study of 20 patients. *Cancer* 1992;69: 717.
183. D'Incan M, Souteyrand P, Bignon YJ, et al. Hydantoin-induced cutaneous pseudolymphoma with clinical pathologic, and immunologic aspects of Sezary syndrome. *Arch Dermatol* 1992;128:1371.
184. Magro CM, Crowson AN. Drugs with antihistaminic properties as a cause of atypical cutaneous lymphoid hyperplasia. *J Am Acad Dermatol* 1995;32:419.
185. Gibney MD. Cutaneous eruption of lymphocyte recovery mimicking mycosis fungoides in a patient with acute myelocytic leukemia. *J Cutan Pathol* 1995;22:472.
186. Metzman MS. A clinical and histologic mycosis fungoides simulant occurring as a T-cell infiltrate coexisting with B-cell leukemia cutis. *J Am Acad Dermatol* 1995;33:341.
187. Gordon KB, Guitart J, Kuzel T, et al. Pseudo-mycosis fungoides in a patient taking clonazepam and fluoxetine. *J Am Acad Dermatol* 1996;34:304.
188. Magro CM, Crowson AN, Schapiro BL. The interstitial granulomatous drug reaction: a distinctive clinical and pathological entity. *J Cutan Pathol* 1998;25:72–78.
189. Sanchez JL, Ackerman AB. The patch stage of mycosis fungoides: criteria for histologic diagnosis. *Am J Dermatopathol* 1979;1:5–26.
190. Haeffner AC, Smoller BR, Zepter K, et al. Differentiation and clonality of lesional lymphocytes in small plaque parapsoriasis. *Arch Dermatol* 1995;131:321–324.
191. Siddiqui J, Hardman DL, Misra M, et al. Clonal dermatitis: a potential precursor of CTCL with varied clinical manifestations. *J Invest Dermatol* 1997;108:584.
192. Orbaneja G, Diez LI, Lozano JL, et al. Lymphomatoid contact dermatitis. *Contact Dermatitis* 1976;2:139.
193. Ackerman AB, Breza TS, Capland L. Spongiotic stimulants of mycosis fungoides. *Arch Dermatol* 1974;109:218.
194. Toonstra J, Henquet CJM, Weelden HV, et al. Actinic reticuloid: a clinical, photobiologic, histopathologic, and follow-up study of 16 patients. *J Am Acad Dermatol* 1989;21:205–214.
195. Ive FA, Magnus IA, Warin RP, et al. "Actinic reticuloid": a chronic dermatosis associated with severe photosensitivity and the histologic resemblance to lymphoma. *Br J Dermatol* 1969;81:469.
196. Gonzalez E, Gonzales S. Drug photosensitivity, idiopathic photodermatoses, and sunscreens. *J Am Acad Dermatol* 1996;35:871.
197. Lim HW, Buchness MR, Ashinoff R, Soter NA. Chronic actinic dermatitis. *Arch Dermatol* 1990;126:317.
198. Chu AC, Robinson D, Hawk JLM, et al. Immunologic differentiation of the Sezary syndrome due to cutaneous T-cell lymphoma and chronic actinic dermatitis. *J Invest Dermatol* 1986;86:134–137.
199. Ralfkiaer E, Lange WG, Stein H, et al. Photosensitive dermatitis with actinic reticuloid syndrome: an immunohistological study of the cutaneous infiltrate. *Br J Dermatol* 1986;114:47–56.
200. Bakels V, van Oostveen JW, Preesman AH, et al. Differentiation between actinic reticuloid and cutaneous T cell lymphoma by T cell receptor gamma gene rearrangement analysis and immunophenotyping. *J Clin Pathol* 1998;51:154–158.
201. Rietschel R. Chronic actinic dermatitis and sesquiterpene lactone sensitivity. *J Watch Dermatol* 1997;5:105.
202. Ashinoff R. Lymphoma in a black patient with actinic reticuloid treated with PUVA: possible etiologic considerations. *J Am Acad Dermatol* 1989;21:1134.
203. Suchi T, Lennert K, Tu LY, et al. Histopathology and immunochemistry of peripheral T-cell lymphomas: a proposal for their classification. *J Clin Pathol* 1987;40:995–1015.
204. Wood GS, Hoppe RT, Warnke RA, et al. Evidence that mycosis fungoides and transformed MF arise from the same T-cell clone. *J Cutan Pathol* 1998;18:397.
205. Stefanato CM, Tallini G, Crotty P. Histologic and immunophenotypic features prior to transformation in patients with transformed cutaneous T-cell lymphoma: is CD25 expression in skin biopsy samples predictive of large cell transformation in cutaneous T-cell lymphoma? *Am J Dermatopathol* 1998;20:1–6.
206. Li G, Chooback L, Wolfe JT, et al. Overexpression of p53 protein in cutaneous T-cell lymphoma: relationship to large cell transformation and disease progression. *J Invest Dermatol* 1998;110:767–770.
207. Ackerman AB. *Histologic diagnosis of inflammatory skin diseases*. Philadelphia: Lea and Febiger, 1978.
208. Wood GS, Strickler JG, Abel EA, et al. The immunohistology of pityriasis lichenoides et varioliformis acuta and pityriasis lichenoides chronica: evidence for their interrelationship with lymphomatoid papulosis. *J Am Acad Dermatol* 1987;16:559–570.
209. Black MM. Lymphomatoid papulosis and pityriasis lichenoides: are they related? *Br J Dermatol* 1982;106:717–721.
210. Kerl H, Ackerman AB. Cutaneous pseudolymphomas. In: Fitzpatrick TB, eds. *Dermatology in general medicine,* 3rd ed. New York: McGraw-Hill, 1987;1118–1130.
211. LeBoit P. Lymphomatoid papulosis and cutaneous $CD30^+$ lymphoma. *Am J Dermatopathol* 1996;18:221–235.
212. Wood GS. Inflammatory diseases that simulate lymphomas: cutaneous pseudolymphomas. In: Freedberg IM, Eisen AZ, Wolff K, et al, eds. *Dermatology in general medicine*. New York: McGraw-Hill, 1998.
213. Fortson JS, Schroeter AL, Esterley NB. Cutaneous T-cell lymphoma (parapsoriasis en plaque): an association with pityriasis lichenoides et varioliformis acuta in young children. *Arch Dermatol* 1990;126: 1449–1453.
214. Muhlbauer JE, Bhan AK, Harrist TJ, et al. Immunopathology of pityriasis lichenoides acuta. *J Am Acad Dermatol* 1984;10:783–795.
215. Shieh S, Mikkola D, Wood GS. Differentiation and clonality of lesional lymphocytes in pityriasis lichenoides chronica. *J Invest Derm* 2000;114:833.
216. Parks JD, Synovec MS, Masih AS, et al. Immunophenotypic and genotypic characterization of lymphomatoid papulosis. *J Am Acad Dermatol* 1992;26:968–975.
217. Willemze R, Meyer CJL, van Vloten WA, et al. The clinical and histological spectrum of lymphomatoid papulosis. *Br J Dermatol* 1982;107:131–144.
218. Sexton FM, Maize JC. Follicular lymphomatoid papulosis. *Am J Dermatopathol* 1986;8:496–500.
219. Willemze R, Scheffer E, Ruiter DJ, et al. Immunological, cytochemical and ultrastructural studies in lymphomatoid papulosis. *Br J Dermatol* 1983;108:381–394.
220. Kadin M, Nasu K, Sako D, et al. Lymphomatoid papulosis: a cutaneous proliferation of activated helper T-cells expressing Hodgkin's disease-associated antigens. *Am J Pathol* 1985;119:315–325.
221. Espinoza CG, Erkman-Balis B, Fenske NA. Lymphomatoid papulosis: premalignant T-cell disorder. *J Am Acad Dermatol* 1985;13:736–743.
222. Ralfkiaer E, Stein H, Wantzin GL, et al. Lymphomatoid papulosis: characterization of skin infiltrates by monoclonal antibodies. *Am J Clin Pathol* 1985;84:587–593.
223. Willemze R, Beljaards RC. Spectrum of primary cutaneous CD30(Ki-1)–positive lymphoproliferative disorders: a proposal for classification and guidelines for management and treatment. *J Am Acad Dermatol* 1993;28:973.

224. Karp DL, Horn TD. Lymphoid papulosis. *J Am Acad Dermatol* 1994; 30:379.
225. Yagi H, Tokura Y, Furukawa F, et al. Th2 cytokine mRNA expression in primary cutaneous CD30-positive lymphoproliferative disorders: successful treatment with recombinant interferon-γ. *J Invest Dermatol* 1996;107:827–832.
226. Weiss LM, Wood GS, Trela M, et al. Clonal T cell populations in lymphomatoid papulosis: evidence for a lymphoproliferative etiology in a clinically benign disease. *N Engl J Med* 1986;315:475–479.
227. Kadin ME, Vonderheid EC, Sako D, et al. Clonal composition of T-cells in lymphomatoid papulosis. *Am J Pathol* 1987;126:13–17.
228. Wood GS, Crooks CF, and Uluer AZ. Lymphomatoid papulosis and associated cutaneous lymphoproliferative disorders exhibit: a common clonal origin. *J Invest Dermatol* 1995;105:51–55.
229. Davis TH, Morton CC, Miller-Cassman R. Hodgkin's disease, lymphomatoid papulosis, and cutaneous T-cell lymphoma derived from a common clone. *N Engl J Med* 1992;326:1115.
230. Henghold W, Purvis SF, Schaffer J, et al. Kaposi sarcoma–associated herpesvirus/human herpesvirus type 8 and Epstein-Barr virus in iatrogenic Kaposi sarcoma. *Arch Dermatol* 1997;133:109–111.
231. Wood GS. Analysis of the t(2;5)(p23;q35) translocation in CD30$^+$ primary cutaneous lymphoproliferative disorders and Hodgkin's disease. *Leuk Lymphoma* 1998;29:93–101.
232. Sanchez NP, Pittelkow MR, Muller SA, et al. The clinicopathologic spectrum of lymphomatoid papulosis: study of 31 cases. *J Am Acad Dermatol* 1983;8:81–94.
233. Chott A, Vonderheid EC, Olbricht S, et al. The same dominant T-cell clone is present in multiple regressing skin lesions and associated T-cell lymphomas of patients with lymphomatoid papulosis. *J Invest Dermatol* 1996;106:696.
234. McGregor JM, Crook T, Ng B, et al. P53 gene mutations in cutaneous T-cell lymphoma. *J Invest Dermatol* 1996;106:855.
235. Knaus PI, Lindeman D, DeCoteau JF, et al. A dominant inhibitory mutant of the type II transforming growth factor β receptor in the malignant progression of a cutaneous T-cell lymphoma. *Mol Cell Biol* 1996;16:3480–3489.
236. Macauley WL. Lymphomatoid papulosis. *Int J Dermatol* 1978;17: 204–212.
237. Wood GS. Unpublished data, 2000.
238. McLeod WA, Winkelmann RK. Eosinophilic histiocytosis: a variant form of lymphomatoid papulosis or a disease sui generis? *J Am Acad Dermatol* 1985;13:952–958.
239. Helton J, Maize JC. Eosinophilic histiocytosis: histopathology and immunohistochemistry. *Am J Dermatopathol* 1996;18:111–117.
240. Headington JT, Roth MS, Ginsburg D, et al. T-cell receptor gene rearrangement in regressing atypical histiocytosis. *Arch Dermatol* 1987;123:1183–1187.
241. Sioutis N. Primary cutaneous Hodgkin's disease. *Am J Dermatopathol* 1994;16:2.
242. Cerroni L, Beham-Schmid C, Kerl H. Cutaneous Hodgkin's disease: an immunohistochemical analysis. *J Cutan Pathol* 1995;22:229.
243. Vonderheid EC, Sajjadian A, Kadin ME. Methotrexate is effective therapy for lymphomatoid papulosis and other primary cutaneous CD30-positive lymphoproliferative disorders. *J Am Acad Dermatol* 1996;34:470–481.
244. Beljaards RC, Kaudewitz P, Berti E, et al. Primary cutaneous CD30-positive large cell lymphoma: definition of a new type of cutaneous lymphoma with a favorable prognosis. A European multicenter study on 47 cases. *Cancer* 1993;71:2097.
245. van Haselen CW, Vermeer MH, Toonstra J, et al. P53 and bcl-2 expression do not correlate with prognosis in primary cutaneous large T-cell lymphomas. *J Cutan Pathol* 1997;24:462–467.
246. Beljaards RC, Meijer CJLM, van der Putte SCJ, et al. Primary cutaneous T-cell lymphomas: clinicopathologic features and prognostic parameters of 35 cases other than mycosis fungoides and CD30-positive large cell lymphoma. *J Pathol* 1994;172:53.
247. Sterry W, Siebel A, Mielke V. HTLV1–negative pleomorphic T-cell lymphoma of the skin: the clinicopathologic correlations and natural history of 15 patients. *Br J Dermatol* 1992;126:456.
248. Friedmann D, Wechsler J, Farcet JP, et al. Primary cutaneous pleomorphic small T-cell lymphoma. *Arch Dermatol* 1995;131:1009.
249. Gonzalez CL, Medeiros LJ, Braziel RM, et al. T-cell lymphoma involving subcutaneous tissue: a clinicopathologic entity commonly associated with hemophagocytic syndrome. *Am J Surg Pathol* 1991;15: 17.
250. Wang CE, Su WPD, Kurtin PJ. Subcutaneous panniculitic T-cell lymphoma. *Int J Dermatol* 1996;35:1.
251. Mehregan DA, Su WP, Kurtin PJ. Subcutaneous T-cell lymphoma: a clinical, histopathologic, and immunohistochemical study of six cases. *J Cutan Pathol* 1994;21:110–117.
252. Crotty C, Winkelmann R. Cytophagic histiocytic panniculitis with fever cytopenia, liver failure, and terminal hemorrhagic diathesis. *J Am Acad Dermatol* 1981;4:181–194.
253. Burg G, Dummer R, Wilhelm M, et al. A subcutaneous delta-positive T-cell lymphoma that produces interferon gamma. *N Engl J Med* 1991; 325:1078–1081.
254. Chan JKC, Tsang WYW, Lo ESF. Cutaneous angiocentric T-cell lymphoma and subcutaneous panniculitic T-cell lymphoma are distinct entities. *Mod Pathol* 1996;9:109.
255. Avinoach I, Halevy S, Argov S, et al. $\gamma\delta$ T-cell lymphoma involving the subcutaneous tissue and associated with a hemophagocytic syndrome. *Am J Dermatopathol* 1994;16:426.
256. Hull PR, Gibson LE, Triffet M, et al. Panniculitic T-cell lymphoma. *J Cutan Pathol* 1998;25:499.
257. Crosti L, Roscetti E, Berti E. Delta chain-positive T-cell lymphoma of the skin. *Dermatol Clin* 1994;12:391–397.
258. Gould JW, Eppes RB, Gilliam AC, et al. Solitary primary cutaneous CD30-positive large cell lymphoma of natural killer cell phenotype bearing the t(2;5)(p23;q35) and presenting in a child. *J Invest Dermatol*, in press.
259. Emile JF, Boulland ML, Haioun C, et al. CD5$^-$ CD56$^+$ T-cell receptor silent peripheral T-cell lymphomas are natural killer cell lymphomas. *Blood* 1996;87:1466–1473.
260. Bastian BC, Ott G, Muller-Deubert S, et al. Primary cutaneous natural killer/T-cell lymphoma. *Arch Dermatol* 1998;134:109–111.
261. Tanaka T, Takahashi K, Ideyama S. Demonstration of clonal proliferation of T-lymphocytes in early neoplastic disease: studies with probes for the β-chain of the T-cell receptor and human T-cell lymphotropic virus type I. *J Am Acad Dermatol* 1989;21:218–223.
262. Dosaka N, Tanaka T, Miyachi Y, et al. Examination of HTLV-I integration in the skin lesions of various types of adult T-cell leukemia. *J Invest Dermatol* 1991;96:196–200.
263. Su IJ, Wu YC, Chen YC, et al. Cutaneous manifestations of postthymic T-cell malignancies: description of five clinicopathologic subtypes. *J Am Acad Dermatol* 1990;23:653–662.
264. Whittaker S, Smith N. Clinical, pathological and molecular features of HTLV-1 associated cutaneous lymphoma. *J Cutan Pathol* 1990; 17:325.
265. Cann AJ, Chen ISY. Human T-cell leukemia virus types I and II. In: Fields BN, Knipe DM, eds. *Virology*. New York: Raven Press, 1501–1527.
266. Seiki M, Eddy R, Shows TB, et al. Nonspecific integration of the HTLV provirus genome into adult T-cell leukemia cells. *Nature* 1984; 309:640–642.
267. Wood GS, Salvekar A, Schaffer J, et al. Evidence against a role for HTLV-I in the pathogenesis of American cutaneous T-cell lymphoma. *J Invest Dermatol* 1996;107:301–307.
268. Li G, Vowels BR, Benoit BM, et al. Failure to detect human T lymphotropic virus type-I (HTLV-I) proviral DNA in cell lines and tissues from patients with cutaneous T-cell lymphoma. *J Invest Dermatol* 1996;107:308–313.
269. Weiss LM, Wood GS, Nickoloff BF, et al. Gene rearrangement studies in lymphoproliferative disorders of skin. *Adv Dermatol* 1988;3: 141–160.
270. Weiss LM, Strickler JG, Dorfman RF, et al. Clonal T-cell populations in angioimmunoblastic lymphadenopathy and angioimmunoblastic lymphadenopathy-like lymphoma. *Am J Pathol* 1986;122:392–397.
271. Frizzera G, Moran EM, Rappaport H, et al. Angioimmunoblastic lymphadenopathy: diagnosis and clinical course. *Am J Med* 1975;59:803.
272. Lukes RJ, Tindle BH. Immunoblastic lymphadenopathy. *N Engl J Med* 1975;292:1.
273. Ohshima K, Kikuchi M, Hashimoto M, et al. Genetic changes in atypical hyperplasia and lymphoma with angioimmunoblastic lymphadenopathy and dysproteinaemia in the same patients. *Virchows Arch* 1994;425:25.
274. Schlegelberger B, Zhang Y, Weber-Matthiesen K, et al. Detection of aberrant clones in nearly all cases of angioimmunoblastic lymphadenopathy with dysproteinemia-type T-cell lymphoma by combined interphase and metaphase cytogenetics. *Blood* 1994;84:2640–2648.

275. Feller A, Griesser H, Schilling CV, et al. Clonal gene rearrangement patterns correlate with immunophenotype and clinical parameters in patients with angioimmunoblastic lymphadenopathy. *Am J Pathol* 1988;133:549.
276. Su IJ, Hsieh HC, Lin KH, et al. Aggressive peripheral T-cell lymphomas containing Epstein-Barr viral DNA: a clinicopathologic and molecular analysis. *Blood* 1991;77:799.
277. Kon S. Detection of Epstein-Barr virus DNA and EBV-determined nuclear antigen in angioimmunoblastic lymphadenopathy with dysproteinemia T-cell lymphoma. *Pathol Res Pract* 1993;189:1137.
278. Anagnostopoulos I, Hummel ML, Finn T, et al. Heterogeneous Eptein-Barr virus infection patterns in peripheral T-cell lymphoma of angioimmunoblastic lymphadenopathy type. *Blood* 1992;80:1904.
279. Weiss L, Jaffe ES, Liu XF, et al. Detection and localization of Epstein-Barr viral genomes in angioimmunoblastic lymphadenopathy and antioimmunoblastic lymphadenopathy-like lymphomas. *Blood* 1992; 79:1789–1795.
280. Foss HD, Anagnostopoulos I, Herbst H. Patterns of cytokine gene expression in peripheral T-cell lymphoma of angioimmunoblastic lymphadenopathy type. *Blood* 1995;85:2862.
281. Jaffe ES, Chan JKC, Su IJ, et al. Report of the workshop on nasal and related extranodal angiocentric T/natural killer cell lymphomas: definitions, differential diagnosis, and epidemiology. *Am J Surg Pathol* 1996;20:103–111.
282. Jaffe ES. Classification of NK-cell and NK-like T-cell malignancies. *Blood* 1996;87:1207.
283. Wechsler J, Willemze R, van der Brule A, et al. Differences in Epstein-Barr virus expression between primary and secondary cutaneous angiocentric lymphomas. *Arch Dermatol* 1998;1334:479–484.
284. DiGiuseppe JA, Louie DC, Williams JE, et al. Blastic natural killer cell leukemia/lymphoma: a clinicopathologic study. *Am J Surg Pathol* 1997;21:1223–1230.
285. Ichinohasama R, Endoh K, Ishizawa K, et al. Thymic lymphoblastic lymphoma of committed natural killer cell precursor origin: a case report. *Cancer* 1996;77:2592–2603.
286. Koita H, Suzumiya J, Ohshima K, et al. Lymphoblastic lymphoma expressing natural killer cell phenotype with involvement of the mediastinum and nasal cavity. *Am J Surg Pathol* 1997;21:242–248.
287. Scott AA, Head DR, Kopecky KJ, et al. HLA-DR$^-$, CD33$^+$, CD56$^+$, CD16$^-$ myeloid/natural killer cell acute leukemia: a previously unrecognized form of acute leukemia potentially misdiagnosed as French-American-British acute myeloid leukemia-M3. *Blood* 1994;84: 244–255.
288. Suzuki R, Yamamoto K, Seto M, et al. CD7$^+$ and CD56$^+$ myeloid/natural killer cell precursor acute leukemia: a distinct hematolymphoid disease entity. *Blood* 1997;90:2417–2428.
289. Imamura N, Kusunoki Y, Kawa-Ha K, et al. Aggressive natural killer cell leukemia/lymphoma: report of four cases and review of literature. Possible existence of a new clinical entity originating from the third lineage of lymphoid cells. *Br J Haematol* 1990;75:49.
290. Chan JKC, Sin VC, Wong KF, et al. Nonnasal lymphoma expressing the natural killer cell marker CD56: a clinicopathologic study of 49 cases of an uncommon aggressive neoplasm. *Blood* 1997;89: 4501–4513.
291. Matutes E, Brito-Babapulle V, Swansbury J, et al. Clinical and laboratory features of 78 cases of T-prolymphocytic leukemia. *Blood* 1991; 78:3269.
292. Sander CA, Medeiros LJ, Abruzzo LV, et al. Lymphoblastic lymphoma presenting in cutaneous sites: a clinicopathologic analysis of six cases. *J Am Acad Dermatol* 1991;25:1023.
293. Willemze R, Meijer CJL, Scheffer E, et al. Diffuse large cell lymphomas of follicular center cell origin presenting in the skin: a clinicopathologic and immunologic study of 16 patients. *Am J Pathol* 1987; 126:325–333.
294. Burg G. Cutaneous B-cell lymphomas. *J Dermatol Surg Oncol* 1984; 10:229–328.
295. Burg G, Braun-Falco O, Kerl H, et al. Cutaneous lymphomas, pseudolymphomas, and related disorders. Berlin: Springer-Verlag, 1983.
296. Willemze R, Meijer CJLM, Sentis HJ, et al. Primary cutaneous large cell lymphomas of follicular center cell origin. *J Am Acad Dermatol* 1987;16:518.
297. Berti E, Alessi E, Caputo R, et al. Reticulohistiocytoma of the dorsum. *J Am Acad Dermatol* 1988;19:259.
298. Santucci M, Pimpinelli N, Arganini L. Primary cutaneous B-cell lymphoma—a unique type of low-grade lymphoma: clinicopathologic and immunologic study of 83 cases. *Cancer* 1991;67:2311.
299. Ruben BS, Medeiros LJ, McCalmont TH, et al. Unexpected CD20 expression in cutaneous clonal T-cell proliferations: a pitfall in the assessment of lineage. *J Cutan Pathol* 1998;25:511.
300. Wirt DP, Grogan TM, Jolley CS, et al. The immunoarchitecture of cutaneous pseudolymphoma. *Hum Pathol* 1985;16:493–510.
301. Knowles DM, Halper JP, Jakobiec FA. The immunologic characterization of 40 extranodal lymphoid infiltrates. *Cancer* 1982;49: 2321–2335.
302. Jaffe ES, Longo DL, Cossman J, et al. Diffuse B-cell lymphomas with T-cell predominance in patients with follicular lymphoma or "pseudo T-cell lymphoma." *Lab Invest* 1984;50:27–28.
303. Pimpinelli N, Santucci M, Romagnoli P, et al. Dendritic cells in T- and B-cell proliferation in the skin. *Dermatol Clin* 1994;12:255–270.
304. Cleary ML, Sklar J. Nucleotide sequence of a t(14;18) chromosomal breakpoint in follicular lymphoma and demonstration of a breakpoint-cluster region near a transcriptionally active locus on chromosome 18. *Proc Natl Acad Sci USA* 1985;82:7439–7443.
305. Siegelman M, Cleary ML, Warnke R, et al. Frequent bioclonality and immunoglobulin gene alterations among B-cell lymphomas that show multiple histologic forms. *J Exp Med* 1985;161:850–863.
306. Vermeer MH, Geelen FAMJ, van Haselen CW, et al. Primary cutaneous large B-cell lymphomas of the legs: a distinct type of cutaneous B-cell lymphoma with an intermediate prognosis. *Arch Dermatol* 1996;132:1304.
307. Geelen FAMJ, Beljaards RC, van der Putte SCJ, et al. Differences in the expression of bcl-2 protein and adhesion molecules between prognostically different groups of primary cutaneous large B-cell lymphomas. *Ann Oncol* 1996;7:132.
308. Rijlaarsdam JU, Bakels V, van Oostveen JW, et al. Demonstration of clonal immunoglobulin gene rearrangements in cutaneous B-cell lymphomas and pseudo-B-cell lymphomas: differential diagnostic and pathogenetic aspects. *J Invest Dermatol* 1992;99:749.
309. Cerroni L, Volkenandt M, Rieger E, et al. Bcl-2 protein expression and correlation with the inter chromosomal 14;18 translocation in cutaneous lymphomas and pseudo lymphomas. *J Invest Dermatol* 1994;102:231.
310. Chimenti S, Cerroni L, Zenahlik P, et al. The role of MT2 and anti-bcl-2 protein antibodies in the differentiation of benign from malignant cutaneous infiltrates of B-lymphocytes with germinal center formation. *J Cutan Pathol* 1998;23:319–322.
311. Garbe C, Stein H, Dienemann D, et al. *Borrelia burgdorferi* associated cutaneous B cell lymphoma: clinical and immunohistochemical characterization of four cases. *J Am Acad Dermatol* 1991;24:584.
312. Cerroni L, Zochling N, Putz B, et al. Infection by *Borrelia burgdorferi* and cutaneous B-cell lymphoma. *J Cutan Pathol* 1997;24:457–461.
313. Willemze R, Meijer CJLM, Rijlaarsdam JU. Are most primary cutaneous B-cell lymphomas "marginal cell lymphomas"? *Br J Dermatol* 1995;133:950.
314. Rutz S, Gellrich S, Lorenz P, et al. Primary cutaneous B-cell lymphomas are descended from germinal center B cells a molecular biological characterization on the single cell level. *J Invest Dermatol* 1999;112:630.
315. Cerroni L, Arzberger E, Putz B, et al. Laser-based microdissection and molecular analysis of germinal center and interfollicular lymphocytes in primary cutaneous follicular lymphoma (follicle center lymphoma, follicular type). *J Invest Dermatol* 1999;112:528.
316. Rijlaarsdam JU, van der Putte SCJ, Berti E, et al. Cutaneous immunocytomas: a clinicopathologic study of 26 cases. *Histopathology* 1993; 23:117.
317. Guggenberger K, Burg G, Schmoeckel C, et al. Follow-ups in cutaneous immunocytomas. In: Goos M, Christophers E, eds. *Lymphoproliferative diseases of the skin.* Berlin: Springer-Verlag, 1982;192.
318. Van der Putte SCJ, de Kreck EJ, Go DMDS, et al. Primary cutaneous lymphoplasmacytoid lymphoma (immunocytoma). *Am J Dermatopathol* 1984;6:15.
319. Braun-Falco O, Guggenberger K, Burg G. Immunonozytom unter dem Bild einer Acrodermatitis chronica atrophicans. *Hautartz* 1978;29: 644.
320. Mayou SC, Cotter FE, Norton AJ, et al. A cutaneous B-cell lymphoma of novel immunophenotype. *Br J Dermatol* 1991;125:373.
321. Bailey EM, Ferry JA, Harris NL, et al. Marginal zone lymphoma (low-grade B-cell lymphoma) of mucosa-associated lymphoid tissue

type) of skin and subcutaneous tissue. *Am J Surg Pathol* 1996;20: 1011.
322. Tomaszewski M-M, Abbondanzo SL, Lupton G. Extranodal marginal zone B-cell lymphoma of the skin: a morphologic and immunophenotypic study of eight cases. *J Cutan Pathol* 1998;25:516.
323. Cerroni L, Signoretti S, Hofler G, et al. Primary cutaneous marginal zone B-cell lymphoma: a recently described entity of low-grade malignant cutaneous B-cell lymphoma. *Am J Surg Pathol* 1997;21: 1307–1315.
324. Baldassano MF, Harris NL, Ferry JA, et al. The presence of MadCAM-1 in cutaneous endothelium and $\alpha_4\beta_7$ expression by marginal zone lymphoma (MZL) suggest that MZL of the skin and gastrointestinal tract may be related tumors. *J Cutan Pathol* 1998;25:487.
325. Kasper R, LeBoit P. Anetoderma associated with cutaneous B cell lymphoma, marginal zone type: cause or coincidence? *J Cutan Pathol* 1998;25:500.
326. Kamath N, Wood GS. Unpublished data, 2000.
327. Kurtin PJ, DiCaudo DJ, Habermann TM, et al. Primary cutaneous large cell lymphomas: morphologic, immunophenotypic, and clinical features of 20 cases. *Am J Surg Pathol* 1994;18:1183.
328. Busschots AM, Geerts ML, Mecucci C, et al. A translocation (8;14) in a cutaneous large B-cell lymphoma. *Am J Clin Pathol* 1993;99: 615–621.
329. Link MP, Roper M, Dorfman RF, et al. Cutaneous lymphoblastic lymphoma with pre-B markers. *Blood* 1983;61:838–841.
330. Vandersteen D, Gibson LE. Post-transplant lymphoproliferative disorders presenting in skin: a report of three cases. *J Cutan Pathol* 1998; 25:517.
331. Schuneman R, Winfield J, Ahmed I, et al. Cutaneous T-cell post-transplant lymphoproliferative disorder clinically masquerading as cellulitis and presenting with subcutaneous lesions. *J Cutan Pathol* 1998;25:512.
332. Cerroni L, Zenahlik P, Hofler G, et al. Specific cutaneous infiltrates of B-cell chronic lymphocytic leukemia: a clinicopathologic and prognostic study of 42 patients. *Am J Surg Pathol* 1996;20:1000–1010.
333. Schultz-Ehrenburg U, Lammer D. Primary centrocytic lymphoma of the skin: diagnosis, course and therapy [author's translation]. *Dermatologica* 1981;162:350–361.
334. Geerts ML, Burg G, Schmoeckel C, et al. Alkaline phosphatase activity in non-Hodgkin's lymphomas and pseudolymphomas of the skin. *J Dermatol Surg Oncol* 1984;10:306–312.
335. Geerts ML, Busschots AM. Mantle-cell lymphomas of the skin. *Dermatol Clin* 1994;12:409.
336. Ellison DJ, Turner RR, van Antwerp R, et al. High-grade mantle zone lymphoma. *Cancer* 1987;60:2717.
337. Raffeld M, Jaffe ES. Bcl-1, t(11;14), and mantle cell derived neoplasms. *Blood* 1991;78:259.
338. Kumar S, Krenacs L, Otsuki T, et al. Bcl-1 rearrangement and cyclin D1 protein expression in multiple lymphomatous polyposis. *Am J Clin Pathol* 1996;105:737.
339. Yang WI, Zukerberg LR, Motokura T, et al. Cyclin D1 (Bcl-1, PRAD1) protein expression in low-grade B-cell lymphomas and reactive hyperplasia. *Am J Pathol* 1994;145:86.
340. Sheibani K, Battifora H, Winberg CD, et al. Further evidence that "malignant angioendotheliomatosis" is an angiotropic large-cell lymphoma. *N Engl J Med* 1986;314:943–948.
341. Wick MR, Rocamora A. Reactive and malignant "angioendotheliomatosis": a discriminant clinicopathological study. *J Cutan Pathol* 1988;15:260–271.
342. Pfleger L, Tappeiner J. Zur kenntnis der systimisierten Ensotheliomatolse der cutanen Blutgefasse. *Hautarzt* 1959;10:359–363.
343. Wick MR, Mills SE. Intravascular lymphomatosis: clinicopathologic features and differential diagnosis. *Semin Diagn Pathol* 1991;8: 91–101.
344. Kutzner H, Englert W, Hellenbroich D, et al. Systemic proliferative angioendotheliomatosis: a cutaneous manifestation of malignant B-cell lymphomas—histologic and immunohistologic studies of two cases. *Hautarzt* 1991;42:384–390.
345. Petroff N, Koger OW, Fleming MG, et al. Malignant angioendotheliomatosis: an angiotropic lymphoma. *J Am Acad Dermatol* 1989;21: 727–733.
346. Walker E, Robertson AG, Boorman JG, et al. Primary cutaneous plasmacytoma: the use of in situ hybridization to detect monoclonal immunoglobulin light chain mRNA. *Histopathology* 1992;20:135.
347. Llamas-Martin R, Postigo-Llorente C, Vanaclocha-Sebastian F, et al. Primary cutaneous extramedullary plasmacytoma secreting λ IgG. *Clin Exp Dermatol* 1993;18:351.
348. Chang YT, Wong CK. Primary cutaneous plasmacytomas. *Clin Exp Dermatol* 1994;19:177.
349. Wiltshaw E. The natural history of extramedullary plasmacytoma and its relation solitary myeloma of bone and myelomatosis. *Medicine (Baltimore)* 1976;553:217.
350. Canlas MS, Dillon ML, Loughrin JJ. Primary cutaneous plasmacytoma: report of case and review of the literature. *Arch Dermatol* 1979; 115:722–724.
351. Patterson JW, Parsons JM, White RM, et al. Cutaneous involvement of multiple myeloma and extramedullary plasmacytoma. *J Am Acad Dermatol* 1988;19:879–890.
352. Liebow AA, Carrington CRB, Friedman PJ. Lymphomatoid granulomatosis. *Hum Pathol* 1972;3:457–558.
353. Madison JF, Cooper D, Howe G, et al. Lymphomatoid granulomatosis of the skin and lung: an angiocentric T-cell rich B-cell lymphoproliferative disorder. *Arch Dermatol* 1996;132:1464.
354. Colby TV. Central nervous system lymphomatoid granulomatosis in AIDS? *Hum Pathol* 1989;20:301–302.
355. Kessler S, Lund HZ, Leonard DD. Cutaneous lesions of lymphomatoid granulomatosis: comparison with lymphomatoid papulosis. *Am J Dermatopathol* 1981;3:115–127.
356. James WD, Odom RB, Katzenstein AL. Cutaneous manifestations of lymphomatoid granulomatosis. *Arch Dermatol* 1981;117:196–202.
357. Jaffe ES, Lipford EH, Margolick JB, et al. Lymphomatoid granulomatosis and angiocentric lymphoma: a spectrum of post-thymic T-cell proliferations. *Semin Respir Med* 1989;10:167–172.
358. Zinberg M, Heilman E, Glickman F. Cutaneous pseudolymphoma resulting from a tattoo. *J Dermatol Surg Oncol* 1982;8:955–958.
359. Caro WA, Helwig EB. Cutaneous lymphoid hyperplasia. *Cancer* 1969;24:487.
360. Picken RN, Strle F, Ruzic-Sabljic E, et al. Molecular subtyping of *Borrelia burgdorferi sensu lato* isolates from five patients with solitary lymphocytoma. *J Invest Dermatol* 1997;108:92–97.
361. Hammer E, Sangueza O, Suwanjindar P, et al. Immunophenotypic and genotypic analysis in cutaneous lymphoid hyperplasia. *J Am Acad Dermatol* 1993;28:426.
362. Griesser H, Feller AC, Sterry W. T-cell receptor and immunoglobulin gene rearrangements in cutaneous T-cell–rich pseudolymphomas. *J Invest Dermatol* 1990;95:292–295.
363. Bendelac A, Lesavre P, Boitard C, et al. Cutaneous pleomorphic T-cell lymphoma. *J Am Acad Dermatol* 1986;15:657–664.
364. Wood GS, Ngan BY, Tung R, et al. Clonal rearrangements of immunoglobulin genes and progression to B-cell lymphoma in cutaneous lymphoid hyperplasia. *Am J Pathol* 1989;135:13–19.
365. El-Shabrawi L, Kerl K, Cerroni L, et al. Inflammatory Pseudotumor of the skin. *J Cutan Pathol* 1998. 25:494.
366. Duncan SC, Evans HL, Winklemann RK. Large cell lymphocytoma. *Arch Dermatol* 1980;116:1142–1146.
367. English JSC, Smith NP, Wilson-Jones E, et al. Large cell lymphocytoma 3/4 a follow-up study. *J Cutan Pathol* 1986;13:441.
368. Braddock SW, Harrington D, Vose J. Generalized nodular cutaneous pseudolymphoma associated with phenytoin. *J Am Acad Dermatol* 1992;27:337.
369. Ramsay B, Dahl MC, Malcolm AJ, et al. Acral pseudolymphomatous angiokeratoma of children. *Arch Dermatol* 1990;126:1524.
370. Enzinger FM, Weiss SW. *Soft tissue tumors.* St. Louis: CV Mosby, 1983;391–397.
371. Urabe A, Tsuneyoshi M, Enjoji M. Epithelioid hemangioma versus Kimura's disease. *Am J Surg Pathol* 1987;11:758–766.
372. Googe PB, Harris NL, Mihm MCJ. Kimura's disease and angiolymphoid hyperplasia with eosinophilia: two distinct histopathological entities. *J Cutan Pathol* 1987;14:263–271.
373. Chun S, Ji HG. Kimura's disease and angiolymphoid hyperplasia with eosinophilia: clinical and histopathologic differences. *J Am Acad Dermatol* 1992;27:954.
374. Keller AR, Hochholzer L, Castleman B. Hyaline-vascular and plasma cell types of giant lymph node hyperplasia of the mediastinum and other locations. *Cancer* 1972;29:670.
375. Grossin M, Crickx B, Aitken G, et al. Subcutaneous forms of the Castleman's benign lymphoma. *Ann Dermatol Venereol* 1985;112: 497–506.

376. Kubota Y, Noto S, Takakuwa T, et al. Skin involvement in giant lymph node hyperplasia (Castleman's disease). *J Am Acad Dermatol* 1993;29[5 Pt 1]:778.
377. Skelton HG, Smith KJ, Tuur S, et al. Castleman's disease in the skin: a rare lymphoid hyperplasia not previously reported in the skin. *J Cutan Pathol* 1997;24:125.
378. Gherardi RK, Belec L, Fromont G, et al. Elevated levels of interleukin-1 beta (IL-1 beta) and IL-6 serum and increased production of IL-1 beta mRNA in lymph nodes patients with polyneuropathy, organomegaly, endocrinopathy, M protein, and skin changes (POEMS) syndrome. *Blood* 1994;83:2587.
379. Ishiyama T, Nakamura S, Akimoto Y, et al. Immunodeficiency and IL-6 production by peripheral blood monocytes in multicentric Castleman's disease. *Br J Heamatol* 1994;86:483.
380. Kinney MC, Hummell DS, Villiger PM, et al. Increased interleukin-6 (IL-6) production in a young child with clinical and pathologic features of multicentric Castleman's disease. *J Clin Immunol* 1994; 14:382.
381. Cesarman E, Chang Y, Moore PS, et al. Kaposi's sarcoma–associated herpesvirus-like DNA sequences in AIDS-related body-cavity-based lymphomas. *N Engl J Med* 1995;332:1186.
382. Jessner M, Kanof NB. Lymphocytic infiltration of the skin. *Arch Dermatol* 1953;68:447.
383. Guillaume JC, Moulin G, Dieng MT, et al. Crossover study of thalidomide vs placebo in Jessner's lymphocytic infiltration of the skin. *Arch Dermatol* 1995;131:1032.
384. Cerio R, Oliver GF, Jones EW, et al. The heterogeneity of Jessner's lymphocytic infiltration of the skin. *J Am Acad Dermatol* 1990;23: 63.
385. Willemze R, Vermeer BJ, Meijer CJL. Immunohistochemical studies in lymphocytic infiltration of the skin (Jessner) and discoid lupus erythematosus. *J Am Acad Dermatol* 1984;11:832–840.
386. Ashworth J, Turbitt ML, MacKie RM. A comparison of the dermal lymphoid infiltrates in discoid lupus erythematosus and Jessner's lymphocytic infiltrate of the skin using the monoclonal antibody Leu 8. *J Cutan Pathol* 1987;14:198–201.
387. Nelson CE, Dahl MV, Goltz RW. Arcuate dermal erythema in a carrier of granulomatous disease. *Arch Dermatol* 1977;113:798.
388. Silverman CL, Strayer DS, Wasserman TH. Cutaneous Hodgkin's disease. *Arch Dermatol* 1982;118:918–921.
389. Cerroni L, Rieger E, Kerl H. Histologic and immunophenotypic analysis of cutaneous Hodgkin's disease. *J Cutan Pathol* 1990;17:289.
390. Nickoloff BJ, Wood GS, Chu M, et al. Disseminated dermal dendrocytomas: a new cutaneous fibrohistiocytic proliferative disorder? *Am J Surg Pathol* 1990;14:867–871.
391. Wood GS, Beckstead JH, Turner RR, et al. Malignant fibrous histiocytoma tumor cells resemble fibroblasts. *Am J Surg Pathol* 1986;10: 323–335.
392. Gray MH, Smoller BR, McNutt NS, et al. Giant dermal dendrocytoma of the face: a distinct clinicopathologic entity. *Arch Dermatol* 1990; 126:689–690.
393. Koizumi H, Kumakiri M, Yamanaka K, et al. Dermal dendrocyte hamartoma with stubby white hair: a novel connective tissue hamartoma of infancy. *J Am Acad Dermatol* 1995;32:318–321.
394. Soloeta R, Yanguas I, Saracibar N, et al. Multiple clustered histiocytofibroma: apropos of a case with immunohistochemical study. *Ann Dermatol Venereol* 1994;121:482–484.

CHAPTER 33

Gastrointestinal Lymphomas and Lymphoid Hyperplasias

Peter G. Isaacson

In view of the frequency with which nodal lymphoma involves the gastrointestinal tract as a secondary phenomenon, strict criteria have been formulated for the definition of primary gastrointestinal lymphoma (1):

1. Absence of superficial lymphadenopathy
2. A normal white blood cell count
3. Absence of mediastinal lymph node involvement
4. No grossly demonstrable involvement at the time of surgical treatment beyond the involved segments of the gastrointestinal tract and its regional lymph nodes
5. A normal liver and spleen

With the advent of staging procedures, these criteria have become somewhat restrictive, particularly with regard to the relevance of the detection of small foci of disease in the liver, spleen, and bone marrow. There is general, if tacit, agreement that a case can be regarded as an example of primary gastrointestinal lymphoma when the lesion has been the presenting focus of disease, necessitating the direction of treatment primarily to that site.

The gastrointestinal tract is the most common site of primary extranodal lymphoma (2). The lymphomas are almost exclusively of non-Hodgkin's type, and primary gastrointestinal Hodgkin's disease is vanishingly rare. Gastrointestinal lymphoma is an uncommon disease in Western countries, accounting for 4% to 18% of all non-Hodgkin's lymphomas, although there is some evidence that the incidence is rising (3,4). Considerable geographic variation exists in the incidence of primary gastrointestinal lymphoma best illustrated by the extraordinarily high incidence in the Middle East. Here, excluding skin tumors, lymphoma is the most common malignancy, and 25% of these lymphomas occur primarily in the gastrointestinal tract (5). Geographic differences extend also to the site of involvement. In the West, gastric lymphoma is the most common site followed by the small intestine, whereas the reverse is true in the Middle East. In both geographic areas, esophageal, colonic, and rectal lymphomas account for a minority of cases.

Advances in the understanding of the clinical and histologic features of lymphomas have paralleled studies of the properties of normal lymph nodes. There are, however, important structural and functional differences between the lymphoid tissue of peripheral lymph nodes and so-called gut-associated lymphoid tissue, which itself shares common features with the lymphoid tissue of other mucosae—hence, the collective term *mucosa-associated lymphoid tissue* (MALT).

MUCOSA-ASSOCIATED LYMPHOID TISSUE

MALT is a specially adapted component of the immune system that has evolved to protect the freely permeable surface of the gastrointestinal tract and other mucosae directly exposed to the external environment. In the mucosa itself, MALT is divided into three mucosal lymphoid compartments, with the mesenteric lymph nodes constituting a fourth compartment. The principal mucosal compartment consists of unencapsulated organized nodules of lymphoid tissue that are distributed throughout the intestine but concentrated in the terminal ileum to form Peyer's patches. The remaining two mucosal compartments are accounted for by the lamina propria lymphocytes and plasma cells and the intraepithelial lymphocytes (IELs).

The lymphoid nodules, or Peyer's patches (Fig. 33.1), are unencapsulated structures that bear a superficial resemblance to lymph nodes. The B-cell component of these nodules consists of a follicle (i.e., follicle center and mantle zone) and a surrounding marginal zone that is particularly

P. G. Isaacson: Department of Histopathology, Royal Free and University College Medical School, University College, London WC1E 6JJ, United Kingdom

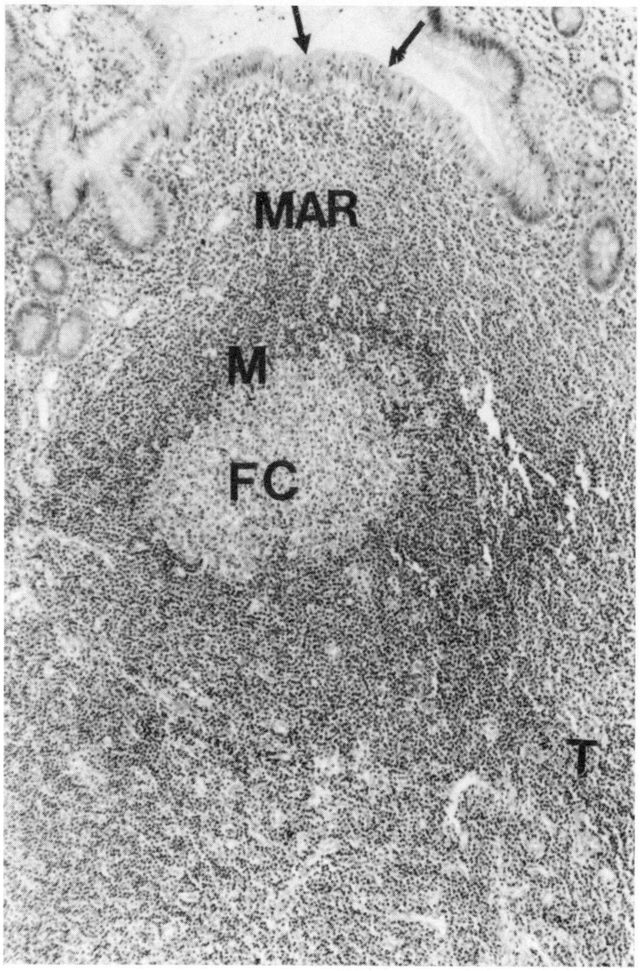

FIG. 33.1. Ileal Peyer's patch. There is a follicle center (FC) surrounded by a narrow mantle zone (M); beyond this is a broad B-cell marginal zone (MAR). Intraepithelial B cells *(arrows)* are seen in the dome epithelium. The T-cell zones (T) are situated toward the serosal aspect between the more prominent B-cell areas.

prominent in Peyer's patches (6). The dome epithelium that covers the lymphoid nodules contains small aggregates of these marginal zone B cells, resulting in the formation of the so-called lymphoepithelium that is a defining feature of MALT. This should be distinguished from the predominantly T-cell IEL population. The lymphoid nodules also contain a small T-cell zone, similar to the lymph node paracortex, which is situated on the inferior aspect that abuts the muscularis mucosae. Immunohistochemical studies of Peyer's patches (7) have shown that the immunophenotype of the B-cell follicles is identical to that in lymph nodes. The immunophenotype of the marginal zone B cells is the same as that of splenic marginal zone cells (Table 33.1). The immunophenotype of the Peyer's patch T-cell zone is the same as that of the lymph node paracortex. The intestinal lamina propria is diffusely infiltrated by plasma cells, most of which are synthesizing IgA. Memory B cells are also present, but most of the lymphocytes in the lamina propria are T cells that are principally CD4 positive ($CD4^+$). Large numbers of macrophages and other accessory cells are also present in the lamina propria.

TABLE 33.1. *Phenotype of marginal zone B cells and centrocyte-like cells of MALT lymphomas*

Antibody	Splenic MZ	Peyer's patch MZ	MALT CCL
Anti-Ig	M, A	M, A	M, A, (G)[a]
CD5	–	–	–
CD10	–	–	–
CD21	+	+	+
CD35	+	+	+
CD23	–	–	–
CD43	–	–	±

MZ, marginal zone; CCL, centrocyte-like; M, IgM; A, IgA; MALT, mucosa-associated lymphoid tissue.
[a] Occasional case expresses IgG.

The entire surface epithelium of the intestine contains an infiltrate of lymphocytes. These IELs are a phenotypically heterogeneous population that, although made up predominantly of $CD8^+$ cytotoxic T cells, also include $CD4^-CD8^-$ $\gamma\delta$ T cells (8,9). Intraepithelial T cells, together with 50% of lamina propria T cells, express CD103 that distinguishes them from T-cell populations elsewhere.

Mesenteric lymph nodes differ marginally from other peripheral lymph nodes. The cortex and paracortex tend to be less well developed, and the sinuses are more prominent. A marginal B-cell zone is often present in mesenteric lymph nodes, whereas this is rarely the case in peripheral lymph nodes.

THE MALT LYMPHOMA CONCEPT

In 1983, Isaacson and Wright (10) observed that, just as nodal lymphomas recapitulated the histologic features of normal nodal lymphoid tissue, certain low-grade B-cell gastrointestinal lymphomas recapitulated the features of Peyer's patches or MALT. These observations were later extended to include a wide variety of extranodal lymphomas (11), many of which arose in mucosal sites other than the gastrointestinal tract. The lymphomas were characterized by reactive, nonneoplastic B-cell follicles around which, in the distribution of the marginal zone, were the neoplastic B cells that extended into the mucosa invading individual glands. The resulting lymphoepithelial lesions were thought to be the neoplastic counterpart of the lymphoepithelium that characterizes MALT. The immunophenotype of these lymphomas closely resembles that of the marginal zone B cells in the spleen and Peyer's patches (Table 33.1). The distinctive nature of this group of lymphomas has found recognition in the Revised European and American Lymphoma (REAL) classification (12), in which they are specifically listed as *extranodal marginal zone B-cell lymphomas of the MALT type*.

An inherent paradox in the MALT lymphoma concept

is that almost all sites where MALT lymphomas occur are normally devoid of lymphoid tissue. The stomach, which is the most common site of MALT lymphoma, is a good example. This paradox has been explained by the observation that the development of MALT lymphoma is invariably preceded by a chronic inflammatory condition such as *Helicobacter pylori* gastritis that results in the acquisition of MALT.

CLASSIFICATION OF PRIMARY GASTROINTESTINAL LYMPHOMAS

The classification of gastrointestinal lymphomas given in Table 33.2 is essentially a regrouping of lymphomas listed in the REAL classification to reflect their occurrence in the gastrointestinal tract. B-cell lymphomas account for the majority, and most of these are of the MALT type. Gastric MALT lymphomas are the paradigm for this group, but MALT lymphomas may arise anywhere in the gastrointestinal tract. Immunoproliferative small intestinal disease (IPSID) is a special subtype of intestinal MALT lymphoma distinguished by its epidemiology and association with the synthesis of an abnormal immunoglobulin (Ig) α heavy chain. By definition, MALT lymphoma is histologically low grade, but transformation to a high-grade lymphoma may occur. In many apparently primary high-grade gastrointestinal B-cell lymphomas, foci of residual low-grade MALT lymphoma may be present. It remains problematic whether those high-grade B-cell gastrointestinal lymphomas in which no low-grade MALT component can be detected are biologically different. Of the other gastrointestinal B-cell lymphomas, mantle cell lymphoma and Burkitt's lymphoma are the most important. Other types of B-cell lymphoma that commonly occur in lymph nodes, such as follicular lymphoma, may arise in the gastrointestinal tract but do so infrequently. The gastrointestinal tract is also a favored site for the origin of lymphomas associated with immunodeficiency (see Chapters 16 and 28).

Primary gastrointestinal T-cell lymphomas are much less common than B-cell tumors and do not show the same epidemiologic features. Enteropathy-associated T-cell lymphoma (EATL) is the only distinctive T-cell tumor and, in some ways, is the equivalent of B-cell MALT lymphoma in that it appears to arise from a gut-committed T cell. A variety of other T-cell lymphomas may occur in the gastrointestinal tract but are infrequent.

TABLE 33.2. *Classification of primary gastrointestinal non-Hodgkin's lymphomas*

B cell

1. Mucosa-associated lymphoid tissue (MALT) type, including immunoproliferative small intestinal disease (IPSID)
   a. Low-grade type
   b. High-grade type, with or without a low-grade component
2. Mantle cell (lymphomatous polyposis)
3. Burkitt's
4. Other types corresponding to peripheral lymph node equivalents
5. Immunodeficiency related

T cell

1. Enteropathy associated
2. Other types unassociated with enteropathy

LOW-GRADE B-CELL GASTRIC LYMPHOMA OF THE MALT TYPE

The formulation and evolution of the MALT lymphoma concept has been largely based on observations of gastric MALT lymphomas. The stomach is the most common site of these tumors, and until recently, gastrectomy was the preferred treatment of this lymphoma. The operation offered specimens with adequate material for pathologic and biologic analysis. The paradox of lymphoma arising in the gastric mucosa, where there is normally no lymphoid tissue, can be explained by the fact that MALT is commonly acquired by the stomach as the result of *H. pylori* infection.

Helicobacter pylori and Gastric MALT Lymphoma

Several groups (13–15) have shown that infection of the stomach by *H. pylori* leads to the accumulation of lymphoid tissue in the gastric mucosa within which B-cell follicles are characteristically present. This acquired gastric lymphoid tissue is accompanied by a lymphoepithelium that defines it as MALT (16). Although other conditions such as Sjögren's syndrome can lead to MALT accumulation in the gastric mucosa, *H. pylori* infection is the most common. There are several lines of evidence that suggest that gastric lymphoma arises from this acquired MALT. The first is that *H. pylori* can be demonstrated in the gastric mucosa of most cases of gastric MALT lymphoma (16). Second, in at least one geographic area, the Veneto region of Italy, where there is a remarkably high incidence of primary gastric lymphoma, there is an accompanying high prevalence of *H. pylori* infection (17). A case-control study has shown an association between previous *H. pylori* infection and the development of primary gastric lymphoma (18).

More direct evidence confirming the importance of *H. pylori* in the pathogenesis of gastric lymphoma has been obtained from a series of *in vitro* studies (19,20). These have shown that the growth of gastric MALT lymphoma B cells can be stimulated by contact with *H. pylori* specific T cells that are present within the lymphoma. In keeping with these observations, numerous patients with low-grade gastric MALT lymphoma have been successfully treated by eradication of *H. pylori* using appropriate antibiotics (21–28).

Clinical Presentation

Low-grade gastric lymphoma occurs predominantly in persons older than 50 years, but cases have been reported in patients as young as 7 years. The male to female ratio

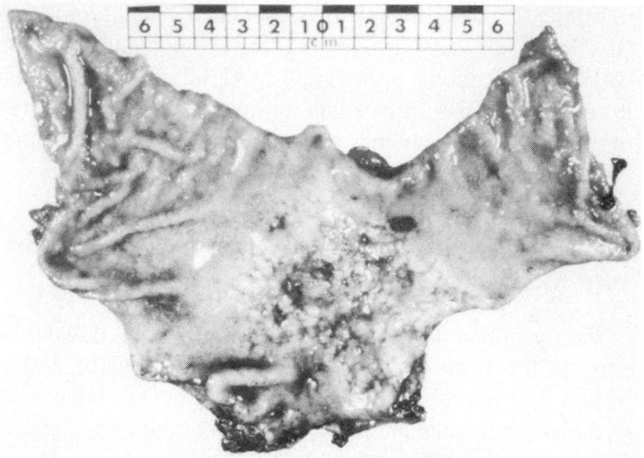

FIG. 33.2. Gastrectomy specimen of a primary low-grade B-cell gastric lymphoma. There is a flat, irregular, nodular, and ulcerating area on the lesser curve in the antrum.

is 1.5:1. The symptoms usually are those of nonspecific dyspepsia; severe abdominal pain and the presence of an abdominal mass are rare. The findings at endoscopy usually are those of nonspecific gastritis or a peptic ulcer, and the presence of a mass is unusual (29). The depth of invasion is difficult to assess from endoscopic examination alone and endosonography is indicated as part of the full staging procedure. Staging infrequently reveals any extraabdominal dissemination.

Macroscopic Appearance

Like carcinoma, gastric lymphoma most often involves the antrum but may occur in any part of the stomach. Consonant with the endoscopic appearances, lymphoma usually appears as a flat, infiltrative lesion sometimes associated with one or more ulcers (Fig. 33.2). Larger masses are less common.

Histology

The histologic features of low-grade MALT lymphoma (30–32) closely simulate those of Peyer's patches. Reactive, nonneoplastic follicles are an integral component and may influence the appearance of the tumor greatly, as discussed later. In most cases, the lymphoma infiltrates around the follicles in the region that corresponds to the Peyer's patch marginal zone, spreading diffusely into the surrounding mucosa (Fig. 33.3). The tumor cells are small to medium, with moderately abundant cytoplasm and nuclei that have an irregular outline that bears a close resemblance to the nuclei of centrocytes (i.e., small cleaved cells). The detailed cytology of these centrocyte-like (CCL) cells covers a spectrum; some are closer in appearance to small lymphocytes, and others show the features of so-called monocytoid B cells with abundant, rather clear cytoplasm and well-defined cell borders (Fig. 33.4). A small number of transformed blasts are characteristically present.

A central feature of low-grade MALT lymphomas is the

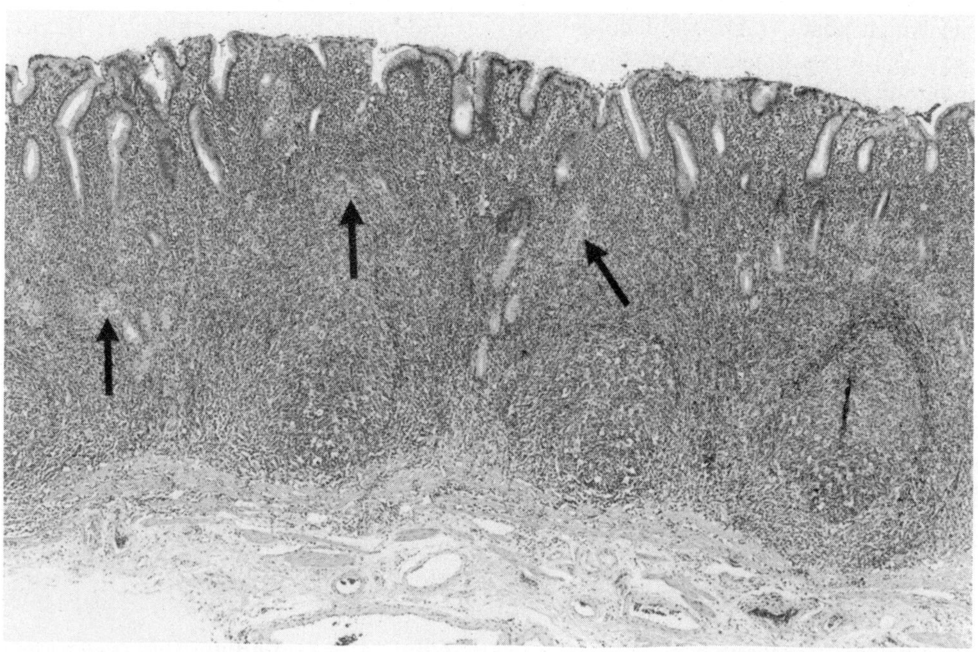

FIG. 33.3. Low-grade gastric lymphoma of mucosa-associated lymphoid tissue (MALT) type that shows infiltration around reactive follicles that extend into the mucosa and produce lymphoepithelial lesions *(arrows)*.

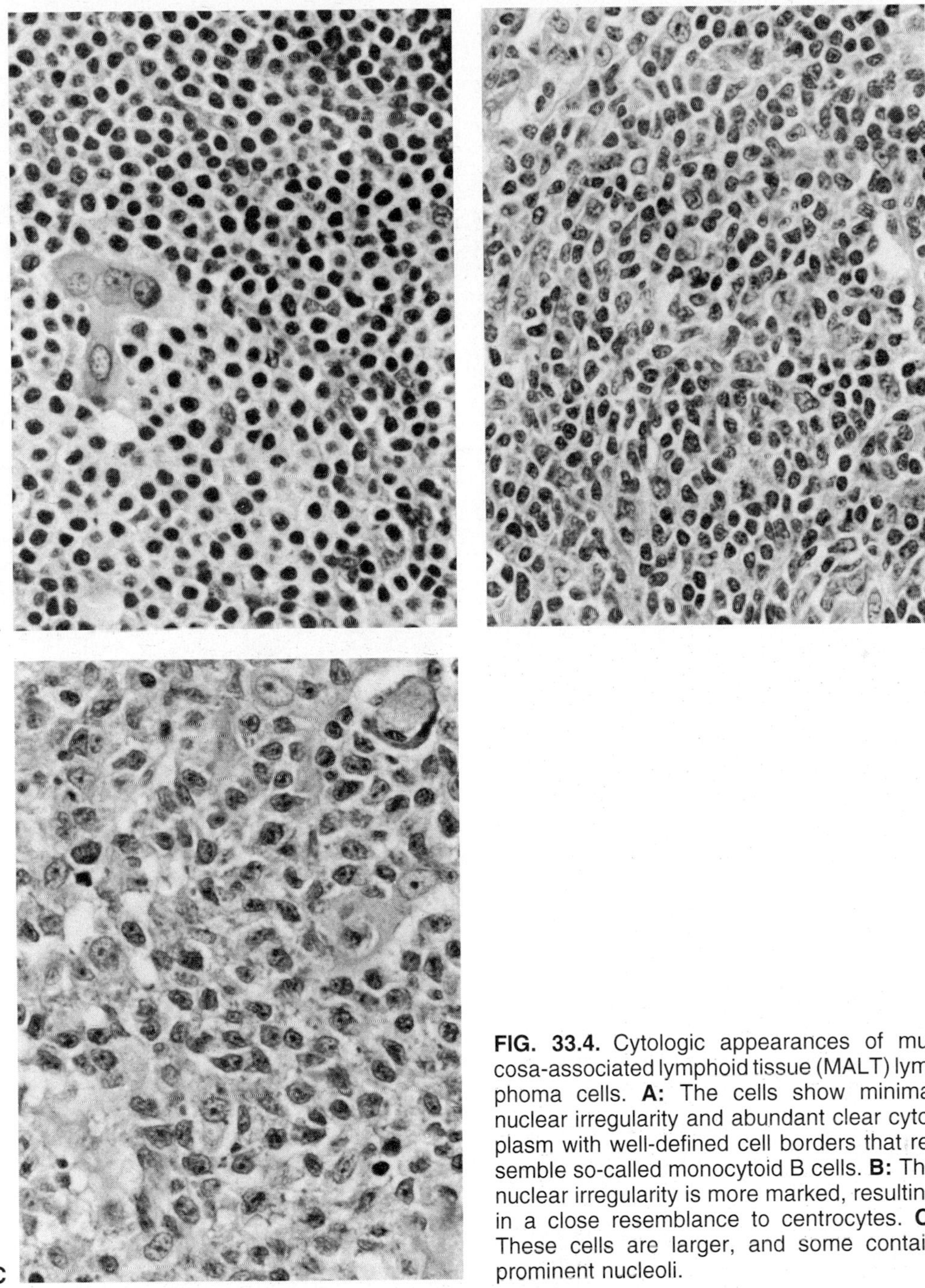

A B C

FIG. 33.4. Cytologic appearances of mucosa-associated lymphoid tissue (MALT) lymphoma cells. **A:** The cells show minimal nuclear irregularity and abundant clear cytoplasm with well-defined cell borders that resemble so-called monocytoid B cells. **B:** The nuclear irregularity is more marked, resulting in a close resemblance to centrocytes. **C:** These cells are larger, and some contain prominent nucleoli.

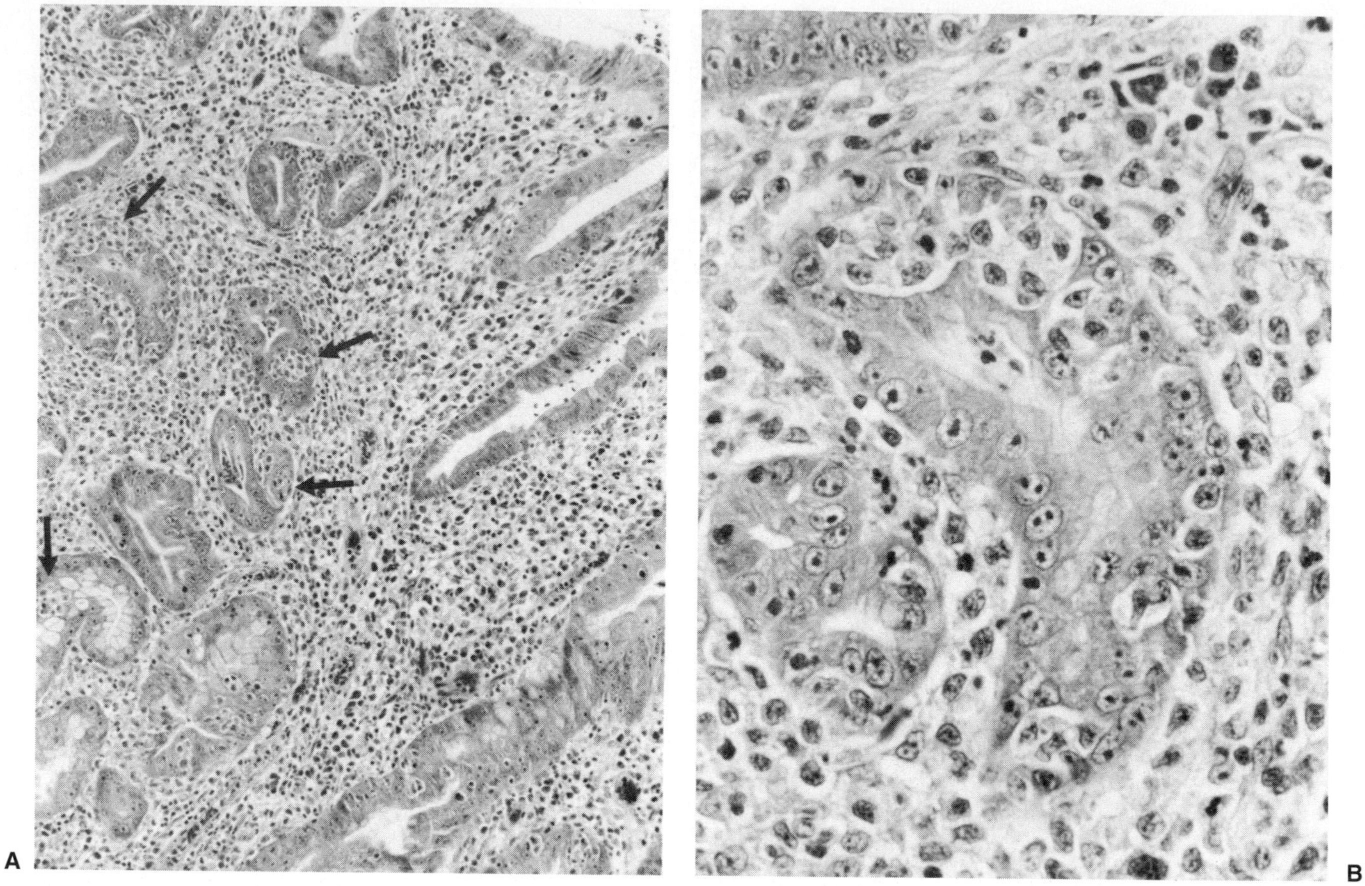

FIG. 33.5. **A:** Mucosal infiltrate from a case of gastric mucosa-associated lymphoid tissue (MALT) lymphoma with numerous lymphoepithelial lesions *(arrows)*. **B:** Detail of lymphoepithelial lesion shows clusters of centrocyte-like cells that displace and destroy glandular epithelium.

presence of lymphoepithelial lesions formed by invasion by aggregates of lymphoma cells of individual gastric glands, which is associated with eosinophilic degeneration or destruction of glandular epithelium (Fig. 33.5). Immunohistochemical staining for cytokeratin is a useful means of highlighting lymphoepithelial lesions (Fig. 33.6).

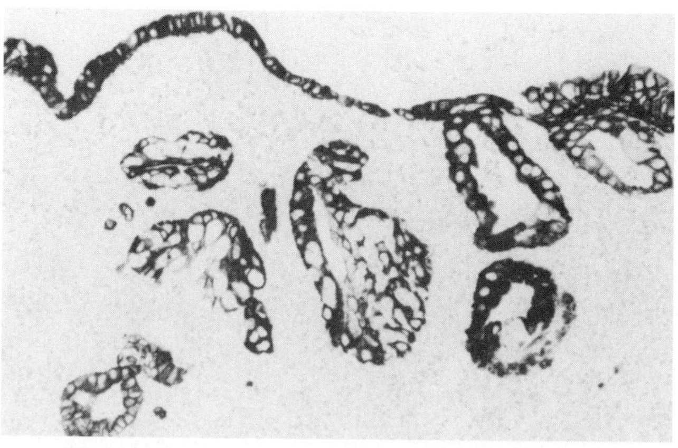

FIG. 33.6. Lymphoepithelial lesions are highlighted by staining with anticytokeratin (immunoperoxidase stain).

Another epithelial change that is seen in some cases is goblet cell metaplasia of gastric epithelium that may lead to confusion with signet ring cell carcinoma (33). Plasma cell differentiation is present to a variable degree in approximately one third of gastric MALT lymphomas and tends to be maximal beneath the surface epithelium (Fig. 33.7). At one extreme, there may be only moderate numbers of plasma cells, and immunocytochemistry is necessary to determine whether these are part of the neoplastic clone (i.e., show light chain restriction) or constitute a reactive population. At the other extreme, plasma cell differentiation may be so extreme that it suggests a diagnosis of plasmacytoma, and many reported cases of gastrointestinal plasmacytoma may be examples of this type of MALT lymphoma. In a significant number of cases, the plasma cells are distorted by accumulations of immunoglobulin, which may be crystalline and occasionally may be found as extracellular tissue deposits.

B-Cell Follicles in MALT Lymphoma

Reactive nonneoplastic follicles are an important component of low-grade B-cell MALT lymphomas and, although especially prominent in the mucosa, may be present throughout the lymphomatous infiltrate. Even the smallest intramu-

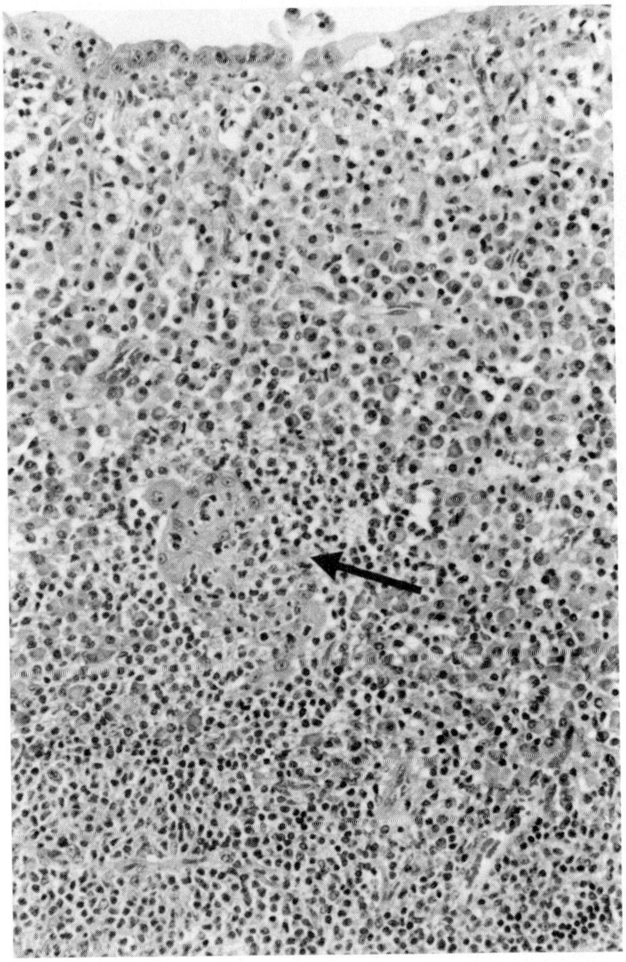

FIG. 33.7. Plasma cell differentiation in a case of gastric mucosa-associated lymphoid tissue (MALT) lymphoma. The mucosa is infiltrated by centrocyte-like cells, which produce a lymphoepithelial lesion *(arrow)*. Beyond this and extending to the surface epithelium, the infiltrate consists predominantly of plasma cells.

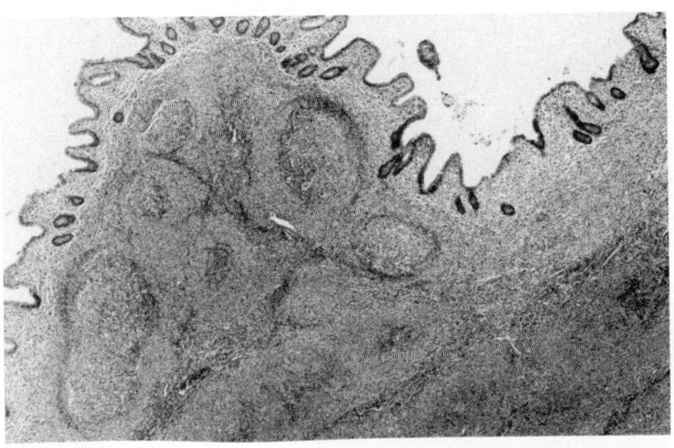

FIG. 33.8. Mucosa-associated lymphoid tissue (MALT) lymphoma, showing a perifollicular infiltrate in the mucosa. A nodular pattern is produced in the deeper infiltrate as follicles are selectively overrun by the centrocyte-like cell infiltrate.

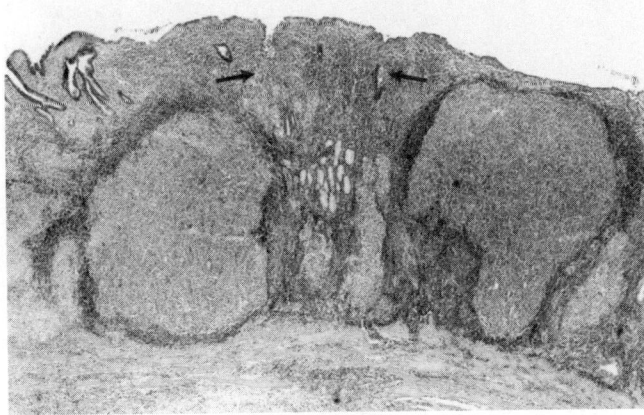

FIG. 33.9. A case of low-grade gastric mucosa-associated lymphoid tissue (MALT) lymphoma that shows a diffuse mucosal infiltrate with lymphoepithelial lesions *(arrows)* and selective colonization of reactive follicle centers resulting in greatly expanded follicles.

cosal focus of lymphoma tends to be accompanied by an underlying lymphoid follicle. The tumor cells interact with these reactive follicles in a complex way (34) that may lead to an appearance that closely resembles follicular lymphoma. This may be enhanced by immunohistochemical studies that show light-chain restriction of the cells that comprise the follicles. The appearances of the follicles that result from the interaction between reactive follicles and CCL cells can be divided into three broad types.

In the first type (Fig. 33.8), reactive follicles are overrun and virtually replaced by CCL cells, resulting in confluent but poorly defined follicles in which fragmented residues of follicle center cells and small, darkly staining mantle zone cells are dispersed. In the second type (Fig. 33.9), follicle centers are selectively replaced, wholly or partly, by CCL lymphoma cells in the presence of an intact mantle zone. The CCL cells within the follicle centers are usually slightly larger than those of the surrounding lymphomatous infiltrate and may show frank blastic transformation. In the third type, the intrafollicular lymphoma cells show plasma cell differentiation (Fig. 33.10). The number of colonized follicles in MALT lymphomas is variable but, at one extreme, results in an appearance almost indistinguishable from follicular lymphoma. Immunohistochemistry is useful in distinguishing the colonized follicles from those of follicular lymphoma.

Multifocality of MALT Lymphoma

Small foci of lymphoma are often present at remote distances from the main tumor mass. The smallest of these consists of a single reactive follicle surmounted by an infiltrate of CCL cells that form lymphoepithelial lesions and can easily be dismissed as nonneoplastic lymphoid nodules (Fig. 33.11). The significance of this has been investigated in a small series of cases (35) in which the Swiss roll technique was used to embed the entire gastrectomy specimen;

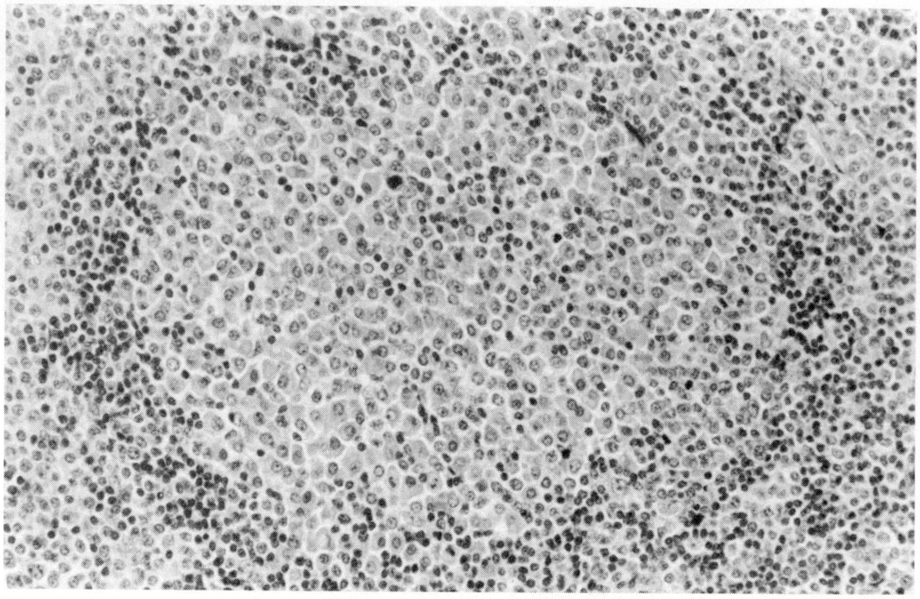

FIG. 33.10. This follicle center from a case of gastric mucosa-associated lymphoid tissue (MALT) lymphoma is composed almost entirely of plasma cells.

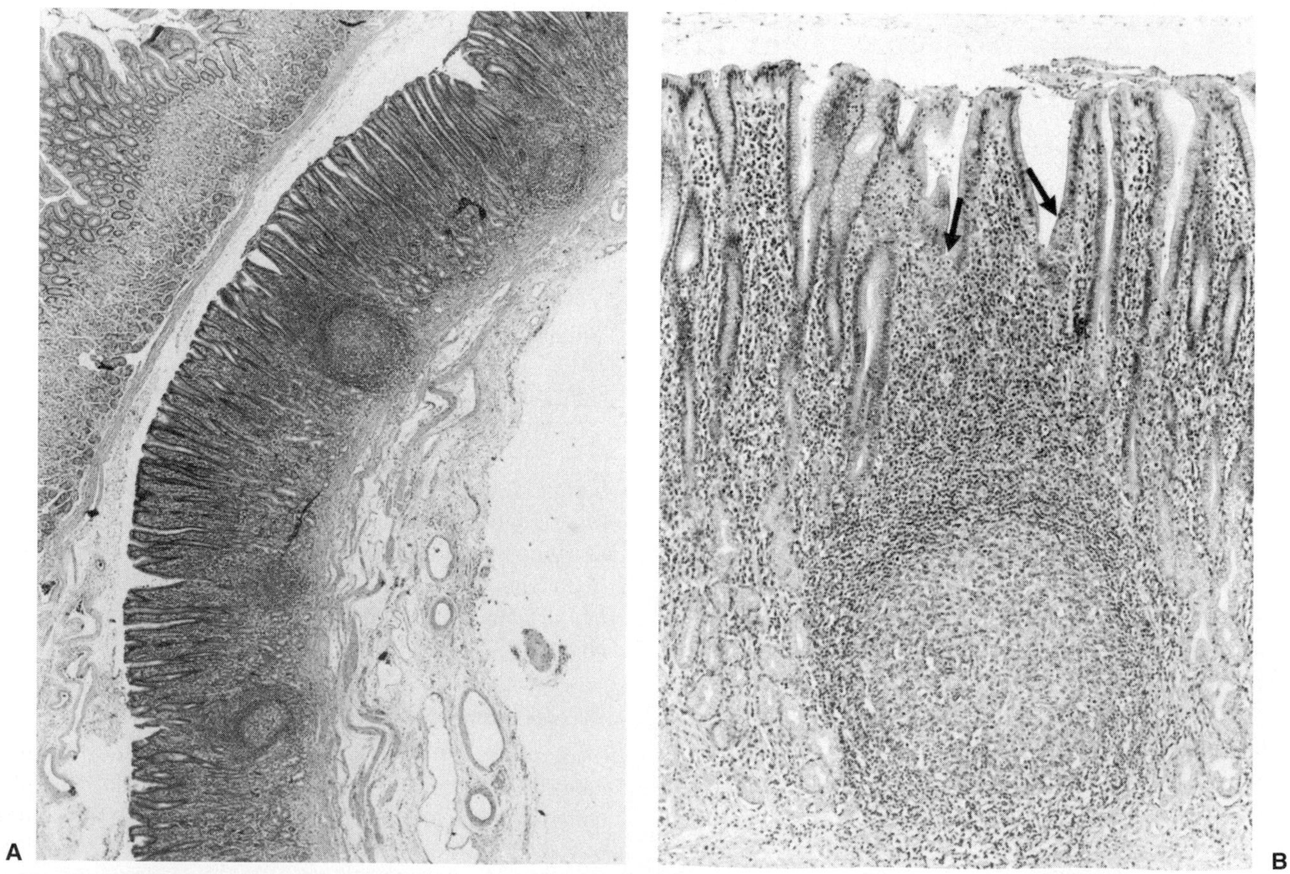

FIG. 33.11. A: Mucosa remote from the main focus of lymphoma, showing four lymphoid aggregates, each of which represents a microscopic focus of lymphoma. **B:** Detail of one of the lymphoid aggregates illustrated in **A**. A reactive B-cell follicle is surmounted by mucosa-associated lymphoid tissue (MALT) lymphoma cells that form lymphoepithelial lesions *(arrows)*.

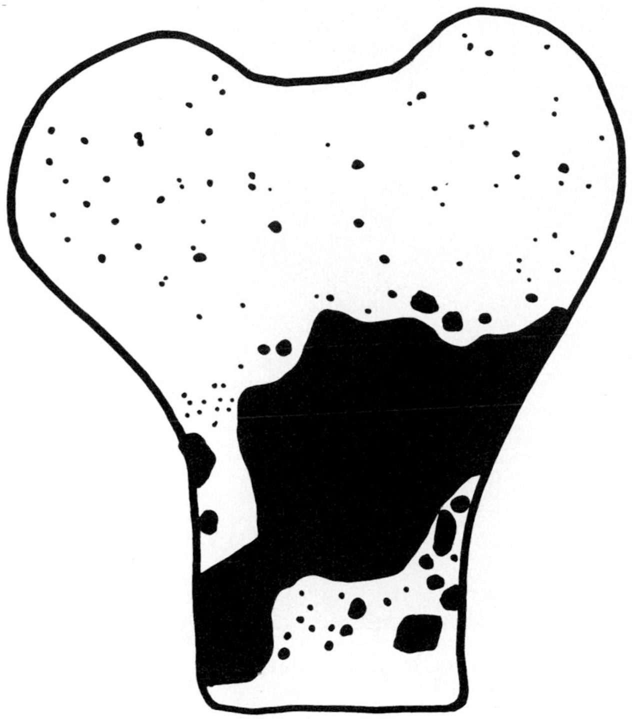

FIG. 33.12. Map of a gastric lymphoma *(black areas)* constructed after total embedding of the gastrectomy specimen by using the Swiss roll technique. Notice the multifocality of the tumor.

this permitted the construction of a map of the distribution of the lymphomas in the gastrectomy specimen. Such a map is shown in Figure 33.12. In some cases, the lymphoma is strikingly multifocal, and clear resection margins are not necessarily evidence that the lesion has been eradicated completely. Molecular studies have shown that the same neoplastic clone is present in each of these lymphomatous foci.

Lymph Node Involvement

The characteristic pattern of lymph node involvement consists of an interfollicular infiltrate of CCL cells that surrounds the follicles in the area corresponding to the marginal zone (Fig. 33.13). This infiltrate extends to form broad, confluent sheets and eventually replaces the entire node. There may be selective colonization of lymph node follicles, leading to an appearance that can be confused with follicular lymphoma.

Distant Spread

Although relatively uncommon, dissemination to the bone marrow (26), liver, and spleen has been recorded for gastric MALT lymphoma. In the spleen, there is a tendency for the lymphoma cells to localize in the marginal zone (36).

Immunophenotype of Gastric MALT Lymphoma

The cells of MALT lymphoma express surface and, to a lesser extent, cytoplasmic immunoglobulin and show light-chain, usually κ, restriction. Most cases express IgM and a few IgA, but IgG expression is rare. In well-fixed immunostained paraffin sections, the immunoglobulin is visible in the perinuclear space, and there may be light staining of the cytoplasm (Fig. 33.14). The more detailed phenotype of these cells is given in Table 33.1, where it is compared with that of Peyer's patch and splenic marginal zone B cells. Neoplastic CCL cells share morphologic features with Peyer's patch marginal zone B cells, and both show tropism for mucosal epithelium. This combined with their immunophenotype suggests the normal cell counterpart of MALT lymphoma is the marginal zone B cell.

In cases where follicular colonization is a feature, the follicles typically show light chain restriction and are often BCL-2 protein positive. However, they do not express CD10 or BCL-6, which can often be seen marking remnants of reactive follicle center cells.

Molecular Genetics

Genotypic investigations of MALT lymphoma using Southern blotting and the polymerase chain reaction (PCR) have confirmed the presence of clonal immunoglobulin heavy (H) and light-chain gene rearrangements, the pattern of which corresponds to the immunohistochemical findings with respect to immunoglobulin heavy chain expression and light-chain restriction (37). Sequence analysis of the IgH genes has shown ongoing mutations and evidence of antigen selection (38,39). The *BCL2* gene is not rearranged in low-grade MALT lymphoma, even in cases showing follicular colonization (40). Microsatellite instability has been demonstrated in MALT lymphoma (41), and *MYC* and *TP53* gene mutations have been demonstrated in 15% to 20% of cases (42,43). Cytogenetic studies have shown trisomy 3 in 55% of cases (44) together with a significant frequency of t(11; 18) (45).

Clinical Behavior

Striking differences exist between the behavior of low-grade MALT lymphoma and comparable lymphomas that occur in peripheral lymph nodes. Low-grade B-cell lymphomas, as recognized in current classifications of non-Hodgkin's lymphomas, all behave in a similar fashion. At diagnosis, these tumors often are already widely disseminated, and in most cases, the bone marrow is involved. Treatment is initially effective, but most patients die within 7 to 10 years, often after transformation of the lymphoma to a higher grade. In contrast, low-grade MALT lymphomas are seldom disseminated at the time of diagnosis. Local recurrences and limited dissemination, often to other mucosal sites, characterize their clinical course. Although relapse-free survival is similar to that of nodal low-grade lymphomas, relatively few patients with gastric MALT lymphoma die of their disease. Ninety percent are alive 5 years after diagnosis and 75% after 10 years (46,47).

A
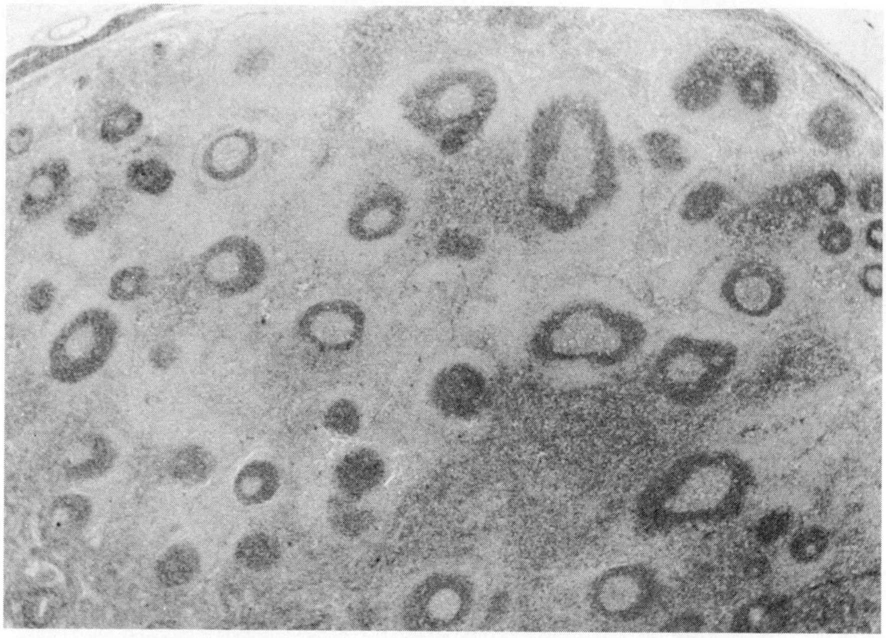

B
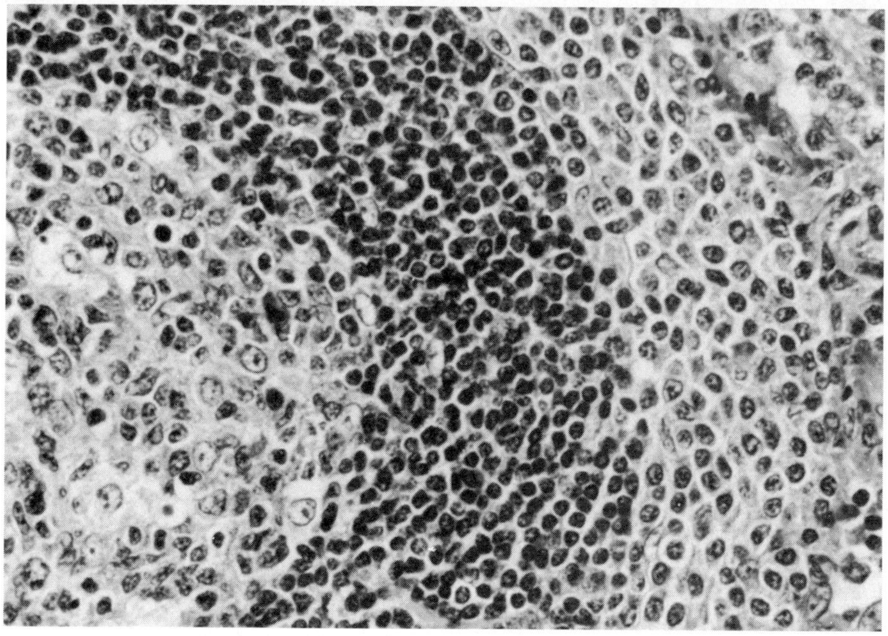

FIG. 33.13. A: Lymph node involvement in a case of gastric mucosa-associated lymphoid tissue (MALT) lymphoma that shows the perifollicular (marginal zone) distribution of the infiltrate. **B:** Higher power shows centrocyte-like cells in the marginal zone of a B-cell follicle.

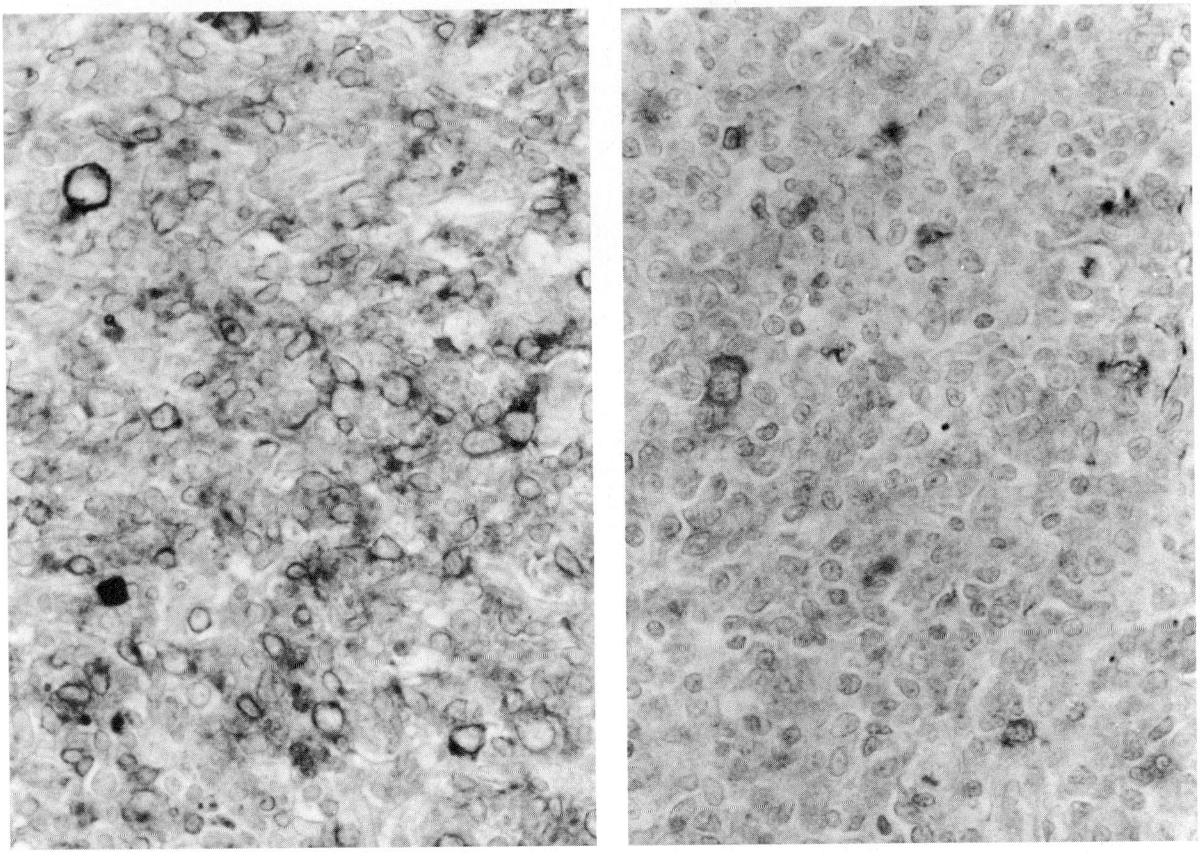

FIG. 33.14. Mucosal infiltrate from a case of gastric mucosa-associated lymphoid tissue (MALT) lymphoma stained by the immunoperoxidase technique for κ light chain **(A)** and for λ light chain **(B)**. There is κ light-chain restriction with staining of the cells in the perinuclear space and, in some cells, the cytoplasm. Only occasional cells stain for λ light chain.

DIFFERENTIAL DIAGNOSIS

Chronic Gastritis Associated with *Helicobacter pylori*

Given that most cases of gastric MALT lymphoma develop from MALT that has accumulated as a result of *H. pylori* infection, it is not surprising that there is a histologic continuum between the two conditions. This can lead to difficulty in the differential diagnosis between florid *H. pylori*–associated gastritis, sometimes known as follicular gastritis, and MALT lymphoma. This presents a particular problem in assessing gastric biopsies that contain a heavy lymphoid infiltrate, and for this reason, a scoring system has been devised (Table 33.3).

In borderline cases (score 3), reactive B-cell follicles are surrounded by a poorly formed marginal zone, the cells of which infiltrate adjacent gastric glandular epithelium (Fig.

TABLE 33.3. *Histologic scoring for the diagnosis of MALT lymphoma*

Score	Description	Histologic features
0	Normal	Scattered plasma cells in lamina propria; no lymphoid follicles
1	Chronic active gastritis	Small clusters of lymphocytes in lamina propria; no lymphoid follicles; no LELs
2	Chronic active gastritis with florid lymphoid follicle formation	Prominent lymphoid follicles with surrounding mantle zone and plasma cells; no LELs
3	Suspicious lymphoid infiltrate in lamina propria, probably reactive	Lymphoid follicles surrounded by small lymphocytes that infiltrate diffusely in lamina propria and occasionally into epithelium
4	Suspicious lymphoid infiltrate in lamina propria, probably lymphoma	Lymphoid follicles surrounded by CCL cells that infiltrate diffusely in lamina propria and into epithelium in small groups
5	Low-grade B-cell lymphoma of MALT	Presence of dense diffuse infiltrate of CCL cells in lamina propria with prominent LELs

LEL, lymphoepithelial lesion; CCL, centrocyte-like, MALT, mucosa-associated lymphoid tissue.

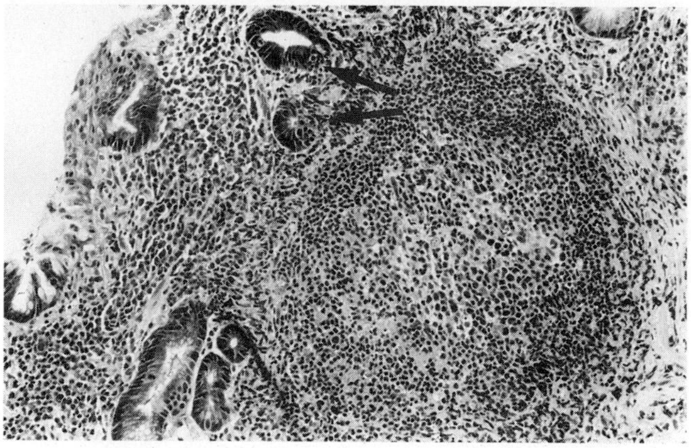

FIG. 33.15. Mucosal biopsy from a case of *H. pylori*–associated chronic gastritis showing a B-cell follicle with lymphocytic infiltration of adjacent glands *(arrows).*

33.15). Unlike MALT lymphoma, there is no eosinophilic degeneration or necrosis of the epithelium, and the lymphoid infiltrate does not extend beyond the immediate confines of the follicles although other chronic inflammatory cells are present throughout the lamina propria. In these difficult lesions, demonstration of immunoglobulin light-chain restriction is extremely useful in confirming a diagnosis of MALT lymphoma, but this presents technical problems, especially in small, often crushed biopsy specimens. A popular approach to this problem is to extract DNA from the biopsy material and use PCR to demonstrate the presence or absence of monoclonal IgH gene rearrangement. This technique is useful only to support histologic findings because false-negative and false-positive results may be obtained. Two studies (48,49) shed some light on the finding of monoclonality in cases of *H. pylori*–associated chronic gastritis. Both showed that a dominant clone can emerge in *H. pylori*–associated chronic gastritis and that this same clone may be detected in subsequent lymphoma. The larger, retrospective study of Nakamura and colleagues (49) showed that, whereas B-cell clones destined to become lymphoma persist in repeated biopsies, those associated with uncomplicated gastritis are transient.

Lymphoid Hyperplasia Associated with Chronic Peptic Ulcer

Numerous lymphoid follicles may be present in the base of a chronic peptic ulcer and in the adjacent mucosa (Fig. 33.16). The follicles are typically surrounded by scar tissue, and neither marginal zones nor lymphoepithelial lesions are present.

Other Low-Grade Lymphomas

With the exception of mantle cell lymphoma, other low-grade lymphomas only rarely arise in the stomach. However,

A

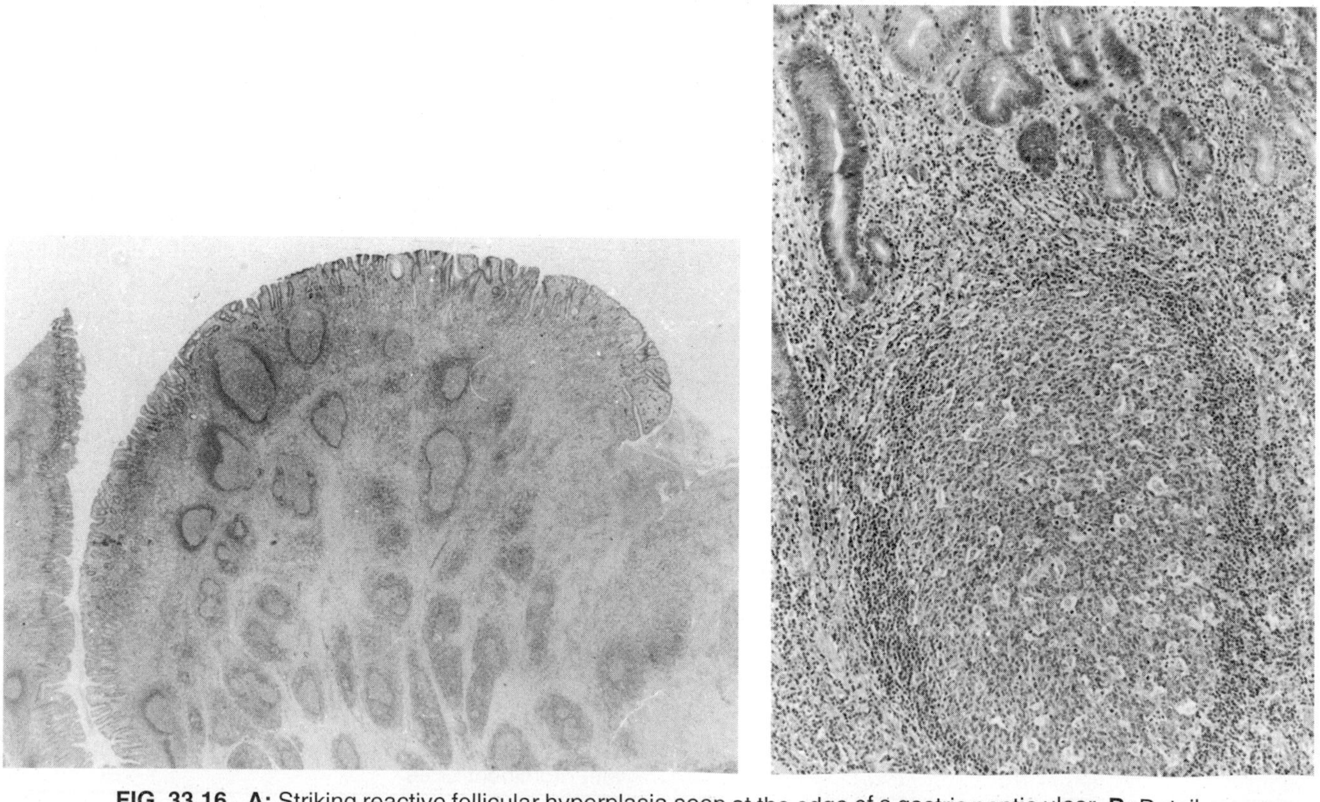

B

FIG. 33.16. A: Striking reactive follicular hyperplasia seen at the edge of a gastric peptic ulcer. **B:** Detail of intramucosal follicle, which is reactive in nature. Notice the absence of any lymphoid infiltrate in the marginal zone. Compare with Figure 33.11B.

secondary gastric involvement is common, and these lymphomas may be encountered in gastric biopsies. The differential diagnosis between mantle cell lymphoma and MALT lymphoma is most important because this aggressive disease may closely resemble MALT lymphoma. Primary or, more commonly, secondary follicular and lymphocytic lymphoma (e.g., chronic lymphocytic leukemia) may be encountered in gastric biopsies and can be difficult to distinguish from MALT lymphoma. The differential diagnosis between these lymphomas is addressed subsequently.

HIGH-GRADE TRANSFORMATION OF MALT LYMPHOMA AND DIFFUSE LARGE B-CELL LYMPHOMA OF THE STOMACH

Scattered large transformed cells are a feature of gastric MALT lymphomas. These cells are more prominent in some cases, and it has been suggested that when they increase to constitute 5% to 10% of the population, although the lymphoma is still designated low grade, the prognosis is slightly worse (47). Frank high-grade transformation is signified by sheets or clusters of more than 20 transformed cells that may increase to constitute the dominant component of the tumor within which a low-grade component can still be identified (48). When no low-grade component can be identified, it is preferable to classify the tumor as a *diffuse large B-cell lymphoma* although survival curves suggest that there is no biologic difference between this group and the transformed MALT lymphomas (46,47).

Clinical Presentation

The mean age of patients presenting with high-grade gastric lymphoma is higher than that of those presenting with low-grade MALT lymphoma (64 versus 55 years). The symptoms are essentially similar to those of gastric carcinoma and include pain, weight loss, and bleeding. Endoscopy usually shows an obvious tumor mass. The stage of these cases is equally divided between IE and IIE. Evidence of distant spread is uncommon.

Macroscopic Appearance and Histology

Most high-grade gastric lymphomas are bulky exophytic tumors. The cells of high-grade gastric lymphoma infiltrate the gastric mucosa as solid sheets between surviving gastric glands (Figs. 33.17, 33.18). Lymphoepithelial lesions are present in some cases. The cells are large with moderately abundant eosinophilic cytoplasm and vesicular nuclei with prominent nucleoli. Bizarre, multinucleated cells may be present.

Immunohistochemistry

The cells usually contain abundant, easily stained immunoglobulin, usually IgM, and show light-chain restriction.

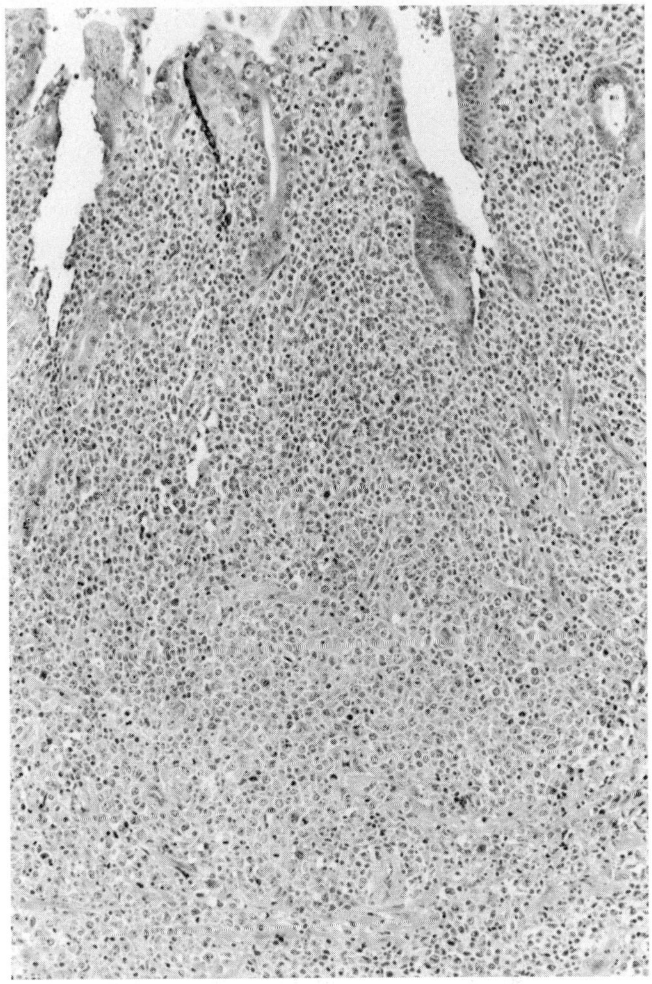

FIG. 33.17. Low-grade B-cell mucosa-associated lymphoid tissue (MALT) lymphoma of stomach *(above)* merging with a high-grade lymphoma *(below)*.

The proliferation fraction in sections stained with Ki-67 is usually about 50%.

Molecular Genetics

Analysis of immunoglobulin genes in cases of high-grade transformation of MALT lymphoma confirm clonal identity between the low- and high-grade components. However, ongoing mutations are not present in the high-grade tumors. *TP53* gene mutations with loss of heterozygosity and expression of the protein are present in approximately 30% of cases (43), and the loss of p16 (49) and *MYC* gene rearrangement [t(8;14)] (45) have been described.

Clinical Behavior

Some investigators have suggested that grade is not an independent variable in the prognosis of gastric lymphoma, but others have argued to the contrary. Cogliatti and colleagues (46) and De Jong and associates (47) found a decreased survival in high-grade compared with low-grade

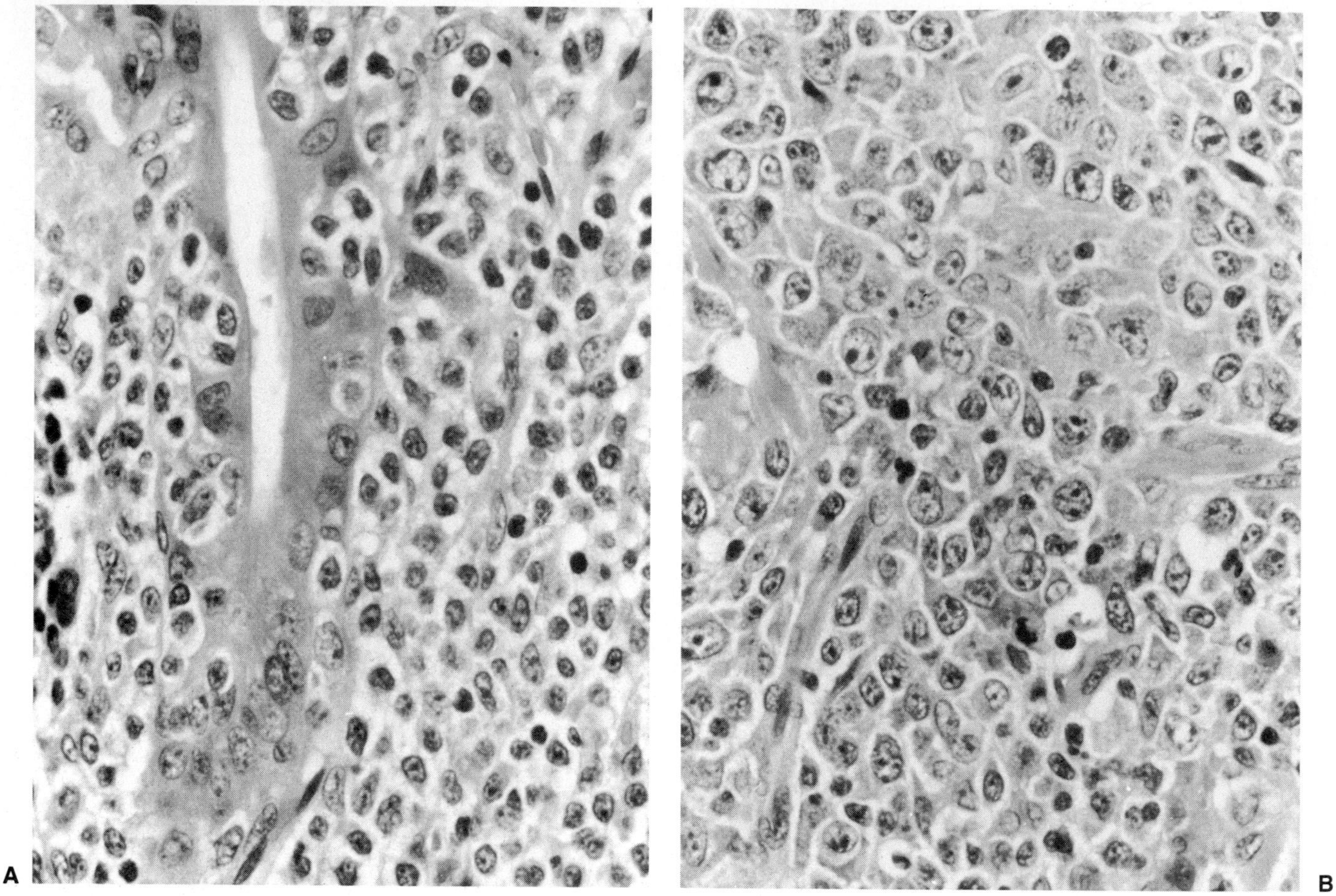

FIG. 33.18. A: Detail of low-grade area illustrated in Figure 33.17. Notice the lymphoepithelial lesion. **B:** Detail of the high-grade area illustrated in Figure 33.17.

gastric lymphoma of 75% versus 91% and 46% versus 95%, respectively.

Gastric MALT Lymphoma and Carcinoma

There are numerous reports of synchronous gastric carcinoma and lymphoma (50). In a series of 190 MALT lymphomas, Nakamura and coworkers found 9 (5%) carcinomas (51). Given that both conditions are linked with *H. pylori* infection, this finding is not surprising.

INTESTINAL MALT LYMPHOMA OF THE USUAL TYPE

A distinction must be drawn between usual (sometimes called Western) intestinal lymphoma and IPSID, which is a special type of MALT lymphoma with a restricted geographic distribution and is discussed separately. The same spectrum of low-grade MALT-type lymphoma, high-grade B-cell lymphoma with a low-grade MALT component, and diffuse large B-cell lymphoma that occurs in the stomach also characterizes lymphomas that arise in the intestine (52). Among these tumors, however, diffuse large B-cell lymphoma is the most common. Most intestinal lymphomas arise in the small intestine and colorectal lymphomas are infrequent.

Clinical Presentation

Most usual MALT lymphomas occur in elderly patients and manifest with bleeding or obstruction. Inflammatory bowel disease is a risk factor for colorectal but not small intestinal B-cell lymphoma (53). These lymphomas usually occur as single ulcerating or polypoid tumors, but occasionally they are multiple and may even result in a variant of intestinal polyposis (54). Mesenteric lymph node involvement is common (stage IIE), but extraabdominal spread is not characteristic.

Histology

The histologic features are the same as those of gastric B-cell lymphomas described previously (52,55). In the low-grade lesions, however, lymphoepithelial lesions may be a much less prominent feature. There are no reports of molecular genetic studies on intestinal B-cell lymphomas.

Clinical Behavior

The clinical behavior is not as favorable as that of gastric B-cell lymphoma. Histologic grade, stage, and resectability have all been shown to affect the prognosis (52,55). Five-year survival rates of 44% to 75% have been reported for low-grade MALT lymphoma and 25% to 37% for high-grade disease.

IMMUNOPROLIFERATIVE SMALL INTESTINAL DISEASE

IPSID, first described by Ramot in 1965 (56), is a variant of MALT lymphoma characterized by a diffuse lymphoplasmacytic (predominantly plasmacytic) infiltrate in the upper small intestine. It occurs almost exclusively in the Middle East, but significant numbers of cases have also been reported from the Cape region of South Africa (57), with sporadic cases from elsewhere. An important distinguishing feature of IPSID is the synthesis of α heavy chain, without light chain, by the plasma cells; this can be detected in the serum or duodenal juice in approximately two thirds of cases—hence the term α-chain disease that is sometimes used for this condition. In the remaining one third of cases, the α chain protein is synthesized but not secreted (58). The α chain is almost always of the α_1 subclass and shows inconstant deletions of the variable portion, which renders preparation of antiidiotypes not feasible.

Clinical Features

IPSID attacks young adults and usually manifests with profound malabsorption. It runs a prolonged course and rarely spreads out of the abdomen until the terminal stages, when high-grade transformation may occur. There are numerous reports describing remissions or even cure of IPSID in its early stages after the use of broad-spectrum antibiotics (59). There is little doubt that the removal of specific or nonspecific immune stimulants from the gut lumen can have a profound effect on some cases of early-stage IPSID. Given the natural history of the disease, however, prolonged follow-up is needed before the term *cure* can be used with confidence. The fact that this type MALT lymphoma is antigen responsive suggests that its relationship with a luminal, unidentified bacterium is similar to that between gastric MALT lymphoma and *H. pylori.*

Macroscopic Appearance

The macroscopic appearance of IPSID depends on the stage. In most cases, there is diffuse, even thickening of the upper jejunum together with enlarged mesenteric lymph nodes. Circumscribed lymphomatous masses may be present and these may be multiple, sometimes producing multiple, small intestinal polyps. The stomach is sometimes involved, but spread to other abdominal organs is rare.

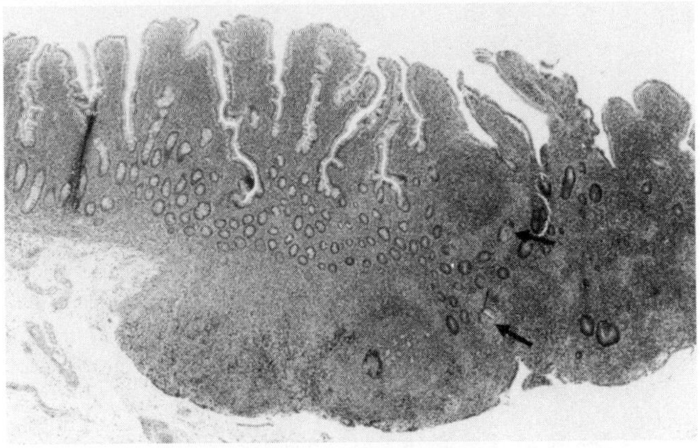

FIG. 33.19. Immunoproliferative small intestinal disease, showing expansion of villi by a lymphoplasmacytic infiltrate extending into the submucosa (i.e., stage B). Notice the follicles and lymphoepithelial lesions *(arrows).*

Histology

The histology of IPSID exemplifies all the features of low-grade B-cell lymphoma of the MALT type (Figs. 33.19–33.21) with marked plasma cell differentiation. Three stages of IPSID are recognized (60). In stage A, the lymphoplasmacytic infiltrate is confined to the mucosa and mesenteric lymph nodes; in stage B, nodular mucosal lymphoid infiltrates are present and the infiltrate extends below the muscularis mucosae; and stage C is characterized by the presence of lymphomatous masses and transformation to high-grade lymphoma (Fig. 33.22). The plasma cell infiltrate in the mucosa causes broadening, but not shortening, of the villi. These cells are not invasive and show no evidence of mitotic division. Already present in stage A IPSID and increasing in prominence in stage B are aggregates of CCL B cells that cluster around epithelial crypts and form lymphoepithelial lesions. Reactive follicles vary in number, and it is colonization of these by CCL cells that results in the lymphoid nodules of stage B IPSID (61) and the so-called follicular lymphoma variant (61,62).

Intrafollicular blast transformation and plasma cell differentiation also occur. Transformation to high-grade lymphoma may occur in the same way as in gastric lymphoma, except that the high-grade cells more frequently show bizarre cytologic features. The mesenteric lymph nodes are involved early in the course of IPSID. Initially, mature plasma cells fill the sinuses, but later CCL or monocytoid lymphoma cells invade the marginal zone. Colonization of follicle centers by plasma cells is a frequent finding.

Immunohistochemistry and Molecular Genetics

Immunohistochemical studies of IPSID (57,61) confirm the synthesis of α heavy chain, without light chain, by the plasma cells, centrocyte-like cells, and transformed blasts (Fig. 33.23). Synthesis of immunoglobulin light chain with

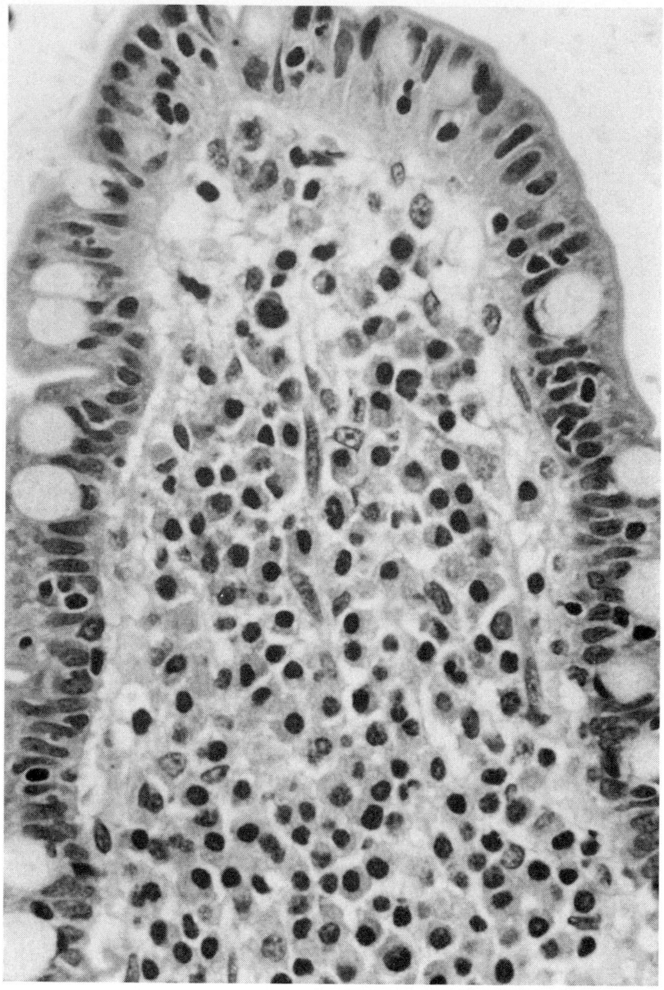

FIG. 33.20. Immunoproliferative small intestinal disease, showing plasma cell infiltration of villi.

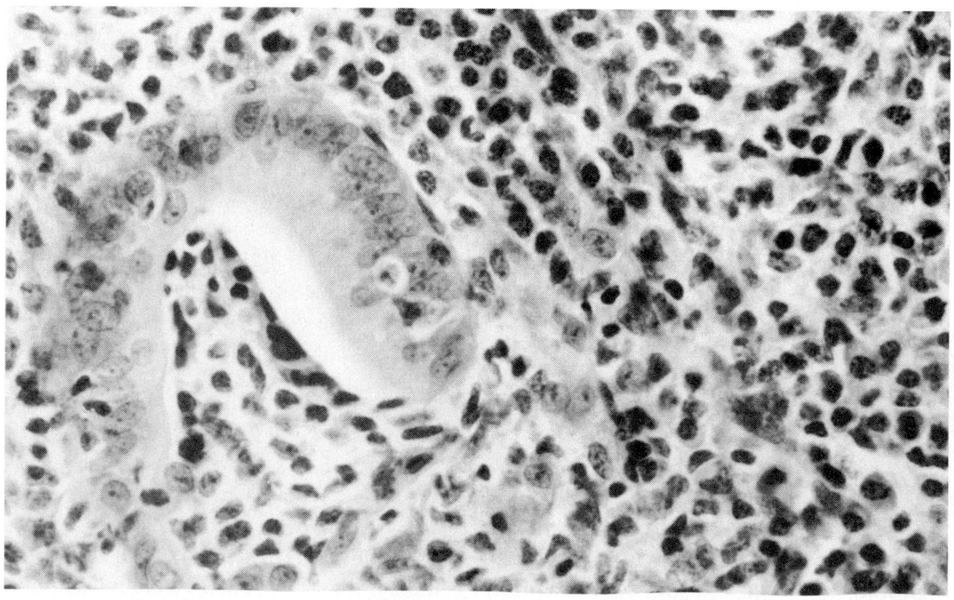

FIG. 33.21. Immunoproliferative small intestinal disease, showing centrocyte-like cells that produce a lymphoepithelial lesion.

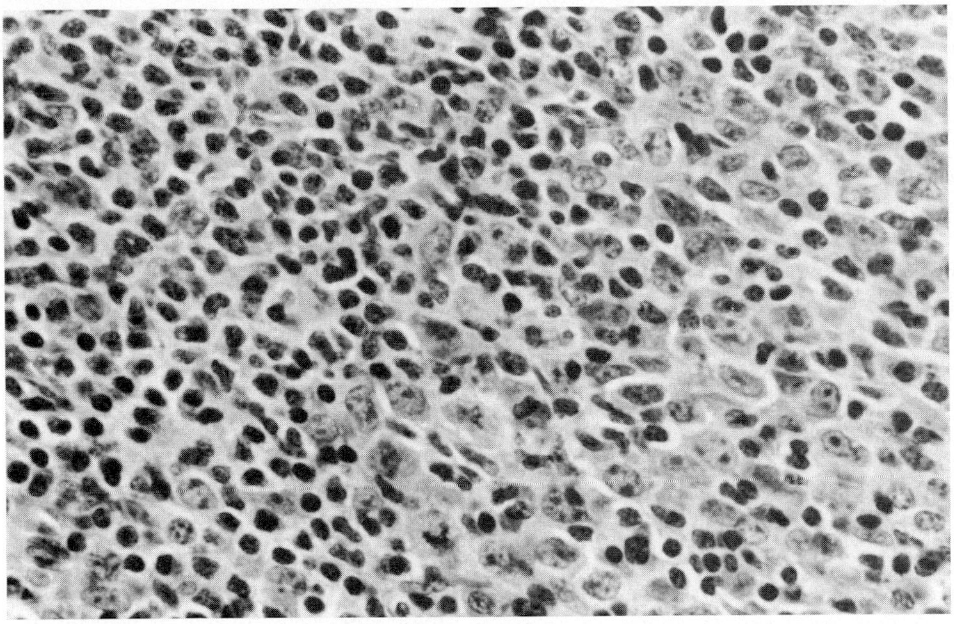

FIG. 33.22. Immunoproliferative small intestinal disease, showing low-grade mucosal infiltrate composed of centrocyte-like cells merging with a high-grade lymphoma.

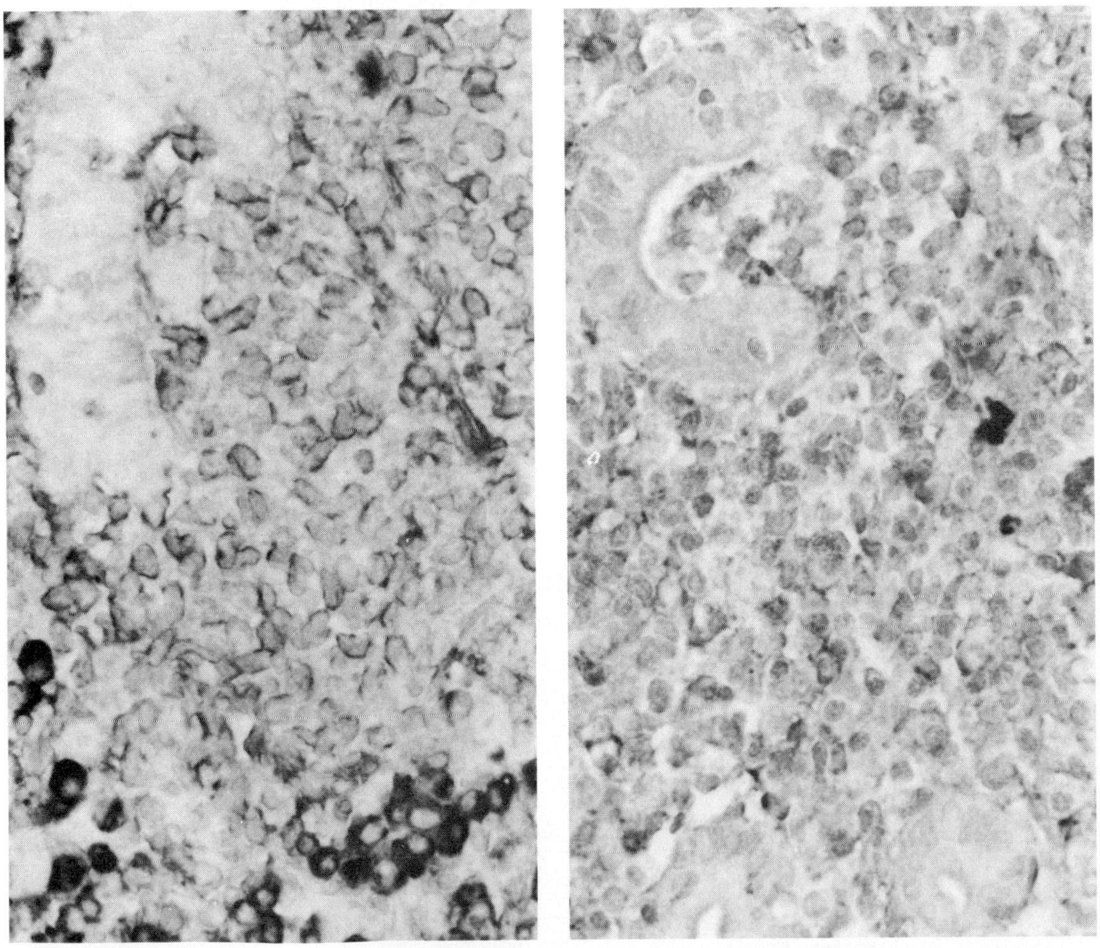

A B

FIG. 33.23. Mucosal infiltrate in immunoproliferative small intestinal disease stained for α chain **(A)** and for κ light chain **(B)**. Plasma cells are heavily stained for α chain, and there is perinuclear space staining of centrocyte-like cells, which are forming a lymphoepithelial lesion. These cells failed to stain for κ light chain, and stains for λ light chain were similarly negative.

light-chain restriction has been demonstrated in a few cases (63). Southern blotting has shown that the lymphoplasmacytic proliferation in IPSID is monoclonal (64). Cytogenetic analysis has been performed in a few cases and has shown a variety of abnormalities.

Immunoproliferative small intestinal disease is in many ways the prototype of MALT lymphomas, exemplifying the prolonged natural history and the tendency of the lymphoma to remain localized in the abdomen with only few documented cases of spread to the periphery. Histologically, the centrocyte-like morphology of the lymphoid cells, the formation of lymphoepithelial lesions, plasma cell differentiation, and follicular colonization place IPSID firmly in the MALT category. The clinical indolence and response of some cases of stage A IPSID to broad-spectrum antibiotics has led to the common view that, at this stage, IPSID is a hyperplastic, nonneoplastic, but prelymphomatous condition. Observations of light-chain restriction and monoclonal immunoglobulin gene rearrangement in stage A IPSID (63,64) show that IPSID is neoplastic *de novo.*

MANTLE CELL LYMPHOMA

Cases of gastrointestinal lymphoma characterized by multiple lymphomatous polyps were first described in 1961 (65). Subsequently, it was established that a specific type of lymphoma, now known as mantle cell lymphoma, was responsible for the formation of the polyps in this disorder (66,67). However, there have been reports of polyposis caused by other types of lymphoma.

Clinical Features

Most cases of LP have been reported in patients older than 50 years, and there is no established sex preponderance. Presenting symptoms are those of abdominal pain, sometimes accompanied by melena, and barium studies or endoscopy reveal multiple polyps. Any part of the gastrointestinal tract may be involved, but in many of the cases, the largest tumors are in the ileocecal region. Like its nodal counterpart, gastrointestinal mantle cell lymphoma disseminates widely early in its course. Although histologically low grade, it is an extremely aggressive tumor, and patients have a median survival of only 3 years (68).

Macroscopic Features

Typically, the intestinal mucosa is peppered with multiple white, fleshy polyps that are 0.5 to 2 cm in diameter; much larger tumors may be present, especially in the ileocecal region (Fig. 33.24). The mesenteric lymph nodes usually are obviously involved.

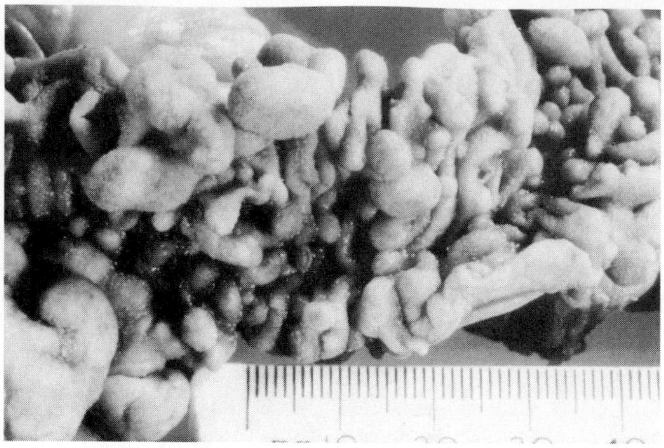

FIG. 33.24. Macroscopic appearances of the ileum in a case of lymphomatous polyposis.

Histology

The smallest lesions consist of a mucosal lymphoid nodule formed by lymphomatous replacement of a single lymphoid follicle. The larger polyps are formed by coalescence of these single polyps and, as a result, frequently manifest a nodular or follicular growth pattern. In some cases, this leads to a close resemblance to follicular lymphoma. Characteristically, residual reactive follicle centers are trapped in the lymphomatous infiltrate, which appears to replace the mantle zones selectively (Fig. 33.25). Intestinal glands are displaced and obliterated, and isolated lymphoepithelial lesions may be present. The lymphomatous cells are small and typically contain nuclei with an irregular outline that resemble centrocytes (Fig. 33.26). Transformed blasts are not usually seen but residual centroblasts may sometimes confuse the picture.

Immunohistochemistry

The tumor cells express pan-B-cell markers, CD5, and CD43. There is strong perinuclear space expression of IgM and IgD, usually with λ light-chain restriction. $CD21^+$ follicular dendritic cell meshworks are prominent. Nuclear expression of cyclin D1 is present in almost all cases (69).

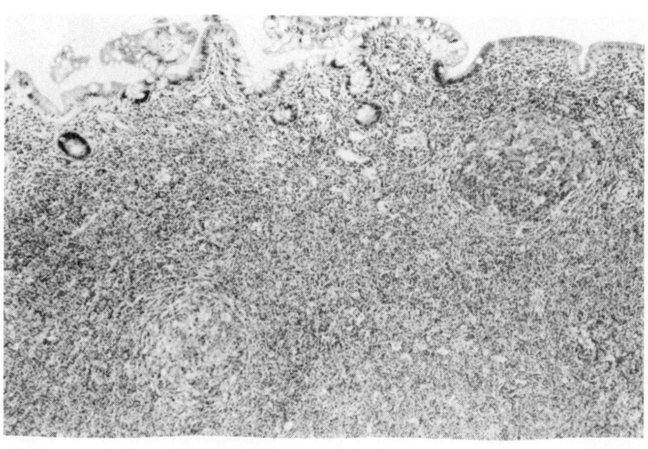

FIG. 33.25. Lymphomatous polyposis that shows mucosal infiltrate with entrapped follicle centers.

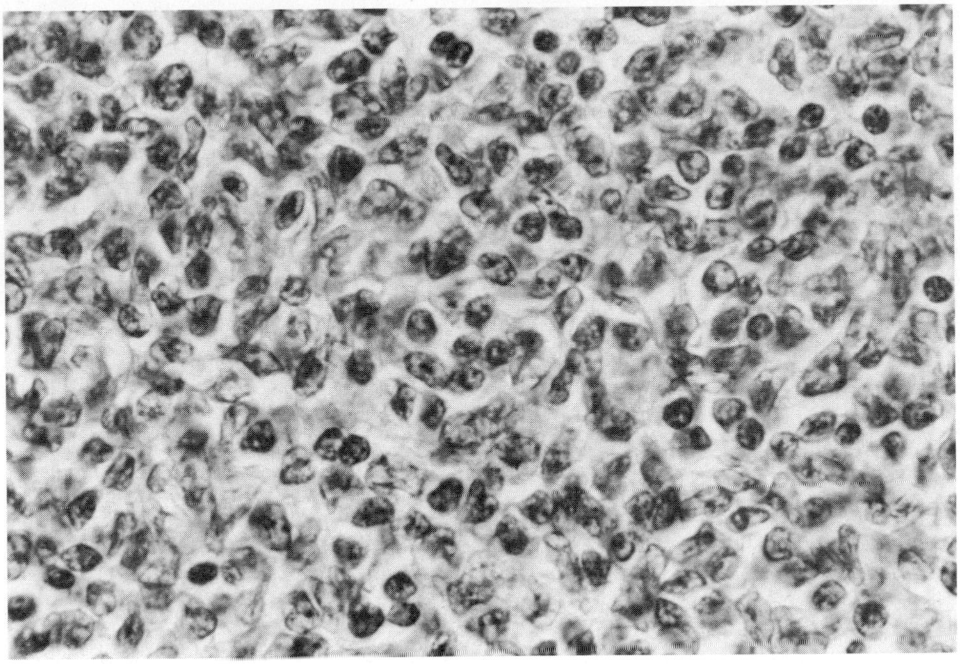

FIG. 33.26. Detail of infiltrate in lymphomatous polyposis that shows a uniform population of small lymphoid cells with irregularly shaped (cleaved) nuclei.

Molecular Genetics

The normal cell counterpart of mantle cell lymphoma is thought to be the naive B cell of the follicular mantle, and in keeping with this, the immunoglobulin genes are in germline configuration. Almost all cases show the translocation t(11; 14) that juxtaposes the cyclin D1 gene to the IgH gene, resulting in overexpression of cyclin D1 protein in the nucleus (69).

BURKITT'S LYMPHOMA

In the Middle East, primary gastrointestinal Burkitt's lymphoma is a common disease of children. It has been studied comprehensively in Algeria (70,71), where Burkitt's lymphoma accounts for 46.5% of all childhood non-Hodgkin's lymphomas, and 60% of these cases occur primarily in the intestine. The cytogenetic alterations in this form of Burkitt's lymphoma are the same as those seen in the classic African form, as is the association with the Epstein-Barr virus (EBV). The disease is more common in boys and shows a peak incidence between 4 and 5 years of age. There is a predilection for the terminal ileum, but any part of the small intestine may be involved. Burkitt's lymphoma is the most common childhood gastrointestinal lymphoma in the West, where it also occurs in teenagers. It is not so closely associated with EBV as in the Middle East.

Macroscopic Features

The lesions vary from localized obstructing tumors to huge masses that involve long segments of the intestine. Extension into the retroperitoneum is common, although the mesenteric lymph nodes are often not involved.

Histology

There is effacement of the mucosa by sheets of monomorphic blasts interspersed with phagocytic histiocytes. The blasts have a narrow rim of cytoplasm and round nuclei with several nucleoli. Lymphoepithelial lesions are not present. In Western Burkitt's, the histologic appearances may be identical but more commonly show slightly greater cytologic variability.

OTHER TYPES OF PRIMARY B-CELL LYMPHOMA THAT CORRESPOND TO PERIPHERAL LYMPH NODE EQUIVALENTS

There is no reason why any type of lymphoma cannot result from MALT, but in practice, those entities common in peripheral lymph nodes only rarely occur in the gastrointestinal tract. The reasons for this are obscure.

Follicular Lymphoma

Although the gastrointestinal tract is frequently secondarily involved by follicular lymphoma, primary follicular lymphoma is distinctly uncommon. When it occurs, it usually does so in the ileocecal region. Cases characterized by the formation of numerous polyps have been described. The histology is the same as that of nodal follicular lymphoma with infiltration of the mucosa by neoplastic follicles. In endoscopic biopsies the differential diagnosis from other small B-cell lymphomas can be difficult.

Lymphocytic Lymphoma

The gastrointestinal tract is commonly involved by chronic lymphocytic leukemia (i.e., lymphocytic lymphoma), and occasionally, endoscopic biopsy may be the first diagnostic procedure. The biopsies show diffuse infiltration by small round lymphocytes without follicle formation. Lymphoepithelial lesions are not characteristic.

DIFFERENTIAL DIAGNOSIS OF GASTROINTESTINAL B-CELL LYMPHOMA

Because of their different clinical behaviors, distinction between the various primary and secondary gastrointestinal lymphomas is of paramount importance. Certain nonneoplastic lymphoid hyperplasias also may be confused with B-cell lymphoma.

Small B-Cell Lymphomas

The differential diagnosis of lymphomas comprising small B cells poses special problems, especially in small endoscopic biopsies. The distinctions between MALT and mantle cell lymphoma and between MALT lymphoma with follicular colonization and follicular lymphoma are especially difficult areas. Immunophenotyping plays a particularly important role. The principal histologic and immunophenotypic features that help to distinguish these lymphomas are listed in Table 33.4.

Focal Lymphoid Hyperplasia

Focal lymphoid hyperplasia in the small intestine (72) is a condition of the terminal ileum and can be subdivided into a more common form seen in children and young adults and a rarer form seen in older persons. In the case of young patients, the condition is known by several names, including enteritis follicularis, cobblestone ileum, nonsclerosing ileitis, pseudopolyposis lymphatica, and terminal lymphoid ileitis. It occurs more frequently in males and may present as ileocecal intussusception (an appendicitis-like illness) or with bleeding. Because the diagnosis usually is made clinically, there are few histologic descriptions of this condition, but published reports describe marked hyperplasia of Peyer's patches with sharply defined follicles and submucosal edema. There is no disorganization of lymphoid tissue or infiltration of the muscularis, and there is little resemblance to lymphoma. In the adult form (73), the clinical presentation is one of weeks to years of abdominal pain, which may be associated with a mass in the right iliac fossa. The histologic features (Fig. 33.27) include follicular hyperplasia of the mucosa, which is frequently associated with ulceration, and a diffuse lymphoplasmacytic infiltrate that extends deeply into the wall of the ileum, often involving the serosa. Eosinophils may be a prominent component of the infiltrate. The normal marginal zone cell component of Peyer's patches participates in the hyperplastic process that leads to exaggeration of the normal association of these cells with dome epithelium. Structures that resemble lymphoepithelial lesions (Fig. 33.28) may be seen in tangentially cut sections. The result is a picture that may closely simulate MALT lym-

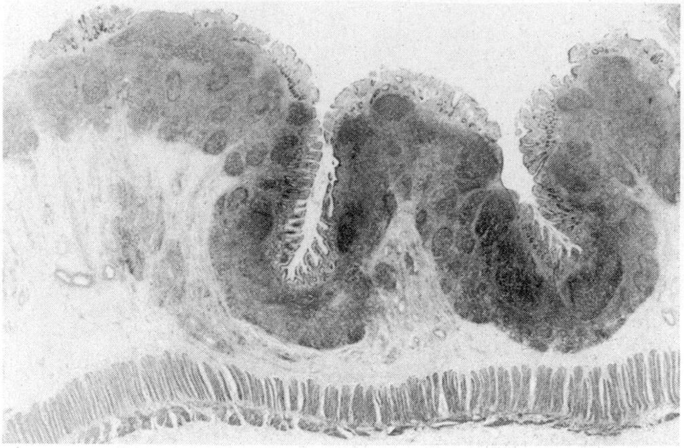

FIG. 33.27. Focal lymphoid hyperplasia of the terminal ileum, showing follicular hyperplasia and lymphoid infiltration extending into the submucosa.

TABLE 33.4. *Differential diagnoses of gastrointestinal small B-cell lymphoma*

Histology	MALT	Mantle cell	Follicular	Lymphocytic
Follicles	±	±	+	−
LEL	+	±	−	−
Cytology	CCL/monocytoid	CCL	CB/CC	Lymphocytic
Phenotype				
CD20	+	+	+	+
CD5	−	+	−	+
CD10	−	−	+	−
Cyclin D1	−	+	−	−

LEL, lymphoepithelial lesions; CB/CC, centroblastic/centrocytic; MALT, mucosa-associated lymphoid tissue.

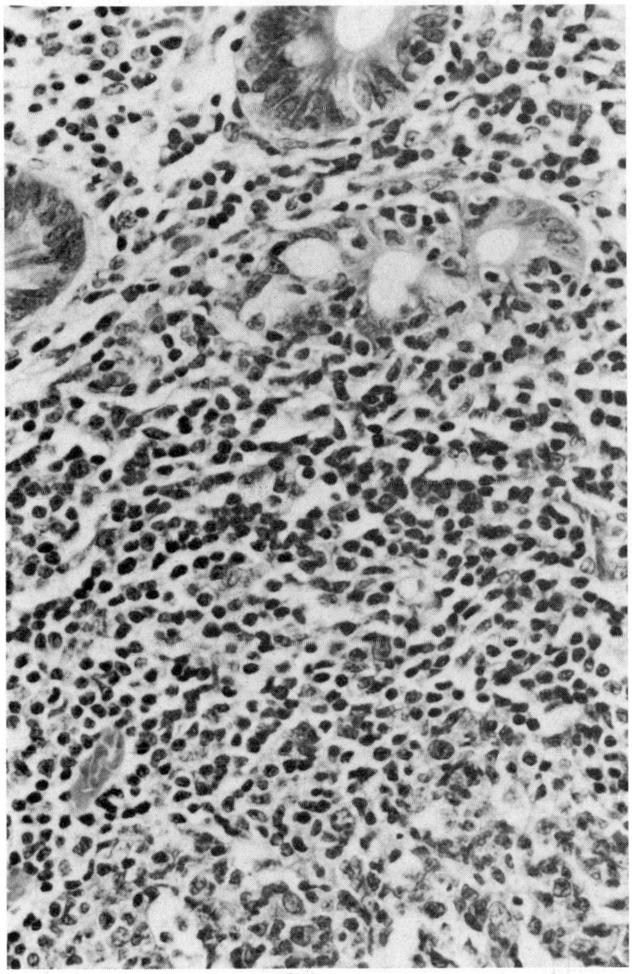

FIG. 33.28. Lymphoid infiltration of epithelium from a case of focal lymphoid hyperplasia of the terminal ileum with the formation of a structure resembling a lymphomatous lymphoepithelial lesion.

phoma, from which it can be distinguished by its polyclonal nature.

Diffuse Nodular Lymphoid Hyperplasia

Diffuse nodular lymphoid hyperplasia of the small intestine, colon, or both is a rare condition that involves long segments of bowel and occurs in two forms. The best recognized of these is associated with congenital or acquired hypogammaglobulinemia, which is only rarely associated with lymphoma (74). Histologically, there is enlargement of the mucosal B-cell follicles caused by hyperplasia of follicle centers. These hyperplastic follicles are confined to the mucosa and surrounded by a normal appearing mantle zone (Fig. 33.29). The marginal zone is inconspicuous, and there is no associated interfollicular infiltrate. In the second form (75), in which immunoglobulin deficiency does not occur, there is a well-documented association with malignant lymphoma. The lymphoma is of the MALT type and is related to the hyperplastic follicles already described.

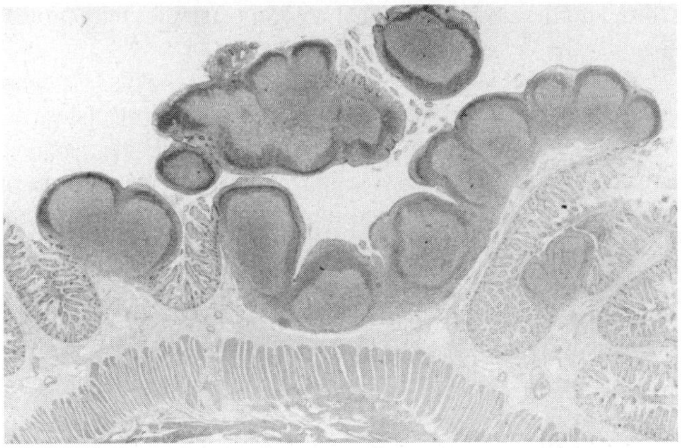

FIG. 33.29. Diffuse nodular lymphoid hyperplasia of the small intestine.

ENTEROPATHY-ASSOCIATED T-CELL LYMPHOMA

An association between malabsorption and intestinal lymphoma was first reported in 1937 (76), at which time it was thought that the lymphoma was in some way responsible for the malabsorption. It subsequently became clear that the reverse is true (77) and that intestinal lymphoma, in common with various other tumors, is a complication of celiac disease or gluten-sensitive enteropathy. In 1978, Isaacson and Wright characterized celiac-associated lymphoma as a single entity, a variant of malignant histiocytosis (78). Later, Isaacson and colleagues showed that the phenotype and genotype of this disease were those of T cells rather than histiocytes (79), and the EATL designation was coined by O'Farrelly and associates in recognition of the phenotype and some doubt that the associated malabsorption state was caused by celiac disease (80).

Clinical Features

EATL may complicate established long-standing celiac disease but more usually follows a short history of adult celiac disease or dermatitis herpetiformis. In a proportion of cases, no history of malabsorption occurs, but jejunal villous atrophy and crypt hyperplasia are found when the tumor is excised. In a minority of cases, the jejunum appears normal or near normal; studies of latency in celiac disease (81) provide an explanation for this finding that previously was thought to argue against a strict association of celiac disease and EATL. Evidence in favor of the enteropathy in EATL being caused by celiac disease includes the identical distribution and histologic appearances of the mucosal lesion, the close similarity of HLA types (82), signs of gluten sensitivity

(83), and the observation that a gluten-free diet may protect against the development of lymphoma (84).

The sex incidence of EATL is equal and the disease characteristically occurs in the sixth and seventh decades, although sporadic reports exist of cases in younger persons. The most common presentation is that of reappearance of malabsorption accompanied by abdominal pain in a patient who has a history of adult or childhood celiac disease and who is responding to a gluten-free diet. Other patients may present with the sudden onset of severe, usually gluten-insensitive malabsorption or as an abdominal emergency. There is another group in whom there is a long, latent interval characterized by severe malabsorption that is not responsive to a gluten-free diet, so-called nonresponsive celiac disease. In yet another group, there is a preceding history of intestinal ulceration with or without stricture formation, an entity known as ulcerative jejunitis.

The clinical course of EATL usually is extremely unfavorable, except for a few cases in which resection of a localized tumor is followed by long remission. In most cases, the lymphoma involves multiple segments of the intestine and already has disseminated at the time of diagnosis. Common sites of dissemination include mesenteric lymph nodes, liver, spleen, bone marrow, lung, and skin. Rarely, the lymphoma

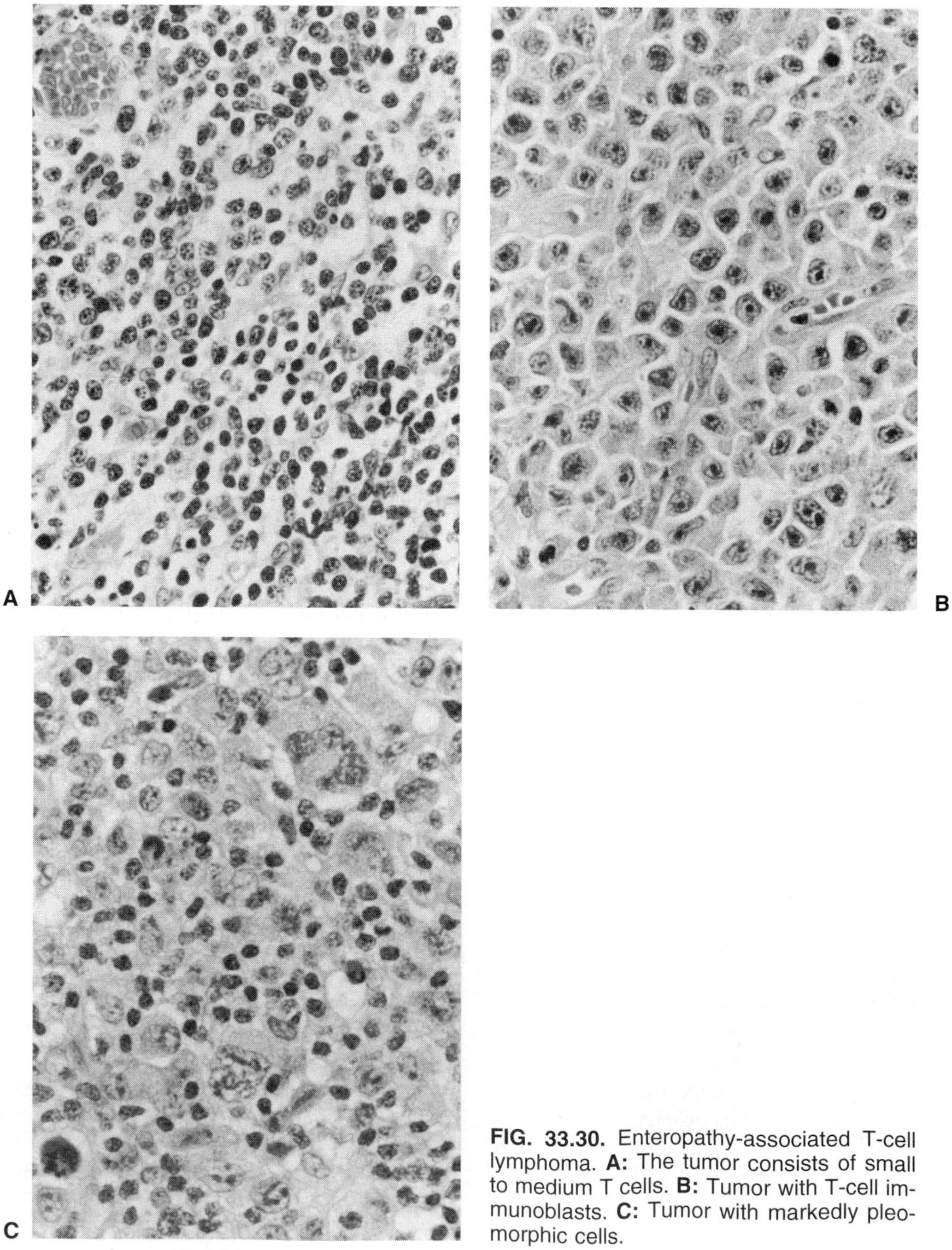

FIG. 33.30. Enteropathy-associated T-cell lymphoma. **A:** The tumor consists of small to medium T cells. **B:** Tumor with T-cell immunoblasts. **C:** Tumor with markedly pleomorphic cells.

presents at one of these sites and intestinal involvement is apparent only later.

Macroscopic Features

EATL may involve any part of the small intestine and occasionally involves other parts of the gastrointestinal tract, but most cases occur in the jejunum. The tumor is usually multifocal and forms ulcerating nodules or large masses that may be accompanied by benign appearing ulcers and strictures. The mesentery and mesenteric lymph nodes are commonly involved.

Histology

The histologic features of EATL show great variation between cases and within any single case (Fig. 33.30). The tumor cells may be only slightly larger than normal small lymphocytes, or they may resemble immunoblasts. The most characteristic appearance, however, is that of a highly pleomorphic tumor with numerous bizarre, multinucleated forms. Intraepithelial tumor cells may be prominent (Fig. 33.31). Interpretation of the histology is complicated even more by the heavy inflammatory component that often contains many eosinophils and extensive necrosis that, together, may mask the neoplastic infiltrate (Fig. 33.32).

The intervening uninvolved small intestinal mucosa usually shows villous atrophy and crypt hyperplasia to a variable degree. In some cases, however, the mucosa is normal, especially if the patient is on a gluten-free diet or the resection is from the ileum, because the villous atrophy of celiac disease improves distally. IELs are nearly always increased, even when villous atrophy is not apparent, and may be quite spectacular, almost obscuring the epithelium and spilling over into the lamina propria where they may merge with the lymphoma (Fig. 33.33).

Immunohistochemistry

The most commonly reported phenotype of the cells in EATL is $CD3^+CD4^-CD8^-CD7^+CD103^+$ (85). The cells contain cytotoxic granules recognized by the TIA-1 monoclonal antibody (86). Although the cells are $CD4^-CD8^-$, they are not $\gamma\delta$ T cells. Cases of EATL composed of large anaplastic cells are usually $CD30^+$. A small round cell subtype of EATL has been described (87) in which the cells are $CD8^+CD56^+$. The IELs in the adjacent nonlymphomatous small intestine typically share the immunophenotype of the lymphoma cells.

Molecular Genetics

There is clonal rearrangement of the T-cell receptor β and γ genes (88). A clonally identical population is also present in the adjacent nonlymphomatous enteropathic mucosa and this appears to reside in the IEL compartment (89,90). No distinctive genetic abnormality has been associated with EATL.

Nonresponsive Celiac Disease and Ulcerative Jejunitis

Both of these conditions (90,91) are grave complications of celiac disease that can precede the onset of EATL. More-

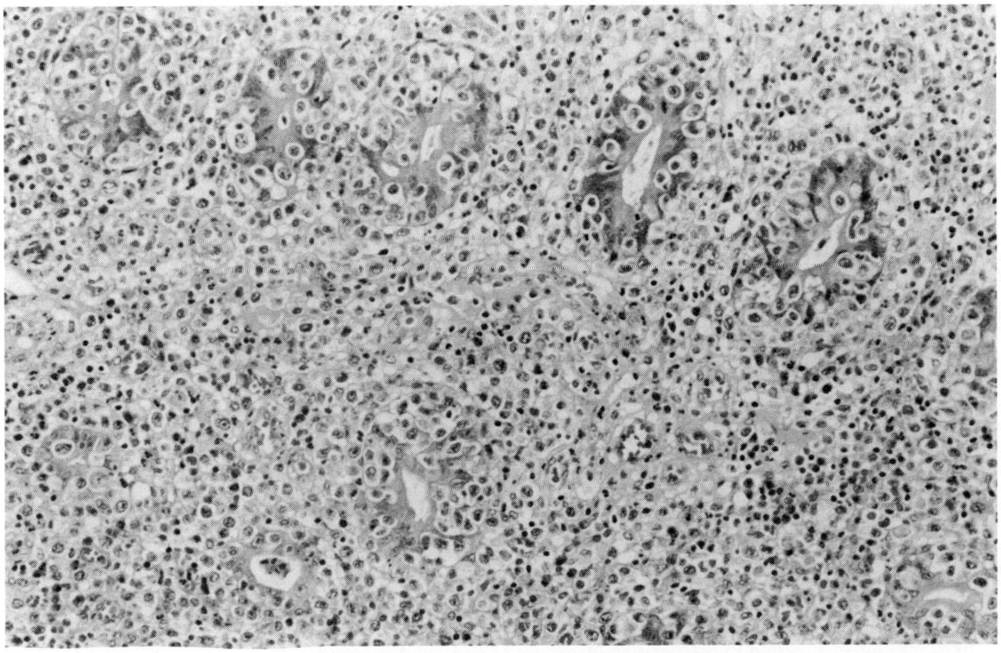

FIG. 33.31. Mucosal infiltrate from a case of enteropathy-associated T-cell lymphoma (EATL) that shows intraepithelial tumor cells.

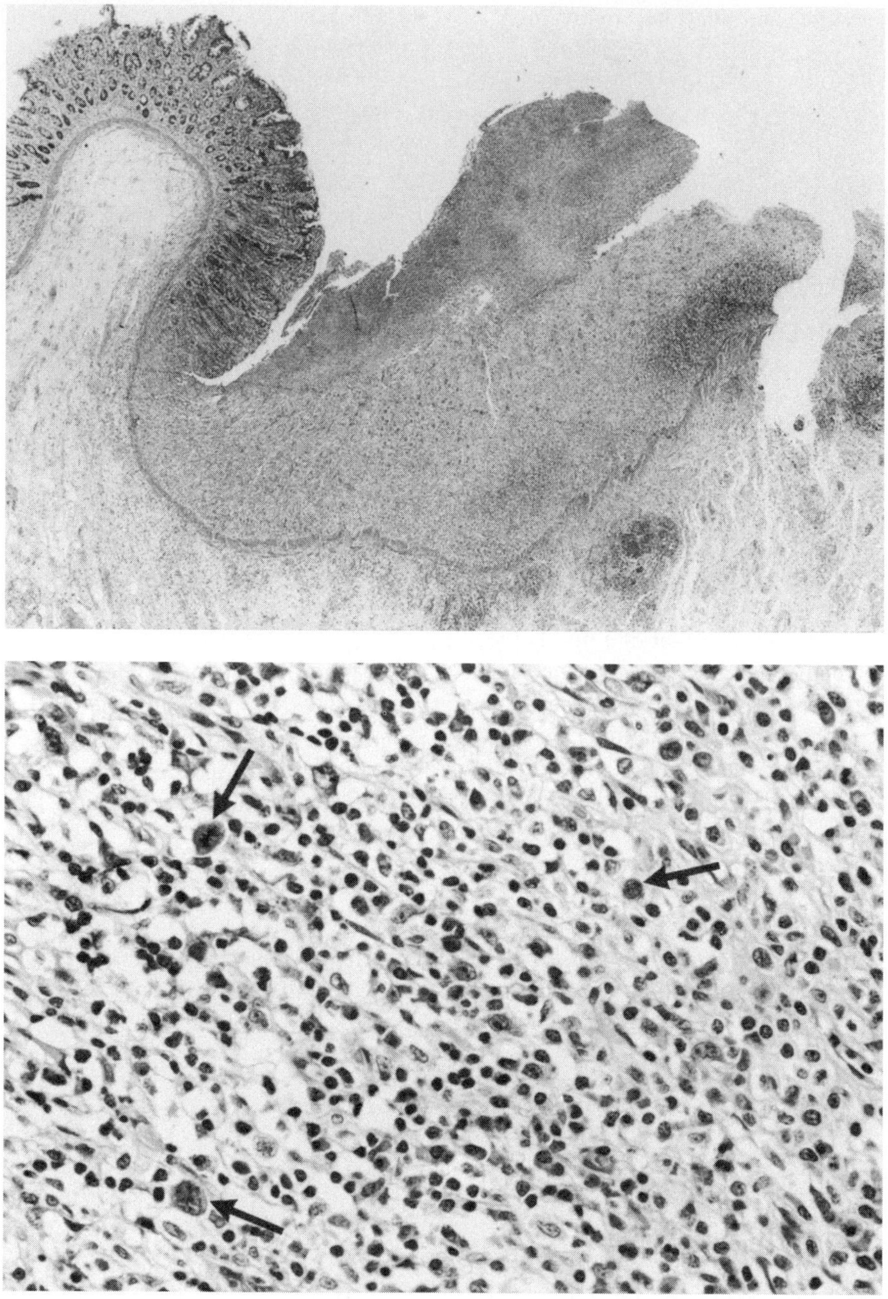

A

B

FIG. 33.32. A: Extensive necrosis with ulceration in a case of enteropathy-associated T-cell lymphoma (EATL). **B:** Detail of ulcer base that shows a chronic inflammatory infiltrate in which there are scattered large tumor cells *(arrows)*.

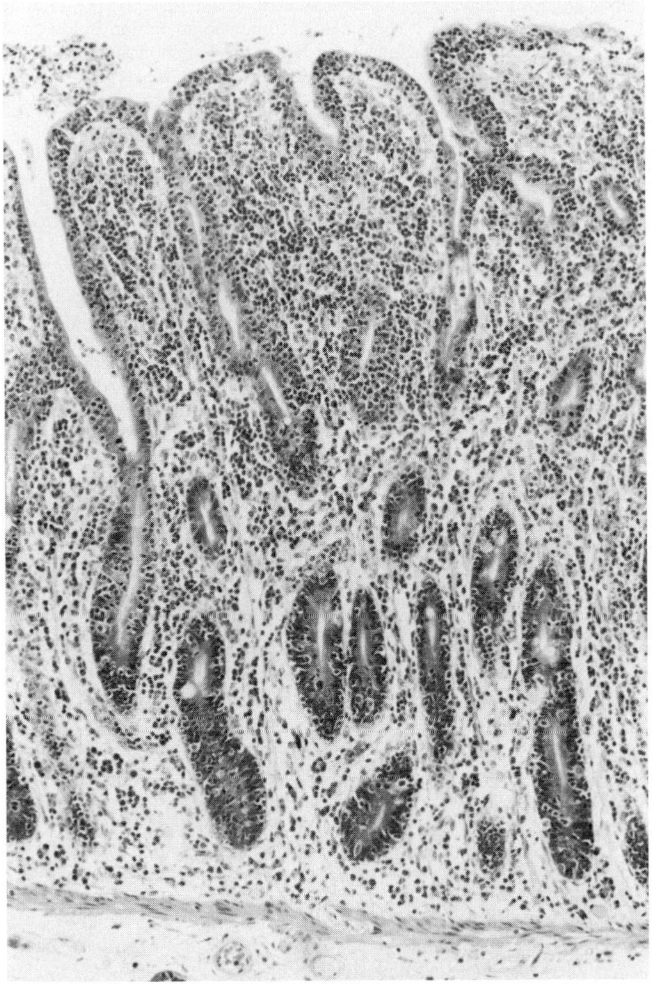

FIG. 33.33. Small intestinal mucosa from a case of enteropathy-associated T-cell lymphoma (EATL) that shows intense intraepithelial lymphocytosis. Intraepithelial lymphocytes have spilled out into the lamina propria.

over, the enteropathy in ulcerative jejunitis and EATL typically fails to respond to a gluten-free diet, and nonspecific inflammatory ulcers, which characterize ulcerative jejunitis, are often present in EATL. Studies have shown that the IELs in nonresponsive celiac disease (91) and ulcerative jejunitis (90) share the immunophenotype of EATL and constitute a monoclonal population. These two conditions are therefore neoplastic, although not overtly lymphomatous.

HISTIOCYTIC AND MYELOPROLIFERATIVE LESIONS OF THE GASTROINTESTINAL TRACT

The histiocytic and myeloproliferative disorders are discussed elsewhere in this volume. Histiocytic tumors (92) have a special predilection for the intestinal tract and should always be considered when faced with an unusual "lymphoma." To a lesser extent, the same is true of granulocytic sarcoma (93), which is more likely to occur in the stomach than the intestine (see Chapters 47, 49, and 51).

SUMMARY AND CONCLUSIONS

As an important immunologic organ in its own right, it is not surprising that the gastrointestinal tract is the most common site of extranodal lymphoma. However, the relative incidence and the subtypes of gastrointestinal lymphoma are sharply different from lymphomas of peripheral lymphoid tissues. It is likely that there are important biologic lessons to be learned from these differences. As new treatments specific for gastrointestinal, as opposed to nodal, lymphomas emerge, it becomes increasingly important that these disorders are diagnosed with a high degree of precision.

REFERENCES

1. Dawson IMP, Cornes JS, Morson BC. Primary malignant tumour of the intestinal tract. *Br J Surg* 1961;49:80–89.
2. Greiner TC, Medeiros LJ, Jaffe ES. Non-Hodgkin's lymphoma. *Cancer* 1995;75:370–380.
3. Azab MB, Henry-Amar M, Rougier P, et al. Prognostic factors in primary gastrointestinal non-Hodgkin's lymphoma: a multivariate analysis, report of 106 cases and review of the literature. *Cancer* 1989;64: 1208–1217.
4. Hayes J, Dunn E. Has the incidence of primary gastric lymphoma increased? *Cancer* 1989;63:2073–2076.
5. Salem P, El-Hashimi L, Anaissie E, et al. Primary small intestinal lymphoma in adults: a comparative study of IPSID in the Middle East. *Cancer* 1987;59:1670–1676.
6. Spencer J, Finn T, Pulford KAF, et al. The human gut contains a novel population of B-lymphocytes which resemble marginal zone cells. *Clin Exp Immunol* 1985;62:607–612.
7. Spencer J, Finn T, Isaacson PG. Human Peyer's patches: an immunohistochemical study. *Gut* 1986;27:405–410.
8. Cerf-Bensussan N, Guy-Grand D, Griscelli C. Intraepithelial lymphocytes of human gut: isolation, characterisation and study of natural killer activity. *Gut* 1985;26:81–88.
9. Spencer J, Isaacson PG, Diss TC, et al. Expression of disulphide linked and non-disulphide linked forms of the T-cell receptor gamma/delta heterodimer in human intestinal intraepithelial lymphocytes. *Eur J Immunol* 1989;19:1335–1338.
10. Isaacson PG, Wright DH. Malignant lymphoma of mucosa-associated lymphoid tissue: a distinctive type of B-cell lymphoma. *Cancer* 1983; 52:1410–1416.
11. Isaacson PG, Wright DH. Extranodal malignant lymphoma arising from mucosa associated lymphoid tissue. *Cancer* 1984;53:2515–2524.
12. Harris NL, Jaffe ES, Stein H, et al. A revised European-American classification of lymphoid neoplasms: a proposal from the International Lymphoma Study Group. *Blood* 1994;84:1361–1392.
13. Wyatt JL, Rathbone BJ. Immune response of the gastric mucosa to *Campylobacter pylori. Scand J Gastroenterol* 1988;[Suppl 142]: 44–49.
14. Stolte M, Eidt S. Lymphoid follicles in antral mucosa: immune response to *Campylobacter pylori*? *J Clin Pathol* 1989;42:1269–1271.
15. Genta RM, Hamner HW, Graham DY. Gastric lymphoid follicles in *Helicobacter pylori* infection: frequency, distribution and response to triple therapy. *Hum Pathol* 1993;24:577–583.
16. Wotherspoon AC, Ortiz-Hidalgo C, Falzon MR, et al. *Helicobacter pylori*–associated gastritis and primary B-cell gastric lymphoma. *Lancet* 1991;338:1175–1176.
17. Doglioni C, Wotherspoon AC, Moschini A, et al. High incidence of primary gastric lymphoma in North Eastern Italy. *Lancet* 1992;339: 834–835.
18. Parsonnet J, Freidman GD, Vandersteen DP, et al. *Helicobacter pylori* infection and the risk of gastric carcinoma. *N Engl J Med* 1991;325: 1127–1131.
19. Hussell T, Isaacson PG, Crabtree JE, et al. The response of cells from low grade B-cell gastric lymphomas of mucosa-associated lymphoid tissue to *Helicobacter pylori. Lancet* 1993;342:571–574.
20. Hussell T, Isaacson PG, Crabtree JE, et al. *Helicobacter pylori*–specific tumour infiltrating T-cells provide contact dependent help for the

growth of malignant B-cells in low grade gastric lymphoma of mucosa-associated lymphoid tissue. *J Pathol* 1996;178:122–127.
21. Wotherspoon AC, Doglioni C, Diss TC, et al. Regression of primary low grade B-cell gastric lymphoma of mucosa-associated lymphoid tissue after eradication of *Helicobacter pylori*. *Lancet* 1993;342: 575–577.
22. Wotherspoon AC, Doglioni C, de Boni M, et al. Antibiotic treatment for low grade gastric MALT lymphoma. *Lancet* 1994;343:1503.
23. Weber DM, Dimopoulos MA, Anandu MA, et al. Regression of gastric lymphoma of mucosa-associated lymphoid tissue with antibiotic therapy for *Helicobacter pylori*. *Gastroenterology* 1994;107:1835–1838.
24. Roggero E, Zucca E, Pinotti G, et al. Eradication of *Helicobacter pylori* infection in primary low grade gastric lymphoma of mucosa-associated lymphoid tissue. *Ann Intern Med* 1995;122:767–769.
25. Bayerdorffer E, Neubauer A, Rudolph B, et al. Regression of primary gastric lymphoma of mucosa-associated lymphoid tissue type after cure of *Helicobacter pylori* infection. *Lancet* 1995;345:1591–1594.
26. Montalban C, Castrillo JM, Abraira V, et al. Gastric B-cell mucosa-associated lymphoid tissue (MALT) lymphoma: clinicopathological study and evaluation of the prognostic factors in 143 patients. *Ann Oncol* 1995;6:355–362.
27. Blecker U, McKeithan TW, Hart J, et al. Resolution of *Helicobacter pylori*–associated gastric lymphoproliferative disease in a child. *Gastroenterology* 1995;109:973–977.
28. Savio A, Franzin G, Wotherspoon AC, et al. Diagnosis and post-treatment follow-up of *Helicobacter pylori*–positive gastric lymphoma of mucosa-associated lymphoid tissue: histology, polymerase chain reaction, or both? *Blood* 1996;87:1255–1260.
29. Taal BG, Boot H, van Heerde P, et al. Primary non-Hodgkin's lymphoma of the stomach: endoscopic pattern and prognosis in low versus high grade malignancy in relation to the MALT concept. *Gut* 1996; 39:556–561.
30. Isaacson PG, Spencer J. Malignant lymphoma of mucosa-associated lymphoid tissue. *Histopathology* 1987;11:445–462.
31. Myhre MJ, Isaacson PG. Primary B-cell gastric lymphoma—a reassessment of its histogenesis. *J Pathol* 1987;152:1–11.
32. Isaacson PG, Norton AJ. *Extra nodal lymphomas*. Edinburgh: Churchill Livingstone, 1994.
33. Zamboni G, Franzin G, Scarpa A, et al. Carcinoma-like signet-ring cells in gastric mucosa-associated lymphoid tissue (MALT) lymphoma. *Am J Surg Pathol* 1996;20:588–598.
34. Isaacson PG, Wotherspoon AC, Diss TC, et al. Follicular colonization in B-cell lymphoma of mucosa-associated lymphoid tissue. *Am J Surg Pathol* 1991;15:819–828.
35. Wotherspoon AC, Doglioni C, Isaacson PG. Low grade gastric B-cell lymphoma of mucosa-associated lymphoid tissue (MALT) a multifocal disease. *Histopathology* 1992;20:29–34.
36. Du MQ, Peng HZ, Diss TC, et al. Preferential dissemination of B-cell mucosa associated lymphoid tissue (MALT) to the splenic marginal zone. *Blood* 1997;90:4071–4077.
37. Spencer J, Diss TC, Isaacson PG. Primary B-cell gastric lymphoma and ''pseudolymphoma'': a genotypic analysis. *Am J Pathol* 1989;135: 557–564.
38. Qin Y, Greiner A, Trunk MJF, et al. Somatic hypermutation in low grade mucosa-associated lymphoid tissue-type B-cell lymphoma. *Blood* 1995;86:3528–3534.
39. Du M, Diss TC, Xu C, et al. Ongoing mutation in MALT lymphoma immunoglobulin gene suggests that antigen stimulation plays a role in the clonal expansion. *Leukaemia* 1996;10:1190–1197.
40. Pan L, Diss TC, Cunningham D, et al. The bcl-2 gene in primary B-cell lymphomas of mucosa associated lymphoid tissue (MALT). *Am J Pathol* 1989;135:7–11.
41. Peng H, Chen G, Du M, et al. Replication error phenotype and p53 gene mutation in lymphomas of mucosa-associated lymphoid tissue. *Am J Pathol* 1996;148:643–648.
42. Peng HZ, Diss TC, Isaacson PG, et al. C-myc gene abnormalities in mucosa-associated lymphoid tissue (MALT) lymphomas. *J Pathol* 1997;181:381–386.
43. Du M, Peng H, Singh N, et al. The accumulation of p53 abnormalities is associated with progression of mucosa-associated lymphoid tissue lymphoma. *Blood* 1995;86:4587–4593.
44. Wotherspoon AC, Finn TM, Isaacson PG. Trisomy 3 in low grade B-cell lymphomas of mucosa-associated lymphoid tissue. *Blood* 1995; 85:2000–2004.
45. Ott G, Katzenberger T, Greiner A, et al. The (11;8)(q21;q21) chromosome translocation is a frequent and specific aberration in low grade but not high grade malignant non-Hodgkin's lymphomas if the mucosa-associated lymphoid tissue (MALT-) type. *Cancer Res* 1997;57: 3944–3948.
46. Cogliatti SB, Schmid U, Schumacher U, et al. Primary B-cell gastric lymphoma: a clinicopathological study of 145 patients. *Gastroenterology* 1991;101:1159–1170.
47. De Jong D, Boot H, Van Heerde P, et al. Histological grading in gastric lymphoma: pre-treatment criteria and clinical relevance. *Gastroenterology* 1997;112:1466–1474.
48. Zucca E, Bertoni F, Roggero E, et al. Molecular analysis of the progression from *Helicobacter pylori*–associated chronic gastritis to mucosa-associated lymphoid-tissue lymphoma of the stomach. *N Engl J Med* 1998;338:804–810.
49. Nakamura S, Aoyagi K, Furuse M, et al. B-cell monoclonality precedes the development of gastric MALT lymphoma in *Helicobacter pylori*–associated chronic gastritis. *Am J Pathol* 1998;152:1271–1279.
50. Wotherspoon AC, Isaacson PG. Synchronous adenocarcinoma and low grade B-cell lymphoma of mucosa associated lymphoid tissue (MALT) of the stomach. *Histopathology* 1995;27:325–331.
51. Nakamura A, Akazawa K, Yao T, et al. Primary gastric lymphoma: a clinicopathological study of 233 cases with special reference to evaluation with the MIB-1 index. *Cancer* 1995;76:1313–1324.
52. Domizio P, Owen RA, Shepherd NA, et al. Primary lymphoma of the small intestine: a clinicopathological study of 119 cases. *Am J Surg Pathol* 1993;17:429–432.
53. Greenstein AJ, Mullin GE, Strauchen JA, et al. Lymphoma in inflammatory bowel disease. *Cancer* 1992;69:1119–1123.
54. Schmid C, Vazquez JJ, Diss TC, et al. Primary B-cell mucosa-associated lymphoid tissue lymphoma presenting as a solitary colorectal polyp. *Histopathology* 1994;24:357–362.
55. Radaszkiewicz T, Dragosics B, Bauer P. Gastrointestinal malignant lymphomas of the mucosa-associated lymphoid tissue: factors relevant to prognosis. *Gastroenterology* 992;102:1628–1638.
56. Ramot B, Shahin N, Bubis JJ. Malabsorption syndrome in lymphoma of small intestine: a study of 13 cases. *Isr J Med Sci* 1965;1:221–226.
57. Price SK. Immunoproliferative small intestinal disease: a study of 13 cases with alpha heavy-chain disease. *Histopathology* 1990;17:7–17.
58. Rambaud JC, Modigliani R, Nguyen Phuoc BK, et al. Non-secretory alpha-chain disease in intestinal lymphoma. *N Engl J Med* 1980;303: 53.
59. Ben-Ayed F, Halphen M, Najjar T, et al. Treatment of alpha chain disease—results of a prospective study in 21 Tunisian patients by the Tunisian-French intestinal lymphoma study group. *Cancer* 1989;63: 1251–1256.
60. Galian A, Lecester MJ, Scott J, et al. Pathological study of alpha-chain disease, with special emphasis on evolution. *Cancer* 1977;39: 2081–2101.
61. Isaacson PG, Dogan A, Price SK, et al. Immunoproliferative small intestinal disease: an immunohistochemical study. *Am J Surg Pathol* 1989;13:1023–1033.
62. Nemes Z, Thomazy V, Steifert G. Follicular centre cell lymphoma with alpha heavy chain disease: a histopathological and immunohistochemical study. *Virchows Arch* 1981;394:119–132.
63. Isaacson PG, Price SK. Light chains in Mediterranean lymphoma. *J Clin Pathol* 1985;38:601–607.
64. Smith W, Price SK, Isaacson PG. Immunoglobulin gene rearrangement in immunoproliferative small intestinal disease (IPSID). *J Clin Pathol* 1987;40:1291–1297.
65. Cornes JS. Multiple lymphomatous polyposis of the gastrointestinal tract. *Cancer* 1961;14:249–257.
66. Isaacson PG, MacLennan KA, Subbuswamy SG. Multiple lymphomatous polyposis of the gastrointestinal tract. *Histopathology* 1983;8: 641–656.
67. O'Briain DS, Kennedy MJ, Daly PA, et al. Multiple lymphomatous polyposis of the gastrointestinal tract: a clinicopathologically distinctive form of non-Hodgkin's lymphoma of B-cell centrocytic type. *Am J Surg Pathol* 1989;13:691–699.
68. Ruskone-Fourmestraux A, Aegerter P, Delmer A, et al. Primary digestive tract lymphoma: a prospective multicentric study of 91 patients. Groupe de Etude des Lymphomes Digestifs. *Gastroenterology* 1993; 105:1662–1671.
69. Kumar S, Krenacs L, Orsuki T, et al. Bcl-2 rearrangement and cyclin

D-1 protein expression in multiple lymphomatous polyposis. *Am J Clin Pathol* 1996;105:737–743.
70. Ladjadj Y, Philip T, Lenior GM, et al. Abdominal Burkitt-like lymphomas in Algeria. *Br J Cancer* 1984;49:503–512.
71. Anaissie E, Geha S, Allam C, et al. Burkitt's lymphoma in the Middle East: a study of 34 cases. *Cancer* 1985;56:2539–2543.
72. Fieber SS, Schaefer HJ. Lymphoid hyperplasia of the terminal ileum—a clinical entity? *Gastroenterology* 1961;50:83–98.
73. Rubin A, Isaacson PG. Florid reactive lymphoid hyperplasia of the terminal ileum in adults: a condition bearing a close resemblance to low grade malignant lymphoma. *Histopathology* 1990;17:19–26.
74. Matuchansky C, Touchard G, Lemoire M, et al. Malignant lymphoma of the small bowel associated with diffuse nodular lymphoid hyperplasia. *N Engl J Med* 1985;313:166–171.
75. Rambaud JC, Saint-Louvent P, Mati R, et al. Diffuse follicular lymphoid hyperplasia of the small intestine without primary immunoglobulin deficiency. *Am J Med* 1982;73:125–132.
76. Fairley NH, Mackie FP. The clinical and biochemical syndrome in lymphadenoma and allied disease involving the mesenteric lymph glands. *Br Med J* 1937;1:3972–3980.
77. Gough KR, Read Ae, Naish JM. Intestinal reticulosis as a complication of idiopathic steatorrhoea. *Gut* 1962;3:232–239.
78. Isaacson PG, Wright DH. Malignant histiocytosis of the intestine: its relationship to malabsorption and ulcerative jejunitis. *Hum Pathol* 1978;9:661–677.
79. Isaacson PG, Wright DH. Intestinal lymphoma associated with malabsorption. *Lancet* 1978;1:67–70.
80. O'Farrelly C, Feighery C, O'Briain DS, et al. Humoral response to wheat protein in patients with coeliac disease and enteropathy associated T-cell lymphoma. *Br Med J* 1986;292:908–910.
81. O'Mahony S, Vestey JP, Ferguson A. Similarities in intestinal humoral immunity in dermatitis herpetiformis without enteropathy and in coeliac disease. *Lancet* 1990;335:1487–1490.
82. O'Driscoll BRC, Stevens FM, O'Gorman, et al. HLA-type of patients with coeliac disease and malignancy in the west of Ireland. *Gut* 1982; 23:662–665.
83. Swinson CM, Slavin G, Coles EC, et al. Coeliac disease and malignancy. *Lancet* 1983;1:111–115.
84. Holmes GKT, Prior P, Lane MR, et al. Malignancy in coeliac disease—effect of a gluten free diet. *Gut* 1989;30:333–338.
85. Spencer J, Cerf-Bensussan N, Jarry A, et al. Enteropathy associated T-cell lymphoma (malignant histiocytosis of the intestine) is recognised by a monoclonal antibody (HML1) that defines a membrane molecule on human mucosal lymphocytes. *Am J Pathol* 1988;132:1–5.
86. De Bruin PC, Kummer JA, van der Valk P, et al. Granzyme B–expressing peripheral T-cell lymphomas: neoplastic equivalents of activated cytotoxic T-cells with preference for mucosa associated lymphoid tissue localization. *Blood* 1994;84:3785–3791.
87. Chott A, Haedicke W, Mosberger I, et al. Most $CD56^+$ intestinal lymphomas are $CD8^+CD5^-$ T-cell lymphomas of monomorphic small to medium size histology. *Am J Pathol* 1998;153:1483–1490.
88. Isaacson PG, Spencer J, Connolly CE. Malignant histiocytosis of the intestine: a T-cell lymphoma. *Lancet* 1985;28:688–691.
89. Murray A, Cuevas EC, Jones DB, et al. Study of the immunohistochemistry and T-cell clonality of enteropathy associated T-cell lymphoma. *Am J Pathol* 1995;146:509–519.
90. Ashton-Key M, Diss TC, Pan LX, et al. Molecular analysis of T-cell clonality in ulcerative jejunitis and enteropathy associated T-cell lymphoma. *Am J Pathol* 1997;151:493–498.
91. Cellier C, Patey N, Mauvieux L, et al. Abnormal intestinal intraepithelial lymphocytes in refractory sprue. *Gastroenterology* 1998;114: 471–481.
92. Milchgrub S, Kamel OW, et al. Malignant histiocytic neoplasms of the small intestine. *Am J Surg Pathol* 1992;16:11–20.
93. Brugo EA, Marshall RB, Riberi AM, et al. Pre-leukaemic granulocytic sarcomas of the gastrointestinal tract: report of two cases. *Am J Clin Pathol* 1977;68:616–621.

CHAPTER 34

Pulmonary Lymphomas and Lymphoid Hyperplasias

Douglas B. Flieder and Samuel A. Yousem

Lymphoid proliferations of the lung represent a rare and vexing collection of lesions, including primary pulmonary lesions, spanning the gamut from reactive hyperplasia to high-grade malignant lymphoma. Reclassification of many of these entities, such as pseudolymphoma, low-grade lymphoma, and lymphomatoid granulomatosis, by immunohistochemical and molecular techniques and the use of the Revised European-American Lymphoma (REAL) classification has contributed to pathologists' and clinicians' confusion. This chapter aims to clarify the confusion by presenting our current understanding of lymphoid proliferations of the lung within a historical context, with emphasis on recent changes in diagnostic criteria and classification.

GENERAL CONSIDERATIONS

Understanding the pathology of pulmonary lymphoid proliferations requires knowledge of the normal distribution of lymphoid tissue and lymphatics within the pleuropulmonary system. The lymphatics of the lung are divided into two interconnecting drainage systems, one that drains through the visceral pleura around the lung and into the mediastinal lymph nodes and a second system that drains from the parenchyma centrally to the peribronchial and hilar lymph nodes. These two systems can compensate for one another if interrupted. The lymphatic channels usually are not obvious in histologic sections of normal lung but are easily recognized in pathologic states. If distended with malignant cells as in *lymphangitic carcinoma,* lymphatic channels are readily apparent within the visceral pleura, the interlobular septa and the adventitia of arteries, veins and bronchioles. The lymphatics along the bronchovascular bundles are analogous to lymphatics in the portal tracts of the liver. Small submucosal aggregates of lymphoid cells are prominent at bronchial bifurcations and near distal respiratory bronchioles (''pulmonary microtonsils'').

Whether these sparse lymphoid aggregates truly represent a specialized secondary lymphoid system—bronchus-associated lymphoid tissue (BALT)—remains controversial (1,2). In children, ''microtonsils'' are readily identified suggesting these lymphoid aggregates are part of the normal development of the pulmonary local immune system. The lung can, in certain chronic inflammatory states such as obstructive pneumonia, viral infections, connective tissue diseases and acquired immunodeficiency syndrome (AIDS), develop peribronchial lymphoid aggregates consisting of B lymphocytes, T lymphocytes, HLA-DR^{+} interdigitating cells, follicular dendritic cells and often times lymphoid follicles with an overlying flattened and attenuated specialized epithelium analogous to intestinal Peyer's patches (3–5). These lesions are referred to as acquired BALT.

It is believed that BALT plays a role in immunologic responses to inhaled antigens that land on airway mucosa. Conceptually, BALT and its better developed analogue in the gastrointestinal tract, the gut-associated lymphoid tissue (GALT), can be considered as parts of the mucosa-associated lymphoid tissue (MALT), which may be distinct but not necessarily exclusive of the lymph node and spleen-based somatic system (see Chapters 33 and 35). Mucosa-associated lymphoid tissue synthesizes IgA and other immunoglobulins in response to mucosal surface antigens. Approximately 60% of the lymphoid cells of the BALT are B cells, with the remainder being T cells. The B cells are mostly small lymphocytes with a centrocyte-like appearance. As demonstrated in other MALT sites, these lymphoid cells circulate but return to the lung, perhaps through an organ-specific receptor involving the high endothelial venules present within BALT (6). This is also the case with neoplastic MALT lymphoid proliferations (7) (see Chapter 23).

D. B. Flieder: Assistant Professor of Pathology, Weill Medical College of Cornell University, New York, New York, 10021

S. A. Yousem: Department of Pathology, University of Pittsburgh Medical Center, Pittsburgh, Pennsylvania 15213

EVALUATION OF LYMPHOID PROCESSES OF LUNG

Clinical history and radiographic studies are essential in rendering a complete interpretation of any pulmonary lymphoid process. Toxic symptoms, including fever, chills and night sweats, paraneoplastic syndromes, and pleural effusions, usually indicate an aggressive lymphoma. Radiographic studies are necessary for localization and delineation of the process (Table 34.1). Some light microscopic diagnostic considerations can be excluded purely on the radiographic findings. For example, while pulmonary lymphomas can be localized or multifocal, diffuse lymphoid hyperplasia/lymphocytic interstitial pneumonitis is always bilateral and diffuse. Nodular lymphoid hyperplasia/pseudolymphoma is typically solitary; therefore, diffuse hyperplasia and nodular hyperplasia should never be confused. The radiographic presence of hilar adenopathy should dissuade one from making a diagnosis of nodular lymphoid hyperplasia instead of low-grade lymphoma (8). Those lymphoid infiltrates occurring in the setting of chronic lymphocytic leukemia (CLL) or monoclonal gammopathy are most likely clonal proliferations.

More often than not, diagnoses of pulmonary lymphoid processes require open lung biopsies. Given the architectural and cytologic variability of these lesions, secondary changes in adjacent lung parenchyma and biopsy artifacts, transbronchial biopsies may only be diagnostic in processes with distinctive cytology (e.g., large cell lymphoma) or in patients with established diagnoses of malignant lymphoma. Although molecular studies improve the rate of diagnosis, such studies are not routinely performed and are limited by sample size and fixation (9–11). The diagnosis of lymphoma by fine needle aspiration or bronchoalveolar lavage, supplemented with ancillary studies, including polymerase chain reaction (PCR) and Southern blot analysis, is rare (12,13).

Low-magnification pattern recognition is the single most important step in evaluating a pulmonary lymphoid process. A ''lymphatic distribution'' may be seen in nonlymphoid processes such as sarcoidosis but is most striking in lymphoproliferative lesions and reflects the homing of lymphoid cells to the endogenous pulmonary lymphatic routes. This pattern is typically seen with lymphomas of lung as the primary pattern of lung infiltration or at the periphery of a mass lesion. The lymphangitic pattern may leave large amounts of normal intervening lung parenchyma intact, which contrasts with the effacement of architecture that helps in the identification of lymphoma in lymph nodes. Only when large masses are present in the lung is a morphologic analogy with lymph nodes useful (14). In contrast, processes that diffusely involve alveolar septa without a beaded lymphangitic pattern at scanning magnification tend to be inflammatory rather than neoplastic. Lymphocytic interstitial pneumonitis is an example of a process that diffusely involves alveolar septa in a nonlymphangitic distribution.

TABLE 34.1. *Reactive lymphoid proliferations*

Solitary nodule	Diffuse disease
Intraparenchymal lymph node	Follicular bronchitis/bronchiolitis
Pulmonary hyalinizing granuloma	Diffuse lymphoid hyperplasia
Plasma cell granuloma	Lymphocytic interstitial pneumonitis
Castleman's disease-hyaline vascular type (?)	Multicentric Castleman's disease
Nodular amyloidosis/light-chain deposition disease	
Nodular lymphoid hyperplasia	

Cellular monotony is not the sole criterion for malignancy. Whereas sheets of centrocyte-like cells or atypical large lymphoid cells are diagnostic of MALT-type lymphoma and large cell lymphoma respectively, lymphomatoid granulomatosis, T-cell lymphomas and Hodgkin's disease may be polymorphous with atypical large and small cells admixed with eosinophils, plasma cells, histiocytes and even granulomas (15). Such benign polymorphous infiltrates may obscure the malignant cellular infiltrate. Intraepithelial lymphocytes are a normal component of BALT and lymphoepithelial lesions are not always indicative of a malignant process (16), as suggested in the past. Germinal centers are frequently seen in reactive and malignant lymphoid lesions of the lung and have little or no diagnostic value. Primary malignant lymphomas of lung involve hilar and mediastinal lymph nodes in up to 30% of cases, and the absence of thoracic nodal involvement does not necessarily exclude a diagnosis of lymphoma (8,17,18).

Because many pulmonary lymphomas preserve underlying lung parenchymal architecture, secondary changes in uninvolved lung can create diagnostic difficulties. Lymphomatous involvement of airways can lead to airway obstruction with consequent bacterial or postobstructive pneumonias. Involvement of blood vessels may lead to parenchymal infarction or necrosis. In such instances, transbronchial biopsies may demonstrate nonspecific findings and multiple tissue sections from open biopsies may be required to identify diagnostic foci of lymphoma amidst largely necrotic nodules. Palisaded histiocytes in aggressive lymphomas and lymphomatoid granulomatosis may suggest infection (19).

Lymphoid processes of lung may be closely mimicked by or may have superimposed infections. The two prototypes are *Pneumocystis carinii* pneumonia, which in its classic form is rich in interstitial lymphocytes and plasma cells, and Epstein-Barr virus–related lymphoproliferative processes in transplant recipients. Both infections have prominent lymphoid components and can be misdiagnosed as lymphoma. These distinctions are especially difficult when these processes occur in individuals with lymphoma or altered immune systems such as collagen vascular disease. Histochemical and immunohistochemical studies can aid in diagnosis.

The ever-improving era of immunohistochemistry greatly alters the diagnostic approach to extranodal lymphoid proliferations. Because frozen tissue is no longer required to perform necessary cell surface and immunoglobulin studies, unsuspected lymphoid lesions can be characterized and monoclonality assessed on formalin-fixed, paraffin-embedded tissue sections. Demonstration of immunoglobulin light-chain restriction by flow cytometry or immunoperoxidase techniques is almost universally accepted as a criterion of malignancy, whereas demonstration of aberrant antigen expression (i.e., aberrant phenotypes such as CD5 and CD43 coexpression) supports a diagnosis of B-cell lymphoma (20). Although the number of markers continues to expand, depending on the differential diagnosis, cytokeratin, CD3, CD5, CD10, CD20, CD21, CD23, CD43, CD45, cyclin D1, BCL-2, κ, and λ usually suffice for diagnostic purposes. In the 20% to 30% of cases in which immunostains for immunoglobulin light chains are negative or weak, PCR may be used as an adjunct to show rearrangement of the immunoglobulin heavy-chain gene joining region (J_H) or the T-cell receptor γ-chain gene (TCR-γ) (21); however, this modality should not be interpreted outside the context of morphologic and immunophenotypic data. Chromosomal abnormalities recognized by highly sensitive PCR techniques can on occasion support the diagnosis of pulmonary low-grade lymphoma; however, the role of specific markers such as t(11; 18), t(14;18), and BCL-2 immunoglobulin heavy-chain gene translocation remains to be defined.

Although clonality indicates malignancy, clonality in pulmonary lymphoid lesions may not predict clinical outcome. Many low-grade B-cell lymphomas have long indolent courses with 10-year survival rates of more than 80% (8,18,22), and diffuse lymphoid hyperplasia or lymphocytic interstitial pneumonitis may be progressive, with up to one third of affected individuals dying of end-stage honeycomb fibrosis (23).

REACTIVE OR INFLAMMATORY LYMPHOID PROCESSES

Inflammatory processes in the lung can be divided into nodular and diffuse forms with specific clinicopathologic entities restricted to one or the other category (Table 34.1). The discussion of these reactive proliferations is divided along these lines.

Reactive Lymphoid Processes, Nodular

Intrapulmonary Lymph Nodes

Although once regarded as an incidental finding in up to 18% of autopsy lungs (24), widespread use of chest computed tomography (CT) has made the intrapulmonary lymph node (IPL) a significant radiographic lesion not to be mistaken for a malignancy. Intrapulmonary lymph nodes are found in all ages; in children the nodules are usually found during evaluation for metastases from nonpulmonary primary tumors such as osteosarcoma, while in adults the nodules are identified in routine chest roentgenograms and lung cancer screening CT scans. Up to 80% of reported cases occur in men with histories of tobacco use. More than 50% of individuals also have a history of exposure to asbestos, nonfibrous silicates or both (25). Radiographically, IPLs are usually sharply circumscribed homogeneous subpleural opacities located inferior to the carina and measure less than 2.0 cm in diameter (25–27). Thirty-five percent of cases are multiple. Histologically, IPNs are seen in subpleural areas, along interlobular septa or within the major or minor fissures of the lung. Intrapulmonary lymph nodes resemble normal lymph nodes; they are encapsulated and have recognizable nodal architecture (Fig. 34.1). Sinus histiocytes frequently contain abundant anthracosilicotic pigment, and, if this material is excessive, silicotic nodules may form and even calcify. Consequently, IPNs may appear radiographically as solitary calcified nodules. The cortices and medullas may demonstrate prominent germinal centers or paracortical hyperplasia after percutaneous needle biopsies. In patients with chronic lymphocytic leukemia, IPLs may be involved and, rarely, primary lung carcinoma or carcinoma from a nonpulmonary site can metastasize to IPLs. Most importantly, IPLs can be clinically, radiographically and cytologically mistaken for malignant processes. Although fine-needle aspiration specimens should exclude the possibility of carcinoma and obviate thoracotomies, these specimens can yield an erroneous diagnosis of lymphoma. Clinical information should be obtained before such a diagnosis is made.

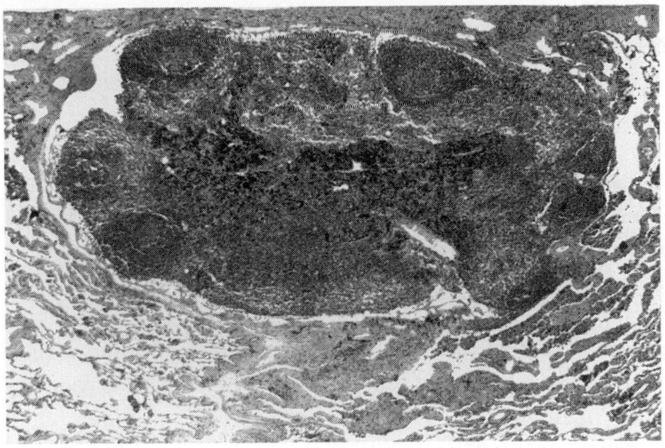

FIG. 34.1. Intrapulmonary lymph node. Intrapulmonary lymph nodes have the same architectural features as extrapulmonary lymph nodes: a prominent subcapsular sinus, corticomedullary differentiation, and primary and secondary follicles. Sinusoidal macrophages may be rich in anthracosilicotic pigment (hematoxylin and eosin stain, original magnification: 40× magnification).

Pulmonary Hyalinizing Granuloma

Pulmonary hyalinizing granuloma (PHG) is a unique fibrosing process that shares clinicopathologic and morphologic features with sclerosing mediastinitis, inflammatory pseudotumor of the orbit, Riedel thyroiditis and idiopathic retroperitoneal fibrosis (28). Almost a fourth of reported series observed concomitant mediastinal or retroperitoneal disease (29,30). PHG has also been reported in a patient with Castleman's disease and in a patient with malignant lymphoma who subsequently developed multiple myeloma (31,32). Pulmonary nodules occur twice as often in women. Age at presentation ranges from 24 to 77 years and most patients present with mild or nonspecific symptoms, including cough, shortness of breath, fever, fatigue, and pleuritic chest pain. Up to 25% of reported individuals are asymptomatic. Laboratory studies show evidence of autoimmune phenomena, including positive antinuclear antibodies, rheumatoid factor, antineutrophil cytoplasmic antibodies, and Coombs'-positive hemolytic anemia (30,33). Skin testing usually demonstrates exposure to *Mycobacterium tuberculosis* or *Histoplasma capsulatum.*

Chest radiographs reveal ill-defined homogeneous nodules that resemble metastatic carcinoma (34). Often bilateral and multilobar, up to one third of the cases in one large series were unilateral and solitary (30). Sequential chest films demonstrate enlargement over years with worsening of pulmonary symptoms, but a sudden increase in size, cavitation and the development of calcification are rare events.

Histologically, PHGs are characterized by well-circumscribed nodules of irregular haphazard or whorl-like deposits of dense eosinophilic lamellar collagen that form around capillary-sized vessels and compress airways (Fig. 34.2). The thick collagen lamellae are separated by a sparse to focally dense lymphoplasmacytic infiltrate composed of mature lymphocytes, predominantly T-cell phenotype, and polytypic plasma cells (Fig. 34.2). Inconspicuous fibroblasts are also interposed between the bands and karyorrhectic and necrotic debris may be present while discrete foci of punctate necrosis or necrotizing granulomatous inflammation are absent. At the periphery, prominent germinal centers and a variably intense lymphoplasmacytic infiltrate are seen. Bronchovascular structures abutting the lesion demonstrate peribronchiolar inflammation and in most cases arterioles at the edge have transmural lymphoplasmacytic infiltrates without fibrinoid necrosis. Adjacent pulmonary parenchyma may feature inflammatory pseudotumor-like changes and diffuse hyperplasia of BALT-like areas (30).

Pulmonary hyalinizing granuloma may represent a peculiar lymphoid and fibrohistiocytic reaction induced by fungal or mycobacterial antigens or an autoimmune phenomenon. Although benign, the prognosis of PHG is difficult to predict. Solitary nodules can be excised and symptoms appear to cease, whereas patients with enlarging or recurrent nodules often experience worsening pulmonary symptoms with eventual respiratory compromise.

Plasma Cell Granuloma

The various terms given to these lesions, such as *plasma cell granuloma, inflammatory myofibroblastic tumor, lymphoid inflammatory pseudotumor, fibrous histiocytoma, inflammatory myofibrohistiocytic proliferation, plasma cell granuloma–histiocytoma complex, xanthoma,* and *xanthogranuloma,* reflect the varied histologic appearances and divergent views concerning their pathogenesis and malignant potential (35–37). Although these tumors demonstrate a morphologic continuum, most lesions belong to two broad categories: postinflammatory subtype and fibrohistiocytic subtype. The fibrohistiocytic lesions are considered low-grade mesenchymal tumors, and evidence of tumor cell monoclonality supports this view (38,39), whereas the postinflammatory subtype probably represents a slowly resolving pneumonic process associated with abundant inflammatory cells (37).

Individuals between 1 and 77 years of age present with

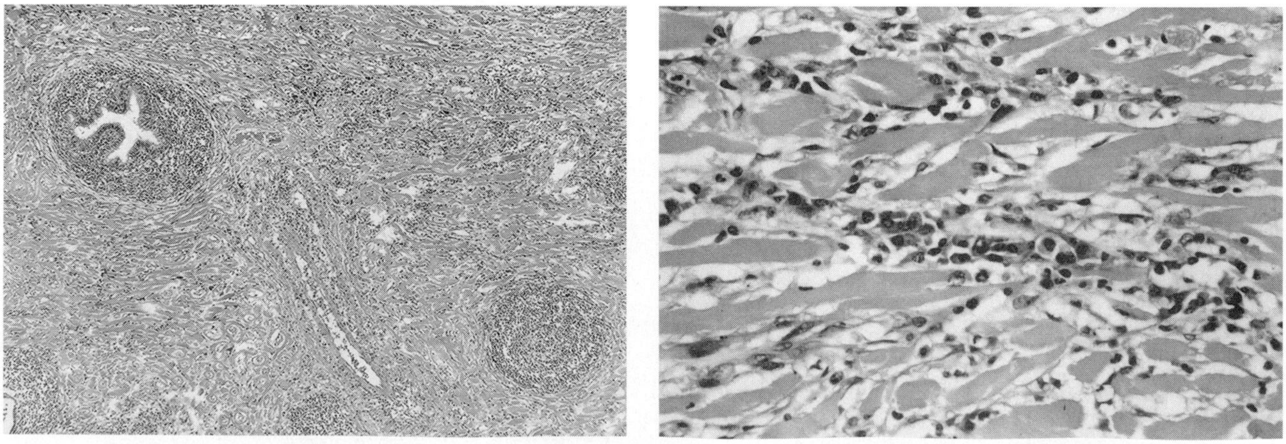

A B

FIG. 34.2. Pulmonary hyalinizing granuloma. **A:** Lung parenchyma is overrun by a fibroinflammatory process. Notice the peribronchiolar lymphoid infiltrate and reactive germinal center (hematoxylin and eosin stain, original magnification: 40× magnification). **B:** Storiform arrays of lamellar collagen are separated by a lymphoplasmacytic infiltrate (hematoxylin and eosin stain, original magnification: 200× magnification).

plasma cell granuloma (PCG). Approximately 60% of patients are younger than 40 years, 25% are younger than 18 years, and 8% are in the first decade of life (40–43). A sex predilection is not seen and these lesions are found mostly in the lung, but also in the mediastinum and retroperitoneum, among other sites (37,41,44).

Although most patients are asymptomatic, the remainder provide a history of previous infections, cough, hemoptysis, or wheeze related to proximal airway involvement. Laboratory tests are normal in almost all individuals; however, hypergammaglobulinemia secondary to interleukin-1β and interleukin-6 production has been reported (45). Chest radiographs most often demonstrate a solitary, well-defined right-sided lower lobe lesion, but poorly circumscribed lesions with spiculation can be seen (46). Two or three separate lesions are seen in up to 5% of cases (41) and radiographic evidence of mediastinal extension has been described (40).

Lesions vary from 0.5 to 36 cm in diameter, with a mean size of 5.5 cm. The parenchymal tumors are typically nonencapsulated but well circumscribed, whereas intrabronchial masses are polypoid. The postinflammatory subtype is more likely to penetrate the pleura and extend into the mediastinum than the fibrohistiocytic subtype (43). Tumor color varies depending on the presence of numerous xanthoma cells (yellow), plasma cells and lymphocytes (tan) or fibrous connective tissue (white) (Fig. 34.3). Small foci of necrosis or calcification may be seen.

Microscopically, the lesion obliterates lung parenchyma with entrapped alveolar septa, bronchioles and vessels seen at tumor margins (Fig. 34.4). Intrabronchial lesions may invade underlying mucosa, surround and partially destroy bronchial cartilage and extend into peribronchial adventitia. The fibrohistiocytic subtype consists of spindled myofibroblasts and fibroblasts arrayed in storiform and fascicular patterns and admixed with macrophages, foamy macrophages (xanthoma cells), multinucleated Touton-type giant cells, lymphocytes and plasma cells (Fig. 34.4). The postinflammatory subtype shows short fascicles of plump myofibroblasts, fibroblasts and abundant plasma cells embedded in a dense collagenous matrix (Fig. 34.4). The spindle cell nuclei are usually oval with small nucleoli and eosinophilic cytoplasm. Mild nuclear atypia and up to 2 mitoses per 50 high-power fields may be seen. A brisker mitotic rate is a parameter of clinical aggressiveness (47). The polytypic plasma cells are mature, and Mott or Russell bodies can be seen. Lymphoid follicles can also be seen at the edge of the lesion and occasional foamy macrophages, neutrophils, eosinophils and mast cells can be found. Necrosis is infrequent, but when present is associated with cholesterol clefts. Spindle cells are usually vimentin, muscle-specific actin, and focally desmin positive, and ultrastructural studies demonstrate fibroblastic and myofibroblastic features.

The postinflammatory subtype can have spindle cells invade pulmonary vessels. In one case, death resulted from extension of the lesion into main pulmonary veins and pericardium (48). Cytologically bland PCG can invade the pleura, chest wall, hilus, spine and mediastinum (43), raising the possibility that this subtype is, as has been shown for the fibrohistiocytic lesions, a low-grade malignancy.

The histologic differential diagnosis for the postinflammatory subtype includes inflammatory fibrosarcoma and plasmacytoma of lung. The former entity demonstrates significant nuclear atypia and is usually extrapulmonary, while solitary plasmacytomas of the lung consist entirely of plasma cells with various degrees of nuclear pleomorphism and a monoclonal immunoglobulin light-chain staining pattern (49).

Castleman's Disease

The three different disorders historically considered under the heading *Castleman's disease* (CD) (i.e., angiofollicular

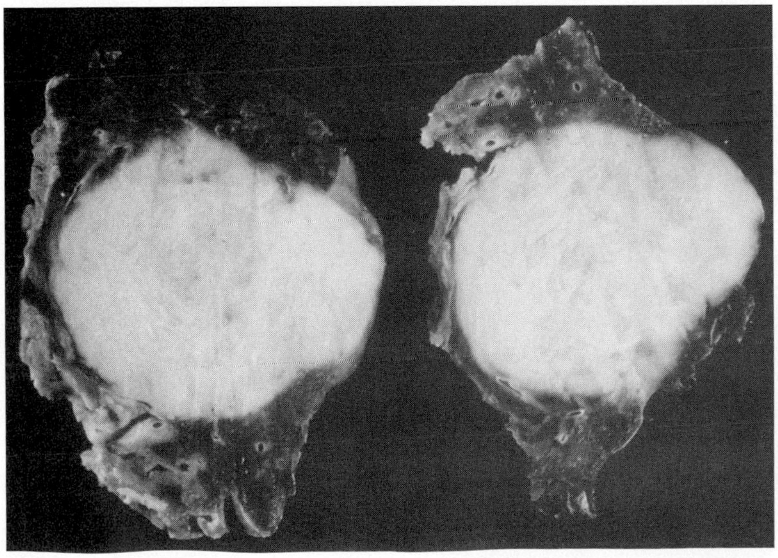

FIG. 34.3. Plasma cell granuloma. Solitary lesions are usually well circumscribed but may invade pleura and mediastinal structures. Tumor color depends on cellular content. This pale lesion was paucicellular.

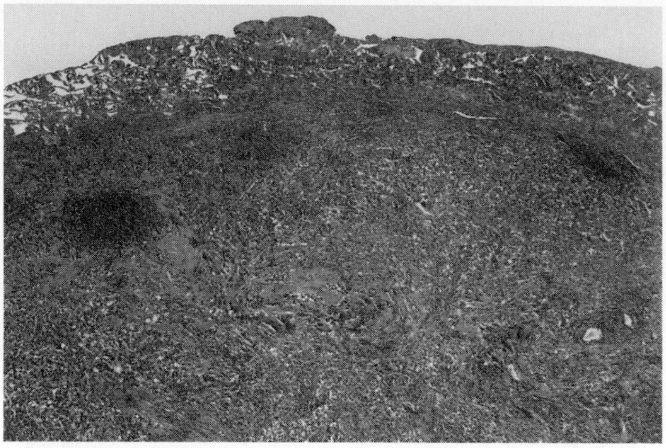

A

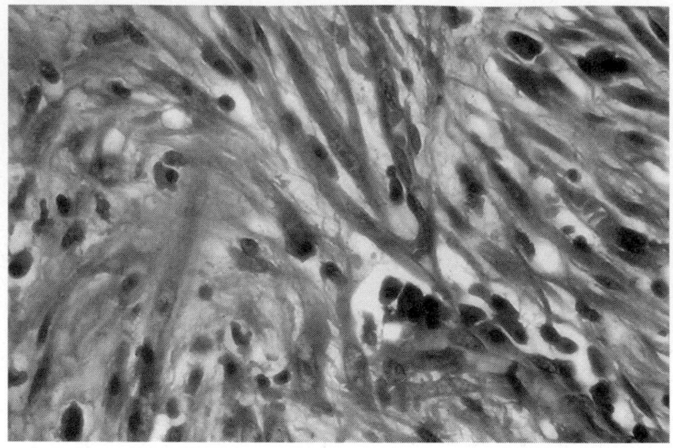

B

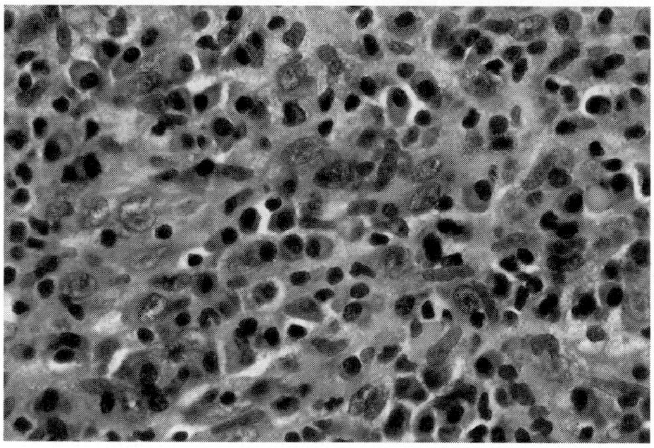

C

FIG. 34.4. Plasma cell granuloma. **A:** Relatively well-circumscribed tumors with lymphoid aggregates obliterate lung parenchyma (hematoxylin and eosin stain, original magnification: 40× magnification). **B:** The fibrohistiocytic variant consists of spindle cells arranged in storiform and fascicular patterns (hematoxylin and eosin stain, original magnification: 400× magnification). **C:** The postinflammatory subtype features abundant plasma cells with many Russell bodies (hematoxylin and eosin stain, original magnification: 400× magnification).

or giant lymph node hyperplasia) are discussed in Chapter 16; however, several comments regarding pulmonary involvement are necessary. Given the propensity for the hyaline-vascular type of CD to involve mediastinal lymph nodes, especially along the tracheobronchial tree, most cases of pulmonary hilar HV-CD probably represent nodal disease rather than true pulmonary disease. Only one of 74 HV-CD cases reviewed in 1973 presented as a pulmonary ''coin lesion'' (50). Given that this lesion is considered a lymph node disorder, rare pulmonary cases with HV-CD morphology may represent involvement of intrapulmonary lymph nodes. Nodal CD-HV is a nonrecurrent lesion cured with excision and should be distinguished from systemic variants of CD, namely CD of plasma cell type and multicentric CD (MCD).

Although solitary HV-CD may exist as a localized lung lesion, the localized plasma cell variant (CD-PC) has not been reported in the lung. However, several cases of pulmonary involvement in MCD or IL-6 syndrome have been reported (51–55). The pathologic findings in these cases are similar and feature peribronchiolar lymphoplasmacytic infiltrates with focal extension into interlobular and alveolar septa (Fig. 34.5). Mild focal interstitial fibrosis and honeycomb change have also been observed, but such findings in the absence of the proper clinical context are nonspecific. In one case, immunohistochemical studies revealed polyclonal plasma cells and lymphocytes (55), whereas in another case, PCR and *in situ* hybridization with a probe specific for Kaposi's sarcoma–associated herpesvirus (KSHV) sequences demonstrated the presence of KSHV in a transbronchial sample (54). Human IL-6 and IL-6 receptor genes introduced into Wistar rats resulted in histopathologic lesions similar to these pulmonary MCD (i.e., IL-6 syndrome) lesions (56).

Nodular Amyloidosis and Light-Chain Deposition Disease

Amyloid is composed of extracellular deposits of chemically diverse proteins that form a three-dimensional, twisted, β-pleated sheet. Clinically recognizable disease in the lung can manifest as tracheobronchial disease, solitary or multiple nodules or in a diffuse interstitial parenchymal pattern (57).

Solitary and multiple amyloidomas are more common in older individuals with an average age of 64 years (57). Solitary lesions present as incidental findings on chest radiographs (58) while multiple nodules can distort airways or visceral pleura leading to cough, hemoptysis or pleuritic chest pain secondary to pleural effusion (57). A radiographic diagnosis can be strongly suggested when calcification or ossification are observed; otherwise, the clinical impression is that of a neoplasm.

Serum or urine monoclonal proteins are found in 10% of patients (57) and a variety of lymphoproliferative diseases

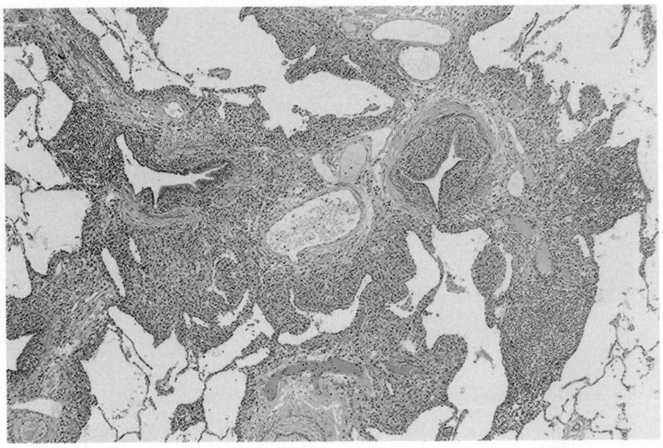

A

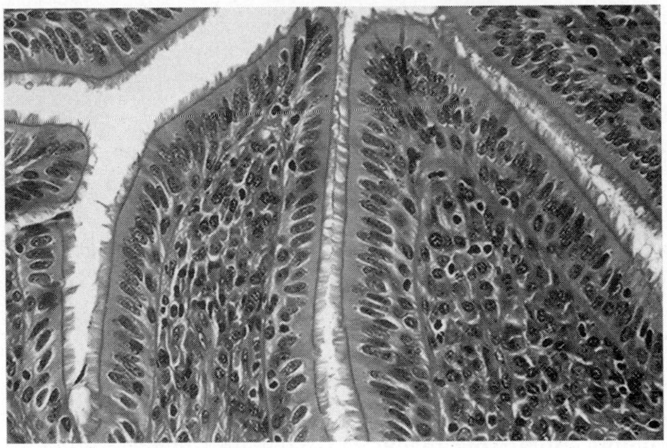

B

FIG. 34.5. Pulmonary involvement in multicentric Castleman's disease (i.e., interleukin-6 syndrome). **A:** Peribronchiolar infiltrates extend into interlobular and alveolar septa (hematoxylin and eosin stain, original magnification: 40× magnification). **B:** Numerous polyclonal plasma cells expand the peribronchiolar submucosa without destroying respiratory epithelium (hematoxylin and eosin stain, original magnification: 200× magnification). (Photomicrographs courtesy of Dr. J. English, Vancouver, British Columbia, Canada.)

can occur in association with nodular amyloid, including benign monoclonal gammopathy (57), Sjögren's syndrome (59), nodular lymphoid hyperplasia (60), lymphocytic interstitial pneumonitis (23), MALT lymphoma (14,61), large cell lymphoma (8,57,61), and multiple myeloma (57).

Nodules range in diameter from 0.6 to 15 cm, with an average of 3.0 cm (57). The lesions are waxy, hard and gritty and yellow to tan-white. Histologically, pulmonary parenchyma is replaced by an irregular mass of amorphous eosinophilic hyaline material that spares many arterioles (Fig. 34.6). Clusters of lymphocytes and plasma cells and multinucleated giant cells occur throughout the lesion, but the cellular infiltrate is most dense at the periphery of the nodules. Calcification and ossification exist in most cases. Congo red staining examined by polarizing microscopy reveals lesional apple-green birefringence. Cases not associated with systemic inflammatory conditions such as collagen-vascular diseases are Congo red positive after potassium permanganate digestion, confirming the nonamyloid A protein nature of the lesion (62).

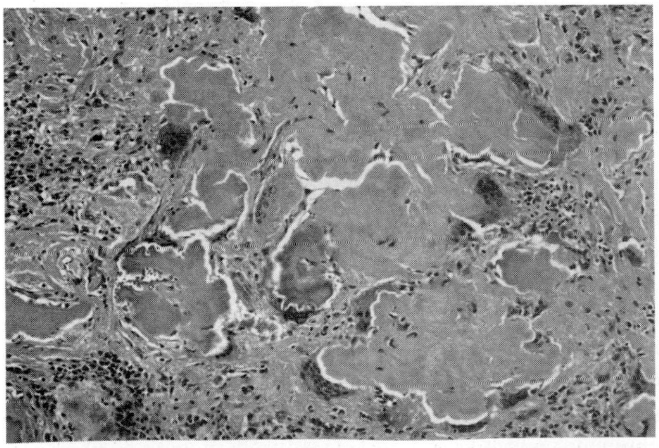

FIG. 34.6. Nodular amyloidosis. Lung parenchyma is replaced by amorphous eosinophilic hyaline material with scattered inflammatory cells, including amyloid-ingesting giant cells (hematoxylin and eosin stain, original magnification: 100× magnification).

Immunohistochemical studies usually demonstrate κ light-chain composition and negative immunoreactivity for amyloid A and transthyretin. Plasma cells are most often polytypic, and probably represent an inflammatory reaction to the amyloid. Ultrastructural examination demonstrates a disorderly arrangement of nonbranching hollow-core 7.5- to 12-nm fibrils.

Most cases of nodular amyloid are diagnosed in resection specimens; however, percutaneous needle biopsies or transbronchial biopsies can also yield a diagnosis as long as reactive epithelial cells are not misinterpreted as carcinoma (63). Although surgical excision is curative, the deposition of AL type amyloid is associated with some form of monoclonal B-cell proliferation. Despite the fact that most individuals with nodular amyloidosis do not have classic multiple myeloma or any other overt B-cell malignancy, they have an underlying B-cell dyscrasia that produces the abnormal protein rather than a tumor.

Although nodular amyloidosis is relatively easy to diagnoses, surgical pathologists should be aware that light-chain deposition disease (LCDD) can also manifest as localized pulmonary nodules. Light-chain deposition disease most commonly affects the kidney with free monoclonal light chains, (IgG, IgA and IgM in decreasing frequency), in the urine or serum of more than 90% of patients (64), but patients may present with hepatic or cardiac symptoms (65–67) as well as asymptomatic pulmonary or pleural nodule(s) (68,69). The frequency of the disease first described in 1976 (70) is difficult to evaluate because light-chain–specific antibodies are not used in a systemic fashion; however, the mean age of patients in reported cases is 57 years, with a 2.5 to 4:1 male to female ratio (68,71,72). These nonamyloidotic deposits of light chains polymerize but do not form β-pleated sheets, resulting in granular deposits focally resembling amyloid and in other areas fibrin. The material is periodic acid–Schiff–positive (PAS^+), diastase resistant, refractile blue on a Giemsa stain; Congo red negative and 80% of LCDD stain for κ light chains with only occasional reports of λ light-chain (71) or combined light-chain and heavy-chain staining (72). IgG, IgM, and IgA staining is absent. Electron microscopy reveals finely granular electron-dense material sometimes containing 11- to 14-nm fibrils (69). It is imperative to exclude this rare entity because an association with multiple myeloma is found in approximately two thirds of the reported cases and a lymphoid malignancy, including solitary plasmacytoma of the lung, in an additional 8% (72,73). The coexistence of LCDD and AL-type amyloidosis and the similarities of both entities suggests that they may represent two poles of the same disease with slightly different manifestations (65,74).

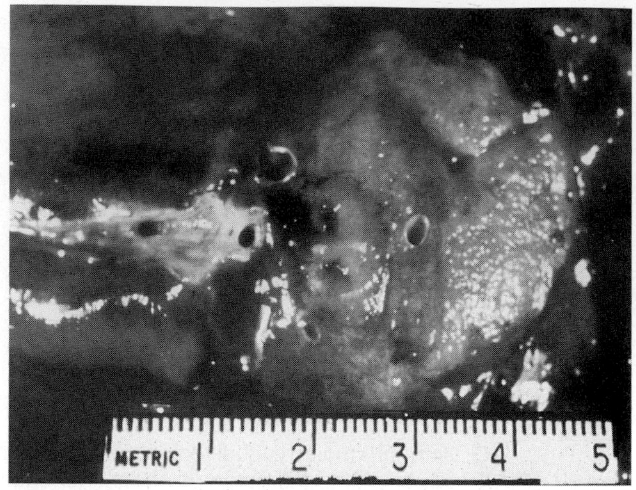

FIG. 34.7. Nodular lymphoid hyperplasia. Excised nodules are 0.6 to 6.0 cm in diameter and are usually well circumscribed, firm, and tan.

Nodular Lymphoid Hyperplasia of Bronchus-Associated Lymphoid Tissue

There is perhaps no pulmonary lesion that has generated as much interest and shift in opinion as nodular lymphoid hyperplasia (NLH) of BALT (i.e., pseudolymphoma). Once considered a common entity (75), then almost a nonexistent lesion (16,17,22,76), NLH is now recognized as a bona fide, albeit rare, reactive lymphoid lesion of the lung. The interesting historical evolution is based in part on careful clinical follow-up of so-called lesions, the development of immunohistochemistry, and greater understanding of extranodal B-cell lymphomas. Initially, NLH was defined as any polymorphous lymphoid condition that did not behave aggressively (76,77), but in the published data from 1963 through 1981, 5 of 33 patients with so-called NLH developed disseminated lymphoma or chronic lymphocytic leukemia (78–81). These results combined with the use of immunohistochemistry to assess for monoclonality has led to a reappraisal of the light microscopic criteria of NLH. And while immunohistochemical evaluation of polymorphous pulmonary lymphoid lesions has led to the belief that B-cell lymphomas of BALT develop within preexisting reactive masses of BALT (17,60), current diagnostic criteria enable surgical pathologists to correctly distinguish between benign and malignant (8,82).

Patients' ages range from the second to the eighth decade, but most are middle aged with a nearly equal gender incidence (8,82). They are typically asymptomatic, and although 10% to 15% of patients were reported to have autoimmune diseases, including systemic lupus erythematosus, Sjögren's syndrome, and transverse myelitis (8,83), one study of 14 cases found no such association (82). Polyclonal hypergammaglobulinemia also occurs.

The most common radiologic presentation is a solitary 2.0- to 5.0-cm nodule. Air bronchograms can be seen, reflecting parenchymal consolidation around patent airways (60). A minority of cases present as a localized infiltrate (84) or several nodules. Such cases emphasize the continuum between nodular and diffuse lymphoid hyperplasia and lymphocytic interstitial pneumonitis. Up to one third of cases feature regional lymphadenopathy (82), but the absence of adenopathy does not exclude a diagnosis of malignant lymphoma.

Excised tan-white and firm nodules may have a central scar and vary from 0.6 to 6.0 cm in the greatest dimension (60,82) (Fig. 34.7). Smaller nodules may be present adjacent to the dominant mass. Histologically, lesions are fairly well demarcated, with slight outward extension along alveolar septa (Fig. 34.8). Most cases feature large reactive germinal centers with well-preserved mantle zones and interfollicular plasma cells admixed with mature noncleaved lymphocytes in a collapsed sclerotic pulmonary parenchyma, but lesions composed almost exclusively of germinal centers can be seen (Figs. 34.8, 34.9). The follicles have reactive light microscopic features, including mitoses, immunoblasts, tingible bodies, central arborizing vessels, and PAS^+ amorphous material. Russell and Mott bodies may be found, but Dutcher bodies are not seen. Scattered giant cells and amyloid are rare findings. Several cases have demonstrated microabscesses and a small foreign body aspiration granuloma, raising the possibility that local inflammatory stimuli are responsible for these lesions (82). Enlarged regional lymph nodes feature benign reactive follicular hyperplasia (60,82).

Immunohistochemical studies demonstrate polytypic immunoglobulin light chains in plasma cells, and germinal center cell expression of CD20 without coexpression of CD5 or CD43. BCL-2 expression is not seen in the germinal centers, but decorates mantle zone cells and interfollicular lymphocytes, while cyclin D1 is entirely negative. One case demonstrated a mixed population of CD4 (helper/inducer) and CD8 (suppressor/cytotoxic) T cells, in keeping with a reactive lesion (60). Molecular genetic analysis by PCR failed to demonstrate rearrangements of the immunoglobulin

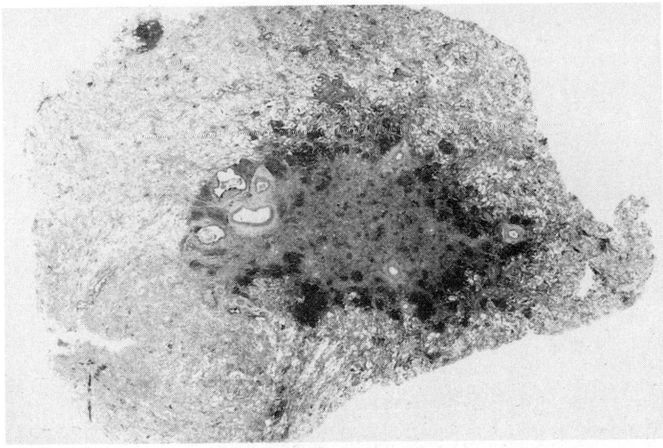

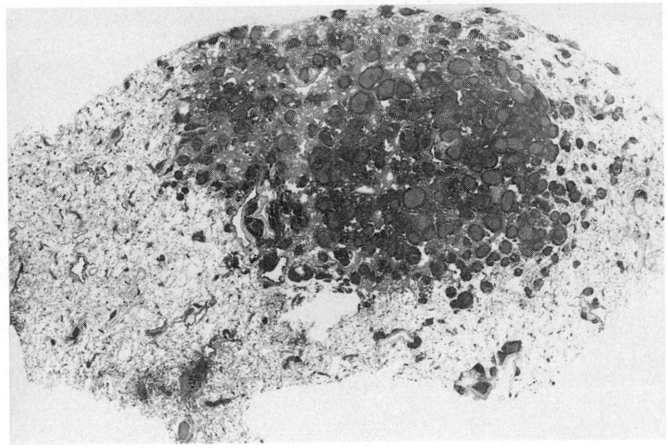

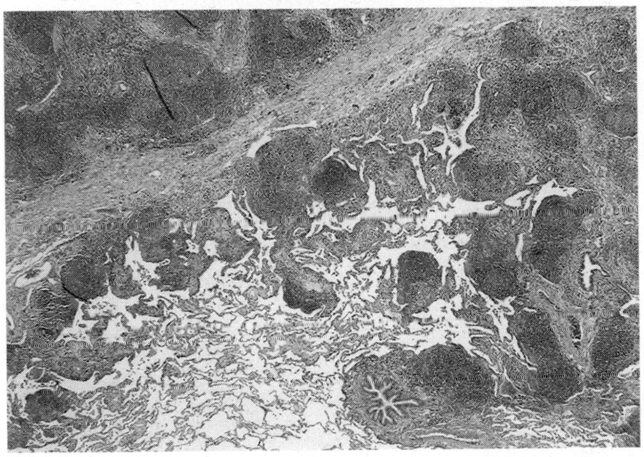

FIG. 34.8. Nodular lymphoid hyperplasia. **A:** Central sclerosis is the most common low-magnification appearance (hematoxylin and eosin stain, original magnification: 4× magnification). **B:** Rare lesions are composed almost exclusively of germinal centers (hematoxylin and eosin stain, original magnification: 4× magnification). **C:** Outward extension along alveolar septa should not be overinterpreted as lymphocytic interstitial pneumonitis (hematoxylin and eosin stain, original magnification: 20× magnification).

heavy-chain gene or major or minor break point regions of the t(14;18) in 10 cases (82).

Although resection of a solitary lesion is usually curative, up to 15% of patients develop local recurrences (8), often at the original surgical site. Neither systemic spread nor death has been reported.

The differential diagnosis of NLH includes diffuse lymphoid hyperplasia (DLH), lymphocytic interstitial pneumonitis (LIP) and B-cell lymphoma. Distinguishing NLH from DLH and LIP is simple as NLH is a localized lesion while DLH and LIP are diffuse bilateral interstitial processes. Differentiating NLH from MALT lymphoma is very

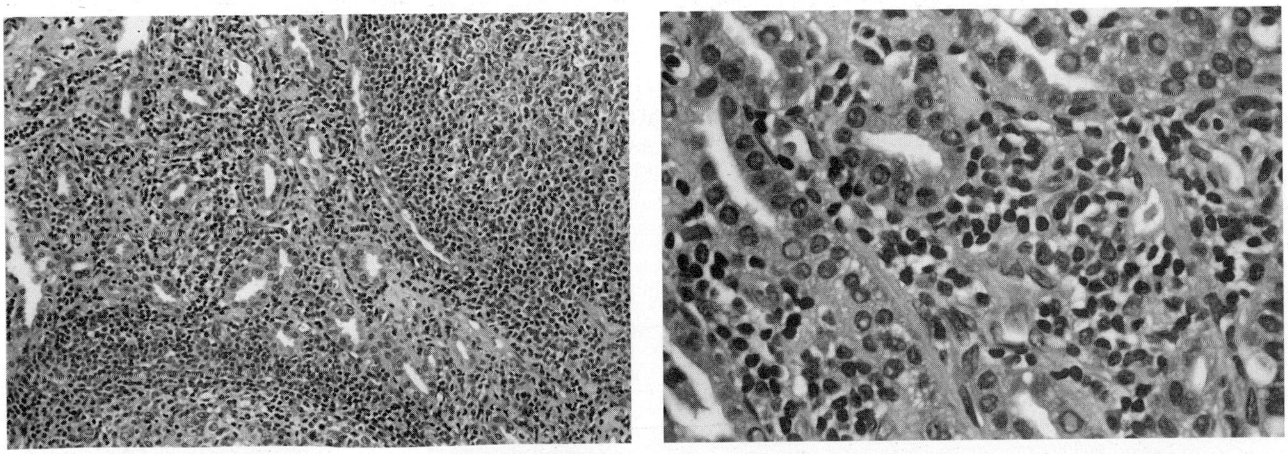

FIG. 34.9. Nodular lymphoid hyperplasia. **A:** Reactive germinal centers embedded in sclerotic parenchyma distort alveolar parenchyma (hematoxylin and eosin stain, original magnification: 200× magnification). **B:** Lymphocytes and plasma cells percolate through sclerotic parenchyma. Notice the reactive pneumocyte atypia (hematoxylin and eosin stain, original magnification: 600× magnification).

A

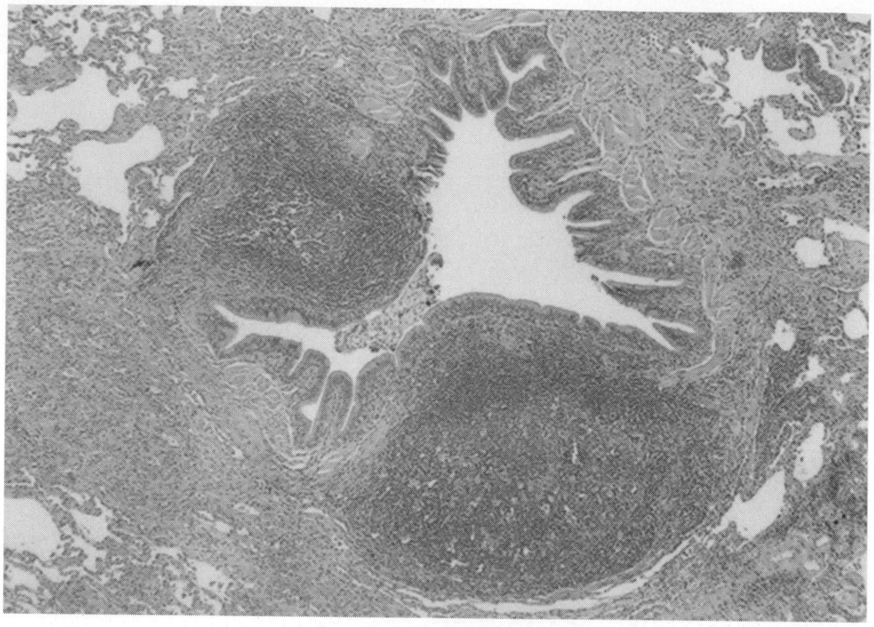

B

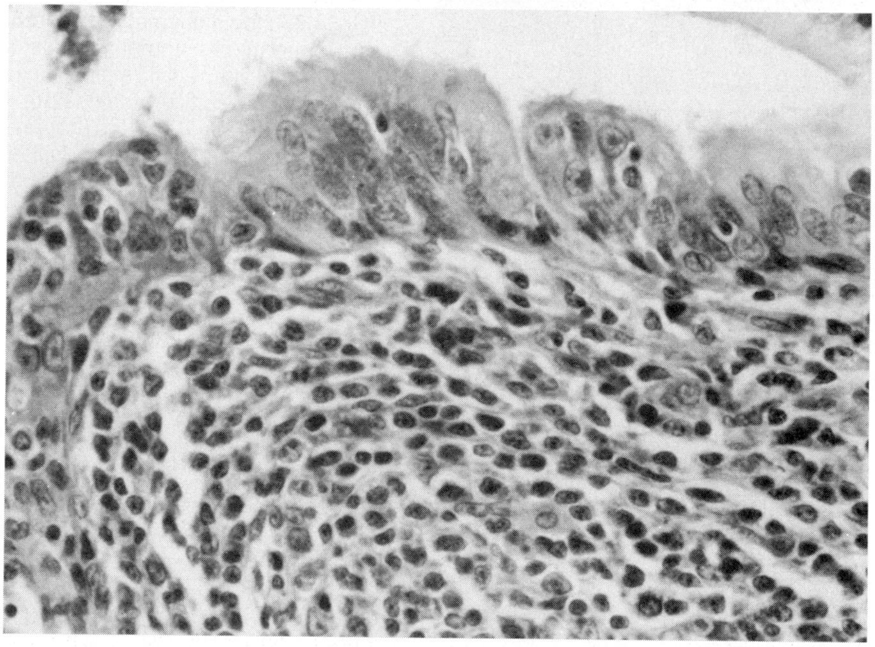

FIG. 34.10. Follicular bronchiolitis. **A:** Airways are distorted by submucosal germinal centers and concentric fibrosis (hematoxylin and eosin stain, original magnification: 40× magnification). **B:** Lymphocytes permeate the respiratory epithelium and may be associated with epithelial necrosis, denudation, and luminal exudates (hematoxylin and eosin stain, original magnification: 400× magnification).

difficult and requires immunohistochemical and, often, molecular studies. Pertinent negative findings in NLH include a lack of pleural invasion (despite the frequent subpleural location of the lesions), destructive vasculitis, necrosis, lymphoepithelial lesions and ill-defined mantle zones. However, it is imperative to recognize that MALT lymphomas can have reactive follicles and polytypic plasma cells with only a focal monotypic cell population or centrocyte-like cells (17), and studies indicate that NLH may evolve into lymphomas (17,85–87) and even solitary plasmacytomas (60). When morphology, immunohistochemistry and molecular studies cannot definitively exclude the presence of lymphoma, a diagnosis of atypical lymphoid infiltrate is warranted (18,82).

Reactive Lymphoid Processes, Diffuse

Diffuse reactive lymphoid processes are best understood within the context of acquired hyperplasia of BALT. Because NLH most likely represents a local response to an extrinsic stimulus, follicular bronchitis/bronchiolitis (FBB), diffuse lymphoid hyperplasia (DLH) and lymphocytic interstitial pneumonitis (LIP) are best considered diffuse patterns of lung reaction to extrinsic stimuli or systemic disease. These are merely descriptive clinicopathologic terms and not diagnostic entities with single causes. Although several hematopathologists (17) recommend separating these lesions into etiologic categories, little work has been pursued toward this reasonable goal.

Follicular Hyperplasia of Bronchus-Associated Lymphoid Tissue

Although investigators debate the presence of BALT in healthy humans (1,2), diffuse lymphoid nodules restricted to the walls of airways and associated peribronchial tissue are seen in many pathologic states and represent follicular hyperplasia of BALT (i.e., follicular bronchitis or bronchiolitis) (60). When relatively common causes such as bronchiectasis and chronic obstructive pulmonary diseases (COPD), including asthma, are excluded, a small number of reported cases called follicular bronchitis/bronchiolitis (FBB) remain that show some overlap with DLH and LIP (16,88).

Follicular bronchitis/bronchiolitis is seen in three clinical settings. First, FBB may be seen as a pulmonary manifestation of connective tissue disease. These patients usually have rheumatoid arthritis or Sjögren's disease and present with dyspnea, cough and obstructive disease on functional studies (89), bilateral interstitial infiltrates on chest radiographs and small centrilobular nodules variably associated with peribronchial nodules and areas of ground-glass opacity on high-resolution CT scans (HRCT) (90). Response to steroid therapy is variable. Second, FBB may be seen as a hypersensitivity reaction that occurs in older persons who have peripheral blood eosinophilia. This subgroup is steroid responsive. Third, FBB may be seen in cases of congenital or acquired immunodeficiency states. The former conditions include severe combined immunodeficiency syndrome, neutrophil chemotaxic defects and other inherited defects. In AIDS, FBB reflects systemic antigenic stimulation. This group of immunodeficiency patients with FBB has a young age at presentation and a poor long term prognosis.

Histologically, enlarged secondary follicles in airway submucosa bulge into the epithelium and disrupt the basal elastica (Fig. 34.10). The B-cell–rich polyclonal follicles distort and compromise the bronchiolar lumens into irregular shapes that predisposes to airway mucostasis, superimposed infectious bronchitis/bronchiolitis and obstructive pneumonia. Rare T cells wander beyond the follicles into adjacent alveolar septa (16). The respiratory epithelium overlying the hyperplastic nodules is attenuated and permeated by lymphocytes but lymphoepithelial lesions are not seen (Fig. 34.10). A concentric ring of lymphocytes and plasma cells may cuff the airways and rare nonnecrotizing granulomas are seen.

Diffuse Lymphoid Hyperplasia of Bronchus-Associated Lymphoid Tissue

Diffuse lymphoid hyperplasia (DLH) of BALT (i.e., diffuse lymphoid hyperplasia and lymphocytic interstitial pneumonitis) represents the pulmonary analogue of reactive follicular hyperplasia of the lymph node demonstrating prominent germinal centers along lymphatic routes and involving pulmonary microtonsils (16,60). This uncommon parenchymal pattern of lymphoid hyperplasia is seen in patients with connective tissue disorders, immunodeficiency disorders and in chronic low-grade infections such as *Mycoplasma, Chlamydia,* or Epstein-Barr virus (4). More commonly, individuals with any of these underlying pathologic states demonstrate clinical, radiographic and histologic evidence of diffuse pulmonary disease not confined to the lymphatic routes, but involving the entire interstitium. This process is called lymphocytic (lymphoid) interstitial pneumonitis (diffuse hyperplasia of BALT).

Lymphocytic interstitial pneumonitis (LIP) was initially described as a chronic interstitial pneumonia rich in lymphocytes and plasma cells with a predilection for transformation into malignant lymphoma (91). It appears, however, that malignant transformation is less frequent than previously believed (23) because, as is the case with NLH, many reported examples of LIP transforming into lymphoma likely represent *de novo* lymphoma (92,93). Immunohistochemical and molecular studies have confirmed the existence of LIP (16,94) and we now recognize LIP within the spectrum of hyperplasia of BALT, including FBB, DLH, and malignant lymphoma (60).

Lymphocytic interstitial pneumonitis histology is found in a number of diseases and reflects these patient populations (Table 34.2). Lymphocytic interstitial pneumonitis usually occurs in women in the fourth through seventh decades of life, with an average age of 56 years. Patients complain of

TABLE 34.2. *Diseases associated with lymphocytic interstitial pneumonitis (diffuse hyperplasia of BALT)*

Autoimmune diseases
Sjögren's syndrome
Primary biliary cirrhosis
Myasthenia gravis
Hashimoto's thyroiditis
Pernicious anemia/agammaglobulinemia
Autoimmune hemolytic anemia
Systemic lupus erythematosus
Immunodeficiency syndromes
Common variable immunodeficiency
Unexplained childhood immunodeficiency
Acquired immunodeficiency syndrome
Virus-associated (excluding HIV infections)
Epstein-Barr virus infection
Chronic active hepatitis
Drug-induced forms
Allogeneic bone marrow transplantation
Dilantin
Miscellaneous
Tuberculosis/Chylamydia/Mycoplasma
Celiac sprue
Familial

From Koss MN. Pulmonary lymphoproliferative disorders. In: Churg A, Katzenstein ALA, eds. *The lung: current concepts.* Philadelphia: Williams & Wilkins, 1993:144–194, with permission.

progressive shortness of breath, dyspnea on exertion and dry cough for months to years, as well as fevers, arthralgias, weight loss, pleuritic chest pain, and hemoptysis (23,95). Sjögren's syndrome accounts for at least 25% of the reported cases (96) and familial cases have also been described (97).

Pulmonary function tests reveal restrictive disease with reduced diffusion capacity. Laboratory studies show dysproteinemias in greater than 60% of patients (23) and can precede the onset of LIP or can occur any time during the clinical course (96). Hypergammaglobulinemia is due to elevation of IgG and IgM or IgG, or IgA and IgM (23). Hypogammaglobulinemia occurs in approximately 10% of adult cases and can be seen in children (98). Serum immunoelectrophoresis should be performed if a monoclonal spike is identified, because this finding suggests a diagnosis of lymphoma rather than LIP.

Chest radiographs show bibasilar and hilar linear infiltrates that may progress to honeycomb lung (84), and HRCT demonstrates ground glass attenuation, poorly defined centrilobular nodules, and thickened perilymphatic interstitium (99). Pleural effusions are rare, but hilar adenopathy has been reported, depending on the underlying disease and imaging modality used (84,99).

Histologically, LIP shows a diffuse, prominent interstitial infiltrate of small noncleaved lymphocytes, immunoblasts, plasma cells, fibroblasts, scattered epithelioid histiocytes, and nonnecrotizing granulomas centered on the airways with infiltration into alveolar and interlobular septa (Fig. 34.11).

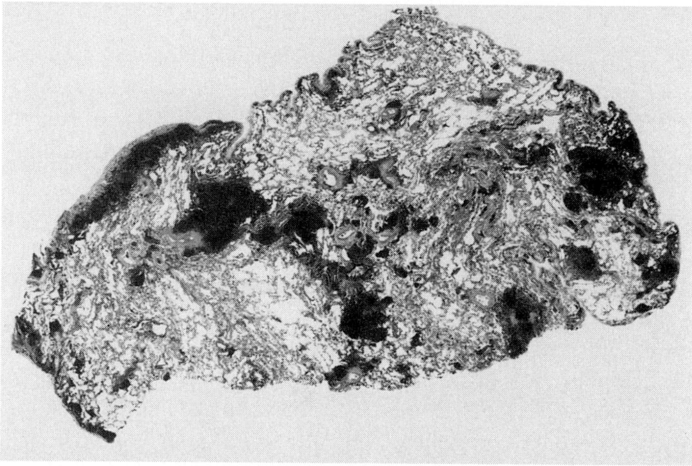
A

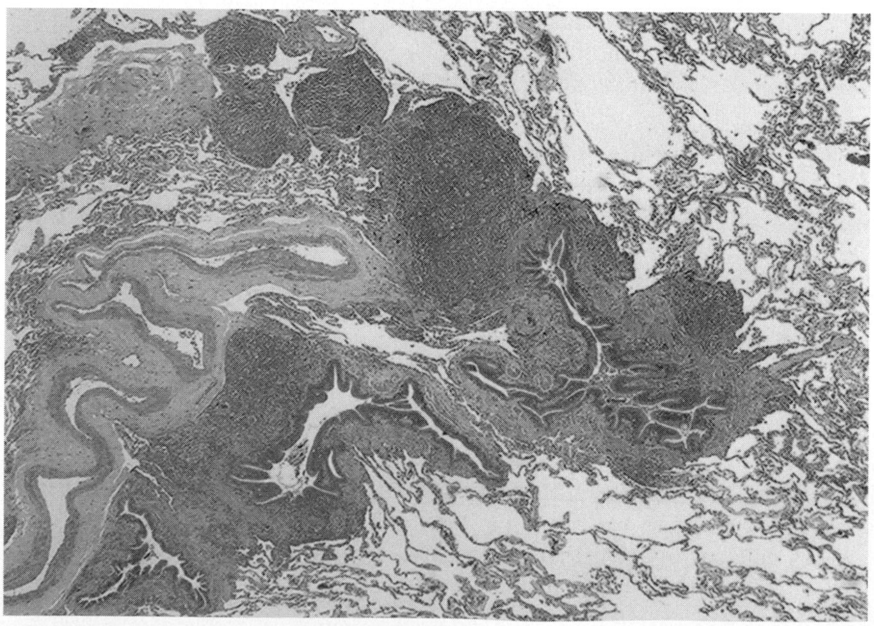
B

FIG. 34.11. Lymphocytic interstitial pneumonitis. **A:** A relatively diffuse interstitial lymphoid process follows pulmonary lymphatic routes with prominent subpleural involvement (hematoxylin and eosin stain, original magnification: 4× magnification). **B:** Peribronchiolar lymphoid follicles illustrate the morphologic continuum between follicular bronchitis or bronchiolitis and lymphocytic interstitial pneumonitis (hematoxylin and eosin stain, original magnification: 20× magnification). *(continued)*

C

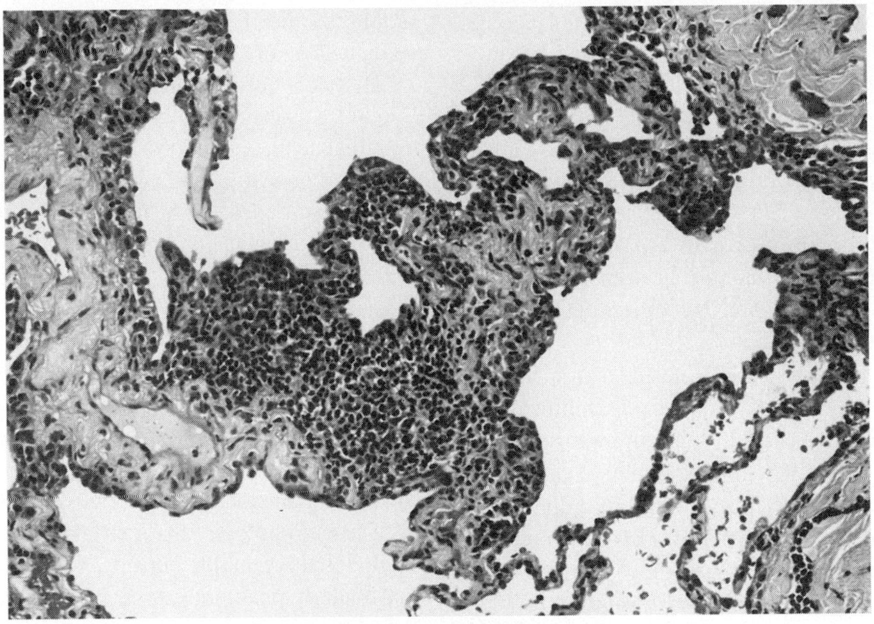

D

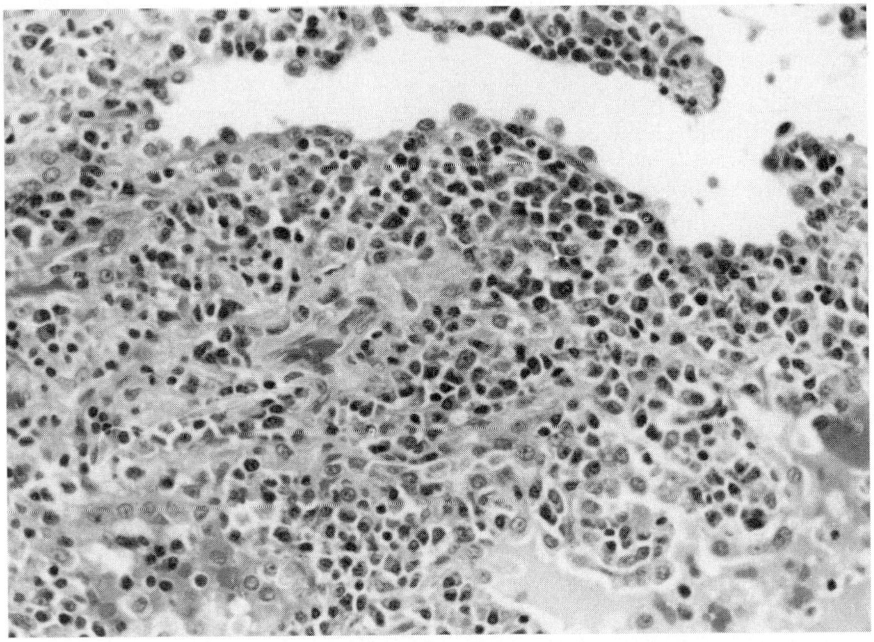

FIG. 34.11. *Continued.* **C:** Long-standing lesions feature alveolar septal fibrosis (hematoxylin and eosin stain, original magnification: 200× magnification). **D:** The polyclonal interstitial lymphoid infiltrate consists of lymphocytes, plasma cells, and macrophages. Notice the intraalveolar fluid accumulation *(bottom right)* (hematoxylin and eosin stain, original magnification: 250× magnification).

Peribronchiolar lymphoid follicles are seen in up to 90% of cases (16,23) illustrating the morphologic continuum between FB/FBB, DLH, and LIP (Fig. 34.11). Intraepithelial lymphocytes are almost always observed, and aggregates can mimic lymphoepithelial lesions (16). Scattered lymphocytes can overflow into alveolar lumens. In long-standing lesions, cords of hyaline and sclerotic collagen (''paramyloid'') or rarely amyloid are deposited within the interstitium and honeycomb fibrosis may evolve (Fig. 34.11). Biopsy material at this stage produces nonspecific findings, and a definitive diagnosis is not possible. Secondary changes include filling of airspaces with foamy macrophages, mucoid or edema fluid within the alveoli and intraalveolar giant cells (Fig. 34.11). Cytologic atypia of the lymphoid infiltrate is not seen and although plasma cells may be binucleated and contain Russell bodies, Dutcher bodies are infrequently identified.

The number of plasma cells correlates with the presence and degree of gammopathy (60). Rare cases with few plasma cells are associated with hypogammaglobulinemia (23,98).

Cases rich in plasma cells and associated with dysproteinemia have been called lymphoplasmacytic pneumonia and plasma cell interstitial pneumonitis, but should be considered variants of LIP rather than distinct entities (100,101).

Immunohistochemical stains reveal a polyclonal population of B cells, particularly within peribronchial lymphoid aggregates, with a cuff of T cells around the germinal centers. The interstitial lymphoid infiltrates are predominantly T cells, and this pattern is similar to that seen in reactive lymph nodes leading some observers to suggest that the lung can function like a giant lymphoid organ (16).

The prognosis of LIP is variable; one third of patients have resolution of the disease, one third have stabilization and the remaining third progresses despite immunosuppressive therapy (23,91,95,102). The nonresponders usually die of therapy-related infections but occasional individuals die of respiratory insufficiency resulting from end-stage pulmonary fibrosis. Blast cell transformation, low-grade T-cell transformation and high-grade B-cell transformation of LIP have been described (16,103,104).

In patients with human immunodeficiency virus (HIV) infection or AIDS, LIP is part of a spectrum of pulmonary lymphoid proliferations referred to as pulmonary lymphoid hyperplasia–lymphocytic interstitial pneumonitis complex (PLH-LIP complex). The anatomic distribution of pulmonary lymphoid infiltrates is similar to that seen in non-AIDS patients and a similar spectrum of lymphoid proliferations ranging from FBB through LIP and possibly, including low-grade lymphoma is observed (105–107).

In patients with HIV infection, LIP is most commonly seen in children (9,108,109) and is a CDC category B indicator condition in children younger than age 13 (110). Up to 17% of children infected with HIV have LIP (111,112). Patients suffer a slowly progressive hypoxia with eventual respiratory failure. The chest radiograph shows a diffuse micronodular or linear interstitial pattern with hilar and mediastinal widening but rarely shows adenopathy (84). These clinicoradiographic findings suggest the diagnosis and open lung biopsy is not usually performed. Other findings include salivary gland enlargement and generalized lymphadenopathy (106). Therapy for AIDS-related LIP is uncertain; poor and irregular responses to steroid therapy have been the norm. Occasional cases manifest dramatic responses. Oral chloroquine therapy has shown clinical promise (113). Nevertheless, the mean survival is 33 months (114).

Whereas LIP can occur in adults infected with HIV, it is far less frequent than in children. The disease usually presents in individuals with AIDS-related complex with generalized lymphadenopathy and polyclonal hypergammaglobulinemia. Unlike in children, the clinicoradiographic findings are not specific and biopsy is often required to exclude more common processes such as *Pneumocystis carinii* pneumonia. Bronchoalveolar lavage specimens feature lymphocytosis, with CD8 lymphocytes comprising up to 90% of the lymphoid cells (115). Unlike the childhood population, adults with LIP rarely die of the pulmonary process, but rather of other AIDS-related diseases.

Histologically, when a polymorphous lymphoid infiltrate extends even minimally from around the airways into the alveolar septa, the process is called LIP (108,116). In distinction to non-AIDS LIP, only rare secondary follicles with follicle lysis are seen. In adults with AIDS, nonspecific interstitial pneumonia/fibrosis is more commonly seen than LIP, but in cases of LIP, the lymphoid infiltrate is less dense than in childhood cases (117).

In AIDS patients with LIP, polyclonal B cells and T cells can be seen (117,118), but most cases show a majority of T cells, usually CD8 (119–121). Similar lymphocytic infiltrates in the salivary glands and an expansion of $CD8^+$ lymphocytes in the peripheral blood often accompany the pulmonary CD8 tissue lymphocytosis (119).

The morphologic differential diagnosis of DLH and LIP includes three major entities. First, exclusion of infection, particularly pneumocystosis, is essential. For this reason, an open lung biopsy is recommended for definitive diagnosis. Unusual microorganisms should also be considered, including Epstein-Barr virus. Hypersensitivity pneumonitis (HP), usually recognized by its triad of bronchiolitis, patchy interstitial infiltrates and granulomas, can be mistaken for DLH or LIP if the interstitial infiltrate is pronounced. In these cases, a clinical history of exposure is helpful. Lymphoma is distinguished by its exquisite lymphatic distribution, pleural infiltration, relatively monomorphous cytology and formation of large nodules. Diffuse lymphoid hyperplasias are polymorphic, whereas lymphomas are monoclonal and may involve hilar or mediastinal lymph nodes. Additional comments about the differential diagnosis with lymphoma are included in the next section.

Recognizing the variety of systemic disorders associated with LIP, the diversity of the cellular components and the variable clinical course, it is not surprising that this process represents a morphologic manifestation of different diseases and does not have a single pathogenetic cause. Although previous investigators focused on autoimmune or immune complex–mediated processes (95,100), the association of HIV infection with pulmonary lymphoid hyperplasias, including LIP, led to studies examining the roles of Epstein-Barr virus (EBV) (117,122–124), HIV (117,125–127) and human T lymphotropic virus type 1 (HTLV-1) (128–130) in the pathogenesis of DLH and LIP. Many intriguing hypotheses remain unproven.

PRIMARY MALIGNANT LYMPHOMAS

Primary pulmonary lymphomas, generally defined as lymphomas involving the lung and sometimes hilar lymph nodes, are both rare lung tumors, comprising 0.3% of all primary pulmonary neoplasms (131) and rare extranodal lymphomas representing less than 10% of extranodal lymphomas (132). Because most of these lymphomas differ clinically, morphologically, and immunohistochemically from most nodal lymphomas and have their origin in mucosa-associated lymphoid tissue (MALT) of the lung (85), these lymphomas are no longer classified according to node-based classification schemes. Hematology and pulmonary pathologists no longer diagnose these lymphomas as well-differentiated lymphocytic lymphoma, plasmacytoid lymphoma or small lymphocytic, plasmacytoid lymphoma, but rather as malignant lymphoma of MALT. In the REAL classification system, these tumors are designated extranodal marginal zone lymphomas (133) (see Chapter 19). It is also apparent that pulmonary lymphomas have a range of morphologic grade and clinical aggressiveness, such that separating these lymphomas into low- and high-grade categories is a potentially dangerous oversimplification that could hinder attempts to further elucidate pathogenesis and therapy (133).

Although almost 80% of primary lung lymphomas are extranodal marginal zone lymphomas of MALT type (22,134), traditional nodal lymphomas such as follicle center lymphoma, mantle cell lymphoma, lymphoplasmacytoid lymphoma/immunocytoma, diffuse large B-cell lymphoma, peripheral T cell lymphoma, $CD30^{+}$ anaplastic large cell lymphoma, and Hodgkin's disease can present as pulmonary primaries. Other entities, including lymphomatoid granulomatosis, also merit discussion.

Extranodal Marginal Zone Lymphomas of the Mucosa-Associated Lymphoid Tissue Type

More than 35 years after the recognition that pulmonary lymphomas had better clinical outcomes than node-based counterparts (75), their histologic appearance and clinical behavior have been linked to that of lymphomas occurring in other mucosal sites such as the gastrointestinal tract and salivary glands (malignant lymphomas of MALT) (see Chapter 33). Although there are no lymphoid structures comparable to Peyer's patches in the lung, progenitor centrocyte-like cells are present in the marginal zones of reactive follicles in BALT (135). This hypothesis suggests that some degree of lymphoid hyperplasia is a necessary precondition to the development of these lymphomas and explains the common finding of reactive germinal centers in lymphomas of the BALT. This single observation had led to erroneous diagnoses of malignant lymphomas as pseudolymphomas for many years (17,75,86).

Patients range in age from the second to the ninth decades with an average age of 58 years (8,22,136). The incidence in men and women is approximately equal (136). Up to 10% of patients have preexisting diseases associated with hyperplasia of BALT such as systemic lupus erythematosus and Sjögren's syndrome (137). BALT lymphomas also occur in children with AIDS (9,18,107).

Individuals are usually asymptomatic and are identified on the basis of a routine chest radiograph; however, dyspnea, cough, hemoptysis, and shortness of breath reflect extensive disease causing airway constriction, poor compliance, and atelectasis (136). Rare individuals present with B symptoms (22). Laboratory findings are often nonspecific, but may be helpful in diagnosis. Mean lymphocyte counts are typically normal and the peripheral blood lacks evidence of a leukemic phase (22). Sedimentation rates are elevated in many patients. Bone marrow involvement has been reported in only 16% of cases (18), but bone marrow examination is not mentioned in several of the larger studies (8,22,136). Nevertheless, a serum monoclonal IgM or less frequently IgG or IgA spike is present in up to 30% of patients (8,22,136).

Chest radiographs demonstrate peripheral and perihilar consolidations and solitary or multiple nodules while CT scans feature solitary or multifocal, round or irregular, central or peripheral parenchymal consolidations with air bronchograms. Cavitation is rare and these lymphomas do not calcify and are rarely associated with pleural effusions (138,139). Hilar adenopathy is observed in less than 25% of cases (8,18).

The defining clinical feature of these tumors is their tendency to remain localized in the lung for prolonged periods. The interval between the finding of a radiographic abnormality and the definitive pathologic diagnosis has been reported to be between 1.5 and 21 years, with a mean of 5.3 years (136), and up to 80% of patients present with stage I disease (22).

On gross examination, lymphomatous nodules range in size from 2.0 to 20 cm, are tan, and have a fleshy consistency (Fig. 34.12). Single or multiple lesions are ill-defined while pulmonary architecture may be maintained (140). Necrosis and hemorrhage are not seen.

Scanning microscopy is often diagnostic of malignant lymphoma given the dense and monotonous masses that centrally collapse the architectural framework of the lung or consolidate the airspaces and feature a lymphangitic bead-like arrangement of lymphoid nodules in the visceral pleura,

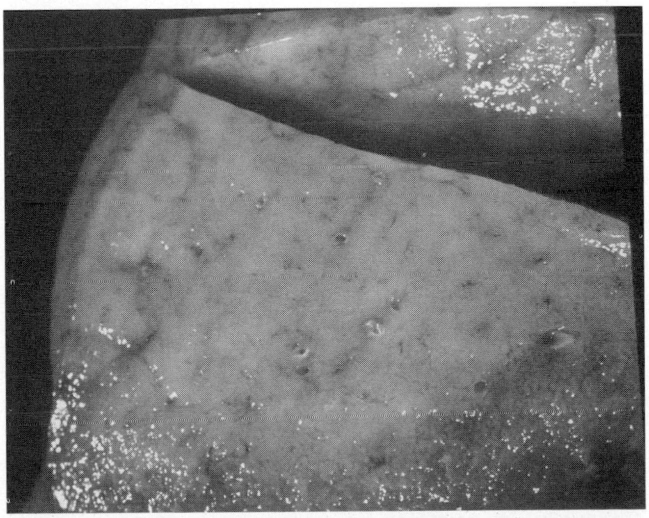

FIG. 34.12. Extranodal marginal zone B-cell lymphoma. The tan, fleshy tumoral consolidation spares underlying lung architecture. Pulmonary lobules, airways, and vessels are preserved.

A 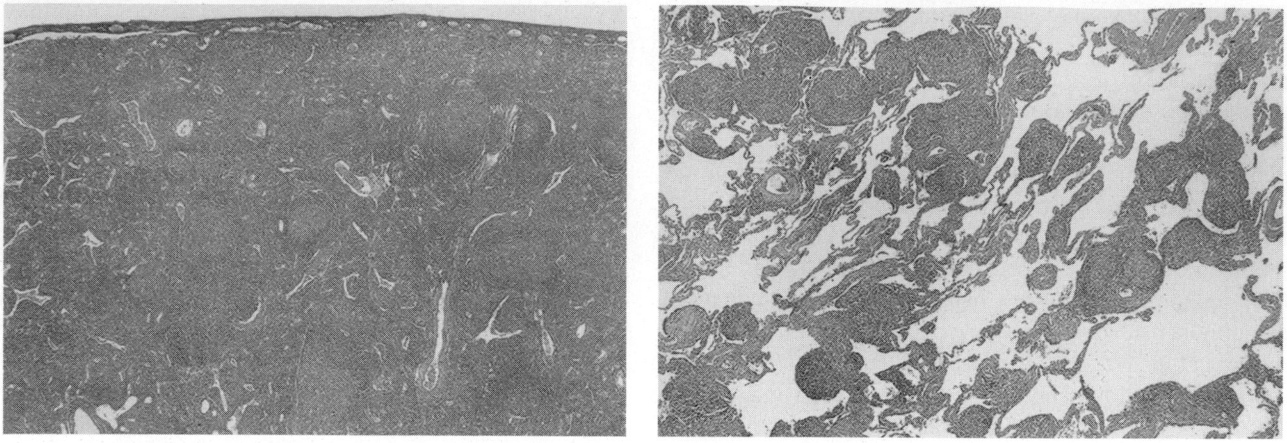 B

FIG. 34.13. Extranodal marginal zone B-cell lymphoma. **A:** Parenchymal consolidation with scattered germinal centers is most often seen. Notice the pleural involvement (hematoxylin and eosin stain, original magnification: 20× magnification). **B:** A lymphangitic pattern may be difficult to discern from reactive lymphoid processes (hematoxylin and eosin stain, original magnification: 20× magnification).

interlobular septa, and along bronchovascular bundles (Fig. 34.13). Additional microscopic nodules are not uncommon in adjacent pulmonary lobules. Sometimes, the dominant growth pattern is interstitial with prominent perivascular and peribronchiolar expansion. In many cases, the lymphoid infiltrate spills over into the air spaces to form a lymphomatous pneumonia and often invades normal pulmonary structures, including the visceral pleura and bronchial cartilage (Fig. 34.14). Malignant cells often infiltrate and may obliterate small veins, but they rarely affect arterial walls and rarely have fibrinoid change.

Another striking low-magnification feature is the presence of reactive-appearing germinal centers in most of these lymphomas (8,11,17,18,22,134) (Fig. 34.13). The germinal centers may be scattered throughout the tumor or may be seen at the periphery. These germinal centers lack well-developed mantle zones and more often feature compressed or absent mantle zones with only small collections of centrocytes (Fig. 34.15). Most of these follicles are polytypic, but up to a quarter may be monotypic secondary to neoplastic colonization of reactive follicles (Fig. 34.15). This follicular colonization is not always apparent on hematoxylin and eosin stained tissue sections, but is easily demonstrated with immunohistochemical staining for CD21, which highlights the follicular dendritic cells (21,22).

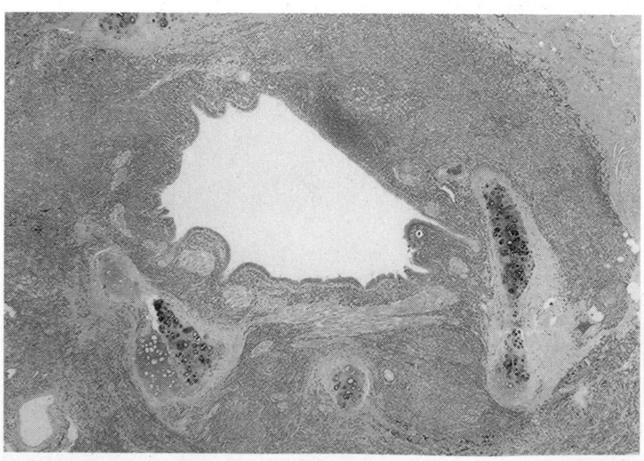

FIG. 34.14. Extranodal marginal zone B-cell lymphoma. Conducting airways can be extensively involved leading to pulmonary symptoms. The dense infiltrate and bronchial cartilage involvement favor a diagnosis of malignancy (hematoxylin and eosin stain, original magnification: 20× magnification).

Although not often emphasized, extranodal marginal zone lymphomas of the lung are heterogeneous displaying the same degree of cytologic variation as other MALT lymphomas. The most characteristic cells are small to medium sized, with a moderate amount of cytoplasm, often pale staining, and they have a nucleus with an irregular outline (Fig. 34.16). Because of their resemblance to centrocytes (small cleaved cells), these cells have been called centrocyte-like (CCL) cells (141); however, this should not be taken to mean that all pulmonary MALT lymphomas are only composed of such cells. Cytologic heterogeneity is almost always seen within a single lesion. Cells may have a less irregular nuclear outline and resemble small lymphocytes or may contain abundant clear cytoplasm resembling monocytoid B cells (Fig. 34.16). Plasma cell differentiation is common and these plasmacytoid lymphocytes may have Russell or Dutcher bodies; the latter are rarely seen in reactive proliferations (Fig. 34.16). The plasmacytic cells may be compartmentalized beneath the bronchiolar epithelium. Occasional larger cells with irregularly shaped nuclei and medium to large nucleoli (immunoblasts) may also be present (Fig. 34.16) while malignant cells colonizing the germinal centers frequently feature nuclear enlargement and increased mitotic activity (21). This polymorphous microscopic appearance differs from that of the usual node-based lymphomas, although some have suggested a morphologic similarity to monocytoid B-cell lymphomas (142).

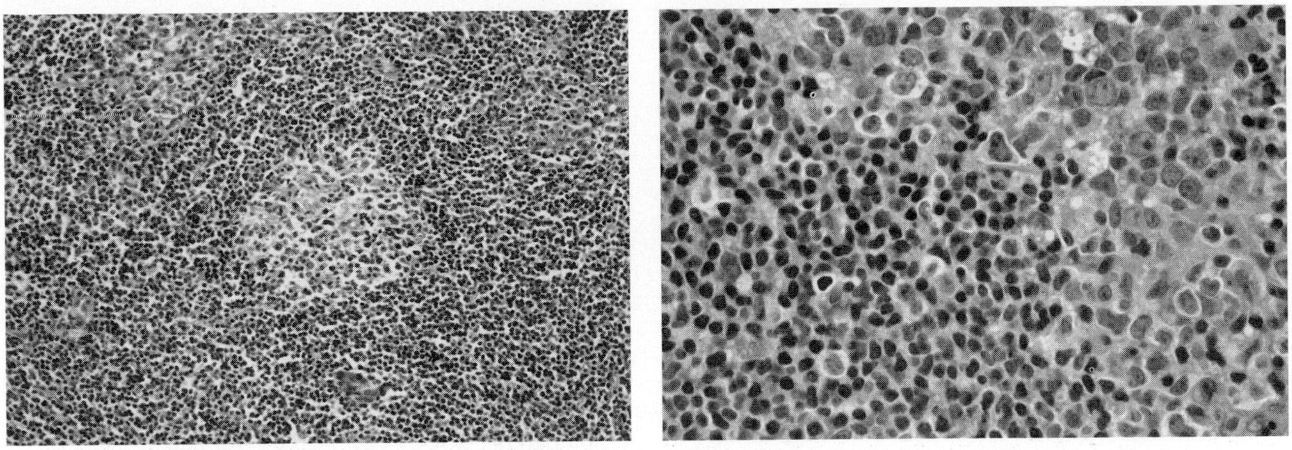

A B

FIG. 34.15. Extranodal marginal zone B-cell lymphoma. **A:** Germinal centers lack well-developed mantle zones (hematoxylin and eosin stain, original magnification: 100× magnification). **B:** Reactive germinal centers are infiltrated by smaller neoplastic lymphocytes. Follicular colonization can be highlighted with an immunohistochemical stain for CD21 (hematoxylin and eosin stain, original magnification: 600× magnification).

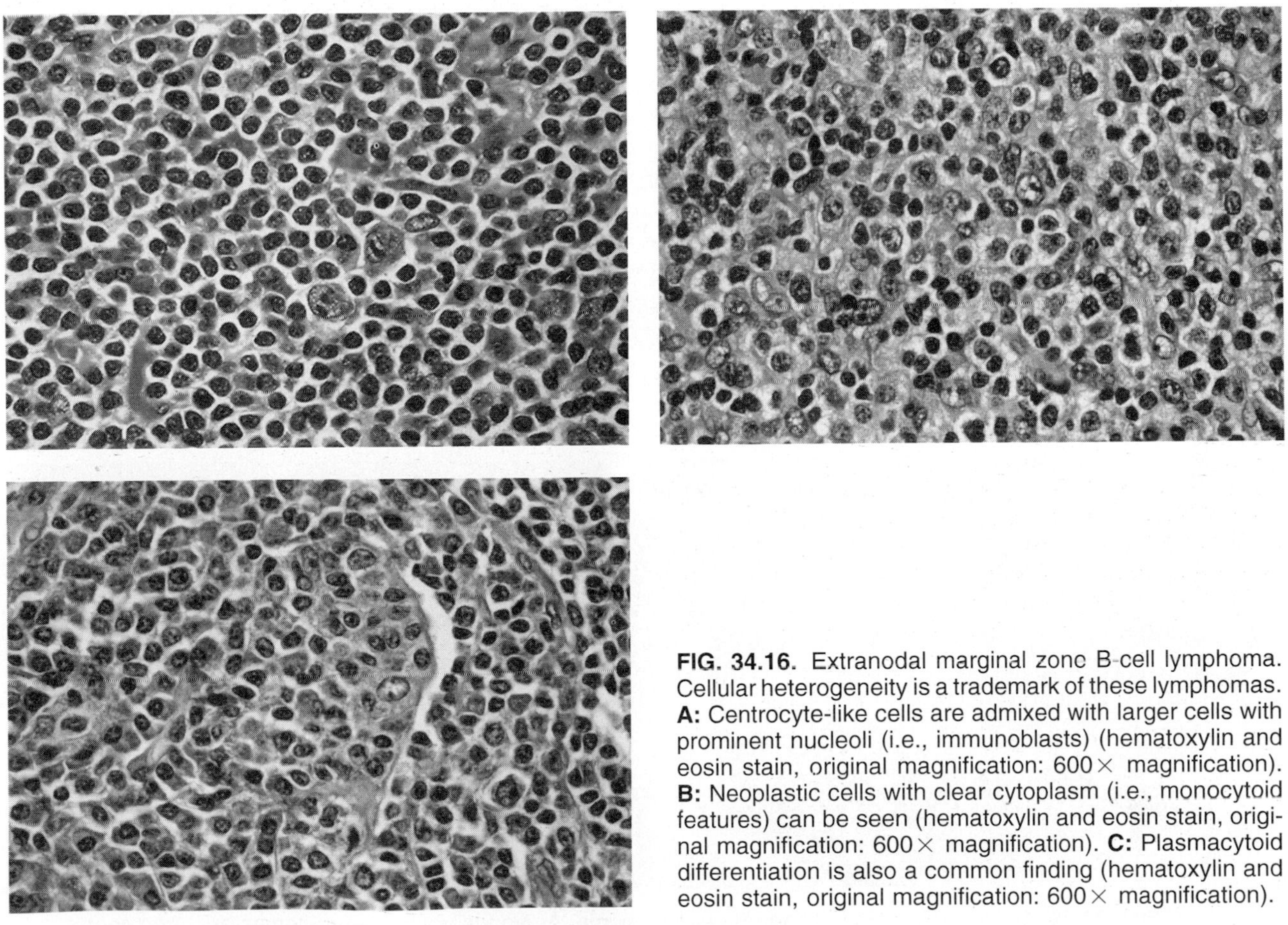

A B C

FIG. 34.16. Extranodal marginal zone B-cell lymphoma. Cellular heterogeneity is a trademark of these lymphomas. **A:** Centrocyte-like cells are admixed with larger cells with prominent nucleoli (i.e., immunoblasts) (hematoxylin and eosin stain, original magnification: 600× magnification). **B:** Neoplastic cells with clear cytoplasm (i.e., monocytoid features) can be seen (hematoxylin and eosin stain, original magnification: 600× magnification). **C:** Plasmacytoid differentiation is also a common finding (hematoxylin and eosin stain, original magnification: 600× magnification).

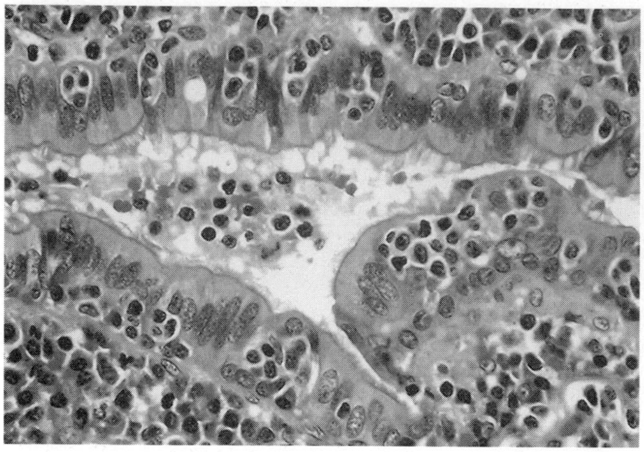

FIG. 34.17. Extranodal marginal zone B-cell lymphoma. Lymphoepithelial lesions are seen in up to 90% of pulmonary mucosa-associated lymphoid tissue (MALT) lymphomas; however, they are not diagnostic of malignant lymphoma. Lymphocyte transmigration of respiratory epithelium can lead to epithelial necrosis and obstructive symptoms (hematoxylin and eosin stain, original magnification: 400× magnification).

Invasion of bronchiolar epithelium (i.e., lymphoepithelial lesion [LEL]) is a common feature of BALT lymphomas, seen in up to 90% of cases and highlighted by cytokeratin stains (Fig. 34.17). Unlike some other MALT sites, LELs are not a useful diagnostic criteria of pulmonary malignancy (16,22).

Secondary features often seen in these lymphomas include fibrosis, sclerosis and rarely necrosis at the center of nodules, foci of organizing pneumonia, nodular or diffuse alveolar septal amyloid deposition, interstitial multinucleated giant cells, sarcoidal granulomas and even granulomatous vasculitis (8) (Fig. 34.18). These findings are entirely nonspecific and can also be seen in lymphoid hyperplasias of the lung and in nonneoplastic processes, including hypersensitivity pneumonitis and granulomatous infections. Giant lamellar bodies, possibly composed of surfactant and necrotic pneumocytes and seen in sclerosing hemangiomas of the lung and pulmonary alveolar proteinosis, are occasionally seen in pulmonary MALT lymphomas (143,144) (Fig. 34.18).

Immunohistochemical studies performed on paraffin-embedded tissue sections of extranodal marginal zone lymphomas of the lung demonstrate light-chain restriction in 50% to 70% of cases. Percentages with κ and λ light-chain restriction are equal. Most cases feature heavy-chain IgM staining with rare plasma cell cytoplasmic and lymphoid cell surface IgA and IgG immunoreactivity (11,22). In the nonmarking cases, PCR can be performed on tissue dissected from the paraffin block to evaluate for clonal rearrangement of the joining region of the immunoglobulin heavy-chain gene (145). In one study, seven out of 13 cases of lymphoma without immunohistochemical evidence of light-chain restriction demonstrated clonally rearranged alleles (11). Extranodal marginal zone lymphomas of the lung are $CD19^+$, $CD20^+$, and $CD79a^+$ with rare scattered $CD45RO^+$ cells and most often, but not always, demonstrate a $CD5^-CD10^-CD23^-CD43^-$cyc lin $D1^-$ immunophenotypic profile (146,147), but scattered $CD45RO^+$ T cells may also be found. No rearrangements of *BCL2* are seen (148). Trisomy 3 or t(11;18) have been reported in extranodal cases (149,150), while only a single report of a t(1;14)(p2;q32) translocation has been demonstrated in a pulmonary lesion (151). This profile helps discern this lymphoma from B-cell chronic lymphocytic leukemia (B-CLL)/small lymphocytic lymphoma (B-SLL) ($CD5^+CD23^+CD43^+$), mantle cell lymphoma ($CD5^+CD43^+$cyclin $D1^+$), and follicle center lymphoma ($CD10^+$BCL-2^+).

This immunophenotype is not specific, and some investigators consider these extranodal MALT lymphomas a diag-

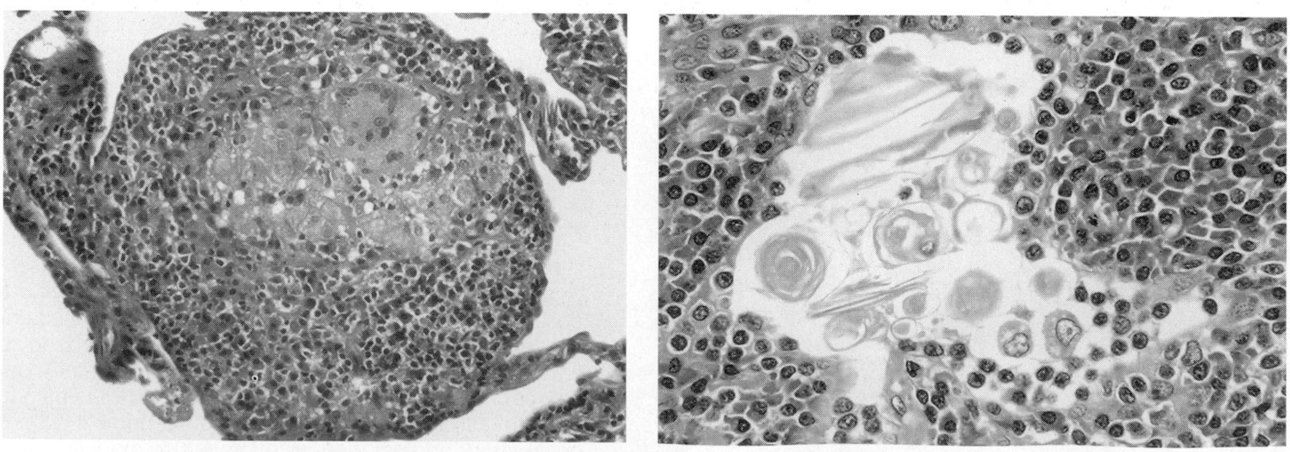

A B

FIG. 34.18. Extranodal marginal zone B-cell lymphoma. **A:** Nonnecrotizing granulomas are often seen in pulmonary lymphoid lesions, including mucosa-associated lymphoid tissue (MALT) lymphomas (hematoxylin and eosin stain, original magnification: 200× magnification). **B:** Intraalveolar giant lamellar bodies have been reported in MALT lymphomas of the lung and may be diagnostically helpful in fine needle aspiration specimens (hematoxylin and eosin stain, original magnification: 400× magnification).

nosis of exclusion requiring morphologic features (e.g., lymphoepithelial lesions, germinal centers, marginal zone or monocytoid B cells, small lymphocytes with or without plasma cells and scattered transformed blasts), and CD5 and cyclin D1 negativity. When lymphoepithelial lesions or germinal centers are lacking and are positive for CD5, a diagnosis of *consistent with MALT-type lymphoma* can be made, with the reservation that CLL/SLL cannot be excluded (152). Ocular and tongue $CD5^{+}CD23^{-}$ extranodal lymphomas with morphologic features of MALT lymphoma have been reported that do not share the relatively indolent clinical course of most extranodal marginal zone lymphomas (147).

Although many cases of pulmonary marginal zone lymphoma of BALT and of CLL/SLL feature plasmacytoid cells or plasma cells, lymphoplasmacytoid lymphoma/immunocytoma appears to be a separate distinct tumor (146) showing maturation to plasma cells and corresponding to most but not all cases of Waldenstrom's macroglobulinemia. Although many cases of lymphoplasmacytic or lymphoplasmacytoid lymphoma (Kiel classification) or plasmacytoid lymphocytic lymphoma (Lukes-Collins classification) have been included in large series (8,153), most probably represent extranodal marginal zone lymphomas.

The principal concern of the general surgical pathologist evaluating a pulmonary lymphoid mass is to decide whether a lesion is a malignant lymphoma or a reactive lymphoid hyperplasia (Table 34.3). Although central areas of lymphomas may resemble NLH and the periphery of lymphomas may resemble LIP, the physician should approach these cases with the understanding that most lymphoid masses composed of small lymphocytes are extranodal marginal zone lymphomas rather than reactive processes. Involvement of regional lymph nodes or of parietal pleura by tumor and the demonstration of a monotypic cell population support a diagnosis of malignancy. Plaquelike involvement of visceral pleura, invasion of bronchial cartilage, broad areas of a relatively uniform small lymphoid population between reactive follicles and thinning of mantle zones around reactive follicles are additional light microscopic features strongly suggestive of malignant lymphoma (8). Microscopic multifocality, lymphoepithelial lesions, germinal centers and interstitial granulomas are nonspecific findings. Although such a guide to diagnosing malignancy seems straightforward, it is imperative to realize that monotypic cells may occur in small aggregates or around polytypic lymphoid follicles and may not demonstrate light-chain restriction by immunohistochemcal studies. When light microscopic features favor a diagnosis of malignant lymphoma, all available ancillary studies, including PCR, should be used to make a correct diagnosis. Within this context, it behooves the surgical pathologist to recognize that the diagnosis of extranodal marginal zone lymphoma of the lung is often difficult on thoracoscopic biopsies or lobectomy specimens, and even more difficult on transbronchial or core biopsies. Bronchoscopic biopsies from patients with diffuse mucosal thickening or bronchial stenosis are more likely to yield a definitive diagnosis, yet these small biopsies with dense lymphoid infiltrates and lymphoepithelial lesions often require concomitant bronchoalveolar lavage specimens and ancillary immunohistochemical stains demonstrating a monotypic immunophenotype (154). It is not surprising to note that a definitive diagnosis of lymphoma can be made in less than 10% of these cases.

TABLE 34.3. *Extranodal marginal zone lymphoma of the BALT: useful diagnostic features*

Architectural features
Consolidation and destruction of architecture
Lymphatic tracking with perivascular nodular infiltrates
Germinal centers with thinned mantle zones (highlighted by CD21)
Invasion of visceral pleura
Destruction of bronchial cartilage
Vasculitis
Necrosis
Cytologic features
+/− Cellular monotony or heterogeneity
centrocyte-like cells +/− monocytoid cells +/− plasmacytoid cells
+/− immunoblast-like cells
+/− Airspace lymphoid infiltration
+/− Dutcher bodies
+/− Amyloid
Other
Involvement of peribronchial or hilar lymph nodes
Immunoglobulin light chain restriction and heavy chain gene rearrangements
$CD5^{-}$, $CD10^{-}$, $CD23^{-}$, $CD43^{+/-}$, cyclin $D1^{-}$, BCL-2^{-}
Involvement of other extrathoracic sites (especially MALT sites)

Extranodal marginal zone lymphomas of the lung are indolent with 85% to 94% 5- and 10-year survival in several large series (8,22,153), while other studies did not reach median survival at 10 years (18,136). In several studies, there was no statistical difference between the survival of patients with lymphoma and that of the normal population at the same age (22) and outcome did not vary depending on whether surgical excision was complete, or whether patients received adjunct radiation therapy, chemotherapy, or both (22,136). For these reasons, aggressive chemotherapy is avoided and limited staging is suggested. One group of investigators noticed that patients with stage IE or IIE disease without systemic symptoms had a favorable prognosis and did not die of the lymphoma while those with B symptoms had a statistically worse prognosis (22). There is conflicting data regarding the prognostic significance of a monoclonal gammopathy (18,22).

Tumor recurrences and transformations do occur. In up to 50% of cases, tumors recur in the lung, in other mucosal sites such as salivary gland or gastrointestinal tract, or rarely in lymph nodes and bone marrow within 30 months (8,22). This fascinating homing of malignant cells to other MALT sites is similar to that reported in malignant B-cell lymphomas of the GALT (see Chapter 33). Thirteen percent of these so-called indolent lymphomas have been reported to transform into more aggressive forms, including diffuse large cell lymphoma within, by one report, 78 months (22).

Other Non-Hodgkin's Lymphomas

Non-Hodgkin's lymphomas other than extranodal marginal zone B-cell lymphomas do originate in the lung, but as a group are approximately one fourth as common as marginal zone lymphomas of BALT (8,11,22,134,155,156). These lymphomas are a heterogeneous group consisting primarily of diffuse large B-cell lymphoma (8,11,22,134,156), with fewer cases of follicle center cell lymphoma (8) and rare examples of mantle cell lymphoma (156), lymphoplasmacytoid lymphoma/immunocytoma (8,157), Burkitt's lymphoma (22), peripheral T-cell lymphomas (22,155), anaplastic large cell lymphoma, and T- and null cell types (158) reported. AIDS-related non-Hodgkin's lymphomas are overwhelmingly of B-cell origin and most often diffuse large B-cell lymphomas and Burkitt's lymphomas (159). Rare AIDS-related primary pulmonary lymphomas with the morphologic and immunohistochemical features of anaplastic large cell lymphoma but lacking t(2;5) and associated with KSHV and EBV (160) have been described. AIDS-related primary pulmonary lymphomas that do not disseminate have also been described (161,162). These B-cell and T-cell lymphomas appear to be related to severe immunodeficiency and contain EBV RNA (161).

Follicle center cell lymphomas, lymphoplasmacytoid lymphomas/immunocytomas, and mantle cell lymphomas may share architectural and cytologic features with marginal zone lymphomas of the lung (157). However, clinical findings combined with light microscopy, immunohistochemical results, and molecular studies allow proper diagnoses.

Several comments regarding the pulmonary presentation, morphology and differential diagnosis of aggressive lymphomas are warranted. Most patients are adults, but there is a wide age range, including children, especially with immunodeficiency states. Although 5% to 10% of patients infected with HIV have non-Hodgkin's lymphoma, only 10% of this patient population presents with stage IE primary lung disease (159,161,162). In contrast to patients with extranodal marginal zone lymphomas, most individuals with aggressive lymphomas, including HIV-infected individuals, present with shortness of breath, fever, chest pain, and hemoptysis and often develop extrapulmonary lesions shortly after diagnosis, as well as paraneoplastic syndromes. Chest radiographs reveal solitary nodules and infiltrates that may involve one or more lobes. Cavitation and pleural effusions are commonly seen, and rapidly developing infiltrates can suggest acute infection, including tuberculosis (163,164). Regional lymph node involvement is seen in up to 50% of cases.

B-cell and rarely reported T-cell large cell lymphomas have several common histologic features. Large masses are usually predominantly necrotic and multiple tissue sections may be required to identify viable malignant cells (Fig. 34.19). Scattered benign lymphocytes, plasma cells and histiocytes should not be mistaken for malignancy. Diffuse lesions feature a lymphangitic pattern, and in such cases close attention to pleural and perivascular infiltrates can aid in making a diagnosis because peribronchiolar infiltrates tend to be a mixture of reactive and neoplastic lymphoid cells (Fig. 34.20). Some large cell lymphomas, especially T-cell lymphomas, are truly polymorphous and can be misinterpreted as reactive lymphoid hyperplasia. Vascular invasion by malignant cells or reactive cells with mural necrosis is often seen; however, vessel wall necrosis in the absence of parenchymal necrosis is rare (165). Large areas of infarction

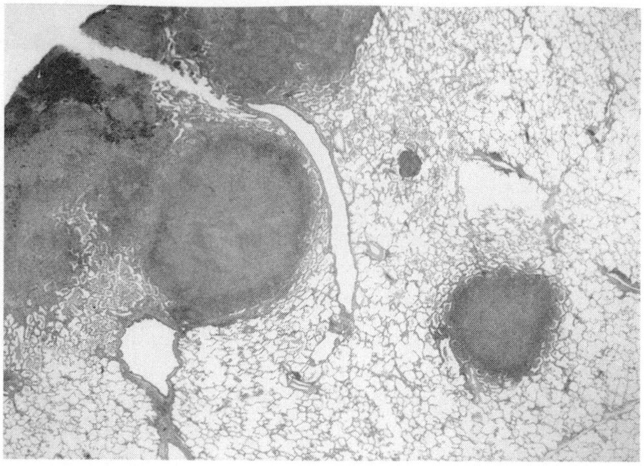

FIG. 34.19. $CD30^+$ anaplastic large cell lymphoma of the lung. Multiple centrally necrotic subpleural and paraseptal masses usually progress to form a large lesion. Identifying viable malignant cells may be difficult (hematoxylin and eosin stain, original magnification: 7.5× magnification). (Photomicrograph courtesy of Dr. W. Rush, Washington, D.C.)

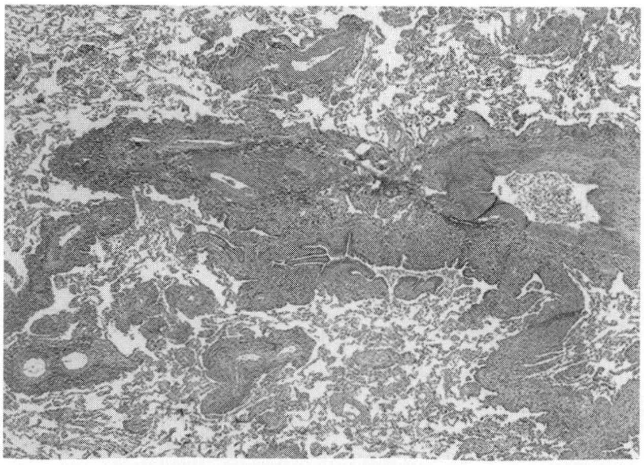

FIG. 34.20. T-cell lymphoma of the lung. This primary pulmonary lymphoma tracks along lymphatic pathways without nodule formation. A malignant process in such cases is usually not clinically suspected (hematoxylin and eosin stain, original magnification: 20× magnification).

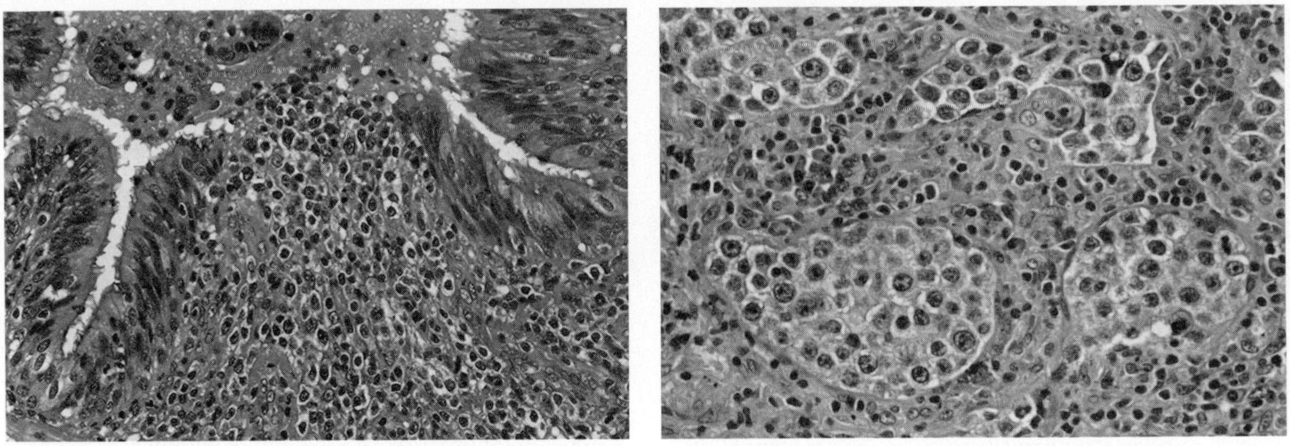

A B

FIG. 34.21. T-cell lymphoma of the lung. **A:** Neoplastic cells infiltrate and destroy airways leading to pneumonia. The reactive inflammatory infiltrate can obscure the malignant process (hematoxylin and eosin stain, original magnification: 200× magnification). **B:** Aggressive lymphomas can also produce so-called tumoral pneumonia (hematoxylin and eosin stain, original magnification: 400× magnification).

can be seen. Destruction of airways results in distal obstructive changes, including bacterial or postobstructive pneumonia with intraalveolar macrophages, granulomatous inflammation, alveolar septal infiltrates, and reactive pneumocytes (166) (Fig. 34.21). In most cases, mitotically active malignant cells and fibrin fill alveoli producing a ''tumoral pneumonia'' (8,22) (Fig. 34.21). There are fewer germinal centers than in the marginal zone lymphomas (18), but foci of coexistent marginal zone lymphoma can be seen (11,22,134).

Although the cytologic atypia and necrosis in these lymphomas make it relatively easy to distinguish them from benign lymphoid processes and marginal zone lymphomas, confusion with Hodgkin's disease or poorly differentiated epithelial tumors can occur. Immunohistochemical studies can aid in making a correct diagnosis, but one should consider $CD45^-CD30^+$ anaplastic large cell lymphoma in the differential diagnosis and remember that CD15 and rarely CD45 can be expressed in sarcomas and carcinomas (167).

Although localized lymphomas are potentially curable with surgery and adjunct therapy, reported 5-year survival for individuals with pulmonary large cell lymphoma is only 44% to 60%, with a median survival of 3 years (22,134,153). Only 50% of patients with HIV infection and non-Hodgkin's lymphoma achieve clinical remission and the average duration of such remissions is only 6 months (161,162,168).

Lymphomatoid Granulomatosis

Since its description in 1972 as an angiocentric lymphoproliferative process with prominent pulmonary involvement, lymphomatoid granulomatosis (LYG) has puzzled physicians and scientists alike. The original investigators could not decide whether lesions with a polymorphic lymphoid infiltrate, angiitis and necrosis were a form of malignant lymphoma or Wegener's granulomatosis and settled on the term LYG (169). Although these investigators were hesitant to label the disease malignant, they recognized the capability of the process to progress to an ''atypical lymphoma'' and observed that most patients lacked nodal, bone marrow, and splenic involvement, that some patients improved without therapy, and that the lymphoid infiltrate did not fulfill the then-current morphologic criteria for a diagnosis of malignancy. During the past decades, it was proposed that LYG was a B-cell lymphoma (170) or T-cell lymphoma (171,172), whereas others noticed that LYG shared clinical and pathologic features with nasal and nasal type natural killer (NK)/T-cell lymphoma (i.e., angiocentric lymphoma) and considered LYG part of the clinicopathologic entity angiocentric immunoproliferative lesion/angiocentric lymphoma (AIL) (173,174). Immunologic and molecular biologic studies have provided new insights into the nature and pathogenesis of this disease process, and LYG is currently viewed as a T-cell–rich EBV^+ B-cell immunoproliferative disorder with a propensity toward multiorgan involvement and death (175–180).

Given the complexities of the disease and the many different opinions regarding its true nature, it is not surprising that nomenclature remains problematic. Pulmonary pathologists use the terms *LYG* and *LYG-lymphoma* while hematopathologists favor the designation *angiocentric lymphoma*. The REAL classification published in 1994 places the entity in the T-cell angiocentric lymphoma category but notes that in at least some pulmonary lesions, clonal Ig gene rearrangements have been detected (133). Another designation has been proposed (180).

Although rare, LYG has characteristic clinical features. Patients usually present in the fifth or sixth decade of life, although disease in children and the elderly has been reported (181). Men are affected two to three times as often as women (182,183). The disease also occurs sporadically in individuals with immunodeficiency states such as Wiskott-Aldrich syndrome (184), HIV infection (185), and secondary

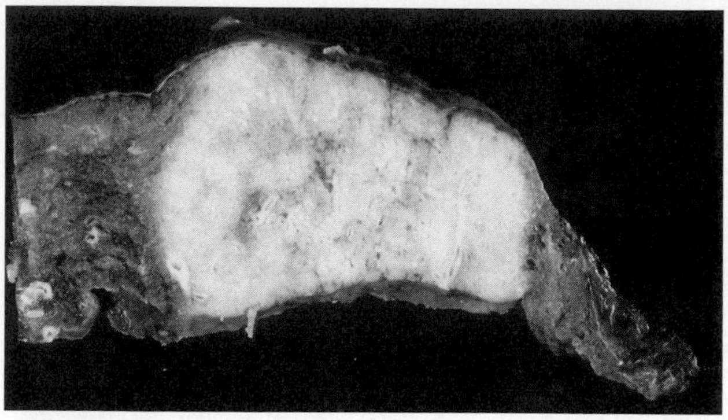

FIG. 34.22. Lymphomatoid granulomatosis. Large, well-circumscribed nodules grossly feature foci of necrosis. Thoracoscopic or open lung biopsies are required for diagnosis.

immunodeficiences related to chemotherapy and organ transplantation (186,187). These associations suggest that patients with LYG have altered immune status, and studies have demonstrated impaired humoral and cell-mediated responses to EBV (188), as well as decreased numbers of CD4 helper and CD8 cytotoxic cells (180).

The lungs are the most commonly involved organ, and most patients complain of cough, dyspnea, chest pain, fever, malaise, and weight loss. Between 30% and 40% of patients also present with skin nodules, ulcers, rashes, peripheral neuropathies, or symptoms referable to central nervous system involvement. Less than 20% initially present with gastrointestinal, musculoskeletal, or nodal involvement. Lymphomatoid granulomatosis rarely presents as an asymptomatic solitary lung nodule on a routine chest radiograph (169,182,183).

Laboratory findings can include a leukocytosis or leukopenia and nonspecific abnormalities in serum immunoglobulins, including elevated IgG and IgM, can be seen (182).

TABLE 34.4. *Histologic criteria for diagnosing lymphomatoid granulomatosis*

Polymorphic lymphoid infiltrate
Large atypical cells along with lymphocytes, plasma cells, histiocytes
Vascular infiltration without fibrinoid necrosis
Parenchymal necrosis without granuloma formation

Cerebrospinal fluid (CSF) often has abnormal protein and glucose levels with increased numbers of mature T cells. Only in rare instances does the CSF contain monoclonal B cells (176). Despite the presence of angiitis, serologic tests for autoimmune diseases, including antinuclear antibody and rheumatoid factor, are negative. In keeping with our current understanding of the disease, serologic evidence of EBV infection has been reported (180,189).

Chest radiographs most often demonstrate bilateral noncavitating peripheral nodules in the middle and lower lung fields measuring up to 10.0 cm (83). Nonspecific reticulonodular infiltrates are also seen in a minority of patients and pleural effusions have been reported in up to one third of patients (84). With disease progression, nodules enlarge and cavitate.

Grossly, nodules are tan-yellow, round, and often show central necrosis (Fig. 34.22). Microscopically, LYG is composed of nodular lymphoid infiltrates centered on lymphatic routes, including bronchovascular bundles (Fig. 34.23, Table 34.4). Perivascular nodules expand into alveoli and as the nodules enlarge, central necrosis and cavitation occur (Fig. 34.23). Large vessels within the necrotic center and peripheral smaller vessels are infiltrated by the lymphoid infiltrate (Fig. 34.24). These findings may be highlighted by elastic tissue stains. Although vascular and airway infiltration are distinctive light microscopic features of LYG, and rare cases

A

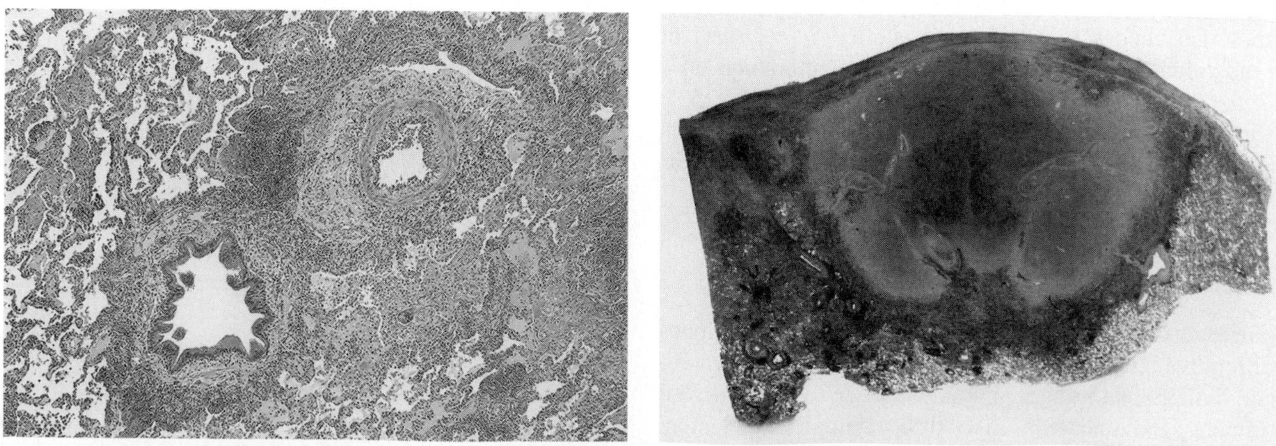

B

FIG. 34.23. Lymphomatoid granulomatosis. **A:** The earliest lesions feature nodular lymphoid aggregates centered on bronchovascular bundles. Notice the surrounding airspace involvement (hematoxylin and eosin stain, original magnification: 20× magnification). **B:** Eventually, the process forms large necrotic masses (hematoxylin and eosin stain, original magnification: 4× magnification).

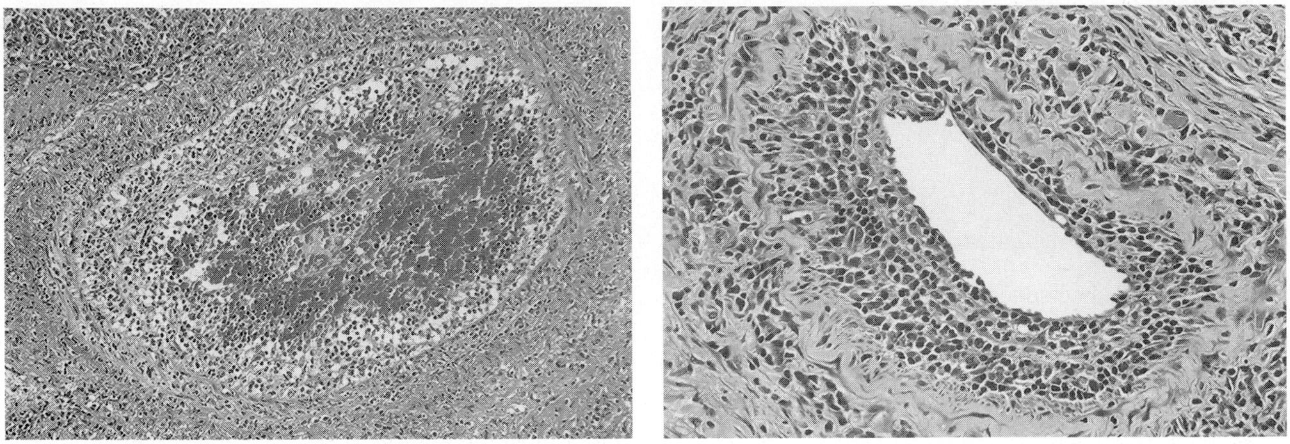

A B

FIG. 34.24. Lymphomatoid granulomatosis. **A:** Vessels within necrotic nodules almost always demonstrate neoplastic infiltration (hematoxylin and eosin stain, original magnification: 100× magnification). **B:** Not all involved vessels feature necrosis (hematoxylin and eosin stain, original magnification: 200× magnification).

demonstrate exquisite preferential vascular involvement, the angiocentric nature of the infiltrate is the result of the true lymphatic distribution of the process. That is to say, vessels and airways are simply overrun as nodules expand.

The nodules and infiltrates are composed of a heterogeneous population with field to field variation, including small, intermediate, and large lymphocytes; plasma cells; and histiocytes (Fig. 34.25). Whereas the small- and intermediate-sized lymphocytes can feature ''twisted'' nuclei and irregular nuclear chromatin, large cells can resemble immu-

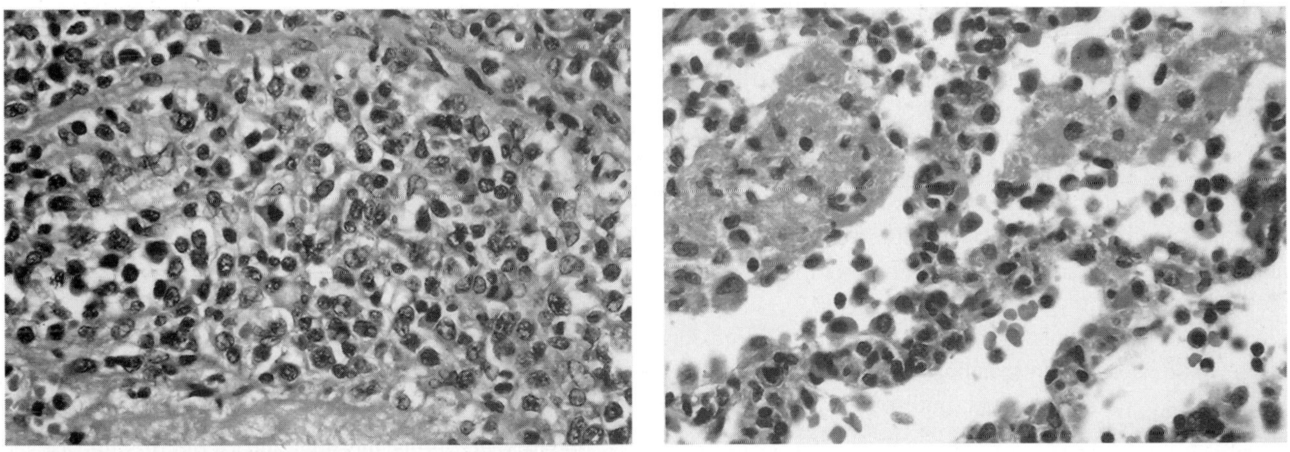

A B

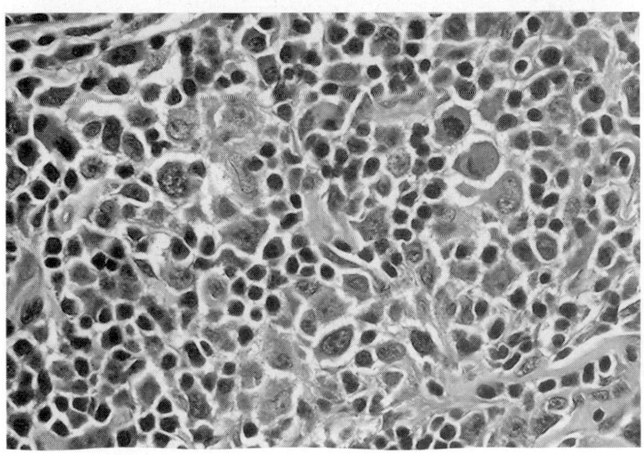

C

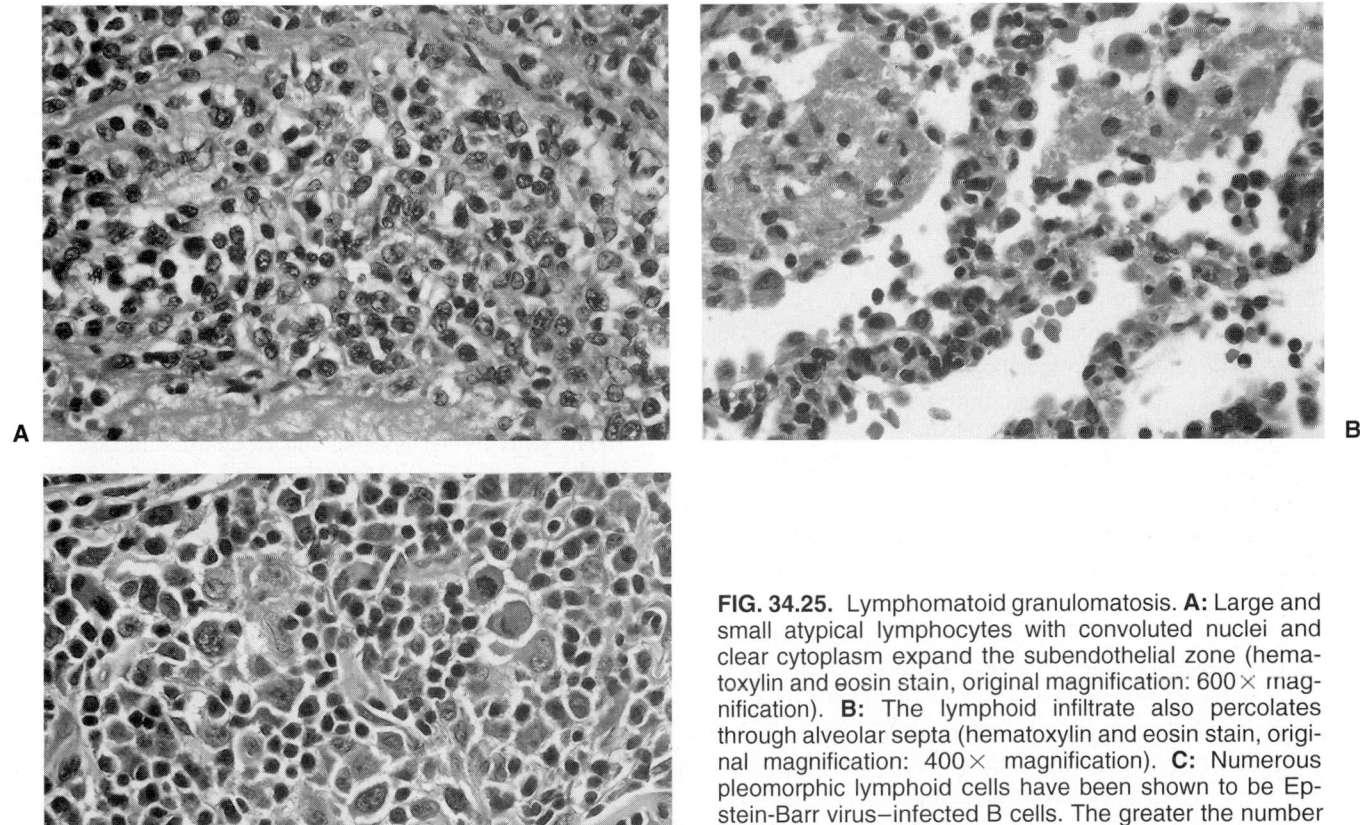

FIG. 34.25. Lymphomatoid granulomatosis. **A:** Large and small atypical lymphocytes with convoluted nuclei and clear cytoplasm expand the subendothelial zone (hematoxylin and eosin stain, original magnification: 600× magnification). **B:** The lymphoid infiltrate also percolates through alveolar septa (hematoxylin and eosin stain, original magnification: 400× magnification). **C:** Numerous pleomorphic lymphoid cells have been shown to be Epstein-Barr virus–infected B cells. The greater the number of large atypical cells, the more readily the lesion is recognizable as a malignant lymphoma (hematoxylin and eosin stain, original magnification: 600× magnification).

TABLE 34.5. *Histologic and in situ hybridization grading of lymphomatoid granulomatosis*

Grade 1/Pure LYG
- Angiocentric polymorphous infiltrate without atypia or necrosis
- Rare Epstein-Barr virus (EBV) infected cells

Grade 2/LYG-lymphoma, focal (LYG-LF)
- Angiocentric predominantly polymorphous infiltrate with occasional large or atypical lymphoid cells and parenchymal necrosis
- Scattered EBV-infected cells but fewer than 100/high-power field

Grade 3/LYG-lymphoma, diffuse (LYG-LD)
- Angiocentric and destructive monomorphous infiltrate with widespread necrosis
- Sheets of EBV-infected cells in excess of 100/high-power field

noblasts, pleomorphic cells or even multinucleated Reed-Sternberg–like cells. Occasional mitotic figures are seen in all cases, but lesions with many atypical cells have a higher proliferation index (190). Diagnostic foci composed of atypical intermediate and large cells are found in larger nodules, while many microscopic fields are composed of a bland collection of small lymphocytes, histiocytes and plasma cells. Epithelioid cell clusters and minute nonnecrotizing granulomas are rarely seen, and neutrophils and eosinophils are usually absent.

Given the complex histologic features of LYG and the variety of nonspecific findings in adjacent lung, including mild interstitial lymphoplasmacytic infiltrates, intraalveolar macrophages, pneumocyte hyperplasia, and foci of organizing pneumonia, large tissue samples are almost always required for diagnosis. Transbronchial biopsies are rarely diagnostic, whereas open lung biopsies have a high diagnostic yield (174).

Correlation between varied histopathologic features and prognosis has led to two grading systems for LYG (Table 34.5). These grading schemes, both of which are tripartite, are based on the degree of cytologic atypia, extent of necrosis, and retention of the polymorphous cellular infiltrate. Lesions are classified as grade 1 through 3 or pure LYG, LYG-lymphoma, focal, and LYG-lymphoma, diffuse (172,173,182,191). Grade 1 lesions are polymorphous with little or no atypia or necrosis. This category probably includes cases of so-called *benign lymphocytic angiitis* and *granulomatosis* (192,193). Grade 2 lesions are also polymorphous but have scattered atypical cells with enlarged nuclei, prominent nucleoli, and foci of necrosis. This grade includes most cases of LYG. Grade 3 lesions are monomorphous with prominent atypia and widespread necrosis. These lesions are essentially large cell lymphomas and include clinical relapses after observation or single agent chemotherapy. It has been demonstrated that the spectrum of B-cell proliferation (i.e., proliferation index) and quantification of EBV-infected B cells correlate with this histologic grading scheme (176,190). However, the potential for biologic aggressiveness is equivalent in all grades.

Immunohistochemical and molecular studies appear to have clarified the nature of LYG. As initially suggested in 1972, LYG is associated with EBV (191), and further studies suggest that vascular damage and necrosis are caused by the cellular infiltration of vessels and by chemokines upregulated by EBV latent membrane protein (194). Although most lymphocytes, including those within vessel walls, are T cells, the large, atypical cells are EBV-infected B cells (175,177,178,195) with an immunophenotypic profile similar to that reported in T-cell–rich B-cell lymphomas (196). PCR has demonstrated in a large proportion of cases, including cases with histologic progression, that the EBV-infected B cells are monoclonal (175,178,180). Some studies reported that several cases of ''LYG'' still feature large atypical T cells (not B cells) lacking EBV RNA (177,178).

Although LYG shares clinical and histologic features with angiocentric nasal NK/T-cell lymphoma, evidence demonstrates that the process is an EBV^+ B-cell proliferation with an exuberant T-cell reaction. Lymphomatoid granulomatosis may also have features resembling PTLPDs (see Chapter 16). Both processes may occur in immunocompromised patients and contain EBV-infected polyclonal, oligoclonal, or monoclonal B cells (197), which over the course of the disease proliferate in different organs (180,198). However, LYG features a striking angiocentric T-cell reaction with vasculitis, whereas most PTLPDs are composed of plasmacytoid B cells with few T cells and rare necrotizing vasculitis (199). It has been suggested that LYG should be called T-cell–rich, EBV-associated, B-cell lymphoproliferative disorder (T-RELD) to distinguish it from EBV-associated PTLPDs (T-cell–poor, EBV-associated, B-cell lymphoproliferative disorder [T-PELD]) and from EBV-associated angiocentric NK/T-cell lymphomas (180).

The morphologic differential diagnosis also includes necrotizing and inflammatory conditions, nonlymphoid malignancies, aggressive pulmonary lymphomas, lymphomas secondarily involving the lung and Hodgkin's disease.

The natural history of LYG varies greatly and its clinical behavior ranges from indolent to aggressive. Some patients experience spontaneous remission, others achieve therapy-induced remissions but more than 60% die with a median survival of 14 months. Although LYG most often manifests with pulmonary involvement, during its course multiple organs are involved, including the skin (up to 50% of cases), central and peripheral nervous systems (≤30% of cases), the kidneys (30% to 40%), and the liver, adrenal glands, bladder, prostate, and pancreas (<10% of cases) (169,182,183). Lymphoid tissue including the spleen is rarely involved except in the 25% of patients who develop grade 3 lesions/diffuse large B-cell lymphomas. Bone marrow involvement is rare, but cases of hemophagocytic syndrome related to systemic EBV infection have been reported (200).

Because of the rarity of LYG, the paucity of clinical trials and the variable clinical course, the most effective treatment is not known. Asymptomatic patients or those with minimal disease and grade 1 or 2 histology may be observed, and patients with symptomatic grade 1 or 2 LYG require treatment with corticosteroids or single or multiagent chemotherapy. Patients with aggressive grade 1 or 2 disease and all patients with grade 3 disease are treated with combination chemotherapy such as CHOP (cyclophosphamide, doxorubicin hydrochloride, vincristine sulfate and prednisone). Additional therapies targeting the EBV-bearing B cells (i.e., interferon-α2b) or reactive T cells (i.e., cyclosporine), as well as high-dose chemotherapy and stem cell transplantation, have been reported (176,180,201), but further studies are necessary.

Intravascular Lymphomatosis

Intravascular lymphomatosis (IVL), also called *angiotropic lymphoma* or *malignant angioendotheliomatosis,* is a rare non-Hodgkin's lymphoma characterized by intravascular proliferation and dissemination of malignant lymphoid cells without solid organ involvement (202,203). Although IVL most often manifests with neurologic or dermatologic manifestations (see Chapter 32), pulmonary presentations are also well described (203–206). Most individuals are in their fifth to seventh decades, and those with pulmonary presentations demonstrate fever, dyspnea, cough, chest pain, or respiratory failure (203–205). Arterial blood gases reveal moderate hypoxia and pulmonary function tests indicate a decreased diffusion capacity (204,207). Radiographs demonstrate reticulonodular infiltrates while CT scans can show diffuse or patchy ground glass opacities (i.e., mosaic pattern) (204,206,207). Histologically, low magnification demonstrates a diffuse interstitial process superficially resembling cellular interstitial pneumonia (Fig. 34.26) and higher magnification reveals large neoplastic cells with vesicular nuclei, prominent eosinophilic nucleoli and moderate amounts of pale cytoplasm confined to the intravascular component (i.e., arteries, veins, lymphatics and especially capillaries) (Fig. 34.26). Mitoses, including atypical forms, are frequently seen. Vascular intimal fibroelastosis and adjacent interstitial lymphoplasmacytic infiltrates are also observed (203).

Although most reported cases of IVL are B-cell lymphomas (208), rare cases of T-cell IVL associated with EBV have been described (204,209,210). EBV-associated IVL within Kaposi's sarcoma (KS) in a patient with AIDS has also been reported (211), but further studies into the roles of EBV and KSHV in the pathogenesis of IVL are needed.

The intravascular nature of this process is also an enigma, but a study demonstrated tumor cell negativity for CD29 (β_1 integrin) and CD54 (ICAM-1) (212). Perhaps the impairment of multiple adhesion molecules prevents neoplastic cell–endothelial cell interactions and subsequent extravascular spread.

Almost 50% of cases of IVL are diagnosed at autopsy (213), but a definitive antemortem diagnosis is possible on thoracoscopic and even transbronchial biopsy (206,207). And despite the distinctive architectural and cytologic features of the disease, the morphologic differential diagnosis includes many primary and metastatic lesions involving the lung, including carcinoma, LYG-like and other aggressive primary and secondary NHL, leukemia, and angiosarcoma. The absence of an extravascular component discerns this entity from LYG-like and other aggressive NHLs involving

A
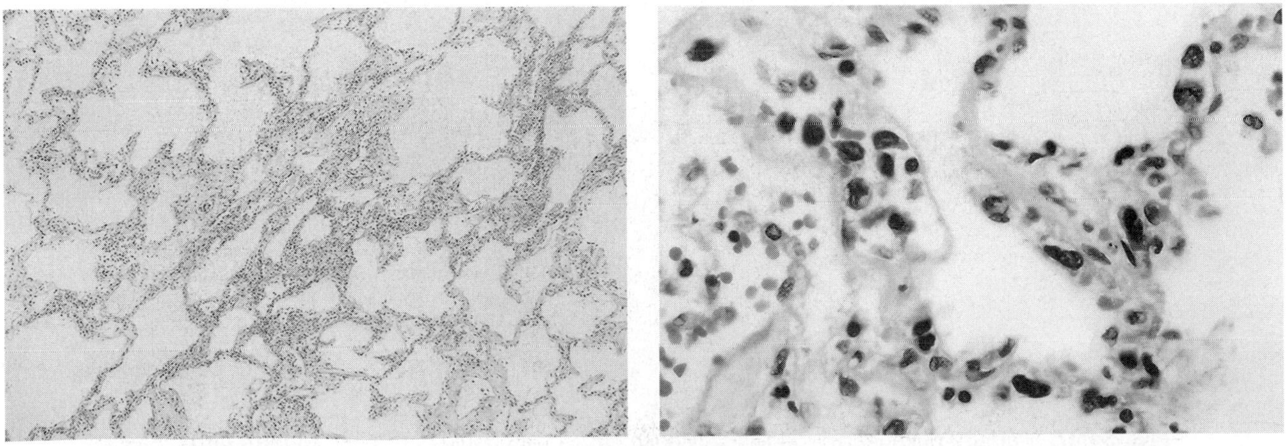
B

FIG. 34.26. Intravascular lymphomatosis. **A:** Low magnification demonstrates a diffuse interstitial process (hematoxylin and eosin stain, original magnification: 40× magnification). **B:** Alveolar septal capillaries are engorged with large, atypical lymphoid cells (hematoxylin and eosin stain, original magnification: 400× magnification).

the lung, which permeate and consolidate lung parenchyma. Leukemic infiltrates also form small perivascular aggregates. Metastatic cancers, including renal cell carcinoma; adenocarcinomas of breast, prostate, bladder, and lung; and malignant melanoma, may require histochemical and immunohistochemical studies to separate these from IVL, whereas the spindle cell appearance of most angiosarcomas and CD45 negativity allow for distinction.

Although prognosis appears relatively poor in the small number of cases reported, complete remission and long-term survival can be achieved with aggressive combination chemotherapy (202).

Hodgkin's Disease

More than 13% of patients with Hodgkin's disease (HD) have lung involvement at presentation (214), 50% have relapses in the lung, and almost 60% are found to have pulmonary involvement at autopsy (215). Primary pulmonary HD is a rare but well-documented process (216–218). Unlike primary pulmonary NHL where regional nodal involvement is seen in up to 30% of cases, diagnostic criteria for primary pulmonary HD include radiographic or morphologic absence of hilar lymph node involvement.

Primary pulmonary HD shows the usual bimodal age distribution of systemic HD; however, mean age is skewed

A

B

C

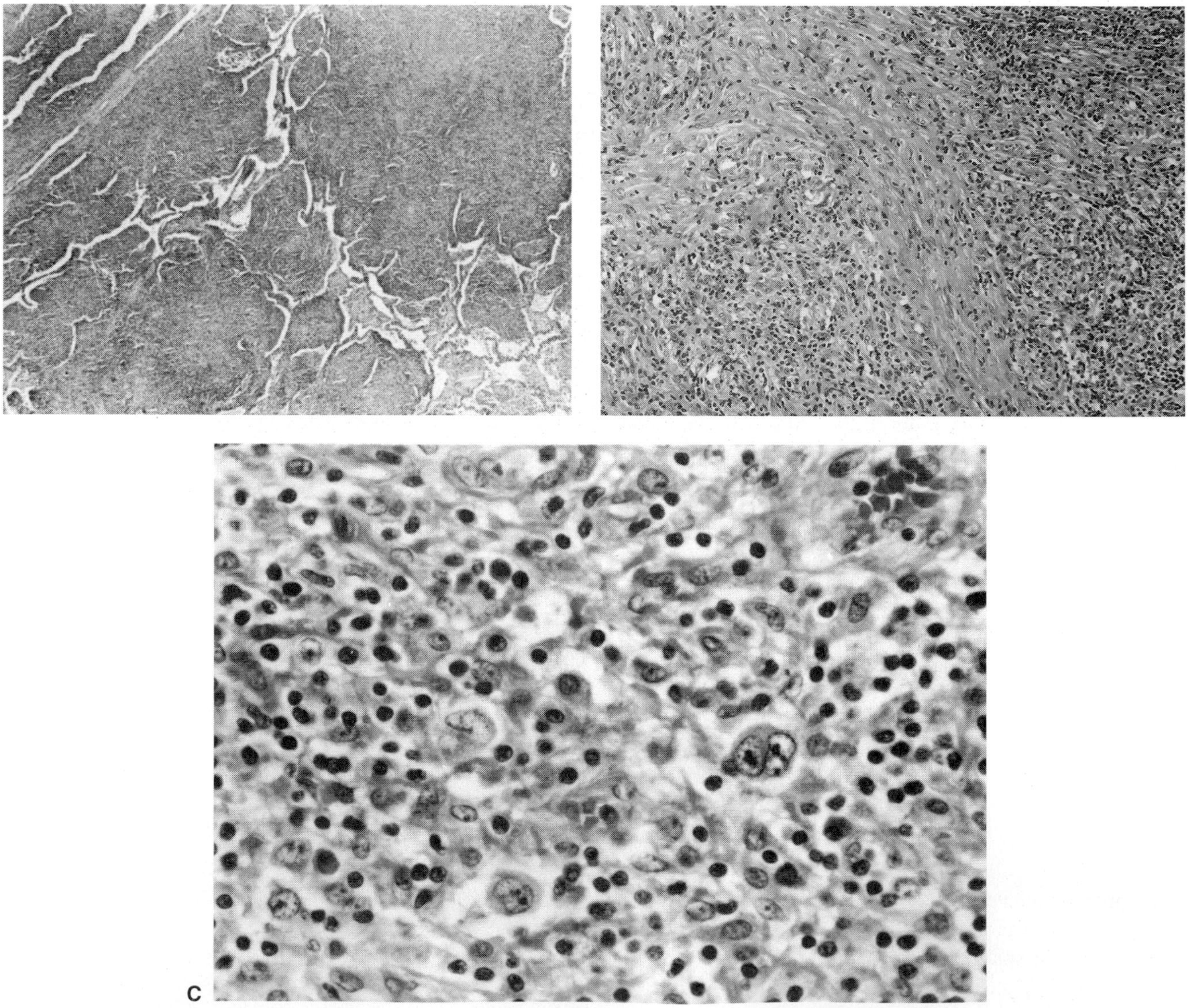

FIG. 34.27. Primary pulmonary Hodgkin's disease. **A:** Small nodules coalesce to form large masses (hematoxylin and eosin stain, original magnification: 40× magnification). **B:** Irregular fibrous bands suggest the nodular sclerosis subtype of Hodgkin's disease (hematoxylin and eosin stain, original magnification: 100× magnification). **C:** Reed-Sternberg cells are easily identified in a polymorphous inflammatory background (hematoxylin and eosin stain, original magnification: 400× magnification).

toward an older population (mean age, 42 years; range, 12 to 82 years), and women outnumber men by almost 1.5 to 1. Symptoms include cough, dyspnea, hemoptysis, and chest pain, and B symptoms are observed in one third of patients (217). Up to 15% of patients are asymptomatic and diagnosed after the detection of a radiographic abnormality (217). Chest radiographs and CT scans usually demonstrate multiple nodular lesions, with one half involving more than one lobe, but solitary nodules and pneumonic consolidation, with or without air bronchograms, are also seen (217,219). Upper lobe involvement is twice as common as lower lobe disease, and cavitation is found in nearly one third of cases (220).

Large tumors often demonstrate a multinodular appearance, and nodular sclerosis and mixed cellularity subtypes are more common than lymphocyte predominance (paragranuloma). Lymphocyte depletion has not been reported in primary pulmonary HD (216,217). Although small nodules distributed along the lymphatic routes coalesce to form large masses, satellite lesions are often seen (Fig. 34.27). Large nodules may cavitate because of central necrosis or may be associated with crisscrossing bands of birefringent collagen (Fig. 34.27). In many cases the infiltrate invades overlying visceral pleura. Peritumoral lung and rare cases of pneumonic HD feature fibrin and fibroblast proliferation (i.e., organizing pneumonia), admixed with neoplastic and background cells. The cellular infiltrates are identical to nodal HD and central necrosis, granulomatous inflammation and vascular permeation of arteries and veins by the polymorphous infiltrate are commonly seen (Fig. 34.27). However, fibrinoid necrosis and Reed-Sternberg cells have not been reported in vessel walls. Bronchial involvement can result in a polypoid endobronchial mass, mural permeation, and destruction of the cartilaginous plates, with resulting bronchostenosis or multiple plaquelike nodules with focal involvement of acquired BALT.

The differential diagnosis of primary pulmonary HD includes benign/inflammatory and malignant processes. Infectious processes, sarcoidosis and Wegener's granulomatosis can be separated on the basis of light microscopic findings. Poorly differentiated carcinomas such as pleomorphic giant cell carcinoma, LYG and pulmonary NHL, including B-cell lymphoma, T-cell lymphoma and anaplastic large cell lymphoma, require immunohistochemical and molecular studies to separate them from HD with certainty (221) (see Chapter 17).

The prognosis for patients with primary pulmonary HD is variable, with approximately 50% 2-year disease-free periods reported in small patient groups. The extent of lung involvement (multiple lobe involvement or bilateral involvement), pleural invasion, and cavitary disease, as well as the presence of B symptoms, appear to portend a worse outcome. It is uncertain whether age, histologic subtype, presence of pleural effusions, or peripheral versus central tumor location are prognostically relevant (216,217).

SECONDARY LYMPHOMA INVOLVING THE LUNG

Primary nodal and extranodal lymphomas frequently involve the lungs. More often than not, patients present with synchronous nodal and lung disease or relapse in the lung. Almost 60% and 50% of patients with HD and NHL, respectively, have pulmonary involvement at autopsy (215,222). Clinical and radiographic findings may suggest an infectious process and histologic findings vary from patchy infiltrates to endobronchial masses (223) and large necrotic nodules. A lymphangitic pattern of disease is usually seen. Because the morphology of these malignancies, including disseminated marginal zone and T-cell lymphomas, are indistinguishable from primary pulmonary MALT lymphoma and some cases of LYG, respectively, clinical history and review of previous tissue samples are imperative for reaching the proper diagnosis. Secondary lymphomas involving the lung may also transform to aggressive histology with increased numbers of large cells. Secondary changes in the lung include fibrinous, postobstructive, and organizing pneumonia.

Mycosis fungoides (MF) may involve the lung after dissemination of cutaneous disease or as part of the Sezary syndrome (224). The lung is the second most commonly involved extracutaneous site after lymph nodes (224,225). Clinical and radiographic features may simulate pneumonia with nodular and diffuse disease and patients may present in respiratory distress (226). Lung specimens demonstrate airspace and interstitial infiltrates extending along lymphatic routes while granulomas, extensive vascular infiltration and necrosis may be seen (227) (Fig. 34.28). The cytology of the infiltrate ranges from small cells with cerebriform nuclei to large cells with prominent nucleoli (Fig. 34.28).

The lungs are also frequently involved with angioimmunoblastic T-cell lymphoma. This entity warrants brief mention only to emphasize the malignant nature of what was originally described as a reactive process (angioimmunoblastic lymphadenopathy with dysproteinemia) (228). Pulmonary findings can be easily mistaken for an interstitial pneumonia given the associated mediastinal adenopathy and pleural effusion, but the lymphatic distribution of the infiltrate should lead one to consider malignant lymphoma (229,230). Clusters of atypical "clear" cells with slightly indented nuclei and abundant pale cytoplasm admixed with immunoblasts, plasma cells, histiocytes and occasional eosinophils must also be distinguished from pulmonary involvement with HD. Immunohistochemical studies can facilitate this distinction.

Hodgkin's disease relapsing in the lung most often features a lymphatic distribution with infiltrates dispersed along the visceral pleura, interlobular septa and bronchovascular bundles. Large nodules are less often seen than in primary pulmonary HD. Infiltrates often rim vessels with central necrosis and may feature greater numbers of atypical cells and fewer numbers of inflammatory cells than in primary HD.

A

B

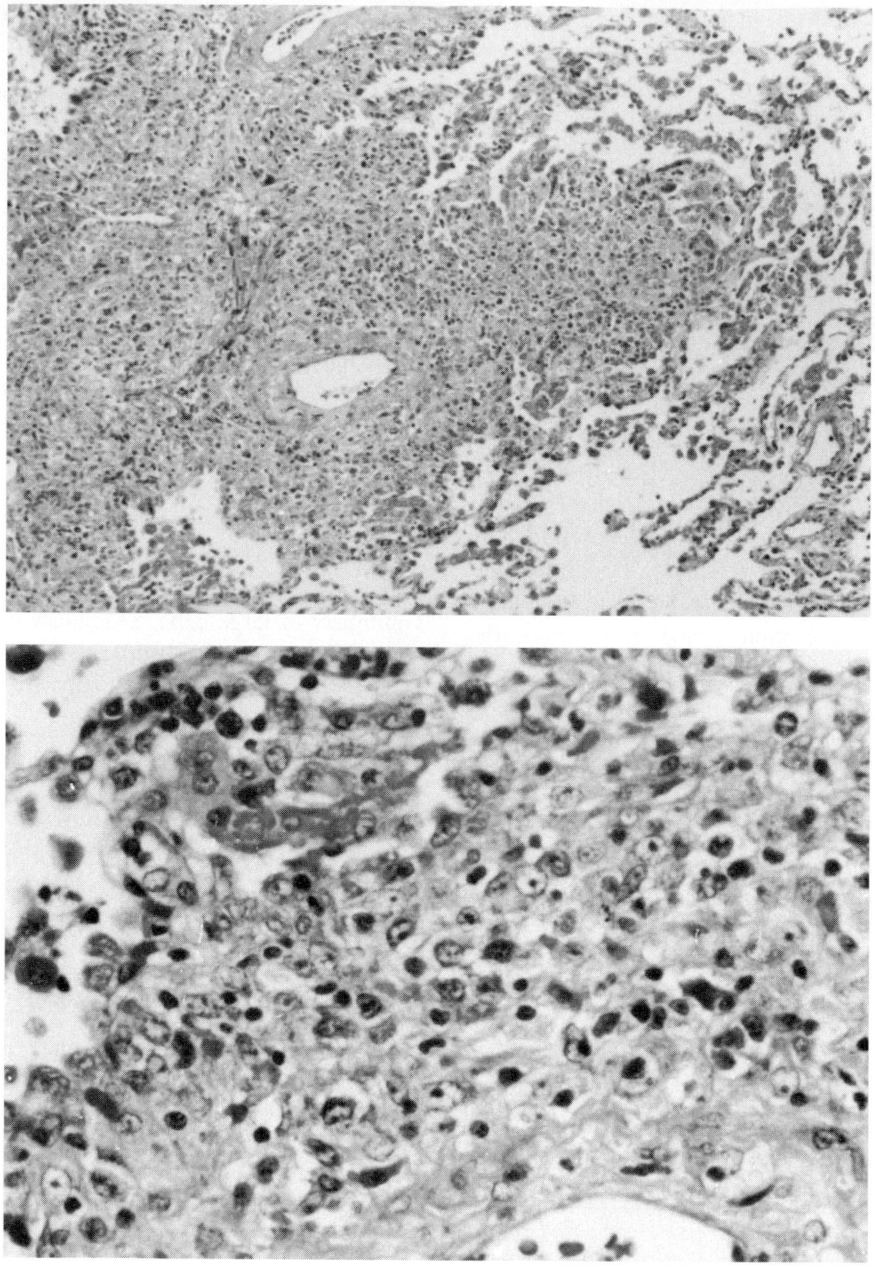

FIG. 34.28. Mycosis fungoides. **A:** Airspace and interstitial infiltrates extend along lymphatic routes (hematoxylin and eosin stain, original magnification: 100× magnification). **B:** Malignant cells feature vesicular nuclei and prominent nucleoli. Clinical history is necessary to make a specific diagnosis (hematoxylin and eosin stain, original magnification: 400× magnification).

LEUKEMIC INFILTRATES INVOLVING THE LUNG

Whereas leukemic infiltration of the lung at autopsy is seen in up to 65% of patients (231), clinically significant involvement during life occurs in less than 7% of patients (232–234). Most patients with leukemia suffer from secondary effects of the leukemia or its therapy including infections, intravascular thrombosis and leukostasis, hemorrhage, leukemic cell lysis pneumonopathy, alveolar proteinosis, and chemotherapy effects. Most cases of leukemic lung infiltration occur in patients with active leukemia and may represent an incidental finding adjacent to a life-threatening infection or the cause of significant respiratory symptoms.

Pulmonary symptoms secondary to leukemia are usually only seen in patients with high (40% or greater) blast counts; however, several reports of patients with T-cell leukemias found a large percentage of patients with subacute pulmonary symptoms for months to years before tissue diagnosis (235,236). Radiographic findings run the gamut from localized and diffuse infiltrates to nodules.

All subtypes of leukemia can involve the lung, and acute

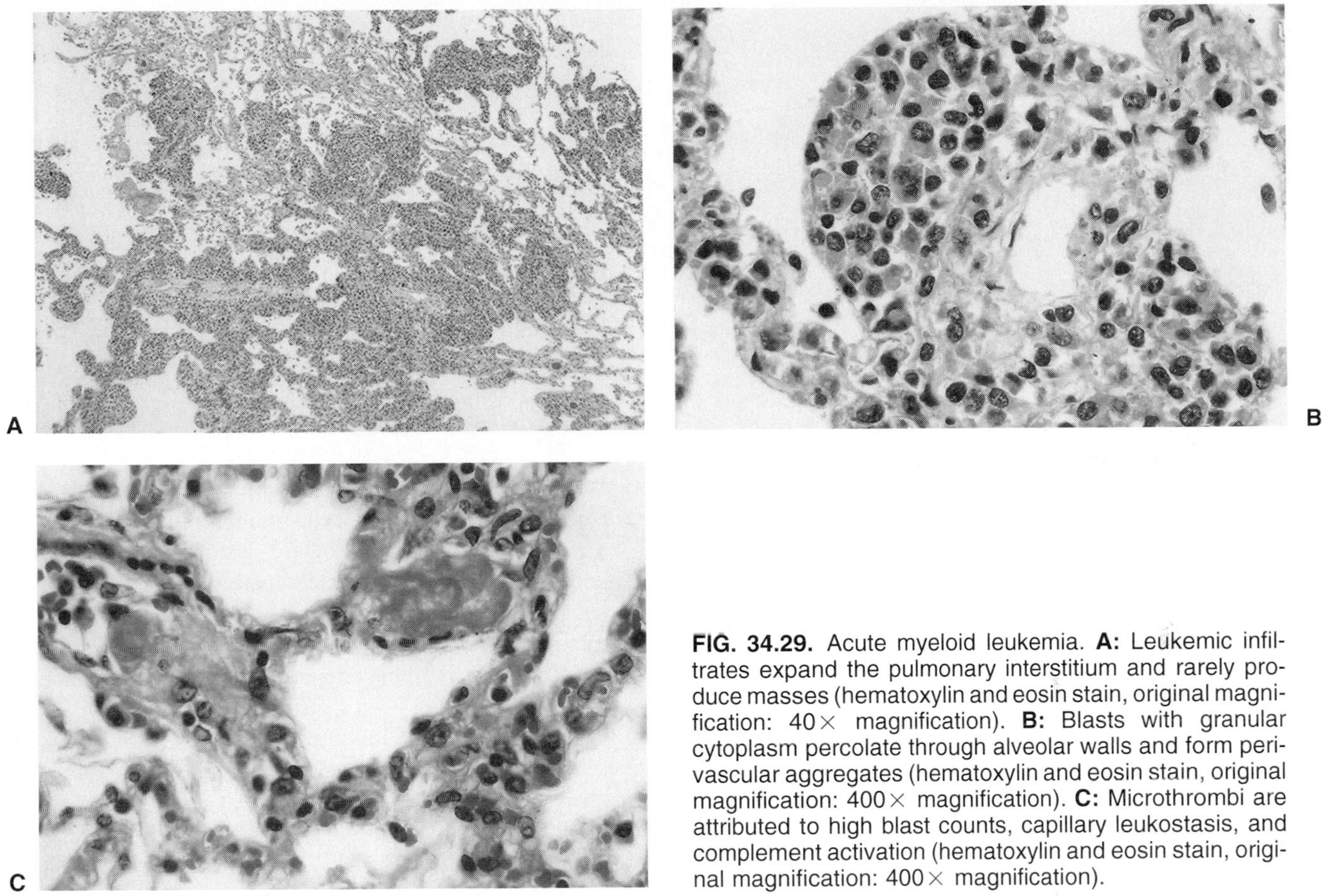

FIG. 34.29. Acute myeloid leukemia. **A:** Leukemic infiltrates expand the pulmonary interstitium and rarely produce masses (hematoxylin and eosin stain, original magnification: 40× magnification). **B:** Blasts with granular cytoplasm percolate through alveolar walls and form perivascular aggregates (hematoxylin and eosin stain, original magnification: 400× magnification). **C:** Microthrombi are attributed to high blast counts, capillary leukostasis, and complement activation (hematoxylin and eosin stain, original magnification: 400× magnification).

myeloid leukemia, acute lymphoblastic leukemia, and chronic lymphocytic leukemia (CLL) are most often encountered in biopsy material. Morphologically, leukemic infiltrates are restricted to the pulmonary lymphatic distribution and rarely form nodules (237,238) (Fig. 34.29). The infiltrates can be subtle, and ancillary studies, including chloroacetate esterase and myeloperoxidase stains, can highlight and help subtype the leukemia. Transformation of CLL (i.e., Richter's syndrome) in the lung (239), CLL mimicking idiopathic bronchiolitis obliterans organizing pneumonia (236), and bronchiolar involvement producing asthma-like symptoms (240) have been reported.

Agnogenic myeloid metaplasia (myelofibrosis) (241,242) occasionally involves the lungs and pleura. Diffuse and nodular foci of extramedullary hematopoiesis usually follow lymphatic channels, whereas associated reactive fibrous tissue can form large nodules. The process can progress to widespread interstitial fibrosis, which may be mistaken for a primary chronic fibrosing interstitial pneumonitis.

Secondary effects relating to leukemia and treatment, including infection, hemorrhage, and infarction, are responsible for more morbidity and mortality than pulmonary leukemic infiltrates in patients with leukemia (232). When leukemic counts rise to more than 200,000/μm, capillary leukostasis with thrombosis can occur (243). Low deformability of blasts and complement activation (244) result in compact fibrin and cellular plugs (Fig. 34.29). If treated with chemotherapy, blast lysis with liberation of cell contents precipitates interstitial edema, hemorrhage, small infarcts, and diffuse alveolar damage. This leukemic cell lysis pneumonopathy manifests with severe hypoxia within 48 hours of initial chemotherapy (245). Thrombocytopenia associated with marrow replacement by leukemic infiltrates or therapy also plays a role in alveolar hemorrhage. An alveolar proteinosis-like reaction is seen in up to 10% of patients with myeloid leukemias. Usually ascribed to an underlying infection, often *Nocardia,* it has been suggested that the process is caused by macrophage dysfunction and might be reversible with successful treatment of the underlying leukemia (246).

PLASMACYTOMAS AND MULTIPLE MYELOMA

Primary plasmacytomas of the lung are exceptionally rare tumors with less than 25 *bona fide* cases reported in the world literature (49,72,247). Like their counterparts with extramedullary plasmacytomas from other sites (49,248), patients are usually in their fifth and sixth decades of life, with an approximately equal sex ratio. Most patients are asymptomatic, although cough, dyspnea, and hemoptysis are

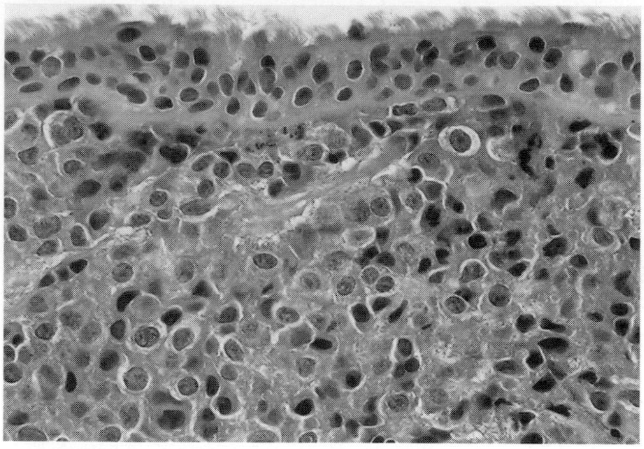

FIG. 34.30. Pulmonary plasmacytoma. This endobronchial lesion does not destroy overlying respiratory epithelium (hematoxylin and eosin stain, original magnification: 400× magnification).

reported symptoms. The radiographic appearance is that of a solitary mass in the midlung or hilar area, yet peripheral lesions also occur that are amenable to transthoracic needle aspiration biopsy diagnosis (249). Unlike multiple myeloma, patients can lack a serum M-protein or Bence Jones light chains in the urine (49). The presence or absence and amount of M-protein may mirror tumor burden and clinical course while an increase or decrease in levels may be associated with recurrence or complete treatment (250,251).

Tumors range from 2.5 to 8.0 cm in diameter and usually involve a major bronchus with occasional involvement of peribronchial, hilar or mediastinal lymph nodes. Histologically, sheets of plasma cells destroy lung parenchyma and bronchial cartilage and scattered fibrous bands course through the neoplasm (Fig. 34.30). Binucleate plasma cells with nuclear pyknosis and anisonucleosis usually lack appreciable mitotic activity or necrosis; however, poorly differentiated cases with nuclear pleomorphism and mitotic activity have been reported. Mott and Russell bodies can be seen, but Dutcher bodies have not been reported. Scattered macrophages with paraprotein crystalloids have been described in these tumors (252). Nodular or broad bands of amyloid are often associated with the tumor or in regional lymph nodes while light-chain deposition disease is a rare finding (72,253). The κ and λ light chains and IgG, IgA, and IgD can be expressed immunohistochemically or produced as M-proteins by pulmonary plasmacytomas. Discerning this tumor from PCG or even marginal zone lymphoma of the lung (254) may require immunohistochemical studies.

Although little can be surmised about the natural history of pulmonary plasmacytomas, it appears that cases can evolve into multiple myeloma or can be cured with surgical excision or radiation therapy (49). Overall 2- and 5-year survivals of 66% and 40%, respectively, have been reported (49).

Although rare, pulmonary involvement with multiple myeloma is more common than pulmonary plasmacytoma. The myeloma infiltrate presents as nodules of mature and immature plasma cells, occasionally with nodular or diffuse septal amyloid or light-chain deposits (68,255,256), or as an interstitial pneumonitis. A lymphangitic pattern with venular wall penetration and amyloid deposits or bronchial mucosal infiltration (257) can be seen in the latter. This pattern of disease must be clinically distinguished from infectious processes (258). Intracytoplasmic crystalline casts akin to those seen in the kidneys, have also been reported in lungs involved with multiple myeloma (259).

HISTIOCYTIC INFILTRATES INVOLVING THE LUNG

Whereas macrophages are ubiquitous in the lung, localized and systemic histiocytic proliferations rarely involve the lung. Reactive histiocytic lesions, including malakoplakia and Whipple's disease, are often seen in immunocompromised individuals (260–262) while Gaucher's disease and diffuse pulmonary parenchymal sinus histiocytosis with massive lymphadenopathy (Rosai-Dorfman disease) (SHML) have also been described (263,264) (Fig. 34.31).

Langerhans cell histiocytosis (LCH) can involve the lung in the multifocal, multisystem disease that includes many cases of Letterer-Siwe syndrome but more commonly presents in adults as a unique tobacco-related entity separate from other forms of LCH (265). These lesions are alternatively designated *pulmonary eosinophilic granuloma, pulmonary Langerhans cell granulomatosis or pulmonary histiocytosis X* (see Chapter 51).

Pulmonary LCH (PLCH) usually affects women in the third to fourth decades of life and virtually all cases occur in cigarette smokers (265,266). Although up to 25% of patients are asymptomatic at diagnosis, most present with nonproductive cough, dyspnea, chest pain and spontaneous pneumothorax. Chest radiographs demonstrate diffuse bilateral midzonal reticulonodular infiltrates while HRCT scans show thin-walled cysts and nodules, often limited to the upper lung fields (267).

At low magnification, PLCH are discrete nodular infiltrates centered on bronchioles with a stellate border extending into the surrounding interstitium (Fig. 34.32). As the disease progresses, lesions cavitate and become fibrotic. Fibrotic scars maintain the stellate configuration and eventual honeycomb fibrosis results. The historical term eosinophilic granuloma is a misnomer because lesions are neither eosinophilic nor granulomatous, but rather composed of large round to oval cells with cerebriform nuclei and inconspicuous nucleoli, such as Langerhans cells (LCs), admixed with various numbers of lymphocytes, eosinophils, and macrophages (Fig. 34.32). Cellular lesions can contain numerous mitotic figures raising the possibility of malignancy. Diagnosis rests on the demonstration of LCs, which express CD1a and S-100 protein (268). Adjacent lung often features marked accumulations of pigmented macrophages (smoker's

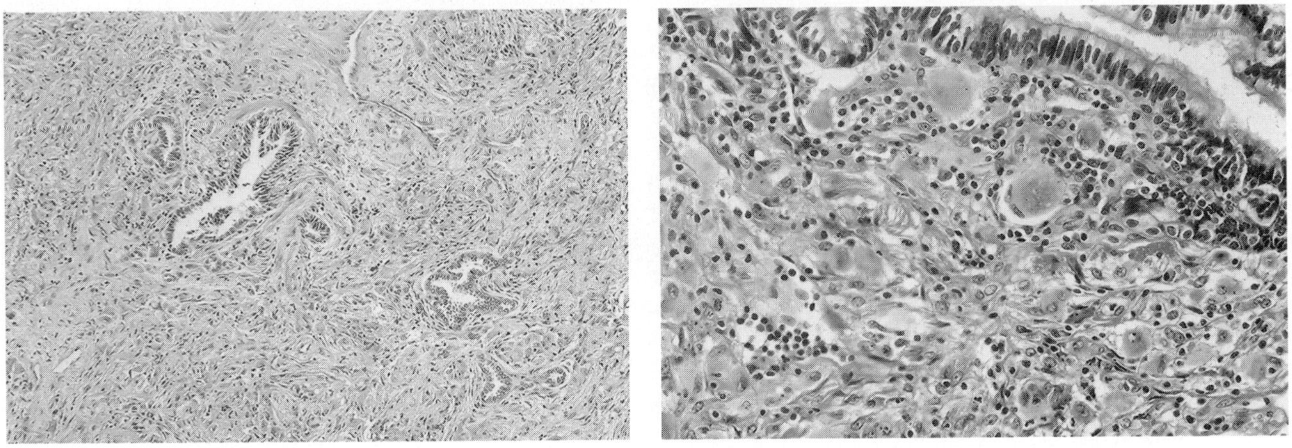

A B

FIG. 34.31. Sinus histiocytosis with massive lymphadenopathy involving the lung. **A:** Pulmonary lobules are encircled and infiltrated by a fibroinflammatory process (hematoxylin and eosin stain, original magnification: 100× magnification). **B:** Histiocytes with abundant cytoplasm and scattered lymphocytes expand bronchiolar submucosa (hematoxylin and eosin stain, original magnification: 200× magnification).

macrophages). Radiographic findings can suggest the diagnosis, but open lung biopsy or rarely transbronchial biopsy provide a definitive diagnosis.

Although some studies have demonstrated clonality of LCs in the multisystem, multiorgan diseases (269–272), such work has not been undertaken with solitary lung lesions. The fact that progression of PLCH can be halted with smoking cessation argues in favor of a nonneoplastic immunologic etiology (273). Symptomatic patients are also treated with steroids with resolution of symptoms. Treatment leads to fibrosis of active lesions and less than 20% of patients develop progressive fibrotic lung disease (265,266). Lung transplantation is a viable treatment option for patients with end-stage pulmonary fibrosis, but disease relapse after transplantation has been reported (274).

In marked distinction to PLCH, lung involvement in multifocal, multisystem histiocytosis can have nodular lesions, flooding of airspaces with LCs or a lymphangitic pattern. Mitotic figures are more commonly seen than in PLCH and background inflammatory cells can be sparse.

Pulmonary involvement in Erdheim-Chester disease, a rare non-Langerhans cell histiocytosis characterized by symmetric sclerosis involving the diametaphyseal aspects of the long bones, occurs in approximately 15% of patients and plays a significant role in the disease's overall morbidity and mortality (275–278). Patients present with dry cough and exertional dyspnea. Skeletal radiographs show symmetrical sclerotic or mixed sclerotic/lytic lesions of the metaphyseal and diaphyseal regions and chest radiographs demonstrate interstitial markings and pleural thickening. HRCT scans show diffuse interlobular septal thickening and patchy regions of ground glass attenuation (277,278).

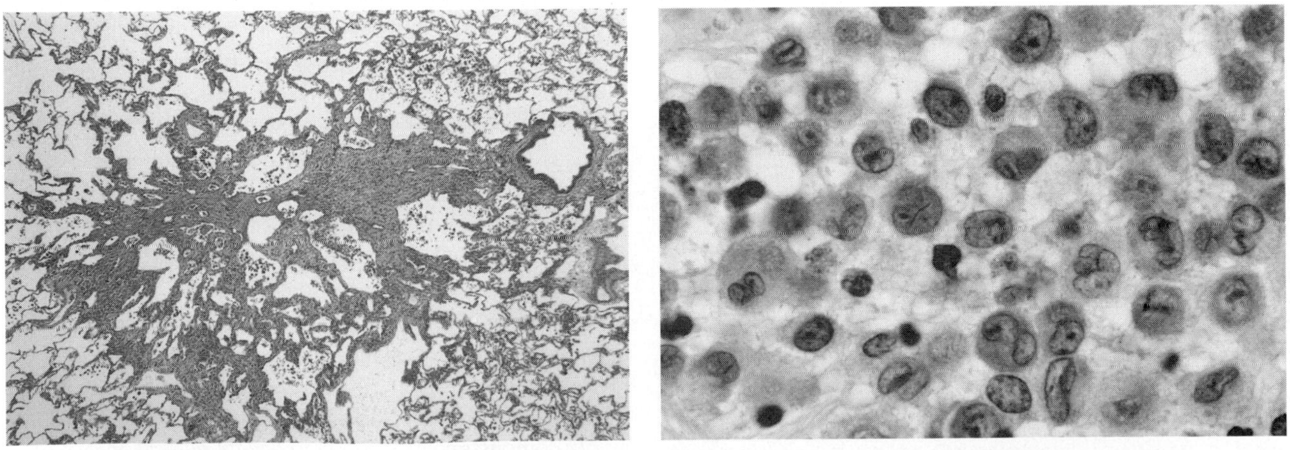

A B

FIG. 34.32. Pulmonary Langerhans cell histiocytosis. **A:** Peribronchiolar infiltrates with fibrosis extend out in a stellate manner along alveolar septa (hematoxylin and eosin stain, original magnification: 40× magnification). **B:** Diagnostic Langerhans cells feature convoluted nuclei and pale cytoplasm. These cells are positive for S-100 protein and CD1a (hematoxylin and eosin stain, original magnification: 600× magnification).

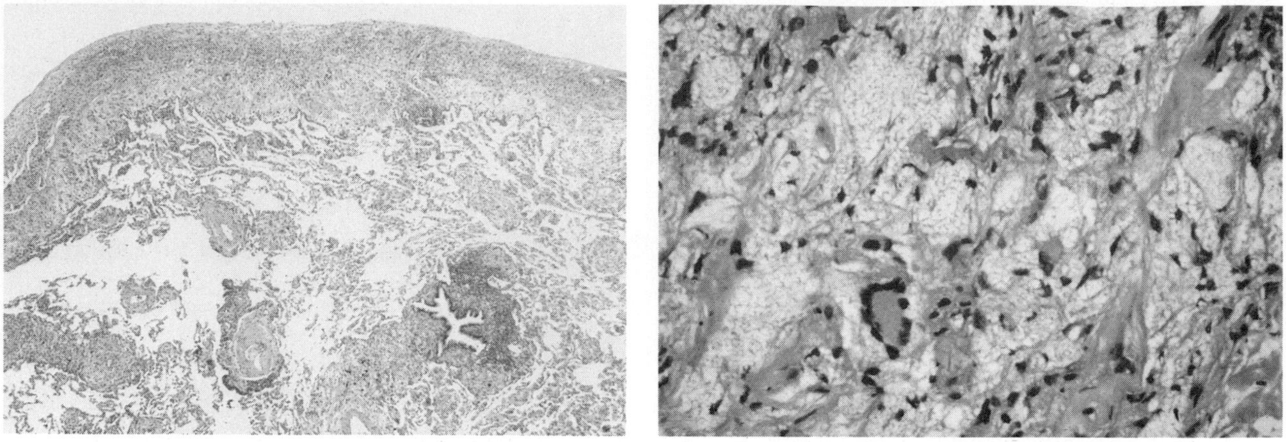

A B

FIG. 34.33. Erdheim-Chester disease. **A:** Pulmonary involvement features a lymphangitic pattern of fibrosis and inflammatory cell infiltrates. Notice the strikingly thickened visceral pleura (hematoxylin and eosin stain, original magnification: 40× magnification). **B:** Foamy histiocytes lack nuclear features of Langerhans cells. Rare scattered Touton giant cells can also be seen (hematoxylin and eosin stain, original magnification: 400× magnification).

Histologically, lung biopsies feature interstitial thickening with a striking lymphangitic distribution at low magnification (Fig. 34.33). The visceral pleura, interlobular septa and bronchovascular bundles to a lesser degree are expanded by collagen and large histiocytes with round to oval nuclei and abundant pale staining and foamy cytoplasm (Fig. 34.33). Scattered plasma cells, lymphocytes and Touton giant cells, but no granulomas, are seen. The histiocytes express CD68, and occasionally S-100 protein and lack CD1a. Birbeck granules are not observed on ultrastructural examination (276–278). One study demonstrated factor XIIIa staining in the lesional cells, suggesting that Erdheim-Chester disease is a dendritic cell process (278) while another group has demonstrated clonality (279). Perhaps Erdheim-Chester disease is the dendritic cell counterpart of LCH in the spectrum of histiocytosis. Erdheim-Chester disease with pulmonary involvement associated with eosinophilic granuloma of the mandible and vulva have been described (279,280).

Given the progressive cardiopulmonary decline in patients with pulmonary Erdheim-Chester disease, distinction from PLCH and other histiocytic entities, including SHML, is of paramount importance and requires clinical and radiographic correlation.

So-called malignant histiocytosis was reported to involve the lung (281), but these cases most likely represent anaplastic large cell lymphoma or T-cell lymphoma (see Chapter 51). Reevaluation of the cases with immunohistochemical stains not available at the time of the original publication demonstrates CD30 positivity in three of the five malignant tumors (282).

PLEURAL LYMPHOMAS/LEUKEMIAS

Primary pulmonary and disseminated lymphoproliferative processes involve the visceral pleura and the pleural cavity. Non-Hodgkin's lymphomas often invade the visceral pleura while pleural effusions are more commonly seen at presentation of HD because of mediastinal nodal involvement and secondary lymphatic obstruction. Leukemia and multiple myeloma can rarely manifest with pleural disease (255). Effusion cytology and parietal pleural biopsies with immunohistochemical studies can yield definitive diagnoses, but infectious, inflammatory and carcinomatous processes must be excluded.

Primary pleural lymphomas are much less common, and two distinct clinicopathologic malignancies have been described. Primary effusion lymphomas (PEL), seen in AIDS patients and associated with infection by KSHV, also called human herpesvirus-8 (283), are discussed in Chapter 28, and pyothorax-associated lymphomas (PALs) are reviewed here.

Pyothorax-associated lymphomas develop in the pleural cavities of immunocompetent patients with chronic suppurative pleuritis. First described as a clinicopathologic entity in 1987 in three Japanese patients who developed pleural lymphomas after long-standing artificial pneumothorax for treatment of tuberculosis (284), more than 40 additional cases have been reported in others, including Westerners with chronic tuberculous pleuritis (285–289) and pleuritis secondary to pulmonary asbestosis (290). Up to 2.2% of patients with chronic pyothorax may develop PAL (286).

Patients are usually in their sixth to eight decades of life and typically present with chest pain, back pain or shoulder pain and dyspnea, while elevated serum lactic dehydrogenase levels, sedimentation rate and hypergammaglobulinemia have been reported (287,289). Radiographic studies invariably demonstrate a visceral or parietal pleural mass with direct invasion into the chest wall, lung, pericardium, or diaphragm in more than 50% of cases (291). Adjacent pleural fibrosis and calcification are also observed.

Biopsy and resection specimens show mass lesions com-

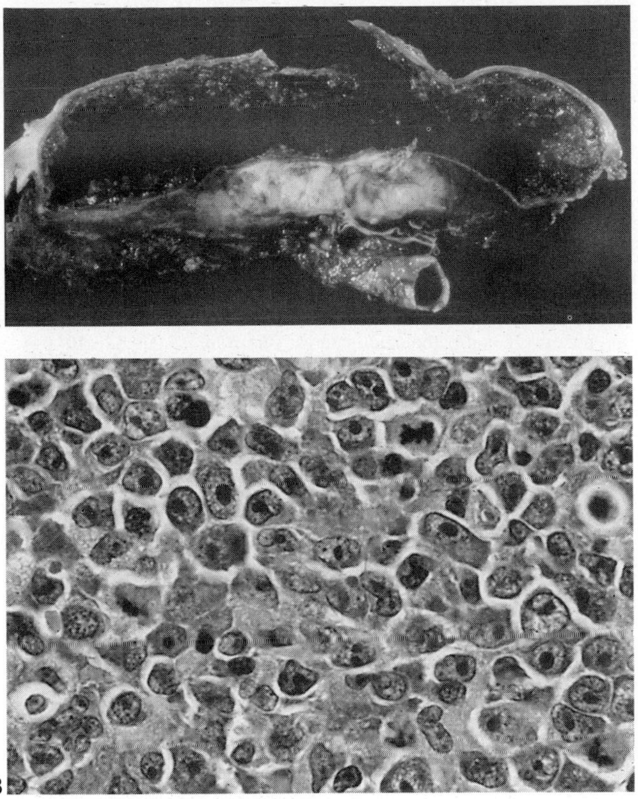

A

B

FIG. 34.34. Pyothorax-associated lymphoma. **A:** This pleural resection demonstrates a fleshy, partially necrotic mass arising in the pleural rind and infiltrating into adjacent lung. Notice the thickened pleural cavity with adherent exudate (i.e., pyothorax). (Photomicrograph courtesy of Dr. K. Aozasa, Suita, Japan) **B:** Sheets of mitotically active large atypical cells with basophilic cytoplasm and prominent nucleoli resemble nodal diffuse large B-cell lymphoma (hematoxylin and eosin stain, original magnification: 600× magnification).

posed of sheets of uninucleate to multinucleate lymphoid cells with prominent nucleoli and clear to basophilic cytoplasm (i.e., immunoblastic or plasmablastic morphology) (Fig. 34.34). Mitoses abound. Scattered histiocytes, small lymphocytes and eosinophils are also seen. Most cases are of B-cell lineage (i.e, diffuse large B-cell lymphomas [286]) and T-cell phenotypes (286), including anaplastic large cell lymphoma (289), a single example with biphenotypic characteristics of B and T cells (292), and a case that evolved from a T- and B-cell phenotype to a B-cell phenotype (293) have all been reported.

The EBV genome has been detected in almost all PALs suggesting an etiologic role for this virus in the development of PAL (294,295). Unlike PELs, KSHV has not been identified in these tumors (287,294,296). Although the precise mechanisms of lymphomagenesis remains to be demonstrated, the presence of EBV latent membrane protein-1 (LMP-1) and EBV-associated nuclear antigen-2 (EBNA-2), oncogenic and immunogenic proteins known to induce a T-cell–mediated reaction with destruction of infected cells (297), suggests that immunocompetent cells cannot enter the diseased pleural cavity resulting in local immunodepression (295). Interleukin-10 has also been postulated to play a role in the development of PAL (298). PAL shares many features with AIDS-related lymphomas and PTLPDs where a depressed immune system favors the clonal evolution of EBV-infected B cells.

Patients with PAL are treated with combination chemotherapy and radiation therapy, but the prognosis is dismal, with most deaths occurring within 8 months of diagnosis (286,287). At autopsy, malignant lymphoma is localized to the thorax in approximately one half of the cases, with dissemination to the liver, spleen, stomach, kidney, adrenal glands, intestine, pancreas, central nervous system, or superficial and deep lymph nodes in the remaining cases (286,287,298).

SUMMARY AND CONCLUSIONS

Pulmonary and pleural lymphomas and reactive processes are uncommon entities that have been described with a bewildering array of terms. Various investigations and the use of the REAL classification scheme have clarified nomenclature and elucidated the pathogenesis of many lesions. Although peculiar lung lesions such as pulmonary hyalinizing granuloma and plasma cell granuloma are not likely to be confused with lymphomas, pulmonary lymphoid hyperplasias, currently viewed within the context of acquired BALT, may still pose diagnostic difficulties. Nodular lymphoid hyperplasia, diffuse lymphoid hyperplasia and lymphocytic interstitial pneumonitis are often associated with autoimmune diseases and should be considered descriptive diagnoses rather than clinicopathologic entities. These rare, localized, and diffuse hyperplasias can be reproducibly separated from extranodal marginal zone lymphomas on the basis of architectural, cytologic, immunohistochemical, and molecular findings; however, an unknown percentage evolve into MALT lymphomas. Although many cases of extranodal marginal zone lymphoma, the most common pulmonary lymphoma, had been considered pseudolymphomas or lymphocytic interstitial pneumonia in the recent past, these relatively indolent malignancies can recur in the lung or other MALT sites and occasionally transform into aggressive lymphomas. Primary pulmonary non-Hodgkin's lymphomas other than marginal zone lymphomas and Hodgkin's disease also arise in the lung, but more commonly involve the lung secondarily. Large B-cell and Burkitt's lymphomas are the most common AIDS-related primary pulmonary lymphomas. Lymphomatoid granulomatosis is a T-cell–rich EBV^+ B-cell lymphoproliferative process with a propensity for multiorgan involvement and death. Recognizing the angiocentric nature of the process along with often subtle cytologic atypia in the lymphoid cells raises the diagnostic possibility and demonstrating EBV DNA in the atypical B cells confirms the diagnosis. Leukemias, intravascular lymphomatosis, plasma cell malignancies, and a wide variety of histiocytic processes can also involve the lung. Pyothorax-associated lymphoma is most likely an Epstein-Barr virus–related malignancy seen in individuals with long-standing pyothorax or pleuritis.

In conclusion, the spectrum and interpretation of pulmonary lymphoid hyperplasias and neoplasms continues to evolve. The use of more sophisticated techniques will undoubtedly lead to refined diagnostic criteria and a greater understanding of these lesions. Such advances will hopefully improve therapies and lower patient morbidity and mortality.

REFERENCES

1. Pabst R, Gehrke I. Is the bronchus-associated lymphoid tissue (BALT) an integral structure of the lung in normal mammals, including humans? *Am J Respir Cell Mol Biol* 1990;3:131–135.
2. Pabst R. Is BALT a major component of the immune system? *Immunol Today* 1992;13:119–122.
3. Sato A, Hayakawa H, Uchiyama H, et al. Cellular distribution of bronchus-associated lymphoid tissue in rheumatoid arthritis. *Am J Respir Crit Care Med* 1996;154:1903–1907.
4. Meuwissen HJ, Hussain M. Bronchus-associated lymphoid tissue in human lung: correlation of hyperplasia with chronic pulmonary disease. *Clin Immunol Immunopathol* 1982;23:548–561.
5. Richmond I, Pritchard GE, Ashcroft T, et al. Bronchus associated lymphoid tissue (BALT) in human lung: its distribution in smokers and non-smokers. *Thorax* 1993;48:1130–1134.
6. Sminia T, van der Brugge-Gamelkoorn GJ, Jeurissen SHM. Structure and function of bronchus-associated lymphoid tissue (BALT). *Crit Rev Immunol* 1989;9:119–150.
7. Hernandez JA, Sheehan WW. Lymphomas of the mucosa-associated lymphoid tissue. *Cancer* 1985;55:592–597.
8. Koss MN, Hochholzer L, Nichols PW, et al. Primary non-Hodgkin's lymphoma and pseudolymphoma of lung: a study of 161 patients. *Hum Pathol* 1983;14:1024–1038.
9. Koss MN. Pulmonary lymphoproliferative disorders. In: Churg A, Katzenstein ALA, eds. *The lung: current concepts.* Philadelphia: Williams & Wilkins, 1993:144–194.
10. Kurosu K, Yumoto N, Mikata A, et al. Monoclonality of B-cell lineage in primary pulmonary lymphoma demonstrated by immunoglobulin heavy chain gene sequence analysis of histologically non-definitive transbronchial biopsy specimens. *J Pathol* 1996;178:316–322.
11. Nicholson AG, Wotherspoon AC, Diss TC, et al. Pulmonary B-cell non-Hodgkin's lymphomas: the value of immunohistochemistry and gene analysis in diagnosis. *Histopathology* 1995;26:395–403.
12. Pisani RJ, Witzig TE, Li CY, et al. Confirmation of lymphomatous pulmonary involvement by immunophenotypic and gene rearrangement analysis of bronchoalveolar lavage fluid. *Mayo Clin Proc* 1990; 65:651–656.
13. Philippe B, Delfau-Larue MH, Epardeau B, et al. B-cell pulmonary lymphoma: gene rearrangement analysis of bronchoalveolar lymphocytes by polymerase chain reaction. *Chest* 1999;115:1242–1247.
14. Colby TV, Carrington CB. Pulmonary lymphomas: current concepts. *Hum Pathol* 1983;14:884–887.
15. Turner RR, Colby TV, Doggett RS. Well differentiated lymphocytic lymphoma; a study of 47 cases with primary manifestations of the lung. *Cancer* 1994;54:2088–2096.
16. Nicholson AG, Wotherspoon AC, Diss TC, et al. Reactive pulmonary lymphoid disorders. *Histopathology* 1995;26:405–412.
17. Addis BJ, Hyjek E, Isaacson PG. Primary pulmonary lymphoma: a reappraisal of its histogenesis and its relationship to pseudolymphoma and lymphoid interstitial pneumonia. *Histopathology* 1988;13:1–17.
18. Kennedy JL, Nathwani BN, Burke J, et al. Pulmonary lymphomas and lymphoid lesions. A clinicopathologic and immunologic study of 64 patients. *Cancer* 1985;56:539–552.
19. Safadi R, Berkman N, Haviv YS, et al. Primary non-Hodgkin's lymphoma of the lung presenting as bronchiolitis obliterans organizing pneumonia. *Leuk Lymphoma* 1997;28:209–213.
20. Picker L, Weiss L, Medeiros L, et al. Immunophenotypic criteria for the diagnosis of non-Hodgkin's lymphoma. *Am J Pathol* 1987;128: 181–201.
21. Isaacson PG, Wotherspoon AC, Pan L. Follicular colonization in B-cell lymphoma of mucosa-associated lymphoid tissue. *Am J Surg Pathol* 1991;15:819–828.
22. Li G, Hansmann ML, Zwingers T, et al. Primary lymphoma of the lung: Morphological, immunohistochemical and clinical features. *Histopathology* 1990;16:519–531.
23. Koss MN, Hochholzer L, Langloss JM, et al. Lymphoid interstitial pneumonia: clinicopathologic and immunopathologic findings in 18 cases. *Pathology* 1987;19:178–185.
24. Trapnell DH. Recognition and incidence of intrapulmonary lymph nodes. *Thorax* 1964;19:44–50.
25. Kradin RL, Spirn PW, Mark EJ. Intrapulmonary lymph nodes: clinical, radiologic, and pathologic features. *Chest* 1985;87:662–667.
26. Miyake H, Yamada Y, Kawagoe T, et al. Intrapulmonary lymph nodes: CT and pathologic features. *Clin Radiol* 1999;54:640–643.
27. Bankoff MS, McEniff NJ, Bhadelia RA, et al. Prevalence of pathologically proven intrapulmonary lymph nodes and their appearance on CT. *Am J Roentgenol* 1996;167:629–630.
28. Flieder DB, Suster S, Moran CM. Idiopathic fibroinflammatory (fibrosing/sclerosing) lesions of the mediastinum: a study of 30 cases with emphasis on morphologic heterogeneity. *Mod Pathol* 1999;12: 257–264.
29. Engleman P, Liebow AA, Gmelich J, et al. Pulmonary hyalinizing granuloma. *Am Rev Respir Dis* 1977;115:997–1008.
30. Yousem SA, Hochholzer L. Pulmonary hyalinizing granuloma. *Am J Clin Pathol* 1987;87:1–6.
31. Atagi S, Sakatani M, Akira M, et al. Pulmonary hyalinizing granuloma with Castleman's disease. *Ann Intern Med* 1994;33:689–91.
32. Drasin H, Blume MR, Rosenbaum EH, et al. Pulmonary hyalinizing granulomas in a patient with malignant lymphoma, with development nine years later of multiple myeloma and systemic amyloidosis. *Cancer* 1979;44:215–220.
33. Gorini M, Forloni F, Pezzoli A, et al. Pulmonary hyalinizing granuloma: a limited form of Wegener's granulomatosis? *Ann Ital Med Int* 1998;13:176–179.
34. Chalaoui J, Gregoire P, Sylvester J, et al. Pulmonary hyalinizing granuloma: a cause of pulmonary nodules. *Radiology* 1984;152:23–26.
35. Bahadori H, Liebow A. Plasma cell granulomas of the lung. *Cancer* 1973;31:191–208.
36. Spencer H. The pulmonary plasma cell/histiocytoma complex. *Histopathology* 1984;8:903–916.
37. Matsubara O, Tan LN, Kenney RM, et al. Inflammatory pseudotumors of the lung. Progression from organizing pneumonia to fibrous histiocytoma or to plasma cell granuloma in 32 cases. *Hum Pathol* 1988; 19:807–814.
38. Snyder CS, DellAquila M, Haghighi P, et al. Clonal changes in inflammatory pseudotumor of the lung: a case report. *Cancer* 1995;76: 1545–154.
39. Su LD, Atayde-Perez A, Sheldon S, et al. Inflammatory myofibroblastic tumor: cytogenetic evidence supporting clonal origin. *Mod Pathol* 1998;11:364–368.
40. Berardi R, Lee S, Chen H, et al. Inflammatory pseudotumors of the lung. *Surg Gynecol Obstet* 1983;156:89–96.
41. Pettinato G, Manivel J, De Rosa N, et al. Inflammatory myoblastic tumor (plasma cell granuloma): clinicopathologic study of 20 cases with immunohistochemical and ultrastructural observations. *Am J Clin Pathol* 1990;94:538–546.
42. Cerfolio RJ, Allen MS, Nascimento AG, et al. Inflammatory pseudotumors of the lung. *Ann Thorac Surg* 1999;67:933–936.
43. Koss MN. Unusual tumor-like conditions of the lung. *Adv Pathol Lab Med* 1994:7:123–150.
44. Tang TT, Segura AD, Oechler HW, et al. Inflammatory myofibrohistiocytic proliferation simulating sarcoma in children. *Cancer* 1990;65: 1626–1634.
45. Rohrlich P, Peuchmaur M, Cocci SN, et al. Interleukin-6 and interleukin-1β production in a pediatric plasma cell granuloma of the lung. *Am J Surg Pathol* 1995;19:590–595.
46. Agrons GA, Rosado-de-Christenson ML, Kirejczyk WM, et al. Pulmonary inflammatory pseudotumor: radiologic features. *Radiology* 1998;206:511–518.
47. Gal AA, Koss MN, McCarthy WF, et al. Prognostic factors in pulmonary fibrohistiocytic lesions. *Cancer* 1994;73:1817–1824.
48. Warter A, Satge D, Roeslin N. Angioinvasive plasma cell granulomas of the lung. *Cancer* 1987;59:435–443.

49. Koss MN, Hochholzer L, Moran CA, et al. Pulmonary plasmacytomas: a clinicopathologic and immunohistochemical study of five cases. *Ann Diagn Pathol* 1998;2:1–11.
50. Keller AR, Hochholzer L, Castleman B. Hyaline-vascular and plasma-cell types of giant lymph node hyperplasia of the mediastinum and other locations. *Cancer* 1972;29:670–683.
51. Frizzera G, Banks PM, Massarelli G, et al. A systemic lymphoproliferative disorder with morphologic features of Castleman's disease: pathologic findings in 15 patients. *Am J Surg Pathol* 1983;7:211–231.
52. Barrie JR, English JC, Müller N. Castleman's disease of the lung: radiographic, high-resolution CT, and pathologic findings. *Am J Roentgenol* 1996;166:1055–1056.
53. Johkoh T, Müller NL, Ichikado K, et al. Intrathoracic multicentric Castleman disease: CT findings in 12 patients. *Radiology* 1998;209: 477–481.
54. Hayashi M, Aoshiba K, Shimada M, et al. Kaposi's sarcoma-associated herpesvirus infection in the lung in multicentric Castleman's disease. *Intern Med* 1999;38:279–282.
55. Torii K, Ogawa Y, Kawabata Y, et al. Lymphoid interstitial pneumonia as a pulmonary lesion of idiopathic plasmacytic lymphadenopathy with hyperimmunoglobulinemia. *Ann Intern Med* 1994;33:237–241.
56. Yoshida M, Sakuma J, Hayashi S, et al. A histologically distinctive interstitial pneumonia induced by overexpression of the interleukin 6, transforming growth factor β-1, or platelet-derived growth factor B gene. *Proc Natl Acad Sci USA* 1995;10:9570–9574.
57. Hui AN, Koss MN, Hochholzer L, et al. Amyloidosis presenting in the lower respiratory tract: clinicopathologic, radiologic, immunohistochemical and histochemical studies on 48 cases. *Arch Pathol Lab Med* 1986;110:212–218.
58. Chen TKT. Amyloidosis presenting in the respiratory tract. *Pathol Annu* 1989;24:253–273.
59. Kobayashi H, Matsuoka R, Kitamura S, et al. Sjögren's syndrome with multiple bullae and pulmonary nodular amyloidosis. *Chest* 1988; 94:438–440.
60. Kradin R, Mark E. Benign lymphoid disorders of the lung, with a theory regarding their development. *Hum Pathol* 1983;14:857–867.
61. Davis CJ, Butchart EG, Gibbs AR. Nodular pulmonary amyloidosis occurring in association with pulmonary lymphoma. *Thorax* 1991;46: 217–218.
62. Laden SA, Cohen ML, Harley RA. Nodular pulmonary amyloidosis with extrapulmonary involvement. *Hum Pathol* 1984;15:594–597.
63. Halliday BE, Silverman JF, Finley JL. Fine-needle aspiration cytology of amyloid associated with nonneoplastic and malignant lesions. *Diagn Cytopathol* 1998;18:270–275.
64. Gallo GR, Feiner HD, Katz LA, et al. Nodular glomerulopathy associated with nonamyloidotic kappa light chain deposits and excess immunoglobulin light chain synthesis. *Am J Pathol* 1980;99:621–644.
65. Ganeval D, Noel LH, Preud'homme JL, et al. Light chain deposition disease: its relation with AL-type amyloidosis. *Kidney Int* 1984;26: 1–9.
66. Preud'homme JL, Morel-Maroger L, Brouet JC, et al. Synthesis of abnormal immunoglobulins in lymphoplasmacytic disorders with visceral light chain deposition. *Am J Med* 1980;69:703–710.
67. Gallo G, Goni F, Boctor F, et al. Light chain cardiomyopathy. Structural analysis of the light chain tissue deposits. *Am J Pathol* 1996; 148:1397–1406.
68. Kijner CH, Yousem SA. Systemic light chain deposition disease presenting as multiple pulmonary nodules. A case report and review of the literature. *Am J Surg Pathol* 1988;12:405–413.
69. Linder J, Crocker BP, Vollmer RT, Shelburne J. Systemic kappa light-chain deposition. An ultrastructural and immunohistochemical study. *Am J Surg Pathol* 1983;7:85–93.
70. Randall RE, Williamson WCJ, Mullinax F, et al. Manifestations of systemic light chain deposition. *Am J Med* 1976;60:293–299.
71. Ganeval D, Noel LH, Droz D, et al. Systemic lambda light chain deposition in a patient with myeloma. *Br Med J* 1981;282:681–683.
72. Piard F, Yaziji N, Jarry O, et al. Solitary plasmacytoma of the lung with light chain extracellular deposits: a case report and review of the literature. *Histopathology* 1998;32:356–361.
73. Morinaga S, Watanabe H, Gemma A, et al. Plasmacytoma of the lung associated with nodular deposits of immunoglobulin. *Am J Surg Pathol* 1987;11:989–995.
74. Stokes MB, Jagirdar J, Burchstin O, et al. Nodular pulmonary immunoglobulin light chain deposits with coexistent amyloid and nonamyloid features in an HIV-infected patient. *Mod Pathol* 1997;10: 1059–1065.
75. Salzstein SL. Pulmonary malignant lymphomas and pseudolymphomas: classification, therapy and prognosis. *Cancer* 1963;16: 928–955.
76. Herbert A, Wright DH, Isaacson PG, Smith JL. Primary malignant lymphoma of the lung. *Hum Pathol* 1984;15:415–422.
77. Salzstein SL. Extranodal malignant lymphomas and pseudolymphomas. *Pathol Annu* 1969;4:159–184.
78. Fisher C, Grubb C, Kenning B, et al. Pseudolymphoma of the lung: a rare cause of a solitary nodule. A case report and review of the literature. *J Thorac Cardiovasc* 1980;11–16.
79. Greenberg SD, Heisler JG, Gyorkey F, et al. Pulmonary lymphoma vs. pseudolymphoma: a perplexing problem. *South Med J* 1972;65: 775–784.
80. McNamara JJ, Kingsley WB, Paulson DB, et al. Primary lymphosarcoma of the lung. *Ann Surg* 1969;169:133–140.
81. Reich NE, McCormack LJ, Van Ordstrand HS. Pseudolymphoma of the lung. *Chest* 1974;65:424–427.
82. Abbondanzo SL, Rush W, Bijwaard KE, et al. Nodular lymphoid hyperplasia of the lung: a clinicopathologic study of 14 cases. *Am J Surg Pathol* 2000:24:587–597.
83. Yum MN, Ziegler JR, Walker PD, et al. Pseudolymphoma of the lung in a patient with systemic lupus erythematosus. *Am J Med* 1979;66: 172–176.
84. Bragg DG, Chor PJ, Murray KA, et al. Lymphoproliferative disorders of the lung: histopathology, clinical manifestations, and imaging features. *Am J Roentgenol* 1994:163:273–281.
85. Isaacson PG, Wright DH. Extranodal malignant lymphoma arising from mucosa associated lymphoid tissue. *Cancer* 1984;53: 2515–2524.
86. Isaacson PG, Spencer J. Malignant lymphoma of mucosa-associated lymphoid tissue. *Histopathology* 1987;11:445–462.
87. Marchevsky A, Padilla M, Kaneko M, et al. Localized lymphoid nodules of the lung: a reappraisal of the lymphoma versus pseudolymphoma dilemma. *Cancer* 1983;51:2070–2077.
88. Yousem SA, Colby TV, Carrington CB. Follicular bronchitis/bronchiolitis. *Hum Pathol* 1985;16:70–706.
89. Yousem SA, Colby TV, Carrington CB. Lung biopsy in rheumatoid arthritis. *Am Rev Respir Dis* 1985;131:770–777.
90. Howling SJ, Hansell DM, Wells AU, et al. Follicular bronchiolitis: thin-section CT and histologic findings. *Radiology* 1999;212: 637–642.
91. Liebow AA, Carrington CB. Diffuse pulmonary lymphoreticular infiltrates associated with dysproteinemia. *Med Clin North Am* 1973;57: 809–843.
92. Herbert A, Walters MT, Cawley MI, et al. Lymphocytic interstitial pneumonia identified as lymphoma of mucosa associated lymphoid tissue. *J Pathol* 1985;146:129–138.
93. Kurosu K, Yumoto N, Furukawa M, et al. Third complementarity-determining-region sequence analysis of lymphocytic interstitial pneumonia: most cases demonstrate a minor monoclonal population hidden among normal lymphocyte clones. *Am J Respir Crit Care Med* 1997;155:1453–1460.
94. Kawabuchi B, Tsuchiya S, Nakagawa K, et al. Immunophenotypic and molecular analysis of a case of lymphocytic interstitial pneumonia. *Acta Pathol Jpn* 1993;43:260–264.
95. Strimlan CV, Rosenow EC, Divertie MB, et al. Pulmonary manifestations of Sjögren's syndrome. *Chest* 1976;70:354–361.
96. Schwartz MI. Lymphoplasmacytic interstitial pneumonias. In: Schwarz MI, King TJ, eds. *Interstitial lung disease*. St. Louis: Mosby–Year Book, 1992:405–412.
97. O'Brodovich HM, Moser MM, Lu L. Familial lymphoid interstitial pneumonia: a long term follow-up. *Pediatrics* 1980;65:523–528.
98. Church JA, Hart I, Saxon A, et al. Lymphoid interstitial pneumonitis and hypogammaglobulinemia in children. *Am Rev Respir Dis* 1981; 124:491–496.
99. Johkoh T, Müller NL, Pickford HA, et al. Lymphocytic interstitial pneumonia: Thin-section findings in 22 patients. *Radiology* 1999;212: 567–572.
100. Greenberg SD, Haley MD, Jendkins DE, et al. Lymphoplasmacytic pneumonia with accompanying dysproteinemia. *Arch Pathol* 1973; 96:73–80.
101. Moran TJ, Totten RS. Lymphoid interstitial pneumonia with dyspro-

teinemia; report of two cases with plasma cell predominance. *Am J Clin Pathol* 1970;54:747–756.
102. Fishback N, Koss M. Update on lymphoid interstitial pneumonitis. *Curr Opin Pulmonol Med* 1996;2:429–433.
103. Kradin RL, Young RH, Kradin LA, Mark EJ. Immunoblastic lymphoma arising in chronic lymphoid hyperplasia of the pulmonary interstitium. *Cancer* 1982;50:1339–1343.
104. Schuurman HJ, Gooszen HCH, Tan IWN, et al. Low-grade lymphoma of immature T-cell phenotype in a case of lymphocytic interstitial pneumonia and Sjögren's syndrome. *Histopathology* 1987;11: 1193–1204.
105. Joshi VV. Pathology of childhood AIDS. *Pedriatr Clin North Am* 1991;38:97–120.
106. Joshi VV, Gagnon GA, Chadwick EG, et al. The spectrum of mucosa-associated lymphoid tissue lesions in pediatric patients infected with HIV: a clinicopathologic study of six cases. *Am J Clin Pathol* 1997; 107:592–600.
107. Teruya-Feldstein J, Temeck BK, Sloas MM, et al. Pulmonary malignant lymphoma of mucosa-associated lymphoid tissue (MALT) arising in a pediatric HIV-positive patient. *Am J Surg Pathol* 1995;19: 357–363.
108. Joshi VV, Oleske JM, Minnefor AB, et al. Pathologic pulmonary findings in children with the acquired immunodeficiency syndrome. *Hum Pathol* 1985;16:241–246.
109. Klassen MK, Lewin-Smith M, Frankel SS, et al. Pathology of human immunodeficiency virus infection: noninfectious conditions. *Ann Diagn Pathol* 1997;1:57–64.
110. Centers for Disease Control and Prevention (CDC). 1994 Revised classification system for Human Immunodeficiency Virus infection in children less than 13 years of age. *Morb Mortal Wkly Rep* 1994; 43:1–10.
111. Scott GB, Hutto C, Makuch RW, et al. Survival in children with perinatally acquired immunodeficiency virus type 1 infection. *N Engl J Med* 1989;321:1791–1796.
112. Moran CA, Suster S, Pavlova Z, et al. The spectrum of pathological changes in the lung of children with the acquired immunodeficiency syndrome: an autopsy study of 36 cases. *Hum Pathol* 1994;25: 877–882.
113. Waters KA, Bale P, Isaacs D, et al. Successful chloroquine therapy in a child with lymphoid interstitial pneumonitis. *J Pediatr* 1991;119: 989–991.
114. Saldana MJ, Mones JM. Lymphoid interstitial pneumonia in HIV infected individuals. *Prog Surg Pathol* 1992;12:181–215.
115. Wallace JM, Barbers RG, Oishi JS, et al. Cellular and T-lymphocyte subpopulation profiles in bronchoalveolar lavage fluid from patients with acquired immunodeficiency syndrome and pneumonitis. *Am Rev Respir Dis* 1984;130:768–790.
116. Saldana MJ, Mones JM. Pulmonary pathology in AIDS; atypical *Pneumocystis carinii* infection and lymphoid interstitial pneumonia. *Thorax* 1994;49:S46–S55.
117. Travis WD, Fox CH, Devaney KO, et al. Lymphoid pneumonitis in 50 adult patients infected with the human immunodeficiency virus: lymphocytic interstitial pneumonitis versus nonspecific interstitial pneumonitis. *Hum Pathol* 1992;23:529–541.
118. Anderson VM, Lee H. Lymphocytic interstitial pneumonitis in pediatric AIDS. *Pediatr Pathol* 1988;8:417–421.
119. Itescu S, Brancato LJ, Buxbaum J, et al. A diffuse infiltrative CD8 lymphocytosis syndrome in human immunodeficiency virus (HIV) infection: a host immune response associated with HLA-DR5. *Ann Intern Med* 1990;112:3–10.
120. Kornstein MJ, Pietra GG, Hoxie JA, et al. The pathology and treatment of interstitial pneumonitis in two infants with AIDS. *Am Rev Respir Dis* 1986;133:1196–1198.
121. Morris JC, Rosen MJ, Marchevesky A, et al. Lymphocytic interstitial pneumonia in patients at risk for the acquired immune deficiency syndrome. *Chest* 1987;91:63–67.
122. Malamou-Mitsi V, Tsai MM, Gal AA, et al. Lymphoid interstitial pneumonia not associated with HIV infection: role of Epstein-Barr virus. *Mod Pathol* 1992;5:487–491.
123. Barbera JA, Hayashi S, Hegele RG, et al. Detection of Epstein-Barr virus in lymphocytic interstitial pneumonia by in situ hybridization. *Am Rev Respir Dis* 1992;145:940–946.
124. Kann PM, Hegele RG, Hayashi S, et al. Expression of bcl-2 and Epstein-Barr virus LMP1 in lymphocytic interstitial pneumonia. *Thorax* 1997;52:12–16.
125. Brodie SJ, de la Rosa C, Howe JG, et al. Pediatric AIDS-associated lymphocytic interstitial pneumonia and pulmonary arterio-occlusive disease: role of VCAM-1/VLA-4 adhesion pathway and human herpesviruses. *Am J Pathol* 1999;154:1453–1464.
126. Fitzpatrick EA, Avdiushko M, Kaplan AM, et al. Role of virus replication in a murine model of AIDS-associated interstitial pneumonitis. *Exp Lung Res* 1999;25:647–461.
127. Couderc LJ, Brun-Vezinet F, Rey MA, et al. Lymphoid interstitial pneumonitis and infection with human immunodeficiency virus type 2 [Letter]. *Chest* 1991;99:1320.
128. Kawakami K, Miyazato A, Iwakura Y, et al. Induction of lymphocytic inflammatory changes in lung interstitium by human T lymphotropic virus type I. *Am J Respir Crit Care Med* 1999;160:995–1000.
129. Kompoliti A, Gage B, Sharma L, et al. Human T-cell lymphotropic virus type 1–associated myelopathy, Sjögren syndrome, and lymphocytic pneumonitis. *Arch Neurol* 1996;53:940–942.
130. Setoguchi Y, Takahashi S, Kira S. Detection of human T-cell lymphotropic virus type I-related antibodies in patients with lymphocytic interstitial pneumonia. *Am Rev Respir Dis* 1991;144:1361–1365.
131. Miller DL, Allen MS. Rare pulmonary neoplasms. *Mayo Clin Proc* 1993;68:492–498.
132. Colby TV, Yousem SA. Pulmonary lymphoid neoplasms. *Semin Diagn Pathol* 1985;2:183–196.
133. Harris NL, Jaffe ES, Stein H, et al. A revised European-American classification of lymphoid neoplasms: a proposal from the international lymphoma study group. *Blood* 1994;84:1361–1392.
134. Fiche M, Capron F, Berger F, et al. Primary pulmonary non-Hodgkin's lymphomas. *Histopathology* 1995;26:529–537.
135. Kurosu K, Yumoto N, Furukawa M, et al. Low-grade pulmonary mucosa-associated lymphoid tissue lymphoma with or without intraclonal variation. *Am J Respir Crit Care Med* 1998;158:1613–1619.
136. Cordier JF, Chailleux E, Lauque D, et al. Primary pulmonary lymphomas: a clinical study of 70 cases in nonimmunocompromised patients. *Chest* 1993;103:201–208.
137. Hansen LA, Prakash UBS, Colby TV. Pulmonary lymphoma in Sjögren's syndrome. *Mayo Clin Proc* 1989;64:920–931.
138. O'Donnell PG, Jackson SA, Tung KT, et al. Radiological appearances of lymphomas arising from mucosa-associated lymphoid tissue (MALT) in the lung. *Clin Radiol* 1998;53:258–263.
139. Knisely BL, Mastey LA, Mergo PJ, et al. Pulmonary mucosa-associated lymphoid tissue lymphoma: CT and pathologic findings. *Am J Roentgenol* 1999;172:1321–1326.
140. Elenitoba-Johnson KE, Medeiros LJ, Khorsand J, et al. Lymphoma of the mucosa-associated lymphoid tissue of the lung: a multifocal case of common clonal origin. *Am J Clin Pathol* 1995;103:341–345.
141. Isaacson PG, Norton AJ. Mucosa-associated lymphoid tissue (MALT) and the MALT lymphoma concept. In: *Extranodal lymphomas.* Edinburgh: Churchill Livingstone, 1994:5–14.
142. Harris NL. Low-grade B-cell lymphoma of mucosa-associated lymphoid tissue and monocytoid B-cell lymphoma: related entities that are distinct from other low-grade B-cell lymphomas. *Arch Pathol Lab Med* 1993:117:771–775.
143. Guccion JG, Rohatgi PK, Patterson RH, et al. Giant lamellar bodies in a pulmonary MALT lymphoma: a case report with ultrastructural and immunohistochemical studies. *Ultrastruct Pathol* 1998;22: 101–107.
144. Hirokawa M, Kanahara T, Ariyasu S, et al. Giant lamellar bodies in pulmonary MALT lymphoma: a case report. *Acta Cytol* 1999;43: 1159–1162.
145. Tashiro K, Ohshima K, Suzumiya J, et al. Clonality of primary pulmonary lymphoproliferative disorders: using in situ hybridization and polymerase chain reaction for immunoglobulin. *Leuk Lymphoma* 1999;36:157–167.
146. Zukerberg LR, Medeiros LJ, Ferry JA, et al. Diffuse low-grade B-cell lymphomas: four clinically distinct subtypes defined by a combination of morphologic and immunophenotypic features. *Am J Clin Pathol* 1993;100:373–385.
147. Ferry JA, Yang WI, Zukerberg LR, et al. $CD5^+$ extranodal marginal zone B-cell (MALT) lymphoma: a low grade neoplasm with a propensity for bone marrow involvement and relapse. *Am J Clin Pathol* 1996;105:31–37.
148. Wotherspoon AC, Pan L, Diss TC, et al. A genotypic study of low

grade B-cell lymphomas, including lymphomas of mucosa associated lymphoid tissue (MALT). *J Pathol* 1990;162:135–140.
149. Finn T, Isaacson P, Wotherspoon AC. Numerical abnormality of chromosomes 3, 7, 12, and 18 in low grade lymphomas of MALT-type and splenic marginal zone lymphomas detected by interphase cytogenetics on paraffin embedded tissue. *J Pathol* 1993;170:335a.
150. Wotherspoon AC, Pan L, Diss TC, et al. Cytogenetic study of B-cell lymphoma of mucosa-associated lymphoid tissue. *Cancer Genet Cytogenet* 1992;58:35–38.
151. Wotherspoon AC, Soosay GN, Diss TC, et al. Low-grade primary B-cell lymphoma of the lung: an immunohistochemical, molecular and cytogenetic study of a single case. *Am J Clin Pathol* 1990;94:655–660.
152. Harris NL, Isaacson PG. What are the criteria for distinguishing MALT from non-MALT lymphoma at extranodal sites? *Am J Clin Pathol* 1999;111:S126–S132.
153. L'Hoste RJ, Filippa DA, Lieberman PH, et al. Primary pulmonary lymphomas: a clinicopathologic analysis of 36 cases. *Cancer* 1984; 54:1397–1406.
154. Philippe B, Delfau-Larue MH, Epardeau B, et al. B-cell pulmonary lymphoma: gene rearrangement analysis of bronchoalveolar lymphocytes by polymerase chain reaction. *Chest* 1999;115:1242–1247.
155. Toh HC, Ang PT. Primary pulmonary lymphoma—clinical review from a single institution in Singapore. *Leuk Lymphoma* 1997;27: 153–163.
156. Weiss LM, Yousem SA, Warnke RA. Non-Hodgkin's lymphoma of the lung: a study of 19 cases emphasizing the utility of frozen section immunologic studies in differential diagnosis. *Am J Surg Pathol* 1985; 9:480–490.
157. Prasad ML, Charney DA, Sarlin J, et al. Pulmonary immunocytoma with massive crystal storing histiocytosis: a case report with review of literature. *Am J Surg Pathol* 1998;22:1148–1153.
158. Rush WL, Andriko JAW, Taubenberger JK, et al. Primary anaplastic large cell lymphoma (ALCL) of the lung: a clinicopathologic study of 5 cases. *Mod Pathol* (in press).
159. Eisner MD, Kaplan LD, Herndier B, et al. The pulmonary manifestations of AIDS-related non-Hodgkin's lymphoma. *Chest* 1996;110: 729–736.
160. Katano H, Suda T, Morishita Y, et al. Human herpesvirus 8–associated solid lymphomas that occur in AIDS patients take anaplastic large cell morphology. *Mod Pathol* 2000;13:77–85.
161. Ray P, Antoine M, Mary-Krause M, et al. AIDS-related primary pulmonary lymphoma. *Am J Respir Crit Care Med* 1998;158:1221–1229.
162. Kohler CA, Rowley P, Malamud F, et al. Primary pulmonary T-cell lymphoma associated with AIDS: the syndrome of the indolent pulmonary mass lesion. *Am J Med* 1995;99:324–326.
163. Chechani V, Allam AA, Kamholz SL. Pulmonary non-Hodgkin's lymphoma mimicking infection. *Respir Med* 1990;84:401–405.
164. Close PM, Macrae MB, Hammond JM, et al. Anaplastic large-cell Ki-1 lymphoma: pulmonary presentation mimicking miliary tuberculosis. *Am J Clin Pathol* 1993;99:631–636.
165. Colby TV, Carrington CB. Malignant lymphoma simulating lymphomatoid granulomatosis. *Am J Surg Pathol* 1982;6:19–32.
166. Colby TV, Carrington CB. Lymphoreticular tumors and infiltrates of the lung. *Pathol Annu* 1983;18:27–70.
167. Nandedkar MA, Palazzo J, Abbondanzo SL, et al. CD45 (leukocyte common antigen) immunoreactivity in metastatic undifferentiated and neuroendocrine carcinoma: a potential diagnostic pitfall. *Mod Pathol* 1998;11:1204–1210.
168. Lynch JW. AIDS-related non-Hodgkin's lymphoma: useful techniques for diagnosis. *Chest* 1996;110:585–586.
169. Liebow AA, Carrington CRB, Friedman PJ. Lymphomatoid granulomatosis. *Hum Pathol* 1972;3:457–558.
170. Bender BL, Jaffe R. Immunoglobulin production in lymphomatoid granulomatosis and relation to other "benign" lymphoproliferative disorders. *Am J Clin Pathol* 1980;73:41–47.
171. Nichols PW, Koss M, Levine AM, et al. Lymphomatoid granulomatosis: a T-cell disorder? *Am J Med* 1982;72:467–471.
172. Lipford EH, Margolick JB, Longo DL, et al. Angiocentric immunoproliferative lesions: a clinicopathologic spectrum of post-thymic T-cell proliferations. *Blood* 1988;72:1674–1681.
173. Jaffe ES, Lipford EH, Margolick JB, et al. Lymphomatoid granulomatosis and angiocentric lymphoma: a spectrum of post-thymic T-cell proliferations. *Semin Respir Med* 1989;10:167–172.
174. Pisani RJ, DeRemee RA. Clinical implications of the histopathologic diagnoses of pulmonary lymphomatoid granulomatosis. *Mayo Clin Proc* 1990;65:151–163.
175. Guinee DG Jr, Jaffe E, Kingman D, et al. Pulmonary lymphomatoid granulomatosis: evidence for a proliferation of Epstein-Barr virus infected B-lymphocytes with a prominent T-cell component and vasculitis. *Am J Surg Pathol* 1994;18:753–764.
176. Jaffe ES, Wilson WH. Lymphomatoid granulomatosis: Pathogenesis, pathology and clinical implications. *Cancer Surv* 1997;30:233–248.
177. Myers JL, Kurtin PJ, Katzenstein ALA, et al. Lymphomatoid granulomatosis: evidence of immunophenotypic diversity and relationship to Epstein-Barr virus infection. *Am J Surg Pathol* 1995;19:1300–1312.
178. Nicholson AG, Wotherspoon AC, Diss TC, et al. Lymphomatoid granulomatosis: evidence that some cases represent Epstein-Barr virus-associated B-cell lymphoma. *Histopathology* 1996:29:317–324.
179. McNiff JM, Cooper D, Howe G, et al. Lymphomatoid granulomatosis of the skin and lung: an angiocentric T-cell–rich B-cell lymphoproliferative disorder. *Arch Dermatol* 1996;132:1464–1470.
180. Wilson WH, Kingma DW, Raffeld M, et al. Association of lymphomatoid granulomatosis with Epstein-Barr viral infection of B lymphocytes and response to interferon α2b. *Blood* 1996;87:4531–4537.
181. Karnak I, Ciftci AO, Talim B, et al. Pulmonary lymphomatoid granulomatosis in a 4 year old. *J Pediatr Surg* 1999;1033–1035.
182. Katzenstein AL, Carrington CB, Liebow AA. Lymphomatoid granulomatosis: a clinicopathologic study of 152 cases. *Cancer* 1979;43: 360–373.
183. Koss MN, Hochholzer L, Langloss JM, et al. Lymphomatoid granulomatosis: a clinicopathologic study of 42 cases. *Pathology* 1986;18: 283–288.
184. Ilowite NT, Fligner CL, Ochs HD, et al. Pulmonary angiitis with atypical lymphoreticular infiltrates in Wiskott-Aldrich syndrome: possible relationship of lymphomatoid granulomatosis and EBV infection. *Clin Immunol Immunopathol* 1986;41:479–484.
185. Haque AK, Myers JL, Hudnall SD, et al. Pulmonary lymphomatoid granulomatosis in acquired immunodeficiency syndrome: lesions with Epstein-Barr virus infection. *Mod Pathol* 1998;11:347–356.
186. Michaud J, Banerjee D, Kaufmann J. Lymphomatoid granulomatosis involving the central nervous system: complication of a renal transplant with terminal monoclonal B-cell proliferation. *Acta Neuropathol* 1983;61:141–147.
187. Troussard X, Galateau F, Gaulard P, et al. Lymphomatoid granulomatosis in a patient with acute myeloblastic leukemia in remission. *Cancer* 1990;65:107–111.
188. Parkhurst JB, Kuhls TL, Elrod JP, et al. Lymphomatoid granulomatosis in a child with familial chronic active Epstein-Barr virus infection. *Int J Pediatr Haematol Oncol* 1994;1:299–304.
189. Veltri RW, Raich PC, McClung JE, et al. Lymphomatoid granulomatosis and Epstein-Barr virus. *Cancer* 1982;50:1513–1517.
190. Guinee DG Jr, Perkins SL, Travis WD, et al. Proliferation and cellular phenotype in lymphomatoid granulomatosis: implications of a higher proliferation index in B cells. *Am J Surg Pathol* 1998;22:1093–1100.
191. Katzenstein ALA, Peiper SC. Detection of Epstein-Barr virus genomes in lymphomatoid granulomatosis: analysis of 29 cases by the polymerase chain reaction technique. *Mod Pathol* 1990;3:435–441.
192. Israel HI, Patchefsky AS, Saldana MJ. Wegener's granulomatosis, lymphomatoid granulomatosis and benign lymphocytic angiitis and granulomatosis of lung: recognition and treatment. *Ann Intern Med* 1977;87:691–699.
193. Saldana MJ, Patchefsky AS, Israel HI, et al. Pulmonary angiitis and granulomatosis: the relationship between histologic features, organ involvement, and response to treatment. *Hum Pathol* 1977;8:391–409.
194. Teruya-Feldstein J, Jaffe ES, Burd PR, et al. The role of Mig, the monokine induced by interferon γ, and IP-10, the interferon γ-inducible protein 10, in tissue necrosis and vascular damage associated with Epstein-Barr virus–positive lymphoproliferative disease. *Blood* 1997; 10:4099–4105.
195. Taniere P, Thivolet-Bejui F, Vitrey D, et al. Lymphomatoid granulomatosis—a report on four cases: evidence for B phenotype of the tumoral cells. *Eur Respir J* 1998;12:102–106.
196. Chang C, Guinee D, Koss MN, et al. The immunohistochemical profile of neoplastic B-cells and background T cells in pulmonary lymphomatoid granulomatosis is similar to that of T-cell rich B-cell lymphoma. *Mod Pathol* 2000;1:145a(abst).
197. Khoor A, Kurtin PJ, AL Katzenstein, et al. Pulmonary post-transplant lymphoproliferative disorders (PTLD) and lymphomatoid granuloma-

tosis (LYG): histologically and immunophenotypically overlapping entities. *Mod Pathol* 1997;10:166a(abst).
198. Chadburn A, Cesarman E, Liu YF, et al. Molecular genetic analysis demonstrates that multiple posttransplantation lymphoproliferative disorders occurring in one anatomic site in a single patient represent distinct primary lymphoid neoplasms. *Cancer* 1995;75:2747–2756.
199. Knowles DM, Cesarman E, Chadburn A, et al. Correlative morphologic and molecular genetic analysis demonstrates three distinct categories of posttransplant lymphoproliferative disorders. *Blood* 1995; 85:552–565.
200. Reisman RP, Greco MA. Virus-associated hemophagocytic syndrome due to Epstein-Barr virus. *Hum Pathol* 1984;15:290–293.
201. Raez LE, Temple JD, Saldana M. Successful treatment of lymphomatoid granulomatosis using cyclosporin-A after failure of intensive chemotherapy. *Am J Hematol* 1996;53:192–195.
202. DiGiuseppe JA, Nelson WG, Seifter EJ, et al. Intravascular lymphomatosis: a clinicopathologic study of 10 cases and assessment of response to chemotherapy. *J Clin Oncol* 1994;12:2573–2579.
203. Yousem SA, Colby TV. Intravascular lymphomatosis presenting in the lung. *Cancer* 1990;65:349–353.
204. Ko YH, Han JH, Go JH, et al. Intravascular lymphomatosis: a clinicopathological study of two cases presenting as an interstitial lung disease. *Histopathology* 1997;31:555–562.
205. Gabor EP, Sherwood T, Mercola KE. Intravascular lymphomatosis presenting as adult respiratory distress syndrome. *Am J Hematol* 1997; 56:155–160.
206. Walls JG, Hong G, Cox JE, et al. Pulmonary intravascular lymphomatosis. Presentation with dyspnea and air trapping. *Chest* 1999;115: 1207–1210.
207. Takamura K, Nasuhara Y, Mishina T, et al. Intravascular lymphomatosis diagnosed by transbronchial lung biopsy. *Eur Respir J* 1997; 10:955–957.
208. Ferry JA, Harris NL, Picker LJ, et al. Intravascular lymphomatosis (malignant angioendotheliomatosis): a B-cell neoplasm expressing surface homing receptors. *Mod Pathol* 1988;1:444–452.
209. Ip M, Chan KW, Chan IK. Systemic inflammatory response syndrome in intravascular lymphomatosis. *Intensive Care Med* 1997;23: 783–786.
210. Au WY, Shek WH, Nicholls J, et al. T-cell intravascular lymphomatosis: association with Epstein-Barr virus infection. *Histopathology* 1997;31:563–567.
211. Hsiao CH, Su IJ, Hsieh SF, et al. Epstein-Barr virus-associated intravascular lymphomatosis within Kaposi's sarcoma in an AIDS patient. *Am J Surg Pathol* 1999;23:482–487.
212. Ponzoni M, Arrigoni G, Gould V, et al. Lack of CD29 (β_1 integrin) and CD54 (ICAM-1) adhesion molecules in intravascular lymphomatosis. *Hum Pathol* 2000;31:220–226.
213. Domizio P, Hall PA, Cotter F, et al. Angiotropic large cell lymphoma (ALCL): morphological, immunohistochemical and genotypic studies with analysis of previous reports. *Hematol Oncol* 1989;7:195–206.
214. Colby TV, Hoppe RT, Warnke RA. Hodgkin's disease: a clinicopathologic study of 659 cases. *Cancer* 1981;48:1848–1858.
215. Colby TV, Hoppe RT, Warnke RA. Hodgkin's disease at autopsy, 1972–1977. *Cancer* 1981;47:1852–1862.
216. Yousem SA, Weiss LM, Colby TV. Primary pulmonary Hodgkin's disease: a clinicopathologic study of 15 cases. *Cancer* 1986;57: 1217–1224.
217. Radin AI. Primary pulmonary Hodgkin's disease. *Cancer* 1990;65: 550–563.
218. Chetty R, Slavin JL, O'Leary JJ, et al. Primary Hodgkin's disease of the lung. *Pathology* 1995;27:111–114.
219. Pik A, Cohen N, Weissgarten J, et al. Primary pulmonary Hodgkin's disease with air bronchogram. *Respiration* 1986;50:226–229.
220. Cartier Y, Johkoh T, Honda O, et al. Primary pulmonary Hodgkin's disease: CT findings in three patients. *Clin Radiol* 1998;54:182–184.
221. Harris NL. Hodgkin's disease: classification and differential diagnosis. *Mod Pathol* 1999;12:159–176.
222. Risdall R, Hoppe RT, Warnke R. Non-Hodgkin's lymphoma: a study of the evolution of the disease based upon 92 autopsied cases. *Cancer* 1979;44:529–544.
223. Hardy K, Nicholson DP, Schaefer RF, et al. Bilateral endobronchial non-Hodgkin's lymphoma. *South Med J* 1995;88;367–370.
224. Wolfe JD, Trevor ED, Kjeldsberg CR. Pulmonary manifestations of mycosis fungoides. *Cancer* 1980;46:2648–2653.
225. Rubin DL, Blank N. Rapid pulmonary dissemination in mycosis fungoides simulating pneumonia: a case report and review of the literature. *Cancer* 1985;56:649–651.
226. Miller KS, Sahn SA. Mycosis fungoides presenting as ARDS and diagnosed by bronchoalveolar lavage: radiographic and pathologic pulmonary manifestations. *Chest* 1986;89:312–314.
227. Kitching PA, Gibbs AR. Pulmonary involvement by mycosis fungoides: a case showing angiocentric lesions and granulomas. *Pathol Res Pract* 1993;189:594–596.
228. Frizzera G, Moran E, Rappaport H. Angio-immunoblastic lymphadenopathy with dysproteinemia. *Lancet* 1974;1:1070–1073.
229. Iseman MD, Schwarz MI, Stanford RE. Interstitial pneumonia in angioimmunoblastic lymphadenopathy with dysproteinemia. *Ann Intern Med* 1976;85:752–755.
230. Starke ID, Elkon KB, Hermer CL, et al. Pulmonary involvement in angioimmunoblastic lymphadenopathy following autoimmune disease. *Respiration* 1983;44:136–142.
231. Klatte EC, Yardley J, Smith ED, Rohn R, Campbell JA. The pulmonary manifestations and complications of leukemia. *Am J Roentgenol* 1963;89:598–609.
232. Hildebrand FL Jr, Rosenow ED, Habermann TM, et al. Pulmonary complications of leukemia. *Chest* 1990;98:1233–1239.
233. Tenholder MF, Hooper RG. Pulmonary infiltrates in leukemia. *Chest* 1980;78:468–473.
234. Rosenow EC, Wilson WR, Cockerill FR. Pulmonary disease in the immunocompromised host. *Mayo Clin Proc* 1985;60:473–487.
235. Yoshioka R, Yamaguchi K, Ysohinaga T, et al. Pulmonary complications in patients with adult T-cell leukemia. *Cancer* 1985;55: 2491–2494.
236. Vaiman E, Odeh M, Attais D, et al. T-cell chronic lymphocytic leukaemia with pulmonary involvement and relapsing BOOP. *Eur Respir J* 1999;14:471–474.
237. Doran HM, Sheppard MN, Collins PW, et al. Pathology of the lung in leukaemia and lymphoma: a study of 87 autopsies. *Histopathology* 1991;18:211–219.
238. Callahan M, Wall S, Askin F, et al. Granulocytic sarcoma presenting as pulmonary nodules and lymphadenopathy. *Cancer* 1987;60: 1902–1904.
239. Snyder LS, Cherwitz DL, Dykoski RK, et al. Endobronchial Richter's syndrome: a rare manifestation of chronic lymphocytic leukemia. *Am Rev Respir Dis* 1988;138:980–983.
240. Palosaari D, Colby TV. Bronchiolocentric chronic lymphocytic leukemia. *Cancer* 1986;58:1695–1698.
241. Beckman EN, Oehrle JS. Fibrous hematopoietic tumors arising in angiogenic myeloid metaplasia. *Hum Pathol* 1982;13:804–810.
242. Asakura S, Colby TV. Two cases of agnogenic myeloid metaplasia with extramedullary hematopoiesis and fibrosis in the lung. *Chest* 1994;105:1866–1668.
243. Lester RJ, Johnson JW, Cuttner J. Pulmonary leukostasis is the single worst prognostic factor in patients with acute myelocytic leukemia and hyperleukocytosis. *Am J Med* 1985;79:43–48.
244. van Buchem MA, Levelt CN, Hogendoorn PC, et al. Involvement of the complement systemic in the pathogenesis of pulmonary leukostasis in experimental myelocytic leukemia. *Leukemia* 1993;10: 1608–1614.
245. Myers TJ, Solon RC, Klatsky AU, et al. Respiratory failure due to pulmonary leukostasis following chemotherapy of acute nonlymphocytic leukemia. *Cancer* 1983;51:1808–1813.
246. Cordonnier C, Fleury-Feith J, Escudier E, et al. Secondary alveolar proteinosis is a reversible cause of respiratory failure in leukemic patients. *Am J Respir Crit Care Med* 1994;149:788–794.
247. Wang J, Pandha HS, Treleaven J, et al. Metastatic extramedullary plasmacytoma of the lung. *Leuk Lymphoma* 1999;35:423–425.
248. Joseph G, Pandit M, Korfhage L. Primary pulmonary plasmacytoma. *Cancer* 1993;71:721–724.
249. Husain M, Nguyen G-K. Primary pulmonary plasmacytoma diagnosed by transthoracic needle aspiration cytology and immunocytochemistry. *Acta Cytol* 1996;40:622–624.
250. Amin R. Extramedullary plasmacytoma of the lung. *Cancer* 1985;56: 15–156.
251. Wile A, Olinger G, Peter JB, et al. Solitary intraparenchymal pulmonary plasmacytoma associated with production of an M-protein: report of a case. *Cancer* 1976;37:2338–2342.

252. Kazzaz B, Dewar A, Corrin B. An unusual pulmonary plasmacytoma. *Histopathology* 1992;21:285–287.
253. Morinaga S, Watanabe H, Gemma A, et al. Plasmacytoma of the lung with nodular deposits of immunoglobulin. *Am J Surg Pathol* 1987; 11:989–995.
254. Hussong JW, Perkins SL, Schnitzer B, et al. Extramedullary plasmacytoma: a form of marginal zone cell lymphoma? *Am J Clin Pathol* 1999;111:11–116.
255. Garewal H, Durie BG. Aggressive phase of multiple myeloma with pulmonary plasma cell infiltrates. *JAMA* 1982;248:1875–1876.
256. Scully RE, Mark EJ, McNeely WF, et al. Case records of the Massachusetts General Hospital: weekly clinicopathologic exercises. Case 20-1987. *N Engl J Med* 1987;316:1259–1267.
257. Gilchrist D, Chan CK, LaRoye GJ, et al. Bronchial mucosal infiltration and unilateral lung collapse: an unusual complication of multiple myeloma. *Am J Med* 1988;85:740–741.
258. Weber CK, Friedrich JM, Merkle E, et al. Reversible metastatic pulmonary calcification in a patient with multiple myeloma. *Ann Hematol* 1996;72:329–332.
259. Chejfec G, Natarelli J, Gould VE. ''Myeloma lung''—a previously unreported complication of multiple myeloma. *Hum Pathol* 1983;14: 558–561.
260. Kelly C, Egan M, Rawlinson J. Whipple's disease presenting with lung involvement. *Thorax* 1996;51:343–344.
261. Lambert C, Gansler T, Mansour KA, et al. Pulmonary malakoplakia diagnosed by fine needle aspiration: case report. *Acta Cytol* 1997;41: 1833–1838.
262. Kwon KY, Colby TV. Rhodococcus equi pneumonia and pulmonary malakoplakia in acquired immunodeficiency syndrome: pathologic features. *Arch Pathol Lab Med* 1994;118:744–748.
263. Schneider EL, Epstein CJ, Kaback MJ, et al. Severe pulmonary involvement in adult Gaucher's disease: report of three cases and review of the literature. *Am J Med* 1977;63:475–480.
264. Zander DS, Mergo PJ, Foster RA, et al. Pulmonary parenchymal sinus histiocytosis with massive lymphadenopathy (Rosai-Dorfman disease): report of a case with immunohistochemical studies. *Mod Pathol* 1997;10:174a(abst).
265. Travis WD, Borok Z, Roum JH, et al. Pulmonary Langerhans cell granulomatosis (histiocytosis X): a clinicopathologic study of 48 cases. *Am J Surg Pathol* 1993;17:971–986.
266. Colby TV, Lombard C. Histiocytosis X in the lung. *Hum Pathol* 1983; 14:847–856.
267. Müller NL, Miller RR. Computed tomography of chronic diffuse infiltrative lung disease (parts I and II). *Am Rev Respir Dis* 1990; 1206–1215.
268. Emile JF, Wechsler J, Brousse N, et al. Langerhans' cell histiocytosis: definitive diagnosis with the use of monoclonal antibody O10 on routinely paraffin-embedded samples. *Am J Surg Pathol* 1995;19: 636–641.
269. Lu RC, Chu C, Buluwela L, et al. Clonal proliferation of Langerhans cells in Langerhans cell histiocytosis. *Lancet* 1994;343:767–768.
270. Cotter FE, Pritchard J. Clonality in Langerhans' cell histiocytosis [Editorial; see comments]. *BMJ* 1995;310:74–75.
271. Willman CL, Busque L, Griffith BB, et al. Langerhans'-cell histiocytosis (histiocytosis X)—a clonal proliferative disease [see comment]. *N Engl J Med* 1994;331:154–160.
272. Willman CL, McClain KL. An update on clonality, cytokines, and viral etiology in Langerhans cell histiocytosis. *Hematol Oncol Clin North Am* 1998;12:407–416.
273. Lieberman PH, Jones CR, Steinman RM, et al. Langerhans cell (eosinophilic) granulomatosis—a clinicopathologic study encompassing 50 years. *Am J Surg Pathol* 1996;20:519–552.
274. Etienne B, Bertocchi M, Gamondes JP, et al. Relapsing pulmonary Langerhans cell histiocytosis after lung transplantation. *Am J Respir Crit Care Med* 1998;157:288–291.
275. Veyssier-Belot C, Cacoub P, Caparros-Lefebvre D, et al. Erdheim-Chester disease. Clinical and radiologic characteristics of 59 cases. *Medicine (Baltimore)* 1996;75:157–169.
276. Devouassoux G, Lantuejoul S, Chatelain P, et al. Erdheim-Chester disease: a primary macrophage cell disorder. *Am J Respir Crit Care Med* 1998;157:650–653.
277. Egan AJM, Boardman LA, Tazelaar HD, et al. Erdheim-Chester disease: clinical, radiologic, and histopathologic findings in five patients with interstitial lung disease. *Am J Surg Pathol* 1999;23:17–26.
278. Rush WL, Andriko JAW, Galateau-Salle F, et al. Pulmonary pathology of Erdheim-Chester disease. *Mod Pathol* 2000;13:747–754.
279. Chetritt J, Paradis V, Dargere D, et al. Chester-Erdheim disease: a neoplastic disorder. *Hum Pathol* 1999;30:1093–1096.
280. Kambouchner M, Colby TV, Domenge C, et al. Erdheim-Chester disease with prominent pulmonary involvement associated with eosinophilic granuloma of mandibular bone. *Histopathology* 1997;30: 353–358.
281. Colby TV, Carrington CB, Mark GJ. Pulmonary involvement in malignant histiocytosis: a clinicopathologic spectrum. *Am J Surg Pathol* 1981;5:61–73.
282. Colby TV, Koss MN, Travis WD. Tumors of the Lower Respiratory Tract. In: *Armed Forces Institute of Pathology atlas of tumor pathology,* 3rd series, fascicle 13. Washington, DC: Armed Forces Institute of Pathology, 1995.
283. Cesarman R, Chang Y, Moore PS, et al. Kaposi's sarcoma-associated herpesvirus-like DNA sequences in AIDS-related body-cavity-based lymphomas. *N Engl J Med* 1995;332:1186–1191.
284. Iuchi K, Ichimiya A, Akashi A, et al. Non-Hodgkin's lymphoma of the pleural cavity developing from longstanding pyothorax. *Cancer* 1987;60:1771–1775.
285. Luther VR, Schoefer G, Sporman H, et al. Malignes immunoblastisches lymphom unter einer pneumolysenschwarte mit pleuraempyem. *Z Gesamte Inn Med* 1984;39:399–402.
286. Iuchi K, Aozasa K, Yamamoto S, et al. Non-Hodgkin's lymphoma of the pleural cavity developing from long-standing pyothorax. Summary of clinical and pathological findings in 37 cases. *Jpn J Clin Oncol* 1989;19:249–257.
287. Molinie V, Pouchot J, Navratil E, et al. Primary Epstein-Barr virus-related non-Hodgkin's lymphoma of the pleural cavity following long-standing tuberculous empyema. *Arch Pathol Lab Med* 1996;120: 288–291.
288. Martin A, Capron F, Liguory-Brunaud MD, et al. Epstein-Barr Virus-associated primary malignant lymphomas of the pleural cavity occurring in longstanding pleural chronic inflammation. *Hum Pathol* 1994; 25:1314–1318.
289. Nakamura S, Sasajima Y, Koshikawa T, et al. Ki-1 (CD30) positive anaplastic large cell lymphoma of T-cell phenotype developing in association with long-standing tuberculous pyothorax: report of a case with detection of Epstein-Barr virus genome in the tumor cells. *Hum Pathol* 1995;26:1382–1385.
290. Parisio E, Bianchi C, Rovej R, et al. Pulmonary asbestosis associated to pleural non-Hodgkin lymphoma. *Tumori* 1999;85:75–77.
291. Kanno H, Ohsawa M, Iuchi K, et al. Appearance of a different clone of Epstein-Barr virus genome in recurrent tumor of pyothorax-associated lymphoma (PAL) and a mini-review of PAL. *Leukemia* 1998;12: 1288–1294.
292. Mori N, Yatabe Y, Narita M, et al. Pyothorax-associated lymphoma. An unusual case with biphenotypic character of T and B cells. *Am J Surg Pathol* 1996;20:760–766.
293. Ibuka T, Fukayama M, Hayashi Y, et al. Pyothorax-associated pleural lymphoma. A case evolving from T-cell–rich lymphoid infiltration to overt B-cell lymphoma in association with Epstein-Barr virus. *Cancer* 1994;73:738–744.
294. Taniere P, Manai A, Charpentier R, et al. Pyothorax-associated lymphoma: relationship with Epstein Barr virus, human herpes virus-8 and body cavity-based high grade lymphomas. *Eur Respir J* 1998;11: 779–783.
295. Fukayama M, Ibuka T, Hayashi Y, et al. Epstein-Barr virus in pyothorax-associated pleural lymphoma. *Am J Pathol* 1993;143:1044–1049.
296. Cesarman E, Nador RG, Aozasa K, et al. Kaposi's sarcoma-associated herpesvirus in non-AIDS related lymphomas occurring in body cavities. *Am J Pathol* 1996;149:53–57.
297. Rickinson AB, Murray RJ, Brooks J, et al. T cell recognition of Epstein-Barr virus associated lymphomas. *Cancer Surv* 1992;13:53–80.
298. Kanno H, Naka N, Yasunaga Y, et al. Role of an immunosuppressive cytokine, interleukin-10, in the development of pyothorax-associated lymphoma. *Leukemia* 1997;11:525–526.

CHAPTER 35

Malignant Lymphomas and Lymphoid Hyperplasias That Occur in the Ocular Adnexa (Orbit, Conjunctiva, and Eyelids)

Daniel M. Knowles

Lymphoid infiltrates occurring in the ocular adnexa (i.e., orbit, conjunctiva, and eyelid) have traditionally posed a formidable clinical and histopathologic dilemma. In the past, the rate of error in accuracy of histopathologic diagnosis and ability to predict clinical outcome were estimated to lie between 20% and 50% (1,2). Some patients diagnosed with malignant lymphoma of the ocular adnexa enjoyed disease-free survivals despite minimal therapy, whereas some patients diagnosed with lymphoid hyperplasia of the ocular adnexa developed systemic lymphoma (1–5). Several factors contributed to diagnostic errors and inaccurate prognostication:

1. Difficulties inherent in the histopathologic evaluation of extranodal lymphoid proliferations, particularly those predominantly composed of small lymphocytes (3–8)
2. Reliance on histopathologic criteria (9,10) that failed to recognize the existence of extranodal diffuse small lymphocytic lymphomas (11), including those containing plasmacytoid cells (11) and pseudofollicular proliferation centers (12,13), mantle cell lymphomas (14–16), and the occasional benign follicles and reactive germinal centers in extranodal malignant lymphomas (7)
3. Indiscriminate consideration of all lymphoid proliferations that occur in or about the eye together, disregarding the fact that the conjunctiva contains indigenous lymphoid tissue, whereas the orbit normally does not (17,18)
4. Lack of a large clinical series of patients whose lesions were diagnosed and categorized according to an acceptable standard histopathologic classification and who were systematically evaluated using modern staging practices
5. Lack of access to immunologic and molecular biologic techniques capable of delineating lymphoid cell subpopulations and determining their monoclonal or polyclonal nature

D. M. Knowles: Department of Pathology, Weill Medical College of Cornell University, New York, New York 10021

Almost 20 years ago, Knowles and Jakobiec demonstrated that the diagnostic dilemma posed by ocular adnexal and other extranodal lymphoid infiltrates often may be resolved by immunophenotypic analysis of their constituent lymphoid subpopulations (5,19,20). Immunophenotypic analysis is capable of determining the immunologic polyclonality or B-cell monoclonality and presumably the benign or malignant nature of lymphoid proliferations that cannot be deciphered morphologically (21) (see Chapter 3). The inclusion of these immunologic criteria in the evaluation of ocular adnexal and other extranodal lymphoid infiltrates substantially altered many of the traditional beliefs concerning these lymphoid proliferations. In particular, multiple investigators demonstrated by immunophenotypic analysis that most extranodal diffuse, monomorphic small lymphoid cell infiltrates are monoclonal B-cell proliferations (5,19,20,22–32). Application of immunologic criteria resulted in the reclassification as small B-cell lymphomas many ocular adnexal lymphoid proliferations formerly classified as benign lymphoid hyperplasia by traditional morphologic criteria (8). Lymphoid hyperplasias of the ocular adnexa occur far less commonly than previously believed (8,24,25,27,31,32). This reclassification also resulted in a dramatic shift in the distribution of ocular adnexal malignant lymphomas according to histopathologic category. We know that most ocular adnexal malignant lymphomas belong to the small B-cell lymphoma categories (24,25,27,31,32). The correlative histopathologic and immunophenotypic analysis of ocular adnexal lymphoid proliferations occurring in a large cohort of patients that had been systematically evaluated clinically (32) resulted in important clinicopathologic correlations with therapeutic and prognostic relevance not obvious or predictable by morphologic criteria alone.

Nonetheless, results of some studies suggested that immunophenotypic analysis also might be limited in its ability to prognosticate reliably for patients who have ocular adnexal lymphoid proliferations (8,32). In the early 1980s, several scientists discovered that the antigen recognition molecules of B and T cells, immunoglobulin and T-cell receptors were encoded by genetic loci that undergo somatic recombination (i.e., rearrangement) to become functionally active in mature lymphocytes (33–35). Clonal rearrangements of the immunoglobulin and T-cell receptor genes have proved to be accurate and objective molecular genetic markers of the lineage and clonality of B and T cells, respectively (21). The demonstration of clonal immunoglobulin and T-cell receptor gene rearrangements by Southern blot hybridization analysis and by polymerase chain reaction analysis has been used successfully to determine the lineage and clonality of lymphoproliferative disorders and has become an important adjunct in the diagnosis, classification, and investigation of lymphoid neoplasia (see Chapter 7). This approach is capable of determining the presence of clonal B- and T-cell populations that are not detectable by morphologic examination or by immunophenotypic analysis (36–38). Southern blot hybridization and polymerase chain reaction analysis are also capable of detecting viral sequences, chromosomal translocations, and structural alterations of protooncogenes and tumor suppressor genes, and thereby investigating pathogenetic mechanisms of neoplasia as well (see Chapters 8 and 9).

Correlative multiparametric clinical, morphologic, immunophenotypic, and molecular genetic analysis has provided considerable insight into the origin, nature, and natural history of the ocular adnexal lymphoid proliferations, transcending what was historically attainable by light microscopic examination alone. This chapter is largely devoted to a review of our current knowledge and understanding of the clinical, morphologic, and biologic characteristics of the ocular adnexal lymphoid proliferations. Other hematopoietic disorders involve the eye and the ocular adnexa less commonly; these are summarized briefly here as well.

TERMINOLOGY

The often indiscriminate use of a wide variety of terms to refer to the lymphoid proliferations that involve the orbit, conjunctiva, and eyelid over the years contributed significantly to the long-standing failure to delineate the clinical, pathologic, and biologic features of these lesions. It also engendered confusion about these entities among ophthalmologists and pathologists alike, much of which remains to this day.

The term *pseudotumor* was originally introduced to designate the wide spectrum of local and systemic inflammatory conditions affecting the orbital contents that produce proptosis and the false clinical impression of a neoplasm (39). Orbital reactive lymphoid hyperplasia was initially thought to be a specific hypercellular type of orbital pseudotumor (40,41) and was referred to as *orbital lymphoid pseudotumor* (42,43) by Hogan and Zimmerman (44). In 1963, the term *pseudolymphoma* was introduced by Saltzstein (9) to designate the extranodal benign lymphoid infiltrates that mimic malignant lymphoma clinically and histopathologically. Consequently, orbital reactive lymphoid hyperplasias and orbital pseudotumors came to be categorized as benign lymphoid tumors (45,46) and called orbital pseudolymphomas (4,19). The terms orbital pseudotumor, orbital lymphoid pseudotumor, orbital reactive lymphoid hyperplasia, and orbital pseudolymphoma often were used interchangeably (42,45,47–52).

The term *pseudolymphoma,* generally considered to be confusing and misleading, has been largely abandoned. The equally ambiguous term *lymphoid pseudotumor* similarly should be discarded (53). It is further recommended that the term *lymphoid hyperplasia* replace the term *reactive lymphoid hyperplasia,* because the word reactive implies a response to an exogenous stimulus, which may not be the case. It is widely recognized that the generally hypocellular, lymphoid cell-poor orbital pseudotumors and the usually hypercellular, lymphoid cell–rich lymphoid hyperplasias represent distinct entities. They differ with respect to clinical presentation, natural history, histopathology, treatment, management, and prognosis, as well as pathogenesis (32,53–57) and should therefore be clearly distinguished from one another. It is recommended that the term *orbital pseudotumor* be used to denote those benign, hypocellular, lymphoid cell-poor orbital inflammatory conditions that are without evidence of a specific local or systemic cause and that the term *lymphoid hyperplasia* be used to denote those hypercellular, lymphoid cell–rich lesions that mimic malignant lymphomas clinically and histopathologically.

The term *histologically indeterminate* has been used by some investigators (25,31,58,59) to refer to those lesions that cannot be assigned with certainty to the category of lymphoid hyperplasia or malignant lymphoma. This term is acceptable only when the morphology of such lesions has been studied, and they are truly indeterminate histologically. However, use of this term is inappropriate if such a lesion still defies classification after immunophenotypic or molecular genetic analysis. In these instances, the term *atypical lymphoid hyperplasia,* recommended by Knowles and Jakobiec (4,32), is clearly more appropriate.

The term *ocular adnexal lymphoid proliferation* is used to encompass all the hypercellular, lymphoid cell–rich lymphoid hyperplasias, atypical lymphoid hyperplasias, and malignant lymphomas that occur in the ocular adnexa (i.e., the orbit, conjunctiva, and eyelids). The intraocular lymphoid proliferations include the same categories but involving the choroid, retina, and vitreous body. In addition to the orbital pseudotumors, the other hematopoietic disorders, such as plasmacytomas, granulocytic sarcomas, and Langerhans cell histiocytosis, that involve the ocular adnexa represent distinct clinicopathologic entities. They exhibit fundamental clinical, pathologic, and biologic differences from the ocular adnexal lymphoid proliferations (53) and therefore should be distinguished from them.

ORBITAL PSEUDOTUMOR

Birch-Hirschfeld is credited with coining the term *inflammatory orbital pseudotumor* in 1905 to describe the instance of a mysterious orbital mass believed clinically to be a benign or malignant neoplasm that was discovered instead to be inflammatory in nature (39). Inflammatory orbital pseudotumor soon became a diagnostic term used to encompass a wide array of poorly understood inflammatory disorders that are now recognized as specific disease entities (60). Unfortunately, the term *inflammatory orbital pseudotumor* also was sometimes used for poorly understood lymphoid proliferations, probably even including some malignant lymphomas (60). Older studies and literature reports of inflammatory orbital pseudotumors include examples of numerous, well-defined disease conditions, such as syphilis, tuberculosis, sarcoidosis, infectious cellulitis, Graves' ophthalmopathy, polyarteritis nodosa, and Wegener's granulomatosis (60). Over time, conditions with a known infectious or immune cause were recognized and separated, and misuse of the term *inflammatory orbital pseudotumor* gradually diminished (60). As a result, the definition of inflammatory orbital pseudotumor has evolved to denote the benign, nonspecific, orbital inflammatory processes that have no evidence of a specific local or systemic origin (57,61).

The term *pseudotumor* has been attacked over the years, because it defines what this entity is not, rather than what it is (62). Many investigators have proposed alternative names for this entity in an effort to label it more appropriately, based on an evolving appreciation for its histopathologic characteristics and presumed pathogenesis. Unfortunately, this practice often merely engendered further confusion surrounding the definition of orbital pseudotumor. Some of the recommended names in the older literature include orbital granuloma, nonspecific orbital granuloma, and orbital lipogranuloma (60). Hogan and Zimmerman (44) called it inflammatory nonneoplastic orbital pseudotumor. Jakobiec and colleagues initially proposed the term *idiopathic inflammatory orbital pseudotumor* (40) but later suggested that the term *idiopathic orbital inflammation* is more appropriate (61). Henderson initially called it lymphocytic inflammatory orbital pseudotumor (41) and later called it nonvasculitic inflammatory orbital tumor (57). Kennerdell and Dresner (63) and Rootman and colleagues (64) preferred the term *nonspecific orbital inflammation*. Despite these and numerous other attempts to replace it, the term *orbital pseudotumor* remains in widespread use (60). Unfortunately, the interpretation of older studies of orbital pseudotumor is complicated by these terminologic difficulties. Moreover, the multiple early descriptions and subclassifications of orbital pseudotumor are largely unhelpful in delineating a histopathologic spectrum of orbital pseudotumor in the modern sense of the term.

Among orbital disorders, pseudotumor, after Grave's disease and lymphoid proliferations, is a common ophthalmologic disease. Orbital pseudotumor accounts for approximately 5% of all orbital disorders (63,65). Orbital pseudotumor usually occurs in adults but may also affect children. Pediatric orbital pseudotumor encompasses about 6% to 16% of orbital pseudotumors (66,67). Men and women are affected (57). Orbital pseudotumor is protean in its clinical and radiologic presentation (40). Except for myositic pseudotumor, only one orbit is almost always affected (57). The clinical presentation ranges from that of orbital inflammation with an abrupt onset of periocular discomfort or pain accompanied by epibulbar injection, erythema of the lid skin, chemosis, ptosis, and diplopia to that of a space-occupying or infiltrating orbital lesion with proptosis, motility disturbances, and optic nerve compression, varying according to the location and extent of the mass in the orbit (65) and to the extent of the fibrotic component of the lesion (64,68). Symptoms usually develop over the course of days (acute pseudotumor) to weeks (subacute pseudotumor) but sometimes occur insidiously over a period of months (chronic pseudotumor). The patient may complain of generalized malaise but is usually afebrile (53,63,65,66,68) (Fig. 35.1).

Orbital pseudotumor may manifest as a focal or diffuse mass, which is poorly demarcated and enhances with con-

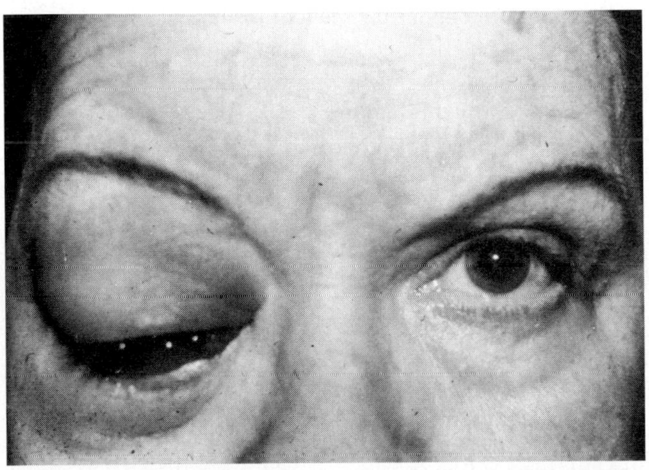

FIG. 35.1. Orbital pseudotumor. This 66-year-old woman initially developed painful external ophthalmoplegia mimicking the Tolosa-Hunt syndrome; it evolved into an orbital pseudotumor with proptosis and eyelid erythema. The histologic appearance of the lesion is shown in Figure 35.2. The patient was treated with systemic steroids and remained alive and well without recurrence 123 months after presentation. (From Knowles DM, Jakobiec FA, Halper JP. Immunologic characterization of ocular adnexal lymphoid neoplasms. *Am J Ophthalmol* 1979;87:603–619, with permission.)

trast on computed tomography (CT) (69,70). Lesions located anteriorly may have sharply defined borders (57). Sinus involvement (71,72) or intracranial extension (73,74), with or without bone erosion, is seen rarely. This clinicoradiologic picture is shared with a number of other orbital disorders, however (75).

Orbital pseudotumor is a benign lesion and is believed to be a self-limited disorder (41,76). However, the natural history and evolution of orbital pseudotumor is unknown. It is generally believed that orbital pseudotumors are sensitive to systemic corticosteroids (61,76). A prompt favorable clinical response within days of corticosteroid administration has been advocated as evidence for orbital pseudotumor, even in the absence of histopathologic confirmation (61,77). Consequently, the working diagnosis of orbital pseudotumor based on clinical and radiologic findings and a favorable response to corticosteroids, without histopathologic support (70,77), has been widely adopted. However, steroid nonresponsive orbital pseudotumors have been described in many series (51,70,78,79). Many orbital lesions, including malignant lymphomas, may be steroid responsive transiently (75,78,79). Consequently, steroid responsiveness may not in itself represent a valid criterion for the reliable diagnosis of orbital pseudotumor (75,78,79). A biopsy is necessary for a definitive diagnosis of orbital pseudotumor and to exclude many other entities from consideration (60). A biopsy should be obtained in all cases of suspected orbital pseudotumor (46,74,75,79,80), except in pure myositic locations in which the clinicoradiologic picture is distinctive and a surgical biopsy may damage the muscle (46,81,82) and except in posterior locations in which the optic nerve may be at risk during surgery (46,65,79). Fine needle aspiration biopsy is not helpful in the differential diagnosis of orbital pseudotumor, because a nonspecific cytologic smear of inflammatory cells does not exclude an underlying malignancy (83–85).

Although orbital pseudotumors are benign, they may pursue a malignant clinical course in which the eye, extraocular muscles and optic nerve are endangered (57). Therapy is advised to relieve discomfort during the active phase to preserve visual and motility functions and to prevent sequelae in a later stage (60). Systemic corticosteroids are the popular first choice for treating orbital pseudotumors; the acute form of the disease is especially responsive to high doses of systemically administered prednisone (61,63,65,68,77,86). Corticosteroids may not always be effective, however (52,70,78, 79). Low-dose irradiation has been administered with various degrees of success in steroid-dependent and steroid-nonresponsive cases (49,52,77,87). Combined therapy with other immunosuppresive drugs, including cyclosporine, cyclophosphamide, azathioprine, or methotrexate, may be successful in the case of some aggressive orbital pseudotumors (64,88,89). The wide spectrum in clinical behavior, therapeutic responsiveness, and prognosis among orbital pseudotumors has prompted attempts to relate these features to anatomic location (65), to particular histopathologic patterns (41,51,64), and to duration of disease (76).

Grossly, orbital pseudotumors appear as firm, rubbery, yellowish gray to pink lesions (57). Pseudotumors can affect any orbital structure. The lesion may be confined to one structure, such as the lacrimal gland, the orbital fat, or extraocular muscle (i.e., myositic pseudotumor), but often more than one of these structures are involved in a localized or diffuse pattern (63,76), thereby simulating a tumor mass. They are generally hypocellular, lymphoid cell-poor lesions that consist of a variably dense connective tissue stroma (57). The stromal changes range from edema to proliferative fibrosis and sclerosis to marked hyalinization (61) (Figs. 35.2, 35.3). Eosinophil degranulation has been found in the areas of fibrosis and contributes to fibrosis formation in orbital pseudotumors (90). It had been long assumed that the fibrosis and sclerosis that develops in orbital pseudotumors is the result of long-standing inflammation (57,61,67,68). However, it has been suggested that fibrosis formation in orbital pseudotumors is an immune-mediated process and that the fibrosis forms early in the development of the lesion (64). Orbital pseudotumors contain a variable but generally sparse polymorphous cellular infiltrate that may be diffuse or multifocal. It is primarily composed of chronic inflammatory cells (i.e., small lymphocytes and plasma cells) accompanied by variable numbers of immunoblasts, histiocytes, and eosinophils and sometimes by neutrophils (57,61,68,76). Most of the lymphocytes are T cells, with helper T cells predominating over suppressor or cytotoxic T cells (91). The B cells are polyclonal (19,57). Mitotic figures are infrequent (Fig. 35.4). Variable numbers of lymphoid follicles, some containing germinal centers, may be present (57,91). They are usually surrounded by abundant, dense, fibrous connective tissue (Fig. 35.5). In some pediatric orbital pseudotumors, eosinophils sometimes represent the majority cell population (67). Orbital pseudotumors may be highly vascularized because of capillary proliferation (57). The endothelial cells are increased in number and swollen and hypertrophic (57). The most common vascular change is perivasculitis presenting as angiocentric lymphocytic cuffing (57). The hypocellular and inflammatory histopathologic appearance of these lesions nearly always allows them to be readily distinguished from ocular adnexal lymphoid hyperplasias and malignant lymphomas.

The involvement of specific orbital structures (i.e., orbital fat, lacrimal gland, and extraocular muscle) by orbital pseudotumor is associated with additional histopathologic changes (60). For example, orbital pseudotumor involving the orbital fat appears as a mixed inflammatory cell infiltrate with increased supportive fibrous tissue. The delicate interlobular septa of the adipose tissue become thickened and accentuated and become confluent (67). Lipogranuloma formation may occur (57,61,92). Involvement of the lacrimal gland by pseudotumor results in periductal and periacinar fibrosis, ductal dilatation and acinar atrophy (61). When ex-

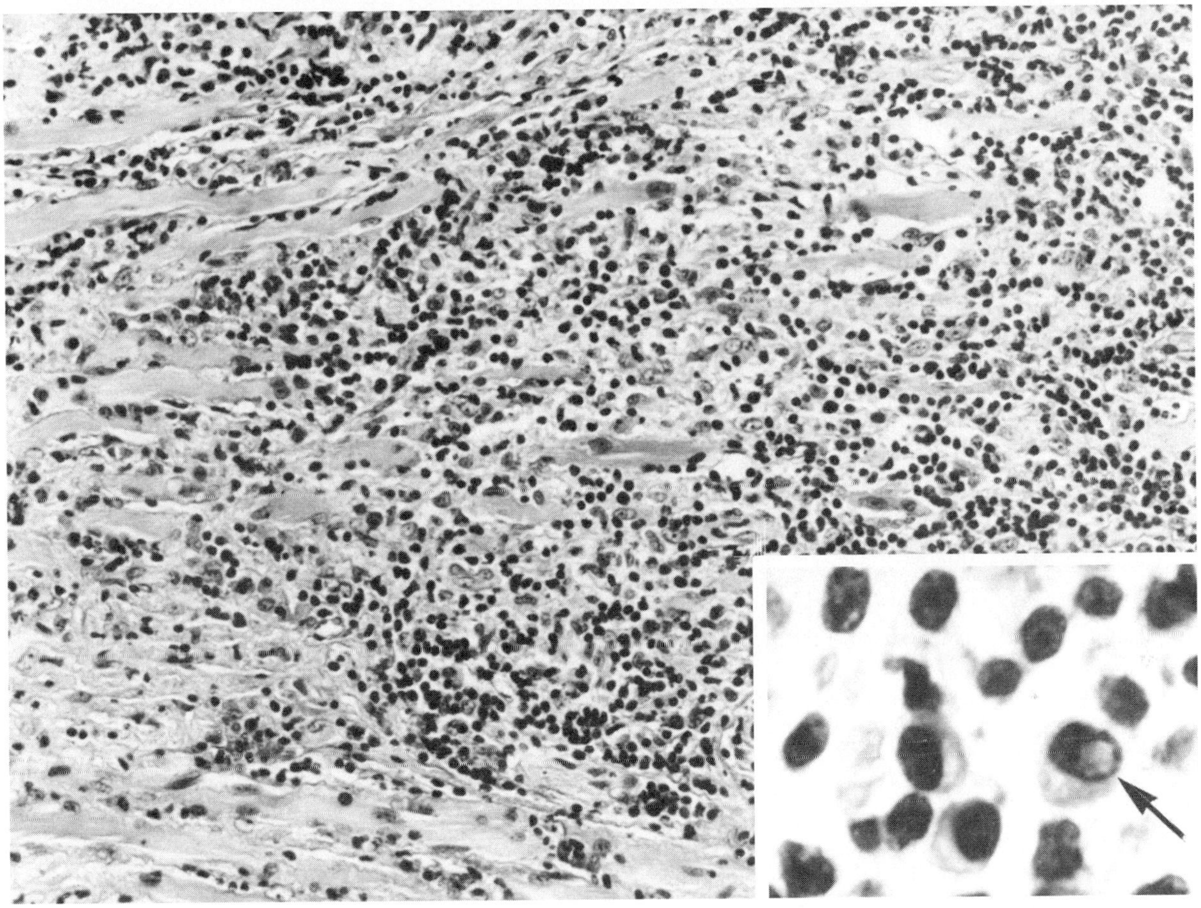

FIG. 35.2. Skeletal muscle infiltration by an orbital pseudotumor. The connective tissue stroma is focally edematous. High-power magnification reveals the polymorphous nature of the cellular infiltrate, including the presence of many plasma cells, one of which contains a Dutcher body *(arrow)*. These intranuclear immunoglobulin inclusions are seen commonly in mucosa-associated lymphoid tissue lymphomas and plasmacytoid small lymphocytic lymphomas but only rarely in pseudotumors (hematoxylin and eosin stain, original magnifications: 176× magnification; **Inset:** 1,100× magnification). (From Knowles DM, Jakobiec FA, Halper JP. Immunologic characterization of ocular adnexal lymphoid neoplasms. *Am J Ophthalmol* 1979;87:603–619, with permission.)

traocular muscle is involved by orbital pseudotumor the muscle fibers become swollen, the normal striations are lost and the fibers degenerate; they become separated by edema and fibrosis (60).

Occasionally, the stromal, cellular, or vascular component of orbital pseudotumor deviates significantly from the classic histopathologic pattern (60). This has led to the recognition of four histopathologic subtypes of orbital pseudotumor: sclerosing, granulomatous, vasculitic, and eosinophilic (60). The principal features of these lesions are summarized only briefly here; they have been reviewed in detail elsewhere (60).

If the amount of interstitial connective tissue is disproportionately great and the inflammatory infiltrate is paucicellular or nearly absent, the pseudotumor is designated fibrotic (41), sclerotic (44), or idiopathic sclerosing (nonspecific) orbital inflammation (64,93). Although fibrosis and sclerosis differ histologically, fibrosing and sclerosing orbital pseudotumors are often equated (51,72,91,93,94). In the past, extensive sclerosis was believed to be the result of chronic, recurrent or severe inflammation (51,61,95). However, Henderson observed that the amount of fibrosis in orbital pseudotumor was not always related to disease duration (41). In a series of 16 patients who had sclerosing orbital pseudotumor, Rootman and colleagues found that the clinical presentation was dominated by mild chronic inflammation and cicatricial entrapment of orbital structures (64). They discovered that the amount of fibrosis correlated poorly with duration of symptoms; significant sclerosis was present in some cases in which symptoms were present for only a short time (64). Rootman and colleagues hypothesized that the development of fibrosis in these cases, as in retroperitoneal fibrosis (96), was mediated by inflammation (64). Systemic corticosteroids and irradiation often have been found to be unsatisfac-

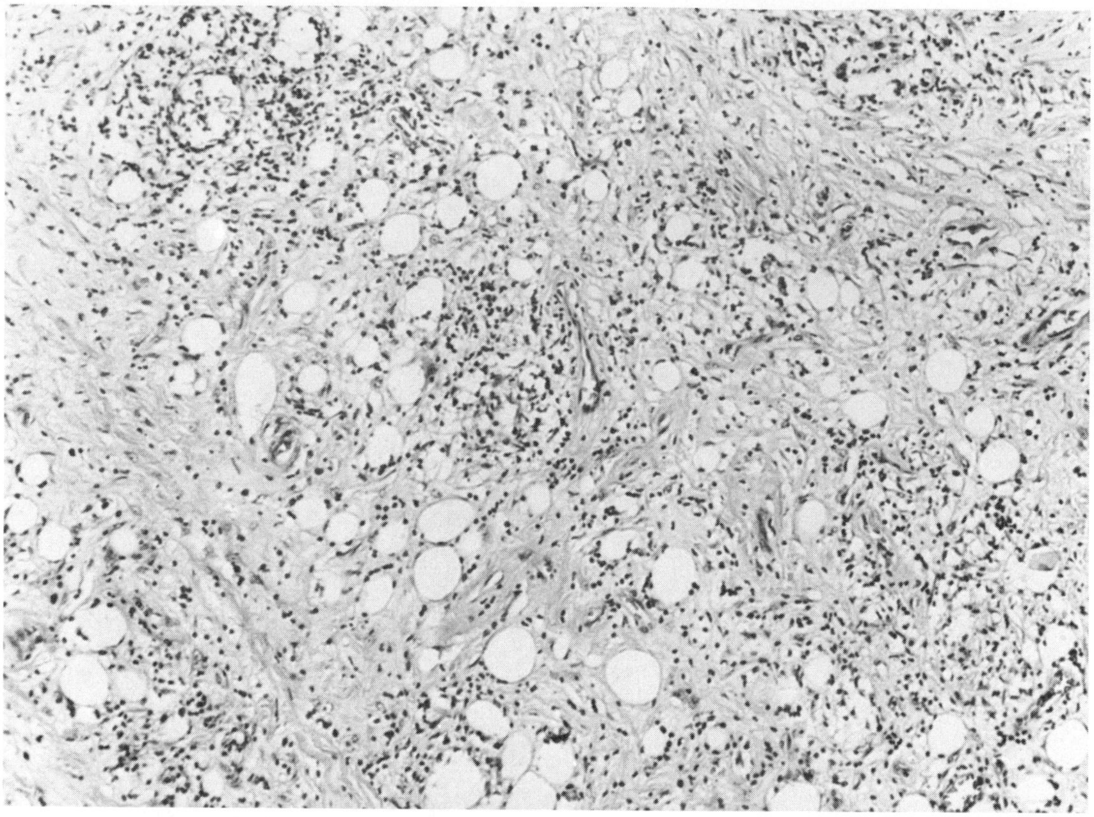

FIG. 35.3. Orbital pseudotumor containing a dense connective tissue stroma and a sparsely cellular inflammatory cell infiltrate that incompletely replaces the soft tissues of the orbit, simulating a tumor mass clinically (hematoxylin and eosin stain, original magnification: 24× magnification).

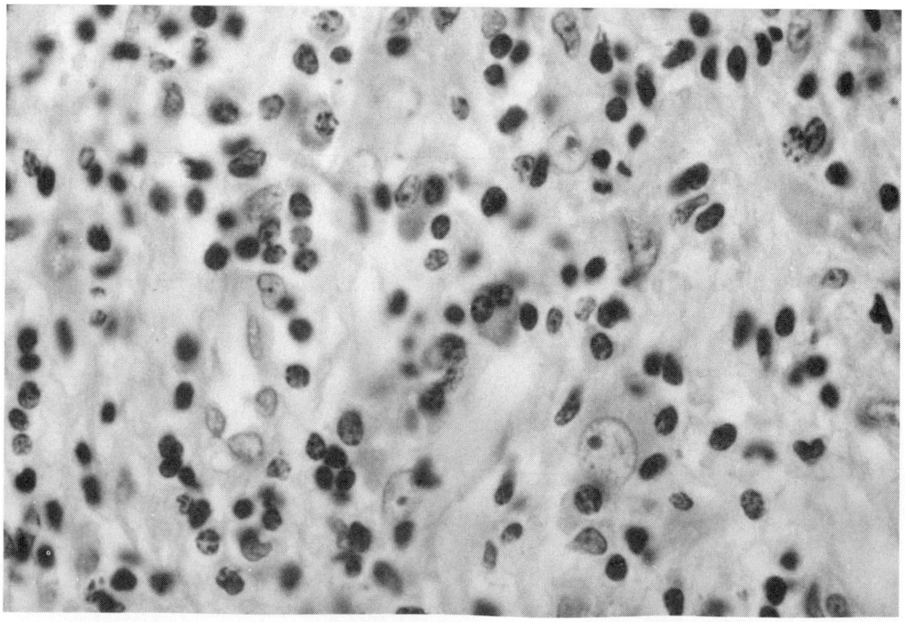

FIG. 35.4. Orbital pseudotumors are generally composed of a sparse, polymorphous cellular infiltrate containing predominantly small lymphocytes, plasma cells, immunoblasts, and histiocytes. Eosinophils and neutrophils also may be present. Mitotic figures are uncommon (hematoxylin and eosin stain, original magnification: 400× magnification).

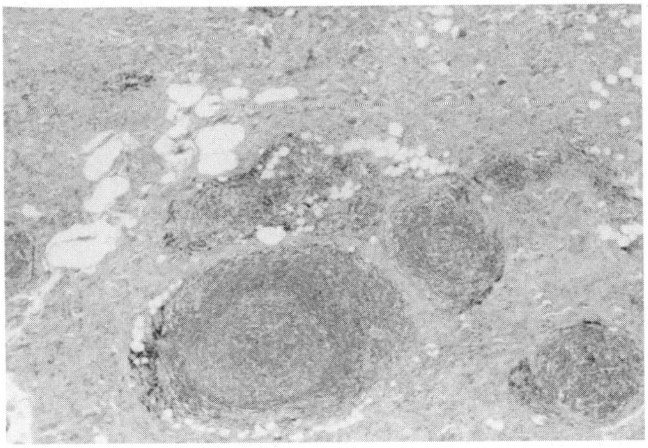

FIG. 35.5. Orbital pseudotumors may contain lymphoid follicles that are surrounded and separated by abundant, dense fibrous connective tissue (hematoxylin and eosin stain, original magnification: 40× magnification).

tory therapeutically in these patients (51,64,93). However, the interpretation of studies concerning sclerosing orbital pseudotumor has been hampered by the inconsistent use of criteria to distinguish these cases from classic orbital pseudotumor (60).

Approximately 30 cases of granulomatous orbital pseudotumor have been described (51,57,76,97–99). The lesion is characterized histopathologically by infiltration by histiocytes and multinucleated giant cells, which sometimes form well-developed, noncaseating granulomas and is not associated with vasculitis and tissue necrosis. Systemic granulomatous disorders, such as sarcoidosis, tuberculosis, and Wegener's granulomatosis, foreign bodies, and fungal and parasitic organisms must be excluded (60). The clinical presentation of these cases is the same as classic orbital pseudotumor and most patients are managed adequately with systemic corticosteroids (51,57,97–99).

Rarely, primary vasculitis of the small vessels is observed in orbital pseudotumor (41,61). Only a few cases of nongranulomatous vasculitic orbital pseudotumor without systemic involvement have been reported (57,87,100). In these cases, lymphocytes and granulocytes attack the vessel wall, resulting in destruction of the muscularis and elastic lamina and extravasation of red blood cells (60). Systemic vasculitis of the granulomatous or nongranulomatous type must be excluded (57). It is critically important that Wegener's granulomatosis be ruled out (101). The clinical presentation of vasculitic orbital pseudotumor is often that of classic orbital pseudotumor but the prognosis appears to be worse (57,87,100).

Rarely, orbital pseudotumor displays significant tissue eosinophilia without vasculitis (67,68). This pattern was observed in one-half of children who had orbital pseudotumor. Eosinophils are scattered throughout the proliferating fibroblastic tissue, are localized in cuffs around small blood vessels, and infiltrate fat lobules (68). Eosinophilic orbital pseudotumor may be accompanied by peripheral blood eosinophilia (67). Because of the limited number of these cases that have been described, conclusions cannot be drawn concerning therapy and prognosis.

The etiology and pathogenesis of orbital pseudotumor are unknown. Many theories have been suggested but none have been substantiated (60). Originally, it was thought that orbital pseudotumor is infectious in origin. The onset of orbital myositis has been reported after upper respiratory tract infection (102,103) or a flulike viral illness (104). Cell wall–deficient bacteria have been detected ultrastructurally in leukocytes present in some orbital pseudotumors (105). However, an infectious cause appears inconsistent with the fact that orbital pseudotumor may improve with immunosuppressive therapies. Many years ago, Easton and Smith suggested an autoimmune pathogenesis for orbital pseudotumor (106). This theory fits with the occasional observation of a coexistent autoimmune disorder, such as diabetes mellitus, rheumatoid arthritis, or systemic lupus erythematosus, in patients who have orbital pseudotumor (61,64). That an immunologic process is central to the pathogenesis of orbital pseudotumor is also strongly supported by the fact that these lesions are often treated successfully with corticosteroids and other immunosuppressive agents (60). The fact that orbital pseudotumor is commonly unilateral seems incongruous with an autoimmune basis, however. Orbital pseudotumor shares histopathologic similarities with idiopathic mediastinal fibrosclerosis (107) and idiopathic retroperitoneal fibrosis (91). For this reason, Barrett proposed many years ago that orbital pseudotumors result from a fibroproliferative disorder (107). Studies by McCarty and Rootman and colleagues (64,91) support this theory by providing evidence that fibrosis formation in at least some orbital pseudotumors is an immunologically mediated process. Orbital pseudotumor has been rarely reported to occur in association with retroperitoneal fibrosis (94,108,109), mediastinal fibrosclerosis (110), and other fibroproliferative disorders (111–113). It has been suggested that all of these entities may be a manifestation of a single generalized disorder called multifocal fibrosclerosis (92). It has been suggested that development of orbital pseudotumor should be considered a form of aberrant wound healing with cytokine driven fibroblast proliferation and collagen synthesis as a final common pathway provoked by damage (e.g., infectious, autoimmune) (60).

OCULAR ADNEXAL LYMPHOID PROLIFERATIONS

Background

Between 1977 and 1987, Knowles and Jakobiec prospectively evaluated 108 patients who had lymphoid proliferations (i.e., lymphoid hyperplasia, atypical lymphoid hyperplasia, and malignant lymphoma) that originated or presented in the ocular adnexa (32). Patients who had an orbital pseudotumor, plasmacytoma or multiple myeloma, or an intraocular lymphoid proliferation were excluded for the reasons cited earlier. They examined the histopathology and analyzed the immunophenotypic characteristics of 117 ocular adnexal and 9 nonocular lymphoid proliferations obtained from these 108 patients during that time. After these studies were completed, the patients were referred to a hematologist-oncologist for systemic evaluation, including radiologic survey and bone marrow examination, before therapy. The patients were followed carefully and periodically underwent reexamination. Complete clinical information concerning each patient was collected; this included age, sex, past medical history, presenting complaints, duration of symptoms, principal clinical findings, precise anatomic location of the lesion, results of laboratory and radiologic studies, extent of disease, type and extent of therapy, therapeutic response, duration of survival, and outcome. In 1988, Knowles and Jakobiec correlated the clinical, histopathologic, and immunophenotypic findings and critically reviewed them. The results of this prospective multiparametric analysis (32) and the numerous other studies performed by Knowles and Jakobiec during the 1980s (4,5,19,20,22,29, 37,55,114–119) have served as the basis for much of our modern understanding of the ocular adnexal lymphoid proliferations.

However, since the time of those studies, two important developments have taken place that have contributed significantly to our further understanding of lymphoid neoplasia, especially that involving the ocular adnexa. The first is the recognition of mucosa-associated lymphoid tissue (MALT) and the special characteristics of MALT and the malignant lymphomas that arise within MALT (120); the second is the development of the Revised European-American Lymphoma (REAL) classification, the only standard lymphoma classification that is relevant for nodal and extranodal lymphomas, by the International Lymphoma Study Group in 1994 (121). These two highly significant contributions provided the scientific underpinnings to support and extend many of the notions of Knowles and Jakobiec, but they also challenged many others, especially the classification of ocular adnexal malignant lymphomas. Other large clinicopathologic studies of the ocular adnexal lymphoid proliferations that have incorporated these two developments (59,122) have built on the classic studies of Knowles and Jakobiec to provide us with a better understanding of these lesions.

Definition

Nearly every malignant lymphoid neoplasm originating in the ocular adnexa and most that involve the ocular adnexa secondarily are B-cell lymphomas. These are predominately small B-cell lymphomas but also include large B-cell and follicular lymphomas (31,32,59,122). High-grade (immunoblastic and Burkitt's) lymphomas may arise or manifest in the ocular adnexa of adults in the setting of the acquired immunodeficiency syndrome (AIDS) (123,124) (see Chapter 28). Rarely, sporadic (Western) Burkitt's lymphoma may involve the ocular adnexa in children (125,126) (see Chapter 27). Peripheral T-cell lymphomas frequently involve the ocular adnexa and nearly always represent systemic disease (59,127); very few cases of primary ocular adnexal T-cell lymphoma have been described (128,129). Mycosis fungoides occasionally involves the skin of the eyelid (130), and much less commonly, other adnexal locations (131), usually in the late plaque or tumor stage of the disease. Rarely, the ocular adnexa may serve as the initial site of presentation of disseminated mycosis fungoides (132). Lastly, Hodgkin's disease of the ocular adnexa is extraordinarily rare (133). All of these lymphoid neoplasms differ clinically and biologically from conventional ocular adnexal B-cell lymphomas. Consequently, the discussion that follows concerning the clinical, radiologic, histopathologic, immunophenotypic, immunogenotypic, and molecular genetic features of ocular adnexal lymphoid proliferations excludes the B-cell neoplasms arising in association with AIDS and other immunodeficiency states, T-cell neoplasms, and Hodgkin's disease.

Mucosa-Associated Lymphoid Tissue

In the mid-1980s, Isaacson and colleagues brought attention to the characteristic arrangement of lymphoid tissue underlying certain mucosal surfaces, for which the term *mucosa-associated lymphoid tissue* (MALT) was employed (134). The arrangement of MALT consists of the following characteristic histologic and immunologic features: submucosal B-cell follicles composed of reactive germinal centers containing a network of CD21-positive ($CD21^+$) follicular dendritic cells and a surrounding mantle zone of small $CD20^+$ B cells expressing immunoglobulin M (IgM) and IgD, and a region of larger, centrocyte-like $CD20^+$ B cells expressing IgM, which extend from the mantle zone into the overlying epithelium to form a characteristic lymphoepithelium. Scattered plasma cells may be observed around and above the lymphoid follicles. $CD3^+$ T cells are seen within and around the germinal centers, condensing at the base of the follicle farthest from the surface epithelium (135,136).

In humans, most of the organized MALT is located in the terminal ileum, whereas other mucosal sites are apparently normally devoid of organized MALT (135). However, MALT may be acquired in these other mucosal sites, particularly the bronchus, stomach, salivary gland, and thyroid gland, as a result of antigenic stimulation (135,137). Bronchus-associated lymphoid tissue is absent in the newborn but is acquired in early childhood in response to antigenic stimulation (138–140). In the stomach, MALT is acquired specifically in response to local infection by *Helicobacter pylori* (141). In the case of the salivary and thyroid glands, the antigenic stimulation may be a component of autoimmune disease, Sjögren's syndrome (142) and Hashimoto's thyroiditis (143), respectively. Once acquired, subsequent oncogenic events, occurring in a small number of cases, may eventually result in the development of a distinctive type of

B-cell non-Hodgkin's lymphoma that morphologically and immunologically resembles the MALT from which it arises (120).

Morphologic and functional studies in animals suggest that MALT is variably present in the conjunctiva of normal turkey, rabbit, mouse, rat, and guinea pig (144–148). In the guinea pig, MALT displays structural organization similar to that of the human Peyer's patch (148). Examination of conjunctival MALT in animals raised in a bacteria-free environment shows that fornix follicle size and the number of lymphocytes in the conjunctival lamina propria, although present, remain lower than in animals reared conventionally (144). Other experimental studies performed in animals suggest that conjunctival MALT can be induced and stimulated by external antigenic stimuli (146,147).

Knowles and colleagues showed that the lamina propria of the normal human conjunctiva contains a mixed lymphoid cell infiltrate in which T cells outnumber B cells and occasional intraepithelial T cells are present (18). This was later confirmed by Wotherspoon and coworkers (135). Jakobiec and associates also described the presence of organized MALT, including the formation of lymphoid follicles, in the forniceal region of the apparently normal conjunctiva of some individuals (149). In a carefully conducted investigation of representative strips of superior and inferior forniceal conjunctiva obtained during the autopsy examination of 90 individuals with no known history of ocular or conjunctival disease, Wotherspoon and colleagues found organized MALT in about 30% of the cases, the youngest one being 28 years old (135). This finding suggests that conjunctival MALT, like that of other mucosal surfaces, is not found in the normal human conjunctiva but is acquired during life in response to external antigenic stimulation (135). In support of these findings and this conclusion, it is known that conjunctival folliculosis, a common childhood condition of limited clinical significance (150), has an appearance consistent with that of exuberant MALT (135). In adults, follicular conjunctivitis may be observed in response to infection by *Chlamydia,* adenovirus, and Epstein-Barr virus or a chemically induced allergic reaction (135). Regardless of the natural history of conjunctival MALT, once acquired, it provides the cellular milieu from which primary conjunctival B-cell MALT lymphomas may arise, analogous to MALT in other locations.

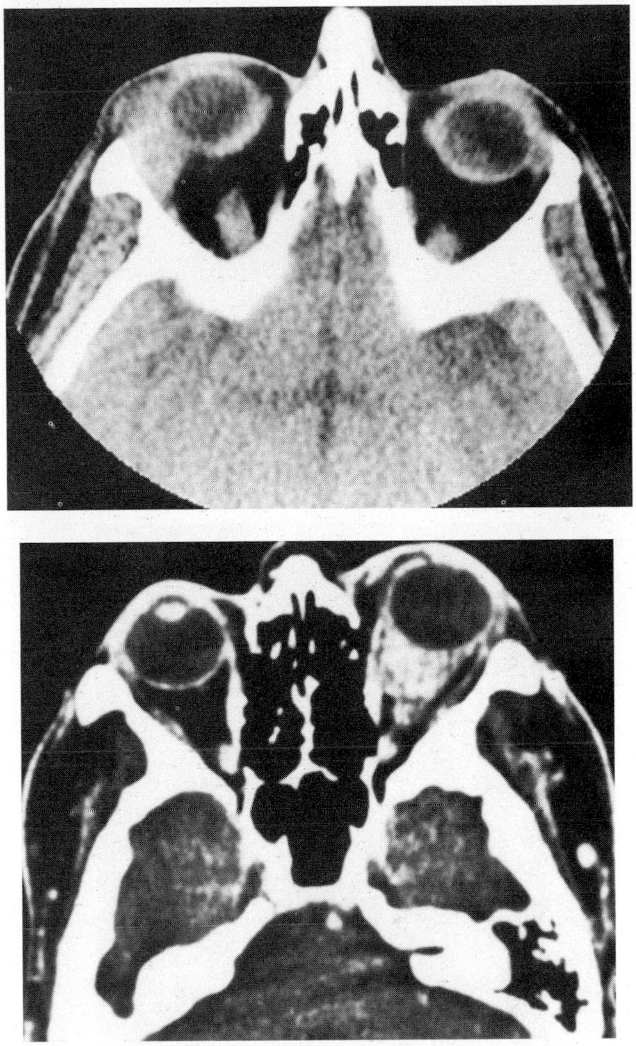

FIG. 35.6. CT scan of orbital lymphoid proliferation. **A:** A lymphoid proliferation occupies the lacrimal gland on the left. Approximately 45% of orbital lymphoid proliferations involve the lacrimal gland. **B:** A lymphoid proliferation molded to the posterior sclera occurs in the retrobulbar orbital soft tissues on the right. (From Knowles DM, Jakobiec FA, McNally L, et al. Lymphoid hyperplasia and malignant lymphoma occurring in the ocular adnexa [orbit, conjunctiva, and eyelids]: a prospective multiparametric analysis of 108 cases during 1977–1987. *Hum Pathol* 1990;21:959–973, with permission.)

Anatomic Location

Knowles and Jakobiec suggested that the proportion of ocular adnexal lymphoid proliferations classified as lymphoid hyperplasia and malignant lymphoma and their natural history, including the development of systemic lymphoma, varies according to their location within the ocular adnexa (i.e., orbit, conjunctiva, or eyelid) (32). Although not all investigators agree (58,59), it is important that the patient who has an ocular adnexal lymphoid proliferation receive a careful clinical ocular examination, usually in conjunction with imaging studies, so that the precise anatomic location of the lesion can be determined. The following guidelines can be used in this determination.

Lesions should be designated as orbital if the lacrimal gland is involved or if any aspect of the retroorbital soft tissue, including the muscles, is involved (Fig. 35.6). Lesions that manifest subconjunctivally or in the lids whose epicenters obviously are within the orbit also should be categorized among the orbital lesions (Fig. 35.7). Most orbital lesions occur superiorly or in the retrobulbar tissues; fewer than 5% are located predominantly in the inferior orbit. Orbital lesions frequently cause proptosis, ocular displacement, and

A

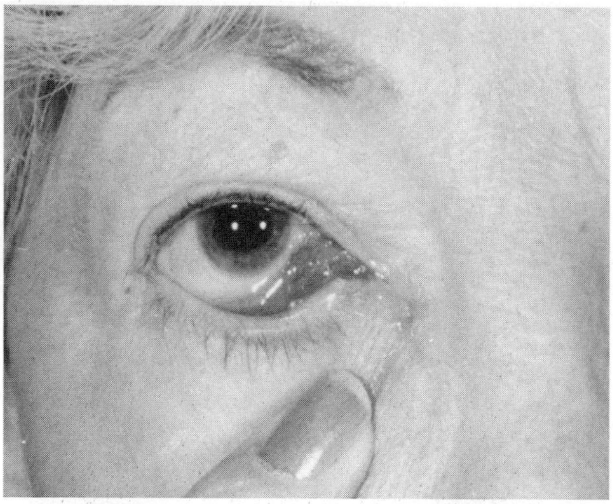

B

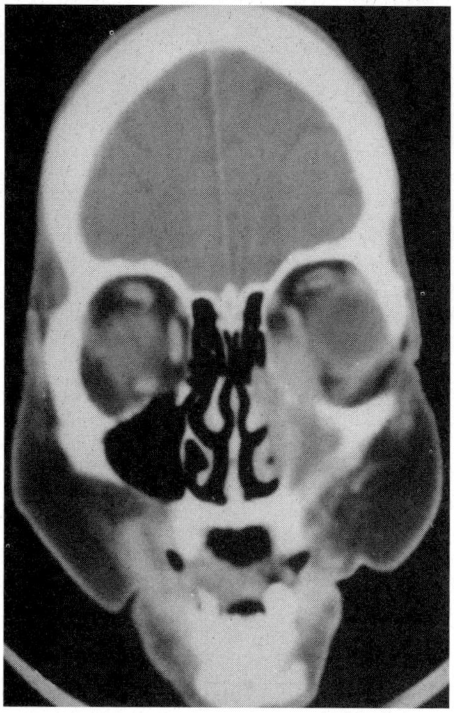

FIG. 35.7. An orbital monoclonal large B-cell lymphoma is beneath the nasal conjunctiva. **A:** There is some displacement of the globe, suggesting that the lesion extends beyond the conjunctiva. **B:** CT scan of the patient shown in **A**. The lesion involved the inferonasal orbit and caused bone destruction inferonasally by extending into the contiguous maxillary sinus. The patient had no evidence of systemic lymphoma. Local radiation therapy was administered, with resolution of the process.

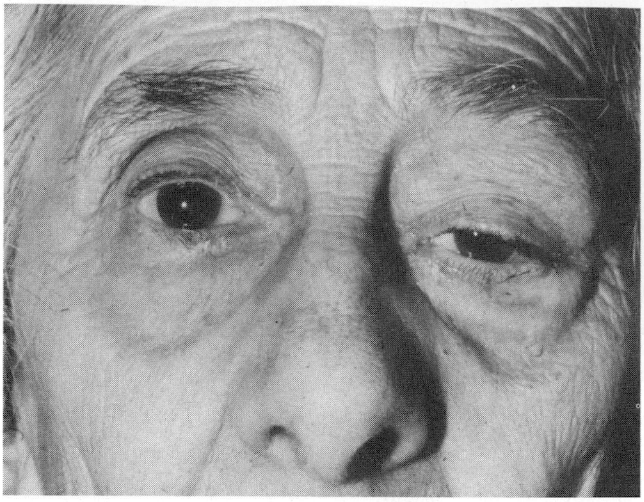

FIG. 35.8. Orbital malignant lymphoma. This 84-year-old woman presented with a 36-month history of painless, increasing left-sided proptosis. A rubbery superolateral mass was palpated. Incisional biopsy demonstrated a monoclonal B-cell lymphoma of the mucosa-associated lymphoid tissue type. The patient received localized radiation therapy, and the lesion regressed. The patient died 8 years later without evidence of orbital or systemic lymphoma. (From Knowles DM, Jakobiec FA, Halper JP. Immunologic characterization of ocular adnexal lymphoid neoplasms. *Am J Ophthalmol* 1979; 87:603–619, with permission.)

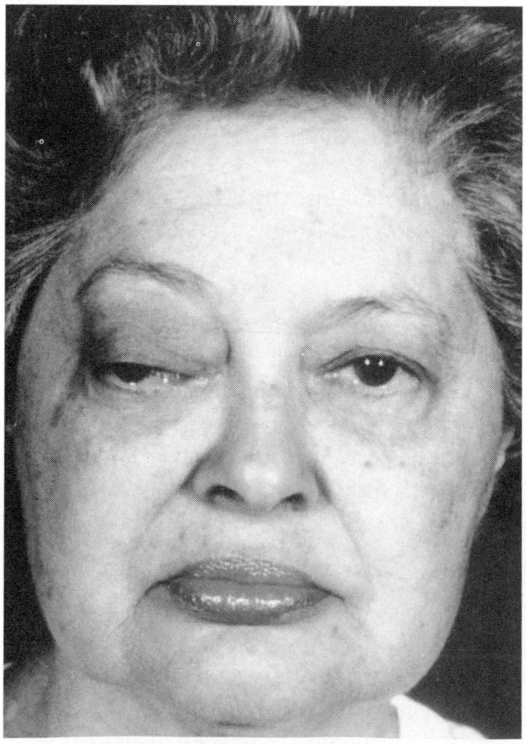

FIG. 35.9. Orbital malignant lymphoma. This woman presented with a superior and superonasal orbital monoclonal B-cell lymphoma that caused proptosis and lateral displacement of the globe. On evaluation, the patient was found to have no evidence of systemic lymphoma. The lesion was treated with local radiation therapy and regressed.

diplopia (Figs. 35.8, 35.9). Lesions should be designated as conjunctival if they occur as freely movable salmon patches on the epibulbar, forniceal, caruncular, or palpebral surfaces without infiltrating the eyelid skin or encroaching on the orbit. These lesions do not cause ptosis or orbital signs such as proptosis or diplopia (Fig. 35.10, 35.11). Lesions should be designated as occurring primarily in the eyelids if the dermis or orbicularis muscle of the anterior eyelid skin is

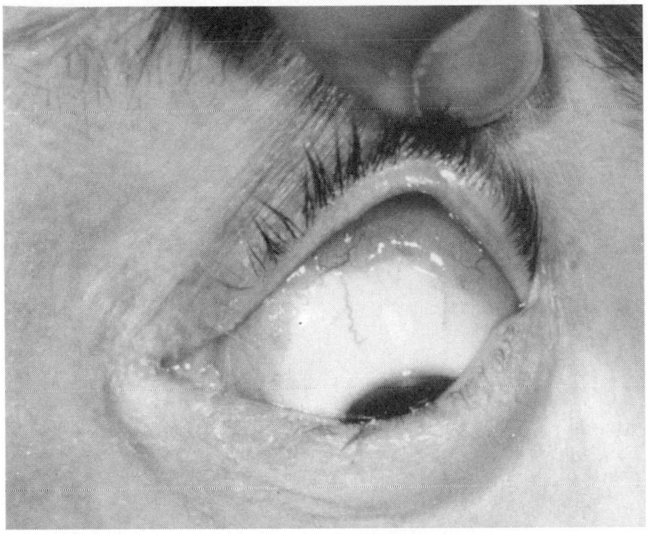

FIG. 35.10. Conjunctival lymphoid proliferation. A typical sausage-shaped swelling of the superofornix occurred in a patient with a lymphoid lesion confined to the substantia propria of the conjunctiva. These lesions are sometimes referred to as salmon patches by clinical ophthalmologists. (From Knowles DM, Jakobiec FA, McNally L, et al. Lymphoid hyperplasia and malignant lymphoma occurring in the ocular adnexa [orbit, conjunctiva, and eyelids]: a prospective multiparametric analysis of 108 cases during 1977–1987. *Hum Pathol* 1990;21:959–973, with permission.)

infiltrated and if they are located anterior to the orbital septum (found by physical examination or imaging studies). These lesions occur predominantly in the superior eyelids, where they nearly always cause ptosis. They almost never cause ocular displacement or proptosis (32) (Figs. 35.12, 35.13).

Clinical Characteristics

Patients who have ocular adnexal lymphoid proliferations, regardless of histopathology (i.e., lymphoid hyperplasia, atypical lymphoid hyperplasia, or malignant lymphoma) or bilaterality, do not appear to differ significantly with respect to age, sex, presenting complaints, duration of symptoms, or ophthalmic findings (3–5,32,53,118). The one exception is pain associated with bone erosion on radiologic examination, which apparently is only observed in malignant lymphoma (4,59,151), primarily large B-cell lymphomas (59,152). Otherwise, clinical evaluation alone usually is of little value in distinguishing benign and malignant ocular adnexal lymphoid proliferations. For this reason, these proliferations are grouped together for the purpose of discussing their clinical characteristics (Table 35.1).

In the experience of Knowles and Jakobiec (32), these patients range in age from 17 to 93 years. About 85% of patients are 50 years of age or older, and the median age is 61 years, regardless of the anatomic site of disease. Other investigators agree. For example, Coupland and colleagues

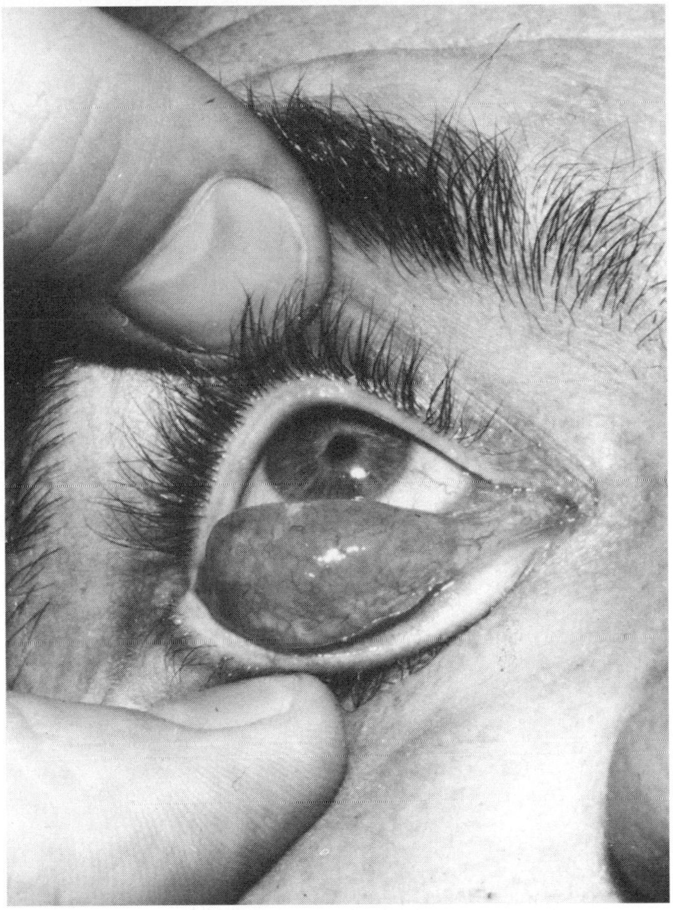

FIG. 35.11. Conjunctival lymphoid proliferation. This 39-year-old man presented with a 2-month history of increasing fullness of the right lower lid unaccompanied by diplopia, proptosis, or displacement of the globe. The lymphoid lesion is exposed by eversion of the right lower eyelid. The lesion is restricted to the tarsal and inferior forniceal conjunctiva, making this a conjunctival rather than an eyelid lymphoid proliferation. Excisional biopsy demonstrated a polyclonal follicular lymphoid hyperplasia. No additional therapy was administered. The patient was alive and well without evidence of ocular adnexal or systemic lymphoma 115 months later. (From Knowles DM, Jakobiec FA, Halper JP. Immunologic characterization of ocular adnexal lymphoid neoplasms. *Am J Ophthalmol* 1979;87:603–619, with permission.)

reported that 112 patients collected from Germany and Scotland ranged in age from 14 to 91 years (median, 61 years) (59). Ocular adnexal lymphoid proliferations occur very uncommonly in children. Many of the childhood orbital ''histiocytic lymphomas'' reported many years ago probably represent granulocytic sarcomas, embryonal rhabdomyosarcomas, or other neoplasms and not malignant lymphomas (53). Knowles and Jakobiec (32) and Coupland and colleagues (59) reported a male to female ratio of 1:1.4 and 1:2.5, respectively, for all lymphoid proliferations occurring in all adnexal locations. Ocular adnexal lymphoid proliferations occur primarily in the sixth and seventh decades of life, and more often affect women than men.

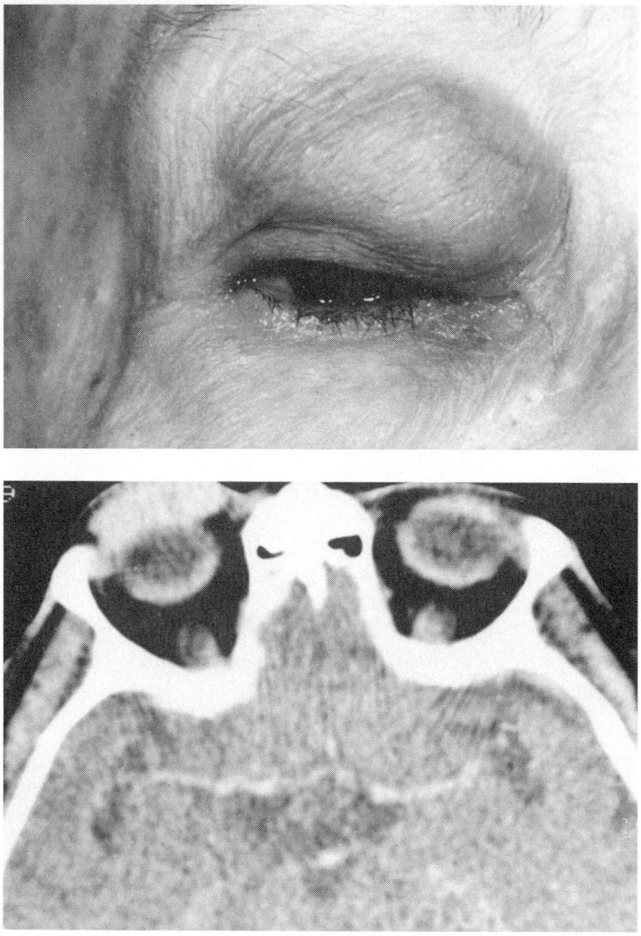

A

B

FIG. 35.12. Eyelid lymphoid proliferation. **A:** The clinical appearance of an elderly patient presenting with a lymphoid proliferation of the upper eyelid that infiltrated the dermis of the eyelid skin and the orbicularis striated muscle. **B:** The CT scan indicates that the mass is confined to the lid tissues and occupies the lid space anterior to the orbital septum. The retroseptal orbital tissues are not infiltrated, and there were no orbital findings on physical examination (e.g., absence of proptosis, ocular displacement or diplopia). The patient was discovered to have systemic lymphoma on further evaluation. (From Knowles DM, Jakobiec FA, McNally L, et al. Lymphoid hyperplasia and malignant lymphoma occurring in the ocular adnexa [orbit, conjunctiva, and eyelids]: a prospective multiparametric analysis of 108 cases during 1977–1987. *Hum Pathol* 1990;21:959–973, with permission.)

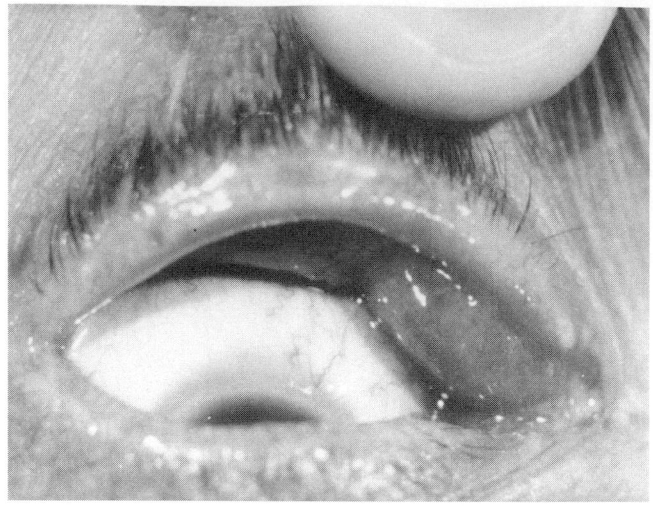

FIG. 35.13. Eyelid lymphoid proliferation. This lymphoid tumor with a rounded appearance affected the upper eyelid and penetrated through the tarsus to beneath the palpebral conjunctiva. The lesion was a monoclonal diffuse large B-cell lymphoma. Systemic evaluation revealed evidence of systemic malignant lymphoma.

In the experience of Knowles and Jakobiec (32), lymphoid proliferations occurring within the ocular adnexa are distributed as follows: orbit, 64%; conjunctiva, 28%; and eyelids, 8%. Coupland and colleagues reported a slightly lower proportion of orbital, a slightly higher proportion of eyelid, and an identical proportion of conjunctival lesions (59). Among persons who have orbital lesions, about 46% have lacrimal gland involvement and 54% have involvement of the non–lacrimal gland orbital soft tissues. All orbital lesions may be considered together, however, because their clinical and other characteristics are virtually identical (32).

Lymphoid proliferations involve the right and left adnexa about equally and are bilateral in about 15% of cases. Approximately 80% of patients with bilateral ocular adnexal lymphoid proliferations have simultaneous bilateral disease; the remaining patients initially present with a unilateral lesion and subsequently develop a lesion in the contralateral eye. Equal proportions of patients with orbital, conjunctival, and eyelid lesions develop bilateral disease (32,118). In most cases, bilateral orbital, bilateral conjunctival, or bilateral eyelid lesions occur (32,118). Rarely, for example, does a bilateral lesion develop that involves the conjunctiva in one eye and the orbit in the other eye (153).

Approximately 90% of patients who present with an orbital lymphoid proliferation complain of a mass or swelling, proptosis or ocular displacement, diplopia, or ptosis. Less common secondary complaints include redness, irritation, and pain. Nearly all of these patients have a palpable mass, proptosis, ocular displacement, diplopia or decreased ocular motility on physical examination. The mass usually is firm to rubbery (Figs. 35.8, 35.9). About 20% of patients are discovered to have a history or concurrent evidence of extraocular lymphoma (32,152).

Approximately 80% of patients who present with a conjunctival lymphoid proliferation complain of a mass or swelling. These lesions are situated in the substantia propria of the conjunctiva and do not infiltrate the anterior orbital tissues or the anterior eyelid skin. They do not cause orbital signs and symptoms, namely proptosis, ocular displacement, or diplopia. Essentially every patient is discovered to have a palpable mass on physical examination, by palpating a fullness through the lid or by everting the eyelid and finding the typical thickening on the forniceal, epibulbar, or palpebral conjunctiva. The mass typically is salmon or pink to

TABLE 35.1. *Clinical characteristics of 108 patients presenting with ocular adnexal lymphoid proliferations*

Parameter	Orbit	Conjunctiva	Eyelid	Total
Patients (no.)	69	30	9	108
Age range (yr)	17–93	29–89	48–85	17–93
Median (yr)	63	60	63	61
Male–female ratio	35:34	7:23	3:6	45:63
Location				
Right	29	12	7	48
Left	31	12	1	44
Bilateral	9	6	1	16
Chief complaint				
Mass/swelling	59	24	9	92
Ptosis	6	1	9	16
None—incidental finding	0	3	0	3
Other	4	2	0	6
Secondary complaints				
Diplopia	9	0	0	9
Ptosis	5	0	0	5
Pain	1	0	0	1
Other	3	4	0	7
Duration of symptoms				
Range (mo)	1–72	0.25–120	2–36	0.25–120
Median (mo)	4	4	4	4
Physical findings				
Ocular				
Palpable mass	56	30	9	95
Proptosis	34	0	0	34
Ptosis	13	1	9	23
Diplopia	9	0	0	9
Decreased motility	8	0	0	8
Other	1	0	0	1
Extraocular				
Negative	56	27	7	90
Lymphadenopathy	11	2	2	15
Hepatomegaly	3	0	0	3
Splenomegaly	4	1	0	5
Other	1	0	0	1
Number of patients with concurrent extraocular lymphoma	13	3	4	20
Locations				
Lymph nodes	12	2	4	18
Bone marrow	8	1	0	9
Peripheral Blood	2	1	0	3
Other	6	2	1	9

From Knowles DM, Jakobiec FA, McNally FA, et al. Lymphoid hyperplasia and malignant lymphoma occurring in the ocular adnexa (orbit, conjunctiva, and eyelids): a prospective multiparametric analysis of 108 cases during 1977–1987. *Hum Pathol* 1990;21:959–973, with permission.

flesh colored, sausage shaped, and freely movable (Figs. 35.10, 35.11). Only about 10% of patients are discovered to have a history or concurrent evidence of extraocular lymphoma (32).

Essentially all patients who present with an eyelid lymphoid proliferation complain of ptosis and a mass or swelling of the eyelid. These lesions represent infiltrations of the dermis and orbicularis muscle of the anterior eyelid skin in front of the orbital septum. This results in a palpable mass with a firm to rubbery consistency that causes ptosis. These patients do not develop orbital signs and symptoms (Figs. 35.12, 35.13). They frequently are discovered to have a history or concurrent evidence of extraocular lymphoma (32).

The duration of symptoms varies markedly, from as short as 1 week to as long as 10 years. The median duration of symptoms is approximately 4 months, however, regardless of the anatomic location of the lesion within the ocular adnexa (32).

The nonophthalmic findings discovered on general physical examination depend on the presence or absence of systemic malignant lymphoma and vary according to the anatomic location of the lesion within the ocular adnexa. Knowles and Jakobiec found that 90% of patients with con-

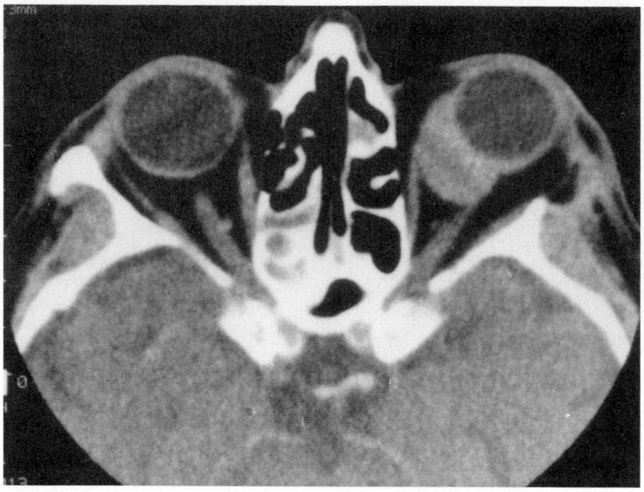

FIG. 35.14. CT scan of an orbital lymphoid proliferation. A retrobulbar nasal lymphoid proliferation molded to the posterior sclera of the globe. Despite its size, this lesion produced only minimal proptosis.

junctival, 81% with orbital, and 78% with eyelid lymphoid proliferations have a negative nonophthalmic physical examination. Most of the remaining patients have lymphadenopathy, hepatomegaly, or splenomegaly (32). However, biopsy examination often reveals that the lymphadenopathy is merely reactive and not the result of involvement by malignant lymphoma (32,154). Fewer than 10% of patients are found to have peripheral blood or bone marrow involvement by malignant lymphoma (32,152). A small subset of lymphoplasmacytic lymphomas, histologically indistinguishable from the nodal lymphomas observed in Waldenström's macroglobulinemia, may be associated with a monoclonal gammopathy and systemic disease (27,59). These lymphomas also may be associated with the local or systemic deposition of amyloid (24,155–157).

Radiologic Characteristics

CT greatly assists in the preoperative evaluation of patients who have orbital lesions, including determination of the location, size and extent of a lesion, which are essential

A

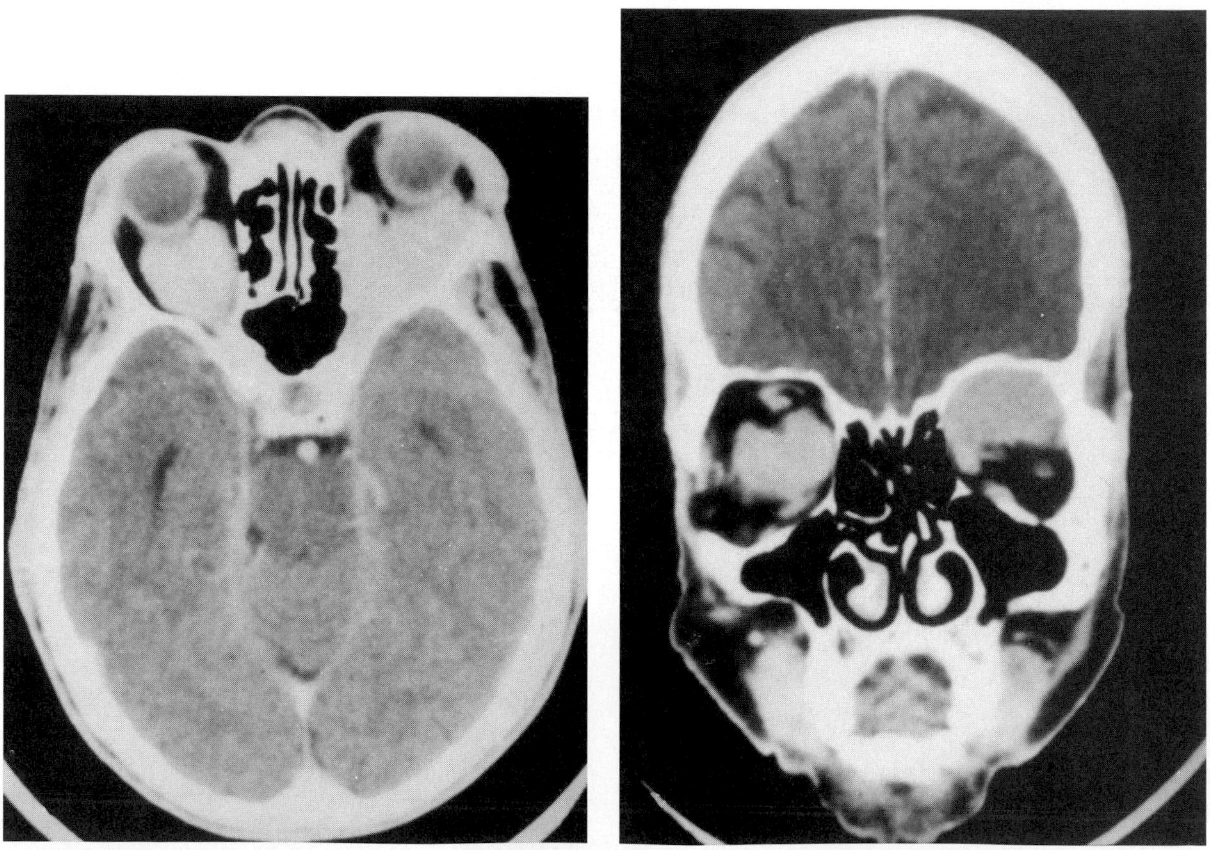

B

FIG. 35.15. CT scan of a bilateral orbital malignant lymphoma. **A:** Bilateral orbital malignant lymphoma occurring in an elderly patient surrounds the optic nerve bilaterally, conferring a bilobed appearance. Particularly on the left, the negative optic nerve shadow can be seen running down the middle of the lesion. Despite the presence of tumor tissue surrounding the optic nerve, vision was well preserved because of absence of compression as a result of the stroma-free nature of the lymphoid proliferation. **B:** A coronal projection of the axial depiction of the lesion shown in **A**. There is no bone destruction, which is typical of most orbital lymphoid proliferations. There is also molding of the lesional tissue to the bone of the roof of the orbit.

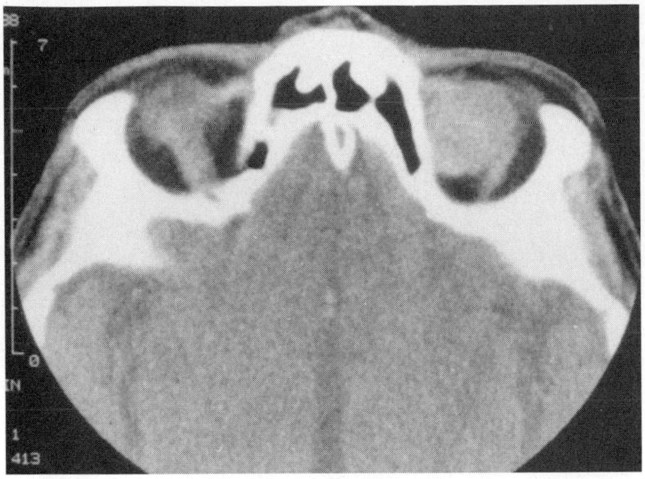

FIG. 35.16. CT scan of an orbital lymphoid proliferation. A superior orbital lymphoid proliferation molding as a straight line to the bone of the medial orbital wall without bone destruction.

factors in planning the surgical approach and treatment (158,159) (Figs. 35.6, 35.7, 35.12). CT also can provide a strong presumptive diagnosis of a lymphoid proliferation within the orbit. However, CT reveals no known characteristic features that permit this technique to discriminate reliably, much less definitively, between benign and malignant orbital lymphoid proliferations (53,151,158,160).

Orbital lymphoid hyperplasias and malignant lymphomas are nearly always unifocal mass lesions, in contrast to orbital pseudotumors, which frequently are multifocal. Most are located in the orbital fat and soft tissues. Most of the remaining lesions are represented by diffuse, oblong, molded expansions of the lacrimal gland (53). Rarely, a lymphoid proliferation may be situated predominantly within an extraocular muscle (158,161).

CT demonstrates the distinctive tendency of orbital lymphoid proliferations to mold or plaster themselves along preexisting orbital structures (158). They may contour to the globe, lacrimal gland, optic nerve, extraocular muscles, and orbital bones, but they do not enlarge the orbit and only rarely cause bone destruction. Arclike contours are seen in coronal planes in which the lesions abut against orbital bones and sclera. Straight lines and unusually angulated patterns may be seen on CT soft tissue analysis. These are caused by abutments against the orbital bones, optic nerve, or fascial planes or by delimitations caused by fibrous connective tissue strands. Irregular margins are seen in the orbital soft tissue because of a lack of encapsulation and the irregular replacement of lobules of orbital fat (53,158) (Figs. 35.14–35.16).

Lymphoid proliferations involving the lacrimal gland generally create a diffuse expansion of the gland, exaggerating its normally oblong and pancake character in axial and coronal computed tomograms. The lesions mold to the globe and to the adjacent bone without producing a fossa in the bone. The anterior aspect of the lesion may extend beyond the orbital rim, indicating involvement of the palpebral lobe. The posterior aspect of the lesion that abuts against the orbital fat often gives the appearance of a straight line (53).

Histopathology

Classification

Previously, Knowles and Jakobiec proposed a histopathologic classification system for the ocular adnexal lymphoid proliferations that divided them into three broad categories: lymphoid hyperplasia (follicular or diffuse), atypical lymphoid hyperplasia, and malignant lymphoma (162) (Table 35.2). The term *lymphoid hyperplasia* was used to designate the hypercellular, lymphoid cell–rich lesions that mimic malignant lymphoma clinically and histopathologically (Figs. 35.17–35.19). The term *atypical lymphoid hyperplasia* was used to designate those lymphoid proliferations that cannot be categorized unequivocally as lymphoid

TABLE 35.2. *Histopathologic classification of ocular adnexal lymphoid proliferations*

Former classification (162)	Current classification
Lymphoid hyperplasia	Lymphoid Hyperplasia
Diffuse	Diffuse
Follicular	Follicular
Atypical lymphoid hyperplasia	Atypical lymphoid hyperplasia
Malignant lymphoma subclassified according to the Working Formulation (60)	Malignant lymphoma subclassified according to the REAL classification (121)[a]
Small lymphocytic, diffuse	B-cell chronic lymphocytic leukemia/small lymphocytic lymphoma
Small lymphocytic, plasmacytoid, diffuse	Lymphoplasmacytoid lymphoma
Intermediate lymphocytic, diffuse	Mantle cell lymphoma
Small cleaved cell, diffuse or follicular	Follicle center lymphoma
Mixed small and large cell, diffuse or follicular	Extranodal marginal zone (MALT) lymphoma
Large cell, diffuse or follicular	Diffuse large B-cell lymphoma
Lymphoblastic	
Small, noncleaved cell, diffuse	
Plasmacytoma, including myeloma	

[a] Chapter 19 provides additional categories of the REAL classification.

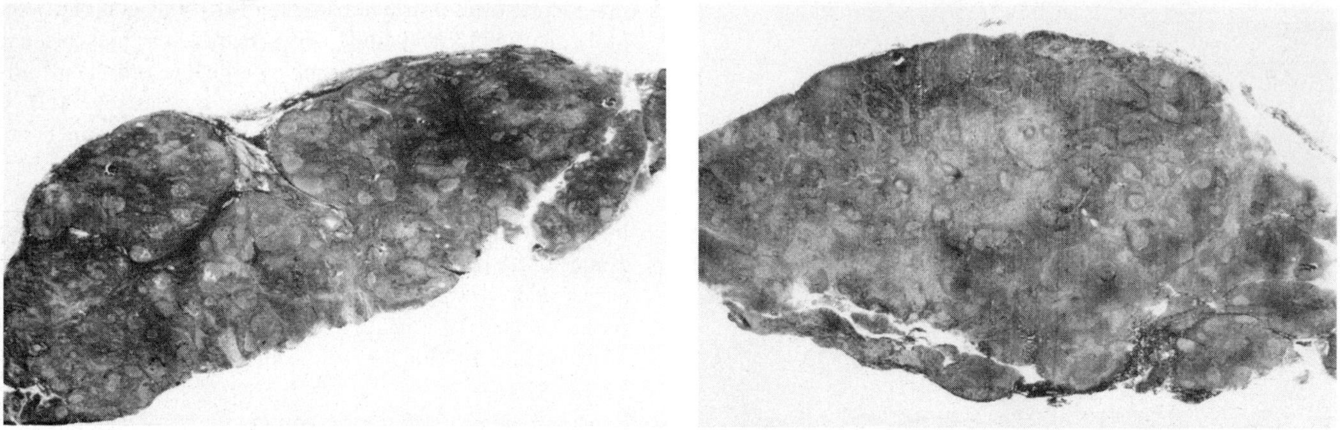

FIG. 35.17. Bilateral lacrimal gland follicular lymphoid hyperplasia. Each lacrimal gland shows extensive and dense lymphoid infiltration. Numerous, well-formed germinal centers are present. Immunophenotypic analysis demonstrated a polyclonal cell marker profile. Immunoglobulin gene rearrangement studies failed to demonstrate evidence for a clonal B-cell proliferation (hematoxylin and eosin stain, original magnification: 5× magnification). (From McNally L, Jakobiec FA, Knowles DM. Clinical, morphologic, immunophenotypic, and molecular genetic analysis of bilateral ocular adnexal lymphoid neoplasms in 17 patients. *Am J Ophthalmol* 1987;103:555–568, with permission.)

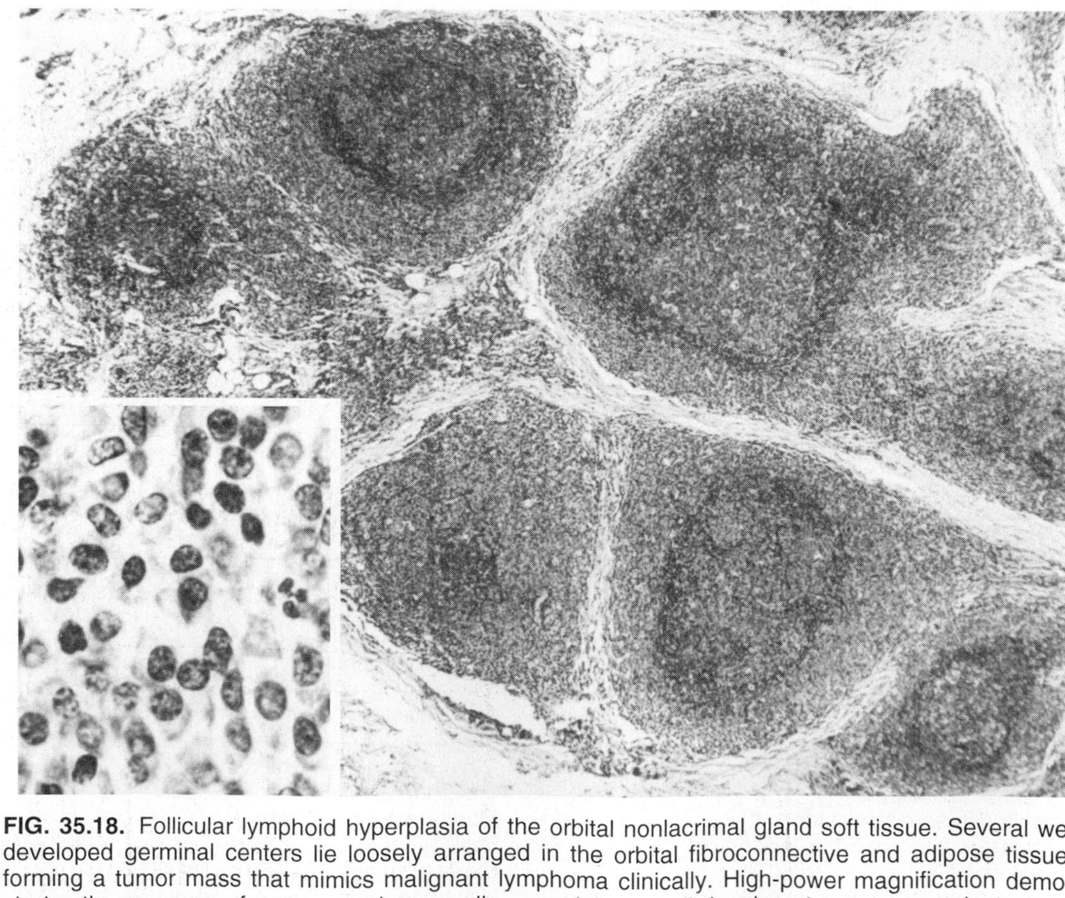

FIG. 35.18. Follicular lymphoid hyperplasia of the orbital nonlacrimal gland soft tissue. Several well-developed germinal centers lie loosely arranged in the orbital fibroconnective and adipose tissues, forming a tumor mass that mimics malignant lymphoma clinically. High-power magnification demonstrates the presence of numerous plasma cells around these well-developed reactive germinal centers (hematoxylin and eosin stain, original magnifications: 37× magnification; **Inset:** 600× magnification). (From Knowles DM, Jakobiec FA, Halper JP. Immunologic characterization of ocular adnexal lymphoid neoplasms. *Am J Ophthalmol* 1979;87:603–619, with permission.)

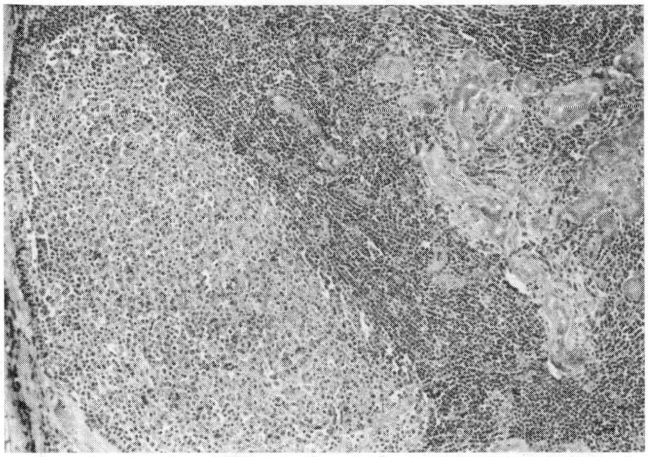

FIG. 35.19. Higher-power magnification of the lacrimal gland follicular lymphoid hyperplasia illustrated in Figure 35.17. A large reactive germinal center is easily distinguished from a neoplastic follicle by its polymorphous cell population, large numbers of mitotic figures, and numerous tingible body macrophages. This reactive germinal center also is surrounded by a polymorphous cell population and numerous large vessels lined by hypertrophic endothelial cells. Islands of residual lacrimal gland acini also are present (hematoxylin and eosin stain, original magnification: 100× magnification). (From McNally L, Jakobiec FA, Knowles DM. Clinical, morphologic, immunophenotypic, and molecular genetic analysis of bilateral ocular adnexal lymphoid neoplasms in 17 patients. *Am J Ophthalmol* 1987;103:555–568, with permission.)

hyperplasia or malignant lymphoma. Knowles and Jakobiec subclassified the malignant lymphomas according to the then widely accepted Working Formulation (163), recognizing the additional entities intermediate lymphocytic lymphoma (14,15) and mantle zone lymphoma (16) that were not included in that classification.

It is recommended that the terms *lymphoid hyperplasia* and *atypical lymphoid hyperplasia* be retained but that the malignant lymphomas be classified according to the REAL classification (121) (Table 35.2). This is especially important because such a large proportion of the ocular adnexal malignant lymphomas have been shown to represent MALT (extranodal marginal zone) lymphomas (59,122,164) and because of the greater prognostic value of the REAL classification when applied to ocular adnexal malignant lymphomas (59,122).

Lymphoid Hyperplasia

In 1978, based solely on morphologic examination, Sigelman and Jakobiec (154) suggested that the small lymphocytic proliferations of the conjunctiva represent hyperplasia of the indigenous conjunctival lymphoid tissue, which we now know represents MALT (135). This assessment led to the belief that lymphoid hyperplasias outnumber malignant lymphomas in the conjunctiva by 5 to 1 (5,154). Later, Knowles and Jakobiec demonstrated by immunophenotypic analysis that most of these conjunctival small lymphocytic proliferations represent monoclonal small B-cell lymphomas (32). They suggested that approximately 27% and 70% of ocular adnexal lymphoid proliferations, unilateral and bilateral, are lymphoid hyperplasias and malignant lymphomas, respectively; they considered the remaining 3% of cases unclassifiable (e.g., atypical lymphoid hyperplasias) (32,118). According to their analysis, approximately equivalent proportions of the lymphoid proliferations occurring in the orbit and conjunctiva are lymphoid hyperplasias, whereas most of those occurring in the eyelid are malignant lymphomas. In summary, according to Knowles and Jakobiec, 30% of orbital and 26% of conjunctival, but only 10% of eyelid lymphoid proliferations are lymphoid hyperplasias (32). Regardless of location, most lymphoid hyperplasias are follicular (i.e., contain reactive germinal centers) (32).

In some studies, lymphoid hyperplasias constitute an even lower proportion of ocular adnexal lymphoid proliferations, however. For example, Coupland and colleagues (59) classified only 12 of 102 (12%) and White and coworkers (165) classified even fewer ocular adnexal lymphoid proliferations as lymphoid hyperplasia. It is likely that patient referral patterns or case selection bias account in part for this discrepancy. However, the lower percentage of lymphoid hyperplasias in recent series also reflects increased histopathologic sophistication, an awareness of MALT lymphomas, and an enhanced ability to detect clonality because of technologic advances in immunohistochemical, flow cytometric, and molecular genetic methods. Fifteen years ago, Knowles and Jakobiec (37,119) and, later, other investigators (166,167) detected small clonal B-cell populations by molecular genetic techniques in some ocular adnexal lymphoid proliferations that were otherwise considered to be lymphoid hyperplasias (primarily diffuse) morphologically and immunophenotypically. Today, many investigators would interpret at least some of those lesions as malignant lymphomas, primarily belonging to the MALT category.

Lymphoid hyperplasias are hypercellular, lymphoid cell–rich lesions that can mimic malignant lymphomas clinically and histopathologically, sometimes to an extraordinary degree (Fig. 35.17). In contrast to pseudotumors but like malignant lymphomas, they lack a significant connective tissue stroma. The term *follicular* is used for lymphoid hyperplasias that contain prominent reactive germinal centers, and the term *diffuse* is used for lymphoid hyperplasias devoid of reactive germinal centers. Some follicular lymphoid hyperplasias are composed predominantly of reactive germinal centers that lie almost back to back (Fig. 35.18). Reactive germinal centers usually are easily distinguished from neoplastic follicles by their polymorphous cell population, high mitotic rate, and numerous tingible body macrophages (Fig. 35.19). The diffuse lymphoid hyperplasias are composed largely of a densely cellular, sometimes seemingly monomorphous, infiltrate of small lymphocytes. Dutcher bodies are absent. Occasional immunoblasts, plasma cells, and histiocytes are almost invariably present, however, im-

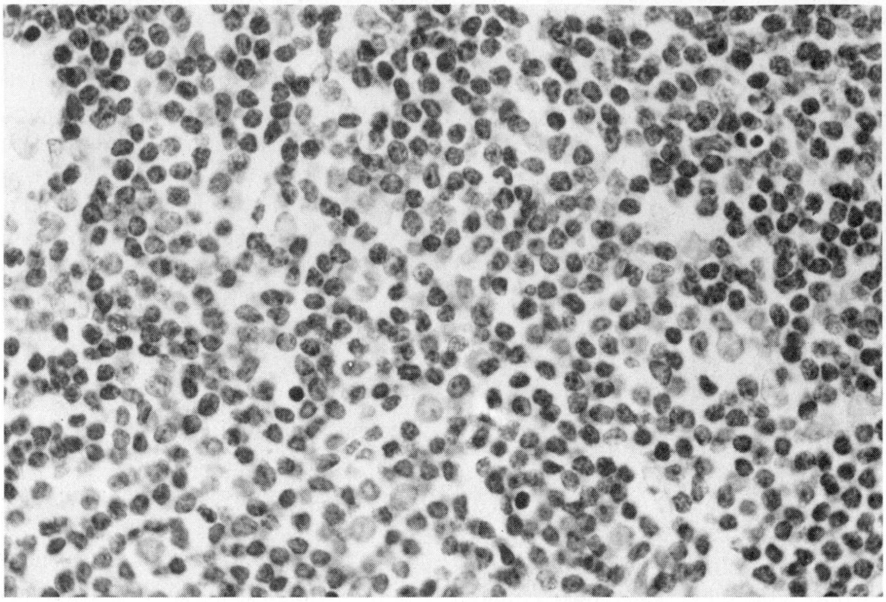

FIG. 35.20. Diffuse lymphoid hyperplasia of the orbit. Diffuse lymphoid hyperplasias tend to be less densely cellular than small B-cell lymphomas. They also are composed of small lymphocytes admixed with a few plasma cells, immunoblasts, and histiocytes. This subtle cellular polymorphism is helpful in distinguishing diffuse lymphoid hyperplasia from small B-cell lymphomas (hematoxylin and eosin stain, original magnification: 500× magnification).

parting a subtle yet detectable polymorphous appearance (Fig. 35.20). This cellular polymorphism greatly assists in distinguishing diffuse lymphoid hyperplasias from small B-cell lymphomas that usually are monomorphic. Neutrophils and eosinophils are absent. Mitotic figures are infrequent. Numerous vessels lined by prominent hypertrophic endothelial cells are often present. Hemosiderin may be present (32,162). The lymphoepithelial lesions characteristically seen in MALT lymphomas (120) are absent (32,59).

Atypical Lymphoid Hyperplasia

Atypical lymphoid hyperplasias are those lymphoid proliferations that cannot be categorized unequivocally as lymphoid hyperplasia or malignant lymphoma. Most are predominantly diffuse, densely cellular lymphoid proliferations that fail to display a sufficiently obvious degree of cellular polymorphism or monomorphism to permit definitive classification as lymphoid hyperplasia or malignant lymphoma. At one time, Knowles and Jakobiec classified as many as 10% of all ocular adnexal lymphoid proliferations as atypical lymphoid hyperplasia (4). Since then, extensive correlative histopathologic and immunophenotypic studies, many supported by antigen receptor gene rearrangement analyses, have taught us that the diffuse, densely cellular, monomorphic ocular adnexal small lymphocytic proliferations, including those cases that contain reactive germinal centers or in which most of the cells display plasmacytoid differentiation, represent small B-cell lymphomas (5,19,20,23,29,31, 32,37,38,55,58,59,116,136,152,165,168). Most ocular adnexal lymphoid proliferations not readily categorized as lymphoid hyperplasia or malignant lymphoma by morphologic criteria alone usually can be classified after immunophenotypic or molecular genetic analysis. Only about 5% or less of ocular adnexal lymphoid proliferations are classified as atypical lymphoid hyperplasia at the present time (59,122,165).

Malignant Lymphoma

Most malignant lymphomas occurring in the ocular adnexa are diffuse, densely cellular proliferations composed predominantly of small lymphoid cells superimposed on a sparse connective tissue stroma (Fig. 35.21). Based on the Working Formulation (163) and the prevailing criteria for classifying malignant lymphomas in the mid-1980s, Knowles and Jakobiec categorized 82 ocular adnexal malignant lymphomas as follows: small lymphocytic (38%), intermediate lymphocytic (mantle cell) (18%), plasmacytoid small lymphocytic (10%), diffuse small cleaved cell (10%), follicular, predominantly small cleaved cell (9%), follicular, mixed small cleaved and large cell (6%), diffuse large cell (6%), diffuse mixed small and large cell (2%), and follicular large cell (1%) (32). According to their studies, 84% of malignant lymphomas occurring in the ocular adnexa, apparently irrespective of adnexal site, exhibit a diffuse pattern, and the remaining 16% exhibit a follicular growth pattern (32). Small lymphocytic, plasmacytoid small lymphocytic, and mantle cell lymphomas account for two thirds and follicle center and large cell lymphomas account for the remain-

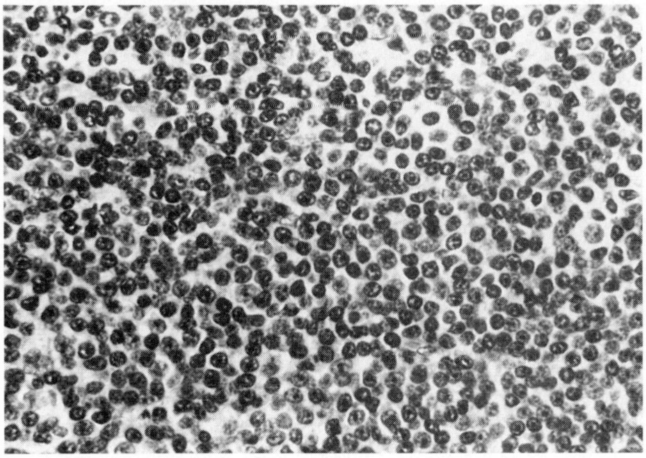

FIG. 35.21. Most malignant lymphomas occurring in the ocular adnexa are diffuse, densely cellular proliferations composed predominately of small lymphoid cells superimposed on a sparse connective tissue stroma.

ing one third of ocular adnexal malignant lymphomas (32). Other investigators generally agree with this distribution when employing the Working Formulation (31,163).

MALT lymphomas were initially recognized by Isaacson and Wright in the gastrointestinal tract in 1983 and in the lung, salivary gland, and thyroid gland shortly thereafter (169,170). Over time, the breadth of distribution and the frequency of occurrence of MALT lymphomas became increasingly appreciated. In the early to mid-1990s investigators began to recognize that the clinicopathologic features of some malignant lymphomas arising in the ocular adnexa resemble those of MALT lymphomas arising at other extranodal sites (29,31,136,152,168,171). It is now known that MALT lymphomas are ubiquitous and comprise a significant proportion of the malignant lymphomas arising in the gastrointestinal tract and in all other extranodal locations where MALT is acquired. This includes the skin, breast, urinary bladder, kidney, and many other sites in addition to the ones already mentioned (172). In the Non-Hodgkin's Lymphoma Classification Project, MALT lymphomas ranked third, constituting almost 8% of all non-Hodgkin's lymphomas, behind diffuse large B-cell and follicle center lymphomas (173). Most ocular adnexal malignant lymphomas arise in MALT, represent MALT lymphomas, and display the morphologic spectrum observed in MALT lymphomas originating in other extranodal sites (122,152,164).

The essential morphologic characteristics of MALT lymphomas is their emulation of normal MALT as exemplified by Peyer's patches found in the terminal ileum (120). MALT lymphomas are characterized by the presence of neoplastic centrocyte-like cells distributed in a marginal zone pattern around reactive follicles and frequently attenuated rims of mantle zone lymphocytes (174). (Figs. 35.22, 35.23). The neoplastic cells are believed to originate from benign equivalents that normally reside in the marginal zone around the mantle zone and the germinal centers (175). The neoplastic centrocyte-like cells may infiltrate into the follicles, at times entirely overtaking them, a process called *follicle colonization* (176). Sometimes, the neoplastic proliferation may be sufficiently extensive to result in architectural obliteration and masking of the residual benign germinal centers. In these instances, the preexisting benign follicles can be highlighted by the immunohistochemical demonstration of $CD21^{+}$ follicular dendritic cells (120). The neoplastic cells also infiltrate the surrounding tissue where they characteristically invade the overlying epithelium to form lymphoepithelial lesions (174), which are associated with epithelial destruction (177) (Fig. 35.24). Their presence can be highlighted by the immunohistochemical demonstration of cytokeratin-positive epithelium in which the neoplastic lymphoid cells lie (120). Coupland and colleagues found lymphoepithelial lesions in the conjunctival or lacrimal gland epithelium in

A

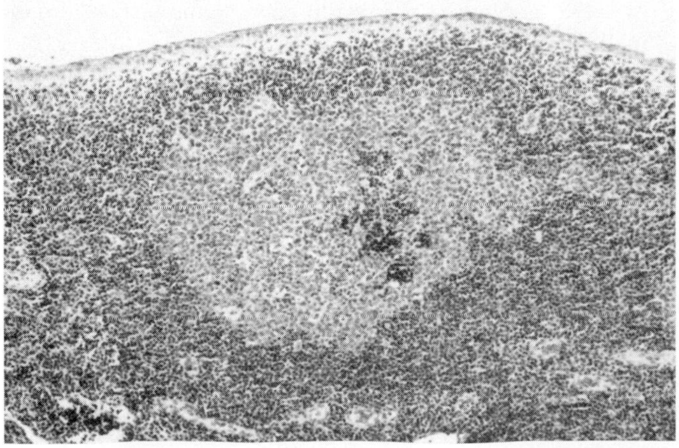

B

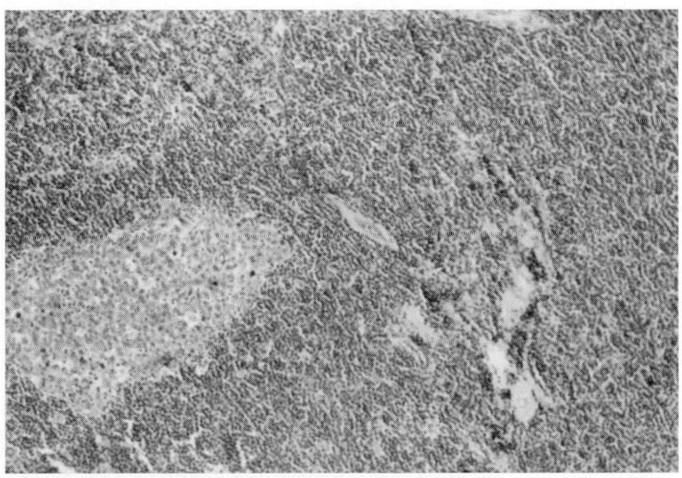

FIG. 35.22. Mucosa-associated lymphoid tissue lymphoma arising in the conjunctiva **(A)** and the orbit **(B)**. In each instance, a benign germinal center is surrounded by a dense, monomorphic small lymphocytic proliferation (hematoxylin and eosin stain, original magnifications: 100× and 40× magnification).

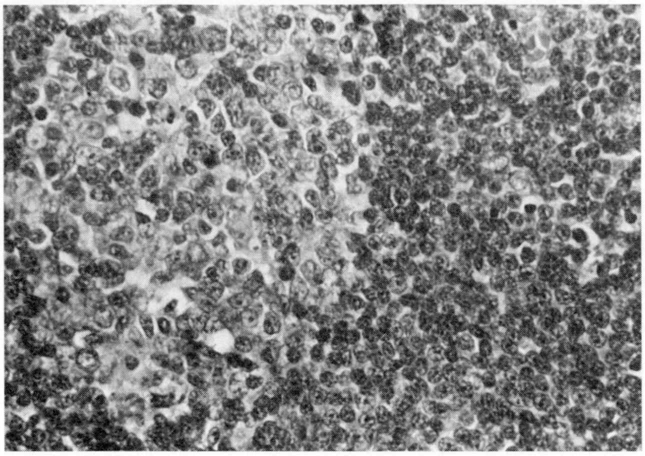

FIG. 35.23. Conjunctival mucosa-associated lymphoid tissue (MALT) lymphoma. MALT lymphomas are characterized by the presence of a dense, monomorphic proliferation of neoplastic centrocyte-like cells distributed in a marginal zone pattern around benign germinal centers (hematoxylin and eosin stain, original magnification: 400× magnification).

70% of the ocular adnexal MALT lymphomas in their series (59). The neoplastic cells may also migrate into the same organ at different locations or into other mucosal sites (172). These properties probably account for the high frequency of multiple localizations of MALT lymphoma in the same organ (i.e., the stomach, at diagnosis [178,179]) as well as recurrences in other organs that harbor MALT (169,180). The latter explains the synchronous and dysynchronous occurrence of MALT lymphoma in the ocular adnexa and other mucosal sites (152,164,181,182).

The neoplastic cells of MALT lymphoma have been called centrocyte-like because of their resemblance to follicle center centrocytes. These cells characteristically are small to medium-sized and contain moderately abundant cytoplasm and irregularly shaped nuclei that bear a close resemblance to those of centrocytes (small cleaved cells) (120) (Fig. 35.25). They exhibit greater cytologic variability than centrocytes, however. Sometimes, they have minimal nuclear membrane irregularities and closely resemble small lymphocytes (Fig. 35.26). Other times, they contain abundant pale-staining to clear cytoplasm and resemble monocytoid B cells. They frequently exhibit plasmacytoid differentiation (120,172,174) (Fig. 35.27). Coupland and colleagues identified Dutcher bodies in more than 20% of the ocular adnexal MALT lymphomas in their series (59). The latter finding suggests that many cases formerly classified as lymphoplasmacytic lymphomas and immunocytomas represent MALT lymphomas. They are capable of undergoing large cell transformation, which is associated with more aggressive clinical behavior (120,137,172).

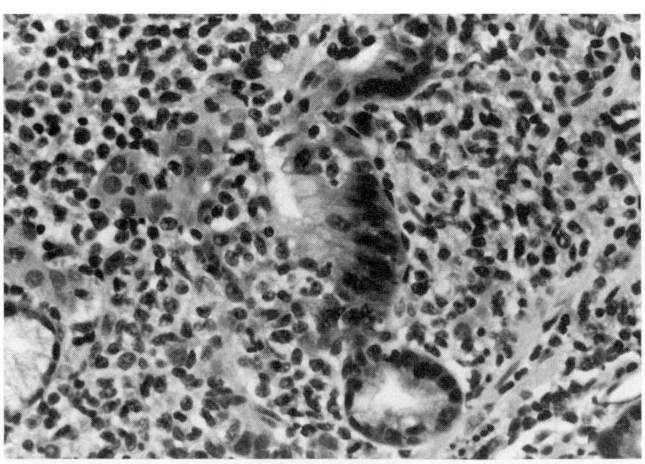

FIG. 35.24. Orbital mucosa-associated lymphoid tissue lymphoma. The neoplastic cells invade the lacrimal gland epithelium, forming so-called lymphoepithelial lesions (hematoxylin and eosin stain, original magnification: 400× magnification).

The MALT lymphomas are classified among the marginal zone B-cell lymphomas in the REAL classification (121). The Working Formulation (163) was developed before the identification of the MALT lymphomas; consequently, they are not specifically included in the Working Formulation (163). MALT lymphomas can be found principally in the small lymphocytic category of the Working Formulation (163) (see Chapter 19). This explains why small lymphocytic lymphoma was the most common category of ocular adnexal malignant lymphoma (27,31,32,152) before the REAL classification (121). However, because of their cytologic variability, MALT lymphomas may also be found included among the plasmacytoid small lymphocytic, diffuse small cleaved, and diffuse mixed small and large cell categories of the Working Formulation (163) (see Chapter 19). MALT lymphomas may be confused with mantle cell lymphomas because of the presence of residual benign reactive follicles (120) and with follicular lymphomas because of their tendency to colonize preexisting benign reactive follicles (176). The wide cytologic spectrum of MALT lymphomas and their consequent misclassification among numerous histologic categories before their recognition accounts for the multiple additional diagnostic categories used by Knowles and Jakobiec (32) and others (31,58) to classify the ocular adnexal malignant lymphomas in the past.

As already discussed, it is not generally recognized that a large proportion of ocular adnexal malignant lymphomas previously classified otherwise instead represent MALT lymphomas. Three large clinicopathologic studies of ocular adnexal lymphoid proliferations (59,122,152) have used the REAL classification (121). All of them included secondary as well as primary ocular adnexal lymphomas, however. Nonetheless, MALT lymphomas comprised approximately 50%, 70%, and 80% of the classifiable ocular adnexal B-cell lymphomas, respectively, in these series (59,122,152). In contrast, small lymphocytic, plasmacytoid small lymphocytic, and mantle cell lymphomas in aggregate comprised only about 5% of the cases in these series (59,122,152). The Working Formulation categories diffuse small cleaved and diffuse mixed small and large cell were not represented at all

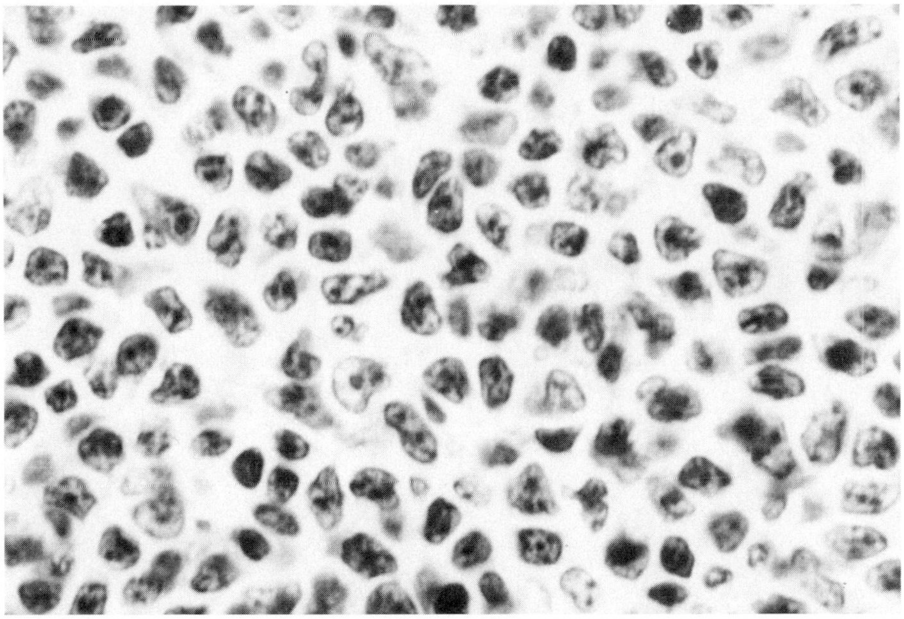

FIG. 35.25. Ocular adnexal mucosa-associated lymphoid tissue (MALT) lymphoma. The malignant lymphoid cells that make up MALT lymphomas have been called centrocyte-like because of their close resemblance to follicle center centrocytes (small cleaved cells). These cells characteristically are small to medium sized and contain moderately abundant cytoplasm and irregularly shaped nuclei (hematoxylin and eosin stain, original magnification: 1,000× magnification).

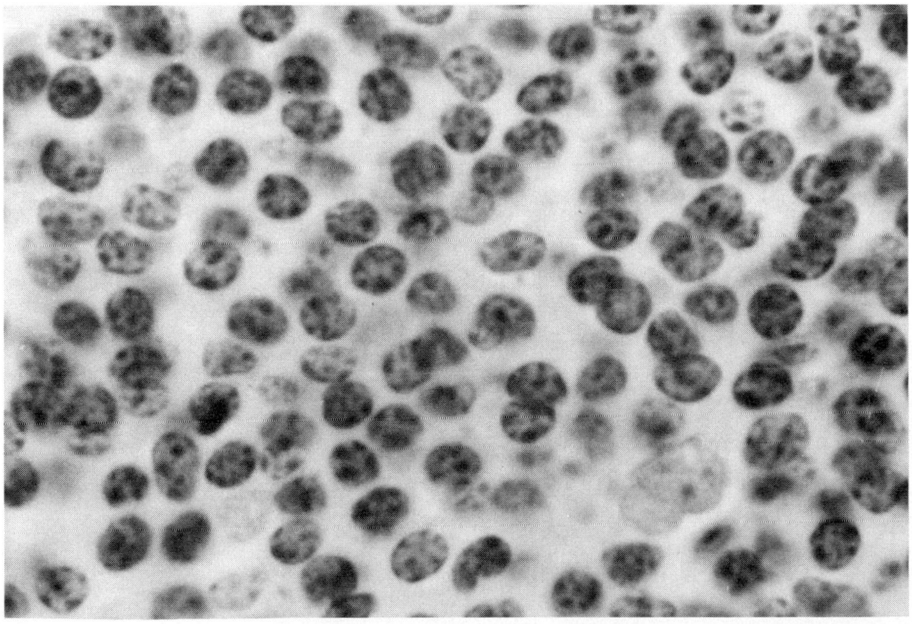

FIG. 35.26. Ocular adnexal mucosa-associated lymphoid tissue (MALT) lymphoma. The centrocyte-like neoplastic cells that make up MALT lymphomas exhibit greater cytologic variability than centrocytes. Sometimes, as in this case, they possess minimal nuclear membrane irregularities and closely resemble the neoplastic cells of small lymphocytic lymphoma. For this reason, many MALT lymphomas were previously included within the small lymphocytic lymphoma category of the Working Formulation (hematoxylin and eosin stain, original magnification: 1,000× magnification).

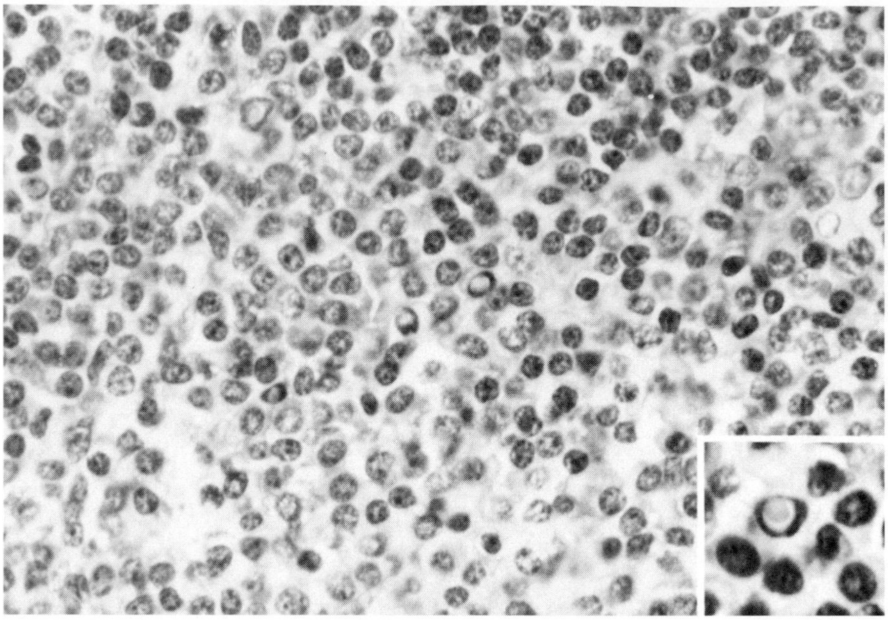

FIG. 35.27. Ocular adnexal mucosa-associated lymphoid tissue (MALT) lymphoma. The centrocyte-like neoplastic cells that make up some MALT lymphomas exhibit plasmacytoid differentiation, including the presence of Dutcher bodies, as in this case. Many such lymphomas were formerly classified as lymphoplasmacytic lymphomas (hematoxylin and eosin stain, original magnifications: 630× magnification; **Inset:** 1,000× magnification).

(59,122,152). Follicular lymphomas (Fig. 35.28) and diffuse large B-cell lymphomas comprised the remainder of the classifiable B-cell lymphomas in these series, ranging between 0% and 20% and between 10% and 23%, respectively (59,122,152). The follicular lymphomas were grade I (mixed small and large cell) or grade II (predominantly small cleaved cell) lesions (59,152). In conclusion, the widespread recognition that MALT lymphomas represent a distinct clinicopathologic entity and the rapidly increasing appreciation for their broad morphologic spectrum has resulted in a dramatic shift in the histopathologic classification of the ocular adnexal malignant lymphomas.

Differential Diagnosis

The histopathologic criteria that traditionally have been used to distinguish between benign and malignant extranodal lymphoid infiltrates emphasize that minimal architectural effacement, the presence of germinal centers, and cytologic maturity and polymorphism favor benignancy, whereas ex-

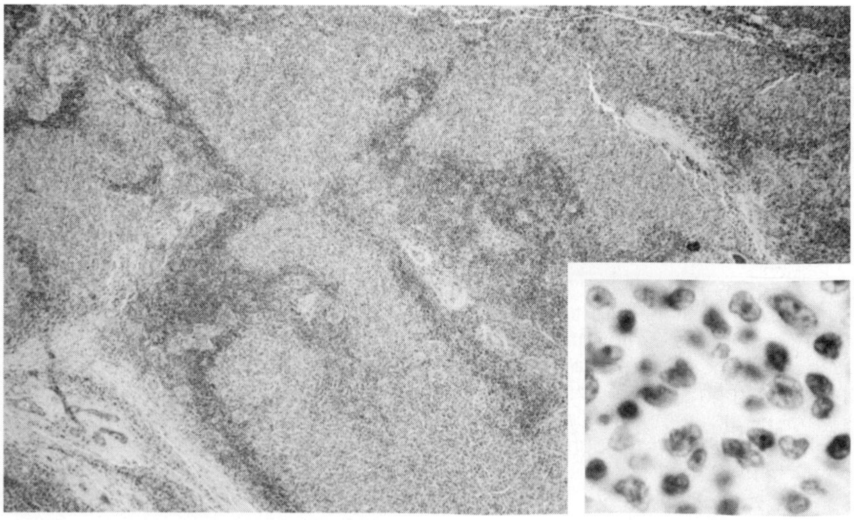

FIG. 35.28. Follicular lymphoma, cytologic grade II, of the lacrimal gland. The lacrimal gland is replaced by lymphoid follicles of variable size and shape. The follicles consist of a mixture of small neoplastic lymphoid cells with irregular, cleaved nuclei and larger neoplastic lymphoid cells with cleaved or noncleaved nuclei (hematoxylin and eosin stain, original magnifications: 50× magnification; **Inset:** 800× magnification).

tensive architectural effacement, the absence of germinal centers, cytologic atypia, and monomorphism favor malignancy (9,10). These criteria often are not only not helpful in evaluating ocular adnexal small lymphocytic proliferations but may be misleading in some instances (6–8). Criteria that sometimes are useful in evaluating nodal lymphoid proliferations, such as effacement of the preexisting lymph node architecture and capsular invasion, are not useful in evaluating ocular adnexal lymphoid proliferations. Lymphoid hyperplasias and malignant lymphomas may infiltrate into the adipose and fibrous connective tissue of the ocular adnexa without regard for anatomic boundaries (4–7). Definitive diagnosis usually depends on careful evaluation of the cytomorphology of the cell populations that comprise the lymphoid proliferation, despite the shortcomings inherent in the application of solely cytologic criteria to proliferations of small lymphocytic cells with a relatively bland cytologic appearance occurring in an extranodal location. For these reasons, some investigators have suggested that ocular adnexal lymphoid proliferations should be designated as small lymphocytic proliferations (183) and others have designated them as atypical (24) or histologically indeterminate (2,25,31,58,184). The latter approach does not truly help patients clinically, nor does it assist in improving our understanding of the natural history and pathobiology of these lesions.

The several parameters that are important to evaluate in the differential diagnosis of ocular adnexal lymphoid proliferations include the presence or absence of reactive germinal centers and pseudofollicular proliferation centers, the rela-

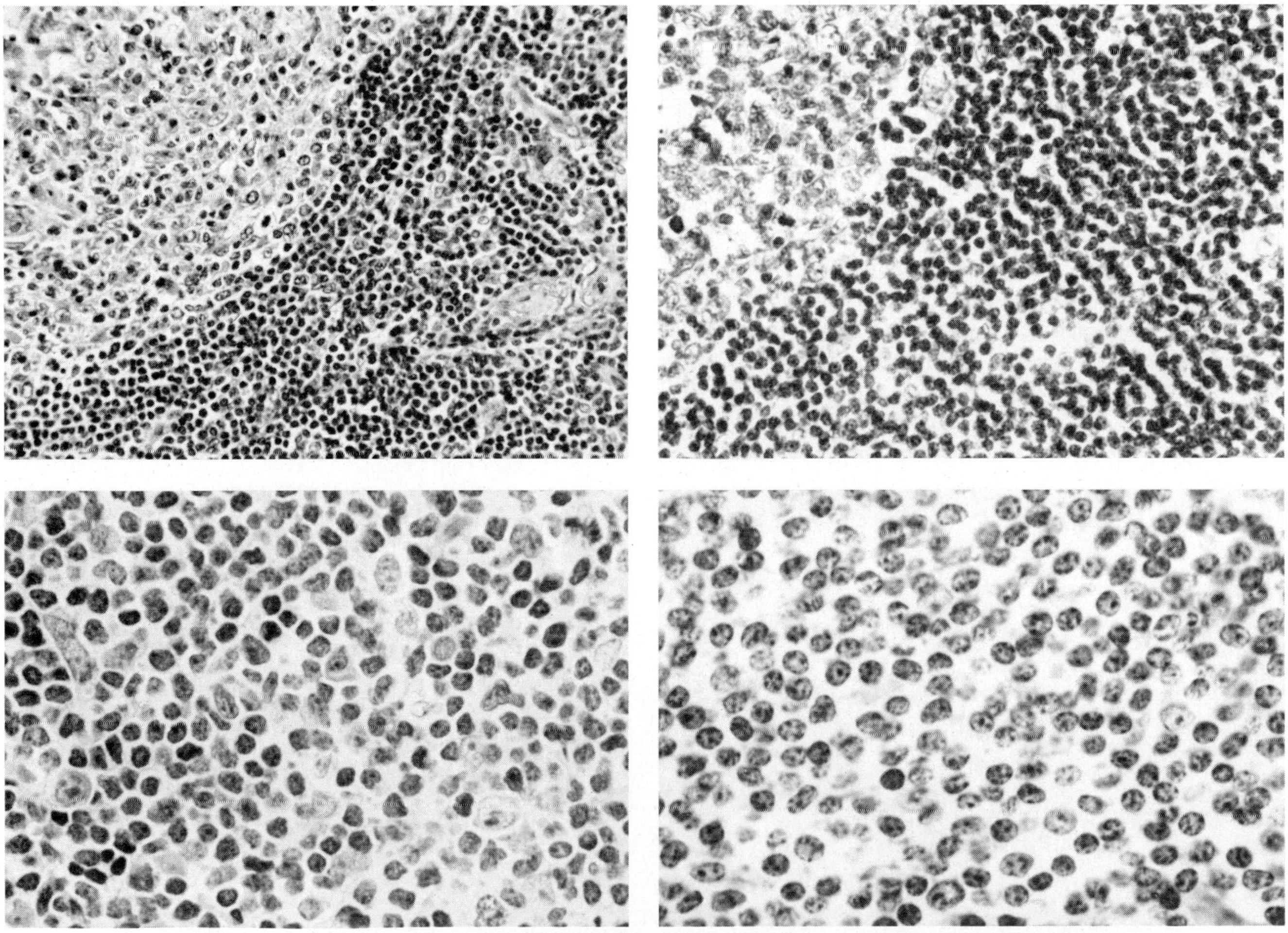

A B C D

FIG. 35.29. Follicular lymphoid hyperplasia **(A)** and mucosa-associated lymphoid tissue (MALT) lymphoma containing a benign germinal center **(B)**. In the follicular lymphoid hyperplasia, the benign germinal center is surrounded by a polymorphous lymphoid proliferation that includes small lymphocytes, plasma cells, immunoblasts, and histiocytes. Numerous prominent vessels lined by hypertrophic endothelial cells also are present **(C)**. The benign germinal center in the midst of a MALT lymphoma is surrounded by a dense proliferation of monomorphic small lymphocytes **(D)**. These two entities usually can be distinguished easily by immunophenotypic analysis (hematoxylin and eosin stain, original magnifications: 250×, 400×, 630×, and 800× magnification).

tionship between the germinal centers and the interfollicular cells, the density, monomorphic versus polymorphic nature, the degree of cytologic atypia of the cellular proliferation, and the presence or absence of lymphoepithelial lesions and Dutcher bodies.

Lymphoid hyperplasias generally contain one to several reactive germinal centers. These usually are surrounded by well-defined mantle zones of small lymphocytes and are separated by an interfollicular polymorphous cell population (32,162) (Fig. 35.29). MALT lymphomas also may contain reactive germinal centers. These may be circumscribed by a thin zone of mantle cells but are characteristically surrounded by a diffuse, relatively monomorphic proliferation of centrocyte-like cells, which sometimes may infiltrate and even colonize the follicles (120) (Fig. 35.29). Mantle cell lymphomas similarly may contain reactive germinal centers, which may range from small and atrophic to large and hyperplastic. They usually are devoid of mantle zones and characteristically are surrounded and separated by a dense, monotonous, small to medium-sized lymphoid cell proliferation exhibiting variable but obvious cytologic atypia (14–16). The reactive germinal centers in lymphoid hyperplasias, MALT lymphomas, and mantle cell lymphomas are distinguishable from the neoplastic follicles of follicular lymphoma by their polymorphous cell population, numerous tingible body macrophages, and high mitotic index (Figs. 35.18, 35.19, 35.22, 35.29). Some lymphoid hyperplasias are diffuse. These usually are less densely cellular than small B-cell lymphomas and nearly always exhibit polymorphous cytomorphology because of the admixture of distinct cell populations, namely, cytologically benign small lymphocytes, mature plasma cells, immunoblasts, and histiocytes (32,162) (Fig. 35.20). In contrast, small lymphocytic lymphomas are strikingly monomorphic because of the presence of a dense, diffuse proliferation of monotonous-appearing small lymphoid cells. Plasmacytoid small lymphocytic lymphomas, also referred to as lymphoplasmacytic lymphomas (26,155,157), often retain this homogeneous appearance because of the presence of a diffuse proliferation of small lymphocytes, plasmacytoid lymphocytes and plasma cells. A variable proportion of the neoplastic cells in these cases contain Dutcher bodies, eosinophilic periodic acid–Schiff–positive, diastase-resistant intranuclear inclusions of immunoglobulin or Russell bodies, cytoplasmic globules of immunoglobulin (26,155,157) (Figs. 35.30, 35.31). Lymphoid hyperplasias lack the pseudofollicular proliferation centers comprising large, variably transformed lymphoid cells that are characteristically observed in small lymphocytic lymphomas (11–13,121,163). Lymphoepithelial lesions are present in most MALT lymphomas (120,174) (Fig. 35.24). However, they are less relevant as a diagnostic criterion outside of the stomach because they may be observed in nonlymphomatous extranodal lymphocytic infiltrates (185). Dutcher bodies are only rarely, if ever, identified in lymphoid hyperplasias, but they are found relatively frequently in MALT lymphomas (Fig. 35.27) and plasmacytoid small lymphocytic lymphomas (31,59). Recognition of these subtle morphologic differences usually permits most ocular adnexal lymphoid hyperplasias and malignant lymphomas to be distinguished from one another. However, im-

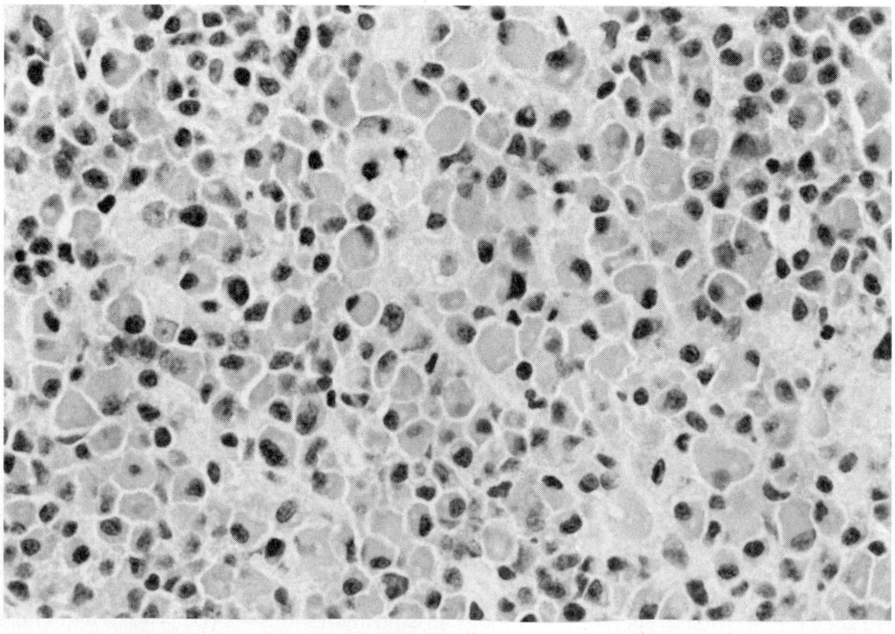

FIG. 35.30. Plasmacytoid small lymphocytic lymphoma of the orbit. In this instance, many of the neoplastic cells contain abundant cytoplasmic globules of immunoglobulin, so-called Russell bodies (hematoxylin and eosin stain, original magnification: 400× magnification).

A 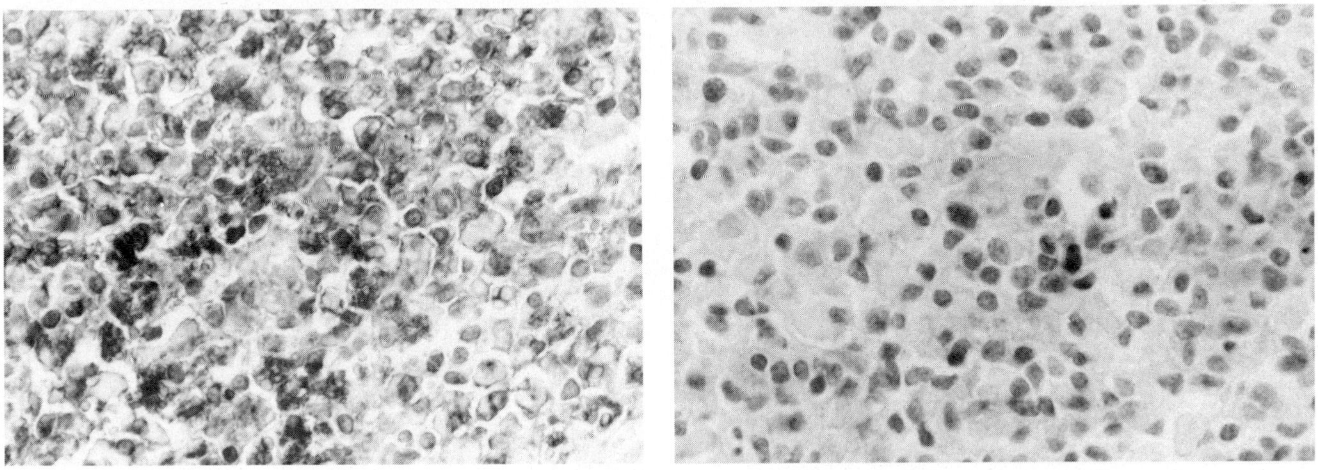 B

FIG. 35.31. Paraffin sections of the orbital plasmacytoid small lymphocytic lymphoma illustrated in Figure 35.30 stained for cytoplasmic immunoglobulin by immunoperoxidase. This technique demonstrates that most of these immunoglobulin inclusions are κ light-chain positive **(A)** and λ light-chain negative **(B)**, consistent with a clonal B-cell derivation (original magnification: 630× magnification).

munophenotypic and, if necessary, molecular analysis serve as the final arbiters for morphologically insolvable cases.

Immunophenotypic Characteristics

More than 90% of all ocular adnexal lymphoid proliferations can be categorized as polyclonal lymphoid hyperplasias or monoclonal B-cell lymphomas based on the results of immunophenotypic analysis; the remaining cases generally are considered indeterminate because of various technical problems encountered during immunophenotypic analysis (32,122,152).

Immunophenotypic analysis of isolated cells in suspension by flow cytometry offers the advantage of precise quantitation of lymphoid cell subpopulations and the ability to perform preferential gated and rare event analysis, sometimes permitting the detection of a small clonal B-cell population in the middle of a large polyclonal cell population (see Chapter 5). Immunohistochemical analysis of frozen and paraffin tissue sections allows precise localization of lymphoid cell subpopulations *in situ* and avoids the possible loss of selected cell populations during cell isolation (see Chapter 4). Maximum information is derived by performing flow cytometric and immunohistochemical analysis in each case and then correlating the results in conjunction with morphologic examination of the histologic sections. Knowles and Jakobiec collected immunophenotypic data on more than 150 ocular adnexal lymphoid proliferations analyzed in this manner during the 1980s (5,32,116–118). They based many of their conclusions concerning the ocular adnexal lymphoid proliferations on these data, which are subsequently described.

In the experience of Knowles and Jakobiec (5,32,116, 117), diffuse and follicular lymphoid hyperplasias of the ocular adnexa contain between 38% and 73% (mean, 55%) T cells based on the enumeration of sheep erythrocyte (E) rosette-forming cells or the flow cytometric detection of cells that express pan-T-cell antigens CD3, CD5, CD2, or some combination. The one case of lymphoid hyperplasia that contained only 38% T cells was the only one they encountered in which T cells accounted for less than 40% of the total cell population. In tissue sections, T cells usually appear to represent between 50% and 75% of the total cell population. This varies, however, with the number and size of the reactive germinal centers (B-cell zones) present in the lesion. The ratio of CD4 (helper) to CD8 (suppressor or cytotoxic) T cells ranges from 2.2 to 14.4 (mean, 5.6) based on flow cytometric analysis. Polyclonal lymphoid hyperplasias contain from 4% to 57% (mean, 35%) B cells based on the flow cytometric detection of cells that express pan-B-cell–associated antigens CD20 or CD22. The ratio of κ to λ light-chain–positive B cells ranges from 0.3 to 6.3 (mean, 2.0). Most of the remaining cells express HLA-DR (Ia) antigens and represent small numbers of surface immunoglobulin–negative B cells and tissue monocytes (32). Ocular adnexal polyclonal lymphoid hyperplasias recapitulate the immunophenotypic profiles of benign and reactive lymph nodes, except for a generally higher CD4 to CD8 ratio (Fig. 35.32).

Knowles and Jakobiec (5,32,116,117) found that the ocular adnexal B-cell lymphomas contain 48% to 96% (mean, 78%) B cells based on the flow cytometric detection of cells that express surface immunoglobulin or B-cell–associated antigen CD20. B cells comprised less than 60% of the total cell population in only 3 of 65 B-cell lymphomas that they examined. In tissue sections, B cells always appear to represent the majority cell population, comprising from about 60% to 90% of the total cell population. Approximately 95% of these B-cell lymphomas express monotypic surface im-

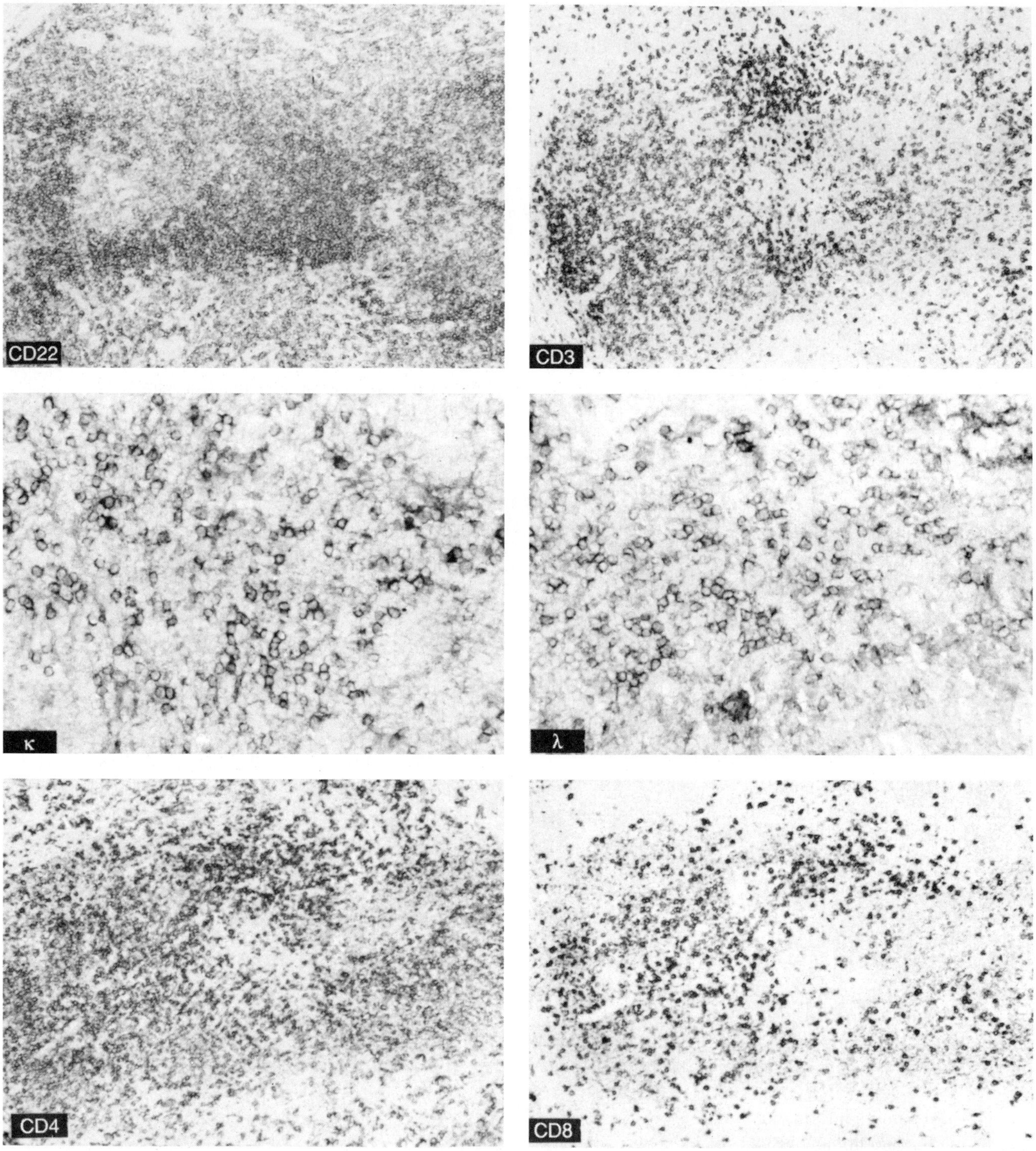

FIG. 35.32. Immunostaining of an orbital polyclonal lymphoid hyperplasia. Immunoperoxidase staining of frozen tissue sections of this orbital lymphoid proliferation shows that approximately 60% of the cells are B cells based on the expression of CD22. In this case the number of B cells is large because of the presence of several large germinal centers (B-cell zones). The B cells are polyclonal with respect to light-chain determinants, because numerous κ light-chain– and λ light-chain–positive B cells are identified. Approximately 40% of the cells are T cells based on the expression of CD3. The CD4$^+$ T cells outnumber the CD8$^+$ T cells. The number of CD4$^+$ cells is large because macrophages and helper T cells express CD4.

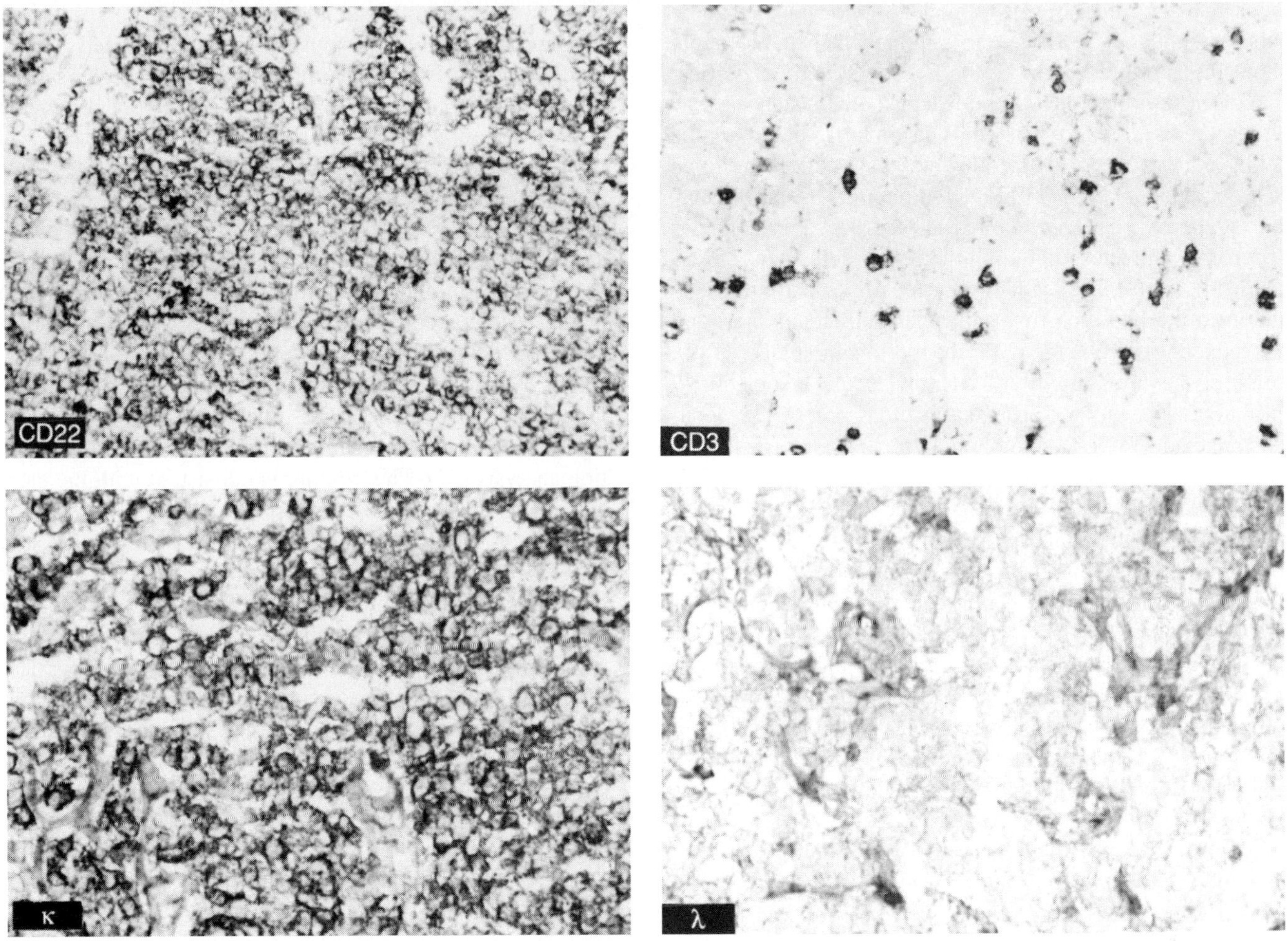

FIG. 35.33. Immunostaining of an orbital monoclonal B-cell lymphoma. Immunoperoxidase staining of frozen tissue sections of an orbital monoclonal B-cell lymphoma demonstrates that approximately 90% of the cells are B cells, based on the expression of CD22, and that fewer than 10% of the cells are T cells, based on the expression of CD3. Most of the B cells express κ light chains in high density. In contrast, almost no λ light-chain–positive cells are identified. There is, however, slight background staining because of nonspecific binding to collagen.

munoglobulin (Fig. 35.33). The most common surface immunoglobulin isotypes are IgMκ, IgMDκ, IgMλ, and IgMDλ; these account for about 85% of the immunoglobulin isotypes expressed by ocular adnexal B-cell lymphomas. Ocular adnexal lymphomas infrequently express IgA, even though IgA B cells, IgA plasma cells, and IgA secretory antibody are present in the MALT of the conjunctiva (18) and lacrimal gland (186). The ratio of κ to λ light-chain–positive B cells was $\leq$0.1 or $\geq$13.8 in 56 (92%) of 61 B-cell lymphomas and between 6.9 and 9.5 in the remaining 5 cases that they studied. The intensity of staining for surface immunoglobulin is sometimes faint, as in the case of B-cell chronic lymphocytic leukemia, but usually is moderate to bright, as in the case of most B-cell non-Hodgkin's lymphomas (21). Monoclonal B-cell lymphomas contain 1% to 46% (mean, 18%) T cells. Only 3 of 65 monoclonal B-cell lymphomas that Knowles and Jakobiec studied contained greater than 40% T cells. In contrast with lymphoid hyperplasias, the CD4 to CD8 ratio among monoclonal B-cell lymphomas ranges from 0.8 to 5.7 (mean, 2.5) and is virtually identical to that of systemic B-cell lymphomas (187).

The neoplastic cells of MALT lymphoma, which represent most primary ocular adnexal malignant lymphomas, express B-cell–associated antigens CD19, CD20, CD22, and CD79a, and monotypic surface immunoglobulin, usually IgM (172). They usually also express CD21 and CD35 and usually lack CD5, CD10, and CD23 (172). They also usually exhibit a low proliferation index based on monoclonal antibody Ki-67 reactivity (172). Ocular adnexal MALT lymphomas display these same immunophenotypic characteristics (122,152,188).

In this regard, it may be considered somewhat surprising that Knowles and Jakobiec found variable populations of CD5$^+$ neoplastic B cells in 22% of their cases, primarily those that they classified as small lymphocytic or mantle cell lymphoma (32). However, although there is no doubt about the appropriateness of the histopathologic classification of most of these lesions, at least in some instances, they represented systemic lymphomas secondarily involving the ocular adnexa. Ferry and colleagues have since described cases of apparent CD5$^+$ MALT lymphoma (189). They further suggested that CD5 expression in MALT lymphomas occurring in all sites, including the ocular adnexa, is a prognostic marker for persistent or recurrent disease, for dissemination to the bone marrow and other extranodal sites, and for leukemic involvement of the peripheral blood (189). Some of the cases reported by Knowles and Jakobiec may fall into this category. Rarely, cases of apparent CD5$^+$ ocular adnexal MALT lymphoma have been described (59,122,152). Some of the latter patients, uncharacteristically for MALT lymphoma, also had advanced stage disease and died from their disease within 5 years after diagnosis (59). Further studies are necessary to determine the prognostic value of CD5 expression among ocular adnexal and other MALT lymphomas.

These results provide some useful guidelines for employing immunophenotypic analysis as an adjunct in the differential diagnosis of lymphoid hyperplasia versus malignant lymphoma in the ocular adnexa. First, Knowles and Jakobiec found that 24 (96%) of 25 polyclonal lymphoid hyperplasias contained more than 40% T cells and fewer than 60% B cells, whereas 62 (95%) of 65 monoclonal B-cell lymphomas contained more than 60% B cells and fewer than 40% T cells. Merely determining the proportion of T and B cells resulted in accurately predicting the histopathologic diagnosis and the polyclonal or monoclonal B-cell nature of 86 of 90 (96%) ocular adnexal lymphoid proliferations. Second, they found that the κ to λ light-chain ratio ranged between 0.3 and 6.3 (mean, 2.0) among 25 polyclonal lymphoid hyperplasias but was ≤ 0.1 and ≥ 13.8 among 56 (92%) of 61 B-cell lymphomas and between 6.9 and 9.5 in the remaining 5 cases. Precise quantitation of the ratio of κ to λ light chains by flow cytometric analysis of isolated cells in suspension is extremely useful for distinguishing reliably between lymphoid hyperplasia and malignant lymphoma. Third, they found that approximately 25% of B-cell lymphomas express anomalous immunophenotypic profiles (i.e., CD5 expression or absence of surface immunoglobulin) (32). In conclusion, the judicious application of these immunophenotypic criteria usually permits an ocular adnexal lymphoid proliferation to be classified as polyclonal lymphoid hyperplasia or monoclonal B-cell lymphoma.

Immunogenotypic Characteristics

Antigen receptor gene rearrangement (immunogenotypic) analysis by Southern blot hybridization and especially by polymerase chain reaction is a considerably more sensitive, objective, and accurate approach than morphologic examination and immunophenotypic analysis in determining the lineage and clonality of lymphoid neoplasms (21) (see Chapter 7). Immunogenotypic analysis has demonstrated that the ocular adnexal lymphoid proliferations classified as B-cell lymphomas by histopathologic and immunophenotypic criteria consistently display clonal immunoglobulin heavy- and light-chain gene rearrangements (37,59,165) (Fig. 35.34) and are monoclonal B-cell proliferations at the molecular level. This includes the diffuse, monomorphic small lymphocytic infiltrates that exhibit immunoglobulin light-chain isotypic exclusion and are limited to the ocular adnexa. The latter lesions represent monoclonal B-cell lymphomas (37,59,165).

The ocular adnexal B-cell lymphomas consistently exhibit monoallelic or biallelic clonal immunoglobulin heavy- and light-chain gene rearrangements by Southern blot hybridization analysis (37). This finding is consistent with the clonal expansion of a mature B-cell population (21). The hybridization signals usually are clear and intense because the clonal B-cell population nearly always represents at least 60% of the total cell population in the lesion. The presence of more than two new hybridizing bands—suggesting biclonality, somatic mutation, or clonal evolution—is uncommon (Fig. 35.34). They almost never are bigenotypic (i.e., exhibit clonal T-cell receptor gene and clonal immunoglobulin gene rearrangements) (37).

Simultaneous bilateral ocular adnexal B-cell lymphomas usually exhibit identical clonal immunoglobulin gene rearrangements (37,118,136,168) (Fig. 35.35). This finding strongly suggests that, in these instances, both lesions are derived from the identical B-cell clone and represent the same B-cell neoplasm. In these cases, it would appear that the lymphoma arose on one side and subsequently spread to the other side. That this can occur without systemic dissemination is a property of mucosal B lymphocytes and reflects their known behavior to home back to their parent tissue after passage through the general circulation (190). Such a pattern of spread is observed in MALT lymphomas in other sites, resulting, for example, in multifocal deposits in primary gastric lymphoma (178) and the high incidence of bilateral involvement in cases of parotid gland MALT lymphoma (120). Ocular adnexal and extraocular lymphomas that occur concurrently in the same patient may exhibit identical clonal immunoglobulin gene rearrangements, suggesting that they are derived from the identical B-cell clone, or distinct clonal immunoglobulin gene rearrangements, suggesting that they are derived from the identical B-cell clone but have undergone clonal evolution or somatic mutation or, alternatively, are derived from unique B-cell clones and represent the synchronous occurrence of separate B-cell neoplasms (37,118).

Immunogenotypic analysis has demonstrated that some unilateral and bilateral ocular adnexal polyclonal lymphoid hyperplasias are polyclonal at the molecular genetic level (37,118,119,165). These lesions appear to represent truly reactive proliferations of lymphoid cells, perhaps occurring in response to an as yet unidentified antigenic stimulus. An unanticipated finding, however, was the demonstration

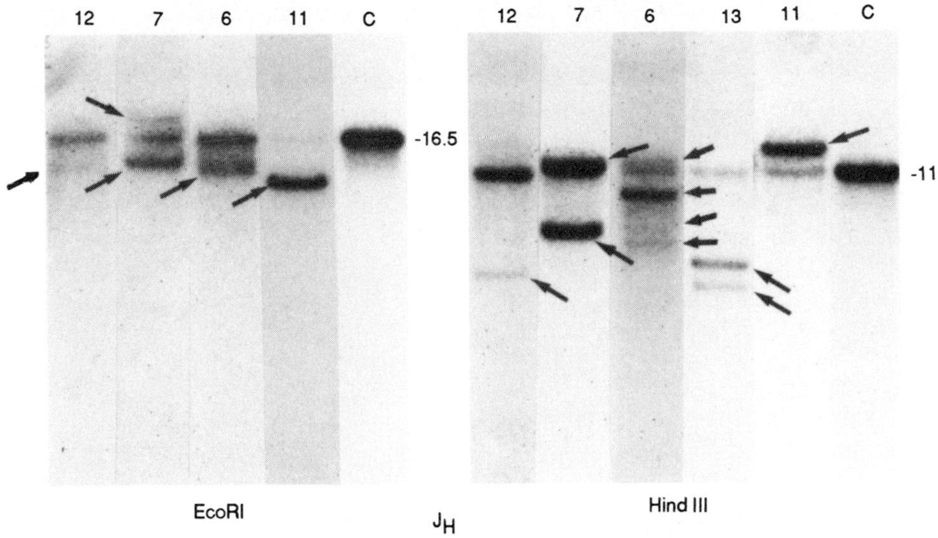

FIG. 35.34. Southern blot hybridization analysis of ocular adnexal lymphoid proliferations for immunoglobulin gene rearrangements. The DNA extracted from ocular adnexal lymphoid proliferations classified as B-cell lymphomas according to histopathologic and immunophenotypic criteria and from human fibroblasts (control [C]) were digested with *Eco*RI or *Hin*dIII and hybridized to an immunoglobulin heavy-chain joining region (J_H) probe. Rearrangement bands are indicated by arrows. Lane C displays the immunoglobulin gene germline configuration. Each ocular adnexal lymphoid proliferation exhibits clonal Immunoglobulin heavy-chain gene rearrangements consistent with a clonal B-cell derivation. (Modified from Neri A, Jakobiec FA, Pelicci PG, et al. Immunoglobulin and T cell receptor beta chain gene rearrangement analysis of ocular adnexal lymphoid neoplasms: clinical and biologic implications. *Blood* 1987;70:1519–1529, with permission.)

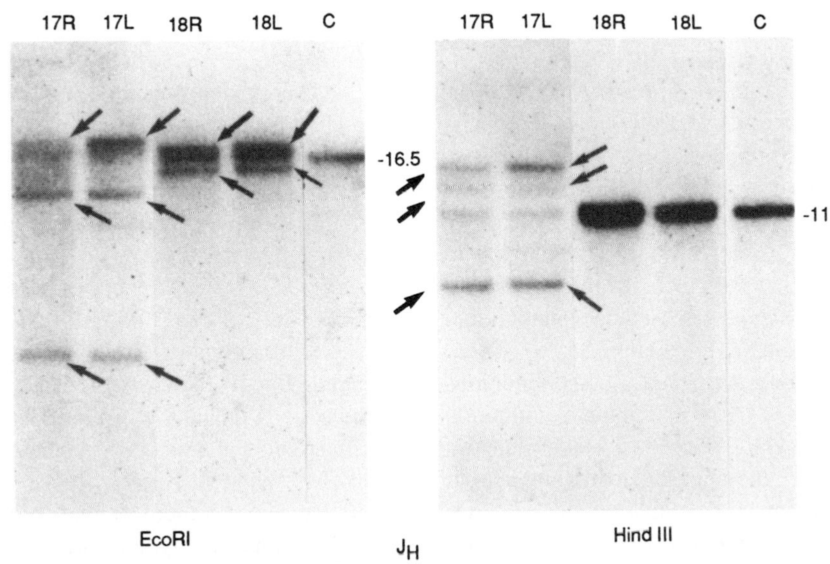

FIG. 35.35. Southern blot hybridization analysis of two pairs of bilateral ocular adnexal monoclonal B-cell lymphomas for immunoglobulin gene rearrangements. The DNA extracted from the right (R)- and left (L)-sided neoplasms occurring in two patients (lanes 17 and 18) and from human fibroblasts (control [C]) were digested with *Eco*RI or *Hin*dIII and were hybridized to an immunoglobulin heavy-chain joining region (J_H) probe. Rearrangement bands are indicated by arrows. Lane C shows the immunoglobulin heavy-chain gene germline configuration. The bilateral ocular adnexal monoclonal B-cell lymphomas that occur simultaneously in each patient exhibited identical clonal immunoglobulin heavy-chain gene rearrangement patterns. This finding suggests that the two neoplasms were derived from the same B-cell clone and do not represent separate primary neoplasms. (Modified from Neri A, Jakobiec FA, Pelicci PG, et al. Immunoglobulin and T cell receptor beta chain gene rearrangement analysis of ocular adnexal lymphoid neoplasms: clinical and biologic implications. *Blood* 1987;70:1519–1529, with permission.)

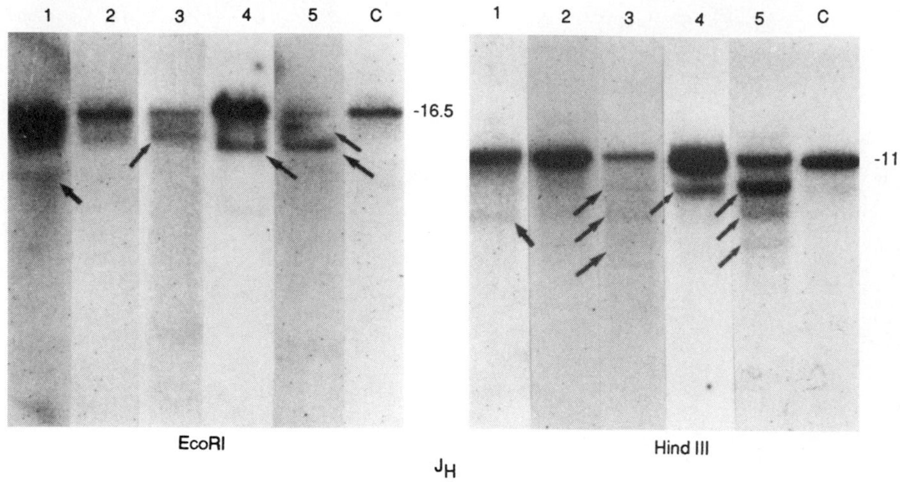

FIG. 35.36. Southern blot hybridization analysis of ocular adnexal lymphoid proliferations exhibiting seemingly benign histopathology and a polyclonal cell marker profile for immunoglobulin gene rearrangements. The DNA extracted from the indicated cases (lanes 1–5) and human fibroblasts (control [C]) were digested with *Eco*RI or *Hin*dIII and hybridized to an immunoglobulin heavy-chain joining region (J_H) probe. Arrows indicate rearrangement bands. Lane C displays the immunoglobulin heavy-chain gene germline configuration. Four of the five apparently benign polyclonal ocular adnexal lymphoid proliferations exhibit one or more rearrangement bands. The hybridization patterns include solitary to multiple faint and barely perceptible bands, solitary clearly visible bands, and a solitary clearly visible band associated with multiple faint bands. These findings suggest the presence of monoclonal and oligoclonal B-cell populations that have escaped recognition by morphologic examination and immunophenotypic analysis. At least some of these lesions probably represent mucosa-associated lymphoid tissue lymphomas whose histopathologic features were not appreciated in the past and whose monoclonal nature cannot be determined immunophenotypically because of numerous benign polyclonal lymphoid cells or for various technical reasons. (Modified from Neri A, Jakobiec FA, Pelicci PG, et al. Immunoglobulin and T cell receptor beta chain gene rearrangement analysis of ocular adnexal lymphoid neoplasms: clinical and biologic implications. *Blood* 1987;70:1519–1529, with permission.)

many years ago by Knowles and Jakobiec that many ocular adnexal lymphoid proliferations classified as polyclonal lymphoid hyperplasias histopathologically exhibit clonal immunoglobulin gene rearrangements (37,38,119). Among these cases, the patterns of immunoglobulin gene rearrangement included solitary and multiple, barely perceptible to faint bands, solitary clear and easily recognizable bands, and solitary high-intensity bands superimposed on a background of multiple less intense bands (37,38) (Fig. 35.36). These lesions contain oligoclonal or monoclonal B-cell populations that have escaped recognition by morphologic examination and immunophenotypic analysis. These lesions consistently lack clonal T-cell receptor gene rearrangements, indicating that the constituent T cells are truly polyclonal (37,38,118, 119). Similar results have been obtained when immunogenotypic analysis has been applied to lymphoid hyperplasias occurring in other extranodal sites in which B-cell lymphomas frequently arise, such as the salivary gland, gastrointestinal tract, and skin (38,191–193). These findings suggest that extranodal lymphoid hyperplasias and B-cell lymphomas are pathogenetically related. They suggest that the ocular adnexal and other extranodal lymphoid hyperplasias represent a continuous and progressive spectrum of B-cell neoplasia, up to and including the earliest identifiable stages of malignant lymphoma (38).

These molecular genetic findings help to explain certain previously unexplainable clinical observations concerning ocular adnexal and other extranodal lymphoid proliferations. First, the common occurrence of occult clonal B-cell populations in lesions classified as polyclonal lymphoid hyperplasias helps to explain their frequent association with the prior, concurrent, or subsequent development of extraocular lymphoma (32). At least some of these seemingly polyclonal lymphoid hyperplasias represent malignant lymphomas obscured by a brisk polyclonal inflammatory host response—an anomalous deposit of systemic lymphoma or a primary ocular adnexal malignant lymphoma that already has disseminated. Second, these findings also explain the apparent development of malignant lymphoma after polyclonal lymphoid hyperplasia in the same anatomic site (165,194,195). It is reasonable to speculate that the initial lesion contained an occult malignant lymphoma below the threshold of morphologic and immunophenotypic detection that eventually manifested clinically. Alternatively, some occult clonal B-cell expansions may be transformed incompletely but are susceptible to additional genetic alterations that permit transformation and development into malignant lymphoma.

The frequent detection of clonal immunoglobulin gene rearrangements in ocular adnexal lymphoid proliferations otherwise classified as polyclonal lymphoid hyperplasias has also raised important practical questions concerning the role of immunogenotypic analysis in the diagnosis and classification of these and other extranodal lymphoid proliferations. In this regard, it is important to remember that the molecular determination of clonality does not necessarily imply malignancy or aggressive clinical behavior. Clonal immunoglobulin and T-cell receptor gene rearrangements have been detected in many lymphoproliferative disorders that are not overt malignant lymphomas and are not inevitably associated with the development of malignant lymphoma (21,36,38,191–193,196–198). Most patients who have apparently morphologically benign and immunophenotypically polyclonal ocular adnexal and other extranodal lymphoid proliferations but contain immunogenotypically detectable clonal B-cell populations do not develop disseminated lymphoma despite conservative therapy (37,38,119, 191). For these reasons, Knowles and Jakobiec recommended against classifying ocular adnexal lymphoid proliferations as malignant lymphomas merely based on the detection of occult clonal B-cell populations by immunogenotypic analysis. However, many of these lesions represent MALT lymphomas whose histopathologic features were not appreciated in the past and whose monoclonal nature sometimes cannot be determined immunophenotypically because of the presence of large numbers of benign polyclonal lymphoid cells or for various technical reasons (59,136,165,168).

Molecular Genetic and Cytogenetic Characteristics

Specific structural alterations involving a variety of protooncogenes and tumor suppressor genes are highly associated with the development and progression of lymphoid malignancy (see Chapter 8). These genetic alterations are often associated with recurring chromosomal abnormalities that occur nonrandomly in conjunction with specific clinicopathologic entities (see Chapter 10). The principal genes involved among the major clinicopathologic categories of B-cell non-Hodgkin's lymphomas, and therefore believed to play a role in their pathogenesis, are *BCL1, BCL2, BCL6, MYC,* and *TP53* (see Chapter 8). The MALT lymphomas characteristically lack rearrangements of the *BCL1, BCL2, BCL6,* and *MYC* genes (199,200); a *MYC* gene rearrangement has only been described in some high-grade MALT lymphomas (201). However, later cytogenetic studies have revealed a recurring translocation, t(11;18)(q21;q21) (202), or a trisomy 3 (203) in a significant proportion of MALT lymphomas.

Only a few investigators have studied the molecular genetic characteristics of the ocular adnexal lymphoid proliferations. Knowles and coworkers failed to detect evidence of *BCL1, BCL2,* or *MYC* gene rearrangements among more than 20 primary ocular adnexal malignant lymphomas that they studied (unpublished observations). Wotherspoon and colleagues similarly failed to detect rearrangements of these genes among several primary conjunctival malignant lymphomas (136,168), as did Baldini and associates (188). The latter investigators also failed to detect *BCL6* gene rearrangements among these cases (188). These negative findings reflect the fact that most of the cases studied by all these investigators are MALT lymphomas. Unfortunately, only very few additional studies have been performed. Coupland and colleagues, for example, identified p53 protein overexpression in occasional malignant cells in 11% of their ocular adnexal MALT lymphomas (59). Although p53 protein overexpression does not consistently correlate with *TP53* gene mutation (204), this finding may have prognostic significance. Further insight into the pathogenesis of the ocular adnexal malignant lymphomas awaits more extensive investigation of their molecular genetic basis.

Therapy and Management

Knowles and Jakobiec found that extraocular lymphoma is most frequently discovered during the initial staging evaluation or within 6 months after presentation of a patient who has an ocular adnexal lymphoid proliferation (32). Every patient should be referred to a hematologist/oncologist for systemic evaluation, including bone marrow examination, at the time of presentation. Occasionally, patients develop extraocular lymphoma as long as 4 years and sometimes even later after presentation (32). It is further recommended that systemic evaluation be repeated every 6 months for a minimum of 5 years and ideally indefinitely after diagnosis.

If the patient is found to have a lymphoid proliferation limited to the ocular adnexa (unilateral or bilateral) after a careful and thorough systemic evaluation, local radiation therapy is recommended (59,87,122,152,159,164,184,188, 205). A surgical approach is not recommended because of the infiltrative nature of lymphoid proliferations. Complete surgical excision of these lesions usually is not possible without causing severe functional deficiencies (53). Some physicians have adopted a ''watch and wait'' policy and have treated patients who have asymptomatic MALT lymphoma restricted to the ocular adnexa with ''observation only'' after excisional biopsy (122). However, disease recurs locally or develops systemically in a significant proportion of these individuals (152,164,188,206). For these reasons, surgery alone is suboptimal. Even polyclonal lymphoid hyperplasias are capable of recurrence (59,165) and therefore should be ablated by radiation therapy (53,207). Systemic corticosteroids usually are only useful in treating orbital pseudotumors. They generally produce only a temporary clinical suppression of ocular adnexal lymphoid proliferations that rebound on cessation of the drug (53). There is no consensus on the optimal radiation dose for treating ocular adnexal lymphomas (159,205). It has been recommended that doses of 1,500 to 2,000 rad in a fractionated schedule be delivered to polyclonal lymphoid hyperplasias and low-grade lymphomas (e.g., MALT lymphomas) and that 2,000 to 3,000 rad in divided doses be delivered to follicular lymphomas and diffuse large B-cell lymphomas (162). The eyeball should be protected with a metallic shield to reduce radiation-induced keratopathy, cataractogenesis, and vasculopathy of the retina and optic nerve (207). The specifics of ocular radiation therapy are discussed in detail elsewhere (159,205). Most patients who have stage IE disease treated only with local radiation therapy undergo complete remission (59,152,159,164,188,205,208). Some patients require repeated radiation therapy to achieve total tumor eradication and complete remission (59). Ocular recurrence is rare and systemic dissemination occurs uncommonly among patients who have stage IE disease and are treated in this manner (59,159,164,188,205,208). However, the contralateral eye is a potential site of relapse (205).

It may be argued that local radiation therapy alone is too limited to treat effectively bilateral ocular adnexal small B-cell lymphomas and unilateral ocular adnexal diffuse large B-cell lymphomas, even those classified as stage IE lesions. However, the incidence of past, concurrent, or subsequent development of extraocular lymphoma is virtually identical among patients who have unilateral and bilateral ocular adnexal lymphoid proliferations (32,118,184). In other words, systemic lymphoma is not more likely to develop in patients who have bilateral than in patients who have unilateral ocular adnexal malignant lymphoma (165). Bilateral ocular adnexal involvement by malignant lymphoma in the absence of systemic dissemination is considered stage IE disease (152,205). Moreover, most of these lesions are MALT lymphomas (136,168). In the experience of Knowles and Jabobiec, only 2 of 14 patients who had stage IE ocular adnexal non–small B-cell malignant lymphomas treated by ocular radiation therapy alone developed extraocular lymphoma (32). Similarly, White and colleagues found that five of six patients who had stage IE ocular adnexal diffuse large B-cell lymphoma treated with radiation therapy alone achieved complete remission and were disease free at a mean follow-up of more than 5 years (152). The presence of bilateral adnexal lesions or of follicular or diffuse large B-cell lymphoma in the ocular adnexa does not necessarily imply the existence or the eventual development of systemic disease. A few of these lesions appear to represent truly localized disease. Perhaps some of the large B-cell lymphomas arise from low-grade MALT lymphomas. Some data suggest that high-grade MALT lymphomas arising in other sites are associated with a better prognosis than for non-MALT types (209). For these reasons, it is recommended that patients who have lymphoid proliferations—even follicular and large B-cell lymphomas limited to the ocular adnexa (unilateral or bilateral)—be subjected to local ocular radiation therapy, which may be curative, rather than to systemic chemotherapy.

If extraocular lymphoma is discovered, systemic chemotherapy can be administered and the effect on the ocular adnexal lymphoid proliferation awaited. Generally, ocular adnexal malignant lymphoma is sensitive to radiation therapy and systemic chemotherapy and so only one and not both modalities are necessary (164,210). The patient should be carefully followed (e.g., by repeat CT scanning) by an ophthalmologist to determine the adequacy of local ocular regression. If the ocular response to chemotherapy is suboptimal, adjunctive local ocular radiation therapy can be administered. If the ocular adnexal lesion is bulky or causing a threat to vision, radiation therapy can be administered when systemic chemotherapy is given (32).

Natural History and Outcome

Effect of Anatomic Location

Knowles and Jakobiec suggested that the precise anatomic location of a lymphoid proliferation within the ocular adnexa has a significant bearing on its natural history, including the development of extraocular lymphoma. They found that approximately 35%, 20%, and 67% of patients who present with lymphoid proliferations of the orbit, conjunctiva, and eyelids, respectively, have prior, concurrent, or subsequent extraocular lymphoma (statistical significance, $p < 0.03$) (32). Based on these findings, Knowles and Jakobiec concluded that the conjunctiva is the most favorable prognostic location within the ocular adnexa (32). White and colleagues confirmed that extraocular lymphoma is significantly more likely to develop in patients who have orbital rather than conjunctival lymphoma (165). Knowles and Jakobiec postulated that this is because the conjunctiva, unlike the orbit, contains its own indigenous lymphoid tissue that is capable of undergoing hyperplasia or developing primary localized malignant lymphoma (53). We now know that the conjunctiva contains MALT (135), that most malignant lymphomas originating in the conjunctiva arise in this MALT (59,122,152,164) and that MALT lymphomas characteristically tend to remain localized to the mucosal surface where they develop and do not disseminate systemically (120,173,211). Wotherspoon and colleagues also found that malignant lymphomas arising in the conjunctiva are MALT lymphomas and tend not to disseminate, even when they are bilateral (136,168).

In contrast, some other investigators have failed to identify prognostic differences among adnexal locations (58,59). However, most of these series included cases of secondary and primary ocular adnexal malignant lymphoma. In part, these differences may be explained by differing patient referral patterns and case selection bias. It is important to point out that the precise anatomic site of origination of an ocular adnexal lymphoid proliferation often may not be appreciated clinically by the examining ophthalmologist. In one series, no effort was even made to distinguish between eyelid and conjunctival lesions, for example, and so they were lumped together for purposes of analysis (122). It is important that the precise anatomic location of a lymphoid proliferation occurring within the ocular adnexa be determined. For this reason, the patient should receive a careful clinical ocular examination in conjunction with orbital imaging studies. This was done in all of the patients included in the series reported by Knowles and Jakobiec (32).

Relation of Histopathology and Immunophenotype

Knowles and Jakobiec found that approximately one third of all patients who had a lymphoid proliferation originating or manifesting in the ocular adnexa (unilateral or bilateral) developed extraocular lymphoma before, concurrent with, or after ocular adnexal manifestation. This included similar percentages (29% and 35%) of patients who had lesions that they had determined to be polyclonal lymphoid hyperplasia and monoclonal B-cell lymphoma, respectively. Based on these findings, they raised the possibility that classifying ocular adnexal lymphoid proliferations into benign and malignant categories according to histopathologic criteria and into polyclonal and monoclonal B-cell categories according to immunophenotypic criteria may not be useful for predicting eventual outcome (32). However, Knowles and Jakobiec detected clonal B-cell populations, albeit small, in several ocular adnexal lymphoid proliferations that were thought to be lymphoid hyperplasias morphologically (37,38). Almost 15 years later, at least some of those lesions would be classified as malignant lymphomas today. This conclusion is based in part on an increased awareness of the histopathologic spectrum of MALT lymphomas, including the features that may cause them to be misinterpreted as lymphoid hyperplasia. The study by Coupland and associates in which they failed to find evidence of dissemination among 12 patients with lymphoid hyperplasia supports this conclusion (59). Their follow-up period (median, 31 months) was too brief to be definitive, however. Moreover, sampling errors, especially in the case of small ocular adnexal biopsies, have to be considered in the interpretation of such studies. Further studies are probably necessary to clarify fully this issue.

Knowles and Jakobiec also found that the further histopathologic subclassification of ocular adnexal monoclonal B-cell lymphomas is helpful in predicting eventual outcome. They reported that although identical proportions (27%) of patients who had ocular adnexal lymphoid proliferations that they classified as lymphoid hyperplasia and small lymphocytic or intermediate lymphocytic lymphoma developed extraocular lymphoma, a significantly higher proportion (46%) of patients who had lesions that they classified as follicle center and large cell lymphomas developed extraocular lymphoma ($p < 0.09$) (32). Based on these findings, they suggested that the prior, concurrent, or future development of extraocular lymphoma varies according to the histopathologic category of the ocular adnexal lymphoid proliferation (32).

In retrospect, we now know that most of the small B-cell lymphomas classified in this manner represented MALT lymphomas. The behavior of MALT lymphomas is distinctly nonaggressive and differs from that of all other extranodal B-cell lymphomas (173,211). MALT lymphomas generally remain localized to the mucosal surface where they originate and do not disseminate systemically (120,173,211). Patients who have MALT lymphomas usually do not have adverse prognostic factors such as high tumor burden, disseminated disease, bone marrow involvement, poor performance status or high lactate dehydrogenase (LDH) levels (212). Patients who have MALT lymphoma have a high response rate with local treatment (i.e., surgery or radiotherapy) or with single agent chemotherapy, and enjoy a long survival. These patients have a better prognosis than patients who have a non-MALT lymphoma arising at the same site (209). This accounts for the indolent clinical behavior and excellent prognosis of a subset of cases classified as ''well-differentiated lymphocytic lymphoma'' by Knowles and Jakobiec (29). For these reasons, the accurate identification of MALT lymphoma at all anatomic sites, including the ocular adnexa, and its distinction from other forms of non-Hodgkin's lymphoma is clinically significant. Recurrences may appear several years after therapy (212,213) in the same organ or in other extranodal sites (214). Histologic transformation to a more aggressive lymphoma may occur in association with recurrence (137,172).

Role of Systemic Evaluation and Relationship with Clinical Stage

Knowles and Jakobiec uncovered a documented past history of extraocular lymphoma in 13% of patients who presented with an ocular adnexal lymphoid proliferation (13% orbital, 0% conjunctival, and 33% eyelid). About 60% of these patients and 15% of the remaining patients were found to have evidence of extraocular lymphoma within 6 months of presentation and were considered to have concurrent ocular and extraocular lymphoma. In summary, about 24% of patients overall who presented with an ocular adnexal lymphoid proliferation (20% orbital, 10% conjunctiva, and 44% eyelid) were discovered to have had prior or concurrent extraocular lymphoma. The remaining 76% of patients did not have a past history of lymphoma and did not develop evidence of extraocular lymphoma within 6 months after ocular presentation (32). Coupland and colleagues similarly found that 76% of their patients who had ocular adnexal B-cell lymphoma had disease limited to the ocular adnexa (e.g., had stage IE disease) (59).

The results of these studies (32,59) suggest that patients who present with ocular adnexal lymphoid proliferations should be subdivided into two broad categories: those with and those without a past history or evidence of extraocular lymphoma within 6 months after ocular presentation. Many, if not the majority, of the approximately 25% of patients who belong to the former category probably already had disseminated extraocular lymphoma with secondary involvement of the ocular adnexa at the time of presentation. Most of the approximately 75% of patients who belong to the latter category probably have stage IE primary ocular adnexal lymphoid proliferations.

According to Knowles and Jakobiec, these two patient groups exhibit several important clinical differences. First, the anatomic sites of involvement appear to differ. They found that approximately 90% of patients who have conjunctival, but only 74% who have orbital, and 44% who have eyelid, lymphoid proliferations have stage IE disease. Second, the histopathology apparently differs. They found that approximately 32% and 66% of stage IE ocular adnexal lymphoid proliferations are polyclonal lymphoid hyperplasias and monoclonal B-cell lymphomas, respectively. In contrast, 14% and 86% of ocular adnexal lymphoid proliferations associated with past and concurrent extraocular lymphoma are polyclonal lymphoid hyperplasias and monoclonal B-cell lymphomas, respectively. Among the patients who had stage IE disease, they classified 72% of the lesions as small B-cell lymphomas and the remaining 28% as follicle center or diffuse large B-cell lymphomas. In contrast, among patients who had past or concurrent extraocular lymphoma, they classified 52% of the lesions as small B-cell lymphomas and the remaining 48% as follicle center cell or large B-cell lymphomas (32). Coupland and colleagues reported similar findings (59), albeit employing the REAL classification (121). Among patients who had stage IE ocular adnexal B-cell lymphomas, they classified 88% as small B-cell lymphomas (predominantly MALT lymphomas) and the remaining 12% as follicular lymphomas. Among patients who had concurrent extraocular B-cell lymphoma (stages II, II, or IV), Coupland and associates classified 67% as small B-cell lymphomas and the remaining 33% as follicle center and diffuse large B-cell lymphomas (59). This is consistent with studies showing that most malignant lymphomas involving the ocular adnexa secondarily are follicle center and large cell lymphomas (152,210). Third, and most important, prognosis and outcome apparently differ according to stage at the time of ocular presentation ($p < 0.001$). In the experience of Knowles and Jakobiec, approximately 86% of patients who presented with a stage IE ocular adnexal lymphoid proliferation, unilateral or bilateral (78% with polyclonal lymphoid hyperplasia and 90% with monoclonal B-cell lymphoma), remained alive and well and were disease free, despite conservative therapy, at a median follow-up of 51 months. In contrast, only 20% of patients who presented with an ocular adnexal lymphoid proliferation and who had past or current extraocular lymphoma remained alive and well and were disease free at a mean follow-up of 57 months after ocular presentation. The remaining 80% of these patients were alive with disease or had died from progressive lymphoma with a median survival of only 19 months (32). Knowles and Jakobiec found that the single most important and statistically significant prognostic factor among patients who present with ocular adnexal lymphoid proliferations is the extent of disease determined after a thorough clinical staging. In their experience, most patients who present with a lymphoid proliferation limited to the ocular adnexa (stage IE), regardless of histopathology, immunophenotype, or bilaterality, have a benign indolent clinical course (32) (Table 35.3). Coupland and associates arrived at the same conclusion (59) and other investigators have reported a similar experience (24,122,184).

Other Prognostic Factors

Studies have identified a number of additional parameters that may have prognostic value among the ocular adnexal malignant lymphomas. For example, Coupland and associates suggested that the immunohistochemical demonstration of MIB-1 (Ki-67) and p53 have prognostic significance (59). They found that high proliferation rates, as determined by MIB-1 positivity, within the ocular adnexal malignant lymphomas corresponded significantly with their subdivision into high- and low-grade malignancy according to the REAL classification (121) ($p < 0.001$) and into MALT versus other

TABLE 35.3. *Eventual outcome of 108 patients presenting with ocular adnexal lymphoid proliferations*

Characteristic	Orbit	Conjunctiva	Lid	Total
No evidence of disease				
Patients (no.)	50[a]	24	3[c]	77
Follow-up, range (mo)	4–113	8–115	11–46	4–115
Follow-up, median (mo)	54	56	21	53
Alive with disease				
Patients (no.)	14[b]	3	2	19
Follow-up, range (mo)	6–108	18–62	22–42	6–108
Follow-up, median (mo)	58	43	32	51
Dead because of lymphoma				
Patients (no.)	4	2	2	8
Follow-up, range (mo)	12–28	8–67	23–79	8–79
Follow-up, median (mo)	15	38	51	19
Lost to follow-up	1	1	2	4
Patients (total)	69	30	9	108

[a] Two patients died of other causes and had no evidence of lymphoma at the time of death.
[b] One patient died of carcinoma but had systemic lymphoma at the time of death.
[c] One patient died of carcinoma and had no evidence of lymphoma at the time of death.
From Knowles DM, Jakobiec FA, McNally FA, et al. Lymphoid hyperplasia and malignant lymphoma occurring in the ocular adnexa (orbit, conjunctiva and eyelids): a prospective multiparametric analysis of 108 cases during 1977–1987. *Hum Pathol* 1990;21:959–973, with permission.

categories of malignant lymphoma ($p < 0.05$). They found the average MIB-1 proliferation rate for the MALT lymphomas to be 15%, which correlated with stage IE disease. They also found that 14 of the 15 cases that had a MIB-1 proliferation rate greater than 20% had at least stage II disease. They further found that high proliferation rates corresponded positively with stage of disease at presentation, stage of disease at final follow-up and the occurrence of lymphoma-related death ($p < 0.001$). They observed similar statistically significant correlations with respect to tumor subdivision, stage of disease at presentation and at final follow-up, and occurrence of lymphoma-related death with tumor cell p53 positivity. Multivariate analysis showed that the MIB-1 proliferation rate had the highest risk rates for predicting persistence of disease at follow-up and lymphoma-related deaths (59).

Nakata and colleagues analyzed the survival data of 57 patients who had ocular adnexal malignant lymphoma with a median follow-up period of 5.0 years (122). Univariate analysis of the prognostic factors influencing the cause-specific survival of these patients revealed that histopathology, LDH levels, and clinical stage were statistically significant. The 5-year cause-specific survival rate of patients with MALT lymphoma compared with those with non-MALT lymphoma was 100% versus 25% ($p < 0.0001$); with normal LDH versus abnormal LDH values was 98% versus 68% ($p < 0.0001$); and with stage I versus more advanced stage disease was 96% versus 67% ($p = 0.001$). Multivariate analysis demonstrated that the histologic subtype according to the REAL classification ($p = 0.01$) and the serum LDH level ($p = 0.015$) were independent significant predictors of cause-specific survival (122). These findings largely reflect the fact that most ocular adnexal lymphomas are MALT lymphomas, which are usually localized lesions unassociated with adverse prognostic factors.

OTHER HEMATOPOIETIC DISORDERS

Sinus Histiocytosis with Massive Lymphadenopathy

Sinus histiocytosis with massive lymphadenopathy (SHML), also called Rosai-Dorfman disease, is a rare histiocytic proliferative disorder that exhibits distinctive clinical and pathologic features and usually resolves spontaneously (215). Reports by Rosai and Dorfman in 1969 (216) and 1972 (217) established SHML as a distinct entity, hence the alternative designation of Rosai-Dorfman disease. Unfortunately, almost 30 years later, the cause and pathogenesis of this disease remains obscure (218). SHML is discussed in detail in Chapter 51. This discussion is limited primarily to ocular adnexal and ocular globe involvement by SHML.

SHML occurs in individuals belonging to all racial groups, regardless of socioeconomic status, worldwide. It occurs in all age groups; the youngest reported patient had congenital SHML and the oldest reported patient was 74 years old. The mean age at onset of symptoms is 21 years. The male to female ratio is about 1.5:1. Rarely, SHML occurs among family members (218).

Lymph node involvement occurs in nearly all cases. Approximately 87% of patients have cervical lymphadenopathy, which is usually bilateral. Axillary, inguinal and mediastinal lymph nodes are commonly affected as well. Typically, it is bulky, nontender and painless. The lymphadenopathy is accompanied by fever in about 25% of cases and sometimes by constitutional symptoms such as malaise, weight loss and night sweats as well. Most patients have a mild anemia and an elevated erythrocyte sedimentation rate. About 13% of cases are associated with or preceded by an immune-mediated disease (218).

Although SHML is considered a lymph node-based disease, at least one extranodal site is involved in about 43% of cases. Extranodal SHML may occur as part of a generalized disease process involving lymph nodes or may involve extranodal sites independent of lymph node involvement. The most common site of extranodal involvement is the head and neck region; other sites include the skin, soft tissues, and bones. Within the head and neck region, SHML has a predilection for the nasal cavity and paranasal sinuses. However, virtually all head and neck sites may be affected, in association with or independent of lymph node disease (218). Among 423 well-documented cases of SHML collected by Rosai and Dorfman over a 20-year period, orbital or eyelid involvement was described in 36 cases (8.5%), and ocular globe involvement was described in 6 cases (1.4%) (218). Of the 36 cases, 22 had only orbital, 5 had only eyelid, and 9 had orbital and eyelid involvement. In two of the cases, involvement of all four eyelids was described (218). Since then, two additional patients with SHML involving all four eyelids but not the orbits have been described (219,220).

Among persons who have SHML involving the orbit or eyelids, approximately 67% are men and 75% are black. The mean age of onset of symptoms is 17 years. Most patients present with an orbital or eyelid mass or swelling associated with proptosis, ocular displacement, decreased ocular motility, or ptosis. The masses usually are firm and rubbery to palpation. Bilateral disease exists in 22% of patients. Approximately 57% of patients have additional sites of extranodal involvement, most commonly the nasal cavity and paranasal sinuses. Lymphadenopathy is absent in 17% of patients, suggesting that the disease is entirely extranodal in some individuals (218).

The ocular globe is very rarely involved by SHML. The mean age of onset of symptoms is 6 years. Males outnumber females by 2 to 1. Blacks are affected more often than whites. The patients present with conjunctivitis, photophobia, and loss of visual acuity. Nearly all of them have additional sites of extranodal disease, and most of them have lymph node involvement as well (218).

The pathology of SHML occurring in extranodal sites, including the ocular adnexa, is highly distinctive (218,221,222) and is remarkably similar to that of SHML occurring in lymph nodes (216,217). Grossly, the lesions may be polypoid, nodular, or exophytic, depending on the site of origin, and are tan-white to yellow. Microscopically, nests, clusters and sheets of loosely aggregated histiocytes alternate with trabecular collections of mature plasma cells and small, benign and mature-appearing lymphocytes, mimicking the dilated sinuses and medullary cords, respectively, of lymph nodes involved by SHML. In some instances, the lymphocytes and especially the plasma cells dominate, obscuring the histiocytes. Germinal centers are generally absent. The histiocytes are usually large and contain abundant pale eosinophilic cytoplasm with indistinct borders. Sometimes, the histiocytes possess glassy eosinophilic cytoplasm with well-defined cell membranes. Birbeck granules, characteristic of Langerhans cells (223), are absent. Most nuclei are round to oval, vesicular, and contain a single small nucleolus, but some contain a prominent nucleolus or multiple nucleoli. Nuclear atypia and mitotic figures within the histiocytes are infrequent. Foamy histiocytes may be present. Well-formed granulomas and multinucleated giant cells are absent and histochemical stains for microorganisms are negative. A variable number of the histiocytes contain well-preserved lymphocytes and, occasionally, plasma cells, neutrophils, and erythrocytes in their cytoplasm, a phenomenon called emperipolesis (218,221,222). The histiocytes characteristically strongly express S-100 protein, CD11c, CD14, CD33, and CD68, variably express lysozyme, CD11b and CD36, and generally lack CD1a and HLA-DR (221,224–226). The lymphoid cells and plasma cells are polyclonal (222,224,225). In general, extranodal SHML exhibits more fibrosis (sometimes imparting the appearance of a nodular proliferation), fewer typical histiocytes, and smaller numbers of histiocytes displaying emperipolesis than lymph nodal SHML (218,222). Consequently, the diagnosis of SHML is often more difficult when it occurs in an extranodal site.

Most patients remain alive with stable, persistent disease or eventually enter remission; progression to death is uncommon. Consequently, therapy is not necessary for most patients. However, patients who have immunologic abnormalities and involvement of multiple or critical extranodal sites (i.e., the lower respiratory tract, the kidneys, liver, and the central nervous system) fare worse; some of these individuals may have a fatal outcome. When the manifestations of the disease are severe or progressive, therapeutic intervention in the form of corticosteroids in conjunction with cytotoxic drugs is often offered, although the response is not always dramatic. Although some patients who have massive ocular adnexal disease may require enucleation, involvement of the orbit or eyelid *per se* does not have an adverse effect on prognosis. In contrast, all known patients who have ocular globe involvement have died from their disease or are alive with persistent disease (218).

Langerhans Cell Histiocytosis

Langerhans cell histiocytosis (i.e., histiocytosis X) is an uncommonly occurring multisystem disease that has a broad spectrum of clinical and pathologic presentations (227). Lichtenstein introduced the generic term histiocytosis X in 1953 to encompass three clinicopathologic syndromes: eosinophilic granuloma of bone, Hand-Schüller-Christian syndrome (i.e., triad of exophthalmos, diabetes insipidus, and osteolytic bone lesions), and Letterer-Siwe disease (228). Lichtenstein believed that these syndromes represented a spectrum of related inflammatory histiocytoses ranging from least to most aggressive, but was uncertain of their pathogenesis (228). Later, Nezelof and coworkers (229) appreciated that the lesions of histiocytosis X are the result of the proliferation and tissue infiltration by cells that are morphologically and immunologically similar to Langerhans cells. For this reason, the Histiocyte Society has recommended use of the term *Langerhans cell histiocytosis* instead of histiocytosis X since 1985 (230,231).

The disease is further described clinically as unifocal or multifocal, localized or disseminated, and with or without systemic involvement (230,231). The prevailing opinion has been that Langerhans cell histiocytosis is nonneoplastic (230,231); it had been suggested that it is a disorder of immune regulation (232). However, it has been shown that all forms of Langerhans cell histiocytosis represent clonal proliferative processes (233) and probably represent true neoplasms exhibiting variable clinical behavior. These disorders are discussed in detail in Chapter 51. They are summarized briefly here, primarily as they relate to the ocular adnexa.

In general, the younger the patient who has Langerhans cell histiocytosis, the greater is the likelihood of multifocal disease (228,232). Letterer-Siwe disease is the acute disseminated form of Langerhans cell histiocytosis; it accounts for approximately 10% of all cases. Letterer-Siwe disease occurs in infants and very young children (<2 years). It is characterized by fever, anemia, thrombocytopenia, failure to thrive, and multisystem (i.e., cutaneous, lymph node, and visceral) involvement. Death usually occurs within 2 years after diagnosis (234). Hand-Schüller-Christian disease is the chronic disseminated form of Langerhans cell histiocytosis. It occurs in children and is characterized by chronic, progressive, remitting and relapsing lesions of the skull bones, especially the orbit, jaw, and mastoid, and frequently is accompanied by skin and pulmonary involvement (232). Eosinophilic granuloma is the localized form of Langerhans cell histiocytosis. It usually occurs in older children and adolescents and rarely in adults. It occurs primarily as solitary osseous lesions or in the lungs. This is the most common form of the disease and carries the best prognosis (232). No satisfactory explanation exists to account for the various clinical courses observed among patients who have Langerhans cell histiocytosis, but young age, multifocal disease, and organ dysfunction appear to indicate a poor prognosis (235,236).

Intraocular involvement by Langerhans cell histiocytosis is rare; it usually occurs as part of the acute disseminated form of the disease (i.e., Letterer-Siwe disease) (236). In these cases, the uveal tract, particularly the choroid, is affected (237–239), although involvement of the retina and sclera also has been described (240,241). Orbital involvement occurs in about 25% of cases of Langerhans cell histiocytosis, overall (236). It is rare in Letterer-Siwe disease but is a common component of the chronic disseminated form of the disease, but this comprises only 10% to 15% of patients who have Langerhans cell histiocytosis (230,231). The most common form of Langerhans cell histiocytosis involving the orbit is the localized form (i.e., eosinophilic granuloma), which usually is associated with an osteolytic lesion of the orbit (236). Eosinophilic granuloma is said to have a distinct predilection for the superotemporal orbital bone at the rim of the orbit (242); however, the lateral wall is frequently involved (243). Orbital soft tissue involvement without a bony defect is uncommon and should raise the suspicion of an alternative disease process, such as a pseudotumor or granulocytic sarcoma (53).

Orbital involvement by Langerhans cell histiocytosis accounts for less than 1% of all orbital tumors (236). The most common sign and symptom is proptosis; other signs and symptoms include erythema of the eyelids, edema, ptosis and periorbital pain (236,244). Typical findings include a unifocal osteolytic lesion of the frontal bone or the lateral wall of the orbit with erosion of the greater wing of the sphenoid bone accompanied by a large soft tissue mass that extends into the extraconal space of the orbit, the infratemporal fossa, middle cranial fossa and the ocular adnexa. Intraocular and brain parenchymal involvement are rare (236,245). Occasionally, additional osteolytic lesions may be present in the region, but the radiographic skeletal survey is usually otherwise normal (245,246). The osteolytic lesions display irregular, serrated margins radiographically and may be confused with clinically more aggressive neoplasms. Calcification and periosteal new bone formation are absent (245). Radiologic evidence of disease may be present without clinical signs (236). Nonophthalmic findings and laboratory studies are generally unremarkable (245). These unifocal lesions often respond well to curettage with or without low-dose irradiation or corticosteroids (228,236,243,246, 247); they also may heal completely without treatment (236,248).

Grossly, the lesions are described as soft, friable, hemorrhagic tan-yellow tissue. The unifying histopathologic feature of Langerhans cell histiocytosis is the presence of organ infiltration by dendritic cells related to the normally occurring Langerhans cell population. Langerhans cells are weakly phagocytic, antigen presenting dendritic cells (see Chapters 2 and 3). These cells are large and contain abundant, ill-defined acidophilic cytoplasm. Peculiar cytoplasmic organelles called Birbeck (Langerhans) granules may be identified in the cytoplasm of many, although not all, of these cells by electron microscopy (223). The nuclei are pale, vesicular, and oval to irregular in shape, often having an indented, folded, or creased appearance. Many nuclei exhibit a longitudinal groove resulting in a "coffee-bean" appearance. They contain stippled chromatin and nucleoli are inconspicuous. Phagocytosis is not seen and mitoses are uncommon. Some of the cells may become foamy. Multinucleated giant cells containing "coffee bean" nuclei may be present. The cells characteristically express S-100 protein, CD45, CD1a, HLA-DR, ATPase, and α-D-mannosidase and lack CD68, nonspecific esterase, lysozyme, and α_1-antichymotrypsin, analogous to normal Langerhans cells. Variable numbers of inflammatory cells, especially eosinophils, usually are present in the lesions (53,227,231,232,249, 250) (Fig. 35.37). There are no obvious histopathologic differences among lesions occurring in patients who have localized disease compared with multisystem involvement (250). The histopathologic features cannot be used to predict clinical behavior or determine prognosis (249,250).

Multiple Myeloma and Plasmacytoma

Multiple myeloma is a systemic malignant plasma cell proliferation. It is characterized by the presence of multiple "punched-out" osteolytic lesions, particularly in the skull and vertebrae, caused by tumor-like collections of neoplastic plasma cells within the bone and bone marrow. Myeloma plasma cells are monoclonal. They synthesize and secrete a specific monoclonal immunoglobulin composed of one heavy and one light chain (e.g., IgGκ, IgAκ, IgDλ) or free light chains. This myeloma (M) protein often is detectable in the urine, where it is known as Bence Jones protein, or in the serum. Some cases of multiple myeloma are nonsecretory (251,252). Cases of multiple myeloma comprise most plasma cell neoplasms (251,252) (see Chapter 42).

A plasmacytoma is a solitary, localized tumor-like collection of clonal neoplastic plasma cells that are similarly capable of synthesizing and secreting a specific monoclonal immunoglobulin. In these instances, however, the M protein often is produced in too small a quantity to be detected in the serum or urine. Plasmacytomas comprise less than 10% of all plasma cell tumors (251,252). Plasmacytomas may occur within bone (i.e., solitary plasmacytoma of bone [osseous plasmacytoma]) or outside of bone (i.e., extramedullary plasmacytoma) (251). Solitary osseous plasmacytomas manifest as lytic bone lesions, most commonly in the femur, pelvis and spine. These patients have no evidence of bone marrow disease and radiologic surveys of the skeleton are otherwise normal. However, solitary osseous plasmacytomas generally represent an early manifestation of multiple myeloma with dissemination occurring within 3 years in most cases (251,253). Solitary extramedullary plasmacytomas are soft tissue plasma cell tumors. They occur most frequently in the head and neck, especially in the sinonasal or nasopharyngeal regions (251,252,254). These patients similarly have no evidence of bone marrow disease and radiologic surveys of the skeleton are normal, except perhaps for erosion of bone adjacent to the plasmacytoma (251,253). Dissemination is far less common than with solitary osseous plasmacytomas. Solitary extramedullary plasmacytomas are considered to be a separate disease process, whereas solitary

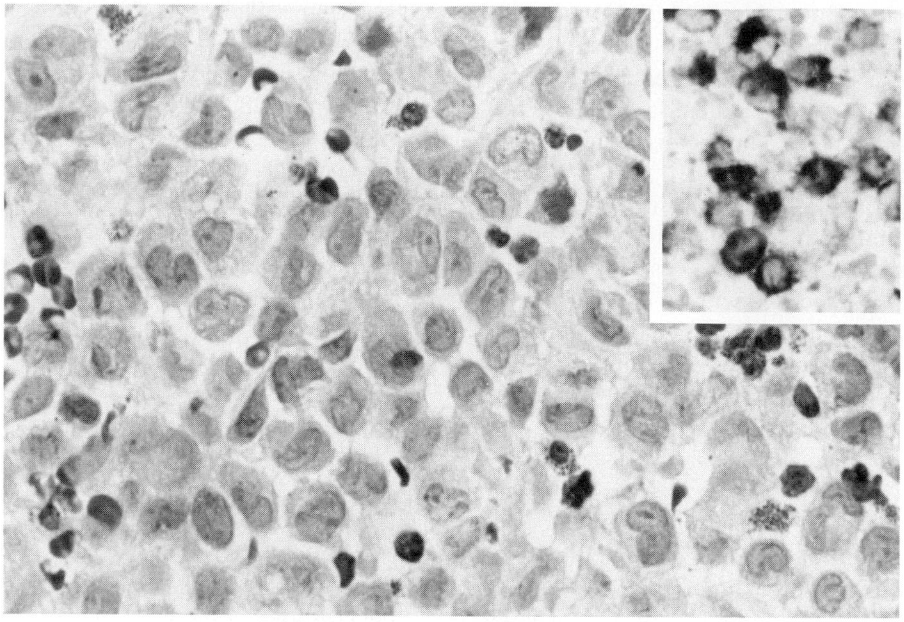

FIG. 35.37. Langerhans cell histiocytosis (i.e., histiocytosis X) manifesting as an orbital tumor mass in a 7-year-old boy. The lesion is composed of large histiocytoid cells containing abundant, ill-defined acidophilic cytoplasm and pale nuclei that often have an indented, folded, or creased appearance. Eosinophils are scattered throughout. Immunoperoxidase staining demonstrates that many of these large histiocytoid cells contain S-100 protein (hematoxylin and eosin stain, original magnification: 630× magnification; **Inset:** immunostain, original magnification: 400× magnification).

osseous plasmacytomas are probably in a continuum toward multiple myeloma (251,253).

The ocular adnexa rarely is the site of involvement by systemic multiple myeloma, a solitary osseous plasmacytoma, or an extramedullary plasmacytoma. In a compilation of four series of orbital tumors, only 4 of almost 2,000 such tumors were plasmacytomas (255). Orbital involvement may be the initial clinical manifestation of multiple myeloma or may occur sometime during the course of the disease. The orbital roof and frontal bones are most often affected; occasionally, tumors erode upward from the floor of the orbit. A solitary plasmacytoma of bone unassociated with systemic disease may arise in the same locations. In both instances, secondary infiltration of the orbital contents may occur. Extramedullary plasmacytomas unassociated with bone destruction arise only rarely in the orbit and conjunctiva (256–259). As of 1997, fewer than 20 cases of solitary extramedullary plasmacytoma of the ocular adnexa had been reported (260). Rarely, orbital myeloma plasma cell infiltrates and plasmacytomas are associated with the local deposition of amyloid (261,262).

Most patients who have orbital involvement present with slowly progressive proptosis over weeks to months, often accompanied by vision loss, diplopia, disturbances in ocular motility, and sometimes by ptosis, similar to patients who present with orbital lymphoid proliferations. Patients also may complain of pain, particularly if there is bone destruction (257,258,263). The presence of one or more osteolytic lesions is helpful in the differential diagnosis because inflammatory pseudotumors are not associated and lymphoid proliferations rarely are associated with bone destruction (32,53,66,67).

Systemic multiple myeloma, solitary plasmacytoma of bone, and extramedullary plasmacytoma display the same morphologic spectrum. The lesions consist of a diffuse, sheetlike proliferation of neoplastic plasma cells supported by a sparse fibrous connective tissue stroma. The neoplastic plasma cells may be small and well differentiated, approximating normal plasma cells in appearance, or they may be variably sized and exhibit cytologic atypia or may be poorly differentiated, even anaplastic, and difficult to recognize as plasma cells (264). The immunohistochemical demonstration of monotypic cytoplasmic immunoglobulin within the cells confirms their plasma cell lineage, clonal origin and neoplastic nature (21,256). This and other immunohistochemical studies are also useful in excluding other entities such as undifferentiated carcinomas, malignant melanoma, and neuroectodermal tumors from consideration.

It is important to distinguish a solitary extramedullary plasmacytoma from multiple myeloma because of the difference in therapy, management and prognosis. Most patients found to have a malignant plasma cell tumor involving the orbit or orbital bones are discovered to have multiple myeloma on systemic evaluation or develop disseminated disease shortly thereafter (53,256,258,265). All such patients should be referred to a hematologist-oncologist for evaluation that includes a skeletal survey, bone marrow biopsy, and immunoelectrophoretic studies of the serum and urine.

Patients who have solitary plasmacytomas of bone without evidence of systemic disease remain at increased risk of developing systemic disease for many years (251). Extramedullary plasmacytomas eventuate into multiple myeloma far less frequently (251) but may do so (254). For this reason, these patients must be followed carefully and reevaluated periodically (251). Solitary osseous and extramedullary plasmacytomas are highly radiosensitive and usually can be managed successfully with localized radiation therapy; surgery and chemotherapy are generally reserved for recurrent or persistent disease (251,257,258). Systemic disease generally is treated with chemotherapy (251,252).

Granulocytic Sarcoma

Granulocytic sarcoma is a localized extramedullary tumor comprised of malignant cells of myeloid-lineage derivation (266). Granulocytic sarcomas were initially described in 1811 (267); their association with acute leukemia was recognized in 1893 (268). Initially, these tumors were called chloromas (269) because some of them have a characteristic grossly green color attributable to the presence of the enzyme myeloperoxidase (270). Because not all myeloid tumors are green, the term *granulocytic sarcoma,* recommended by Rappaport in 1966 (264), has been widely adopted and is the prevailing term used today. Granulocytic sarcoma occurs in four clinical situations:

1. As a localized tissue manifestation in patients who have acute myeloid leukemia
2. As a sign of impending blast crisis in chronic myelogenous leukemia or leukemic transformation in patients who have myelodysplastic disorders
3. As a forerunner of acute myeloid leukemia in nonleukemic patients (266)
4. Less commonly, as an isolated neoplasm without progression to acute myeloid leukemia (271)

Granulocytic sarcoma is observed in only about 3% to 7% of cases of myeloid leukemia overall (272). Among adults, granulocytic sarcomas are most frequently associated with those acute myeloid leukemias classified as M2 according to the French-American-British (FAB) classification (273). They sporadically occur in other morphologic subtypes, including acute myelomonocytic leukemia (FAB M4, M5), acute promyelocytic leukemia (FAB M3), and acute megakaryoblastic leukemia (FAB M7) (273).

Granulocytic sarcomas have been described in many locations but occur most frequently in the soft tissues, lymph nodes, and skin and as isolated lytic bone lesions (266). They also may arise in the orbital bones or the soft tissues of the orbit and eyelids (274). The most common presentation is that of a tumor confined to a single location (266). A disproportionate number of ophthalmic and nonophthalmic granulocytic sarcomas appear to occur in individuals from Asia, the South Pacific and Africa (275). The incidence of ophthalmic granulocytic sarcoma also appears to be remarkably high among Turkish children (276).

Granulocytic sarcomas may involve the ocular adnexa of persons of all ages, but predominantly occur in the pediatric population. Among 33 patients reported by Zimmerman and Font (274), the age range was 1 to 61 years. However, 75% of the patients were in the first decade, the median age being 7 years (274). Males predominate over females by a ratio of about 1.5:1. Unlike nonophthalmic cases, when granulocytic sarcoma occurs in the orbit or eyelids, it usually represents the initial clinical manifestation of an as yet undiagnosed underlying leukemia (274). Most patients have simultaneous evidence of bone marrow and peripheral blood involvement by acute myeloid leukemia or their leukemia manifests itself within 6 months after the ocular presentation (274,275). Occasionally, however, granulocytic sarcoma occurs late in the course of disease. Most patients present with an orbital or eyelid mass or swelling associated with proptosis, ocular displacement, diplopia, or ptosis. Often, patients have bilateral disease (274,275,277). Other patients have diffuse disease, including involvement of the paranasal sinuses and other skull bones (274). Consequently, granulocytic sarcoma should be strongly considered when an intraorbital mass, especially if bilateral, is encountered in a child.

The differential diagnosis of a retrobulbar orbital soft tissue mass in a child includes, in addition to granulocytic sarcoma, inflammatory pseudotumor, African Burkitt's lymphoma, rhabdomyosarcoma, and metastatic neuroblastoma (275). Inflammatory pseudotumors more commonly present as extraocular polymyositis or optic nerve inflammation rather than as a focal orbital tumor mass (275). African Burkitt's lymphoma characteristically involves the maxillary bone, and orbital involvement is secondary. Other non-Hodgkin's lymphomas of the orbit and eyelids generally occur in older persons (32). Moreover, unlike orbital lymphomas, orbital granulocytic sarcomas frequently are associated with destruction of the bony walls of the orbit (275). Granulocytic sarcomas have a predilection for the lateral orbit (277), which differs from the more common location of rhabdomyosarcoma in the superior orbit (275). Bilateral disease or multiple intraorbital and extraorbital soft tissue masses mitigates strongly against rhabdomyosarcoma (275). Metastatic neuroblastoma more commonly causes concomitant osteolytic defects (275). Radiographically, granulocytic sarcoma lesions tend to mold to contiguous structures, including the sclera and the orbital bones, in patterns that mimic orbital lymphomas in adults (32,158,160), and only the medial wall is likely to show dissolution with sinus involvement (275). The lesional tissue has a magnetic resonance signal intensity different from that of the contiguous heavily collagenized sclera because leukemic masses generally are devoid of a significant fibrous stroma (275).

Granulocytic sarcomas exhibit a spectrum of histopathologic features. Approximately 50% of cases contain occasional to numerous eosinophilic myelocytes, characterized by immature unilobar nuclei and eosinophilic cytoplasmic granules, which indicate myeloid differentiation (266,271). The presence of these cells is considered practically diagnostic of granulocytic sarcoma (278). Consequently, these are the easiest cases to identify correctly in routine histologic sections. The remaining approximately 50% of cases lack eosinophilic myelocytes and are primarily composed of myeloblasts, characterized by the presence of immature and round, ovoid, or reniform blastlike nuclei that possess finely stippled chromatin and one or two small nucleoli (266,271). These cells may be mistaken for those comprising diffuse large B and T lymphomas, Burkitt's lymphoma, or lymphoblastic lymphoma (266,271). Consequently, granulocytic sarcomas are frequently misinterpreted as non-Hodgkin's lymphomas. Alternatively, especially in children, these lesions sometimes may be misinterpreted histopathologically as rhabdomyosarcoma, neuroblastoma or various other nonhematopoietic neoplasms (274).

The histopathologic differential diagnosis of granulocytic sarcoma from malignant lymphoma and nonhematopoietic neoplasms is greatly aided by histochemical and immunohistochemical studies. The first significant advance in this regard was the introduction in 1964 of the Leder stain for naphthol ASD-chloroacetate esterase, whose expression is indicative of myeloid lineage derivation (279). Approximately 75% of granulocytic sarcomas stain positively with the Leder stain (266). However, the number of positive cells varies considerably among cases; some cases contain as few as 10% positive cells (280,281). Mast cells stain positively with the Leder stain, which may cause diagnostic confusion. A higher proportion of granulocytic sarcomas contain lysozyme (266); therefore, the immunohistochemical demonstration of lysozyme can be very helpful in diagnosis, especially in those cases in which the Leder stain is negative. However, tissue histiocytes contain lysozyme. The combined absence of naphthol-ASD-chloroacetate esterase and lysozyme does not exclude a diagnosis of granulocytic sarcoma (271,281). The immunohistochemical demonstration of monoclonal antibody-defined cell surface antigens in routinely prepared paraffin tissue sections is the most helpful approach. Approximately 90% or more of granulocytic sarcomas express CD45 (leukocyte common antigen) (282), indicative of their hematopoietic origin, which greatly assists in distinguishing them from various nonhematopoietic neoplasms. The immunohistochemical demonstration of myeloid-associated antigens (i.e., CD13, CD14, CD15, CD33, and CD68) in the absence of B- and T-cell–associated antigens, is most helpful in the immunodiagnosis of granulocytic sarcoma and its differential from B- and T-cell non-Hodgkin's lymphomas (281,282). In this regard it is important to remember that CD43, commonly thought of as a T-cell–associated antigen, is expressed by myeloid cells (see Chapter 3). Approximately 50% of granulocytic sarcomas express CD43 (282); these cases should not be misdiagnosed as T-cell lymphoma. For all these reasons, the immunodiagnosis of granulocytic sarcoma should be based on the constellation of histochemical and immunohistochemical findings.

A translocation between chromosomes 8 and 21, t(8;21), occurs in approximately 7% of all acute myeloid leukemias and in 18% of those classified as M2 according to the FAB classification (283,284). Characteristic clinical features of these patients include a younger age of onset, frequently splenomegaly, a high complete remission rate, and among the longest relapse-free survival durations (285,286). A subgroup of patients who have acute myeloid leukemia and t(8;21) develop granulocytic sarcomas (273,287–293). Investigators have reported incidences of 17%, 21%, and 22% of granulocytic sarcomas among patients who have acute myeloid leukemia exhibiting t(8;21) (288,290,292). Among 53 patients with M2 acute myeloid leukemia seen at one institution between 1980 and 1992, 8 (15%) had t(8;21) (273). Three (38%) of these eight patients and none of those with the M2 acute myeloid leukemias lacking t(8;21) developed granulocytic sarcoma (273). Among the literature cases of granulocytic sarcoma in which karyotypic analyses were performed, most of the abnormal karyotypes were t(8;21) (273). Although other chromosomal abnormalities have been reported (288,294–296), granulocytic sarcoma is believed to occur most frequently in association with t(8;21) (273). The pathogenesis of extramedullary tumor formation in t(8;21) acute myeloid leukemia is unclear.

The prognosis of patients who have granulocytic sarcoma depends on the initial context in which it occurs (266). Most cases of granulocytic sarcoma occurring in nonleukemic patients progress to acute myeloid leukemia within months (266). The median interval from diagnosis to acute myeloid leukemia has been reported to be about 10 months and the median survival 22 months (266,297). Among patients who have orbital granulocytic sarcoma, the interval to death secondary to overt leukemia has been reported to vary from 1 to 30 months after the onset of tumor symptoms (274). The prevailing opinion is that granulocytic sarcoma should be treated as acute myeloid leukemia, even in the absence of clinically detectable leukemia (298). Patients who receive induction chemotherapy that includes cytosine arabinoside appear to have a significantly lower probability of developing acute leukemia and therefore a longer survival (297,299). Some nonleukemic patients have remained disease free for several years after discontinuation of treatment (271). Among those patients who have overt acute myeloid leukemia, the presence of granulocytic sarcoma does not alter the rate of remission after chemotherapy (276). However, among those patients who have acute myeloid leukemia exhibiting t(8;21), those who develop granulocytic sarcoma may have a less favorable prognosis (273).

SUMMARY AND CONCLUSIONS

Lymphoid infiltrates occurring in the ocular adnexa have traditionally posed a formidable clinical and histopathologic dilemma. In the past, the rate of error in accuracy of histopathologic diagnosis and ability to predict clinical outcome were estimated to lie between 20% and 50%. Significant advances in our understanding of these lesions has occurred during the past 15 years because of improvements in histopathologic criteria; the development of immunodiagnostic criteria; the correlative clinical, histopathologic, and immunophenotypic analysis of large patient cohorts; and the application of molecular genetic techniques. The recognition of MALT lymphomas and the development of the REAL classification have contributed to our further understanding of the ocular adnexal lymphoid proliferations.

The term *ocular adnexal lymphoid proliferation* is employed to encompass all of the hypercellular, lymphoid cell–rich lymphoid hyperplasias, atypical lymphoid hyperplasias, and malignant lymphomas that occur in the ocular adnexa. The term *orbital pseudotumor* is used to denote those benign, hypocellular, lymphoid cell-poor orbital inflammatory conditions that are without evidence of a specific local or systemic cause. In addition to the orbital pseudotumors, other hematopoietic disorders, such as SHML, Langerhans cell histiocytosis, plasmacytomas, and granulocytic sarcomas, involve the ocular adnexa. These disorders represent distinct clinicopathologic entities that exhibit fundamental clinical, pathologic, and biologic differences from the ocular adnexal lymphoid proliferations and should be distinguished from them.

Patients who have ocular adnexal lymphoid proliferations, regardless of histopathology (i.e., lymphoid hyperplasia, atypical lymphoid hyperplasia, or malignant lymphoma), or bilaterality, do not appear to differ significantly with respect to age, sex, presenting complaints, duration of symptoms, or ophthalmic findings, with the possible exception of orbital bone erosion, which is highly associated with malignant lymphoma. Clinical evaluation alone usually is of little value in distinguishing benign and malignant ocular adnexal lymphoid proliferations. CT similarly reveals no known characteristic features that permit this technique to discriminate reliably between benign and malignant orbital lymphoid proliferations. Consequently, the accurate diagnosis of ocular adnexal lymphoid proliferations requires histopathologic examination assisted by ancillary techniques such as immunophenotypic and molecular genetic analysis.

Lymphoid hyperplasias are hypercellular, lymphoid cell–rich lesions that mimic malignant lymphoma clinically and histopathologically, sometimes to an extraordinary degree. The fact that a significantly lower proportion of ocular adnexal lymphoid proliferations represent lymphoid hyperplasias than was previously believed is a reflection of increased histopathologic sophistication, the awareness of MALT lymphomas and our enhanced ability to detect clonality because of technologic advances, especially in molecular genetic techniques. Atypical lymphoid hyperplasias are lymphoid proliferations that cannot be categorized unequivocally as lymphoid hyperplasia or malignant lymphoma. These lesions comprise only about 5% or less of ocular adnexal lymphoid proliferations.

Most lymphoid proliferations occurring in the ocular adnexa are malignant lymphomas. Most of these lesions are diffuse, densely cellular proliferations comprised predominantly of small lymphoid cells superimposed on a sparse connective tissue stroma. Before the development of the REAL classification, the ocular adnexal malignant lymphomas were subclassified among multiple categories in the Working Formulation, particularly the small lymphocytic, plasmacytoid small lymphocytic, diffuse small cleaved cell, and diffuse mixed small and large cell categories, with lesser numbers of follicular and diffuse large cell lymphomas. However, it is widely recognized that most ocular adnexal malignant lymphomas arise in MALT, represent MALT lymphomas, and display the morphologic spectrum observed in MALT lymphomas originating in other extranodal sites. The MALT lymphomas share common histopathologic characteristics that include a marginal zone-type distribution and a variable cytologic composition, dominated by centrocyte-like cells, monocytoid cells, small lymphocytes, or plasmacytoid cells. The neoplastic cells often surround, and sometimes infiltrate into, benign reactive follicles and infiltrate the overlying epithelium, resulting in so-called lymphoepithelial lesions. MALT lymphomas and nearly all other categories of malignant lymphoma occurring in the ocular adnexa are B-cell neoplasms. Consequently, they express a variety of pan-B-cell–associated antigens and monotypic surface immunoglobulin and exhibit clonal immunoglobulin heavy- and light-chain gene rearrangements. The molecular genetic and cytogenetic features of the ocular adnexal malignant lymphomas is largely unknown, although they do not apparently exhibit *BCL1, BCL2,* or *MYC* gene rearrangements.

If a patient is found to have a lymphoid proliferation limited to the ocular adnexa, unilateral or bilateral, after a careful and thorough systemic evaluation, local radiation therapy is recommended. The disease recurs locally or develops systemically in a significant proportion of patients who are treated by observation only or surgery alone. Even polyclonal lymphoid hyperplasias are capable of recurrence and similarly should be ablated by radiation therapy, and not simply treated with systemic corticosteroids. The latter approach is usually reserved for orbital pseudotumors. Most patients who have stage IE disease treated only with local radiation therapy undergo complete remission. This is also true for patients who have bilateral disease and many patients who have stage IE diffuse large B-cell lymphoma. The single most important and statistically significant prognostic factor among individuals who present with ocular adnexal lymphoid proliferations appears to be the extent of disease determined after a thorough clinical staging. Most patients who present with a lymphoid proliferation limited to the ocular adnexa (stage IE), regardless of the histopathology, immunophenotype, or bilaterality, have a benign, relatively indolent clinical course.

ACKNOWLEDGMENTS

The author thanks his longtime friend and colleague, Dr. Frederick Jakobiec, for his collaborative participation in many of the studies cited here. The author also thanks Ida Nathan and Al Lamme for preparing the excellent photomicrographs.

REFERENCES

1. Morgan G. Lymphocytic tumors of the orbit. In: *Modern problems in ophthalmology: orbit disorders.* Basel: Karger, 1975:14:35–38.
2. Morgan G, Harry J. Lymphocytic tumors of indeterminate nature: a 5 year follow-up of 98 conjunctival and orbital lesions. *Br J Ophthalmol* 1978;62:381–383.
3. Jakobiec FA, McLean I, Font R. Clinicopathologic characteristics of orbital lymphoid hyperplasia. *Ophthalmology* 1979;86:948–966.
4. Knowles DM, Jakobiec FA. Orbital lymphoid neoplasms: a clinicopathologic study of 60 patients. *Cancer* 1980;46:576–589.
5. Knowles DM, Jakobiec FA. Ocular adnexal lymphoid neoplasms: clinical, histopathologic, electron microscopic and immunologic characteristics. *Hum Pathol* 1982;13:148– 162.
6. Knowles DM. The extranodal lymphoid infiltrate: a diagnostic dilemma. *Semin Diagn Pathol* 1985;2:147–151.
7. Burke JS. Histologic criteria for distinguishing between benign and malignant extranodal lymphoid infiltrates. *Semin Diagn Pathol* 1985; 2:151–162.
8. Knowles DM, Jakobiec FA. Cell marker analysis of extranodal lymphoid infiltrates: to what extent does the determination of mono- or polyclonality resolve the diagnostic dilemma of malignant lymphoma *v* pseudolymphoma in an extranodal site? *Semin Diagn Pathol* 1985;2:163–168.
9. Saltzstein SL. Pulmonary malignant lymphomas and pseudolymphomas: classification, therapy and prognosis. *Cancer* 1963;16: 928–955.
10. Saltzstein SL. Extranodal malignant lymphomas and pseudolymphomas. *Pathol Annu* 1969;4:159–184.
11. Pangalis GA, Nathwani BN, Rappaport H. Malignant lymphoma, well differentiated lymphocytic: its relationship with chronic lymphocytic leukemia and macroglobulinemia of Waldenström. *Cancer* 1977;39: 999–1010.
12. Lennert K, Mohri N, Stein H, et al. The histopathology of malignant lymphoma. *Br J Haematol* 1975;31[Suppl]:193–203.
13. Lukes RJ, Collins RD. A functional classification of malignant lymphomas. In: Rebuk JW, Berard CW, Abell MR, eds. *The reticuloendothelial system.* Baltimore: Williams & Wilkins, 1975:213–242.
14. Berard CW, Jaffe ES, Braylan RC, et al. Immunologic aspects and pathology of the malignant lymphoma. *Cancer* 1978;32:911–921.
15. Weisenburger DD, Nathwani BN, Diamond LW, et al. Malignant lymphoma, intermediate lymphocytic type: a clinicopathologic study of 42 cases. *Cancer* 1981;48:1415–1425.
16. Weisenburger DD, Kim H, Rappaport H. Mantle-zone lymphoma: a follicular variant of intermediate lymphocytic lymphoma. *Cancer* 1982;49:1429–1438.
17. Jakobiec FA, Iwamoto T. The ocular adnexa: introduction to lids, conjunctiva, and orbit. In: Jakobiec FA, ed. *Ocular anatomy, embryology and teratology.* Philadelphia: Harper and Row, 1982:677–732.
18. Sachs E, Wieczorek R, Jakobiec FA, et al. Lymphocyte subpopulations in the normal human conjunctiva: a monoclonal antibody study. *Ophthalmology* 1986;93:1276–1283.
19. Knowles DM, Jakobiec FA, Halper JP. Immunologic characterization of ten ocular adnexal lymphoid neoplasms. *Am J Ophthalmol* 1979; 87:603–619.
20. Knowles DM, Halper JP, Jakobiec FA. The immunologic characterization of 40 extranodal lymphoid infiltrates: usefulness in distinguishing between benign pseudolymphoma and malignant lymphoma. *Cancer* 1982;49:2321–2335.
21. Knowles DM. Immunophenotypic and immunogenotypic approaches useful in distinguishing benign and malignant lymphoid proliferations. *Semin Oncol* 1993;20:583–610.
22. Jakobiec FA, Iwamoto T, Knowles DM. Ocular adnexal lymphoid tumors: correlative ultrastructural and immunologic marker studies. *Arch Ophthalmol* 1982;100:84–98.
23. Harmon DC, Aisenberg AC, Harris NL, et al. Lymphocyte surface markers in orbital lymphoid neoplasms. *J Clin Oncol* 1984;2: 856–860.
24. Turner RR, Egbert P, Warnke R. Lymphocytic infiltrates of the conjunctiva and orbit: immunohistochemical staining of 16 cases. *Am J Clin Pathol* 1984;81:447–452.
25. Harris NL, Harmon DC, Pilch BZ, et al. Immunohistologic diagnosis of orbital lymphoid infiltrates. *Am J Surg Pathol* 1984;8:83–91.
26. Turner RR, Colby TV, Doggett RS. Well-differentiated lymphocytic lymphoma: a study of 47 patients with primary manifestation in the lung. *Cancer* 1984;54:2088–2096.
27. Ellis JH, Banks PM, Campbell J, et al. Lymphoid tumors of the ocular adnexa: clinical correlation with the Working Formulation classification and immunoperoxidase staining of paraffin sections. *Ophthalmology* 1985;92:1311–1324.
28. Kennedy JL, Nathwani BN, Burke JS, et al. Pulmonary lymphomas and other lymphoid lesions: a clinicopathologic and immunologic study of 64 patients. *Cancer* 1985;56:539–552.
29. Jakobiec FA, Iwamoto T, Patell M, et al. Ocular adnexal monoclonal lymphoid tumors with a favorable prognosis. *Ophthalmology* 1986; 93:1547–1557.
30. Burke JS, Sheibani K, Nathwani BN, et al. Monoclonal small (well-differentiated) lymphocytic proliferations of the gastrointestinal tract resembling lymphoid hyperplasia: a neoplasm of uncertain malignant potential. *Hum Pathol* 1987;18:1238–1245.
31. Medeiros LJ, Harris NL. Lymphoid infiltrates of the orbit and conjunctiva: a morphologic and immunophenotypic study of 99 cases. *Am J Surg Pathol* 1989;13:459–471.
32. Knowles DM, Jakobiec FA, McNally FA, et al. Lymphoid hyperplasia and malignant lymphoma occurring in the ocular adnexa (orbit, conjunctiva and eyelids): a prospective multiparametric analysis of 108 cases during 1977–1987. *Hum Pathol* 1990;21:959–973.
33. Seidman JG, Leder P. The arrangement and rearrangement of antibody genes. *Nature* 1978;276:790–796.
34. Tonegawa S. Somatic generation of antibody diversity. *Nature* 1983; 302:575–581.
35. Yanagi Y, Yoshikai Y, Legett K, et al. A human T cell specific cDNA clone encodes a protein having extensive homology to immunoglobulin chains. *Nature* 1984;308:145–149.
36. Pelicci PG, Knowles DM, Arlin ZA, et al. Multiple monoclonal B cell expansions and c-myc oncogene rearrangements in acquired immune deficiency syndrome-related lymphoproliferative disorders. *J Exp Med* 1986;164:2049–2060.
37. Neri A, Jakobiec FA, Pelicci PG, et al. Immunoglobulin and T cell receptor β chain gene rearrangement analysis of ocular adnexal lymphoid neoplasms: clinical and biologic implications. *Blood* 1987; 70:1519–1529.
38. Knowles DM, Athan E, Ubriaco A, et al. Extranodal non-cutaneous lymphoid hyperplasias represent a continuous spectrum of B-cell neoplasia: demonstration by molecular genetic analysis. *Blood* 1989;73: 1635–1645.
39. Birch-Hirschfeld A. Zur Diagnostik und Pathologie der Orbital-tumoren. *Berl Dtsch Ophthalmol Ges* 1905;32:127–135.
40. Jakobiec FA, Jones IS. Orbital inflammations. In: Jones IS, Jakobiec FA, eds. *Diseases of the orbit.* Hagerstown, MD: Harper & Row, 1979:187–205.
41. Henderson JW. *Orbital* tumors. New York: Decker, Thieme-Statton, 1980:513–546.
42. Garner A, Chavis RM. Lymphoid pseudotumor of the orbit. *Trans Ophthalmol Soc UK* 1979;99:231–233.
43. Garner A, Rahi AHS, Wright JE. Lymphoproliferative disorders of the orbit: an immunological approach to diagnosis and pathogenesis. *Br J Ophthalmol* 1983;67:561–569.
44. Hogan MJ, Zimmerman LE. *Ophthalmic pathology: an atlas and textbook.* Philadelphia: WB Saunders, 1962:727–771.
45. Chavis RM, Garner A, Wright JE. Inflammatory orbital pseudotumor: a clinicopathologic study. *Arch Ophthalmol* 1978;96:1817–1822.
46. Char DH. *Clinical ocular oncology.* New York: Churchill Livingstone, 1989:349–366.
47. Kelly AG, Rosas-Uribe A, Kraus ST. Orbital lymphomas and pseudolymphomas: a clinicopathologic study of eleven cases. *Am J Clin Pathol* 1977;68:377–386.
48. Kennerdell JS, Johnson BL, Deutsch M. Radiation treatment of orbital lymphoid hyperplasia. *Ophthalmology* 1979;86:942–947.
49. Sergott RC, Glaser JS, Charyulu K. Radiotherapy for idiopathic inflammatory orbital pseudotumor: indications and results. *Arch Ophthalmol* 1981;99:853–856.

50. Fitzpatrick PJ, Macko S. Lymphoreticular tumors of the orbit. *Int J Radiat Oncol Biol Phys* 1984;10:333–340.
51. Fuji H, Fujisada H, Kondo T, et al. Orbital pseudotumor: histopathological classification and treatment. *Ophthalmalogica* 1985;190: 230–242.
52. Lanciano R, Fowblc B, Sergott RC, et al. The results of radiotherapy for orbital pseudotumor. *Int J Radiat Oncol Biol Phys* 1990;18: 407–411.
53. Jakobiec FA, Font RL. Orbit: lymphoid tumors. In: Spencer WH, Font RL, Green WR, et al, eds. *Ophthalmic pathology: an atlas and textbook,* 3rd ed. Philadelphia: WB Saunders, 1986:2663–2737.
54. Mauriello JA, Flanagan JC. Pseudotumor and lymphoid tumor: distinct clinicopathologic entities. *Surv Ophthalmol* 1989;34:142–148.
55. Jakobiec FA, Knowles DM. An overview of ocular adnexal lymphoid tumors. *Trans Am Ophthalmol Soc* 1989;137:420–444.
56. Garner A. Orbital lymphoproliferative disorders. *Br J Ophthalmol* 1992;76:47–48.
57. Henderson JW. *Orbital tumors.* New York: Raven Press, 1994: 317–411.
58. Medeiros LJ, Harmon DC, Linggood RM, et al. Immunohistologic features predict clinical behavior of orbital and conjunctival lymphoid infiltrates. *Blood* 1989;74:2121–2129.
59. Coupland SE, Krause L, Delecluse H-J, et al. Lymphoproliferative lesions of the ocular adnexa: analysis of 112 cases. *Ophthalmology* 1998;105:1430–1441.
60. Mombaerts I, Goldschmeding R, Schlingermann RO, et al. What is orbital pseudotumor? *Surv Ophthalmol* 1996;41:66–78.
61. Jakobiec FA, Font RL. Noninfectious orbital inflammations. In: Spencer WH, ed. *Ophthalmic pathology: an atlas and textbook,* vol 3, 3rd ed. Philadelphia: WB Saunders, 1986:2777–2795.
62. Garner A. Pathology of pseudotumors of the orbit: a review. *J Clin Pathol* 1973;26:639–648.
63. Kennerdell JS, Dresner SC. The nonspecific orbital inflammatory syndromes. *Surv Ophthalmol* 1984;29:93–103.
64. Rootman J, McCarthy M, White V, et al. Idiopathic sclerosing inflammation of the orbit: a distinct clinicopathologic entity. *Ophthalmology* 1994;101:570–584.
65. Rootman J, Nugent R. The classification and management of acute orbital pseudotumors. *Ophthalmology* 1982;89:1040–1048.
66. Mottow LS, Jakobiec FA. Idiopathic inflammatory orbital pseudotumor in childhood: I. Clinical characteristics. *Arch Ophthalmol* 1978; 96:1410–1417.
67. Mottow-Lippa L, Jakobiec FA, Smith M. Idiopathic inflammatory orbital pseudotumor in childhood: II. Results of diagnostic tests and biopsies. *Ophthalmology* 1981;88:565–574.
68. Snebold NG. Noninfectious orbital inflammations and vasculitis. In: Albert DM, Jakobiec FA, eds. *Principles and practice of ophthalmology: clinical practice,* vol 3. Philadelphia: WB Saunders, 1994: 1923–1942.
69. Nugent RA, Rootman J, Robertson WD, et al. Acute orbital pseudotumors: classification and CT features. *Am J Neuroradiol* 1981;2: 431–436.
70. McNicholas MM, Power WJ, Griffin JF. Idiopathic inflammatory pseudotumor of the orbit: CT features correlated with clinical outcome. *Clin Radiol* 1991;44:3–7.
71. Edwards MK, Zauel DW, Gilmor RL, et al. Invasive orbital pseudotumor: CT demonstration of extension beyond orbit. *Neuroradiology* 1982;23:215–217.
72. Weissler MC, Miller E, Fortune MA. Sclerosing orbital pseudotumor: a unique clinicopathologic entity. *Ann Otol Rhinol Laryngol* 1989; 98:496–501.
73. Frohman LP, Kupersmith MJ, Lang J, et al. Intracranial extension and bone destruction in orbital pseudotumor. *Arch Ophthalmol* 1986; 104:380–384.
74. Clifton AG, Borgstein RL, Moseley IF, et al. Intracranial extension of orbital pseudotumor. *Clin Radiol* 1992;45:23–26.
75. Moseley IF, Wright JE. Orbital pseudotumor. *Clin Radiol* 1992;45: 67–68.
76. Rootman J, Robertson W, Lapointe JS. Inflammatory diseases. In: Rootman J, ed. *Diseases of the orbit: a multidisciplinary approach.* Philadelphia: JB Lippincott, 1988:159–179.
77. Leone CR Jr, Lloyd WC III. Treatment protocol for orbital inflammatory disease. *Ophthalmology* 1985;92:1325–1333.
78. Char DH, Miller T. Orbital pseudotumor: fine-needle aspiration biopsy and response to therapy. *Ophthalmology* 1993;100:1702–1710.
79. Mombaerts I, Schlingemann RO, Goldschmeding R, et al. Are systemic corticosteroids useful in the management of orbital pseudotumors? *Ophthalmology* 1996;103:521–528.
80. Wright JE, Stewart WB, Krobel GB. Clinical presentation and management of lacrimal gland tumors. *Br J Ophthalmol* 1979;63: 600–606.
81. Bullen CL, Younge BR. Chronic orbital myositis. *Arch Ophthalmol* 1982;100:1749–1751.
82. Mauriello JA, Flanagan JC. Management of orbital inflammatory disease: a protocol. *Surv Ophthalmol* 1984;29:104–116.
83. Van der Gaag R, Koornneef L, van Heerde P, et al. Lymphoid proliferations in the orbit: malignant or benign? *Br J Ophthalmol* 1984;68: 892–900.
84. Kennerdell JS, Slamovits TL, Dekker A, et al. Orbital fine-needle aspiration biopsy. *Am J Ophthalmol* 1985;99:547–551.
85. Tijl JWM, Koornneef L. Fine needle aspiration biopsy in orbital tumors. *Br J Ophthalmol* 1991;75:491–492.
86. Brown DH, MacRae DL, Allen LH. Orbital pseudotumors. *J Otolaryngol* 1988;17:164–168.
87. Austin-Seymour MM, Donaldson SS, Egbert PR, et al. Radiotherapy of lymphoid diseases of the orbit. *Int J Radiat Oncol Biol Phys* 1985; 11:371–379.
88. Paris GL, Waltuch GF, Egbert PR. Treatment of refractory orbital pseudotumors with pulsed chemotherapy. *Ophthalmic Plast Reconstr Surg* 1990;6:96–101.
89. Shah SS, Lowder CY, Schmitt MA, et al. Low-dose methotrexate therapy for ocular inflammatory disease. *Ophthalmology* 1992;99: 1419–1423.
90. Noguchi H, Kephart GM, Campbell J, et al. Tissue eosinophilia and eosinophil degranulation in orbital pseudotumor. *Ophthalmology* 1991;98:928–932.
91. McCarthy JM, White VA, Harris G, et al. Idiopathic sclerosing inflammation of the orbit: immunohistologic analysis and comparison with retroperitoneal fibrosis. *Mod Pathol* 1993;6:581–587.
92. Comings DE, Skubi KB, Van Eyes J, et al. Familial multifocal fibrosclerosis: findings suggesting that retroperitoneal fibrosis, mediastinal fibrosis, sclerosing cholangitis, Riedel's thyroiditis, and pseudotumor of the orbit may be different manifestations of a single disease. *Ann Intern Med* 1967;66:884–892.
93. Kennerdell JS. The management of sclerosing nonspecific orbital inflammation. *Ophthalmic Surg* 1991;22:512–518.
94. Levine MR, Kaye L, Mair S, et al. Multifocal fibrosclerosis: report of a case of bilateral idiopathic sclerosing pseudotumor and retroperitoneal fibrosis. *Arch Ophthalmol* 1993;111:841–843.
95. Henderson JW. *Orbital tumors.* Philadelphia: WB Saunders, 1973: 555–587.
96. Hughes D, Buckley PJ. Idiopathic retroperitoneal fibrosis is a macrophage-rich process: implications for its pathogenesis and treatment. *Am J Surg Pathol* 1993;17:482–490.
97. Collison JM, Miller NR, Green WR. Involvement of orbital tissues by sarcoid. *Am J Ophthalmol* 1986;102:302–307.
98. Satorre J, Antle CM, O' Sullivan R, et al. Orbital lesions with granulomatous inflammation. *Can J Ophthalmol* 1991;26:174–195.
99. Raskin EM, McCormick SA, Maher EA, et al. Granulomatous idiopathic orbital inflammation. *Ophthalmic Plast Reconstr Surg* 1995; 11:131–135.
100. Garrity JA, Kennerdell JS, Johnson BL, et al. Cyclophosphamide in the treatment of orbital vasculitis. *Am J Ophthalmol* 1986;102: 97–102.
101. Kalina PH, Lie JT, Campbell J, et al. Diagnostic value and limitations of orbital biopsy in Wegener's granulomatosis. *Ophthalmology* 1992; 99:120–124.
102. Purcell JJ, Taulbee WA. Orbital myositis after upper respiratory tract infection. *Arch Ophthalmol* 1981;99:437–438.
103. Weinstein GS, Dresner SC, Slamovits Tl, et al. Acute and subacute orbital myositis. *Am J Ophthalmol* 1983;96:209–217.
104. Slavin ML, Glaser JS. Idiopathic orbital myositis. *Arch Ophthalmol* 1982;100:1261–1265.
105. Wirostko E, Johnson L, Wirostko B. Chronic orbital inflammatory disease: parasitisation of orbital leucocytes by mollicute-like organisms. *Br J Ophthalmol* 1989;73:865–870.

106. Easton JA, Smith WT. Non-specific granuloma of orbit (''orbital pseudotumor''). *J Pathol Bacteriology* 1961;82:345–354.
107. Barrett NR. Idiopathic mediastinal fibrosis. *Br J Surg* 1958;46: 207–218.
108. Richards AB, Skalka HW, Roberts FJ, et al. Pseudotumor of the orbit and retroperitoneal fibrosis: a form of multifocal fibrosclerosis. *Arch Ophthalmol* 1980;98:1617–1620.
109. Schonder AA, Clift RC, Brophy JW, et al. Bilateral recurrent orbital inflammation associated with retroperitoneal fibrosclerosis. *Br J Ophthalmol* 1985;69:783–787.
110. DuPont HL, Varco RL, Winchell CP. Chronic fibrous mediastinitis simulating pulmonic stenosis associated with inflammatory pseudotumor of the orbit. *Am J Med* 1968;44:447–452.
111. Andersen SR, Seedorff HH, Halberg P. Thyroiditis with myxoedema and orbital pseudotumor. *Acta Ophthalmol* 1963;41:120–125.
112. Arnott EJ, Greaves DP. Orbital involvement in Riedel's thyroiditis. *Br J Ophthalmol* 1965;49:1–5.
113. Wenger J, Gingrich JW, Mendeloff J. Sclerosing cholangitis: a manifestation of systemic disease. *Arch Intern Med* 1965;116:509–514.
114. Jakobiec FA, Gibralter RA, Knowles DM, et al. Lymphoid tumor of the lid. *Ophthalmology* 1980;87:1058–1064.
115. Knowles DM, Jakobiec FA. Quantitative determination of T cells in ocular lymphoid infiltrates: an indirect method for distinguishing between pseudolymphomas and malignant lymphomas. *Arch Ophthalmol* 1981;99:309–316.
116. Knowles DM, Jakobiec FA. The expression of surface antigen Leu 1 by ocular adnexal lymphoid neoplasms. *Am J Ophthalmol* 1982;94: 246–254.
117. Knowles DM, Jakobiec FA. Identification of T lymphocytes in ocular adnexal lymphoid neoplasms by hybridoma monoclonal antibodies. *Am J Ophthalmol* 1983;95:233–242.
118. McNally L, Jakobiec FA, Knowles DM. Clinical, morphologic, immunophenotypic, and molecular genetic analysis of bilateral ocular adnexal lymphoid neoplasms in 17 patients. *Am J Ophthalmol* 1987; 103:55–68.
119. Jakobiec FA, Neri A, Knowles DM. Genotypic monoclonality in immunophenotypically polyclonal orbital lymphoid tumors: a model of tumor progression in the lymphoid system. *Ophthalmology* 1987;94: 980–994.
120. Isaacson PG, Norton AJ. *Extranodal lymphomas.* Edinburgh: Churchill Livingstone, 1994:5–14.
121. Harris NL, Jaffe ES, Stein H, et al. A Revised European-American Classification of Lymphoid Neoplasms: a proposal from the International Lymphoma Study Group. *Blood* 1994;84:1361–1392.
122. Nakata M, Matsumo Y, Katsumata N, et al. Histology according to the Revised European-American lymphoma classification significantly predicts the prognosis of ocular adnexal lymphoma. *Leuk Lymphoma* 1999;32:533–543.
123. Knowles DM, Chaumulak GA, Subar M, et al. Lymphoid neoplasia associated with AIDS: the New York University Medical Center experience with 105 cases (1981–1986). *Ann Intern Med* 1988;108: 744–753.
124. Reifler DM, Warzynski MJ, Blount WR, et al. Orbital lymphoma associated with acquired immune deficiency syndrome (AIDS). *Surv Ophthalmol* 1994;38:371–380.
125. Weisenthal RW, Streeten BW, Dubansky AS, et al. Burkitt lymphoma presenting as a conjunctival mass. *Ophthalmology* 1995;102: 129–134.
126. Edelstein C, Shields JA, Shields CL, et al. Non-African Burkitt lymphoma presenting with oral thrush and an orbital mass in a child. *Am J Ophthalmol* 1997;124:859–861.
127. Sherman MD, Van Dalen JTW, Conrad K. Bilateral orbital infiltration as the initial sign of a peripheral T cell lymphoma presenting in a leukemic phase. *Ann Ophthalmol* 1990;22:93–95.
128. Henderson JW, Banks PM, Yeatts BP. T-cell lymphoma of the orbit. *Mayo Clin Proc* 1989;64:940–944.
129. Leidenix MJ, Mamalis N, Olson RJ, et al. Primary T cell immunoblastic lymphoma of the orbit in a pediatric patient. *Ophthalmology* 1993; 100:998–1002.
130. Stenson S, Ramsay DL. Ocular findings in mycosis fungoides. *Arch Ophthalmol* 1981;99:272–277.
131. Zucker JL, Doyle MF. Mycosis fungoides metastatic to the orbit. *Arch Ophthalmol* 1991;109:668–691.
132. Meekins B, Proia AD, Klintworth GK. Cutaneous T-cell lymphoma presenting as a rapidly enlarging ocular adnexal tumor. *Ophthalmology* 1985;92:1288–1293.
133. Jakobiec FA. Orbital Hodgkin's disease: clinicopathologic conference. *N Engl J Med* 1989;320:447–457.
134. Spencer J, Finn T, Isaacson P. Gut-associated lymphoid tissue: a morphological and immunocytochemical study of the human appendix. *Gut* 1985;26:672–679.
135. Wotherspoon AC, Hardman-Lea S, Isaacson PG. Mucosa-associated lymphoid tissue (MALT) in the human conjunctiva. *J Pathol* 1994; 174:33–37.
136. Hardman-Lea S, Kerr-Muir M, Wotherspoon AC, et al. Mucosa-associated lymphoid tissue lymphoma of the conjunctiva. *Arch Ophthalmol* 1994;112:1207–1212.
137. Isaacson PG. The MALT lymphoma concept updated. *Ann Oncol* 1995;6:319–320.
138. Emery JL, Dinsdale F. The perinatal development of lymphoreticular aggregates and lymph nodes in infants' lungs. *J Clin Pathol* 1973; 26:539–545.
139. Pabst R, Gehrke J. Is the bronchus-associated lymphoid tissue (BALT) an integral structure of the lung in normal mammals including humans? *Am J Respir Cell Mol Biol* 1990;3:131–135.
140. Gould SJ, Isaacson PG. Bronchus-associated lymphoid tissue (BALT) in human fetal and infant lung. *J Pathol* 1993;180:229–234.
141. Wotherspoon AC, Ortiz-Hidalgo C, Falzon MR, et al. *Helicobacter pylori*-associated gastritis and primary B cell gastric lymphoma. *Lancet* 1991:338:1175–1176.
142. Hyjck E, Smith WJ, Isaacson PG. Primary B cell lymphoma of salivary glands and its relationship to myoepithelial sialadenitis. *Hum Pathol* 1988;19:766–776.
143. Hyjek E, Isaacson PG. Primary B cell lymphoma of the thyroid and its relationship to Hashimoto's thyroiditis. *Hum Pathol* 1988;19: 1315–1326.
144. McMaster PRB, Aronson SB, Bedford MJ. Mechanisms of the host response in the eye: the anterior eye in germ-free animals. *Arch Ophthalmol* 1967;77:392–399.
145. Franklin RM, Remus LE. Conjunctival-associated lymphoid tissue: evidence for a role in the secretory immune system. *Invest Ophthalmol Vis Sci* 1984;25:181–187.
146. Fix AS, Arp LH. Conjunctiva-associated lymphoid tissue (CALT) in normal and *Bordetella avium*-infected turkeys. *Vet Pathol* 1989;26: 222–330.
147. Khatami M, Donnelly JJ, Haldar JP, et al. Massive follicular lymphoid hyperplasia in experimental allergic conjunctivitis: local antibody production. *Arch Ophthalmol* 1989;107:433–438.
148. Latkovic S. Ultrastructure of M cells in the conjunctival epithelium of the guinea pig. *Curr Eye Res* 1989;8:751–755.
149. Jakobiec FA, Lefkowitch J, Knowles DM. B- and T-lymphocytes in ocular disease. *Ophthalmology* 1984;91:635–654.
150. Duke-Elder S, ed. *Disease of the outer eye, part 1. System of ophthalmology.* London: Henry Kempton, 1965:102–103.
151. Westacott S, Garner A, Moseley IF, et al. Orbital lymphoma versus reactive lymphoid hyperplasia: an analysis of the use of computed tomography in differential diagnosis. *Br J Ophthalmol* 1991;75: 722–725.
152. White WL, Ferry JA, Harris NL, et al. Ocular adnexal lymphoma: a clinicopathologic study with identification of mucosa-associated lymphoid tissue type. *Ophthalmology* 1995;102:1994–2006.
153. Mamalis N, Mackman G, Hoids JB, et al. Simultaneous bilateral conjunctival and orbital lymphoma presenting as a conjunctival lesion. *Ophthalmic Surg* 1988;19:662–663.
154. Sigelman J, Jakobiec FA. Lymphoid lesions of the conjunctiva: relation of histopathology to clinical outcome. *Ophthalmalogica* 1978; 85:819–843.
155. Jampol LM, Marsh JC, Albert DM, et al. IgA associated lymphoplasmacytic tumor involving the conjunctiva, eyelid, and orbit. *Am J Ophthalmol* 1975;79:279–284.
156. Knowles DM, Jakobiec FA, Rosen M, et al. Amyloidosis of the orbit and adnexa. *Surv Ophthalmol* 1975;19:367–384.
157. Brisbane JU, Lessell S, Finkel HE, et al. Malignant lymphoma presenting in the orbit: a clinicopathologic study of a rare immunoglobulin-producing variant. *Cancer* 1981;47:548–553.
158. Yeo JH, Jakobiec FA, Abbott GF, et al. Combined clinical and computed tomographic diagnosis of orbital lymphoid tumors. *Am J Ophthalmol* 1982;94:235–245.

159. Chao CKS, Lin H-S, Devineni R, et al. Radiation therapy for primary orbital lymphoma. *Int J Radiat Oncol Biol Phys* 1995;31:929–934.
160. Jakobiec FA, Yeo JH, Trokel SL, et al. Combined clinical and computed tomographic diagnosis of primary lacrimal fossa lesions. *Am J Ophthalmol* 1982;94:785–807.
161. Hornblass A, Jakobiec FA, Reifler DM, et al. Orbital lymphoid tumors located predominantly within extraocular muscles. *Ophthalmology* 1987;94:688–697.
162. Knowles, DM, Jakobiec FA. Malignant lymphomas and lymphoid hyperplasias that occur in the ocular adnexa (orbit, conjunctiva and eyelids). In: Knowles DM, ed. *Neoplastic hematopathology*. Baltimore: Williams & Wilkins, 1992:1009–1046.
163. The Non-Hodgkin's Lymphoma Pathologic Classification Project. National Cancer Institute sponsored study of classification of non-Hodgkin's lymphomas: summary and description of a working formulation for clinical usage. *Cancer* 1982;49:2112–2135.
164. Galieni P, Polito E, Leccisotti A, et al. Localized orbital lymphoma. *Haematologica* 1997;82:436–439.
165. White VA, Gascoyne RD, McNeil BK, et al. Histopathologic findings and frequency of clonality detected by the polymerase chain reaction in ocular adnexal lymphoproliferative lesions. *Mod Pathol* 1996;9: 1052–1061.
166. Chen P, Lin J, Lin S, et al. Rearrangements of immunoglobulin genes and oncogenes in ocular adnexal pseudolymphoma. *Curr Eye Res* 1991;10;547.
167. Ohshima K, Kikuchi M, Sumiyoshi Y, et al. Clonality of benign lymphoid hyperplasia in orbit and conjunctiva. *Pathol Res Pract* 1994; 190:436–443.
168. Wotherspoon AC, Dias TC, Pan LX, et al. Primary low grade B cell lymphoma of the conjunctiva: a mucosa-associated lymphoid tissue type lymphoma. *Histopathology* 1993;23:417–424.
169. Isaacson PG, Wright DH. Malignant lymphoma of mucosal-associated lymphoid tissue: a distinctive type of B cell lymphoma. *Cancer* 1983; 52:1410–1416.
170. Isaacson PG, Wright DH. Extranodal malignant lymphoma arising from mucosa-associated lymphoid tissue. *Cancer* 1984;53: 2515–2524.
171. Petrella T, Bron A, Foulet A, et al. Report of a primary lymphoma of the conjunctiva: a lymphoma of MALT origin? *Pathol Res Pract* 1991;187:78–84.
172. Thieblemont C, Berger F, Coiffier B. Mucosa-associated lymphoid tissue lymphomas. *Curr Opin Oncol* 1995;7:415–420.
173. The Non-Hodgkin's Lymphoma Classification Project. A clinical evaluation of the International Lymphoma Study Group classification of non-Hodgkin's lymphoma. *Blood* 1997;89:3909–3918.
174. Isaacson PG. Gastrointestinal lymphoma. *Hum Pathol* 1994;25: 1020–1029.
175. Spencer J, Finn T, Pulford KA, et al. The human gut contains a novel population of B lymphocytes which resemble marginal zone cells. *Clin Exp Immunol* 1985;62:607–612.
176. Isaacson PG, Wotherspoon AC, Diss T, et al. Follicular colonization in B-cell lymphoma of mucosa-associated lymphoid tissue. *Am J Surg Pathol* 1991;15:819–828.
177. Papadaki L, Wotherspoon AC, Isaacson PG. The lymphoepithelial lesions of gastric low-grade B cell lymphoma of mucosa-associated lymphoid tissue (MALT): an ultrastructural study. *Histopathology* 1992;21:415–421.
178. Wotherspoon AC, Doglioni C, Isaacson PG. Low-grade gastric B cell lymphoma of mucosa-associated lymphoid tissue (MALT): a multifocal disease. *Histopathology* 1992;20:29–34.
179. Morel P, Quiquandon I, Janin A. Involvement of minor salivary glands in gastric lymphomas. *Lancet* 1994;344:139–140.
180. Hernandez J, Sheenan W. Lymphomas of the mucosa-associated lymphoid tissue: signet ring cell lymphomas presenting in mucosal lymphoid organs. *Cancer* 1985;55:592–597.
181. Kurz-Levin MM, Flury R, Bernauer W. Diagnosis of MALT lymphoma by conjunctival biopsy: A case report. *Graefes Arch Clin Exp Ophthalmol* 1997;235:606–609.
182. Cahill MT, Moriarty PA, Kennedy SM. Conjunctival "MALToma" with systemic recurrence. *Arch Ophthalmol* 1998;116:97–99.
183. Evans HL. Extranodal small lymphocytic proliferation: a clinicopathologic and immunocytochemical study. *Cancer* 1982;49:84–96.
184. Bessell EM, Henk JM, Wright JE, et al. Orbital and conjunctival lymphoma treatment and prognosis. *Radiother Oncol* 1988;13: 237–244.
185. Isaacson PG. Lymphomas of mucosa-associated lymphoid tissue (MALT). *Histopathology* 1990;16:617–619.
186. Wieczorek R, Jakobiec FA, Sacks EH, et al. The immunoarchitecture of the normal human lacrimal gland: relevancy for understanding pathologic conditions. *Ophthalmology* 1988;95:100–109.
187. Knowles DM, Halper JP, Jakobiec FA: T lymphocyte subpopulations in B cell derived non-Hodgkin's lymphomas and Hodgkin's disease. *Cancer* 1984;54:644–651.
188. Baldini L, Blini M, Guffant A, et al. Treatment and prognosis in a series of primary extranodal lymphomas of the ocular adnexa. *Ann Oncol* 1998;9:779–781.
189. Ferry JA, Yang WI, Zukerberg LR, et al. $CD5^+$ extranodal marginal zone B-cell (MALT) lymphoma: a low grade neoplasm with a propensity for bone marrow involvement and relapse. *Am J Clin Pathol* 1996;105:31–37.
190. Goudie RB, McFarlane PS, Lindsay MK. Homing of lymphocytes to non-lymphoid tissues. *Lancet* 1974;1:292–293.
191. Fishleder A, Tubbs R, Hessie B, et al. Uniform detection of immunoglobulin gene rearrangement in benign lymphoepithelial lesions. *N Engl J Med* 1987;316:1118–1121.
192. Wood GS, Ngan BY, Tung R, et al. Clonal rearrangements of immunoglobulin genes and progression to B cell lymphoma in cutaneous lymphoid hyperplasia. *Am J Pathol* 1989;135:13–19.
193. Spencer J, Diss TC, Isaacson PG. Primary B cell gastric lymphoma: a genotypic analysis. *Am J Pathol* 1989;135:557–564.
194. Alper MG, Bray M. Evolution of a primary lymphoma of the orbit. *Br J Ophthalmol* 1984;68:255–260.
195. Scoazec JY, Brousse N, Potet F, et al. Focal malignant lymphoma in gastric pseudolymphoma: histologic and immunohistochemical study of a case. *Cancer* 1986;57:1330–1336.
196. Weiss LM, Woods GS, Trela M, et al. Clonal T cell populations in lymphomatoid papulosis: evidence of a lymphoproliferative origin for a clinically benign disease. *N Engl J Med* 1986;315:475–479.
197. Kadin ME, Vonderheid EC, Sako D, et al. Clonal composition of T cells in lymphomatoid papulosis. *Am J Pathol* 1987;126:13–17.
198. Hanson CA, Frizzera G, Patton DF, et al. Clonal rearrangement of immunoglobulin and T-cell receptor genes in systemic Castleman's disease: association with Epstein-Barr virus. *Am J Pathol* 1988;131: 84–91.
199. Pan LX, Diss TC, Cunningham D, et al. Isaacson PG. The bcl-2 gene in primary B-cell lymphoma of mucosa-associated lymphoid tissue (MALT). *Am J Pathol* 1989;135:7–11.
200. Wotherspoon AC, Pan LX, Diss TC, et al. A genotypic study of low grade B-cell lymphomas, including lymphomas of mucosa-associated lymphoid tissue (MALT). *J Pathol* 1990;162:135–140.
201. Raghoebier S, Kramer MHH, Vankrieken JHJM, et al. Essential differences in oncogene involvement between primary nodal and extranodal large cell lymphoma. *Blood* 1991;78:2680–2685.
202. Ott G, Katzenberger T, Greiner A, et al. The t(11;18)(q21;q21) chromosome translocation is a frequent and specific aberration in low-grade but not high-grade malignant non-Hodgkin's lymphomas of the mucosa-associated lymphoid tissue (MALT) type. *Can Res* 1997;57: 3944–3948.
203. Wotherspoon AC, Finn TM, Isaacson PG. Trisomy 3 in low-grade B-cell lymphomas of mucosa-associated lymphoid tissue. *Blood* 1995; 85:2000–2004.
204. Cesarman E, Inghirami G, Chadburn A, et al. High levels of p53 protein expression do not correlate with p53 gene mutations in CD30 (Ki-1) positive anaplastic large cell lymphoma. *Am J Pathol* 1993; 143:1–12.
205. Smitt MC, Donaldson SS. Radiotherapy is successful treatment for orbital lymphoma. *Int J Radiat Oncol Biol Phys* 1993;26:59–66.
206. Bennett CL, Putterman AP, Bitran JD, et al. Staging and therapy of orbital lymphomas. *Cancer* 1986;57:1204–1208.
207. Jereb B, Lee H, Jakobiec FA, et al. Radiation therapy of conjunctival and orbital lymphoid tumors. *Int J Radiat Oncol Biol Phys* 1984;10: 1013–1019.
208. Platanias LC, Putterman AM, Vijayakumar S, et al. Treatment and prognosis of orbital non-Hodgkin's lymphomas. *Am J Clin Oncol* 1992;15:79–83.
209. Cogliatti SB, Schmid U, Schumacher U, et al. Primary B cell gastric

lymphoma: a clinicopathological study of 145 patients. *Gastroenterology* 1991;101:1159–1170.
210. Bairey O, Kremer I, Rakowsky E, et al. Orbital and adnexal involvement in systemic non-Hodgkin's lymphoma. *Cancer* 1994;73:2395–2399.
211. Thieblemont C, Bastion Y, Berger F, et al. Mucosa-associated lymphoid tissue gastrointestinal and non-gastrointestinal lymphoma behavior: analysis of 108 patients. *J Clin Oncol* 1997;15:1624–1630.
212. Berger B, Pelman P, Soner A, et al. Nonfollicular small B cell lymphomas: a heterogeneous group of patients with distinct clinical features and outcome. *Blood* 1994;83:2829–2835.
213. Montalban C, Castrillo JM, Abraira V, et al. Gastric B cell mucosa-associated lymphoid tissue (MALT) lymphoma: clinicopathological study and evaluation of the prognostic factors in 143 patients. *Ann Oncol* 1995;6:355–362.
214. Radaszkiewicz T, Dragosics B, Bauer P. Gastrointestinal malignant lymphomas of the mucosa-associated lymphoid tissue: factors relevant to prognosis. *Gastroenterology* 1992;102:1628–1638.
215. Foucar E, Rosai J, Dorfman RF, eds. Sinus histiocytosis with massive lymphadenopathy (Rosai-Dorfman disease). *Semin Diagn Pathol* 1990;7:1–86.
216. Rosai J, Dorfman RF. Sinus histiocytosis with massive lymphadenopathy: a newly recognized benign clinicopathologic entity. *Arch Pathol* 1969;87:63–70.
217. Rosai J, Dorfman RF. Sinus histiocytosis with massive lymphadenopathy: a pseudolymphomatous benign disorder with massive lymphadenopathy. Analysis of 34 cases. *Cancer* 1972;30:1171–1188.
218. Foucar E, Rosai J, Dorfman R. Sinus histiocytosis with massive lymphadenopathy (Rosai-Dorfman disease): review of the entity. *Semin Diagn Pathol* 1990;7:19–73.
219. Zimmerman LE, Hidayat AA, Grantham RL, et al. Atypical cases of sinus histiocytosis (Rosai-Dorfman disease) with ophthalmological manifestations. *Trans Am Ophthalmol Soc* 1988;86:113–135.
220. Levinger S, Pe'er J, Aker M, et al. Rosai-Dorfman disease involving four eyelids. *Am J Ophthalmol* 1993;116:382–384.
221. Sacchi S, Artusi T, Torelli U, et al. Sinus histiocytosis with massive lymphadenopathy. *Leuk Lymphoma* 1992;7:189–194.
222. Wenig BM, Abbondanzo SL, Childers EL, et al. Extranodal sinus histiocytosis with massive lymphadenopathy (Rosai-Dorfman disease) of the head and neck. *Hum Pathol* 1993;24:483–492.
223. Mierau GW, Favara BE, Brenman JM. Electron microscopy in histiocytosis X. *Ultrastruct Pathol* 1982;3:137–142.
224. Bonetti F, Chilosi M, Menestrina F, et al. Immunohistological analysis of Rosai-Dorfman histiocytosis: a disease of S-100$^+$ CD1$^-$ histiocytes. *Virchows Arch A Pathol Anat* 1987;411:129–135.
225. Eisen RN, Buckley PJ, Rosai J. Immunophenotypic characterization of sinus histiocytosis with massive lymphadenopathy (Rosai-Dorfman disease). *Semin Diagn Pathol* 1990;7:74–82.
226. Paulli M, Russo R, Kindl S, et al. Immunophenotypic characterization of the cell infiltrate in five cases of sinus histiocytosis with massive lymphadenopathy. *Hum Pathol* 1992;23:647–654.
227. Cline MJ. Histiocytes and histiocytosis [Review]. *Blood* 1994;84:2840–2853.
228. Lichtenstein L. Histiocytosis X: integration of eosinophilic granuloma of bone, "Letterer-Siwe disease," and "Hand-Schüller-Christian disease" as related manifestations of a single nosologic entity. *Arch Pathol* 1953;56:84–102.
229. Nezelof C, Basset F, Rousseau MF. Histiocytosis X: histogenetic arguments for a Langerhans' cell origin. *Biomedicine* 1973;18:365–371.
230. McClelland J, Pritchard J, Chu AC. Current controversies. *Hematol Oncol Clin North Am* 1987;1:147–162.
231. Favara BE, Jaffe R. Pathology of Langerhans' cell histiocytosis. *Hematol Oncol Clin North Am* 1994;1:75–97.
232. Favara BE, McCarthy RC, Mierau GW. Histiocytosis X. *Hum Pathol* 1983;14:663–676.
233. Willman CL, Busque L, Griffith BB, et al. Langerhans' cell histiocytosis (histiocytosis X): a clonal proliferative disease. *N Engl J Med* 1994;331:154–160.
234. Raney RB, D'Angio OJ. Langerhans' cell histiocytosis: experience at the Children's Hospital of Philadelphia, 1970–1984. *Med Pediatr Oncol* 1989;17:20–28.
235. Nezelof C, Frileux-Herbet F, Cronier-Sachot J. Disseminated histiocytosis X: analysis of prognostic factors based on a retrospective study of 50 cases. *Cancer* 1979;44:1824–1838.
236. Moore AT, Pritchard J, Taylor DSI. Histiocytosis X: an ophthalmological review. *Br J Ophthalmol* 1985;69:7–14.
237. Mittelman D, Apple DJ, Goldberg MF. Ocular involvement in Letterer-Siwe disease. *Am J Ophthalmol* 1973;75:261–265.
238. Lahav M, Albert DM. Unusual ocular involvement in acute disseminated histiocytosis X. *Arch Ophthalmol* 1974;91:455–458.
239. MacCumber MW, Hoffman P, Wand GS, et al. Ophthalmic involvement in aggressive histiocytosis X. *Ophthalmology* 1990;97:22–27.
240. Heath P. The ocular features of a case of acute reticuloendotheliosis (Letterer-Siwe type). *Trans Am Ophthalmol Soc* 1959;57:290–302.
241. Mozziconacci P, Offret G, Forest A, et al. Histiocytose "X" avec lesions oculaires: etude anatomique. *Ann Pediatr* 1966;13:348–355.
242. Bilaniuk LT, Atlas SW, Zimmerman RA. The orbit. In: Lee SH, Rao KCVC, Zimmerman RA, eds. *Cranial MRI and CT.* San Francisco: McGraw-Hill, 1992;178.
243. Feldman RB, Moore DM, Hood CI, et al. Solitary eosinophilic granuloma of the lateral orbital wall. *Am J Ophthalmol* 1985;100:318–323.
244. Hidayat AA, Mafee MF, Laver NV, et al. Langerhans' cell histiocytosis and juvenile xanthogranuloma of the orbit: clinicopathologic, CT and MR imaging features. *Radiol Clin North Am* 1998;36:1229–1240.
245. Erly WK, Carmody RF, Dryden RM. Orbital histiocytosis X. *Am J Neuroradiol* 1994;16:1258–1261.
246. LaBorwit SE, Karesh JW, Hirschbein MJ, et al. Multifocal Langerhans' cell histiocytosis involving the orbit. *J Pediatr Ophthalmol Strabismus* 1998;35:234–236.
247. Mickelson MR, Bonfiglio M. Eosinophilic granuloma and its variations. *Orthop Clin North Am* 1977;8:933–945.
248. Glover AT, Grove AS. Eosinophilic granuloma of the orbit with spontaneous healing. *Ophthalmology* 1987;94:1008–1012.
249. Favara BE. Langerhans' cell histiocytosis pathobiology and pathogenesis. *Semin Oncol* 1991;18:3–7.
250. Malone M. The histiocytoses of childhood. *Histopathology* 1991;19:105–119.
251. Kyle RA. Diagnosis and management of multiple myeloma and related disorders. *Prog Hematol* 1987;14:257–282.
252. Osserman EF, Merlini G, Butler VP. Multiple myeloma and related plasma cell dyscrasias. *JAMA* 1987;258:2930–2937.
253. Knowling MA, Harwood AR, Bergsagel DE. Comparison of extramedullary plasmacytomas with solitary and multiple plasma cell tumors of bone. *J Clin Oncol* 1983;1:255–262.
254. Miller FR, Lavertu P, Wanamaker JR, et al. Plasmacytomas of the head and neck. *Otolaryngol Head Neck Surg* 1998;119:614–618.
255. Mewis-Levin L, Garcia CA, Olson JD. Plasma cell myeloma of the orbit. *Ann Ophthalmol* 1981;13:477–481.
256. Knowles DM, Halper J, Trokel S, et al. Immunofluorescent and immunoperoxidase characteristics of IgDλ myeloma involving the orbit. *Am J Ophthalmol* 1978;85:485–494.
257. De Smet MD, Rootman J. Orbital manifestations of plasmacytic lymphoproliferations. *Ophthalmology* 1987;94:995–1003.
258. Knapp AJ, Gartner S, Henkind P. Multiple myeloma and its ocular manifestations. *Surv Ophthalmol* 1987;31:343–351.
259. Aboud N, Sullivan T, Whitehead K. Primary extramedullary plasmacytoma of the orbit. *Aust N Z J Ophthalmol* 1995;23:235–239.
260. Adkino JW, Shields JA, Shields CL, et al. Plasmacytoma of the eye and orbit. *Int Ophthalmol* 1997;20:339–343.
261. Levine ME, Buckman G. Primary localized orbital amyloidosis. *Ann Ophthalmol* 1986;18:165–167.
262. Yakulis R, Dawson RR, Wang SE, et al. Fine needle aspiration diagnosis of orbital plasmacytoma with amyloidosis: a case report. *Acta Cytol* 1995;39:104–110.
263. Rodman HI, Font RL. Orbital involvement in multiple myeloma. *Arch Ophthalmol* 1972;87:30–35.
264. Rappaport H. Tumors of the hematopoietic system. *In: Atlas of tumor pathology.* Washington, DC: Armed Forces Institute of Pathology, 1966.
265. Ryder C, Naclerio RM. Multiple myeloma presenting as proptosis. *Ann Otol Rhinol Laryngol* 1999;108:211–213.
266. Neiman RS, Barcos M, Berard C, et al. Granulocytic sarcoma: a clinicopathologic study of 61 biopsied cases. *Cancer* 1981;48:1426–1437.
267. Burns A. *Observations on surgical anatomy of head and neck.* Edinburgh: Thomas Bryce, 1811:364–366.
268. Dock G. Chloroma and its relation to leukemia. *Am J Med Sci* 1893;106:152–185.

269. King A. Case of chloroma. *Monthly J Med* 1853;17:97–104.
270. Anger K. Verdoperoxidase. *Adv Enzymol* 1943;3:137–148.
271. Meis JM, Butler JJ, Osborne BM, et al. Granulocytic sarcoma in nonleukemic patients. *Cancer* 1986;58:2697–2709.
272. Liu PI, Ishimaru T, McGregor DH, et al. Autopsy study of granulocytic sarcoma (chloroma) in patients with myelogenous leukemia: Hiroshima-Nagasaki 1949–1969. *Cancer* 1973;31:948–955.
273. Tallman MS, Hakimian D, Shaw JM, et al. Granulocytic sarcoma is associated with the 8;21 translocation in acute myeloid leukemia. *J Clin Oncol* 1993;11:690–697.
274. Zimmerman LE, Font RL. Ophthalmologic manifestations of granulocytic sarcoma (myeloid sarcoma or chloroma). *Am J Ophthalmol* 1975;80:975–990.
275. Jakobiec FA. Granulocytic sarcoma. *Am J Neuroradiol* 1991;12: 263–264.
276. Cavdar AD. Ocular granulocytic sarcoma (chloroma) with acute myelomonocytic leukemia in Turkish children. *Cancer* 1978;41: 1606–1609.
277. Banna M, Aur R, Akkad S. Orbital granulocytic sarcoma. *Am J Neuroradiol* 1991;12:255–258.
278. Jaffe ES. *Surgical pathology of the lymph nodes and related organs.* Philadelphia: WB Saunders, 1985:430.
279. Leder LD. The origin of blood monocytes and macrophages. *Blut* 1967;16:86–98.
280. Castella A, Davey RF, Elbadawi A, et al. Granulocytic sarcoma of the hard palate: report of the first case. *Hum Pathol* 1984;15:1190–1192.
281. Fellbaum C, Hansmann M-L. Immunohistochemical differential diagnosis of granulocytic sarcomas and malignant lymphomas on formalin-fixed material. *Virchows Archiv A Pathol Anat* 1990;416:351–353.
282. Davey FR, Olson S, Kurec AS, et al. The immunophenotyping of extramedullary myeloid cell tumors in paraffin-embedded tissue sections. *Am J Surg Pathol* 1988;12:699–707.
283. Bennett JM, Catovsky D, Daniel MT, et al. The French-American-British (FAB) Cooperative Group proposals for the classification of the acute leukemias. *Br J Haematol* 1976;33:451–458.
284. Fourth International Workshop on Chromosomes in Leukemia. *Cancer Genet Cytogenet* 1984;11:284–287.
285. Second International Workshop on Chromosomes in Leukemia 1979. Cytogenetic, morphologic and clinical correlations in acute nonlymphocytic leukemia with t(8q – ,21q +). *Cancer Genet Cytogenet* 1980;2:99–102.
286. Arthur DC, Berger R, Golomb HM, et al. The clinical significance of karyotype in acute myelogenous leukemia. *Cancer Genet Cytogenet* 1989;40:203–216.
287. Kaneko Y, Sakurai M, Hattori M. Childhood acute myelogenous leukemia with an 8;21 chromosome translocation. *J Pediatr* 1978;93: 1066–1067.
288. Swirsky DM, Li YS, Matthews JG, et al. 8;21 Translocation in acute granulocytic leukemia: cytological, cytochemical and clinical features. *Br J Haematol* 1984;56:199–213.
289. Rajantie J, Tarkkanen A, Rapola J, et al. Orbital granulocytic sarcoma as a presenting sign in acute myelogenous leukemia. *Ophthalmalogica* 1984;189:158–161.
290. Abe R, Umezu H, Uchida T, et al. Myeloblastoma with an 8;21 chromosome translocation in acute myeloblastic leukemia. *Cancer* 1986; 58:1260–1264.
291. Wodzinski MA, Collin R, Winfield DA, et al. Epidural granulocytic sarcoma in acute myeloid leukemia with a 8;21 translocation. *Cancer* 1988;62:1299–1300.
292. Hagihara M, Kobayashi H, Miyachi H, et al. Clinical heterogeneity in acute myelogenous leukemia with the 8;21 translocation. *Keio J Med* 1991;40:90–93.
293. Frappez D, Bertheas MF, Vasselon C, et al. Retro-orbital chloroma in children with t(8;21) acute myeloblastic leukemia of M2 type. *Am J Pediatr Hematol Oncol* 1998;10:134–138.
294. Russell SJ, Giles FJ, Thompson DS, et al. Granulocytic sarcoma of the small intestine preceding acute myelomonocytic leukemia with abnormal eosinophils and inv (16). *Cancer Genet Cytogenet* 1988; 35:231–235.
295. Adams LR, Angus B, Carey P, et al. Cytogenetic analysis of granulocytic sarcoma in a patient without systemic leukemia. *J Clin Pathol* 1991;44:81–82.
296. Cavdar AO, Bokesoy I, Sunguroglu A, et al. Orbito-ocular granulocytic sarcoma (OOGS) and acute myeloblastic leukemia (AML) with duplication of Philadelphia chromosome. *Cancer Genet Cytogenet* 1993;69:38–40.
297. Imrie KR, Kovacs MJ, Selby D, et al. Isolated chloroma: the effect of early antileukemic therapy. *Ann Intern Med* 1995;123:351–353.
298. Hutchison RE, Kurec AS, Davey FR. Granulocytic sarcoma. *Clin Lab Med* 1990;10:889–901.
299. Beck TM, Day JC, Smith CE, et al. Granulocytic sarcoma treated as an acute leukemia. *Cancer* 1984;53:1764–1766.

CHAPTER 36

Waldeyer's Ring, Sinonasal Region, Salivary Gland, Thyroid Gland, Central Nervous System, and Other Extranodal Lymphomas and Lymphoid Hyperplasias

Jerome S. Burke

The incidence of extranodal lymphomas in various anatomic sites is relatively consistent. Most extranodal lymphomas occur in the gastrointestinal tract, predominantly stomach and small intestine, and in most studies, are followed in frequency by lymphomas of the head and neck region (1,2); involvement of other sites is highly variable (3) (see Chapter 31). Despite the relative rarity of primary extranodal lymphomas in some of these sites, they form a fascinating group of neoplasms and are interesting to epidemiologists, pathologists, immunologists, and oncologists. This interest stems in some cases from the prevalence of extranodal lymphomas at one specific site in a specific geographic region; in other cases, the interest stems from the association of extranodal lymphomas with autoimmune disorders and immunodeficiency states; in still other cases, the interest revolves around the relationship to an infectious agent, as for example Epstein-Barr virus (EBV). In all sites, extranodal lymphomas represent a challenge in the establishment of an accurate diagnosis, specifically in the distinction of extranodal lymphoma from undifferentiated carcinoma, an extramedullary myeloid tumor (granulocytic sarcoma), or extranodal florid lymphoid hyperplasia. The general principles of extranodal lymphomas and the differential diagnosis are discussed in Chapter 31. The characteristics of lymphomas of skin, gastrointestinal tract, lung, and ocular adnexa are described in Chapters 32 through 35. In this chapter, lymphomas and lymphoid hyperplasias of other extranodal sites are reviewed. Table 36.1 provides a summary of the predominant lymphomas and their immunophenotypes that occur in these different extranodal sites.

J. S. Burke: Department of Anatomic Pathology, Alta Bates Medical Center, Berkeley, California 94705

WALDEYER'S RING

Waldeyer's ring refers to the lymphoid tissues of the faucial tonsils, nasopharynx, base of tongue, and oropharyngeal wall (4). Lymphomas of Waldeyer's ring are omitted from some series of extranodal non-Hodgkin's lymphomas because, by strict definition, Waldeyer's ring is an "extranodal" but not an "extralymphatic" site (1). Nonetheless, Waldeyer's ring is included in most studies and is mainly second to the gastrointestinal tract in the incidence of extranodal non-Hodgkin's lymphomas (1,2,5).

A curious link between Waldeyer's ring lymphomas and those of the gastrointestinal tract exists in 3% to 11% of patients, despite the lack of direct lymphatic communication between these two sites (6). There is greater than expected incidence of gastrointestinal involvement in patients who have lymphomas of Waldeyer's ring, and conversely, there is an increased risk of involvement of Waldeyer's ring in patients who have gastrointestinal lymphomas (4–7). The association between lymphomas of Waldeyer's ring and the gastrointestinal tract is considered a result of the homing tendency of common gut-associated lymphoid tissue (GALT) or mucosa-associated lymphoid tissue (MALT) (7,8). This homing pattern is offered as an explanation for the tendency of some lymphomas that originate in extranodal sites to relapse in other extranodal sites, such as Waldeyer's ring and the gastrointestinal tract (8). Paradoxically, the incidence of low-grade lymphomas of MALT in Waldeyer's ring is low (3.6%), but it has been proposed that many of the

TABLE 36.1. *Predominant histologic type and immunophenotype of various extranodal lymphomas*

Site	Predominant lymphoma	Immunophenotype
Waldeyer's ring	Large cell	B
Sinonasal region	Large cell/polymorphous	NK/T
Salivary gland	MALT (MESA/BLEL-associated)	B
	Follicular (non-MESA/BLEL)	B
Thyroid gland	Large cell	B
Central nervous system	Large cell	B
Testis	Large cell	B
Ovary	Burkitt/large cell	B
Cervix	Large cell/follicular	B
Bone	Large cell (multilobated)	B
Breast	Large cell/Burkitt	B
Miscellaneous	Large cell/MALT	B

MESA, myoepithelial sialadenitis; BLEL, benign lymphoepithelial lesion; B, B cell; T, T cell; NK, natural killer cell; MALT, mucosa-associated lymphoid tissue.

more prevalent high-grade B-cell lymphomas of Waldeyer's ring may be of MALT type (9,10).

Patients who have lymphomas that arise in Waldeyer's ring generally are in their sixth and seventh decades of life, and they frequently present with symptoms of local swelling, pain, or the sensation of a foreign body in the throat (4,6,11, 12). A fleshy, tan tumor mass usually is discovered on clinical examination (Fig. 36.1).

All varieties of non-Hodgkin's lymphomas, including follicular lymphomas, are seen in Waldeyer's ring, but up to 85% of the lymphomas are diffuse (4,5,11–13). Most diffuse lymphomas of Waldeyer's ring are the large B-cell type (13,14) (Fig. 36.2). Florid immunoblastic hyperplasia in the tonsils, such as infectious mononucleosis, may simulate a large cell lymphoma, but these two conditions generally can be differentiated by the clinical setting and the orderly range of lymphocytic transformation found in the hyperplastic conditions (Fig. 36.3). A more common problem is found in cases of large cell lymphoma, which may be difficult to

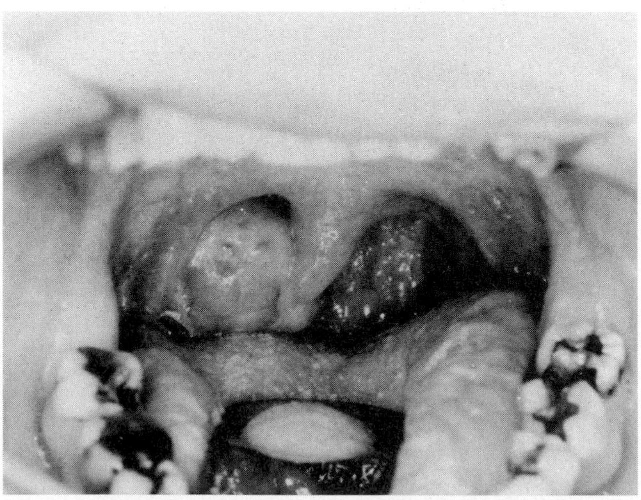

FIG. 36.1. Malignant lymphoma of the tonsil results in a flesh-like, tan tumor mass that often is associated with pain and the sensation of a foreign body in the throat.

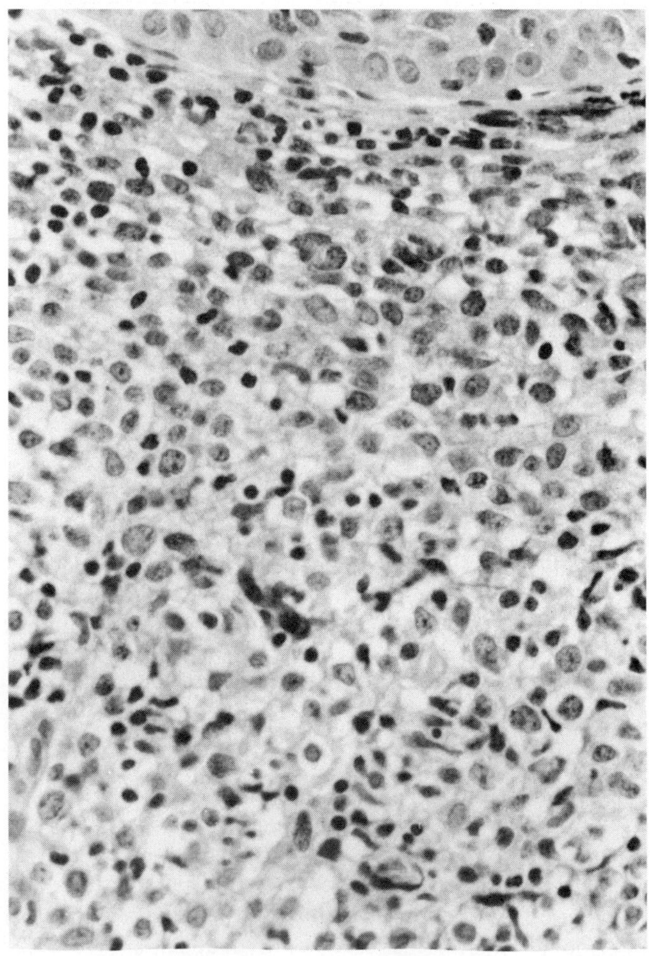

FIG. 36.2. Malignant lymphoma, diffuse large B-cell type, is found adjacent to tonsillar squamous epithelium *(top)*. This lymphoma may be difficult to distinguish from poorly differentiated squamous carcinoma (hematoxylin and eosin stain, original magnification: 480× magnification).

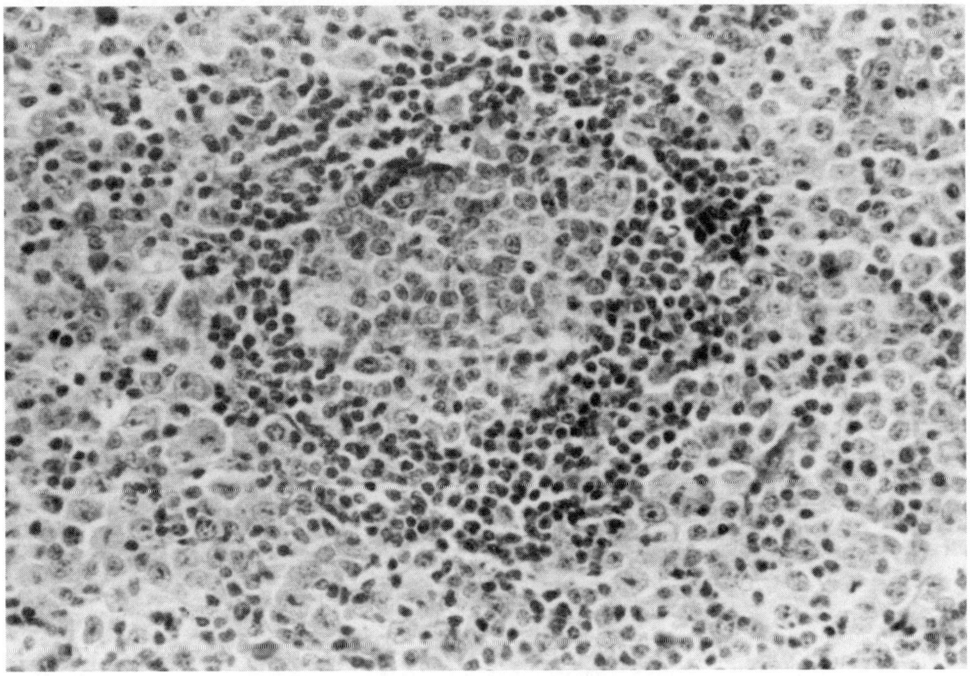

FIG. 36.3. Florid lymphoid hyperplasia of the tonsil in infectious mononucleosis. Surrounding the germinal center, there is a polymorphous proliferation of lymphocytes dominated by immunoblasts. Unlike malignant lymphoma, there is a relatively orderly range of lymphocytic transformation (hematoxylin and eosin stain, original magnification: 375× magnification).

distinguish from poorly differentiated squamous carcinoma of the lymphoepithelial type (4,14). Histologically, the distinction of carcinoma from large cell lymphoma relies on the observation of cellular cohesion or a syncytial growth pattern in carcinoma; however, the lymphoepithelial type of squamous carcinoma occasionally occurs in diffuse sheets and is accompanied by inflammation and fibrosis. This results in difficulty in the distinction of carcinoma from lymphoma. Immunohistochemical studies that use antibodies directed against cytokeratin and pan-B-cell and pan-T-cell antigens almost always resolve this diagnostic problem (see Chapter 30).

Mantle cell lymphoma is another type that may be encountered in Waldeyer's ring, as a primary malignant lymphoma or as a manifestation of disseminated disease (13,15). The gastrointestinal tract and Waldeyer's ring are involved in 20% to 30% of patients who have mantle cell lymphoma and are the most common extranodal sites found in this type (15). In the Working Formulation study of non-Hodgkin's lymphomas, the mantle cell cases probably comprised most lymphomas that were classified as diffuse small cleaved cell type (16); the latter subtype was found more commonly among the malignant lymphoma cases that were derived from Milan, with a large number of these cases involving Waldeyer's ring. In general, Europeans have a higher incidence of non-Hodgkin's lymphoma of Waldeyer's ring compared with patients from the United States, Hong Kong, and Japan (1,11,14,17,18). The explanation for this observation is not clear, but it probably reflects various environmental factors.

Hodgkin's disease that manifests in Waldeyer's ring is uncommon and most such cases likely represent examples of peripheral T-cell lymphoma with a high content of epithelioid histiocytes (Lennert's lymphoma) (Fig. 36.4), or T-cell/histiocyte–rich B-cell lymphoma (4,5,19–21). Lennert's lymphoma and T-cell/histiocyte–rich B-cell lymphoma seem to have a predilection to involve the tonsils and Lennert's lymphoma proves an exception, together with lymphoblastic lymphoma, to the general consensus that most lymphomas in Waldeyer's ring are B-cell–derived (11–14,18,22).

In the Far East, where T-cell lymphomas are common, more than 70% of lymphomas of Waldeyer's ring are found to be of B-cell origin (14,18,22). In one study from Japan, all 25 cases of non-Hodgkin's lymphoma of Waldeyer's ring from an adult T-cell leukemia/lymphoma (ATLL) nonendemic area were B-cell malignancies and, with one exception, were of diffuse large cell type (22). Of 37 cases from an ATLL endemic area, 20 (54%) also were B-cell lymphomas (75% large cell) with the remaining 17 cases exhibiting a T-cell phenotype. As expected, the human T-cell leukemia virus type I proviral genome was present in 85% of the T-cell cases; however, the EBV genome was uncommon among the T- and B-cell Waldeyer's ring lymphoma cases (22).

The most important prognostic factor for patients who have malignant lymphomas that manifest in Waldeyer's ring

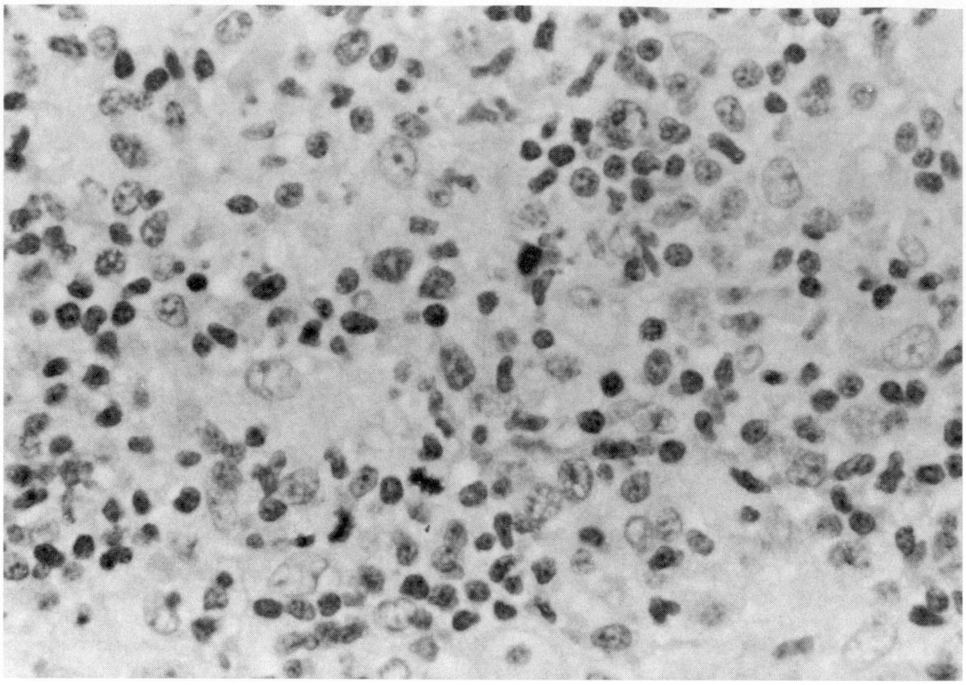

FIG. 36.4. Diffuse lymphoma with epithelioid histiocytes (Lennert's lymphoma) mimics Hodgkin's disease in the tonsil. Immunohistochemical studies demonstrated that this lymphoma was of T-cell lineage and was composed mainly of $CD4^+$ lymphocytes (hematoxylin and eosin stain, original magnification: 600× magnification).

is clinical stage. Patients who have diffuse large cell lymphoma and stage IE disease have a good prognosis with a reported 5-year survival rate ranging from 60% to 86% (4–6,11); patients who are stage IIE have a significantly worse prognosis and have a 5-year survival rate of 30% (5,6). Poor prognostic factors include not only advanced clinical stage at presentation, but also a T-cell phenotype and lesions of the base of the tongue (6,18,23).

SINONASAL REGION

Non-Hodgkin's lymphomas of the sinonasal region are an extraordinary group of extranodal lymphomas because they are more prevalent in specific geographic regions, mainly the Far East and Latin America; they predominately are of natural killer (NK)/T-cell immunophenotype; and the NK/T-cell cases almost always are associated with EBV (24). As corroboration of their uniqueness, sinonasal malignant lymphomas comprise a separate category, referred to as *angiocentric lymphomas,* among the T- and NK-lineage malignant lymphomas in the Revised European-American Lymphoma classification (25). In the proposed World Health Organization classification of malignant lymphomas, they are coded as *nasal type of extranodal NK/T-cell lymphomas* in recognition of the observation that angiocentric growth is not always present in some nasal type NK/T-cell malignant lymphomas and that angiocentric growth is not absolutely specific and may be seen in other types of malignant lymphoma (26).

Malignant lymphomas of the sinonasal region, including those in the hard palate, are uncommon neoplasms in the United States and Europe and account for only 0.17% to 1.5% of non-Hodgkin's lymphomas (27,28). In contrast, sinonasal malignant lymphomas are much more widespread in the Far East, particularly China, where such neoplasms comprise up to 10.7% of all non-Hodgkin's lymphomas (29,30). They also are more frequent in Latin America, for example in Peru, Guatemala, and Mexico, where they primarily affect individuals of Native American descent (31–34). The apparent shared susceptibility to sinonasal lymphomas among Asians and Latin Americans of Native American origin indicates that racial disposition may be a possible factor in the pathogenesis of these lymphomas (31–34).

Sinonasal malignant lymphomas form a fascinating, and often confusing, group because many cases are included in the clinical spectrum of the midline granuloma syndrome (35). This unusual clinical syndrome is characterized by slowly progressive ulceration and destruction of the nose and paranasal sinuses, with frequent erosion of the soft tissues, bone, and cartilage. The differential diagnosis of the midline granuloma syndrome includes infectious diseases, whether bacterial, fungal, or parasitic, inflammatory diseases of unknown cause, particularly Wegener's granulomatosis and idiopathic midline destructive disease, but most cases are regarded currently as malignant lymphomas of NK/T-cell type (30,35,36). The major clinical symptom associated with malignant lymphomas of the sinonasal region is nasal obstruction; however, depending on the extent of the disease, epistaxis, nasal discharge, repeated infections, ozena, facial swelling, and cranial nerve palsy may ensue (6,29,37).

Pathologic assessment of a biopsy specimen from the sinonasal region frequently is problematic, particularly in the setting of severe inflammation. With extensive inflammatory changes, it always is speculative whether the biopsy specimen is truly representative or whether neoplastic cells have been obscured by the inflammation and the commonly accompanying necrosis. A diagnosis of lymphoma depends on the recognition of atypical lymphoid cells against the background of severe inflammation, necrosis, and cellular degeneration (Fig. 36.5). To identify the frequently obscure neoplastic lymphoid cells in this environment, the biopsy must be not only of sufficient size but also of adequate technical quality. If all cultures have been negative and if atypical lymphocytes are not evident, the lesion may be idiopathic midline destructive disease, a localized, destructive inflammatory process confined to the upper respiratory tract and responsive to radiation therapy (36).

The NK/T-cell lymphomas associated with the midline granuloma syndrome frequently exhibit a wide morphologic spectrum with a mixed or polymorphous cellular composition including immunoblasts and occasional epithelioid histiocytes (24,38,39) (Fig. 36.6). In the past, the polymorphous and diffuse, mixed NK/T-cell lymphomas of the sinonasal region were described under various designations, for example polymorphic reticulosis and midline malignant reticulosis (37,40,41). These terms reflect the frequent difficulty in establishing and recognizing these polymorphous NK/T-cell malignant lymphomas with their associated extensive inflammation and coagulative necrosis. The necrosis often has a zonal distribution to suggest a vascular cause (24). Many polymorphous NK/T-cell lymphomas in the sinonasal region encircle vessels and frequently are angioinvasive, raising the spectrum of Wegener's granulomatosis (24,28,38) (Fig. 36.7). An absolute diagnosis of Wegener's granulomatosis requires the presence of granulomatous inflammation, necrosis, and vasculitis (42). In contrast, the NK/T-cell malignant lymphomas do not exhibit granulomatous angiitis or fibrinoid necrosis, but rather concentrate around and within blood vessels with lymphomatous infiltration and destruction of the vessel walls (24). In addition to frequent necrosis and an angiocentric growth pattern, NK/T-cell malignant lymphomas may exhibit epitheliotropism similar to that seen in the skin in mycosis fungoides (Fig. 36.8), and in Wright-Giemsa–stained touch imprint preparations, azurophilic granules often are observed in tumor cells (38,43,44).

The polymorphous NK/T-cell lymphomas of the sinonasal region share many pathologic features with lymphomatoid granulomatosis of the lung, including the tendency to be angiocentric and angiodestructive with associated necrosis (45,46). The designation *angiocentric immunoproliferative lesion* was devised for these cases, as they were thought to represent a spectrum of postthymic T-cell proliferations, involving a common association with EBV (24,47–49). Current studies demonstrate that lymphomatoid granulomatosis is an EBV-linked B-cell lymphoma with a vigorous T-cell reaction (50). Nevertheless, cases of bona fide nasal type

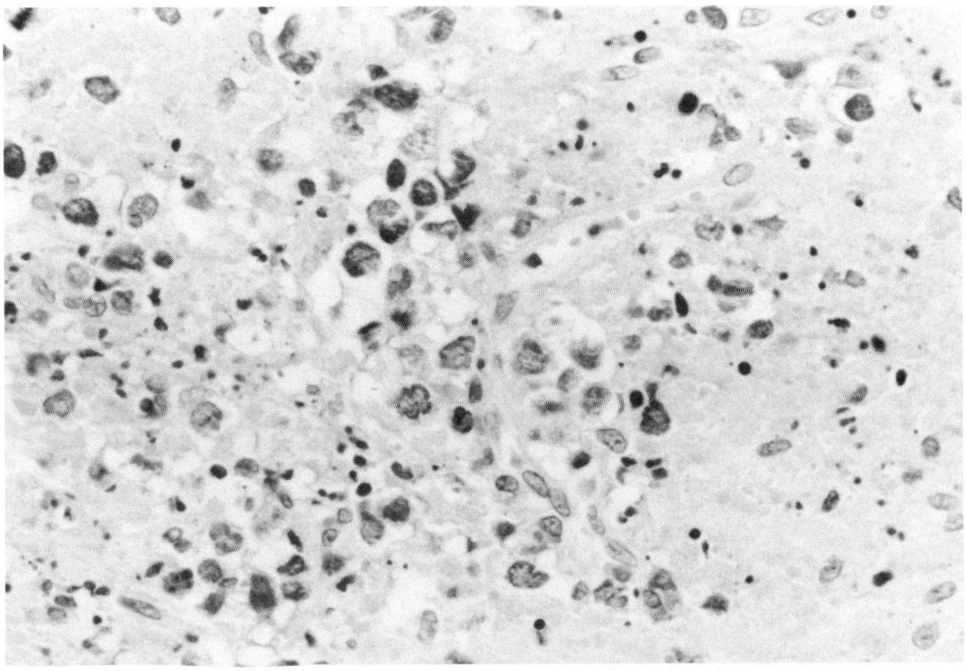

FIG. 36.5. Extensive necrosis is common in malignant lymphoma of the nasal cavity and may mask a large cell lymphoma of polymorphous cell type. The large cells expressed the T-cell antigen CD45RO (UCHL1) (hematoxylin and eosin stain, original magnification: 480× magnification).

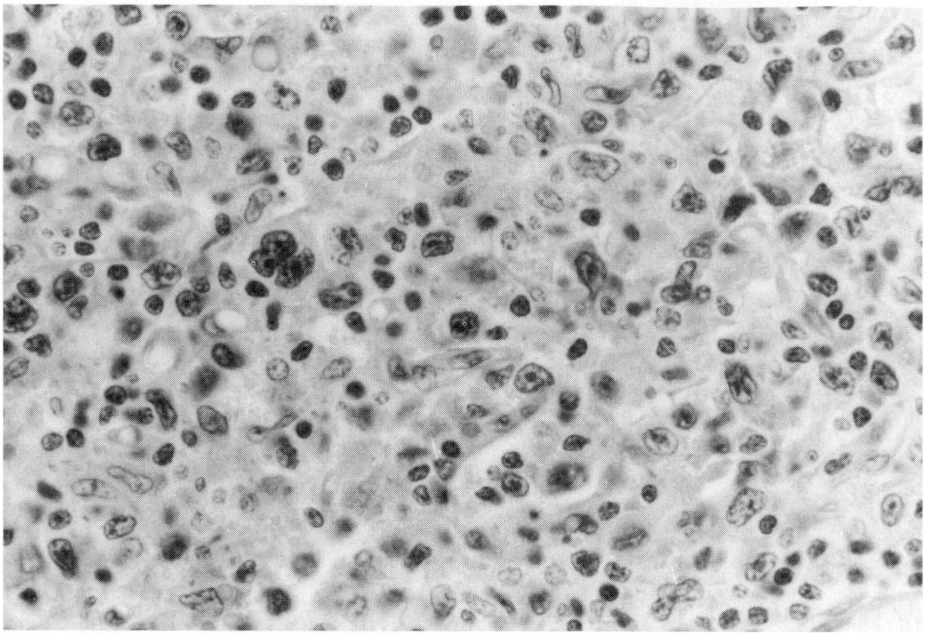

FIG. 36.6. Large cell polymorphous lymphoma of natural killer (NK)/T-cell lineage. NK/T-cell lymphomas are prevalent in the sinonasal region (hematoxylin and eosin stain, original magnification: 600× magnification).

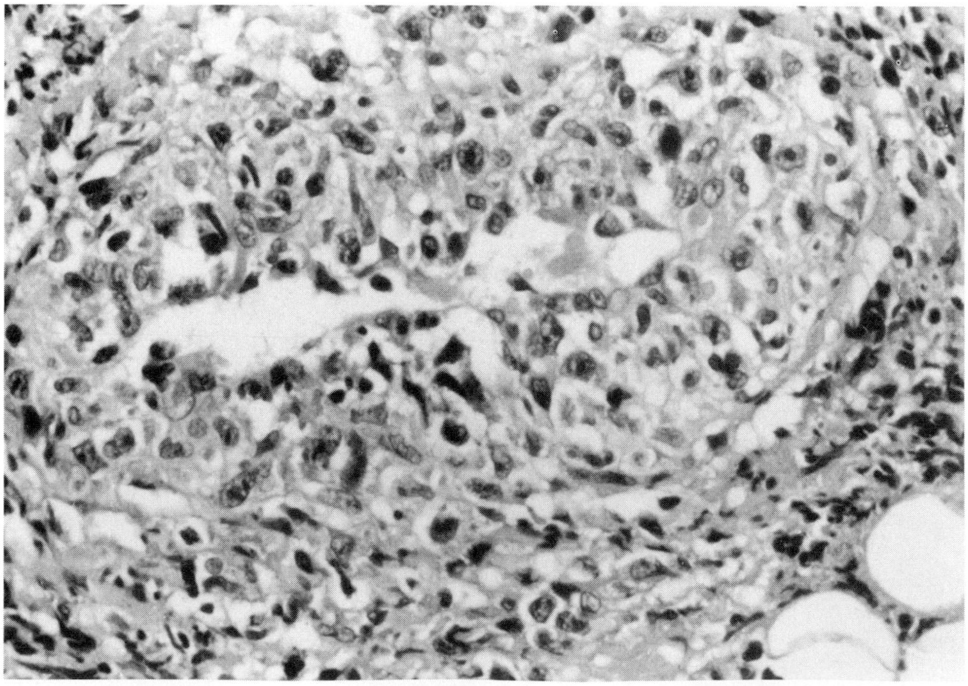

FIG. 36.7. Angioinvasion by malignant lymphoma in the sinonasal region is a common occurrence and may be confused with Wegener's granulomatosis (hematoxylin and eosin stain, original magnification: 480× magnification).

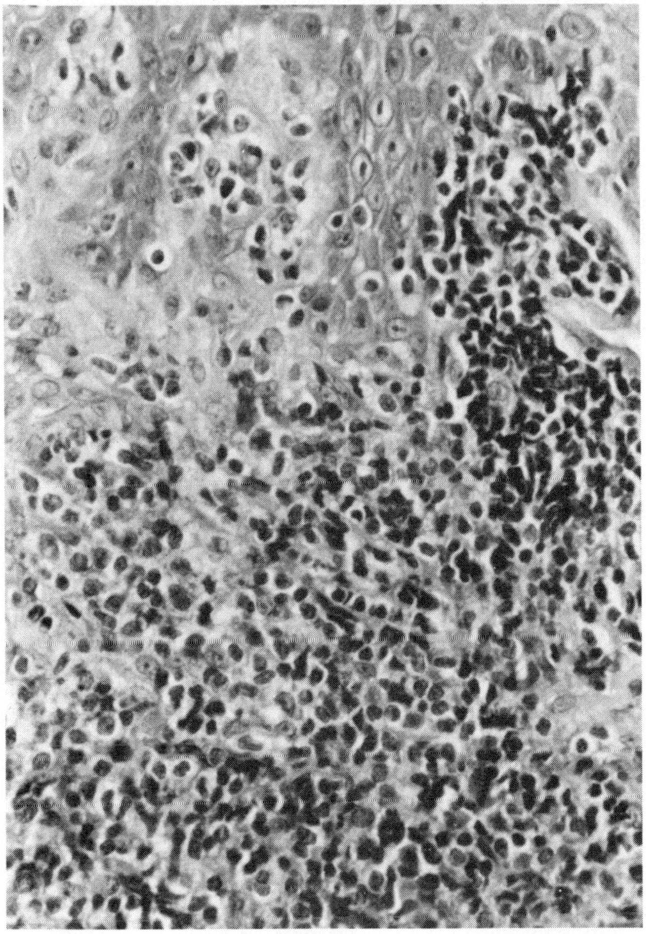

FIG. 36.8. A natural killer (NK)/T-cell lymphoma of the palate invades the overlying squamous mucosa (epitheliotropism) and parallels the epidermotropism common in mycosis fungoides (hematoxylin and eosin stain, original magnification: 375× magnification).

NK/T-cell malignant lymphomas can arise external to the sinonasal region, especially in extranodal sites such as skin, upper respiratory tract, testis, soft tissue, gastrointestinal tract, and spleen (51); curiously, NK/T-cell sinonasal lymphomas tend to disseminate to these same sites. The nonnasal NK/T-cell malignant lymphomas are morphologically and phenotypically identical to the cases in the sinonasal region and they also harbor EBV (see Chapter 29).

Immunophenotypic studies have confirmed the NK/T-cell nature of most malignant lymphomas of the sinonasal region. In one study of 113 Chinese patients with sinonasal malignant lymphoma from Hong Kong, 45.1% had a NK/T-cell (CD56-positive [$CD56^+$]) immunophenotype, 21.3% were peripheral T-cell lymphomas ($CD56^-$), and 33.6% were B-cell lymphomas (30). Although there is heterogeneity, the commonest immunophenotype of NK/T-cell sinonasal malignant lymphomas is $CD2^+$, membranous $CD3^-$, cytoplasmic $CD3\epsilon^+$, and $CD56^+$ (24,30,32,44,52–54). This immunophenotypic profile is found not only in the Far East and Latin America, but also in sinonasal malignant lymphoma cases originating in patients from Europe and the United States (55–58). The malignant lymphomas with the $CD2^+$, membranous $CD3^-$, cytoplasmic $CD3\epsilon^+$, and $CD56^+$ immunophenotype may express other T cell–associated antigens, such as CD43 and CD45RO and occasionally CD4, but they generally lack CD5 expression, as well as βF1 and TCR-δ1 (24,32,34,37,44,55). Notwithstanding that these sinonasal malignant lymphomas are usually negative for NK cell markers CD16 and CD57, the reactivity for CD56 in frozen and paraffin-embedded tissues with lack of expression of surface membranous CD3, but presence of cytoplasmic CD3ϵ and sporadic expression of T lineage antigens other than CD2, connotes that the $CD56^+$ sinonasal malignant lymphomas probably are derived from NK cells rather than T cells (30,32,44,56). In concert with the putative NK lineage, such sinonasal malignant lymphomas do not exhibit clonal T-cell receptor (TCR) gene rearrangements (44,55,57,59,60).

Other immunophenotypes among the overall group of NK/T-cell sinonasal malignant lymphomas include $CD2^+CD3^-CD56^-$; $CD2^+CD3^+CD56^-$; $CD2^-CD3^-CD56^+$; and $CD2^-CD3^-CD56^-$ (30,44,52,56,60). Supporting the T-cell derivation of a minority of the sinonasal malignant lymphoma cases, clonal TCR gene rearrangements have been reported and some cases originate from $\gamma\delta$ T cells (55,60–62). The sinonasal $\gamma\delta$ T-cell cases are similar to the NK-cell cases in that they are pleomorphic tumors with frequent angiocentricity and epitheliotropism (62).

The NK and the $\gamma\delta$ T-cell cases express cytotoxic proteins TIA-1 and granzyme B, as well as perforin (34,53,54,56,62,63). The NK/T-cell malignant lymphomas, including those in the sinonasal region, also express CD95 (FAS) and CD95 ligand (54,64). The release of cytotoxic proteins probably leads to zonal tumor cell death and likely contributes to the necrosis seen in cases of NK/T-cell sinonasal malignant lymphomas that are without an angiocentric growth pattern (63). It is postulated that the cytotoxic proteins that are manufactured by the malignant lymphoma also may damage endothelial cells to further the effects of ischemia and lead to additional tumor cell death (63). Activation of the CD95/CD95 ligand apoptotic pathways, however, may not be a major factor in tumor cell death in NK/T-cell malignant lymphomas, but EBV-induced pathways, mediated by the chemokines Mig and IP-10, may provide another mechanism for the necrosis and tissue damage in the sinonasal region (64,65).

EBV is a significant and consistent discovery among NK/T-cell sinonasal malignant lymphomas (48). In virtually every study and regardless of geographic origin, EBV can be demonstrated in more than 95% of NK/T-cell sinonasal malignant lymphoma cases, including those of $\gamma\delta$ T-cell type (31,32,34,55–58,61,62,66–68). For example, in one report all 21 cases with a $CD56^+CD3^-$ immunophenotype were EBV positive employing *in situ* hybridization to detect EBV-encoded RNA (EBER) (68). Moreover, the finding of $EBER^+$ cells may be beneficial in diagnosis, particularly in cases with small numbers of lymphomatous cells and in the distinction of NK/T-cell malignant lymphoma from Wegener's granulomatosis (24,69); EBER positivity is not found in Wegener's granulomatosis. EBER transcripts also are rarely present in B-cell malignant lymphomas of the sinonasal region (68,70). The virtual restriction of EBER to NK/T-cell lymphomas of the sinonasal region has suggested the etiologic role of EBV in the pathogenesis of these lymphomas (61,68,70). The significance of EBV also is implied by the presence of low numbers of EBV^+ cells in nasal polyps (71). The latter observation indicates that the nasal mucosa could be one of the sites of EBV persistence with low levels of infected reactive lymphocytes and represent a nidus for the development of EBV-associated neoplasms. The P-ala subtype of EBV is found in most sinonasal malignant lymphomas and this subtype accumulates multiple mutations consistent with the generation of variant species of EBER-1 (72). The nonrandom distribution of EBV subtypes is additional evidence pointing to an etiologic role for EBV in the lymphomagenesis of NK/T-cell sinonasal malignant lymphomas.

Overexpression of p53 is seen in most NK/T-cell sinonasal malignant lymphoma cases, and although *TP53* may be mutated, the precise cause of p53 overexpression in this form of malignant lymphoma has not been established (32); however, a cytogenetic study of sinonasal malignant lymphomas revealed frequent DNA loss of chromosome 17p, consistent with loss of p53 (32,73). The most frequent recurrent cytogenetic abnormalities among NK/T-cell sinonasal malignant lymphomas involve deletions of chromosome 6 at around the q21-23 region and fluorescence *in situ* hybridization studies have confirmed the existence of deletions at 6q22-23 in the $CD56^+CD3^-$ lymphoma cells (74).

Studies from Europe and the United States have documented cases of sinonasal malignant lymphomas that are of NK/T-cell lineage (38,43,55–58,75). Most reports from these areas, however, have shown a preponderance of sinonasal malignant lymphomas that are of B-cell lineage (27,39,58,76); moreover, B-cell lymphomas constitute almost a third of the sinonasal malignant lymphomas in Hong Kong (30). The B-cell sinonasal malignant lymphomas, regardless of origin, tend to be large cell malignant lymphomas and usually are composed of relatively monomorphous noncleaved lymphocytes (27,30,39,43,58,76) (Fig. 36.9). The

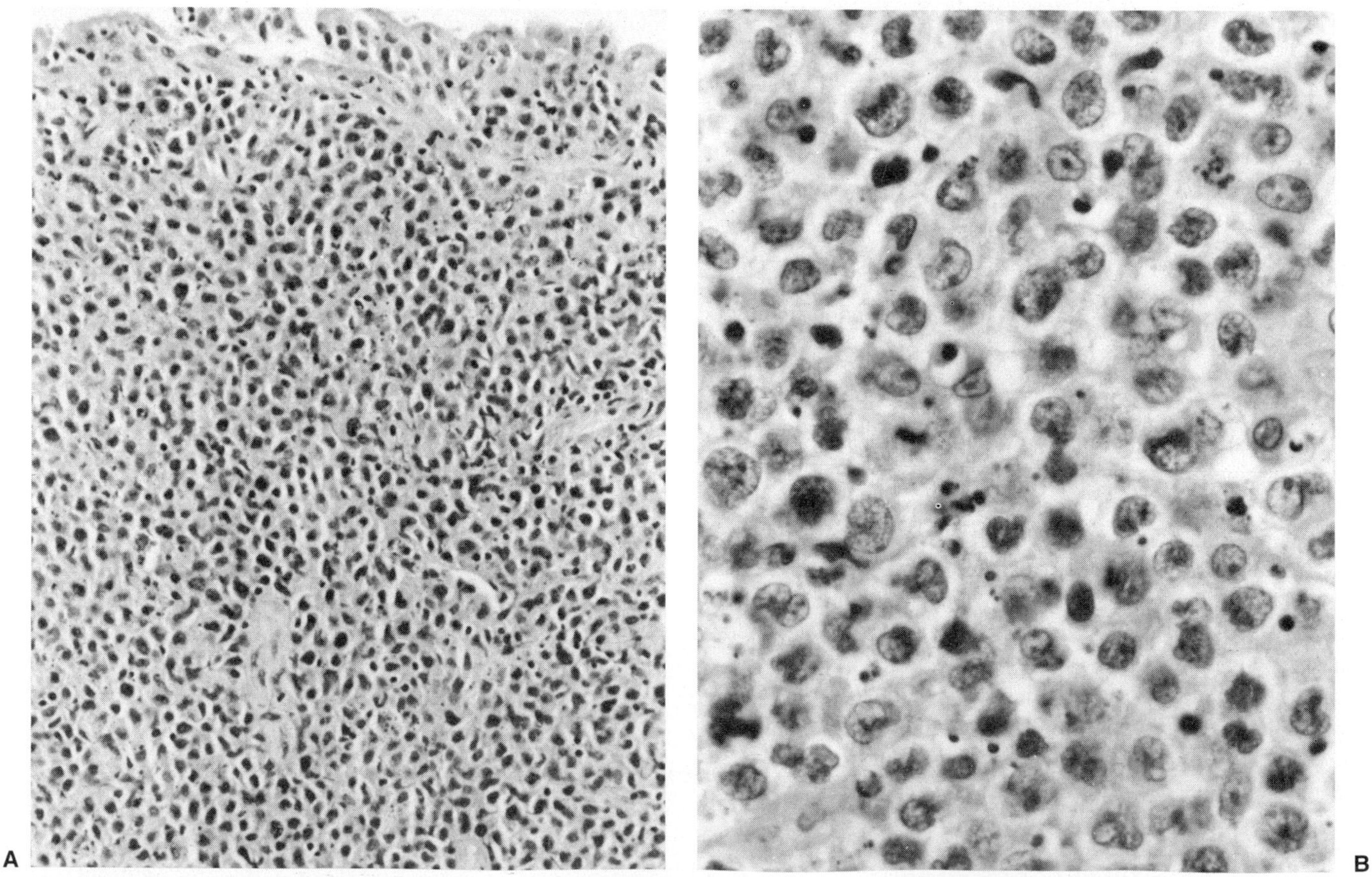

FIG. 36.9. A: A "conventional" lymphoma of diffuse large cell type completely replaces the submucosa and partially infiltrates the mucosa of a paranasal sinus (hematoxylin and eosin stain, original magnification: 240× magnification). **B:** Detail of the large cells of mainly noncleaved cell type in the sinus. Despite degeneration, the large cells expressed B-cell antigens (hematoxylin and eosin stain, original magnification: 720× magnification).

large B-cell lymphomas predominately involve the paranasal sinuses, whereas those limited to the nasal cavity are mainly the NK/T-cell malignant lymphomas (58).

The clinical prognosis of patients who have sinonasal malignant lymphomas is variable and difficult to evaluate, possibly because the polymorphous forms of NK/T-cell lymphoma are unrecognized for prolonged periods, and many patients are not treated according to conventional lymphoma protocols. In one study of 70 patients who were treated between 1947 and 1993 at the M. D. Anderson Cancer Center, the 5-year overall survival rate was 52% (77); patients who had stage IE and IIE disease receiving combined modality therapy had a better prognosis and had an actuarial 5-year freedom from progression and overall survival of 83% and 67%, respectively. Most patients (86%) were diagnosed with diffuse large cell lymphoma, but immunophenotypic data were not provided (77). In the Far East, where patients who have sinonasal lymphomas mainly have those of NK/T-cell type, between 67% and 80% of patients present with stage IE or IIE disease (6,29,30,78). One series of 90 patients with stage IE or IIE lymphoma demonstrated a complete response rate of 75% and a 2-year overall survival of approximately 50% (30). Combined modality therapy did not improve outcome and patients with NK/T-cell ($CD56^+$) malignant lymphomas fared worse. In another large series, a high 5-year overall survival of 90% was reported for patients who had stage IE disease limited to the nasal cavity (29); however, a lower survival rate of 57% was found among stage IE patients who had lymphomas that extended from the nasal cavity to the paranasal sinuses. Prognostic factors that predict for better overall survival include stage IE disease, age less than 60 years, no B symptoms, and a non–NK/T-cell ($CD56^+$) immunophenotype (30,78). Sinonasal malignant lymphomas tend to relapse in other extranodal sites such as the skin, lung, liver, gastrointestinal tract, testis, and brain (6,29,30,75). Some patients develop a terminal hemophagocytic syndrome (24).

SALIVARY GLAND

Malignant lymphomas that manifest initially in salivary glands are uncommon and are estimated to constitute only 1.7% of all reported salivary gland tumors (79). The parotid gland is the salivary gland most frequently involved by malignant lymphoma; malignant lymphoma is discovered in 4% of patients who undergo parotid gland surgery (80,81). In the Non-Hodgkin's Lymphoma Classification Project, the salivary gland was the primary site of involvement in 5% of patients who were diagnosed with marginal zone lymphoma of extranodal MALT type (82).

It is convenient to separate lymphomas of the salivary gland that develop in patients who have no prior history of antecedent disease from those that develop in patients who have a history of Sjögren's syndrome, another autoimmune disease, or myoepithelial sialadenitis/benign lymphoepithelial lesion (MESA/BLEL) (83,84) (Table 36.2). The term *lymphoepithelial sialadenitis* (LESA) was proposed as a replacement for MESA and BLEL to reflect the fact that the cells in epimyoepithelial islands may be exclusively of basal epithelial origin and that many cases that formerly were coded as BLEL may represent low-grade malignant lymphomas (85). However, because MESA and BLEL are best known and most ingrained in the literature, MESA and BLEL are the idioms of choice in this section.

Sjögren's syndrome, or sicca syndrome, is a multisystem autoimmune disorder in which the salivary and lacrimal glands are damaged, resulting in keratoconjunctivitis sicca, xerostomia, lymphoid infiltrates in the minor salivary glands of the lip, and bilateral parotid enlargement (6). Classic Sjögren's syndrome is indistinguishable from MESA/BLEL; patients with Sjögren's syndrome all have MESA/BLEL, although not all patients with MESA/BLEL have Sjögren's syndrome. In MESA/BLEL, there is a histologic spectrum that ranges from focal lymphocytic infiltrates associated with mild acinar atrophy to a fully developed reactive process in which the lymphocytic infiltrates are dense and con-

TABLE 36.2. *Comparison of malignant lymphomas of salivary glands that develop in patients with or without myoepithelial sialadenitis or benign lymphoepithelial lesion*

Characteristic	MESA/BLEL	Non-MESA/BLEL
Age/sex	Elderly/female	Elderly/female
Antecedent disease	With or without Sjögren's syndrome or other autoimmune disorder	None
Symptoms	Pain, swelling, not fixed to adjacent tissues	Pain, mass, often fixed to adjacent tissues
Lymphoma type	Low grade—MALT (monocytoid and plasmacytic variants)	All types—follicular (most common)
Lymphoma extent	Often focal	Usually diffuse replacement of gland
Immunophenotype	B cell	B cell
BCL2 rearrangements	No	Yes
Clinical course	Indolent, potential for extrasalivary presentation (lymph nodes, lungs) and histologic transformation	Similar to nodal counterpart

MALT, mucosa-associated lymphoid tissue; MESA, myoepithelial sialadenitis; BLEL, benign lymphoepithelial lesion.

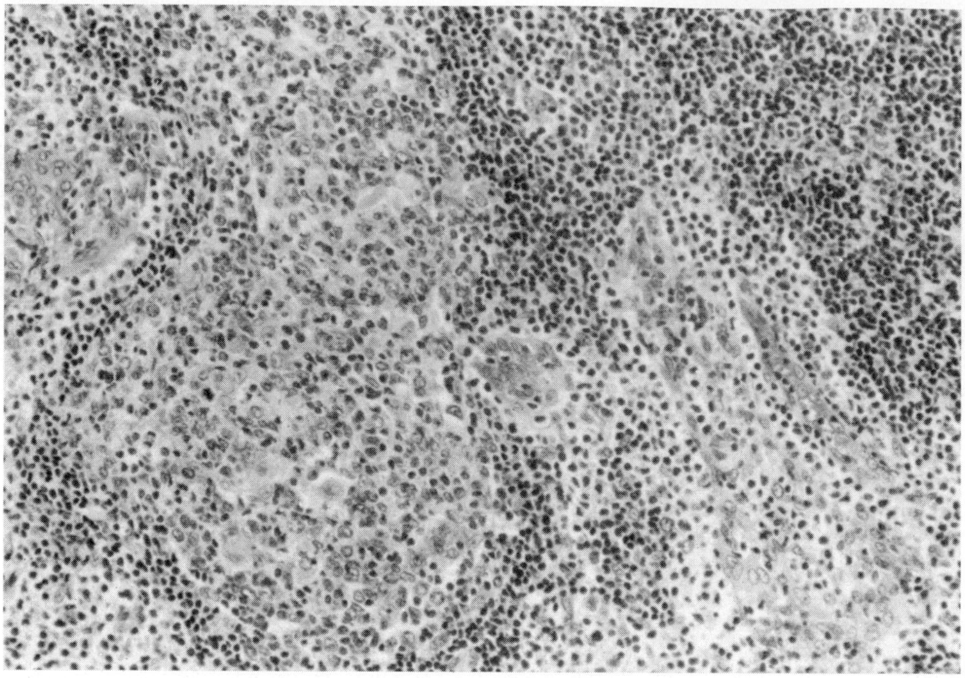

FIG. 36.10. In myoepithelial sialadenitis (MESA)/benign lymphoepithelial lesion (BLEL), there frequently is florid lymphoid hyperplasia associated with germinal centers, dense lymphocytic infiltrates, atrophy of salivary gland acini, and the formation of epimyoepithelial islands (hematoxylin and eosin stain, original magnification: 240× magnification).

fluent and are associated with germinal center formation, extensive acinar atrophy, disruption of ducts, and the presence of numerous epimyoepithelial islands (Fig. 36.10); monocytoid B cells often are in the epimyoepithelial islands (85). The lymphocytes between the germinal centers are mainly small lymphocytes with scattered plasma cells, immunoblasts, and occasional monocytoid B cells. Morphologic changes similar to MESA/BLEL have been described in salivary glands and intrasalivary gland lymph nodes in patients who have the acquired immunodeficiency syndrome (AIDS) and in intravenous drug users (86–88); cystically dilated salivary gland ducts with squamous metaplasia and that are filled with keratin are observed in these cases (88,89) (see Chapter 28) (Fig. 36.11). The lymphoepithelial cysts probably form secondary to the obstruction of salivary ducts by the florid reactive lymphocytic infiltrate (90). Occasionally, in the salivary gland from a patient with AIDS, the degree of lymphoid and immunoblastic hyperplasia may be so prolific as to mimic a malignant lymphoma (Fig. 36.12).

Like patients who have AIDS, patients who have actual Sjögren's syndrome have a predisposition to develop malignant lymphoma, which has been reported to occur 43.8 times more than expected in the general population (91). Cases of MESA/BLEL are characterized by a predominance of T helper cells, and it has been proposed that the increased risk of malignant lymphoma in Sjögren's syndrome is a consequence of chronic simulation of B cells by T helper cells with eventual immunoglobulin gene hypermutation and escape of a malignant B-cell clone (92,93). The growth of early clones in MESA/BLEL is thought to initiate as nonmalignant antigen selected expansions (94). Genotypic studies have documented rearrangement of immunoglobulin genes in salivary gland tissues from patients who have MESA/BLEL, including patients who show none of the usual morphologic characteristics of malignant lymphoma (95–98); these findings also help explain the increased incidence of malignant lymphoma

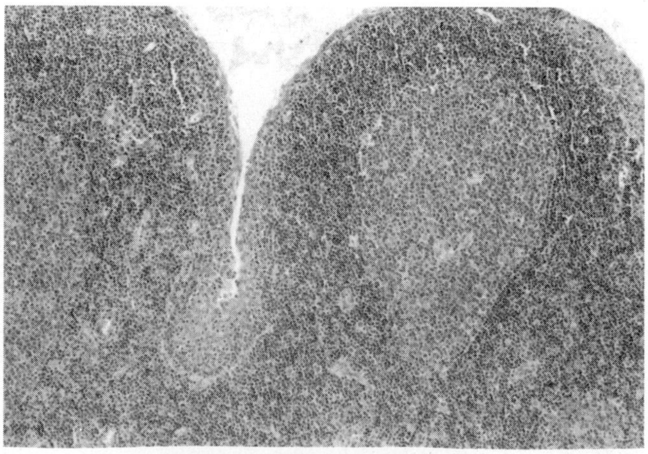

FIG. 36.11. Lymphoid hyperplasia with cyst formation may mimic myoepithelial sialadenitis (MESA)/benign lymphoepithelial lesion (BLEL) in the salivary gland and intrasalivary gland lymph nodes of patients infected with the human immunodeficiency virus (HIV) (hematoxylin and eosin stain, original magnification: 120× magnification).

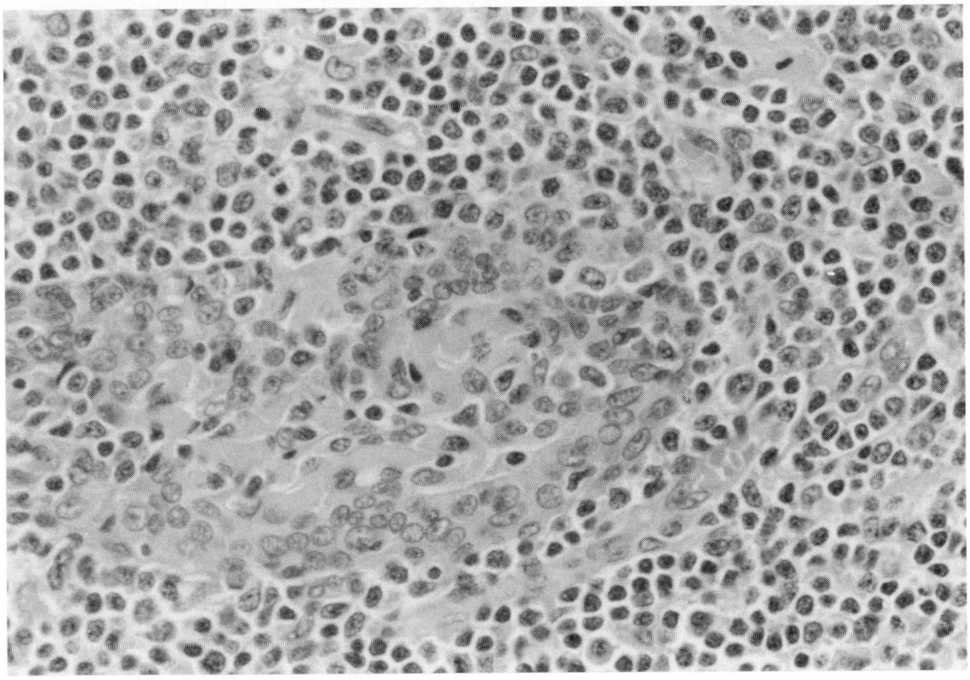

FIG. 36.12. Florid immunoblastic hyperplasia in the salivary gland of a patient infected with the human immunodeficiency virus (HIV) is indistinguishable from myoepithelial sialadenitis (MESA)/benign lymphoepithelial lesion (/BLEL). Notice the invasion of the epimyoepithelial islands by the proliferating small lymphocytes and immunoblasts despite the reactive nature of this process (hematoxylin and eosin stain, original magnification: 480× magnification).

associated with Sjögren's syndrome. It is unlikely that EBV plays a role in the pathogenesis of malignant lymphoma occurring in the setting of Sjögren's syndrome, but, in some cases, hepatitis C virus may be involved (96,99–101). Curiously, although patients who have Sjögren's syndrome may develop clinically overt lymphoma in the salivary gland, most patients who do have this syndrome evince their lymphoma clinically in extrasalivary gland sites, particularly marginal zone lymphomas in lymph nodes and lung (79,99,102–104).

Most patients who have Sjögren's syndrome and who develop symptoms related to their salivary gland frequently complain of local pain, tenderness, and swelling without apparent fixation to superficial or deep structures (81,102); there usually is no associated cervical lymphadenopathy.

Despite the fact that clinically obvious malignant lymphoma is relatively uncommon in the salivary glands of patients who have Sjögren's syndrome, immunophenotypic and genotypic studies have served to refine the histologic criteria of MESA/BLEL and have led to the discovery of subtle malignant lymphoma in this setting (84,96–98,104, 105). Frequently, a histologic and immunologic continuum develops from areas of benign polyclonal lymphocytic infiltrates to monoclonal B-cell lymphoma (84,96–98,105,106); this continuum has implied that malignant lymphomas of salivary gland form part of the spectrum of lymphomas of MALT (105). The MALT lymphomas of salivary gland conform to the general morphologic features of MALT lymphomas with the exception that their centrocyte-like cells have a distinct monocytoid or clear cell appearance or have plasmacytic characteristics (98,104,105). The neoplastic monocytoid B cells in the salivary gland have a marginal zone–type distribution, encircling reactive follicles and the adjacent rims of attenuated mantle zone lymphocytes. The unequivocal salivary gland MALT lymphomas exhibit coalescence of monocytoid cells to form broad, interconnecting strands that surround and invade epimyoepithelial islands, displace germinal centers, and eventually produce sheetlike masses resulting in destruction of the acinar architecture of the gland (98,104,105,107–109). In contrast to a reactive process, these low-grade MALT lymphomas usually are dense and have monotonous cytologic features (Fig. 36.13). The presence of wide strands of coalescing monocytoid B cells correlates with monoclonality and the development of extrasalivary gland malignant lymphomas, all of which exhibit the same light-chain restriction as the corresponding neoplastic monocytoid B cells in the salivary gland (84,104). The immunophenotypic profile of salivary gland MALT lymphomas that are dominated by monocytoid B cells replicates the established B-cell immunophenotype of MALT lymphomas in other extranodal sites and in many cases the neoplastic monocytoid B cells coexpress CD43 (8,98,104, 107). In the salivary gland, the neoplastic monocytoid B cells may express BCL-2 protein, but they almost never exhibit the t(14;18) chromosomal translocation as determined by molecular studies (96,99,107).

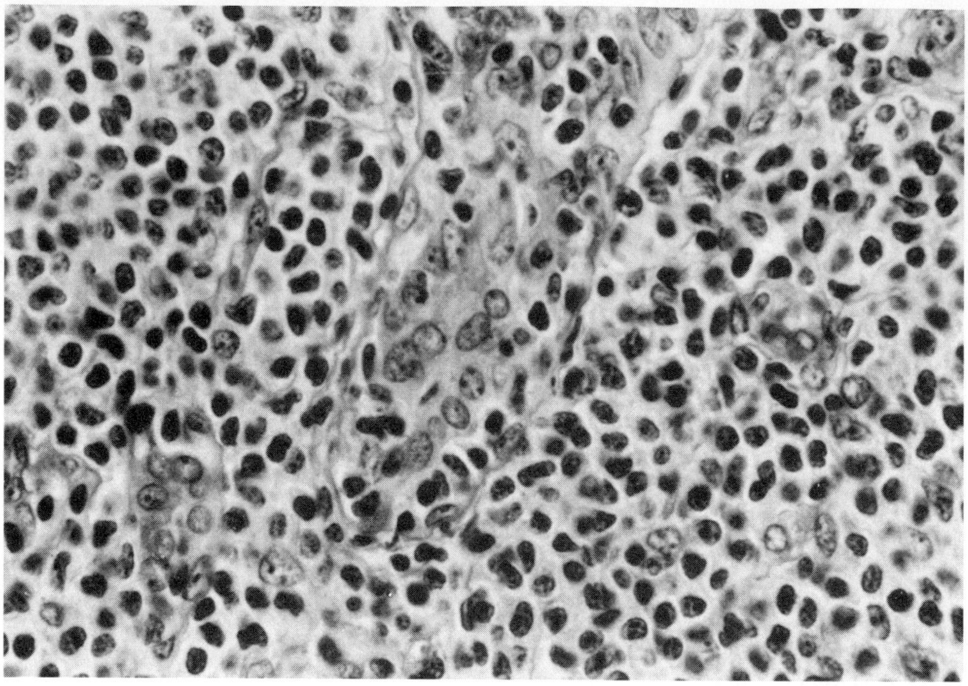

FIG. 36.13. Mucosa-associated lymphoid tissue (MALT) lymphoma in a salivary gland is characterized by a dense, monotonous pattern of infiltration with invasion of residual salivary gland ducts. The neoplastic lymphocytes are monocytoid with slight nuclear membrane irregularities and abundant lucent cytoplasm. Immunophenotypic studies demonstrated κ light-chain restriction (hematoxylin and eosin stain, original magnification: 600× magnification).

The main contention in salivary gland MALT lymphomas concerns the morphologic threshold for interpreting cases as malignant lymphoma (109). With polymerase chain reaction (PCR) techniques, for example, clonality has been demonstrated across the full spectrum of lymphoid infiltrates in the salivary gland including cases regarded as reactive MESA/BLEL, cases with halos of monocytoid cells surrounding epimyoepithelial islands, and cases with unequivocal confluent-type MALT lymphomas (96–98). The difficulty concerns the cases containing monocytoid or clear cell halos (Fig. 36.14). In some instances, cases with focal or halo-type monocytoid B-cell proliferations in the salivary gland are ignored or simply misconstrued as hyperplastic and as variants of MESA/BLEL because of their juxtaposition to benign reactive areas, including germinal centers and mantle zone cells. Nonetheless, the abundant, pale, often clear cytoplasm with well-defined cytoplasmic borders of the monocytoid cells in the halos is morphologically distinct and should assist in distinguishing them from the adjacent reactive small lymphocytes and associated germinal centers (Fig. 36.15). The monocytoid halos that are recognized in salivary glands with MESA/BLEL are analogous to the circumscribed pale-staining ''proliferation areas'' that previously were reported and some investigators consider clonal halo-type cases as examples of early MALT lymphoma, whereas others regard the halo-type cases as indeterminate, borderline, or perhaps as examples of disorders of ''uncertain malignant potential'' (84,96,98,105,110).

This issue is not readily resolved because clonality does not appear to predict progression of lymphoid lesions in the salivary gland to clinically overt lymphoma (97). For example, Quintana and associates examined 61 salivary gland specimens with lymphoid infiltrates and histologically classified them as equivalent to MESA/BLEL, MESA/BLEL with monocytoid B-cell halos, unequivocal low-grade malignant lymphomas of the MALT type with confluent monocytoid B-cell zones, low-grade MALT lymphomas with monoclonal plasma cells, and high-grade B-cell lymphomas of MALT type (98). As demonstrated by others, CD43 coexpression on monocytoid B cells did not correlate with the histologic category, clonality, or with extrasalivary gland malignant lymphoma (104). Employing a PCR technique, clonal B cells were identified across the entire morphologic spectrum of salivary gland lymphoid infiltrates, including 42% of the cases that were regarded as histologically classic benign MESA/BLEL and 65% of the cases with halos of monocytoid B cells (98); yet, most patients pursued an indolent clinical course. The investigators concluded that two types of borderline lesions exist within the context of salivary gland lymphoid infiltrates (98) (Table 36.3). One has the morphologic appearance of benign MESA/BLEL but with demonstrable B-cell clonality, and the other is MESA/BLEL that has halos of monocytoid B cells that extend beyond the confines of the epimyoepithelial islands or lymphoepithelial lesions. With either of these lesions, the term *borderline* portends that there is morphologic or clonal

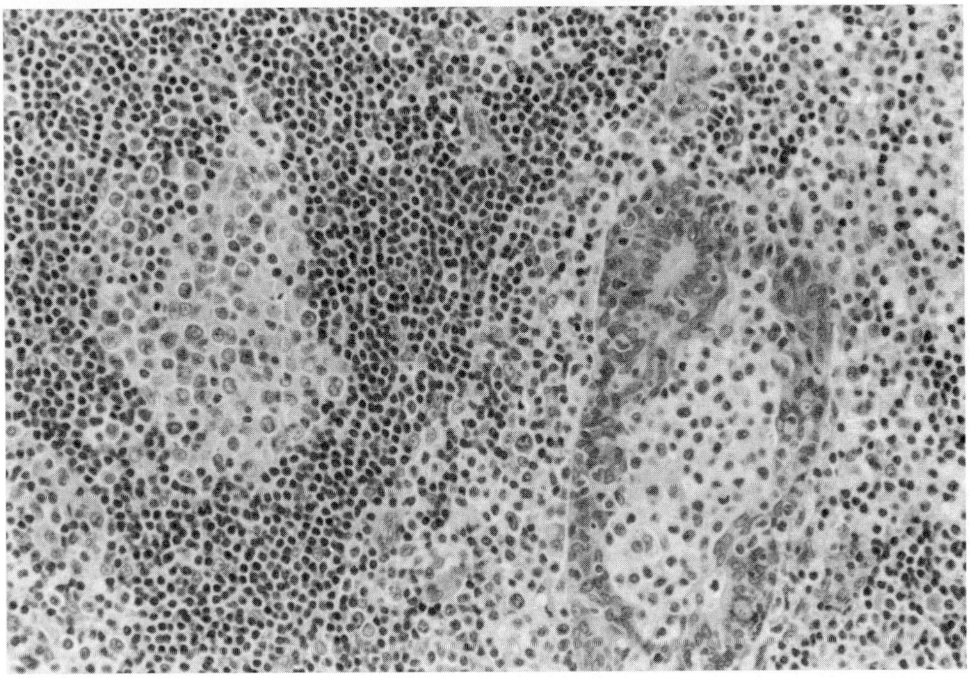

FIG. 36.14. Monocytoid B cells concentrate around and invade epimyoepithelial islands to form a halo pattern. The pale-staining cytoplasm of the monocytoid cells contrasts with the darker-staining small lymphocytes of the adjacent mantle zone surrounding a germinal center. Despite the presence of frequent monoclonality, there is no agreement on whether cases with monocytoid halos are an early form of mucosa-associated lymphoid tissue (MALT) lymphoma or a borderline lesion (hematoxylin and eosin stain, original magnification: 240× magnification).

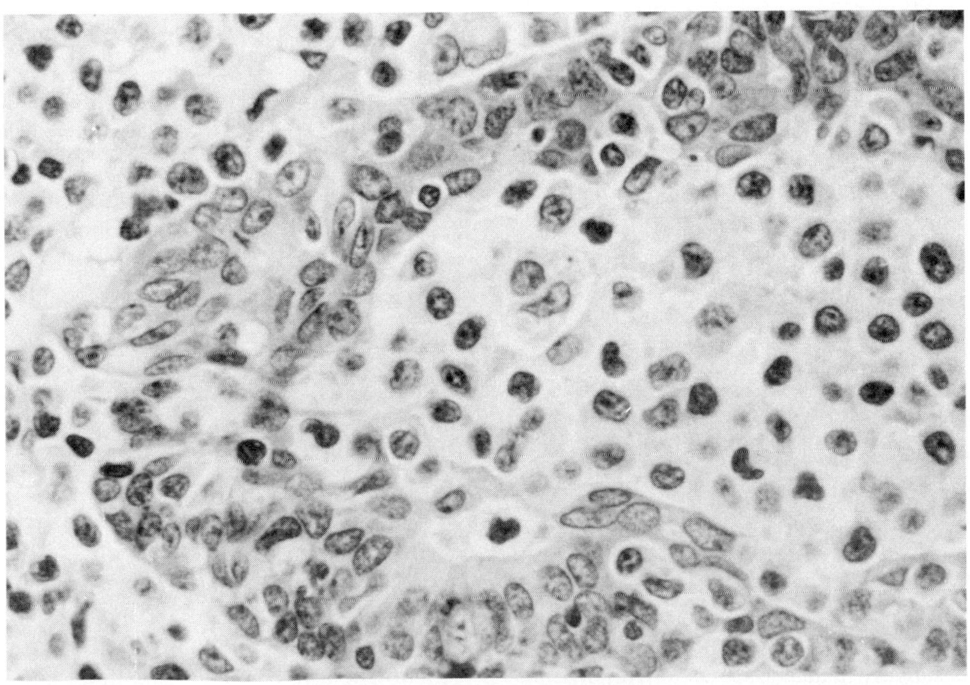

FIG. 36.15. Detail of the neoplastic monocytoid cells with disruption of an epimyoepithelial island in the parotid salivary gland. The cytoplasm is characteristically pale staining and the nuclei frequently are reniform (hematoxylin and eosin stain, original magnification: 720× magnification).

TABLE 36.3. *Synopsis of lymphoid infiltrates of the salivary gland associated with myoepithelial sialadenitis and benign lymphoepithelial lesion*

Benign
MESA/BLEL, polyclonal
Borderline (clonal or morphologic features suggesting malignant lymphoma but with little risk of dissemination)
MESA/BLEL, monoclonal
MESA/BLEL with halos of monocytoid B cells
Low-grade lymphoma (risk for spread to extrasalivary lymph nodes)
MALT-type (MESA/BLEL with wide interconnecting strands of monocytoid B cells, with or without plasmacytic differentiation)
High-grade lymphoma (primary or secondary to low-grade lymphoma of MALT)
Large B-cell type

MALT, mucosa-associated lymphoid tissue; MESA, myoepithelial sialadenitis; BLEL, benign lymphoepithelial lesion.

Adapted from Quintana PG, Kapadia SB, Bahler DW, et al. Salivary gland lymphoid infiltrates associated with lymphoepithelial lesions: a clinicopathologic, immunophenotypic, and genotypic study. *Hum Pathol* 1997;28:850–861, with permission.

documentation that is suggestive of malignant lymphoma, but that there is limited chance of dissemination unless histologic progression develops (98). However, this viewpoint is contentious and others signify that the emergence of a monoclonal B-cell population in a setting of MESA/BLEL with monocytoid B-cell halo-type lesions heralds the onset of frank malignant lymphoma, although genetic alterations may be required for progression and dissemination (96). Regardless of whether clonality is interpreted as tantamount to malignant lymphoma in cases of MESA/BLEL with halos, patients with such lesions require careful clinical monitoring. Patients who have a salivary gland low-grade MALT lymphoma are at risk to develop a synchronous or a subsequent high-grade lymphoma (98,107,108) (Fig. 36.16).

Malignant lymphomas of salivary gland associated with Sjögren's syndrome or MESA/BLEL, specifically the low-grade malignant lymphomas of MALT, usually are relatively indolent (105). Although some patients may develop extrasalivary gland lymphomas in months instead of years, most patients behave similarly to patients who have equivalent extranodal marginal zone lymphomas of MALT and have a predilection for localized disease (8,84,96,104). The onset of progressive malignant lymphoma can vary from 3 to 19 years and if extrasalivary gland lymphoma does develop, it usually exhibits the identical histologic and immunohistochemical features of the initial low-grade lymphoma in the salivary gland (96,111).

The management of patients who have a low-grade MALT lymphoma in the salivary gland associated with MESA/BLEL is uncertain, but, at the very least, the patients should be staged appropriately and followed, with, perhaps, involved-field radiation therapy for those with symptomatic disease (6,112). However, because many cases of MALT lymphoma of the salivary gland are discovered after retrospective review of cases originally regarded as benign MESA/BLEL, and because these patients have not received therapy except for surgical biopsy, they may not require any therapy and need only careful follow-up (98,105).

Malignant lymphomas that arise in the salivary glands of patients who have no history of antecedent disease are, paradoxically, more common than the often publicized lymphomas of salivary glands that develop in patients who have Sjögren's syndrome or MESA/BLEL (79,102,113). Patients who have overt lymphoma that arise in the salivary gland generally present with a firm, bulging mass that may be fixed to superficial or deep structures and occasionally is associated with nerve palsy (79). Grossly, malignant lymphomas of the salivary gland appear gray-tan to pink, bulge on cut section, and often are circumscribed (113).

In contrast to the diffuse, low-grade MALT lymphomas characteristic of the salivary gland in patients who have Sjögren's syndrome or MESA/BLEL, patients who have no autoimmune disorder develop all histologic types of salivary gland non-Hodgkin's lymphomas, but follicular lymphomas are the most common (79,81,83,102) (Fig. 36.17). Many lymphomas, including those with a follicular architectural pattern, probably originate in lymph nodes attached to the capsule or entrapped within the involved gland, for example, intraparotid lymph nodes (81,85). Diagnosis in these cases is usually not a problem, although occasional follicular large cell lymphomas may be difficult to differentiate from florid reactive follicular hyperplasia with so-called giant follicles (114). The distinction of follicular lymphoma from reactive follicular hyperplasia with giant follicles in the salivary gland depends on the application of criteria identical to those used to separate these two lesions in lymph nodes. The same criteria are equally applicable to the diagnosis of rare follicular lymphomas that arise in salivary glands involved by Warthin's tumor (102,115).

Histologically and immunologically, no differences are apparent between a follicular lymphoma that arises in a salivary gland and one in a lymph node. For example, studies have demonstrated that follicular lymphomas that present in the salivary gland have molecular evidence of the t(14;18) translocation (116). This contrasts with the MALT lymphomas of salivary gland that lack *BCL2* gene rearrangements (96,99,107).

Although most primary malignant lymphomas of the salivary gland are B-cell malignancies, rare cases of T-cell lymphoma, including $CD30^+$ anaplastic large cell lymphoma, and $CD56^+$ NK/T-cell lymphoma, also may primarily involve the salivary glands (117). The T-cell and NK/T-cell malignant lymphomas are characterized by polymorphous infiltrates of small, medium-sized, or large lymphocytes and by invasion of salivary gland ducts and acini to form lymphoepithelial lesions; angioinvasion also may develop. Similar to NK/T-cell malignant lymphomas of the sinonasal region, the $CD56^+$ cases in the salivary gland exhibit reactivity for EBER (117).

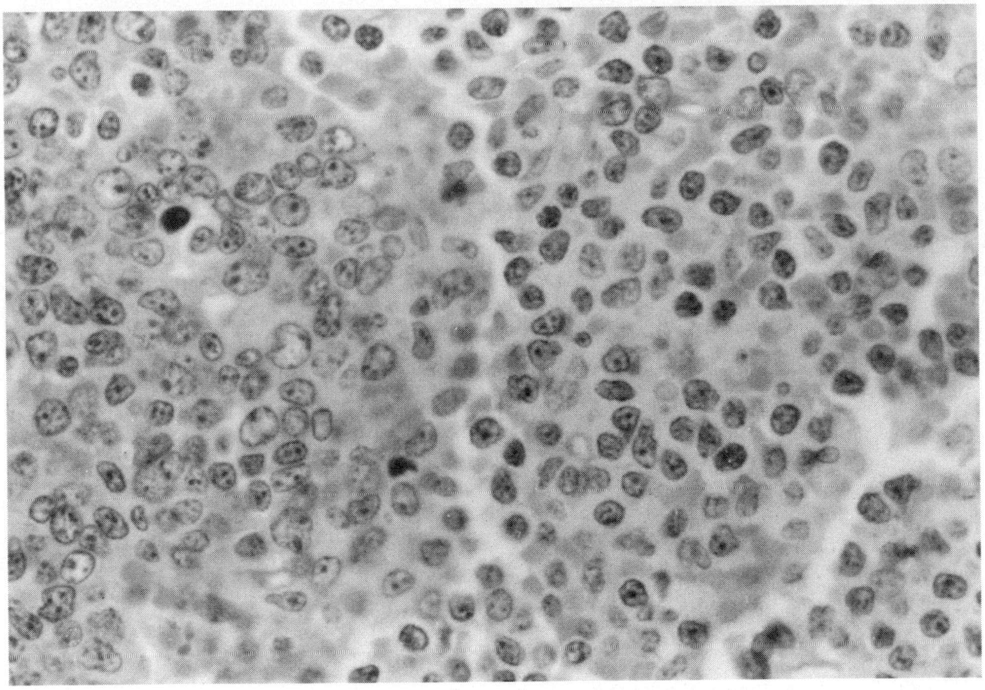

FIG. 36.16. Interface of large cell lymphoma on the left and a mucosa-associated lymphoid tissue (MALT) lymphoma composed of monocytoid B cells on the right. The large cell lymphoma was focal and developed in a background of a low-grade lymphoma of MALT type in the parotid gland. The monocytoid B cells and the large cells expressed identical immunoglobulin heavy and light chains (IgM λ) (hematoxylin and eosin stain, original magnification: 720× magnification).

The prognosis of patients who have salivary gland lymphomas that are unrelated to Sjögren's syndrome or to MESA/BLEL also is similar to patients who have histologically identical malignant lymphomas that present in lymph nodes or other extranodal sites (79,83,102,113,117). For example, patients who have T-cell or NK/T-cell lymphomas of the salivary gland have an aggressive clinical behavior, whereas patients who have follicular lymphomas of the salivary gland have a favorable clinical course that is likely attributable to the follicular properties of the lymphoma instead of to any unique biologic properties indigenous to the salivary gland.

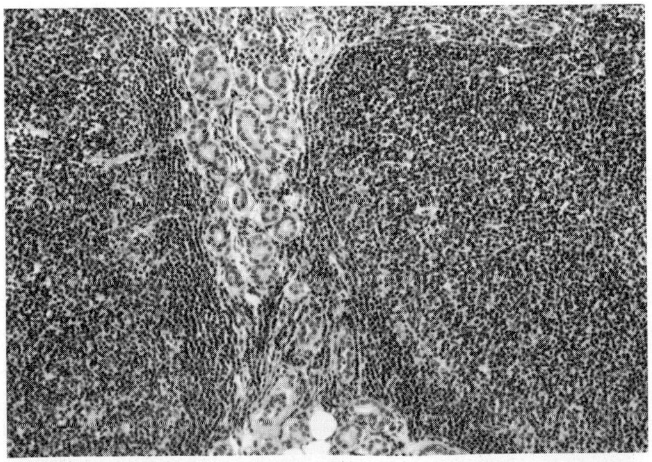

FIG. 36.17. Follicular, predominantly small cleaved cell lymphoma is the most common malignant lymphoma that occurs in the salivary gland of patients who do not have Sjögren's syndrome or myoepithelial sialadenitis (MESA)/benign lymphoepithelial lesion (BLEL) (hematoxylin and eosin stain, original magnification: 150× magnification).

THYROID GLAND

Malignant lymphomas of the thyroid gland share many features with those that manifest in the salivary glands in that they almost always are associated with an immunologically mediated, extranodal lymphoid infiltrate, specifically chronic lymphocytic thyroiditis or Hashimoto's thyroiditis (118–123). Between 80% and 100% of patients who have malignant lymphoma of the thyroid exhibit chronic lymphocytic thyroiditis in the adjacent tissue and 67% to 80% have thyroid antibodies (121,124). The chance of developing malignant lymphoma of the thyroid gland in patients who have chronic lymphocytic thyroiditis is greatly increased, with an estimated relative risk of 67, and in Japan, the frequency of thyroid lymphomas in patients with Hashimoto's thyroiditis is 80 times greater than expected (125,126). The predisposition among patients who have chronic lymphocytic thyroiditis to develop malignant lymphoma is analogous to the proposed pathways in patients with Sjögren's syndrome. As in Sjögren's syndrome, the lymphocytes infiltrating the thyroid in chronic lymphocytic thyroiditis are mainly activated T helper cells that are specific for thyroid antigens (124). The T helper cells stimulate autoreactive B cells. The onset of malignant lymphoma likely is a consequence of the chronic antigenic stimulation of B lymphocytes that take place in this autoimmune disorder; this chronic stimulation probably leads to a population of lymphocytes that are more susceptible to neoplastic transformation, possibly as a result of a disorder of immune surveillance related to B cells with probable associated cytogenetic changes that triggers histologic progression (124,125,127). Activation of EBV is uncommon in chronic lymphocytic thyroiditis and malignant lymphomas of the thyroid (4% to 9% of cases), and EBV probably is not a significant factor in the pathogenesis of the malignant lymphomas (128,129). Mutations of *TP53* also are not found in malignant lymphomas of the thyroid (130).

Unlike patients who have morphologically benign MESA/BLEL, clonal immunoglobulin gene rearrangements usually are not detected in patients who have chronic lymphocytic thyroiditis with only occasional exceptions (131–134). Most cases that have immunoglobulin gene rearrangements in chronic lymphocytic thyroiditis probably are malignant lymphomas at the outset and the low frequency of monoclonality in chronic lymphocytic thyroiditis compared with MESA/BLEL reflects the relative rarity of malignant lymphomas of the thyroid as opposed to those in the salivary gland (134). Notwithstanding, histologic studies have demonstrated that there is a histologic gradation between chronic lymphocytic thyroiditis (Fig. 36.18), low-grade lymphomas of MALT that resemble chronic lymphocytic thyroiditis, and the more common high-grade lymphomas of the thyroid (120,122,123). This morphologic spectrum between reactive and neoplastic lymphoid infiltrates has suggested that thyroid lymphomas are derived from MALT (120,122,123,135). In some cases where a follicular architecture is present, however, the follicles are massive and often there is the impression of a subtle transition from coalescing large reactive germinal centers in chronic lymphocytic thyroiditis to follicular lymphoma (118). Whether the malignant lymphomas of the thyroid are of MALT or of follicle center cell lineage, immunologic studies have demonstrated that almost all lymphomas of the thyroid gland are B-cell derived (120,122,123,136–138).

Like patients who have Hashimoto's thyroiditis, patients who have malignant lymphoma of the thyroid gland are predominantly female and in the sixth and seventh decades of life (118,139,140). Patients generally present with complaints of a painless neck mass. They also may have a history of rapid growth of the mass and compression symptoms, including dysphagia, dyspnea, pain, and hoarseness (118–120,123,140). The clinical diagnosis generally is a possible primary thyroid malignancy, but malignant lymphoma usually is not suspected except in patients with a history of Hashimoto's thyroiditis who have rapid thyroid enlargement (140). In cases of malignant lymphoma, the use of fine needle aspiration (FNA) of the thyroid has yielded mixed results with a correct diagnosis found in 50% to 80% of patients (129,140). Because almost every malignant lymphoma of the thyroid evolves out of chronic lymphocytic thyroiditis, the distinction of a low-grade malignant lymphoma of MALT from chronic lymphocytic thyroiditis is problematic in FNA specimens. Molecular methods, such as PCR, can be used to detect monoclonality in a FNA cytology specimen from the thyroid, but most cases generally are diagnosed by an open biopsy or surgical resection (141). On gross examination, the resected thyroid gland often is replaced by a fleshy, pink-tan tumor mass similar to a lymphoma in a lymph node (Fig. 36.19).

Malignant lymphoma usually is morphologically distinguishable from chronic lymphocytic thyroiditis with the exception of cases of florid thyroiditis in which there is an absence of germinal centers and there is associated destruc-

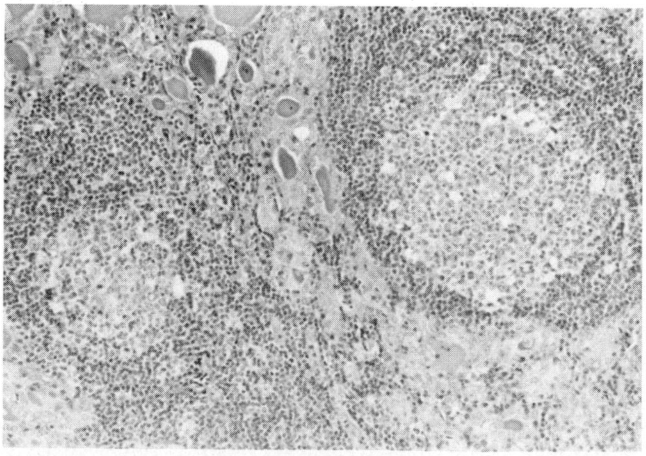

FIG. 36.18. Fully developed chronic lymphocytic thyroiditis is characterized by reactive lymphoid follicles with germinal center formation and Hürthle cell change in the thyroid follicles. These lesions often are encountered adjacent to malignant lymphomas in the thyroid gland (hematoxylin and eosin stain, original magnification: 150× magnification).

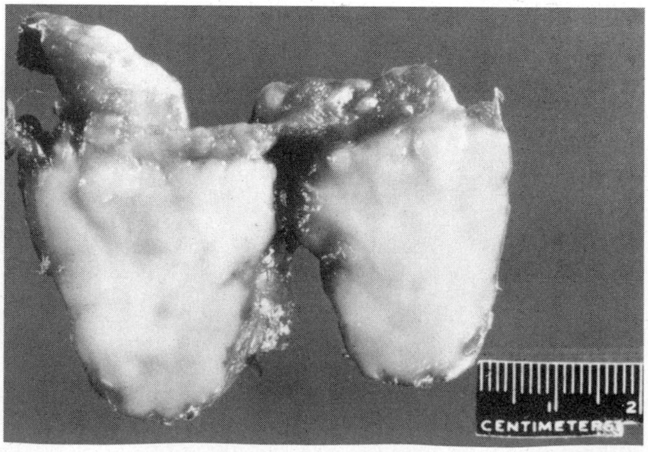

FIG. 36.19. Diffuse large cell lymphoma of the thyroid gland forms a large, fleshy mass and virtually replaces the thyroid parenchyma.

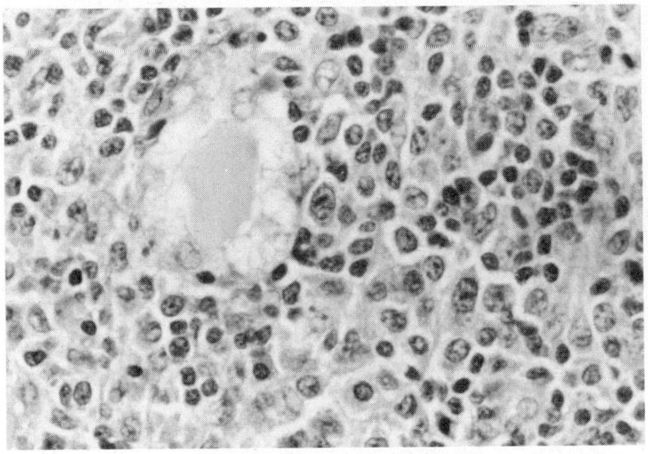

FIG. 36.20. In florid chronic lymphocytic thyroiditis, diffuse lymphocytes proliferate, including numerous immunoblasts. This results in obliteration of thyroid follicles. The heterogeneity of the lymphocytic population and the relatively regular sequence of lymphocytic transformation differ from what is seen in malignant lymphoma (hematoxylin and eosin stain, original magnification: 720× magnification).

tion of normal thyroid follicles because of a diffuse proliferation of small lymphocytes together with plasma cells and immunoblasts (Fig. 36.20). In these cases, an unequivocal diagnosis of reactive lymphoid hyperplasia or chronic lymphocytic thyroiditis depends on an awareness of the reactive nature of the infiltrate by the absence of cellular atypia, the polymorphous nature of the infiltrate, and the orderly transformation of small lymphocytes to immunoblasts (142). With florid chronic lymphocytic thyroiditis, clusters of reactive immunoblasts are easily mistaken for focal large cell lymphoma. Immunophenotypic and immunoglobulin gene rearrangement studies are valuable in supporting this distinction, especially when the histologic diagnosis is equivocal (143).

There are some morphologic features that are specifically thought to aid in the differentiation of chronic lymphocytic thyroiditis from malignant lymphoma in the thyroid gland. Invasion of blood vessel walls and extension of the lymphocytic infiltrate beyond the thyroid capsule into the surrounding perithyroidal soft tissues are more common to lymphoma (118,119). Invasion by lymphocytes into the lumens of residual thyroid follicles that result in lymphoepithelial lesions is another morphologic feature thought to be important in the distinction of malignant lymphoma from thyroiditis (Fig. 36.21) (122,144); a cytokeratin stain can accentuate lymphoid infiltration of thyroid follicles (122,134,142,144). The finding of thyroid follicular infiltration by lymphocytes, however, is not an absolute diagnostic criterion for malignancy because a similar infiltration by benign, reactive B lymphocytes has been described in cases of chronic lymphocytic thyroiditis (122,145) (Fig. 36.22). Nonetheless, there are quantitative and qualitative differences in so far as the lymphoepithelial lesions in low-grade MALT lymphomas of the thyroid are more common, larger, and more destructive (134).

The problem of whether a lymphocytic infiltrate is benign

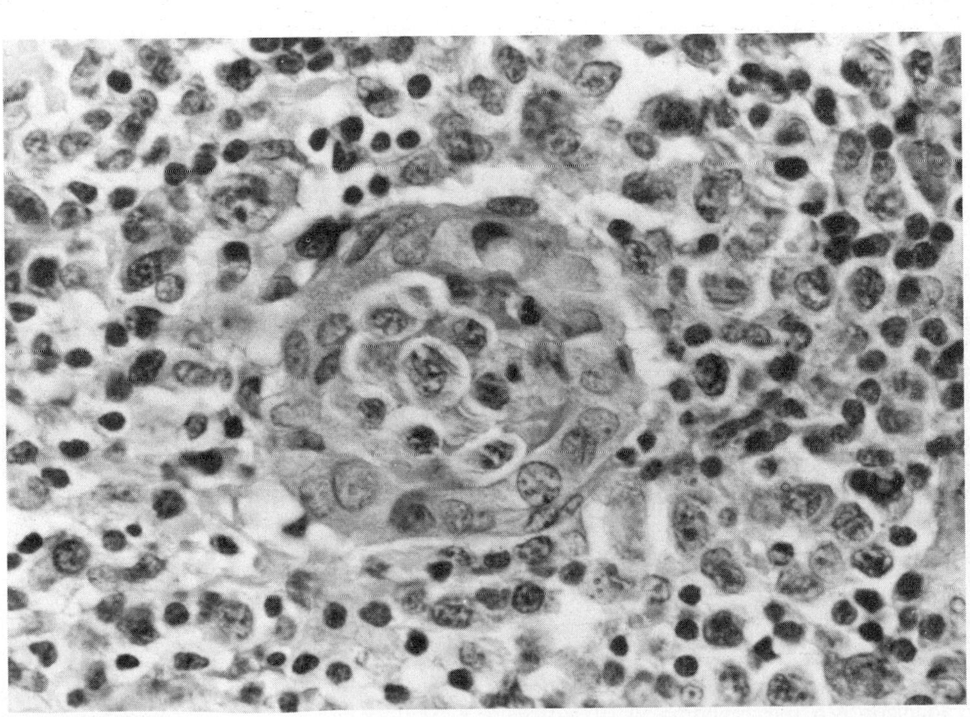

FIG. 36.21. Malignant lymphoma, large B-cell type. Invasion of residual thyroid follicles is a frequent observation in malignant lymphomas of the thyroid gland (hematoxylin and eosin stain, original magnification: 600× magnification).

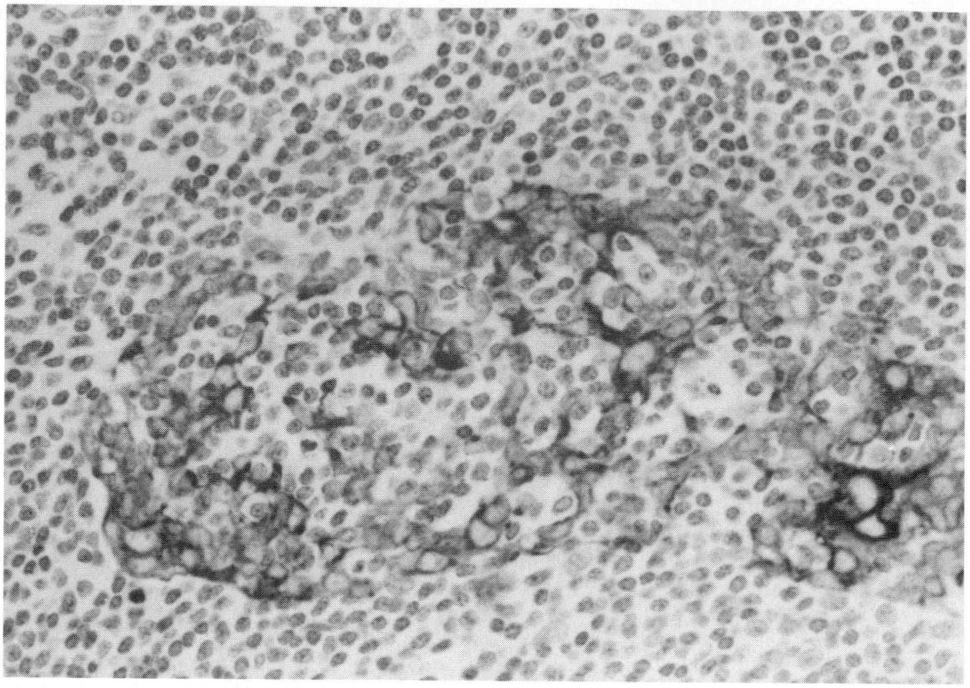

FIG. 36.22. An immunoperoxidase stain for cytokeratin highlights the invasion of residual thyroid follicles by small lymphocytes in chronic lymphocytic thyroiditis and reinforces the tenet that epithelial invasion is not a conclusive diagnostic criterion for extranodal malignant lymphoma (immunoperoxidase stain, original magnification: 480× magnification).

or malignant generally is not a major issue because low-grade lymphomas of the thyroid, including the marginal zone lymphomas of MALT, are relatively uncommon (119,122). In three series of primary malignant lymphomas of the thyroid comprising 23, 47, and 53 patients, low-grade lymphomas of MALT represented 4 (17.3%), 8 (17%), and 3 (5.6%) of the cases, respectively (123,129,139). When present, the low-grade MALT lymphomas of the thyroid recapitulate the morphologic features of MALT lymphomas in other sites with confluent dense lymphocytic infiltrates surrounding residual germinal centers resulting in effacement of the thyroid architecture, except for scattered residual thyroid follicles with Hürthle-cell changes (109,122) (Fig. 36.23). Follicular colonization of the germinal centers may be florid and impart a follicular-like pattern (146). The cytologic features of MALT lymphomas of the thyroid can be variable,

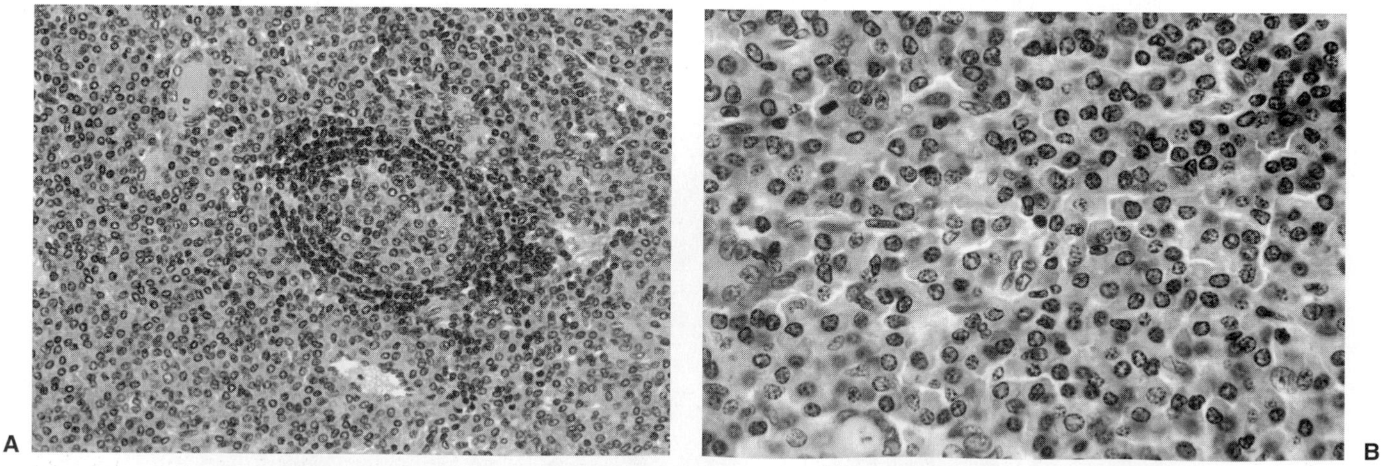

FIG. 36.23. A: The thyroid parenchyma is practically obliterated by a low-grade mucosa-associated lymphoid tissue (MALT) lymphoma, which surrounds a germinal center and attenuated corona of mantle cells (hematoxylin and eosin stain, original magnification: 300× magnification). **B:** The neoplastic cells of MALT lymphomas in the thyroid often display plasmacytic features (hematoxylin and eosin stain, original magnification: 600× magnification).

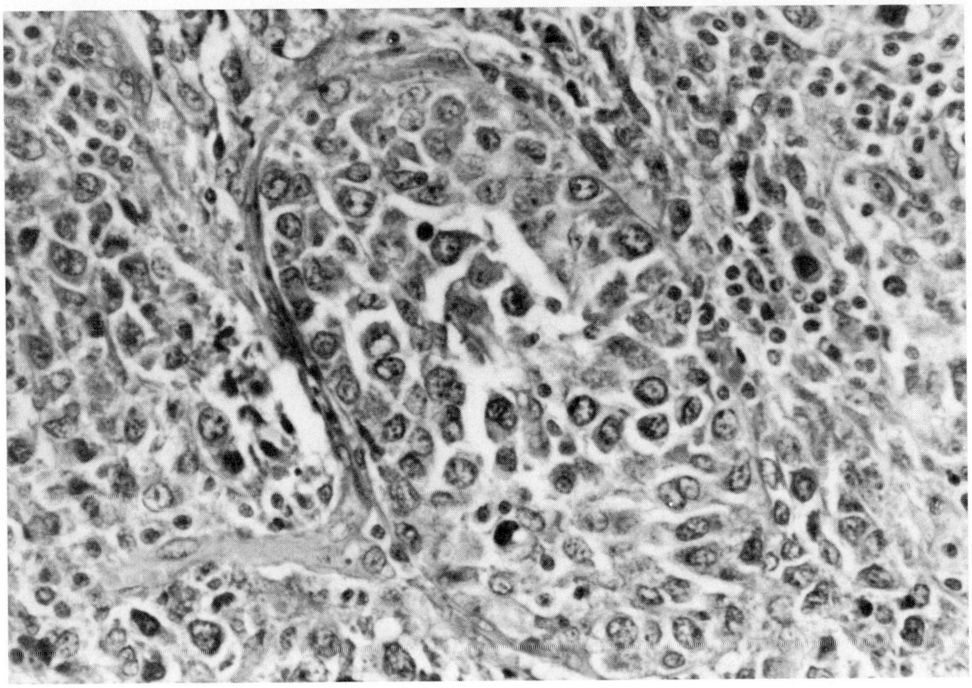

FIG. 36.24. Large B-cell lymphomas form the major histologic category of lymphomas in the thyroid gland. The infiltration and replacement of thyroid follicles by the large cells may be misinterpreted as carcinoma (hematoxylin and eosin stain, original magnification: 375× magnification).

but most cases have a plasmacytic appearance (122). Most cases that formerly were classified as plasmacytoma of the thyroid likely are MALT lymphomas, as are the cases that formerly were classified as intermediate lymphocytic lymphoma (119,147,148).

Most lymphomas of the thyroid gland are high-grade lymphomas, particularly large B-cell (Fig. 36.24) and immunoblastic types (118,120,121,129,138,139). Some large B-cell lymphoma cases are thought to be high-grade lymphomas of MALT based on a residual low-grade component (129,139,144). The high-grade cases are not difficult to separate from lymphocytic thyroiditis, but they may be difficult to distinguish from carcinomas, specifically cases interpreted as ''small cell'' carcinoma of thyroid. Small cell undifferentiated or anaplastic carcinoma of the thyroid is very rare and most investigators have questioned the existence of such an entity, because almost all cases diagnosed as small cell carcinoma in the thyroid have been reclassified retrospectively as lymphoma (118,149,150). The question of whether a thyroid neoplasm is carcinoma or lymphoma can be resolved readily with a combination of appropriate immunohistochemical studies that use antibodies directed against cytokeratin, B-cell (CD20), and T-cell (CD3) lineage antigens (Fig. 36.25).

Immunophenotypic analysis of malignant lymphomas of the thyroid gland on fresh tissue clearly demonstrates a preponderance of B-cell lymphomas with monoclonal immunoglobulin light-chain restriction (136). Cases of thyroid lymphoma that do not express detectable immunoglobulin in fixed tissue usually react with monoclonal antibodies directed against B cell–associated antigens, such as CD20 and CD79a (120,122,123,129,136–138,150). Most low-grade marginal zone lymphomas of MALT in the thyroid can be differentiated from other B-cell lymphomas of small lymphocytes by using an immunohistochemical panel incorporating antibodies to CD5, CD10, CD20, CD23, CD43, and cyclin D1 (151). With this panel, the lymphomas of MALT consistently only express CD20 and have variable expression of CD43, whereas other lymphomas, such as small lymphocytic lymphomas express CD5 and CD23, mantle cell lymphomas express CD5 and cyclin D1, and follicular lymphomas express CD10. T-cell lymphomas of the thyroid gland are uncommon, even in ATLL endemic areas in Japan (123,152); a case of $\gamma\delta$ T-cell lymphoma of the thyroid has been reported (153).

Patients who have low-grade malignant lymphomas of the thyroid gland have a relatively good prognosis. Evidence of MALT histology was the only significant prognostic factor for overall survival in one series of thyroid lymphomas (154); the cause specific survival at 5 years for patients who had lymphomas of MALT type in the thyroid was 90% compared with 55% for patients who had no evidence that their lymphoma had originated in MALT. Radiation therapy is recommended for patients who have stage IE small bulk MALT and other low-grade lymphomas of the thyroid (140). For patients who have the more common aggressive high-grade large B-cell lymphomas of thyroid, combined modality therapy is the treatment of choice (129,140,155). Prog-

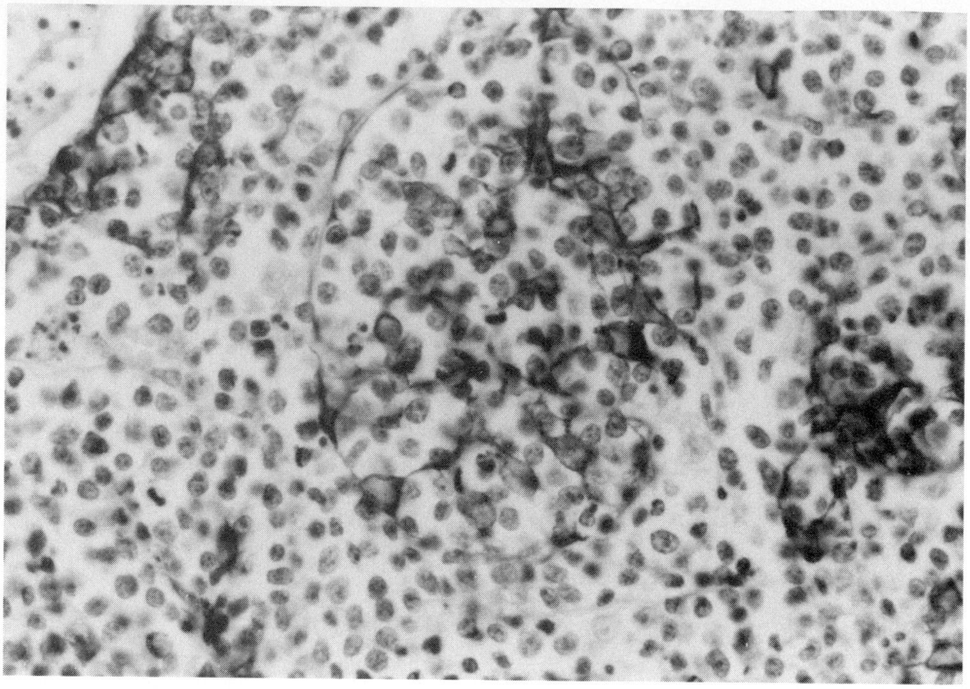

FIG. 36.25. A cytokeratin stain serves to distinguish malignant lymphoma of the thyroid from small cell undifferentiated carcinoma. Only the residual thyroid follicular cells express cytokeratin. In contrast, the neoplastic lymphoid cells express B-cell antigen CD20 (not shown) (immunoperoxidase stain, original magnification: 480× magnification).

nostic factors include tumor bulk, presence of retrosternal extension, and extracapsular spread (118,138,140,154,155). In most studies, survival has not been correlated consistently with age, sex, thyroid status, regional lymph node involvement, or even with histologic type, probably because of the absence of heterogeneity in these variables because most patients are older than 55 years of age and have large B-cell lymphomas (140). The large B-cell lymphomas of the thyroid that disseminate often involve the gastrointestinal tract and this pattern of spread likely is another example of the homing tendency of lymphomas of MALT (8,120,140, 155).

CENTRAL NERVOUS SYSTEM

Malignant lymphomas that originate in the central nervous system (CNS) are relatively uncommon and represent from 2% to 6.6% of all primary brain tumors (156,157). Although there is no trend toward an increasing incidence of non-AIDS related primary CNS lymphomas in Denmark, for unknown reasons the incidence of primary brain lymphomas is increasing among men and women alike in the immunocompetent population of the United States (158,159). Data from the Surveillance, Epidemiology, and End Results (SEER) program of the National Cancer Institute demonstrate a more than 10-fold increase in primary brain lymphoma from 2.5 cases in 1973 to 30 cases per 10 million population in 1991 to 1992 (159); it is projected that by the year 2000, the incidence rate of malignant lymphomas of the brain will continue to increase. The AIDS epidemic is an obvious contributor to this trend, but the increased incidence rates are independent of age and gender and are found in immunocompetent patients who have no overt risk factors for the onset of malignant lymphoma. Immunocompromise, however, is a predisposing factor for the development of primary CNS lymphoma including those who have AIDS, congenital immunodeficiency syndromes, and organ transplantation (160–163). After the gastrointestinal tract, the CNS is the next most frequent extranodal site for the presentation of malignant lymphoma in patients who have AIDS (164) (see Chapter 28). Lymphoma of the CNS develops late in the course of AIDS with a reported incidence of 2% to 6% (162); the incidence has increased as supportive care for patients with AIDS has improved and patients survive longer with CD4 counts below 50/mm^3. EBV is implicated in the pathogenesis of CNS lymphomas in immunocompromised patients, including those who have AIDS (160,163,165,166). Employing *in situ* hybridization techniques, EBV sequences are detected in almost all CNS lymphomas from immunocompromised patients and are discovered far less commonly in immunocompetent patients who have CNS lymphomas (166). Non-Hodgkin's lymphomas of the CNS also have been reported in patients after therapy for Hodgkin's disease, and this also may be related to immunosuppression and, possibly, to EBV (167,168). The AIDS-related lymphomas of the CNS do not express p53 or exhibit rearrangements of the *BCL2* or *MYC* oncogenes (163).

The typical immunocompetent patient with CNS lymphoma is from 42 to 60 years of age. The patients often present with nonfocal and nonspecific symptoms related to elevated intracranial pressure and there frequently are general complaints of headache, lethargy, nausea, confusion, personality changes, and seizures (162). Antemortem diagnosis of lymphoma in the brain has been facilitated greatly by computerized tomographic (CT) scans that demonstrate an isodense or hyperdense intracranial space-occupying lesion and by CT-guided stereotactic needle biopsies coupled with the use of immunohistochemistry to demonstrate cell lineage and clonality (162,169,170); immunocytochemical studies and molecular genetic analysis of cerebrospinal fluid lymphocytes using the PCR technique also may complement conventional cytology and be able to detect occult CNS lymphoma (171). In one study, the incidence of leptomeningeal tumor was 42% at the time of diagnosis of primary CNS lymphoma (172).

Most CNS lymphomas are supratentorial, but they also are infratentorial, including involvement of the cerebellum (161,169,173). They tend to have a periventricular distribution, usually involving corpus callosum, basal ganglia, or thalamus (169). Most primary lymphomas of the CNS are bulky tumors, immediately adjacent to the meningeal or the ventricular surfaces, and with indistinct margins that merge with the surrounding normal or edematous brain (156). Many lymphomas that are associated with AIDS have a multifocal distribution in the brain and the lesions are dark to pale gray with indistinct borders and a granular texture (163,169,173).

On microscopic examination, there often is dense, concentric cuffing of lymphocytes in the perivascular spaces with diffuse centrifugal invasion into the adjacent parenchyma (Fig. 36.26) (156,173). There frequently is associated necrosis and there may be extensive areas of confluent malignant lymphoma with no perivascular relationship (156). Lymphomas also may invade dura and blood vessels, and at the periphery, a glial reaction may ensue. Large B-cell lymphomas and variants, including immunoblastic lymphomas, constitute the most common primary CNS lymphomas and comprise up to 86% of cases (156,157,161,174). The large B-cell lymphomas of the CNS commonly have a polymorphous appearance and exhibit striking variability in nuclear size and shape (157,175). Some cases of primary large cell lymphoma in the CNS are purely intravascular (156,176,177); the patients with intravascular lymphomatosis have neurologic manifestations that reflect a vascular occlusive disease. In addition to large B-cell lymphomas, the Burkitt and Burkitt-like lymphomas also occur in the CNS, but Hodgkin's disease rarely is encountered as a primary malignancy in the CNS (156,157,175,178). T-cell lymphomas also are uncommon (156,157,174,179); rare cases of primary anaplastic large cell lymphoma of the CNS have been reported in children (180).

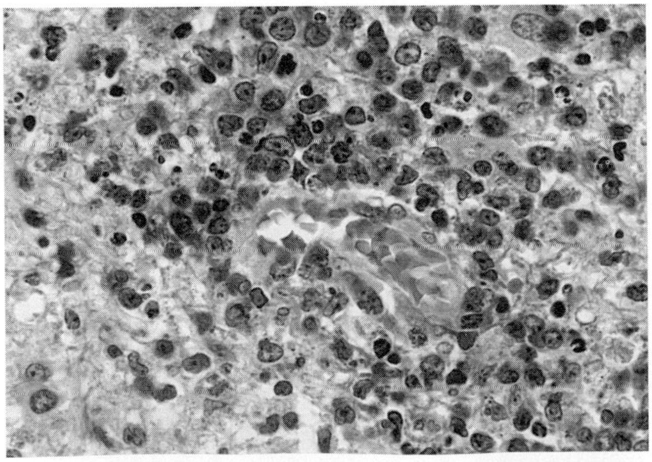

FIG. 36.26. Malignant lymphoma, large B-cell type in the cerebellum concentrates around blood vessels. This is a characteristic feature of many central nervous system lymphomas (hematoxylin and eosin stain, original magnification: 600× magnification).

Almost all primary CNS lymphomas, including cases reported from Japan, are of B-cell lineage (156,157,174,175, 181). Immunoglobulin gene rearrangement studies have confirmed the B-cell nature of primary cerebral lymphomas (182). A minority of primary CNS lymphomas from immunocompetent patients have detectable p53 overexpression and BCL-2 reactivity, but none show *MYC* gene overexpression (181). In one study, BCL-6 protein and hMSH2 (a nuclear located protein selectively expressed by follicle center B cells) were found in almost all primary CNS lymphomas from immunocompetent patients to suggest that primary lymphomas of the CNS may be related to germinal center B cells (183). Moreover, analysis of the immunoglobulin variable region genes in cases of primary CNS lymphoma demonstrate high levels of somatic mutations with intraclonal heterogeneity, which also indicates that primary CNS lymphomas are derived from germinal center B lymphocytes (184). The chromosomal abnormalities of primary lymphomas of the CNS are similar to those of diffuse large B-cell lymphomas at other nodal and extranodal sites and probably are not related to cerebral presentation (185).

Low-grade B-cell lymphomas of the CNS are uncommon; however, MALT lymphomas of the dura have been described (186,187). Morphologically, the cases in the dura are similar to MALT lymphomas in other regions (Fig. 36.27). They mainly are composed of lymphoplasmacytic cells with admixed centrocyte-like or monocytoid cells. Germinal centers are variable, but there are no evident lymphoepithelial lesions (186,187). Cases that were reported as meningeal-restricted small lymphocytic lymphomas and plasmacytomas also are thought to be lymphomas of MALT type, although the current fashion to group these cases with MALT lymphomas may be excessive (109,188,189). Primary MALT-type lymphomas of the dura clinically are limited to females who present with localized intracranial masses. Like other MALT lymphomas, the prognosis seems favorable with no evident recurrence or extracranial spread (186,187).

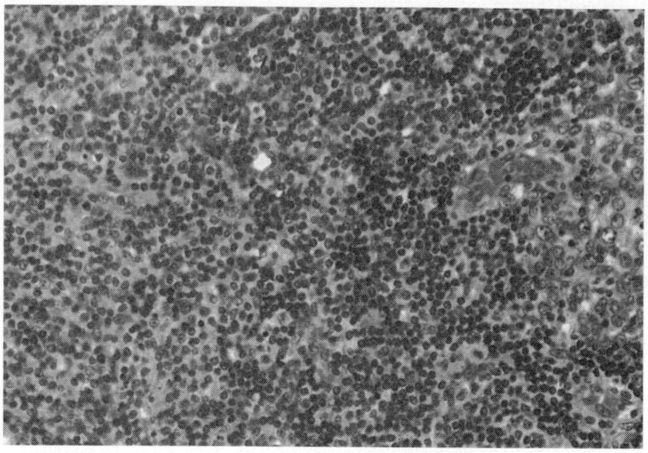

FIG. 36.27. In the dura, a lymphoma of mucosa-associated lymphoid tissue (MALT) forms a dense infiltrate. Notice the germinal center on the right (hematoxylin and eosin stain, original magnification: 300× magnification).

Although primary lymphomas of the CNS are increasing in frequency, secondary lymphomatous involvement in patients who have systemic lymphoma is more common (190). Secondary lymphomas of the CNS tend to infiltrate the leptomeninges, but otherwise their distribution is similar to that of primary CNS lymphomas. Almost all secondary lymphomas are aggressive forms of malignant lymphoma and the risk is greatest for patients who have lymphoblastic lymphoma and for patients with stage IV disease and B symptoms (190,191). In one study of 605 patients with large cell (including immunoblastic) lymphoma, the probability of CNS recurrence at 1 year after diagnosis was 4.5% (192). By multivariate analysis, an elevated serum lactate dehydrogenase and involvement of more than one extranodal site proved to be independent risk factors for CNS recurrence among patients who had large cell lymphoma. The predictability of increased risk of CNS dissemination in patients who have large cell lymphoma and extranodal disease has been verified in a study of primary mediastinal large B-cell lymphomas (193); among 23 patients who had primary mediastinal large B-cell lymphoma, six patients (26%) developed CNS involvement and all had extranodal disease. Spread to the CNS also may occur in patients who have mantle cell lymphoma, especially those patients who have blastic cytology and advanced disease (194). The prognosis of primary and secondary CNS lymphomas is dismal. Despite intracranial radiation therapy, most patients die of the disease in less than 2 years (162). The addition of intrathecal and systemic chemotherapy results in an improvement in mean survival from 16 to 29 months, compared with radiation therapy alone, but the optimal chemotherapy regimen remains undefined (162,169). Telomerase activity may be a novel factor that correlates with the prognosis of patients with primary lymphomas of the CNS (195).

TESTIS

Malignant lymphomas of the testis represent up to 9% of testicular neoplasms, but they are the most common testicular malignancy after the age of 60 years (196). Although many patients who have testicular lymphoma are discovered to have widespread disease at the time of presentation, there are a significant number of patients who have localized stage IE and IIE testicular lymphoma (197–201). Approximately 20% of patients have initial involvement of both testes (196). The most common presenting symptom is painless testicular enlargement of generally short duration (196,201). Some patients present with constitutional symptoms at the time of diagnosis and this is associated with more aggressive disease (197). There are no known predisposing causes for primary lymphomas of the testis, including no known association with an undescended testis.

Testicular lymphomas range from less than 1 to 16 cm in diameter with an average of 4 to 6 cm (197,199,201). The tumors are almost always covered by an attenuated but intact tunica vaginalis. Involvement of the epididymis is common, as is invasion of the tunica albuginea, and in some patients, the lymphomas extend to the spermatic cord (197,201). On cut section, the testicular parenchyma is diffusely replaced by a circumscribed tumor mass that varies from gray to light tan; in some cases, there may be foci of hemorrhage and necrosis (Fig. 36.28).

Usually, no difficulty arises in distinguishing a lymphoma in the testis from reactive lymphoid hyperplasia because testicular low-grade lymphomas are uncommon, and most reactive lymphocytic infiltrates conform to the appearance of granulomatous or nongranulomatous lymphocytic orchitis. Lymphocytic orchitis is an unusual inflammatory lymphocytic infiltrate composed of small lymphocytes with scattered germinal centers that involves the testis (202). Like most reactive lymphoid proliferations and inflammatory pseudotumors, nongranulomatous lymphocytic orchitis is

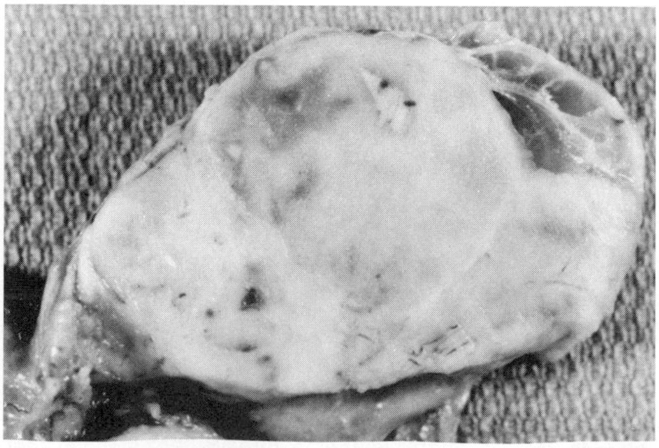

FIG. 36.28. Diffuse large cell lymphoma of the testis forms a large, bulky tumor mass and destroys the testicular stroma. The variegated appearance is the result of tumor necrosis.

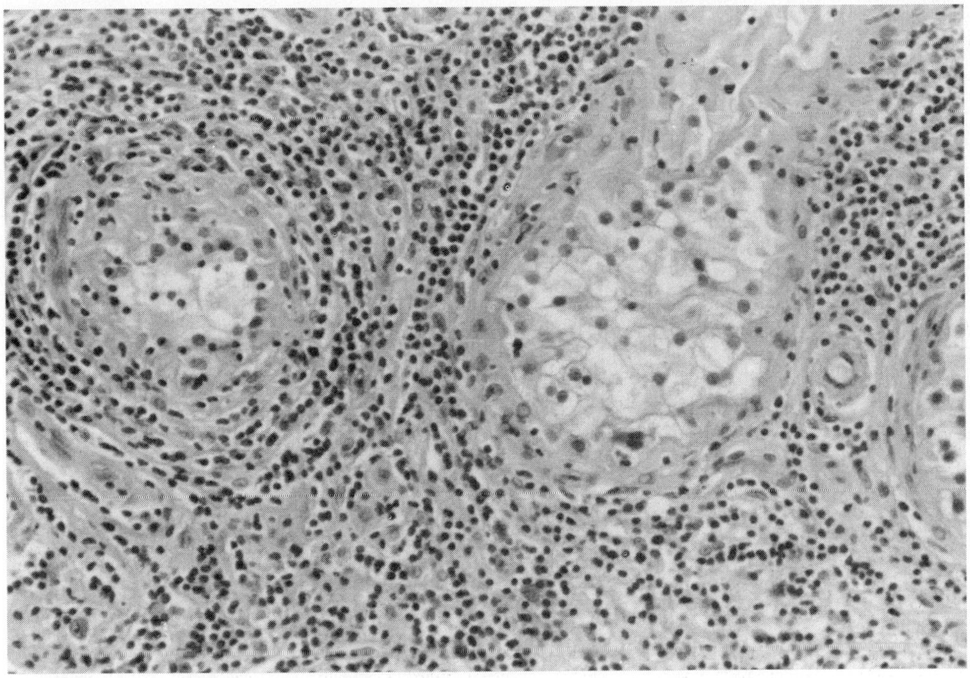

FIG. 36.29. Lymphocytic orchitis of the nongranulomatous type forms a dense infiltrate and surrounds seminiferous tubules (hematoxylin and eosin stain, original magnification: 240× magnification).

associated with a polymorphous cell population, including plasma cells and macrophages, and with fibrosis. The fibrosis tends to be in the interstitium and the infiltrate encases the seminiferous tubules (202) (Fig. 36.29).

Most malignant lymphomas of the testis display large cell (including immunoblastic) histologies and are of B-cell origin (197–201,203). Although an extramedullary myeloid tumor (granulocytic sarcoma) and perhaps plasmacytoma should be considered in the diagnosis, the main differential diagnosis is seminoma (196,201,204,205). In contrast with seminoma, the margins of an aggressive lymphoma are infiltrative and without a pushing border. The large B-cell lymphomas and immunoblastic variants exhibit a diffuse intertubular growth pattern and tend to surround and invade seminiferous tubules with frequent disruption of the basement membranes (199–201) (Fig. 36.30). Sclerosis and tubular atrophy are common and vascular invasion by lymphoma can be highlighted with the use of an elastic stain or an appropriate marker for endothelial cells, such as factor VIII–related antigen (197). Often, the periphery of the lymphoma contains a benign-appearing lymphocytic infiltrate composed of small lymphocytes and plasma cells.

Testicular large B-cell lymphomas express the usual complement of B-cell antigens, such as CD20 (201,203). They are not associated with EBV or the Kaposi's sarcoma–associated herpesvirus (KSHV/HHV-8) and do not exhibit t(14; 18) or t(11;14) translocations (203). However, most testicular large B-cell lymphomas demonstrate molecular evidence of ongoing mutations, as indicated by intraclonal variation in immunoglobulin heavy-chain gene sequences (203); this observation has suggested that the large B-cell lymphomas of the testis are related to other antigen exposure, or post–germinal center cell lymphocytes, such as found in extranodal marginal zone lymphoma of MALT type.

In addition to the more prevalent large B-cell lymphomas, a variety of other non-Hodgkin's lymphomas also manifest in the testis. One report described four children who had primary follicular large cell lymphoma of the testis (206). All were B-cell malignancies, and despite the follicular architecture, none of the malignant lymphomas expressed BCL-2 protein or had demonstrable *BCL2* gene rearrangements; the cases also did not express p53. In contrast, the childhood testicular lymphoma cases showed BCL-6 protein reactivity and a *BCL6* gene rearrangement, implying that there is a different molecular pathogenesis for pediatric follicular lymphoma in the testis (206). Occasionally, T-cell lymphomas primarily occur in the testis, comprising anaplastic large cell lymphoma and aggressive NK/T-cell ($CD56^+$) types (51,207,208). The NK/T-cell lymphomas of the testis are histologically and immunophenotypically similar to those in the sinonasal region, including the tendency for angiocentric growth and necrosis (208). They also have an aggressive clinical course.

Sclerosis is thought to have a favorable impact on prognosis, but among patients who have testicular lymphoma clinical stage is the best recognized prognostic factor (196,198,199,201). Nonetheless, patients who have stage IE lymphoma of the testis frequently exhibit progressive disease, often within 12 months of diagnosis, and this probably is a reflection of clinically occult lymphoma (197,209). Tes-

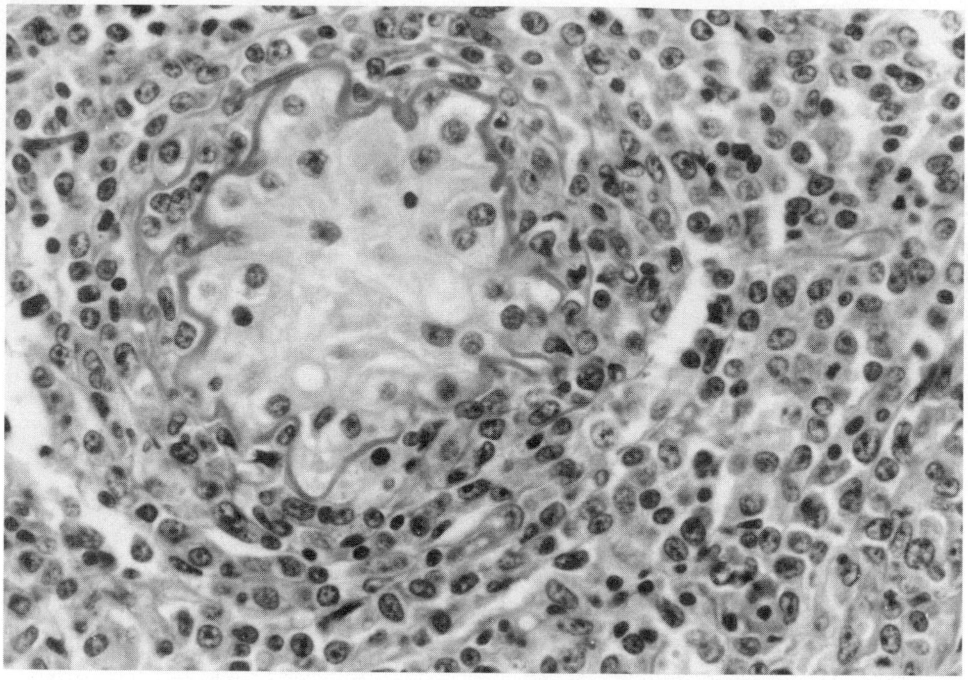

FIG. 36.30. Large B-cell lymphoma of the testis encircles and invades seminiferous tubules, leading to disruption of the basement membranes (hematoxylin and eosin stain, original magnification: 480× magnification).

ticular lymphomas spread to retroperitoneal lymph nodes, CNS, Waldeyer's ring, skin, lung, and the contralateral testis (196,209,210). In some centers, early chemotherapy, in addition to orchiectomy with or without regional radiation therapy, has altered the natural history of testicular lymphomas by preventing many relapses and has improved the survival to as high as 93% and 79% at 4 and 5 years, respectively (211,212). Despite chemotherapy, however, other major centers continue to report a poor prognosis with actuarial disease-free survivals of 40% for patients who have stage I testicular lymphoma (209,210).

FEMALE GENITAL TRACT

Malignant lymphomas that manifest in the ovary are exceedingly unusual. In a study from the Armed Forces Institute of Pathology, only 19 of 9500 women (0.2%) who had lymphoma initially manifested the disease in the ovary (213). An exception to the rarity of lymphomas in the ovary is found in African countries in which Burkitt's lymphoma is endemic; in these areas, the ovaries are second only to the jaw in frequency of presentation (214). Involvement of the ovary by lymphoma can be a result of primary ovarian lymphoma, the initial manifestation of clinically occult disease in lymph nodes, or as a late complication of widespread lymphoma (197).

An ovary involved by lymphoma may be massive and measure more than 20 cm in diameter and frequently there is bilateral ovarian lymphoma (197,215). The capsule usually is intact, but, on the cut surface, the ovarian stroma is replaced by a lobulated, often bosselated gray-tan fleshy mass with frequent areas of necrosis and cystic degeneration (197,213,216) (Fig. 36.31). Although low-grade lymphomas, such as follicular lymphomas, can manifest in the ovary, most are diffuse aggressive lymphomas, including large B-cell and Burkitt-type lymphomas (197,215,216) (Fig. 36.32); the latter tend to predominate in patients younger than 20 years of age. A starry-sky pattern is ob-

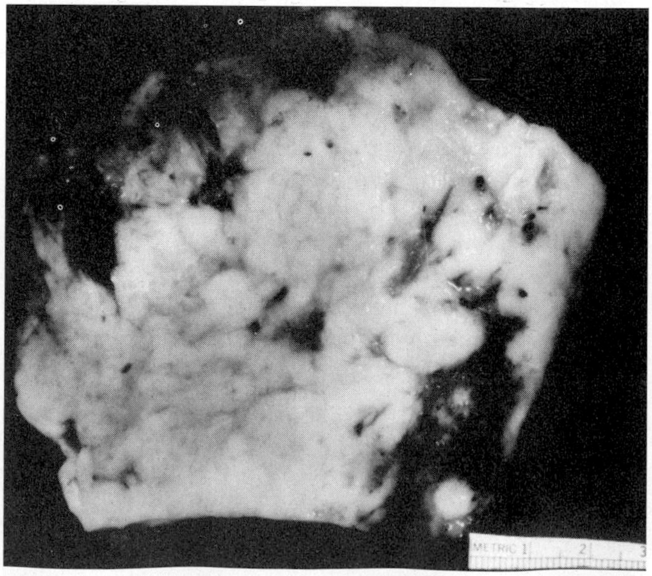

FIG. 36.31. Malignant lymphoma in the ovary forms a large fleshy mass with areas of hemorrhage and degeneration.

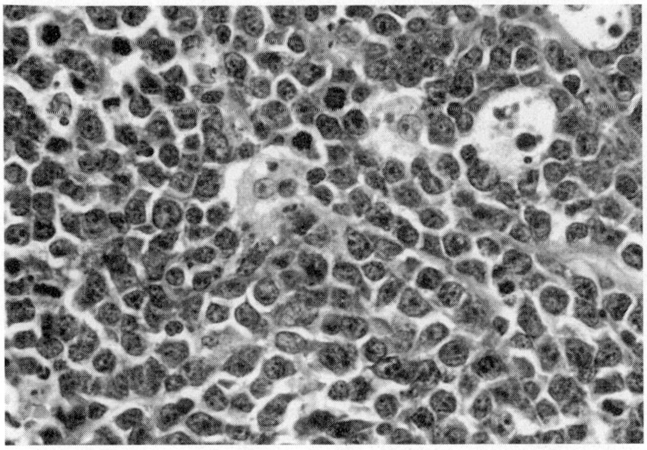

FIG. 36.32. Burkitt-type lymphoma is the most common malignant lymphoma to involve the ovary in young women (hematoxylin and eosin stain, original magnification: 600× magnification).

served frequently in cases of diffuse large cell lymphoma and in the Burkitt type (197,215). The corpora lutea and albicantes often are spared and the lymphomas surround rather than replace these structures (197,213). Lymphomas in the ovary have a curious tendency to grow in cords with almost a linear pattern of infiltration (213,215,217) (Fig. 36.33). This linear pattern raises the differential diagnosis of an extramedullary myeloid tumor (granulocytic sarcoma), which also may manifest initially in the ovary (213,216,218); the recognition of eosinophilic myelocytes is helpful in the diagnosis, but most cases do not exhibit myeloid differentiation histologically and are characterized by primitive, blastlike nuclear features. The use of the naphthol-ASD-chloracetate esterase stain (NASDCA) and immunoperoxidase stains for B- and T-cell antigens, as well as reactivity for myeloperoxidase, lysozyme, CD68, or CD43 are valuable in

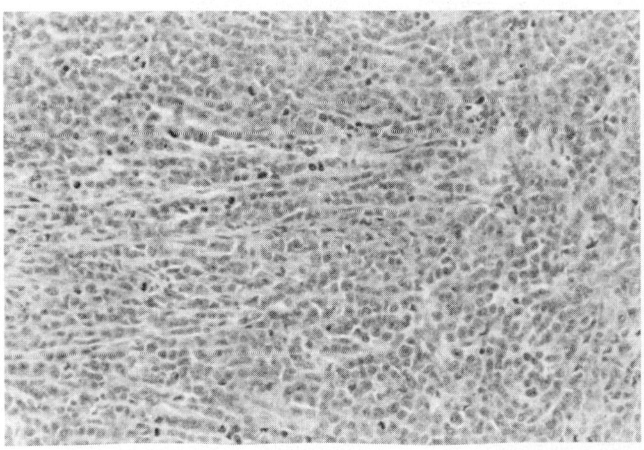

FIG. 36.33. Ovarian lymphomas occasionally have a cordlike pattern of infiltration and resemble an epithelial malignancy or an extramedullary myeloid tumor (hematoxylin and eosin stain, original magnification: 240× magnification).

separating malignant lymphoma from extramedullary myeloid tumors (218). Immunologic studies on lymphomas of the ovary have demonstrated that almost all the lymphomas have a B-cell immunophenotype (215,219). In addition to an extramedullary myeloid tumor, the major differential diagnosis of ovarian lymphomas includes dysgerminoma, undifferentiated carcinoma, metastatic carcinoma, especially those from the breast, primary small cell carcinoma, and adult granulosa cell tumor (217). Careful examination of the morphologic characteristics of the neoplasm and employment of immunohistochemical studies, such as antibodies against B- and T-cell antigens, as well as cytokeratin, should resolve this differential diagnosis.

Up to 90% of patients who have lymphomas that manifest in the ovary have disseminated disease at the time of diagnosis (215,216). In addition to the opposite ovary, other extranodal sites that are involved include the fallopian tubes and omentum. The median survival is less than 3 years (197,216). Favorable prognostic factors are unilateral ovarian involvement, stage IE disease, and the rare instance of a follicular architecture (215,216).

Malignant lymphomas that arise in other sites of the female genital tract, including vagina, cervix, and uterine corpus, are even less common than those in the ovary, although these sites frequently are involved in cases of disseminated lymphoma (220). Patients regularly present with vaginal bleeding and the cervix is engaged more often than the other genital sites. In the cervix, the tumors may appear sessile or polypoid or may manifest as diffuse circumferential enlargement to assume a barrel shape, without evident mucosal abnormalities (220–222). Large B-cell lymphomas predominate, but, unlike primary lymphomas of the ovary, lymphomas in the cervix, uterine corpus, and vagina may be low-grade types, specifically follicular lymphomas and probable lymphomas of MALT type (220–225). For example, unusual low-grade lymphomas were discovered as incidental microscopic findings in the endometrium of three patients (225); none formed grossly evident tumors and the lymphomas in all cases were confined to the endometrium. Although germinal centers and marginal zone patterns were not observed, the lymphomas were composed of centrocyte-like B cells and displayed CD43 coexpression to suggest that they were low-grade MALT lymphomas. Moreover, these low-grade lymphomas presumably arose from endometrial lymphatic tissue or MALT (225).

The low-grade lymphomas of the cervix, uterine corpus, and vagina must be separated from chronic inflammatory reactions in the lower female genital tract, including chronic endometritis, severe chronic cervicitis, and follicular cervicitis (217). Occasionally, the reactive lesions are characterized by a marked proliferation of immunoblasts and there is accompanying erosion and ulceration of cervical squamous mucosa (226); some cervical and vulvar lesions are associated with infectious mononucleosis (Fig. 36.34). Unlike malignant lymphomas, florid reactive lymphoid hyperplasias in the lower female genital tract are superficial and do not form

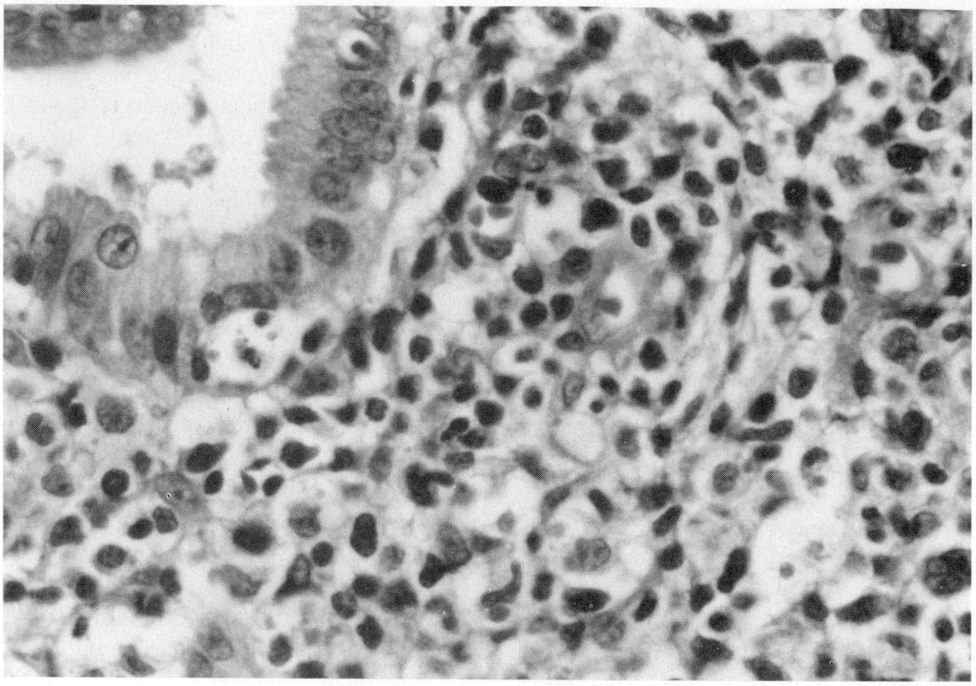

FIG. 36.34. Biopsy of a weeping lesion of the uterine cervix in a 19-year-old patient with known infectious mononucleosis. The reactive immunoblasts are difficult to distinguish from malignant lymphoma (hematoxylin and eosin stain, original magnification: 480× magnification).

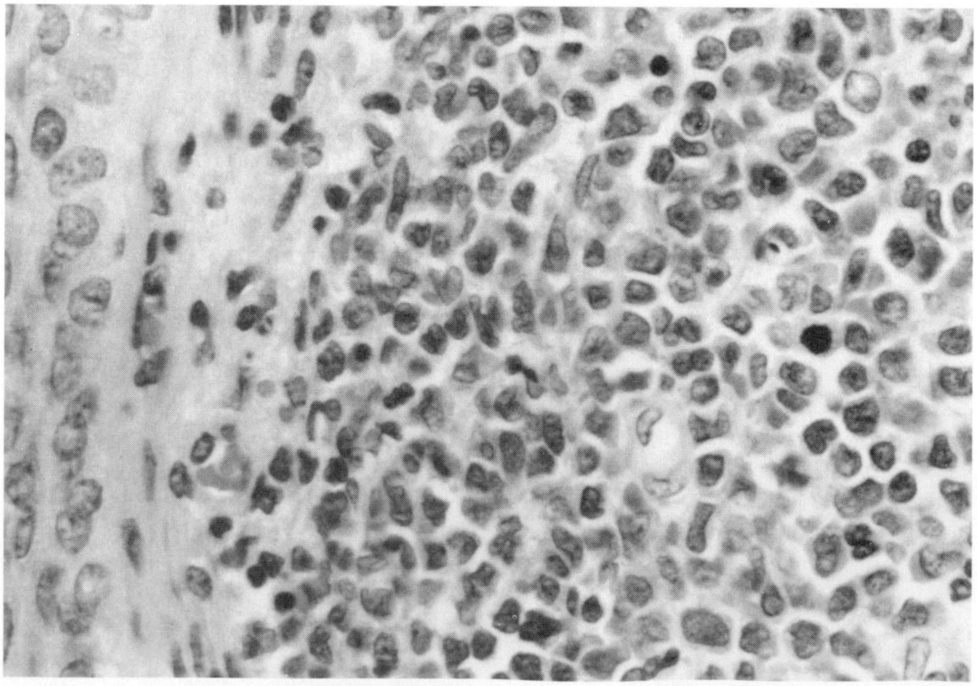

FIG. 36.35. This mononuclear cell infiltrate adjacent to uterine cervical squamous mucosa resembles malignant lymphoma; however, immunohistochemical stains demonstrated that the mononuclear cells were myeloid in origin and diagnostic of an extramedullary myeloid tumor (granulocytic sarcoma) (hematoxylin and eosin stain, original magnification: 720× magnification).

tumor masses. The infiltrates are polymorphous and similar to other extranodal reactive lymphoid proliferations. Extramedullary myeloid tumors also may manifest in the lower female genital tract (218) (Fig. 36.35). These are distinguished from malignant lymphoma by employing the same morphologic criteria, histochemical stains, and immunologic techniques used to separate an extramedullary myeloid tumor from lymphoma in the ovary.

Many patients who have lymphomas of the cervix have stage IE disease; in one review, there was only one treatment failure among 28 patients whose treatment included radiation therapy and whose cases were followed for at least 2 years (222). This experience suggests that most patients who have stage IE lymphomas of the cervix are amenable to cure.

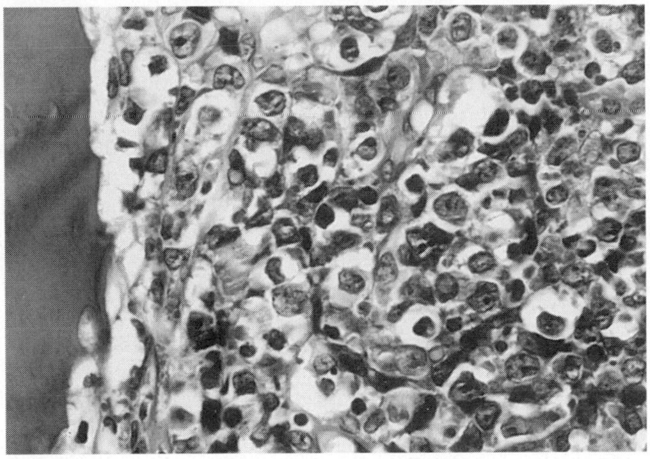

FIG. 36.36. Large B-cell lymphoma is the most common type of primary lymphoma of bone. Although it is not obvious in this case, osseous large cell lymphomas often have irregular nuclear contours, including cleaved or multilobated shapes (hematoxylin and eosin stain, original magnification: 600× magnification).

BONE

Malignant lymphomas that arise in bone are uncommon neoplasms, and any one institution requires long periods to accumulate sufficient cases for morphologic and clinical analysis. In the largest published series, 422 cases were collected over a 76-year span (227). On review, the largest group (42%) had apparent primary lymphoma of bone, but other patients had multifocal osseous lymphoma, and others had evidence of extraosseous lymphoma. There is a peak incidence in the fifth decade, but the age range is wide and bone lymphomas can occur in pediatric patients as well (227–229). Various sites are involved, with the most prevalent being the femur and other tubular long bones, maxilla and mandible, pelvic bones, and spine (227–230). The most common symptoms are local pain with occasional associated soft tissue swelling, a mass, or both (227). Radiologic studies show variable changes, including lytic lesions or blastic lesions (228,230). Magnetic resonance imaging (MRI) registers significant variability in imaging characteristics and often displays minimal cortical changes despite an accompanying soft tissue mass (228,231). An explanation for this phenomenon is offered by one study in which MRI of primary intramedullary lymphomas of bone demonstrated penetrating channels that extended through the cortex in proximity to osteoclastic bone resorption (232). By immunoperoxidase, the osseous lymphomas had reactivity for cytokine mediators that stimulate osteoclastic activation. Such observations suggest that tumor activation of osteoclastic resorption and production of lymphomatous tumor channels through the cortex may account for the escape of intramedullary lymphoma and the formation of soft tissue masses without cortical destruction (232).

Most bone lymphomas are classified as large cell lymphoma (227,229,230,233–237) (Fig. 36.36). A curious feature of large cell lymphomas of bone, which has not been widely described in large cell lymphomas that occur in other extranodal sites, is the presence of complex nuclear contours; the large cells frequently are portrayed as cleaved or multilobated (230,233,234,237). Most large cell lymphomas of bone are associated with fibrosis that ranges from delicate reticulin fibrosis to dense sclerosis with osteoid formation (227). The lymphoma cells often are entrapped within the fibrous connective tissue and may appear spindled or may form small clusters that resemble carcinoma. An accurate diagnosis often is hampered not only because of the fibrosis, but also because of decalcification and crush artifact (238); therefore, to establish the diagnosis more than one biopsy procedure may be required (228).

Immunologic studies indicate that most large cell lymphomas of bone are of B-cell lineage (234,235,237,239). In addition to large B-cell lymphomas, anaplastic large cell lymphomas may manifest in bone, as can cases of Hodgkin's disease (see Chapter 17), and precursor B-cell lymphoblastic lymphomas (237,240–243). The cases of osseous precursor B-cell lymphoblastic lymphoma often manifest as a lytic lesion and must be differentiated from other small round cell tumors of bone including Ewing's sarcoma. A comprehensive immunohistologic panel is required to certify the diagnosis including antibodies directed against CD10, CD20, CD43, CD79a, CD99, and terminal deoxynucleotidyl transferase (242,243) (see Chapter 26). Peripheral T-cell lymphomas occasionally arise in bone and have been reported in the mandible (235,237); in Japan, 10% of primary lymphomas of bone have a T-cell phenotype (244). Cases classified as small lymphocytic lymphoma with plasmacytoid features (lymphoplasmacytic lymphoma) also are more common in Japan than in the West (244).

The observation of cleaved-cell and multilobated-cell lymphomas of bone correlates with absence of CD30 expression and long-term survival in comparison to patients who have osseous large noncleaved cell and anaplastic $CD30^+$ lymphomas (230,233,237). General agreement prevails that clinical stage is the single most important prognostic variable in predicting overall survival in patients with malignant lymphoma of bone (227,230). In the M.D. Anderson Cancer Center series of 37 primary lymphomas of bone, 73% of patients who had localized lymphoma were long-term survivors in contrast to 9% of those who had disseminated disease (230). Although the current trend is to treat patients with combined modality therapy, it remains unclear whether chemotherapy, radiation therapy, or a combination of both is the best treatment for stage IE lymphoma of bone (228,236,245).

BREAST

Although well recognized, primary malignant lymphomas of breast are infrequent and comprise less than 0.5% of primary malignant mammary tumors and fewer than 2.5% of all primary extranodal lymphomas (2,238,246–251). One major issue concerns the definition of primary malignant lymphomas of the breast. Some investigators include all cases in which the breast is the first site of presentation, even if subsequent staging procedures reveal stage IIIE or IVE disease (246–249). Other investigators exclude cases in which staging procedures demonstrate more advanced disease despite an initial presentation in the breast (251–254); these cases are designated as secondary lymphomas of breast (250,255).

Patients who have lymphomas in the breast range from teenagers to those in their ninth decade; the median age is between 40 and 67 years (247,249,251,252,255). Most patients present with a breast mass and are diagnosed clinically as possible carcinoma of breast. Inexplicably, the right breast often is reported to be more commonly involved than the left (246,247,249,256). Some patients have bilateral tumor masses and some are pregnant (246,247,256).

Lymphomas of the breast usually are well circumscribed on gross examination and are composed of white or gray-white firm tissue (250,251,253). Microscopically, most lymphomas of the breast are large cell lymphomas (Fig. 36.37) and, to a lesser extent, Burkitt or Burkitt-like lymphomas (246–257). Cases of lymphoblastic lymphoma also have been described as originating in the breast, and there are reports of follicular lymphomas in the breast (247, 249–252,254,256). Except for the lymphoblastic lymphomas, virtually all lymphomas in the breast have a B-cell immunophenotype (249–257). Low-grade malignant lymphomas are far less common, and some series do not contain any cases of low-grade malignant lymphomas, including those of MALT type (254,255). Nonetheless, cases of primary lymphoma of breast classified as lymphomas of MALT type or monocytoid B-cell lymphoma are described (223,249,256,258). The incidence of MALT lymphomas among the breast lymphoma cases ranges between 8.5% and 35% (259). Mammary MALT lymphomas contain randomly scattered germinal centers and are composed mainly of monocytoid-appearing cells with admixed plasma cells (258); Dutcher bodies are present and follicular colonization can occur. Lymphoepithelial lesions are observed in ductal epithelium, but these may not be conspicuous because the tumor often is extensive leading to architectural obliteration of the normal breast lobules (Fig. 36.38) (223,258); some intraepithelial lymphocytes are reactive T cells (258).

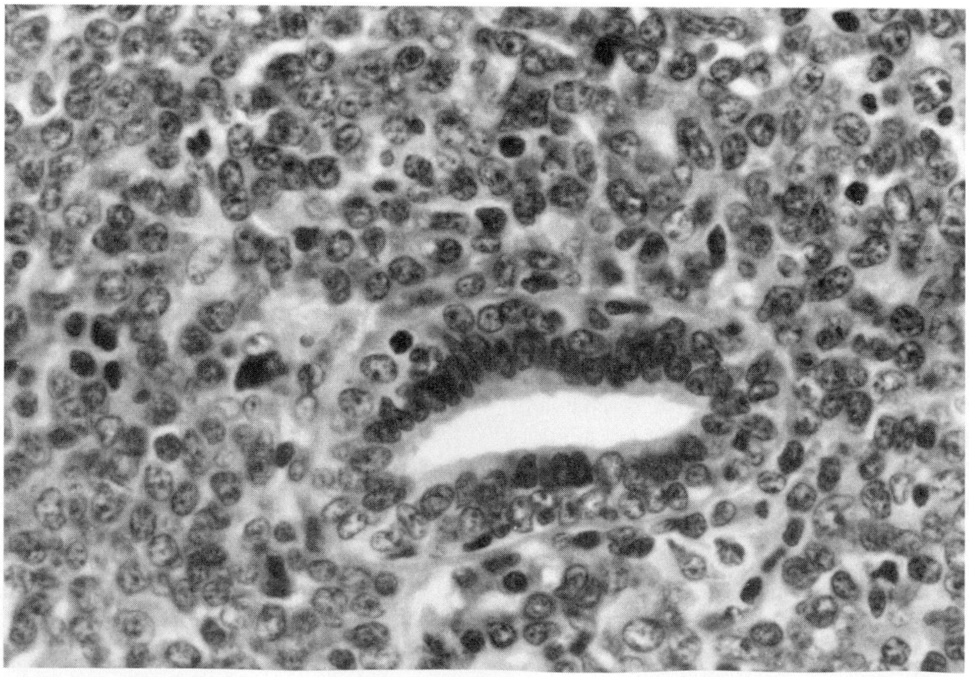

FIG. 36.37. In the breast, most lymphomas are aggressive types, such as this diffuse large B-cell lymphoma. Lymphomas of the breast frequently surround and encase residual ducts (hematoxylin and eosin stain, original magnification: 720× magnification).

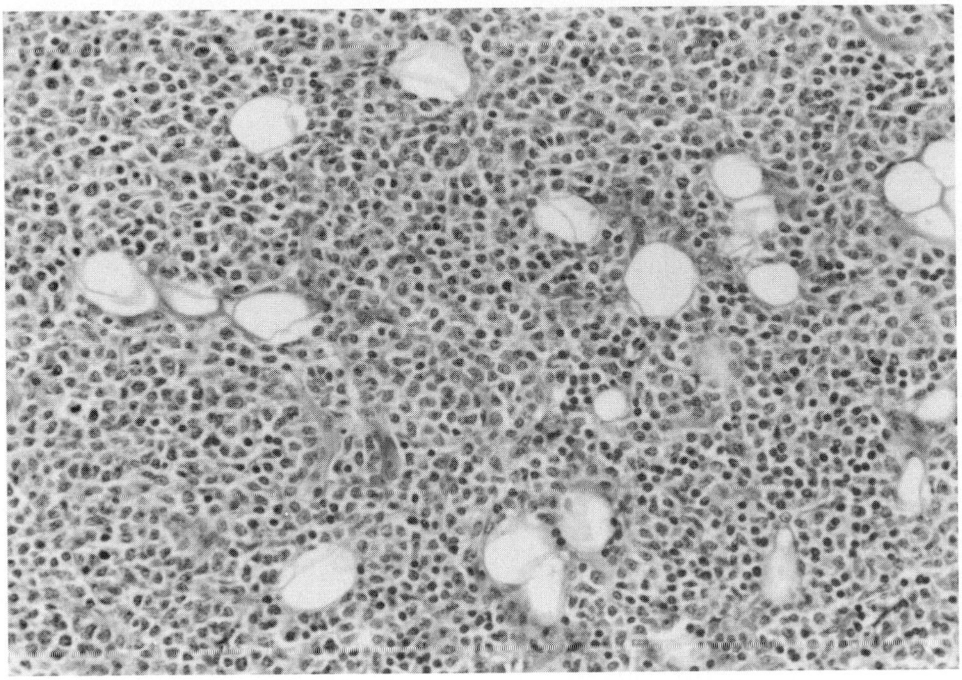

FIG. 36.38. Low-grade lymphomas dominated by monocytoid B cells may occur in the breast. The monocytoid cells are recognizable on low-power magnification by the wide separation of the nuclei caused by the relatively abundant, pale-staining cytoplasm (hematoxylin and eosin stain, original magnification: 240× magnification).

Like lymphomas of MALT, some large B-cell breast lymphomas invade and disrupt breast ducts to create lymphoepithelial lesions (248–251,255–257). Frequently, lymphomas of the breast infiltrate the lobules or surround and separate individual ducts and lobules that may not be infiltrated but are compressed; this pattern of infiltration may impart a targetoid arrangement (247,255). The presence of a targetoid configuration and a frequent single file pattern of infiltration with accompanying sclerosis or lymphomatous signet ring cells mimics infiltrating lobular carcinoma. Unlike lobular carcinoma, lymphomas of breast do not exhibit carcinoma *in situ*, cellular cohesion, or syncytial aggregation but may display lymphoepithelial lesions and associated karyorrhexis (255). Malignant lymphomas in the breast also may be confused with an extramedullary myeloid tumor (i.e., granulocytic sarcoma) because these cases may manifest as a solitary mass in the breast (255). The use of histochemical stains for NASDCA; a battery of immunoperoxidase stains for myeloperoxidase, lysozyme, CD43, CD68, and B- and T-cell antigens; and the detection of eosinophilic myelocytes should distinguish an extramedullary myeloid tumor from malignant lymphoma (218,255).

There usually is no problem in distinguishing lymphoid hyperplasia in the breast from malignant lymphoma. Lymphoid hyperplasia in the breast is uncommon and is differentiated from lymphoma by the innocuous cytologic features (Fig. 36.39), the polymorphous cell population, and the finding of germinal centers (260). If the histologic features are ambiguous, demonstration of polyclonality by immunoperoxidase techniques, flow cytometry, or molecular analysis may be required (259). Some cases of mammary lymphoma , including those of MALT type, may be preceded by a form of lymphoid hyperplasia referred to as *lymphocytic mastopathy* or *sclerosing lymphocytic lobulitis* (261,262). Lymphocytic mastopathy and sclerosing lymphocytic lobulitis are morphologically similar to a process known as *diabetic mastopathy* that has been described in patients with diabetes mellitus (259,263). In these conditions, the breast develops dense intralobular, perilobular, and perivascular lymphocytic infiltrates associated with germinal center formation, lymphoepithelial-type lesions, lobular atrophy, and stromal keloid-like fibrosis (261–263). Diabetic or lymphocytic mastopathy with sclerosing lobulitis may represent an autoimmune disease because of morphologic and immunologic similarities to MESA/BLEL of salivary glands or Hashimoto's thyroiditis.

Analysis of breast lymphomas in the literature suggests that there are two clinicopathologic types of primary lymphoma of the breast (238,249,253,256,259). One type affects younger patients (<40 years), who frequently are pregnant and often have bilateral diffuse disease. These patients have a higher proportion of Burkitt lymphomas and a rapidly fatal clinical course (median survival, 9.5 months). The second and more common group, which represents up to 80% of cases, involves a broad age range of patients but is mainly limited to older women who have unilateral breast lymphoma. These patients have a variable clinical course (median survival, 47 months) that may be affected by the histo-

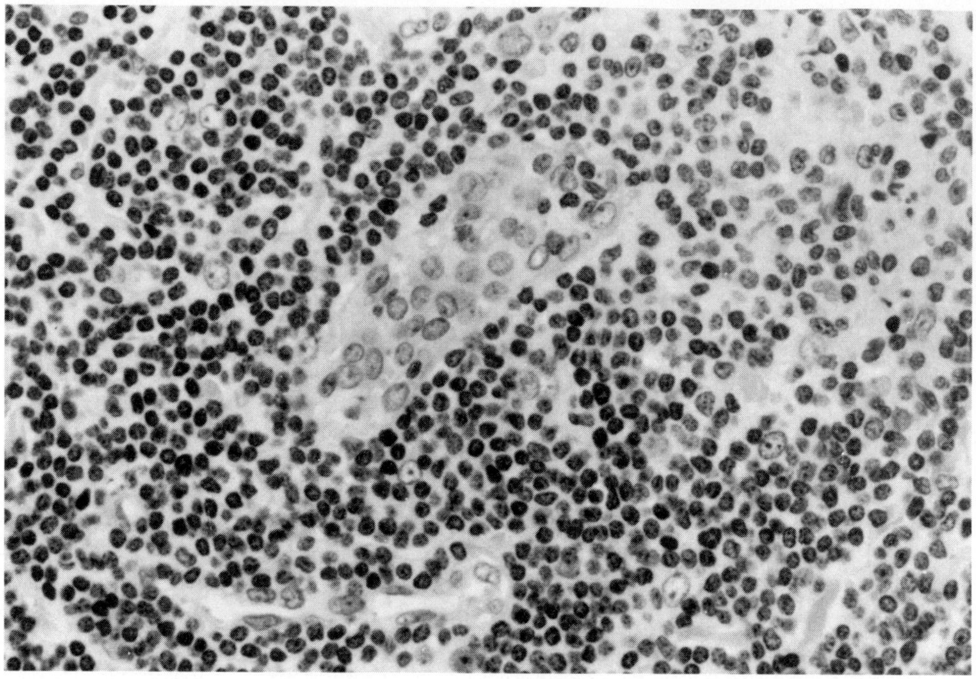

FIG. 36.39. Lymphoid hyperplasia of the breast is a relatively infrequent pathologic finding but is distinguished from malignant lymphoma by the bland cytologic features of the lymphocytes and the variation in cellular density. Despite the benign infiltrate, there is focal invasion of ductal epithelium (hematoxylin and eosin stain, original magnification: 480× magnification).

logic grade of lymphoma and the clinical stage (249). Treatment of breast lymphomas has been highly variable, but generally treatment parallels that given for systemic lymphomas of similar morphologic type. For example, patients who have large B-cell lymphomas of the breast receive chemotherapy or radiation therapy (257). In one retrospective study, the 5-year overall survival and relapse-free survival for 17 patients with primary diffuse large cell lymphoma of the breast was 65% and 70%, respectively (264). Stage and the International Prognostic Index were statistically significant factors in overall survival and it appears that patients who have localized primary large cell lymphomas of the breast have a similar prognosis to patients who have large cell lymphomas in other sites. Patients who have low-grade MALT lymphomas of the breast are treated by surgical excision, radiation therapy, or both (259). Although there are too few reported cases of mammary MALT lymphomas to render meaningful statements concerning prognosis, it is implied that MALT lymphomas of the breast may be relatively innocent tumors with a potential for prolonged disease-free survival (109,223,258)

MISCELLANEOUS SITES

Primary malignant lymphomas may involve virtually any anatomic site, but, with the exception of the extranodal lymphomas discussed in this and previous chapters, primary extranodal lymphomas that involve other organs are relatively uncommon (2,3). Lymphomas that apparently arise in the adrenals, ampulla of Vater, urethra, peripheral nerve, and spinal cord are considered pathologically novel and generally are the subject of single case reports or review of cases gleaned from the literature (265–269); in many instances the lymphoma in these extranodal sites are encountered in patients who develop rapid progression of disease within 3 to 6 months after diagnosis. The incidence of primary lymphomas that affects these exotic and miscellaneous sites is increasing, however, probably because of the AIDS epidemic (164) (see Chapter 28). For example, malignant lymphomas of the heart rarely are diagnosed antemortem and almost always are restricted to case reports (270). Nonetheless, one study described nine cardiac lymphoma cases found in a single institution over an 8-year period (271); four of the patients fulfilled the criteria for AIDS. Primary effusion (body cavity–based) lymphoma is another unusual AIDS-related and morphologically pleomorphic large B-cell lymphoma that is found in the pleural, pericardial, or peritoneal cavities of patients who do not have an affiliated tumor mass and are without lymphadenopathy or organomegaly (272) (see Chapter 28). Kaposi's sarcoma–associated herpes virus and EBV have been identified in cases of primary effusion lymphoma and these lymphomas share some features with another group of EBV-associated extranodal lymphomas of the pleural cavity known as pyothorax-associated lymphoma (273,274). Pyothorax-associated lymphomas arise in the pleural cavity after a prolonged (20 years and longer) history of pyothorax resulting from therapeutic artificial pneumothorax for pleural or pulmonary tuberculosis. Unlike primary

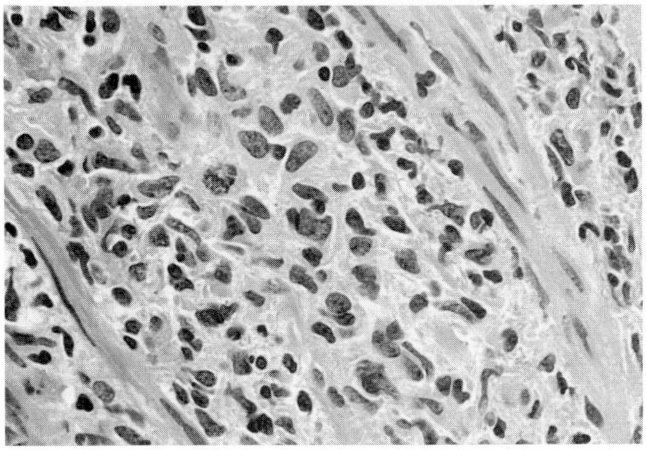

FIG. 36.40. In the urinary bladder, a large B-cell lymphoma infiltrates between smooth muscle bundles. Patients who present with large cell lymphoma in the urinary bladder usually have disseminated disease (hematoxylin and eosin stain, original magnification: 600× magnification).

effusion lymphomas, pyothorax-associated lymphomas are accompanied by contiguous tumor masses and are not related to AIDS or KSHV/HHV-8 (275).

In addition to AIDS-related lymphomas of uncommon sites, several series have been published of non–AIDS-related lymphomas that arise clinically in other uncommon extranodal sites including the liver, kidney, urinary bladder (Fig. 36.40), prostate, spinal epidural space, larynx, and soft tissues (276–289) (Fig. 36.41). A subset of primary hepatic large B-cell lymphomas was associated with the hepatitis C virus, and two patients had malignant lymphoma in soft tissues that arose in the context of chronic postmastectomy lymphedema (279,290). The stage IE primary lymphomas of the urinary bladder are low-grade lymphomas of MALT type, whereas those lymphomas that manifest in the urinary bladder and that subsequently are discovered in patients who have stage IIE or disseminated disease usually are large B-cell lymphomas (282,283). Occasionally, lymphomas of the urinary bladder may contain signet ring cells to simulate carcinoma, and conversely, carcinomas of the urinary bladder may have an associated lymphocytic infiltrate to simulate malignant lymphoma (291,292). The mediastinum is another site of extranodal lymphoma, although many cases likely originate in lymph nodes that are obliterated by the lymphoma, whereas others begin in the thymus (293,294); some cases in the thymus have features of low-grade B-cell lymphomas of MALT (295). MALT lymphomas also have been described in other unusual sites, such as kidney, prostate, gallbladder, uterine cervix, trachea, ampulla of Vater, and liver (223,266,296,297).

Immunophenotypic analysis of the lymphomas that involve these miscellaneous sites have demonstrated that they are predominantly of B-cell lineage (265,267,268,271–273, 279-287,289,290). This includes the extranodal large cell lymphomas confined to the lumens of small blood vessels, diagnostic of intravascular lymphoma (Fig. 36.42); intravascular large cell lymphomas have been reported in the CNS, skin, adrenal, lung, pituitary, gallbladder, prostate, and kidney (177,298).

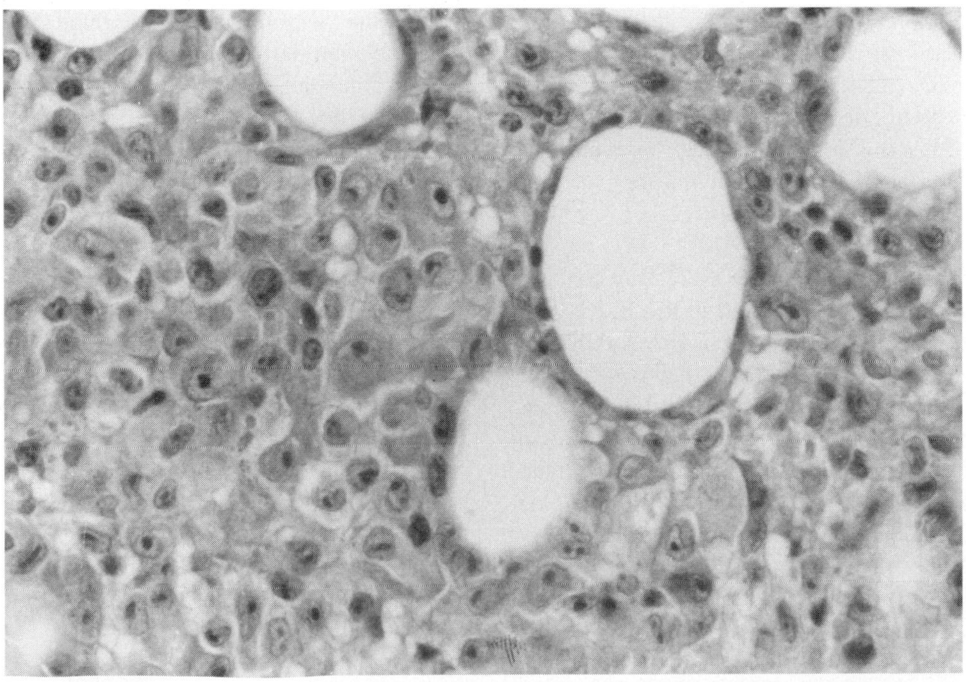

FIG. 36.41. Large cell lymphoma composed of plasmacytoid immunoblasts, discovered after biopsy of a soft tissue mass. Patients who have stage IE lymphoma of soft tissues frequently respond to therapy and have a favorable prognosis (hematoxylin and eosin stain, original magnification: 480× magnification).

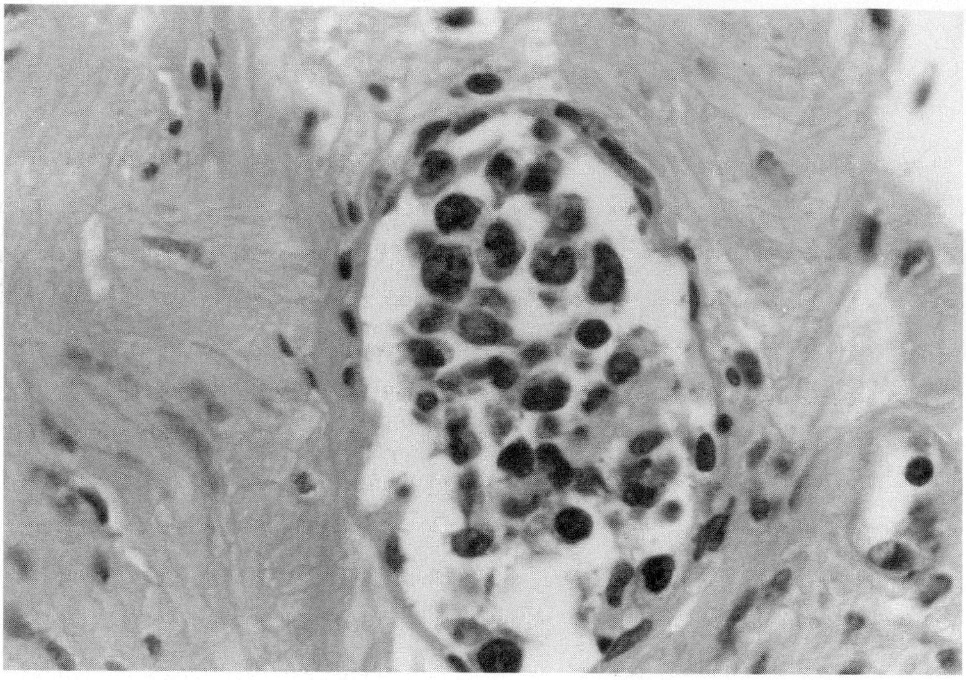

FIG. 36.42. Intravascular large cell lymphoma in the prostate is characterized by the intraluminal proliferation of neoplastic lymphoid cells within blood vessels. The large cells were shown to be of B-cell origin and did not express factor VIII–related antigen (hematoxylin and eosin stain, original magnification: 720× magnification).

Despite a standard history of rapid dissemination of disease among many patients who have lymphoma of unusual sites, probably because of occult lymphoma, patients who have lymphoma that manifests in the liver, kidney, urinary bladder, spinal epidural space, larynx, or soft tissues often have stage IE disease, respond to therapy, and have a favorable prognosis (276,277,280,281,283,285,287,288). The favorable prognosis occurs despite the classification of most extranodal lymphomas that originate in these extraordinary sites as large cell lymphomas.

SUMMARY AND CONCLUSIONS

The extranodal lymphomas discussed in this chapter are relatively uncommon malignant tumors compared with other neoplasms or even other lymphomas, but they provide provocative insights into the pathogenesis of extranodal lymphomas and perhaps lymphomas in general. For example, many malignant lymphomas that arise in the salivary gland, and almost all of those in the thyroid gland, are closely linked to autoimmune disorders, namely Sjögren's syndrome or MESA/BLEL and Hashimoto's or chronic lymphocytic thyroiditis (91,125,126). In these conditions, the lymphomas are of B-cell origin and are thought to evolve secondary to chronic antigenic stimulation of B lymphocytes, because of unrestricted T helper activity leading to immunoglobulin gene hypermutation or because of a disorder of immune surveillance with subsequent onset of cytogenetic aberrations (92,93,124,127). Curiously, the malignant lymphomas that develop from these altered immune states are morphologically and clinically distinctive. In patients who have Sjögren's syndrome or MESA/BLEL, the lymphomas commonly appear clinically in extrasalivary gland lymph nodes rather than within the salivary gland. When lymphomas do occur within the salivary gland, they usually are clinically and pathologically occult lymphomas of low-grade MALT type and they often require verification by immunologic and molecular genetic techniques (96,98,105,107,108). In contrast, lymphomas of the thyroid gland associated with Hashimoto's or chronic lymphocytic thyroiditis generally are clinically obvious malignancies and usually are morphologically aggressive lymphomas of large B-cell type that occur within the thyroid gland. No evident explanation is available for these clinical and histologic discrepancies between those lymphomas of the salivary and the thyroid glands that are associated with a predisposing autoimmune disorder.

EBV also plays a role in the pathogenesis of some extranodal lymphomas and has been implicated particularly in lymphomas of the sinonasal region and CNS (48,55-58,61, 66–68,163,165,166). Like salivary and thyroid glands, however, differences in histology and immunophenotype occur between the EBV-related lymphomas in these two sites. Lymphomas of the sinonasal region associated with EBV are polymorphous lymphomas of NK/T or T-cell lineage (24,30,32,39,44). These cases are found in the United States and Europe but are relatively more prevalent in the Far East and Latin America, and almost half or more of the cases exhibit NK/T ($CD56^+$) cell markers (30,37,44,52–54). In comparison, EBV has been identified in lymphomas of the CNS that occur in immunocompromised patients, including patients who have AIDS (160,163,165,166); however, these CNS lymphomas, although also aggressive and mainly of large cell type, are of B-cell lineage (156,157,174,275). Almost all malignant lymphomas of extranodal sites discussed in this chapter express B-cell markers, with the exception of those in the sinonasal region. Moreover, the B-cell lymphomas are virtually all high-grade malignancies of large cell or immunoblastic and Burkitt or Burkitt-like types. The extranodal low-grade lymphomas covered in this chapter, especially the marginal zone lymphomas of MALT, are prevalent only in salivary glands associated with MESA/BLEL or are found occasionally in the thyroid gland and breast and in a variety of miscellaneous organs, such as urinary bladder (98,105,122,129,223,249,258,282,283). The extranodal marginal zone lymphomas of MALT reflect a continuum of neoplastic evolution from polyclonal reactive hyperplasia to monoclonal malignant lymphoma (8,109) (see Chapter 31).

The clinical course of extranodal lymphomas varies, but, in general, the extranodal low-grade lymphomas have a relatively good prognosis and often are clinically occult, whereas the more common extranodal large B-cell lymphomas are clinically aggressive but are responsive to therapy, particularly if the lesion is confined to the extranodal site (stage IE).

REFERENCES

1. Paryani S, Hoppe RT, Burke JS, et al. Extralymphatic involvement in diffuse non-Hodgkin's lymphoma. *J Clin Oncol* 1983;1:682–688.
2. Gospodarowicz MK, Sutcliffe SB. The extranodal lymphomas. *Semin Radiat Oncol* 1995;4:281–300.
3. Greiner TC, Medeiros JL, Jaffe ES. Non-Hodgkin's lymphoma. *Cancer* 1995;75:370–380.
4. Barton JH, Osborne BM, Butler JJ, et al. Non-Hodgkin's lymphoma of the tonsil: a clinicopathologic study of 65 cases. *Cancer* 1984;53:86–95.
5. Saul SH, Kapadia SB. Primary lymphoma of Waldeyer's ring: clinicopathologic study of 68 cases. *Cancer* 1985;56:157–166.
6. Yuen A, Jacobs C. Lymphomas of the head and neck. *Semin Oncol* 1999;26:338–345.
7. Ree HJ, Rege VB, Knisley RE, et al. Malignant lymphoma of Waldeyer's ring following gastrointestinal lymphoma. *Cancer* 1980;46:1528–1535.
8. Isaacson PG. Mucosa-associated lymphoid tissue lymphoma. *Semin Hematol* 1999;36:139–147.
9. Paulsen J, Lennert K. Low-grade B-cell lymphoma of mucosa-associated lymphoid tissue type in Waldeyer's ring. *Histopathology* 1994;24:1–11.
10. Wright DH. Lymphomas of Waldeyer's ring. *Histopathology* 1994;24:97–99.
11. Hoppe RT, Burke JS, Glatstein E, Kaplan HS. Non-Hodgkin's lymphoma: involvement of Waldeyer's ring. *Cancer* 1978;42:1096–1104.
12. Shima N, Kobashi Y, Tsutsui K, et al. Extranodal non-Hodgkin's lymphoma of the head and neck: a clinicopathologic study in the Kyoto-Nara area of Japan. *Cancer* 1990;66:1190–1197.
13. Menárguez J, Mollejo M, Carrión R, et al. Waldeyer ring lymphomas: a clinicopathological study of 79 cases. *Histopathology* 1994;24:13–22.
14. Chan JKC, Ng CS, Lo STH. Immunohistological characterization of malignant lymphomas of the Waldeyer's ring other than the nasopharynx. *Histopathology* 1987;11:885–899.
15. Weisenburger DD, Armitage JO. Mantle cell lymphoma: an entity comes of age. *Blood* 1996;87:4483–4494.
16. The Non-Hodgkin's Lymphoma Pathologic Classification Project. National Cancer Institute sponsored study of classifications of non-Hodgkin's lymphomas: summary and description of a working formulation for clinical usage. *Cancer* 1982;49:2112–2135.
17. Banfi A, Bonadonna G, Ricci SB, et al. Malignant lymphomas of Waldeyer's ring: natural history and survival after radiotherapy. *Br Med J* 1972;3:140–143.
18. Yamanaka N, Harabuchi Y, Sambe S, et al. Non-Hodgkin's lymphoma of Waldeyer's ring and nasal cavity: clinical and immunologic aspects. *Cancer* 1985;56:768–776.
19. Kapadia SB, Roman LN, Kingma DW, et al. Hodgkin's disease of Waldeyer's ring: clinical and histoimmunophenotypic findings and association with Epstein-Barr virus in 16 cases. *Am J Surg Pathol* 1995;19:1431–1439.
20. Burke JS, Butler JJ. Malignant lymphoma with a high content of epithelioid histiocytes (Lennert's lymphoma). *Am J Clin Pathol* 1976;66:1–9.
21. Dargent J-L, Roufosse C, Remmelink M, et al. Primary T-cell–rich B-cell lymphoma of the Waldeyer's ring: a pathologic condition more frequent than presupposed? [Letter]. *Am J Surg Pathol* 1998;22:638–640.
22. Tomita Y, Ohsawa M, Mishiro Y, et al. Non-Hodgkin's lymphoma of Waldeyer's ring as a manifestation of lymphoproliferative diseases associated with human T-cell leukemia virus type 1 in southwestern Japan. *Mod Pathol* 1997;10:933–938.
23. Harabuchi Y, Tsubota H, Ohguro S, et al. Prognostic factors and treatment outcome in non-Hodgkin's lymphoma of Waldeyer's ring. *Acta Oncol* 1997;36:413–420.
24. Jaffe ES, Chan JKC, Su IH, et al. Report of the workshop on nasal and related extranodal angiocentric T/natural killer cell lymphomas: definitions, differential diagnosis, and epidemiology. *Am J Surg Pathol* 1996;20:103–111.
25. Harris NL, Jaffe ES, Stein H, et al. A revised European-American classification of lymphoid neoplasms: a proposal from the International Lymphoma Study Group. *Blood* 1994;84:1361–1392.
26. Jaffe ES, Harris NL, Diebold J, et al. World Health Organization classification of lymphomas: a work in progress. *Ann Oncol* 1998;9[Suppl 5]:S25–S30.
27. Fellbaum C, Hansmann M-L, Lennert K. Malignant lymphoma of the nasal cavity and paranasal sinuses. *Virchows Arch Path Anat* 1989;414:399–405.
28. Frierson HF, Mills SE, Innes DJ. Non-Hodgkin's lymphomas of the sinonasal region: histologic subtypes and their clinicopathologic features. *Am J Clin Pathol* 1984;81:721–727.
29. Li Y-X, Coucke PA, Li J-Y, et al. Primary non-Hodgkin's lymphoma of the nasal cavity: prognostic significance of paranasal extension and the role of radiotherapy and chemotherapy. *Cancer* 1998;83:449–456.
30. Cheung MMC, Chan JKC, Lau WH, et al. Primary non-Hodgkin's lymphoma of the nose and nasopharynx: clinical features, tumor immunophenotype, and treatment outcome in 113 patients. *J Clin Oncol* 1998;16:70–77.
31. Arber DA, Weiss LM, Alb-jar PF, et al. Nasal lymphomas in Peru: high incidence of T-cell immunophenotype and Epstein-Barr virus infection. *Am J Surg Pathol* 1993;17:392–399.
32. Quintanilla-Martinez L, Franklin JL, Guerrero I, et al. Histological and immunophenotypic profile of nasal NK/T cell lymphomas from Peru: high prevalence of p53 overexpression. *Hum Pathol* 1999;30:849–855.
33. van de Rijn M, Bhargava V, Molina-Kirsch H, et al. Extranodal head and neck lymphomas in Guatemala: high frequency of Epstein-Barr virus-associated sinonasal lymphomas. *Hum Pathol* 1997;28:834–839.
34. Elenitoba-Johnson KSJ, Zarate-Osorno A, Meneses A, et al. Cytotoxic granular cell protein expression, Epstein-Barr virus strain type, and latent membrane protein-1 oncogene deletions in nasal T-lymphocyte/natural killer cell lymphomas from Mexico. *Mod Pathol* 1998;11:754–761.
35. Costa J, Delacretaz F. The midline granuloma syndrome. *Pathol Annu* 1986;21:159–171.
36. Tsokos M, Fauci AS, Costa J. Idiopathic midline destructive disease (IMDD): a subgroup of patients with the "midline granuloma" syndrome. *Am J Clin Pathol* 1982;77:162–168.

37. Ho FCS, Choy D, Loke SL, et al. Polymorphic reticulosis and conventional lymphomas of the nose and upper aerodigestive tract: a clinicopathologic study of 70 cases and immunophenotypic studies of 16 cases. *Hum Pathol* 1990;21:1041–1050.
38. Ratech H, Burke JS, Blayney DW, et al. A clinicopathologic study of malignant lymphomas of the nose, paranasal sinuses, and hard palate, including cases of lethal midline granuloma. *Cancer* 1989;64: 2525–2531.
39. Abbondanzo SL, Wenig BM. Non-Hodgkin's lymphoma of the sinonasal tract: a clinicopathologic and immunophenotypic study of 120 cases. *Cancer* 1995;75:1281–1291.
40. Kassel SH, Echevarria RA, Guzzo FP. Midline malignant reticulosis (so-called lethal midline granuloma). *Cancer* 1969;23:920–935.
41. Strickler JG, Meneses MF, Habermann TM, et al. Polymorphic reticulosis: a reappraisal. *Hum Pathol* 1994;25:659–665.
42. Colby TV, Tazelaar HD, Specks U, et al. Nasal biopsy in Wegener's granulomatosis. *Hum Pathol* 1991;22:101–104.
43. Campo E, Cardesa A, Alos L, et al. Non-Hodgkin's lymphomas of nasal cavity and paranasal sinuses: an immunohistochemical study. *Am J Clin Pathol* 1991;96:184–190.
44. Chan JKC, Ng CS, Tsang WYW. Nasal/nasopharyngeal lymphomas: an immunohistochemical analysis of 57 cases on frozen tissues. *Mod Pathol* 1993;6:87A(abst).
45. DeRemee RA, Weiland LH, McDonald TJ. Polymorphic reticulosis, lymphomatoid granulomatosis: two diseases or one? *Mayo Clin Proc* 1978;53:634–640.
46. Colby TV, Carrington CB. Pulmonary lymphoma simulating lymphomatoid granulomatosis. *Am J Surg Pathol* 1982;6:19–32.
47. Lipford EH, Margolick JB, Longo DL, et al. Angiocentric immunoproliferative lesions: a clinicopathologic spectrum of post-thymic T-cell proliferations. *Blood* 1988;72:1674–1681.
48. Harabuchi Y, Yamanaka N, Kataura A, et al. Epstein-Barr virus in nasal T-cell lymphomas in patients with lethal midline granuloma. *Lancet* 1990;335:128–130.
49. Katzenstein ALA, Peiper SC. Detection of Epstein-Barr virus genomes in lymphomatoid granulomatosis: analysis of 29 cases by the polymerase chain reaction technique. *Mod Pathol* 1990;3:435–441.
50. Guinee D, Jaffe E, Kingma D, et al. Pulmonary lymphomatoid granulomatosis: evidence for a proliferation of Epstein-Barr virus infected B-lymphocytes with a prominent T-cell component and vasculitis. *Am J Surg Pathol* 1994;18:753–764.
51. Chan JKC, Sin VC, Wong KF, et al. Nonnasal lymphoma expressing the natural killer cell marker CD56: a clinicopathologic study of 49 cases of an uncommon aggressive neoplasm. *Blood* 1997;89: 4501–4513.
52. Suzumiya J, Takeshita M, Kimura N, et al. Expression of adult and fetal natural killer cell markers in sinonasal lymphomas. *Blood* 1994; 83:2255–2260.
53. Mori N, Yatabe Y, Oka K, et al. Expression of perforin in nasal lymphoma: additional evidence of its natural killer cell derivation. *Am J Pathol* 1996;149:699–705.
54. Ohshima K, Suzumiya J, Shimazaki K, et al. Nasal T/NK cell lymphomas commonly express perforin and Fas ligand: important mediators of tissue damage. *Histopathology* 1997:31:444–450.
55. Kanavaros P, Lescs M-C, Brière J, et al. Nasal T-cell lymphoma: a clinicopathologic entity associated with peculiar phenotype and with Epstein-Barr virus. *Blood* 1993;81:2688–2695.
56. Van Gorp J, De Bruin PC, Sie-Go DMDS, et al. Nasal T-cell lymphoma: a clinicopathological and immunophenotypic analysis of 13 cases. *Histopathology* 1995;27:139–148.
57. Petrella T, Delfau-Larue M-H, Caillot D, et al. Nasopharyngeal lymphomas: further evidence for a natural killer cell origin. *Hum Pathol* 1996;27:827–833.
58. Cuadra-Garcia I, Proulx GM, Wu CL, et al. Sinonasal lymphoma: a clinicopathologic analysis of 58 cases from the Massachusetts General Hospital. *Am J Surg Pathol* 1999;23:1356–1369.
59. Weiss LM, Picker LJ, Grogan TM, et al. Absence of clonal beta and gamma T-cell receptor gene rearrangements in a subset of peripheral T-cell lymphomas. *Am J Pathol* 1988;130:436–442.
60. Chiang AKS, Srivastava G, Lau PWF, et al. Differences in T-cell-receptor gene rearrangement and transcription in nasal lymphomas of natural killer and T-cell types: implications on cellular origin. *Hum Pathol* 1996;27:701–707.
61. Harabuchi Y, Imai S, Wakashima J, et al. Nasal T-cell lymphoma causally associated with Epstein-Barr virus: clinicopathologic, phenotypic, and genotypic studies. *Cancer* 1996;77:2137–2149.
62. Arnulf B, Copie-Bergman C, Delfau-Larue M-H, et al. Nonhepatosplenic $\gamma\delta$ T-cell lymphoma: a subset of cytotoxic lymphomas with mucosal or skin localization. *Blood* 1998;91:1723–1731.
63. Ng C-S, Lo STH, Chan JKC, et al. $CD56^+$ putative natural killer cell lymphomas: production of cytolytic effectors and related proteins mediating tumor cell apoptosis? *Hum Pathol* 1997;28:1276–1282.
64. Ng C-S, Lo STH, Chan JKC. Peripheral T and putative natural killer cell lymphomas commonly coexpress CD95 and CD95 ligand. *Hum Pathol* 1999;30:48–53.
65. Teruya-Feldstein J, Jaffe ES, Burd PR, et al. The role of Mig, the monokine induced by interferon-γ, and IP-10, the interferon-γ-inducible protein-10, in tissue necrosis and vascular damage associated with Epstein-Barr virus–positive lymphoproliferative disease. *Blood* 1997; 90:4099–4105.
66. Weiss LM, Gaffey MJ, Chen Y-Y, et al. Frequency of Epstein-Barr viral DNA in ''Western'' sinonasal and Waldeyer's ring non-Hodgkin's lymphomas. *Am J Surg Pathol* 1992;16:156–162.
67. Borisch B, Hennig I, Laeng RH, et al. Association of the subtype 2 of the Epstein-Barr virus with T-cell non-Hodgkin's lymphoma of the midline granuloma type. *Blood* 1993;82:858–864.
68. Chan JKC, Yip TTC, Tsang WYW, et al. Detection of Epstein-Barr viral RNA in malignant lymphomas of the upper aerodigestive tract. *Am J Surg Pathol* 1994;18:938–946.
69. Dictor M, Cervin A, Kalm O, et al. Sinonasal T-cell lymphoma in the differential diagnosis of lethal midline granuloma using in situ hybridization for Epstein-Barr virus RNA. *Mod Pathol* 1996;9:7–14.
70. Kanavaros P, Briere J, Lescs MC, et al. Epstein-Barr virus in non-Hodgkin's lymphomas of the upper respiratory tract: association with sinonasal localization and expression of NK and/or T-cell antigens by tumor cells. *J Pathol* 1996;178:297–302.
71. Tao Q, Srivastava G, Dickens P, et al. Detection of Epstein-Barr virus-infected mucosal lymphocytes in nasal polyps. *Am J Pathol* 1996; 149:1111–1118.
72. Gutiérrez MI, Spangler G, Kingma D, et al. Epstein-Barr virus in nasal lymphomas contains multiple ongoing mutations in the EBNA-1 gene. *Blood* 1998;92:600–606.
73. Cheng RZ, Guan XY, Lau G, et al. Chromosome 1p terminal deletion and loss of chromosomes 17p and 16p are common findings in nasal NK/T cell lymphoma by comparative genomic hybridization. *Mod Pathol* 1998;11:126A(abst).
74. Wong KF, Zhang YM, Chan JK. Cytogenetic abnormalities in natural killer cell lymphoma/leukemia: is there a consistent pattern? *Leuk Lymphoma* 1999;34:241–250.
75. Chott A, Rappersberger K, Schlossarek W, et al. Peripheral T cell lymphoma presenting primarily as lethal midline granuloma. *Hum Pathol* 1988;19:1093–1101.
76. Frierson HF, Innes DJ, Mills SE, et al. Immunophenotypic analysis of sinonasal non-Hodgkin's lymphomas. *Hum Pathol* 1989;20:636–642.
77. Logsdon MD, Ha CS, Kavadi VS, et al. Lymphoma of the nasal cavity and paranasal sinuses: improved outcome and altered prognostic factors with combined modality therapy. *Cancer* 1997;80:477–488.
78. Liang R, Todd D, Chan TK, et al. Treatment outcome and prognostic factors for primary nasal lymphoma. *J Clin Oncol* 1995;13:666–670.
79. Gleeson MJ, Bennett MH, Cawson RA. Lymphomas of salivary glands. *Cancer* 1986;58:699–704.
80. Mehle ME, Kraus DH, Wood BG, et al. Lymphoma of the parotid gland. *Laryngoscope* 1993;103:17–21.
81. Barnes L, Myers EN, Prokopakis EP. Primary malignant lymphoma of the parotid gland. *Arch Otolaryngol Head Neck Surg* 1998;124: 573–577.
82. Nathwani BN, Anderson JR, Armitage JO, et al. Marginal zone B-cell lymphoma: a clinical comparison of nodal and mucosa-associated lymphoid tissue types. *J Clin Oncol* 1999;17:2486–2492.
83. Schmid U, Helbron D, Lennert K. Primary malignant lymphomas localized in salivary glands. *Histopathology* 1982;6:673–687.
84. Schmid U, Helbron D, Lennert K. Development of malignant lymphoma in myoepithelial sialadenitis (Sjögren's syndrome). *Virchows Arch Path Anat* 1982;395:11–43.
85. Harris NL. Lymphoid proliferations of the salivary glands. *Am J Clin Pathol* 1999;111[Suppl 1]:S94–S103.
86. Ulirsch RC, Jaffe ES. Sjögren's syndrome-like illness associated with

the acquired immunodeficiency syndrome-related complex. *Hum Pathol* 1987;18:1063–1068.
87. Smith FB, Rajdeo H, Panesar N, et al. Benign lymphoepithelial lesion of the parotid gland in intravenous drug users. *Arch Pathol Lab Med* 1988;112:742–745.
88. Ioachim HL, Ryan JR, Blaugrund SM. Salivary gland lymph nodes: the site of lymphadenopathies and lymphomas associated with human immunodeficiency virus infection. *Arch Pathol Lab Med* 1988;112: 1224–1228.
89. Elliott JN, Oertel YC. Lymphoepithelial cysts of the salivary glands: histologic and cytologic features. *Am J Clin Pathol* 1990;93:39–43.
90. Maiorano E, Favia G, Viale G. Lymphoepithelial cysts of salivary glands: an immunohistochemical study of HIV-related and HIV-unrelated lesions. *Hum Pathol* 1998;29:260–265.
91. Kassan SS, Thomas TL, Moutsopoulos HM, et al. Increased risk of lymphoma in sicca syndrome. *Ann Intern Med* 1978;89:888–892.
92. Fox RI, Adamson TC, Fong S, et al. Lymphocyte phenotype and function in pseudolymphoma associated with Sjögren's syndrome. *J Clin Invest* 1983;72:52–62.
93. Bahler DW, Miklos JA, Swerdlow SH. Ongoing Ig gene hypermutation in salivary gland mucosa-associated lymphoid tissue-type lymphomas. *Blood* 1997;89:3335–3344.
94. Bahler DW, Swerdlow SH. Clonal salivary gland infiltrates associated with myoepithelial sialadenitis (Sjögren's syndrome) begin as nonmalignant antigen-selected expansions. *Blood* 1998;91:1864–1872.
95. Fishleder A, Tubbs R, Hesse B, et al. Uniform detection of immunoglobulin-gene rearrangement in benign lymphoepithelial lesions. *N Engl J Med* 1987;316:1118–1121.
96. Diss TC, Wotherspoon AC, Speight P, et al. B-cell monoclonality, Epstein Barr virus, and t(14;18) in myoepithelial sialadenitis and low-grade B-cell MALT lymphoma of the parotid gland. *Am J Surg Pathol* 1995;19:531–536.
97. Hsi ED, Siddiqui J, Schnitzer B, et al. Analysis of immunoglobulin heavy chain gene rearrangement in myoepithelial sialadenitis by polymerase chain reaction. *Am J Clin Pathol* 1996;106:498–503.
98. Quintana PG, Kapadia SB, Bahler DW, et al. Salivary gland lymphoid infiltrates associated with lymphoepithelial lesions: a clinicopathologic, immunophenotypic, and genotypic study. *Hum Pathol* 1997; 28:850—861.
99. Royer B, Cazals-Hatem D, Sibilia J, et al. Lymphomas in patients with Sjögren's syndrome are marginal zone B-cell neoplasms, arise in diverse extranodal and nodal sites, and are not associated with viruses. *Blood* 1997;90:766–775.
100. Scott CA, Avellini C, Desinan L, et al. Chronic lymphocytic sialoadenitis in HCV-related chronic liver disease: comparison with Sjögren's syndrome. *Histopathology* 1997;30:41–48.
101. DeVita S, Sacco C, Sansonno D, et al. Characterization of overt B-cell lymphomas in patients with hepatitis C virus infection. *Blood* 1997;90:776–782.
102. Colby TV, Dorfman RF. Malignant lymphomas involving the salivary glands. *Pathol Annu* 1979;14:307–324.
103. McCurley TL, Collins RD, Ball E, et al. Nodal and extranodal lymphoproliferative disorders in Sjögren's syndrome: a clinical and immunopathologic study. *Hum Pathol* 1990;21:482–492.
104. Hsi ED, Zukerberg LR, Schniker B, et al. Development of extrasalivary gland lymphoma in myoepithelial sialadenitis. *Mod Pathol* 1995; 8:817–824.
105. Hyjek E, Smith WJ, Isaacson PG. Primary B-cell lymphoma of salivary glands and its relationship to myoepithelial sialadenitis. *Hum Pathol* 1988;19:766–776.
106. Zulman J, Jaffe R, Talal N. Evidence that the malignant lymphoma of Sjögren's syndrome is a monoclonal B-cell neoplasm. *N Engl J Med* 1978;299:1215–1220.
107. Ngan B-Y, Warnke RA, Wilson M, et al. Monocytoid B-cell lymphoma: a study of 36 cases. *Hum Pathol* 1991;22:409–421.
108. Shin SS, Sheibani K, Fishleder A, et al. Monocytoid B-cell lymphoma in patients with Sjögren's syndrome: a clinicopathologic study of 13 patients. *Hum Pathol* 1991;22:422–430.
109. Burke JS. Are there site-specific differences among the MALT lymphomas—morphologic, clinical? *Am J Clin Pathol* 1999;111[Suppl 1]:S133–S143.
110. Collins RD. Is clonality equivalent to malignancy: specifically, is immunoglobulin gene rearrangement diagnostic of malignant lymphoma? *Hum Pathol* 1997;28:757–759.
111. Falzon M, Isaacson PG. The natural history of benign lymphoepithelial lesion of the salivary gland in which there is a monoclonal population of B cells: a report of two cases. *Am J Surg Pathol* 1991;15: 59–65.
112. Aviles A, Delgado S, Huerta-Guzman J. Marginal zone B cell lymphoma of the parotid glands: results of a randomized trial comparing radiotherapy to combined therapy. *Eur J Cancer B Oral Oncol* 1996; 32B:420–422.
113. Hyman GA, Wolff M. Malignant lymphomas of the salivary glands: review of the literature and report of 33 new cases, including four cases associated with the lymphoepithelial lesion. *Am J Clin Pathol* 1976;65:421–438.
114. Osborne BM, Butler JJ, Variakojis D, et al. Reactive lymph node hyperplasia with giant follicles. *Am J Clin Pathol* 1982;78:493–499.
115. Medeiros LJ, Rizzi R, Lardelli P, et al. Malignant lymphoma involving a Warthin's tumor: a case with immunophenotypic and gene rearrangement analysis. *Hum Pathol* 1990;21:974–977.
116. Kerrigan DP, Irons J, Chen I-M. Bcl-2 gene rearrangement in salivary gland lymphoma. *Am J Surg Pathol* 1990;14:1133–1138.
117. Chan JKC, Tsang WYW, Hui P-K, et al. T- and T/natural killer-cell lymphomas of the salivary gland: a clinicopathologic, immunohistochemical and molecular study of six cases. *Hum Pathol* 1997;28: 238–245.
118. Burke JS, Butler JJ, Fuller LM. Malignant lymphomas of the thyroid: a clinical pathologic study of 35 patients including ultrastructural observations. *Cancer* 1977;39:1587–1602.
119. Compagno J, Oertel JE. Malignant lymphoma and other lymphoproliferative disorders of the thyroid gland: a clinicopathologic study of 245 cases. *Am J Clin Pathol* 1980;74:1–11.
120. Anscombe AM, Wright DH. Primary malignant lymphoma of the thyroid—a tumour of mucosa-associated lymphoid tissue: review of seventy-six cases. *Histopathology* 1985;9:81–97.
121. Aozasa K, Inoue A, Tajima K, et al. Malignant lymphomas of the thyroid gland: analysis of 79 patients with emphasis on histologic prognostic factors. *Cancer* 1986;58:100–104.
122. Hyjek E, Isaacson PG. Primary B cell lymphoma of the thyroid and its relationship to Hashimoto's thyroiditis. *Hum Pathol* 1988;19: 1315–1326.
123. Pedersen RK, Pedersen NT. Primary non-Hodgkin's lymphoma of the thyroid gland: a population based study. *Histopathology* 1996;28: 25–32.
124. Dayan CM, Daniels GH. Chronic autoimmune thyroiditis. *N Engl J Med* 1996;335:99–107.
125. Holm L-E, Blomgren H, Löwhagen T. Cancer risks in patients with chronic lymphocytic thyroiditis. *N Engl J Med* 1985;312:601–604.
126. Kato I, Tajima K, Suchi T, et al. Chronic thyroiditis as a risk factor for B-cell lymphoma in the thyroid gland. *Jpn J Cancer Res* 1985; 76:1085–1090.
127. Matsubayashi S, Tamai H, Morita T, et al. Possible disorder of B-cell related surveillance and malignant lymphoma of the thyroid. *Cancer* 1989;64:2259–2261.
128. Tomita Y, Ohsawa M, Kanno H, et al. Sporadic activation of Epstein-Barr virus in thyroid lymphoma. *Leuk Lymphoma* 1995;19:129–134.
129. Lam KY, Lo CY, Kwong DLW, et al. Malignant lymphoma of the thyroid: a 30-year clinicopathologic experience and an evaluation of the presence of Epstein-Barr virus. *Am J Clin Pathol* 1999;112: 263–270.
130. Iyota K, Takeda K, Matsuzuka F, et al. Absence of p53 mutation in Japanese patients with malignant thyroid lymphoma. *J Endocrinol Invest* 1994;17:775–782.
131. Katzin WE, Fishleder AJ, Tubbs RR. Investigation of the clonality of lymphocytes in Hashimoto's thyroiditis using immunoglobulin and T-cell receptor gene probes. *Clin Immunol Immunopathol* 1989;51: 264–274.
132. Ben-Ezra J, Wu A, Sheibani K. Hashimoto's thyroiditis lacks detectable clonal immunoglobulin and T cell receptor gene rearrangements. *Hum Pathol* 1988;19:1444–1448.
133. Knowles DM, Athan E, Ubriaco A, et al. Extranodal noncutaneous lymphoid hyperplasias represent a continuous spectrum of B-cell neoplasia: demonstration by molecular genetic analysis. *Blood* 1989;73: 1635–1645.
134. Hsi ED, Singleton TP, Svoboda SM, et al. Characterization of the lymphoid infiltrate in Hashimoto's thyroiditis by immunohistoche-

mistry and polymerase chain reaction for immunoglobulin heavy chain gene rearrangement. *Am J Clin Pathol* 1998;110:327–333.
135. Isaacson PG, Spencer J. Malignant lymphoma and autoimmune disease. *Histopathology* 1993;22:509–510.
136. Aozasa K, Ueda T, Katagiri S, et al. Immunologic and immunohistochemical analysis of 27 cases with thyroid lymphomas. *Cancer* 1987; 60:969–973.
137. Faure P, Chittal S, Woodman-Memeteau F, et al. Diagnostic features of primary malignant lymphomas of the thyroid with monoclonal antibodies. *Cancer* 1988;61:1852–1861.
138. Mizukami Y, Michigishi T, Nonomura A, et al. Primary lymphoma of the thyroid: a clinical, histological and immunohistochemical study of 20 cases. *Histopathology* 1990;17:201–209.
139. Skacel M, Ross CW, Hsi ED. Primary malignant lymphoma of the thyroid gland. *Mod Pathol* 1999;12:146A(abst).
140. Ansell SM, Grant CS, Habermann TM. Primary thyroid lymphoma. *Semin Oncol* 1999;26:316–323.
141. Lovchik J, Lane MA, Clark DP. Polymerase chain reaction–based detection of B-cell clonality in the fine needle aspiration biopsy of a thyroid mucosa-associated lymphoid tissue (MALT) lymphoma. *Hum Pathol* 1997;28:989–992.
142. Burke JS. Histologic criteria for distinguishing between benign and malignant extranodal lymphoid infiltrates. *Semin Diagn Pathol* 1985; 2:152–162.
143. Matsuzuka F, Fukata S, Kuma K, et al. Gene rearrangement of immunoglobulin as a marker of thyroid lymphoma. *World J Surg* 1998;22: 558–561.
144. Bateman AC, Wright DH. Epitheliotropism in high-grade lymphomas of mucosa-associated lymphoid tissue. *Histopathology* 1993;23: 409–415.
145. Matias-Guiu X, Esquius J. Lymphoepithelial lesion in the thyroid: a non-specific histological finding. *Pathol Res Pract* 1991;187: 296–300.
146. Isaacson PG, Androulakis-Papachristou A, Diss TC, et al. Follicular colonization in thyroid lymphoma. *Am J Pathol* 1992;41:43–52.
147. Aozasa K, Inoue A, Yoshimura H, et al. Plasmacytoma of the thyroid gland. *Cancer* 1986;58:105–110.
148. Aozasa K, Inoue A, Yoshimura H, et al. Intermediate lymphocytic lymphoma of the thyroid: an immunologic and immunohistologic study. *Cancer* 1986;57:1762–1767.
149. Tobler A, Maurer ATR, Hedinger CE. Undifferentiated thyroid tumors of diffuse small cell type: histological and immunohistochemical evidence for their lymphomatous nature. *Virchows Arch Path Anat* 1984; 404:117–126.
150. Wolf BC, Sheahan K, DeCoste D, et al. Immunohistochemical analysis of small cell tumors of the thyroid gland: an Eastern Cooperative Oncology Group study. *Hum Pathol* 1992;23:1252–1261.
151. Diaz de Leon E, Alkan S, Huang JC, et al. Usefulness of an immunohistochemical panel in paraffin-embedded tissues for the differentiation of B-cell non-Hodgkin's lymphomas of small lymphocytes. *Mod Pathol* 1998;11:1046–1051.
152. Ohsawa M, Noguchi S, Aozasa K. Immunologic type of thyroid lymphoma in an adult T-cell leukemia endemic area in Japan. *Leuk Lymphoma* 1995;17:341–344.
153. Yamaguchi M, Ohno T, Kita K. $\gamma\delta$ T-cell lymphoma of the thyroid gland [Letter]. *N Engl J Med* 1997;336:1391–1392.
154. Laing RW, Hoskin P, Hudson BV, et al. The significance of MALT histology in thyroid lymphoma: a review of patients from the BNLI and Royal Marsden Hospital. *Clin Oncol (R Coll Radiol)* 1994;6: 300–304.
155. Tsang RW, Gospodarowicz MK, Sutcliffe SB, et al. Non-Hodgkin's lymphoma of the thyroid gland: prognostic factors and treatment outcome. The Princess Margaret Hospital Lymphoma Group. *Int J Radiat Oncol Biol Phys* 1993;27:599–604.
156. Miller DC, Hochberg FH, Harris NL, et al. Pathology with clinical correlations of primary central nervous system non-Hodgkin's lymphoma: the Massachusetts General Hospital experience 1958–1989. *Cancer* 1994;74:1383–1397.
157. Camilleri-Broët S, Martin A, Moreau A, et al. Primary central nervous system lymphomas in 72 immunocompetent patients: pathologic findings and clinical correlations. *Am J Clin Pathol* 1998;110:607–612.
158. Krogh-Jensen M, D'Amore F, Jensen MK, et al. Clinicopathological features, survival and prognostic factors of primary central nervous system lymphomas: trends in incidence of primary central nervous system lymphomas and primary malignant brain tumors in a well-defined geographical area. Population-based data from the Danish lymphoma registry, LYFO, and the Danish Cancer Registry. *Leuk Lymphoma* 1995;19:223–233.
159. Corn BW, Marcus SM, Topham A, et al. Will primary central nervous system lymphoma be the most frequent brain tumor diagnosed in the year 2000? *Cancer* 1997;79:2409–2413.
160. Hochberg FH, Miller DC. Primary central nervous system lymphoma. *J Neurosurg* 1988;68:835–853.
161. Helle TL, Britt RH, Colby TV. Primary lymphoma of the central nervous system: clinicopathological study of experience at Stanford. *J Neurosurg* 1984;60:94–103.
162. Maher EA, Fine HA. Primary CNS lymphoma. *Semin Oncol* 1999; 26:346–356.
163. Camilleri-Broët S, Davi F, Feuillard J, et al. AIDS-related primary brain lymphomas: histopathologic and immunohistochemical study of 51 cases. *Hum Pathol* 1997;28:367–374.
164. Knowles DM, Chamulak GA, Subar M, et al. Lymphoid neoplasia associated with the acquired immunodeficiency syndrome (AIDS): the New York University Medical Center experience with 105 patients (1981–1986). *Ann Intern Med* 1988;108:744–753.
165. Bashir RM, Hochberg FH, Harris NL, et al. Variable expression of Epstein-Barr virus genome as demonstrated by in situ hybridization in central nervous system lymphomas in immunocompromised patients. *Mod Pathol* 1990;3:429–434.
166. Chang KL, Flaris N, Hickey WF, et al. Brain lymphoma of immunocompetent and immunocompromised patients: study of the association with Epstein-Barr virus. *Mod Pathol* 1993;6:427–432.
167. Davenport RD, O'Donnell LR, Schnitzer B, et al. Non-Hodgkin's lymphoma of the brain after Hodgkin's disease. *Cancer* 1991;67: 440–443.
168. DeAngelis LM. Primary central nervous system lymphoma as a secondary malignancy. *Cancer* 1991;67:1431–1435.
169. Fine HA, Mayer RJ. Primary central nervous system lymphoma. *Ann Intern Med* 1993;119:1093–1104.
170. Sherman ME, Erozan YS, Mann RB, et al. Stereotactic brain biopsy in the diagnosis of malignant lymphoma. *Am J Clin Pathol* 1991:95: 878–883.
171. Rhodes CH, Glantz MJ, Glantz L, et al. A comparison of polymerase chain reaction examination of cerebrospinal fluid and conventional cytology in the diagnosis of lymphomatous meningitis. *Cancer* 1996; 77:543–548.
172. Balmaceda C, Gaynor JJ, Sun M, et al. Leptomeningeal tumor in primary central nervous system lymphoma: recognition, significance, and implications. *Ann Neurol* 1995:38:202–209.
173. Henry JM, Heffner RR, Dillard SH, et al. Primary malignant lymphomas of the central nervous system. *Cancer* 1974;34:1293–1302.
174. Ferracini R, Pileri S, Bergmann M, et al. Non-Hodgkin's lymphomas of the central nervous system: clinico-pathologic and immunohistochemical study of 147 cases. *Pathol Res Pract* 1993;189:249–260.
175. Schwechheimer K, Braus DF, Schwarzkopf G, et al. Polymorphous high-grade B cell lymphoma is the predominant type of spontaneous primary cerebral malignant lymphomas: histological and immunomorphological evaluation of computed tomography-guided stereotactic brain biopsies. *Am J Surg Pathol* 1994;18:931–937.
176. Glass J, Hochberg FH, Miller DC. Intravascular lymphomatosis: a systemic disease with neurologic manifestations. *Cancer* 1993;71: 3156–3164.
177. DiGiuseppe JA, Nelson WG, Seifter EJ, et al. Intravascular lymphomatosis: a clinicopathologic study of 10 cases and assessment of response to chemotherapy. *J Clin Oncol* 1994;12:2573–2579.
178. Ashby MA, Barber PC, Holmes AE, et al. Primary intracranial Hodgkin's disease: a case report and discussion. *Am J Surg Pathol* 1988; 12:294–299.
179. Villegas E, Villa S, Lopez-Guillermo A, et al. Primary central nervous system lymphoma of T-cell origin: description of two cases and review of the literature. *J Neurooncol* 1997;34:157–161.
180. Abdulkader I, Cameselle-Teijeiro J, Fraga M, et al. Primary anaplastic large cell lymphoma of the central nervous system. *Hum Pathol* 1999; 30:978–981.
181. Nozaki M, Tada M, Mizugaki Y, et al. Expression of oncogenic molecules in primary central nervous system lymphomas in immunocompetent patients. *Acta Neuropathol* 1998;95:505–510.
182. Smith WJ, Garson JA, Bourne SP, et al. Immunoglobulin gene rear-

rangement and antigenic profile confirm B cell origin of primary cerebral lymphoma and indicate a mature phenotype. *J Clin Pathol* 1988; 41:128–132.
183. Larocca LM, Capello D, Rinelli A, et al. The molecular and phenotypic profile of primary central nervous system lymphoma identifies distinct categories of the disease and is consistent with histogenetic derivation from germinal center-related B cells. *Blood* 1998;92: 1011–1019.
184. Thompsett AR, Ellison DW, Stevenson FK, et al. V_H gene sequences from primary central nervous system lymphomas indicate derivation from highly mutated germinal center B cells with ongoing mutational activity. *Blood* 1999;94:1738–1746.
185. Rickert CH, Dockhorn-Dworniczak B, Simon R, et al. Chromosomal imbalances in primary lymphomas of the central nervous system. *Am J Pathol* 1999;155:1445–1451.
186. Kumar S, Kumar D, Kaldjian EP, et al. Primary low-grade B-cell lymphoma of the dura: a mucosa associated lymphoid tissue-type lymphoma. *Am J Surg Pathol* 1997;21:81–87.
187. Kambham N, Chang Y, Matsushima AY. Primary low-grade B-cell lymphoma of mucosa-associated lymphoid tissue (MALT) arising in dura. *Clin Neuropathol* 1998;17:311–317.
188. Nguyen D, Nathwani BN. Primary meningeal small lymphocytic lymphoma. *Am J Surg Pathol* 1989;13:67–70.
189. Mancardi GL, Mandybur TI. Solitary intracranial plasmacytoma. *Cancer* 1983;51:2226–2233.
190. Mackintosh FR, Colby TV, Podolsky WJ, et al. Central nervous system involvement in non-Hodgkin's lymphoma: an analysis of 105 cases. *Cancer* 1982;49:586–595.
191. Keldsen N, Michalski W, Bentzen SM, et al. Risk factors for central nervous system involvement in non-Hodgkin's lymphoma: a multivariate analysis. *Acta Oncol* 1996;35:703–708.
192. van Besien K, Ha CS, Murphy S, et al. Risk factors, treatment, and outcome of central nervous system recurrence in adults with intermediate-grade and immunoblastic lymphoma. *Blood* 1998;91: 1178–1184.
193. Bishop PC, Wilson WH, Pearson D, et al. CNS involvement in primary mediastinal B-cell lymphoma. *J Clin Oncol* 1999;17: 2479–2485.
194. Montserrat E, Bosch F, López-Guillermo A, et al. CNS involvement in mantle-cell lymphoma. *J Clin Oncol* 1996;14:941–944.
195. Harada K, Kurisu K, Arita K, et al. Telomerase activity in central nervous system malignant lymphoma. *Cancer* 1999;86:1050–1055.
196. Shahab N, Doll DC. Testicular lymphoma. *Semin Oncol* 1999;26: 259–269.
197. Paladugu RR, Bearman RM, Rappaport H. Malignant lymphoma with primary manifestation in the gonad: a clinicopathologic study of 39 patients. *Cancer* 1980;45:561–571.
198. Duncan PR, Checa F, Gowing NFC, et al. Extranodal non-Hodgkin's lymphoma presenting in the testicle: a clinical and pathologic study of 24 cases. *Cancer* 1980;45:1578–1584.
199. Turner RR, Colby TV, MacKintosh FR. Testicular lymphomas: a clinicopathologic study of 35 cases. *Cancer* 1981;48:2095–2102.
200. Wilkins BS, Williamson JMS, O'Brien CJ. Morphological and immunohistological study of testicular lymphomas. *Histopathology* 1989; 15:147–156.
201. Ferry JA, Harris NL, Young RH, et al. Malignant lymphoma of the testis, epididymis, and spermatic cord: a clinicopathologic study of 69 cases with immunophenotypic analysis. *Am J Surg Pathol* 1994; 18:376–390.
202. Agarwal V, Li JKH, Bard R. Lymphocytic orchitis: a case report. *Hum Pathol* 1990;21:1080–1082.
203. Hyland J, Lasota J, Jasinski M, et al. Molecular pathological analysis of testicular diffuse large cell lymphomas. *Hum Pathol* 1998;29: 1231–1239.
204. Ferry JA, Srigley JR, Young RH. Granulocytic sarcoma of the testis: a report of two cases of a neoplasm prone to misinterpretation. *Mod Pathol* 1997;10:320–325.
205. Ferry JA, Young RH, Scully RE. Testicular and epididymal plasmacytoma: a report of 7 cases, including three that were the initial manifestation of plasma cell myeloma. *Am J Surg Pathol* 1997;21:590–598.
206. Finn LS, Viswanatha DS, Belasco JB, et al. Primary follicular lymphoma of the testis in childhood. *Cancer* 1999;85:1626–1635.
207. Akhtar M, Al-Dayel F, Siegrist K, et al. Neutrophil-rich Ki-1–positive anaplastic large cell lymphoma presenting as a testicular mass. *Mod Pathol* 1996;9:812–815.
208. Chan JKC, Tsang WYW, Lau W-H, et al. Aggressive T/natural killer cell lymphoma presenting as testicular tumor. *Cancer* 1996;77: 1198–1205.
209. Touroutoglou N, Dimopoulos MA, Younes A, et al. Testicular lymphoma: late relapses and poor outcome despite doxorubicin-based therapy. *J Clin Oncol* 1995;13:1361–1367.
210. Tondini C, Ferreri AJM, Siracusano L, et al. Diffuse large-cell lymphoma of the testis. *J Clin Oncol* 1999;17:2854–2858.
211. Connors JM, Klimo P, Voss N, et al. Testicular lymphoma: improved outcome with early brief chemotherapy. *J Clin Oncol* 1988;6: 776–781.
212. Zeitman AL, Coen JJ, Ferry JA, et al. The management and outcome of stage IAE non-Hodgkin's lymphoma of the testis. *J Urol* 1996; 155:943–946.
213. Chorlton I, Norris HJ, King FM. Malignant reticuloendothelial disease involving the ovary as a primary manifestation: a series of 19 lymphomas and 1 granulocytic sarcoma. *Cancer* 1974;34:397–407.
214. Berard CW, O'Connor GT, Thomas LB, et al. Histopathologic definition of Burkitt's tumor. *Bull World Health Organ* 1969;40:601–607.
215. Monterroso V, Jaffe ES, Merino MJ, et al. Malignant lymphomas involving the ovary: a clinicopathologic analysis of 39 cases. *Am J Surg Pathol* 1993;17:154–170.
216. Osborne BM, Robboy SJ. Lymphomas or leukemia presenting as ovarian tumors: an analysis of 42 cases. *Cancer* 1983;52:1933–1943.
217. Ferry JA, Young RH. Malignant lymphoma, pseudolymphoma, and hematopoietic disorders of the female genital tract. *Pathol Annu* 1991; 26:227–263.
218. Oliva E, Ferry JA, Young RH, et al. Granulocytic sarcoma of the female genital tract: a clinicopathologic study of 11 cases. *Am J Surg Pathol* 1997;21:1156–1165.
219. Linden MD, Tubbs RR, Fishleder AJ, et al. Immunotypic and genotypic characterization of non-Hodgkin's lymphomas of the ovary. *Am J Clin Pathol* 1988;89:156–162.
220. Chorlton I, Karnei RF, Norris HJ. Primary malignant reticuloendothelial disease involving the vagina, cervix, and corpus uteri. *Obstet Gynecol* 1974;44:735–748.
221. Harris NL, Scully RE. Malignant lymphoma and granulocytic sarcoma of the uterus and vagina: a clinicopathologic analysis of 27 cases. *Cancer* 1984;53:2530–2545.
222. Muntz HG, Ferry JA, Flynn D, et al. Stage IE?? primary malignant lymphomas of the uterine cervix. *Cancer* 1991;68:2023–2032.
223. Pelstring RJ, Essell JH, Kurtin PJ, et al. Diversity of organ site involvement among malignant lymphomas of mucosa-associated tissues. *Am J Clin Pathol* 1991;96:738–745.
224. Aozasa K, Saeki K, Ohsawa M, et al. Malignant lymphoma of the uterus: report of seven cases with immunohistochemical study. *Cancer* 1993;72:1959–1964.
225. van de Rijn M, Kamel OW, Chang PP, et al. Primary low-grade endometrial B-cell lymphoma. *Am J Surg Pathol* 1997;21:187–194.
226. Young RH, Harris NL, Scully RE. Lymphoma-like lesions of the lower female genital tract: a report of 16 cases. *Int J Gynecol Pathol* 1985;4:289–299.
227. Ostrowski ML, Unni KK, Banks PM, et al. Malignant lymphoma of bone. *Cancer* 1986;58:2646–2655.
228. Baar J, Burkes RL, Gospodarowicz M. Primary non-Hodgkin's lymphoma of bone. *Semin Oncol* 1999;26:270–275.
229. Suryanarayan K, Shuster JJ, Donaldson SS, et al. Treatment of localized primary non-Hodgkin's lymphoma of bone in children: a Pediatric Oncology Group study. *J Clin Oncol* 1999;17:456–459.
230. Clayton F, Butler JJ, Ayala AG, et al. Non-Hodgkin's lymphoma in bone: pathologic and radiologic features with clinical correlates. *Cancer* 1987;60:2494–2501.
231. Haussler MD, Fenstermacher MJ, Johnston DA, et al. MRI of primary lymphoma of bone: cortical disorder as a criterion for differential diagnosis. *J Magn Reson Imaging* 1999;9:93–100.
232. Hicks DG, Gokan T, O'Keefe RJ, et al. Primary lymphoma of bone: correlation of magnetic resonance imaging features with cytokine production by tumor cells. *Cancer* 1995;75:973–980.
233. Dosoretz DE, Raymond AK, Murphy GF, et al. Primary lymphoma of bone: the relationship of morphologic diversity to clinical behavior. *Cancer* 1982;50:1009–1014.
234. Pettit CK, Zukerberg LR, Gray MK, et al. Primary lymphoma of bone:

a B-cell neoplasm with a high frequency of multilobated cells. *Am J Surg Pathol* 1990;14:329–334.
235. Pileri SA, Montanari M, Falini B, et al. Malignant lymphoma involving the mandible: clinical, morphologic, and immunohistochemical study of 17 cases. *Am J Surg Pathol* 1990;14:652–659.
236. Baar J, Burkes RL, Bell R, et al. Primary non-Hodgkin's lymphoma of bone: a clinicopathologic study. *Cancer* 1994;73:1194–1199.
237. Jones D, Kraus MD, Dorfman DM. Lymphoma presenting as a solitary bone tumor. *Am J Clin Pathol* 1999;111:171–178.
238. Mann RB. Are there site-specific differences among extranodal aggressive B-cell neoplasms? *Am J Clin Pathol* 1999;111[Suppl 1]:S144–S150.
239. Radaszkiewicz T, Hansmann M-L. Primary high-grade malignant lymphomas of bone. *Virchows Arch Path Anat* 1988;413:269–274.
240. Chan JKC, Ng C-S, Hui P-K, et al. Anaplastic large cell Ki-1 lymphoma of bone. *Cancer* 1991;68:2186–2191.
241. Ostrowski ML, Inwards CY, Strickler JG, et al. Osseous Hodgkin's disease. *Cancer* 1999;85:1166–1178.
242. Ozdemirli M, Fanburg-Smith JC, Hartmann D-P, et al. Precursor B-lymphoblastic lymphoma presenting as a solitary bone tumor and mimicking Ewing's sarcoma: a report of four cases and review of the literature. *Am J Surg Pathol* 1998;22:795–804.
243. Iravani S, Singleton TP, Ross CW, et al. Precursor B-lymphoblastic lymphoma presenting as lytic bone lesions. *Am J Clin Pathol* 1999; 112:836–843.
244. Ueda T, Aozasa K, Ohsawa M, et al. Malignant lymphomas of bone in Japan. *Cancer* 1989;64:2387–2392.
245. Christie DR, Barton MB, Bryant G, et al. Osteolymphoma (primary bone lymphoma): an Australian review of 70 cases. *Aust NZ Med* 1999;29:214–219.
246. Wiseman C, Liao KT. Primary lymphoma of the breast. *Cancer* 1972; 29:1705–1712.
247. Mambo NC, Burke JS, Butler JJ. Primary malignant lymphomas of the breast. *Cancer* 1977;39:2033–2040.
248. Brustein S, Filippa DA, Kimmel M, et al. Malignant lymphoma of the breast: a study of 53 patients. *Ann Surg* 1987;205:144–150.
249. Hugh JC, Jackson FI, Hanson J, et al. Primary breast lymphoma: an immunohistologic study of 20 new cases. *Cancer* 1990;66: 2602–2611.
250. Cohen PL, Brooks JJ. Lymphomas of the breast: a clinicopathologic and immunohistochemical study of primary and secondary cases. *Cancer* 1991;67:1359–1369.
251. Giardini R, Piccolo C, Rilke F. Primary non-Hodgkin's lymphomas of the female breast. *Cancer* 1992;69:725–735.
252. Aozasa K, Ohsawa M, Saeki K, et al. Malignant lymphoma of the breast: immunologic type and association with lymphocytic mastopathy. *Am J Clin Pathol* 1992;97:699–704.
253. Jeon HJ, Akagi T, Hoshida Y, et al. Primary non-Hodgkin's malignant lymphoma of the breast: an immunohistochemical study of seven patients and literature review of 152 patients with breast lymphoma in Japan. *Cancer* 1992;70:2451–2459.
254. Borbrow LG, Richards MA, Happerfield LC, et al. Breast lymphomas: a clinicopathologic review. *Hum Pathol* 1993;24:274–278.
255. Lin Y, Govindan R, Hess JL. Malignant hematopoietic breast tumors. *Am J Clin Pathol* 1997;107:177–186.
256. Arber DA, Simpson JF, Weiss LM, et al. Non-Hodgkin's lymphoma involving the breast. *Am J Surg Pathol* 1994;18:288–295.
257. Abbondanzo SL, Seidman JD, Lefkowitz M, et al. Primary diffuse large B-cell lymphoma of the breast: a clinicopathologic study of 31 cases. *Pathol Res Pract* 1996;192:37–43.
258. Mattia AR, Ferry JA, Harris NL. Breast lymphoma: a B-cell spectrum including the low grade B-cell lymphoma of mucosa associated lymphoid tissue. *Am J Surg Pathol* 1993;17:574–587.
259. Brogi E, Harris NL. Lymphomas of the breast: pathology and clinical behavior. *Semin Oncol* 1999;26:357–364.
260. Lin JJ, Farha GJ, Taylor RJ. Pseudolymphoma of the breast: I. In a study of 8,654 consecutive tylectomies and mastectomies. *Cancer* 1980;45:973–978.
261. Schwartz IS, Strauchen JA. Lymphocytic mastopathy: an autoimmune disease of the breast? *Am J Clin Pathol* 1990;93:725–730.
262. Lammie GA, Bobrow LG, Staunton MDM, et al. Sclerosing lymphocytic lobulitis of the breast: evidence for an autoimmune pathogenesis. *Histopathology* 1991;19:13–20.
263. Tomaszewski JE, Brooks JSJ, Hicks D, et al. Diabetic mastopathy: a distinctive clinicopathologic entity. *Hum Pathol* 1992;23:780–786.
264. Ha CS, Dubey P, Goyal LK, et al. Localized primary non-Hodgkin's lymphoma of the breast. *Am J Clin Oncol* 1998;21:376–380.
265. Ohsawa M, Tomita Y, Hashimoto M, et al. Malignant lymphoma of the adrenal gland: its possible correlation with the Epstein-Barr virus. *Mod Pathol* 1996;9:534–543.
266. Pawade J, Lee CS, Ellis DW, et al. Primary lymphoma of the ampulla of Vater. *Cancer* 1994;73:2083–2086.
267. Ohsawa M, Mishima K, Suzuki A, et al. Malignant lymphoma of the urethra: report of a case with detection of Epstein-Barr virus genome in the tumour cells. *Histopathology* 1994;24:525–529.
268. Eusebi V, Bondi A, Cancellieri A, et al. Primary malignant lymphoma of sciatic nerve: report of a case. *Am J Surg Pathol* 1990;14:881–885.
269. Schild SE, Wharen RE, Menke DM, et al. Primary lymphoma of the spinal cord. *Mayo Clin Proc* 1995;70:256–260.
270. Ceresoli GL, Ferreri AJM, Bucci E, et al. Primary cardiac lymphoma in immunocompetent patients: diagnostic and therapeutic management. *Cancer* 1997;80:1497–1506.
271. Gill PS, Chandraratna AN, Meyer PR, et al. Malignant lymphoma: cardiac involvement at initial presentation. *J Clin Oncol* 1987;5: 216–224.
272. Nador RG, Cesarman E, Chadburn A, et al. Primary effusion lymphoma: a distinct clinicopathologic entity associated with the Kaposi's sarcoma–associated herpesvirus. *Blood* 1996;88:645–656.
273. Martin A, Capron F, Liguory-Brunaud M-D, et al. Epstein-Barr virus-associated primary malignant lymphomas of the pleural cavity occurring in longstanding pleural chronic inflammation. *Hum Pathol* 1994; 25:1314–1318.
274. Aozasa K. Pyothorax-associated lymphoma. *Int J Hematol* 1996;65: 9–16.
275. Cesarman E, Nador RG, Aozasa K, et al. Kaposi's sarcoma-associated herpesvirus in non-AIDS–related lymphomas occurring in body cavities. *Am J Pathol* 1996;149:53–57.
276. Osborne BM, Butler JJ, Guarda LA. Primary lymphoma of the liver: ten cases and a review of the literature. *Cancer* 1985;56:2902–2910.
277. Ryan J, Straus DJ, Lange C, et al. Primary lymphoma of the liver. *Cancer* 1988;61:370–375.
278. Harris AC, Ben-Ezra JM, Contos MJ, et al. Malignant lymphoma can present as hepatobiliary disease. *Cancer* 1996;78:2011–2019.
279. Ohsawa M, Tomita Y, Hashimoto M, et al. Hepatitis C virus genome in a subset of primary hepatic lymphomas. *Mod Pathol* 1998;11: 471–478.
280. Ferry JA, Harris NL, Papanicolaou N, et al. Lymphoma of the kidney: a report of 11 cases. *Am J Surg Pathol* 1995;19:134–144.
281. Okuno SH, Hoyer JD, Ristow K, et al. Primary renal non-Hodgkin's lymphoma: an unusual extranodal site. *Cancer* 1995;75:2258–2261.
282. Pawade J, Banerjee SS, Harris M, et al. Lymphomas of mucosa-associated lymphoid tissue arising in the urinary bladder. *Histopathology* 1993;23:147–151.
283. Kempton CL, Kurtin PJ, Inwards DJ, et al. Malignant lymphoma of the bladder: evidence from 36 cases that low-grade lymphoma of the MALT-type is the most common primary bladder lymphoma. *Am J Surg Pathol* 1997;21:1324–1333.
284. Bostwick DG, Iczkowski KA, Amin MB, et al. Malignant lymphoma involving the prostate: report of 62 cases. *Cancer* 1998;83:732–738.
285. Lyons MK, O'Neill BP, Kurtin PJ, et al. Diagnosis and management of primary spinal epidural non-Hodgkin's lymphoma. *Mayo Clin Proc* 1996;71:453–457.
286. Schwechheimer K, Hashemian A, Ott G, et al. Primary spinal epidural manifestation of malignant lymphoma. *Histopathology* 1996;29: 265–269.
287. Morgan K, MacLennan KA, Narual A, et al. Non-Hodgkin's lymphoma of the larynx (stage IE). *Cancer* 1989;64:1123–1127.
288. Lanham GR, Weiss SW, Enzinger FM. Malignant lymphoma: a study of 75 cases presenting in soft tissue. *Am J Surg Pathol* 1989;13:1–10.
289. Salomao DR, Nascimento AG, Lloyd RV, et al. Lymphoma in soft tissue: a clinicopathologic study of 19 cases. *Hum Pathol* 1996:27: 253–257.
290. d'Amore ESG, Wick MR, Geisinger KR, et al. Primary malignant lymphoma arising in postmastectomy lymphedema: another facet of the Stewart-Treves syndrome. *Am J Surg Pathol* 1990;14:456–463.
291. Siegel RJ, Napoli VM. Malignant lymphoma of the urinary bladder:

a case with signet-ring cells simulating urachal adenocarcinoma. *Arch Pathol Lab Med* 1991;115:635–637.
292. Zukerberg LR, Harris NL, Young RL. Carcinomas of the urinary bladder simulating malignant lymphoma: a report of five cases. *Am J Surg Pathol* 1991;15:569–576.
293. Perrone T, Frizzera G, Rosai J. Mediastinal diffuse large-cell lymphoma with sclerosis: a morphologic and immunologic study of 60 cases. *Am J Surg Pathol* 1986;10:176–191.
294. Aisenberg AC. Primary large cell lymphoma of the mediastinum. *Semin Oncol* 1999;26:251–258.
295. Yamasaki S, Matsushita H, Tanimura S, et al. B-cell lymphoma of mucosa-associated lymphoid tissue of the thymus: a report of two cases with a background of Sjögren's syndrome and monoclonal gammopathy. *Hum Pathol* 1998;29:1021–1024.
296. Kaplan MA, Pettit CL, Zukerberg LR, et al. Primary lymphoma of the trachea with morphologic and immunophenotypic characteristics of low-grade B-cell lymphoma of mucosa-associated lymphoid tissue. *Am J Surg Pathol* 1992;16:71–75.
297. Isaacson PG, Banks PM, Best PV, et al. Primary low-grade hepatic B-cell lymphoma of mucosa-associated lymphoid tissue (MALT)-type. *Am J Surg Pathol* 1995;19:571–575.
298. Wick MR, Mills SE. Intravascular lymphomatosis: clinicopathologic features and differential diagnosis. *Semin Diagn Pathol* 1991;8:91–101.

CHAPTER 37

Bone Marrow Specimen Processing

LoAnn C. Peterson and Richard D. Brunning

The techniques used to obtain and process bone marrow biopsies are critical to the evaluation of these specimens. A major emphasis in bone marrow pathology is the study of cytologic detail, which can only be accomplished with optimal processing of an adequate biopsy specimen. An artifactually distorted or inadequate biopsy or improper processing can lead to serious difficulties in interpretation and possibly to erroneous conclusions. Because the bone marrow specimen optimally includes the trephine biopsy and the fluid aspiration, this chapter describes processing of both components of the bone marrow specimen.

PROCUREMENT OF THE SPECIMEN

Several instruments are available for procuring bone marrow biopsy specimens; the most widely used are patterned on the needle introduced by Jamshidi and Swaim in 1971 (1). These needles are available in several sizes designed for adult and pediatric patients and in disposable and reusable types. They yield high-quality specimens and have a wide margin of safety when properly used. Biopsy with these instruments involves relatively little discomfort to the patient if careful attention is given to accurate positioning of the needle and infiltration of the biopsy site with local anesthetic. Proper use cannot be overemphasized; improper technique often results in increased discomfort for the patient and poor-quality biopsy specimens. If a patient experiences severe discomfort during the initial part of the biopsy procedure, the needle may be misdirected and should be withdrawn. The effectiveness of the local anesthetic should also be reevaluated before redirecting the needle. Detailed instructions for use of these needles are provided in the manufacturers' brochures.

The posterior superior iliac spine is the most common biopsy site for trephine biopsies in adults and children. This site provides a large area for placement of the needle and access to the medullary cavity. The posterior superior iliac spine is relatively remote from vital areas, minimizing the potential for complications. It is desirable to obtain the trephine biopsy before the fluid portion of the marrow is aspirated. Aspirating marrow with the trephine biopsy needle and then advancing the needle for the biopsy, a procedure advocated by some, may result in hemorrhage into the area of the biopsy site, leading to difficulties in interpretation.

The optimal size of a trephine biopsy is at least 1.0 to 2.0 cm; specimens should be free of distortion and crush artifact. Before placing the biopsy in fixative, several touch imprint preparations should be made for routine Wright-Giemsa staining and other procedures, such as cytochemistry and immunocytochemistry. Less damage to the biopsy specimen results when the imprint is made by gently touching a glass slide to the specimen rather than by squeezing the specimen with a forceps and touching it to a slide. The imprint preparations of the biopsy occasionally may serve as the single most important resource for the evaluation of cytologic, cytochemical, and immunocytochemical characteristics.

After obtaining the trephine biopsy, the aspiration is performed through a separate puncture; aspiration needles, such as the Illinois needle or modifications of this instrument, are ideal for aspiration of the fluid portion of the specimen and cause less discomfort to the patient than the larger trephine biopsy needles. The aspiration needle can be inserted through the same skin incision used for the trephine biopsy and placed on the periosteal surface at a distance of approximately 1 cm from the trephine biopsy site. Approximately 1.0 mL of fluid should be aspirated for morphologic studies. Additional fluid should be aspirated for other studies including cytogenetic analysis, immunophenotyping by flow cytometry, and molecular studies, as indicated.

FIXATION AND PROCESSING OF THE TREPHINE BIOPSY

Several choices of fixative (2) are available for bone marrow trephine biopsies. Because of the overriding importance

L. C. Peterson: Department of Pathology, Northwestern University Medical School, Chicago, Illinois 60611

R. D. Brunning: Department of Laboratory Medicine and Pathology, University of Minnesota, Minneapolis, Minnesota 55455

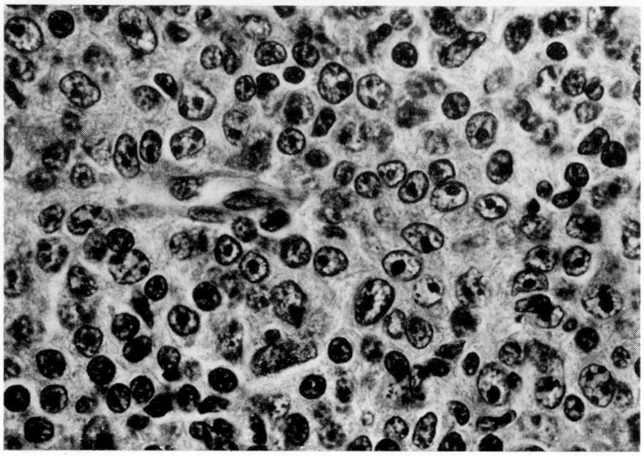

FIG. 37.1. Bone marrow trephine biopsy from a patient with B-cell chronic lymphocytic leukemia with proliferation centers. There are numerous prolymphocytoid cells with single prominent nucleoli and small lymphocytes with condensed chromatin without evident nucleoli. This biopsy was fixed in Zenker's fixative (hematoxylin and eosin stain).

of cytologic detail (Fig. 37.1) in the evaluation of hematopoietic tumors, the choice of fixative is one of the most crucial steps in the processing of marrow biopsies. In laboratories that are dedicated to the processing of hematopoietic tissues, the mercury-based fixatives are generally preferred. In laboratories in which bone marrow biopsies are processed with other tissues, neutral buffered formalin is sometimes used. Because of restrictions on the disposal of mercury-based fixatives such as Zenker's and B5 solutions, neutral buffered formalin or other fixatives such as zinc-formalin are being increasingly used. A core biopsy of 1 to 2 cm in length should be placed in approximately 15 to 20 mL of fixative.

B5, a mercury-based fixative, is prepared by mixing 45 mL of B5 base solution with 5 mL of 37% formaldehyde immediately before use. The optimal fixation period for bone marrow biopsies in B5 is 2 to 4 hours; specimens exposed to B5 for longer than 6 hours may become hard and brittle resulting in difficulty in sectioning.

Zenker's is prepared by adding 5 mL of glacial acetic acid to 95 mL of stock Zenker's solution. The solution should be prepared each day. The biopsy should be allowed to fix in the Zenker's for a minimum of 4 hours; overnight and over the weekend fixation in Zenker's has no adverse effect on the tissue. Specimens in neutral buffered formalin should be in fixative for at least 18 to 24 hours. Specimens in zinc-formalin should be fixed for 3 to 4 hours.

The following steps in the processing of marrow trephine biopsies are generally applicable to tissues fixed in the above fixatives. After removal from the fixative, use the following procedure:

1. Decalcify for a period appropriate to the size of the biopsy. Decalcification in RDO (APB Engineering Products Corporation, Plainfield, IL 60544), a commercially available dilute solution of hydrochloric acid in coal tar base, gives satisfactory results within 30 to 60 minutes. Decalcification in Surgipath decalcifier (Surgipath Medical Industries, Grayslake, IL 60030) for 90 minutes or in a hydrochloric acid (HCl) and formic acid solution for 2 hours is also satisfactory.
2. Wash 60 to 90 minutes with several changes of water. Avoid washing in running tap water because this may damage the specimen.
3. Process tissue in automatic tissue processor.
4. Embed in paraffin or Surgipath embedding medium.
5. The biopsies should be sectioned at 3 to 4 μm with a knife blade that is free of defects. If the biopsy is performed for determination of marrow involvement by lymphoma, metastatic tumor, granulomatous inflammation, or other process that may be focal, it is advantageous to section the biopsy completely with step-wise mounting of serial sections.

The hematoxylin and eosin (H&E) stain is the most widely used routine stain for bone marrow trephine biopsies. It is familiar to pathologists and yields the most information. Several other stains are important in diagnostic hematopathology and, although not used for all specimens, are applied with sufficient frequency to be detailed. These are the periodic acid–Schiff (PAS) and Giemsa stains and stains for reticulin and collagen. PAS stain is useful in the identification of maturing granulocytes and megakaryocytes and may also be used as an initial screening procedure for the detection of fungal organisms. The Giemsa stain may be used to accentuate granules in maturing neutrophils, eosinophils and basophils; it also highlights the mast cells in the lesions of mastocytosis. The reticulin and the collagen stains are used to determine the degree of fibrosis in marrow sections. The reticulin stain is invaluable for demonstrating an increase in reticulin fibers. Frank collagen fibrosis is uncommon in hematopoietic disorders but occurs frequently in marrows involved by metastatic tumor.

PROCESSING THE BONE MARROW ASPIRATION SPECIMEN

Various techniques can be used to prepare satisfactory smears of the aspirated portion of the bone marrow specimen (3). This chapter discusses three common methods used in making smears, and using more than one of these techniques for an individual case can optimize the available material for examination. The three methods are direct smears of the aspirate, buffy coat smears from a centrifuged, anticoagulated aspirate, and particle crush smears of particles from the aspirate. Techniques for making particle clot sections are also included in this section.

Direct smears of the bone marrow aspirate should be made as soon as possible before clotting occurs. One drop of the marrow aspirate is placed at one end of a slide and smeared with a pusher slide, as illustrated in Figure 37.2. The smear is immediately air dried. These smears, which are free of

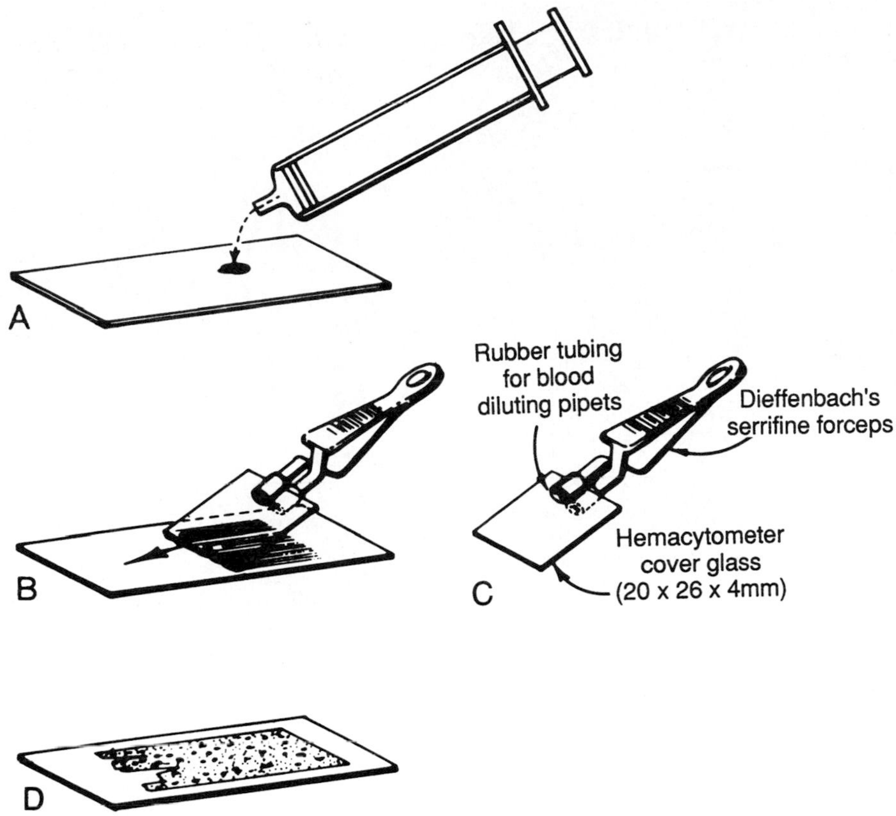

FIG. 37.2. **A:** A single drop of the marrow aspirate from the syringe is placed on a clean slide. **B:** The drop is smeared by using a pusher slide. **C:** The pusher slide is prepared by placing a hemacytometer coverglass held in a Dieffenbach's serrefine forceps. **D:** The result is a thin smear that is narrower than the width of the slide. The slide should be dried immediately after being made.

anticoagulant artifact and result in well-spaced cells, usually result in excellent preservation of nuclear and cytoplasmic detail. Several slides can be prepared from each aspirate.

When making *buffy coat smears,* most of the aspirated fluid is transferred immediately from the syringe to a paraffin-coated vial that contains powdered disodium EDTA (about 1 mg/1 mL of fluid marrow); the vial is inverted gently several times to ensure mixing of the fluid with the anticoagulant. The smaller portion (about 0.1 mL) of the specimen remaining in the syringe can be used to make direct smears. The anticoagulated specimen should be transferred as soon as possible after aspiration to the laboratory for processing. On arrival, the specimen is poured into a clean glass Petri dish; the fluid from the specimen is then aspirated into a Pasteur pipette and transferred to a Wintrobe hematocrit tube. The particles that remain in the Petri dish after this step can be used for two purposes: particle crush preparations and particle sections.

The Wintrobe tube containing the aspirate is centrifuged at 850 *g* (2,800 rpm) for 8 minutes in a table-top centrifuge. After centrifugation of the aspirated fluid, the marrow specimen is layered into four major components, the relative amounts of which can be determined from the markings on the Wintrobe tube. The four layers (Fig. 37.3), from top to bottom, are as follows:

1. Fat and perivascular (F-PV) layer
2. Plasma (P) layer
3. Myeloid-erythroid (M-E) layer, which is essentially the buffy coat of nucleated cells of the bone marrow
4. Erythrocyte (E) layer.

The relative proportion of the F-PV and M-E layers usually reflects the cellularity of the marrow. The F-PV layer from a normal marrow is usually 1% to 3%, and the M-E layer is 5% to 8%. An increase in the M-E layer and a decrease in the F-PV layer usually reflects marrow hypercellularity (Fig. 37.4). An increase in the F-PV layer and a decrease in the M-E layer indicates a hypocellular marrow (Fig. 37.5). A marrow aspirate diluted with sinusoidal blood is reflected by a decrease in the F-PV and M-E layers.

After examination of the individual layers, the F-PV component is gently aspirated from the Wintrobe tube with a pipette and can be smeared onto one to three slides. Because of the rich component of macrophages in the perivascular tissue, these preparations are ideal for staining with Prussian blue for the evaluation of iron stores. Using a clean pipette, the P layer is then aspirated and set aside in a 12 $\times$ 75 mm tube. The M-E (buffy coat) layer is then aspirated from the tube and transferred onto a clean watch glass. A small portion of the plasma is then added to the M-E layer in a portion

A 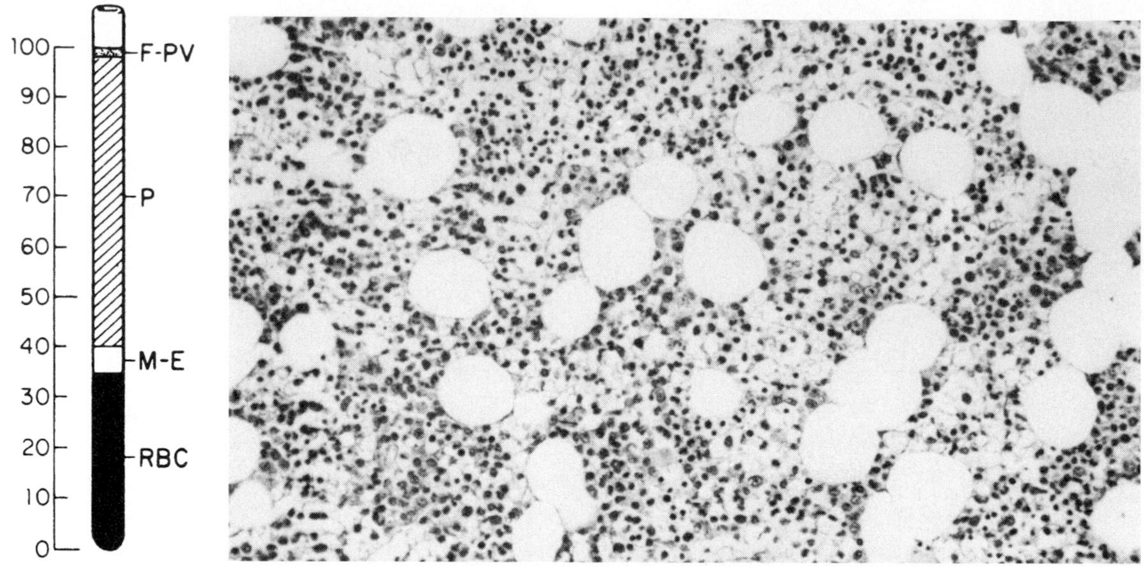 B

FIG. 37.3. A: Normal anticoagulated bone marrow specimen after centrifugation in a Wintrobe tube. The fat and perivascular (F-PV) layer is approximately 1% to 3%. The myeloid-erythroid (M-E) or nucleated cell layer is approximately 5% to 8%. **B:** The cellularity of the marrow as shown in the trephine biopsy from the patient is within normal limits for an adult.

equal to twice the volume of the M-E layer. These two layers are then mixed thoroughly but gently. Using a Pasteur pipette, one drop of this mixture is then placed on a slide and smeared using a second pusher slide (Fig. 37.2); the slides are immediately air dried. Approximately 10 to 15 slides can be prepared if sufficient specimen is available.

Particle crush smears are made from the particles in the bone marrow aspirate. The smears are made by picking up and gently crushing particles between two slides with a small amount of liquid from the aspirate. Using a flat, push-pull motion for smear preparation ensures that most cellular elements remain intact. The slides are immediately air dried.

A 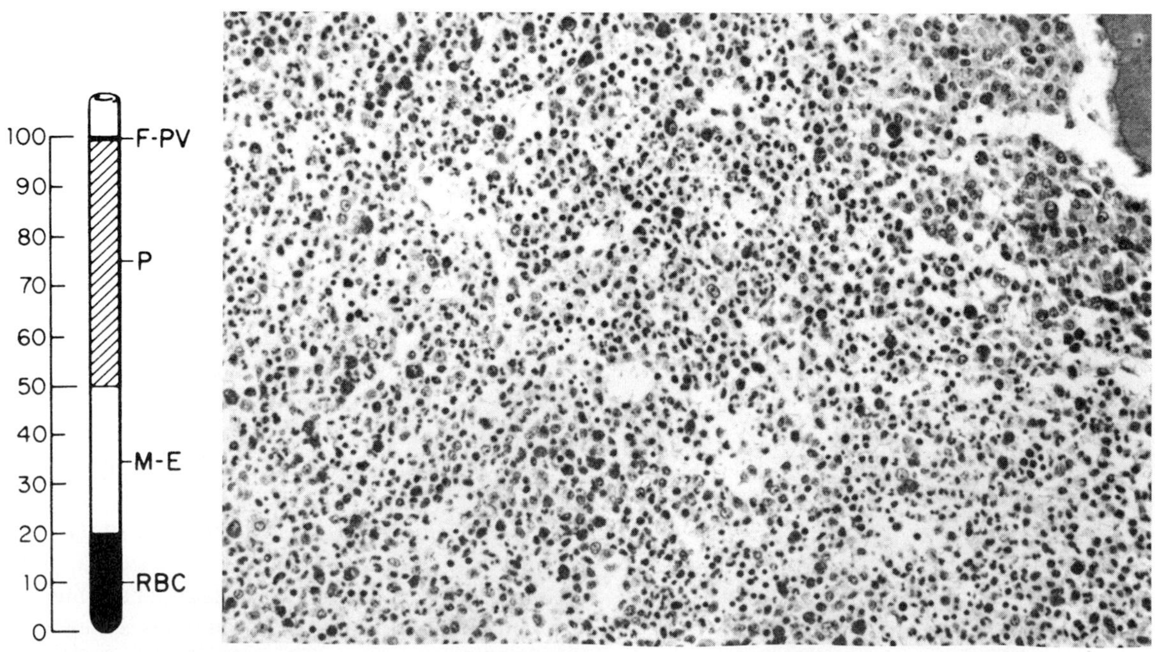 B

FIG. 37.4. A: Spun anticoagulated marrow specimen from a patient who has a hypercellular marrow showing a fat and perivascular (F-PV) layer of approximately 1% and a myeloid-erythroid (M-E) layer of 30%, indicating a hypercellular specimen. **B:** The marrow trephine biopsy from this patient confirms the hypercellularity.

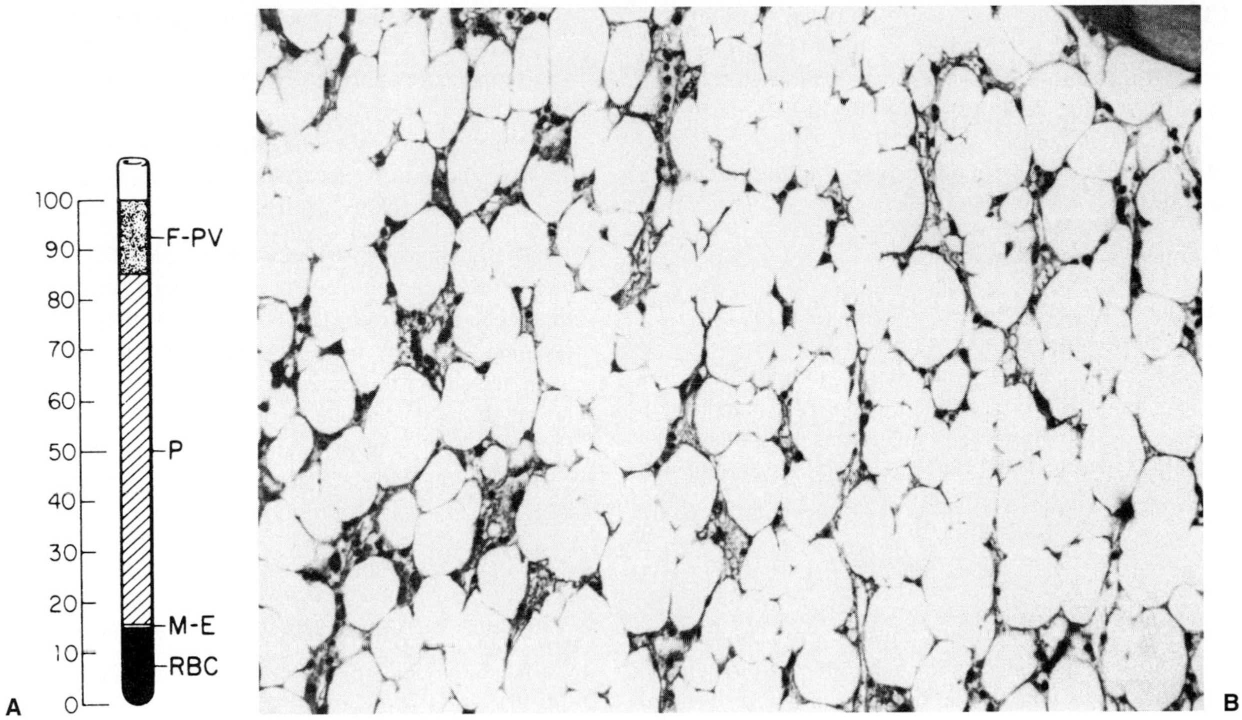

FIG. 37.5. A: Spun anticoagulated marrow specimen shows a marked increase in the fat and perivascular (F-PV) layer and a marked decrease in the myeloid-erythroid (M-E) layer, suggesting a hypocellular marrow. **B:** This suspicion was confirmed by the trephine biopsy specimen.

Particle clot sections are made by aggregating the remaining particles and placing them into a fixative. If the specimen is anticoagulated, clotting of the particles is aided by the addition of 2 to 3 drops of 0.015 M $CaCl_2$. With the exception of the decalcification step, these particles are processed and cut into sections similar to the trephine biopsy.

Air dried smears are routinely stained using a Romanowsky-type stain. Iron stains are also performed, as indicated. An adequate number of slides should be reserved for any cytochemical and immunocytochemical reactions that are appropriate to the disease process.

STANDARD STAINING PROCEDURES

Gill's Hematoxylin and Eosin Stain

Gill's procedure for the H&E stain (4) may be used for bone marrow biopsies in all fixatives, but if a non–mecuric-based fixative is used, omit steps 5 and 6. Alternatively, automated stainers may be used for H&E staining. Put mounted sections in a 58°C to 62°C oven for 40 minutes, cool, and then process:

1. Xylol: two changes, 3 to 5 minutes each.
2. 100% alcohol: two changes, 3 to 5 minutes each.
3. 95% alcohol: two changes, 3 to 5 minutes each.
4. 70% alcohol: 3 to 5 minutes.
5. Dilute alcohol solution of iodine: 10 minutes (medium amber color of iodine solution in 70% alcohol).
6. 5% aqueous solution of sodium thiosulfate: 10 minutes.
7. Wash in running tap water for 5 to 10 minutes.
8. Bluing solution: 1 minute.
9. Deionized H_2O: two changes, 10 dips each.
10. Gill's hematoxylin: 5 minutes for particles and 10 to 15 minutes for trephine biopsies. Some trephine sections require a longer staining time.
11. Rinse in running water for 5 minutes.
12. Differentiate in diluted acid alcohol with one dip.
13. Rinse in two changes of tap or deionized water.
14. Wash in running tap water for at least 20 minutes.
15. Bluing solution: 2 minutes and two changes deionized H_2O, 10 dips each.
16. 70% alcohol: 3 to 5 minutes; check intensity of hematoxylin color, and if the hematoxylin is too light, place back into the water for 2 minutes and hematoxylin for 10 to 20 minutes or longer. Then repeat steps 11 to 16. If the stain is too dark, repeat steps 12 to 16.
17. Stain with eosin for 2 to 5 seconds, depending on the age of the eosin, dilution of the solution, and intensity of counterstain desired. Dip several times before allowing them to remain in solution. Usually, formalin and B5 fixatives need a longer time in eosin.
18. 70% alcohol: two to three changes, 4 dips each.
19. 95% alcohol: two changes, 15 dips each.
20. 100% alcohol: two changes, 3 to 5 minutes each.
21. 100% alcohol plus equal amount of xylol: 3 to 5 minutes.
22. Xylol: three changes, 3 to 5 minutes each (or longer).

Check eosin in the first xylol solution. If too light, dip back through the solutions of eosin, and repeat steps 17 to 22. If the stain is too dark, dip back through solutions to the first 95% alcohol step (or 70% if very dark), and repeat steps 19 to 22.

23. Mount with Permount or other solvent-soluble mounting medium.

Solutions include the following:

Acid alcohol: 1% HCl in 70% alcohol (950 mL of 70% ethanol and 9.5 mL of concentrated HCl)
Dilute acid alcohol: 1% HCl mixed 1 : 1 with 70% alcohol
Bluing reagent (0.2% sodium bicarbonate, 1.0% magnesium sulfate): 2 g of sodium bicarbonate plus 10 g of magnesium sulfate, diluted to 1,000 mL with deionized or distilled water.

Wright-Giemsa Stain

For air-dried smears and touch imprints, a Romanovsky staining procedure yields consistently high-quality cellular detail and clear distinction of each cell type, which is essential for bone marrow interpretation (Fig. 37.6). High-quality staining can be obtained with Wright-Giemsa stain using a rack or dip method. The dip method can be performed manually or can be automated. Automated stainers using previously made stains are also widely available. If these are used, careful attention should be given to the quality and consistency of the stain on bone marrow smears.

The staining procedure uses the dip method:

1. Fix slides in absolute methanol for 2 minutes.
2. Quickly blot off excess methanol and stain slides with Wright-Giemsa stock solution for 4 to 5 minutes.
3. Stain slides in the freshly prepared Wright-Giemsa/buffer working solution for 20 to 30 minutes.

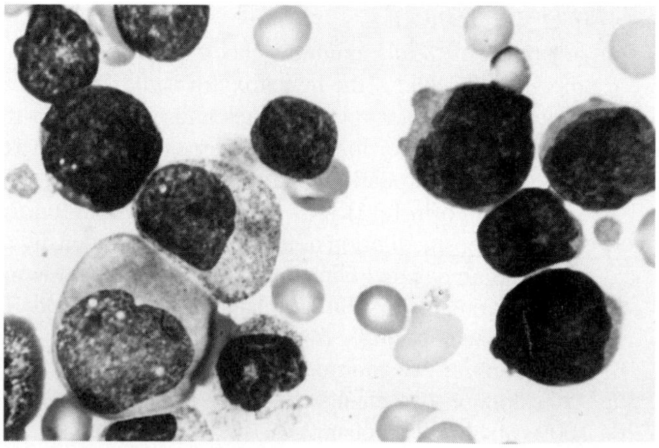

FIG. 37.6. Bone marrow smear from a patient with follicular center cell lymphoma. The lymphoma cells are intermixed with normal myeloid cells (Wright-Geimsa stain).

4. Quickly dip slides in a freshly prepared solution of 50% methanol.
5. Immediately rinse through three changes of deionized water.
6. Wipe the back of each slide with methanol soaked gauze to remove any excess stain if necessary and place into a vertical rack to air dry.

The staining intensity may be increased or decreased by altering the staining time. If the red cells appear too blue or the nuclei appear too deeply stained, it may be because of prolonged staining time, inadequate rinsing or excessively alkaline stain or buffer. Excessive redness in the slides may be caused by inadequate staining time, excessive rinsing, or increased acidity of the stain or buffer.

Several solutions are needed. Use the following for the Wright-Giemsa stock solution:

15.8 g of Wright stain (powder)
0.35 g of Giemsa stain (powder)
3,500 mL of absolute methanol (acetone free).

Mix the powdered Wright and Giemsa stains in a 2000-mL Erlenmeyer flask. Add 250 mL of methanol to the stain using 50-mL aliquots, mixing well between each addition. Transfer the solution into a brown glass jug. Use additional 125-mL aliquots of methanol to rinse any remaining stain from the flask and transfer to the jug. Add any remaining methanol directly to the brown jug. Place the 4-L jug onto a magnetic stirrer, and allow the stain to mix for approximately 2 hours. Transfer the staining solution to a 37°C incubator for 24 hours. Allow the stain to remix on the magnetic stirrer for approximately 2 hours. Store at room temperature. Filter before use.

Use the following for the phosphate buffer (pH 6.4):

23.1 g of KH_2PO_4
9.1 g of Na_2HPO_4
3,500 mL of deionized water.

Combine the KH_2PO_4 and Na_2HPO_4 in a clean plastic jug. Add 3,500 mL of deionized water, and mix well to dissolve. Store at room temperature.

Use the following for the Wright-Giemsa/buffer working solution:

Wright/Giemsa stock stain, 5 mL
Giemsa stain (original azure blend), 5 mL
Phosphate buffer (pH 6.4), 40 mL.

Mix well before use. Discard after 1 hour.

Iron Stain

The iron stain (5,6) can be used for air-dried smears using the following procedure:

1. Air-dried smears of peripheral blood or bone marrow are fixed with absolute methanol for 15 to 20 minutes.
2. Incubate the slides for 10 minutes in a 1% potassium

ferrocyanide solution at 50°C to 56°C. (*Note:* Excessive heat or prolonged incubation can alter the reaction.)

3. Rinse with distilled or deionized water, wash in running tap water for 20 minutes, and rinse again in distilled or deionized water. Do not dry. Drying before the counterstain may cause artifact.
4. Weakly counterstain with 0.1% aqueous safranin or 0.1% aqueous eosin for 5 to 10 seconds. Safranin is preferred.
5. Rinse briefly with distilled or deionized water. Air dry. Coverslip with a solvent-soluble mounting medium if desired. (*Note:* A smear with a previously determined increase in siderocytes or sideroblasts should be processed as a control with each batch of slides.)

The iron stain can be used for smears of fat and the perivascular layer using the following procedure:

1. Air dry the specimen.
2. Fix with formalin by allowing to stand in weak formalin vapors (10% formalin) for 10 minutes. A piece of filter paper is placed in the top of a Coplin jar, and one drop of 10% formalin is placed on the filter paper. The cover is replaced and the slides are allowed to fix in the formalin vapor for 10 minutes. Do not wash. Excess formalin causes black granular precipitate.
3. Immerse in Prussian blue reagent.
4. Wash thoroughly with deionized or distilled water and then with running tap water for 2 minutes. Air dry.
5. Coverslip with Permount or other solvent-soluble mounting medium if desired. Do not put oil directly on noncoverslipped preparations. The tissue on the slide is removed when xylol is used to remove oil.

The iron stain can be used for sections using the following procedure:

1. Deparaffinize the slide and bring to distilled or deionized water. Run Zenker's solution–fixed tissue through iodine and sodium thiosulfate in the usual manner.
2. Stain for 30 minutes with the Prussian blue reagent.
3. Wash in distilled or deionized water and then with running tap water for 20 minutes.
4. Counterstain with eosin for 8 to 10 seconds.
5. Dehydrate through 70%, 95%, and 100% ethanol to xylol.
6. Coverslip with Permount or other solvent-soluble mounting medium.

Iron may be leached out of the sections during the decalcification procedure. As a result of this procedure, diffuse and particulate iron in all specimens is colored a vivid blue or blue-green.

Solutions include the following:

2% potassium ferrocyanide (crystals). This solution is good for 1 week and should be stored in the dark. The solution is a pale to moderate yellow.

0.5% HCl

1% potassium ferrocyanide. Mix equal volumes of 2% potassium ferrocyanide and 0.2 N HCl (30 mL of each for Coplin jar). The solution of 1% potassium ferrocyanide should be made up just before using and can be used only once. The solution is a pale yellow.

Prussian blue reagent. Mix 15 mL of 2% potassium ferrocyanide and 45 mL 0.5% HCl (1:3 mixture) for 10 minutes. This solution is good for 1 hour.

Giemsa Stain for Sections

Giemsa stain can be used for sections (4) using the following procedure:

1. Process the biopsy as for H&E through step 7.
2. Place slides into Giemsa stain immediately after making the solution. Leave sections 2 to 4 hours (or overnight) in the staining solution.
3. Place sections individually into deionized or distilled water for 8 to 10 dips.
4. Differentiate each slide individually in 95% ethyl alcohol for 2 quick dips. Section should turn a purplish pink color. (*Note:* 95% ethyl alcohol is preferred to the originally described solution of 95% ethyl alcohol plus a few drops of 10% rosin solution in absolute alcohol.)
5. Dehydrate sections in absolute alcohol for three to four quick dips.
6. Clear in xylol, and mount in solvent-soluble mounting medium.

If the sections are not differentiated enough, dip quickly back through the alcohols to water and then back through the alcohols to xylol. If overdifferentiated (i.e., too light), slides must go back to water and then into fresh Giemsa solution for 2 to 4 hours.

Solutions include the following:

Giemsa stain stock solution: Dissolve 0.5 g of powdered Giemsa's blood stain in 33 mL of glycerin at 55°C to 60°C for 1.5 to 2 hours. Add 33 mL of absolute methanol, and filter the solution.

Working solution (make fresh each time): 1.25 mL of stock Giemsa stain, 1.5 mL of methanol, and 50 mL of deionized water.

Periodic Acid–Schiff Reaction

The PAS stain (4) can be used for sections with the following procedure:

1. Remove paraffin from sections in usual manner, and take the slides through the alcohols to distilled or deionized water. Run Zenker's- or B5-fixed tissue through iodine and sodium thiosulfate in the usual manner.
2. Place slides in 0.5% periodic acid for 5 minutes. The periodic acid can be reused the same day.
3. Wash for 5 minutes in running water.

4. Stain for 30 minutes in Schiff reagent. This solution may be used several times during the day but should be prepared fresh each day.
5. Wash in tap water in a staining dish for 5 to 10 minutes.
6. Rinse in distilled or deionized water. (*Note:* For section counterstain see step 7 below; for smear counterstain, see step 4 under smear procedures.)
7. Counterstain with hematoxylin for 8 minutes.
8. Wash in running water for 5 minutes.
9. Agitate up and down in acid alcohol (1% hydrochloric acid in 70% ethanol) for 4 to 5 seconds.
10. Wash in running water for 10 minutes.
11. 95% alcohol: 2 minutes, two changes.
12. 100% alcohol: 2 minutes, two changes.
13. 100% alcohol plus equal amount of xylol: 2 minutes.
14. Xylol: 2 minutes, three changes.
15. Mount with Permount or other solvent-soluble mounting medium.

The PAS stain can be used for smears using the following procedure:

1. Fix smear in strong formalin fumes for 10 minutes; allow slides to air dry; and wipe off excess formalin.
2. Place in methanol for 10 minutes.
3. Rinse in running water for 10 minutes, and place into 0.5% periodic acid solution. Process in same manner as sections until counterstain. See step 2 in the previous list.
4. Counterstain with hematoxylin for 6 to 8 minutes.
5. Rinse in running water for 5 to 10 minutes.
6. Rinse in distilled or deionized water, and air dry.
7. Cover slip with Permount or other solvent-soluble mounting medium.

The results of PAS staining differ according to the substrate:

Glycogen: dark red to purple
Amyloid: light red
Mucin: dark red to purple
Fibrinoid: red
Some fungi: red
Basement membrane and reticulin: red
Loose collagen: light red
Nuclei: blue.

The solutions include Schiff reagent and periodic acid. For the Schiff reagent

Combine 32.0 g of basic fuchsin (pararosanilin) 60.8 g of sodium metabisulfite, 480 mL of 1 N hydrochloric acid, 2,720 mL of distilled or deionized water.
Mix on magnetic stirrer for 2 to 3 hours.
Add approximately 32 g of fresh powdered decolorizing charcoal.
Mix on magnetic stirrer for about 1 hour.
Filter, using double thickness of extra fine filter paper.
Refrigerate.
The filtered solutions must be colorless or pale straw colored. Return of pink color is a sign of age. The solutions have a usable period of approximately 1 month.

For 0.5% periodic acid:

Combine 10 g of periodic acid with 2,000 mL of distilled or deionized water.
The solution is good for approximately 2 weeks.

Reticulin Stain

Reticulin stain (i.e., Wilder's stain) (3) can be used with the following procedure:

1. Process as for H&E through step 7.
2. Wash well in distilled or deionized water.
3. Phosphomolybdic acid solution for 1 minute; this should be prepared fresh each time.
4. Rinse well in running water for at least 1 minute.
5. Dip in 1% aqueous uranium nitrate for 1 minute or less.
6. Wash in distilled or deionized water for 10 to 20 seconds.
7. Place in ammoniacal silver solution for 1 minute.
8. Dip very quickly in 95% alcohol and go immediately to step 9.
9. Reducing solution for 1 minute.
10. Rinse well in distilled water; dip several times.
11. Tone in gold chloride solution for 30 seconds or until sections lose their yellow color and turn lavender. Too much toning makes sections red. Check individually under microscope.
12. Dip once or twice in distilled or deionized water and then check.
13. Place in 5% sodium thiosulfate solution for 5 minutes.
14. Wash well in tap water.
15. If desired, counterstain with nuclear fast red or 0.1% aqueous safranin for 3 to 5 seconds. Rinse well in distilled water.
16. Dehydrate in 70%, 95%, and 100% alcohols to xylol. Mount in Permount or other solvent-soluble mounting medium.

The results of reticulin staining differ according to the substrate:

Reticulin fibers: black
Collagen: rose
Other tissue elements: depends on counterstain used.

Solutions include the following:

Phosphomolybdic acid solution: Combine 10 g of phosphomolybdic acid (do not use metal spatula) and 100 mL of deionized water.The unused solution is good for 2 months; use fresh each time.
Uranium nitrate solution (1%): Combine 1.0 g of uranium nitrate and 100 mL of deionized water. Dispose of the

solution the same as radioactive waste. The solution is good for approximately 3 months.

Ammoniacal silver solution: To 5 mL of a 10.2% aqueous solution of silver nitrate add 28% ammonia water, drop by drop, until the precipitate that forms is almost dissolved. Add 5 mL of 3.1% sodium hydroxide, and dissolve the resulting precipitate with a few drops of ammonia water. Make the solution up to 50 mL with distilled or deionized water. For the 10.2% aqueous solution of silver nitrate (10.2 g of $AgNO_3$/100 mL of H_2O), combine 28% (concentrated) ammonia water and 3.1% sodium hydroxide. Use the solution at once.

Reducing solution: Combine 50.0 mL of deionized or distilled water, 0.5 mL of 40% neutral formaldehyde, calcium carbonate in excess (1 g/10 mL 40% formaldehyde), and 1.5 mL of a 1% aqueous solution of uranium nitrate. Dispose of this solution the same as for radioactive waste. Make this solution fresh just before use.

Gold chloride working solution: Combine 10 mL of 1% gold chloride solution and 40 mL of deionized or distilled water. Make this solution fresh each time.

Sodium thiosulfate (hypo) solution: Combine 5.0 g of sodium thiosulfate and 100 mL of deionized or distilled water.

Optional counterstain: nuclear fast red (kernechtrot) stain: Dissolve 0.1 g of nuclear fast red in 100 mL of a 5% solution of aluminum sulfate with the aid of heat. Cool, filter, and add a grain of thymol as a preservative.

Masson's Trichrome Stain for Collagen

Masson's trichrome stain can be used for collagen (4) with the following procedure:

1. Dehydrate sections to distilled or deionized water. Carry Zenker's- or B5-fixed tissue through sodium thiosulfate and iodine in the usual manner.
2. Mordant in Bouin's fixative for 1 hour at 56°C or overnight at room temperature. Do not reuse the solution.
3. Cool and wash in running water until the yellow color disappears. With bone marrow sections, the yellow disappears in 3 to 5 minutes; however, washing for at least 15 minutes is recommended (7).
4. Place in Weigert's iron hematoxylin solution for 10 minutes. Wash in running water for 10 minutes.
5. Rinse in distilled or deionized water.
6. Place in Biebrich scarlet–acid fuchsin solution for 15 seconds. If a more intense red stain is desired, the slides can be left in the solution longer. Save the solution.
7. Rinse in running water for 3 minutes, and then rinse with deionized or distilled water.
8. Place in aqueous phosphotungstic acid 5% for 5 minutes. Do not wash. Discard the solution.
9. Place in light green solution for 25 minutes. Save the solution.
10. Dip once quickly in distilled or deionized water.
11. Dip twice quickly in 1% acetic water. Discard the solution.
12. Dip two to three times in 95% alcohol.
13. Dip 4 to 5 times in absolute alcohol.
14. Place in xylene for two changes.
15. Mount in Permount or other organic solvent mounting media.

The results of Masson's trichrome staining differ according to the substrate:

Nuclei: black
Cytoplasm, keratin, muscle fibers, intracellular fibers: red
Collagen, mucus: blue or green

Solutions include the following:

Light green solution: Combine 5.0 g of light green, 250 mL of distilled or deionized water, and 2.0 mL of glacial acetic acid. Heat the water, dissolve the light green, filter, and add the acid. The stain is stable.

Acetic water solution (1%): Combine 1.0 mL of glacial acetic acid and 100 mL of distilled or deionized water.

Weigert's iron hematoxylin: For solution A, combine 1.0 g of hematoxylin and 100 mL of 95% alcohol. For solution B, combine 4.0 mL of 29% aqueous ferric chloride (which heats up and fumes when water is added), 95 mL of distilled or deionized water, and 1.0 mL of concentrated hydrochloric acid.

Working solution: Combine equal parts of solution A and solution B. Solutions A and B are stable and can be made up in larger quantities. The working solution is good for 3 weeks.

Biebrich scarlet–acid fuchsin solution: Combine 90 mL of 1% aqueous Biebrich scarlet, 10.0 mL of 1% aqueous acid fuchsin, and 1.0 mL of glacial acetic acid. The Biebrich scarlet is difficult to dissolve, but the completed stain is extremely stable.

IMMUNOHISTOCHEMISTRY

As in other disciplines of pathology, immunohistochemistry is used increasingly in the evaluation of bone marrow biopsies (8–13). Although immunohistochemistry is most commonly used for paraffin-embedded bone marrow trephine biopsies, this method can also be applied to other types of bone marrow specimens including plastic-embedded trephine biopsies, cryostat sections, air-dried smears, touch imprints, and cytospin preparations. The application of immunohistochemical methods has been facilitated by the commercial availability of monoclonal antibodies that react in paraffin-embedded biopsies. Immunostaining can be performed manually using commercially available kits or by using an automated immunochemistry instrument. Antigen retrieval methods such as microwave heat or enzyme treatment can be applied to the tissue to enhance reactivity with selected antigens (14,15). Each laboratory must determine the reactivity pattern of the various monoclonal antibodies in the specimens processed in that laboratory. Differences in fixatives and decalcification procedures may lead to different results from those published in the literature or specified by the manufacturer. The most common problem is the loss of antigen reactivity because of the type of fixative or decalcification solution. When a new antibody is introduced into a laboratory, the reactivity must be authenticated. This is accomplished by testing tissues of known antigenicity.

One of the most useful roles of immunocytochemistry for bone marrow sections is the application of antibodies to κ and λ light chains to determine relative proportions of κ and λ reacting cells in multiple myeloma and other lymphoproliferative disorders (16,17). Although the antibodies to κ and λ polypeptide chains react well in fixed, decalcified sections, the reactivity is usually restricted to cells that contain intracytoplasmic immunoglobulin such as plasma cells; the technique is generally not sufficiently sensitive to determine clonality in lymphoproliferative disorders characterized by the presence of only surface immunoglobulin. It is uncommon for the lymphocytes in a B-cell lymphoma to exhibit sufficient cytoplasmic immunoglobulin to be detected.

Several antibodies directed against lymphocyte-asssociated antigens such as CD20, a B-cell antigen (Fig. 37.7), and CD3, a marker of T cells, can be applied to bone marrow biopsies (8–11,18–20). These antibodies are discussed in Chapters 3 and 38. Other antibodies relevant to lymphoid processes in the bone marrow include those that react against protein products of lymphoid cells such as BCL-2 and cyclin D1 (21–23); enzymes, including terminal deoxynucleotidyl transferase (TdT) (24); activation markers such as CD30 (25); and nonlymphoid markers that may be expressed in lymphoid cells in specific diseases such as CD15 in the Reed-Sternberg cells in Hodgkin's disease. Immunohistochemistry using these antibodies has several applications: determining the immunophenotype of individual cells or the immunophenotypic profile of a proliferative process involving the bone marrow, evaluating the extent of marrow involvement, highlighting processes that may be difficult to identify on routinely stained sections (20,25,26), aiding in the classification of lymphoid lesions in the bone marrow (18–21), and evaluating the bone marrow for minimal residual disease after therapy (27) or early relapse (28). Because these antibodies are not a determinant of clonality, their utility in distinguishing a malignant from a reactive process is limited. The histologic pattern of the process and the morphology of the individual cells in the bone marrow sections must be used in conjunction with the antibody studies to distinguish a benign from a malignant process. It is also important that the immunophenotypic evaluation of a lymphoproliferative disorder include a panel of antibodies to other cell lineages and not just the suspected immunophenotype.

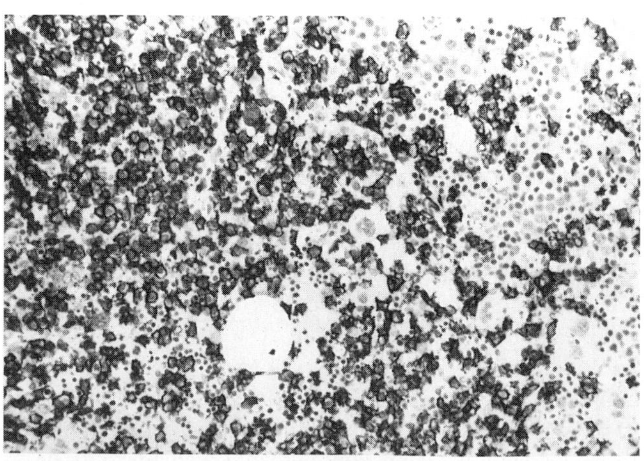

FIG. 37.7. Bone marrow biopsy from a patient with hairy cell leukemia reacted with antibody L26 (anti-CD20). The numerous hairy cells show intense reactivity. There are residual nonreacting normal hematopoietic cells, principally erythroid precursors (peroxidase–anti-peroxidase stain).

Antibodies reactive against myeloid cells in paraffin-embedded tissue are also applicable to bone marrow biopsies (29–31). Particularly useful antibodies are those to myeloperoxidase, lysozyme, and CD68. The antibody to myeloperoxidase reacts with neutrophils; antibodies to lysozyme and CD68 react with neutrophils and monocytes. A limitation of these antibodies is failure to react with myeloblasts in some cases of acute myeloblastic leukemia without maturation (M0 and M1). Antibodies to hemoglobin A can be used to identify the erythroblast series, although they may not react with very early erythroblasts. Antibodies to factor VIII antigen and CD41 can be used to highlight megakaryocytes; antibodies to factor VIII may not identify primitive megakaryocytes. Antibodies to CD34 highlight hematopoietic progenitor cells; this may aid in identifying blasts in acute leukemias in which the blasts express CD34 (28). Antibodies against tryptase are sensitive and specific markers for mast cells in bone marrow sections (30).

In addition to the antibodies to hematopoietic cells that are reactive with paraffin-embedded marrow biopsies, several antibodies are available that react with tumors that commonly metastasize to the bone marrow (32).

Additional aspects of cell markers, flow cytometry, and immunocytochemistry with relevance to bone marrow specimens are discussed in Chapters 3, 4, 5, 11, and 38.

PLASTIC EMBEDDING

Paraffin embedding is the most widely used routine method for the processing of bone marrow. In certain instances, when it is desirable to perform cytochemical reactions that are ablated in the decalcification process used for paraffin-embedded specimens, it may be preferable to use a plastic embedding procedure that bypasses decalcification or a decalcification process that uses a nonrapid acid decalcifier such as EDTA. Virtually any enzymatic reaction can be performed on plastic-embedded tissue if it is properly processed. The processing includes the avoidance of the mercury-based fixatives, which interfere with most enzymatic reactions, and the performance of the major steps at 4°C. Neutral buffered formalin is the preferred fixative for this method. With the introduction of newer resins for plastic embedding, the processing, although more time consuming than paraffin embedding, has been improved and allows for excellent morphologic detail; some laboratories prefer plastic embedding to paraffin for routine biopsies (33).

Plastic Sections for Routine Stains and Cytochemistry

Plastic sections for routine stains and cytochemistry (34,35) can be prepared using the following procedure:

1. Place specimen in cold, 10% buffered formalin fixative overnight. Omit steps 2 and 3 for specimens not decalcified.
2. Rinse with EDTA decal for a few seconds. EDTA or saturated versonate solution remains good for several months. It is prepared by combining 10 g of EDTA (versonate) with 100 mL of phosphate buffer (pH 6.4; combine 6.63 g of potassium monobasic phosphate with 2.56 g of sodium dibasic phosphate and dilute to 1,000 mL with distilled or deionized water), which is shaken well (does not dissolve completely) and then refrigerated.
3. Put in fresh Decal solution (EDTA) for 4 hours.
4. Wash with cold 0.1 M phosphate buffer (pH 7.3) for 1 hour; change the solution after 30 minutes. The buffer (pH 7.3) is made by combining 0.272 g of potassium monobasic phosphate and 1.135 g of sodium dibasic phosphate, which is diluted to 100 mL with distilled or deionized water and kept in a refrigerator.
5. Place in acetone and buffer (1:1) for 10 minutes.
6. Place in acetone and buffer (3:1) for 10 minutes.
7. Place in acetone for 10 minutes.
8. Place in acetone and JB-4 component A + catalyst (1:1) for 10 minutes. Make the solution under the hood by combining 50 mL of JB-4 component A (kept in the refrigerator) and one-half scoop catalyst (approximately 0.45 g). Mix on an automatic mixer with a magnet, and keep covered with parafilm for 15 minutes until dissolved. Refrigerate for 15 minutes before using.
9. Place in the JB-4 component A + catalyst for 10 minutes and then in fresh JB-4 component A + catalyst overnight and 1 more day and night or over the weekend. Use the hood for the rest of the procedure. Combine 25 mL of the JB-4 component A (kept in refrigerator) and one-fourth scoop of the catalyst (about 0.23 g). Mix on automatic mixer with a magnet and keep covered with parafilm for 15 minutes until dissolved. Refrigerate for 15 minutes before using.
10. To 25 mL of JB-4 component A + catalyst, add 1 mL of JB-4 component B, and mix well with applicator stick. Keep the beaker on a cold plate while preparing.
11. Pipette 1.5 mL of JB-4 component A + catalyst and JB-4 component B mixture into plastic block mold; drop the section in and position. Keep the plastic mold on a cold plate. The solution does not thicken for 15 minutes or longer; the specimen may be manipulated during this time.
12. Place the metal block holder on top.
13. Place in the refrigerator overnight; place the embedded section into an open slide box, and set in the refrigerator. When ready to remove, gently loosen the embedded tissue from the plastic mold. There may be fluid around specimen; this can be ignored if the face of the block is hard. Cut within 48 hours, because the tissue becomes dry and hard after that time.
14. After cutting, float sections out in weak ammonia water (approximately 4 to 5 drops concentrated ammonia per 200 mL of water). Do not use hot plate or oven for special stains. Dry; this may take 30 to 60 minutes. For H&E and Wright-Giemsa stains, place in an oven for 30 to 60 minutes; cool before staining.

Gill's Hematoxylin and Eosin for Plastic Sections

Gill's H&E stain can be used for plastic sections. Fix mounted sections in an oven of 58°C to 62°C for 0.5 hour, and then use the following procedure:

1. Gill's hematoxylin (#2 or #3 or equal amounts) for 1 hour
2. Water: two changes, 10 dips each
3. Bluing solution: 2 minutes
4. Water: two changes, 10 dips each
5. 70% ethanol: 10 dips
6. Eosin Y alcoholic: 6 to 7 minutes
7. Absolute ethyl alcohol: two changes, 10 dips each
8. Xylene: three changes, 3 to 5 minutes each
9. Coverslip with solvent-soluble mounting media.

The bluing reagent (0.2% sodium bicarbonate, 1.0% magnesium sulfate) is made by combining 2 g of sodium bicarbonate and 10 g of magnesium sulfate, which is diluted to 1,000 mL with deionized water.

Plastic Embedded Sections for Immunohistochemistry

Plastic embedding procedures have been developed for immunocytochemistry (11,26). The following method for plastic embedding by Casey and colleagues can be used for routine H&E-stained sections and for cytochemical and immunocytochemical procedures (13,36):

1. Collect bone marrow trephine biopsies or other specimen (2-to 3-mm sections) in 4°C acetone. Keep a vial with acetone on ice while transporting the specimen.
2. Place the acetone and specimen in the freezer (−20°C) immediately on receipt in the laboratory for overnight fixation.
3. The fixed samples are infiltrated the next day in 5 to 10

mL of JB-4 component A with 5% methyl benzoate for 3 to 8 hours at 4°C.
4. After infiltration, the specimen is embedded in catalyzed JB-4 component A with JB-4 component B, which is prepared by adding 2.5 mL of catalyzed JB-4 component A to 0.063 mL of JB-4 component B. Pipette 1.5 mL of the solution into plastic molding cups, add the specimen, and cover with appropriate plastic block holder. Polymerize overnight at 4°C in a desiccator. After polymerization, the block can be stored at −20°C until needed.

The sectioning procedure follows:

1. Allow blocks to come to room temperature in a desiccator.
2. Tissue sections are cut at 2 μm using a glass knife and a histology microtome.
3. Sections are collected on an appropriate water bath. Sections to be used for H&E staining or cytochemistry are collected on plain water bath. Sections to be used for immunocytochemistry are collected on a water bath prepared by adding 25 mL of acetone to 600 mL of distilled or deionized water (total volume = 625 mL), adding 5 to 10 drops ammonium hydroxide and allowing the sections to float on the above mixture for 15 minutes before transferring sections to coverslips. Discard the mixture at the end of each day.
4. Transfer sections to labeled coverslips, and allow to air dry overnight at room temperature. Sections should be collected 1 day before staining.

The immunohistochemistry procedure follows:

1. Using a fine tweezers, place the labeled coverslips that contain tissue sections into a staining rack; align sections to face in the same direction.
2. Place staining rack into beaker containing 0.05 M Tris buffered saline (TBS) (pH 7.6) for 10 to 30 minutes at room temperature.
3. Blot the coverslip vertically onto absorbent paper, and place the section side down onto a parafilmed slide tray containing 100 μL of 2% normal swine serum for 30 minutes in a moist, 37°C chamber. The 2% normal swine serum is prepared by adding 0.06 mL of normal swine serum to 2.94 mL of TBS (total volume = 3.00 mL). This amount is adequate for 25 coverslips. The solution should be discarded at the end of the day.
4. Blot the coverslip vertically, and place the section side down on 100 μL of appropriate dilutions of mouse monoclonal antibody on a parafilmed slide tray. Incubate for 2 hours at 37°C. Dilutions are prepared using a solution of 95.0 mL of TBS, 5 mL of 2% sodium azide, and 100 mg of bovine serum albumin. This should be stored at 4°C. Discard dilutions at the end of the day.
5. Blot the coverslips, and perform two 5-minute washes by gently dipping staining rack into beaker containing TBS.
6. Blot the coverslip, and place the section side down onto a parafilmed slide tray containing 100 μL of 0.1% sodium azide with 3% H_2O_2 for 10 minutes at room temperature. Prepare the solution by adding 0.25 mL of 2% sodium azide and 0.05 mL of 30% H_2O_2 to 4.70 mL distilled or deionized water (total volume = 5.00 mL).
7. Blot coverslips, and perform two 5-minute washes in TBS.
8. Blot the coverslip, and place the section side down on a parafilmed slide tray containing 100 μL of a $\frac{1}{40}$ dilution of horseradish peroxidase–conjugated rabbit antimouse with 2.5% human AB serum for 1 hour at 37°C. For the 2.5% human AB serum in TBS, add 0.175 mL of human AB serum to 6.825 mL of TBS (total volume = 7.000 mL). This volume is sufficient for 25 coverslips. Discard any remaining solution. For the $\frac{1}{40}$ dilution of horseradish peroxidase–conjugated rabbit antimouse antibody with 2.5% human AB serum, add 0.075 mL of peroxidase conjugated rabbit antimouse to 2.925 mL of 2.5% human AB serum in TBS (total volume = 3.000 mL). This is sufficient for 25 coverslips. Discard any remaining solution.
9. Blot the coverslips, and perform two 5-minute washes in TBS.
10. Blot the coverslips, and place the section side down on a parafilmed slide tray containing 100 μL of $\frac{1}{40}$ dilution of horseradish peroxidase–conjugated swine anti-rabbit with 2.5% human AB serum for 1 hour at 37°C. Make the $\frac{1}{40}$ dilution of horseradish peroxidase–conjugated antibody with 2.5% human AB by adding 0.075 mL of peroxidase-conjugated swine anti-rabbit antibody to 2.925 mL of 2.5% human AB serum in TBS (total volume = 3.000 mL). This is sufficient for 25 coverslips. Discard any remaining solution.
11. Blot the coverslips, and perform two 5-minute washes in TBS.
12. Wash the coverslips in 0.1 M acetate buffer (pH 5.2) for 5 minutes.
13. Incubate the coverslips in small Coplin jars filled with aminoethylcarbizole in formamide for 15 minutes at 37°C. Prepare immediately before use by adding 2.034 mL of aminoethylcarbizole (AEC) in formamide and 0.030 mL of 3% H_2O_2 to 28.5 mL of 0.1 M acetate buffer.
14. Wash the coverslips with distilled or deionized water two or three times; collect excess AEC and all washings for proper disposal.
15. Counterstain with Gill's hematoxylin for 10 to 15 minutes at room temperature.
16. Wash the coverslips in running tap water for 5 minutes.
17. Air dry the coverslips, and mount with Glycergel or other water-based mounting media onto an appropriately labeled glass slide.

Embedding Materials

Embedding molds included Sorvall plastic block holder and molding for use on the Sorvall microtome. Coverslips (catalog #M6050-2) were supplied by Scientific Products. The JB-4 Embedding kit (catalog #0226) was supplied by Polysciences Inc. Individual components included JB-4 Component A (catalog #0226A), JB-4 Component B (catalog #0226B), and JB-4 Catalyst (catalog #02618). The procedure uses acetone, ammonium hydroxide, and methyl benzoate (all American Chemical Society certified).

Reagents

The JB-4 component A with 5% methyl benzoate was made by adding 5 mL of methyl benzoate to 95 mL of JB-4 component A (total volume = 100 mL). The solution is stored at 4°C and expires in 3 to 4 weeks.

The catalyzed JB-4 component A is made by adding 0.15 g of JB-4 catalyst to 40 mL of JB-4 component A. Add a magnet, and place the solution on a magnetic mixer for 15 minutes or until the catalyst is dissolved. Store at 4°C. The solution expires in 3 to 4 weeks.

CRYOSTAT SECTIONS

Cryostat sections have limited use in diagnostic bone marrow pathology, but they do have an advantage over paraffin-embedded sections for immunohistochemical procedures in that there is complete preservation of surface and cytoplasmic antigens. However, in most proliferative processes involving the bone marrow, immunophenotyping can be performed by flow cytometry on aspirated bone marrow; alternatively, touch imprint slides prepared from the core biopsy can be used for immunocytochemical studies. For uncommon occasions when detailed immunophenotyping is required and no specimens can be obtained by these methods, cryostat sections of a trephine core biopsy can be prepared (11,37).

Cryostat sections have the disadvantages of suboptimal morphology. It is difficult to section cryostat tissue with such dense bone structure, and architectural distortion results from compression or tearing of the specimen. Sections of one-cell thickness are difficult to achieve. This may lead to considerable difficulties in interpretation, and caution must be exercised in the evaluation of these specimens.

The trephine for cryostat sections is obtained in the same manner as for conventional processing. Immediately after it is obtained, the biopsy is placed on a saline-soaked gauze and is transported to the laboratory. Before freezing of the biopsy specimen, it should be examined with a magnifying glass to determine whether there is substantial cortical bone present. If cortical bone is present, it should be carefully dissected away and processed in a routine manner. The presence of cortical bone in a biopsy causes greater difficulty in sectioning and may lead to increased tissue distortion. The specimen to be frozen is then placed in a plastic specimen holder that is filled with OCT embedding compound (Tissue Tek II; Lab Tek Products Division, Miles Laboratories, Inc., Naperville, IL). The specimen holder is grasped with a long pair of tongs and gradually is immersed in liquid nitrogen or isopentane. After immersion for a few minutes, the specimen is withdrawn, wrapped in aluminum foil, and stored at −70°C until sectioning is performed.

When the specimen is to be sectioned, it should be placed in the cryostat for approximately 15 to 20 minutes before the actual cutting. The chuck on which the specimen is mounted should be placed so that the long axis of the specimen is oriented vertically or at a diagonal to the cutting edge of the knife. The knife blade should be moved frequently because dulling of the blade occurs after only a few cuts. Because of damage to the knife blade, disposable knife blades should be used. The specimens should be picked up on albumin-coated slides that are placed in the cryostat 30 minutes before use. The sections are air dried for approximately 18 to 24 hours. After drying, the specimens are fixed in acetone at room temperature for approximately 10 minutes. The slides may then be immunostained by standard immunoperoxidase or immunoalkaline phosphatase methods. If the specimens are to be immunostained at a later time, they should be wrapped in aluminum foil and stored at −20°C until used.

PREPARATION OF BONE MARROW SPECIMENS FOR ELECTRON MICROSCOPY

If electron microscopic (EM) studies are anticipated, an additional 1.0 to 2.0 mL of marrow should be aspirated. An anticoagulated specimen of marrow, using powdered EDTA or heparin, is spun in a Wintrobe tube in the same way as the anticoagulated routine marrow aspirate. After the tube has been spun and the separated layers are identified, the F-PV and plasma layers are drawn off with a Pasteur pipette. Cold 2.5% glutaraldehyde fixative is layered over the M-E layer without disrupting this layer. After 10 minutes of fixation, the Wintrobe tube is scored at the level of the interface of the M-E and erythrocyte layer. The tube is cracked and the portion of the tube with the M-E layer is placed in a vial of fresh cold glutaraldehyde so that the exposed portion of the M-E layer is in contact with the fixative. After an additional 10 minutes of fixation, the M-E layer is ejected gently from the Wintrobe tube into a vial of fresh cold glutaraldehyde using a Pasteur pipette. After another 10 minutes of fixation, the M-E pellet is diced into 1-mm portions with a sharp razor blade. These portions are then placed into fresh cold glutaraldehyde and allowed to fix for at least 30 minutes. The particles are then processed for EM by standard techniques. The specimen may remain in fixative for up to 2 weeks at 4°C before processing.

As an alternative to using an M-E layer for EM, particles from the aspirated anticoagulated specimen can be separated from the fluid portion of the specimen and placed directly into cold glutaraldehyde for 1 hour. If the particles are large or clumped, they should be cut into 1-mm cubes.

If no aspirate can be obtained because of fibrosis, portions of the trephine biopsy specimen can be used. The biopsy specimen should be placed on saline-soaked gauze and transferred to the laboratory immediately after the biopsy procedure. Small portions of the biopsy should be cut away with a sharp scalpel blade. These should be placed in cold glutaraldehyde for approximately 10 minutes. The specimens should then be cut into 1-mm cubes and placed in fresh cold glutaraldehyde.

ULTRASTRUCTURAL PLATELET PEROXIDASE

The diagnosis of acute megakaryoblastic leukemia (French-American-British M7) is based on the demonstration of reactivity of cells with antibodies to platelet glycoproteins or platelet peroxidase at the ultrastructural level (38).

The blood or marrow specimen is prepared in the same manner as for routine transmission electron microscopy. If the primary purpose of the study is the demonstration of platelet peroxidase, tannic acid fixative is substituted for glutaraldehyde. The tannic acid is added gently over the nucleated cell layer (M-E) of the spun specimen; a fixation time of 10 minutes is optimal. The Wintrobe tube is then scored at the lower margin of the nucleated cell layer and broken. The tube is then placed into a fresh vial of tannic acid with the exposed M-E layer down for 10 minutes. The slightly solidified M-E layer is gently ejected into the fixative and allowed to fix for an additional 5 minutes. The specimen is diced into 1-mm cubes that are placed in a vial of fresh tannic acid for 5 minutes. After the 5-minute fixation, the specimen is washed three times in 0.05 M Tris-HCl buffer.

The specimen is incubated in platelet peroxidase reaction mixture for 1 to 1.5 hours at room temperature; the specimen is gently agitated during the incubation. After this incubation, the specimen is washed three times in 0.05 M Tris-HCl buffer. After this, the specimen is fixed in 1% buffered OsO_4 for 1 hour at room temperature. Next, the specimen is processed in the same manner as for routine electron microscopy.

If the processing cannot be completed during one period, it may be interrupted at two points. The fixed cells can be held overnight in Tris wash buffer at 4°C and incubated with the platelet peroxidase reaction mixture the next day, or after incubation, they can be held overnight in the Tris-HCl buffer at 4°C.

Reagents are made as follows:

Tannic acid fixative: Stock (2% formaldehyde and 0.5% glutaraldehyde in 0.1 M phosphate buffer) is made by adding 25 mL of 16% formaldehyde to 4 mL of 25% glutaraldehyde, which is diluted up to 100 mL with 0.1 M phosphate buffer (pH 7.4). Store in a refrigerator. On the day of use, add 0.25 g of tannic acid to 25 mL of stock fix, and adjust pH to 7.3 with 1 N NaOH. Filter and use the same day.

Platelet peroxidase (PPO) medium: Dissolve 20 mg of diaminobenzidine tetrahydrochloride (DAB) in 10 mL of 0.05 M Tris-HCl buffer (pH 7.5), and add 0.033 mL of 3% H_2O_2. (*Note:* Make up 3% H_2O_2 fresh from 30% H_2O_2.) Adjust the pH to 7.6 with 1 N NaOH. For the control, make up the medium without the 3% H_2O_2. Use the PPO medium the same day it is prepared.

SUMMARY AND CONCLUSIONS

Proper processing of bone marrow specimens is critical for obtaining the optimal cytologic detail necessary for the study of hematopoietic diseases. Excellent results can be obtained with trephine biopsies fixed in mercury-based or other fixatives. Paraffin-embedded biopsies can be used for routine H&E stains, several histochemical techniques, and immunocytochemical studies with an increasing number of antibodies. When studies not applicable to paraffin-embedded sections are necessary, bone marrow biopsies may be embedded in plastic embedding medium or snap frozen for cryostat sections. The bone marrow aspirate specimen should be used to make smears for routine staining and, when appropriate, cytochemical and immunocytochemical studies. A peripheral blood smear made at the time of the bone marrow biopsy often contributes important information about disorders that affect the bone marrow. Other techniques, including immunophenotyping by flow cytometry, cytogenetic analysis, and molecular genetic analysis, are integral components of bone marrow interpretation and should be used when indicated and correlated with the morphologic findings of the bone marrow. Application of these techniques is discussed in Chapters 3-5, 7-11, and 38.

REFERENCES

1. Jamshidi K, Swaim WR. Bone marrow biopsy with unaltered architecture: a new biopsy device. *J Lab Clin Med* 1971;77:335–342.
2. Carson FL. Fixation. In: *Histotechnology: a self-instructional text.* Chicago: ASCP Press, 1997:1–24.
3. Brynes RK, McKenna RW, Sundberg RD. Bone marrow aspiration and trephine biopsy. *Am J Clin Pathol* 1978;70:753–759.
4. Luna LG, ed. *Manual of histologic staining methods of the Armed Forces Institute of Pathology,* 3rd ed. New York: McGraw-Hill, 1958.
5. Sundberg RD, Broman H. The application of the Prussian blue stain to previously stained films of blood and bone marrow. *Blood* 1955;10:160–166.
6. Dacie JV, Lewis SM. *Practical haematology.* London: J & A Churchill, 1966:85.
7. Lillie RD. *Histopathologic technic and practical histochemistry,* 3rd ed. New York: McGraw-Hill, 1965:194.
8. Bluth RF, Casey TT, McCurley TL. Differentiation of reactive from neoplastic small-cell lymphoid aggregates in paraffin-embedded marrow particle preparations using L-26 (CD20) and UCHL-1 (CD45RO) monoclonal antibodies. *Am J Clin Pathol* 1993;99:150–156.
9. Horny HP, Wehrmann M, Grisser H, et al. Investigation of bone marrow lymphocyte subsets in normal, reactive, and neoplastic states, using paraffin-embedded biopsy specimens. *Am J Clin Pathol* 1993;99:142–149.
10. O'Donnell LR, Adler SL, Balis UJ, et al. Immunohistochemical refer-

ence ranges for B lymphocytes in bone marrow biopsy paraffin sections. *Am J Clin Pathol* 1995;104:517–523.
11. Thaler J, Dietze O, Denz H, et al. Bone marrow diagnosis in lymphoproliferative disorders: comparison of results obtained from conventional histomorphology and immunohistology. *Histopathology* 1991; 18:495–504.
12. Kubic VL, Brunning RD. Immunohistochemical evaluation of neoplasms in bone marrow biopsies using monoclonal antibodies reactive in paraffin-embedded tissue. *Mod Pathol* 1989;77:335–342.
13. Casey TT, Olson SJ, Cousar JB, et al. Plastic section immunohistochemistry in the diagnosis of hematopoietic and lymphoid neoplasms. *Clin Lab Med* 1990;10:199–213.
14. Erbor WN, Gibbs TA, Ivey JG. Antigen retrieval by microwave oven heating for immunohistochemical analysis of bone marrow trephine biopsies. *Pathology* 1996;28:45–50.
15. Erbor WN, Willis JI, Hoffman GJ. An enhanced immunocytochemical method for staining bone marrow trephine sections. *J Clin Pathol* 1997; 50:389–393.
16. Peterson LL, Brown BA, Crosson JT, et al. Application of the immunoperoxidase technic to bone marrow trephine biopsies in the classification of patients with monoclonal gammopathies. *Am J Clin Pathol* 1986;85:688–693.
17. Thiry A, Delvenne P, Fontaine MA, et al. Comparison of bone marrow sections, smears and immunohistological staining for immunoglobulin light chains in the diagnosis of benign and malignant plasma cell proliferations. *Histopathology* 1993;22: 423–428.
18. Skinnider BF, Connors JM, Gascoyne RD. Bone marrow involvement in T-cell–rich B-cell lymphoma. *Am J Clin Pathol* 1997;108:570–578.
19. Gaulard P, Kanavaros P, Farcet JP, et al. Bone marrow histologic and immunohistochemical findings in peripheral T-cell lymphoma. *Hum Pathol* 1991;22:331–338.
20. Franco V, Florena AM, Campesi G. Intrasinusoidal bone marrow infiltration: a possible hallmark of splenic lymphoma. *Histopathology* 1996; 29:571–575.
21. Vasef MA, Medeiros LJ, Koo C, et al. Cyclin D1 immunohistochemical staining is useful in distinguishing mantle cell lymphoma from other low grade B-cell neoplasms in bone marrow. *Am J Clin Pathol* 1997; 108:302–307.
22. Ben-Ezra JM, King BE, Harris AC, et al. Staining for Bcl-2 protein helps to distinguish benign from malignant lymphoid aggregates in bone marrow biopsies. *Mod Pathol* 1994;7:560–563.
23. Lai R, Arber DA, Chang KL, et al. Frequency of bcl-2 expression in non-Hodgkin's lymphoma: a study of 778 cases with comparison of marginal zone lymphoma and monocytoid B-cell hyperplasia. *Mod Pathol* 1998;2:864–869.
24. Orazi A, Cotton J, Cattoretti G, et al. Terminal deoxynucleotidyl transferase staining in acute leukemia and normal bone marrow in routinely processed paraffin sections. *Am J Clin Pathol* 1994;102:640–645.
25. Fraga M, Brousset P, Schlaifer D, et al. Bone marrow involvement in anaplastic large cell lymphoma. *Am J Clin Pathol* 1994;103:82–89.
26. Hakimian D, Tallman MS, Kiley C, et al. Detection of minimal residual disease by immunostaining of bone marrow biopsies after 2-chlorodeoxyadenosine for hairy cell leukemia. *Blood* 1993;82:1798–1802.
27. Wheaton S, Tallman MS, Hakimian D, et al. Minimal residual disease may predict bone marrow relapse in patients with hairy cell leukemia treated with 2-chlorodeoxyadenosine. *Blood* 1996;87:1556–1560.
28. Rimsza LM, Viswanatha DS, Winter SS, et al. The presence of $CD34^+$ cell clusters predicts impending relapse in children with acute lymphoblastic leukemia receiving maintenance chemotherapy. *Am J Clin Pathol* 1998;110:313–320.
29. Chuang SS, Li CY. Useful panel of antibodies for the classification of acute leukemia by immunohistochemical methods in bone marrow trephine biopsy specimens. *Am J Clin Pathol* 1996;107:410–418.
30. Li WV, Kapadia SB, Sonmez-Alpan E, et al. Immunohistochemical characterization of mast cell disease in paraffin sections using tryptase, CD68, myeloperoxidase, lysozyme, and CD20 antibodies. *Mod Pathol* 1996;9:982–988.
31. Davey RF, Olson S, Kurec AS, et al. The immunophenotyping of extramedullary myeloid cell tumors in paraffin-embedded tissue sections. *Am J Surg Pathol* 1988;12:699–707.
32. Brunning RD. Bone marrow. In: Rosai J, ed. *Ackerman's surgical pathology.* St. Louis: CV Mosby, 1989:1379–1454.
33. Frisch B, Bartl R. Atlas of bone marrow pathology. In: Gresham GA, ed. *Current histopathology,* vol 15. Boston: Kluwer Academic Publishers, 1990.
34. Brinn NT, Pickett JP. Glycol methacrylate for routine, special stains, histochemistry, enzyme histochemistry and immunohistochemistry: a simplified method for surgical biopsy tissue. *J Histotechnol* 1979;2: 125–130.
35. Beckstead JH, Bainton DF. Enzyme histochemistry on bone marrow biopsies. Reactions useful in the differential diagnosis of leukemia and lymphoma applied to 2-micron plastic sections. *Blood* 1980;55: 386–394.
36. Casey TT, Olson SJ, Cousar JB, et al. Plastic section immunohistochemistry in the diagnosis of hematopoietic and lymphoid neoplasms. *Clin Lab Med* 1990;10:199–213.
37. Kronland R, Grogan T, Spier C, et al. Immunotopographic assessment of lymphoid and plasma cell malignancies of the bone marrow. *Hum Pathol* 1985;16:1247–1254.
38. Breton-Gorius J, Reyes F, Duhamel G, et al. Megakaryoblastic acute leukemia: identification by the ultrastructural demonstration of platelet peroxidase. *Blood* 1978;51: 45–60.

CHAPTER 38

Cytochemical, Histochemical, and Immunohistochemical Analysis of the Bone Marrow

Chin-Yang Li and Lung T. Yam

Continuous advances in therapy for neoplastic diseases necessitate accurate diagnosis and classification to provide the most effective treatment. Because neoplastic diseases are generally classified according to cell type and degree of differentiation of the malignant cells, their accurate identification is a prerequisite for making the correct diagnosis. Traditional morphologic diagnoses made on the basis of conventional stains, such as hematoxylin and eosin or Wright-Giemsa stains, are sometimes difficult, and opinions may vary among observers, especially about poorly differentiated neoplasms. Over the years, many cell type–specific chemical constituents, enzymes, differentiation antigens, and surface receptors have been identified and characterized. These cell type–specific markers are used successfully for cell identification in the diagnosis and classification of neoplastic diseases. To best use these specific cell markers in bone marrow specimens, it is important to carefully collect and process the bone marrow specimen to preserve these individual cell markers. The techniques for demonstrating cell markers include selective dye binding or enzyme cytochemistry, flow cytometry, and enzyme immunocytochemistry using polyclonal or monoclonal antibodies. The cytochemical methods and enzyme immunocytochemical techniques applicable to various common laboratory specimens (including smears, cytospin preparation, tissue imprints, frozen, and paraffin or plastic sections) are most practical for clinical application and the easiest to correlate with morphology.

C.-Y. Li: Department of Laboratory Medicine and Pathology, Mayo Clinic, Rochester, Minnesota 55905

L. T. Yam: Department of Medicine, University of Louisville, School of Medicine, Louisville, Kentucky 40292 and VA Medical Center, Louisville, Kentucky 40206

TECHNICAL CONSIDERATIONS

Preparation of Specimens

Handling of the marrow biopsy for morphologic studies is discussed in Chapter 37. The discussions that follow are limited to the preparation of the marrow for special diagnostic studies by cytologic or histologic methods.

The marrow materials useful for studies include the aspirate and the biopsy core. The marrow aspirate may be used to prepare cell suspensions, smears, and clot sections. The biopsy core is useful for the preparation of sections and imprints. The cytologic materials should be properly prepared and fixed before staining. The histologic materials may be used fresh (unfixed) or fixed and embedded in gelatin, paraffin, or plastic before sectioning.

Fixation

Fixatives commonly used for the processing of clinical specimens include aldehyde fixatives (e.g., formalin), metallic ions (e.g., chromium, mercury, zinc), alcohol, and acetone. Overfixation tends to block most reactive groups, leading to reduced stainability by basic and acid dyes and to denaturation of enzymes. It also often masks many antigenic determinants. Alcohol and acetone are protein precipitants. They preserve the reactive groups of enzymes and the antigenic sites very well. The fixatives most often used for cytochemical and histochemical studies include acetone and buffered formalin (1,2). For immunochemical stains, the useful fixatives that preserve morphology and common cell type-specific antigens include buffered formalin for tissues processed for paraffin sections, B5 (i.e., formalin and mercury chloride) for bone marrow biopsies processed for paraffin sections (1), brief (5 minutes) fixation with cold acetone for fresh frozen sections and imprints (3,4), and short (30 seconds) fixation with cold buffered formalin-acetone for smears and imprints (5).

Problems in Plastic Sections

Plastic embedding provides excellent preservation of morphologic details of cells in sections, but it also causes difficulties for histochemical and immunohistochemical studies. Because of the slow penetration of reagents in the plastic matrix, it requires at least twice as much time as other preparations for most histochemical and immunohistochemical stains. Water-soluble plastics such as glycol-methacrylate bind to the amino-terminal portions of proteins during polymerization and mask antigenic epitopes. This masking phenomenon may be reversed by trypsin or protease treatment of sections (6–8).

Cytochemistry and Histochemistry

In general, cytochemical methods are simple and can be applied easily to air-dried aspirate smears, cytospin preparations, or tissue imprints. They are most useful for identification of granulocytes, monocytes-macrophages, hairy cells, and mast cells (Table 38.1). Clinically useful cytochemical stains can be divided into two general categories. The first is selective dye-binding stains, including Sudan black, toluidine blue, chlorazol–fast pink, periodic acid–Schiff (PAS) reaction, and stains for iron and reticulin fibers. The second is cell type–specific enzymatic reactions, including myeloperoxidase, cyanide-resistant peroxidase, alkaline phosphatase, acid phosphatase, tartrate-resistant acid phosphatase, chloroacetate esterase, butyrate esterase, acetate esterase, and aminocaproate esterase.

Histochemical studies of tissue sections of the marrow clot and the biopsy core are similar to those of cytochemical studies. They are most useful in disease processes with marrow lesions that are difficult to obtain or difficult to see on cytologic preparations. Examples of these diseases include the paratrabecular lesions and fibrosis seen in lymphomas, hairy cell leukemia (HCL), systemic mast cell disease, and metastatic tumors. The best results of histochemical studies can be achieved only when the technical details of a number of essential tissue processing steps are followed closely. These include fixation, decalcification of bony tissue, and embedding in the proper matrix for sectioning.

Conventional frozen tissue sectioning of the marrow biopsy tends to have excessive artifact with compression and displacement of bone trabeculae and hematopoietic tissue, making morphologic correlation very difficult. The processing method for traditional paraffin tissue sections involves formalin fixation, prolonged heating, and repeated exposure to organic solvents. These steps inactivate most enzymes (except chloroacetate esterase) and eliminate some essential substances, including metachromatic substances in basophils and mast cells. The processing methods suitable for histochemical study of the marrow biopsy include fixation in cold (4°C) buffered formalin at neutral pH, decalcifying in cold chelating agent (e.g., ethylene diamine tetraacetic acid), and sectioning in a cryostat (9) and fixation in cold buffered formalin and embedding in glycol methacrylate at low temperature with a reduced amount of catalyst for plastic sections (9–11).

Immunocytochemistry and Immunohistochemistry

Immunocytochemistry is the application of immunochemical procedures to cytologic materials, including fresh cells in suspension, prefixed smears, and tissue imprints. Immunohistochemistry usually denotes immunochemical studies of tissue sections. Immunocytochemistry and immunohistochemistry involve the use of visible indicators to identify cell or tissue antigens through the binding of a specific antibody to a particular antigen. With light microscopy, fluorochrome and enzymatic indicators are most commonly used. The enzyme indicators that are frequently used include horseradish peroxidase (12,13), intestinal alkaline phosphatase (14,15), glucose oxidase (16), and β-galactosidase (17). Linkage between the antigen and the indicator-antibody conjugate may be direct, indirect, or a series of steps (Figs. 38.1, 38.2). Careful selection of the appropriate procedure

TABLE 38.1. *Useful cytochemical stains for identifying hematopoietic cells in smears, frozen sections, and plastic sections*

Cytochemical stains	Cellular distribution and staining pattern
Sudan black B	Granulocytes, monocytes
Peroxidase	Granulocytes, monocytes
Cyanide-resistant peroxidase	Eosinophils
Chlorazol-fast pink	Eosinophils
Toluidine blue	Basophils, mast cells
Chloroacetate esterase	Neutrophils, mast cells
Aminocaproate esterase	Mast cells
α-Naphthyl butyrate esterase	Monocytes/histiocytes (diffuse), helper T lymphocytes (focal)
α-Naphthyl acetate esterase	Helper T lymphocytes (focal), monocytes/histiocytes (diffuse), megakaryocytes (diffuse), plasma cells (diffuse)
Acid phosphatase	T lymphoblasts/transformed T lymphocytes (focal), monocytes/histiocytes (diffuse)
Tartrate-resistant acid phosphatase	Hairy cells, histiocytes in lipid storage diseases, osteoclasts, mast cells

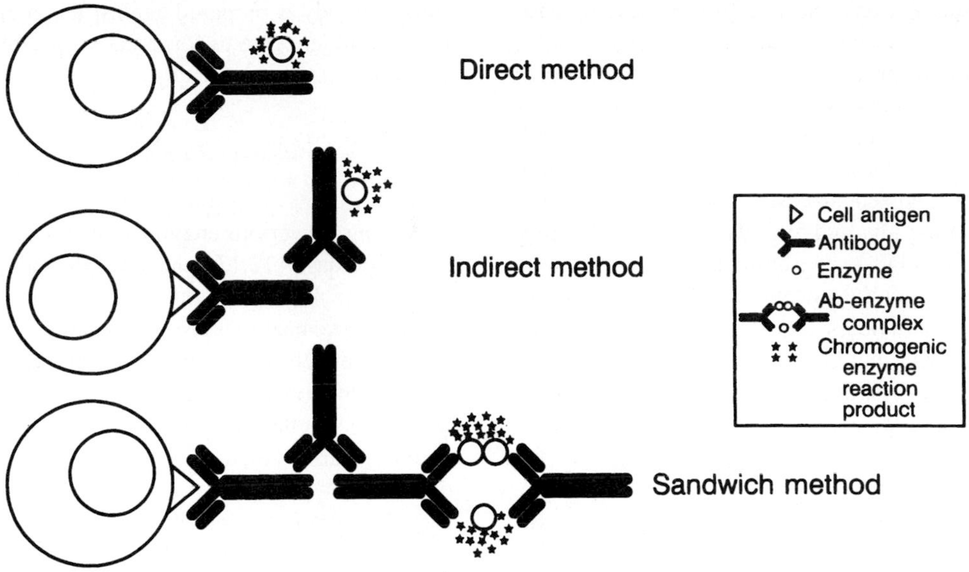

FIG. 38.1. Conventional enzyme immunochemical techniques.

is necessary to ensure the sensitivity and specificity needed for studying clinical specimens.

Effect of Detergents

In smear preparations, pretreatment with detergent (0.25% Triton X-100) may enhance the immunocytochemical staining of intracellular antigens (e.g., keratin), presumably because of the increased membrane permeability for reagents (18). The addition of detergent (Brij or Tween 20) in the rinsing solution for immunostaining of paraffin tissue sections increases sensitivity and specificity of the reaction, presumably by reducing the background staining caused by hydrophobic interactions between tissue and protein reagents (19).

Antigen Retrieval for Immunohistochemistry

Immunohistochemistry grew out of frozen section applications in which antigens remain unfixed and entirely native. Formalin fixation and paraffin embedding often alters antigen structure or severely cross-links antigens in tissue, rendering them unreactive or inaccessible to antibodies.

Growing interest in immunohistochemical techniques for clinical diagnosis and research has stimulated efforts to develop suitable procedures for routine formalin-fixed, paraf-

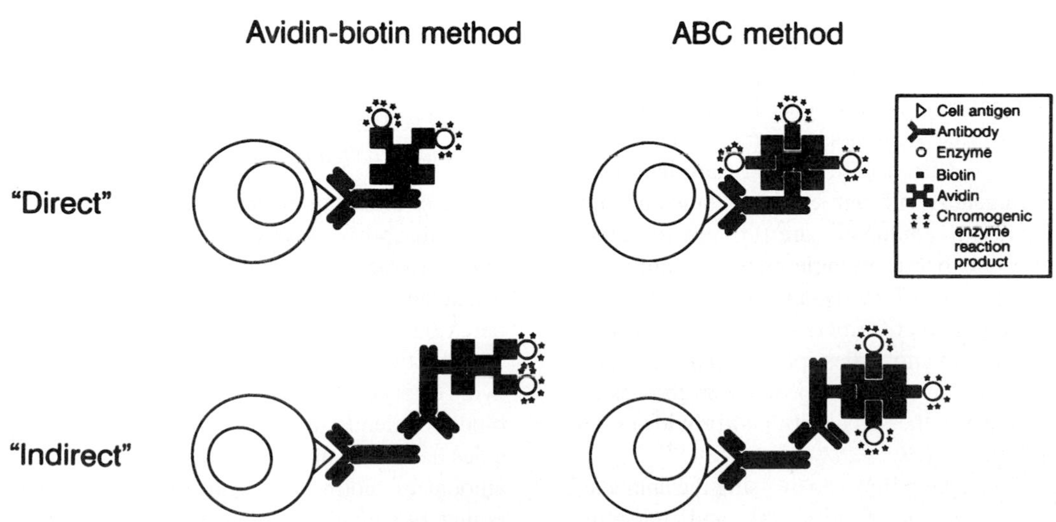

FIG. 38.2. Immunochemical techniques using avidin-biotin enzyme complex (ABC) or enzyme-labeled avidin.

fin-embedded tissue sections. Initial efforts to develop antibodies that recognize formalin-resistant epitopes (20–23) and the introduction of protease digestion of formalin-fixed sections to unmask antigenic sites had limited success, confined to only a small number of antigens (24–26). From what we have learned about the chemistry of formalin fixation, crosslinking can be reversed, at least in part, by high-temperature heating or strong alkaline hydrolysis (27,28). By pretreating sections by high-temperature heating in alkaline buffer solutions, many antigens can be made reactive again with their specific antibodies (29–31). Microwave ovens were used initially, but other heating methods, including autoclaves, pressure cookers, and steamers, have been shown to yield similar results. Most studies indicate an inverse correlation between heating temperature and heating time for optimal antigen retrieval.

Another important factor is the pH of the antigen retrieval solution. Although some antigens are satisfactorily unmasked by heating in distilled water, others require heating in a buffer of specific pH to obtain the strongest intensity of staining. Optimization of the antigen retrieval system should include consideration of the pH of the retrieval solution in addition to time and temperature. Commonly used solutions include 10 mM citrate buffer (pH 6.0) and 1 mM EDTA (pH 8.0). For many antigens, optimal antigen retrieval enhances the sensitivity of immunohistochemical stains on paraffin tissue sections to levels observed in frozen sections.

''Nonspecific'' background staining may also be reduced in paraffin tissue sections after antigen retrieval. Although the list of antigens to which antigen retrieval has been successfully applied grows steadily, some antigens are not unmasked by this method, particularly the cell surface antigens, including many markers of hematopoietic cells.

Selection of Staining Methods

Direct and Indirect Methods

In direct immunochemical procedures, the primary antibody reacting with antigen bears the indicator (Fig. 38.1). Although the procedure is simple, this direct approach is seldom used for enzyme immunochemistry because of its low sensitivity and because it requires that each individual antibody be conjugated with an enzyme indicator. Enzyme–primary antibody conjugates are difficult to obtain. It is more convenient to use a single enzyme–conjugated reagent for the detection of many antigens. This can be achieved by using an indirect format, in which enzyme conjugates are prepared from antibodies specific to the immunoglobulin of the species in which the primary antibodies are produced. This increases the sensitivity and provides more versatility for the techniques.

Sensitivity can be further improved by using the unlabeled antibody sandwich technique of Sternberger and colleagues (12). In this three-step procedure, the second antibody is unlabeled and used in excess to allow free combining sites for a third antibody of the same species as the primary. The final antibody is prepared against the enzyme indicator and mixed with enzyme to form stable, soluble complexes with multiple enzyme molecules.

Immunoperoxidase and Immunoalkaline Phosphatase Methods

Among the various enzyme indicators available, horseradish peroxidase (12,13) and intestinal alkaline phosphatase (14,15) are most commonly used. Methods for demonstrating these two enzymes are simple, and the reaction end products are very chromogenic. However, there are shortcomings in the immunoperoxidase and the immunoalkaline phosphatase methods; the most troublesome is endogenous enzyme activity. Various methods have been described for inhibiting endogenous peroxidase (32–35) or alkaline phosphatase (36,37), but none is entirely satisfactory. However, an effective method using azide and hydrogen peroxide has been developed for inhibition of endogenous peroxidase activity. This method makes possible better application of immunoperoxidase techniques for immunocytochemical evaluation of cells in blood and marrow (38).

Antibody Linkage and Avidin-Biotin Binding

The methods of avidin-biotin enzyme complex (ABC) or enzyme-labeled avidin or streptavidin (Fig. 38.2) are also useful for immunochemical studies (13,39). Where the antigen concentration or the antibody concentration is low, these methods may be more sensitive than the conventional immunochemical methods (40). However, these ABC methods may be plagued by the problems of background staining in tissues with endogenous avidin-binding activity. Although a number of technical maneuvers have been developed to circumvent these problems (41), it is still necessary to deal with background staining with the comprehensive use of rigid controls. The method using streptavidin instead of avidin may improve the specificity by lowering the background staining (39).

Tyramine Amplification Technique for Immunohistochemistry

The tyramine amplification technique is based on the characteristic ability of tyramine to become nonspecifically reactive to tissues after oxidation (42). The antigen of interest is labeled with peroxidase enzymes by any suitable immunoperoxidase technique. The labeled tissue is then incubated with biotinylated tyramine and H_2O_2. The peroxidase enzyme catalyzes the oxidation of tyramine, which then rapidly binds covalently to free amino groups in nearby tissue molecules before it can diffuse, thereby effectively increasing the amount of biotin at the site of antigen. The biotin on the bound tyramine is visualized by peroxidase- or other enzyme-labeled streptavidin or the ABC technique (Fig. 38.3) and disclosed cytochemically as usual. Heat-induced epitope retrieval and tyramine amplification techniques represent

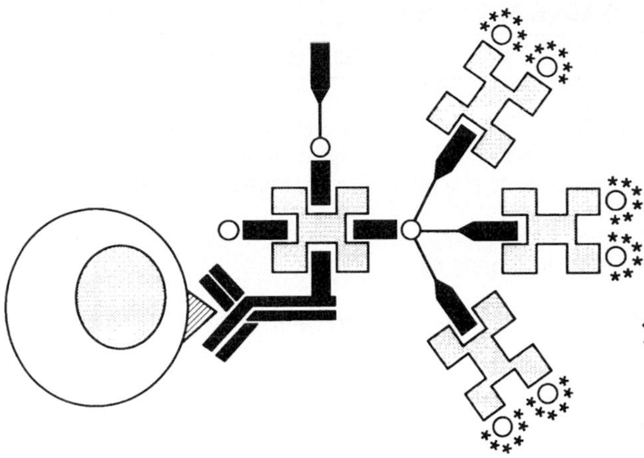

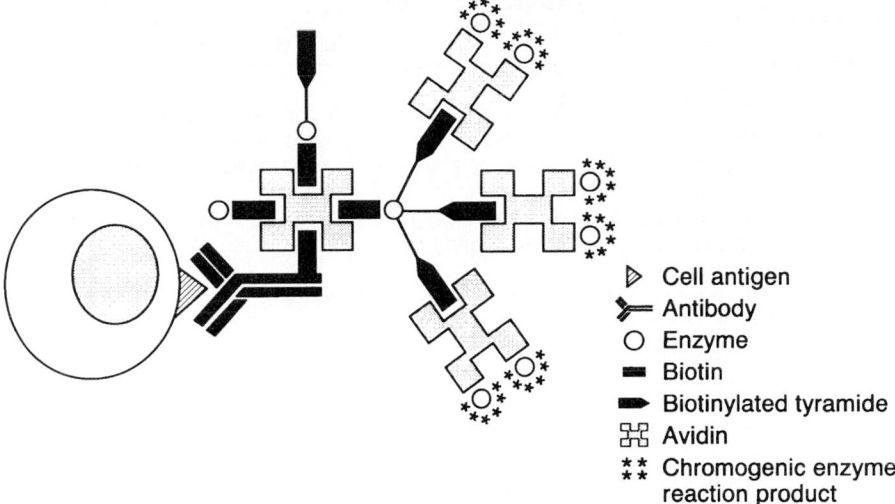

FIG. 38.3. Tyramine amplification technique.

technical advances in immunohistochemistry that greatly increase the range of antibodies that can be used and their sensitivity to study formalin-fixed, paraffin-embedded tissues (43–45).

Staining of Fresh Cell Suspensions and Air-Dried Smears

The cell suspension technique labels living cells in suspension with antibodies before making the smear, fixation, and staining of enzyme indicator (46). This technique is generally more sensitive than the immunostaining of air-dried smears and provides excellent morphologic detail and little or no background staining. However, it is labor intensive and requires large numbers of cells to compensate for loss during the incubation and washing steps. This technique is best reserved for special use such as demonstrating surface immunoglobulin or extremely labile surface antigens. Some of the shortcomings of this technique may be avoided by using air-dried smears. In most instances, the air-dried smears can be stored without fixation for at least 1 week before staining. The technique using air-dried smears is particularly valuable when the need for immunochemical studies is not realized until after routine cytologic examination.

Useful Immunochemical Markers

Many commercially available polyclonal and monoclonal antibodies have been shown to be of value in recognizing certain cell or tissue antigens. These immunochemical markers may be divided into those suitable for fresh cells or frozen sections (Table 38.2) and paraffin-embedded sections (Table 38.3) (see Chapter 3).

TABLE 38.2. *Useful immunocytochemical markers for identifying hematopoietic cells in smears and frozen tissue sections*

Immunocytochemical markers	Cellular distribution
Common leukocyte antigen	Immature hematopoietic cells
Lymphoid markers	
TdT	B and T lymphoblasts and subsets of myeloblasts
CD7	T lymphoblasts and lymphocytes
CD5	T lymphoblasts and lymphocytes, B-cell subsets
CD2	T lymphocytes
CD3	T lymphocytes
CD4	Helper T lymphocytes
CD8	Cytotoxic/suppressor T lymphocytes
CD56	Natural killer (NK) cells
CD57	NK cells, brain
CD10	Progenitor B lymphocytes and follicle center cells
CD19	Progenitor and mature B lymphocytes
CD20	B lymphocytes
CD21	B lymphocytes
CD22	Progenitor, mature, and activated B lymphocytes
CD23	B cell subsets and follicular dendritic cells
CD30	Activated T and B lymphocytes, Reed-Sternberg cells, anaplastic large cells (T or null cells)

(continued)

TABLE 38.2. *Continued.*

Immunocytochemical markers	Cellular distribution
Surface Ig	B lymphocytes
Cytoplasmic Ig	Plasma cells, pre-B lymphocytes, activated B lymphocytes
CD38	Plasma cells, pre-B lymphocytes, thymocytes, activated T and B lymphocytes
HLA-DR	B lymphocytes, monocytes, activated T cells, immature granulocytes
Granulocytic/monocytic markers	
CD11b	Monocytes, granulocytes
CD13	Monocytes, granulocytes, early myeloid cells
CD14	Monocytes
CD15	Monocytes, granulocytes, Reed-Sternberg cells
CD33	Early myeloid cells
CD34	Stem cells
Erythroid markers	
RC 82.4	Erythroblasts
Glycophorin	Erythroblasts and erythrocytes
Megakaryocytic markers	
CD41	Megakaryoblasts, megakaryocytes, platelets
CD42b	Megakaryocytes, platelets

TABLE 38.3. *Useful immunohistochemical markers for paraffin sections*

Immunohistochemical markers	Cell distribution
Lymphoid markers	
CD45	Lymphocytes, histiocytes
Cytoplasmic CD3	Precursor T, T lymphocytes
CD5	T lymphocytes, B-cell subset
CD45RO	T lymphocytes
CD43	T lymphocytes, granulocytes, monocytes
CD15	Reed-Sternberg cells, granulocytes
CD30	Reed-Sternberg cells, anaplastic large cells (T, B, or null cells)
CD8	Cytotoxic/suppressor T lymphocytes
CD56	Natural killer (NK) cells
TIA-1	Cytotoxic T/NK cells, granulocytes
CD79a	Precursor B, B lymphocytes
CD10	Precursor B, follicular center cells
CD20	B lymphocytes, activated B lymphocytes
Cytoplasmic Ig	Activated B lymphocytes, plasma cells
CD23	B-cell subsets, follicular dendritic cells
Hairy cell markers	
DBA.44	Hairy cells, B-cell subset
TRAP (9C5)	Hairy cells, osteoclasts, histiocytes
Granulocytic/monocytic markers	
Myeloperoxidase	Granulocytes, monocytes
Lysozyme	Granulocytes, monocytes/histiocytes
CD68 (PG-M1)	Monocytes/histiocytes
CD34	Stem cells, endothelial cells
Erythroid markers	
Hemoglobin	Erythroblasts, erythrocytes
TGF-β1	Erythroblasts
Megakaryocytic marker	
Factor VIII antigen	Megakaryocytes, endothelial cells
Mast cell marker	
Tryptase	Mast cells
Epithelial markers	
Keratin	Epithelial cells
Epithelial membrane antigen	Epithelial cells, plasma cells
Prostate-specific antigen	Prostatic epithelial cells
Prostatic acid phosphatase	Prostatic epithelial cells
Others	
Chromogranin	Neuroendocrine cells
Synaptophysin	Neuron
Desmin	Muscle cells
Muscle actin	Muscle cells
CD99	Ewing's sarcoma, lymphoblasts

SPECIAL STUDIES AND INTERPRETATIONS

Cytochemistry and Histochemistry

Peroxidase

Cytochemical demonstration of myeloperoxidase activity is used for the identification of granulocytes and therefore is useful in the diagnosis of acute leukemia. The method using 3,3′-diaminobenzidine as the color reagent with Giemsa counterstain has proven to be the most satisfactory (47,48) (Fig. 38.4; see also Color Plate 2, between pp. 1446–1447). Methods using 3-amino-9-ethylcarbazole also provide excellent results (48). Eosinophils, neutrophils, and monocytes have peroxidase activity, and basophils have very weak or equivocal activity. The enzyme in eosinophils is resistant to cyanide inhibition and is a helpful marker for the diagnosis of acute myeloid leukemia with eosinophilic differentiation (49,50) (Fig. 38.5; see also Color Plate 3, between pp. 1446–1447). The enzyme in platelets is also fairly characteristic, which may be useful as a marker for megakaryocytes but can only be demonstrated reliably ultrastructurally (51,52). In interpreting the peroxidase stain for the differential diagnosis of acute leukemias, the examiner assesses only the enzyme activity in the leukemic blasts. The test is meaningful only when it is positive, indicating acute granulocytic or myelomonocytic or monocytic leukemia. Cases in which the leukemic blasts are negative for peroxidase stain may represent acute lymphoblastic, monocytic, megakaryoblastic, erythroblastic, or undifferentiated leukemia. The presence of peroxidase-negative cytoplasmic granules in leukemic blasts may suggest the possibility of acute myeloid leukemia with basophilic or megakaryocytic differentiation (53). The presence of many mature neutrophils with negative peroxidase staining may indicate congenital or acquired deficiency of myeloperoxidase (54,55).

Peroxidase is fairly sensitive to heat and storage and is not used in tissue sections as often as chloroacetate esterase for diagnostic purposes. The clinical usefulness of the histochemical demonstration of myeloperoxidase is rather limited.

Alkaline Phosphatase

The alkaline phosphatases are a group of enzymes capable of hydrolyzing phosphoesters in alkaline medium. They are most often classified according to their tissue origin (56). Only the enzyme from the leukocytes is used for hematologic diagnosis. This enzyme is present in juvenile and mature neutrophils but not in eosinophils, basophils, or neutrophilic metamyelocytes and the more immature forms (57,58). It is also present in osteoblasts, vascular endothelial cells, and lymphocytes derived from the mantle zone of the spleen and lymph nodes (2,59–61). The cytochemical method using naphthol AS-BI phosphate and fast red-violet LB salt is used most often (58), although the method using naphthol AS phosphate and fast blue BBN is equally satisfactory (62).

Neutrophilic alkaline phosphatase activity is increased in polycythemia vera, infections, and inflammatory reactions. It is decreased in chronic myelocytic leukemia, paroxysmal nocturnal hemoglobinuria, and sickle cell anemia. In secondary erythrocytosis, agnogenic myeloid metaplasia, and essential thrombocytosis, neutrophil alkaline phosphatase ac-

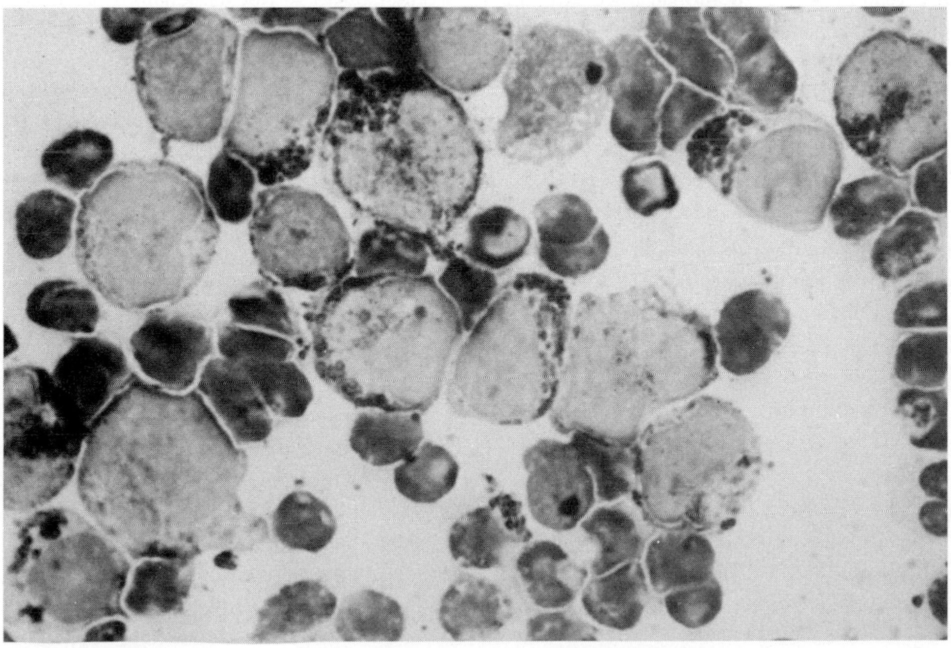

FIG. 38.4. Acute granulocytic leukemia (M2) with positive myeloperoxidase stain, as evidenced by the dark brownish cytoplasmic granules (peroxidase stain with diaminobenzidine, original magnification: 320× magnification). See Color Plate 2, between pp. 1446–1447.

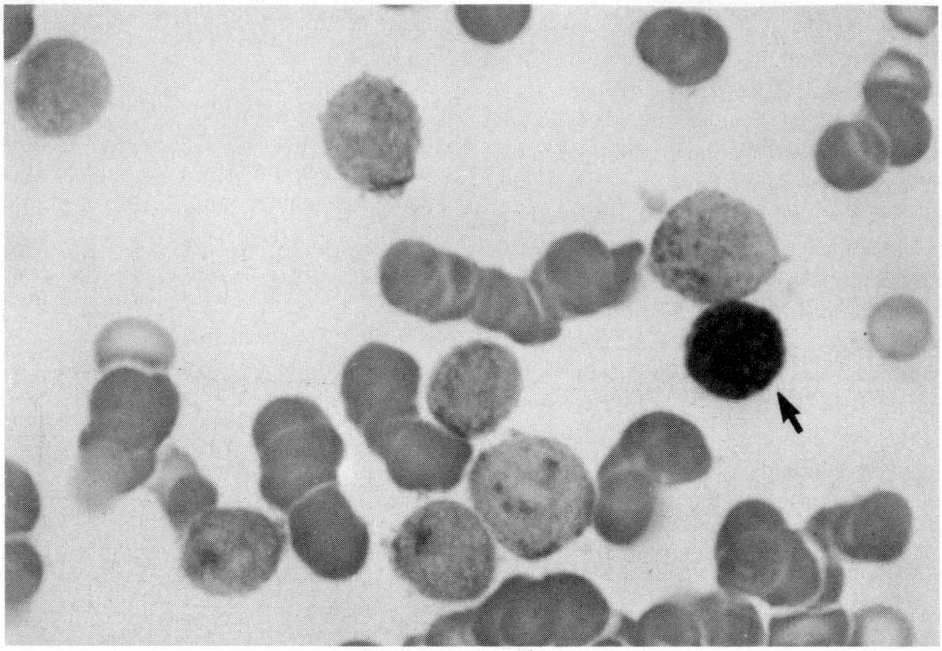

FIG. 38.5. Acute eosinophilic leukemia with positive cyanide-resistant peroxidase stain (brownish cytoplasmic granules and rods) and negative chloroacetate esterase (bright red cytoplasmic granules). A neutrophil *(arrow)* with positive chloroacetate esterase stain is at the right side of the field (combined stains for cyanide-resistant peroxidase and chloroacetate esterase, original magnification: 320× magnification). See Color Plate 3, between pp. 1446–1447.

tivity is usually normal (59). Semiquantitative assessment of neutrophil alkaline phosphatase activity (i.e., leukocyte alkaline phosphatase test) is a useful diagnostic adjunct to differentiate reactive leukocytosis from chronic myelocytic leukemia and erythrocytosis from polycythemia vera.

With the possible exceptions of demonstrating enzyme activity in the neoplastic lymphoid cells of mantle cell lymphoma (61), histochemical demonstration of alkaline phosphatase activity in tissue sections is of limited practical significance.

Esterases

The esterases useful for hematologic diagnosis include chloroacetate esterase for granulocytes, α-naphthyl butyrate esterase (i.e., nonspecific esterase) for monocytes or histiocytes, α-naphthyl acetate esterase (ANAE) for T lymphocytes, and aminocaproate esterase for mast cells.

Chloroacetate Esterase

This stain probably demonstrates the elastase and the chymotrypsin-like enzyme (63,64). Several cytochemical methods are available for chloroacetate esterase on smears of blood or marrow aspirate (48,49,65,66). The method using naphthol AS-D chloroacetate and hexazotized new fuchsin at pH 7.4 (48,49) provides precise localization of enzyme activity without any noticeable background staining or cross-reactivity with other esterases that may be demonstrable by other methods (67) (Fig. 38.6; see also Color Plate 4, between pp. 1446–1447). In human blood cells, chloroacetate esterase activity is predominantly in neutrophilic granulocytes and mast cells (65). In rare instances, it may be present in leukemic eosinophils (68–70).

Chloroacetate esterase is useful as a marker for neutrophils, but it is not as sensitive as the peroxidase or Sudan black B stains in identifying primitive myeloblasts. Nevertheless, the combined method for α-naphthyl butyrate esterase and chloroacetate esterase (48,59) provides an objective means for demonstrating monocytes and granulocytes simultaneously in cytologic preparations and is useful for the diagnosis of acute myeloblastic (FAB M1-3), myelomonocytic (FAB M4), and monocytic (FAB M5) leukemias (Figs. 38.7–38.9; see also Color Plates 5–7, between pp. 1446–1447). A combination of chloroacetate esterase and cyanide-resistant peroxidase stains is also helpful in the diagnosis of acute eosinophilic leukemia, which is characteristically negative for chloroacetate esterase and positive for cyanide-resistant peroxidase (50) (Fig. 38.5).

Chloroacetate esterase is unusually stable and withstands storage and tissue processing. Enzyme activity can be demonstrated in the myeloid cells in formalin-fixed and paraffin-embedded tissues that have been stored for many years (66). However, fixatives containing mercury chloride (e.g., B5) inactivate the enzyme completely. The histochemical demonstration of chloroacetate esterase in myeloid cells is useful for the diagnosis of myeloid metaplasia or granulocytic sarcoma (71). Because of the low sensitivity of this enzyme for the early myeloblasts in tissues of such disorders, immunohistochemical staining for myeloperoxidase or lysozyme

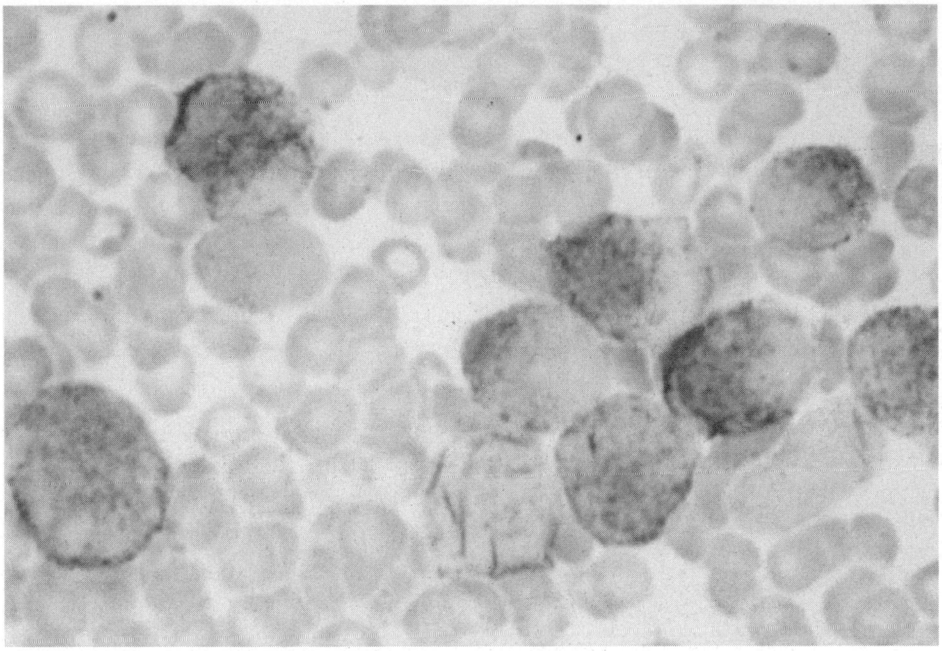

FIG. 38.6. Acute progranulocytic leukemia (M3) with strong chloroacetate esterase stain as shown by the bright red cytoplasmic granules and rods (chloroacetate esterase stain, original magnification: 320× magnification). See Color Plate 4, between pp. 1446–1447.

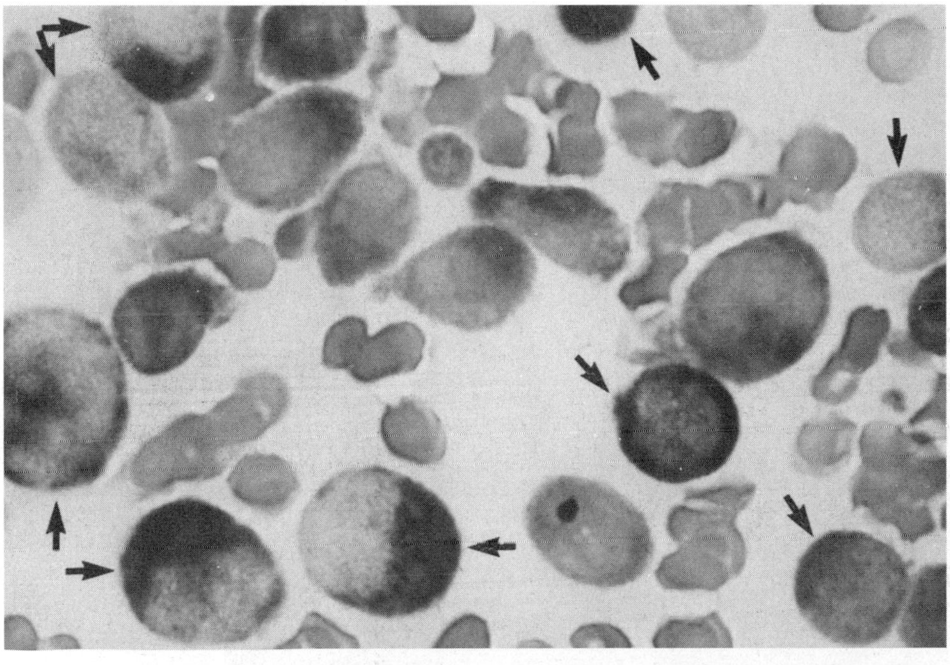

FIG. 38.7. Acute myelomonocytic leukemia (M4): monocytic cells with positive butyrate esterase stain and granulocytic cells with positive chloroacetate esterase stain. Darker staining cells, mostly at the left lower corner of the field *(arrows)*, represent cells with chloroacetate esterase activity (combined butyrate esterase and chloroacetate esterase stains, original magnification: 320× magnification). See Color Plate 5, between pp. 1446–1447.

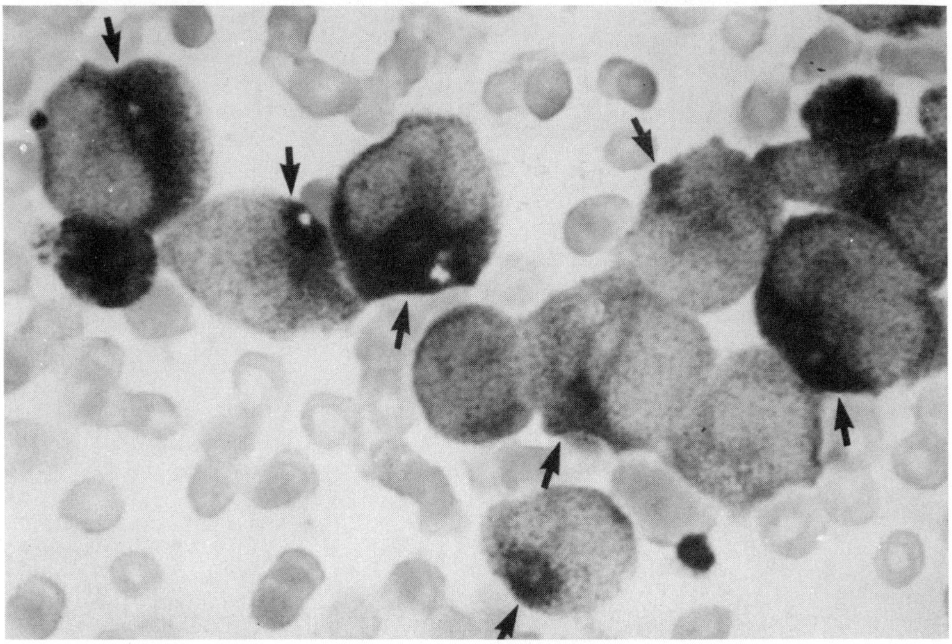

FIG. 38.8. Variant acute myelomonocytic leukemia (M4 variant). Many leukemic cells are positive for both butyrate esterase and chloroacetate esterase. Darker staining at Golgi areas *(arrows)* represents chloroacetate esterase activity (combined butyrate esterase and chloroacetate esterase stains, original magnification: 320× magnification). See Color Plate 6, between pp. 1446–1447.

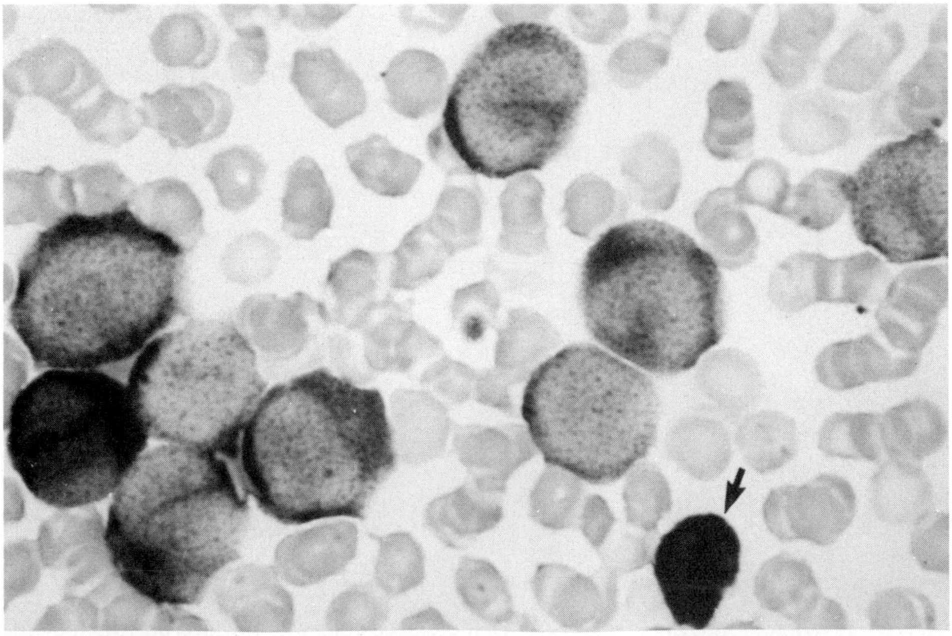

FIG. 38.9. Acute monocytic leukemia (M5b) with positive butyrate esterase stain in the cytoplasm of leukemic cells. A normal neutrophil at right lower corner *(arrow)* shows positive chloroacetate esterase activity (combined butyrate esterase and chloroacetate esterase stains, original magnification: 320× magnification). See Color Plate 7, between pp. 1446–1447.

may offer additional diagnostic assistance (71–74). In tissue sections containing many cells positive for chloroacetate esterase, it is important to remember that mast cells also possess this enzyme and that the possibility of mast cell disease should be considered.

α-Naphthyl Acetate Esterase

ANAE was initially used for the cytochemical identification of monocytes (49). This was replaced by the α-naphthyl butyrate esterase method (75). ANAE also gives distinctive focal staining in mature lymphocytes and can be used as a marker for these cells. Although several methods for the cytochemical demonstration of lymphocytic esterase (76–78) had been developed for this purpose, the original method (49), using α-naphthyl acetate as substrate and hexazotized pararosanilin as a coupler at pH 6.3, remains the simplest method for demonstrating monocyte and lymphocyte esterases. The incubation time can be prolonged to 2 hours if necessary for enhancement of focal staining in the mature T lymphocytes.

In human blood cells, ANAE activity is present in monocytes, macrophages, megakaryocytes, plasma cells, hairy cells, and lymphocytes (49,75). Lymphocytes with dotlike ANAE activity have been correlated to T lymphocytes with sheep erythrocyte receptors (CD2), receptors for IgM (T_μ or T_m cell), pan-T (CD3) antigen, and helper T antigen (CD4) (79–82) (Figs. 38.10–38.12). In contrast, T lymphocytes with surface receptors for IgG (T_γ or T_g-cells) display a more diffuse reaction pattern with a paranuclear localization (80,83,84). B lymphocytes are generally negative for ANAE activity.

When using ANAE staining for identification of monocytes or macrophages, megakaryocytes may also show intense diffuse cytoplasmic staining and plasma cells show reactions that may vary from diffuse to coarse and granular (75). Positive acetate esterase and weak or negative butyrate esterase staining have been considered characteristic of megakaryoblasts in acute myeloid leukemia (AML-M7) (85,86). The ANAE stain is more commonly used for the identification of mature helper T lymphocytes. It is particularly useful for distinguishing helper T-cell chronic lymphocytic leukemia from other lymphoproliferative disorders of mature cell type (87–91) (Fig. 38.11).

α-Naphthyl Butyrate Esterase

In human blood cells, α-naphthyl butyrate esterase (i.e., nonspecific esterase) activity is seen in monocytes, macrophages, megakaryocytes, and mature helper T lymphocytes. Monocytes and macrophages usually exhibit intense diffuse cytoplasmic staining. Megakaryocytes may also show diffuse weak cytoplasmic staining. Reactivity in lymphocytes is usually localized in one to three discrete dots in the cytoplasm.

α-Naphthyl butyrate esterase staining is most useful for identifying cells in the monocyte-macrophage lineage. In the typing of leukemias on blood or marrow smears, it is used to identify the monocytic or monoblastic subtypes of leukemia (M5a and M5b) and to identify the monocytic component in acute myelomonocytic leukemias (M4) and in chronic myelomonocytic leukemia (48,92–94) (Figs. 38.7–38.9).

The histochemical demonstration of α-naphthyl butyrate esterase is useful for identifying monocytes and histiocytes

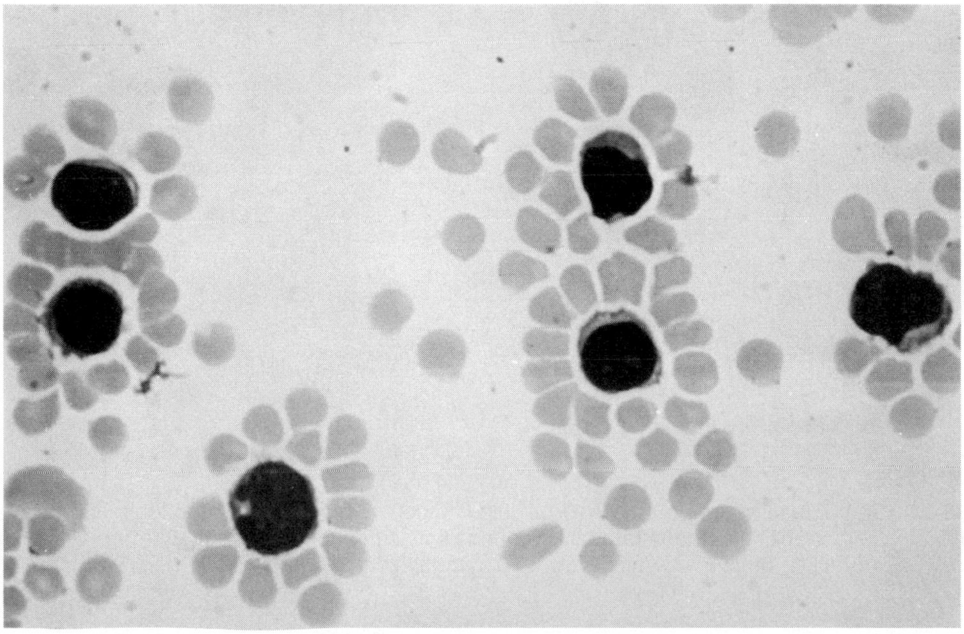

FIG. 38.10. Helper T-cell chronic lymphocytic leukemia with sheep erythrocyte rosette (E-rosette) formation (original magnification: 320× magnification).

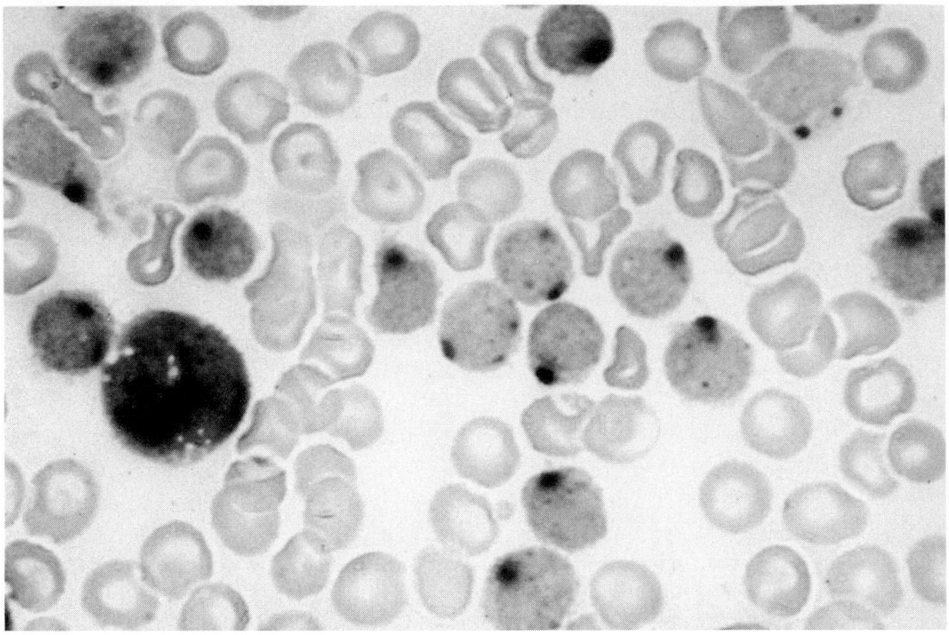

FIG. 38.11. Same case as in Figure 38.10 of helper T-cell chronic lymphocytic leukemia with strong focal α-naphthyl acetate esterase activity in the leukemic cells. A monocyte with strong diffuse acetate esterase activity is also present at the left lower corner of the field (α-naphthyl acetate esterase stain, original magnification: 320× magnification).

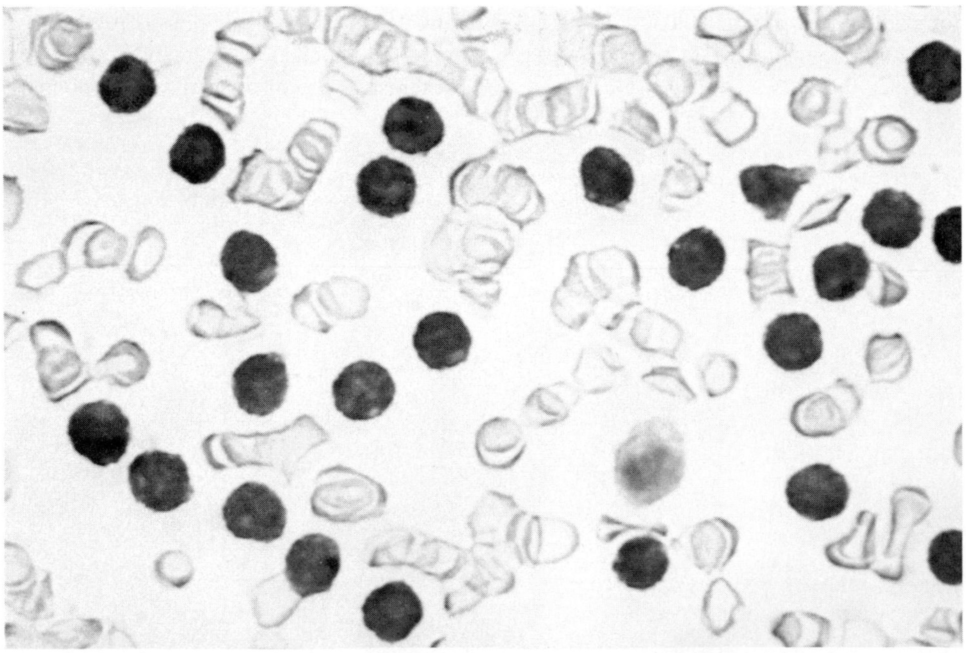

FIG. 38.12. Same case as in Figure 38.10 of helper T-cell chronic lymphocytic leukemia with strong helper T-cell antigen (CD4) demonstrated by immunoalkaline phosphatase stain (immunoalkaline phosphatase stain for CD4, original magnification: 320× magnification).

and for the diagnosis of true histiocytic lymphoma or malignant histiocytosis (95–97). In this context, it is important to keep in mind that some epithelial or carcinoma cells may also show significant staining for esterase activity (98,99). When sodium fluoride is added to the staining solution, enzyme activity in the monocytes and many tissue histiocytes and epithelial cells is inhibited; however, enzyme activity may be retained in the specialized or differentiated histiocytes, such as the Gaucher cells and epithelioid cells in granulomas (2).

Aminocaproate Esterase

Aminocaproate esterase is a specific enzyme marker for mast cells. The method using naphthol AS ϵ-aminocaproate as substrate and hexazotized new fuchsin or fast blue BB as a coupler at pH 7.4 is the most satisfactory (75,100–102). Normal mast cells show intense diffuse cytoplasmic staining (Fig. 38.13; see also Color Plate 8, between pp. 1446–1447), and the abnormal mast cells seen in mast cell disease usually show similar, but weaker, staining (Fig. 38.14). Other blood cells do not show significant staining, except very weak reactivity in occasional immature granulocytes after prolonged staining.

This enzyme is fairly sensitive to heat and tissue processing and is not demonstrable in paraffin-embedded tissue sections. Histochemical staining can be done on frozen sections but is most satisfactory on properly prepared plastic sections, which preserves morphology and enzyme activity nicely. The histochemical demonstration of aminocaproate esterase is most useful for the identification or confirmation of mast cell diseases (102) (Fig. 38.15; see also Color Plate 9, between pp. 1446–1447).

Acid Phosphatase and Tartrate-Resistant Acid Phosphatase

The acid phosphatases are a group of enzymes capable of hydrolyzing phosphate ester in an acid pH. Seven acid phosphatase isoenzymes (0, 1, 2, 3, 3b, 4, and 5) are present in human leukocytes and other tissues (103,104). Some of these isoenzymes are cell specific, such as isoenzymes 2 and 4 in neutrophils and epithelial cells of the prostate gland, 4 in monocytes, 3 in lymphocytes and platelets, 3b in primitive blasts, and 5 in HCL cells, epithelioid histiocytes, lipid storage cells (e.g., Gaucher cells), and osteoclasts (105). Isoenzyme 5 differs from the other isoenzymes in its resistance to L(+)-tartaric acid treatment. The method using naphthol AS-BI phosphoric acid and fast garnet GBC is most satisfactory for the cytochemical demonstration of acid phosphatase activity in smear preparations, and the method using naphthol AS-BI phosphoric acid and hexazotized pararosanilin is best for tissue sections (106,107).

The acid phosphatases are present in all types of blood cells. Enzyme activity is strong in monocytes and moderate to weak in granulocytes, lymphocytes, and platelets. Various stages of transformed T cells in lectin-stimulated lymphocytic cultures have strong acid phosphatase activity that is largely confined to the Golgi region. This focal acid phosphatase activity in the Golgi area has also been demonstrated in various T-cell–derived malignancies, including T-cell acute lymphoblastic leukemia (T-ALL) (Fig. 38.16), lymphoblastic lymphoma, cutaneous T-cell lymphomas, and large T-cell lymphomas (95,108–110). In contrast, the various stages of transformed B cells seen in reactive follicular cen-

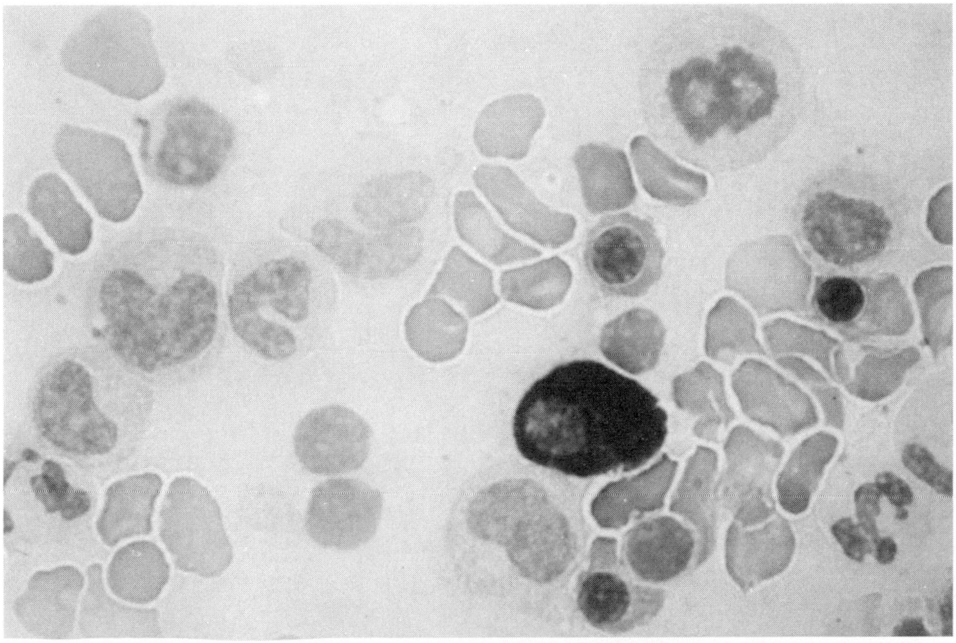

FIG. 38.13. A normal mast cell in the marrow aspirate smear with strong aminocaproate esterase activity is illustrated by bright red granules in the cytoplasm (aminocaproate esterase stain, original magnification: 320× magnification). See Color Plate 8, between pp. 1446–1447.

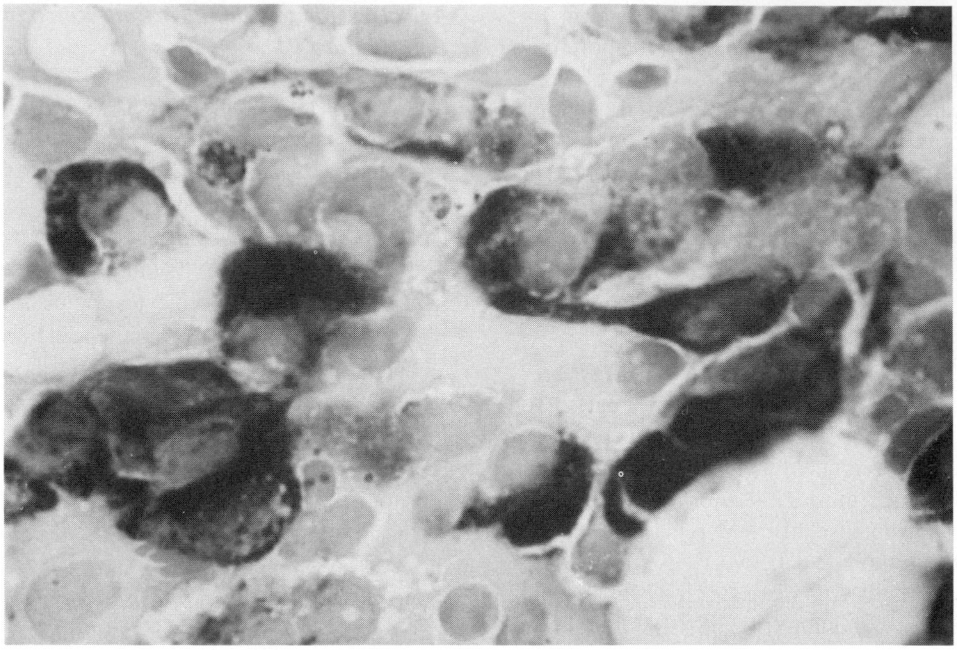

FIG. 38.14. Bone marrow aspirate smear from patient with systemic mast cell disease shows an aggregate of atypical mast cells with elongated nuclei and positive aminocaproate esterase activity (aminocaproate esterase stain, original magnification: 320× magnification).

ters and various B-cell–derived leukemias and lymphomas have very weak and diffuse cytoplasmic acid phosphatase activity. The acid phosphatase reaction can be useful for differentiating T-ALL from non-T-ALL. However, erythroblasts and early myeloblasts may also show similar focal acid phosphatase staining features. In classifying acute leukemia, the acid phosphatase stain is best used in combination with peroxidase and butyrate esterase stains to ensure the distinction of lymphoblastic leukemia from the myeloblastic or monoblastic type.

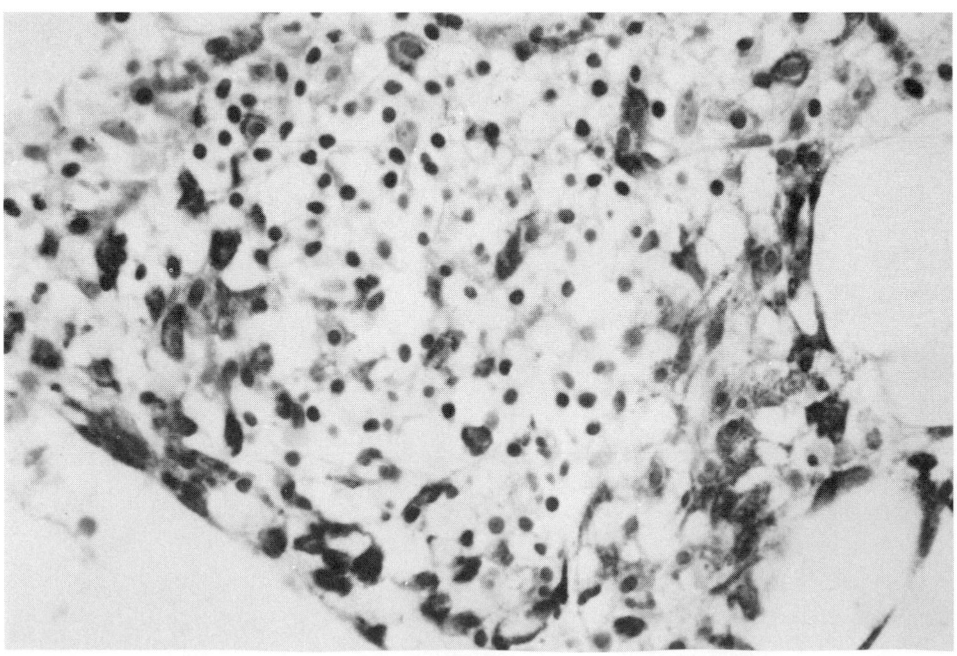

FIG. 38.15. Plastic section of bone marrow biopsy from patient with systemic mast cell disease showing aminocaproate esterase positive atypical mast cells infiltrating around a lymphoid follicle (aminocaproate esterase stain, original magnification: 128× magnification). See Color Plate 9, between pp. 1446–1447.

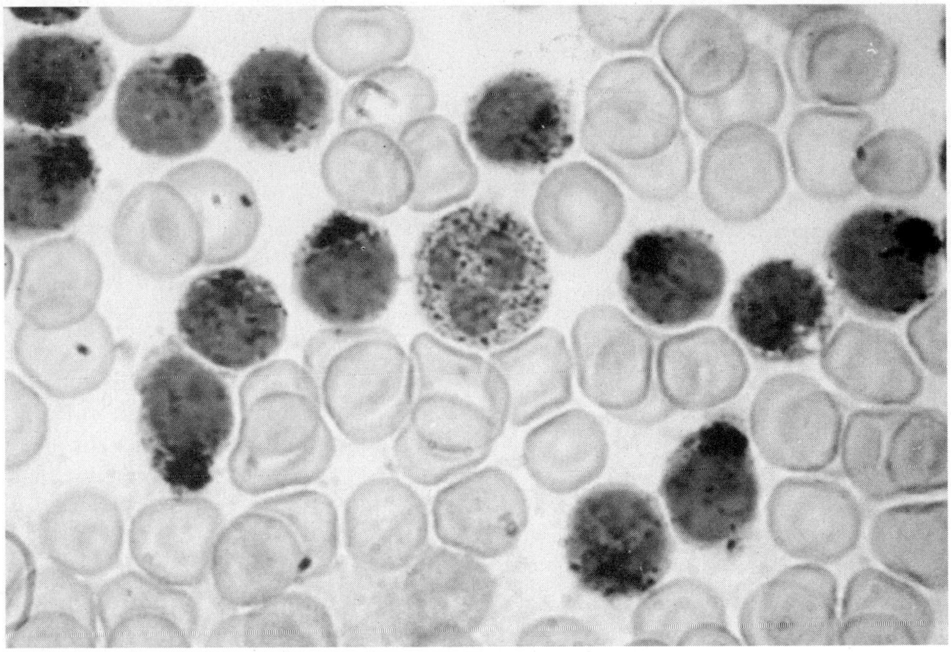

FIG. 38.16. T-cell acute lymphoblastic leukemia with strong focal acid phosphatase activity confined to the Golgi areas (acid phosphatase stain, original magnification: 320× magnification).

In myeloma, activity of acid phosphatase in the plasma cells is significantly higher than in those of other diseases (111,112).

Cytochemical demonstration of the tartrate-resistant acid phosphatase (isoenzyme 5) (TRAP) is used for identifying the hairy cells of HCL (113,114) (Fig. 38.17; see also Color Plate 10, between pp. 1446–1447). This method is particularly useful when there are only a few leukemic cells in a leukopenic patient. As few as two or more cells with strong enzyme activity (i.e., more than 40 dark red granules in the cytoplasm) in blood or buffy coat smears are sufficient to establish the diagnosis of this disease. Strong TRAP activity is also present in other cells, such as epithelioid cells, lipid storage cells, osteoclasts, and mast cells (115,116). The mor-

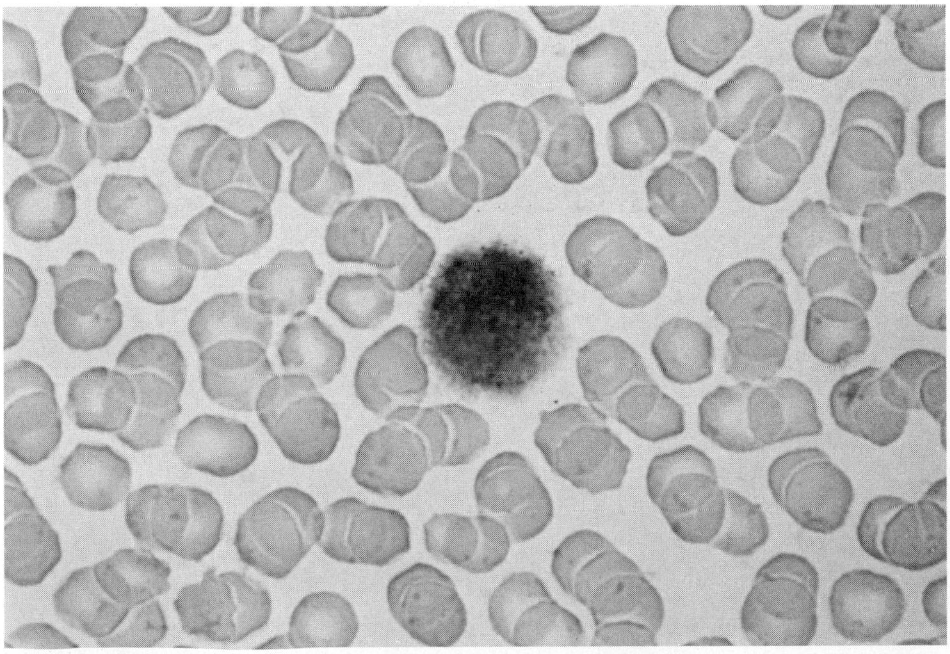

FIG. 38.17. Hairy cell leukemia with strong tartrate-resistant acid phosphatase activity (tartrate-resistant acid phosphatase stain, original magnification: 320× magnification). See Color Plate 10, between pp. 1446–1447.

phologic appearance of these cells is easily distinguished from that of hairy cells. Weak to moderate TRAP activity (i.e., less than 40 granules in the cytoplasm) may be seen in some activated lymphocytes and has been observed in prolymphocytic leukemia and Sezary cells (117,118).

The histochemical demonstration of acid phosphatase for focal enzyme activity at the Golgi region is useful for identifying transformed T lymphocytes. It may be useful for the diagnosis of T-cell lymphomas or leukemias. In other lesions containing many lipid storage cells, epithelioid cells, osteoclasts, and some phagocytic histiocytes, histochemical studies with TRAP stain also are helpful. Mast cells also have significant TRAP activity, and the morphology of abnormal mast cells on tissue sections is similar to that of hairy cells. Additional histochemical stains, including aminocaproate esterase and toluidine blue, are helpful in distinguishing mast cells from hairy cells (53).

Sudan Black B Stain

Sudan black B stain is a fat-soluble dye with very high affinity for phospholipids in the granules of granulocytes and is useful for identifying granulocytes. The method of Sheehan and Storey (119) is most widely used. Sudan black B is comparable to that of the peroxidase stain in its staining pattern of leukocytes. It may be preferred over the peroxidase stain for smears more than 2 weeks old. Because of its fat solubility, Sudan black B may also stain the marrow fat and some cytoplasmic vacuoles of transformed lymphocytes such as the L3 lymphoblasts in B-cell acute lymphoblastic leukemia or Burkitt's lymphoma (120,121). Histochemical studies of tissue sections with Sudan black B are of little clinical value.

Toluidine Blue Stain

Toluidine blue O dye can bind with acid mucopolysaccharides to give metachromatic staining. The granules in basophils and mast cells stain reddish violet because of the strong metachromatic effect of the inorganic sulfuric acid esterified in heparin. All other elements are stained pale blue. The toluidine blue stain is useful for identifying basophils and mast cells and helpful in the diagnosis of acute myeloid leukemia with basophilic differentiation (Fig. 38.18; see also Color Plate 11, between pp. 1446–1447) and mast cell diseases (49,53,122).

Histochemical studies with toluidine blue for metachromatic substances are best performed in plastic sections of tissue without decalcification. They may be done on frozen tissue sections and, to a limited extent, on paraffin tissue sections (123).

Chlorazol–Fast Pink Stain

Chlorazol–fast pink selectively stains eosinophilic granules bright red and is useful in tissue sections for the identification of eosinophils (2). However, the chlorazol–fast pink only stains well-formed eosinophilic granules and is not as effective as the cyanide-resistant peroxidase for cells in the cases of acute myeloid leukemia with eosinophilic differentiation (50).

Iron Stain

The Prussian blue stain for iron can be done in smears, imprints, and tissue sections. It is used for identifying the ringed sideroblasts in myelodysplastic syndromes (MDS) and in erythroleukemia.

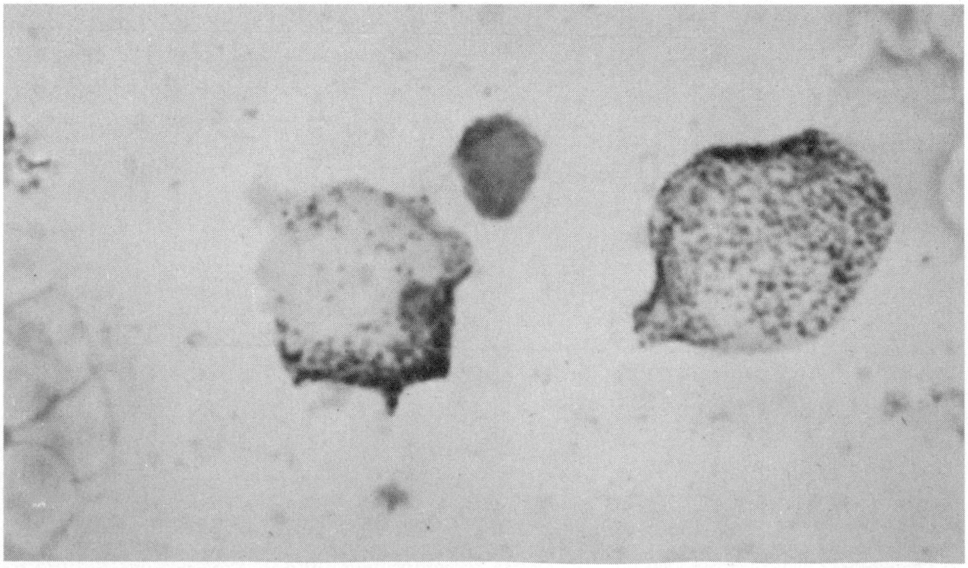

FIG. 38.18. Acute basophilic leukemia with metachromatic cytoplasmic granules (toluidine blue stain, original magnification: 640× magnification). See Color Plate 11, between pp. 1446–1447.

Periodic Acid–Schiff Reaction

In the PAS reaction, the periodic acid serves as the oxidizing agent to furnish the aldehyde groups, and the Schiff reagent (leucofuchsin) stains tissues containing aldehyde groups bright red. Many compounds in tissues stain with the PAS reaction. The stainable compound in the blood cells is primarily glycogen. Although the mature granulocytes, platelets, megakaryocytes, and monocytes are stained positively with the PAS reaction, early myeloid cells, erythroid cells, and many lymphoid cells are not (124,125). "Blocks" of PAS-positive material in these cells may indicate a disturbance in glycogen metabolism that may be useful for diagnostic purposes (126). In acute lymphoblastic leukemia, the PAS reaction is frequently seen in the $CD10^+$ lymphoblasts but not in the B-cell lymphoblasts with L3 morphology (127). The PAS reaction may therefore be used as a marker for common acute lymphoblastic leukemia. In dysplastic or neoplastic disorders involving erythroid cells, block staining is seen in the early erythroblasts and diffuse staining in the late erythroblasts (128). The PAS reaction, especially when coupled with the iron stain, is useful for the diagnosis of these disorders. In bone marrow sections, the PAS reaction is useful for outlining the fibrous tissues and the marrow framework. It also stains the cytoplasm of the megakaryocytes and is useful for the identification of these cells.

Reticulin Stain

The reticulin fibers form the supporting framework of the bone marrow. These fibers may increase when there is hyperplasia of the marrow. In pathologic conditions such as myelofibrosis, these fibers are increased, and their growth patterns become distorted (129). Although reticulin fibers are stainable by the PAS reaction, many cells in the marrow also may be extensively stained, obscuring the staining pattern of the reticulin fibers. Silver staining methods for reticulin are more suitable (130). When the reticulin stains are performed properly, the reticulin fibers stain intensely, but the nuclei of many hematopoietic cells stain only weakly or not at all. The finding of reticulin fibrosis with distorted growth patterns is seen in disorders such as myelofibrosis with myeloid metaplasia and the late stages of a number of disorders, including polycythemia vera, chronic myelocytic leukemia, essential thrombocythemia, HCL, and mast cell diseases. It is also seen in carcinoma with metastasis to the bone marrow.

Immunocytochemistry and Immunohistochemistry

Lymphoid Markers

Lymphocytes are functionally heterogeneous but are morphologically similar. They are derived from pluripotent stem cells of the marrow that differentiate into mature B or T lymphocytes. This differentiation process is accompanied by significant alterations in nuclear, cytoplasmic, and surface antigens in addition to some morphologic changes. T and B cells recirculate between blood and lymph, but within lymphoid tissue, they are selectively compartmentalized into T- or B-cell dominant zones. On contact with specific antigens, mature T or B lymphocytes may transform from small, resting lymphocytes into large, activated cells. The excess number of abnormal lymphoid cells seen in lymphoproliferative disorders is thought to result from maturation arrest at certain levels of lymphoid differentiation or transformation (131,132). The immunochemical characteristics of these abnormal cells are often the same as their normal counterparts. Immunochemical studies with a number of lymphoid markers (Tables 38.2, 38.3) can identify the lymphoid cells, disclose their stage of differentiation and transformation, and determine their clonality (133,134) (Fig. 38.19). Most of the markers in Table 38.2 (5,133,135) can be demonstrated in smears, cell suspensions, and fresh frozen tissue sections (5,38,46,136–140) but not in paraffin-embedded tissue sections without epitope retrieval or signal amplification.

Several antibodies, including CD45 (leukocyte common antigen), CD20 (L26), CD3, CD45RO (UCHL-1), LN1, LN2, LN3, MB2, MT1, and CD30 (BER-H2) (141–143), have been developed to react with lymphoid antigens in paraffin-embedded tissues. Only a few are specific enough for identifying all lymphocytes (CD45), B lymphocytes (CD20 and cytoplasmic immunoglobulin), T lymphocytes (CD3), and natural killer (NK) cells (CD57) (Table 38.3). CD45 has been used to distinguish lymphoid cells and histiocytes from nonlymphoid cells (144). Cytoplasmic immunoglobulin light chains have been used to determine the clonality of B lymphocytes and plasma cells (95,145). CD20 is the most specific and sensitive marker for identifying B lymphocytes, including transformed (activated) B lymphocytes (146–147). UCHL-1 is mainly immunoreactive with small mature T lymphocytes and usually only very weakly or not at all with large activated T lymphocytes (148). CD43 (Leu-22) is sensitive for the identification of large activated T lymphocytes in lymph node sections; however, its cross-reactivity with granulocytes and monocytes limits its ability to delineate T-cell lesions in marrow sections (149). With the improvement of immunohistochemical methods using effective antigen retrieval and signal amplification techniques, the number of lymphoid antigens that can be demonstrated in paraffin-embedded tissues increased significantly. These include cytoplasmic CD3 for T and precursor T cells, CD79a for B and precursor B cells, CD8 for cytotoxic T cells, CD56 for NK cells, TIA-1 for cytotoxic T and NK cells, and CD5 and CD23 for subsets of B cells (29–31,43–45,150) (see Chapter 3).

Myeloid Markers

Many immunochemical markers specific for granulocytes and monocytes have been identified, including CD11, CD13, CD14, CD15, and CD33 (151). Most of these markers, although identifiable by immunocytochemical techniques, are

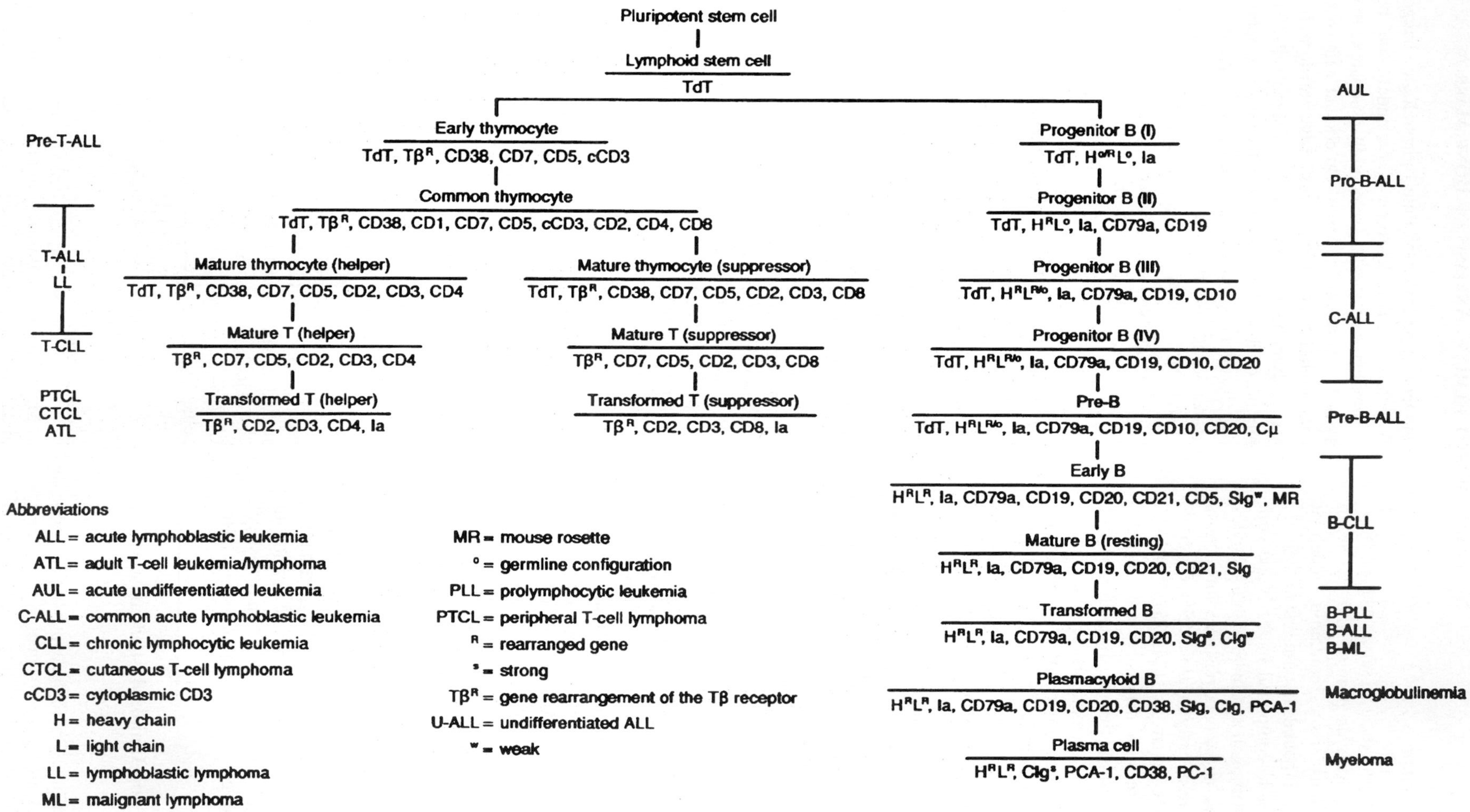

FIG. 38.19. Presumptive levels of maturation arrest in lymphoproliferative diseases and immunochemical characteristics of cells at each level of differentiation.

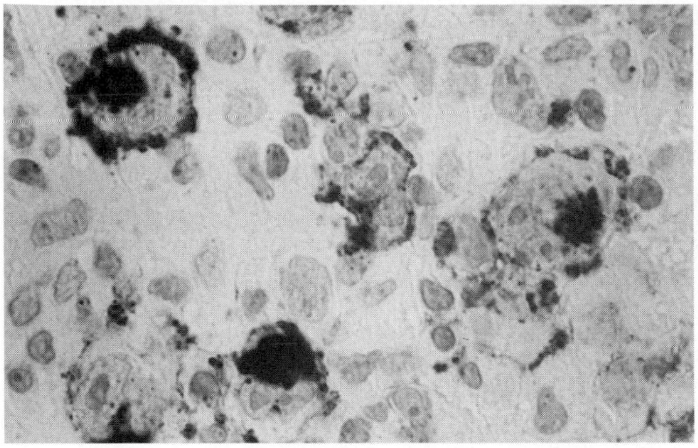

FIG. 38.20. Paraffin section of a bone marrow biopsy for Hodgkin's lesion, showing characteristic surface and paranuclear immunostaining of CD15 in Reed-Sternberg cells (indirect immunoperoxidase staining for CD15 using monoclonal antibody Leu-M1, original magnification: 320× magnification).

less sensitive than a simple peroxidase stain for identifying early myeloblasts (152) or a butyrate esterase stain for identifying monocytes. However, some of these markers may be a useful alternative in identifying myeloblasts (CD13) with myeloperoxidase deficiency or monocytes (CD14) with esterase deficiency.

In paraffin-embedded marrow sections, myeloperoxidase, lysozyme, and CD68 (PG-M1) are useful markers for identifying immature granulocytes, monocytes, or histiocytes (71–74,95,97,153). CD15 (Leu-M1) and CD43 are strongly expressed by mature granulocytes. CD15 also shows rather characteristic paranuclear and surface membrane expression in the Reed-Sternberg cells of Hodgkin's lesions and is commonly used for confirming the diagnosis of Hodgkin's disease (154,155) (Fig. 38.20) (see Chapter 3).

Erythroid Markers

For cells in smears, suspensions, and fresh tissue, glycophorin present in erythroblasts and erythrocytes has been considered the erythroid-specific cell surface marker of choice (156). However, the sensitivity and specificity of the antibodies for glycophorin may vary according to the sources of these antibodies (157). Epitopes immunologically related to glycophorin A are also present in a variety of nonerythroid cell types (158). Other monoclonal antibodies such as RC82.4 and EP-1 have specificity for yet uncharacterized surface antigens on erythroblasts and erythroid progenitors (159,160). Monoclonal antibody RC82.4 has been used successfully to confirm the diagnosis of poorly differentiated erythroleukemia (159) (Fig. 38.21; see also Color Plate 12, between pp. 1446–1447).

For paraffin-embedded tissues, hemoglobin and transforming growth factor-β1 are sensitive and specific markers for erythroblasts (161,162). They are useful in distinguishing diseases associated with left-shifted erythropoiesis from other neoplastic diseases involving bone marrow, such as nonerythroid acute leukemia or malignant lymphomas (163). However, the sensitivity of this marker for the primitive erythroblasts of erythroid leukemia remains to be determined.

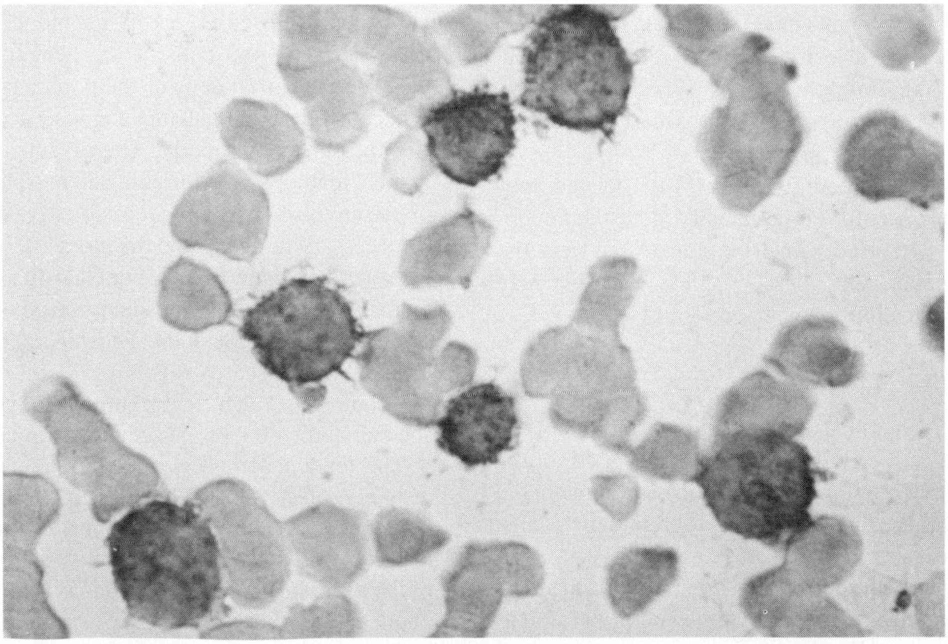

FIG. 38.21. Poorly differentiated acute erythroblastic leukemia with strong red cell antigen demonstrated by immunoperoxidase technique (indirect immunoperoxidase stain for red cell antigen using monoclonal antibody RC-82.4, original magnification: 320× magnification). See Color Plate 12, between pp. 1446–1447.

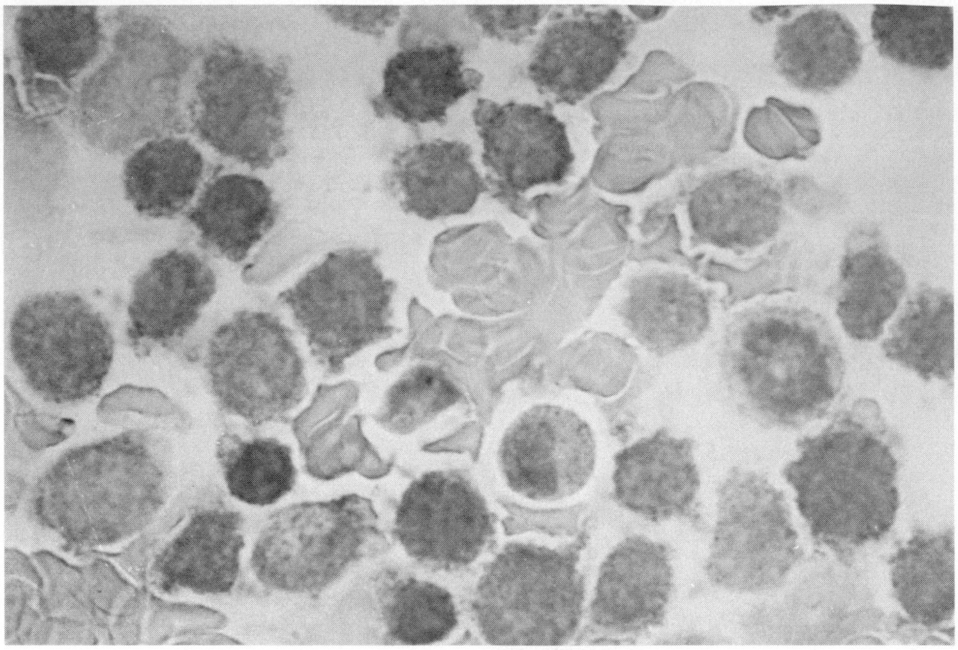

FIG. 38.22. Acute megakaryocytic leukemia (M7) with strong CD41 (glycoprotein IIb/IIIa) complex demonstrated by immunoalkaline phosphatase stain (immunoalkaline phosphatase stain for CD41 using monoclonal antibody HP1-1D, original magnification: 320× magnification). See Color Plate 13, between pp. 1446–1447.

Megakaryocytic Markers

Several immunochemical markers, including CD41 and CD42b have been used to identify megakaryocytes and platelets in smears (164–167); the CD41 (glycoprotein IIb/IIIa complex) is particularly suitable for this purpose. Immunocytochemical studies of this marker are helpful in identifying early megakaryocytic cells in acute megakaryocytic leukemia (Fig. 38.22; see also Color Plate 13, between pp. 1446–1447). It has definite advantages over the more tedious method of demonstrating platelet peroxidase by electron microscopy for the same purpose (165).

In paraffin-embedded sections, factor VIII–related antigen can be used for identifying megakaryocytes and endothelial cells (163,164,168). In air-dried smears and fresh tissue sections, however, this marker is less sensitive than CD41 in the identification of megakaryoblasts.

Epithelial and Other Markers

The immunohistochemical demonstration of keratin or epithelial membrane antigen (EMA) is commonly used for the identification or confirmation of metastatic carcinoma in the marrow. In using EMA as a marker for epithelial cells, plasma cells in the marrow may also show significant staining. Careful morphologic correlation is important in interpreting immunostaining to be sure that the activity is associated with malignant cells. Prostate-specific antigen and prostatic acid phosphatase can be used as markers for metastatic prostatic carcinoma (169,170). Other useful markers include chromogranin and synaptophysin for neuroendocrine or neurogenic tumors (i.e., undifferentiated small cell carcinoma, neuroblastoma, and medulloblastoma) (171–173) and desmin and muscle actin for muscle tumors (i.e., rhabdomyosarcoma) (173–176) (see Chapter 30).

CLINICAL APPLICATION

Neoplastic diseases involving blood or marrow include those derived from cells of the hematopoietic system and those derived from cells of the nonhematopoietic system. It is necessary to establish the diagnosis accurately and to classify the subtype properly. The diagnosis is often based on clinical features of the disease and morphologic examination of the involved tissues. Occasionally, special studies may be necessary to determine the clonality of the cells involved to ensure the diagnosis. Proper classification is always based on recognition of cell type and its stage of maturation, which often require special study. The general diagnostic approach to neoplastic diseases involving blood or marrow is to use morphologic studies for accurate diagnosis and to rely on special studies for proper classification.

The tendency to perform a complete battery of special tests nonselectively for diagnostic purposes is highly desirable in research environments; it is cost prohibitive in clinical practice. A more practical approach is to take advantage of the available technology and to select the simplest method applicable to the available specimen.

The choice of techniques for clinical diagnosis is often determined by the type of specimens available. The specimens available are often determined by the disease. In leukemias, for example, smears or cell suspensions prepared from

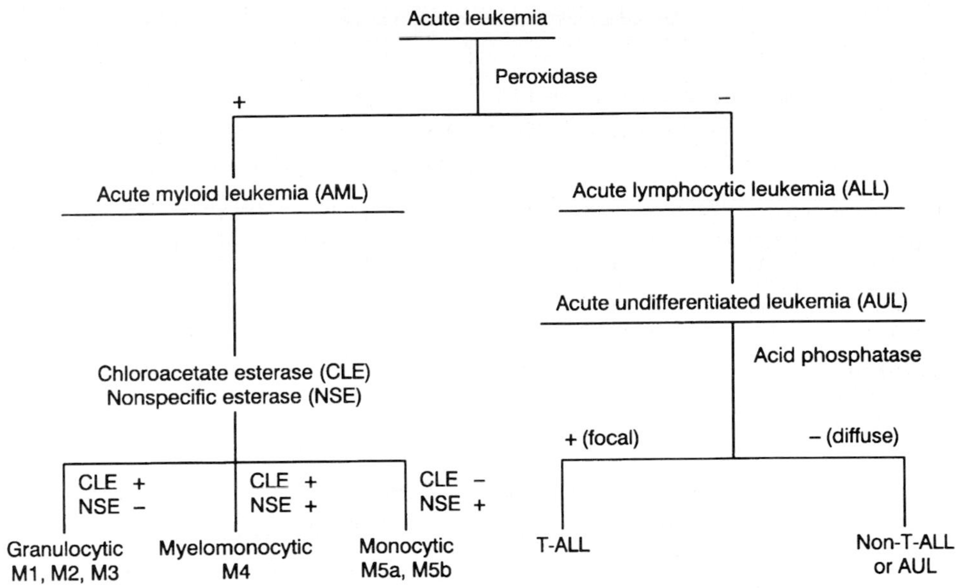

FIG. 38.23. Classification of acute leukemia using four cytochemical stains.

blood and marrow are often available, whereas in lymphomas or metastatic tumors, imprints and tissue sections from marrow biopsies are often used for diagnostic purposes. The general indications for special studies include

A difficult differential diagnosis between atypical reactive hyperplasia and neoplastic disease

Subclassification of neoplastic diseases in which the morphologic distinction is difficult, such as for acute leukemias, chronic lymphoproliferative disorders, non-Hodgkin's lymphomas, round cell tumors

Confirmation of the diagnosis in an unusual disease such as HCL or systemic mast cell disease

Confirmation of a diagnosis in a patient with an unusual clinical presentation, such as chronic lymphocytic leukemia or multiple myeloma in a person younger than 40 years

Acute Myeloid Leukemias

The French-American-British (FAB) classification scheme has the acute myeloid leukemias (AMLs) classified according to the type of cell involved and degree of differentiation into M1 through M7 (177,178). Cytochemical techniques help classify M1 through M5 in most instances (Figs. 38.4, 38.6–38.9, 38.23). They also help to recognize cases with blasts in early eosinophilic (50) or basophilic differentiation (122) (Figs. 38.5, 38.18). The use of erythroid and megakaryocytic immunologic markers helps to identify these respective elements in M6 and M7 subtypes of AML (Table 38.4; Figs. 38.21, 38.22, 38.24). The use of other myeloid and lymphoid markers offers little additional information except in recognizing undifferentiated (M0) or biphenotypic cases (179–183).

If only the marrow biopsy or clot sections are available,

TABLE 38.4. *Cytochemical and immunocytochemical characteristics of acute leukemia*

Marker	M0	M1	M2	M3	M4	M5	M6	M7	T-ALL	Non-T-ALL
Peroxidase	0	1–3+	3+	4+	1–3+	0–1+	1–3+	0	0	0
Sudan black B	0	1–3+	3+	4+	1–3+	0–2+	1–3+	0	0	0
Chloroacetate esterase	0	0–2+	1–3+	1–3+	1–3+	0	1–3+	0	0	0
α-Naphthyl butyrate esterase	0	0	0	0–2+	1–2+ (D)	2–4+ (D)	0–1+ (D)	0–1+ (D)	0–1+ (F)	0
Acid phosphatase	0–1+ (D)	1–2+ (D)	1–2+ (D)	3+ (D)	1–3+ (D)	1–3+ (D)	1–3+ (D+F)	1–2+ (D)	1–3+ (F)	0–1+ (D)
Prussian blue	0	0	0	0	0	0	+	0	0	0
Megakaryocytic marker (CD41)	0	0	0	0	0	0	0	+	0	0
Red cell antigen (RC 82.4)	0	0	0	0	0	0	+	0	0	0
Myeloid markers (CD13)	+	+	+	+	+	+	+	0	0	0
Lymphoid markers (TdT)	±	0	0	0	0	0	0	0	+	+

ALL, acute lymphoblastic leukemia; D, diffuse cytoplasmic staining; F, focal staining confined to Golgi area; T, T cell.

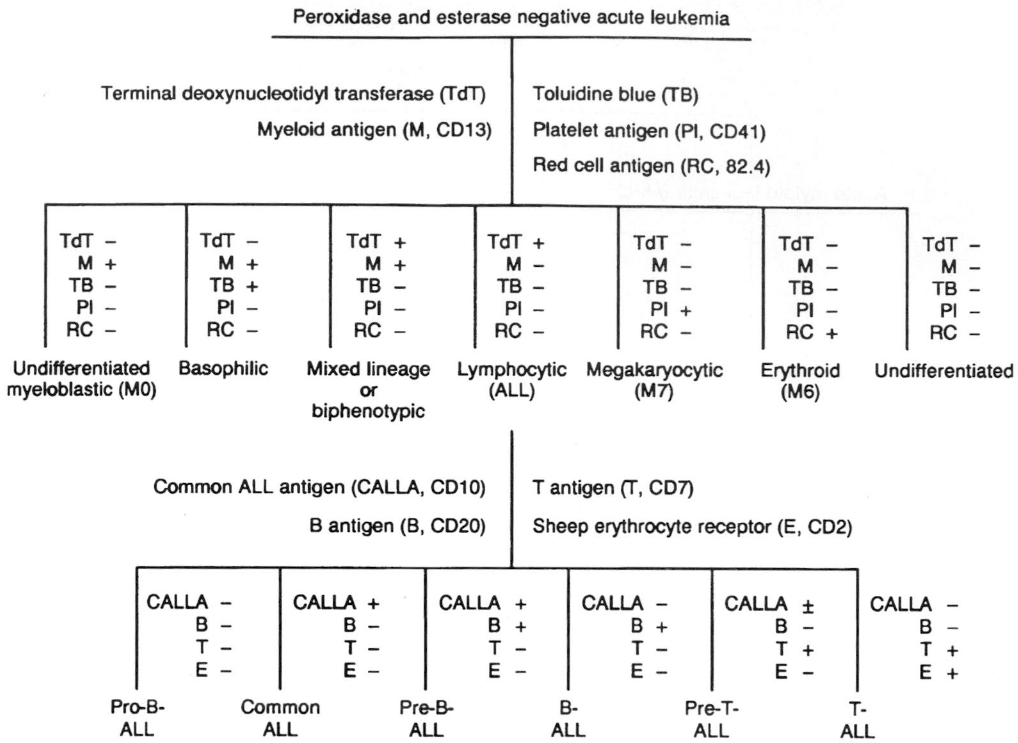

FIG. 38.24. Classification of peroxidase- and esterase-negative acute leukemia using immunocytochemical methods.

immunohistochemical studies of myeloperoxidase, CD68 (PG-M1), hemoglobin, and factor VIII antigen may be helpful for confirming granulocytic, monocytic, erythroid, and megakaryocytic cell types, respectively (163,184) (see Chapter 47).

Acute Lymphoid Leukemias

Although the diagnosis and classification of acute lymphoid leukemias had been established by morphologic criteria according to the FAB scheme (177), the use of immunocytochemical techniques can attain better diagnostic accuracy (Tables 38.4, 38.5; Figs. 38.23–38.27; see also Color Plate 14, between pp. 1446–1447). Cytochemical studies are of limited value except in demonstrating focal enzyme activity of acid phosphatase and ANAE in T lymphoblasts (Fig. 38.16). For paraffin tissue sections of marrow specimens, immunohistochemical studies for CD3, CD79a, and CD20 are helpful for confirming precursor-T-cell, precursor-B-cell, and B-cell immunophenotypes respectively (163,184) (see Chapter 46).

Myelodysplastic Syndromes

The cytochemical and immunocytochemical markers for AML are also useful for MDS. Ringed sideroblasts (i.e., iron stain) and the PAS reaction for blocks of PAS-positive cytoplasmic glycogen are useful markers for dysplastic erythroblasts and immature megakaryocytes (185). Many immature myeloid cells with activities of chloroacetate esterase and α-naphthyl butyrate esterase are also commonly seen in MDS (185,186). In secondary MDS, the morphology of the dysplastic myeloid cells is frequently bizarre, and involvement of the erythroid and megakaryocytic cells is common. In some cases, it is necessary to perform immunocytochemical studies to identify these cells with specific markers (185–187) (see Chapter 48).

Chronic Myelocytic Leukemias

In more than 90% of chronic myelocytic leukemia (CML) cases, the leukocyte alkaline phosphatase (LAP) activity is decreased, and a Philadelphia chromosome can be detected in the myeloid and the erythroid cells in the marrow (188). However, normal LAP activity may be found in the early phase of CML. In the remaining atypical cases, the Philadelphia chromosome may not be detectable in the marrow cells and the LAP activity may be normal. In chronic myelomonocytic leukemia, the LAP activity in neutrophils may be normal, and many monocytes are detectable by cytochemical studies with α-naphthyl butyrate esterase (94). In chronic neutrophilic leukemia, the LAP activity is markedly increased, and the Philadelphia chromosome is invariably absent (189). The marrow biopsy in CML usually reveals hypercellularity and granulocytic hyperplasia; these features are

TABLE 38.5. *Characteristics of leukemic cells in ALL subtypes*

	Precursor B-cell ALL				Precursor T-cell ALL	
Characteristics	Pro-B-ALL	cALL	Pre-B-ALL	B-ALL	Pre-T-ALL	T-ALL
Conventional						
SIg	−	−	−	+	−	−
Cμ	−	−	+	−	−	−
E-rosette	−	−	−	−	−	+
Monoclonal antibodies						
HLA-DR (Ia)	+	+	+	+	−	−
CD79a	+	+	+	+	−	−
CD19	±	+	+	+	−	−
CD10	−	+	±	−	−	−
CD20	−	−	+	+	−	−
CD7	−	−	−	−	+	+
CD3 (cytoplasmic)	−	−	−	−	+	+
CD2	−	−	−	−	−	+
Enzyme						
TdT	+	+	+	−	+	+
FAcP	−	−	−	−	+	+
FAB	L1, L2	L1, L2	L1, L2	L3	L1, L2	L1, L2

ALL, acute lymphoblastic leukemia; FAB, French-American-British leukemia classification; FAcP, focal acid phosphatase; TdT, terminal deoxynucleotidyl transferase.

not diagnostic. Demonstration of many basophils in the biopsy by toluidine blue staining, however, strongly favors CML over reactive granulocytic hyperplasia. In cases of CML in the accelerated phase or in blastic transformation, the LAP score is frequently increased and many primitive, bizarre cells are seen. Cytochemical and immunocytochemical studies show that these may be myeloid, lymphoid, erythroid, or megakaryocytic precursors. Marrow biopsies often exhibit myelofibrosis that is best demonstrated by a reticulin stain (see Chapter 49).

Myeloproliferative Disorders

Traditionally, the myeloproliferative disorders include chronic myelocytic leukemia, myelofibrosis with myeloid metaplasia, polycythemia vera, essential thrombocythemia,

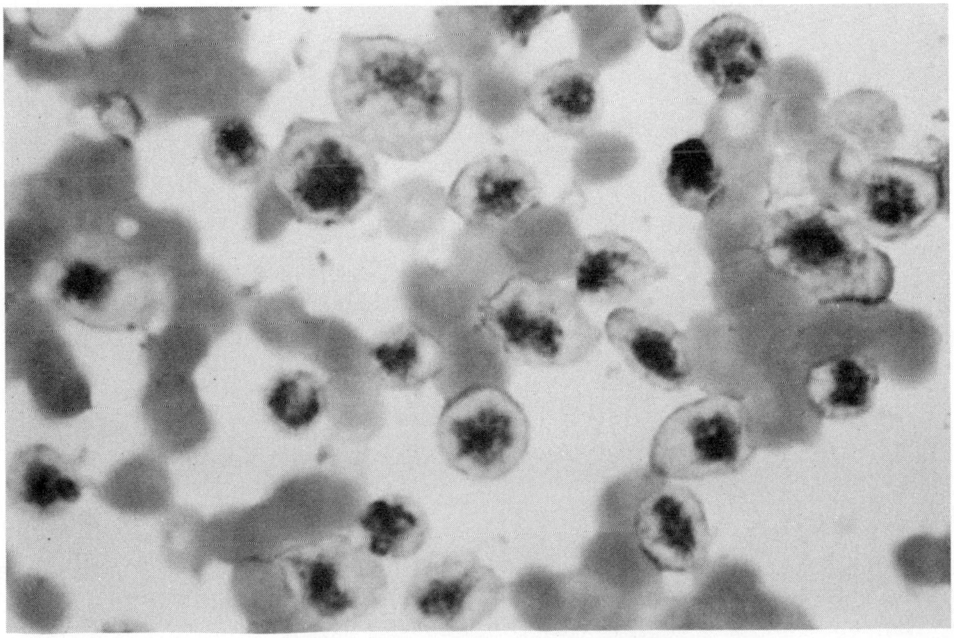

FIG. 38.25. Acute lymphoblastic leukemia strongly positive for nuclear terminal deoxynucleotidyl transferase (TdT) (granules on the nuclei) is demonstrated by immunoperoxidase stain (PAP immunoperoxidase stain for TdT, original magnification: 320× magnification).

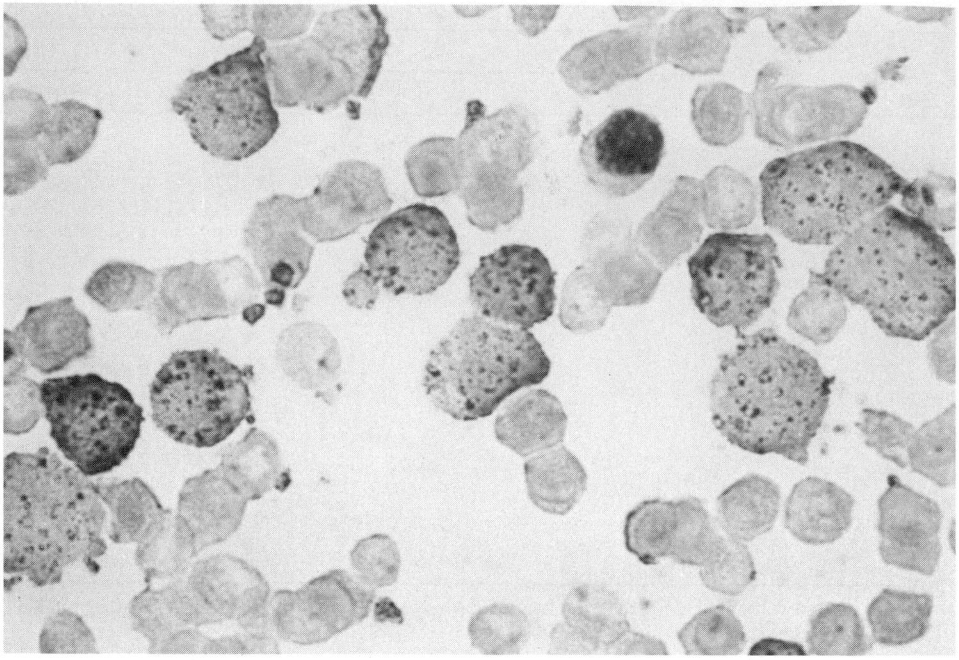

FIG. 38.26. Common acute lymphoblastic leukemia with strong common acute lymphoblastic leukemia antigen (CALLA, CD10) demonstrated by immunoperoxidase stain (indirect immunoperoxidase stain for CALLA, original magnification: 320× magnification). See Color Plate 14, between pp. 1446–1447.

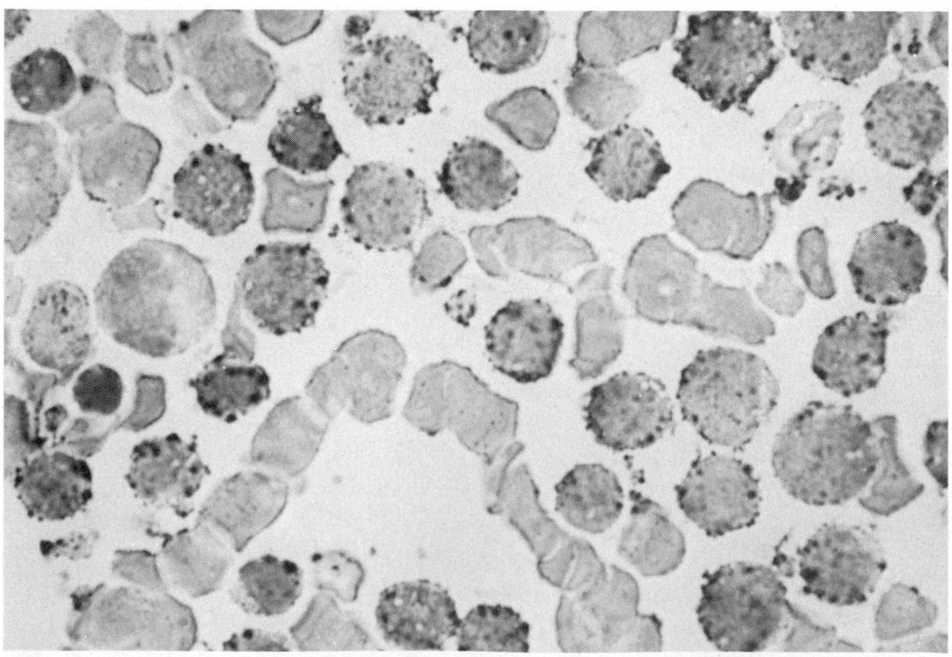

FIG. 38.27. B-cell acute lymphocytic leukemia (L3) with strong B-cell antigen (CD20) demonstrated by immunoperoxidase stain (indirect immunoperoxidase stain for B-cell antigen, original magnification: 320× magnification).

and DiGuglielmo's syndrome (190). Cases of DiGuglielmo's syndrome are frequently included in the MDS or the M6 subtype of AML.

Myelofibrosis with myeloid metaplasia is characterized by marked fibrosis and atypical megakaryocytic hyperplasia in the marrow. The fibrosis can be demonstrated by a reticulin stain and the megakaryocytes by specific cell markers. In the early phase of the disease, the marrow may be hyperplastic, and reticulin fibrosis may be inconspicuous, rendering it difficult to be differentiated from the other disorders of the group. Studies for LAP and for Philadelphia chromosome, in addition to close clinical observation, are helpful. In the terminal phase of this disorder, some cases may exhibit increased numbers of blasts in the marrow and may eventually transform into AML. Some of these patients may have many megakaryoblasts in their blood and marrow.

Polycythemia vera is characterized by pancytosis in the marrow. The LAP activity in the neutrophils is increased, and the marrow cells do not possess a Philadelphia chromosome. Essential thrombocythemia is characterized by hyperplasia of the marrow with a striking proliferation of clusters of normal and abnormal-appearing megakaryocytes. In both disorders, myelofibrosis may appear and the number of primitive cells in the marrow increases as the disorder progresses. These findings may be indistinguishable from those of myelofibrosis with myeloid metaplasia (see Chapter 49).

Granulocytic and Monocytic Sarcomas

In patients with myeloid disorders, the abnormal cells may proliferate locally, giving rise to tumor masses in the marrow that may extend into the surrounding area. Sometimes these myeloid cell tumors or granulocytic sarcomas may occur in tissues away from the marrow. In some instances, the tumor may acquire a greenish hue because of the high content of myeloperoxidase in the tumor cells; these are called chloroma. In other instances, the tumor may appear so dysplastic as to be indistinguishable from lymphomas or anaplastic carcinoma. When cytologic materials are available, the diagnosis can be established by cytochemical staining for myeloid cells. If only tissue sections are available, a careful examination of plastic sections stained with Giemsa frequently discloses the presence of basophils and immature eosinophils. Additional cytochemical studies to identify these cells and the immature myeloid cells usually suffice to establish the diagnosis. In paraffin-embedded tissue sections, the diagnosis must rely on histochemical study for chloroacetate esterase and immunohistochemical studies for myeloperoxidase, lysozyme, and other myeloid markers (71–74).

In rare instances, monocytes and histiocytes may proliferate to form localized tumors inside or outside of the marrow (191,192). The diagnosis of such disorders depends on the disclosure of cell-specific cytochemical and immunochemical markers.

Chronic Lymphoproliferative Disorders

Chronic lymphoproliferative disorders (CLPDs) are a group of slowly progressive disorders involving the mature or nearly mature lymphocytes of the B- or T-cell subtypes. The diagnosis of CLPD is based on the morphologic examination of blood and marrow. The classification of CLPD is based on morphologic, cytochemical, and immunochemical characteristics of the leukemic cells (5,193) (Table 38.6; Fig.

TABLE 38.6. *Characteristics of leukemic cells in chronic lymphoproliferative disorders*

Markers	B-CLL	MCL	B-SCL	MZL	B-PLL	PCL	HCL	T_H-CLL	T_S-CLL	T_M-CLL	T-LL
Conventional											
SIg (CIg)	±	+	+	+	+	(+)	+	−	−	−	−
E-rosette	−	−	−	−	−	−	−	+	+	+	+
Monoclonal antibodies											
CD2	−	−	−	−	−	−	−	+	+	+	+
CD5	+	+	−	−	−	−	−	+	+	+	+
CD3	−	−	−	−	−	−	−	+	+	+	+
CD4	−	−	−	−	−	−	−	+	−	±	±
CD8	−	−	−	−	−	−	−	−	+	+	±
HLA-DR (Ia)	+	+	+	+	+	−	+	−	−	−	+
CD10	−	−	+	−	−	−	−	−	−	−	−
CD20	±	+	+	+	+	−	+	−	−	−	−
CD23	+	−	±	−	−	−	−	−	−	−	−
Enzyme											
FANAE	−	−	−	−	−	−	−	+	−	±	±
FAcP	−	−	−	−	−	−	−	±	−	±	+
TRAP	−	−	−	−	±	−	+	−	−	−	−
Morphology											
Nuclei	Round	Irregular	Clefted	Round	Round	Round	Oval	Convoluted	Round	Convoluted	Convoluted
Large nucleolus	−	−	±	−	+	±	−	−	−	−	±
Azurophilic granules	−	−	−	−	−	−	−	−	+	−	−

CLL, chronic lymphocytic leukemia; MCL, mantle cell lymphoma/leukemia; SCL, small cleaved cell lymphoma/leukemia; MZL, marginal zone lymphoma/leukemia; PLL, prolymphocytic leukemia; PCL, plasma cell leukemia; HCL, hairy cell leukemia; LL, lymphoma/leukemia; T_H, helper T cell; T_S, suppressor T cell; T_M, mixed T cell; FANAE, focal α-naphthyl acetate esterase; FAcP, focal acid phosphatase; TRAP, tartrate-resistant acid phosphatase.

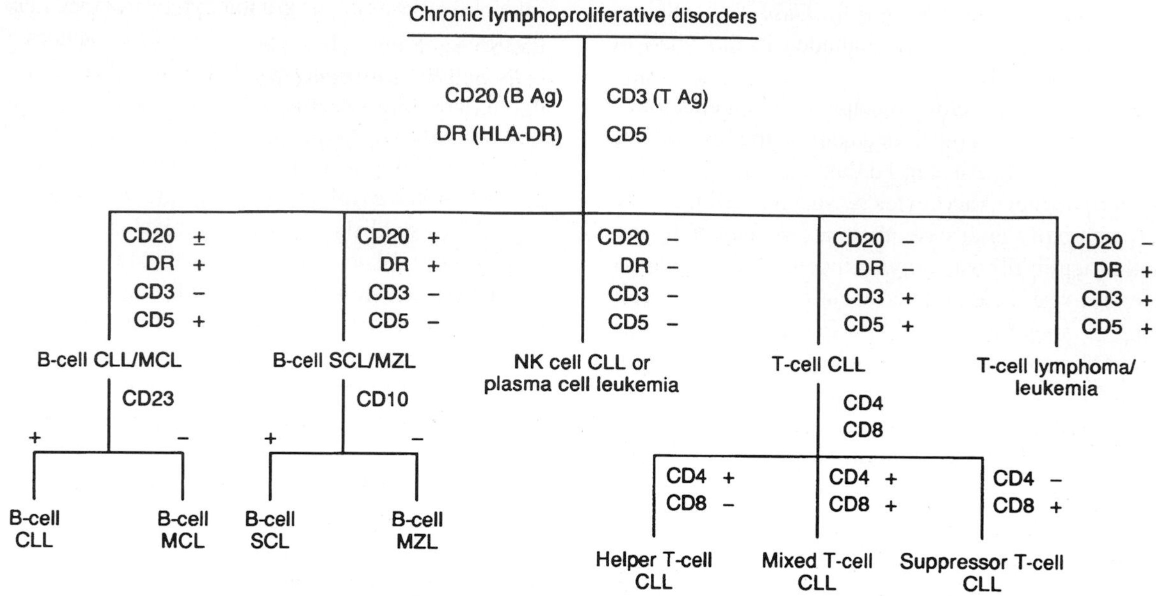

FIG. 38.28. Classification of chronic lymphoproliferative disorders using immunocytochemical methods. CLL, chronic lymphocytic leukemia; MCL, mantle cell lymphoma/leukemia; MZL, marginal zone lymphoma/leukemia; SCL, small cleaved, follicular center cell lymphoma/leukemia.

38.28). Approximately 90% to 95% of CLPD cases are of the B-cell type, mostly chronic lymphocytic leukemia (B-CLL), and 1% to 3% are of T-cell type (194). The leukemic B-CLL cells are small, mature-appearing cells exhibiting strong HLA-DR surface antigen and weak monotypic surface immunoglobulin light chains, CD20, CD5, and CD23 surface antigens. These characteristics are different from the neoplastic cells of B-cell lymphoma in the leukemic phase (i.e., small cleaved cell leukemia). In the latter disorder, the neoplastic cells are the small cleaved follicle center cells that often vary in nuclear size and shape and have abundant surface immunoglobulin light chains and strong CD20 and weak CD10 surface antigens.

Other subtypes of B-cell chronic lymphoproliferative disorders include the leukemic phase of mantle cell lymphoma (MCL) and marginal zone lymphoma (MZL), including MZL of the spleen and mucosa-associated lymphoid tissue or nodal origin (195–199). Morphologic distinction between these subtypes of lymphoma cells can be difficult and often requires immunophenotyping for accurate classification. Besides the strong CD20 surface antigen positivity, the neoplastic cells of MCL are usually cyclin $D1^+$, $CD5^+$, $CD23^-$, and $CD10^-$, and the neoplastic cells of MZL are usually cyclin $D1^-$, $CD5^-$, $CD23^-$, and $CD10^-$.

The T-cell CLLs can be further subdivided according to phenotypic characteristics into the helper, (Figs. 38.10–38.12), suppressor, and NK variants (87,194, 200–205). As the leukemia progresses, some patients may develop concomitant large cell lymphoma (i.e., Richter syndrome) in which the newly arising lymphoma cells and the leukemic CLL share the same or different phenotypic characteristics (206,207). Other cases may have many prolymphocytes and eventually transform into prolymphocytic leukemia (208). A rare case of CLL may convert into ALL (209,210) (see Chapters 40 and 43).

Hairy Cell Leukemia

The hairy cells are best recognized in a bone marrow aspirate by their characteristic morphologic features and abundance of cytoplasmic tartrate-resistant acid phosphatase (113,114) (Fig. 38.17). They also have the phenotypic features of the monotypic B lymphocytes and are positive for CD11c, CD20, CD22, CD25, CD103, and CD45 (211–215). T-cell HCL is rare (216,217). For aspirates with few marrow particles, it is often necessary to prepare buffy coat smears for morphologic and special studies. Histochemical studies for TRAP can be done on fresh frozen section or plastic-embedded tissue. In cases after interferon therapy, the hairy cells often lose their cytoplasmic hairy processes and TRAP activity. It may be difficult to evaluate the effect of interferon therapy in some of these cases. In bone marrow biopsies, the diagnosis of HCL may be established by the typical morphologic features of the disease and immunohistochemical characteristics of hairy cells with strong expression of CD20, DBA.44, and TRAP (using monoclonal antibody 9C5) (218–220) (see Chapter 41).

Hodgkin's Disease

Hodgkin's disease seldom involves the marrow. However, in cases with advanced disease or in those with poor histology subtypes, the marrow may become involved. The lesions in the marrow are frequently atypical, and Reed-Sternberg cells usually are not seen. The epithelioid cells in the granuloma may be easily identified by tartrate-resistant acid phosphatase or fluoride-resistant α-naphthyl butyrate esterase stains on fresh or plastic-embedded tissue sections (221). The Reed-Sternberg cells may be identified by positive immunochemical staining for CD30 (BER-H2) or CD15 (Leu-M1) (143,154) and negative staining for CD45 (Fig. 38.20). CD15 and CD30 also stain some epithelial carcinoma cells. The diagnosis of Hodgkin's disease with marrow involvement should be established cautiously by morphologic and special studies (see Chapters 17 and 39).

Non-Hodgkin's Lymphomas

The frequency of marrow involvement is related to the types of diseases in this group. Lymphomas of the small lymphocytic cells or small cleaved follicle center cells involve the marrow frequently while those of the large cells do so only seldomly. The diagnosis and classification of the non-Hodgkin's lymphomas by morphologic and immunochemical studies have been described in detail elsewhere in this book. Only the tactical approach of dealing with problems of marrow involvement by these diseases is considered here (95) (Table 38.7). In marrow specimens with many small lymphocytes, the primary concern is to distinguish benign hyperplasia (i.e., benign lymph follicles in the marrow) from that of focal neoplasia (i.e., focal or nodular involvement). Immunochemical studies for surface and cytoplasmic immunoglobulin light chains are most useful in determining the clonality and therefore the nature of the proliferation of these cells. In marrow specimens with involvement by large lymphoid cells, it may be necessary to use the appropriate cell markers to determine whether these cells are lymphoid (Fig. 38.29), histiocytic, granulocytic, epithelial, or sarcoma cells. After the lymphoid nature of these cells has been recognized, immunochemical studies should be done to determine the phenotypic features and the clonality of the cells (see Chapter 39).

Plasma Cell Dyscrasias

Included in the group of plasma cell dyscrasias are diseases such as Waldenström's macroglobulinemia, multiple myeloma, and amyloidosis. Studies of cytoplasmic immunoglobulin are important for the diagnosis of these diseases. Because of the large amount of immunoglobulin in the plasma or tissue fluids surrounding the cells, it is necessary to wash the adsorbed immunoglobulins from the cells before the immunocytochemical studies are done. With tissue sections, it is necessary to practice rigid quality control to ensure proper interpretation (145).

In macroglobulinemia, the neoplastic cells are small, mature lymphocytes or lymphocytes with plasmacytoid features. These cells are monoclonal B cells with monotypic cytoplasmic but few or no surface immunoglobulins. The diagnosis of macroglobulinemia is established by correlating the morphologic and immunochemical studies of the lymphoid cells with the clinical features of the patient.

In myeloma, the marrow involvement by the neoplastic plasma cells may be focal or diffuse. In marrow specimens, particularly in those containing relatively few plasma cells, immunohistochemical studies of the marrow clot or biopsy can demonstrate monotypic cytoplasmic immunoglobulin in the plasma cells (145) (Fig. 38.30).

In amyloidosis, Congo red staining to demonstrate the congophilic deposits exhibiting green birefringence when viewed under polarization microscopy is useful in confirmation of amyloidosis. Immunohistochemical methods using

TABLE 38.7. *Histochemical and immunohistochemical characteristics of histiocytes, transformed B and T lymphocytes, and granulocytes*

Stains	Suitable tissue	Histiocytes	B lymphocytes	T lymphocytes	Granulocytes
Acid phosphatase	S, FS, PI	4+ (D)	0–2+ (D)	2–3+ (F)	2+ (D)
Butyrate esterase	S, FS, PA	4+ (D)	0	0–1+ (F)	0
Chloroacetate esterase	S, FS, PI, PA	0	0	0	4+
Myeloperoxidase	PA	0	0	0	4+
Lysozyme	PA	1–3+	0	0	4+
CD68 (PG-M1)	PA	4+	0	0	0
Surface Ig (SIg)	FS	0	1–3+	0	0
Cytoplasmic Ig (CIg)	FS, PA	0–1+	0–3+[a]	0	0–1+
T antigens (CD2, CD3)	S, FS	–	–	+	–
(cytoplasmic CD3)	PA	–	–	+	–
B antigens (CD20)	S, FS, PA	–	+	–	–

S, smears; FS, frozen sections; PI, plastic sections; PA, paraffin sections; D, diffuse cytoplasmic staining; F, focal staining confined to Golgi area.

[a] Monotypic in lymphoma cells

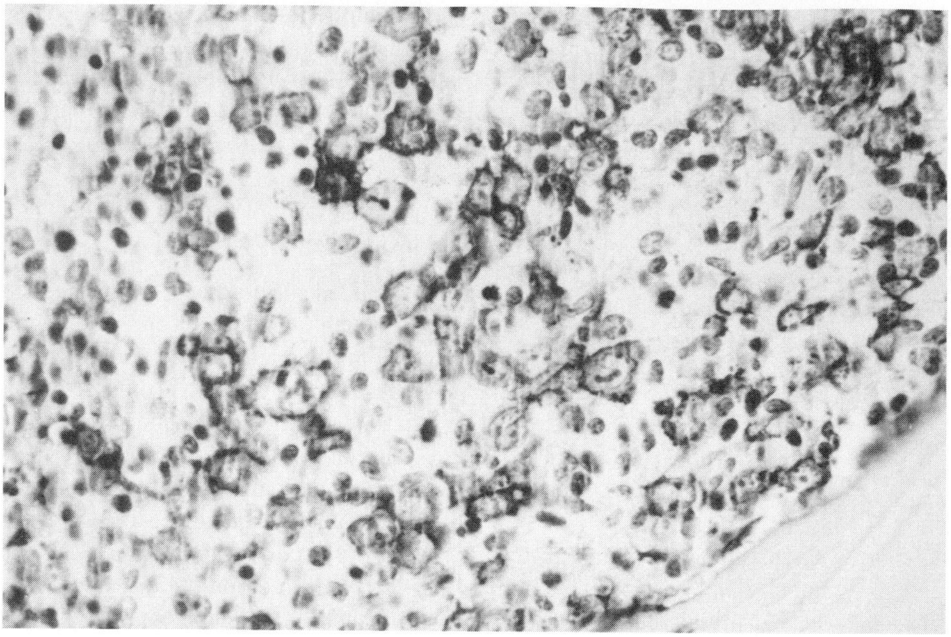

FIG. 38.29. Paraffin section of bone marrow biopsy shows interstitial infiltration by large B-lymphoma cells with strong B-cell antigen (CD20) demonstrated by immunoperoxidase stain (indirect immunoperoxidase stain for CD20 using monoclonal antibody L26, original magnification: 128× magnification).

A

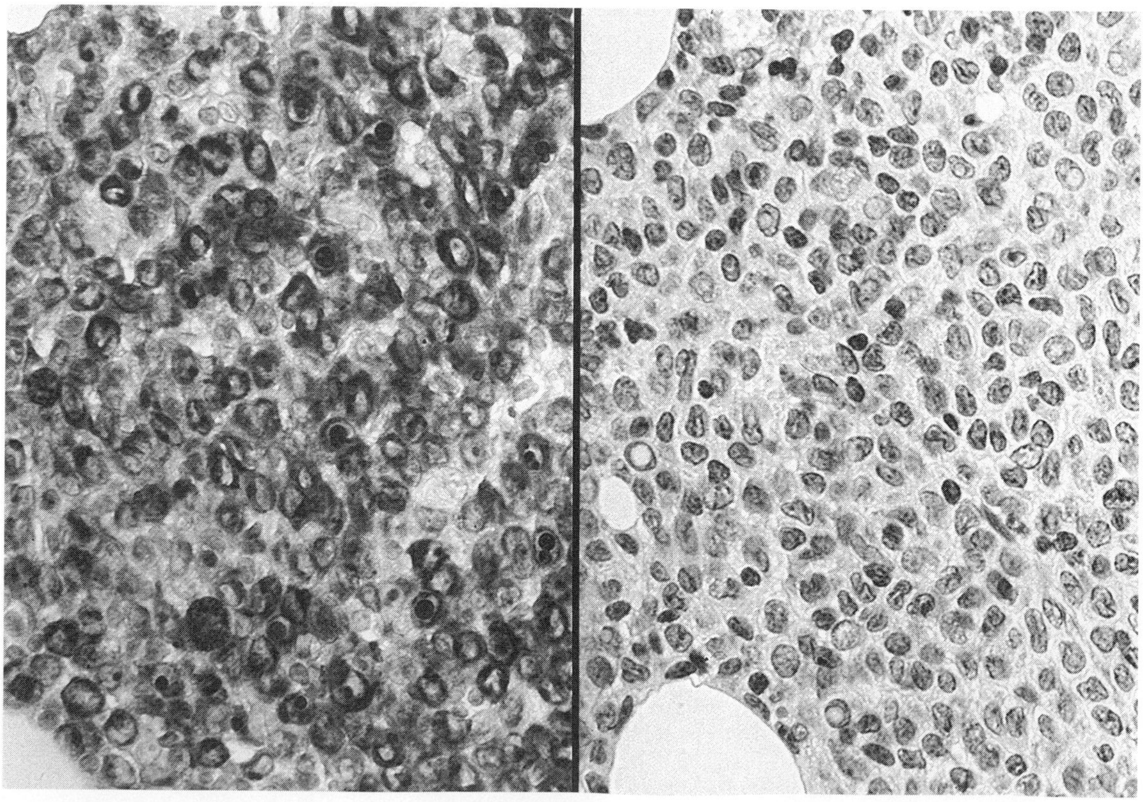

B

FIG. 38.30. A: Paraffin section of bone marrow biopsy shows strong cytoplasmic κ light-chain immunoglobulin in myeloma cells (indirect immunoperoxidase stain for κ light chains, original magnification: 128× magnification). **B:** Paraffin section of bone marrow biopsy from the same patient shows negative staining for cytoplasmic λ light chains in myeloma cells (indirect immunoperoxidase stain for λ light chains, original magnification: 128× magnification).

TABLE 38.8. *Immunohistochemical characterization of amyloid deposits in paraffin sections*

Protein type	Related protein	Clinicopathologic form
AL	Immunoglobulin light chain (κ or λ)	Primary and myeloma-associated
AA	Amyloid A protein	Secondary, familial Mediterranean fever
AS	Prealbumin (transthyretin)	Senile
AF	Prealbumin (transthyretin)	Heredofamilial
	β_2-microglobulin	Hemodialysis associated
AP	Amyloid P component	All amyloid

antibodies against different types of amyloid related proteins (e.g., AL, AA, prealbumin, β_2-microglobulin) are helpful in distinguishing primary, secondary, senile, familial, and dialysis-associated amyloidosis (222–224) (Table 38.8) (see Chapter 42).

Mast Cell Diseases

Mast cell diseases include urticaria pigmentosa, mastocytoma, systemic mast cell disease (SMCD), and mast cell leukemia (225). The one that often involves the marrow is SMCD. The marrow in SMCD is often hypercellular, showing increased numbers of mast cells. Many of these cells exhibit abnormal nuclear features and few cytoplasmic granules (Fig. 38.14). The marrow biopsies frequently show granulocytic hyperplasia and paratrabecular, perivascular, or parafollicular lesions. These lesions are frequently composed of many eosinophils and mast cells that appear as elongated fibroblast-like cells (101,226) (Figs. 38.14, 38.15). The mast cells can be demonstrated in fresh or plastic-embedded marrow sections with histochemical markers such as aminocaproate esterase, toluidine blue, Giemsa stain, and chloroacetate esterase (9,101). The immunohistochemical stain for tryptase is the most practical for confirming mast cell lineage paraffin tissue sections (227). In some cases of SMCD, the marrow hyperplasia may result from concomitant myelodysplasia or leukemia (226–228) (see Chapter 52).

Round Cell Tumors

The group of round cell tumors that commonly involves the marrow and can cause difficulty in the morphologic differential diagnosis includes malignant lymphoma, small cell carcinoma of lung, neuroblastoma, rhabdomyosarcoma, and Ewing's sarcoma. Among the many immunohistochemical markers that have been evaluated, those most useful include leukocyte common antigen for identification of malignant lymphoma, EMA and cytokeratin for small cell carcinoma, chromogranin and synaptophysin for neuroblastoma, and muscle actin and desmin for rhabdomyosarcoma (173) and CD99 for Ewing's sarcoma (229). Although some of these markers are not unique to a specific cell type, the combined use of them as a panel serves as a practical approach to the differential diagnosis of round cell tumors in routinely processed biopsy specimens (Table 38.9) (see Chapter 30).

Metastatic Carcinomas

The morphologic identification of metastatic carcinoma in the marrow is not difficult in most cases. Occasionally, the proliferation of atypical megakaryocytes associated with myelofibrosis as seen in agnogenic myeloid metaplasia or acute megakaryocytic leukemia may mimic metastatic carcinoma or *vice versa.* In these situations, the immunohistochemical demonstration of factor VIII–related antigen is helpful in confirming the megakaryocytic nature of atypical cells and the presence of keratin or EMA is helpful in confirming the epithelial nature of carcinoma cells (168,173). Among the metastatic carcinomas, identification of prostatic carcinoma is important for proper management. Prostatic acid phosphatase and prostate specific antigen are fairly specific immunohistochemical markers for identification or confirmation of metastatic prostatic carcinoma (169,170,230).

SUMMARY AND CONCLUSIONS

Morphologic study of the bone marrow is traditionally the cornerstone for the diagnosis of many hematologic disorders. Special studies with cytochemical, histochemical, and immunochemical procedures have been used with increasing frequency for the same purpose. Occasionally, these special

TABLE 38.9. *Immunohistochemical characteristics of round cell tumors in paraffin sections*

Tumor	LCA	EMA	Chromogranin	Muscle actin	Desmin	CD99	Vimentin
Lymphoma	+	−	−	−	−	±[a]	−
Small cell carcinoma	−	+	+	−	−	−	−
Neuroblastoma	−	−	+	−	−	−	−
Rhabdomyosarcoma	−	−	±	+	+	−	+
Ewing's sarcoma	−	−	−	−	−	+	+

EMA, epithelial membrane antigen; LCA, leukocyte common antigen.
[a] Lymphoblastic lymphoma is positive for CD99, and other lymphomas are negative.

techniques have been used in lieu of morphologic studies for hematologic diagnosis. Many of the special procedures have been well established and are well known to many workers in the field. However, the key to their successful use is appropriate selection of these procedures for the diagnosis of a particular hematologic disorder. A clear understanding of these special procedures ensures their successful application to clinical medicine, and misunderstanding them leads to confusion and waste.

Cytologic materials of the bone marrow are generally most useful for the diagnosis of leukemia, particularly the acute leukemias. Histologic materials are most useful for the diagnosis of the malignant lymphomas, metastatic tumors, and disorders associated with fibrosis in the marrow. The cytologic materials are easy to obtain and to prepare for morphologic, cytochemical, and immunocytochemical studies. The histologic materials are more restricted to those that have been properly prepared and processed.

The cytochemical and histochemical procedures are technically simple; their practical usefulness and limitations are well understood. They are most useful for disorders involving the myeloid cells but are of limited value for disorders of the lymphoid cells. The immunochemical procedures are more costly and technically more difficult than the cytochemical and histochemical procedures. They are most valuable for the diagnosis of lymphoid disorders. In these disorders, the immunochemical techniques can help to identify the cell type (i.e., T or B cells) and the maturation and the clonality of the lymphoid cells. The immunochemical techniques are also useful for the diagnosis of nonhematologic malignancies with marrow metastasis. Although the immunochemical techniques are also capable of identifying the myeloid cells, they often cannot accurately distinguish monocytes from granulocytes nor determine maturation or clonality of the myeloid cells. In this regard, the immunochemical techniques offer little significant advantage over the cytochemical and, to a lesser extent, the histochemical techniques for the diagnosis of myeloid disorders of the bone marrow.

There is a tendency to place too much emphasis on the immunochemical techniques and to overlook the practical value of the cytochemical and histochemical techniques in the hematopathologic diagnosis of disorders of the marrow. The immunochemical studies are frequently done as a battery, often on bone marrow sections. Sometimes, the immunochemical studies have taken the place of morphologic studies in the diagnosis of disorders of the bone marrow. Such high expectations for special studies, particularly the immunochemical studies, that are improperly performed are hardly justified. We believe that morphologic studies are for the diagnosis of hematologic disorders of the marrow and that special procedures are for identification of the cells involved and for classification of the disorder. The best diagnostic results can be obtained when the morphologic and special studies are interpreted in the context of the clinical features of the patients.

ACKNOWLEDGMENTS

The authors thank Sara Brackett for typing this manuscript and Drs. Anthony J. Janckila, Patrick C. Roche, and Paul J. Kurtin for their critiques of the manuscript.

APPENDIX 1. RECOMMENDED CYTOCHEMICAL STAINING PROCEDURES

Peroxidase Reaction

Principle

The peroxidase enzyme in the granules of the cells releases the oxygen from H_2O_2. The oxygen oxidizes the diaminobenzidine to form an insoluble golden brown compound deposited at the sites of peroxidase activity.

Reagents and Preparation of Solutions

1. Fixative is cold buffered formalin acetone, pH 6.6: Dissolve 20 mg of Na_2HPO_4 and 100 mg of KH_2PO_4 in 30 mL of distilled water. Add 45 mL of acetone and 25 mL of 37% formaldehyde solution. Mix well, and store at 4 to 10°C.
2. 0.067 M phosphate buffer, pH 7.4: Dissolve 7.572 g of Na_2HPO_4 and 1.814 g of KH_2PO_4 in 1,000 mL of distilled water.
3. 0.1% H_2O_2.
4. 3,3-diaminobenzidine tetrahydrochloride
5. Incubation solution: Dissolve 30 mg of 3,3-diaminobenzidine tetrahydrochloride in 40 mL of phosphate buffer. Add 0.4 mL of 0.1% H_2O_2, and use immediately.

Procedure

1. Fix smears in cold buffered formalin acetone for 30 seconds.
2. Rinse briefly with water.
3. Place in the incubation mixture for 15 minutes at room temperature.
4. Rinse briefly in running water.
5. Counterstain with Giemsa stain for 40 minutes.
6. Rinse with water, air dry, and mount with Permount.

Results

Enzyme activity appears as dark brown granules in the cytoplasm of granulocytes and monocytes. Red blood cells also stain brown because of the pseudoperoxidase activity of hemoglobin. The abnormal fusiform particles (phi bodies) and rods with hydroperoxidase activity in leukemic cells of acute myelogenous leukemia may be easily identified by this method.

REFERENCE

1. Hanker JS, Lazlo J, Moore JO. The light microscopic demonstration of hydroperoxidase positive phi bodies and rods in leukocytes in acute myeloid leukemia. *Histochemistry* 1978:58:241–252.

Neutrophil Alkaline Phosphatase: Azo Dye Method; Naphthol AS Phosphate

Reagents and Preparation of Solutions

1. Fixative is cold 10% formalin in absolute methanol.
2. 0.2 M Tris buffer, pH 9.1: Dissolve 48.44 g of Trizma base in 200 mL of distilled water. Adjust the pH to 9.1 with hydrochloric acid.
3. Substrate solution: Dissolve 30 mg of naphthol AS phosphate in 0.5 mL of *N,N*-dimethyl formamide. Add 100 mL of 0.2 M Tris buffer, pH 9.1. Store refrigerated.
4. Fast blue BBN.
5. Incubation solution: Dissolve 40 mg of fast blue BBN in 40 mL of substrate solution. Filter before use.

Procedure

1. Fix smears in cold 10% formalin methanol for 30 seconds.
2. Rinse briefly with water.
3. Place in the incubation mixture for 20 minutes at room temperature.
4. Rinse in water.
5. Counterstain with 0.1% aqueous solution of neutral red for 3 minutes.
6. Rinse in water, and air dry.

Results

Enzyme activity is seen as discrete bright blue granules in the cytoplasm of segmented and stab forms of neutrophils. Nuclei stain brilliant red-orange. A rare lymphocyte may show a weak reaction. All other types of cells in the blood are not stained.

Scoring Procedures and Interpretations

One hundred consecutive segmented or stab forms of neutrophils are rated 0 to 4 + on the basis of the intensity of the precipitating dye:

0 = no granules
1 + = few blue granules
2 + = moderate number of granules
3 + = moderate to numerous granules
4 + = cytoplasm of the neutrophils is saturated by closely approximated granules.

The sum of ratings in 100 neutrophils is the score of the test. The leukocyte alkaline phosphatase score for normal adults ranges from 40 to 100. Because the scoring of enzyme activity is influenced by technique and reagents used, the normal range should be determined in each laboratory. An abnormally low score is seen in untreated chronic granulocytic leukemia, paroxysmal nocturnal hemoglobinuria, and hereditary hypophosphatasia. A marked increase of enzyme activity is seen in infections and in inflammatory leukocytosis, polycythemia vera, pregnancy or use of oral contraceptives, and active Hodgkin's disease.

REFERENCE

1. Rutenburg AM, Rosales CL, Bennett JM. An improved histochemical method for the demonstration of leukocyte alkaline phosphatase activity: clinical application. *J Lab Clin Med* 1965:65:698–705.

Neutrophil Alkaline Phosphatase: Azo Dye Method; Naphthol AS-BI Phosphate

Principle

The substrate is hydrolyzed to phosphate and arylnaphtholamide by leukocyte enzyme at pH 9.5. The arylnaphtholamide is coupled to a diazonium salt, forming an insoluble dye.

Reagents and Preparation of Solutions

1. Fixative is 60% acetone in citrate buffer: Add 168 mL of 0.03 M citric acid (6.3 g/L) to 32 mL of 0.03 M sodium citrate (8.8 g/L), and then add slowly, while stirring, 300 mL of absolute acetone. The final pH should be 4.2 to 4.5. Store at room temperature.
2. Stock buffer solution (0.2 M propanediol): Dissolve 21 g of 2-amino-2-methyl-1,3-propanediol in distilled water, and dilute to 1,000 mL with distilled water. Store refrigerated.
3. Stock working buffer (0.05 M propanediol, pH 9.4 to 9.6): Add 70 mL of 0.1 N HCl to 250 mL of stock buffer solution and dilute to 1,000 mL with distilled water. Store refrigerated, but warm to room temperature before use.
4. Fast violet B salt.
5. Incubation solution: Dissolve 5 mg of sodium naphthol AS-BI phosphate and 40 mg of fast violet B salt in 60 mL of the working propanediol buffer. Mix well. Filter into a Coplin jar. Use immediately after preparation.

Procedure

1. Fix smears in buffered acetone solution at room temperature for 10 seconds.
2. Rinse briefly with water, and air dry.

3. Place in the freshly prepared incubation solution for 15 minutes at room temperature.
4. Rinse in water.
5. Counterstain with Mayer's hematoxylin solution for 2 to 8 minutes.
6. Wash in running tap water. Mount in a drop of water, and examine with oil immersion lens.
7. Remove coverslip after examination. Wash, dry, and store slide unmounted.

Results

Enzyme activity is seen as bright red granules in the cytoplasm of segmented and stab forms of neutrophils. An occasional lymphocyte may be weakly stained. All other types of cells in blood are not stained.

Scoring Procedures and Interpretations

One hundred segmented or stab forms of neutrophils are rated from 0 to 4 + on the basis of the intensity of the precipitating dye:

0 = no granules
1 + = very few granules
2 + = moderate number of granules
3 + = moderate to numerous granules
4 + = cytoplasm of the neutrophils is saturated by closely approximated granules.

The sum of ratings in 100 neutrophils is the score of the test. The leukocyte alkaline phosphatase score in normal adults is about 60, with a range of 30 to 130.

REFERENCE

1. Shibuta A, Bennett JM, Castoldi GL, et al. Recommended methods for cytologic procedures in haematology. *Clin Lab Haematol* 1985:7:55-74.

Chloroacetate Esterase

Reagents and Preparation of Solutions

1. Fixative is cold buffered formalin acetone, pH 6.6: Dissolve 20 mg of Na_2HPO_4 and 100 mg of KH_2PO_4 in 30 mL of distilled water. Add 45 mL of acetone and 25 mL of 37% formaldehyde solution. Store refrigerated at 4°C.
2. Substrate solution: Dissolve 10 mg of naphthol AS-D chloroacetate in 5 mL of *N,N*-dimethylformamide. Store refrigerated.
3. M/15 phosphate buffer, pH 7.73: Dissolve 8.52 g of Na_2HPO_4 and 0.9 g of KH_2PO_4 in 1,000 mL of distilled water.
4. New fuchsin solution: Dissolve 1 g of new fuchsin in 25 mL of warm 2 N hydrochloric acid. Allow to cool and then filter. Store at room temperature away from direct sunlight. The solution is stable for 2 months.
5. 4% sodium nitrite solution: Dissolve 1 g of sodium nitrite in 25 mL of distilled water. Store refrigerated, and prepare fresh weekly.
6. Hexazotized new fuchsin: Mix equal volumes of new fuchsin solution and 4% sodium nitrite solution for 1 minute before use.
7. Incubation solution: Add together 38 mL of M/15 phosphate buffer (pH 7.73), 0.2 mL of hexazotized new fuchsin, and 2 mL (4 mg) of naphthol AS-D chloroacetate solution. Use immediately without filtration.

Procedure

1. Fix smears in cold buffered formalin acetone for 30 seconds.
2. Rinse briefly with water.
3. Place in the incubation mixture for 10 minutes at room temperature.
4. Rinse in water.
5. Counterstain with Mayer's hematoxylin for 10 minutes.
6. Rinse in running water for 10 minutes, and air dry.
7. Mount in a synthetic mounting medium.

Results

Enzyme activity is seen as bright red granules in the cytoplasm of mast cells and neutrophilic granulocytes.

REFERENCES

1. Yam LT, Li CY, Crosby WH. Cytochemical identification of monocytes and granulocytes. *Am J Clin Pathol* 1971:55:283–290.
2. Shibata A, Bennett JM, Castoldi GL, et al. Recommended methods for cytological procedures in haematology. *Clin Lab Haematol* 1985:7: 55–74.

α-Naphthyl Butyrate Esterase

Reagents and Preparation of Solutions

1. Fixative is cold buffered formalin acetone, pH 6.6: Dissolve 20 mg of Na_2HPO_4 and 100 mg of KH_2PO_4 in 30 mL of distilled water. Add 45 mL of acetone and 25 mL of 37% formaldehyde solution. Store refrigerated at 4°C.
2. Substrate solution: Dissolve 250 mg of α-naphthyl butyrate in 12.5 mL of ethylene glycol monomethyl ether (20 mg/mL). Store refrigerated.
3. M/15 phosphate buffer, pH 6.64: Dissolve 3.786 g of Na_2HPO_4 and 5.443 g of KH_2PO_4 in 1,000 mL of distilled water.
4. Pararosanilin solution: Dissolve 1 g of pararosanilin in 25 mL of warm 2 N hydrochloric acid solution. Filter

when cool, and store at room temperature away from direct sunlight. The solution is stable for 2 months.

5. 4% sodium nitrite solution: Dissolve 1 g of sodium nitrite in 25 mL of distilled water. Store refrigerated, and prepare fresh weekly.
6. Hexazotized pararosanilin: Mix equal volumes of pararosanilin solution and 4% sodium nitrite solution for 1 minute before use.
7. Incubation solution: Mix together 38 mL of M/15 phosphate buffer (pH 6.64), 0.4 mL of hexazotized pararosanilin, and 2 mL (40 mg) of the α-naphthyl butyrate solution. Filter before use.

Procedure

1. Fix smears in cold buffered formalin acetone for 30 seconds.
2. Rinse briefly with water.
3. Place in the incubation mixture for 45 minutes at room temperature.
4. Rinse in water.
5. Counterstain with Mayer's hematoxylin for 10 minutes.
6. Rinse in running water for 10 minutes, and air dry.
7. Mount in a synthetic mounting medium.

Results

Enzyme activity is indicated as dark red precipitates in the cytoplasm of monocytes and histiocytes.

REFERENCES

1. Li CY, Lam KW, Yam LT. Esterases in human leukocytes. *J Histochem Cytochem* 1973:21:1–12.
2. Shibata A, Bennett JM, Catoldi GL, et al. Recommended methods for cytological procedures in haematology. *Clin Lab Haematol* 1985:7: 55–74.

Combined Butyrate Esterase and Chloroacetate Esterase

Reagents and Preparation of Solutions

1. Fixative is cold buffered formalin acetone, pH 6.6.
2. Substrate solution #1: Dissolve 250 mg of α-naphthyl butyrate in 12.5 mL of ethylene glycol monomethyl ether (20 mg/mL). Store refrigerated.
3. Substrate solution #2: Dissolve 10 mg of naphthol AS-D chloroacetate in 5 mL of *N,N*-dimthylformamide. Store refrigerated.
4. M/15 phosphate buffer, pH 6.64
5. M/15 phosphate buffer, pH 7.4: Dissolve 7.572 g of Na_2HPO_4 and 1.814 g of KH_2PO_4 in 1,000 mL of distilled water.
6. Pararosanilin solution
7. 4% sodium nitrite solution
8. Hexazotized pararosanilin
9. Fast blue BBN
10. Incubation solution #1: Mix together 38 mL of M/15 phosphate buffer (pH 6.64), 0.4 mL of hexazotized pararosanilin, and 2 mL (40 mg) of α-naphthyl butyrate solution. Filter before use.
11. Incubation solution #2: Mix together 38 mL of M/15 phosphate buffer (pH 7.4), 20 mg of fast blue BBN, and 2 mL (4 mg) of naphthol AS-D chloroacetate solution. Use immediately without filtration.

Procedure

1. Fix smears in cold buffered formalin acetone for 30 seconds.
2. Rinse briefly in water.
3. Place in incubation mixture #1 for 45 minutes at room temperature.
4. Rinse in water.
5. Place in incubation mixture #2 for 10 minutes at room temperature.
6. Rinse in water.
7. Counterstain with Mayer's hematoxylin for 10 minutes.
8. Rinse in running water for 10 minutes, and air dry.
9. Mount in a synthetic mounting medium.

Results

Butyrate esterase activity is seen as dark red precipitate in the cytoplasm of monocytes. Chloroacetate esterase activity is seen as blue granular precipitate in the cytoplasm of neutrophilic granules.

REFERENCES

1. Li CY, Lam KW, Yam LT. Esterases in human leukocytes. *J Histochem Cytochem* 1973:21:1–12.
2. Yam LT, Li CY, Crosby WH. Cytochemical identification of monocytes and granulocytes. *Am J Clin Pathol* 1971:55:283–290.

α-Naphthyl Acetate Esterase

Reagents and Preparation of Solutions

1. Fixative is cold buffered formalin acetone, pH 6.6.
2. Substrate solution: Dissolve 100 mg of α-naphthyl acetate in 5 mL of ethylene glycol monomethyl ether (20 mg/mL). Store refrigerated.
3. M/15 phosphate buffer, pH 6.64
4. Pararosanilin solution
5. 4% sodium nitrite solution
6. Hexazotized pararosanilin
7. Incubation solution: Mix together 38 mL of M/15 phos-

phate buffer (pH 6.64), 0.4 mL of hexazotized pararosanilin, and 2 mL (40 mg) of the α-naphthyl acetate solution. Filter before use.

Procedure

1. Fix smears in cold buffered formalin acetone for 30 seconds.
2. Rinse briefly with water.
3. Place in the incubation mixture for 60 to 20 minutes at room temperature.
4. Rinse in water.
5. Counterstain with Mayer's hematoxylin for 10 minutes.
6. Rinse in running water for 10 minutes, and air dry.
7. Mount in a synthetic mounting medium.

Results

Enzyme activity is seen as diffuse cytoplasmic staining in monocytes and focal staining (dot type) in helper T lymphocytes.

REFERENCES

1. Li CY, Lam KW, Yam LT. Esterases in human leukocytes. *J Histochem Cytochem* 1973:21:1–12.
2. Knowles DM, Halper JP, Machin GA, et al. Acid alpha naphthyl acetate esterase activity in human neoplastic lymphoid cells: usefulness as a T cell marker. *Am J Pathol* 1979:96:257–278.

Aminocaproate Esterase

Reagents and Preparation of Solutions

1. Fixative is cold buffered formalin acetone, pH 6.6.
2. Substrate solution: Dissolve 10 mg of naphthyl AS ϵ-aminocaproate in 5 mL of ethylene glycol monomethyl ether (2 mg/mL). Store refrigerated.
3. M/15 phosphate buffer, pH 7.73: Dissolve 8.52 g of Na_2HPO_4 and 0.9 g of KH_2PO_4 in 1,000 mL of distilled water.
4. New fuchsin solution
5. 4% sodium nitrite solution
6. Hexazotized new fuchsin
7. Incubation solution: Mix together 36 mL of M/15 phosphate buffer (pH 7.73), 0.4 mL of hexazotized new fuchsin, and 4 mL (8 mg) of the naphthol AS ϵ-aminocaproate solution. Filter before use.

Procedure

1. Fix smears in cold buffered formalin acetone for 30 seconds.
2. Rinse briefly with water.
3. Place in the incubation mixture for 30 minutes at room temperature.
4. Rinse in water.
5. Counterstain with Mayer's hematoxylin for 10 minutes.
6. Rinse in running water for 10 minutes, and air dry.
7. Mount in a synthetic mounting medium.

Results

Enzyme activity is seen as bright red granules in the cytoplasm of mast cells.

REFERENCE

1. Li CY, Lam KW, Yam LT. Esterases in human leukocytes. *J Histochem Cytochem* 1973:21:1–12.

Acid Phosphatase (Fast Garnet GBC Method)

Reagents and Preparation of Solutions

1. Fixative is cold buffered methanol-acetone mixture: Dissolve 630 mg of citric acid in 30 mL of distilled water. Add 60 mL of acetone and 10 mL of methanol. Adjust the pH of this mixture to 5.4 with concentrated NaOH solution. Store at 4°C.
2. 0.1 M acetate buffer, pH 5.2: Dissolve 10.75 g of sodium acetate · 3 H_2O in 21 mL of 1 N acetic acid, and bring the volume to 1 L with distilled water. Store at 4°C.
3. Substrate solution: Dissolve 10 mg of naphthol AS-BI phosphoric acid in 0.5 mL of *N,N*-dimethylformamide. Add 0.1 M of acetate buffer (pH 5.2) to 100 mL. Store at 4°C.
4. Incubation solution: Dissolve 5 mg of fast garnet GBC in 50 mL of substrate solution, and filter before use. Tartrate-containing medium is prepared by adding 375 mg of L(+)-tartaric acid and 5 mg of fast garnet GBC in 50 mL of substrate solution. Adjust the pH of this solution to 5.2 with concentrated NaOH solution. Filter and use immediately.

Procedure

1. Fix smears in cold buffered methanol-acetone mixture for 30 seconds.
2. Rinse briefly with water.
3. Place in the incubation mixture with or without tartaric acid at 37°C for 45 minutes.
4. Rinse in water.
5. Counterstain with Mayer's hematoxylin for 15 to 20 minutes.
6. Wash with water, and dry.
7. Mount with glycerin jelly.

Results

Acid phosphatase activity is indicated as discrete dark red granules in the cytoplasm of the blood cells. Tartrate in the incubation solution almost completely inhibits enzyme activity in all types of blood cells. The hairy cells and lipid storage cells have strong tartrate-resistant acid phosphatase activity.

REFERENCES

1. Li CY, Yam LT, Lam KW. Acid phosphatase isoenzyme in human leukocytes in normal and pathologic conditions. *J Histochem Cytochem* 1970:18:473–481.
2. Janckila AJ, Li CY, Lam KW, et al. The cytochemistry of tartrate-resistant acid phosphatase. *Am J Clin Pathol* 1978:70:45–55.

REFERENCES

1. Lillie RD, Fullmer HM, eds. *Histopathologic technic and practical histochemistry,* 4th ed. New York: McGraw-Hill, 1976.
2. Li CY, Yam LT, Crosby WH. Histochemical characterization of cellular and structural elements of the human spleen. *J Histochem Cytochem* 1972;20:1049–1058.
3. Warnke R, Levy R. Detection of T and B cell antigens with hybridoma monoclonal antibodies: a biotin–avidin–horseradish peroxidase method. *J Histochem Cytochem* 1980;28:771–776.
4. Banks PM, Caron BL, Morgan TW. Use of imprints for monoclonal antibody studies: suitability of air-dried preparations from lymphoid tissues with an immunohistochemical method. *Am J Clin Pathol* 1983; 79:438–442.
5. Li CY, Ziesmer SC, Yam LT, et al. Practical immunocytochemical identification of human blood cells. *Am J Clin Pathol* 1984;81: 204–212.
6. Takamiya H, Batsford S, Vogt A. An approach to postembedding staining of protein (immunoglobulin) antigen embedded in plastic: prerequisites and limitations. *J Histochem Cytochem* 1980;28: 1041–1049.
7. Beckstead JH. Optimal antigen localization in human tissues using aldehyde-fixed plastic-embedded sections. *J Histochem Cytochem* 1985;33:954–958.
8. Casey TT, Cousar JB, Collins RD. A simplified plastic embedding and immunohistologic technique for immunophenotypic analysis of human hematopoietic and lymphoid tissues. *Am J Pathol* 1988;131: 183–189.
9. Li CY, Travis WD, Van Hale PC, et al. Useful cytochemical stains for the diagnosis of systemic mast cell disease (SMCD). *J Histochem Cytochem* 1986;34:1355(abst).
10. Beckstead JH, Bainton DF. Enzyme histochemistry on bone marrow biopsies: reactions useful in the differential diagnosis of leukemia and lymphoma applied to 2 micron plastic sections. *Blood* 1980;55: 386–394.
11. Beckstead JH, Halverson PS, Ries CA, et al. Enzyme histochemistry and immunohistochemistry on biopsy specimens of pathologic human bone marrow. *Blood* 1981;57:1088–1098.
12. Sternberger LA, Hardy PH, Cuculis JJ, et al. The unlabeled antibody enzyme method of immunohistochemistry. *J Histochem Cytochem* 1970;18:315–333.
13. Hsu SM, Raine L, Fanger H. Use of avidin-biotin peroxidase complex (ABC) in immunoperoxidase techniques: a comparison between ABC and unlabeled antibody (PAP) procedures. *J Histochem Cytochem* 1981;29:577–580.
14. Cordell JL, Falini B, Erber WN, et al. Immunoenzymatic labeling of monoclonal antibodies using immune complexes of alkaline phosphatase and monoclonal anti-alkaline phosphatase (APAAP complexes). *J Histochem Cytochem* 1984;32:219–229.
15. Yam LT, Janckila AJ, Li CY. The immuno-alkaline phosphatase methods. In: DeLellis RA, ed. *Advances in immunohistochemistry.* New York: Raven Press, 1988:1–29.
16. Clark CA, Downs EC, Primus FJ. An unlabeled antibody method using glucose oxidase-anti-glucose oxidase complexes (GAG): a sensitive alternative to immunoperoxidase for the detection of tissue antigens. *J Histochem Cytochem* 1982;30:27–34.
17. Porstmann B, Porstman T, Nugle E, et al. Which of the commonly used marker enzymes gives the best results in colorimetric and fluorometric immunoassays: horseradish peroxidase, alkaline phosphatase, or beta galactosidase? *J Immunol Methods* 1985;79:27–37.
18. Li CY, Lazcano-Villareal O, Pierre RV, et al. Immunocytochemical identification of cells in serous effusions. *Am J Clin Pathol* 1987;88: 696–706.
19. Wasdahl DA, Li CY, Morris MA. Paraffin section immunoperoxidase (IP) lymph node staining methodology for use with the Fisher Automated Stainer (FAS). *J Histochem Cytochem* 1989;37:939(abst).
20. Mason DY, Krissansen GW, Davey FR, et al. Antisera against epitopes resistant to denaturation on T3 (CD3) antigen can detect reactive and neoplastic T cells in paraffin embedded tissue biopsy specimens. *J Clin Pathol* 1988;41:121–127.
21. Mason DY, Cordell J, Brown M, et al. Detection of T cells in paraffin wax embedded tissue using antibodies against a peptide sequence from the CD3 antigen. *J Clin Pathol* 1989;42:1194–1200.
22. Mason DY, Cordell JL, Gaulard P, et al. Immunohistological detection of human cytotoxic/suppressor T cells using antibodies to a CD8 peptide sequence. *J Clin Pathol* 1992;45:1084–1088.
23. Steward M, Bishop R, Piggott NH, et al. Production and characterization of a new monoclonal antibody effective in recognizing the CD3 T-cell associated antigen in formalin-fixed embedded tissue. *Histopathology* 1997;30:16–22.
24. Curran RC, Gregory J. The unmasking of antigens in paraffin sections of tissue by trypsin. *Experimentia* 1977;33:1400–1401.
25. Denk H, Radaszkiewicz T, Weirich E. Pronase pretreatment of tissue sections enhances sensitivity of the unlabelled antibody-enzyme (PAP) technique. *J Immunol Methods* 1977;15:163–167.
26. Reading M. A digestion technique for the reduction of background staining in the immunoperoxidase method. *J Clin Pathol* 1977;30: 88–90.
27. Fraenkel-Conrat H, Brandon BA, Olcott HS. The reaction of formaldehyde with proteins. IV. Participation of indole groups: gramicidin. *J Biol Chem* 1947;168:99–118.
28. Fraenkel-Conrat H, Olcott HS. The reaction of formaldehyde with proteins. V. Cross-linking between amino and primary amide or quanidyl groups. *J Am Chem Soc* 1948;70:2673–2684.
29. Shi S-R, Key MC, Kalra KL. Antigen retrieval in formalin-fixed, paraffin-embedded tissues: an enhancement method for immunohistochemical staining based on microwave oven heating of tissue sections. *J Histochem Cytochem* 1991;39:741–748.
30. Shi S-R, Cote RJ, Taylor CR. Antigen retrieval immunohistochemistry: past, present and future. *J Histochem Cytochem* 1997;43:327–343.
31. Taylor CR, Shi SR, Cote RJ. Antigen retrieval for immunohistochemistry: status and need for greater standardization. *Appl Immunohistochem* 1996;4:144–166.
32. Streefkerk JG. Inhibition of erythrocyte pseudoperoxidase activity by treatment with hydrogen peroxide following methanol. *J Histochem Cytochem* 1972;20:829–831.
33. Weir EE, Pretlow TG II, Pitts A, et al. Destruction of endogenous peroxidase activity in order to locate cellular antigens by peroxidase-labeled antibodies. *J Histochem Cytochem* 1974;22:51–54.
34. Jasani B, Hallam LA, Newman GR, et al. Non-deleterious inhibition of endogenous peroxidase in immunolocalization studies involving the use of monoclonal antibodies. *Histochem J* 1983;15:1257–1258.
35. Köller U, Stockinger H, Majdic O, et al. A rapid and simple immunoperoxidase staining procedure for blood and bone marrow samples. *J Immunol Method* 1986;86:75–81.
36. Janckila AJ, Yam LT, Li CY. Immunoalkaline phosphatase cytochemistry: technical considerations of endogenous phosphatase activity. *Am J Clin Pathol* 1985;84:476–480.
37. Yam LT. Endogenous phosphatase activity in tumor cells in a liver aspirate: a potential problem for immunocytodiagnosis using immunoalkaline phosphatase methods. *Acta Cytol* 1989;33:505–510.
38. Li CY, Ziesmer SC, Lazcano-Villareal O. Use of azide and hydrogen peroxide as an inhibitor for endogenous peroxidase in the immunoperoxidase method. *J Histochem Cytochem* 1987;35:1457–1460.
39. Shi ZR, Itzkowitz SH, Kim YS. A comparison of three immunoperoxidase techniques for antigen detection in colorectal carcinoma tissues. *J Histochem Cytochem* 1988;36:317–322.

40. Sternberger LA, Sternberger NH. The unlabeled antibody method: comparison of peroxidase-antiperoxidase with avidin-biotin complex by a new method of quantification. *J Histochem Cytochem* 1986;34: 599–605.
41. Wood GS, Warnke R. Suppression of endogenous avidin-binding activity in tissues and its relevance to biotin-avidin detection systems. *J Histochem Cytochem* 1981;29:1196–1204.
42. Gross AJ, Sizer IW. The oxidation of tyramine, tyrosine and related compounds by peroxidase. *J Biol Chem* 1959;234:1611–1614.
43. von Wasielewski R, Mengel M, Gignac S, et al. Tyramine amplification technique in routine immunohistochemistry. *J Histochem Cytochem.* 1997;45:1455–1459.
44. Erber WN, Willis JI, Hoffman GJ. An enhanced immunocytochemical method for staining bone marrow trephine sections. *J Clin Pathol* 1997;50:389–393.
45. Malisius R, Merz H, Heinz B, et al. Constant detection of CD2, CD3, CD4, and CD5 in fixed and paraffin-embedded tissue using the peroxidase-mediated deposition of biotin-tyramide. *J Histochem Cytochem* 1997;45:1665–1672.
46. Yam LT, English MC, Janckila AJ, et al. Immunocytochemical characterization of human blood cells. *Am J Clin Pathol* 1983;80:314–321.
47. Graham RC Jr, Karnovsky MJ. The early stages of absorption of injected horseradish peroxidase in the proximal tubules of mouse kidney: ultrastructural cytochemistry by a new technique. *J Histochem Cytochem* 1966;14:291–302.
48. Shibata A, Bennett JM, Castoldi GL, et al. Recommended methods for cytological procedures in hematology. *Clin Lab Haematol* 1985; 7:55–74.
49. Yam LT, Li CY, Crosby WH. Cytochemical identification of monocytes and granulocytes. *Am J Clin Pathol* 1971;55:283–290.
50. Gabbas AG, Li CY. Acute non-lymphocytic leukemia with eosinophilic differentiation. *Am J Hematol* 1986;21:29–38.
51. Breton-Gorius J, Daniel MT, Flandrin G, et al. Fine structure and peroxidase activity of circulating micromegakaryoblasts and platelets in a case of acute myelofibrosis. *Br J Haematol* 1973;25:331–339.
52. Bain BJ, Catovsky D, O'Brien M, et al. Megakaryoblastic leukemia presenting as acute myelofibrosis: a study of 40 cases with platelet peroxidase reaction. *Blood* 1981;58:206–213.
53. Li CY, Yam LT. Cytochemical characterization of leukemic cells with numerous cytoplasmic granules. *Mayo Clin Proc* 1987;62:978–985.
54. Catovsky D, Gatton DAG, Robinson J. Myeloperoxidase deficient neutrophils in acute myeloid leukemia. *Scand J Haematol* 1972;9: 142–148.
55. Breton-Gorius J, Coquin Y, Vilde JL, et al. Cytochemical and ultrastructural studies of aberrant granules in the neutrophils of two patients with myeloperoxidase deficiency during a preleukemic state. *Blood Cells* 1976;2:187–209.
56. Fishman WH. Perspectives on alkaline phosphatase isoenzymes. *Am J Med* 1974;56:617–650.
57. Hayhoe FGJ, Quaglino D. Cytochemical demonstration and measurement of leukocyte alkaline phosphatase activity in normal and pathological states by a modified azo-dye coupling technique. *Br J Haematol* 1958;4:375–389.
58. Kaplow LS. Cytochemistry of leukocyte alkaline phosphatase: use of complex naphthol phosphatase in azo dye coupling techniques. *Am J Clin Pathol* 1963;39:439–449.
59. Kaplow LS. Leukocyte alkaline phosphatase: applications and methods. *Ann NY Acad Sci* 1968;155:911–947.
60. Kaplow LS. Alkaline phosphatase activity in peripheral blood lymphocytes. *Arch Pathol* 1969;88:69–72.
61. Nanba K, Jaffe ES, Braylan RC, et al. Alkaline phosphatase–positive malignant lymphoma: a subtype of B cell lymphoma. *Am J Clin Pathol* 1977;68:535–542.
62. Rutenburg AM, Rosales CL, Bennett JM. An improved histochemical method for the demonstration of leukocyte alkaline phosphatase activity: clinical application. *J Lab Clin Med* 1965;65:698–705.
63. Gomori G. Chloracyl esters as histochemical substrates. *J Histochem Cytochem* 1953;1:469–470.
64. Sweetman F, Ornstein L. Electrophoresis of elastase-like esterases from human neutrophils. *J Histochem Cytochem* 1974;22:327–339.
65. Moloney WC, McPherson K, Fliegelman L. Esterase activity in leukocytes demonstrated by the use of naphthol AS-D chloroacetate substrate. *J Histochem Cytochem* 1960;8:200–207.
66. Leder LD. Über die seleketive fermentcytochemische darstellung Von neutrophilen myeloischen zellen und gavebsmastzellen im paraffinschnitt. *Klin Wochenschr* 1964;42:553.
67. Keifer J, Abromowitch M, Stass SA. Chloroacetate esterase positivity in acute lymphoblastic leukemia. *Am J Clin Pathol* 1985;83:647–649.
68. Schaefer VHE, Hellriegel KP, Hennekeuser HH, et al. Eosinophilenleukämie, eine unreifzellige Myelose mit Chloroacetatesterasepositiver Eosinophilie. *Blut* 1973;26:7–19.
69. Liso V, Troccoli G, Specchia G, et al. Cytochemical "normal" and "abnormal" eosinophils in acute leukemias. *Am J Hematol* 1977;2: 123–131.
70. Leder LD. Akute myelo-monozytäre Leukämie mit atypischen Naphthol-AS-D-Chloracetat-Esterase-positiven Eosinophilen. *Acta Haematol* 1970;44:52–62.
71. Neiman RS, Barcos M, Berard C, et al. Granulocytic sarcoma: a clinicopathologic study of 61 biopsied cases. *Cancer* 1981;48:1426–1437.
72. Storr J, Dolan G, Coustan-Smith E, et al. Value of monoclonal antimyeloperoxidase (MPO7) for diagnosing acute leukemia. *J Clin Pathol* 1990;43:847–849.
73. Buccheri V, Shetly V, Yoshida N, et al: The role of an anti-myeloperoxidase antibody in the diagnosis and classification of acute leukemia: a comparison with light and electron microscopy cytochemistry. *Br J Haematol* 1992;80:62–68.
74. Furebring-Fredén M, Martinsson U, Sundström C. Myelosarcoma without acute leukaemia: immunohistochemical and clinicopathologic characterization of eight cases. *Histopathology* 1990;16:243–250.
75. Li CY, Lam KW, Yam LT. Esterases in human leukocytes. *J Histochem Cytochem* 1973;21:1–12.
76. Mueller J, Brien Delré G, Buerk H, et al. Non-specific esterase activity: a criterion for differentiation of T and B lymphocytes in mouse lymph nodes. *Eur J Immunol* 1975;5:270–274.
77. Higgy KE, Burns GF, Hayhoe FGJ. Discrimination of B, T, and null lymphocytes by esterase cytochemistry. *Scand J Haematol* 1977;18: 437–448.
78. Knowles DM, Holck S. Tissue localization of T lymphocytes by the histochemical demonstration of acid a naphthyl acetate esterase. *Lab Invest* 1978;39:70–76.
79. Horwitz DA, Allison AC, Ward P, et al. Identification of human mononuclear leucocyte population by esterase staining. *Clin Exp Immunol* 1977;30:289–298.
80. Grossi CE, Webb SR, Zicca A, et al. Morphological and histochemical analysis of two human T-cell subpopulations bearing receptors for IgM or IgG. *J Exp Med* 1978;147:1405–1417.
81. Bernard J, Dufer J. Cytochemical analysis of human peripheral blood lymphocyte subsets defined by monoclonal antibodies. *Scand J Immunol* 1983;17:89–93.
82. Zicca A, Leprini A, Candoni A, et al. Ultrastructural localization of alpha-naphthyl acid esterase in human TM lymphocytes. *Am J Pathol* 1981;105:40–46.
83. Beran A, Burns CF, Gray L, et al. Cytochemistry of human T cell subpopulations. *Scand J Immunol* 1980;11:223–233.
84. Ferrarini M, Cadoni A, Franzi AT, et al. Ultrastructure and cytochemistry of human peripheral blood lymphocytes. Similarities between the cells of the third population and T_γ lymphocytes. *Eur J Immunol* 1980;10:562–570.
85. Bennett JM, Catovsky D, Daniel MT, et al. Criteria for the diagnosis of acute leukemia of megakaryocyte lineage (M7): a report of the French-American-British Cooperative Group. *Ann Intern Med* 1985; 103:460–462.
86. de Oliveira MSP, Gregory C, Matutes E, et al. Cytochemical profile of megakaryoblastic leukaemia: a study with cytochemical methods, monoclonal antibodies and ultrastructural cytochemistry. *J Clin Pathol* 1987;40:663–669.
87. Witzig TE, Phyliky RL, Li CY, et al. T-cell chronic lymphocytic leukemia with a helper/inducer membrane phenotype: a distinct clinicopathologic subtype with a poor prognosis. *Am J Hematol* 1986;21: 139–155.
88. Crockard A, Chambers D, Matutes E, et al. Cytochemistry of acid hydrolases in chronic B and T cell leukemias. *Am J Clin Pathol* 1982; 78:437–444.
89. Yang K, Bearman RM, Pangalis GA, et al. Acid phosphatase and alpha naphthyl acetate esterase in neoplastic and non-neoplastic lymphocytes: a statistical analysis. *Am J Clin Pathol* 1982;78:141–149.
90. Crockard AD. Cytochemistry of lymphoid cells: a review of findings in the normal and leukemic state. *Histochem J* 1984;16:1027–1050.

91. Boesen AM, Hokland P, Jensen M. Acid phosphatase and acid esterase activity in neoplastic and non-neoplastic lymphoid cells: a semiquantitative evaluation related to immunological markers in 112 cases. *Scand J Haematol* 1984;32:313–322.
92. Li CY. Leukemia cytochemistry. *Mayo Clin Proc* 1981;56:712–713.
93. Li CY, Phyliky RL, Yam LT: Acute myelomonocytic leukemia: an unusual variant with both granulocytic and monocytic esterases in the leukemic cells. *Mayo Clin Proc* 1986;61:104–109.
94. Geary CG, Catovsky D, Wiltshaw E, et al. Chronic myelomonocytic leukaemia. *Br J Haematol* 1975;30:289–302.
95. Li CY, Harrison EG. Histochemical and immunohistochemical study of diffuse large-cell lymphomas. *Am J Clin Pathol* 1978;70:721–732.
96. Carbone A, Micheau C, Caillaud JM, et al. A cytochemical and immunohistochemical approach to malignant histiocytosis. *Cancer* 1981; 47:2862–2871.
97. Risdall RJ, Sibley RK, McKenna RW, et al. Malignant histiocytosis: a light- and electron-microscopic and histochemical study. *Am J Surg Pathol* 1980;4:439–450.
98. Tubbs RR, Savage RA, Crabtree RH, et al. Expression of monocytic histiocytic cytochemical markers in epithelial neoplasia. *Am J Clin Pathol* 1979;72:789–794.
99. Yam LT, Janckila AJ, Winkler CF. Non-specific esterase activity in cancer cells in the marrow. *Hum Pathol* 1980;11:689–690.
100. Yam LT, Yam CF, Li CY. Eosinophilia in systemic mastocytosis. *Am J Clin Pathol* 1980;73:48–54.
101. Webb TA, Li CY, Yam LT. Systemic mast cell disease: a clinical and hematopathologic study of 26 cases. *Cancer* 1982;49:927–938.
102. Sun T, Li CY, Yam LT. *Atlas of cytochemistry and immunocytochemistry of hematologic neoplasms.* Chicago: ASCP Press, 1985.
103. Kaplow LS, Burstone MS. Cytochemical demonstration of acid phosphatase in haematopoietic cells in health and in various hematological disorders using azo dye techniques. *J Histochem Cytochem* 1964;12: 805–811.
104. Li CY, Yam LT, Lam KW. Acid phosphatase isoenzyme in human leukocytes in normal and pathologic conditions. *J Histochem Cytochem* 1970;18:473–481.
105. Li CY, Yam LT, Lam KW. Studies of acid phosphatase isoenzymes in human leukocytes: demonstration of isoenzyme cell-specificity. *J Histochem Cytochem* 1970;18:901–910.
106. Barka T, Anderson PJ. Histochemical methods for acid phosphatase using hexazonium pararosanilin as coupler. *J Histochem Cytochem* 1962;10:741–753.
107. Janckila AJ, Li CY, Lam KW, et al. The cytochemistry of tartrate-resistant acid phosphatase: technical considerations. *Am J Clin Pathol* 1978;70:45–55.
108. Catovsky D, Greaves MF, Pain C, et al. Acid phosphatase reaction in acute lymphoblastic leukemia. *Lancet* 1978;1:749–751.
109. Smithson WA, Li CY, Pierre RV, et al. Acute lymphoblastic leukemia in children: immunologic, cytochemical, morphologic, and cytogenetic studies in relation to pretreatment risk factors. *Med Pediatr Oncol* 1979;7:83–93.
110. Krishnan J, Li CY, Su WPD. Cutaneous lymphomas: correlation of histochemical and immunohistochemical characteristics and clinicopathologic features. *Am J Clin Pathol* 1983;79:157–165.
111. Bataille R, Durie BG, Sany J, et al. Myeloma bone marrow acid phosphatase staining: a correlative study of 38 patients. *Blood* 1980; 55:82–85.
112. Tontarolo M, Cantore N, Grande M, et al. Plasma cell acid phosphatase as an adjunct in the differential diagnosis of monoclonal immunoglobulinemias. *Acta Haematol* 1981;65:103–107.
113. Yam LT, Li CY, Lam KW. Tartrate-resistant acid phosphatase isoenzyme in the reticulum cells of leukemic reticuloendotheliosis. *N Engl J Med* 1971;284:357–360.
114. Yam LT, Janckila AJ, Li CY, et al. Cytochemistry of tartrate-resistant acid phosphatase: fifteen years' experience. *Leukemia* 1987;1: 285–288.
115. Mover S, Li CY, Yam LT. Semiquantitative evaluation of tartrate-resistant acid phosphatase activity in human blood cells. *J Lab Clin Med* 1972;80:711–717.
116. Radzun HJ, Kreipe H, Paswaresch MR. Tartrate resistant acid phosphatase as a differentiation marker for the human mononuclear phagocyte systems. *Hematol Oncol* 1983;1:321–327.
117. Leder LD. Alkaline phosphatase and tartrate-resistant acid phosphatase in cells of prolymphocytic leukemia. *Klin Wochenschr* 1978;56: 313–314.
118. Naeim F, Capostagno VJ, Johnson CE, et al. Sézary syndrome: tartrate-resistant acid phosphatase in the neoplastic cells. *Am J Clin Pathol* 1979;71:528–533.
119. Sheehan HL, Storey GW. An improved method of staining leukocyte granules with Sudan black B. *J Pathol Bacteriol* 1947;59:336–337.
120. Tricot G, Broechoert-van Orshoren T, van Hoof A, et al. Sudan black B positivity in acute lymphoblastic leukaemia. *Br J Haematol* 1982; 51:615–621.
121. Stass SA, Prie CH, Melvin S, et al. Sudan black B positive acute lymphoblastic leukaemia. *Br J Haematol* 1984;57:413–421.
122. Wick MR, Li CY, Pierre RV. Acute nonlymphocytic leukemia with basophilic differentiation. *Blood* 1982;60:38–45.
123. Yam LT, Chan CH, Li CY. Hepatic involvement in systemic mast cell disease. *Am J Med* 1986;80:819–826.
124. Wislocki BG, Rheingold JJ, Dempsey EW. The occurrence of the periodic acid–Schiff reaction in various normal cells of blood and connective tissues. *Blood* 1949;4:562–568.
125. Mitus MJ, Bergna LJ, Mednicoff IB, et al. Cytochemical studies of glycogen content of lymphocytes in lymphocytic proliferations. *Blood* 1958;13:748–756.
126. Humphrey GB, Nesbit ME, Brunning RD. Prognostic value of the periodic acid–Schiff (PAS) reaction in acute lymphoblastic leukemia. *Am J Clin Pathol* 1974;61:393–397.
127. Lilleyman JS, Scott CS. PAS and acid phosphatase cytochemistry in acute lymphoblastic leukemia. In: Scott SC, ed. *Leukemia cytochemistry.* Chichester, UK: Ellis Harwood, 1989:103–120.
128. Quaglino D, Hayhoe FGJ. Periodic acid–Schiff positivity in erythroblasts with special reference to DiGuglielmo disease. *Br J Haematol* 1960;6:26–33.
129. Roberts BE, Miles DW, Wood CG. Polycythaemia vera and myelosclerosis: a bone marrow study. *Br J Haematol* 1969;16:75–85.
130. Luna LG, ed. *Manual of histologic staining methods of the Armed Forces Institute of Pathology,* 3rd ed. New York: McGraw-Hill, 1968.
131. Lukes RJ. The immunologic approach to the pathology of malignant lymphomas. *Am J Clin Pathol* 1979;72:657–669.
132. Aisenberg AC. Cell-surface markers in lymphoproliferative disease. *N Engl J Med* 1981;304:331–336.
133. Foon KA, Todd RF III. Immunologic classification of leukemia and lymphoma. *Blood* 1986;68:1–31.
134. Van Der Valk P, Meijer CJLM. The non-Hodgkin's lymphomas: old and new thinking. *Histopathology* 1988;13:367–384.
135. Knapp W, Dörken B, Rieber P, et al. CD antigens, 1989. *Blood* 1989; 74:1448–1450.
136. Pizzolo G, Chilosi M, Fiore-Donati L, et al. Immunohistological analysis of bone marrow involvement in lymphoproliferative disorder: the use of cryostat sections from trephine biopsies. *Haematologia* 1984; 17:247–257.
137. Falini B, Martelli F, Tarallo F, et al. Immunohistological analysis of human bone marrow trephine biopsies using monoclonal antibodies. *Br J Haematol* 1984;56:365–386.
138. Kronland R, Grogan T, Spier C, et al. Immunotopographic assessment of lymphoid and plasma cell malignancies in the bone marrow. *Hum Pathol* 1985;16:1247–1254.
139. Thaler J, Denz H, Gattringer C, et al. Diagnostic and prognostic value of immunohistological bone marrow examination: results in 212 patients with lymphoproliferative disorders. *Blut* 1987;54:213–222.
140. Nash JRG, Smith SR, Mackie MJ. An immunocytochemical study of lymphocyte and macrophage populations in the bone marrow of patients with non-Hodgkin's lymphoma. *J Pathol* 1988;154:141–149.
141. Epstein AL, Marder RJ, Winter JN, et al. Two new monoclonal antibodies (LN-1, LN-2) reactive in B5 formalin-fixed, paraffin-embedded tissues with follicular center and mantle zone human B lymphocytes and derived tumors. *J Immunol* 1984;133:1028–1036.
142. Linder J, Ye Y, Armitage JO, et al. Monoclonal antibodies marking B-cell non-Hodgkin's lymphoma in paraffin-embedded tissue. *Mod Pathol* 1988;1:29–34.
143. van der Valk P, Mullink H, Huijgens PC, et al. Immunohistochemistry in bone marrow diagnosis: value of a panel of monoclonal antibodies on routinely processed bone marrow biopsies. *Am J Surg Pathol* 1989; 13:97–106.
144. Kurtin PJ, Pinkus GS. Leukocyte common antigen—a diagnostic discriminant between hematopoietic and nonhematopoietic neoplasms in

paraffin sections using monoclonal antibodies: correlation with immunologic studies and ultrastructural localization. *Hum Pathol* 1985;16: 353–365.
145. Hitzman JL, Li CY, Kyle RA. Immunoperoxidase staining of bone marrow sections. *Cancer* 1981;48:2438–2446.
146. Cartun RW, Coles FB, Pastuszak WT. Utilization of monoclonal antibody L26 in the identification and confirmation of B cell lymphomas: a sensitive and specific marker applicable to formalin- and B5-fixed, paraffin-embedded tissues. *Am J Pathol* 1987;129:415–421.
147. Mason DY, Comans-Bitter WM, Cordell JL, et al. Antibody L26 recognizes an intracellular epitope on the B-cell–associated CD20 antigen. *Am J Pathol* 1990;136:1215–1222.
148. Linder J, Ye Y, Harrington DS, et al. Monoclonal antibodies marking T lymphocytes in paraffin-embedded tissue. *Am J Pathol* 1987;127: 1–8.
149. Said JW, Stoll PN, Shintaku P, et al. Leu-22: a preferential marker for T-lymphocytes in paraffin sections. Staining profile in T- and B-cell lymphomas, Hodgkin's disease, other lymphoproliferative disorders, myeloproliferative diseases and various neoplastic processes. *Am J Clin Pathol* 1989;91:542–549.
150. Tsang WYW, Chan JKC, Ng CS, et al. Utility of a paraffin section-reactive CD56 antibody (123C3) for characterization and diagnosis of lymphoma. *Am J Surg Pathol* 1996;20:202–210.
151. Merle-Beral H, Duc LNC, Leblond V, et al. Diagnostic and prognostic significance of myelomonocytic cell surface antigens in acute myeloid leukaemia. *Br J Haematol* 1989;73:323–330.
152. van der Schoot CE, Daams GM, Pinkster J, et al. Monoclonal antibodies against myeloperoxidase are valuable immunological reagents for the diagnosis of acute myeloid leukaemia. *Br J Haematol* 1990;74: 173–178.
153. Falini B, Flengh L, Pileri S, et al. PG-M1: a new monoclonal antibody directed against a fixative-resistant epitope on the macrophage-restricted form of the CD68 molecule. *Am J Pathol* 1993;142: 1359–1372.
154. Pinkus GS, Thomas P, Said JW. Leu-M1—a marker for Reed-Sternberg cells in Hodgkin's disease: an immunoperoxidase study of paraffin-embedded tissues. *Am J Pathol* 1985;119:244–252.
155. Hall PA, D'Ardenne AJ. Value of CD15 immunostaining in diagnosing Hodgkin's disease: a review of published literature. *J Clin Pathol* 1987;40:1298–1304.
156. Greaves MF, Sieff C, Edwards PAW. Monoclonal antiglycophorin as a probe for erythroleukemias. *Blood* 1983;61:645–651.
157. Liszka K, Majdic O, Bettelheim P, et al. Glycophorin A expression in malignant hematopoiesis. *Am J Hematol* 1983;15:219–226.
158. Barsoum AL, Czuczman MS, Bhavanandan VP, et al. Epitopes immunologically related to glycophorin A on human malignant and non-malignant cells in culture. *Int J Cancer* 1984;34:789–795.
159. Solberg LA, Oles KJ, Kimlinger TK, et al. A new murine monoclonal antibody for the diagnosis of erythroleukemia. *Am J Clin Pathol* 1990;93:387–390.
160. Yokochi T, Brice M, Rabinovitch PS, et al. Monoclonal antibodies detecting antigenic determinants with restricted expression on erythroid cells: from the erythroid committed progenitor level to the mature erythroblast. *Blood* 1984;63:1376–1384.
161. Crocker J, Gyde O, Jenkins R. Demonstration of normoblasts in tissue sections by means of an immunohistochemical technique for haemoglobin. *J Clin Pathol* 1984;37:1312–1313.
162. Chuang SS, Li C-Y. Distribution of three transforming growth factor-β isoforms on hematopoietic cells and possible feedback inhibition role in hematopoietic regulation. *Cell Vision* 1996;3:429–433.
163. Chuang SS, Li C-Y. Useful panel of antibodies for the classification of acute leukemia by immunohistochemical methods in bone marrow trephine biopsy specimens. *Am J Clin Pathol* 1997;107:410–418.
164. Huang MJ, Li CY, Nichols WL, et al. Acute leukemia with megakaryocytic differentiation: a study of 12 cases identified immunocytochemically. *Blood* 1984;64:427–439.
165. Breton-Gorius J, Vanhaeke D, Pryzwansky KB, et al. Simultaneous detection of membrane markers with monoclonal antibodies and peroxidatic activities in leukaemia: ultrastructural analysis using a new method of fixation preserving the platelet peroxidase. *Br J Haematol* 1984;58:447–458.
166. Erber WN, Breton-Gorius J, Villeral JL, et al. Detection of cells of megakaryocyte lineage in haematological malignancies by immunoalkaline phosphatase labelling cell smears with a panel of monoclonal antibodies. *Br J Haematol* 1987;65:87–94.
167. Windebank KP, Tefferi A, Smithson WA, et al. Acute megakaryocytic leukemia (M7) in children. *Mayo Clin Proc* 1989;64:1339–1351.
168. Innes DJ Jr, Mills SE, Walker GK. Megakaryocytic leukemia: identification utilizing anti-factor VIII immunoperoxidase. *Am J Clin Pathol* 1982;77:107–110.
169. Li CY, Lam WKW, Yam LT. Immunohistochemical diagnosis of prostatic cancer with metastasis. *Cancer* 1980;46:706–712.
170. Lam KWL, Li CY, Yam LT, et al. Improved immunohistochemical detection of prostatic acid phosphatase by a monoclonal antibody. *Prostate* 1989;15:13–21.
171. Walts AE, Said JW, Shintaku IP, et al. Chromogranin as a marker of neuroendocrine cells in cytologic material—an immunocytochemical study. *Am J Clin Pathol* 1985;84:273–277.
172. Gould VE, Lee I, Wiedenmann B, et al. Synaptophysin: a novel marker for neurons, certain neuroendocrine cells, and their neoplasms. *Hum Pathol* 1986;17:979–983.
173. Chang TK, Li CY, Smithson WA. Immunocytochemical study of small round cell tumors in routinely processed specimens. *Arch Pathol Lab Med* 1989;113:1343–1348.
174. Schmidt RA, Cone R, Haas JE, et al. Diagnosis of rhabdomyosarcomas with HHF35, a monoclonal antibody directed against muscle actins. *Am J Pathol* 1988;131:19–28.
175. Azumi N, Ben-Ezra J, Battifora H. Immunophenotypic diagnosis of leiomyosarcomas and rhabdomyosarcomas with monoclonal antibodies to muscle-specific actin and desmin in formalin-fixed tissue. *Mod Pathol* 1988;1:469–474.
176. Cho KR, Olson JL, Epstein JI. Primitive rhabdomyosarcoma presenting with diffuse bone marrow involvement: an immunohistochemical and ultrastructural study. *Mod Pathol* 1988;1:23–28.
177. Bennett JM, Catovsky D, Daniel MT, et al. French-American-British (FAB) Cooperative Group: proposals for the classification of acute leukemias. *Br J Haematol* 1976;33:451–458.
178. Bennett JM, Catovsky D, Daniel MT, et al. Criteria for the diagnosis of acute leukemia of megakaryocytic lineage (M7): a report of the French-American-British Cooperative Group. *Ann Intern Med* 1985; 103:460–462.
179. Cuttner J, Seremetis S, Najfield V, et al. TdT-positive acute leukemia with monocytoid characteristics: clinical, cytochemical, cytogenetic, and immunologic findings. *Blood* 1984;64:237–243.
180. Chan LC, Greaves MF. Acute leukaemia with mixed lymphoid and myeloid phenotype. *Br J Haematol* 1984;58:203–205.
181. Gale RP, Ben-Basset I. Hybrid acute leukemia [Annotation]. *Br J Haematol* 1987;65:261–264.
182. Griffin JD, Davis R, Nelson DA, et al. Use of surface marker analysis to predict outcome of adult acute myeloblastic leukemia. *Blood* 1986; 68:1232–1241.
183. Browman GP, Neame PB, Soamboonsrup P. The contribution of cytochemistry and immunophenotyping to the reproducibility of the FAB classification in acute leukemia. *Blood* 1986;68:900–905.
184. Arber DA, Jenkins KA. Paraffin section immunophenotyping of acute leukemia in bone marrow specimens. *Am J Clin Pathol* 1996;106: 462–468.
185. Seo IS, Li CY, Yam LT. Myelodysplastic syndrome: diagnostic implications of cytochemical and immunocytochemical studies. *Mayo Clin Proc* 1993;68:47–53.
186. Scott CS, Cahill A, Bynoe AG, et al. Esterase cytochemistry in primary myelodysplastic syndromes and megaloblastic anemias: demonstration of abnormal staining patterns associated with dysmyelopoiesis. *Br J Haematol* 1983;55:414–418.
187. Erber WN, Jacobs A, Oscier DG, et al. Circulating micromegakaryocytes in myelodysplasia. *J Clin Pathol* 1987;40:1349–1352.
188. Koeffler JP, Golde DW. Chronic myelogenous leukemia: new concepts. *N Engl J Med* 1981;304:1201–1209.
189. Rubin H. Chronic neutrophilic leukemia. *Ann Intern Med* 1966;65: 93–100.
190. Dameshek W. Some speculation on myeloproliferative syndromes [Editorial]. *Blood* 1951;6:372–375.
191. Darbyshire PJ, Smith JHF, Oakhill A, et al. Monocytic leukemia in infancy: a review of eight children. *Cancer* 1985;56:1584–1589.
192. Mongkonsritragoon W, Letendre L, Qian J, et al. Nodular lesions of monocytic component in myelodysplastic syndrome. *Am J Clin Pathol* 1998;110:154–162.

193. Li CY. Immunocytochemical techniques for identifying leukemias. *Mayo Clin Proc* 1984;59:185–188.
194. Tefferi A, Li CY, Phyliky RL. Role of immunotyping in chronic lymphocytosis: review of the natural history of the condition in 145 adult patients. *Mayo Clin Proc* 1988;63:801–806.
195. Harris NL, Jaffe ES, Stein H, et al. A revised European-American classification of lymphoid neoplasms: a proposal from the International Lymphoma Study Group. *Blood* 1994;84:1361–1392.
196. Weisenburger DD, Armitage JO. Mantle cell lymphoma: an entity comes of age. *Blood* 1996;87:4483–4494.
197. Pittaluga S, Verhoef G, Criel A, et al. ''Small'' B-cell non-Hodgkin's lymphomas with splenomegaly at presentation are either mantle cell lymphoma or marginal zone lymphoma: a study based on histology, cytology, immunohistochemistry and cytogenetic analysis. *Am J Surg Pathol* 1996;20:211–223.
198. Mollejo M, Menarguez J, Lloret E, et al. Splenic marginal zone lymphoma: a distinctive type of low-grade B-cell lymphoma. A clinicopathological study of 13 cases. *Am J Surg Pathol* 1995;19:1146–1157.
199. Vasef MA, Medeiros LJ, Koo C, et al. Cyclin D1 immunohistochemical staining is useful in distinguishing mantle cell lymphoma from other low-grade B-cell neoplasms in bone marrow. *Am J Clin Pathol* 1997;108:302–307.
200. Hoyer JD, Ross CW, Li C-Y, et al. True T-cell chronic lymphocytic leukemia: a morphologic and immunophenotypic study of 25 cases. *Blood* 1995;86:1163–1169.
201. Phyliky RL, Li CY, Yam LT. T-cell chronic lymphocytic leukemia with morphologic and immunologic characteristics of cytotoxic/suppressor phenotype. *Mayo Clin Proc* 1983;58:709–720.
202. Pandolfi F, Loughran TP, Starkebaum G, et al. Clinical course and prognosis of the lymphoproliferative disease of granular lymphocytes: a multicenter study. *Cancer* 1990;65:341–348.
203. Staven P, Førre O, Brandtzeg P, et al. T-lymphocytes with both helper and suppressor markers on the same cell in chronic lymphocytic leukemia. *Scand J Haematol* 1983;30:177–182.
204. Dhodapkar MV, Li C-Y, Lust JA, et al. Clinical spectrum of clonal proliferations of T-large granular lymphocytes: a T-cell clonopathy of undetermined significance? *Blood* 1994;84:1620–1627.
205. Tefferi A, Li C-Y, Witzig TE, et al. Chronic natural killer cell lymphocytosis: a descriptive clinical study. *Blood* 1994;84:2721–2725.
206. Foucar K, Rydell R. Richter's syndrome in chronic lymphocytic leukemia. *Cancer* 1980;46:118–134.
207. Ansell SM, Li C-Y, Phyliky RL. Epstein-Barr virus infection in patients with chronic lymphocytic leukemia and Richter's transformation. *Hematol Cell Ther* 1997;39[Suppl 1]:S91–S92.
208. Melo JV, Catovsky D, Galton DAG. The relationship between chronic lymphocytic leukaemia and prolymphocytic leukaemia. II. Patterns of evolution in ''prolymphocytoid'' transformation. *Br J Haematol* 1986;64:77–86.
209. Evidani S, Parry H, Glass U, et al. Acute lymphoblastic leukemia supervening in a case of chronic lymphocytic leukemia after continuous 3-year treatment with chlorambucil. *Cancer* 1984;54:397–399.
210. Archimbaud E, Charrin C, Gentihomme O, et al. Initial clonal acute lymphoblastic transformation of chronic lymphocytic leukemia with (11;14) and (8;12) chromosome translocations and acquired homozygosity. *Acta Haematol* 1988;79:168–173.
211. Hsu SM, Yang K, Jaffe ES. Hairy cell leukemia: a B cell neoplasia with unique antigenic phenotype. *Am J Clin Pathol* 1983;80:421–428.
212. Schwarting R, Stein H, Wang CY. The monoclonal antibodies a S-HCL1 (a Leu-14) and a S-HCL3 (a Leu-M5) allow the diagnosis of hairy cell leukemia. *Blood* 1985;65:974–983.
213. Korsmeyer SJ, Greene WC, Waldmann TA. Cellular origin of hairy cell leukemia: malignant B cells that express receptors for T cell growth factor. *Semin Oncol* 1984;11:394–400.
214. Martin JME, Boras VF, Houwen B, et al. Hairy cell leukemia and anti-leukocyte common antigen. *Am J Clin Pathol* 1988;90:412–420.
215. Cordone I, Annino L, Masi S, et al. Diagnostic relevance of peripheral blood immunocytochemistry in hairy cell leukemia. *J Clin Pathol* 1995;48:955–960.
216. Saxon A, Stevens RH, Golde DW. T-lymphocyte variant of hairy-cell leukemia. *Ann Intern Med* 1978;88:323–326.
217. Burns GF, Worman CP, Cawley JC. Fluctuations in the T and B characteristics of two cases of T-cell hairy-cell leukemia. *Clin Exp Immunol* 1980;39:76–82.
218. Janckila AJ, Cardwell EM, Yam LT, et al. Hairy cell identification by immunohistochemistry of tartrate-resistant acid phosphatase. *Blood* 1995;85:2839–2844.
219. Hoyer JD, Li C-Y, Yam LT, et al. Immunohistochemical demonstration of acid phosphatase isoenzyme 5 (tartrate-resistant) in paraffin sections of hairy cell leukemia and other hematologic disorders. *Am J Clin Pathol* 1997;108:308–315.
220. Li C-Y, Wang CYE, Phyliky RL, et al. Evaluation of methods for immunohistochemical identification of hairy cell leukemia on paraffin sections. *Histochem Cytochem* 1996;29[Suppl]:1080–1081.
221. Yam LT, Li CY. Histogenesis of splenic lesions in Hodgkin's disease. *Am J Clin Pathol* 1976;66:976–985.
222. Shirahama T, Cohen AS, Skinner M. Immunohistochemistry of amyloid. In: DeLellis RA, ed. *Advances in immunohistochemistry*. New York: Masson Publishing, 1984:277–302.
223. Fujihara S, Balow JE, Costa JC, et al. Identification and classification of amyloid in formalin-fixed, paraffin-embedded tissue sections by the unlabeled immunoperoxidase method. *Lab Invest* 1980;43:358–365.
224. Shirahama T, Skinner M, Cohen AS, et al. Histochemical and immunohistochemical characterization of amyloid associated with chronic hemodialysis as β_2-microglobulin. *Lab Invest* 1985;53:705–709.
225. Travis WD, Li CY, Hoagland HC, et al. Mast cell leukemia: report of a case and review of the literature. *Mayo Clin Proc* 1986;61:957–966.
226. Travis WD, Li CY, Bergstralh EJ, et al. Systemic mast cell disease. Analysis of 58 cases and literature review. *Medicine (Baltimore)* 1988; 67:345–368.
227. Hughes DM, Kurtin PJ, Hanson CA, et al. Identification of normal and neoplastic mast cells by immunohistochemical demonstration of tryptase in paraffin sections. *J Surg Pathol* 1995;1:87–96.
228. Travis WD, Li CY, Yam LT, et al. Significance of systemic mast cell disease with associated hematologic disorders. *Cancer* 1988;62: 965–972.
229. Ramani P, Rampling D, Link M. Immunocytochemical study of 12E7 in small round-cell tumours of childhood: an assessment of its sensitivity and specificity. *Histopathology* 1993;23:557–561.
230. Papsidero LD, Croghan GA, Asirwatham J, et al. Immunohistochemical demonstration of prostate-specific antigen in metastases with the use of monoclonal antibody F5. *Am J Pathol* 1985;121:451–454.

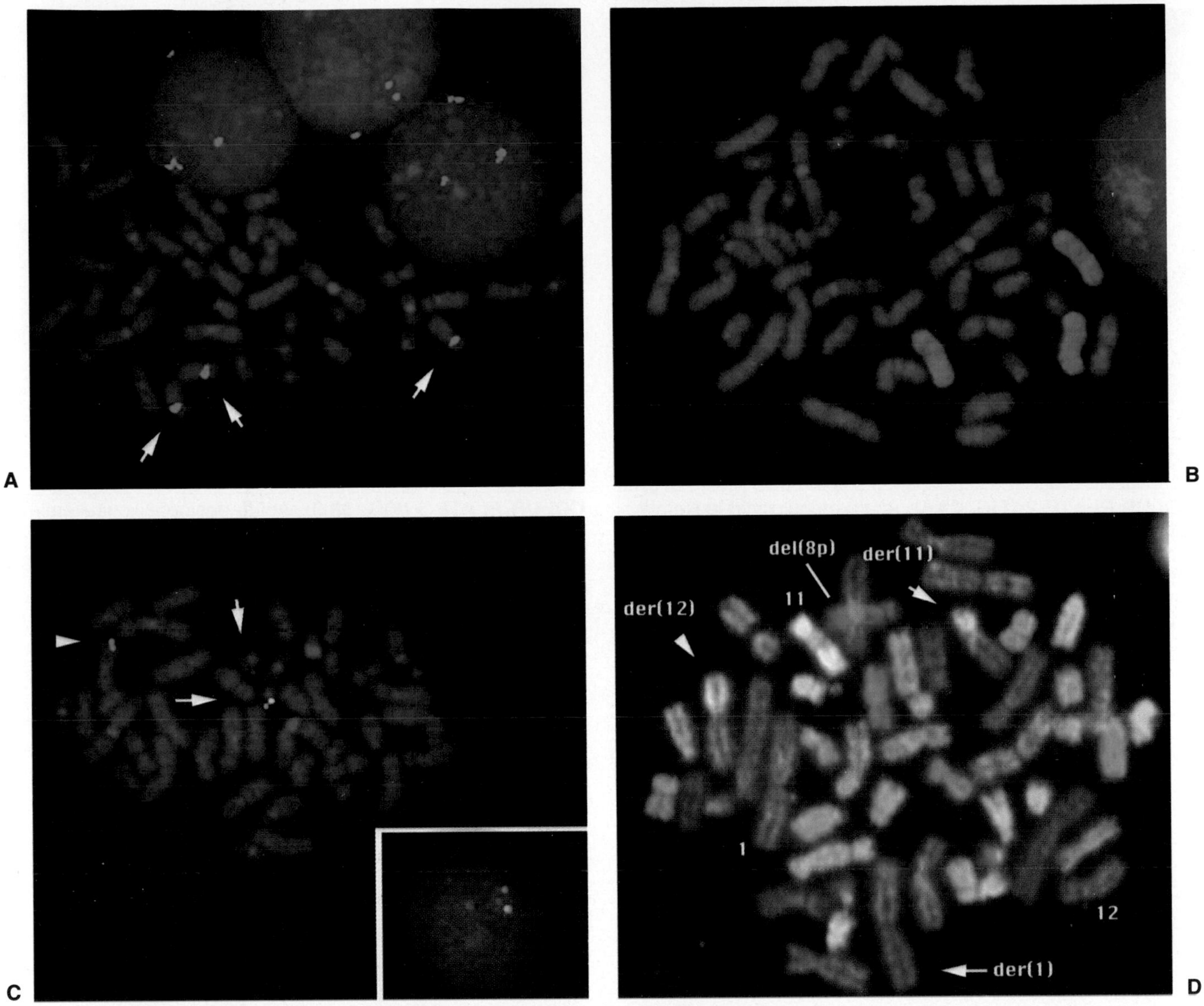

COLOR PLATE 1 (FIG. 10.4). Photomicrographs of metaphase and interphase cells after fluorescence *in situ* hybridization (FISH). In **A** through **C**, the cells are counterstained with 4,6-diamidino-2-phenylindole-dihydrochloride (DAPI). **A:** Hybridization of a directly labeled centromere-specific probe for chromosome 8 (CEP8 Spectrum Green, Vysis, Inc. Downers Grove, IL) to metaphase and interphase cells with trisomy 8 from a bone marrow aspirate of a patient with acute myeloid leukemia (AML). Centromere-specific probes hybridize to the repetitive DNA sequences that are present at the centromeres of human chromosomes. The chromosome 8 homologues are identified with arrows. **B:** Hybridization of a directly labeled chromosome 8–specific painting probe (WCP8 Spectrum Green, Vysis, Inc.) to a metaphase cell with trisomy 8 from a bone marrow aspirate of a patient with AML. **C:** Hybridization of a locus-specific probe for the detection of a recurring translocation, the t(9;22)(q34;q11.2) in chronic myelogenous leukemia (CML). The probe is a mixture of digoxigenin-labeled DNA probes (detected with rhodamine-labeled antibodies) for the major breakpoint cluster region of the *BCR* gene at 22q11.2 and biotin-labeled probes (detected with fluorescein-labeled avidin) for the *ABL* gene at 9q34 (M-bcr/abl probe, Ventana Medical Systems, Tucson, AZ). In cells with the t(9;22), only one green signal *(arrowhead)* and one red signal *(short arrow)* are observed on the normal 9 and 22 homologues, and a yellow fusion signal *(long arrow)* is observed on the Ph chromosome as a result of the juxtaposition of the *ABL* and *BCR* sequences. **D:** Spectral karyotyping analysis of a metaphase cell from a case of AML-M7. Twenty-four differentially labeled probes representing each human chromosome were cohybridized, and imaging analysis software assigned a unique color to each. A complex karyotype was identified by conventional cytogenetic analysis, including a derivative chromosome 1 with additional material of unknown origin on 1p, a deletion of 8p, a derivative chromosome 11 resulting from an unbalanced translocation involving 1 and 11, and a derivative chromosome 12 consisting of 11q and 12q. The results of spectral karyotyping confirmed the identity of the rearranged chromosome 12 *(arrowhead)* but clarified the other abnormalities. The additional material on 1p was derived from chromosome 8 (*long arrow,* blue signal), and the der(11) actually consisted of material from chromosomes 1, 11, and 12 (*short arrow,* 11p white signal; chromosome 12, brown signal; 1p, blue-pink signal).

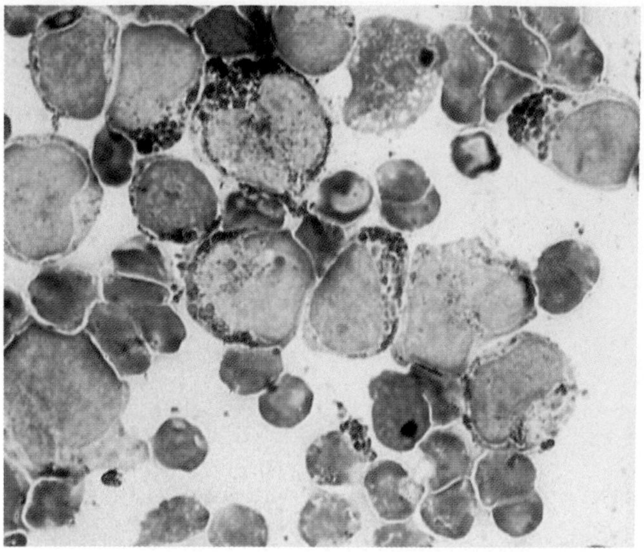

COLOR PLATE 2 (FIG. 38.4). Acute granulocytic leukemia (M2) with positive myeloperoxidase stain, as evidenced by the dark brownish cytoplasmic granules (peroxidase stain with diaminobenzidine, original magnification: 320× magnification).

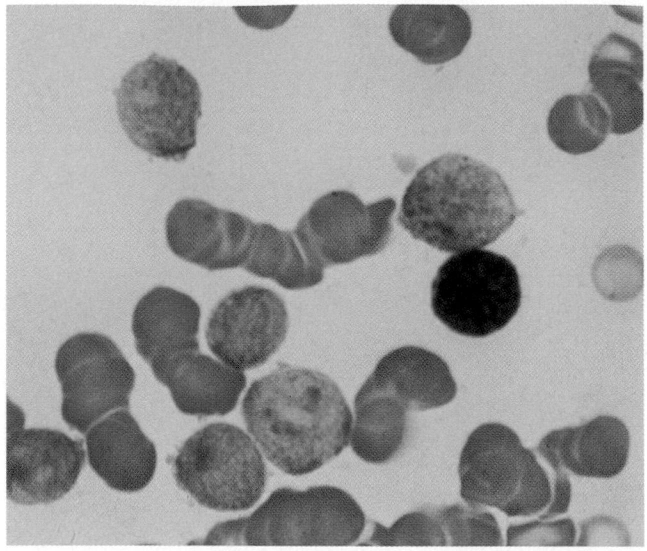

COLOR PLATE 3 (FIG. 38.5). Acute eosinophilic leukemia with positive cyanide-resistant peroxidase stain (brownish cytoplasmic granules and rods) and negative chloroacetate esterase (bright red cytoplasmic granules). A neutrophil *(red)* with positive chloroacetate esterase stain is at the right side of the field (combined stains for cyanide-resistant peroxidase and chloroacetate esterase, original magnification: 320× magnification).

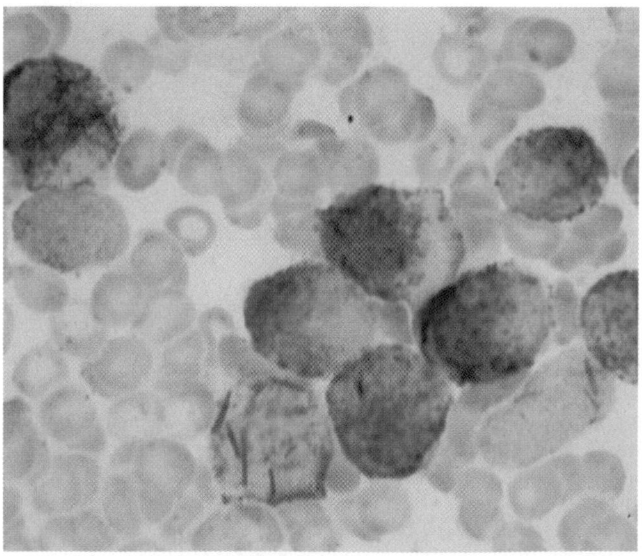

COLOR PLATE 4 (FIG. 38.6). Acute progranulocytic leukemia (M3) with strong chloroacetate esterase stain as shown by the bright red cytoplasmic granules and rods (chloroacetate esterase stain, original magnification: 320× magnification).

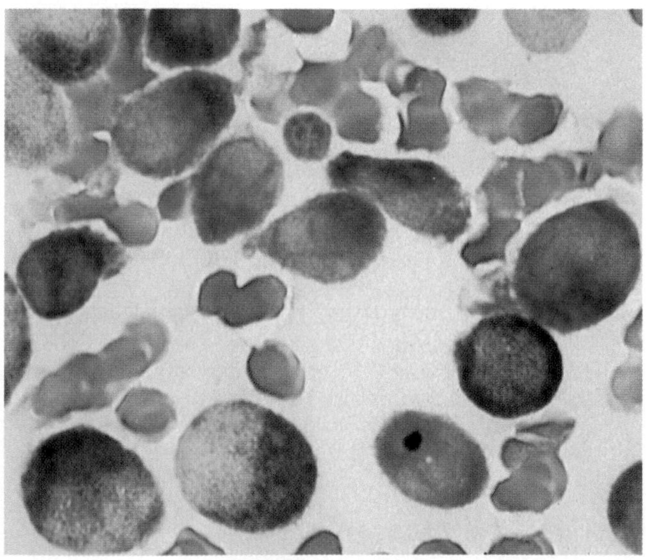

COLOR PLATE 5 (FIG. 38.7). Acute myelomonocytic leukemia (M4): monocytic cells with positive butyrate esterase stain *(red)* and granulocytic cells with positive chloroacetate esterase stain *(blue)*. Darker staining cells, mostly at the left lower corner of the field *(blue)*, represent cells with chloroacetate esterase activity (combined butyrate esterase and chloroacetate esterase stains, original magnification: 320× magnification).

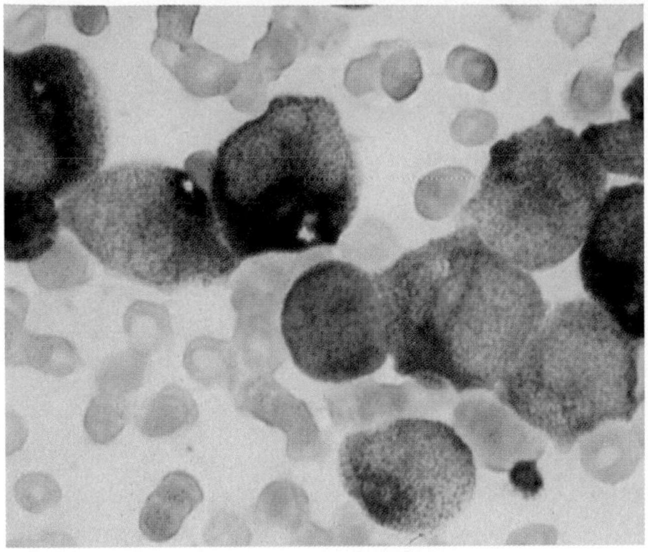

COLOR PLATE 6 (FIG. 38.8). Variant acute myelomonocytic leukemia (M4 variant). Many leukemic cells are positive for both butyrate esterase and chloroacetate esterase. Darker staining at Golgi areas *(blue)* represents chloroacetate esterase activity (combined butyrate esterase and chloroacetate esterase stains, original magnification: 320× magnification).

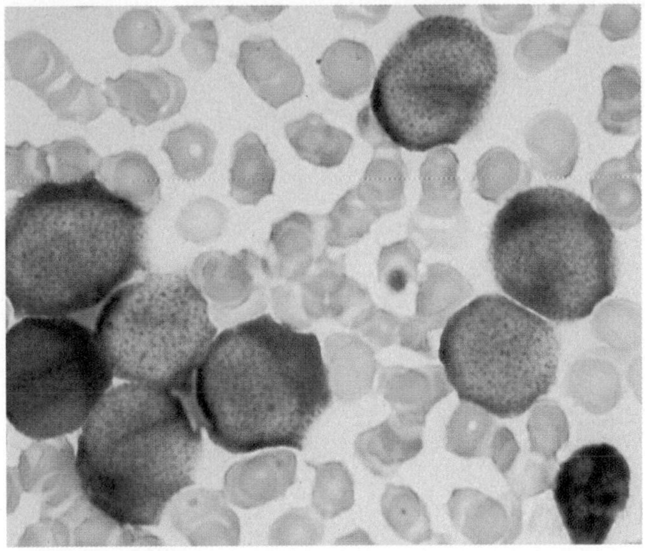

COLOR PLATE 7 (FIG. 38.9). Acute monocytic leukemia (M5b) with positive butyrate esterase stain *(red)* in the cytoplasm of leukemic cells. A normal neutrophil at right lower corner shows positive chloroacetate esterase activity *(blue)* (combined butyrate esterase and chloroacetate esterase stains, original magnification: 320× magnification).

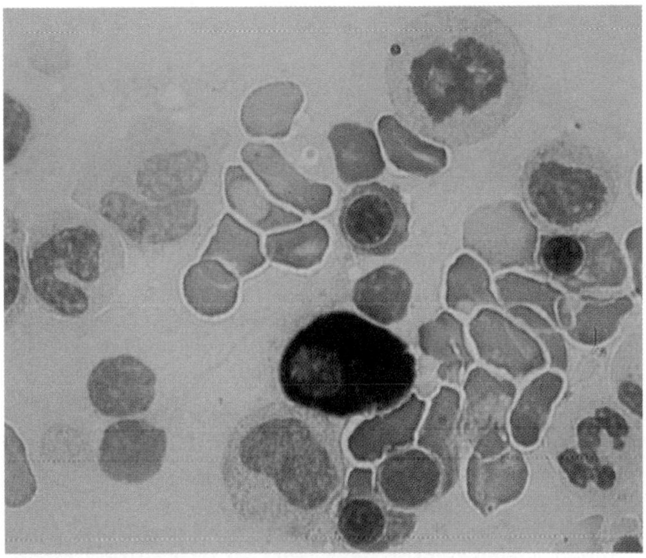

COLOR PLATE 8 (FIG. 38.13). A normal mast cell in the marrow aspirate smear with strong aminocaproate esterase activity is illustrated by bright red granules in the cytoplasm (aminocaproate esterase stain, original magnification: 320× magnification).

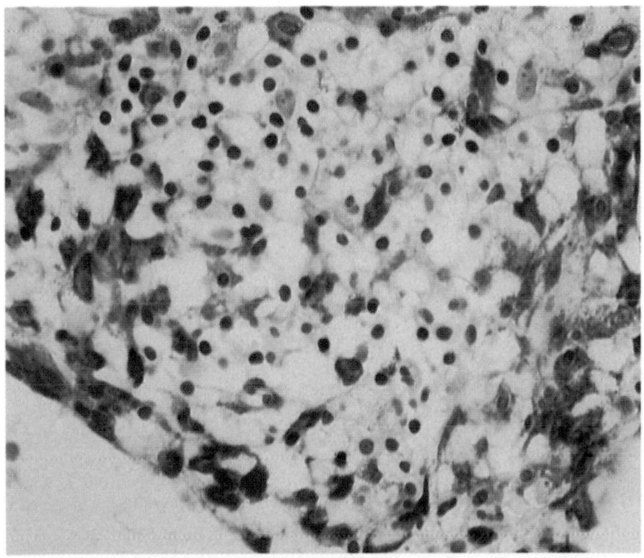

COLOR PLATE 9 (FIG. 38.15). Plastic section of bone marrow biopsy from patient with systemic mast cell disease showing aminocaproate esterase positive atypical mast cells infiltrating around a lymphoid follicle (aminocaproate esterase stain, original magnification: 128× magnification).

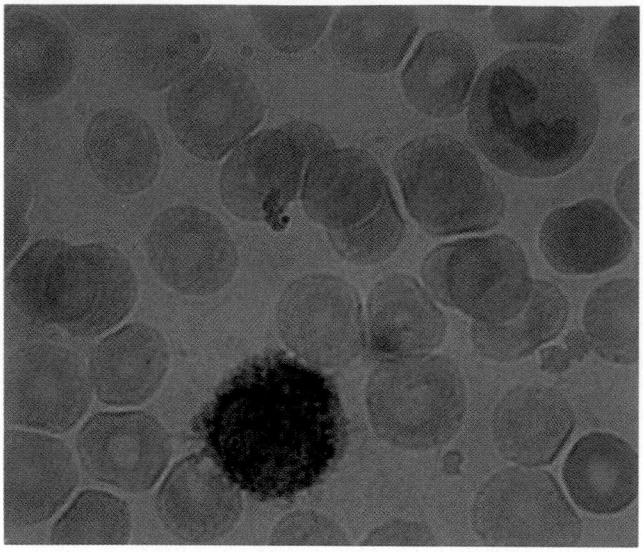

COLOR PLATE 10 (FIG. 38.17). Hairy cell leukemia with strong tartrate-resistant acid phosphatase activity (tartrate-resistant acid phosphatase stain, original magnification: 320× magnification).

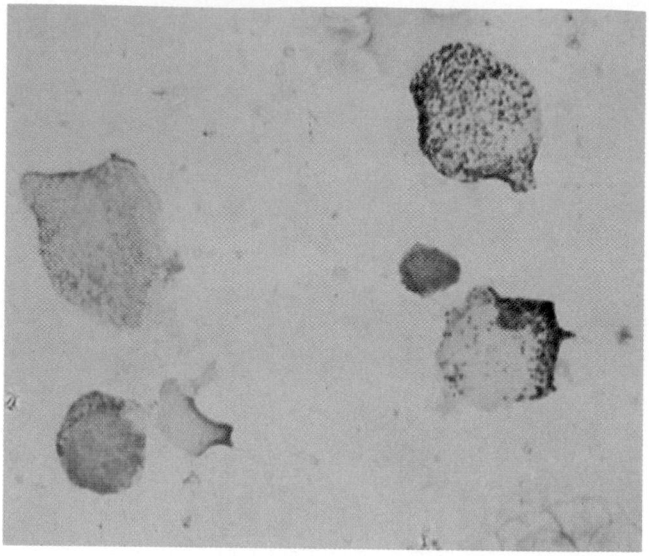

COLOR PLATE 11 (FIG. 38.18). Acute basophilic leukemia with metachromatic cytoplasmic granules (toluidine blue stain, original magnification: 640× magnification).

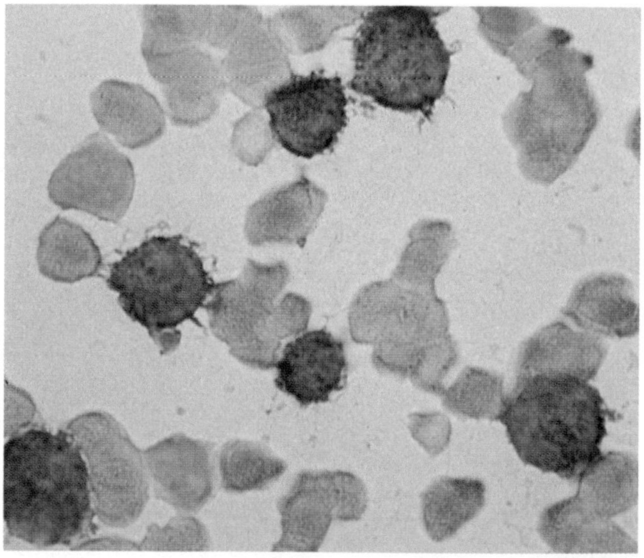

COLOR PLATE 12 (FIG. 38.21). Poorly differentiated acute erythroblastic leukemia with strong red cell antigen demonstrated by immunoperoxidase technique (indirect immunoperoxidase stain for red cell antigen using monoclonal antibody RC-82.4, original magnification: 320× magnification).

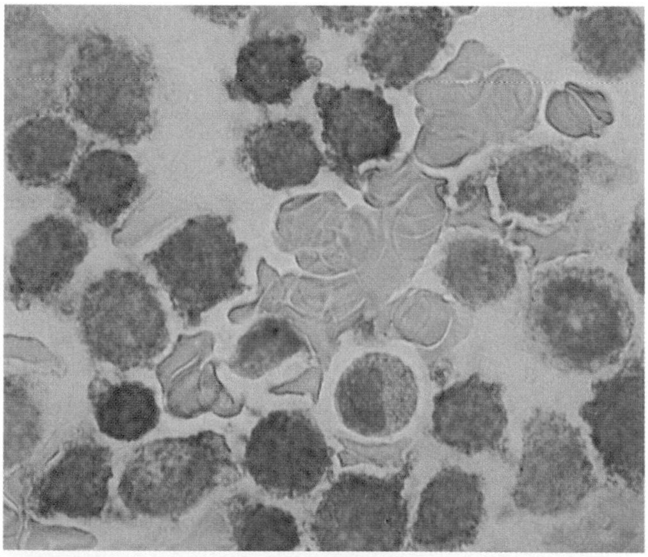

COLOR PLATE 13 (FIG. 38.22). Acute megakaryocytic leukemia (M7) with strong CD41 (glycoprotein IIb/IIIa) complex demonstrated by immunoalkaline phosphatase stain (immunoalkaline phosphatase stain for CD41 using monoclonal antibody HP1-1D, original magnification: 320× magnification).

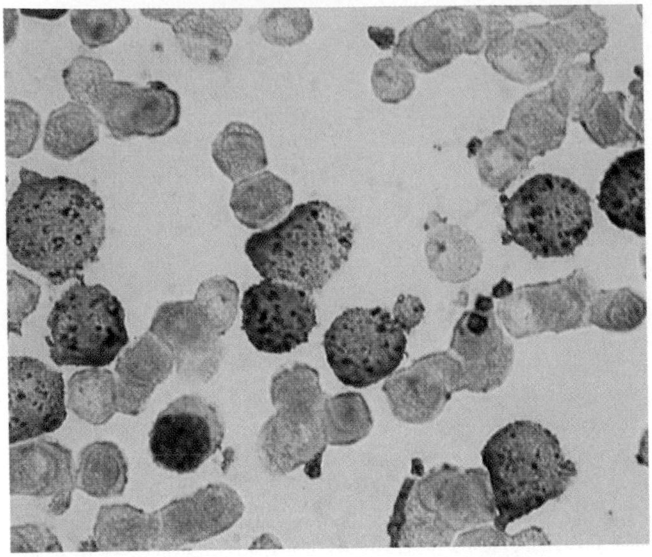

COLOR PLATE 14 (FIG. 38.26). Common acute lymphoblastic leukemia with strong common acute lymphoblastic leukemia antigen (CALLA, CD10) demonstrated by immunoperoxidase stain (indirect immunoperoxidase stain for CALLA, original magnification: 320× magnification).

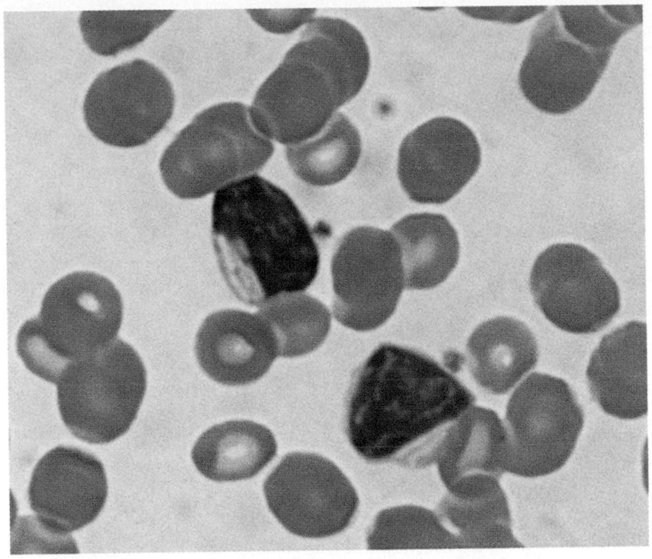

COLOR PLATE 15 (FIG. 40.2). The peripheral blood smear illustrates crystals within the cytoplasm of chronic lymphocytic leukemia cells (Wright stain, original magnification: 1,000× magnification).

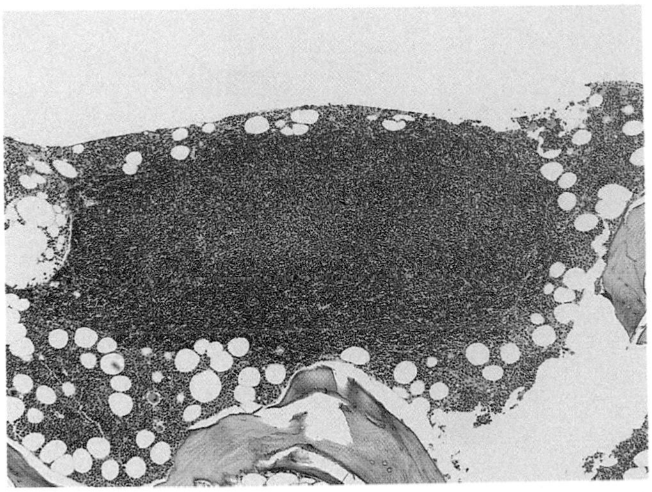

COLOR PLATE 16 (FIG. 40.3). This low-power photomicrograph of a bone marrow biopsy illustrates a large chronic lymphocytic leukemia nodule with several pale proliferation foci (hematoxylin and eosin stain, original magnification: 200× magnification).

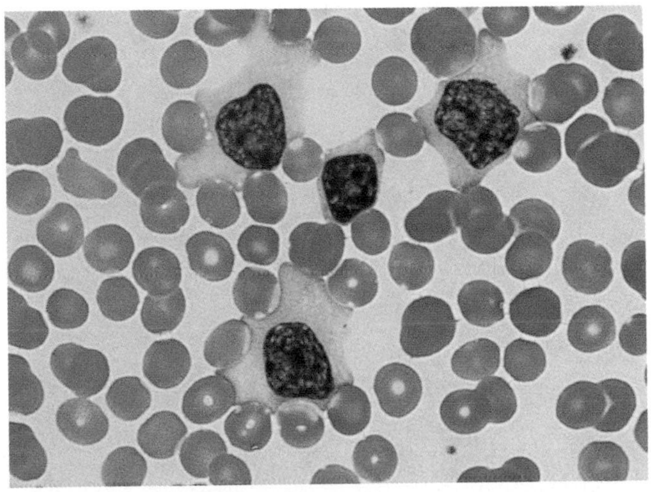

COLOR PLATE 17 (FIG. 40.13). This peripheral blood smear from a patient with prolymphocytic leukemia illustrates the morphologic and ultrastructural features of these cells. Notice the central prominent nucleoli and the moderately condensed nuclear chromatin patterns (Wright's stain, original magnification: 1,000× magnification).

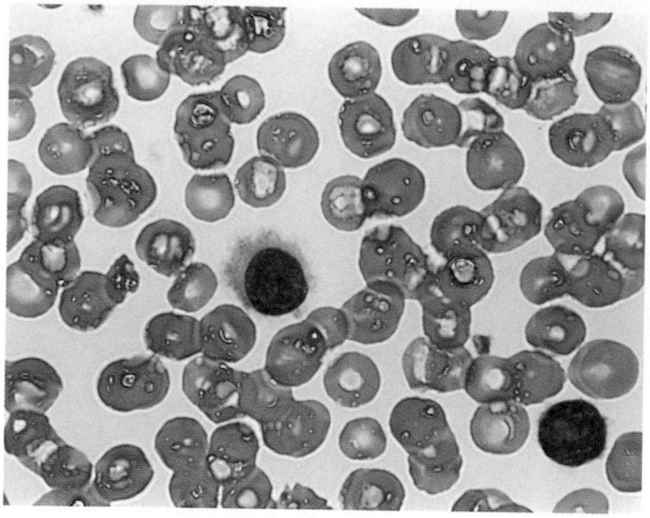

COLOR PLATE 18 (FIG. 41.1). Hairy cell in a peripheral blood film (Wright's stain, original magnification: 1,000× magnification).

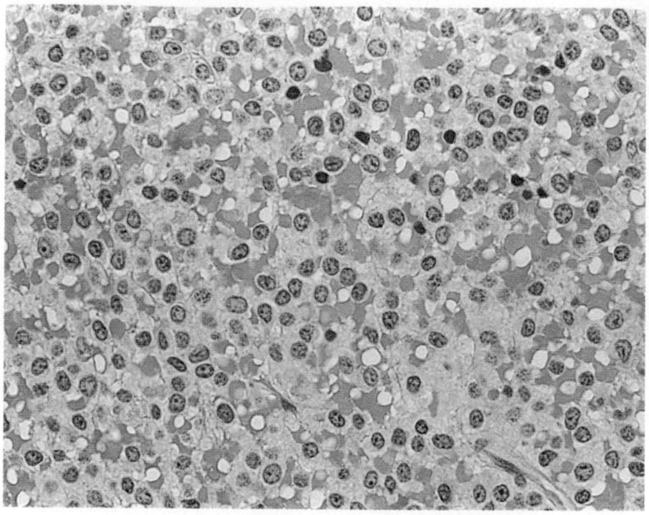

COLOR PLATE 19 (FIG. 41.4B). Hypercellular bone marrow with complete replacement of normal hematopoietic elements by hairy cells (hematoxylin and eosin stain, original magnification: 1,500× magnification).

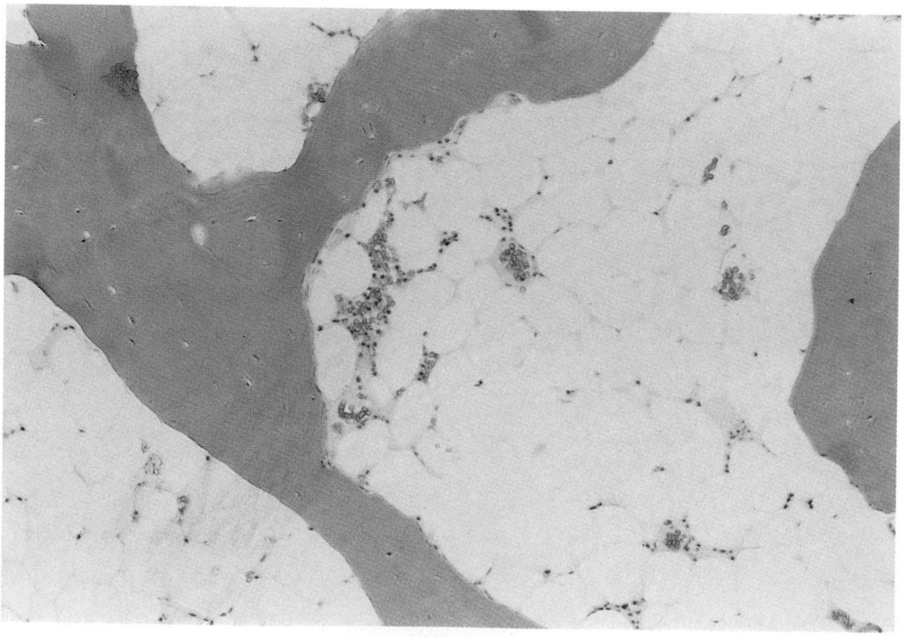

COLOR PLATE 20 (FIG. 41.6). Markedly hypocellular bone marrow with sparse infiltration by hairy cells. **A:** Low magnification (hematoxylin and eosin stain, original magnification: 100× magnification).

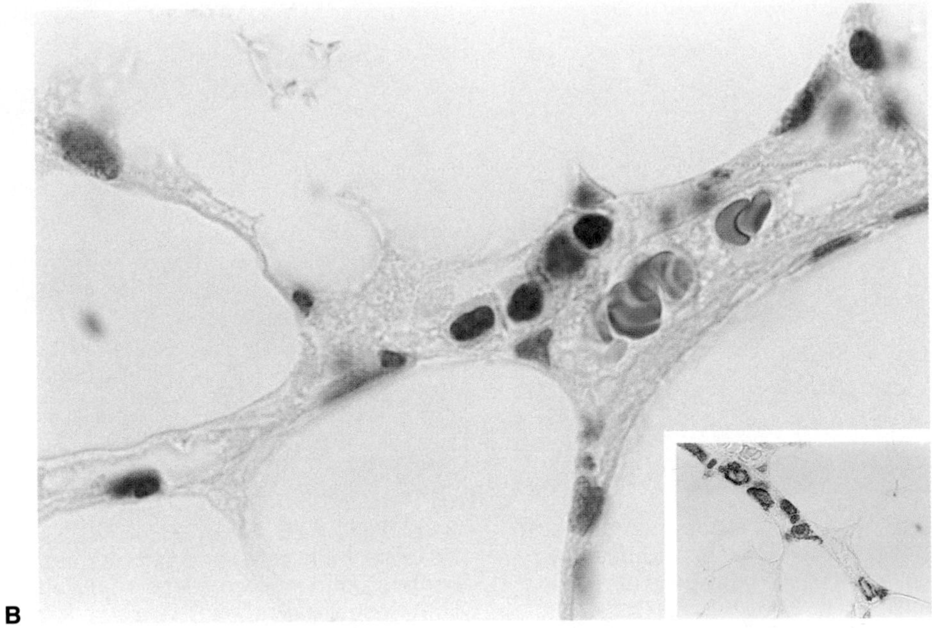

COLOR PLATE 20 (FIG. 41.6). Markedly hypocellular bone marrow with sparse infiltration by hairy cells. **B:** High magnification (original magnification: 800× magnification) shows hairy cells with abundant cytoplasm infiltrating between adipocytes. CD20 immunostain **(Inset)** reveals membrane positivity with ruffled border (immunoperoxidase stain, original magnification: 1,000× magnification).

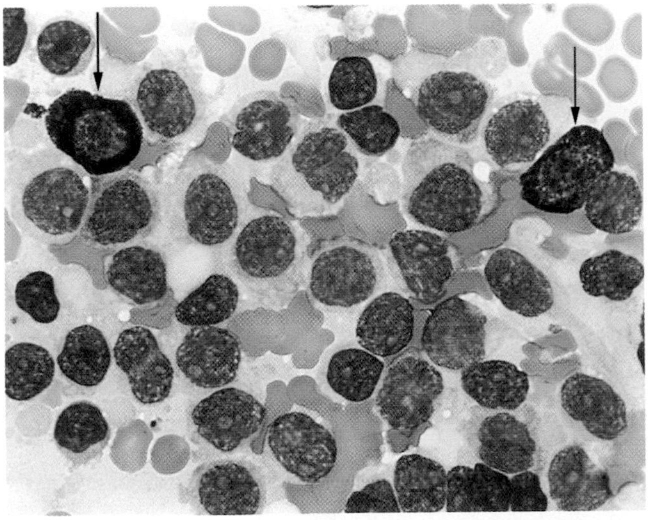

COLOR PLATE 21 (FIG. 41.9). Bone marrow aspirate from a patient with hairy cell leukemia. Hairy cells in marrow aspirates often show a more "smudgy" chromatin than those in the peripheral blood. Hairy projections are difficult to appreciate, and the background often is littered with cytoplasmic fragments. Mast cells are indicated by *arrows* (Wright stain, original magnification: 1,000× magnification).

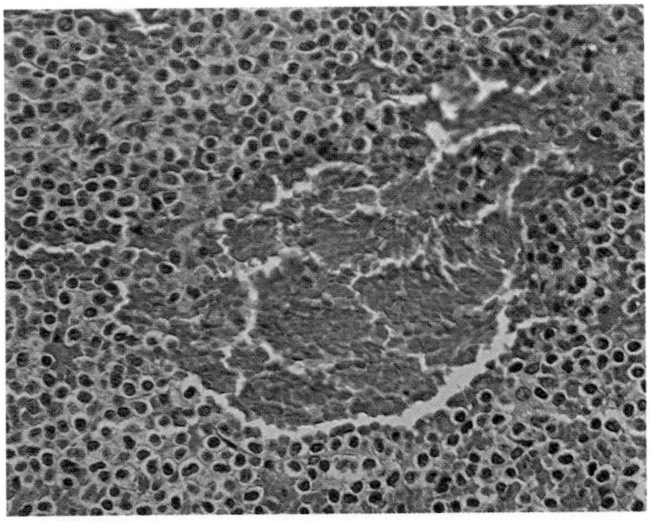

COLOR PLATE 22 (FIG. 41.11). Hairy cell leukemia infiltrating the spleen. A well-formed pseudosinus is present (hematoxylin and eosin stain, original magnification: 250× magnification).

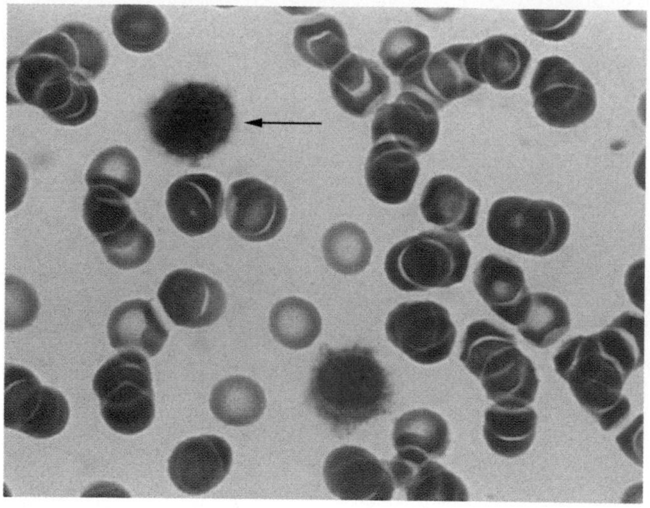

COLOR PLATE 23 (FIG. 41.15A). Tartrate-resistant acid phosphatase staining of hairy cell leukemia. Diffuse cytoplasmic staining is seen in one of two hairy cells (*arrow*) in a blood film (original magnification: 2,000× magnification).

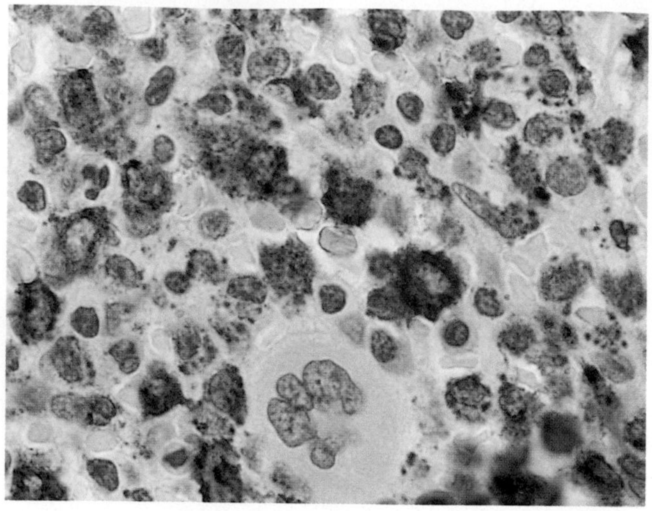

COLOR PLATE 24 (FIG. 41.17). DBA.44 in hairy cell leukemia. Hairy cells show cytoplasmic staining with irregular borders (immunoperoxidase stain, original magnification: 500× magnification).

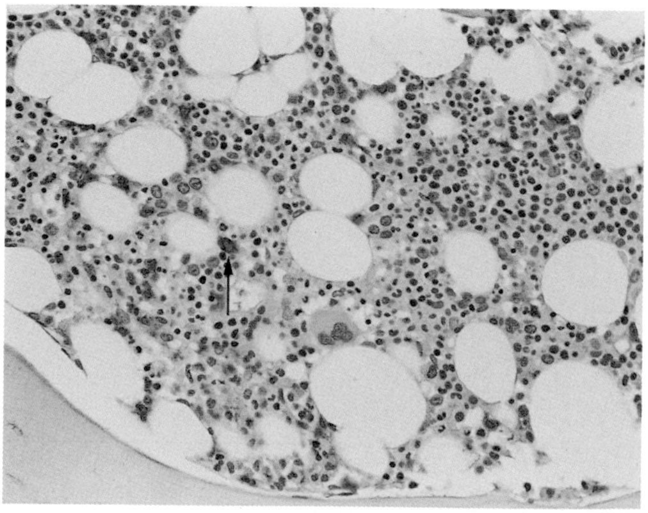

COLOR PLATE 25 (FIG. 41.20). Residual hairy cell leukemia after therapy with 2-chlorodeoxyadenosine (cladrabine). Hairy cells are positive for CD20 (immunoperoxidase stain, original magnification: 100× magnification).

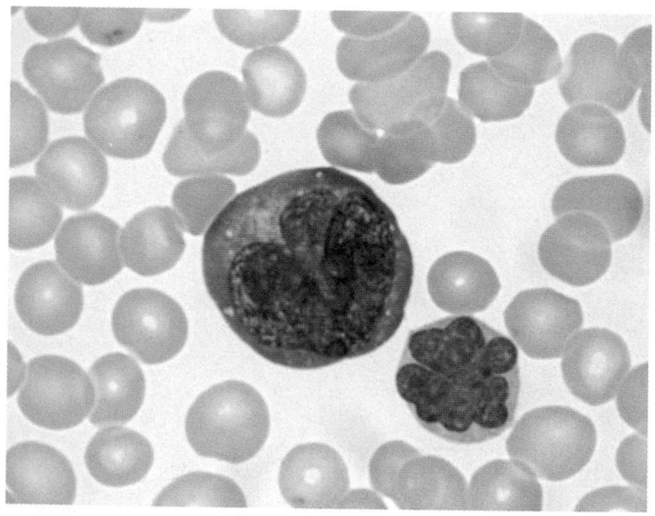

COLOR PLATE 26 (FIG. 44.3). Peripheral blood of a patient with adult T-cell leukemia/lymphoma. Deep indentation of nuclei appears as a flower-like figure (May-Giemsa stain, original magnification: 1,000× magnification).

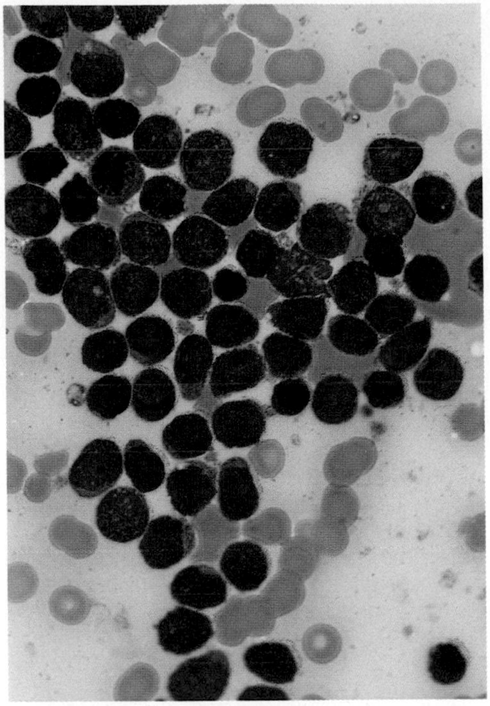

A

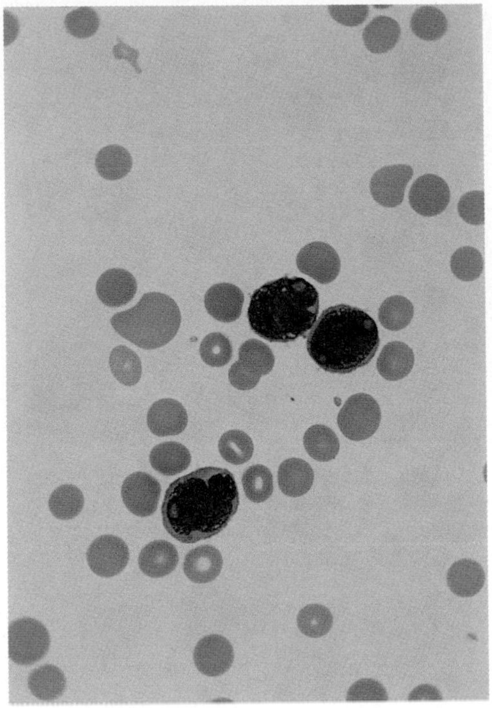

B

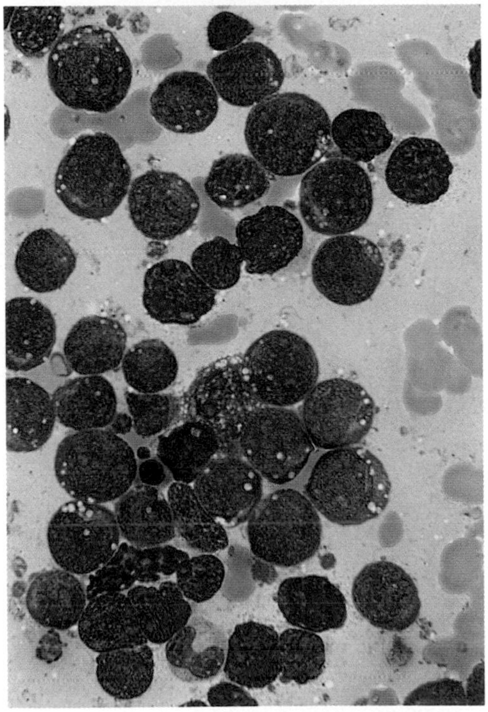

C

COLOR PLATE 27 (FIG. 46.1A, C, and D). French–American–British classification of acute lymphoblastic leukemia (ALL). **A (Fig 46.1A):** In L1 ALL, blasts are small with homogeneous dark chromatin and scant cytoplasm. Some size heterogeneity, as seen here, is acceptable. **B (Fig 46.1C):** Some patients with L2 ALL are more polymorphous with size heterogeneity and highly convoluted nuclei. **C (Fig 46.1D):** L3 ALL has uniform cells with distinct cytoplasm with prominent vacuolization. Mitoses and apoptotic bodies often are seen (Wright-Giemsa stain, original magnification: 1,000× magnification).

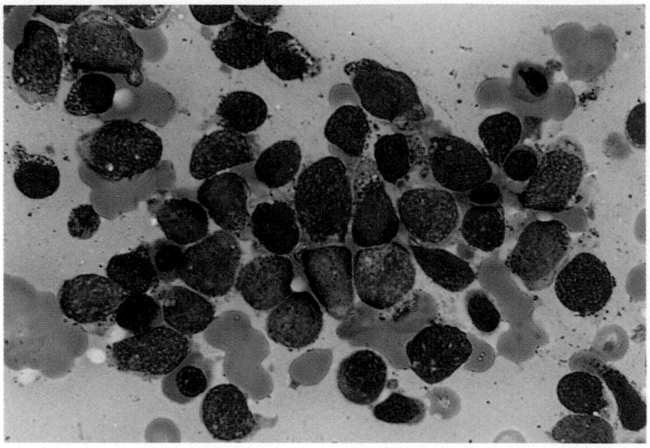

COLOR PLATE 28 (FIG. 46.4). Granular acute lymphoblastic leukemia. Note blasts with smooth chromatin and striking coarse granularity in many cells (Wright-Giemsa stain, original magnification: 1,000× magnification).

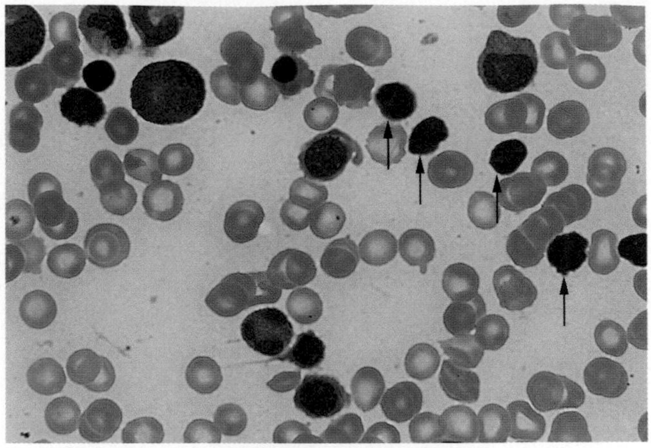

COLOR PLATE 29 (FIG. 46.7). Increased normal B-cell precursors ("hematogones"). These lymphoid cells (*arrows*) are generally smaller than normal elements and even L1 leukemic blasts. They have very high nuclear:cytoplasmic ratios, so that cytoplasmic rims often are not seen (Wright-Giemsa, original magnification: 1,000× magnification).

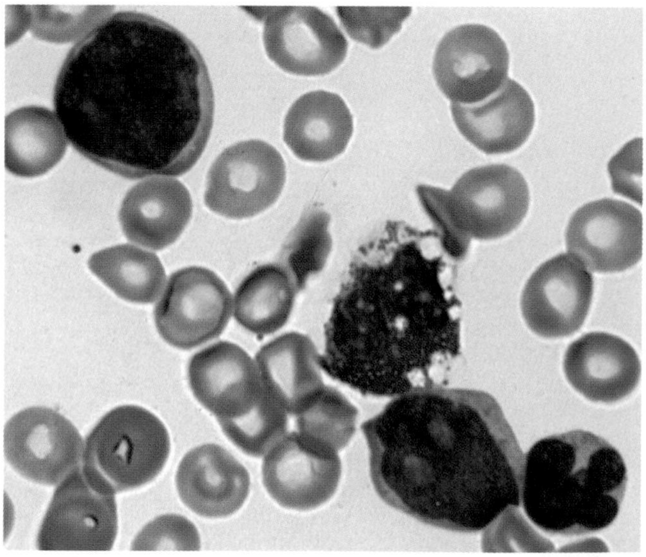

COLOR PLATE 30 (FIG. 47.1). Type I and type II myeloblasts. Bone marrow smear showing a type I myeloblast (**top**) with scant, agranular, basophilic cytoplasm and distinct nucleoli and a type II myeloblast (**bottom**) with the same features and a few azurophilic granules (Wright-Giemsa stain, original magnification: 400× magnification).

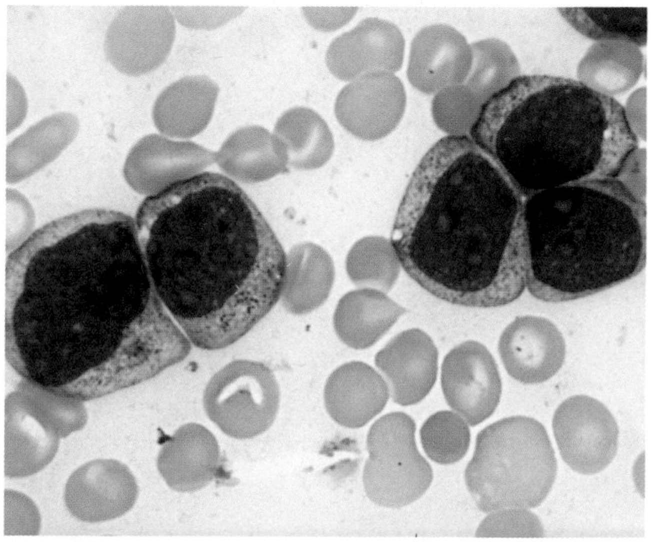

COLOR PLATE 31 (FIG. 47.2). Type III myeloblasts. Blood smear with numerous type III myeloblasts with numerous azurophilic granules (Wright-Giemsa stain, original magnification: 640× magnification).

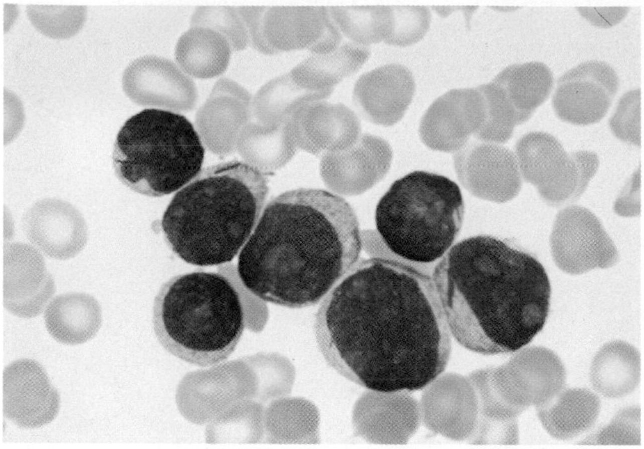

COLOR PLATE 32 (FIG. 47.3). Acute myeloblastic leukemia without maturation (M1). Bone marrow smear showing myeloblasts, several of which contain Auer rods (Wright-Giemsa stain, original magnification: 400× magnification).

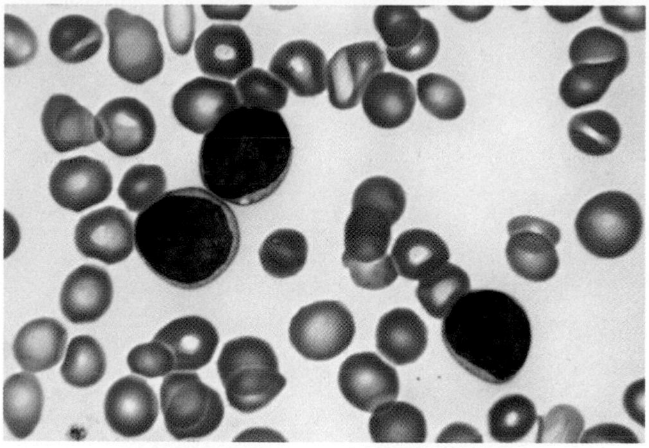

COLOR PLATE 33 (FIG. 47.4). Acute myeloblastic leukemia, minimally differentiated (M0). Blood smear with three blasts without differentiating features. The blasts were myeloperoxidase- and Sudan black B–negative but expressed CD13 and CD33 (Wright-Giemsa stain, original magnification: 400× magnification).

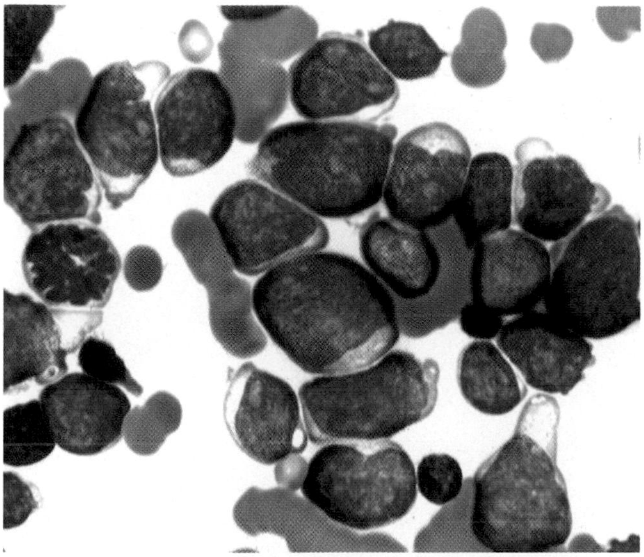

COLOR PLATE 34 (FIG. 47.5). Acute myeloid leukemia, minimally differentiated (M0). Bone marrow smear showing blasts that lack differentiating features and are myeloperoxidase- and Sudan black B–negative. The cells are CD33-positive (Wright-Giemsa stain, original magnification: 256× magnification).

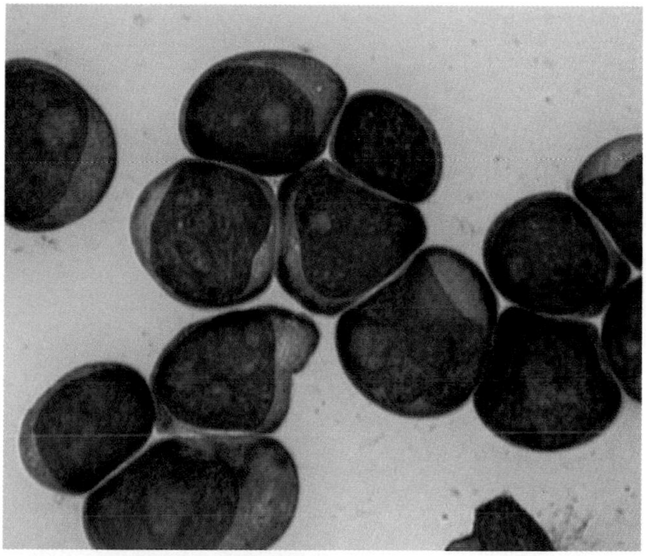

COLOR PLATE 35 (FIG. 47.6). Acute myeloblastic leukemia without maturation (M1). Bone marrow smear showing myeloblasts with a moderate amount of cytoplasm. More than 3% blasts reacted for myeloperoxidase (Wright-Giemsa stain, original magnification: 400× magnification).

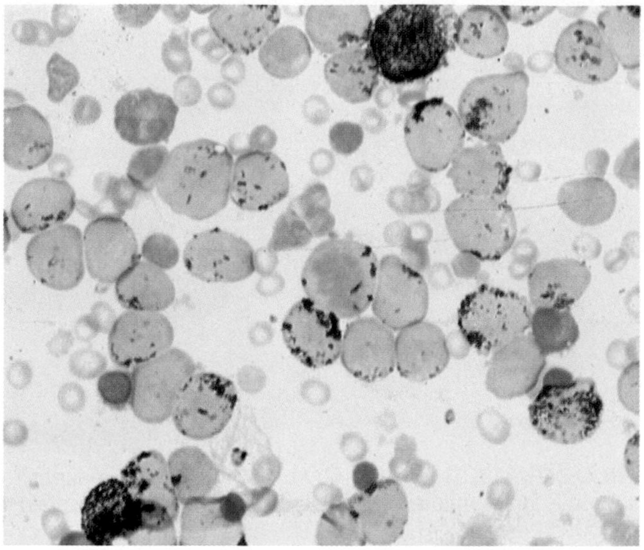

COLOR PLATE 36 (FIG. 47.8). Acute myeloblastic leukemia without maturation (M1). Bone marrow smear showing myeloblasts with uniform but varying degrees of reactivity for myeloperoxidase. The more mature cells are intensely positive (myeloperoxidase stain, original magnification: 256× magnification).

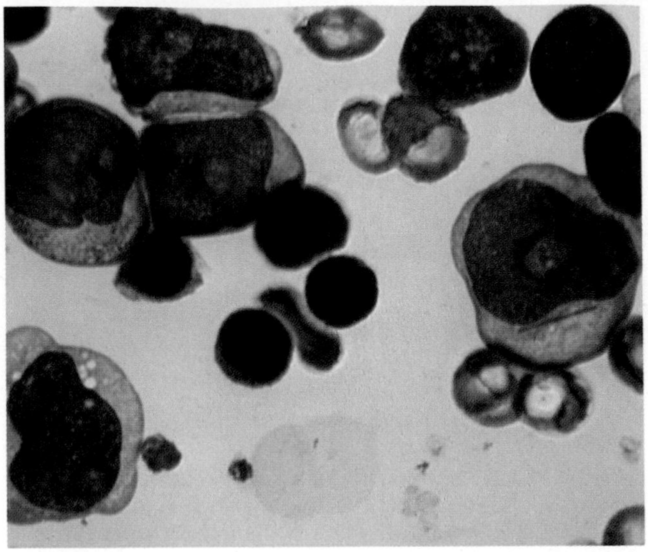

COLOR PLATE 37 (FIG. 47.10). Acute myeloblastic leukemia with maturation (M2). Bone marrow smears showing myeloblasts and more mature neutrophils. Two myeloblasts in the right portion of the field contain long, slender Auer rods (Wright-Giemsa stain, original magnification: 400× magnification).

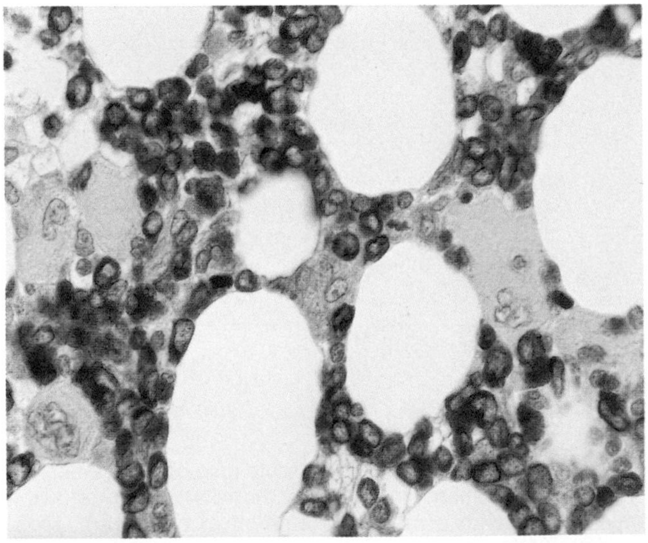

COLOR PLATE 38 (FIG. 47.12). Acute myeloblastic leukemia with maturation (M2). Bone marrow section reacted with antibody to myeloperoxidase; there are numerous reactive immature hematopoietic cells, some with striking cytoplasmic positivity (immunoperoxidase stain, original magnification: 256× magnification).

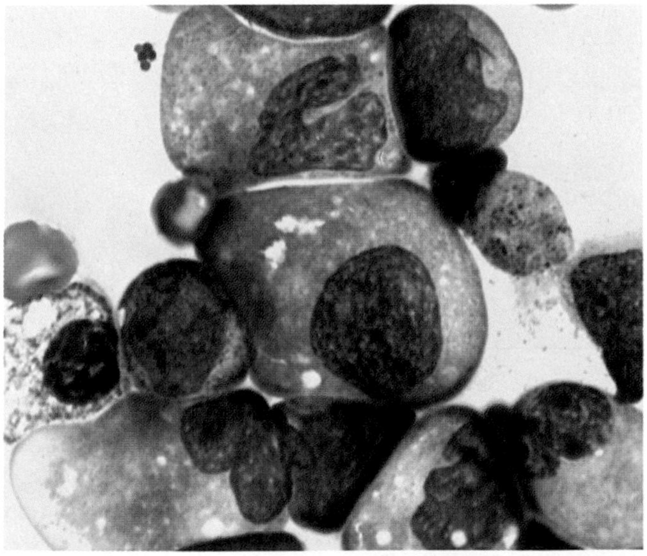

COLOR PLATE 39 (FIG. 47.13). Acute myeloblastic leukemia with maturation (M2) with a t(8;21)(q22;q22) cytogenetic abnormality. Bone marrow smear showing abnormal neutrophil precursors with abundant cytoplasm and prominent specific granulation, which appears slightly smudgy in some cells. The myeloblast in the center shows an Auer rod (Wright-Giemsa stain, original magnification: 400× magnification).

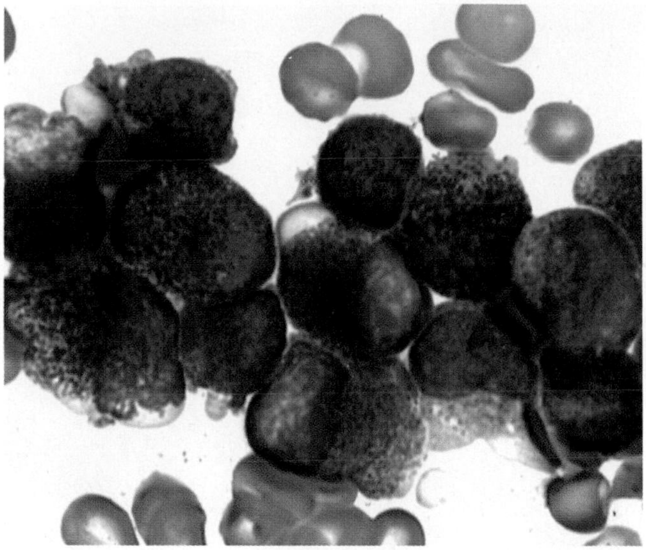

COLOR PLATE 40 (FIG. 47.14). Hypergranular acute promyelocytic leukemia (M3). Bone marrow smear showing leukemic promyelocytes that have abundant coarse azurophilic granules partially obscuring the nuclear outline (Wright-Giemsa stain, original magnification: 400× magnification).

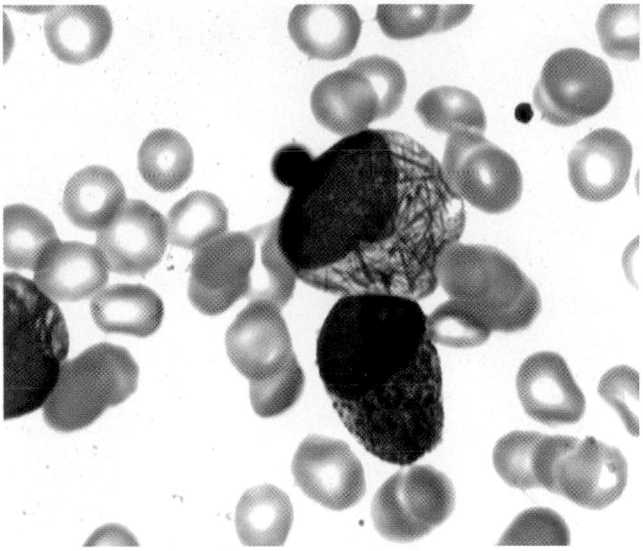

COLOR PLATE 41 (FIG. 47.15). Hypergranular acute promyelocytic leukemia (M3). Bone marrow smear showing a "faggot" cell with numerous intertwining Auer rods. The adjacent cell is an abnormal hyperbasophilic, hypergranular neutrophil promyelocyte (Wright-Giemsa stain, original magnification: 400× magnification).

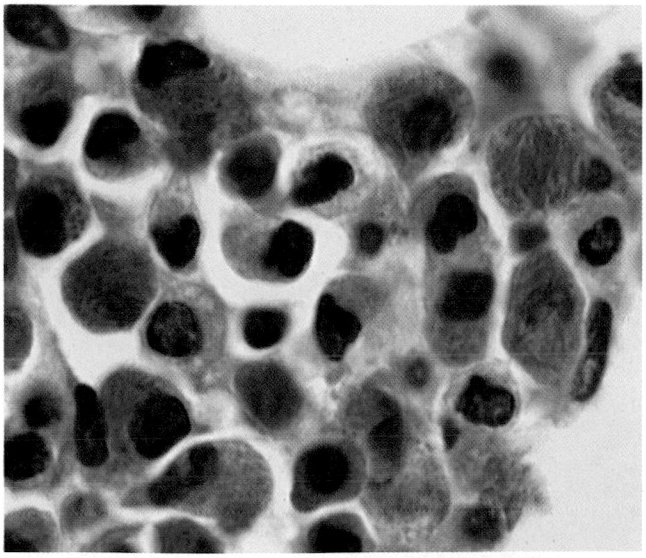

COLOR PLATE 42 (FIG. 47.18). Hypergranular acute promyelocytic leukemia (M3). Bone marrow section showing faggot cells with numerous Auer rods (hematoxylin and eosin stain, original magnification: 400× magnification).

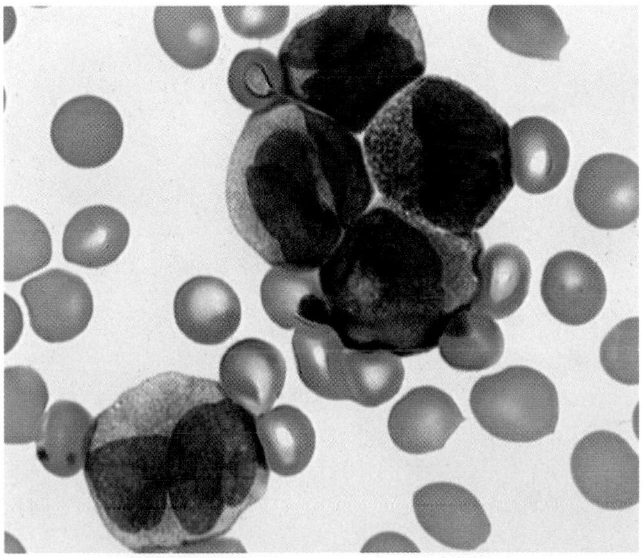

COLOR PLATE 43 (FIG. 47.19). Acute promyelocytic leukemia, microgranular variant (M3V). Blood smear showing leukemic promyelocytes with markedly folded and lobulated nuclei. The cytoplasm of the majority of cells contains numerous delicate azurophilic granules (Wright-Giemsa stain, original magnification: 400× magnification).

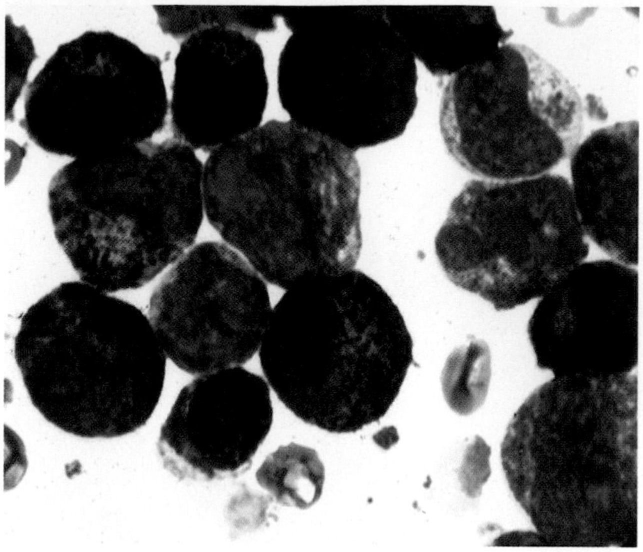

COLOR PLATE 44 (FIG. 47.20). Hypergranular acute promyelocytic leukemia (M3). Bone marrow smear showing numerous leukemic promyelocytes with markedly basophilic cytoplasm, "hyperbasophilic" cells. A centrally located faggot cell is present (Wright-Giemsa stain, original magnification: 400× magnification).

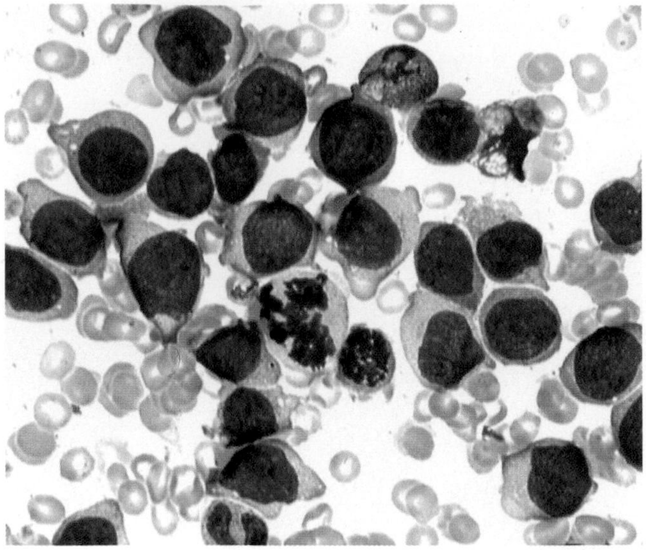

COLOR PLATE 45 (FIG. 47.21). Acute monoblastic leukemia (M5A). Bone marrow smear showing monoblasts that have abundant cytoplasm and scattered fine azurophilic granules. The majority of cells have round nuclei. Two mitotic figures are noted in the center (Wright-Giemsa stain, original magnification: 256× magnification).

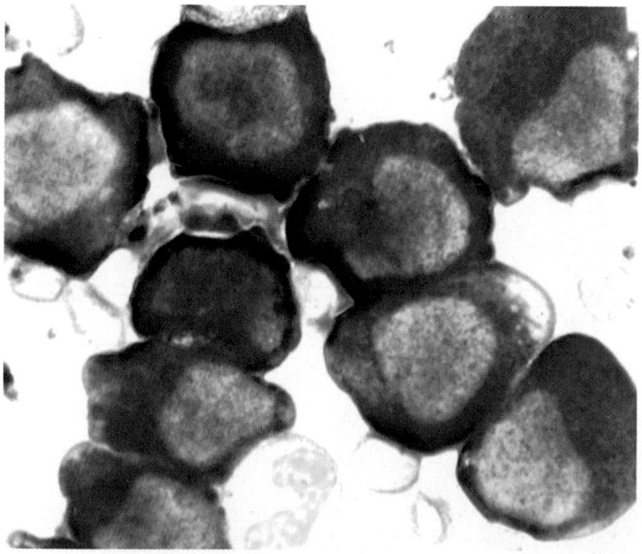

COLOR PLATE 46 (FIG. 47.22). Acute monoblastic leukemia (M5A). Bone marrow smear showing monoblasts with intense cytoplasmic positivity for nonspecific esterase (nonspecific esterase stain, original magnification: 400× magnification).

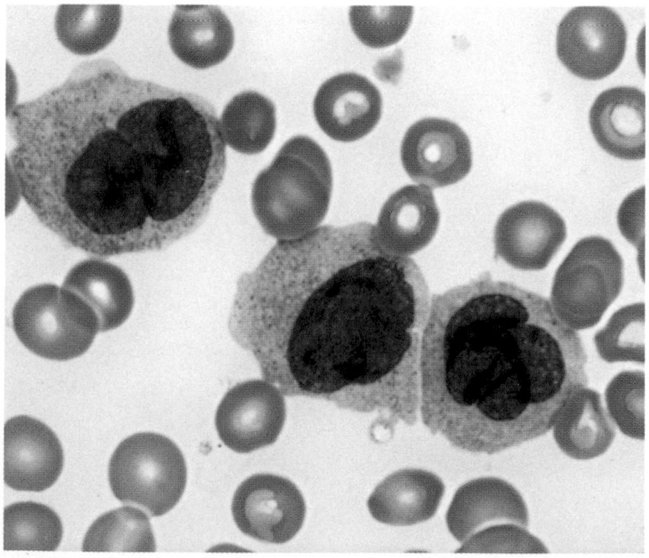

COLOR PLATE 47 (FIG. 47.24). Acute monocytic leukemia (M5B). Blood smear showing three promonocytes. The cells have abundant cytoplasm with numerous fine azurophilic granules. The nuclei show delicate nuclear folding with nuclear creasing imparting a cerebriform appearance (Wright-Giemsa stain, original magnification: 640× magnification).

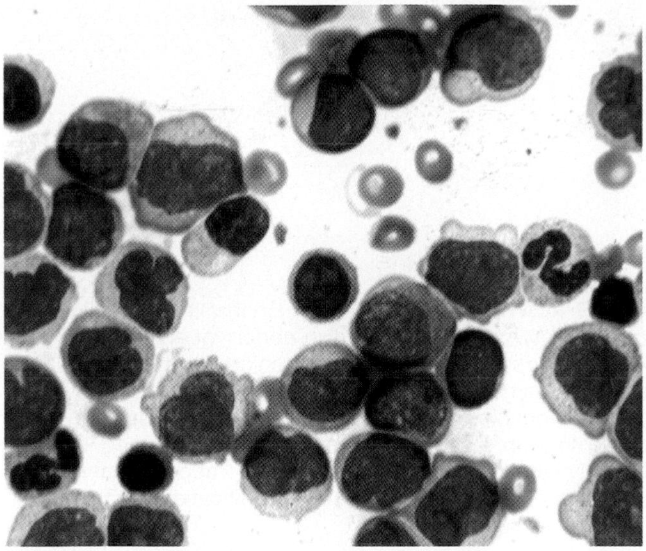

COLOR PLATE 48 (FIG. 47.26). Acute myelomonocytic leukemia (M4). Bone marrow smear showing myeloblasts, maturing neutrophils, and monocytes (Wright-Giemsa stain, original magnification: 256× magnification).

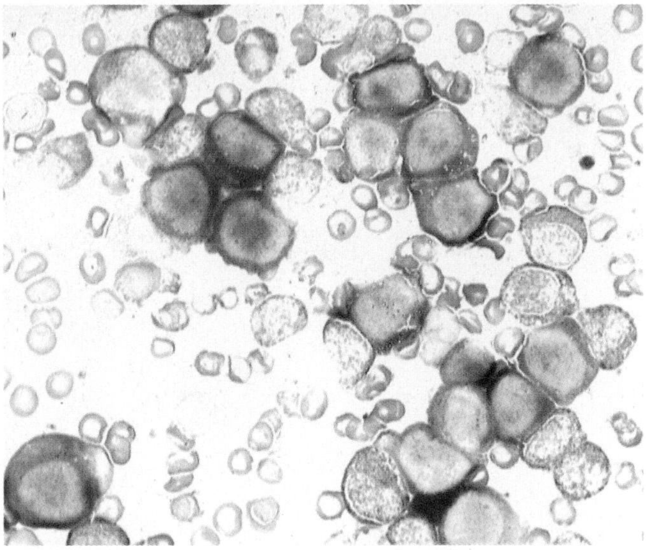

COLOR PLATE 49 (FIG. 47.27). Acute myelomonocytic leukemia (M4). Bone marrow smear stained with combined nonspecific esterase (red-brown staining) and chloroacetate esterase (blue staining), showing numerous nonspecific esterase–positive cells interpreted as monoblasts and promonocytes and chloroacetate esterase–positive cells interpreted as neutrophil precursors. Several of these cells manifest dual staining (chloroacetate esterase–nonspecific esterase staining, original magnification: 256× magnification).

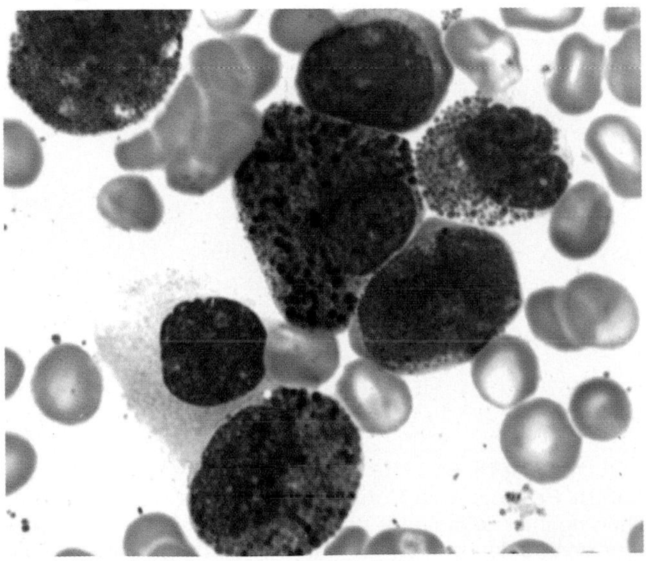

COLOR PLATE 50 (FIG. 47.28). Acute myelomonocytic leukemia with increased bone marrow eosinophils (M4E0). Bone marrow smear showing four eosinophils, two of which contain a mixture of eosinophilic and basophilic granules. This case is associated with an inversion of chromosome 16 (Wright-Giemsa stain, original magnification: 400× magnification).

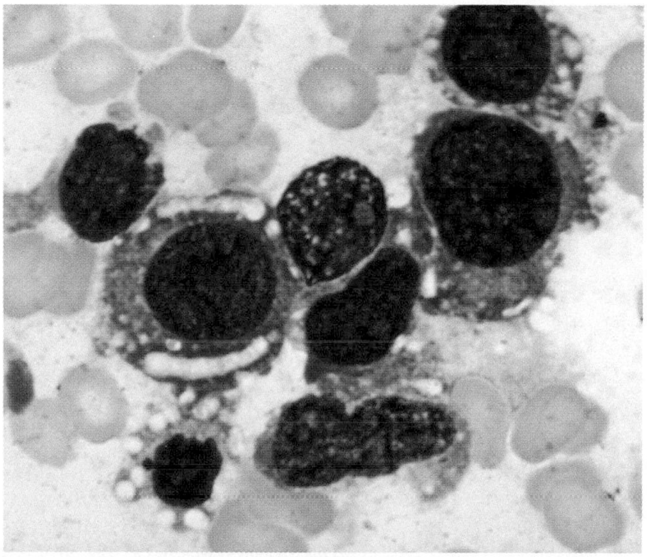

COLOR PLATE 51 (FIG. 47.30). Erythroleukemia (M6A). Bone marrow smear showing abnormal erythroblasts and two myeloblasts, one with an Auer rod. The erythroblasts have megaloblastoid nuclei and cytoplasmic vacuoles (Wright-Giemsa stain, original magnification: 400× magnification).

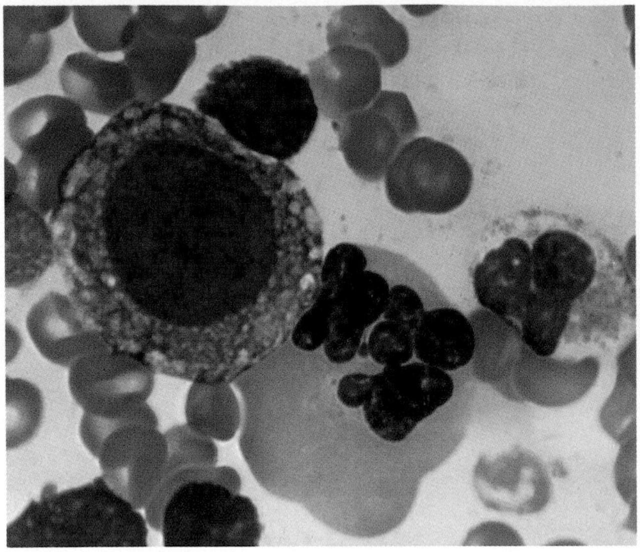

COLOR PLATE 52 (FIG. 47.31). Erythroleukemia (M6A). Bone marrow smear showing two abnormal erythroblasts at different stages of maturation. The enlarged proerythroblast has abundant basophilic cytoplasm with numerous poorly demarcated vacuoles and a prominent single nucleolus; the late polychromatophilic erythroblast is macrocytic and has a markedly lobulated nucleus and several Pappenheimer bodies (Wright-Giemsa stain, original magnification: 400× magnification).

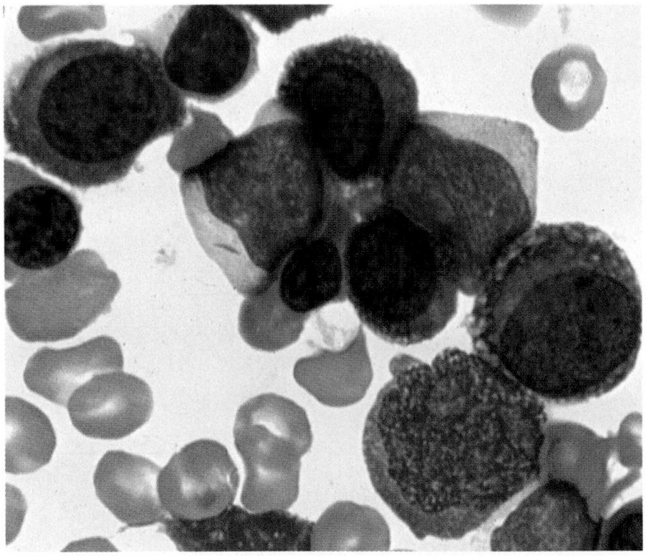

COLOR PLATE 53 (FIG. 47.32). Pure erythroid leukemia (M6B). Bone marrow smear showing a predominant population of proerythroblasts with markedly vacuolated cytoplasm; the larger vacuoles result from coalescence of the smaller vacuoles (Wright-Giemsa stain, original magnification: 400× magnification).

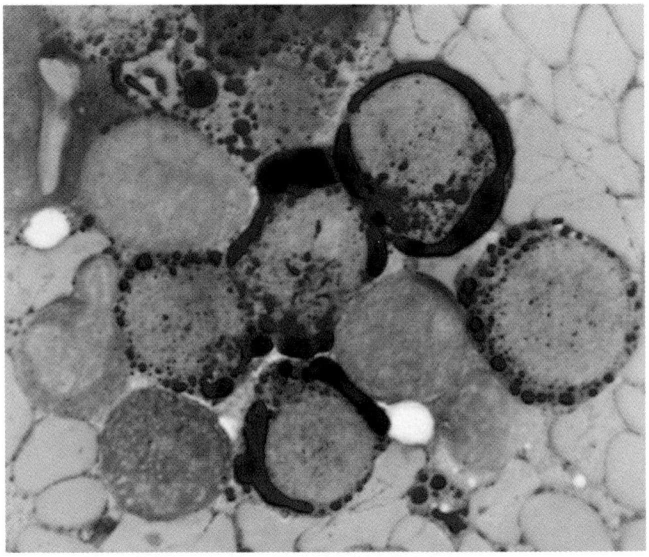

COLOR PLATE 54 (FIG. 47.33). Pure erythroid leukemia (M6B). Periodic acid-Schiff stain of bone marrow smear showing intense globular positivity in the vacuoles of immature erythroblasts (original magnification: 400× magnification).

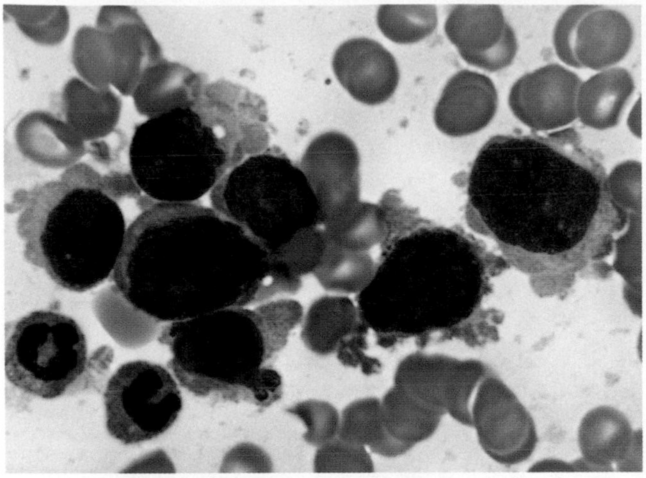

A

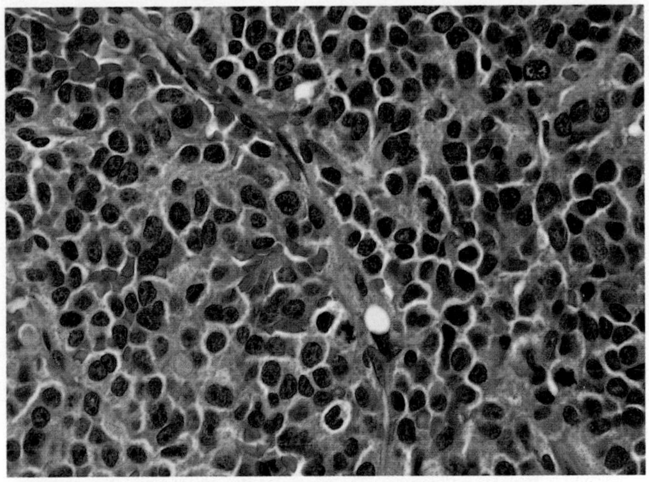

B

COLOR PLATE 55 (FIG. 47.34). A: Acute megakaryoblastic leukemia (M7). Bone marrow smear from a 22-month-old girl. The blasts vary in appearance; they may have abundant basophilic cytoplasm with pseudopod formation. The blasts express CD41 and CD61 and show evidence of platelet peroxidase on electron microscopy (Wright-Giemsa stain, original magnification: 640× magnification). **B:** Bone marrow trephine biopsy section from the specimen illustrated in **A**. The marrow is replaced extensively by blasts that show no clear evidence of maturation to more mature megakaryocytes (hematoxylin and eosin, original magnification: 400× magnification).

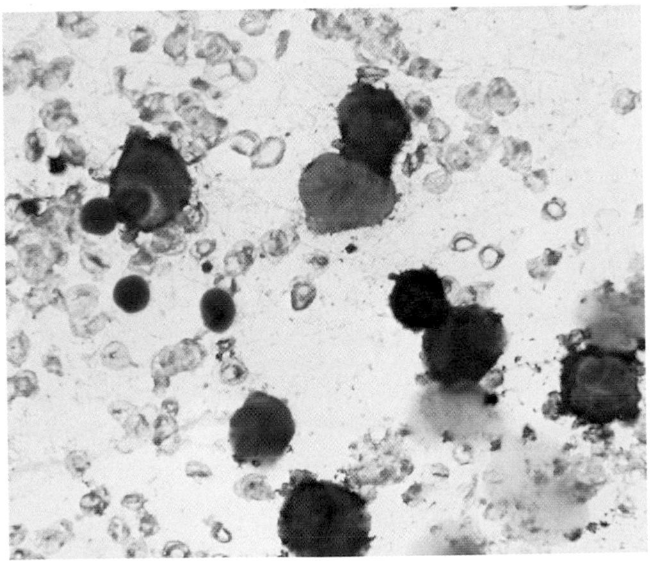

COLOR PLATE 56 (FIG. 47.35). Bone marrow smear from a patient with acute megakaryoblastic leukemia reacted with a monoclonal antibody to platelet glycoprotein (IIIa), CD61. The blasts are intensely reactive (alkaline phosphatase, anti-alkaline phosphatase [APAAP], original magnification: 400× magnification).

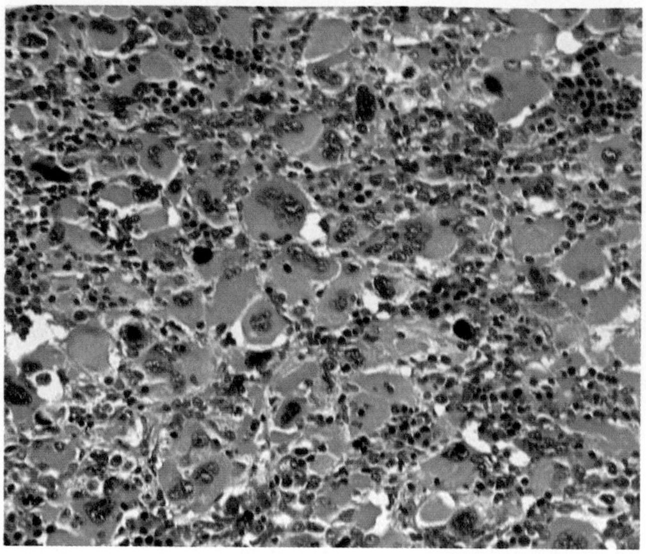

A

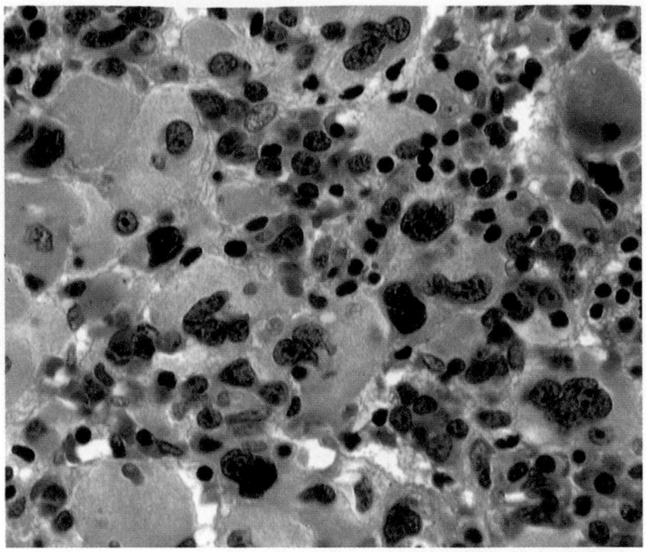

B

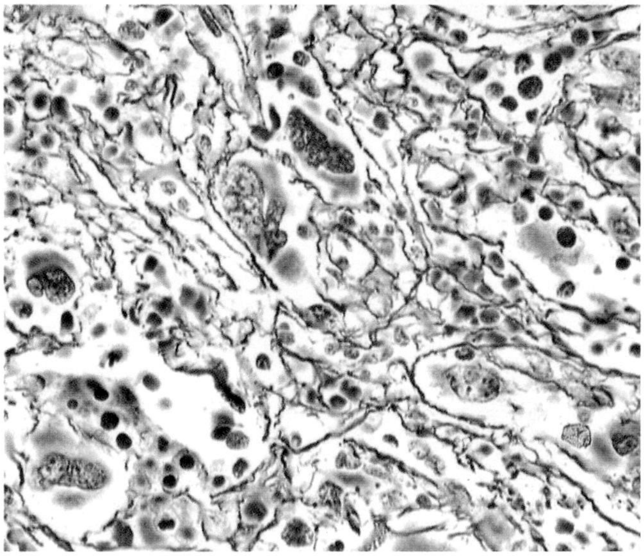

C

COLOR PLATE 57 (FIG. 47.37). Acute megakaryoblastic leukemia (M7). **A:** Bone marrow section showing replacement of normal marrow architecture by a prominent proliferation of megakaryoblasts, micromegakaryocytes, and atypical megakaryocytes. Erythroblasts are numerous (hematoxylin and eosin stain, original magnification: 160× magnification). **B:** High magnification of bone marrow section illustrated in **A**. Numerous atypical megakaryocytes, uninucleate micromegakaryocytes, and blasts can be noted. Erythroblasts are present (hematoxylin and eosin stain, original magnification: 256× magnification). **C:** Reticulin stain of bone marrow section illustrated in **A** and **B** showing diffuse increase in reticulin fibers (Wilder's reticulin stain, original magnification: 256× magnification).

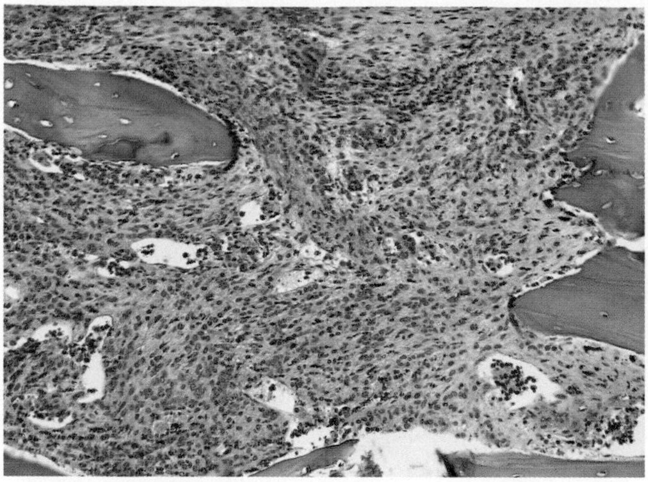

A

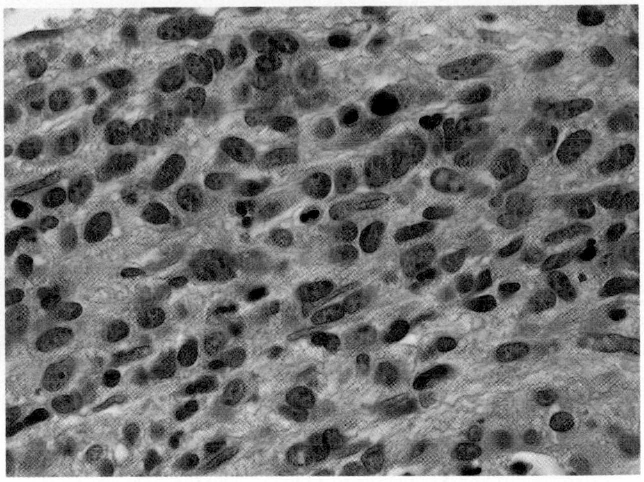

B

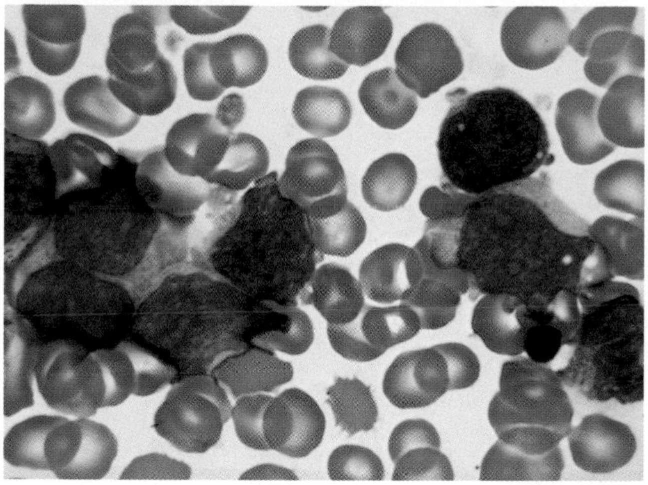

C

COLOR PLATE 58 (FIG. 47.38). Acute megakaryoblastic leukemia associated with a t(1;22)(p13;q13)cytogenetic abnormality. **A:** This bone marrow biopsy specimen shows extensive replacement by intertwining bundles of blasts; several of the sinuses are patent (hematoxylin and eosin stain, original magnification: 240× magnification). **B:** Higher magnification of the specimen in **A** showing blast cells without differentiating features. The specimen showed a moderate increase in reticulin fibers (hematoxylin and eosin stain, original magnification: 400× magnification). **C:** Bone marrow smear from the specimen illustrated in **A** and **B**. Several blasts without differentiating features are present. One cell resembling a promegakaryocyte is present (Wright-Giemsa stain, original magnification: 400× magnification).

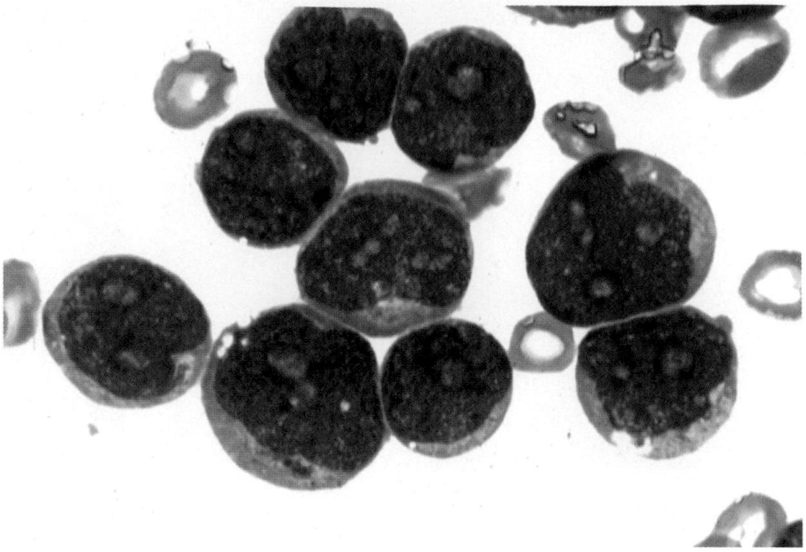

COLOR PLATE 59 (FIG. 47.39). Acute myeloid leukemia associated with Down syndrome. Bone marrow smear from a 3-year-old girl who has Down syndrome showing myeloblasts with reticular chromatin pattern, prominent nucleoli, a moderate amount of basophilic cytoplasm, and focal coarse azurophilic granulation (Wright-Giemsa stain, original magnification: 400× magnification).

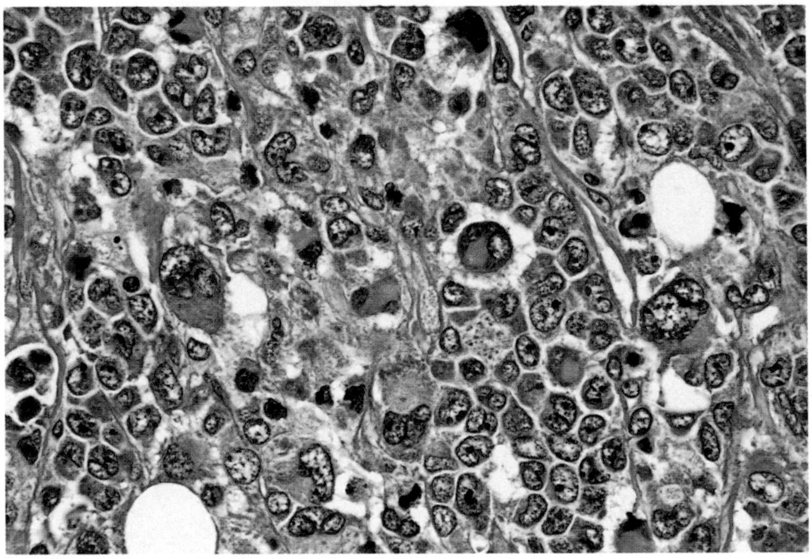

COLOR PLATE 60 (FIG. 47.40). Acute megakaryoblastic leukemia associated with Down syndrome. One of numerous enlarged abdominal lymph nodes from a 2-year-old child with Down syndrome and acute megakaryoblastic leukemia. The node is replaced completely; the cells are predominantly blasts, with several mature megakaryocytes and occasional small megakaryocytes with hypolobated nuclei (hematoxylin and eosin stain, original magnification: 400× magnification).

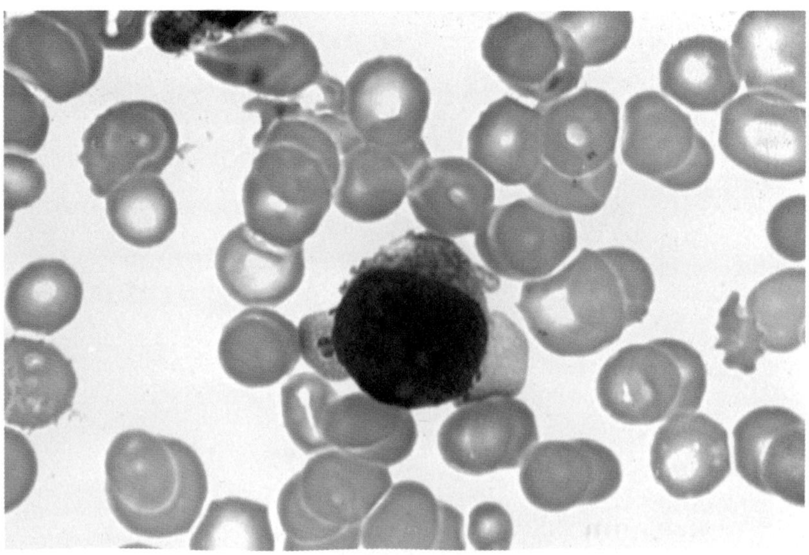

COLOR PLATE 61 (FIG. 47.47). A micromegakaryocyte in the blood smear of a patient who has a therapy-related myelodysplastic syndrome. The nucleus is round with condensed chromatin; irregular platelet budding is present (Wright-Giemsa stain, original magnification: 400× magnification).

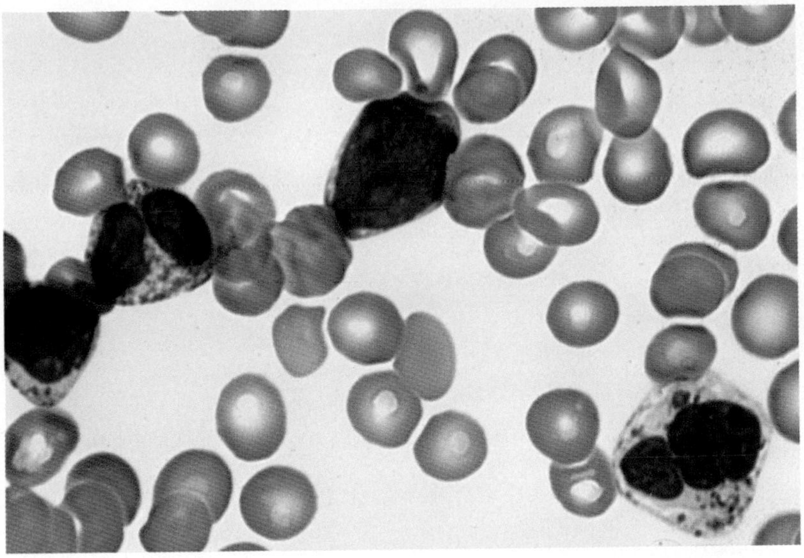

COLOR PLATE 62 (FIG. 47.48). Blood smear from a patient who has a therapy-related myelodysplastic syndrome presenting with 22% basophils. This field shows three basophils, two with decreased granules, and one blast (Wright-Giemsa stain, original magnification: 400× magnification).

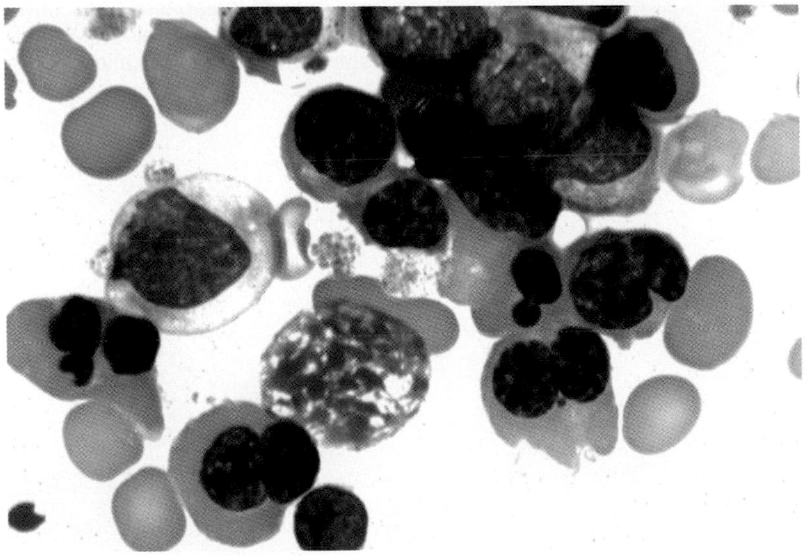

COLOR PLATE 63 (FIG. 47.49). Smear of a bone marrow specimen from an adult who has a therapy-related myelodysplastic syndrome. The nuclei of the red blood cell precursors have a slightly open chromatin and show marked lobulation (Wright-Giemsa stain, original magnification: 256× magnification).

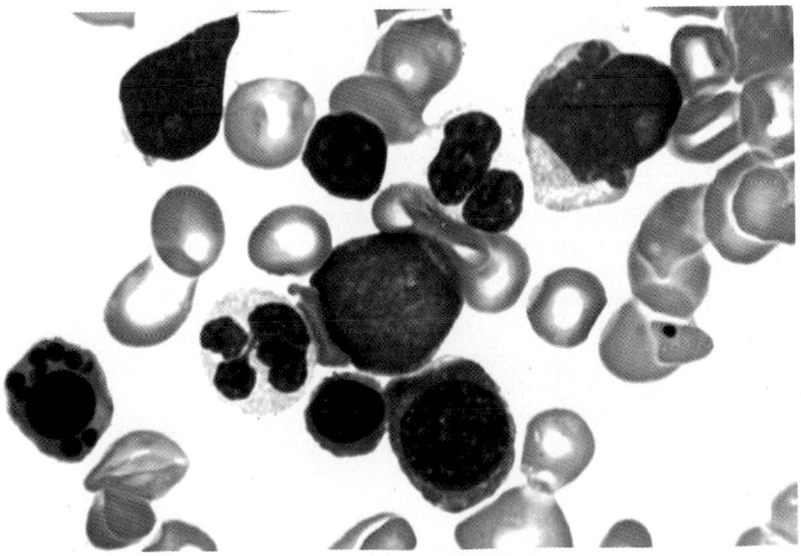

COLOR PLATE 64 (FIG. 47.50). Bone marrow smear from a 17-year-old man who has a myelodysplastic syndrome related to therapy for Hodgkin's disease. Two markedly hypogranular neutrophils, a red cell precursor with multiple nuclear fragments, and two myeloblasts are present in this field (Wright-Giemsa stain, original magnification: 400× magnification).

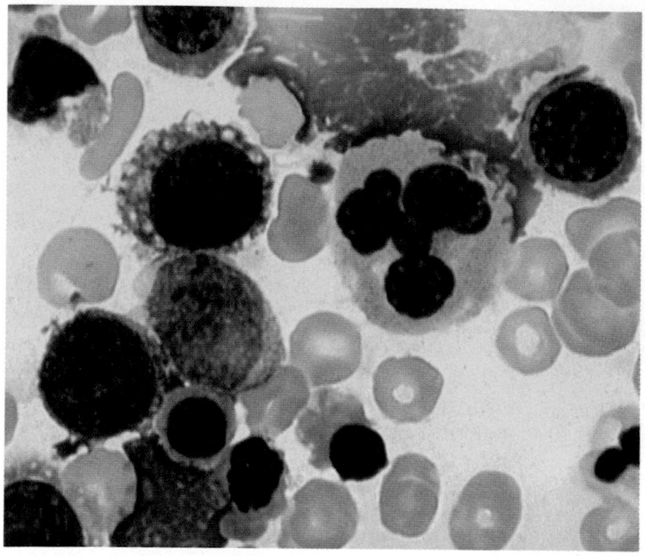

COLOR PLATE 65 (FIG. 47.51). Bone marrow smear from an adult who has a therapy-related myelodysplastic syndrome. The large red cell precursor in the center shows marked nuclear lobation. One erythroblast on the left shows numerous cytoplasmic vacuoles (Wright-Giemsa stain, original magnification: 400× magnification).

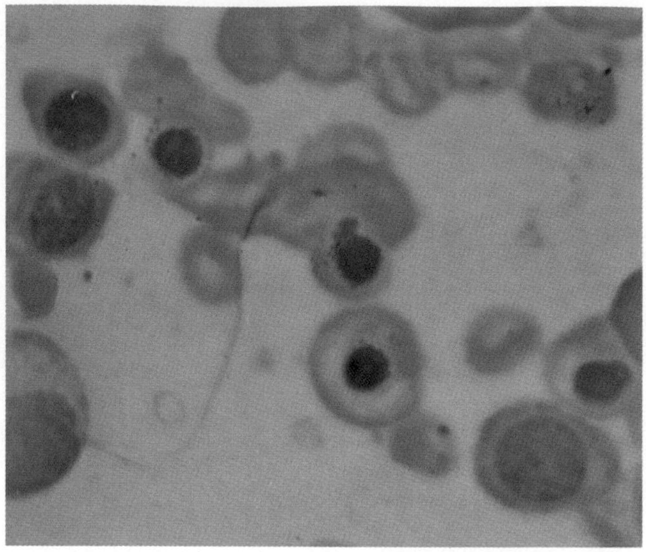

COLOR PLATE 66 (FIG. 47.52). Iron stain of a bone marrow smear from a 24-year-old woman who developed a myelodysplastic syndrome following therapy for Hodgkin's disease. This specimen from the initial diagnostic specimen shows several ringed sideroblasts (Prussian blue stain followed by Safranin counterstain, original magnification: 400× magnification).

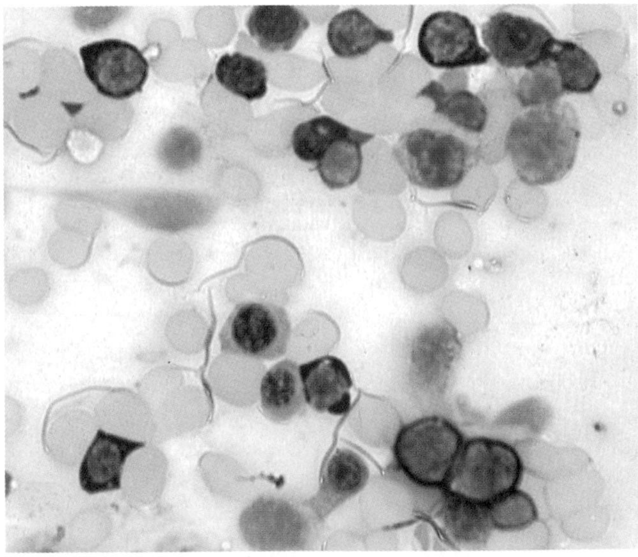

COLOR PLATE 67 (FIG. 47.53). Bone marrow smear stained with periodic acid–Schiff stain from a woman with a therapy-related myelodysplastic syndrome following chemotherapy for multiple myeloma. Numerous red cell precursors are intensely positive (original magnification: 256× magnification).

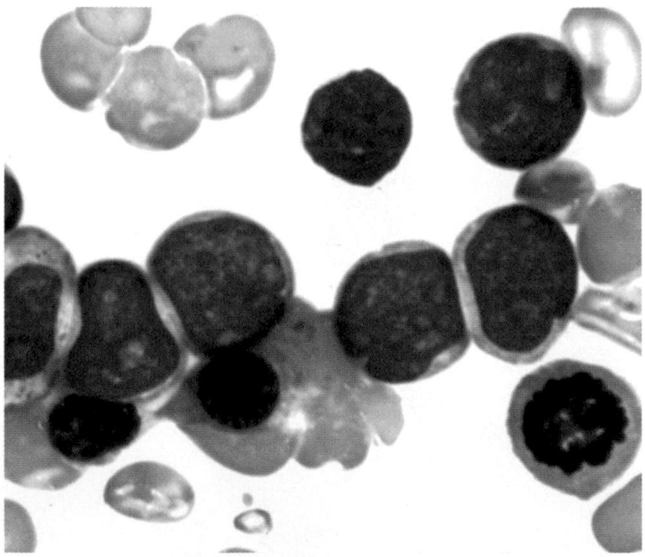

COLOR PLATE 68 (FIG. 47.55). Bone marrow smear from a man who has an M2 acute myeloid leukemia related to treatment for Hodgkin's disease (Wright-Giemsa stain, original magnification: 400× magnification).

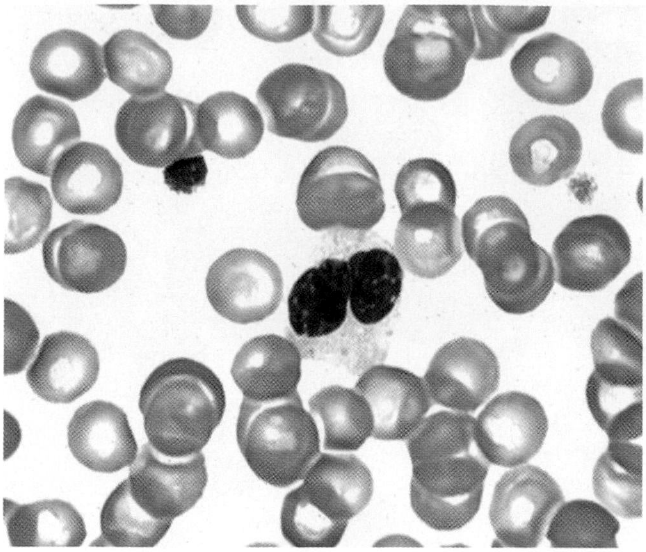

COLOR PLATE 69 (FIG. 48.1). Mature neutrophil in the blood smear of a patient who has refractory anemia with excess blasts, type 1. The cytoplasm is pale because of a marked decrease in specific granules. The nucleus appears hypolobated because of overlapping nuclear segments (Wright-Giemsa stain, original magnification: 400× magnification).

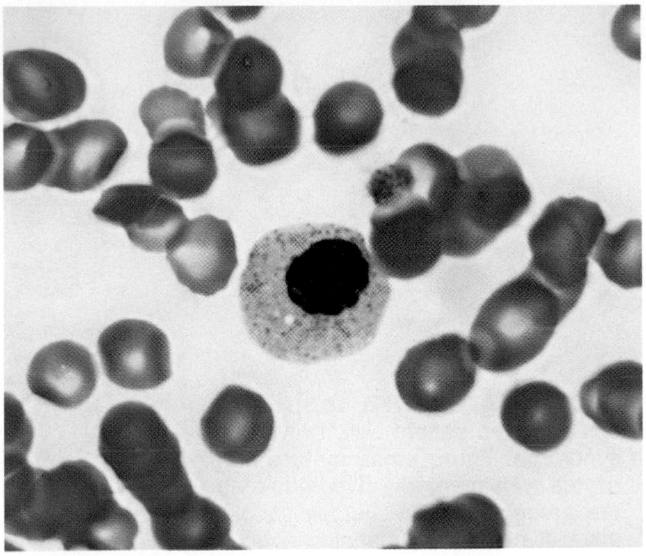

COLOR PLATE 70 (FIG. 48.4). Blood smear from a 68-year-old woman with refractory anemia with excess blasts, type 1 associated with del(17p). The blood contained numerous neutrophils with nonlobated nuclei similar to this cell (Wright-Giemsa stain, original magnification: 400× magnification).

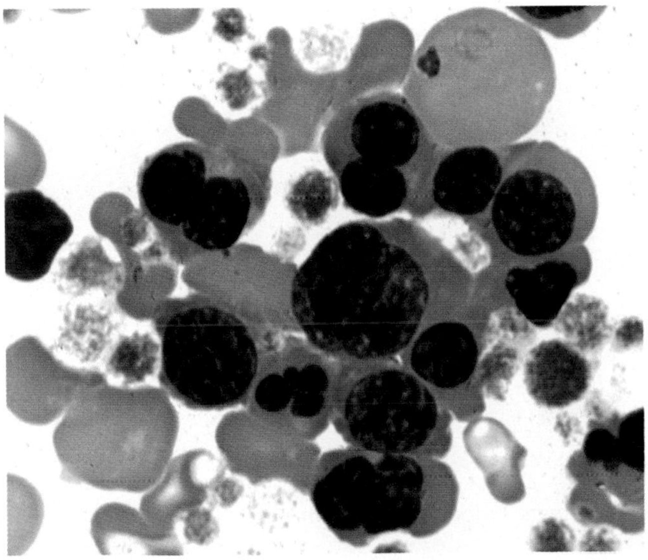

COLOR PLATE 71 (FIG. 48.5). Bone marrow smear from a patient who has an unclassified myelodysplastic syndrome showing marked dyserythropoiesis. The erythroid cells show nuclear lobulation and slightly open chromatin (Wright-Giemsa stain, original magnification: 256× magnification).

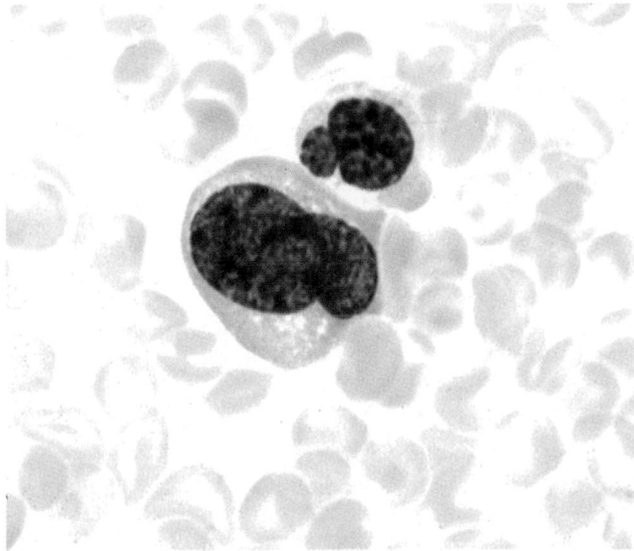

COLOR PLATE 72 (FIG. 48.6). Two large erythroblasts in a bone marrow smear from a patient who has refractory anemia. The nucleus of the larger cell is lobated and the chromatin has the features of a megaloblast (Wright-Giemsa stain, original magnification: 400× magnification).

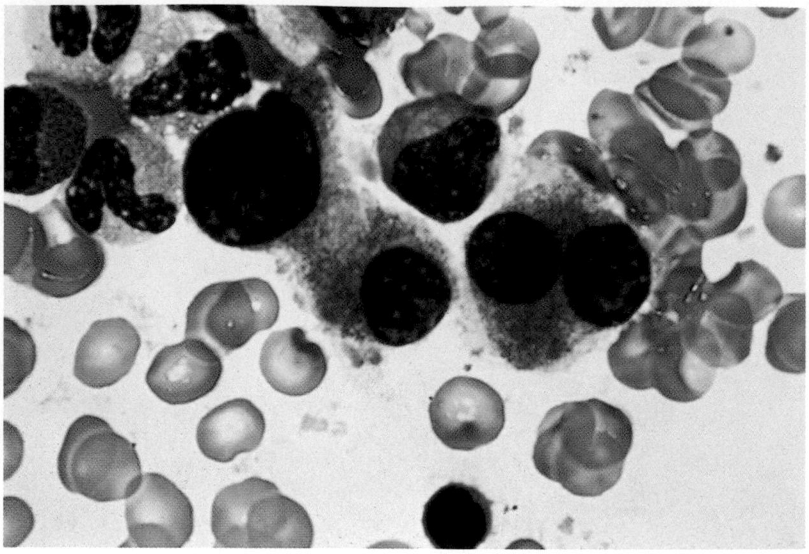

COLOR PLATE 73 (FIG. 48.8). Bone marrow smear from a patient with a myelodysplastic syndrome. Three small mature megakaryocytes with markedly hypolobulated nuclei are present (Wright-Giemsa stain, original magnification: 400× magnification).

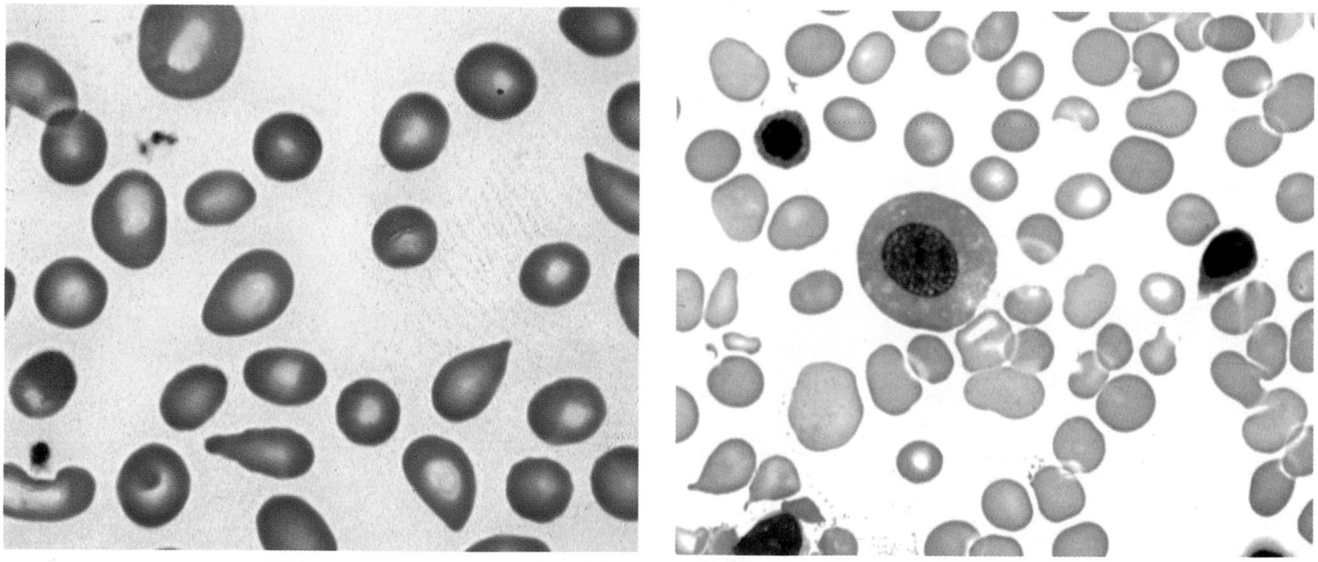

A B

COLOR PLATE 74 (FIG. 48.10). A: Blood smear from a patient with an 8-year history of refractory anemia. There is marked anisocytosis with numerous dacryocytes. Anisocytosis is slight to moderate. **B:** Bone marrow smear from the same patient showing a polychromatic megaloblastic erythroblast (Wright-Giemsa stain, original magnification: 400× magnification).

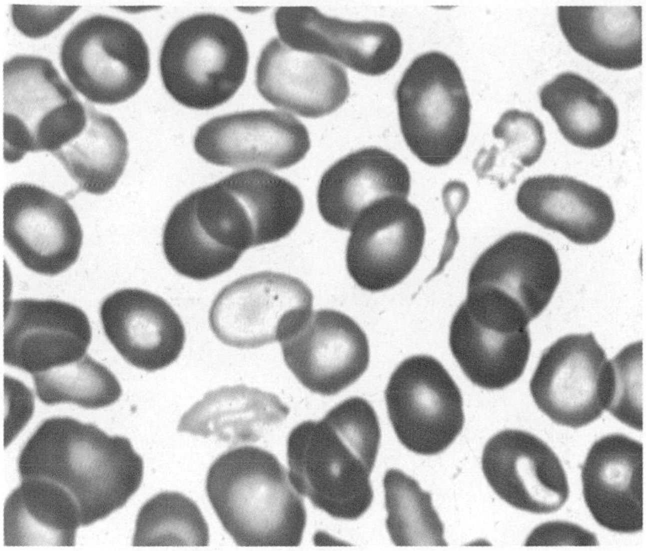

A

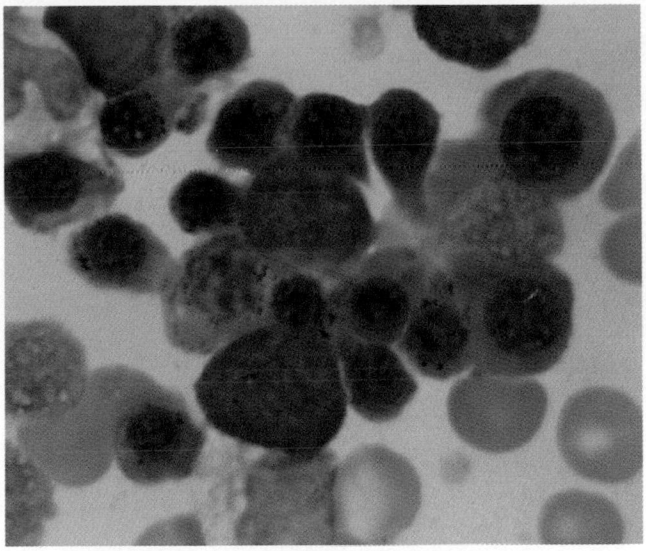

B

COLOR PLATE 75 (FIG. 48.12). A: Blood smear from a 42-year-old man who has RARS. The predominant red blood cells are normochromic with a minor population of red blood cells that is hypochromic dimorphic. There is increased poikilocytosis in both the normochromic and hypochromic populations. Some of the normochromic cells are macrocytic (Wright-Giemsa stain, original magnification: 400× magnification). **B:** Iron stain of a bone marrow smear from the patient illustrated in **A** showing numerous ringed, type III sideroblasts (Prussian blue stain followed by Safranin counterstain, original magnification: 256× magnification).

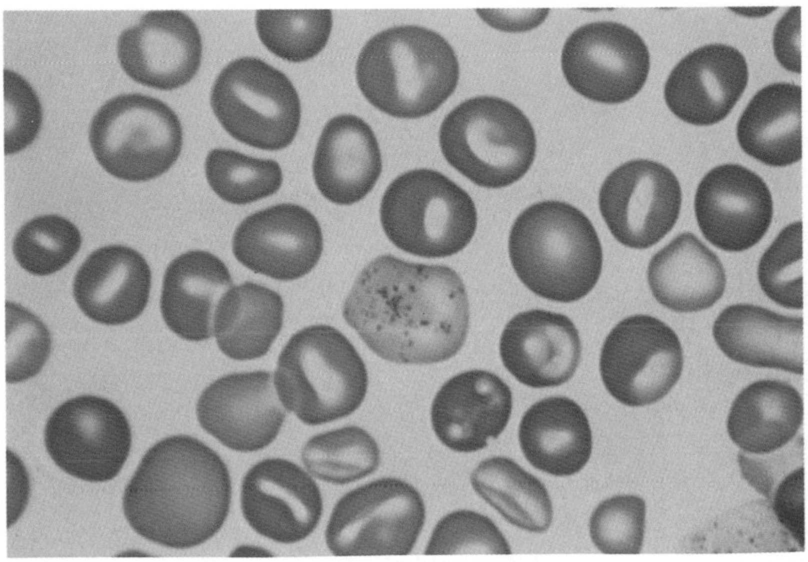

COLOR PLATE 76 (FIG. 48.13). Blood smear from a patient who has RARS. The red blood cells are predominantly normochromic macrocytic. The red blood cell in the center contains numerous Pappenheimer bodies (Wright-Giemsa stain, original magnification: 400× magnification).

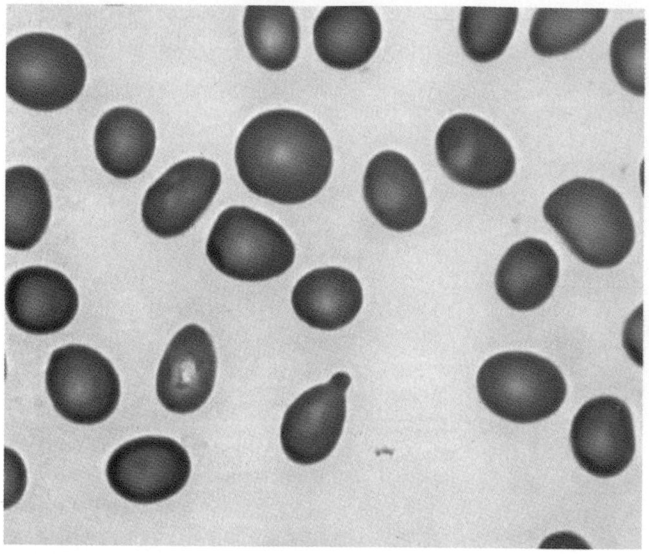

COLOR PLATE 77 (FIG. 48.14). Blood smear from a man who has refractory anemia with excess blasts, type 1. The red blood cells show increased anisocytosis and poikilocytosis with macrocytes, including oval macrocytes, and dacrocytes (Wright-Giemsa stain, original magnification: 400× magnification).

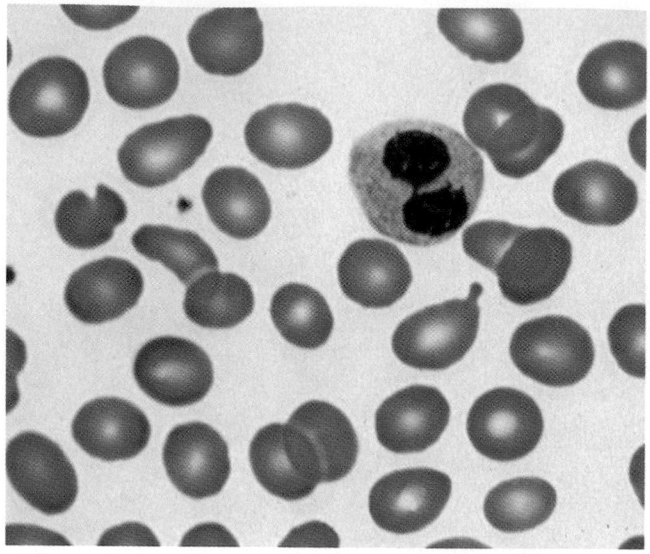

COLOR PLATE 78 (FIG. 48.15). Blood smear from a man who has refractory anemia with excess blasts, type 1, showing a mature neutrophil with a bilobed, pseudo–Pelger-Huet nucleus. The red blood cells show minimal anisocytosis and slight poikilocytosis (Wright-Giemsa stain, original magnification: 400× magnification).

A

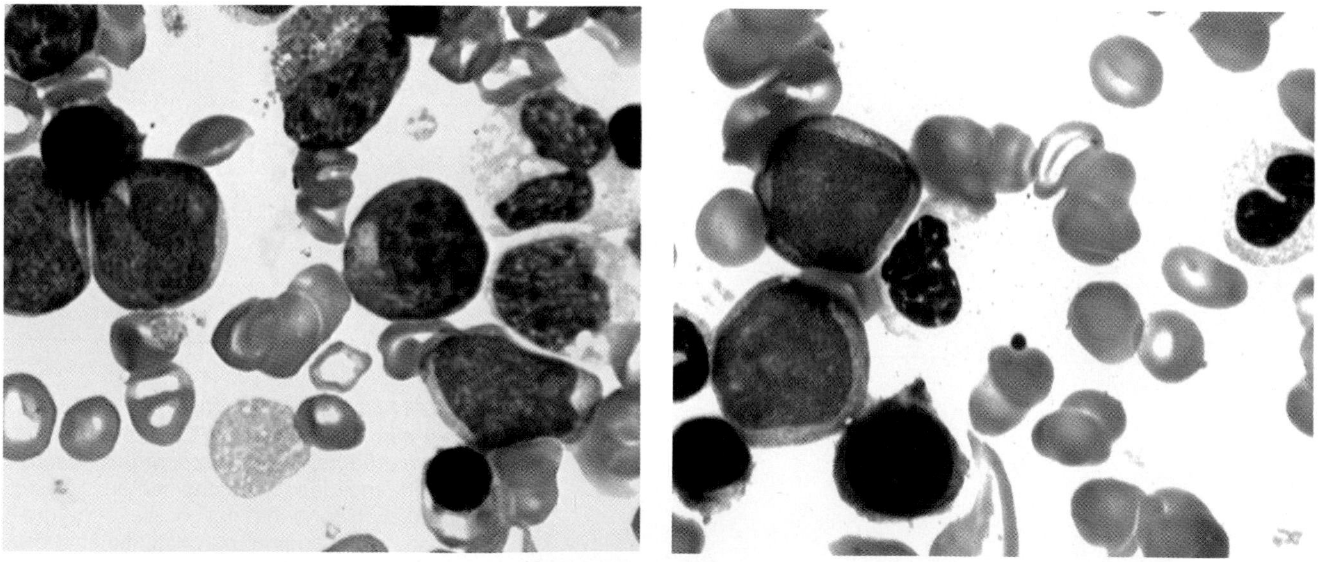

B

COLOR PLATE 79 (FIG. 48.16). A: Bone marrow smear from a patient who has refractory anemia with excess blasts, type 2, showing three myeloblasts. **B:** The same specimen as **A**, showing three mature neutrophils with hyposegmented nuclei. Two early promyelocytes are also present (Wright-Giemsa stain, original magnification: 400× magnification).

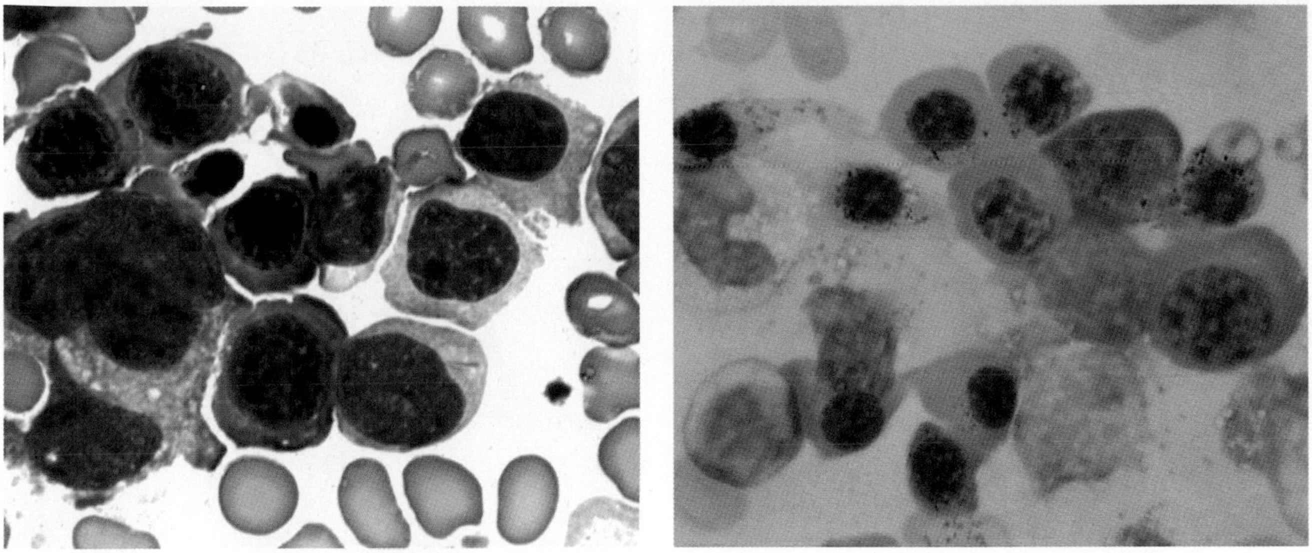

A B

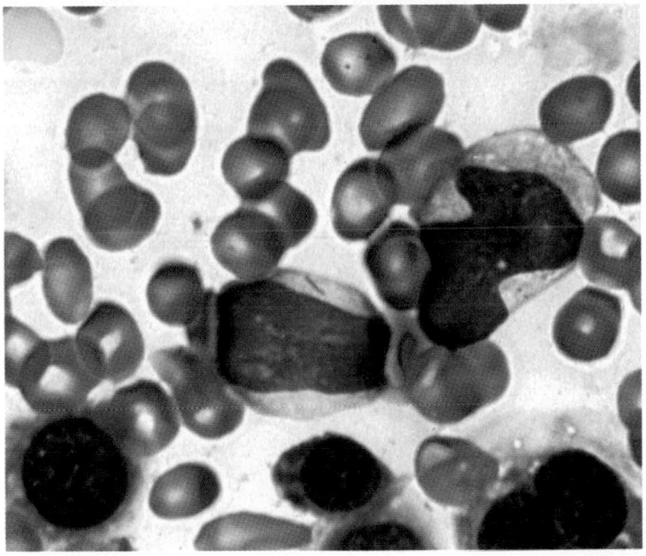

C

COLOR PLATE 80 (FIG. 48.17). A: Bone marrow smear from a 72-year-old man who has refractory anemia with excess blasts, type 2, and who presented with a 1-year history of macrocytic anemia, neutropenia, and thrombocytopenia. This marrow specimen showed 62% erythroblasts and 4% myeloblasts. A myeloblast with a delicate Auer rod is present in the lower right. A megakaryocyte with a phagocytosed red cell is also present (Wright-Giemsa stain, original magnification: 400× magnification). **B:** An iron stain of the specimen illustrated in **A** shows numerous ringed sideroblasts (Prussian blue stain followed by Safranin counterstain, original magnification: 400× magnification). **C:** High-magnification view of the specimens in **A** and **B** showing a myeloblast with a distinct Auer rod. Several normoblasts are present (Wright-Giemsa stain, original magnification: 256× magnification).

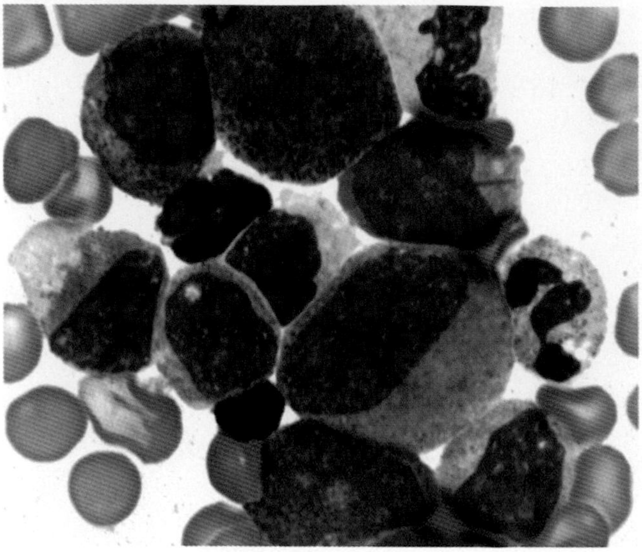

COLOR PLATE 81 (FIG. 48.18). Bone marrow smear from a 27-year-old man who has pancytopenia and refractory anemia with excess blasts, type 2. There is a full spectrum of neutrophil maturation. This specimen showed 8% myeloblasts, several of which contained Auer rods, as shown in the only blast in this field (Wright-Giemsa stain, original magnification: 256× magnification).

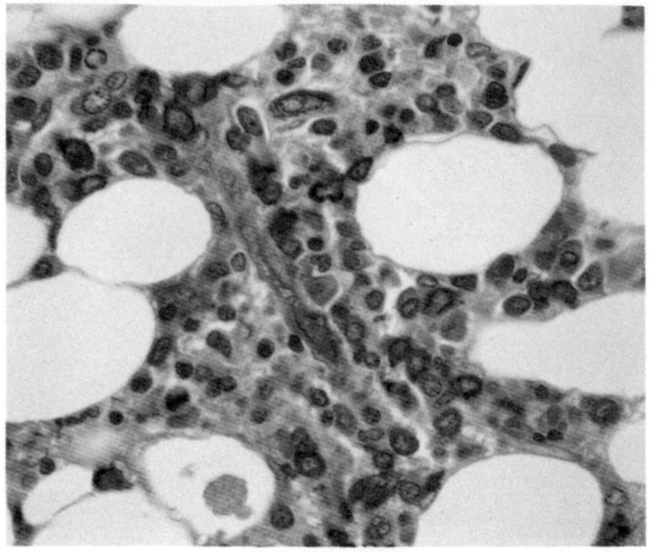

COLOR PLATE 82 (FIG. 48.22). Hypocellular marrow biopsy from a patient with refractory anemia with excess blasts, type 1, reacted with antibody to CD34. Several immature cells expressing CD34 are present (immunoperoxidase stain, original magnification: 400× magnification).

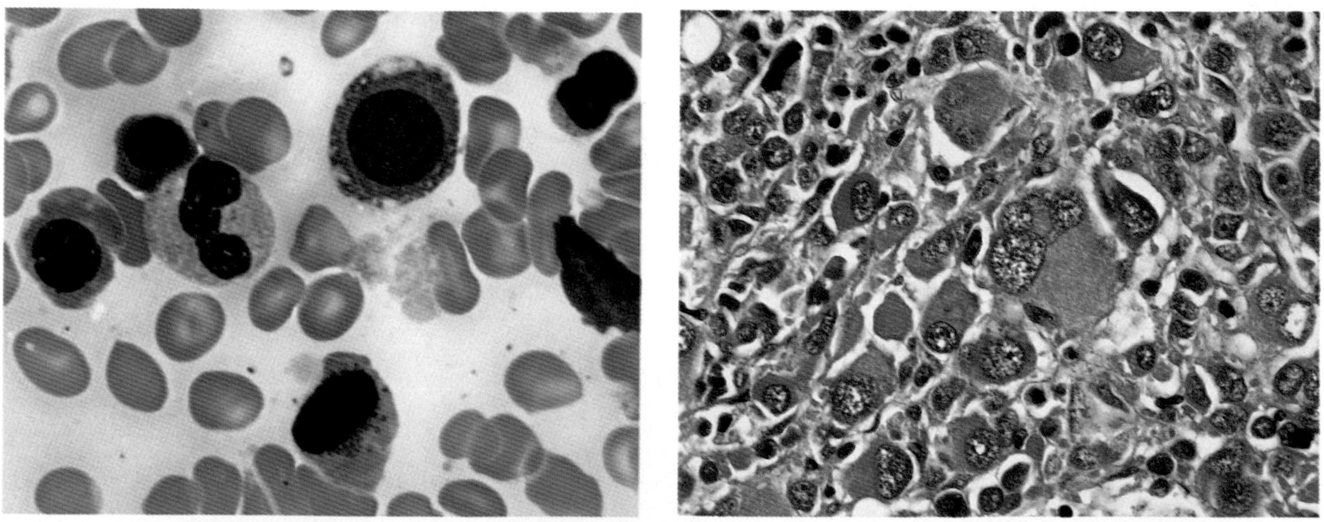

A **B**

COLOR PLATE 83 (FIG. 48.23). A: Bone marrow smear from a 38-year-old male with refractory cytopenia with multilineage dysplasia. A basophilic erythroblast with a megaloblastic nucleus and cytoplasmic vacuoles and a polychromatic ringed sideroblast are present. The blasts were less than 2%. Cytogenetic analysis of this specimen showed complex abnormalities, including deletion of chromosomes 5 and 7 (Wright-Giemsa stain, original magnification: 400× magnification). **B:** Bone marrow biopsy from the same specimen as illustrated in **A**. There is a marked increase in megakaryocytes with dysplastic features, including small size and hypolobulated nuclei (hematoxylin and eosin stain, original magnification: 240× magnification).

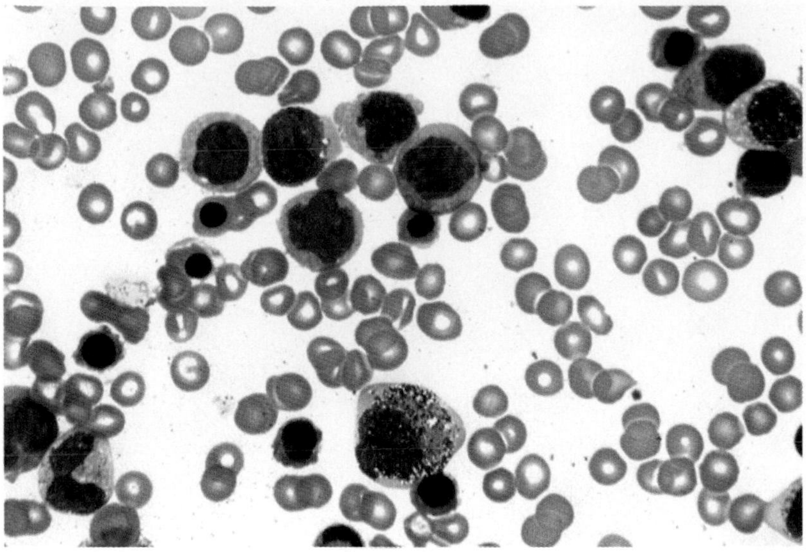

COLOR PLATE 84 (FIG. 48.26). Bone marrow smear from a 3.5-year-old boy who has a myelodysplastic syndrome associated with an isolated 7− chromosome abnormality. There are scattered monocytes and neutrophil precursors (Wright-Giemsa stain, original magnification: 256× magnification).

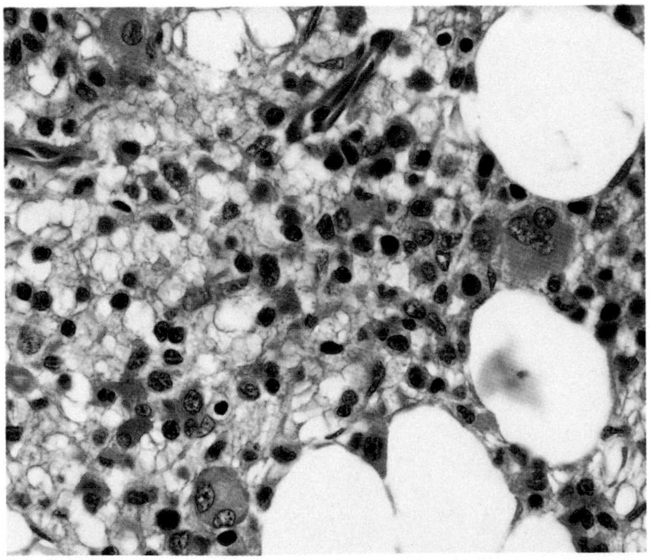

COLOR PLATE 85 (FIG. 48.28). Bone marrow biopsy from a 2-year-old male with a myelodysplastic syndrome associated with an isolated monosomy 7 cytogenetic abnormality. The marrow interstitium shows marked cellular depletion (hematoxylin and eosin stain, original magnification: 240× magnification).

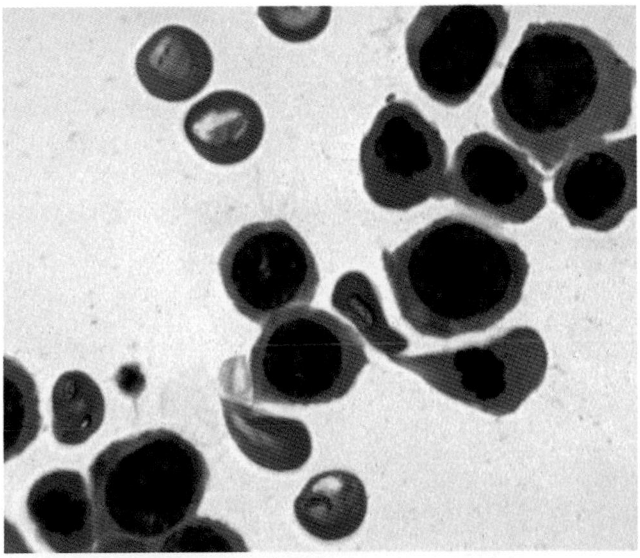

COLOR PLATE 86 (FIG. 48.29). Bone marrow smear from a 42-year-old man admitted to the hospital with a depressed sensorium and pancytopenia. The red blood cell precursors show marked dysplastic changes, including megaloblastoid nuclear chromatin and nuclear hyperlobulation and karyorrhexis. The cells were slightly positive on periodic acid–Schiff staining. Five days after this specimen was obtained, the patient's spouse admitted lacing his evening meals with arsenic. The patient was treated with dimercaprol and recovered completely (Wright-Giemsa stain, original magnification: 400× magnification).

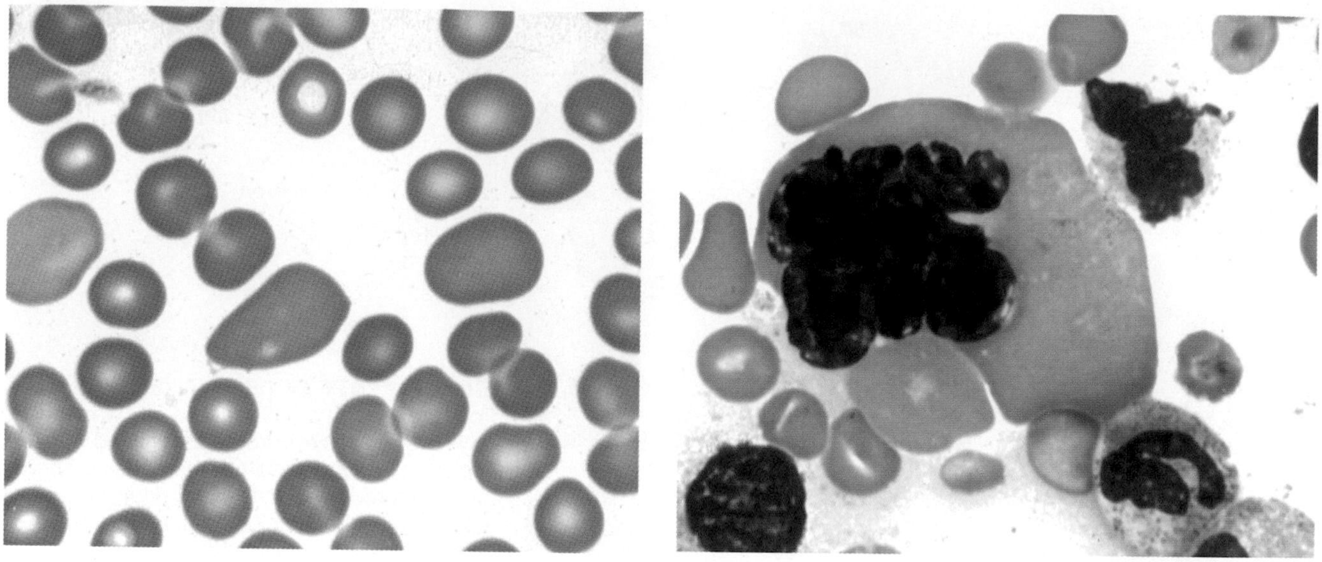

A B

COLOR PLATE 87 (FIG. 48.30). A: Blood smear from a 22-year-old man with a hemoglobin of 13.7 g/dL and a slight reticulocytosis. Very macrocytic red blood cells are noted. The platelet count and leukocyte count were normal. Similar findings were present in the blood smear of his 14-month-old daughter. **B:** Giant polychromatic erythroblast with marked nuclear hyperlobulation in the bone marrow specimen from the patient in **A**. The granulocytes and megakaryocytes were normal in number and appearance. The morphologic findings were classified as congenital dyserythropoietic anemia, type III (Wright-Giemsa stain, original magnification: 400× magnification).

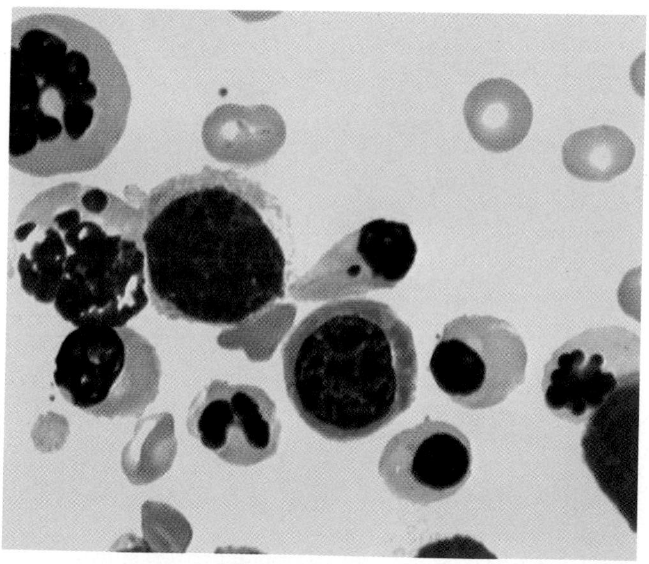

COLOR PLATE 88 (FIG. 48.31). Bone marrow from an 11-month-old boy with congenital dyserythropoietic anemia. The red blood cell precursors show marked dysplastic changes, including hyperlobulation, megaloblastoid chromatin, and karyorrhexis. The serologic and morphologic studies were not definitive for a specific subtype of congenital dyserythropoietic anemia (Wright-Giemsa stain, original magnification: 400× magnification).

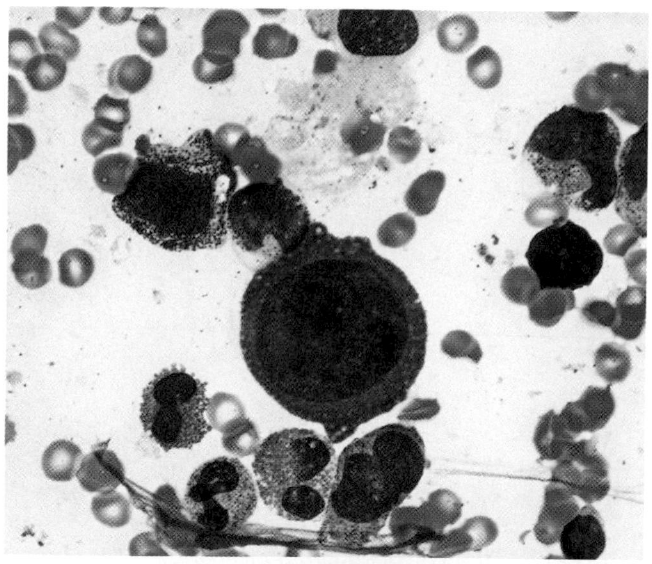

COLOR PLATE 89 (FIG. 48.32). Giant erythroblast in a marrow smear from a 17-year-old male with parvovirus B19 infection. The cytoplasm contains numerous very small vacuoles (Wright-Giemsa stain, original magnification: 400× magnification).

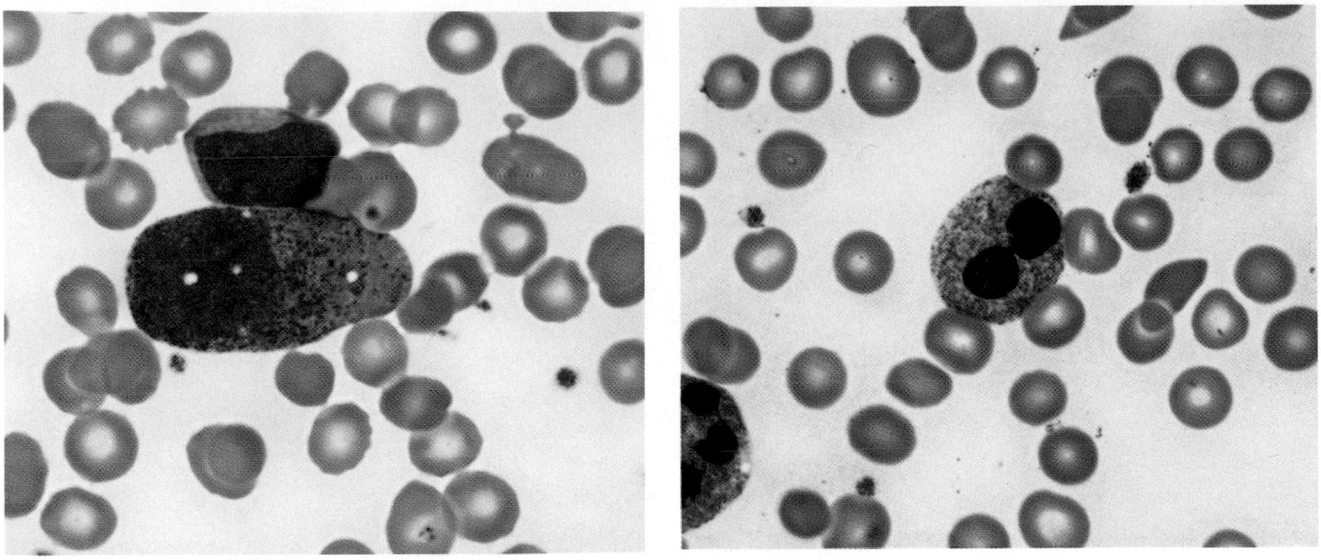

A B

COLOR PLATE 90 (FIG. 48.33). Blood smear from a 7-year-old male being treated with granulocyte colony stimulating factor following bone marrow transplantation. **A:** A myeloblast and a very large promyelocyte with markedly increased azurophilic granulation. **B:** A mature neutrophil with a bilobed (pseudo–Pelger-Huet) nucleus and increased azurophilic granulation (Wright-Giemsa stain, original magnification: 640× magnification).

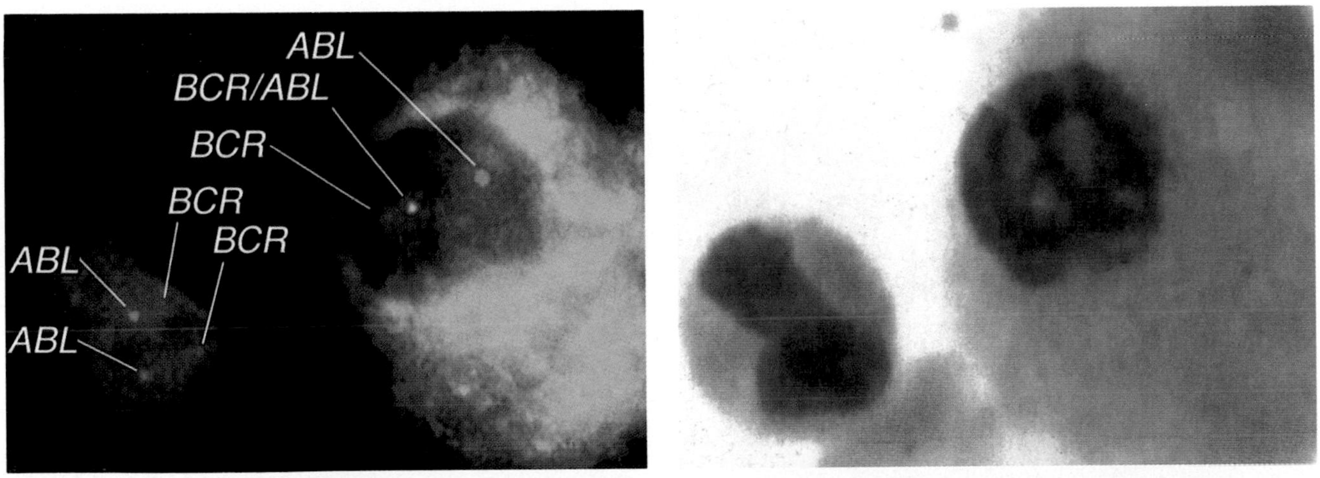

A B

COLOR PLATE 91 (FIG. 49.3). Illustration of fluorescence *in situ* hybridization analysis for the *BCR-ABL* fusion in interphase nuclei (**A**), performed on a previously Wright-stained smear (**B**). In a normal cell (**left**), there are two (red) signals, one for each of the *BCR* genes, and there are two (green) signals, one for each of the *ABL* genes. In a cell with the translocation t(9;22) and *BCR-ABL* (**right**), there is one (red) signal for *BCR*, one (green) for *ABL*, and a (yellow) fusion signal from the juxtaposition of *BCR* with *ABL*. The cells were from a patient with chronic myelogenous leukemia who had been transplanted a year earlier, but who continued to test positive with polymerase chain reaction assay for *BCR-ABL* transcripts. The normal granulocyte likely arose from the transplanted cells, but the pseudo-Gaucher cell likely persisted from the original chronic myelogenous leukemia clone.

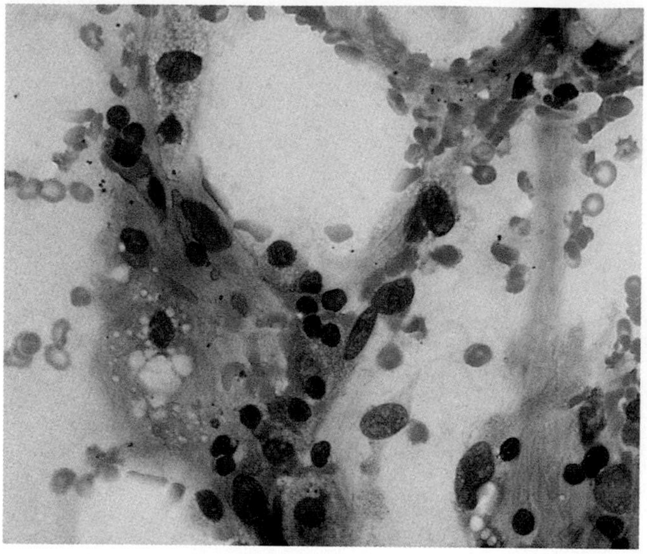

COLOR PLATE 92 (FIG. 50.3). Markedly hypocellular bone marrow particles are evident from a patient status postinduction chemotherapy for relapsed acute leukemia. Occasional macrophages contain ingested material. Endothelial cells line aspirated portions of blood vessels (Wright stain, original magnification: 1,000× magnification).

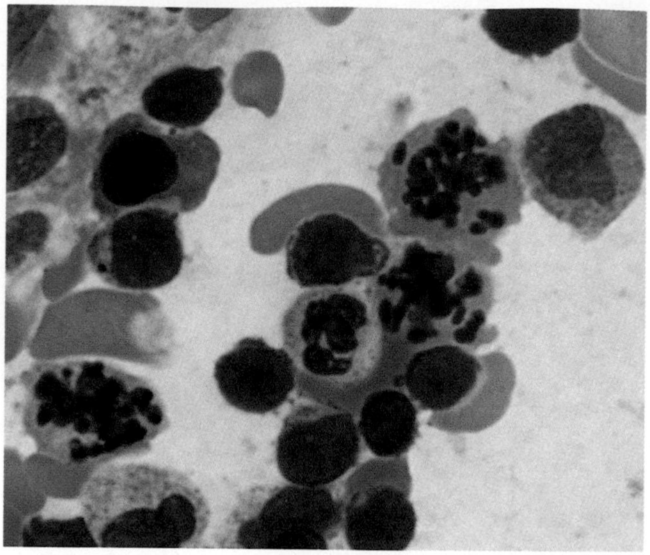

COLOR PLATE 93 (FIG. 50.5). Prominent dyserythropoiesis with apoptosis is evident on this bone marrow aspirate smear from a child receiving aggressive therapy for high risk T-cell acute lymphoblastic leukemia (Wright stain, original magnification: 1000× magnification).

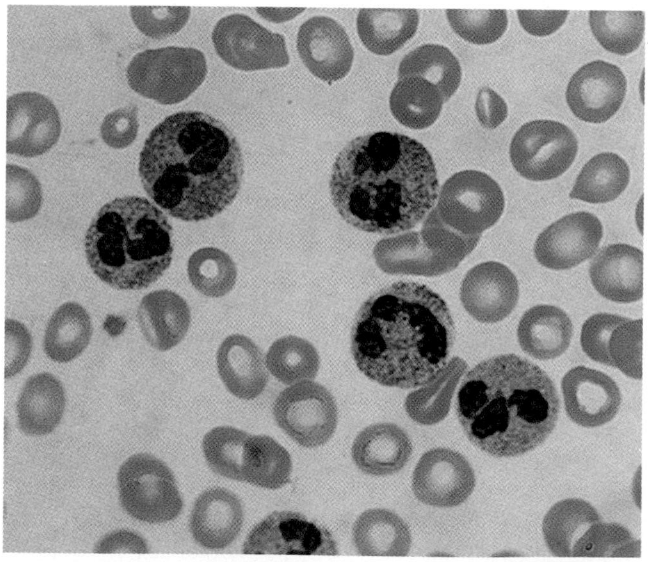

COLOR PLATE 94 (FIG. 50.11). Peripheral blood smear illustrating the prominent toxic neutrophilia that occurs in patients receiving sustained granulocyte colony-stimulating factor therapy (Wright stain, original magnification: 1,000× magnification).

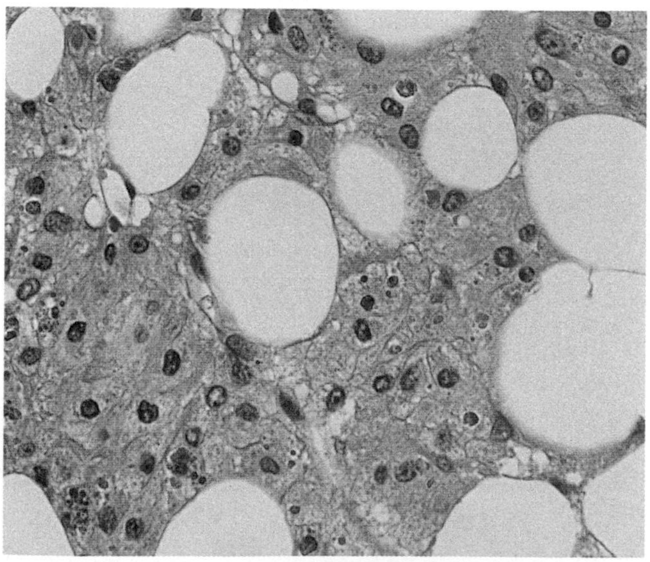

COLOR PLATE 95 (FIG. 50.18). Bone marrow biopsy specimen from a bone marrow transplant recipient shows prominent histiocytic hyperplasia; note failure of engraftment (hematoxylin and eosin stain, original magnification: 400× magnification). (Courtesy of N. Rosenthal, M.D., Department of Pathology, University of Iowa.)

CHAPTER 39

Bone Marrow Manifestations of Hodgkin's and Non-Hodgkin's Lymphomas and Lymphoma-Like Disorders

Steven H. Kroft and Robert W. McKenna

Hodgkin's lymphoma (HL), the non-Hodgkin's lymphomas (NHLs), and many of the lymphoma-like lesions have been discussed in detail elsewhere in this text. This chapter focuses on the manifestations of these disorders in bone marrow. The details of morphologic and immunologic classification and methods of diagnosis as they apply to lymph nodes and other tissues are not repeated here.

The bone marrow examination is a valuable procedure in the diagnosis and management of patients who have HL or NHL. It is commonly used to define the extent of disease in the initial staging protocol. Posttherapy bone marrow examination is useful for assessing a patient's response to chemotherapy and for monitoring previously treated patients for evidence of recurrent disease. In some instances, the primary diagnosis of HL or NHL is made from a bone marrow biopsy performed in the evaluation of a fever of unknown origin, blood cytopenias, or a mass lesion in the chest or abdomen.

The bone marrow examination should include trephine biopsy sections, trephine imprints, aspiration smears, and blood smears (1–4) (see Chapter 37). All of these preparations should be studied by the same pathologist. The diagnostic contributions provided by the different specimens and preparations frequently complement one another. The combination of clues obtained from the composite examination of the bone marrow preparations and blood smears often leads to the correct diagnosis when any single component would not. By performing a thorough bone marrow examination initially, the most information is gathered and the necessity for a repeat biopsy is reduced (1,3–6).

S. H. Kroft and R. W. McKenna: Department of Pathology, University of Texas Southwestern Medical School, Dallas, Texas 75390-9073

Comparative studies have shown the relative value of trephine biopsy sections and aspirate smears in the assessment of the bone marrow for lymphoma (4–6). Trephine biopsy sections generally provide the most useful morphologic information. In patients who have Hodgkin's disease, bone marrow aspirate smears rarely show definitive evidence of involvement even when there is extensive disease in the trephine biopsy. Trephine biopsies are more often positive for NHL as well, but, in most cases, disease is found in the biopsy and aspirate smears alike. In a minority of cases of NHL, the aspirate smears are diagnostic when the sections are negative or equivocal (4,7–11) (Table 39.1). In addition to the morphologic evaluation, the aspirated marrow is the best material for several important supplemental studies for characterization of NHLs, including immunophenotyping by flow cytometry, cytogenetics, most molecular studies, and microbiologic cultures.

Bone marrow involvement with lymphoma usually is generalized throughout the hematopoietic marrow. However, lymphoma infiltrates are often focal with normal uninvolved marrow intervening between lesions. Focal lesions can be missed if the volume of the biopsy specimen is insufficient. For this reason, bilateral posterior iliac crest trephine biopsies are preferred. They provide more tissue for examination and sample two separate sites. The yield of demonstrable marrow involvement with HL and NHLs is significantly increased when bilateral biopsies are performed(3,9,10, 12–15) (Fig. 39.1). Specimens of at least 2 cm long from each iliac crest, taken with an 11-gauge biopsy needle, are recommended as a minimum (1). Trephine biopsies that consist largely of periosteum, cortical bone, and subcortical marrow are usually inadequate, and repeat biopsies should be obtained. Stepwise serial sectioning is desirable in clinical settings in which focal lesions are anticipated. Samples can

TABLE 39.1. *Non-Hodgkin's lymphoma on trephine biopsy sections and aspirate smears in 93 patients with bone marrow involvement by non-Hodgkin's lymphoma*

Sample	Adults (84 patients)	Children (9 patients)	Total (93 patients)
Lymphoma only on trephine sections	19%	0	17%
Lymphoma only on aspirate smears	0	33%	3%
Lymphoma on trephine sections and aspirate smears	81%	67%	80%

From Foucar F, McKenna RW, Frizzera G, et al. Bone marrow and blood involvement by lymphoma in relationship to the Lukes-Collins classification. *Cancer* 1982;49:888–897, with permission.

be mounted for examination at various levels through the entire specimen to avoid missing small lesions. The previously cut ribbon can be used if additional sections are required for further morphologic assessment or for histochemical or immunohistochemical stains (1,16,17).

Some laboratories routinely process bone marrow trephine biopsies for plastic embedding and thin sectioning. When these techniques are used, decalcification is not required and the cytology of the sections is often superior, allowing for more accurate identification of cell types (18,19). In most instances, however, thin, well-prepared paraffin-embedded marrow sections that have been fixed in B5 or Zenker's solutions, combined with marrow aspirate and blood smears are adequate for identifying and characterizing lymphomas.

Immunohistochemistry is a valuable tool in the diagnosis and differential diagnosis of HL and NHLs in the bone marrow. The yield of positive biopsies can be increased and the lymphoma can be more specifically characterized by appropriate application of immunohistochemistry (20–27).

In addition to morphologic and immunohistochemical assessment, it often is important to perform supplementary diagnostic studies on lymphoma tissue obtained from the bone marrow or blood. These include immunophenotyping

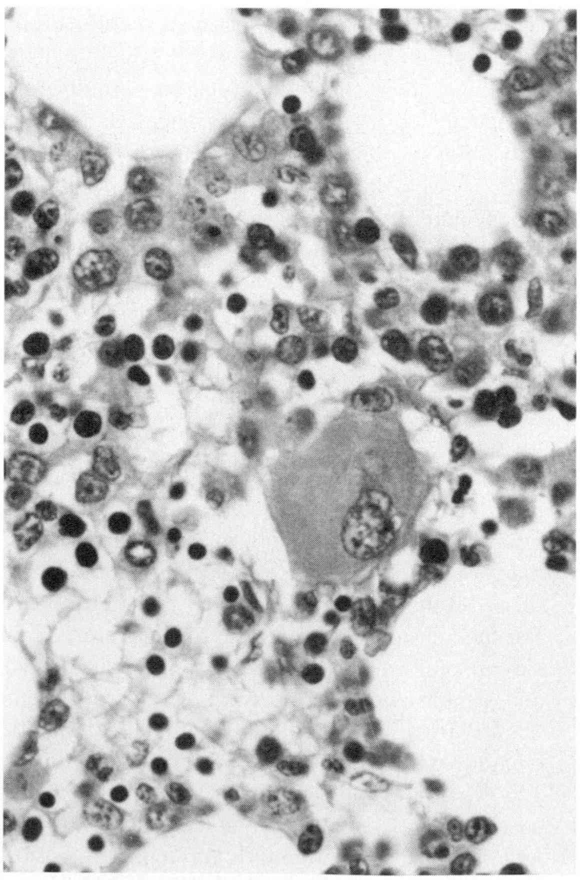

A

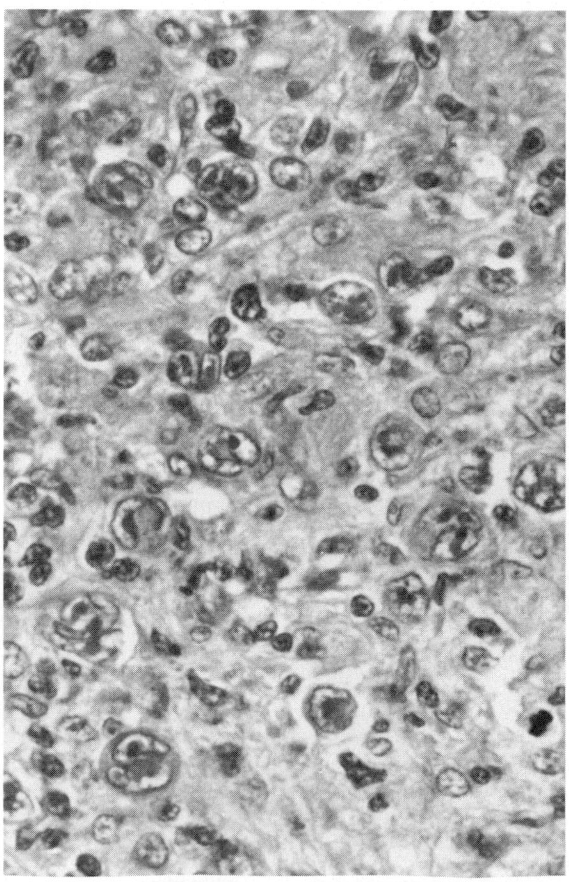

B

FIG. 39.1. Bilateral posterior iliac crest trephine biopsies were performed on a 51-year-old man who had mixed cellularity Hodgkin's lymphoma (HL). **A:** The biopsy from the left iliac crest was negative for HL and showed a normocellular marrow. **B:** The biopsy from the right iliac crest was diffusely infiltrated with Hodgkin's tissue (hematoxylin and eosin stain, original magnification: 400× magnification).

by flow cytometry, cytogenetics, and molecular analysis. These additional studies may provide important diagnostic, prognostic and therapeutic information (28–34). The methods and applications of these techniques for characterization of lymphomas are detailed in Chapters 3 through 10 and in Chapter 38.

HODGKIN'S LYMPHOMA

Infiltration of the bone marrow by HL results from widely disseminated disease in nearly all cases; rarely, the marrow is involved because of direct extension from contiguously involved lymph nodes (35). The trephine biopsy is the preferred specimen for identifying HL involvement in the marrow. Evidence of HL rarely is found in aspiration smears, as the fibrosis that invariably is associated with HL prevents aspiration of Hodgkin's cells (Fig. 39.2). When marrow disease is extensive, attempts at aspiration may yield a "dry tap."

The bone marrow is involved with HL at diagnosis in 5% to 15% of cases overall (8,25,36–44). Asymptomatic patients with clinical stages I or II disease have a very low incidence, whereas patients with an advanced clinical stage or constitutional symptoms are far more likely to have bone marrow involvement. In patients with the acquired immunodeficiency syndrome (AIDS), the incidence of marrow involvement is approximately 50% (45–47). If a thorough evaluation for bone marrow HL is negative, it is uncommon to find other extranodal disease when a laparotomy is performed (8).

Typically patients with marrow involvement have clinical stage III or IV disease, are older than average for HL, and have constitutional symptoms (8,36,39,40,48). Organomegaly and lymphadenopathy are often present. Rarely, an altered immune state leads to infectious manifestations as a presenting complaint. Thrombocytopenia, leukopenia, and osseous lesions are highly specific for bone marrow involvement (8,44). Most patients with marrow involvement are also anemic, but this is a nonspecific finding. Biochemical abnormalities like those associated with other disseminated neoplasms are found with advanced HL (40).

The value of performing bone marrow biopsies routinely in staging HL has been questioned in some studies (41,44,49, 50). It has been suggested that the marrow examination should be reserved for patients who have clinically advanced disease or constitutional symptoms (41,44,49,50). This ap-

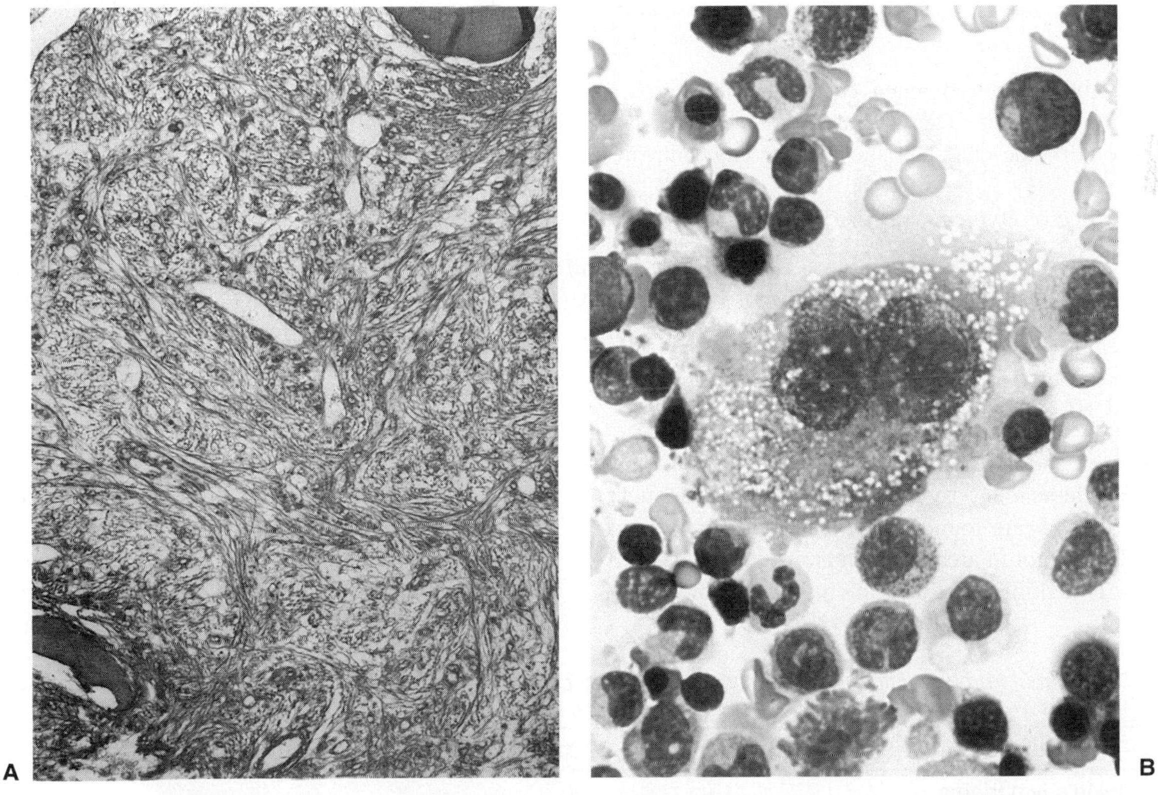

FIG. 39.2. A: A reticulin stain on a trephine biopsy from a 38-year-old woman with diffuse marrow replacement by Hodgkin's lymphoma (HL). There is a marked increase in reticulin. Reticulin or collagen fibrosis invariably is present in marrow Hodgkin's tissue (Wilder's reticulin stain, original magnification: 100× magnification). **B:** A classic Reed-Sternberg cell is depicted in this bone marrow aspiration smear from a 49-year-old man with advanced HL. This is a rare finding. The reticulin fibrosis associated with Hodgkin's lesions usually inhibits aspiration of Hodgkin's cells (Wright-Giemsa stain, original magnification: 400× magnification).

proach is supported by several studies showing that patients who have clinical stage IA or IIA rarely exhibit bone marrow involvement (40,41,44,49). Still other data discount the prognostic significance of marrow involvement in stage IV disease (40). These observations, together with the success of bone marrow imaging techniques for identifying HL, have led to discontinuance of marrow biopsies as a component of the staging protocols in some treatment centers (40,51–54). Despite these findings, the bone marrow biopsy remains a standard component of the evaluation of patients who have newly diagnosed HL in most institutions. In several studies bone marrow involvement has been the most significant factor in predicting an unfavorable course (36,42,55,56).

In addition to its utility in staging, the marrow biopsy may be the primary diagnostic tissue in cases of HL that manifest with blood cytopenias or an abdominal or chest mass without peripheral lymphadenopathy (25,57–59). This presentation is particularly common in patients with AIDS (60).

Histopathologic criteria for diagnosis of bone marrow involvement in patients with proven HL in a lymph node biopsy were recommended by the Committee on Histopathological Criteria Contributing to Staging of Hodgkin's Disease at the Ann Arbor Symposium in 1971 (61). A summary of the committee's recommendations is shown subsequently. Criteria similar to those defined at the Ann Arbor symposium have been suggested by other investigators (62,63).

1. HL may be diagnosed when typical Reed-Sternberg cells or their mononuclear variants are found in the marrow in one of the characteristic cellular environments of HL.
2. The presence of atypical cells that lack the nuclear features of Reed-Sternberg cells in one of the characteristic polycellular environments of HL or in focal or diffuse areas of fibrosis is strongly suggestive of marrow involvement.
3. Fibrosis or necrosis alone should be considered suspicious for HL in a previously diagnosed patient.

In most cases, Hodgkin's cells can be identified in marrow lesions when adequate biopsy material is available for study (8). Hodgkin's cells are found in a stromal reaction characteristic of HL and not in areas of normal marrow. However, occasionally Hodgkin's cells may intermix with normal hematopoietic cells at the edge of a lesion (64). The trephine biopsy should be repeated in cases that have lesions suspicious for HL in which Hodgkin's cells are not identified in serial sections unless other unequivocal evidence of pathologically advanced disease is present.

In cases in which the initial diagnosis of HL is made from a bone marrow biopsy it is essential that typical Reed-Sternberg cells are identified and that the other characteristic histologic features of HL are present. Caution must be exercised when interpreting marrow lesions that resemble HL histologically but lack typical Hodgkin's cells. Some NHLs, and other bone marrow lesions, may mimic HL histologically (2,65,66). Reed-Sternberg–like cells have been described in several types of lesions other than HL (67–71). The use of immunohistochemical stains for the Hodgkin's cell–associated antigens CD15 and CD30, together with other appropriate immunohistochemical stains has made the diagnosis of HL in bone marrow more precise. Table 39.2 lists the usual immunohistochemical staining profile for the neoplastic cells in HL and the NHLs that are most likely to mimic HL in bone marrow.

In early studies the highest incidence of bone marrow involvement was found with lymphocyte depletion HL (8,57). Many cases formerly diagnosed as lymphocyte depletion HL were examples of NHL, especially anaplastic large cell lymphomas. In most studies, mixed cellularity HL has the highest incidence of BM involvement, approximately 20%. Fewer than 10% of patients with nodular sclerosis HL have marrow disease at diagnosis, and only rare cases of bone marrow involvement in lymphocyte predominance HL have been reported (8,25,35,38,40,41,44,72).

The extent of bone marrow involvement in trephine biopsy specimens varies from small lesions that occupy less than 10% of the marrow space to complete replacement of the marrow biopsy (Figs. 39.3–39.8). The pattern of infiltration may be focal or diffuse. Focal involvement is found in 20% to 30% of cases and is characterized by small, isolated lesions that are encircled completely by normal marrow tissue or that are in a paratrabecular location. A polycellular infiltrate with a uniform admixture of cells throughout the lesion is most common (8). Diffuse involvement is observed in 70% to 80% of cases. Hodgkin's tissue occupies entire areas between bone trabeculae and usually replaces large contiguous portions of marrow. The cellular infiltrate in dif-

TABLE 39.2. *Usual immunohistochemical profile of neoplastic cells in Hodgkin's lymphoma and non-Hodgkin's lymphoma that may simulate Hodgkin's lymphoma in bone marrow*

Lymphoma type	CD15	CD30	LCA	CD3	CD20	EMA
Classic Hodgkin's lymphoma	+	+	−	−	±	−
Lymphocyte predominance, Hodgkin's lymphoma	−	−	+	−	+	+
Anaplastic large cell lymphoma	−	+	+	+	−	+
T-cell–rich and histiocyte-rich large B-cell lymphomas	−	−	+	−	+	−
Peripheral T-cell lymphoma, NOS	−	−	+	+	−	−

LCA, leukocyte common antigen; EMA, epithelial membrane antigen; NOS, not otherwise specified; +, detected; −, not detected; ±, sometimes detected.

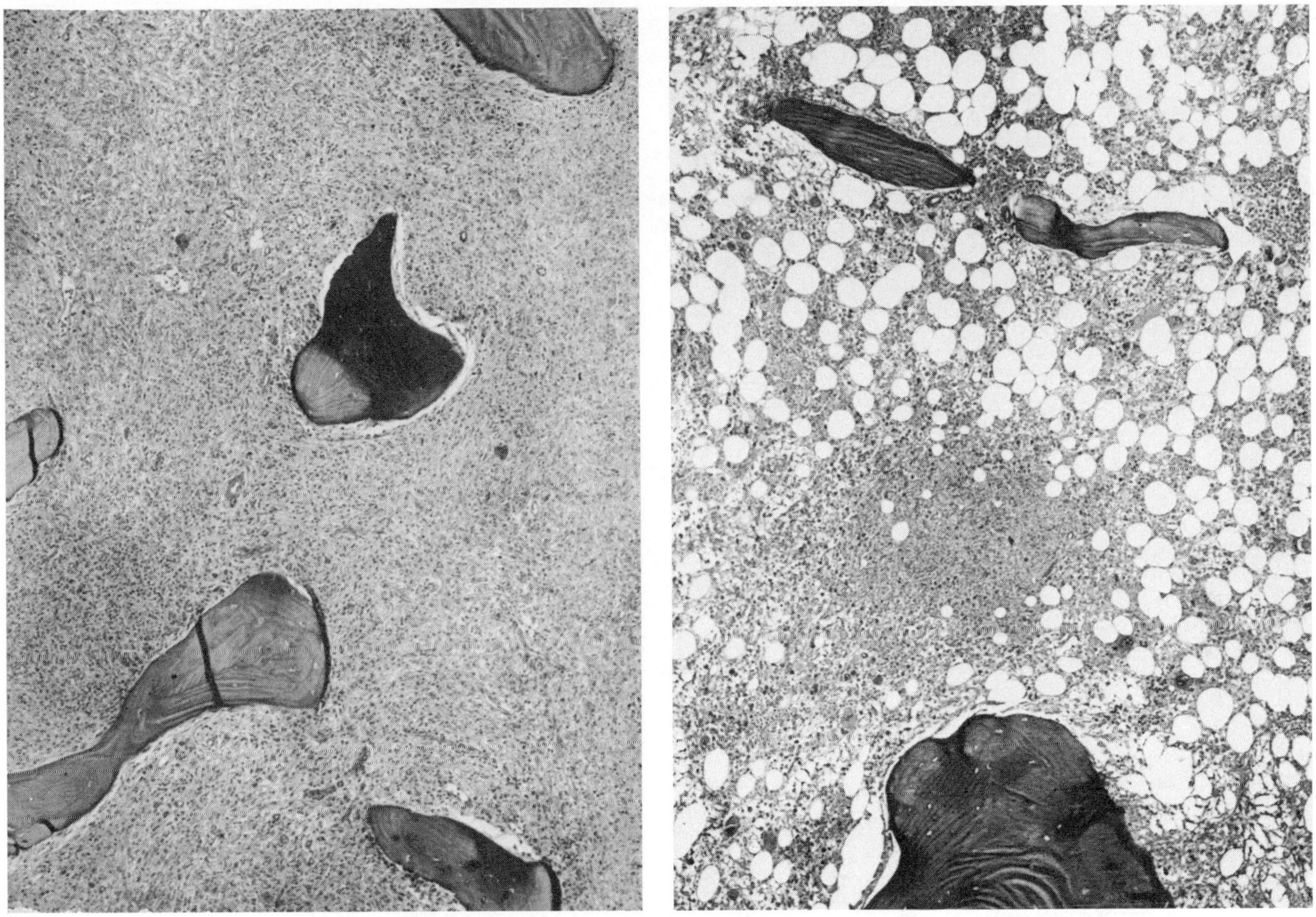

A B

FIG. 39.3. A: A trephine biopsy section from a 59-year-old man with Hodgkin's lymphoma (HL). The marrow is diffusely replaced with Hodgkin's tissue. **B:** This trephine biopsy section shows a focal Hodgkin's lesion. The lesion is surrounded by normal hematopoietic tissue (hematoxylin and eosin stain, original magnification: 40× magnification).

fuse lesions is distributed uniformly or localized between broad areas of sparsely cellular loose or dense connective tissue (Fig. 39.8). Diffuse and focal lesions may be found in the same biopsy. Reticulin or collagen invariably is present in the bone marrow lesions and is often extensive. Fibrosis is most profound when there is diffuse involvement (8) (Figs. 39.2, 39.3).

Marked variation occurs in the cellular composition of the marrow lesions in HL. Any of the histologic patterns of infiltrate found in lymph nodes may be observed in the bone marrow. The infiltrate most often is polycellular, with large and small lymphocytes, histiocytes, plasma cells, eosinophils, neutrophils, and Hodgkin's cells (Figs. 39.4, 39.6–39.8). In some cases, a relatively uniform cell proliferation that consists of lymphocytes or histiocytes is observed (Fig. 39.5). Hodgkin's cells are the predominant cell types in some cases (Figs. 39.4, 39.6); in others, serial sections are required to find a single diagnostic cell.

Classification of HL should not be attempted from a bone marrow biopsy alone. The small size of the marrow biopsy precludes evaluation of the complete histologic pattern; nodular sclerosis HL may have the features of mixed cellularity or lymphocyte depletion in the marrow (63). The histopathology of HL may differ significantly in lymph nodes and bone marrow from the same patient.

The areas of marrow adjacent to Hodgkin's tissue often show nonspecific changes, such as granulocytic and megakaryocytic hyperplasia (8,57). Hypoplasia may be particularly prominent in some cases (Fig. 39.5) (36). Increased plasma cells, erythroid hyperplasia, eosinophilic and granulocytic hyperplasia and increased megakaryocytes may be observed in HL patients who have no evidence of marrow involvement (73). These nonspecific changes are not generally related to pathologic stage of disease. However, one study showed a significantly poorer prognosis in patients with various types of noninfiltrative changes in the bone marrow (74). The changes included necrosis, increased reticulin, stromal damage, disturbed hematopoiesis, and alterations in cellularity. The several types of noninfiltrative changes were analyzed in composite in this study, and it is not clear which of these may have a significant relationship to prognosis. The nature of some of the changes (e.g., bone

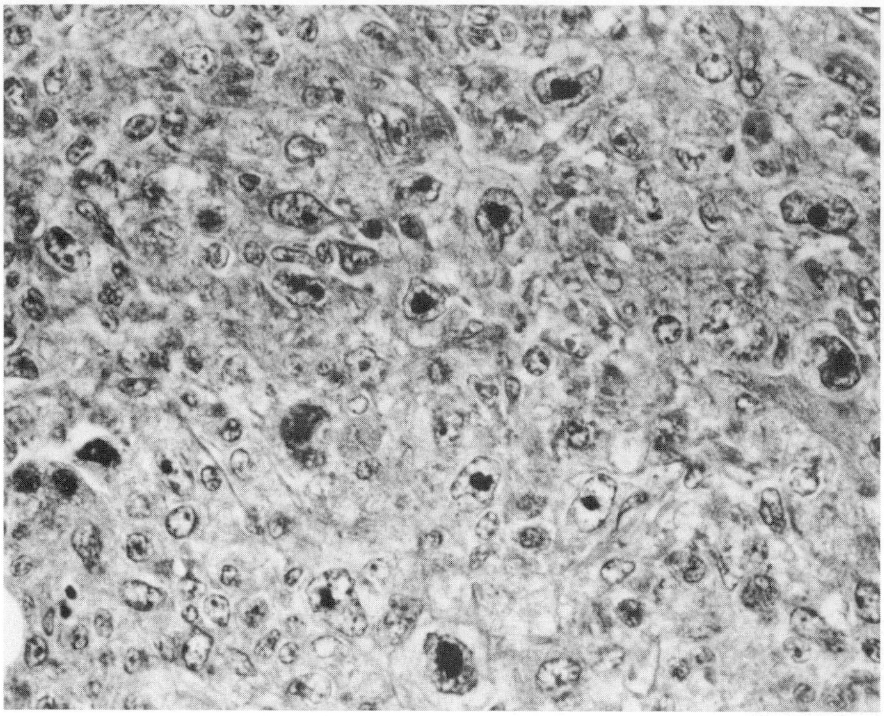

FIG. 39.4. A high-magnification view of the focal bone marrow lesion illustrated in Figure 39.3. It consists primarily of mononuclear Hodgkin's cells (hematoxylin and eosin stain, original magnification: 400× magnification).

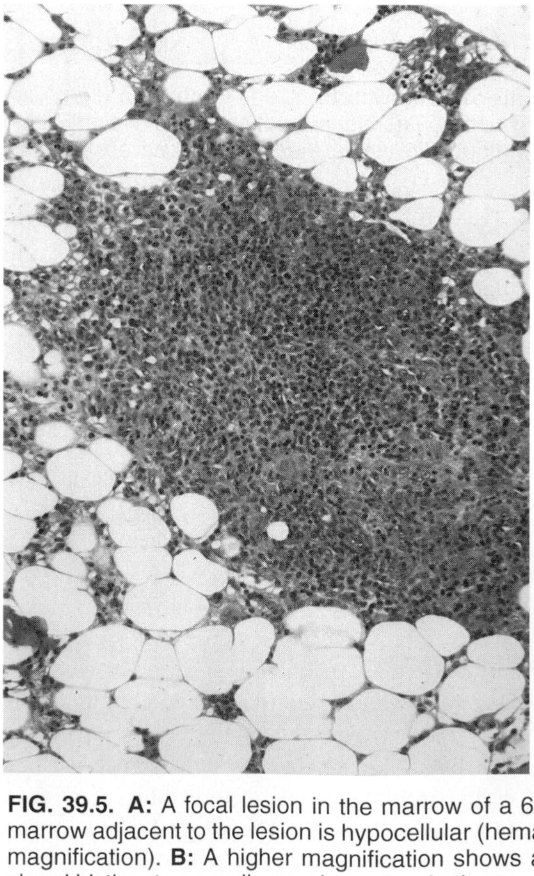

A

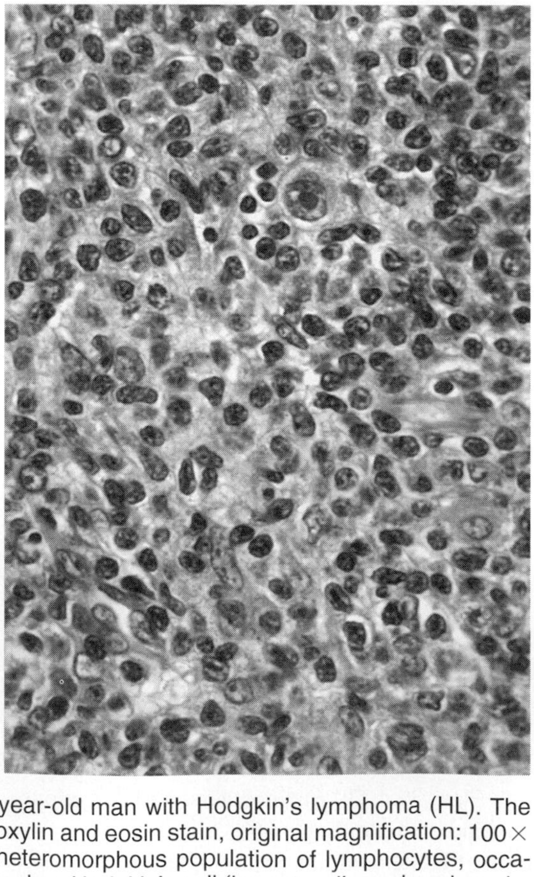

B

FIG. 39.5. A: A focal lesion in the marrow of a 62-year-old man with Hodgkin's lymphoma (HL). The marrow adjacent to the lesion is hypocellular (hematoxylin and eosin stain, original magnification: 100× magnification). **B:** A higher magnification shows a heteromorphous population of lymphocytes, occasional histiocytes, small vessels, and a single mononuclear Hodgkin's cell (hematoxylin and eosin stain, original magnification: 400× magnification).

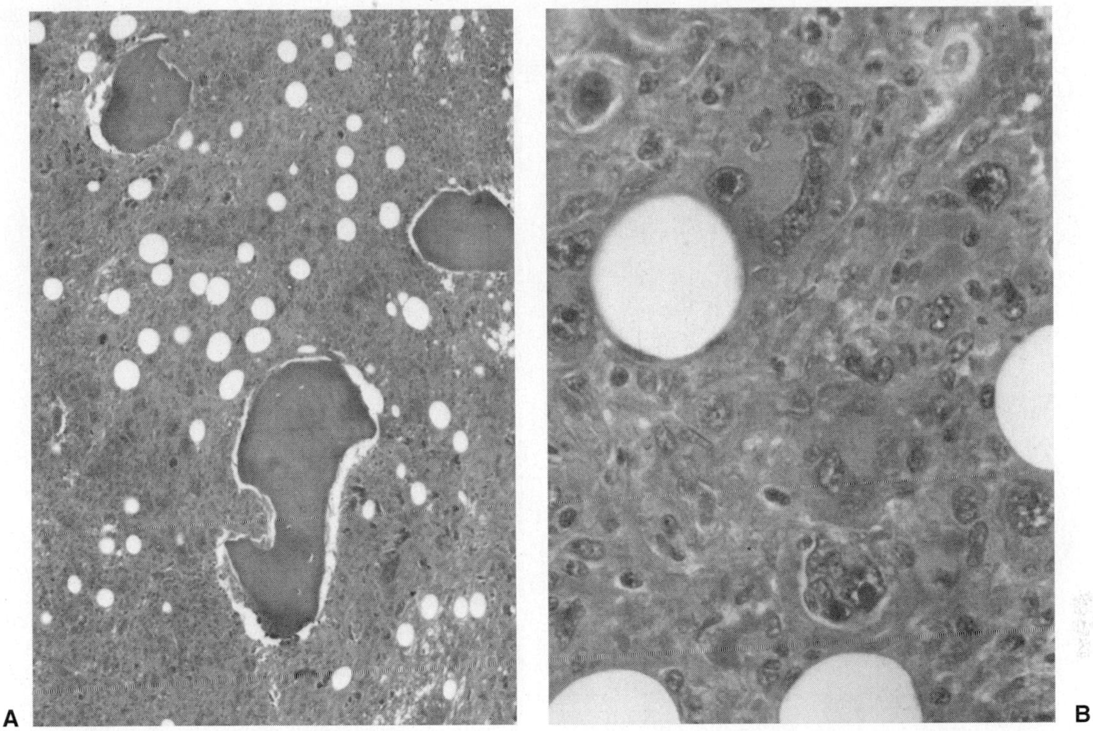

FIG. 39.6. Intermediate-magnification (A) and high-magnification (B) views of a trephine biopsy section with diffuse involvement by Hodgkin's lymphoma (HL). The lesion is depleted of lymphocytes and contains numerous Hodgkin's cells (hematoxylin and eosin stain, original magnifications: 250× and 400× magnification).

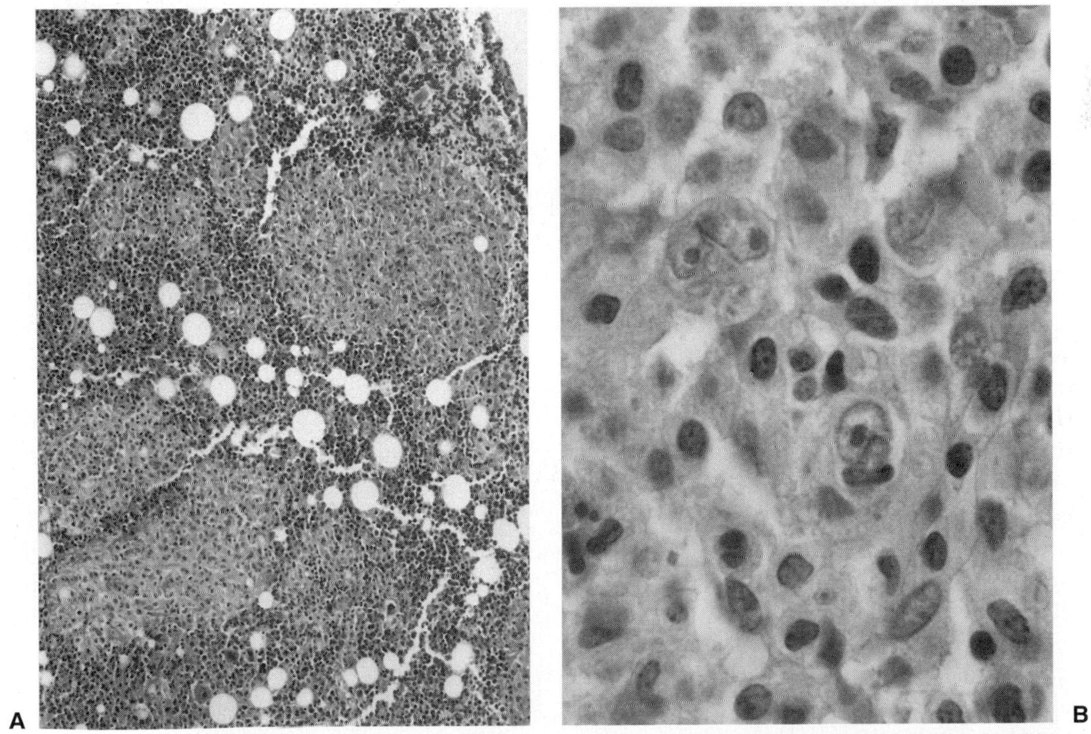

FIG. 39.7. Bone marrow aspirate clot section from a 23-year-old man with clinical stage IIIB nodular sclerosis Hodgkin's lymphoma (HL). **A:** Several focal lesions strongly resembling epithelioid granulomas at low power. These lesions were present in the clot section but not in the core biopsy, an unusual finding (hematoxylin and eosin stain, original magnification: 100× magnification). **B:** High-power examination reveals scattered Hodgkin's cells within the granulomatous infiltrate (hematoxylin and eosin stain, original magnification: 1,000× magnification).

A

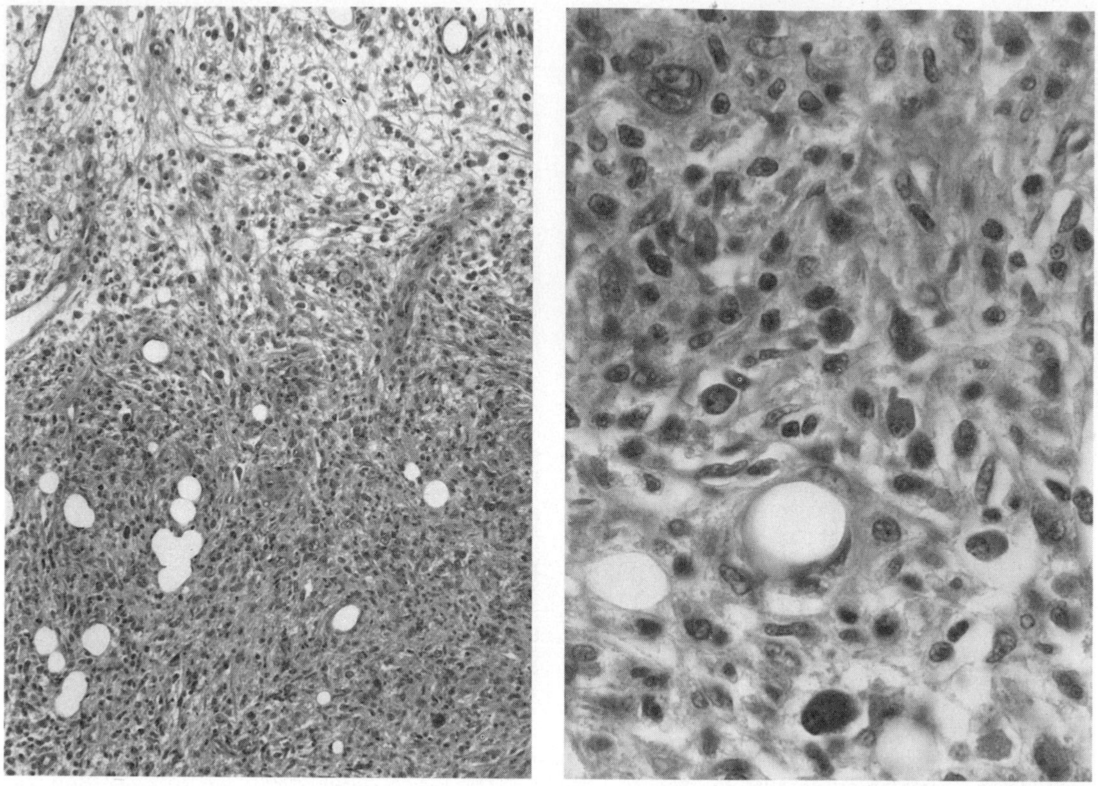

B

FIG. 39.8. A trephine biopsy from a 42-year-old man with stage IV Hodgkin's lymphoma (HL) shows diffuse marrow involvement (**A** and **B**). Most of the lesion is composed of loose fibrous connective tissue and a polycellular infiltrate. There are foci of greater cellularity. Rarely were Reed-Sternberg cells encountered in this case (hematoxylin and eosin stain, original magnifications: 40× and 250× magnification).

marrow necrosis, stromal damage) suggests that more extensive evaluation would have revealed definitive evidence of marrow HL in these cases.

Posttreatment Biopsies

The histopathology of posttreatment residual disease and relapse of HL in the bone marrow generally is similar to that of pretreatment lesions. Evolution to lesions with larger numbers of Hodgkin's cells occurs in some cases. Similar changes have been described in serial lymph node biopsies (75). Posterior iliac crest trephine biopsies taken from patients who have received radiotherapy to the iliac lymph nodes usually are markedly hypocellular or aplastic. These changes may persist even several years after therapy.

Necrosis of Hodgkin's tissue in bone marrow may be observed at diagnosis but is more often found in patients on chemotherapy (8). Usually only part of the Hodgkin's tissue is necrotic; patches of amorphous eosinophilic material with karyorrhectic and karyolytic cells may be found. The pattern of cellular infiltrate of the nonnecrotic tissue is otherwise similar to pretreatment lesions. The myelofibrotic component of Hodgkin's tissue is reversible with successful chemotherapy and often shows complete resolution (39). Occasionally, granulomas secondary to opportunistic infections such as cryptococcosis are observed separately or in association with HL lesions (see Chapter 50).

Blood Findings

Hodgkin's cells are not found on blood smears. Leukemoid and exudative reactions in the blood of patients who have HL have been associated with poor prognosis. Lymphocytopenia is an indicator of poor prognosis in patients who have advanced stage disease (36,55). In untreated patients, pancytopenia, neutropenia, or thrombocytopenia rarely are encountered unless the bone marrow is involved with HL or obvious hypersplenism is present. Neutrophilia, eosinophilia, thrombocytosis, and anemia are relatively common findings and are generally not considered reliable indicators of bone marrow involvement or prognosis (38,39,76). However, elevated sedimentation rates and thrombocytosis adversely affected treatment outcome in one series of advanced HL treated with chemotherapy (43).

Differential Diagnosis

Some of the NHLs may resemble HL in bone marrow sections. Peripheral T-cell lymphomas with a polymorphous cell proliferation and epithelioid histiocytes are particularly

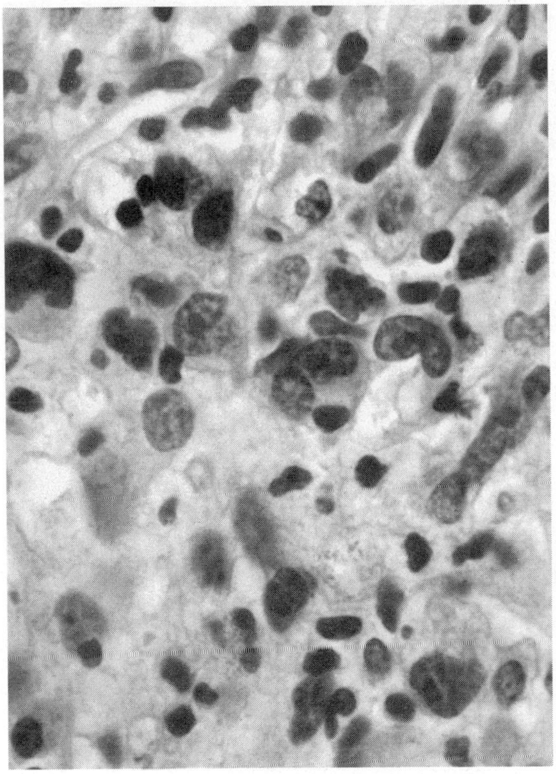

FIG. 39.9. Trephine biopsy from a 56-year-old man with peripheral T-cell lymphoma. The marrow infiltrate is heteromorphous, with a mixture of small lymphocytes, histiocytes, and large lobulated cells with prominent nucleoli, resembling Hodgkin's cells. However, some of the smaller cells are also irregular and hyperchromatic (hematoxylin and eosin stain, original magnification: 1,000× magnification).

problematic (Fig. 39.9) (65). The pattern of marrow involvement in T-cell– and histiocyte-rich large B-cell lymphomas, and occasionally follicular lymphomas, may manifest histologic features similar to HL (Fig. 39.10). Reed-Sternberg–like cells have been observed in the marrow of patients with NHL (65,70). In cases of NHL, the cytology of the lymphoma cells on marrow smears or trephine imprints may help distinguish the process from HL (65,77,78). A panel of antibodies to Hodgkin's cell–associated antigens and antigens of the major lymphocyte subsets can be applied to biopsy sections and usually clarify the diagnosis in problematic cases (16,17,79) (Table 39.2, Fig. 39.11). In some cases, biopsy of lymph node or other tissue may be necessary to resolve a differential diagnosis.

Reactive lymphoid lesions and granulomas are commonly found in bone marrow sections from patients with negative-staining marrow biopsies (8) (Fig. 39.12). Potentially, these can be misinterpreted as HL. Importantly, occasional HL lesions may closely resemble reactive epithelioid granulomas (Fig. 39.7). Other disorders that may resemble the bone marrow lesions of HL include myelofibrosis, Richter's syndrome, eosinophilic granuloma, and systemic mast cell disease. The features that distinguish these lesions from HL

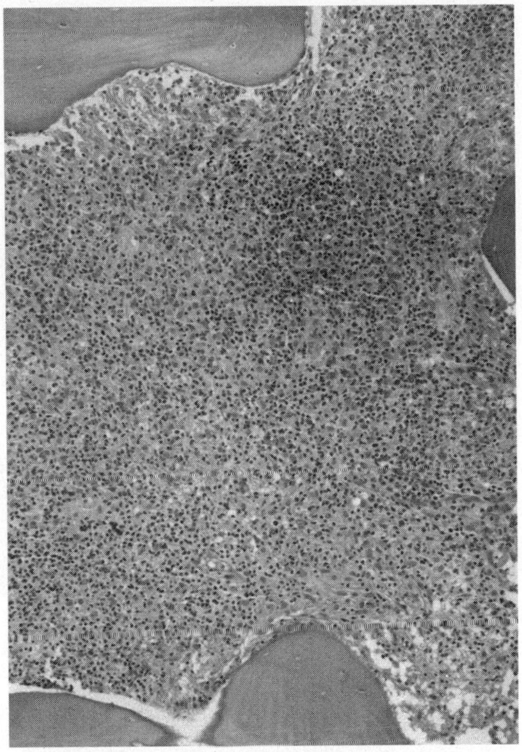

A

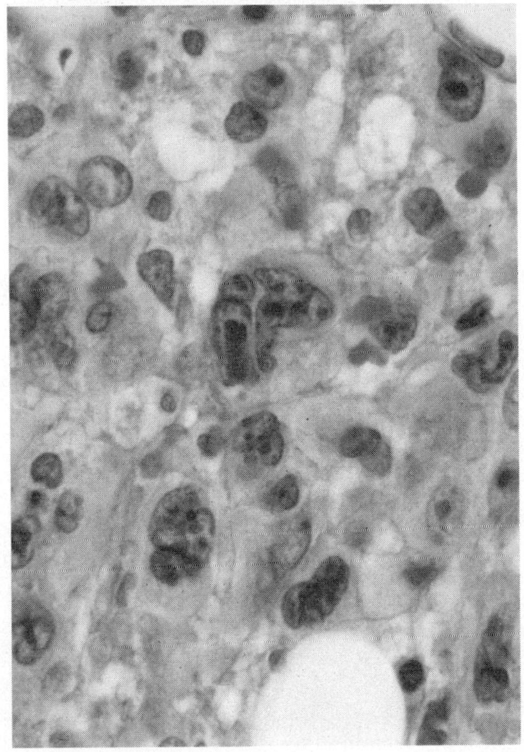

B

FIG. 39.10. Trephine biopsy from a 44-year-old man with a T-cell and histiocyte-rich large B-cell lymphoma diagnosed on a lymph node biopsy. **A:** This polymorphous infiltrate rich in histiocytes and small reactive lymphocytes diffusely involves the biopsy (hematoxylin and eosin stain, original magnification: 100× magnification). **B:** The neoplastic cells were relatively few in number and closely resembled Hodgkin's cells (hematoxylin and eosin stain, original magnification: 1,000× magnification).

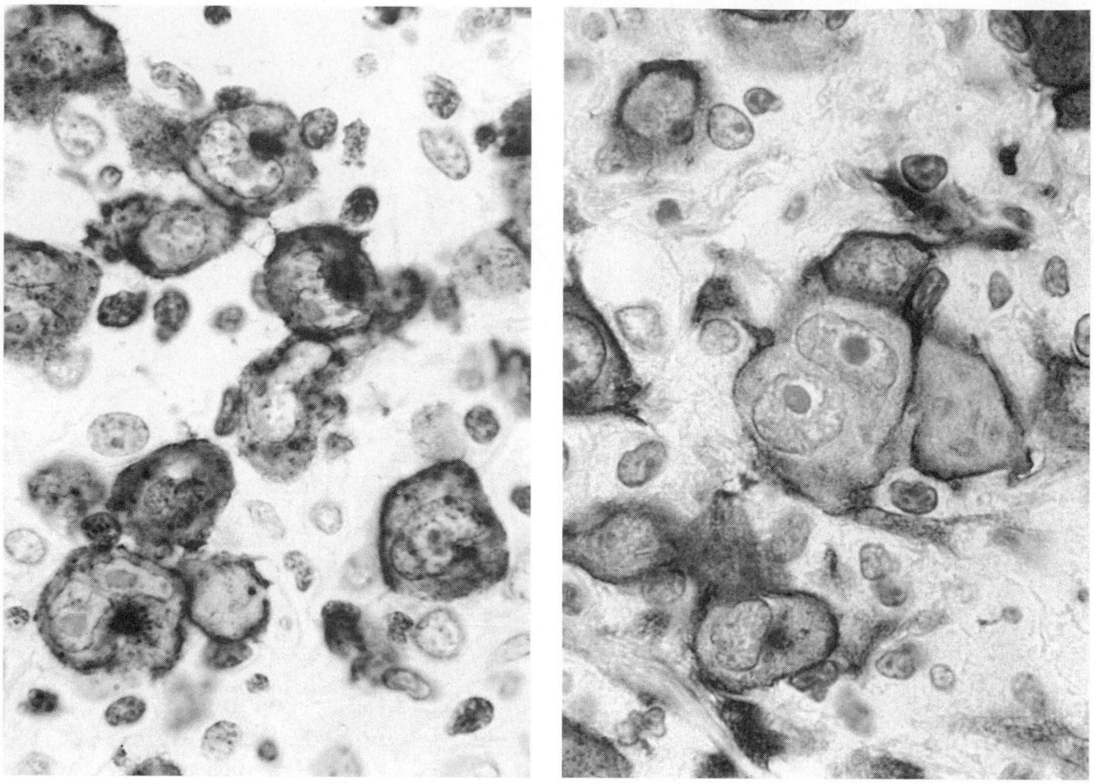

FIG. 39.11. **A:** A CD15 (Leu-M1) stain demonstrates membrane and Golgi-region staining in a lesion rich in Hodgkin's cells. **B:** A CD30 (BER-H2) stain demonstrates a similar pattern, although the Golgi staining is less prominent (hematoxylin and eosin stain, original magnification: 1,000× magnification).

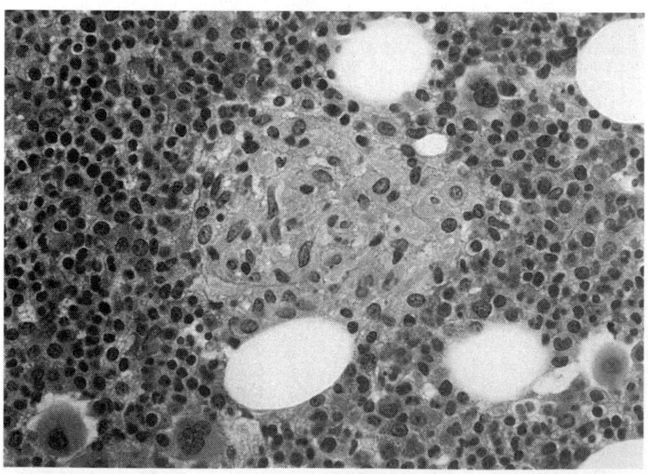

FIG. 39.12. A small, compact, epithelioid granuloma in negative-staging bone marrow in a patient with Hodgkin's lymphoma (HL). There was no evidence of HL in any of the marrow sections. Stains and cultures for microorganisms were negative. Nonspecific granulomas commonly are found in hematopoietic tissues of patients with HL, and these potentially can be mistaken for Hodgkin's tissue. The absence of Hodgkin's cells and sometimes the presence of Langhans' giant cells help distinguish the two (hematoxylin and eosin stain, original magnification: 400× magnification).

in bone marrow and other tissues are discussed later in this chapter and in other chapters.

Secondary myelodysplastic syndromes (MDS) and acute myeloid leukemias (AML) may follow treatment for HL with alkylating agent chemotherapy or radiotherapy. These therapy related myeloid disorders are associated with blood cytopenias and, in some instances, with fibrosis or reactive lymphocytic infiltrates (8,80,81). These changes may raise suspicion of recurrent HL. The absence of Hodgkin's cells and the presence of dysplastic changes or increased myeloblasts in blood smears, bone marrow smears, or trephine imprints should alert the pathologist to the correct diagnosis (2,81,82).

NON-HODGKIN'S LYMPHOMA

The utility of the bone marrow biopsy in patients who have NHL has been demonstrated in several studies (7,13,37, 83–87). Its importance in pathologic staging of patients who have clinical stages I and II disease and in monitoring patients with advanced disease for response to therapy is well documented (88). Some data suggest that the bone marrow biopsy findings may not contribute significantly to management decisions or provide useful prognostic information for patients who have advanced clinical stages of some categories of NHL (89). Despite this, bone marrow biopsies are presently performed routinely at diagnosis for most types of NHL (88).

Several detailed reports have addressed the incidence and morphologic features of marrow involvement in relationship to the Rappaport, Lukes-Collins, Kiel, or the International Working Formulation classifications (2,4,7,13,65,77,85–87, 90–93). The International Lymphoma Study Group (ILSG) has proposed a new classification of NHL, the ILSG classification (also known as the Revised European and American Lymphoma [REAL] Classification) (94) (see Chapters 19 and 20). Although no systematic studies of bone marrow lymphoma specifically using the ILSG classification have been published, translation between lymphoma subtypes in the various classifications is possible for many of the NHLs (94). The following discussion is organized according to the ILSG classification (94) (Table 39.3). Although this classification spans the entire spectrum of lymphoid neoplasia, only those diseases commonly regarded as lymphomas are addressed. The bone marrow manifestations of the other lymphoproliferative diseases are discussed in other chapters (Chapters 40, 41, 42, and 43).

Incidence of Marrow Involvement

The incidence of marrow involvement at the time of diagnosis of NHL (excluding chronic lymphocytic leukemia) is 30% to 53% (4,7,10,85–87,92,95–97). The NHLs that involve the bone marrow most frequently are subtypes primarily composed of small cells (small lymphocytic, follicle center lymphoma grade I, mantle cell lymphomas), high-grade lymphomas of lymphoblastic and Burkitt's types, and the various peripheral T-cell lymphomas (4,65,98,99).

Pattern and Extent of Marrow Involvement in Biopsy Sections

There are five patterns of bone marrow infiltration by NHLs, although mixed patterns may occur as well (Table 39.4, Figs. 39.13–39.15):

1. Focal, paratrabecular: Infiltrates that extend along trabeculae, sometimes producing irregularities of the bony surface. Although these may extend away from the trabeculae, one surface of the aggregate is intimately associated with the bone. This does not include random lesions that incidentally abut the bone tangentially.
2. Focal, random (nonparatrabecular): lesions that are surrounded by normal hematopoietic tissue and fat but that focally distort normal architecture.
3. Interstitial: lymphomatous infiltrates between normal adipose tissue without disruption of the overall marrow architecture.
4. Diffuse: infiltrates that efface marrow architecture between adjacent bony trabeculae.

TABLE 39.3. *International lymphoma study group classification of non-Hodgkin's lymphoma*

B-cell neoplasms

I. Precursor B-cell neoplasm: precursor B-lymphoblastic leukemia/lymphoma
II. Peripheral B-cell neoplasms
   1. B-cell chronic lymphocytic leukemia/prolymphocytic leukemia/small lymphocytic lymphoma
   2. Lymphoplasmacytoid lymphoma/immunocytoma
   3. Mantle cell lymphoma
   4. Follicle center lymphoma, follicular
      Provisional cytologic grades: I (small cell), II (mixed small and large cell), III (large cell)
      Provisional subtype: diffuse, predominantly small cell type
   5. Marginal zone B-cell lymphoma
      Extranodal (MALT-type ± monocytoid B cells)
      Provisional subtype: nodal (± monocytoid B cells)
   6. Provisional entity: splenic marginal zone lymphoma (± villous lymphocytes)
   7. Hairy cell leukemia
   8. Plasmacytoma/plasma cell myeloma
   9. Diffuse large B-cell lymphoma
      Subtype: primary mediastinal (thymic) B-cell lymphoma
   10. Burkitt's lymphoma
   11. Provisional entity: high-grade B-cell lymphoma, Burkitt-like

T-cell and putative natural killer cell neoplasms

I. Precursor T-cell neoplasm: precursor T-lymphoblastic lymphoma/leukemia
II. Peripheral T-cell and NK-cell neoplasms
   1. T-cell chronic lymphocytic leukemia/prolymphocytic leukemia
   2. Large granular lymphocyte leukemia (LGL)
      T-cell type
      NK-cell type
   3. Mycosis fungoides/Sezary syndrome
   4. Peripheral T-cell lymphomas, unspecified
      Provisional cytologic categories: medium-sized cell, mixed medium and large cell, large cell, lymphoepithelioid cell
      Provisional subtype: hepatosplenic $\gamma\delta$ T-cell lymphoma
      Provisional subtype: subcutaneous panniculitic T-cell lymphoma
   5. Angioimmunoblastic T-cell lymphoma (AILD)
   6. Angiocentric lymphoma
   7. Intestinal T-cell lymphoma (± enteropathy associated)
   8. Adult T-cell lymphoma/leukemia (ATL/L)
   9. Anaplastic large cell lymphoma (ALCL), CD30$^+$, T- and null-cell types
   10. Provisional entity: anaplastic large-cell lymphoma, Hodgkin-like

From Harris NL, Jaffe ES, Stein H, et al. A revised European-American classification of lymphoid neoplasms: a proposal from the International Lymphoma Study Group. *Blood* 1994;84:1361–1392, with permission.

TABLE 39.4. *Pattern and extent of bone marrow involvement by non-Hodgkin's lymphoma in trephine biopsies*

Marrow involvement	Percent involvement
Focal	≈70
Paratrabecular	≈40
Random	≈30
Diffuse and interstitial	≈30
Intrasinusoidal/intravascular	<5
Extent	
<30% of marrow replaced	≈55
30% to 70% of marrow replaced	≈20
>70% of marrow replaced	≈25

5. Sinusoidal or intravascular: infiltrates confined to endothelium-lined spaces.

Focal lesions are most common (about 70% of cases), with the paratrabecular pattern observed slightly more commonly than random lesions (4). In some cases, both patterns of focal involvement are present in the same specimen. The number of lesions varies from a single focus of involvement to several on each section.

Some categories of NHL manifest a predilection for a particular pattern of marrow infiltration. For example, the bone marrow lesions of grade I and II follicle center lymphomas are predominantly focal and paratrabecular; those of small lymphocytic lymphomas are usually randomly focal; Burkitt's and lymphoblastic lymphomas generally have an interstitial or diffuse pattern of infiltration; and splenic marginal zone, hepatosplenic $\gamma\delta$ T-cell, and angiotropic or intravascular lymphomas show a distinct intrasinusoidal or intravascular distribution (2,4,7,10,77,85,91,99–104).

The degree of bone marrow replacement correlates with the pattern of infiltration, which has been found to correlate with prognosis in some studies (93,105). With focal lesions, there is often considerable marrow sparing, with less than 30% of the marrow space occupied by malignant lymphoma (4). With advanced disease, focal lesions enlarge and may coalesce and occupy a greater proportion of the marrow. With interstitial infiltration, much of the hematopoietic tissue and marrow fat are often spared. Diffuse involvement is associated with extensive replacement of normal marrow

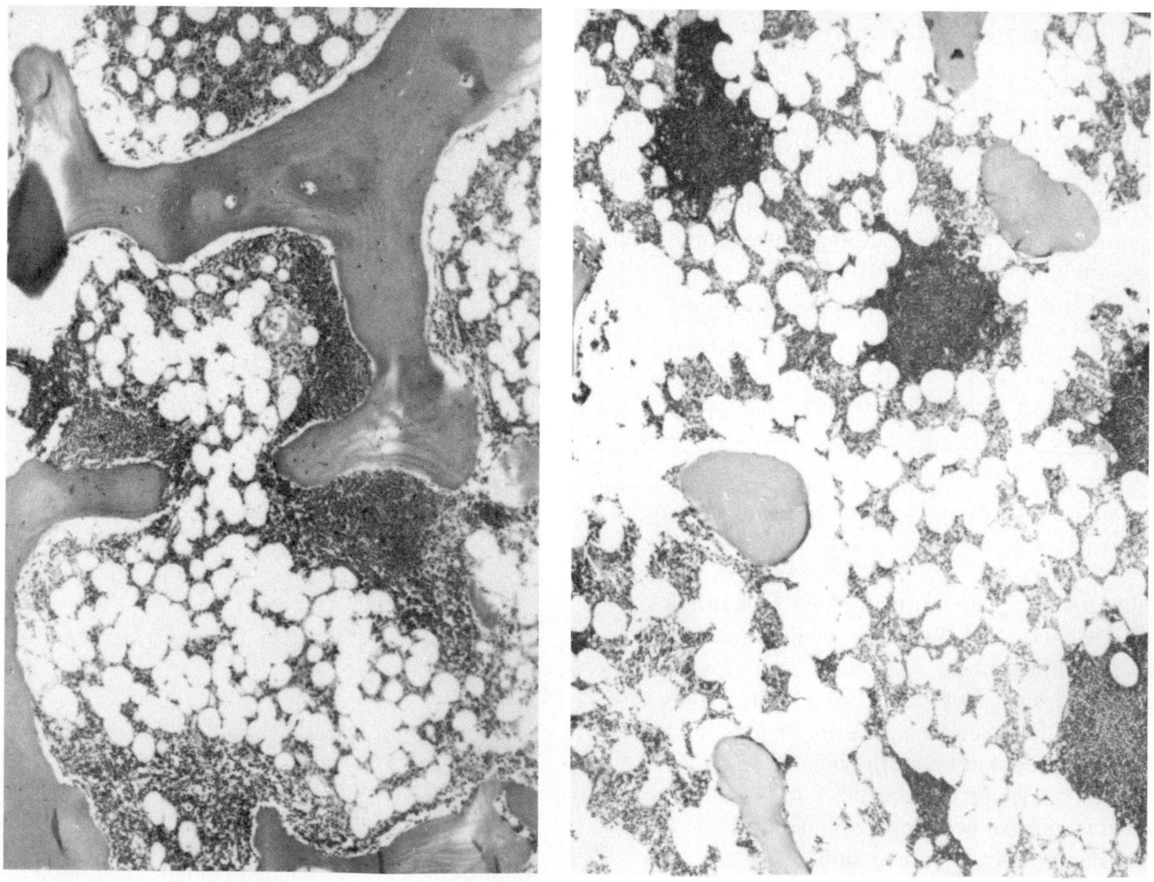

A B

FIG. 39.13. A: A bone marrow trephine biopsy section with a focal paratrabecular pattern of involvement in a patient with grade I follicle center lymphoma (hematoxylin and eosin stain, original magnification: 450× magnification). **B:** A focal random (nonparatrabecular) distribution of lesions in a bone marrow trephine biopsy section from a patient with small lymphocytic lymphoma (hematoxylin and eosin stain, original magnification: 40× magnification).

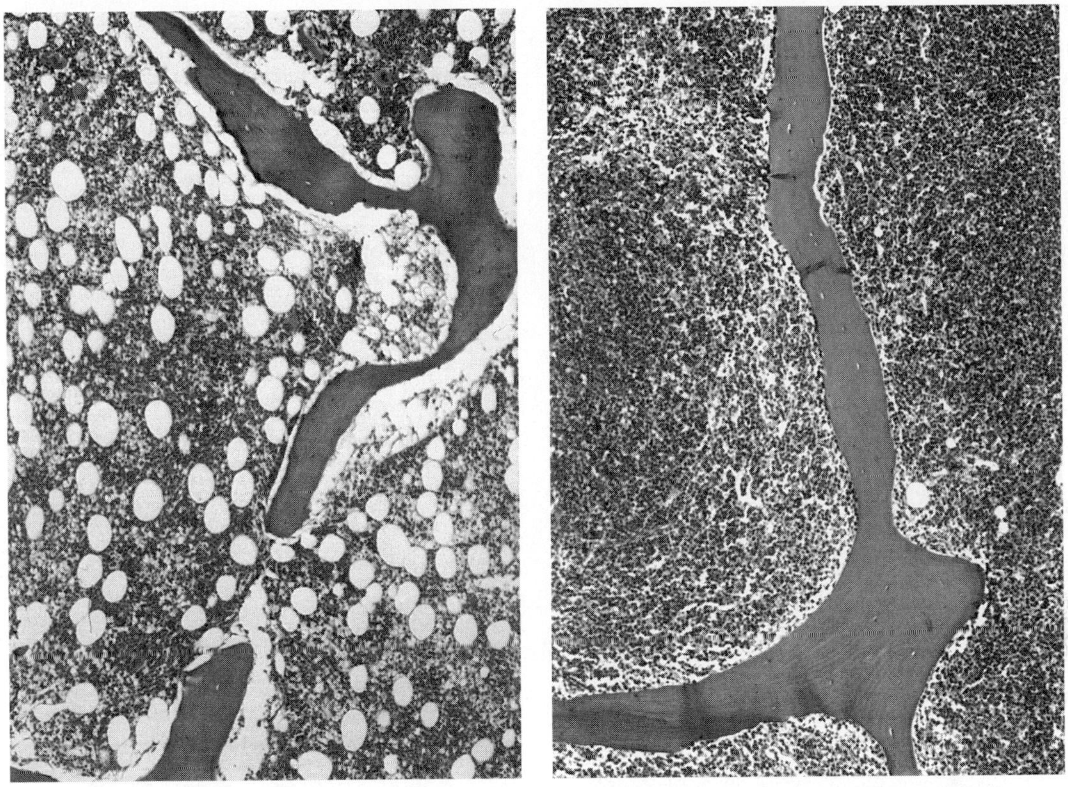

FIG. 39.14. A: Interstitial pattern of involvement in a patient with mantle cell lymphoma. The marrow is normocellular, and the lymphoma infiltrate is barely perceptible at this magnification (hematoxylin and eosin stain, original magnification: 40× magnification). **B:** This trephine biopsy section shows a diffuse pattern of infiltration in a patient with Burkitt's lymphoma. The hematopoietic marrow and fat are completely replaced (hematoxylin and eosin stain, original magnification: 40× magnification).

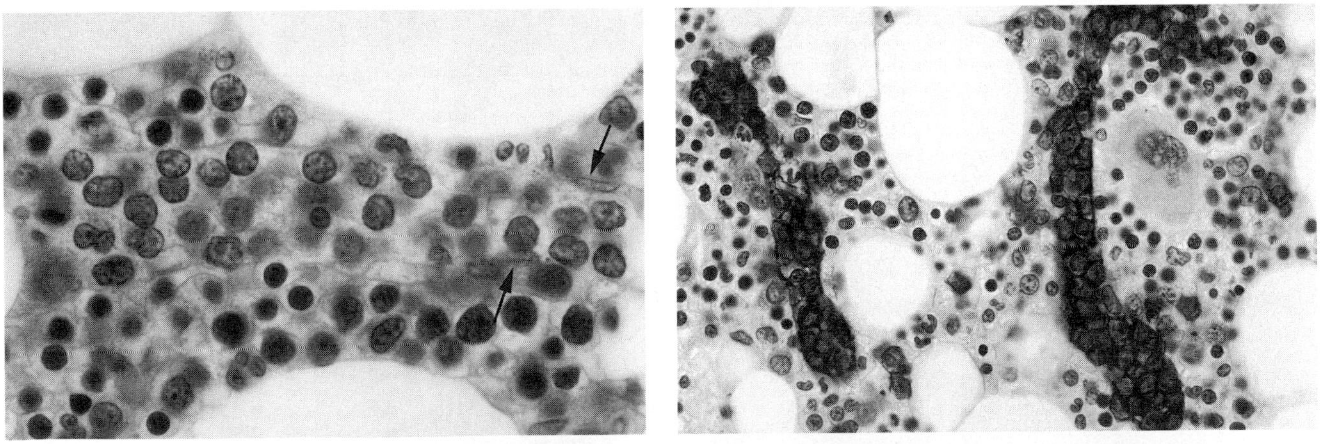

FIG. 39.15. A bone marrow trephine section in a patient with splenic marginal zone lymphoma shows a distinct sinusoidal pattern of marrow infiltration. **A:** A small sinusoid is filled by a population of small lymphoid cells with slightly irregular nuclei, moderately condensed chromatin, and moderate amounts of pale cytoplasm. Endothelial cells *(arrows)* can be seen lining the sinusoid (hematoxylin and eosin stain, original magnification: 400× magnification). **B:** Immunohistochemistry with anti-CD20 (L26) highlights the intrasinusoidal pattern (hematoxylin and eosin stain, original magnification: 400× magnification).

elements. Intrasinusoidal or intravascular involvement spares normal hematopoietic marrow, and is often quite subtle. This pattern may also coexist with other patterns of infiltration.

Morphologic Discordance of Lymph Node and Bone Marrow Histology

Differences in morphologic appearance of lymphomatous infiltrates between lymph node and bone marrow (histologic discordance) is observed in 9% to 40% of cases (4,10,95, 96,106–109). The more aggressive subtype usually is found in the lymph node. Divergent histology is most common with follicle center and diffuse large cell lymphomas (4,95,96,106,107). A typical discordant pattern is a lymph node with a diffuse large cell lymphoma with lesions composed of small cells in the bone marrow (Fig. 39.16) (4,95,107). In fact, in some studies, most lymphomatous bone marrow infiltrates in patients with large cell lymphoma are discordant small cell lesions (96,110). For patients who have large cell lymphomas, bone marrow lesions with histologic features of a low-grade lymphoma do not adversely impact prognosis; median survival for these patients is similar to that of patients who have no marrow involvement (96,106,110). An aggressive histology in the marrow of a patient who has a low-grade lymphoma in a lymph node portends a poor prognosis (107). In most cases, the divergent histologies in lymph node and marrow appear to represent the same neoplastic clone (107).

B-Cell Neoplasms

Precursor-B-Cell Neoplasms

Compared with their more common T-cell counterparts, little information is available regarding manifestations of lymphoblastic lymphoma of precursor-B–lineage (B-LBL) presenting primarily in extramedullary sites. From what little is available, it appears that these tumors have a propensity to manifest in skin or bone, lack mediastinal involvement, and have a high frequency of bone marrow involvement (111–117). As with precursor-T-cell lymphoblastic lymphoma (T-LBL), the distinction from acute lymphoblastic leukemia (ALL) rests on arbitrary criteria, most commonly the percentage of bone marrow lymphoblasts. The morphologic characteristics and differential diagnosis of B-LBL are

A

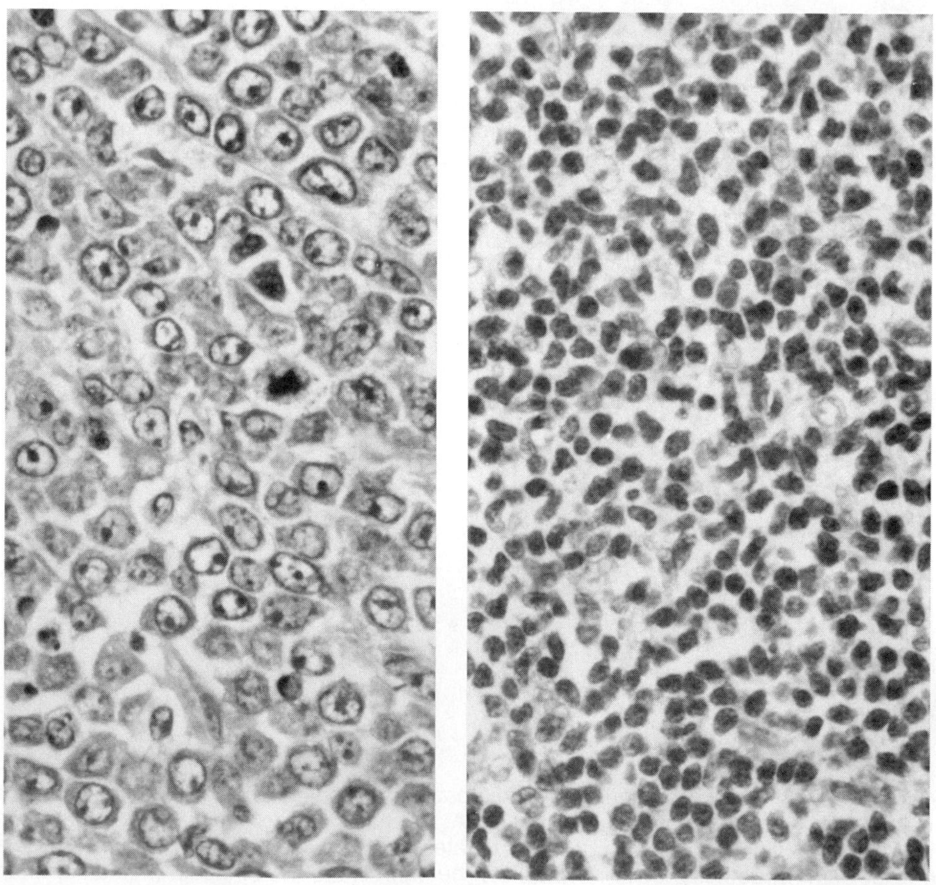

B

FIG. 39.16. Morphologic discordance of lymph node and bone marrow histology. **A:** A lymph node biopsy showed follicular large cell lymphoma (hematoxylin and eosin stain, original magnification: 400× magnification). **B:** The bone marrow trephine biopsy section showed focal paratrabecular lesions that consisted of mostly small cleaved cells (hematoxylin and eosin stain, original magnification: 400× magnification).

essentially the same as for T-LBL, and are discussed in that section. However, one differential diagnosis that bears mentioning is that of nonhematopoietic small blue cell tumors, particularly Ewing's sarcoma, because of the occasional presentation of B-LBL as lytic bone lesions. B-LBLs may show positive immunohistochemical staining for CD99 (MIC2), which is expressed in Ewing's sarcomas and peripheral neuroectodermal tumors. At the same time, they may be negative for CD20 and CD45 in paraffin sections and may be misdiagnosed as Ewing's sarcoma (117–119). Use of a more extensive panel of markers, in particular the addition of CD79a and terminal deoxynucleotidyl transferase (TdT), alleviates diagnostic difficulties in these lesions (117) (see Chapter 26).

Peripheral B-Cell Neoplasms

Small lymphocytic lymphoma (SLL) is the term used for lymphomas that are morphologically and immunophenotypically indistinguishable from chronic lymphocytic leukemia (CLL), but lack peripheral lymphocytosis (94,120–122). The proportion of SLL cases that subsequently develop lymphocytosis is somewhat controversial (94,120,121); clonal B cells may be present in the blood even in the absence of absolute lymphocytosis (123).

Small lymphocytic lymphoma involves the bone marrow in 58% to 89% of cases (4,10,121,122). In trephine biopsy sections, the proliferative lymphocytes generally are cytologically uniform with mature features. The nuclei are generally round with clumped chromatin and small nucleoli (Fig. 39.17). Occasionally, the nuclear contours are slightly irregular. Prolymphocytes are generally not prominent, and proliferation centers are uncommon. The pattern of involvement in trephine biopsy sections is randomly focal or interstitial in most cases (Fig. 39.18). A diffuse pattern or combination of focal and interstitial infiltration may be observed with extensive marrow replacement. Focal lesions are round, oval, or irregular in shape with sharply or poorly circumscribed margins (Fig. 39.18). Paratrabecular aggregates are essentially never encountered, although extensive infiltrates can abut trabeculae. An increase in small lymphocytes may be seen in areas between foci of lymphoma. Considerable preservation of normal marrow usually is observed even with relatively extensive marrow infiltration.

The bone marrow smears are usually diagnostic, generally

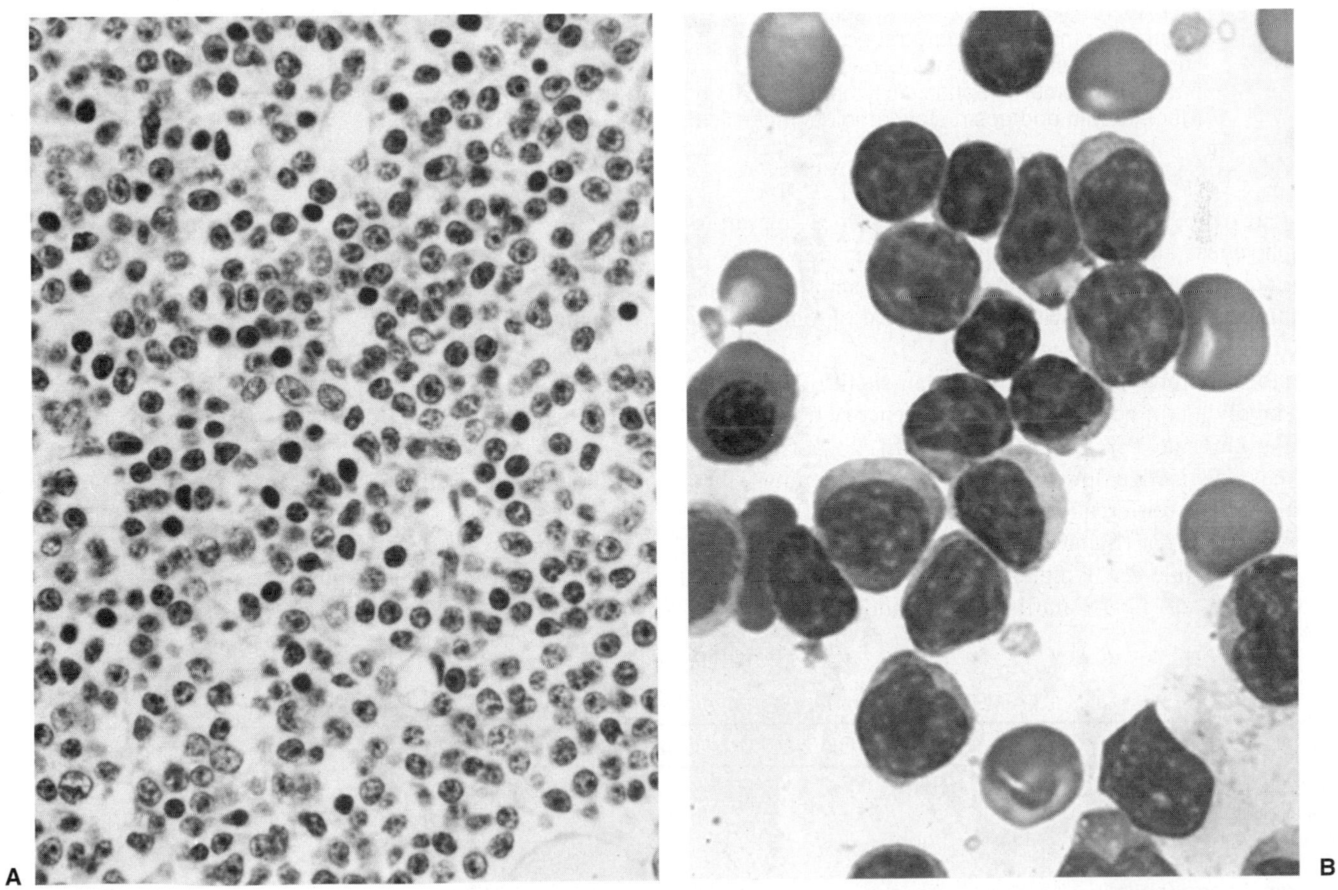

FIG. 39.17. A: Trephine biopsy section of a focal marrow lesion in a patient who has a small lymphocytic lymphoma (hematoxylin and eosin stain, original magnification: 400× magnification). **B:** A bone marrow aspirate smear from the same case shows numerous small lymphocytes with round nuclei, clumped chromatin, inconspicuous nucleoli, and scant cytoplasm (Wright-Giemsa stain, original magnification: 1,000× magnification).

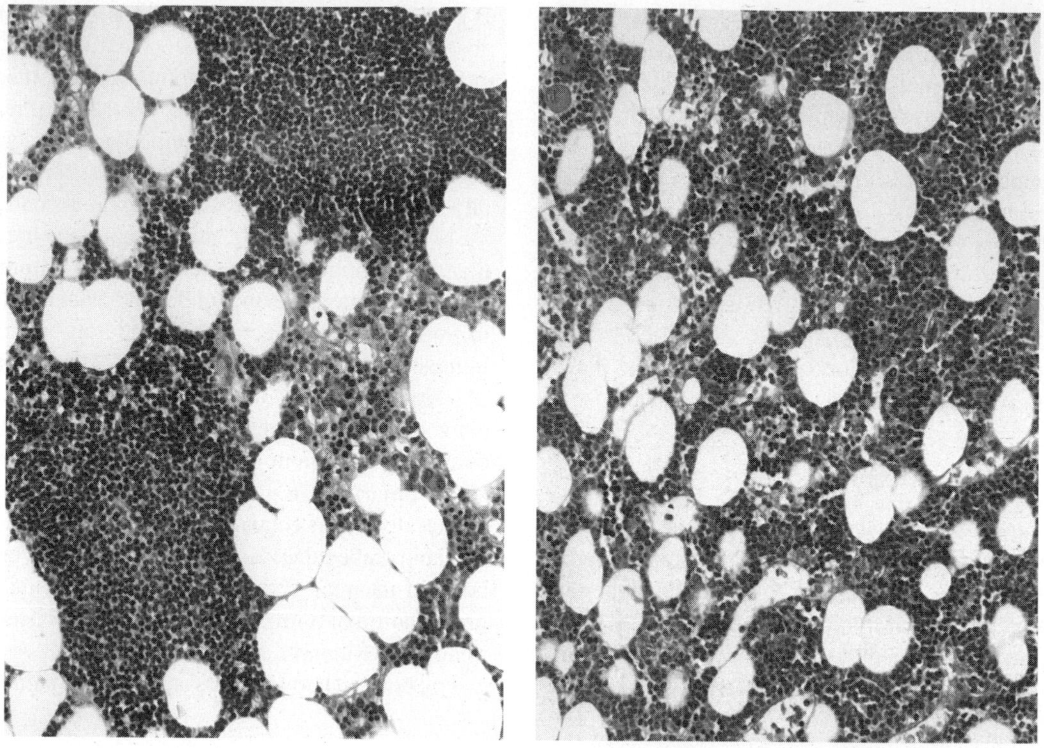

A B

FIG. 39.18. **A:** Trephine biopsy section from a 67-year-old man who has a small lymphocytic lymphoma. There is a random (nonparatrabecular) focal pattern of lymphoma involvement in the marrow (hematoxylin and eosin stain, original magnification: 100× magnification). **B:** A trephine biopsy section from another patient with small lymphocytic lymphoma. The pattern of bone marrow involvement is largely interstitial (hematoxylin and eosin stain, original magnification: 100× magnification).

showing a moderate or marked increase in mature-appearing lymphocytes, although occasionally a case shows only a minimal increase. The cells have sparse to moderate cytoplasm and round nuclei with coarse nuclear chromatin; nucleoli generally are lacking (Fig. 39.17).

In the differential diagnosis with other small B-cell disorders involving the bone marrow, the presence of true paratrabecular infiltrates essentially excludes SLL/CLL. CLL/SLL also has a distinctive flow cytometric immunophenotype that usually allows differentiation from other small B-cell processes (124–128) (Table 39.5). In paraffin sections, SLL/CLL and mantle cell lymphomas usually coexpress CD20 and CD43 (129–131). Paraffin-reactive antibodies to CD23 (expressed in CLL/SLL but not in mantle cell lymphoma) and cyclin D1 (expressed in mantle cell lymphoma but not CLL/SLL) have also proved to be useful in the differential diagnosis (26,130–136).

Lymphoplasmacytoid lymphoma or immunocytoma (LpL) is the term used to describe lymphoproliferations composed of a maturational spectrum ranging from small mature lymphocytes to plasma cells (94). Because plasmacytoid differentiation is not restricted to this lymphoma subtype, lesions showing features of other NHLs should not be designated LpL. This is particularly relevant to marginal zone lymphomas, in which plasmacytoid differentiation is relatively common. Since the recognition of marginal zone subtypes

TABLE 39.5. *Immunophenotypic features of small B-cell malignancies*

B-cell malignancies	CD19	CD20	CD5	CD10	CD23	FMC7	sIg	CD43	CD22	CD11c	CD103
Small lymphocytic	+	+ (dim)	+	−	+	± (dim)	Dim	+	±	±	−
Lymphoplasmacytoid	+	+	−	−	±	±	+	±	+	±	−
Mantle cell	+	+ (bright)	+	−	−	+	+	+	+	−	−
Follicle center	+	+	−	+	±	+	+	−	+	−	−
Marginal zone (nodal and extranodal)	+	+	−	−	−	+	+	±	+	±	−
Splenic marginal zone	+	+	−	−	±	+	+	−	+	±	± (dim)
Hairy cell leukemia	+	+	−	−	−	+	+	−	+ (bright)	+ (bright)	+ (bright)

of lymphoma, diagnoses of LpL have become distinctly uncommon; most that do receive this designation are accompanied by monoclonal immunoglobulin M gammopathy and satisfy clinicopathologic criteria for Waldenström's macroglobulinemia (WM) (94).

The bone marrow is involved in WM in 80% of patients at presentation, and in virtually all patients at some point during the clinical course (137). In contrast, lymphocytosis is uncommon (121,137,138). The cells of LpL in aspirate smears demonstrate a spectrum of morphology, including small lymphocytes resembling those of SLL; plasmacytoid lymphocytes with more abundant, deeply basophilic cytoplasm and eccentric nuclei; plasma cells, which may show morphologic abnormalities; and in occasional cases, substantial numbers of immunoblasts (137,139). A similar heterogeneous population is seen in trephine biopsy sections. These forms are present in various proportions, and the distribution of cell types forms the basis of proposed subclassifications of LpL into lymphoplasmacytoid, lymphoplasmacytic, and polymorphous subtypes (137,139,140). These have been related to pattern of bone marrow invasion and prognosis (137). All subtypes may contain intranuclear, periodic acid–Schiff–positive immunoglobulin inclusions (Dutcher bodies). These inclusions may also be seen in extranodal marginal zone lymphomas, multiple myeloma, and occasionally in reactive proliferations. The patterns of bone marrow involvement, in decreasing frequency, are focal, random; mixed focal and interstitial; and diffuse. Occasional paratrabecular infiltrates may be seen (137).

The differential diagnosis of LpL in bone marrow includes SLL/CLL, multiple myeloma, and other subtypes of lymphoma demonstrating plasmacytoid differentiation. The immunophenotype of LpL is shown in Table 39.5 (94,138,141). The lack of CD5 is a useful differential diagnostic feature with CLL, although CD5 expression is occasionally encountered in otherwise typical WM (personal observation). However, CLL, when strictly defined, almost never shows true plasmacytoid differentiation morphologically. LpL is usually negative for CD23 (141,142). The neoplastic cells may show phenotypic evidence of plasmacytoid differentiation, such as diminished expression of pan-B-cell markers and surface immunoglobulin, and increased expression of CD38. Clonal plasma cells may be present as well. Occasional myelomas are composed of relatively small cells with little cytoplasm, imparting a deceptively lymphoid appearance in aspirate smears and sections (Fig. 39.19). In paraffin sections, the

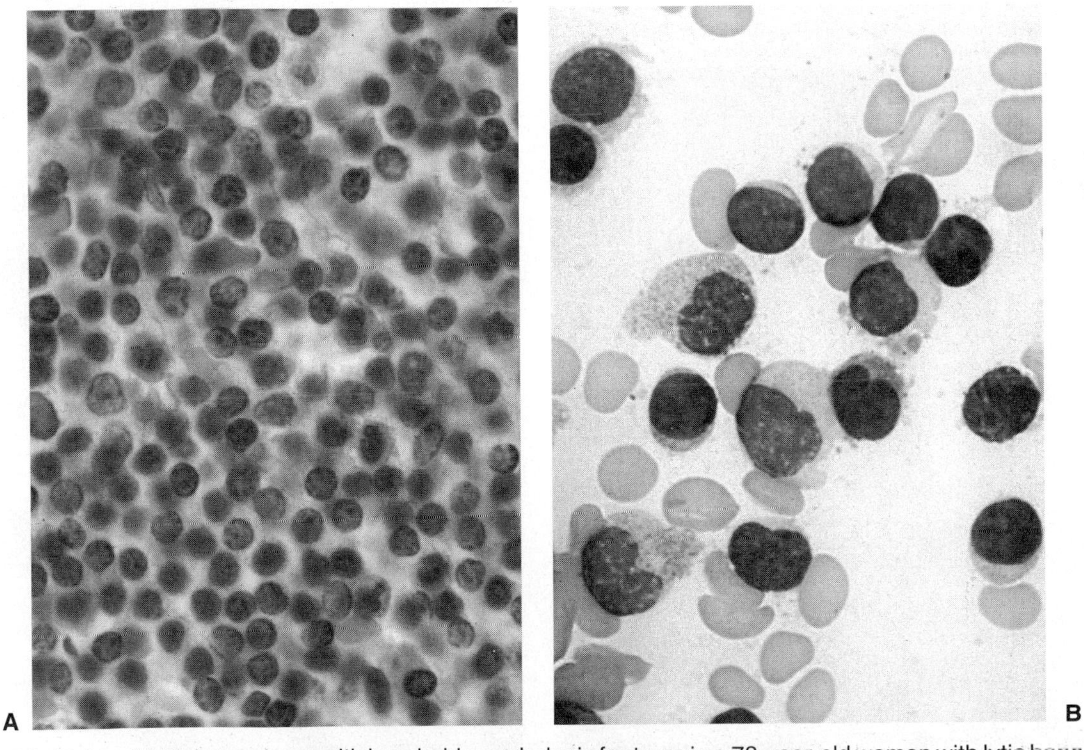

FIG. 39.19. Multiple myeloma with lymphoid morphologic features in a 78-year-old woman with lytic bone lesions and renal failure. **A:** The bone marrow trephine biopsy section demonstrates a monomorphous population of small round cells with little evident plasmacytoid differentiation (hematoxylin and eosin stain, original magnification: 1,000× magnification). **B:** The bone marrow aspirate smear demonstrates multiple abnormal plasma cells. These have round or indented nuclei with smooth to clumped chromatin, inconspicuous nucleoli, and little cytoplasm. A few of the cells have slightly more cytoplasm with eccentric nuclear placement. However, without other clinical and laboratory data these cells are extremely difficult to recognize as plasma cells (Wright-Giemsa stain, original magnification: 1,000× magnification).

presence of light-chain restricted cytoplasmic immunoglobulin and lack of significant CD20 and CD45 expression is strongly suggestive of myeloma.

Mantle cell lymphoma is a term that encompasses lymphomas previously designated as centrocytic, intermediately differentiated lymphocytic lymphoma, and mantle zone lymphoma (143). Three architectural patterns in tissue biopsies have been described: mantle zone, nodular, and diffuse, with the last generally found to be most common (144–154).

Mantle cell lymphoma is usually disseminated at presentation, with involvement of the bone marrow in 53% to 93% of cases (145,146,148,150,154–158). The bone marrow may be the initial diagnostic tissue biopsy. The frequency of bone marrow involvement is highest in cases with a diffuse pattern and lowest in those with a mantle zone pattern in extramedullary tissues (145). Occasionally, patients who have a mantle cell lymphoma present with spleen and marrow involvement, without peripheral lymphadenopathy (159). Peripheral blood involvement is detected morphologically at presentation in as many as 80% of patients, although fewer than one third have an absolute lymphocytosis (149,150,154,157). Leukemic involvement portends a poor prognosis (144,149,154).

Traditionally, mantle cell lymphoma cells have been described as being cytologically intermediate between small lymphocytic and small cleaved lymphoma cells (Fig. 39.20) (151,160–163), but a wide morphologic spectrum exists (147,150,164–167). The individual nuclei in sections and smears may be round, resembling SLL/CLL cells; slightly irregular; frankly cleaved, resembling small cleaved follicle center cells; highly irregular; or blastoid, resembling lymphoblasts (Fig. 39.21). Plasmacytoid differentiation is essentially never seen. The chromatin tends to be more coarse than in follicle center cells. Rarely, the cells are large with prominent nucleoli, mimicking large cell lymphoma. The cells often are quite pleomorphic in smears of blood or marrow, more than would be expected from the appearance in sections, and may contain distinct nucleoli (167,168). Most cases demonstrate a combination of infiltration patterns in trephine biopsies, with about three fourths showing areas of focal random infiltration, one half to two thirds showing an interstitial pattern, and a diffuse pattern in one fourth to one third of cases (150,157,167). About half of cases show areas of paratrabecular localization. Another characteristic feature, although not uniformly present, is the presence of large ''pink'' histiocytes within the neoplastic infiltrates (157).

Mantle cell lymphoma may be difficult to distinguish from other small B-cell lesions in bone marrow. The pattern of bone marrow involvement may be useful, in that a focal

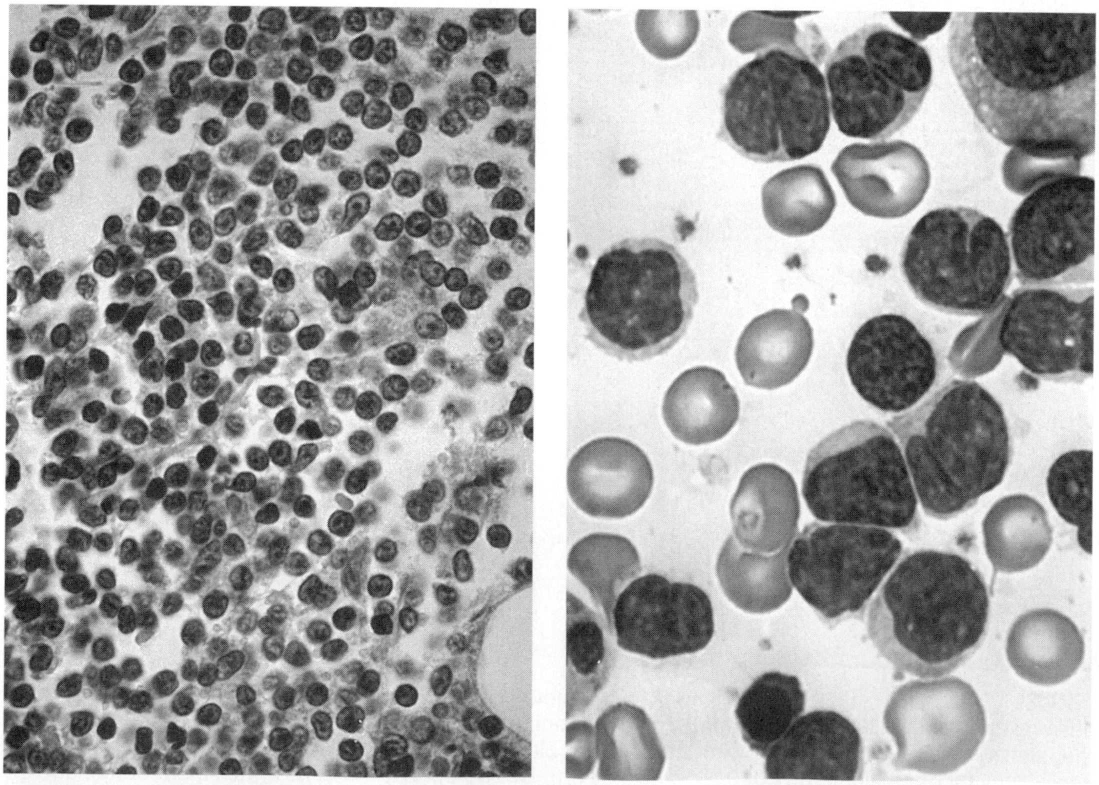

A B

FIG. 39.20. A: High-magnification view of a trephine biopsy section from a patient with mantle cell lymphoma. The nuclei range from round to slightly irregular and have relatively condensed nuclear chromatin (hematoxylin and eosin stain, original magnification: 400× magnification). **B:** A marrow aspirate smear from the same patient shows lymphocytes with coarse nuclear chromatin and indented or partially cleaved nuclei (Wright-Giemsa stain, original magnification: 1,000× magnification).

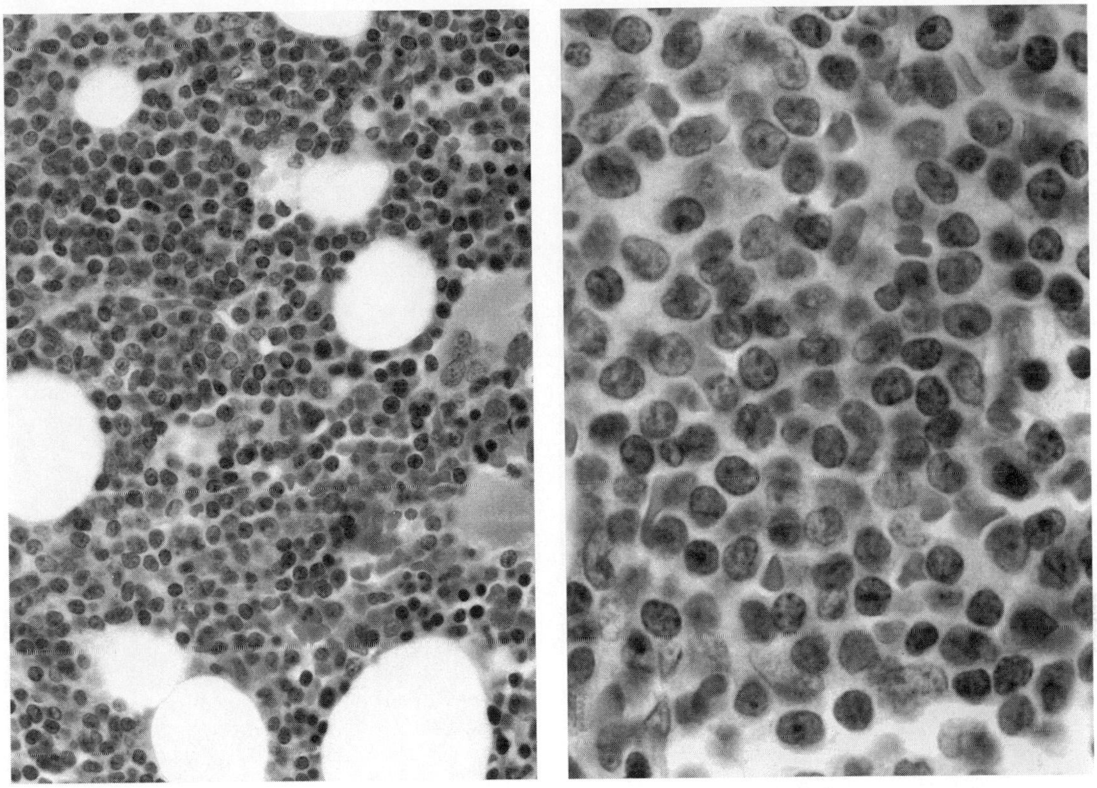

FIG. 39.21. Bone marrow trephine biopsy section containing blastoid mantle cell lymphoma. **A:** Interstitial infiltration of neoplastic cells. This pattern heightened the resemblance to lymphoblastic lymphoma (hematoxylin and eosin stain, original magnification: 400× magnification). **B:** The cells are small to intermediate in size with fine chromatin, round to irregular nuclei, and indistinct cytoplasm (hematoxylin and eosin stain, original magnification: 1,000× magnification).

paratrabecular pattern is often evident, ruling out CLL/SLL. Mantle cell lymphomas have a characteristic immunophenotype by flow cytometry, which allows distinction from SLL/CLL (124,127,130–132,141,144,149,169,170) (Table 39.5). Mantle cell lymphomas lack CD23 expression in paraffin sections, in contrast to CLL/SLL. Cases of blastoid mantle cell lymphoma may closely mimic acute lymphoblastic leukemia/lymphoblastic lymphoma (LBL/ALL) (Fig. 39.21). However, despite the blastoid cytology, the lesions in the trephine biopsy usually have areas of focal infiltration, a pattern that is not seen in cases of LBL/ALL. Immunohistochemistry is also useful, because mantle cell lymphoma shows strong CD20 expression and lacks TdT. LBL/ALL of B or T lineage expresses TdT; in addition T-LBL/ALL expresses T-cell antigens, and B-LBL/ALL generally have weak or absent expression of CD20.

Ultimately, the most important distinguishing feature of mantle cell lymphoma is overexpression of cyclin D1, often in association with a t(11;14)(q13;q32) and rearrangements of the *BCL1* gene (135,136,171–177). Cyclin D1 may be detected in paraffin sections, including decalcified bone marrow sections, in most mantle cell lymphomas, whereas it is not overexpressed in normal lymphoid cells and only rarely found in other lymphoma types (26,131,134,178–181) (see Chapter 22).

Follicle center lymphomas, grades I and *II* (follicular predominantly small cleaved cell and mixed small cleaved and large cell lymphomas), have a high incidence (50% to 60%) of marrow involvement at diagnosis when bilateral trephine biopsies are performed (4,7,10,77). Immunohistochemistry for B-cell markers may highlight subtle infiltrates that are not evident on routine preparations (21). In trephine biopsy sections the predominant pattern of marrow infiltration is focal with a distinctly paratrabecular distribution (77,85) (Figs. 39.13, 39.22). Even when the marrow is heavily infiltrated and individual lesions coalesce, the paratrabecular concentration of lymphoma still can be appreciated. In most instances, the lymphoma cells are predominantly small cleaved cells regardless of the lymph node histology (4,77) (Fig. 39.22). In a minority of cases, a broad morphologic spectrum of lymphocytes is observed, including large cleaved and noncleaved cells, small cleaved cells, and small mature appearing lymphocytes (77). Transformation of bone marrow lesions from predominantly small cleaved to large cleaved or noncleaved cells may occur in some instances. Transformed lymphoma cells that resemble Reed-Sternberg cells occasionally are found in these cases (70).

Marrow lesions that resemble germinal centers occasionally are seen. These consist of a central concentration of large cleaved and noncleaved lymphocytes with small

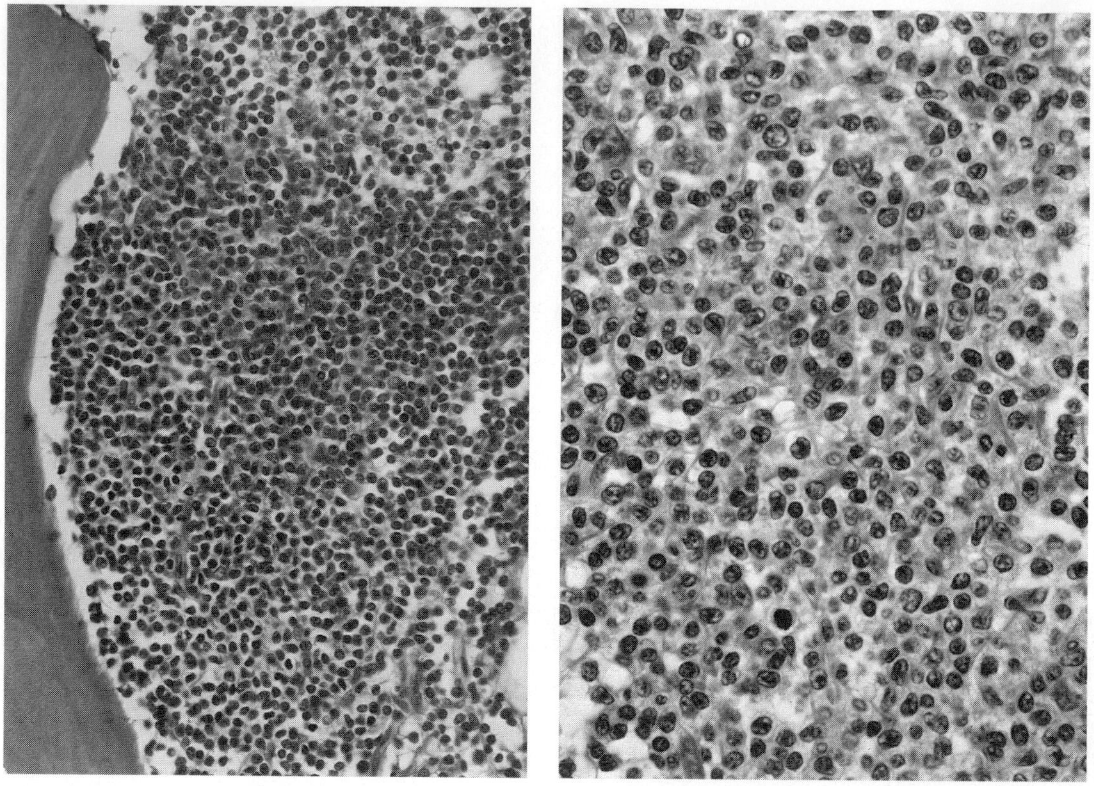

FIG. 39.22. Focal paratrabecular infiltrate in a patient with grade I follicle center lymphoma. **A:** Although the infiltrate does extend away from the bone trabecula somewhat, one surface is closely associated with the trabecula. Slight bony irregularity is evident (hematoxylin and eosin stain, original magnification: 200× magnification). **B:** A higher-magnification view demonstrates small mature cells, some with irregular, elongate, or twisted-appearing nuclei (hematoxylin and eosin stain, original magnification: 400× magnification).

cleaved cells at the periphery. Careful examination of the cytology of the lymphocytes usually allows distinction of these lesions from a reactive process. Clusters of histiocytes are a component of some follicular lymphomas in the marrow and may impart the appearance of a granuloma (2). Morphologic distinction of these infiltrates from granulomas, HL, or a peripheral T-cell lymphoma may be difficult; immunophenotyping studies on frozen or paraffin embedded sections may resolve this differential diagnosis (16,182).

In many cases, a diagnosis of follicle center lymphoma is made from marrow aspirate smears. The cytology of the lymphoma cells encompasses a wide morphologic spectrum that includes small cleaved lymphocytes, small round lymphocytes, and large transformed lymphocytes. In most instances, the predominant cell is the small cleaved cell, characterized in smear preparations by sparse or no recognizable cytoplasm and a smooth, uniformly staining nucleus that frequently is deeply indented or cleaved (77,78,85,183). (Fig. 39.23). Smear preparations often contain few or no obvious lymphoma cells, because of a sparsity of marrow lesions or because reticulin fibrosis interferes with collection of a representative aspirate.

Follicle center lymphoma, grade III (i.e., follicular, predominantly large cell lymphoma) appears to demonstrate bone marrow involvement less frequently than grades I and II (one third or less of patients) (83,96,184,185). In most cases the infiltrates are composed of small cells (histologic discordance) (96,185), with similar histologic features as grade I and II. When the marrow involvement is composed of large cells, the histologic features are those described for diffuse large cell lymphoma (see Chapter 24).

Marginal zone B-cell lymphoma (MZL) (nodal and extranodal) is a term that encompasses lesions previously known as monocytoid B-cell lymphoma and low-grade B-cell lymphoma of mucosa-associated lymphoid tissue (MALT) (94). Whereas extranodal proliferations (MALT lymphomas) are well characterized, the nodal MZLs are a more controversial issue. Many, or perhaps most, nodal MZLs represent spread from an extranodal site, but a minority may represent a distinct entity (94,186–193). These tumors have in common proliferations of two cell types in varying proportions: cells resembling splenic marginal zone cells with slightly irregular nuclei, slightly more open chromatin than mature lymphocytes, and moderate amounts of pale chromatin and cells closely resembling reactive monocytoid B cells, with larger, more irregular nuclei with more dispersed chromatin, often small but distinct nucleoli, and more abundant pale cytoplasm. Plasmacytoid differentiation may be seen, and ad-

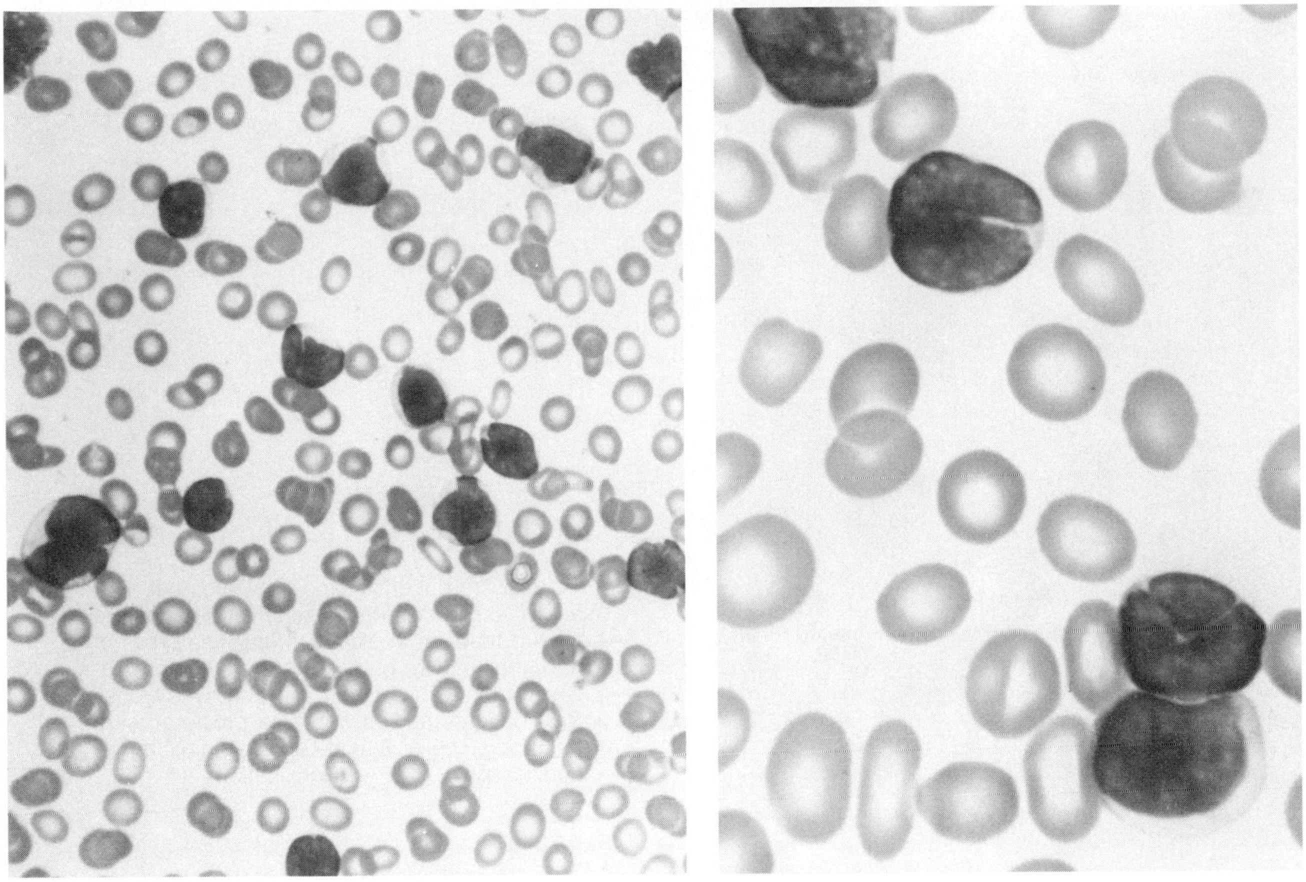

A B

FIG. 39.23. A blood smear from a patient with a grade I follicle center lymphoma. **A:** There is marked leukocytosis that consists of small cleaved lymphoma cells (Wright-Giemsa stain, original magnification: 400× magnification). **B:** A higher-magnification view illustrates the typical cytologic features of small cleaved cells. Cases of grade I follicle center lymphoma with blood involvement may simulate chronic lymphocytic leukemia. The identification of typical small cleaved cells serves to distinguish the two processes in most instances (Wright-Giemsa stain, original magnification: 1,000× magnification).

mixed transformed lymphocytes are common (188,189). The immunophenotype of MZLs is shown in Table 39.5 (129,141,189,193,194). Several cases of CD5-positive ($CD5^+$) MALT lymphoma have been reported (195,196), potentially complicating the differential diagnosis with mantle cell lymphoma and SLL/CLL.

Extranodal MZLs, in contrast to other B-cell lymphomas composed of small lymphocytes, tend to remain localized to the primary site or local lymph nodes for prolonged periods of time (197). When dissemination does occur, it tends to be to other extranodal (MALT) sites (198–201). Bone marrow involvement by extranodal MZL has been only occasionally reported (195,202–205). Based on the few reports that have systematically addressed the incidence of bone marrow involvement in these lesions, the frequency appears to be approximately 10% (187,195,206,207). Peripheral blood involvement is rare (195,203,205,206). Nodal marginal zone lymphomas, as opposed to their extranodal counterparts, appear to manifest more commonly with disseminated disease. Advanced stage has been reported in 76% and bone marrow involvement in 32% at presentation (187). However, leukemic forms are rarely encountered (208–210) (Fig. 39.24).

The morphologic features of MZL in bone marrow have not been well described. In smears and imprints the cells are medium-sized with folded or irregular nuclei, condensed chromatin, generally small but distinct nucleoli, and moderate amounts of basophilic to gray cytoplasm (189,203,208, 210,211) (Fig. 39.24). Plasmacytoid differentiation may be seen. In the few reported cases, MZLs manifest focal lesions in trephine biopsies (Fig. 39.25) that are often paratrabecular (193,195,202,203,210). In general, the cytologic features appear to be similar to those seen in primary sites (Fig. 39.25). However, in some cases, the infiltrating cells may have scanty cytoplasm, and thereby mimic SLL/CLL or follicle center lymphoma (212) (see Chapter 23).

Splenic marginal zone lymphoma (SMZL) is another entity that is distinct from nodal and extranodal MZLs (159,213–216). This is a tumor that closely recapitulates the cytologic, immunophenotypic, and architectural features of the normal splenic marginal zone. It is generally felt that SMZL comprises most of the tumors previously described as

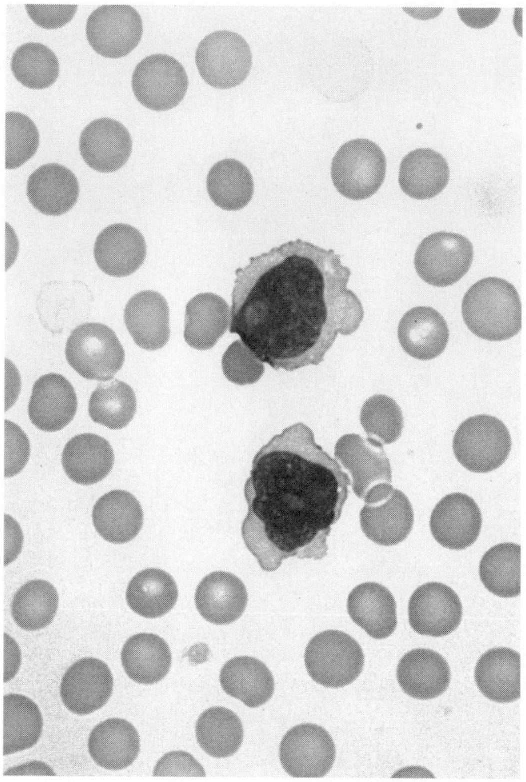

FIG. 39.24. Leukemic blood involvement in a man with a nodal marginal zone lymphoma. The cells are medium in size with large amounts of pale cytoplasm, irregular nuclei, mature chromatin, and prominent nucleoli. A lymph node biopsy in this patient showed a diffuse proliferation of monocytoid B cells (Wright-Giemsa stain, original magnification: 1,000× magnification).

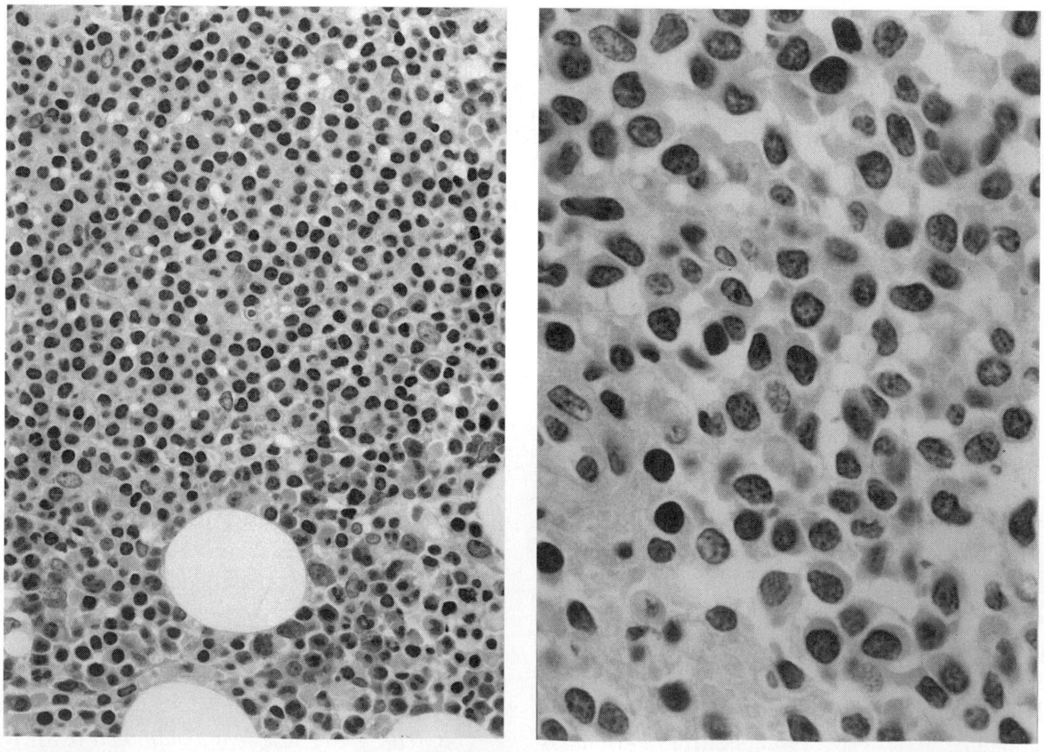

A B

FIG. 39.25. Bone marrow trephine biopsy involvement in a 51-year-old man with a conjunctival extranodal marginal zone lymphoma. **A:** The lesions in this patient were focal and nonparatrabecular. Normal hematopoietic elements are seen at the bottom of the field (hematoxylin and eosin stain, original magnification: 400× magnification). **B:** A higher-magnification view shows slightly irregular cells with condensed chromatin, absent nucleoli, and moderately abundant pale cytoplasm. Plasmacytoid differentiation is evident in some of the cells (hematoxylin and eosin stain, original magnification: 1,000× magnification).

splenic lymphoma with villous lymphocytes (SLVL) (217). SMZL usually manifests with prominent splenomegaly, cytopenias, and lack of significant peripheral lymphadenopathy . This is a disseminated disease at presentation, with bone marrow involvement in greater than 80% of patients, atypical circulating cells in about 80%, and frank leukemic manifestations in about 50% (159,213–216). Occasional patients present without splenomegaly, so this diagnosis should be entertained in patients with a lymphoproliferative disorder in blood and bone marrow with compatible morphology and immunophenotype, but lacking splenomegaly (218,219).

The morphologic appearance of SMZL cells in smears of peripheral blood and bone marrow is fairly consistent (Fig. 39.26). The cells are small to medium in size with round to slightly irregular nuclei, condensed chromatin and often small but distinct nucleoli. Occasional larger cells with prominent nucleoli are seen. The cytoplasm is scant to moderate in amount and has increased basophilia compared with mature lymphocytes and CLL/SLL cells. In some cases, the cytoplasm demonstrates irregularly distributed cytoplasmic projections, as described in SLVL (220,221). In trephine sections, the infiltrates most commonly take the form of focal, random aggregates, although the infiltrates may be interstitial (Fig. 39.27), diffuse, and occasionally paratrabe-

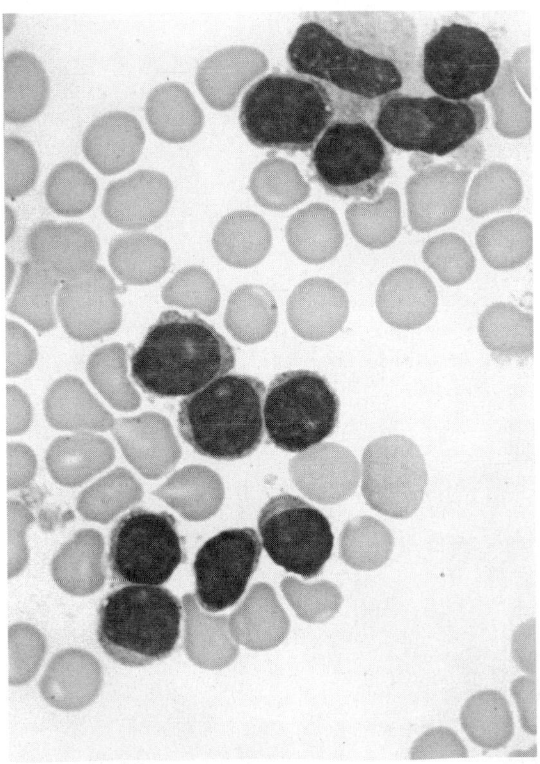

FIG. 39.26. Splenic marginal zone lymphoma in a bone marrow aspirate smear. The cells are small with condensed chromatin, small but distinct nucleoli, and scant to moderate amounts of basophilic cytoplasm that in some cells has an irregular border (Wright-Giemsa stain, original magnification: 1,000× magnification).

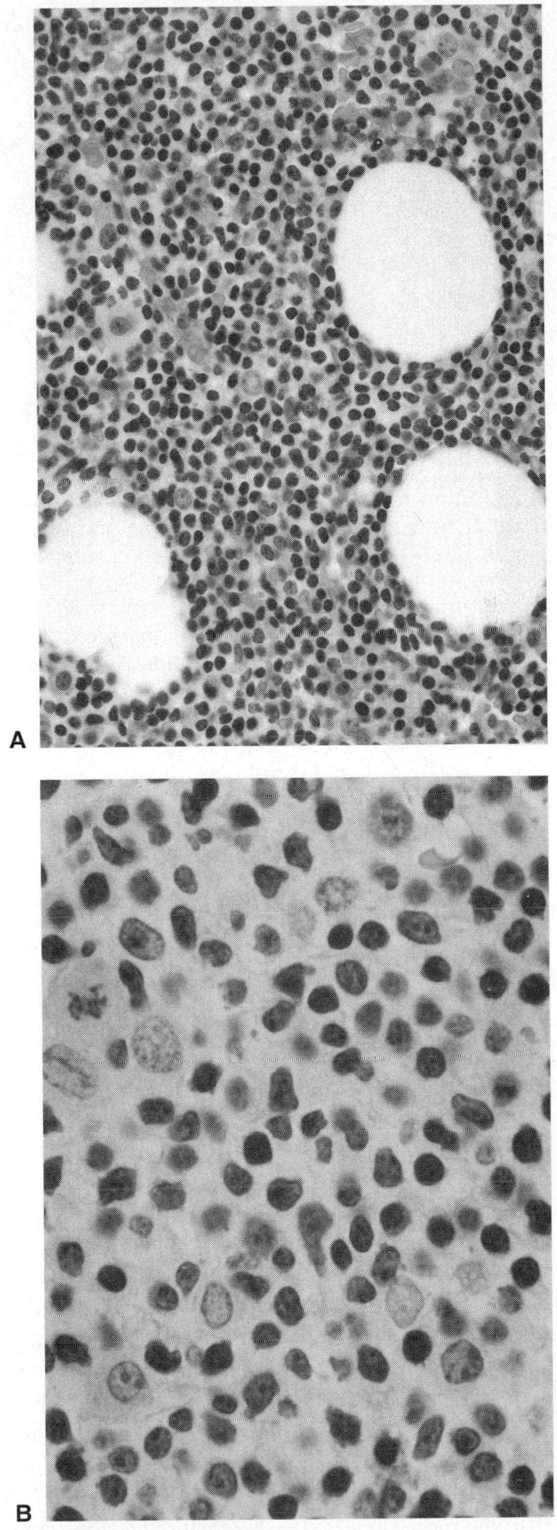

FIG. 39.27. Bone marrow trephine section from a 42-year-old woman with splenic marginal zone lymphoma. **A:** An interstitial pattern of infiltration is present. Other areas of the biopsy showed focal random infiltrates (hematoxylin and eosin stain, original magnification: 400× magnification). **B:** The infiltrating cells have a marginal zone appearance with slightly irregular nuclei, mature chromatin, and moderately abundant pale cytoplasm (hematoxylin and eosin stain, original magnification: 1,000× magnification).

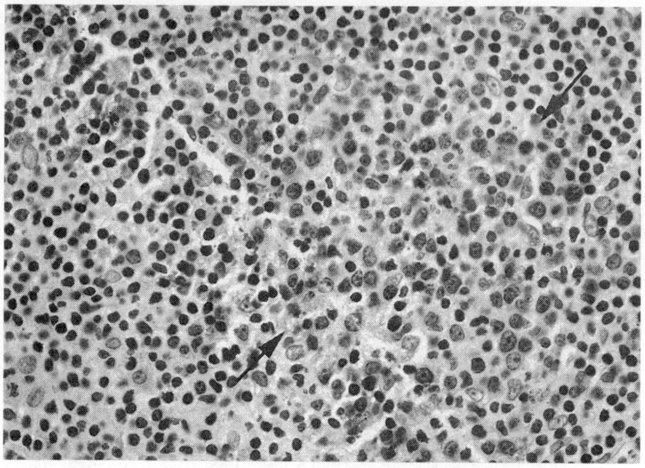

FIG. 39.28. Bone marrow trephine section in a 42-year-old woman with splenic marginal zone lymphoma (same patient as in Figure 39.27). This focal infiltrate, along with several others in this trephine biopsy, contained a benign germinal center. The germinal center is surrounded and eroded by marginal zone cells and lacks a discernible mantle zone (hematoxylin and eosin stain, original magnification: 400× magnification).

cular (213,214,216). A peculiar pattern of intrasinusoidal infiltration has been observed (Fig. 39.15) (103,104). This may be subtle, and at times occurs in the absence of obvious lymphoid lesions in the sections. Immunohistochemistry may be useful to highlight this intrasinusoidal pattern of infiltration. Reactive germinal centers are occasionally encountered within the lymphoma aggregates, mimicking the architectural pattern in the spleen (Fig. 39.28) (215). Cytologically, the infiltrating cells resemble splenic marginal zone cells, with slightly irregular nuclei, occasional small nucleoli, and moderately abundant pale cytoplasm.

Hairy cell leukemia (HCL) is an important differential diagnosis in cases of SMZL, especially those with villous morphology. In smears, SLVL has been described to have polar processes compared with the circumferential villi of HCL; however, this is not a reliable distinguishing feature. Instead, the character of the chromatin (condensed in SMZL vs. reticulated in HCL), the cytoplasmic staining qualities (basophilic in SMZL vs. gray in HCL), and the often distinct nucleoli of SMZL facilitate the distinction in Wright-Giemsa stained smears. The infiltrates of SMZL in trephine biopsies more closely resemble those of other small B-cell processes, producing fairly compact aggregates of small lymphocytes, rather than the more diffuse, loosely textured lesions characteristic of HCL.

The immunophenotype of SMZL resembles that of normal splenic marginal zone cells and is listed in Table 39.5 (213,214,216). CD11c and CD22 may be coexpressed, complicating the differential diagnosis with HCL. CD103 may be dimly expressed. However, the intensity of expression of these markers is generally less than in HCL. A useful differential diagnostic feature in these tumors is the uniform lack of CD43 expression (213,214), in contrast to CLL/SLL and mantle cell lymphoma (see Chapters 23 and 53).

Diffuse large B-cell lymphomas (DLBCL) have a relatively low incidence of marrow involvement at diagnosis (25%) (4,10,92,96). DLBCL cells may be seen on occasion in the peripheral blood, but frank leukemic involvement is uncommon (4,222) (Fig. 39.29). The incidence is higher late in the course of disease in patients who fail treatment. Although many of the lymphomatous infiltrates in cases of DLBCL are composed of small cells, the following discussion concerns only large cell marrow infiltrates. The pattern and extent of such infiltrates is highly variable, ranging from minimal small foci to total replacement of the marrow (Figs. 39.30–39.32). In some patients who have minimal involvement, the lymphoma may only be detected by identification of lymphoma cells in smears or imprints.

The lesions in trephine sections usually are readily recognized by the abnormal cytologic characteristics of the lymphocytes (Fig. 39.33). In some cases, they are composed of fairly uniform, large cells with large round nuclei, prominent nucleoli, and a moderate amount of cytoplasm. In other cases, there is striking pleomorphism (Fig. 39.32); the cells may have contorted nuclei and abundant cytoplasm. In most instances, reticulin is increased and a profound desmoplastic reaction is sometimes observed (85).

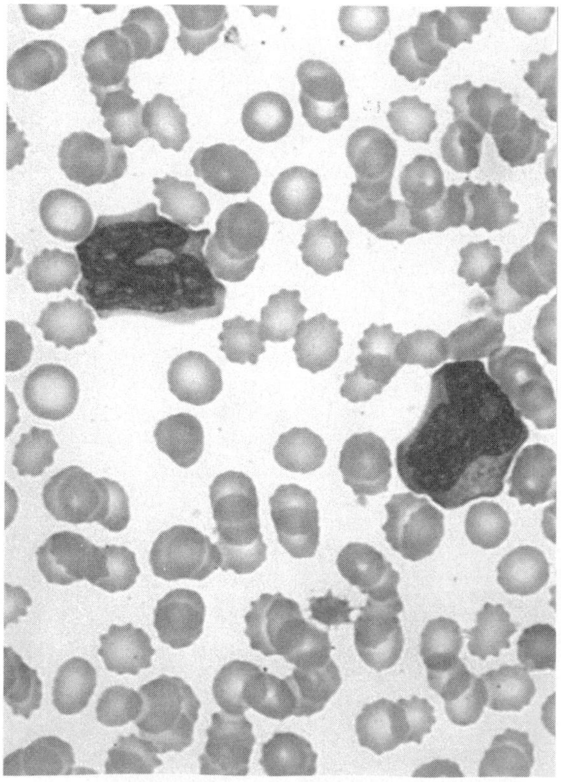

FIG. 39.29. Peripheral blood in a 61-year-old man with advanced large B-cell lymphoma. The leukemic lymphoma cells are large with irregular nuclei, coarse chromatin, prominent nucleoli, and moderate amounts of basophilic cytoplasm. The bone marrow also was involved in this patient (Wright-Giemsa stain, original magnification: 1,000× magnification).

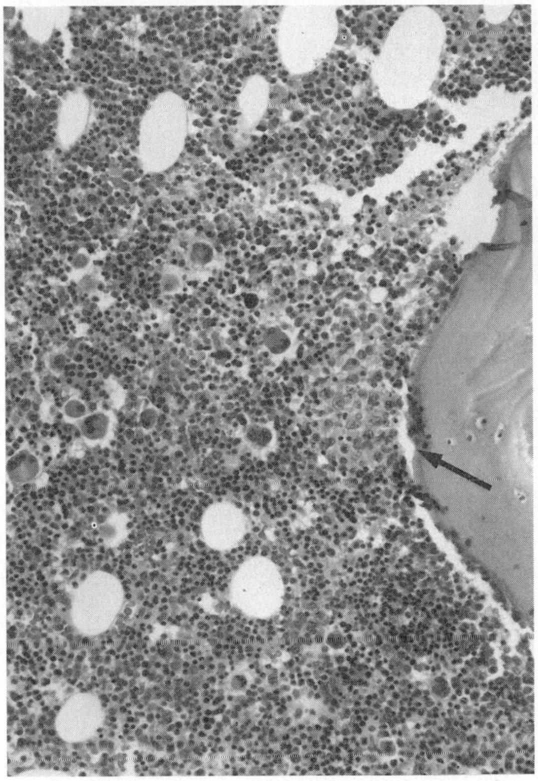

FIG. 39.30. Bone marrow trephine biopsy with a minute paratrabecular focus of large B-cell lymphoma *(arrow)* (hematoxylin and eosin stain, original magnification: 100× magnification).

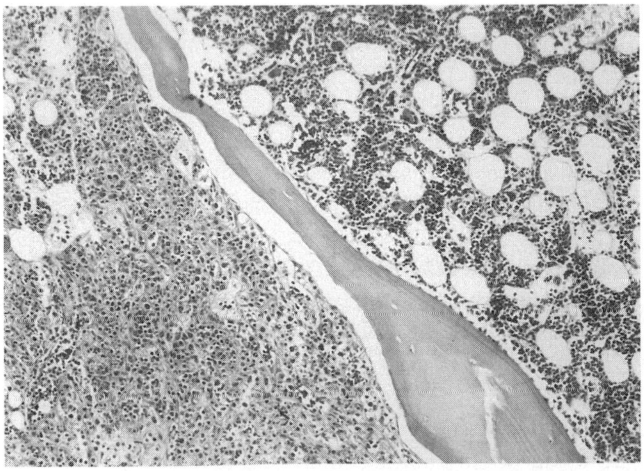

FIG. 39.31. Bone marrow trephine biopsy demonstrating a diffuse pattern of infiltration involving a portion of the marrow *(left)* separated from intact marrow *(right)* by a bony trabecula (hematoxylin and eosin stain, original magnification: 100× magnification).

A

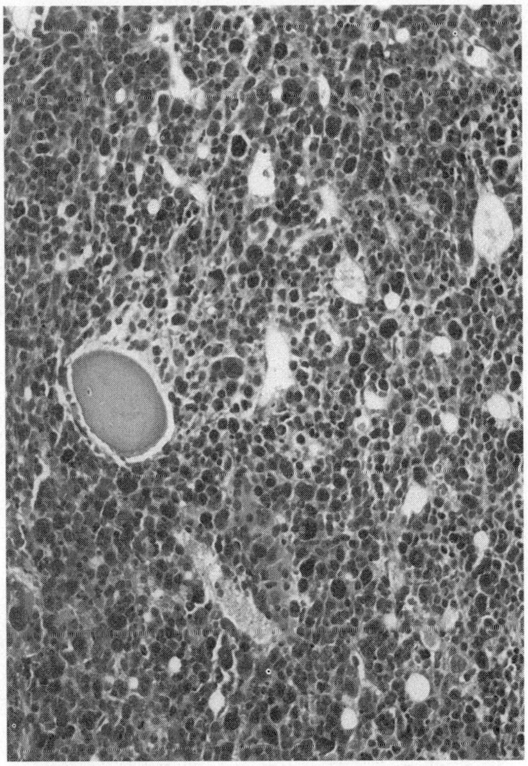

B

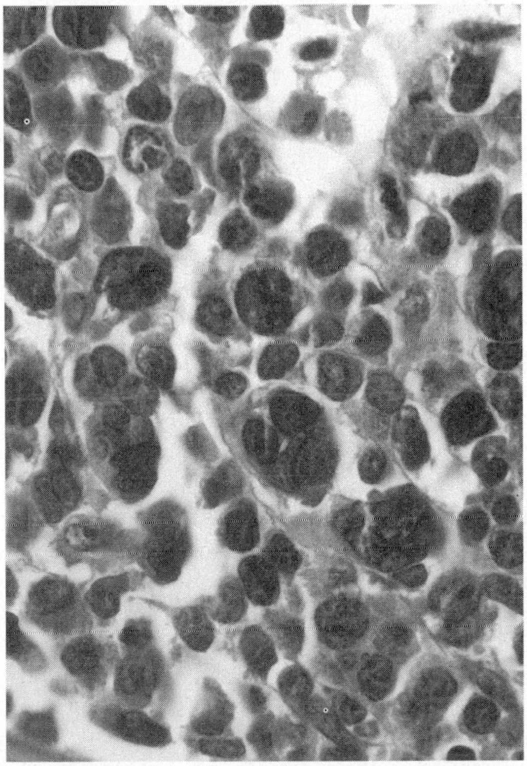

FIG. 39.32. Trephine biopsy in a 50-year-old man with extensive adenopathy. **A:** The bone marrow was completely replaced by a highly pleomorphic neoplastic population (hematoxylin and eosin stain, original magnification: 100× magnification). **B:** The cells showed marked variability in size and shape, including many multilobulated and multinucleated forms (hematoxylin and eosin stain, original magnification: 1,000× magnification).

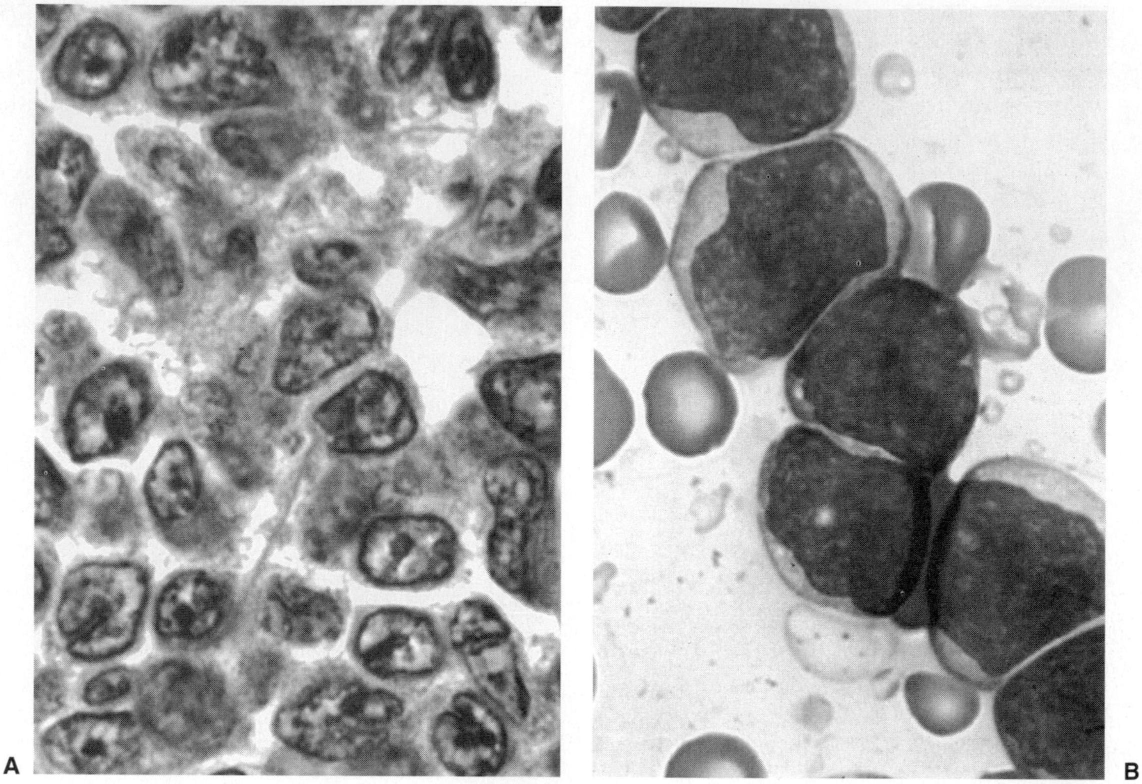

FIG. 39.33. **A:** High-magnification view of a trephine biopsy section from a patient with extensive marrow involvement by diffuse large cell lymphoma (hematoxylin and eosin stain, original magnification: 1,000× magnification). **B:** The aspirate smears from the same patient consisted primarily of large lymphoma cells with basophilic cytoplasm, coarsely reticular chromatin, and prominent nucleoli (Wright-Giemsa stain, original magnification: 1,000× magnification).

The cytology of the large cell lymphomas in smear and imprint preparations can be extremely pleomorphic. The spectrum of cell types includes large transformed lymphocytes with large nuclei (1) and abundant, often vacuolated, cytoplasm (2). The nucleus may be round or slightly monocytoid with a delicate reticular chromatin pattern; nucleoli are prominent and may be single or multiple (Fig. 39.33). In some cases, extremely large cells with abundant basophilic, vacuolated cytoplasm are observed. Some of these large cells contain fine azurophilic granules; cytoplasmic projections or fragmentation may be present (2,85).

Among the DLBCLs, only one subtype is provisionally recognized by the ILSG classification: *primary mediastinal large B-cell lymphoma* (94). Although the biologic distinctiveness of this lesion is a matter of some debate (223), it appears to possess a relatively distinct clinicopathologic profile (224–227). Bone marrow involvement is only seen at presentation in about 1% of patients (224,225,227–229). The pathologic features of mediastinal large B-cell lymphoma in bone marrow have not been described, except for one patient who was reported to have a small lymphocytic marrow infiltrate (227).

Although not recognized as a distinct entity in the ILSG classification, the category of *T-cell–rich large B-cell lymphoma* (TCRBCL) bears mentioning because of the potential for confusing bone marrow infiltrates of this lesion with other types of lymphoma. Most studies have concluded that the category of TCRBCL is composed of a heterogeneous group of disorders having a minority of neoplastic large B cells with a prominent infiltrate of reactive T cells and should be considered morphologic variants of diffuse large B-cell lymphoma (94,230–233). However, within this group there may be a distinct entity that has been called histiocyte-rich B-cell lymphoma (234,235). This particular subtype, in addition to having a reactive T-cell infiltrate, possesses a prominent population of reactive histiocytes, and morphologically resembles lymphocyte predominance Hodgkin's disease (234,236,237). These tumors have a high incidence of bone marrow involvement (>70%) (234,236,237). The infiltrates are focal, often paratrabecular, and demonstrate the same distribution of cell types as seen in the primary lesions. The lesions are pale appearing at low power because of the prominent histiocytic population, and because of the heterogeneity of the infiltrate and the small numbers of neoplastic cells, the lesions closely mimic Hodgkin's disease or peripheral T-cell lymphoma (Fig. 39.10). The similarity to Hodgkin's disease is heightened by the frequent resemblance of the neoplastic cells to Hodgkin's variants. Immunohistochemistry is essential in the differential diagnosis—the large cells stain for B-cell markers and CD45, and they lack CD15 and usually CD30 (see Chapter 25).

Angiotropic (intravascular) large B-cell lymphoma is a subtype of large cell lymphoma with unique clinical and pathologic features that is not recognized in the ILSG classification. It manifests with varied, nonspecific systemic manifestations and lack of mass disease, such that lymphoma is usually not suspected clinically (238–241). Pathologically it manifests as an intravascular proliferation of large atypical B cells in a wide variety of organ systems. Although bone marrow involvement is generally not observed on routine histologic preparations (33), when the marrow is overtly involved, the intravascular distribution is maintained, producing a distinct histologic appearance (Fig. 39.34). A variant of angiotropic lymphoma has been described in Japanese patients who present with hepatosplenomegaly and bone marrow involvement (102). Even when no histologic evidence of marrow involvement is present, molecular methods detect minimal clonal populations (33). The diagnosis is easily confirmed with the application of antibodies to B-cell markers in paraffin sections (Fig. 39.34), with the exception of the occasional angiotropic lymphomas with a T-cell phenotype (240,242–244) (see Chapters 25, 32, and 34).

Burkitt's lymphoma involves the bone marrow in up to 57% of cases (4,86,87,97,245). Many patients who have no initial involvement manifest marrow invasion later in their course. The pattern is nearly always diffuse or interstitial, and the extent of involvement varies from occasional scattered lymphoma cells to complete replacement of the marrow (83,246) (Fig. 39.14). Even with extensive involvement, the starry-sky pattern, commonly observed in lymph nodes, is infrequent (246). There may be small foci or expansive areas of necrosis; in some cases, the entire section consists of necrotic tissue. In bone marrow sections, the cells have round or oval nuclei with two to four small nucleoli. There is a distinct rim of cytoplasm, and cell borders are sharply defined (Fig. 39.35). Mitotic figures often are numerous (see Chapter 27). In patients with acquired immunodeficiency syndrome the cells may have atypical morphology that is intermediate between that of Burkitt's and large cell or immunoblastic lymphoma (see Chapter 28).

Aspirate smears generally are diagnostic because of the characteristic cytology of the lymphoma cells. In fact, in contrast to most other types of lymphoma, aspirate smears may be more sensitive than trephine biopsy in the detection of Burkitt's lymphoma cells (245). They are medium to large sized, with a round or oval nucleus that contains reticular or slightly condensed chromatin. Nucleoli may be multiple but generally are small. There is a moderate amount of

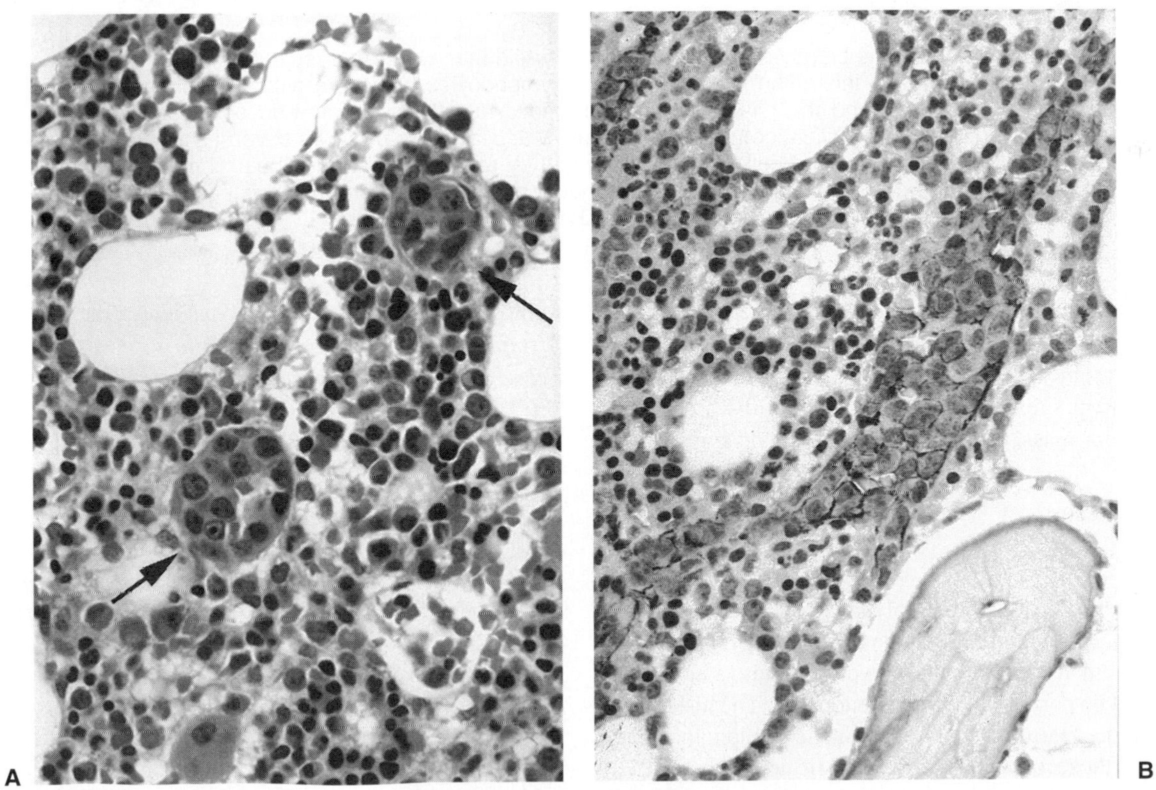

FIG. 39.34. Bone marrow trephine biopsy from a patient with angiotropic large B-cell lymphoma. **A:** Two small blood vessels *(arrows)* are filled with large lymphoid cells (hematoxylin and eosin stain, original magnification: 400× magnification). **B:** A CD20 (L26) stain highlights the intravascular infiltrate (immunoperoxidase stain, original magnification: 400× magnification).

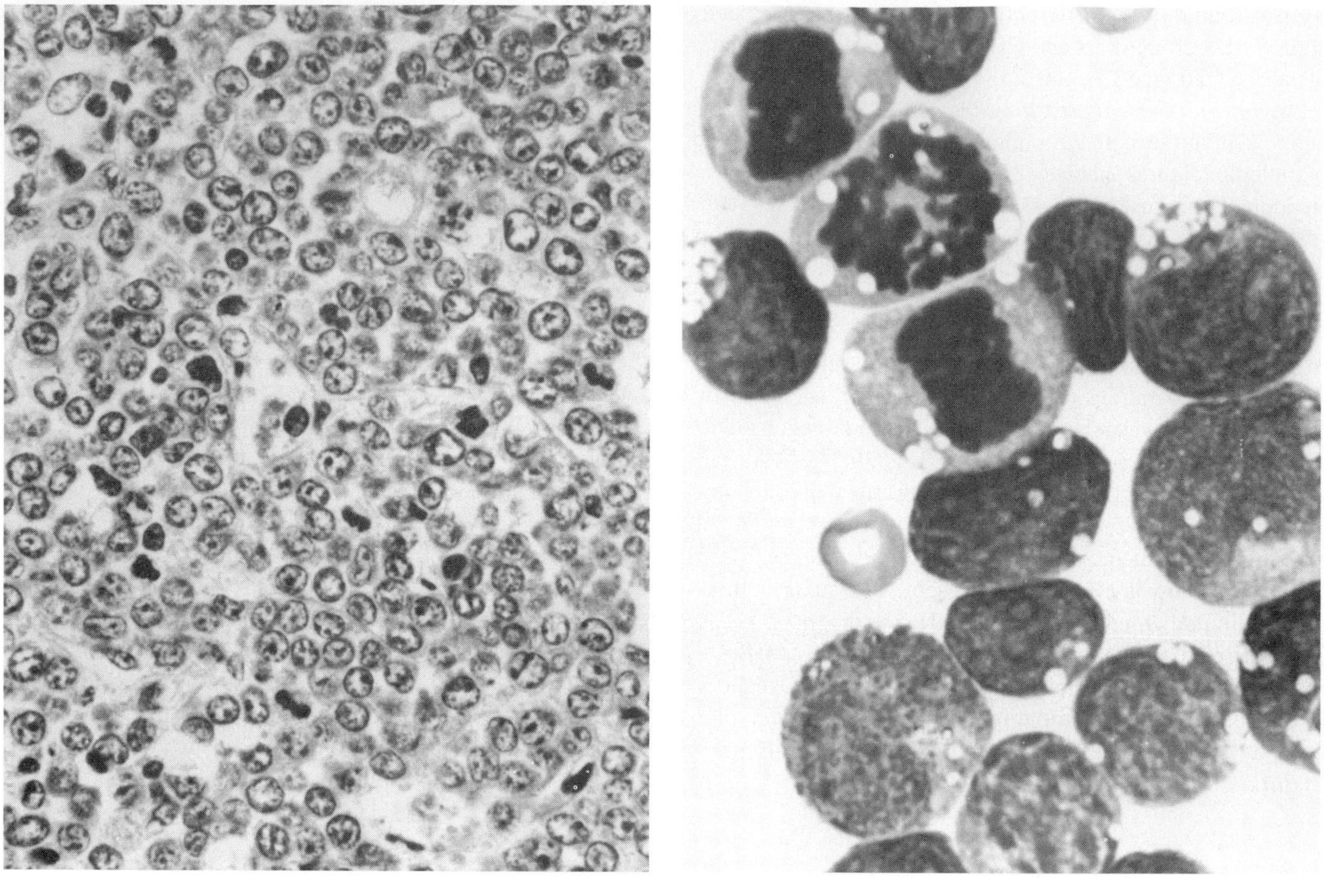
A B

FIG. 39.35. **A:** Trephine biopsy section from a 19-year-old man with a paraspinal Burkitt's lymphoma. The pattern of marrow infiltration was diffuse. The lymphocytes show the typical cytologic features of Burkitt's lymphoma and the characteristic high mitotic rate (hematoxylin and eosin stain, original magnification: 400× magnification). **B:** A bone marrow aspirate smear shows several lymphoma cells, including three in mitosis. The cells are characterized by relatively coarse nuclear chromatin, one to three nucleoli, and deeply basophilic cytoplasm that contains several sharply defined, clear vacuoles (Wright-Giemsa stain, original magnification: 1,000× magnification).

deeply basophilic cytoplasm, which in most cases contains a variable number of sharply defined vacuoles (Fig. 39.35).

In some instances, the bone marrow is the most obvious or only apparent site of involvement. A careful search often reveals a tumor mass, usually in the abdominal cavity (246).

T-Cell Neoplasms

Precursor-T-Cell Neoplasms

The incidence of marrow involvement by T-LBL is 50% to 60% (4,7). Bone marrow may be the primary tissue available for examination in patients who present with a mediastinal mass and no peripheral lymphadenopathy. The histologic and cytologic features of lymphoblastic lymphomas are identical to those of acute lymphoblastic leukemia (ALL) (247–252). The distinction is arbitrary, but usually is based on the percentage of lymphoblasts in the marrow at the time of diagnosis; 25% or greater is a commonly used criterion for ALL. The high incidence of marrow involvement for lymphoblastic lymphomas and the morphologic and immunologic uniformity with ALL has led to the use of the term *lymphoblastic lymphoma/leukemia* in cases with mass disease and a T-cell immunophenotype (114).

The pattern of marrow infiltration is nearly always interstitial or diffuse in trephine biopsies (4,7) (Fig. 39.36). The degree of involvement varies from occasional lymphoma cells, recognizable only in smear preparations, up to 25% of the bone marrow cells. Nuclear convolution and a high mitotic rate are prominent features (248). Nonconvoluted types have round or oval nuclei and are more cytologically uniform (249).

In bone marrow smears the cells are identical to those of French-American-British (FAB) L1 or L2 acute lymphoblastic leukemia (251) (Fig. 39.36). Identification of lymphoblasts in smears is essential to the diagnosis when there is minimal involvement not recognizable in the trephine sections.

The differential diagnosis of T-LBL in marrow sections includes such diverse entities as B-LBL, blastoid mantle cell lymphoma, Burkitt's lymphoma, and nonhematopoietic tu-

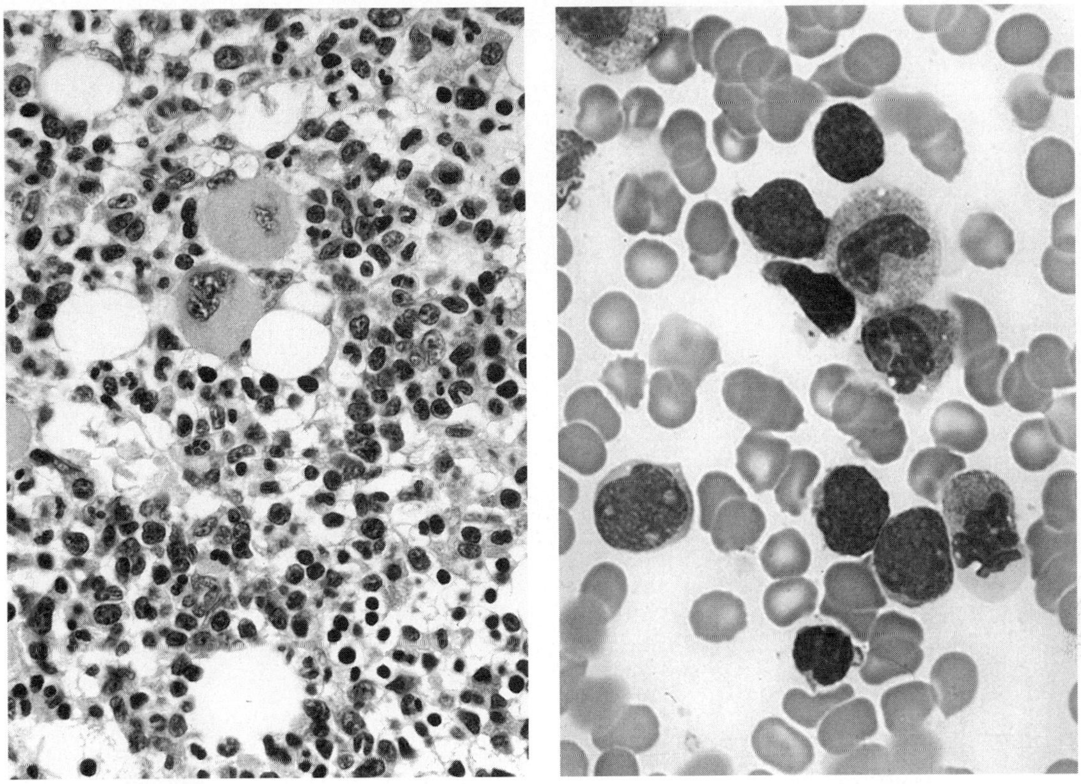

FIG. 39.36. Bone marrow from a patient with lymphoblastic lymphoma. **A:** The trephine biopsy section shows a fairly subtle interstitial infiltrate of medium-sized cells with variably irregular nuclear contours and scant cytoplasm (hematoxylin and eosin stain, original magnification: 400× magnification). **B:** The aspirate smear showed scattered cells with typical features of lymphoblasts; several are present in this field (Wright-Giemsa stain, original magnification: 1,000× magnification).

mors. The differential diagnosis with B-LBL rests on immunophenotyping data and cannot be made reliably on morphology. Most cases of T-LBL express CD3 and TdT in paraffin sections; UCHL1 (CD45RO) is positive in roughly one half of cases (119,253–256). Although essentially all T-LBLs are positive for CD43 in paraffin sections, so are most B-LBLs, Burkitt's lymphomas, and acute myeloid leukemias, so positivity for this marker should not be construed as evidence of T lineage (119,254,257). T-LBL, like B-LBL, usually shows positivity for CD99 (MIC2) (118) and may be confused with Ewing's sarcoma or peripheral neuroectodermal tumor; panels including CD43 and TdT should allow distinction (see Chapter 26).

Peripheral T-Cell and Natural Killer Cell Neoplasms

Mycosis fungoides involves the bone marrow in approximately 25% of cases during the course of disease (258,259). Although bone marrow involvement is more common in patients late in the course of advanced clinical stages, a significant minority of patients have involvement within 3 months of diagnosis or have early clinical stage disease (258,259). Nodules or interstitial infiltrates of lymphocytes with cerebriform nuclei are characteristic (Fig. 39.37). Paratrabecular infiltration may be seen, but diffuse marrow involvement is uncommon. The lesions often are subtle without increased cellularity, and immunohistochemistry for T-cell markers may be useful to highlight these infiltrates (258). Some cases contain large transformed cells admixed with the small cerebriform cells (259). Marrow eosinophilia is seen in the bone marrows of 38% of patients with mycosis fungoides, with or without lymphomatous marrow involvement (259).

The presence of bone marrow involvement has an adverse impact on survival (258,259). Among patients with bone marrow involvement, those with infiltrative disease or large transformed cells appear to fare more poorly (258). Circulating cerebriform lymphocytes are nearly always identified in blood smears in cases that have an infiltrative interstitial pattern and are absent in those cases that have focal marrow disease (Fig. 39.37) (258). Patients with peripheral blood involvement commonly demonstrate marrow involvement. Blood involvement varies from rare lymphoma cells to a marked lymphocytosis. Large and small cytologic variants have been described (Fig. 39.37). Traditionally these cells have been quantitated morphologically; flow cytometric analysis has been proposed as a more accurate alternative (260,261).

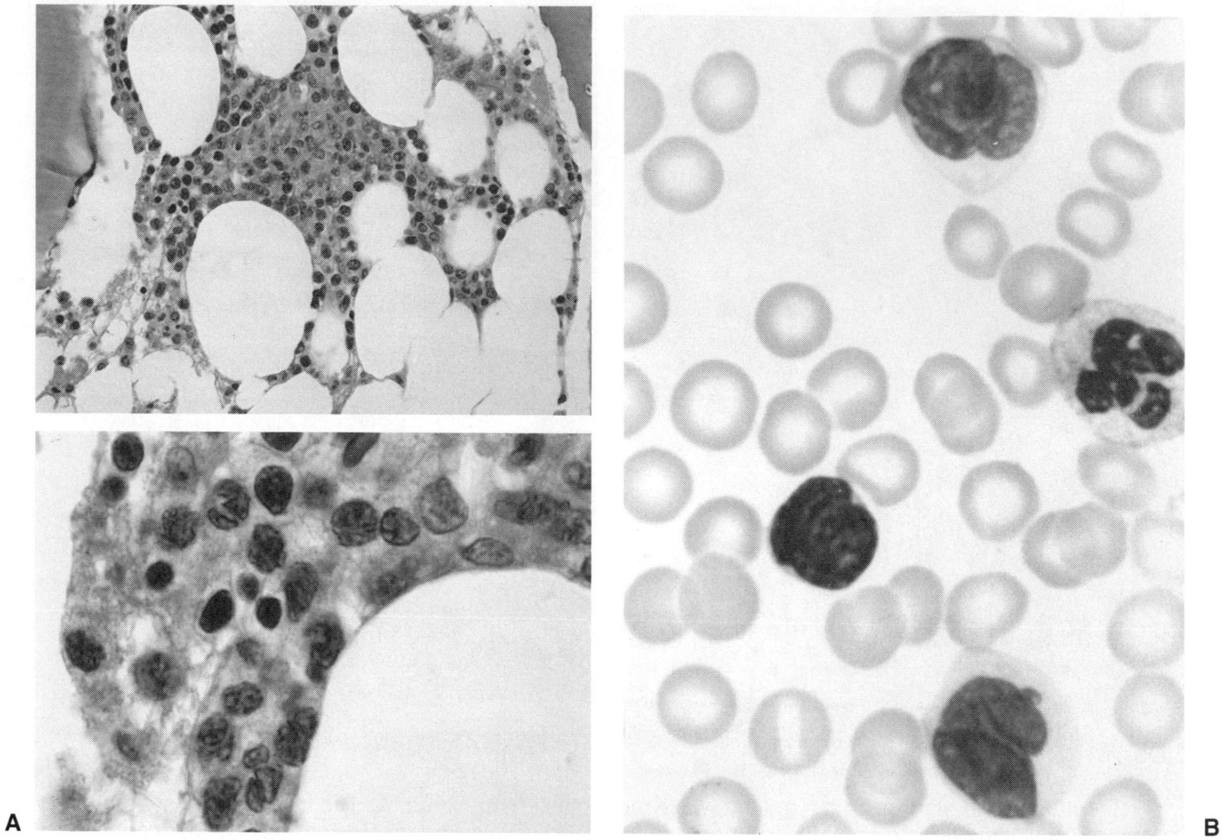

FIG. 39.37. A: Top: Trephine biopsy section from a patient with advanced Sezary syndrome. Despite extensive organ infiltration and an elevated blood leukocyte count, there were only a few small foci of cerebriform lymphocytes in the marrow sections (hematoxylin and eosin stain, original magnification: 400× magnification). **Bottom:** A higher-magnification view shows several markedly convoluted lymphocytes (hematoxylin and eosin stain, original magnification: 1,000× magnification). **B:** A blood smear from the same patient depicts three Sezary cells with cerebriform nuclei (Wright-Giemsa stain, original magnification: 1,000× magnification).

Peripheral T-cell lymphomas, unspecified (PTCL-U), are a heterogeneous group of diseases that have defied satisfactory classification (94) (see Chapter 29). Although two provisional subtypes within this category have been identified, the remainder demonstrate a wide range of cytologic and clinical features. Several provisional cytologic categories are proposed by the ILSG: medium-sized cell, mixed medium and large cell, large cell, and lymphoepithelioid cell (94) (see Chapter 19).

Overall, bone marrow involvement occurs in 50% to 80% of cases of PTCL-U, and is strongly associated with a poor prognosis (65,96,99,262). The morphologic characteristics of PTCL-U in trephine sections are similar in any given case to those seen in extramedullary tissues (65,99,262). Often a spectrum of cell sizes and shapes is encountered, producing a polymorphous cellular appearance (Figs. 39.9, 39.38). Nuclei tend to be hyperchromatic with prominent nuclear irregularity and coarse chromatin. Larger cells with vesicular chromatin and prominent nucleoli may also be seen, some mimicking Hodgkin's cells (Fig. 39.9). Occasional cases show monomorphic proliferations of large cells that are morphologically similar to B immunoblasts (65).

The pattern of marrow involvement of PTCL-U is split about equally between diffuse and randomly focal; rarely focal paratrabecular lesions are encountered (65,79). Lesions commonly are accompanied by a polycellular infiltrate of eosinophils, plasma cells, neutrophils, endothelial cells, and epithelioid histiocytes (Figs. 39.38, 39.39). The reactive cell component is mixed with lymphoma cells. This reactive cell infiltrate is least commonly seen in neoplasms composed primarily of large immunoblastic cells. There is often prominent vascularity and reticulin fibrosis. The fibrosis is confined to the lymphoma lesions and does not extend to the uninvolved adjacent marrow. Epithelioid histiocytes may be found in clusters; detection of atypical lymphocytes is necessary to distinguish these lesions from reactive granulomas (Fig. 39.39). Foci of necrosis may be observed, primarily in cases consisting of immunoblast-like cells (65).

In some cases of PTCL-U, diffuse bone marrow infiltrates may blend uniformly with the normal hematopoietic cells. Reticulin fibrosis generally is a component of these lesions, and the overall picture may suggest a myeloproliferative disorder (65,99,263). With this pattern of infiltration, the lymphoma may be difficult to discern even with rather extensive

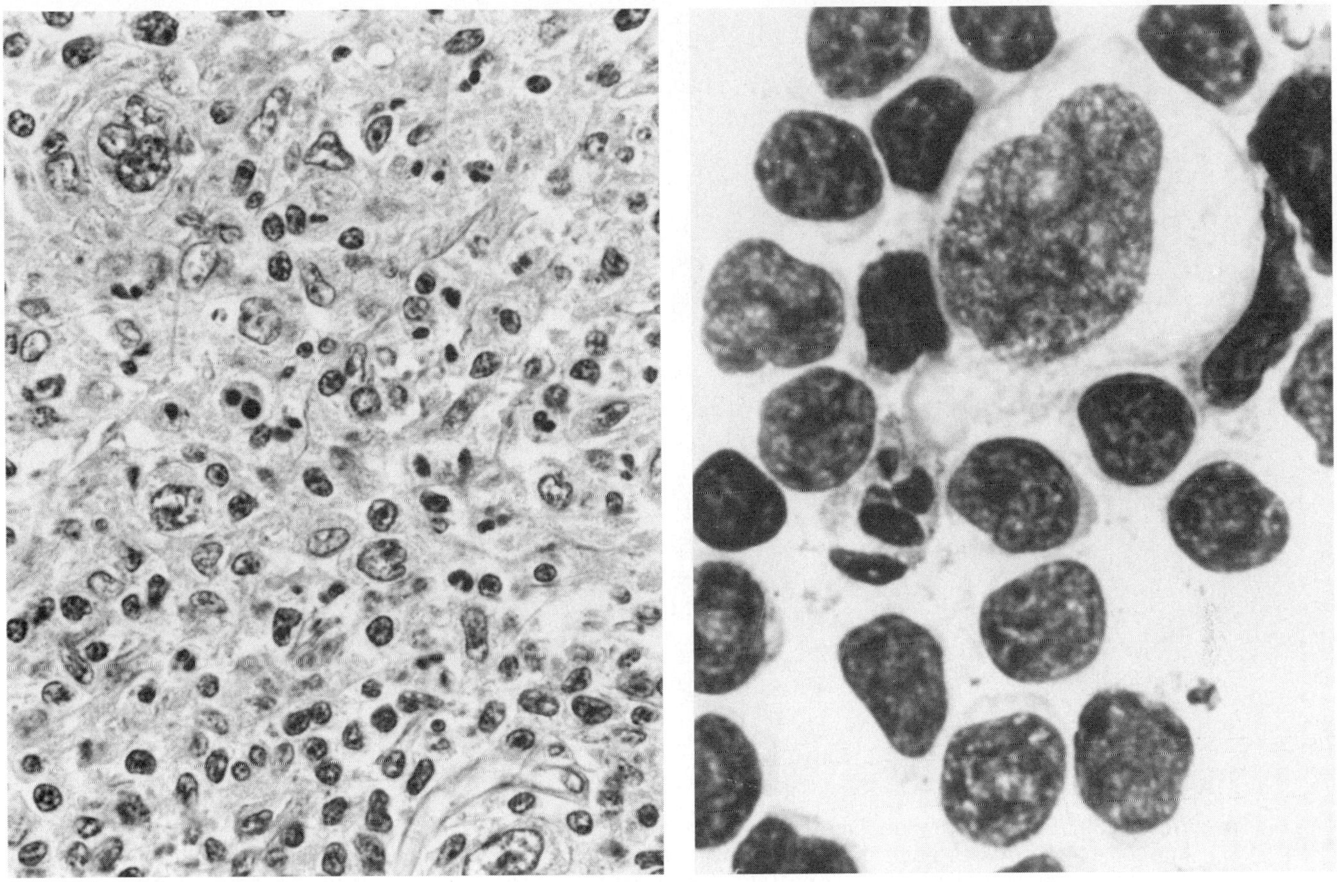

A B

FIG. 39.38. A: High-magnification view of a peripheral T-cell lymphoma in a trephine biopsy section. The pattern is of mixed small and large cells and resembles Hodgkin's lymphoma (HL) (hematoxylin and eosin stain, original magnification: 400× magnification). **B:** A bone marrow trephine biopsy touch preparation shows a spectrum of lymphoma cells. The majority are medium-sized lymphocytes with condensed chromatin. Some have a slightly irregular nuclear border or visible nucleoli. A single large cell comparable to those in the trephine section is present. This cell has condensed chromatin, a prominent nucleolus, and abundant cytoplasm (Wright-Giemsa stain, original magnification: 1,000× magnification).

marrow disease. In the absence of a confirmatory lymph node biopsy, the diagnosis may be problematic.

A marrow aspirate often is difficult to obtain because of the fibrosis associated with many of the peripheral T-cell lymphomas. Despite this, lymphoma cells are found in aspirate smears in at least 50% of cases with bone marrow disease (65). Interpretation of the smears may be difficult, however, because of the heteromorphous lymphocyte populations, many of which exhibit cytologic features of mature or reactive lymphocytes (65). The number of lymphoma cells in the smears varies from rare to greater than 90% of the bone marrow cells. The morphologic spectrum of cells generally reflects the heterogeneity of the lesions in the trephine sections (Fig. 39.38). The large immunoblastic cells have lightly to deeply basophilic cytoplasm and sometimes are finely vacuolated. The contour of the nucleus varies but usually is convoluted. The chromatin is dispersed, and prominent nucleoli are present. The cytoplasm of the small- and medium-sized lymphocytes ranges from sparse to moderately abundant and is lightly to deeply basophilic. The nuclear chromatin is coarse and nucleoli are indistinct; convolutions often are not as obvious in the smear preparations as in the sections.

The differential diagnosis of PTCL-U in bone marrow may be very difficult, and includes a diverse group of disorders. Pleomorphic focal lesions are distributed randomly and usually are poorly circumscribed, and may be difficult to distinguish from lymphohistiocytic reactive lesions, particularly those commonly encountered in patients who have AIDS or an autoimmune disease (Fig. 39.40) (65,99,264). Careful attention to the cytologic features of the lymphocytes may suggest the correct diagnosis, but in some cases, ancillary techniques may be necessary to establish the presence of an abnormal T-cell process. Although frozen section immunohistochemistry may demonstrate aberrant T-cell antigen expression (79,99), this technique is rarely employed currently in bone marrow trephine biopsies. Unfortunately, paraffin section immunohistochemistry is unlikely to be helpful in this differential diagnosis, with the possible exception of demonstrating subtle infiltrative bone marrow lesions

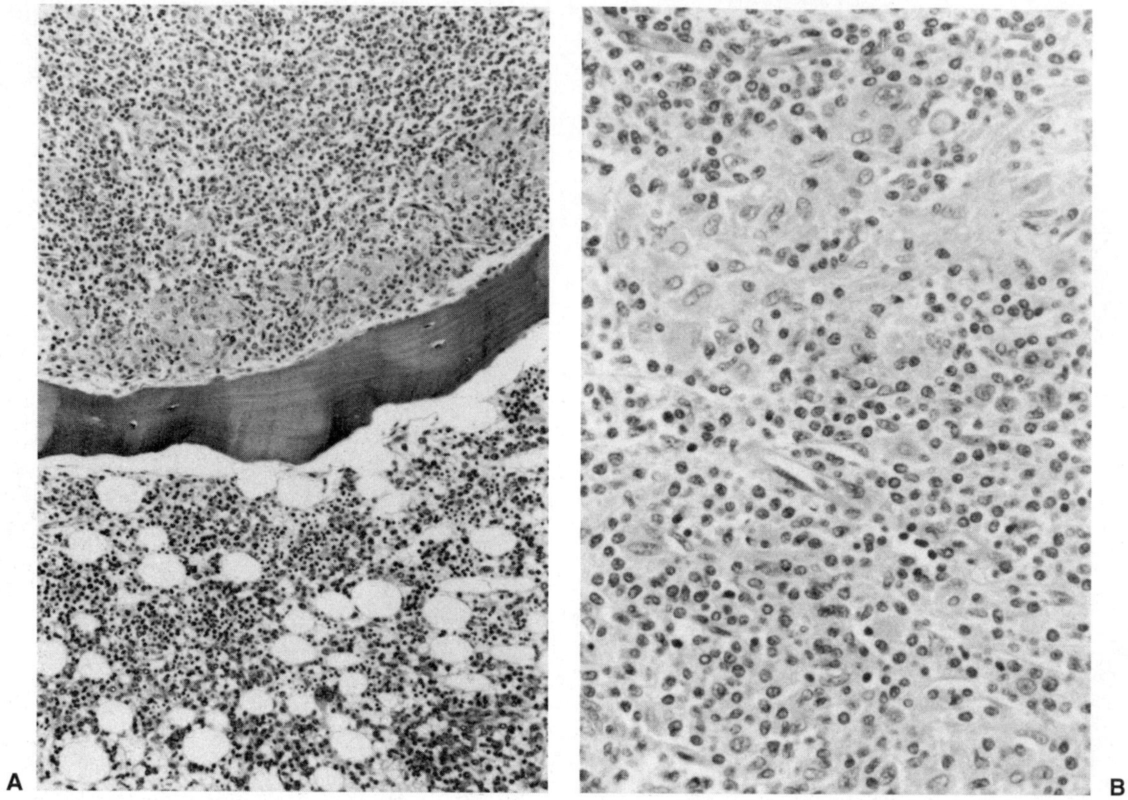

FIG. 39.39. Bone marrow trephine section from a 72-year-old man with peripheral T-cell lymphoma. **A:** A bone trabecula separates a lymphoma infiltrate *(top)* from normal hematopoietic tissue (hematoxylin and eosin stain, original magnification: 100× magnification). **B:** The lymphoma is composed of a heteromorphous population of lymphocytes, clusters of epithelioid histiocytes, and small vessels and endothelial cells (hematoxylin and eosin stain, original magnification: 250× magnification).

that were inapparent in routine sections. Most T-cell lymphomas demonstrate aberrant levels of expression of one or more T-cell antigens by flow cytometry (unpublished data), although abnormal results must be interpreted with caution. The demonstration of clonal T-cell antigen receptor gene rearrangements provides definitive evidence of clonality.

Because of the polymorphous cellular background and occasional presence of Reed-Sternberg–like cells, PTCL-U may closely mimic Hodgkin's disease morphologically (Figs. 39.9, 39.38). Immunohistochemistry usually discriminates between these tumors, with PTCL-U demonstrating CD45 and T-cell markers and Hodgkin's disease lacking these antigens but expressing CD15, CD30, or both (265) (Table 39.2). Large cells of PTCL-U may express CD30, so this marker alone does not provide reliable discrimination (266).

One rather treacherous differential diagnosis with PTCL-U is T-cell–rich large B-cell lymphoma (TCRBCL). This entity may bear a strong resemblance to PTCL-U in bone marrow and other tissues, and a high index of suspicion is required to avoid misdiagnosis in polymorphous lesions. Lack of significant atypia in the smaller lymphocytes may provide a diagnostic clue that the lesion is a TCRBCL. Immunohistochemical techniques of good quality on well-fixed material demonstrate the B-cell nature of the large neoplastic cells in this disease; poor immunohistochemical technique or poorly fixed tissue may produce incorrect diagnoses.

Two provisional subtypes are recognized within the category of PTCL-U, and both require specific discussion because of distinctive clinical and pathologic features. Hepatosplenic $\gamma\delta$ T-cell lymphoma is a distinct neoplasm that manifests primarily with sinusoidal involvement of spleen and liver (100,267–269). The bone marrow is involved in most cases, as is the blood, although frank lymphocytosis is uncommon (100). As in the spleen and liver, the bone marrow involvement usually is distinctly sinusoidal (Fig. 39.41) (99–101), although diffuse marrow involvement has also been reported (270). In sections, the neoplastic cells are medium sized with regular nuclear contours, moderately dispersed chromatin and moderate amounts of cytoplasm (100). Marrow involvement may be subtle, and immunohistochemical stains for T-cell markers are useful (101,271). Immunophenotypic analysis is helpful in identifying this tumor: the cells express the $\gamma\delta$ T-cell receptor, express weak CD8 or are dual $CD4^-CD8^-$, demonstrate cytotoxicity antigens, and generally have weak or absent CD5. Cytogenetic analysis reveals isochromosome 7q and trisomy 8 in most cases (267–269).

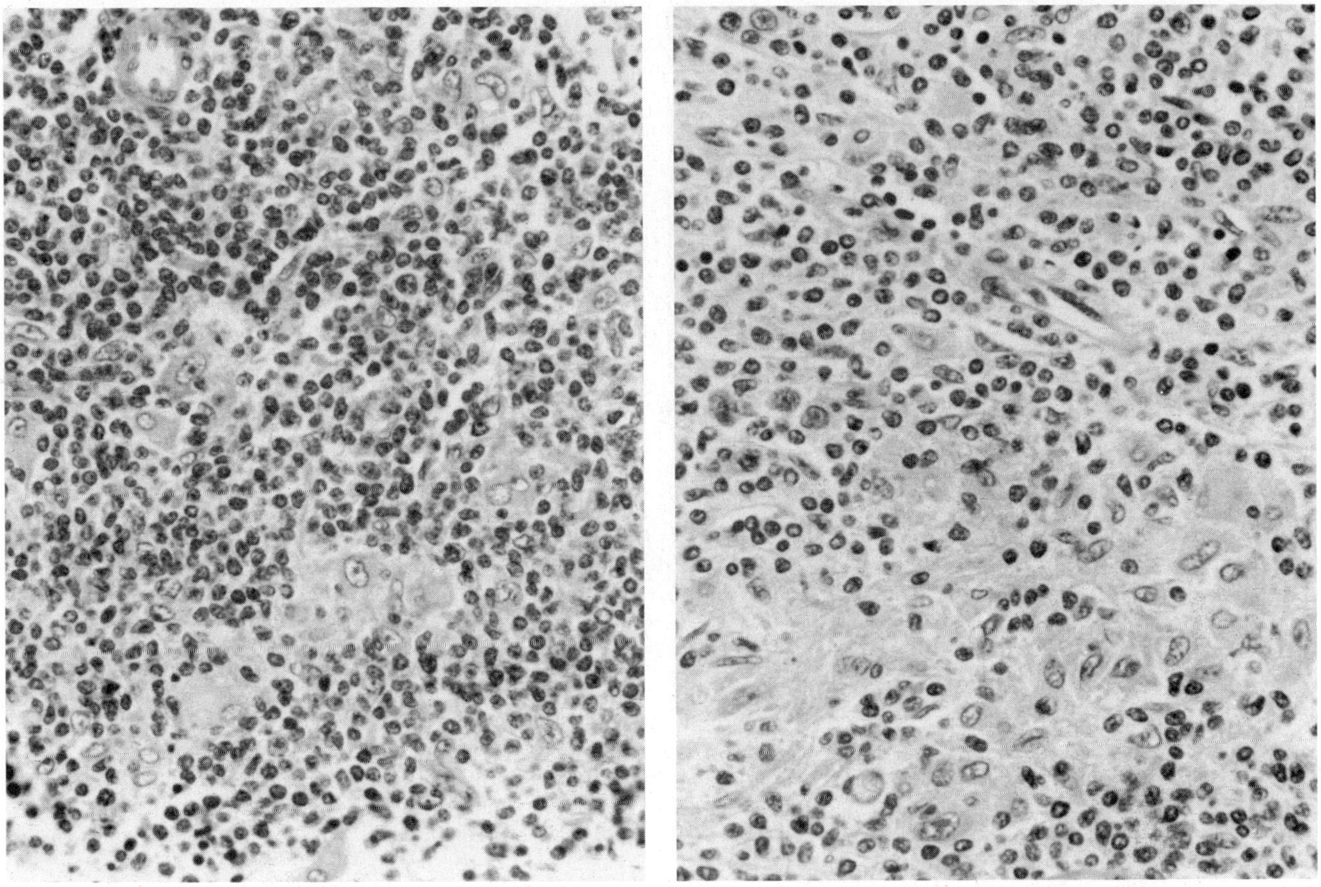

A B

FIG. 39.40. A: A reactive lymphohistiocytic lesion from the bone marrow of a patient with acquired immunodeficiency syndrome (AIDS) (hematoxylin and eosin stain, original magnification: 250× magnification). **B:** A lesion from the bone marrow of a patient with peripheral T-cell lymphoma with epithelioid histiocytes. There may be considerable morphologic similarity between the reactive lesions in the bone marrow of patients with AIDS and the infiltrates of peripheral T-cell lymphomas (hematoxylin and eosin stain, original magnification: 250× magnification).

Subcutaneous panniculitic T-cell lymphoma is a rare tumor of cytotoxic T lymphocytes that manifests in and remains localized to subcutaneous adipose tissue, clinically and pathologically mimicking panniculitis (272–274). Although the bone marrow does not become involved by tumor directly, a common and frequently fatal feature of this neoplasm is the development of a systemic hemophagocytic syndrome at some point during the clinical course (273). Bone marrow smears and trephine sections demonstrate histiocytes containing numerous phagocytized red blood cells (see Chapter 32).

Angioimmunoblastic T-cell lymphoma involves the bone marrow in 50% to 80% of cases (275–278). The lesions in trephine biopsy sections vary in their composition but generally are similar to those in the lymph nodes. Immunoblasts, plasmacytoid immunoblasts, and plasma cells proliferate. A vascular proliferation that consists of numerous small arborizing vessels and a deposition of amorphous pale eosinophilic interstitial material usually are observed (2,275,279–282). Marrow involvement may be focal or diffuse; focal lesions are paratrabecular or are randomly distributed. In addition to immunoblasts and plasma cells, the infiltrate often contains histiocytes, eosinophils, a heteromorphous population of lymphocytes, and occasionally, large multinucleated cells. Reticulin is increased and a fibroblastic proliferation that replaces large areas of marrow has been observed in some cases. Uninvolved marrow is usually hypercellular. Erythroid hyperplasia secondary to hemolytic anemia may be found. In marrow aspirate smears, mature lymphocytes often are increased, and immunoblasts may be observed. Circulating immunoblasts and plasma cells are seen in blood smears in some cases and rarely cause a profound leukocytosis (281).

Infiltrates similar to those seen in angioimmunoblastic T-cell lymphoma may be observed in marrow biopsies from patients who have immune cytopenias, viral infections, and AIDS and, occasionally, in other conditions associated with lymphocytic hyperplasia.

Angiocentric lymphomas are aggressive lesions, most commonly with a true natural killer cell phenotype, with a propensity for angioinvasion and tissue necrosis. Although classically seen in the upper airways, similar lesions may

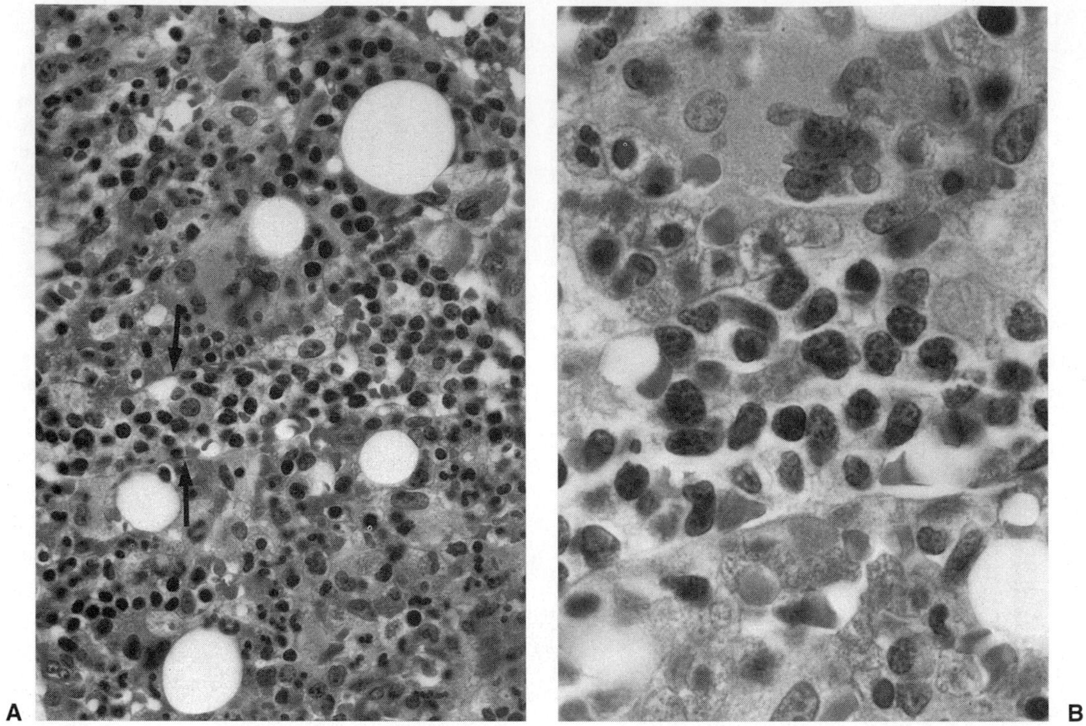

FIG. 39.41. Bone marrow trephine section from a patient with hepatosplenic $\gamma\delta$ T-cell lymphoma. **A:** A sinusoid is filled with lymphoma cells *(arrows)* (hematoxylin and eosin stain, original magnification: 400× magnification). **B:** A higher-power view demonstrates medium-sized cells with coarse chromatin and inconspicuous nucleoli (hematoxylin and eosin stain, original magnification: 1,000× magnification).

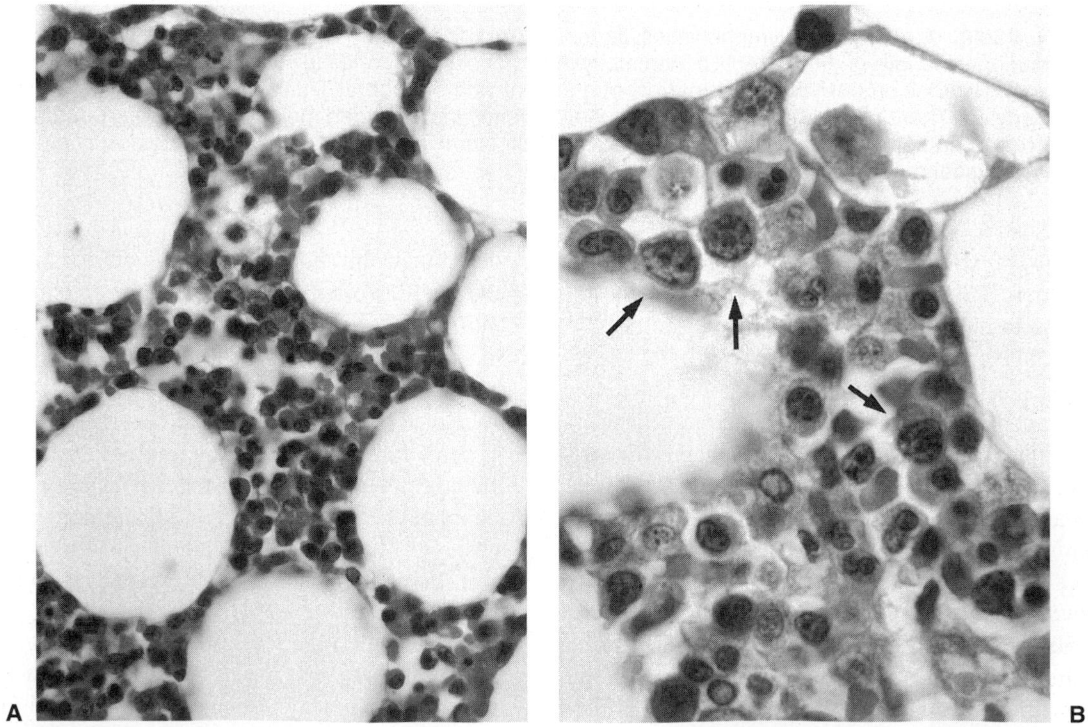

FIG. 39.42. Bone marrow trephine biopsy in a 63-year-old man with enteropathy-associated T-cell lymphoma. **A:** The neoplastic infiltrate is very difficult to discern in this architecturally intact marrow (hematoxylin and eosin stain, original magnification: 400× magnification). **B:** A higher-power view shows single neoplastic cells infiltrating among normal hematopoietic elements *(arrows)*. The cells are large with clumped chromatin, one to two small nucleoli, and moderate amounts of amphophilic cytoplasm (hematoxylin and eosin stain, original magnification: 1,000× magnification).

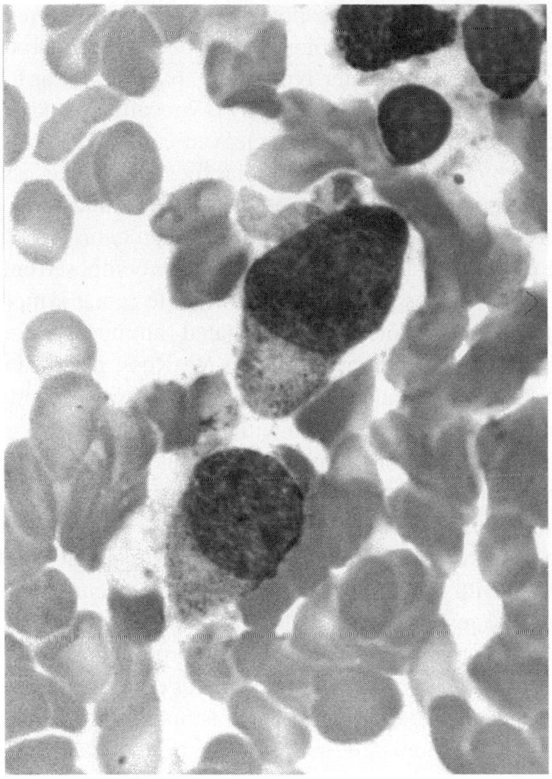

FIG. 39.43. Bone marrow aspirate smear from the same patient with enteropathy-associated T-cell lymphoma illustrated in Figure 39.42. The cells are large with coarse chromatin, somewhat indistinct nucleoli, and moderate amounts of pale basophilic cytoplasm containing azurophilic granulation (Wright-Giemsa stain, original magnification: 1,000× magnification).

occur in a variety of sites (283–290). It appears that the bone marrow is involved in these lesions in roughly 20% of cases (284,286–288,291). Descriptions of features of marrow involvement are not available. In primary sites these tumors have a wide cytologic spectrum (283). Tumor cells demonstrate azurophilic cytoplasmic granulation in air-dried, Giemsa-stained smears and imprints (284,286). An important diagnostic feature of these lesions is the expression of CD56, which may be detected in paraffin sections (292), and most contain Epstein-Barr viral sequences (286,293). However, these tumors do not contain T-cell antigen receptor gene rearrangements. As in the case of subcutaneous panniculitic T-cell lymphoma, angiocentric lymphoma may be accompanied by a reactive hemophagocytic syndrome (286,294) (see Chapter 29).

No data are available in the literature for incidence or pathologic features of *intestinal T-cell lymphoma* (with or without associated enteropathy) in the bone marrow. A case in our laboratory demonstrated a subtle interstitial pattern of infiltration. Medium to large cells with coarse chromatin, one to several distinct nucleoli, and moderately abundant eosinophilic cytoplasm percolated among normal hematopoietic elements (Fig. 39.42). In the aspirate smears the cells had coarse chromatin and moderately abundant pale blue cytoplasm with distinct azurophilic granulation; nucleoli were not readily visible (Fig. 39.43).

Adult T-cell lymphoma/leukemia (i.e., HTLV-1–related lymphoma/leukemia) involves the bone marrow in more than half of cases; all patients with marrow infiltration also demonstrate peripheral blood involvement (295). Involvement varies from sparse interstitial infiltration among normal hematopoietic cells (295) to extensive, diffuse replacement (65,296). Typically, the neoplastic cells in smears and sections are composed of a monomorphic population of medium-sized lymphocytes with prominent, exophytic nuclear convolutions, coarse chromatin, and inconspicuous or absent nucleoli (65,296) (Fig. 39.44). However, this neoplasm may also be composed of large cells with prominent nucleoli and without prominent nuclear convolutions or of mixtures of small and large cells (295). Trephine biopsies from patients with hypercalcemia demonstrate increased osteoclastic activity (295).

Immunophenotypic analysis demonstrates a characteristic, although not pathognomonic phenotype: $CD3^+$, $CD4^+$, $CD5^+$, $CD7^-$, and $CD25^+$. The diagnosis should be confirmed in all cases by identification of antibodies to HTLV-1 (in nonendemic areas) or, preferably, the demonstration of HTLV-1 viral sequences in the neoplastic cells (see Chapter 44).

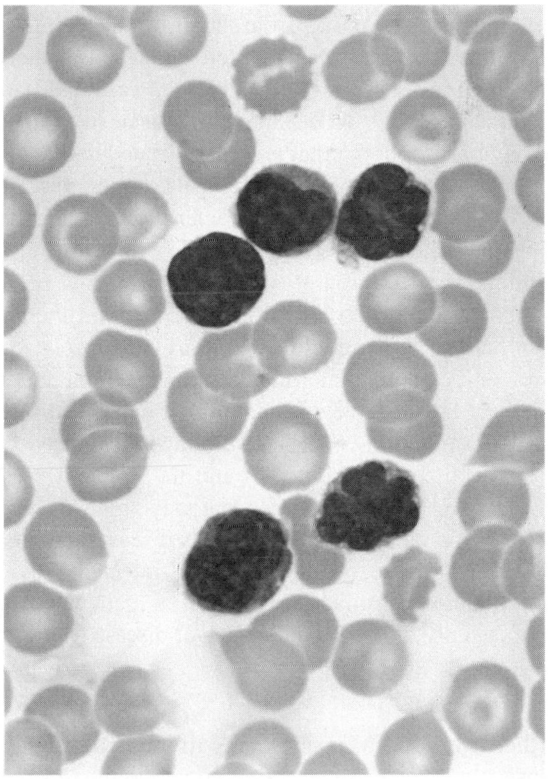

FIG. 39.44. Adult T-cell lymphoma/leukemia in peripheral blood. The cells have the characteristic convoluted, flower-shaped nuclei with coarse chromatin (Wright-Giemsa stain, original magnification: 1,000× magnification).

Anaplastic large cell lymphoma (ALCL) involves the bone marrow in approximately 20% of cases (297–303). Infiltrating cells are generally large, but vary considerably in size. A similar cytologic spectrum may be seen as in primary sites; cells often have lobulated or embryoid nuclei, abundant cytoplasm, a pale paranuclear zone, and prominent nucleoli. Involvement may take the form of diffuse, massive infiltration, scattered focal cell clusters, or singly scattered cells (298–300,304,305). This last pattern may be extremely difficult to appreciate on routine histology; detection is facilitated by immunohistochemistry for CD30 or epithelial membrane antigen (297,299) (see Chapter 25).

ALCL may also be detected in bone marrow aspirate smears (298,302,305). Peripheral blood involvement is uncommonly observed (298,305,306). The cells are large, with folded nuclei, prominent nucleoli, and abundant basophilic cytoplasm that may contain clear vacuoles (298,302,305). The neoplastic cells may be difficult to distinguish from immature megakaryocytes (302).

Primary Bone Marrow Lymphoma

Occasionally, a clinically unsuspected NHL or HL is diagnosed initially on bone marrow examination (307–309). Although in most patients careful investigation reveals involvement of extramedullary tissue sites, some patients apparently have disease localized to the bone marrow at presentation. Pathologically, this group of "primary" marrow lymphomas is heterogeneous, ranging from small cell to pleomorphic large cell proliferations, with B-cell and T-cell phenotypes. Common clinical features include fever, weakness, fatigue, and cytopenias (307–309). Although it seems likely that rare examples of lymphoma that are truly isolated to the marrow exist, it is important to rule out unusual tumors that do not generally have lymph node involvement, such as angiotropic lymphoma or hepatosplenic $\gamma\delta$ T-cell lymphoma.

Within this discussion of lymphoma presenting primarily in the bone marrow, it is important to mention the special case of human immunodeficiency virus (HIV)–related lymphoma. These patients are more likely than immunocompetent individuals to have lymphoma first diagnosed on bone marrow examination because of the high incidence of marrow involvement (45,310–312) and the frequent presence of systemic HIV manifestations that may obscure the initial signs of malignancy. Even Hodgkin's disease may initially be diagnosed on marrow biopsy in HIV-infected individuals (60), although, similar to non-AIDS patients, clinical workup usually discloses other sites of disease (see Chapter 28).

Posttherapy Bone Marrow and Minimal Residual Disease

Changes after chemotherapy vary for the different types of NHL. For low-grade lymphomas, the lesions diminish in size with response to chemotherapy, but in many cases, complete resolution does not occur; detection of residual disease is relatively common. With some therapy protocols for grade I follicle center lymphoma, paratrabecular foci of lymphoma become progressively hypocellular and sometimes contain few or no small cleaved cells (313). Presence of these hypocellular paratrabecular foci does not necessarily indicate remission and has no predictive value for longer survival or cure (313). An unusual phenomenon is the presence of discrete paratrabecular aggregates composed entirely of T lymphocytes in patients with follicle center lymphoma treated with radioisotope-conjugated antibodies directed against the CD20 antigen (Charles W. Ross, personal communication). Reticulin fiber content is not significantly decreased in focal lesions, even with response to therapy (314). Complete resolution of marrow lesions may be observed with effective response to chemotherapy for high-grade lymphomas. Areas of necrotic tumor may be seen in the marrow biopsy shortly after induction therapy. Repopulation of the marrow with normal hematopoietic tissue occurs relatively soon after resolution of the lymphoma.

Bone marrow relapse usually is morphologically similar to the original lymphoma. In some cases of lymphoma, transformation to a more aggressive histopathologic type may occur. Morphologically undetectable or equivocal early relapse or minimal residual disease (MRD) may be identified using immunophenotypic, cytogenetic, molecular, or culture methods (31,206,315–325). Polymerase chain reaction has emerged as a sensitive and useful assay for the detection of MRD, particularly when clone-specific primers are used. It has become apparent that detection of MRD in blood or bone marrow after therapy or in bone marrow or peripheral blood stem cell harvests before transplantation is associated with increased risk of relapse and decreased disease-free survival (316–319,324).

Blood Involvement by Lymphomas

Circulating lymphoma cells are found in blood smears in 40% to 50% of cases with bone marrow involvement and rarely in cases without marrow disease (4,7) (Table 39.6). The degree of blood involvement generally is related to the extent of marrow disease (7). The incidence of circulating lymphoma cells is highest for the low-grade lymphomas, small lymphocytic and follicle center grade I, but virtually every category may manifest blood involvement in some cases (326).

TABLE 39.6. *Blood involvement at diagnosis of non-Hodgkin's lymphoma*

Patients with blood involvement	10–25%
Marrow-positive patients with blood involvement	40–50%
Extent of blood involvement	
Slight	≈40%
Moderate	≈40%
Marked	≈20%

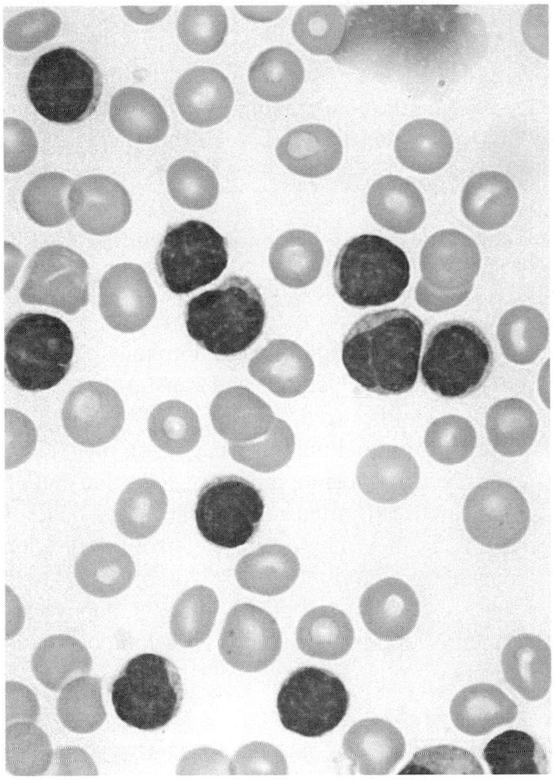

FIG. 39.45. Leukemic phase of mantle cell lymphoma in a 70-year-old woman; the absolute lymphocyte count was 28 $\times$ 10^9 cells/L. The cells have folded, cleaved, or indented nuclei with coarse chromatin and absent nucleoli (Wright-Giemsa stain, original magnification: 1,000$\times$ magnification).

Usually, only a small or moderate number of lymphoma cells is identified on scanning the blood smears and the total leukocyte count and differential are unaffected (Fig. 39.29). In some cases of follicle center, mantle cell, and peripheral T-cell lymphomas (adult T-cell leukemia/lymphoma), an elevated leukocyte count may be the first recognizable manifestation of disease. A frankly leukemic picture may be encountered in some cases (Figs. 39.23, 39.24, 39.45). The blood smear findings in these disorders must be distinguished from chronic lymphocytic leukemia (CLL) (77,78,327). The cytologic features, immunophenotype of the circulating lymphoma cells, and the pattern of distribution in the bone marrow usually serve to characterize properly the lymphoproliferative disorder. A lymph node biopsy confirms the diagnosis of follicle center or mantle cell lymphoma. Even with markedly elevated leukocyte counts, patients who have low-grade lymphomas may have normal or only slightly decreased hemoglobin, platelet, and neutrophil counts.

The incidence of circulating lymphoma cells probably is significantly higher than has been reported in morphologic studies of blood smears. Patients who have small lymphocytic lymphoma, follicle center lymphoma, mantle cell lymphoma, and mycosis fungoides may have a low number of morphologically undetectable circulating lymphoma cells that can be identified by flow cytometry or molecular analysis (206,260,315,321,328–333).

LYMPHOMA-LIKE DISORDERS

There are several bone marrow lesions that may mimic lymphomas histologically. Their presence in trephine biopsies may be particularly problematic in patients being staged or followed for HL or NHL. Lymphoma-like lesions also present differential diagnosis considerations when discovered in patients undergoing assessment of blood cytopenias or constitutional symptoms. This section focuses on reactive lesions and a few neoplastic disorders that are commonly encountered or particularly difficult. These include reactive lymphoid lesions, increased normal B-cell precursors (i.e., hematogones), granulomas, myelofibrosis, Langerhans cell histiocytosis, mast cell disease, and metastatic nonhematopoietic tumors. Several other disorders that may potentially cause difficulties in differential diagnosis, including other hematopoietic neoplasms, are covered in the previous discussion of individual types of lymphoma in bone marrow.

Reactive Lymphoid Lesions

Benign reactive lymphoid lesions have been identified in 18% to 47% of bone marrow biopsy specimens in different studies (334–338). They appear to be more frequent in women and are particularly common in older age groups; they increase in frequency with age after approximately 50 years. In geriatric populations they are not associated with any particular disease process and are of unknown clinical significance. Reactive lymphoid lesions are found in association with a spectrum of unrelated diseases and in healthy persons (336,339,340). In young individuals, they often are associated with an inflammatory process or immune disorder (336,340,341).

Reactive lymphoid lesions range from 50 to 1,000 μm in diameter and vary in number from a solitary focus in one section to several foci on every section of a trephine biopsy specimen. They are generally distributed randomly in the marrow without a predilection for a paratrabecular location, although they may abut on a trabecula (342). This discussion includes four general morphologic types of bone marrow reactive lymphoid lesions. They differ in some histologic features and in the clinical conditions in which they are encountered.

Lymphocytic Aggregates

The most common benign lymphoid lesions in bone marrow are lymphocytic aggregates. They are relatively small, round to oval, well circumscribed and clearly demarcated from the surrounding marrow (Fig. 39.46). Small blood vessels or endothelial cells often are identified in these lesions. The cellular component consists of generally loosely arranged, well-differentiated lymphocytes of various sizes;

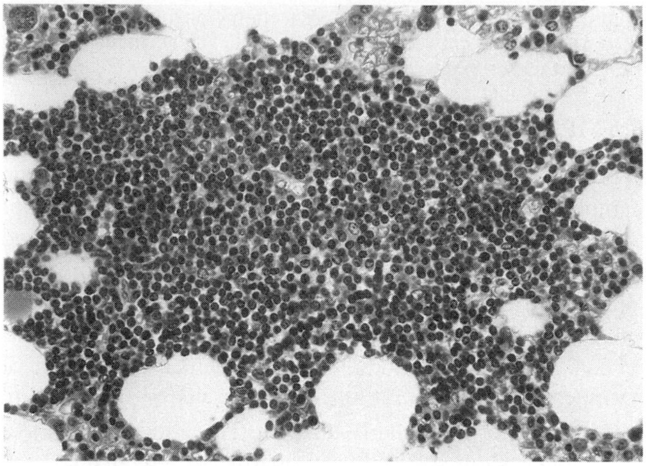

FIG. 39.46. Trephine biopsy section showing a reactive lymphocytic aggregate in the bone marrow of a 72-year-old woman with carcinoma of the breast. The lesion is well circumscribed and is composed of apparently mature lymphocytes (hematoxylin and eosin stain, original magnification: 250× magnification).

histiocytes, plasma cells, mast cells, and eosinophils also may be observed (2,334–336,343). These lymphoid lesions are most commonly seen in bone marrow biopsies from older patients, but may be found at any age. They are not associated with a particular disease process and their significance is unknown.

Reactive Polymorphous Lymphohistiocytic Lesions

Reactive polymorphous lymphohistiocytic lesions are less common than lymphocytic aggregates. They consist of a polycellular infiltrate with a heteromorphous population of lymphocytes that includes small and transformed cells; some of the nuclei may be irregular (Fig. 39.47). These lesions are often rich in epithelioid and phagocytic histiocytes and contain plasma cells, eosinophils, mast cells, and endothelial cells. The lesions are often multiple and may have poorly defined borders; they may occupy relatively large portions of the bone marrow biopsy (344). Polymorphous lymphohistiocytic lesions differ histologically from lymphocytic aggregates by their size, prominent histiocytic component, a more heteromorphous population of cells, and generally more

A 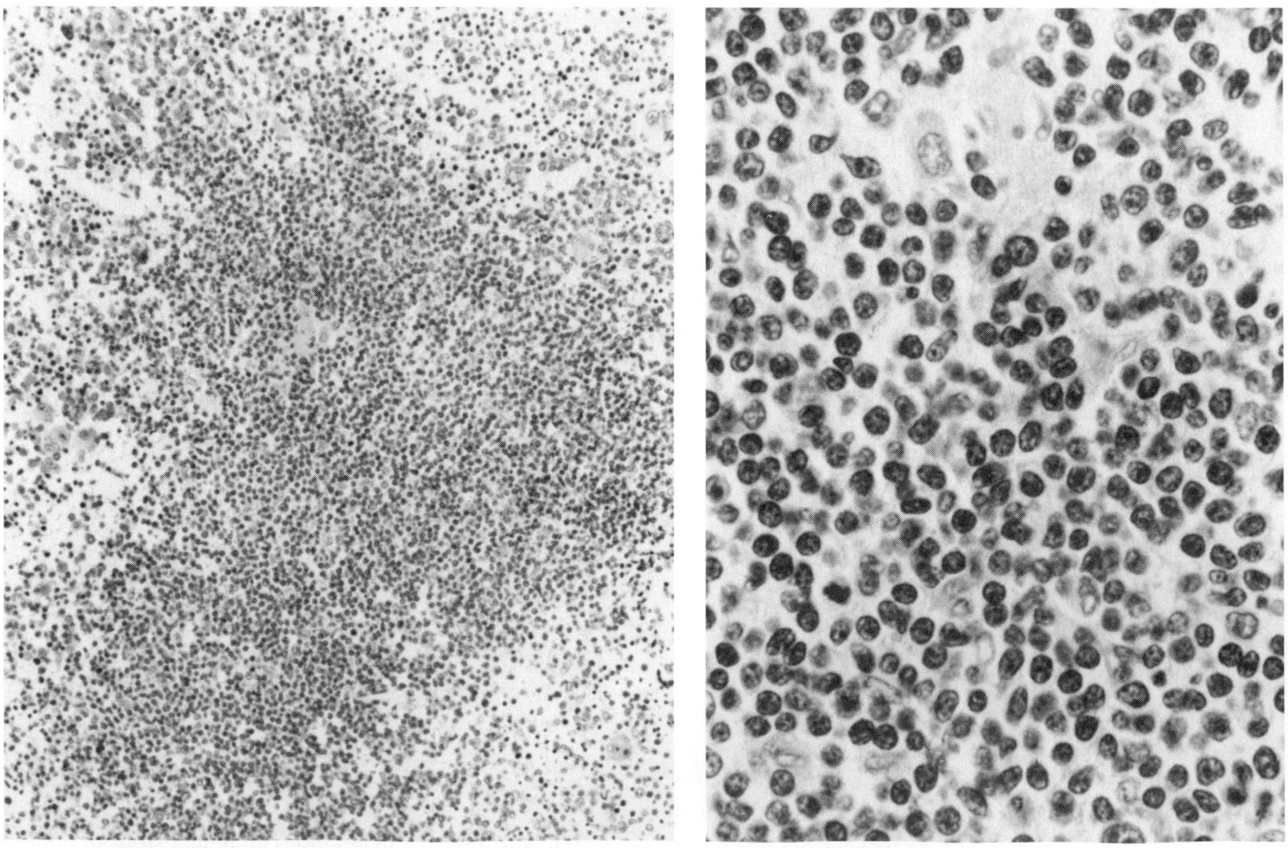 B

FIG. 39.47. A: A reactive lymphocytic lesion from the bone marrow of a 26-year-old man with immune neutropenia and thrombocytopenia. The lesion is large and has an irregular shape (hematoxylin and eosin stain, original magnification: 100× magnification). **B:** A higher-magnification view shows predominantly small lymphocytes with scattered transformed lymphocytes and histiocytes. The lymphocytes did not exhibit clonality by immunophenotypic and immunogenotypic analysis. Florid reactive lesions of this type often are mistaken for neoplastic proliferations (hematoxylin and eosin stain, original magnification: 400× magnification).

poorly defined margins; however, morphologic overlap between these two types of lesions exists. Florid polymorphous lymphohistiocytic lesions are commonly observed in patients with an immune deficiency or collagen-vascular disease, such as the acquired immunodeficiency syndrome or rheumatoid arthritis (340,344–346).

Reactive Follicles with Germinal Centers

Reactive follicles with germinal centers, alone or as a component of the florid reactive lesions previously described, are occasionally observed in bone marrow biopsies (2,347) (Fig. 39.48). They are randomly distributed and are often single on a biopsy section. They consist of a variably prominent mantle zone encircling a distinct germinal center. Reactive follicles with germinal centers vary in size and are composed of small and large cleaved and noncleaved lymphocytes, often with frequent mitotic figures and scattered histiocytes. These lesions are generally associated with an immune or inflammatory disorder and may be encountered in patients of any age, perhaps most commonly in young adults and children. These lesions are most problematic when they are poorly developed or bisected on the edge of a section (Fig. 39.49). Importantly, germinal centers may rarely be seen within neoplastic bone marrow infiltrates (Fig. 39.28).

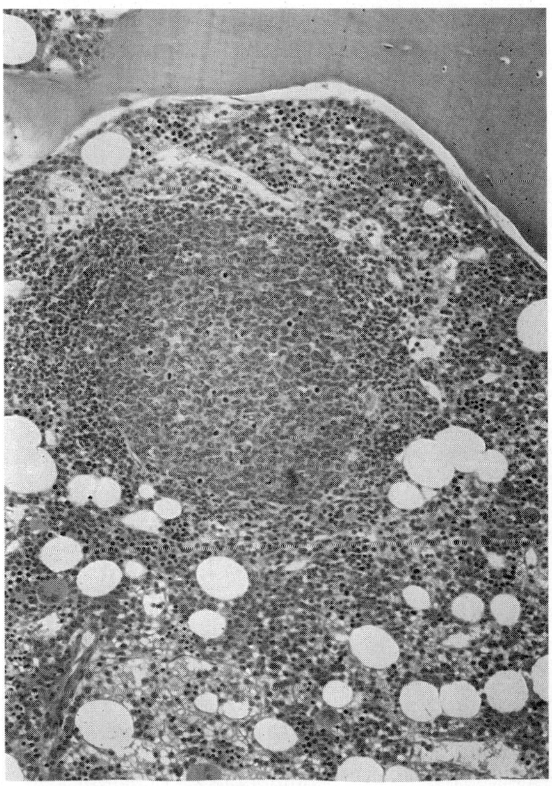

FIG. 39.48. A bone marrow trephine biopsy section from a child with juvenile rheumatoid arthritis. The biopsy contains a reactive lymphoid nodule with a germinal center (hematoxylin and eosin stain, original magnification: 100× magnification).

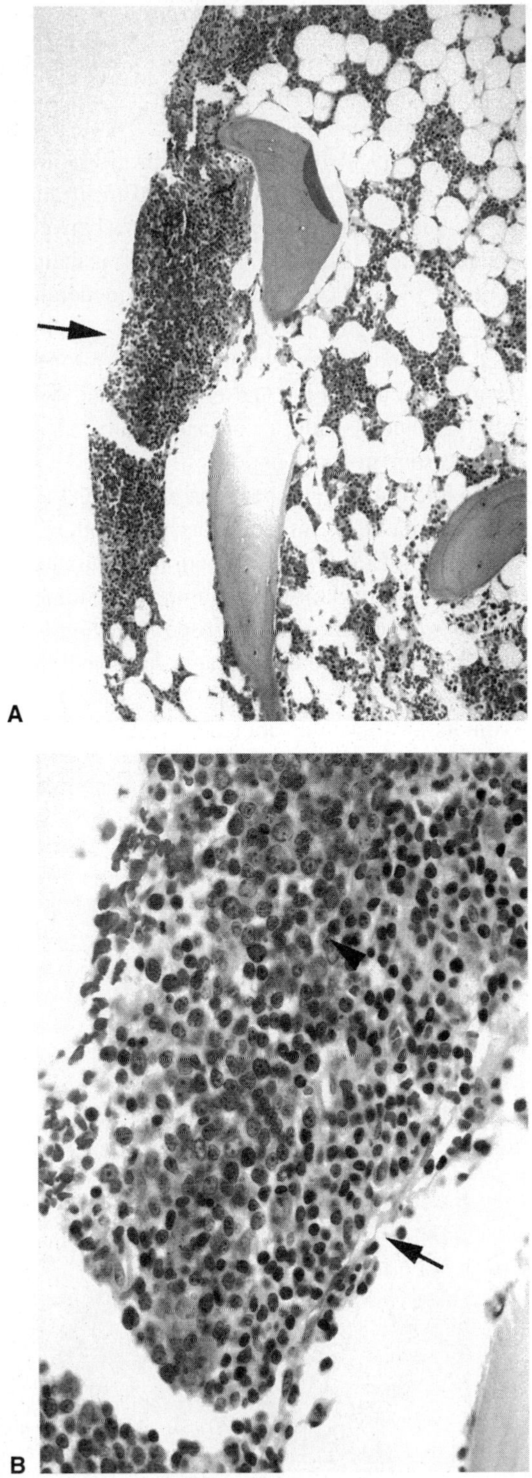

FIG. 39.49. A bone marrow trephine biopsy with a bisected reactive germinal center in a 38-year-old man previously treated for large cell lymphoma. The patient was being evaluated before bone marrow transplantation. **A:** Large lymphoid infiltrate on the edge of the core biopsy *(arrow)* (hematoxylin and eosin stain, original magnification: 100× magnification). **B:** Higher power demonstrates a mantle zone composed of small cells *(arrow)* and a germinal center composed of a fairly uniform population of larger cells *(arrowhead)*. CD20 demonstrated positive staining in small and large cells (hematoxylin and eosin stain, original magnification: 400× magnification).

Polyclonal Immunoblastic Proliferations

The least common but potentially most problematic reactive lymphoid lesions involving bone marrow are polyclonal immunoblastic proliferations (348–350). These are poorly circumscribed, atypical immunoblastic proliferations (Fig. 39.50). There are areas of loose interstitial infiltration with lymphocytes, plasma cells, and immunoblasts between more dense focal lesions. Multiple lesions are usually found throughout the biopsy. Cytologic atypia is generally not a feature.

Patients with polyclonal immunoblastic proliferations present with an acute illness and constitutional symptoms, often with lymphadenopathy or organomegaly; blood cytopenias are present in most patients. The blood leukocyte count is variable but usually is at least mildly elevated with circulating plasma cells, immunoblasts, and other reactive cells. The cause of these florid reactions is unknown, but the patients frequently exhibit autoimmune phenomena such as immune hemolytic anemia and respond to high doses of steroids. Some of these reactions have followed infections or have been an early manifestation of a collagen vascular disease; others have been attributed to severe drug or other allergic reactions.

Differential Diagnosis of Reactive Lymphoid Lesions

Reactive lymphoid lesions in bone marrow are problematic because of their morphologic similarity to some types of lymphoma. Reactive lymphoid lesions of various type have been identified in bone marrow trephine biopsies from 6% and 9% of patients at the time of staging for HL and NHL, respectively (8,96). When the typical features are present, recognition of reactive lymphoid lesions, especially lymphocytic aggregates, and their distinction from lymphoma generally is not difficult (Fig. 39.51). The usual small size, well-defined borders, random distribution in the marrow, prominent vascularity, and polymorphous cell proliferation of reactive lymphocytic aggregates help to distinguish them from lymphoma (Table 39.7). When lymphocytic aggregates are present in large numbers or are of unusually large size they may be confused with a low-grade lymphoma.

Reactive lymphoid hyperplasia may be particularly striking in patients who have immune disorders such as rheumatoid arthritis or AIDS (264,336,340,345,346,351–353). The lesions in these disorders may be particularly difficult to distinguish from lymphoma and caution must be exercised. The reactive polymorphous lymphohistiocytic lesions found in the marrow of patients with AIDS may be multiple and have poorly defined margins (264,345,346,351–353). These

A

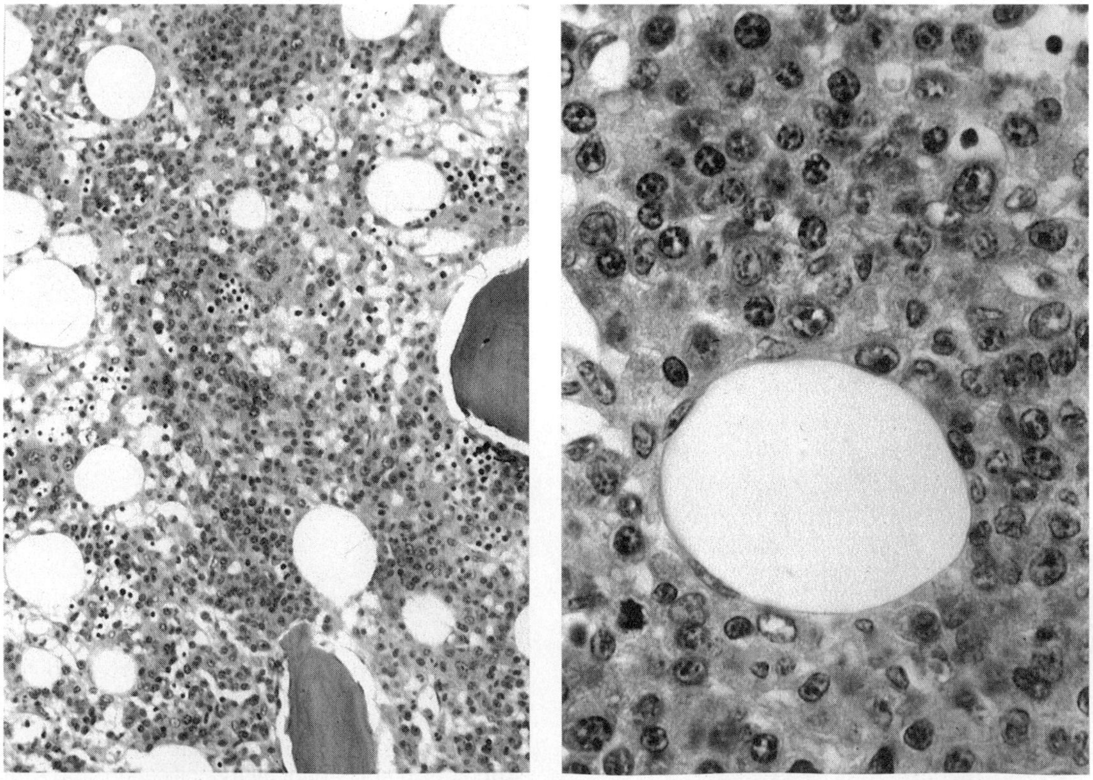

B

FIG. 39.50. Bone marrow trephine section in a patient with systemic polyclonal immunoblastic proliferation. **A:** The marrow architecture is altered by a polymorphous infiltrate (hematoxylin and eosin stain, original magnification: 250× magnification). **B:** High-power view shows a mixture of plasma cells, plasmacytoid lymphocytes, and immunoblasts (hematoxylin and eosin stain, original magnification: 1,000× magnification).

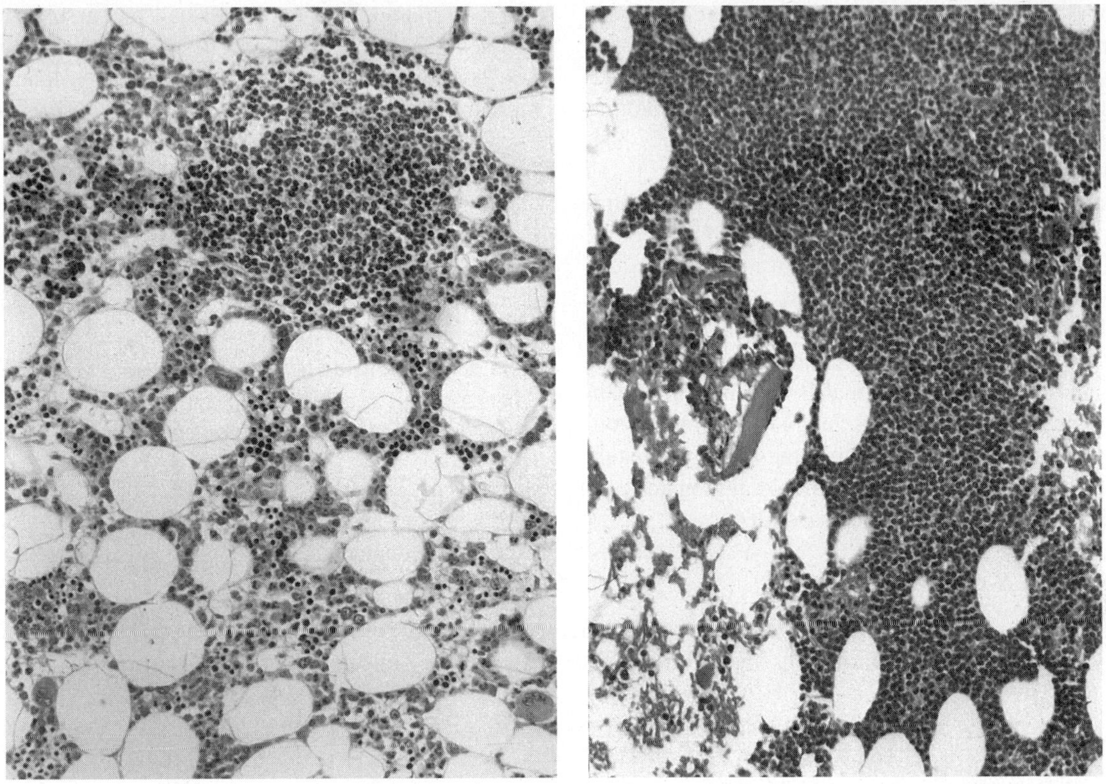

A B

FIG. 39.51. Comparison of benign and malignant lymphoid aggregates in trephine sections. **A:** This benign aggregate is small with well-defined borders and a somewhat loose texture. The cells vary somewhat in size, and a few histiocytes and endothelial cells are present (hematoxylin and eosin stain, original magnification: 100× magnification). **B:** This aggregate in a patient with small lymphocytic lymphoma/chronic lymphocytic leukemia (SLL/CLL) is large with infiltrating borders and a compact, monomorphous proliferation of small round lymphocytes (hematoxylin and eosin stain, original magnification: 100× magnification).

TABLE 39.7. *Distinction between reactive lymphoid lesions and lymphoma in marrow sections*

Reactive	Malignant
Random distribution	Frequently paratrabecular
Usually well-circumscribed	Often irregular shape with infiltration into adjacent marrow
Polymorphous cellularity with small lymphocytes, plasma cells, transformed lymphocytes, immunoblasts, histiocytes, and endothelial cells	Usually homogeneous, may be foci of transformation in small lymphocytic lymphomas; cellular atypia (e.g., cleaved or convoluted nuclei, nucleoli)
Vascularity frequently is prominent	Vascularity is not usually prominent (except in Hodgkin's lymphoma and peripheral T-cell lymphomas)
Germinal centers occasionally present	Germinal centers rarely present
No lymphoma cells present in marrow smears and imprints	Lymphoma cells may be present in smear and imprints

florid proliferations can occupy relatively large portions of the marrow. Histologic distinction of these lesions from peripheral T-cell lymphomas, T-cell–rich large B-cell lymphomas or HL may be difficult (65,99,264,345,351) (Fig 39.40). Any of these diagnoses should be considered very cautiously in patients with AIDS in the absence of a lymph node biopsy or other confirmatory studies.

The histologic distinction of polyclonal systemic immunoblastic reactions from lymphoplasmacytic or immunoblastic lymphoma or from plasma cell myeloma is difficult in some cases. Careful clinical history and recognition of the polyclonal nature of the proliferation by immunohistochemical stains for κ and λ light chains can generally distinguish these unusual lesions from lymphoma.

Immunohistochemistry, immunophenotyping by flow cytometry, cytogenetic studies, or molecular analysis may help in distinguishing between reactive lymphoid lesions and malignant lymphoma (16,22,23,45,99,109,182,206,328,341, 354–357). On immunohistochemical stains of bone marrow sections, mixtures of B and T lymphocytes with a majority of T lymphocytes is typical of reactive lymphocytic aggregates and polymorphous lymphohistiocytic lesions. In B-cell lymphomas consisting predominantly of small cells, there is an excess of B lymphocytes, although a substantial number of T cells may be present. BCL-2 staining has been reported in some studies to distinguish B-cell lymphomas from reactive bone marrow lymphoid lesions; most B-cell lymphomas are positive and reactive lesions are negative (21,22,27,341, 358). Identification of a clonal immunoglobulin or T-cell receptor gene rearrangement is strong evidence for lymphoma.

The finding of lymphoid aggregates in marrow sections may be associated with eventual progression to a neoplastic lymphoproliferative disorder. Some lymphoid lesions that are benign by histologic and immunophenotypic criteria have been shown to contain a clonal B lymphocyte expansion by immunogenotypic analysis and may progress to malignant lymphomas (356,359). In one study, approximately one third of patients with benign lymphoid aggregates progressed to a lymphoproliferative disease (360).

Increased Normal B-Cell Precursors

Bone marrow aspirate specimens from young children and occasionally from adolescents and adults may contain increased numbers of normal B-cell precursors (i.e., hematogones) (361–363). Many of these have morphologic features in common with the lymphoblasts of lymphoblastic lymphoma or acute lymphoblastic leukemia. They range in size from 10 to 20 μm and have smudged, homogeneous nuclear chromatin. The nucleus may be indented but usually lacks a nucleolus. Cytoplasm is sparse, deeply basophilic, and devoid of granules or vacuoles (Fig. 39.52). A morphologic spectrum may be observed from immature-appearing cells to cells morphologically approaching mature lymphocytes. In trephine biopsy sections they are diffusely dispersed as single cells, and are never seen as clusters (364). They resemble small or medium-sized lymphocytes but with slightly less dense and more homogeneous nuclear chromatin (Fig. 39.52).

B-cell precursors are found in bone marrow smears in large numbers in normal infants and in older children and adults with several diverse disorders (361–363,365,366). These include various cytopenias (iron deficiency, congenital neutropenia, congenital red cell aplasia, idiopathic thrombocytopenic purpura); neoplasms (neuroblastoma,

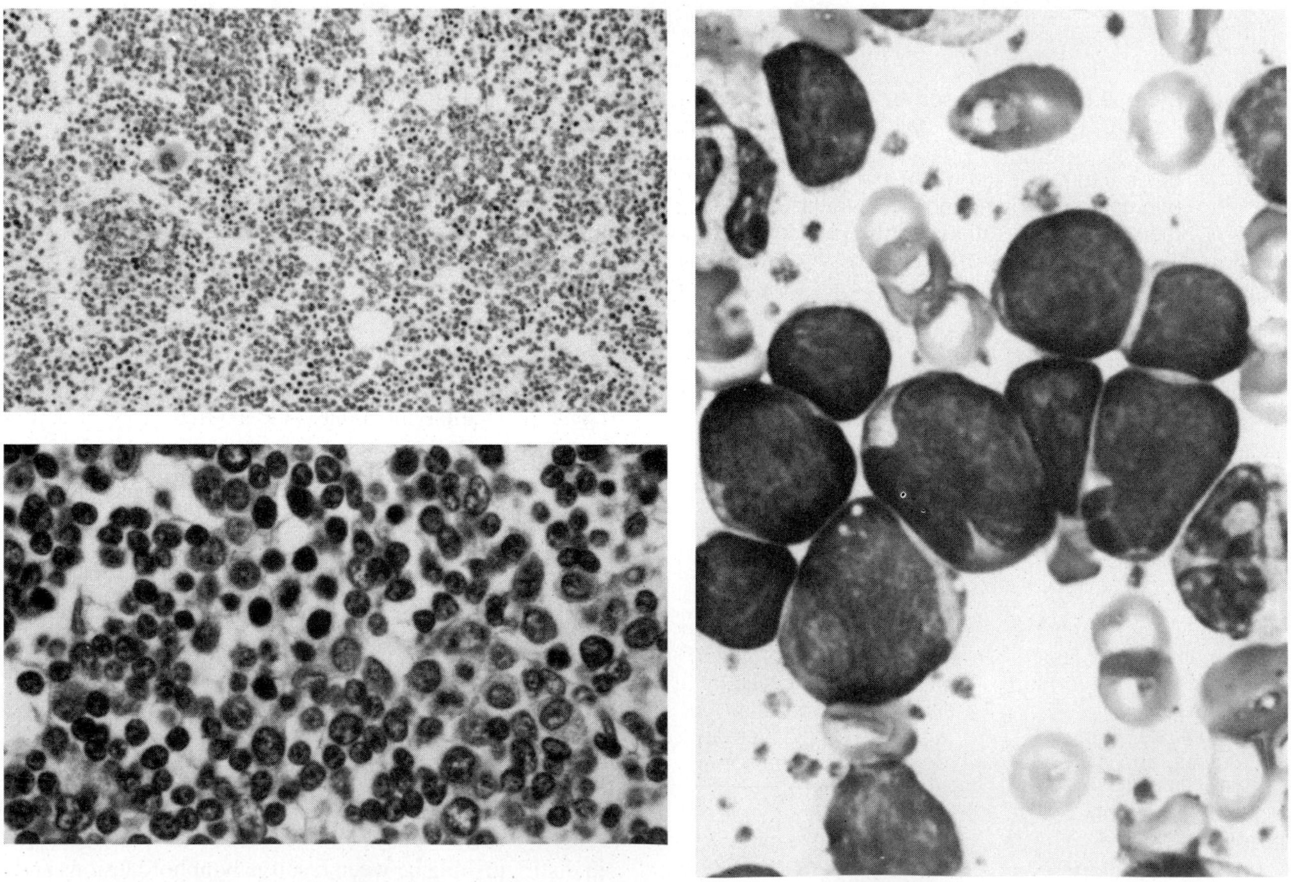

A B

FIG. 39.52. Bone marrow trephine biopsy and aspirate from a 2.5-year-old boy who was a bone marrow transplant donor for an older sibling who had aplastic anemia. **A:** The trephine section shows a highly cellular marrow with a marked increase in lymphoid cells (hematoxylin and eosin stain, original magnifications: **(top)** 100× and **(bottom)** 400× magnification). **B:** The aspirate smear contained approximately 50% lymphocytes and lymphoid progenitor cells (i.e., hematogones). Some of these cells bear resemblance to lymphoblasts. In the appropriate clinical context, a marrow with increased numbers of these cells could be mistaken for lymphoblastic lymphoma (Wright-Giemsa stain, original magnification: 1,000× magnification).

retinoblastoma, lymphoma); HIV infection; and after chemotherapy or bone marrow transplantation (361,362, 367–369). Occasionally B-cell precursors may represent as many as 50% to 60% of the bone marrow cells. When present in increased numbers in the bone marrow of children being evaluated for cytopenias or organomegaly, a diagnosis of lymphoblastic lymphoma or ALL may be considered. Normal B-cell precursors may express an antigen profile similar to malignant lymphoblasts, such as expression of TdT, CD34, CD10, and various pan-B-cell antigens (361,362,367, 368,370). However, by flow cytometric immunophenotyping, they differ from malignant lymphoblasts by demonstrating a continuous maturational spectrum of antigen expression and lacking aberrant antigen expression. In contrast, malignant lymphoblasts generally exhibit an incomplete maturational spectrum and phenotypic aberrancy (364,371–373). Normal B-cell precursors have a diploid DNA content, and clonal abnormalities are not demonstrable by cytogenetic or molecular analysis (362). Pathologists must be aware of the conditions in which normal B-cell precursors may be increased to avoid an erroneous diagnosis of lymphoblastic lymphoma or leukemia.

Granulomas

Granulomas may be found in bone marrow biopsies in the course of a directed search in patients being evaluated for an infectious disease or fever of unknown origin, but more commonly they are encountered as an incidental finding (374,375). Most bone marrow granulomas have no demonstrable infectious cause. These nonspecific granulomas often are found in hematopoietic tissues of patients who have HL or NHL (Fig. 39.12) (8,374–380). Granulomas have been observed in the bone marrow in approximately 7% of patients whose marrow biopsies were negative for HL at the time of staging. They appear to be slightly less common in patients who have NHL (8,374,375,378–380).

The granulomas generally are nonnecrotic, sarcoid-like, and consist of epithelioid histiocytes, occasional Langhans giant cells, lymphocytes, and eosinophils (8,376,377). They usually are small focal lesions and may be present in only one of two or more trephine biopsy specimens.

When bone marrow granulomas are unusually large or confluent, lack giant cells, and have an eosinophil component, they may resemble HL, a peripheral T-cell lymphoma, or histiocyte-rich large B-cell lymphoma. They are distinguished from Hodgkin's lesions by the usual predominance of epithelioid histiocytes, Langhans giant cells, and the absence of Hodgkin's cells. The cytologic features of the lymphocytes and comparison with lymphoma tissue from lymph nodes are important in distinguishing marrow granulomas from NHLs. Immunohistochemical stains for Hodgkin's cells and appropriate B- and T-lymphocyte subsets usually clarify a particularly problematic differential diagnosis.

The significance of nonspecific granulomas in patients who have a lymphoma is not clear. It has been suggested that the granulomas in HL are a manifestation of altered, delayed hypersensitivity (376). Evidence also exists, however, to suggest that the granulomas reflect a host response to the tumor and their presence may be indicative of a favorable prognosis (381,382). Bone marrow granulomas in some patients who have NHL have been intimately associated with lymphoma infiltrates and may represent a direct immune response (379,380).

The presence of granulomas in the marrow should always be considered carefully, particularly in patients receiving immunosuppressive chemotherapy. Appropriate special stains and microbiologic cultures should be performed. Opportunistic infections such as cryptococcosis, histoplasmosis, and the like may be first identified by bone marrow biopsy in these patients (8).

Langerhans Cell Histiocytosis

Langerhans cell histiocytosis (LCH) may be unifocal, multifocal, or disseminated (383,384). The distinction between these forms is made by clinical and radiologic findings; the histologic characteristics of the lesions are similar. In trephine biopsy sections, the lesions range from focal and randomly distributed to large and confluent, occupying most of the marrow space (Fig. 39.53 and 39.54). The lesions in most cases consist of a mixture of Langerhans cells with distinct nuclear folding, reactive histiocytes, multinucleated giant cells, eosinophils, plasma cells, lymphocytes, and neutrophils (Fig. 39.53). In some cases, there is a predominance of Langerhans cells (Fig. 39.54). The lesions often resemble granulomas (Fig. 39.53).

Because of their polycellular nature, these lesions may resemble HL or occasionally an NHL. The characteristic nuclear indentation of the Langerhans cells histiocytes, lack of exceptionally prominent nucleoli, and the lipid and pigment often contained in their cytoplasm should distinguish these cells from Hodgkin's cells. When the histopathology is equivocal, positive immunohistochemical stains for S-100 and CD1a are essentially diagnostic of LCH (385–390). Rarely it may be necessary to perform electron microscopy to identify diagnostic Birbeck granules (391).

The single bone lesions of localized Langerhans cell histiocytosis (eosinophilic granuloma) are theoretically the most likely to be problematic in the differential diagnosis of HL (392,393). In addition to the distinguishing features discussed previously, the clinical presentation of eosinophilic granulomas and their radiographic appearance should serve to distinguish these lesions from HL (see Chapter 51).

Systemic Mast Cell Disease

Systemic mast cell disease (i.e., mastocytosis) is a disseminated proliferation of abnormal mast cells that may involve several organs. Bone marrow involvement can be demonstrated in biopsy specimens in approximately 90% of cases and is the most common diagnostic tissue (394,395).

The distribution of mast cell lesions in trephine biopsy sections is focal in approximately 80% of cases and diffuse

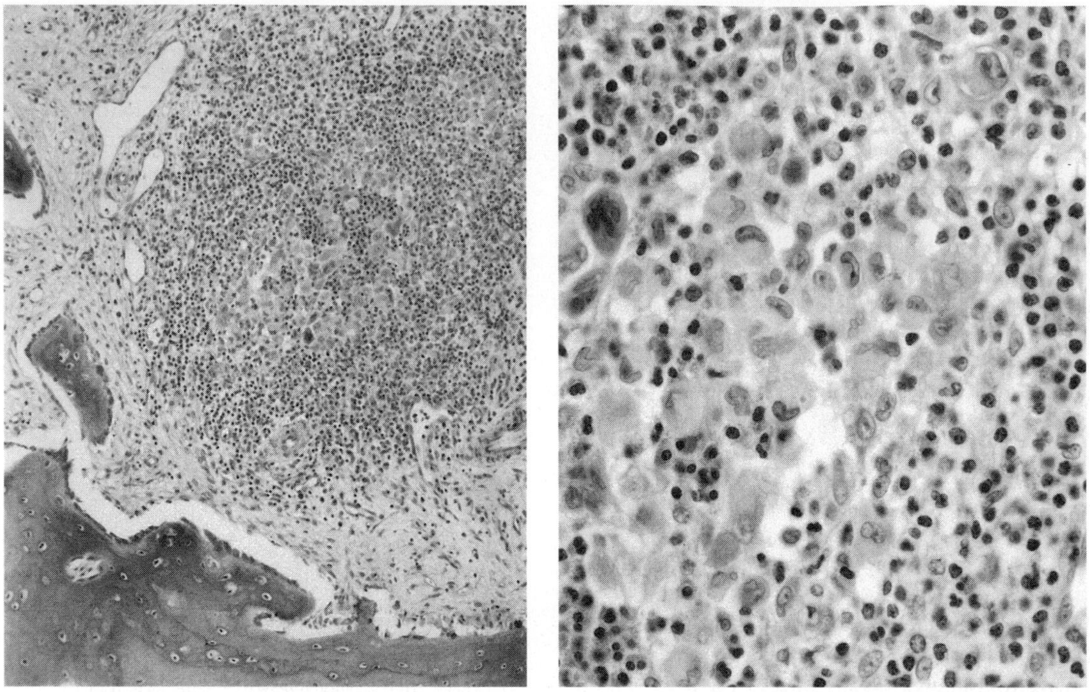

A B

FIG. 39.53. Focal lesion in a 12-year-old girl with multifocal Langerhans' cell histiocytosis. **A:** This polymorphous lesion consists of a central concentration of large pale Langerhans' cells surrounded by lymphocytes, neutrophils, and eosinophils. The marrow surrounding the lesion is densely fibrotic (hematoxylin and eosin stain, original magnification: 100× magnification). **B:** Higher-power view demonstrates cells with the characteristic feature of Langerhans' cells: large cells with abundant pale cytoplasm and bent, grooved, or irregular nuclei with pale chromatin and inconspicuous nucleoli (hematoxylin and eosin stain, original magnification: 400× magnification).

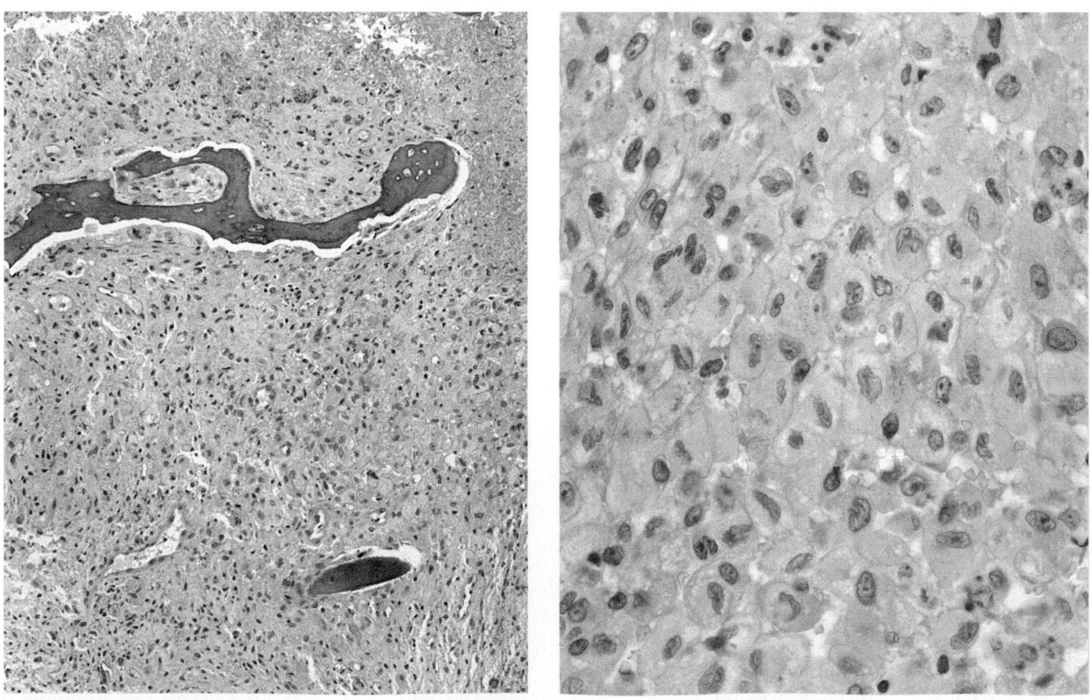

A B

FIG. 39.54. Bone marrow trephine biopsy in a small child with disseminated, aggressive Langerhans' cell histiocytosis. **A:** The bone marrow is diffusely replaced by sheets of pale-staining cells. An area of necrosis is present at the top of the field (hematoxylin and eosin stain, original magnification: 100× magnification). **B:** A higher-power view reveals a monomorphous proliferation of cells with the morphologic features of Langerhans' cells and few other reactive cellular elements (hematoxylin and eosin stain, original magnification: 400× magnification).

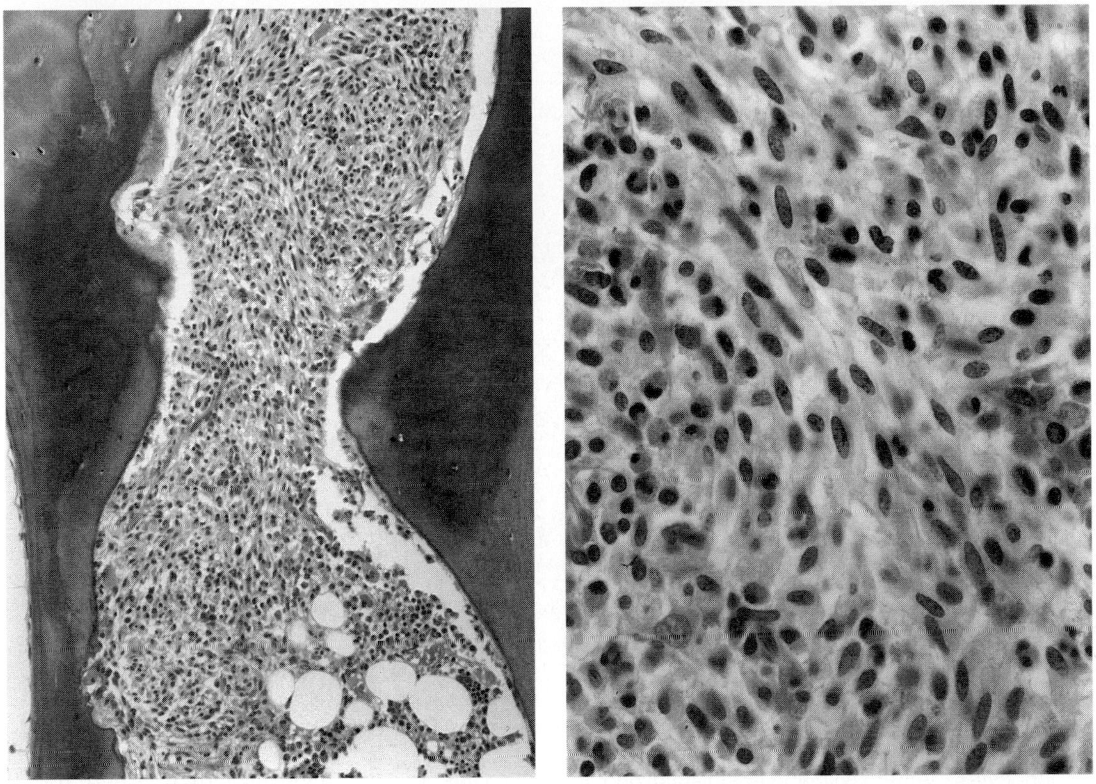

A B

FIG. 39.55. Bone marrow trephine biopsy with a paratrabecular mast cell lesion. **A:** Notice the thickened and irregular bony trabeculae (hematoxylin and eosin stain, original magnification: 250× magnification). **B:** Higher-power view reveals proliferation of spindled mast cells with bland nuclei, inconspicuous nucleoli, and moderate amounts of pale cytoplasm (hematoxylin and eosin stain, original magnification: 400× magnification).

in the remainder (394–396). Focal lesions may be monomorphic or polymorphic and are paratrabecular, perivascular, or randomly distributed; all patterns may be observed in the same biopsy specimen (394,397). The paratrabecular lesions usually are associated with fibrosis and thickened, mottled, irregular bone trabeculae (Fig. 39.55). Perivascular lesions manifest prominent medial and adventitial hypertrophy with layers of mast cells encircling the vessel. The randomly distributed focal lesions are usually polymorphic and consist of mast cells, lymphocytes, eosinophils, neutrophils, histiocytes, endothelial cells, and fibroblasts in varying proportions.

In some lesions there is a central focus of lymphocytes encircled by mast cells (Fig. 39.56). In others, the various cell types appear randomly mixed. Eosinophils frequently are scattered among the mast cells or concentrated at the periphery of the lesion. The mast cells in these lesions are round with abundant eosinophilic cytoplasm, closely resembling histiocytes in trephine sections (398,399).

Monomorphic focal lesions are composed predominantly of mast cells with scattered lymphocytes and eosinophils (Fig. 39.57). In some of these, the mast cells are spindle-shaped with round, oval, elongated, or monocytoid nuclei (Fig. 39.55). They resemble collections of histiocytes or fibroblasts.

Diffuse lesions replace large portions of the marrow. They generally consist of scattered mast cells in fibrous connective tissue; lymphocytes and other reactive cells may be present (394).

The distinction of mast cell disease in bone marrow from a large B-cell lymphoma, peripheral T-cell lymphoma, or HL occasionally may be problematic. In large B-cell lymphomas and peripheral T-cell lymphomas, the proliferative cells generally exhibit greater nuclear pleomorphism, more prominent nucleoli, and a distinctly higher mitotic rate than in mast cell disease. HL in bone marrow may be associated with loosely structured fibrosis and a polycellular infiltrate similar to mast cell disease, but HL is distinguished by the presence of Hodgkin's cells (2,91).

Mast cell lesions are uncommon, and may be easily overlooked or mistaken for other processes unless the pathologist is familiar with the characteristic features of these infiltrates, and includes this entity in broad differential diagnoses. Immunohistochemical stains definitively establish a diagnosis of mast cell disease. Antibodies to mast cell tryptase are most sensitive and specific for identifying mast cells in trephine

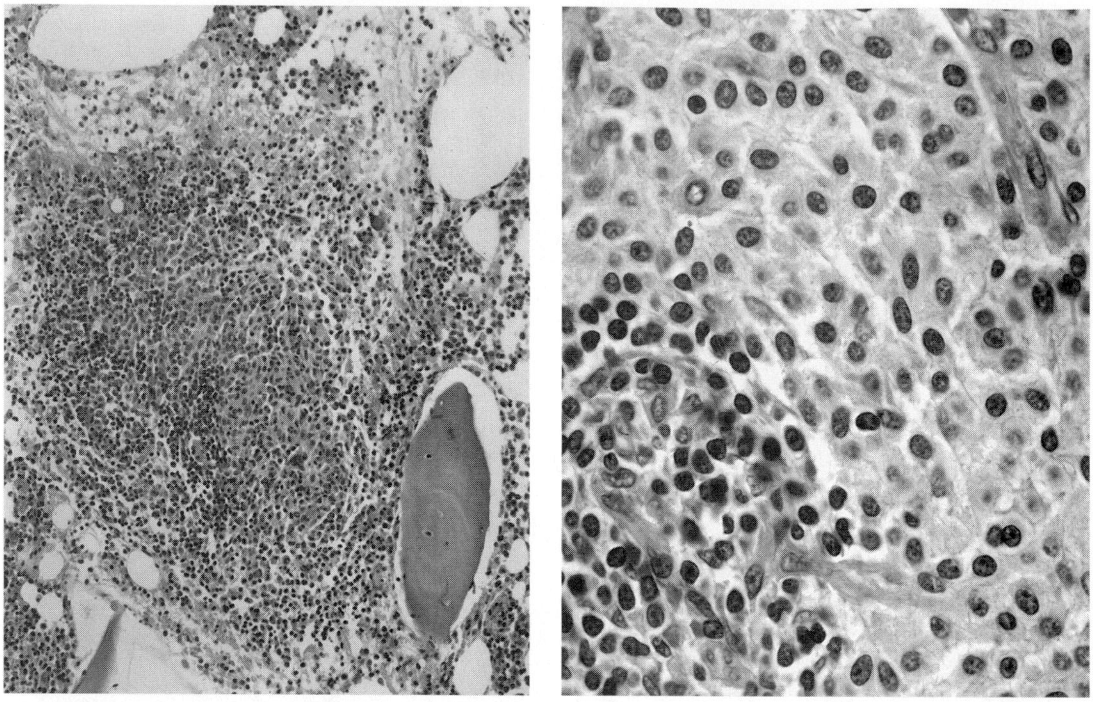

A B

FIG. 39.56. A targetoid mast cell lesion in a bone marrow trephine section from a patient with systemic mastocytosis. **A:** The lesion has a central zone of pale-staining mast cells surrounded by a cuff of lymphocytes (hematoxylin and eosin stain, original magnification: 250× magnification). **B:** Higher-power view demonstrates the characteristic cytologic features of mast cell infiltrates in sections (hematoxylin and eosin stain, original magnification: 400× magnification).

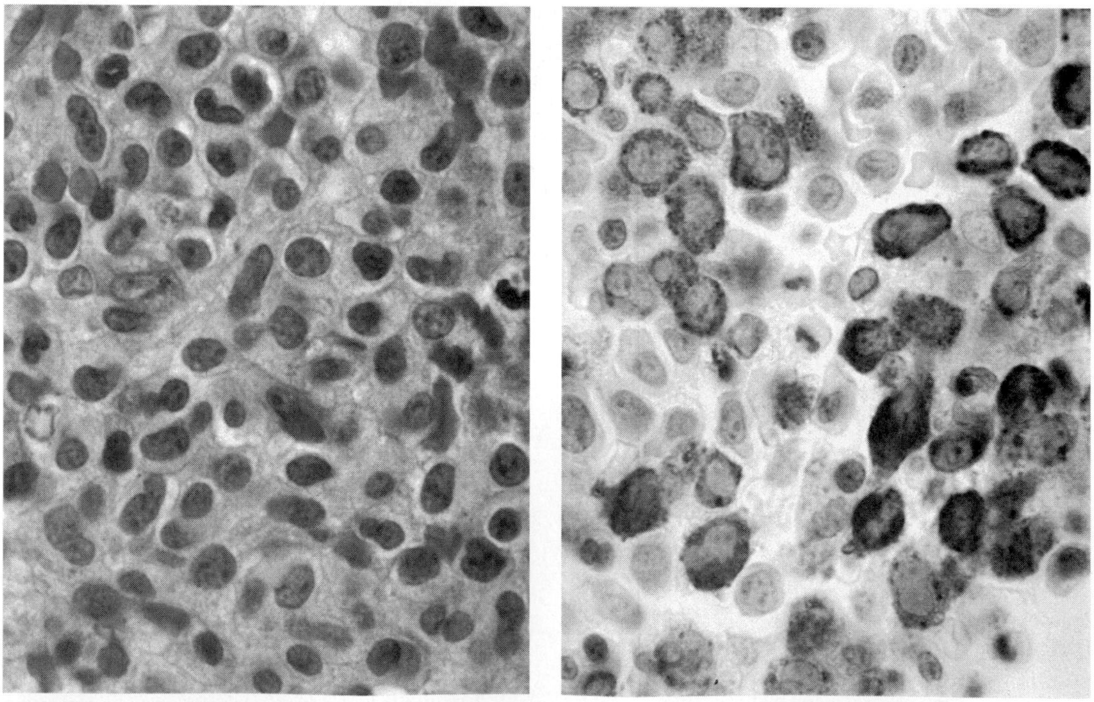

A B

FIG. 39.57. Trephine biopsy from a 73-year-old patient who had a history of refractory anemia with excess blasts who developed systemic mastocytosis. The bone marrow was extensively infiltrated by mast cells. **A:** Monomorphous infiltrate of mast cells showing elongate, bean-shaped, or monocytoid nuclei with delicate chromatin and abundant pale cytoplasm (hematoxylin and eosin stain, original magnification: 1,000× magnification). **B:** A mast cell tryptase immunohistochemical stain showing distinct granular cytoplasmic reactivity in the mast cells. The negatively staining cells are residual hematopoietic elements (mast cell tryptase stain, original magnification: 1,000× magnification).

biopsy sections (Fig. 39.57) (400). This procedure has effectively replaced the traditional demonstration of metachromatic staining using Giemsa or toluidine blue stains. Mast cells also stain positively for leukocyte common antigen, lysozyme, and α_1-antichymotrypsin (2,344,394–397,400) (see Chapter 52).

Myelofibrosis

Chronic idiopathic myelofibrosis (CIM) with myeloid metaplasia (primary myelofibrosis) is a chronic myeloproliferative disorder in which fibrosis of the marrow and extramedullary hematopoiesis are prominent features (401,402). Patients generally present with splenomegaly and blood count abnormalities. As the disease advances, the marrow is replaced increasingly by fibrous connective tissue and occasionally by osteosclerosis (402) (see Chapter 49).

Myelofibrosis rarely simulates HL (65,99,263). In unusual cases, the clusters of megakaryocytes in CIM could potentially be misinterpreted as Hodgkin's cells in suboptimally prepared trephine sections, but should be distinguished readily in technically good preparations (Fig. 39.58). Negative immunohistochemical stains for Hodgkin's cells aid in ruling out HL. Lymphoid infiltrates are present in some cases of CIM and potentially may present a differential diagnostic problem with NHL (401). Examination of blood smears for the characteristic blood cell abnormalities associated with CIM and familiarity with the patient's clinical manifestations aid in the differential diagnosis (402).

Metastatic Tumors

Several metastatic tumors may present with bone marrow involvement. Rarely, the initial tissue available for diagnosis is a marrow biopsy (403–405). The cytologic features of some metastatic solid tumors may resemble lymphoma in marrow smears and occasionally in trephine biopsy sections. In children, the clinical presentation and morphology of neuroblastoma, embryonal rhabdomyosarcoma, retinoblastoma, Ewing's sarcoma, and medulloblastoma may simulate lymphoblastic lymphoma or, occasionally, Burkitt's lymphoma. In adults, small cell carcinoma and, less commonly, other carcinomas may resemble lymphoma in marrow biopsies.

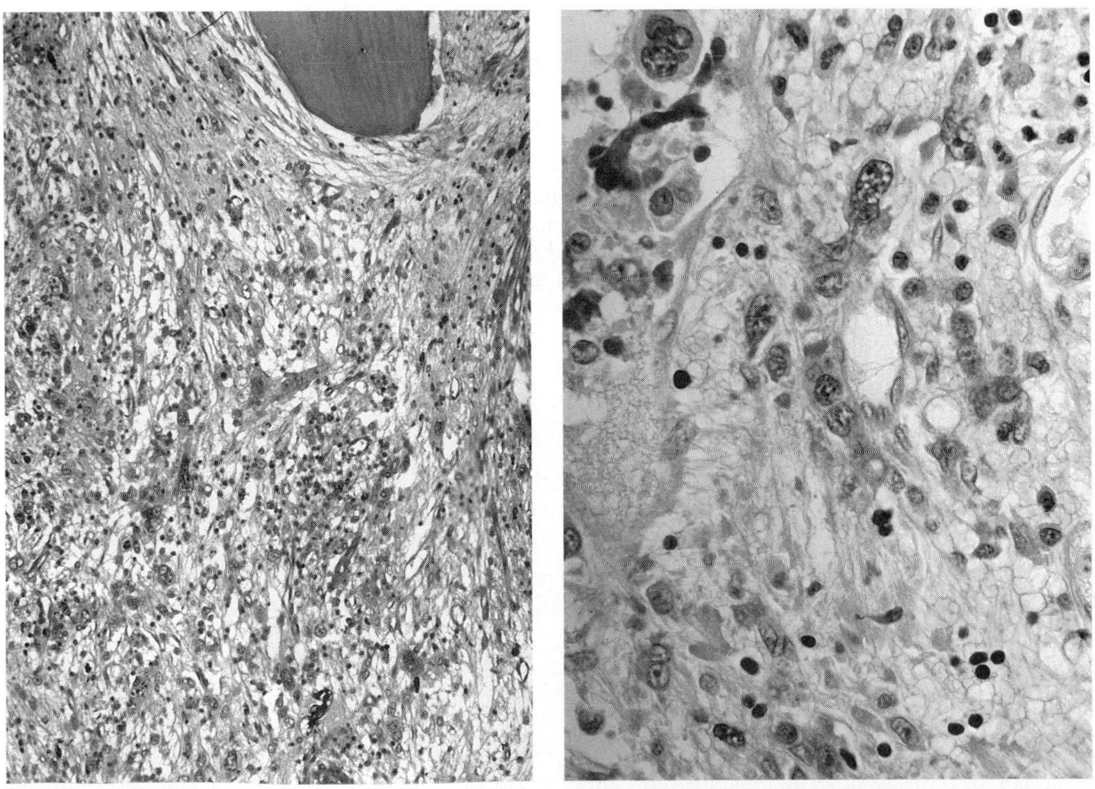

A B

FIG. 39.58. Primary idiopathic myelofibrosis in bone marrow trephine section. **A:** Low-power view demonstrates diffuse fibrosis containing scattered large cells (hematoxylin and eosin stain, original magnification: 100× magnification). **B:** Higher-magnification view reveals that the large cells are atypical megakaryocytes that lack the inclusion-like nucleoli of Hodgkin's cells. This differential may be problematic in poorly prepared sections (hematoxylin and eosin stain, original magnification: 400× magnification).

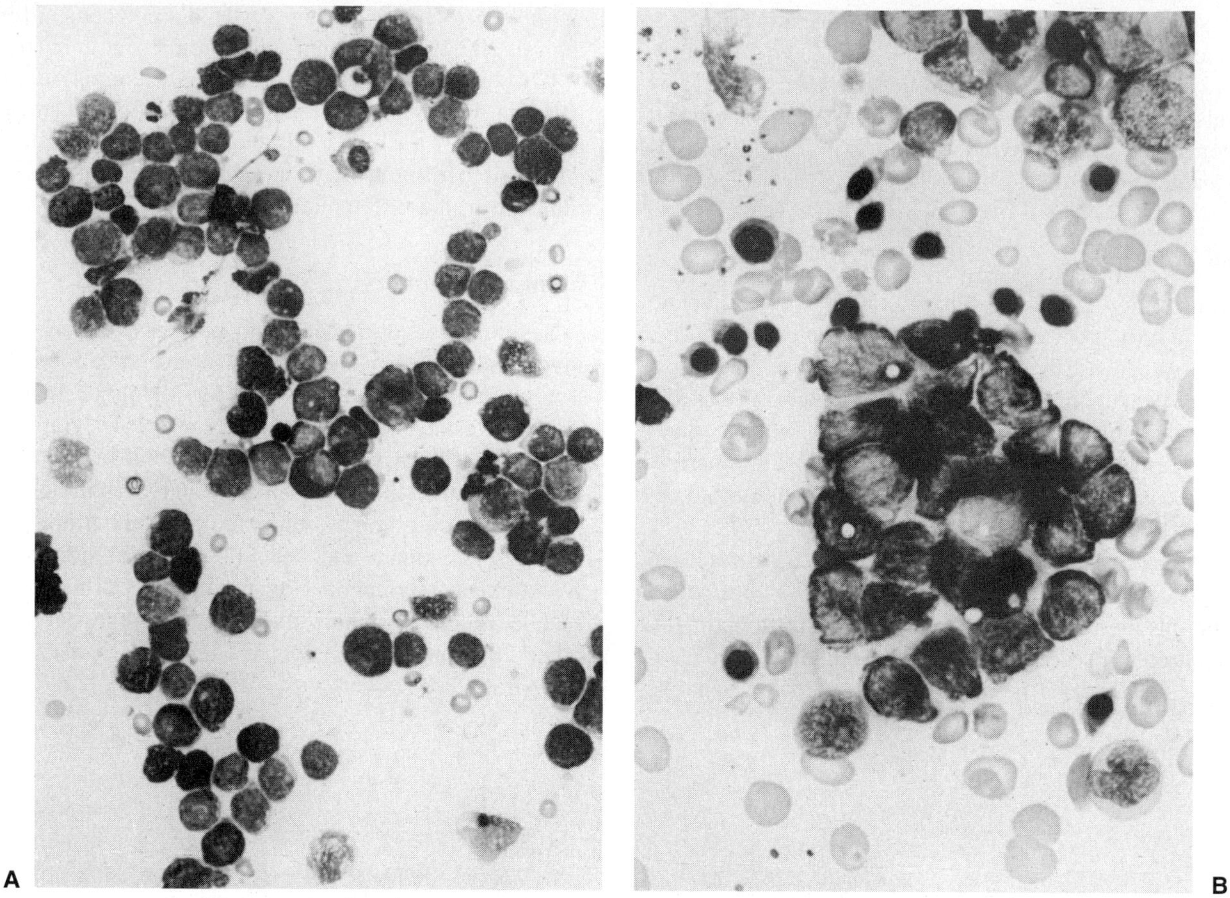

FIG. 39.59. A: A bone marrow aspirate smear from a 3-year-old girl with an abdominal mass. The marrow was involved extensively with neuroblastoma. For the most part, tumor cells were spread randomly and individually throughout the smear. Rare tumor clusters were identified. The size and cytologic features of these tumor cells resemble those of lymphoblasts. In cases with ambiguous cytology in aspirate smears, the trephine biopsy sections usually allow for distinction between metastatic small cell tumors and lymphomas (Wright-Giemsa stain, original magnification: 250× magnification). **B:** A cluster of tumor cells in a bone marrow aspirate smear from a patient who has small cell carcinoma of the lung. The presence of clumps and clusters of metastatic tumor cells helps distinguish between metastatic small cell tumors and lymphomas (Wright-Giemsa stain, original magnification: 250× magnification).

The necessity to distinguish one of these tumors from lymphoma usually arises when a primary tissue mass is not identified and the patient initially is evaluated for blood cytopenias or a leukemoid reaction. In marrow aspirate smears metastatic tumor cells are usually found in clumps or clusters; large numbers of damaged tumor cells and bare nuclei may be observed throughout the smear. Occasionally, the neoplastic cells in small cell tumors in children are spread evenly on the smear as single cells with few or no clumps (Figs. 39.59, 39.60). When this occurs, the morphologic distinction from lymphoma or leukemia may be difficult. The trephine biopsy sections may show histologic features distinctive for the metastatic tumor. In equivocal cases, immunohistochemistry, immunophenotyping by flow cytometry, and , rarely, electron microscopy may be necessary to resolve the differential diagnosis. Immunohistochemistry using panels that include antibodies to lymphocyte-associated antigens, as well as those for specific metastatic tumors is particularly helpful. By flow cytometry, a bright $CD56^+$ small blue cell tumor is occasionally encountered that is negative for all other leukocyte markers; these generally represent small cell undifferentiated carcinoma or other tumors of neuroectodermal origin.

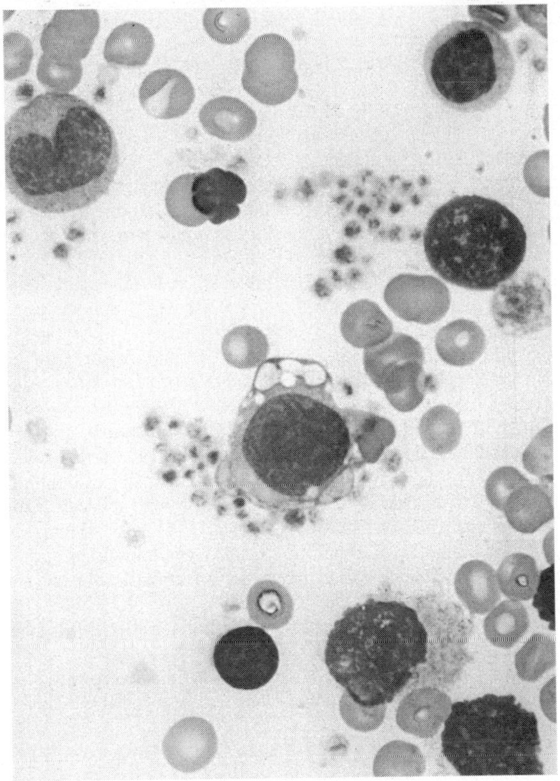

FIG. 39.60. Bone marrow aspirate smear from a 28-year-old man with metastatic rhabdomyosarcoma. The neoplastic cells in this aspirate smear were distributed almost entirely as single cells. Only very rare cell clusters were present. The cells had blastoid chromatin and varying amounts of lightly basophilic cytoplasm. Notice the irregular but sharply defined cytoplasmic vacuoles; these contain glycogen and stain positively with periodic acid–Schiff stain (Wright-Giemsa stain, original magnification: 1,000× magnification).

SUMMARY AND CONCLUSIONS

Bone marrow examination is a valuable procedure in the diagnosis and management of patients who have HL or NHL. The optimal bone marrow morphologic assessment for lymphoma includes examination of trephine biopsy sections and touch imprints, aspiration smears, and blood smears. The trephine biopsy is the specimen that is most commonly diagnostic of bone marrow involvement in HL and NHLs alike. Aspirated bone marrow provides the best material for assessment of cytology in some neoplasms, and is optimal for immunophenotyping by flow cytometry, cytogenetics, and many molecular studies.

The NHLs involve the bone marrow more commonly than does HL. The NHLs that involve the bone marrow most frequently are those primarily composed of small cells (i.e., small lymphocytic, follicle center, and mantle cell lymphomas), high-grade lymphomas of lymphoblastic and Burkitt's types, and the various categories of peripheral T-cell lymphoma. For HLs, the mixed cellularity type has the highest incidence of bone marrow disease. The pattern of marrow infiltration in trephine biopsy sections is most commonly diffuse in HL and focal in NHL. There is a predilection for focal paratrabecular infiltrates in follicle center lymphomas and for focal random (nonparatrabecular) infiltrates in the small lymphocytic lymphomas. Diffuse or interstitial patterns of involvement predominate in lymphoblastic and Burkitt's lymphomas. An intrasinusoidal or intravascular pattern is observed in splenic marginal zone, hepatosplenic $\gamma\delta$ T-cell, and angiotropic large B-cell lymphomas.

Morphologic discordance of lymph node and bone marrow histology may be observed in 9% to 40% of cases. Divergent histology is most common in follicle center lymphomas; the more aggressive histologic subtype is most commonly found in the lymph node.

Lymphoma cells frequently are observed in blood smears of patients who have lymphomas composed of small cells; in some cases, there is a frankly leukemic blood picture. Lymphoma cells are less commonly observed in blood smears from patients with more aggressive subtypes, but any of the NHL categories may involve the blood. The blood is never involved in HL.

Several benign lymphoma-like lesions may simulate lymphoma in the bone marrow. The most common and problematic of these are the reactive lymphoid lesions. They must be distinguished from several categories of NHL and occasionally from HL. In children who have increased bone marrow B-cell precursors (i.e., hematogones), an erroneous diagnosis of lymphoblastic lymphoma is possible if the pathologist is not familiar with these cells and the conditions in which they are commonly increased. Pathologists must be familiar with the bone marrow manifestations of the several reactive and neoplastic proliferations that may simulate lymphoma in the bone marrow.

Appropriate use of immunohistochemistry, immunophenotyping by flow cytometry, and molecular techniques is essential for the diagnosis and classification in many cases of NHL and in some cases of HL in bone marrow. These studies are often particularly important in distinguishing lymphoma from lesions simulating lymphoma.

REFERENCES

1. Brynes RK, McKenna RW, Sundberg RD. Bone marrow aspiration and trephine biopsy: an approach to a thorough study. *Am J Clin Pathol* 1978;70:753–759.
2. Brunning RD, McKenna RW. Bone marrow manifestations of malignant lymphoma and lymphoma-like conditions. *Pathol Annu* 1979; 14:1–59.
3. Barekman CL, Fair KP, Cotelingam JD. Comparative utility of diagnostic bone-marrow components: a 10-year study. *Am J Hematol* 1997;56:37–41.
4. Foucar K, McKenna RW, Frizzera G, et al. Bone marrow and blood involvement by lymphoma in relationship to the Lukes-Collins classification. *Cancer* 1982;49:888–897.
5. Grann V, Pool JL, Mayer K. Comparative study of bone marrow aspiration and biopsy in patients with neoplastic disease. *Cancer* 1966; 19:1898–1900.
6. Vinciguerra V, Silver RT. The importance of bone marrow biopsy in the staging of patients with lymphosarcoma. *Blood* 1973;41:913–920.

7. Lai HS, Tien HF, Hsieh HC, et al. Bone marrow involvement in non-Hodgkin's lymphoma. *Taiwan I Hsueh Hui Tsa Chih* 1989;88:114–121.
8. O'Carroll DI, McKenna RW, Brunning RD. Bone marrow manifestations of Hodgkin's disease. *Cancer* 1976;38:1717–1728.
9. Haddy TB, Parker RI, Magrath IT. Bone marrow involvement in young patients with non-Hodgkin's lymphoma: the importance of multiple bone marrow samples for accurate staging. *Med Pediatr Oncol* 1989;17:418–423.
10. Juneja SK, Wolf MM, Cooper IA. Value of bilateral bone marrow biopsy specimens in non-Hodgkin's lymphoma. *J Clin Pathol* 1990;43:630–632.
11. Horlyck A, Thorling K. Bone marrow examination in non-Hodgkin's lymphoma: comparison of the diagnostic value of marrow aspirations and trephine biopsy [Letter]. *Eur J Haematol* 1991;46:54–56.
12. Brunning RD, Bloomfield CD, McKenna RW, et al. Bilateral trephine bone marrow biopsies in lymphoma and other neoplastic diseases. *Ann Intern Med* 1975;82:365–366.
13. Coller BS, Chabner BA, Gralnick HR. Frequencies and patterns of bone marrow involvement in non-Hodgkin lymphomas: observations on the value of bilateral biopsies. *Am J Hematol* 1977;3:105–119.
14. Luoni M, Declich P, De Paoli AP, et al. Bone marrow biopsy for the staging of non-Hodgkin's lymphoma: bilateral or unilateral trephine biopsy? *Tumori* 1995;81:410–413.
15. Ebie N, Loew JM, Gregory SA. Bilateral trephine bone marrow biopsy for staging non-Hodgkin's lymphoma: a second look. *Hematol Pathol* 1989;3:29–33.
16. Andrade RE, Wick MR, Frizzera G, et al. Immunophenotyping of hematopoietic malignancies in paraffin sections. *Hum Pathol* 1988;19:394–402.
17. Kubic VL, Brunning RD. Immunohistochemical evaluation of neoplasms in bone marrow biopsies using monoclonal antibodies reactive in paraffin-embedded tissue. *Mod Pathol* 1989;2:618–629.
18. Beckstead JH, Halverson PS, Ries CA, et al. Enzyme histochemistry and immunohistochemistry on biopsy specimens of pathologic human bone marrow. *Blood* 1981;57:1088–1098.
19. Block M, Trenner L, Ruegg P, et al. Glycol methacrylate embedding technique emphasizing cost containment, ultrarapid processing, and adaptability to a variety of staining techniques. *Laboratory Medicine* 1982;13:290–298.
20. Thaler J, Denz H, Gattringer C, et al. Diagnostic and prognostic value of immunohistological bone marrow examination: results in 212 patients with lymphoproliferative disorders. *Blut* 1987;54:213–222.
21. Chetty R, Echezarreta G, Comley M, et al. Immunohistochemistry in apparently normal bone marrow trephine specimens from patients with nodal follicular lymphoma. *J Clin Pathol* 1995;48:1035–1038.
22. Bluth RF, Casey TT, McCurley TL. Differentiation of reactive from neoplastic small-cell lymphoid aggregates in paraffin-embedded marrow particle preparations using L-26 (CD20) and UCHL-1 (CD45RO) monoclonal antibodies. *Am J Clin Pathol* 1993;99:150–156.
23. Ben-Ezra JM, King BE, Harris AC, et al. Staining for Bcl-2 protein helps to distinguish benign from malignant lymphoid aggregates in bone marrow biopsies. *Mod Pathol* 1994;7:560–564.
24. Schwonzen M, Pohl C, Steinmetz T, et al. Bone marrow involvement in non-Hodgkin's lymphoma: increased diagnostic sensitivity by combination of immunocytology, cytomorphology and trephine histology. *Br J Haematol* 1992;81:362–369.
25. Lambertenghi-Deliliers G, Annaloro C, Soligo D, et al. Incidence and histological features of bone marrow involvement in malignant lymphomas. *Ann Hematol* 1992;65:61–65.
26. Vasef MA, Medeiros LJ, Koo C, et al. Cyclin D1 immunohistochemical staining is useful in distinguishing mantle cell lymphoma from other low-grade B-cell neoplasms in bone marrow. *Am J Clin Pathol* 1997;108:302–307.
27. Horny HP, Wehrmann M, Griesser H, et al. Investigation of bone marrow lymphocyte subsets in normal, reactive, and neoplastic states using paraffin-embedded biopsy specimens. *Am J Clin Pathol* 1993;99:142–149.
28. Fineberg S, Marsh E, Alfonso F, et al. Immunophenotypic evaluation of the bone marrow in non-Hodgkin's lymphoma. *Hum Pathol* 1993;24:636–642.
29. Stelzer GT, Shults KE, Wormsley SB, et al. Detection of occult lymphoma cells in bone marrow aspirates by multi-dimensional flow cytometry. *Prog Clin Biol Res* 1992;377:629–635.
30. Coad JE, Olson DJ, Christensen DR, et al. Correlation of PCR-detected clonal gene rearrangements with bone marrow morphology in patients with B-lineage lymphomas. *Am J Surg Pathol* 1997;21:1047–1056.
31. Hetu F, Coutlee F, Roy DC. A non-isotopic nested polymerase-chain reaction method to quantitate minimal residual disease in patients with non-Hodgkin's lymphoma. *Mol Cell Probes* 1994;8:449–457.
32. Lambrechts AC, de Ruiter PE, Dorssers LC, et al. Detection of residual disease in translocation (14;18) positive non-Hodgkin's lymphoma, using the polymerase chain reaction: a comparison with conventional staging methods. *Leukemia* 1992;6:29–34.
33. DiGiuseppe JA, Hartmann DP, Freter C, et al. Molecular detection of bone marrow involvement in intravascular lymphomatosis. *Mod Pathol* 1997;10:33–37.
34. Chen PM, Fan S, Lin SH, et al. Study of bone marrow cells in non-Hodgkin's lymphoma by DNA analysis. *Leuk Res* 1991;15:1097–1106.
35. Musshoff K. Prognostic and therapeutic implications of staging in extranodal Hodgkin's disease. *Cancer Res* 1971;31:1814–1827.
36. Bartl R, Frisch B, Burkhardt R, et al. Assessment of bone marrow histology in Hodgkin's disease: correlation with clinical factors. *Br J Haematol* 1982;51:345–360.
37. Bartl R, Frisch B, Burkhardt R, et al. Lymphoproliferations in the bone marrow: identification and evolution, classification and staging. *J Clin Pathol* 1984;37:233–254.
38. Rosenberg SA. Hodgkin's disease of the bone marrow. *Cancer Res* 1971;31:1733–1736.
39. Myers CE, Chabner BA, De Vita VT, et al. Bone marrow involvement in Hodgkin's disease: pathology and response to MOPP chemotherapy. *Blood* 1974;44:197–204.
40. Munker R, Hasenclever D, Brosteanu O, et al. Bone marrow involvement in Hodgkin's disease: an analysis of 135 consecutive cases. German Hodgkin's Lymphoma Study Group. *J Clin Oncol* 1995;13:403–409.
41. Doll DC, Ringenberg QS, Anderson SP, et al. Bone marrow biopsy in the initial staging of Hodgkin's disease. *Med Pediatr Oncol* 1989;17:1–5.
42. Straus DJ, Gaynor JJ, Myers J, et al. Prognostic factors among 185 adults with newly diagnosed advanced Hodgkin's disease treated with alternating potentially noncross-resistant chemotherapy and intermediate-dose radiation therapy. *J Clin Oncol* 1990;8:1173–1186.
43. Longo DL, Duffey PL, DeVita VT Jr, et al. Treatment of advanced-stage Hodgkin's disease: alternating noncrossresistant MOPP/CABS is not superior to MOPP. *J Clin Oncol* 1991;9:1409–1420.
44. Ellis ME, Diehl LF, Granger E, et al. Trephine needle bone marrow biopsy in the initial staging of Hodgkin disease: sensitivity and specificity of the Ann Arbor staging procedure criteria. *Am J Hematol* 1989;30:115–120.
45. Knowles DM, Chamulak GA, Subar M, et al. Lymphoid neoplasia associated with the acquired immunodeficiency syndrome (AIDS): the New York University Medical Center experience with 105 patients (1981–1986). *Ann Intern Med* 1988;108:744–753.
46. Tirelli U, Vaccher E, Rezza G, et al. Hodgkin's disease in association with acquired immunodeficiency syndrome (AIDS): a report on 36 patients. Gruppo Italiano Cooperativo AIDS and Tumori. *Acta Oncol* 1989;28:637–639.
47. Serrano M, Bellas C, Campo E, et al. Hodgkin's disease in patients with antibodies to human immunodeficiency virus: a study of 22 patients. *Cancer* 1990;65:2248–2254.
48. Jacquillat C, Auclerc G, Auclerc MF, et al. Hodgkin's disease: characteristics and prognosis of forms with initial bone marrow involvement [Author's translation]. *Nouv Presse Med* 1981;10:95–100.
49. Macintyre EA, Vaughan Hudson B, Linch DC, et al. The value of staging bone marrow trephine biopsy in Hodgkin's disease. *Eur J Haematol* 1987;39:66–70.
50. Moormeier JA, Williams SF, Golomb HM. The staging of Hodgkin's disease. *Hematol Oncol Clin North Am* 1989;3:237–251.
51. Shields AF, Porter BA, Churchley S, et al. The detection of bone marrow involvement by lymphoma using magnetic resonance imaging. *J Clin Oncol* 1987;5:225–230.
52. Dohner H, Guckel F, Knauf W, et al. Magnetic resonance imaging of bone marrow in lymphoproliferative disorders: correlation with bone marrow biopsy. *Br J Haematol* 1989;73:12–17.

53. Linden A, Zankovich R, Theissen P, et al. Malignant lymphoma: bone marrow imaging versus biopsy. *Radiology* 1989;173:335–339.
54. Barbu RR, Port JL, Elkowitz SS, et al. Marrow space imaging in Hodgkin's disease: MRI prior to biopsy for improved accuracy. *Am J Pediatr Hematol Oncol* 1993;15:343–345.
55. Specht L, Nissen NI. Prognostic factors in Hodgkin's disease stage IV. *Eur J Haematol* 1988;41:359–367.
56. Hurd DD, Haake RJ, Lasky LC, et al. Treatment of refractory and relapsed Hodgkin's disease: intensive chemotherapy and autologous bone marrow or peripheral blood stem cell support. *Med Pediatr Oncol* 1990;18:447–453.
57. Neiman RS, Rosen PJ, Lukes RJ. Lymphocyte-depletion Hodgkin's disease: a clinicopathological entity. *N Engl J Med* 1973;288: 751–755.
58. Sobrinho-Simoes M, Paiva ME, Goncalves V, et al. Hodgkin's disease with predominant infradiaphragmatic involvement and massive invasion of the bone marrow: a necroscopic study of nine cases. *Cancer* 1983;52:1927–1932.
59. Kinney MC, Greer JP, Stein RS, et al. Lymphocyte-depletion Hodgkin's disease: histopathologic diagnosis of marrow involvement. *Am J Surg Pathol* 1986;10:219–226.
60. Karcher DS. Clinically unsuspected Hodgkin disease presenting initially in the bone marrow of patients infected with the human immunodeficiency virus. *Cancer* 1993;71:1235–1238.
61. Rappaport H, Berard CW, Butler JJ, et al. Report of the Committee on Histopathological Criteria Contributing to Staging of Hodgkin's Disease. *Cancer Res* 1971;31:1864–1865.
62. Webb DI, Ubogy G, Silver RT. Importance of bone marrow biopsy in the clinical staging of Hodgkin's disease. *Cancer* 1970;26:313–317.
63. Lukes RJ. Criteria for involvement of lymph node, bone marrow, spleen, and liver in Hodgkin's disease. *Cancer Res* 1971;31: 1755–1767.
64. Brunning R, McKenna R. Bone marrow lymphomas: tumors of the bone marrow. Washington DC: Armed Forces Institute of Pathology, 1994:369–408.
65. Hanson CA, Brunning RD, Gajl-Peczalska KJ, et al. Bone marrow manifestations of peripheral T-cell lymphoma: a study of 30 cases. *Am J Clin Pathol* 1986;86:449–460.
66. Colon-Otero G, McClure SP, Phyliky RL, et al. Peripheral T-cell lymphoma simulating Hodgkin's disease with initial bone marrow involvement. *Mayo Clin Proc* 1986;61:68–71.
67. Strum SB, Park JK, Rappaport H. Observation of cells resembling Sternberg-Reed cells in conditions other than Hodgkin's disease. *Cancer* 1970;26:176–190.
68. Wright DH. Reed-Sternberg–like cells in recurrent Burkitt lymphomas. *J Pathol* 1970;101:xv.
69. Schnitzer B. Reed-Sternberg–like cells in lymphocytic lymphoma and chronic lymphocytic leukaemia. *Lancet* 1970;1:1399–1400.
70. McKenna RW, Brunning RD. Reed-Sternberg–like cells in nodular lymphoma involving the bone marrow. *Am J Clin Pathol* 1975;63: 779–785.
71. Nakanuma Y, Kurumaya H, Kurashima K. An autopsy case of malignant histiocytosis with Reed-Sternberg–like cells. *Acta Pathol Jpn* 1989;39:79–83.
72. Abrahamsen AF, Jakobsen E, Langholm R, et al. Bone marrow examination in Hodgkin's disease. *Acta Oncol* 1992;31:41–42.
73. Te Velde J, Den Ottolander GJ, Spaander PJ, et al. The bone marrow in Hodgkin's disease: the non-involved marrow. *Histopathology* 1978; 2:31–46.
74. Anwar M, Nur S, Saleem M, et al. Bone marrow involvement in Hodgkin's disease: the significance of non-infiltrative changes. *JPMA J Pak Med Assoc* 1997;47:110–113.
75. Strum SB, Rappaport H. Interrelations of the histologic types of Hodgkin's disease. *Arch Pathol* 1971;91:127–134.
76. Weiss RB, Brunning RD, Kennedy BJ. Hodgkin's disease in the bone marrow. *Cancer* 1975;36:2077–2083.
77. McKenna RW, Bloomfield CD, Brunning RD. Nodular lymphoma: bone marrow and blood manifestations. *Cancer* 1975;36:428–440.
78. Spiro S, Galton DA, Wiltshaw E, et al. Follicular lymphoma: a survey of 75 cases with special reference to the syndrome resembling chronic lymphocytic leukaemia. *Br J Cancer* 1975;31:60–72.
79. White DM, Smith AG, Whitehouse JM, et al. Peripheral T cell lymphoma: value of bone marrow trephine immunophenotyping. *J Clin Pathol* 1989;42:403–408.
80. Michels SD, McKenna RW, Arthur DC, et al. Therapy-related acute myeloid leukemia and myelodysplastic syndrome: a clinical and morphologic study of 65 cases. *Blood* 1985;65:1364–1372.
81. Gottlieb CA, Maeda K, Hawley RC, et al. Myelodysplasia with bone marrow lymphocytosis and fibrosis mimicking recurrent Hodgkin's disease. *Am J Clin Pathol* 1989;91:6–11.
82. McKenna RW, Brunning RD. Myelodysplasia and acute leukemia following treatment for Hodgkin's disease. *Am J Clin Pathol* 1989; 92:127–128.
83. Foucar K, McKenna RW, Frizzera G, et al. Incidence and patterns of bone marrow and blood involvement by lymphoma in relationship to the Lukes-Collins classification. *Blood* 1979;54:1417–1422.
84. Cousar JB, Glick AD, York JC, et al. Peripheral blood and bone marrow involvement by non-Hodgkin's lymphoma: morphological, immunological and cytochemical features. *Prog Clin Pathol* 1984;9: 173–196.
85. Dick F, Bloomfield CD, Brunning RD. Incidence cytology, and histopathology of non-Hodgkin's lymphomas in the bone marrow. *Cancer* 1974;33:1382–1398.
86. Jones SE, Rosenberg SA, Kaplan HS. Non-Hodgkin's lymphomas: I. Bone marrow involvement. *Cancer* 1972;29:954–960.
87. Stein RS, Ultmann JE, Byrne GE Jr, et al. Bone marrow involvement in non-Hodgkin's lymphoma: implications for staging and therapy. *Cancer* 1976;37:629–636.
88. Pond GD, Castellino RA, Horning S, et al. Non-Hodgkin lymphoma: influence of lymphography, CT, and bone marrow biopsy on staging and management. *Radiology* 1989;170:159–164.
89. Bennett JM, Cain KC, Glick JH, et al. The significance of bone marrow involvement in non-Hodgkin's lymphoma: the Eastern Cooperative Oncology Group experience. *J Clin Oncol* 1986;4:1462–1469.
90. The Non-Hodgkin's Lymphoma Pathologic Classification Project. National Cancer Institute sponsored study of classifications of non-Hodgkin's lymphomas: summary and description of a working formulation for clinical usage. *Cancer* 1982;49:2112–2135.
91. McKenna RW, Hernandez JA. Bone marrow in malignant lymphoma. *Hematol Oncol Clin North Am* 1988;2:617–635.
92. Lee WI, Lee JH, Kim IS, et al. Bone marrow involvement by non-Hodgkin's lymphoma. *J Korean Med Sci* 1994;9:402–408.
93. Bartl R, Frisch B, Burkhardt R, et al. Assessment of bone marrow histology in the malignant lymphomas (non-Hodgkin's): correlation with clinical factors for diagnosis, prognosis, classification and staging. *Br J Haematol* 1982;51:511–530.
94. Harris NL, Jaffe ES, Stein H, et al. A revised European-American classification of lymphoid neoplasms: a proposal from the International Lymphoma Study Group. *Blood* 1994;84:1361–1392.
95. Bartl R, Hansmann ML, Frisch B, et al. Comparative histology of malignant lymphomas in lymph node and bone marrow. *Br J Haematol* 1988;69:229–237.
96. Conlan MG, Bast M, Armitage JO, et al. Bone marrow involvement by non-Hodgkin's lymphoma: the clinical significance of morphologic discordance between the lymph node and bone marrow. Nebraska Lymphoma Study Group. *J Clin Oncol* 1990;8:1163–1172.
97. Brunning RD. Bone marrow and peripheral blood involvement in non-Hodgkin's lymphomas. *Geriatrics* 1975;30:75–80.
98. Burkhardt R, Bartl R, Jager K, et al. Chronic myeloproliferative disorders (CMPD). *Pathol Res Pract* 1984;179:131–186.
99. Gaulard P, Kanavaros P, Farcet JP, et al. Bone marrow histologic and immunohistochemical findings in peripheral T-cell lymphoma: a study of 38 cases. *Hum Pathol* 1991;22:331–338.
100. Cooke CB, Krenacs L, Stetler-Stevenson M, et al. Hepatosplenic T-cell lymphoma: a distinct clinicopathologic entity of cytotoxic gamma delta T-cell origin. *Blood* 1996;88:4265–4274.
101. Farcet JP, Gaulard P, Marolleau JP, et al. Hepatosplenic T-cell lymphoma: sinusal/sinusoidal localization of malignant cells expressing the T-cell receptor gamma delta. *Blood* 1990;75:2213–2219.
102. Murase T, Nakamura S, Tashiro K, et al. Malignant histiocytosis-like B-cell lymphoma, a distinct pathologic variant of intravascular lymphomatosis: a report of five cases and review of the literature. *Br J Haematol* 1997;99:656–664.
103. Franco V, Florena AM, Campesi G. Intrasinusoidal bone marrow infiltration: a possible hallmark of splenic lymphoma. *Histopathology* 1996;29:571–575.
104. Labouyrie E, Marit G, Vial JP, et al. Intrasinusoidal bone marrow

involvement by splenic lymphoma with villous lymphocytes: a helpful immunohistologic feature. *Mod Pathol* 1997;10:1015–1020.
105. Bartl R, Frisch B, Diem H, et al. Bone marrow histology and serum beta 2 microglobulin in multiple myeloma: a new prognostic strategy. *Eur J Haematol Suppl* 1989;51:88–98.
106. Fisher DE, Jacobson JO, Ault KA, et al. Diffuse large cell lymphoma with discordant bone marrow histology: clinical features and biological implications. *Cancer* 1989;64:1879–1887.
107. Kluin PM, van Krieken JH, Kleiverda K, et al. Discordant morphologic characteristics of B-cell lymphomas in bone marrow and lymph node biopsies. *Am J Clin Pathol* 1990;94:59–66.
108. Mead GM, Kushlan P, O'Neil M, et al. Clinical aspects of non-Hodgkin's lymphomas presenting with discordant histologic subtypes. *Cancer* 1983;52:1496–1501.
109. Crisan D, Mattson JC. Discordant morphologic features in bone marrow involvement by malignant lymphomas: use of gene rearrangement patterns for diagnosis. *Am J Hematol* 1995;49:299–309.
110. Hodges GF, Lenhardt TM, Cotelingam JD. Bone marrow involvement in large-cell lymphoma: prognostic implications of discordant disease. *Am J Clin Pathol* 1994;101:305–311.
111. Borowitz MJ, Croker BP, Metzgar RS. Lymphoblastic lymphoma with the phenotype of common acute lymphoblastic leukemia. *Am J Clin Pathol* 1983;79:387–391.
112. Sander CA, Medeiros LJ, Abruzzo LV, et al. Lymphoblastic lymphoma presenting in cutaneous sites: a clinicopathologic analysis of six cases. *J Am Acad Dermatol* 1991;25:1023–1031.
113. Cheng AL, Su IJ, Tien HF, et al. Characteristic clinicopathologic features of adult B-cell lymphoblastic lymphoma with special emphasis on differential diagnosis with an atypical form probably of blastic lymphocytic lymphoma of intermediate differentiation origin. *Cancer* 1994;73:706–710.
114. Cossman J, Chused TM, Fisher RI, et al. Diversity of immunological phenotypes of lymphoblastic lymphoma. *Cancer Res* 1983;43:4486–4490.
115. Sheibani K, Nathwani BN, Winberg CD, et al. Antigenically defined subgroups of lymphoblastic lymphoma: relationship to clinical presentation and biologic behavior. *Cancer* 1987;60:183–190.
116. Grogan T, Spier C, Wirt DP, et al. Immunologic complexity of lymphoblastic lymphoma. *Diagn Immunol* 1986;4:81–88.
117. Ozdemirli M, Fanburg-Smith J, Hartmann D-P, et al. Precursor B-lymphoblastic lymphoma presenting as a solitary bone tumor and mimicking Ewing's sarcoma: a report of four cases and review of the literature. *Am J Surg Pathol* 1998;22:795–804.
118. Soslow RA, Bhargava V, Warnke RA. MIC2, TdT, bcl-2, and CD34 expression in paraffin-embedded high-grade lymphoma/acute lymphoblastic leukemia distinguishes between distinct clinicopathologic entities. *Hum Pathol* 1997;28:1158–1165.
119. Arber DA, Jenkins KA. Paraffin section immunophenotyping of acute leukemias in bone marrow specimens. *Am J Clin Pathol* 1996;106:462–468.
120. Batata A, Shen B. Relationship between chronic lymphocytic leukemia and small lymphocytic lymphoma: a comparative study of membrane phenotypes in 270 cases. *Cancer* 1992;70:625–632.
121. Pangalis GA, Nathwani BN, Rappaport H. Malignant lymphoma, well differentiated lymphocytic: its relationship with chronic lymphocytic leukemia and macroglobulinemia of Waldenstrom. *Cancer* 1977;39:999–1010.
122. Adelstein DJ, Henry MB, Bowman LS, et al. Diffuse well differentiated lymphocytic lymphoma: a clinical study of 22 patients. *Oncology* 1991;48:48–53.
123. Batata A, Shen B. Chronic lymphocytic leukemia with low lymphocyte count. *Cancer* 1993;71:2732–2738.
124. Kilo MN, Dorfman DM. The utility of flow cytometric immunophenotypic analysis in the distinction of small lymphocytic lymphoma/chronic lymphocytic leukemia from mantle cell lymphoma. *Am J Clin Pathol* 1996;105:451–457.
125. Bennett JM, Catovsky D, Daniel MT, et al. Proposals for the classification of chronic (mature) B and T lymphoid leukaemias. French-American-British (FAB) Cooperative Group. *J Clin Pathol* 1989;42:567–584.
126. Batata A, Shen B. Immunophenotyping of subtypes of B-chronic (mature) lymphoid leukemia: a study of 242 cases. *Cancer* 1992;70:2436–2443.
127. Matutes E, Owusu-Ankomah K, Morilla R, et al. The immunological profile of B-cell disorders and proposal of a scoring system for the diagnosis of CLL. *Leukemia* 1994;8:1640–1655.
128. Moreau EJ, Matutes E, A'Hern RP, et al. Improvement of the chronic lymphocytic leukemia scoring system with the monoclonal antibody SN8 (CD79b). *Am J Clin Pathol* 1997;108:378–382.
129. Contos MJ, Kornstein MJ, Innes DJ, et al. The utility of CD20 and CD43 in subclassification of low-grade B-cell lymphoma on paraffin sections. *Mod Pathol* 1992;5:631–633.
130. Kumar S, Green GA, Teruya-Feldstein J, et al. Use of CD23 (BU38) on paraffin sections in the diagnosis of small lymphocytic lymphoma and mantle cell lymphoma. *Mod Pathol* 1996;9:925–929.
131. Singh N, Wright DH. The value of immunohistochemistry on paraffin wax embedded tissue sections in the differentiation of small lymphocytic and mantle cell lymphomas. *J Clin Pathol* 1997;50:16–21.
132. Dorfman DM, Pinkus GS. Distinction between small lymphocytic and mantle cell lymphoma by immunoreactivity for CD23. *Mod Pathol* 1994;7:326–331.
133. Yang WI, Zukerberg LR, Motokura T, et al. Cyclin D1 (Bcl-1, PRAD1) protein expression in low-grade B-cell lymphomas and reactive hyperplasia. *Am J Pathol* 1994;145:86–96.
134. Zukerberg LR, Yang WI, Arnold A, et al. Cyclin D1 expression in non-Hodgkin's lymphomas: detection by immunohistochemistry. *Am J Clin Pathol* 1995;103:756–760.
135. Swerdlow SH, Yang WI, Zukerberg LR, et al. Expression of cyclin D1 protein in centrocytic/mantle cell lymphomas with and without rearrangement of the BCL1/cyclin D1 gene. *Hum Pathol* 1995;26:999–1004.
136. de Boer CJ, Schuuring E, Dreef E, et al. Cyclin D1 protein analysis in the diagnosis of mantle cell lymphoma. *Blood* 1995;86:2715–2723.
137. Bartl R, Frisch B, Mahl G, et al. Bone marrow histology in Waldenstrom's macroglobulinaemia: clinical relevance of subtype recognition. *Scand J Haematol* 1983;31:359–375.
138. Harris NL, Bhan AK. B-cell neoplasms of the lymphocytic, lymphoplasmacytoid, and plasma cell types: immunohistologic analysis and clinical correlation. *Hum Pathol* 1985;16:829–837.
139. Reed M, McKenna RW, Bridges R, et al. Morphologic manifestations of monoclonal gammopathies. *Am J Clin Pathol* 1981;76:8–23.
140. Gerard-Marchant R, Hamlin I, Lennert K, et al. Classification of non-Hodgkin's lymphomas. *Lancet* 1974;2:406–408.
141. Zukerberg LR, Medeiros LJ, Ferry JA, et al. Diffuse low-grade B-cell lymphomas: four clinically distinct subtypes defined by a combination of morphologic and immunophenotypic features. *Am J Clin Pathol* 1993;100:373–385.
142. Murray PG, Janmohamed RM, Crocker J. CD23 expression in non-Hodgkin lymphoma: immunohistochemical demonstration using the antibody BU38 on paraffin sections. *J Pathol* 1991;165:125–128.
143. Banks PM, Chan J, Cleary ML, et al. Mantle cell lymphoma: a proposal for unification of morphologic, immunologic, and molecular data. *Am J Surg Pathol* 1992;16:637–640.
144. Pittaluga S, Wlodarska I, Stul MS, et al. Mantle cell lymphoma: a clinicopathological study of 55 cases. *Histopathology* 1995;26:17–24.
145. Majlis A, Pugh WC, Rodriguez MA, et al. Mantle cell lymphoma: correlation of clinical outcome and biologic features with three histologic variants. *J Clin Oncol* 1997;15:1664–1671.
146. Duggan MJ, Weisenburger DD, Ye YL, et al. Mantle zone lymphoma: a clinicopathologic study of 22 cases. *Cancer* 1990;66:522–529.
147. Lardelli P, Bookman MA, Sundeen J, et al. Lymphocytic lymphoma of intermediate differentiation: morphologic and immunophenotypic spectrum and clinical correlations. *Am J Surg Pathol* 1990;14:752–763.
148. Fisher RI, Dahlberg S, Nathwani BN, et al. A clinical analysis of two indolent lymphoma entities: mantle cell lymphoma and marginal zone lymphoma (including the mucosa-associated lymphoid tissue and monocytoid B-cell subcategories). A Southwest Oncology Group study. *Blood* 1995;85:1075–1082.
149. Argatoff LH, Connors JM, Klasa RJ, et al. Mantle cell lymphoma: a clinicopathologic study of 80 cases. *Blood* 1997;89:2067–2078.
150. Cohen PL, Kurtin PJ, Donovan KA, et al. Bone marrow and peripheral blood involvement in mantle cell lymphoma. *Br J Haematol* 1998;101:302–310.
151. Weisenburger DD, Kim H, Rappaport H. Mantle-zone lymphoma: a follicular variant of intermediate lymphocytic lymphoma. *Cancer* 1982;49:1429–1438.
152. Gascoyne R, Diebold J, Muller-Hermelink K, et al. Non-Hodgkin's

lymphoma classification project (NHLCP): diffuse small B-cell lymphomas. *Lab Invest* 1998;78:129A(abst).
153. Bookman MA, Lardelli P, Jaffe ES, et al. Lymphocytic lymphoma of intermediate differentiation: morphologic, immunophenotypic, and prognostic factors. *J Natl Cancer Inst* 1990;82:742–748.
154. Decaudin D, Bosq J, Munck JN, et al. Mantle cell lymphomas: characteristics, natural history and prognostic factors of 45 cases. *Leuk Lymphoma* 1997;26:539–550.
155. Velders GA, Kluin-Nelemans JC, De Boer CJ, et al. Mantle-cell lymphoma: a population-based clinical study. *J Clin Oncol* 1996;14: 1269–1274.
156. Norton AJ, Matthews J, Pappa V, et al. Mantle cell lymphoma: natural history defined in a serially biopsied population over a 20-year period. *Ann Oncol* 1995;6:249–256.
157. Pittaluga S, Verhoef G, Criel A, et al. Prognostic significance of bone marrow trephine and peripheral blood smears in 55 patients with mantle cell lymphoma. *Leuk Lymphoma* 1996;21:115–125.
158. Zucca E, Roggero E, Pinotti G, et al. Patterns of survival in mantle cell lymphoma. *Ann Oncol* 1995;6:257–262.
159. Pittaluga S, Verhoef G, Criel A, et al. ''Small'' B-cell non-Hodgkin's lymphomas with splenomegaly at presentation are either mantle cell lymphoma or marginal zone cell lymphoma: a study based on histology, cytology, immunohistochemistry, and cytogenetic analysis. *Am J Surg Pathol* 1996;20:211–223.
160. Weisenburger DD, Nathwani BN, Diamond LW, et al. Malignant lymphoma, intermediate lymphocytic type: a clinicopathologic study of 42 cases. *Cancer* 1981;48:1415–1425.
161. Jaffe ES, Bookman MA, Longo DL. Lymphocytic lymphoma of intermediate differentiation—mantle zone lymphoma: a distinct subtype of B-cell lymphoma. *Hum Pathol* 1987;18:877–880.
162. Perry DA, Bast MA, Armitage JO, et al. Diffuse intermediate lymphocytic lymphoma: a clinicopathologic study and comparison with small lymphocytic lymphoma and diffuse small cleaved cell lymphoma. *Cancer* 1990;66:1995–2000.
163. Carbone A, Poletti A, Manconi R, et al. Intermediate lymphocytic lymphoma encompassing diffuse and mantle zone pattern variants: a distinct entity among low-grade lymphomas? *Eur J Cancer Clin Oncol* 1989;25:113–121.
164. Zoldan MC, Inghirami G, Masuda Y, et al. Large-cell variants of mantle cell lymphoma: cytologic characteristics and p53 anomalies may predict poor outcome. *Br J Haematol* 1996;93:475–486.
165. Swerdlow SH, Zukerberg LR, Yang WI, et al. The morphologic spectrum of non-Hodgkin's lymphomas with BCL1/cyclin D1 gene rearrangements. *Am J Surg Pathol* 1996;20:627–640.
166. Swerdlow SH, Saboorian MH, Pelstring RJ, et al. Centrocytic lymphoma: a morphometric study with comparison to other small cleaved follicular center cell lymphomas and genotypic correlates. *Am J Pathol* 1993;142:329–337.
167. Wasman J, Rosenthal NS, Farhi DC. Mantle cell lymphoma: morphologic findings in bone marrow involvement. *Am J Clin Pathol* 1996; 106:196–200.
168. Pombo de Oliveira M. Leukaemic phase of mantle zone (intermediate) lymphoma: its characterisation in 11 cases. *J Clin Pathol* 1989;42: 962–972.
169. Weisenburger DD, Sanger WG, Armitage JO, et al. Intermediate lymphocytic lymphoma: immunophenotypic and cytogenetic findings. *Blood* 1987;69:1617–1621.
170. Swerdlow SH, Habeshaw JA, Murray LJ, et al. Centrocytic lymphoma: a distinct clinicopathologic and immunologic entity. A multiparameter study of 18 cases at diagnosis and relapse. *Am J Pathol* 1983;113:181–197.
171. Weisenburger DD. Non-Hodgkin's lymphomas of primary follicle/ mantle zone origin. *Leukemia* 1991;5:26–29.
172. Medeiros LJ, Van Krieken JH, Jaffe ES, et al. Association of bcl-1 rearrangements with lymphocytic lymphoma of intermediate differentiation. *Blood* 1990;76:2086–2090.
173. Rimokh R, Berger F, Delsol G, et al. Detection of the chromosomal translocation t(11;14) by polymerase chain reaction in mantle cell lymphomas. *Blood* 1994;83:1871–1875.
174. Rimokh R, Berger F, Delsol G, et al. Rearrangement and overexpression of the BCL-1/PRAD-1 gene in intermediate lymphocytic lymphomas and in t(11q13)-bearing leukemias. *Blood* 1993;81: 3063–3067.
175. Williams ME, Westermann CD, Swerdlow SH. Genotypic characterization of centrocytic lymphoma: frequent rearrangement of the chromosome 11 bcl-1 locus. *Blood* 1990;76:1387–1391.
176. Williams ME, Swerdlow SH, Rosenberg CL, et al. Characterization of chromosome 11 translocation breakpoints at the bcl-1 and PRAD1 loci in centrocytic lymphoma. *Cancer Res* 1992;52:5541s–5544s.
177. Rimokh R, Berger F, Cornillet P, et al. Break in the BCL1 locus is closely associated with intermediate lymphocytic lymphoma subtype. *Genes Chromosomes Cancer* 1990;2:223–226.
178. Yatabe Y, Nakamura S, Seto M, et al. Clinicopathologic study of PRAD1/cyclin D1 overexpressing lymphoma with special reference to mantle cell lymphoma: a distinct molecular pathologic entity. *Am J Surg Pathol* 1996;20:1110–1122.
179. Nakamura S, Yatabe Y, Kuroda H, et al. Immunostaining of PRAD1/ cyclin D1 protein as a marker for the diagnosis of mantle cell lymphoma. *Leukemia* 1997;11:536–537.
180. Soslow RA, Zukerberg LR, Harris NL, et al. BCL-1 (PRAD-1/cyclin D-1) overexpression distinguishes the blastoid variant of mantle cell lymphoma from B-lineage lymphoblastic lymphoma. *Mod Pathol* 1997;10:810–817.
181. Savilo E, Campo E, Mollejo M, et al. Absence of cyclin D1 protein expression in splenic marginal zone lymphoma. *Mod Pathol* 1998; 11:601–606.
182. Chilosi M, Pizzolo G, Fiore-Donati L, et al. Routine immunofluorescent and histochemical analysis of bone marrow involvement of lymphoma/leukaemia: the use of cryostat sections. *Br J Cancer* 1983;48: 763–775.
183. Rosenthal N, Dreskin D, Vural I, et al. The significance of hematogones in blood, bone marrow and lymph node aspiration in giant follicular lymphoblastoma. *Acta Haematol* 1952;8:368–377.
184. Wendum D, Sebban C, Gaulard P, et al. Follicular large-cell lymphoma treated with intensive chemotherapy: an analysis of 89 cases included in the LNH87 trial and comparison with the outcome of diffuse large B-cell lymphoma. Groupe d'Etude des Lymphomes de l'Adulte. *J Clin Oncol* 1997;15:1654–1663.
185. Kantarjian HM, McLaughlin P, Fuller LM, et al. Follicular large cell lymphoma: analysis and prognostic factors in 62 patients. *J Clin Oncol* 1984;2:811–819.
186. Campo E, Miquel R, Krenacs L, et al. Primary nodal marginal zone lymphomas of splenic and MALT type. *Am J Surg Pathol* 1999;23: 59–68.
187. Nathwani B, Anderson J, Armitage J, et al. A clinicopathologic comparison of 21 patients with nodal marginal zone lymphoma and 72 patients with MALT type lymphoma. *Lab Invest* 1998;78:137A(abst).
188. Harris NL. Low-grade B-cell lymphoma of mucosa-associated lymphoid tissue and monocytoid B-cell lymphoma: related entities that are distinct from other low-grade B-cell lymphomas. *Arch Pathol Lab Med* 1993;117:771–775.
189. Nizze H, Cogliatti SB, von Schilling C, et al. Monocytoid B-cell lymphoma: morphological variants and relationship to low-grade B-cell lymphoma of the mucosa-associated lymphoid tissue. *Histopathology* 1991;18:403–414.
190. Cogliatti SB, Lennert K, Hansmann ML, et al. Monocytoid B cell lymphoma: clinical and prognostic features of 21 patients. *J Clin Pathol* 1990;43:619–625.
191. Shin SS, Sheibani K, Fishleder A, et al. Monocytoid B-cell lymphoma in patients with Sjögren's syndrome: a clinicopathologic study of 13 patients. *Hum Pathol* 1991;22:422–430.
192. Ngan BY, Warnke RA, Wilson M, et al. Monocytoid B-cell lymphoma: a study of 36 cases. *Hum Pathol* 1991;22:409–421.
193. Sheibani K, Burke JS, Swartz WG, et al. Monocytoid B-cell lymphoma: clinicopathologic study of 21 cases of a unique type of low-grade lymphoma. *Cancer* 1988;62:1531–1538.
194. Kroft S, Hsi E, Ross C, et al. Evaluation of CD23 expression in paraffin-embedded gastric MALT lymphoma. *Mod Pathol* 1998;11: 967–970.
195. Ferry JA, Yang WI, Zukerberg LR, et al. $CD5^+$ extranodal marginal zone B-cell (MALT) lymphoma: a low grade neoplasm with a propensity for bone marrow involvement and relapse. *Am J Clin Pathol* 1996;105:31–37.
196. Ballesteros E, Osborne BM, Matsushima AY. $CD5^+$ low-grade marginal zone B-cell lymphomas with localized presentation. *Am J Surg Pathol* 1998;22:201–207.
197. Isaacson PG, Spencer J. Malignant lymphoma of mucosa-associated lymphoid tissue. *Histopathology* 1987;11:445–462.
198. Bailey EM, Ferry JA, Harris NL, et al. Marginal zone lymphoma

(low-grade B-cell lymphoma of mucosa-associated lymphoid tissue type) of skin and subcutaneous tissue: a study of 15 patients. *Am J Surg Pathol* 1996;20:1011–1023.

199. Hsi ED, Zukerberg LR, Schnitzer B, et al. Development of extrasalivary gland lymphoma in myoepithelial sialadenitis. *Mod Pathol* 1995; 8:817–824.
200. Mattia AR, Ferry JA, Harris NL. Breast lymphoma: a B-cell spectrum including the low grade B-cell lymphoma of mucosa associated lymphoid tissue. *Am J Surg Pathol* 1993;17:574–587.
201. Kempton CL, Kurtin PJ, Inwards DJ, et al. Malignant lymphoma of the bladder: evidence from 36 cases that low-grade lymphoma of the MALT-type is the most common primary bladder lymphoma. *Am J Surg Pathol* 1997;21:1324–1333.
202. Graziadei G, Pruneri G, Carboni N, et al. Low-grade MALT lymphoma involving multiple mucosal sites and bone marrow. *Ann Hematol* 1998;76:81–83.
203. Griesser H, Kaiser U, Augener W, et al. B-cell lymphoma of the mucosa-associated lymphatic tissue (MALT) presenting with bone marrow and peripheral blood involvement. *Leuk Res* 1990;14: 617–622.
204. Blazquez M, Haioun C, Chaumette MT, et al. Low grade B cell mucosa associated lymphoid tissue lymphoma of the stomach: clinical and endoscopic features, treatment, and outcome. *Gut* 1992;33: 1621–1625.
205. White WL, Ferry JA, Harris NL, et al. Ocular adnexal lymphoma: a clinicopathologic study with identification of lymphomas of mucosa-associated lymphoid tissue type. *Ophthalmology* 1995;102: 1994–2006.
206. Liang R, Chan VV, Chan TK, et al. Immunoglobulin gene rearrangement in the peripheral blood and bone marrow of patients with lymphomas of the mucosa-associated lymphoid tissues. *Acta Haematol* 1990;84:19–23.
207. Pinotti G, Zucca E, Roggero E, et al. Clinical features, treatment and outcome in a series of 93 patients with low-grade gastric MALT lymphoma. *Leuk Lymphoma* 1997;26:527–537.
208. Carbone A, Gloghini A, Pinto A, et al. Monocytoid B-cell lymphoma with bone marrow and peripheral blood involvement at presentation. *Am J Clin Pathol* 1989;92:228–236.
209. Traweek ST, Sheibani K. Regarding the article entitled ''Monocytoid B-cell lymphoma with bone marrow and peripheral blood involvement at presentation'' (Letter). *Am J Clin Pathol* 1990;94:117–118.
210. Fend F, Kraus-Huonder B, Muller-Hermelink HK, et al. Monocytoid B-cell lymphoma: its relationship to and possible cellular origin from marginal zone cells. *Hum Pathol* 1993;24:336–339.
211. Sheibani K, Sohn CC, Burke JS, et al. Monocytoid B-cell lymphoma: a novel B-cell neoplasm. *Am J Pathol* 1986;124:310–318.
212. Nathwani BN, Mohrmann RL, Brynes RK, et al. Monocytoid B-cell lymphomas: an assessment of diagnostic criteria and a perspective on histogenesis. *Hum Pathol* 1992;23:1061–1071.
213. Hammer RD, Glick AD, Greer JP, et al. Splenic marginal zone lymphoma: a distinct B-cell neoplasm. *Am J Surg Pathol* 1996;20: 613–626.
214. Mollejo M, Menarguez J, Lloret E, et al. Splenic marginal zone lymphoma: a distinctive type of low-grade B-cell lymphoma. *Am J Surg Pathol* 1995;19:1146–1157.
215. Schmid C, Kirkham N, Diss T, et al. Splenic marginal zone lymphoma. *Am J Surg Pathol* 1992;16:455–466.
216. Pawade J, Wilkins BS, Wright DH. Low-grade B-cell lymphomas of the splenic marginal zone: a clinicopathological and immunohistochemical study of 14 cases. *Histopathology* 1995;27:129–137.
217. Isaacson PG, Matutes E, Burke M, et al. The histopathology of splenic lymphoma with villous lymphocytes. *Blood* 1994;84:3828–3834.
218. Rosso R, Neiman RS, Paulli M, et al. Splenic marginal zone cell lymphoma: report of an indolent variant without massive splenomegaly presumably representing an early phase of the disease. *Hum Pathol* 1995;26:39–46.
219. Dunphy CH, Bee C, McDonald JW, et al. Incidental early detection of a splenic marginal zone lymphoma by polymerase chain reaction analysis of paraffin-embedded tissue. *Arch Pathol Lab Med* 1998; 122:84–86.
220. Melo JV, Hegde U, Parreira A, et al. Splenic B cell lymphoma with circulating villous lymphocytes: differential diagnosis of B cell leukaemias with large spleens. *J Clin Pathol* 1987;40:642–651.
221. Melo JV, Robinson DS, Gregory C, et al. Splenic B cell lymphoma with ''villous'' lymphocytes in the peripheral blood: a disorder distinct from hairy cell leukemia. *Leukemia* 1987;1:294–298.
222. Bain B, Matutes E, Robinson D, et al. Leukaemia as a manifestation of large cell lymphoma. *Br J Haematol* 1991;77:301–310.
223. Abou-Elella A, Vose J, Anderson J, et al. Primary mediastinal large B-cell lymphoma: a clinicopathologic study of 50 cases. *Lab Invest* 1997;77:119A(abst).
224. Cazals-Hatem D, Lepage E, Brice P, et al. Primary mediastinal large B-cell lymphoma: a clinicopathologic study of 141 cases compared with 916 nonmediastinal large B-cell lymphomas. A GELA (''Groupe d'Etude des Lymphomes de l'Adulte'') study. *Am J Surg Pathol* 1996; 20:877–888.
225. Lamarre L, Jacobson JO, Aisenberg AC, et al. Primary large cell lymphoma of the mediastinum: a histologic and immunophenotypic study of 29 cases. *Am J Surg Pathol* 1989;13:730–739.
226. Perrone T, Frizzera G, Rosai J. Mediastinal diffuse large-cell lymphoma with sclerosis: a clinicopathologic study of 60 cases. *Am J Surg Pathol* 1986;10:176–191.
227. Jacobson JO, Aisenberg AC, Lamarre L, et al. Mediastinal large cell lymphoma: an uncommon subset of adult lymphoma curable with combined modality therapy. *Cancer* 1988;62:1893–1898.
228. Chim CS, Liang R, Chan AC, et al. Primary B cell lymphoma of the mediastinum. *Hematol Oncol* 1996;14:173–179.
229. Falini B, Venturi S, Martelli M, et al. Mediastinal large B-cell lymphoma: clinical and immunohistological findings in 18 patients treated with different third-generation regimens. *Br J Haematol* 1995;89: 780–789.
230. Krishnan J, Wallberg K, Frizzera G. T-cell-rich large B-cell lymphoma: a study of 30 cases, supporting its histologic heterogeneity and lack of clinical distinctiveness. *Am J Surg Pathol* 1994;18:455–465.
231. Macon WR, Williams ME, Greer JP, et al. T-cell-rich B-cell lymphomas: a clinicopathologic study of 19 cases. *Am J Surg Pathol* 1992;16:351–363.
232. Rodriguez J, Pugh WC, Cabanillas F. T-cell-rich B-cell lymphoma. *Blood* 1993;82:1586–1589.
233. Greer JP, Macon WR, Lamar RE, et al. T-cell-rich B-cell lymphomas: diagnosis and response to therapy of 44 patients. *J Clin Oncol* 1995; 13:1742–1750.
234. Delabie J, Vandenberghe E, Kennes C, et al. Histiocyte-rich B-cell lymphoma: a distinct clinicopathologic entity possibly related to lymphocyte predominant Hodgkin's disease, paragranuloma subtype. *Am J Surg Pathol* 1992;16:37–48.
235. De Wolf-Peeters C, Pittaluga S. T-cell rich B-cell lymphoma: a morphological variant of a variety of non-Hodgkin's lymphomas or a clinicopathological entity? *Histopathology* 1995;26:383–385.
236. Chittal SM, Brousset P, Voigt JJ, et al. Large B-cell lymphoma rich in T-cells and simulating Hodgkin's disease. *Histopathology* 1991; 19:211–220.
237. Skinnider BF, Connors JM, Gascoyne RD. Bone marrow involvement in T-cell-rich B-cell lymphoma. *Am J Clin Pathol* 1997;108:570–578.
238. Domizio P, Hall PA, Cotter F, et al. Angiotropic large cell lymphoma (ALCL): morphological, immunohistochemical and genotypic studies with analysis of previous reports. *Hematol Oncol* 1989;7:195–206.
239. Wick MR, Mills SE, Scheithauer BW, et al. Reassessment of malignant ''angioendotheliomatosis'': evidence in favor of its reclassification as ''intravascular lymphomatosis.'' *Am J Surg Pathol* 1986;10: 112–123.
240. Stroup RM, Sheibani K, Moncada A, et al. Angiotropic (intravascular) large cell lymphoma: a clinicopathologic study of seven cases with unique clinical presentations. *Cancer* 1990;66:1781–1788.
241. Ferry JA, Harris NL, Picker LJ, et al. Intravascular lymphomatosis (malignant angioendotheliomatosis): a B-cell neoplasm expressing surface homing receptors. *Mod Pathol* 1988;1:444–452.
242. Sheibani K, Battifora H, Winberg CD, et al. Further evidence that ''malignant angioendotheliomatosis'' is an angiotropic large-cell lymphoma. *N Engl J Med* 1986;314:943–948.
243. Sepp N, Schuler G, Romani N, et al. ''Intravascular lymphomatosis'' (angioendotheliomatosis): evidence for a T-cell origin in two cases. *Hum Pathol* 1990;21:1051–1058.
244. Au WY, Shek WH, Nicholls J, et al. T-cell intravascular lymphomatosis (angiotropic large cell lymphoma): association with Epstein-Barr viral infection. *Histopathology* 1997;31:563–567.
245. Subira M, Domingo A, Santamaria A, et al. Bone marrow involvement

in lymphoblastic lymphoma and small non-cleaved cell lymphoma: the role of trephine biopsy. *Haematologica* 1997;82:594–595.
246. Brunning RD, McKenna RW, Bloomfield CD, et al. Bone marrow involvement in Burkitt's lymphoma. *Cancer* 1977;40:1771–1779.
247. Smith JL, Clein GP, Barker CR, et al. Characterisation of malignant mediastinal lymphoid neoplasm (Sternberg sarcoma) as thymic in origin. *Lancet* 1973;1:74–77.
248. Barcos MP, Lukes RJ. Malignant lymphoma of convoluted lymphocytes: a new entity of possible T-cell type. In: Sinks LF, Godden JO, eds. *Conflicts in childhood cancer: an evaluation of current management.* New York: Liss, 1975;4:147–178.
249. Nathwani BN, Kim H, Rappaport H. Malignant lymphoma, lymphoblastic. *Cancer* 1976;38:964–983.
250. McKenna RW, Parkin J, Brunning RD. Morphologic and ultrastructural characteristics of T-cell acute lymphoblastic leukemia. *Cancer* 1979;44:1290–1297.
251. Bennett JM, Catovsky D, Daniel MT, et al. Proposals for the classification of the acute leukaemias. French-American-British (FAB) cooperative group. *Br J Haematol* 1976;33:451–458.
252. Bennett JM, Catovsky D, Daniel MT, et al. The morphological classification of acute lymphoblastic leukaemia: concordance among observers and clinical correlations. *Br J Haematol* 1981;47:553–561.
253. Chadburn A, Knowles DM. Paraffin-resistant antigens detectable by antibodies L26 and polyclonal CD3 predict the B- or T-cell lineage of 95% of diffuse aggressive non-Hodgkin's lymphomas. *Am J Clin Pathol* 1994;102:284–291.
254. Hall PA, d'Ardenne AJ, Stansfeld AG. Paraffin section immunohistochemistry: I. Non-Hodgkin's lymphoma. *Histopathology* 1988;13: 149–160.
255. Orazi A, Cattoretti G, John K, et al. Terminal deoxynucleotidyl transferase staining of malignant lymphomas in paraffin sections. *Mod Pathol* 1994;7:582–586.
256. Suzumiya J, Ohshima K, Kikuchi M, et al. Terminal deoxynucleotidyl transferase staining of malignant lymphomas in paraffin sections: a useful method for the diagnosis of lymphoblastic lymphoma. *J Pathol* 1997;182:86–91.
257. Poppema S, Hollema H, Visser L, et al. Monoclonal antibodies (MT1, MT2, MB1, MB2, MB3) reactive with leukocyte subsets in paraffin-embedded tissue sections. *Am J Pathol* 1987;127:418–429.
258. Salhany KE, Greer JP, Cousar JB, et al. Marrow involvement in cutaneous T-cell lymphoma: a clinicopathologic study of 60 cases. *Am J Clin Pathol* 1989;92:747–754.
259. Graham SJ, Sharpe RW, Steinberg SM, et al. Prognostic implications of a bone marrow histopathologic classification system in mycosis fungoides and the Sezary syndrome. *Cancer* 1993;72:726–734.
260. Bogen SA, Pelley D, Charif M, et al. Immunophenotypic identification of Sezary cells in peripheral blood. *Am J Clin Pathol* 1996;106: 739–748.
261. Kuchnio M, Sausville EA, Jaffe ES, et al. Flow cytometric detection of neoplastic T cells in patients with mycosis fungoides based on levels of T-cell receptor expression. *Am J Clin Pathol* 1994;102: 856–860.
262. Caulet S, Delmer A, Audouin J, et al. Histopathological study of bone marrow biopsies in 30 cases of T-cell lymphoma with clinical, biological and survival correlations. *Hematol Oncol* 1990;8:155–168.
263. Auger MJ, Nash JR, Mackie MJ. Marrow involvement with T cell lymphoma initially presenting as abnormal myelopoiesis. *J Clin Pathol* 1986;39:134–137.
264. Mead JH, Mason TE. Lymphoma versus AIDS [Letter]. *Am J Clin Pathol* 1983;80:546–547.
265. Tosi P, Leoncini L, Del Vecchio MT, et al. Phenotypic overlaps between pleomorphic malignant T-cell lymphomas and mixed-cellularity Hodgkin's disease. *Int J Cancer* 1992;52:202–207.
266. Nakamura S, Koshikawa T, Koike K, et al. Phenotypic analysis of peripheral T cell lymphoma among the Japanese. *Acta Pathol Jpn* 1993;43:396–412.
267. Alonsozana EL, Stamberg J, Kumar D, et al. Isochromosome 7q: the primary cytogenetic abnormality in hepatosplenic gammadelta T cell lymphoma [Letter]. *Leukemia* 1997;11:1367–1372.
268. Jonveaux P, Daniel MT, Martel V, et al. Isochromosome 7q and trisomy 8 are consistent primary, non-random chromosomal abnormalities associated with hepatosplenic T gamma/delta lymphoma. *Leukemia* 1996;10:1453–1455.
269. Wang CC, Tien HF, Lin MT, et al. Consistent presence of isochromosome 7q in hepatosplenic T gamma/delta lymphoma: a new cytogenetic-clinicopathologic entity. *Genes Chromosomes Cancer* 1995;12: 161–164.
270. Sallah S, Smith SV, Lony LC, et al. Gamma/delta T-cell hepatosplenic lymphoma: review of the literature, diagnosis by flow cytometry and concomitant autoimmune hemolytic anemia. *Ann Hematol* 1997;74: 139–142.
271. Gaulard P, Bourquelot P, Kanavaros P, et al. Expression of the alpha/beta and gamma/delta T-cell receptors in 57 cases of peripheral T-cell lymphomas: identification of a subset of gamma/delta T-cell lymphomas. *Am J Pathol* 1990;137:617–628.
272. Kumar S, Krenacs L, Medeiros J, et al. Subcutaneous panniculitic T-cell lymphoma is a tumor of cytotoxic T lymphocytes. *Hum Pathol* 1998;29:397–403.
273. Gonzalez CL, Medeiros LJ, Braziel RM, et al. T-cell lymphoma involving subcutaneous tissue. A clinicopathologic entity commonly associated with hemophagocytic syndrome. *Am J Surg Pathol* 1991; 15:17–27.
274. Salhany K, Macon W, Choi J, et al. Subcutaneous panniculitis-like T-cell lymphoma: clinicopathologic, immunophenotypic, and genotypic analysis of alpha/beta and gamma/delta subtypes. *Am J Surg Pathol* 1998;22:881–893.
275. Schnaidt U, Vykoupil KF, Thiele J, et al. Angioimmunoblastic lymphadenopathy: histopathology of bone marrow involvement. *Virchows Arch A Path Anat* 1980;389:369–380.
276. Ohsaka A, Saito K, Sakai T, et al. Clinicopathologic and therapeutic aspects of angioimmunoblastic lymphadenopathy-related lesions. *Cancer* 1992;69:1259–1267.
277. Ghani AM, Krause JR. Bone marrow biopsy findings in angioimmunoblastic lymphadenopathy. *Br J Haematol* 1985;61:203–213.
278. Diebold J, Tulliez M, Vercelli-Retta G, et al. [Histopathologic aspects of bone marrow in angioimmunoblastic lymphadenopathy]. *Ann Pathol* 1984;4:339–348.
279. Frizzera G, Moran EM, Rappaport H. Angio-immunoblastic lymphadenopathy: diagnosis and clinical course. *Am J Med* 1975;59:803–818.
280. Lukes RJ, Tindle BH. Immunoblastic lymphadenopathy: a hyperimmune entity resembling Hodgkin's disease. *N Engl J Med* 1975;292: 1–8.
281. Pangalis GA, Moran EM, Rappaport H. Blood and bone marrow findings in angioimmunoblastic lymphadenopathy. *Blood* 1978;51:71–83.
282. Nathwani BN, Rappaport H, Moran EM, et al. Malignant lymphoma arising in angioimmunoblastic lymphadenopathy. *Cancer* 1978;41: 578–606.
283. Jaffe ES, Chan JK, Su IJ, et al. Report of the Workshop on Nasal and Related Extranodal Angiocentric T/Natural Killer Cell Lymphomas: definitions, differential diagnosis, and epidemiology. *Am J Surg Pathol* 1996;20:103–111.
284. Nakamura S, Suchi T, Koshikawa T, et al. Clinicopathologic study of CD56 (NCAM)-positive angiocentric lymphoma occurring in sites other than the upper and lower respiratory tract. *Am J Surg Pathol* 1995;19:284–296.
285. Chan JK, Ng CS, Lau WH, et al. Most nasal/nasopharyngeal lymphomas are peripheral T-cell neoplasms. *Am J Surg Pathol* 1987;11: 418–429.
286. Chan JK, Sin VC, Wong KF, et al. Nonnasal lymphoma expressing the natural killer cell marker CD56: a clinicopathologic study of 49 cases of an uncommon aggressive neoplasm. *Blood* 1997;89: 4501–4513.
287. Wong KF, Chan JK, Ng CS, et al. CD56 (NKH1)-positive hematolymphoid malignancies: an aggressive neoplasm featuring frequent cutaneous/mucosal involvement, cytoplasmic azurophilic granules, and angiocentricity. *Hum Pathol* 1992;23:798–804.
288. Chott A, Rappersberger K, Schlossarek W, et al. Peripheral T cell lymphoma presenting primarily as lethal midline granuloma. *Hum Pathol* 1988;19:1093–1101.
289. Lorenzen J, Liu WP, Gi GD, et al. Nasal T/NK cell lymphoma: a clinicopathologic study of 30 West Chinese patients with special reference to proliferation and apoptosis. *Leuk Lymphoma* 1996;23: 593–602.
290. Nakamura S, Katoh E, Koshikawa T, et al. Clinicopathologic study of nasal T/NK-cell lymphoma among the Japanese. *Pathol Int* 1997; 47:38–53.
291. Emile JF, Boulland ML, Haioun C, et al. $CD5^{-}CD56^{+}$ T-cell receptor

silent peripheral T-cell lymphomas are natural killer cell lymphomas. *Blood* 1996;87:1466–1473.
292. Tsang WY, Chan JK, Ng CS, et al. Utility of a paraffin section-reactive CD56 antibody (123C3) for characterization and diagnosis of lymphomas. *Am J Surg Pathol* 1996;20:202–210.
293. Chan JK, Yip TT, Tsang WY, et al. Detection of Epstein-Barr viral RNA in malignant lymphomas of the upper aerodigestive tract. *Am J Surg Pathol* 1994;18:938–946.
294. Chan JK, Ng CS. Malignant lymphoma, natural killer cells and hemophagocytic syndrome [Letter]. *Pathology* 1989;21:154–155.
295. Jaffe ES, Blattner WA, Blayney DW, et al. The pathologic spectrum of adult T-cell leukemia/lymphoma in the United States: human T-cell leukemia/lymphoma virus-associated lymphoid malignancies. *Am J Surg Pathol* 1984;8:263–275.
296. Foucar K, Carroll TJ Jr, Tannous R, et al. Nonendemic adult T-cell leukemia/lymphoma in the United States: report of two cases and review of the literature. *Am J Clin Pathol* 1985;83:18–26.
297. Delsol G, Al Saati T, Gatter KC, et al. Coexpression of epithelial membrane antigen (EMA), Ki-1, and interleukin-2 receptor by anaplastic large cell lymphomas: diagnostic value in so-called malignant histiocytosis. *Am J Pathol* 1988;130:59–70.
298. Kinney M, Greer J, Macon W, et al. Peripheral blood and marrow involvement in Ki-1$^+$ anaplastic large cell malignant lymphoma. *Lab Invest* 1990;62:52A(abst).
299. Fraga M, Brousset P, Schlaifer D, et al. Bone marrow involvement in anaplastic large cell lymphoma: immunohistochemical detection of minimal disease and its prognostic significance. *Am J Clin Pathol* 1995;103:82–89.
300. Chott A, Kaserer K, Augustin I, et al. Ki-1-positive large cell lymphoma: a clinicopathologic study of 41 cases. *Am J Surg Pathol* 1990;14:439–448.
301. Tilly H, Gaulard P, Lepage E, et al. Primary anaplastic large-cell lymphoma in adults: clinical presentation, immunophenotype, and outcome. *Blood* 1997;90:3727–3734.
302. Wong KF, Chan JK, Ng CS, et al. Anaplastic large cell Ki-1 lymphoma involving bone marrow: marrow findings and association with reactive hemophagocytosis. *Am J Hematol* 1991;37:112–119.
303. Longo G, Federico M, Pieresca C, et al. Anaplastic large cell lymphoma (CD30$^+$/Ki-1$^+$): analysis of 35 cases followed at GISL centres. *Eur J Cancer* 1995;31A:1763–1767.
304. Delsol G, Laurent G, Kuhlein E, et al. Richter's syndrome: evidence for the clonal origin of the two proliferations. *Am J Clin Pathol* 1981;76:308–315.
305. Anderson MM, Ross CW, Singleton TP, et al. Ki-1 anaplastic large cell lymphoma with a prominent leukemic phase. *Hum Pathol* 1996;27:1093–1095.
306. Chhanabhai M, Britten C, Klasa R, et al. t(2;5)-Positive lymphoma with peripheral blood involvement. *Leuk Lymphoma* 1998;28:415–422.
307. Ponzoni M, Li CY. Isolated bone marrow non-Hodgkin's lymphoma: a clinicopathologic study. *Mayo Clin Proc* 1994;69:37–43.
308. Wong KF, Chan JK, Ng CS, et al. Large cell lymphoma with initial presentation in the bone marrow. *Hematol Oncol* 1992;10:261–271.
309. Barton JC, Conrad ME, Vogler LB, et al. Isolated marrow lymphoma: an entity of possible T-cell derivation. *Cancer* 1980;46:1767–1774.
310. Ioachim HL, Dorsett B, Cronin W, et al. Acquired immunodeficiency syndrome-associated lymphomas: clinical, pathologic, immunologic, and viral characteristics of 111 cases. *Hum Pathol* 1991;22:659–673.
311. Lowenthal DA, Straus DJ, Campbell SW, et al. AIDS-related lymphoid neoplasia: the Memorial Hospital experience. *Cancer* 1988;61:2325–2337.
312. Rubio R. Hodgkin's disease associated with human immunodeficiency virus infection: a clinical study of 46 cases. Cooperative Study Group of Malignancies Associated with HIV Infection of Madrid. *Cancer* 1994;73:2400–2407.
313. Osborne BM, Butler JJ. Hypocellular paratrabecular foci of treated small cleaved cell lymphoma in bone marrow biopsies. *Am J Surg Pathol* 1989;13:382–388.
314. Thiele J, Langohr J, Skorupka M, et al. Reticulin fibre content of bone marrow infiltrates of malignant non-Hodgkin's lymphomas (B-cell type, low malignancy): a morphometric evaluation before and after therapy. *Virchows Arch A Path Anat* 1990;417:485–492.
315. Ligler FS, Smith RG, Kettman JR, et al. Detection of tumor cells in the peripheral blood of nonleukemic patients with B-cell lymphoma: analysis of "clonal excess." *Blood* 1980;55:792–801.
316. Lopez-Guillermo A, Cabanillas F, McLaughlin P, et al. The clinical significance of molecular response in indolent follicular lymphomas. *Blood* 1998;91:2955–2960.
317. Gribben JG, Neuberg D, Freedman AS, et al. Detection by polymerase chain reaction of residual cells with the bcl-2 translocation is associated with increased risk of relapse after autologous bone marrow transplantation for B-cell lymphoma. *Blood* 1993;81:3449–3457.
318. Corradini P, Astolfi M, Cherasco C, et al. Molecular monitoring of minimal residual disease in follicular and mantle cell non-Hodgkin's lymphomas treated with high-dose chemotherapy and peripheral blood progenitor cell autografting. *Blood* 1997;89:724–731.
319. Andersen NS, Donovan JW, Borus JS, et al. Failure of immunologic purging in mantle cell lymphoma assessed by polymerase chain reaction detection of minimal residual disease. *Blood* 1997;90:4212–4221.
320. Chan DW, Liang R, Kwong YL, et al. Detection of T-cell receptor delta gene rearrangement in T-cell malignancies by clonal specific polymerase chain reaction and its application to detect minimal residual disease. *Am J Hematol* 1996;52:171–177.
321. Kurokawa T, Kinoshita T, Murate T, et al. Complementarity determining region-III is a useful molecular marker for the evaluation of minimal residual disease in mantle cell lymphoma. *Br J Haematol* 1997;98:408–412.
322. Nylund SJ, Ruutu T, Saarinen U, et al. Detection of minimal residual disease using fluorescence DNA in situ hybridization: a follow-up study in leukemia and lymphoma patients. *Leukemia* 1994;8:587–594.
323. Lee MS, Chang KS, Cabanillas F, et al. Detection of minimal residual cells carrying the t(14;18) by DNA sequence amplification. *Science* 1987;237:175–178.
324. Sharp JG, Joshi SS, Armitage JO, et al. Significance of detection of occult non-Hodgkin's lymphoma in histologically uninvolved bone marrow by a culture technique. *Blood* 1992;79:1074–1080.
325. Gribben JG, Freedman A, Woo SD, et al. All advanced stage non-Hodgkin's lymphomas with a polymerase chain reaction amplifiable breakpoint of bcl-2 have residual cells containing the bcl-2 rearrangement at evaluation and after treatment. *Blood* 1991;78:3275–3280.
326. Bain BJ, Catovsky D. The leukaemic phase of non-Hodgkin's lymphoma. *J Clin Pathol* 1995;48:189–193.
327. Uchiyama T, Yodoi J, Sagawa K, et al. Adult T-cell leukemia: clinical and hematologic features of 16 cases. *Blood* 1977;50:481–492.
328. Ellison DJ, Hu E, Zovich D, et al. Immunogenetic analysis of bone marrow aspirates in patients with non-Hodgkin lymphomas. *Am J Hematol* 1990;33:160–166.
329. Horning SJ, Galili N, Cleary M, et al. Detection of non-Hodgkin's lymphoma in the peripheral blood by analysis of antigen receptor gene rearrangements: results of a prospective study. *Blood* 1990;75:1139–1145.
330. Brada M, Mizutani S, Molgaard H, et al. Circulating lymphoma cells in patients with B and T non-Hodgkin's lymphoma detected by immunoglobulin and T-cell receptor gene rearrangement. *Br J Cancer* 1987;56:147–152.
331. Hiorns LR, Nicholls J, Sloane JP, et al. Peripheral blood involvement in non-Hodgkin's lymphoma detected by clonal gene rearrangement as a biological prognostic marker. *Br J Cancer* 1994;69:347–351.
332. Muche JM, Lukowsky A, Asadullah K, et al. Demonstration of frequent occurrence of clonal T cells in the peripheral blood of patients with primary cutaneous T-cell lymphoma. *Blood* 1997;90:1636–1642.
333. Berinstein NL, Reis MD, Ngan BY, et al. Detection of occult lymphoma in the peripheral blood and bone marrow of patients with untreated early-stage and advanced-stage follicular lymphoma. *J Clin Oncol* 1993;11:1344–1352.
334. Maeda K, Hyun BH, Rebuck JW. Lymphoid follicles in bone marrow aspirates. *Am J Clin Pathol* 1977;67:41–48.
335. Rywlin A. *Histopathology of the bone marrow.* Boston: Little, Brown, 1976:110–113.
336. Rywlin AM, Ortega RS, Dominguez CJ. Lymphoid nodules of bone marrow: normal and abnormal. *Blood* 1974;43:389–400.
337. Liu PI, Takanari H, Yatani R, et al. Comparative studies of bone marrow from the United States and Japan. *Ann Clin Lab Sci* 1989;19:345–351.
338. Kemona A, Dzieciol J, Sulik M, et al. [Lymphocytic aggregations in the bone marrow: their occurrence and morphologic analysis]. *Patol Pol* 1989;40:219–225.

339. Cervantes F, Pereira A, Marti JM, et al. Bone marrow lymphoid nodules in myeloproliferative disorders: association with the nonmyelosclerotic phases of idiopathic myelofibrosis and immunological significance. *Br J Haematol* 1988;70:279–282.
340. Rosenthal NS, Farhi DC. Bone marrow findings in connective tissue disease. *Am J Clin Pathol* 1989;92:650–654.
341. Franco V, Florena AM, Aragona F, et al. Immunohistochemical evaluation of bone marrow lymphoid nodules in chronic myeloproliferative disorders. *Virchows Arch A Path Anat* 1991;419:261–266.
342. Salisbury JR, Deverell MH, Seaton JM, et al. Three-dimensional reconstruction of non-Hodgkin's lymphoma in bone marrow trephines. *J Pathol* 1997;181:451–454.
343. Crocker J, Jones EL, Curran RC. Study of nuclear sizes in the centres of malignant and benign lymphoid follicles. *J Clin Pathol* 1983;36: 1332–1334.
344. Brunning RD, McKenna RW. *Lesions simulating lymphoma and miscellaneous tumor-like lesions in the bone marrow: Tumors of the bone marrow.* Washington, DC: Armed Forces Institute of Pathology, 1994: 409–438.
345. Osborne BM, Guarda LA, Butler JJ. Bone marrow biopsies in patients with the acquired immunodeficiency syndrome. *Hum Pathol* 1984; 15:1048–1053.
346. Karcher DS, Frost AR. The bone marrow in human immunodeficiency virus (HIV)-related disease: morphology and clinical correlation. *Am J Clin Pathol* 1991;95:63–71.
347. Farhi DC. Germinal centers in the bone marrow. *Hematol Pathol* 1989;3:133–136.
348. Peterson LC, Kueck B, Arthur DC, et al. Systemic polyclonal immunoblastic proliferations. *Cancer* 1988;61:1350–1358.
349. Poje EJ, Soori GS, Weisenburger DD. Systemic polyclonal B-immunoblastic proliferation with marked peripheral blood and bone marrow plasmacytosis. *Am J Clin Pathol* 1992;98:222–226.
350. Peterson L, Marcelli A, Arthur D, et al. Systemic polyclonal immunoblastic proliferation: a distinct atypical lymphoproliferative disorder. *Lab Invest* 1998;78:138A(abst).
351. Castella A, Croxson TS, Mildvan D, et al. The bone marrow in AIDS: a histologic, hematologic, and microbiologic study. *Am J Clin Pathol* 1985;84:425–432.
352. Danova M, Riccardi A, Brugnatelli S, et al. Bone marrow morphology and proliferative activity in acquired immunodeficiency syndrome. *Haematologica* 1989;74:365–369.
353. Sandhaus LM, Scudder R. Hematologic and bone marrow abnormalities in pediatric patients with human immunodeficiency virus (HIV) infection. *Pediatr Pathol* 1989;9:277–288.
354. Benjamin D, Magrath IT, Douglass EC, et al. Derivation of lymphoma cell lines from microscopically normal bone marrow in patients with undifferentiated lymphomas: evidence of occult bone marrow involvement. *Blood* 1983;61:1017–1019.
355. Sangster G, Crocker J, Nar P, et al. Benign and malignant (B cell) focal lymphoid aggregates in bone marrow trephines shown by means of an immunogold-silver technique. *J Clin Pathol* 1986;39:453–457.
356. Sandhaus LM, Voelkerding KV, Dougherty J, et al. Combined utility of gene rearrangement analysis and flow cytometry in the diagnosis of lymphoproliferative disease in the bone marrow. *Hematol Pathol* 1990;4:135–148.
357. Horny HP, Ruck P, Xiao JC, et al. Immunoreactivity of normal and neoplastic human tissue mast cells with macrophage-associated antibodies, with special reference to the recently developed monoclonal antibody PG-M1. *Hum Pathol* 1993;24:355–358.
358. Ben-Ezra J, Burke JS, Swartz WG, et al. Small lymphocytic lymphoma: a clinicopathologic analysis of 268 cases. *Blood* 1989;73: 579–587.
359. Knowles DM, Athan E, Ubriaco A, et al. Extranodal noncutaneous lymphoid hyperplasias represent a continuous spectrum of B-cell neoplasia: demonstration by molecular genetic analysis. *Blood* 1989;73: 1635–1645.
360. Faulkner-Jones BE, Howie AJ, Boughton BJ, et al. Lymphoid aggregates in bone marrow: study of eventual outcome. *J Clin Pathol* 1988; 41:768–775.
361. Muehleck SD, McKenna RW, Gale PF, et al. Terminal deoxynucleotidyl transferase (TdT)-positive cells in bone marrow in the absence of hematologic malignancy. *Am J Clin Pathol* 1983;79:277–284.
362. Longacre TA, Foucar K, Crago S, et al. Hematogones: a multiparameter analysis of bone marrow precursor cells. *Blood* 1989;73:543–552.
363. Motley D, Meyer MP, King RA, et al. Determination of lymphocyte immunophenotypic values for normal full-term cord blood. *Am J Clin Pathol* 1996;105:38–43.
364. Rimza L, Viswanatha D, Winter S, et al. The presence of CD34$^+$ cell clusters predicts impending relapse in children with acute lymphoblastic leukemia receiving maintenance chemotherapy. *Am J Clin Pathol* 1998;110:313–320.
365. Davis RE, Longacre TA, Cornbleet PJ. Hematogones in the bone marrow of adults: immunophenotypic features, clinical settings, and differential diagnosis. *Am J Clin Pathol* 1994;102:202–211.
366. Richard G, Brody J, Sun T. A case of acute megakaryocytic leukemia with hematogones. *Leukemia* 1993;7:1900–1903.
367. van den Doel LJ, Pieters R, Huismans DR, et al. Immunological phenotype of lymphoid cells in regenerating bone marrow of children after treatment for acute lymphoblastic leukemia. *Eur J Haematol* 1988;41:170–175.
368. Kobayashi SD, Seki K, Suwa N, et al. The transient appearance of small blastoid cells in the marrow after bone marrow transplantation. *Am J Clin Pathol* 1991;96:191–195.
369. Leitenberg D, Rappeport JM, Smith BR. B-cell precursor bone marrow reconstitution after bone marrow transplantation. *Am J Clin Pathol* 1994;102:231–236.
370. Stass SA, McGraw TP, Folds JD, et al. Terminal transferase in acute lymphoblast leukemia in remission. *Am J Clin Pathol* 1981;75: 838–840.
371. Washington L, Ansari M, Picker L, et al. Immunophenotypic analysis of B cell precursors in 661 bone marrow specimens by 4-color flow cytometry. *Mod Pathol* 1999;12:148A(abst).
372. Wells DA, Sale GE, Shulman HM, et al. Multidimensional flow cytometry of marrow can differentiate leukemic from normal lymphoblasts and myeloblasts after chemotherapy and bone marrow transplantation. *Am J Clin Pathol* 1998;110:84–94.
373. Farahat N, Lens D, Zomas A, et al. Quantitative flow cytometry can distinguish between normal and leukaemic B-cell precursors. *Br J Haematol* 1995;91:640–646.
374. Bodem CR, Hamory BH, Taylor HM, et al. Granulomatous bone marrow disease: a review of the literature and clinicopathologic analysis of 58 cases. *Medicine (Baltimore)* 1983;62:372–383.
375. Bhargava V, Farhi DC. Bone marrow granulomas: clinicopathologic findings in 72 cases and review of the literature. *Hematol Pathol* 1988; 2:43–50.
376. Kadin ME, Donaldson SS, Dorfman RF. Isolated granulomas in Hodgkin's disease. *N Engl J Med* 1970;283:859–861.
377. Brincker H. Sarcoid reactions and sarcoidosis in Hodgkin's disease and other malignant lymphomata. *Br J Cancer* 1972;26:120–123.
378. Kim H, Dorfman RF. Morphological studies of 84 untreated patients subjected to laparotomy for the staging of non-Hodgkin's lymphomas. *Cancer* 1974;33:657–674.
379. Yu NC, Rywlin AM. Granulomatous lesions of the bone marrow in non-Hodgkin's lymphoma. *Hum Pathol* 1982;13:905–910.
380. Kahn LB, King H, Jacobs P. Florid epithelioid cell and sarcoid-type reaction associated with non-Hodgkin's lymphoma. *S Afr Med J* 1977; 51:341–347.
381. O'Connell MJ, Schimpff SC, Kirschner RH, et al. Epithelioid granulomas in Hodgkin disease: a favorable prognostic sign? *JAMA* 1975; 233:886–889.
382. Sacks EL, Donaldson SS, Gordon J, et al. Epithelioid granulomas associated with Hodgkin's disease: clinical correlations in 55 previously untreated patients. *Cancer* 1978;41:562–567.
383. Favara BE, McCarthy RC, Mierau GW. Histiocytosis X. *Hum Pathol* 1983;14:663–676.
384. Risdall RJ, Dehner LP, Duray P, et al. Histiocytosis X (Langerhans' cell histiocytosis): prognostic role of histopathology. *Arch Pathol Lab Med* 1983;107:59–63.
385. Ide F, Iwase T, Saito I, et al. Immunohistochemical and ultrastructural analysis of the proliferating cells in histiocytosis X. *Cancer* 1984;53: 917–921.
386. Hage C, Willman CL, Favara BE, et al. Langerhans' cell histiocytosis (histiocytosis X): immunophenotype and growth fraction. *Hum Pathol* 1993;24:840–845.
387. Dehner LP. Morphologic findings in the histiocytic syndromes. *Semin Oncol* 1991;18:8–17.
388. Favara BE. Langerhans' cell histiocytosis pathobiology and pathogenesis. *Semin Oncol* 1991;18:3–7.

389. Mierau GW, Favara BE. S-100 protein immunohistochemistry and electron microscopy in the diagnosis of Langerhans cell proliferative disorders: a comparative assessment. *Ultrastruct Pathol* 1986;10: 303–309.
390. Emile JF, Wechsler J, Brousse N, et al. Langerhans' cell histiocytosis: definitive diagnosis with the use of monoclonal antibody O10 on routinely paraffin-embedded samples. *Am J Surg Pathol* 1995;19: 636–641.
391. Birbeck M. An electron microscopic study of basal melanocytes and high-level clear cells (Langerhans' cells) in vitiligo. *J Invest Dermatol* 1961;37:51–58.
392. Ochsner SF. Eosinophilic granuloma of bone; experience with 20 cases. *Am J Roentgenol Radium Ther Nucl Med* 1966;97:719–726.
393. Nauert C, Zornoza J, Ayala A, et al. Eosinophilic granuloma of bone: diagnosis and management. *Skeletal Radiol* 1983;10:227–235.
394. Brunning RD, McKenna RW, Rosai J, et al. Systemic mastocytosis: extracutaneous manifestations. *Am J Surg Pathol* 1983;7:425–438.
395. Travis WD, Li CY, Bergstralh EJ, et al. Systemic mast cell disease: analysis of 58 cases and literature review. *Medicine (Baltimore)* 1988; 67:345–368.
396. Horny HP, Parwaresch MR, Lennert K. Bone marrow findings in systemic mastocytosis. *Hum Pathol* 1985;16:808–814.
397. Horny HP, Kaiserling E. Lymphoid cells and tissue mast cells of bone marrow lesions in systemic mastocytosis: a histological and immunohistological study. *Br J Haematol* 1988;69:449–455.
398. Rywlin AM, Hoffman EP, Ortega RS. Eosinophilic fibrohistiocytic lesion of bone marrow: a distinctive new morphologic finding, probably related to drug hypersensitivity. *Blood* 1972;40:464–472.
399. te Velde J, Vismans FJ, Leenheers-Binnendijk L, et al. The eosinophilic fibrohistiocytic lesion of the bone marrow: a mastocellular lesion in bone disease. *Virchows Arch A Path Anat* 1978;377:277–285.
400. Li WV, Kapadia SB, Sonmez-Alpan E, et al. Immunohistochemical characterization of mast cell disease in paraffin sections using tryptase, CD68, myeloperoxidase, lysozyme, and CD20 antibodies. *Mod Pathol* 1996;9:982–988.
401. Jager K, Burkhardt R, Bartl R. Lymphoid infiltrates in chronic myeloproliferative disorders (MPD). *Verh Dtsch Ges Pathol* 1983;67:239.
402. Hasselbalch H. Idiopathic myelofibrosis: a clinical study of 80 patients. *Am J Hematol* 1990;34:291–300.
403. Frisch B, Bartl R, Mahl G, et al. Scope and value of bone marrow biopsies in metastatic cancer. *Invasion Metastasis* 1984;4:12–30.
404. Gale P, McKenna R. Monitoring metastasis in bone marrow. In: Stoll B, ed. *Screening and monitoring of cancer.* Chichester: John Wiley and Sons, 1985:265–283.
405. Brunning R, McKenna R. *Metastatic tumors involving bone marrow: tumors of the bone marrow.* Washington, DC: Armed Forces Institute of Pathology, 1994:457–472.

CHAPTER 40

B-Cell Chronic Lymphocytic Leukemia and Prolymphocytic Leukemia

M. Kathryn Foucar

The chronic lymphoid neoplasms that manifest with a dominant leukemic blood and bone marrow picture encompass a broad spectrum of disorders with relatively distinct clinical, morphologic, and immunophenotypic features. The focus of this chapter is to review two of these chronic leukemias: B-cell chronic lymphocytic leukemia (CLL) and B-cell prolymphocytic leukemia (PLL). The types and relative frequencies of chronic lymphoid leukemias are listed in Table 40.1 (1–3). CLL is by far the most common of these disorders. Other relatively common types of chronic lymphoid leukemia include hairy cell leukemia (see Chapter 41) and PLL (1–4). The remaining chronic lymphoid leukemias account for less than 5% of cases. Even though the clinicopathologic features of all these chronic lymphoid leukemias have been delineated, it is occasionally difficult to determine a definitive diagnosis. This chapter emphasizes the importance of integrating clinical features, morphology, and immunophenotypic findings to subclassify chronic lymphoid leukemias optimally to facilitate therapeutic decision making and assessment of prognosis.

B-CELL CHRONIC LYMPHOCYTIC LEUKEMIA

Definition

CLL is an acquired clonal lymphoproliferative disorder, usually of B-cell origin, manifested by the accumulation of uniform, immunologically incompetent mature lymphocytes that are generally characterized by a low cell proliferation rate and prolonged cell survival (2,5,6). Molecular and glucose-6-phosphate dehydrogenase studies indicate that the neoplastic clone consists exclusively of these neoplastic B lymphocytes, without involvement of hematopoietic elements or other lymphocyte populations (5,6). These clonal B lymphocytes generally demonstrate a characteristic hematologic, morphologic, immunophenotypic, and genotypic profile.

Epidemiology and Incidence

CLL is the most common leukemia of adults in the West, with an incidence of up to 50 cases per 100,000 persons older than 80 years of age (5,7–10). In contrast, the incidence of CLL in some other parts of the world, notably Japan and China, is much lower (9). In the West, men are affected more often than women, and an increased risk of CLL has been demonstrated in farmers, rubber manufacturing and asbestos workers, and persons exposed to benzene (5,7,8,10). Unlike many other types of leukemia, CLL is not linked to prior radiation exposure (8). Genetic factors play a role in the development of this leukemia, because CLL is the most common of the familial leukemias (10–12).

CLL typically affects middle-aged to elderly patients and occurs only rarely before the fourth decade (5,7,13–16). Despite its rarity, well-characterized case reports of CLL in young adults and children have been published (17–21) (Table 40.2). Several of the documented cases of CLL in children have been associated with a unique karyotypic abnormality, t(2;14). The clinical course of CLL in young patients is variable, and the staging systems that segregate older

TABLE 40.1. *Chronic lymphoid leukemias*

Type	Frequency (%)
B-cell chronic lymphocytic leukemia	>80
Hairy cell leukemia	10
B-cell prolymphocytic leukemia	<5
Peripheralized lymphomas	<5
All T-cell leukemias	<5

Data from references 1 through 4.

M. K. Foucar: Department of Pathology, University of New Mexico Health Sciences Center, Albuquerque, New Mexico 87131

TABLE 40.2. *Chronic lymphocytic leukemia in children and young adults*

Age (yr)	Morphology/ALC	Immunophenotype	Comments	References
<20	Small mature lymphocytes; ALC >22.9 × 10^9/L	Monoclonal sIg when studied	Several cases exhibit t(2;14)	17–19
20–30	Small mature lymphocytes; ALC 7.5–136 × 10^9/L	Monoclonal sIg and CD5 expressed, TdT negative	Clinical course similar to CLL in older patients	20
31–50	Small mature lymphocytes; ALC broad range, always exceeded 5 × 10^9/L	Monoclonal sIg on all cases studied (20% of total)	133 cases; most important prognostic factor is extent of bone marrow lymphocytosis	21

ALC, absolute lymphocyte count; CLL, chronic lymphocytic leukemia; sIg, surface immunoglobulin; TdT, terminal deoxynucleotidyl transferase.

patients into prognostic groups are not useful in young patients (21).

Pathologic Features

Peripheral Blood

Although a monotonous lymphocyte population generally predominates, the morphologic spectrum of CLL is fairly broad, overlapping with various reactive disorders and with other B-cell lymphoproliferative disorders (1,2,4,6,7,13,16). In typical cases of CLL, the blood contains a relatively homogeneous lymphocyte population characterized by cells with a high nuclear to cytoplasmic ratio, scant to moderate nongranular cytoplasm, and round nuclei with highly condensed chromatin and inconspicuous nucleoli (Fig. 40.1). The exaggerated chromatin clumping results in a characteristic ''blocky'' separation of chromatin and parachromatin. Admixed with these mature-appearing lymphocytes may be prolymphocytes or lymphocytes with nuclear irregularity, which generally account for less than 10% of the lymphocyte population, respectively (1,2,13,16). Prolymphocytes are distinguished from prototypic CLL cells by their greater amounts of cytoplasm, less condensed chromatin, and prominent central nucleoli (Fig. 40.1). The nuclear irregularity described in some cases of CLL typically occurs in only a minority of lymphocytes and is characterized by prominent nuclear clefting and notching (1,2,13,16). However, in some cases, the lymphocyte population is substantially more heterogenous with fair numbers of clefted lymphocytes, larger cells with more cytoplasm, or prolymphocytes; these cases are often designated as atypical or mixed-type CLL (1,22).

In about 5% to 10% of cases of CLL, cytoplasmic inclusions, such as rodlike bodies, crystals, and vacuoles, are

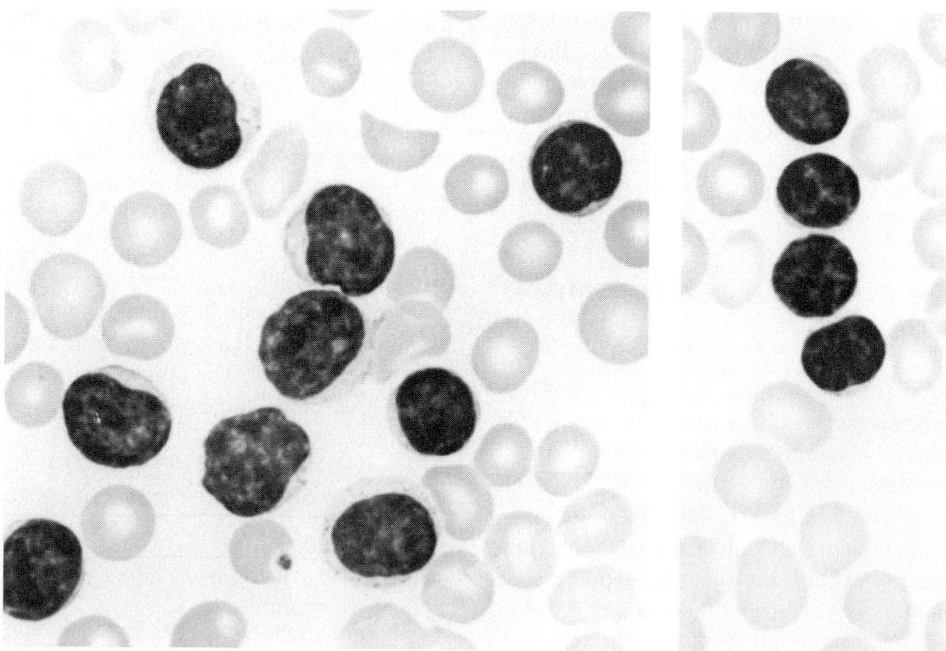

FIG. 40.1. This composite of circulating chronic lymphocytic leukemia cells from two patients shows the highly condensed chromatin with scant cytoplasm that is characteristic of this leukemia (Wright stain, original magnification: 1,000× magnification).

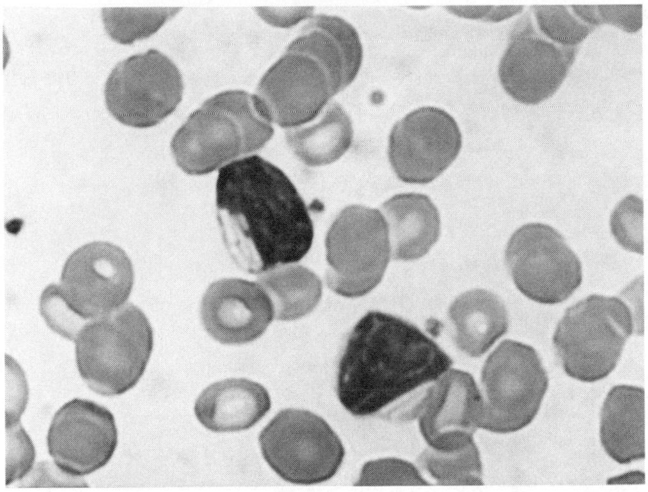

FIG. 40.2. The peripheral blood smear illustrates crystals within the cytoplasm of chronic lymphocytic leukemia cells (Wright stain, original magnification: 1,000× magnification). See Color Plate 15, between pp. 1446–1447.

identified (Fig. 40.2; see also Color Plate 15, between pp. 1446–1447) (23). These inclusions generally are derived from immunoglobulin and, when present, are found in a variable percentage of the CLL cells (23,24).

In addition to evaluating the morphology and absolute lymphocyte count, assessment of normal hematopoietic elements is essential in CLL patients, and this information is used in staging these patients, as discussed later. At presentation, most CLL patients demonstrate intact hematopoiesis (i.e., normal erythrocyte, platelet, and neutrophil counts) or modest hematopoietic compromise such as mild anemia.

Bone Marrow

Because peripheral blood involvement is a defining feature of CLL, bone marrow examination is generally not required to establish the diagnosis of CLL. Aspirate smears typically reveal a mature lymphocytosis that exceeds 30% of the differential cell count. These cells are similar to those present in the blood, although foci of transformed cells may rarely be evident (16). Mast cells may be increased and plasma cells are often decreased.

The patterns of bone marrow infiltration in biopsy sections are helpful in distinguishing CLL infiltrates from benign lymphoid aggregates and in offering significant prognostic information (2,4,6,13,16,25–28). Benign lymphoid nodules are generally well circumscribed, nonparatrabecular, and surround a blood vessel (29–32) (Table 40.3). In contrast, the infiltrates of CLL may be nodular (i.e., focal), interstitial, or diffuse, and various combinations of these patterns have been described (2,6,16,27) (Figs. 40.3, 40.4; see also Color Plate 16, between pp. 1446–1447). Nodular infiltrates are characterized by dense, localized aggregations of CLL cells that are nonparatrabecular, have infiltrative margins, and may be confluent. In contrast, interstitial infiltrates of CLL

TABLE 40.3. *Bone marrow biopsy: distinction between chronic lymphocytic leukemia and benign lymphoid infiltrates*

Chronic lymphocytic leukemia	Benign lymphoid nodules
Nodular, diffuse, and interstitial patterns described	Nodules well-circumscribed, nonparatrabecular, often associated with blood vessels
Nodules have infiltrative margins and may be confluent	Nodules usually few in number and widely separated
Germinal centers absent	Germinal centers may be present
Small lymphocytes predominate	Small lymphocytes predominate, plasma cells and macrophages may be admixed

Data from references 4 and 29 through 32.

cells are admixed with fat cells and hematopoietic elements, whereas bone marrow architecture is completely effaced in the packed diffuse infiltrates. The designation of *mixed infiltrates* has been applied inconsistently by researchers and sometimes refers to mixed nodular and diffuse infiltrates, whereas other investigators use this term to describe admixed nodular and interstitial infiltrates (2,16,27).

A frequent observation is the link between diffuse bone marrow infiltration in CLL and worse prognosis (25–27). This can be especially important in patients who have low-stage CLL, in whom a diffuse pattern of bone marrow infiltration is associated with rapid disease progression (26,27).

Other Organs

Although CLL infiltrates have been identified in numerous organ systems, lymph nodes and spleen are the most

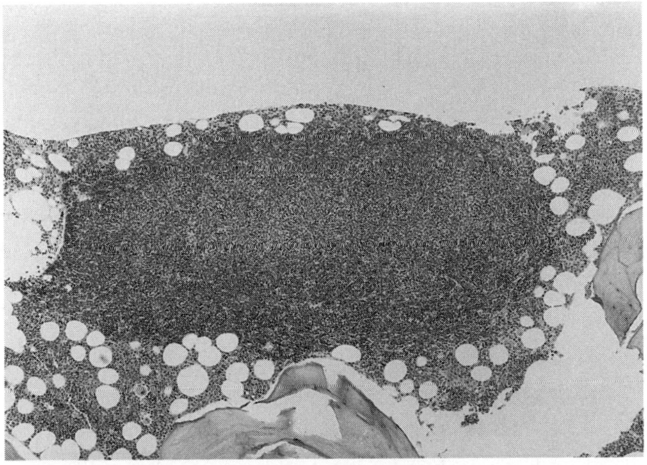

FIG. 40.3. This low-power photomicrograph of a bone marrow biopsy illustrates a large chronic lymphocytic leukemia nodule with several pale proliferation foci (hematoxylin and eosin stain, original magnification: 200× magnification). See Color Plate 16, between pp. 1446–1447.

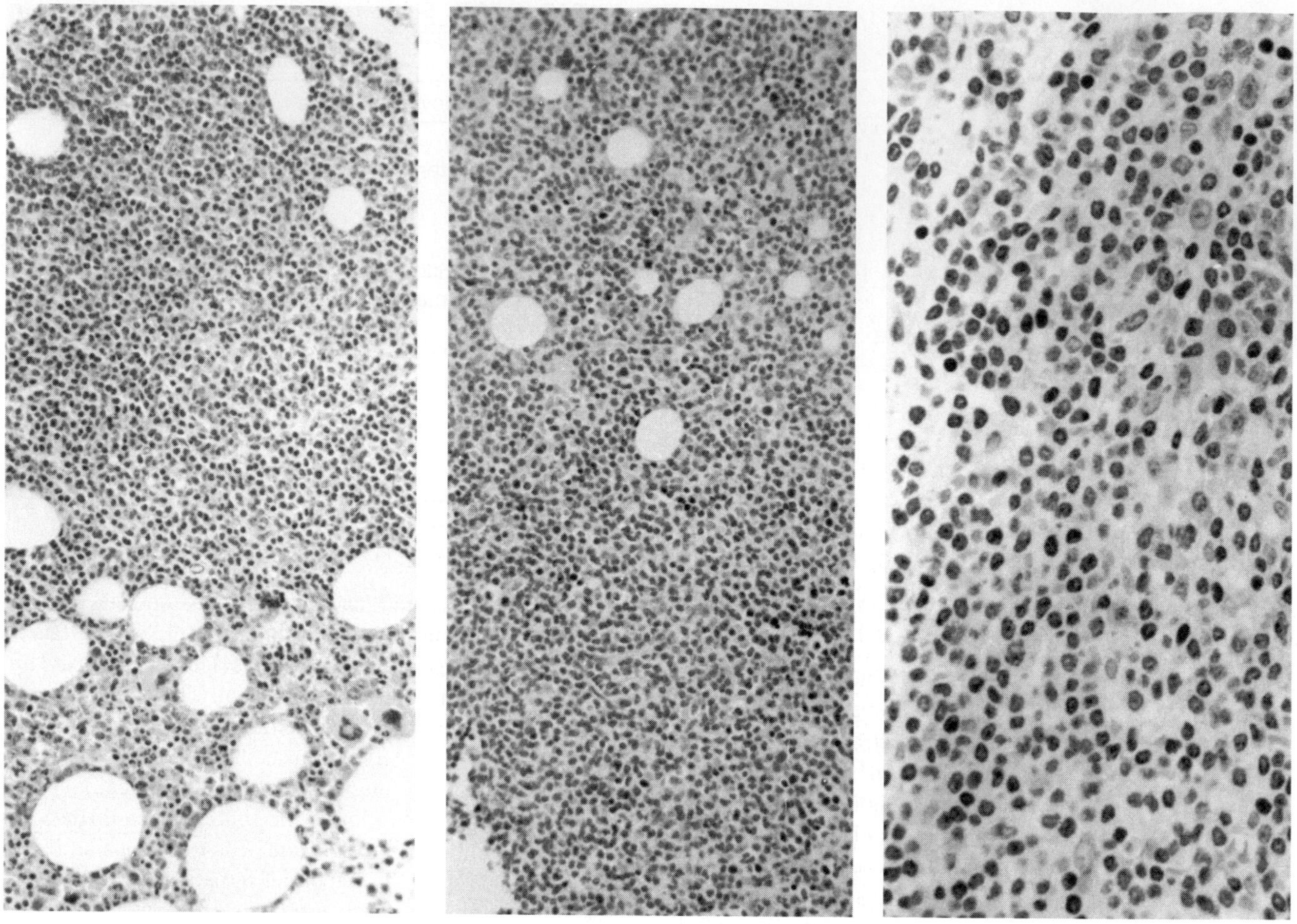

FIG. 40.4. This composite of bone marrow biopsies from three patients with chronic lymphocytic leukemia (CLL) shows a nodule of CLL (**A**), an interstitial infiltrate of CLL (**B**), and a diffuse infiltrate of CLL with replacement of all hematopoietic and fat elements (**C**) (hematoxylin and eosin stain, original magnification: 400× magnification).

commonly evaluated extramedullary sites (Table 40.4) (see Chapters 21 and 53). Several distinct lymph node patterns of CLL involvement have been defined (6,7,13,33,34). In ''stable phase'' CLL, lymph nodes generally exhibit diffuse architectural effacement by a monotonous infiltrate of small lymphocytes with round nuclear contours, inconspicuous nucleoli, and scant cytoplasm (Fig. 40.5). Proliferation foci (i.e., pseudofollicles or growth centers) that consist of intermediate-sized cells with more cytoplasm and more readily apparent mitotic activity frequently are identified. These larger cells are thought to comprise the proliferative component of the neoplasm. Occasionally, the intermediate-sized cells are admixed diffusely with the small lymphocytes of CLL, but if they account for more than 30% of the total cells, there is no adverse impact on clinical course (33). Different lymph node histology has been described in patients with atypical CLL (34). In these cases the proliferation foci are larger, more distinct, and contain large transformed cells. Greater nuclear irregularity of the small lymphocytes may be evident. Although infiltration by small lymphocytes is the most common morphologic pattern at presentation, nodal morphology may change during the course of CLL, and the lymph node may be the initial site of transformation of CLL to large cell lymphoma (Fig. 40.6).

Splenomegaly caused by leukemic infiltration is a common clinical finding in CLL (6,35–38). Although the leukemic cells infiltrate the white and red pulp, white pulp disease usually dominates, creating a miliary nodular pattern grossly (Fig. 40.7). The larger cells tend to be concentrated in the white pulp and form proliferation foci like those seen in lymph nodes. These cells express proliferation markers such as Ki-67, whereas ''resting'' B cells are concentrated in the red pulp cords (38). Spleens from CLL patients may also demonstrate trabecular, subendothelial, and prominent sinus involvement (35).

Table 40.4 details the patterns of CLL infiltration in other organ systems, including liver, skin, lung, gastrointestinal tract, bone, central nervous system, heart, adrenal, and kidney. In all of these sites, CLL infiltrates may be associated with fibrosis (37). Even though widespread multiorgan system infiltrates of CLL are commonly documented at autopsy, these infiltrates may not cause organ dysfunction.

TABLE 40.4. *Extramedullary organ involvement in chronic lymphocytic leukemia*

Site	Usual pattern of infiltration	Comments	References
Lymph node (see Chapter 21)	Small lymphocytic lymphoma, diffuse; pseudofollicles (growth centers) present; immature cells may be diffusely admixed with small lymphocytes.	May see variation in morphology with disease progression, duration, and in cases of atypical chronic lymphocytic leukemia	6, 7, 13, 33, 34
Spleen (see Chapter 53)	May see white pulp predominant or red pulp predominant patterns, but infiltration of both sites generally present	Splenomegaly in majority of patients, usually mild	6, 35–38
Liver	Usually portal tract involvement predominates; may be associated with fibrosis	Liver involvement common; may be associated with cholestatic jaundice or other liver function abnormalities	6, 37
Skin	Dermal infiltrates	Clinical spectrum including localized or generalized papules, plaques, nodules, or large tumor masses	6, 178
Lung	Variable	Generally involves hilar nodes with resulting bronchial compression or lymphatic obstruction causing effusions	6
Gastrointestinal tract	Mucosal infiltrates described in stomach, small bowel, and large bowel	May cause malabsorption (small bowel infiltrates)	6, 179
Bone	Variable	Diffuse demineralization (<5% patients); rare patient develops osteolytic lesions with hypercalcemia	6
Central nervous system	Variable	Less than 2% of patients develop CNS symptoms that range from meningeal signs to tumor masses[a]	6, 180–182
Heart, adrenal, kidney	Diffuse infiltrates of small lymphocytes	Usually subclinical but may be associated with fibrosis	37

[a] CNS tumor mass is usually associated with transformation to large cell lymphoma.

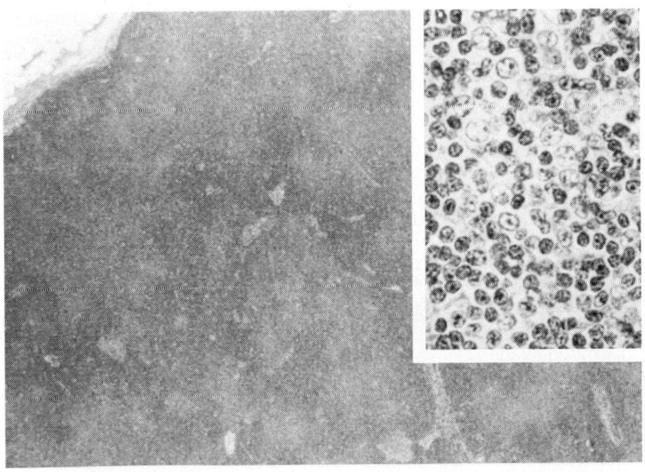

FIG. 40.5. This composite illustrates low- and high-power lymph node morphology from a patient with chronic lymphocytic leukemia (CLL) (hematoxylin and eosin stain). At low power, a diffuse infiltrate with pale proliferative foci, capsular attenuation, and occasional patent sinuses is evident (original magnification: 25× magnification). High-power **(inset)** shows round lymphocytes with admixed larger lymphoid cells from proliferative foci (original magnification: 400× magnification).

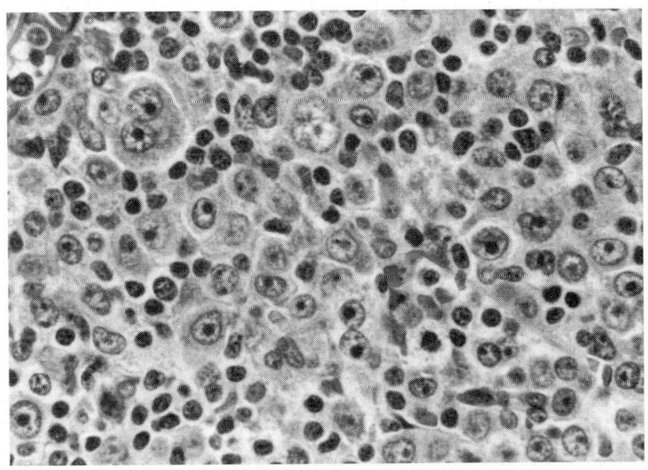

FIG. 40.6. In this lymph node section from a patient with chronic lymphocytic leukemia, large cells exceed 30%, indicating transformation (i.e., evolving Richter's syndrome) (hematoxylin and eosin stain, original magnification: 400× magnification).

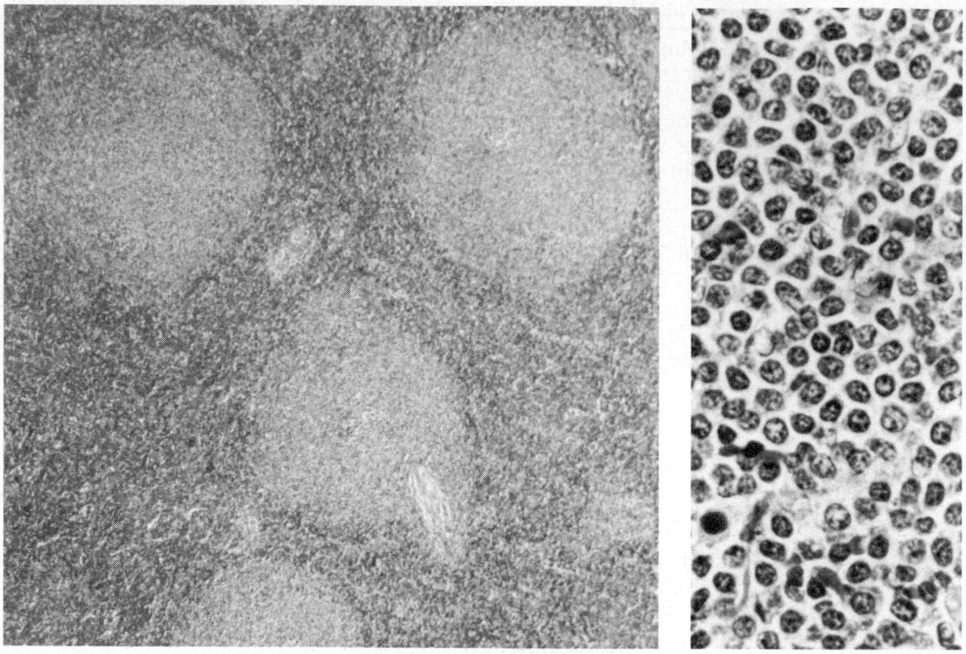

FIG. 40.7. Photomicrographs from a spleen removed for chronic lymphocytic leukemia (CLL). The prominent white pulp with some red pulp infiltration is illustrated at low power (**left**) (original magnification: 25× magnification), and the monotonous infiltrate of small, round lymphocytes is evident at higher magnification (**right**) (original magnification: 400× magnification).

Immunologic Features

A wealth of immunologic research has been performed on CLL cells, ranging from pioneering mouse erythrocyte rosette studies to sophisticated multicolor flow cytometric analyses. Using these studies, a B-cell origin for most cases of CLL has been documented. By applying a battery of monoclonal antibodies, a spectrum of immunophenotypic characteristics has been delineated that generally can be used to distinguish CLL from other B-lymphoproliferative disorders (2,4,6,7,13,16,39–42) (Table 40.5).

The comprehensive surface antigenic profile of prototypic B-CLL entails expression of weak monotypic immunoglobulin (usually IgM, but also IgM plus IgD or IgG), CD19, CD23, CD5, and weak (or absent) CD20, CD22, FMC7, and CD11c, but neither CD79b nor CD10 is expressed (2,6,13, 39,40,42). By using this broad antigenic fingerprint of the leukemic clone, CLL can usually be distinguished from other mature B-cell neoplasms such as peripheralizing mantle cell lymphoma/follicle center cell lymphoma, splenic lymphoma with villous lymphocytes, hairy cell leukemia, and PLL (Table 40.5). Antigens of particular utility in segregating chronic leukemias and lymphomas of B-cell origin include CD5, CD20, CD22, CD23, CD79b, and CD10 (Fig. 40.8). Multicolor flow cytometric immunophenotyping is also useful in identifying early cases of CLL in which only a modest absolute lymphocytosis is present (43). Likewise, paraffin immunoperoxidase techniques are now available for assessment of cyclin D1 (in mantle cell lymphomas) and CD23 (in CLL) for cases in which viable cell suspensions are not available (44,45).

Investigators have studied the role of adhesion molecule expression in the pathophysiology of CLL (46). The migra-

TABLE 40.5. *Typical immunophenotypic features of B-chronic leukemias or lymphomas*

Disorder	sIg	CD19	CD20	CD22	CD23	CD25	CD5	FMC7	CD11c	CD10	CD79b
CLL	W	+	W	W	+	−	+	−	W	−	−
PLL	+	+	+	+	−	−	±	+	−	−	+
HCL	+	+	+	+	−	+	−	+	+	−	−
MCL	+	+	+	+	−	−	+	+	−	−	+
FCC	+	+	+	+	−	−	−	+	−	+	+
SLVL	+	+	+	+	−	−	±	+	±	±	+

CLL, chronic lymphocytic leukemia; PLL, prolymphocytic leukemia; HCL, hairy cell leukemia; MCL, mantle cell lymphoma; FCC, small cleaved follicle center cell lymphoma; SLVL, splenic lymphoma with villous lymphocytes; +, expressed; −, not expressed; ±, variable expression; W, weakly expressed.

Data from references 2, 4, 6, 7, 13, and 39 through 43.

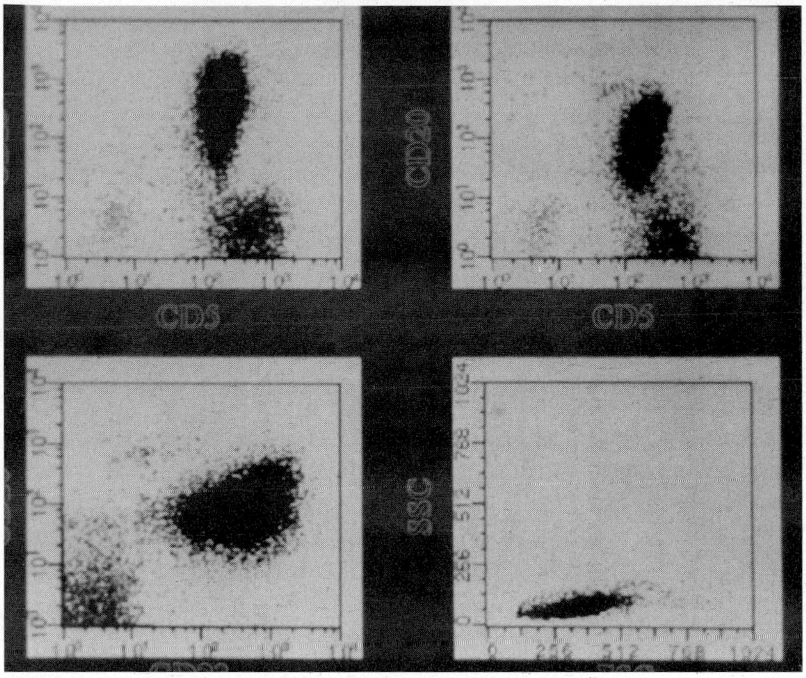

FIG. 40.8. This flow histogram illustrates classic immunophenotypic features of chronic lymphocytic leukemia in which the small lymphocytes coexpress CD5, weak CD20, and CD23. Admixed normal T cells ($CD5^+$) are also present.

tion of CLL cells probably is linked to patterns of adhesion molecule expression, and it is postulated that clinical features at presentation and disease progression are impacted by these adhesion molecules (47,48). These adhesion receptors include L-selectins, integrins, CD54, and CD44. Although initial studies indicate different adhesion molecule profiles among the various types of chronic lymphoproliferative disorders, further studies are needed to determine how these adhesion pathways influence lymphocyte trafficking and clinical disease manifestations (46–48).

A substantial body of literature has documented a whole spectrum of T-cell and natural killer (NK) cell abnormalities in patients who have B-CLL. Some of these are detailed in Table 40.6 (6,7,49–62). Numeric and functional abnormalities of these cells have been described, and several investigators state that the T-cell and NK cell defects contribute to immunologic impairment of patients who have B-CLL. Some investigators propose that the clonal B lymphocytes produce substances that suppress NK cell and T-cell activity, whereas others suggest that B-CLL patient serum contains a factor that promotes NK cell–like growth (56,59). In contrast, some investigators suggest that earlier reports of major T-cell abnormalities in CLL may be incorrect or at least are exaggerated because of their less specific methods of analyzing T-cell function (57). To further complicate this confusing area of investigation, investigators have observed different patterns of phenotypic and functional alterations of T and NK cells that were linked to the morphologic features of the CLL (i.e., typical versus atypical morphology) (63). In another study, increased cytoplasmic interleukin-4 was detected in CD8-positive ($CD8^+$) suppressor cells in patients with B-CLL, suggesting a link between this T-cell aberration and modulation of the B-cell clone (64). Other

TABLE 40.6. *T-cell and natural killer cell abnormalities in B-cell chronic lymphocytic leukemia*

Type of defect or abnormality	References
Inversion of helper/suppressor ratio	6, 7, 13
Helper cell dysfunction, increased suppressor effector cells	49–51
Helper cell production of CD40 may drive B-CLL proliferation in subset of cases	62
Abnormal mitogen response	6
Excess suppressor cell activity	6, 49
Multiple T-cell defects impair T-cell proliferation	52
Clonal T-cell proliferations identified	61
Defect in induction of B-cell differentiation	6
Decreased IL-2 production[a]	6, 52, 53
Secreted IL-2 rapidly removed by CLL cells	54
Large granular lymphocytes may suppress B-cell proliferation	55
B-CLL cells secrete, shed substance that suppresses NK and T-cell activity	56
Sera from B-CLL patients contain factor that promotes NK cell–like LAK cell growth	59
Defective LAK function	58
Increased cytoplasmic IL-4 in CD8 T cells	64

B-CLL, B-cell chronic lymphocytic leukemia; IL, interleukin; LAK, lymphokine-associated killer; NK, natural killer.

[a] Some studies found no defect in IL-2 response with production of normal numbers of helper and cytotoxic T cells (57).

associations between helper T-cell activity and B-CLL cell proliferation have also been reported (62). Studies document clonal T-cell proliferations in the bone marrow of patients with B-CLL (61).

Cytogenetic Features

Historically, cytogenetic studies of CLL cells have been technically difficult to perform because of their low proliferative rate. These early studies were hindered by scant leukemia cell metaphases, and in some instances, the mitoses analyzed probably were from admixed nonneoplastic T cells. With the development of potent B-cell mitogens, great progress has been made in this field, and studies indicate that cytogenetic abnormalities are common in CLL, occurring in more than 50% of cases (3–6,22,42,65–74). An even higher proportion of cytogenetic abnormalities is identified by fluorescence *in situ* hybridization (FISH) studies because this technique can be applied to interphase cells and does not require mitotic activity. Likewise, molecular studies also yield a higher abnormality rate than standard cytogenetics (6,42,65). Karyotypic evolution occurs in a minority of cases and may or may not be associated with morphologic transformation (5,42).

Key associations between karyotype, morphology, immunophenotype, and clinical findings are presented in Table 40.7. Trisomy 12 is the most frequent numeric karyotypic abnormality; one half of these cases exhibit an isolated trisomy 12, and the other half demonstrate complex cytogenetic abnormalities. Reports describe frequent structural abnormalities of chromosome 13, often involving the site of the retinoblastoma gene, a known tumor suppressor gene (74). Structural abnormalities of chromosome 14 are also common in B-CLL, although translocations involving this site are rare. In general, a normal karyotype is associated with lower disease stage and good prognosis, single abnormalities are linked to an intermediate disease course, whereas complex chromosome abnormalities are associated with advanced disease, morphologic transformation, or refractoriness to treatment.

Molecular Features

A synopsis of molecular analyses in B-CLL is presented in Table 40.8 (5,6,75–81). As predicted, clonal immunoglobulin heavy- and light-chain gene rearrangement is evident in virtually all cases. By sequencing studies, limited selection of V_H and V_L gene segments has been identified and this finding has been linked to autoimmunity (6,76). CLL cells generally express the multidrug resistance phenotype by mRNA studies (77,82). Except for decreased B29 or *B29* mutations by mRNA analyses, all other types of molecular abnormalities assessed are infrequent in B-CLL (78). Although rare, *BCL3* gene rearrangement in B-CLL is associated with distinctive clinical and morphologic features and an aggressive disease course (79). Similarly, *TP53* mutations in B-CLL are linked to progressive disease and poor outcome (5,83).

TABLE 40.7. *Cytogenetic features of B-cell lymphocytic leukemia*

Karyotype	Comments and associations	References
Normal	Linked to longest survival time and typical morphology	5, 6, 67, 72
tri 12	Identified in 10–20% of cases by cytogenetics and 20–30% by FISH Linked to atypical morphology, strong CD20 expression, bright surface immunoglobulin, absent CD23, higher stage, and more aggressive disease course May be a secondary event; not found in all clonal cells	5, 6, 22, 42, 65, 66, 71, 73
13q deletion or translocation	Identified in 15–20% of cases by standard cytogenetics, >30% by FISH (band q14 affected) May find single allelic deletion or translocation of retinoblastoma gene (tumor suppressor gene); presumed mutation of other allele May be a secondary event; not found in all clonal cells Linked to typical morphology, typical immunophenotypic profile, and more favorable outcome than other cytogenetic abnormalities	3, 5, 6, 42, 65–71, 74
14q+	Identified in about 20% of cases Usually late event, linked to transformation	5, 6
11q deletion or translocation	Deletion or structural abnormality in 5–15% of cases Usually involves 11q23 Linked to typical or atypical morphology, but high stage and aggressive disease course	22, 42, 69, 72
t(11;14)(q13;q32)	*BCL1* gene rearrangement; rarely reported in CLL (3%) and it is possible that these cases represent leukemic mantle cell lymphoma	3, 5, 6, 42, 66
t(14;18)(q32;q21)	*BCL2* gene rearrangement rare in CLL (1–2%)	3, 42, 66
t(14;19)(q32;q13)	*BCL3* gene rearrangement rare in CLL (<2 %)	3, 42, 66
17q13 deletion or translocation	Inactivation of *TP53* in 10–15% of cases Correlated with advanced stage, resistance to chemotherapy, and short survival	13, 42, 66

FISH, fluorescence *in situ* hybridization; CLL, chronic lymphocytic leukemia.

TABLE 40.8. *Molecular studies of B-cell chronic lymphocytic leukemia*

Study	Comments	References
Immunoglobulin gene rearrangement	Limited selection of V_H and V_L gene segments Present in virtually all cases Incidence of somatic mutations variable and linked to karyotype	6, 76, 81
T-cell receptor gene rearrangement	Rare in B-CLL; TCR-β, GR linked to deletion of chromosome 6q	5
Retinoblastoma gene (*RB*)	Abnormalities of *RB* rarely detected by Southern blot analysis, although hemizygous *RB* gene deletion detected in 30% of cases by FISH	5
MDR-1 expression	Cells express multidrug resistance phenotype	77, 82
Decreased B29 mRNA or mutations of *B29* gene (*CD79B*)	Linked to reduced or absent surface immunoglobulin; encodes CD79b	78
BCL1, BCL2, BCL3 gene rearrangements	*BCL1* GR rare; some cases may represent leukemic mantle cell lymphoma	5, 42
	BCL2 GR rare; BCL2 protein expression not linked to *in vitro* drug resistance	80
	BCL3 GR occurs in <2% of B-CLL and is linked to younger age, atypical morphology, aberrant immunophenotype and short survival time	79
TP53 mutations	Present in about 15% of cases; linked to refractoriness to therapy, progressive disease, advanced stage, atypical morphology, and poor outcome	5, 83

CLL, chronic lymphocytic leukemia; GR, gene rearrangement; FISH, fluorescence *in situ* hybridization; TCR, T-cell receptor.

Cell of Origin

CLL is thought to represent the neoplastic counterpart of a normal peripheral blood B lymphocyte usually present in very low numbers (14,84). Normal B cells with an immunophenotypic pattern similar to CLL also have been identified in mantle zones of lymph node, tonsil, and blood, whereas abundant $CD5^+$ B cells are present in fetal lymph node, spleen, and blood (14,84,85).

The expression of CD5 by a unique subpopulation of B cells reflects one of the phenotypic changes after B-cell activation with certain antigens (86). On these B cells, CD5 antigen is coexpressed along with activation antigens such as B5, CD25, and CD23 (86). Likewise, studies of $CD5^+$ B cells from cord blood reveal coexpression of CD23, CD25, CD71 (transferrin receptor), and the cell cycle–associated antigen Ki-67 (85). With lymphokine stimulation, these $CD5^+$ B lymphocytes can be induced to differentiate into $CD5^-$ follicle center cell–like B lymphocytes (85).

In addition to CD5 expression, several other unique properties are attributed to B-CLL lymphocytes, including production of natural autoantibodies, expression of autoantibody-associated cross-reactive idiotypes, and biased V_H gene expression (6,14,87–90). From hybridoma studies, researchers have documented the frequent production of autoantibodies by $CD5^+$ B-cell CLL lymphocytes, similar to the previously noted production of autoantibodies by normal $CD5^+$ B cells (87). Similar results have been obtained by using murine monoclonal antibodies specific for immunoglobulin cross-reactive idiotypes (88). A substantial portion of B-cell CLL cells reacted with this monoclonal antibody against this cross-reactive idiotype on IgM autoantibodies (88). Because the non-Hodgkin's lymphomas (NHL) studied did not express these cross-reactive idiotypes, the investigators postulate molecularly distinct (in terms of immunoglobulin [Ig] variable region genes) cells of origin for B-cell CLL and B-cell NHL (88). This was confirmed by molecular studies of immunoglobulin V_H gene expression in various B-cell lines (derived from adult and fetal tissues) and B-cell CLL cells (89). Although normal cell lines use V_H genes roughly in proportion to estimated family size, V_H gene expression in B-cell CLL cells is highly biased (89).

By correlating immunologic and molecular features of B-CLL cells with the known stages of the normal humoral immune response, some investigators propose that CLL is derived from a relatively immature virgin (prefollicular) B-cell that is activated and intermediately differentiated, and committed to the production of natural autoantibodies (14,84,90–92). This cell corresponds immunologically to the major population of fetal B cells that migrate from the bone marrow to primary follicles in lymph node and spleen (92). A similar cell of origin is proposed for B-cell small lymphocytic lymphoma, whereas PLL, NHL, Waldenström's macroglobulinemia, and myeloma are derived from more mature B cells (84,92).

Diagnostic Criteria

When an elderly patient presents with a markedly elevated, mature, monotonous lymphocytosis, the diagnosis of CLL is not difficult. The criteria for diagnosing CLL in patients who have relatively low absolute lymphocyte counts vary substantially, and confirmatory immunophenotypic evi-

TABLE 40.9. *Proposed minimal diagnostic criteria in published reports for B-cell chronic lymphocytic leukemia*

Blood[a]	Comments	Bone marrow	Comments	References
Minimal ALC = 5–10 × 10^9/L	Predominance of small mature appearing lymphocytes; prolymphocytes ≤10%; sustained lymphocytosis	20–50% lymphocytes	Bone marrow cellularity normal or increased	1, 7, 15, 93–96

ALC, absolute lymphocyte count.
[a] When ALC ≤10 × 10^9/L, weak monoclonal surface immunoglobulin is required; also helpful to confirm other immunophenotypic characteristics and karyotype.

dence usually is required. Proposed minimal blood and bone marrow requirements for the diagnosis of CLL are detailed in Table 40.9 (1,7,15,93–96). The recommended minimal absolute lymphocyte count ranges from 5 × 10^9/L to 10 × 10^9/L, and when the absolute lymphocyte count in the blood is only mildly increased over normal range, additional diagnostic information such as immunophenotype, bone marrow findings, and clinical data are often required to establish the diagnosis of CLL (1,43,96).

In 1989, French-American-British (FAB) morphologic and immunophenotypic diagnostic criteria were proposed for CLL and various other chronic B- and T-lymphoproliferative disorders in which leukemic manifestations were dominant (1) (Table 40.10). The disorders encompassed in this FAB proposal include diseases in which a leukemic blood picture is a defining criterion (e.g., CLL and PLL), as well as NHLs that commonly demonstrate blood involvement, usually as a manifestation of advanced disease. The World Health Organization (WHO) has commissioned a comprehensive classification system for all hematolymphoid neoplasms (97). Although not finalized, in this classification system, leukemias and lymphomas are integrated and segregated into B and T categories, as well as mature (i.e., peripheral) and immature (i.e., acute leukemia) categories. It is likely that some diagnostic entities proposed by the FAB group, such as CLL/PL, will not be included in the WHO proposal (97).

Differential Diagnosis

When evaluating an absolute lymphocytosis in blood or bone marrow, the diagnostic challenge for pathologists is to identify reactive disorders successfully and to subcategorize neoplastic processes. When all causes of blood and bone marrow lymphocytoses are considered, the differential diagnosis of CLL is extensive (1,2,14,16,40,98–105) (Table 40.11). The difficulty in distinguishing CLL from reactive lympho-

TABLE 40.10. *FAB Proposals for chronic B lymphoid leukemias*

Subtype[a]	Definition	Comments
CLL	Persistent lymphocytosis >10 × 10^9/L; <10% prolymphocytes	IP: weak sIg, >30% mouse rosettes, >50% CD5+, <30% FMC7+; lower ALC acceptable with IP
CLL/PL[b]	Mixed type with 10–55% prolymphocytes	Includes cases formerly called prolymphocytoid transformation of CLL Morphologic and immunophenotypic spectrum More heterogenous than *de novo* PLL
PLL	>55% of cells are prolymphocytes	Strong sIg, low mouse rosettes, low CD5, >30% FMC7+
HCL	Predominance of characteristic hairy cells (see Chapter 41)	Monoclonal B-cell phenotype with coexpression of selected T and myeloid antigens
HCL variant	Blastic variant with prominent nucleoli	See Chapter 41
Splenic lymphoma with circulating villous lymphocytes	Lymphoid cells with short cytoplasmic projections	White pulp infiltration predominates over red pulp involvement Immunophenotypically distinct from HCL
Leukemic phase of NHL	Heterogeneous cell population; nuclear clefting often prominent; lymphoplasmacytoid cells may be present	Includes follicular, intermediate, lymphoplasmacytic, and mantle zone lymphomas (note original 1989 terminology used)
Plasma cell leukemia[b]	Blood shows predominance of plasmablasts in some cases; other cases exhibit spectrum of lymphocytes and plasma cells	

CLL, chronic lymphocytic leukemia; CLL/PL, chronic lymphocytic leukemia with prolymphocytes; HCL, hairy cell leukemia; IP, immunoperoxidase staining; NHL, non-Hodgkin's lymphoma; PLL, prolymphocytic leukemia; sIg, surface immunoglobulin.
[a] Diagnosis is based on integration of clinical, morphologic, histologic, and immunophenotypic data.
[b] Although included within the FAB classification, it is not included as a distinct clinicopathologic entity in more recently proposed classification systems.

TABLE 40.11. *Differential diagnosis of chronic lymphocytic leukemia*

Disorder	Principle distinguishing features	Immunophenotypic characteristic[a]	References
Reactive lymphocytoses	Morphologic heterogeneity; association with infection or drug treatments; usually not sustained; very transient lymphocytosis common in severe trauma; sustained lymphocytosis may occur after surgery Rarely, adult females develop sustained atypical lymphocytoses with binucleate forms.	Polyclonal, often T cells predominate	98–100
Benign lymphoid aggregates in bone marrow	Generally well circumscribed and nonconfluent More common among women and elderly patients Associated with collagen vascular diseases Some patients eventually develop lymphoproliferative disorder (often NHL).	T cells predominate; B cells polyclonal	30–32
Prolymphocytic leukemia	Predominant cell has moderate amounts of cytoplasm and a nucleus with condensed chromatin and a prominent central nucleolus. Splenomegaly may be prominent.	Monoclonal Ig, bright intensity. Other antigens expressed are pan-B cell antigens, including CD22, FMC7 and CD79b.	2, 14, 16, 40, 96
Hairy cell leukemia (see Chapter 41)	Variable morphology but typical hairy cell has abundant cytoplasm with numerous thin cytoplasmic projections and a round to oval nucleus with spongy chromatin and inconspicuous nucleoli. Prominent splenomegaly Strong tartrate-resistant acid phosphatase activity Red pulp infiltration in spleen	Monoclonal Ig, bright intensity. Other antigens coexpressed include pan-B cell antigens CD22, CD11c, CD25 (IL-2 receptor), and FMC7	2, 14, 16, 40
Splenic lymphoma with villous lymphocytes (see Chapter 53)	Villous projections of cytoplasm Splenomegaly with predominant white but also red pulp infiltration; may show plasmacytoid differentiation	Monoclonal Ig, moderate intensity CD5 negative. Other antigens expressed are pan-B cell antigens including CD22, FMC7, and CD79b	2, 14, 16, 40, 102
Peripheralizing lymphoma	Several morphologic subtypes may mimic CLL, including small cleaved follicle center cell and mantle cell lymphomas.		14, 40, 101, 103, 104
FCC (see Chapter 24)	Small cleaved cell characterized by scant cytoplasm and nuclei with highly condensed chromatin and deep nuclear clefts	Monoclonal Ig, bright intensity. Cells also express pan-B cell antigens CD10, FMC7, and CD79b.	
Mantle cell lymphoma (see Chapter 22)	Cells morphologically heterogeneous with variable amounts of cytoplasm and moderate nuclear irregularity	Monoclonal Ig, moderate to strong intensity. Other antigens expressed are CD5, CD22, FMC7, and CD79b. Cyclin D1 positive by immunoperoxidase.	
Large granular lymphocytosis (see Chapter 43)	Cells have moderate to abundant cytoplasm with coarse granules. Nuclei are generally round, and chromatin is condensed. Interstitial bone marrow infiltrates similar to HCL	Polyclonal or monoclonal T suppressor cells or, less commonly, NK cells	2, 16, 105

CLL, chronic lymphocytic leukemia; FCC, follicle center cell lymphoma; HCL, hairy cell leukemia; Ig, immunoglobulin; NHL, non-Hodgkin's lymphoma; NK, natural killer.

[a] See Table 40.5.

cytoses and other lymphoproliferative disorders varies considerably from case to case. Often, a morphologic review of the blood smear is all that is required, whereas sophisticated immunologic and even molecular techniques may be necessary for successful diagnosis. In general, reactive lymphocytoses in blood exhibit morphologic heterogeneity, have a predominance of T cells, and are associated with a specific underlying cause, such as infection or drug treatment. Rare cases of sustained atypical lymphocytoses in adult women have been described, and in these patients, no underlying cause of the lymphocytosis is identified (98–100).

Although benign lymphoid aggregates are common in the bone marrow, especially in elderly women, these lymphoid aggregates are also found in young patients who have various collagen vascular diseases. When these young patients with benign lymphoid aggregates are followed for many years, a substantial number of them eventually develop a lymphoproliferative disorder, often NHL (30–32). Benign lymphoid aggregates consist predominantly of T cells, and the B cells present are polyclonal. The morphologic distinction between benign lymphoid aggregates and CLL is detailed in Table 40.3.

Beside CLL, the chronic lymphoproliferative disorders that can present with an elevated absolute lymphocyte count in blood include PLL, hairy cell leukemia, splenic lymphoma with circulating villous lymphocytes, peripheralizing lymphoma, large granular lymphocytosis, and several other rare T-cell disorders. All these disorders, except large granular lymphocytosis and the other rare T-cell disorders, are composed of monoclonal B cells. Various morphologic and immunologic features can be used to distinguish these disorders from B-CLL (Tables 40.5, 40.11).

The disorder that shows the greatest morphologic and immunologic overlap with CLL is PLL. Recent FAB proposals suggest that the percentage of prolymphocytes should be used to segregate disorders into CLL (<10% prolymphocytes), CLL/PL (10% to 55% prolymphocytes), or PLL (>55% prolymphocytes) (Fig. 40.9). Table 40.10 illustrates the FAB proposals for these disorders (1). In the proposed WHO classification, CLL/PL is not recognized as a distinct clinicopathologic entity, and terms such as mixed-type CLL may be more appropriate (97).

Clinical Features

In patients who have B-CLL, peripheral blood abnormalities range from isolated leukocytosis to lymphocytosis with severe cytopenias. The white blood cell count varies widely, and although absolute lymphocyte counts usually are lower than 100×10^9/L, about 5% of patients who have CLL have hyperleukocytosis exceeding 500×10^9/L, which may be associated with hyperviscosity or leukostasis (2,6,7,16,106). About one half of CLL patients are mildly anemic at presentation, whereas anemia and mild thrombocytopenia are demonstrated in one fourth of patients (6,7). More severe thrombocytopenia can occur at presentation or later in the disease course as the spleen enlarges and the bone marrow is progressively replaced by the neoplastic infiltrate (6). Although

A,B
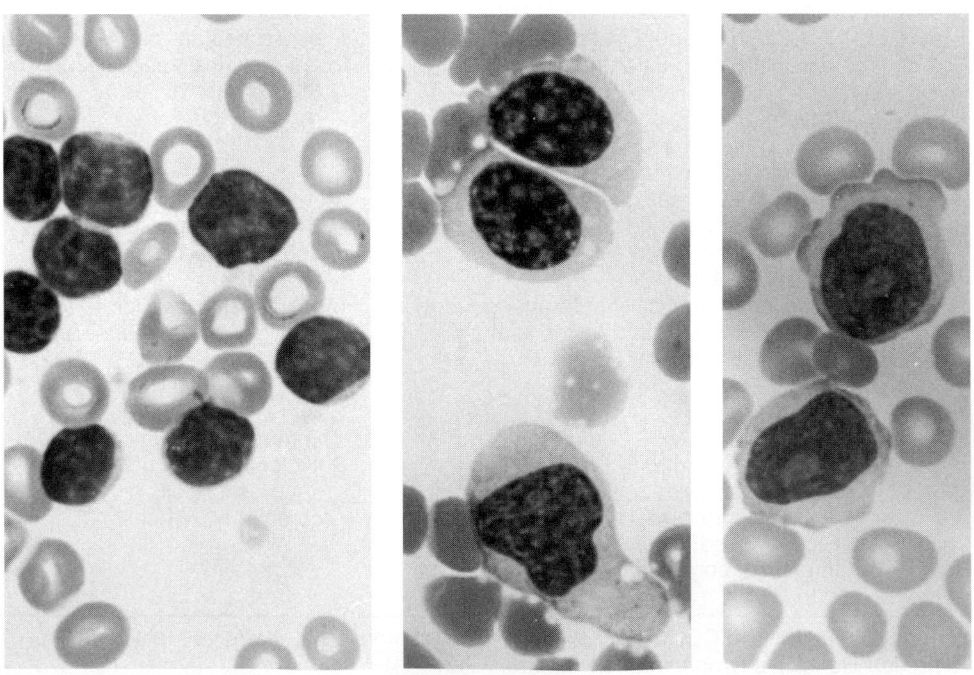
C

FIG. 40.9. This composite illustrates the morphologic features of typical chronic lymphocytic leukemia (CLL) (**A**), mixed-type CLL (**B**), and prolymphocytic leukemia (**C**). Notice the differences in amount of cytoplasm, nuclear chromatin condensation, and nucleoli (Wright's stain, original magnification: 1,000× magnification).

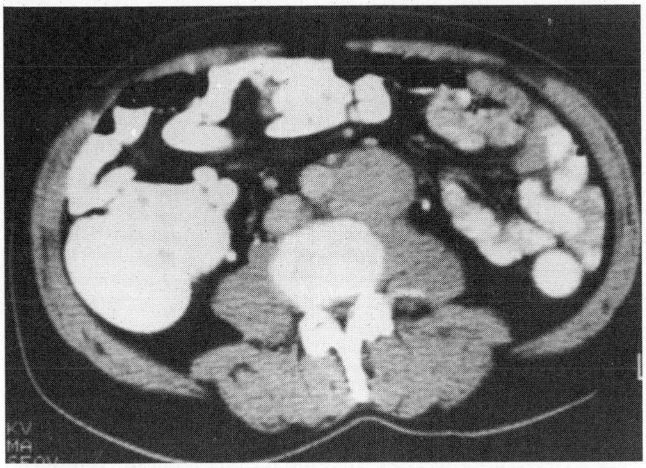

FIG. 40.10. This CT scan from a patient with advanced chronic lymphocytic leukemia shows prominent retroperitoneal lymphadenopathy.

anemia generally is caused by deficient production, Coombs-positive hemolytic anemia may develop in patients who have CLL. Neutropenia generally is not evident at presentation, but severe neutropenia can occur as a consequence of extensive bone marrow replacement (6,14). The development of a leukoerythroblastic blood picture usually indicates that a large cell transformation of the CLL has occurred or that the patient has developed a second bone marrow neoplasm (6).

Although CLL is an incidental finding in some patients, the clinical manifestations generally are related to the consequences of infiltration of bone marrow, lymph node, and spleen. Common presenting features include weakness, night sweats, weight loss, and bleeding. Some studies reveal that CLL cells produce tumor necrosis factor, which may mediate some of these symptoms (107). Although generally mild, lymphadenopathy and splenomegaly are evident in most patients (Fig. 40.10). Several other less frequent and unique complications of CLL are detailed in Table 40.12, including autoimmune disease, hypogammaglobulinemia, monoclonal gammopathy, and pure red cell aplasia (2,6,14, 16,60,88,108–115). Autoimmune hemolytic anemia is the most common type of autoimmune disorder described in patients who have CLL, but some patients develop immune thrombocytopenic purpura, neutropenia, or thyroid disease (6,14,108). Hypogammaglobulinemia is common in CLL, occurring in up to one half of patients, and this complication is implicated in increased risk of infection. Various mechanisms for this hypogammaglobulinemia have been proposed, including B, T, and NK cell defects (6,60,109). At the other extreme, almost 50% of CLL patients have a monoclonal gammopathy. The amount of monoclonal immunoglobulin usually is low and may require highly sensitive techniques for detection (110). This monoclonal antibody is not linked with the autoimmune disorders.

The association of red cell aplasia with CLL is well known and can occur at any time during the disease course (6,16,61, 112–114). The cause of red cell aplasia may be an autoantibody directed against erythropoietin or red blood cell precursors, although infection with parvovirus or a T-cell defect with excessive suppression of red cell development could also produce aplasia. A clonal T-cell proliferation with associated red cell aplasia was observed in a patient with B-CLL (61). Various drugs, including immune modulating and chemotherapeutic agents, have been used to successfully treat red cell aplasia (Table 40.12).

Staging

As in all neoplasms, the purpose of staging CLL patients is to segregate them into good-, intermediate-, and poor-risk categories. This is especially relevant to CLL because the clinical course is so variable, ranging from indolent disease that remains stable for decades to steadily progressive organ-

TABLE 40.12. *Unique clinicopathologic manifestations of chronic lymphocytic leukemia*

Disorder	Features	References
Autoimmune disorders	Autoimmune hemolytic anemia in 10% (Coombs' reactivity in up to 25% of patients) Immune thrombocytopenic purpura in <10% patients Rare cases of immune neutropenia, Graves' disease, and neurologic disease Cause unknown, may be related to T-cell dysfunction	6, 7, 14, 16, 108, 115
Hypogammaglobulinemia	Occurs in 50% of patients, associated with increased infectious complications Attributed to B, T, and NK cell defects, leading to excessive suppression of Ig secretion by B cells; normal B cells decreased	2, 6, 7, 14, 16, 109
Monoclonal gammopathy	With more sensitive techniques, detected in <50% of patients (5–10% with conventional techniques) Rare cases of biclonal gammopathy described	6, 7, 110, 111
Pure red cell aplasia	Rare complication of CLL that may occur anytime during disease course Variety of mechanisms proposed, including autoantibody directed against erythropoietin or red cell precursors; T-cell abnormality with excessive suppression of red cell growth; parvovirus infection of erythroid precursors Successful treatment with variety of agents: cyclosporin, cytotoxic drugs, antithymocyte globulin, corticosteroids, methotrexate	6, 16, 112–114

TABLE 40.13. *Two most commonly used staging systems for chronic lymphocytic leukemia*

Rai system		Binet system	
0	Lymphocytosis only (ALC >15 × 10^9/L)	A	No anemia, no thrombocytopenia, involvement of fewer than 3 lymphoid areas[a]
I	Lymphocytosis plus enlarged lymph nodes	B	No anemia, no thrombocytopenia, involvement of 3 or more lymphoid areas[a]
II	Lymphocytosis plus enlarged spleen or liver	C	Anemia (<10 g/dL) or thrombocytopenia (<100 × 10^9/L)
III	Lymphocytosis with anemia (Hgb <11 g/dL)		
IV	Lymphocytosis with thrombocytopenia (<100 × 10^9/L)		

ALC, absolute lymphocyte count.
[a] Cervical, axillary, inguinal node groups, spleen, and liver comprise the "lymphoid areas."
Data from references 6, 14, 16, 93, 96, and 116 through 120.

omegaly and cytopenias. Although several researchers have proposed classification systems that attempt to stratify CLL patients, the two most commonly used systems in clinical medicine are those proposed by Rai and Binet (6,14,16, 116–120) (Table 40.13). In 1975, Rai and coworkers proposed a five-stage classification system for CLL, based on the extent of anatomic involvement of lymphoid organs and the presence or absence of anemia and thrombocytopenia. Although the clinical relevance of the Rai Staging System for CLL is well established, the five categories proved difficult to use in clinical trials, prompting several groups to recommend a combination of stages to include low-risk (stage 0), intermediate-risk (stages I and II), and high-risk patients (stages III and IV) (93).

Median survival times have been determined for patients categorized by the Rai staging system (118):

Rai stage 0: 120 to 180 months
Rai stage I: 60 to 130 months
Rai stage II: 40 to 100 months
Rai stage III: 9 to 60 months
Rai stage IV: 18 to 60 months

Subsequently, Binet and coworkers proposed a more simplified staging system, designating stages A, B, and C (117,120) (Table 40.13). In this staging system, lymphoid areas relevant to classification include three lymph node groups (cervical, axillary, and inguinal) plus the spleen and liver. Patients are categorized according to the number of these lymphoid areas that are enlarged and the degree of anemia or thrombocytopenia. The clinical relevance of the Binet classification system also has been established in clinical trials. Because both classification systems are successful in segregating patients into broad prognostic groups, the International Workshop on CLL recommended that patients be staged using a combined Rai-Binet classification system. For example, patients who had Binet stage A disease would be categorized as Rai stage 0, I, or II (96); however, the complexity of this combined staging system has been emphasized by subsequent investigators, and it has not been widely used.

Even though the Rai and Binet classification systems segregate groups of patients into general survival groups, many other parameters impact on individual patient survival time (2,6,14,15,22,25,118,120–123) (Table 40.14). These prognostic variables include hemogram and morphologic features, other laboratory parameters, and clinical variables such as sex and age. All variables listed in Table 40.14 have been established as independent prognostic variables, al-

TABLE 40.14. *Prognostic variables in B-cell chronic lymphocytic leukemia*

Hemogram variables	Other laboratory variables	Clinical variables
Lymphocytosis >50,000	Diffuse pattern of bone marrow infiltration	Age
Anemia	Extent of bone marrow replacement	Sex
Thrombocytopenia	Cytogenetic studies: normal karyotype versus any abnormal karyotype	Binet stage
Number of prolymphocytes	Cytogenetic studies: simple versus complex karyotypic abnormality	International Workshop stage
Typical or atypical lymphocyte morphology	Cytogenetic studies: 13q versus trisomy 12 versus 14q abnormalities	Performance status
	FISH: *TP53* gene deletions	Lymphadenopathy, extent
	Thymidine kinase level	Static or progressive disease
	β_2-microglobulin level	Response to therapy; immunophenotypic documentation of CR
	Lymphocyte doubling time ≤12 months	
	LDH level	
	Soluble CD23 level	

CR, complete response; FISH, fluorescence *in situ* hybridization; LDH, lactate dehydrogenase.
Data from references 2, 6, 14, 15, 22, 25, and 121 through 123.

though the number of patients evaluated and the number of studies that have confirmed the prognostic significance of these individual variables varies substantially. The integration of these significant prognostic variables into an "ideal" staging system is a goal for hematology-oncology.

Transformation and Progression

It has been known for decades that the cells that comprise CLL can undergo morphologic changes during the course of the disease. When morphologic, clinical, and immunophenotypic data are correlated, the types of CLL transformation can be separated roughly into five categories. These include prolymphocytoid transformation, Richter's syndrome, blastic transformation, plasmacytoid transformation, and an infrequently described paraimmunoblastic variant of small lymphocytic lymphoma/CLL (Table 40.15). The most common transformation of CLL is prolymphocytoid transformation (or CLL/PL in the proposed FAB classification), which occurs in about 15% of all CLL patients (2,5,7,91,121–129) (Fig. 40.9). These patients develop gradually progressive cytopenias and organomegaly and become more refractory to treatment. The defining morphologic feature is an increasing proportion of prolymphocytes. The lymphocytes in the blood tend to be more heterogeneous than those seen in *de novo* PLL, and they may retain the immunophenotypic characteristics of the earlier CLL or demonstrate brighter surface immunoglobulin, as well as variable CD5 and FMC7 positivity. After prolymphocytoid transformation has occurred, the median survival is generally about 1 year.

The next most frequent type of transformation is Richter's syndrome, which occurs in 3% to 10% of patients and is characterized by the abrupt onset of fever, weight loss, and increasing organomegaly (2,5,130–146) (Figs. 40.11, 40.12; Table 40.15). Often rapidly enlarging tumor masses develop in nodal and other sites. Biopsy of these tumor masses reveals a pleomorphic large cell lymphoma that can exhibit multinucleated cells with prominent nucleoli that resemble Reed-Sternberg cells. Although some exceptions have been reported, most molecular or immunologic studies confirm the clonal relationship between Richter's syndrome (i.e., large cell lymphoma or Hodgkin's disease) and the underlying CLL (131,137,139,141,142,146). However, a fraction of cases of Richter's syndrome appear to represent secondary neoplasms that have arisen in a background of immunosuppression, the consequence of CLL (144). The clinical course of Richter's syndrome is that of a rapidly progressive, high-grade neoplasm with generally short median survivals.

The other types of CLL transformation are all rare and include the development of a blood and bone marrow picture that resembles acute leukemia, a plasmacytoid/myelomatous transformation, and a nodal disorder called *paraimmunoblastic variant of small lymphocytic lymphoma/CLL* (2,5,7,147–156) (Table 40.15).

Treatment and Survival

Because of the highly variable clinical course of CLL, determining optimal therapy and the appropriate time to initiate therapy in these patients is a major problem

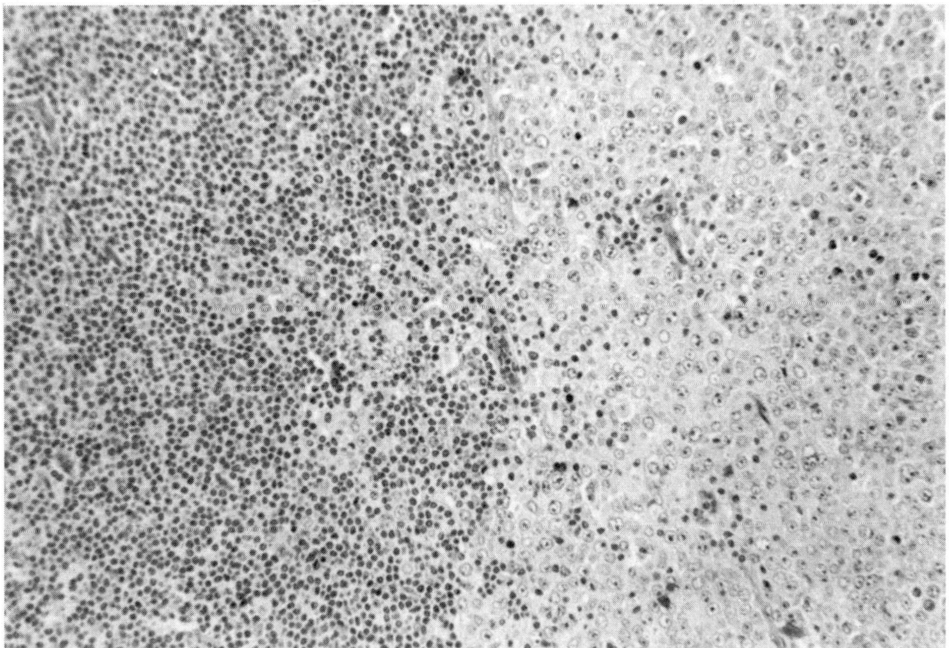

FIG. 40.11. This lymph node shows a discrete area of large cell transformation in a patient with underlying chronic lymphocytic leukemia (hematoxylin and eosin stain, original magnification: 250× magnification).

TABLE 40.15. *Proposed types of transformation of chronic lymphocytic leukemia*

Morphology	Incidence (%)	Clinical features	Pathologic features	Immunophenotype	Comments and additional studies	References
Prolymphocytoid transformation (FAB CLL/PL)	15	Gradual onset of progressive cytopenias Increasing lymphocytosis, lymphadenopathy and splenomegaly Progressive refractoriness to therapy Median survival about 1 year, especially if stage III, IV	Increasing percentage of prolymphocytes Morphology more heterogeneous than *de novo* PLL	Monoclonal Ig same as initial CLL; variable intensity of sIg Prolymphocytes may express FMC7 May see dual population by IP studies	Originally described in 1979 Some cases originally termed "blast crisis" represent prolymphocytoid transformation Neither morphology nor phenotype consistently predictive of outcome No correlation between percentage of prolymphocytes and survival	2, 5, 7, 94, 124–129
Richter's syndrome (RS)	3–10	Abrupt onset of fever, weight loss, increasing organomegaly and lymphadenopathy Large tumor masses may develop GI tract involvement common Rapid downhill course, median survival usually $<$1 year Rare cases involve CNS	Lymph node tends to be primary site of transformation Bone marrow often involved, but circulating transformed cells rare Very heterogeneous morphology resembling pleomorphic large cell lymphoma or even Hodgkin's disease Most cases currently thought to be NHL, although a few CLL patients develop bonafide HD	Controversial, some cases show same isotype on CLL and Richter's cells; others are different CD5 antigen not expressed on lymphoma cells	Clonality of RS with prior CLL confirmed in most cases; occasional case is secondary NHL in background of immunodeficiency Even when isotype difference occurs, some cases still clonal by molecular analyses Isotype switch may be associated with transformation Underlying CLL generally evident but exceptions reported Usually develops after years of CLL but may be initial manifestation of CLL	2, 5, 130–146

Blastic transformation	<1	Acute leukemic blood and bone marrow picture develops in rare CLL patient	Morphology usually ALL L2 or L3 type; some cases of AML described	Usually monoclonal sIg of same isotype as CLL; may be TdT positive	AML cases may be secondary to cytotoxic therapy ALL linked to prior CLL by IP and cytogenetic studies Rare ALL-L3 associated with t(8;14)	2, 5, 7, 147–152
Plasmacytoid transformation	<1	Development of myeloma during course of CLL is most frequent type of plasmacytoid transformation Rare CLL patient develops acute leukemia picture with plasmacytoid blasts	Variable, myeloma or plasmacytoma exhibit typical spectrum of plasma cell morphology Plasmablastic leukemia characterized by predominance of blasts in blood	Some reports indicate same isotype for CLL and MM, others report differences	Clonality of CLL and MM determined by several idiotype and isotype studies Karyotype of single case of plasmablastic transformation showed +12, t(14;17)	2, 7, 153–155
Paraimmunoblastic variant of small lymphocytic lymphoma/CLL	<1	2/16 patients with prior diagnosis of CLL, others had lymphocytosis at time of presentation with nodal disease Median survival, 28 months	Diffuse nodal proliferation of cells similar to those usually confined to growth centers Bone marrow contains predominantly mature lymphocytes with no increase in prolymphocytes	B-cell phenotype with CD5 expression	May be analogous to prolymphocytoid transformation of CLL that is primarily node based	2, 156

ALL, acute lymphoblastic leukemia; AML, acute myelogenous leukemia; CLL/PL, chronic lymphocytic leukemia with prolymphocytes; CNS, central nervous system; GI, gastrointestinal tract; HD, Hodgkin's disease; IP, immunoperoxidase; MM, multiple myeloma; NHL, non-Hodgkin's lymphoma; PLL, prolymphocytic leukemia; sIg, surface immunoglobulin; TdT, terminal deoxynucleotidyl transferase.

A 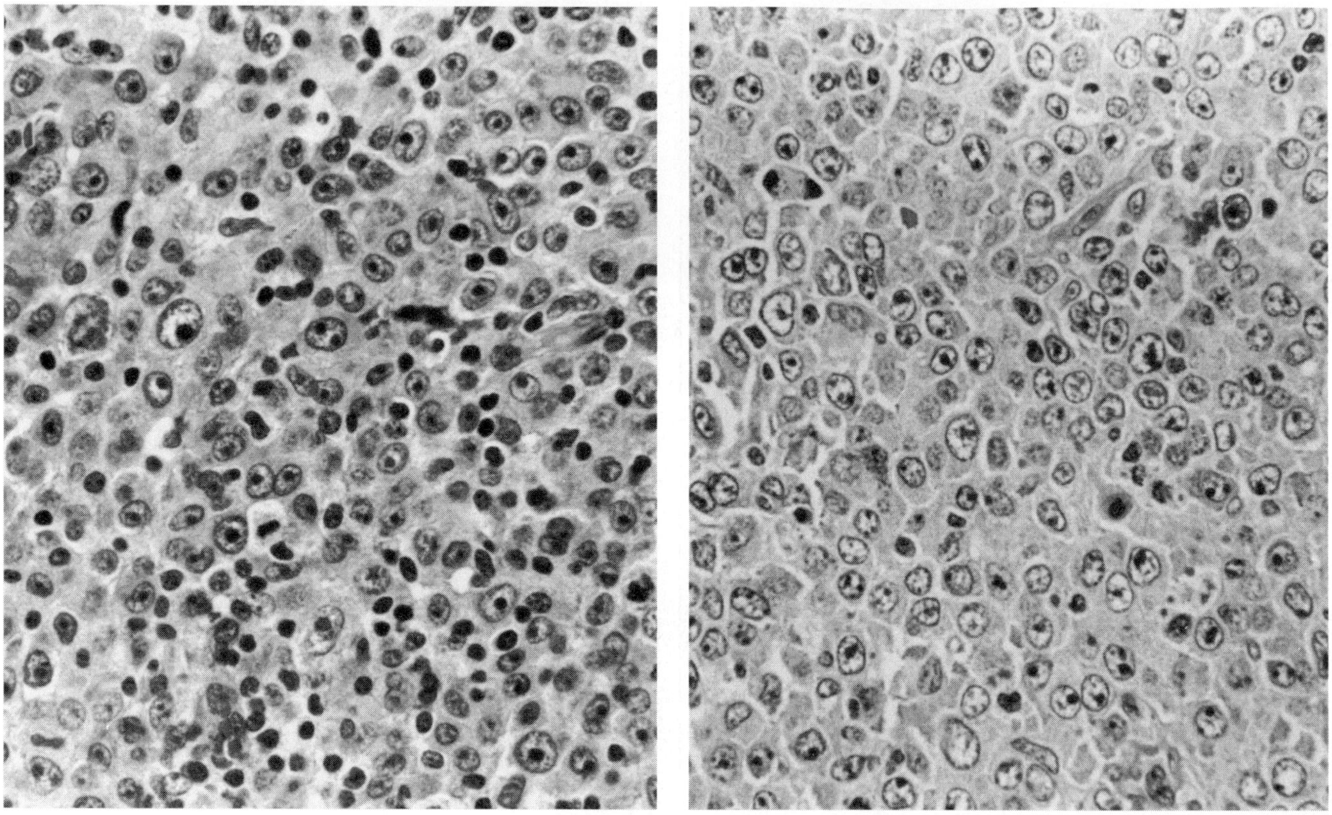 B

FIG. 40.12. This composite of two patients with Richter's syndrome illustrates the morphologic heterogeneity of this transformation. **A:** Pleomorphic large lymphoma cells are admixed with abundant residual, small lymphoid cells. **B:** A monomorphic population of large lymphoma cells is evident (hematoxylin and eosin stain, original magnification: 400× magnification).

(5–7,157–163). Studies on the natural history of CLL have shown that, although overall 5-year survival exceeds 80%, about 10% of untreated low-stage CLL patients experience disease progression (157,164). To better assess the rate of disease progression in each patient who has CLL, some investigators suggest an observation period during which the absolute lymphocyte count is monitored. A stable absolute lymphocyte count may indicate indolent disease, whereas a rising absolute lymphocyte count may be associated with disease progression (7,158). It also is important to evaluate the bone marrow at diagnosis to determine the extent and pattern of bone marrow infiltration. The stability or progression of organomegaly and lymphadenopathy, as well as the patient's performance status, all may be parameters used to determine indolent versus progressive disease. Although the appropriate time to initiate therapy in patients who have CLL is controversial, some indications for therapy include increasing disease-related symptoms, pattern of bone marrow infiltration, bone marrow failure, autoimmune manifestations, karyotype abnormalities, massive splenomegaly, massive lymphadenopathy, progressive hyperlymphocytosis, and increasing infections (5–7,26).

The treatments used in patients who have CLL are detailed in Table 40.16 (5–7,75,157–164) and include various agents, ranging from traditional chemotherapy to mono-

TABLE 40.16. *Treatment modalities in B-cell chronic lymphocytic leukemia*

Therapy[a]	Comments
Alkylating agents (single agent or combination chemotherapy)	Chlorambucil, cyclophosphamide, COP (cyclophosphamide, vincristine, prednisone), CHOP (COP plus doxorubicin)
Nucleoside analogues	Fludarabine 2-deoxycoformycin 2-chlorodeoxyadenosine
Biologic response modifiers	Interferon-α
Monoclonal antibodies	Toxin-conjugated anti-CD19, CD5, CD23
Bone marrow transplantation	Allogeneic for patients <55 years Autologous for older patients
Radiation	Local for isolated symptomatic lymphadenopathy or splenomegaly Total body irradiation (with or without combination chemotherapy)

[a] Treatment for autoimmune combinations and pure red cell aplasia include prednisone and cyclosporin.

Data from references 5 through 7, 75, and 157 through 164.

clonal antibodies and biologic response modifiers. Nucleoside analogues have demonstrated potent antileukemic activity in clinical trials (6,160,161). Prednisone, androgens, and cyclosporine have been used to improve the patient's hemoglobin level, whereas granulocyte-macrophage colony-stimulating factor may be useful in increasing neutrophil and monocyte levels. Although experience is limited, allogeneic bone marrow transplantation may have a role in the treatment of CLL in younger patients, and autologous bone marrow or stem cell transplantation has been occasionally used in older patients (5,6,162,163).

B-CELL PROLYMPHOCYTIC LEUKEMIA

Definition

The clinical and pathologic features of PLL, originally described in 1974 by Galton and coworkers, have been well delineated (165). The prototypic patient who has B-PLL is an elderly man who presents with striking splenomegaly and marked hyperleukocytosis (1,2,6,13,16,94,166–169). Adenopathy usually is absent or minimal, although rare patients present with pronounced lymphadenopathy (168). The marked leukocytosis present at diagnosis in at least three fourths of patients who have B-PLL is characterized by absolute lymphocyte counts that exceed 100 × 10^9/L. There is also evidence of substantial bone marrow failure in that thrombocytopenia, anemia, and neutropenia are common at presentation.

As with any chronic leukemia, however, a spectrum of clinical and pathologic features is encountered in patients who have B-PLL. PLL is substantially less common than CLL, with an incidence of less than 5% that of CLL in my experience, and about 70% to 80% of PLL cases are B cell in type (2,6,13,16,167,170,171).

Pathologic and Cytochemical Features

Peripheral Blood

The prolymphocyte has distinct morphologic features, including moderate to abundant pale blue agranular cytoplasm and a round nucleus with moderately condensed chromatin that contains a large, prominent central vesicular nucleolus (Figs. 40.9, 40.13; see also Color Plate 17, between pp. 1446–1447). Although the nuclear morphology of prolymphocytes shows some variation, the chromatin generally is less condensed than that of typical CLL but not as finely dispersed as that seen in lymphoblasts (1,2,4,6,13,16, 165–171).

Bone Marrow

B-cell prolymphocytic leukemia (B-PLL) patients who present with a marked lymphocytosis generally also exhibit extensive and diffuse infiltration of the bone marrow (4,16,167). In some patients with less advanced disease, however, a mixed nodular and diffuse pattern is identified

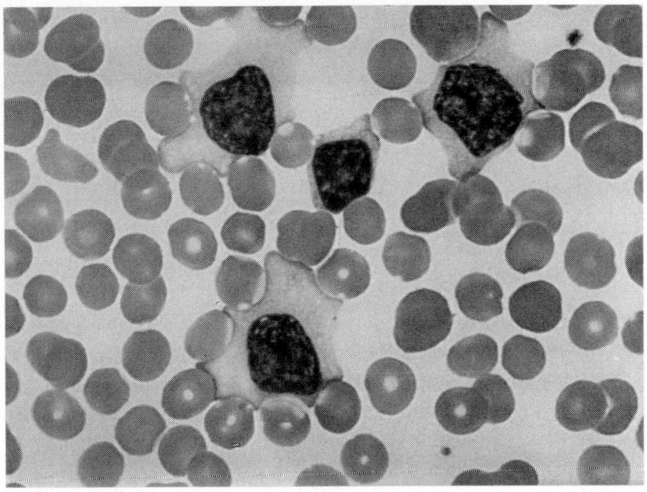

FIG. 40.13. This peripheral blood smear from a patient with prolymphocytic leukemia illustrates the morphologic and ultrastructural features of these cells. Notice the central prominent nucleoli and the moderately condensed nuclear chromatin patterns (Wright's stain, original magnification: 1,000× magnification). See Color Plate 17, between pp. 1446–1447.

(2,13,16). The nodular infiltrates are nonparatrabecular, and nodular and diffuse infiltrates alike are frequently associated with increased reticulin fibrosis (167). On histologic sections, the distinct nucleoli, intermediate cell size, and moderate amounts of cytoplasm are readily apparent.

Other Organs

Much like CLL, the most common extramedullary sites evaluated in patients who have B-PLL are lymph nodes and spleen. Even though lymphadenopathy is not generally a prominent feature of PLL, replacement of nodal architecture by neoplastic prolymphocytes is frequently identified in lymph node sections (166,168,169). The pattern of lymph node effacement is diffuse and pseudofollicular growth centers composed of cells with distinct nucleoli are usually present. Occasional cases have a distinct mantle zone pattern of infiltration with nodules of prolymphocytes that surround reactive germinal centers (169). The typical morphology of prolymphocytes is evident on imprint smears of these lymph nodes.

Massive splenic involvement by PLL is a characteristic feature of this disease. Because of prominent white pulp involvement, a miliary nodular pattern can be appreciated grossly. Microscopic examination reveals extensive white pulp and red pulp infiltration. The larger cells tend to be concentrated in the white pulp, often forming an inverse pseudofollicular pattern with a central collection of small lymphocytes surrounded by a broad cuff of pale prolymphocytes (16,36).

Within the liver, a sinusoidal pattern of infiltration can be appreciated, especially in patients who show high numbers of circulating prolymphocytes. Although not a major site of disease involvement, skin infiltrates of prolymphocytes can be identified in some patients at diagnosis (172).

Immunologic, Cytogenetic, and Molecular Features

Even though most cases of PLL represent monoclonal B-cell processes such as CLL, important immunophenotypic differences exist between these two disorders (Table 40.5). In contrast to CLL, the surface immunoglobulin expressed in B-PLL is brightly intense, CD23 is absent, expression of CD5 is variable, and bright CD22 and FMC7 expression are evident (2,6,13,16,165,167,170,173–175) (Fig. 40.14).

The most common karyotype abnormality is 14q + with a breakpoint at the site of the immunoglobulin heavy-chain gene, sometimes involving a reciprocal translocation with chromosome 11 [t(11;14)] (1,2,13,167,170,174–177). Other cytogenetic abnormalities identified in low numbers of cases include del(3), t(17;21), t(6;12), and trisomy 12 (167,174–177). Karyotypic evolution has been described in some patients who have B-PLL (1). Molecular findings in B-PLL include the predicted consistent detection of clonal immunoglobulin heavy and light-chain gene rearrangements, as well as frequent *TP53* mutations, and infrequent *BCL1* gene rearrangement (166,174,175). However, distinction between B-PLL and a peripheralizing mantle cell lymphoma may be an issue in cases with *BCL1* gene rearrangement (169).

Diagnostic Criteria

Although most cases of *de novo* B-PLL demonstrate a monotonous population of circulating prolymphocytes, the specific FAB requirement is that prolymphocytes exceed 55% (1).

Differential Diagnosis

The reactive and neoplastic disorders that overlap with CLL also are in the differential diagnosis of PLL (Table 40.11). The criteria to distinguish CLL, CLL/PL, and PLL generally involve the percentage of blood prolymphocytes, and these are detailed in Table 40.10. In clinical practice, the most difficult diagnostic dilemmas involve the distinction of PLL from hairy cell leukemia or prolymphocytoid transformation of CLL (FAB designation is CLL/PL). For both dilemmas, a constellation of clinical, pathologic, and immunologic features needs to be integrated. Even then, occasional cases of the blastic variant of hairy cell leukemia can be

A

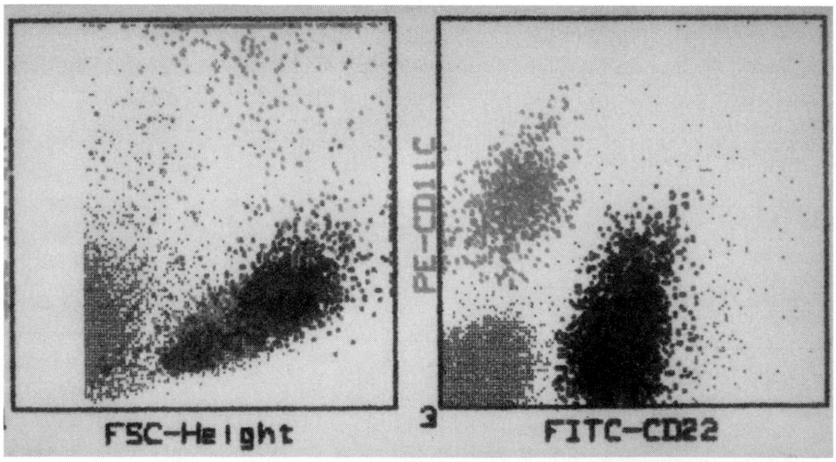

B

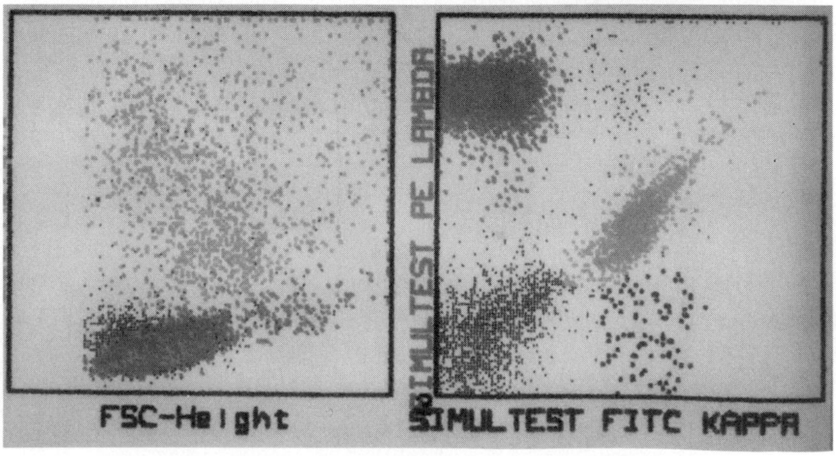

FIG. 40.14. A, B: This composite of flow cytometric data shows histograms illustrating cell size and strong expression of CD22 and λ light chain in this case of B-cell prolymphocytic leukemia. Admixed normal monocytes ($CD11c^+$) are present.

impossible to distinguish from PLL, and some investigators believe that variant hairy cell leukemia is closer to B-PLL than typical hairy cell leukemia. In my experience, the characteristic multicolor immunophenotyping by flow cytometry of hairy cells for CD22, CD11c, and CD25 can be a valuable discriminator of cases in which a diagnosis of hairy cell leukemia should be strongly considered. In our desire to assign disorders into discrete categories, we must not forget that lymphoid neoplasms mimic the tremendous continuum of dynamic normal lymphocyte populations.

Staging, Clinical Course, Treatment, and Survival

Because of its relative rarity, studies of staging of large numbers of cases of PLL have not been undertaken. When the Rai or Benet staging classification systems is applied to PLL, most patients have advanced-stage disease (i.e., Rai stage IV or Benet's stage C) (1). Unlike patients who have CLL, most patients who have PLL have a steady downhill course, with median survivals in the range of 2 or 3 years (12,166). Rare patients who have PLL, however, have experienced a prolonged, indolent disease course.

Treatment options for PLL are not clear-cut. Many of the therapeutic regimens effective in treating CLL are not efficacious in treating PLL. The types of therapies that have been applied to patients who have PLL include splenic irradiation, splenectomy, leukapheresis, multiagent chemotherapy (e.g., CHOP regimen), L-asparaginase, deoxycoformycin, and interferon-α (1,166–168). The p53 abnormalities detected in most cases may explain the poor treatment response encountered in these patients (175).

SUMMARY AND CONCLUSIONS

During the past three decades, substantial progress has been made in improving our understanding of CLL and PLL. This knowledge has impacted on the diagnosis, treatment, and prognosis prediction of patients who have these diseases. The application of specialized immunophenotypic, cytogenetic, and molecular techniques has expanded substantially our knowledge of these cell types and, when correlated with the morphologic and clinical features, has greatly facilitated diagnostic decision making. These specialized techniques also are useful in monitoring response to treatment and in detecting residual disease. Evidence that relates B-cell lymphoproliferative disorders to their normal counterpart lymphoid cells has been obtained from multiparameter immunologic and molecular studies, advancing even more our knowledge of these chronic lymphoid leukemias.

Progress has been made in determining optimal staging systems and in identifying laboratory and clinical variables that impact on survival. Recently developed drugs that exhibit potent antileukemic activity have improved the outlook for CLL patients who have advanced disease. Improvements in the therapy of PLL also are likely as causes of resistance to standard therapeutic regimens become better understood.

ACKNOWLEDGMENTS

The author is grateful for the excellent assistance of Jerri A. Lusk.

REFERENCES

1. Bennett JM, Catovsky D, Daniel MT, et al. Proposals for the classification of chronic (mature) B and T lymphoid leukaemias. French-American-British (FAB) Cooperative Group. *J Clin Pathol* 1989;42: 567–584.
2. Foucar K. Chronic lymphoproliferative disorders. In: Foucar K, ed. *Bone marrow pathology,* 1st ed. Chicago: ASCP Press, 1995: 275–314.
3. Greaves MF, Grossi CE, Ferrarini M. Lymphoproliferative disorders. In: Zucker-Franklin D, Greaves MF, Grossi CE, et al., eds. *Atlas of blood cells: function and pathology,* vol 2. Philadelphia: Lea & Febiger, 1988:445–548.
4. Foucar K. Chronic lymphoid leukemias and lymphoproliferative disorders. *Mod Pathol* 1999;12:141–150.
5. O'Brien S, del Giglio A, Keating M. Advances in the biology and treatment of B-cell chronic lymphocytic leukemia. *Blood* 1995;85: 307–318.
6. Jandl JH. Chronic lymphatic leukemia. In: Jandl JH, ed. *Blood—textbook of hematology.* Boston: Little, Brown, 1996:991–1018.
7. Keating MJ. Chronic lymphocytic leukemia. In: Henderson ES, Lister TA, Greaves MF, eds. *Leukemia,* 6th ed. Philadelphia: WB Saunders, 1996:554–586.
8. Linet MS, Blattner WA. The epidemiology of chronic lymphocytic leukemia. In: Polliack A, Catovsky D, eds. *Chronic lymphocytic leukemia.* New York: Harwood Academic Publishers, 1988:11–32.
9. Chan LC, Lam CK, Yeung TC, et al. The spectrum of chronic lymphoproliferative disorders in Hong Kong: a prospective study. *Leukemia* 1997;11:1964–1972.
10. Fernhout F, Dinkelaar RB, Hagemeijer A, et al. Four aged siblings with B cell chronic lymphocytic leukemia. *Leukemia* 1997;11: 2060–2065.
11. Neuland CY, Blattner WA, Mann DL, et al. Familial chronic lymphocytic leukemia. *J Natl Cancer Inst* 1983;71:1143–1150.
12. Conley CL, Misiti J, Laster AJ. Genetic factors predisposing to chronic lymphocytic leukemia and to autoimmune disease. *Medicine (Baltimore)* 1980;59:323–334.
13. Kroft SH, Finn WG, Peterson LC. The pathology of the chronic lymphoid leukaemias. *Blood Rev* 1995;9:234–250.
14. Rozman C, Montserrat E. Chronic lymphocytic leukemia [published erratum appears in *N Engl J Med* 1995;30;333:1515] [see comments]. *N Engl J Med* 1995;333:1052–1057.
15. Brittinger G, Hellriegel KP, Hiddemann W. Chronic lymphocytic leukemia and hairy-cell leukemia—diagnosis and treatment: results of a consensus meeting of the German CLL Co-operative Group [Editorial]. *Leukemia* 1997;11[Suppl 2]:S1–S3.
16. Brunning RD, McKenna RW. Small lymphocytic leukemias and related disorders. In: Brunning RD, McKenna RW, eds. *Tumors of the bone marrow.* Washington: Armed Forces Institute of Pathology, 1993:255–322.
17. Sonnier JA, Buchanan GR, Howard-Peebles PN, et al. Chromosomal translocation involving the immunoglobulin kappa-chain and heavy-chain loci in a child with chronic lymphocytic leukemia. *N Engl J Med* 1983;309:590–594.
18. Yoffe G, Howard-Peebles PN, Smith RG, et al. Childhood chronic lymphocytic leukemia with (2;14) translocation. *J Pediatr* 1990;116: 114–117.
19. Fell HP, Smith RG, Tucker PW. Molecular analysis of the t(2;14) translocation of childhood chronic lymphocytic leukemia. *Science* 1986;232:491–494.
20. Spier CM, Kjeldsberg CR, Head DR, et al. Chronic lymphocytic leukemia in young adults. *Am J Clin Pathol* 1985;84:675–678.
21. De Rossi G, Mandelli F, Covelli A, et al. Chronic lymphocytic leukemia (CLL) in younger adults: a retrospective study of 133 cases. *Hematol Oncol* 1989;7:127–137.
22. Criel A, Verhoef G, Vlietinck R, et al. Further characterization of morphologically defined typical and atypical CLL: a clinical, immu-

nophenotypic, cytogenetic and prognostic study on 390 cases. *Br J Haematol* 1997;97:383–391.
23. Peters O, Thielemans C, Steenssens L, et al. Intracellular inclusion bodies in 14 patients with B cell lymphoproliferative disorders. *J Clin Pathol* 1984;37:45–50.
24. Ralfkiaer E, Hou-Jensen K, Geisler C, et al. Cytoplasmic inclusions in lymphocytes of chronic lymphocytic leukaemia: a report of 10 cases. *Virchows Arch Pathol Anat* 1982;395:227–236.
25. Rozman C, Montserrat E, Rodriguez-Fernandez JM, et al. Bone marrow histologic pattern—the best single prognostic parameter in chronic lymphocytic leukemia: a multivariate survival analysis of 329 cases. *Blood* 1984;64:642–648.
26. Pangalis GA, Roussou PA, Kittas C, et al. B-chronic lymphocytic leukemia: prognostic implication of bone marrow histology in 120 patients experience from a single hematology unit. *Cancer* 1987;59: 767–771.
27. Montserrat E, Villamor N, Reverter JC, et al. Bone marrow assessment in B-cell chronic lymphocytic leukaemia: aspirate or biopsy? A comparative study in 258 patients [see comments]. *Br J Haematol* 1996; 93:111–116.
28. Bartl R, Frisch B, Burkhardt R, et al. Assessment of marrow trephine in relation to staging in chronic lymphocytic leukaemia. *Br J Haematol* 1982;51:1–15.
29. Foucar K. Reactive lymphoid proliferations in blood and bone marrow. In: Foucar K, ed. *Bone marrow pathology,* 1st ed. Chicago: ASCP Press, 1995:255–274.
30. Faulkner-Jones BE, Howie AJ, Boughton BJ, et al. Lymphoid aggregates in bone marrow: study of eventual outcome. *J Clin Pathol* 1988; 41:768–775.
31. Rywlin AM, Ortega RS, Dominguez CJ. Lymphoid nodules of bone marrow: normal and abnormal. *Blood* 1974;43:389–400.
32. Navone R, Valpreda M, Pich A. Lymphoid nodules and nodular lymphoid hyperplasia in bone marrow biopsies. *Acta Haematol* 1985; 74:19–22.
33. Dick FR, Maca RD. The lymph node in chronic lymphocytic leukemia. *Cancer* 1978;41:283–292.
34. Bonato M, Pittaluga S, Tierens A, et al. Lymph node histology in typical and atypical chronic lymphocytic leukemia. *Am J Surg Pathol* 1998;22:49–56.
35. Edelman M, Evans L, Zee S, et al. Splenic microanatomical localization of small lymphocytic lymphoma/chronic lymphocytic leukemia using a novel combined silver nitrate and immunoperoxidase technique. *Am J Surg Pathol* 1997;21:445–452.
36. Lampert IA, Thompson I. The spleen in chronic lymphocytic leukemia and related disorders. In: Polliack A, Catovsky D, eds. *Chronic lymphocytic leukemia.* New York: Harwood Academic Publishers, 1988:193–208.
37. Schwartz JB, Shamsuddin AM. The effects of leukemic infiltrates in various organs in chronic lymphocytic leukemia. *Hum Pathol* 1981; 12:432–440.
38. Lampert IA, Hegde U, Van Noorden S. The splenic white pulp in chronic lymphocytic leukaemia: a microenvironment associated with CR2 (CD21) expression, cell transformation and proliferation. *Leuk Lymphoma* 1990;1:319–326.
39. Jennings CD, Foon KA. Recent advances in flow cytometry: application to the diagnosis of hematologic malignancy. *Blood* 1997;90: 2863–2892.
40. Moreau EJ, Matutes E, A'Hern RP, et al. Improvement of the chronic lymphocytic leukemia scoring system with the monoclonal antibody SN8 (CD79b). *Am J Clin Pathol* 1997;108:378–382.
41. Davis BH, Foucar K, Szczarkowski W, et al. U.S.-Canadian Consensus recommendations on the immunophenotypic analysis of hematologic neoplasia by flow cytometry: medical indications. *Cytometry* 1997;30:249–263.
42. Hamblin TJ, Oscier DG. Chronic lymphocytic leukaemia: the nature of the leukaemic cell. *Blood Rev* 1997;11:119–128.
43. Schleiffenbaum BE, Ruegg R, Zimmermann D, et al. Early diagnosis of low grade malignant lymphoma and chronic lymphocytic leukaemia: verification of morphologically suspected malignancy in blood lymphocytes by flow cytometry. *Eur J Haematol* 1996;57:341–348.
44. Dunphy CH, Wheaton SE, Perkins SL. CD23 expression in transformed small lymphocytic lymphomas/chronic lymphocytic leukemias and blastic transformations of mantle cell lymphoma. *Mod Pathol* 1997;10:818–822.
45. Vasef MA, Medeiros LJ, Koo C, et al. Cyclin D1 immunohistochemical staining is useful in distinguishing mantle cell lymphoma from other low-grade B-cell neoplasms in bone marrow. *Am J Clin Pathol* 1997;108:302–307.
46. Lucio PJ, Faria MT, Pinto AM, et al. Expression of adhesion molecules in chronic B-cell lymphoproliferative disorders. *Haematologica* 1998;83:104–111.
47. Behr SI, Korinth D, Schriever F. Differential adhesion pattern of B cell chronic lymphocytic leukemia cells. *Leukemia* 1998;12:71–77.
48. Csanaky G, Matutes E, Vass JA, et al. Adhesion receptors on peripheral blood leukemic B cells: a comparative study on B cell chronic lymphocytic leukemia and related lymphoma/leukemias. *Leukemia* 1997;11:408–415.
49. Foon KA, Rai KR, Gale RP. Chronic lymphocytic leukemia: new insights into biology and therapy. *Ann Intern Med* 1990;113:525–539.
50. Kunicka JE, Platsoucas CD. Defective helper function of purified T4 cells and excessive suppressor activity of purified T8 cells in patients with B-cell chronic lymphocytic leukemia: T4 suppressor effector cells are present in certain patients. *Blood* 1988;71:1551–1560.
51. Velardi A, Prchal JT, Prasthofer EF, et al. Expression of NK-lineage markers on peripheral blood lymphocytes with T-helper ($Leu3^+/T4^+$) phenotype in B cell chronic lymphocytic leukemia. *Blood* 1985;65: 149–155.
52. Kay NE, Kaplan ME. Defective T cell responsiveness in chronic lymphocytic leukemia: analysis of activation events. *Blood* 1986;67: 578–581.
53. Ayanlar-Batuman O, Ebert E, Hauptman SP. Defective interleukin-2 production and responsiveness by T cells in patients with chronic lymphocytic leukemia of B cell variety. *Blood* 1986;67:279–284.
54. Foa R, Giovarelli M, Jemma C, et al. Interleukin 2 (IL 2) and interferon-gamma production by T lymphocytes from patients with B-chronic lymphocytic leukemia: evidence that normally released IL 2 is absorbed by the neoplastic B cell population. *Blood* 1985;66: 614–619.
55. Perri RT, Kay NE. Large granular lymphocytes from B-chronic lymphocytic leukemia patients inhibit normal B cell proliferation. *Am J Hematol* 1989;31:166–172.
56. Burton JD, Weitz CH, Kay NE. Malignant chronic lymphocytic leukemia B cells elaborate soluble factors that down-regulate T cell and NK function. *Am J Hematol* 1989;30:61–67.
57. Janssen O, Nerl C, Kabelitz D. T cells in B-cell chronic lymphocytic leukemia: quantitative assessment of cytotoxic and interleukin-2–producing lymphocyte precursors by limiting dilution analysis. *Blood* 1989;73:1622–1626.
58. Foa R, Fierro MT, Raspadori D, et al. Lymphokine-activated killer (LAK) cell activity in B and T chronic lymphoid leukemia: defective LAK generation and reduced susceptibility of the leukemic cells to allogeneic and autologous LAK effectors. *Blood* 1990;76:1349–1354.
59. Santiago-Schwarz F, Panagiotopoulos C, Sawitsky A, et al. Distinct characteristics of lymphokine-activated killer (LAK) cells derived from patients with B-cell chronic lymphocytic leukemia (B-CLL): a factor in B-CLL serum promotes natural killer cell–like LAK cell growth. *Blood* 1990;76:1355–1360.
60. Kay NE, Perri RT. Evidence that large granular lymphocytes from B-CLL patients with hypogammaglobulinemia down-regulate B-cell immunoglobulin synthesis [published erratum appears in *Blood* 1989; 73:2232]. *Blood* 1989;73:1016–1019.
61. Yamada O, Yun-Hua W, Motoji T, et al. Clonal T-cell proliferation causing pure red cell aplasia in chronic B-cell lymphocytic leukaemia: successful treatment with cyclosporine following in vitro abrogation of erythroid colony-suppressing activity. *Br J Haematol* 1998;101: 335–337.
62. Schattner EJ, Mascarenhas J, Reyfman I, et al. Chronic lymphocytic leukemia B cells can express CD40 ligand and demonstrate T-cell type costimulatory capacity. *Blood* 1998;91:2689–2697.
63. Reyes E, Prieto A, Carrion F, et al. Morphological variants of leukemic cells in B chronic lymphocytic leukemia are associated with different T cell and NK cell abnormalities. *Am J Hematol* 1997;55:175–182.
64. Mu X, Kay NE, Gosland MP, et al. Analysis of blood T-cell cytokine expression in B-chronic lymphocytic leukaemia: evidence for increased levels of cytoplasmic IL-4 in resting and activated CD8 T cells. *Br J Haematol* 1997;96:733–735.
65. Garcia-Marco JA, Price CM, Catovsky D. Interphase cytogenetics

in chronic lymphocytic leukemia. *Cancer Genet Cytogenet* 1997;94:52–58.
66. Crossen PE. Genes and chromosomes in chronic B-cell leukemia. *Cancer Genet Cytogenet* 1997;94:44–51.
67. Kroft SH, Finn WG, Kay NE, et al. Isolated 13q14 abnormalities and normal karyotypes are associated with typical lymphocyte morphology in B-cell chronic lymphocytic leukemia. *Am J Clin Pathol* 1997;107:275–282.
68. Garcia-Marco JA, Caldas C, Price CM, et al. Frequent somatic deletion of the 13q12.3 locus encompassing BRCA2 in chronic lymphocytic leukemia. *Blood* 1996;88:1568–1575.
69. Neilson JR, Auer R, White D, et al. Deletions at 11q identify a subset of patients with typical CLL who show consistent disease progression and reduced survival. *Leukemia* 1997;11:1929–1932.
70. Dohner H, Stilgenbauer S, Fischer K, et al. Cytogenetic and molecular cytogenetic analysis of B cell chronic lymphocytic leukemia: specific chromosome aberrations identify prognostic subgroups of patients and point to loci of candidate genes. *Leukemia* 1997;11[Suppl 2]:S19–S24.
71. Finn WG, Thangavelu M, Yelavarthi KK, et al. Karyotype correlates with peripheral blood morphology and immunophenotype in chronic lymphocytic leukemia. *Am J Clin Pathol* 1996;105:458–467.
72. Bigoni R, Cuneo A, Roberti MG, et al. Chromosome aberrations in atypical chronic lymphocytic leukemia: a cytogenetic and interphase cytogenetic study. *Leukemia* 1997;11:1933–1940.
73. Su'ut L, O'Connor SJ, Richards SJ, et al. Trisomy 12 is seen within a specific subtype of B-cell chronic lymphoproliferative disease affecting the peripheral blood/bone marrow and co-segregates with elevated expression of CD11a. *Br J Haematol* 1998;101:165–170.
74. Merup M, Jansson M, Corcoran M, et al. A FISH cosmid "cocktail" for detection of 13q deletions in chronic lymphocytic leukaemia: comparison with cytogenetics and Southern hybridization. *Leukemia* 1998;12:705–709.
75. O'Brien S. Clinical challenges in chronic lymphocytic leukemia. *Semin Hematol* 1998;35:22–26.
76. Efremov DG, Ivanovski M, Siljanovski N, et al. Restricted immunoglobulin VH region repertoire in chronic lymphocytic leukemia patients with autoimmune hemolytic anemia. *Blood* 1996;87:3869–3876.
77. Wall DM, el-Osta S, Tzelepis D, et al. Expression of mdr1 and mrp in the normal B-cell homologue of B-cell chronic lymphocytic leukaemia. *Br J Haematol* 1997;96:697–707.
78. Thompson AA, Talley JA, Do HN, et al. Aberrations of the B-cell receptor B29 (CD79b) gene in chronic lymphocytic leukemia. *Blood* 1997;90:1387–1394.
79. Michaux L, Dierlamm J, Wlodarska I, et al. t(14;19)/BCL3 rearrangements in lymphoproliferative disorders: a review of 23 cases. *Cancer Genet Cytogenet* 1997;94:36–43.
80. Morabito F, Filangeri M, Callea I, et al. Bcl-2 protein expression and p53 gene mutation in chronic lymphocytic leukemia: correlation with in vitro sensitivity to chlorambucil and purine analogs. *Haematologica* 1997;82:16–20.
81. Oscier DG, Thompsett A, Zhu D, et al. Differential rates of somatic hypermutation in V(H) genes among subsets of chronic lymphocytic leukemia defined by chromosomal abnormalities. *Blood* 1997;89:4153–4160.
82. Webb M, Brun M, McNiven M, et al. MDR1 and MRP expression in chronic B-cell lymphoproliferative disorders. *Br J Haematol* 1998;102:710–717.
83. Cordone I, Masi S, Mauro FR, et al. P53 expression in B-cell chronic lymphocytic leukemia: a marker of disease progression and poor prognosis. *Blood* 1998;91:4342–4349.
84. Freedman AS, Nadler LM. The relationship of chronic lymphocytic leukemia to normal activated B cells. *Leuk Lymphoma* 1990;1:293–300.
85. Caligaris-Cappio F, Riva M, Tesio L, et al. Human normal CD5$^+$ B lymphocytes can be induced to differentiate to CD5$^-$ B lymphocytes with germinal center cell features. *Blood* 1989;73:1259–1263.
86. Freedman AS, Freeman G, Whitman J, et al. Studies of in vitro activated CD5$^+$ B cells. *Blood* 1989;73:202–208.
87. Borche L, Lim A, Binet JL, et al. Evidence that chronic lymphocytic leukemia B lymphocytes are frequently committed to production of natural autoantibodies. *Blood* 1990;76:562–569.
88. Kipps TJ, Carson DA. Autoantibodies in chronic lymphocytic leukemia and related systemic autoimmune diseases. *Blood* 1993;81:2475–2487.
89. Logtenberg T, Schutte ME, Inghirami G, et al. Immunoglobulin VH gene expression in human B cell lines and tumors: biased VH gene expression in chronic lymphocytic leukemia. *Int Immunol* 1989;1:362–366.
90. Caligaris-Cappio F. B-chronic lymphocytic leukemia: a malignancy of anti-self B cells. *Blood* 1996;87:2615–2620.
91. Gottardi D, Alfarano A, De Leo AM, et al. In leukaemic CD5$^+$ B cells the expression of BCL-2 gene family is shifted toward protection from apoptosis. *Br J Haematol* 1996;94:612–618.
92. Weisenburger DD, Harrington DS, Armitage JO. B-cell neoplasia: a conceptual understanding based on the normal humoral immune response. *Pathol Annu* 1990;25:99–115.
93. Rai KR, Han T. Prognostic factors and clinical staging in chronic lymphocytic leukemia. *Hematol Oncol Clin North Am* 1990;4:447–456.
94. Melo JV, Catovsky D, Galton DAG. Chronic lymphocytic leukemia and prolymphocytic leukemia: a clinicopathological reappraisal. *Blood Cells* 1987;12:339–353.
95. Cheson BD, Bennett JM, Grever M, et al. National Cancer Institute–sponsored Working Group guidelines for chronic lymphocytic leukemia: revised guidelines for diagnosis and treatment. *Blood* 1996;87:4990–4997.
96. International Workshop on Chronic Lymphocytic Leukemia. Chronic lymphocytic leukemia: recommendations for diagnosis, staging, and response criteria. International Workshop on Chronic Lymphocytic Leukemia. *Ann Intern Med* 1989;110:236–238.
97. Harris NL. Peripheral B-cell neoplasms. *Am J Surg Pathol* 1997;21:114–121.
98. Thommasen HV, Boyko WJ, Montaner JS, et al. Absolute lymphocytosis associated with nonsurgical trauma. *Am J Clin Pathol* 1986;86:480–483.
99. Perreault C, Boileau J, Gyger M, et al. Chronic B-cell lymphocytosis. *Eur J Haematol* 1989;42:361–367.
100. Wilkinson LS, Tang A, Gjedsted A. Marked lymphocytosis suggesting chronic lymphocytic leukemia in three patients with hyposplenism. *Am J Med* 1983;75:1053–1056.
101. Foucar K. Non-Hodgkin's lymphoma and Hodgkin's disease in bone marrow. In: Foucar K, ed. *Bone marrow pathology*, 1st ed. Chicago: ASCP Press, 1995:343–378.
102. Melo JV, Hegde U, Parreira A, et al. Splenic B cell lymphoma with circulating villous lymphocytes: differential diagnosis of B cell leukaemias with large spleens. *J Clin Pathol* 1987;40:642–651.
103. Argatoff LH, Connors JM, Klasa RJ, et al. Mantle cell lymphoma: a clinicopathologic study of 80 cases. *Blood* 1997;89:2067–2078.
104. Wasman J, Rosenthal NS, Farhi DC. Mantle cell lymphoma: morphologic findings in bone marrow involvement. *Am J Clin Pathol* 1996;106:196–200.
105. Agnarsson BA, Loughran TP Jr, Starkebaum G, et al. The pathology of large granular lymphocyte leukemia [see comments]. *Hum Pathol* 1989;20:643–651.
106. Baer MR, Stein RS, Dessypris EN. Chronic lymphocytic leukemia with hyperleukocytosis: the hyperviscosity syndrome. *Cancer* 1985;56:2865–2869.
107. Foa R, Massaia M, Cardona S, et al. Production of tumor necrosis factor-alpha by B-cell chronic lymphocytic leukemia cells: a possible regulatory role of TNF in the progression of the disease. *Blood* 1990;76:393–400.
108. Haubenstock A, Zalusky R. Autoimmune hyperthyroidism and thrombocytopenia developing in a patient with chronic lymphocytic leukemia. *Am J Hematol* 1985;19:281–283.
109. Rozman C, Montserrat E, Vinolas N. Serum immunoglobulins in B-chronic lymphocytic leukemia: natural history and prognostic significance. *Cancer* 1988;61:279–283.
110. Deegan MJ, Abraham JP, Sawdyk M, et al. High incidence of monoclonal proteins in the serum and urine of chronic lymphocytic leukemia patients. *Blood* 1984;64:1207–1211.
111. Schaffner KF, Krause JR, Kelly RH. Biclonal IgM gammopathy in chronic lymphocytic leukemia. *Arch Pathol Lab Med* 1988;112:206–208.
112. Radosevich CA, Gordon LI, Weil SC, et al. Complete resolution of pure red cell aplasia in a patient with chronic lymphocytic leukemia following antithymocyte globulin therapy. *JAMA* 1988;259:723–725.

113. Chikkappa G, Pasquale D, Phillips PG, et al. Cyclosporin-A for the treatment of pure red cell aplasia in a patient with chronic lymphocytic leukemia. *Am J Hematol* 1987;26:179–189.
114. Vashi P, Patel B, Musson P, et al. Corticosteroid-responsive pure red cell aplasia in chronic lymphatic leukemia. *Am J Hematol* 1987;26: 279–284.
115. Jonsson V, Svendsen B, Vorstrup S, et al. Multiple autoimmune manifestations in monoclonal gammopathy of undetermined significance and chronic lymphocytic leukemia. *Leukemia* 1996;10:327–332.
116. Rai KR. The different staging systems proposed in chronic lymphocytic leukemia. In: Polliack A, Catovsky D, eds. *Chronic lymphocytic leukemia.* New York: Harwood Academic Publishers, 1988:105–110.
117. Binet J-L. Clinical classifications and treatment of chronic lymphocytic leukemia: the experience of the French Cooperative Group trials. In: Polliack A, Catovsky D, eds. *Chronic lymphocytic leukemia.* New York: Harwood Academic Publishers, 1988:123–140.
118. Montserrat E, Rozman C. Prognostic factors in chronic lymphocytic leukemia. In: Polliack A, Catovsky D, eds. *Chronic lymphocytic leukemia.* New York: Harwood Academic Publishers, 1988:111–122.
119. Rai KR, Sawitsky A, Cronkite EP, et al. Clinical staging of chronic lymphocytic leukemia. *Blood* 1975;46:219–234.
120. Binet JL, Auquier A, Dighiero G, et al. A new prognostic classification of chronic lymphocytic leukemia derived from a multivariate survival analysis. *Cancer* 1981;48:198–206.
121. Hallek M, Kuhn-Hallek I, Emmerich B. Prognostic factors in chronic lymphocytic leukemia. *Leukemia* 1997;11[Suppl 2]:S4–S13.
122. Brugiatelli M, Claisse JF, Lenormand B, et al. Long-term clinical outcome of B-cell chronic lymphocytic leukaemia patients in clinical remission phase evaluated at phenotypic level [see comments]. *Br J Haematol* 1997;97:113–118.
123. Sarfati M, Chevret S, Chastang C, et al. Prognostic importance of serum soluble CD23 level in chronic lymphocytic leukemia [see comments]. *Blood* 1996;88:4259–4264.
124. Ghani AM, Krause JR, Brody JP. Prolymphocytic transformation of chronic lymphocytic leukemia: a report of three cases and review of the literature. *Cancer* 1986;57:75–80.
125. Kjeldsberg CR, Marty J. Prolymphocytic transformation of chronic lymphocytic leukemia. *Cancer* 1981;48:2447–2457.
126. Economopoulos T, Fotopoulos S, Hatzioannou J, et al. ''Prolymphocytoid'' cells in chronic lymphocytic leukaemia and their prognostic significance. *Scand J Haematol* 1982;28:238–242.
127. Enno A, Catovsky D, O'Brien M, et al. ''Prolymphocytoid'' transformation of chronic lymphocytic leukaemia. *Br J Haematol* 1979;41: 9–18.
128. Roberts JD, Tindle BH, MacPherson BR. Prolymphocytic transformation of chronic lymphocytic leukemia: a case report of lengthy survival after intensive chemotherapy. *Am J Hematol* 1989;31:131–132.
129. Scott CS, Stark AN, Head C, et al. Diagnostic features and survival in typical and prolymphocytoid variants of chronic lymphocytic leukemia. *Hematol Oncol* 1989;7:175–179.
130. Flandrin G. Richter's syndrome. In: Polliack A, Catovsky D, eds. *Chronic lymphocytic leukemia.* New York: Harwood Academic Publishers, 1988:209–218.
131. Bertoli LF, Kubagawa H, Borzillo GV, et al. Analysis with antiidiotype antibody of a patient with chronic lymphocytic leukemia and a large cell lymphoma (Richter's syndrome). *Blood* 1987;70:45–50.
132. Bayliss KM, Kueck BD, Hanson CA, et al. Richter's syndrome presenting as primary central nervous system lymphoma: transformation of an identical clone. *Am J Clin Pathol* 1990;93:117–123.
133. Richter MN. Generalized reticular cell sarcoma of lymph nodes associated with lymphatic leukemia. *Am J Pathol* 1928;4:285–292.
134. Foucar K, Rydell RE. Richter's syndrome in chronic lymphocytic leukemia. *Cancer* 1980;46:118–134.
135. Strauchen JA, May MM, Crown J. Large cell transformation of subclinical small lymphocytic leukemia/lymphoma: a variant of Richter's syndrome. *Hematol Oncol* 1987;5:167–174.
136. Brecher M, Banks PM. Hodgkin's disease variant of Richter's syndrome: report of eight cases. *Am J Clin Pathol* 1990;93:333–339.
137. Michiels JJ, van Dongen JJ, Hagemeijer A, et al. Richter's syndrome with identical immunoglobulin gene rearrangements in the chronic lymphocytic leukemia and the supervening non-Hodgkin lymphoma. *Leukemia* 1989;3:819–824.
138. Lane PK, Townsend RM, Beckstead JH, et al. Central nervous system involvement in a patient with chronic lymphocytic leukemia and non-Hodgkin's lymphoma (Richter's syndrome), with concordant cell surface immunoglobulin isotypic and immunophenotypic markers. *Am J Clin Pathol* 1988;89:254–259.
139. Cherepakhin V, Baird SM, Meisenholder GW, et al. Common clonal origin of chronic lymphocytic leukemia and high-grade lymphoma of Richter's syndrome. *Blood* 1993;82:3141–3147.
140. Momose H, Jaffe ES, Shin SS, et al. Chronic lymphocytic leukemia/small lymphocytic lymphoma with Reed-Sternberg–like cells and possible transformation to Hodgkin's disease: mediation by Epstein-Barr virus [see comments]. *Am J Surg Pathol* 1992;16:859–867.
141. Nakamine H, Masih AS, Sanger WG, et al. Richter's syndrome with different immunoglobulin light chain types: molecular and cytogenetic features indicate a common clonal origin. *Am J Clin Pathol* 1992;97:656–663.
142. Miyamura K, Osada H, Yamauchi T, et al. Single clonal origin of neoplastic B cells with different immunoglobulin light chains in a patient with Richter's syndrome. *Cancer* 1990;66:140–144.
143. Sun T, Susin M, Desner M, et al. The clonal origin of two cell populations in Richter's syndrome. *Hum Pathol* 1990;21:722–728.
144. Matolcsy A, Inghirami G, Knowles DM. Molecular genetic demonstration of the diverse evolution of Richter's syndrome (chronic lymphocytic leukemia and subsequent large cell lymphoma). *Blood* 1994;83:1363–1372.
145. Fayad L, Robertson LE, O'Brien S, et al. Hodgkin's disease variant of Richter's syndrome: experience at a single institution. *Leuk Lymphoma* 1996;23:333–337.
146. Ohno T, Smir BN, Weisenburger DD, et al. Origin of the Hodgkin/Reed-Sternberg cells in chronic lymphocytic leukemia with ''Hodgkin's transformation.'' *Blood* 1998;91:1757–1761.
147. Torelli UL, Torelli GM, Emilia G, et al. Simultaneously increased expression of the c-myc and mu chain genes in the acute blastic transformation of a chronic lymphocytic leukaemia. *Br J Haematol* 1987; 65:165–170.
148. Zarrabi MH, Grunwald HW, Rosner F. Chronic lymphocytic leukemia terminating in acute leukemia. *Arch Intern Med* 1977;137:1059–1054.
149. Laurent G, Gourdin MF, Flandrin G, et al. Acute blast crisis in a patient with chronic lymphocytic leukemia: immunoperoxidase study. *Acta Haematol* 1981;65:60–66.
150. Frenkel EP, Ligler FS, Graham MS, et al. Acute lymphocytic leukemic transformation of chronic lymphocytic leukemia: substantiation by flow cytometry. *Am J Hematol* 1981;10:391–398.
151. Januszewicz E, Cooper IA, Pilkington G, et al. Blastic transformation of chronic lymphocytic leukemia. *Am J Hematol* 1983;15:399–402.
152. Asou N, Osato M, Horikawa K, et al. Burkitt's type acute lymphoblastic transformation associated with t(8;14) in a case of B cell chronic lymphocytic leukemia [Letter]. *Leukemia* 1997;11:1986–1988.
153. Fermand JP, James JM, Herait P, et al. Associated chronic lymphocytic leukemia and multiple myeloma: origin from a single clone. *Blood* 1985;66:291–293.
154. Brouet JC, Fermand JP, Laurent G, et al. The association of chronic lymphocytic leukaemia and multiple myeloma: a study of eleven patients. *Br J Haematol* 1985;59:55–66.
155. Saltman DL, Ross JA, Banks RE, et al. Molecular evidence for a single clonal origin in biphenotypic concomitant chronic lymphocytic leukemia and multiple myeloma. *Blood* 1989;74:2062–2065.
156. Pugh WC, Manning JT, Butler JJ. Paraimmunoblastic variant of small lymphocytic lymphoma/leukemia. *Am J Surg Pathol* 1988;12: 907–917.
157. French Cooperative Group on Chronic Lymphocytic Leukaemia. Natural history of stage A chronic lymphocytic leukaemia untreated patients. French Cooperative Group on Chronic Lymphocytic Leukaemia. *Br J Haematol* 1990;76:45–57.
158. Han T, Ozer H, Gavigan M, et al. Benign monoclonal B cell lymphocytosis—a benign variant of CLL: clinical, immunologic, phenotypic, and cytogenetic studies in 20 patients. *Blood* 1984;64:244–252.
159. Vadhan-Raj S, Velasquez WS, Butler JJ, et al. Stimulation of myelopoiesis in chronic lymphocytic leukemia and in other lymphoproliferative disorders by recombinant human granulocyte-macrophage colony-stimulating factor. *Am J Hematol* 1990;33:189–197.
160. Tallman MS, Hakimian D. Purine nucleoside analogs: emerging roles in indolent lymphoproliferative disorders [published erratum appears in *Blood* 1996 Mar 1;87(5):2093]. *Blood* 1995;86:2463–2474.
161. Pott C, Hiddemann W. Purine analogs in the treatment of chronic lymphocytic leukemia. *Leukemia* 1997;11[Suppl 2]:S25–S28.

162. Khouri IF, Przepiorka D, van Besien K, et al. Allogeneic blood or marrow transplantation for chronic lymphocytic leukaemia: timing of transplantation and potential effect of fludarabine on acute graft-versus-host disease. *Br J Haematol* 1997;97:466–473.
163. Keating MJ. Chronic lymphocytic leukemia in the next decade: where do we go from here? *Semin Hematol* 1998;35:27–33.
164. Keating MJ, O'Brien S, Lerner S, et al. Long-term follow-up of patients with chronic lymphocytic leukemia (CLL) receiving fludarabine regimens as initial therapy. *Blood* 1998;92:1165–1171.
165. Galton DA, Goldman JM, Wiltshaw E, et al. Prolymphocytic leukaemia. *Br J Haematol* 1974;27:7–23.
166. Stone RM. Prolymphocytic leukemia. *Hematol Oncol Clin North Am* 1990;4:457–471.
167. Catovsky D. Prolymphocytic and hairy cell leukemia. In: Henderson ES, Lister TA, eds. *Leukemia,* 5th ed. Philadelphia: WB Saunders, 1990:639–660.
168. Owens MR, Strauchen JA, Rowe JM, et al. Prolymphocytic leukemia: histologic findings in atypical cases. *Hematol Oncol* 1984;2:249–257.
169. Pallesen G, Madsen M, Pedersen BB. B-prolymphocytic leukaemia: a mantle zone lymphoma? *Scand J Haematol* 1979;22:407–416.
170. Jandl JH. Prolymphocytic and hairy cell leukemias. In: Jandl JH, ed. *Blood: textbook of hematology.* Boston: Little, Brown, 1996: 1019–1039.
171. Melo JV, Catovsky D, Gregory WM, et al. The relationship between chronic lymphocytic leukaemia and prolymphocytic leukaemia: IV. Analysis of survival and prognostic features. *Br J Haematol* 1987; 65:23–29.
172. Logan RA, Smith NP. Cutaneous presentation of prolymphocytic leukaemia. *Br J Dermatol* 1988;118:553–558.
173. Berrebi A, Bassous-Guedj L, Vorst E, et al. Further characterization of prolymphocytic leukemia cells as a tumor of activated B cells [see comments]. *Am J Hematol* 1990;34:181–185.
174. Davi F, Maloum K, Michel A, et al. High frequency of somatic mutations in the VH genes expressed in prolymphocytic leukemia. *Blood* 1996;88:3953–3961.
175. Lens D, De Schouwer PJ, Hamoudi RA, et al. P53 abnormalities in B-cell prolymphocytic leukemia. *Blood* 1997;89:2015–2023.
176. Juliusson G, Robert KH, Ost A, et al. Del(3)(p13) in B-prolymphocytic leukemia: a new nonrandom chromosomal aberration possibly related to the c-ras oncogene. *Cancer Genet Cytogenet* 1985;14: 191–195.
177. Brito-Babapulle V, Pittman S, Melo JV, et al. Cytogenetic studies on prolymphocytic leukemia: 1. B-cell prolymphocytic leukemia. *Hematol Pathol* 1987;1:27–33.
178. Cerroni L, Zenahlik P, Hofler G, et al. Specific cutaneous infiltrates of B-cell chronic lymphocytic leukemia: a clinicopathologic and prognostic study of 42 patients. *Am J Surg Pathol* 1996;20:1000–1010.
179. Kuse R, Lueb H. Gastrointestinal involvement in patients with chronic lymphocytic leukemia. *Leukemia* 1997;11[Suppl 2]:S50–S51.
180. O'Neill BP, Habermann TM, Banks PM, et al. Primary central nervous system lymphoma as a variant of Richter's syndrome in two patients with chronic lymphocytic leukemia. *Cancer* 1989;64:1296–1300.
181. Miller K, Budke H, Orazi A. Leukemic meningitis complicating early stage chronic lymphocytic leukemia. *Arch Pathol Lab Med* 1997;121: 524–527.
182. Garicochea B, Cliquet MG, Melo N, et al. Leptomeningeal involvement in chronic lymphocytic leukemia identified by polymerase chain reaction in stored slides: a case report. *Mod Pathol* 1997;10:500–503.

CHAPTER 41

Hairy Cell Leukemia and Related Disorders

Mitchell A. Bitter

Bouroncle, Wiseman, and Doan, in their 1958 report entitled "Leukemic Reticuloendotheliosis," are generally credited with establishing what is now called hairy cell leukemia (HCL) as a distinct clinical entity (1). The descriptive name *hairy cell leukemia* was coined 6 years later by Schreck and Donnelly (2).

In the 20 years after its initial description, much information was gathered regarding the clinical findings, histopathology, and cytochemistry of HCL. During this time, much debate centered on the cell of origin of the hairy cell. In the early 1980s, the hairy cell was confirmed to be a B lymphocyte (3–11). During the 1980s, the immunophenotype of the hairy cell was defined further; however, whether a normal counterpart to the hairy cell exists and, if so, which cell it is remain unsettled issues. During the past 15 years, several effective therapeutic agents have become available that have markedly prolonged the survival of patients who have this disorder, although it is still uncertain whether any patients may be cured of this leukemia (12–18).

Despite much progress in our ability to accurately diagnose and to effectively treat this disorder, relatively little is known about the basic mechanisms involved in the pathogenesis of HCL. In contrast to some other hematopoietic neoplasms, neither a specific chromosomal abnormality nor a characteristic molecular genetic alteration has been uncovered. Scant information exists regarding alterations in the expression of growth-regulating DNA sequences.

Although it is an uncommon lymphoproliferative disorder, many pathologists, particularly those in large centers, encounter patients who have HCL. Moreover, HCL must be considered in the differential diagnosis for many other patients who have cytopenias and splenomegaly. Accurate diagnosis of HCL rests on careful morphologic examination of well-prepared peripheral blood films and on biopsy specimens of bone marrow, spleen, and other tissues. Immunophenotypic and cytochemical studies serve as valuable adjuncts. The emphasis in this chapter is on the cytologic and histopathologic features, together with the immunophenotypic and cytochemical findings that permit the diagnosis of HCL and distinguish it from other hematologic disorders. Pertinent clinical information and immunologic, cytogenetic, and molecular genetic findings are summarized.

M. A. Bitter: Department of Pathology, University of Colorado Health Sciences Center, Denver, Colorado 80262

INCIDENCE AND EPIDEMIOLOGY

Six hundred new cases of HCL are recognized in the United States each year; HCL accounts for 2% of all leukemias (19). The mean age at diagnosis is approximately 54 years (range, 20 to 80 years), with a male to female ratio of about 4:1 (20–23) (Table 41.1). It is primarily a disease of Caucasians; Jewish men are overrepresented (19). Several families that have two or more affected members have been reported (24–30); however, most cases are sporadic. There is no clear association between HCL and exposure to mutagens.

CLINICAL AND LABORATORY FEATURES AT DIAGNOSIS

Most patients who have HCL initially seek medical attention because of complaints related to cytopenias. These include fatigue, infection, or less commonly, bleeding (20–23). Some have symptoms referable to splenomegaly. A minority of patients are asymptomatic at the time of diagnosis (20–23). The frequency of asymptomatic presentations may increase as more people undergo routine screening blood counts. Splenomegaly, sometimes massive, is present in about 85% of patients, and hepatomegaly occurs in 40% of patients (Table 41.1). Peripheral lymphadenopathy (>2 cm) is seen in only 5% to 15% of patients and is localized when present (20–23).

Pancytopenia is observed at the time of diagnosis in more than half of all patients, and most others show various combinations of cytopenias (Table 41.1) (20–23). Normochromic,

TABLE 41.1. *Clinical and peripheral blood findings in patients who have hairy cell leukemia*

Findings	Frassoldati et al (23) study of 725 patients
Clinical findings	
Age (yr)	
Mean	54
Range	23–85
Male to female ratio	3.9:1
Performance status	
0–1	85.8%
2–4	14.2%
Splenomegaly (cm below costal margin)	
Not palpable	14.2%
1–4	26.3%
5–10	34.4%
>10	25.1%
Liver size (cm below costal margin)	
Not palpable	27.4%
1–2	32.4%
3–4	27.0%
>4	13.2%
Peripheral lymphadenopathy	
Absent	86.6%
Present	13.4%
Peripheral blood findings	
Hemoglobin (g/dL)	
<8.5	28.4%
8.5–12	48.5%
>12	23.1%
WBC ($\times 10^9$/L)	
<1.0	5.1%
1.0–3.5	57.3%
3.5–7.0	18.8%
>7.0	18.8%
Neutrophils ($\times 10^9$/L)	
<0.5	39%
0.5–1.5	40.9%
>1.5	20.1%
Monocytes ($\times 10^9$/L)	
Not detected	55.5%
0.0–0.15	33.5%
0.15–0.5	8.8%
>0.5	2.2%
Hairy cells ($\times 10^9$/L)	
Not detected	15%
0.01–0.5	38%
0.5–5.0	34%
>50	13%
Platelets ($\times 10^9$/L)	
<50	30.6%
50–100	42.6%
>100	26.8%

normocytic anemia (hemoglobin < 12 g/dL), thrombocytopenia (< 150 $\times$ 10^9/L), and neutropenia (absolute neutrophil count [ANC] < 2 $\times$ 10^9/L) are each observed in 75% to 90% of patients. Severe thrombocytopenia (<50 $\times$ 10^9/L) or severe neutropenia (ANC < 0.5 $\times$ 10^9/L) affects 30% to 40% of patients (20–23).

It is often helpful in the diagnosis of HCL to know that monocytopenia is nearly always observed in untreated patients (23,31), although this may not be the case in patients with hairy cell variants. It is wise to proceed with caution in the diagnosis of HCL in the face of normal or increased numbers of monocytes. Lymphocytes generally are present in normal numbers; however, the number of large granular lymphocytes may be reduced (32). Platelets may show morphologic and functional abnormalities (33,34).

CYTOMORPHOLOGY AND HISTOPATHOLOGY

Peripheral Blood

At diagnosis, the number of hairy cells present in the peripheral blood is variable (20,21,23). Most patients are leukopenic; however, 10% to 20% of patients have ''leukemic'' presentations (white blood cell [WBC] count > 10 $\times$ 10^9/L, with >50% hairy cells), and a few patients have WBC counts that exceed 100 $\times$ 10^9/L (20–23). Hairy cells may be identified in Wright's stained peripheral blood films in about 90% of patients, although a diligent search may be required (20,21,23). Some reports have emphasized the importance of phase contrast microscopy in preparations of living cells, which preferably are supravitally stained (1,35). However, a correct diagnosis may be made with confidence by an experienced observer on the basis of the characteristic morphology of hairy cells in air dried Wright's stained blood films (Fig. 41.1; see also Color Plate 18, between pp. 1446–1447).

Hairy cells are generally 1.5 to 2 times the size of small lymphocytes (10 to 20 μm) (36–38). The cells generally have eccentrically located round, oval, or dumbbell-shaped nuclei (37,38). Occasionally, cells with convoluted, or even multilobated (39) nuclei may be seen (Fig. 41.2, *top row*). The chromatin is stippled, in contrast to the clumped chromatin of the normal lymphocyte, and nucleoli are absent or inconspicuous. The pale blue cytoplasm has a ''fluffy'' texture, and the cell border is shaggy (36–38). Cytoplasmic

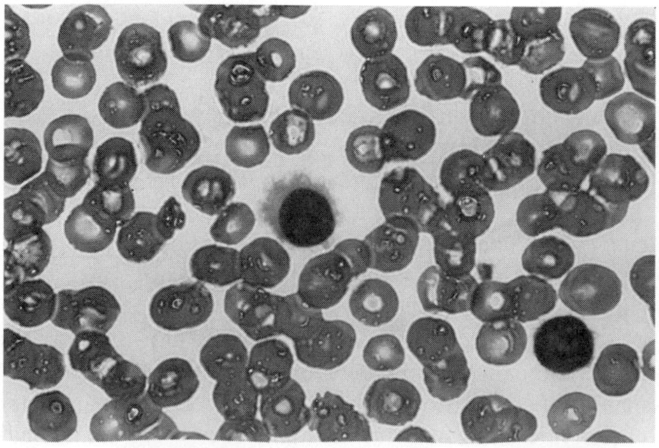

FIG. 41.1. Hairy cell in a peripheral blood film (Wright's stain, original magnification: 1,000× magnification). See Color Plate 18, between pp. 1446–1447.

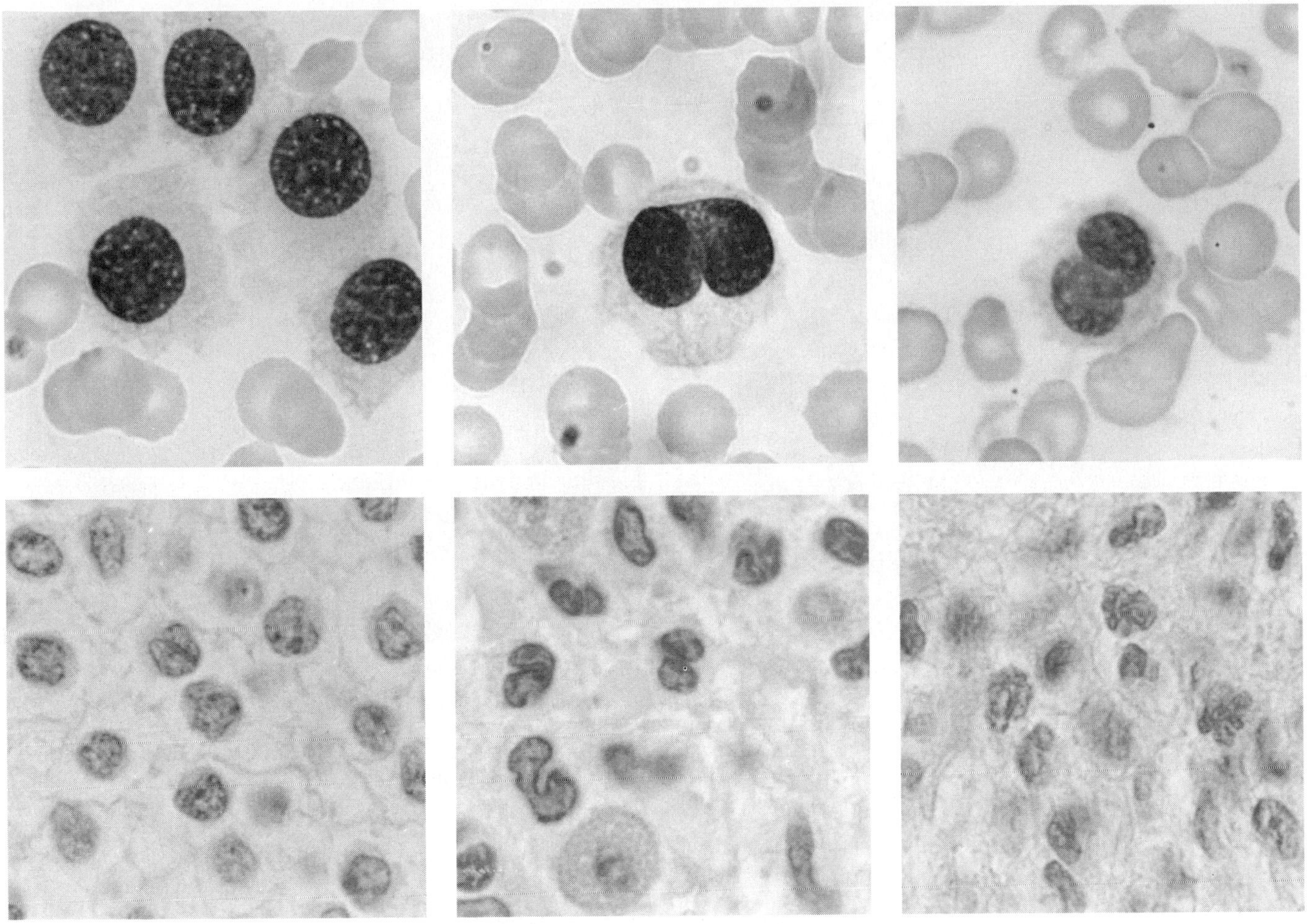

FIG. 41.2. Varied nuclear morphology of hairy cells is demonstrated in Wright-stained peripheral blood (original magnification: 2,000× magnification) *(top row)* and hematoxylin and eosin–stained, plastic-embedded sections (original magnification: 1,500× magnification) *(bottom row)*. Left to right: round to oval nuclei, reniform nuclei, convoluted nuclei.

granules are present occasionally (37,38). Rarely, rod-shaped inclusions may be seen; these correspond to the ribosome-lamellar complexes, which are observed ultrastructurally in approximately 50% of cases. These ribosome-lamellar complexes appear in cross section as target-shaped structures that consist of a hollow central core surrounded by concentric lamellae that alternate with parallel rows of ribosomes (40) (Fig. 41.3). These structures are not specific for HCL (41,42). Ultrastructural examination of the hairy cell emphasizes the irregular shape of the nuclei. The cell membrane is ruffled, with numerous microvilli 50 to 150 Å wide and 0.6 to 1.4 μm long (40), which corresponds to the ''hairy'' projections (Fig. 41.3).

Bone Marrow

Examination of the bone marrow is the cornerstone of the diagnosis of HCL (43,44). With rare exceptions (45,46), the bone marrow is involved at the time of initial examination in all patients who have HCL. Because the bone marrow is inaspirable in more than half the patients (36,38,47), and because it may be difficult to recognize hairy cells in aspirates, a bone core biopsy should be performed. The initial biopsy specimen generally is diagnostic. However, HCL may be overlooked in small specimens and in specimens that are not optimally fixed, processed, and thinly sectioned (47).

As in the peripheral blood, the extent of involvement of the bone marrow by HCL at the time of diagnosis varies. Most patients have a hypercellular marrow (36,38,47) (Fig. 41.4; see also Color Plate 19, between pp. 1446–1447). In some patients, the marrow is completely effaced; other patients show a patchy infiltration of hairy cells. In the latter group, the hairy cell infiltrates show no preference for paratrabecular locations (43,47). The bone marrow is normocellular in some patients (Fig. 41.5). The diagnosis may be difficult in instances in which only small aggregates of hairy cells blend subtly with adjacent hematopoietic cells or in hypocellular marrows (in 10% to 20% of patients) (48) in which small numbers of hairy cells infiltrate between fat cells (47,48). The latter cases may be diagnosed incorrectly as aplastic anemia (47,48) (Fig. 41.6; see also Color Plate

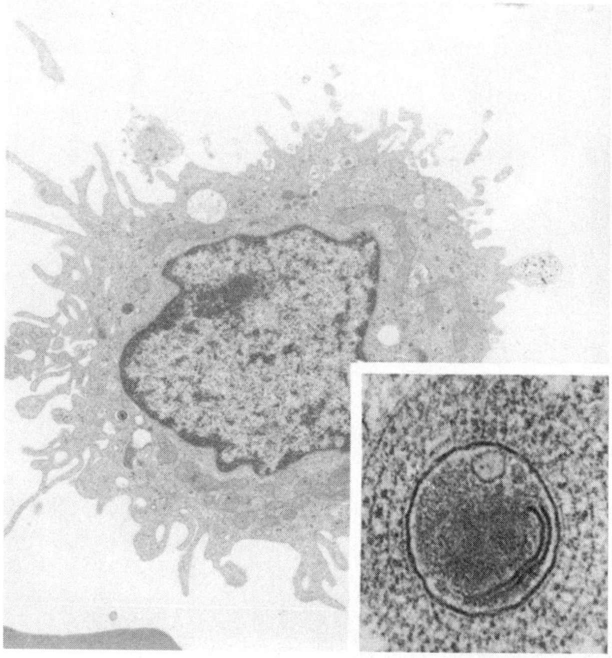

A

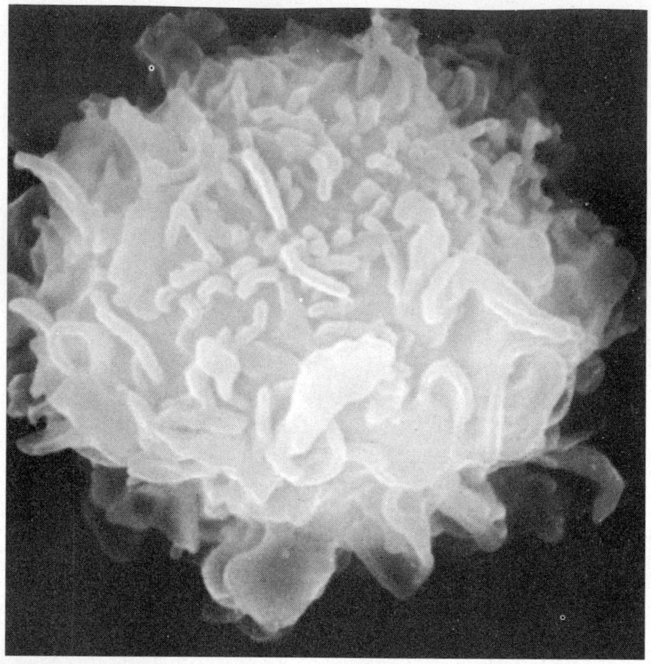

B

FIG. 41.3. Transmission and scanning electron micrographs of hairy cells. **A:** Transmission electron micrograph of a hairy cell demonstrates prominent surface projections (original magnification: 9,000× magnification). A ribosome-lamella complex **(inset)** from the cytoplasm of another hairy cell shows the typical concentric lamellae that alternate with rows of ribosomes (original magnification: 72,000× magnification). (Courtesy of Wilbur A. Franklin, M.D., University of Colorado, and Cosimo Sciotto, M.D., Penrose Hospital, Colorado Springs, CO.) **B:** Scanning electron micrograph of a hairy cell with ruffles and microvilli (original magnification: 15,000× magnification). (Courtesy of Haim Gamliel, M.D., and Harvey M. Golomb, M.D., Department of Medicine, University of Chicago Medical Center, Chicago, IL.)

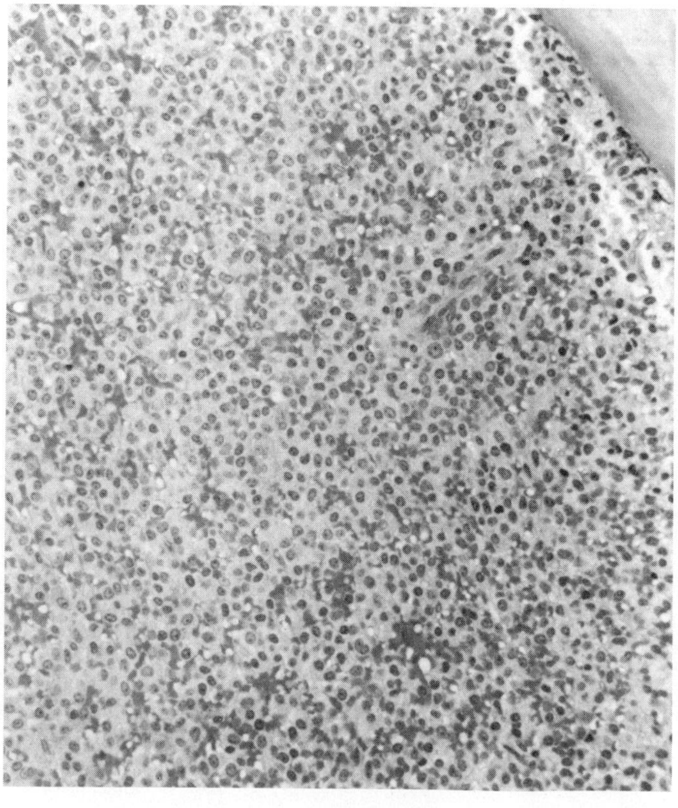

A

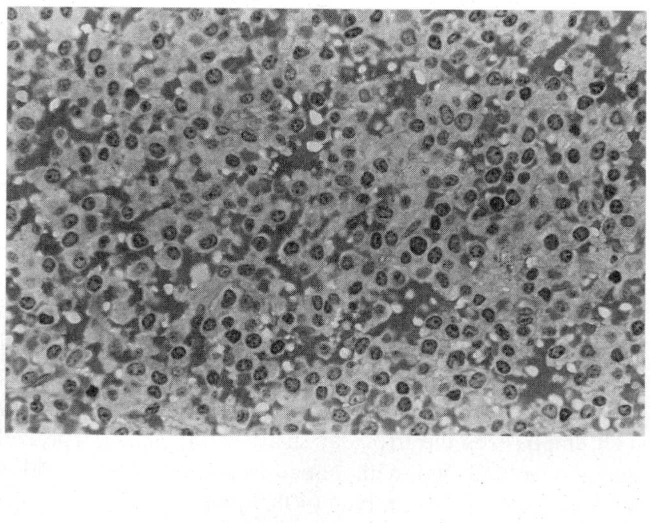

B

FIG. 41.4. Hypercellular bone marrow with complete replacement of normal hematopoietic elements by hairy cells (**A**,**B**) (hematoxylin and eosin stain, original magnifications: 250× and 1,500× magnification). See Color Plate 19, between pp. 1446–1447.

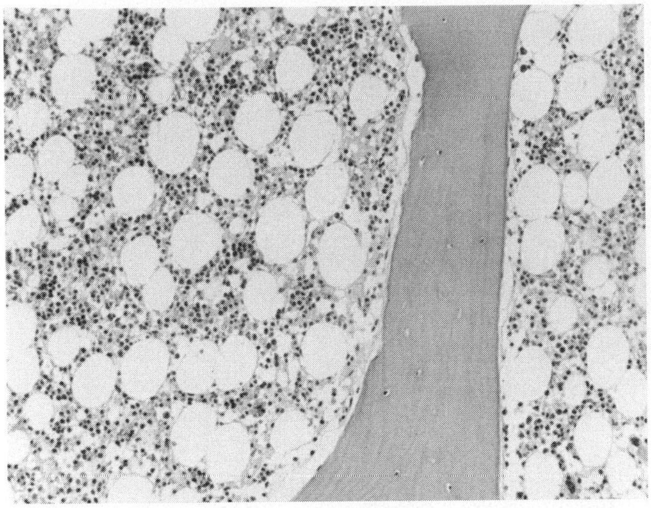

FIG. 41.5. Normocellular bone marrow infiltrated by hairy cells. Residual erythroid islands show darkly stained, regular nuclei (hematoxylin and eosin stain, original magnification: 200× magnification).

20, between pp. 1446–1447). Immunohistochemical stains may be helpful in such cases (Fig. 41.6B, *inset*).

At low power, collections of hairy cells have a characteristic appearance. In hematoxylin and eosin–stained tissue, the cells possess abundant water clear to lightly eosinophilic cytoplasm, so that, in thin sections, the individual nuclei are well spaced and generally do not touch (Fig. 41.4B). At high power, the hairy cell nuclei appear to be bland and are slightly larger than those of lymphocytes (43,47). They may be oval, indented, bilobed, or convoluted (47,49) (Fig. 41.2, *bottom row*). Nucleoli usually are inconspicuous (47). Mitoses are rare or absent (38,47). Lymphocytes and plasma cells are admixed with the hairy cell infiltrate. Mast cells often are prominent (49) (Fig. 41.2, *middle of bottom row*).

The extent of hairy cell involvement may be quantified. The hairy cell index is derived from the bone marrow cellularity and the percentage of hairy cells [(% cellularity × % hairy cells)/10^4], yielding a number between 0 and 1 (50).

Variable numbers of residual hematopoietic elements may be identified at diagnosis in the bone marrow of patients who have HCL. In general, the numbers of megakaryocytes and erythroid cells are reduced less severely than are those of granulocytes (32). In marrows that are almost completely involved by HCL, residual hematopoietic activity often consists of only scattered megakaryocytes and clusters of erythroid cells, which typically show a shift toward immaturity (Fig. 41.7); granulocytes are usually scant. In marrows that show a patchy hairy cell infiltration, granulocytes are more severely reduced than are megakaryocytes and erythroid cells. The granulocyte to erythroid ratio is rarely greater than 1:1 (32).

Bone marrow reticulin is almost always increased (Fig. 41.8); however, collagen fibrosis is typically absent (38). The increased reticulin probably accounts for the high frequency of ''dry taps'' in patients who have this disorder (40), although interdigitation of hairy cell projections may also be important. When an aspirate can be obtained, a ''dirty background'' often is present because of the traumatic fragmentation of the hairy cell cytoplasm. Many of the hairy cells are represented by naked nuclei. Hairy projections are difficult to discern even in those cells that have intact cytoplasm, and the chromatin often appears smudgy (Fig. 41.9; see also Color Plate 21, between pp. 1446–1447).

A

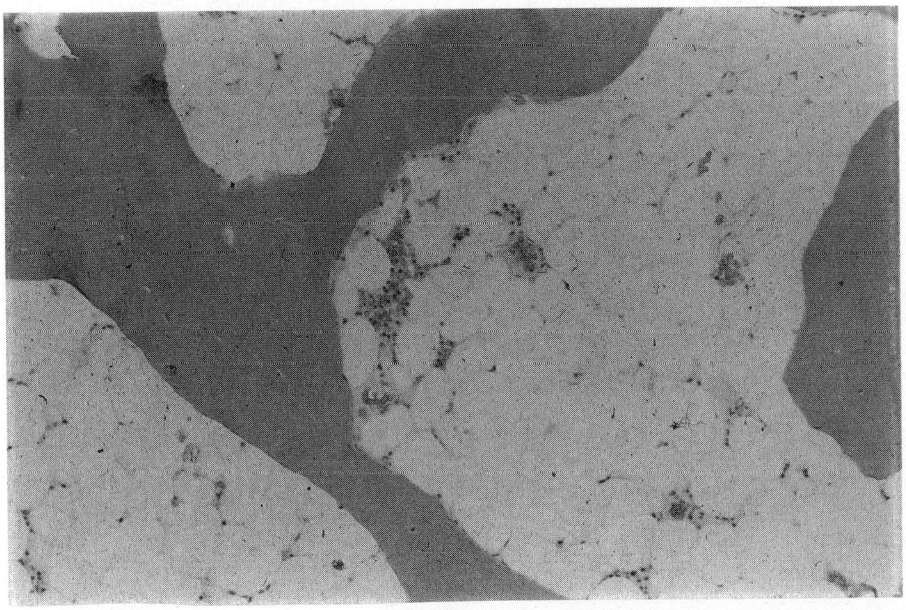

FIG. 41.6. Markedly hypocellular bone marrow with sparse infiltration by hairy cells. **A:** Low magnification (hematoxylin and eosin stain, original magnification: 100× magnification). See Color Plate 20A, between pp. 1446–1447. *(continued)*

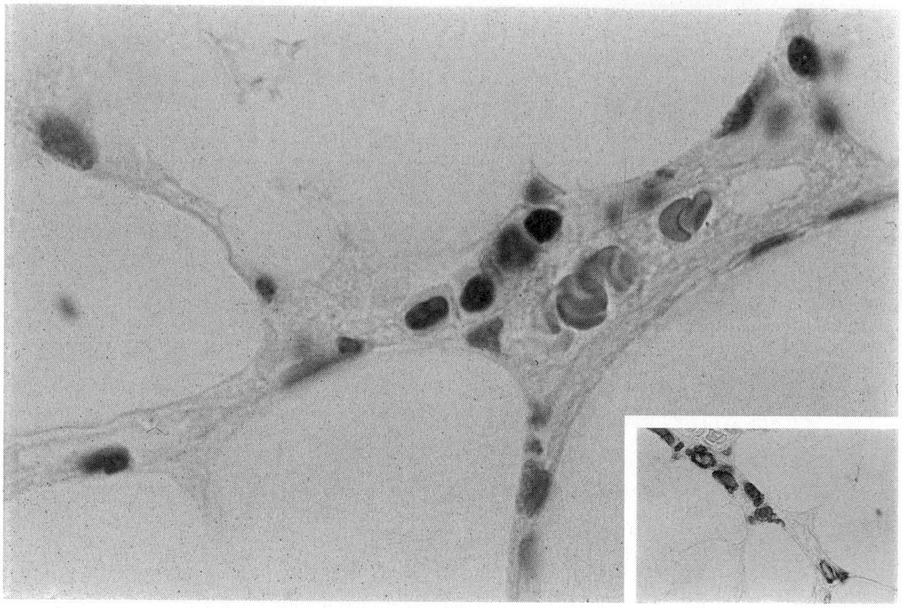

B

FIG. 41.6. *Continued.* **B:** High magnification (original magnification: 800× magnification) shows hairy cells with abundant cytoplasm infiltrating between adipocytes. CD20 immunostain **(inset)** reveals membrane positivity with ruffled border (immunoperoxidase stain, original magnification: 1,000× magnification). See Color Plate 20B, between pp. 1446–1447.

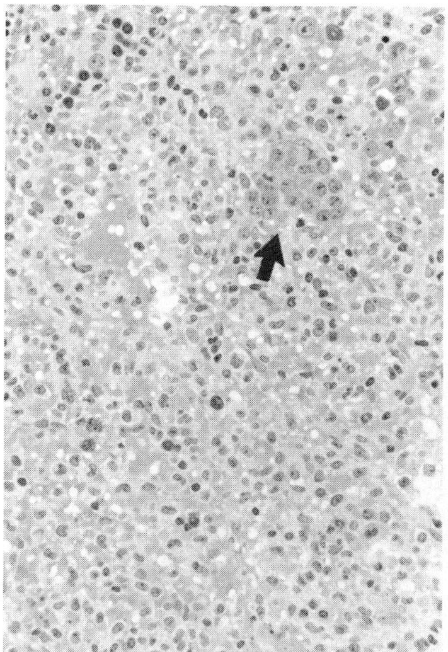

FIG. 41.7. Hypercellular marrow with hairy cell leukemia shows a cluster of immature erythroid cells *(arrow)* (hematoxylin and eosin stain, original magnification: 4,000× magnification).

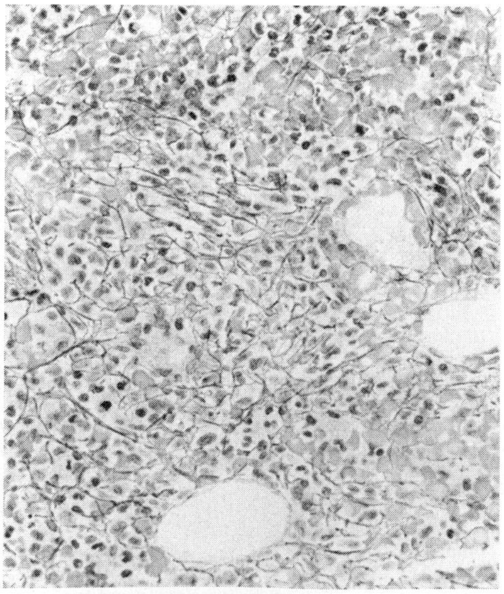

FIG. 41.8. Increased reticulin fibers in a bone marrow infiltrated by hairy cell leukemia (reticulin stain, original magnification: 350× magnification).

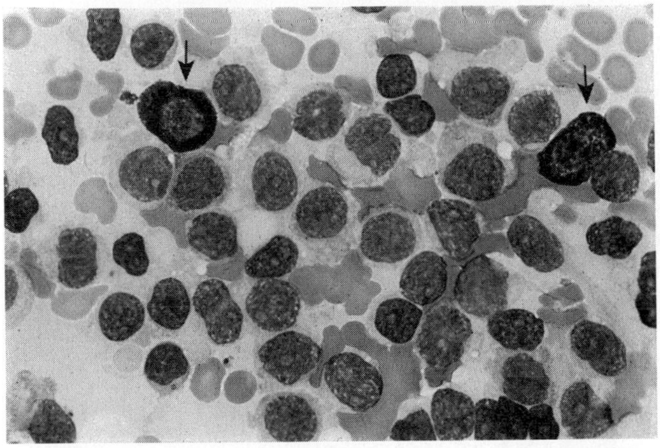

FIG. 41.9. Bone marrow aspirate from a patient with hairy cell leukemia. Hairy cells in marrow aspirates often show a more "smudgy" chromatin than those in the peripheral blood. Hairy projections are difficult to appreciate, and the background often is littered with cytoplasmic fragments. Mast cells are indicated by *arrows* (Wright stain, original magnification: 1,000× magnification). See Color Plate 21, between pp. 1446–1447.

In some patients, the hairy cell infiltrate within the marrow displays a spindled appearance (38,47) (Fig. 41.10). This may be caused by the admixture of increased numbers of fibroblasts with the hairy cells (47). Extravasated red cells often are associated with foci of HCL and may be helpful in calling attention to them (47). Occasionally, blood lakes, similar to those seen in the spleen, may be observed in bone core biopsy specimens.

Spleen

A palpably enlarged spleen is present at diagnosis in 80% to 90% (20,21,23) of patients who have HCL. It appears that the absence of splenomegaly does not indicate that the disease is in an early stage in these patients (22). In rare instances in which bone marrow involvement is not demonstrated, the diagnosis of HCL rests on examination of the spleen (45,46).

Cytopenias in HCL are considered to result from splenic sequestration of blood cells as well as from underproduction by the bone marrow (50). Before the advent of effective pharmacologic therapy, splenectomy generally was accepted as first-line treatment for patients who had clinically significant cytopenias. Presently, with effective drug therapy the role of splenectomy in the treatment of patients who have HCL has diminished greatly; however, it continues to be recommended in occasional clinical circumstances (12,35). The extent of bone marrow infiltration appears to be a better predictor than spleen size for the correction of cytopenias, particularly thrombocytopenia, by splenectomy (50).

In one large study (50), the weight of splenectomy specimens in cases of HCL ranged from 250 to 4600 g (median, 1,300 g). Evidence of rupture is rare. The cut surface of the spleen is beefy red, because HCL involves the red pulp (47). Microscopically, involvement of the red pulp is usually diffuse, and the white pulp is atrophied (47). In small spleens, infiltration by hairy cells may be patchy and occasionally may be subtle (51,52). In specimens with sparse infiltration, hairy cells often can be identified adjacent to trabeculae and as subendothelial infiltrates within trabecular veins (52). In such cases, the use of immunohistochemical and cytochemical studies may be helpful (52).

The morphologic appearance of HCL in the spleen, as in the marrow, is that of a lymphoid infiltrate of bland cells with abundant cytoplasm. In thin sections, the hairy cell nuclei do not appear to touch one another (47) (Fig. 41.11; see also Color Plate 22, between pp. 1446–1447). On closer inspec-

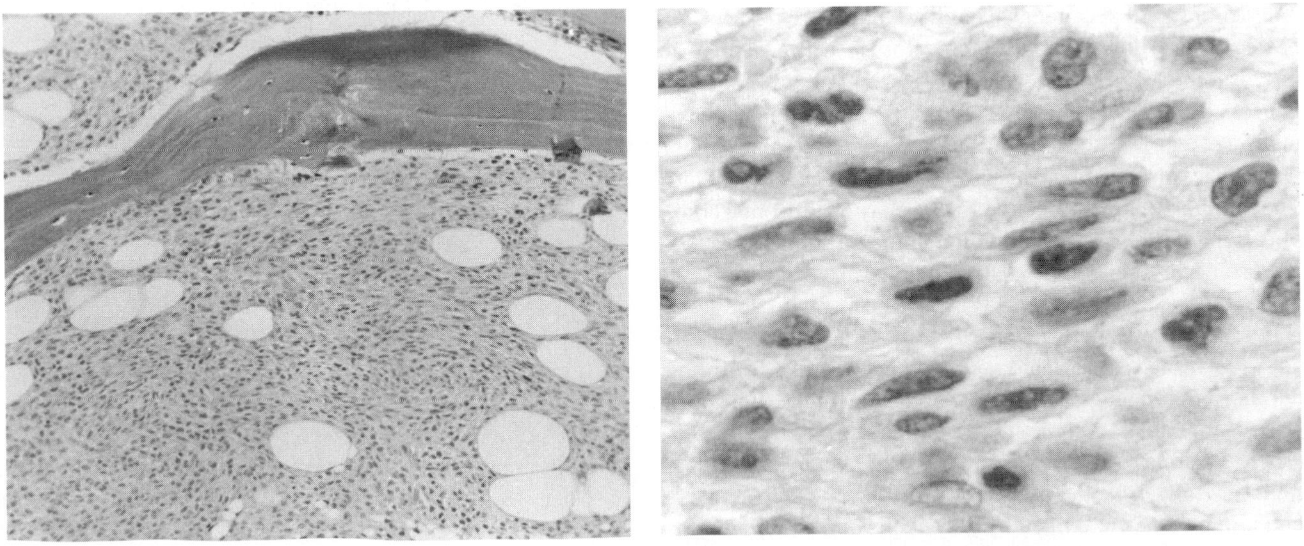

A B

FIG. 41.10. Hairy cell leukemia in a bone core biopsy **(A)** shows a spindled pattern. At higher magnification **(B)**, it is difficult to distinguish individual hairy cells from accompanying connective tissue cells (hematoxylin and eosin stain, original magnifications: 200× and 1,200× magnification).

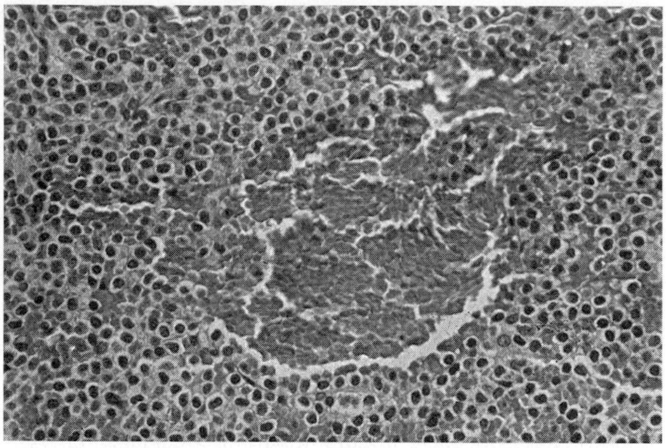

FIG. 41.11. Hairy cell leukemia infiltrating the spleen. A well-formed pseudosinus is present (hematoxylin and eosin stain, original magnification: 250× magnification). See Color Plate 22, between pp. 1446–1447.

tion, and by electron microscopy, hairy cells infiltrate the cords and adhere to the endothelial lining of the sinuses, possibly damaging the sinus wall (53). This may result in the formation of blood-filled pseudosinuses lined by hairy cells that often are a prominent finding (54) (Fig. 41.11) but are not limited to HCL. Similar blood-filled spaces have been observed in chronic lymphocytic leukemia (CLL), chronic myelogenous leukemia, and multiple myeloma (47). Extramedullary hematopoiesis may be evident (47).

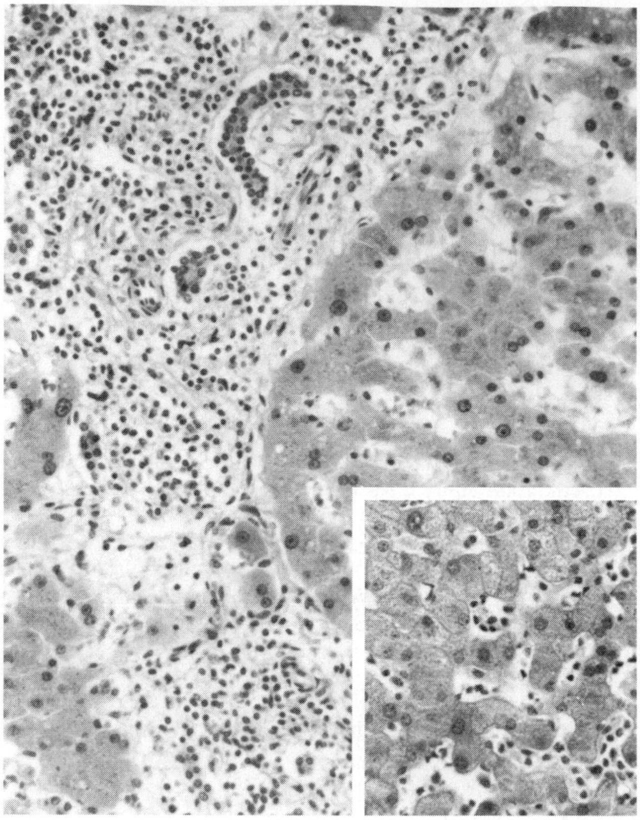

FIG. 41.12. Hairy cell leukemia infiltrating the liver. Portal involvement is prominent. Sinusoidal infiltrate (**inset**) is also seen (hematoxylin and eosin stain, original magnification: 250× magnification).

Liver

Hepatomegaly is noted on physical examination in 20% to 40% of patients who have HCL (20–22). In an autopsy series, livers ranged in weight from 1,630 to 4,500 g (mean, 2,690 g) (55). Microscopic involvement has been observed in essentially all specimens examined at autopsy (55) or biopsied at the time of splenectomy (56,57). The degree of microscopic infiltration by HCL varies, and it does not seem to be well correlated with liver size (56). Biochemical abnormalities such as elevated transaminases and alkaline phosphatase levels are seen in a small percentage of patients. They are most often unrelated to HCL or result from a complication of HCL such as granulomatous inflammation (56).

Portal and sinusoidal infiltration by hairy cells may be present (55–58) (Fig. 41.12). Portal infiltration may be associated with fibrosis; however, cirrhosis is rare (56). Sinusoidal involvement is variable and does not correlate with the number of circulating hairy cells (56). Sinusoids can be congested and dilated, sometimes mimicking peliosis hepatis (56). Angiomatoid lesions are seen in half of patients (54,55,57,58). Like the pseudosinusoids of the spleen, angiomatoid channels are lined by hairy cells and contain erythrocytes and hairy cells. As originally described by Namba (54), the angiomatoid channels are located primarily in the portal areas; however, other investigators (57) have described apparently similar lesions randomly distributed within the lobules. These lesions appear to result from hairy cell adherence to, and subsequent destruction of, the sinusoidal wall (57,58). Occasionally, they may be recognized as red nodules on gross inspection of the liver (57).

Lymph Nodes

Peripheral lymphadenopathy of 2 cm or more is observed in only 5% to 15% of patients who have HCL (20,22,23). In contrast, retroperitoneal, abdominal, and mediastinal adenopathy are frequently observed at autopsy (55) and may be detected during life (59–61). When present, abdominal lymphadenopathy may be massive and appears to be more common in patients with longstanding disease and those who have had splenectomy (60,62).

Histologically, lymph nodes may be totally or, more commonly, partially effaced (Fig. 41.13). In the latter circumstance, hairy cells infiltrate through the paracortex and medulla in a leukemic pattern, and they often surround residual lymphoid follicles (36,55). The hairy cell infiltrate may extend outside the capsule of the lymph node (36,55).

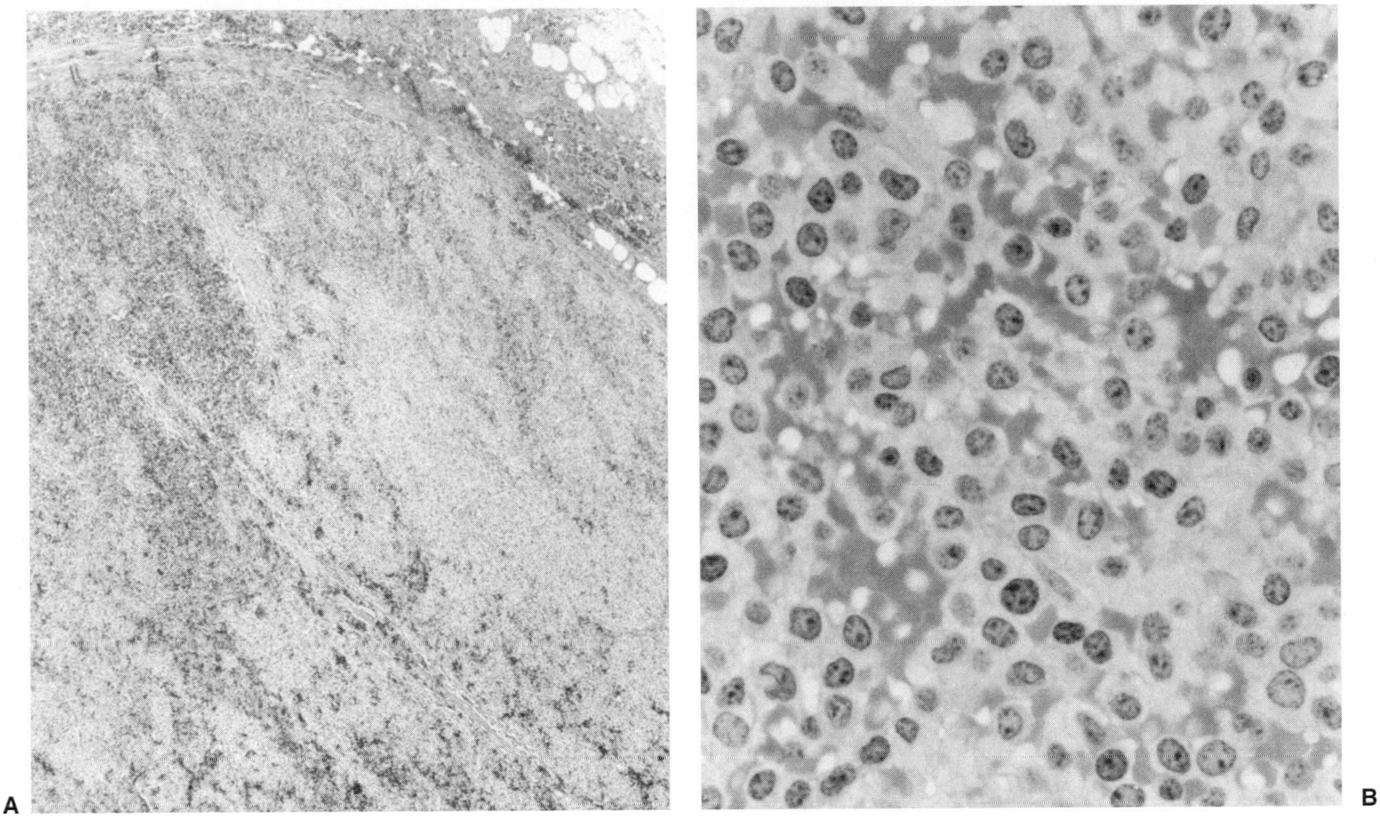

FIG. 41.13. Lymph node involvement by hairy cell leukemia, shown at low magnification (original magnification: 50×) **(A)** and at high magnification (original magnification: 600×) **(B)**. In this specimen, there is complete effacement by hairy cells. Hairy cells infiltrate through the capsule into the perinodal fat *(left)* (hematoxylin and eosin stain).

Additional Findings

Hairy Cell Leukemia in Other Tissues

Hairy cell infiltrates have been noted at autopsy in numerous tissues including kidneys, colon, stomach, myocardium, meninges, adrenals, pancreas, and in the connective tissue as well as in the fat that invests these organs (55). These infiltrates are rarely symptomatic.

Bone complications are observed in approximately 3% of patients who have HCL (63). Patients most often complain of pain related to osteolytic lesions of the axial skeleton, with the proximal femur being the most common site (63–66). Biopsies show hairy cell infiltrates within the cortical bone (65). Generalized osteoporosis or osteosclerosis may be seen occasionally (64,67).

Lung biopsy was commonly performed in the past to investigate fever and respiratory insufficiency in neutropenic patients with HCL. Focal hairy cell infiltrates frequently are observed in these specimens, but they rarely are sufficient to account for the patient's hypoxemia, which is usually caused by infection (55).

Skin lesions are common in patients who have HCL; however, they are rarely caused by infiltration by hairy cells (68–70). When present, hairy cell infiltrates typically involve the reticular dermis and are distributed around vessels and adnexa, often leaving a grenz zone. In some patients, the infiltrate may be more extensive (68,69). Historically, nearly half the skin lesions in patients with HCL are caused by infections. Other causes include drug reactions and vasculitis (69).

Infections

Granulocytopenia, monocytopenia, and various immunologic defects predispose patients who have HCL to develop infections. Infection is observed in one third of patients at diagnosis (20–22,71). Historically, infection has been the major cause of morbidity and mortality in patients who have HCL, accounting for about two thirds of the deaths (20,21,55). However, the incidence of infectious complications in HCL has decreased markedly with the availability of effective therapy. The types of infections may change as well.

Eighty percent of fatalities from infections are the result of septicemia and pneumonia, most commonly caused by gram-negative bacilli such as *Pseudomonas aeruginosa* and *Escherichia coli* (20,21,71–73). Fungal infections, which account for about 7% of deaths, are most often caused by *Aspergillus* and *Candida* (pulmonary) or *Cryptococcus* (meningitis) (21,72). Mycobacterial infections, particularly with *Mycobacterium kansasii* are seen in 5% to 10% of patients (72,74). Because patients with HCL form granulomas poorly, stains for acid-fast and fungal organisms should be performed on tissues from febrile patients who have HCL, regardless of the presence or absence of granulomas. Viral hepatitis is the cause of death in fewer than 5% of patients (72). In contrast to other immunosuppressed patients, HCL patients rarely are infected with *Pneumocystis carinii* (55).

Vasculitis

Vasculitis is observed in fewer than 10% of patients who have HCL (75–77) (Fig. 41.14). It may affect small vessels, resulting in arthralgias and skin lesions (76–79). A syndrome of polyarteritis nodosa may occur (77,80–83). In some, this may be related to hepatitis B virus or other infectious disorders (77). Vasculitis has improved or resolved in some patients with successful therapy for HCL (77).

Other Tumors

There is evidence that HCL patients, like those who have another chronic B-cell leukemia, chronic lymphocytic leukemia (CLL), may have an increased incidence of other malignancies (19). The reported incidence of second cancers has ranged from 4% to 21% (19,23,84–88). There are a number of anecdotal reports of various nonhematopoietic tumors such as cancers of the lung (84), colon (19,84,85), pancreas (84), kidney (84,85), breast (19), prostate (19), and testis (86), as well as Kaposi's sarcoma (19). Patients who have HCL also have been reported to develop therapy-related myelodysplastic syndrome (84), Hodgkin's disease (89,90), multiple myeloma (91), Sezary syndrome (92), and large cell non-Hodgkin's lymphomas (56,93–96).

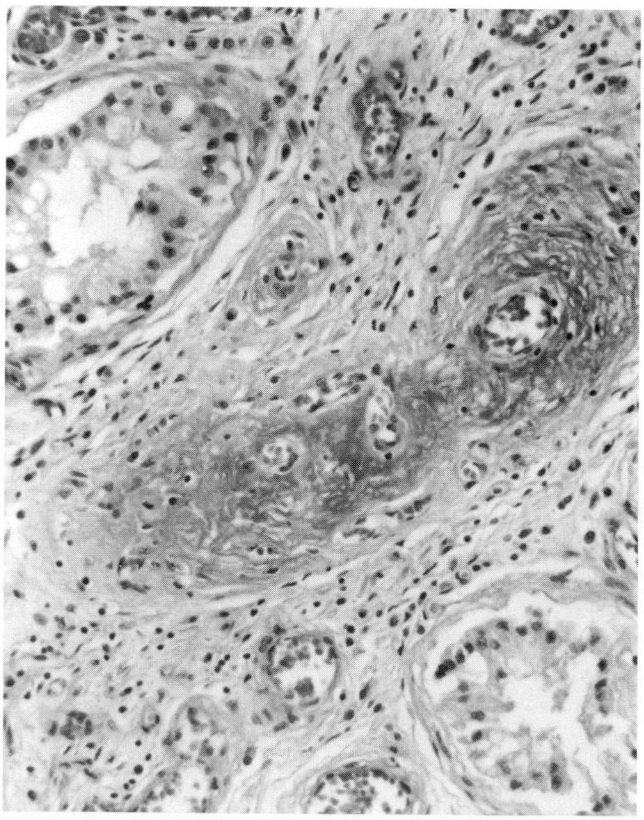

FIG. 41.14. Vasculitis in hairy cell leukemia. A section of testis shows fibrinoid necrosis of a vessel (hematoxylin and eosin stain, original magnification: 250× magnification).

A few studies compared the observed incidence of second malignancies in cohorts of patients with HCL compared with the expected incidence (85,87,88,97). Results varied. Two studies found no increase in the incidence of second tumors (88,97). A study of 350 patients (87) found no statistically significant increase in solid tumors but an excess of lymphomas and myelomas among their patients. Another study found an excess of all tumors, particularly hematopoietic neoplasms (85). Yet another study reported an increased frequency of second tumors, primarily solid tumors (98).

It is uncertain whether the myelomas and large cell lymphomas seen in these patients are derived from the same clone as in HCL. If there is an increased incidence of second malignancies, it is uncertain whether this is related to an underlying genetic susceptibility to neoplasia, immunodeficiency or therapy for HCL.

CYTOCHEMICAL FINDINGS

Acid Phosphatase

The presence of acid phosphatase activity resistant to inhibition by L(+)-tartaric acid (i.e., tartrate-resistant acid phosphatase [T-AcP] positivity) is a widely used test to confirm the diagnosis of HCL. With careful attention to technical details, the T-AcP reaction, despite certain limitations, remains a valuable tool in the diagnosis of HCL. However, the availability of sensitive and specific combinations of immunophenotypic markers has eroded the importance of T-AcP in the diagnosis of HCL.

In the hairy cell, T-AcP activity resides in isoenzyme 5, which is one of seven acid phosphatase isoenzymes present in human leukocytes (99–101). Although a cDNA encoding this isoenzyme has been cloned and the resultant amino acid sequence has been deduced, its function is unknown (102).

The T-AcP reaction is most commonly performed on blood films, buffy coat preparations, marrow aspirates, and imprints of bone marrow, spleen, or other tissues. Freshly prepared specimens are preferred; however, air-dried smears may retain their enzyme activity for up to two weeks at room temperature (103). Naphthol-AS-BI is the preferred substrate, and fast garnet GBC provides maximum sensitivity as the coupler (104). When these reagents are used, the red granular reaction product is present diffusely within the

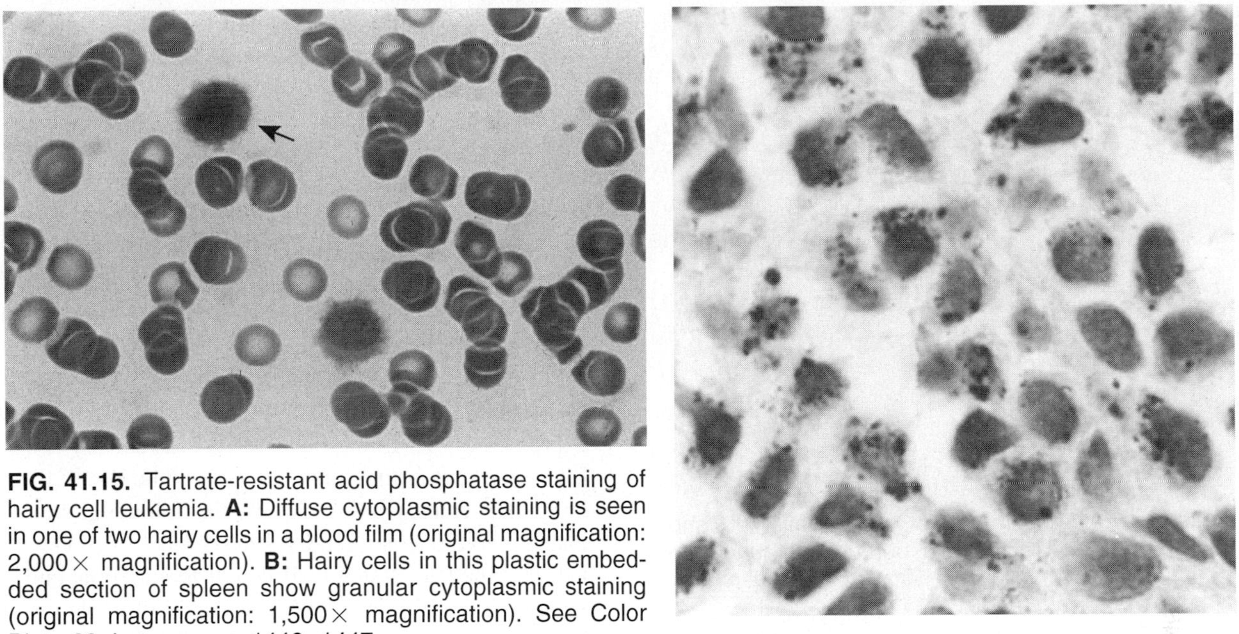

A

B

FIG. 41.15. Tartrate-resistant acid phosphatase staining of hairy cell leukemia. **A:** Diffuse cytoplasmic staining is seen in one of two hairy cells in a blood film (original magnification: 2,000× magnification). **B:** Hairy cells in this plastic embedded section of spleen show granular cytoplasmic staining (original magnification: 1,500× magnification). See Color Plate 23, between pp. 1446–1447.

cytoplasm of hairy cells (Fig. 41.15; see also Color Plate 23, between pp. 1446–1447). Neutrophils, monocytes, and platelets that have AcP activity sensitive to tartrate may serve as internal controls.

Cytochemical staining for T-AcP in formalin-fixed and paraffin-embedded specimens is not reliable (105). Frozen sections or specially processed, plastic-embedded sections are recommended. In frozen sections, the coupler pararosaniline may be preferred because of its superior localization (104). Generally, T-AcP activity can be demonstrated in tissues that have been fixed in cold 1% paraformaldehyde, embedded in glycol methacrylate, and polymerized in the cold (106). This procedure may be useful in confirming the diagnosis of HCL in severely hypocellular marrows (48). An antibody to T-AcP has been described that may be used in paraffin-embedded tissues (107–109).

Strongly T-AcP–positive cells are observed in the peripheral blood in as many as 99% of HCL patients if multiple blood films or buffy coat preparations are scanned at low power (104). If the stain is technically adequate, the most common cause for a ''negative'' T-AcP stain in HCL is the absence of sufficient numbers of hairy cells to evaluate. In most studies, fewer than 5% of cases of HCL have been T-AcP negative (104,110,111). The percentage of hairy cells that are T-AcP positive varies greatly among patients (111) (Fig. 41.16). Over time, the percentage of hairy cells that are T-AcP positive tends to decline, particularly in interferon-treated patients (104,112). It is generally agreed that the presence of as few as one or two intensely staining cells is sufficient to confirm a morphologic diagnosis of HCL.

Hairy cells are not the only ones that may display T-AcP activity (104). In tissue imprints, certain cells derived from the mononuclear phagocytic system may be positive. These include some bone marrow macrophages, osteoclasts, epithelioid cells from granulomas, Gaucher cells, and lipid-laden macrophages in idiopathic thrombocytopenic purpura (104). Caution must be used in interpreting the significance of small numbers of T-AcP–positive cells in a tissue imprint. Positive cells must have morphologic features consistent with hairy cells for the diagnosis of HCL to be confirmed.

In neoplasms, T-AcP activity has been reported in occasional cases of CLL (104,110,113), prolymphocytic leukemia (114), Waldenström's macroglobulinemia (104,115), ''malignant histiocytosis'' (104), large cell lymphoma (104),

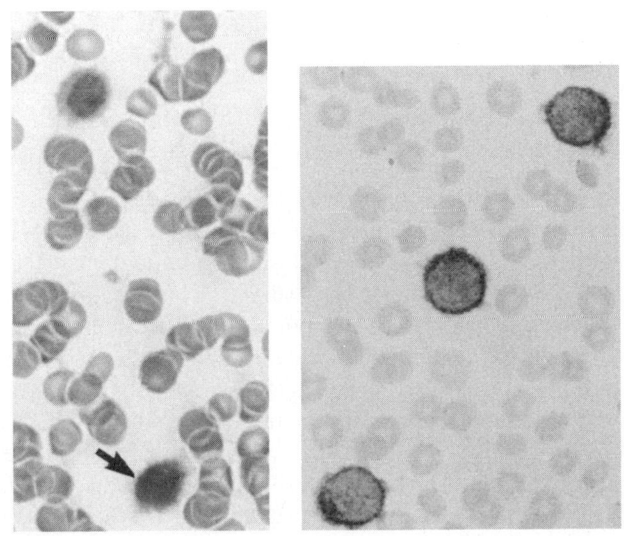

A,B

FIG. 41.16. CD11c in a case of hairy cell leukemia. Strong CD11c expression is observed in virtually all hairy cells in patients who have hairy cell leukemia. Each of three hairy cells shows CD11c expression in a blood film from the same patient (original magnification: 700× magnification).

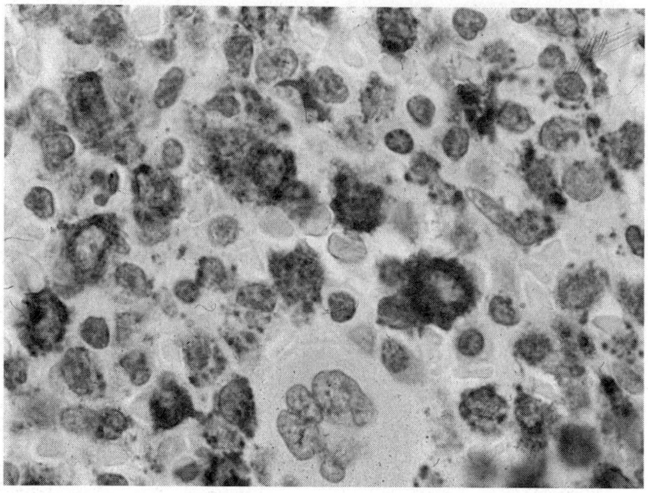

FIG. 41.17. DBA.44 in hairy cell leukemia. Hairy cells show cytoplasmic staining with irregular borders (immunoperoxidase stain, original magnification: 500× magnification). See Color Plate 24, betweeen pp. 1446–1447.

acute lymphoblastic leukemia (113), Sezary syndrome (104,116), and adult T-cell leukemia/lymphoma (113). In some of these disorders, staining may be focal in the region of the Golgi apparatus rather than diffuse, which is characteristic of HCL. Cells in systemic mast cell disease are often T-AcP positive (117), and in histologic sections of bone marrow and spleen, systemic mast cell disease can mimic HCL closely (118) (Fig. 41.17; see also Color Plate 24, between pp. 1446–1447). Because the reaction may occasionally be negative in cases of HCL and cells other than hairy cells may be positive, the T-AcP stain should be used as a confirmatory test and not as a substitute for careful morphologic examination.

IMMUNOLOGIC FINDINGS

Lineage and Immunophenotype of the Hairy Cell

Lineage of HCL was controversial for years after the 1958 publication by Bouroncle and associates of their paper "Leukemic Reticuloendotheliosis" (1). Initially, it was believed that HCL represented a neoplasm of "reticulum cells." Later, the debate focused on whether the hairy cell was a B lymphocyte or was derived from a cell of the mononuclear phagocytic system. Properties favoring the latter concept included the weak phagocytic capability of the hairy cell, its ability to adhere to glass, and the presence on the cell surface of receptors for the Fc portion of the immunoglobulin molecule (119,120). The presence of surface immunoglobulin (sIg), and the demonstration that this sIg was light chain restricted indicated that HCL is a B-cell malignancy (3–5). The cells in HCL often bear multiple immunoglobulin heavy chain isotypes on their surface (6). The most common isotype is IgG, usually of the IgG3 subclass (121). The B lymphocyte origin in virtually all cases of HCL has been confirmed by studies with lineage-restricted monoclonal antibodies (6–9) and by the demonstration of clonal rearrangements of immunoglobulin heavy- and light-chain genes (10,11). Only occasional cases of T-cell HCL have been reported (122), and in rare cases, sIg and T-cell markers have been described on the same cells (123).

Hairy cells display immunophenotypic features suggestive of a middle- to late-stage B cell, sometimes referred to as a preplasma cell (7,8). The small amount of somatic mutation in rearranged immunoglobulin genes suggests a cell that has not undergone antigenic selection (124).

The CD45 antigen (leukocyte common antigen) and pan-B-cell antigens such as CD19, CD20, CD22, and CD79a are expressed (6–9). Expression of CD24 is usually absent (6). Like CLL, but unlike most other leukemic B-cell disorders, hairy cells usually fail to express the immunoglobulin-associated membrane antigen CD79b (B29) (125). CD21, which is lost in the later stages of B-cell differentiation, and CD10, which is seen in precursor B cells and in follicle center cell lymphomas, also are absent (6,8,9). FMC-7 is expressed on hairy cells (126). The plasma cell associated-antigen PCA-1 is usually present (8).

Several other antigens expressed by hairy cells are not clearly associated with a preplasma cell stage of differentiation. Hairy cells consistently express the low affinity p55 receptor for interleukin-2 (CD25) (127). The S-100 protein has been demonstrated in fresh preparations of hairy cells (128,129), however, reports of S-100 protein positivity in paraffin sections are conflicting (125,128–130).

Several monoclonal antibodies have been raised with hairy cells used as the immunogen. These include anti-HC1 (131) and anti-HC2 (131,132), CD22 (SHCL-1) (133), CD11c (SHCL-3) (133), and CD103 (B-ly7) (134). These reagents have various specificities for HCL. Anti-HC1 is positive in 40% to 70% of cases of HCL and is positive in some epithelial and endothelial cells (9,135); anti-HC2 is positive in 80% to 100% of cases of HCL. It may also react with some B-cell lymphoproliferative disorders other than HCL, with an human T-cell lymphotrophic virus type 1 (HTLV-1)–infected T-cell line, and with some myeloid leukemias (9,131,135). CD22 (SHCL-1), shows a wide spectrum of reactivity with nonneoplastic B cells and a variety of B lymphoproliferative processes (133).

Originally raised against hairy cells, CD11c recognizes the α chain of the leukocyte adhesion molecule, p150,95, which is also present on monocytes, macrophages, granulocytes, some activated T cells, and in some T-lymphoproliferative disorders (133,136). It is strongly expressed by virtually all hairy cells in essentially all cases of HCL (137) (Fig. 41.16). Although it is frequently positive in CLL, it is generally of low intensity (138).

CD103 (B-ly7, HML-1, Ber-ACT8, LF61) recognizes an integrin subunit β_7 (139). It is expressed on intramucosal T cells in the intestines. For B-cell lymphoproliferative disorders, it is the most specific commercially available marker for HCL (134,139–141). However, it has been reported to be positive in a minority of patients with so-called splenic lymphoma with villous lymphocytes (142). These cases should be distinguished from hairy cells by morphology and other immunologic markers (142).

In paraffin sections, hairy cells react, in various proportions, with several antibodies that recognize fixation-resistant epitopes. These include CD20 (L26), CD68 (KP1), CD74 (LN2), CDw75 (LN1), MB2, and CD45RA (MT2, MB1, 4KB5) (105,130,143,144). None of these shows any degree of specificity for hairy cells. Like many other low-grade lymphoproliferative disorders, HCL is positive for BCL-2 (145).

The monoclonal antibody DBA.44 stains follicle mantle cells in routinely fixed and decalcified paraffin-embedded tissues. In the normal bone marrow, this antigen is expressed by only scattered small lymphocytes. It is positive in more than 90% of cases of HCL and in a generally lower percentage of cases of low-grade and high-grade B-lymphoproliferative disorders (146). In a given case of HCL, the number of cells expressing DBA.44 is generally lower than the number of $CD20^+$ cells. Although this antibody is not specific, when combined with assessment of the morphology of the positive cells, it is useful in the initial diagnosis and detection of minimal residual leukemia after therapy in patients with HCL (145) (Fig. 41.17).

Normal Counterpart of the Hairy Cell

Based on morphologic, cytochemical, and immunophenotypic similarities, several cell types have been proposed as normal counterparts to the hairy cell. These include marginal zone cells, which surround the lymphoid follicles of the spleen (147); monocytoid B cells, which are prominent in the sinuses of lymph nodes in certain reactive and neoplastic processes (130,148,149); and small subsets of peripheral blood B cells (150–152).

The marginal zone cells of the spleen are morphologically similar to hairy cells. Like hairy cells, they are FMC-7–positive B cells (153). Unlike hairy cells, however, they are negative for CD11c (153) and T-AcP (146) and positive for CD21 (154,155). Investigators differ about whether CD25 (IL2R) is expressed on marginal zone cells (153–155).

Monocytoid B cells show striking morphologic similarities to hairy cells (149). Like hairy cells, they are CD11c positive, and most are PCA-1 positive (149). In contrast to hairy cells, however, they do not express CD25 (149).

Some investigators have suggested that small subsets of circulating B cells may be the normal counterparts of hairy cells (134,150–152). A subset of IgG-bearing B cells has been shown to have cytoplasmic processes and T-AcP activity (150). The HCL-restricted antibody CD103 is reactive with a small population of peripheral blood B cells, including cells that express CD11c, CD25, PCA-1, and HC2 (134). It is still uncertain whether a normal counterpart to the hairy cell exists; however, these cells may be the most attractive candidates.

Practical Issues in the Immunophenotypic Diagnosis of Hairy Cell Leukemia

In many laboratories, immunophenotypic studies have replaced cytochemical staining for T-AcP as the most important confirmatory test in the diagnosis of HCL. As in the case of all hematopoietic neoplasms, immunophenotypic information must be correlated closely with morphologic findings in the diagnosis of HCL.

The most specific markers for HCL generally require fresh or frozen tissue. Peripheral blood and touch imprints of bone marrow cores (aspirates are usually not available at the time of diagnosis) are most commonly used, although frozen bone core biopsies may be studied. Touch imprints and frozen bone cores are used for immunocytochemical techniques. Peripheral blood may be studied by immunocytochemistry or flow cytometry. Both techniques are reliable in experienced laboratories. Flow cytometry offers multiparameter capabilities. Immunocytochemistry allows for examination of the morphology of the positive and negative staining cells, or "visual gating."

Flow cytometry panels should include reagent combinations such as CD19/CD11c and CD19/CD103 so that B cells may be evaluated for the coexpression of these hairy cell–associated antigens. Hairy cells typically have higher forward and wide angle light scatter than do normal lymphocytes. The percentage of positive cells and the fluorescence intensity should be evaluated for surface immunoglobulin, CD11c, CD20, and CD22 to help distinguish hairy cells from CLL. CD11c and CD103 positive B cells may be detected in low percentage in normal peripheral blood. Small numbers of circulating hairy cells may often be discriminated from these rare normal cells by higher intensity and more uniform staining of the neoplastic population (138).

Immunocytochemical stains of peripheral blood for B-cell markers, CD11c, and CD103 may be performed on routine peripheral blood films, buffy coat preparations, or cytospins of mononuclear cells after density gradient centrifugation. Methods using centrifugation disturb cell morphology, but hairy cells may still be recognized (156). In each of these preparations, hairy cells, even when present in small numbers, may be detected if close attention is paid to the morphology of the positive cells.

Immunologic Abnormalities in Patients Who Have Hairy Cell Leukemia

Reversal of the helper to suppressor T-cell ratio is common in patients who have HCL, particularly in those who have active disease or have had a splenectomy (157–159). Decreased numbers of memory T cells have been observed in the peripheral blood (160), and abnormally activated T cells have been observed in the spleen in HCL (161). Natural killer (NK) cell activity is decreased in patients who have active HCL (162–166). Up to 30% of patients may demonstrate some abnormality in serum immunoglobulins (20); a polyclonal hypergammaglobulinemia is most common (20). Up to 16% of patients have a monoclonal gammopathy demonstrated in serum or urine, which is usually of low concentration (167). In many cases, this is produced by a separate clone of immunosecretory cells rather than by the patient's hairy cells (167,168).

Some investigators have suggested that the bone marrow failure seen in patients who have HCL may be caused in part by cytokines released by or in response to hairy cells (169,170). Hairy cell–conditioned medium has been shown by some investigators (169), but not by others (171), to suppress CFU-C formation. High levels of tumor necrosis factor-α, which suppresses hematopoiesis, has been detected in the bone marrow serum by one group (170) but not detected in hairy cell–conditioned medium by other investigators (169). Some believe myelosuppression may be exacerbated by an inadequate supply of growth factors, perhaps in part because of monocytopenia (172,173).

CYTOGENETIC, MOLECULAR GENETIC, AND VIROLOGIC STUDIES

Cytogenetic Studies

Cytogenetic studies in HCL have been limited by the low proliferative index of hairy cells. When unstimulated cultures are analyzed, mitoses are seen infrequently. In mitogen-stimulated cultures, various nonclonal as well as clonal abnormalities have been observed (174–176). Although characteristic patterns have been described in some studies (177), it appears that there is no specific cytogenetic change in HCL.

Molecular Genetic Studies

In HCL, clonal rearrangement of immunoglobulin heavy- and light-chain genes are present (10,11). Somatic mutation is rare in Vκ genes (124). The T-β locus has been in a germline configuration (10,11,178).

Nothing is known about molecular genetic abnormalities that may be important in leukemogenesis in this disorder. A characteristic molecular genetic alteration, analogous to those observed in Burkitt's lymphoma or follicular lymphomas, has not been discovered. Few data are available concerning the expression of various protooncogenes and other DNA sequences important in cell proliferation. In one study, investigators observed expression of FOS; however, MYC expression was not observed in typical HCL cells (179). Investigators have demonstrated that *PRAD1/CCND1*, the gene which encodes cyclin D1, is expressed in HCL (180,181).

Cyclin D1 is a protein that plays an important role in cell cycle regulation. It is highly expressed in mantle cell lymphoma, often associated with the t(11;14) (182–184). This translocation results in juxtaposition of the immunoglobulin heavy-chain locus (14q32) and *PRAD1/CCND1*, mapped to chromosome 11q13. PRAD1/CCND1 is expressed in most cases of HCL, and in about one third of cases, expression is high, approaching levels observed in mantle cell lymphoma (180,181). Overexpression in HCL appears to be caused by mechanisms other than the t(11; 14). Protein is detected by Western blotting (180); however, positive staining by immunohistochemical techniques is infrequent in routinely fixed and paraffin-embedded tissues (185,186).

Virologic Studies

Some investigators have examined the role of certain viruses in the pathogenesis of HCL. Two patients have been reported in whom an atypical T-cell HCL was believed to be associated with infection by the retrovirus human T-cell lymphotrophic virus type 2 (HTLV-2) (122,187). More detailed analysis of one of these patients revealed that he actually had two distinct lymphoproliferative processes: B-cell HCL and a CD8$^+$ T-cell leukemia. The HTLV-2 genome was found to be oligoclonally integrated into the DNA of the leukemic T cells but not into the hairy cells (188). The HTLV-2 genome is not present in typical B-cell HCL (189).

In one study, Epstein-Barr virus genome was detected in hairy cells by *in situ* hybridization techniques (190). This finding was not confirmed by other investigators (191).

DIFFERENTIAL DIAGNOSTIC CONSIDERATIONS

General Comments

Depending on the tissue being examined, numerous disorders can enter into the differential diagnosis of HCL. These include lymphoproliferative disorders other than HCL (192), certain myeloproliferative disorders, and even nonhematopoietic malignancies (193). Based on morphologic, cytochemical, and immunophenotypic similarities to "typical" HCL, several lymphoproliferative disorders have been designated as *variants.*

Peripheral Blood

A number of neoplastic disorders characteristically show pancytopenia and splenomegaly despite minimal lymphadenopathy. These include myelosclerosis with myeloid metaplasia (194), some forms of CLL (195), prolymphocytic leukemia (114,196–198), T-cell lymphoproliferative disorders such as hepatosplenic $\gamma\delta$ T-cell lymphoma (199–201), and splenic B-cell lymphomas, including so-called splenic lymphoma with villous lymphocytes (SLVL) (202–204). In most instances, these disorders may be differentiated from

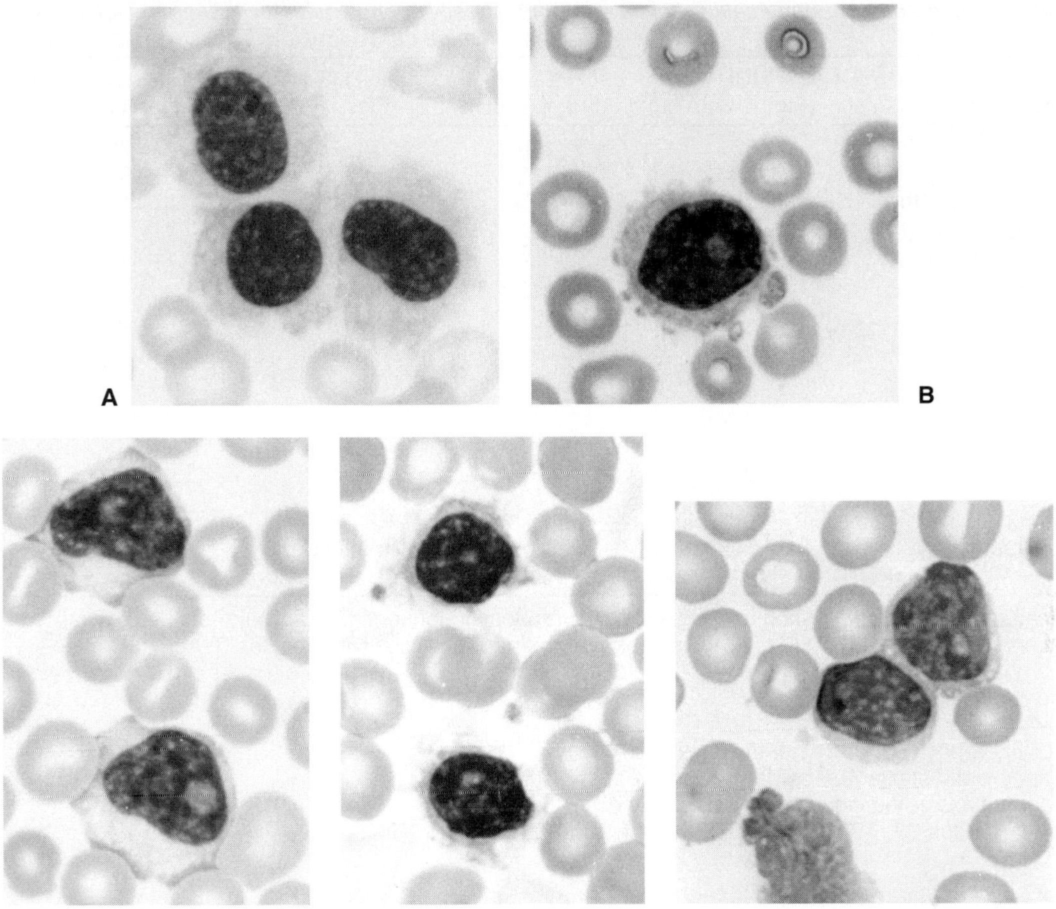

FIG. 41.18. Wright-stained peripheral blood films from patients with B-lineage lymphoproliferative disorders that may be associated with cytopenias and splenomegaly demonstrate hairy cell leukemia **(A)**, hairy cell variant **(B)**, prolymphocytic leukemia **(C)**, splenic B-cell lymphoma with circulating "villous" lymphocytes **(D)**, and chronic lymphocytic leukemia **(E)** (original magnification: 1,200× magnification). (From Paoletti M, Bitter MA, Vardiman JW. Hairy cell leukemia: morphologic, cytochemical, and immunologic features. *Clin Lab Med* 1988;8:179–195, with permission.)

HCL by examination of the peripheral blood film (Fig. 41.17).

CD11c^{+} Chronic Lymphocytic Leukemia

Occasionally, CLL cells may show hairy projections, particularly in smears made from aged blood. Cells of CLL may be distinguished from hairy cells by their more clumped chromatin (Fig. 41.18E); T-AcP negativity; expression of CD5; weak expression of sIg, CD20, and CD22; and absence of staining for CD103 (138) (Table 41.2).

Some cases of CD5^{+}, CD11c^{+} lymphoproliferative disorders were reported showing morphology most consistent with CLL. They were postulated to result from malignant transformation of lymphocytes at a stage of differentiation between CLL and HCL (205). CD11c expression had been thought to be extremely unusual in CLL (206). Some studies have found that most cases of CLL express CD11c, albeit at intensities generally lower than observed in HCL (138). This is probably because of methodologic improvements resulting in increased sensitivity. The expression of CD11c should not deter one from making a diagnosis of CLL in a case showing clinical, morphologic and other immunophenotypic markers typical of that disorder.

Splenic Marginal Zone Lymphoma with or without Villous Lymphocytes and Splenic Lymphoma with Villous Lymphocytes

Another disorder that may be associated with cytopenias, splenomegaly, and the presence in the peripheral blood of neoplastic lymphoid cells with hairy projections is an entity called SLVL (142,202–204,207) (Table 41.2; Fig. 41.18D). This disorder overlaps with splenic marginal zone lymphoma (see Chapters 23 and 53), and the two are tentatively grouped as ''splenic marginal zone lymphoma with or without villous lymphocytes,'' a provisional entity in the Revised European-American Lymphoma classification scheme of the International Lymphoma Study Group (208).

Splenic lymphoma with villous lymphocytes was de-

TABLE 41.2. *Comparison of hairy cell leukemia and other B-cell lymphoproliferative disorders with splenomegaly and circulating malignant cells*

Characteristic	HCL (Fig. 41.18A)	HCL-V (Fig. 41.18B)	B-PLL (Fig. 41.18C)	SLVL (Fig. 41.18C)	CLL (Fig. 41.18E)
Mean or median age	52	69	70	72	60
Male:female ratio	4:1	2:1	1.6:1	1.9:1[a]	2:1
Palpable lymphadenopathy	10%	10%	50%	20%	>80%
Peripheral blood					
Mean WBC ($\times 10^9$/L)	5	116	176	17	96
Monocytopenia	Present	Absent	Absent	Absent	Absent
T-AcP	+	–[b]	–[c]	–[d]	–
Immunophenotype[e]					
CD5	–	–	+/–	–/+	+
CD10 (CALLA)	–	–	–	–/+	–
CD11c	+	+	–	+/–	+/–(wk)
CD19	+	+	+	+	+
CD25	+	–	–	–/+	–
CD103	+	–/+	–	–/+	–
M protein	16%	0%	30%	28–60%	5%
Spleen involvement	Red pulp	Red pulp	White pulp ± Red pulp	White pulp	White pulp ± Red pulp

B-PLL, B-cell prolymphocytic leukemia; CLL, chronic lymphocytic leukemia; HCL, hairy cell leukemia; HCL-V, prolymphocytoid variant of HCL; SLVL, splenic lymphoma with villous lymphocytes; T-AcP, tartrate-resistant acid phosphatase, wk, weak; +/–, >30% of cases positive; –/+, <30% of cases positive.
[a] Varies between reports.
[b] May show focal activity (224).
[c] T-AcP activity reported in occasional cases (100).
[d] Several apparently similar cases demonstrated T-AcP activity (209).
[e] Immunophenotype of individual cases may vary.
Data from references 23, 192, 196, 202, 207, 224, and 234.

scribed in 1987 (202–204); however, similar patients may have been included in earlier studies (209,210). It is an uncommon lymphoproliferative disorder in which patients may have cytopenias and splenomegaly with minimal lymphadenopathy, as well as circulating lymphoid cells with hairy projections (202). Patients, on average, are two decades older than those who have HCL, with a male predominance in most series but with a lower male to female ratio than observed in HCL. The WBC count is mildly elevated (mean, 17×10^9/L). The peripheral blood film is characterized by a proliferation of cells that are slightly smaller than hairy cells and have a more clumped chromatin. Short villous projections are seen, often concentrated at one pole of the cell (Fig. 41.18D). A portion of the malignant cells often have plasmacytoid features, and a monoclonal protein in serum or urine is observed in 28% to 60% of cases (202,207).

Staining with T-AcP is reported as negative (202,203). Several patients who were described in an earlier report (209), however, may have had a similar disorder; their leukemic cells were T-AcP positive. The lymphoma cells in most cases of SLVL are reported to express CD22, FMC-7, and DBA.44. One half of cases express CD11c; CD25, CD103, and HC2 are expressed in 25% or fewer cases (142,207).

It is of particular importance that SLVL, unlike HCL, generally involves the white pulp of the spleen, with red pulp involvement to some degree (203,211). Bone marrow involvement is inconsistently observed (203). When it is present, it is patchy and in most cases is readily distinguished from HCL based on the more abundant cytoplasm in the latter.

Because the pattern of splenic involvement described in SLVL resembles that reported in splenic marginal zone lymphoma (211–216), several investigators have reviewed the morphology of the spleen and lymph nodes in cases diagnosed as SLVL or reviewed the peripheral blood films in patients with splenic marginal zone lymphoma. The histopathology of the spleen in cases of SLVL was found to be indistinguishable from splenic marginal zone lymphoma (211). Moreover, some patients with splenic marginal zone lymphoma had lymphocytosis with the leukemic cells showing villous projections indistinguishable from those described in SLVL (211,214–216). Immunophenotypic features in the two disorders are similar (142,213–215). Overall, it appears that series of patients reported to have SLVL and splenic marginal zone lymphoma are composed of largely overlapping populations.

Bone Marrow

A diagnosis of HCL most commonly is made by bone marrow examination (43). Hairy cells are distinguished eas-

A,B

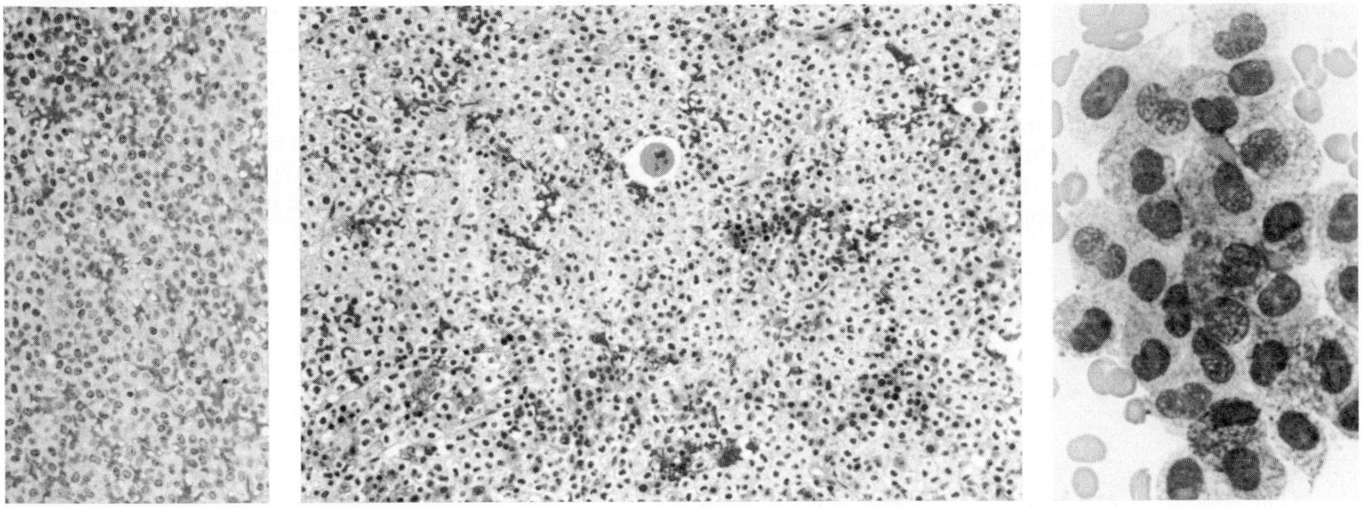

C

FIG. 41.19. Rare cases of mast cell leukemia may mimic hairy cell leukemia in bone core biopsies. **A:** Hairy cell leukemia (hematoxylin and eosin stain, original magnification: 250× magnification). **B:** Mast cell leukemia in bone core biopsy (hematoxylin and eosin stain, original magnification: 250× magnification). **C:** Mast cell leukemia in bone marrow aspirate (Wright stain, original magnification: 800× magnification).

ily from cells of CLL at low power by their abundant clear to pale eosinophilic cytoplasm. Hairy cell nuclei, unlike those in CLL, are evenly spaced apart and tend not to touch one another in thin sections. Bone marrow involvement in splenic marginal zone lymphoma with or without villous lymphocytes or SLVL is generally manifested as aggregates of small lymphocytes (215); however, occasional cases may mimic HCL. Unlike the infiltrates in follicle center cell lymphoma (217), hairy cell infiltrates are not found preferentially in a paratrabecular location. Prolymphocytic leukemia cells may be distinguished by their large central nucleoli and heterogeneity (114,197,198). The lymphoplasmacytic infiltrates in bone marrows from patients who have Waldenström's macroglobulinemia may simulate HCL, and they are occasionally positive for T-AcP (104).

In most cases, mast cell disease is easily distinguished from HCL. Unlike hairy cells, the neoplastic cells in mastocytosis often form tight aggregates or nodules that tend to lie adjacent to trabeculae. There is usually an associated infiltrate of eosinophils and small lymphocytes (118). In a few cases in which there is more widespread marrow involvement, the infiltrate in mastocytosis may bear a striking resemblance to HCL (47) (Fig. 41.19). In these cases, a proper diagnosis may be made by examination of Wright stained aspirates or imprints, by means of metachromatic stains, and by the naphthol-ASD-chloroacetate esterase reaction, which is positive in mast cells, or antibodies to tryptase. Mast cells, like hairy cells, may be positive for T-AcP (117).

Spleen

In the spleen, lymphomas, including splenic marginal zone lymphoma with or without villous lymphocytes, may be distinguished from HCL by their primary involvement of the white pulp rather than the red pulp (Table 41.2) (218). CLL expands the white pulp but with more extensive involvement may extend into the red pulp, so that a more diffuse pattern results (218). In the latter cases, cytologic features, particularly the scant cytoplasm of CLL, are the most helpful in the distinction of CLL from HCL. Prolymphocytic leukemia may involve red and white pulp alike. It often forms a pseudonodular pattern, and the infiltrates are composed of a mixture of cells, including some with large nucleoli (198). T-cell leukemias and lymphomas that involve the red pulp of the spleen may simulate HCL closely in tissue sections. These include large granular lymphocyte proliferations (219) and hepatosplenic $\gamma\delta$ T-cell lymphoma (200). Like HCL, histiocytic proliferations, infectious mononucleosis, and acute leukemias involve the red pulp, but they differ from HCL in their cytologic features (220). As in the bone marrow, mastocytosis in the spleen may occasionally mimic HCL; however, it tends to be distributed in and around splenic trabeculae and often is associated with an intense fibrous reaction (221).

Variants of Hairy Cell Leukemia

A few B-cell lymphoproliferative disorders have been described that are similar to ''typical'' HCL, but they display various differences in clinical presentation, morphology, immunophenotype, and response to therapy. Whether these disorders are truly HCL variants or distinct lymphoproliferative processes is mainly a matter of semantics; nevertheless, they should be distinguished from typical HCL because of possible differences in response to therapy.

Prolymphocytoid Variant

Patients who have the rare prolymphocytoid variant of HCL (HCL-V, also known as type II or variant HCL) show many of the clinical features of typical (type I) HCL (222–224). They often are middle-aged or elderly and have prominent splenomegaly with minimal lymphadenopathy. Unlike patients who have typical HCL, however, they generally have elevated WBC counts without neutropenia or monocytopenia. The cytologic features and immunophenotype of the neoplastic cells have been described as being intermediate between those of HCL and those of prolymphocytic leukemia (PLL) (223). The HCL-V cells have prominent hairy projections, but compared with typical hairy cells, their nucleus is positioned more centrally, chromatin is slightly more condensed, nucleoli are prominent, the nuclear to cytoplasmic ratio is higher, and the cytoplasm exhibits more basophilic staining (Fig. 41.18). Ribosome-lamellar complexes have not been observed. Bone marrows are typically aspirable, with preservation of hematopoiesis. As in typical HCL, the red pulp of the spleen is involved (222). The T-AcP reaction may be positive, but the reaction product tends to be localized at one pole of the cell. FMC-7 and CD11c are positive, CD103 is expressed in one third of cases, and antibodies to HC2 and CD25 are generally negative (224,225). Patients who have the prolymphocytoid variant do not respond as well to interferon, 2′-deoxycoformycin, or 2-chlorodeoxyadenosine therapy as those who have typical HCL (224,226).

Blastic Variant

Three elderly patients have been reported who had pancytopenia and splenomegaly that resulted from a neoplastic proliferation of T-AcP$^+$ B cells with villous projections and blastic features (227). The splenic red pulp was involved (227). Unlike patients who had typical HCL, these patients had prominent adenopathy, the neoplastic cells had fine chromatin and prominent nucleoli, cytoplasmic granules were observed, and erythrophagocytosis was seen in two of the patients (227). A rare patient has been reported with what the investigators believed to represent blastic transformation of HCL accompanied by loss of CD11c, CD25, and T-AcP positivity (228).

Japanese Variant

A disorder with similarities to HCL in the West is observed occasionally in Japan (229–231). In Japanese HCL patients, unlike those in the West, WBC counts are elevated, and neutropenia is typically absent (229,230). Although hairy projections are seen on the neoplastic cells by phase contrast microscopy, the cell border is smooth in blood films (231). In Japanese patients, T-AcP staining is less frequently positive (229,231), and immunophenotypic differences from Western HCL have been observed (230,232,233). Like HCL in Western populations, the neoplastic cells in this variant are positive for CD11c, CD20, and CD22. Results for CD103 are not reported (232,233). In contrast to Western HCL, CD25 is negative, and immunoglobulin is weak (232,233). Earlier reports suggested frequent expression of CD5 and CD10 (228,230). Preliminary evidence suggests that these patients may not respond as well to interferon therapy as do Western patients (231).

RESPONSE TO THERAPY

General Comments

In about 10% of patients, HCL is indolent, and therapy is not required, particularly in older patients with low tumor burden (12). Until effective treatments became available in the mid-1980s, splenectomy had been the mainstay of therapy for HCL, providing improvement of cytopenias in most patients and a normalization of blood counts in 40% to 60% (12). In a minority of cases, this improvement may be long lasting; however, most patients eventually develop progressive disease (12). In general, the initial response to splenectomy and the duration of that response depend on the extent of bone marrow involvement and on the total cellularity of the marrow, not on the spleen size (50,234). Splenectomy is most effective in patients who have significant cytopenias despite only patchy bone marrow involvement.

Beginning in 1984, effective medical therapies became available for HCL that abruptly changed the outlook for patients who have this disease. Several agents have been shown to control HCL in most patients, but it remains uncertain if any patients are truly cured of their disease. Active agents include the interferons and the adenosine deaminase inhibitor 2′-deoxycoformycin (pentostatin). Since the first edition of this text was published in 1992, the purine analogue 2-chlorodeoxyadenosine has emerged as the treatment of choice in HCL.

With effective therapy, many HCL bone marrows are now obtained to assess the patient's response to therapy. When the tumor burden is low, it becomes challenging to identify small numbers of residual hairy cells, even in ideally processed specimens. Immunohistochemical studies of the bone marrow may be helpful in this regard, although the clinical significance of detecting minimal residual disease is uncertain. Several noninvasive tests may be useful.

Interferon-α

In 1984, Quesada first reported on the effectiveness of partially purified interferon-α in the treatment of HCL (13,235). Later, recombinant interferon-α2 products were shown to be effective, and these became the most commonly used preparations.

The overall response rate for HCL patients treated with interferon-α varies from 38% to 82% (236–238). Complete remissions (239) (hemoglobin > 12 g/dL; platelets > 100

$\times$ 10^9/L; neutrophils > 1.5 $\times$ 10^9/L; no circulating hairy cells; bone marrow without identifiable hairy cells; regression to normal of organomegaly) are achieved in fewer than 15% of patients (12,237,240) because residual hairy cells almost always can be demonstrated in the bone marrow (32). However, most patients can achieve a good partial remission.

After an initial decline in the first weeks of therapy, improvement or normalization of blood counts is seen at 3 to 6 months along with elimination of hairy cells from the blood. Bone marrow morphology is often quite variable from area to area. Hairy cells gradually decline and hematopoiesis increases over the course of a year. Granulopoiesis lags behind erythroid recovery, and the myeloid to erythroid ratio seldom exceeds 1:1 (12,241). Lymphoid nodules are frequent. It is not clear whether interferon achieves its effects in HCL by a direct antiproliferative action on the hairy cells (242,243), by activation of elements of the immune system such as NK cells (244), or by another mechanism.

With the discontinuation of interferon-α therapy, hematopoietic activity decreases progressively, and the hairy cell infiltrate increases slowly. Despite the worsening histologic appearance of the bone marrow, blood counts usually remain stable for some time (32,241).

2′-Deoxycoformycin

An adenosine deaminase inhibitor, 2′-deoxycoformycin (dCF, pentostatin), has proved to be an extremely effective agent in the treatment of HCL. It is given as a rapid intravenous infusion every 2 weeks until maximum response is achieved.

Nearly all patients respond to dCF therapy, and approximately 50% to 85% achieve a durable complete remission (14,16,17,237,245). A large randomized study comparing dCF with interferon showed a significantly higher complete response rate and greater durability of responses in patients treated with the former agent (237). The response to dCF is rapid. After an initial decrease, blood counts improve within a few weeks from the start of therapy. By 3 to 6 months, hairy cells and reticulin fibrosis generally disappear from the marrow (14,16). Treatment is associated with lymphopenia that may persist for several years (246).

Although responses are more durable than in interferon treated patients, over time, relapses do occur. In studies with median follow-up times of 6 to 8 years, 25% to 50% of complete responders have relapsed (247,248). However, even with bone marrow relapse, blood counts remain stable, and retreatment may be delayed for months or years (14).

2-Chlorodeoxyadenosine

In 1990 Piro and colleagues (15) described 12 patients with HCL treated with a single 7-day infusion of the purine analogue 2-chlorodeoxyadenosine (2-CdA, cladrabine). Remarkably, 11 of the 12 achieved complete remissions. No relapses were seen initially, with patients followed as long as 3.8 years.

Since that report, large series with up to several hundred patients who were treated with this regimen have been reported, and it has emerged as the treatment of choice in HCL. This is based on the high rates and relative durability of response to this agent coupled with the relative ease of administration and manageable toxicity (18). The 2-CdA therapy is associated with a near 100% response rate. Complete response is obtained in 75% to 91% of patients (249–251), usually within 3 months.

Toxicity includes fever, neutropenia, infection and lymphopenia (245). Fever is observed in 40%. In most patients, infection cannot be documented, and fever is thought to be related to cytokines liberated as the hairy cells are eliminated (245). Neutrophil counts reach a nadir at 1 to 2 weeks and rebound to normal within 2 to 3 months (245). Lymphopenia, particularly of CD4 cells, may last for 1 to 2 years or longer (245,252,253).

Even in patients in so-called complete remission, small numbers of residual hairy cells may be demonstrated in the marrow by immunohistochemical techniques or molecular genetic studies. Of patients who enter complete remission, an estimated 16% relapse within 4 years (250,254) and 28% within 7 years (251), based on the reappearance of morphologically identifiable hairy cells in the bone core. Because there is no evident plateau in the curve for progression free survival, it is still uncertain whether any patients are cured or whether all patients who are followed for a long enough period eventually relapse (250). Up to 50% of patients in morphologic complete remission show evidence of minimal residual disease by immunohistochemical methods (255,256).

Reappearance of hairy cells in the marrow is generally not associated with deterioration of blood counts for many months or years. Retreatment is generally not required initially at relapse. A second course of 2-CdA therapy results in complete remission in about 40% to 60% of patients (250,254).

Detection of Minimal Residual Disease

In most studies of HCL, the definition of complete remission requires the absence of morphologically identifiable hairy cells in bone cores and aspirates (239). Pathologists often are asked to detect and quantify small numbers of residual hairy cells in bone marrows from treated patients. This task requires excellent histologic sections. However, even in optimally processed and sectioned bone cores examined by experienced observers, hairy cells in the range of 5% or fewer are extremely difficult to identify. Even if adequate Wright-stained aspirates are obtained, hairy cells are extremely difficult to identify when present in small percentages. The observation that relapse of HCL occurs over time in various proportions of patients treated with the therapeutic agents discussed previously suggests that hairy cells persist

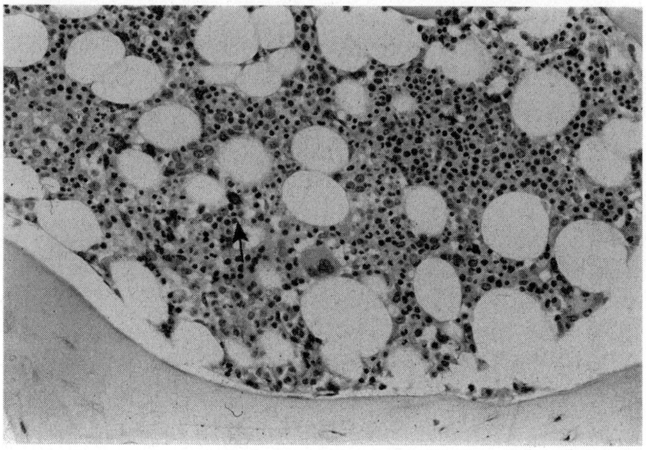

FIG. 41.20. Residual hairy cell leukemia after therapy with 2-chlorodeoxyadenosine (cladrabine). Hairy cells are positive for CD20 (immunoperoxidase stain, original magnification: 100× magnification). See Color Plate 25, between pp. 1446–1447.

in the bone marrow in many, if not all, treated patients at levels below the threshold of identification by morphologic examination. Investigators have identified minimal residual HCL in paraffin embedded bone cores by the staining of cells showing morphologic features of hairy cells with antibodies such as CD20 and DBA.44 (255,256) (Fig. 41.20; see also Color Plate 25, between pp. 1446–1447). These antibodies are not specific for hairy cells, and it is not always possible to be certain if an individual positive cell shows the morphology of a hairy cell in the bone core. Various groups have devised different criteria to define the presence of minimal residual HCL in 2-CdA treated patients. For this reason and others, the incidence of minimal residual HCL obtained by different groups is not comparable, but it ranges from 13% to 50% (255,256).

In cryostat sections, certain monoclonal antibodies such as anti-HC2 and CD103 that are more specific for hairy cells may be useful in detecting minimal residual disease (257,258). A small study using molecular techniques, including the polymerase chain reaction with clonospecific probes, reported minimal residual HCL in each of seven patients in ''complete remission'' after therapy with 2-CdA (259). Because of the slow rate of proliferation of hairy cells, the clinical significance of detection of minimal residual disease is uncertain.

Noninvasive Monitoring of Disease

Noninvasive studies may be helpful in assessing the extent of bone marrow involvement in HCL. The neutrophil alkaline phosphatase (NAP) score is elevated in most patients who have HCL, regardless of the presence or absence of infection (32,260). The NAP scores parallel the hairy cell index (32,241). With response to therapy, the NAP score falls, but it rises after treatment is discontinued, and the number of hairy cells in the bone marrow begins to increase (32,241).

Serum levels of soluble interleukin-2 receptor (IL-2R) are markedly elevated when enzyme-linked immunosorbent assays are used in patients who have HCL (261–263). It is believed that IL-2R is derived from the shedding of membrane interleukin-2 receptors from the surface of hairy cells (263). The level of IL-2R correlates with the extent of bone marrow involvement and with spleen size (262), falls in patients who respond to therapy (261,262,264), and may become normal in a few patients who achieve a complete remission (265,266). Magnetic resonance imaging has been used as a noninvasive way to measure the extent of bone marrow infiltration (267,268).

SUMMARY AND CONCLUSIONS

HCL is an uncommon chronic lymphoproliferative disorder that primarily affects middle-aged to elderly white men who often have cytopenias and enlarged spleens, without peripheral lymphadenopathy. The hallmark of HCL is the presence in the peripheral blood, bone marrow, and other tissues of characteristic malignant cells that, in stained peripheral blood films, using phase contrast microscopy or electron microscopy, have prominent villous projections. Immunophenotypic studies have shown hairy cells to be B cells at a middle to late stage of differentiation, and characteristic patterns of staining with combinations of monoclonal antibodies have proven helpful in confirming the diagnosis. Little is known about the basic mechanisms involved in the pathogenesis of HCL. During the past several years, a number of therapeutic agents have proven to be extremely effective in controlling this disorder and have improved greatly the prognosis for patients who have HCL.

ACKNOWLEDGMENTS

I am indebted to Drs. James Vardiman and Maria Paoletti for their valuable contributions in the preparation of this chapter, Drs. Sanford Peck and Randy McMurtry for helpful suggestions, and Ms. Nancy Hart for typing the manuscript.

REFERENCES

1. Bouroncle BA, Wiseman BK, Doan CA. Leukemic reticuloendotheliosis. *Blood* 1958;13:609–630.
2. Schreck R, Donnelly WJ. ''Hairy'' cells in blood in lymphoreticular neoplastic disease and ''flagellated'' cells of normal lymph nodes. *Blood* 1966;27:199–211.
3. Catovsky D, Pettit JE, Galetto J, et al. The B-lymphocyte nature of the hairy cell of leukaemic reticuloendotheliosis. *Br J Haematol* 1974; 26:29–37.
4. Golde DW, Stevens RH, Quan SG, et al. Immunoglobulin synthesis in hairy cell leukemia. *Br J Haematol* 1977;35:359–365.
5. Golomb HM, Vardiman J, Sweet DL, et al. Hairy cell leukaemia: evidence for the existence of a spectrum of functional characteristics. *Br J Haematol* 1978;38:161–170.
6. Jansen J, Schuit HRE, Meijer CJLM, et al. Cell markers in hairy cell leukemia studied in cells from 51 patients. *Blood* 1982;59:52–60.

7. Jansen J, denOttolander GJ, Schuit HRE, et al. Hairy cell leukemia: its place among the chronic B cell leukemias. *Semin Oncol* 1984;11: 386–393.
8. Anderson KC, Boyd AW, Fisher DC, et al. Hairy cell leukemia: a tumor of pre-plasma cells. *Blood* 1985;65:620–629.
9. Falini B, Schwarting R, Erber W, et al. The differential diagnosis of hairy cell leukemia with a panel of monoclonal antibodies. *Am J Clin Pathol* 1985;83:289–300.
10. Korsmeyer SJ, Greene WC, Cossman J, et al. Rearrangement and expression of immunoglobulin genes and expression of Tac antigen in hairy cell leukemia. *Proc Natl Acad Sci USA* 1983;80:4522–4526.
11. Cleary ML, Wood GS, Warnke R, et al. Immunoglobulin gene rearrangements in hairy cell leukemia. *Blood* 1984;64:99–104.
12. Doane LL, Ratain MJ, Golomb HM. Hairy cell leukemia: current management. *Hematol Oncol Clin North Am* 1990:4:489–502.
13. Quesada JR, Reuben J, Manning JT, et al. Alpha interferon for induction of remission in hairy cell leukemia. *N Engl J Med* 1984;310: 15–18.
14. Kraut EH, Bouroncle BA, Grever MR. Pentostatin in the treatment of advanced hairy cell leukemia. *J Clin Oncol* 1989;7:168–172.
15. Piro LD, Carrera CJ, Carson DA, et al. Lasting remissions in hairy cell leukemia induced by a single infusion of 2-chlorodeoxyadenosine. *N Engl J Med* 1990;322:1117–1121.
16. Spiers ASD, Moore D, Cassileth PA, et al. Remissions in hairy cell leukemia with pentostatin (2′-deoxycoformycin). *N Engl J Med* 1987; 316:825–830.
17. Johnston JB, Eisenhauer E, Corbett WEN, et al. Efficacy of 2′-deoxycoformycin in hairy cell leukemia: a study of the National Cancer Institute of Canada Clinical Trials Group. *J Natl Cancer Inst* 1988; 80:765–769.
18. Piro LD, Ellison DJ, Saven A. The Scripps Clinic experience with 2-chlorodeoxyadenosine in the treatment of hairy cell leukemia. *Leuk Lymphoma* 1994;13:121–125.
19. Bernstein L, Newton P, Ross RK. Epidemiology of hairy cell leukemia in Los Angeles County. *Cancer Res* 1990;50:3605–3609.
20. Golomb HM, Catovsky D, Golde DW. Hairy cell leukemia: a clinical review based on 71 cases. *Ann Intern Med* 1978;89:677–683.
21. Bouroncle B. Leukemic reticuloendotheliosis (hairy cell leukemia). *Blood* 1979;53:412–436.
22. Flandrin G, Sigaux F, Sebahoun G, et al. Hairy cell leukemia: clinical presentation and follow-up of 211 patients. *Semin Oncol* 1984;11: 458–471.
23. Frassoldati A, Lamparelli T, Federico M, et al. Hairy cell leukemia: a clinical review based on 725 cases of the Italian Cooperative Group (ICGHCL). *Leuk Lymphoma* 1994;13:307–316.
24. Ramseur WL, Golomb HM, Vardiman JW, et al. Hairy cell leukemia in father and son. *Cancer* 1981;48:1825–1829.
25. Wylin RF, Greene MH, Palutke M, et al. Hairy cell leukemia in three siblings: an apparent HLA-linked disease. *Cancer* 1982;49:538–542.
26. Milligan DW, Stark AN, Bynoe AG. Case reports: Hairy cell leukaemia in two brothers. *Clin Lab Haematol* 1987;9:321–325.
27. Begley CG, Tait B, Crapper RM, et al. Familial hairy cell leukemia. *Leuk Res* 1987;11:1027–1029.
28. Ward FT, Baker J, Krishnan J, et al. Hairy cell leukemia in two siblings: a human leukocyte antigen-linked disease? *Cancer* 1990;65: 319–321.
29. Egli FL, Koller B, Furrer J. Hairy cell leukemia and glucose-6-phosphate dehydrogenase deficiency in two brothers. *N Engl J Med* 1990; 322:1159.
30. Gramatovici M, Bennett JM, Hiscock JG, et al. Three cases of familial hairy cell leukemia. *Am J Hematol* 1993;42:337–339.
31. Seshadri RS, Brown EJ, Zipursky A. Leukemic reticuloendotheliosis: a failure of monocyte production. *N Engl J Med* 1976;295:181–184.
32. Bardawil RG, Ratain MJ, Golomb HM, et al. Changes in peripheral blood and bone marrow specimens during and after α 2b interferon therapy for hairy cell leukemia. *Leukemia* 1987;1:340–343.
33. Levine PH, Katayama I. The platelet in leukemic reticuloendotheliosis: functional and morphological evidence of a qualitative disorder. *Cancer* 1975;36:1353–1358.
34. Zuzel M, Cawley JC, Paton RC, et al. Platelet function in hairy cell leukemia. *Am J Clin Pathol* 1979;32:814–821.
35. Bouroncle BA. Thirty-five years in the progress of hairy cell leukemia. *Leuk Lymphoma* 1994;14:1–12.
36. Burke JS, Byrne GE, Rappaport H. Hairy cell leukemia (leukemic reticuloendotheliosis): a clinical pathologic study of 21 patients. *Cancer* 1974;33:1399–1410.
37. Katayama I, Finkel HE. Leukemic reticuloendotheliosis: a clinicopathologic study with review of the literature. *Am J Med* 1974;57: 115–126.
38. Naeim F, Smith GS. Leukemic reticuloendotheliosis. *Cancer* 1974; 34:1813–1821.
39. Hanson CA, Ward PCJ, Schnitzer B. A multilobular variant of hairy cell leukemia with morphologic similarities to T-cell lymphoma. *Am J Surg Pathol* 1989;13:671–679.
40. Katayama I, Schneider GB. Further ultrastructural characterization of hairy cells of leukemic reticuloendotheliosis. *Am J Pathol* 1977;86: 163–182.
41. Brunning RD, Parkin J. Ribosome-lamella complexes in neoplastic hematopoietic cells. *Am J Pathol* 1975;79:565–578.
42. Tubbs RR, Savage RA. Occurrence of ribosome-lamella complexes. *N Engl J Med* 1983;309:616.
43. Burke JS. The value of the bone-marrow biopsy in the diagnosis of hairy cell leukemia. *Am J Clin Pathol* 1978;70:876–884.
44. Katayama I. Bone marrow in hairy cell leukemia. *Hematol Oncol Clin North Am* 1988;2:585–602.
45. Ng J-P, Hogg RB, Cumming RLC, et al. Primary splenic hairy cell leukaemia: a case report and review of the literature. *Eur J Haematol* 1987;39:349–352.
46. Myers TJ, Ikeda Y, Schwartz S, et al. Primary splenic hairy cell leukemia remission for 21 years following splenectomy. *Am J Hematol* 1981;11:299–303.
47. Burke JS, Rappaport H. The diagnosis and differential diagnosis of hairy cell leukemia in bone marrow and spleen. *Semin Oncol* 1984; 11:334–346.
48. Lee WMF, Beckstead JH. Hairy cell leukemia with bone marrow hypoplasia. *Cancer* 1982;50:2207–2210.
49. Paoletti M, Bitter MA, Vardiman JW. Hairy cell leukemia: morphologic, cytochemical, and immunologic features. *Clin Lab Med* 1988; 8:179–195.
50. Golomb HM, Vardiman JW. Response to splenectomy in 65 patients with hairy cell leukemia: an evaluation of spleen weight and bone marrow involvement. *Blood* 1983;61:349–352.
51. Bouroncle BA. Unusual presentations and complications of hairy cell leukemia. *Leukemia* 1987;1:288–293.
52. Burke JS, Sheibani K, Winberg CD, et al. Recognition of hairy cell leukemia in a spleen of normal weight: the contribution of immunohistologic studies. *Am J Clin Pathol* 1987;87:276–281.
53. Pilon VA, Davey FR, Gordon GB, et al. Splenic alterations in hairy cell leukemia: II. An electron microscopic study. *Cancer* 1982;49: 1617–1623.
54. Nanba K, Soban EJ, Bowling MC, et al. Splenic pseudosinuses and hepatic angiomatous lesions: distinctive features of hairy cell leukemia. *Am J Clin Pathol* 1977;67:415–426.
55. Vardiman JW, Golomb HM. Autopsy findings in hairy cell leukemia. *Semin Oncol* 1984;11:370–380.
56. Yam LT, Janckila AJ, Chan CH, et al. Hepatic involvement in hairy cell leukemia. *Cancer* 1983;51:1497–1504.
57. Roquet ML, Zafrani ES, Farcet JP, et al. Histopathological lesions of the liver in hairy cell leukemia: a report of 14 cases. *Hepatology* 1985; 5:496–500.
58. Zafrani ES, Degos F, Guigui B, et al. The hepatic sinusoid in hairy cell leukemia: an ultrastructural study of 12 cases. *Hum Pathol* 1987; 18:801–807.
59. Malik STA, Amess J, D'Ardenne AJ, et al. Hairy cell leukemia—mediastinal involvement. A report of two cases and review of the literature. *Hematol Oncol* 1989;7:303–306.
60. Hakimian D, Tallman MS, Hogan DK, et al. Prospective evaluation of internal adenopathy in a cohort of 43 patients with hairy cell leukemia. *J Clin Oncol* 1994;12:268–272.
61. Mercieca J, Matutes E, Moskovic E. Massive abdominal lymphadenopathy in hairy cell leukemia: a report of 12 cases. *Br J Haematol* 1992;82:547–554.
62. Mercieca J, Puga M, Matutes E, et al. Incidence and significance of abdominal lymphadenopathy in hairy cell leukaemia. *Leuk Lymphoma* 1994;14:79–83.
63. Lembersky BC, Ratain MJ, Golomb HM. Skeletal complications in hairy cell leukemia: diagnosis and therapy. *J Clin Oncol* 1988;6: 1280–1284.

64. Herold CJ, Wittich GR, Schwarzinger I, et al. Skeletal involvement in hairy cell leukemia. *Skel Radiol* 1988;17:171–175.
65. Arkel YS, Lake-Lewin D, Savopoulos AA, et al. Bone lesions in hairy cell leukemia: a case report and response of bone pains to steroids. *Cancer* 1984;53:2401–2403.
66. DeManes DJ, Lane N, Beckstead JH. Bone involvement in hairy cell leukemia. *Cancer* 1982;49:1697–1701.
67. VanderMolen LA, Urba WJ, Longo DL, et al. Diffuse osteosclerosis in hairy cell leukemia. *Blood* 1989;74:2066–2069.
68. Lawrence DM, Sun NCJ, Mena R, et al. Cutaneous lesions in hairy cell leukemia: case report and review of the literature. *Arch Dermatol* 1983;119:322–325.
69. Finan MC, Su WP, Li C-Y. Cutaneous findings in hairy cell leukemia. *J Am Acad Dermatol* 1984;11:788–797.
70. Ari E, Ikeda S, Itoh S, et al. Specific skin lesions as the presenting symptom of hairy cell leukemia. *Am J Clin Pathol* 1988;90:459–464.
71. Bouza E, Burgaleta C, Golde DW. Infections in hairy cell leukemia. *Blood* 1978;51:851–859.
72. Cawley JC, Gordon FB, Hayhoe FGJ. *Hairy cell leukemia*. New York: Springer-Verlag, 1980.
73. Golomb HM, Hadad L. Infectious complications in 127 patients with hairy cell leukemia. *Am J Hematol* 1984;16:393–401.
74. Bennett C, Vardiman J, Golomb H. Disseminated atypical mycobacterial infection in patients with hairy cell leukemia. *Am J Med* 1986; 80:891–896.
75. Gabriel SE, Conn DL, Phyliky RL, et al. Vasculitis in hairy cell leukemia: review of literature and consideration of possible pathogenic mechanisms. *J Rheumatol* 1986;13:1167–1172.
76. Farcet J-P, Weschsler J, Wirquin V, et al. Vasculitis in hairy cell leukemia. *Arch Intern Med* 1987;147:660–664.
77. Hasler P, Kistler H, Gerber H. Vasculitides in hairy cell leukemia. *Semin Arthritis Rheum* 1995;25:134–142.
78. Westbrook CA, Golde DW. Autoimmune disease in hairy cell leukaemia: clinical syndromes and treatment. *Br J Haematol* 1985;61: 349–356.
79. Spann CR, Callen JP, Yam LT, et al. Cutaneous leukocytoclastic vasculitis complicating hairy cell leukemia (leukemic reticuloendotheliosis). *Arch Dermatol* 1986;122:1057–1059.
80. Hughes GRV, Elkon KB, Spiller R, et al. Polyarteritis nodosa and hairy cell leukemia. *Lancet* 1979;1:678.
81. Elkon KB, Hughes GRV, Catovsky D, et al. Hairy cell leukemia with polyarteritis nodosa. *Lancet* 1979;2:280–282.
82. Goedert JJ, Neefe JR, Smith FR, et al. Polyarteritis nodosa, hairy cell leukemia and splenosis. *Am J Med* 1981;71:323–326.
83. Lie JT. Isolated polyarteritis of testis in hairy cell leukemia. *Arch Pathol Lab Med* 1988;112:646–647.
84. Jacobs RH, Vokes EE, Golomb HM. Second malignancies in hairy cell leukemia. *Cancer* 1985;56:1462–1467.
85. Kampmeier P, Spielberger R, Dickstein J, et al. Increased incidence of second neoplasms in patients treated with interferon α-2b for hairy cell leukemia: a clinicopathologic assessment. *Blood* 1994;83: 2931–2938.
86. Huang T-Y, Yam LT. Coexistence of testicular carcinoma and hairy cell leukemia. *Urology* 1991;37:135–137.
87. Kurzrock R, Strom SS, Estey E, et al. Second cancer risk in hairy cell leukemia: analysis of 350 patients. *J Clin Oncol* 1997;15:1803–1810.
88. Troussard X, Henry-Amar M, Flandrin G. Second cancer risk after interferon therapy? *Blood* 1994;84:3242–3243.
89. Vokes EE, Bitter MA, Prystowsky MB, et al. Hairy cell leukemia associated with Hodgkin's disease: a case report. *Am J Hematol* 1985; 18:413–419.
90. Nakamine H, Okamoto Y, Tsuda T, et al. Hodgkin's disease in hairy cell leukemia: phenotypic characterization of neoplastic cells. *Cancer* 1987;60:1751–1756.
91. Catovsky D, Costello C, Loukopoulos D, et al. Hairy cell leukemia and myelomatosis: chance association or clinical manifestations of the same B-cell disease spectrum. *Blood* 1981;57:758–763.
92. Crump M, Sutton DM, Pantalony D. Sézary syndrome in a patient with hairy cell leukemia in remission. *Cancer* 1991;68:829–833.
93. Franssila KO. Coincidental hairy cell leukemia and large cell malignant lymphoma. *Arch Pathol Lab Med* 1979;103:437–439.
94. Downing JR, Grossi CE, Smedberg CT, et al. Diffuse large cell lymphoma in a patient with hairy cell leukemia: immunoglobulin gene analysis reveals separate clonal origins. *Blood* 1986;67:739–744.
95. Arnalich F, Camacho J, Jimenez C, et al. Occurrence of immunoblastic B-cell lymphoma in hairy cell leukemia. *Cancer* 1987;59:1161–1164.
96. Abbondanzo SL, Sulak LE. Ki-1–positive lymphoma developing 10 years after the diagnosis of hairy cell leukemia. *Cancer* 1991;67: 3117–3122.
97. Pawson R, A'Hern RA, Catovsky D. Second malignancy in hairy cell leukaemia: no evidence of increased incidence after treatment with interferon alpha. *Leuk Lymphoma* 1996;22:103–106.
98. Au WY, Klassa RJ, Gallagher R, et al. Second malignancies in patients with hairy cell leukemia in British Columbia: a 20-year experience. *Blood* 1998;92:1160–1164.
99. Li CY, Yam LT, Lam KW. Studies of acid phosphatase isoenzymes in human leukocytes: demonstration of isoenzyme cell specificity. *J Histochem Cytochem* 1970;18:901–910.
100. Li CY, Yam LT, Lam KW. Acid phosphatase isoenzyme in human leukocytes in normal and pathologic conditions. *J Histochem Cytochem* 1970;18:473–481.
101. Yam LT, Li CY, Lam KW. Tartrate-resistant acid phosphatase isoenzyme in the reticulum cells of leukemic reticuloendotheliosis. *N Engl J Med* 1971;284:357–360.
102. Ketcham CM, Roberts RM, Simmen RCM, et al. Molecular cloning of the type 5, iron-containing, tartrate-resistant acid phosphatase from human placenta. *J Biol Chem* 1989;264:557–563.
103. Janckila AJ, Li C-Y, Lam KW, et al. The cytochemistry of tartrate-resistant acid phosphatase: technical considerations. *Am J Clin Pathol* 1978;70:45–55.
104. Yam LT, Janckila AJ, Li C-Y, et al. Chemistry of tartrate-resistant acid phosphatase: 15 years' experience. *Leukemia* 1987;1:285–288.
105. Strickler JG, Schmidt CM, Wick MR. Methods in pathology: immunophenotype of hairy cell leukemia in paraffin sections. *Mod Pathol* 1990;3:518–523.
106. Beckstead JH, Halverson PS, Ries CA, et al. Enzyme histochemistry and immunohistochemistry on biopsy specimens of pathologic human bone marrow. *Blood* 1981;57:1088–1098.
107. Janckila AJ, Cardwell EM, Yam LT, et al. Hairy cell identification by immunohistochemistry of tartrate-resistant acid phosphatase. *Blood* 1995;85:2839–2844.
108. Janckila AJ, Lear SC, Martin AW, et al. Epitope enhancement for immunohistochemical demonstration of tartrate-resistant acid phosphatase. *J Histochem Cytochem* 1996;44:235–244.
109. Hoyer JD, Li C-Y, Yam LT, et al. Immunohistochemical demonstration of acid phosphatase isoenzyme 5 (tartrate-resistant) in paraffin sections of hairy cell leukemia and other hematologic disorders. *Am J Clin Pathol* 1997;108:308–315.
110. Katayama I, Yang JPS. Reassessment of a cytochemical test for differential diagnosis of leukemic reticuloendotheliosis. *Am J Clin Pathol* 1977;68:268–272.
111. Variakojis D, Vardiman JW, Golomb HM. Cytochemistry of hairy cells. *Cancer* 1980;45:72–77.
112. Naeim F, Jacobs AD. Bone marrow changes in patients with hairy cell leukemia treated by recombinant alpha$_2$-interferon. *Hum Pathol* 1985;16:1200–1205.
113. Usui T, Konishi H, Sawada H, et al. Existence of tartrate-resistant acid phosphatase activity in differentiated lymphoid leukemic cells. *Am J Hematol* 1982;12:47–54.
114. Katayama I, Motohiko A, Pechet L, et al. B-lineage prolymphocytic leukemia as a distinct clinicopathologic entity. *Am J Pathol* 1980;99: 399–412.
115. Drexler HG, Gaedicke G, Minowada J. Isoenzyme studies in human leukemia-lymphoma cell lines: II. Acid phosphatase. *Leuk Res* 1985; 9:537–548.
116. Naeim F, Capostagno VJ, Johnson CE Jr, et al. Sézary syndrome: tartrate-resistant acid phosphatase in the neoplastic cells. *Am J Clin Pathol* 1979;71:528–533.
117. Yam LT, Yam C-F, Li C-Y. Eosinophilia in systemic mastocytosis. *Am J Clin Pathol* 1980;73:48–54.
118. Webb TA, Li C-Y, Yam LT. Systemic mast cell disease: a clinical and hematopathologic study of 26 cases. *Cancer* 1982;49:927–938.
119. Jaffe ES, Shevach EM, Frank MM, et al. Leukemic reticuloendotheliosis: presence of a receptor for cytophilic antibody. *Am J Med* 1974; 57:108–114.
120. King GW, Hurtubise PE, Sagone AL, et al. Leukemic reticuloendotheliosis: a study of the origin of the malignant cell. *Am J Med* 1975; 59:411–416.

121. Kluin-Nelemans HC, Krouwels MM, Jansen JH, et al. Hairy cell leukemia preferentially expresses the IgG3-subclass. *Blood* 1990;75: 972–975.
122. Kalyanaraman VS, Sarngadharan MG, Robert-Guroff M, et al. A new subtype of human T-cell leukemia virus (HTLV-II) associated with a T-cell variant of hairy cell leukemia. *Science* 1982;218:571–573.
123. Armitage RJ, Worman CP, Galvin MC, et al. Hairy cell leukemia with hybrid B-T features: a study with a panel of monoclonal antibodies. *Am J Hematol* 1985;18:335–344.
124. Wagner SD, Martinelli V, Luzzatto L. Similar patterns of Vκ gene usage but different degrees of somatic mutation in hairy cell leukemia, prolymphocytic leukemia, Waldenström's macroglobulinemia, and myeloma. *Blood* 1994;83:3647–3653.
125. Zomas AP, Matutes E, Morilla R, et al. Expression of the immunoglobulin-associated protein B29 in B cell disorders with the monoclonal antibody SN8 (CD79b). *Leukemia* 1996;10:1966–1970.
126. Melo JV, San Miguel JF, Moss VE, et al. The membrane phenotype of hairy cell leukemia: a study with monoclonal antibodies. *Semin Oncol* 1984;11:381–385.
127. Hsu S-M, Yang K, Jaffe ES. Hairy cell leukemia: a B cell neoplasm with a unique antigenic phenotype. *Am J Clin Pathol* 1983;80: 421–428.
128. Naeim F, Hoon DSB, Cheng L, et al. Reactivity of neoplastic cells of hairy cell leukemia with antisera to S-100 protein. *Am J Clin Pathol* 1987;88:86–91.
129. Sansoni P, Rowden G, Manara GC, et al. Immunoelectron microscopic demonstration of S-100 protein in hairy cell leukemia cells. *Am J Clin Pathol* 1988;89:374–377.
130. Stroup R, Sheibani K. Antigenic phenotypes of hairy cell leukemia and monocytoid B-cell lymphoma: an immunohistochemical evaluation of 66 cases. *Hum Pathol* 1992;23:172–177.
131. Posnett DN, Chiorazzi N, Kunkel HG. Monoclonal antibodies with specificity for hairy cell leukemia cells. *J Clin Invest* 1982;70: 254–261.
132. Berman E, Posnett DN. Diagnosis and monitoring in patients with hairy cell leukemia using the monoclonal antibody anti-HC2. *Leukemia* 1987;1:305–307.
133. Schwarting R, Stein H, Wang C-Y. The monoclonal antibodies αS-HCL 1 (αLeu-14) and αS-HCL 3 (αLeu-M5) allow the diagnosis of hairy cell leukemia. *Blood* 1985;65:974–983.
134. Visser L, Shaw A, Slupsky J, et al. Monoclonal antibodies reactive with hairy cell leukemia. *Blood* 1989;74:320–325.
135. Posnett DN, Marboe CC. Differentiation antigens associated with hairy cell leukemia. *Semin Oncol* 1984;11:413–415.
136. Chadburn A, Inghirami G, Knowles DM. Hairy cell leukemia-associated antigen LeuM5 (CD11c) is preferentially expressed by benign activated and neoplastic CD8 T cells. *Am J Pathol* 1990;136:29–37.
137. Vardiman JW, Gilewski TA, Ratain MJ, et al. Bradlow BA, Golumb HM. Evaluation of leu-M5 (CD11c) in hairy cell leukemia by the alkaline phosphatase anti-alkaline phosphatase technique. *Am J Clin Pathol* 1988;20:250–256.
138. Robbins BA, Ellison DJ, Spinosa JC, et al. Diagnostic application of two-color flow cytometry in 161 cases of hairy cell leukemia. *Blood* 1993;82:1277–1287.
139. Micklem KJ, Dong Y, Willis A, et al. HML-1 antigen on mucosa-associated T cells, activated cells, and hairy leukemic cells is a new integrin containing the β7 subunit. *Am J Pathol* 1991;139:1297–1301.
140. Mulligan SP, Travade P, Matutes E, et al. B-LY-7, a monoclonal antibody reactive with hairy cell leukemia, also defines an activation antigen on normal $CD8^+$ T cells. *Blood* 1990;76:959–964.
141. Möller P, Mielke B, Moldenhauer G. Monoclonal antibody HML-1, a marker for intraepithelial T cells and lymphomas derived thereof, also recognizes hairy cell leukemia and some B-cell lymphomas. *Am J Pathol* 1990;136:509–512.
142. Matutes E, Morilla R, Owusu-Ankomah K, et al. The immunophenotype of splenic lymphoma with villous lymphocytes and its relevance to the differential diagnosis with other B-cell disorders. *Blood* 1994; 83:1558–1562.
143. Chilosi M, Pizzolo G. Immunophenotypical diagnosis and monitoring of hairy cell leukemia. *Leukemia* 1990;4:168–169.
144. Kreft A, Büsche G, Bernhards J, et al. Immunophenotype of hairy cell leukaemia after cold polymerization of methyl-methacrylate embeddings from 50 diagnostic bone marrow biopsies. *Histopathology* 1997;30:145–151.
145. Zaja F, Di Loreto C, Amoroso V, et al. BCL-2 immunohistochemical evaluation in B-cell chronic lymphocytic leukemia and hairy cell leukemia before treatment with fludarabine and 2-chloro-deoxy-adenosine. *Leuk Lymphoma* 1998;28:567–572.
146. Hounieu H, Chittal SM, Saati TA, et al. Hairy cell leukemia: diagnosis of bone marrow involvement in paraffin-embedded sections with monoclonal antibody DBA.44. *Am J Clin Pathol* 1992;98:26–33.
147. van den Oord JJ, de Wolf-Peters C, Desmet VJ. Hypothesis. Hairy cell leukemia: a B-lymphocytic disorder derived from splenic marginal zone lymphocytes? *Blut* 1985;50:191–194.
148. Sheibani K, Sohn CC, Burke JS, et al. Monocytoid B-cell lymphoma: a novel B-cell neoplasm. *Am J Pathol* 1986;124:310–318.
149. Burke JS, Sheibani K. Hairy cells and monocytoid B lymphocytes: are they related? *Leukemia* 1987;1:298–300.
150. Machii T, Kitani T. Similarities between IgG-bearing lymphocytes and hairy cells: cytologic and cytochemical studies. *Blood* 1984;64: 166–172.
151. Posnett DN, Wang C-Y, Chiorazzi N, et al. An antigen characteristic of hairy cell leukemia cells is expressed on certain activated B cells. *J Immunol* 1984;133:1635–1640.
152. Robinson DSF, Posnett DN, Zola H, et al. Normal counterparts of hairy cells and B-prolymphocytes in the peripheral blood: an ultrastructural study with monoclonal antibodies and the immunogold method. *Leuk Res* 1985;9:335–348.
153. Hsu S-M. Phenotypic expression of B lymphocytes: III. Marginal zone B cells in the spleen are characterized by the expression of tac and alkaline phosphatase. *J Immunol* 1985;135:123–130.
154. van Krieken JHJM, von Schilling C, Kluin M, et al. Splenic marginal zone lymphocytes and related cells in the lymph node: a morphologic and immunohistochemical study. *Hum Pathol* 1989;20:320–325.
155. Timens W, Poppema S. Lymphocyte compartments in human spleen: an immunohistologic study in normal spleens and noninvolved spleens in Hodgkin's disease. *Am J Pathol* 1985;120:443–454.
156. Cordone I, Annino A, Masi, et al. Diagnostic relevance of peripheral blood immunocytochemistry in hairy cell leukaemia. *J Clin Pathol* 1995;48:955–960.
157. Cawley JC, Armitage RJ, Worman CP. T cell subsets in hairy cell leukemia. *Semin Oncol* 1984;11:405–408.
158. Lauria F, Foà R, Matera L, et al. Membrane phenotype and functional behavior of T lymphocytes in hairy cell leukemia. *Semin Oncol* 1984; 11:409–412.
159. Foà R, Fierro MT, Lusso P, et al. Effect of α-interferon on the immune system of patients with hairy cell leukemia. *Leukemia* 1987;1: 377–379.
160. Van der Horst FAL, van der Marel A, den Ottolander GJ, et al. Decrease of memory T helper cells ($CD4^+CD45RO^+$) in hairy cell leukemia. *Leukemia* 1993;7:46–50.
161. Kluin-Nelemans JC, Kester MGD, Oving I, et al. Abnormally activated T lymphocytes in the spleen of patients with hairy cell leukemia. *Leukemia* 1994;8:2095–2101.
162. Ruco LP, Procopio A, Maccallini V, et al. Severe deficiency of natural killer activity in the peripheral blood of patients with hairy cell leukemia. *Blood* 1983;61:1132–1137.
163. Nielson B, Hokland P, Ellegaard J, et al. Whole blood assay for NK activity in splenectomized and non-splenectomized hairy cell leukemia patients during IFN-α treatment. *Leuk Res* 1989;13:451–456.
164. Trentin L, Zambello R, Agostini C, et al. Mechanisms accounting for the defective natural killer activity in patients with hairy cell leukemia. *Blood* 1990;75:1525–1530.
165. Demeter J, Paloczi K, Lehoczky D, et al. Hairy cell leukemia: observations on natural killer activity in different clinical stages of the disease. *Br J Haematol* 1989;71:239–244.
166. Hooper WC, Barth RF, Shah NT. Lack of natural killer cell activity in hairy cell leukemia patients and partial restoration with interleukin-2. *Cancer* 1986;57:988–993.
167. Hansen DA, Robbins BA, Bylund DJ, et al. Identification of monoclonal immunoglobulins and quantitative immunoglobulin abnormalities in hairy cell leukemia and chronic lymphocytic leukemia. *Am J Clin Pathol* 1994;102;580–585.
168. Giardina SL, Schroff RW, Woodhouse CS, et al. Detection of two distinct malignant B cell clones in a single patient using anti-idiotype monoclonal antibodies and immunoglobulin gene rearrangement. *Blood* 1985;86:1017–1021.
169. Taniguchi N, Kuratsune H, Kanamaru A. Inhibition against CFU-C

and CFU-E colony formation by soluble factor(s) derived from hairy cells. *Blood* 1989;73:907–913.
170. Lindemann A, Ludwig W-D, Oster W, et al. High-level secretion of tumor necrosis factor-alpha contributes to hematopoietic failure in hairy cell leukemia. *Blood* 1989;73:880–884.
171. Richman CM, Golomb HM. Hairy cell leukemia: effect of hairy cells on normal granulopoiesis in vitro. *Exp Hematol* 1979;7:411–415.
172. Schwarzmeier JD, Gaschè CG, Hilgarth MF, et al. Myelosuppression in HCL: role of hairy cells, T cells and haematopoietic growth factors. *Br J Haematol* 1994;55:257–262.
173. Schwarzmeier JD, Hilgarth M, Nguyen ST, et al. Inadequate production of hematopoietic growth factors in hairy cell leukemia: up-regulation of interleukin 6 by recombinant IFN-α in vitro. *Cancer Res* 1996; 56:4679–4685.
174. Golomb HM, Lindgren V, Rowley JD. Chromosome abnormalities in patients with hairy cell leukemia. *Cancer* 1978;41:1374–1380.
175. Ueshima Y, Alimena G, Rowley JD, et al. Cytogenetic studies in patients with hairy cell leukemia. *Hematol Oncol* 1983;1:215–226.
176. Ohyashiki K, Ohyashiki JH, Takeuchi J, et al. Cytogenetic studies in hairy cell leukemia. *Cancer Genet Cytogenet* 1987;24:109–117.
177. Haglund U, Juliusson G, Stellan B, et al. Hairy cell leukemia is characterized by clonal chromosome abnormalities clustered to specific regions. *Blood* 1994;83:2637–2645.
178. Migone N, Giubellino MC, Casorati G, et al. Configuration of the immunoglobulin and T cell receptor gene regions in hairy cell leukemia and B-chronic lymphocytic leukemia. *Leukemia* 1987;1:393–394.
179. Lehn P, Sigaux F, Grausz D, et al. c-Myc and c-fos expression during interferon-α therapy for hairy cell leukemia. *Blood* 1986;68:967–970.
180. Bosch F, Campo E, Jares P, et al. Increased expression of the PRAD-1/CCND1 gene in hairy cell leukemia. *Br J Haematol* 1995;91: 1025–1030.
181. DeBoer CJ, van Krieken JHJM, Kluin-Nelemans HC, et al. Cyclin D1 messenger RNA overexpression as a marker for mantle cell lymphoma. *Oncogene* 1995;10:1833–1840.
182. Motokura T, Bloom T, Kim HG, et al. A novel cyclin encoded by a bcl1-linked candidate oncogene. *Nature* 1991;350:512–515.
183. Williams ME, Meeker TC, Swerdlow SH. Rearrangement of the chromosome 11 bcl-1 locus in centrocytic lymphoma: analysis with multiple breakpoint probes. *Blood* 1991;78:493–498.
184. Rimokh R, Berger F, Delsol G, et al. Rearrangement and overexpression of the BCL-1/PRAD-1 gene in intermediate lymphocytic lymphomas and in t(11q13)-bearing leukemias. *Blood* 1993;81: 3063–3067.
185. Ukerberg LR, Yand W-I, Arnold A, et al. Cyclin D1 expression in non-Hodgkin's lymphomas: detection by immunohistochemistry. *Am J Clin Pathol* 1995;103:756–760.
186. Medeiros LJ, Koo C, McCourty A, et al. Cyclin D1 immunohistochemical staining is useful in distinguishing mantle cell lymphoma from other low-grade B-cell neoplasms in bone marrow. *Am J Clin Pathol* 1997;108:302–307.
187. Rosenblatt JD, Golde DW, Wachsman W, et al. A second isolate of HTLV-II associated with atypical hairy cell leukemia. *N Engl J Med* 1986;315:372–377.
188. Rosenblatt JD, Giorgi JV, Golde DW, et al. Integrated human T-cell leukemia virus II genome in $CD8^+$ T cells from a patient with "atypical" hairy cell leukemia: evidence for distinct T and B cell lymphoproliferative disorders. *Blood* 1988;71:363–369.
189. Lion T, Razvi N, Golomb M, et al. B-lymphocytic hairy cells contain no HTLV-II DNA sequences. *Blood* 1988;72:1428–1430.
190. Wolf BC, Martin AW, Neiman RS, et al. The detection of Epstein-Barr virus in hairy cell leukemia cells by in situ hybridization. *Am J Pathol* 1990;136:717–723.
191. Chang KL, Chen Y-Y, Weiss LM. Lack of evidence of Epstein-Barr virus in hairy cell leukemia and monocytoid B-cell lymphoma. *Hum Pathol* 1993;24:58–61.
192. Bennett JM, Catovsky D, Daniel M-T, et al. Proposals for the classification of chronic (mature) B and T lymphoid leukaemias. *J Clin Pathol* 1989;42:567–584.
193. Yam LT, Phyliky RL, Li C-Y. Benign and neoplastic disorders simulating hairy cell leukemia. *Semin Oncol* 1984;11:353–361.
194. Ward HP, Block MH. The natural history of agnogenic myeloid metaplasia (AMM) and a critical evaluation of its relationship with the myeloproliferative syndrome. *Medicine (Baltimore)* 1971;60: 357–420.
195. Dighiero G, Charron D, Debre P, et al. Identification of a pure splenic form of chronic lymphocytic leukaemia. *Br J Haematol* 1979;41: 169–176.
196. Melo JV, Catovsky D, Galton DAG. The relationship between chronic lymphocytic leukaemia and prolymphocytic leukaemia. *Br J Haematol* 1986;63:377–387.
197. Galton DAG, Goldman JM, Wiltshaw E, et al. Prolymphocytic leukaemia. *Br J Haematol* 1974;27:7–23.
198. Bearman RM, Pangalis GA, Rappaport H. Prolymphocytic leukemia: clinical, histopathological, and cytochemical observations. *Cancer* 1978;42:2360–2372.
199. Sohn CC, Blayney DW, Misset JL, et al. Leukopenic chronic T cell leukemia mimicking hairy cell leukemia: association with human retroviruses. *Blood* 1986;67:949–956.
200. Greenberg BR, Grogan TM, Takasugi BJ, et al. A unique malignant T-cell lymphoproliferative disorder with neutropenia simulating hairy cell leukemia. *Cancer* 1985;56:2823–2830.
201. Cooke CB, Krenacs L, Stetler-Stevenson M, et al. Hepatosplenic T-cell lymphoma: a distinct clinicopathologic entity of cytotoxic $\gamma\delta$ T-cell origin. *Blood* 1996;88:4265–4274.
202. Melo JV, Robinson DSF, Gregory C, et al. Splenic B cell lymphoma with "villous" lymphocytes in the peripheral blood: a disorder distinct from hairy cell leukemia. *Leukemia* 1987;1:294–299.
203. Melo JV, Hegde U, Parreira A, et al. Splenic B cell lymphomas with circulatory villous lymphocytes: differential diagnosis of B cell leukemias with large spleens. *J Clin Pathol* 1987;40:642–651.
204. Mulligan SP, Matutes E, Dearden C, et al. Splenic lymphoma with villous lymphocytes: natural history and response to therapy in 50 cases. *Br J Haematol* 1991;78:206–209.
205. Hanson CA, Gribbin TE, Schnitzer B, et al. CD11c (LEU-M5) expression characterizes a B-cell chronic lymphoproliferative disorder with features of both chronic lymphocytic leukemia and hairy cell leukemia. *Blood* 1990;76:2360–2367.
206. Palutke M, Tabaczka P, Gingrich D. CD11C expression in chronic lymphocytic leukemia. *Blood* 1992;80:2685.
207. Troussard X, Valensi F, Duchayne E, et al. Splenic lymphoma with villous lymphocytes: clinical presentation, biology and prognostic factors in a series of 100 patients. *Br J Haematol* 1996;93:731–736.
208. Harris NL, Jaffe ES, Stein H, et al. A revised European-American classification of lymphoid neoplasms: a proposal from the International Lymphoma Study Group. *Blood* 1994;84:1361–1392.
209. Neiman RS, Sullivan AL, Jaffe R. Malignant lymphoma stimulating leukemic reticuloendotheliosis: a clinicopathologic study of ten cases. *Cancer* 1979;43:329–342.
210. Palutke M, Tabaczka P, Mirchandani ILA, et al. Lymphocytic lymphoma simulating hairy cell leukemia: a consideration of reliable and unreliable diagnostic features. *Cancer* 1981;48:2047–2055.
211. Isaacson PG, Matutes E, Burke M, et al. The histopathology of splenic lymphoma with villous lymphocytes. *Blood* 1994;84:3828–3834.
212. Schmid C, Kirkham N, Diss T, et al. Splenic marginal zone cell lymphoma. *Am J Surg Pathol* 1992;16:455–466.
213. Hammer RD, Glick AD, Greer JP, et al. Splenic marginal zone lymphoma: a distinct B-cell neoplasm. *Am J Surg Pathol* 1996;20: 613–626.
214. Wu CD, Jackson CL, Medeiros J. Splenic marginal zone cell lymphoma: an immunophenotypic and molecular study of five cases. *Am J Clin Pathol* 1996;105:277–285.
215. Mollejo M, Menárguez J, Lloret E, et al. Splenic marginal zone lymphoma: a distinctive type of low grade B-cell lymphoma. A clinicopathological study of 13 cases. *Am J Surg Pathol* 1995;19:1146–1157.
216. Pittaluga S, Verhoef G, Criel A, et al. "Small" B-cell non-Hodgkin's lymphomas with splenomegaly at presentation are either mantle cell lymphoma or marginal zone cell lymphoma: a study based on histology, cytology, immunohistochemistry, and cytogenetic analysis. *Am J Surg Pathol* 1996;20:211–223.
217. Foucar K, McKenna RW, Frizzera G, et al. Incidence and patterns of bone marrow and blood involvement by lymphoma in relationship to the Lukes-Collins classification. *Blood* 1979;54:1417–1422.
218. Burke JS. Surgical pathology of the spleen: an approach to the differential diagnosis of splenic lymphomas and leukemias. Part I: diseases of the white pulp. *Am J Surg Pathol* 1981;5:551–563.
219. Agnarsson BA, Loughran TP, Starkebaum G, et al. The pathology of large granular lymphocyte leukemia. *Hum Pathol* 1989;20:643–651.
220. Burke JS. Surgical pathology of the spleen: an approach to the differ-

ential diagnosis of splenic lymphomas and leukemias. Part II: diseases of the red pulp. *Am J Surg Pathol* 1981;5:681–694.
221. Travis WD, Li C-Y. Pathology of the lymph node and spleen in systemic mast cell disease. *Mod Pathol* 1988;1:4–14.
222. Cawley JC, Burns GF, Hayhoe FGJ. A chronic lymphoproliferative disorder with distinctive features: a distinct variant of hairy cell leukaemia. *Leuk Res* 1980;4:547–559.
223. Catovsky D, O'Brien M, Melo JV, et al. Hairy cell leukemia (HCL) variant: an intermediate disease between HCL and B prolymphocytic leukemia. *Semin Oncol* 1984;11:362–369.
224. Sainati L, Matutes E, Mulligan S, et al. A variant form of hairy cell leukemia resistant to α-interferon: clinical and phenotypic characteristics of 17 patients. *Blood* 1990;76:157–162.
225. De Totero D, Tazzari PL, Lauria F, et al. Phenotypic analysis of hairy cell leukemia: "variant" cases express the interleukin-2 receptor β chain, but not the α chain (CD25). *Blood* 1993;82:528–535.
226. Blasinska-Morawiec M, Robak T, Krykowski E, et al. Hairy cell leukemia: variant treated with 2-chlorodeoxyadenosine. A report of three cases. *Leuk Lymphoma* 1997;25:381–385.
227. Diez Martin JL, Li C-Y, Banks PM. Blastic variant of hairy cell leukemia. *Am J Clin Pathol* 1987;87:576–583.
228. Nazeer T, Burkart P, Dunn H, et al. Blastic transformation of hairy cel leukemia. *Arch Pathol Lab Med* 1997;121:707–713.
229. Katayama I, Mochino T, Honma T, et al. Hairy cell leukemia: a comparative study of Japanese and non-Japanese patients. *Semin Oncol* 1984;11:486–492.
230. Katayama I, Hirashima K, Maruyama K, et al. Hairy cell leukemia in Japanese patients: a study with monoclonal antibodies. *Leukemia* 1987;1:301–305.
231. Tominaga K, Sho S. α-Interferon therapy for Japanese patients with hairy cell leukemia. *Leukemia* 1988;2:554–555.
232. Machii T, Tokumine Y, Inoue R, et al. Predominance of a distinct subtype of hairy cell leukemia in Japan. *Leukemia* 1993;7:181–186.
233. Yamaguchi M, Machii T, Shibayama H, et al. Immunophenotypic features and configuration of immunoglobulin genes in hairy cell leukemia—Japanese variant. *Leukemia* 1996;10:1390–1394.
234. Ratain MJ, Vardiman JW, Barker CM, et al. Prognostic variables in hairy cell leukemia after splenectomy as initial therapy. *Cancer* 1988; 62:2420–2424.
235. Quesada JR, Lepe-Zuniga JL, Gutterman JU. Mid-term observations on the efficacy of α-interferon in hairy cell leukemia and status of the interferon system of patients in remission. *Leukemia* 1987;1:317–319.
236. Rai KR, Davey F, Peterson B, et al. Recombinant alpha-2b-interferon in therapy of previously untreated hairy cell leukemia: long-term follow-up results of study by Cancer and Leukemia Group B. *Leukemia* 1995;9:1116–1120.
237. Grever M, Kopecky K, Foucar MK, et al. Randomized comparison of pentostatin versus interferon alfa 2a in previously untreated patients with hairy cell leukemia: an intergroup study. *J Clin Oncol* 1995;13: 974–982.
238. Gollard R, Lee TC, Piro LD, et al. The optimal management of hairy cell leukaemia. *Drugs* 1995;49:921–931.
239. Consensus resolution: proposed criteria for evaluation of response to treatment in hairy cell leukemia. *Leukemia* 1987;1:405–408.
240. Golomb HM, Fetor, A, Golde DW, et al. Sequential evaluation of alpha-2b-interferon treatment in 128 patients with hairy cell leukemia. *Semin Oncol* 1987;14[Suppl 2]:13.
241. Ratain MJ, Golomb HM, Bardawil RG, et al. Durability of responses to interferon alfa-2b in advanced hairy cell leukemia. *Blood* 1987;69: 872–877.
242. Paganelli KA, Evans SS, Han T, et al. B cell growth factor-induced proliferation of hairy cell lymphocytes and inhibition by type 1 interferon in vitro. *Blood* 1986;67:937–942.
243. Griffiths SD, Cawley JC. The beneficial effects of α-interferon in hairy cell leukemia are not attributable to NK cell-mediated cytotoxicity. *Leukemia* 1987;4:372–376.
244. Semenzato G, Pizzolo G, Agostini C, et al. α-Interferon activates the natural killer system in patients with hairy cell leukemia. *Blood* 1986; 68:293–296.
245. Saven A, Piro L. Newer purine analogues for the treatment of hairy cell leukemia. *N Engl J Med* 1994;10:691–697.
246. Urba WJ, Baseler MW, Kopp WC, et al. Deoxycoformycin-induced immunosuppression in patients with hairy cell leukemia. *Blood* 1989; 73:38–46.
247. Kraut EH, Grever MR, Bouroncle BA. Long-term follow-up of patients with hairy cell leukemia after treatment with 2′-deoxycoformycin. *Blood* 1994;84:4061–4063.
248. Catovsky D. Clinical experience with 2′-deoxycoformycin. *Hematol Cell Ther* 1996;38 (Suppl) 2:S103–S107.
249. Rondelli D, Zinzani PL, Bocchia M, et al. Long-lasting complete remission in patients with hairy cell leukemia treated with 2-CdA: a 5-year survey. *Leukemia* 1997;11:629–632.
250. Saven A, Burian C, Koziol JA, et al. Long-term follow-up of patients with hairy cell leukemia after cladribine treatment. *Blood* 1998;92: 1918–1926.
251. Fayad L, Kurzrock R, Keating M, et al. Treatment of hairy cell leukemia (HCL) with 2-CdA: long term follow-up at M.D. Anderson Cancer Center. *Blood* 1997;90[Suppl 1]:530a(abst).
252. Juliusson G, Lenkei R, Liliemark J. Flow cytometry of blood and bone marrow cells from patients with hairy cell leukemia: phenotype of hairy cells and lymphocyte subsets after treatment with 2-chlorodeoxyadenosine. *Blood* 1994;83:3672–3681.
253. Seymour JF, Kurzrock R, Freireich EJ, et al. 2-Chlorodeoxyadenosine induces durable remissions and prolonged suppression of $CD4^+$ lymphocyte counts in patients with hairy cell leukemia. *Blood* 1994;83: 2906–2911.
254. Tallman MS, Hakimian D, Rademaker AW, et al. Relapse of hairy cell leukemia after 2-chlorodeoxyadenosine: long-term follow-up of the Northwestern University experience. *Blood* 1996;88:1954–1959.
255. Ellison DJ, Sharpe RW, Robbins BA, et al. Immunomorphologic analysis of bone marrow biopsies after treatment with 2-chlorodeoxyadenosine for hairy cell leukemia. *Blood* 1994;84:4310–4315.
256. Wheaton S, Tallman MS, Hakimian D, et al. Minimal residual disease may predict bone marrow relapse in patients with hairy cell leukemia treated with 2-chlorodeoxyadenosine. *Blood* 1996;87:1556–1560.
257. Thaler J, Dietze O, Faber V, et al. Monoclonal antibody B-ly7: a sensitive marker for detection of minimal residual disease in hairy cell leukemia. *Leukemia* 1990;4:170–176.
258. Matutes E, Meeus P, McLennan K, et al. The significance of minimal residual disease in hairy cell leukaemia treated with deoxycoformycin: a long-term follow-up study. *Br J Haematol* 1997;98:375–383.
259. Filleul B, Delannoy A, Ferrant A, et al. A single course of 2-chlorodeoxyadenosine does not eradicate leukemic cells in hairy cell leukemia patients in complete remission. *Leukemia* 1994;8:1153–1156.
260. Aiba M, Raffa PP, Katayama I. Significance of leukocyte alkaline phosphatase in hairy cell leukemia. *Am J Clin Pathol* 1980;74: 297–300.
261. Chilosi M, Semenzato G, Cetto G, et al. Soluble interleukin-2 receptors in the sera of patients with hairy cell leukemia: relationship with the effect of recombinant α-interferon therapy on clinical parameters and natural killer in vitro activity. *Blood* 1987;5:1530–1535.
262. Steis RG, Marcon L, Clark J, et al. Serum soluble IL-2 receptor as a tumor marker in patients with hairy cell leukemia. *Blood* 1988;71: 1304–1309.
263. Ambrosetti A, Semenzato G, Prior M, et al. Serum levels of soluble interleukin-2 receptor in hairy cell leukemia: a reliable marker of neoplastic bulk. *Br J Haematol* 1989;73:181–186.
264. Chrobak L, Podzimek K, Pliskova L, et al. Serum soluble IL-2 receptor as a reliable and noninvasive marker of disease activity in patients with hairy cell leukemia. *Neoplasma* 1996;43:321–325.
265. Ho AD, Grobmann M, Knauf W, et al. Plasma levels of soluble CD8 antigen and interleukin-2 receptor antigen in patients with hairy cell leukemia: relationship with splenectomy and with clinical response to therapy. *Leukemia* 1989;10:718–723.
266. Ambrosetti A, Corato A, Nadali V, et al. Response to purine analogues in hairy cell leukemia is assessable by soluble CD25. *Blood* 1997; 90[Suppl 1]:91a(abst).
267. Thompson JA, Shields AF, Porter BA, et al. Magnetic resonance imaging of bone marrow in hairy cell leukemia: correlation with clinical response to α-interferon. *Leukemia* 1987;1:315–316.
268. Silingardi V, Davolio-Marani S, Federico M, et al. Bone marrow infiltration in hairy cell leukemia after interferon therapy detected by magnetic resonance imaging. *Eur J Cancer Clin Oncol* 1989;25: 209–213.

CHAPTER 42

B-Cell Immunoproliferative Disorders, Including Multiple Myeloma and Amyloidosis

Thomas M. Grogan and Catherine M. Spier

Plasma cell dyscrasias are a group of related disorders, each of which is associated with the expansion of a single clone of immunoglobulin-secreting cells. These monoclonal plasma cell proliferations are characterized by secretion of a single homogeneous immunoglobulin product known as an M-component or monoclonal component. The prominence of the M-component in serum and urine electrophoresis profiles has led to a variety of designations for these disorders, including dysproteinemia, paraproteinemia, and monoclonal gammopathy. M-components, although monoclonal, may be seen in both malignant plasma cell conditions (i.e., multiple myeloma and Waldenström's macroglobulinemia) and benign or premalignant disorders (e.g., monoclonal gammopathy of unknown significance [MGUS]). Among these gammopathies are found a number of clinicopathologic entities, including multiple and solitary myeloma, extramedullary plasmacytoma, Waldenström's macroglobulinemia, heavy-chain disease, secondary amyloidosis, and MGUS. Each of these entities are discussed after a general discussion of monoclonal gammopathies. The plasma cell malignancies may be seen as far more complex than a simple proliferation of end-stage B cells.

MULTIPLE MYELOMA

Multiple myeloma (i.e., plasma cell myeloma) is a lethal plasma cell proliferation involving the bone marrow and extraosseous tissues in a multifocal fashion. The unique triad of osteolytic lesions, atypical marrow plasmacytosis, and a monoclonal gammopathy is characteristic (Figs. 42.1–42.6). The disease spans a spectrum from localized, indolent to disseminated, aggressive forms. Generally, patients have significant bone pain, hypercalcemia, anemia, renal failure, and recurrent infections. Nearly all patients die after a median of 3 years, with 10% survival at 10 years (1).

T. M. Grogan: Department of Hematology and Immunology, University of Arizona, Tucson, Arizona 85274

C. M. Spier: Department of Pathology, University of Arizona, Tucson, Arizona 85274

Incidence

Multiple myeloma accounts for more than 1% of all malignancies in Caucasians and more than 2% in blacks (2). The higher incidence in blacks mirrors the finding of a higher immunoglobulin level in blacks relative to whites, suggesting a larger B-cell population at risk for malignant change. Myeloma is the most common lymphoid malignancy in blacks and the second most common in whites, representing 15% of all hematopoietic malignancies (3,4). From 1940 through the 1970s, the incidence of myeloma has shown a net increase of 45% (5). Characteristically, the incidence of myeloma increases with age, beginning with a very low incidence in patients younger than 40 years (<2% of myeloma patients) and with a peak in the eighth decade (2). The median age at diagnosis is 68 years for men and 70 for women (2). A similar ascending incidence is described for Waldenström's macroglobulinemia and MGUS (6).

Etiology

The exact cause of human multiple myeloma is largely unknown. There are no obvious environmental causes, although an increased risk (three to four times) of myeloma is described in cosmetologists, farmers, and petroleum, wood, leather, and asbestos workers, as well as in laxative takers (7–10). Specific exposure agents include pesticides, petroleum products, asbestos, rubber, plastic, and wood products (7–10). High-dose irradiation (100 cGy) of survivors of the atomic bomb at Hiroshima and Nagasaki resulted in a myeloma rate 4.7 times greater than controls (11). Low-level radiation exposure has been implicated as a risk factor by

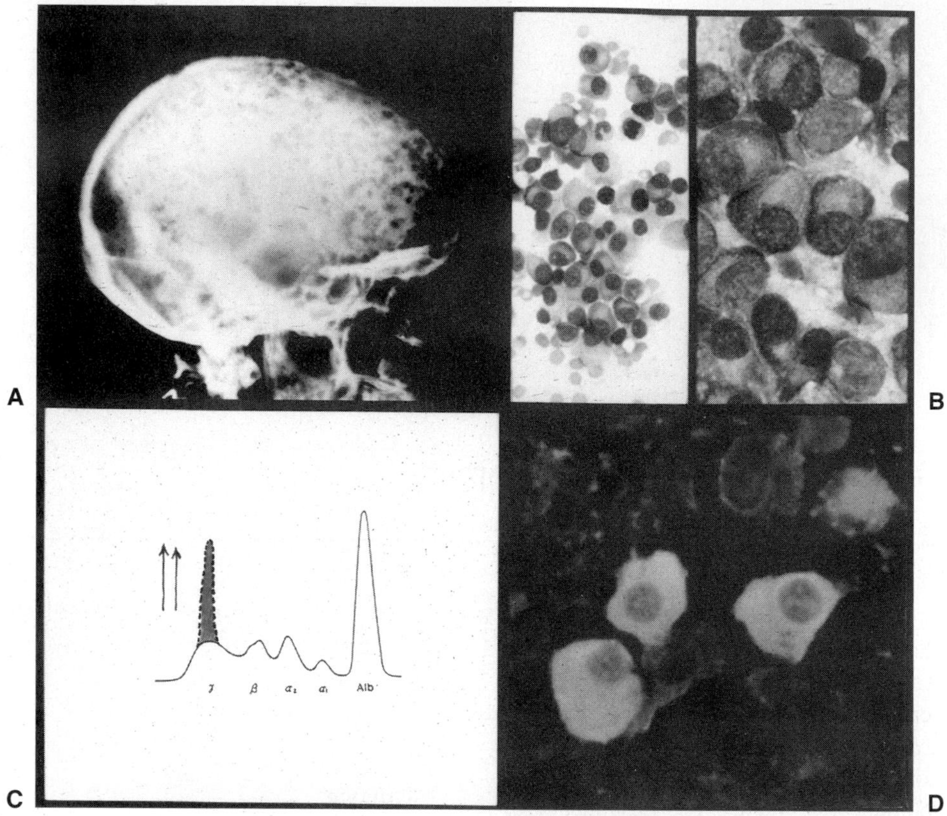

FIG. 42.1. This composite illustrates the salient features of plasma cell myeloma pathology: discrete osteolytic lesions **(A)**, aggregates of immature plasma cells **(B)**, monotypic cytoplasmic immunoglobulin expression shown by immunofluorescence **(C)**, and a monoclonal gammopathy evidenced by a "spike" in the γ region of a serum protein electrophoresis densitometry profile **(D)**.

virtue of the increased incidence of myeloma among radiologists (12) and nuclear plant workers (13). Historically, longstanding, chronic infection or chronic antigenic stimulation of the reticuloendothelial system has been considered a predisposing factor (14). Osteomyelitis and rheumatoid arthritis are two examples among many (15). A possible role for virus has been postulated with the finding of the Kaposi's sarcoma–associated human herpesvirus-8 (HHV-8) in myeloma marrow samples (16). Intriguingly, HHV-8 was localized to marrow dendritic antigen presenting cells; viral interleukin-6 (vIL-6) may stimulate plasma cell growth and pathogenesis. This finding remains controversial because some have and others have not confirmed this result (17). Although not all data support a role for HHV-8 in the cause of myeloma, the possibility of a related KS330-containing virus has been raised (18).

The occurrence of multiple myeloma in human immunodeficiency virus (HIV)–infected patients also suggests a possible etiologic association. In some instances, the HIV-mediated suppression of immunosurveillance may result in emergence of Epstein-Barr virus–infected B-cell clones (19). In other instances, the effect is more direct; the HIV

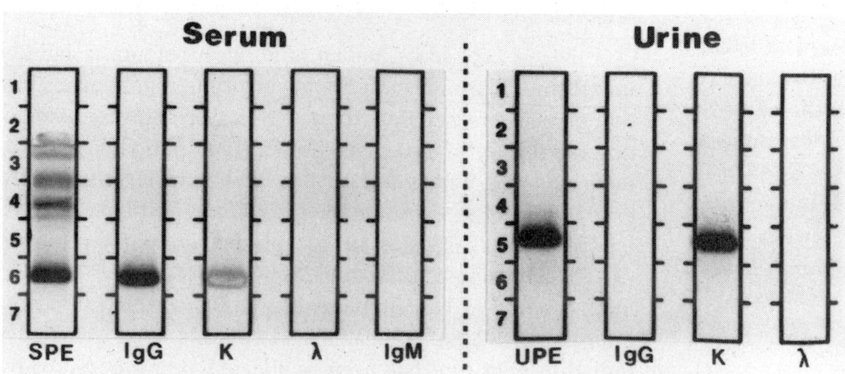

FIG. 42.2. Demonstration of serum and urine M-component using the immunofixation technique. The patient has an immunoglobulin G (IgG) κ serum M-component and a κ Bence Jones proteinuria.

A

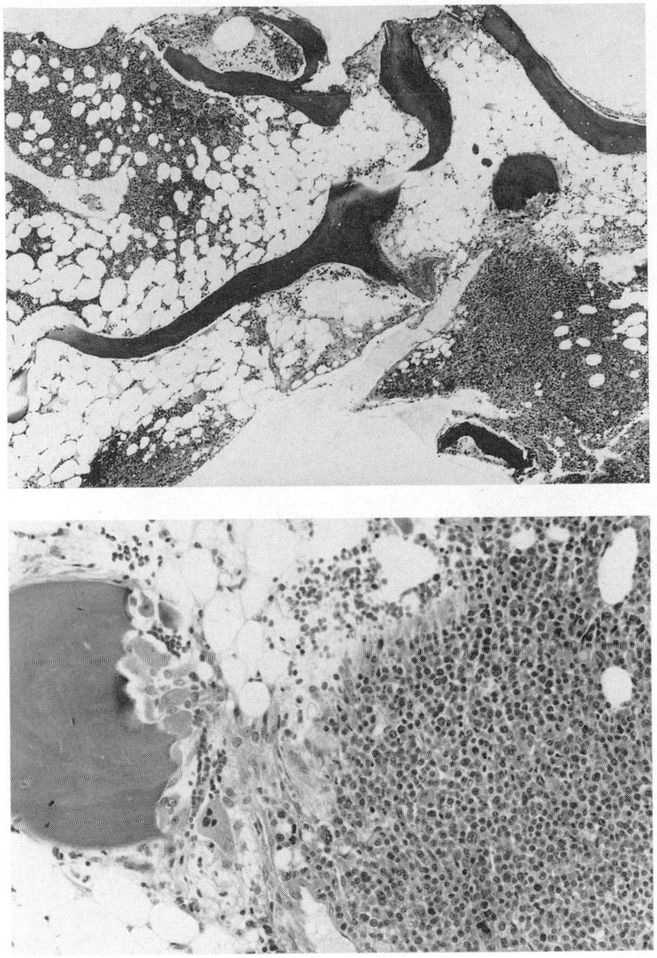

B

FIG. 42.3. Histologic appearance of plasma cell myeloma in a bone marrow biopsy. **A:** A discrete plasma cell mass *(lower right)* displaces normal marrow fat cells and hematopoietic elements. This displacing mass contrasts with the normal fat cell pattern in a focus of normal hematocytopoiesis *(upper left).* Above the myeloma mass is prominent osteoclastic activity, which is shown in detail in **B** (hematoxylin and eosin stain, original magnifications: 40× and 100× magnification).

patient with myeloma may produce an M-component directed against the HIV-1 p24 antigen (20).

Pathogenesis

Development of multiple myeloma is said to follow the *two-hit hypothesis*: an initial antigenic stimulus giving rise to multiple benign clones and a second hit representing an ''accident'' or mutagenic event causing malignant transformation (21). The importance of the initial antigenic stimulus is reinforced by the Balb/c mouse model for plasma cell neoplasia induced by mineral oil injections (22). Although the initial antigenic stimulus may be well established in some instances (e.g., mineral oil, petroleum, asbestos, laxatives), in most cases of myeloma, the initial antigenic stimulus is unknown. Most myeloma proteins lack specificity for foreign antigen. Among the rare documented instances are the

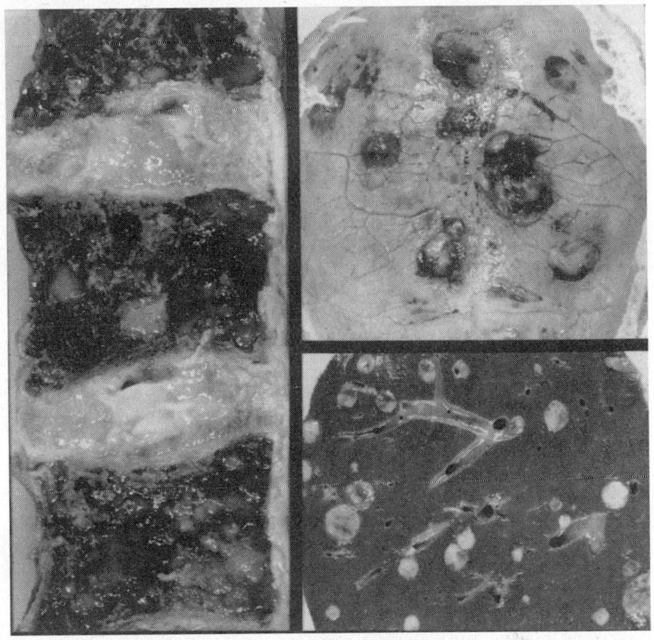

A B C

FIG. 42.4. Illustrated is the gross appearance of plasma cell myeloma and extramedullary plasmacytoma in the vertebral marrow **(A)**, calvarium **(B)**, and liver **(C)**. The lesional tissue has a soft, white-tan, fish-flesh appearance with associated hemorrhage and osteolysis. Associated osteoporosis and compression or pathologic fractures of bone are common.

remarkable case of the M-component in a canary breeder related to canary droppings (23) and the M-component to horse α-macroglobulin 30 years after passive serotherapy with horse serum for tetanus (24). The very oddity of these circumstances indicates the obvious difficulty of ascribing foreign antigen specificity to myeloma proteins. Nonetheless, the perception that myeloma immunoglobulin is largely of nonforeign specificity has led to another speculation regarding pathogenesis: autoreactivity (25–27). This theory suggests that myeloma proteins may be autoantibodies directed against immunoregulatory autoantibodies. This suggests that myeloma may arise from B cells within the idiotypic network of Jerne (27). In Jerne's hierarchy, anti-idiotype antibodies may lack specificity for the original stimulating antigen serving an immunoregulatory function (27). This hypothesis suggests that myeloma is a malignancy of differentiated autoimmunoregulatory B cells (27).

Following the two-hit hypothesis, the second event in myeloma is surmised to be a mutagenic or transforming genetic event. Relevant to this hypothesis is abundant evidence regarding genetic and molecular defects in plasma cell neoplasia.

Chromosomal and Molecular Alterations

Malignant progression in plasma cell neoplasms is triggered by a variety of genetic changes, including chromosomal translocations, deletions, and alterations; gene rear-

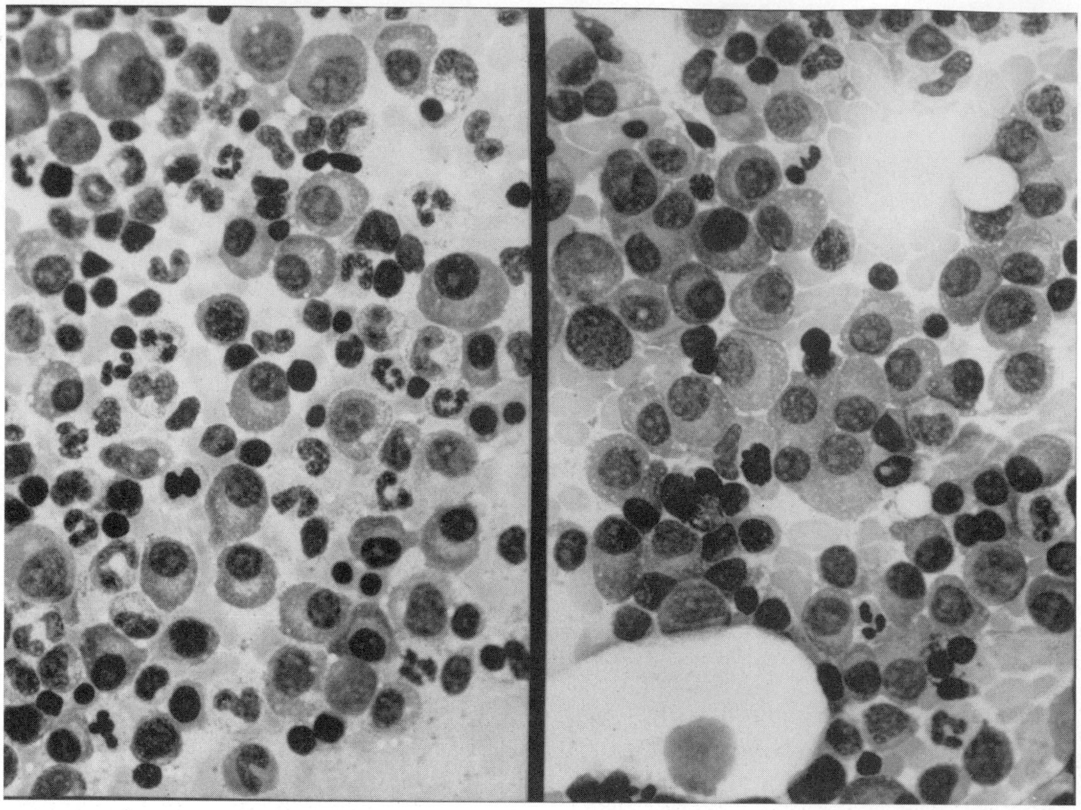

FIG. 42.5. Shown is the cytologic appearance of plasma cell myeloma in bone marrow aspirates representing 20% and 65% atypical plasmacytosis. The designation "atypical" stems from the nuclear immaturity evidenced by prominent nucleoli and fine chromatin patterning (Wright-Giemsa stain, original magnification 400× magnification).

A

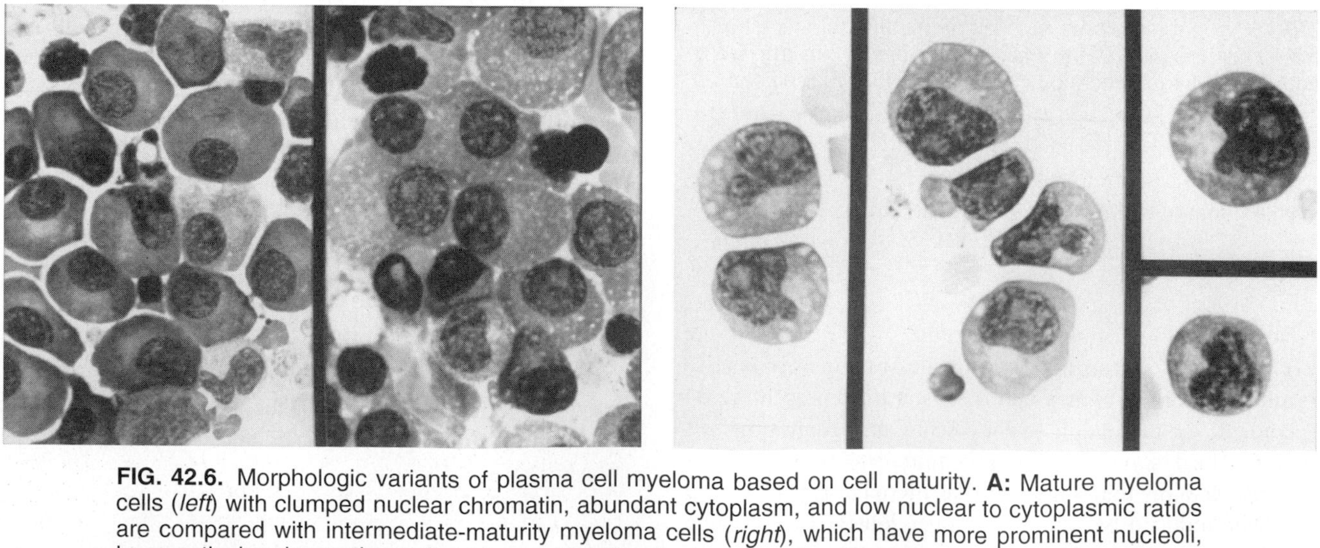

B

FIG. 42.6. Morphologic variants of plasma cell myeloma based on cell maturity. **A:** Mature myeloma cells (*left*) with clumped nuclear chromatin, abundant cytoplasm, and low nuclear to cytoplasmic ratios are compared with intermediate-maturity myeloma cells (*right*), which have more prominent nucleoli, loose reticular chromatin, and moderate nuclear-cytoplasmic ratios. **B:** Immature plasmablasts from a plasmablastic myeloma demonstrate prominent nucleoli, reticular chromatin, and high nuclear-cytoplasmic ratios (Wright-Giemsa stain, original magnification: 630× magnification).

rangements; and mutations. These alterations frequently involve alteration of oncogenes, suppressor genes, or both (28–30). The most common structural abnormalities are described in chromosomes 1, 11, and 14, with an 11;14 translocation being the most common (28–30). Abnormalities of chromosome 11 could relate to the known 11q23 localization of neuronal cell adhesion molecule (NCAM) said to be relevant to myeloma tumorigenicity (31,32). The chromosome 11 break point is also near the *HRAS* gene location. An inverse relationship between p21 (HRAS) levels and trisomy 11 has been noted, with an effect on myeloma survival (33,34). An abnormal chromosome 6 has been associated with increased tumor necrosis factor (TNF) secretion and linked to increased osteoclast activation and bone disease (35). Deletion of the long arm of chromosome 7 has also been related to alteration of the multidrug resistance gene conferring an increased clinical drug resistant phenotype relevant to myeloma survival (36). Structural and numeric chromosomal abnormalities are described in 18% of newly diagnosed patients and in 63% of aggressive disease patients, indicating an ascending scale of chromosomal aberration in pathogenesis (28) (see Chapter 10). Similar genetic alterations of growth factor genes could affect the autocrine and paracrine growth characteristic of myeloma cells.

Molecular studies of immunoglobulin (Ig) genes commonly reveal the expected hierarchy of J_H, C_κ, and C_λ rearrangements (Fig. 42.7). Although a single, monoclonal rearranged Ig band is the rule in myeloma, multiple rearranged Ig bands characterize 5% of myeloma patients and may reflect clonal evolution into oligoclonal or biclonal myeloma (37). Ig genetic deletion characterizes some myeloma patients. Patients with light chain only disease or Bence Jones proteinuria are especially likely to lose J_H segments or parts or all of chromosome 14 (Fig. 42.7). Consistent with the sometimes multilineage, stem cell origin of late progressive myeloma, some myeloma samples with γ T-cell receptor rearrangements are described (37).

Studies of *MYC* indicate high levels of MYC RNA expression in 25% of myeloma patients, particularly in those of IgA isotype and among those with a t(8;14) translocation, as described in Burkitt's lymphoma (38,39). In general, high MYC expression occurs without DNA rearrangement, without change of DNA transcript size, and without DNA amplification (38,39). Mutant *MYC* in myeloma has been described (40), suggesting that *MYC* point mutations and *HRAS* alteration may be major mechanisms of abnormal growth in myeloma.

In myeloma, mutations of the *TP53* gene are rare events. However, *TP53* gene deletion identified by interphase fluorescence *in situ* hybridization occurs in one third of newly diagnosed myeloma cases and predicts poor survival (41). The poor survival is related to drug resistance caused by a loss of p53 function. Because cytotoxic drugs act through induction of apoptosis, and apoptosis requires a functional p53, myeloma cells with impaired p53 function may have blocked apoptosis leading to drug resistance. Alternatively,

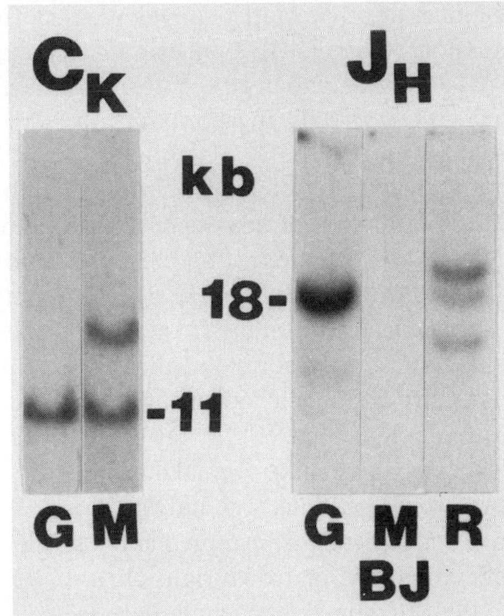

FIG. 42.7. Immunoglobulin gene rearrangements in plasma cell myeloma. Southern blot analyses in myeloma (M) reveal rearrangement of C κ gene relative to germline (G). The same patient proved to have Bence Jones (BJ) proteinuria. This patient's (M) light chain–only disease is explained by the absent heavy chain rearrangement (JH), in contrast with germline (G) and a rearranged (R) form in another myeloma patient. This patient with C κ rearranged, JH absent, light chain only, Bence Jones proteinuria showed a deleted chromosome 14 on karyotypic analysis, indicating structural absence of the heavy chain locus. Bence Jones proteinuria in this case relates to structural gene loss.

an altered *TP53* gene may lose its function as "guardian of the genome" and as a consequence complex cytogenetic abnormalities may develop as detailed previously (41). A case in point is the altered expression of the *PAX5* gene in myeloma, which results in the loss of CD19 expression characteristic of the transition from normal $CD19^+$ plasma cells to $CD19^-$ myeloma cells (42). This PAX-5–mediated pathogenic effect on plasma cells is probably a critical factor in myeloma pathogenesis. With regard to initial myeloma pathogenesis the dysregulation of cyclin D1 by translocation (t11;14 into an IgH γ switch region) is also a notable factor in myeloma cell immortalization (43).

Monoclonal Gammopathy

Plasma cell neoplasms are characterized by synthesis and secretion of monoclonal Ig that appears as an electrophoretically homogeneous band or "spike" in the γ or β region of a serum protein electrophoresis profile (Figs. 42.1, 42.2) (44,45). The term M-component referred initially to "malignant" or "myeloma" protein but now connotes "monoclonal," recognizing that some M-components occur in benign conditions known as MGUS (46,47). Although the pathologically increased M-component may lead to red blood cell rouleaux formation, the normal nonneoplastic Ig-producing clones are characteristically depressed. Concomitant suppression of normal Ig synthesis is characteristic of myeloma (44–46). Immunoelectrophoresis indicates that the monoclonal protein is IgG in approximately 50% of myeloma cases, IgA in 20%, IgD in less than 1%, and IgM and IgE rarely (44), with the remainder being light-chain only disease. This distribution of heavy chains among myeloma patients reflects the synthetic fractions of normal serum polyclonal Igs (51% IgG, 37% IgA, 1% IgD, <1% IgE). This correspondence between the frequency of Ig isotype in plasma cell neoplasia and normal serum suggests myeloma neoplastic transformation may occur at random among available plasma cell clones (except for IgM) (48). The reduced IgA incidence may reflect the normal dual sites for IgA synthesis: IgA1 from bone marrow and IgA2 from gut. Myeloma derivation typically is restricted to the former subtype of IgA, reflecting bone marrow origin (49).

Because the M-component accurately reflects tumor burden, serial quantitative Ig determinations are useful in monitoring the course of disease and the effect of therapy (46). The M-component on serum electrophoresis may be discriminated from normal Ig levels at 0.5 g/dL or greater, representing more than 10^9 neoplastic plasma cells (50). As few as 10^3 neoplastic plasma cells may produce a detectable M-component by the more sensitive but less clinically practical radioimmunoassay method (51). The incidence of monoclonal Igs in unselected populations is approximately 1%, ranging from 0.16% at 25 to 49 years to 9.2% at 80 to 89 years (52). The M-component in one half to two thirds of these patients is related directly to multiple myeloma or Waldenström's macroglobulinemia (53). The latter neoplastic circumstances, in contrast to MGUS, typically have higher M-component expression with depressed normal Igs, differing quantitatively and qualitatively (45).

An M-component is found in serum or urine in 99% of myeloma patients (48). The 1% nonsecretory myelomas are discussed subsequently. The secreted M-component generally is in the form of the whole Ig molecule with balanced expression of heavy and light chains (51). Some patients manifest "unbalanced" excess light-chain secretion in addition to the whole Ig molecule (45). Approximately 10% to 25% of myeloma patients secrete only light chains (i.e., Bence Jones protein) (45,48). Because of their low molecular weight, light chains normally pass through the renal glomerulus, are reabsorbed, are partially catabolized, and then are excreted in the renal tubule and into the urine. This loss of urinary light chains results in hypogammaglobulinemia. In light chain–only disease, the M-component may only be detectable in the urinary protein electrophoresis (44,51) (Fig. 42.2). Excreted light chains may result in inspissated tubular protein, tubular obstruction, loss of nephrons, and renal insufficiency known as myeloma kidney (51) (Fig. 42.8).

Detection of M-components generally entails sampling of serum and urine. Serum M-components generally appear as a "spike" on serum protein electrophoresis (SPE). Immunoelectrophoresis (IEP) or immunofixation (IMF) employing

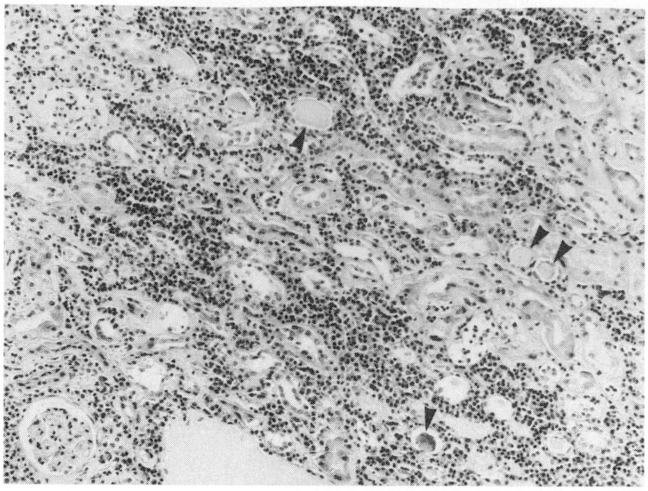

FIG. 42.8. Bence Jones nephropathy. Plasma cells infiltrate the kidney. Scattered renal tubules are plugged with dense protein-forming inspissated casts (*arrowheads*). Adjacent tubular epithelioid cells may be devitalized, and foreign body giant cells may form (hematoxylin and eosin stain, original magnification: 100× magnification).

anti-Ig reagents ensures identification of specific monoclonal isotypes (45) (Fig. 42.2). The technique of immunofixation in particular (Fig. 42.2) is rapidly replacing SPE in the clinical laboratory because of its speed, sensitivity, and ease of interpretation. With the immunofixation method samples of patient serum or urine are subjected to electrophoresis in a high-resolution gel, followed by application of monospecific antisera. Urinary M-components are usually detected in concentrates of 24-hour urine collections. The specificity and sensitivity of the immunofixation method is especially useful with the rare IgD and IgE myelomas, in which the M-component can be quantitatively very small (45). Immunofixation may also be critical in determining a minor monoclonal IgA or IgM component hidden within a broad γ-globulin band, giving an umbrella effect.

Different M-component isotypes are associated with different clinicopathologic syndromes (54). In particular, patients with light chain–only disease (54) and with IgD myeloma (55,56) have a poor prognosis, probably related to prominent myeloma nephropathy. IgE myeloma also has a poor prognosis related to a high incidence of plasma cell leukemia (57). Prognosis is particularly poor among those who have λ light-chain disease; the 10-month median survival is one-third that of patients with κ-only light-chain disease (58,59). IgM, and some IgA with high carbohydrate content, and rare IgG components may take aberrant aggregated form, resulting in the hyperviscosity syndrome causing visual, central nervous system, or bleeding symptoms (46). Some myeloma proteins show increased molecular affinities at low (cryoglobulins) or high (pyroglobulins) temperatures (46). Myeloma proteins (usually IgM or IgG) that form precipitates on cooling result in Raynaud's phenomenon, purpura, or cold urticaria.

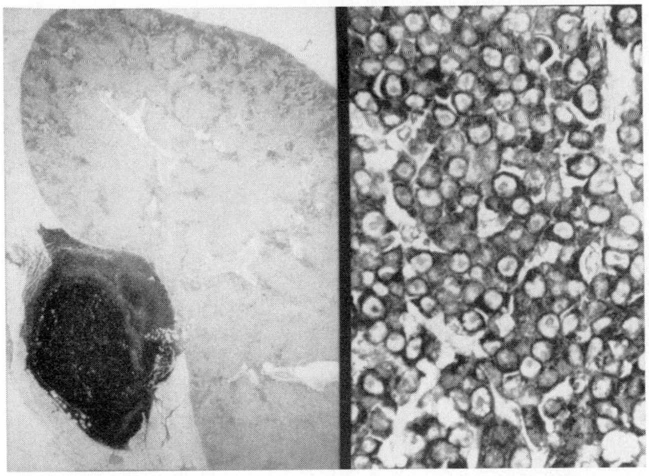

FIG. 42.9. Perirenal extramedullary plasmacytoma. Immunohistochemical assay reveals λ light chain–bearing perirenal plasmacytoma. Some patchy renal λ deposition reflects renal tubal Bence Jones protein reabsorption (immunoperoxidase anti-λ light chain stain, original magnifications: 4× and 250× magnification).

Morphology

Ultimately, the diagnosis of multiple myeloma and dyscrasias requires the morphologic identification of abnormal sheets or clusters of plasma cells (60) (Figs. 42.3, 42.9, 42.10). Because plasma cell neoplasms may be composed of mature plasma cells indistinguishable cytologically from reactive plasma cells, the finding of plasma cells in sheets or aggregates indicates displacement of normal tissue through plasma cell infiltration and invasion, evidencing the uncontrolled growth of a malignant clone (60,61). This pathologic microanatomic property contrasts with the usually randomly dispersed, nonaggregated plasma cells in a benign reactive plasmacytosis (Figs. 42.11, 42.12). Beyond tissue section evidence of a mass effect, additional cytologic properties favor a neoplastic rather than a hyperplastic proliferation. Specifically, these include the findings of multinucleated plasma cells and plasma cell immaturity or anaplasia (Fig. 42.13) (62,63). Because 1% to 5% of reactive plasma cells may be binucleate or, rarely, trinucleate, it is the finding of bizarre multinucleate (greater than trinucleate) forms that is considered pathologic (64,65) (Fig. 42.13). Immaturity may include findings of dispersed nuclear chromatin and a high nuclear to cytoplasmic ratio and prominent nucleoli, giving a ''blastic'' appearance indicative of plasmablasts (63) (Figs. 42.5, 42.6). Because nuclear-cytoplasmic asynchrony and immaturity rarely occur in reactive circumstances, they are reliable indicators of atypical or pleomorphic plasmacytosis, greatly favoring neoplasia (61). Even given this atypicality, it is said that no single morphologic feature distinguishes between normal and malignant plasma cells (61). Nevertheless, a constellation of findings including cytologic pleomorphism and tissue evidence of a displacing mass or abnormal aggregates strongly favors neoplasia. Beyond diagnosis,

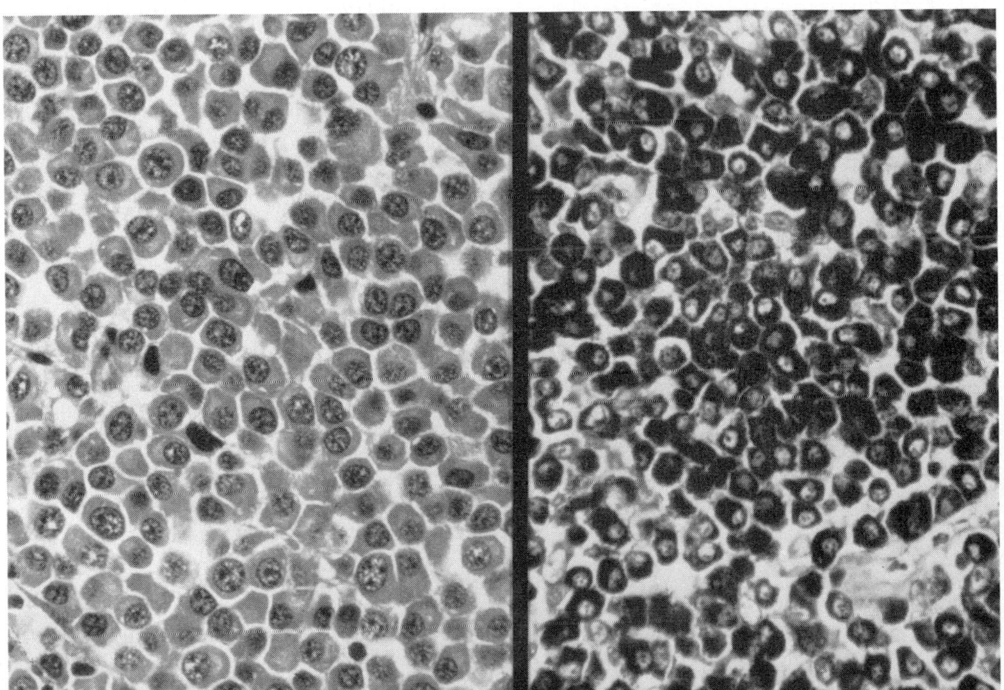

A B

FIG. 42.10. Morphologic and immunologic features of an extramedullary plasmacytoma. **A:** This plasmacytoma shows intermediate chromatin with abundant cytoplasm (hematoxylin and eosin stain, original magnification: 400× magnification). **B:** Immunoperoxidase (anti-κ) stain reveals monotypic cytoplasmic κ light chain expression (original magnification: 400× magnification).

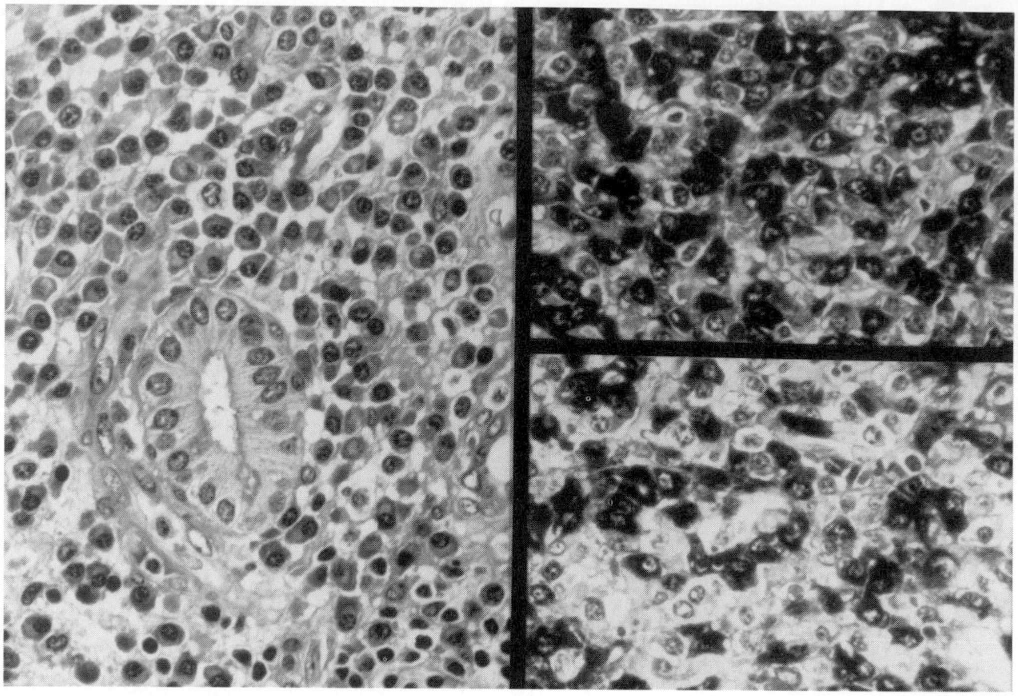

A B

FIG. 42.11. Allergic nasal polyp with reactive plasmacytosis. **A:** The central nasal mucosal gland is surrounded by scattered mature reactive plasma cells with "clock-face" chromatin and abundant cytoplasm (hematoxylin and eosin stain, 400× magnification). **B:** Immunoperoxidase stain indicates a polyclonal cytoplasmic proliferation with plasma cells containing κ (*top*) and λ (*bottom*) immunoglobulin (original magnification: 400× magnification).

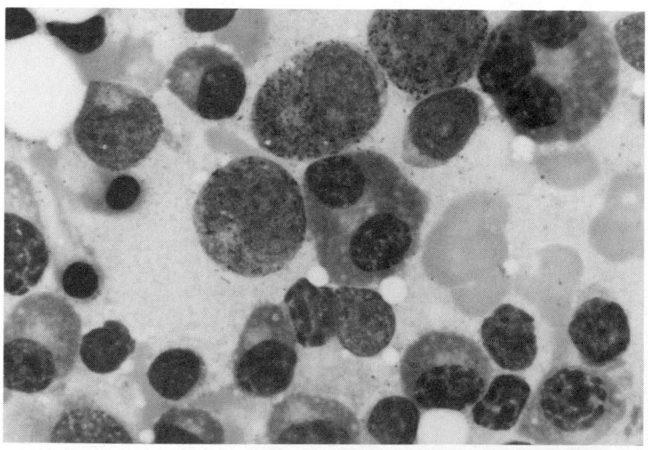

FIG. 42.12. Reactive marrow plasmacytosis as seen in the marrow aspirate. This striking plasmacytosis (>50% plasma cells) occurred in the recovery phase of marrow agranulocytosis related to drug therapy. Notice the mature "block clock-face" chromatin and inapparent nuclei heralding a typical plasmacytosis. Notice also the binucleate and trinucleate plasma cells in a benign circumstance. The prominent promyelocytes reflect the recovery from agranulocytosis. On the basis of this and other extreme reactive cases, the numeric plasma cell count alone does not establish a diagnosis of myeloma (Wright-Giemsa stain, original magnification: 630× magnification).

plasma cell immaturity, in the form of variants resembling lymphoid precursors and plasmablasts, has been highly associated with an adverse prognosis (63) (Fig. 42.6).

In contrast with the frequent telltale nuclear changes, the cytoplasmic features of neoplastic plasma cells may greatly simulate normalcy. The round or egg-shaped plasma cell with eccentrically placed nucleus contains abundant basophilic cytoplasm with a paranuclear clear zone. Electron microscopy reveals highly developed endoplasmic reticulum specialized for Ig synthesis (61). The blue of Romanowsky-type stains reflects high RNA content, and the paranuclear clear zone reflects the Golgi apparatus, where Ig is processed and glycosylated for secretion (66). A great variety of cytoplasmic appearances may be found, including multiple pale bluish white, grapelike accumulations (i.e., Mott cells or Morula cells) (Fig. 42.14), cherry red round bodies (i.e., Russell bodies) (Fig. 42.14), vermilion-staining patterns (i.e., flame cells), cells ''overstuffed'' with ''silky fibrils'' (i.e., Gaucher-like cells and thesaurocytes), cells with hairy cell–like appearance, and crystalline rods (Fig. 42.14) (67–70). These inclusions all represent aggregated, altered, retained, phagocytosed, condensed, or crystallized cytoplasmic Ig or glycoproteins (67–70). Although morphologically remarkable, these cytoplasmic changes are not pathognomonic of myeloma or plasma cell neoplasia because they may also be seen in reactive plasma cells, particularly in inflammatory disorders of chronicity (61). These disorders

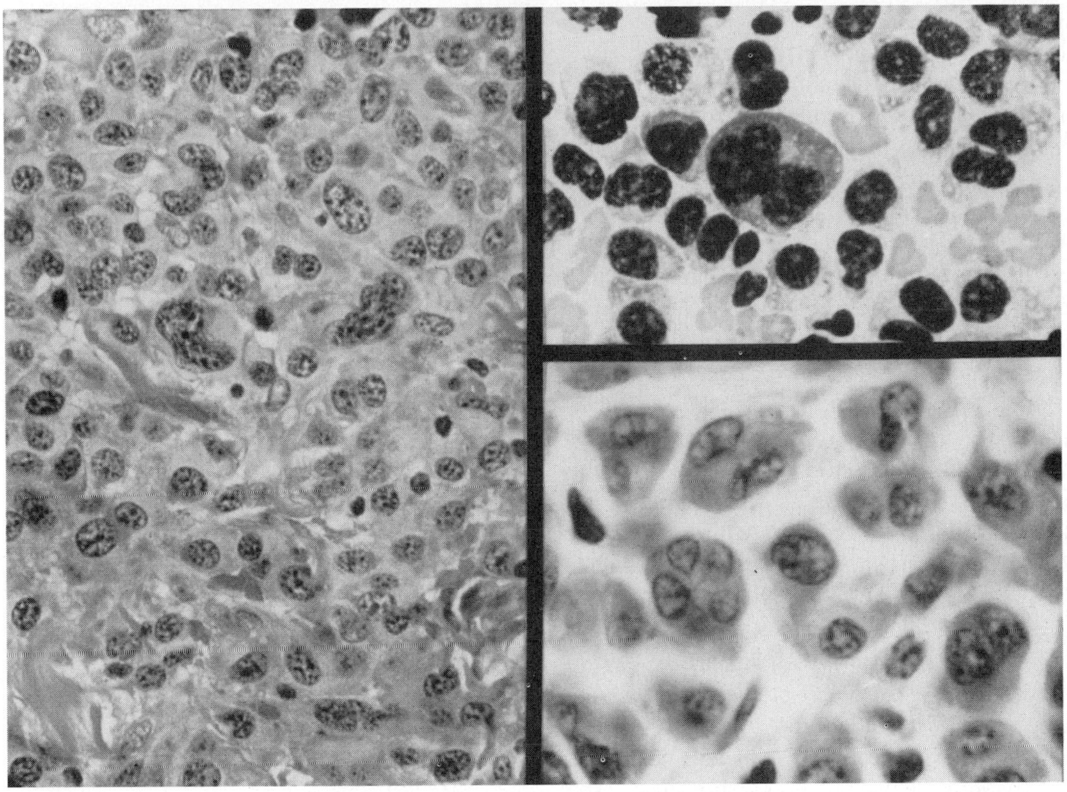

FIG. 42.13. Anaplastic plasmacytoma. This composite illustrates both histologic and cytologic features of immature, pleomorphic, polylobated, and multinucleate "anaplastic" plasmacytomas. A combination of vestigial "clock-face" chromatin, the presence of eccentric nuclei, the low nuclear-cytoplasmic ratio, and abundant cytoplasm with occasional Golgi structures combined with an immunoperoxidase demonstration of cytoplasmic immunoglobulin but without pan-B antigens leads to the diagnosis of plasmacytoma, even in the face of substantial morphologic "immaturity" (hematoxylin and eosin stain, original magnifications: 400× and 630× magnification).

A

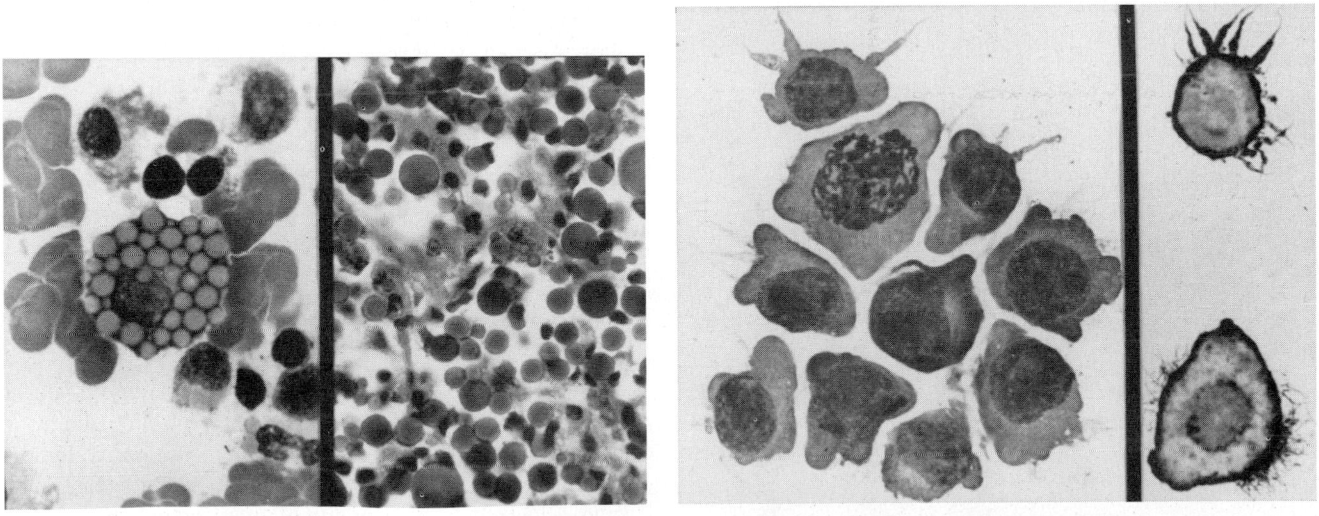

B

FIG. 42.14. Plasma cell morphologic variants based on cytoplasmic features. **A:** A Mott cell with abundant grapelike cytoplasmic inclusions of immunoglobulin (*left:* original magnification: 630× magnification) and the presence of Russell bodies representing both cytoplasmic and extracellular inclusions seen in bone marrow biopsy (*right:* original magnification: 250× magnification). **B:** An unusual "hairy cell" variant of plasma cell myeloma with prominent cytoplasmic extensions appearing as "hirsutism" (original magnification: 630× magnification).

include syphilis, rheumatoid arthritis, tuberculosis and secondary amyloidosis in particular (71).

The morphologic diagnosis of multiple myeloma almost invariably is made by bone marrow aspiration or biopsy. The scattered, focal bony disease may pose sampling difficulties such that failure to demonstrate marrow plasmacytosis does not rule out multiple myeloma. Other sites should be aspirated, especially at specific sites of bony tenderness or radiologic evidence of osteolysis (72). Involved marrow usually contains more than 10% plasma cells (normal marrow has less than 5% plasma cells), with 20% and 30% of samples, respectively, meeting minor and major diagnostic criteria (73–75). Core biopsy reveals diffuse and nodular involvement (Fig. 42.3). Characteristically, there is displacement of normal hematopoietic cells with adjacent areas of bony erosion or resorption due to osteoclastic activity (Fig. 42.3). Clumped osteoblasts found in children with active bone growth should not be confused with clumped plasma cells (Fig. 42.15).

The degree of marrow plasma cell infiltration has prognostic value. Three stages (stage I, <20%; stage II, 20% to 50%; stage III, >50% plasma cells) predict progressively poorer prognoses (76). When the latter staging is coupled with cytologic features (plasmacytic versus plasmablastic), there is strong predictive power of good-, moderate-, and poor-risk groups representing median survivals of 72, 23, and 6 months, respectively (Fig. 42.6) (62). The main constraint on this strict morphologic predictive system is the common observation that the percent of plasma cells in the marrow varies greatly with the sample and is not always a reliable measure of the total amount of disease present (72). A similar caveat regards the qualitative judgment of the plasmacytic versus plasmablastic morphology. The subjectivity and heterogeneity within a given sample preclude full acceptance by all observers.

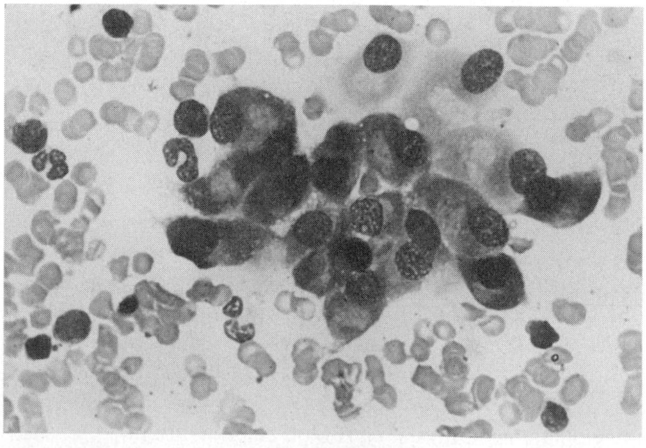

FIG. 42.15. A clump of osteoblasts in a bone marrow aspirate. The prominent Golgi structures, eccentric nuclei, abundant cytoplasm, and a "clumped" appearance may falsely suggest plasma cell myeloma (Wright-Giemsa stain, original magnification: 400× magnification).

Immunophenotypic Properties of Myeloma Cells

Multiple myeloma as a malignancy of plasma cells, the most mature cell in the B-cell series, expectedly manifests expression of monotypic cytoplasmic Ig- and plasma cell–associated antigens (PCA, PC, CD38) with the unexpected absence of most pan-B-cell antigens except for the Ig-associated pan-B antigen (CD79a) (Fig. 42.16) (77–79). In contrast with normal plasma cells that express CD19 and lack the adhesion molecules CD56 and CD58, malignant plasma cells lack CD19 and express CD56 and CD58 (80,81). The latter adhesion molecules are thought relevant to bone marrow localization. Besides CD56 and CD58, the collagen-1 binding proteoglycan, syndecan-1 (CD138), found on myeloma and normal plasma cells is also relevant to plasma cell marrow anchoring (82).

Besides the marrow plasma cells, the neoplastic clone includes circulating monoclonal idiotype-identical B lymphocytes, which may represent the myeloma stem cell (83,84). These circulating B cells express the same idiotype and isotype as the paraprotein secreted by the malignant plasma cells. Occasionally, both components, lymphoid and plasma cells, may manifest immature B-cell antigen expression (e.g., common acute lymphoblastic leukemia antigen [CALLA], CD10) (85–87). This has been referred to as CALLA$^+$ myeloma, representing a clinically significant finding portending a poor prognosis (86). Some CALLA$^+$ myeloma cells have a pre-B-cell phenotype (88–90) with cytoplasmic μ chain and nuclear terminal deoxynucleotidyl transferase (TdT) expression (Fig. 42.17). These highly proliferative myeloma pre-B cells could represent a significant component of the self-renewal or stem cell population of myeloma (77). The view that myeloma may begin with normal precursor pre-B cells is questioned by the novel nature of the myeloma pre-B cells that coexpress immature B-cell and plasma cell antigens. They may represent myeloma cells with aberrant or disorganized gene expression that produce novel phenotypes (88,89). Malignant myeloma cells may not express antigens in the normal one-way progressive, sequential fashion found in normal B-cell differentiation (89). Clinically, CALLA$^+$ myeloma survival appears favorably altered by therapy directed at the immature acute lymphoblastic leukemia-like component (88).

Myeloid and T-Cell Antigens

Occasionally (13%), myeloma may present with aberrant coexpression of myelomonocytic antigens preceding overt leukemia (Fig. 42.18) (91,92). Because many myelomonocytic myelomas express IgA, a possible receptor for granulocyte-macrophage colony-stimulating factor, the potential role of cytokine modulation is envisioned (49). These myeloid ''lineage infidelities'' or phenotypic ''platypuses'' question the true cell of origin in certain cases. Myelomonocytic myeloma, as an obvious contradiction in terms, suggests that myeloma clonal origin may entail the concept of

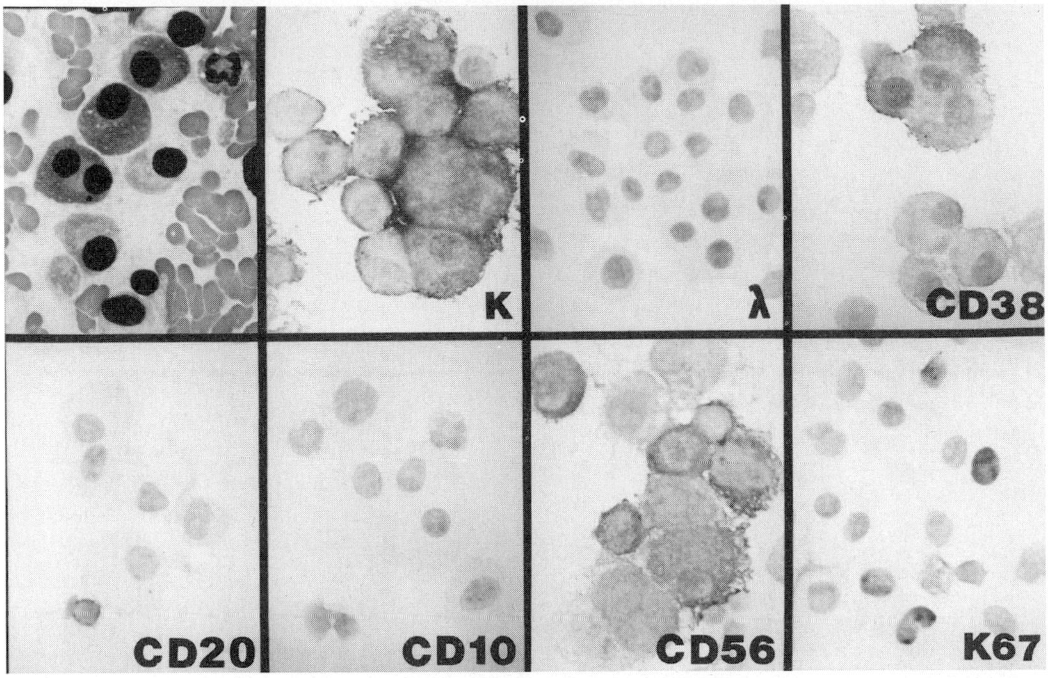

FIG. 42.16. Typical plasma cell myeloma phenotype. Immunohistochemical assay reveals monotypic immunoglobulin expression, evidenced by κ expression and absent λ; plasma cell antigen expression (CD38); absent mature (CD20) and immature (CALLA, CD10) B-cell antigens; cell adhesion molecule (CAM) expression (N-CAM, CD56); and nuclear proliferation antigen as detected by Ki-67 (K67) (immunoperoxidase stain, original magnification: 400× magnification).

sequential lineage commitment during hematopoiesis rather than a stochastic model of development (93). The rare occurrence of T-cell antigen coexpression in myeloma adds fuel to this speculative model (94). Demonstration by multiparameter flow cytometry studies of erythroid or megakaryocytic antigens on myeloma cells further favors the presence of a myeloma stem cell early in hematopoietic development as in chronic myelogenous leukemia (CML) (92,95). The analogy to CML may also have clinical relevance as CML-like myeloma has a long initial stable period followed by a terminal blastic phase (95).

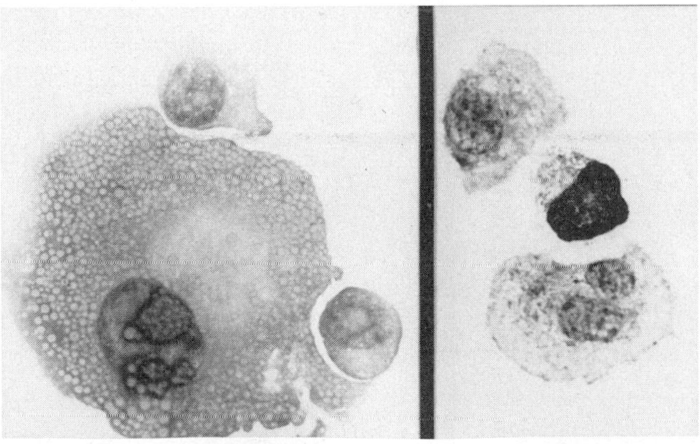

FIG. 42.17. Pre-B-cell lymphoid component associated with plasma cell myeloma. **Left:** Notice the large plasma cell with cytoplasmic inclusions (Mott cell) and nuclear inclusions (Dutcher body). **Right:** Adjacent are two small lymphoblasts with an immature pre-B-cell phenotype: cytoplasmic mu^{+}, light chain^{-}, CD10^{+}, nuclear TdT^{+} (Wright-Giemsa and immunoperoxidase stains; original magnification: 1,000× magnification).

These aberrantly acquired, mutated lineage infidelities may directly herald myeloma progression. A case in point is the emergence of CD28^{+} myeloma cells (96). This T-cell antigen initially lacking in myeloma presentation is commonly expressed in myeloma relapse and extramedullary spread. CD28 doubly adds to myeloma aggressiveness by facilitating myeloma cell survival (by overexpression of BCL-X) and proliferation (by increased labeling index) (96).

Drug Resistance Protein

Resistance to cytotoxic chemotherapy is a major problem in the treatment of patients with multiple myeloma. This phenomenon of multidrug resistance is associated with a variety of molecular mechanisms including P-glycoprotein and the lung resistance protein (LRP-56). P-glycoprotein is a surface efflux pump that removes toxic substances from plasma cells protecting them from chemotherapy (36,97,98) (Fig. 42.19). P-glycoprotein overexpression is induced specifically by known doses of Adriamycin (>300 mg) and of vincristine (>20 mg), resulting in clinical resistance to the vincristine-Adriamycin-dexamethasone (VAD) regimen (99). Although P-glycoprotein–mediated drug resistance

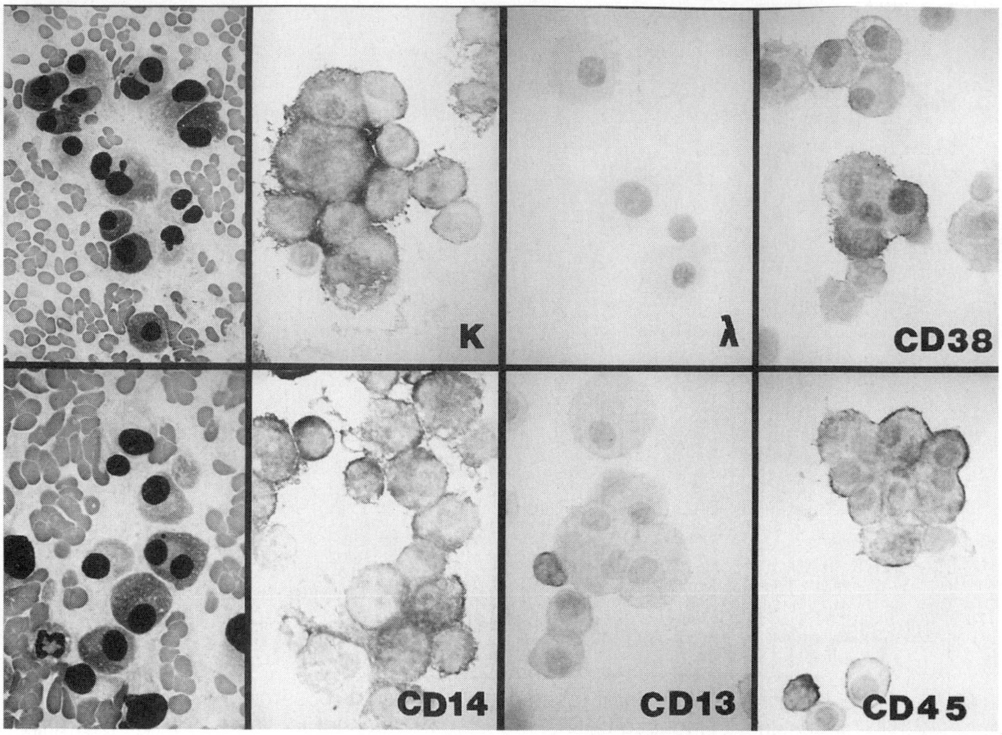

FIG. 42.18. Myelomonocytic myeloma phenotype. Immunocytochemical assay of this myeloma variant reveals monotypic immunoglobulin expression (κ^+, λ^-); plasma cell antigen expression ($CD38^+$); myeloid antigen expression ($CD14^+$, $CD13^+$); and leukocyte common antigen expression ($CD45^+$) (immunoperoxidase stain, original magnification: 400× magnification).

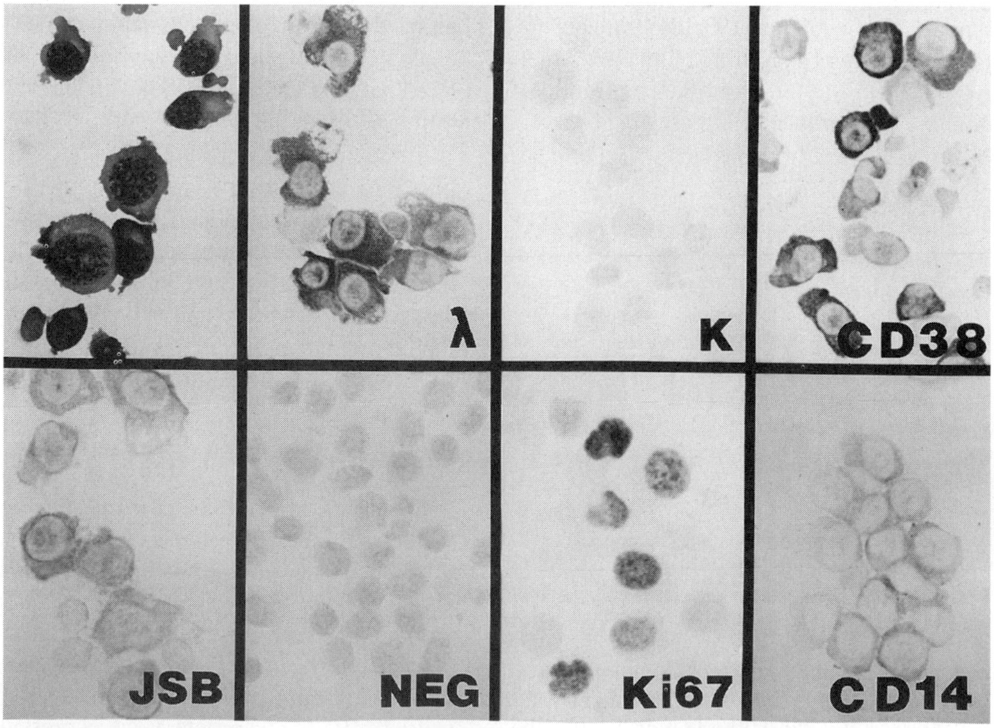

FIG. 42.19. Plasma cell leukemia with expression of drug resistance protein (P-glycoprotein). Immunocytochemical assay reveals monotypic immunoglobulin, plasma cell antigens, P-glycoprotein (as measured by JSB1), a high proliferative rate (Ki-67), and coexpressed myeloid antigen (CD14). Collectively, these findings suggest combined phenotypic escape, including myeloid and P-glycoprotein escape (immunoperoxidase stain, original magnification: 400× magnification).

could be favorably modulated by chemomodifiers (100), the clinical benefit to patients was limited because other drug-resistance mechanisms emerged (e.g., LRP56) (101,102). The multifactorial nature of multidrug-resistant glycoproteins is a factor explaining the current incurability of myeloma (101,103,104).

Proliferation Antigens

Tritiated thymidine labeling, DNA S-phase assay and bromodeoxyuridine immunofluorescence are all measures of cell kinetics that have previously proven valuable predictors of myeloma outcome (105–107). Although most myeloma patients at presentation typically show low proliferative activity, more symptomatic, progressive myeloma patients demonstrate higher plasma cell labeling indices associated with shorter survival (65,102,107) (Figs. 42.16, 42.19, 42.20). The utility of these proliferative assays has been greatly facilitated by monoclonal antibodies to nuclear proliferation antigens (e.g., Ki-67, PCNA) (102,108,109). A Ki-67 index of 20% predicts poor prognosis as illustrated in Fig. 42.20 (102,108,109). Ki-67 has also demonstrated high proliferative activity in myeloma pre-B cells, adding to the impression that the pre-B-cell may be the stem cell accounting for myeloma self-renewal (89).

Survival-Related Antigens

Myeloma cell immortalization may be, firstly, a consequence of unending proliferation or secondly because of prolonged survival through a failure to die (i.e., loss of death control) (110–112). In myeloma, death avoidance probably is a more important factor, because myeloma is characterized by a latent accumulation of "resting" plasma cells that are not in cycle and typically display very low proliferative activity (<1% Ki-67 in 90% of myeloma patients). In the pathogenesis of myeloma, the key event is not loss of growth control but enhanced myeloma cell survival through loss of death control. Myeloma cell death (apoptosis) is determined by a complex balance of survival versus contravailing death specific factors. Survival factors (e.g., BCL-2, NF-κB) confer long-term cell survival by blocking programmed cell death. Dexamethasone-induced cytotoxicity in myeloma cells is thought to be the consequence of decreased BCL-2 expression (110). Regarding proapoptotic death factors the CD95 (FAS) antigen by its ligand FASL or anti-FAS antibodies triggers the cascade of signals for apoptosis in myeloma cells (111). As myeloma progresses, suppression of FAS antigen expression on tumor cells renders them resistant to the FASL on tumor-infiltrating T cells (T-TIL) averting any antitumor immunosurveillance (111). Remarkably, the finding of constitutive expression of FASL on myeloma cells presents another potential mechanism of tumor-induced suppression of immunosurveillance (112). The FASL^{+} myeloma cells foil immunosurveillance by triggering secretion of granzyme and perforin, resulting in cytotoxic T-cell death (112).

Infiltrating Accessory Cells and Cell Adhesion Molecules

Contrary to the view that myeloma is an entirely autonomous growth, findings suggest that the host accessory cell response (e.g., T lymphocytes, monocytes, natural killer cells) can modulate the disease (113–115). Specifically, study of T-TILs suggests that immunosurveillance is a major factor in myeloma containment. Methodologies that preserve tumor-host immunoarchitectural relationships have proven pivotal in delineating these relationships (Fig. 42.21) (116). Suppressor or cytotoxic T cells within the myeloma tumor have been associated with immunosurveillance (113–115).

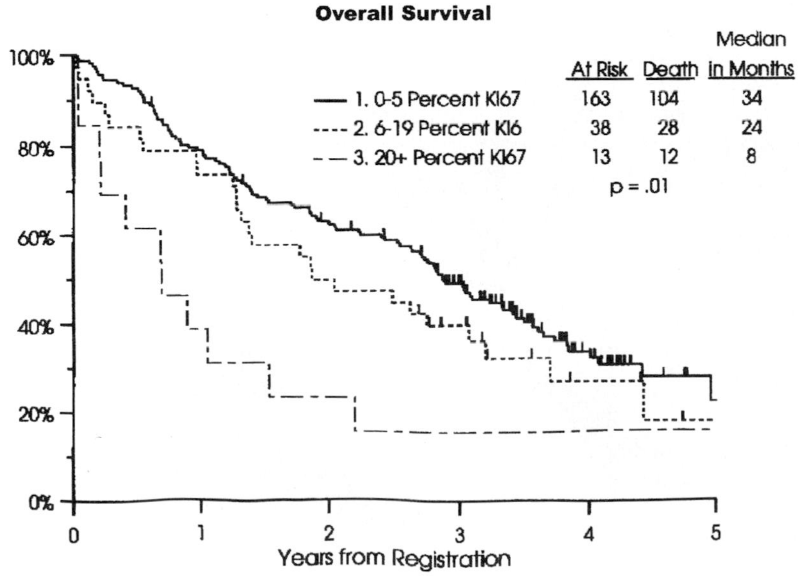

FIG. 42.20. Survival of plasma cell myeloma related to proliferative rate as measured by Ki-67 (102).

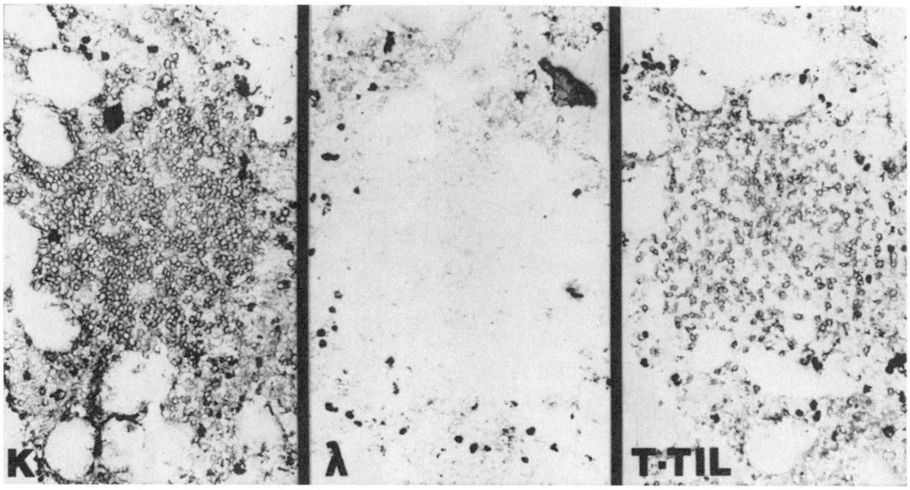

FIG. 42.21. Immunotopography of marrow myeloma. Snap-frozen sections reveal a discrete monotypic immunoglobulin-bearing tumor with striking tumor-infiltrating lymphocytes of T-cell type (T-TIL), representing idiotype-specific suppressor/cytotoxic T cells (immunoperoxidase stain, original magnification: 100× magnification).

In vitro culture studies have demonstrated enhanced growth of myeloma cells with removal of suppressor or cytotoxic T lymphocytes before plating (37). Myeloma protein stimulates idiotypic specific suppressor T-cell activity relevant to tumor containment (113–115). T-TIL in myeloma is likely subject to cytokine modulation (e.g., T-TIL adaptive immunotherapy). Knowing that myeloma is a malignancy of immunoregulatory cells leads to consideration of immunoregulatory mechanisms of containment. FASL has been identified on cytotoxic T cells and its activation by FAS on adjacent myeloma cells results in attachment of cytotoxic T cells to myeloma cells with subsequent cytotoxic T-cell secretion of granzyme and perforin resulting in myeloma cell apoptosis. FAS status and FASL status may be important to ascertain not only in myeloma cells but in myeloma infiltrating T-TILs (111,112).

Adhesion cell molecules are important in plasma cell homing and anchoring in the bone marrow (Fig. 42.22). Normal plasma cells use a repertoire of adhesion molecules, including ICAM-1 (CD54); the homing receptor (CD44); fibronectin receptors (VLA-4, VLA-5); and the collagen-binding proteoglycan, syndecan-1 (CD138) (82,84). Malignant plasma cells have a similar repertoire (Fig. 42.22), except for overexpression of CD44v variant isoforms (e.g., CD44v9) (117); overexpression of LFA-3 (CD58) (81); and overexpression of CD56, the neuronal cell adhesion mole-

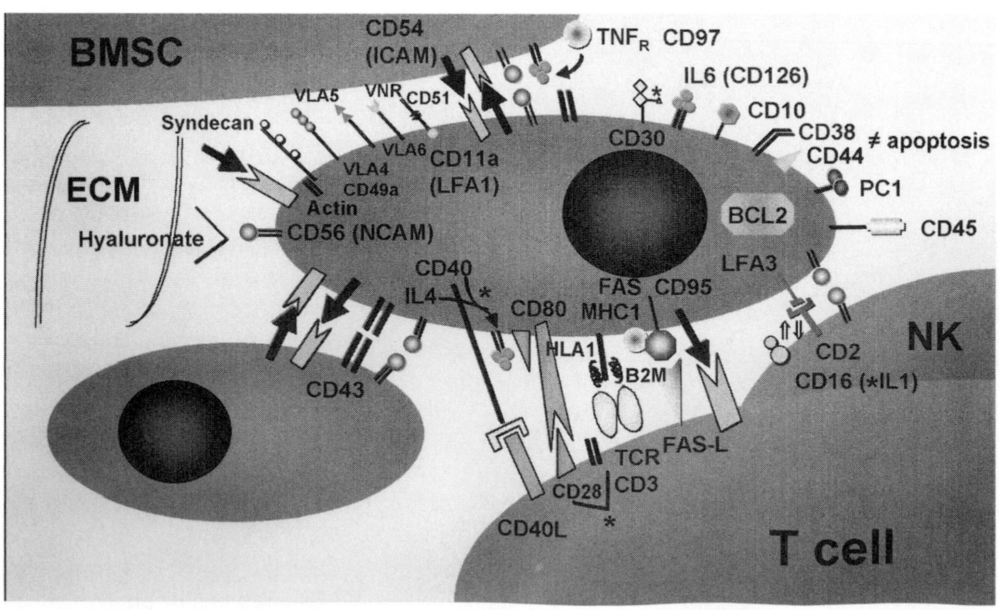

FIG. 42.22. Repertoire of cell adhesion and recognition molecules on myeloma-associated plasma cells.

cule NCAM (118,119) (Fig. 42.16). Because CD56 in particular is uniquely myeloma associated, serum levels of NCAM are especially useful in distinguishing myeloma from benign paraproteinemias (e.g., MGUS) (120). Although CD44, CD56, and CD58 are initial landmarks of beginning myeloma relevant to initial myeloma localization, later in the disease there is downregulation of CD56 and CD58, resulting in lost marrow stromal anchoring, enhanced extravasation and extramedullary dissemination (118,121). Tumor progression in myeloma is also associated with overexpression of CD44v9 variant isoforms known to facilitate tumor metastasis in other tumor types (122).

In conclusion, myeloma is not simply a malignancy of end-stage plasma cells. It is a proliferation of a complex immunoregulatory cell with a myriad of phenotypic aberrancies begging explanation and yielding rational strategies for alternative therapy.

Angiogenesis

Angiogenesis is well established as an obligatory factor in the growth, invasion, and metastasis of solid tumors (123). Angiogenesis has also been associated with progression of myeloma (124). Specific vascular growth factor receptors (e.g., VEGF, FLT-1) have been isolated in myeloma, suggesting specific antiangiogenesis agents (e.g., anti-VEGF, anti-FLT-1) (125).

Cytokines

Myeloma cells express receptors for a great variety of growth factors (e.g., vitamin D_3, glucocorticoids, estrogen, progesterones) (126,127) and lymphokines (e.g., IL-1, IL-4, IL-5, IL-6) (128–130). Growth and lymphokine receptors probably play an important role in sustaining growth and differentiation in myeloma. The therapeutic response to glucocorticoids and interferon-α could correlate with specific receptor expression (131). Myeloma cells constitutively produce a variety of cytokines (IL-4 through IL-6) that may have autostimulatory effects by means of complementary (IL-4 through IL-6) receptors (128–130). This autostimulatory loop would characterize the autonomous growth phase of myeloma (129). This may be preceded or supplemented by a paracrine growth mechanism whereby cytokines (e.g., IL-6) produced by marrow-adherent accessory cells (e.g., fibroblasts, monocytes, T cells) provide growth regulation of myeloma cells (130). Mouse plasmacytoma related to intraperitoneal injections of pristane or mineral oil may relate to cytokine expression by stimulated macrophages (22). In early phase myeloma, bone marrow derived monocytes, fibroblasts and T cells may account for growth-stimulating effects and may facilitate myeloma cell localization in bone marrow by peripheral blood precursors. According to the three-signal Kishimoto model, B-cell activation, proliferation, stimulation, and differentiation of plasma cells depend on the respective effects of IL-4, IL-5, and IL-6 (128,131,132). Paracrine and autocrine effects in particular are the critical last steps in ensuring plasma cell morphology and phenotype (128,132).

Besides autostimulatory signals plasma cells may produce cytokines with effects on other cells, accounting for a variety of remote disease effects. A case in point would be the constitutive expression by myeloma cells of TNF-β (lymphotoxin) and IL-1, which represent osteoclast-activating factors that stimulate osteoclasts and cause osteolytic bone lesions (133–135).

An ascending scale of regulatory aberrancies could account for the pathogenesis of myeloma: initial marrow localization or anchoring of immature lymphoid pre-B-cell precursors may be caused by marrow paracrine stimulations (128–130) and cell adhesion molecule expressions (e.g., NCAM) (118,119); subsequent autocrine growth by plasma cells may lead to self-sustained growth (128); or subsequent abnormal gene expression through rearrangement, mutation, or loss of suppressor gene activity because of deletion or alteration of critical antioncogenes (increased *MYC*, increased *HRAS, TP53*) could result in myeloma progression (33,34,40).

Tumor Cells in the Peripheral Blood

In a reactive plasmacytosis and in malignant myeloma, circulating mature plasma cells are not generally found in the peripheral blood. Rather, circulating tumor cells take the form of lymphoid B-cell precursors, frequently of B-cell and pre-B-cell phenotypes. This fact is evidenced by findings of circulating DNA-aneuploid lymphoid cells (136), concordant Ig gene rearrangement between blood and marrow lymphoid and plasma cells (137), plasma cell antigens on peripheral B cells (83,89,138), and idiotype-identical, isotype-concordant surface Ig on circulating lymphoid and marrow-bound plasma cells (83,85,139,140). Several of these peripheral blood phenotypic alterations have been associated with poor survival, including increased peripheral blood lymphocytes expressing plasma cell antigen ($CD38^+$, $PCA1^+$) (138); increased suppressor to helper T-cell ratio (138); increased CD10 $(CALLA)^+$ lymphoid cells (85,88,89); and loss of light-chain isotype concordant lymphoid suppression (141). The increased $CD38^+$ and $CD10^+$ and isotype specific cells reflect increased neoplastic precursor activity (138), and the increased suppressor T cells are thought to represent attempted suppression of tumor clone expression (114,115). As reflected by electrophoresis, decreased nonneoplastic γ-globulins indicates a reduction of normal peripheral blood B cells. This immunodeficiency and consequent hypogammopathy are concomitants of the monoclonal gammopathy and account for frequent recurrent bacterial infections common among myeloma patients. Suppression of normal B cells in myeloma is thought to occur by a combination of suppressor T-cell effect (114,115) and an Ig-binding factor similar to Ig-FMC receptor shed by T cells (142). Myeloma precursor lymphoid cells are thought to displace other B-cell precursors (83).

Phenotypic Escape

Analogous to CML, terminal myeloma progression is characterized by tumor cell phenotypic transformation. In some cases, this takes the form of a lymphoma-like transition with a high lactate dehydrogenase (LDH) level and lymphoid features with disease in lymph nodes, liver, blood, and brain. This phenomenon is sometimes accompanied by loss of the myeloma M-component and has been referred to as *phenotypic escape.* Analogous to CML, myeloma in this instance has escaped into a lymphoma-like phenotype. Besides lymphoma-like escape, other modes of escape include:

Acute lymphoid leukemia escape (pre-B and $CD10^+$ phenotypes)
Transition to acute myelomonocytic leukemia (20% of cases at 5 years)
Drug-resistant escape (P-glycoprotein found in 75% of drug refractory myeloma in VAD-resistant cases)
Proliferative escape (high Ki-67 or labeling indices characterize many terminal myeloma states)
Immunosurveillance escape related to loss of effective immunoregulation

This suggests multiple modes whereby a myeloma tumor escapes, causing therapeutic failure. Any effective therapeutic strategy necessarily must overcome this multifactorial problem.

In the end, the value of phenotyping myeloma is twofold: in selecting poor prognosis patients as potential candidates for newly proposed aggressive chemotherapy regimens or alternative therapies such as allogeneic bone marrow transplantation and in identifying new cellular targets for therapy (e.g., P-glycoprotein, VEGF, cyclin D1).

Diagnosis and Staging

Plasma cell proliferative disease ranges from asymptomatic patients with an incidental monoclonal gammopathy known as MGUS to highly symptomatic myeloma patients with generalized multifocal destructive bone lesions throughout the skeletal system. Between these extremes are a variety of clinical phases representing a spectrum of diseases, including indolent myeloma, smoldering myeloma, and solitary plasmacytoma of bone or soft tissue (143–145). In the case of MGUS with only monoclonal protein in the serum or urine, the major diagnostic focus has been on distinction of MGUS from early multiple myeloma. Between 20% and 30% of MGUS patients develop myeloma over 10 years, indicating that MGUS is a ''premyelomatous'' condition (47,146). The puzzle remains: which patients will convert?

With overt generalized myeloma, the patients commonly present with bone pain, anemia, and infection (e.g., pneumococcal). Some may also have hypercalcemia, renal failure, or spinal cord compression (147). In all of the aforementioned conditions, diagnosis is based on finding an increase in plasma cells, as described previously. A serum or urinary M-component is found in 99% of patients (147). In the case of multiple myeloma, skeletal x-ray films reveal multiple ''punched-out'' osteolytic bony lesions. Radiographically, the lesions appear as 1- to 4-cm punched-out defects without sclerosis. The most common sites of involvement are in areas of active hematocytopoiesis, including (in order of frequency) vertebrae, ribs, skull, pelvis, femur, clavicle, and scapula. The bony defects on gross examination are filled with a soft gelatinous, fish-flesh, hemorrhagic tissue (148) (Fig. 42.4). A combination of findings leads to the diagnosis of multiple myeloma, including a marrow plasmacytosis of more than 10%, osteolytic lesions and a plasma or urinary monoclonal protein (147). Given the difficulty of sampling spotty disease, a mixture of criteria has been established to diagnose myeloma and its various phases (147). These criteria are shown in Tables 42.1 and 42.2 (73,143,144,147). In the case of diagnostic uncertainty, the ultimate diagnosis of plasma cell myeloma rests on finding evidence of uncontrolled plasma cell growth as evidenced by plasma cell sheets, osteolytic lesions, or a progressive increase in the concentration of monoclonal protein (149,150).

Different schemes have evolved to define the extent of myeloma based on clinical features and direct measurement of myeloma mass. A useful clinical staging system using a combination of tumor mass and renal function was devised at the Arizona Cancer Center by Durie and Salmon (147,151,152). In this scheme (Table 42.3), increased tumor burden and poor renal function are associated with shorter survival time. As confirmed by other investigations, median survival strongly relates to stage, with stage I survival of more than 60 months, stage II survival of 41 months, and stage III survival of 23 months determined for more than 1,400 patients (147). Similarly, myeloma patients with normal renal function experienced a 37-month median survival,

TABLE 42.1. *Diagnostic criteria for multiple myeloma*

A. The diagnosis of myeloma requires a minimum of one major and one minor criteria or three minor criteria, which must include (1) and (2). These criteria must manifest in a symptomatic patient with progressive disease.
B. Major criteria
   1. Plasmacytoma on biopsy
   2. Marrow plasmacytosis (>30%)
   3. M-component: Serum: IgG > 3.5 g/dL, IgA >2 g/dL Urine ≥1 g/24 hr of κ or λ (Bence Jones [BJ] protein) without amyloidosis
C. Minor criteria
   1. Marrow plasmacytosis (10–30%)
   2. M-component: present but less than above
   3. Lytic bone lesions
   4. Reduced normal immunoglobulins (<50% normal): IgG <600 mg/dL, IgA <100 mg/dL, IgM <50 mg/dL

Data from references 73, 143, 144, and 147.

TABLE 42.2. *Diagnostic criteria for monoclonal gammopathy of undetermined significance, indolent and smoldering myeloma*

A. Monoclonal gammopathy of undetermined significance
   1. M-component present but less than Table 42. 1 B myeloma levels
   2. Marrow plasmacytosis <10%
   3. *No* lytic bone lesions
   4. *No* myeloma-related symptoms
B. Indolent myeloma: criteria as for myeloma (Table 42.1) except
   1. Absent or rare bone lesions (≤3 lytic lesions), without compression fractures
   2. M-component: IgG <7 g/dL, IgA <5 g/dL
   3. Normal hemoglobin, serum calcium and creatinine
   4. *No* infection
C. Smoldering myeloma: same as indolent except
   1. *No* bone lesions
   2. Marrow plasmacytosis (10–30%)

Data from references 73, 143, 144, and 147.

compared with 8 months for the renally impaired (147,151,152). Other factors used include hemoglobin, serum calcium, assessment of lytic lesions, and amount of the M-component. Serum level of β_2-microglobulin has also been used as a discriminating factor, with a higher β_2-microglobulin level (76 mg/dL) associated with poor survival (153). The β_2-microglobulin level is thought to reflect tumor mass and renal function, giving in a single assay clear separation of risk groups (153).

Differential Diagnosis

The unique triad of osteolytic lesions, atypical marrow plasmacytosis, and monoclonal gammopathy generally makes the diagnosis of plasma cell myeloma straightforward. Together, the findings are pathognomonic and unambiguous. However, each finding may occur independent of myeloma, leading to diagnostic confusion.

TABLE 42.3. *Myeloma staging system*

Stage I
   1. Low M-component levels: IgG <5 g/dL, IgA <3 g/dL; urine Bence Jones (BJ) protein <4 g/24 hr.
   2. Absent or solitary bone lesions.
   3. Normal hemoglobin, serum calcium, Ig levels (non-M component).

Stage III: any one or more of the following:
   1. High M-component: IgG >7 g/dL, IgA >5 g/dL; urine BJ 12/24 hr
   2. Advanced, multiple lytic bone lesions
   3. Hemoglobin <8.5 g/dL, serum calcium >12 mg/dL

Stage II: overall values between I and III

Subclassification: based on renal function
   A = serum creatinine <2 mg/dL
   B = serum creatinine >2 mg/dL

Examples
   Stage IA = low myeloma mass (<$0.6 \times 10^{12}/m^2$) with normal renal function
   Stage IIIB = high myeloma mass (<$1.2 \times 10^{12}/m^2$) with abnormal renal function

Data from references 147, 151, and 152.

Osteolytic lesions independent of myeloma may occur in hyperparathyroidism, metastatic carcinoma, or primary bone neoplasia (154). Although the constellation of lytic lesions, hypercalcemia, and renal disease in secondary hyperparathyroidism may be clinically confusing initially, the absence of a marrow plasmacytosis and of a monoclonal gammopathy coupled with the usual elevated serum alkaline phosphatase allow unambiguous distinction (154). Although the bone marrow biopsy shows osteoclastic activity, there is also striking osteoblastic activity unlike myeloma. Direct marrow biopsy reveals the true nature of osteolysis related to metastatic carcinoma and primary bone tumors. Because isolated monoclonal gammopathy has been described in metastatic cancer, direct marrow biopsy and serial assessment of gammopathy are necessary (155). The M-component in metastatic carcinoma is not produced by the neoplasm but rather thought to be a host response to the neoplasm or, in some cases, a second incipient neoplasm (154).

Marrow plasmacytosis of striking proportions may occur in a number of inflammatory conditions, chronic infections, autoimmune diseases, and hypersensitivity states (Figs. 42.11, 42.12). Marrow plasmacytosis may be associated with liver cirrhosis, syphilis, agranulocytosis, rheumatoid arthritis, Hodgkin's disease, and aplastic or hypoplastic anemia (146,155,156). These reactive plasmacytoses, although sometimes striking (e.g., more than 50% plasma cells in recovery from agranulocytosis) (Fig. 42.12), are generally composed of scattered, not aggregated, plasma cells. Although binucleate or rare trinucleate plasma cells may be seen, pleomorphic, anaplastic, dyssynchronous plasma cells with prominent nucleoli are usually not found in reactive states (Fig. 42.12). In these reactive plasmacytoses, electrophoresis generally reveals a broad-based polyclonal hypergammaglobulinemia (146,155,156). Although scattered, not sheetlike, plasma cells are the general rule in reactive plasmacytoses, a few exceptional circumstances are worthy of note. Hashimoto's thyroiditis and plasma cell granuloma are examples of benign conditions that may produce a displacing mass or tumor suggesting neoplasia (157). In the case of plasma cell granuloma a primary plasmacytoma is suggested clinically (157). In this circumstance of nonneoplastic tumorous reactive plasmacytosis, there are three important differential properties: lack of plasma cell pleomorphism, dyssynchrony, or anaplasia; lack of a monoclonal gammopathy; and direct phenotypic evidence of cytoplasmic plasma cell polyclonal Ig through immunohistochemistry (Fig. 42.11). These three specific criteria are highly applicable in the head and neck or nasopharyngeal region, where most extramedullary plasmacytomas occur, but there is also a high incidence of chronic mucosa-associated plasmacytosis related to hypersensitivity or allergic states (Fig. 42.11) (158). Comparable confusion may occur in Felty's syndrome, in which the splenomegaly associated with rheumatoid arthritis is largely the consequence of splenic plasmacytosis. The sheer extent of the latter may suggest neoplasia, but the previously mentioned morphologic and phenotypic criteria, coupled with knowledge of the clinical circumstance, make the diagnosis unambiguous.

The differential diagnosis of extramedullary plasmacytoma may be difficult in two circumstances of differentiation. In the first case, that of a ''well-differentiated plasmacytoma,'' the morphologic criteria of pleomorphism and anaplasia may be absent, making distinction from plasma cell granuloma moot. In this instance, serologic or urinary evidence of a monoclonal gammopathy plus phenotypic evidence of clonality by immunohistochemistry are pivotal (Figs. 42.9, 42.10). In the second case, that of an ''anaplastic'' plasmacytoma, the lack of obvious plasma cell differentiation begs distinction from an immunoblastic lymphoma with plasmacytic features (159–161) or even a poorly differentiated carcinoma (Fig. 42.13).

The distinction between anaplastic plasmacytoma and immunoblastic lymphoma has important clinical implications (159). Extramedullary solitary plasmacytomas (EPCs) may experience prolonged survival (median, >10 years) with simple local excision, radiotherapy, or both, whereas immunoblastic lymphoma (IBL), a high-grade lymphoma, has a more aggressive course (median survival, 16 months) and requires combined chemotherapy (159,162) to ensure favorable results (154). Major differences in therapy and outcome hinge on the morphologic distinction of EPC from IBL. However, anaplastic myeloma may lack the obvious plasma cell differentiation found in some IBLs, making morphologic distinction uncertain at best (Fig. 42.13). In this difficult circumstance a combination of nuclear features and phenotypic properties are said to be discriminating (160). EPCs have variegated chromatin, less conspicuous nucleoli, and eccentrically placed nuclei, whereas IBL nuclei generally have clear chromatin and prominent nucleoli (Fig. 42.13) (160). Although useful in many cases, the anaplastic EPCs can defy ready categorization by this morphologic scheme. In this circumstance, further diagnostic assertion may be gained by phenotyping as immunophenotypic differences between EPC and IBL are described (160,161). Plasmacytomas more commonly express γ or α Ig heavy chains; have plasma cell-associated antigens (e.g., CD38, PC, PCA); lack Ia, pan-B-cell antigens (except CD79a), pan-T-cell antigens, and leukocyte common antigen (LCA, CD45); and have a low proliferative rate (Ki-67) (161). Immunoblastic lymphomas more frequently express μ Ig, CD45 (LCA), and pan-B-cell (CD19, CD20, CD22, CD79a) or T-cell antigens; express Ia; and have a high Ki-67 index with absent plasma cell–associated antigen (161).

A battery of phenotypic findings generally strongly supports EPC or IBL immunohistochemically. Exceptionally, true phenotypic hybrids with a complete admixture of myeloma-like and lymphoma-like markers occur. These plasmacytoma-lymphoma hybrids appear as a phenotypic platypus, not fitting into the usual therapy schemes. The occurrence of these phenotypic hybrids, although confusing the therapeutic choice, should not be seen as surprising given our knowledge of phenotypic escape as a complication of myeloma (162). This lymphoma-like complication of myeloma is characterized by a high LDH, lymphorecticular system involvement (lymph nodes, spleen, liver [Fig. 42.4], bone marrow), and a rapid downhill course—a constellation associated with IBL (163). The sometimes lymphoma-like properties of plasmacytoma and myeloma may be inherent in plasma cell neoplastic pathogenesis. In this context, the finding of complete phenotypic hybrids is fully understandable. Further study may establish that this variant warrants lymphoma-like combined chemotherapy rather than localized therapy, given its present poor outcome (163).

Besides lymphoma-like EPCs, myeloma may also present with leukemia-like features. Sometimes, this is in the form of circulating plasma cells, as in plasma cell leukemia (discussed subsequently), or sometimes this takes the form of myeloid or lymphoid leukemia (88,89,91,92). Much as a multilineage blast crisis may complicate CML terminally, myeloma may eventuate (and rarely manifest) as acute myeloid or lymphoid leukemia (164,165). Approximately 20% of myeloma patients develop acute myelomonocytic leukemia by 5 years (164,165). Although in many cases this is probably a second neoplasm complicating the primary myeloma, in numerous instances, the neoplastic cells are true hybrids of myeloid and plasma cell antigens, suggesting a multilineage stem cell (89,92). This has been referred to as *myelomonocytic myeloma*, and it sometimes occurs at presentation, before therapy, indicating that it may be inherently part of myeloma and not necessarily a complication of therapy (89) (Fig. 42.18). This implies, as with CML, an early stem cell lineage in some myeloma cases and in any discussion of differential diagnosis begs the question of certain distinction between myelomonocytic myeloma and AML (89,92). Rare cases of myelomonocytic leukemia with a cytoplasmic M-component in the neoplastic myeloid cells may be explained by the multilineage origin (166). As with lymphoma-like myeloma, the distinction is moot in some cases and may suggest a rationale for alternative leukemia-like adapted therapy—a matter for future research.

Acute lymphoblastic leukemia-like myeloma has been described in the context of some myeloma cases with prominent pre-B-cell phenotypes (Fig. 42.17) (88,89). It has been referred to as $CALLA^{+}$ myeloma (86). As with lymphoma-like and myeloid leukemia-like myeloma, this form of myeloma, although clinically not separable, may be readily recognized phenotypically by the presence of coexpressed plasma cell (CD38) and pre-B-cell antigens (89).

Besides osteolytic lesions and plasmacytosis, the final triad member, a monoclonal gammopathy, may also occur independent of myeloma (Table 42.4). It may occur in the context of other immunoproliferative disorders: Waldenström's macroglobulinemia or heavy-chain disease (167). The former diseases are distinguished by their morphology, which is more lymphocytic than plasmacytic, and by their

TABLE 42.4. *Diseases associated with monoclonal gammopathy of undetermined significance*

Disease category (examples)	Incidence (%)
None:	26
Cardiac/cerebrovascular: myocardial infarction, atherosclerosis	13
Inflammatory/infections: "FUO," phlebitis, cholelithiasis, second-degree amyloidosis, bronchitis, pyelonephritis, parasitic disease	11
Malignant: malignant lymphoma, CLL, CML, AMML; carcinoma of colon, breast, prostate	7
Connective tissue: rheumatoid arthritis, ankylosing spondylitis, lupus erythematosus, scleroderma, Sjögren's syndrome	6
Neurologic: peripheral neuropathy/ myopathy	6
Benign tumor: thyroid nodules and colon polyps	3
Hematologic: agnogenic myeloid metaplasia, polycythemia vera, ITP, red cell aplasia, Gaucher's disease	3.5
Endocrine: hyperparathyroidism, osteoporosis	3.5
Miscellaneous: lichen myxedematous, cirrhosis, cryoglobulinuria, cold agglutinin disease, sarcoid, renal acidosis	21

AMML, acute myelomonocytic leukemia; CLL, chronic lymphocytic leukemia; CML, chronic myelogenous leukemia; FUO, fever of unknown origin; ITP, idiopathic thrombocytopenic purpura.

Data from references 47, 146, 155, 156, and 168.

organ distribution, which is usually also more lymphoid (e.g., reticuloendothelial system). Monoclonal gammopathies in the form of monoclonal serum proteins or light-chain proteinuria may occur independent of a plasma cell dyscrasia in nonmyelomatous neoplasia (i.e., metastatic carcinoma) and in benign conditions (Table 42.4) (47,146,155,156,168). The latter circumstance has been referred to as benign monoclonal gammopathy (BMG) (156) or as MGUS (47,146) (defined in Table 42.2). As implied by the former term, a variety of inflammatory, infectious, and neoplastic features (Table 42.4) may have an M-component as an incidental or transient secondary circumstance (47,146,155,156,168). This non-neoplastic M-component or spike, benign monoclonal gammopathy, is characterized by a serum Ig level of less than 1 to 1.5 g/dL, with no serial increase over several years and without marrow plasmacytosis (146). The term BMG emphasizes that a transition to myeloma is not a necessary circumstance. The term MGUS emphasizes the obverse circumstance, whereby transition to myeloma or macroglobulinemia or to related disorders occurs at the rate of 2% per year, resulting in a nearly 30% conversion to neoplasia by 5 years (47,146). The MGUS term emphasizes the unpredictable ''unknown'' but nonetheless possible conversion to neoplasia (''significance'') (47,146). The ''unpredictable'' conversion necessitates regular serum/urine electrophoresis for MGUS patients over long intervals, because conversions may occur even two to three decades later and transition may be sudden (47,146). Because the incidence of MGUS increases with age to 3% to 5% by the seventh decade, many disorders said to be associated with a monoclonal gammopathy could merely represent chance associations (47). A case in point is the sometimes-associated atherosclerotic heart disease and MGUS (Table 42.4) (155,156), a likely chance association without a parallel control group of comparable age. In the differential diagnosis of myeloma, the frequent occurrence of MGUS poses the most common entity requiring distinction. The absolute criteria are listed in Tables 42.1 and 42.2, but fundamentally it is systemic evidence of progressive uncontrolled plasma cell growth in the form of x-ray proof of lytic lesions and electrophoretic proof of progressive monoclonal gammopathy that allows distinction of myeloma from MGUS.

VARIANT FORMS OF MULTIPLE MYELOMA

Solitary Plasmacytoma of Bone

Truly solitary skeletal plasmacytomas are a rare localized expression of multiple myeloma with an unpredictable natural history (169–176). By definition, it is a clonal plasma cell malignancy that appears solitary on a radiologic skeletal survey (169,170). Away from the solitary lesion, the marrow is initially free of plasmacytosis, and lytic lesions are absent. Consistent with low overall tumor burden many patients (75%) with solitary osseous myeloma (SOM) lack an M-component. The 25% with serum spikes typically have low-level gammopathies (e.g., >1.5 g/dL) with normal or near-normal nonclonal Ig levels (176). Although the vertebral bodies are the most common (60%) site of involvement, other central hematopoietically active sites (e.g., pelvis, femur, humerus) are also described, with rare involvement possible anywhere in the skeletal system (169–172,176). The radiologic appearance of the solitary bone lesion is typically purely osteolytic, without a blastic component, and may resemble a primary giant cell tumor of bone (169). Although some plasmacytomas develop singly and remain solitary (30%), most spread within 3 years and become typically disseminated multiple myeloma (70%) (169–175). The solitary lesions independent of myeloma may recur locally or as a new solitary lesion at a distant site (175,176). This unpredictable amalgam of outcomes nonetheless leads to a median survival of more than 10 years for SOM (170,175,176). Rare cases of SOM without dissemination as long as 15 to 35 years after initial diagnosis are described, suggesting ''a true solitary plasmacytoma is one whose growth is slow enough for the patient to die of some other disease'' (169).

Besides occasional long-term survival, the median age of onset for SOM is 50 years, compared with the median age for multiple myeloma of 63 years. There is also a higher male incidence of SOM relative to multiple myeloma, suggesting a different clinical profile compared with multiple myeloma (174–176).

Treatment for solitary plasmacytoma is appropriately localized, consisting of either or both surgical excision and supervoltage irradiation (40 to 50 Gy), which generally eradicates the myeloma tumor, although subsequent multiple myeloma remains an unpredictable possibility. Unlike typical multiple myeloma, the SOM-related gammopathy often disappears completely after surgical excision or local irradiation of the tumor (169–175).

Extramedullary Plasmacytoma

Extraosseous myelomas constitute 3% to 5% of all plasma cell neoplasms (158). These neoplasms may occur in virtually any location around the body, including unusual sites like the foot, thigh, testes, vocal cords, salivary glands, vagina, spleen, kidney, skin, and liver (158,169,173,177) (Figs. 42.4, 42.9, 42.10).

Unusual sites aside, the most common (>80%) site of extramedullary plasmacytomas is the upper respiratory tract, including the oropharynx, nasopharynx, nasal cavities and sinuses, and larynx (158,178). These head and neck plasmacytomas tend to occur primarily in mucosa-associated sites and secondarily involve the lymph nodes draining these sites (179). Many extramedullary plasmacytomas (EMP) tend to remain localized and surgical excision with localized radiotherapy (30 to 50 Gy) is frequently curative (162,180). Specifically, 70% of EMP patients are alive at 10 years, with a median survival of more than 100 months (162,180). Because secondary spread is through regional lymph nodes, regional radiotherapy is a rational form of therapy. Occasionally, EMPs are not localized and may represent metastasis from multiple myeloma or may disseminate to produce widespread disease with a less favorable disease course (169,170). A complete skeletal survey and clinical staging are important for predicting outcome. As with solitary plasmacytoma, a monoclonal gammopathy is found in 25% of cases and therapy may prove curative with disappearance of the M-component (180).

Nonsecretory Myeloma

Between 1% and 4% of patients with multiple myeloma may lack a demonstrable monoclonal protein in the serum or urine (181–183). In most cases, immunohistochemical studies demonstrate the presence of light- or heavy-chain restricted Ig expression within the neoplastic plasma cells, indicating a functional failure to secrete despite intact Ig synthesis (184). In rare cases, no Ig synthesis may be detected (185). The lack of a serum or urine monoclonal gammopathy can make nonsecretory myeloma difficult to detect. A case in point is a rare variant known as *oncocytic nonsecretory myeloma* (181), which is doubly difficult to diagnose because the neoplastic cells are large, polygonal, eosinophilic, and packed with mitochondria not looking like plasma cells, and the patient lacks an M-component. In this difficult diagnostic circumstance, immunohistochemical evaluation of tissue generally reveals unequivocal monoclonality (186) (Figs. 42.10, 42.11). Survival of nonsecretory myeloma has variously been said to be worse than, similar to, or better than secretory myeloma (182,187). The past reports which have indicated a more favorable survival (medians of 39 and 46 months versus 21 months for secretory myeloma) reflect a lower tumor burden. Nonsecretory myeloma of a stage comparable to classic secretory myeloma showed a disease course and natural history identical to classic myeloma (183).

Plasma Cell Leukemia

Plasma cell leukemia (PCL) is generally a rare (1%), terminal complication of multiple myeloma characterized by increased numbers of plasma cells in the peripheral blood (Fig. 42.19) (188–191). Specifically, PCL is diagnosed when more than 20% of peripheral blood white blood cells are plasma cells or their absolute number exceeds 2×10^9/L (188). More infrequently, PCL may present *de novo* without preceding myeloma. With primary *de novo* or secondary multiple myeloma–related cases this peripheral blood plasmacytosis usually heralds rapid disease progression (median survival of less than 6 months) with massive (>90%) marrow replacement, hepatosplenomegaly, anemia, and bleeding (188–191). Only rare long-term survivors (>4 years) are described (192,193). Osteolytic lesions and consequent bone pain are less frequent than in typical multiple myeloma (188–191). There is also a lower incidence of monoclonal gammopathy. Plasma cell leukemia is a more frequent complication of IgE (>25%) and IgD (75%) myeloma and less frequently related to IgG or IgA (188,194). Frequently, PCL patients secrete unassembled or half molecules of Ig indicating aberrant Ig synthesis (190). The blast cells of PCL have a more immature phenotype than classic myeloma (e.g., PCL $CD20^+$, MM $CD20^-$) and a higher proliferative rate. The latter would explain the poor outcome of PCL. The lack of CD56 expression in PCL compared with multiple myeloma is thought to explain the loss of anchoring to marrow stroma (191).

OTHER PLASMA CELL NEOPLASMS

Waldenström's Macroglobulinemia

This immunoproliferative disorder presents with an amalgam of lymphoma-like and myeloma-like features (195–197). Commonly, there is simultaneous enlargement of lymph nodes, liver and spleen and bone marrow involvement, without osteolysis, consistent with a lymphocytic lymphoma-like tissue distribution (195–197). The myeloma-like property, consistent with derivation from an Ig secretory B-cell, is the characteristic M-component composed of high-molecular-weight IgM, which often causes a hyperviscosity syndrome, bleeding manifestations, and cryoglobulinemia (195).

This hybrid lymphoma-myeloma quality is also manifested morphologically and immunologically. Morphologically, the tissue infiltrates are composed of a mixture of small ovoid lymphocytes, plasmacytoid lymphocytes, and plasma cells (198) (Figs. 42.21, 42.22). The distinctive cell in this disorder, the plasmacytoid lymphocyte, is sometimes referred to as a *plymph.* Characteristically, Dutcher bodies, representing PAS positive IgM inclusions, are often seen in the nucleus or cytoplasm of these cells (Figs. 42.23, 42.24) (198). Tissue mast cells are commonly admixed. Marrow effacement is common with initial ''nodular'' and subsequent diffuse involvement (198). In general, the proliferative index of the neoplastic lymphoid and plasma cells is low and explains the indolent ''low-grade'' natural history with a 50-month median survival (196). Some Waldenström's infiltrates initially, and others eventually, show a polymorphous pattern with admixed immunoblastic and plasmablastic cells, heralding a more proliferative lesion (198). A histologic staging scheme has been proposed entailing three cytologic categories: lymphocyte predominant, plasma cell predominant, and mixed ''polymorphous'' with numerous plasmablasts (198). A histologic scheme details the degree of marrow lymphocytosis. Median survival of patients with Waldenström's macroglobulinemia has specifically been related to the degree of marrow involvement: 55, 21, and 8 months, respectively, for marrow involvement of less than 20%, 20% to 50%, and more than 50%. Marrow morphologic assessments then are useful in prognostic judgments of Waldenström's macroglobulinemia.

Waldenström's macroglobulinemia cells show phenotypic properties consistent with late stage B-cell development with transition into plasma cell differentiation (199). Specifically, the lymphoid cells show pan-B antigen and surface IgM coexpressions, while the plasmacytoid and plasma cells contain cytoplasmic IgM (199). The serum M-component often exceeds 10 g/dL with frequent consequent hyperviscosity (200,201). The patient's reduced visual acuity is thought to reflect rouleaux formation or ''sludging'' in ocular vessels (201,202). The frequent peripheral neuropathies are thought to reflect specificity or cross-reactivity of the IgM with myelin sheath antigens (203). The frequent bleeding problems are related to coagulopathies caused by IgM binding to clotting factors, platelets, and fibrin (204,205). Cutaneous bullous disease may result from IgM paraprotein directed to epidermis (206). Unlike the pattern in myeloma, only 10% of macroglobulinemia patients have Bence Jones proteins, and depression of normal Igs, while evident, is less pronounced (207). Renal disease is also less common, perhaps reflecting reduced Bence Jones proteinuria (208). The usual serum protein electrophoresis and immunofixation IgM M-

A

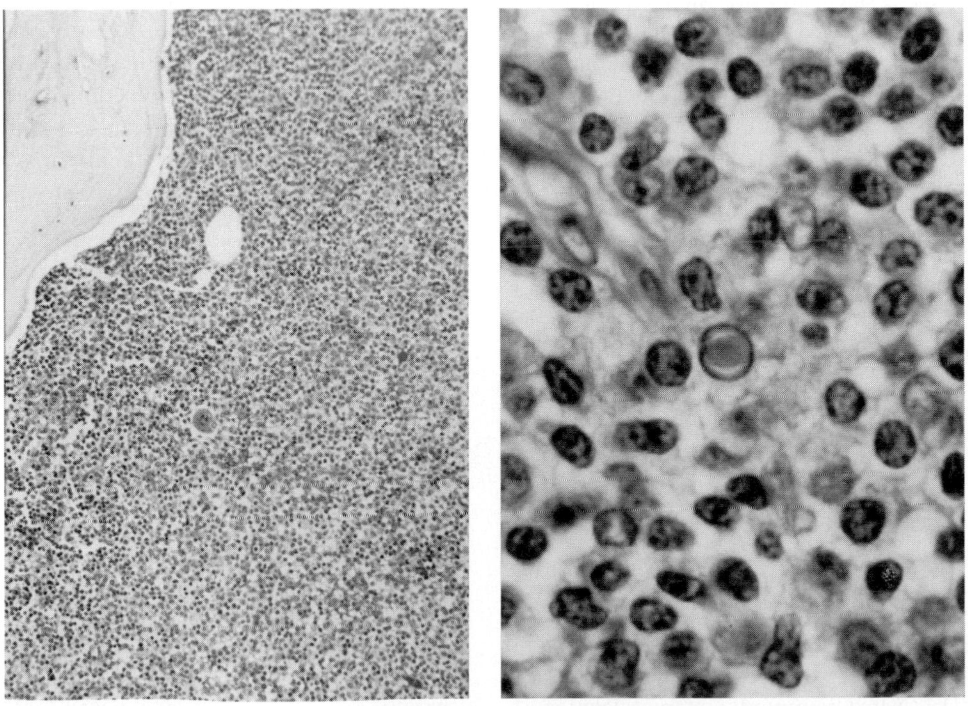

B

FIG. 42.23. Waldenström's macroglobulinemia in the marrow. **A:** The marrow core biopsy reveals complete effacement by small, round lymphoid cells and lymphoplasmacytic cells (hematoxylin and eosin stain, original magnification: 40× magnification). **B:** At higher magnification, a lymphoid cell with a nuclear inclusion (Dutcher body) stands out centrally among mature lymphoid cells (hematoxylin and eosin stain, original magnification: 630× magnification).

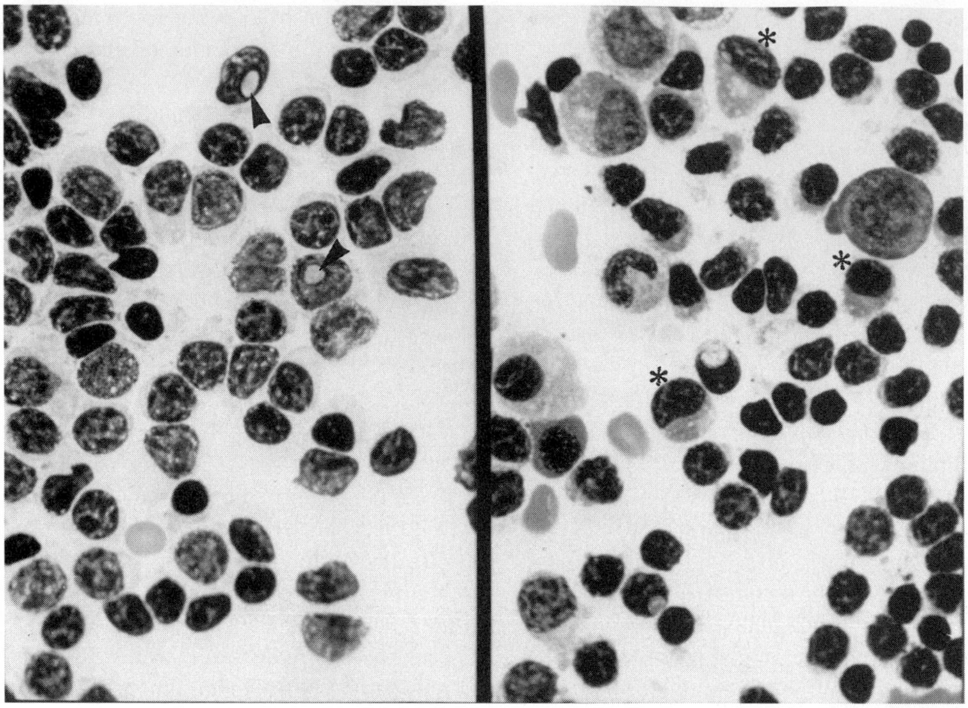

FIG. 42.24. Cytologic features of Waldenström's macroglobulinemia. These cytologic preparations reveal small, ovoid lymphocytes with "block" chromatin (i.e., pachychromia). The nuclear inclusions are Dutcher bodies (*arrows*). Admixed are characteristic plasmacytoid lymphocytes (*asterisk*). Not shown but frequently seen are admixed mast cells (Wright-Giemsa stain, original magnification: 630× magnification).

component is not solely associated with macroglobulinemia, because other entities with IgM secretion include chronic lymphocytic leukemia, small lymphocytic lymphoma, cold hemagglutinin syndrome, and MGUS (208). Only 25% of patients with IgM M-components ultimately prove to have macroglobulinemia (208). Rarely, the IgM M-component occurs in patients with marrow plasmacytosis and osteolytic lesions, representing IgM myeloma (209). Unlike myeloma, the age-adjusted incidence of Waldenström's macroglobulinemia is considerably lower (3.4 per 10^6 males, 1.7 per 10^6 females), and it occurs twice as often among whites as blacks (210). Chronic antigenic stimulation, including viral infections (e.g., hepatitis C), has been suspected to play an etiologic role in Waldenström's macroglobulinemia (211).

Heavy-Chain Diseases

Rare lymphoplasmacytic neoplasms produce monoclonal heavy chain–only Ig fragments that typically are defective at the Ig gene level (212–220). This defect usually results in aberrant RNA processing and truncated heavy-chain protein that cannot assemble with light chains or fails to produce light chain (214–216). Most commonly, internal deletion of the variable region of the heavy chain produces Ig heavy chain of one-half to three-fourths the usual Ig size (214–216). These truncated, aberrant Ig forms tend to polymerize, producing variably sized Ig molecules with different net charges (214–216). This diversity of Ig molecular forms can cause detection difficulties as the variably charged and sized Ig may yield a broad serum protein electrophoresis band or even a normal SPE band rather than a characteristic ''spike'' (214–216). This difficulty necessitates use of immunoelectrophoresis or immunofixation to establish heavy-chain–specific reactivity.

γ Heavy-Chain Disease

The γ heavy-chain disease is a rare disorder characterized by systemic symptoms (e.g., anorexia, weakness, weight loss and recurrent bacterial infections), lymphadenopathy, and hepatosplenomegaly (217). This constellation of symptoms and findings makes clinical distinction between an infectious or inflammatory process and an indolent lymphoproliferative disorder difficult. This uncertainty is compounded by the sometimes difficult detection of γ heavy chain because of the broad band or near-normal serum protein electrophoresis pattern for reasons cited previously (217).

Although indolent, this lymphoplasmacytic disorder is progressive, and lymphadenopathy and bone marrow involvement with consequent anemia, leukopenia, and thrombocytopenia become more evident over time (218). Involvement of Waldeyer's ring is characteristic of γ heavy-chain

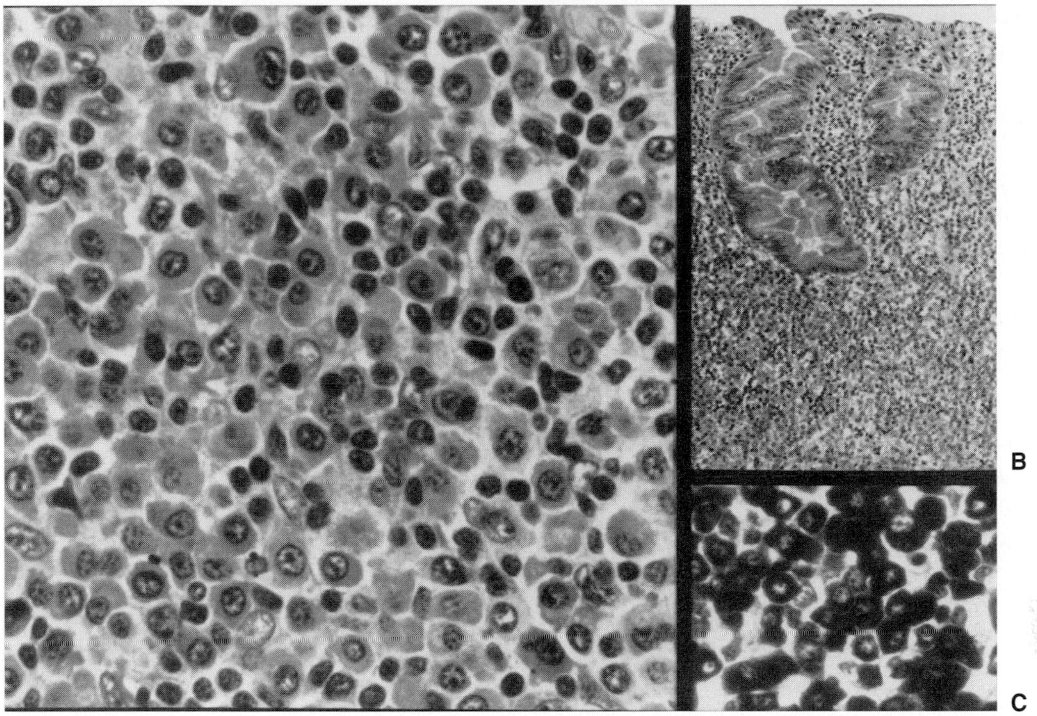

FIG. 42.25. Example of γ heavy chain disease. **A, B:** This polymorphous lymphoplasmacytic proliferation is comprised of admixed plasma cells, plasmacytoid lymphocytes, and lymphoid cells infiltrating the jejunum (original magnifications: 100× and 400× magnification). **C:** Immunohistologic assay reveals monotypic staining with anti-immunoglobulin G, without additional light or heavy chain staining (original magnification: 400× magnification).

disease with associated edema and erythema of the uvula and soft palate (217–220); also characteristic is an associated eosinophilia (218). The patients generally have no lytic bone lesions, no Bence Jones proteinuria, and no renal failure. Monotypic Ig of less than 1 g/day is sometimes found in the urine (217). The diagnosis is made by showing that serum protein reacts on immunoelectrophoresis with antisera to γ chains and not to light chains (217). Atypical circulating plasma cells sometimes herald termination in plasma cell leukemia (219,220). Morphologically, lesions are polymorphous with admixed lymphocytes, plasmacytoid lymphs, plasma cells, immunoblasts, and eosinophils, as shown in Figure 42.25 (218). Clinical outcome is variable with a median survival of 12 months (219,220).

μ Heavy-Chain Disease

This rare entity is characterized as a chronic lymphocytic leukemia (CLL)–like illness (221,222). Admixed with CLL-like lymphoid cells, particularly in the bone marrow, are characteristic vacuolated plasma cells, as shown in Figure 42.26 (221,222). Occasional μ heavy-chain disease cases are more myeloma-like with lytic bone lesions. Most μ heavy-chain disease cases present as slowly progressive CLL with prominent hepatosplenomegaly without peripheral lymphadenopathy (221,222). For reasons stated previously, routine serum protein electrophoresis is frequently normal. Immunoelectrophoresis reveals reactivity to anti-μ in polymers of diverse sizes. Although μ chain is not found in the urine, Bence Jones light chains, particularly κ chains, are commonly (50%) found in the urine (221,222). The latter

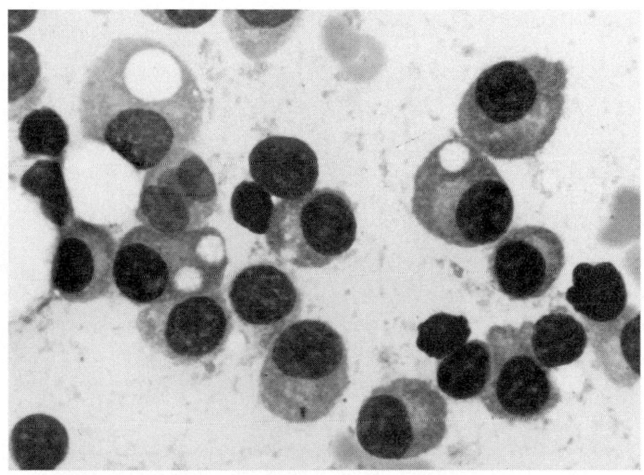

FIG. 42.26. Example of μ heavy chain disease. This marrow monoclonal immunoglobulin proliferation is comprised primarily of atypical, nucleolated plasma cells showing prominent cytoplasmic vacuolation (Wright-Giemsa stain, original magnification: 630× magnification).

are still produced in μ heavy-chain disease but are not assimilable because of heavy-chain structural deletions.

α Heavy-Chain Disease

The α heavy-chain disease is common, unlike the other forms, and it involves a younger age group, representing individuals in their second or third decades who are frequently of low socioeconomic groups with poor hygiene, malnutrition, and intestinal infections (223–225). Typically, α heavy-chain disease, otherwise known as Mediterranean lymphoma or immunoproliferative small intestine disease, manifests with small bowel involvement resulting in malabsorption, diarrhea, hypocalcemia, abdominal pain, wasting, fever, and steatorrhea (223–225). The bowel typically reveals a massive lymphoplasmacytic infiltration of the intestinal mucosa with consequent separation of the crypts of Lieberkühn and villous atrophy (223–225). Usually, bone marrow and nonintestinal lymphoid organs are not involved, although in a few patients the respiratory tract may be involved (224). In early phases, α heavy-chain disease may completely remit with antibiotic therapy, suggesting an initial premalignant state (223–225). However, most patients experience ''immune escalation'' with transformation to frank lymphoma (e.g., immunoblastic sarcoma). In the latter circumstance, a fatal outcome is usual. For reasons cited previously, the serum protein electrophoresis in α heavy-chain disease is usually normal or decreased with hypogammaglobulinemia (223–225). Typically, specific anti-IgA is required to detect aberrant IgA (see Chapter 33).

AMYLOIDOSIS

Amyloid is a fibrillary protein that may accumulate systemically and cause damage to infiltrated vital organs such as the heart and kidneys (226–230). This accumulative, destructive process, known as amyloidosis, complicates 10% to 20% of myeloma cases and frequently constitutes a significant lethal complication (228). Amyloid grossly has a dense, white, porcelain-like appearance, but histologically, it stains pink with hematoxylin and eosin (Fig. 42.27). Characteristically, when stained with Congo Red, it shows apple-green birefringence on polarization microscopy (Fig. 42.27). The apple-green birefringence relates to the β-pleated sheets of polypeptide seen as feltlike mats on electron microscopy. The gold standard for the diagnosis of amyloidosis has been tissue biopsy demonstration with hematoxylin and eosin and Congo red. Amyloid detection is now also possible by immunohistochemical assay or thioflavin T (231). The diagnostic biopsy site is generally the gingivae, rectum, or abdominal subcutaneous fat pad tissue (227,228).

Biochemical and clinical classifications of amyloidosis

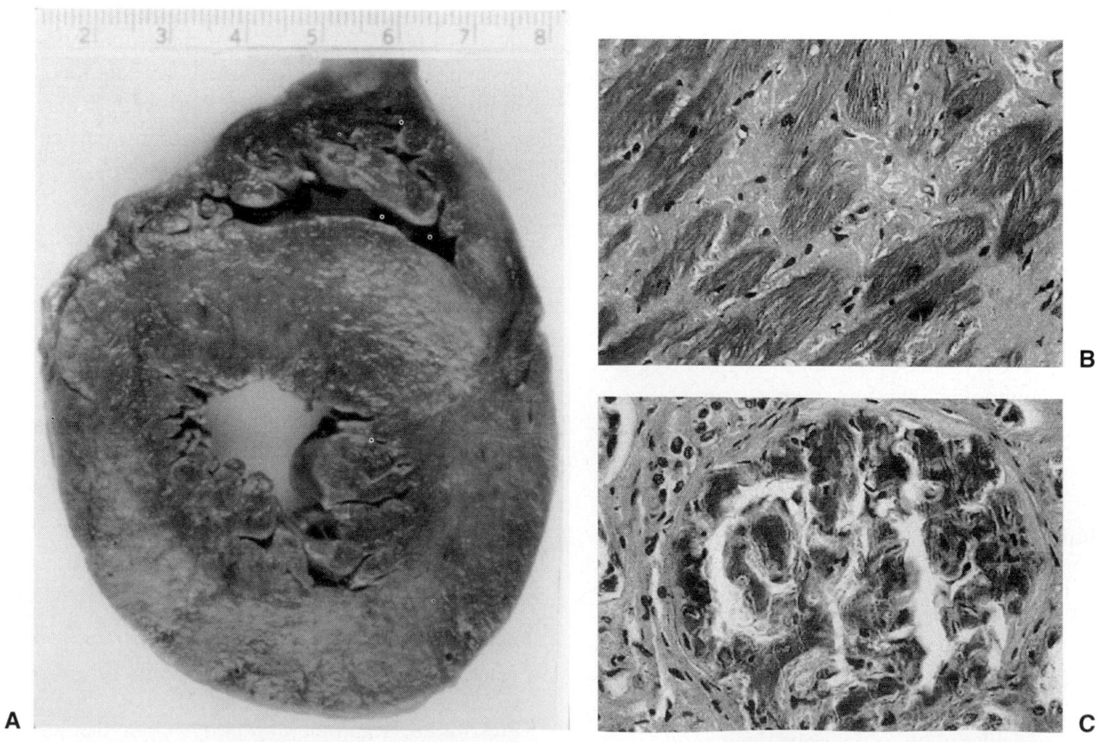

FIG. 42.27. Amyloidosis related to myeloma. **A:** This section of the heart shows the diffuse enlargement characteristic of amyloid deposition, especially notable in the left ventricle. It is pale and has a waxy consistency. **B:** The hematoxylin and eosin stain of section of myocardium demonstrates the interstitial replacement of myofibers by amorphous amyloid. **C:** Congo Red stain of kidney shows the extracellular deposition of amyloid within the glomerulus (original magnification: 250× magnification).

exist (232–234). There are 15 biochemically distinct forms known by chemical composition; the three most common types of amyloid are amyloid light chain (AL), amyloid-associated (AA), and amyloid in Alzheimer's disease (AB).

The chemical composition of amyloid is fibril protein (95%) with P-component and other glycoproteins (5%) (234). The AL type is made up of Ig light chain; sequencing demonstrates this protein to have an N-terminal amino acid residue identical to that of the variable regions of the light chain. In AL, there is a 2:1 predominance of λ light chain (usually L VI), which is opposite to the myeloma and physiologic 2:1 predominance of κ light chain (234). A case of heavy chain (AH)–related amyloidosis has been reported (235). Myeloma-related AL protein derives from intact Ig light chains that accumulate and polymerize in myeloma cells and that are secreted, ingested, processed, and discharged by adjacent macrophages into the extracellular matrix (230). This process, beyond simple light-chain secretion, may involve accessory cell function (230).

The chemical composition of the AA type of amyloid shows it to be a unique protein, with a molecular mass of 8,400 kd and with 76 amino acid residues in a single chain unrelated to Ig (234). Serum amyloid A (SAA) protein, synthesized in the liver, is its precursor; this circulates complexed to an high-density lipoprotein. Although SAA is commonly elevated in chronic inflammation, that alone does not generate amyloid deposition; another factor (e.g., monocyte enzyme) may be required (234).

The AB amyloid is present in Alzheimer's disease cerebral plaques and cerebral blood vessels. It has a molecular mass of 4,000 daltons (234).

By clinical designation, amyloidosis is considered to be

Primary: Also known as systemic amyloidosis, this is exclusive to patients with a monoclonal plasma cell proliferation.

Secondary: Also called reactive, this form is secondary to a chronic inflammatory or infectious process.

Familial: Disease is usually inherited in an autosomal dominant fashion and shows mainly cardiopathy, neuropathy, or nephropathy. Familial Mediterranean fever also belongs in this category, although its inheritance pattern is autosomal recessive (236,237).

The clinical designation of amyloidosis follows its cause. Primary (AL) amyloidosis requires an increase in plasma cells. However straightforward this may seem, the plasma cell proliferation is at times elusive, small, and even extramedullary. The classic plasma cell dyscrasia, multiple myeloma, has only a 10% to 20% incidence of amyloidosis (238). Most patients have an increase in marrow plasma cells, however modest. All patients, however, have an increase in serum or urinary monoclonal proteins, with the presence of Bence Jones proteinuria. Regardless of the number of plasma cells, the diagnosis of primary systemic (AL) amyloidosis is serious, with a median survival of 13 months (239). One study showed long-term (>10 years) survival of only 30 of 810 patients, and those survivors had been treated with alkylating agents (240). Patients with multiple myeloma and AL amyloidosis have a poor prognosis as well, with survival average of 6 months (238). The amyloid deposits are generalized but found most frequently in the heart, kidney, gastrointestinal tract, peripheral nerves, tongue, and skin (241,242). Other sites include the joints (243) and even the fingernails (244). There is a propensity to small blood vessel involvement and clotting abnormalities that may result in bilateral periorbital purpura or ''raccoon eyes'' after proctoscopy (229).

Reactive (AA) amyloidosis, resulting from chronic inflammation or chronic infection, is also systemic. Rheumatoid arthritis is the most frequently associated chronic inflammatory disease, with an estimated 1% of those patients having clinically significant amyloid deposition. Other diseases where secondary amyloidosis is a complication include inflammatory bowel disease, systemic lupus erythematosus, ankylosing spondylitis, jejunoileal bypass, myelofibrosis, and chronic ''skin popping'' of heroin by addicts (245–247). Chronic infections such as osteomyelitis and tuberculosis are less common causes because they are now more successfully eradicated by antibiotic therapy. Renal cell carcinoma and Hodgkin's disease are malignancies associated with this type of amyloid. Organ involvement may be severe and frequently involving the kidneys, lymph nodes, spleen (sago spleen or lardaceous spleen are appropriate gross descriptions), liver, adrenals, and thyroid (233,241).

The gene for familial Mediterranean fever has been cloned, and its product, pyrin, appears to regulate the severe inflammation characteristic of this disease (236,237). This disorder is found in those of Arabic, Armenian, and Sephardic Jewish origin. Clinical findings are the same as described for other secondary types of amyloidosis.

Familial syndromes of amyloidosis are autosomal dominant in their inheritance and show fibrils composed of mutated transthyretin (ATTR) (236). It differs from normal transthyretin by just one amino acid, the substitution of methionine for valine at position 30. Kinships in Portugal, Japan, Sweden, and the United States are known to be affected and demonstrate neuropathic changes including peripheral and autonomic neuropathy, postural hypotension, inability to sweat, and poor sphincter tone (236).

Other notable types of amyloidosis include the $\alpha\beta_2$-microglobulin amyloidosis seen in patients on chronic hemodialysis, which produces synovial, joint, and tendon sheath deposits (248); localized amyloidosis, which may occur as a discrete mass (242,249); amyloid associated with endocrine disorders, especially medullary carcinoma of the thyroid; and senile amyloidosis, found in some people in their eighth and ninth decades, which is systemic but most often dominated by cardiac amyloidosis with its restrictive cardiomyopathy and arrhythmias (250).

IMMUNOGLOBULIN DEPOSITION DISEASES

There are rare monoclonal Ig deposition diseases (MIDD) with prominent tissue monoclonal Ig deposits of a nonamyloid, nonfibrillary, amorphous nature that do not bind Congo red nor contain amyloid P-component (251–254). These deposits seen by electron microscopy are typically discrete, dense, punctate, granular, nonfibrillary deposits with an absence of the β-pleated sheet structure seen by x-ray diffraction. These disorders include light-chain deposition disease (LCDD) (251,252), heavy-chain deposition disease (HCDD) (253,254), and light and heavy-chain deposition disease (LHCDD) (254). These nonamyloid MIDDs usually occur in association with MGUS or overt myeloma. HCDD differs from more common heavy-chain disease by the prominence of tissue Ig deposition in the former resulting in compromised organ function (e.g., renal failure) (254). In contrast to primary amyloidosis with a predominance of λ light chain with over representation of the VλVI variable region, LCDD has prevalence of κ light chains (80%) with overrepresentation of the VκIV variable region (252). Typically, the κ chains are demonstrated by immunofluorescence in the renal glomerular basement membrane. Deposition in LCDD may involve many organs including the joints resulting in an arthropathy or the liver resulting in a failure to produce procoagulants resulting in a coagulopathy (251). In HCDD the critical event is deletion of the CH1 constant domain (254). When a mutant heavy chain lacks CH1 domain, it fails to associate with heavy-chain binding protein (BiP) resulting in premature secretion into the circulation (254). In HCDD the variable regions contain amino acid substitutions that cause an increased propensity for tissue deposition and for binding blood elements. In particular, HCDD of IgG3 or IgG1isotypes result in hypocomplementemia because the G3 and G1 subclasses most readily fix complement. In contrast with HCDD, the heavy-chain disease lack of tissue deposition reflect the presence of an intact CH1 domain and deletion of the variable region (254).

SUMMARY AND CONCLUSIONS

The morphologic and phenotypic complexities of neoplastic plasma cells as discussed and illustrated in this chapter challenge the common perception that the plasma cell malignancies are merely proliferations of end stage B cells. As shown throughout, the great range of phenotypic and biologic properties suggests that neoplastic plasma cells may not simply mimic normal B-cell differentiation and proliferation. They may not always be frozen in one stage of B-cell development. Rather, in many instances they acquire aberrant phenotypic properties reflecting unique malignancy-related genetic alterations or possible ''dedifferentiation'' to a primitive stem cell. This phenotypic dedifferentiation or drift frequently corresponds with a loss of paracrine effects, the emergence of autocrine tumor growth, the occurrence of oncogene activation, and increased chromosomal abnormality. The ultimate aneuploid, oncogenic transformed state may herald phenotypic escape and a lethal outcome. Although the latter circumstance seems futile, some of the newly identified surface receptors and oncogenic events may serve as future therapeutic targets providing new rationales for phenotype-adapted therapy.

REFERENCES

1. Alexanian R. Ten-year survival in multiple myeloma. *Arch Intern Med* 1985;145:2073–2074.
2. Young JL, Percy CL, Asire AJ. *Surveillance, epidemiology, and end results: incidence and mortality data, 1973–1977.* National Cancer Institute monograph 57, publication (NIH) 81:2330. Bethesda: Department of Health and Human Services, 1981.
3. Silverberg E. Cancer statistics, 1985. *CA Cancer J Clin* 1985;35:19–35.
4. Culter SJ, Young JL. *Third national cancer survey: incidence data.* Washington, DC: US Government Printing Office, 1975.
5. Devesa SS, Silverman DT, Young JL Jr, et al. Cancer incidence and mortality trends among whites in the United States, 1947–84. *J Natl Cancer Inst* 1988;79:701–770.
6. Blattner WA. Multiple myeloma and macroglobulinemia. In: Schottenfeld D, Fraumeni JF, eds. *Cancer epidemiology and prevention.* Philadelphia: WB Saunders, 1982:722.
7. Nandakumar A, Armstrong BK, DeKlerk NH. Multiple myeloma in Western Australia: a case-control study in relation to occupation, father's occupation, socioeconomic status and country of birth. *Int J Cancer* 1986;37:223–226.
8. Alberts SR, Lanier AP. Leukemia, lymphoma, and multiple myeloma in Alaskan natives. *J Natl Cancer Inst* 1987;78:831–837.
9. Linet MS, Sioban DH, McLaughlin JK. A case-control study of multiple myeloma in whites with chronic antigenic stimulation, occupation and drug use. *Cancer Res* 1987;47:2978–2981.
10. Kagan E, Jacobson RJ, Yeung K-Y, et al. Asbestos-associated neoplasms of B cell lineage. *Am J Med* 1979;67:325–330.
11. Ichimaru M, Ishimaru T, Mikami M, et al. *Multiple myeloma among atomic bomb survivors, Hiroshima and Nagasaki, 1950–1976.* Radiation Effects Research Foundation Technical Report No. 9-79. Hiroshima: , 1979.
12. Lewis EB. Leukemia, multiple myeloma and aplastic anemia in American radiologists. *Science* 1963;142:1492–1494.
13. Mancuso TF, Stewart A, Kneale G. Radiation exposures of Hanford workers dying from cancer and other causes. *Health Phys* 1977;33:369–385.
14. Penny R, Hughes S. Repeated stimulation of the reticuloendothelial system and the development of plasma cell dyscrasias. *Lancet* 1970;1:77–78.
15. Wohlenberg H. Osteomyelitis and plasmacytomas. *N Engl J Med* 1970;283:822–823.
16. Said J, Rettig M, Heppner K, et al. Localization of Kaposi's-associated herpesvirus in bone marrow biopsy samples from patients with multiple myeloma. *Blood* 1997;90:4278–4282.
17. Corbellino M, Pizzuto M, Bestetti G, et al. Absence of Kaposi's sarcoma-associated herpes virus DNA sequences in multiple myeloma. *Blood* 1999;93:1110–1111.
18. Tisdale J, Stewart K, Dickstein B, et al. Molecular and serological examination of the relationship of human herpesvirus 8 to multiple myeloma: orf 26 sequences in bone marrow stroma are not restricted to myeloma patients and other regions of the genome are not detected. *Blood* 1998; 92:2681–2687.
19. Voelkerding K, Sandhaus L, Kim H, et al. Plasma cell malignancy in the acquired immune deficiency syndrome. *Am J Clin Pathol* 1989;92:222–228.
20. Konrad R, Kricka L, Goodmam D, et al. Myeloma-associated paraprotein directed against the HIV-1 p24 antigens in an HIV-1 seropositive patient. *N Engl J Med* 1993;328:1817–1819.
21. Salmon SE, Seligmann M. B-cell neoplasia in man. *Lancet* 1974;2:1230–1233.
22. Potter M, Boyce CR. Induction of plasma cell neoplasms in strain BALB/C mice with mineral oil and mineral oil adjuvants. *Nature* 1962;193:1086–1087.
23. James JM, Brouet JC, Orudenfrija, et al. Waldenström's macroglobulinemia in a bird breeder: a case history with pulmonary involvement and antibody activity of the monoclonal IgM to canary droppings. *Clin Exp Immunol* 1987;68:397–401.

24. Seligmann M, Sassy C, Chevalier A. A human IgG myeloma protein with anti-alpha 2 macroglobulin antibody activity. *J Immunol* 1973; 110:85–90.
25. Durie BGM. Plasma cell disorders: recent advances in the biology and treatment. In: *Recent advances in hematology.* New York: Churchill Livingstone, 1988.
26. Zouali M, Fine JM, Eyquem A. Anti-DNA autoantibody activity and idiotypic relationships of human monoclonal proteins. *Eur J Immunol* 1984;14:1085–1089.
27. Jerne NK. Towards a network theory of the immune system. *Ann Immunol* 1974;125c:373–389.
28. Dewald GW, Kyle RA, Hicks GA, et al. The clinical significance of cytogenetic studies in 100 patients with multiple myeloma, plasma cell leukemia, or amyloidosis. *Blood* 1985;66:380–390.
29. Gould J, Alexanian K, Goodacre A, et al. Plasma cell karyotype in multiple myeloma. *Blood* 1988;71:453–456.
30. Linet MS, Harlow SD, McLaughlin JK. A case-control study of multiple myeloma in whites: chronic antigenic stimulation, occupation, and drug use. *Cancer Res* 1987;47:2978–2981.
31. Grogan TM. Altered cell adhesion molecule (CAM) expression associated with tumorigenicity in plasma cell myeloma. In: Pileri A, Boccadoro M, eds. *Multiple myeloma from biology to therapy: Abstracts book of III international workshop.* Turino, Italy, April 10, 1991.
32. McConville CM, Formstone CJ, Hernandez D, et al. Fine mapping of the chromosome 11q22-23 region using PFGE, linkage and haplotype analysis: localization of the gene for ataxia telangiectasia to a 5 cM region flanked by NCAM/DRD2 and STMy/CJ52.75, ϕ2.22. *Nucleic Acids Res* 1990;18:4335–4343.
33. Tsuchiya H, Epstein J, Selvanayagam P, et al. Correlated flow cytometric analysis of H-ras p21 and nuclear DNA in multiple myeloma. *Blood* 1988;72:796–800.
34. Harris H: The analysis of malignancy by cell fusion: the position in 1988. *Cancer Res* 1988;48:3302–3306.
35. Durie BGM, Baum VE, Vela E, et al. Abnormalities of chromosome 6q and osteoclast activating factor production in multiple myeloma. *Blood* 1986;68:208A.
36. Dalton WS, Durie BGM, Alberts DS et al. Characterization of a new drug resistant human myeloma cell line which expresses P-glycoprotein. *Cancer Res* 1986;45:5125–5130.
37. Barlogie B, Epstein J, Selvanayagam P, et al. Plasma cell myeloma: new biological insights and advances in therapy. *Blood* 1989;73: 865–879.
38. Selvanayagam P, Blick M, Narni F, et al. Alteration and abnormal expression of the c-myc oncogene in human multiple myeloma. *Blood* 1988;71:30–35.
39. Sümegi J, Hedberg T, Björkholm M, et al. Amplification of the c-myc oncogene in human plasma cell leukemia. *Int J Cancer* 1985; 36:367–371.
40. Meltzer P, Shadle K, Durie B. Somatic mutation alters a critical region of the c-myc gene in multiple myeloma. *Blood* 1987;70:985A.
41. Drach J, Ackermann J, Fritz E, et al. Presence of a p53 gene deletion in patients with multiple myeloma predicts for short survival after conventional-dose chemotherapy. *Blood* 1998;92:802–809.
42. Mahmoud M, Huang N, Nobuyoshi M, et al. Altered expression of PAX-5 gene in human myeloma cells. *Blood* 1996;87:4311–4315.
43. Chesi M, Bergsagel L, Brents L, et al. Dysregulation of cyclin D1 by translocation into an IgH gamma switch region in two multiple myeloma cell lines. *Blood* 1996;88:647–681.
44. Salmon SE. Plasma cell disorders. In: Wyngaarden JB, Smith LH, eds. *Cecil textbook of medicine,* 18th ed. Philadelphia: WB Saunders, 1988:1026–1036.
45. Richardo MJ, Romar RH. Humoral immunity: antibodies and immunoglobulins. In: Henry JB, ed. *Clinical diagnosis and management by laboratory methods,* 18th ed. Philadelphia: WB Saunders, 1991: 824–829.
46. Bergsagel DE. Plasma cell neoplasms: general consideration. In: Williams WJ, Beutler E, Erslev AJ, et al., eds. *Hematology,* 3rd ed. New York: McGraw-Hill, 1983:1071–1075.
47. Kyle RA. Monoclonal gammopathy of undetermined significance (MGUS): a review. *Clin Hematol* 1982;11:123–150.
48. Jandl J. Multiple myeloma and other differentiated B cell malignancies. In: *Blood: textbook of hematology.* Boston: Little, Brown, 1987: 810.
49. Weisbart RH, Kascena A, Schuh A, et al. GM-CSF induces human neutrophil IgA-mediated phagocytosis by an IgA Fc receptor activation mechanism. *Nature* 1988;332:647–648.
50. Salmon SE. Immunoglobulin synthesis and tumor kinetics of multiple myeloma. *Semin Hematol* 1973;10:136–147.
51. Salmon SE, Cassady JR. Plasma cell neoplasms. In: DeVita VT, Hellman S, Rosenberg S, eds. *Cancer: principles and practice of oncology.* Philadelphia: JB Lippincott, 1988:1854.
52. Axelsson U, Hällén J. Review of fifty-four subjects with monoclonal gammopathy. *Br J Haematol* 1968;15:417–420.
53. Kelly RH, Tardy TJ, Shah PM. Benign monoclonal gammopathy: a reassessment of the problem. *Immunol Invest* 1985;14:183–197.
54. Hobbs JR. Immunochemical classes of myelomatosis. *Br J Haematol* 1969;16:599–606.
55. Pruzanski W, Rother I. IgD plasma cell neoplasia: clinical manifestations and characteristic features. *Can Med Assoc J* 1970;102: 1061–1065.
56. Jancelewicz Z, Takatsuki K, Sugae S, et al. IgD multiple myeloma: review of 133 cases. *Arch Intern Med* 1975;135:87–93.
57. Ogawa M, Kochwa S, Smith C, et al. Clinical aspects of IgE myeloma. *N Engl J Med* 1969;281:1217–1220.
58. Shustik C, Bergsagel DE, Pruzanski W. Kappa and lambda light chain disease: survival rates and clinical manifestations. *Blood* 1976;48: 41–51.
59. Alexanian R, Haut A, Khan AU, et al. Treatment for multiple myeloma: combination chemotherapy with different melphalan dose regimens. *JAMA* 1969;208:1680–1685.
60. Buss DH, Prichard RW, Hartz JW, et al. Initial bone marrow findings in multiple myeloma: significance of plasma cell nodules. *Arch Pathol Lab Med* 1986;110:30–33.
61. Zucker-Franklin D. The pathology of multiple myeloma and related disorders. In: Wiernik P, Cannellos GP, Kyle R, et al., eds. *Neoplastic diseases of the blood.* New York: Churchill Livingstone, 1985:462.
62. Fritz E, Ludwig H, Kundi M. Prognostic relevance of cellular morphology in multiple myeloma. *Blood* 1984;63:1072–1079.
63. Greipp R, Raymond NM, Kyle RA, et al. Multiple myeloma: significance of plasmablastic subtype in morphological classification. *Blood* 1985;65:305–310.
64. Azar HA. Pathology of multiple myeloma. In: Azar HA, Potter M, eds. *Multiple myeloma and related disorders,* vol 1. New York: Harper & Row, 1973:5.
65. Greipp PR, Kyle RA. Clinical morphological and cell kinetic differences among multiple myeloma, monoclonal gammopathy of undetermined significance and smoldering multiple myeloma. *Blood* 1983; 62:166–171.
66. Farquhar MG, Palade GE. The Golgi apparatus (1954–1981) from artifact to center stage. *J Cell Biol* 1981;91[Suppl]:77–103.
67. Maldonado JE, Brown AL Jr, Bayrd ED, et al. Cytoplasmic and intranuclear electron-dense bodies in the myeloma cell. *Arch Pathol* 1966; 81:484–500.
68. Pavelta M, Ludwig H. Ultrastructural studies of myeloma cells: observations concerning the Golgi apparatus and intermediate-size filaments. *Am J Hematol* 1983;15:237–251.
69. Blom J, Mansa B, Wiik A. A study of Russell bodies in human monoclonal plasma cells by means of immunofluorescence and electron microscopy. *Acta Pathol Microbiol Scand A* 1976;84A:335–349.
70. Maldonado JE, Bayrd ED, Brown AL Jr. The flaming cell in multiple myeloma: a light and electron microscopy study. *Am J Clin Pathol* 1965;44:605–612.
71. Jandl J. Multiple myeloma and other differentiated B cell malignancies. In: *Blood: textbook of hematology.* Boston: Little, Brown, 1987: 831.
72. Bergsagel DE. Plasma cell myeloma. In: Williams WJ, Beutler E, Erslev AJ, et al., eds. *Hematology,* 3rd ed. New York: McGraw-Hill, 1983:831.
73. Durie BGM, Salmon SE. Multiple myeloma, macroglobulinemia and monoclonal gammopathies. In: Hoffbrand AV, Brian MC, Hirsh J, eds. *Recent advances in hematology.* Edinburgh: Churchill Livingstone, 1977:243.
74. Durie BGM. Staging and kinetics of multiple myeloma. *Semin Oncol* 1986;13:300–309.
75. Salmon SE, Cassady JR: Plasma cell neoplasms. In: DeVita VT, Hellman S, Rosenberg S, eds. *Cancer: principles and practice of oncology.* Philadelphia: JB Lippincott, 1988:1864.
76. Bartl R, Frisch B, Burkhardt R, et al. Bone marrow histology in my-

eloma: its importance in diagnosis, prognosis, classification and staging: *Br J Haematol* 1982;51:361–375.
77. Anderson KC, Bates MP, Slaughenhoupt B, et al. A monoclonal antibody with reactivity restricted to normal and neoplastic plasma cells. *J Immunol* 1984;132:3172–3179.
78. Ling NR, MacLennan ICM, Mason DY. B-cell and plasma cell antigens: new and previously defined clusters. In: McMichael AJ, Beverley PCL, Cobbold S, et al., eds. *Leukocyte typing III: white cell differentiation antigens.* Oxford: Oxford University Press, 1987:302.
79. San Miguel JF, Caballero MD, Gonzalez M, et al. Immunological phenotype of neoplasms involving the B cell in the last step of differentiation. *Br J Haematol* 1986;62:75–83.
80. Harada H, Kawano M, Huang N, et al. Phenotypic difference of normal plasma cells from mature myeloma cells. *Blood* 1993;81: 2658–2663.
81. Barker H, Hamilton M, Ball J, et al. Expression of adhesion molecules LFA-3 and N-CAM on normal and malignant human plasma cells. *Br J Haematol* 1992;81:331–335.
82. Ridley R, Xiao H, Hata H, et al. Expression of syndecan regulates human myeloma plasma cell adhesion to type 1 collagen. *Blood* 1993; 81:767–774.
83. Kubagawa J, Vogler LB, Capra JD, et al. Studies on the clonal origin of multiple myeloma: use of individually specific (idiotype) antibodies to trace the oncogenic event to its earliest point of expression in B-cell differentiation. *J Exp Med* 1979;150:792–807.
84. Van Riet I, Vanderkerken K, De Greef C, et al. Homing behaviour of the malignant cell clone in multiple myeloma. *Med Oncol* 1998; 15:1554–1564.
85. Ruiz-Arüelles GJ, Katzmann JA, Greipp PR, et al. Multiple myeloma: circulating lymphocytes that express plasma cell antigens. *Blood* 1984;64:352–356.
86. Durie BGM, Grogan TM. CALLA-positive myeloma: an aggressive subtype with poor survival. *Blood* 1985;66:229–232.
87. Caligaris-Cappio F, Berui L, Tesio L, et al. Identification of malignant plasma cell precursors in the bone marrow of multiple myeloma. *J Clin Invest* 1985;76:1243–1251.
88. Epstein J, Barlogie B, Katzmann J, et al. Phenotypic heterogeneity in aneuploid multiple myeloma indicates pre-B cell involvement. *Blood* 1988;71:861–865.
89. Grogan TM, Durie BGM, Lomen C, et al. Delineation of a novel pre-B cell component in plasma cell myeloma: immunochemical, immunophenotypic, genotypic, cytologic, cell culture and kinetic features. *Blood* 1987;70:932–942.
90. Pilarski LM, Mant MJ, Reuther BA. Pre-B cells in peripheral blood of multiple myeloma patients. *Blood* 1985;66:416–422.
91. Grogan TM, Durie BGM, Spier CM, et al. Myelomonocytic antigen positive multiple myeloma. *Blood* 1989;73:763–769.
92. Epstein J, Xiao H, He X-Y. Markers of multiple hematopoietic cell lineages in multiple myeloma. *N Engl J Med* 1990;322:664–668.
93. Brown G, Bunce CM, Howie AJ, et al. Stochastic or ordered lineage commitment during hemopoiesis [Editorial]. *Leukemia* 1987;2: 150–153.
94. Spier CS, Grogan TM, Durie BGM, et al. T cell antigen-positive multiple myeloma. *Mod Pathol* 1990;3:302–307.
95. Buchsbaum RJ, Schwartz RS. Cellular origins of hematologic neoplasms. *N Engl J Med* 1990;322:694–696.
96. Robillard N, Jego G, Pellat-Deceunynck, et al. CD28, a marker associated with tumoral expansion in multiple myeloma. *Clin Cancer Res* 1998;4:1521–1526.
97. Dalton WS, Grogan T, Rybski J, et al. Immunohistochemical detection and quantitation of P-glycoprotein in multiple drug-resistant human myeloma cells: association with level of drug resistance and drug accumulation. *Blood* 1989;73:747–752.
98. Grogan T, Dalton W, Rybski J, et al. Optimization of immunocytochemical P-glycoprotein assessment in multidrug-resistant plasma cell myeloma using 3 antibodies. *Lab Invest* 1990;63:815–824.
99. Grogan T, Spier C, Salmon S, et al. P-glycoprotein expression in human plasma cell myeloma: correlation with prior chemotherapy. *Blood* 1993;81:490–495.
100. Durie BGM, Dalton WS. Reversal of drug-resistance in multiple myeloma with verapamil. *Br J Haematol* 1988;68:203–206.
101. Wyler B, Shao Y, Schneider E, et al. Intermittent exposure to doxorubicin *in vitro* selects for multifactorial non-P-glycoprotein-associated multidrug resistance in RPMI 8226 human myeloma cells. *Br J Haematol* 1997;97:65–75.
102. Rimsza L, Dalton W, Campbell K, et al. In multiple myeloma the non-P-glycoprotein multidrug resistance protein LRP is frequently expressed and an increased proliferative rate (Ki67 >5%) is associated with a significantly shorter survival. *Leuk Lymphoma* 1999;10: 123–126.
103. Dalton WS, Grogan TM, Meltzer PS, et al. Drug-resistance in multiple myeloma and non-Hodgkin's lymphoma: detection of P-glycoprotein and potential circumvention by addition of verapamil to chemotherapy. *J Clin Oncol* 1990;7:415–424.
104. Miller TP, Grogan TM, Dalton WS, et al. P-glycoprotein expression in malignant lymphoma and reversal of clinical drug resistance with chemotherapy plus high-dose verapamil. *J Clin Oncol* 1991;9:17–24.
105. Gratzner H. Monoclonal antibody to 5-bromo- and 5-iododeoxyuridine: a new reagent for detection of DNA replication. *Science* 1982; 218:474–475.
106. Dolbeare F, Gratzner H, Pallavicini M, et al. Flow cytometric measurement of total DNA content and incorporated bromodeoxyuridine. *Proc Natl Acad Sci USA* 1983;80:5573–5577.
107. Durie BGM, Salmon SE. Staging, kinetics and flow cytometry of multiple myeloma. In: Wiernik P, Cannellos, Kyle R, et al., eds. *Neoplastic diseases of the blood.* New York: Churchill Livingstone, 1985: 513.
108. Gerdes J, Dallenbach F, Lennert K. Growth fractions in malignant non-Hodgkin's lymphomas (NHL) as determined in situ with the monoclonal antibody Ki67. *Hematol Oncol* 1984;2:365–371.
109. Grogan TM, Lippman SM, Spier CM, et al. Independent prognostic significance of a nuclear proliferative antigen in diffuse large cell lymphomas as determined by the monoclonal antibody Ki67. *Blood* 1988;71:1157–1160.
110. Tosi P, Pellacani A, Visani G, et al. In vitro treatment with retinoids decreases bcl-2 protein expression and enhances dexamethasone-induced cytotoxicity and apoptosis in multiple myeloma cells. *Eur J Haematol* 1999;62:143–148.
111. Landowski T, Gleason-Guzman M, Dalton W. Selection for drug resistance to fas-mediated apoptosis. *Blood* 1997;89:1854–1861.
112. Villunger A, Egle A, Marschitz I, et al. Constitutive expression of Fas (Apo-1/CD95) ligand on multiple myeloma cells: a potential mechanism of tumor-induced suppression of immune surveillance. *Blood* 1997;90:12–20.
113. Lynch RG, Rohrer JM, Odermatt B, et al. Immunoregulation of murine myeloma cell growth and differentiation: a monoclonal model of B cell differentiation. *Immunol Rev* 1979;48:45–80.
114. Broder S, Humphrey R, Durm, M et al. Impaired synthesis of polyclonal (non-paraprotein) immunoglobulin by circulating lymphocytes from patients with multiple myeloma: role of suppressor cells. *N Engl J Med* 1975;293:887–892.
115. Dianzani U, Pileri A, Boccadoro M, et al. Activated idiotype-reactive cells in suppressor/cytotoxic subpopulations of monoclonal gammopathies: correlation with diagnosis and disease status. *Blood* 1988;72: 1064–1068.
116. Kronland R, Grogan T, Spier C, et al. Immunotopographic assessment of lymphoid and plasma cell malignancies in the bone marrow. *Hum Pathol* 1985;16:1247–1254.
117. Stauder R, Van Driel M, Schwarzler C, et al. Different CD44 splicing patterns define prognostic subgroups in multiple myeloma. *Blood* 1996;88:3101–3108.
118. Van Camp B, Durie BGM, Spier C, et al. Plasma cells in multiple myeloma express a natural killer cell-associated antigen: CD56 (NKH-1; Leu 19). *Blood* 1990;76:377–382.
119. Drach J, Gattringer C, Huber H. Expression of the neural cell adhesion molecule (CD56) by human myeloma cells. *Clin Exp Immunol* 1991; 83:418–422.
120. Ong F, Kaiser U, Seelen P, et al. Serum neural cell adhesion molecule differentiates multiple myeloma from paraproteinemias due to other causes. *Blood* 1996;87:712–716.
121. Pellat-Deceunynck C, Barille S, Jego G, et al. The absence of CD56 (NCAM) on malignant plasma cells is a hallmark of plasma cell leukemia and of a special subset of multiple myeloma. *Leukemia* 1998;12: 1977–1982.
122. Van Driel M, Gunthert U, Stauder R, et al. CD44 isoforms distinguish between bone marrow plasma cells from normal individuals and pa-

tients with multiple myeloma at different stages of disease. *Leukemia* 1998;12:1821–1828.
123. Folkman J. Clinical applications of research on angiogenesis. *N Engl J Med* 1995;333:1757–1763.
124. Ribatti D, Vacca A, Nico B, et al. Bone marrow angiogenesis and mast cell density increase simultaneously with progression of human multiple myeloma. *Br J Cancer* 1999;79:451–455.
125. Bellamy W, Richter L, Frutiger Y, et al. Expression of vascular endothelial growth factor and its receptors in hematopoietic malignancies. *Cancer Res* 1999;59:728–733.
126. Rossi J-F, Durie BGM, Duperray C, et al. Phenotypic and functional analysis of 1,25-dihydroxyvitamin D_3 receptor mediated modulation of the human myeloma cell line RPMI 8226. *Cancer Res* 1988;48:1213–1216.
127. Danel L, Menouni M, Cohen JH, et al. Distribution of androgen and estrogen receptors among lymphoid and haemopoietic cell lines. *Leuk Res* 1985;9:1373–1378.
128. Kishimoto T. Factors affecting B-cell growth and differentiation. *Annu Rev Immunol* 1985;3:133–157.
129. Kawano M, Hirano T, Matsudat, et al. Autocrine generation and requirement of BSF-2/Il-6 for human multiple myelomas. *Nature* 1988; 332:83–85.
130. Klein B, Zhang X-G, Jourdan M, et al. Paracrine rather than autocrine regulation of myeloma-cell growth and differentiation by interleukin-6. *Blood* 1989;73:517–526.
131. Alexanian R, Barlogie B, Dixon D. High-dose glucocorticoid treatment of resistant myeloma. *Ann Intern Med* 1986;105:8–11.
132. Kishimoto T. B-cell stimulating factors (BSFs): Molecular structure, biological function, and regulations of expression. *J Clin Immunol* 1987;7:343–355.
133. Garrett LR, Durie BGM, Nedwin GE, et al. Production of the bone resorbing cytokine lymphotoxin by cultured human myeloma cells. *N Engl J Med* 1987;317:526–532.
134. Cozzolino F, Torcia M, Aldinucci D, et al. Production of interleukin-1 by bone marrow myeloma cells: its role in the pathogenesis of lytic bone lesions. *Blood* 1989;74:380–387.
135. Kawano M, Yamamoto I, Iwato K, et al. Interleukin-1 beta rather than lymphotoxin as the major bone resorbing activity in human multiple myeloma. *Blood* 1988;74:380–387.
136. Barlogie B, Latreille J, Swartzenchuber D, et al. Quantitative cytology in myeloma research. In: *Clinics in hematology.* London: WB Saunders, 1982:19.
137. Berenson J, Wong R, Kim K, et al. Evidence for peripheral blood B lymphocyte but not T lymphocyte involvement in multiple myeloma. *Blood* 1987;70:1550–1553.
138. Omede P, Boccadoro M, Gallone G, et al. Multiple myeloma: increased circulating lymphocytes carrying plasma cell-associated antigens as an indicator of poor survival. *Blood* 1990;76:1375–1379.
139. Mellstedt H, Hammarström S, Holm G. Monoclonal lymphocyte population in human plasma cell myeloma. *Clin Exp Immunol* 1974;17: 371–384.
140. Bast E, Van Camp B, Reynaert P, et al. Idiotypic peripheral blood lymphocytes in monoclonal gammopathy. *Clin Exp Immunol* 1982; 47:677–682.
141. Ruiz-Arüelles GJ, Katzmann JA, Greipp PR, et al. Multiple myeloma: circulating lymphocytes that express plasma cell antigens. *Blood* 1984;64:352–356.
142. Ullrich S, Zolla-Pazner S. Immunoregulatory circuits in myeloma. *Clin Hematol* 1982;11:87–111.
143. Alexanian R. Localized and indolent myeloma. *Blood* 1980;56: 521–525.
144. Kyle RA, Greipp R: Smouldering multiple myeloma. *N Engl J Med* 1980;302:1347–1349.
145. Knowling MA, Harwood AR, Bergsagel DE. Comparison of extramedullary plasmacytomas with solitary and multiple plasma cell tumors of the bone. *J Clin Oncol* 1983;1:255–262.
146. Kyle RA. Monoclonal gammopathy of undetermined significance: natural history in 241 cases. *Am J Med* 1978;64:814–826.
147. Salmon S, Cassady JR. Plasma cell neoplasms. In: DeVita VT, Hellman S, Rosenberg S, eds. *Cancer: principles and practice of oncology.* Philadelphia: JB Lippincott, 1988:1862.
148. Azar HA. Pathology of multiple myeloma. In: Azar HA, Potter M, eds. *Multiple myeloma and related disorders,* vol 1. New York: Harper & Row, 1973:8.
149. Kyle RA, Greipp PR. "Idiopathic" Bence Jones proteinuria: long term follow-up in seven patients. *N Engl J Med* 1982;306:564–567.
150. Bergsagel DE. Plasma cell myeloma. In: Williams WJ, Beutler E, Erslev AJ, et al, eds. *Hematology,* 3rd ed. New York: McGraw-Hill, 1983:1090.
151. Durie BGM, Salmon SE. A clinical staging system for multiple myeloma: correlation of measured myeloma cell mass with presenting clinical features, response to treatment and survival. *Cancer* 1975;36: 842–852.
152. Durie BGM. Staging and kinetics of multiple myeloma. *Semin Oncol* 1986;13:300–309.
153. Bataille R, Grenier J, Sany J. Beta-2 microglobulin in myeloma: optimal use for staging, prognosis and treatment. A prospective study of 160 patients. *Blood* 1984;63:468–476.
154. Bergsagel DE. Plasma cell myeloma. In: Williams WJ, Beutler E, Erslev AJ, et al., eds. *Hematology,* 3rd ed. New York: McGraw-Hill, 1983:1089.
155. Isobe T, Osserman EF. Pathologic conditions associated with plasma cell dyscrasias: a study of 806 cases. *Ann N Y Acad Sci* 1972;190: 507–518.
156. Williams RC, Bailly RC, Howe RB. Studies of "benign" serum M-components. *Am J Med Sci* 1969;257:275–293.
157. Azar HA. Pathology of multiple myeloma. In: Azar HA, Potter M, eds. *Multiple myeloma and related disorders,* vol 1. New York: Harper & Row, 1973:10.
158. Kapadia S, Desai U, Cheng U. Extramedullary plasmacytoma of the head and neck: a clinicopathologic study of 20 cases. *Medicine (Baltimore)* 1982;61:317–329.
159. Bergsagel DE, Rider W: Plasma cell neoplasms. In: DeVita VT, Hellman S, Rosenberg S, eds. *Cancer: principles and practice of oncology.* Philadelphia: JB Lippincott, 1988:1753–1795.
160. Strand W, Banks P, Kyle R. Anaplastic plasma cell myeloma and immunoblastic lymphoma: clinical, pathologic and immunologic comparison. *Am J Med* 1984;76:861–867.
161. Strickler J, Audel M, Copehaven C, et al. Immunophenotypic difference between plasmacytoma/multiple myeloma and immunoblastic lymphoma. *Cancer* 1988;61:1782–1786.
162. Knowling M, Harwood A, Bergsagel D. Comparison of extramedullary plasmacytomas with solitary and multiple plasma cell tumors of bone. *J Clin Oncol* 1983;1:255–262.
163. Barlogie B, Smallwood L, Smith T, et al. High serum levels of lactic dehydrogenase identify a high grade lymphoma-like myeloma. *Ann Intern Med* 1989;110:521–525.
164. Bergsagel DE. Plasma cell neoplasms and acute leukemia. *Clin Hematol* 1982;11:221–234.
165. Bergsagel DE, Bailey AJ, Langley GR, et al. The chemotherapy of plasma-cell myeloma and the incidence of acute leukemia. *N Engl J Med* 1979;301:743–748.
166. Barnard D, Burns G, Gordon J, et al. Chronic myelomonocytic leukemia with paraproteinemia but no detectable plasmacytosis. *Cancer* 1979;44:927–936.
167. Kyle RA, Garton JP. The spectrum of IgM monoclonal gammopathy in 430 cases. *Mayo Clin Proc* 1987;62:719–731.
168. Salmon S, Cassady JR. Plasma cell neoplasms. In: DeVita VT, Hellman S, Rosenberg S, eds. *Cancer: principles and practice of oncology.* Philadelphia: JB Lippincott, 1988:1854.
169. Kyle RA, Bayrd ED. Multiple myeloma: variant forms. *In: The monoclonal gammopathies, multiple myeloma and related plasma cell disorders.* Springfield, IL: Charles C Thomas, 1976:141–145.
170. Azar HA, Potter M. Pathology of multiple myeloma. In: Azar HA, Potter M, eds. *Multiple myeloma and related disorders.* New York: Harper & Row, 1973:13–18.
171. Wiltshaw E. The natural history of extramedullary plasmacytoma and its relation to solitary myeloma of bone and myelomatosis. *Medicine (Baltimore)* 1976;55:217–238.
172. Corwin J, Lindberg RD. Solitary plasmacytoma of bone vs extramedullary plasmacytoma and their relationship to multiple myeloma. *Cancer* 1979;43:1007–1013.
173. Woodruff RK, Whittle JM, Malpas JS. Solitary plasmacytoma: I. Extramedullary soft tissue plasmacytoma. *Cancer* 1979;43:2340–2343.
174. Woodruff RK, Malpas JS, White FE. Solitary plasmacytoma: II. Solitary plasmacytoma of bone. *Cancer* 1979;43:2344–2347.
175. Bataille R, Sany J. Solitary myeloma: clinical and prognostic features of a review of 114 cases. *Cancer* 1981;48;845–851.

176. Bataille R. Localized plasmacytomas. *Clin Hematol* 1982;11: 113–122.
177. Kyle RA, Bayrd ED. Multiple myeloma: variant forms. *In: The monoclonal gammopathies, multiple myeloma and related plasma cell disorders.* Springfield, IL: Charles C Thomas, 1976:145–148.
178. Castro EB, Lewis JS, Strong EW. Plasmacytoma of paranasal sinuses and nasal cavity. *Arch Otolaryngol* 1973;97:326–329.
179. Addis BJ, Isaacson P, Billings JA. Plasmacytoma of lymph nodes. *Cancer* 1980;46:340–346.
180. Wollersheim HCH, Holdrinet RSG, Haanen C. Clinical course and survival in 16 patients with localized plasmacytoma. *Scand J Haematol* 1984;32:423–428.
181. Bosman C, Fusilli S, Bisceglia M, et al. Oncocytic nonsecretory multiple myeloma. *Acta Haematol* 1996;96:50–56.
182. Dreicer R, Alexanian R. Non-secretory multiple myeloma. *Am J Hematol* 1982;13:313–318.
183. Bourantas K. Nonsecretory multiple myeloma. *Eur J Haematol* 1996; 56:109–111.
184. Preud'homme JL, Hurez D, Danon F, et al. Intracytoplasmic and surface-bound immunoglobulins in nonsecretory and Bence Jones myeloma. *Clin Exp Immunol* 1976;25:428–436.
185. River GL, Tewksbury DA, Gudenberg HH. "Non-secretory" multiple myeloma. *Blood* 1972;40:204–206.
186. Papadimitriou CS, Schwarze EW. Extramedullary non-gastrointestinal plasmacytomas: an immunohistochemical study of sixteen cases. *Pathol Res Pract* 1983;176:306–312.
187. Smith DB, Harris M, Gowland F, et al. Non-secretory multiple myeloma: a report of 13 cases with a review of the literature. *Hematol Oncol* 1986;4:307–313.
188. Kyle RA, Maldonado JE, Bayrd ED. Plasma cell leukemia: report on 17 cases. *Arch Intern Med* 1974;133:813–818.
189. Woodruff RK, Malpas JS, Paxton AM, et al. Plasma cell leukemia (PCL): a report on 15 patients. *Blood* 1978;52:839–845.
190. Bernier GM, Berman JH, Fanger MW. Plasma cell leukemia with excretion of half-molecules of immunoglobulin A ($\alpha 1\ \lambda 1$). *Ann Intern Med* 1977;86:572–575.
191. Garcia-Sanz R, Orfao A, Gonzalez M, et al. Primary plasma cell leukemia: clinical, immunophenotypic, DNA ploidy, and cytogenetic characteristics. *Blood* 1999;93:1032–1037.
192. Gailani S, Seon BK, Henderson ES. Plasma cell leukemia: response to conventional myeloma therapy. *J Med* 1977;8:403–414.
193. Osanto S, Müller HP, Schuit HRE, et al. Primary plasma cell leukemia: a case report and a review of the literature. *Acta Haematol* 1983;70: 122–129.
194. West NC, Smith AM, Ward R. IgE myeloma associated with plasma cell leukemia. *Post Grad Med J* 1983;59:784–785.
195. Waldenström J. Macroglobulinemia. *Adv Metab Dis* 1965;2:115–158.
196. Krajny M, Pruzanski W. Waldenström's macroglobulinemia: review of 45 cases. *Can Med Assoc J* 1976;114:899–905.
197. Stein RS, Ellman L, Bloch KJ. The clinical correlates of IgM M-components: an analysis of thirty-four patients. *Am J Med Sci* 1975; 269:209–216.
198. Bartl R, Frisch B, Mahl G, et al. Bone marrow histology in Waldenström's macroglobulinemia: clinical relevance of subtype recognition. *Scand J Haematol* 1983;31:359–375.
199. Kucharska-Pulczvnska M, Ellegaard J, Hokland P. Analysis of leukocyte differentiation antigens in blood and bone marrow from patients with Waldenström's macroglobulinemia. *Br J Haematol* 1987;65: 395–399.
200. Carter P, Koval JJ, Hobbs JR. The relation of clinical and laboratory findings to the survival of patients with macroglobulinemia. *Clin Exp Immunol* 1977;28:241–249.
201. Bloch KJ, Maki DG. Hyperviscosity syndromes associated with immunoglobulin abnormalities. *Semin Hematol* 1973;10:113–124.
202. Giarelli L, Melato M, Galconieri G. Eye involvement in Waldenström's macroglobulinemia. *Opthalmologica* 1982;185:214–219.
203. Julien J, Vital C, Ballat J-M, et al. Polyneuropathy in Waldenström's macroglobulinemia: deposition of M-component on myelin sheaths. *Arch Neurol* 1978;35:423–425.
204. Lackner H. Hemostatic abnormalities associated with dysproteinemias. *Semin Hematol* 1973;10:125–133.
205. Coleman M, Vigliano EM, Weksler ME, et al. Inhibition of fibrin monomer polymerization by lambda myeloma globulins. *Blood* 1972; 39:210–223.
206. Whittaker S, Bhogal B, Black M. Acquired immunobullous disease: a cutaneous manifestation of IgM macroglobulinaemia. *Br J Dermatol* 1996;135:283–286.
207. Ameis A, Ko HS, Pruzanski W. M-components: a review of 1242 cases. *Can Med Assoc J* 1976;114:889–895.
208. Morel-Maroger L, Basch A, Danon F, et al. Pathology of the kidney in Waldenström's macroglobulinemia: study of 16 cases. *N Engl J Med* 1970;283;123–129.
209. Takahashi K, Yamamura F, Motoyama H. IgM multiple myeloma—its distinction from Waldenström's macroglobulinemia. *Acta Pathol Jpn* 1986;36:1553–1563.
210. Groves F, Travis L, Devesa S, et al. Macroglobulinemia: incidence patterns in the United States, 1988–1994. *Cancer* 1998;82: 1078–1081.
211. Silvestri F, Barillari G, Fanin R, et al. Risk of hepatitis C virus infection, Waldenström's macroglobulinemia, and monoclonal gammopathies. *Blood* 1996;88:1125–1126.
212. Franklin EC, Kyle R, Seligmann M, et al. Correlation of protein structure and immunoglobulin gene organization in the light of two new deleted heavy chain disease proteins. *Mol Immunol* 1979;16:919–921.
213. Frangione B, Franklin EC. Heavy-chain diseases: clinical features and molecular significance of the disordered immunoglobulin structure. *Semin Hematol* 1973;10:53–64.
214. Bakhshi A, Guglielmi P, Coligan JE. A pre-translational defect in a case of human mu heavy hain disease. *Mol Immunol* 1986;23: 725–732.
215. Bakhshi A, Guglielmi P, Siebenlist U, et al. A DNA insertion/deletion necessitates an aberrant RNA splice accounting for a mu heavy chain disease protein. *Proc Natl Acad Sci USA* 1986;83:2689–2693.
216. Levo Y, Recht B, Michaelsen T, et al. The interaction of immunoglobulin heavy and light chains in the absence of the VH domain. *J Immunol* 1977;119:635–640.
217. Franklin EC, Lowenstein J, Bigelow B, et al. Heavy chain disease: a new disorder of serum gamma-globulins: report of the first case. *Am J Med* 1964;37:332–350.
218. Kyle RA, Greipp PR, Banks PM. The diverse picture of gamma heavy-chain disease: report of seven cases and review of literature. *Mayo Clin Proc* 1987;56:439–451.
219. Kyle RA. The heavy-chain diseases. In: Wiernik P, Cannellos GP, Kyle R, Schiffer C, eds. *Neoplastic diseases of the blood.* New York: Churchill Livingstone, 1985:593–605.
220. Seligmann M, Mihaesco E, Preud'homme JL, et al. Heavy chain diseases: current findings and concepts. *Immunol Rev* 1979;48:145–167.
221. Ballard HS, Hamilton LM, Marcus AJ, et al. A new variant of heavy-chain disease (mu-chain) disease). *N Engl J Med* 1970;282: 1060–1062.
222. Forte FA, Prelli F, Yount WJ, et al. Heavy chain disease of the mu (γM) type: report of the first case. *Blood* 1970;36:137–144.
223. Westin J, Eyrich R, Falsen E, et al. Gamma heavy chain disease: reports of three patients. *Acta Med Scand* 1972;192:281–292.
224. Seligmann M. Immunochemical, clinical, and pathological features of alpha-heavy chain disease. *Arch Intern Med* 1975;135:78–82.
225. Galian A, Lecestre MJ, Scotto J, et al. Pathological study of alpha-chain disease, with special emphasis on evolution. *Cancer* 1977; 39,2081–2101.
226. Glenner GG. Amyloid deposits and amyloidoses: the beta-fibrilloses. *N Engl J Med* 1980;302:1283–1292.
227. Glenner GG. Amyloid deposits and amyloidosis: the beta-fibrilloses (second of two parts). *N Engl J Med* 1980;302:1333–1343.
228. Kyle RA. Amyloidosis. *Clin Hematol* 1982;11:151–180.
229. Kyle RA, Bayrd ED. Amyloidosis: review of 236 cases. *Medicine (Baltimore)* 1975;54:271–299.
230. Durie BGM, Salmon SE, Peasky E, et al. Amyloid production in human myeloma stem-cell culture with morphologic evidence of amyloid secretion by associated macrophages. *N Engl J Med* 1982;307: 1689–1692.
231. Larson RS, Sukpanichnant S, Greer JP, et al. The spectrum of multiple myeloma: diagnostic and biological implications. *Hum Pathol* 1997; 28:1336–1347.
232. Bellotti V, Merlini G. Current concepts on the pathogenesis of systemic amyloidosis. *Nephrol Dial Transplant* 1996;11[Suppl 9]:53–62.
233. Buxman J. The amyloidoses. *Mt Sinai J Med* 1996;63:16–23.
234. Serpell LC, Sunde M, Blake CCF. The molecular basis of amyloidosis. *Cell Mol Life Sci* 1997;53:871–887.

235. Herzenberg AM, Lien J, Magil AB. Monoclonal heavy chain (immunoglobulin G3) deposition disease: report of a case. *Am J Kidney Dis* 1996;28:128–131.
236. Benson MD. Inherited amyloidosis. *J Med Genet* 1991;28:73–78.
237. Kastner DL. Familial Mediterranean fever: the genetics of inflammation. *Hosp Pract* 1998;33:131–158.
238. Nair DR, Mehta A, Milhaildis DP, et al. Multiple myeloma with primary amyloidosis. *J R Soc Med* 1997;90:502.
239. Kyle RA. High-dose therapy in multiple myeloma and primary amyloidosis: an overview. *Semin Oncol* 1999;26:74–83.
240. Kyle RA, Gertz MA, Greipp PR, et al. Long-term survival (10 years or more) in 30 patients with primary amyloidosis. *Blood* 1999;93:1062–1066.
241. Kyle RA, Gertz MA. Systemic amyloidosis. *Crit Rev Oncol Hematol* 1990;10:49–87.
242. Hagari Y, Mihara M, Konohana I, et al. Nodular localized cutaneous amyloidosis: further demonstration of monoclonality of infiltrating plasma cells in four additional Japanese patients. *Br J Dermatol* 1998;138:652–654.
243. Shim J-C, Lee YW, Lee GJ, et al. MR finding of primary amyloid arthropathy associated with multiple myeloma. *J Comput Assist Tomogr* 1997;21:800–802.
244. Mancuso G, Fanti PA, Berdondini RM. Nail changes as the only skin abnormality in myeloma-associated systemic amyloidosis. *Br J Dermatol* 1997;137:471–472.
245. Queffeulou G, Berentbaum F, Michel C, et al. AA amyloidosis in systemic lupus erythematosus: an unusual complication. *Nephrol Dial Transplant* 1998;13:1846–1848.
246. Korzets Z, Smorjik Y, Zahavi T, et al. Renal AA amyloidosis: a long-term sequela of jejuno-ileal bypass. *Nephrol Dial Transplant* 1998;13:1843–1845.
247. Ferhanoglu B, Erzin Y, Baslar Z, et al. Secondary amyloidosis in the course of idiopathic myelofibrosis. *Leuk Res* 1997;21:897–898.
248. Campistol JM, Argiles A. Dialysis-related amyloidosis: visceral involvement and protein constituents. *Nephrol Dial Transplant* 1996;11[Suppl 3]:142–145.
249. Prayson RA. Amyloid myopathy: clinicopathologic study of 16 cases. *Hum Pathol* 1998;29:463–468.
250. Cornwell GG II, Johnson KH, Westermark P. The age related amyloids: a growing family of unique biochemical substances. *J Clin Pathol* 1995;48:984–989.
251. Randall RE, Williamson WL, Mullinax F, et al. Manifestations of systemic light chain deposition. *Am J Med* 1976;60:293–299.
252. Preudhomme J, Aucouturier P, Touchard G, et al. Monoclonal immunoglobulin deposition disease (Randall type): relationship with structural abnormalities of immunoglobulin chains. *Kidney Int* 1994;46:965–972.
253. Aucouturier P, Khamlichi AA, Touchard G, et al. Heavy-chain deposition disease. *N Engl J Med* 1993;329:1389–1393.
254. Kambham N, Markowitz G, Appel G, et al. Heavy chain deposition disease: the disease spectrum. *Am J Kidney Dis* 1999;33:954–962.

CHAPTER 43

Leukemias of Mature T Cells

Daniel Catovsky and Estella Matutes

With the recognition in the 1970s of membrane markers that distinguish B and T lymphocytes, it became apparent that, although most chronic lymphoid leukemias are of B-cell origin, a distinct minority display T-cell characteristics. Greater diagnostic precision followed the use of monoclonal antibodies, which help to identify lymphocyte subsets according to their maturation stage and function.

Since that time, immunologic studies together with cell morphology have formed the basis for the classification of lymphoid malignancies. Within T-cell disorders, the broad division between thymus-derived (or immature) and postthymic (or mature) types has biologic and clinical implications (Table 43.1). Thymus-derived leukemias and lymphomas comprise lymphoblastic proliferations that occur more frequently in children and young adults. The lymphoblasts always express the nuclear enzyme terminal deoxynucleotidyl transferase (TdT) and have other immature phenotypic features such as expression of CD1a, coexpression of CD4 and CD8, lack of expression of membrane CD3 (mCD3), and in the very immature cells, absence of CD2, the receptor for sheep erythrocytes. Cells in the mature T-cell malignancies, in contrast, lack TdT and CD1a, express as a rule CD2 and mCD3, and rarely coexpress CD4 and CD8.

Within the diseases of mature T cells, the only two primary leukemias are T-cell prolymphocytic leukemia (T-PLL) and large granular lymphocytic (LGL) leukemia. This chapter is concerned with these leukemias and makes only passing reference to other T-cell disorders better defined as lymphoma/leukemia syndromes, such as Sezary syndrome and adult T-cell leukemia/lymphoma (ATLL) (1). Sezary syndrome and its related disorder, mycosis fungoides, are cutaneous T-cell lymphomas and are described in Chapter 32. ATLL, a disease with distinct epidemiology and association with the retrovirus human T-cell lymphotrophic virus type 1 (HTLV-1), is described in Chapter 44.

In the past, T-PLL and LGL leukemia were reported as T-cell chronic lymphocytic leukemia (T-CLL), particularly since the paper by Brouet and colleagues (2) in 1975 that described the findings in nine cases of LGL leukemia and two T-PLL cases. Two years earlier, we reported a case of T-PLL (3) and included it within the disease described by Galton and associates (4) as prolymphocytic leukemia, in which most cases are the B-cell type. B-PLL and T-PLL have morphologic similarities and common clinical features, such as splenomegaly and high white blood cell (WBC) count (usually $>100 \times 10^9$/L) but can be distinguished by their different cell lineage, precisely defined by immunologic tests, and subtle morphologic features, which were not recognized in the early publications.

Initially, we retained the term T-CLL for cases of LGL leukemia, a disease also described under various other designations, and T-PLL for cases with the morphology originally described as PLL (4). Unfortunately, some confusion remained because investigators tended to describe all cases of mature T-cell leukemia under the broad designation of T-CLL without distinguishing between the two disorders, which is now possible by considering cell morphology and membrane phenotype. This problem was addressed by the French-American-British Cooperative Group (FAB) (5), which recognized T-PLL as an entity distinct from LGL leukemia. Studies by our group and others have fully justified the separation of these two types of mature T-cell leukemia in humans: T-PLL and LGL leukemia (1,6). Despite this statement, a degree of phenotypic heterogeneity is seen in both disorders, although it is also possible to recognize in each a predominant or characteristic membrane phenotype, $CD4^+CD8^-$ in T-PLL and $CD4^-CD8^+$ in LGL leukemia. This apparent heterogeneity does not correlate in T-PLL with any special clinical or biologic features. For example, the consistently progressive course and the high frequency of specific chromosome abnormalities that involve chromosome 14 with breakpoints at 14q11 and 14q13 (7,8) seem to override any morphologic or immunologic differences between groups of T-PLL cases. The common form of LGL

D. Catovsky and E. Matutes: Academy of Hematology, Royal Marsden Hospital, London, United Kingdom

TABLE 43.1. *Comparison of the two main types of T-cell malignancy*

Feature	Thymic (immature)	Postthymic (mature)
Age	Adolescents and young adults	Adults
Clinical manifestations	Anterior mediastinal mass (50%); CNS involvement; high WBC	Variable: spleen, lymph nodes, and skin involvement
Disease prototypes	T-ALL; T lymphoblastic lymphoma	T-PLL, LGL leukemia, Sezary syndrome, ATLL
Phenotype		
TdT	++	−
CD1a	±	−
CD2	±	+
CD3 (membrane)	− (rare +)	+ (rare −)
CD4 and CD8 (coexpression)	+	− (rare +)
CD7	++	±
Therapy	All protocols; CNS prophylaxis	Variable: single agent or combinations; pentostatin; CAMPATH-1H

ALL, acute lymphoblastic leukemia; ATLL, adult T-cell leukemia/lymphoma; CAMPATH-1H, a monoclonal antibody; CNS, central nervous system; LGL, large granular lymphocytic; T-PLL, T-cell prolymphocytic leukemia; TdT, terminal deoxynucleotidyl transferase; WBC, white blood cell count.

leukemia with a $CD4^-CD8^+$ membrane phenotype is associated, however, with distinct clinical and laboratory features such as isolated cytopenias and a chronic clinical course. The rare cases of LGL leukemia with atypical or unusual phenotypes, with cells expressing natural killer (NK) cell antigens, often run a more progressive course than the $CD8^+$ cases and tend to have more overt leukemic characteristics (1).

T-PROLYMPHOCYTIC LEUKEMIA

Background

Prolymphocytic leukemia was described by Galton and associates (4) in a series of 15 patients with an enlarged spleen, a high WBC count, and a predominant population of medium-sized nucleolated lymphocytes in the peripheral blood films. The presence of a prominent nucleolus suggested immaturity—hence, the designation *prolymphocyte*. Few of the cases in the original series had cell markers performed, and these suggested a B-cell nature. Shortly afterward, we identified a case with similar clinical and morphologic characteristics but in which the cells were mature T lymphocytes (3).

We hold the view that B- and T-cell PLL are distinct entities. The retention of the term prolymphocyte is justified on historical and practical grounds because no better name has emerged (5). With the systematic use of membrane markers for all cases of leukemia, it has been possible in the past few years to recognize subtle morphologic differences between B and T prolymphocytes (1,9).

Although both diseases are relatively rare, if we consider all cases of B- and T-cell leukemia (excluding acute leukemias), B-PLL represents 1.5% of cases and T-PLL accounts for 2%. In the past 20 years, we have collected clinical and laboratory data on 135 patients with T-PLL, and they form the basis of this report.

Clinical Features

Most of our patients were adults older than 50 years of age. The main presenting symptoms are anemia, sweating, malaise, weight loss, skin lesions, lymphadenopathy, and shortness of breath caused by pleural effusions. The disease is discovered by chance on a laboratory test and may run an indolent course in some patients before giving rise to symptoms (10,11). Physical findings are summarized in Table 43.2. Splenomegaly is common, with the spleen extending more than 10 cm below the costal margin in most patients. Generalized lymphadenopathy, which includes en-

TABLE 43.2. *Clinical and laboratory features of T-cell prolymphocytic leukemia*

Feature	Incidence[a]
Organomegaly	
Spleen	79%
Lymph nodes	46%
Liver	39%
Other tissues	
Skin[b]	23%
Effusions[c]	15%
Blood counts	
Hemoglobin (<10 g/dL)	25%
WBC (>100 × 10^9/L)	72%
Platelets (<100 × 10^9/L)	44%

[a] From a series of 135 cases studied in our laboratory.
[b] Generalized maculopapular rash or nodular lesions; erythroderma seen in two patients. Skin biopsy shows characteristic involvement of the dermis and the appendages without epidermotropism.
[c] Pleural most common; ascites in some.

larged abdominal and mediastinal nodes as detected by computed tomography (CT) scan investigations, is frequent in T-PLL and rare in B-PLL, in which it is seen only in advanced stages of the disease. Histologically, the spleen shows diffuse infiltration of the red pulp or both red and white pulps (12,13). The lymph node histology is less well characterized, but it tends to infiltrate diffusely from the paracortical areas (12). Skin deposits, often seen as small nodules or a generalized rash, are frequent at presentation or later in the course of the disease. Erythroderma, as in Sezary syndrome, is rare, but when present, it is not associated with epidermotropism in the skin biopsies. The histology of the skin lesions is characterized by dense infiltrates around the blood vessels and appendages in the dermis. Pleural effusions or ascites correlate with disease activity and high WBC counts and often constitute a major clinical problem. Central nervous system involvement is infrequent but may occur during the course of the disease.

Laboratory Findings

The major abnormality is the very high WBC count (Table 43.2). Leukocyte counts in T-PLL tend to be higher than in B-PLL, with two thirds of patients having WBC counts greater than 200×10^9/L (1,10). Anemia and thrombocytopenia are also frequent (Table 43.2) but less marked than in B-PLL. Serum immunoglobulins are normal and so are absolute numbers of neutrophils and monocytes; monoclonal bands are not detected in the serum of T-PLL patients. Liver function test results are only moderately abnormal but can deteriorate in later stages of the disease, correlating with greater infiltration.

Morphology of T Prolymphocytes

The examination of well-spread, peripheral blood films is the main diagnostic test in PLL. Most cells are prolymphocytes with a well-defined central nucleolus. In 40% to 50% of T-PLL cases, the cells may look identical to B prolymphocytes. Differences between these cell types have been recognized, however, with greater experience in many cases (1,9). These are chiefly the following: T prolymphocytes (Figs. 43.1, 43.2) tend to be smaller and have less cytoplasm than B prolymphocytes; in half of the cases, the nuclear outline is irregular, but nuclei are rarely polylobed as in ATLL or deeply convoluted with deep indentations as in Sezary cells. Other characteristic features of T-PLL cells are deeply basophilic cytoplasm and cytoplasmic protrusions (10). In 20% of cases, the T prolymphocytes are small, with more condensed nuclear chromatin than usual and a nucleolus is not readily apparent by light microscopic examination. These cases, also called small cell variant of T-PLL (9,10), may present diagnostic problems mainly because the cells are not readily recognized morphologically as prolymphocytes. Electron microscopic examination (Fig. 43.3) is useful to identify these small prolymphocytes and to visualize the nu-

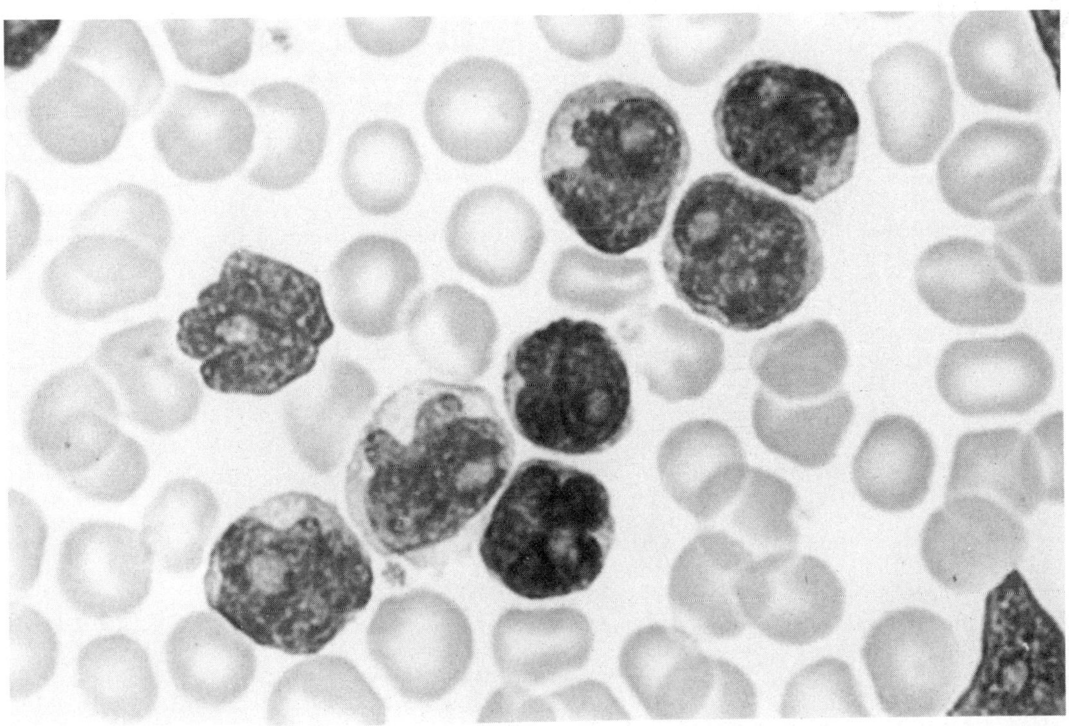

FIG. 43.1. Peripheral blood film from a case of T-cell prolymphocytic leukemia. The cells have an irregular nuclear outline and prominent nucleolus.

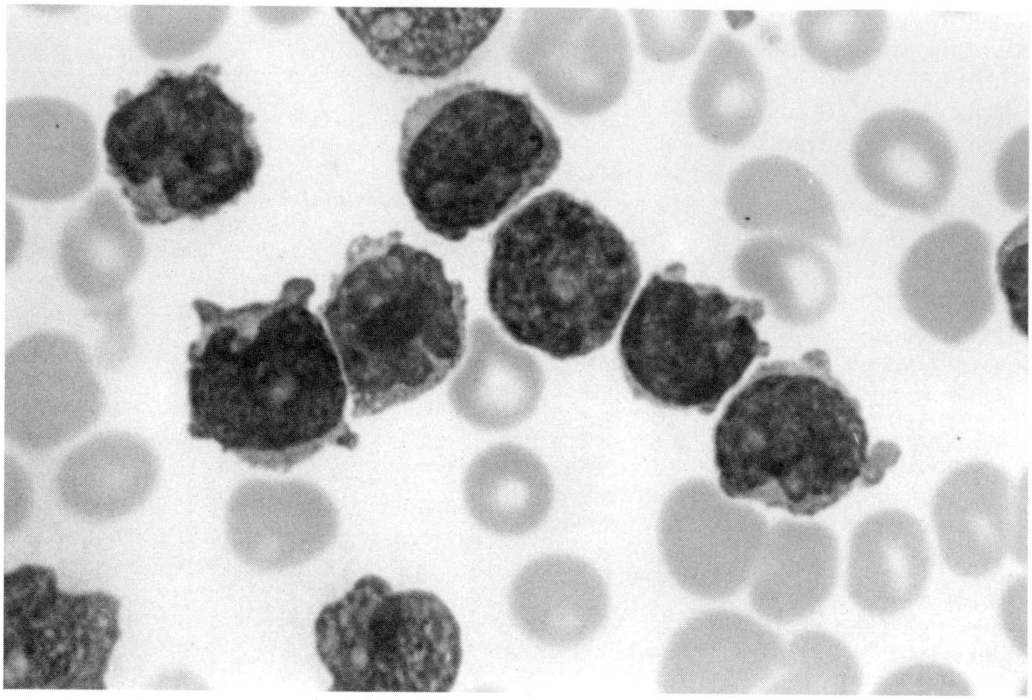

FIG. 43.2. Peripheral blood film from another patient with T-cell prolymphocytic leukemia. The cells have basophilic cytoplasm (seen on the original slide) and cytoplasmic protrusions.

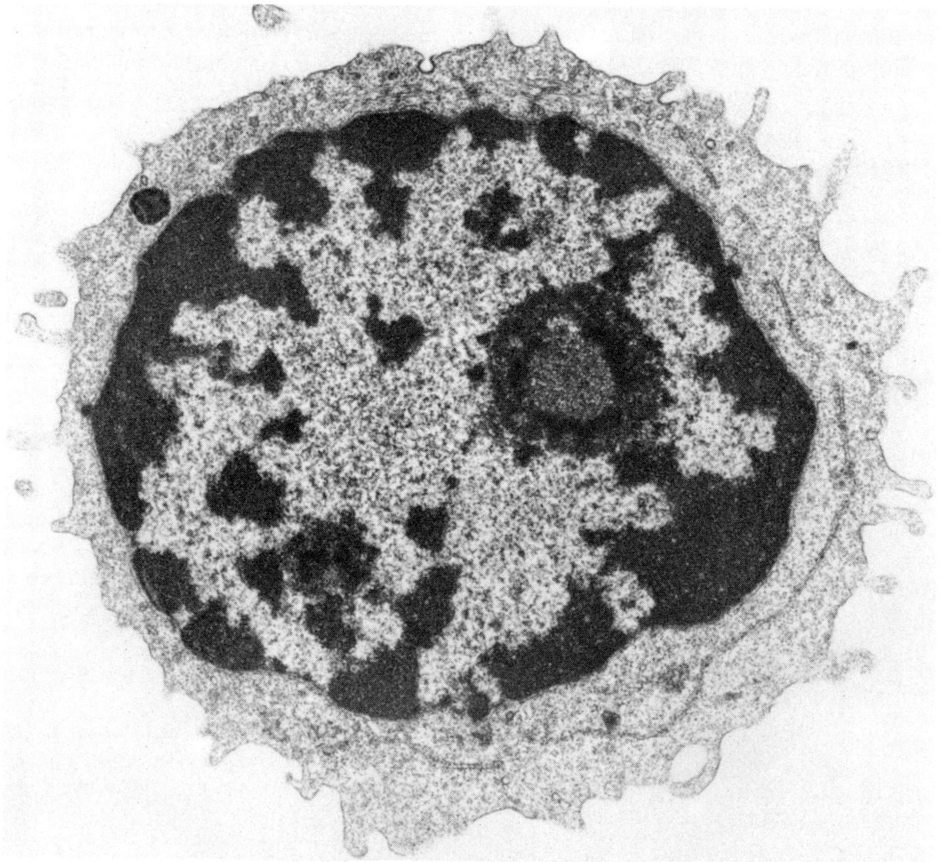

FIG. 43.3. Electron micrograph from a case of small cell variant of T-cell prolymphocytic leukemia shows the typical features of peripheral nuclear chromatin condensation, a prominent nucleolus, and abundant ribosomes in the cytoplasm.

cleolus (9). In rare instances, the differential diagnosis is with Sezary syndrome or Sezary cell leukemia, and this also can be resolved by ultrastructural analysis (6). Abundant clusters of ribosomes and strands of endoplasmic reticulum are prominent in T prolymphocytes and account for the cytoplasmic basophilia seen at light microscopy. Another cell feature more noticeable by electron microscopy is the lysosomal granules and the Gall bodies that are large and dense in T-PLL cells (9) and have a high content of acid hydrolases. Studies by our group have shown that the rare cases previously described as Sezary cell leukemia (14) represent a variant form of T-PLL (cerebriform variant) based on similarities in clinical features, disease course, and cytogenetic abnormalities (15,16).

One major difference between malignant B and T cells is the different content of lysosomal enzymes, which is always higher in T cells (1). In common with other T-cell leukemias, T-PLL cells are rich in acid hydrolases. The content of α-naphthyl acetate esterase (ANAE), localized in the Gall bodies, is much greater than in other types of T cells. In contrast to findings for other T-cell leukemias, T prolymphocytes are always positive for all the cytochemical reactions for acid hydrolases (1) and characteristically show a dotlike pattern with the cytochemical reactions, particularly ANAE, which may be seen in other $CD4^+$ leukemias (1,17).

Bone Marrow

Bone marrow aspirates are not critical for the diagnosis of T-PLL, because the characteristic morphology of prolymphocytes is better seen in blood films. The bone marrow shows heavy infiltration, which is confirmed on trephine biopsies. The latter show roughly similar features in B-PLL and T-PLL (18). The most frequent patterns of infiltration are mixed, interstitial and nodular, and diffuse. The content of bone marrow reticulin fibers is always increased. There are no specific histologic features in T-PLL that distinguish this disorder from other T-cell leukemias except that the degree of involvement is greater and more consistent than in Sezary syndrome, ATLL, and LGL leukemia, conditions in which the bone marrow may be partially or significantly spared.

Membrane Markers

In common with other postthymic T-cell disorders, T-PLL cells are TdT and CD1a negative (Table 43.1); in two thirds of cases the main phenotype is $CD4^+CD8^-$, whereas in 25%, cells coexpress CD4 and CD8. A comparison between the findings in T-PLL and the other types of $CD4^+$ T-cell disorders is shown in Table 43.3. One of the main differences is the consistent strong reactivity with anti-CD7 reagents in T-PLL (19) and the lack or weak expression of CD25 (Table 43.3). Studies with monoclonal antibodies should be performed routinely in lymphoid leukemias as a prerequisite for the correct diagnosis and classification (5). Prolymphocytic leukemia is a good example of this concept because with morphology alone the type of disease (B or T) can not easily be discerned.

TABLE 43.3. *Membrane phenotype of T-cell prolymphocytic leukemia and comparison with other $CD4^+$ disorders*

Monoclonal antibody	T-PLL	ATLL	Sezary syndrome
CD2	++	++	++
mCD3[a]	++	++	++
CD4	++	++	++
CD5	++	++	++
CD7	++	±	+
CD8	+[b]	−	−
CD25	±	++	±

ATLL, adult T-cell leukemia/lymphoma; T-PLL, T-cell prolymphocytic leukemia; ++, 80% of cases; +, 30–80% positive; ±, <30% positive; −, negative or occasionally (<10% of cases) positive.

[a] Membrane staining in cell suspensions; about 20% of cases are mCD3 negative but are always cytoplasmic CD3 positive.

[b] In most cases, CD8 is coexpressed with CD4; about 12% of cases are $CD4^-$ $CD8^+$.

Chromosome Abnormalities and Molecular Genetics

The main cytogenetic information derives from studies from our laboratory (7,8,10,20), and this is summarized in Table 43.4. The most consistent findings are translocations with breakpoints at 14q11 (locus for the T-cell receptor α and δ genes) and at 14q32. The most frequent chromosomal abnormality in T-PLL is inv(14)(q11;q32.1) (or the equivalent t(14;14)(q11;q32.1)). This juxtaposes T-cell receptor-α (TCR-α) in 14q11 to a region in 14q32.1 that lies about 10 Mb centromeric of the immunoglobulin heavy-chain (IgH) locus. This 350-kb region in 14q32.1 contains two CpG islands. An oncogene called *TCL1* has been identified and cloned from within this region (21,22). A second gene of the *TCL1* family, *TCL1B*, has been cloned and characterized (23).

TABLE 43.4. *Chromosome abnormalities in T-cell prolymphocytic leukemia*

Abnormality	Frequency[a]
Inversion 14 (q11;q32)	60–70%[b]
Translocations with breakpoints 14q11-q32, including t(X;14)(q28;q11)	10–20%[b]
Other translocations with breakpoint 14q32	4%
Trisomy 8q	50–80%[b]
Normal or random changes	2%

[a] Results from our laboratory in 54 cases (7,8,10,16,20).

[b] A higher proportion of these abnormalities is found by the systematic use of fluorescence *in situ* hybridization (FISH) analysis (20).

The nonrandom chromosome abnormalities of T-PLL are also seen in the small cell and cerebriform variants (15,16) confirming that these morphologic subtypes are part of the same disease spectrum, but they are rare in other T-cell leukemias.

Transgenic mice expressing human TCL1 by means of a T-cell lineage-specific promoter display late onset of a T-cell leukemia with morphology and immunophenotype similar to T-PLL (24). Breakpoints up to approximately 200 kb on either side of *TCL1* have been cloned from T-PLL cases. These breakpoint clones have been used to screen a panel of 40 T-PLL cases for rearrangement. None was detected, despite the high frequency of 14q32 breakpoints in T-PLL. The breakpoints in 14q32 do not show clustering around known breakpoints. When *TCL1* cDNA was used as a probe, however, one case showed a rearrangement that is currently being cloned (M. Yuille, personal communication).

Although *TCL1* has been shown to be rearranged in only a few cases, most have expression of transcripts of this gene (24). It is likely that this oncogene is involved in the development of T-cell leukemias in man. The discovery of *TCL1B* would explain cases of T-cell leukemia with an amplification at 14q32 without activation of *TCL1* (23).

Rare cases that lack a 14q32.1 breakpoint are usually observed to carry t(X;14)(q28;q11) or, rarely, t(X;7)(q28;q33-35) (20). Cloning of such cases has revealed a clustering of breakpoints in exon I and 5′-UTR of the *MTCP1* gene, another member of the *TCL1* gene family, at Xq28 (25,26).

Abnormalities of chromosome 11q23 are not rare in T-PLL, although not necessarily at the cytogenetic level. The 11q23 region contains the ataxia telangiectasia mutated *(ATM)* gene, and mutations and disruptions of *ATM* or its inactivation have been documented in a high proportion of cases of T-PLL; this has been considered a key event in the development of this disease (27–29). Cytogenetic findings similar to those of T-PLL have been documented in peripheral blood T-cell clones of patients who have ataxia telangiectasia (AT) (8,26), including expression of *TCL1* transcripts, even when they have not developed leukemia. The similarities between T-PLL and AT are even more striking if we consider that patients with AT develop a T-cell leukemia identical to T-PLL (8,26), confirming that *TCL1* (14q32) and *ATM* (11q23) may be relevant to the pathogenesis of this T-cell leukemia. Abnormalities of chromosome 8 are common, particularly iso8q or trisomy 8, which are seen in more than one half of the cases and probably represent a secondary event. DNA analysis has not shown rearrangement of *MYC*, but cases with an extra copy of 8q tend to show overexpression of the MYC oncoprotein demonstrated by flow cytometry (30).

Natural History and Prognosis

T-prolymphocytic leukemia is an aggressive T-cell malignancy with a median survival of 7 months in our historical series (10); T-PLL progresses more rapidly than B-PLL and responds less well to therapy. Some clinical features, chiefly hepatomegaly but not variations in phenotype, may be associated with a worse prognosis; lymphadenopathy appears to be slightly favorable. There is no correlation of prognosis with the WBC count, and this may be explained by the fact that the prolymphocyte count is high in most patients. In a few patients in whom the diagnosis was made by chance at an early stage, the disease progressed over the next 18 months until they became symptomatic and then died shortly afterward. Another report also described a group of patients who experienced an initial indolent course with relatively stable lymphocytosis but ultimately the disease progressed and median survival after progression is similar to those presenting with an aggressive course (11). The overall prognosis of T-PLL is similar to that of ATLL, although we have no serologic or molecular evidence in any of the 27 T-PLL cases investigated of a relationship with HTLV-1 (31).

Treatment and Survival

A summary of our experience is given in Table 43.5. Complete remissions (CRs) were rare and were occasionally seen with the combination CHOP regimen (10) and with pentostatin (2′-deoxycoformycin) using weekly doses of 4 mg/m^2 (1,10,32). Responses are rare with alkylating agents used alone. Our results with pentostatin in the treatment of T-cell leukemias suggests that this adenosine deaminase inhibitor is useful in T-PLL, particularly in cases with a CD4$^+$CD8$^-$ phenotype (10), in which an overall response rate (partial and complete) has been achieved in 45% of cases, and in Sezary syndrome, where 62% of patients treated benefited with improvement of the erythroderma (32). The CRs in T-PLL lasted unmaintained for up to 1 year, but second remissions with the same agent are difficult to obtain.

Dramatically improved CR rates have been documented with the humanized monoclonal antibody CAMPATH-1H (33). The use of CAMPATH-1H has revolutionized the treatment of T-PLL with promising results, in particular a high CR rate in patients who are resistant to pentostatin (Table

TABLE 43.5. *Response to treatment in T-cell prolymphocytic leukemia*

Modality used[a] (no. of patients)	Remission rate	
	Partial	Complete
Alkylating agents (32)	28%	
CHOP[b] (15)	27%	
Pentostatin (55)	36%	9%
CAMPATH-1H (22)[c]	18%	59%

[a] Some patients treated with more than one modality are counted twice.

[b] Cyclophosphamide, doxorubicin, vincristine (Oncovin), and prednisolone regimen.

Adapted from Pawson R, Dyer MJS, Barge R, et al. Treatment of T-cell prolymphocytic leukemia with human CD52 antibody. *J Clin Oncol* 1997;15:2667–2672, with permission.

43.5). This antibody should now be considered as first-line treatment, with the aim of achieving CR. Such a strategy allows proceeding with high-dose therapy and an autologous transplant. We have carried out such procedures in three T-PLL patients. One of them treated in first CR is alive, well, and free of disease 1 year after transplantation. The other two had prolonged CR after CAMPATH-1H, but the autograft was carried out late, when the disease relapsed, and after a further reinduction with CAMPATH-1H. They both eventually relapsed and died. It is possible that combinations of the various approaches listed in Table 43.5 or new ones will be necessary to improve the outlook of patients with T-PLL. It seems, however, that high-dose therapy should be carried out soon after a first CR is achieved. One possible rationale to explain the high CR rate with CAMPATH-1H is the high density of the CAMPATH antigen (CD52) shown by quantitative flow cytometry in T prolymphocytes (34).

LARGE GRANULAR LYMPHOCYTIC LEUKEMIA

Background

Two problems that beset the recognition of LGL leukemia as a distinct disease entity are the benign and chronic clinical course in many patients and the inability, in the pre-DNA analysis era, to demonstrate T-cell clonality.

The early reports (2,35–38) clearly established the basic components of the disease: persistent lymphocytosis with granular lymphocytes associated with cytopenias that affect one or more of the three bone marrow lineages but more frequently neutropenia. The demonstration of clonality, sometimes by karyotype (35,38–40) and more frequently by rearrangement of the TCR genes (41–44), no longer justifies the use of the term T-cell lymphocytosis, which should be reserved for the rare (nonclonal) reactive cases. Numerous other designations have been used in the past 15 years that reflected the prevailing uncertainties about the nature of the disease. All of them include one or more of the main laboratory findings in the description (38,44,45).

Although it is always advisable to demonstrate T-cell clonality, DNA analysis is only essential in cases with borderline features. Using simple clinical and laboratory guidelines, it is possible to establish the diagnosis of LGL leukemia in most instances. There are several diagnostic features:

1. Lymphocytosis, usually more than 5×10^9/L, sometimes more than 4×10^9/L, and only rarely lower, persisting for 6 months or longer without an obvious cause
2. Morphology of the peripheral blood lymphocytes (>80% granular)
3. Neutropenia or any other cytopenia in the absence of heavy bone marrow infiltration
4. Predominance of a discrete T-cell subset by membrane marker analysis (e.g., $CD8^+$, $CD56^+$, $CD57^+$), often with features infrequent in normal blood lymphocytes

We have found that investigations of patients with these characteristics nearly always correlate with clonality by TCR gene analysis (6,42,43).

Clinical Features

The age of presentation is variable and includes young and old patients. Most are adults; the median age in our series is 63 years, with a range of 19 to 84 years (6). Rarely, the disease can be seen in children. The symptoms are related to the manifestations of cytopenias, such as recurrent mouth ulcers or other infections in neutropenic patients. Pure red cell aplasia may be the only presenting symptom (45,46). Many patients are asymptomatic and are discovered by routine blood examination. Some patients complain of tiredness, and in a few, this seems to be unrelated to the degree of anemia.

Organomegaly is not a major feature, with moderate splenomegaly being the most common finding (Table 43.6). The splenic involvement is mainly in the red pulp. Because of the slightly abundant cytoplasm of the LGLs, this pattern of infiltration could be confused with that of hairy cell leukemia. Erythematous or papular skin rashes occur but they are often nonspecific in nature. In some cases, infiltration by lymphocytes in the deep dermis has been demonstrated (2).

In up to 30% of patients, there is serologic and clinical evidence of rheumatoid arthritis (RA) (35,37,47). The peripheral polyarthritis involves the proximal interphalangeal and metatarsophalangeal joints. RA precedes in most patients the discovery of T-cell lymphocytosis. The association of splenomegaly, neutropenia, and RA suggests a diagnosis of Felty's syndrome. Although lymphocytosis is not a feature of RA or Felty's, it is possible that there is a causal relationship in a minority of patients. A distinct possibility for a minority of RA patients is the development of T-cell clones that result eventually in LGL leukemia. Alternatively,

TABLE 43.6. *Clinical and laboratory features of large granular lymphocytic leukemia*

Feature	Incidence (%)[a]
Organomegaly	
Spleen[b]	50
Liver	20
Lymph nodes	10
Other tissues	
Skin rash	20
Blood counts	
Hemoglobin (<10 g/dL)	30
Lymphocytes (>5×10^9/L)	95
Neutrophils (<0.5×10^9/L)	50
Platelets (<100×10^9/L)	20
Hypogammaglobulinemia	5

[a] Based on our own cases (1,6) and others reported in the literature (2,35,44,45,50).
[b] Moderately enlarged, rarely >10 cm below the costal margin.

T-cell clones may have a causative role in the pathogenesis of RA (47,48). Regardless of the exact mechanism, it seems that, in patients who have RA, the association may result in a distinct form of LGL leukemia. The new techniques of DNA analysis may help clarify the relationship between these two disorders. The study by Loughran and associates (47) has shown clonal TCR-β chain rearrangement in four patients who had LGL leukemia associated with RA and neutropenia but failed to show clonality in six patients who had Felty's syndrome with neutropenia but no increase in LGLs.

Laboratory Findings

The main features are normal or mildly elevated WBC with lymphocytosis and neutropenia (Table 43.6). Anemia or thrombocytopenia can be seen alone or associated with neutropenia. These latter manifestations may result from hypersplenism and can be corrected by splenectomy, but the neutropenia usually persists. Anemia caused by pure red cell aplasia is also a well-recognized manifestation of LGL leukemia (45,46).

Lymphocytosis of 5 to 15 $\times$ 10^9/L is seen in most cases; counts higher than 15 $\times$ 10^9/L are infrequent, but high counts often follow splenectomy (36). In a few patients who have large spleens, the WBC and lymphocyte counts are low, but the lymphocytosis becomes apparent after a splenectomy is performed, usually for diagnostic purposes. Hypogammaglobulinemia is rarely seen, and in these patients, the T lymphocytes suppress B-cell differentiation and secretion of immunoglobulins (1,49). Autoimmune hemolytic anemia and thrombocytopenia have been reported in a few cases (50). Although there have been several reports documenting the presence of antibodies to HTLV-1, HTLV-2, or both in LGL patients by enzyme-linked immunoabsorbent assay, more specific serologic tests such as Western blot did not confirm these findings and instead showed negative or indeterminate serologic patterns. Our own data on 28 cases of LGL leukemia, which included extensive serologic and molecular tests for HTLV-1 and HTLV-2, offered further support that these retroviruses are not involved in the pathogenesis of this disease (31).

Morphology of Large Granular Lymphocytic Leukemia Cells

As described in the original report by Brouet and colleagues (2), the lymphocytes have abundant cytoplasm and prominent azurophilic granules. The morphology of the LGLs in these patients is not different from LGLs seen in normal persons. As in T-PLL, peripheral blood films are the best material to establish a diagnosis and to recognize the morphologic features of LGL leukemia.

Large granular lymphocytes have mature (condensed) nuclear chromatin and an eccentric nucleus with a round or slightly indented nuclear outline (Fig. 43.4). The cytoplasm contains several prominent azurophilic granules. If the quality of the stain is suboptimal, LGL cells can still be recog-

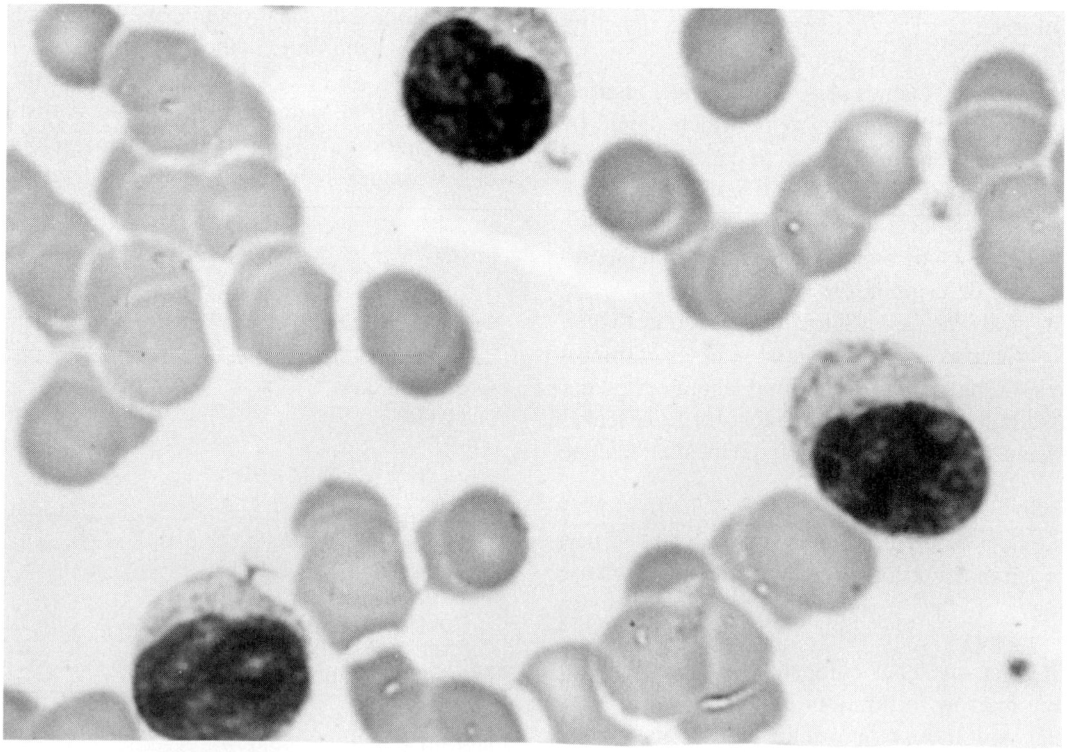

FIG. 43.4. Peripheral blood film from a case of large granular lymphocytic leukemia with eccentric nucleus and cytoplasmic granules.

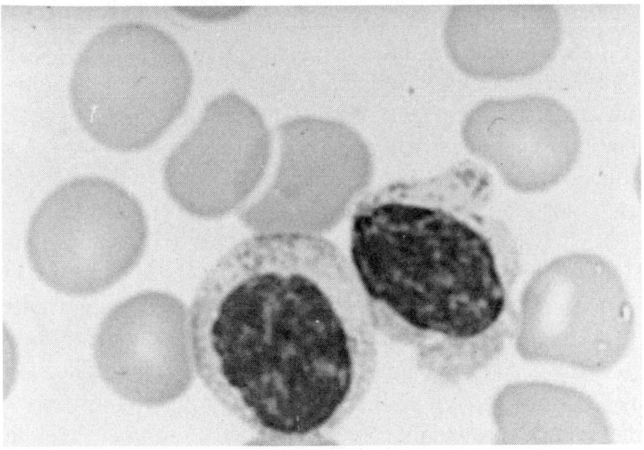

FIG. 43.5. Two cells from another case of large granular lymphocytic leukemia. These lymphocytes are slightly larger than those of Figure 43.4 and have a more open nuclear chromatin pattern.

nized by the relatively abundant cytoplasm, even if the granules are not clearly visible. Ultrastructural analysis confirms these features (1,35). The more prominent azurophil granules correspond to bundles of microtubules that contain acid hydrolases described as parallel tubular arrays (PTAs) (51). These structures are not unique to LGL leukemia and are also seen in normal $CD8^+$ lymphocytes (52) and in lymphocytes in several pathologic conditions, including RA and infectious mononucleosis (35). In a few patients who have a more aggressive clinical course, the leukemia LGLs look less mature and are slightly larger (Fig. 43.5). In one such patient, the cytoplasmic granules were not PTAs but resembled the scrolls that are a type of granular structure seen in mast cells.

Bone Marrow and Spleen

In the early stages of the disease, the bone marrow shows little or no evidence of lymphocytic infiltration, with fewer than 30% lymphocytes in the aspirates and mild interstitial infiltration in the trephine biopsies, which often needs to be highlighted by immunohistochemistry. In more advanced cases, there is nodular or moderately diffuse involvement but the percentage of lymphocytes is rarely greater than 50%. These cells have the same morphology as those in the peripheral blood. In general, bone marrow aspirates are less useful than peripheral blood films for diagnostic purposes.

The pattern of spleen involvement in LGL leukemia is characterized by expansion of the red pulp with atrophy or some preservation of the white pulp, resembling that of hairy cell leukemia. The pattern of infiltration of the liver, when involved, is preferentially sinusoidal, although it may spread to the portal tracts in cases with marked involvement.

Membrane Markers

Based on the membrane phenotype, LGL leukemias are divided into two groups: T-cell LGL leukemia ($CD3^+$) and

TABLE 43.7. *Membrane phenotypes in large granular lymphocytic leukemia*

Most cases
$CD1a^-$, $CD2^+$, $CD3^+$, $CD5^{+(-)}$, $CD7^{-(+)}$, TdT^-
Common phenotype
$CD4^-$, $CD8^+$, $CD57^+$, $CD11b^{-(+)}$, $CD16^{+(-)}$, $CD56^{-(+)}$
Infrequent phenotypes
$CD4^+$, $CD8^-$, $CD11b^{+(-)}$, $CD16^{-(+)}$, $CD57^{+(-)}$
$CD4^+$, $CD8^+$, $CD11b^{+(-)}$, $CD16^-$, $CD57^+$
$CD3^-$, $CD4^-$, $CD8^-$, $CD11b^{+(-)}$, $CD16^+$, $CD56^+$, $CD57^{-(+)}$

Signs in parentheses: occasionally positive (+) or occasionally negative (−)

NK LGL leukemia ($CD3^-$) (50). The cells of LGL leukemia show a mature (postthymic) phenotype (Table 43.7). About 90% of cases have the immunophenotype $CD3^+$ $CD4^-CD8^+$, which can be defined as the common phenotype. Using a range of monoclonal antibodies that characterize T lymphocyte subsets, there is a degree of variability in the results. Table 43.7 lists several of the infrequent phenotypes that may be quite variable, perhaps reflecting the many discrete subsets of LGLs in normal persons. From a diagnostic point of view, the less frequent phenotypes (reflecting cell populations hardly represented in normal peripheral blood) are more easily recognized as pathologic (leukemic) because of their unusual nature. Such are the cases that express markers of NK cells, such as CD11b and CD16 in $CD4^+$ cells.

The group of NK LGL leukemias is rare, and they have been reported more frequently in Japan than elsewhere (44,45,53). The cells express CD2 and NK markers, but they are negative with anti-T-cell monoclonal antibodies.

One of the clinical scenarios in which there may be a persistent increase in LGLs that may resemble LGL leukemia is after splenectomy (36,54). The main difference is that in the latter condition there is a polyclonal increase of T-cell subsets, not just a single subset, although there is a tendency toward a greater increase of $CD8^+$ lymphocytes. Rarely is the absolute number of lymphocytes greater than 4×10^9/L, and only one third of them are LGLs (54).

Normal and neoplastic LGLs are two of the few cell types that express the interleukin-2 receptor (IL-2R) of intermediate affinity (p75), recognized by the monoclonal antibodies TU27 and MIK-B1 but not the low-affinity IL-2R (p55), identified by its reactivity with the monoclonal antibody anti-Tac or CD25 (44). Both peptides form an heterodimer p55/p75, which is the high-affinity IL-2R highly expressed on ATLL lymphocytes but not on LGL leukemia cells. Most LGL leukemia cases are also TIA-1 positive, a monoclonal antibody that detects intragranular structures on cytotoxic T cells, and this contrasts with the few cases of $CD8^+$ T-PLL and Sezary syndrome that are TIA-1 negative (55). Leukemic LGL cells but not normal T and NK lymphocytes, constitutively express FAS ligand on the membrane and have high serum levels of the soluble form (sFASL) of this tumor necrosis factor (56). This release of sFASL may be involved in the pathogenesis of the systemic tissue damage, such as liver function abnormalities, and cytopenias often seen in patients with LGL leukemia.

T Functional Subsets

The cells of LGL leukemia that represent clonal expansions of cells poorly represented in the peripheral blood have provided a unique opportunity to gain greater knowledge of the functional properties of T lymphocyte subsets. These studies are also relevant to the pathogenesis of some manifestations of LGL leukemia, such as neutropenia, red cell aplasia, or hypogammaglobulinemia. There is no clear-cut correlation between phenotypic changes and function because few membrane antigens are uniquely specific to certain cell types. Some of these studies have been reviewed in detail elsewhere (1,44). The common form of the disease has $CD3^+CD4^-CD8^+$ cells, and these often have been shown to function *in vitro* in antibody-mediated cellular cytotoxicity (ADCC) assays, whereas the rare cases with $CD3^-CD4^-CD8^-CD16^+$ cells show NK function (i.e., non–major histocompatibility complex [MHC]–restricted cytotoxicity). Some $CD3^+CD8^+$ cells can suppress immunoglobulin synthesis *in vitro* (1,44,49). Paradoxically, in a few instances, $CD3^+CD4^-CD8^+$ lymphocytes were shown to act as helper cells (57). Another rare clone of $CD4^+CD11b^+CD16^+$ cells was found to have only ADCC activity (58).

The role of LGLs in suppressing granulopoiesis has been more difficult to prove, although data that support an inhibitory activity on colony-forming unit–granulocyte-macrophage colonies have been published (1,44). Inhibition of erythroid colonies (burst-forming unit–erythroid [BFU-E] and colony-forming unit–erythroid) has been more convincing. Removal of T cells from bone marrow samples of LGL leukemia patients who have pure red cell aplasia has been shown to enhance significantly BFU-E colony growth, which was shown in separate experiments to be inhibited by the patient's T lymphocytes (44,59,60). In a patient with LGL leukemia and pure red cell aplasia, the LGLs expressed killer cell inhibitory receptors and were able to kill selectively erythroid precursors in an MHC-unrestricted manner, as the expression of class I human leukocyte antigen (HLA) molecules in erythroid cells is reduced (61).

Chromosome Abnormalities

Although it is possible in T-PLL to obtain analyzable metaphases in most cases and these are almost always abnormal, results in LGL leukemia have been less consistent. One of the main reasons is the poor response *in vitro* to T-cell mitogens like phytohemagglutinin (PHA) of $CD3^+CD8^+$ lymphocytes. By extending the culture to 5 days, it was possible for us to demonstrate clonal karyotypic abnormalities in five cases (40,62). One of the cases was a proliferation of T cells bearing TCR-$\gamma\delta$, as demonstrated by DNA analysis (43). Another case had the translocation t(8;14)(q24;q32), characteristic of Burkitt's lymphoma but, surprisingly, without evidence of clonality by TCR gene rearrangement (62). The presence of karyotypic abnormalities may also have a clinical impact as it seems that patients respond poorly to immunosuppressive drugs when these are present (46).

Technical considerations may be critical in obtaining divisions of leukemic LGLs. We have used peripheral blood samples stimulated with PHA and IL-2 (40). Normal results were reported by Oshimi (44) in all 10 cases studied; however, this analysis was performed on bone marrow cells with a low content of lymphocytes. It is likely that in those cases the metaphases examined corresponded to normal myeloid progenitor cells.

T-Cell Clonality of Large Granular Lymphocytic Leukemia

The uncertainty about the neoplastic nature of this disease has been clarified with the availability of techniques to demonstrate clonality by DNA analysis. Even with optimal techniques, it is not possible to obtain chromosome preparations in all cases. In cases with the NK membrane phenotype $CD3^-CD16^+CD56^+$, however, DNA analysis demonstrates TCR genes in the germline configuration (44,53,63, 64). Most cases defined by the guidelines for LGL leukemia already outlined show evidence of T-cell clonality by DNA analysis (41–44,53,64,65) or, rarely, by the karyotype (40,57,62). The techniques for T-cell clonality by DNA analysis are Southern blotting and PCR. Probes for the TCR-β, -γ, and -δ chains are used to cover all the possibilities and exclude a germline configuration (42,43). In our earlier series, clonality was documented by gene rearrangement or by chromosome abnormalities in all 15 cases studied (6). It is generally agreed that failure to show clonality by using all the appropriate techniques favors a reactive T-cell proliferation in cases in which the clinical and laboratory data do not suggest malignancy and would indicate that a cause for the lymphocytosis should be investigated further (1).

Animal Model for Large Granular Lymphocytic Leukemia

Extensive studies in the 1980s have characterized a spontaneous LGL lymphoproliferative disease in aged Fischer (F344) rats (66). Clinical, morphologic, and histochemical features show a striking similarity with the human disease counterpart, except for the absence of PTAs, which are not seen in rat LGLs. Experiments using splenectomy have reduced the incidence of the leukemia and suggest that the source of progenitors for this leukemia may be a radiosensitive cell that resides in the spleen. The possible early involvement of the spleen in human LGL leukemia and the relative sparing of the bone marrow would also suggest an analogy with possible therapeutic implications, such as early splenectomy.

Natural History and Prognosis

Most cases of LGL leukemia have a protracted clinical course without much evidence of progression. The symptoms depend on the nature and severity of the cytopenias. Patients who have severe neutropenia have frequent infections, and this marks the course and often determines the outcome. Some patients have no evidence of cytopenia or organ enlargement, and in this respect, they resemble patients with stage 0 (Rai system) B-cell CLL who may remain with stable asymptomatic disease for many years and who commonly die of unrelated causes.

Evidence of chromosome abnormalities and an unusual membrane phenotype does not necessarily indicate a worse outcome, as illustrated by one of our patients, a 44-year-old woman with circulating $CD4^+CD56^+CD57^+$ lymphocytes, a translocation t(4;17)(p15-16;q23) (25), and TCR-β rearrangement who has remained clinically well with a lymphocytosis ranging between 7 and 8 $\times$ 10^9/L for the past 7 years. Except for this case, our experience and that of other published cases tend to show a correlation between rare phenotypes and disease progression and poor prognosis.

A typical example of $CD3^+CD8^+$ LGL leukemia is illustrated in Figure 43.6, which corresponds to a patient in whom the anemia was caused by red cell hypoplasia, one of the main problems associated with this T lymphoproliferative disorder. After splenectomy, the lymphocytosis became more manifest, as it does in most patients (36), but transfusion requirements continued unchanged. A similar example is illustrated elsewhere (1) from another of our patients in whom neutropenia rather than anemia was the main problem.

There are not enough large series of cases to enable us to estimate the median survival of this disease. In an earlier series (6), the median was 4 years, but two of the patients had died of unrelated causes. It is likely that in the more benign $CD3^+CD8^+$ cases this figure could extend to 8 or 10 years. Problems may arise from three sources: infectious complications leading to morbidity and mortality; leukemic progression with rising WBC and organ infiltration; and transformation to an immunoblastic or large cell lymphoma (i.e., Richter-like syndrome). None of these three possibilities is common, but all have been well documented. Some patients who have severe neutropenia have compensatory levels of monocytes, which seem to convey a degree of protection. Progression characterizes some patients who include most of those with infrequent phenotypes.

Transformation to a large cell lymphoma with the same karyotypic abnormality in both tissues (the lymphocytes and the large cells) was reported by Nowell and colleagues (67) in a patient originally described during the chronic phase

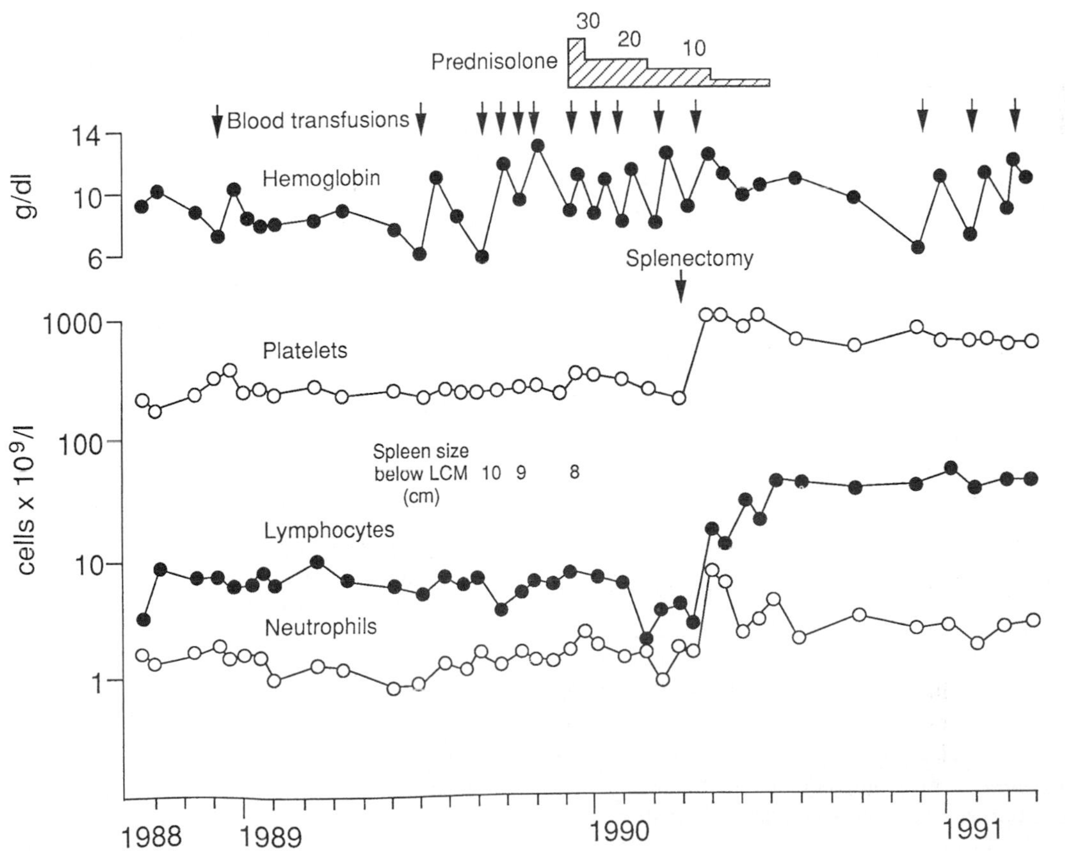

FIG. 43.6. Hematologic chart of a patient with large granular lymphocytic leukemia illustrating the lymphocytosis postsplenectomy and the lack of response of the anemia.

(68). We have reported a young patient with t(8;14) in whom the small and large transformed cells were found to have PTAs in the cytoplasm (62). We have subsequently documented two other patients with LGL leukemia in immunoblastic transformation. The disease in all of them was characterized by hepatosplenomegaly and pancytopenia (6). The transformation event occurred at 8 months, 12 months, and 7 years from diagnosis, and two of the patients barely survived 1 month from transformation.

Treatment and Survival

The various modalities that we and others have used are summarized in Table 43.8. A good rule for the management of these patients is first to assess the tempo of the disease and then evaluate carefully whether treatment is indicated and may be beneficial. Spontaneous remissions are rare. Indications for treatment are twofold: to correct cytopenias and to treat progressive disease. Chlorambucil and cyclophosphamide have been effective in reducing the lymphocyte count. This approach has induced prolonged remissions in some of our patients (1). Remissions also have been observed with courses of corticosteroids. Therapeutic combinations such as the CHOP regimen have been used in aggressive forms of the disease, although with limited success.

Splenectomy has often been performed, in some patients only for the purpose of diagnosis when a tissue diagnosis is not easily apparent and in others in an attempt to correct the cytopenias. Although anemia and thrombocytopenia can be corrected, neutropenia rarely improves, suggesting that hypersplenism is not its main pathogenic mechanism. Hemopoietic growth factors such as granulocyte-macrophage colony-stimulating factor (GM-CSF) or granulocyte colony-stimulating factor (G-CSF) seem to be ineffective in the long term, although a few patients may exhibit a response. We have used G-CSF to facilitate the use of cyclophosphamide in a severely neutropenic patient who eventually achieved CR.

We have also experienced moderate success with pentostatin; several CRs were documented in rare patients with a $CD4^+CD11b^+$ phenotype but less frequently in others with $CD4^-CD8^+$ cells (32). A more recent development has been the use of the immunosuppressive agent cyclosporine, which has been associated with correction of the cytopenia, anemia (69), or agranulocytosis or even complete clinical remission in patients resistant to immunosuppressive drugs and splenectomy (70). We have documented a long-term remission (>5 years) in a patient with LGL leukemia associated with RA and neutropenia ($>0.2 \times 10^9$/L). In this patient, cyclosporine was given at low doses continuously, resulting in neutrophil counts of greater than 1.0×10^9/L and a reduction of spleen size. Because cyclosporine is not a cytotoxic agent, its effect in improving the cytopenias supports the view that the inhibition of granulopoiesis and erythropoiesis is mediated by an immune mechanism.

TABLE 43.8. *Treatment modalities in large granular lymphocytic leukemia*

Treatment may not be necessary in a high proportion of cases. When indicated, the following have been of use with variable success:
Splenectomy
Corticosteroids (e.g., prednisone)
Alkylating agents ± prednisolone
CHOP: cyclophosamide, doxorubicin, vincristine (Oncovin), prednisolone regimen
Pentostatin
Cyclosporin

SUMMARY AND CONCLUSIONS

We have described the main disease features of the two primary leukemias that arise from mature (postthymic) T lymphocytes. For the most part, T-PLL is clinically and morphologically homogeneous, with florid leukemic manifestations and short survival. In our experience, T-PLL is the most common malignancy of mature T cells. Advances in the pathogenesis may be forthcoming as a result of the demonstration of nonrandom abnormalities that involve chromosome 14 with breakpoints at q11 and q32 in over 70% of cases and the reported abnormalities of the *ATM* gene. These changes are identical to those reported in ataxia telangiectasia, a disease that may evolve to T-cell leukemia with features of T-PLL. LGL leukemia usually is a more complex disorder, with greater clinical and immunologic heterogeneity. The most common form of the disease has a relatively benign course associated with cytopenias, chiefly neutropenia, which may be mediated by an immunologic mechanism. Despite its chronic course, there is evidence of clonality in almost all cases, provided they are defined according to clear guidelines. These guidelines are also useful to distinguish true LGL leukemia from rare cases with reactive T-cell lymphocytosis.

REFERENCES

1. Catovsky D, Foa R. *The lymphoid leukaemias.* London: Butterworths, 1990.
2. Brouet J-C, Flandrin G, Sasportes M, et al. Chronic lymphocytic leukaemia of T-cell origin: immunological and clinical evaluation in eleven patients. *Lancet* 1975;2:890–893.
3. Catovsky D, Galetto J, Okos A, et al. Prolymphocytic leukaemia of B and T cell type. *Lancet* 1973;2:232–234.
4. Galton DAG, Goldman JM, Wiltshaw E, et al. Prolymphocytic leukaemia. *Br J Haematol* 1974;27:7–23.
5. Bennett JM, Catovsky D, Daniel M-T, et al. Proposals for the classification of chronic (mature) B and T lymphoid leukaemias. *J Clin Pathol* 1989;42:567–584.
6. Matutes E, Catovsky D. Mature T-cell leukemias and leukemia/lymphoma syndromes: review of our experience in 175 cases. *Leuk Lymphoma* 1991;4:81–91.
7. Brito-Babapulle V, Pomfret M, Matutes E, et al. Cytogenetic studies on prolymphocytic leukemia: II. T-cell prolymphocytic leukemia. *Blood* 1987;70:926–931.
8. Brito-Babapulle V, Catovsky D. Inversions and tandem translocations involving chromosome 14q11 and 14q32 in T-prolymphocytic leuke-

mia and T-cell leukemias in patients with ataxia telangiectasia. *Cancer Genet Cytogenet* 1991;55:1–9.
9. Matutes E, Garcia-Talavera J, O'Brien M, et al. The morphological spectrum of T-prolymphocytic leukaemia. *Br J Haematol* 1986;64: 111–124.
10. Matutes E, Brito-Babapulle V, Swansbury J, et al. Clinical and laboratory features of 78 cases of T-prolymphocytic leukemia. *Blood* 1991; 78:3269–3274.
11. Garand R, Goasguen J, Brizard A, et al. Indolent course as a relatively frequent presentation in T-prolymphocytic leukaemia. Groupe Francais d'Hematologie Cellulaire. *Br J Haematol* 1998;103:488–494.
12. Bearman RM, Pangalis GA, Rappaport H. Prolymphocytic leukemia: clinical, histopathological and cytochemical observations. *Cancer* 1978;42:2360–2372.
13. Lampert I, Catovsky D, Marsh GW, et al. The histopathology of prolymphocytic leukaemia with particular reference to the spleen: a comparison with chronic lymphocytic leukaemia. *Histopathology* 1980;4: 3–19.
14. Matutes E, Keeling DM, Newland AC, et al. Sézary cell-like leukemia: a distinct type of mature T-cell malignancy. *Leukemia* 1990;4:262–266.
15. Pawson R, Matutes E, Brito-Babapulle V, et al. Sézary cell leukemia: a distinct T-cell disorder or a variant form of T-prolymphocytic leukaemia? *Leukemia* 1997;11:1009–1013.
16. Brito-Babapulle V, Maljaie SH, Matutes E, et al. Relationship of T leukaemias with cerebriform nuclei to T-prolymphocytic leukaemia: a cytogenetic analysis with in situ hybridization. *Br J Haematol* 1997; 96:724–732.
17. Crockard AD, Chalmers D, Matutes E, et al. Cytochemistry of acid hydrolases in chronic B and T cell leukemias. *Am J Clin Pathol* 1982; 78:437–444.
18. Hernandez-Nieto L, Lampert IA, Catovsky D. Bone marrow histological patterns in B-cell and T-cell prolymphocytic leukemia. *Hematol Pathol* 1989;3:79–84.
19. Ginaldi L, Matutes E, Farahat N, et al. Differential expression of CD3 and CD7 in T-cell malignancies: a quantitative study by flow cytometry. *Br J Haematol* 1996;93:921–927.
20. Maljaie SH, Brito-Babapulle V, Hiorns LR, et al. Abnormalities of chromosomes 8, 11, 14 and X in T-prolymphocytic leukemia studied by fluorescence in situ hybridization. *Cancer Genet Cytogenet* 1998; 103:110–116.
21. Virgilio L, Isobe M, Narducci MG, et al. Chromosome walking on the TCL-1 locus involved in T-cell neoplasia. *Proc Natl Acad Sci USA* 1993;90:9275–9279.
22. Virgilio L, Narducci MG, Isobe M, et al. Identification of the TCL1 gene involved in T-cell malignancies. *Proc Natl Acad Sci USA* 1994; 91:12530–12534.
23. Pekarsky Y, Hallas C, Isobe M, et al. Abnormalities at 14q32.1 in T cell malignancies involve two oncogenes. *Proc Natl Acad Sci USA* 1999;96:2949–2951.
24. Virgilio L, Lazzeri C, Bichi R, et al. Deregulated expression of TCL1 causes T cell leukemia in mice. *Proc Natl Acad Sci USA* 1998;95: 3885–3889.
25. Fisch P, Forster A, Sherrington PD, et al. The chromosomal translocation t(X;14)(q28;q11) in T-cell pro-lymphocytic leukaemia breaks within one gene and activates another. *Oncogene* 1993;8:3271–3276.
26. Thick J, Mak Y-F, Metcalfe J, et al. A gene on chromosome Xq28 associated with T-cell prolymphocytic leukaemia in two patients with ataxia telangiectasia. *Leukemia* 1994;8:564–573.
27. Vorechovsky I, Luo L, Dyer MJS, et al. Clustering of missense mutations in the ataxia-telangiectasia gene in a sporadic T-cell leukaemia. *Nat Genet* 1997;17:96–99.
28. Stilgenbauer S, Schaffner C, Litterst A, et al. Biallelic mutations in the ATM gene in T-prolymphocytic leukemia. *Nat Med* 1997;3: 1155–1159.
29. Stoppa-Lyonnet D, Soulier J, Laugé A, et al. Inactivation of the ATM gene in T-cell prolymphocytic leukemias. *Blood* 1998;91:3920–3926.
30. Maljaie HS, Brito-Babapulle V, Matutes E, et al. Expression of c-myc oncoprotein in chronic T cell leukemias. *Leukemia* 1995;9:1694–1699.
31. Pawson R, Schulz TF, Matutes E, et al. The human T-cell lymphotropic viruses types I/II are not involved in T-prolymphocytic leukemia and large granular lymphocytic leukemia. *Leukemia* 1997;11:1305–1311.
32. Mercieca J, Matutes E, Dearden C, et al. The role of pentostatin in the treatment of T-cell malignancies: analysis of response rate in 145 patients according to disease subtype. *J Clin Oncol* 1994;12:2588–2593.
33. Pawson R, Dyer MJS, Barge R, et al. Treatment of T-cell prolymphocytic leukemia with human CD52 antibody. *J Clin Oncol* 1997;15: 2667–2672.
34. Ginaldi L, De Martinis M, Matutes E, et al. Levels of expression of CD52 in normal and leukemic B and T cells: correlation with in vivo therapeutic responses to CAMPATH-1H. *Leuk Res* 1998;22:185–191.
35. McKenna RW, Parkin J, Kersey JH, et al. Chronic lymphoproliferative disorder with unusual clinical, morphologic, ultrastructural and membrane surface marker characteristics. *Am J Med* 1977;62:588–596.
36. Newland AC, Catovsky D, Linch D, et al. Chronic T-cell lymphocytosis: a review of 21 cases. *Br J Haematol* 1984;58:433–446.
37. Wallis WJ, Loughran TP Jr, Kadin ME, et al. Polyarthritis and neutropenia associated with circulating large granular lymphocytes. *Ann Intern Med* 1985;103:357–362.
38. Loughran TP Jr, Starkebaum G. Large granular lymphocytic leukemia: report of 38 cases and review of the literature. *Medicine (Baltimore)* 1987;66:397–405.
39. Loughran TP Jr, Kadin ME, Starkebaum G, et al. Leukemia of large granular lymphocytes: association with clonal chromosomal abnormalities and autoimmune neutropenia, thrombocytopenia, and hemolytic anemia. *Ann Intern Med* 1985;102:169–175.
40. Brito-Babapulle V, Matutes E, Parreira L, et al. Abnormalities of chromosome 7q and Tac expression in T cell leukemias. *Blood* 1986;67: 516–521.
41. Rambaldi A, Pelicci PG, Allavena P, et al. T-cell receptor β chain rearrangement in lymphoproliferative disorders of large granular lymphocytes/natural killer cells. *J Exp Med* 1985;162:2156–2162.
42. Foroni L, Matutes E, Foldi J, et al. T cell leukemias with rearrangement of the δ but not β T cell receptor genes. *Blood* 1988;71:356–362.
43. Foroni L, Laffan M, Boehm T, et al. Rearrangement of the T-cell receptor δ genes in human T-cell leukemias. *Blood* 1989;73:559–565.
44. Oshimi K. Granular lymphocyte proliferative disorders: report of 12 cases and review of the literature. *Leukemia* 1988;2:617–627.
45. Oshimi K, Yamada O, Kaneko T, et al. Laboratory findings and clinical courses of 33 patients with granular lymphocyte-proliferative disorders. *Leukemia* 1992;7:782–788.
46. Lacy MQ, Kurtin PJ, Tefferi A. Pure red cell aplasia: association with large granular lymphocyte leukemia and the prognostic value of cytogenetic abnormalities. *Blood* 1996;87:3000–3006.
47. Loughran TP Jr, Starkebaum G, Kidd P, et al. Clonal proliferation of large granular lymphocytes in rheumatoid arthritis. *Arthritis Rheum* 1988;31:31–36.
48. Goudie RB, Lee FD. Is rheumatoid arthritis really a consequence of benign T cell neoplasia? *J Pathol* 1990;160:3.
49. Thien SL, Catovsky D, Oscier D, et al. T-chronic lymphocytic leukaemia presenting as primary hypogammaglobulinaemia: evidence of a proliferation of T-suppressor cells. *Clin Exp Immunol* 1982;47: 670–676.
50. Loughran TP. Clonal diseases of large granular lymphocytes. *Blood* 1993;82:1–14.
51. Matutes E, Crockard AD, O'Brien M, et al. Ultrastructural cytochemistry of chronic T-cell leukaemias: a study with four acid hydrolases. *Histochem J* 1983;15:895–909.
52. Matutes E, Catovsky D. The fine structure of normal lymphocyte subpopulations: a study with monoclonal antibodies and the immunogold technique. *Clin Exp Immunol* 1982;50:416–425.
53. Hara J, Yumura-Yagi K, Tagawa S, et al. Molecular analysis of T cell receptor and CD3 genes in CD3 − large granular lymphocytes (LGLs): evidence for the existence of $CD3^-$ LGLs committed to the T cell lineage. *Leukemia* 1990;4:580–583.
54. Kelemen E, Gergely P, Lehoczky D, et al. Permanent large granular lymphocytosis in the blood of splenectomized individuals without concomitant increase of in vitro natural killer cell cytotoxicity. *Clin Exp Immunol* 1986;63:696–702.
55. Matutes E, Coelho E, Aguado MJ. Expression of TIA-1 and TIA-2 in T-cell malignancies and T-cell lymphocytosis. *J Clin Pathol* 1996;49: 154–158.
56. Tanaka M, Suda T, Haze K, et al. Fas ligand in human serum. *Nat Med* 1996;2:317–322.
57. Siegal FP, Rambotti P, Siegal M, et al. Helper cell function of leukemic $Leu\text{-}2a^+$, histamine $receptor^+$, T gamma lymphocytes. *J Immunol* 1982;129:1775–1781.

58. Moss VE, Miedema F, Matutes E, et al. An unusual variant of T-CLL: evidence for the existence of a hitherto unrecognized T-cell subset. *Clin Exp Immunol* 1986;63:303–311.
59. Linch DC, Cawley JC, MacDonald SM, et al. Acquired pure red cell aplasia associated with an increase of T cells bearing receptors for the Fc of IgG. *Acta Haematol* 1981;65:270–274.
60. Nagasawa T, Abe T, Nakagawa T. Pure red cell aplasia and hypogammaglobulinemia associated with T-cell chronic lymphocytic leukemia. *Blood* 1981;57:1025–1031.
61. Handgretinger R, Geiselhart A, Moris A, et al. Pure red-cell aplasia associated with clonal expansion of granular lymphocytes expressing killer-cell inhibitory receptors. *N Engl J Med* 1999;340:278–284.
62. Brito-Babapulle V, Matutes E, Foroni L, et al. A t(8;14)(q24;q32) in a T-lymphoma/leukemia of $CD8^+$ large granular lymphocytes. *Leukemia* 1987;1:789–794.
63. Pelicci P-G, Allavena P, Subar M, et al. T cell receptor (α, β, γ) gene rearrangements and expression in normal and leukemic large granular lymphocytes/natural killer cells. *Blood* 1987;70:1500–1508.
64. Foa R, Pelicci P-G, Migone N, et al. Analysis of T-cell receptor beta chain (Tβ) gene rearrangements demonstrates the monoclonal nature of T-cell chronic lymphoproliferative disorders. *Blood* 1986;67:247–250.
65. Loughran TP, Starkebaum G, Aprile JA. Rearrangement and expression of T-cell receptor genes in large granular lymphocyte leukemia. *Blood* 1988;71:822–824.
66. Reynolds CW. Large granular lymphocyte (LGL) lymphoproliferative diseases: naturally cytotoxic tumors in man and experimental animals. *Crit Rev Oncol Hematol* 1985;2:185–208.
67. Nowell P, Finan J, Glover D, et al. Cytogenetic evidence for the clonal nature of Richter's syndrome. *Blood* 1981;58:183–186.
68. Nowell P, Jensen J, Winger L, et al. T cell variant of chronic lymphocytic leukaemia with chromosome abnormality and defective response to mitogens. *Br J Haematol* 1976;33:459–468.
69. Tura S, Finelli C, Bandini G, et al. Cyclosporin A in the treatment of CLL associated PRCA and bone marrow hypoplasia. *Nouv Rev Fr Hematol* 1988;30:479–481.
70. Brinkman K, van Dongen JJM, van Lom K, et al. Induction of clinical remission in T-large granular lymphocyte leukemia with cyclosporin A, monitored by use of immunophenotyping with Vβ antibodies. *Leukemia* 1998;12:150–154.

CHAPTER 44

Adult T-Cell Leukemia/Lymphoma

Shaw Watanabe

Adult T-cell leukemia (ATL) is the first human malignancy shown to be caused by a retrovirus. An antibody reacting with an established ATL cell line (1) was found in the sera of ATL patients (2), and a retrovirus later was isolated from the same ATL cell line and characterized (3). A retrovirus had been isolated independently from an ATL patient in the United States that had been previously diagnosed as mycosis fungoides (4). Comparison of these two viruses revealed the same DNA sequence (5). At a joint meeting, researchers from Japan and the United States proposed the designation ATL for the disease and human T lymphotropic virus type 1 (HTLV-1) for the virus (6). After the discovery of HTLV-1, studies on viral carcinogenesis opened up an entirely new field of research that has contributed significantly to the study of human immunodeficiency virus (HIV).

Leukemias with special characteristics, different from those of ordinary leukemia, had long been recognized in the southwestern part of Japan, especially Kyushu Island (7). After the introduction of immunologic techniques for characterizing neoplastic lymphoid cells, concepts of lymphatic leukemia and malignant lymphoma changed dramatically (8,9). A special type of lymphocytic leukemia of T lymphocyte origin with a very poor prognosis was characterized by Takatsuki and his colleagues as ATL (10,11). These investigators described the clustering of ATL patients in the Kyushu district; the peculiar morphologic features of the leukemic cells, such as their polymorphic appearance with lobulated nuclei; the peculiar clinical manifestations, such as hepatosplenomegaly, cutaneous involvement, and absent thymic mass; and poor prognosis, mostly because of progressive disease. Histopathologic examination of these cases revealed varied morphology, but typical cases were characterized by the pleomorphic appearance of the neoplastic cells (8,12,13). Because these neoplasms do not have the monomorphic composition of B-cell lymphomas, atypical chronic lymphocytic leukemia, malignant reticulosis, or reticulosis frequently had been the diagnosis.

Several clinical subtypes of HTLV-1–related T-cell malignancy can be distinguished. Because the lymphoma stage often evolves into a leukemic stage, this neoplasm usually is designated *adult T-cell leukemia/lymphoma* (ATLL). After the discovery of ATLL and HTLV-1, the same disease was recognized in other HTLV-1 endemic areas, such as West Africa and the Caribbean Islands (14,15). Further seroepidemiologic studies contribute to make a phylogenetic tree of HTLV-1 in relation to the other simian leukemia virus (16–22) (Fig. 44.1).

Another problem related to HTLV-1 infection is HTLV-1–associated myelopathy (HAM) or tropical spastic paresis (TSP) (23–25). Although a causal connection between HTLV-1 and the occurrence of ATLL and HAM/TSP is not questioned, little is known about the natural history of this infection or about the role of cofactors in the induction of these diseases (26).

This chapter addresses the incidence and epidemiology; the diagnosis; the pathologic, immunologic, cytogenetic, molecular, and clinical features; leukemogenesis; and the treatment and survival of ATLL.

DIAGNOSIS

The diagnosis of ATLL is based on determining the presence of integrated viral DNA of HTLV-1, because the variety of clinical and pathologic features of ATLL cannot be combined without the viral parameter. A form of HTLV-1–negative ATLL also has been reported, but it appears to be rare (27). Four clinical subtypes of ATLL are recognized: acute, chronic, lymphomatous, and smoldering (11,28,29). Definition of the smoldering type is still under debate, but several different preceding manifestations, such as cutaneous infiltration, lung infiltration, or incipient lymphade-

S. Watanabe: Department of Applied Bioscience, Tokyo University of Agriculture, Tokyo, Japan

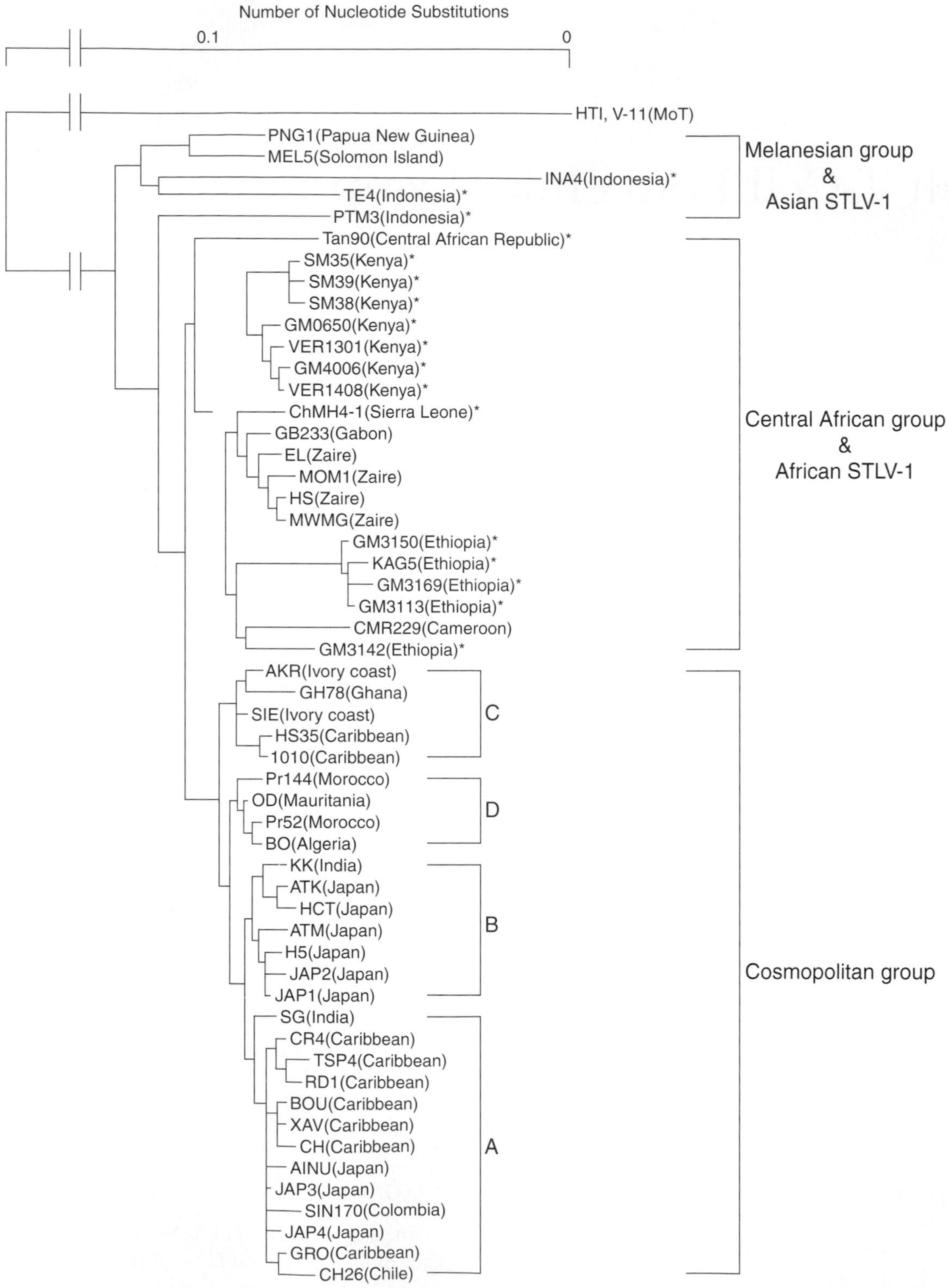

FIG. 44.1. Phylogenetics of human T-cell lymphotropic virus type 1 (HTLV-1) and simian T-cell lymphotropic virus type 1 (STLV-1). HTLV is classified into Melanesian type, central African type, and Cosmopolitan type. Similarity with STLV suggests the presence of interspecies infection in the past. Bifurcation of Asian STLV-1 seems to be older than that of African STLV-1. It has more variety and involves the Melanesian type. The Central African type makes a close cluster with STLV-1. Analysis of the long terminal repeats (LTR) region of HTLV-1 further divided Cosmopolitan type into transcontinental subtype (A), Japanese subtype (B), West African subtype (C), and North American subtype (D).

TABLE 44.1. *Categories of adult T-cell leukemia/lymphoma*

	Flower cells in PB	CLL-like cells	Skin rash	Lymph-adenopathy	Hepato-splenomegaly	Hypercalcemia LDH	Prognosis
ATLL Acute type	+ + +	−	+/−	+	+ +	+ + +	Few mos
Crisis	+ + +	−	+/−	+	+ +	+ + +	Few mos
Chronic type	+	+ + +	+/−	+	+	−	1–5 yrs
Lymphoma type	+/−	−	−	+ + +	−	−	1–2 yrs
Smoldering type							
Cutaneous type	+/−	+/−	+ + +	−	−	−	Up to 10 yrs
Pulmonary type	+/−	+/−	−	−	−	−	Several yrs
Incipient type	−	−	−	+	−	−	Several yrs
Pre-ATLL	+	+	−	−	−	−	10 or more yrs
Carrier	−	−	−	−	−	−	Some evolved to leukemia

LDH, Lactate dehydrogenase.

nopathy, are distinguished (Table 44.1). International collaborative study on the diagnostic criteria of ATLL was proposed in 1994 (Table 44.2). In almost all cases, infection by HTLV-1 can be confirmed by detecting the presence of circulating antibodies specific for HTLV-1 antigens (ATLAs) or by the demonstration of monoclonally integrated HTLV-1 proviral DNA into the host genome by Southern blot hybridization analysis (30,31). Clonal expansions of T cells also can be determined by showing a distinct band caused by the rearrangement of the T-cell receptor gene (Fig. 44.2).

TABLE 44.2. *Diagnostic criteria of adult T-cell leukemia*

Criteria	Points
Clinical/routine laboratory criteria	
Hypercalcemia	1
Skin lesions (lymphomatous cells documented morphologically)	1
Leukemic phase (more than 2% abnormal lymphocytes)	1
Research/laboratory criteria	
T-cell lymphoma or leukemia	2
HTLV-1 antibody	2
TAC-positive tumor cells	1
HTLV-1–positive tumors	2
ATLL classification	
Classic	>7
Probable	5 or 6
Possible	3 or 4
Inconsistent with ATLL	<3
Exclusion data	
B-cell positivity, nodular or follicular lymphoma	
Lymphoblastic lymphoma	
Small lymphocytic lymphoma	

From the International collaborative study on the diagnostic criteria of ATLL.

Registry criteria for definition of ATLL. *Int J Cancer* 1994; 59:491–493.

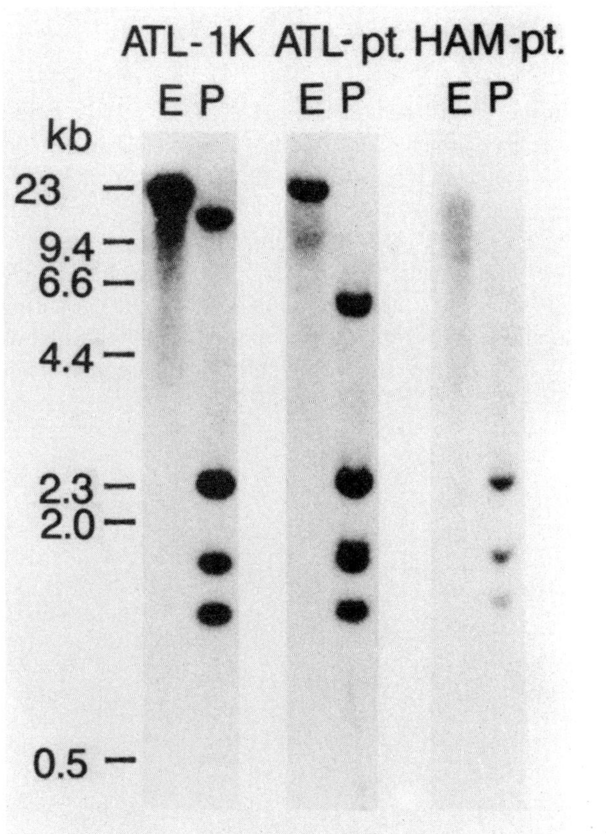

FIG. 44.2. Provirus DNA in adult T-cell leukemia/lymphoma (ATLL) cells by Southern blotting. The ATLL cell line (ATL-1K), ATLL leukemic cells, and lymphocytes from a patient with human T-cell lymphotropic virus type 1 (HTLV-1)–associated myelopathy show three bands, at 2.4, 1.7 and 1.3 kb, which are produced from proviral DNA by the restriction enzyme *Pst*I (P). A band at 6 kb produced by *Eco*RI (E) suggests monoclonal integration of HTLV-1 only in ATLL cells.

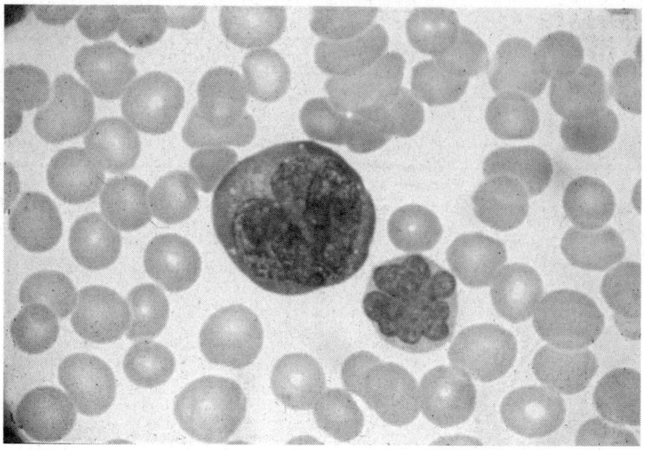

FIG. 44.3. Peripheral blood of a patient with adult T-cell leukemia/lymphoma. Deep indentation of nuclei appears as a flower-like figure (May-Giemsa stain, original magnification: 1,000× magnification). See Color Plate 26, between pp. 1446–1447.

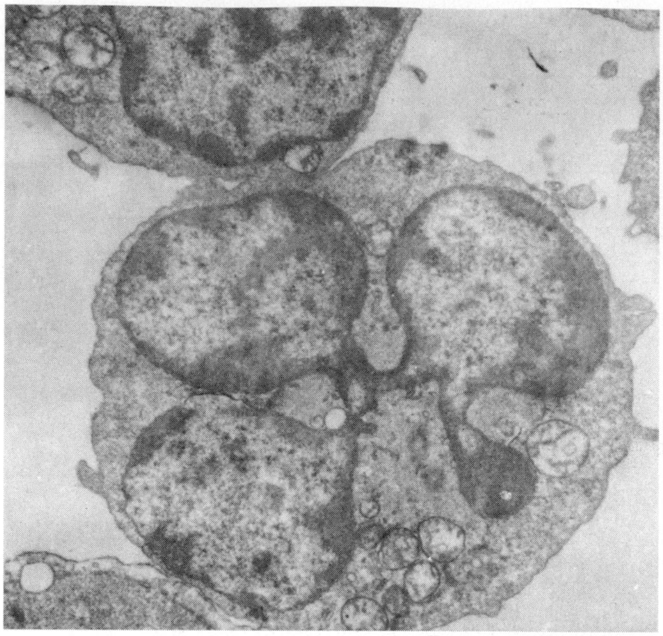

FIG. 44.4. Ultrastructure of the flower cell. Cytoplasmic organelles are scanty (original magnification: 3,000× magnification).

PATHOLOGIC FEATURES

Peripheral Blood

In the typical acute form of ATLL or in crisis, the leukemic cells are characterized by deep nuclear indentation or lobulation and prominent nucleoli. These cells often are called *flower cells* (Figs. 44.3, 44.4; see also Color Plate 26, between pp. 1446–1447). Azurophilic granules are rare. The flower-like appearance of the lobulated nuclei, the thickness of the nuclear membrane, and the coarser nuclear chromatin distinguish them from the convoluted nuclei of lymphoblastic lymphoma/leukemia. Nucleoli usually are inconspicuous in smaller cells. In the chronic type, the leukemic cells have less atypism and often resemble T-cell chronic lymphocytic leukemia. In the smoldering type, only one to a few percent of abnormal cells are present. Nuclear and cellular atypism is inconspicuous, with only mild indentation or buttock-like folding of the nuclei. These cells are occasionally recognized in the peripheral blood of HTLV-1 carriers.

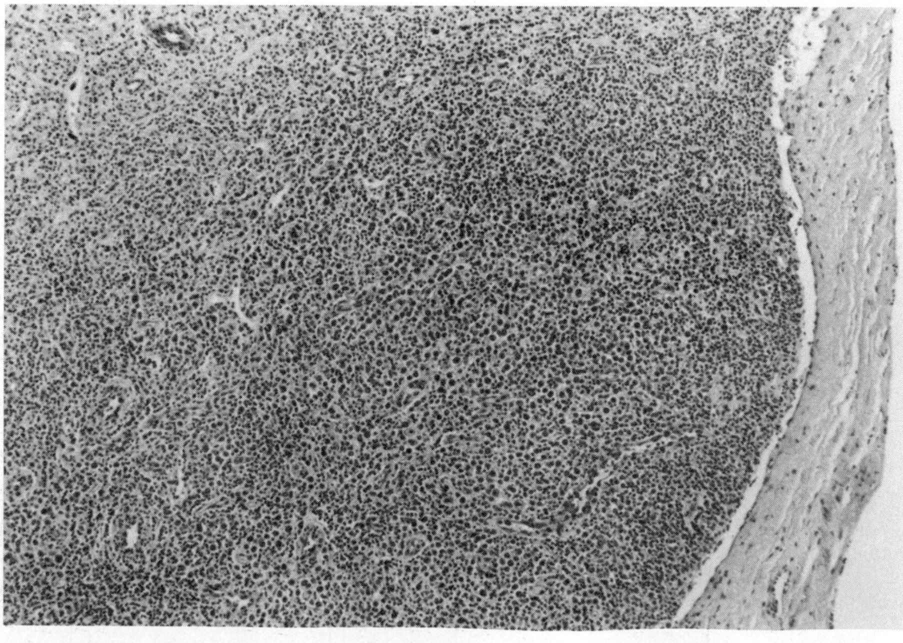

FIG. 44.5. Lymph node of adult T-cell leukemia/lymphoma. Diffuse infiltration by neoplastic cells destroys the architecture of the lymph node but saves the peripheral sinus (hematoxylin and eosin stain, original magnification: 100× magnification).

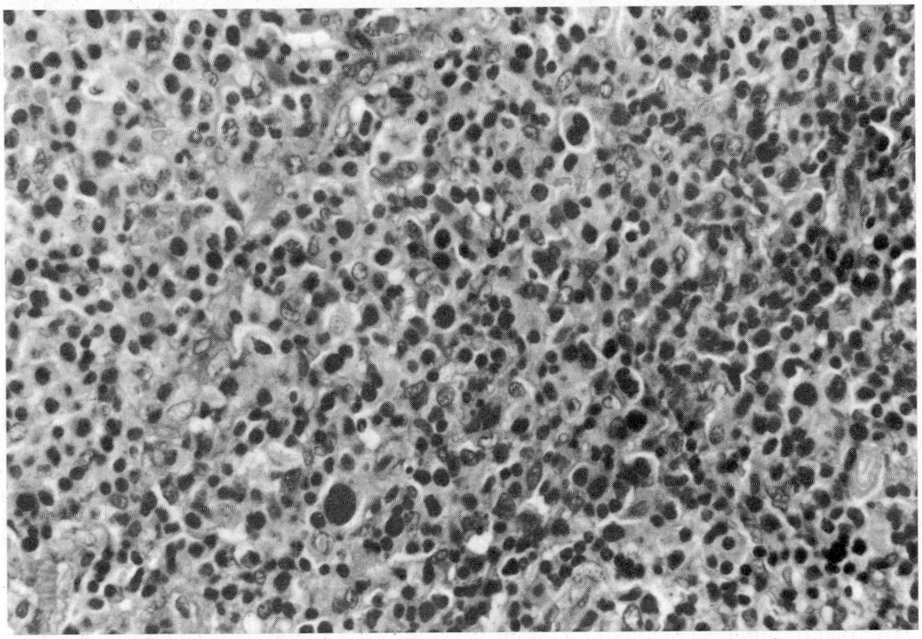

FIG. 44.6. Pleomorphic type lymphoma of adult T-cell leukemia/lymphoma is composed of various-sized neoplastic cells, such as giant cells, large cells, medium cells, and small cells. Giant cells usually have bizarre nuclei more than four times the diameter of small lymphocytic nuclei (hematoxylin and eosin stain, original magnification: 400× magnification).

Lymph Nodes

In the typical ATLL case, the normal architecture of the lymph node is entirely destroyed, although the vascular arrangement and the peripheral sinus usually remain intact (Fig. 44.5). Germinal centers and lymphoid follicles disappear entirely, because of the diffuse proliferation of polymorphic or pleomorphic cells (Fig. 44.6). These are large cells with prominent ovoid, vesicular nuclei, conspicuous nucleoli, and abundant pyroninophilic but periodic

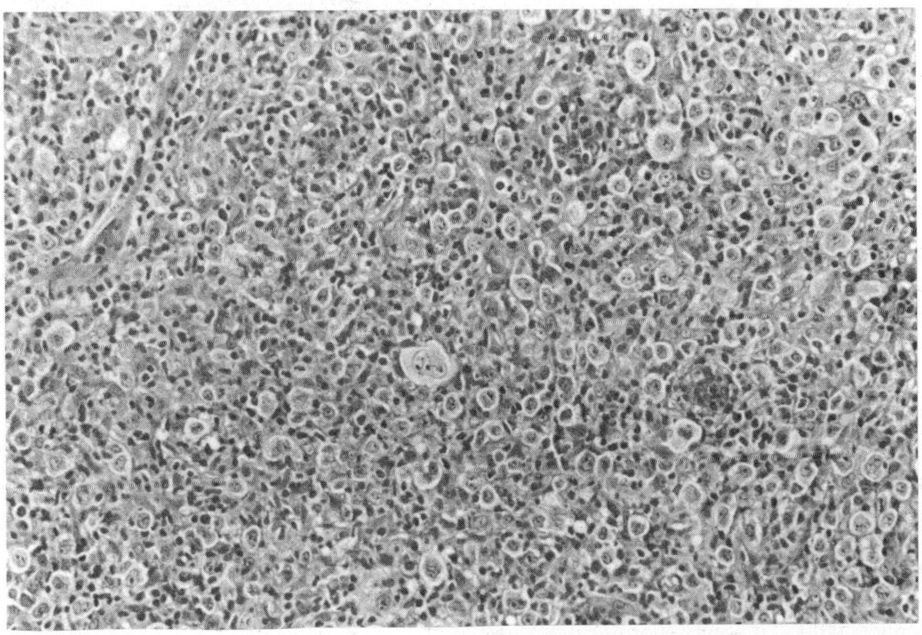

FIG. 44.7. Giant cell in lymph node of adult T-cell leukemia/lymphoma. Reed-Sternberg-like giant cells are often present (hematoxylin and eosin stain, original magnification: 400× magnification).

TABLE 44.3. *Histologic variety of adult T-cell leukemia/lymphoma*

	Hanaoka (12), Kikuchi (13), Yunoki (71), Kinoshita (72)					
			ATL	ML	ATL	ML
Small cell type	2			1	4	0
Medium cell type	38	14	6	13	24	16
Mixed large and medium cell[a]	9		7	9	1	3
Large cell type	9	10	1	6	9	27
Pleomorphic type	43	15	10	24	30	7
TOTAL	101	39	24	53	77	56

Frequent findings: preserved peripheral sinus, 82%; compartmentalization, 43%; residual lymph follicle, 18%; eosinophils, 11%; plasma cells, 4%

[a] Including immunoblastic lymphadenopathy-like and Lennert lymphoma.

acid–Schiff (PAS)–negative cytoplasm. Medium-sized cells with smaller, round, or occasionally cerebriform nuclei and small cells with irregular, dark, and pyknotic nuclei are also seen. These are not infrequently intermingled with multinucleated giant cells that resemble Reed-Sternberg cells and that contain basophilic or amphophilic cytoplasm by Giemsa stain (Fig. 44.7). The diameter of the giant cells usually is more than four times that of the small lymphocyte, and if giant cells and a mixed lymphoid cell proliferation are present, the diagnosis of pleomorphic lymphoma is made. Eosinophils, plasma cells, histiocytes, and vascular proliferation are rarely seen, in contrast with the immunoblastic lymphadenopathy–like T-cell lymphoma or T-zone lymphoma (8,32–34). A fine reticulin network is usually found by silver impregnation (Table 44.3).

In the lymphomatous type, local tumor growth is characteristic, although it often becomes leukemic, or systemic lymph node enlargement appears within a short period. This type is composed predominantly of large neoplastic cells (Fig. 44.8). Destructive growth is usual. Focal necrosis or eosinophilic infiltration is present in some cases.

Skin

Cutaneous involvement by neoplastic cells is one of the characteristics of ATLL. The skin lesions are sometimes

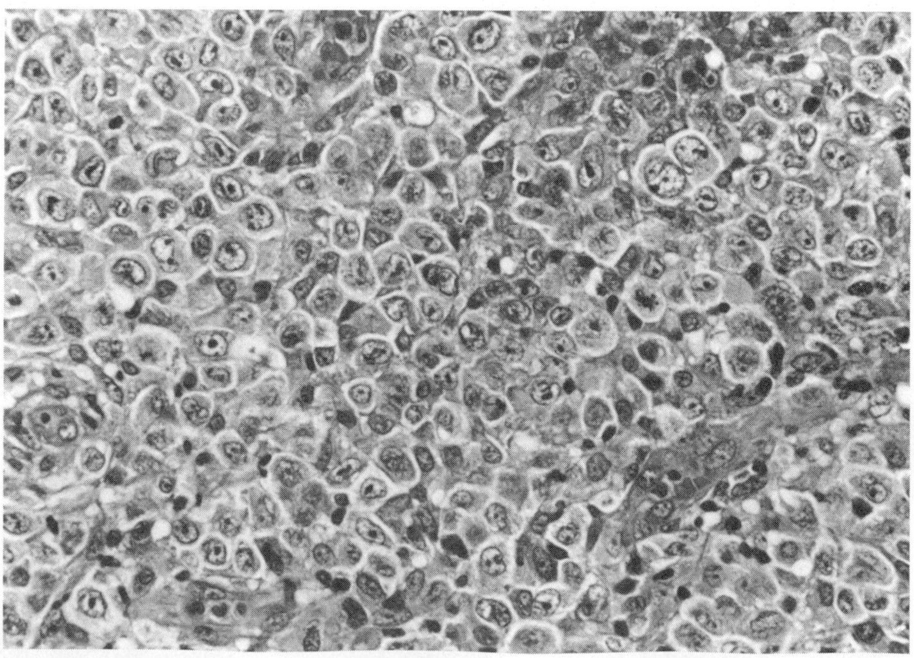

FIG. 44.8. Large cell adult T-cell leukemia/lymphoma. A monomorphic proliferation of large cells produces a diffuse lesion. Some cells have conspicuous nucleoli (hematoxylin and eosin stain, original magnification: 400× magnification).

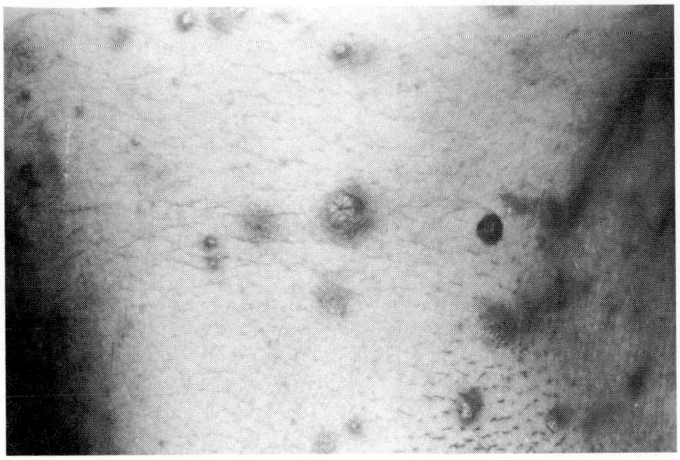

FIG. 44.9. Cutaneous lesions of smoldering adult T-cell leukemia/lymphoma. Papules and erythematous nodules are scattered on the chest.

indistinguishable from those of mycosis fungoides, because they look like various eruptions, tumorous, nodular, plaque, papular, or erythematous forms (Fig. 44.9). Only the papular form of ATLL has attained consensus as an ATLL-specific eruption. Infiltration around the perivascular space in the upper dermis by neoplastic cells is usual. Pautrier's microabscesses are present in more than one half of the skin lesions of ATLL cases (Fig. 44.10). Plasma cells and other reactive cells are rare, unlike the cutaneous lesions of mycosis fungoides. Immunostaining with monoclonal antibody to the pX portion of HTLV-1 clarifies directly the cells infected by HTLV-1 (35).

Infiltration by pleomorphic T cells is also characteristic of the $CD30^+$ anaplastic large cell lymphoma (36). Expression of the CD30 antigen, epithelial membrane antigen, and CD3 or CD8 and a self-healing tendency with scar formation are points that favor anaplastic large cell lymphoma in the differential diagnosis. Lymphomatoid papulosis is distinguished by the typical, seemingly bizarre cells and its clinical course.

Other Organs

The liver, spleen, and bone marrow are frequent sites of infiltration by ATLL cells. Only a slight infiltration is noticed in the bone marrow in some cases. This indicates proliferation of leukemic cells in extramedullary sites. The cellular characteristics are the same as those in the lymph nodes and skin. The lung is also one of the target organs,

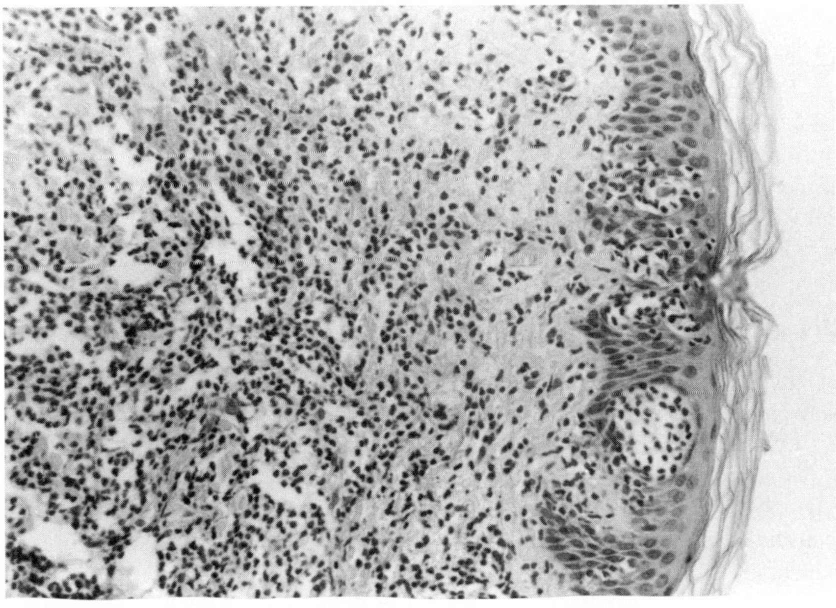

FIG. 44.10. Pautrier's microabscess of the cutaneous lesion of adult T-cell leukemia/lymphoma. Neoplastic cells in the cutaneous lesions usually are smaller than those in the lymph nodes, except in the terminal stage (hematoxylin and eosin stain, original magnification: 200× magnification).

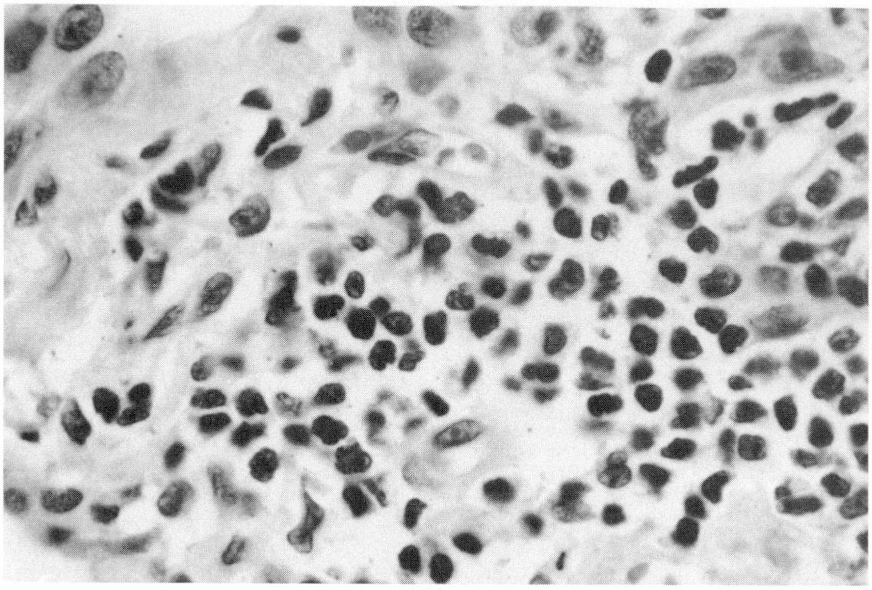

FIG. 44.11. Pulmonary biopsy of smoldering adult T-cell leukemia/lymphoma (ATLL). This specimen was obtained 5 years before the typical ATLL. Only small cell infiltration is recognized in the peribronchial region, but a review of the slide indicates nuclear atypism (hematoxylin and eosin stain, original magnification: 1,000× magnification).

with lesions that resemble lymphomatoid granulomatosis (Fig. 44.11).

IMMUNOLOGIC FEATURES

The surface phenotype of ATLL cells is predominantly that of helper T cells that express interleukin-2 receptor (IL-2R) γ chain (CD25) (37); CD2, CD3, and CD4 are commonly expressed, but CD8 is usually absent. Soluble IL-2R levels in the serum are usually elevated (38). In tissue sections, immunostaining with monoclonal antibodies to surface antigens shows abundant infiltration by reactive suppressor T cells, unlike mycosis fungoides (39). The significant phenotypic difference between ATLL cells and mycosis fungoides cells is the expression of Leu 8 (lymph node homing receptor) and CD25 and the lack of CD7 antigens on the cell surface. The ATLL cells that infiltrate the skin are different from those that infiltrate the peripheral blood or lymph nodes in that they lack CD29 and CD45RA expression (40).

CYTOGENETIC AND MOLECULAR FEATURES

More than 80% of cases of ATLL exhibit DNA aneuploidy. The acute type shows more complicated chromosomal abnormalities than the chronic type. Since 1985, Japanese cytogeneticists have collected clinical and cytogenetic data on 114 cases of ATLL and on 52 T-cell lymphomas from the principal cytogenetic laboratories in Japan and have reviewed the karyotypes in detail. Higher frequencies of chromosomal abnormalities are observed in chromosome segments 1p, 3q, 6q, 9q, 12q, and 14q (41,42). The most commonly rearranged chromosome regions among these cases were 6q21, 14q32, 11p21-25, and 1p36. Karyotypes of 107 cases with ATLL were reviewed by a panel of cytogeneticists (42). In addition to the trisomies for chromosomes 3 (21%), 7 (10%), and 21 (9%), monosomy for X chromosomes in females (38%), and loss of a Y chromosome in males (17%), translocations involving 14q32 (28%) or 14q11 (14%) and deletion of 6q (23%), 10p (9%), 3q (8%), 5q, 9q, and 13q (7%) each) and of 1p and 7p (6% each) were determined. Presence of aneuploid clones and higher frequency of numerical and structural abnormalities are more frequent in aggressive acute type and lymphoma type.

INCIDENCE AND EPIDEMIOLOGY

The standardized mortality ratio of malignant lymphomas and leukemias in the western part of Japan has been known to be significantly elevated (43). The T- and B-cell Lymphoma Study Group has collected malignant lymphomas from major hospitals in Japan (44,45) and determined the frequency of T- and B-cell lymphomas in various districts, showing local aggregation of T-cell lymphoma in the southwestern part of Japan, Kyushu, and Shikoku (Fig. 44.12). The endemic area of HTLV-1 is coincident with the area of ATLL (46). The population seropositive for HTLV-1 is estimated to be 1 million on Kyushu Island (47).

Transmission of HTLV-1 occurs primarily by two routes: perinatal and sexual. The transmission rate among children born to HTLV-1–infected mothers is up to 10% to 20%. A study of 311 mother-child pairs conducted over 18 years

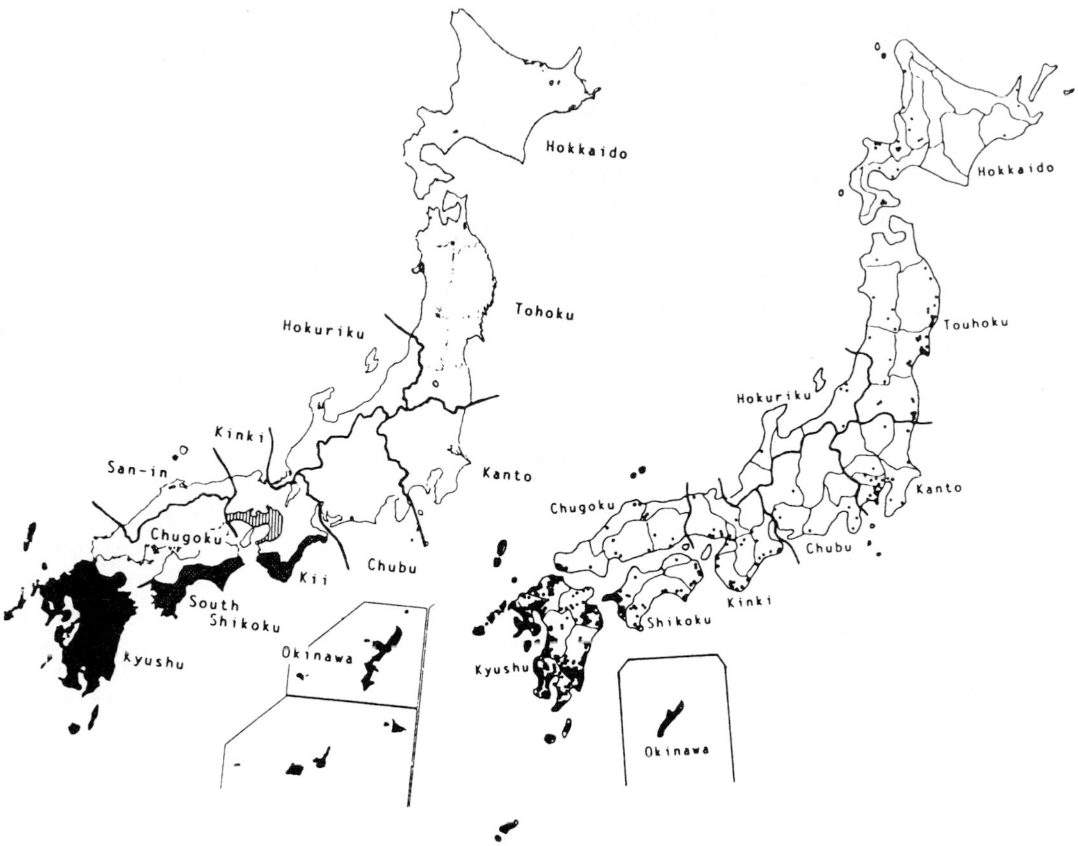

FIG. 44.12. Left: Seropositivity to human T-cell lymphotropic virus type 1 (HTLV-1) in Japan. **Right:** Distribution of T- and B-cell lymphoma by birthplace. Highest prevalence (6%) is recognized in Kyushu and then in Kii and South Shikoku (3%), around Osaka (1.5%), and in Tohoku and Hokkaido (1%). The background rate is less than 0.5%. The birthplaces of 656 adult T-cell leukemia/lymphoma (ATLL) patients were collected by the fourth nationwide survey. Each dot corresponds to one patient. (From Tajima K. The 4th nation-wide study of adult T-cell leukemia/lymphoma in Japan. *Int J Cancer* 1990; 45:237–243, with permission.)

revealed that no children, other than those infected perinatally, seroconverted by the age of 18 years (48). Beginning in young adulthood, however, a very slow increase in prevalence becomes evident in the HTLV-1 carrier state. The average risk of infection by sexual exposure is likely to be low during the most sexually active years, accounting for the gradual increase in seroprevalence in young adulthood. High concordance of anti-HTLV-1 antibody status in couples suggests that seroconversion is five times more likely to occur among wives of carriers than among husbands (49). The mature age-specific seroprevalence curve for HTLV-1 antibodies begins at less than 5% from birth to adolescence, gradually increases to 25% to 30% from age 20 to the mid-fifties in both sexes, and then continues to increase to 35% to 50% among elderly women. Among older persons, seropositivity is greater among women than men (50). The lifelong rate of ATLL occurrence among HTLV-1 carriers has been estimated to be not more than a few percent (47).

Patients who have ATLL or persons seropositive for HTLV-1 have not been found in Korea and China, although both countries have had close relations with the Japanese (51,52). Some Chinese in Formosa were infected with HTLV-1 and had resultant ATLL, but these infections were probably contracted in the southern parts of Japan, such as Okinawa and Kyushu. Japanese immigrants in Hawaii and Brazil retain the same high seropositive rates as native inhabitants, such as those people who live in the southern part of Japan (53,54). In other areas, ATLL patients were found among Caribbean immigrants to London (55). Sporadic cases occurred in the Florida peninsula and in the northern part of South America (53). Prevalence of HTLV-1 at levels of 1% or higher has been reported in Barbados, Trinidad, Panama, Venezuela, Colombia, and Brazil (56–61). Most of these patients were black, and their origins could be traced to West Africa, which is considered to be one of the HTLV-1–endemic areas (62,63) (Fig. 44.13). What connects these three endemic areas—Southern Japan, West Africa, and the Caribbean islands? A survey for HTLV-1 seropositivity in various primates revealed that the virus, with some diversity by evolution, is maintained only among Old World monkeys, such as the green monkey, rhesus monkey, and bonnet monkey, and only in the chimpanzee among anthropoid apes

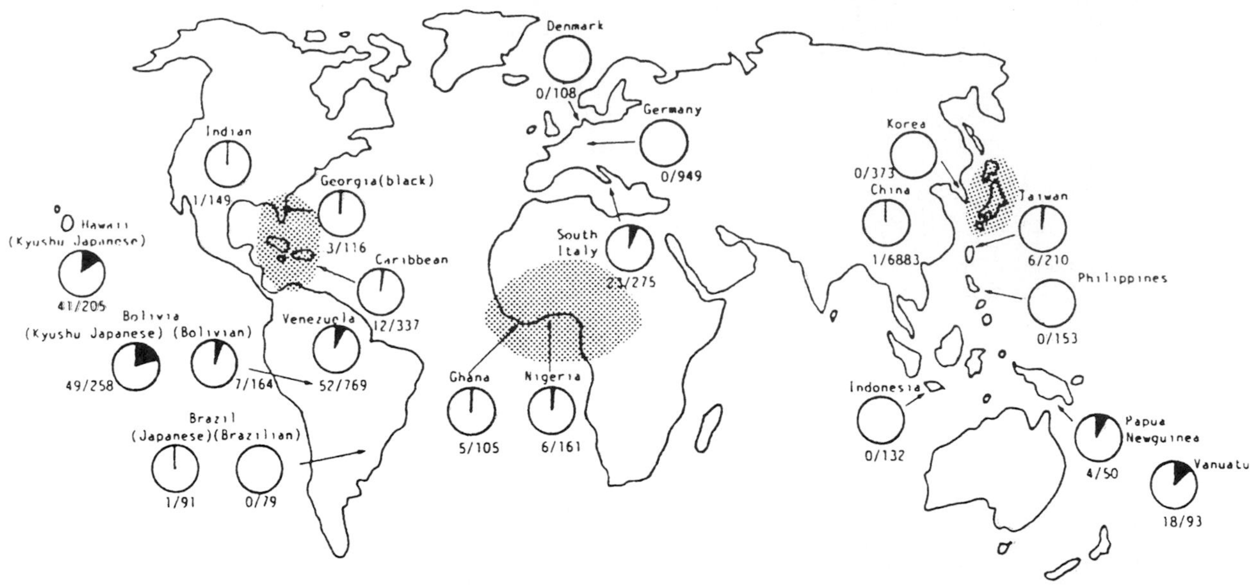

FIG. 44.13. Seropositive areas of the world. Geographic distribution of carriers of human T-cell lymphotropic virus type 1 (HTLV-1) and areas of endemic adult T-cell leukemia/lymphoma (ATLL) *(shadowed)*. Circles and numbers indicate seropositive rates and positive-tested subjects, respectively. (From Tajima K, et al. Malignant lymphomas in Japan: Epidemiologic analysis of ATLL. *Cancer Metastasis Rev* 1988; 7:223, with permission.)

(16,64). This may be a missing link. We should consider the evolution of primates in the Old World and their movement in addition to human movement during the prehistorical period.

LEUKEMOGENESIS

The HTLV-1 contains dual long terminal repeats (LTRs) as well as *GAG, POL,* and *ENV* structural genes (Fig. 44.14) (3). Generally, HTLV-1 does not appear to transform T cells by integrating at specific sites in the host genome. The pX region of the virus encodes at least two distinct nonstructural proteins through the translation of a doubly spliced, polycitronic mRNA (65). The two proteins are referred to as Tax

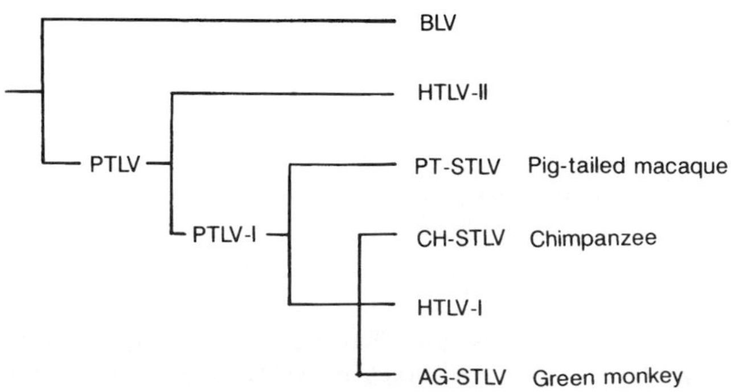

FIG. 44.14. Suggested evolution of human T-cell lymphotropic virus type 1 (HTLV-1) virus. Close similarity is present between HTLV-1 and simian T-cell lymphotropic virus. These viruses are detected only among the Old World monkeys.

(formerly p40x or tat-1) and Rex (formerly p27) (65–68). The Tax protein may act early in the process, facilitating polyclonal proliferation of the T cells. Tax also activates the HTLV-1 LTR. The Rex protein facilitates the nuclear export of structural gene mRNAs by acting through a Rex response element located in the 3′LTR of HTLV-1. These transactivating proteins may turn on cellular growth promoting genes such as those for FOS, IL-2, and the IL-2R. The step-wise process of clonal evolution leads to eventual malignancy (69). After the process has been initiated, continued viral transcription apparently is not required, because virus-specific RNAs are not detected in mononuclear cells from the blood or from tumor cells of HTLV-1–infected humans (66).

Considering the long latent period and low incidence of ATLL among HTLV-1 carriers (about 1 per 1,500 to 2,000), a mathematical model for leukemogenesis is informative. My colleagues and I attempted to clarify the possible nature of the events by fitting them to the Weibull distribution, in which the ‘‘shape parameter’’ could be regarded as the number of ‘‘hits’’ or ‘‘steps’’ in which normal cells would give rise to leukemia (70). Cumulative ATLL occurrence could be expressed as a single straight line on the Weibull plot (Fig. 44.15). The distribution of both sexes was identical. Based on this stochastic model, it is assumed that age-dependent accumulation of leukemogenic events consists most likely of somatic mutations, and that only carriers infected at birth may develop leukemia.

The probability density function for the Weibull model, f(t), expressed as a function of time (t, in years), was described as

$$f(t) = a/b\ t^{a-1}\exp^{(-ta/b)}$$

where a, the shape parameter, was 5.03 and b, the "scale parameter," was 8.00×10^8. The hazard rate, (t), expressed as a function of time can be written as

$$(t) = f(t) = a/b\ t^{a-1}/t(x)dx$$

The risk of ATLL development at each age therefore is approximately proportional to the fourth power of the age, suggesting that at least five events, each of which occurs spontaneously and independently, may be required for development of the disease (Fig. 44.16).

CLINICAL FEATURES

The clinical features of ATLL have been described by several investigators (10,28,71,72). The white blood cell (WBC) count in acute ATLL ranges from 25,000 to 463,000/mm^3, with an average of 96,700/mm^3. In chronic ATLL, an increased number of WBCs is also found, similar to the acute type, but hypercalcemia and hyperbilirubinemia are lacking. Leukemia invariably terminates in a rapidly progressive malignant course to crisis. It is frequently associated with lymphadenopathy and hepatosplenomegaly, disseminated skin lesions, and invasion into the lungs, gastrointestinal tract, and central nervous system (Table 44.4). Acute ATLL usually has hypercalcemia up to 6.0 mEq/L and a high lactate dehydrogenase (LDH) level (>1,000), whereas, in chronic ATLL, calcium and LDH levels remain within normal limits. The lymphoma type starts as ordinary lymphoma, but leukemic changes occur after a relatively short period of local growth. The smoldering type includes various forms, such as long-lasting cutaneous lesions with recurrent self-healing and progression for many years, pulmonary infiltration of small lymphocytes (like lymphomatoid granulomatosis), and a small percentage of atypical lymphocytes present in the peripheral blood.

In addition to leukemia, a paraneoplastic state that includes hypercalcemia, unexplained rashes, hepatic dysfunction, and encephalopathy in the more terminal stages of illness is frequently associated with ATLL. These multiple clinical conditions may be induced by various cytokines, such as IL-2 and IL-2R-γ, IL-3, IL-4, parathyroid hormone-

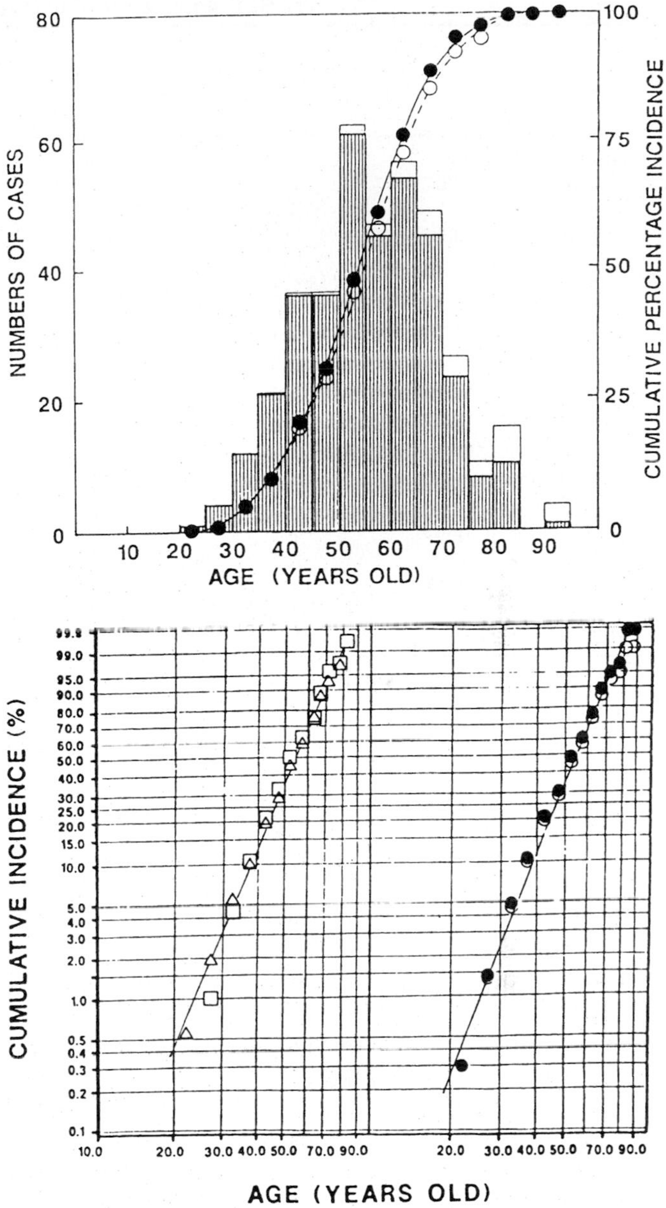

FIG. 44.16. Top: Distribution of age at onset of disease of patients with adult T-cell leukemia/lymphoma (ATLL). The observed number in each 5-year age category is shown in the shadowed columns. White columns represent corrected death rates according to the national population survey in Japan conducted in 1985. The cumulative percentages of ATLL are shown by circles and lines, respectively. **Bottom:** Cumulative occurrence of ATLL by age plotted on the Weibull model. Good fitness is obtained for men *(open box)* and women *(open triangle)* and by observed *(closed circle)* and corrected *(open circle)* incidences (cf1611).

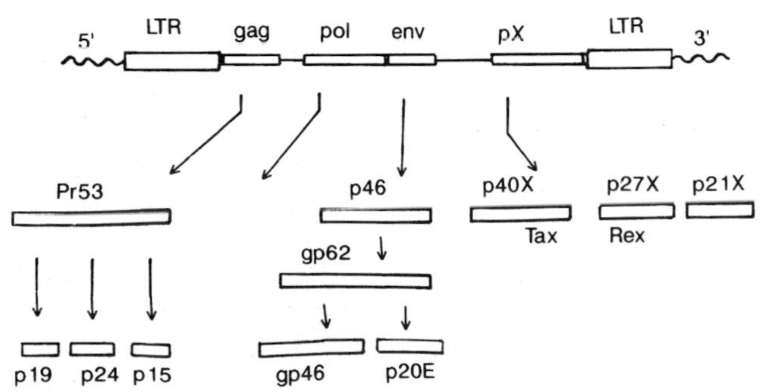

FIG. 44.15. Structure of human T-cell lymphotropic virus type 1 virus and its gene products.

related protein, granulocyte-macrophage colony-stimulating factor, tumor necrosis factor, lymphotoxin, and vimentin (Table 44.4). The altered regulation of such cellular genes by viral transactivation may have profound consequences and account for the subverted cellular physiology associated with HTLV-1 infection (73).

TABLE 44.4. *Clinical features of adult T cell leukemia/lymphoma*

	Uchiyama (10) (1977)	Yunoki (71) Kagoshima (1982)		Kinoshita (72) Nagasaki (1982)		Yamaguchi[a] (1990)
	n = 16	ATL n = 55	T-ML n = 44	ATL n = 84	T-ML n = 54	n = 187
Chief Complaints						
Lymphadenopathy	25%			26.2%	73.5%	
Skin rash	43.7			23.8	2.0	
Abdominal pain		23.6	18.0			
Malaise				23.8	8.2	
Weakness	31.2					
Fever		45.5	48.3			
Cough	18.7	10.9	1.6			
Findings						
Lymphadenopathy	93.7	74.6	93.4	88.1	87.7	72
Splenomegaly	56.2	36.4	12.0	28.6	12.2	26
Hepatomegaly	75.0	50.9	37.9	66.7	36.7	47
Skin rash	56.2	23.6	6.6	51.2	12.2	53
Leukemia change	100	100		100		
Mediastinal mass	0	0	0	0	2.0	
Hypercalcemia		35.3		4.8	0	28
Average age range	56	58.5	56.3	54.8	57.0	
	30–67	25–76	33–79	16–82	18–85	
Male/Female ratio	1.0	1.4	2.8	1.5	1.0	

[a] personal communication

Cellular and humoral immune responses are markedly impaired in patients who have ATLL. Abnormalities in ATLL patients include disordered helper and suppressor T-cell function, mitogen responsiveness, killer cell induction, and B-cell immunoglobulin synthesis (74,75). Delayed hypersensitivity by skin testing routinely reveals anergy in ATLL patients. Altered regulation of the immune response in ATLL manifests clinically by the frequent occurrence of opportunistic infections, which include *Pneumocystis carinii* and cytomegalovirus pneumonia, cryptococcal meningitis, fungal and bacterial sepsis, and parasitic gastroenteritis. These are causes of death in more than one half of the cases of ATLL.

TREATMENT AND SURVIVAL

A poor prognosis is predicted by elevated serum LDH levels, hypercalcemia, performance status, number of involved sites, and age (76). The results of ATLL treatment have been unfavorable in the past (77). In general, patients who have acute and lymphomatous ATLL should be treated with combination chemotherapy. Patients who have hypercalcemia, high LDH levels, and an abnormal increase in WBC counts have a 50% survival rate of less than 6 months. Aggressive combination chemotherapy such as CHOP, VEPA, or MACOP-B did not improve the prognosis. Deoxycoformycin was used successfully as a single agent to treat patients who had acute ATLL, and a phase II clinical trial has been ongoing in Japan since 1988.

Regardless of treatment, chronic, cutaneous, and other smoldering types of ATLL have longer courses. It is not unusual for patients who have cutaneous ATLL to show repetitive remission and progression for more than 10 years.

SUMMARY AND CONCLUSIONS

ATLL was first discovered in Japan, but isolation of the HTLV-1 retrovirus opened up a broad and virgin field of research in human leukemogenesis. It also influenced histologic diagnosis, because a spectrum of morphologically diverse lymphomas and leukemias are now unified by the presence of the HTLV-1 proviral genome. Clarification of viral transmission has been translated into the primary prevention of ATLL. In addition to the prevention of neonatal transmission by heating mother's milk or avoiding breast-feeding by the carrier (78), viral transmission by transfusion has been prevented by routine checks for ATL virus-associated antigen since 1986. The ATLL story is a good example of the success of a multidisciplinary collaborative approach by clinicians, pathologists, epidemiologists, and molecular biologists.

REFERENCES

1. Miyoshi I, Kubonishi I, Sumida M, et al. Characterization of a leukemic T-cell line derived from adult T-cell leukemia. *Jpn J Clin Oncol* 1979; 9[Suppl 1]:485–494.
2. Hinuma Y, Nagata K, Hanaoka M, et al. Adult T-cell leukemia: antigen in a ATL cell line and detection of antibodies to the antigen in human sera. *Proc Natl Acad Sci USA* 1981;78:6476–6480.
3. Yoshida M, Miyoshi I, Hinuma Y. Isolation and characterization of retrovirus from cell lines of human adult T-cell leukemia and its implication in the disease. *Proc Natl Acad Sci USA* 1982;79:2031–2035.
4. Poiesz BJ, Ruscetti FW, Gazdar AF, et al. Detection and isolation of type C retrovirus particles from fresh and cultured lymphocytes of a

patient with cutaneous T-cell lymphoma. *Proc Natl Acad Sci USA* 1980; 77:7415–7419.
5. Seiki M, Hattori S, Hirayama Y, et al. Human adult T-cell leukemia virus: complete nucleotide sequence of the provirus genome integrated in leukemic cell DNA. *Proc Natl Acad Sci USA* 1983;80:3618–3622.
6. Blattner WA, Takatsuki Y, Steele PE, et al. Human T-cell leukemia/lymphoma virus and adult T-cell leukemia. *JAMA* 1981;250: 1074–1080.
7. Itoga K, Ohki K. Statistical study on lymphatic leukemia and lymphosarcoma in Nagasaki and PAS reaction of leukemia lymphoid cells. *Nagasaki Med J* 1963;38:154–161.
8. Watanabe S, Shimosato Y, Shimoyama M. Lymphoma and leukemia of T-lymphocytes. In: Sommers SC, Rosen PP, eds. *Pathology annual 1981,* part 2. New York: Appleton-Century-Crofts, 1981:155–204.
9. Watanabe S. Malignant lymphomas: immunologic aspects. In: Brunson KW, ed. *Cancer growth and progression.* Boston: Kluwer Academic Publishers, 1989:177–178.
10. Uchiyama T, Yodoi J, Sagawa K, et al. Adult T-cell leukemia: clinical and hematologic features of 16 cases. *Blood* 1977;50:481–492.
11. Takatsuki K, Uchiyama T, Ueshima Y, et al. Adult T-cell leukemia: further clinical observations and cytogenetic and functional studies of leukemic cells. *Jpn J Clin Oncol* 1979;9[Suppl 1]:317–324.
12. Hanaoka M. Disease entity of adult T-cell leukemia: cytological aspects and geographic pathology. In: Hanaoka M, Takatsuki K, Shimoyama M, eds. *Adult T cell leukemia and related diseases.* Tokyo: Japan Scientific Societies Press, 1982:1–12.
13. Kikuchi M, Mitsui T, Eimoto T. Biopsy of adult T-cell leukemia. In: Hanaoka M, Takatsuki K, Shimoyama M, eds. *Adult T cell leukemia and related diseases.* Tokyo: Japan Scientific Societies Press, 1982: 37–50.
14. Blattner WA, Kalynaraman VS, Robert-Guroff M, et al. The human type-C retrovirus HTLV in blacks from the Caribbean region, and relationship to adult T-cell leukemia/lymphoma. *Int J Cancer* 1982;30: 257–264.
15. Hunsmann G, Schneider J, Schmitt J, et al. Detection of serum antibodies to adult T-cell leukemia virus in non-human primates and in people from Africa. *Int J Cancer* 1983;32:329–332.
16. Shimotohno K. Human T cell leukemia virus type-II. *Gann Monogr Cancer Res* 1992;39:237–246.
17. Tajima K, Hinuma Y. Epidemiology of HTLV-1/II in Japan and the world. *Gann Monogr Cancer Res* 1992;39:129–150.
18. Ido E, Yamashita M, Hayami M. Ethnic variation of HTLV in the world. *Gann Monogr Cancer Res* 1996;44:107–122.
19. Gabbai AA, Bordin JO, Vieira-Filho JP, et al. Selectivity of human T lymphotropic virus type-1 (HTLV-1) and HTLV-2 infection among different populations in Brazil. *Am J Trop Med Hyg* 1993;49: 664–671.
20. Song KJ, Nerurkar VR, Pereira-Cortez AJ, et al. Sequence and phylogenetic analyses of human T-cell lymphotropic virus type 1 from a Brazilian woman with adult T cell leukemia: comparison with virus strains from South America and the Caribbean basin. *Am J Trop Med Hyg* 1995;52:101–108.
21. Houston S, Thornton C, Emmanuel J, et al. Human T-cell lymphotropic virus type 1 in Zimbabwe. *Trans R Soc Trop Med Hyg* 1994;88: 170–172.
22. Tajima K. HTLV-I/II related diseases with special reference to the distribution among mongoloids. *Gann Monogr Cancer Res* 1996;44: 123–136.
23. Osame M, Usuku K, Izumo S, et al. HTLV-I associated myelopathy, a new clinical entity. *Lancet* 1986;1:1031–1032.
24. Furukawa Y, Fujisawa J, Osame M, et al. Frequent clonal proliferation of human T-cell leukemia virus type I (HTLV-I)–infected T cells in HTLV-1–associated myelopathy (HAM-TSP). *Blood* 1992;80: 1012–1016.
25. Elovaara I, Koenig S, Brewah AY, et al. High human T cell lymphotropic virus type 1 (HTLV-1)–specific precursor cytotoxic T lymphocyte frequencies in patients with HTLV-1–associated neurological disease. *J Exp Med* 1993;1993:1567–1573.
26. Sonoda S, Fujiyoshi T. HTLV-I infection and HLA. *Gann Monogr Cancer Res* 1996;44:207–218.
27. Shimoyama M, Kagami Y, Shimotono K, et al. Adult T-cell leukemia/lymphoma not associated with human T-cell leukemia virus type I. *Proc Natl Acad Sci USA* 1986;83:4524–4528.
28. Shimoyama M, Minato K, Saito H, et al. Comparisons of clinical, morphologic and immunologic characteristics of adult T-cell leukemia-lymphoma and cutaneous T-cell lymphoma. *Jpn J Clin Oncol* 1979; 9[Suppl 1]:357–372.
29. Yamaguchi K, Nishimura H, Kohrogi H, et al. A proposal for smoldering T-cell leukemia: a clinicopathologic study of 5 cases. *Blood* 1983; 62:758–766.
30. Yoshida M, Seiki M, Yamaguchi K, et al. Monoclonal integration of HTLV in all primary tumors of adult T cell leukemia suggests causative role of HTLV in the disease. *Proc Natl Acad Sci USA* 1984;81: 2534–2537.
31. Yamaguchi K, Seiki M, Yoshida M, et al. The detection of human T-cell leukemia virus proviral DNA and its application for classification and diagnosis of T-cell malignancy. *Blood* 1984;63:1235–1240.
32. Watanabe S, Shimosato Y, Shimoyama M, et al. Adult T cell lymphoma with hypergammaglobulinemia. *Cancer* 1980;46:2472–2483.
33. Watanabe S, Sato Y, Shimoyama M, et al. Immunoblastic lymphadenopathy, angioimmunoblastic lymphadenopathy, and IBL-like T-cell lymphoma: a spectrum of T-cell neoplasia. *Cancer* 1986;58: 2224–2232.
34. Suchi T, Ueda R, Suzuki H, et al. T-zone dysplasia with hyperplastic follicles: an incipient T-cell lymphoma. In: Hanaoka M, et al., eds. *Lymphoid malignancy: immunocytology and cytogenetics.* New York: Field and Wood, 1990:155–164.
35. Watanabe S, Sato Y, Shima H, et al. Monoclonal antibody NCC-pX-1G reactive with gene products coded from X-regions of human T-cell leukemia virus. *Jpn J Cancer Res* 1986;77:338–341.
36. Kadin ME, Sako D, Berliner N, et al. Childhood Ki-1 lymphoma presenting with skin lesions and peripheral lymphadenopathy. *Blood* 1986; 68:1041–1049.
37. Uchiyama T, Hori T, Tsudo M, et al. Interleukin-2 receptor (Tac antigen) expressed on adult T-cell leukemia cells. *J Clin Invest* 1985;76: 446–453.
38. Greene WC, Leonard WJ, Depper JM, et al. The interleukin-2 receptor: normal and abnormal expression in T cells and leukemia induced by the human T-lymphotropic retroviruses. *Ann Intern Med* 1986;105: 560–572.
39. Watanabe S. Peripheral T-cell lymphomas and leukemias. *Hematol Oncol* 1986;4:45–58.
40. Nagatani T, Matsuzaki T, Iemoto G, et al. Comparative study of cutaneous T-cell lymphoma and adult T-cell leukemia/lymphoma: clinical, histopathological and immunohistochemical analyses. *Cancer* 1990; 66:2380–2386.
41. Kamada N, Tanaka K, Sakatani K, et al. Chromosome aberrations in lymphoid malignancies and transforming gene in adult T-cell leukemia. In: Hanaoka M, et al, eds. *Lymphoid malignancy: immunocytology and cytogenetics.* New York: Field & Wood, 1990:57–66.
42. Kamada N, Sakurai M, Miyamoto K, et al. Chromosome abnormalities in adult T cell leukemia/lymphoma: a karyotype review committee report. *Cancer Res* 1992;52:1481–1493.
43. Watanabe S, Arimoto H. Standardized mortality ratio of cancer by prefecture in Japan. *Jpn J Clin Oncol* 1990;20:316–337.
44. The T- and B-cell Malignancy Study Group. Statistical analysis of immunologic, clinical and histopathologic data on lymphoid malignancies in Japan. *Jpn J Clin Oncol* 1981;11:15–38.
45. Tajima K, The T- and B-cell Malignancy Study Group. The 4th nationwide study of adult T-cell leukemia/lymphoma in Japan: estimates of risk of ATL and its geographical and clinical features. *Int J Cancer* 1990;45:237–243.
46. Hinuma Y, Komoda H, Chosa T, et al. Antibodies on adult T-cell leukemia-virus-associated antigen (ATLA) in sera from patients with ATL and controls in Japan: a nationwide seroepidemiologic study. *Int J Cancer* 1982;29:631–636.
47. Tajima K. Malignant lymphomas in Japan: epidemiological analysis of adult T-cell leukemia/lymphoma (ATL). *Cancer Metastasis Rev* 1988;7:223–241.
48. Kusuhara K, Sonoda S, Takahashi K, et al. Mother-to-child transmission of human T-cell leukemia virus type I (HTLV-I): a fifteen year follow-up study in Okinawa, Japan. *Int J Cancer* 1987;40:755–757.
49. Tajima K, Tominaga S, Suchi T, et al. Epidemiological analysis of the distribution of antibody to adult T-cell leukemia-virus-associated antigen (ATLA): possible horizontal transmission of adult T-cell leukemia virus. *Gann* 1982;73:893–901.
50. Mueler N, Tachibana N, Stuver SO, et al. Epidemiologic perspectives of HTLV-I. In: Blattner WA, ed. *Human retrovirology: HTLV.* New York: Raven Press, 1990:281–293.

51. Hinuma Y, Chosa T, Komoda H, et al. Sporadic retrovirus (ATLV)-seropositive individuals outside Japan. *Lancet* 1983;1:824–825.
52. Zeng Y, Lan XY, Fang J, et al. HTLV antibody in China. *Lancet* 1984; 1:799–800.
53. Blattner WA, Clark JW, Gibbs WN, et al. HTLV: epidemiology and relationship to disease. In: *Retrovirus in human lymphoma/leukemia.* Proceedings of the 15th International Symposium Princess Takamatsu Cancer Fund. , 1984;93–108.
54. Tsugane S, Watanabe S, Sugimura H, et al. Infectious states of human T lymphotropic virus type I and hepatitis B virus among Japanese immigrants in the Republic of Bolivia. *Am J Epidemiol* 1988;128: 1153–1161.
55. Catovsky D, Greavges MF, Rose M, et al. Adult T-cell lymphoma-leukemia in blacks from the West Indies. *Lancet* 1982;1:639–643.
56. Riedel DA, Evans AS, Saxinger C, et al. A historical study of human T-lymphotropic virus type I transmission in Barbados. *J Infect Dis* 1989;159:603–609.
57. Blattner WA, Saxinger C, Cleghorn F, et al. *HTLV-I: associated risk factors in Trinidad and Tobago.* IV International Conference on AIDS. Stockholm: , 1988.
58. Reeves WC, Saxinger C, Brenes M, et al. Human T-cell lymphotropic virus type I (HTLV-I) seroepidemiology and risk factors in metropolitan Panama. *Am J Epidemiol* 1988;127:532–539.
59. Merino F, Robert-Guroff M, Clark J, et al. Natural antibodies to human T-cell leukemia/lymphoma virus in healthy Venezuelan populations. *Int J Cancer* 1984;34:501–506.
60. Maloney EM, Ramirez H, Levin A, et al. A survey of the human T-cell lymphotrophic virus type I (HTLV-I) in Southwestern Colombia. *Int J Cancer* 1989;44:419–423.
61. Cortes E, Detels R, Aboulafia D, et al. HIV-1, HIV-2, and HTLV-1 in high-risk groups in Brazil. *N Engl J Med* 1989;320:953–958.
62. Fleming AF, Yamamoto N, Bhesnurmath SR, et al. Antibodies to ATLV (HTLV) in Nigerian blood donors and patients with chronic lymphocytic leukemia or lymphoma. *Lancet* 1983;2:334–335.
63. Biggar RJ, Saxinger C, Gardiner C. Type 1 HTLV antibody in urban and rural Ghana, West Africa. *Int J Cancer* 1984;34:215–219.
64. Hayami M, Komuro A, Nozawa K, et al. Prevalence of anti-adult T-cell leukemia virus (ATLV) antibody in Japanese monkeys and other non-human primates. *Int J Cancer* 1984;33:179–183.
65. Chou KS, Okayama A, Tachibana N, et al. Nucleotide sequence analysis of a full-length human T-cell leukemia virus type I from adult T-cell leukemia cells: a prematurely terminated Px open reading frame II. *Int J Cancer* 1995;60:701–706.
66. Greene WC, Ballard DW, Bohnlein E, et al. The trans-regulatory proteins of HTLV-I: analysis of Tax and Rex. In: Blattner WA, ed. *Human retrovirology HTLV.* New York: Raven Press, 1990:35–43.
67. Yoshida M, Fujisawa J. Positive and negative regulation of HTLV-I gene expression and their roles in leukemogenesis in ATL. *Gann Monogr Cancer Res* 1992;39:217–236.
68. Caputo A, Haseltine WA. Reexamination of the coding potential of the HTLV-1 pX region. *Virology* 1992;188:618–627.
69. Seiki M, Inoue J-I, Hidaka M, et al. Two cis-acting elements responsible for posttranscriptional trans-regulation of gene expression of human T-cell leukemia virus type I. *Proc Natl Acad Sci USA* 1988;85: 7174–7128.
70. Okamoto T, Ohno Y, Tsugane S, et al. Multi-step carcinogenesis model for adult T-cell leukemia. *Jpn J Cancer Res* 1989;80:191–195.
71. Yunoki K, Matsumoto M, Matsumoto T, et al. Adult T-cell leukemia in Kagoshima: its clinical features and skin lesions. In: Hanaoka M, Takatsuki K, Shimoyama M, eds. *Adult T cell leukemia and related diseases.* Tokyo: Japan Scientific Societies Press, 1982:151–166.
72. Kinoshita K, Kamihira S, Yamada Y, et al. Adult T cell leukemia-lymphoma in the Nagasaki District. In: Hanaoka M, Takatsuki K, Shimoyama M, eds. *Adult T cell leukemia-lymphoma in the Nagasaki District.* Tokyo: Japan Scientific Societies Press, 1982:167–184.
73. Greenberg SJ, Tendler CL, Mann A, et al. Altered cellular gene expression in human retroviral-associated leukemogenesis. In: Blattner WA, ed. *Human retrovirology: HTLV.* New York: Raven Press, 1990: 87–104.
74. Uchiyama T, Sagawa K, Takatsuki K, et al. Effect of adult T-cell leukemia cells on pokeweed mitogen-induced normal B-cell differentiation. *Clin Immunol Immunopathol* 1978;10:23–24.
75. Shaw GM, Broder S, Essex M, et al. Human T-cell leukemia virus: its discovery and role in leukemogenesis and immunosuppression. *Ann Intern Med* 1984;30:1–27.
76. Lymphoma Study Group, Shimoyama M, et al. Major prognostic factors of patients with adult T-cell leukemia/lymphoma: a cooperative study. *Leuk Res* 1991;15:81–90.
77. Shimoyama M, Ota K, Kikuchi M, et al. Major prognostic factors of adult patients with advanced T-cell lymphoma/leukemia. *J Clin Oncol* 1988;6:1088–1097.
78. Kajiyama W, Kashiwaga S, Ikematsu H, et al. Intrafamilial transmission of adult T-cell leukemia virus. *J Infect Dis* 1986;154:851–857.

CHAPTER 45

Application of Molecular Genetics to the Diagnosis and Classification of Acute Leukemia

James R. Downing and Frederick G. Behm

The advances made in molecular genetics over the past decade have had a major impact on our understanding of the pathogenesis of cancer and on our ability to diagnose, treat, and monitor a patient's response to therapy. Nowhere has this been more evident than in the medical management of patients with acute leukemias. During the past decade, molecular-based approaches have led to the identification of the genes targeted by each of the major chromosomal rearrangements associated with the acute leukemias. This information has provided fundamental knowledge about the underlying cause of these leukemias and has provided insights into the significant clinical variability that is observed among patients. Molecular genetic data are starting to provide the outlines for a clinically useful classification of acute leukemias. Moreover, molecular-based approaches have provided a means to accurately monitor a patient's response to therapy. These latter efforts offer the hope of individually modifying a patient's therapy to provide the optimal chance for cure. Elucidation of the intracellular pathways involved in the control of normal and malignant hematopoiesis has resulted in the identification of rational molecular targets against which highly specific antileukemic drugs can be developed. Taken together, these advances have significantly changed our approach to the diagnosis and management of patients with acute leukemia.

In this chapter, we describe the molecular-based assays that have proven clinical utility in the evaluation of patients with acute leukemia. To facilitate the practical application of this information, we organized our presentation around the distinct clinical settings in which these assays are used, including the initial diagnostic workup and monitoring a patient's therapeutic response.

J. R. Downing and F. G. Behm: Department of Pathology, St. Jude Children's Research Hospital, Memphis, Tennessee 38105

INITIAL DIAGNOSTIC WORKUP

Because acute leukemia usually manifests as a fulminate malignant process, the issue of malignancy is rarely in question at the time of initial diagnosis. Nevertheless, molecular-based approaches to assess clonality have figured prominently in the acute leukemia literature, equating clonal hematopoietic proliferations with a malignant process. The most common assays used to determine the presence of a clonal lymphoid proliferation are detection of clonal immunoglobulin (Ig) and T-cell receptor (TCR) gene rearrangements by Southern blot analysis or polymerase chain reaction (PCR). These assays are described in detail in Chapters 7 and 9. Although these approaches are only infrequently used in the initial workup of patients with acute leukemia, in rare situations, their use can help to clarify the nature of a hematopoietic proliferation. Moreover, the sensitive detection of clonal Ig and TCR gene rearrangements by PCR-based assays has assumed a prominent role in evaluating a patient's response to therapy. This latter use is subsequently described.

After a diagnosis of leukemia has been made and the specific leukemia subtype defined, it is essential to determine the appropriate risk group to which the patient should be assigned. Modern leukemia therapy is based on the concept of risk stratification, with patients having a low risk of relapse treated with low-intensity or targeted chemotherapy and patients predicted to have a high risk of relapse treated with high-intensity therapy or experimental approaches. Although a variety of clinical and laboratory-based parameters help to define a patient's risk group, the presence or absence of specific molecular genetic lesions have been shown to play an important role in making these assignments. In particular, the presence of certain specific molecular genetic lesions appear to accurately predict the susceptibility of leukemic blasts to therapeutic agents such as all-*trans* retinoic acid (ATRA), high-dose cytarabine (AraC), anthracyclines, and L-asparaginase (1–4).

TABLE 45.1. *Genetic lesions in acute leukemia*

Chromosomal abnormality	Molecular target	Overall frequency	
		Adult	Pediatric
Acute lymphoblastic leukemia			
B-lineage			
t(9;22)(q34;q11)	*BCR-ABL*	25%	5%
t(1;19)(q23;p13)	*E2A-PBX1*	<1%	5%
t(17;19)(q23;p13)	*E2I-HLF*	<1%	<1%
t(4;11)(q21;q23)	*MLL-AF4*	<1%	2%
t(11;19)(q23;p13;3)	*MLL-ENL*	<1%	<1%
t(9;11)(p21;q23)	*MLL-AF9*	<1%	<1%
t(12;21)(p12;q22)	*TEL-AMLI*	<1%	20%
t(8;14)(p24;q32)	*MYC-IgH*	<1%	<1%
Hyperdiploid	?	<2%	25%
del(6)	?	<1%	10%
T-lineage			
t(11;14)(p13;q11)	*LM02-TCR8*	<1%	1%
t(10;14)	*HOX11-TCR8*	<1%	1%
t(1;14)	*TALI-TCR8*	<1%	<1%
t/del(9)(p21)	*INK4A*, $p19^{ARF}$	<1%	10%
Acute myeloid leukemia			
t(15;17)(q21;q21)	*PML-RAR*α	8%	8%
t(11;17)(q23;q21)	*PLZF-RAR*α	<1%	<1%
t(5;17)(q32;q21)	*NPM-RAR*α	<1%	<1%
t(8;21)(q22;q22)	*AML1-ETO*	12%	12%
inv(16)(p13;q22)	*CBFb-MYH11*	10%	10%
t(9;11)(p21;q23)	*MLL-AF9*	2%	7%
t(10;11)(pq21;q23)	*MLL-AF10*	<1%	<1%
t(11;19)(q23;p13.3)	*MLL-ENL*	<1%	<1%
t(11;19)(q23;p13.1)	*MLL-ELL*	<1%	<1%
t(6;9)(p23;q34)	*DEK-CAN*	<1%	<1%
t(7;11)(p15;p15)	*NUP98-HOXA9*	<1%	<1%

During the past two decades, the nature of many of the genetic lesions underlying the acute leukemias has been revealed through the routine use of cytogenetics. These studies have identified a large number of recurrent clonal chromosomal abnormalities including deletions, whole chromosome gains or losses, and translocations (see Chapter 10). The more prevalent of these recurrent chromosomal translocations have been cloned and the involved genes identified. The genes targeted by some of the recurrent deletions have been identified (5) (Table 45.1). This information has allowed the development of molecular-based strategies for the accurate and sensitive identification of these underlying molecular lesions. With the application of these molecular-based approaches, it has become clear that routine cytogenetics, even in the best of hands, is incapable of accurately identifying these lesions. Molecular-based approaches have become the gold standard for the identification of these prognostic markers.

Although a variety of different molecular-based approaches are available to identify chromosomal translocations or their underlying genetic lesions, the most reliable methods have proven to be reverse transcription–polymerase chain reaction (RT-PCR), fluorescence *in situ* hybridization (FISH) of metaphase or interphase chromosomes, and for a subset of lesions, Southern blot analysis (Fig. 45.1). Detailed descriptions of these methodologies can be found in several published reviews (6–8). Briefly, RT-PCR involves the isolation of mRNA, its reverse transcription into cDNA, and its amplification using oligonucleotide primers that bracket the region of interest. Because most of the acute leukemia-associated translocations result in the formation of chimeric genes, amplification primers are typically designed to be complementary to sequences 5′ and 3′ to the fusion breakpoint within the chimeric mRNA. This allows the specific amplification of the chimeric message only from cells in which it is expressed. The identity of the amplified product can be verified by a second round of amplification with internal "nested primers" or by hybridization of the amplified product with an oligonucleotide probe that is complementary to sequences contained within the PCR product. Individual primer sets are needed for each translocation, however, multiplex reactions containing multiple primer pairs against the individual chimeric messages may be combined in a single amplification reaction to screen for the more common translocations in acute leukemia.

FISH uses fluorescence-labeled chromosome-specific DNA (i.e., chromosome painting) or genomic DNA clones that are from defined regions of a particular chromosome. Typically for a translocation, painting probes from the two

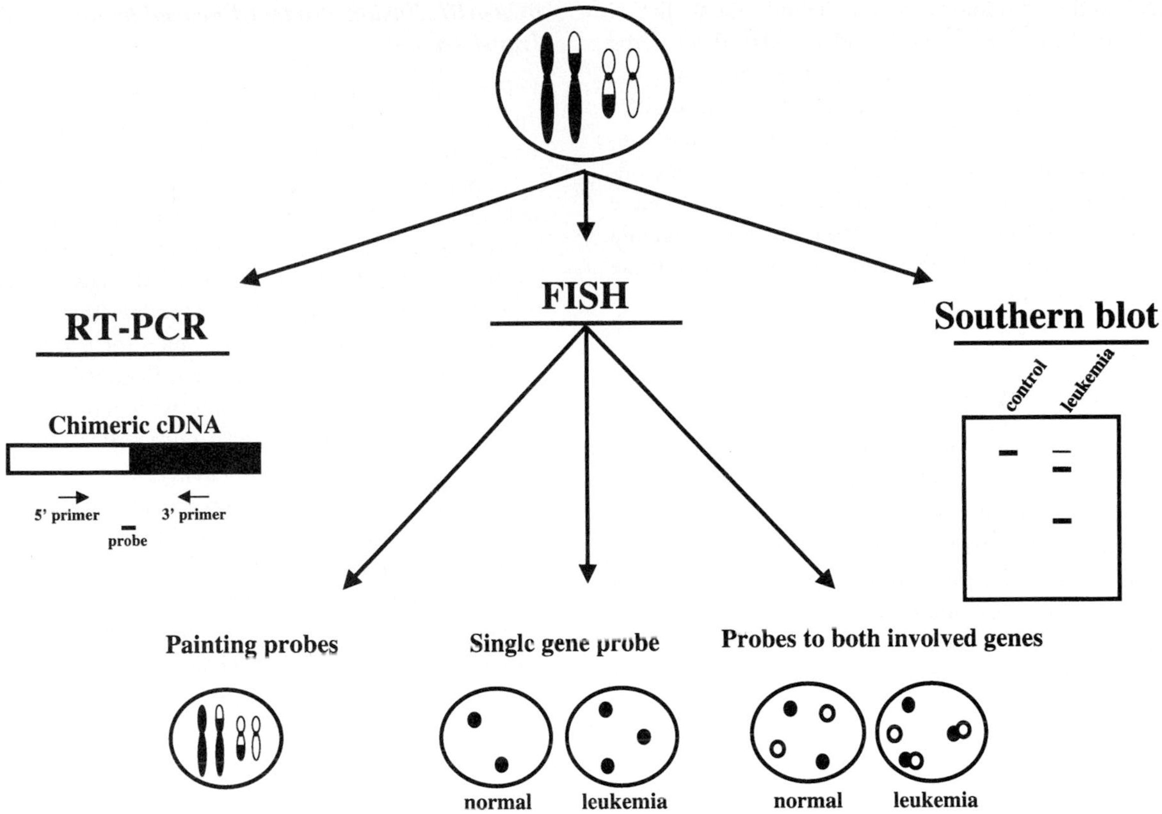

FIG. 45.1. Schematic representation of reverse transcription–polymerase chain reaction (RT-PCR), fluorescence *in situ* hybridization (FISH), and Southern blot analysis.

involved chromosomes or individual probes from one or both of the genes involved in the translocation are labeled with fluorescent dyes and hybridized to metaphase spreads prepared from leukemic cells. If a translocation is present that involves the chromosomes to which the painting probes hybridize (Fig. 45.1), derivative chromosomes composed of a portion of each of the involved chromosomes are visible. In contrast, when individual gene probes are used, the pattern differs depending on whether probes to a single gene or both genes are used and whether the probe crosses the breakpoint. With a single-gene probe that hybridizes to portions of the gene on either side of the breakpoint, a translocation results in splitting of the hybridization signal so that it is localized to both derivative chromosomes (Fig. 45.1). If two probes are used, the translocation results in the juxtaposition of the probes from the different genes onto each of the derivative chromosomes. The individual gene probes can also be used on interphase cells, significantly simplifying the ability to perform this type of analysis (Fig. 45.1). In interphase cells, the use of a single probe results in two signals in a normal cell (i.e., corresponding to the two normal chromosomes) and three signals in a leukemic cell containing this translocation (i.e., one normal chromosome and two signals resulting from the probe hybridizing to the portion of the split gene on each derivative chromosome). Use of two probes results in four independent signals in a normal cell (i.e., two from each probe). In contrast, in a leukemic cell containing this translocation, one normal signal can be detected for each probe, along with one or two fused signals resulting from the cohybridization of the probes for each gene on the derivative chromosomes. Two fused signals are seen if the individual gene probes cross the breakpoint, whereas only a single fused signal is seen if the individual gene probes hybridize to only one side of the breakpoint within the involved genes.

Southern blot analysis can be used to assess the genomic structure of genes involved in chromosomal rearrangements (Fig. 45.1). In this procedure, the DNA from leukemic cells is isolated and digested with a restriction endonuclease that cleaves the DNA in defined regions within the gene of interest. The restricted DNA is then size fractionated by electrophoresis through an agarose gel and transferred to a nylon membrane. The membrane is hybridized with a DNA probe that is specific to a defined region within the gene of interest. The pattern of restriction fragments obtained is then compared between DNA isolated from normal and leukemic cells. The presence of a restriction fragment with an altered size in the leukemic sample is consistent with a chromosomal rearrangement involving the gene. However, before definitive diagnosis of a gene rearrangement can be made, it is essential to ensure that the altered fragment does not represent a normal restriction fragment length polymorphism within the gene.

The preferred methodology used in the individual clinical settings is stressed where useful, and we also discuss the advantages and disadvantages of alternative methodologies. We point out where controversies exist and introduce alternative strategies that may help to resolve these issues. Because the specific molecular genetic lesions that provide important clinical information differ between acute lymphoblastic leukemia (ALL) and acute myeloid leukemia (AML), we discuss the molecular diagnostic workup of these leukemic subtypes separately.

ACUTE LYMPHOBLASTIC LEUKEMIA

ALL is the most common malignancy in childhood and accounts for approximately 80% of acute leukemias in this age group (1). In contrast, ALL accounts for only 20% of cases in older patients (9) (see Chapter 46). The spectrum of molecular genetic lesions differs significantly between adults and children, suggesting that ALL is fundamentally a different disease in these two age groups (1,9) (Table 45.1). Despite these differences, some genetic lesions portend the same clinical significance regardless of a patient's age. For example, the presence of a t(9;22)(q34;q11) within the leukemic blasts defines a leukemia as having a high probability of failing standard therapeutic approaches. Screening for this molecular lesion should be performed in all patients irrespective of their age. Conversely, other molecular lesions provide prognostic information only within certain age groups. Moreover, the molecular genetic lesions that need to be identified also differ between B and T lineage ALLs (Table 45.1). At the time of diagnosis, the age of a patient and the lineage of the leukemic blasts dictate which molecular diagnostic assays should be performed.

B-Lineage Acute Lymphoblastic Leukemia

A number of different molecular genetic lesions provide critical prognostic information for B-lineage ALL (Table 45.1). Chromosomal rearrangements in pediatric patients that define a high risk of relapse include t(9;22)(q34;q11), t(1;19)(q23;p13), and t(4;11)(q21;q13) or other 11q23 translocations involving the *MLL* gene. In contrast, the presence of the t(12;21)(p21;q22) or a hyperdiploid DNA content within the leukemic blasts defines a group of patients with an excellent prognosis, with 5-year event-free survivals approaching 90% (1). Because in pediatric patients the therapeutic approaches for these two groups differ significantly, it is essential in this age group to know whether the leukemic blasts contain one of these genetic lesions. In adult patients, only the t(9;22) and t(4;11) provide clear prognostic information (9). Screening for the other lesions in adult patients has not proven to be of clinical benefit, because they occur at exceedingly low frequencies or fail to provide clear prognostic information.

BCR-ABL Fusion Product Encoded by the t(9;22) Translocation

The Philadelphia chromosome was the first recurrent chromosomal abnormality identified in a human malignancy, and since its auspicious beginnings, it has remained an important diagnostic criteria for chronic myelogenous leukemia (CML) (10–12). The identical chromosomal translocation is seen in approximately 25% of adults and 3% to 5% of pediatric ALL cases. In ALL, it defines an exceedingly poor prognostic group, with 5-year event-free survival rates of less than 25% (13). However, data for pediatric patients suggest that prognosis is further influenced by a patient's peripheral white blood cell count, with patients with counts less than 25,000 faring significantly better after treatment with intensive chemotherapy (14).

The t(9;22)(q34;q11) encodes a chimeric gene consisting of the 5′ portion of *BCR* gene fused to the 3′ portion of *ABL* gene (15–18). Two different BCR-ABL fusion proteins can result from this rearrangement, depending on the site of the chromosomal break within the BCR gene (16,19). Breaks within the major breakpoint cluster region (M-BCR) occur in most CML patients and up to 25% of adult ALL patients. This chimeric gene encodes a 210-kd BCR-ABL fusion protein (Fig. 45.2) (18). In contrast, breaks in the remaining adult ALL patients and most pediatric ALL patients occur further 5′ in *BCR*, in the so-called minor breakpoint cluster regions (m-bcr) (16,19,20). This rearrangement results in the formation of a 190-kd BCR-ABL oncogenic fusion kinase (Fig. 45.2). In both fusion proteins, the N-terminal sequences of ABL are removed and replaced with BCR sequences. These alterations result in a constituitively active cytoplasmic tyrosine kinase that induces aberrant oncogenic signaling by activating multiple pathways (12). Expression of either chimeric protein results in the transformation of hematopoietic cells in murine experimental systems; however, the development of a full leukemic phenotype appears to require the acquisition of cooperating mutations in other cellular regulatory pathways (21–23).

RT-PCR or FISH-based assays have become the standard diagnostic approach for the identification of this molecular genetic lesion. For RT-PCR analysis, a common 3′ *ABL* primer is coupled with one of two distinct 5′ *BCR* oligonucleotide primers to amplify the ALL- and CML-type *BCR-ABL* chimeric messages (24,25) (Fig. 45.2). An individual amplification reaction with the different primer sets allows direct determination of whether the chimeric *BCR-ABL* message results from breaks within M-BCR or m-bcr, respectively. Alternatively, amplification can be carried out in the presence of all three primers and then the nature of the amplified product defined by hybridizing with a type-specific probe or setting up the oligonucleotide primers so that the size of the ALL- and CML-type *BCR-ABL*–encoded messages differ. Although in most clinical settings this distinction is not important, occasionally the identification of a CML-type *BCR-ABL* chimeric message may be suggestive of a CML making its initial presentation in a blast phase.

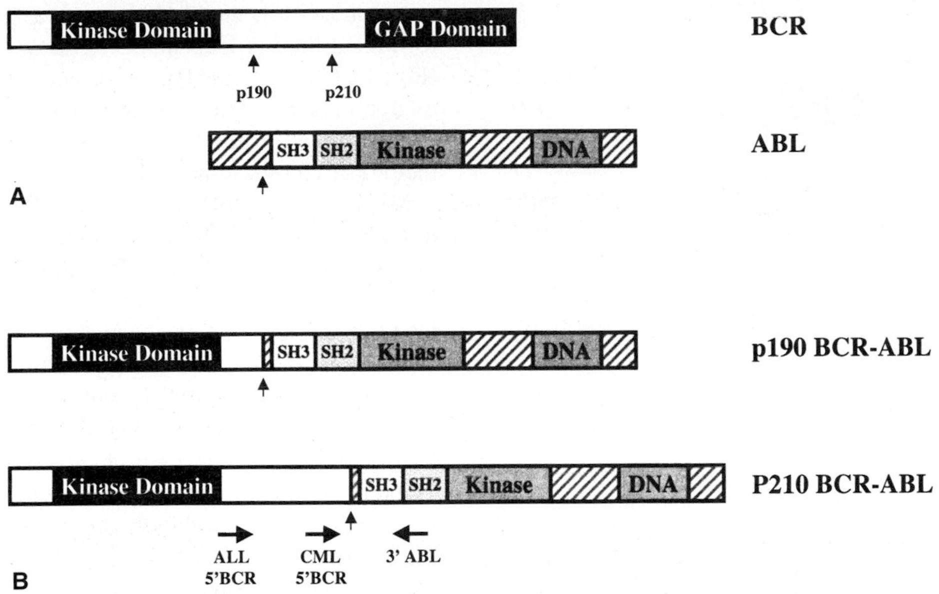

FIG. 45.2. Schematic representation of BCR, ABL, and the BCR-ABL fusion proteins. The positions of the breakpoints in BCR that result in formation of the p190 and p210 chimeric proteins are indicated. The ABL protein contains SH2 and SH3 domains, a central tyrosine kinase domain, and a C-terminal DNA-binding domain. The polymerase chain reaction (PCR) amplification primers are indicated.

The t(9;22) translocation can also be accurately detected by FISH (26). In the most commonly used assay, differentially labeled *BCR* and *ABL* genomic probes are simultaneously hybridized to metaphase or interphase cells and the location of the hybridizing signals detected by fluorescent microscopy. This is a highly accurate and efficient method for the identification of the t(9;22). Moreover, it provides a semi-quantitative estimate of the number of leukemic cells within the analyzed sample.

RT-PCR and FISH-based methods significantly enhance the ability to identify the t(9;22) compared with classic cytogenetic approaches. The choice of which method to use in an individual laboratory depends on the availability of equipment and technical expertise.

E2A-PBX1 Product Encoded by the t(1;19) Translocation

The t(1;19)(q23;p13) is found in the leukemic blasts of 5% of pediatric ALL patients and a much smaller percentage of adult cases. Typically, the t(1;19) is found in cases having a pre-B immunophenotype (cytoplasmic Ig but not surface Ig), with up to 25% of these cases in the pediatric population containing this translocation (27–29). This genetic lesion targets the genes encoding the E2A transcription factor on chromosome 19 and the PBX1 homeodomain containing transcription factor on chromosome 1 (30–32) (Fig. 45.3A). The resulting E2A-PBX1 fusion protein contains the transcriptional activation domains of E2A linked to the DNA-binding domain of PBX1. This chimeric transcription factor is predicted to activate the transcription of genes normally regulated by PBX1. PBX1 functions as a transcriptional regulator and is required for critical steps in the development of the proximal limb, axial skeleton, and spleen (33–35). The critical downstream pathways through which E2A-PBX1 induces the transformation of hematopoietic cells remain to be identified.

Although in initial studies the presence of a t(1;19) defined a subgroup of patients with a poor prognosis, later studies demonstrate that this adverse effect is overcome by more aggressive therapy (29). Patients whose leukemic blasts contain the t(1;19) are now classified as high risk and are treated accordingly. This approach has resulted in a cure rate as high as 90% (1).

A second but rarer ALL-associated translocation, t(17;19), also involves the *E2A* gene (36,37). In this chromosomal rearrangement, *E2A* is fused to the gene encoding hepatic leukemia factor *(HLF)* (Fig. 45.3B). The E2A-HLF fusion protein contains the transcriptional activation domains of E2A linked to the DNA-binding and protein-protein interaction motifs of HLF, a basic leucine zipper (bZIP) transcription factor that is normally expressed in the brain, liver, and kidney (38). Studies suggest that E2A-HLF causes leukemia by inducing a gene that inhibits apoptosis (39). This leukemic subtype is associated with high peripheral counts, frequent coagulation abnormalities, and a poor outcome even when treated with aggressive multiagent chemotherapy (29).

RT-PCR–based assays have been developed for the identification of each of these molecular lesions. In the t(1;19), the location of breakpoints in the *E2A* and *PBX1* genes is variable (40,41). Despite this variability, a single set of amplification primers can detect the presence of this chimeric

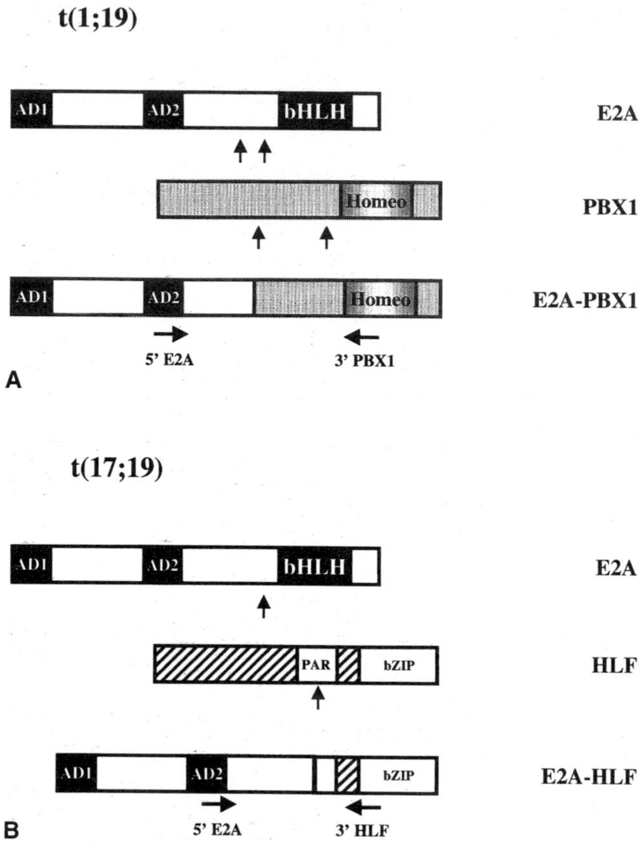

FIG. 45.3. Structure of the t(1;19) and t(17;19) encoded fusion proteins. **A:** Schematic diagram of E2A, PBX1, and the E2A-PBX1 fusion protein. The positions of the breakpoints and amplification primers are indicated. E2a is characterized by two activation domains (AD1 and AD2) and a basic helix-loop-helix (bHLH) DNA-binding domain. **B:** Schematic of E2A, hepatic leukemia factor (HLF), and the E2A-HLF fusion protein. HLF is a member of the proline and acidic amino acid-rich (PAR) domain family of basic leucine zipper (bZIP) transcription factors. The positions of the breakpoints and amplification primers are indicated.

message within a leukemic sample. This approach provides the highest level of diagnostic accuracy. A similar RT-PCR assay can also be used for the identification of the *E2A-HLF* chimeric message (37). Although a FISH-based assay should be able to identify either of these genetic lesions, no reliable genomic probes have been developed against the involved genes. This situation is likely to change with the completion of the human genome project.

Rearrangements of MLL *Induced by 11q23 Translocations*

Structural alterations involving chromosome 11, band q23, are detected in 6% to 8% of ALLs and are the most frequent cytogenetic abnormality in infant ALL (42). It is estimated that more than 30 different chromosomal loci can participate in these 11q23 translocations. The molecular cloning of a number of these translocations has demonstrated that in most cases the 11q23 target is a gene designated *MLL* for mixed-lineage leukemia (i.e., *HRX*, *ALL1*, and *HTRX1*) (Fig. 45.4A) (43–48). These translocations result in the formation of a chimeric message consisting of the 5′ portion of *MLL* fused to the 3′ portion of a gene encoded on the reciprocal chromosome.

MLL is a large molecule with several regions of homology to the *Drosophila* trithorax protein, including two centrally placed zinc finger–like motifs and a C-terminal region referred to as the SET domain (49). Each of these regions mediates protein-protein interactions that are required for the normal function of MLL. In addition to these regions of homology to trithorax, MLL contains three AT hook motifs that mediate binding to AT-rich sequences within the minor groove of DNA, a cysteine-rich domain that is homologous to the noncatalytic domain of DNA methyltransferase, and a lysine-rich region with homology to the C-terminal tail of the late histone H1.

MLL normally functions to maintain expression of specific *HOX* genes (50). This function is mediated through MLL binding to DNA and functioning in part to maintain chromatin in an open conformation so that it is accessible to transcriptional activators. In addition to interacting with DNA, MLL also interacts through its SET domain with an anti-phosphatase called Sbf1 (51,52). Sbf1 acts as a positive regulator of kinase signaling pathways, inducing sustained signaling through tyrosine and serine kinase pathways leading to transformation.

The most frequent 11q23 abnormality in ALL is the t(4;11) (47). This translocation results in the formation of a chimeric gene that encodes a MLL-AF-4 fusion protein that contains the N-terminal portion of MLL, including the AT hooks and methyltransferase domains linked in frame to the C-terminal portion of AF-4 (Fig. 45.4B). This structure is typical of translocation-encoded MLL fusion proteins and results in an alteration in the ability of MLL to regulate *HOX* gene expression and to interact with Sbf1.

Clinical studies in pediatric patients suggest that the presence of an *MLL* gene rearrangement is predictive of an extremely poor prognosis (53,54). At the time of diagnosis, it is essential to employ a screening method that is able to identify the presence of any *MLL* gene fusion. Initial studies focused on the use of Southern blot analysis to detect rearrangement of the *MLL* gene (55,56). These studies demonstrated that, regardless of the fusion partner, most *MLL* breakpoints occur within a single breakpoint cluster region that is encompassed by exons 5 through 11 (56). Because of this clustering of breakpoints, *MLL* gene rearrangements can be accurately identified by Southern blot analysis of *Bam*HI and *Hind*III digested genomic DNA hybridized with an *MLL* probe that contains the exons surrounding the breakpoint cluster region (Fig. 45.4A). Using this approach it has been shown that rearrangements of *MLL* occur in greater than 98% of cases with 11q23 translocations. Southern blot analysis has become the gold standard for detecting *MLL* gene alterations.

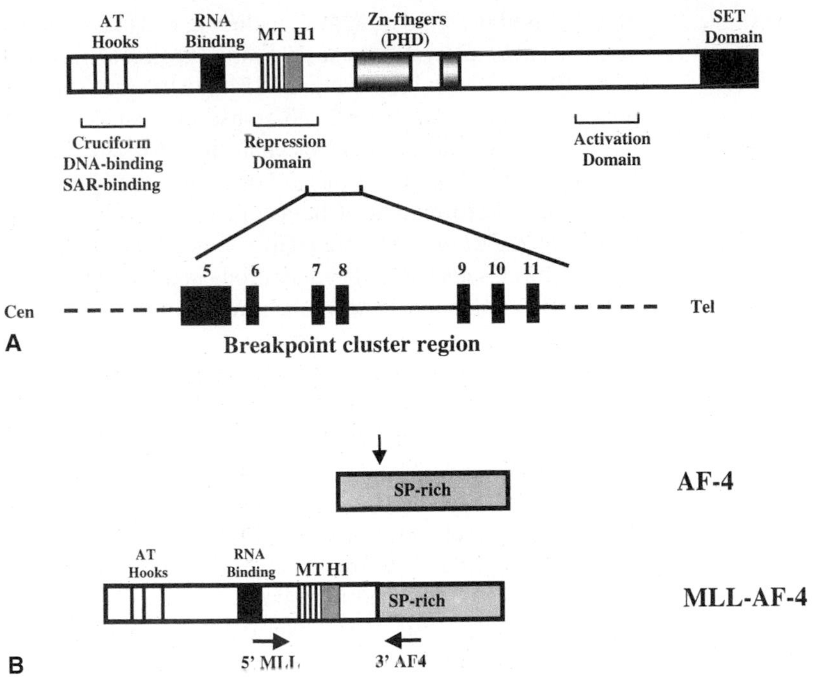

FIG. 45.4. Normal and leukemia-associated MLL proteins. **A:** MLL is organized into domains that include an N-terminal AT hook region, RNA-binding domain, DNA methyltransferase (MT) and histone H1 homology regions, two PHD-type zinc (Zn) fingers, and a C-terminal SET domain. The breakpoint cluster region containing exons 5 through 11 is drawn. **B:** Schematic representation of AF4 and the t(4;11)-encoded MLL-AF4 fusion protein. The positions of the amplification primers are indicated.

In parallel to these studies, RT-PCR–based assays have been developed for most of the cloned *MLL* translocations (Fig. 45.4B) (54,57,58). Although these assays provide a highly sensitive and specific approach for identifying individual translocations, they are of restricted clinical utility at the time of diagnosis because of the diversity of *MLL* partners. This limitation can be partially overcome by combining individual assays into a single multiplex reaction. For example, by combining RT-PCR assays for the four to six most common 11q23 translocation-encoded fusion messages, more than 90% of lesions can be identified. Negative cases can then be screened by Southern blot analysis to detect the rarer *MLL* translocations.

FISH-based assays have been developed for the identification of 11q23 translocations involving the *MLL* gene (59,60). These assays use *MLL* genomic clones that encompass the gene and hybridize as a single signal to each allele. In contrast, in leukemic cells containing an 11q23 translocation, the probe hybridizes to each derivative chromosome, resulting in splitting of one of the hybridization signals in both metaphase and interphase cells. In a head-to-head comparison with Southern blot analysis, FISH was able to identify more than 85% of cases with confirmed *MLL* rearrangements (60,61). Although not perfect, the ease with which this assay can be performed has resulted in its incorporation into our diagnostic armamentarium.

No consensus has been reached on the best strategy for identifying MLL alterations at the time of diagnosis. Typically, various combinations of the three established approaches are used. In infants, among whom the frequency of this lesion is greater than 70%, it is reasonable to analyze all cases by RT-PCR for *MLL-AF4* [t(4;11)], *MLL-ENL* [t(11;19)], and *MLL-AF9* [t(9;11)]. These three chimeric messages account for approximately 90% of the 11q23 translocations in this patient population. Negative cases can then be screened by Southern blot or FISH-based methods. This combination provides a rapid, accurate, and cost-efficient diagnostic approach. In older patients, the frequency of these lesions decreases with age. Moreover, controversy exists over the prognostic significance of these lesions in adolescents and adults. No consensus has been reached over the need to identify this group of molecular lesion in these older patients. If treatment will be altered because of an *MLL* rearrangement, an exhaustive screen identical to that used in infants can be performed. Alternatively, screening by FISH can provide a rapid and relatively accurate means of identifying this genetic lesion.

TEL-AML1 Product Encoded by the t(12;21) Translocation

Abnormalities of the short arm of chromosome 12, including translocations, inversion, insertions, and deletions, are seen in more than 10% of childhood ALLs, in 2% of adult ALLs, and in occasional cases of myelodysplastic syndrome (62). The genetic target of a substantial number of these chromosomal rearrangements was initially identified by the cloning of a t(5;12) in a case of chronic myelomonocytic leukemia (63). In this translocation, the 5′ portion of the *TEL* gene (also known as *ETV6*), a member of the ETS family of transcription factors, is fused to the 3′ portion of the gene for the platelet-derived growth factor receptor-β (PDGFR-β). The resultant chimeric gene encodes a fusion protein consisting of the N-terminal region of TEL fused to the cytoplasmic kinase domain of PDGFR-β. Subsequent studies on other 12p21 rearrangements demonstrated that *TEL* is rear-

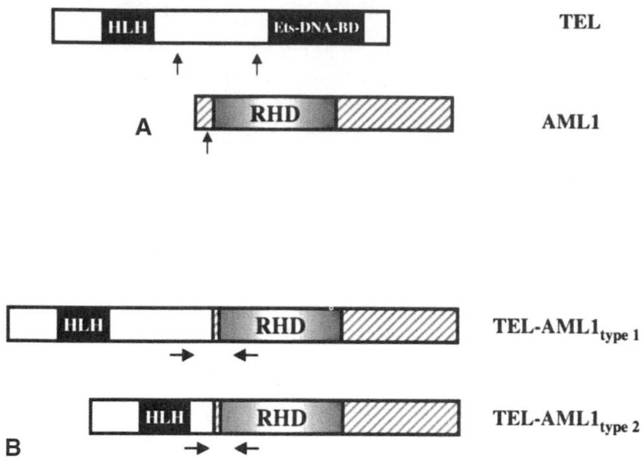

FIG. 45.5. Schematic representation of TEL, acute myeloid leukemia 1 (AML1), and the t(12;21)-encoded TEL-AML1 fusion proteins. **A:** Structure of the normal TEL and AML1 proteins. TEL is organized into an N-terminal helix-loop-helix or pointed domains and a C-terminal ETS-like DNA-binding domain. AML1 contains a central region DNA-binding domain that has a high degree of homology to the *Drosophila* runt protein. **B:** Structure of the TEL-AML1 fusion proteins. Alternative breakpoints in TEL result in formation of the two different fusion proteins. The positions of the amplification primers are indicated.

ranged to a variety of other partner genes. As a result of the t(12;21) in pediatric ALL, the 5′ portion of *TEL* is fused to almost the complete *AML1* gene, resulting in the formation of a TEL-AML fusion protein (Fig. 45.5) (64,65). Based on routine cytogenetic analysis the t(12;21) was felt to be an exceedingly rare translocation. Surprisingly, FISH analysis demonstrated a cryptic t(12;21) in a substantial number of ALL cases (66). Through the subsequent use of RT-PCR and Southern blot analysis, this translocation has been shown to be the most common genetic abnormality in pediatric ALL, accounting for approximately 20% of cases (67,68). In pediatric patients, more than one half of 12p chromosomal abnormalities are the result of a cryptic t(12;21) that encode a TEL-AML1 fusion protein (69). This molecular lesion occurs rarely in adult patients.

TEL contains an N-terminal helix-loop-helix or pointed domain and a C-terminal ETS DNA-binding domain and functions as a sequence specific DNA-binding transcription regulator. TEL is widely expressed in hematopoietic and nonhematopoietic tissues, and gene targeting experiments have demonstrated an essential role in yolk sac angiogenesis, in neuronal development, and in the establishment of bone marrow hematopoiesis (70,71). The other target of the t(12;21), AML1, was initially cloned as the chromosome 21q22 target of the AML-associated t(8;21). *AML1* encodes a transcription factor that binds the enhancer core sequence, TGT/cGGT (72). AML1 binds DNA as a heterodimer with CBFβ and is essential for the development of definitive hematopoiesis of all lineages (73,74). The t(12;21)-encoded TEL-AML1 fusion protein contains the N-terminal HLH domain of TEL fused in frame to AML1, including its DNA-binding domain and its C-terminal transactivation region (Fig. 45.5). As predicted from its structure, TEL-AML1 actively represses normal AML1-mediated transcriptional activation through a dominant negative mechanism (75). This inhibition of normal AML1 functions is thought to directly contribute to the transformation of hematopoietic cells. The nontranslocated *TEL* allele is frequently deleted in ALL cases with t(12;21), suggesting that alterations in the normal function of TEL also contributes to the process of leukemogenesis (76).

The detection of the t(12;21) or its encoded RNA message requires the use of a molecular-based assay. In large published series, a cytogenetically detectable t(12;21) is seen in less than 2% to 3% of cases that are confirmed to express the TEL-AML1 chimeric product (62). The inability to detect this chromosomal translocation by routine chromosomal banding methods results from the exchange of similar appearing regions between chromosomes 12 and 21. As a result of this exchange, the derivative chromosomes that are formed appear identical to their normal counterparts. To overcome this, Southern blot, RT-PCR, and FISH-based approaches must be used to identify this genetic lesion (67,68). Each approach provides a reliable clinical assay, with the choice of which assay to use dictated by a laboratory's expertise and the availability of equipment. We routinely screen cases for this lesion using the RT-PCR assay illustrated in Figure 45.5 (77).

Several laboratories have focused their efforts on developing a single RT-PCR screening assay that is able to identify each of the risk-stratifying abnormalities described previously (77,78). These so-called multiplex assays use combinations of oligonucleotide primers that allow efficient amplification of any fusion transcript present within the leukemic blasts. Multiplex reactions that combine the individual RT-PCR assays into a single reaction can result in significant savings in labor and reagent costs and are therefore ideal for the routine diagnostic evaluation of patients. A multiplex RT-PCR assay that is able to detect chimeric messages encoding the *E2A-PBX1*, *TEL-AML1*, *MLL-AF4*, and the ALL- and CML-type *BCR-ABL* has been developed (77,78). Combining this multiplex assay with rapid and accurate methods to detect the presence of specific PCR product results in an ideal assay for the screening of pediatric ALL patients for the major risk-stratifying lesions. Methods to detect the amplified PCR products have included reverse dot blot or plate-based assays, in which a specific detection probe is coupled to either a membrane or an enzyme-linked immunoabsorbent assay (ELISA) plate.

Real-time PCR assays have been developed in which a detection probe is incorporated into the amplification reaction (79,80). This approach provides a quantitative measure of the amount of a chimeric message present within a sample and eliminates the need for postamplification detection steps. Real-time PCR-based assays, however, require individual reactions for each chimeric message.

Hyperdiploid Acute Lymphoblastic Leukemia

Chromosomal hyperdiploidy defines another distinct genetic subgroup of ALLs that are characterized by leukemic blasts with a modal chromosomal number of 50 or greater, an early pre-B-cell immunophenotype, and in the pediatric population, an excellent prognosis with cure rates of greater than 80% (81–84). This leukemic subgroup accounts for 25% of pediatric ALL cases but is rarely seen in adult patients. Although this subgroup has been recognized for more than 15 years, little is known about its underlying molecular pathology. The simple duplication of a whole chromosome may contribute to the process of cellular transformation, however, the variability in chromosomes duplicated between cases makes this an unlikely scenario (82). The hyperdiploid karyotype is typically stable throughout the course of the leukemia, suggesting that global genetic instability is not a part of the pathogenesis. Approximately 50% of hyperdiploid cases have additional structural chromosomal abnormalities within the leukemic blasts, including duplications of 1q and isochromosome of 17q; however, no consistent structural abnormalities have been identified. Similarly, no specific areas of interstitial deletion have been detected using fine resolution genotypic mapping (85). These observations suggest that a cryptic genetic abnormality may exist within the leukemic blasts that explains the transformed phenotype, the hyperdiploid karyotype, and the unique susceptibility of these cells to antimetabolite-based chemotherapy (86). This subgroup of patients can be easily identified by measuring the modal chromosome number by flow cytometry methods or cytogenetics. Because of its strong predictive value, identification of this subgroup of pediatric ALL patients is essential before initiating treatment on most contemporary protocols.

T-Cell and Mature B-Cell Lymphoblastic Malignancies

Chromosomal translocations in leukemias with a T-lineage or mature B-cell immunophenotype typically result from errors in antigen receptor gene rearrangements. As a result of these alterations, genes that are not normally expressed in mature differentiated lymphoid cells or that have tightly regulated patterns of expression become inappropriately expressed as a result of their juxtaposition next to enhancer or promoter elements of the antigen receptor genes. The prototype of this type of rearrangement is the t(8;14) translocation or its variants, t(2;8) and t(8;22), seen in Burkitt's lymphoma and B-lineage ALL (87). As a result of these rearrangements, the expression of the *MYC* protooncogene is dysregulated, resulting in alterations in cell proliferation, survival, and senescence. Dysregulated *MYC* expression in mice results in the generation of B-lineage leukemia/lymphoma; however, similar to what has been observed with chimeric oncogenes, cooperating mutations are required for full malignant transformation (88–90) (see Chapter 8). Clinically, the morphologic and immunophenotypic diagnosis of Burkitt's lymphoma or its leukemic phase is sufficient for the clinical management of these patients. Identification of the chromosomal rearrangements or the underlying molecular lesions does not provide any additional prognostic information.

Genes that are dysregulated in T-lineage ALLs include *SCL (TAL-1)*, *LMO1 (TTG-1)*, *LMO2 (TTG-2)*, and *HOX11*. *SCL* encodes a transcription factor that is essential for the commitment of mesoderm to form hematopoietic stem cells (91–93). As a result of the t(1;14) seen in approximately 3% of T-lineage ALL cases, *SCL* is rearranged into the TCR-δ gene on chromosome 14, resulting in deregulation of normal SCL expression (94). An internal deletion in the 5′ untranslated region of *SCL* has been identified in an additional 25% of T-ALL cases (95,96). This deletion juxtaposes a locus called *SIL* next to the *SCL* coding region and results in the expression of a fused *SIL-SCL* transcript that encodes a normal SCL protein (95). Together these genetic changes implicate aberrant SCL expression in almost 30% of T-lineage ALLs.

The t(11;14)(p15;q11) results in rearrangement of *LMO1* into the TCR-$\alpha\delta$ locus, whereas the t(11;14)(p13;q11) results in rearrangement of *LMO2* into this locus (93,97–99). These translocations result in inappropriate expression of LMO1/2. The LMO1/2 proteins contain two zinc-binding domains and function as part of a multiprotein DNA binding complex. LMO2, like SCL, has been demonstrated to play an essential role in the development of primitive and definitive hematopoiesis (100,101). The mechanism through which this occurs involves the formation of LMO2-SCL heterodimers (102,103). In T-lineage ALL a substantial proportion of cases contain chromosomal translocations that target the SCL/LMO2 transcriptional regulatory complex that is known to be essential for the development of the hematopoietic system. The targeting of critical regulators of normal hematopoiesis by the leukemia-associated chromosomal rearrangements is a theme that is repeated in translocations that alter the core-binding transcription factor complex in AML.

An additional alteration that has been detected in a substantial percentage of T-lineage ALLs is deletion of the *INK4A* and *INK4B* genes on chromosome 9p21, which encodes the $p16^{INK4a}$ and $p15^{INK4b}$ inhibitors of the CDK4 cyclin D–dependent kinase (104). Deletion of this locus occurs in more than 50% of T-lineage cases and has been suggested to predict a poor prognosis, although this latter finding has not been uniformly observed (105–107). Analysis of a large number of cases suggests that the target of these deletions is *INK4A*; however, this locus encodes a second cell cycle regulatory protein, $p19^{ARF}$, which functions to arrest cell cycle progression through p53 (108,109). Because both of these proteins function as tumor suppressors, it is important to determine whether alterations in $p19^{ARF}$ can also lead to leukemia. Alterations of this genetic locus are not restricted to T-lineage ALL; they also occur in precursor B-cell ALLs, although at a lower frequency (110–112).

Moreover, silencing of this locus has also been shown to occur through hypermethylation of the transcriptional regulatory region of these genes (104).

None of the abnormalities identified in T-lineage ALL has been shown to provide clinically useful information over that provided by lineage determination. Screening for these molecular lesions remains a research tool and is not recommended as part of the routine workup of these patients.

ACUTE MYELOGENOUS LEUKEMIA

The incidence of AML increases with age and accounts for more than 80% of acute leukemias in adult patients. In contrast, AML is much rarer in pediatric patients, accounting for less than 20% of acute leukemias (see Chapter 47). Regardless of a patient's age, AML can be divided conceptually and clinically into *de novo* disease, AML arising in the setting of myelodysplasia, and secondary AML occurring as a consequence of prior exposure to a mutagenic agent (3,113). Secondary AML is a nearly incurable disease and therefore must be distinguished from the other entities. In contrast, *de novo* AML and myelodysplastic syndrome (MDS)–related AML, although arising from different pathogenic mechanisms, overlap significantly in clinical characteristics and therapeutic responses. Recent treatment approaches have shown that the response of these diseases may depend more on the presence or absence of specific chromosomal abnormalities than on their morphologic appearance (114,115). For example, within *de novo* AML, a good prognostic subgroup is identified by the presence of the t(15;17), t(8; 21), or inv(16) (115–118). In contrast, a poor prognosis is associated with the presence of −5, 5q−, −7, 7q−, +8, or a normal karyotype, regardless of whether the disease was classified as *de novo* AML, or AML arising in the setting of MDS (114). Cytogenetic or direct molecular genetic methods have become an essential part of the routine diagnostic workup of patients with AML. This approach allows the physician to modify therapy according to the treatment sensitivity of biologically defined subsets of cases and provides unique markers with which to accurately monitor a patient's response to therapy. We describe the molecular-based assays for the major risk-stratifying lesions identified in AML. Although FISH-based assays are available for the clinically relevant chromosomal deletions and duplications, these are not discussed in this chapter, because routine cytogenetics is still the predominant approach used for their identification.

Acute Promyelocytic Leukemia

Acute promyelocytic leukemia (APL) is characterized by the expansion of a clonal population of malignant myeloid cells blocked at the promyelocyte stage of differentiation. In greater than 95% of the cases a t(15;17)(q22;q11) chromosomal translocation is identified within the leukemic promyelocytes. This chromosomal rearrangement results in a fusion between a previously unidentified gene called promyelocytic leukemia *(PML)* on chromosome 15, and the retinoic acid receptor-α *(RARA)* on chromosome 17, resulting in the formation of a PML-RARα fusion protein (4) (Fig. 45.6A).

The RARα is a member of the nuclear hormone receptor superfamily and functions as a ligand-dependent transcription factor that regulates the expression of a large number of target genes, some of which are critical for normal myeloid cell differentiation (119). In contrast, less is known about the normal biologic function of PML. Sequence analysis has revealed that PML contains a unique cysteine and histidine-rich zinc-binding domain called a RING finger, followed by two cysteine/histidine-rich regions known as B-boxes, an α-helical coiled-coil domain, and a C-terminal serine/proline rich region (Fig. 45.6A) (120). Each of these regions appear to play roles in protein-protein interactions. PML is ubiquitously expressed and resides in unique subnuclear organelles referred to as PML nuclear bodies (NBs) or PML oncogenic domains (PODs) (121,122). Approximately 10 to 30 PML NBs exist within each cell. Overexpression of PML has been shown to have growth-suppressive effects, suggesting that PML may normally function in the NBs to limit the proliferative potential of cells. Data supporting this interpretation have come from gene-targeting experiments in which loss of PML results in enhanced cellular proliferation and an increase in the frequency of chemically induced tumors, raising the possibility that PML is a true tumor suppressor (123). Terminal myeloid cell differentiation was impaired, suggesting that PML may be required for appropriate retinoic acid signaling.

In the PML-RARα chimeric product, the N-terminal portion of PML, including the RING finger, B-boxes, and a variable amount of the α-helical coiled-coil domain, is fused in frame to most of RARα (Fig. 45.6A). This fusion protein contains nearly all of the key functional domains of each molecule, including the protein-protein interaction motifs of PML and the DNA-binding, dimerization, ligand-binding and transcriptional activation domains of RARα. This structure suggests that the PML-RARα fusion protein functions to disrupt the normal biologic activities of RARα and PML. Consistent with this interpretation, PML-RARα continues to bind retinoic acid response elements (RARE) in target genes; however, instead of inducing the transcriptional activation of these genes in response to retinoic acid, this fusion protein functions as a constitutive transcriptional repressor, blocking normal retinoic acid–induced differentiation signals (124,125).

In the absence of retinoic acid, normal RARα is bound to RARE in a complex with RXR, the nuclear co-repressors N-CoR/SMRT and Sin3A/B, and a histone deacetylase (HDAC) (126–128). This complex induces deacetylation of lysine residues in histone proteins, resulting in transcriptional repression. Addition of physiologic levels of retinoic acid induces a conformational change in the RARα subunit, resulting in the release of co-repressors and their replacement

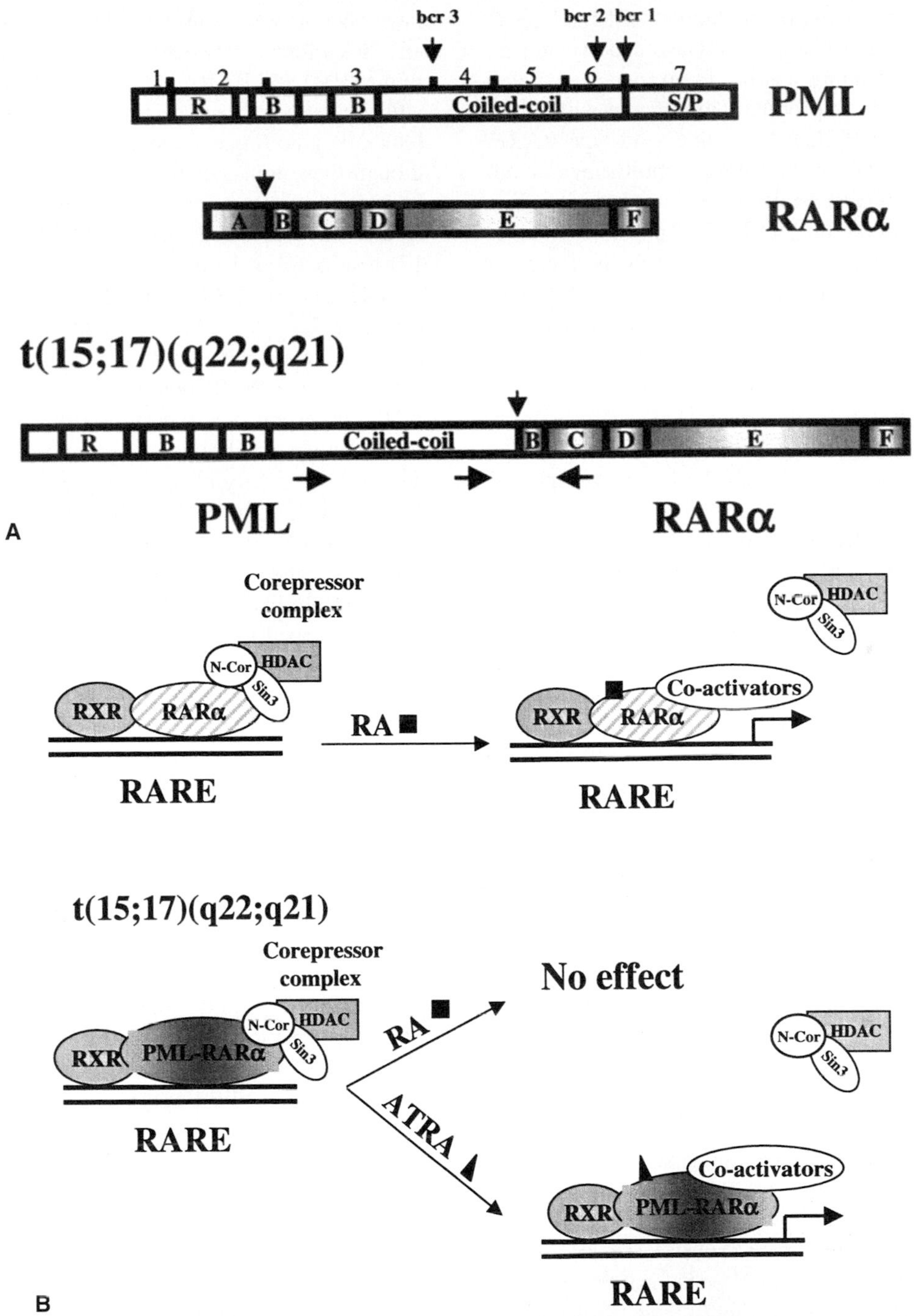

FIG. 45.6. Structure and molecular mechanisms of the t(15;17)-encoded promyelocytic leukemia (PML)–retinoic acid receptor (RARα) fusion protein. **A:** PML is organized into an N-terminal RING finger domain followed by two B-box domains (B), a coiled-coil region, and a C-terminal serine and proline (S/P)-rich region. RARα is organized into domains A through F, which correspond to a ligand-independent transactivation domain (A/B), a DNA-binding domain that contains two zinc-finger motifs (C), a region containing a nuclear localization signal (D), a large domain responsible for ligand-binding and heterodimerization (E), and a C-terminal domain (F). The positions of the breakpoint cluster regions 1 through 3, are indicated, as are the positions of the amplification primers. **B:** The retinoic acid receptor binds DNA as a heterodimer with RXR and in the absence of retinoic acid (RA) interacts with the nuclear corepressors N-Cor, Sin3, and a histone deacetylase (HDAC). Addition of physiologic doses of RA results in release of the corepressor complex and its replacement by transcriptional coactivators. Like the normal receptor, PML-RARα binds the corepressor complex; however, this is not released by addition of RA. By contrast, addition of all-*trans* retinoic acid (ATRA) results in release of the corepressor complex and its replacement by transcriptional coactivators.

by transcriptional coactivators, including CBP and p300. These coactivators have histone acetylase activity and induce nucleosome unfolding leading to an increased ability of transcription factors to productively interact with DNA. The t(15;17)-encoded PML-RARα, like wild-type RARα, directly binds to the nuclear co-repressor multisubunit complex, resulting in the repression of gene transcription (Fig. 45.6B). However, unlike normal RARα, physiologic doses of retinoic acid fail to induce the release of the co-repressor complex from the chimeric molecule (126,129,130). This inability to respond to the normal levels of retinoic acid results in a dominant inhibition of ligand-responsive RARα-induced transcriptional activation. In contrast to retinoic acid, pharmacologic doses of ATRA lead to a conformational change in PML-RARα, resulting in the release of the co-repressors and their replacement by transcriptional coactivators (121,122).

In addition to its effects on retinoid signaling, PML-RARα also induces the disruption of normal PML NBs into a microparticulate pattern within the nucleus (121,122,131). This change in nuclear localization is believed to result in an inhibition of the normal growth regulatory activity of PML. This activity of the PML-RARα fusion protein is also reversed by treatment with ATRA. Treatment with ATRA reverses the inhibitory activity of PML-RARα on RARα and PML and results in the specific growth arrest of leukemic promyelocytes and their terminal differentiation.

Studies from China have demonstrated that ATRA-responsive and -resistant APL cases are also sensitive to treatment with arsenic trioxide (As_2O_3) (132). This therapy leads to apoptosis of the leukemic blasts without induction of their terminal differentiation (133–135), suggesting that As_2O_3 blocks an antiapoptotic effect of the chimeric product. Future protocols combining the use of ATRA, As_2O_3, and standard chemotherapeutic agents should provide improvements over presently used approaches (136).

The breakpoint in the RARα gene *(RARA)* always occurs within the second intron of the gene, suggesting that a recombination hot spot exists within this stretch of DNA. In contrast, breakpoints in PML vary, with three breakpoint cluster regions (bcr) identified (Fig. 45.6A). In most patients, the breakpoint in *PML* occurs in the 3′ portion of the gene, in intron 6 (bcr1) or within exon 6 (bcr2). These breakpoints result in fusion products that contain the N-terminal portion of PML, including most of the α-helical coiled-coil domain. In approximately one third of APL patients, however, the *PML* breakpoint occurs within intron three (bcr3), resulting in deletion of most of the α-helical coiled-coil domain. This variation in the amount of PML contained in the chimeric product is likely to lead to functional alterations. Consistent with this prediction, data have shown a correlation between the type of PML-RARα fusion protein expressed, and the clinical or laboratory features of the leukemia (137). In contrast, no consistent correlation has been found between the type of fusion and a patient's response to treatment.

Two variant translocations that involve the RARα gene have been identified in APL. These include the t(5;17) that encodes a fusion between the nucleolar protein nucleophosmin (NPM) and RARα (138) and the t(11;17) that encodes a fusion between the transcriptional repressor promyelocytic leukemia zinc finger protein (PLZF) and RARα (139). Although these translocations result in APL morphology, the leukemias are unresponsive to ATRA therapy. Mechanistic studies have revealed that this latter property in the t(11; 17) results from the direct binding of nuclear co-repressor complexes to the RARα and PLZF portions of the chimeric protein (126–128,140). The PLZF-RARα protein contains an ATRA responsive co-repressor complex bound through RARα, and a PLZF bound co-repressor complex that is ATRA unresponsive. Experimentally, this unresponsiveness can be reversed through direct inhibition of the histone deacetylase activity of the co-repressor complex.

Only APLs that contain the t(15;17) are responsive to ATRA, and before initiation of therapy, it is essential to determine whether this molecular lesion is present within the leukemic blasts. RT-PCR and FISH-based assays have been developed for the rapid and accurate identification of this lesion (4). Because of the variability in the location of PML breakpoints, RT-PCR assays require a combination of two different 5′ PML oligonucleotide primers coupled with a single 3′ RARα primer (Fig. 45.6A). This assay provides an efficient method to identify this molecular lesion and can define the breakpoint cluster region involved in the rearrangement. The clinical features of the leukemia appear to differ depending on the breakpoint region involved. However, whether a difference in prognosis exists among the various groups remains a somewhat controversial issue. FISH-based assays have also proven to be of clinical utility in the identification of this genetic lesion. The ease with which these FISH assays can be performed has resulted in their incorporation into the routine workup of leukemia patients at many medical centers.

Acute Myeloid Leukemia Affecting the Core-Binding Factor Complex

The two most common chromosomal rearrangements in *de novo* AML, t(8;21) and inv(16), each result in an alteration in the heterodimeric AML1/CBFβ core-binding factor transcription complex (72,141) (Fig. 45.7). The t(8;21) targets the *AML1* gene on chromosome 21q22 and encodes an AML1-ETO fusion protein (142–145), whereas the inv(16) targets the CBFβ gene *(CBFB)* on chromosome 16q22 and results in the formation of a CBFβ-MYH11 fusion protein (146). Although these leukemias include a range of different French-American-British (FAB) morphologic subtypes, they are linked by a common underlying molecular pathogenesis. This unifying feature correlates closely with a relatively good response to conventional multiagent chemotherapy. For example, among the different subtypes of *de novo* AML, cases with an alteration of AML1/CBFβ have the best 5-year event-free survival times (115,118,147). The excel-

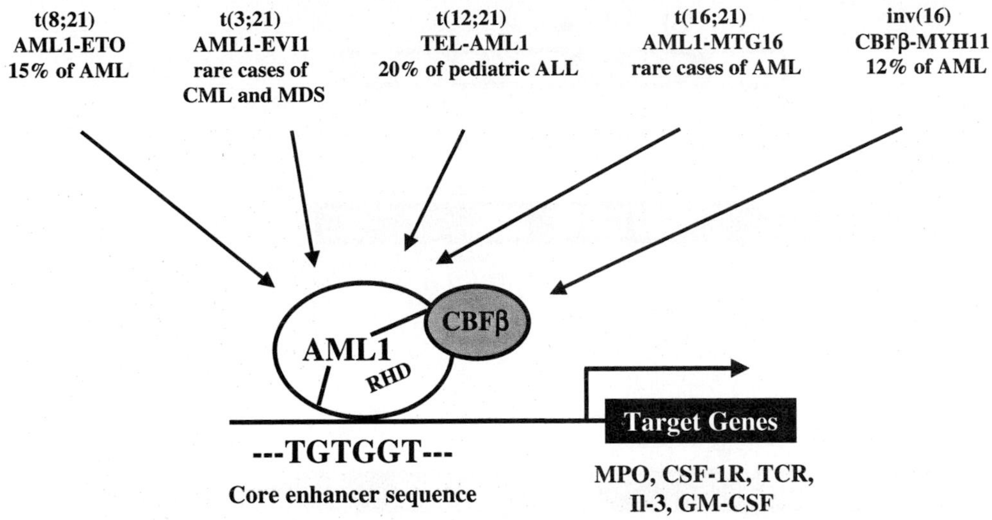

FIG. 45.7. The acute myeloid leukemia 1 (AML1)/CBFβ transcription factor complex is the most common target of chromosomal rearrangement in acute leukemia. AML1/CBFβ functions as a transcriptional organizer activating the transcription of target genes through the core enhancer sequence. DNA binding is mediated through the runt homology domain (RHD). Target genes regulated by this complex include myeloperoxidase (MPO), the receptor for colony-stimulating factor-1 (CSF-1R), and the subunits of the T-cell antigen receptor (TCR), interleukin 3 (IL-3), and granulocyte macrophage colony-stimulating factor (GM-CSF).

lent outcome in these patients appears to require treatment with conventional or high-dose AraC.

The AML1/CBFβ transcription factor complex is essential for the normal development of all hematopoietic lineages (73,74,148,149) and is the most common target of chromosomal rearrangements in human acute leukemia. It is targeted not only by the t(8;21) and inv(16), but also by the t(16;21) *(AML1-MTG16)* in rare cases of AML (150), the t(3;21) *(AML1-EVI1)* in myelodysplasia and rare cases of blast transformation of CML (151), a variety of uncloned translocations in therapy-related AML (152), and the t(12; 21) *(TEL-AML1)*, the most common chromosomal rearrangement in pediatric ALL (64,65) (Fig. 45.7). The AML1/CBFβ transcription factor binds to the enhancer core sequence in the transcriptional regulatory region of target genes and mediates transcriptional activation. DNA binding occurs through the AML1 subunit and its DNA-binding affinity is increased through heterodimerization with CBFβ. *AML1* is a member of a family containing three closely related genes: *AML1, AML2,* and *AML3.*

AML1/CBFβ is critical for the tissue specific expression of a number of different hematopoietic specific genes, including myeloperoxidase, the receptor for colony stimulating factor-1 (CSF-1), the subunits of the T-cell antigen receptor (TCR), neutrophil elastase, and the cytokines interleukin-3 (IL-3) and granulocyte macrophage-colony stimulating factor (GM-CSF) (141) (Fig. 45.7). Although the core enhancer sequence is important for the hematopoietic specific expression of these genes, expression also depends on the presence of adjacent binding sites for lineage-restricted transcription factors such as MYB, LEF-1 C/EBPα, and ETS family members (153–157). This observation suggests that AML1/CBFβ functions as a transcriptional organizer that recruits tissue-specific factors to form an enhancesome that stimulates lineage-restricted transcription.

Consistent with a critical role in normal hematopoiesis, gene-targeting experiments have demonstrated that both AML1 and CBFβ are essential for the formation of the definitive hematopoietic system (73,74,148,149). Null mutations in either gene results in an embryonic lethal phenotype with embryos dying during the midpoint of development from a complete absence of fetal liver-derived hematopoiesis and lethal central nervous system hemorrhages. The hematopoietic defect that results from the loss of AML1 is intrinsic to the definitive hematopoietic stem cell, suggesting that AML1/CBFβ functions as a master regulatory switch that establishes a transcriptional cascade necessary for the development of the definitive hematopoietic system.

The t(8;21)(q22;q22) translocation is seen almost exclusively in cases of AML with FAB M2 morphology and accounts for more than 40% of these cases (158). This translocation results in the formation of an AML1-ETO fusion protein (Fig. 45.8A) (142–145). This product consists of the N-terminal portion of AML1, including its entire DNA-binding domain, fused in frame to the C-terminal portion of ETO. *ETO* is the mammalian homologue of the *Drosophila* gene *nervy*, and although its normal function is unknown, two *ETO*-related genes, *MTGX* and *MTG16,* have been identified. MTG16 was identified as part of a chimeric AML1-MTG16 product that formed as a result of a t(16;21)(q24; q22) translocation seen in rare cases of therapy-related AML or MDS (150).

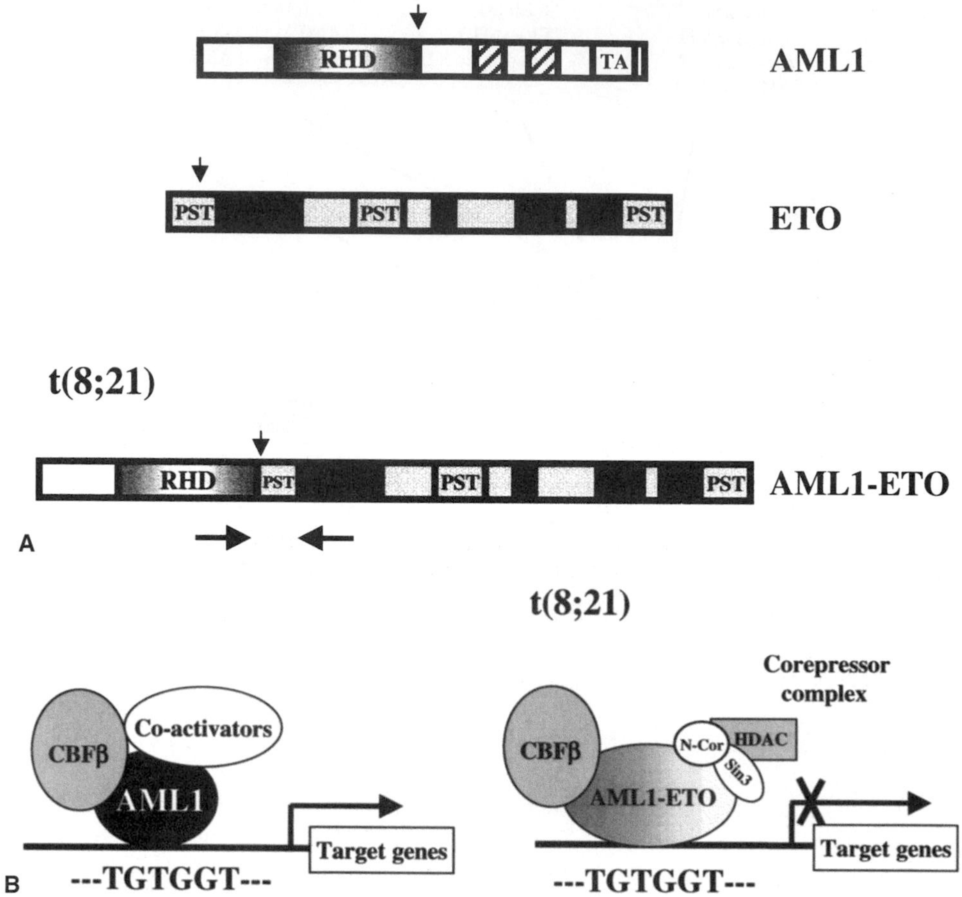

FIG. 45.8. Structure and function of the t(8;21)-encoded acute myeloid leukemia 1 (AML1)-ETO fusion protein. **A:** Schematic diagram of AML1, ETO, and AML1-ETO. The central runt homology domain (RHD) and C-terminal transcriptional activation domain (TA) of AML1 are indicated, as are the proline/serine/threonine-rich (PST) domains of ETO. The positions of the breakpoints and amplification primers are indicated. **B:** AML1/CBFβ activates transcription by interacting with transcriptional coactivators that induce the acetylation of histones. By contrast, AML1-ETO directly interacts with the transcriptional repressors, N-Cor and Sin3, and a histone deacetylase (HDAC) acts to repress AML1-mediated transcriptional activation.

As predicted from its structure, AML1-ETO retains the ability to bind the enhancer core sequence and to interact with CBFβ (Fig. 45.8B). However, AML1-ETO does not function to activate transcription, but instead acts to dominantly repress normal AML1-mediated transcriptional activation (159). This function depends on the DNA-binding domain of AML1 and on sequences contained within ETO. Transcriptional repression appears to be mediated through the direct interaction of ETO to the nuclear co-repressor complex (160–163) (Fig. 45.8B). ETO directly binds N-CoR and through formation of the co-repressor complex, leading to the deacetylation of histones and the repression of transcription of normal AML1/CBFβ transcription targets.

Direct proof of the role of AML1-ETO in hematopoietic cell transformation has come from gene targeting experiments in which an *AML1-ETO* chimeric gene was created by knocking ETO into the *AML1* genomic locus (164,165). Expression of AML1-ETO resulted in an embryonic lethal phenotype almost identical to that observed from the loss of AML1 or CBFβ. However, in contrast to AML1- or CBFβ-deficient embryos, fetal livers from AML1-ETO–expressing embryos contained dysplastic multilineage hematopoietic progenitors (165). These cells had an abnormally high self-renewal capacity and readily established immortal cell lines in culture. However, these cells were not leukemic when transplanted into syngeneic or immunocompromised recipients. The full leukemic transformation requires additional genetic mutations that cooperate with the signals generated through AML1-ETO. The nature of these cooperating mutations remains to be defined.

The inv(16)(p13;q22) and the variant translocation t(16;16)(p13;q22) result in the fusion of *CBFB* and the smooth muscle myosin heavy-chain gene *MYH11* (166) (Fig. 45.9A). This chimeric gene encodes a fusion protein consisting of the N-terminal portion of CBFβ fused in frame to a variable amount of the C-terminal α-helical rod domain of

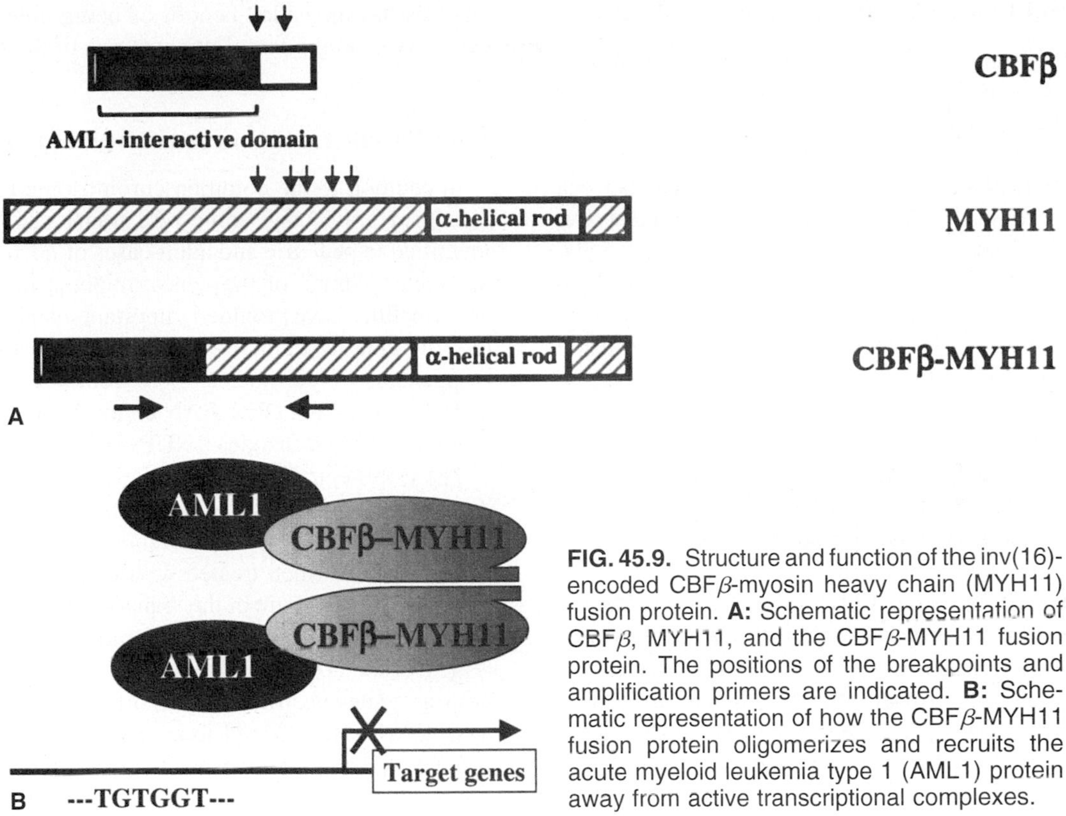

FIG. 45.9. Structure and function of the inv(16)-encoded CBFβ-myosin heavy chain (MYH11) fusion protein. **A:** Schematic representation of CBFβ, MYH11, and the CBFβ-MYH11 fusion protein. The positions of the breakpoints and amplification primers are indicated. **B:** Schematic representation of how the CBFβ-MYH11 fusion protein oligomerizes and recruits the acute myeloid leukemia type 1 (AML1) protein away from active transcriptional complexes.

MYH11. Breakpoint diversity occurs in *CBFB* and *MYH11;* however, in every case, the AML1-binding domain of CBFβ is retained, and the chimeric product is able to bind to normal AML1 (167). The portion of MYH11 contained within the fusion protein is capable of forming oligomers through intermolecular interactions of the MYH11 rod domains. Through these interactions, CBFβ-MYH11 directly represses AML1-mediated transcriptional activation. Although the exact mechanism of transcriptional repression is at present unclear, it appears, at least in part, to involve sequestration of normal AML1 into functionally inactive complexes within the nucleus (Fig. 45.9B). Direct evidence that the CBFβ-MYH11 fusion product functions in a dominant negative fashion comes from experiments in which a *CBFB-MYH11* allele was created by targeting the *MYH11* gene into the murine CBFβ locus (168). Embryos heterozygous for the *CBFB-MYH11* allele died during embryogenesis from a phenotype nearly identical to that observed after the loss of AML1 or CBFβ. Like the *AML1-ETO* knockin allele, *CBFB-MYH11* on its own failed to induce leukemia, but treatment of these chimeric mice with chemical mutagens resulted in a high frequency of AML (169). These results suggest that CBFβ-MYH11 requires cooperating mutations to induce a full leukemic phenotype.

Because of the unique sensitivity of the core-binding factor leukemias to high-dose cytarabine, it is now thought to be essential to accurately identify this leukemic subgroup before initiation of therapy. Although in most cases the t(8;21) translocation is easily identified by routine cytogenetics, some cases have been shown to express the AML1-ETO fusion message but to lack an identifiable translocation (170). A molecular-based approach is required to ensure the appropriate categorization of every case. Because of the large size of the AML1 gene, Southern blot analysis has proven inadequate to accurately identify evidence of this rearrangement. In contrast, RT-PCR–based assays for AML1-ETO accurately identify this lesion in all cases containing the t(8;21) (171). Because of the consistency of breakpoints in AML1 and ETO, only a single set of amplification primers is needed (Fig. 45.8A). A FISH-based assay for t(8;21) that uses genomic probes against AML1 and ETO has been developed (172). This assay works efficiently on metaphase spreads or interphase cells and is therefore an effective screening tool for the identification of this lesion.

In contrast to the t(8;21), the routine cytogenetic detection of the inv(16) is very difficult, even in the best of hands. A molecular-based assay is essential for the accurate identification of this leukemic subtype. RT-PCR–based assays have been developed and provide a rapid and accurate means to detect the CBFβ-MYH11 mRNA (146,167,173) (Fig. 45.9A). Similarly, a FISH-based assay has been developed (174). A polyclonal antibody directed against a junctional epitope of the most common type of CBFβ-MYH11 has been used to identify cases containing this molecular lesion (175). The choice of assay to use depends on the equipment and expertise available within the testing laboratory.

Acute Myeloid Leukemia with Alterations of *MLL*

Structural alterations involving chromosome 11, band q23 occur in approximately 6% to 8% of *de novo* AMLs and in up to 85% of secondary AMLs that develop after exposure to topoisomerase II inhibitors (53,176–178). It has been estimated that more than 30 different chromosomal loci can participate in these 11q23 translocations. The most frequently involved sites in AML include 1p32, 1q21, 6q27, 9p22, 10p12, 16p13.3, 17q21, 19p13.1, 19p13.3, and 22q13 (Table 45.1). Like the ALL 11q23 translocations previously described, most AML translocations target *MLL* and result in the formation of chimeric genes that consist of the 5′ portion of *MLL* fused to the 3′ portion of a gene encoded on the reciprocal chromosome. In addition to these translocation-induced alterations in *MLL,* this gene has been found to undergo partial internal duplications in rare cases of AML that have a normal karyotype or trisomy of chromosome 11 (179).

The major AML-associated 11q23 translocations include the t(6;11) *(MLL-AF6)*, t(9;11) *(MLL-AF9)*, t(11;19) *(MLL-ENL)*, and t(10;11) *(MLL-A10)* (54). RT-PCR–based assays have been developed for each of these chimeric messages. However, because of the large number of potential partner genes, the identification of *MLL* gene rearrangements is better accomplished through the use of Southern blot or FISH-based approaches as described previously. Southern blot analysis has the added benefit of being able to also detect cases containing internal duplications of *MLL.*

Rare Genetic Lesions in Acute Myeloid Leukemia

In addition to the common chromosome rearrangements discussed previously, some rare translocations have been identified in pediatric and adult cases of *de novo* AML. The molecular cloning of the genes involved in some of these abnormalities have provided important insights into the biology of acute leukemia. Two of these translocations affect components of the nuclear pore complex, the t(6;9)(p23;q34) that encodes a DEK-CAN chimeric protein and the t(7;11)(p15;p15) that encodes a NUP98-HOXA9 fusion protein.

The t(6;9)-containing leukemia is seen primarily in children and young adults and accounts for approximately 1% of AML patients (180). This subgroup as a whole has a poor prognosis when treated with conventional therapeutic approaches. As a result of this translocation, almost the entire DEK protein is linked to the C-terminal two thirds of CAN (Fig. 45.10A) (180,181). DEK is a nuclear protein that functions as a site-specific DNA-binding protein (182). In contrast, CAN, also referred to as NUP214, is a nuclear pore complex (NPC) protein, or nucleoporin, that functions in the transport of RNA and protein across the nuclear membrane (183–185). The DEK-CAN fusion protein is thought to in-

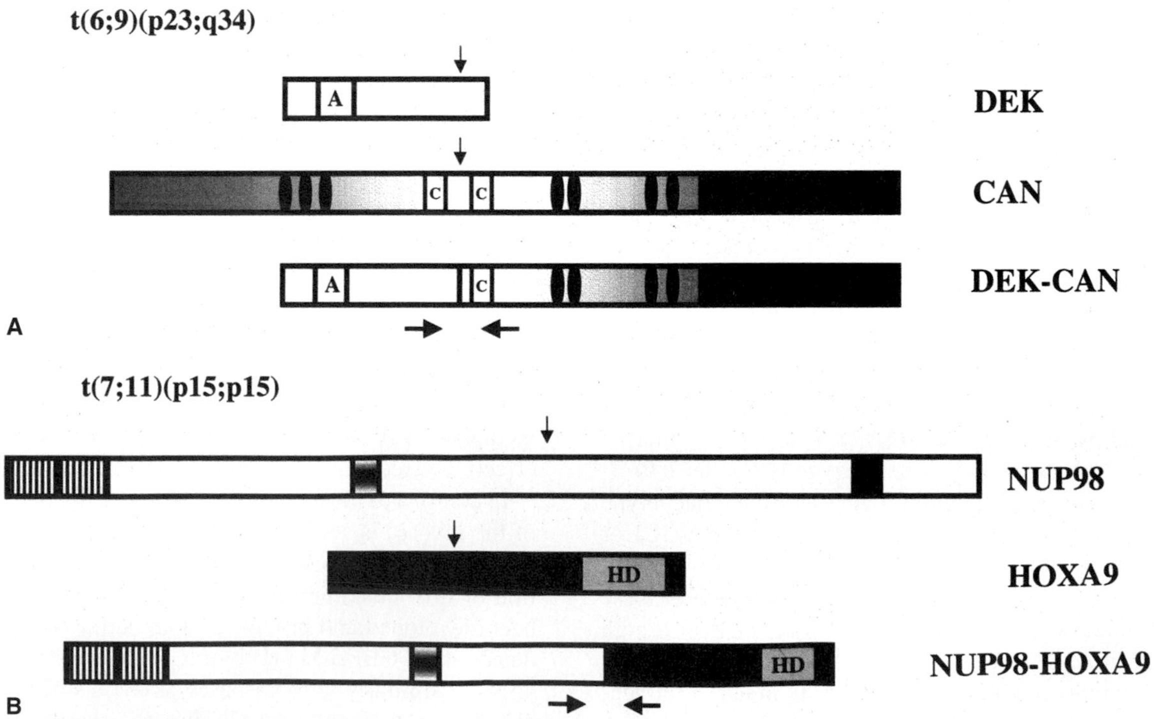

FIG. 45.10. Schematic representation of the chimeric proteins formed as a result of the t(6;9) and t(7;11) translocations. **A:** DEK contains an activation domain (A). The positions of the breakpoints and amplification primers are indicated. **B:** HOXA9 contains a homeobox DNA-binding domain (HD) that is retained in the NUP98-HOXA9 fusion protein. The positions of the breakpoints and amplification primers are indicated.

duce alterations in the structure of the NPC, resulting in changes in nuclear-cytoplasmic transport that are likely to contribute directly to hematopoietic cell transformation. Alteration in the transcriptional activity of the DEK protein induced by its fusion to functional domains in CAN is also likely to play a role in the development of leukemia.

A second nucleoporin, NUP98, was identified as the target of the AML-associated t(7;11)(p15;p15) (186). As a result of this translocation, a NUP98-HOXA9 fusion protein is formed. In this chimeric protein the FG repeats of NUP98 are fused in frame to the homeobox DNA-binding domain of HOXA9 (Fig. 45.10B). As a result, the NUP98-HOXA9 fusion protein functions as an activated transcription factor that directly contributes to cellular transformation (187).

Only RT-PCR–based assays have been developed for the identification of these molecular lesions. However, identification of these lesions has not yet provided clinically useful information, and these tests remain investigational.

Another distinct molecular subgroup of AMLs are those with alteration at 3q26 that target the *EVI1* and fused *MDS1 EVI1* genes. EVI1 and MDS1-EVI1 are DNA-binding proteins that bind to a sequence that includes the binding site for GATA transcriptional activators. Functional studies suggest that these EVI1-containing proteins inhibit GATA-mediated transcriptional activation, but EVI1 and MDS1-EVI1 show subtle differences in their ability to repress in a promoter specific fashion. Normally, EVI1 is not expressed in hematopoietic tissue, but instead plays a critical role in the development of the peripheral nervous system and the heart (188,189). Expression of EVI1 is induced in hematopoietic cells as a result of a variety of leukemia-associated chromosomal rearrangements including the t(3;21) encoding an AML1-EVI1 or AML1-MDS1-EVI1 fusion protein (151), a t(3;12)(q26;p13) encoding a TEL-EVI1 or TEL-MDS1-EVI1 fusion protein (190,191), and a number of other leukemia-associated 3q26 rearrangements, including the inv(3)(q21;q26), t(3;3)(q21;q26), and insertions (3;3) (192–194). These latter rearrangements do not generate EVI1-containing fusion proteins but instead lead to the aberrant expression of wild-type EVI1. Abnormal EVI1 expression is also detected in rare cases of AML that lack any detectable alteration of chromosome 3q26 (194). In these latter cases, there appear to be alterations in sequences 5′ or 3′ of the *EVI1* genes, resulting in alterations in the pattern of expression of EVI1. The aberrant expression of EVI1 or the fused MDS1-EVI1 protein appears to result in the repression of normal GATA-mediated transcriptional activation. Leukemia appears to result, at least in part, from the inhibition of GATA-mediated signals that are required for normal hematopoietic cell differentiation. Although these leukemias have a common underlying mechanism, they do not represent a distinct therapeutic or prognostic group. Identification of these lesions is not required for the clinical management of these patients.

Summary of Diagnostic Testing and Future Perspective

The application of the molecular-based assays described previously is rapidly becoming a required part of the diagnostic workup of patients with acute leukemia. The results of these assays dictate the type of therapy to be used and provide prognostic information that can help a patient and their family to better cope with these diseases. Although traditional cytogenetics still remains the most commonly used method to detect these genetic lesions, it is rapidly being supplanted by molecular-based approaches. These latter assays have already proven to improve accuracy over that achieved with traditional chromosome banding analysis. In the near future, it is likely that they will also prove to be more cost effective.

The molecular lesions described previously account for only approximately one half of ALL and AML patients. The underlying molecular lesions in the other patients remain to be defined. Several experimental approaches have been developed to assist in the identification of these lesions. Spectral karyotyping (SKY), a global screening method developed to identify chromosomal rearrangements, has shown great promise (195). This is a modified FISH-based assay in which metaphase spreads are simultaneously hybridized with 24 chromosome-specific painting probes labeled with different combinations of fluorochromes. Measurement of the unique emission spectra of each chromosome allows assignment of a different color to each chromosome, greatly assisting the detection of rearrangements that are not visible by traditional banding methods. The application of SKY to ALL and AML cases with normal karyotypes, complex chromosomal rearrangements, or marker chromosomes should provide critical insights into the underlying pathogenesis in these cases. However, although SKY is an important complement to standard cytogenetics, it fails to detect chromosome rearrangements involving fewer than 1.5 Mb of DNA. Detection of small interstitial rearrangements or deletions requires alternative approaches such as loss of heterozygosity (LOH) analysis or FISH with well-defined, locus-specific probes.

MONITORING A PATIENT'S THERAPEUTIC RESPONSE

In treating ALL and AML, the goal of induction therapy is to achieve a complete remission (CR). This has traditionally been defined by the presence of less than 5% blasts within a bone marrow aspirate as assessed by morphology. Although this is a clinically useful definition, it fails to identify the substantial subset of patients in CR who subsequently relapse. This is in part thought to result from the relative insensitivity of morphology in detecting residual disease. Patients defined as being in CR based on the morphologic analysis of a single bone marrow aspirate may have no residual disease or may have as many as 10^{10} undetectable leukemic cells circulating within the body, and the predicted outcomes of patients at these two extremes probably are quite different. A working premise has been that, if we could use a more sensitive approach to detect the presence of so-called minimal residual disease (MRD), we could improve our ability to identify patients who will subsequently relapse. Many studies performed over the past several years have validated this concept (196,197). Through the application of a variety of different methods, including conventional and molecular-based cytogenetics, immunologic methods, and PCR-based assays, it has been shown that patients who lack evidence of disease by these sensitive approaches have a much lower incidence of relapse. Moreover, the reappearance of MRD in a patient after documented molecular remission is strongly correlated with impending relapse. Because of these results, molecular-based MRD assays are rapidly being added to the studies used to monitor leukemic patients during therapy.

PCR-based assays provide an exceptional level of sensitivity, being able to identify the presence of one leukemic cell in 10^5 to 10^6 normal cells. Because of this, PCR has moved to the forefront in the evaluation of MRD. For PCR-based studies to accurately measure the level of MRD, it is essential that the expression of the target sequence is limited to leukemia cells. Leukemia-specific targets that are used include chimeric transcripts encoded by chromosomal translocations and clone-specific Ig and T-cell receptor gene rearrangements (see Chapters 7 and 9). Because of the exceptionally high level of sensitivity inherent in PCR methods, it is essential to eliminate the possibility of sample cross-contamination. This requires close attention to techniques and to the separation of pre- and post-PCR reagents.

RT-PCR assays for translocation-encoded chimeric messages were described previously. Within an individual leukemia, the sequence of a translocation-encoded fusion transcript is stable over time and therefore provides a specific and constant marker for the identification of leukemic cells. The major limitation of this approach, however, is that specific chimeric transcripts only exist within the leukemic blasts of a minority of ALL and AML patients. Less than 50% of patients can be analyzed by this approach. In contrast, unique Ig or TCR gene rearrangements exist in more than 90% of ALL cases, regardless of the lineage of the lymphoblasts. The junctional regions of rearranged Ig and TCR genes are unique fingerprints of each leukemic clone and therefore are ideal targets for the specific and sensitive detection of leukemic blasts. Rearrangements of the Ig heavy-chain gene are seen in 80% to 90% of B-lineage ALLs, whereas TCR-β, -γ, and -δ rearrangements are found in up to 95% of T-lineage cases and a significant proportion of B-lineage cases (197). Amplification of the V-D-J junction region of rearranged IgH and TCR genes is accomplished by using V and J region consensus primers for the respective genes. The amplified products are then sequenced and a unique junction-specific probe is generated. This probe is then used to specifically detect the presence of the leukemia-specific rearrangement in subsequent samples from this patient. Two major limitations are inherent in this method. First, the approach is labor intensive, requiring the generation of a unique junction-specific probe for each patient. Second, Ig and TCR genes can continue to undergo rearrangements during the growth of the leukemic blasts. This process involves the continued rearrangement of V or J regions and results in the modification of the junction sequence so that it no longer hybridizes to the initial junction-specific probe. The clonal evolution of the leukemic population can result in false-negative results. The incidence of clonal evolution increases with time from diagnosis.

In ALL, most clinical studies have focused on the use of Ig and TCR gene rearrangements to detect MRD. These studies have shown that, after induction therapy, low or undetectable levels of MRD are highly predictive of a good outcome, whereas high levels of MRD tightly correlate with eventual relapse. The reappearance of MRD after a disease-free period is a strong predictor of impending relapse. However, the absence of MRD, so-called molecular remission, does not ensure that a patient is cured. False-negative results can result from clonal evolution. Moreover, MRD assays only screen a small fraction of the total marrow and therefore can miss the presence of minor levels of residual disease.

The MRD status of ALL patients has also been assessed using RT-PCR assays for translocation-encoded fusion messages. Extensive studies have been performed using a RT-PCR assay for BCR-ABL transcripts (198,199). These studies have shown that this transcript is rarely detectable in long-term disease survivors. In contrast, in patients treated with bone marrow transplantation, the reemergence of *BCR-ABL*–encoded mRNA is predictive of relapse. Frequently, this finding results in the initiation of additional therapy, including the use of donor lymphocytes that can induce a graft-versus-leukemia effect (200,201). Additional RT-PCR reactions that have been used to detect MRD include assays for *MLL-AF4, TEL-AML1, SIL-TAL,* and *E2A-PBX1*. Although there is usually a good correlation between the results obtained using Ig or TCR rearrangements and RT-PCR assays for chimeric messages, some differences have been observed. A low level of some of the chimeric transcripts can be detected in normal bone marrow, typically from elderly patients (202). This suggests that the simple presence of a chimeric transcript may not equate with persistent leukemia. This concept is consistent with experimental data for mice, in which expression of these chimeric genes is insufficient by themselves to induce leukemia. Moreover, detection of MRD by amplification of *E2A-PBX1* at the end of consolidation therapy failed to provide prognostic information (203). The reason for this remains to be determined. Although these data demonstrate that MRD studies can provide information that can alter the therapeutic approach for an individual patient with ALL, significant controversy still exists over the type of assay to use and the timing of analysis.

In AML, extensive studies have been done using RT-PCR assays for t(15;17)-encoded PML-RARα, t(8;21)-encoded

AML1-ETO, inv(16)-encoded CBFβ-MYH11, and a variety of MLL chimeric transcripts. In APL, RT-PCR negativity is now regarded as a goal in the clinical management of these patients (4). Persistence of PML-RARα after consolidation therapy is considered to be highly predictive of subsequent relapse, whereas repeated negative assays are associated with long-term disease-free survival in most patients. In contrast, testing earlier during therapy fails to provide prognostic information, because many cases that are positive at this time point eventually become PCR negative. The timing of MRD analysis appears critical in the analysis of APL patients. In core-binding factor leukemias, some studies have detected persistence of the AML1-ETO and CBF AML–MYH11 fusion transcripts in patients in clinical remission for up to 12 years (204–208). However, later studies demonstrated the absence of RT-PCR detectable disease in some patients, suggesting that eventual elimination of AML1-ETO–expressing cells is possible (209,210). The significance of a positive result in patients with core-binding factor leukemias remains to be defined. The possibility exists that these patients have persistence of a clone that contains the translocation that encodes the AML1 or CBFβ chimeric protein but lack cooperating mutations necessary for the development of the full leukemic phenotype. This possibility is supported by the data obtained from expression of these fusion proteins in murine experimental systems (165, 168,169). The data suggest that these patients may have a preleukemic clone that is incapable of producing leukemia. Treatment of these patients at this time may be ill advised in that it may not lead to the eradication of the clonal population but instead may induce secondary mutations that could result in the development of a fully leukemic population.

Although significant controversies exist over the type of assay to use, the time to perform the test, and the importance of a positive result, it is clear that PCR-based assays provide a powerful method to closely monitor a patients response to therapy. In some clinical settings, this information can provide critical prognostic information that can influence whether a change in therapy should be undertaken. One of the major limitations of PCR-based assays is their qualitative nature. Typically, they provide a positive or negative result but fail to define the relative level of disease present. Further improvements in the clinical value of MRD studies are likely to come through the development of quantitative assays that can accurately measure the level of disease present. This type of analysis can define the presence or absence of disease and permit assessment of the rate of disappearance of disease in response to therapy. This latter measurement has already been shown to be an important predictor of a patient's prognosis. Although a variety of semi-quantitative RT-PCR assays have been developed, most are labor intensive and are therefore not suitable for routine clinical applications. One promising approach is real-time PCR (Fig. 45.11) (211). In this approach, PCR amplification is carried out in the presence of a hybridization-specific oligonucleotide probe that contains a reporter fluorescence dye at the 5′ end and a quencher dye attached to the 3′ end. While the probe is intact, the quencher reduces the fluorescence emitted by the reporter dye. In contrast, during the extension phase of PCR, the 5′exonuclease activity of *Taq* DNA polymerase cleaves the probe, resulting in the release of the reporter dye and an increase in its signal intensity. The amount of signal generated is directly proportional to the amount of the amplicon produced. This approach provides a sensitive, reproducible, and quantitative measure of the level of MRD present. Moreover, real-time PCR uses a closed system so that the chance of sample cross-contamination is greatly reduced. In the future, it is likely that real-time PCR will become one of the standard approaches used for diagnosis and monitoring of patients during treatment.

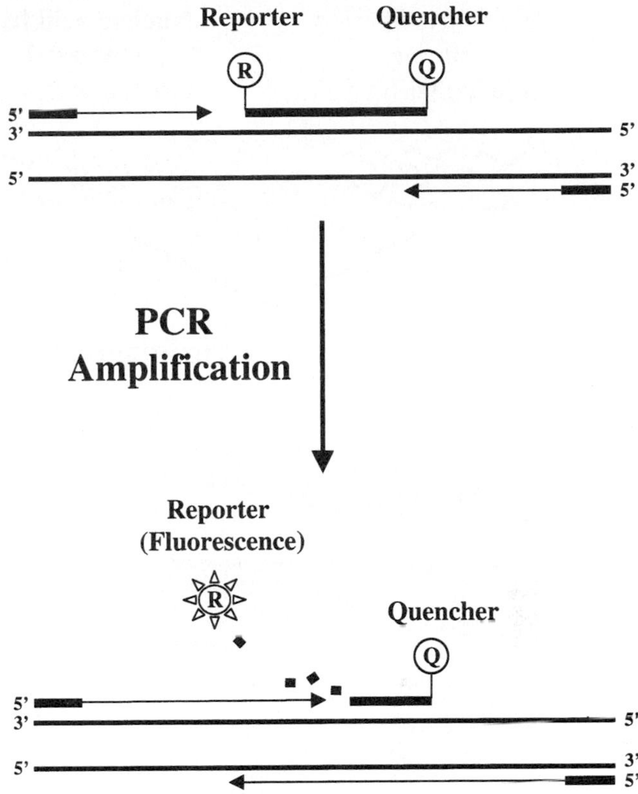

FIG. 45.11. Real-time quantitative polymerase chain reaction (PCR) using the TaqMan technology.

SUMMARY AND CONCLUSIONS

The human genome project has placed within reach the detailed characterization of each of the 70,000 to 100,000 human genes. Estimates have suggested that a working draft of the human DNA sequence will be completed sometime in 2000 (212). With this information in hand, we can begin the task of trying to understand at a genomic level the variability in leukemia phenotypes, a patient's response to therapy, and the risk of therapy-induced complications, including organ toxicity, infection, and secondary malignancies (213,214). Data that are likely to shed light on these issues

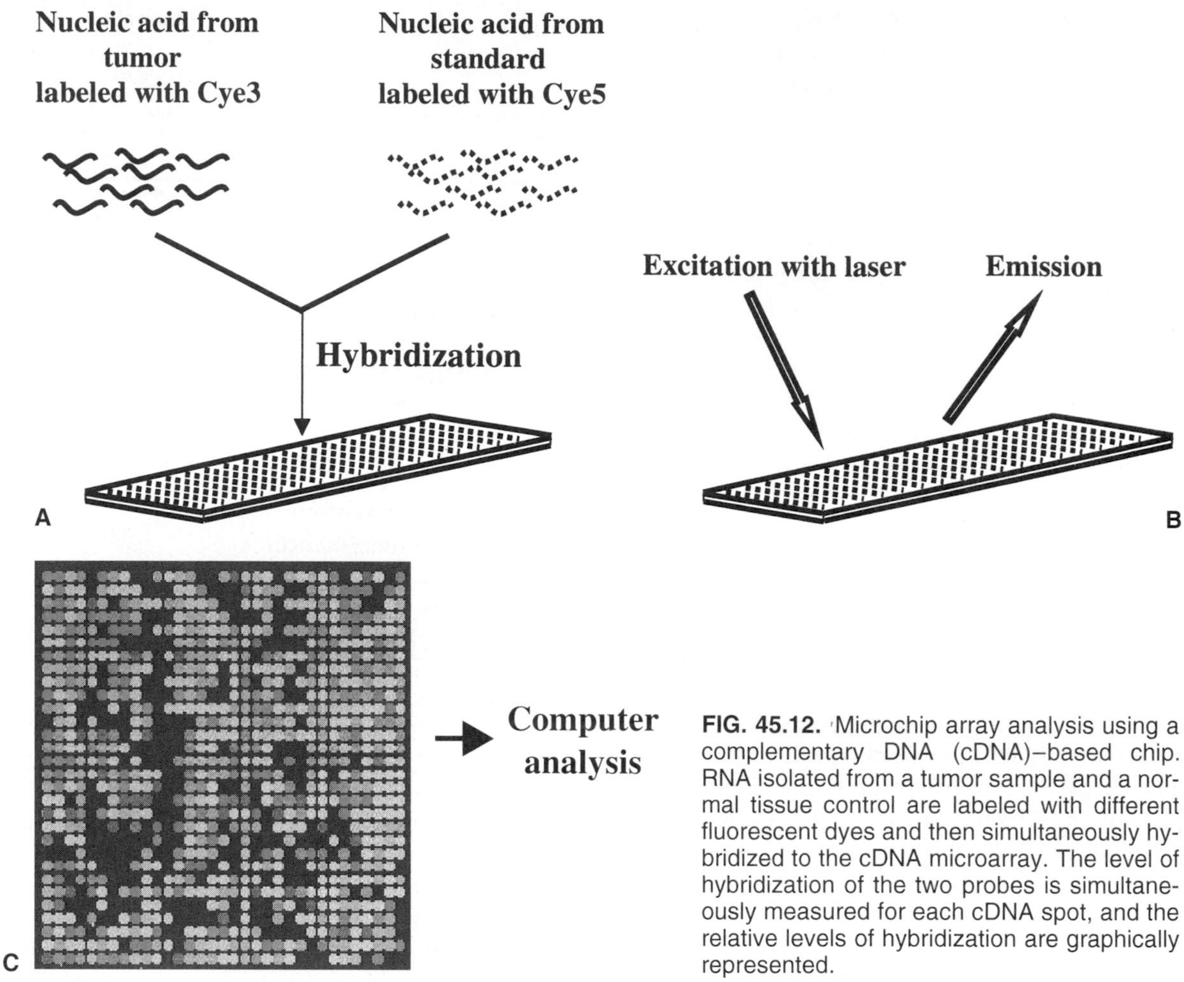

FIG. 45.12. Microchip array analysis using a complementary DNA (cDNA)–based chip. RNA isolated from a tumor sample and a normal tissue control are labeled with different fluorescent dyes and then simultaneously hybridized to the cDNA microarray. The level of hybridization of the two probes is simultaneously measured for each cDNA spot, and the relative levels of hybridization are graphically represented.

will include analysis of gene expression patterns within tumor samples, the detection of mutations within causative genes, and the identification of polymorphisms within genes that influence the response to therapeutic agents. The development of microarray technology has provided a platform for the rapid acquisition of this type of data across the entire genome (215). Microarrays have been developed for the simultaneous and quantitative measurement of the level of expression of the complete set of transcripts in a human tissue sample. An example of this approach is illustrated in Fig. 45.12. Similarly, microarray-based methods have been developed for the rapid detection of mutations and polymorphisms within a wide range of human genes and the genomes of infectious organisms (215). Microarray-based comparative genomic hybridization methods have significantly improved our ability to detect gene deletions or amplifications (216). Although these methods are extremely expensive, it is likely that minor modifications will allow them to rapidly find their way into the routine clinical laboratory. The application of these assays to patients with acute leukemia will revolutionize our ability to rationally individualize therapy so that each patient can be given the highest possible chance for a cure.

REFERENCES

1. Pui CH, Evans WE. Acute lymphoblastic leukemia. *N Engl J Med* 1998;339:605–615.
2. Burnett AK. Tailoring the treatment of acute myeloid leukemia. *Curr Opin Hematol* 1999;6:247–252.
3. Lowenberg B, Downing JR, Burnett A. Acute myeloid leukemia. *N Engl J Med* 1999;341:1051–1062.
4. Lo CF, Diverio D, Falini B, et al. Genetic diagnosis and molecular monitoring in the management of acute promyelocytic leukemia. *Blood* 1999;94:12–22.
5. Look AT. Oncogenic transcription factors in the human acute leukemias. *Science* 1997;278:1059–1064.
6. Baumforth KR, Nelson PN, Digby JE, et al. Demystified . . . the polymerase chain reaction. *Mol Pathol* 1999;52:1–10.
7. Nath J, Johnson KL. Fluorescence in situ hybridization (FISH): DNA probe production and hybridization criteria. *Biotech Histochem* 1998; 73:6–22.
8. Coad JE, Olson DJ, Lander TA, et al. Molecular assessment of clonality in lymphoproliferative disorders: I. Immunoglobulin gene rearrangements. *Mol Diagn* 1996;1:335–355.
9. Finiewicz KJ, Larson RA. Dose-intensive therapy for adult acute lymphoblastic leukemia. *Semin Oncol* 1999;26:6–20.
10. Nowell PC, Hungerford DA. A minute chromosome in human chronic granulocytic leukemia. *Science* 1960;132:1497.
11. Rowley JD. A new consistent chromosomal abnormality in chronic myelogenous leukaemia identified by quinacrine fluorescence and Giemsa staining [Letter]. *Nature* 1973;243:290–293.
12. Faderl S, Talpaz M, Estrov Z, et al. The biology of chronic myeloid leukemia. *N Engl J Med* 1999;341:164–172.

13. Uckun FM, Nachman JB, Sather HN, et al. Poor treatment outcome of Philadelphia chromosome–positive pediatric acute lymphoblastic leukemia despite intensive chemotherapy. *Leuk Lymphoma* 1999;33: 101–106.
14. Ribeiro RC, Broniscer A, Rivera GK, et al. Philadelphia chromosome–positive acute lymphoblastic leukemia in children: durable responses to chemotherapy associated with low initial white blood cell counts. *Leukemia* 1997;11:1493–1496.
15. de Klein A, van Kessel AG, Grosveld G, et al. A cellular oncogene is translocated to the Philadelphia chromosome in chronic myelocytic leukaemia. *Nature* 1982;300:765–767.
16. Groffen J, Stephenson JR, Heisterkamp N, et al. Philadelphia chromosomal breakpoints are clustered within a limited region, bcr, on chromosome 22. *Cell* 1984;36:93–99.
17. Heisterkamp N, Stam K, Groffen J, et al. Structural organization of the bcr gene and its role in the Ph^1 translocation. *Nature* 1985;315: 758–761.
18. Ben-Neriah Y, Daley GQ, Mes-Masson AM, et al. The chronic myelogenous leukemia-specific P210 protein is the product of the bcr/abl hybrid gene. *Science* 1986;233:212–214.
19. Clark SS, McLaughlin J, Crist WM, et al. Unique forms of the abl tyrosine kinase distinguish Ph1-positive CML from Ph1-positive ALL. *Science* 1987;235:85–88.
20. Fainstein E, Marcelle C, Rosner A, et al. A new fused transcript in Philadelphia chromosome positive acute lymphocytic leukaemia. *Nature* 1987;330:386–388.
21. Daley GQ, Van Etten RA, Baltimore D. Induction of chronic myelogenous leukemia in mice by the P210bcr/abl gene of the Philadelphia chromosome. *Science* 1990;247:824–830.
22. Heisterkamp N, Jenster G, ten Hoeve J, et al. Acute leukaemia in bcr/abl transgenic mice. *Nature* 1990;344:251–253.
23. Pear WS, Miller JP, Xu L, et al. Efficient and rapid induction of a chronic myelogenous leukemia-like myeloproliferative disease in mice receiving P210 bcr/abl-transduced bone marrow. *Blood* 1998; 92:3780–3792.
24. Wells SJ, Phillips CN, Farhi DC. Detection of bcr/abl in acute leukemia by molecular and cytogenetic methods. *Mol Diagn* 1996;1: 305–313.
25. Kawasaki ES, Clark SS, Coyne MY, et al. Diagnosis of chronic myeloid and acute lymphocytic leukemias by detection of leukemia-specific mRNA sequences amplified in vitro. *Proc Natl Acad Sci USA* 1988;85:5698–5702.
26. Cuneo A, Bigoni R, Emmanuel B, et al. Fluorescence in situ hybridization for the detection and monitoring of the Ph-positive clone in chronic myelogenous leukemia: comparison with metaphase banding analysis. *Leukemia* 1998;12:1718–1723.
27. Crist WM, Carroll AJ, Shuster JJ, et al. Poor prognosis of children with pre-B acute lymphoblastic leukemia is associated with the t(1; 19)(q23;p13): a Pediatric Oncology Group study. *Blood* 1990;76: 117–122.
28. Raimondi SC, Behm FG, Roberson PK, et al. Cytogenetics of pre-B-cell acute lymphoblastic leukemia with emphasis on prognostic implications of the t(1;19). *J Clin Oncol* 1990;8:1380–1388.
29. Hunger SP. Chromosomal translocations involving the E2A gene in acute lymphoblastic leukemia: clinical features and molecular pathogenesis. *Blood* 1996;87:1211–1224.
30. Kamps MP, Murre C, Sun XH, et al. A new homeobox gene contributes the DNA binding domain of the t(1;19) translocation protein in pre-B ALL. *Cell* 1990;60:547–555.
31. Nourse J, Mellentin JD, Galili N, et al. Chromosomal translocation t(1;19) results in synthesis of a homeobox fusion mRNA that codes for a potential chimeric transcription factor. *Cell* 1990;60:535–545.
32. Hunger SP, Galili N, Carroll AJ, et al. The t(1;19)(q23;p13) results in consistent fusion of E2A and PBX1 coding sequences in acute lymphoblastic leukemias. *Blood* 1991;77:687–693.
33. Lu Q, Kamps MP. Heterodimerization of Hox proteins with Pbx1 and oncoprotein E2a-Pbx1 generates unique DNA-binding specificities at nucleotides predicted to contact the N-terminal arm of the Hox homeodomain: demonstration of Hox-dependent targeting of E2a-Pbx1 in vivo. *Oncogene* 1997;14:75–83.
34. Chang CP, De Vivo I, Cleary ML. The Hox coooperativity motif of the chimeric oncoprotein E2a-Pbx1 is necessary and sufficient for oncogenesis. *Mol Cell Biol* 1997;17:81–88.
35. Selleri L, Jacobs Y, Choe S, et al. The Hox-cofactor PBX1 is required for normal development of proximal limb and axial skeleton and for spleen morphogenesis. *Blood* 1998;92[Suppl 1]:308(abst).
36. Hunger SP, Ohyashiki K, Toyama K, et al. Hlf, a novel hepatic bZIP protein, shows altered DNA-binding properties following fusion to E2A in t(17;19) acute lymphoblastic leukemia. *Genes Dev* 1992;6: 1608–1620.
37. Inaba T, Roberts WM, Shapiro LH, et al. Fusion of the leucine zipper gene HLF to the E2A gene in human acute B-lineage leukemia. *Science* 1992;257:531–534.
38. Look AT. E2A-HLF chimeric transcription factors in pro-B cell acute lymphoblastic leukemia. *Curr Top Microbiol Immunol* 1997;220: 45–53.
39. Inaba T, Inukai T, Yoshihara T, et al. Reversal of apoptosis by the leukaemia-associated E2A-HLF chimaeric transcription factor. *Nature* 1996;382:541–544.
40. Numata S, Kato K, Horibe K. New E2A/PBX1 fusion transcript in a patient with t(1;19)(q23;p13) acute lymphoblastic leukemia. *Leukemia* 1993;7:1441–1444.
41. Izraeli S, Kovar H, Gadner H, et al. Unexpected heterogeneity in E2A/PBX1 fusion messenger RNA detected by the polymerase chain reaction in pediatric patients with acute lymphoblastic leukemia. *Blood* 1992;80:1413–1417.
42. Kaneko Y, Maseki N, Takasaki N, et al. Clinical and hematologic characteristics in acute leukemia with 11q23 translocations. *Blood* 1986;67:484–491.
43. Rowley JD, Diaz MO, Espinosa R, et al. Mapping chromosome bank 11q23 in human acute leukemia with biotynylated probes: identification of 11q23 translocation breakpoints with a yeast artificial chromosome. *Proc Natl Acad Sci USA* 1990;87:9358–9362.
44. Ziemin-van dP, McCabe NR, Gill HJ, et al. Identification of a gene, MLL, that spans the breakpoint in 11q23 translocations associated with human leukemias [published erratum appears in *Proc Natl Acad Sci USA* 19921;89:4220]. *Proc Natl Acad Sci USA* 1991;88: 10735–10739.
45. Cimino G, Moir DT, Canaani O, et al. Cloning of ALL-1, the locus involved in leukemias with the t(4;11)(q21;q23), t(9;11)(p22;q23), and t(11;19)(q23;p13) chromosome translocations. *Cancer Res* 1991; 51:6712–6714.
46. Tkachuk DC, Kohler S, Cleary ML. Involvement of a homolog of *Drosophila* trithorax by 11q23 chromosomal translocations in acute leukemias. *Cell* 1992;71:691–700.
47. Gu Y, Nakamura T, Alder H, et al. The t(4;11) chromosome translocation of human acute leukemias fuses the ALL-1 gene, related to *Drosophila* trithorax, to the AF-4 gene. *Cell* 1992;71:701–708.
48. McCabe NR, Burnett RC, Gill HJ, et al. Cloning of cDNAs of the MLL gene that detect DNA rearrangements and altered RNA transcripts in human leukemic cells with 11q23 translocations. *Proc Natl Acad Sci USA* 1992;89:11794–11798.
49. Waring PM, Cleary ML. Disruption of a homolog of trithorax by 11q23 translocations: leukemogenic and transcriptional implications. *Curr Top Microbiol Immunol* 1997;220:1–23.
50. Yu BD, Hess JL, Horning SE, et al. Altered Hox expression and segmental identity in Mll-mutant mice. *Nature* 1995;378:505–508.
51. Cui X, De Vivo I, Slany R, et al. Association of SET domain and myotubularin-related proteins modulates growth control. *Nat Genet* 1998;18:331–337.
52. Hunter T. Anti-phosphatases take the stage. *Nat Genet* 1998;18: 303–305.
53. Pui CH, Frankel LS, Carroll AJ, et al. Clinical characteristics and treatment outcome of childhood acute lymphoblastic leukemia with the t(4;11)(q21;q23): a collaborative study of 40 cases. *Blood* 1991; 77:440–447.
54. Rubnitz JE, Behm FG, Downing JR. 11q23 rearrangements in acute leukemia. *Leukemia* 1996;10:74–82.
55. Stock W, Thirman MJ, Dodge RK, et al. Detection of MLL gene rearrangements in adult acute lymphoblastic leukemia: a Cancer and Leukemia Group B study. *Leukemia* 1994;8:1918–1922.
56. Thirman MJ, Gill HJ, Burnett RC, et al. Rearrangement of the MLL gene in acute lymphoblastic and acute myeloid leukemias with 11q23 chromosomal translocations. *N Engl J Med* 1993;329:909–914.
57. Downing JR, Head DR, Raimondi SC, et al. The der(11)-encoded MLL/AF-4 fusion transcript is consistently detected in t(4;11)(q21; q23)-containing acute lymphoblastic leukemia. *Blood* 1994;83: 330–335.

58. Hilden JM, Chen CS, Moore R, et al. Heterogeneity in MLL/AF-4 fusion messenger RNA detected by the polymerase chain reaction in t(4;11) acute leukemia. *Cancer Res* 1993;53:3853–3856.
59. Kobayashi H, Espinosa R, Thirman MJ, et al. Variability of 11q23 rearrangements in hematopoietic cell lines identified with fluorescence in situ hybridization. *Blood* 1993;81:3027–3033.
60. Kobayashi H, Espinosa R, Thirman MJ, et al. Heterogeneity of breakpoints of 11q23 rearrangements in hematologic malignancies identified with fluorescence in situ hybridization. *Blood* 1993;82:547–551.
61. Mathew S, Behm FG, Dalton J, et al. Comparison of cytogenetics, Southern blotting, and fluorescence in situ hybridization (FISH) as methods for detecting MLL gene rearrangements in children with acute leukemias and 11q23 abnormalities. *Leukemia* 1999;13: 1713–1720.
62. Rubnitz JE, Pui CH, Downing JR. The role of TEL fusion genes in pediatric leukemias. *Leukemia* 1999;13:6–13.
63. Golub TR, Barker GF, Lovett M, et al. Fusion of PDGF receptor beta to a novel ets-like gene, tel, in chronic myelomonocytic leukemia with t(5;12) chromosomal translocation. *Cell* 1994;77:307–316.
64. Golub TR, Barker GF, Bohlander SK, et al. Fusion of the TEL gene on 12p13 to the AML1 gene on 21q22 in acute lymphoblastic leukemia. *Proc Natl Acad Sci USA* 1995;92:4917–4921.
65. Romana SP, Mauchauffe M, Le Coniat M, et al. The t(12;21) of acute lymphoblastic leukemia results in a tel-AML1 gene fusion. *Blood* 1995;85:3662–3670.
66. Romana SP, Le Coniat M, Berger R. t(12;21): a new recurrent translocation in acute lymphoblastic leukemia. *Genes Chromosomes Cancer* 1994;9:186–191.
67. Romana SP, Poirel H, Leconiat M, et al. High frequency of t(12;21) in childhood B-lineage acute lymphoblastic leukemia. *Blood* 1995; 86:4263–4269.
68. Shurtleff SA, Buijs A, Behm FG, et al. TEL/AML1 fusion resulting from a cryptic t(12;21) is the most common genetic lesion in pediatric ALL and defines a subgroup of patients with an excellent prognosis. *Leukemia* 1995;9:1985–1989.
69. Raimondi SC, Shurtleff SA, Downing JR, et al. 12p abnormalities and the TEL gene (ETV6) in childhood acute lymphoblastic leukemia. *Blood* 1997;90:4559–4566.
70. Wang LC, Kuo F, Fujiwara Y, et al. Yolk sac angiogenic defect and intra-embryonic apoptosis in mice lacking the Ets-related factor TEL. *EMBO J* 1997;16:4374–4383.
71. Wang LC, Swat W, Fujiwara Y, et al. The TEL/ETV6 gene is required specifically for hematopoiesis in the bone marrow. *Genes Dev* 1998; 12:2392–2402.
72. Downing JR. The AML1-ETO chimaeric transcription factor in acute myeloid leukaemia: biology and clinical significance. *Br J Haematol* 1999;106:296–308.
73. Okuda T, van Deursen J, Hiebert SW, et al. AML1, the target of multiple chromosomal translocations in human leukemia, is essential for normal fetal liver hematopoiesis. *Cell* 1996;84:321–330.
74. Wang Q, Stacy T, Binder M, et al. Disruption of the Cbfa2 gene causes necrosis and hemorrhaging in the central nervous system and blocks definitive hematopoiesis. *Proc Natl Acad Sci USA* 1996;93: 3444–3449.
75. Hiebert SW, Sun W, Davis JN, et al. The t(12;21) translocation converts AML-1B from an activator to a repressor of transcription. *Mol Cell Biol* 1996;16:1349–1355.
76. Romana SP, Le Coniat M, Poirel H, et al. Deletion of the short arm of chromosome 12 is a secondary event in acute lymphoblastic leukemia with t(12;21). *Leukemia* 1996;10:167–170.
77. Scurto P, Hsu RM, Kane JR, et al. A multiplex RT-PCR assay for the detection of chimeric transcripts encoded by the risk-stratifying translocations of pediatric acute lymphoblastic leukemia. *Leukemia* 1998;12:1994–2005.
78. Viehmann S, Borkhardt A, Lampert F, et al. Multiplex PCR: a rapid screening method for detection of gene rearrangements in childhood acute lymphoblastic leukemia. *Ann Hematol* 1999;78:157–162.
79. Heid CA, Stevens J, Livak KJ, et al. Real time quantitative PCR. *Genome Res* 1996;6:986–994.
80. Wang T, Brown MJ. mRNA Quantification by real time TaqMan polymerase chain reaction: validation and comparison with RNase protection. *Anal Biochem* 1999;269:198–201.
81. Look AT, Roberson PK, Williams DL, et al. Prognostic importance of blast cell DNA content in childhood acute lymphoblastic leukemia. *Blood* 1985;65:1079–1086.
82. Harris MB, Shuster JJ, Carroll A, et al. Trisomy of leukemia cell chromosomes 4 and 10 identifies children with B-progenitor cell acute lymphoblastic leukemia with a very low risk of treatment failure: a Pediatric Oncology Group study. *Blood* 1992;79:3316–3324.
83. Whitehead VM, Vuchich MJ, Lauer SJ, et al. Accumulation of high levels of methotrexate polyglutamates in lymphoblasts from children with hyperdiploid (greater than 50 chromosomes) B-lineage acute lymphoblastic leukemia: a Pediatric Oncology Group study. *Blood* 1992;80:1316–1323.
84. Chessels JM, Swansbury GJ, Reeves B, et al. Cytogenetics and prognosis in childhood lymphoblastic leukaemia: results of MRC UKALL X. Medical Research Council Working Party in Childhood Leukaemia. *Br J Haematol* 1997;99:93–100.
85. Chambon-Pautas C, Cave H, Gerard B, et al. High-resolution allelotype analysis of childhood B-lineage acute lymphoblastic leukemia. *Leukemia* 1998;12:1107–1113.
86. Kaspers GJ, Smets LA, Pieters R, et al. Favorable prognosis of hyperdiploid common acute lymphoblastic leukemia may be explained by sensitivity to antimetabolites and other drugs: results of an in vitro study. *Blood* 1995;85:751–756.
87. Gaidano G, Pastore C, Volpe G. Molecular pathogenesis of non-Hodgkin lymphoma: a clinical perspective. *Haematologica* 1995;80: 454–472.
88. Adams JM, Harris AW, Pinkert CA, et al. The c-myc oncogene driven by immunoglobulin enhancers induces lymphoid malignancy in transgenic mice. *Nature* 1985;318:533–538.
89. Harris AW, Pinkert CA, Crawford M, et al. The E mu-myc transgenic mouse: a model for high-incidence spontaneous lymphoma and leukemia of early B cells. *J Exp Med* 1988;167:353–371.
90. Sidman CL, Denial TM, Marshall JD, et al. Multiple mechanisms of tumorigenesis in E mu-myc transgenic mice. *Cancer Res* 1993;53: 1665–1669.
91. Uckun FM, Sensel MG, Sun L, et al. Biology and treatment of childhood T-lineage acute lymphoblastic leukemia. *Blood* 1998;91: 735–746.
92. Baer R, Hwang LY, Bash RO. Transcription factors of the bHLH and LIM families: synergistic mediators of T cell acute leukemia? *Curr Top Microbiol Immunol* 1997;220:55–65.
93. Rabbitts TH. LMO T-cell translocation oncogenes typify genes activated by chromosomal translocations that alter transcription and developmental processes. *Genes Dev* 1998;12:2651–2657.
94. Chen Q, Cheng JT, Tasi LH, et al. The tal gene undergoes chromosome translocation in T cell leukemia and potentially encodes a helix-loop-helix protein. *EMBO J* 1990;9:415–424.
95. Brown L, Cheng JT, Chen Q, et al. Site-specific recombination of the tal-1 gene is a common occurrence in human T cell leukemia. *EMBO J* 1990;9:3343–3351.
96. Bash RO, Hall S, Timmons CF, et al. Does activation of the TAL1 gene occur in a majority of patients with T-cell acute lymphoblastic leukemia? A Pediatric Oncology Group study. *Blood* 1995;86: 666–676.
97. Boehm T, Baer R, Lavenir I, et al. The mechanism of chromosomal translocation t(11;14) involving the T-cell receptor C delta locus on human chromosome 14q11 and a transcribed region of chromosome 11p15. *EMBO J* 1988;7:385–394.
98. McGuire EA, Hockett RD, Pollock KM, et al. The t(11;14)(p15;q11) in a T-cell acute lymphoblastic leukemia cell line activates multiple transcripts, including Ttg-1, a gene encoding a potential zinc finger protein. *Mol Cell Biol* 1989;9:2124–2132.
99. Royer-Pokora B, Loos U, Ludwig WD. TTG-2, a new gene encoding a cysteine-rich protein with the LIM motif, is overexpressed in acute T-cell leukaemia with the t(11;14)(p13;q11). *Oncogene* 1991;6: 1887–1893.
100. Warren AJ, Colledge WH, Carlton MB, et al. The oncogenic cysteine-rich LIM domain protein rbtn2 is essential for erythroid development. *Cell* 1994;78:45–57.
101. Porcher C, Wojciech S, Rockwell K, et al. The T cell leukemia oncoprotein SCl/tal-1 is essential for development of all hematopoietic lineages. *Cell* 1996;86:47–57.
102. Wadman I, Li J, Bash RO, et al. Specific in vivo association between the bHLH and LIM proteins implicated in human T cell leukemia. *EMBO J* 1994;13:4831–4839.

103. Valge-Archer VE, Osada H, Warren AJ, et al. The LIM protein RBTN2 and the basic helix-loop-helix protein TAL1 are present in a complex in erythroid cells. *Proc Natl Acad Sci USA* 1994;91: 8617–8621.
104. Drexler HG. Review of alterations of the cyclin-dependent kinase inhibitor INK4 family genes p15, p16, p18 and p19 in human leukemia-lymphoma cells. *Leukemia* 1998;12:845–859.
105. Yamada Y, Hatta Y, Murata K, et al. Deletions of p15 and/or p16 genes as a poor-prognosis factor in adult T-cell leukemia. *J Clin Oncol* 1997;15:1778–1785.
106. Batova A, Diccianni MB, Yu JC, et al. Frequent and selective methylation of p15 and deletion of both p15 and p16 in T-cell acute lymphoblastic leukemia. *Cancer Res* 1997;57:832–836.
107. Cayuela JM, Madani A, Sanhes L, et al. Multiple tumor-suppressor gene 1 inactivation is the most frequent genetic alteration in T-cell acute lymphoblastic leukemia. *Blood* 1996;87:2180–2186.
108. Sharpless NE, DePinho RA. The INK4A/ARF locus and its two gene products. *Curr Opin Genet Dev* 1999;9:22–30.
109. Sherr CJ, Roberts JM. CDK inhibitors: positive and negative regulators of G_1-phase progression. *Genes Dev* 1999;13:1501–1512.
110. Okuda T, Shurtleff SA, Valentine MB, et al. Frequent deletion of p16INK4a/MTS1 and p15INK4b/MTS2 in pediatric acute lymphoblastic leukemia. *Blood* 1995;85:2321–2330.
111. Rubnitz JE, Behm FG, Pui CH, et al. Genetic studies of childhood acute lymphoblastic leukemia with emphasis on p16, MLL, and ETV6 gene abnormalities: results of St Jude Total Therapy Study XII. *Leukemia* 1997;11:1201–1206.
112. Hayette S, Thomas X, Bertrand Y, et al. Molecular analysis of cyclin-dependent kinase inhibitors in human leukemias. *Leukemia* 1997;11: 1696–1699.
113. Heaney ML, Golde DW. Myelodysplasia. *N Engl J Med* 1999;340: 1649–1660.
114. Estey E, Thall P, Beran M, et al. Effect of diagnosis (refractory anemia with excess blasts, refractory anemia with excess blasts in transformation, or acute myeloid leukemia [AML]) on outcome of AML-type chemotherapy. *Blood* 1997;90:2969–2977.
115. Nevill TJ, Fung HC, Shepherd JD, et al. Cytogenetic abnormalities in primary myelodysplastic syndrome are highly predictive of outcome after allogeneic bone marrow transplantation. *Blood* 1998;92: 1910–1917.
116. Grimwade D, Walker H, Oliver F, et al. The importance of diagnostic cytogenetics on outcome in AML: analysis of 1,612 patients enrolled into the MRC AML 10 trial. *Blood* 1998;92:2322–2333.
117. Bloomfield CD, Lawrence D, Byrd JC, et al. Frequency of prolonged remission duration after high-dose cytarabine intensification in acute myeloid leukemia varies by cytogenetic subtype. *Cancer Res* 1998; 58:4173–4179.
118. Bloomfield CD, Shuma C, Regal L, et al. Long-term survival of patients with acute myeloid leukemia: a third follow-up of the Fourth International Workshop on Chromosomes in Leukemia. *Cancer* 1997; 80:2191–2198.
119. Chambon P. A decade of molecular biology of retinoic acid receptors. *FASEB J* 1996;10:940–954.
120. Borden KL, Boddy MN, Lally J, et al. The solution structure of the RING finger domain from the acute promyelocytic leukaemia proto-oncoprotein PML. *EMBO J* 1995;14:1532–1541.
121. Weis K, Rambaud S, Lavau C, et al. Retinoic acid regulates aberrant nuclear localization of PML-RAR alpha in acute promyelocytic leukemia cells. *Cell* 1994;76:345–356.
122. Dyck JA, Maul GG, Miller WH, et al. A novel macromolecular structure is a target of the promyelocyte-retinoic acid receptor oncoprotein. *Cell* 1994;76:333–343.
123. Wang ZG, Delva L, Gaboli M, et al. Role of PML in cell growth and the retinoic acid pathway. *Science* 1998;279:1547–1551.
124. de The H, Lavau C, Marchio A, et al. The PML-RAR alpha fusion mRNA generated by the t(15;17) translocation in acute promyelocytic leukemia encodes a functionally altered RAR. *Cell* 1991;66:675–684.
125. Kakizuka A, Miller WHJ, Umesono K, et al. Chromosomal translocation t(15;17) in human acute promyelocytic leukemia fuses RAR alpha with a novel putative transcription factor, PML. *Cell* 1991;66: 663–674.
126. Grignani F, De Matteis S, Nervi C, et al. Fusion proteins of the retinoic acid receptor-alpha recruit histone deacetylase in promyelocytic leukaemia. *Nature* 1998;391:815–818.
127. Lin RJ, Nagy L, Inoue S, et al. Role of the histone deacetylase complex in acute promyelocytic leukaemia. *Nature* 1998;391:811–814.
128. He LZ, Guidez F, Tribioli C, et al. Distinct interactions of PML-RARalpha and PLZF-RARalpha with co-repressors determine differential responses to RA in APL. *Nat Genet* 1998;18:126–135.
129. Raelson JV, Nervi C, Rosenauer A, et al. The PML/RAR alpha oncoprotein is a direct molecular target of retinoic acid in acute promyelocytic leukemia cells. *Blood* 1996;88:2826–2832.
130. Hong SH, David G, Wong CW, et al. SMRT corepressor interacts with PLZF and with the PML-retinoic acid receptor alpha (RARalpha) and PLZF-RARalpha oncoproteins associated with acute promyelocytic leukemia. *Proc Natl Acad Sci USA* 1997;94:9028–9033.
131. Koken MHM, Puvion-Dutilleul F, Guillemin MC, et al. The t(15;17) translocation alters a nuclear body in a retinoic acid-reversible fashion. *EMBO J* 1994;13:1073–1083.
132. Shao W, Fanelli M, Ferrara FF, et al. Arsenic trioxide as an inducer of apoptosis and loss of PML/RAR alpha protein in acute promyelocytic leukemia cells. *J Natl Cancer Inst* 1998;90:124–133.
133. Chen GQ, Zhu J, Shi XG, et al. In vitro studies on cellular and molecular mechanisms of arsenic trioxide (As_2O_3) in the treatment of acute promyelocytic leukemia: As_2O_3 induces NB4 cell apoptosis with downregulation of Bcl-2 expression and modulation of PML-RAR alpha/PML proteins. *Blood* 1996;88:1052–1061.
134. Zhu J, Koken MH, Quignon F, et al. Arsenic-induced PML targeting onto nuclear bodies: implications for the treatment of acute promyelocytic leukemia. *Proc Natl Acad Sci USA* 1997;94:3978–3983.
135. Look AT. Arsenic and apoptosis in the treatment of acute promyelocytic leukemia. *J Natl Cancer Inst* 1998;90:86–88.
136. Conrad ME. Treatment of acute promyelocytic leukemia with arsenic trioxide. *N Engl J Med* 1999;340:1043–1045.
137. Gallagher RE, Willman CL, Slack JL, et al. Association of PML-RAR alpha fusion mRNA type with pretreatment hematologic characteristics but not treatment outcome in acute promyelocytic leukemia: an intergroup molecular study. *Blood* 1997;90:1656–1663.
138. Redner RL, Rush EA, Faas S, et al. The t(5;17) variant of acute promyelocytic leukemia expresses a nucleophosmin-retinoic acid receptor fusion. *Blood* 1996;87:882–886.
139. Chen Z, Brand NJ, Chen A, et al. Fusion between a novel Kruppel-like zinc finger gene and the retinoic acid receptor-alpha locus due to a variant t(11;17) translocation associated with acute promyelocytic leukaemia. *EMBO J* 1993;12:1161–1167.
140. Collins SJ. Acute promyelocytic leukemia: relieving repression induces remission. *Blood* 1998;91:2631–2633.
141. Speck NA, Stacy T, Wang Q, et al. Core-binding factor: a central player in hematopoiesis and leukemia. *Cancer Res* 1999;59: 1789s–1793s.
142. Miyoshi H, Shimizu K, Kozu T, et al. t(8;21) breakpoints on chromosome 21 in acute myeloid leukemia are clustered within a limited region of a single gene, AML1. *Proc Natl Acad Sci USA* 1991;88: 10431–10434.
143. Erickson P, Gao J, Chang KS, et al. Identification of breakpoints in t(8; 21) acute myelogenous leukemia and isolation of a fusion transcript, AML1/ETO, with similarity to *Drosophila* segmentation gene, runt. *Blood* 1992;80:1825–1831.
144. Nisson PE, Watkins PC, Sacchi N. Transcriptionally active chimeric gene derived from the fusion of the AML1 gene and a novel gene on chromosome 8 in t(8;21) leukemic cells [published erratum appears in *Cancer Genet Cytogenet* 1993;66:81]. *Cancer Genet Cytogenet* 1992;63:81 88.
145. Miyoshi H, Kozu T, Shimizu K, et al. The t(8;21) translocation in acute myeloid leukemia results in production of an AML1-MTG8 fusion transcript. *EMBO J* 1993;12:2715–2721.
146. Liu P, Tarle SA, Hajra A, et al. Fusion between transcription factor CBF beta/PEBP2 beta and a myosin heavy chain in acute myeloid leukemia. *Science* 1993;261:1041–1044.
147. Ferrant A, Labopin M, Frassoni F, et al. Karyotype in acute myeloblastic leukemia: prognostic significance for bone marrow transplantation in first remission. A European Group for Blood and Marrow Transplantation study. Acute Leukemia Working Party of the European Group for Blood and Marrow Transplantation (EBMT). *Blood* 1997; 90:2931–2938.
148. Wang Q, Stacy T, Miller JD, et al. The CBFbeta subunit is essential for CBFalpha2 (AML1) function in vivo. *Cell* 1996;87:697–708.
149. Sasaki K, Yagi H, Bronson RT, et al. Absence of fetal liver hematopoi-

esis in mice deficient in transcriptional coactivator core binding factor beta. *Proc Natl Acad Sci USA* 1996;93:12359–12363.
150. Gamou T, Kitamura E, Hosoda F, et al. The partner gene of AML1 in t(16;21) myeloid malignancies is a novel member of the MTG8 (ETO) family. *Blood* 1998;91:4028–4037.
151. Nucifora G, Rowley JD. AML1 and the 8;21 and 3;21 translocations in acute and chronic myeloid leukemia. *Blood* 1995;86:1–14.
152. Roulston D, Espinosa R, Nucifora G, et al. CBFA2(AML1) translocations with novel partner chromosomes in myeloid leukemias: association with prior therapy. *Blood* 1998;92:2879–2885.
153. Wotton D, Ghysdael J, Wang S, et al. Cooperative binding of Ets-1 and core binding factor to DNA. *Mol Cell Biol* 1994;14:840–850.
154. Hernandez-Munain C, Krangel MS. c-Myb and core-binding factor/PEBP2 display functional synergy but bind independently to adjacent sites in the T-cell receptor delta enhancer [published erratum appears in *Mol Cell Biol* 1995;15:4659]. *Mol Cell Biol* 1995;15:3090–3099.
155. Zhang DE, Hohaus S, Voso MT, et al. Function of PU.1 (Spi-1), C/EBP, and AML1 in early myelopoiesis: regulation of multiple myeloid CSF receptor promoters. *Curr Top Microbiol Immunol* 1996;211:137–147.
156. Britos-Bray M, Friedman AD. Core binding factor cannot synergistically activate the myeloperoxidase proximal enhancer in immature myeloid cells without c-Myb. *Mol Cell Biol* 1997;17:5127–5135.
157. Erman B, Cortes M, Nikolajczyk BS, et al. ETS-core binding factor: a common composite motif in antigen receptor gene enhancers. *Mol Cell Biol* 1998;18:1322–1330.
158. Berger R, Bernheim A, Daniel MT, et al. Cytologic characterization and significance of normal karyotypes in t(8;21) acute myeloblastic leukemia. *Blood* 1982;59:171–178.
159. Meyers S, Lenny N, Hiebert SW. The t(8;21) fusion protein interferes with AML-1B-dependent transcriptional activation. *Mol Cell Biol* 1995;1974:
160. Wang J, Hoshino T, Redner RL, et al. Novel human nuclear receptor co-repressor: cloning and identification as a binding partner for the ETO proto-oncoprotein. *Blood* 1997;90:244a(abst).
161. Lutterbach B, Westendorf JJ, Linggi B, et al. ETO, a target of t(8;21) in acute leukemia, interacts with the N-CoR and mSin3 corepressors. *Mol Cell Biol* 1998;18:7176–7184.
162. Gelmetti V, Zhang J, Fanelli M, et al. Aberrant recruitment of the nuclear receptor corepressor-histone deacetylase complex by the acute myeloid leukemia fusion partner ETO. *Mol Cell Biol* 1998;18:7185–7191.
163. Wang J, Hoshino T, Redner RL, et al. ETO, fusion partner in t(8;21) acute myeloid leukemia, represses transcription by interaction with the human N-CoR/mSin3/HDAC1 complex. *Proc Natl Acad Sci USA* 1998;95:10860–10865.
164. Yergeau DA, Hetherington CJ, Wang Q, et al. Embryonic lethality and impairment of haematopoiesis in mice heterozygous for an AML1-ETO fusion gene. *Nat Genet* 1997;15:303–306.
165. Okuda T, Cai Z, Yang S, et al. Expression of a knocked-In AML1-ETO leukemia gene inhibits the establishment of normal definitive hematopoiesis and directly generates dysplastic hematopoietic progenitors. *Blood* 1998;91:3134–3143.
166. Prasad R, Zhadanov AB, Sedkov Y, et al. Structure and expression pattern of human ALR, a novel gene with strong homology to ALL-1 involved in acute leukemia and to *Drosophila* trithorax. *Oncogene* 1997;15:549–560.
167. Shurtleff SA, Meyers S, Hiebert SW, et al. Heterogeneity in CBF beta/MYH11 fusion messages encoded by the inv(16)(p13q22) and the t(16;16)(p13;q22) in acute myelogenous leukemia. *Blood* 1995;85:3695–3703.
168. Castilla LH, Wijmenga C, Wang Q, et al. Failure of embryonic hematopoiesis and lethal hemorrhages in mouse embryos heterozygous for a knocked-in leukemia gene CBFB-MYH11. *Cell* 1996;87:687–696.
169. Castilla LH, Garrett L, Adya N, et al. The fusion gene cbfb-MYH11 blocks myeloid differentiation and predisposes mice to acute myelomonocytic leukaemia. *Nat Genet* 1999;23:144–146.
170. Downing JR, Head DR, Curcio-Brint AM, et al. An AML1/ETO fusion transcript is consistently detected by RNA-based polymerase chain reaction in acute myelogenous leukemia containing the (8;21)(q22;q22) translocation. *Blood* 1993;81:2860–2865.
171. Barragan E, Bonanad S, Lopez JA, et al. Comparison of two reverse transcription–polymerase chain reaction methods for detection of AML1/ETO rearrangement in the M2 subtype of acute myeloid leukaemia. *Clin Chem Lab Med* 1998;36:137–142.
172. Harrison CJ, Radford-Weiss I, Ross F, et al. Fluorescence in situ hybridization analysis of masked (8;21)(q22;q22) translocations. *Cancer Genet Cytogenet* 1999;112:15–20.
173. Ritter M, Thiede C, Schakel U, et al. Underestimation of inversion (16) in acute myeloid leukaemia using standard cytogenetics as compared with polymerase chain reaction: results of a prospective investigation. *Br J Haematol* 1997;98:969–972.
174. Dauwerse HG, Smit EM, Giles RH, et al. Two-colour FISH detection of the inv(16) in interphase nuclei of patients with acute myeloid leukaemia. *Br J Haematol* 1999;106:111–114.
175. Viswanatha DS, Chen I, Liu PP, et al. Characterization and use of an antibody detecting the CBFbeta-SMMHC fusion protein in inv(16)/t(16;16)-associated acute myeloid leukemias. *Blood* 1998;91:1882–1890.
176. Raimondi SC, Peiper SC, Kitchingman GR, et al. Childhood acute lymphoblastic leukemia with chromosomal breakpoints at 11q23. *Blood* 1989;73:1627–1634.
177. Pui CH, Behm FG, Raimondi SC, et al. Secondary acute myeloid leukemia in children treated for acute lymphoid leukemia [see comments]. *N Engl J Med* 1989;321:136–142.
178. Pui CH, Ribeiro RC, Hancock ML, et al. Acute myeloid leukemia in children treated with epipodophyllotoxins for acute lymphoblastic leukemia. *N Engl J Med* 1991;325:1682–1687.
179. Schichman SA, Caligiuri MA, Strout MP, et al. ALL-1 tandem duplication in acute myeloid leukemia with a normal karyotype involves homologous recombination between Alu elements. *Cancer Res* 1994;54:4277–4280.
180. Soekarman D, Von Lindern M, Daenen S, et al. The translocation (6;9) (p23;q34) shows consistent rearrangement of two genes and defines a myeloproliferative disorder with specific clinical features. *Blood* 1992;79:2990–2997.
181. Von Lindern M, Poustka A, Lerach H, Grosveld G. The (6;9) chromosome translocation, associated with a specific subtype of acute nonlymphocytic leukemia, leads to aberrant transcription of a target gene on 9q34. *Mol Cell Biol* 1990;10:4016–4026.
182. Fu GK, Grosveld G, Markovitz DM. DEK, an autoantigen involved in a chromosomal translocation in acute myelogenous leukemia, binds to the HIV-2 enhancer. *Proc Natl Acad Sci USA* 1997;94:1811–1815.
183. van Deursen J, Boer J, Kasper L, et al. G2 arrest and impaired nucleocytoplasmic transport in mouse embryos lacking the proto-oncogene CAN/Nup214. *EMBO J* 1996;15:5574–5583.
184. Boer J, Bonten-Surtel J, Grosveld G. Overexpression of the nucleoporin CAN/NUP214 induces growth arrest, nucleocytoplasmic transport defects, and apoptosis. *Mol Cell Biol* 1998;18:1236–1247.
185. Rout MP, Blobel G. Isolation of the yeast nuclear pore complex. *J Cell Biol* 1993;123:771–783.
186. Borrow J, Shearman AM, Stanton VPJ, et al. The t(7;11)(p15;p15) translocation in acute myeloid leukaemia fuses the genes for nucleoporin NUP98 and class I homeoprotein HOXA9. *Nat Genet* 1996;12:159–167.
187. van Deursen J, Kasper LH, Pritchard C, et al. The oncogenic properties of the NUP98-HOXA9 fusion protein: nucleoporin-specific FG repeats as well as the HOXA9 homeodomain and PBCX interaction motif are essential. *Blood* 1997;90:324a(abst).
188. Morishita K, Parganas E, Parham DM, et al. The Evi-1 zinc finger myeloid transforming gene is normally expressed in the kidney and in developing oocytes. *Oncogene* 1990;5:1419–1423.
189. Hoyt PR, Bartholomew C, Davis AJ, et al. The EVI1 proto-oncogene is required at midgestation for neural, heart, and paraxial mesenchyme development. *Mech Dev* 1997;65:55–70.
190. Raynaud SD, Baens M, Grosgeorge J, et al. Fluorescence in situ hybridization analysis of t(3;12)(q26;13): a recurring chromosomal abnormality involving the TEL gene (ETV6) in myelodysplastic syndromes. *Blood* 1996;88:682–689.
191. Peeters P, Wlodarska I, Baens M, et al. Fusion of ETV6 to MDS1/EVI1 as a result of t(3;12)(q26;p13) in myeloproliferative disorders. *Cancer Res* 1997;57:564–569.
192. Morishita K, Parganas E, William CL, et al. Activation of EVI1 gene expression in human acute myelogenous leukemias by translocations spanning 300-400 kilobases on chromosome ban 3q26. *Proc Natl Acad Sci USA* 1992;89:3937–3941.
193. Levy ER, Parganas E, Morishita K, et al. DNA rearrangements proxi-

mal to the EVI1 locus associated with the 3q21q26 syndrome. *Blood* 1994;83:1348–1354.
194. Russell M, List A, Greenberg P, et al. Expression of EVI1 in myelodysplastic syndromes and other hematologic malignancies without 3q26 translocations. *Blood* 1994;84:1243–1248.
195. Schrock E, Veldman T, Padilla-Nash H, et al. Spectral karyotyping refines cytogenetic diagnostics of constitutional chromosomal abnormalities. *Hum Genet* 1997;101:255–262.
196. Campana D, Jacques JM, van Dongen JM, et al. Minimal residual disease. In: Pui CH, ed. *Childhood leukemias.* New York: Cambridge University Press, 1999:413–439.
197. Negrin RS. Minimal residual disease. *Curr Opin Hematol* 1998;5: 488–493.
198. Cross NC. Minimal residual disease in chronic myeloid leukaemia. *Hematol Cell Ther* 1998;40:224–228.
199. Faderl S, Talpaz M, Kantarjian HM, et al. Should polymerase chain reaction analysis to detect minimal residual disease in patients with chronic myelogenous leukemia be used in clinical decision making? *Blood* 1999;93:2755–2759.
200. Falkenburg JH, Wafelman AR, Joosten P, et al. Complete remission of accelerated phase chronic myeloid leukemia by treatment with leukemia-reactive cytotoxic T lymphocytes. *Blood* 1999;94:1201–1208.
201. Falkenburg JH, Smit WM, Willemze R. Cytotoxic T-lymphocyte (CTL) responses against acute or chronic myeloid leukemia. *Immunol Rev* 1997;157:223–230.
202. Bose S, Deininger M, Gora-Tybor J, et al. The presence of typical and atypical BCR-ABL fusion genes in leukocytes of normal individuals: biologic significance and implications for the assessment of minimal residual disease. *Blood* 1998;92:3362–3367.
203. Hunger SP, Fall MZ, Camitta BM, et al. E2A-PBX1 chimeric transcript status at end of consolidation is not predictive of treatment outcome in childhood acute lymphoblastic leukemias with a t(1; 19)(q23;p13): a Pediatric Oncology Group study. *Blood* 1998;91: 1021–1028.
204. Nucifora G, Larson RA, Rowley JD. Persistence of the 8;21 translocation in patients with acute myeloid leukemia type M2 in long-term remission. *Blood* 1993;82:712–715.
205. Guerrasio A, Rosso C, Martinelli G, et al. Polyclonal haemopoieses associated with long-term persistence of the AML1-ETO transcript in patients with FAB M2 acute myeloid leukaemia in continuous clinical remission. *Br J Haematol* 1995;90:364–368.
206. Saunders MJ, Tobal K, Keeney S, et al. Expression of diverse AML1/MTG8 transcripts is a consistent feature in acute myeloid leukemia with t(8;21) irrespective of disease phase. *Leukemia* 1996;10: 1139–1142.
207. Jurlander J, Caligiuri MA, Ruutu T, et al. Persistence of the AML1/ETO fusion transcript in patients treated with allogeneic bone marrow transplantation for t(8;21) leukemia. *Blood* 1996;88:2183–2191.
208. Miyamoto T, Nagafuji K, Akashi K, et al. Persistence of multipotent progenitors expressing AML1/ETO transcripts in long-term remission patients with t(8;21) acute myelogenous leukemia. *Blood* 1996;87: 4789–4796.
209. Satake N, Maseki N, Kozu T, et al. Disappearance of AML1-MTG8(ETO) fusion transcript in acute myeloid leukaemia patients with t(8;21) in long-term remission. *Br J Haematol* 1995;91:892–898.
210. Preudhomme C, Philippe N, Macintyre E, et al. Persistence of AML1/ETO fusion mRNA in t(8;21) acute myeloid leukemia (AML) in prolonged remission: is there a consensus? *Leukemia* 1996;10:186–188.
211. Mensink E, van de Locht A, Schattenberg A, et al. Quantitation of minimal residual disease in Philadelphia chromosome positive chronic myeloid leukaemia patients using real-time quantitative RT-PCR. *Br J Haematol* 1998;102:768–774.
212. Collins FS. Shattuck lecture: medical and societal consequences of the Human Genome Project. *N Engl J Med* 1999;341:28–37.
213. Evans WE, Relling MV. Pharmacogenomics: translating functional genomics into rational therapeutics. *Science* 1999;286:487–491.
214. Golub TR, Slonim D, Tamayo P, et al. Molecular classification of cancer: class discovery and class prediction by gene expression monitoring. *Science* 1999;286:531–537.
215. The chipping forecast. *Nat Genet* 1999;21:1–56.
216. Pollack JR, Perou CM, Alizadeh AA, et al. Genome-wide analysis of DNA copy-number changes using cDNA microarrays. *Nat Genet* 1999;23:41–46.

CHAPTER 46

Acute Lymphoblastic Leukemia

Michael J. Borowitz and Joseph A. DiGiuseppe

Acute lymphoid leukemia (ALL) is a malignant bone marrow disease of lymphocyte precursors. In hematology parlance, these precursors often are referred to as *blasts*, and ALL sometimes is called *acute lymphoblastic leukemia*; these two terms are interchangeable. Although ALL superficially resembles acute myeloid leukemia (AML), and hybrid lymphoid and myeloid leukemias exist, in general the clinical and biologic features of the two diseases are sufficiently distinct to warrant separate discussion.

Acute lymphoblastic leukemia is the most common malignancy in childhood. It accounts for about 80% of cases of acute leukemia in childhood but only about 20% of adult cases. In developed Western nations, the incidence of ALL reaches a peak between ages 2 and 10 years, declines progressively to about age 55 years, and then rises slowly throughout the remainder of life (1). In childhood, the incidence is lower in underdeveloped nations and in Asia, and it is lower among American blacks than whites. Many of these differences can be attributed to a relative underrepresentation of the "common ALL" form of the disease in nonwhites (2).

Little is known about the cause of ALL; indeed, many of the data concerning environmental factors and leukemia have focused on AML, for which much better data are available. Ionizing radiation clearly has been shown to increase the incidence of ALL, particularly among those exposed *in utero* or at an early age (1,3). Genetic predisposition is indicated not only from the racial data but also from the known association with genetic diseases such as Down's syndrome and ataxia telangiectasia (4–7). A sibling of a monozygotic twin who has ALL has a several hundred times increased risk of developing the disease (8).

M. J. Borowitz: Department of Pathology, Johns Hopkins Medical Institutions, Baltimore, Maryland 21287-6417

J. A. DiGiuseppe: Department of Pathology and Laboratory Medicine, Hartford Hospital, Hartford, Connecticut 06102-5037

CLINICAL AND LABORATORY FEATURES

Clinical features of ALL at presentation can be related directly to the replacement of normal bone marrow elements by neoplastic cells. Pallor, weakness, and lassitude attributable to anemia are the most common presenting features, and bleeding in the form of petechial hemorrhage frequently accompanies thrombocytopenia. Bone pain is a common complaint, especially in children, and is related to massive marrow infiltration with leukemic cells. Fever is present in more than one half of patients, but despite granulocytopenia, bacterial infection at diagnosis is not common. Tissue infiltration in the form of hepatosplenomegaly or lymphadenopathy is seen in more than one half of patients, and an anterior mediastinal mass is present in a significant number of patients who have T-cell ALL (although other parenchymal involvement at diagnosis is uncommon). Central nervous system (CNS) leukemia is present at diagnosis in about 5% of patients but is generally occult. None of these features carries any particular diagnostic specificity for leukemia in general, although they do show associations with particular subtypes.

The typical patient who has ALL presents with anemia, thrombocytopenia, and leukocytosis, sometimes to levels greater than 100×10^9 per liter but more commonly less than 50×10^9 per liter. Under such circumstances, the diagnosis of acute leukemia is readily apparent from examination of peripheral blood. "Aleukemic" presentations are common, however, and any person who has unexplained pancytopenia requires a bone marrow examination to exclude leukemia. In patients in whom marrow cannot be aspirated, or in which it is heavily contaminated by uninvolved peripheral blood, a core biopsy may be essential to establish the diagnosis.

MORPHOLOGIC CLASSIFICATION

The relative ease with which blood or bone marrow can be obtained from patients who have leukemia has made morphologic examination the principal tool in leukemia diagnosis. Thin films of peripheral blood or well-spread bone marrow are essential for recognizing the sometimes subtle nuclear characteristics of blasts; diagnostic criteria are described based on staining characteristics with so-called Romanowsky stains, most commonly Wright-Giemsa.

The most commonly used morphologic classification system is the French–American–British (FAB) system, first described in 1976 (9) and subsequently revised (10). In this system, ALL is divided into three types, designated *L1*, *L2*, and *L3* (Fig. 46.1; see also Color Plate 27, between pp. 1446–1447). The first of these is characterized by homogeneous small blasts with very high nuclear:cytoplasmic (N:C) ratios, smooth but often darkly staining chromatin, and inconspicuous nucleoli. By contrast, L2 ALL is characterized by more pleomorphic blasts with lower N:C ratios, highly irregular nuclear contours, and more prominent nucleoli. Of the three types, L3 ALL is the most distinctive, with large homogenous blasts with dispersed nuclear chromatin, multiple nucleoli, and deep-blue cytoplasm that contains numerous vacuoles; the morphology is identical to that of similarly stained Burkitt's lymphoma cells. In classic cases, L1 ALL

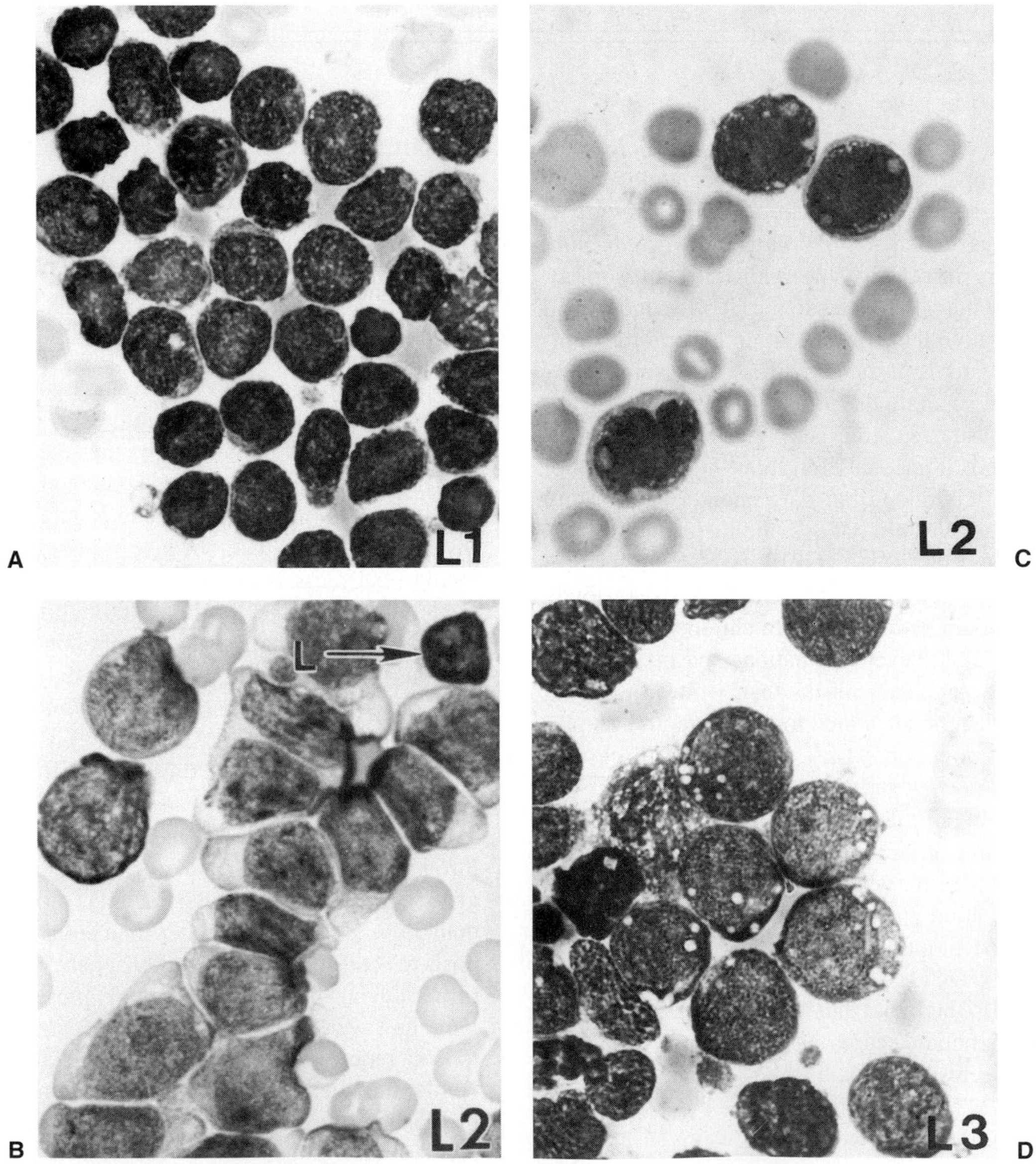

FIG. 46.1. French–American–British classification of acute lymphoblastic leukemia (ALL). **A:** In L1 ALL, blasts are small with homogeneous dark chromatin and scant cytoplasm. Some size heterogeneity, as seen here, is acceptable. **B:** L2 ALL has blasts at least twice the size of a small lymphocyte (*L*) with abundant cytoplasm and distinct nucleoli. **C:** Some patients with L2 ALL are more polymorphous with size heterogeneity and highly convoluted nuclei. **D:** L3 ALL has uniform cells with distinct cytoplasm with prominent vacuolization. Mitoses (*arrow*) and apoptotic bodies often are seen (Wright-Giemsa stain, original magnification: 1,000× magnification). See Color Plate 27, between pp. 1446–1447.

TABLE 46.1. *French–American–British classification of acute lymphoid leukemia*

Feature	Description	Scoring
Nuclear–cytoplasmic ratio	>20% of cell area is cytoplasm in >25% of cells	−1 (Favors L2)
	<20% of cell area is cytoplasm in >75% of cells	+1 (Favors L1)
Nucleoli	One or more prominent in >25% of cells	−1
	Absent or inconspicuous in >75% of cells	+1
Nuclear membrane	Irregular in >25% of cells	−1
Cell size	>50% of large cells (>2× diameter of lymphocyte)	−1

L1: Sum of 4 features is 0 to +2.
L2: Sum of 4 features is −1 to −4.
L3: Scoring not relevant; recognized as homogenous large cells with round nuclei, several prominent nucleoli, and abundant, deeply basophilic cytoplasm that contains numerous vacuoles.

blasts can be confused with normal lymphocytes (in poor preparations), L2 cells resemble AML (FAB M0 or M1) blasts, and L3 morphology suggests either Burkitt's or occasionally other types of non-Hodgkin's lymphomas. In practice, however, concordance rates in classification of L1 compared with L2 ALL for most studies have been in the range of 70% if the criteria presented here are applied (10–12). Because of this, in 1981, the FAB group proposed a scoring system for the distinction of L1 and L2 ALL (Table 46.1). Scoring blasts based on features of N:C ratio, prominence of nucleoli, nuclear membrane irregularity and cell size, concordance rates inproved to close to 90% (10,12). Unlike L3 ALL, however, which identifies B-cell ALL with relative specificity, L1 and L2 ALL morphologies do not specify immunologic, cytogenetic, or molecular entities. Moreover, although patients with L3 ALL fare poorly and require specific therapy, most studies fail to show the distinction between L1 and L2 ALL to be a particularly important prognostic factor, especially if other factors are considered (11–17). In newer classifications of ALL, such as the one proposed in the World Health Organization Classification of Neoplastic Diseases of the Hematopoietic and Lymphoid Tissues, morphologic classification of ALL is supplanted by immunologic classification.

CYTOCHEMISTRY

Unlike the central role it plays in the subclassification of myeloid leukemia, cytochemistry is not as useful for the diagnosis or classification of ALL. Certainly, ALL can be characterized by the absence of myeloperoxidase activity (Fig. 46.2A), but this is also true of megakaryocytic and some monocytic leukemias as well as ''M0'' AML (18). Sudan black B staining, often used as a surrogate for myeloperoxidase, actually can be positive in ALL (19,20). The periodic acid–Schiff reaction commonly is thought to be a marker for ALL; however, positivity of periodic acid–Schiff staining is seen in nearly equal frequency in AML. The char-

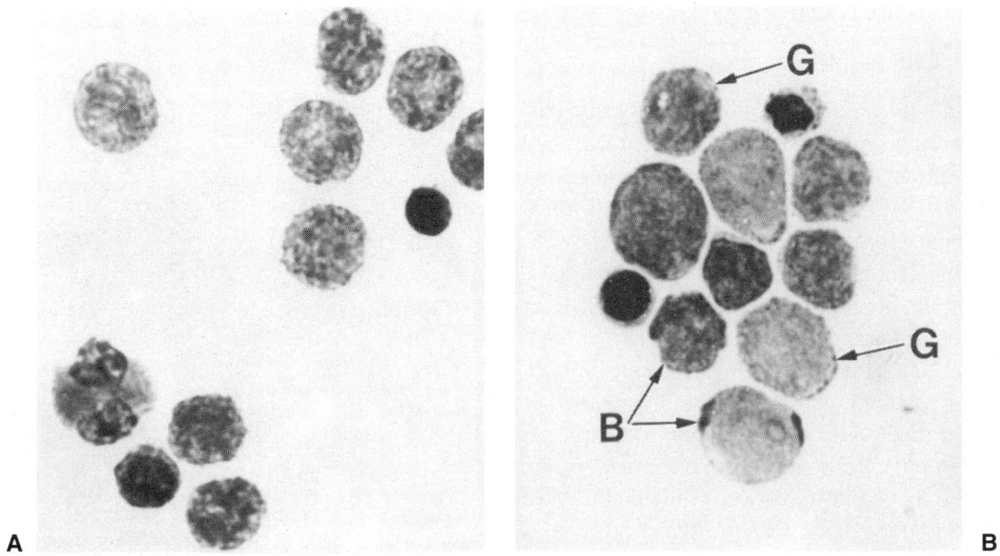

FIG. 46.2. Histochemistry in acute lymphoblastic leukemia. **A:** The myeloperoxidase reaction is negative in the blast population but is positive in a residual segmented granulocyte (original magnification: 1,300× magnification). **B:** The reaction to periodic acid–Schiff staining (original magnification: 1,300× magnification) is positive, with a pattern that ranges from finely granular (*G*) to coarse blocks (*B*).

acteristic "block" positive reaction is much more specific for ALL but is present only in slightly more than 10% of patients (20) (Fig. 46.2B).

Because acid phosphatase expression has been described as a differentiation marker for thymocytes, it has been used widely as a cytochemical indicator of T-cell ALL (21). Focal Golgi acid phosphatase activity is present, however, in about 10% of cases of B-lineage ALL. Although such activity is present more often in T-cell ALL, the relatively low prevalence of T-cell ALL implies that the predictive value of a positive acid phosphatase stain for the T-cell phenotype is only slightly more than 50% (22).

The single most useful cytochemical marker for ALL is terminal deoxynucleotidyl transferase (TdT) (see Chapter 3). Although generally performed by immunocytochemical methods, TdT is detected by a relatively simple slide test that may be done along with conventional cytochemistry. With increasing frequency TdT analysis is being performed as part of flow cytometric evaluation. TdT is absent from patients with L3 ALL but is found in at least 90% to 95% of patients with L1 and L2 ALL, provided freshly prepared smears are used (23). Atypical lymphocytes can be distinguished from L1 lymphoblasts by virtue of TdT expression, and this may be of particular diagnostic value in sites such as the CNS. Expression of TdT is not specific for ALL; it has been reported in variable percentages of patients with AML (24). Recent work suggests, however, that quantitative assessment of TdT expression by flow cytometry may permit distinction between ALL and AML, as TdT expression in AML is significantly weaker than that seen in both precursor B- and T-ALL (25).

MORPHOLOGIC VARIANTS OF ACUTE LYMPHOBLASTIC LEUKEMIA

Hand-Mirror Cell Leukemia

A distinct morphologic variant of acute lymphoblastic leukemia has been described in which blasts are characterized by the presence of an asymmetrical cytoplasmic projection called a *uropod* (26–28) (Fig. 46.3). Although small numbers of hand-mirror cells frequently are seen in ALL, they are the dominant cytologic finding in only about 1% of patients. Because this condition is such a morphologically distinct entity, several early studies suggested that this was a clinical entity as well (25). Hand-mirror lymphocytes can be seen in the circulation of patients who have a number of other benign or malignant diseases. Because immune complexes can cause normal lymphocytes to form uropods *in vitro* (29), it has been suggested that hand-mirror cells in leukemia owe their shapes to an immune response (30). It has been recognized that hand-mirror cells may be seen in L1, L2, and even L3 ALL, and that they are not associated with any particular immunophenotype. Moreover, although there are reports of long-term survival with this disease in spite of failure to

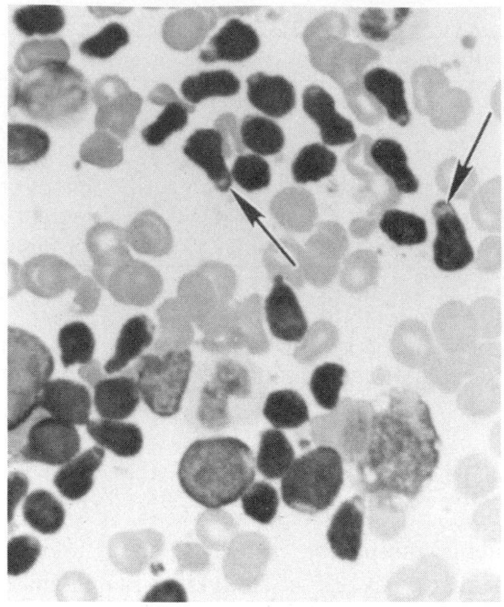

FIG. 46.3. Hand-mirror variant of acute lymphoblastic leukemia. Note small, irregular L1 blasts with eccentric cytoplasmic protuberances (*arrows*) called *uropods* (Wright-Giemsa stain, original magnification: 675× magnification).

achieve remission (31), it generally is conceded that no prognostic significance attends this diagnosis (27,28).

Granular Acute Lymphoblastic Leukemia

In a small percentage of patients who have ALL, blasts contain azurophilic cytoplasmic inclusions that are distinct from myeloid primary granules and do not stain with myeloperoxidase (Fig. 46.4; see also Color Plate 28, between pp. 1446–1447). In some patients, these stain with acid phos-

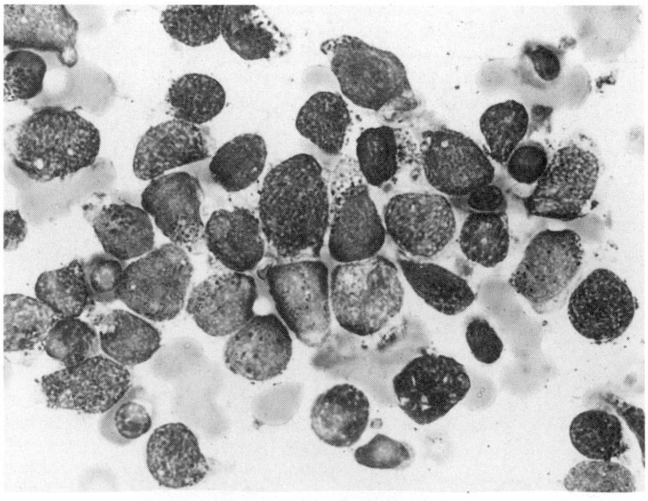

FIG. 46.4. Granular acute lymphoblastic leukemia. Note blasts with smooth chromatin and striking coarse granularity in many cells (Wright-Giemsa stain, original magnification: 1,000× magnification). See Color Plate 28, between pp. 1446–1447.

phatase or acid esterases, suggesting a lysosomal origin. Their presence is not associated with any particular immunophenotype. Although granular ALL accounts for only about 5% of cases in one series of childhood ALLs (32), these patients had distinctly worse outcomes, particularly children with precursor B-cell ALL. There was a much higher incidence of granular ALL among patients classified with FAB L2 than L1 disease, and only among granular cases was there an adverse prognostic impact of FAB classification, suggesting that the higher incidence of granular ALL may be responsible for the poor prognostic effect of L2 ALL reported in many series. Granular ALL also has been noted in adults (33), and recently it was noted that there is a higher incidence of azurophilic granules in ALL blasts that coexpress myeloid and lymphoid antigens (34).

HISTOPATHOLOGY

Bone marrow biopsies in ALL are almost always hypercellular (Fig. 46.5A). In well-fixed material, the diagnosis of acute leukemia is usually obvious, although subclassification is much less reliable. Patients with L1 ALL generally have highly uniform collections of blasts with fine chromatin, inconspicuous nucleoli, and no discernible cytoplasm (Fig. 46.5B); findings in patients with L2 are more heterogeneous, with irregular nuclei and often some cytoplasm (Fig. 46.5C). L3 ALL is the most characteristic, with distinct nucleoli and a rim of frequently squared-off cytoplasm (Fig. 46.5D); in well-prepared material, even vacuoles can be detected. Because of the distinct cytoplasm, care must be taken not to misdiagnose such patients as having AML. Although

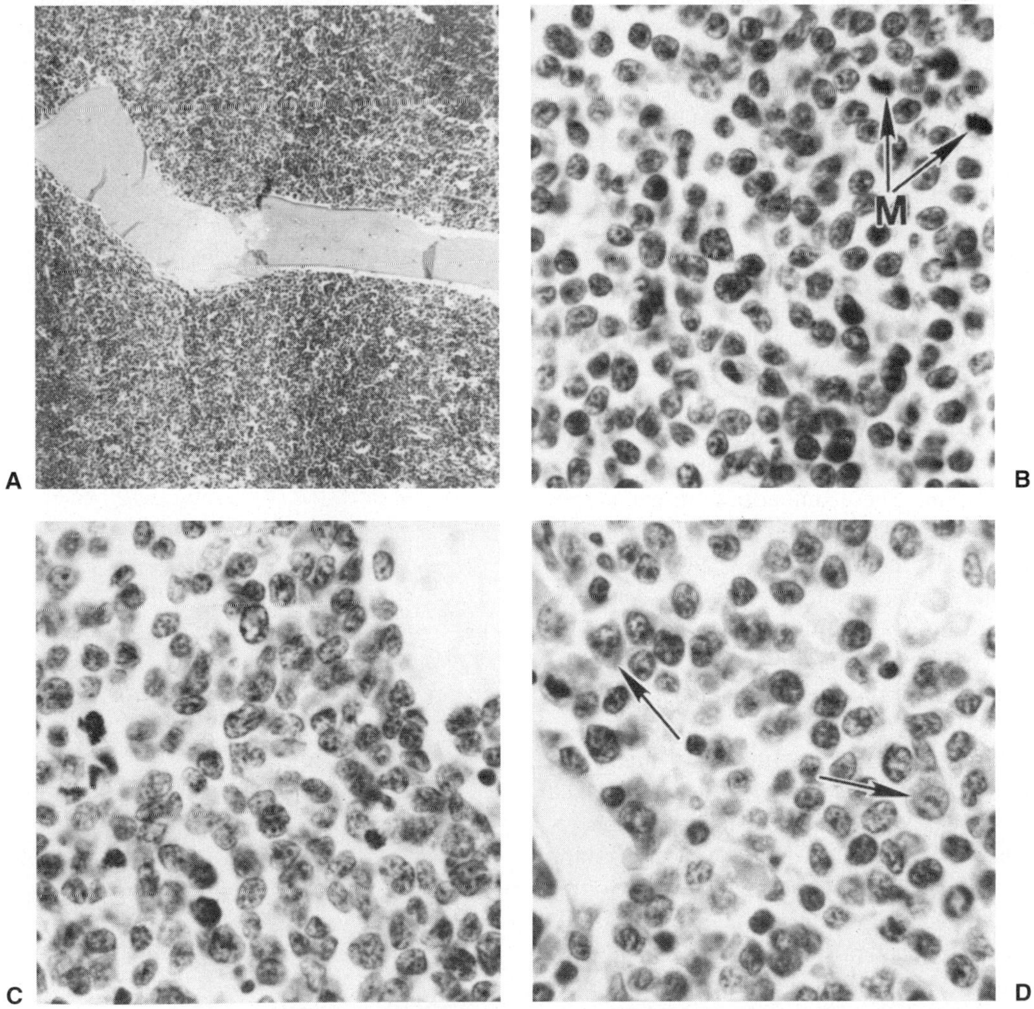

FIG. 46.5. Bone marrow biopsy in acute lymphoblastic leukemia (ALL). **A:** Low-power view showing diffuse and homogeneous replacement of marrow space by lymphoblasts in this patient with L1 ALL (hematoxylin and eosin stain, original magnification: 68× magnification). **B:** High-power appearance of L1 ALL in marrow sections. Note homogeneous population of blasts with stippled chromatin that is fairly darkly staining. Mitoses (*M*) are found easily (hematoxylin and eosin stain, original magnification: 680× magnification). **C:** L2 ALL. Note larger, more polymorphous blasts with less darkly staining cytoplasm (hematoxylin and eosin stain, original magnification: 680× magnification). **D:** L3 ALL. Blasts have distinct nucleoli and a rim of cytoplasm is evident in many cells (*arrows*) (hematoxylin and eosin stain, original magnification: 680× magnification).

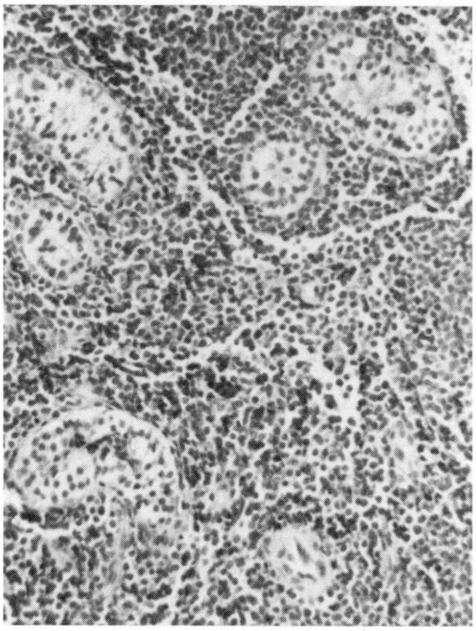

FIG. 46.6. Testicular infiltration in acute lymphoblastic leukemia. Note the dense interstitial infiltration separating residual testicular tubules (hematoxylin and eosin stain, original magnification: 170× magnification).

bone marrow aspirates are obtained easily in most patients with ALL, even in those in whom aspiration is not possible, it is probably best to rely on Wright-Giemsa–stained imprint preparations for leukemia classification.

Morphologically, L1 or L2 ALL is indistinguishable from lymphoblastic lymphoma, and L3 ALL from Burkitt's or Burkitt's-like lymphoma. These similarities present a problem in nomenclature if leukemia presents in its aleukemic phase and a lymph node or tissue biopsy specimen is the first material obtained from a patient. Although sometimes arbitrary criteria are used for definitional purposes for research protocols, increasingly the distinction between the two is not being considered in making treatment decisions (see Chapter 26).

Leukemic infiltrates can involve virtually any organ system, particularly in advanced disease. The spleen, liver, and lymph nodes commonly are affected; outside the lymphoreticular system, the CNS and kidneys are the most common sites of involvement. Special mention should be made of the fact that in boys, the testis may represent a ''protected site'' not fully accessible to chemotherapeutic agents; in early therapeutic protocols, the testis underwent biopsy before therapy was discontinued (35), although with more recent intensification programs this often is not necessary. Testicular involvement is interstitial (Fig. 46.6), and if the degree of involvement is limited, blasts generally form small clusters. In small biopsy specimens of testis or other organs with poorly preserved tissue, clear distinction of L1 lymphoblasts and mature lymphocytes may be difficult. In such cases, immunologic studies on fresh-frozen tissue, including detection of TdT or other markers of immature lymphocytes, may be useful for distinguishing reactive and leukemic infiltrates.

DIFFERENTIAL DIAGNOSIS

Although many diseases can mimic ALL clinically, ALL usually is distinguished readily in pathologic material from almost all other diseases, except for some forms of AML. Unlike AML, ALL almost always presents *de novo*, so that no criteria need be established for distinguishing a preleukemic phase. Many small round cell tumors of childhood, however, may present with bone marrow involvement. If no clinically obvious mass is present, the potential exists for these tumors to be confused with ALL, particularly if only Wright-Giemsa–stained material is examined. Low-power examination of aspirated material for distinct clumps of cells and examination of core biopsy specimens are the most reliable ways of avoiding this pitfall. Rhabdomyosarcoma is probably the most common small round cell tumor misdiagnosed as ALL.

If an adequate amount of material is obtained, few if any nonneoplastic conditions can be confused with ALL. Although much has been written about the need to distinguish lymphoblasts and atypical lymphocytes in viral infections, in practice this is rarely a problem, because the latter have lower N:C ratios, more prominent nucleoli, and a different chromatin pattern from lymphoblasts. Also, marrow replacement by lymphoid cells is not a usual feature of viral disease. One lesser-known condition is the increase in ''hematogones'' seen normally in infants and in some children who have cytopenias (Figure 46.7; see also Color Plate 29, between pp. 1446–1447). These cells represent normal B-cell

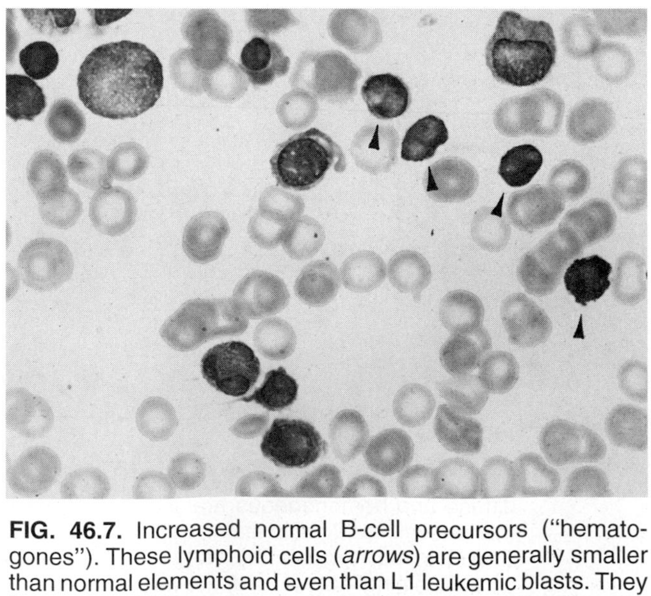

FIG. 46.7. Increased normal B-cell precursors ("hematogones"). These lymphoid cells (*arrows*) are generally smaller than normal elements and even than L1 leukemic blasts. They have very high nuclear:cytoplasmic ratios, so that cytoplasmic rims often are not seen (Wright-Giemsa, original magnification: 1,000× magnification). See Color Plate 29, between pp. 1446–1447.

precursors and differ from L1 lymphoblasts by virtue of relatively more compact nuclear chromatin and a lack of discernible cytoplasm (36,37), although the distinction may present some difficulty in poorly prepared material. Like precursor B-cell ALL, hematogones express an immature phenotype (CD10-positive [$CD10^+$], TdT^+); however, they differ from ALL blasts in that they are much more heterogeneous in their expression of B-lineage antigens and can be distinguished from blasts with multiparameter flow cytometry (36,38).

IMMUNOLOGIC CLASSIFICATION

In the early 1970s it was recognized that a subset of cases of ALL had blasts that formed spontaneous rosettes with sheep red blood cells (39,40). More significantly, it was noted that children whose blasts had this property had a particular constellation of clinical features, most notably high peripheral white blood cell (WBC) counts and, frequently, large anterior mediastinal masses (40). The clinical importance of an immunologic subclassification of ALL was bolstered by the subsequent finding that the highly distinctive L3 lymphoblasts were unique among patients with ALL in that they expressed cell surface immunoglobulin (41). Although the immunologic subdivision of cases of ALL into T-, B-, and ''null''cell varieties lasted well into the 1980s, the availability of an increasing array of monoclonal antibodies led to the discovery that the majority of cases of null cell ALL were, in fact, of B-cell origin (42,43). (Because the term *B-ALL* historically has referred to a leukemia that is surface immunoglobulin–positive, this discussion uses the term *B-lineage ALL* to refer to the larger group of leukemias of B-cell origin. Similarly, the term *pre-B-cell* has referred specifically to those leukemias that express cytoplasmic μ heavy chain without surface immunoglobulin heavy chain; here we use the term *precursor B-cell ALL* to encompass tumors of B-cell origin that lack surface immunoglobulin irrespective of their μ heavy chain status.)

Because acute leukemias are extraordinarily heterogeneous in their expression of surface antigens, and because

TABLE 46.2. *Sensitivity and specificity of commonly used markers in phenotyping of acute lymphoid leukemia (ALL)*

	Sensitivity		Specificity[a]	
Marker	B-cell ALL	T-cell ALL	Lymphoid vs. myeloid	T vs. B lymphoid
Primarily T-cell associated				
CD7	—	High	Low	High
CD5	—	Moderate	Moderate	High
CD3	—	Low	High	High
CD2	—	High	Low	High
CD4	—	Moderate	Low	High
CD8	—	Low	High	High
CD1	—	Low	High	High
cCD3	—	High	High	High
Primarily B-cell associated				
CD19	High	—	Moderate[b]	High
CD22	Moderate	—	High	High
CD20	Low	—	High	High
CD10	Moderate	—	High	Low
CD24	High	—	Moderate	Moderate
CD9	Moderate	—	Low	Low
CD79a	High	—	Moderate	Low
sIg	Very Low	—	High	High
cIg	Low	—	High	High
cCD22	High	—	Moderate	High
Other markers				
TdT	High	High	Moderate	None
HLA-DR	High	Low	None	Moderate[c]
CD45	Moderate	High	Low	Low[d]
CD38	Moderate	High	None	None

[a] "High" specificity implies reactivity with no more than 1% to 2% of cases of the type of leukemia being excluded. "Moderate" vs. "low" specificity is more subjective but markers that react with more than about 10% to 15% of conflicting cases are considered to have "low" specificity. Note that specificity in difficult cases may even be lower.

[b] Bright CD19 positivity has high specificity for B-lineage ALL.

[c] HLA-DR is rare in T-cell ALL in childhood but more common in adult ALL.

[d] Intensity of CD45 expression may be more specific because it is generally much less intense in precursor B-cell ALL than in acute myeloid leukemia or T-cell ALL.

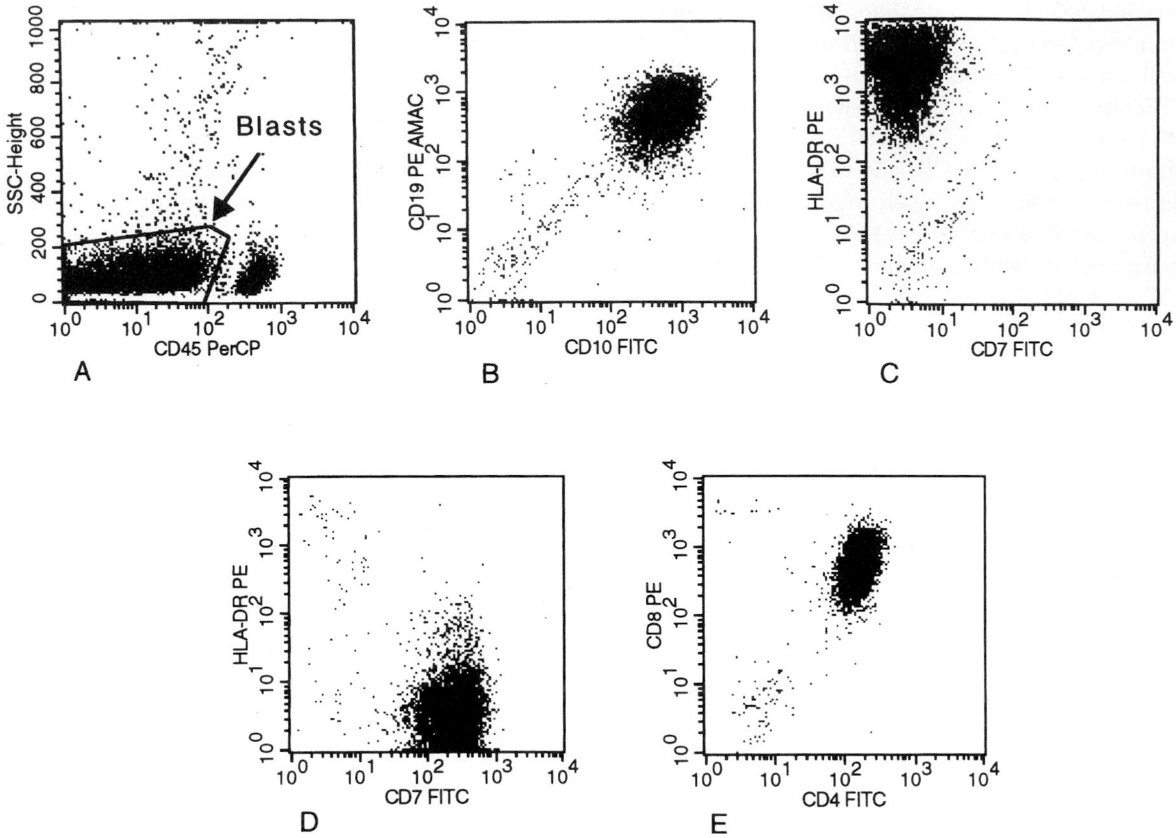

FIG. 46.8. Flow cytometric analysis in acute lymphoblastic leukemia (ALL). **A–C:** Precursor B-cell ALL. Blasts can be identified based on low-density expression of CD45 and low right angle (side) scatter (*SSC*) **(A)**. This is often a useful feature for gating on the blast population. Almost all cells within the blast gate are doubly positive for CD10 and CD19 **(B)**. By contrast, the gated blasts lack the T-cell marker CD7 but are strongly positive for HLA-DR **(C)**. **D,E:** T-cell acute lymphoblastic leukemia. Cells express CD7 but not HLA-DR **(D)**. Cells are doubly positive for CD4 and CD8 in contrast to normal T cells, which would be comprised of a mixture of $CD4^+CD8^-$ and $CD4^-CD8^+$ cells **(E)**.

many markers are relatively rather than absolutely lineage-specific, it is difficult to describe a simple algorithm that accurately classifies all cases of acute leukemia. In some patients, interpretation of lineage is straightforward, based on the reactivity of a relatively small number of antibodies. In more complex cases, however, a larger panel of antibodies may be necessary. Table 46.2 lists some relatively common antibodies used in ALL phenotyping, along with estimates of their relative sensitivities and specificities for various types of leukemia. In those patients in whom surface marker studies are equivocal, flow cytometric evaluation of specific intracellular antigens may be valuable. For example, cytoplasmic expression of CD22 and CD3 is detectable in essentially all patients with B- and T-lineage ALL, respectively, including those patients with absent surface expression of these molecules (44–47). Cytoplasmic CD79a is also a highly sensitive marker of B-cell differentiation, although its specificity has been called into question (see Chapters 3 and 4). Examples of flow cytometry diagrams of B- and T-lineage ALL are illustrated in Figure 46.8.

T-Cell Acute Lymphoblastic Leukemia

Definition

Although E-rosette formation long was considered the standard for defining T-cell ALL, it has become clear that not all patients with T-cell ALL have this capability or possess the receptor (CD2) for sheep red blood cells. Rather, the most sensitive surface marker for T-cell ALL is CD7, which detects all (48–50) or at least the majority of cases (51). This antigen is also present, however, in up to 20% of patients with AML (52), so its utility as a single marker is limited. Virtually all patients with $CD7^+$ AML also express the HLA-DR antigen, whereas $CD7^+$, HLA^- DR^+ T-cell ALL is rare in children and only occasionally found in adults; this combination of antibodies is more useful than CD7 alone. Theoretically, TdT may be useful in distinguishing T-cell ALL and AML, although TdT is present in 10% to 20% of patients of AML (and possibly even a higher percentage of ambiguous cases). The CD5 antigen is a more specific marker for T-cell differentiation than CD7, although not as sensitive, and markers such as CD1, CD3, and CD8, which show high degrees of specificity for T cells, are found in fewer than one half of patients. Conversely, the CD2 antigen, which is fairly sensitive, also is expressed in a significant number of patients with AML (53).

Functionally, the most sensitive and specific marker for T-cell ALL has proved to be CD3 antigen expression in the cytoplasm (cCD3) of lymphoblasts. Although cCD3 is detected readily in frozen sections of lymphoblastic lymphoma (54) and in appropriately fixed cytocentrifuge preparations (55,56), it is not analyzed routinely if live cells are stained by immunofluorescence. Flow cytometric methods for analyzing intracellular constituents are available (44–47,57), however, so that detection of this marker can be used to resolve ambiguous cases. In two of the largest reported series, cCD3 was found in all patients with T-cell ALL tested but was absent in precursor B-cell ALL and AML, including $CD7^{+}$ AML (45,55).

Attempts to use genetic markers as defining characteristics for T-cell ALL have not been successful. Clonal rearrangement of the T-cell receptor (TCR) β chain gene has been shown to be a highly sensitive marker for T-cell ALL. Because this rearrangement occurs very early in the commitment of normal precursor cells to T-cell differentiation, it is not surprising to find a clonal rearrangement in virtually all patients with T-cell ALL (58–63). The specificity of this rearrangement, however, or of rearrangements of the other TCR genes, is low (59,63–67). In fact, the majority of patients with precursor B-cell ALL show rearrangement of at least one of the TCR genes, most often TCRDδ (65); even TCRBβ is rearranged in 20% to 30% of patients with B-lineage ALL (64), as well as in some with AML (64,66). Rearrangements at the TCR loci are ongoing during the clinical evolution of an individual leukemia (68–71). This observation has both theoretic implications for the development of subclones with distinct biologic properties and practical implications regarding molecular monitoring for minimal residual disease. TCR gene rearrangement may also have prognostic significance in B-lineage ALL; in one recent study leukemias with rearrangement of TCR δ were associated with a significantly more favorable event-free survival, independent of other prognostic factors (72).

From a practical standpoint, the definition of T-cell ALL usually rests on interpretation of an overall pattern of reactivity with several immunologic markers. Most cases will express several T-cell-associated markers, so that expression of a single aberrant or unexpected marker can be safely ignored. In some cases, however, particularly those expressing only CD7, it may be difficult to distinguish T-cell ALL and AML, FAB M0. Some such cases may, in fact, represent either mixed-lineage leukemias or true stem cell leukemias (73).

Phenotypic Heterogeneity

When panels of antibodies are used to study T-cell ALL cases, there is considerable variability in the phenotypes encountered (52,74–81). Many investigators have attempted to explain this heterogeneity by relating the phenotypes seen to those described in normal stages of T cell differentiation (69,71,75–77,82). In general, T-cell ALL is a neoplasm of T-cell precursors, and the cells bear some phenotypic resemblance to cells normally found within the thymus. Because discrete stages of thymocyte development have been described, several authors have tried to superimpose the phenotypes encountered in leukemias on these normal stages and have described "early," "mid-," and "late" thymic stages of T-cell ALL (75,77) (see Chapter 26). Unfortunately, precise definition of each of these stages is not standard, and many patients with T-cell ALL express phenotypes that are not easily reconciled with the normal differentiation scheme. The relative frequency of patients in each of the differentiation stages also has varied among series (80).

In addition to heterogeneity of expression of T cell–associated antigens, patients with T-cell ALL often express antigens more commonly associated with other lineages. Thus, 20% to 30% of patients express the common ALL antigen CD10 (83,84), and B cell–associated antigens, including CD24, CD9 and CD21, also may be seen in some patients. Expression of myeloid antigens, especially CD13 and CD33, is not an infrequent occurrence. Diagnosticians should be aware of this and not misclassify an otherwise straightforward T-cell ALL as a mixed-lineage leukemia (85).

Clinical Significance

Although not every patient fits the characteristic clinical picture, a constellation of features has come to be associated with T-cell ALL. Patients who have T-cell ALL are more likely than others to present with elevated WBC counts (often over 50×10^9 per liter) and are more likely to have adenopathy and organomegaly (40,84–90). An anterior mediastinal mass, if present, is a highly specific predictor for T-cell phenotype in patients who have ALL. About 15% of children with ALL have T-cell ALL, compared with 20% to 25% of adults, and in children T-cell ALL is associated with older age at presentation. Because many of these clinical features are associated with poor prognosis, there is some controversy about whether the T-cell phenotype in and of itself confers a poor prognosis or requires different therapy (81–88,91). Adult ALL is a poor prognosis disease, and adult patients who have T-cell ALL in general do not fare differently from those with precursor B-cell ALL (15,16,92, 93). Although the T-cell phenotype probably does not confer a worse prognosis in a child who has a high WBC count, many investigators treat children who have T-cell ALL as having "high-risk" disease, even if other clinical features with poor prognoses are not present (85,86,91).

It is not clear if the immunologic diversity seen within T-cell ALL has particular clinical significance (78,80,81, 94–96). There is some suggestion that the most "immature" type of T-cell ALL, defined on the basis of reactivity with T antibodies but lack of E-rosette formation (and sometimes referred to as *pre-T*-cell ALL) may represent a distinct group (81,94,95). Such patients have clinical characteristics that are intermediate between T- and precursor B-cell ALL patients in terms of age and WBC count and are less likely to present with a mediastinal mass (94,95). More recently, the Children's Cancer Group has demonstrated a significant association between absence of CD2 and adverse clinical outcome in a large series of patients with pediatric T-cell ALL (97). In this study, CD2 status remained an important prognosticator even after stratification of patients on the basis of clinical parameters (97). Likewise, adults with a CD2-negative ($CD2^-$) phenotype fare significantly less well than other patients who have T-cell ALL (81). These data notwithstanding, the immunologic diversity of T-cell ALL has not explained fully the variability in clinical behavior seen among these patients.

B-lineage Acute Lymphoblastic Leukemia

Definition

The majority of cases of B-lineage ALL can be recognized without difficulty. Almost 98% of patients express both CD19 and HLA-DR (85). The CD19 antigen is not present in T-cell ALL, and although it may be seen occasionally in AML, its expression is dim and usually heterogeneous. Moreover, 90% of patients with B-lineage ALL express the common ALL antigen, CD10, which is rarely (and very faintly) expressed in AML. The $CD10^-$ cases may be recognized as B cell–derived in most cases by virtue of expression of other B cell–specific antigens, particularly CD19 and CD22. The CD20 antigen expression is also highly specific, although not as sensitive as either CD22 or CD19 (85). Analogous to cCD3, the CD22 antigen has been detected in the cytoplasm of ALL blasts even if it is not on the surface; it is a very sensitive marker for B-lineage ALL (44,98). In contrast to cCD3, however, cCD22 may be detected in AML, although the CD22 antigen found in AML is actually a cross-reacting protein (99). TdT is present in at least 95% of patients with B-lineage ALL, although its absence from "true" B-ALL (i.e., surface immunoglobulin heavy chain– and light chain–positive) is noteworthy.

Essentially all B-lineage ALLs show clonal rearrangement of the immunoglobulin heavy chain gene (42,100). Analogous to the situation with TCR and T-cell ALL, however, this marker is nonspecific and has been noted in many patients with T-cell ALL and AML alike (101,102). Rearrangement or deletion of immunoglobulin light chain genes is a more specific marker for B-cell differentiation; not surprisingly, it is less sensitive. Patterns of immunoglobulin gene rearrangements are thought to reflect the normal hierarchy of B-cell development (42). Although a high frequency of immunoglobulin gene rearrangements occurs in "immature" leukemias, or those of uncertain lineage (42,103), it is not clear to what extent this can be used as evidence of B-cell differentiation in these tumors.

Phenotypic Heterogeneity

As is the case with T-cell ALL, panels of antibodies tested against B-lineage ALL have demonstrated diversity that has been related to stages of normal B-cell differentiation (43,104) (see Chapter 26). Many phenotypes have been encountered, however, that are not part of the normal models of differentiation, particularly if a large panel of antibodies is used to formulate a fairly detailed model (38,85,105). Whether this is because the normal models are not correct, because the normal counterparts of the leukemic cells are seen only rarely, or because leukemias aberrantly express B-cell differentiation antigens has not been determined.

Additional markers that have been described in B-lineage ALL include CD24, present in the majority of patients (85,106,107); CD34, present in about 75% (85,108–110); and CD9 (111), present in about 90% 85,106). About 20% of patients with childhood B-lineage ALL express cytoplasmic μ heavy chain without surface immunoglobulin and are considered to have pre-B-cell ALL (112). CD45, the common leukocyte antigen, is absent in about 10% to 20% of patients with B-lineage ALL, and if it is present, its intensity varies greatly (113–115). Finally, myeloid antigens, including CD13, CD15, and CD33, are found in 10% to 15% of patients with childhood B-lineage ALL (105) and in more than twice that amount in adult B-lineage ALL (116–119).

Clinical Significance

In contrast to T-cell ALL, there is no single clinical picture associated with all B-lineage ALL. Rather, B-lineage ALL can be divided into distinct clinical subgroups. Some of these are defined on the basis of cytogenetic or molecular abnormalities; others are defined immunologically.

B-Acute Lymphoblastic Leukemia

Although it accounts for fewer than 2% of ALL cases, true B-ALL is recognized easily as the leukemic equivalent of Burkitt's lymphoma. It is associated with L3 morphology, and patients who have B-ALL also have a high incidence of abdominal masses, particularly related to bowel involvement. Historically it was considered to have a notoriously poor prognosis compared with other forms of ALL, and, in childhood at least, it requires specific therapy if a cure is to be attempted. Highly aggressive regimens with multiple chemotherapeutic agents have shown some promise in treating this disease (120). There are occasional cases with L3 morphology and *MYC* rearrangements, which lack surface immunoglobulin expression; these nonetheless are considered functionally equivalent to B-ALL (121). Conversely, rare patients with B-ALL (i.e., those expressing surface heavy and light chains) lack L3 morphology. The experience of the Pediatric Oncology Group with these rare patients suggests a clinical behavior similar to that of the usual type of precursor B-cell ALL.

Transitional Pre-B-Cell Acute Lymphoblastic Leukemia

Recently, a novel immunologic subset of B-lineage ALL with immunophenotypic properties intermediate between B-ALL and pre-B-cell ALL, termed *transitional pre-B-cell ALL*, has been described (120). As in B-ALL, surface IgM is expressed in transitional pre-B-ALL; however, unlike B-ALL, immunoglobulin light chain expression is absent (122). Further distinguishing transitional pre-B-cell ALL from true B-cell ALL is the uniform absence of L3 morphology and translocations involving *MYC*, as well as expression of TdT and, often, CD34, immunophenotypic features characteristically lacking in true B-ALL. Recognition of transitional pre-B-cell ALL, which appears to respond well to antimetabolite-based therapy, requires assessment of both surface heavy and light chain expression, a practice likely to prevent misdiagnosis of these leukemias as B-ALL.

Pre-B-Cell Acute Lymphoblastic Leukemia

Although there is no distinct set of clinical features associated with pre-B-cell ALL, there is a clear association with the presence of a specific t(1;19) translocation (123) involving the *E2A* and *PBX1* genes. Compared with other patients with precursor B-cell ALL, children who have pre-B-cell ALL fare poorly, reflecting a higher incidence of bone marrow and CNS relapse (122–124). Subsequent work, however, has revealed that the poor prognosis associated with pre-B-cell ALL is attributable to its association with the translocation t(1;19); thus, patients with pre-B-cell ALL without such a translocation fared no worse than those with precursor B-cell ALL lacking cytoplasmic μ (c_μ) (early pre-B-cell ALL) (125,126). Patients with early pre-B-cell ALL with the translocation t(1;19) may not have an adverse prognosis (126,127); this likely reflects the fact that such patients generally have translocations involving other genes with the same cytogenetic breakpoint.

Common ALL Antigen-Negative Acute Lymphoblastic Leukemia

The ALL blasts in about 10% of children and in about 25% of adults lack the CD10 antigen (15,16,84–86,89,92, 128–130). The majority of infants with ALL are $CD10^-$ (131). This association explains in part the poor prognosis that has been described for patients who have this phenotype (132). Lack of CD10 expression, however, also has been described as a poor prognostic factor in adults (15,16,92, 130,133) and may be so in children other than infants (92,128,129,134). Some cases of $CD10^-$ ALL described in the early 1980s may represent cases of M0 leukemia, but most are $CD10^-CD19^+$ and clearly of B-cell origin. Absence of CD10 often is associated with high WBC counts, which also helps make it difficult to assess its effect on prognosis.

Other Markers

Several other monoclonal antibody-defined antigens have been studied to determine if their expression can be correlated with outcome. Although CD24 is present in the majority of patients with ALL, its absence helps to define a poor prognostic group (107). The observation that $CD24^-$ blasts show greater resistance to γ irradiation compared with $CD24^+$ blasts provides one possible explanation for this association (135). Early studies also suggested that CD34 expression conveys a good prognosis, at least in childhood, independent of other clinical risk factors (110,136). In long-term follow-up, however, early differences in the event-free survival rate may not persist (115). In adults, CD34 expression has been associated with several adverse risk factors, although an impact on leukemia-free survival has not been demonstrated (137). Controversy abounds about the clinical significance of myeloid antigen expression in ALL. Expression of CD13 or CD33 has been shown to have an adverse effect on outcome in adults with B-lineage ALL (117), although this effect was not seen in patients treated with post-remission intensification therapy and bone marrow transplantation (138). Similarly conflicting data have been reported in childhood ALL (139–142), although the weight of evidence suggests no independent prognostic value attributable to myeloid antigen expression *per se*. Some investigators have suggested that the presence of any myeloid antigen in ALL can be interpreted as indicative of mixed-lineage leukemia, a view we and others do not share (143). Further discussion of mixed-lineage leukemia can be found in Chapter 47. Finally, recent work suggests that density of expression of certain antigens, rather than their traditionally described absence or presence, may demonstrate prognostic value. For example, in a recent large study of childhood precursor B-cell ALL, CD45 expression greater than the 75th percentile, and CD20 expression above the 25th percentile, predicted an adverse outcome independent of other clinical and cytogenetic risk factors (115).

CYTOGENETIC ABNORMALITIES

In addition to the immunologic heterogeneity described previously, it long has been recognized that several different, nonrandom chromosomal abnormalities occur in ALL. Many of these abnormalities not only define clinically distinct subgroups of patients but also help to explain the mechanism by which leukemic transformation occurs. A detailed discussion of cytogenetics and leukemia appears in Chapter 10; because many chromosomal abnormalities help to define

TABLE 46.3. *Common cytogenetic abnormalities in acute lymphoid leukemia (ALL)*

Abnormality	Approximate frequency, %	
	Children	Adults
Hyperdiploidy	30–40	20
Hyperdiploidy >50	20–25	5–10
Hypodiploidy	5	5–10
t(9;22)	3–4	25
t(1;19)	6	rare
t(4;11)	2–3	5–10
t(8;__)(q24;__)[a]	1–2	5–10
t(__;14)(__;q11)[b]	2–3	1–2
del(9p)	5–10	—
del(6q)	10	1–2
abnl 12p12[c]	10	—

[a] Includes t(8;14)(q24;q32), t(2;8), t(8;22) in B-ALL.
[b] Includes t(11;14), t(10;14), t(1;14), t(8;14) and inv(14) in T-cell ALL.
[c] Some of these represent t(12;21) translocations; t(12;21) is the most common translocation in childhood ALL, occurring in 20% to 25% of cases. Although generally cytogenetically silent, they may be detectable by fluorescence *in situ* hybridization.

distinct clinicopathologic subgroups of leukemia, the purpose of this section is to review clinical features associated with particular chromosomal changes. Table 46.3 lists many of the more common abnormalities in ALL.

Abnormalities of Chromosome Number

Hyperdiploid Acute Lymphoblastic Leukemia

Between 30% and 40% of children (144–147) and half or fewer than that number of adults (149–153) with ALL have hyperdiploid blasts. Strictly speaking, hyperdiploidy simply means the presence of more than 46 chromosomes. A distinct clinicopathologic group of children has been described, however, with numbers of chromosomes ranging from about 51 to 65. Such patients account for about 25% of children with ALL; the finding is much less common in adults. Patients who have this form of hyperdiploidy often have simple additions of structurally normal chromosomes and almost invariably have precursor B-cell ALL, usually CALLA-positive. Clinically, hyperdiploidy is rare in infancy, and children who have hyperdiploid ALL often have other associated "good prognosis" findings, such as low WBC count (145,146,154). Despite these associations, hyperdiploidy is a powerful, favorable prognostic factor independent of all others (145,154,155), and children with hyperdiploid ALL have been shown to have a high cure rate even if they possess other poor risk features (155). This group of children also can be recognized by flow cytometry studies (154) (see Chapter 5) and corresponds to samples with a DNA index that ranges from about 1.16 to 1.60 (154,156). The ease of DNA flow cytometry analysis and the higher satisfactory rate compared with cytogenetics has made this the preferred method for defining this group of patients. Recent studies, however, have suggested that the good prognosis with hyperdiploidy rests not in ploidy itself, but in the specific additions of chromosomes 4 and 10 (157); cytogenetic determination of ploidy may still be important.

Other Numeric Abnormalities

Other abnormalities of chromosome number are much less common than hyperdiploidy, and it is less clear that they constitute a distinct syndrome (144,147,158). Hypodiplody is well recognized and ranges from patients with 45 chromosomes to a very small and perhaps distinct subgroup of patients with near-haploid ALL (147,159). At the other extreme, near-tetraploid ALL has been described in about 1% of patients with ALL and appears, unlike the hyperdiploid ALL previously described, to be associated with T-cell ALL (160). Finally, near-diploid cases (i.e., 47–50 chromosomes) are well recognized and should be separated out, simply because they probably do not share the favorable prognostic features of the 51 to 65 group (147,148).

Abnormalities of Chromosome Structure

This group of lesions consists of translocations or other alterations at particular bands of a given chromosome. Most of those that have been characterized at the molecular level have been shown to involve activation of cellular protooncogenes, and many oncogenes have been discovered using cytogenetically characterized leukemic cells. More recently, deletion of a tumor suppressor gene (*P16-INK4A-MTS1*) also has been demonstrated. Several different translocations have been seen with enough frequency that they help to define distinct clinical entities.

t(12;21)(p13;q22)

The single most commonly identified structural abnormality in childhood ALL is also the most recently characterized. A multitude of translocations and deletions involving 12p, together comprising in excess of 10% of cases, had been described in childhood ALL using classical cytogenetics (147). Through the use of fluorescence *in situ* hybridization and reverse transcriptase–polymerase chain reaction, however, a generally cryptic balanced translocation juxtaposing the *TEL* gene at 12p13 and the *AML1* gene at 21q22 was found to be highly prevalent in childhood ALL. The incidence of the *TEL-AML1* translocation in series of patients with childhood B-lineage ALL has ranged from 16% to 29%, and in virtually all patients these translocations have not been detected by conventional cytogenetics (161–165). The presence of this translocation may be predicted by immunophenotypic characteristics of blast cells (166,167). Absence or low expression of CD9 is highly associated with this translocation; expression of the marker KORSA-3544 virtually excludes it (167).

Several groups have reported excellent event-free survival rates among patients with the translocation (162–165,168). The favorable effect of the translocation is independent of the other positive chromosomal risk factor, hyperdiploidy—fewer than 5% of patients with *TEL* rearrangement are also hyperdiploid (162,164,165). Patients with *TEL* rearrangement or hyperdiploid DNA content, who together comprise more than half of all patients with B-lineage ALL in childhood, have a fourfold lower risk of failure compared with those lacking these properties (164). Although fewer cases of adult ALL have been studied appropriately for the translocation t(12;21), in one report, 3% of adults compared with 27% of children were positive for the *TEL-AML1* fusion transcript (163). The lower prevalence of this favorable risk factor among adults with ALL may contribute to the comparatively poor prognosis of adult ALL.

Philadelphia Chromosome

The Philadelphia chromosome, t(9;22)(q34;q11), is found in about 5% of cases of childhood ALL and in up to 30% of cases of adult ALL (144,147,150–152,158). This translocation involves the *ABL* oncogene on chromosome 9 and a gene called *BCR* on chromosome 22. The rearrangement results in the production of a *BCR-ABL* fusion protein with tyrosine kinase activity (169,170). Although the same cytogenetic abnormality is seen in chronic myelogenous leukemia, the breakpoint on chromosome 22 is typically different in Philadelphia chromosome–positive ALL (which involves the so-called minor breakpoint cluster region) and chronic myelogenous leukemia (which involves the "major breakpoint cluster region"), and the resulting fusion protein is approximately 190-kd in most cases of childhood and adult Philadelphia chromosome–positive ALL, compared with 210-kd in chronic myelogenous leukemia (169–171). Of note, p190 has been shown to be a more potent transforming agent than p210 *in vitro* (169,172).

Children who have Philadelphia chromosome–positive ALL are more likely to present with poor prognosis features, including older age, higher WBC count, and high frequency of CNS involvement (173). Even accounting for this, the prognosis in children, and in adults as well, is dismal (149,151,152,173–175). Presence of the Philadelphia chromosome is one of the few indications for considering bone marrow transplantation for children in first remission. The incidence of *BCR-ABL* fusion transcripts among children with ALL at first relapse is threefold higher than that seen at diagnosis (176). The Philadelphia chromosome may be seen in many different immunologic subtypes of ALL, and no specifically associated immunophenotype has been described (173,174, unpublished data).

t(4;11)(q21;q23)

This translocation is seen in about 3% of children who have ALL and in a slightly higher proportion of adults (147,149,151,152,158,177,178). An additional group of patients with ALL has other structural abnormalities that involve chromosome 11q23, including translocations that involve chromosomes 1 (1p32) and 19 (19p13). In contrast, the translocations t(6;11)(q27;q23) and t(9;11)(p21;q23), as well as some instances of t(11;19)(q23;p13.1), are associated with AML. In both ALL and AML, the gene residing at 11q23 that is targeted for translocation has been called *MLL* (mixed-lineage leukemia), *ALL1*, or *HRX* (homologous to *Drosophila trithorax*) (179). Patients with ALL who have *MLL* rearrangements are most commonly infants and present with hyperleukocytosis, often greater than 200×10^9 per liter, hepatosplenomegaly, and often CNS involvement (177,180–183). Several recent studies have demonstrated that a significantly higher frequency of *MLL* rearrangements is found in infant leukemia if molecular methods are used compared with conventional cytogenetics (181–183). These same studies have demonstrated a significantly worse prognosis among infants with *MLL* rearrangements relative to infants with germline *MLL*. The poor prognosis of infant ALL is attributable largely to its high prevalence of *MLL* rearrangements.

Virtually all patients with the translocation t(4;11) have a unique immunophenotype: Blasts are $CD19^+CD10^-$ and, unlike in most patients with ALL, are either negative for CD24 antigen or show heterogeneity in expression of the antigen on blast cells. Many, although not all, patients are $CD15^+$ (177,181,184,185). This phenotype is highly specific although only moderately sensitive for predicting 11q23 abnormalities (177). The unusual nature of this phenotype has led to confusion in the literature in describing this group of leukemias; they have been referred to as *mixed-lineage*, or even *myelomonocytic leukemia* (186). Although in some patients, particularly adults, there may be distinct morphologic evidence of monocytic differentiation, this is generally uncommon, so that "t(4;11) leukemia" probably should be regarded as a clinically and biologically distinct subset of precursor B-cell ALL (93,187).

t(1;19)(q23;p13)

This translocation, which until recently was the most common in childhood ALL, also was among the first to be shown to be associated with a particular immunophenotype (123). It is found in about 25% of patients with pre-B-cell ALL and only rarely in other patients with precursor B-cell ALL. In addition, the composite phenotype: homogeneous $CD9^+$ $CD10^+CD19^+$, partial $CD20^+$, and complete $CD34^-$, which is seen in only 8% of patients with childhood precursor B-cell ALL, identifies all cases harboring the *E2A-PBX1* fusion transcript resulting from the translocation t(1;19) (188). The E2A-PBX1 fusion protein, which is a potent oncogene in experimental models, is likely to act as a transcriptional regulator (189,190). A related but much less common translocation, t(17;19)(q21;p13), which juxtaposes *E2A* and *HLF* (hepatic leukemia factor) genes, has been documented at the molecular level in seven patients, all of whom died from their leukemia (189). The t(1;19) abnormality is responsible for the poor prognosis of patients with pre-B-cell ALL treated with antimetabolite-based therapy (126), although this adverse prognostic effect can be overcome by more intensive therapy (127,191).

MYC *Translocations*

The *MYC* protooncogene on chromosome 8 band q24 is well known to be translocated to immunoglobulin-coding regions on chromosomes 2, 22, and most commonly 14 in some B-cell neoplasms (192,193). The details of this translocation are discussed in Chapter 8. In leukemia, the presence of this translocation is associated highly with L3 morphology and a B-cell (surface immunoglobulin–positive) phenotype (194); its presence clearly helps to define a distinct aggressive form of leukemia.

14q11 Abnormalities

The TCRAα and TCRDδ genes have been mapped to band q11 on chromosome 14, and these loci are involved in several translocations in ALL (147,195–197). Translocations in this region are specific for T-cell ALL and are seen in up to 20% of patients (158,198). The most common partners for the translocation, *RBTN1-TTG1* (rhombotin 1–T-cell translocation gene 1) and *RBTN2-TTG2*, reside on the short arm of chromosome 11, at 11p15 and 11p13, respectively (147,197). A t(10;14)(q24;q11) translocation that involves the homeobox gene, *HOX11*, occurs in 5% to 10% of patients with T-cell ALL or T-cell lymphoblastic lymphoma (147,197,199). Translocations between 14q11 and the *MYC* oncogene on chromosome 8 also have been described in T-cell ALL (200); unlike those described previously, which involve the TCRDδ gene, t(8;14)(q24;q11) involves the TCRα gene (197). Another gene targeted both by translocation and, more commonly, deletion in T-cell ALL is *TAL1* (also known as *TCL5* or *SCL*) (147,201). The translocations t(1;14)(p32;q11) and t(1;7)(p32;q35), which juxtapose *TAL1* and TCRδ and TCRβ, respectively, together account for less than 5% of cases of T-cell ALL (147,197,201,202). Site-specific recombination of upstream *TAL1* sequences, however, yielding cytogenetically cryptic deletions, is detectable in about 25% of patients with pediatric T-cell ALL (201). In general, clinical or laboratory differences among cytogenetically defined groups of patients with T-cell ALL have not been reported, although in one study patients with *TAL1* alterations had relatively higher WBC counts and were more likely to express a CD2$^+$CD10$^-$ phenotype, compared with those lacking such alterations (201).

t(5;14)(q31;q32)

Rare patients with ALL have been described in association with hypereosinophilia and the translocation t(5;14)(q31;q32) (203,204). In half of the cases, hypereosinophilia preceded the diagnosis of B-lineage ALL by several months; in the remainder, hypereosinophilia was noted at or subsequent to the time of diagnosis (203). The translocation fuses the immunoglobulin heavy chain locus with the *IL3* gene; in both cases evaluated, *IL3* mRNA or protein was expressed by the leukemic cells harboring the translocation, but not in controls (204). These findings suggest that *IL3* may function in an autocrine loop in these rare but distinctive cases of ALL (204).

Other Abnormalities

Several other common structural chromosomal changes in ALL are considered here. Deletions of 6q are seen in about 10% of cases of ALL (147,149,153,158), but no clinical or immunophenotypic associations have emerged. Abnormalities of 9p have been described in about 10% of patients with ALL (147). These leukemias have been associated with a number of high-risk features, including older age, higher WBC counts, and greater frequency of splenomegaly and T-cell phenotype (147). As might be expected, this group of patients has a reduced event-free survival rate compared with patients lacking 9p abnormalities (191). In recent years, the molecular basis for 9p abnormalities has become apparent; these typically result in deletions of one or both of the cyclin-dependent kinase inhibitors, *P15* (*INK4B-MTS2*) and *P16* (*INK4A-MTS1*) (205–209). Among patients with pediatric T-cell ALL, *P16* deletions appear to be virtually ubiquitous, with up to 95% of patients demonstrating homozygous deletions if assayed using sensitive molecular techniques (205,209). As with *TEL-AML1* translocations, molecular analysis reveals a substantially higher prevalence of *P16* and *P15* abnormalities than would be predicted on the basis of conventional cytogenetic data. As noted previously, 12p abnormalities of uncertain significance had been described in approximately 10% of patients with B-lineage ALL; these 12p abnormalities now appear to be accounted for largely by *TEL* rearrangements, which are associated with a favorable prognosis (162).

TREATMENT AND SURVIVAL

The treatment of ALL in childhood represents one of the great success stories of chemotherapy. Thirty years ago, it was estimated that fewer than 1% of children who had ALL could be cured (210); with contemporary therapy, about 70% of children can be expected to be long-term survivors (191,211). Several principles have governed chemotherapeutic strategies:

1. Combination chemotherapy is more effective than single-agent therapy.
2. Although induction of remission is usually rapid, chemotherapy must be continued for several years to prevent relapse.

3. The CNS is a likely site of relapse, and CNS prophylaxis is essential.
4. Therapy must be tailored to biologically identifiable subgroups of patients.
5. Chemotherapy and radiotherapy have potentially devastating long-term effects, particularly if given to growing children, and should be limited if possible.

The combination of vincristine and prednisone was shown early on to induce remission in up to 85% of children who had ALL (212). Contemporary therapy adds a third and sometimes a fourth agent, including L-asparaginase, daunorubicin, or cyclophosphamide (89,213,214). Remission—defined as eradication of disease measured by conventional morphologic criteria—is commonly achieved in 95% or more of patients, particularly in childhood. Giving more drugs during remission induction improves the duration of remission (213).

After remission, patients enter consolidation and maintenance phases, in which additional combinations of drugs are used. Other agents used include 6-mercaptopurine, methotrexate, cytosine arabinoside, adriamycin, and, most recently, teniposide (VM26) (191,211,214). It is well known that if additional therapy is not given at the time of remission, relapse is certain, so the principle requiring maintenance therapy is well established. There is no generally accepted regimen, however, and new drug combinations are continually under investigation. Also well established is the need for CNS prophylaxis (211,215). This takes the form of multiagent intrathecal therapy, sometimes with added cranial irradiation, depending on the risk of CNS relapse associated with a particular type of leukemia.

Children who have ALL are divided into at least two, and sometimes three, strata based on clinical and laboratory features, and different therapy is given based on this determination of "risk group." Patients deemed to be at high risk are treated more intensively; those at low risk often are treated to limit unnecessary toxicity. Depending on how they are defined, upwards of 90% of patients with "good risk" ALL can be cured; long-term survival of "poor risk" patients is less than 50%, with some groups, such as infants, faring particularly badly. (Factors that impact on prognosis in ALL are discussed in more detail in the next section.)

Although adult patients who have ALL have seen some improvement in their outlook over the past 15 years, results are not as favorable as in children (15,16,93,216). This reflects both the more frequent occurrence of biologically unfavorable forms of leukemia in adults (e.g., Philadelphia chromosome–positive ALL) and the inability of many adult patients, particularly older ones, to withstand the rigors of the intensive chemotherapy given to children (16,93,216). Principles of therapy are similar, although there is not as much tailoring of therapy to biologically defined risk groups. (In part this may be related to the fact that adult ALL is much less common than childhood ALL, and research protocols that ask questions about drug treatment would need twice the number of patients if "good" and "poor" risk arms were treated separately.) Remission rates are high, although not as high as in children, but the very best studies

TABLE 46.4. *Prognostic factors in childhood acute lymphoid leukemia*

Feature	Unfavorable if	References
Clinical		
Age[a]	<1 or >10	88, 89, 90, 131, 155
Mediastinal mass	Present	88, 89, 90
Hepatosplenomegaly	Marked	88, 89, 90
Lymphadenopathy	Marked	88, 89, 90, 155
Race	Nonwhite	88, 89, 90
Sex	Male[b]	88, 89, 90
Central nervous system disease at diagnosis	Present[b]	88, 89
Response to therapy	Residual leukemia in day 14 marrow	88, 90
Laboratory		
White blood cell count[a]	$>50(>20) \times 10^9$/L	88, 89, 90, 155
Platelet count	50×10^9/L[a]	88, 89, 90
Blast morphology	L2[b]	11, 13, 88, 89, 155
Immunophenotype	T (vs. non-T)[b]	80, 94, 155
	pre-B (vs. early pre-B)	87, 123
	$CD24^-$ or $CD10^-$[b]	84, 88, 107, 110, 128, 129, 133, 134
	CD45 or CD20 bright	114, 115
Ploidy[a]	DNA index <1.16 or <51 chromosomes	145, 146, 149, 154, 214
Cytogenetics[a]	t(9;22)	88, 149, 150, 151, 153, 171, 172
	t(1;19)	126
	t(4;11)	146, 147, 148
	Not t(12;21) (molecular)	162, 163, 164

[a] Generally considered the most important factors in multivariate analyses.
[b] Not found to be significant in all studies.

TABLE 46.5. *Prognostic factors in adult acute lymphoid leukemia*

Feature	Unfavorable if	References
Clinical		
Age	>30 or 35 (or 50)	14, 15, 90, 152
Sex	Male	14, 15
Central nervous system disease	Present	14
Response to therapy	No complete remission at 4 or 5 weeks	15, 90, 152
Laboratory		
White blood cell count	>30 or 35 × 10^9/L	14, 15, 90, 152
Blast morphology	L3	14, 15
Immunophenotype	B	14, 152
	CD10 (CALLA)-negative	15, 90, 129, 152
	Myeloid antigen-positive	117
Cytogenetics	t(9;22); t(4;11)	15, 119, 145, 151, 152

show no better than a 35% to 45% survival rate at 5 years (16), and some of these may not be representative of all adult patients with ALL (93).

PROGNOSTIC FACTORS

The biologic diversity of ALL is linked to diversity in clinical behavior. Over the past 30 years it has become clear, particularly in children, that one can use a constellation of clinical and laboratory features to distinguish patients who are likely to be cured with conventional therapy from those whose outcome is likely to be less favorable. Tables 46.4 and 46.5 list clinical and laboratory features that have been shown to have an impact on prognosis.

In virtually all series of patients, childhood ALL, age, and WBC count have been the most important prognostic factors, and assignment of children to risk groups for therapy purposes have used these three features most frequently (88–91). Another clinical feature that has been used at diagnosis to dictate therapy is the extent of disease, as measured by adenopathy, organomegaly, CNS involvement, or the presence of a mediastinal mass. Platelet count has been associated with outcome in some studies. Certain characteristics of blast cells are also predictive of outcome (11,13,84,87, 90,94,107,110,128,129,133,146,154,155,217–219). Because adults who have ALL generally do not have as good an outcome as children, and because adult ALL is less common, less is known about prognostic factors in this age group. Age, WBC count, sex, blast morphology, and immunophenotype all have been shown to have some effect on prognosis (14–16,92,117,130,149,220). A very powerful predictor of outcome, both in adults and children, is initial response to therapy (15,92,220,221).

Clinical features and biologic features are intertwined closely. Practically, it is easier to measure WBC count than to karyotype blasts, so there is a tendency to discount the use of biologic parameters unless they provide ''independent'' prognostic significance. Although multivariate analyses are useful for determining factors that can be used easily to assign patients to treatment protocols, these analyses often combine dissimilar patients. For example, patients who have T-cell ALL and patients with the translocation t(4;11) are found in the group of patients who have high WBC counts, but these two diseases are very different. Although both groups of patients receive high-risk therapy, there is no *a priori* reason to believe that, as therapy improves, the same changes will prove useful in both diseases. Finally, whether patients with a particular biologic abnormality fare poorly because they have adverse clinical features or patients with adverse clinical features do poorly because they have a biologically unfavorable leukemia is moot. It is the combination of clinical and biologic features that forms the most useful definition of types of leukemia.

EVALUATION OF THE PATIENT WITH ACUTE LYMPHOBLASTIC LEUKEMIA AFTER THERAPY

With the advent of successful therapy for ALL, the pathologist frequently is called on not only to make an initial diagnosis of ALL but also to evaluate a patient's response to treatment. Most therapeutic protocols require assessment of marrow status at 14 to 28 days after chemotherapy for a decision about subsequent management of the patient. At this time, the most important criterion to evaluate is the percentage of blasts: Marrows with fewer than 5% blasts are often referred to as *M1 marrows*; those with 5% to 25% blasts are called *M2*; and those with more than 25% blasts are *M3*. (There is unfortunate confusion of this terminology with the FAB classification.) Patients who have M1 marrows by day 28 usually are switched to ''intensification'' or ''consolidation'' regimens; those who have M2 marrows often are given a second course of induction therapy (15,16,93, 222). Depending on the exact therapeutic protocol, patients who have M3 marrows or those who have M2 marrows following a second round of induction may be considered to have failed treatment and are offered more experimental therapies.

Marrow aspirates are often hypocellular after therapy, and a core biopsy may be essential to evaluate remission status (see Fig. 46.9). Clusters of residual blasts may be difficult to distinguish from early regeneration, although this is not usually as difficult as in the evaluation of AML after therapy. Another pitfall in evaluating marrow biopsies from patients who have received methotrexate is that megaloblastic red cell precursors may be confused with leukemic cells if the pathologist is not alert to this possibility. Because of the well-known increase in TdT^+ and $CD10^+$ cells in marrows after chemotherapy (223,224), routine immunophenotyping—that is, simple enumeration of cells with particular

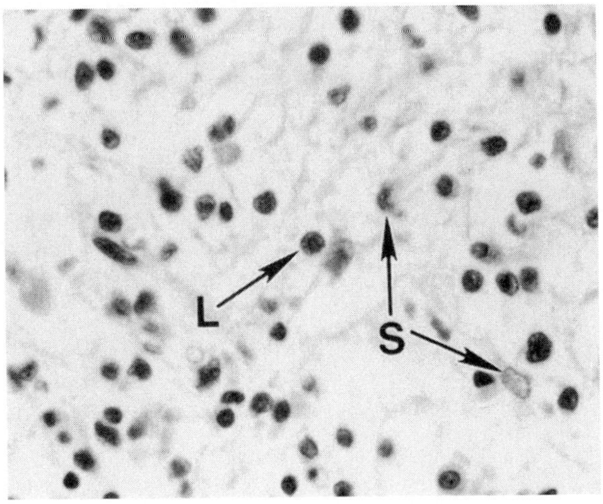

FIG. 46.9. Bone marrow biopsy following chemotherapy for acute lymphoblastic leukemia. Note the edema and strands of fibrin with numerous stromal cells (*S*) visible. There is also a significant increase in residual lymphoblasts (*L*), which, in this patient, have irregular nuclear contours and fine chromatin but no cytoplasm or nucleoli (hematoxylin and eosin stain, original magnification: 520× magnification).

characteristics—fails to distinguish residual leukemia from recovering marrow (see Chapter 50). Multiparameter flow cytometric analysis may be extremely helpful in making this distinction.

In contrast to the initial presentation, patients who have ALL who relapse often show only partial involvement of the bone marrow with leukemia. The marrow at relapse may be hypocellular, normocellular, or hypercellular, and the percentage of blasts may vary from only slightly above normal to 100%.

Although diagnosis of frank relapse is rarely difficult, considerable attention has been given to the much more difficult problem of predicting relapse or detecting minimal residual disease (225). Recent studies, in fact, suggest that this may be a very important new prognostic factor (225–228). Many studies have demonstrated the utility of multiparameter flow cytometric analysis in the detection of minimal residual leukemia (25,227,229–233). Because many patients who have ALL express combinations of antigens on their blasts that differ from those seen in normal cells (e.g., coexpression of B-lineage and myeloid antigens), it is possible to detect rare, phenotypically abnormal cells among predominantly normal marrow elements. Although relatively minor phenotypic changes have been described in relapsed ALL, the composite immunophenotype of ALL at diagnosis appears largely to be retained at relapse (234,235), enabling specific identification of recurrent leukemic cells. For leukemias whose aberrant immunophenotype is not present in normal marrows at detectable levels, flow cytometry may permit detection of as few as 1 in 10,000 cells (225,227,233). One limitation of this approach, especially in B-lineage ALL, is that many leukemias are not immunophenotypically ''aberrant,'' in that their antigenic makeup may be found on small numbers of cells among regenerating marrow elements. In virtually all patients, however, the comparative intensity of expression of multiple antigens differs between leukemic cells and normal elements, and this fact can be exploited to detect small numbers of blast cells using three- or four-color flow cytometry (236).

Molecular approaches to the detection of minimal residual disease have been evaluated. For example, reverse transcriptase–polymerase chain reaction assays to detect leukemia-specific fusion trancripts have been used in cases harboring t(1;19), t(4;11), and t(9;22) translocations (237–240). Overt relapse was heralded by molecular detection of fusion transcripts in four of four patients with t(4;11)-positive ALL, and 12 of 12 with t(9;22)-positive ALL in clinical remission, whereas patients in whom the fusion transcripts could not be detected remained in clinical remission (239,240). Another application of polymerase chain reaction assays in the detection of minimal residual disease is the generation of probes specific for the rearranged immunoglobulin heavy chain of the leukemic clone (226,241–245). Using a variation of this approach, in which clone-specific DNA also was quantified, Brisco and colleagues have demonstrated a significant correlation between detection of minimal residual disease and probability of relapse (246). Moreover, in a later trial employing more aggressive therapy that yielded a better overall survival rate, probability of relapse correlated not only with detection of residual disease but also with the precise quantity of clone-specific DNA detected (246). In two recent multiinstitutional studies, each with nearly 250 patients, the presence and number of molecularly detected residual blasts at the end of induction therapy and early in consolidation therapy were found to be powerful prognostic factors in childhood ALL (226,228). Although these studies illustrate the ability to predict relapse in advance of overt clinical manifestations, whether or not this diagnostic lead time will augment the effect of subsequent therapy remains to be seen.

SUMMARY AND CONCLUSIONS

This chapter focuses on the diversity of what was once thought to be a simple disease. It could be argued that no two cases of ALL are exactly alike. Although taking such an extreme approach is not fruitful, it is fair to say that if clinical, morphologic, immunologic, and cytogenetic and molecular features are taken into account, ALL is not one disease but several. At the same time, therapeutic options in ALL are relatively limited, so precise classification dictates disease-specific therapy only to a limited extent. As therapy continues to improve, clinical advances will be intelligible only in the context of the varied biology of ALL. To a large extent, clinical and biologic factors are able to predict which patients can be cured with conventional therapy and need not be subjected to more toxic, investigational regimens. To detect relapse early, when intervention is more likely to have a favorable impact on outcome, it is essential to understand the biology of the individual patient's leukemia. It is hoped that this chapter gives the reader an indication of how the diversity of ALL can be studied, and why its evaluation is important.

REFERENCES

1. Linet MS, Devesa SS. Descriptive epidemiology of the leukemias. In: Henderson ES, Lister TA, eds. *Leukemia*, 5th ed. Philadelphia: WB Saunders, 1990:207–224.
2. Greaves MF, Pegram SM, Chan LC. Collaborative group study of the epidemiology of acute lymphoblastic leukaemia subtypes: background and first report. *Leuk Res* 1985;9:715–733.
3. Stewart AM, Kneale GW. Age distribution of cancers caused by obstetric X-rays and their relevance to cancer latent periods. *Lancet* 1990;ii:4–8.
4. Rosner F, Lee SL. Down's syndrome and acute leukemia: myeloblastic or lymphoblastic. *Am J Med* 1972;53:203–218.
5. Peterson RDA, Kelly WD, Good RA. Ataxia telangiectasia: its association with defective thymus, immunological deficiency disease, and malignancy. *Lancet* 1964;i:1189–1193.
6. Fraumeni JR Jr, Manning MD, Mitus WJ. Acute childhood leukemia: epidemiologic study by cell type of 1263 cases at the Children's Cancer Research Foundation in Boston, 1947-1965. *J Natl Cancer Inst* 1971;46:461–470.
7. Pui C-H, Raimondi SC, Borowitz MJ, et al. Immunophenotypes and karyotypes of leukemic cells in children with Down syndrome and acute lymphoblastic leukemia. *J Clin Oncol* 1993;11:1361–1367.
8. Litz CE, Davies S, Brunning RD, et al. Acute leukemia and the transient myeloproliferative disorder associated with Down syndrome: morphologic, immunophenotypic and cytogenetic manifestations. *Leukemia* 1995;9:1432–1439.
9. Bennett JM, Catovsky D, Daniel MT, et al. Proposals for the classification of the acute leukaemias. *Br J Haematol* 1976;33:451–458.
10. Bennett JM, Catovsky D, Daniel MT, et al. The morphologic classification of acute lymphoblastic leukaemia: concordance among observers and clinical correlations. *Br J Haematol* 1981;47:553–561.
11. Viana MB, Maurer HS, Ferenc C. Subclassification of acute lymphoblastic leukaemia in children: analysis of the reproducibility of morphologic criteria and prognostic implication. *Br J Haematol* 1980;45: 178–181.
12. Davey FR, Castella A, Lauenstein K, et al. Prognostic significance of the revised French-American-British classification for acute lymphocytic leukaemia. *Clin Lab Haemat* 1983;5:343–351.
13. Miller DR, Leikin S, Albo V, et al. Prognostic importance of morphology (FAB classification) in childhood acute lymphocytic leukemia. *Br J Haematol* 1981;48:199–206.
14. Baccarani M, Corbelli G, Amadori S, et al. Adolescent and adult lymphoblastic leukemia: prognostic features and outcome of therapy: a study of 293 patients. *Blood* 1982;60:677–684.
15. Clarkson B, Ellis S, Little C, et al. Acute lymphoblastic leukemia in adults. *Semin Oncol* 1985;12:160–179.
16. Hoelzer D, Gale RP. Acute lymphoblastic leukemia in adults: recent progress, future directions. *Semin Hematol* 1987;24:27–39.
17. Reed MM, Proctor SJ. Failure of FAB classification to predict relapse-free survival in acute leukaemia. *Lancet* 1982;ii:153–154.
18. Lee EJ, Pollak A, Leavitt RD, et al. Minimally differentiated acute nonlymphocytic leukemia: a distinct entity. *Blood* 1987;70: 1400–1406.
19. Tricot G, Broeckaert Van Orshoven A, Van Hoof A, et al. Sudan black B positivity in acute lymphoblastic leukaemia. *Br J Haematol* 1982;51:615–621.
20. Davey FR, Huntington SJ, MacCallum J, et al. Cytochemical reactions of normal and neoplastic lymphocytes. *J Clin Pathol* 1977;30: 653–660.
21. Catovsky D, Greaves MF, Pan C, et al. Acid phosphatase reaction in acute lymphoblastic leukaemia. *Lancet* 1978;i:749–751.
22. Head DR, Borowitz MJ, Cerezo L, et al. Acid phosphatase positivity in childhood acute lymphocytic leukemia. *Am J Clin Pathol* 1986;86: 650–653.
23. Janossy G, Hoffbrand AV, Greaves MF, et al. Terminal transferase enzyme assay and immunological membrane markers in the diagnosis of leukemia: a multiparameter analysis of 300 cases. *Br J Haematol* 1980;44:221–234.
24. Jani P, Verbi W, Greaves MF, et al. Terminal deoxynucleotidyl transferase in acute myeloid leukemia. *Leuk Res* 1983;7:17–29.
25. Farahat N, Lens D, Morilla R, et al. Differential TdT expression in acute leukemia by flow cytometry: a quantitative study. *Leukemia* 1995;9:583–587.
26. Schumacher HR, Perlin E, Klos JR, et al. Hand-mirror cell leukemia, a new clinical and morphological variant. *Am J Clin Pathol* 1977;68: 531–534.
27. Schumacher HR, Champion JE, Thomas NJ, et al. Acute lymphoblastic leukemia hand-mirror variant: an analysis of a large group of patients. *Am J Hematol* 1979;7:11–17.
28. Glassy EF, Sun NCJ, Okun DB. Hand-mirror cell leukemia: report of 9 cases and a review of literature. *Am J Clin Pathol* 1980;74: 651–656.
29. McFarland W, Schecter GP. The lymphocytes in immunologic reactions in vitro: ultrastructural studies. *Blood* 1970;35:683–688.
30. Schumacher HR, Thomas WJ, Strong M, et al. Acute lymphoblastic leukemia hand-mirror variant: a viral immune interrelationship as demonstrated by ultrastructural studies. *Am J Hematol* 1981;10: 399–403.
31. Mazur EM, Wittles EG, Schiffman E, et al. Hand-mirror cell lymphoid leukemia in adults. *Cancer* 1986;57:92–99.
32. Cerezo L, Shuster JJ, Pullen DJ, et al. Laboratory correlates and prognostic significance of granular acute lymphoblastic leukemia in children: a Pediatric Oncology Group Study. *Am J Clin Pathol* 1990;95: 526–531.
33. Grogan TM, Insalaco SJ, Savage RA, et al. Acute lymphocytic leukemia with prominent azurophilic granulation and punctate acidic nonspecific esterase and phosphatase activity. *Am J Clin Pathol* 1981; 75:716–722.
34. Davey FR, Mick R, Nelson DA, et al. Morphologic and cytochemical characterization of adult lymphoid leukemias which express myeloid antigen. *Leukemia* 1988;2:420–426.
35. Askin FB, Land VJ, Sullivan MP, et al. Occult testicular leukemia: testicular biopsy at three years after continuous complete remission of childhood leukemia. *Cancer* 1981;47:470–475.
36. Longacre TA, Foucar K, Crago S, et al. Hematogones: a multiparameter analysis of bone marrow precursor cells. *Blood* 1989;73:543–552.
37. Vogel P, Enf LA, Rosenthal N. Hematological observations on bone marrow obtained by sternal puncture. *Am J Clin Pathol* 1937;7: 436–447.
38. Loken MR, Shah VO, Dattilio KL, Civin CI. Flow cytometric analysis of human bone marrow: II. Normal B lymphocyte development. *Blood* 1987;70:1316–1324.
39. Kersey JH, Nesbit ME, Luckasen JR, et al. Acute lymphoblastic leukemia and lymphoma cells with thymus derived (T) markers. *Mayo Clin Proc* 1974;49:584–587.
40. Sen L, Borella L. Clinical importance of lymphoblasts with T markers in childhood acute leukemia. *N Engl J Med* 1975;292:828–832.
41. Flandrin G, Abroet JC, Daniel MT, et al. Acute leukemia with Burkitt's tumor cells: a study of six cases with special reference to lymphocyte surface markers. *Blood* 1975;45:183–188.
42. Korsmeyer SJ, Hieter PA, Ravietch JV, et al. A developmental hierarchy of immunoglobulin gene rearrangements in human leukemia preBcells. *Proc Natl Acad Sci USA* 1981;78:7096–7100.
43. Nadler LM, Korsmeyer SJ, Anderson KC, et al. B cell origin of non-T cell acute lymphoblastic leukemia: a model for discrete stages of neoplastic and normal pre-B cell differentiation. *J Clin Invest* 1984; 74:332–340.
44. Janossy G, Coustan-Smith E, Campana D. The reliability of cytoplasmic CD3 and CD22 antigen expression in the immunodiagnosis of acute leukemia: a study of 500 cases. *Leukemia* 1989;3:170–181.
45. Sartor M, Bradstock K. Detection of intracellular lymphoid differentiation antigens by flow cytometry in acute lymphoblastic leukemia. *Cytometry* 1994;18:119–122.
46. Pizzolo G, Vincenzi C, Nadali G, et al. Detection of membrane and intracellular antigens by flow cytometry following ORTHO PermeaFixTM fixation. *Leukemia* 1994;8:672–676.
47. Farahat N, van der Plas D, Praxedes M, et al. Demonstration of cyto-

plasmic and nuclear antigens in acute leukemia using flow cytometry. *J Clin Pathol* 1994;47:843–849.
48. Vodinelich L, Tax W, Bai Y, et al. A monoclonal antibody (WT1) for detecting leukemias of Tcell precursors (T-cell ALL). *Blood* 1983; 62:1108–1113.
49. Link M, Warnke R, Finlay J, et al. A single monoclonal antibody identifies T cell lineage of childhood lymphoid malignancies. *Blood* 1983;62:722–728.
50. Pittaluga S, Raffeld M, Lipford EH, Cossman J. 3A1 (CD7) expression precedes T (gene rearrangements in precursor T (lymphoblastic) neoplasms. *Blood* 1986;68:134–139.
51. Borowitz MJ, Dowell BL, Boyett JM, et al. Monoclonal antibody definition of T cell acute leukemia: a Pediatric Oncology Group study. *Blood* 1985;65:785–788.
52. Greaves MF, Chan LC, Furley AJW, et al. Lineage promiscuity in hematopoietic differentiation and leukemia. *Blood* 1986;67:1–11.
53. Mirro J, Antouin GR, Zipf TF, et al. The E rosette associated antigen of T cells can be identified on blasts from patients with acute myeloblastic leukemia. *Blood* 1985;65:363–367.
54. Link MP, Stewart SJ, Warnke RA, et al. Discordance between surface and cytoplasmic expression of the Leu4 (T3) antigen in thymocytes and blast cells from childhood T lymphoblastic malignancies. *J Clin Invest* 1985;76:248–253.
55. Van Dongen JJM, Krissansen GW, Wolvers Tettero ILM, et al. Cytoplasmic expression of the CD3 antigen as a diagnostic marker for immature T cell malignancies. *Blood* 1988;71:603–612.
56. Campana D, Thompson JS, Amlot T, et al. The cytoplasmic expression of CD3 antigens in normal and malignant cells of the T lymphoid lineage. *J Immunol* 1987;138:648–655.
57. SlaperCortenbach ICM, Admiraal LG, Kerr JM, et al. Flow cytometric detection of terminal deoxynucleotidyl transferase and other intracellular antigens in combination with membrane antigens in acute lymphatic leukemia. *Blood* 1988;72:1639–1644.
58. Knowles DM. Immunophenotypic and antigen receptor gene rearrangement analysis in T cell neoplasia. *Am J Pathol* 1989;134: 761–785.
59. Knowles DM, Pelicci PG, Dalla Favera R. Tcell receptor beta chain gene rearrangements: genetic markers of T cell lineage and clonality. *Human Pathol* 1986;17:546–551.
60. Pittaluga S, Uppenkamp M. Cossman J. Development of T3/T cell receptor gene expression in human preT neoplasms. *Blood* 1987;69: 1062–1067.
61. Waldmann TA, Davis MM, Bongiovanni KF, et al. Rearrangements of genes for the antigen receptor on T cells as markers of lineage and clonality in human lymphoid neoplasms. *N Engl J Med* 1985;313: 776–783.
62. Mirro J Jr, Kitchingman G, Behm FG, et al. T cell differentiation stages identified by molecular and immunologic analysis of the T cell receptor complex in childhood lymphoblastic leukemia. *Blood* 1987; 69:908–912.
63. Minden MD, Mak TW. The structure of the T cell antigen receptor genes in normal and malignant T cells. *Blood* 1986;327–339.
64. Tawa A, Hozumi N, Minden M, et al. Rearrangement of the Tcell receptor β chain gene in non-T cell, non-B cell acute lymphoblastic leukemia of childhood. *N Engl J Med* 1985;313:1033–1037.
65. Griesinger F, Greenberg JM, Kersey JH. T cell receptor gamma and delta rearrangements in hematologic malignancies. *J Clin Invest* 1989; 84:506–516.
66. Foa R, Casorati G, Giubellino MC, et al. Rearrangements of immunoglobulin and T cell receptor β and γ genes are associated with terminal deoxynucleotidyl transferase expression in acute myeloid leukemia. *J Exp Med* 1989;165:879–890.
67. LeBien TW, Elstrom RL, Moseley M, et al. Analysis of immunoglobulin and T cell receptor gene rearrangements in human fetal bone marrow B lineage cells. *Blood* 1990;76:1196–1200.
68. Pui CH, Behm FG, Raimondi SC, et al. Secondary acute myeloid leukemia in children treated for acute lymphoid leukemia. *N Engl J Med* 1989;321:136–142.
69. Beishuizen A, Verhoeven M-AJ, van Wering ER, et al. Analysis of Ig and T-cell receptor genes in 40 childhood acute lymphoblastic leukemias at diagnosis and subsequent relapse: implications for the detection of minimal residual disease by polymerase chain reaction analysis. *Blood* 1994;83:2238–2247.
70. Ghali DW, Panzer S, Fischer S, et al. Heterogeneity of the T-cell receptor δ gene indicating subclone formation in acute precursor B-cell leukemias. *Blood* 1995;85:2795–2801.
71. Steenbergen EJ, Verhagen OJHM, van Leeuwen EF, et al. Frequent ongoing T-cell receptor rearrangements in childhood B-precursor acute lymphoblastic leukemia: implications for monitoring minimal residual disease. *Blood* 1995;86:692–702.
72. Diaz MA, Garcia-Sanchez F, Vicario JL, et al. Clinical relevance of T-cell receptor delta gene rearrangements in childhood B-precursor cell acute lymphoblastic leukemia. *Br J Haematol* 1997;99:308–313.
73. Kurtzberg J, Waldmann TA, Davey MP, et al. CD7+ , CD4-, CD8- acute leukemia: a syndrome of pluripotent lymphohematopoietic cells. *Blood* 1989;73:381–390.
74. Sobol RE, Royston I, LeBien TW, et al. Adult acute lymphoblastic leukemia phenotypes defined by monoclonal antibodies. *Blood* 1985; 65:730–735.
75. Reinherz EL, Kung PC, Goldstein G, et al. Discrete stages of human intrathymic differentiation: analysis of normal thymocytes and leukemic lymphoblasts of T cell lineage. *Proc Natl Acad Sci USA* 1980; 77:1588–1592.
76. Chen PM, Chiang H, Chou CK, et al. Immunological classification of T cell acute lymphoblastic leukaemia using monoclonal antibodies. *Leuk Res* 1983;7:339–348.
77. Roper M, Crist WM, Metzgar RS, et al. Monoclonal antibody characterization of surface antigens in childhood T-cell lymphoid malignancies. *Blood* 1983;61:830–837.
78. Crist WM, Schuster JJ, Falletta J, et al. Clinical features and outcome in childhood T cell leukemialymphoma according to stage of thymocyte differentiation: a Pediatric Oncology Group study. *Blood* 1988; 72:1891–1897.
79. Chan LC, Pegram SM, Greaves MF. Contribution of immunophenotype to the classification and differential diagnosis of acute leukemia. *Lancet* 1985;i:475–479.
80. Borowitz MJ, Falletta JM. Leukemias and lymphomas of thymic differentiation. *Clin Lab Med* 1988;8:119–217.
81. Thiel E, Kranz BR, Raghavachar A, et al. Prethymic phenotype and genotype of preT (CD7+ /ER-) cell leukemia and its clinical significance within adult acute lymphoblastic leukemia. *Blood* 1989;73: 1247–1258.
82. Denning SM, Haynes BF. Differentiation of human T cells. *Clin Lab Med* 1988;8:1–14.
83. Dowell BL, Borowitz MJ, Boyett JM, et al. Immunologic and clinicopathologic features of common acute lymphoblastic leukemia antigen-positive childhood T cell leukemia: a Pediatric Oncology Group study. *Cancer* 1987;59:2020–2026.
84. Greaves MF, Janossy G, Peto J, et al. Immunologically defined subclasses of acute lymphoblastic leukaemia in children: their relationship to presentation features and prognosis. *Br J Haematol* 1981;48: 179–197.
85. Borowitz MJ. Immunologic markers in childhood acute lymphoblastic leukemia. *Hematol Oncol Clin North Am* 1990;4:743–765.
86. Pullen DJ, Crist WM, Falletta JM, et al. A Pediatric Oncology Group classification protocol for acute lymphocytic leukemia: immunologic phenotypes and correlation with treatment results. In: Murphy SB, Gilbert JR, eds. *Leukemia research: advances in cell biology and treatment.* Amsterdam: Elsevier, 1983:221–239.
87. Pullen DJ, Boyett JM, Crist WM, et al. Pediatric Oncology Group utilization of immunologic markers in the designation of acute lymphocytic leukemia: subgroups' influence on treatment response. *Ann NY Acad Sci* 1984;428:26–48.
88. Poplack DG. Acute lymphoblastic leukemia in childhood. *Pediatr Clin North Am* 1985;32:669–697.
89. Miller LP, Miller DR. Acute lymphoblastic leukemia in children: current status, controversies, and future perspectives. *CRC Crit Rev Oncol* 1985;1:129–196.
90. Hammond D, Sather H, Nesbit M, et al. Analysis of prognostic factors in acute lymphoblastic leukemia. *Med Pediatr Oncol* 1986;14: 124–134.
91. Smith M, Arthur D, Camitta B, et al. Uniform approach to risk classifi-

cation and treatment assignment for children with acute lymphoblastic leukemia. *J Clin Oncol* 1996;14:18–24.
92. Hoelzer D, Thiel E, Loffler H, et al. Prognostic factors in a multicenter study for treatment of acute lymphoblastic leukemia in adults. *Blood* 1988;71:123–131.
93. Copelan EA, McGuire EA. The biology and treatment of acute lymphoblastic leukemia in adults. *Blood* 1995;85:1151–1168.
94. Borowitz MJ, Dowell BL, Boyett JM, et al. Clinicopathologic aspects of E rosette negative T cell acute lymphocytic leukemia: a Pediatric Oncology Group Study. *J Clin Oncol* 1986;4:170–177.
95. Thiel E, Rodt H, Huhn D, et al. Multimarker classification of acute lymphoblastic leukemia: evidence for further T subgroups and evaluation of their clinical significance. *Blood* 1980;56:759–772.
96. Shuster JJ, Falletta JM, Pullen DJ, et al. Prognostic factors in childhood T cell ALL: a Pediatric Oncology Group study. *Blood* 1990;75:166–173.
97. Uckun FM, Steinherz PG, Sather HN, et al. CD2 antigen expression on leukemic cells as a predictor of event-free survival after chemotherapy for T-lineage acute lymphoblastic leukemia: a Children's Cancer Group study. *Blood* 1996;88:4288–4295.
98. Campana D, Janossy G, Bofill M, et al. Human B cell development: I. Phenotypic differences of B lymphocytes in the bone marrow and peripheral lymphoid tissue. *J Immunol* 1985;134:1524–1530.
99. Boue DR, LeBien TW. Expression and structure of CD22 in acute leukemia. *Blood* 1988;71:1480–1486.
100. Korsmeyer SJ, Arnold A, Bakahshi A, et al. Immunoglobulin gene rearrangement and cell surface antigen expression in acute lymphocytic leukemias of T cell and B cell origins. *J Clin Invest* 1983;71:301–313.
101. Kitchingman GR, Rovigatti U, Mauer AM, et al. Rearrangement of immunoglobulin heavy chain genes in T cell acute lymphoblastic leukemia. *Blood* 1985;65:725–729.
102. Pugh WC, Stass SA. Immunoglobulin gene rearrangement and its implications for the study of B cell neoplasia. *Clin Lab Med* 1988;8:45–64.
103. Crist WM, Cleary ML, Grossi CE, et al. Acute leukemias associated with the 4;11 chromosome translocation have rearranged immunoglobulin heavy chain genes. *Blood* 1985;66:33–38.
104. Anderson CA, Bates MP, Slaughenhoupt BL, et al. Expression of human B cell associated antigens on leukemias and lymphomas: a model of human B cell differentiation. *Blood* 1984;63:1424–1433.
105. Hurwitz CA, Loken MR, Graham ML, et al. Asynchronous antigen expression in B lineage acute lymphoblastic leukemia. *Blood* 1988;72:299–307.
106. Abramson CS, Kersey JH, LeBien TW. A monoclonal antibody (BA1) reactive with cells of human B lymphocyte lineage. *J Immunol* 1981;126:83–88.
107. Kersey J, Goldman A, Abramson C, et al. Clinical usefulness of monoclonal antibody phenotyping in childhood acute lymphoblastic leukemia. *Lancet* 1982;ii:1419–1423.
108. Civin CI, Strauss LC, Brovall C, et al. Antigenic analysis of hematopoiesis: III. Hematopoietic progenitor cell surface antigen defined by a monoclonal antibody raised against KG1a cells. *J Immunol* 1984;133:157–165.
109. Tindle RW, Nichols RAB, Chan L, et al. A novel monoclonal antibody BI3C5 recognizes myeloblasts and non-B, non-T lymphoblasts in acute leukaemias and CGL blast crises and reacts with immature cells in normal bone marrow. *Leuk Res* 1985;9:1–9.
110. Borowitz MJ, Shuster JJ, Civin CI, et al. Prognostic significance of CD34 expression in childhood B-precursor acute lymphocytic leukemia: a Pediatric Oncology Group study. *J Clin Oncol* 1990;8:1389–1398.
111. Jones NH, Borowitz MJ, Metzgar RS. Characterization of a 24,000 dalton antigen defined by a monoclonal antibody (DU-ALL1) elicited to common acute lymphoblastic leukemia cells. *Leuk Res* 1982;6:449–464.
112. Vogler LB, Crist WM, Bockman DE, et al. Pre-B leukemia: a new phenotype of childhood lymphoblastic leukemia. *N Engl J Med* 1978;298:872–878.
113. Caldwell CW, Patterson WB, Hakami N. Alterations of HLE1 (T200) fluorescence intensity on acute lymphoblastic leukemia cells may relate to therapeutic outcome. *Leuk Res* 1987;11:103–106.
114. Behm FG, Raimondi SC, Schell MJ, et al. Lack of CD45 antigen on blast cells in childhood acute lymphoblastic leukemia is associated with chromosomal hyperdiploidy and other favorable prognostic features. *Blood* 1992;79:1011–1016.
115. Borowitz MJ, Shuster J, Carroll AJ, et al. Prognostic significance of fluorescence intensity of surface marker expression in childhood B-precursor acute lymphoblastic leukemia: a Pediatric Oncology Group study. *Blood* 1997;89:3960–3966.
116. Pui CH, Behm FG, Singh B, et al. Myeloid-associated antigen expression lacks prognostic value in childhood acute lymphoblastic leukemia treated with intensive multiagent chemotherapy. *Blood* 1990;75:198–202.
117. Sobol RE, Mick R, Royston I, et al. Clinical importance of myeloid antigen expression in adult acute lymphoblastic leukemia. *N Engl J Med* 1987;316:1111–1117.
118. Lauria F, Raspadori D, Martinelli G, et al. Increased expression of myeloid antigen markers in adult acute lymphoblastic leukemia patients: diagnostic and prognostic implications. *Br J Haematol* 1994;87:286–292.
119. Boldt DH, Kopecky KJ, Head D, et al. Expression of myeloid antigens by blast cells in acute lymphoblastic leukemia of adults: the Southwest Oncology Group experience. *Leukemia* 1994;8:2118–2126.
120. Sullivan M, Pullen J, Crist W, et al. Clinical and biological heterogeneity of childhood B cell leukemia: implications for clinical trials. *Leukemia* 1990;4:6–11.
121. Navid F, Mosijczuk AD, Head, DR, et al. Acute Lymphoblastic Leukemia with the (8;14) (q24;q32) translocation and FAB L3 morphology associated with a B-precursor immunophenotype: the Pediatric Oncology Group Experience. *Leukemia* 1999;13:135–141.
122. Koehler M, Behm FG, Shuster J, et al. Transitional pre-B-cell acute lymphoblastic leukemia of childhood is associated with favorable prognostic clinical features and an excellent outcome: a Pediatric Oncology Group Study. *Leukemia* 1993;7:2064–2068.
123. Carroll AJ, Crist WM, Parmley RT, et al. Pre-B cell leukemia associated with chromosome translocation (1,19). *Blood* 1984;63:721–724.
124. Crist W, Boyett J, Roper M, et al. Pre B cell leukemia responds poorly to treatment: a Pediatric Oncology Group study. *Blood* 1984;63:407–414.
125. Crist W, Boyett J, Jackson J, et al. Prognostic importance of the pre-B cell immunophenotype and other presenting features in B lineage childhood acute lymphoblastic leukemia. *Blood* 1989;74:1256–1259.
126. Crist WM, Carroll AJ, Shuster JJ, et al. Poor prognosis of children with pre-B acute lymphoblastic leukemia is associated with the t(1;19) (q23;p13): a Pediatric Oncology Group study. *Blood* 1990;76:117–122.
127. Pui C-H, Raimondi SC, Hancock ML, et al. Immunologic, cytogenetic, and clinical characterization of childhood acute lymphoblastic leukemia with the t(1;19)(q23;p13) or its derivative. *J Clin Oncol* 1994;12:2601–2606.
128. Morgan E, Hsu CCS. Prognostic significance of the acute lymphoblastic leukemia (ALL) cell associated antigen in children with null cell ALL. *Am J Pediatr Hematol Oncol* 1980;2:99–102.
129. Chessells JM, Hardisty RM, Rapson NT, et al. Acute lymphoblastic leukemia in children: classification and prognosis. *Lancet* 1977;ii:1307–1309.
130. Hoelzer D, Thiel E, Loffler H, et al. Intensified therapy in acute lymphoblastic and acute undifferentiated leukemia in adults. *Blood* 1984;64:38–47.
131. Crist W, Pullen J, Boyett J, et al. Clinical and biologic features predict a poor prognosis in acute lymphoid leukemias in infants: a Pediatric Oncology Group study. *Blood* 1986;67:135–140.
132. Pui C-H, Rivera GK, Hancock ML, et al. Clinical significance of CD10 expression in childhood acute lymphoblastic leukemia. *Leukemia* 1993;7:35–40.
133. Vannier JP, Bene MC, Faure GC, et al. Investigation of the CD10 (CALLA) negative acute lymphoblastic leukaemia: further description of a group with poor prognosis. *Br J Haematol* 1989;72:156–160.
134. Sallan SE, Ritz J, Pesando J, et al. Cell surface antigens: prognostic implication in childhood acute lymphoblastic leukemia. *Blood* 1980;55:395–402.
135. Uckun FM, Song CW. Lack of CD24 antigen expression in B-lineage

acute lymphoblastic leukemia is associated with intrinsic radiation resistance of primary clonogenic blasts. *Blood* 1993;1323–1332.
136. Pui C-H, Hancock ML, Head DR, et al. Clinical significance of CD34 expression in childhood acute lymphoblastic leukemia. *Blood* 1993; 82:889–894.
137. Thomas X, Archimbaud E, Charrin C, et al. CD34 expression is associated with major adverse prognostic factors in adult acute lymphoblastic leukemia. *Leukemia* 1995;9:249–253.
138. Boucheix C, David B, Sebban C, et al. Immunophenotype of adult acute lymphoblastic leukemia, clinical parameters, and outcome: an analysis of a prospective trial including 562 tested patients (LALA87). *Blood* 1994;84:1603–1612.
139. Wiersma SR, Ortega J, Sorbel E, et al. Clinical importance of myeloid-antigen expression in acute lymphoblastic leukemia of childhood. *N Engl J Med* 1991;324:800–808.
140. Pui C-H, Behm FG, Singh B, et al. Myeloid-associated antigen expression lacks prognostic value in childhood acute lymphoblastic leukemia treated with intensive multiagent chemotherapy. *Blood* 1990;75: 198–202.
141. Borowitz MJ, Shuster JJ, Land VJ, et al. Myeloid-antigen expression in childhood acute lymphoblastic leukemia. *N Engl J Med* 1991;325: 1379–1380.
142. Uckun FM, Sather HN, Gaynon P, et al. Clinical features and treatment outcome of children with myeloid antigen positive acute lymphoblastic leukemia: a report from the Children's Cancer Group. *Blood* 1997; 90:28–35.
143. Pui C-H, Raimondi SC, Head DR, et al. Characterization of childhood acute leukemia with multiple myeloid and lymphoid markers at diagnosis and relapse. *Blood* 1991; 78:1327–1337.
144. Look AT. The cytogenetics of childhood leukemia: clinical and biologic implications. *Pediatr Clin North Am* 1988;35:723–741.
145. Williams DL, Tsiatis A, Brodeur GMG, et al. Prognostic importance of chromosome number in 136 untreated children with acute lymphoblastic leukemia. *Blood* 1982;60:864–871.
146. Secker-Walker LM, Chessells JM, Stewart EL, et al. Chromosomes and other prognostic factors in acute lymphoblastic leukaemia: a long-term followup. *Br J Haematol* 1989;72:336–342.
147. Raimondi SC. Current status of cytogenetic research in childhood acute lymphoblastic leukemia. *Blood* 1993;81:2237–2251.
148. Pui C-H. Childhood leukemia. *N Engl J Med* 1995;332:1618–1630.
149. Bloomfield CD, Secker-Walker LM, Goldman AI, et al. Six year followup of the clinical significance of karyotype in acute lymphoblastic leukemia. *Cancer Genet Cytogenet* 1989;40:171–185.
150. Bloomfield CD, Lindquist LL, Arthur D, et al. Chromosomal abnormalities in acute lymphoblastic leukemia. *Cancer Res* 1981;41: 4838–4843.
151. The Groupe Francais de Cytogenetique Hematologique. Cytogenetic abnormalities in adult acute lymphoblastic leukemia: correlations with hematologic findings and outcome: a collaborative study of the Groupe Francais de Cytogenetique Hematologique. *Blood* 1996;87: 3135–3142.
152. Secker-Walker LM, Prentice HG, Durrant J, et al. Cytogenetics adds independent prognostic information in adults with acute lymphoblastic leukemia on MRC trial UKALL XA. *Br J Haematol* 1997;96: 601–610.
153. Faderl S, Kantarjian WM, Talpaz M, et al. Clinical significance of cytogenetic abnormalities in adult lympholastic leukemia. *Blood* 1998;91:3995–4019.
154. Look AT, Roberson PK, Williams DL, et al. Prognostic importance of blast cell DNA content in childhood acute lymphoblastic leukemia. *Blood* 1985;65:1079–1085.
155. Kalwinsky DK, Roberson P, Dahl G, et al. Clinical relevance of lymphoblast biological features in children with acute lymphoblastic leukemia. *J Clin Oncol* 1985;3:477–484.
156. Trueworthy R, Shuster J, Look T, et al. Ploidy of lymphoblasts is the strongest predictor of treatment outcome in B-progenitor cell acute lymphoblastic leukemia of childhood: a Pediatric Oncology Group study. *J Clin Oncol* 1992;10:606–613.
157. Harris MB, Shuster JJ, Carroll A et al. Trisomy of leukemic cell chromosomes 4 and 10 identifies children with B-progenitor cell acute lymphoblastic leukemia with a very low risk of treatment failure: a Pediatric Oncology Group study. *Blood* 1992; 79:3316–3324.
158. Pui CH, Crist WM, Look AT. Biology and clinical significance of cytogenetic changes in childhood acute lymphoblastic leukemia. *Blood* 1990;76:1449–1463.
159. Pui CH, Carroll AJ, Raimondi SC, et al. Clinical presentation, karyotypic characterization and treatment outcome of childhood acute lymphoblastic leukemia with a near haploid or hypodiploid <45 line. *Blood* 1990;75:1170–1177.
160. Pui CH, Carroll AJ, Head D, et al. Near-triploidy or near-tetraploidy acute lymphoblastic leukemia of childhood. *Blood* 1990;76:590–596.
161. Romana SP, Poirel H, Leconiat M, et al. High frequency of t(12;21) in childhood B-lineage acute lymphoblastic leukemia. *Blood* 1995; 86:4263–4269.
162. Shurtleff SA, Buijs A, Behm FG, et al. TEL/AML1 fusion resulting from a cryptic t(12;21) is the most common genetic lesion in pediatric ALL and defines a subgroup of patients with an excellent prognosis. *Leukemia* 1995;9:1985–1989.
163. McLean TW, Ringold S, Neuberg D, et al. TEL/AML-1 dimerizes and is associated with a favorable outcome in childhood acute lymphoblastic leukemia. *Blood* 1996;88:4252–4258.
164. Rubnitz JE, Downing JR, Pui C-H, et al. TEL gene rearrangement in acute lymphoblastic leukemia: a new genetic marker with prognostic significance. *J Clin Oncol* 1997;15:1150–1157.
165. Borkhardt A, Cazzaniga G, Viehmann S, et al. Incidence and clinical relevance of TEL/AML1 fusion genes in children with acute lymphoblastic leukemia enrolled in the German and Italian multicenter therapy trials. *Blood* 1997;90:571–577.
166. Borowitz MB, Rubnitz J, Nash D, et al. Surface antigen phenotype can predict TEL-AML1 rearrangement in childhood B-precursor ALL: a pediatric oncology group study. *Leukemia* 1998;12:1764–1770.
167. Hrusak O,Trka J, Zuna J. et al. Aberrant expression of KOR-SA3544 antigen in childhood acute lymphoblastic leukemia predicts TEL-AML1 negativity. *Leukemia* 1998;12:1064–1070.
168. Baruchel A, Cayuela JM, Ballerini P, et al. The majority of myeloid-antigen-positive (My +) childhood B-cell precursor acute lymphoblastic leukemias express TEL-AML1 fusion transcripts. *Br J Haematol* 1997;99:101–106.
169. Clark SS, McLaughlin J, Crist WM, et al. Unique forms of the abl tyrosine kinase distinguish Ph1-positive CML from Ph1-positive ALL. *Science* 1987;235:85–88.
170. Lugo TG, Pendergast AM, Muller AJ, et al. Tyrosine kinase activity and transformation potency of bcr-abl oncogene products. *Science* 1990;247:1079–1082.
171. Maurer J, Janssen LWG, Thiel E, et al. Detection of chimeric bcr-abl genes in acute lymphoblastic leukaemia by the polymerase chain reaction. *Lancet* 1991;337:1055–1058.
172. Daley GQ, Van Etten RA, Baltimore D. Induction of chronic myelogenous leukemia in mice by the P210bcr/abl gene of the Philadelphia chromosome. *Science* 1990;247:824–830.
173. Ribeiro RC, Abromowitch M, Raimondi SC, et al. Clinical and biologic hallmarks of the Philadelphia chromosome in childhood acute lymphoblastic leukemia. *Blood* 1987;70:948–953.
174. Crist WM, Carroll A, Shuster J, et al. Philadelphia chromosome positive childhood acute lymphoblastic leukemia: clinical and cytogenetic characteristics and treatment outcome. A Pediatric Oncology Group study. *Blood* 1990;76:489–494.
175. Schlieben S, Borkhardt A, Reinisch I, et al. Incidence and clinical outcome of children with BCR/ABL-positive acute lymphoblastic leukemia (ALL): a prospective RT-PCR study based on 673 patients enrolled in the German pediatric multicenter therapy trials ALL-BFM-90 and CoALL-05-92. *Leukemia* 1996;10:957–963.
176. Beyermann B, Agthe AG, Adams H-P, et al. Clinical features and outcome of children with first marrow relapse of acute lymphoblastic leukemia expressing BCR-ABL fusion transcripts. *Blood* 1996;87: 1532–1538.
177. Pui CH, Frankel LS, Carroll AJ, et al. Clinical characteristics and treatment outcome of childhood acute lymphoblastic leukemia with the t(4;11)(q21;q23): a collaborative study of 40 cases. *Blood* 1991; 77:440–447.
178. Johansson B, Moorman AV, Haas OA, et al. Hematologic malignancies with t(4;11)(q21;q23): a cytogenetic, morphologic, immunophenotypic and clinical study of 183 cases. *Leukemia* 1998;12:779–787.
179. Thirman MJ, Gill HJ, Burnett RC, et al. Rearrangement of the MLL

gene in acute lymphoblastic and acute myeloid leukemias with 11q23 chromosomal translocations. *N Engl J Med* 1993; 329:909–914.
180. Stark B, Umiel T, Mammon Z, et al. Leukemia of early infancy: early B cell lineage associated with t(4;11). *Cancer* 1986;58:1265–1271.
181. Chen C-S, Sorenson PHB, Domer PH, et al. Molecular rearrangements on chromosome 11q23 predominate in infant acute lymphoblastic leukemia and are associated with specific biologic variables and poor outcome. *Blood* 1993;81:2386–2393.
182. Rubnitz JE, Link MP, Shuster JJ, et al. Frequency and prognostic significance of HRX rearrangements in infant acute lymphoblastic leukemia: a Pediatric Oncology Group study. *Blood* 1994;84: 570–573.
183. Cimino G, Rapanotti MC, Rivolta A, et al. Prognostic relevance of ALL-1 gene rearrangement in infant acute leukemias. *Leukemia* 1995; 9:391–395.
184. Arthur DC, Bloomfield CD, Lindquist LL, et al. Translocation 4;11 in acute lymphoblastic leukemia: clinical characteristics and prognostic significance. *Blood* 1982;59:96–99.
185. Parkin JL, Arthur DC, Abramson CS, et al. Acute leukemia associated with the t(4;11) chromosome rearrangement: ultrastructural and immunologic characteristics. *Blood* 1982;60:1321–1331.
186. Childs CC, HirschGinsberg C, Gulbert SJ, et al. Lineage heterogeneity in acute leukemia with the t(4;11) abnormality: implications of acute mixed lineage leukemia. *Hematol Pathol* 1988;2:145–148.
187. Pui C-H, Behm FG, Crist WM. Clinical and biologic relevance of immunologic marker studies in childhood acute lymphoblastic leukemia. *Blood* 1993;82:343–362.
188. Borowitz MJ, Hunger SP, Carroll AJ, et al. Predictability of the t(1; 19)(q23;p13) from surface antigen phenotype: implications for screening cases of childhood acute lymphoblastic leukemia for molecular analysis. A Pediatric Oncology Group Study. *Blood* 1993;82: 1086–1091.
189. Hunger SP. Chromosomal translocations involving the E2A gene in acute lymphoblastic leukemia: clinical features and molecular pathogenesis. *Blood* 1996;87:1211–1224.
190. Mellentin JD, Murre C, Donlon TA, et al. The gene for enhancer binding proteins E12/E47 lies at the t(1;19) breakpoint in acute leukemias. *Science* 1989;246:379–382.
191. Rivera GK, Raimondi SC, Hancock ML, et al. Improved outcome in childhood acute lymphoblastic leukemia with reinforced early treatment and rotational combination chemotherapy. *Lancet* 1991;337: 61–66.
192. Taub R, Kirsch I, Morton C, et al. Translocation of the c-myc gene into the immunoglobulin heavy chain locus in human Burkitt lymphoma and murine plasmacytoma cells. *Proc Natl Acad Sci USA* 1982; 79:7837–7841.
193. DallaFavera R, Bregni M, Erikson J, et al. Human c-myc oncogene is located on the region of chromosome 8 that is translocated in Burkitt lymphoma cells. *Proc Natl Acad Sci USA* 1982;79:7824–7827.
194. Berger R, Bernheim A, Brouet JC, et al. t(8;14) translocation in a Burkitt's type of lymphoblastic leukaemia (L3). *Br J Haematol* 1979; 43:87–90.
195. Le Beau MM, McKeighan TW, Shima EA, et al. T cell receptor α chain gene is split in a human T cell leukemia cell line with a t(11; 14)(p15;q11). *Proc Natl Acad Sci USA* 1986;83:9744–9748.
196. Champagne E, Takihara Y, Sagman U, et al. The T cell receptor delta chain locus is disrupted in the TALL associated t(11;14)(p13;q11) translocation. *Blood* 1989;73:1672–1676.
197. Kersey JH. Fifty years of studies of the biology and therapy of childhood leukemia. *Blood* 1997;90:4243–4251.
198. Raimondi SC, Behm FG, Roberson PK, et al. Cytogenetics of childhood T cell leukemia. *Blood* 1988;72:1560–1566.
199. Zutter M, Hockett RD, Roberts CWM, et al. The t(10;14)(q24;q11) of T cell acute lymphoblastic leukemia juxtaposes the δT cell receptor with TCL3, a conserved and activated locus at 10q24. *Proc Natl Acad Sci USA* 1990;87:3161–3165.
200. Shima EA, Le Beau MM, McKeithan TW, et al. Gene encoding the α chain of the T cell receptor is moved immediately downstream of cmyc in a chromosomal 8;14 translocation in a cell line from a human T cell leukemia. *Proc Natl Acad Sci USA* 1986;83:3439–3443.
201. Bash RO, Crist WM, Shuster JJ, et al. Clinical features and outcome of T-cell acute lymphoblastic leukemia in childhood with respect to alterations at the TAL1 locus: a Pediatric Oncology Group study. *Blood* 1993;81:2110–2117.
202. Chen Q, Cheng JT, Tsai LT, et al. The tal gene undergoes chromosome translocation in T cell leukemia and potentially encodes a helix-loop-helix protein. *EMBO J* 1990;9:415–424.
203. Hogan TF, Koss W, Murgo AJ, et al. Acute lymphoblastic leukemia with chromosomal 5;14 translocation and hypereosinophilia: case report and literature review. *J Clin Oncol* 1987;5:382–390.
204. Meeker TC, Hardy D, Willman C, et al. Activation of the interleukin-3 gene by chromosome translocation in acute lymphocytic leukemia with eosinophilia. *Blood* 1990;76:285–289.
205. Hebert J, Cayuela JM, Berkeley J, et al. Candidate tumor-suppressor genes MTS1 (p16INK4A) and MTS2 (p15INK4B) display frequent homozygous deletions in primary cells from T- but not B-cell lineage acute lymphoblastic leukemias. *Blood* 1994;84:4038–4044.
206. Takeuchi S, Bartram CR, Seriu T, et al. Analysis of family of cyclin dependent kinase inhibitors: p15/MTS2/INK4B, p16/MTS1/INK4A and p18 genes in acute lymphoblastic leukemia of childhood. *Blood* 1995;86:755–760.
207. Quesnel B, Preudhomme C, Philippe N, et al. p16 gene homozygous deletions in acute lymphoblastic leukemia. *Blood* 1995;85:657–663.
208. Okuda T, Shurtleff SA, Valentine MB, et al. Frequent deletion of p16INK4A/MTS1 and p15INK4B/MTS2 in pediatric acute lymphoblastic leukemia. *Blood* 1995;85:2321–2330.
209. Iolascon A, Faienza MF, Coppola B, et al. Homozygous deletions of cyclin-dependent kinase inhibitor genes, p16INK4A and p18, in childhood T cell lineage acute lymphoblastic leukemias. *Leukemia* 1996;10:255–260.
210. Burchenal JH. Long term survivors in acute leukemia and Burkitt's tumor. *Cancer* 1968;21:595–599.
211. Rivera GK, Pinkel D, Simone JV, et al. Treatment of acute lymphoblastic leukemia: 30 years' experience at St. Jude Children's Research Hospital. *N Engl J Med* 1993;329:1289–1295.
212. Holland JF, Glidewell O. Chemotherapy of acute lymphocytic leukemia in childhood. *Cancer* 1972;30:1480–1487.
213. Niemayer CM, Hitchcock-Bryan S, Sallan SE. Comparative analysis of treatment programs for childhood acute lymphoblastic leukemia. *Semin Oncol* 1985;12:122–130.
214. Gaynon PS. Primary treatment of leukemia of non-T cell lineage. *Hematol Oncol Clin North Am* 1990;4:915–936.
215. Pochedly C. Prevention of meningeal leukemia: review of 20 years of research and current recommendations. *Hematol Oncol Clin North Am* 1990;4:951–969.
216. Larson RA, Dodge RK, Burns CP, et al. A five-drug remission induction regimen with intensive consolidation for adults with acute lymphoblastic leukemia: Cancer and Leukemia Group B study 8811. *Blood* 1995;85:2025–2037.
217. Smith M, Arthur D, Camitta B, et al. Uniform approach to risk classification and treatment assignment for children with acute lymphoblastic leukemia. *J Clin Oncol* 1996;14:18–24.
218. Masa-aki K, Manabe A, Pui C-H, et al. Stroma-supported culture of childhood B-lineage acute lymphoblastic leukemia cells predicts treatment outcome. *J Clin Invest* 1996;97:755–760.
219. Goasguen JE, Dossot J-M, Fardel O, et al. Expression of the multidrug resistance-associated P-glycoprotein (P-170) in 59 cases of de novo acute lymphoblastic leukemia: prognostic implications. *Blood* 1993; 81:2394–2398.
220. Gaynor J, Chapman D, Little C, et al. A cause-specific hazard rate analysis of prognostic factors among 199 adults with acute lymphoblastic leukemia: the Memorial Hospital experience since 1969. *J Clin Oncol* 1988;6:1014–1030.
221. Gajjar A, Ribeiro P, Mancock ML, et al. Persistence of circulating blasts after 1 week of multiagent chemotherapy confers a poor prognosis in childhood acute lymphoblastic leukemia. *Blood* 1995;86: 1292–1295.
222. Cortes JE, Kantarjian HM. Acute lymphoblastic leukemia: a comprehensive review with emphasis on biology and therapy. *Cancer* 1995; 76:2393–2417.
223. Greaves MF, Hariri G, Newman RA, et al. Selective expression of the common acute lymphoblastic leukemia (gp100) antigen on immature lymphoid cells and their malignant counterparts. *Blood* 1983;61: 628–639.

224. Janossy G, Bollum FJ, Bradstock KF, et al. Terminal transferase positive human bone marrow cells exhibit the antigenic phenotype of common lymphoblastic leukemia. *J Immunol* 1979;123:1525–1529.
225. Campana D, Pui C-H. Detection of minimal residual disease in acute leukemia: methodologic advances and clinical significance. *Blood* 1995;85:1416–1434.
226. Cave H, ten Bosch JVDW, Suciu S, et al. Clinical significance of minimal residual disease in childhood acute lymphoblastic leukemia. *N Engl J Med* 1998;339:591–598.
227. Coustan-Smith E, Behm FG, Sanchez J, et al. Immunological detection of minimal residual disease in children with acute lymphoblastic leukaemia, *Lancet* 1998;351:550–554.
228. van Dongen JJM, Seriu T, Panzer-Grumayer ER, et al. Prognostic value of minimal residual disease in acute lymphoblastic leukemia in childhood. *Lancet* 1998;352:1731–1738.
229. Campana D, Coustan-Smith E, Janossy G. The immunologic detection of minimal residual disease in acute leukemia. *Blood* 1990;76: 163–171.
230. Campana D, Coustan-Smith E, Behm FG. The definition of remission in acute leukemia with immunologic techniques. *Bone Marrow Transplant* 1991;8:429–437.
231. Drach J, Drach D, Glassl H, et al. Flow cytometric determination of atypical antigen expression in acute leukemia for the study of minimal residual disease. *Cytometry* 1992;13:893–901.
232. Orfao A, Ciudad J, Lopez-Berges MC, et al. Acute lymphoblastic leukemia (ALL): detection of minimal residual disease (MRD) at flow cytometry. *Leuk Lymph* 1994;13(Suppl 1):87–90.
233. Campana D. Applications of cytometry to study acute leukemia: in vitro determination of drug sensitivity and detection of minimal residual disease. *Cytometry* 1994;18:68–74.
234. van Wering ER, Beishuizen A, Roeffen ETJM, et al. Immunophenotypic changes between diagnosis and relapse in childhood acute lymphoblastic leukemia. *Leukemia* 1995;9:1523–1533.
235. Chucrallah AE, Stass SA, Huh YO, et al. Adult acute lymphoblastic leukemia at relapse: cytogenetic, immunophenotypic, and molecular changes. *Cancer* 1995;76:985–991.
236. Weir E, Cowan K, LeBeau P, et al. A limited antibody panel can distinguish B-precursor acute lymphoblastic leukemia from normal B precursors with four color flow cytometry: implications for residual disease detection. *Leukemia* 1998;13:558–567.
237. Devaraj PE, Foroni L, Kitra-Roussos V, et al. Detection of BCR-ABL and E2A-PBX1 fusion genes by RT-PCR in acute lymphoblastic leukemia with failed or normal cytogenetics. *Br J Haematol* 1996; 89:349–355.
238. Devaraj PE, Foroni L, Janossy G, et al. Expression of the E2A-PBX fusion transcripts in t(1;19)(q23;p13) and der(19)t(1;19) at diagnosis and in remission of acute lymphoblastic leukemia with different B lineage immunophenotypes. *Leukemia* 1995;9:821–825.
239. Cimino G, Elia L, Rivolta A, et al. Clinical relevance of residual disease monitoring by polymerase chain reaction in patients with ALL-1/AF-4 positive-acute lymphoblastic leukemia. *Br J Haematol* 1996;92:659–664.
240. Preudhomme C, Henic N, Cazin B, et al. Good correlation between RT-PCR analysis and relapse in Philadelphia (Ph1)-positive acute lymphoblastic leukemia (ALL). *Leukemia* 1997;11:294–298.
241. Katz F, Ball L, Gibbons B, et al. The use of DNA probes to monitor minimal residual disease in childhood acute lymphoblastic leukaemia. *Br J Haematol* 1989;73:173–180.
242. Hansen-Hagge TE, Yokota S, Bartram CR. Detection of minimal residual disease in acute lymphoblastic leukemia by in vitro amplification of rearranged T cell receptor δ chain sequences. *Blood* 1989;74: 1762–1767.
243. Yamada M, Hudson S, Tournay O, et al. Detection of minimal disease in hematopoietic malignancies of the B cell lineage by using third-complementarity-determining region (CDRIII) specific probes. *Proc Natl Acad Sci USA* 1989;86:5123–5127.
244. D'Auriol L, MacIntyre E, Galibert F, et al. In vitro amplification of T cell γ gene rearrangements: a new tool for the assessment of minimal residual disease in acute lymphoid blastic leukemias. *Leukemia* 1989; 3:155–158.
245. Yamada M, Wasserman R, Lange B, et al. Minimal residual disease in childhood B-lineage lymphoblastic leukemia: persistence of leukemic cells during the first 18 months of treatment. *N Engl J Med* 1990; 323:448–455.
246. Brisco MJ, Condon J, Hughes E, et al. Outcome prediction in childhood acute lymphoblastic leukemia by molecular quantification of residual disease at the end of induction. *Lancet* 1994;343:196–200.

CHAPTER 47

Acute Myeloid Leukemia

Richard D. Brunning

The acute myeloid leukemias (AMLs) are a morphologically diverse group of hematopoietic malignancies characterized by a proliferation of immature cells that arise in the myeloid progenitor cells of the bone marrow. For purposes of morphologic classification, these progenitor cells are divided into four major types: granulocytic, which includes neutrophils, eosinophils, and basophils; monocytic; erythroid; and megakaryocytic. AMLs may present with exclusive involvement of one of these cell lines, the most common form of presentation, or with multiple cell types, a panmyelopathy. The proliferation of neoplastic cells usually results in marked replacement of normal marrow cells, and patients with AML frequently present with signs of marrow failure, such as anemia and thrombocytopenia. The manifestation of the leukemic process in the blood varies substantially; patients may present with a marked leukocytosis with a high percentage of leukemic cells, or there may be severe leukopenia with only rare leukemic cells.

The morphologic classification used herein is based on the proposed World Health Organization (WHO) classification of acute leukemias (1). This classification is a modification of the revised French–American–British (FAB) Cooperative Group classification published in 1976 and 1985 with additional changes suggested by a U.S. National Cancer Center Committee in 1990 (2–5). One of the major modifications of the FAB classification in the WHO proposal is the reduction of percentage of blasts from 30% to 20% for a diagnosis of AML; the 20% blasts may be present in the bone marrow or peripheral blood.

Other major considerations in the WHO proposal are the importance of cytogenetics, molecular markers, and evidence of multilineage dysplasia to predicting the biology of these processes; as a result, these factors are integrated into the classification. The proposed WHO classification of AML is shown in Table 47.1.

R. D. Brunning: Professor Emeritus, Department of Laboratory Medicine, University of Minnesota Medical School, Minneapolis, Minnesota 55455

This chapter addresses principally the morphologic classification, that is, AML not otherwise categorized, with brief reference to cytogenetic, molecular, and immunologic studies as they are relevant. The nonmorphologic studies are addressed in more detail in other chapters (see Chapters 3, 10, 38, and 45).

Concurrent or antecedent morphologic evidence of myelodysplastic changes in AML appears to be associated with a more aggressive clinical course (6,7). Because of this, the WHO classification recognizes the acute leukemias with this association as a distinct category. If a case of acute leukemia represents progression from a myelodysplastic syndrome, the diagnostic entity would be AML (of whichever subtype) evolving from a myelodysplastic syndrome. If there is morphologic evidence of multilineage dysplasia at the time of diagnosis of AML, but no antecedent clinical history or morphologic evidence of a myelodysplastic syndrome, the diagnostic terminology should reflect this with the phrase AML (subtype) with evidence of multilineage dysplasia. This necessitates careful evaluation of the blood and marrow smears and sections for evidence of dysplasia. These findings are recognized more readily in leukemias with evidence of maturation than in those processes characterized by a predominant population of blasts.

Another category of AML recognized in the WHO classification is the acute leukemias and myelodysplastic syndromes, which are related to prior therapy, either alkylating agents or topoisomerase II-directed drugs. The therapy-related leukemias and myelodysplastic syndromes are addressed in this chapter after the presentation of the "*de novo*" leukemias.

The classification of the AMLs presented here is primarily morphology- and cytochemistry-based (1–5,8). The role of immunologic markers in the diagnosis and classification is addressed for specific types (9). Cytogenetic and molecular studies are important for the classification and clinical management of the AMLs; the relationship of these studies is noted as relevant (10–14). A more detailed description of

TABLE 47.1. *World Health Organization proposal for the classification of acute myeloid leukemia*

1. Acute myeloid leukemia with recurrent cytogenetic abnormalities Acute myeloid leukemia, t(8;21)(q22;q22) Acute promyelocytic leukemia, t(15;17)(q22;q21) Acute myeloid leukemia, inv(16)(p13;q22) Acute myeloid leukemia, (v;11q23) 2. Acute myeloid leukemia with myelodysplasia-related features Acute myeloid leukemia evolving from myelodysplastic syndrome Acute myeloid leukemia with multilineage dysplasia without prior history of a myelodysplastic syndrome 3. Acute myeloid leukemia, therapy-related Alkylating agent–related type Topoisomerase II–related type	4. Acute myeloid leukemia, not otherwise categorized Acute myeloblastic leukemia, minimally differentiated (M0) Acute myeloblastic leukemia without maturation (M1) Acute myeloblastic leukemia with maturation (M2) Acute promyelocytic leukemia (M3) or microgranular (hypogranular) variant (M3V) Acute myelomonocytic leukemia (M4) or acute myelomonocytic leukemia with increased marrow eosinophils (M4E0) Acute monocytic leukemias Acute monoblastic leukemia (M5A) Acute monocytic leukemia (M5B) Acute erythroid leukemias Erythroleukemia (M6A) Pure acute erythroid leukemia (M6B) Acute megakaryoblastic leukemia (M7) Acute basophilic leukemia Acute panmyelosis with myelofibrosis

the cytogenetic and molecular associations is presented in Chapters 10 and 45.

The morphologic definition of AML is based on the presence of 20% or more myeloblasts or equivalent cells in the bone marrow or peripheral blood smears (1). Two primary types of myeloblasts generally are recognized in AML, types I and II (3). The type I myeloblast is characterized as a cell with a high nuclear:cytoplasmic ratio, lightly basophilic cytoplasm, fine nuclear chromatin, and generally two to four variably prominent nucleoli; these blasts are agranular (Fig. 47.1; see also Color Plate 30, between pp. 1446–1447). The type II myeloblast has the features of a type I myeloblast, with the addition of dispersed delicate azurophilic granules in the cytoplasm; the number of granules generally does not exceed 20. The nuclear:cytoplasmic ratio in the type II myeloblast may be slightly lower and the chromatin slightly more condensed than in a type I myeloblast. The presence of one or more Auer rods classifies a myeloblast as type II.

A third type of myeloblast, type III, occurs most characteristically in M2 AML associated with the cytogenetic abnormality t(8;21) and is marked by the presence of relatively numerous fine azurophilic granules (2,5,12) (Fig. 47.2; see also Color Plate 31, between pp. 1446–1447). It may be the predominant blast in cases of M2 AML not associated with

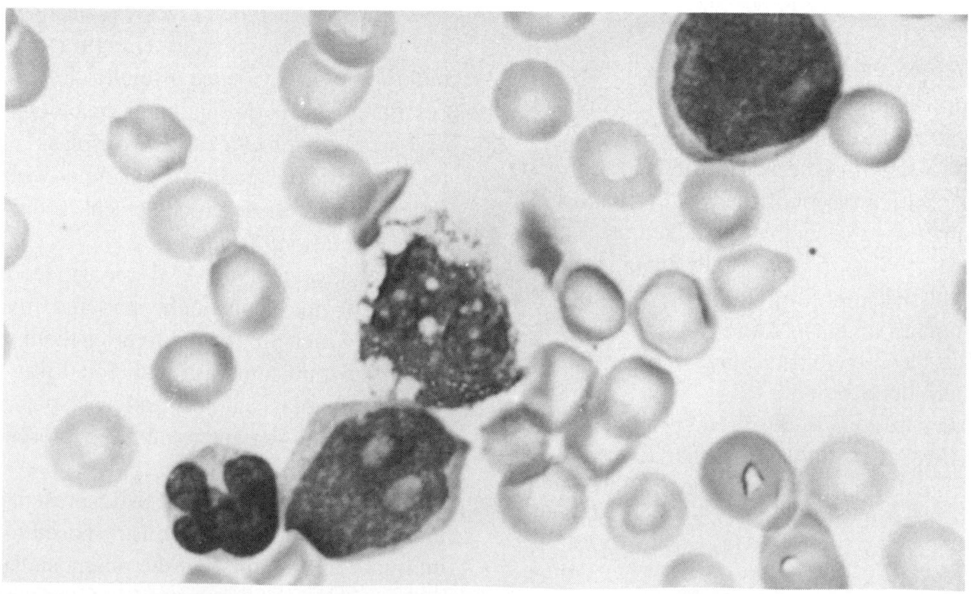

FIG. 47.1. Type I and type II myeloblasts. Bone marrow smear showing a type I myeloblast (**top**) with scant, agranular, basophilic cytoplasm and distinct nucleoli and a type II myeloblast (**bottom**) with the same features and a few azurophilic granules (Wright-Giemsa stain, original magnification: 400× magnification). See Color Plate 30, between pp. 1446–1447.

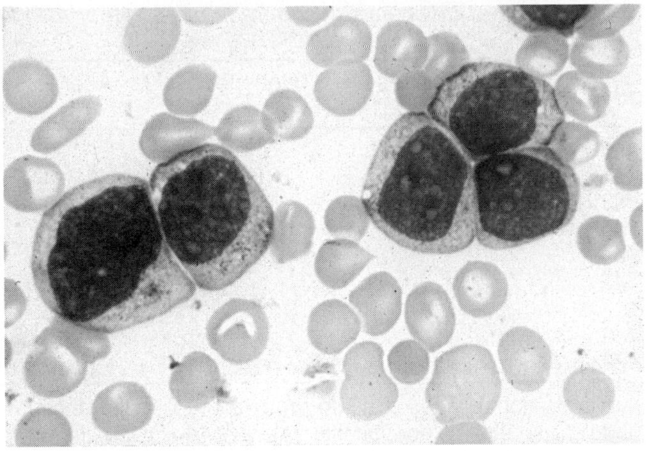

FIG. 47.2. Type III myeloblasts. Blood smear with numerous type III myeloblasts with numerous azurophilic granules (Wright-Giemsa stain, original magnification: 640× magnification). See Color Plate 31, between pp. 1446–1447.

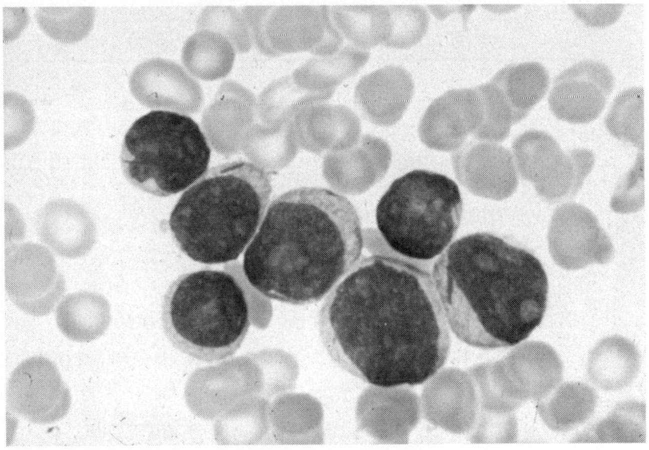

FIG. 47.3. Acute myeloblastic leukemia without maturation (M1). Bone marrow smear showing myeloblasts, several of which contain Auer rods (Wright-Giemsa stain, original magnification: 400× magnification). See Color Plate 32, between pp. 1446–1447.

the translocation t(8;21). The type III myeloblast has the nuclear and cytoplasmic features of the type II myeloblast except for the more abundant azurophilic granules. It is important to distinguish the type III blast from the neutrophil promyelocyte, which is larger, has a lower nuclear: cytoplasmic ratio, a more dense nuclear chromatin, and more coarse azurophilic granules overlying the cytoplasm and nucleus. The promyelocyte normally has a focal pale area in the cytoplasm that corresponds to the Golgi region, which is not apparent in the type III myeloblast.

In practice, distinction of the different types of blasts has little significance, and it is adequate to group all blasts in one category, myeloblasts. The important distinction is distinguishing early-stage promyelocytes from myeloblasts with a few granules.

Forms of AML exist in which the predominant proliferating immature cells are not myeloblasts. These include acute promyelocytic leukemia (APL), characterized by a proliferation of abnormal promyelocytes; acute monocytic leukemia, in which the leukemic cells are predominantly monoblasts and promonocytes; and acute megakaryoblastic leukemia, which is marked by a proliferation of megakaryoblasts. For the purposes of establishing the diagnosis of AML in these instances, these cells are considered equivalent to myeloblasts. A form of acute erythroid malignancy characterized by a proliferation of very immature erythroid precursors, usually more than 80% proerythroblasts and basophilic erythroblasts, is recognized in the proposed WHO classification as pure erythroid leukemia (1). In the other types of AML, proerythroblasts are not considered equivalent to myeloblasts and may not be used to satisfy the requisite 20% blasts.

An important morphologic finding in a significant percentage of AMLs is the Auer rod, an azurophilic linear structure of varying length and width that represents an abnormal alignment and crystallization of azurophilic granules (Fig. 47.3; see also Color Plate 32, between pp. 1446–1447). These structures are seen with myeloperoxidase (MPO) and Sudan black B (SBB) staining (15). The detection of Auer rods in AML varies with the subtype from APL, in which they are virtually always detected, to acute monoblastic leukemia, in which they are uncommonly observed (Table 47.2). The Auer rod generally is found in myeloblasts but also may be detected in more mature cells, including segmented neutrophils; the presence of an Auer rod in an acute leukemia is definitive evidence of myeloid origin.

The morphologic classification of AML is based, to a substantial degree, on cytochemical findings; three cytochemical stains are essential: MPO, SBB, and nonspecific esterase (NSE). The MPO and SBB stains react with cells of neutrophil lineage; monocytes may show scattered positive granules. The presence of MPO reactivity in a blast is evidence of myeloid origin. The MPO reaction usually is sought using cytochemical techniques; however, antibodies to MPO used either in flow cytometry or immunocytochemistry are more sensitive in detecting MPO activity (16). SBB positivity is highly suggestive of myeloid origin; occasional patients with acute lymphoblastic leukemia have coarse, gray-black, SBB-positive granules. Chloroacetate esterase (CAE), which in normal hematopoiesis is present only in neutrophils and mast cells, emerges in the early promyelocyte stage of maturation and usually is not detected in myeloblasts; as a result it does not have the utility of MPO and SBB for determining lineage of blasts. NSE activity is used to identify cells of monocytic lineage.

The lymphoblasts in approximately 90% to 95% of patients with acute lymphoblastic leukemia express the nuclear enzyme terminal deoxynucleotidyl transferase (TdT) (17–20). This nuclear enzyme may be observed in approximately 10% to 15% of patients with AML, most notably those with M2 AML associated with the t(8;21) chromo-

TABLE 47.2. *Summary of bone marrow findings in acute myeloid leukemias (AMLs) (3,8,11)*

AML M0
- ≥20%[a] blasts
- <3% blasts MPO/SBB-positive
- ≥20% Blasts express one or more myeloid-associated antigens (i.e., CD13, CD33)
- Negative for lymphocyte antigens

AML M1
- ≥20% blasts
- ≥3% blasts MPO/SBB-positive
- <10% promyelocytes and more mature neutrophils

AML M2
- ≥20% blasts
- ≥3% blasts MPO/SBB-positive
- ≥10% promyelocytes or more mature neutrophils

AML M3
- ≥20% myeloblasts and abnormal promyelocytes
- Blasts and promyelocytes with multiple Auer rods (faggot cells)
- Intense MPO/SBB positivity

AML M4
- ≥20% myeloblasts, monoblasts and promonocytes
- ≥20% neutrophils
- ≥20% monocytic cells
- Monocytosis: $\geq 5 \times 10^9$/L[b]

AML M5A
- ≥20% myeloblasts, monoblasts, and promonocytes
- ≥80% monocytic cells with ≥80% monoblasts

AML M5B
- >20% myeloblasts, monoblasts and promonocytes
- ≥80% monocytic cells with ≤80% monoblasts
- Predominance of promonocytes

AML M6A
- ≥50% erythroblasts
- ≥20% of nonerythroid cells are myeloblasts
- Myeloblasts may contain Auer rods (Table 47.4)

AML M6B
- ≥80% proerythroblasts and basophilic erythroblasts with dyserythropoiesis
- Myeloblasts may or may not be increased

AML M7
- ≥20% blasts
- ≥50% megakaryocytic cells (megakaryoblasts, promegakaryocytes, and megakaryocytes) by immunologic markers or ultrastructural study

[a] Percentages are of all bone marrow nucleated cells unless otherwise specified.
[b] Relates to blood findings.
MPO, myeloperoxidase; SBB, Sudan black B.

somal abnormality, in whom it may be present in a high percentage of blasts in 60% to 70% of patients (20). In other types of AML that are TdT-positive, the percentage of blasts that is positive generally is significantly lower than in acute lymphoblastic leukemia (17–20).

A peripheral blood and bone marrow differential count is essential to the classification of AML. The differential includes all nucleated marrow cells; in the subclassification of erythroleukemia (M6A), the myeloblast percentage is based on a differential of nonerythroid cells. A practical numeric range of cells to count without forfeiting precision is 500 to 1,000 (21).

TABLE 47.3. *Cytochemistry and frequency of Auer rods in acute myeloid leukemia*

	Myeloperoxidase/ Sudan black B	Nonspecific esterase[a]	Auer Rods (8),[b]%
M0	–	—	0
M1	+	—	49
M2	+	<20%	70
M3	++	—	97
M4	+	>20%	64
M5	–	++	M5A 0, M5B
M6	+	—	58
M7	–	—	0

[a] Occasional cases of acute promyelocytic leukemia show a subpopulation of nonspecific esterase–positive cells. Rare M5 cases are nonspecific esterase–negative. Megakaryocytes can show weak local nonspecific esterase positivity.
[b] No Auer Rods are found in megakaryoblasts.
From Brunning R, McKenna RW. *Tumors of the bone marrow,* 3rd series, fascicle. 9. Washington, DC: Armed Forces Institute of Pathology, 1994, with permission.

The major morphologic features of this classification are summarized in Tables 47.2 and 47.3.

ACUTE MYELOBLASTIC LEUKEMIA, MINIMALLY DIFFERENTIATED (M0)

Acute myeloblastic leukemia, minimally differentiated, is a type of AML in which the blasts lack evidence of myeloid differentiation on conventional morphologic and cytochemical studies; fewer than 3% of the blasts are MPO- or SBB-positive, and Auer rods are not identified (22) (Figs. 47.4, 47.5; see also Color Plates 33 and 34, between pp. 1446–1447). The myeloid origin is recognized by reactivity

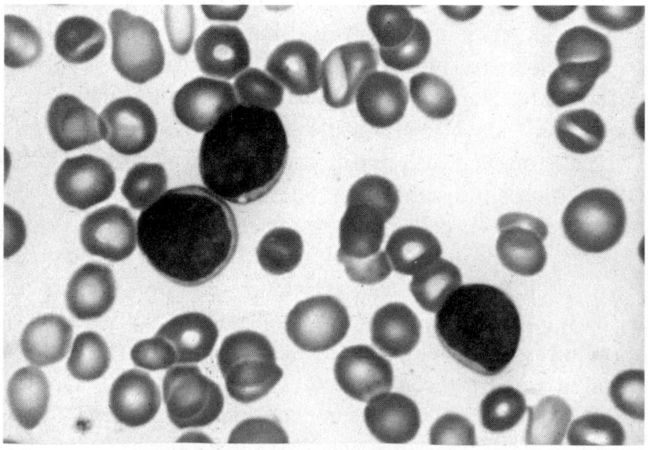

FIG. 47.4. Acute myeloblastic leukemia, minimally differentiated (MO). Blood smear with three blasts without differentiating features. The blasts were myeloperoxidase- and Sudan black B–negative but expressed CD13 and CD33 (Wright-Giemsa stain, original magnification: 400× magnification). See Color Plate 33, between pp. 1446–1447.

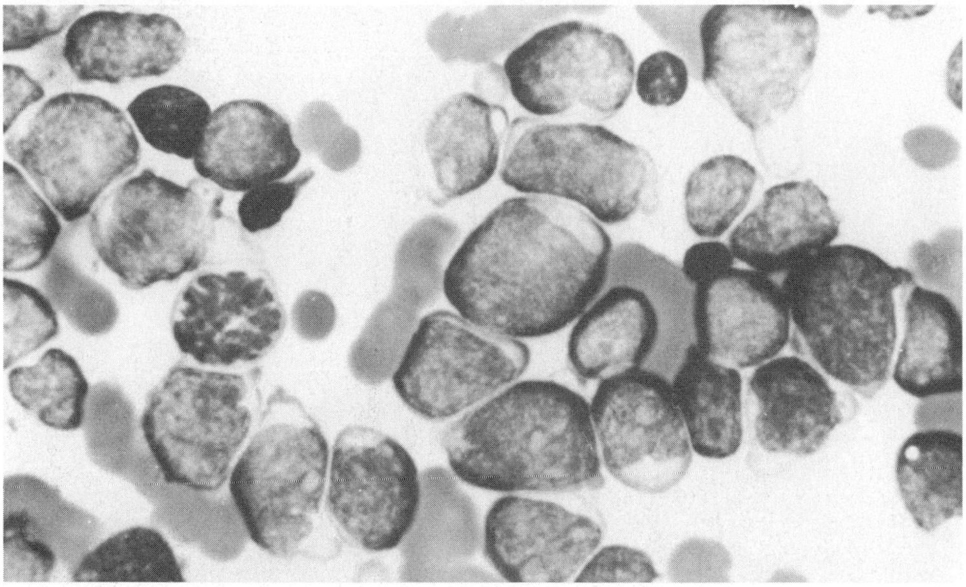

FIG. 47.5. Acute myeloid leukemia, minimally differentiated (M0). Bone marrow smear showing blasts that lack differentiating features and are myeloperoxidase- and Sudan black B–negative. The cells are CD33-positive (Wright-Giemsa stain, original magnification: 256× magnification). See Color Plate 34, between pp. 1446–1447.

of the blasts with antibodies to at least one myeloid-related antigen or ultrastructural demonstration of myeloid features (5,22–26). The blasts do not express lymphocyte antigens (see Chapters 3 and 38).

The blasts in M0 AML usually are agranular (22). Immunophenotypically, at least 20% of the blasts express one or more myeloid-related antigens, such as CD13, CD14, and CD33. Patients with M0 AML frequently express CD34; this antigen lacks specificity and may be present on lymphoblasts (26). Blasts from these patients may express TdT. If the blasts show ultrastructural or immunophenotypic evidence of megakaryocytic differentiation, the patient should be classified as having M7 AML.

Cytogenetic studies in M0 AML have shown a high incidence of abnormalities including complex karyotypes, partial or complete monosomy 5q or 7q + 13, and rearrangements involving 12p12-13 and 2p12-15 (23).

Acute myeloid leukemia of the M0 type accounts for approximately 5% of all acute leukemias in adults; it has been reported to have a less favorable response to combination chemotherapy than other forms of AML (22–24).

In a small percentage of patients with AML, the blasts lack differentiating cytochemical, ultrastructural, and immunophenotypic features; these patients should be classified as having acute leukemia, undifferentiated, and not M0 AML.

ACUTE MYELOBLASTIC LEUKEMIA WITHOUT MATURATION (M1)

Acute myeloid leukemia without maturation (M1) is a form of acute leukemia in which the marrow is composed primarily of myeloblasts; fewer than 10% of the bone marrow cells are promyelocytes and more mature neutrophils. At least 3% of the blasts demonstrate MPO or SBB positivity.

Acute myeloid leukemia of type M1 may present with leukopenia, a normal leukocyte count, or, in approximately 50% of patients, leukocytosis. Virtually all patients are anemic and neutropenic, and most are thrombocytopenic.

Bone marrow aspirates almost always have myeloblast percentages greater than 90%. The blast morphology is variable and may range from small lymphoid-appearing blasts to larger cells with relatively abundant cytoplasm; the blasts are generally type I (Figs. 47.3, 47.6; see also Color Plate 35, between pp. 1446–1447). The nuclei are usually round to oval but, in some patients, may be contorted or lobulated. Myeloblasts with Auer rods are present in approximately 50% of patients. Because the percentage of maturing neutrophils does not exceed 10%, the evidence of dysplastic changes may be minimal. Bone marrow sections are hypercellular in 70% to 80% of patients. Mitotic figures may be numerous (Fig. 47.7). The number of MPO- or SBB-positive blasts is variable, ranging from the minimum criterion of 3% to more than 90% (Fig. 47.8; see also Color Plate 36, between pp. 1446–1447).

The differential diagnosis of M1 AML includes acute lymphoblastic leukemia, acute monoblastic leukemia (M5A), and acute megakaryoblastic leukemia (M7). The TdT determination and MPO and SBB stains distinguish acute lymphoblastic leukemia from M1 AML in most instances. The blasts in acute lymphoblastic leukemia are TdT-positive in more than 90% of patients and MPO- and SBB-negative. TdT positivity may be present in blasts in AML M1; if it is, the median percentage of positive blasts is usually much lower, approximately 35% to 40%, in contrast to

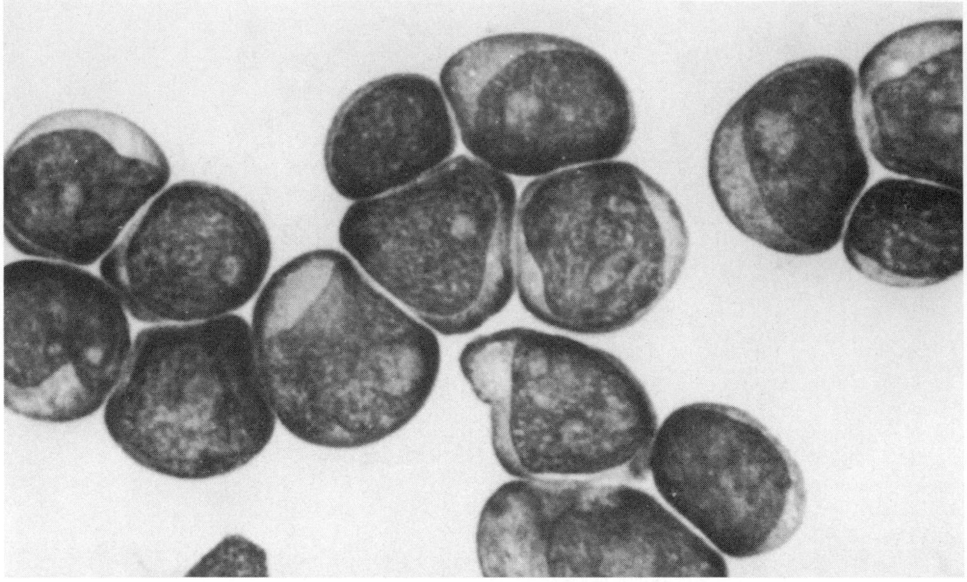

FIG. 47.6. Acute myeloblastic leukemia without maturation (M1). Bone marrow smear showing myeloblasts with a moderate amount of cytoplasm. More than 3% blasts reacted for myeloperoxidase (Wright-Giemsa stain, original magnification: 400× magnification). See Color Plate 35, between pp. 1446–1447.

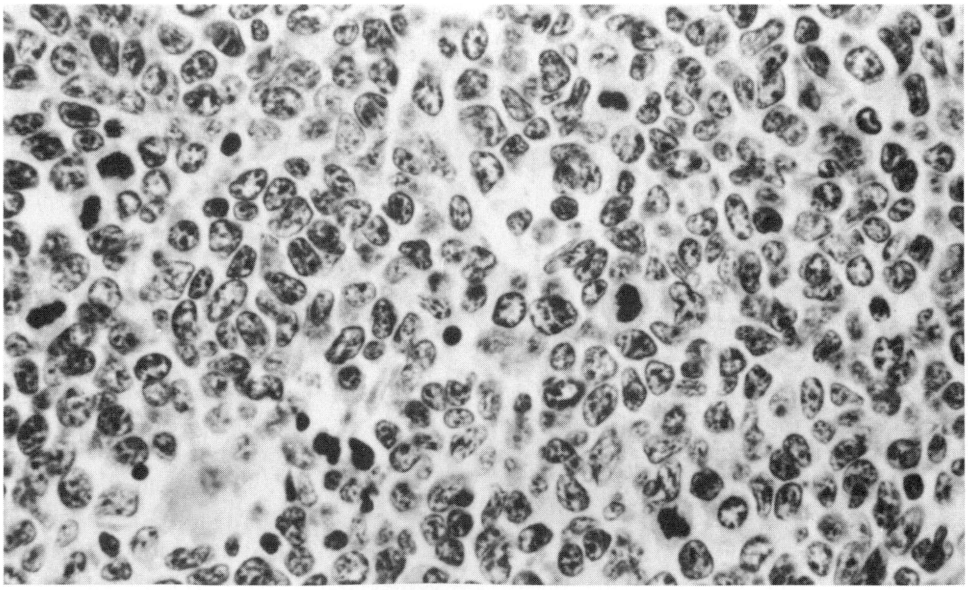

FIG. 47.7. Acute myeloblastic leukemia without maturation (M1). Bone marrow section showing a diffuse proliferation of blasts with a high nuclear: cytoplasmic ratio; numerous mitotic figures are present (hematoxylin and eosin stain, original magnification: 256× magnification).

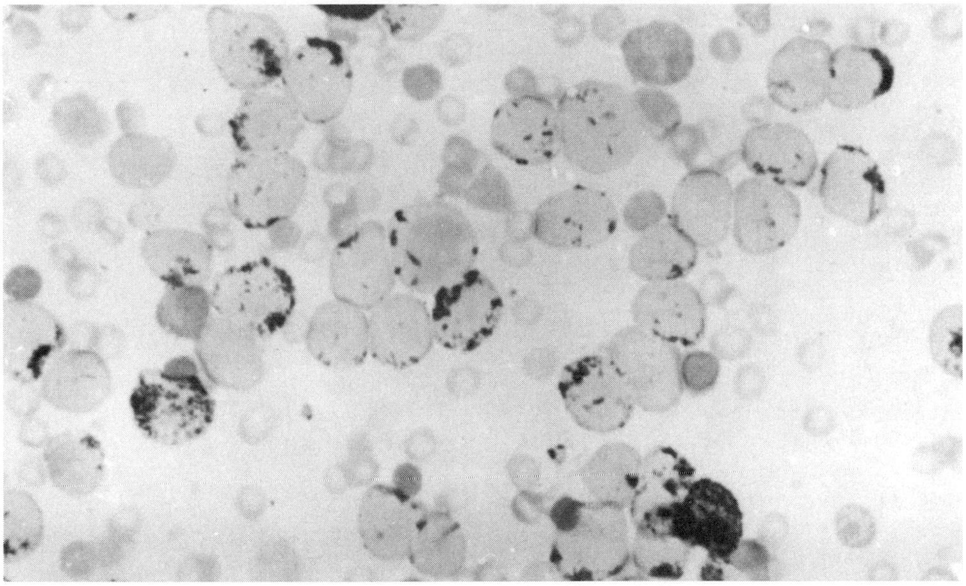

FIG. 47.8. Acute myeloblastic leukemia without maturation (M1). Bone marrow smear showing myeloblasts with uniform but varying degrees of reactivity for myeloperoxidase. The more mature cells are intensely positive (myeloperoxidase stain, original magnification: 256× magnification). See Color Plate 36, between pp. 1446–1447.

acute lymphoblastic leukemia, in which the percent positive blasts exceeds 80%. The monoblasts and promonocytes in AML M5A are NSE-positive in the majority of patients and MPO- and SBB-negative or, at most, slightly positive. The blasts in AML M7 are generally TdT-, MPO-, and SBB-negative; megakaryoblasts are identified by immunoreactivity with antibodies to megakaryocytes (CD41 and CD61) by flow cytometry or immunocytochemistry or by ultrastructural evidence of platelet peroxidase.

ACUTE MYELOBLASTIC LEUKEMIA WITH MATURATION (M2)

Acute myeloid leukemia with maturation (M2) is a form of AML in which the marrow or blood contains 20% or more type I and II myeloblasts. The basic feature distinguishing this type from M1 is evidence of maturation to the promyelocyte or more mature stages in 10% or more of the marrow cells (Fig. 47.9). An alternative criterion for classification as M2 is the presence of 10% or more type II and type III myeloblasts. The peripheral blood in the majority of patients shows leukocytosis, anemia, and thrombocytopenia. An occasional patient presents with a normal or elevated platelet count; this finding has been reported in association with a chromosome inversion, inv(3)(q21;q26), or the translocation t(3;3)(q21;q26) (27–29). There is usually an associated increase in megakaryocytes, some of which may be hypolobate.

The relative proportion of the various types of blasts in the marrow varies. There may be a predominance of type II and III blasts. Myeloblasts with Auer rods are present in approximately 70% of patients; as in M1 AML, the number of blasts with Auer rods and the number of Auer rods per blast varies; some blasts may contain multiple Auer rods (Figs. 47.10, 47.11; see also Color Plate 37, between pp. 1446–1447). Dysplastic changes are frequently present in the neutrophils and precursors. These changes include nuclear hypolobulation (pseudo–Pelger-Huet nuclei), cytoplasmic hypogranularity, pseudo–Chediak-Higashi granules, and bizarre nuclear hypersegmentation. Dyserythropoiesis may be present and is characterized by nuclear multilobulation, nuclear karyorrhexis, nuclear–cytoplasmic asynchrony, basophilic stippling, and cytoplasmic periodic acid-Schiff (PAS) stain positivity. Changes in the megakaryocytes include nuclear hypolobulation and micromegakaryocytes.

The sections generally are hypercellular and reflect the relative proportion of blasts and maturing cells indicated in the aspirate differential count. The neutrophil nature of the proliferating cells may be demonstrated with the immunocytochemical demonstration of MPO (Fig. 47.12; see also Color Plate 38, between pp. 1446–1447). Reticulin fibrosis is observed uncommonly and, if present, frequently is associated with a prominent megakaryocytic component.

Approximately 10% to 30% of patients with M2 AML are associated with a reciprocal translocation that involves chromosomes 8 and 21 (11,30–44). The molecular event involves fusion of the *AML1* gene on chromosome 21q22 and the ETO gene on chromosome 8q22. Patients who have M2 AML associated with a translocation t(8;21) are generally younger and have been reported to have a very favorable prognosis if treated with high-dose cytarabine in the consolidation phase (13,14). Characteristic morphologic features have been reported in this subtype (12,30–44). The blasts may contain numerous azurophilic granules and prominent

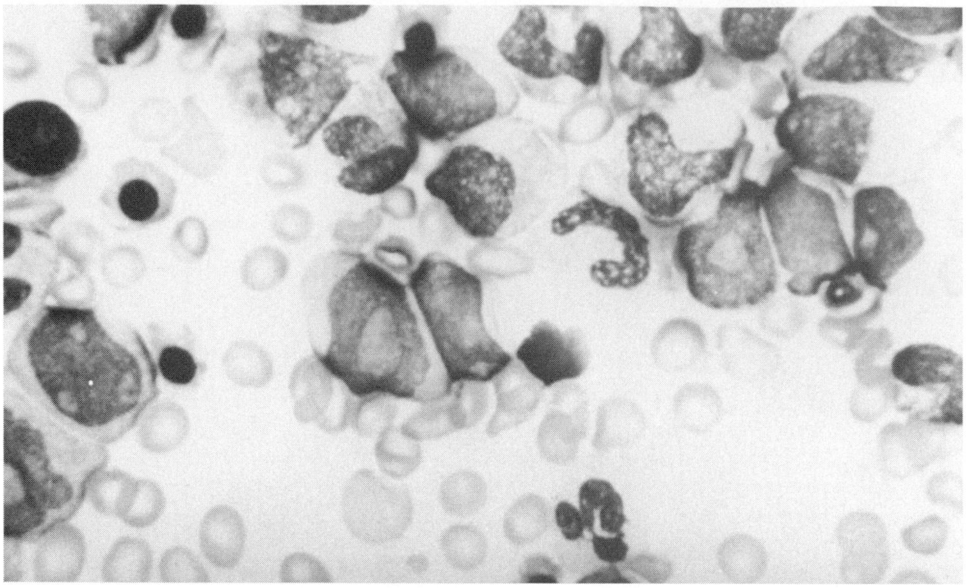

FIG. 47.9. Acute myeloblastic leukemia with maturation (M2). Bone marrow smear showing myeloblasts, maturing neutrophils, and a few erythroid precursors. A long, slender Auer rod is present in the myeloblast in the center of the field (Wright-Giemsa stain, original magnification: 256× magnification).

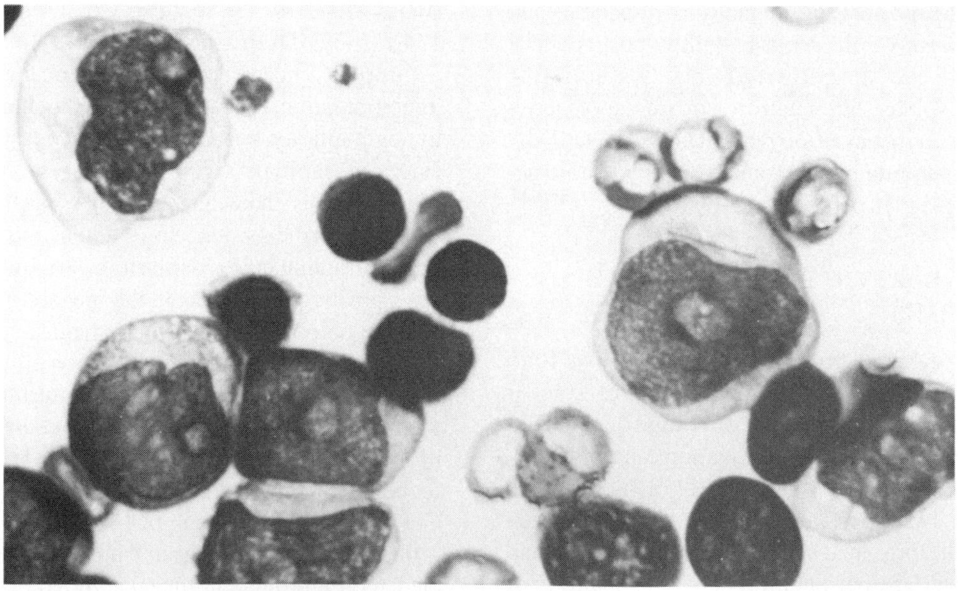

FIG. 47.10. Acute myeloblastic leukemia with maturation (M2). Bone marrow smears showing myeloblasts and more mature neutrophils. Two myeloblasts in the right portion of the field contain long, slender Auer rods (Wright-Giemsa stain, original magnification: 400× magnification). See Color Plate 37, between pp. 1446–1447.

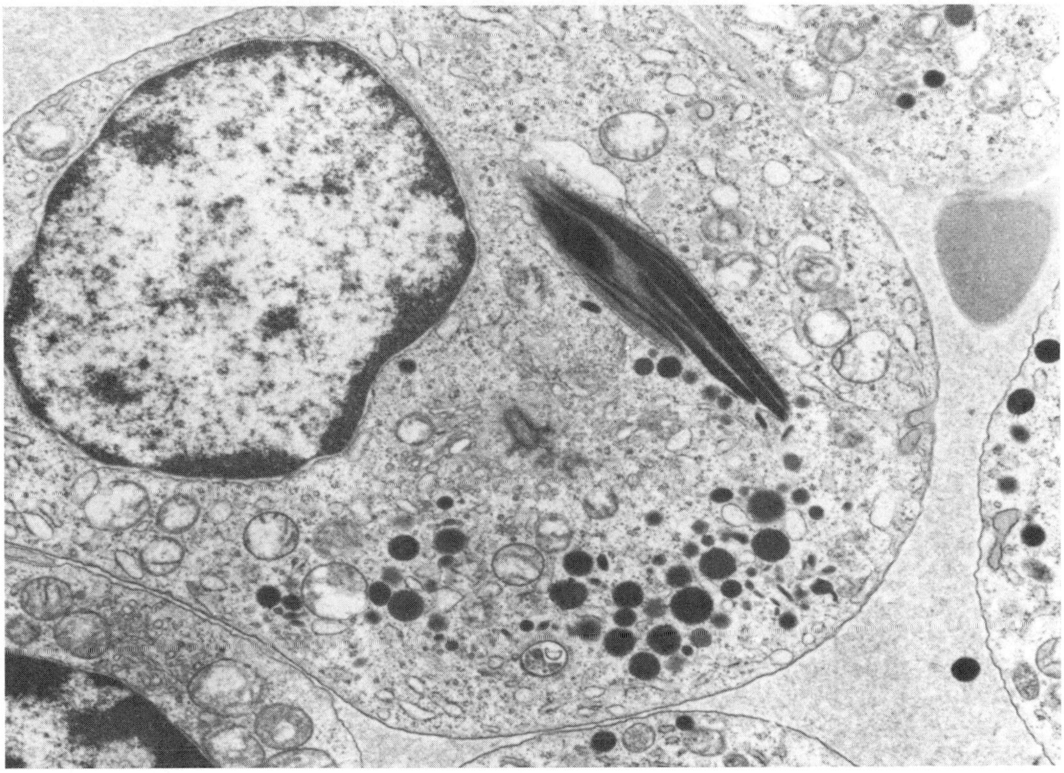

FIG. 47.11. Acute myeloblastic leukemia with maturation (M2). Electron micrograph of a neutrophil precursor from the bone marrow showing numerous primary granules and an Auer rod (uranyl acetate, lead citrate stain, original magnification: 15,000× magnification).

large slender Auer rods with tapered ends. Occasional myeloblasts have two to three Auer rods, and Auer rods may be found in segmented neutrophils. The type III blast is most characteristically observed in this type of AML. The specific granulation in the maturing neutrophils is prominent and may have an orange coalescent smudge-like appearance (Fig. 47.13; see also Color Plate 39, between pp. 1446–1447). Prominent dysplasia is frequently present in the neutrophils. Approximately 25% to 30% of patients with M2 AML with a translocation t(8;21) have increased marrow eosinophils, which are morphologically normal.

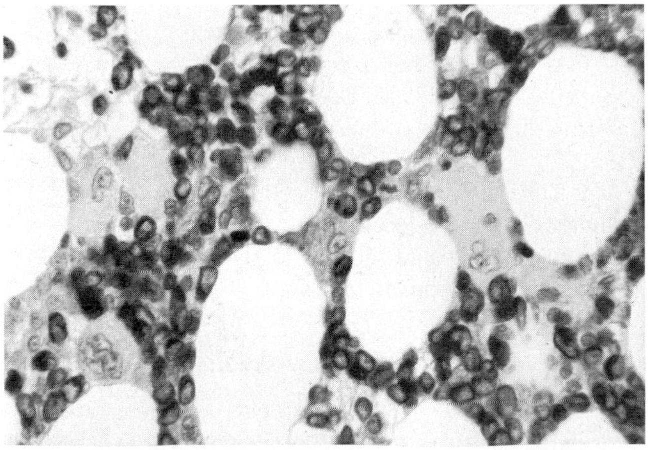

FIG. 47.12. Acute myeloblastic leukemia with maturation (M2). Bone marrow section reacted with antibody to myeloperoxidase; there are numerous reactive immature hematopoietic cells, some with striking cytoplasmic positivity (immunoperoxidase stain, original magnification: 256× magnification). See Color Plate 38, between pp. 1446–1447.

The blasts in M2 AML with the translocation t(8;21)(q22;q22) frequently express the lymphoid-associated antigen CD19; expression of CD34, the stem cell antigen, also may be observed. Coexpression of CD19 and CD56 on the blasts is reported in a pediatric patient population (43). The blasts in M2 AML with or without a translocation t(8;21) may be TdT-positive; up to 68% positive cells have been reported (43).

Acute myeloid leukemia of the M2 type with the translocation t(8;21) has a high association with extramedullary myeloid sarcomas (42,45,46). This constellation of findings has been associated with a less favorable prognosis than in patients with t(8;21)-associated AML without extramedullary involvement in an adult population, and a more favorable prognosis in a group of pediatric patients (45,46).

There is an infrequent association of M2 AML with the translocation t(6;9)(p23;q34) and increased numbers of marrow basophils (47–50). Increased marrow basophils may be observed in M2 AML with deletions or translocations involving 12p. This cytogenetic finding also has been detected in acute myelofibrosis, which has been cited as evidence

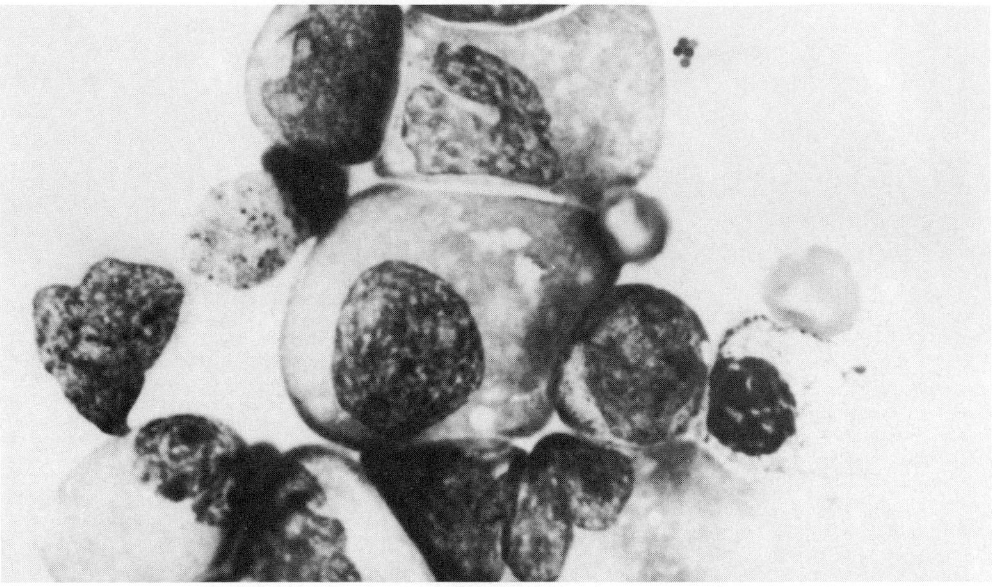

FIG. 47.13. Acute myeloblastic leukemia with maturation (M2) with a t(8;21)(q22;q22) cytogenetic abnormality. Bone marrow smear showing abnormal neutrophil precursors with abundant cytoplasm and prominent specific granulation which appears slightly smudgy in some cells. The myeloblast in the center shows an Auer rod (Wright-Giemsa stain, original magnification: 400× magnification). See Color Plate 39, between pp. 1446–1447.

of multipotent stem cell involvement (48). Both of these associations may be observed in M4 AML.

ACUTE PROMYELOCYTIC LEUKEMIA (M3)

Acute promyelocytic leukemia is characterized principally by a proliferation of abnormal promyelocytes (51,52). In approximately 90% of patients, the number of blasts in the marrow is less than 30%, with the median percentage being approximately 8% (53).

Two morphologic forms of APL are recognized: hypergranular APL and the microgranular (hypogranular) variant, M3V.

Hypergranular Acute Promyelocytic Leukemia

Hypergranular APL comprises approximately 70 to 80% of cases of APL (51–53). Most patients present with leukopenia; the mean leukocyte count is 1.8×10^9 per liter. Thrombocytopenia and anemia generally are present. The bone marrow smear shows a predominant population of abnormal promyelocytes admixed with a minor population of blasts. The promyelocytes are large cells with a relatively low nuclear: cytoplasmic ratio; the cytoplasm contains abundant, coarse azurophilic granules that may obscure the nuclear: cytoplasmic interface. The nuclear outline may be round or irregular with a folded or reniform appearance (51,52) (Fig. 47.14; see also Color Plate 40, between pp. 1446–1447). Blasts and promyelocytes that contain 10 to 20 or more Auer rods, referred to as "faggot" cells, are present in almost all cases (Fig. 47.15; see also Color Plate 41, between pp. 1446–1447). The Auer rods are usually long and slender, frequently with a rust-like color, and often are intertwined. Ultrastructurally, the Auer rods in APL show a unique internal hexagonal tubular structure, with a periodicity of 22 to 25 nm, in contrast to the 8- to 12-nm periodicity of the Auer rods observed in other types of AML (54) (Fig. 47.16). Blasts and promyelocytes with one or two more typical Auer rods also may be noted. Maturing neutrophils may show dysplastic changes and contain Auer rods. Pseudo–Chediak-Higashi inclusions of both azurophilic and specific granules may be prominent. Increased basophils may be increased in some cases.

The abnormal promyelocytes are intensely MPO-, SBB, and CAE-positive. NSE-positive promyelocytes have been reported in 25% to 79% of patients (55,56). Pseudo–Chediak-Higashi granules, if present, usually are very PAS-positive.

The bone marrow trephine sections generally are hypercellular (Fig. 47.17). Occasionally, faggot cells may be identified in well-prepared sections (Fig. 47.18; see also Color Plate 42, between pp. 1446–1447).

Microgranular (Hypogranular) Acute Promyelocytic Leukemia (M3V)

Approximately 20% to 30% of patients with APL are microgranular variants (51,57). The azurophilic granules in this type of APL are very fine, at the threshold of resolution by light microscopy, in contrast to the prominent coarse azurophilic granules of the hypergranular type. Both *hypogranular* and *micrpark* have been used to describe this variant.

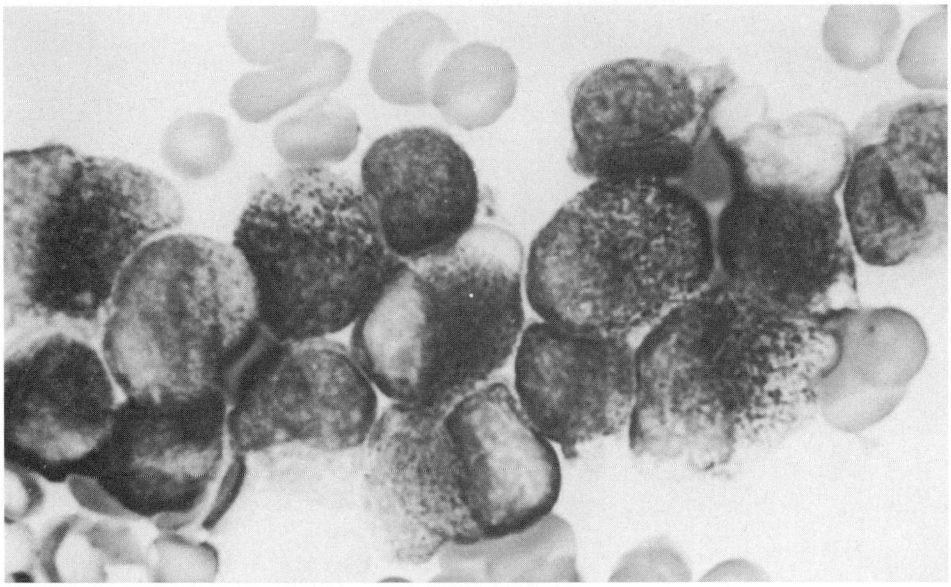

FIG. 47.14. Hypergranular acute promyelocytic leukemia (M3). Bone marrow smear showing leukemic promyelocytes that have abundant coarse azurophilic granules partially obscuring the nuclear outline (Wright-Giemsa stain, original magnification: 400× magnification). See Color Plate 40, between pp. 1446–1447.

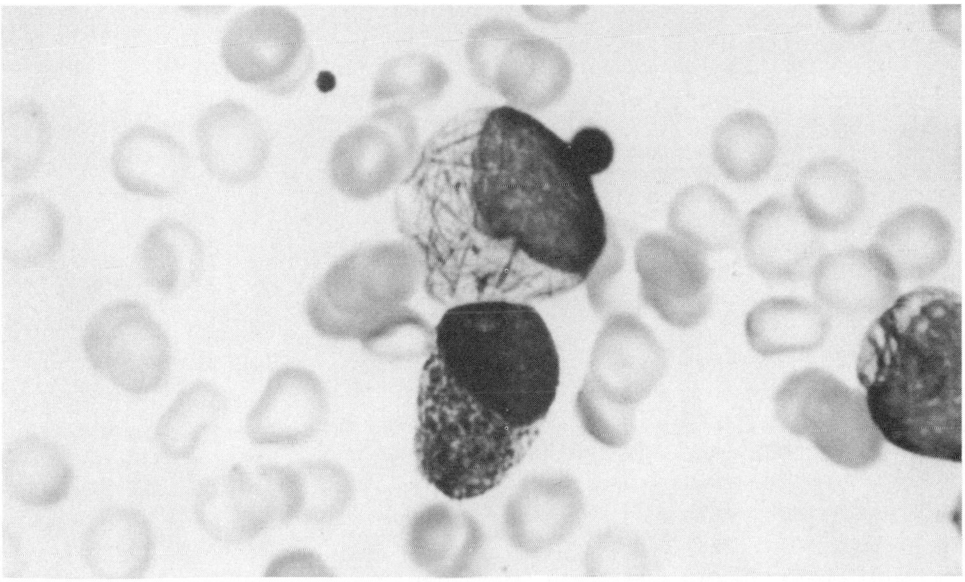

FIG. 47.15. Hypergranular acute promyelocytic leukemia (M3). Bone marrow smear showing a "faggot" cell with numerous intertwining Auer rods. The adjacent cell is an abnormal hyperbasophilic, hypergranular neutrophil promyelocyte (Wright-Giemsa stain, original magnification: 400× magnification). See Color Plate 41, between pp. 1446–1447.

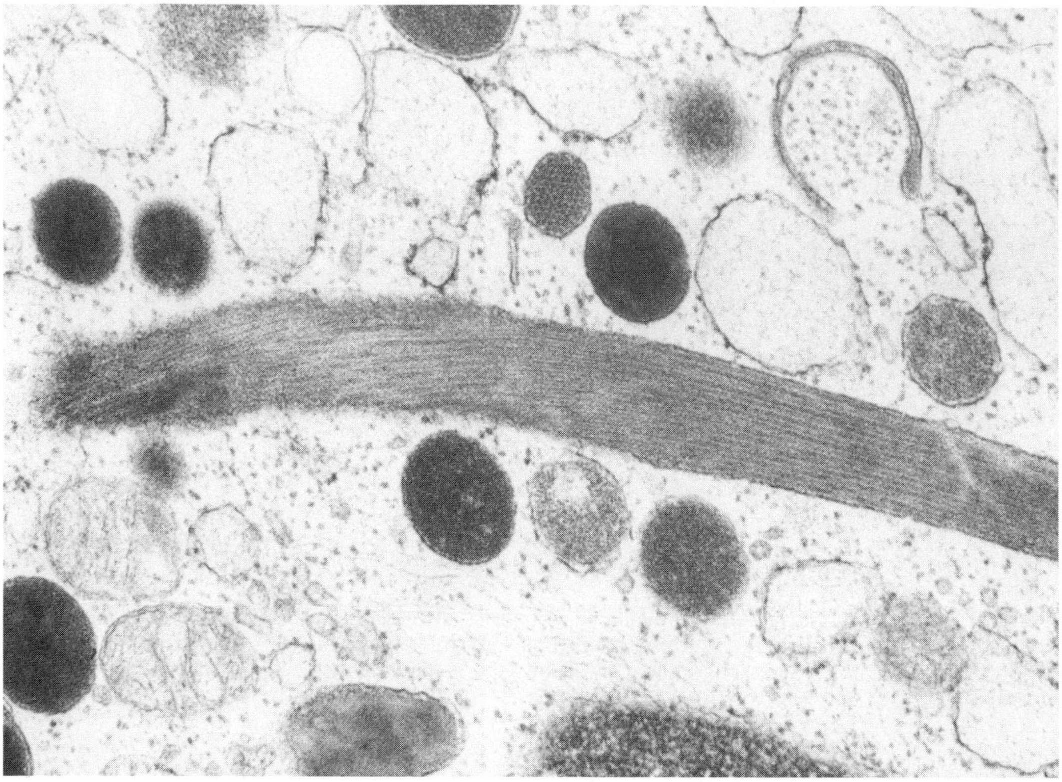

FIG. 47.16. Acute promyelocytic leukemia (M3). Electron micrograph of an Auer rod from a leukemic promyelocyte (Uranyl acetate, lead citrate stain, original magnification: 57,000× magnification).

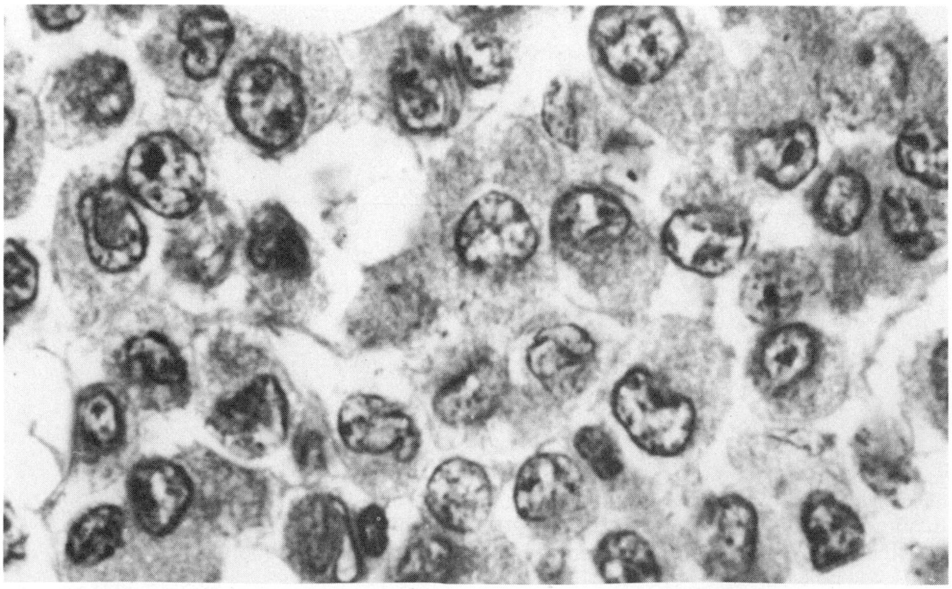

FIG. 47.17. Hypergranular acute promyelocytic leukemia (M3). Bone marrow section showing a uniform population of leukemic promyelocytes with abundant granulated cytoplasm and eccentrically placed nuclei. Occasional nuclei show cytoplasmic invagination (hematoxylin and eosin stain, original magnification: 400× magnification).

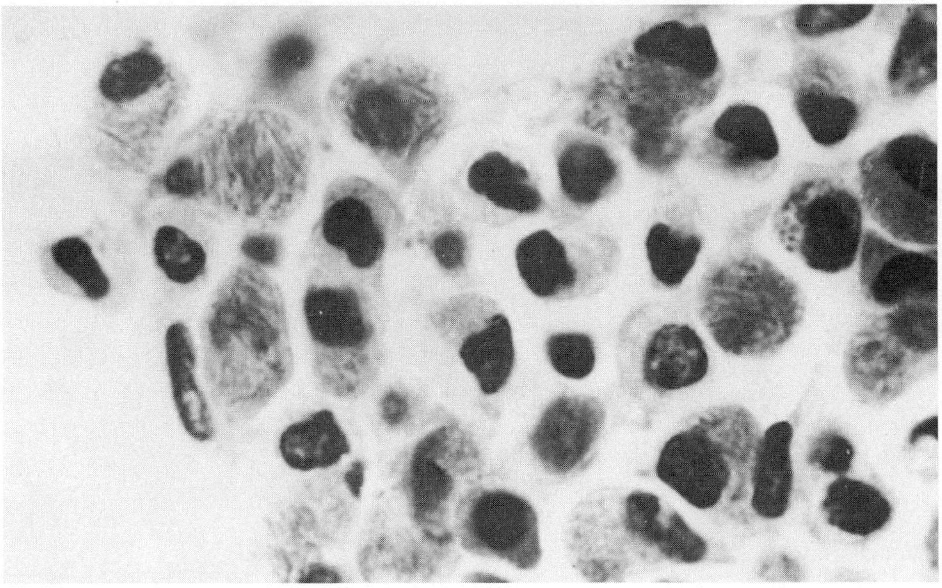

FIG. 47.18. Hypergranular acute promyelocytic leukemia (M3). Bone marrow section showing faggot cells with numerous Auer rods (hematoxylin and eosin stain, original magnification: 400× magnification). See Color Plate 42, between pp. 1446–1447.

As in the hypergranular type, anemia and thrombocytopenia are generally present. In contrast to the hypergranular form, there usually is marked leukocytosis (mean 42 $\times$ 10^9 leukocytes per liter), with a predominance of abnormal promyelocytes. The promyelocytes in the variant are large cells with a relatively low nuclear: cytoplasmic ratio and an unusually lobulated or invaginated nucleus that may resemble a monocyte nucleus. The granules tend to produce a light blush over the invaginated portion of the nucleus (Fig. 47.19; see also Color Plate 43, between pp. 1446–1447). A minor population of typical hypergranular promyelocytes is present in most microgranular cases. Smaller promyelocytes with hyperbasophilic cytoplasm may be present; these cells also may be observed in typical hypergranular APL (51) (Fig 47.20; see also Color Plate 44, between pp. 1446–1447). Faggot cells are almost always present but may not be numerous.

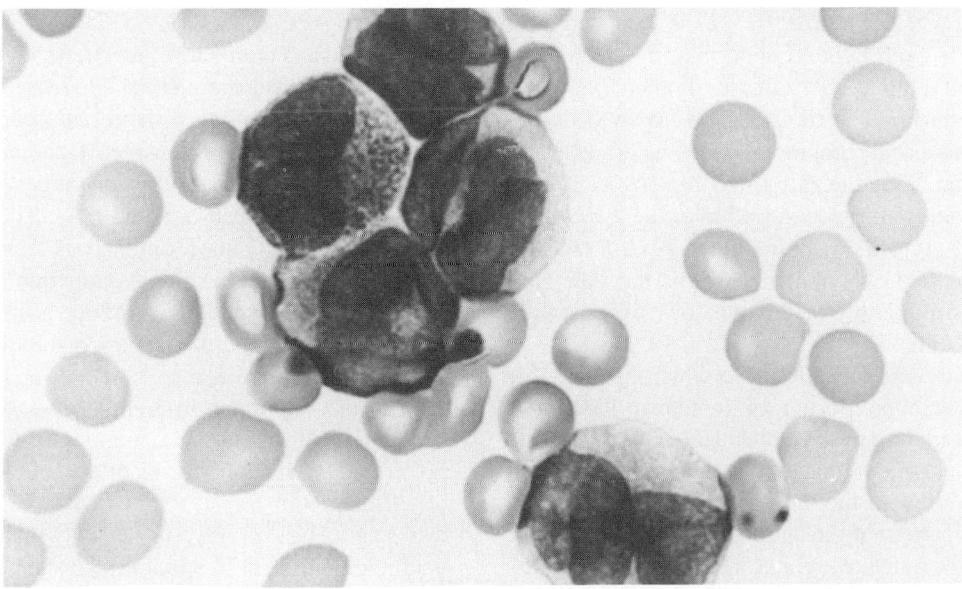

FIG. 47.19. Acute promyelocytic leukemia, microgranular variant (M3V). Blood smear showing leukemic promyelocytes with markedly folded and lobulated nuclei. The cytoplasm of the majority of cells contains numerous delicate azurophilic granules (Wright-Giemsa stain, original magnification: 400× magnification). See Color Plate 43, between pp. 1446–1447.

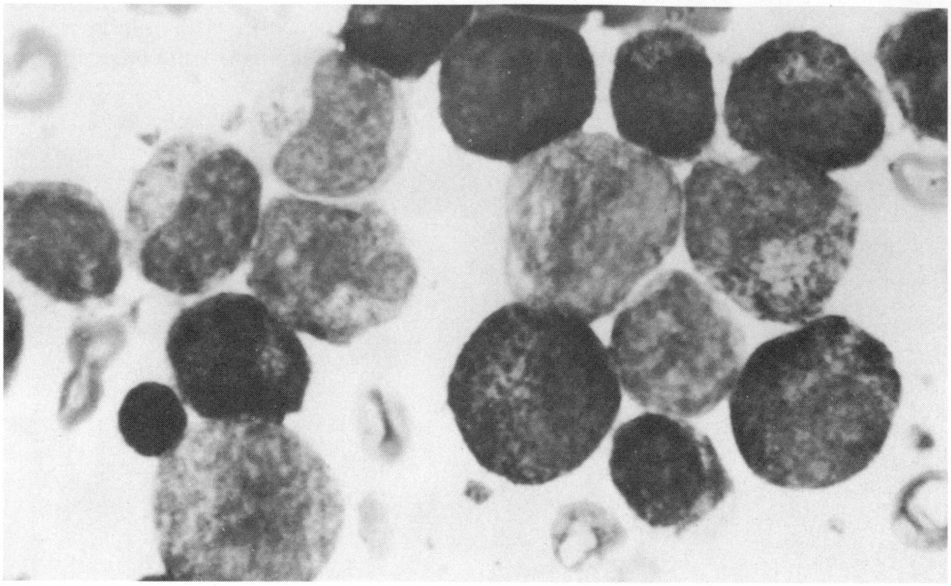

FIG. 47.20. Hypergranular acute promyelocytic leukemia (M3). Bone marrow smear showing numerous leukemic promyelocytes with markedly basophilic cytoplasm, "hyperbasophilic" cells. A centrally located faggot cell is present (Wright-Giemsa stain, original magnification: 400× magnification). See Color Plate 44, between pp. 1446–1447.

Blasts and promyelocytes with one to three Auer rods are usually found. The promyelocytes of M3V AML, similar to the promyelocytes in the hypergranular type, are intensely positive for MPO and SBB. Patients with M3V AML may have NSE-positive cells (56).

The importance of "faggot" cells to the morphologic diagnosis of both morphologic types of APL cannot be overemphasized. In their absence, the diagnosis of APL should be established only if the translocation t(15;17) or molecular evidence is present.

The translocation t(15;17)(q22;q11-12) is considered to be specific to APL, both hypergranular and microgranular types; it is reported in up to 90% of cases, both *de novo* and therapy-related (58–60). The translocation involves fusion of the *RARA* (retinoic acid receptor-α) gene on chromosome 17 with the gene encoding the zinc finger binding transcription factor on chromosome 15, referred to as the *PML* (promyelocytic leukemia) gene, resulting in the *PML-RARA* fusion gene product. This phenomenon forms the basis for the highly successful therapy of this type of leukemia with transretinoic acid (60).

The monoclonal antibody PG-M3, which is directed against the amino-terminal portion of the human PML protein, if combined with immunocytochemical or immunofluorescence techniques, distinguishes the speckled pattern of the antibody reaction with the wild-type PML protein from the microgranular pattern of the antibody reaction characteristic of cells with the translocation t(15;17) (61). The distinctive pattern of reactivity in cells with t(15;17) aids in distinguishing APL from other types of leukemia. The atypical reaction product is not identified in the APLs with variant translocations, t(11;17) and t(5;17).

A cytogenetic variant of APL associated with translocation t(11;17)(q3;q21) and morphologic findings intermediate to M2 AML and typical hypergranular APL has been reported (62). The molecular event in this variant involves fusion of the gene encoding the retinoic acid receptor (*RARA*) on chromosome 17 with a gene encoding a protein with 9 zinc finger motifs named *PZF* (promyelocytic leukemia zinc finger) on chromosome 11. The patients with this variant of APL do not generally respond to differentiating retinoic acid therapy like the patients with typical t(15;17)-associated APL.

A second and more rare cytogenetic variant is APL associated with the translocation t(5;17)(q23;q12), which also does not typically respond to differentiating agent therapy (63).

Clinically, a high percentage of patients who have APL present with a severe coagulopathy or develop one after cytolytic therapy has been initiated (64). The peripheral blood smear occasionally shows numerous fragmented red blood cells consistent with a microangiopathic hemolytic anemia; however, this morphologic finding is not always present, and disseminated intravascular coagulation cannot be excluded by its absence.

The most important differential diagnosis of APL relates to agranulocytosis and acute monocytic leukemia with maturation (M5B). In some forms of agranulocytosis, there may be a "maturation arrest" of the neutrophils at the promyelocyte stage. These promyelocytes may manifest intense azurophilic granulation. In agranulocytosis, however, the megakaryocytic and erythroid precursors are generally normal in number, and no evidence exists of anemia or thrombocytopenia; coagulation studies are normal. In M3 AML the megakaryocytes and erythroid precursors generally are decreased, with an accompanying anemia and thrombocytopenia. The presence of Auer rods is exclusionary for agranulocytosis.

Myeloperoxidase and NSE stains used in combination are definitive in distinguishing AML M3V from AML M5B. The MPO stain is markedly positive in the promyelocytes of AML M3V and negative or only slightly positive in the promonocytes of AML M5B. The promonocytes and monocytes of AML M5B are NSE-positive in the majority of patients. Occasional patients with APL show significant NSE positivity. In M5B AML, Auer rods are identified in the myeloblasts and not in the promonocytes. The presence of ''faggot'' cells excludes the diagnosis of M5B AML.

Occasional cases of M2 AML with numerous promyelocytes may resemble APL; the absence of ''faggot'' cells is evidence against the diagnosis of APL. In some of these instances, cytogenetic and ultrastructural studies may be necessary for definitive classification.

ACUTE MONOCYTIC LEUKEMIA (M5A AND M5B)

Because acute myelomonocytic leukemia (M4) shares morphologic features of AML with maturation (M2) and acute monocytic leukemia (M5), the discussion of acute monocytic leukemia (M5) precedes that of acute myelomonocytic leukemia (M4).

In acute monocytic leukemia (M5 AML), the marrow contains 80% or more monocytic cells, including monoblasts, promonocytes, and monocytes (1,5). The remainder of the cells consist of granulocytes, predominantly neutrophils, erythroid precursors, lymphocytes, and plasma cells. Two types of M5 AML are recognized based on the relative percentage of monoblasts. In acute monoblastic leukemia (acute monocytic leukemia, poorly differentiated; M5A AML), more than 80% of the monocytic cells are monoblasts; in acute monocytic leukemia with differentiation (M5B AML), referred to here as *acute monocytic leukemia,* fewer than 80% of the monocytic cells are monoblasts. The monoblast predominates in M5A AML, and the promonocyte predominates in M5B AML.

Acute Monoblastic Leukemia (M5A)

Acute monoblastic leukemia, M5A AML, generally is a disease of younger individuals and presents with slight to moderate anemia, thrombocytopenia in 60% of patients, and a normal or low leukocyte count in 70%. In this subtype of acute monocytic leukemia, monoblasts predominate in the bone marrow. The monoblasts vary substantially in different patients but generally are large cells (40–50 μm in diameter) with abundant basophilic to lightly basophilic cytoplasm that frequently contains fine to coarse azurophilic granulation (Fig. 47.21; see also Color Plate 45, between pp. 1446–1447). Cytoplasmic projections may be prominent (65). The nucleus is round to oval with finely reticular chromatin and, frequently, one prominent nucleolus; multiple nucleoli may be present. In some instances, the monoblasts resemble myeloblasts with a high nuclear:cytoplasmic ratio. Uncommonly, the monoblasts have vacuolated cytoplasm that may be intensely PAS-positive. Auer rods and myelodysplastic changes generally are not found in M5A AML.

Monoblasts typically react with NSE, but the intensity of the reaction may vary considerably from cell to cell; in approximately 10% to 20% of patients, the monoblasts are

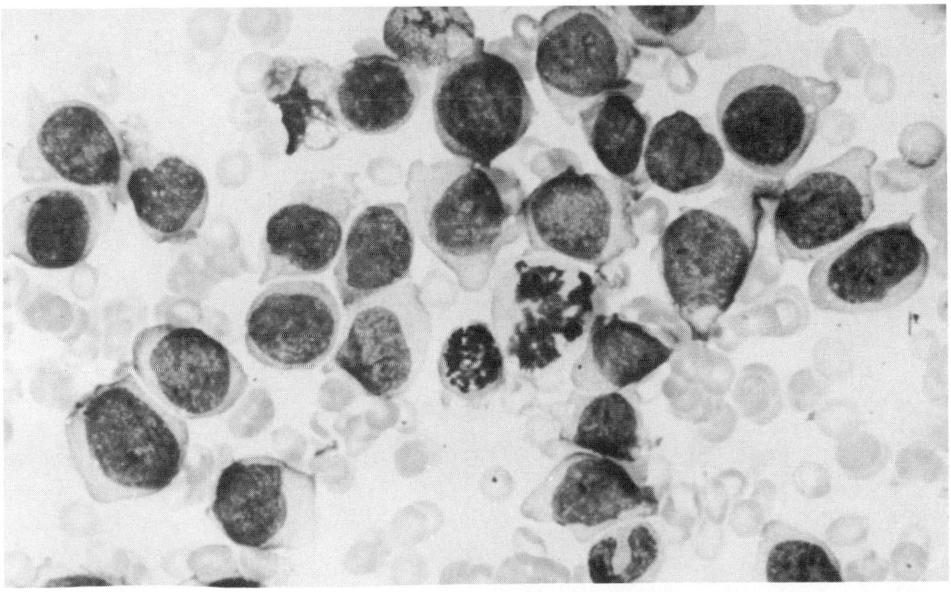

FIG. 47.21. Acute monoblastic leukemia (M5A). Bone marrow smear showing monoblasts that have abundant cytoplasm and scattered fine azurophilic granules. The majority of cells have round nuclei. Two mitotic figures are noted in the center (Wright-Giemsa stain, original magnification: 256× magnification). See Color Plate 45, between pp. 1446–1447.

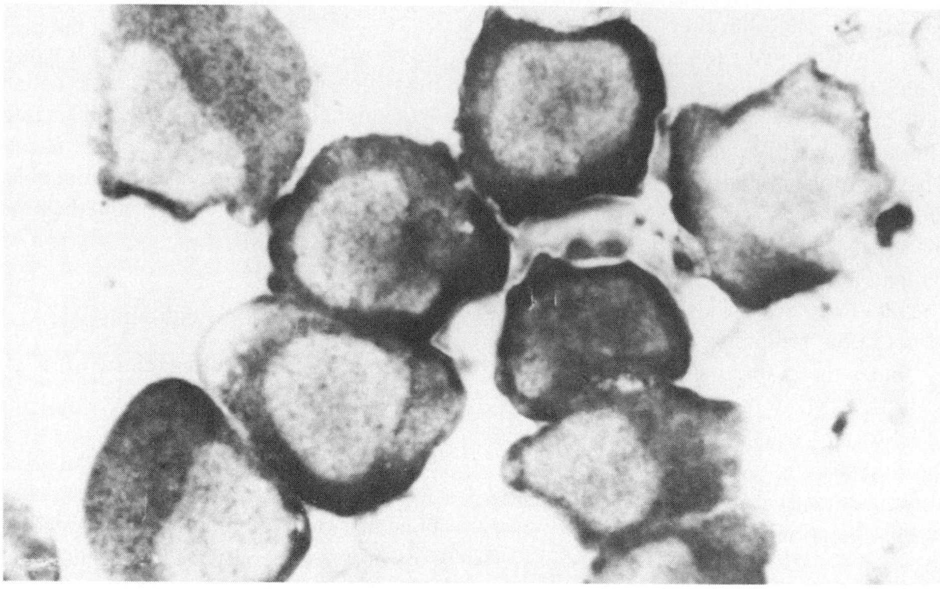

FIG. 47.22. Acute monoblastic leukemia (M5A). Bone marrow smear showing monoblasts with intense cytoplasmic positivity for nonspecific esterase (nonspecific esterase stain, original magnification: 400× magnification). See Color Plate 46, between pp. 1446–1447.

NSE-negative or only very weakly positive (Fig. 47.22; see also Color Plate 46, between pp. 1446–1447). They are usually but not invariably MPO-negative and, with uncommon exception, are negative or slightly positive for PAS. The monoblasts may have slight diffuse reactivity with CAE and tartrate-sensitive acid phosphatase (65). The bone marrow sections generally are hypercellular and are replaced by a proliferation of large blasts with round nuclei, variably prominent nucleoli, and abundant eosinophilic to amphophilic cytoplasm (Fig. 47.23). The monoblasts in section specimens react with antibodies to lysozyme and CD68 (KP-1).

Patients with M5A AML may have extramedullary involvement in lymph nodes, liver, spleen, central nervous system, skin, and rarely other sites; the extramedullary involvement may be the presenting manifestation (66). Partial bone marrow involvement may be present in patients who have a primarily extramedullary presentation. Serum and urine lysozyme may or may not be elevated.

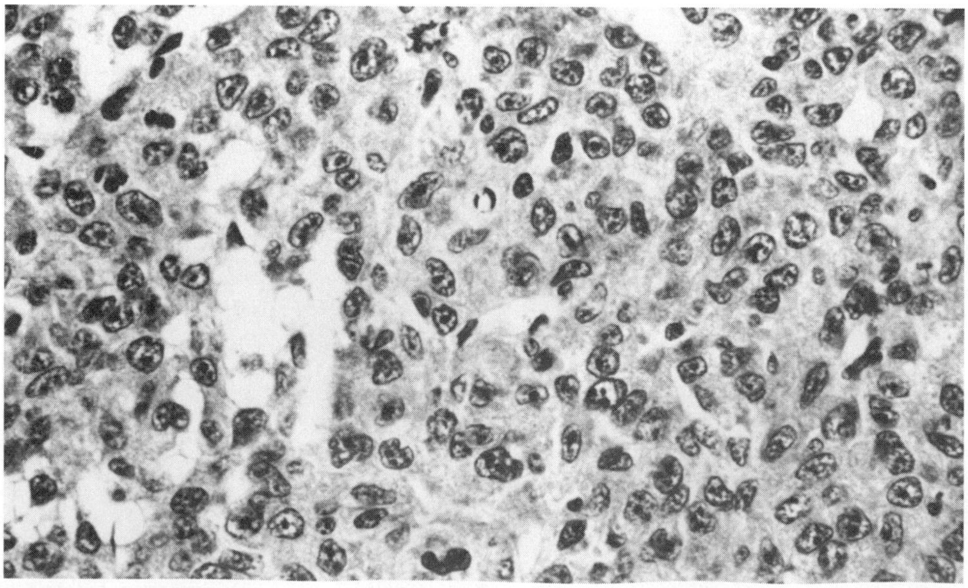

FIG. 47.23. Acute monoblastic leukemia (M5A). Bone marrow section diffusely replaced by monoblasts that have abundant cytoplasm and generally, prominent nucleoli. Note the mitotic figures (hematoxylin and eosin stain, original magnification: 256× magnification).

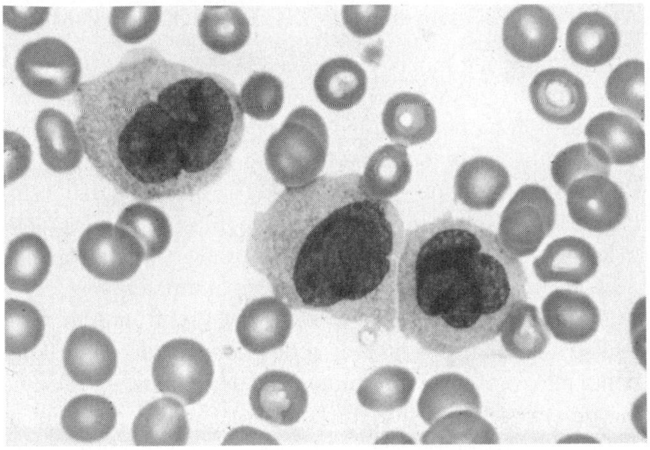

FIG. 47.24. Acute monocytic leukemia (M5B). Blood smear showing three promonocytes. The cells have abundant cytoplasm with numerous fine azurophilic granules. The nuclei show delicate nuclear folding with nuclear creasing imparting a cerebriform appearance (Wright-Giemsa stain, original magnification: 640× magnification). See Color Plate 47, between pp. 1446–1447.

Translocations involving chromosome 11q23 and various partner chromosomes are the most common cytogenetic findings in M5A AML (67).

The differential diagnosis of M5A AML usually includes M1 and M7 AML and acute lymphoblastic leukemia. The myeloblasts in M1 AML are generally MPO-positive and NSE-negative. The blasts in acute lymphoblastic leukemia are TdT-positive and NSE-negative. Megakaryoblasts may show a slight focal NSE reactivity, which contrasts with the diffuse, usually intense positive reaction in the monoblasts. Flow cytometry with antibodies to CD41 and CD61 is necessary to recognize megakaryoblasts definitively (9).

Although monoblasts have been reported to have surface immunoglobulin, this results from adherence of immunoglobulin to the membrane Fc receptors and may be ablated with 24-hour incubation (68). In a small number of patients, the cytochemical and immunophenotypic data is equivocal; ultrastructural studies, including NSE staining, may be definitive.

Acute Monocytic Leukemia (M5B)

Acute monocytic leukemia with maturation (M5B AML) is a relatively uncommon type of acute monocytic leukemia in which fewer than 80% of the monocytic cells are monoblasts. The predominant cell is the promonocyte, a large cell with abundant lightly basophilic to pale cytoplasm that usually contains evenly distributed, fine to coarse azurophilic granulation. In contrast to the monoblast, the nuclei are characterized by nuclear folding with delicate creases of the membrane that impart a somewhat cerebriform appearance; the chromatin is finely stippled to reticular, and two to four inconspicuous nucleoli are present (Fig. 47.24; see also Color Plate 47, between pp. 1446–1447). For purposes of establishing a diagnosis of acute leukemia, the promonocyte is considered to be the equivalent of a blast (1,5).

Leukocytosis generally is present, with a predominance of promonocytes. Most patients are anemic. Thrombocytopenia may or may not be present. The bone marrow aspirate shows varying percentages of monoblasts and promonocytes. Fifty to seventy percent of patients have a combined myeloblast

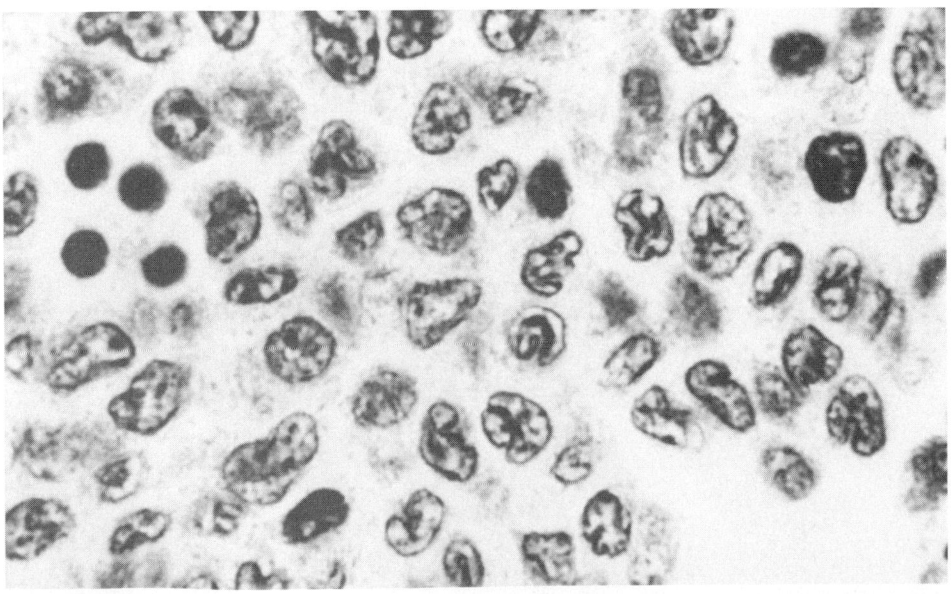

FIG. 47.25. Acute monocytic leukemia with maturation (M5B). Bone marrow section showing a predominant population of monoblasts and promonocytes. The promonocytes are characterized by delicate nuclear lobulation, which, in several instances, imparts a cerebriform appearance to the nucleus (hematoxylin and eosin stain, original magnification: 400× magnification).

and monoblast percentage less than 30%; the promonocytes predominate (53). Auer rods are seen in approximately 30% of patients; the Auer rods are found in the more typical myeloblast component. Most promonocytes are NSE-positive; in some instances, however, the monocytic cells do not react with NSE; the distinctive morphologic features of the promonocyte should suffice for the diagnosis. The promonocytes generally are MPO-negative or weakly positive; the positivity is in the form of evenly distributed granules, which are substantially less numerous than in segmented neutrophils or metamyelocytes. The bone marrow sections in most patients generally are hypercellular and effaced by a population of promonocytes with distinctive lobulated nuclei (Fig. 47.25). Nucleoli are present but not prominent. Serum and urine lysozyme levels are generally elevated.

An uncommon variant of M5B AML associated with a cytogenetic finding of the translocation t(8;16)(p11;p13) is morphologically characterized by monocytes showing hemophagocytosis, most notably erythrophagocytosis, and increased azurophilic granulation. The prognosis may be less favorable than typical M5B AML, and central nervous system involvement appears to be a feature of the disease. Coagulopathy occurs in approximately one third of patients. The monocytes may manifest strong MPO activity and dual reactivity for NSE and CAE (69–71). Similar morphologic findings have been observed with a complex translocation, t(3; 8;17) involving breakpoint 8pll (72).

The major differential diagnoses in M5B AML are the microgranular variant of APL (M3V AML) and M4 AML. The promyelocytes of M3V AML are intensely MPO- and SBB-positive; faggot cells are not found in M5B AML. The distinction between M5B AML and M4 AML involves adherence to the defining criteria; in M4 AML the neutrophil series exceeds 20% in the bone marrow.

ACUTE MYELOMONOCYTIC LEUKEMIA (M4)

In acute myelomonocytic leukemia (M4 AML), the marrow contains 20% or more monocytic cells, including monoblasts, promonocytes, and monocytes, and 20% or more neutrophils and precursors (1,3) (Fig. 47.26; see also Color Plate 48, between pp. 1446–1447). The blast population includes type I and II myeloblasts, monoblasts, and promonocytes. The blood generally, but not in every case, contains 5×10^9 per liter or more monocytes and precursors.

The majority of patients who have M4 AML present with leukocytosis, anemia, and thrombocytopenia; occasional patients may present with normal platelet counts. Myelodysplastic changes in neutrophils and Auer rods are present in a majority of patients. The monocytic series is NSE-positive; the neutrophil series is MPO- and SBB-positive. Occasionally, a population of neutrophils is both NSE- and MPO-positive (Fig. 47.27; see also Color Plate 49, between pp. 1446–1447). The trephine biopsy sections generally are hypercellular.

ACUTE MYELOMONOCYTIC LEUKEMIA WITH INCREASED BONE MARROW EOSINOPHILS (M4 EO)

This variant of M4 AML originally was described in 1983 and was proposed as a distinct type of AML in 1985 (3,73,74). The majority of patients with M4 AML with increased marrow eosinophils have an acquired abnormality of the long arm of chromosome 16, either an inversion or deletion. This variant of M4 AML has a propensity for central nervous system involvement and other forms of extramedullary disease (75). Acute myelomonocytic leukemia with increased marrow eosinophils, with inv(16) or t(16;

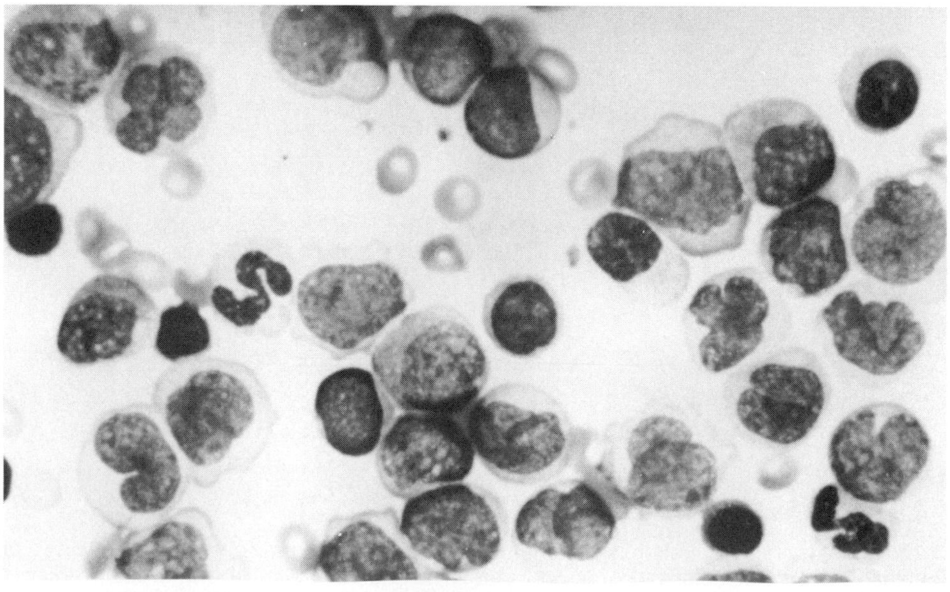

FIG. 47.26. Acute myelomonocytic leukemia (M4). Bone marrow smear showing myeloblasts, maturing neutrophils, and monocytes (Wright-Giemsa stain, original magnification: 256× magnification). See Color Plate 48, between pp. 1446–1447.

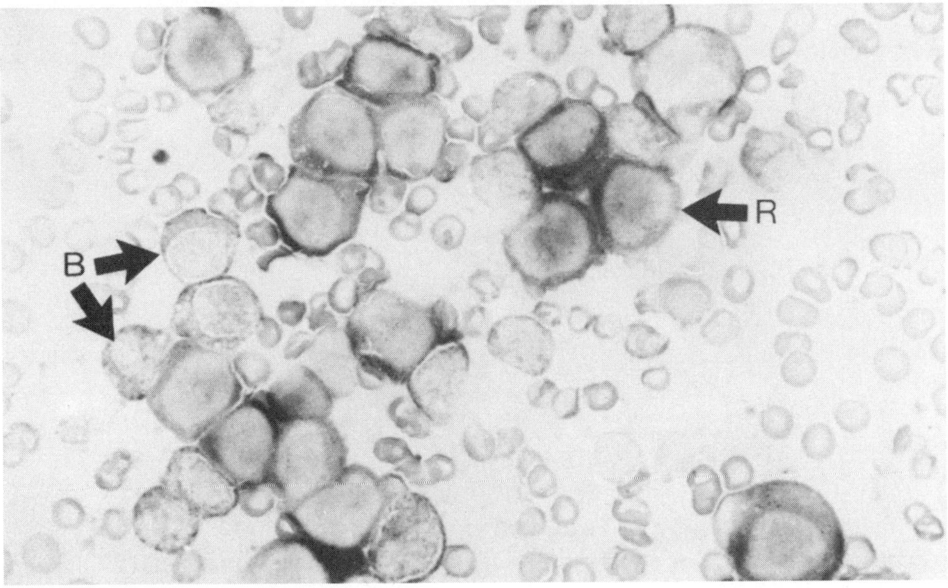

FIG. 47.27. Acute myelomonocytic leukemia (M4). Bone marrow smear stained with combined nonspecific esterase (red-brown staining, *R*) and chloroacetate esterase (blue staining, *B*), showing numerous nonspecific esterase–positive cells interpreted as monoblasts and promonocytes and chloroacetate esterase–positive cells interpreted as neutrophil precursors. Several of these cells manifest dual staining (chloroacetate esterase–nonspecific esterase staining, original magnification: 256× magnification). See Color Plate 49, between pp. 1446–1447.

16), similar to M2 AML with t(8;21), has a very favorable prognosis if treated with high-dosage cytarabine in the consolidation phase (13,14,76).

The peripheral blood generally shows a leukocytosis with the typical findings of M4 AML; an increase in eosinophils is not usually present in the blood, although an occasional patient presents with blood eosinophilia. Anemia and thrombocytopenia usually are present. The bone marrow findings are those of AML M4, with the addition of an increase in eosinophils. The more immature eosinophils, that is, the myelocytes and promyelocytes, are atypical with both eosinophilic- and basophilic-staining granules (Fig. 47.28; see also Color Plate 50, between pp. 1446–1447). The basophilic-staining granules are frequently large and misshapen and react with MPO, CAE, and PAS, which contrasts with normal eosinophil granules, which are positive for MPO but negative for CAE and PAS. The CAE reactivity is usually faint, and not all of the abnormal eosinophils have it (77). The abnormal eosinophil granules generally do not react with toluidine blue staining; this contrasts with basophil granules, which are positive for toluidine blue but negative for MPO. Ultrastructurally, the abnormal granules have the characteristics of eosinophil granules (Fig. 47.29). These abnormal eosinophils are not specific for this variant of leukemia. Similar cells may be observed in conditions with increased numbers of immature marrow eosinophils, such as hypereosinophilic syndrome and chronic myeloid leukemia. Rarely, blast transformation of chronic myeloid leukemia may manifest with the morphologic findings of M4EO AML (8).

The differential diagnosis of M4 AML includes M2 AML and M5B AML. The distinction between these types should be based on the defining criteria for these entities. In M5B AML, 80% or more of the marrow cells are monocytes or monocytic precursors. Patients with AML who have less than 20% monocytic cells in the bone marrow and fewer than 5×10^9 per liter monocytic cells in the peripheral blood are generally classified as having M2 AML. M2 AML with the translocation t(8;21) may have increased marrow eosinophils.

ACUTE ERYTHROID LEUKEMIAS

The proposed WHO classification recognizes two major forms of erythroid leukemia: M6A AML, erythroleukemia, and M6B AML, pure acute erythroid leukemia (1). M6B AML is a newly recognized entity that is marked by a predominant proliferation of erythroid precursors, more than 80%, without a significant increase in myeloblasts; in earlier literature this process was referred to as *erythremic myelosis* (8). The criteria for M6A AML are the same as for erythroleukemia in the FAB classification (3,78–81).

Both types of erythroid leukemia present with some evidence of marrow failure. Anemia is an almost invariant manifestation and may be marked. The peripheral blood frequently shows normoblastemia. Anisopoikilocytosis may be prominent; the erythrocytes may show prominent basophilic stippling, and there may be an increase in polychromatic red blood cells.

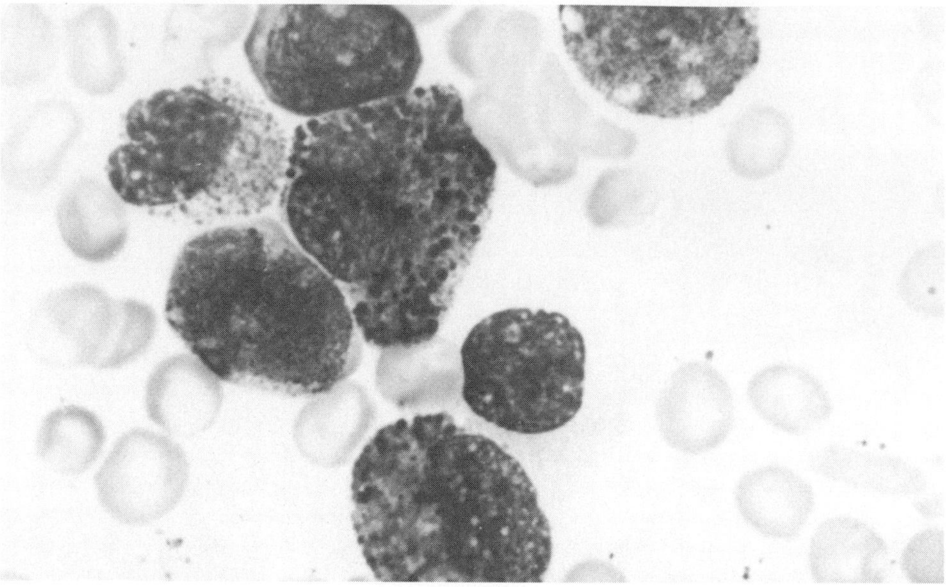

FIG. 47.28. Acute myelomonocytic leukemia with increased bone marrow eosinophils (M4EO). Bone marrow smear showing four eosinophils, two of which contain a mixture of eosinophilic and basophilic granules. This case is associated with an inversion of chromosome 16 (Wright-Giemsa stain, original magnification: 400× magnification). See Color Plate 50, between pp. 1446–1447.

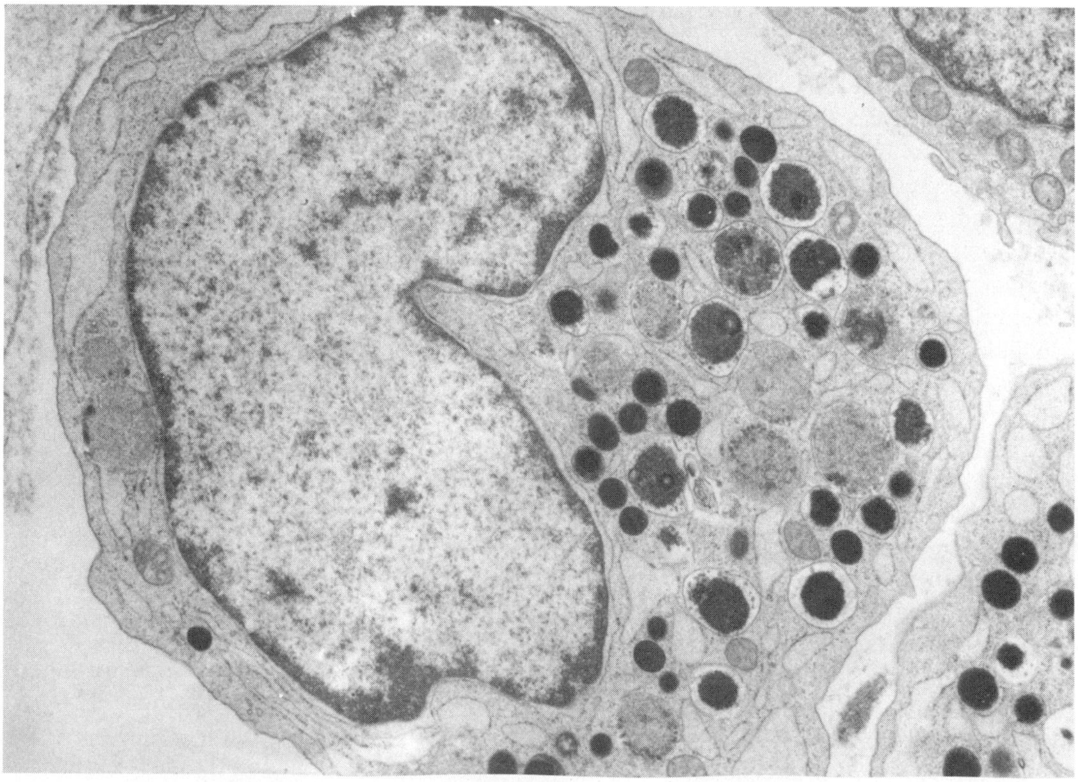

FIG. 47.29. Acute myelomonocytic leukemia with increased bone marrow eosinophils (M4EO). Electron micrograph of an abnormal eosinophil showing electron-dense and abnormal electron-lucent granules; both lack crystalline cores (uranyl acetate, lead citrate stain, original magnification: 13,000× magnification).

TABLE 47.4. *Diagnosis of Erythroleukemia (M6A)*[a]

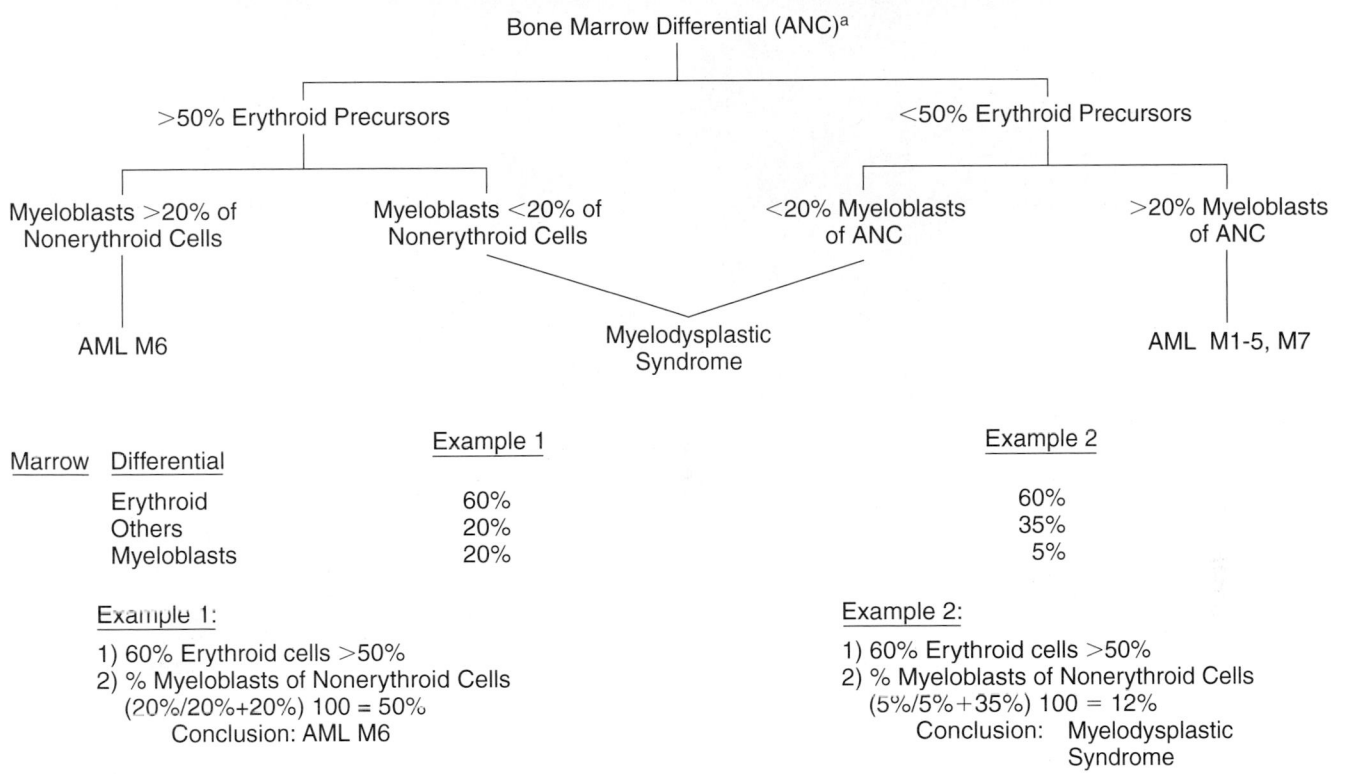

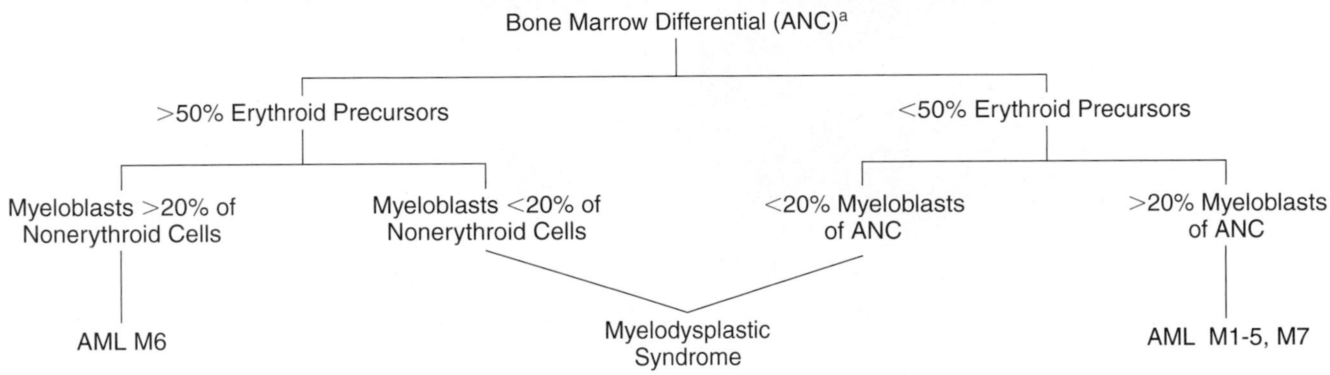

Marrow Differential	Example 1	Example 2
Erythroid	60%	60%
Others	20%	35%
Myeloblasts	20%	5%

Example 1:

1) 60% Erythroid cells >50%
2) % Myeloblasts of Nonerythroid Cells
(20%/20%+20%) 100 = 50%
Conclusion: AML M6

Example 2:

1) 60% Erythroid cells >50%
2) % Myeloblasts of Nonerythroid Cells
(5%/5%+35%) 100 = 12%
Conclusion: Myelodysplastic Syndrome

[a] Modified from Bennett et al. (3)
[b] All nucleated marrow cells

Erythroleukemia (M6A)

Erythroleukemia (M6A) is essentially the entity described in the FAB classification as M6 AML (3). This subtype is defined by two major criteria: 50% or more erythroid precursors in the entire nucleated marrow cell population, and at least 20% myeloblasts in the nonerythroid population (Table 47.4). All the maturation stages of the erythroid precursors are present; the proportions of the different maturation stages vary, but there is generally a shift to more immature forms.

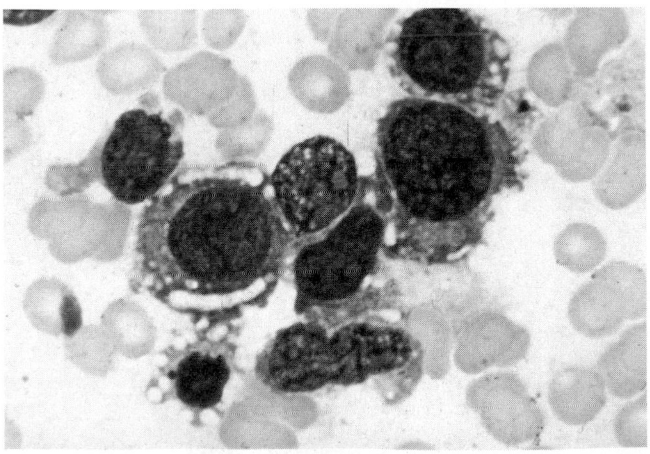

FIG. 47.30. Erythroleukemia (M6A). Bone marrow smear showing abnormal erythroblasts and two myeloblasts, one with an Auer rod. The erythroblasts have megaloblastoid nuclei and cytoplasmic vacuoles (Wright-Giemsa stain, original magnification: 400× magnification). See Color Plate 51, between pp. 1446–1447.

The myeloblasts are similar to the myeloblasts in other types of AML and may contain granules or Auer rods (Fig. 47.30; see also Color Plate 51, between pp. 1446–1447). The erythroid precursors show morphologic changes similar to the findings in M6A AML (Fig. 47.31; see also Color Plate 52, between pp. 1446–1447). The iron stain may show ringed sideroblasts, which in some patients are numerous. The myeloblasts show characteristic reaction patterns for MPO and SBB. Similar to AML-M6A, the vacuoles in the basophilic erythroblasts and proerythroblasts are usually intensely PAS-positive. The polychromatic and orthochromatic erythroid precursors may show a more uniform diffuse PAS reactivity. Dysplastic features may be present in the neutrophils and megakaryocytes and may be marked, suggesting a panmyelopathy.

Pure Acute Erythroid Leukemia (M6B AML)

Pure acute erythroid leukemia may present with or without morphologic features of erythroid differentiation; the defin-

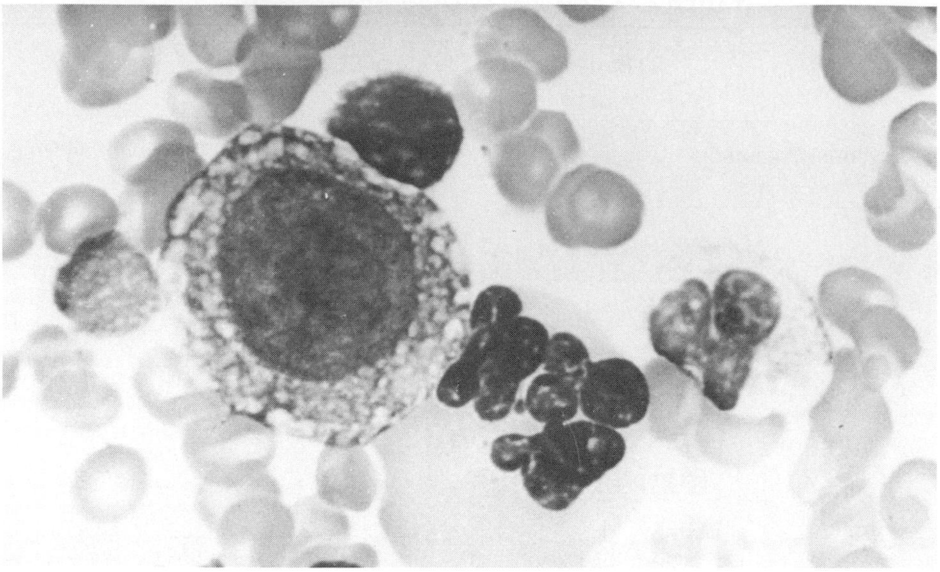

FIG. 47.31. Erythroleukemia (M6A). Bone marrow smear showing two abnormal erythroblasts at different stages of maturation. The enlarged proerythroblast has abundant basophilic cytoplasm with numerous poorly demarcated vacuoles and a prominent single nucleolus; the late polychromatophilic erythroblast is macrocytic and has a markedly lobulated nucleus and several Pappenheimer bodies (Wright-Giemsa stain, original magnification: 400× magnification). See Color Plate 52, between pp. 1446–1447.

ing criterion is at least 80% abnormal proerythroblasts and basophilic erythroblasts (Fig. 47.32; see also Color Plate 53, between pp. 1446–1447). More differentiated erythroid precursors at all stages of maturation may be present. Dyserythropoiesis may be marked, with gigantism, atypical nuclear shapes, multinucleation, multilobulation, nuclear fragmentation, megaloblastic nuclei, and abundant and abnormal mitotic figures. Cytoplasmic vacuoles are frequently present and may be prominent with coalescence, resulting in large clear lacunae; the vacuoles are usually PAS-positive (Fig. 47.33; see also Color Plate 54, between pp. 1446–1447). In occasional patients, with or without vacuoles, the cells are

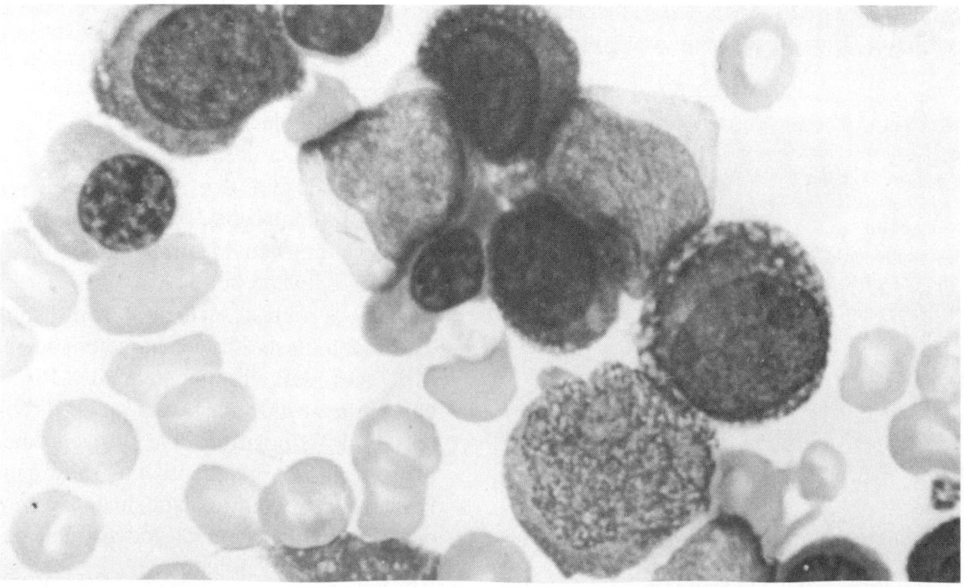

FIG. 47.32. Pure erythroid leukemia (M6B). Bone marrow smear showing a predominant population of proerythroblasts with markedly vacuolated cytoplasm; the larger vacuoles result from coalescence of the smaller vacuoles (Wright-Giemsa stain, original magnification: 400× magnification). See Color Plate 53, between pp. 1446–1447.

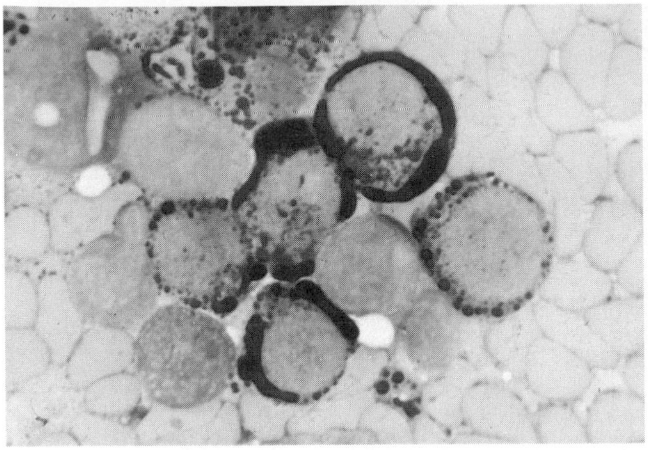

FIG. 47.33. Pure erythroid leukemia (M6B). Periodic acid-Schiff stain of bone marrow smear showing intense globular positivity in the vacuoles of immature erythroblasts (original magnification: 400× magnification). See Color Plate 54, between pp. 1446–1447.

PAS-negative. The erythroblasts are MPO- and SBB-negative; they may show α-naphthyl acetate esterase and acid phosphatase reactivity.

Transmission electron microscopy demonstrates features characteristic of erythroid cells, including free ferritin particles or siderosomes in the cytoplasm and rhopheocytosis.

The neutrophils and megakaryocytes may or may not manifest dysplastic changes. Myeloblasts usually are not increased; even if increased, they represent less than 20% of the nonerythroid cells.

With flow cytometry, erythroblasts are seen to express glycophorin A. The very early erythroid precursors, however, may not express this antigen. The erythroid precursors also may express CD36, which may be present on megakaryoblasts and monocytes. With immunohistochemistry on trephine biopsy and clot sections, it can be shown that the erythroblasts react with antibodies to hemoglobin A. With special handling of the trephine specimen, erythroid precursors may react with antibody to glycophorin A.

There are no cytogenetic findings that are specific to M6 AML. Complex karyotypes with multiple structural abnormalities, frequently involving chromosomes 5 and 7, are common and are generally associated with an unfavorable prognosis (79,80).

The bone marrow sections in M6A and M6B AML are similar; the differences relate to the degree of erythroid hyperplasia. Dysplastic megakaryocytes may be present and prominent.

Patients with AML M6A with the requisite percentage of myeloblasts with Auer rods generally present few diagnostic difficulties. Those with lower absolute numbers of myeloblasts or no increase in myeloblasts and no Auer rods, as occurs in M6A AML, may present serious diagnostic problems. The diagnosis in these instances should be established with extreme caution; vitamin B12 and folate deficiencies, hemolytic anemia, heavy metal intoxication, drug exposure, and congenital dyserythropoietic anemias must be excluded by appropriate laboratory studies and exposure history; marked dyserythropoiesis and intense PAS reactivity in the erythroid precursors is evidence of a malignant process. Recovery from parvovirus B19 infection may be accompanied by marked erythroid hyperplasia with abnormal-appearing erythroid precursors, with cytoplasmic vacuoles similar to the cells observed in M6A AML. Patients with M6B AML with a predominant population of basophilic and proerythroblasts may resemble acute lymphoblastic leukemia or Burkitt's lymphoma that involves the bone marrow. Vacuoles in Burkitt's lymphoma cells are oil red O–positive and PAS-negative, in contrast to the erythroblasts, which are oil red O–negative and PAS-positive. In some patients with M6A AML, the origin of the erythroid cells can be confirmed only with flow cytometry studies (78,80).

ACUTE MEGAKARYOBLASTIC LEUKEMIA (M7)

The diagnosis of acute megakaryoblastic leukemia (M7 AML), is based on two findings: 20% or more blasts in the blood or bone marrow, and evidence of megakaryocytic lineage in at least 50% of the bone marrow cells (1). Megakaryoblasts show a wide morphologic spectrum. In some patients with AML M7, the blasts are small cells with scant cytoplasm and dense chromatin; in other instances, the blasts are large with round nuclei, fine chromatin, one to three prominent nucleoli, and moderate amounts of cytoplasm, sometimes containing fine azurophilic granules (Fig. 47.34A; see also Color Plate 55, between pp. 1446–1447). The blasts in some patients show no distinctive features. Micromegakaryocytes with clumped nuclear chromatin and platelet budding are excluded from the blast percentage. The definitive evidence of megakaryocytic lineage in the blasts is based on immunologic studies for platelet glycoproteins or ultrastructural studies for platelet peroxidase (9,82–85) (Figs. 47.35, 47.36; see also Color Plate 56, between pp. 1446–1447). If it is not possible to perform these studies, clear morphologic evidence of a predominant megakaryocytic component in either smear or section specimens must be present.

The leukocyte count is variable; blasts usually are present in the peripheral blood. The platelet count in M7 AML usually is decreased but may be normal or increased; the hemoglobin generally is decreased. Atypical large, agranular platelets and micromegakaryocytes may be noted. The blasts in the marrow may show morphologic evidence of megakaryocytic differentiation with micromegakaryocytes. Myelodysplastic changes in the granulocytes and erythroid precursors may or may not be present. Cytochemistry is of limited value except for exclusionary purposes. The megakaryoblast is generally SBB-, MPO-, and TdT-negative. Diffuse acid phosphatase and PAS positivity are usually present. There may be variable focal positivity for NSE in the megakaryo-

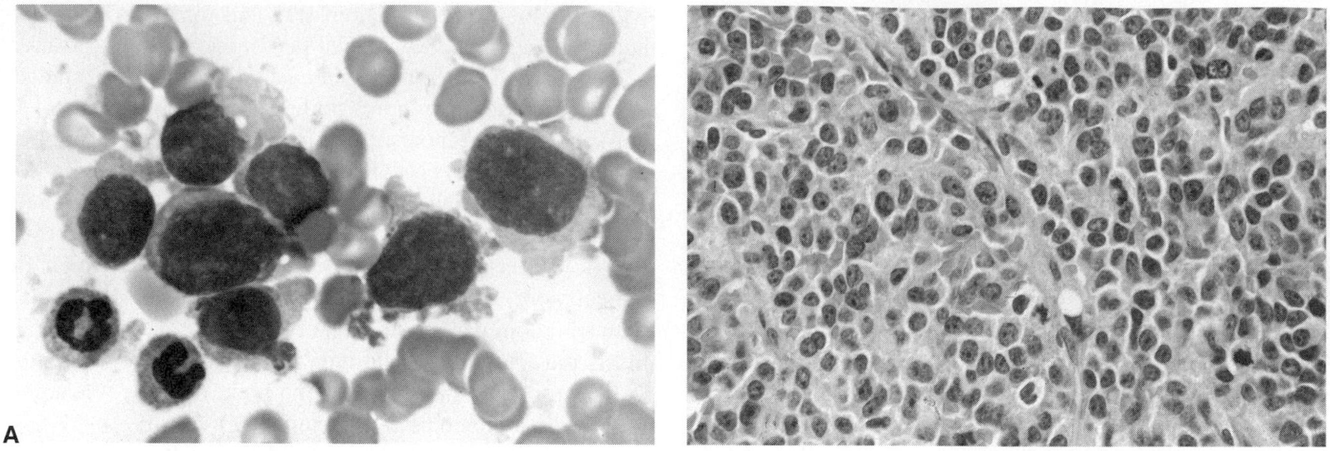

FIG. 47.34. A: Acute megakaryoblastic leukemia (M7). Bone marrow smear from a 22-month-old girl. The blasts vary in appearance; they may have abundant basophilic cytoplasm with pseudopod formation. The blasts express CD41 and CD61 and show evidence of platelet peroxidase on electron microscopy (Wright-Giemsa stain, original magnification: 640× magnification). **B:** Bone marrow trephine biopsy section from the specimen illustrated in **A**. The marrow is replaced extensively by blasts that show no clear evidence of maturation to more mature megakaryocytes (hematoxylin and eosin, original magnification: 400× magnification). See Color Plate 55, between pp. 1446–1447.

blasts (4,82). Typically the bone marrow sections are hypercellular, effaced by a proliferation of blasts with or without evidence of dysplastic megakaryocytes with dispersed chromatin (Figs. 47.34B, 47.37; see also Color Plate 57, between pp. 1446–1447). Micromegakaryocytes may be numerous; these may be identified more readily in PAS-stained sections. In some patients, the sections may be effaced by a population of blasts with no or minimal differentiating features (Fig. 47.34B). The amount of reticulin fibrosis varies substantially among patients from no or minimal increase in reticulin fibers to marked fibrosis; the cases with more fibrosis usually show evidence of differentiation to more mature dysplastic megakaryocytes, frequently small cells with nonlobulated nuclei and dispersed chromatin. Megakaryoblasts may form clusters that resemble metastatic tumor in the aspirate smear, and occasionally metastatic tumor resembles acute megakaryoblastic leukemia.

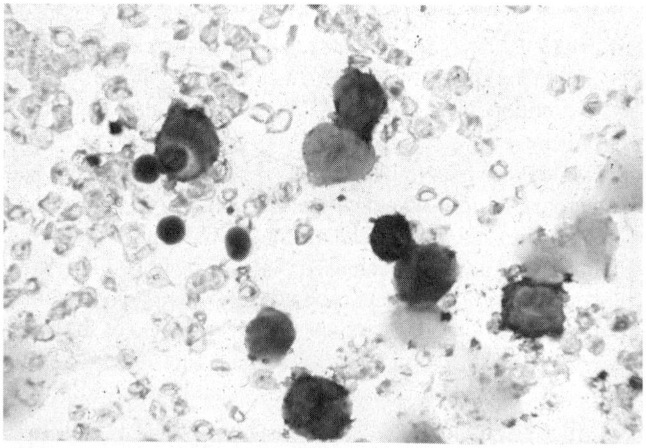

FIG. 47.35. Bone marrow smear from a patient with acute megakaryoblastic leukemia reacted with a monoclonal antibody to platelet glycoprotein (IIIa), CD61. The blasts are intensely reactive (APPAP, original magnification: 400× magnification). See Color Plate 56, between pp. 1446–1447.

Flow cytometry and immunocytochemical methodology with antibodies to platelet glycoproteins have facilitated the recognition of acute megakaryoblastic leukemia (9,84,85). Megakaryoblasts express one or more of the platelet glycoproteins, CD61 (IIIa), CD41 (IIb/IIIa), and CD42 (Ib) (9) (Fig. 47.35). They may express the myeloid markers CD13 and CD31 (82). On bone marrow sections, the megakaryocytes react with antibody to factor VIII; however, megakaryoblasts may not be positive, and a negative reaction with anti-factor VIII does not exclude the diagnosis.

Ultrastructural determination of platelet peroxidase is a sensitive and specific technique for megakaryocytic differentiation; however, rare patients with platelet peroxidase–positive erythroid precursors have been reported (86) (Fig. 47.36).

The application of the described criteria for M7 AML implies the availability of representative marrow aspirate material or an adequate number of blasts in the blood. If reticulin fibrosis precludes marrow aspiration, additional techniques are necessary to obtain cytologic specimens, such as imprint and crush preparations from a fresh trephine biopsy specimen or buffy coat preparations from peripheral blood, which may be used for ultrastructural or immunohistochemical studies (84,85).

In cases in which no cytologic preparations are available, it may be necessary to establish the diagnosis of M7 AML exclusively from section material. This requires the application of the two criteria previously identified. At least 20% of the marrow cells should be blasts; in addition, the sections

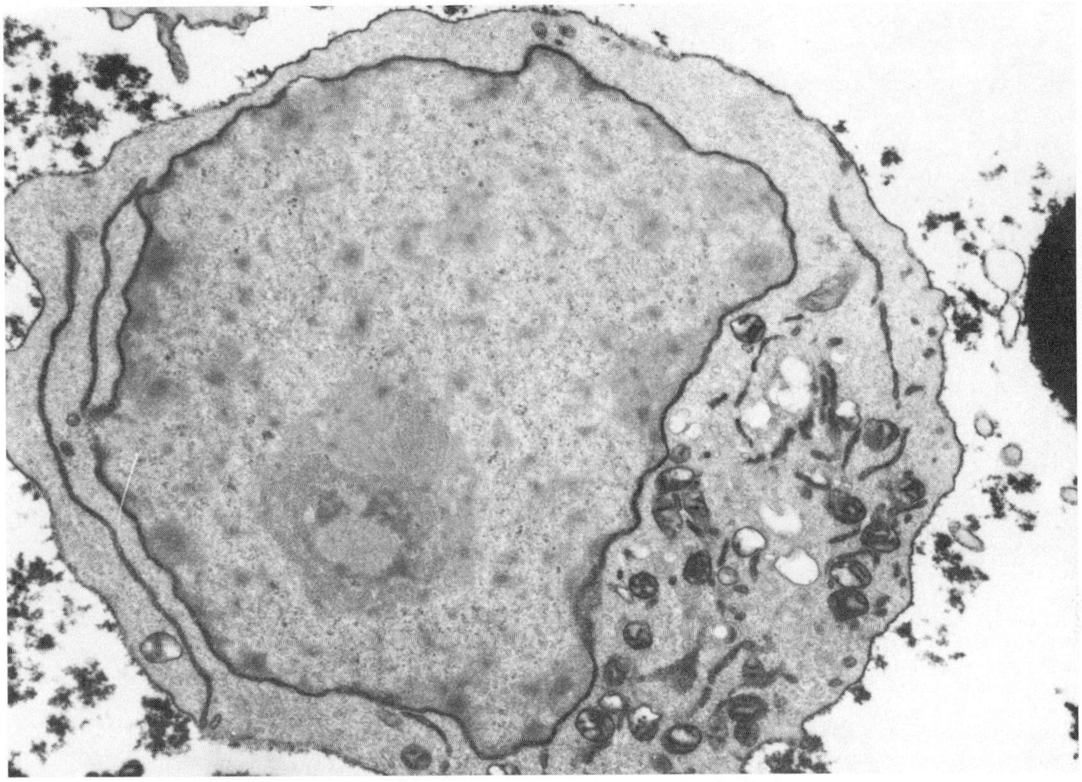

FIG. 47.36. Acute megakaryoblastic leukemia (M7). Electron micrograph of a megakaryoblast reacted for localization of platelet peroxidase. The dense reaction product is localized to the nuclear envelope and rough endoplasmic reticulum; the Golgi and granules are negative (lead citrate stain only, original magnification: 15,000× magnification).

must show clear morphologic, ultrastructural, or immunohistochemical evidence of megakaryocytic differentiation. Sections may show a megakaryocytic hyperplasia with a wide spectrum of abnormal megakaryocytes at all stages of maturation. Although granulocytic and erythroid cells may be present, the megakaryocytic component should predominate. In cases in which the findings are suggestive but equivocal, ultrastructural determination for platelet peroxidase can be carried out on appropriately fixed small portions of a trephine biopsy specimen obtained for this purpose.

The differential diagnosis of M7 AML includes M0, M1, and M5A AML, acute lymphoblastic leukemia, and metastatic tumor. The blasts in M0 AML express myeloid surface antigens such as CD13 and CD33, and are negative for megakaryocyte (platelet) antigens. The blasts of M1 AML are MPO- SBB-positive; the blasts of M7 AML are MPO- and SBB-negative. The monoblasts of AML M5A are NSE-positive and express CD14; megakaryoblasts are negative or weakly positive for NSE, in a focal paranuclear distribution. The lymphoblasts of acute lymphoblastic leukemia are TdT-positive and express pan–B or T cell surface antigens. Megakaryoblasts are TdT-negative.

Although M7 AML usually presents with what appears to be a unilineage proliferation of blasts, there are patients in whom there is evidence of dyserythropoiesis with apparent involvement of the erythroid cells. This differs from acute panmyelosis or acute panmyelosis with myelofibrosis, in which the granulocytes are also a part of the proliferative process.

ACUTE MEGAKARYOBLASTIC LEUKEMIA ASSOCIATED WITH THE TRANSLOCATION T(1;22)(p13;q13)

Acute megakaryoblastic leukemia associated with the chromosome abnormality t(1;22)(p13;q13) may occur in infants (87,88). These children usually present with extensive infiltration of abdominal organs. The bone marrow generally shows prominent reticulin fibrosis and may resemble metastatic tumor (Fig. 47.38; see also Color Plate 58, between pp. 1446–1447). The megakaryoblasts are often cohesive and show sinusoidal and vascular patterns of involvement in extramedullary sites such as the liver and lymph nodes.

ACUTE MYELOID LEUKEMIA AND TRANSIENT MYELOPROLIFERATIVE DISEASE IN DOWN SYNDROME

Children with Down syndrome have a 20-fold increase in the incidence of acute leukemia compared with children without Down syndrome, and a 500-fold increase in a somewhat unique form of acute megakaryoblastic leukemia usu-

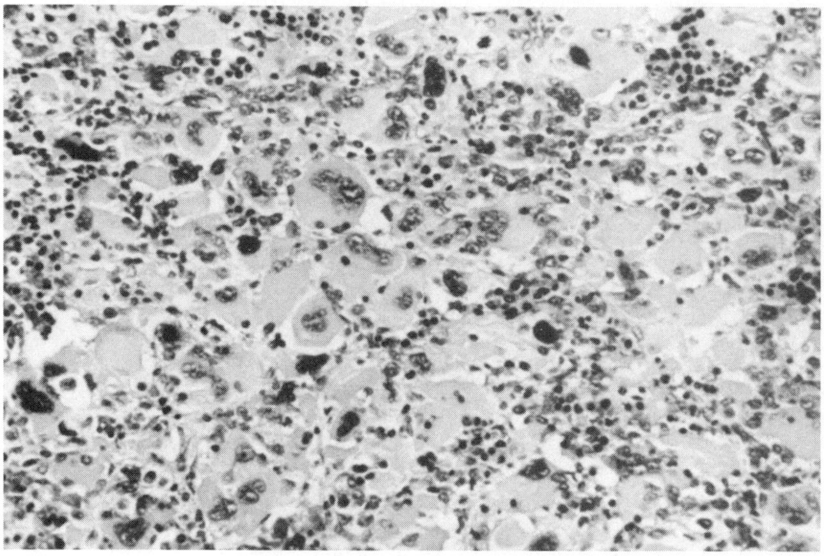

A

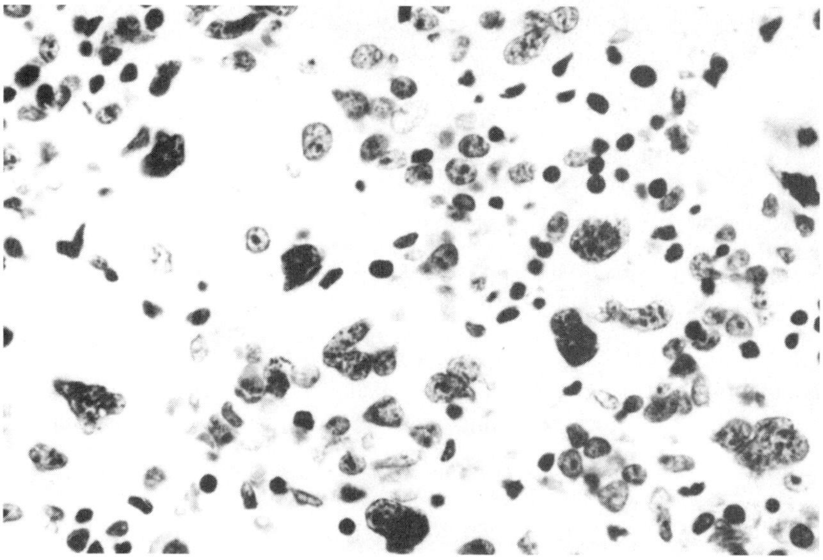

B

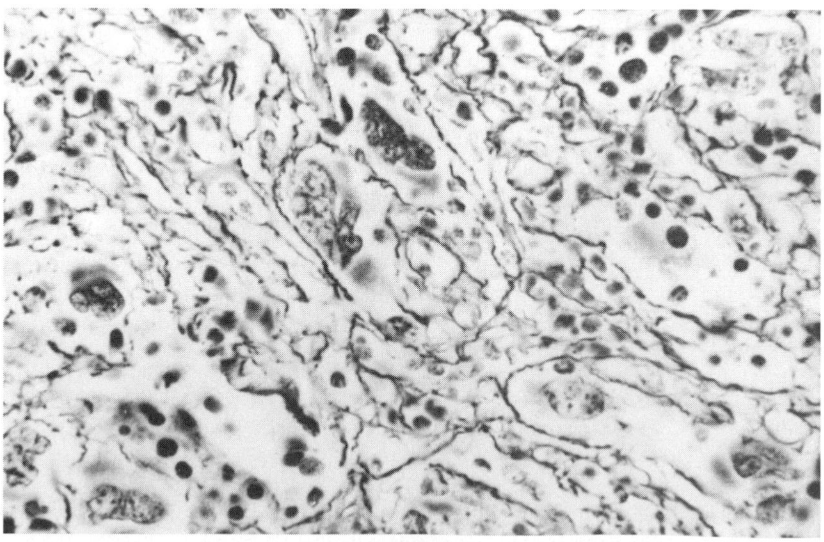

C

FIG. 47.37. A: Acute megakaryoblastic leukemia (M7). Bone marrow section showing replacement of normal marrow architecture by a prominent proliferation of megakaryoblasts, micromegakaryocytes, and atypical megakaryocytes. Erythroblasts are numerous (hematoxylin and eosin stain, original magnification: 160× magnification). **B:** High magnification of bone marrow section illustrated in **A**. Numerous atypical megakaryocytes, uninucleate micromegakaryocytes, and blasts can be noted. Erythroblasts are present (hematoxylin and eosin stain, original magnification: 256× magnification). **C:** Reticulin stain of bone marrow section illustrated in **A** and **B** showing diffuse increase in reticulin fibers (Wilder's reticulin stain, original magnification: 256× magnification). See Color Plate 57, between pp. 1446–1447.

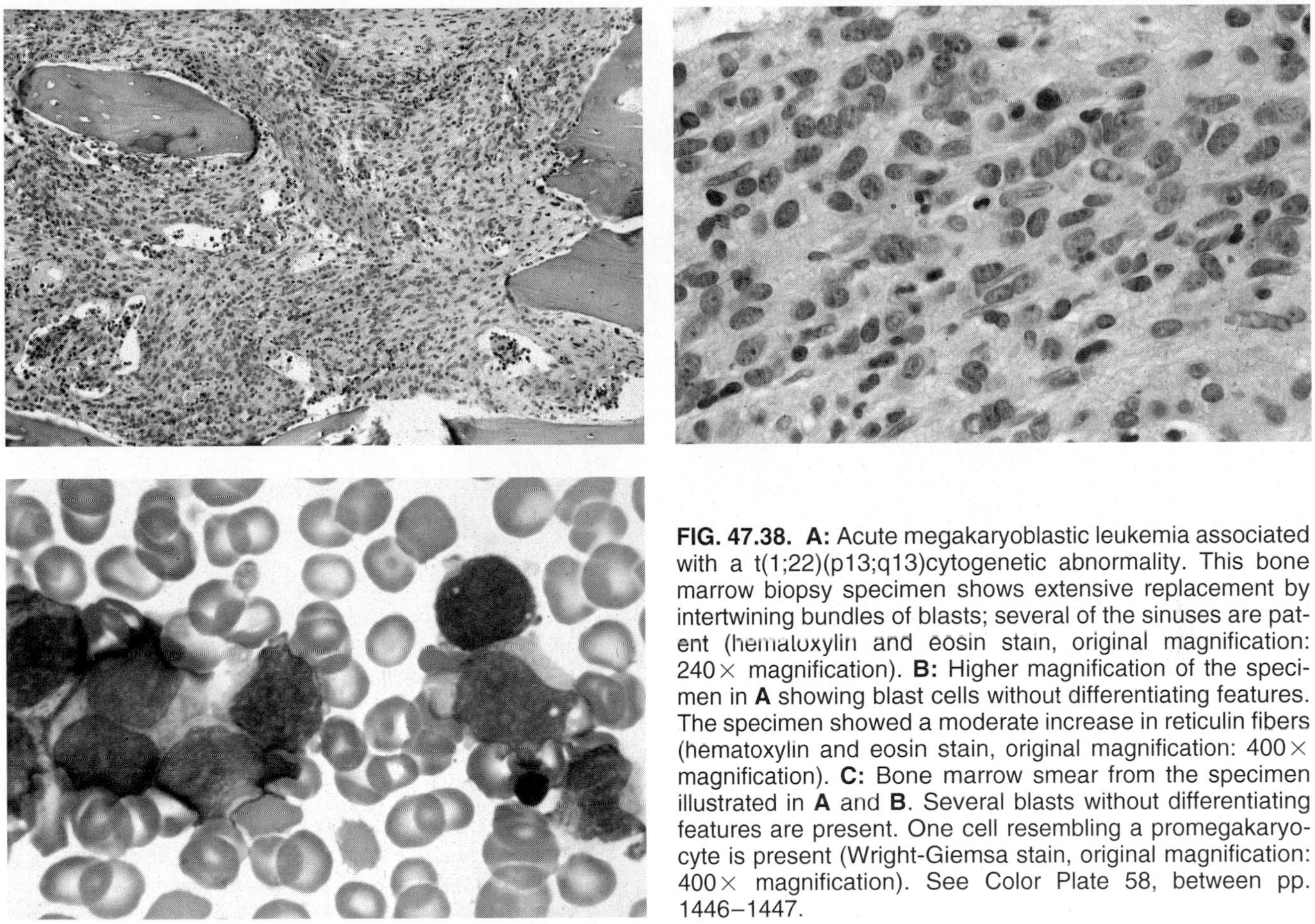

A B C

FIG. 47.38. A: Acute megakaryoblastic leukemia associated with a t(1;22)(p13;q13)cytogenetic abnormality. This bone marrow biopsy specimen shows extensive replacement by intertwining bundles of blasts; several of the sinuses are patent (hematoxylin and eosin stain, original magnification: 240× magnification). **B:** Higher magnification of the specimen in **A** showing blast cells without differentiating features. The specimen showed a moderate increase in reticulin fibers (hematoxylin and eosin stain, original magnification: 400× magnification). **C:** Bone marrow smear from the specimen illustrated in **A** and **B**. Several blasts without differentiating features are present. One cell resembling a promegakaryocyte is present (Wright-Giemsa stain, original magnification: 400× magnification). See Color Plate 58, between pp. 1446–1447.

ally occurring in children younger than 6 years of age (89–97). This type of leukemia may be preceded by a prolonged period of thrombocytopenia. The blasts in this type of leukemia are medium-sized with a moderate amount of basophilic cytoplasm that frequently contains large reddish purple granules that typically cluster (Fig. 47.39; see also Color Plate 59, between pp. 1446–1447). Small megakaryocytes and micromegakaryocytes are usually present. The blasts are MPO- and NSE-negative. There frequently is dyserythropoiesis with nuclear cytoplasmic dyssynchrony and nuclear lobulation. Dysgranulopoiesis usually is not observed. Marrow biopsy sections are hypercellular, with prominent megakaryocyte proliferation; increased fibrosis is usually present. Extramedullary manifestations of leukemia may occur (Fig. 47.40; see also Color Plate 60, between pp. 1446–1447).

The blasts usually express CD7, CD34, and CD36; there is variable expression of CD13, CD33, and CD61. The most common cytogenetic findings in addition to trisomy 21 are trisomy 8 and partial trisomy for the long arm of chromosome 1. The translocation found in some neonates with M7 AML, t(1;22)(p13;q13), is not present.

The major differential diagnosis of this type of acute leukemia in patients with Down syndrome is a transient myeloproliferative disorder that is clinically and hematologically indistinguishable from the described leukemia. The transient disorder virtually always presents in the first year of life and frequently in the neonatal period. Spontaneous remission usually occurs within 2 to 4 weeks of diagnosis (92).

Fluorescent *in situ* hybridization studies and molecular studies have provided evidence for involvement of the erythroid precursors in the M7 AML occurring in patients with Down syndrome, suggesting that the proliferating blast corresponds to an erythroid megakaryocytic precursor cell (96).

Typical acute lymphoblastic leukemia and AML also occur with increased incidence in individuals with Down syndrome. These leukemias have the same immunophenotypic and cytogenetic features and biologic evolution as they do in patients without Down syndrome and are not associated with the transient myeloproliferative disorder.

ACUTE BASOPHILIC LEUKEMIA

Acute basophilic leukemia is a rare type of AML in which the primary differentiation is to basophils (98–103). The acute leukemias with increased numbers of basophils that evolve from various myeloproliferative disorders are not in-

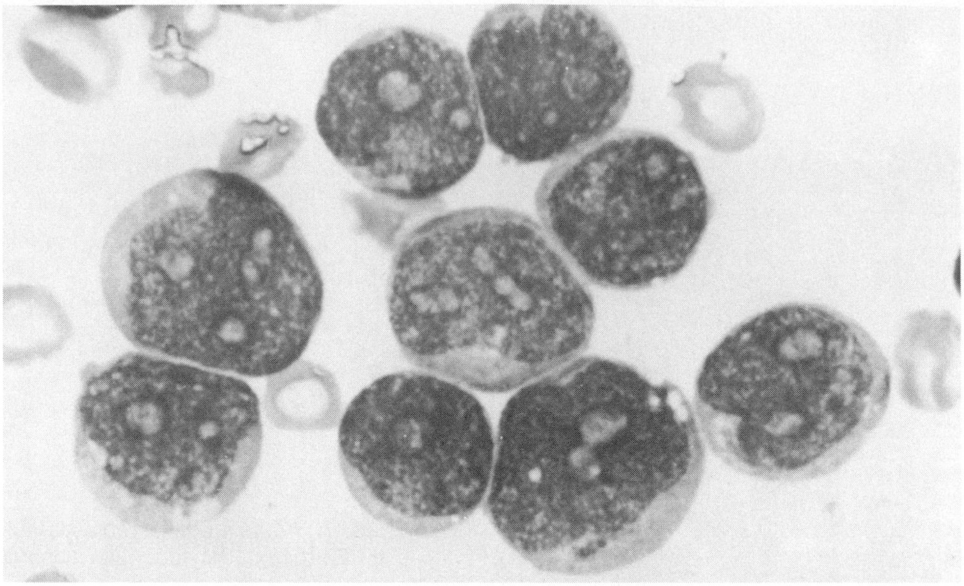

FIG. 47.39. Acute myeloid leukemia associated with Down syndrome. Bone marrow smear from a 3-year-old girl who has Down syndrome showing myeloblasts with reticular chromatin pattern, prominent nucleoli, a moderate amount of basophilic cytoplasm, and focal coarse azurophilic granulation (Wright-Giemsa stain, original magnification: 400× magnification). See Color Plate 59, between pp. 1446–1447.

cluded in this category, although some patients with the features of acute basophilic leukemia have the Philadelphia chromosome and could be viewed as having a basophil blast transformation of chronic myeloid leukemia. The morphologic distinction between *de novo* acute basophilic leukemia and basophil transformation of a previously unrecognized Philadelphia chromosome–related process is not always possible.

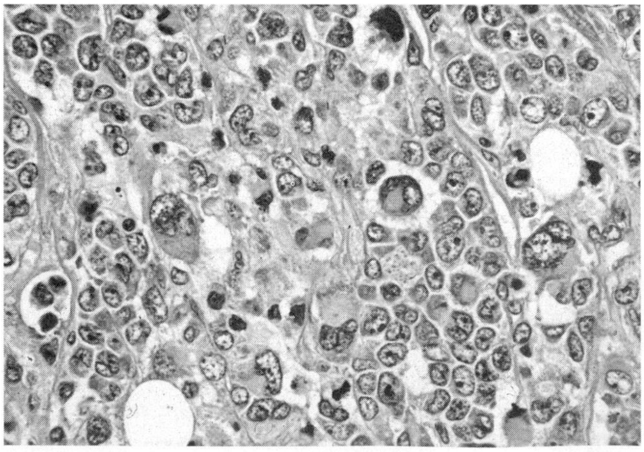

FIG. 47.40. Acute megakaryoblastic leukemia associated with Down syndrome. One of numerous enlarged abdominal lymph nodes from a 2-year-old child with Down syndrome and acute megakaryoblastic leukemia. The node is replaced completely; the cells are predominantly blasts, with several mature megakaryocytes and occasional small megakaryocytes with hypolobated nuclei (hematoxylin and eosin stain, original magnification: 400× magnification). See Color Plate 60, between pp. 1446–1447.

Acute basophilic leukemia usually presents with anemia and thrombocytopenia; the leukocyte count is variable. The blasts in the blood and marrow vary in morphology; the cytoplasm is usually moderately basophilic; there is a variable number of coarse basophilic granules in the cytoplasm and overlying the nucleus. These are variably metachromatic with toluidine blue staining; the granules are usually nonreactive for MPO and SBB. Mature basophils may or may not be present. On ultrastructural examination, the granules contain electron-dense particulate substance and are bisected internally, resembling the Greek letter theta (τ) (90).

The blasts express myeloid antigens such as CD13 and CD33 and usually the early hematopoietic marker CD34. They usually express CD9 and may be TdT-positive.

The major differential diagnoses include basophilic transformation of chronic myeloid leukemia, M2 AML associated with a t(6;9) cytogenetic abnormality, and acute lymphoblastic leukemia with coarse basophilic granules. The distinction between basophilic transformation of chronic myeloid and acute basophilic leukemia is based on the clinical history of chronic myeloid leukemia and cytogenetic studies. Patients presenting *de novo* with a predominance of blasts with basophil differentiation and the Philadelphia chromosome have a condition somewhat analogous to Philadelphia chromosome–positive acute lymphoblastic leukemia. The t(6;9)-associated AML usually has the characteristic findings of M2 AML, with an associated increase in basophils. Cases of acute lymphoblastic leukemia in which the blasts have coarse basophilic granules usually are of the precursor B-cell type with expression of pan–B cell surface antigens and TdT positivity; some of these cases also have the Philadelphia chromosome.

A

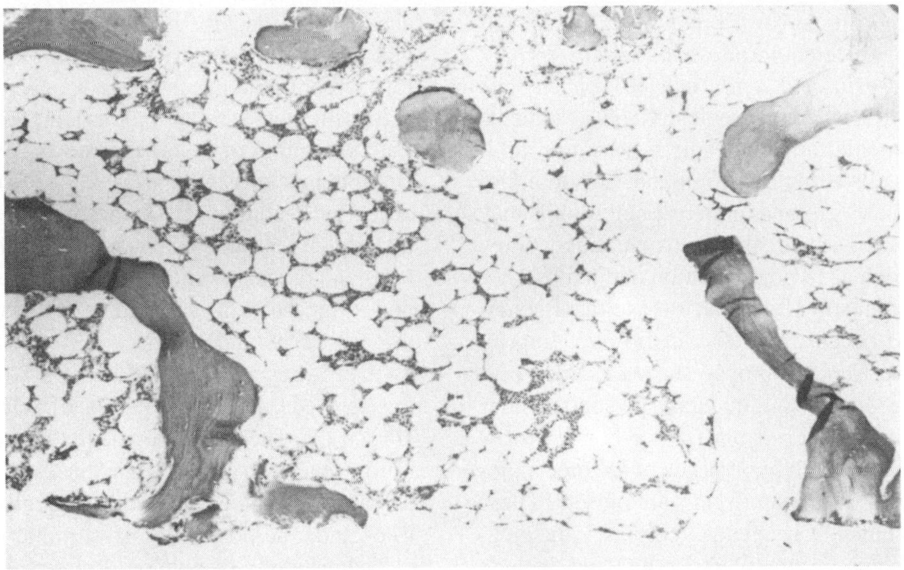

B

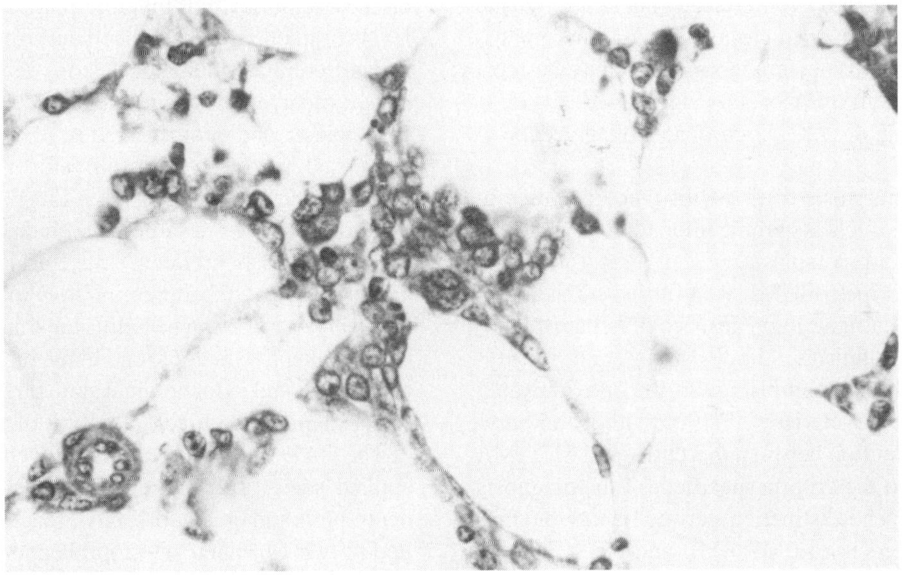

FIG. 47.41. **A:** Hypocellular acute leukemia. Bone marrow section showing markedly hypocellular marrow (hematoxylin and eosin stain, original magnification: 20× magnification). **B:** High magnification of the bone marrow section illustrated in A showing interstitial clusters of blasts (hematoxylin and eosin stain, original magnification: 256× magnification).

HYPOCELLULAR ACUTE LEUKEMIA

Hypocellular acute leukemia is defined as 20% or more blasts in bone marrow that is less than 30% cellular (5,104,105). This should not be viewed as a specific morphologic type of AML; the usual morphologic and immunologic classification criteria should be used in these patients, with *hypocellular* as a qualifying term. In the typical case, the cellularity in the bone marrow sections resembles aplastic anemia; however, on high magnification, the marrow interstitium shows a predominant population of blasts (Fig. 47.41). The blood shows pancytopenia; occasional blasts may be detected. Smears of the bone marrow aspirate show 20% or more blasts. The blasts frequently show no differentiating morphologic features but are cytochemically and immunophenotypically myeloid in the majority of patients—that is, M1 AML. Occasionally the blasts are nonreactive for MPO and SBB and the myeloid origin is documented by demonstration of myeloid surface antigens such as CD13 and CD33—that is, M0. Occasional blasts have large cytoplasmic inclusions that show partial MPO and SBB reactivity.

ACUTE PANMYELOSIS WITH MYELOFIBROSIS (ACUTE MYELOFIBROSIS)

Acute panmyelosis with myelofibrosis has been described as a distinct clinicopathologic entity characterized by an acute panmyelopathy with marrow fibrosis. This disease has been referred to using different terms: *acute myelosclerosis*, *malignant myelosclerosis*, and *acute myelodysplasia with myelofibrosis* (106–108). Hematologically, these patients present with pancytopenia; organomegaly is absent or minimal. The red blood cells show no or minimal anisopoikilocytosis. Occasional blast cells and immature neutrophils may be detected in the blood smear; the neutrophils may show dysplastic changes such as hypogranulation and nuclear hyposegmentation. Diagnostic bone marrow aspirates generally are not obtained because of reticulin fibrosis. Imprint preparations from the trephine biopsy show evidence of a panmyelopathy with significant myelodysplastic changes and an increase in the number of blasts. The bone marrow sections are hypercellular, with hyperplasia of all three major myeloid cell lines. Foci of immature cells are present. There generally is a marked megakaryocytic hyperplasia; the megakaryocytes and precursors are pleomorphic and include small megakaryocytes with hypolobulated nuclei, dysplastic polylobulated forms with open chromatin, and micromegakaryocytes; the megakaryocyte abnormalities may be most readily appreciated with a PAS stain (Fig. 47.42A,B). Reticulin is increased (Fig. 47.42C). Significant collagen deposition is uncommon.

The differential diagnosis of this entity includes myeloproliferative diseases such as chronic idiopathic myelofibrosis (agnogenic myeloid metaplasia) in acute transformation, M7 AML, and other types of AML with fibrosis. The abrupt onset of clinical symptomatology, absence of hepatosplenomegaly, and minimal anisopoikilocytosis in acute panmyelosis with myelofibrosis contrasts with the splenomegaly and chronic course characteristic of chronic idiopathic myelofibrosis. The distinction between this entity and M7 AML requires adherence to the criteria specified for the diagnosis of M7 AML (109). The distinction between acute panmyelosis with myelofibrosis and M7 AML and other types of AML with myelofibrosis is not always possible from morphologic findings. Acute panmyelosis with myelofibrosis is basically a panmyelopathy with significant involvement of all three myeloid cell lines; M7 AML predominantly involves the megakaryocytes. If there is significant involvement of the nonmegakaryocytic lineages, acute panmyelosis with myelofibrosis is the more appropriate diagnostic terminology.

MYELOID SARCOMA (GRANULOCYTIC SARCOMA, CHLOROMA)

Myeloid sarcoma is an extramedullary tumor mass of myeloid precursors. These tumors may be composed of neutrophil precursors or monocytes; rarely, extramedullary tumor masses of megakaryocytes and erythroid precursors occur. Myeloid sarcomas have been referred to as *chloroma*, a name derived from the greenish hue imparted by the peroxidase activity of the freshly cut surface (110). This term has been replaced by *granulocytic sarcoma*, which does not adequately reflect the possible composition of these lesions, which also may consist of monoblasts (67,111–115). Myeloid sarcoma can occur *de novo*, as a manifestation of AML at presentation or relapse, or as a manifestation of the blastic transformation of a myeloproliferative disorder such as chronic myeloid leukemia (112–115). Myeloid sarcomas occur most commonly in the pediatric age group and frequently involve the axial skeleton, with a propensity for the orbit and paranasal sinuses; myeloid sarcomas of the lymph nodes, breast, skin, gastrointestinal, respiratory and genitourinary tracts, and central and peripheral nervous systems have been reported (112–115). *De novo* myeloid sarcomas may precede the manifestation of AML by several months (111–113). They also may be the initial and sole manifestation of relapse in a patient who has AML. The marrow should be carefully evaluated morphologically and cytogenetically to exclude the possibility of minimal involvement.

The histology of myeloid sarcoma is variable, depending on the overall level of myeloid maturation (112,113). Three levels of maturation have been described: blastic, immature, and differentiated. Blastic lesions are composed predominantly of myeloblasts; immature lesions are composed of myeloblasts and promyelocytes; the differentiated type is composed primarily of promyelocytes and cells at later stages of maturation (Figs. 47.43, 47.44). The differential diagnosis of myeloid sarcoma includes large cell lymphoma, lymphoblastic lymphoma, and Burkitt's lymphoma (112). The presence of differentiating myeloid cells such as eosinophilic myelocytes can be helpful in this differential, but these cells frequently are not found in the blastic type. Immunohistochemical and cytochemical stains frequently are necessary to substantiate the myeloid nature of this lesion.

The CAE stain was the first cytochemical reaction to be applied successfully to fixed tissue for the recognition of neutrophils and precursors; CAE reactivity is essentially limited to two cell lines, neutrophils and mast cells. It appears in the early neutrophil promyelocyte stage and is very useful in recognizing myeloid sarcomas with a maturing neutrophil population. The immunohistochemical application of antibodies to very early myeloid precursors largely has supplanted the CAE reaction (8,85,115). The antilysozyme antibody reacts with both neutrophils and monocytes. Anti-MPO is an excellent antibody to neutrophils including the myeloblast stage; this antibody can be used with most fixatives, including mercury-based and most decalcifying agents. Not all myeloid sarcomas, however, are MPO-reactive. Although the myeloblasts in some cases may react with anti-MPO, there may be patients in whom the myeloblasts are nonreactive; immunophenotyping with flow cytometry usually resolves the lineage in these cases.

Acute myeloblastic leukemia M2 associated with the translocation t(8;21) and M4EO AML with inv(16) or t(16;16) are associated with an increased risk of developing myeloid sarcoma (45). Acute monoblastic leukemia with the translocation t(9;11) also is associated with an increased incidence of extramedullary involvement (66). The myeloid

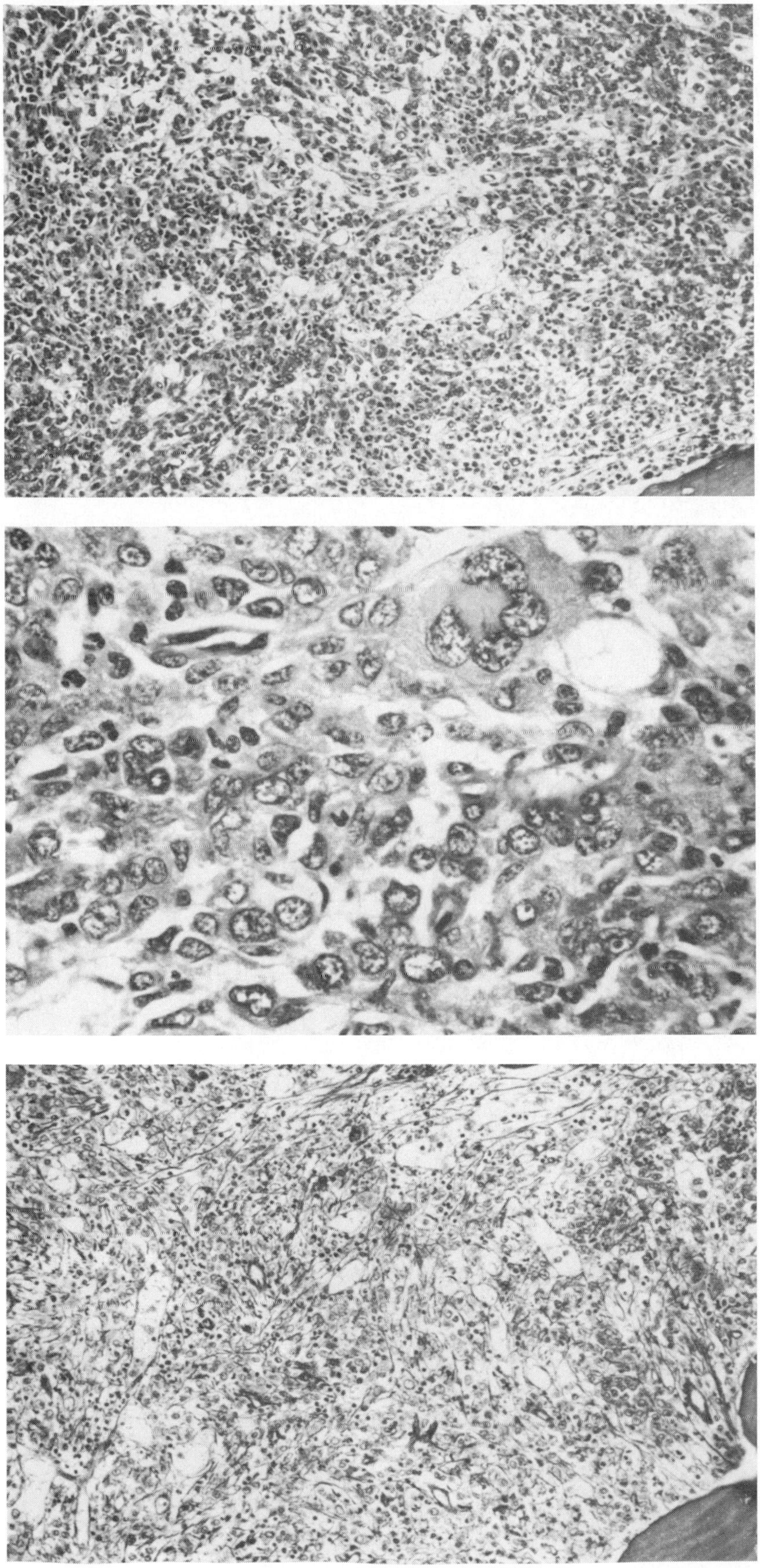

A B C

FIG. 47.42. **A:** Acute panmyelosis with myelofibrosis. Bone marrow section showing hypercellular marrow effaced by a panmyeloid hyperplasia (hematoxylin and eosin stain, original magnification: 40× magnification). **B:** High-magnification view of the bone marrow section illustrated in **A** showing evidence of granulocytic and megakaryocytic differentiation (hematoxylin and eosin stain, original magnification: 256× magnification). **C:** Low-magnification view of the same section as in **A** and **B** stained for reticulin and showing a marked increase in reticulin fibers (Wilder's reticulin stain, original magnification: 40× magnification).

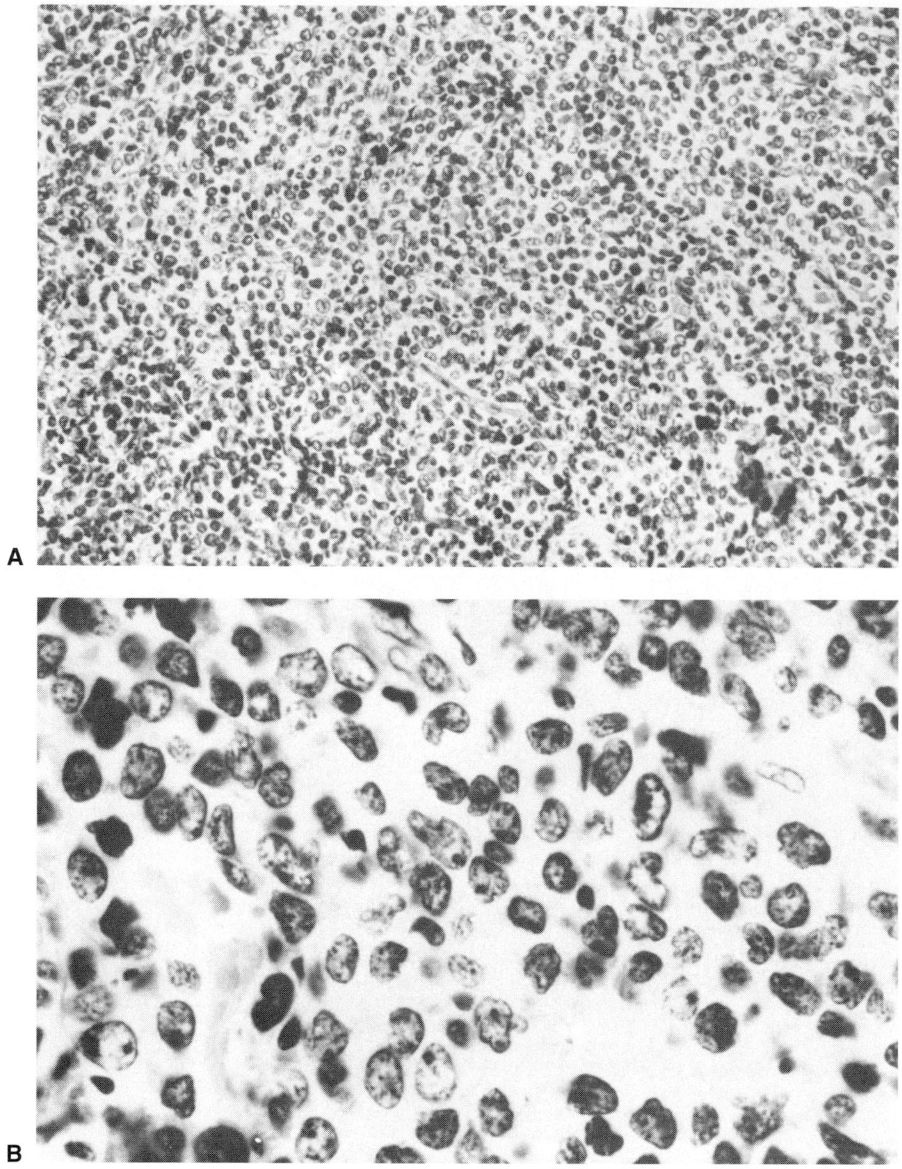

FIG. 47.43. A: Myeloid sarcoma. Lymph node showing diffuse infiltration by immature hematopoietic cells (hematoxylin and eosin stain, original magnification: 64× magnification). B: High magnification of lymph node section illustrated in A. These cells expressed CD7 and CD33 (hematoxylin and eosin stain, original magnification: 256× magnification).

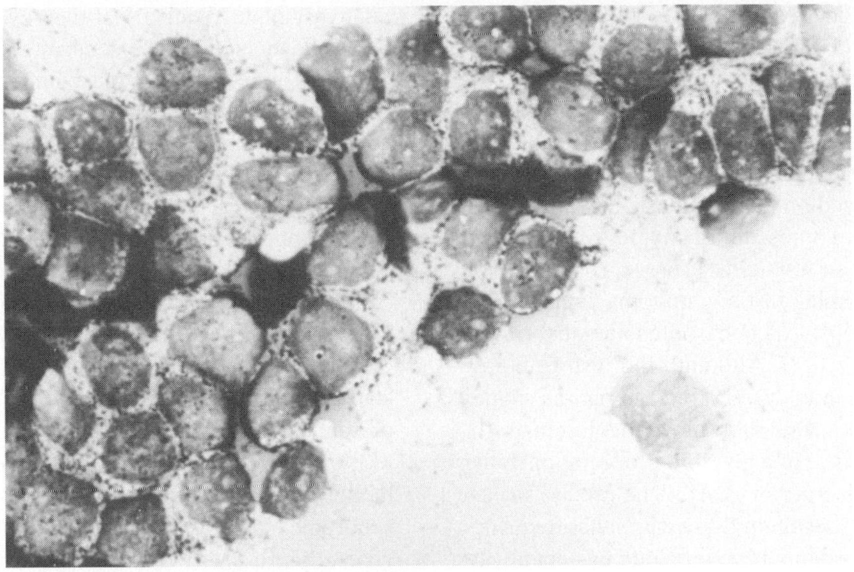

A

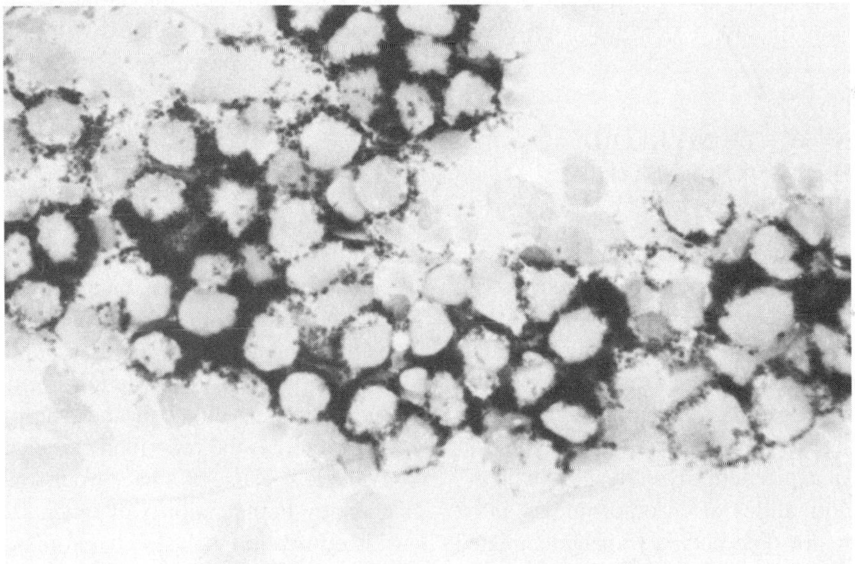

B

FIG. 47.44. A: Myeloid sarcoma. Imprint preparation from a lymph node from a 27-year-old man showing myeloblasts and promyelocytes with prominent azurophilic granulation (Wright-Giemsa stain, original magnification: 256× magnification). **B:** Myeloperoxidase stain on imprint preparation illustrated in **A** showing intense peroxidase reactivity (myeloperoxidase stain, original magnification: 256× magnification).

sarcoma may precede, occur concurrently with the presentation of the leukemic process, or manifest at relapse and may be the only recognizable evidence of relapse.

There is a reported association between CD56 expression on the blasts in AML and extramedullary manifestation. An unusual form of acute myeloid malignancy with prominent extramedullary manifestation, lymphoblast-like morphology and concurrent antigen expression of myeloid markers and CD56 and CD7 has been reported (116).

A syndrome of T-lymphoblastic lymphoma, increased eosinophils, and a t(8;13)(p11;q11) chromosome abnormality has been observed (117,118). Although the histopathology and antigen expression in the presenting lymphoma suggest a lymphoblastic process, the subsequent evolution is frequently more characteristic of a myeloid proliferation, either a myeloproliferative disorder or AML. The precise lineage of the ''lymphoblastic'' lesion in these cases that frequently manifests a prominent eosinophilic infiltrate has not always been studied adequately, and it is possible that some of these tumors represent biphenotypic or myeloblastic processes (117,118).

THERAPY-RELATED ACUTE MYELOID LEUKEMIA AND MYELODYSPLASTIC SYNDROMES

Therapy-related acute myeloid leukemia and myelodysplastic syndromes occur in persons previously treated with cytotoxic agents or radiotherapy. Two major groups of therapy-related processes based on the causative agents, morphologic findings, and cytogenetic abnormalities are recognized (119–128). The first described type occurs in patients treated with alkylating agents or radiotherapy; this type usually is associated with an antecedent myelodysplastic phase, a panmyelosis, and abnormalities of chromosomes 5 and 7 (118–121). The other major type occurs in patients treated with topoisomerase II inhibitors, the topoisomerase II–directed epipodophyllotoxins, and the DNA intercalating agents (59,119,128–130). This type frequently is associated with balanced translocations involving chromosome 11q23 and AMLs with a monocytic component; it may be associated with balanced translocation t(15;17)(q22;q21) and the relatively specific morphologic types of acute leukemia associated with this translocation (119,124–127). Acute lymphoblastic leukemia, frequently with a translocation t(4;11)(q21;q23), also may be observed (131).

The incidence of therapy-related acute myeloid leukemia and myelodysplastic syndromes varies with the different causative agents and ranges up to 15% in patients with Hodgkin's disease treated with MOPP chemotherapy and up to 17% in myeloma patients treated with alkylating agents (132–135). In Hodgkin's disease, the peak risk period appears to occur 6 years after initiation of combined-modality therapy. Risk factors include age of the patient and type, duration, and repetition of exposure to the mutagenic agents. The relationship of drug dosage to risk is recognized in the relatively high frequency of therapy-related AMLs and myelodysplastic syndromes occurring in patients receiving autologous bone marrow transplant for Hodgkin's and non-Hodgkin's lymphomas (136,137). In the alkylating agent–related type, the time interval from initiation of the causative therapy to manifestation of the leukemia or myelodysplastic syndrome is 7 to 133 months; medians of 56, 58, and 71 months are reported in different series (120–122). The therapy-related acute myeloid leukemias occurring in patients treated with DNA-intercalating anthracyclines and topoisomerase II–directed epipodophyllotoxins usually occur after a relatively short interval after the initiation of causative therapy, with a median of 2 to 3 years, and usually present with a distinct morphologic type, such as M5, M2, M3, or M4, without a preceding myelodysplastic phase, although occasional patients present with a myelodysplastic syndrome (130,138,139). This type of therapy-related AML generally presents with a more abrupt onset and higher blast percentage than the alkylating agent–related types. The anthracyclines are associated with a lower incidence of therapy-related leukemia than the epipodophyllotoxins.

Patients with alkylating agent–related acute myeloid leukemia or myelodysplastic syndrome most commonly present with fatigue related to anemia. Because these patients usually are followed for the disorder for which the causative agents were administered, the detection of laboratory abnormalities may precede the onset of clinical symptoms. Cytopenias are common. Anemia virtually always is present, and macrocytosis with ovalocytes is frequent. Thrombocytopenia and neutropenia are present in the majority of patients.

In patients with alkylating agent–related acute myeloid leukemia or myelodysplastic syndrome who have undergone splenectomy, the red blood cell changes may be difficult to evaluate because of a background of postsplenectomy blood changes. In the majority of patients with this type of therapy-related myelodysplastic syndrome or AML, the abnormalities are more marked than found with splenectomy only. The morphologic abnormalities frequently involve multiple myeloid cell lines consistent with a panmyelopathy (140,141).

The myeloid cells in a high percentage of patients with alkylating agent–related acute myeloid leukemia and myelodysplastic syndrome have clonal chromosome abnormalities. The abnormalities tend to be multiple, and approximately 80% involve chromosomes 5 or 7 and include monosomy 5, 5q−, monosomy 7, and 7q−; if a single abnormality is present, it usually involves one of these chromosomes (59,122–124,125). Extreme karyotypic variability may occur. The abnormalities are present in both the leukemia and myelodysplastic phases.

The bone marrow and blood findings in the therapy-related disorders vary, depending on the stage at which the problem initially is diagnosed and the therapeutic agents associated with the process. The disorders related to alkylating agents and radiotherapy are separated into myelodysplastic syndromes and AML based on the percentage of blasts; how-

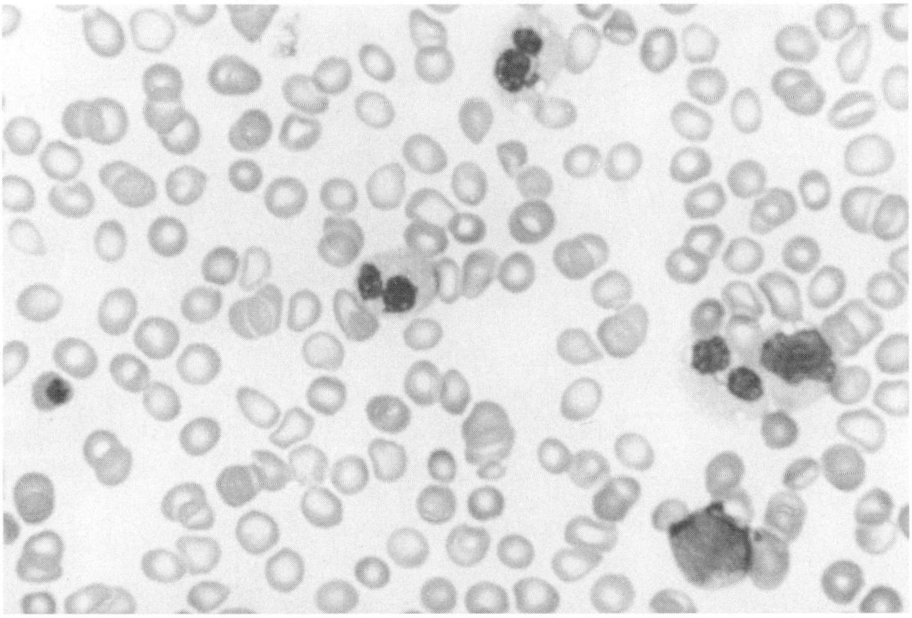

FIG. 47.45. Blood smear from a 77-year-old man who has a therapy-related myelodysplastic syndrome following multiagent chemotherapy for a non-Hodgkin's lymphoma. There are three mature neutrophils with pseudo–Pelger-Huet nuclei, two immature neutrophils, and a normoblast (Wright-Giemsa stain, original magnification: 256× magnification).

ever, these two processes should be viewed as lying on a continuum of the same disease. The majority of patients with alkylating agent-related type are characterized by a panmyelosis that frequently makes precise classification difficult (120–122). The morphologic alterations in the myeloid cells range from subtle alterations to marked abnormalities in size and nuclear and cytoplasmic characteristics (Figs. 47.45–47.50; see also Color Plates 61–64, between pp. 1446–1447). Nuclear hypolobulation and cytoplasmic hypogranulation in the neutrophils are present in a high percentage of patients. Abnormalities of erythroblast nuclei are present in virtually all patients; marked gigantism and hyperlobulated nuclei are frequent (Fig. 47.51; see also Color Plate 65, between pp. 1446–1447). Ringed sideroblasts occur in approximately 60% of patients and range from 1% to approximately 50% of nucleated red blood cells. The presence of ringed sideroblasts or PAS-positive normoblasts may be the initial morphologic manifestation of a therapy-related myelodysplastic syndrome and may be a transient finding in the evolution of the process (Figs. 47.52, 47.53; see also Color Plates 66 and 67, between pp. 1446–1447). Increased marrow or blood basophils occur in approximately 25% of patients and also may be one of the earliest manifestations of the disease (Fig. 47.48).

The marrow is normocellular in approximately 50% of patients; 25% are hypercellular and 25% are hypocellular (Fig. 47.54). The hypercellular marrows generally are characterized by panhyperplasia. Megakaryocytes may be disproportionately increased in number and manifest dysplastic changes and considerable size range, with numerous small megakaryocytes and large megakaryocytes. Clustering of megakaryocytes may be present. Approximately 40% to 50% of marrows show some increase in reticulin fibers; the findings in occasional patients may be those of acute myelofibrosis (140).

The blood and marrow findings in the majority of patients with this type of therapy-related process in the myelodysplastic phase are those of refractory cytopenia with multilineage dysplasia. The therapy-related AMLs of this type are principally of the M2, M4, and M6 subtypes (Figs. 47.55, 47.56; see also Color Plate 68, between pp. 1446–1447). Because of the panmyeloid involvement in many of the leukemias, approximately 40% to 50% of patients cannot be classified (120).

Myyelodysplastic syndromes related to therapy with alkylating agents and AML generally have more aggressive clinical courses than *de novo* AML and myelodysplastic syndromes (Figs. 47.57, 47.58). The overall median duration of survival is 4 to 8 months. Patients with myelodysplastic syndrome have only a slightly longer median duration of survival than patients who have AML (120,121). Several laboratory findings have been associated with a poor prognosis, including more than 5% marrow blasts, hgb less than 10 g/dL, and platelet counts lower than 100×10^9 per liter. Clinical factors associated with an unfavorable prognosis include age older than 65 years, Hodgkin's disease, myeloma or ovarian cancer as the primary tumor, and therapy with the alkylating agents nitrosoureas or procarbazine (121).

The hematologic disorders related to topoisomerase II inhibitor usually manifest as acute leukemia associated with a recurrent chromosome translocation, including t(9;11) or

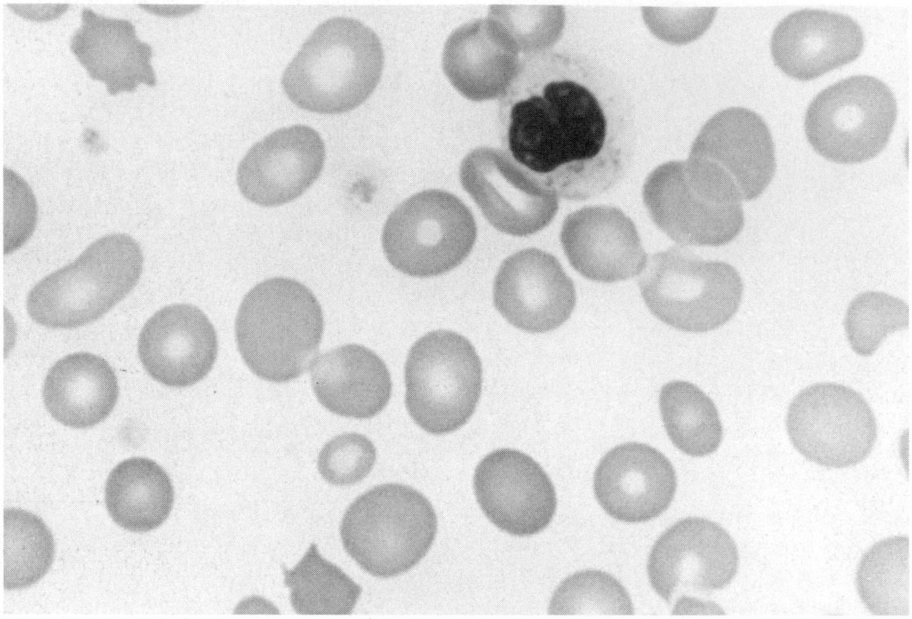

FIG. 47.46. Blood smear from a 21-year-old patient who has a myelodysplastic syndrome related to chemotherapy and radiotherapy for Hodgkin's disease. The patient had undergone splenectomy for staging at the time of diagnosis. The red blood cells show moderate anisocytosis, with macrocytes and increased poikilocytosis; a small neutrophil with a hypolobated nucleus is present (Wright-Giemsa stain, original magnification: 400× magnification).

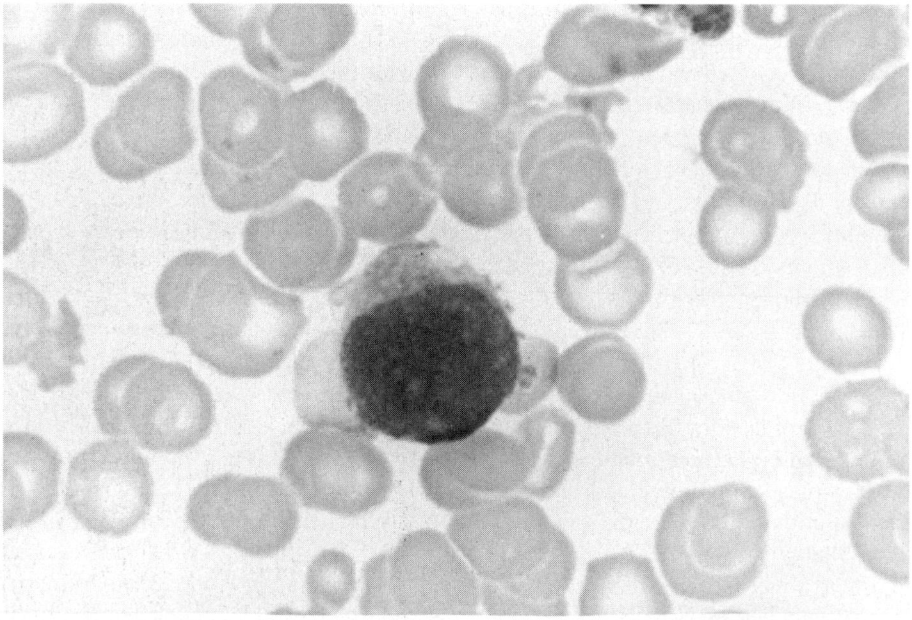

FIG. 47.47. A micromegakaryocyte in the blood smear of a patient who has a therapy-related myelodysplastic syndrome. The nucleus is round with condensed chromatin; irregular platelet budding is present (Wright-Giemsa stain, original magnification: 400× magnification). See Color Plate 61, between pp. 1446–1447.

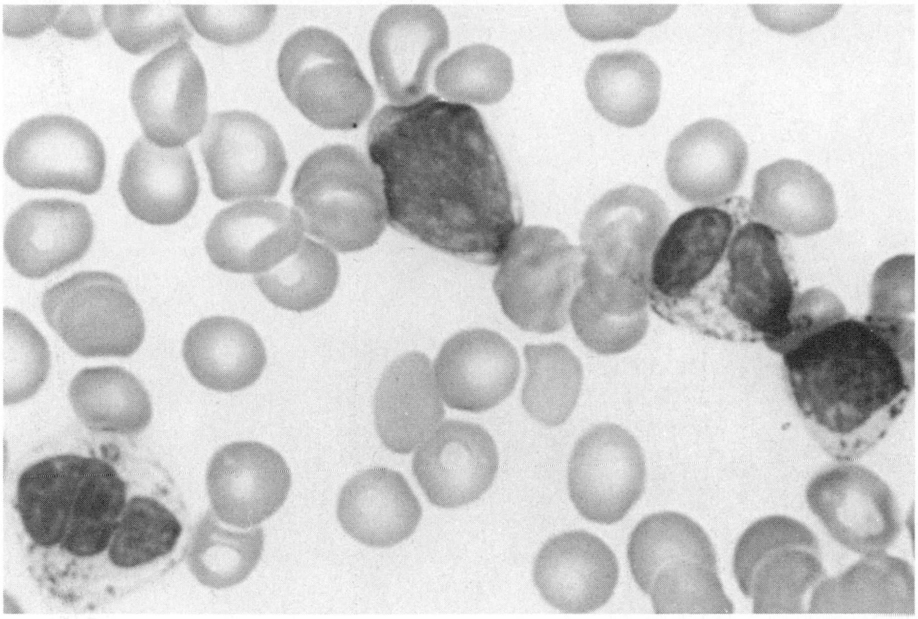

FIG. 47.48. Blood smear from a patient who has a therapy-related myelodysplastic syndrome presenting with 22% basophils. This field shows three basophils, two with decreased granules, and one blast (Wright-Giemsa stain, original magnification: 400× magnification). See Color Plate 62, between pp. 1446–1447.

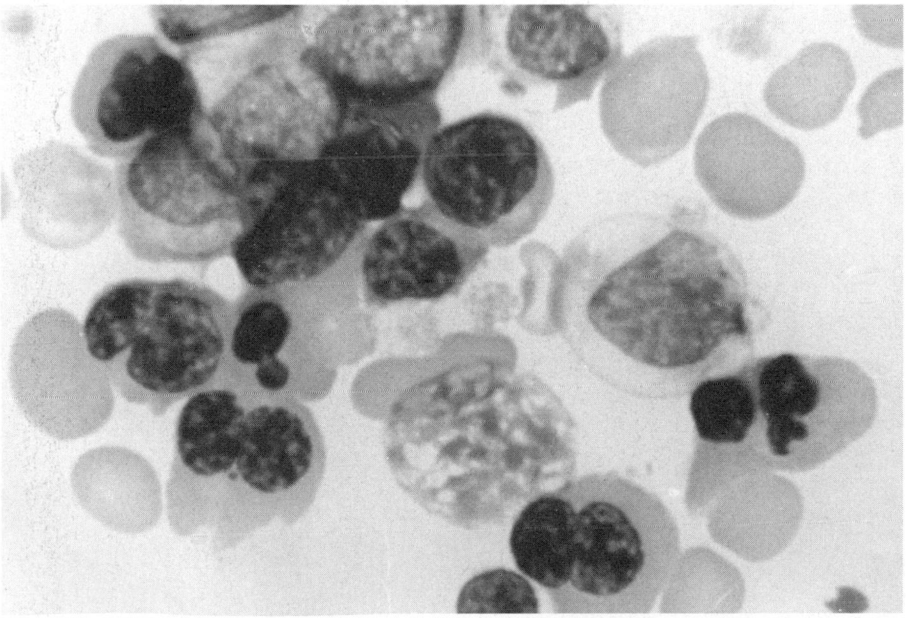

FIG. 47.49. Smear of a bone marrow specimen from an adult who has a therapy-related myelodysplastic syndrome. The nuclei of the red blood cell precursors have a slightly open chromatin and show marked lobulation (Wright-Giemsa stain, original magnification: 256× magnification). See Color Plate 63, between pp. 1446–1447.

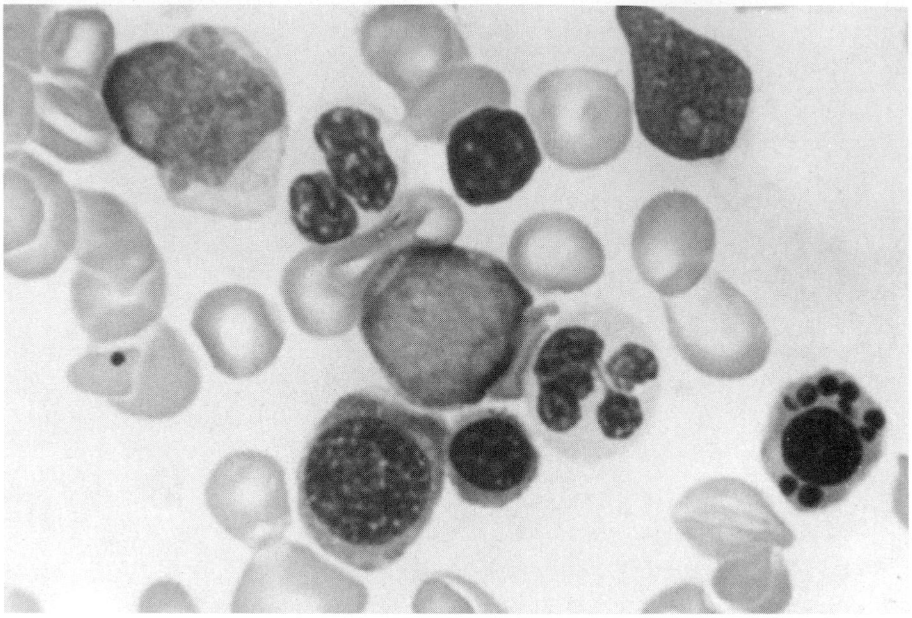

FIG. 47.50. Bone marrow smear from a 17-year-old man who has a myelodysplastic syndrome related to therapy for Hodgkin's disease. Two markedly hypogranular neutrophils, a red cell precursor with multiple nuclear fragments, and two myeloblasts are present in this field (Wright-Giemsa stain, original magnification: 400× magnification). See Color Plate 64, between pp. 1446–1447.

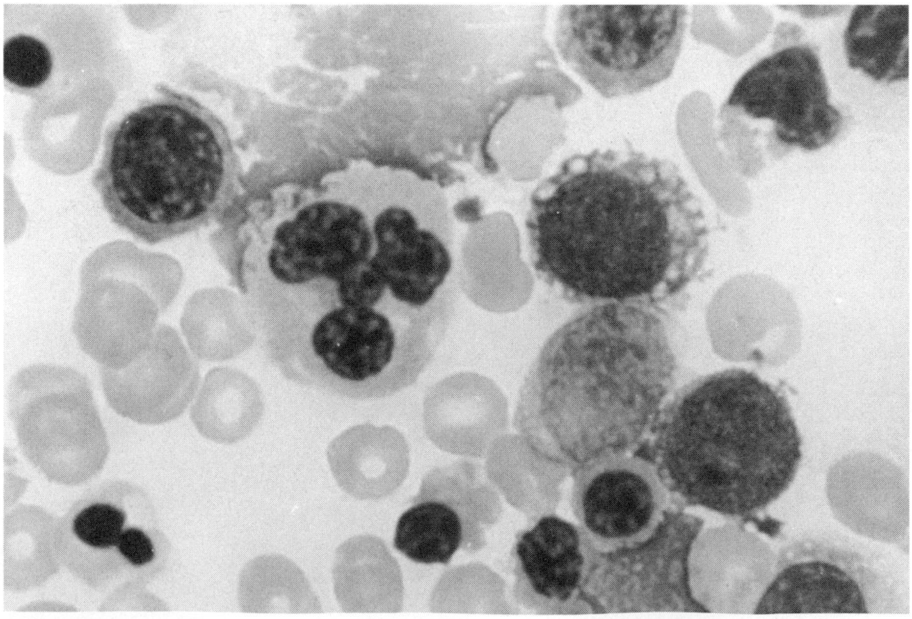

FIG. 47.51. Bone marrow smear from an adult who has a therapy-related myelodysplastic syndrome. The large red cell precursor in the center shows marked nuclear lobation. One erythroblast on the right shows numerous cytoplasmic vacuoles (Wright-Giemsa stain, original magnification: 400× magnification). See Color Plate 65, between pp. 1446–1447.

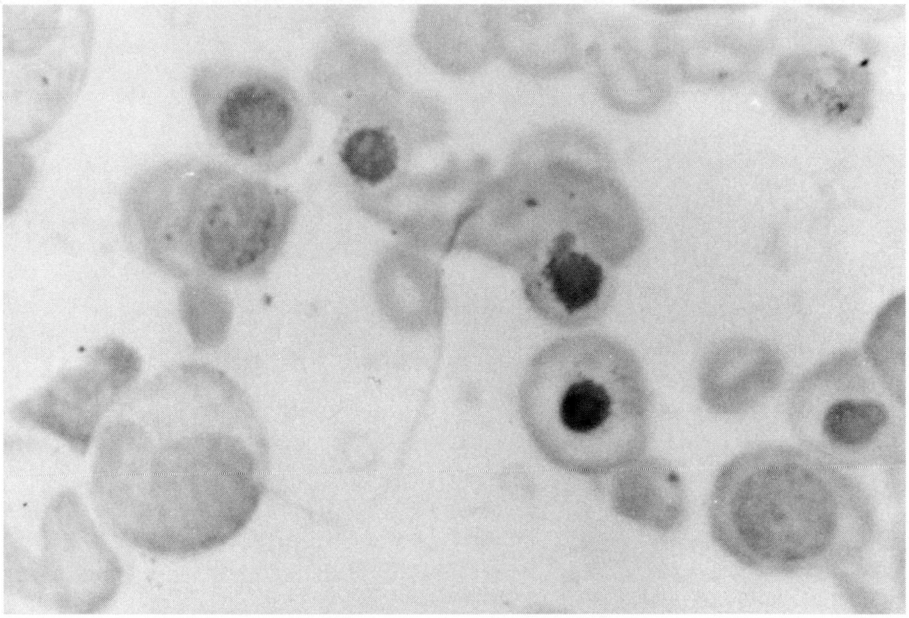

FIG. 47.52. Iron stain of a bone marrow smear from a 24-year-old woman who developed a myelodysplastic syndrome following therapy for Hodgkin's disease. This specimen from the initial diagnostic specimen shows several ringed sideroblasts (Prussian blue stain followed by Safranin counterstain, original magnification: 400× magnification). See Color Plate 66, between pp. 1446–1447.

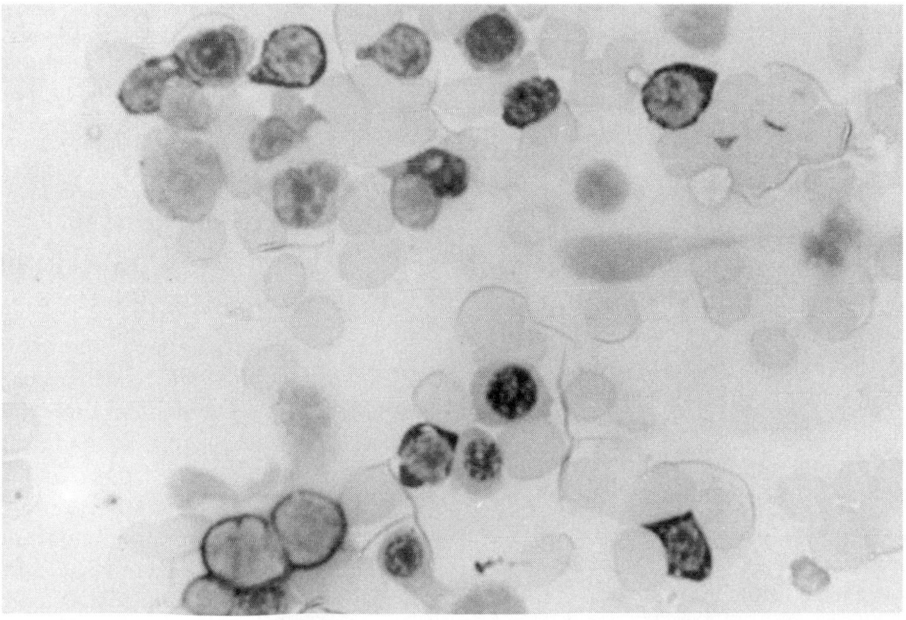

FIG. 47.53. Bone marrow smear stained with periodic acid–Schiff stain from a woman with a therapy-related myelodysplastic syndrome following chemotherapy for multiple myeloma. Numerous red cell precursors are intensely positive (original magnification: 256× magnification). See Color Plate 67, between pp. 1446–1447.

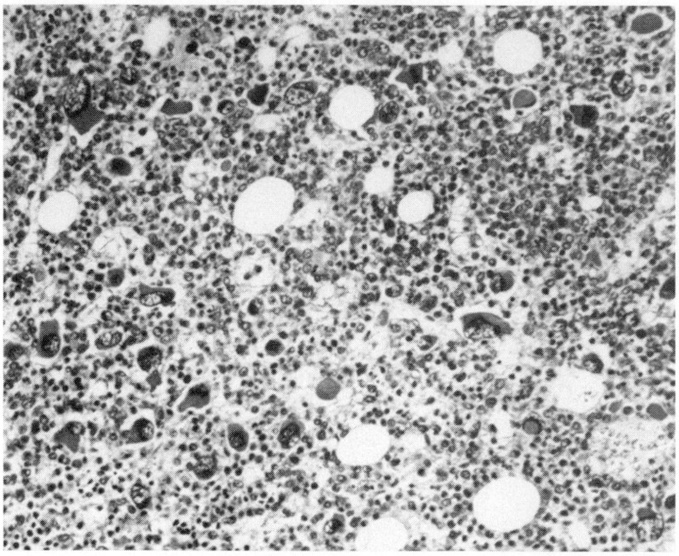
A

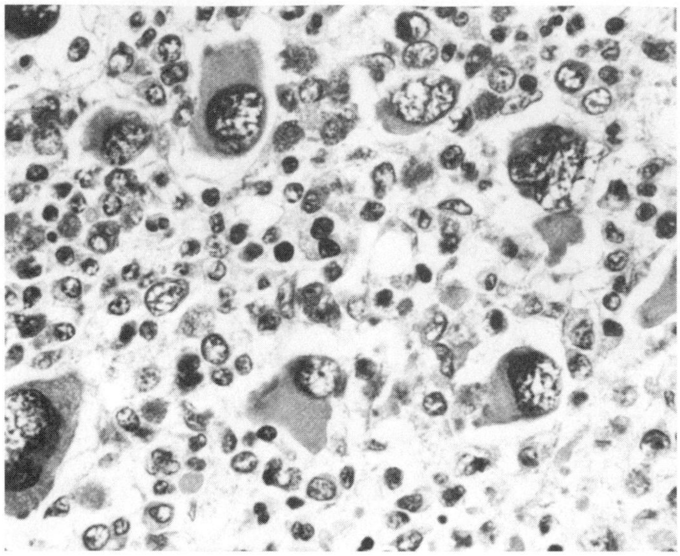
B

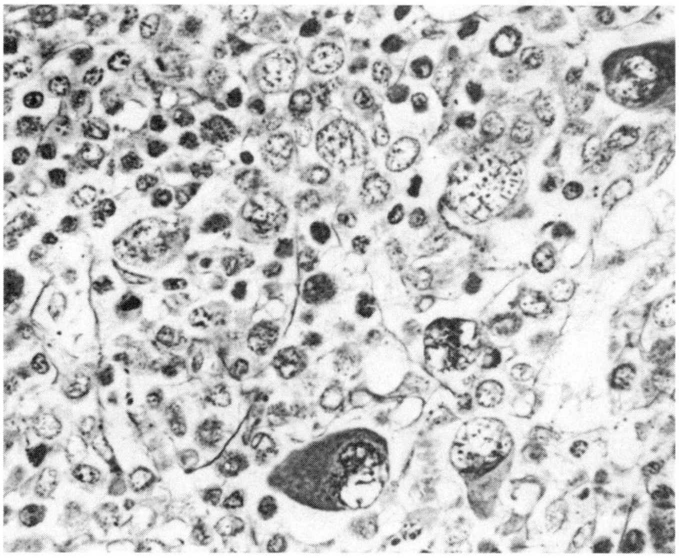
C

FIG. 47.54. A: Bone marrow biopsy from an adult patient who has a myelodysplastic syndrome related to chemotherapy for non-Hodgkin's lymphoma. The marrow is hypercellular with numerous megakaryocytes (hematoxylin and eosin stain, original magnification: 40× magnification). **B:** High magnification of the specimen illustrated in **A** showing dysplastic megakaryocytes with hypolobated and nonlobated nuclei and dispersed nuclear chromatin. Micromegakaryocytes with a high nuclear cytoplasmic ratio are present (hematoxylin and eosin stain, original magnification: 256× magnification). **C:** Reticulin stain of the specimen illustrated in **A** and **B.** There is a slight increase in reticulin fibers (Wilder's reticulin stain, original magnification: 256× magnification).

11q23 translocations associated with partner chromosomes other than number 9, t(8;21), inv(16), and t(15;17). The morphologic subtype is that usually associated with the specific abnormality, for example, M5A with t(9;11), t(8; 21) with M2 AML, and t(15;17) with APL (138). In some patients the initial manifestation may be a myoeldysplastic syndrome with or without a monocytic component (130,135,139).

The topoisomerase II–related leukemias with balanced translocations frequently are characterized by prior therapy for a solid tumor rather than a hematologic malignancy, and prior therapy with a combination of drugs that included an anthracycline and epipodophyllotoxin, agents that target DNA topoisomerase II (59,135). This type of therapy-related leukemia appears to have a response to therapy and prognosis similar to *de novo* acute leukemia with similar cytogenetic and morphologic features.

BONE MARROW EVALUATION FOLLOWING CHEMOTHERAPY: RESPONSE CRITERIA

The evaluation of bone marrow specimens following chemotherapy for AML relates primarily to three findings: the effect of the chemotherapeutic agents on the leukemic process, evidence of regeneration of normal hematopoietic cells, and cellularity. All three findings are considered in the determination of classification of therapeutic response as remission, partial remission, or failure (5).

The classification of complete remission is used if the percentage of blasts in the postchemotherapy marrow specimen is less than 5% and there is evidence of maturation of all myeloid cell lines in a marrow that is more than 20% cellular; the assessment of cellularity should be based on examination of a bone marrow trephine biopsy specimen. Particle crush preparations and smears are not considered reliable for this purpose. The platelet count should be more

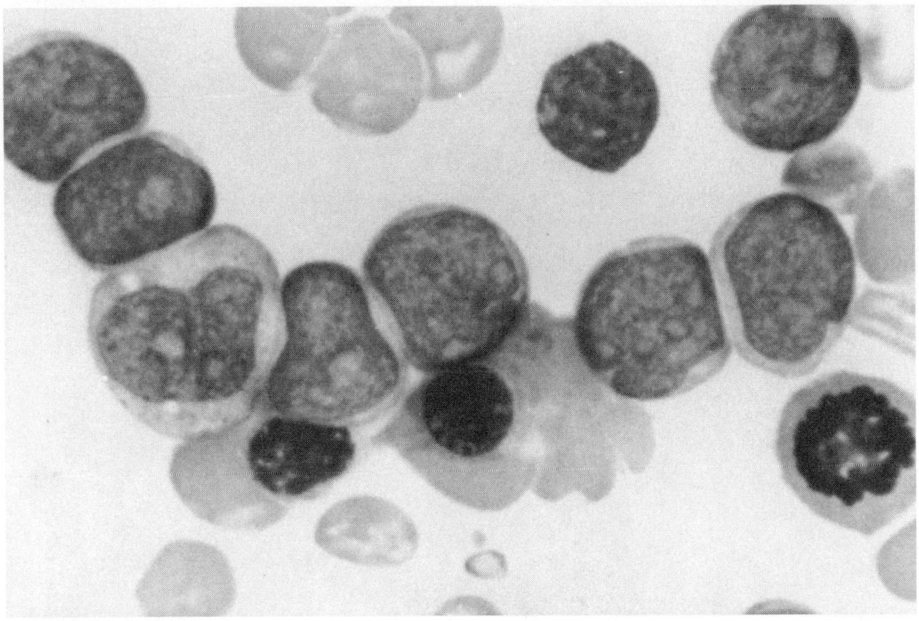

FIG. 47.55. Bone marrow smear from a man who has an M2 acute myeloid leukemia related to treatment for Hodgkin's disease (Wright-Giemsa stain, original magnification: 400× magnification). See Color Plate 68, between pp. 1446–1447.

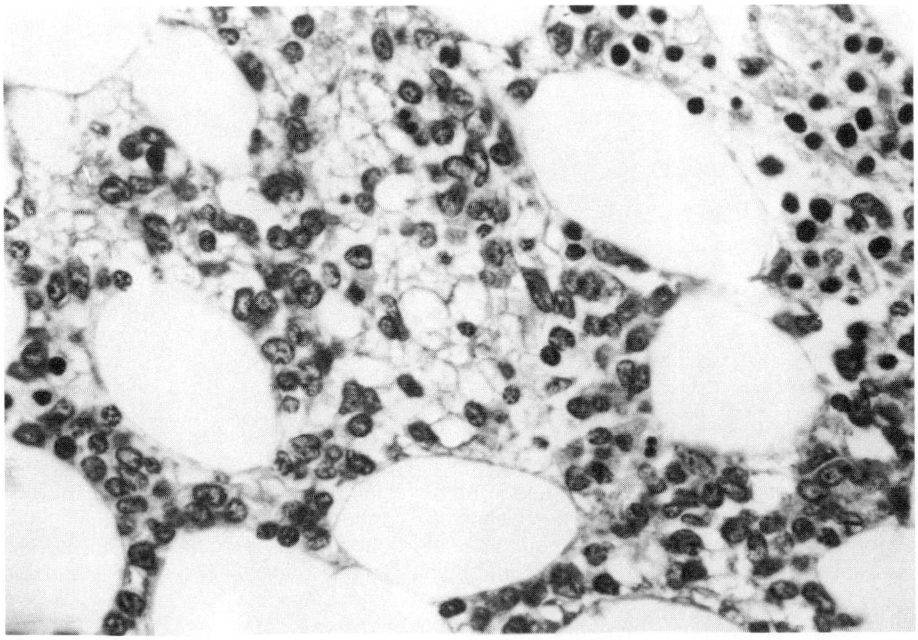

FIG. 47.56. Bone marrow biopsy specimen from a patient who has therapy-related acute myeloid leukemia. Numerous blasts are present. Red cell precursors are present in the upper right quadrant. There is abundant fat, and the interstitium is partially hypocellular (hematoxylin and eosin stain, original magnification: 160× magnification).

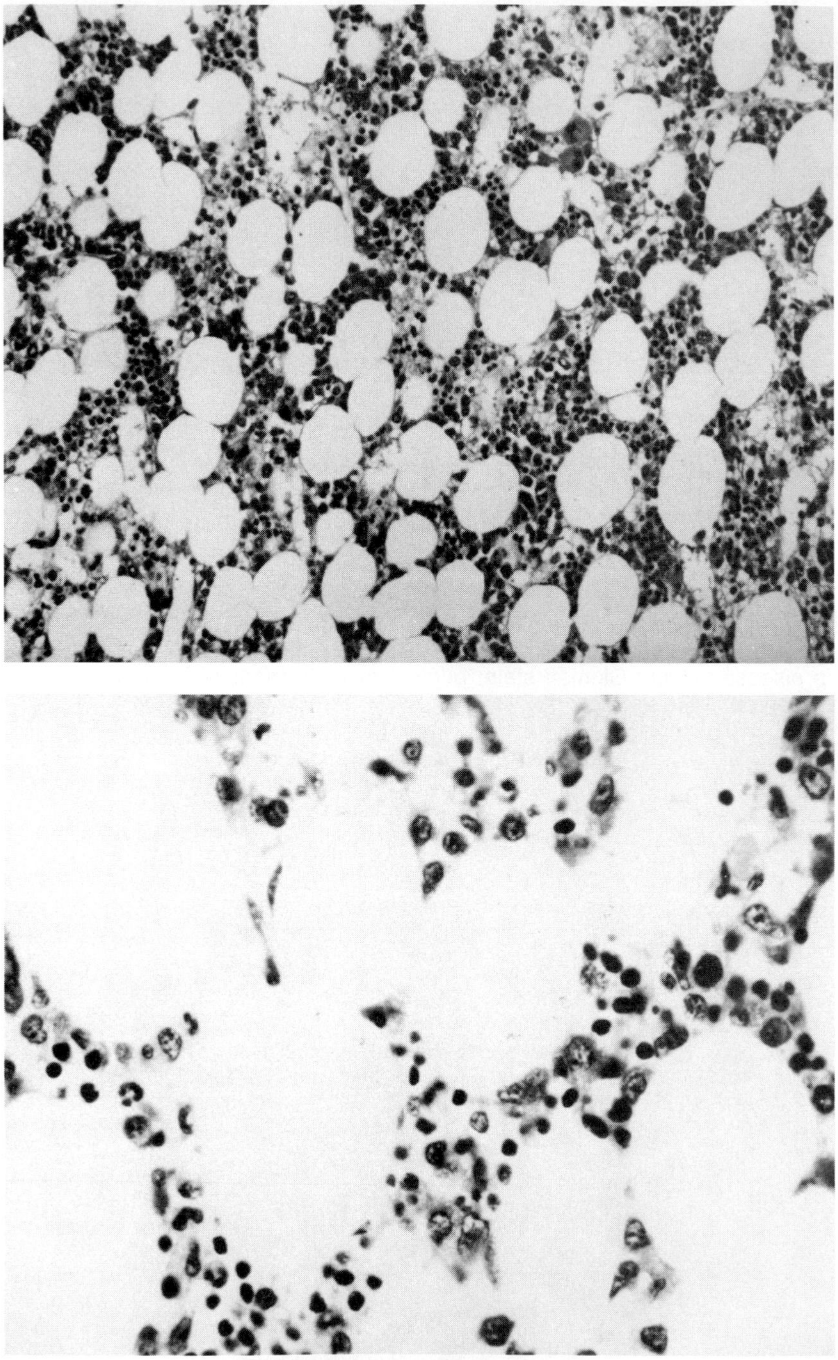

A

B

FIG. 47.57. A: Bone marrow biopsy obtained from a 57-year-old man who has slight pancytopenia; the patient had been treated for Hodgkin's disease 5 years previous. The marrow essentially is normocellular (hematoxylin and eosin stain, original magnification: 40× magnification). **B:** High-magnification view of the specimen in **A** showing normal maturation of neutrophil and erythrocyte precursors. There is no increase in blasts (hematoxylin and eosin stain, original magnification: 256× magnification).

A

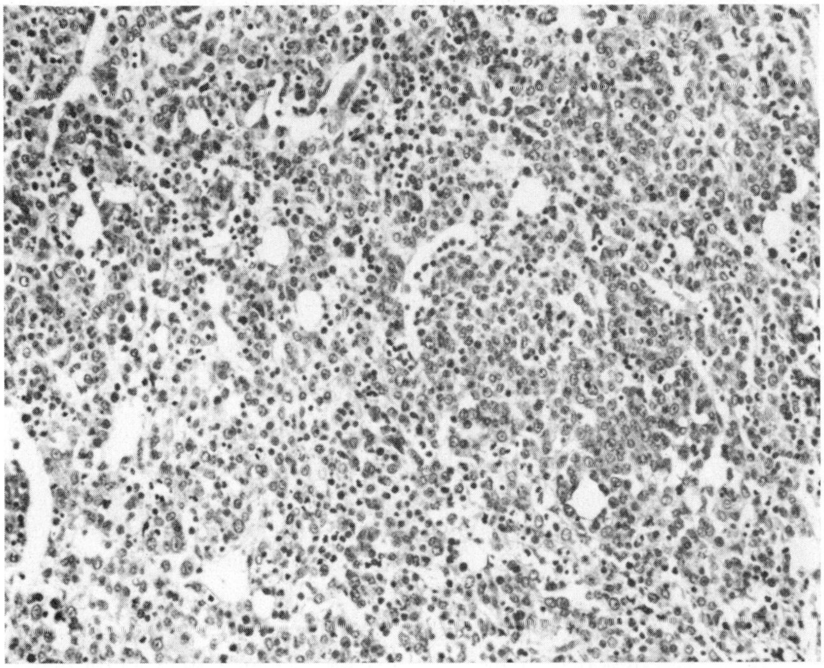

B

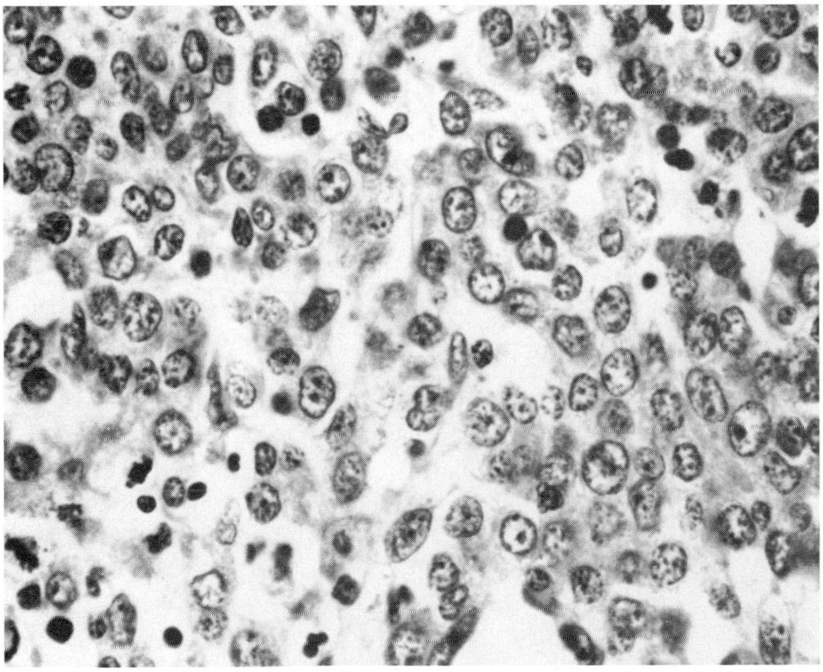

FIG. 47.58. A: Bone marrow biopsy from the same patient as in Figure 47.57, obtained 2 months later, showing a markedly hypercellular marrow (hematoxylin and eosin stain, original magnification: 40× magnification). **B:** High-magnification view of the specimen in **A** showing a high percentage of blasts and promyelocytes. A diagnosis of therapy-related acute myeloid leukemia was established from this specimen (hematoxylin and eosin stain, original magnification: 256× magnification).

than 100×10^9 per liter, and the total neutrophil count more than 1.5×10^9 per liter. A low hemoglobin concentration is acceptable for a remission classification if the other criteria are present. There should be no blasts in the blood, and Auer rods should not be found. The findings should be present for a period of at least 4 weeks. Complete remission is the only response classification that should be used in phase III clinical trials.

Partial remission includes all of the criteria for complete remission, except that the marrow contains 5% to 25% blasts or less than 5% blasts with Auer rods or myeloid cells with abnormalities unrelated to chemotherapy. The classification of partial remission is generally applicable only to patients in phase I or II clinical trials. Occasionally, after treatment, patients who have AML have a normal number of myeloblasts in the marrow, normal platelet and neutrophil counts, normal hemoglobin, and a rare myeloblast in the blood smear. These patients should be classified as essentially in complete remission, with a notation of the reason for the qualification.

It is unusual in AML following chemotherapy to have discrepancies in the number of myeloblasts between smears and biopsy sections. Occasionally, because of poor aspirate sample or other reasons, the smears may show fewer than 5% myeloblasts, and foci of blasts are present in trephine biopsy sections. In these instances, repeat aspirations should be performed at a site removed from the earlier aspiration.

The use of antimetabolites, cytosine arabinoside and 6-thioguanine, in the major treatment protocols for AML results in megaloblastic alterations that may make the interpretation of some posttherapy marrow specimens difficult; this may relate particularly to cases of erythroleukemia that usually are characterized by megaloblastic changes in the erythroid cells (142). The blast percentage and evidence of normal marrow regeneration are helpful features in assessing remission status in these cases. The use of antibiotics in the treatment period may lead to agranulocytosis that is characterized by persistent neutropenia and increased numbers of promyelocytes in the marrow specimen. The promyelocytes in these cases usually have abundant azurophilic granules and are distinguishable from type II myeloblasts.

The use of growth factors in the postchemotherapy period results in changes in neutrophil proliferation and maturation that may cause difficulty in assessing the status of the leukemic process (143). The early effects of both granulocyte and granulocyte-monocyte colony-stimulating factors are reflected by proliferation of neutrophils at the threshold of the promyelocyte–myelocyte stage of maturation; these cells have increased azurophilic granulation. The number of blasts in the marrow is generally in the normal range. Blasts may be present in the blood, usually not exceeding 2% to 3%. In a rare patient without any history of AML, up to 10% blasts may be observed in the blood following growth factor therapy. In a patient with a history of acute leukemia, 10% blasts in the blood following chemotherapy and growth factor therapy is a problem. If a distinction cannot be made between growth factor effect and residual or relapsed leukemia, and a decision on additional therapy is pending, it may be necessary to withdraw growth factor therapy to resolve the issue.

Relapse of AML following complete remission is recognized by the presence of more than 5% blasts in the marrow specimen, detection of Auer rods, or the presence of myeloblasts in the blood smear. If uncertainty exists as to relapse, a repeat marrow aspiration should be performed 1 to 2 weeks later.

CYTOGENETICS

Cytogenetic studies now are viewed as an integral part of most acute leukemia protocols. The impact of these studies relates primarily to two factors: the relationship of specific chromosome abnormalities to morphologic classification, and prognostic significance (13,14,144,145). These relationships are discussed in detail in Chapter 10. In addition, cytogenetic studies may be used to detect evidence of residual leukemia after chemotherapy or recurrent leukemia after a period of remission.

As additional studies of cytogenetic findings in AML are reported, it is becoming apparent that some chromosome abnormalities have an association with well-defined morphologic classifications and biologic course. Other abnormalities appear to be more common in subgroups of morphologically related types of leukemia but lack specificity. The most consistent relation between a chromosome abnormality and morphology is the translocation t(15;17), which appears to be exclusive to APL. Similarly, inv(16) or t(16;16) has a high but not exclusive association with acute myelomonocytic leukemia with increased and abnormal marrow eosinophils.

Table 47.5 lists the nonrandom chromosome abnormalities that have been reported most frequently in *de novo* AML, the frequency of the abnormalities, and the FAB types with which the abnormalities are associated.

Table 47.6 summarizes prognostic categories of AML according to cytogenetic findings. The cytogenetic categories listed are those for which sufficient data are available to suggest a relationship (see Chapter 10).

TABLE 47.5. *Association of nonrandom chromosome abnormalities with French–American–British classification in* de novo *acute myeloid leukemia (144, 145)*

Subgroups	Chromosome abnormality	Frequency, %
M3	t (15;17)(q22;q11–12)	90–100
M4Eo	inv(16)(p13;q22) or t(16;16)(p13;q22)	100
M2	t(8;21)(q22;q22)	18–20
M1,M2	t(9;22)(q34;q11)	8
M1,M2,M4,M5,M6	+8	9
M2,M4,M5	t(V;11)(V;q23)	9
M1,M2,M4	t(6;9)(p23;q34)	2
M1,M2,M4,M6B	inv(3)(q21;q26) or t(3;3)(q21;q26)	2
M1,M2,M4,M6,M7	−7 or del(7q)	9
M1,M2,M4,M6,M7	−5 or del(5q)	6
M1,M2,M4,M5,M6,M7	Complex defects	14

V, various partner chromosomes.

TABLE 47.6. *Prognostic implications of cytogenetic abnormalities in acute myeloid leukemia*

Chromosome findings	Prognostic significance
t(8;21), t(15;17), inv 16	Favorable
normal, +8, 11q23, +21, del(7q) del(9q), +22	Intermediate
complex, −7, abnormal 3, del(5q−), −5	Unfavorable

From Grimwade D, Walker H, Oliver F, et al. The importance of diagnostic cytogenetics on outcome in AML: analysis of 1,612 patients entered into the MRC AML10 trial. Blood 1998;92:2322–2333, with permission.

IMMUNOLOGIC MARKERS IN ACUTE MYELOID LEUKEMIA

Although the FAB classification for most types of AML is based primarily on the morphologic and cytochemical characteristics of the blast population, in two types, minimally differentiated AML (M0) and acute megakaryoblastic leukemia (M7), the diagnosis is established with immunologic markers or electron microscopic studies; in the very poorly differentiated cases of M6B AML, immunologic markers may be necessary to establish cell lineage (4,9,82, 84,85).

In M0 and M7 AML, the blasts are nonreactive for MPO and SBB. The presence of myeloid-related antigen CD13, CD14, or CD33 and the absence of lymphoid markers is evidence of myeloid differentiation. The expression of CD41 (gpIIb/IIIa) or CD61 (gpIIIa) is relatively specific for megakaryocytic differentiation (8,9). The other subclasses of AML (M1–6) also have been characterized immunophenotypically (9) (Table 47.7). Surface antigens HLA-DR and CD14 have been found most commonly in myelomonocytic and monocytic leukemias (M4 and M5 AML), followed in frequency by M1 and M2 AML. The abnormal promyelocytes in APL (M3 AML) do not express CD14 and express HLA-DR only infrequently; CD13 and 33 are expressed commonly in M1 through M5 AML. Because the relative proportion of erythroblasts and myeloblasts may vary substantially in AML M6A, the marker results may show considerable variation; however, the erythroblasts are nonreactive with most panmyeloid antibodies but express glycophorin A and frequently CD36.

Expression of the neural cell adhesion molecule CD56 has been reported in a range of AMLs, myelodysplastic syndromes, and blast crises of chronic myeloid leukemia (146,147). The patients with CD56-positive AML have ranged from those with some cytologic features suggestive of APL to a group with lymphoblast-like features and prominent extramedullay involvement (116).

The reported correlations between myeloid-related antigen expression and FAB classifications are not absolute; the distinct morphologic and cytochemical features, if unequivocal, are definitive in subclassifying AML (see Chapters 3 and 38).

TERMINAL DEOXYNUCLEOTIDYL TRANSFERASE

Terminal deoxynucleotidyl transferase is an enzyme that appears to participate in the determination of antigenic diversity of B- and T-cell antigen receptors at the time of somatic recombination and is a marker of early B- and T-cell differentiation. This enzyme normally is not present in myeloid cells and is useful but not definitive in distinguishing myeloblasts from precursor B- and T-cell lymphoblasts (9). The blasts in AML are generally negative for this enzyme; however, in cases associated with t(8;21) and inv(16), positive blasts may be noted (10–12). The percentage of positive blasts in these patients generally is lower than in those with acute lymphoblastic leukemia, in whom it is usually 90% or higher (see Chapter 3).

SUMMARY AND CONCLUSIONS

The basic requisite for a diagnosis of most forms of AML is the presence of at least 20% blasts in the bone marrow or peripheral blood; this number represents a reduction recommended in the WHO proposals for the classification of hematopoietic disorders. There are exceptions to this generalization: APL, acute monocytic leukemia, erythroleukemia, and acute megakaryoblastic leukemia. In these instances, the diagnosis is based on the percentage of blasts and other imma-

TABLE 47.7. *Immunophenotype of acute myeloid leukemia by French–American–British subgroup*

Surface antigens	M0	M1/M2	M3	M4/M5	M6	M7
HLA-DR	+	+	−	++	−	+
CD11	+	+	+	++	−	−
CD13	I	+	+	++	−	−
CD14	+	+	−	++	−	−
CD33	+	++	+	++	+	+
CD41/61	−	−	−	−	−	++
Glycophorin A	−	−	−	−	++	−

[a] Reactivity of the erythroblasts only. Modified from Bene MC, Castoldi G, Knapp W, et al. European group for the immunological characterization of leukaemias (EGIL); proposal for the immunological classification of acute leukaemias. Leukemia 1995;9:1783–1786, with permission.

ture cells characteristic of the process. Based on morphology, cytochemistry, immunologic, or ultrastructural studies, eight major types of AML are recognized: acute myeloblastic leukemia, minimally differentiated (M0); acute myeloblastic leukemia without maturation (M1); AML with maturation (M2); APL (M3); acute myelomonocytic leukemia (M4); acute monocytic leukemia (M5); erythroleukemia (M6); and acute megakaryoblastic leukemia (M7). A strong association between cytogenetic abnormalities and several of the morphologic types has been recognized, including the translocation t(15;17), which is highly specific for APL; t(8; 21), which is found in approximately 15% to 20% of patients with acute myelocytic leukemia with maturation; inv(16) in acute myelomonocytic leukemia with increased marrow eosinophils; and t(9;11) in acute monocytic leukemia.

REFERENCES

1. Brunning R. Proposed World Heath Organization (WHO) classification of acute leukemia and myelodysplastic syndromes. *Mod Pathol* 1999;12:102.
2. Bennett JM, Catovsky D, Daniel MT, et al. Proposals for the classification of the acute leukaemias. *Br J Haematol* 1976;33:451–458.
3. Bennett JM, Catovsky D, Daniel MT, et al. Proposed revised criteria for the classification of acute myeloid leukemia: a report of the French-American-British cooperative group. *Ann Intern Med* 1985;103: 626–629.
4. Bennett JM, Catovsky D, Daniel MT, et al. Criteria for the diagnosis of acute leukemia of megakaryocytic lineage (M7): a report of the French-American-British cooperative group. *Ann Intern Med* 1985; 103:460–462.
5. Cheson BD, Cassileth PA, Head DR, et al. Report of the National Cancer Institute-sponsored workshop on definitions of diagnosis and response in acute myeloid leukemia. *JClin Oncol* 1990;8:813–819.
6. Gahn B, Unterhalt M, Drescher M, et al. De novo AML with dysplastic hematopoiesis: cytogenetic and prognostic significance. *Leukemia* 1996;10:946–95.
7. Head DR. Revised classification of acute myeloid leukemia. *Leukemia* 1996;10:1826–1831.
8. Brunning R, McKenna RW. *Tumors of the bone marrow*, 3rd series, fasc. 9. Washington, DC: Armed Forces Institute of Pathology, 1994; 19–100.
9. Bene MC, Castoldi G, Knapp W, et al. European group for the immunological characterization of leukaemias (EGIL): proposals for the immunological classification of acute leukaemias. *Leukemia* 1995;9: 1783–1786.
10. Yunis J, Brunning RD, Howe RB, et al. High resolution chromosomes as an independent prognostic indicator in adult acute nonlymphocytic leukemia. *N Engl J Med* 1984;311:812–818.
11. Bitter MA, Le Beau MM, Rowley JD, et al. Associations between morphology, karyotype, and clinical features in myeloid leukemias. *Hum Pathol* 1987;18:211–225.
12. Berger R, Bernheim A, Daniel MT, et al. Cytologic characterization and significance of normal karyotypes in t(8;21) acute myeloblastic leukemia. *Blood* 1982;59:171–178.
13. Grimwade D, Walker H, Oliver F, et al. The importance of diagnostic cytogenetics on outcome in AML: analysis of 1,612 patients entered into the MRC AML10 trial. *Blood* 1998;92:2322–2333.
14. Krzysztof M, Heinonen K, de la Chapalle A, et al. Clinical significance of cytogenetics in acute myeloid leukemia. *Semin Oncol* 1997;24: 17–31.
15. Ackerman GA. Microscopic and histochemical studies on the Auer bodies in leukemic cells. *Blood* 1950;5:847–863.
16. Buccheri V, Shetty V, Yoshida A, et al. The role of an anti-myeloperoxidase antibody in the diagnosis and classification of acute leukaemia: a comparison with light and electron microscopy, cytochemistry. *Br J Haematol* 1992;80:489–498.
17. Bollum FJ. Terminal deoxynucleotidyl transferase as a hematopoietic cell marker. *Blood* 1979;54:1203–1215.
18. Bradstock KF, Hoffbrand AV, Ganeshaguru K, et al. Terminal deoxynucleotidyl transferase expression in acute nonlymphoid leukaemia: an analysis by immunofluorescence. *Br J Haematol* 1981;47: 133–143.
19. Parreira A, PombodeOliveira MS, Matutes E, et al. Terminal deoxynucleotidyl transferase positive acute myeloid leukaemia: an association with immature myeloblastic leukaemia. *Br J Haematol* 1988;69: 219–224.
20. Schachner J, Kantarjian H, Dalton W, et al. Cytogenetic association and prognostic significance of bone marrow blast cell terminal transferase in patients with acute myeloblastic leukemia. *Leukemia* 1988; 2:667–671.
21. Rumke CL. Variability of results in differential counts on blood smears. *Triangle* 1960;4:154–158.
22. Lee EJ, Pollack A, Leavitt RD, et al. Minimally differentiated acute nonlymphocytic leukemia: a distinct entity. *Blood* 1987;70: 1400–1406.
23. Cuneo A, Ferrant A, Michaux JL, et al. Cytogenetic profile of minimally differentiated (FAB-MO) acute myeloid leukemia: correlation with clinicobiologic findings. *Blood* 1995;85:3688–3694.
24. Campos L, Guyotat D, Archimbaud E, et al. Surface marker expression in adult acute myeloid leukaemia: correlations with initial characteristics, morphology and response to therapy. *Br J Haematol* 1989; 72:161–166.
25. Venditti A, Del Peoeta G, Stasi R, et al. Minimally differentiated acute myeloid leukemia (AML-M0): cytochemical, immunophenotypic and cytogenetic analysis of 19 cases. *Br J Haematol* 1994;88:784–793.
26. Borowitz MJ, Gockerman JP, Moore JO, et al. Clinicopathologic and cytogenetic features of CD34 (My10)-positive acute nonlymphocytic leukemia. *Am J Clin Pathol* 1988;91:265–270.
27. Bernstein R, Pinto MR, Behr A, et al. Chromosome 3 abnormalities in acute nonlymphocytic leukemia (ANLL) with abnormal thrombopoiesis: report of three patients with a ''new'' inversion anomaly and a further case of homologous translocation. *Blood* 1982;60:613–617.
28. Bitter MA, Neilly ME, LeBeau MM, et al. Rearrangements of chromosome 3 involving bands 3q21 and 3q26 are associated with normal or elevated platelet counts in acute nonlymphocytic leukemia. *Blood* 1985;60:1362–1370.
29. Fonatsch C, Gudat H, Langfelder E, et al. Correlation of cytogenetic findings with clinical features in 18 patients with in(3)(q21;q26) or t(3;3)(q21;q26). *Leukemia* 1994;8:1318–1326.
30. Nakamura H, Kurigama K, Sadamori N, et al. Morphological subtyping of acute myeloid leukemia with maturation (AML-M2): homogenous pink-colored cytoplasm of mature neutrophils is most characteristic of AML-M2 with t (8;21). *Leukemia* 1997;11:651–655.
31. Galvani DW, Banghar P, Mekawi L. Early identification of M2 AML with the t(8;21) translocation plus myelodysplastic features. *Leuk Res* 1995;19:145.
32. Second International Workshop on Chromosomes in Leukemia: Cytogenetic, morphologic, and clinical correlations in acute nonlymphocytic leukemia with t(8;21q+). *Cancer Genet Cytogenet* 1980;2: 99–102.
33. Andrieu V, Radford-Weiss I, Troussard X, et al. Molecular detection of t(8;21)/AML-ETO in AML M1/M2: correlation with cytogenetics, morphology and immunophenotype. *Br J Haematol* 1995;92: 855–865.
34. Erickson P, Gao J, Chang KS, et al. Identification of breakpoints in t(8; 21) acute myelogenous leukemia and isolation of a fusion transcript, AML1/ETO, with similarity to drosophilia segmentation gene, runt. *Blood* 1992;80:1825–1831.
35. Nucifora G, Dickstein JI, Torbenson V, et al. Correlation between cell morphology and expression of the AML1/ETO chimeric transcript in patients with acute myeloid leukemia with the t(8;21). *Leukemia* 1994;8:1533–1538.
36. Paietta E, Wiernik PH, Andersen J. Eastern Cooperative Oncology Group. Immunophenotypic features of the t(8;21)(q22;q22) acute leukemia in adults. *Blood* 1993;81:1975.
37. Pedersen-Bjergaard J, Philip P. Two different classes of therapy related and de novo acute leukemia? *Cancer Genet Cytogenet* 1991;55: 119–124.
38. Quesnel B, Kantarjian H, Bjefgaard JP, et al. Therapy-related acute

myeloid leukemia with t(8;21), inv(16), and t(8;16): a report of 25 cases and review of the literature. *J Clin Oncol* 1993;12:2370–2379.
39. Xue Y, Yu F, Zhou Z, et al. Translocation (8;21) in oligoblastic leukemia: is this a true myelodysplastic syndrome? *Leukemia* 1994;8: 1780–1784.
40. Caligiuri MA, Strout MP, Gilliland DG. Molecular biology of acute myeloid leukemia. *Semin Oncol* 1997;24:92–102.
41. Haferlach T, Bennett JM, Loffler H, et al. Acute myeloid leukemia with translocation (8;21): cytomorphology, dysplasia and prognostic factors in 41 cases. *Leuk Lymphoma* 1996;23:227–234.
42. Byrd JC, Edenfield J, Shields DJ, et al. Extramedullary myeloid cell tumors in acute non-lymphocytic leukemia: a clinical review. *J Clin Oncol* 1995;13:1800–1816.
43. Hurwitz CA, Raimondi SC, Head D, et al. Distinctive immunophenotypic features of t(8;21)(q22;q22) acute myeloblastic leukemia in children. *Blood* 1992;80:3182–3188.
44. Kita K, Nakase K, Masuya M, et al. Phenotypical characteristics of acute myelomonocytic leukemia with the t(8;21)(q22;q22) chromosomal abnormality: frequent expression of immature B-cell antigen CD19 together with stem cell antigen CD34. *Blood* 1992;80:470–477.
45. Dusenbery KB, Howells WB, Arthur DC, et al. Extramedullary leukemia (EML) in pediatric patients with newly diagnosed acute myeloid leukemia: a report from the Children's Cancer Group. (*in press*).
46. Byrd JC, Weiss RC, Arthur DC, et al. Extramedullary leukemia adversely affects hematologic complete remission rate and overall survival in patients with t(8;21) (q22;q22): results from Cancer and Leukemia Group B 8461. *J Clin Oncol* 1997;15:466–475.
47. Cuneo A, Kerim S, Vandenberghe E, et al. Translocation t(6;9) occurring in acute myofibrosis myelodysplastic syndrome, and acute nonlymphocytic leukemia suggests multipotent stem cell involvement. *Cancer Genet Cytogenet* 1989;54:209–219.
48. Soekarman D, von Lindern M, Daenen S, et al. The translocation (6; 9) (p23; q34) shows consistent rearrangement of two genes and defines a myeloproliferative disorder with specific clinical features. *Blood* 1992;79:2990–2997.
49. Lillington DM, MacCallum PK, Lister TA, et al. Translocation t(6; 9) (p23; q34) in acute myeloid leukemia without myelodysplasia or basophilia: two cases and a review of the literature. *Leukemia* 1993; 7:527–531.
50. Alsabeh R, Brynes RK, Slovak ML, et al. Acute myeloid leukemia with the t (6;9)(p23;q34): association with myelodysplasia, basophilia, and initial CD34 negative immunophenotype. *Am J Clin Pathol* 1997; 107:430–437.
51. McKenna RW, Parkin J, Bloomfield CD, et al. Acute promyelocytic leukaemia: a study of 39 cases with identification of a hyperbasophilic microgranular variant. *Br J Haematol* 1982;50:201–214.
52. Castoldi GL, Liso V, Speccjia G, et al. Acute promyelocytic leukemia: morphological aspects. *Leukemia* 1994;8(Suppl 2):S27–S32.
53. Stanley M, McKenna RW, Ellinger G, et al. Classification of 358 cases of acute myeloid leukemia by FAB criteria: analysis of clinical and morphologic features. In Bloomfield CD, ed. *Chronic and acute leukemias in adults.* Boston: Martinus Nijhoff Publishers, 1985: 147–174.
54. Breton-Gorius J, Houssay D. Auer bodies in acute promyelocytic leukemia: demonstration of their fine structure and peroxidase localization. *Lab Invest* 1973;28:135–141.
55. Tomonaga M, Yoshida Y, Tagawa M, et al. Cytochemistry of acute promyelocytic leukemia (M3): leukemic promyelocytes exhibit heterogenous patterns in cellular differentiation. *Blood* 1985;66:350–357.
56. Davey FR, Davis RB, MacCallum JM, et al. Cancer and leukemia group B, Brookline, Massachusetts: morphologic and cytochemical characteristics of acute promyelocytic leukemia. *Am J Hematol* 1989; 30:221–227.
57. Golomb HM, Rowley J, Vardimann J, et al. ''Microgranular'' acute promyelocytic leukemia: a distinct clinical, ultrastructural, and cytogenetic entity. *Blood* 1980;55:253–259.
58. Raimondi SC, Kalwinsky DK, Hayashi Y, et al. Cytogenetics of childhood acute nonlymphocytic leukemia. *Cancer Genet Cytogenet* 1989; 40:13–27.
59. Karp J, Smith MA. The molecular pathogenesis of treatment-induced (secondary) leukemias: foundations for treatment and prevention. *Semin Oncol* 1997;24:103–113.
60. Fenaux P, Chomienne C, Degus L. Acute promyelocytic leukemia: biology and treatment. *Semin Oncol* 1997;24:92–102.
61. Falini B, Flenghi L, Fagioli M, et al. Immunocytochemical diagnosis of acute promyelocytic leukemia (M3) with the monoclonal antibody PG-M3 (Anti-PML). *Blood* 1997;90:4046–4053.
62. Licht JD, Chomienne C, Goy A, et al. Clinical and molecular characteristics of a rare syndrome of acute promyelocytic leukemia associated with translocation (11;17). *Blood* 1995;85:1083–1094.
63. Redner RL, Rush BA, Faas, S, et al. The t(5;17) variant of acute promyelocytic leukemia expresses a nucleophosphinretinoic acid receptor fusion. *Blood* 1996;87:882–886.
64. Tallman MS, Kwaan HC. Assessing the hemostatic disorder associated with acute promyelocytic leukemia. *Blood* 1992;79:543–553.
65. McKenna RW, Bloomfield CD, Dick F, et al. Acute monoblastic leukemia: diagnosis and treatment of ten cases. *Blood* 1975;46: 481–494.
66. Peterson L, Dehner LP, Brunning RD. Extramedullary masses as presenting features of acute monoblastic leukemia. *Am J Clin Pathol* 1981;75:140–148.
67. Ridge SA, Wiedemann LM. Chromosome 11q23 abnormalities in leukaemia. *Leuk Lymphoma* 1994;14:11–17.
68. Mirchandani I, Tabaczka P, Palutke M. Acute monocytic leukemia: a surface marker study. *Am J Hematol* 1982;12:139–147.
69. Lai JL, Zandecki M, Joulet JP, et al. Three cases of translocation (8; 16) (p11; p13) observed in acute myelomonocytic leukemia: a new specific group? *Cancer Genet Cytogent* 1987;27:101–109.
70. Hanslip JI, Swansbury R, Pinkerton R, et al. The translocation t(8; 16)(p11;p13) defines an AML subtype with distinct cytology and clinical features. *Leuk Lymphoma* 1992;6:479–486.
71. Heim S, Avanzi G, Billstrom R, et al. A new chromosomal rearrangement (t8;16)(p11;p13) in acute monocytic leukemia. *Br J Haematol* 1987;66:323–326.
72. Bertheas MF, Jaubert J, Vasselon C, et al. A complex t(3;8;17) involving breakpoint 8p11 in a case of M5 acute non-lymphoblastic leukemia with erythrophagocytosis. *Cancer Genet Cytogenet* 1989;2:62–73.
73. Arthur DC, Bloomfield CD. Partial deletion of long arm of chromosome 16 and bone marrow eosinophilia in acute nonlymphocytic leukemia: a new association. *Blood* 1983;61:994–998.
74. LeBeau MM, Larson RA, Bitter MA, et al. Association of an inversion of chromosome 16 with abnormal marrow eosinophils in acute myelomonocytic leukemia: a unique cytogenetic-clinicopathological association. *N Engl J Med* 1983;309:630–636.
75. Glass JP, Van Tassel P, Keating MJ, et al. Central nervous system complications of a newly recognized subtype of leukemia: AMML with a pericentric inversion of chromosome 16. *Neurology* 1987;37: 639–644.
76. Larson RA, Williams SF, LeBeau MM, et al. Acute myelomonocytic leukemia with abnormal eosinophils and inv(16) or t(16;16) has a favorable prognosis. *Blood* 1986;68:1242–1249.
77. Bitter MA, LeBeau MM, Larson RA, et al. A morphologic and cytochemical study of acute myelomonocytic leukemia with abnormal marrow eosinophils associated with inv(16)(p13;q22). *Am J Clin Pathol* 1984;81:733–741.
78. Garand R, Duchayne E, Blanchard D, et al. Minimally differentiated erythroleukemia (AML M6 ''variant''): a rare subset of AML distinct from AML M6. *Br J Haematol* 1995;90:868–875.
79. Olopade OI, Thangavelu M, Larson RA, et al. Clinical, morphologic and cytogenetic characteristics of 26 patients with acute erythroblastic leukemia. *Blood* 1992;80:2873–2882.
80. Mazella FM, Kowal-Vern A, Shrit A, et al. Acute erythroleukemia: evaluation of 48 cases with reference to classification proliferation, cytogenetics and prognosis. *Am J Clin Pathol* 1998;110:590–598.
81. Villeval JL, Cramer P, Lemoine F, et al. Phenotype of early erythroblastic leukemias. *Blood* 1986;68:1167–1174.
82. Koike T, Aoki S, Maruyama S, et al. Cell surface phenotyping of megakaryoblasts. *Blood* 1987;69:957–960.
83. Matsuo T, Bennett JM. Acute leukemia of megakaryocytic lineage (M7). *Cancer Genet Cytogenet* 1988;34:1–3.
84. Erber WN, Breton-Gorius J, Villeval JL, et al. Detection of cells of megakaryocyte lineage in haematological malignancies by immunoalkaline phosphatase labeling cell smears with a panel of monoclonal antibodies. *Br J Haematol* 1987;65:87–94.
85. Chuang S-S, Li C-Y. Useful panel of antibodies for the classification of acute leukemia by immunohistochemical methods in bone marrow trephine biopsy specimens. *Am J Clin Pathol* 1977;107:410–418.
86. Breton-Gorius J, Villeval JL, Mitjavila MT, et al. Ultrastructural and

cytochemical characterization of blasts from early erythroblastic leukemias. *Leukemia* 1987;1:173–181.

87. Carroll A, Civin C, Schneider N, et al. The t(1;22)(p13;q13) is nonrandom and restricted to infants with acute megakaryoblastic leukemia: a pediatric oncology group study. *Blood* 1990;76:1704–1709.
88. Lion T, Haas OA, Harbott J, et al. The translocation t(1;22)(p13;q13) is a non random marker specifically associated with acute megakaryocytic leukemia in young children. *Blood* 1992;79:3325–3330.
89. Stiller CA, Kinnier-Wilson LM. Down syndrome and leukemia. *Lancet* 1981;ii:695.
90. Kaneko Y, Rowley JD, Variakojis D, et al. Chromosome abnormalities in Down's syndrome patients with acute leukemia. *Blood* 1981; 58:459–466.
91. Hayashi Y, Eguchi M, Sugita K, et al. Cytogenetic findings and clinical features in acute leukemia and transient myeloproliferative disorder in Down's syndrome. *Blood* 1988;72:15–23.
92. Litz CE, Davies S, Brunning RD, et al. Acute leukemia and the transient myeloproliferative disorder associated with Down syndrome: morphologic, immunophenotypic and cytogenetic manifestations. *Leukemia* 1995;9:1432–1439.
93. Kojima S, Matsuyama T, Sato T, et al. Down's syndrome and acute leukemia in children: an analysis of phenotype by use of monoclonal antibodies and electron microscopic platelet peroxidase reaction. *Blood* 1990;76:2348–2353.
94. Debili N, Kieffer N, Mitjavila MT, et al. Expression of platelet glycoproteins by erythroid blasts in four cases of trisomy 21. *Leukemia* 1989;3:669–678.
95. Yumura-Yagi K, Hara J, Tawa A, et al. Phenotypic characteristics of acute megakaryocytic leukemia and transient abnormal myelopoiesis. *Leuk Lymphoma* 1994;13:393–400.
96. Creutzig U, Ritter J, Vormoor J, et al. Acute myelogenous leukemia in Down's syndrome. *Leukemia* 1996;10:1677–1686.
97. Zipursky A, Thorner P, DeHarven E, et al. Myelodysplasia and acute megakaryoblastic leukemia in Down syndrome. *Leuk Res* 1994;18: 163–171.
98. Peterson LC, Parkin JL, Arthur DC, et al. Acute basophilic leukemia: a clinical, morphologic, and cytogenetic study of eight cases. *Am J Clin Pathol* 1991;96:160–170.
99. Wick MR, CY LI, Pierre RV. Acute nonlymphocytic leukemia with basophilic differentiation. *Blood* 1982;60:38–45.
100. Jennings CV, Dannaher CL, Yam LT. Basophilic leukemia. *South Med J* 1980;73:934–936.
101. Horny HP, Menke DM, Valent P. Criteria for the classification of myelogenous tumors with basophilic differentiation. *Mod Pathol* 1999;139A.
102. Youman JD, Taddeini L, Cooper T. Histamine excess symptoms in basophilic chronic granulocytic leukemia. *Arch Intern Med* 1973;131: 560–562.
103. Rosenthal S, Schwarz JH, Canellos GP. Basophilic chronic granulocytic leukaemia with hyperhistaminaemia. *Br J Haematol* 1977;36: 367–372.
104. Howe RB, Bloomfield CD, McKenna RW. Hypocellular acute leukemia. *Am J Med* 1982;72:391–395.
105. Berdeaux DH, Glasser L, Serokmann R, et al. Hypoplastic acute leukemia: review of 70 cases with multivariate regression analysis. *Hematol Oncol* 1986;4:291–305.
106. Bearman RM, Gerassimas A, Panglis A, et al. Acute (malignant) myelosclerosis. *Cancer* 1979;43:279–293.
107. Hruban RH, Kuhajda FP, Mann RB. Acute myelofibrosis. Immunohistochemical study of four cases and comparison with acute megakaryoblastic leukemia. *Am J Clin Pathol* 1987;88:578–588.
108. Sultan C, Sigaux F, Imbert M, et al. Acute myelodysplasia with myelofibrosis: a report of eight cases. *Br J Haematol* 1981;49:11–16.
109. Bain B, Catovsky D, O'Brien M, et al. Megakaryoblastic leukemia presenting as acute myelofibrosis: a study of four cases with the platelet-peroxidase reaction. *Blood* 1981;58:206–213.
110. King A. A case of chloroma. *Monthly J Med* 1853;17:97.
111. Meis JM, Butler JJ, Osborne BM, et al. Granulocytic sarcoma in nonleukemic patients. *Cancer* 1986;58:2697–2709.
112. Neiman RS, Barcos M, Berard C, et al. Granulocytic sarcoma: clinicopathologic study of 61 biopsied cases. *Cancer* 1981;48:1426–1437.
113. Wiernik PH, Serpick AA. Granulocytic sarcoma (chloroma). *Blood* 1970;35:361–369.
114. Liu PI, Ishimaru T, McGregor DH, et al. Autopsy tudy of granulocytic sarcoma (chloroma) in patients with yelogenous leukemia, Hiroshima-Nagasaki 1949-1969. *Cancer* 1973;31:948–955.
115. Hudock J, Chatten J, Miettinen M. Immunohistochemical evaluation of myeloid leukemia infiltrates (granulocytic sarcomas) in formaldehyde-fixed, paraffin-embedded tissue. *Am J Clin Pathol* 1994;102: 55–60.
116. Suzuki R, Yamamoto K, Seto M, et al. CD7 + and CD56 + myeloid/natural killer cell precursor acute leukemia: a distinct hematolymphoid disease entity. *Blood* 1997;90:2417–2428.
117. Inhorn RC, Aster JC, Roach SA, et al. A syndrome of lymphoblastic lymphoma, eosinophilia, and myeloid hyperplasia/malignancy associated with a t(8;13)(p11;q11): description of a distinctive clinicopathologic entity. *Blood* 1995;85:1881–1887.
118. Aguiar RCT, Chase A, Coulthard S, et al. Abnormalities of chromosome 6 and 8p11 in leukemia: two clinical syndromes can be distinguished on the basis of MO2 involvement. *Blood* 1997;90:3130–3135.
119. Pui C-H, Reiling MV, Rivera GK, et al. Epipodophyllotoxin-related acute myeloid leukemia: a study of 35 cases. *Leukemia* 1995;9: 1990–1996.
120. Michels SD, McKenna RW, Arthur DC, et al. Therapy-related acute myeloid leukemia and myelodysplastic syndrome: a clinical and morphologic study of 65 cases. *Blood* 1985;65:1364–1372.
121. Kantarjian HM, Keating MJ. Therapy-related leukemia and myelodysplastic syndrome. *Semin Oncol* 1987;14:435–443.
122. Le Beau MM, Albain KS, Larson RA, et al. Clinical and cytogenetic correlations in 63 patients with therapy related myelodysplastic syndromes and acute nonlymphocytic leukemia: further evidence for characteristic abnormalities of chromosomes no. 5 and 7. *J Clin Oncol* 1986;4:325–345.
123. Foucar K, McKenna RW, Bloomfield CD, et al. Therapy-related leukemia, a panmyelosis. *Cancer* 1979;43:1285–1296.
124. Pedersen-Bjergaard J, Rowley J. The balanced and the unbalanced chromosome abberations of acute myeloid leukemia may develop in different ways and may contribute differently to malignant transformation. *Blood* 1994;83:2780–2786.
125. Pedersen-Bjergaard J, Preben P, Larsen SO, et al. Therapy-related myelodysplasia and acute myeloid leukemia: cytogenetic characteristics of 115 consecutive cases and risk in seven cohorts of patients treated intensively for malignant diseases in the Copenhagen series. *Leukemia* 1993;7:1975–1986.
126. Van Leeuwen Flora E. Risk of acute myelogenous leukemia and myelodysplasia following cancer treatment. *Baillieres Clin Haematol* 1996;9:57–85.
127. Pedersen-Bjergaard J, Pedersen M, Roulston D, et al. Different genetic pathways in leukemogenesis for patients presenting with therapy-related myelodysplasia and therapy-related acute myeloid leukemia. *Blood* 1995;85:3542–3552.
128. Ratain MJ, Kaminer LS, Bitran JD, et al. Acute nonlymphocytic leukemia following etoposide and cisplatin combination chemotherapy for advanced non-small-cell carcinoma of the lung. *Blood* 1987;70: 1412–1417.
129. Whitlock JA, Greer JP, Lukens JN. Epipodophyllotoxin-related leukemia: identification of a new subset of secondary leukemia. *Cancer* 1991;68:600–604.
130. Winick N, McKenna RW, Shaster JJ, et al. Secondary acute myeloid leukemia in children with acute lymphoblastic leukemia treated with etoposode. *J Clin Oncol* 1993;11:209–217.
131. Secker-Walker LM, Moorman AV, Bain BJ, et al. Secondary acute leukemia and myelodysplastic syndrome with 11q23 abnormalities. *Leukemia* 1998;12:840–844.
132. Tucker MA, Coleman CN, Cox RS, et al. Risk of second cancers after treatment for Hodgkin's disease. *N Engl J Med* 1988;318:76–81.
133. Blayney DW, Longo DL, Young RC, et al. Decreasing risk of leukemia with prolonged follow-up after chemotherapy and radiotherapy for Hodgkin's disease. *N Engl J Med* 1987;316:710–714.
134. Greene MH, Young RC, Merrill JM, et al. Evidence of a treatment dose response in acute nonlymphocytic leukemias which occur after therapy of non-Hodgkin's lymphoma. *Cancer Res* 1983;43: 1891–1898.
135. Ellis M, Ravid M, Lishner M: A comparative analysis of alkylating agent and epipodophyllotoxin-related leukemias. *Leuk Lymphoma* 1993;11:9–13.
136. Miller J, Arthur D, Litz C, et al. Myelodysplastic syndrome after

autologous bone marrow transplantation: an additional late complication of curative cancer therapy. *Blood* 1994;83:3780–3786.
137. Darrington D, Vose J, Anderson J, et al. Incidence and characterization of secondary myelodysplastic syndrome and acute myelogenous leukemia following high-dose chemotherapy and autologous stem-cell transplantation for lymphoid malignancies. *J Clin Oncol* 1994;12: 2527–2534.
138. Kudo K, Yoshida H, Kiyoi H, et al. Etoposide-related acute promyelocytic leukemia. *Leukemia* 1998;12:1171–1175.
139. Bain BJ, Moorman AV, Johansson B, et al. Myelodysplastic syndromes associated with 11q23 abnormalities. *Leukemia* 1998;12: 834–839.
140. Sultan C, Sigaux F, Imbert M, et al. Acute myelodysplasia with myelofibrosis: a report of eight cases. *Br J Haematol* 1981;49:11–16.
141. McKenna RW, Parkin JL, Foucar K, et al. Ultrastructural characteristics of therapy-related acute nonlymphocytic leukemia: evidence for a panmyelosis. *Cancer* 1981;48:725–737.
142. Brunning RD. The effects of leukemia and lymphoma chemotherapy on hematopoietic cells. *Am J Med Technol* 1983;39:165–174.
143. Schmitz LL, McClure JS, Litz CE, et al. Morphologic quantitative changes in blood and marrow cells following growth factor therapy. *Am J Clin Pathol* 1994;101:67–75.
144. Rowley JD. Recurring chromosomal abnormalities in leukemia and lymphoma. *Semin Hematol* 1990;27:122–136.
145. Yunis JJ, Brunning RD. Prognostic significance of chromosomal abnormalities in acute leukemia and myelodysplastic syndromes. *Clin Haematol* 1986;15:597–620.
146. Drexler HG, Thiel E, Ludwig WD. Acute myeloid leukemias expressing lymphoid-associated antigens: diagnosis, incidence, and prognosis significance. *Leukemia* 1993;7:489–498.
147. Seymour JF, Pierce SA, Kantarjian HM, et al. Investigation of karyotypic, morphologic and clinical features in patients with acute myeloid leukemia blast cells expressing the neural adhesion molecule. *Leukemia* 1994;8:823–826.

CHAPTER 48

Myelodysplastic Syndromes

Richard D. Brunning

DEFINITION

The myelodysplastic syndromes (MDSs) are a group of bone marrow disorders characterized by dysplastic changes in one or more myeloid cell lines with or without concurrent increases in myeloblasts in the bone marrow and peripheral blood; in those instances in which the myeloblasts are increased, the number is less than the 20% requisite for a diagnosis of acute myeloid leukemia (1–4). The MDSs occur as primary diseases and as secondary or therapy-related disorders. The therapy-related MDSs occur in patients who have been exposed to chemotherapeutic agents or radiotherapy (5–8). These entities are discussed in Chapter 47.

PRIMARY MYELODYSPLASTIC SYNDROMES

The *de novo* or primary MDSs occur most commonly in persons over the age of 50 years (4,9). MDSs are uncommon in the pediatric population and, in this age group, frequently are associated with specific cytogenetic abnormalities or clinical syndromes such as isolated monosomy 7, juvenile myelomonocytic leukemia, or constitutional hematopoietic disorders such as Fanconi anemia (10,11). Patients who have an MDS generally present with some manifestation of bone marrow failure, most commonly fatigue caused by anemia (12). Bleeding related to thrombocytopenia and infection resulting from decreased neutrophils are frequent features at presentation. Organomegaly and lymphadenopathy are not usually present but may occur in some patients. Some patients with MDSs have autoimmune manifestations (13).

The diagnosis of an MDS is based on quantitative and qualitative alterations in the developing and mature myeloid cells: granulocytes, monocytes, erythroid cells, and megakaryocytes (1,2,14–16). The quantitative changes relate to an increase in type I and II blasts in the marrow and blood. In two of the MDSs, refractory anemia and refractory anemia with ringed sideroblasts, the findings are limited to morphologic changes without an increase in blasts. Refractory cytopenia with multilineage dysplasia is characterized by dysplastic features in more than one cell line and less than 5% blasts in the bone marrow (17).

The morphologic alterations in the neutrophils are characterized by deficient or aberrant granule production, and defects in nuclear segmentation manifest as nuclear hyposegmentation, pseudo–Pelger-Huet changes, and hypersegmentation; unusual nuclear configurations may occur (Figs. 48.1–48.3; see also Color Plate 69, betwen pp. 1446–1447). An association between prominent nuclear hyposegmentation and small and vacuolated neutrophils and deletion 17p has been observed in some patients with acute myeloid leukemia and MDSs (18,19) (Fig.48.4; see also Color Plate 70, between pp. 1446–1447). Erythroid abnormalities include asynchronous nuclear cytoplasmic development with megaloblastoid nuclear chromatin, nuclear lobulation, multinucleate cells, and nuclear karyorrhexis and fragmentation (Figs. 48.5–48.7; see also Color Plates 71 and 72, between pp. 1446–1447). Ringed sideroblasts may be present in all types of MDSs (20). Red blood cells frequently show increased anisopoikilocytosis with oval macrocytes and dacryocytes. Megakaryocytic changes are characterized by abnormally small megakaryocytes with nonlobulated or bilobed nuclei and unusually large megakaryocytes with nonlobulated nuclei and finely dispersed chromatin (Figs. 48.8, 48.9; see also Color Plate 73, between pp. 1446–1447). Atypical, large, agranular platelets may be present. Changes in all the myeloid cells may be present, or the changes may be restricted to one cell line, such as the red cells in refractory anemia or refractory anemia with ringed sideroblasts.

CLASSIFICATION

The *de novo* MDSs may be categorized into six morphologic types based on the World Health Organization proposal for the classification of hematopoietic tumors (21) (Table 48.1).

R. D. Brunning: Department of Laboratory Medicine, University of Minnesota, Minneapolis, Minnesota 55455

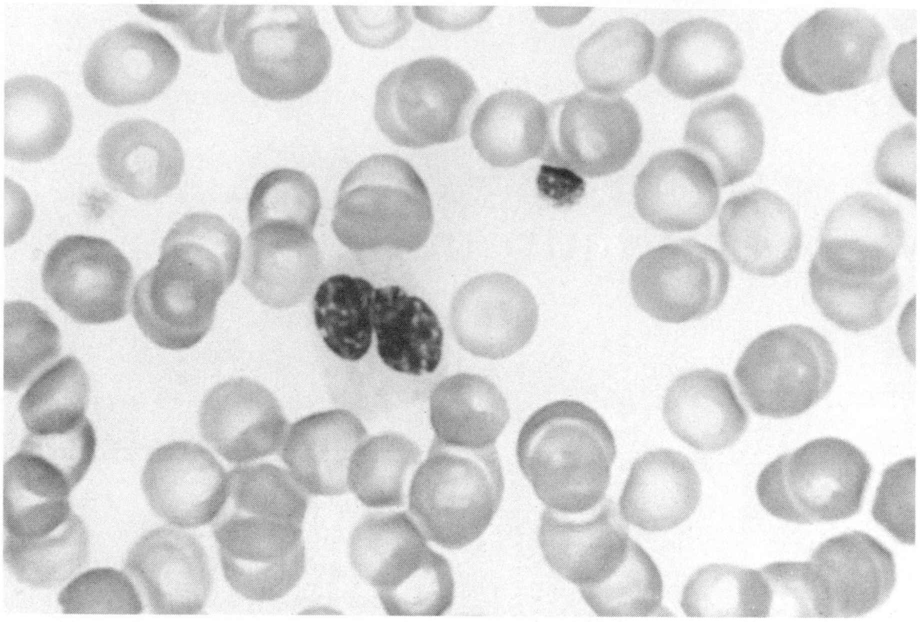

FIG. 48.1. Mature neutrophil in the blood smear of a patient who has refractory anemia with excess blasts, type 1. The cytoplasm is pale because of a marked decrease in specific granules. The nucleus appears hypolobated because of overlapping nuclear segments (Wright-Giemsa stain, original magnification: 400× magnification). See Color Plate 69, between pp. 1446–1447.

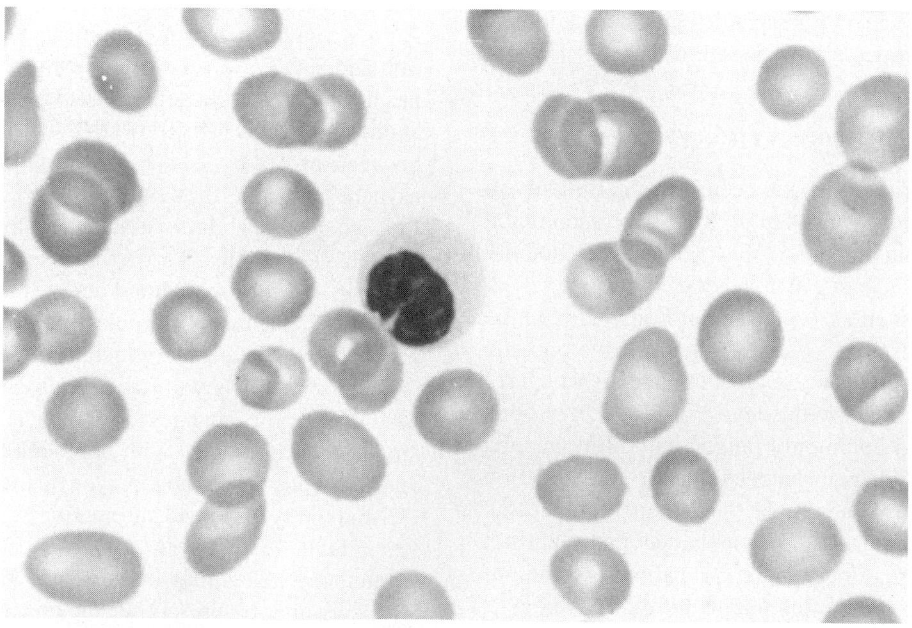

FIG. 48.2. Mature neutrophil with a hyposegmented (pseudo–Pelger-Huet) nucleus in the blood smear of a patient who has refractory anemia with excess blasts, type 1. In addition to the nuclear hyposegmentation, the cell is smaller than a normal mature neutrophil. Granulation is normal (Wright-Giemsa stain, original magnification: 400× magnification).

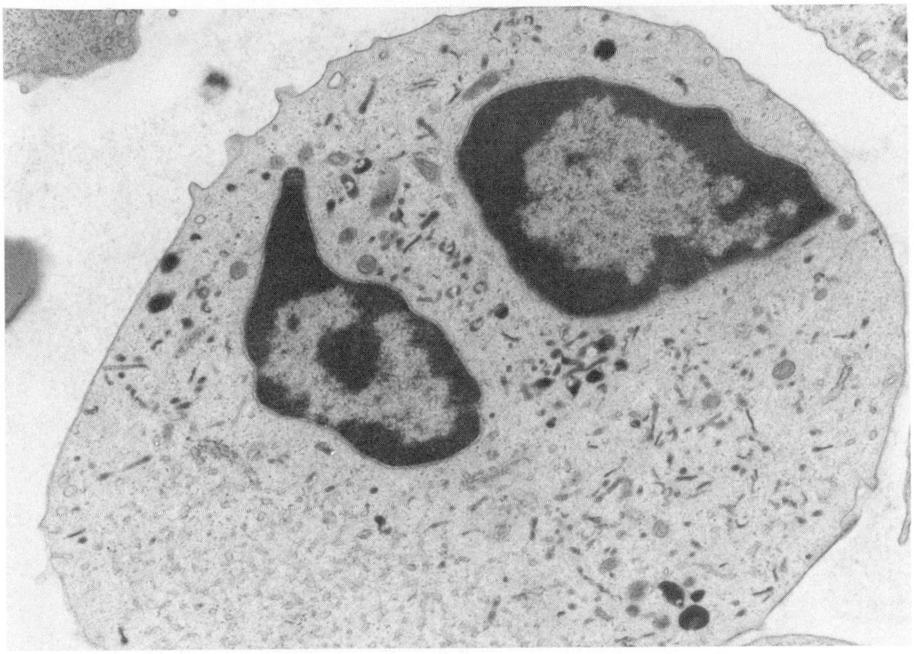

FIG. 48.3. Electron micrograph of a mature neutrophil from the blood of a patient who has refractory anemia with excess blasts, type 1. There is nuclear hyposegmentation, and the cytoplasm is almost devoid of primary and secondary granules (uranyl acetate, lead citrate stain, original magnification: 20,000× magnification).

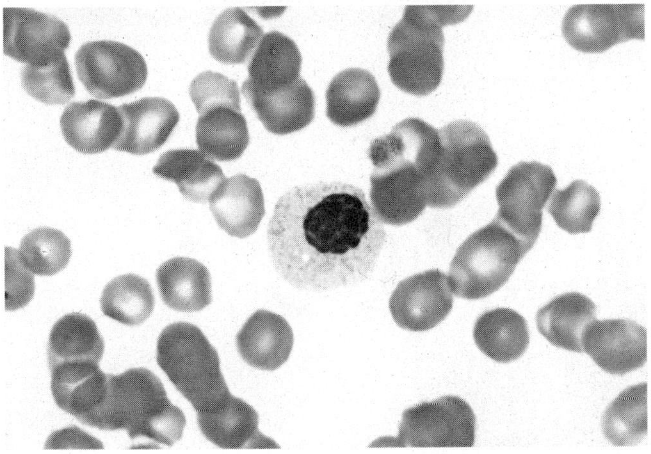

FIG. 48.4. Blood smear from a 68-year-old woman with refractory anemia with excess blasts, type 1 associated with del(17p). The blood contained numerous neutrophils with nonlobated nuclei similar to this cell (Wright-Giemsa stain, original magnification: 400× magnification). See Color Plate 70, between pp. 1446–1447.

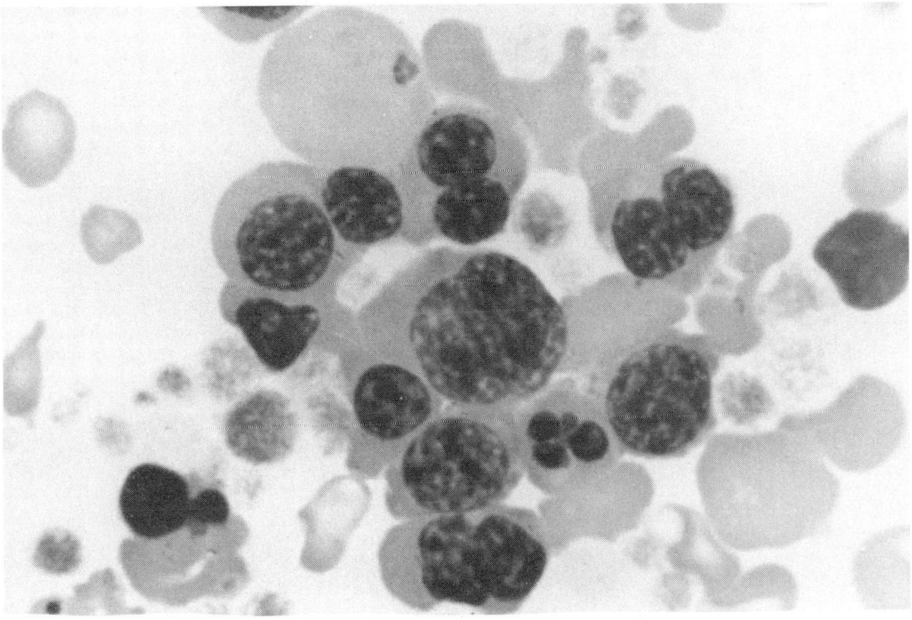

FIG. 48.5. Bone marrow smear from a patient who has an unclassified myelodysplastic syndrome showing marked dyserythropoiesis. The erythroid cells show nuclear lobulation and slightly open chromatin (Wright-Giemsa stain, original magnification: 256× magnification). See Color Plate 71, between pp. 1446–1447.

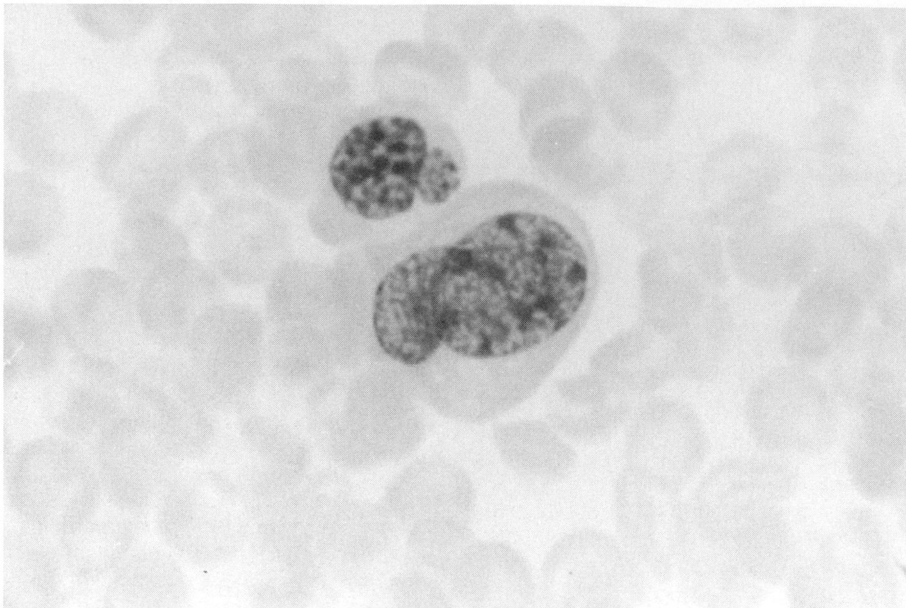

FIG. 48.6. Two large erythroblasts in a bone marrow smear from a patient who has refractory anemia. The nucleus of the larger cell is lobated and the chromatin has the features of a megaloblast (Wright-Giemsa stain, original magnification: 400× magnification). See Color Plate 72, between pp. 1446–1447.

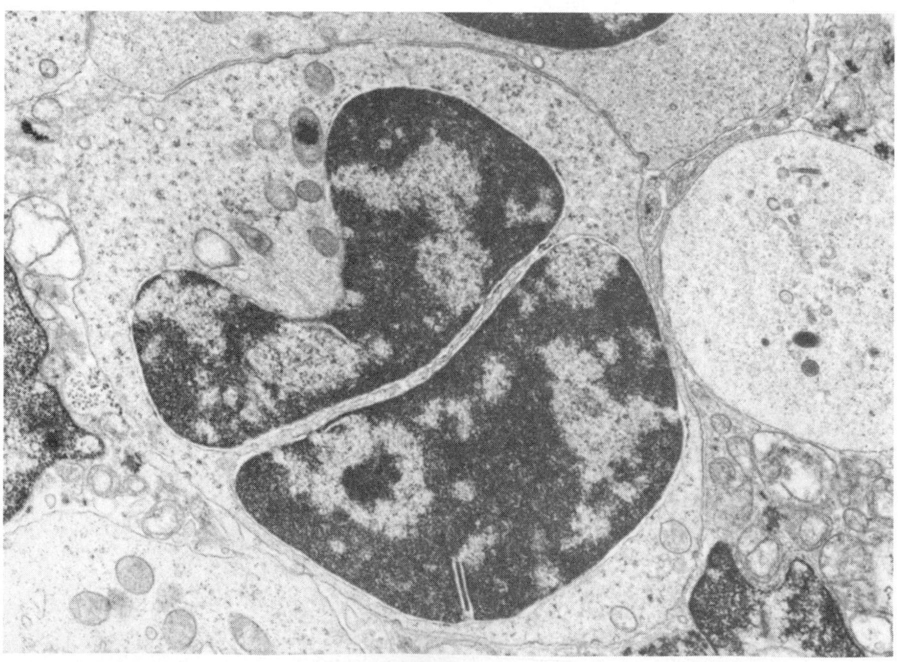

FIG. 48.7. Electron micrograph of an erythroblast in a bone marrow specimen from a patient who has an unclassified MDS. The nucleus shows a cleft and splits (uranyl acetate, lead citrate stain, original magnification: 19,000× magnification).

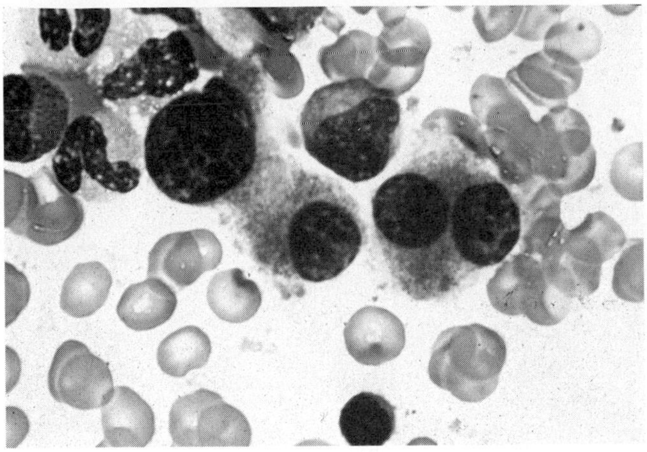

FIG. 48.8. Bone marrow smear from a patient with a myelodysplastic syndrome. Three small mature megakaryocytes with markedly hypolobulated nuclei are present (Wright-Giemsa stain, original magnification: 400× magnification). See Color Plate 73, between pp. 1446–1447.

The *MDS unclassified* category is an appropriate designation for those cases that do not satisfy the criteria for one of the described entities. Many of the cases previously classified as MDS unclassified satisfy the criteria for refractory cytopenia with multilineage dysplasia (17,21).

Chronic myelomonocytic leukemia may have features of both a myeloproliferative process and a MDS. Because of this, it is discussed in Chapter 49 in a category that also includes atypical chronic myeloid leukemia and juvenile myelomonocytic leukemia.

TABLE 48.1. *Proposed World Health Organization classification of myelodysplastic syndromes*

Refractory anemia (RA)
Refractory anemia with ringed sideroblasts (RARS)
Refractory cytopenia with multilineage dysplasia (RCMD)
Refractory anemia with excess blasts-1 (RAEB-1)
Refractory anemia with excess blasts-2 (RAEB-2)
Myelodysplastic syndrome; unclassified (MDS-U)

Refractory Anemia

Anemia refractory to hematenic therapy is the major finding. The red cells usually are normochromic and macrocytic but may be normocytic. The degree of red blood cell anisopoikilocytosis varies and may be marked (Fig. 48.10A; also see Color Plate 74, between pp. 1446–1447). The platelet and neutrophil counts are normal in most patients, but occasional patients have an accompanying neutropenia or thrombocytopenia. Blasts should not be present in the peripheral blood.

In refractory anemia, the bone marrow is usually hypercellular. The bone marrow blasts are less than 5%. The number of erythroid precursors varies from marked erythroid hypoplasia to hyperplasia; erythroid hyperplasia is the predominant pattern. Some degree of dyserythropoiesis usually is evident, and megaloblastoid features may be present (Fig. 48.10B). Ringed sideroblasts may be present, but they make up less than 15% of the nucleated red blood cells. Morphologic abnormalities usually are restricted to the erythroid series.

The bone marrow biopsy specimen in the majority of patients with refractory anemia is hypercellular, usually with

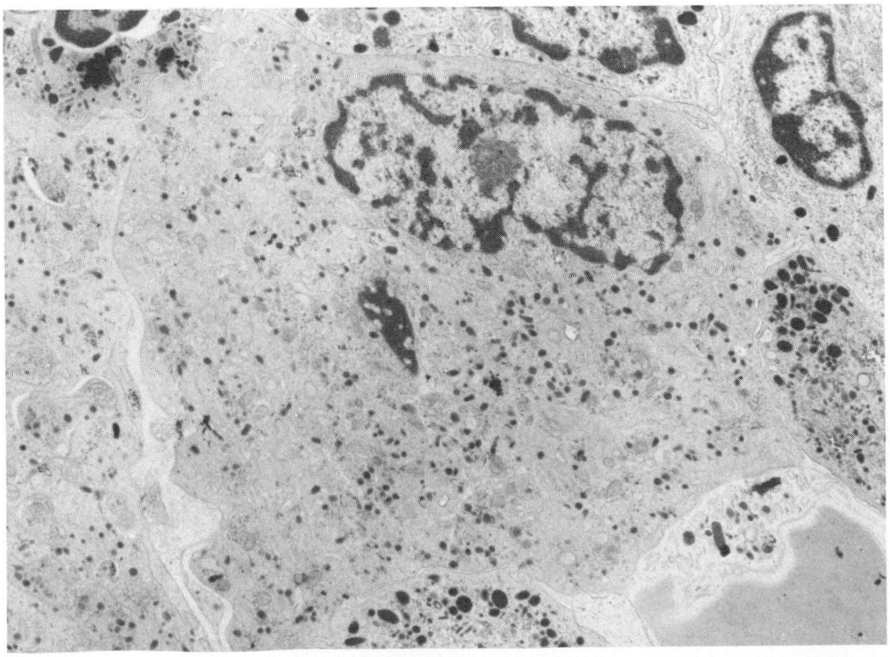

FIG. 48.9. Electron micrograph of a small megakaryocyte in a bone marrow specimen from a patient who has refractory anemia with excess blasts, type 1. The abundant cytoplasm shows decreased granule formation (uranyl acetate, lead citrate stain, original magnification: 8,000× magnification).

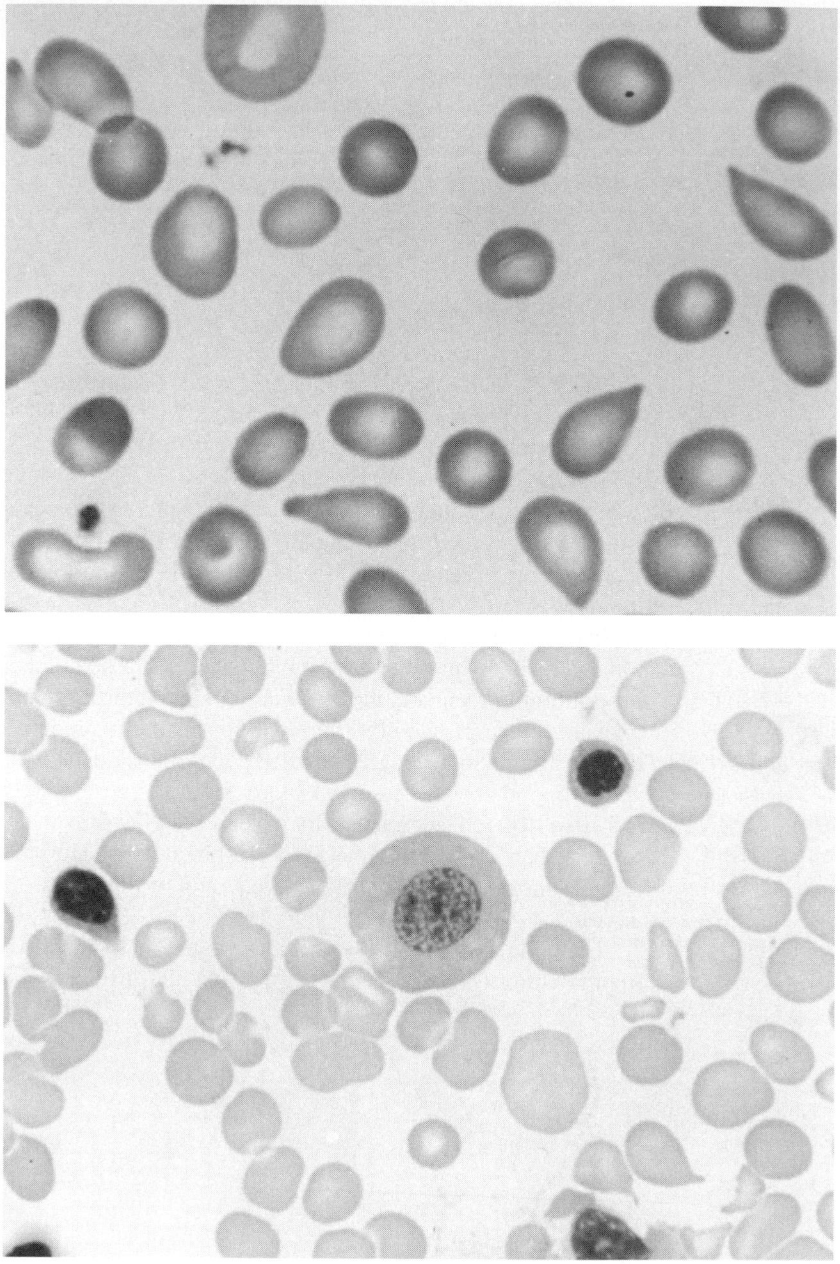

FIG. 48.10. A: Blood smear from a patient with an 8-year history of refractory anemia. There is marked anisocytosis with numerous dacryocytes. Anisocytosis is slight to moderate. **B:** Bone marrow smear from the same patient showing a polychromatic megaloblastic erythroblast (Wright-Giemsa stain, original magnification: 400× magnification). See Color Plate 74, between pp. 1446–1447.

erythroid hyperplasia; in some instances, there is marked erythroid hypoplasia. Neutrophils and megakaryocytes are normal or increased. In approximately 10% to 15% of patients the marrow is hypocellular, and in some instances it may be markedly so, resembling aplastic anemia (22–24). Hypocellular bone marrows also may be observed in other types of MDSs. This finding is more common in older individuals. The distinction from aplastic anemia usually can be made from examination of marrow and blood smears. An additional aid in the distinction is the demonstration of increased numbers of immature cells expressing CD34 and proliferating cell nuclear antigens in hypocellular MDSs and acute leukemia, compared with aplastic anemia (23).

Occasional patients present with anemia refractory to hematenic therapy, with or without thrombocytopenia, or neutropenia, with minimal or no evident dysplastic changes in the myeloid cells and a cytogenetic abnormality associated with an MDS such as 20q− (Fig. 48.11). These patients are classified appropriately as having refractory anemia, based on the cytogenetic findings.

Refractory Anemia with Ringed Sideroblasts

Anemia is always present with this condition, and the hemoglobin level generally is in the range between 9 and 12 g/dL; lower levels may be present (12). The red blood

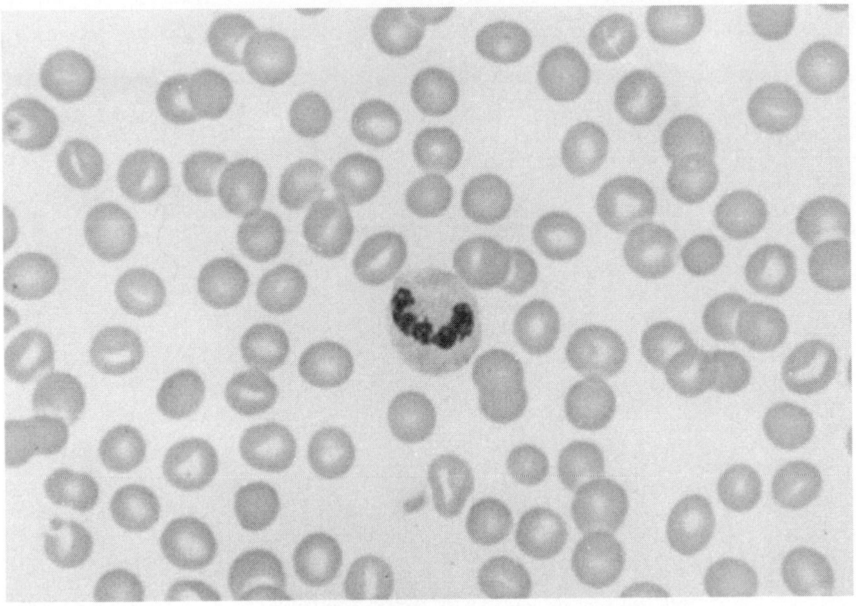

A

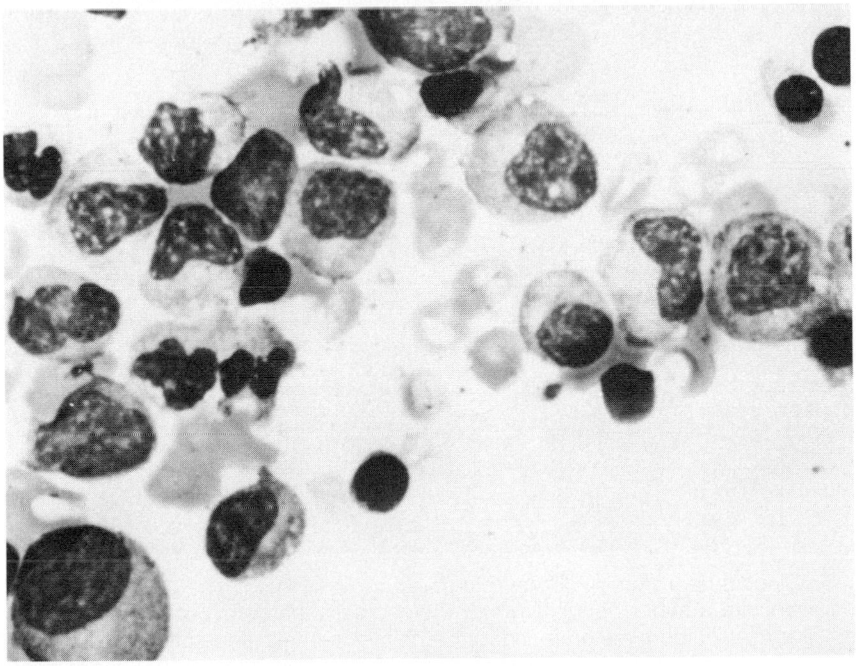

B

FIG. 48.11. A: Blood smear from a 47-year-old woman with anemia refractory to hematenic therapy. The leukocytes and platelets were normal in number (Wright-Giemsa stain, original magnification: 256× magnification). **B:** Bone marrow smear from the same patient showing essentially normal-appearing hematopoiesis. Cytogenetic analysis showed a 20q− clonal chromosome abnormality. A diagnosis of MDS-RA was made on the basis of the cytogenetic finding (Wright-Giemsa stain, original magnification: 205× magnification).

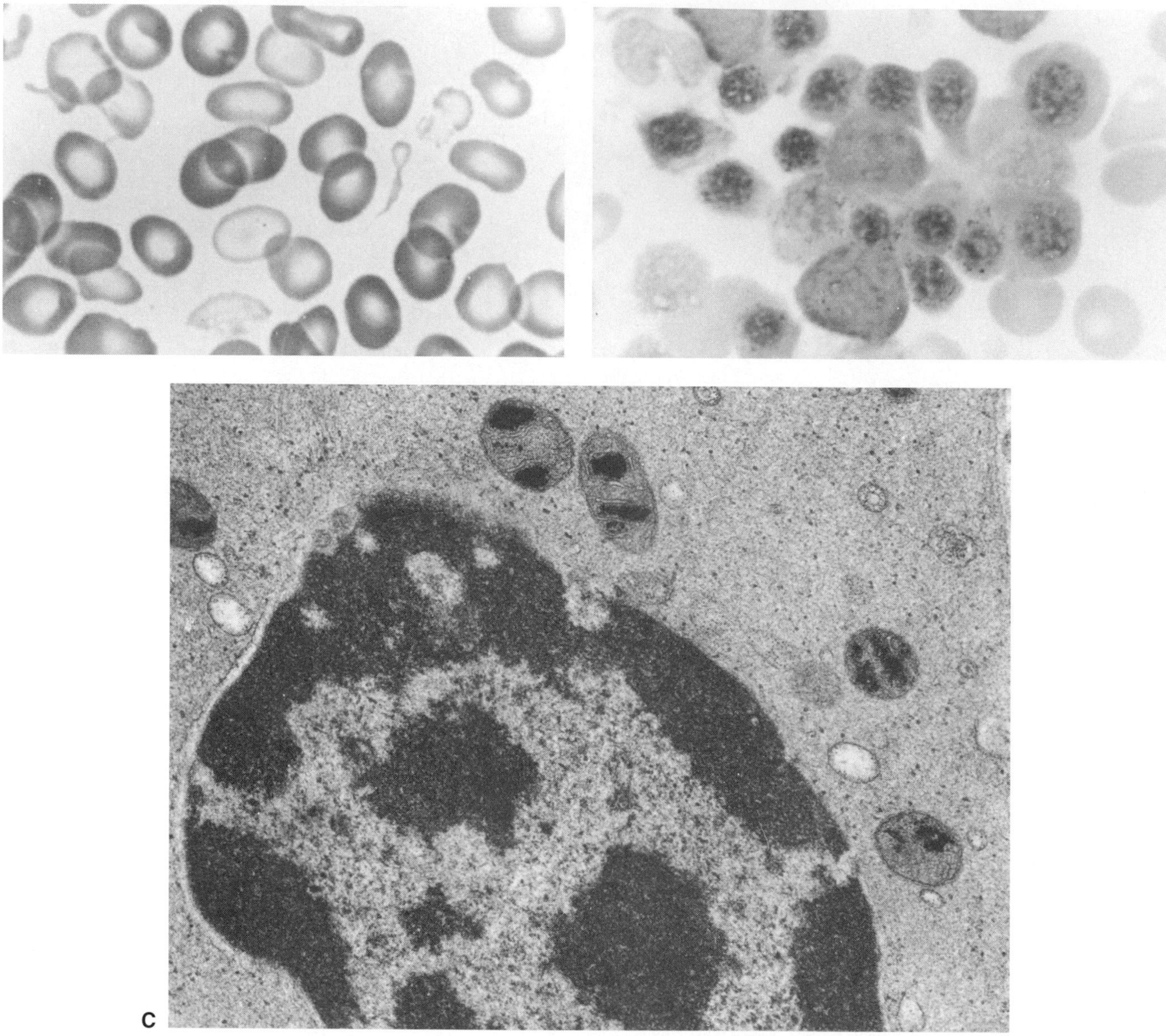

A B C

FIG. 48.12. A: Blood smear from a 42-year-old man who has RARS. The predominant red blood cells are normochromic with a minor population of red blood cells that is hypochromic dimorphic. There is increased poikilocytosis in both the normochromic and hypochromic populations. Some of the normochromic cells are macrocytic (Wright-Giemsa stain, original magnification: 400× magnification). **B:** Iron stain of a bone marrow smear from the patient illustrated in **A** showing numerous ringed, type III sideroblasts (Prussian blue stain followed by Safranin counterstain, original magnification: 256× magnification). **C:** Electron micrograph of an erythroblast from the specimen in **B** showing deposits of iron in the mitochondria of an erythroblast (uranyl acetate, lead citrate stain, original magnification: 40,000× magnification). See Color Plate 75, between pp. 1446–1447.

cells may be dimorphic, with populations of both hypochromic and normochromic cells; in some instances the red blood cells are normochromic and macro- or normocytic (Fig. 48.12A; see also Color Plate 75, between pp. 1446–1447). Pappenheimer bodies may be present in occasional red blood cells (Fig. 48.13; see also Color Plate 76, between pp. 1446–1447). The platelets and neutrophils usually are normal in number and appearance. The bone marrow shows erythroid hyperplasia, sometimes marked, with variable but usually minor degrees of dyserythropoiesis; in occasional patients, prominent dyserythropoiesis with megaloblastoid features is present. In smears stained for iron, 15% or more of the erythroid precursors are ringed (type III) sideroblasts, erythroblasts in which the nucleus is encircled completely or partially by iron granules (Fig. 48.12B). On ultrastructural examination, the perinuclear iron is present in the mitochondria (Fig. 48.12C). Granulopoiesis and megakaryocytopoiesis are essentially normal in most patients.

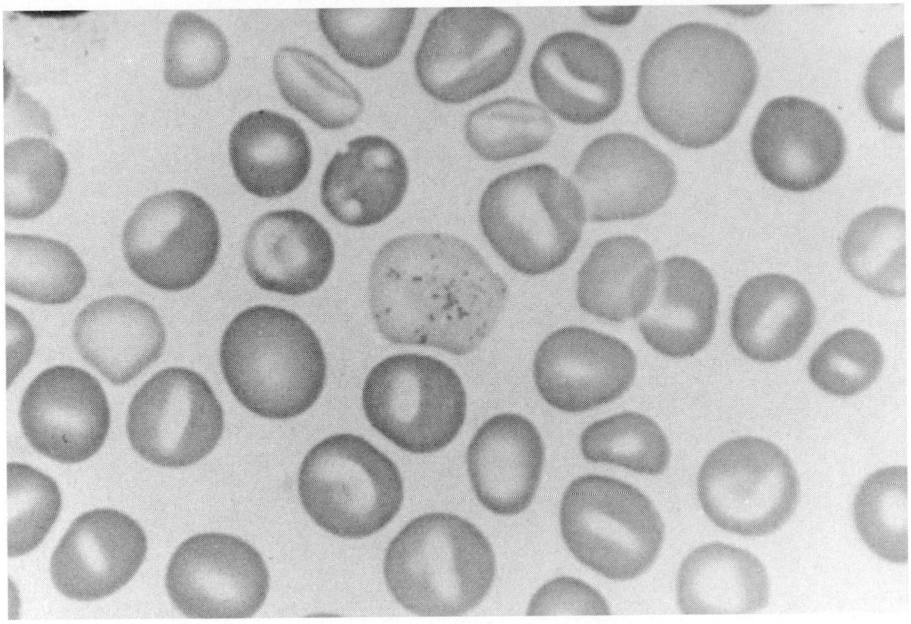

FIG. 48.13. Blood smear from a patient who has RARS. The red blood cells are predominantly normochromic macrocytic. The red blood cell in the center contains numerous Pappenheimer bodies (Wright-Giemsa stain, original magnification: 400× magnification). See Color Plate 76, between pp. 1446–1447.

The bone marrow biopsy shows a hypercellular marrow with prominent erythroid hyperplasia. Megakaryocytes and granulocytes appear to be morphologically and numerically normal. Sections stained for iron show numerous iron-laden macrophages. Ringed sideroblasts may be identified, but this finding is appreciated less readily than in smear or imprint preparations.

Sideroblastic anemia occurs in two forms: a true MDS with eventual evolution to acute myeloid leukemia or a higher grade MDS, and a type that probably results from some inherited or acquired disturbance of iron metabolism (25). The majority of cases appears to fall in the latter category; only approximately 7% to 10% of patients with sideroblastic anemia develop acute leukemia. The morphologic features at initial diagnosis may reflect this potential, in that multilineage dysplasia is an indication that the disorder is not related solely to the erythroid series with a disturbance in iron metabolism. In recognition of this, patients with sideroblastic anemia should receive careful scrutiny for abnormalities in the granulocytic and megakaryocytic lineages; if either of these lineages is involved in addition to the erythroid series, the patient should be considered to have sideroblastic anemia with multilineage dysplasia. Patients with dysplasia only in the erythroid cells should be identified as having sideroblastic anemia with unilineage dysplasia. This is meant to imply not that sideroblastic anemia with unilineage dysplasia may not evolve to a higher-grade MDS or acute myeloid leukemia, but that the potential is higher for those cases with recognizable abnormalities in granulocytes and megakaryocytes.

Refractory Anemia with Excess of Blasts

The defining criterion for refractory anemia with excess blasts (RAEB) is 5% to 19% blasts in the bone marrow. If blasts are present in the peripheral blood they must be less than 20%. Based on data from the International MDS Risk Analysis Workshop, which showed different survival data for patients with RAEB with 5% to 10% and those with 11% to 20% blasts in the marrow, RAEB is divided into RAEB-1 (5–10%) RAEB-2 (11–19%) in the bone marrow (21,26). Patients with blasts in the peripheral blood, but less than 11%, and less than 11% in the bone marrow are classified as having RAEB-1; those with 11% to 19% blasts in the bone marrow or peripheral blood or less than 11% blasts in blood or bone marrow but blasts with Auer rods have RAEB-2 (21,26–28). If the percentage of blasts in the peripheral blood exceeds the bone marrow blast percentage, the blood blast percentage dictates the classification. The criteria for RAEB-1 and RAEB-2 are summarized in Table 48.2.

Anemia is present in virtually all patients; the red blood cells are normochromic and normo- or macrocytic. An in-

TABLE 48.2. *Criteria for refractory anemia with excess blasts (RAEB)*

	RAEB-1	RAEB-2
Bone marrow	5 to 10% blasts	11 to 19% blasts
Peripheral blood	<10% blasts	11 to 19% blasts; Auer rods in blasts but <11% blasts in peripheral blood or bone marrow

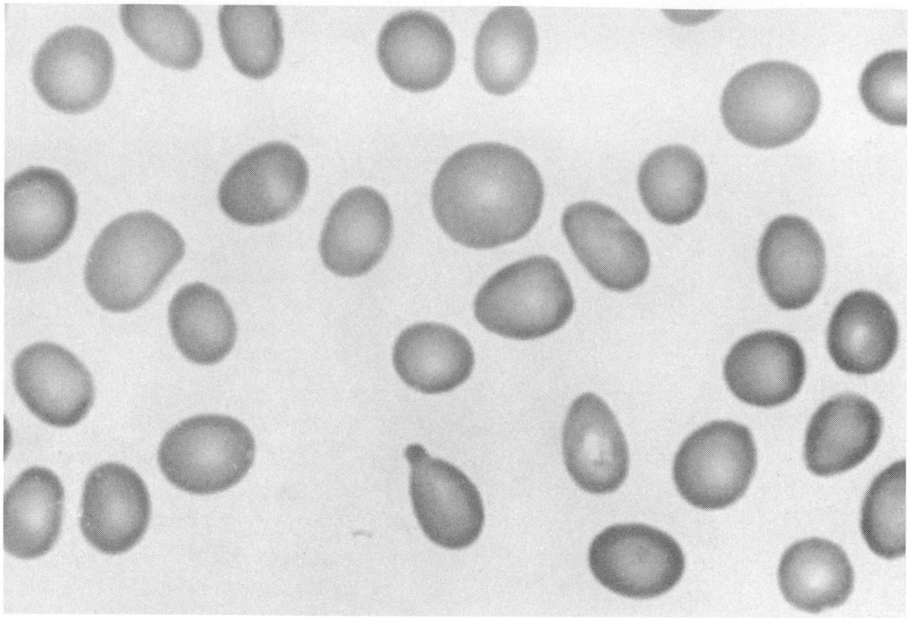

FIG. 48.14. Blood smear from a man who has refractory anemia with excess blasts, type 1. The red blood cells show increased anisocytosis and poikilocytosis with macrocytes, including oval macrocytes, and dacrocytes (Wright-Giemsa stain, original magnification: 400× magnification). See Color Plate 77, between pp. 1446–1447.

creased incidence of anisopoikilocytosis is noted in a high percentage of cases, including macroovalocytes (Fig. 48.14; see also Color Plate 77, between pp. 1446–1447). Nucleated red blood cells may be present. The majority of patients presents with neutropenia and thrombocytopenia; pancytopenia is common. Neutrophil abnormalities include nuclear hyposegmentation, pseudo–Pelger-Huet nuclei, and nuclear hyperlobulation; abnormalities of granulation such as hypogranulation generally are present and frequently are marked (Figs. 48.1, 48.15; see also Color Plate 78, between pp. 1446–1447). Aggregates of granules that resemble the Chediak-Higashi abnormality may be present but are much less

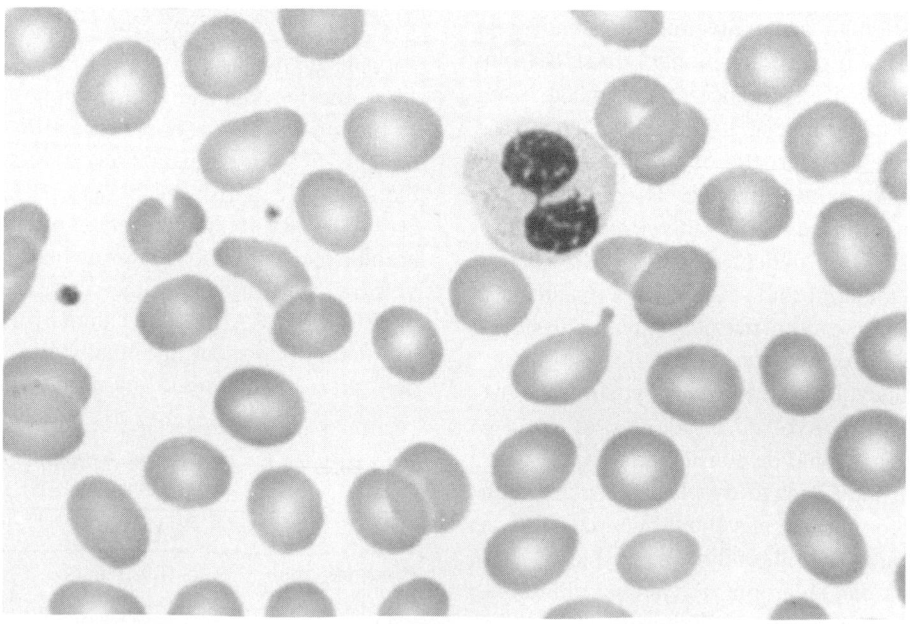

FIG. 48.15. Blood smear from a man who has refractory anemia with excess blasts, type 1, showing a mature neutrophil with a bilobed, pseudo–Pelger-Huet nucleus. The red blood cells show minimal anisocytosis and slight poikilocytosis (Wright-Giemsa stain, original magnification: 400× magnification). See Color Plate 78, between pp. 1446–1447.

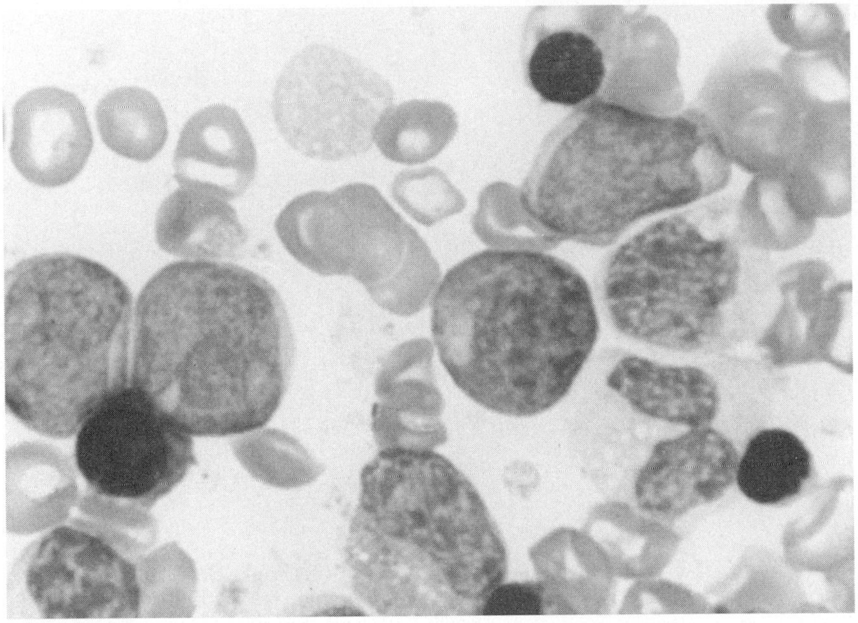

A

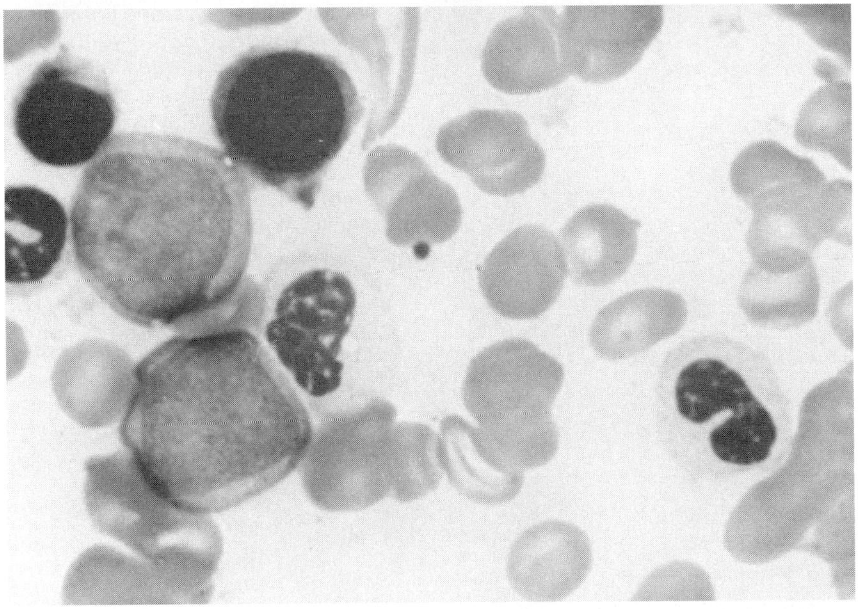

B

FIG. 48.16. **A:** Bone marrow smear from a patient who has refractory anemia with excess blasts, type 2, showing three myeloblasts. **B:** The same specimen as **A**, showing three mature neutrophils with hyposegmented nuclei. Two early promyelocytes are also present (Wright-Giemsa stain, original magnification: 400× magnification). See Color Plate 79, between pp. 1446–1447.

frequent than hypogranulation. Immature neutrophils usually are present in the blood; basophilia is present in some patients. Atypical platelets and micromegakaryocytes may be noted.

The essential finding in the bone marrow is an increase in myeloblasts. In many patients, the increase in blasts is accompanied by an increase in promyelocytes (Fig. 48.16; see also Color Plate 79, between pp. 1446–1447). Abnormalities of nuclear and cytoplasmic development may be present in all the myeloid cell lines. Erythroid abnormalities include megaloblastoid nuclei, nuclear lobulation, karyorrhexis, and multinucleation. Ringed sideroblasts may be present and may exceed 15% of the nucleated red blood cells (20). The increase in blasts or the presence of Auer rods (Fig. 48.17, 48.18; see also Color Plates 80 and 81, between pp. 1446–1447), however, dictates the classification (Table 48.2). Micromegakaryocytes characterized by small size and nonlobulated nuclei may be numerous.

The bone marrow biopsy in the majority of patients is hypercellular with a panmyeloid hyperplasia; in 10% to 20% of patients, the bone marrow is normocellular or hypocellular (22–24) (Figs. 48.19, 48.20). The number of blasts in the

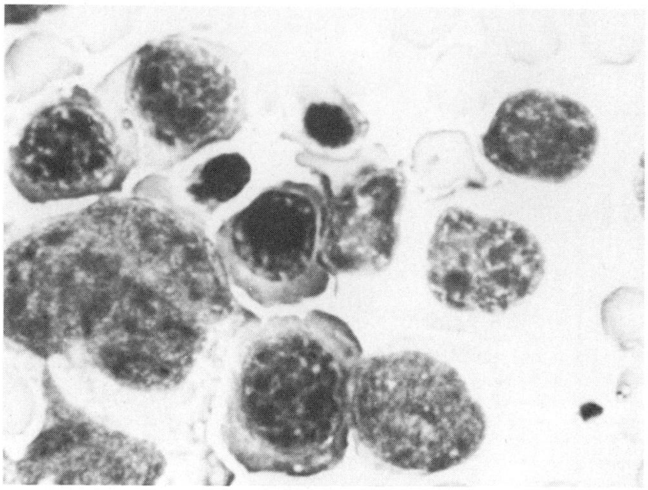

A

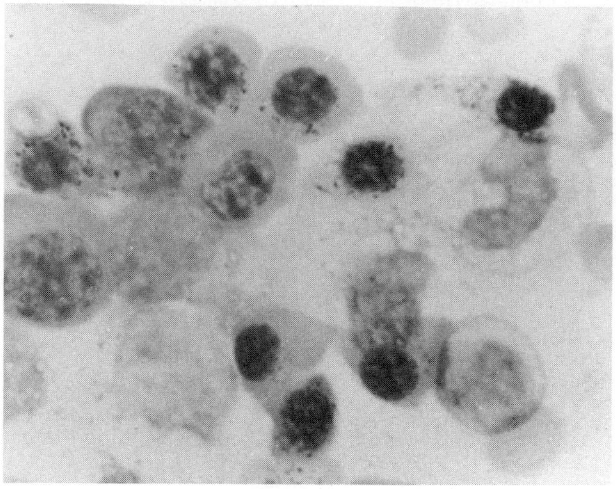

B

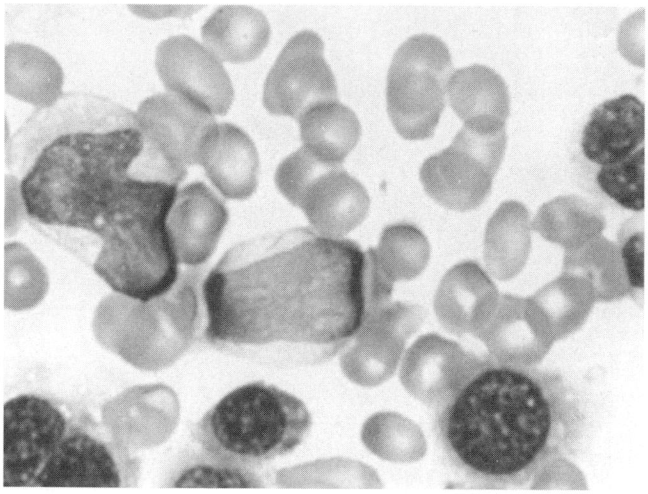

C

FIG. 48.17. **A:** Bone marrow smear from a 72-year-old man who has refractory anemia with excess blasts, type 2, and who presented with a 1-year history of macrocytic anemia, neutropenia, and thrombocytopenia. This marrow specimen showed 62% erythroblasts and 4% myeloblasts. A myeloblast with a delicate Auer rod is present in the lower right. A megakaryocyte with a phagocytosed red cell is also present (Wright-Giemsa stain, original magnification: 400× magnification). **B:** An iron stain of the specimen illustrated in **A** shows numerous ringed sideroblasts (Prussian blue stain followed by Safranin counterstain, original magnification: 400× magnification). **C:** High-magnification view of the specimens in **A** and **B** showing a myeloblast with a distinct Auer rod. Several normoblasts are present (Wright-Giemsa stain, original magnification: 256× magnification). See Color Plate 80, between pp. 1446–1447.

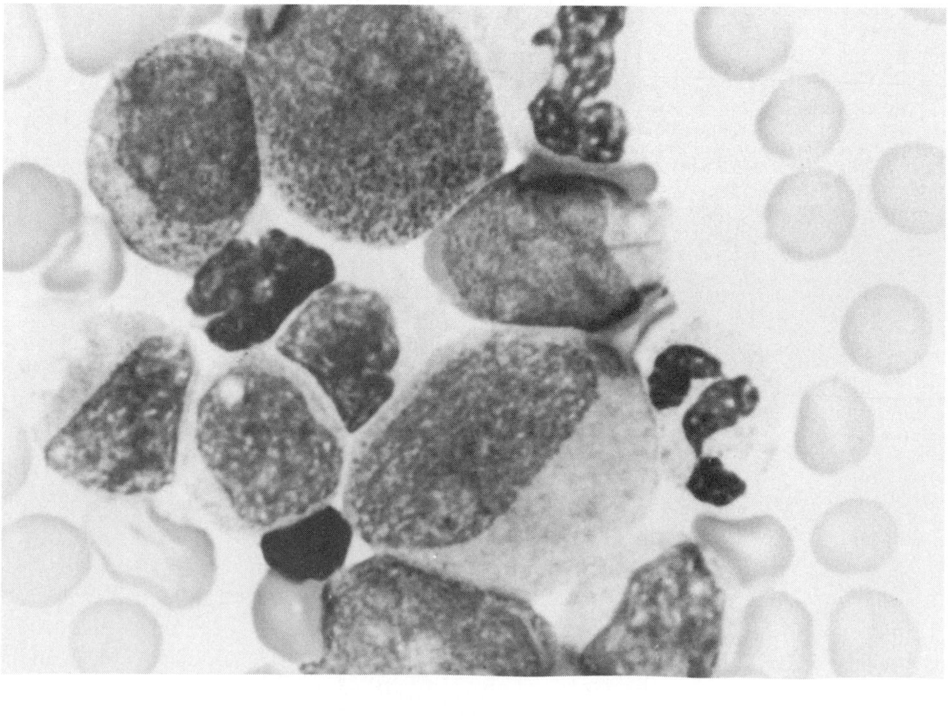

FIG. 48.18. Bone marrow smear from a 27-year-old man who has pancytopenia and refractory anemia with excess blasts, type 2. There is a full spectrum of neutrophil maturation. This specimen showed 8% myeloblasts, several of which contained Auer rods, as shown in the only blast in this field (Wright-Giemsa stain, original magnification: 256× magnification). See Color Plate 81, between pp. 1446–1447.

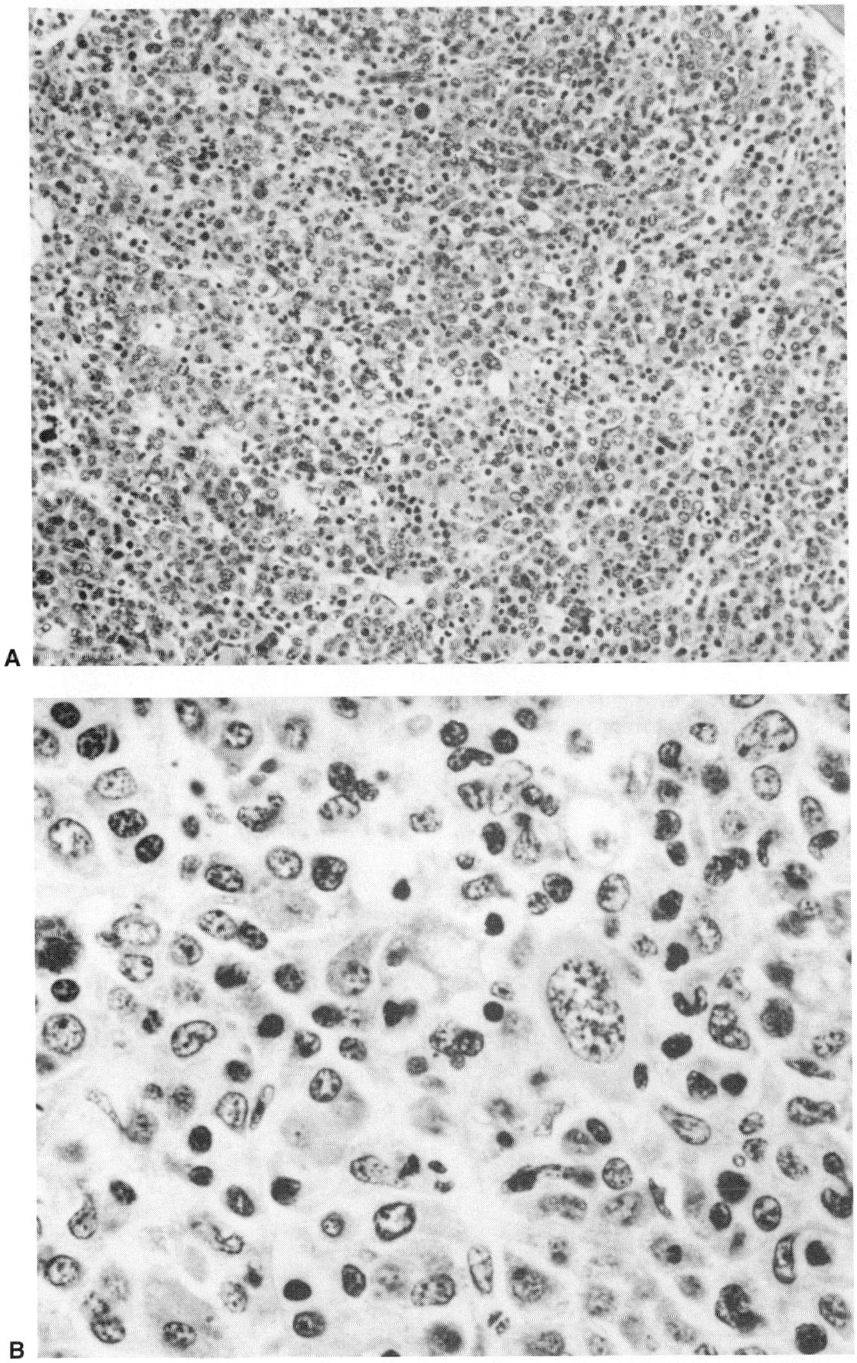

FIG. 48.19. A: Bone marrow biopsy from a 72-year-old woman who has refractory anemia with excess blasts, type 1. The marrow is markedly hypercellular (hematoxylin and eosin stain, original magnification: 40× magnification). **B:** High-magnification view of the specimen in **A**, showing a predominance of granulocytes that predominantly are immature. Erythroblasts are distributed evenly. A large megakaryocyte with a hypolobated nucleus with dispersed chromatin is present (hematoxylin and eosin stain, original magnification: 205× magnification).

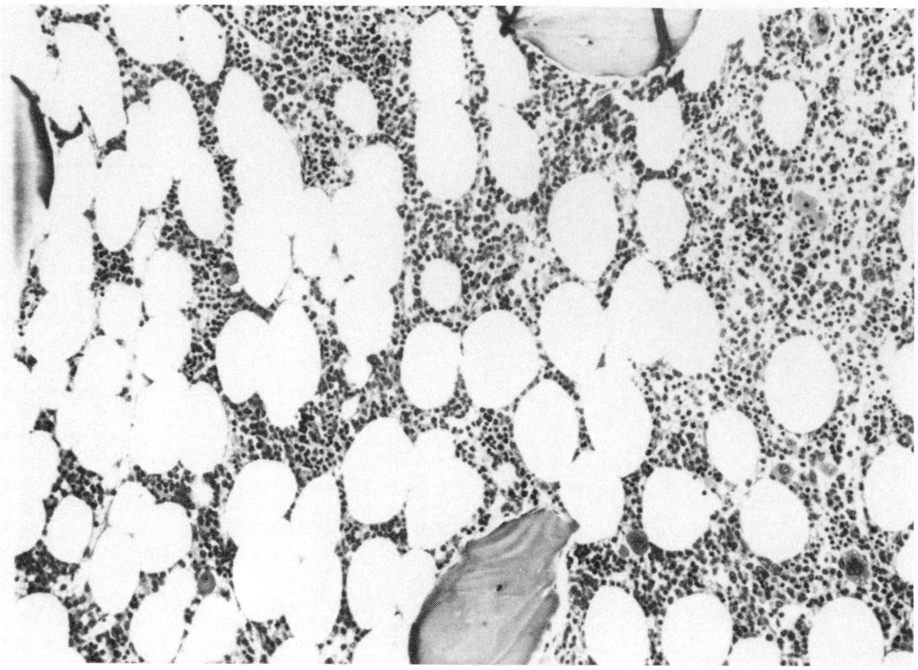

FIG. 48.20. Bone marrow biopsy from a 56 year old woman who has refractory anemia with excess blasts, type 1. The marrow is hypocellular (hematoxylin and eosin stain, original magnification: 40× magnification).

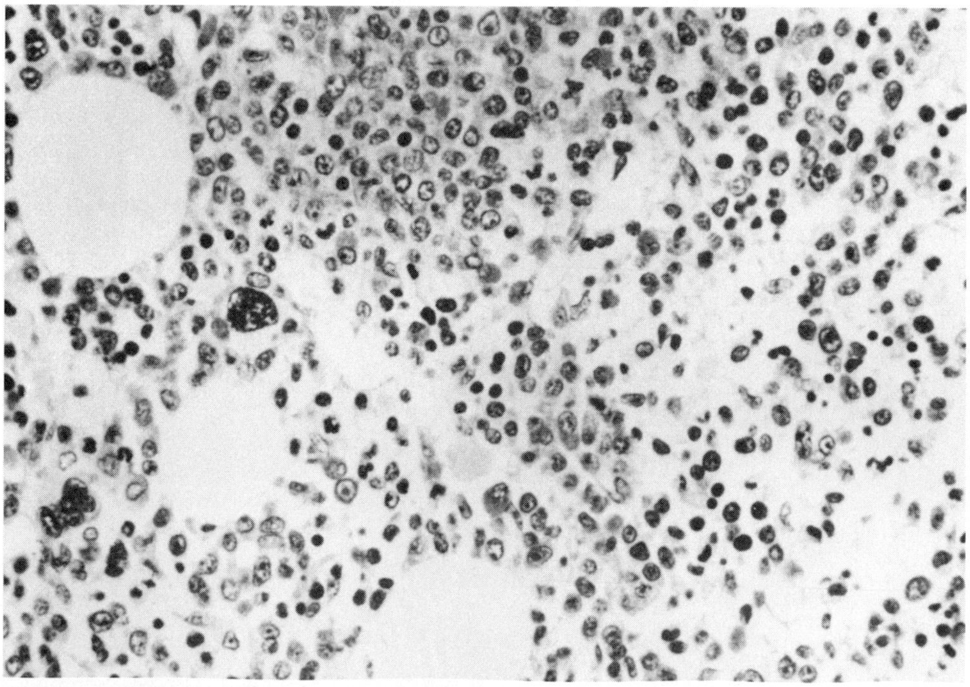

FIG. 48.21. Bone marrow biopsy from a patient who has refractory anemia with excess blasts, type 1, showing a small focal collection of immature cells, unrelated to bone or vascular structure. This is referred to as an abnormal localization of immature precursors (hematoxylin and eosin stain, original magnification: 205× magnification).

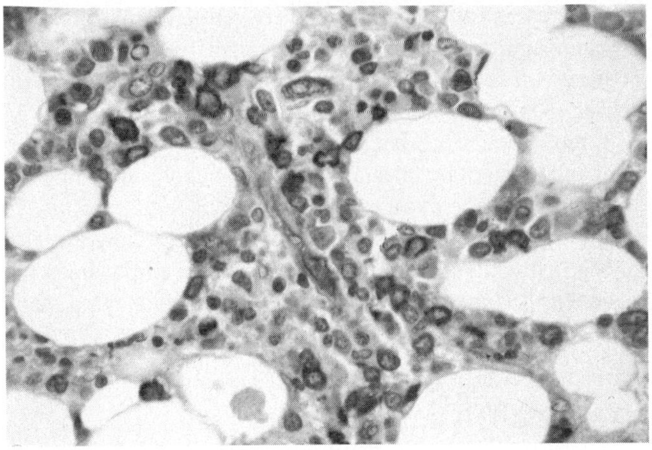

FIG. 48.22. Hypocellular marrow biopsy from a patient with refractory anemia with excess blasts, type 1, reacted with antibody to CD34. Several immature cells expressing CD34 are present (immunoperoxidase stain, original magnification: 400× magnification). See Color Plate 82, between pp. 1446–1447.

sections usually corresponds to the smear or biopsy imprint differential. In some patients, foci of immature cells, blasts, and promyelocytes, spatially unrelated to an endosteal or perivascular location, may be noted (Fig. 48.21). The presence of three or more of these foci in a biopsy specimen, referred to as *abnormal localization of immature precursors*, has been reported to be associated with an increased incidence of leukemic evolution (29,30). Abnormal megakaryocytes, particularly small megakaryocytes and micromegakaryocytes with nuclear hypolobation, may be more apparent in the bone marrow sections than in smears; these cells are accentuated with the periodic acid–Schiff stain and immunohistochemical reactions with antimegakaryocyte antibodies such as factor VIII antibody. A slight degree of reticulin fibrosis is present in the bone marrow in a minority of patients. Marked fibrosis is uncommon but may occur.

In patients with hypocellular bone marrows, the distinction of MDS from aplastic anemia may be aided by immunohistochemical reactions for CD34 and proliferating cell nuclear antigen; positive reactions for these antigens are more compatible with MDS than with aplastic anemia (23) (Fig. 48.22; see also Color Plate 82, between pp. 1446–1447).

Refractory Cytopenia with Multilineage Dysplasia

Some patients with MDS present with bicytopenia or pancytopenia and evidence of multilineage dysplasia without an increase in blasts or monocytes and no Auer rods. The classification of these cases is problematic, because none of the initial French–American–British Cooperative Group classifications is completely satisfactory. The term *MDS unclassified* has been suggested for this type of case but lacks specificity and clinical relevance (16). The term *refractory cytopenia with multilineage dysplasia* was introduced to recognize patients with MDS with multilineage dysplasia and cytopenia, no or minimal increase in blasts or monocytes, and no Auer rods (17). MDSs with similar findings also have been classified as refractory anemia with severe dysplasia (31).

Refractory cytopenia with multilineage dysplasia is characterized by dysplasia of two or more myeloid cell lineages, frequently all myeloid cell types; the degree of dysplasia may be marked. In some patients, one cell lineage, such as the erythroid precursors, is increased, with dysplastic changes, which is the predominant finding. The type and degree of dysplastic change vary substantially from patient to patient, and there is no unifying morphologic feature of this type of MDS (Fig. 48.23; see also Color Plate 83, between pp. 1446–1447). There is no or only a slight increase in myeloblasts in the bone marrow; if increased the percentage is less than 5%. Blasts are not usually present in the peripheral blood. Auer rods are not found. The bone marrow is hypercellular with bilineage or trilineage hyperplasia. Essentially, the findings resemble RAEB without an increase in blasts. There are cytopenias of at least two lineages and frequently there is a pancytopenia.

Bone marrow biopsy may be particularly useful in recognizing the abnormalities in megakaryocytes, particularly small megakaryocytes and micromegakaryocytes with hypolobulated nuclei (Fig. 48.23B).

Many cases of MDS related to therapy with alkylating agents have the morphologic features of this type of MDS, as do some of the cases of MDS associated with the isolated 5q− and 20q− chromosome abnormalities in which both the megakaryocytes and erythroid precursors show morphologic abnormalities (32,33).

Myelodysplastic Syndrome Unclassified

Some patients with MDS present with morphologic features that cannot be classified readily in any of the proposed categories. These patients have no or minimal increase in blasts in the bone marrow and in most instances no blasts in the peripheral blood; in some a rare blast is identified in the peripheral blood (16). Dysplasia, which may be slight or marked, affects a single lineage, in contrast to refractory cytopenia, with multilineage dysplasia. There may be cytopenia of one or more cell lines, including pancytopenia. Because of the lack of categorizing features for other types of MDS, these cases can be designated as MDS unclassified. Some observers might classify some of these cases descriptively according to the major hematologic finding: that is, refractory anemia, refractory neutropenia, or refractory thrombocytopenia. Some patients, however, present with one of these findings without definitive morphologic evidence of dysplasia; the use of myelodysplasia should be restricted to those patients with convincing morphologic evidence of dysplasia.

The unclassified category also may be used for a type of MDS that presents with marked anemia with or without

A

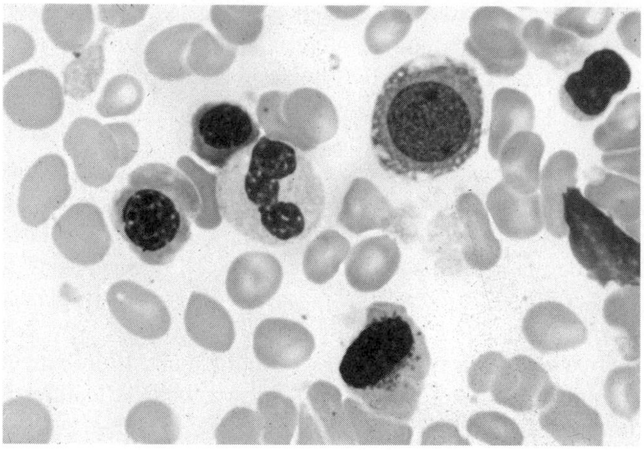

B

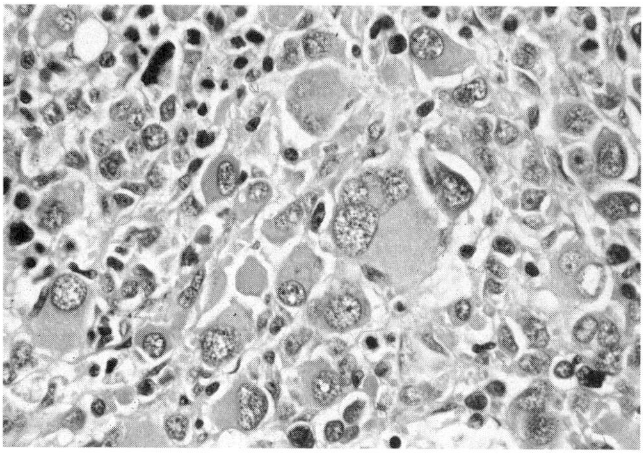

FIG. 48.23. **A:** Bone marrow smear from a 38-year-old male with refractory cytopenia with multilineage dysplasia. A basophilic erythroblast with a megaloblastic nucleus and cytoplasmic vacuoles and a polychromatic ringed sideroblast are present. The blasts were less than 2%. Cytogenetic analysis of this specimen showed complex abnormalities, including deletion of chromosomes 5 and 7 (Wright-Giemsa stain, original magnification: 400× magnification). **B:** Bone marrow biopsy from the same specimen as illustrated in **A**. There is a marked increase in megakaryocytes with dysplastic features, including small size and hypolobulated nuclei (hematoxylin and eosin stain, original magnification: 240× magnification). See Color Plate 83, between pp. 1446–1447.

thrombocytopenia and neutropenia and marked erythroid hyperplasia with marked dyserythropoiesis without an increase in blasts and no evident dysplasia in the neutrophils; the megakaryocytes may or may not show evidence of dysplasia. Such cases have some features of acute myeloid leukemia M6B, pure erythroid malignancy, but the numbers of proerythroblasts and basophilic erythroblasts are less than requisite for that diagnosis. These cases frequently are associated with clonal cytogenetic abnormalities involving chromosome 5 or 7 and may have an aggressive clinical course. The classification of this process is often difficult, because the distinction between acute myeloid leukemia M6 and MDS unclassified or refractory cytopenia with multilineage dysplasia is somewhat arbitrary. The diagnosis of an MDS in these cases rather than acute myeloid leukemia does not preclude aggressive clinical management; this decision must be based on several factors including the age of the patient, degree of marrow failure, and cytogenetic findings.

Some patients present with cytopenias without morphologic evidence of dysplasia but with clonal chromosome abnormalities. If the cytogenetic findings have an established relationship with an MDS, it is appropriate to view the process as MDS unclassified. This approach emphasizes the critical importance of clinical, morphologic, and cytogenetic assessment of MDSs (Fig. 48.11).

CYTOGENETICS

Cytogenetic studies are an essential part of the evaluation of patients with MDS (26,33–41). These studies serve several purposes, including prognosis, the identification of clonality in equivocal cases, and the identification of clinical, morphologic, and cytogenetic syndromes such as the isolated 5q syndrome (33,42–45).

In the International Scoring System for Evaluating Prognosis in Myelodysplastic Syndromes, three prognostic cytogenetic groups are recognized: *good*, with normal chromosomes, 5q− only, or 20q− only; *poor*, with complex chromosome abnormalities (at least three) or chromosome 7 anomalies; and *intermediate*, with other abnormalities (26).

The specific cytogenetic abnormalities in the primary MDSs do not generally have a one-to-one relationship to specific morphologic subtypes. There are some cytogenetic abnormalities, however, that appear to be associated with relatively well-defined morphologic clinical syndromes; these include the isolated 5q− syndrome, monosomy 7 syndrome of childhood, del(17p), and MDS associated with inversion of chromosome 3 (33,43–59). Del(20q) appears to be associated with abnormalities of the megakaryocyte and erythroid lineages (34).

5q− Syndrome

The isolated 5q− syndrome is a *de novo* MDS associated with an interstitial deletion of the long arm of chromosome 5, involving bands q12 through q32 as the sole chromosome abnormality (32,33,42–44). This is an uncommon disorder that occurs in adults, with a female predominance. The blood and bone marrow findings usually are those of refractory anemia, RAEB, or refractory cytopenia with multilineage dysplasia. The clinical course frequently is prolonged; evolution to acute leukemia may occur and usually is accompanied by the occurrence of additional chromosome abnormalities (32,33,42).

The principal hematologic finding is a macrocytic anemia that is moderate to severe; the patient may be transfusion-dependent. The leukocyte count is normal to slightly increased; platelet counts are generally normal to increased (Fig. 48.24). The bone marrow has decreased to normal numbers of erythroid precursors and dysplastic changes in granu-

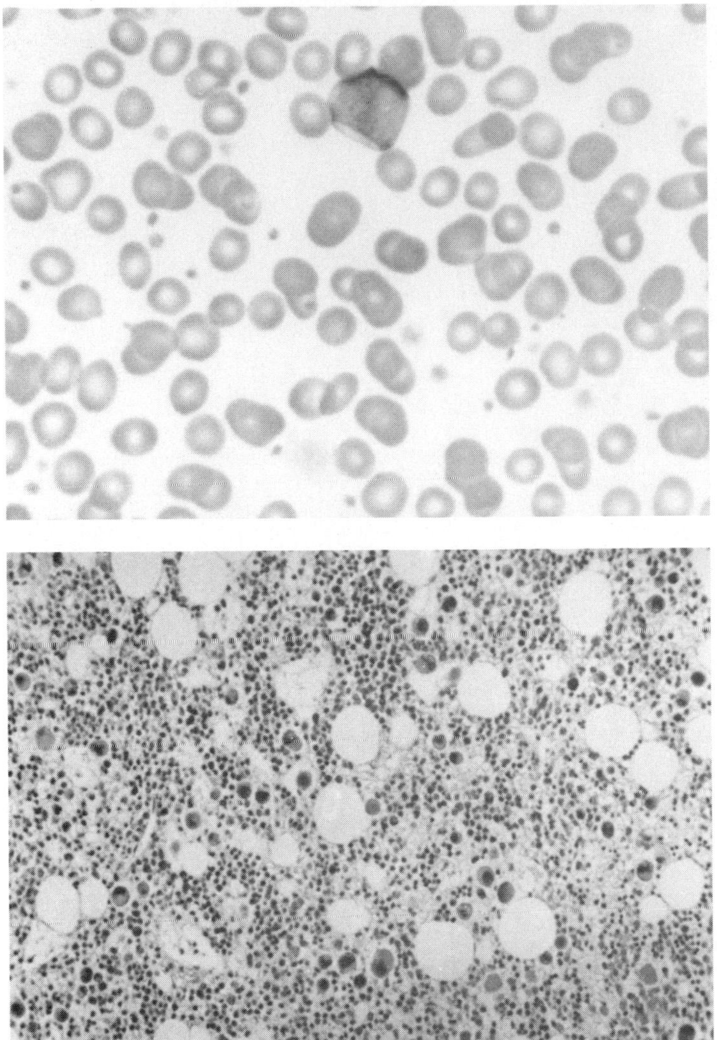

A B C

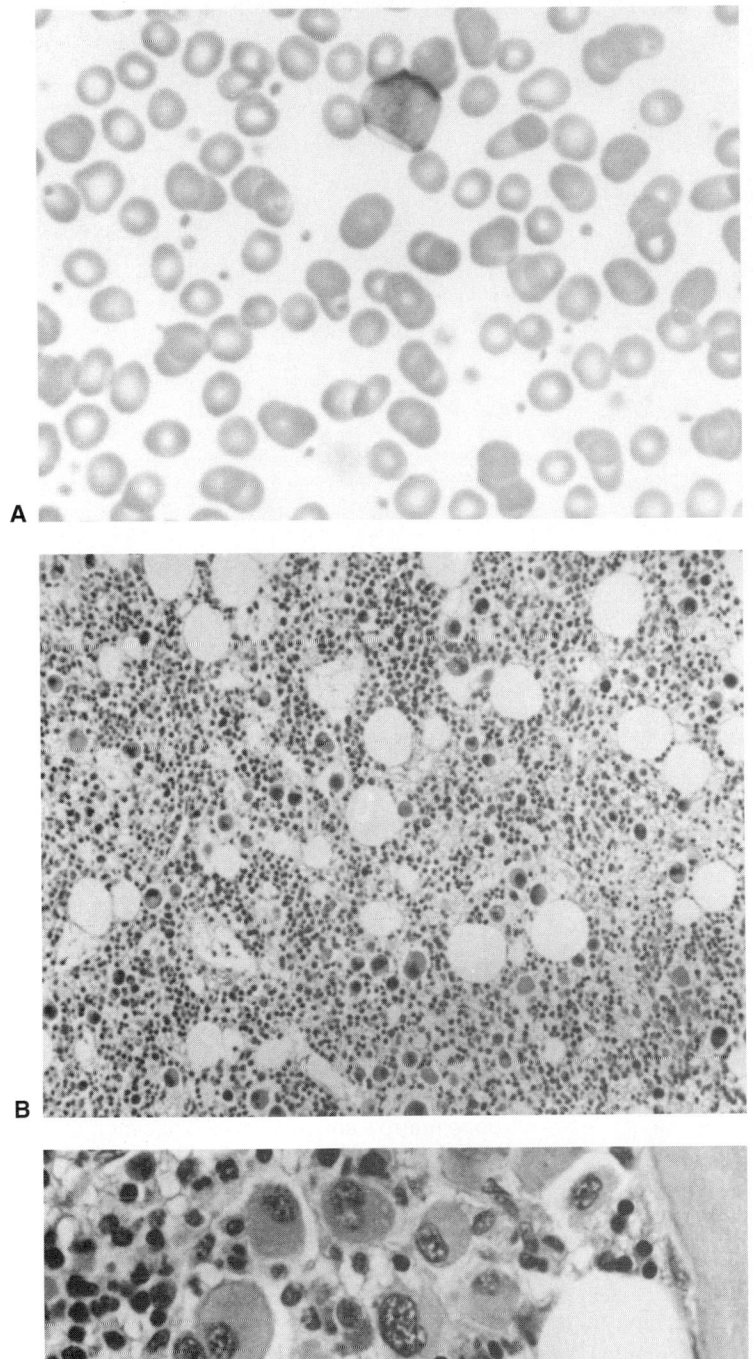

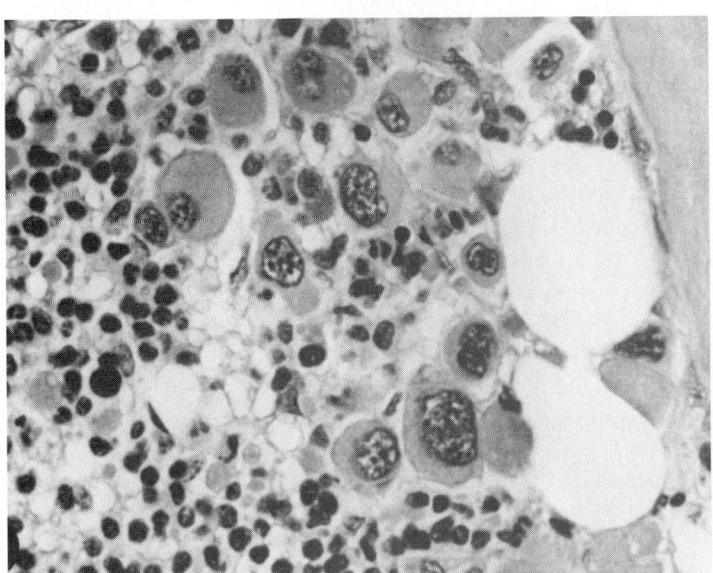

FIG. 48.24. A: Blood smear from a 52-year-old woman who has refractory anemia with excess blasts, type 2, associated with an isolated 5q − chromosome abnormality. The red blood cells are slightly macrocytic, and there is a thrombocytosis. Several myeloblasts similar to the one in this field were present in the blood (Wright-Giemsa stain, original magnification: 256× magnification). **B:** Bone marrow section from the specimen illustrated in **A** showing numerous megakaryocytes (hematoxylin and eosin stain, original magnification: 40× magnification). **C:** High-magnification view of the specimen in **B** showing megakaryocytes with hypolobulated and nonlobulated nuclei; several of the megakaryocytes are smaller than normal (hematoxylin and eosin stain, original magnification: 256× magnification).

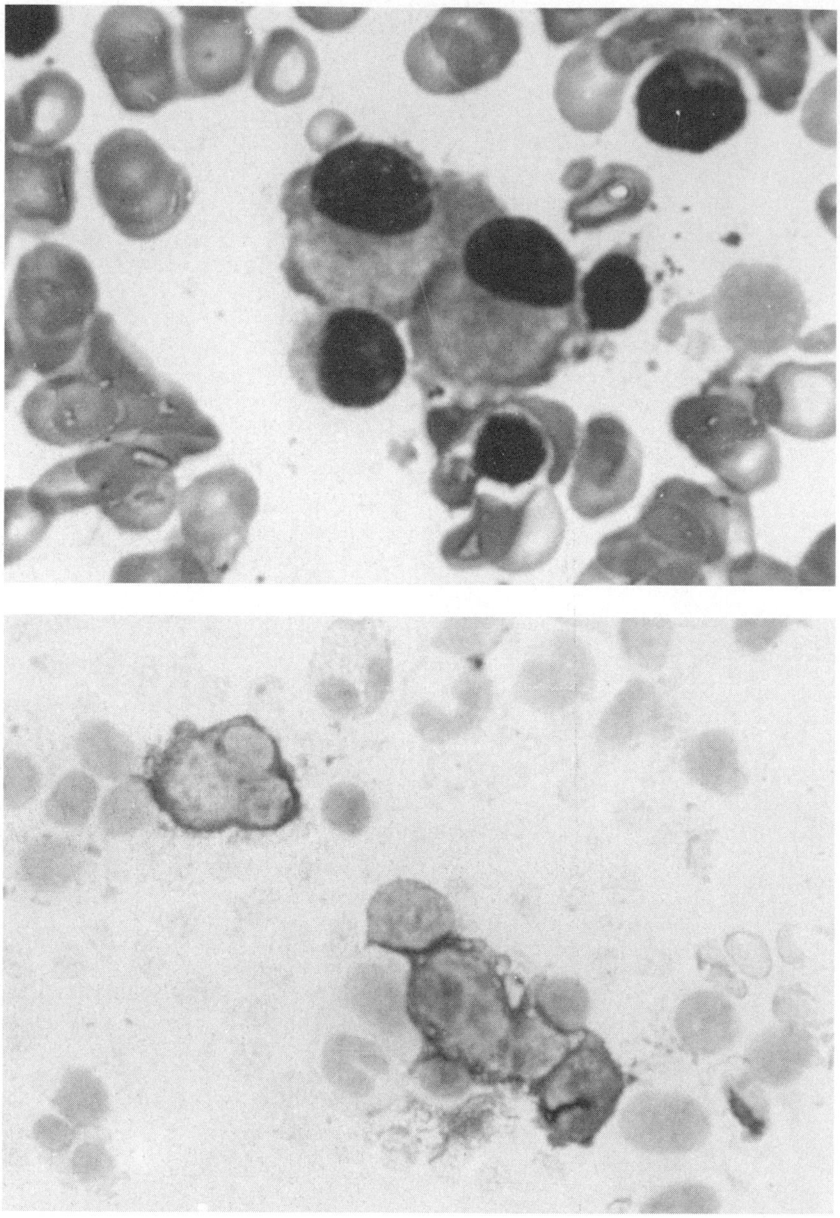

A

B

FIG. 48.25. A: Bone marrow smear from a patient who has refractory anemia with excess blasts, type 1, and an isolated 5q− chromosome abnormality; there are three small micromegakaryocytes with hypolobated nuclei (Wright-Giemsa stain, original magnification: 400× magnification). **B:** Immunoalkaline phosphatase reaction of an antibody to platelet glycoprotein IIIa on a bone marrow smear from the specimen illustrated in **A**. Numerous positively reacting megakaryocytes are present (APAAP, original magnification: 256× magnification).

locytes; myeloblasts may be increased. One of the most prominent features is the presence of an increased number of megakaryocytes, many of which have nonlobulated nuclei (Fig. 48.25). The bone marrow biopsy shows varying degrees of cellularity and reflects the bone marrow smear: Usually, hypoplasia of the erythroid precursors is present. The number of megakaryocytes is increased, and many are smaller than normal with a high percentage with nonlobulated nuclei (Fig. 48.24). In some patients, however, the megakaryocyties show normally lobulated nuclei. There are frequently scattered infiltrates of well-differentiated lymphocytes and plasma cells. Splenomegaly may be observed.

Del(17)

The 17p deletion is associated with cases of acute myeloid leukemia and MDSs that frequently have a particular type of dysgranulopoiesis characterized by small neutrophils with pseudo–Pelger-Huet nuclei and cytoplasmic vacuoles; the nuclei of the mature neutrophils frequently are completely nonlobulated (18,19,45–47) (Fig. 48.4). This constellation of cytogenetic and morphologic findings is accompanied by a high incidence of *P53* mutation and an unfavorable prognosis (46). The del(17p) usually is associated with an unbalance translocation, frequently involving chromosome 5. Approximately half of the patients with del(17p) have a therapy-related process.

Inv(3)(q21-26)

Myelodysplastic syndrome and acute myeloid leukemia with normal to elevated platelet counts have been reported in association with abnormalities of chromosome 3 (48–51). The chromosome abnormalities include a paracentric inv(3q), t(3;3) with breakpoints in q21-26, and ins(5;3). Additional cytogenetic abnormalities frequently are observed, particularly involving chromosomes 5 and 7 (51). The associated findings in these patients usually include increased megakaryocytes with disordered megakaryocytopoiesis, including small megakaryocytes with hypolobulated nuclei. The MDS classification includes RAEB and RARS. The cases of acute leukemia frequently involve more than one myeloid cell line with prominent megakaryocyte proliferation. Patients with acute myeloid leukemia and MDS associated with these abnormalities appear to have an increased incidence of prior exposure to mutagenic or carcinogenic agents. The cytogenetic finding generally is associated with an unfavorable clinical course.

Monosomy 7 Syndrome of Childhood

Monosomy 7 syndrome of childhood as originally described is a myeloid malignancy with morphologic features of MDS associated with an isolated monosomy 7 (10,11,52–59). The syndrome is a rare disorder and constitutes less than 1% of myeloid hematologic malignancies in childhood. The age of presentation ranges from 6 months to 8 years; the median age is 10 months. Some observers restrict the syndrome designation to patients younger than 4 years of age. There is a male predominance, and the disease has been observed in siblings (55). An association of monosomy 7 syndrome and neurofibromatosis type 1, predominantly in young males, has been reported (54).

The patients present with anemia and leukocytosis. Fifty percent of patients are thrombocytopenic. The major clinical findings are a history of recurrent infections and hepatosplenomegaly; lymphadenopathy sometimes is present. The fetal hemoglobin concentration usually is normal but may be slightly elevated; in occasional patients there is a marked elevation in fetal hemoglobin levels. Neutrophil function studies show defective chemotaxis. Chromosome studies show a loss of one chromosome 7 as the only abnormality.

There is a monocytosis and leukoerythroblastosis in the blood. Dysplastic changes may be present in the neutrophils and monocytes. The prevalence of blasts in the blood usually is less than 2% (10,11). The bone marrow shows a slight increase in blasts in most patients; a range of 3% to 11% with a mean of 6% is reported in one series (Fig. 48.26; see also Color Plate 84, between pp. 1446–1447). Dysplastic changes are present in the erythroid cells, granulocytes, and monocytes in approximately 50% of patients. The megakaryocytes usually are morphologically normal but are reduced in number in slightly more than 50% of patients. The bone marrow cellularity in biopsy sections is increased in the majority of patients (Fig. 48.27). In some, the bone marrow is hypocellular with patchy areas of acellular, loosely structured marrow (Fig. 48.28; see also Color Plate 85, between pp. 1446–1447). Slight reticulin fibrosis may be present.

Isolated monosomy 7 may occur with a clinically and morphologically diverse group of *de novo* MDSs and acute

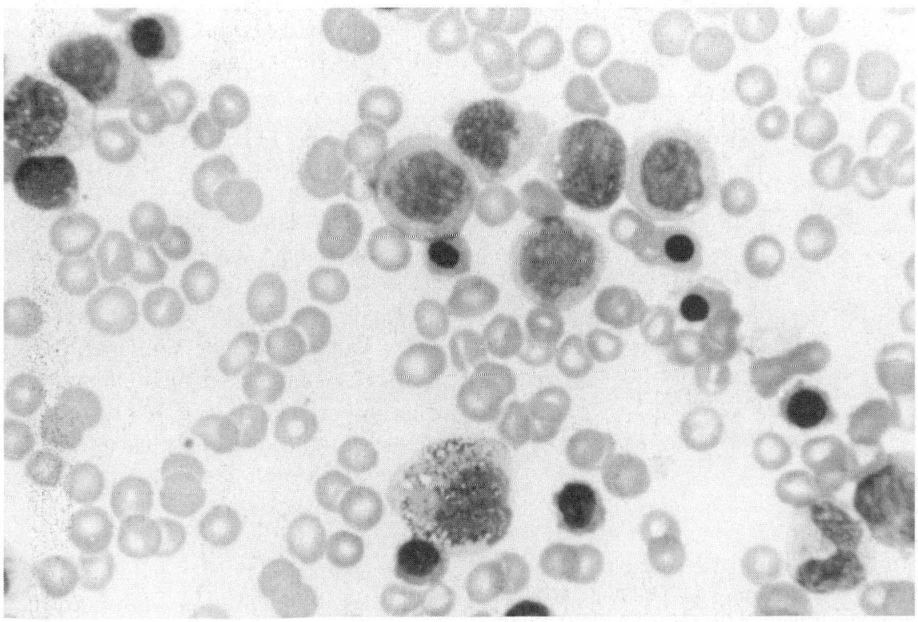

FIG. 48.26. Bone marrow smear from a 3.5-year-old boy who has a myelodysplastic syndrome associated with an isolated 7− chromosome abnormality. There are scattered monocytes and neutrophil precursors (Wright-Giemsa stain, original magnification: 256× magnification). See Color Plate 84, between pp. 1446–1447.

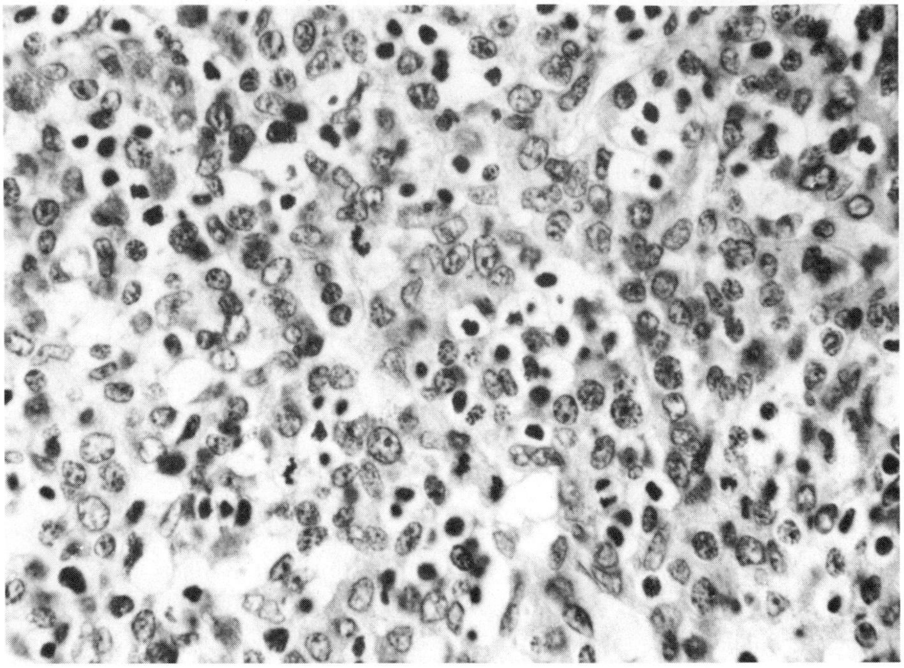

FIG. 48.27. Bone marrow biopsy specimen from the patient in Figure 48.26. The marrow is markedly hypercellular, with increased numbers of immature granulocytes and monocytes. Numerous erythrocyte precursors are present. Occasional mitotic erythroblasts are present; megakaryocytes are reduced (hematoxylin and eosin stain, original magnification: 256× magnification).

myeloid leukemia in children of all ages, and the recognition of an entity distinct from juvenile myelomonocytic leukemia, based on the cytogenetic finding, has been questioned (53,55). The entity described as monosomy 7 syndrome of childhood shares many clinical and hematologic features with juvenile myelomonocytic leukemia; the distinction may not be possible from morphologic findings, and whether these conditions are different points on the spectrum of one entity is not resolved completely (55) (see Chapter 49).

The major differential diagnosis of the isolated monosomy 7 syndrome of childhood is juvenile myelomonocytic leukemia, previously referred to as *juvenile chronic myeloid leukemia*, which is discussed in the chapter on myeloproliferative disorders (see Chapter 49). In some patients, the distinction between these two disorders may not be possible from the morphologic findings.

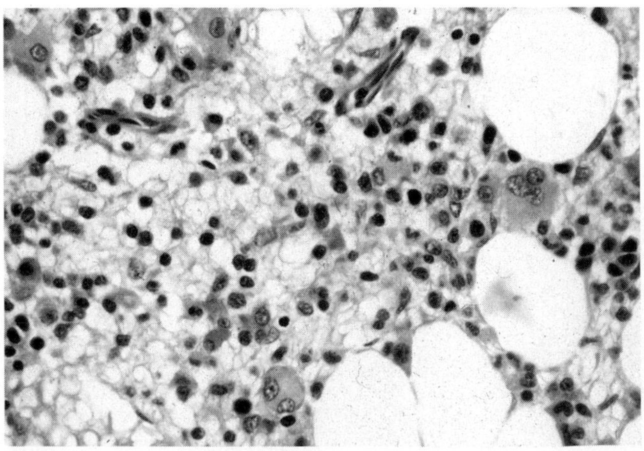

FIG. 48.28. Bone marrow biopsy from a 2-year-old male with a myelodysplastic syndrome associated with an isolated monosomy 7 cytogenetic abnormality. The marrow interstitium shows marked cellular depletion (hematoxylin and eosin stain, original magnification: 240× magnification). See Color Plate 85, between pp. 1446–1447.

DIFFERENTIAL DIAGNOSIS OF MYELODYSPLASTIC SYNDROMES

It is important that the diagnosis of an MDS not be established without knowledge of the patient's clinical history; exposure to drugs, alcohol, or heavy metals can lead to morphologic changes in one or more myeloid cell lines, and these changes may be similar to those observed in MDSs (60). Hematologic examination must include careful evaluation of peripheral blood and bone marrow smears and sections. Chromosome analysis has a crucial role. In patients in whom the morphologic findings are equivocal, cytogenetic studies may be definitive in establishing evidence of a clonal abnormality.

For purposes of differential diagnosis, the MDSs may be considered as two groups: the disorders characterized primarily by morphologic changes without an increase in blasts—refractory anemia, RARS, refractory cytopenia with multilineage dysplasia, MDS unclassified—and the disorders accompanied by an increase in blasts or the presence of Auer rods, RAEB-1 and RAEB-2.

Patients with refractory anemia, RARS, and MDS unclassified may present with hematologic abnormalities similar to those found in patients who have nutritionally related anemias or anemias that result from exposure to toxins. The most important consideration in these processes is megaloblastic anemia caused by vitamin B12 or folate deficiency; red blood cell, serum folate, and serum B12 levels must be assayed before a diagnosis is established. If the sufficiency of the level of any of these vitamins is equivocal, it is advisable to treat patients with the appropriate vitamin. Patients who have macrocytic anemia and neurologic findings suggestive of subacute combined degeneration should be treated with vitamin B12 regardless of serum levels. Patients who have RARS also should receive a therapeutic trial with pyridoxine.

Heavy metal intoxication, most notably arsenic intoxication, can lead to myelodysplastic changes, primarily in the erythroblasts but also in the neutrophils (61,62). Patients may present with pancytopenia, and the morphologic findings may suggest an MDS; nuclear lobulation and megaloblastoid nuclei may be prominent in the erythroid precursors (Fig. 48.29; see also Color Plate 86, between pp. 1446–1447). The red blood cells frequently show coarse basophilic stippling. Exposure to the offending agent may be occupational, accidental, or the result of homicidal intent.

Congenital dyserythropoietic anemia most commonly manifests in childhood but occasionally is recognized initially in the adult years (63) (Fig. 48.30; see also Color Plate 87, between pp. 1446–1447). The erythroid precursors in this group of disorders generally show marked morphologic alterations, including nuclear lobulation, megaloblastoid nuclei, nuclear gigantism, and multinucleation (63) (Figs. 48.30, 48.31; see also Color Plate 88, between pp. 1446–1447). The erythrocytes in the blood smear show varying degrees of anisopoikilocytosis, anisochromasia, and basophilic stippling. The anemia may be severe. The granulocytes and megakaryocytes are normal, and the platelet and leukocyte counts are in the normal range.

The red blood cell precursors in erythropoietic porphyria show subtle nuclear abnormalities that may be mistaken for an MDS.

The myeloid cells of patients who have AIDS may show dysplastic changes, including pseudo–Pelger-Huet nuclei in mature neutrophils, and dyserythropoiesis. Megakaryocytes with sparse cytoplasm or naked nuclei may be prominent in bone marrow sections. The dysplastic changes may occur in the absence of drug therapy (64–66). The cause of these changes is unknown; acute myeloid leukemia has been reported in association with AIDS (65) (see Chapter 28).

Parvovirus B19 infection is associated with erythroblastopenia, with a ''maturation arrest'' of the erythroid precursors at the pronormoblast–basophilic normoblast stage of maturation and giant erythroblasts that may resemble changes found in MDS (67,68) (Fig. 48.32; see also Color Plate 89,

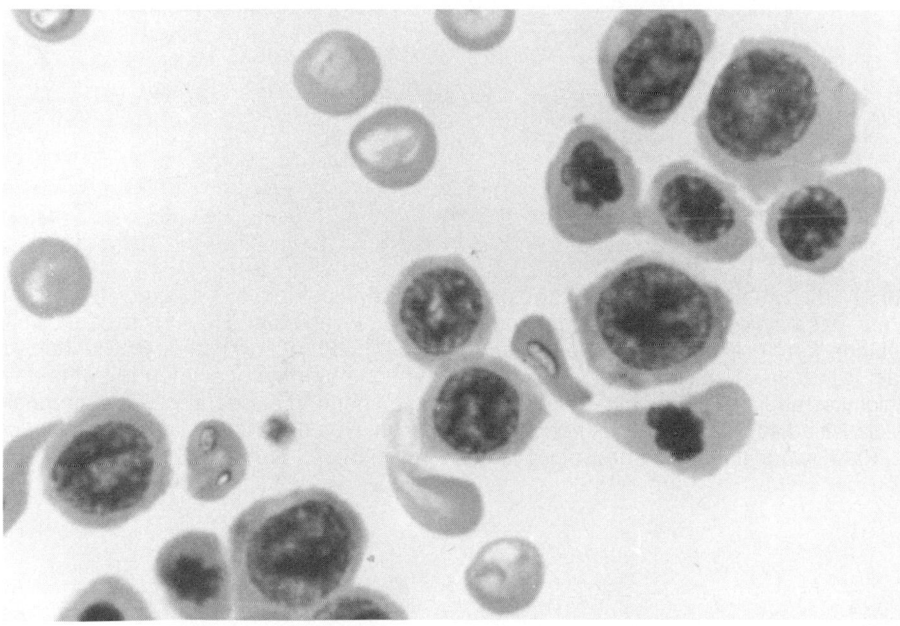

FIG. 48.29. Bone marrow smear from a 42-year-old man admitted to hospital with a depressed sensorium and pancytopenia. The red blood cell precursors show marked dysplastic changes, including megaloblastoid nuclear chromatin and nuclear hyperlobulation and karyorrhexis. The cells were slightly positive on periodic acid–Schiff staining. Five days after this specimen was obtained, the patient's spouse admitted lacing his evening meals with arsenic. The patient was treated with dimercaprol and recovered completely (Wright-Giemsa stain, original magnification: 400× magnification). See Color Plate 86, between pp. 1446–1447.

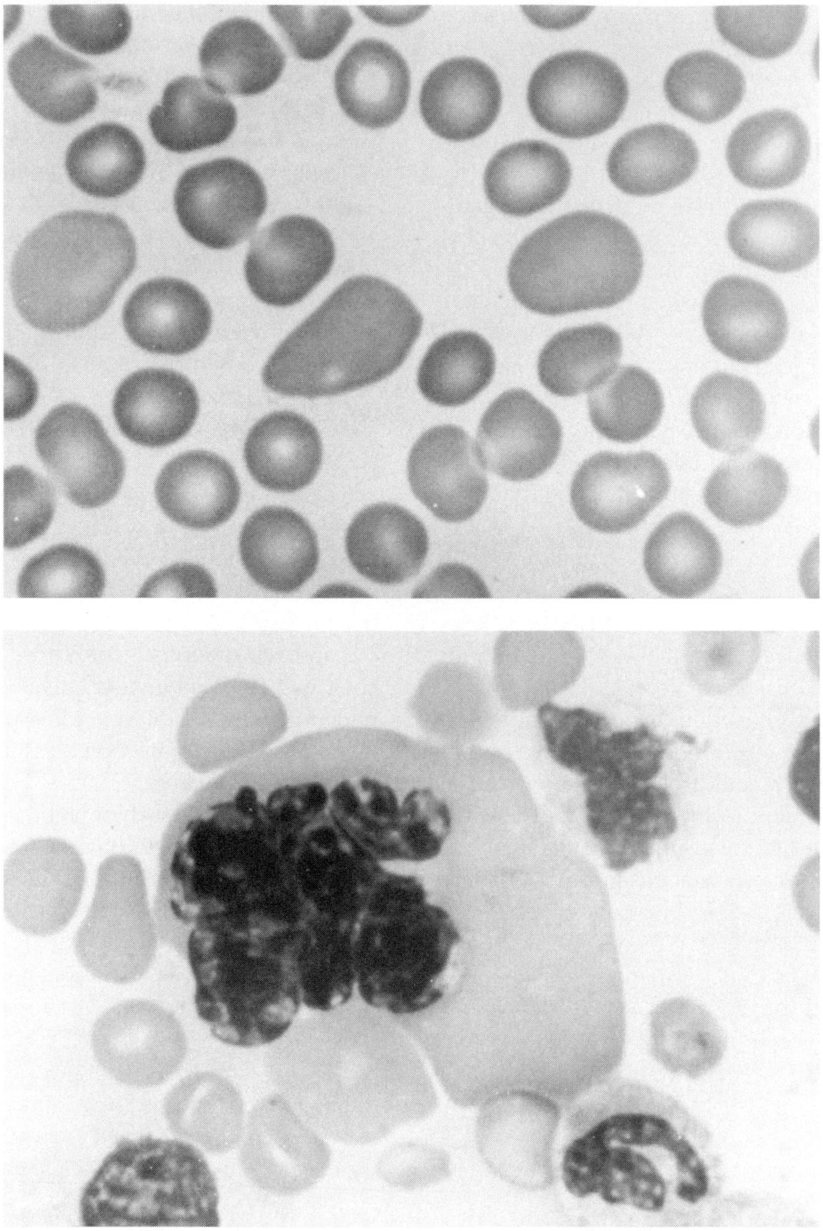

A

B

FIG. 48.30. **A:** Blood smear from a 22-year-old man with a hemoglobin of 13.7 g/dL and a slight reticulocytosis. Very macrocytic red blood cells are noted. The platelet count and leukocyte count were normal. Similar findings were present in the blood smear of his 14-month-old daughter. **B:** Giant polychromatic erythroblast with marked nuclear hyperlobulation in the bone marrow specimen from the patient in **A**. The granulocytes and megakaryocytes were normal in number and appearance. The morphologic findings were classified as congenital dyserythropoietic anemia, type III (Wright-Giemsa stain, original magnification: 400× magnification). See Color Plate 87, between pp. 1446–1447.

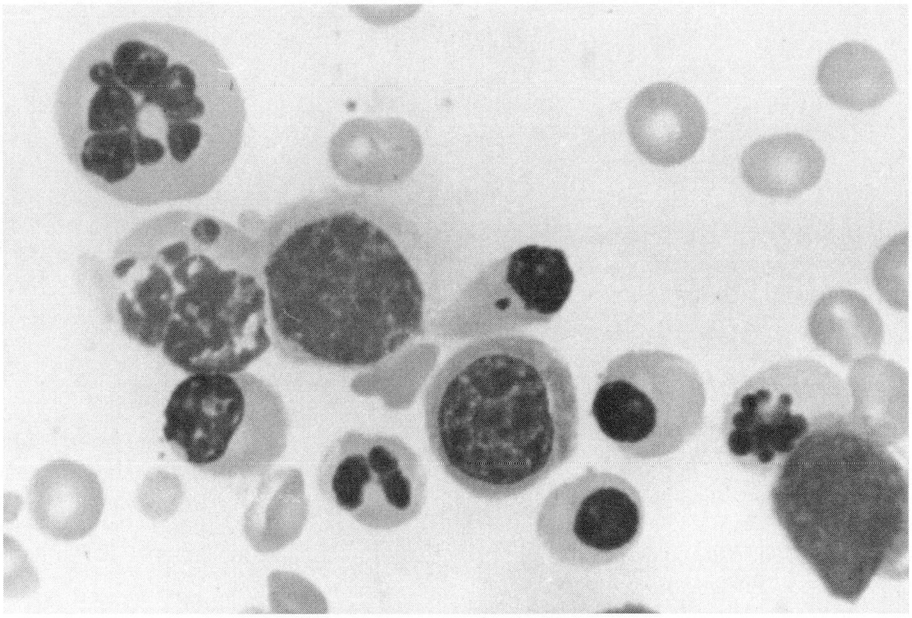

FIG. 48.31. Bone marrow from an 11-month-old boy with congenital dyserythropoietic anemia. The red blood cell precursors show marked dysplastic changes, including hyperlobulation, megaloblastoid chromatin, and karyorrhexis. The serologic and morphologic studies were not definitive for a specific subtype of congenital dyserythropoietic anemia (Wright-Giemsa stain, original magnification: 400× magnification). See Color Plate 88, between pp. 1446–1447.

between pp. 1446–1447). Although MDS occasionally may manifest with erythroblastopenia, it is not generally associated with giant erythroblasts. Serologic or molecular studies for parvovirus B19 infection usually resolves the problem. Most patients with parvovirus B19 infection undergo spontaneous recovery in a few weeks; persistent infection in immunocompromised patients occurs occasionally. DNA analysis is the most reliable method for detecting parvovirus in this group of patients.

Some of the changes that occur with granulocyte-macrophage colony-stimulating factor are virtually indistinguishable from findings that occur in the MDSs; the most notable are the presence of blasts in the peripheral blood and neutrophil nuclear hypolobation or pseudo–Pelger-Huet nuclei (69). The blast percentage in the peripheral blood may reach levels as high as 10% to 15%, and neutrophils with pseudo–Pelger-Huet nuclei may be very numerous (Fig. 48.33; see also Color Plate 90, between pp. 1446–1447). These changes are accompanied by intense azurophilic granulation and numerous Dohle bodies that are suggestive of an inflammatory reaction. These findings may persist for several days following cessation of growth factor administration. The combination of findings, in conjunction with a history of growth factor administration, should minimize the difficulty in distinguishing these changes from a myelodysplastic process.

The differential diagnosis of RAEB-2 primarily relates to M2, M4, or M6 acute myeloid leukemia. The blast percent-

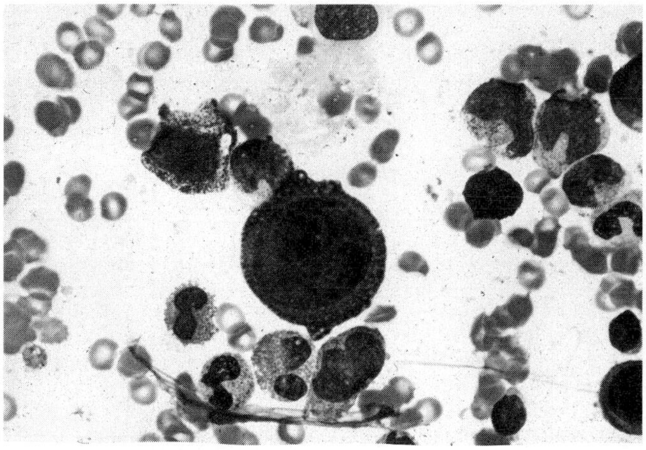

FIG. 48.32. Giant erythroblast in a marrow smear from a 17-year-old male with parvovirus B19 infection. The cytoplasm contains numerous very small vacuoles (Wright-Giemsa stain, original magnification: 400× magnification). See Color Plate 89, between pp. 1446–1447.

A 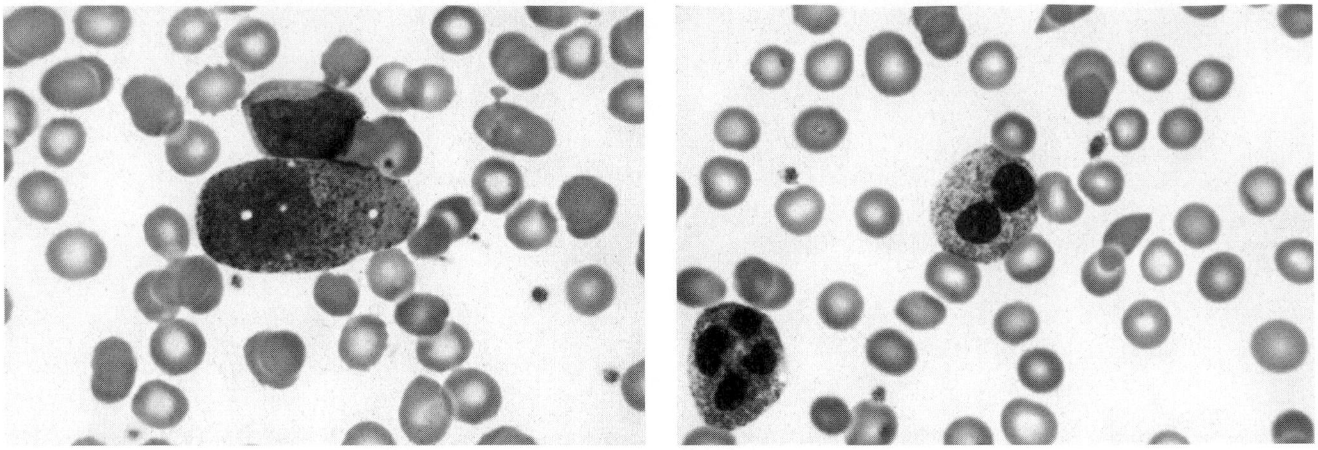 B

FIG. 48.33. Blood smear from a 7-year-old male being treated with granulocyte colony stimulating factor following bone marrow transplantation. **A:** A myeloblast and a very large promyelocyte with markedly increased azurophilic granulation. **B:** A mature neutrophil with a bilobed (pseudo–Pelger-Huet) nucleus and increased azurophilic granulation (Wright-Giemsa stain, original magnification: 640× magnification). See Color Plate 90, between pp. 1446–1447.

age is the defining criterion. If a patient presents with a marrow blast percentage of 10% to 20% and a chromosome abnormality relatively specific to a morphologic type of AML such as t(8;21) or inv(16), it is appropriate to classify the condition as M2 or M4EO acute myeloid leukemia, respectively, if the morphologic findings are consistent with the classification.

EVOLUTION AND PROGNOSIS

The biologic course of the MDSs usually is marked by progressive bone marrow failure with increasing cytopenias or evolution to acute myeloid leukemia (26,70–88). The potential for these events varies with the different types of MDS (Table 48.3). Generally, two types of MDS that are not characterized by an increase in blasts, refractory anemia and RARS, have a low incidence of evolution to acute leukemia and a longer duration of survival than those disorders with increased blasts (26). RAEB-1 and RAEB-2, particularly RAEB-2, are high-grade MDSs, with a high percentage of cases evolving to acute leukemia and short duration of survival. Refractory cytopenia with multilineage dysplasia appears to be intermediate in prognosis (17). The results of the International MDS Risk Analysis Workshop showed median durations of survival of 2.1 years for patients with 5% to 10% marrow blasts and 0.7 years for patients with 11% to 20% marrow blasts (26).

Several scoring systems have been proposed to predict survival and potential for evolution to acute leukemia in the MDSs; these generally are based on blast percentage and degree of cytopenia (75,85,86,89). A study encompassing cytogenetic, morphologic, and clinical data collated from seven studies and evaluated by an International MDS Risk Analysis Workshop identified three major factors impacting risk of evolution to acute myeloid leukemia and survival: type of cytogenetic abnormality, percentage of myeloblasts in marrow, and number of cytopenias. The duration of survival was related to these three variables, and age and gender of the patient (26). As previously noted, three cytogenetic risk groups were identified: poor, intermediate, and good. The median durations of survival for the three groups were 0.8, 3.8, and 2.4 years, respectively.

Based on multivariate analysis of the data evaluated by the workshop, the most significant independent variables for predicting outcome were bone marrow blast percentage, number of cytopenias, cytogenetic subgroup, and age and gender of the patient.

Based on the blast percentage, number of cytopenias, and

TABLE 48.3. *Survival and evolution to acute myeloid leukemia in the myelodysplastic syndromes (original FAB classification) (37)*

Type	Patients, %	Survival range (median), months	Progression to leukemia, %
Refractory anemia	28	18–64 (50)	12
Refractory anemia with ringed sideroblasts	24	14–76+ (51)	8
Refractory anemia with excess of blasts	23	7–16 (11)	44
Refractory anemia with excess of blasts in transformation	16	2.5–11 (5)	60
Chronic myelomonocytic leukemia	9	9–60+ (11)	14

risk scores for the cytogenetic subgroups, four major risk groups for survival and acute myeloid leukemia evolution were proposed: low, intermediate 1, intermediate 2, and high. Patients with complex cytogenetic abnormalities, higher marrow blast percentage, and more cytopenias are at higher risk of evolution to acute leukemia and have a shorter duration of survival then patients in the good cytogenetic risk group, with low marrow blast percentage and less severe cytopenias. These studies emphasize the importance of a multifactorial approach to the prognostic assessment of patients with MDS.

THERAPY

In a discussion of the management of patients who have MDS, it is important to recognize the differences in the biologic course of the different types of the disease (Table 48.3). Patients who have refractory anemia and RARS generally have relatively stable clinical courses for a prolonged period with a low incidence of transformation to acute leukemia (26). Most patients who have RAEB-1 and RAEB-2 have rapidly progressive marrow failure with a high incidence of leukemic evolution; refractory cytopenia with multilineage dysplasia is intermediate. This biologic diversity of the primary MDSs and the occurrence primarily in middle aged and older persons preclude generalizations about therapeutic approaches. The lower-grade MDSs with less potential for transformation to acute leukemia may be managed satisfactorily with supportive therapy if indicated; the use of a biologic response modifier such as granulocyte-macrophage colony-stimulating factor may be efficacious in some patients who have neutropenia. The use of growth-stimulating factors in patients who have increased blast percentages is more problematic, however, because of the potential to stimulate blast proliferation. Older persons are at greater risk for injury or death with aggressive antileukemia therapy, and this approach in these patients must be used with considerable caution.

Combined therapy with topotecan and cytarabine has been shown to be effective in inducing complete remission in patients with primary or therapy-related RAEB or refractory anemia with excess of blasts in transformation, including patients in whom the cytogenetic findings were associated with a poor prognosis; similar results were observed in patients with chronic myelomonocytic leukemia (89).

Preliminary studies with 72-hour continuous infusion of a low dosage (beginning with 50 mg/m^2/d) of 5-aza-2′-deoxycytidine in elderly patients with high-risk MDS, have shown a response in some patients. The major toxicity was myelosuppression with prolonged cytopenias, resulting in a 17% fatality rate (90).

The management of the MDS must be considered carefully, with the important factors including age, overall physical condition, and the presence or absence of the discussed risk factors.

SUMMARY AND CONCLUSIONS

The MDSs are a group of disorders characterized by abnormalities in maturation of one or more myeloid cell lines with or without an increase in blasts; the blast percentage, if increased, is less than the 20% requisite for a diagnosis of acute myeloid leukemia. The MDSs occur as primary or *de novo* processes and as secondary or therapy-related disorders in persons previously treated with chemotherapy or radiotherapy.

The diagnosis and classification of the MDSs are based on peripheral blood and bone marrow findings. The importance of careful examination of blood and marrow specimens in patients suspected of having an MDS cannot be overemphasized. The changes in these disorders often are subtle and may be overlooked with poorly prepared specimens. In addition, improperly prepared specimens from patients who do not have an MDS may exhibit technical artifacts in blood cells, particularly granulocytes, which resemble the findings in the MDS.

Cytogenetic studies are essential to the evaluation of patients with MDS and should be performed in any suspected case. Clonal abnormalities are evidence for the diagnosis in morphologically equivocal cases; the type of abnormality may have substantial prognostic significance. Specific cytogenetic clinical pathologic subtypes such as isolated 5q− or 17p− syndrome will be increasingly recognized.

Cytochemical stains are of limited value and must be interpreted carefully. A decreased neutrophil alkaline phosphatase is strong evidence for a myeloid disorder. A normal or increased neutrophil alkaline phosphatase is not exclusionary for a diagnosis of MDS. Reaction patterns with myeloperoxidase and Sudan black B staining assume importance if a substantial number of neutrophils and precursors is nonreactive.

Morphologic abnormalities of the myeloid cells that resemble the changes in the MDSs may be observed in nutritionally based anemias and congenital dyserythropoietic anemias and may be results of exposure to toxins and drugs. These possibilities should be considered before establishing a diagnosis of MDS, particularly refractory anemia and RARS (79).

The primary MDSs are a biologically heterogenous group of disorders with marked variation in clinical evolution. Refractory anemia and RARS are relatively benign disorders in the majority of patients, with a prolonged clinical course and low incidence of evolution to acute leukemia. RAEB and refractory cytopenia with multilineage dysplasia are variable in clinical evolution, with relatively short median durations of survival.

The MDSs related to therapy with alkylating agents and acute leukemias are panmyelopathies in most instances. The clinical course is marked by rapidly progressive marrow failure in the majority of patients. This hematologic deterioration occurs with the findings of MDS or acute myeloid leukemia. Therapy-related MDS and acute myeloid leukemia each have a high incidence of clonal abnormalities that involve chromosomes 5 and 7, monosomy 5 or 5q −, and monosomy 7 or 7q −. The disorders related to topoisomerase II inhibitor frequently involve chromosome 11 at band q23 but also may manifest as M2 acute myeloid leukemia with the translocation t(8;21), M4EO with inv(16), and acute promyelocytic leukemia.

REFERENCES

1. Bennett JM, Catovsky D, Daniel MT, et al. Proposals for the classification of the acute leukaemias. *Br J Haematol* 1976;33:451–458.
2. Bennett JM, Catovsky D, Daniel MT, et al. Proposals for the classification of the myelodysplastic syndromes. *Br J Haematol* 1982;51:189–199.
3. Bennett JM, Catovsky D, Daniel MT, et al. Proposed revised criteria for the classification of acute myeloid leukemia. *Ann Intern Med* 1985;103:626–629.
4. Dreyfus B. Preleukemic states: I. Definition and classification. II. Refractory anemia with excess of myeloblasts in the bone marrow (smouldering acute leukemia). *Blood Cells* 1976;2:33–45.
5. Foucar K, McKenna RW, Bloomfield CD, et al. Therapy related leukemia, a panmyelosis. *Cancer* 1979;43:1285–1296.
6. Kantarjian HM, Keating MJ, Walters RS, et al. Therapy-related leukemia and myelodysplastic syndrome: clinical, cytogenetic and prognostic features. *J Clin Oncol* 1986;12:1748–1757.
7. LeBeau MM, Albain KS, Larsen RA, et al. Clinical and cytogenetic correlations in 63 patients with therapy-related myelodysplastic syndromes and acute nonlymphocytic leukemia: further evidence for characteristic abnormalities of chromosomes no. 5 and 7. *J Clin Oncol* 1986;4:325–345.
8. Michels SD, McKenna RW, Arthur DC, et al. Therapy related acute myeloid leukemia and myelodysplastic syndrome: a clinical and morphologic study of 65 cases. *Blood* 1985;65:1364–1372.
9. Groupe Francais de Morphologie Hematologique: French Registry of acute leukemia and myelodysplastic syndromes: age distribution and hemogram analysis of the 4496 cases recorded during 1982-1983 and classified according to FAB criteria. *Cancer* 1987;60:1385–1394.
10. Sieff CA, Chessells JM, Harvey BAM, et al. Monosomy 7 in childhood: a myeloproliferative disorder. *Br J Haematol* 1981;49:235–249.
11. Evans JPM, Czepulkowski B, Gibbons B, et al. Childhood monosomy 7 revisited. *Br J Haematol* 1988;69:41–45.
12. Juneja SK, Imbert M, Joualt H, et al. Haematological features of primary myelodysplastic syndromes (PMDS) at initial presentation: a study of 118 cases. *J Clin Pathol* 1983;36:1129–1135.
13. Enright H, Jacob HS, Vercellotti G, et al. Paraneoplastic autoimmune phenomena in patients with myelodysplastic syndromes: response to immunosuppressive therapy. *Br J Haematol* 1995;91:403–408.
14. Koeffler HP. Introduction: myelodysplastic syndromes. *Semin Hematol* 1996;33:87–94.
15. Farhi CD. Myelodysplastic syndromes and acute myeloid leukemia: diagnostic criteria and pitfalls (review). *Pathol Ann* 1995;30:29–57.
16. Brunning RD, McKenna RW. Myelodysplastic syndromes. *In: Tumors of the bone marrow. Atlas of tumor pathology,* 3rd series, fasc 9. Washington, DC: Armed Forces Institute of Pathology, 1994: 143–194.
17. Rosati S, Mick R, Xu F, et al. Refractory cytopenia with multilineage dysplasia: further characterization of an "unclassifiable" myelodysplastic syndrome. *Leukemia* 1996;10:20–26.
18. Jary L, Mossafa H, Fourcase C, et al. The 17-p-syndrome: a distinct myelodysplastic syndrome entity? *Leuk Lymphoma* 1997;25:163–168.
19. Lai H, Preudhomme C, Zandecki M, et al. Myelodysplastic syndromes and acute myeloid leukemia with 17p deletion: an entity characterized by specific dysgranulopoiesis and a high incidence of P53 mutations. *Leukemia* 1995;9:370–381.
20. Juneja SK, Imbert M, Sigaux F, et al. Prevalence and distribution of ringed sideroblasts in primary myelodysplastic syndromes. *J Clin Pathol* 1983;36:566–569.
21. Brunning R. Proposed World Health Organization (WHO) classification of acute leukemia and myelodysplastic syndromes. *Mod Pathol* 1999;12:102.
22. Nand S, Godwin JE. Hypoplastic myelodysplastic syndrome. *Cancer* 1988;62:958–964.
23. Orazi A, Albiter M, Heerema NA, et al. Hypoplastic myelodysplastic syndrome can be distinguished from acquired aplastic anemia by CD34 and PCNA immunostaining of bone marrow biopsy specimens. *Am J Clin Pathol* 1997;107:268–274.
24. Yoshida Y, Oguma H, Maekawa T. Refractory myelodysplastic anaemias with hypocellular bone marrow. *J Clin Pathol* 1995;41: 763–767.
25. Gatterman N, Aul C, Schneider W. Two types of acquired idiopathic sideroblastic anaemia (AISA). *Br J Haematol* 1990;74:45–52.
26. Greenberg P, Cox C, Lebeau M, et al. International scoring system for evaluation prognosis in myelodysplastic syndromes. *Blood* 1997;89:2079–2088.
27. Jacobs RH, Cornbleet MA, Vardiman JW, et al. Prognostic implications of morphology and karyotype in primary myelodysplastic syndromes. *Blood* 1986;67:1765–1772.
28. Seymour JF, Estey EH. The contribution of Auer rods to the classification and prognosis of myelodysplastic syndromes. *Leuk Lymphoma* 1995;17:79–85.
29. Tricot G, De Wolf-Peeters C, Hendrickx B, et al. Bone marrow histology in myelodysplastic syndromes: 1. Histological findings in myelodysplastic syndromes and comparison with bone marrow smears. *Br J Haematol* 1984;57:423–430.
30. Tricot G, Vlietinck R, Boogaers MA, et al. Prognostic factors in the myelodysplastic syndromes: importance of initial data on peripheral blood counts, bone marrow cytology, trephine biopsy and chromosomal analysis. *Br J Haematol* 1985;60:19–32.
31. Matsuda A, Jinnai I, Yagasaki F, et al. Refractory anemia with severe dysplasia: clinical significance of morphological features in refractory anemia. *Leukemia* 1998;12:482–485.
32. Mathew P, Tefferi A, Dewald GW, et al. The 5q-syndrome: a single institution study of 43 consecutive cases. *Blood* 1993;81:1040–1045.
33. Tefferi A, Mathew P, Noel P. The 5q-syndrome: a scientific and clinical update. *Leuk Lymphoma* 1994;14:375–378.
34. Kurtin PJ, DeWald GW, Shields DJ, et al. Hematologic disorders associated with deletions of chromosome 20q-. *Am J Clin Pathol* 1996;106:680–688.
35. Suciu S, Kuse R, Weh H, et al. Results of chromosome studies and their relation to morphology, course, and prognosis in 120 patients with de novo myelodysplastic syndrome. *Cancer Genet Cytogenet* 1990;44:15–26.
36. Fenaux P, Morel P, LucLai J. Cytogenetics in myelodysplastic syndromes. *Semin Hematol* 1996;33:127–138.
37. Third MIC Cooperative Study Group. Recommendations for a morphologic, immunologic, and cytogenetic (MIC) working classification of the primary and therapy related myelodysplastic disorders. *Cancer Genet Cytogenet* 1988;32:1–10.
38. Yunis JJ, Brunning RD. Prognostic significance of chromosomal abnormalities in acute leukemias and myelodysplastic syndromes. *Clin Haematol* 1986;15:597–620.
39. Yunis JJ, Lobell M, Arnesen MA, et al. Refined chromosome study helps define prognostic subgroups in most patients with primary myelodysplastic syndrome and acute myelogenous leukaemia. *Br J Haematol* 1988;68:189–194.
40. Yunis JJ, Rydell RE, Oken MM, et al. Refined chromosome analysis as an independent prognostic indicator in de novo myelodysplastic syndromes. *Blood* 1986;67:1721–1730.
41. Jotterand M, Parlier V. Diagnostic and prognostic significance of cytogenetics in adult primary myelodysplastic syndromes. *Leuk Lymphoma* 1996;23:253–266.
42. Van den Berge H, Vermaelen K, Mecucci C, et al. The 5q-anomaly. *Cancer Genet Cytogenet* 1985;17:189–255.
43. Kerkhofs H, Hagemeijer A, Leeksma CHW, et al. The 5q-chromosome abnormality in haematological disorders: a collaborative study of 34 cases from the Netherlands. *Br J Haematol* 1982;52:365–381.
44. Sokal G, Michaux JL, Van Den Berghe H, et al. A new hematologic syndrome with a distinct karyotype: the 5q-chromosome. *Blood* 1975;46:519–533.
45. Soenen V, Preudhomme C, Roumier C, et al. 17p deletion in acute myeloid leukemia and myelodysplastic syndrome: analysis of breakpoints and deleted segments by fluorescence in situ. *Blood* 1998;91:1008–1015.
46. Lai H, Preudhomme C, Zandecki M, et al. Myelodysplastic syndromes and acute myeloid leukemia with 17p deletion: an entity characterized

by specific dysgranulopoiesis and a high incidence of p53 mutations. *Leukemia* 1995;9:370–381.
47. Sterkers Y, Preudhomme C, Lai J-L, et al. Acute myeloid leukemia and myelodysplastic syndromes following essential thrombocythemia treated with hydroxyurea: high proportion of cases with 17p deletion. *Blood* 1998;91:616–622.
48. Pintado T, Ferro MT, San Roman CL, et al. Clinical correlations of the 3q21;q26 cytogenetic anomaly: a leukemia or myelodysplastic syndrome with preserved or increased platelet production and lack of response to cytotoxic therapy. *Cancer* 1985;55:535–541.
49. Bitter MA, Neilly ME, LeBeau MM, et al. Rearrangements of chromosome 3 involving bands 3q21 and 3q26 are associated with normal or elevated platelet counts in acute nonlymphocytic leukemia. *Blood* 1985; 66:1362–1370.
50. Jenkins RB, Tefferi A, Solberg LA, et al. Acute leukemia with abnormal thrombopoiesis and inversions of chromosome 3. *Cancer Genet Cytogenet* 1989;39:167–179.
51. Fonatsch C, Gudat H, Lengfelder E, et al. Correlation of cytogenetic findings with clinical features in 18 patients with inv(3)(q21;q26) or t(3:3)(q21;q26). *Leukemia* 1994;8:1318–1326.
52. Baranger L, Baruchel A, Leverger G, et al. Monosomy-7 in childhood hemopoietic disorders. *Leukemia* 1990;4:345–349.
53. Hutter JJ, Hecht F, Kaiser-McCaw B, et al. Bone marrow monosomy 7: hematologic and clinical manifestations in childhood and adolescence. *Hematol Oncol* 1984;2:5–12.
54. Shannon KM, Waterson J, Johnson P, et al. Monosomy 7 myeloproliferative disease in children with neurofibromatosis, type 1. epidemiology and molecular analysis. *Blood* 1992;79:1311–1318.
55. Hasle H, Arico M, Basso G, et al. Myelodysplastic syndrome, juvenile myelomonocytic leukemia and acute myeloid leukemia associated with complete or partial monosomy 7. *Leukemia* 1999;13:376–385.
56. Hasle H. Myelodysplastic syndromes in childhood. Classification, epidemiology, and treatment. *Leuk Lymphoma* 1994;13:11–26.
57. Passmore SJ, Hann IM, Stiller CA, et al. Pediatric myelodysplasia: a study of 68 children and a new prognostic scoring system. *Blood* 1995; 85:1742–1750.
58. Luna-Fineman S, Shannon KM, Lange BJ. Childhood monosomy 7: epidemiology, biology, and mechanistic implications. *Blood* 1995;85: 1985–1999.
59. Butcher M, Frenck R, Emperor J, et al. Molecular evidence that childhood monosomy 7 syndrome is distinct from juvenile chronic myelogenous leukemia and other childhood myeloproliferative disorders. *Genes Chromosomes Cancer* 1995;12:50–57.
60. Rosati S, Anastasi J, Vardiman J. Recurring problems in the pathology of the myelodysplastic syndromes. *Semin Hematol* 1996;33:112–126.
61. Kyle RA, Pease GL. Hematologic aspects of arsenic intoxication. *N Engl J Med* 1965;273:18–23.
62. Westhoff DD, Samaha RJ, Barnes A Jr. Arsenic intoxication as a cause of megaloblastic anemia. *Blood* 1975;45:241–246.
63. Lewis SM, Verwilghen RL. Dyserythropoiesis and dyserythropoietic anemias. In: Brown EB, ed. *Progress in hematology*. New York: Grune & Stratton, 1973;99–129.
64. Treacy M, Lai L, Costello C, et al. Peripheral blood and bone marrow abnormalities in patients with HIV related disease. *Br J Haematol* 1987; 65:289–294.
65. Napoli VM, Stein SF, Spira TJ, et al. Myelodysplasia progressing to acute myeloblastic leukemia in an HTLV-III virus positive homosexual man with AIDS-related complex. *Am J Clin Pathol* 1986;86:788–791.
66. Kaloutsi V, Kohlmeyer U, Maschek H, et al. Comparison of bone marrow and hematologic findings in patients with human immunodeficiency virus infection and those with myelodysplastic syndromes and infectious diseases. *Am J Clin Pathol* 1994;101:123.
67. Young N. B19 parvovirus. *Baillieres Clin Haematol* 1995;8:25–27.
68. Brown K, Young N. Parvovirus B19 infection and hematopoiesis. *Blood Rev* 1995;9:176–182.
69. Schmitz LL, McClure JS, Litz CE, et al. Morphologic and quantitative changes in blood and marrow cells following growth factor therapy. *Am J Clin Pathol* 1994;101:67–75.
70. Tricot G, Boogaerts MA, De Wolf-Peeters C, et al. The myelodysplastic syndromes: different evolution patterns based on sequential morphological and cytogenetic investigations. *Br J Haematol* 1985;59: 659–670.
71. Fenaux P, Jouet JP, Zandecki M, et al. Chronic and subacute myelomonocytic leukaemia in the adult: a report of 60 cases with special reference to prognostic factors. *Br J Haematol* 1987;65:101–106.
72. Coiffier B, Adeleine P, Viala TJ, et al. Dysmyelopoietic syndromes: a search for prognostic factors in 193 patients. *Cancer* 1983;52:83–90.
73. Foucar K, Langdon RM, Armitage JO, et al. Myelodysplastic syndromes: a clinical and pathologic analysis of 109 cases. *Cancer* 1985; 56:553–561.
74. Joseph AS, Cinkotai KI, Hunt L, et al. Natural history of smouldering leukaemia. *Br J Cancer* 1982;46:160–166.
75. Kerkhofs H, Hermans J, Haak HL, et al. Utility of the FAB classification for myelodysplastic syndromes: investigation of prognostic factors in 237 cases. *Br J Haematol* 1987;65:73–81.
76. Solal-Celigny P, Desaint B, Herrera A, et al. Chronic myelomonocytic leukemia according to the FAB classification: analysis of 35 cases. *Blood* 1984;63:634–638.
77. Mufti GJ, Stevens JR, Oscier DG, et al. Myelodysplastic syndromes: a scoring system with prognostic significance. *Br J Haematol* 1985; 59:425–433.
78. Vallespi T, Torrabadella M, Julia A, et al. Myelodysplastic syndromes: a study of 101 cases according to the FAB classification. *Br J Haematol* 1985;61:83–92.
79. Varella BL, Chuang C, Woll JE, et al. Modifications in the classification of primary myelodysplastic syndromes: the addition of a scoring system. *Hematol Oncol* 1985;3:55–63.
80. Weisdorf DJ, Oken MM, Johnson GJ, et al. Chronic myelodysplastic syndrome: short survival with or without evolution to acute leukaemia. *Br J Haematol* 1983;55:691–700.
81. Coiffier B, Adeleine P, Gentilhomme O, et al. Myelodysplastic syndromes: a multi-parametric study of prognostic factors in 336 patients. *Cancer* 1987;60:3029–3032.
82. Guillermo F, Sanz MA, Vallespi T, et al. Two regression models and a scoring system for predicting survival and planning treatment in myelodysplastic syndromes: a multivariate analysis of prognostic factors in 370 patients. *Blood* 1989;74:395–408.
83. Kerkhofs H, Hermans J, Haak HL, et al. Utility of the FAB classification for myelodysplastic syndromes: investigation of prognostic factors in 237 cases. *Br J Haematol* 1987;65:73–81.
84. Ribera J, Cervantes F, Rozman C. A multivariate analysis of prognostic factors in chronic myelomonocytic leukaemia according to the FAB criteria. *Br J Haematol* 1987;65:307–311.
85. Tricot G, Vlietinck R, Verwilghen RL, et al. Prognostic factors in the myelodysplastic syndromes: a review. *Scand J Haematol* 1986; 36(S45):107–113.
86. Worsley A, Oscier DG, Stevens J, et al. Prognostic features of chronic myelomonocytic leukaemia: a modified Bournemouth score gives the best prediction of survival. *Br J Haematol* 1988;68:17–21.
87. Sanz GF, Sanz MA, Vallespi T, et al. Two regression models and a scoring system for predicting survival and planning treatment in myelodysplastic syndromes: a multivariable analysis of prognostic factors in 370 patients. *Blood* 1989;74:395–408.
88. List AF, Harinder S, Garewal S, et al. The myelodysplastic syndromes: biology and implications for management. *J Clin Oncol* 1990;8: 1424–1441.
89. Beran M, Estey E, O'Brien S, et al. Topotecan and cytarabine is an active combination regimen in myelodysplastic syndromes and chronic myelomonocytic leukemia. *J Clin Oncol* 1999;17:2819–2830.
90. Wijermans PW, Krulder JWM, Huijgens PC, et al. Continuous infusion of low-dose 5-Aza-2′-deoxycytidine in elderly patients with high-risk myelodysplastic syndrome. *Leukemia* 1997;11:1–5.

CHAPTER 49

Chronic Myelogenous Leukemia and the Chronic Myeloproliferative Diseases

John Anastasi and James W. Vardiman

It has been nearly half a century since William Dameshek, in a now-classic editorial in *Blood*, speculated that chronic myelogenous leukemia (CML), polycythemia vera (PV), chronic idiopathic myelofibrosis with myeloid metaplasia (CIMF), and essential thrombocythemia (ET) were related myeloproliferative disorders in which the bone marrow elements proliferate excessively as a unit in response to an unknown myelostimulatory factor (1). This concept, he believed, could explain why the hyperplasia in the marrow in these disorders often simultaneously involves the erythroid, granulocytic, and megakaryocytic lineages, and apparently, because marrow fibrosis is often present, the fibroblasts as well. The overlap of clinical and laboratory features in CML, PV, CIMF, and ET, such as an insidious onset and an indolent clinical course, hepatosplenomegaly, leukocytosis, and thrombocytosis, as well as the reports of "transitions" from one disorder to another, seemed further justification for uniting these entities into a single disease family, the chronic myeloproliferative diseases (CMPDs).

In the 50 years since the proposal of this hypothesis, numerous clinical, laboratory, and morphologic studies have supported Dameshek's notion that these diseases are similar. One major feature shared by the CMPDs is their clonal origin in a bone marrow stem cell. Even though one cell line may have a proliferative advantage, multiple lineages may be derived from the abnormal stem cell. The first direct evidence for this was the discovery that in CML not only granulocytes but also erythroid precursors and megakaryocytes have the Philadelphia (Ph) chromosome (2,3). Subsequently, the Ph chromosome was demonstrated in mononuclear phagocytes and in some lymphocytes (4–7). Further support for the origin of CML in a pluripotent stem cell was derived from the demonstration that, in women with CML who were heterozygous for the isoenzymes of glucose-6-phosphate dehydrogenase (G6PD), the same G6PD isoenzyme was found in multiple hematopoietic lineages, indicating that they were derived from the neoplastic transformation of a single progenitor cell (8,9). G6PD studies were soon extended to PV, ET, and CIMF (10–12) and provided evidence that these, too, had clonal origins in multipotent marrow stem cells. Other strategies, such as molecular analyses of restriction fragment length polymorphisms of X-linked genes, identification of *RAS* gene mutations, and fluorescence *in situ* hybridization (FISH), have confirmed the clonal and multilineage nature of CML, PV, CIMF, and ET (13–17).

Another unifying feature among the CMPDs is that, initially, there is relatively normal maturation of the progeny of the neoplastic clone. Hematopoiesis is effective and results in increased numbers of mature cells in the blood and marrow that have few morphologic or functional abnormalities. It is usually the increased numbers of one or more elements in the blood, often accompanied by enlargement of the spleen or liver, that produce the clinical signs and symptoms of the CMPDs.

Each CMPD is progressive and may transform to an aggressive phase with ineffective hematopoiesis and marrow failure, or to a blast phase that resembles acute leukemia. Marrow fibrosis is common in the transformed stages, and its appearance may account for some of the "transitions" that have been reported to occur among the various entities. In the CMPDs, marrow fibrosis initially may be demonstrated as an increase in the number and thickness of reticulin fibers, which are composed principally of type III collagen and are detected best by silver staining techniques. Collagen fibrosis, caused by an increase in type I collagen fibers, can be recognized with trichrome stains and is a later manifestation of the process (18,19). Although Dameshek (1) postulated that the fibroblasts in the CMPDs belonged to the neoplastic clone, there is now considerable evidence to the

J. Anastasi and J. W. Vardiman: Department of Pathology, University of Chicago, Chicago, Illinois 60637 contrary (12,20,21). The fibrosis is most likely caused by the abnormal production and release by megakaryocytes of cytokines and growth factors, such as platelet-derived growth factor and transforming growth factor-β (TGF-β) (19,22–24). Platelet-derived growth factor induces proliferation and growth of fibroblasts; TGF-β regulates extracellular matrix synthesis by increasing the expression of genes that code for fibronectin and collagens type I, II, and IV. The abnormal release from megakaryocytes of factors that stimulate deposition of connective tissue is an attractive hypothesis that explains the often-observed relationship between atypical megakaryocytic proliferation and marrow fibrosis, not only in the CMPDs but in some myelodysplastic syndromes (MDSs) and acute megakaryoblastic leukemia as well.

Despite the similarities among the CMPDs (clonality, effective hematopoiesis, maturation of the neoplastic clone, organomegaly, and progressive disease), some fundamental biologic differences exist between individual entities. For example, even though the CMPDs are clonally derived from an abnormal stem cell, the level of stem cell involvement may vary. The finding in CML that the Ph chromosome is present in some lymphoid cells as well as in the myeloid elements (granulocytes, erythroid cells, and megakaryocytes) supports the idea that the neoplastic event in CML involves a pluripotent stem cell (2–9). Data from G6PD isoenzyme, FISH, and restriction fragment length polymorphism studies, however, suggest that in the other CMPDs lineage involvement is more heterogeneous. For example, in PV, most data indicate that the lymphocytes infrequently are derived from the neoplastic clone, and occasionally even the granulocytes may not be derived clonally (13–16). Furthermore, there is no evidence for a single genetic abnormality that is common to all of the entities. The Ph chromosome is unique to CML, and although recurring chromosomal abnormalities are found in the other CMPDs, none are specific or consistently present (25). This does not exclude that the pathways for cellular expansion or transformation may be similar among the various diseases, but the genetic events initiating the process are likely to be different. Finally, there are differences in the clinical, laboratory, and morphologic findings. Each CMPD is a unique entity, and merely assigning a patient's disease to the CMPD family is not sufficient for understanding the clinical behavior or the underlying biology of the disorder.

Over the past several years, some authors have suggested that the list of CMPD entities should be expanded to include atypical CML (aCML), chronic myelomonocytic leukemia (CMML), chronic neutrophilic leukemia (CNL), and juvenile myelomonocytic leukemia (JMML). There is a debate as to whether aCML and CMML are myeloproliferative or myelodysplastic in nature, and whether all cases of CNL are even clonal. The CMPDs are listed in Table 49.1. Also listed are those disorders that have features of both CMPDs and MDSs, which, for ease of presentation, are discussed in this chapter.

TABLE 49.1. *Chronic myeloproliferative diseases and related entities*

Chronic myeloproliferative diseases
Chronic myelogenous leukemia (CML)
Chronic neutrophilic leukemia (CNL)
Hypereosinophilic syndrome/chronic eosinophilic leukemia (CEL)
Polycythemia vera (PV)
Essential thrombocythemia (ET)
Chronic idiopathic myelofibrosis with extramedullary hematopoiesis (CIMF)
Chronic myeloproliferative disorder, unclassifiable
Myeloproliferative/myelodysplastic diseases
Atypical chronic myeloid leukemia (aCML)
Chronic myelomonocytic leukemia (CMML)
Juvenile myelomonocytic leukemia (JMML)

DIAGNOSIS OF CHRONIC MYELOPROLIFERATIVE DISEASES

The evaluation of a patient suspected to have a CMPD requires the careful correlation of clinical, laboratory, and morphologic data. Because there is overlap of features among the various entities, if the findings from only one study are considered without knowledge of other studies, a correct diagnosis may not be achieved. The morphologic examination requires inspection of a well-made peripheral blood smear and of a well-processed bone marrow biopsy specimen that is stained for assessment of cellular detail as well as for detection of marrow fibrosis. The biopsy also provides material for immunohistochemical analysis of a number of antigens that may aid in establishing the diagnosis or in predicting the prognosis. It may not be possible to obtain aspirate smears if there is marrow fibrosis, but in such cases, marrow touch preparations can provide material for cytologic evaluation. The smears and biopsy specimens should be examined together and interpreted in the context of the clinical features and other laboratory data. Cytogenetic studies should be performed if a CMPD is suspected, and material should be saved for molecular genetic studies, should they be required for a diagnosis.

CHRONIC MYELOGENOUS LEUKEMIA

Chronic myelogenous leukemia is the most common of the myeloproliferative disorders and is, arguably, the most studied of all the leukemic disorders. This entity also holds a unique place in the history of medical discovery, because it is associated with a number of "firsts." CML was the first disorder for which the term *leukemia* was used; it was the first malignancy associated with a recurring chromosomal aberration; and it was the first disease in which the associated chromosomal abnormality was found to be a result of a translocation of genetic material from one chromosome to another. In addition, CML was the first disease in which a molecular rearrangement was recognized as giving rise to a fusion gene and a fusion protein, which subsequently were shown to be fundamental to its pathogenesis.

In publications that appeared only a few weeks apart in 1845, Bennett in Scotland (26) and Virchow in Germany (27) were the first to describe patients with the disorder. It was Virchow (28) who introduced the term *leukaemie* (leukemia) in 1865, and it was Neumann (29) who proposed the term *myelogene* (myelogenous) because of his concept that the disease originated in the bone marrow. After years of refinements in the description of the clinical and laboratory features of the disease, Nowell and Hungerford (30) began the inquiry into its molecular and cellular pathogenesis when they recognized an abnormal G-group chromosome with a deletion of part of its long arm in metaphase preparations from patient specimens. This abnormal chromosome later became known as the Philadelphia chromosome, in reference to the city in which it was described. Although there was some debate as to the origin of the Ph chromosome, it was eventually recognized as chromosome 22, after the introduction of banding techniques permitted identification of the individual chromosomes in the early 1970s (31). Banding also permitted Rowley to show, in 1973 (32), that the abnormality was not a deletion but a balanced reciprocal translocation involving the distal deleted segment of the long arm of chromosome 22 and the distal portion of the long arm of chromosome 9 (Fig. 49.1A). The reciprocal nature of the translocation was clarified further in the 1980s, when molecular studies established that the protooncogene *ABL*, normally located on chromosome 9, was transferred to a specific region on chromosome 22 named the breakpoint cluster region (*BCR*), and that a reciprocal exchange occurred between chromosomes 22 and 9 (33,34). The resulting hybrid gene on chromosome 22 (*BCR-ABL*) later was shown to be capable of being transcribed to mRNA and then translated into a chimeric protein, which eventually was shown to have abnormal tyrosine kinase activity and oncogenic potential (35,36).

CML has been a disease model of particular interest to students of molecular pathogenesis, but also to hematologists, hematopathologists, and students of normal and malignant hematopoiesis. CML is a disorder of the hematopoietic stem cell, and as such it affects all formed elements of the blood and bone marrow. It is a disease that has a relatively long chronic phase, which shares features with the other myeloproliferative disorders, and an accelerated and rapidly fatal blast phase, which has similarities to acute leukemia. The disorder serves as a model not only for molecular pathogenesis but also for stem cell biology, hematopoiesis, hematopoietic lineage commitment, and chronic and acute leukemia. Although inroads have been made in therapy for CML, the disorder still remains fatal for most patients. A pathologist's accurate initial diagnosis is of key importance, and his or her evaluation of the effect of therapy and of disease progression and transformation is equally critical. Because there is still a gap in the understanding of how the molecular fusion leads to the clinical disease, insightful interpretation of experimental pathologic findings is paramount in linking the underlying molecular and cellular pathology with the clinical disease.

Epidemiology and Etiology

Chronic myelogenous leukemia has an incidence between 1 and 1.5 cases per 100,000 population, and this has not changed over the past 50 years (37,38). Although the disease can occur in all age groups, the median age at diagnosis is somewhere between 46 and 53 years (39). This represents a younger age than cited in earlier reports (40,41) and probably reflects both earlier detection of the disease and more accurate diagnosis, with exclusion of patients with CMML, aCML, and other myeloproliferative disorders, who tend to be older. There is a slight male predominance in CML, with the male : female ratio ranging from 1.4 : 1 to 2.2 : 1 (38,42). There is no specific ethnic or geographic group in which the disease is more or less common.

The cause of CML is largely unknown. There does not appear to be a genetic disposition, because offspring of patients with CML are not at higher risk (43). There also is not a higher incidence in paired twins of monozygotic twins with CML (44). Survivors of radiation exposure from the atomic blasts in Japan (45) and patients treated with radiation for a chronic disease, such as ankylosing spondylitis (46), do have higher incidences of CML. This correlates with the more recent experimental finding of the development of the *BCR-ABL* fusion in some cell lines exposed to radiation (47). In most patients, however, radiation is not believed to be a major contributor to the development of CML. Exposure to drugs or chemicals also is not known to be a major risk factor, and there is no evidence of a link to a virus.

Molecular and Cellular Pathogenesis

Although the molecular fusion of the *BCR* gene on chromosome 9 with the protooncogene *ABL* on chromosome 22 generally is considered to be the initiating event in CML, there are some intriguing data suggesting that the fusion develops in a stem cell population that is already abnormal and already clonally expanded. Fialkow and coworkers (48), and later other groups (49,50), used G6PD isoenzyme studies in heterozygous individuals with CML, and they were able to generate an excess of B-lymphoid cell lines without the Ph chromosome but with the same G6PD isoenzyme as the CML clone. The presumption is that these cell lines arose from a clone of stem cells that was abnormal and that gave rise to the *BCR-ABL* clone in CML as a secondary subclonal expansion. This hypothesis could be of great significance for detection of residual disease or autologous transplantation of Ph-negative (Ph^-) stem cells, although the hypothesis has yet to be investigated more completely.

Whether there is an initial *BCR-ABL* negative clonal expansion or not, the specific genetic rearrangement generally is considered the underlying molecular event in the pathogenesis of the disorder. Transfection experiments have

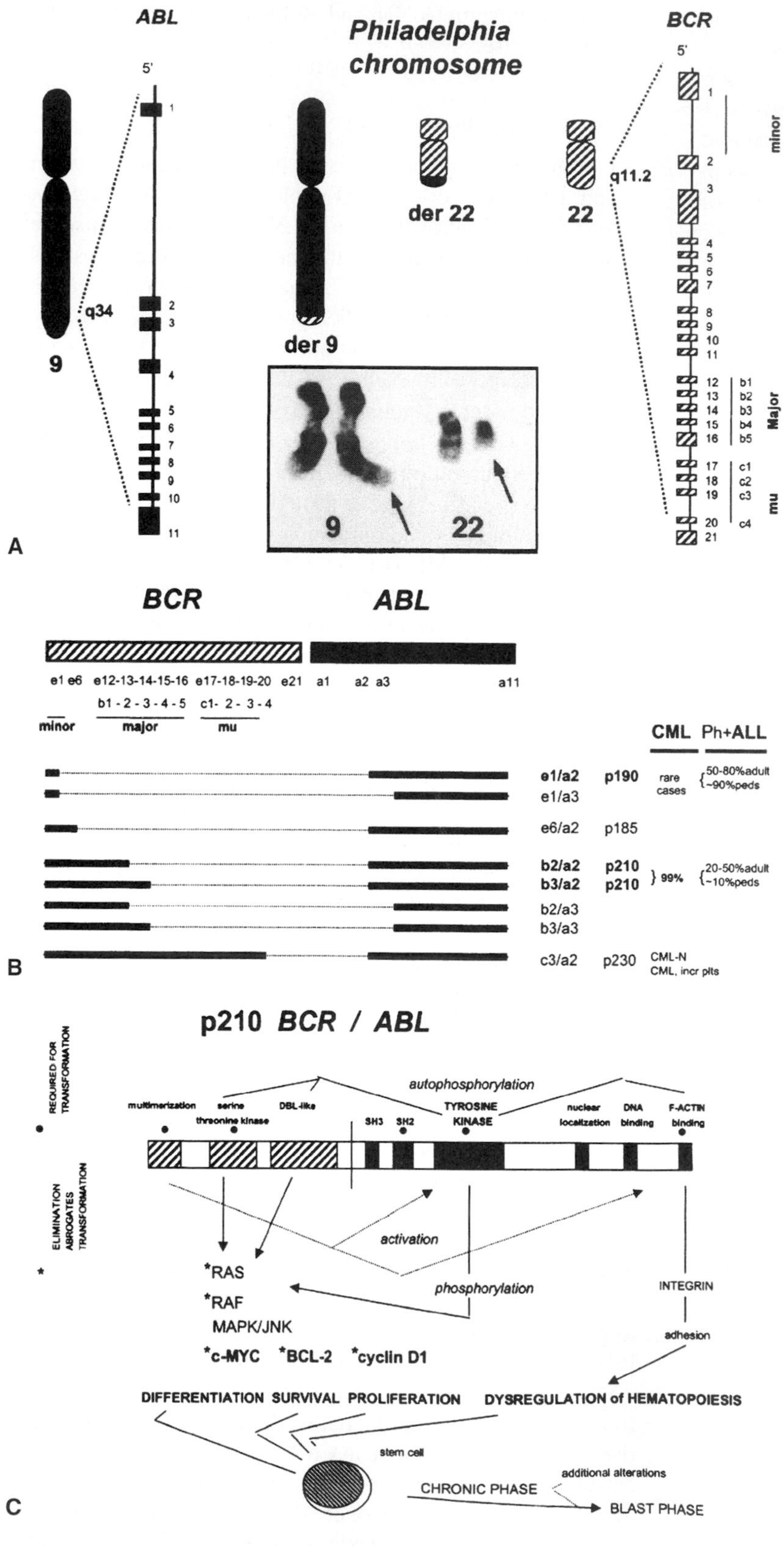

FIG. 49.1. A: Partial karyotype of a typical translocation t(9;22) (**inset**), and a schematic of t(9;22) with specific illustration of *BCR* and *ABL* genes. The *ABL* gene on chromosome 9 has 11 exons, and the *BCR* gene on chromosome 22 has more than 20. Specific areas on *BCR* are designated "minor," "major" and "mu" breakpoint regions. The Philadelphia chromosome is the derivative 22 with the translocated material from 9q. The **inset** illustrates the partial karyotype of a typical t(9;22), with arrows indicating der(9) and der(22). **B:** Illustration of the various *BCR-ABL* fusions. The most common fusions involve the major breakpoint region of *BCR* (exons e12–e16, alternatively called *b1–b5*) and a break in exon a2 of the *ABL* gene. The resulting b3a2 or b2a2 fusions give rise to a p210 protein, referred to as p210BCR-ABL . This is seen in over 99% of patients with chronic myelogenous leukemia but also in 20 to 50% of adult and 10% of pediatric patients with Philadelphia chromosome–positive acute lymphoid leukemia. Another common fusion involves the minor breakpoint of *BCR*, and the same a2 region of *ABL*, resulting in an e1a2 fusion and a p190BCR-ABL protein. This is seen only in rare patients with CML but is present more commonly in Philadelphia chromosome–positive acute lymphoid leukemia. Other rare fusions of the *BCR* and *ABL* genes also are illustrated. One of note is that giving rise to a p230BCR-ABL protein, which is associated with chronic myelogenous leukemia with excessive neutrophilia or with marked thrombocytosis. **C:** Schematic of the p210BCR-ABL protein and pathways involved by its action (61). Multimerization affected by the initial region of the BCR protein causes activation of the tyrosine kinase and actin-binding domains on ABL. Activated tyrosine kinase results in autophosphorylation of a number of sites on the fusion protein and phosphorylation of other proteins, with resulting activation of the indicated pathways affecting cell differentiation, survival, and proliferation. The activation of the actin-binding domain acts through altering integrin and related receptor functions and is believed to result in an abnormal reduced adhesion of the affected stem cell to stroma. This is believed to result in dysregulation of hematopoiesis.

shown that the fusion protein is necessary and sufficient for transformation. Cells transfected with *BCR-ABL* cDNA have tumorigenicity *in vivo* and *in vitro* growth that is independent of growth factors (51). Mice transplanted with stem cells transduced with *BCR-ABL* cDNA develop a CML-like syndrome, although not in all instances (52,53).

The *BCR-ABL* fusion occurs in a pluripotent stem cell in CML. This initially was deduced from the fact that the blast phase of the disease could be of myeloid or lymphoid lineage (54). Later, G6PD isoenzyme studies more directly demonstrated the clonal nature of different types of hematopoietic cells derived from the neoplastic clone (8,9). More recently, studies with FISH have demonstrated the *BCR-ABL* fusion in all mature hematopoietic cell types, including all myeloid elements, B and T cells, and even natural killer cells (7,55–57). The stem cell nature of the disorder also has been verified by the direct finding of *BCR-ABL* in primitive hematopoietic stem cells themselves (58).

How the *BCR-ABL* fusion and the reciprocal *ABL-BCR* come about in the stem cell is not known entirely, although it is believed to occur during late synthesis or metaphase through a reciprocal breakage and rejoining of genetic material on chromosomes 9 and 22. Whether the two regions normally are juxtaposed during some phase of the cell cycle has not been illustrated clearly, although FISH experiments have shown a possible nonrandom localization of the *BCR* and *ABL* regions in the central region of the interphase nucleus (59).

The fusion of *BCR* and *ABL* occurs in distinct regions of each of the genes (60,61). In the *BCR* gene, the breakage almost always occurs within the so-called major breakpoint region that spans exons e12 through e16, which are known otherwise as b1 through b5. The break commonly occurs in the b2 or b3 area (62). In the *ABL* gene, the break occurs in a region represented as a2 at the beginning of the gene, so that most of the *ABL* gene is transferred to chromosome 22 (63). The typical fusion is denoted as *b3a2* or *b2a2*, and there seems to be little significant difference between the two. Both of these particular breakpoints and fusions give rise to mRNA and then to a protein with a molecular weight of 210 kd, which is referred to as p210BCR-ABL. This is present in more than 99% of patients with CML, but it also can be seen in Ph-positive (Ph^+) acute lymphoblastic leukemia (ALL) (in 20–50% of adult and 10% of pediatric cases) (64–66).

Other fusions in the *BCR* and *ABL* genes occur, giving rise to other *BCR-ABL* proteins (67) (Fig. 49.1B). A breakage in the so-called minor breakpoint region gives rise to a p190 protein; this is associated with rare cases of CML (68) and more commonly with Ph^+ ALL (in 50–80% of adult cases and 90% of pediatric cases) (64–66). In other patients with CML, a fusion occurs, giving rise to an e6a2 fusion and a p185 protein (69,70). An e19a2 fusion (also noted as *c3a2*), which gives rise to a p230 protein, is believed by some to be associated with the disorder CNL (71), although leukemias with this fusion probably should be referred to as *CML with excessive neutrophilia*. Others have reported this fusion in a type of CML with marked thrombocytosis that mimics ET (72,73). The issue of whether these other fusions, and particularly that associated with p190BCR-ABL, also arise in the pluripotent stem cell, or a more committed cell, is being debated and further investigated (74,75).

Studies of the structure and function of the normal BCR and ABL proteins have given some insight into the complexity of the cellular pathogenesis of the disease, which is not well understood (60,61) . The BCR protein has a number of domains, including a coiled motif that allows for multimerization, a serine threoine kinease domain that plays a role in signal transduction and cell regulation, a domain that has homology to the *DBL* protooncogene, and a carboxyl-terminal domain (RAC-GAP) that has a GTP-ase–activating function for RAC. The *ABL* gene encodes for an important tyrosine kinase that is highly conserved over evolution. The *ABL* gene also has motifs for actin and DNA binding, and a domain for nuclear localization. The amino terminus has domains with SRC homology, and one of the two isoforms contains a myristoylation domain that causes retention of the protein in the nucleus.

The b2a2 or b3a2 fusion between *BCR* and *ABL* (Fig 49.1C) results in an elimination of the myristoylation site in *ABL*, and this elimination causes a cytoplasmic localization of the hybrid protein. This may allow it to be exposed to substrates, which it usually does not encounter. The fusion also causes the normal tyrosine kinase activity to be dysregulated, resulting in increased phosphorylation and autophosphorylation. This is linked to activation of the RAS and RAF pathways, which function to control cell proliferation. The fusion also causes activation of the actin-binding function, which results in abnormal reduced adhesion, migration, and signal transformation of the *BCR-ABL*-positive cells. Other pathways have been shown to be involved, in experiments evaluating the transforming ability of the oncoprotein after manipulations targeting the various pathways. The other pathways include the *MYC* pathway, which if activated causes increased gene transcription; the cyclin D1 pathway, which controls cell proliferation and growth factor independence, and the *BCL2* pathway, which causes decreased cell death. Although the actual links between the molecular fusion and these different pathways have not been completely elucidated, it appears that the fusion protein may act by increasing cell proliferation, decreasing cell death, inducing independence from growth factors, and causing reduced adhesion of the affected cell to stromal elements, which may disrupt regulation of hematopoiesis.

Futher clarification of the molecular and cellular pathogenesis may come from experimental disease models and studies of cell lines established from patients with the disease. Transgenic (76), transduction (52), and transplantation models have been developed. In the newest transplantation model, cells from patients with the chronic phase are engrafted in sublethally irradiated, nonobese diabetic, severe combined immunodeficient mice (77). The cells persist for up to 7 months and provide the best model to date for the chronic phase of the disease. Approximately three dozen lines have been established from patients with CML, and essentially all were derived from blast crises (78). Most cell lines have the Ph chromosome associated with a complex karyotype, and many have been characterized at a molecular level. The cell lines have quite varied lineage characteristics reflecting the totipotential nature of the primary disease. Some of the cell lines also have been shown to undergo lineage switching if induced by certain biomodulators.

Clinical and Laboratory Findings

Although there is still a gap in the understanding of precisely how the molecular fusion leads to cellular dysfunction, proliferation of the myeloid component, and eventually the transformation to a terminal phase, the clinical and laboratory manifestations of the disease have been described clearly for many years. These are discussed subsequently here in relation to the chronic, accelerated, and blast phases of the disease. Although most patients are diagnosed in chronic phase, occasional patients present in accelerated or even in blast phase. Also, although many patients progress from chronic phase through accelerated to blast phase, some progress directly from chronic to blast phase.

Chronic Phase

Most patients are diagnosed in chronic phase, and the majority experience symptoms related to the expansion of granulocytic elements in the blood, marrow, or extramedullary sites (79). The number of asymptomatic patients has been rising recently and now accounts for between 20 and 40% of all patients (80,81). Such patients are diagnosed based on blood counts performed during routine medical examinations. For patients with symptoms, the most common complaints are fatigue and lethargy, which may be related in part to a chronic and insidious anemia. Bleeding, mild to moderate weight loss, and symptoms related to splenic enlargement are also relatively common. Less common symptoms include sweats, bone pain, and infection. Unusual symptoms at diagnosis include those related to hyperviscosity. The most common physical findings at presentation are those of pallor and splenomegaly, and other findings include lymphadenopathy, purpura, bone tenderness, and stigmata of thyrotoxicosis caused by a hypermetabolic state.

Peripheral Blood Findings

The findings in the peripheral blood represent a hallmark of CML and not infrequently are diagnostic of the disease in themselves (Fig. 49.2A). In essentially all patients, there is leukocytosis with white blood cell count (WBC) ranging from 20 to 500 $\times$ 10^9 per liter, with a mean of between 134 and 225. Asymptomatic patients with an incidental diagnosis tend to have lower counts (81,82). The leukocytes are mostly neutrophilic elements that are present in all stages of maturation. Segmented and band forms constitute the majority of the cells. There are generally few blasts (1–2%) and few promyelocytes, but there is a relative increase in myelocytic forms, particularly in relation to metamyelocytes (the percentage of myelocytes is greater than that of metamyelocytes). This is referred to as a ''myelocyte bulge'' and is notable because it generally is not seen in reactive conditions. The neutrophilic elements in the blood in CML appear normal, although occasional cells show hypersegmentation. Dysplastic features usually are not observed, and if present they suggest an incorrect diagnosis or progression of the disease (83). Studies with electron microscopy have demonstrated that the leukemic neutrophils are indistinguishable from normal cells ultrastructurally, although some abnormalities such as the presence of bundles of microfilaments and an increased frequency of nuclear bodies may be seen in mature forms (84).

Mild functional and biochemical abnormalities have been described in the neutrophils. The best known is a low level of neutrophil alkaline phosphatase (NAP) or leukocyte alkaline phosphatase activity (82,85). This is sometimes helpful at diagnosis in distinguishing CML from a leukemoid reaction, in which this activity is very high. In addition to low NAP, CML neutrophils have decreased adhesiveness to glass slides (86), delayed emigration to extravascular sites (87), abnormal degranulation (88), and decreased levels of lactoferrin and lysozyme activity (89). Despite these abnormalities, patients in chronic phase do not have an increased risk for infections (41).

There is always an absolute basophilia in CML, although in some patients the percentage of basophils is low. In approximately 90% of patients there is also eosinophilia (82). Many of the basophils and eosinophils are morphologically normal, but some of the cells, particularly the basophils, appear hypogranular and may be difficult to recognize. This is the case especially in less than optimally stained smears. The number of monocytes usually is low and accounts for less than 3% of the leukocytes; however, because of the high WBC, there is usually a mild absolute monocytosis (79). The lymphocyte count can be variable; it can be elevated because of an expanded number of T cells (90), or it may be decreased with reduced numbers of CD4 T cells (82,91).

Most patients exhibit mild to moderate normochromic, normocytic anemia, but in some patients the hemoglobin concentration is normal or increased. In still other patients, particularly in those untreated for a long time period, there can be severe anemia (79,82). The red blood cell (RBC) morphology is usually normal. Platelet counts are usually elevated and can be increased to more than 1,000 $\times$ 10^9 per liter. Thrombocytopenia is uncommon. Functional disorders of platelets can be seen, the most common of which is a decrease in the secondary wave with epinephrine-induced aggregation. The platelet functional abnormalities are not associated with spontaneous bleeding (92).

A,B 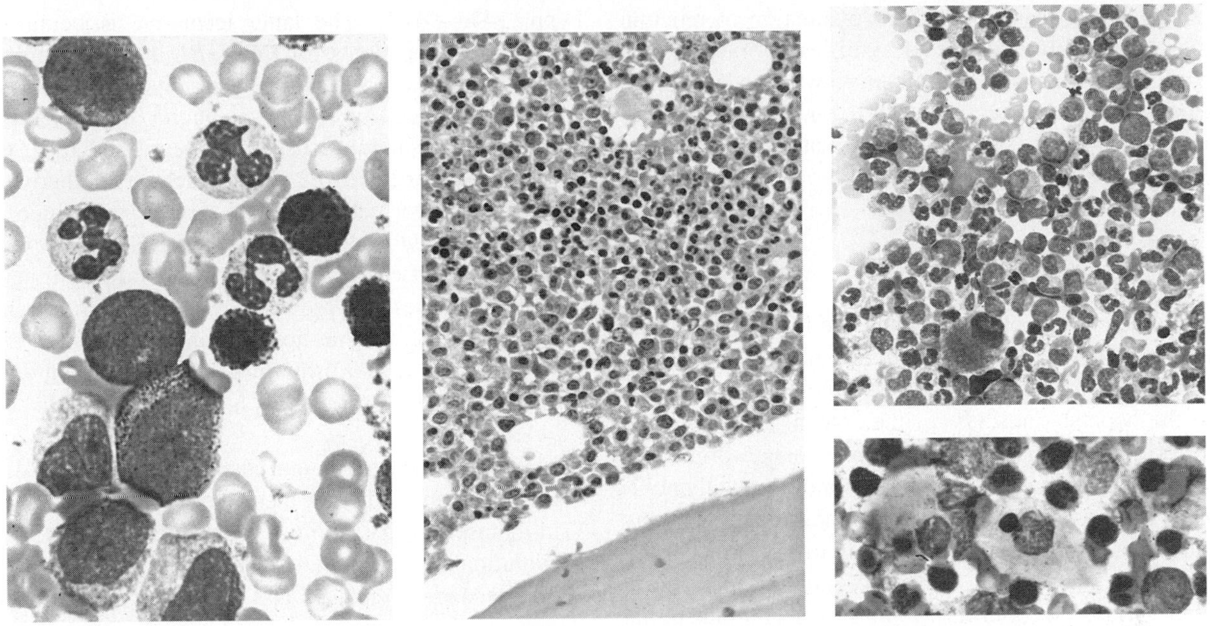 C D

FIG. 49.2. Chronic phase of chronic myelogenous leukemia. **A:** Peripheral blood smear illustrating a marked leukocytosis resulting from a spectrum of granulocytic forms and basophilia. **B:** Bone marrow biopsy specimen illustrating a markedly hypercellular marrow resulting from a proliferation of maturing granulocytic elements. Note the widened cuff of immature granulocytes along the bony trabeculum. In a normal bone marrow biospy this cuff of immature cells would be only two or three cells thick. **C:** Bone marrow aspirate showing the immature and maturing granulocytic elements and small megakaryocyte. **D:** Pseudo-Gaucher cells are also sometimes seen.

Bone Marrow Findings

Although the peripheral blood findings may be sufficient for a diagnosis, the bone marrow aspirate and biopsy results are useful for supporting the diagnosis and for more completely excluding other conditions (93). The bone marrow biopsy specimen is also useful for providing the best material for cytogenetic studies, and for use as a baseline for comparisons with subsequent material. Examination of the biopsy specimen also may pick up focal accumulations of blasts that are not apparent in the aspirate.

During the chronic phase of CML, the bone marrow is hypercellular because of granulocytic expansion and usually the cellularity approaches 100% (Fig. 49.2B). In the marrow aspirate, features similar to those noted in the peripheral blood are found, with the neutrophilic proliferation and ''myelocyte bulge'' but low blast and promyelocyte counts (93–96) (Fig. 49.2C). In chronic phase, the blast count is generally less than 5%, and blasts and promyelocytes combined make up less than 10%. Basophilia and eosinophilia commonly are seen. Erythroid elements can vary and may be present in reduced, normal, or even increased numbers. Rare patients with RBC aplasia, which apparently is immunologically mediated, have been reported (97). An interesting feature in 40% and possibly up to 70% of patients is the presence in the aspirate of abnormal macrophages (98–100). These are of three types: macrophages with blue cytoplasm with the characteristic ''tissue paper'' appearance caused by birefringent crystals called *pseudo-Gaucher cells* or *Gaucher-like cells* (Fig. 49.2D); macrophages with sea-blue granules, referred to as *sea-blue histiocytes*; and macrophages with grey-green nonbirefringent crystals. A recent study demonstrated the *BCR-ABL* fusion in pseudo-Gaucher cells (101), indicating that they are clearly a part of the neoplastic clone. This is the case regarding other macrophage/histiocytic elements, including those outside the marrow such as pulmonary macrophages (102).

The bone marrow biopsy sections in CML show a number of diagnostically useful histologic features. The biopsy specimen reveals a periosteal and perivascular cuff of immature granulocytic elements that is 5 to 10 cells deep, in contrast to the two- or three-cell layer normally seen (Fig. 49.2B). Maturation occurs outward from these cuffs (93–95). There are increased numbers of megakaryocytes, which frequently are small and hypolobated and occur in clusters in the central, intertrabecular regions near marrow sinuses. The megakaryocytes of the other myeloproliferative disorders are larger and more atypical (93,96). The small CML megakaryocytes, however, are usually not as small as the micromegakaryocytes seen in the myelodysplastic disorders. Some patients have prominent or even predominant megakaryocytic proliferations, causing some investigators to refer to these as the *megakaryocytic* or *megakaryocytic predominance* type of CML, in comparison to the other two subtypes, the more common *granulocytic–megakaryocytic* type and the *granulocytic* type (103). Whether such a subclassification has clinical relevance is debatable. The marrow biopsy specimen in CML also can be used for evaluation of reticulin fibrosis, which, some believe, if significantly increased at diagnosis has prognostic significance, with an associated shortened duration of survival (104,105). Some degree of fibrosis can be seen in close to 50% of patients at diagnosis (105).

Extramedullary Manifestations

During the chronic phase of CML, the leukemic cells are minimally invasive, and their proliferation remains confined primarily to the hematopoietic tissues, including the spleen, and to the hepatic sinusoids. In the spleen, the pulp cords are infiltrated by granulocytes in different stages of maturation, and the white pulp is compressed and eventually obliterated. A few erythroid precursors and megakaryocytes may be found in the splenic sinusoids (94). In the liver, distension of the hepatic sinusoids by leukemic granulocytes is common, but variably sized infiltrates may be seen in the portal tracts (94). Evidence of extensive tissue infiltration outside the hematopoietic system, particularly of lymphadenopathy, should be regarded with suspicion, for this finding often is associated with blast crisis (106).

Other Laboratory Features

Commonly there is increased production of uric acid with hyperuricemia and hyperuricosuria. Serum B12 levels and the serum binding capacity of B12 are increased.

Molecular and Cytogenetic Features

Although a firm diagnosis can be made morphologically by examination of peripheral blood and bone marrow specimens, cytogenetic or molecular studies are used for confirmation of the diagnosis. Cytogenetic analysis is also useful for establishing a baseline karyotype for comparison with subsequent studies; karyotypic evolution is thought to be prognostically significant.

At diagnosis, 90 to 95% of patients with CML have the characteristic t(9;22)(q34;q11.2), which is usually present in 100% of the metaphase cells. The remaining patients have variant translocations or a submicroscopic translocation that cannot be identified by visual evaluation of the chromosomes (107). The variant translocations are mostly "complex" in that they involve a third or sometimes even a fourth chromosome, for example, t(9;14;22). In some patients, the involvement of 9q34 is cryptic, giving rise to a translocation that does not seem to involve 9q34. These originally were considered "simple variants," but by *in situ* hybridization they have been shown to involve 9q34 (108). The Ph^- cases, if they truly are CML, have a *BCR* rearrangement or a *BCR-ABL* fusion identified through molecular studies or through the use of FISH (Fig. 49.3; see also Color Plate 91, between pp. 1446–1447). The latter technique is being used for screening of patients for *BCR-ABL* in routine preparations of interphase cells (109). It generally is thought, however, that a complete karyotype evaluation is needed at diagnosis. Molecular techniques used for identifying the *BCR* rearrangements or *BCR-ABL* fusions include Southern blot analysis, and reverse transcriptase–polymerase chain reaction (PCR) (110,111). PCR analysis of DNA, however, is not accomplished easily, and analysis of mRNA transcripts is required. A test for the actual *BCR-ABL* protein has been developed, but this has not yet gained widespread use (112). An antibody to the fusion protein also has been developed, although its diagnostic utility has not been established firmly (113).

Secondary chromosomal changes can be seen at diagnosis. It is debatable whether these have prognostic significance in themselves; it is more generally thought that karyotypic evolution is more predictive of worsening disease (114,115). The secondary changes and karyotypic evolution are discussed subsequently.

Accelerated Phase

Although some patients progress directly from chronic phase CML to a terminal phase, many pass through an accelerated phase, which generally is defined as a stage in the disease at which the clinical and pathologic features are no longer stable and the patient is no longer responsive to the initial therapy. Although well accepted, the accelerated phase does not have well-defined or well-accepted clinical or pathologic criteria (106,116).

Among the clinical features associated with disease progression in CML are worsening of overall performance status, fevers, sweats, weight loss, bone pain, progressive splenomegaly, and loss of responsiveness to therapy. In a recent multivariant analysis, however, only the development of bone pain was a predictor of blast crisis within 3 months of the onset of symptoms (117). Progressive splenomegaly and the new onset of fever and sweats were associated with a significantly increased risk of development of blast phase after between 3 months and 1 year.

Peripheral Blood and Bone Marrow

General peripheral blood parameters evaluated in CML patients for progression of disease include increasing leukocytosis, increasing numbers of blood basophils, a rising percentage of circulating promyelocytes and blasts, falling hemoglobin levels, the appearance of circulating erythroblasts, and changes in platelet counts. Bone marrow parameters include changes in the sum of promyelocytes and blasts and an increase in reticulin fibrosis (117). Which of these parameters must change, and the specific amount of change required, for the diagnosis of the accelerated phase have not been determined precisely or accepted uniformly. In one study, percentage of peripheral blasts more than or equal to

A 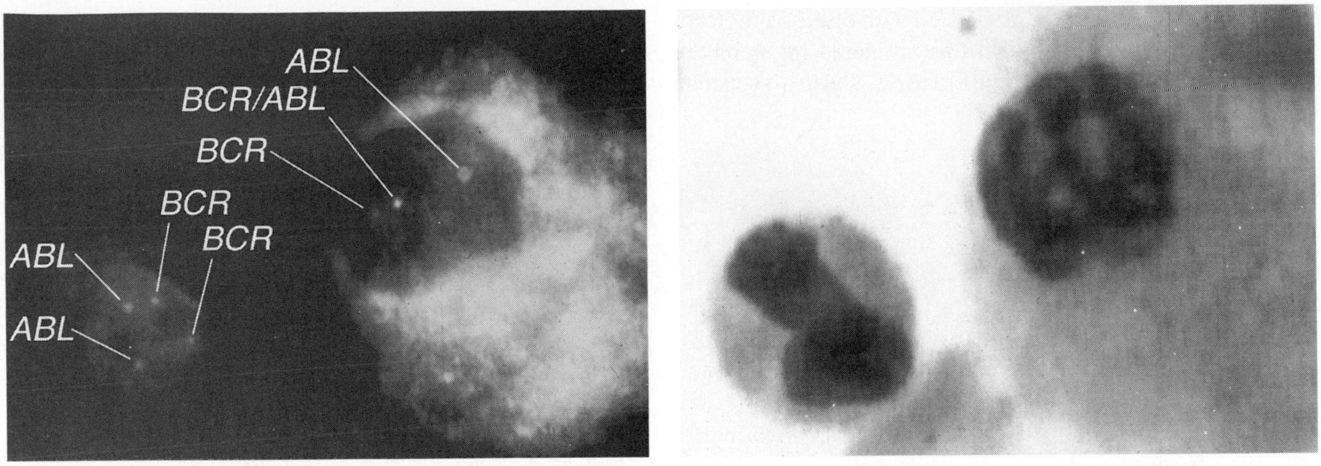 B

FIG. 49.3. Illustration of fluorescence *in situ* hybridization analysis for the *BCR-ABL* fusion in interphase nuclei (**A**), performed on a previously Wright-stained smear (**B**). In a normal cell (**left**), there are two (red) signals, one for each of the *BCR* genes, and there are two (green) signals, one for each of the *ABL* genes (see color illustration). In a cell with the t(9;22) and *BCR-ABL* (**right**), there is one (red) signal for *BCR*, one (green) for *ABL*, and a (yellow) fusion signal from the juxtaposition of *BCR* with *ABL*. The cells were from a patient with chronic myelogenous leukemia who had been transplanted a year earlier, but who continued to test positive with polymerase chain reaction assay for *BCR-ABL* transcripts. The normal granulocyte likely arose from the transplanted cells, but the pseudo-Gaucher cell likely persisted from the original chronic myelogenous leukemia clone (101). See Color Plate 91, between pp. 1446–1447.

15%, peripheral basophilia greater than or equal to 20%, the sum of peripheral blasts and promyelocytes greater than or equal to 30% (Fig. 49.4), and thrombocytopenia each had independent prognostic significance for an ensuing blast phase (118). In another study, however, only the presence of circulating blasts at a level of 6 to 12% and basophila of 20% or higher were found to be major predictors of blast phase (117). In this latter study, more than 12% circulating blasts was associated with bone marrow blast counts above 20%, which, in this study, were considered to indicate blast phase. Other blood or marrow parameters such as increasing reticulin fibrosis, decreasing NAP score, and increasing my-

A,B 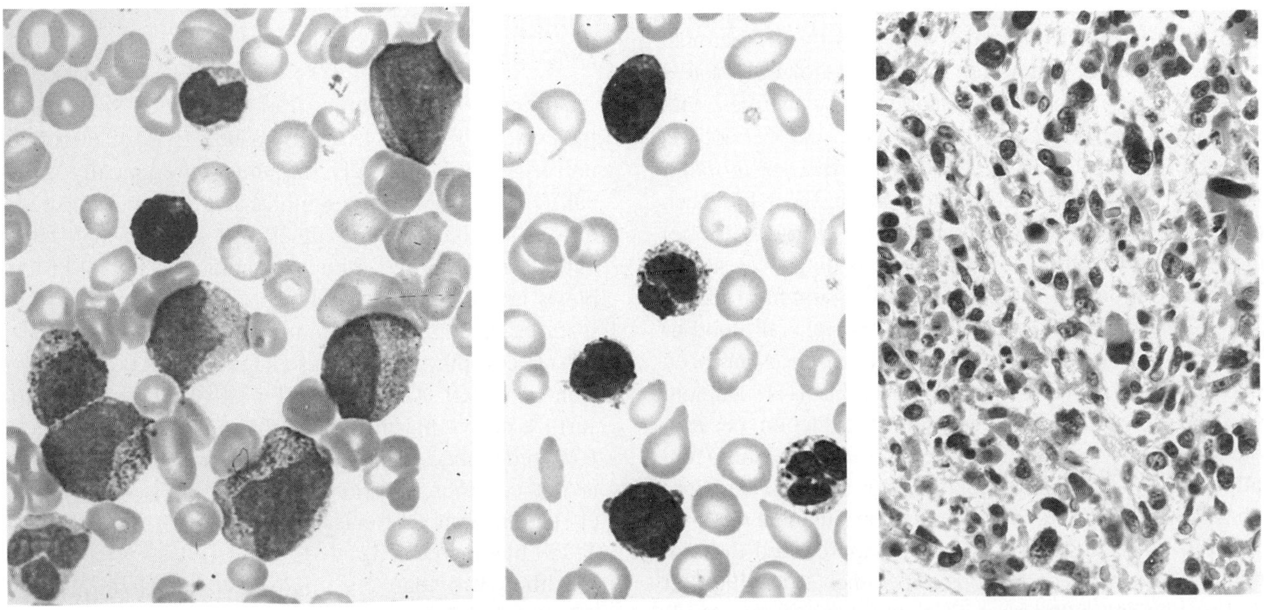 C

FIG. 49.4. In the accelerated phase of chronic myelogenous leukemia one can see "left-shifted" granulocytic elements with increased immature forms including increased promyelocytes and blasts (**A**), increased basophils (**B**), and increased marrow fibrosis with a proliferation of atypical small megakaryocytes and a shift toward immature granulocytic forms (**C**).

elodysplasia also have been associated with disease progression. A recent study has shown that an increasing number of CD34-positive cells in the bone marrow is also associated with disease progression (119).

Cytogenetic Findings

A change in the karyotype is a sign of acceleration or impending blast crisis (114,115,120,121). The most frequently seen secondary changes in CML are a gain of an additional copy of the Ph chromosome, an additional copy of chromosome 8 (+8), and an isochromosome for the long arm of 17, i(17q). Trisomy 19 also is common. These changes occur in 71% of patients with secondary abnormalities. They frequently are seen together, with a gain of the Ph chromosome and +8 being the most common combination. The less common secondary abnormalities include −7, −17, +17, +21, and −Y. Other changes are seen exclusively in blast phase.

The importance of cytogenetic change in identifying the accelerated phase has been recognized in the criteria proposed by the World Health Organization (122). The criteria require identifying one or more of the following: 10 to 19% blasts in the blood or bone marrow; peripheral basophilia more than 20%; persistent thrombocytopenia with platelets less than 100×10^9 per liter, not related to therapy; increasing WBC count and increasing spleen size unresponsive to therapy; and evidence of clonal evolution. Dysplasia and fibrosis alone are not considered sufficient for the diagnosis of accelerated phase.

Blast Phase

Almost all patients with CML progress, after about 4 to 5 years, to a terminal phase that is refractory to treatment and associated with a duration of survival of only a few months (123,124). This phase shares many features with acute myeloid leukemia (AML) or ALL and variably is called *acute phase*, *blast phase*, *blast crisis*, or *terminal phase* CML. As for the accelerated phase, there has been some discussion about uniformly acceptable criteria for defining the process. Because blast phase is diagnosed solely on pathologic grounds, however, the discussion has focused on the required number of blasts in the peripheral blood or bone marrow. Most recently, the general consensus has been that 20% peripheral blood or bone marrow blasts is sufficient for the diagnosis (122). This represents a reduction, because in the past some types of blast phase CML required the identification of at least 30% blasts (96). It should be noted that blast phase can be focal in the marrow, and that recognition of this focal blast process is best appreciated through evaluation of a bone core biopsy specimen (Fig. 49.5). It should also be noted that blast phase can occur in extramedullary sites (125,126), making it important to recommend biopsy of any new masses and particularly of enlarging lymph nodes. Rare patients present in blast phase after an absent, unrecognized, or very short chronic phase (127,128). These cases must be distinguished from AML or ALL and lymphoblastic lymphoma.

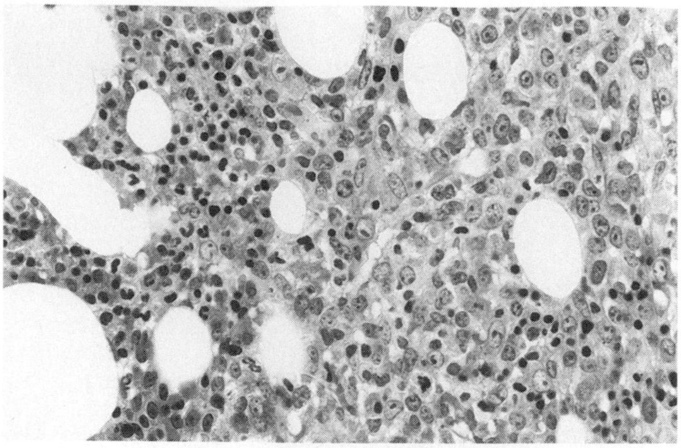

FIG. 49.5. Blast phase of chronic myelogenous leukemia can sometimes be focal (right side) and may be recognized only through evaluation of bone marrow biopsy sections.

Reflecting the fact that CML is a stem cell disorder, the blasts in acute phase can be of any hematopoietic cell lineage or of almost any combinations of cell lineages. This makes it difficult to divide the entire group into well-defined subgroups. For the sake of the following discussion, CML blast phase is divided into lymphoid blast phase (L-BP), myeloid blast phase (M-BP) (including a mixed myeloid type), and other rare types of blast phase including predominant erythroid or megakaryocytic blast phase, true biphenotypic (lymphoid–myeloid) or bilineal blast phase, and blast phase presenting at extramedullary sites.

Lymphoid-Blast Phase

Although L-BP occurs in only between 16 and 30% of patients with CML, it seems to be the most distinctive or uniform morphologically, immunophenotypically, and clinically (129,130). L-BP resembles acute lymphoblastic leukemia. Blasts have smudgy nuclear chromatin and scant blue cytoplasm, usually without granulation (Fig. 49.6A). The blasts in most patients in L-BP display immunophenotypic features of common precursor B cells, with expression of pan–B cell markers such as CD19 or CD20, and coexpression of CD10. They are TdT-positive, lack expression of surface or cytoplasmic immunoglobulin, and show a clonal *IGH* gene rearrangement. Coexpression of myeloid markers is not common, particularly in comparison to Ph^+ ALL (131). Only rare patients with L-BP CML have a precursor T-cell phenotype (132).

Although cytogenetic findings are not entirely lineage-specific, L-BP is more frequently associated with a gain of the Ph chromosome or −7, and less commonly with +8, i(17q), or trisomy 19, than is nonlymphoid blast phase (133). Rare patients with L-BP show secondary changes associated

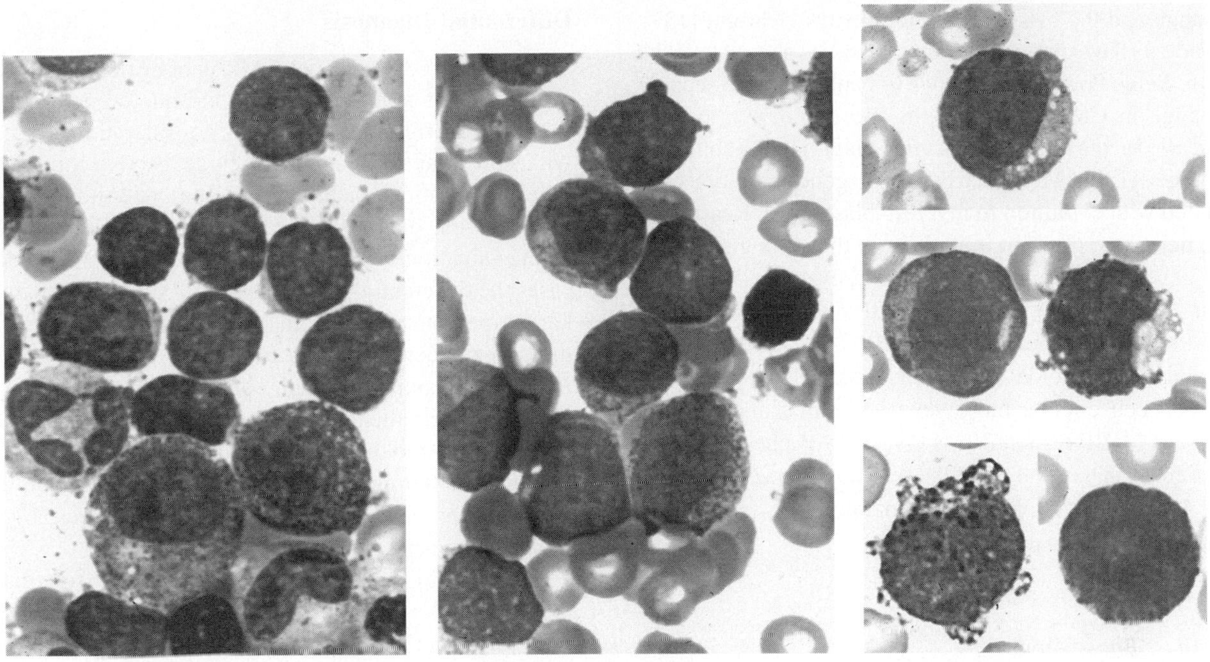

A,B C

FIG. 49.6. Different types of blast phases of chronic myelogenous leukemia. **A:** In lymphoid blast phase, the blasts (in the top portion of the figure) resemble the blasts seen in acute lymphoblastic leukemia. **B:** In myeloid blast phase, the blasts resemble myeloblasts of acute myeloid leukemia. **C:** A mixed myeloid blast phase has blasts of different types, including immature blasts, typical myeloblasts, megakaryoblasts, and immature basophils and or mast cells.

with ALL *de novo,* such as del(9p). Little is known about the underlying molecular basis of L-BP. One study has shown that there is clonal instability leading the blast transformation. Apparently, multiple clonal rearrangements of the *IGH* gene occur prior to the eventual blast transformation, which is associated with an *IGH* gene rearrangement different from those occurring earlier (134).

From a clinical standpoint, L-BP usually occurs in younger individuals who have had less splenomegaly, less anemia, and lower WBC counts than those who develop a nonlymphoid acute phase (130). The lymphoblastic transformation is more abrupt and usually is not associated with a preceding accelerated phase. If patients have L-BP, they tend to have higher bone marrow blast counts but lower levels of lactate dehydrogenase. Central nervous system involvement may be more common than in other types of blast phase. L-BP has a more favorable response to therapy than the nonlymphoid types, and it frequently is treated with drug regimens established for ALL. Although the survival rate is somewhat better than in non L-BP cases, it is rather poor at only 12 months.

Myeloid Blast Phase (including Mixed Myeloid Blast Phase)

Blast phase with a granulocytic or granulocytic–monocytic lineage occurs with about equal frequency as a so-called mixed myeloid phenotype, and together these types account for blast phase in about 50 to 60% of patients with CML (135,136). Morphologically, the granulocytic or granulocytic–monocytic cases generally resemble AML of the French–American–British (FAB) classification scheme, M1, M2, or M4 type, although sometimes in a background still recognizable as CML. Blasts tend to have a fine chromatin and cytoplasm with granules and varying degrees of differentiation to granulocytic or monocytic elements, as in M2 or M4 AML (Fig. 49.6B). Auer rods are not common. Although cytochemical reactions are often positive, they tend to be less intense than in *de novo* AML. Immunophenotypically, blasts express CD13, CD33, and sometimes CD14 along with CD34 (135,136).

The mixed myeloid cases are more unusual because the blasts are varied (Fig. 49.6C). In addition to the more typical myeloblasts, these patients have blasts with features of megakaryoblasts, erythroblasts, and some with primitive features, which, on close inspection or in ultrastructural studies, sometimes can be shown to be primitive basophils or even primitive mast cells (135). These patients also tend to have severe dysplasia in the differentiating cells. Cytochemical reactions of the blasts for myeloperoxidase or nonspecific esterase may be negative, and imunophenotypic markers are mixed with erythroid and megakaryocytic markers in addition to more usual myeloid or monocytic markers.

Cytogenetically, patients who experience M-BP more commonly have +8, i(17q), and trisomy 19 as secondary changes (133), although the relationship between the secondary change and the blast type is not always clear-cut (137). Rare patients have cytogenetic abnormalities associated with AML *de novo*. For example, inv(16) can occur as a secondary change in CML and have the morphology associated with *de novo* acute myelomonocytic leukemia with abnormal eosinophils (138). Molecularly, *TP53* gene alterations are associated with evolution to myeloid blast crisis. Rearrangements, deletions, or point mutations in the coding sequence of the gene have been identified. These generally are not seen in patients who progress to L-BP (139).

M-BP is more common than L-BP after an accelerated phase and is seen in older patients who have had high peripheral blood cell counts, more severe anemia, and a larger spleen size. M-BP responds less favorably to chemotherapy, and patients can have an overall duration of survival as short as 3 or 4 months (130). Newer treatment strategies are being evaluated for these patients (140).

Other Blast Phase Types

Blast phase with a predominant erythroid component (E-BP) has been described, and in one series such patients accounted for close to 10% of all cases in blast crisis (141). In other series, E-BP has been much less frequent (135,136,142). Although E-BP resembles erythroleukemia (M6 AML in the FAB classification), the criteria for classifying a patient as having such have not been established firmly. In some of the reported patients with E-BP, the erythroid proliferation was associated with blasts and immature cells of other lineages, suggesting that they would better fit the mixed myeloid lineage blast phase. A predominant megakaryocytic blast phase also has been reported, but such patients appear to be exceedingly rare (143).

Some patients with CML may have a truly biphenotypic blast phase, with expression of multiple myeloid and multiple lymphoid markers on the blasts (144). Occasional case reports have noted the presence of dual (bilineal) blast phases of myeloid and lymphoid type (145). These have been reported to occur concurrently or sequentially. The finding of more than one distinct secondary clone by cytogenetic analysis in some of the patients supports the notion that there can be more than one clonal evolution.

Although blast phase usually occurs in the bone marrow or peripheral blood, in approximately 5 to 10% of patients it occurs at extramedullary sites (125,126). The most common site is the lymph nodes, but other areas of involvement include soft tissue and the central nervous system. Extramedullary blast phase presentation can be of myeloid or lymphoid type, although in most series the former is more common (126). L-BP at extramedullary sites respond more favorably to therapy than the M-BP, just as in the more typical bone marrow and peripheral blood transformation. Bone marrow involvement may be seen simultaneous with or subsequent to the extramedullary presentation.

Differential Diagnosis

The correct diagnosis of CML is of critical importance in the choice of appropriate therapy and for predicting outcome. The differential diagnostic considerations for patients with a presumptive diagnosis include reactive conditions and other neoplastic hematopoietic disorders. Although in most instances the diagnosis of CML can be arrived at reliably from evaluation of blood and bone marrow (146), in difficult cases the differential ultimately must be resolved with either karyotype analysis for the identification of t(9;22), or through molecular studies for *BCR* rearrangements or the *BCR-ABL* fusion. Although some investigators accept that there are rare patients with true CML in which both the Ph chromosome and the *BCR-ABL* fusion are absent (147), most workers, including those in the major cooperative clinical study groups, require either t(9;22) or *BCR* rearrangements in the diagnostic criteria for CML.

A number of confusing issues arise in the differential diagnosis of CML because of ambiguous terms. One such term is *Ph$^-$ CML*. In the older literature, before molecular analyses were available, the term encompassed cases that truly represented CML (i.e., Ph$^-$ but *BCR-ABL*-positive, as would be shown later) and those that were not CML (i.e., Ph$^-$ and *BCR-ABL* negative) (83). Currently, most diagnosticians use the term only to refer to those patients who have true CML (i.e., *BCR-ABL*-positive) but lack recognizable evidence of a Ph chromosome on routine cytogenetic analysis. Such patients account for only a few percent of all patients with CML, and they have clinical features and survival statistics identical to those with CML who have the Ph chromosome (148). Two additional confusing terms are *aCML* and *juvenile CML*. The rare entity aCML is discussed subsequently; by definition such patients do not have the Ph chromosome or *BCR* rearrangement (148). It is unfortunate that another term that does not incorporate *CML* cannot be devised for the disorder. *Juvenile CML* refers to a disorder that is also not truly CML, and is now more correctly referred to as *JMML* (149). Pediatric cases of true Ph$^+$ or *BCR-ABL*-positive CML sometimes are referred to with the awkward term *adult type CML*.

Differential Diagnosis in Patients Presenting in Chronic Phase

A severe leukemoid reaction can simulate CML, because reactive granulocytoses can be associated with WBC as high as 30 and occasionally up to 100 $\times$ 10^9 per liter (96,150). These patients generally lack the myelocyte bulge and basophilia that are characteristic of CML, and they exhibit toxic changes in the granulocytic elements and elevated leukocyte alkaline phosphatase scores that would be unusual for CML. The patients are likely to lack splenomegaly, and an underlying cause of the granulocytic reaction may become obvious. Bone marrow findings are generally less helpful, especially in excluding early CML (151).

TABLE 49.2. *Distinguishing features among the chronic myeloid leukemias (152)*

	Chronic myelogenous leukemia	Atypical chronic myeloid leukemia	Chronic myelomonocytic leukemia
Ph chromosome	Positive (<5% negative)	Negative	Negative
BCR-ABL	Positive (all cases)	Negative	Negative
Monocytes	<3%	≥3 to <10%	Usually >10%
Immature granulocytes	>20%	10–20%	≤10%
Basophils	≥2%	<2%	<2%
Granulocytic dysplasia	Minimal	Strongly positive	Positive
Marrow erythroid precursors	Few	Few	>15%

The borderline myelodysplastic/myeloproliferative disorder CMML also can mimic chronic or accelerated-phase CML. In one series, reported before the availability of molecular analysis for *BCR-ABL*, the largest group of patients initially reported as having Ph^- CML were reevaluated as having CMML (83). The presence of dysplasia and the monocytosis were thought to be the key features useful in ruling out CML. In a more recent report on distinguishing among the different chronic myeloid leukemias, the FAB group noted that CMML also can be distinguished morphologically from CML by its significantly lower WBC counts, lower percentage of immature granulocytes, and higher percentage of circulating monocytes and marrow erythroid precursors (152) (Table 49.2). In difficult cases, however, cytogenetic and molecular analyses are essential.

The other entity addressed in the FAB publication was aCML. This is discussed more completely in the section on myeloproliferative/myelodysplastic disorders later in this chapter. With regard to its distinction from CML, however, the features that differ significantly between CML and aCML are the presence of increased dysplasia in aCML and the higher basophilia in CML. Other features such as the percentage of immature circulating granulocytes, the number of monocytes, and the overall WBC count do not differ between the two. Because, by definition, patients with aCML lack the Ph chromosome and *BCR-ABL*, cytogenetic and molecular studies are key in arriving at the correct diagnosis. A subset of cases that would fall within the spectrum of aCML has i(17q) as the sole cytogenetic abnormality (153,154). This can be confusing, because i(17q) is among the most common secondary chromosomal changes in CML. The finding of i(17q) as a sole abnormality in a chronic myeloid leukemia makes it even more imperative to rule out a Ph^-, *BCR-ABL*-positive case through molecular means (155).

Chronic neutrophilic leukemia is another somewhat rare entity that must be differentiated from CML (156). To distinguish CNL from CML, one must recognize that in CNL the leukemic proliferation is usually of mature granulocytic forms without the left shift and myelocyte bulge seen in CML. Also, the NAP activity in CNL is usually high. Some patients referred to as having CNL have been found to have a variant *BCR-ABL* translocation involving e19 (e19a2 or c3a2) which results in a p230BCR-ABL protein (71). Such patients probably should be considered to have CML with excessive neutrophilia, rather than CNL, which is *BCR-ABL*-negative.

The other myeloproliferative disorders can overlap CML in both clinical and pathologic features. In general, however, one feature that is characteristic, and a helpful clue supporting CML, is the presence of small, hypolobated megakaryocytes. These contrast with the usual large and atypical megakaryocytes of PV, CIMF, and ET (93) and are particularly helpful if the biopsy results show fibrosis and the condition must be distinguished from CIMF (104,105). It may be particularly difficult to distinguish CML with marked thrombocytosis from ET. Some of the difficult cases have been found to have the same e19a2 (c3a2) *BCR-ABL* as seen in CML with excessive neutrophilia (72,73). The presence of a *BCR-ABL* fusion, albeit a variant one, would make one consider CML with thrombocytosis rather than ET in such patients.

Differential Diagnosis in Patients Presenting in Blast Phase

Rare patients with CML present in L-BP with an unrecognized or possibly an absent chronic phase. These patients can present in the peripheral blood and bone marrow or at an extramedullary site. The differential diagnostic considerations are acute lymphoblastic leukemia and lymphoblastic lymphoma, respectively. Most patients with CML presenting as an ALL have, in addition to lymphoblastemia, a prominent granulocyic component in the blood and marrow, that is, the L-BP with CML in the background (Fig. 49.7). This suggests the correct diagnosis. Some patients, however, lack the granulocytic component, and it is impossible to distinguish these patients from those with ALL, even if the Ph chromosome is found. Molecular studies may be a helpful next step, because identification of the minor *BCR-ABL* transcript (p190) would offer strong support for Ph^+ ALL, because CML with p190 is rare. The finding of the major *BCR-ABL* transcript (p210), however, cannot help to distinguish between the entities, because p210 *BCR-ABL* can be seen in either process. Recently, one report claimed that CML presenting in L-BP could be distinguished from Ph^+ ALL by the respective findings of multilineage involvement by

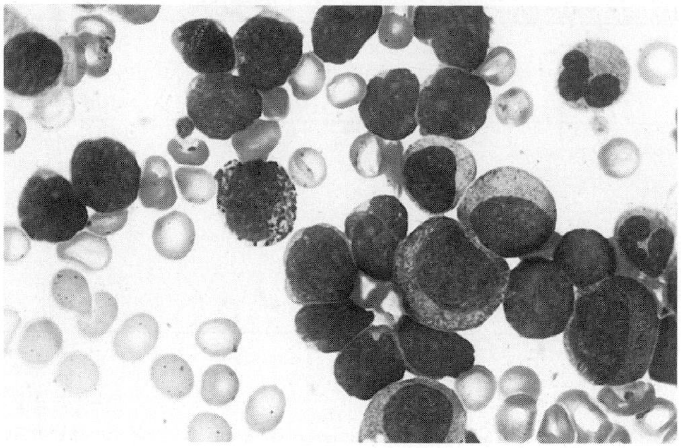

FIG. 49.7. Chronic myelogenous leukemia (CML) can present in blast phase. In the case illustrated, the patient presented with a white blood cell count of 648 $\times$ 10^9 per liter. There were 60% blasts that expressed a common precursor B-cell phenotype. The remainder of the cells were a spectrum of granulocytic precursors and increased basophils typical of CML. After therapy, the patient reverted to chronic phase CML but then relapsed into blast phase and died after 25 months).

the *BCR-ABL* clone *versus* lymphoblastic restricted disease, as evaluated by FISH (74). In another report, however, the conclusion that the two could be so distinguished was challenged (75). Ultimately, it seems that some cases of CML presenting in L-BP may be distinguishable from Ph^+ ALL only if they eventually ''relapse'' or ''revert'' after therapy to a more recognizable form of CML. Although the distinction between CML presenting in L-BP and Ph^+ ALL may seem academic, the duration of survival of patients who present with multilineage disease (L-BP of CML) is quite long compared with that of patients with lymphoblast-restricted disease (Ph^+ ALL) (74,157). Different treatment strategies may be important for the two groups of patients.

If CML presenting in L-BP occurs at an extramedullary site, it is difficult to distinguish the CML from lymphoblastic lymphoma (125,126). The presence of a B-cell phenotype (unexpected in patients with lymphoblastic lymphoma) and the findings of abnormal bone marrow features involving nonlymphoid cells should alert the diagnostician to the possibility of CML in L-BP. The correct diagnosis may not be made until the Ph chromosome, or *BCR-ABL*, is identified or the more typical features of CML become apparent.

Cases of CML presenting as an AML are infrequent, and whether they are truly CML without an actual or recognized chronic phase or they are *de novo* AML has not been resolved entirely (158). The rare cases reported as Ph^+ AML are morphologically heterogeneous (resembling M0, M2, M4, M5, M6, or M7), and they frequently display different types of blasts, as described in the mixed M-BP of CML. They also frequently exhibit lymphoid as well as myeloid markers. The prognosis for such patients is extremely poor.

Prognosis, Therapy, and Disease Monitoring

The median duration of survival of patients with CML in recent reports is 58 to 69 months, but the course of the disease varies widely and the range of survival duration spans 1 to 117 months (39,159). For better evaluation of the prognosis at the time of initial diagnosis, and in an attempt to help direct the selection of optimal therapy, a number of staging systems have been developed (39,159,160). These consider a number of parameters, including patient age, spleen size, basophil count, blast count, platelet count, and eosinophil count, and, with varying degrees of success, are able to stratify patients into low-, intermediate-, and high-risk groups. Other parameters, including degree of bone marrow fibrosis, percentage of CD34 cells in the marrow, and presence of specific cytogenetic abnormalities, also have been shown to have prognostic significance at diagnosis (105,114,119). For some of these parameters, however, an interim change and worsening of the feature are more predictive than the findings from a single observation.

The choice of therapy in CML is dictated not only by the stage of disease but also by a number of factors including the phase of the disease, the availability of a suitable donor for transplantation, and the ability of the patient to tolerate the contemplated regimen. Therapy can be divided into four categories including conventional chemotherapy, interferon-α, hematopoietic transplantation, and newer experimental modalities (161). Splenectomy is no longer a common procedure in routine treatment. If called upon to help evaluate the response to the therapy selected, the pathologist must be acutely aware of the patient's particular treatment history. Although in many situations assessment of the pathologic features seems to be of less importance than the findings from chromosome or molecular studies, a correlation of all types of evaluations can provide more information than a specific evaluation considered separately.

Chemotherapy

Chemotherapy is the most commonly used treatment in CML, and the most frequently used agents are busulfan and hydroxyurea (162). Homoharringtonine is a newer agent that is being evaluated in large clinical trials (163). The chemotherapeutic drugs produce a reduction in the WBC and provide disease control and modest survival prolongation. They do not prevent, however, the transformation to the acute terminal phase.

Patients treated with chemotherapeutic agents usually are evaluated in terms of a reduction in their clinical symptoms, changes in laboratory parameters including the CBC, and peripheral blood and bone marrow findings. The drugs usually do not produce a long-term cytogenetic response; the Ph chromosome continues to be seen in most if not all metaphase cells. Blood and bone marrow changes, however, can be significant, with a reduction in granulocytosis, reduction in cellularity, and increase in erythropoiesis. Usually, however, there are still signs of the disease, as evidenced by persistent basophilia, a persistent left shift, a persistence of small megakaryocytes, and persistent reticulin fibrosis. The increased erythroid activity should not be overinterpreted as normal regeneration, because erythropoiesis can reemerge in CML as disease progresses (164), and erythropoiesis appearing as prominent ''regeneration'' after chemotherapy still may be clonal (165). It is important to recognize that the chemotherapeutic agents commonly cause dysplastic and megaloblastoid changes in the hematopoietic elements. In treated patients, these features should not be relied on for indicating disease progression.

Interferon-α

Interferon-α has been used in the treatment of CML since the 1980s. Unlike chemotherapy, it can modify the course of the disease significantly (166). Interferon-α can produce hematologic responses, but it also can suppress the CML clone and reduce or even eliminate the number of Ph$^+$ metaphase cells seen on routine cytogenetic analysis (167). The mode of action of interferon-α is not entirely known, but it is believed to correct the adhesion abnormalities of the *BCR-ABL*-positive hematopoietic stem cells (168).

Morphologic studies in patients receiving interferon-α have shown that the therapy results in a reduction in cellularity, increases in fat, reduction in the myeloid to erythroid (M:E) ratio, and increases in normal-appearing megakaryocytes (169). Some investigators have reported that, after prolonged therapy (20 months), some patients develop increased reticulin fibrosis (169), but this is not reported in all studies (170). In the absence of other findings, increased reticulin fibrosis in patients treated with interferon-α should not be interpreted as a sign of accelerating disease. In some patients treated with interferon-α, there are no histologic traces of CML. Morphology alone should not be used alone for evaluation of response, however, and the need to correlate the morphologic impression with cytogenetic and molecular findings always should be noted.

Different strategies for evaluating patients on interferon therapy are being developed: In one approach, it is suggested that quantitative Southern blot analysis be used for monitoring of disease in the peripheral blood, and that conventional cytogenetic study be performed on a bone marrow specimen if remission is documented in the blood by Southern blot analysis (171). Although conventional cytogenetic analysis plays an important role in this and most other approaches, some investigators believe that FISH for recognition of the *BCR-ABL* fusion may be more sensitive than routine cytogenetic study. It has been reported that FISH not only identifies a greater proportion of responders to the treatment but also may detect residual Ph$^+$ cells in patients shown to have a complete cytogenetic response by conventional analysis (172,173).

Hematopoietic Cell Transplantation

High-dosage chemotherapy followed by hematopoietic stem cell rescue through either allogeneic bone marrow or peripheral blood stem cell transplantation is the therapy of choice for young patients with suitable donors. This therapy offers the potential for cure, because long-term complete remission can be achieved (174).

Assessment of posttransplant status is undertaken with combined evaluation of morphologic, cytogenetic, and molecular study results. Morphologic findings are similar to those after transplantation for other disorders, but care must be taken to not overinterpret a granulocytic hyperplasia during recovery (175). Cytogenetic studies continue to identify the Ph chromosome for a period of time after a transplant, and early positive cytogenetic results should not be alarming. The results of molecular studies have been somewhat confusing, because *BCR-ABL* transcripts also can be detected by reverse transcriptase–PCR for many months, and even years, after transplantation. How and when positive results can be used for prediction of relapse is a matter of ongoing discussion (176,177). Residual transcripts that are not predictive of relapse may result from residual leukemic cells that are present at the time of analysis but later are removed because of a graft-*versus*-leukemia effect (178). The finding of residual transcripts by PCR also may result from nonclonogenic terminally differentiated cells that linger in the bone marrow. For example, in one study, which correlated morphologic findings with molecular analysis, it was demonstrated that terminally differentiated pseudo-Gaucher histiocytes that persisted in the marrow for up to 1 year after successful transplantation were *BCR-ABL*-positive (101) (Fig. 49.3). Long-lived but nonclonogenic cells are a possible source of *BCR-ABL* transcripts that are not predictive of relapsing disease. Most recently, it has been shown that problems in interpreting qualitative PCR results can be overcome with quantitative PCR. The finding of increasing *BCR-ABL* transcripts in a patient after transplantation appears to be the most sensitive means for predicting a clonal relapse (179).

Experimental Therapies

New experimental modalities for therapy include autologous stem cell harvest with or without expansion of Ph$^-$ stem cells (180), treatment with antisense oligonucleotides for *BCR-ABL* (181), use of tyrosine kinase inhibitors (182), and immunotherapy directed against *BCR-ABL* transcripts or protein (183). Regarding autologous stem cell transplantation, early in the disease there are circulating hematopoietic progenitors without the Ph chromosome. These are actually more numerous than circulating Ph$^+$ stem cells and are increased 50-fold over the number of hematopoietic progenitors in the peripheral blood of normal individuals (184). The Ph$^-$ CD34-positive cells have been shown to be enriched in the fraction of cells adherent to cell culture plastic (185), and they are a potentially good source of normal hematopoietic progenitors . Although some of the new therapies hold great promise, their efficacy still is being evaluated, and the best modalities for evaluating response to these specific treatment approaches have not yet been determined.

CHRONIC NEUTROPHILIC LEUKEMIA

Chronic neutrophilic leukemia is a rare disorder characterized by sustained neutrophilia in the peripheral blood, granulocytic hyperplasia in the bone marrow, and hepatosplenomegaly. There is no Ph chromosome or *BCR-ABL* fusion (156,186,187). CNL frequently resembles a leukemoid reaction, so that underlying disorders which result in granulocytic hyperplasia must be excluded carefully before a diagnosis of CNL is made.

Etiology and Pathogenesis

Fewer than 100 cases of CNL have been reported, and the cause and pathogenesis in most of these is not clear. In nearly 20% of the reported cases, CNL was associated with plasma cell dyscrasia or multiple myeloma; in some others, it preceded the onset of MDS, PV, or CIMF (187–194). Such reports have led to speculation that CNL is not a distinct CMPD but is either a reactive disorder caused by an underlying neoplastic process or an early manifestation of another myeloid disorder. There is evidence in some cases, however, that CNL is a unique, clonal myeloproliferative disease. Cytogenetic studies are normal in most patients, but about 10% are reported to have clonal karyotypic abnormalities that include +8, +9, del(20q), and del(11q) (195–197). In a few patients, neutrophil clonality has been demonstrated by restriction fragment length polymorphism analysis of X-linked polymorphisms or by FISH (197,198). Florescent *in situ* hybridyzation and cytogenetic studies of cells from bone marrow cultures of patients with CNL reportedly have shown that neutrophils and eosinophils are clonal, but that lymphocytes, monocytes, and erythroid cells are not clonal (197,199). These findings indicate that CNL may be a clonal proliferation derived from a progenitor cell with limited lineage potential. Whether CNL associated with a plasma cell dyscrasia is a clonal or a secondary reactive process, however, is not clear. No evidence of neutrophil clonality was detected by restriction fragment length polymorphism analysis in one patient with CNL associated with multiple myeloma (200), and there are no convincing reports of cytogenetic abnormalities in such patients.

Clinical and Laboratory Findings

Clinical Features

The incidence of CNL is unknown, but it is uncommon: There is probably fewer than one case of CNL for every 600 cases of CML (148). CNL is usually a disorder of older adults but has been reported in adolescents as well (201). The sex distribution is nearly even (156,187). Splenomegaly is virtually always present, and nearly 75% of patients also have hepatomegaly. A history of bleeding from mucocutaneous surfaces or from the gastrointestinal tract is not uncommon (156).

Peripheral Blood

Chronic neutrophilic leukemia is characterized by a sustained leukocytosis of 25×10^9 per liter that is comprised primarily of segmented neutrophils (156,187). Bands can account for up to 50% of the leukocyte differential in a few patients, but myelocytes, promyelocytes, and blasts are rarely seen. The neutrophils often contain Döhle bodies and toxic granules, but they may be normal (156,187) (Fig. 49.8). In contrast to CML, in CNL the NAP score is elevated. Anemia may be present, and although platelet counts are generally normal, thrombocytopenia or thrombocytosis is possible (156,187).

Bone Marrow

The bone marrow is hypercellular because of granulocytic hyperplasia, and the M:E ratio often is more than 20:1 (156). Blasts and promyelocytes are not increased in percentage, but myelocytes and mature granulocytes are. Some patients exhibit erythroid or megakaryocytic hyperplasia as well. Although granulocytic, erythroid, and megakaryocytic dysplasia have been reported (192,193), in our opinion, any significant dysplasia should prompt consideration of the diagnosis of aCML rather than CNL. In view of the reported association between CNL and plasma cell dyscrasias, the number and morphology of the plasma cells in the bone marrow, as well as their light chain expression, should be assessed carefully (188–190).

Extramedullary Tissues

Splenomegaly and hepatomegaly result from tissue infiltration by neutrophils. In the spleen, the infiltrate is confined largely to the red pulp; in the liver, the neutrophils may be in the portal areas, sinusoids, or both (156).

Other Laboratory Findings

No Ph chromosome or *BCR-ABL* fusion gene is present. Cytogenetic abnormalities have been reported in about 10% of patients, but none are specific for CNL. Some patients with Ph^+ myeloid leukemias with marked neutrophilia have been reported to have novel breakpoints at e19 in the *BCR* gene that result in a larger fusion protein, p230, than the p210 usually seen in CML (71). Even though such cases may resemble CNL, they probably are better classified as CML with extreme neutrophilia (67).

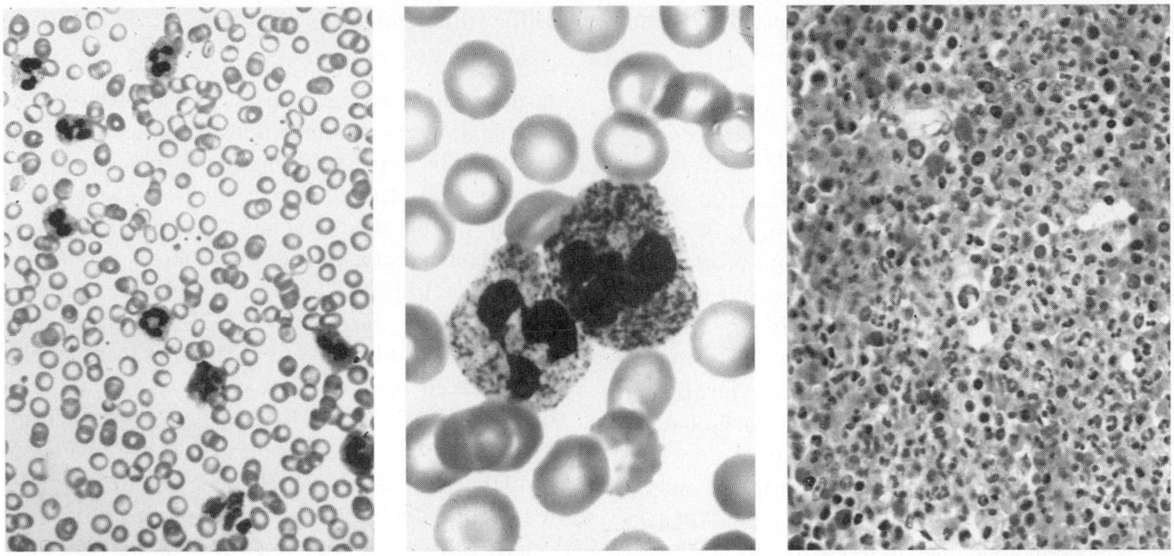

A,B C

FIG. 49.8. In chronic neutrophilic leukemia, the peripheral blood smear shows mainly segmented neutrophils, which often show "toxic" granules (**A,B**). The bone marrow biopsy specimen is hypercellular, with an elevated M:E ratio and a shift towards mature granulocytic elements (**C**). There is no Philadelphia chromosome or *BCR-ABL* fusion gene.

In keeping with the leukocytosis in CNL, there is elevation of serum vitamin B12 and uric acid levels. Indicators of inflammation, such as increased C-reactive protein or an elevated erythrocytic sedimentation rate, are absent (156). Patients with an associated plasma cell lesion may have a paraprotein that often is associated with λ light chain restriction (189).

Differential Diagnosis

Many patients initially suspected to have CNL ultimately are proved to be experiencing leukemoid reactions to infection or an underlying tumor. To exclude CML, all patients should be studied cytogenetically and molecularly for a Ph chromosome or *BCR-ABL* fusion. In view of the reported ''evolution'' of CNL to other myeloproliferative disorders, appropriate studies should be done to rule out the other CMPDs, particularly PV (194). The finding of monocytosis or of any significant dysplasia should prompt consideration of CMML or aCML. The diagnosis of CNL in patients with multiple myeloma should be made only if there is convincing evidence of clonality of the neutrophils.

Prognosis and Prognostic Features

Survival of patients with CNL is variable, ranging from 6 months to more than 20 years (187). In cases associated with myeloma, patients usually die from progression of the plasma cell lesion.

HYPEREOSINOPHILIC SYNDROMES AND CHRONIC EOSINOPHILIC LEUKEMIA

The idiopathic hypereosinophilic syndrome (IHES) is characterized by sustained eosinophilia of unknown origin in the blood and bone marrow that is associated with tissue damage caused by release of eosinophil granules (202–205). It is not yet clear whether most cases of IHES are clonal proliferations of eosinophils or reactive reponses to an undiscovered, underlying disorder that is associated with the abnormal release of cytokines that promote eosinophil proliferation (206). The clinical, laboratory, and morphologic features of IHES, however, overlap or are at times indistinguishable from those reported for chronic eosinophilic leukemia (CEL), which is a clonal process. It is appropriate to consider IHES and CEL as closely related diseases and to include them in this discussion of the CMPDs.

Clinical and Laboratory Findings

Clinical Features

Idiopathic hypereosinophilic syndrome usually occurs in adults but may occur in children (203). The diagnosis requires persistent, unexplained eosinophilia of 1.5×10^9 per liter for at least 6 months. All possible causes for the eosinophilia, such as parasitic infections and underlying tumors, must be excluded, and evidence of organ involvement or damage by the eosinophils must be present (203–205). The initial chief complaint is variable. Weight loss with anorexia and fatigue, fever with night sweats, chest pain accompanied by a nonproductive cough, and congestive heart failure commonly are reported (204). Evidence of central nervous system dysfunction, peripheral neuropathy, cutaneous lesions, and pulmonary infiltrates with fibrosis, arthritis, and gastrointestinal disturbances, however, also may be present initially or develop in the course of the disease. The most common complication is cardiac damage (203–205,207–209).

Splenomegaly is found in 40 to 80% of patients, and hepatomegaly is found in similar percentages (203).

Peripheral Blood

Eosinophilia, ranging from 1.5 to more than 100×10^9 eosinophils per liter, is the most striking finding (208). Most often, the eosinophils are mature, but immature forms may be seen, and cytoplasmic degranulation or vacuolization and nuclear hypersegmentation are frequently reported abnormalities (208,209). Abnormal eosinophil morphology is not a reliable clue as to whether the eosinophils are malignant or benign (205), although demonstration of naphtol-ASD-chloroacetate esterase activity in the eosinophils does suggest a neoplastic origin (210). Absolute neutrophilia and basophilia frequently accompany the eosinophilia. Platelet counts are reduced in about one third of patients, and nearly one half is anemic (204,207).

Bone Marrow

In IHES, the bone marrow aspirate and biopsy specimens may be normocellular to markedly hypercellular (209). Eosinophils at all stages of maturation may account for 60% or more of the marrow elements and show morphologic changes similar to those described in the blood. Macrophages with Charcot-Leyden granules commonly are seen (209). An increase in the number of myeloblasts is not usual, but if present it is reported to be associated with a poor prognosis and may indicate that the process is more likely to be CEL (204,209). In most patients, erythroid precursors are normal, as are the megakaryocytes. Although a slight increase in reticulin fibers has been reported (210), severe myelofibrosis is uncommon.

Cytogenetic and Other Laboratory Findings

Most patients with IHES have normal chromosome findings (204,205). The presence of a Ph chromosome or *BCR-ABL* indicates that the diagnosis is CML rather than IHES or CEL. Trisomy 8 and i(17q) have been reported in occasional patients with IHES. If other myeloproliferative disorders are excluded, a diagnosis of CEL is appropriate if such an abnormality is found, particularly if it can be identified in the eosinophils by FISH or other techniques (205). Demonstration of eosinophil clonality by analyses of X-chromosome inactivation patterns also may provide evidence for considering the patient to have CEL rather than IHES (206). A number of patients with myeloproliferative and MDSs associated with marked eosinophilia have been reported to have the chromosomal translocation t(5;12)(q33;p13) (211–213). Most patients with this cytogenetic abnormality also have signficant monocytosis, however, in which case the diagnosis of CMML with eosinophilia is preferable to CEL.

Differential Diagnosis

To establish a diagnosis of either IHES or CEL, one must exclude all possible causes of secondary eosinophilia (203,204). Parasitic infections, Kimura's disease, angiolymphoid hyperplasia, eosinophilia–myalgia syndrome, hypersensitivity and allergic conditions, and vasculitis are among the conditions that must be considered. It is important to remember that a number of cytokines, including interleukin-2 (IL-2), IL-3, IL-5, and granulocyte-macrophage colony-stimulating factor (GM-CSF), promote eosinophil proliferation and differentiation, and that these cytokines may be produced by normal, reactive, or neoplastic lymphoid or myeloid cells (204,205,207). The eosinophils found in association with some neoplastic processes may not necessarily be malignant but could be stimulated to proliferate by the abnormal production of a cytokine by other neoplastic cells. For example, marked eosinophilia is not uncommon in T-cell lymphoma, mycosis fungoides, Hodgkin's disease, and some patients with acute lymphoblastic leukemia, because of the release of eosinophil-promoting cytokines from the tumor cells (205). A similar mechanism probably accounts for the eosinophilia commonly associated with mast cell disease. Other myeloproliferative disorders and MDS may display prominent eosinophilia, and the distinction among other CMPDs with eosinophilia, IHES, and CEL may be impossible. Evidence of the Ph chromosome or of *BCR-ABL* fusion gene indicates that the correct diagnosis is CML (204,205). The finding of significant dysplasia in the granulocytic, erythroid, or megakaryocytic series is more in keeping with MDS.

Prognosis

Because IHES and CEL are heterogeneous disorders that range from relatively benign proliferations that readily respond to antiinflammatory therapy to aggressive diseases that are therapy-resistant, the prognosis is quite variable. Scoring systems have been proposed for predicting outcome (214), and in general, the finding of advanced cardiac or neurologic disease, evidence of marrow failure, or features that indicate that the disease is leukemic in nature indicate a poorer outcome (208,214). Regardless of the cause, prolonged eosinophilia may lead to severe tissue and organ damage, but if the organ damage inflicted by the eosinophilia can be managed, many patients with IHES have prolonged durations of survival, and nearly 80% are expected to live for 5 years or longer (215).

POLYCYTHEMIA VERA

Polycythemia vera is a neoplastic stem cell disorder associated with the consequences of increased RBC production that is independent of the mechanisms which normally regulate erythropoiesis. It arises in a multilineage stem cell, so that excessive proliferation of lineages in addition to the erythroid series is observed (10,13–16). In the initial ''proliferative'' phase, the increased RBC mass leads to vascular engorgement and circulatory disturbances that may cause thrombosis, tissue infarction, or hemorrhage. Without treatment, patients may die within months. During this stage, the diagnostic challenge is to distinguish PV from ''secondary'' erythrocytosis that is caused by an appropriate or inappropriate increase in erythropoietin (EPO) production. Patients who survive the complications of the proliferative phase of PV may reach a stage in which blood cell counts normalize without further specific therapy. Ultimately, a ''spent phase'' develops, and cytopenias, including anemia, may result from hypersplenism, ineffective hematopoiesis, or bone marrow fibrosis. Acute leukemia also may develop, particularly in patients treated with myelosuppressive agents. With currently available therapy, most patients have an indolent course, and median durations of survival of 10 years or longer are reported commonly (216–218).

Etiology and Pathogenesis

Polycythemia vera has been recognized for more than 100 years, but its cause remains unknown. A genetic predisposition has been postulated, based on the finding of a greater than expected frequency of PV in members of the same family (219–221). Ionizing radiation, occupational exposure to toxins, and viruses also have been suggested as possible causes (222–224).

Despite the lack of knowledge regarding a causative agent in PV, there is considerable information regarding some of the cellular abnormalities. The hormone EPO is one of several important regulators of erythropoiesis and is largely responsible for maintaining the normal balance between RBC mass and tissue oxygenation. Other factors necessary for RBC production include stem cell factor and insulin-like growth factor-1 (IGF-1), which act in synergy with EPO to increase DNA synthesis, prevent apoptosis, and promote maturation of erythroid precursors (225). In patients with PV, serum and urine EPO levels are subnormal; therefore, the erythroid hyperplasia cannot be attributed to excessive EPO production (226,227). In contrast to normal erythroid progenitors, which require exogenous EPO to form colonies in *in vitro* culture systems, those from the blood and bone marrow of patients with PV grow in the absence of exogenous EPO and form *endogenous erythroid colonies* (EECs) (228,229). Initially, there were conflicting notions as to whether the EECs were caused by a population of cells that was hypersensitive to trace amounts of EPO in the culture medium, or by cells that were truly autonomous and independent of the hormone. Recent data have shown that erythroid progenitors from patients with PV have a dose-response curve to EPO similar to that of normal control subjects and thus are not hypersensitive to EPO (230). They are, however, hypersensitive to other growth factors, particularly IGF-1, and it has been postulated that it is trace amounts of IGF-1 in the culture medium that promote the development of the EECs (230,231). The receptor for IGF-1 is a member of the tyrosine kinase receptor family, which is important in mediating the effects of extracellular growth factors on cell proliferation. Mononuclear hematopoietic cells from patients with PV have been shown to have IGF-1 receptors that are hyperresponsive to IGF-1 (231,232). IGF-1 also inhibits apoptosis of erythroid precursors, although the mechanism by which this is accomplished is not clear (225). BCL-X is another protein that inhibits apoptosis and is abnormally expressed in erythroid cells from patients with PV (233). Whether the IGF-1 and BCL-X pathways are interrelated in PV has not been clarified. Other growth factors, including IL-3, GM-CSF, and stem cell factor, promote excessive proliferation not only of erythroid cells but also of granulocytes and megakaryocytes in PV, so that the pathways that lead to cellular expansion are likely to be complex (234).

The genetic events that underlie the cellular abnormalities are not known, nor is there a consistent cytogenetic abnormality that provides a clue to genes that might be involved (25). Furthermore, in contrast to CML, which seems to be always of pluripotent stem cell origin, in PV the level of hematopoietic stem cell commitment at which the oncogenic event occurs is not clear. There is conflicting data as to whether only myeloid lineages or myeloid and lymphoid lineages are involved, or whether lineage involvement may vary from patient to patient (13–16).

Clinical and Laboratory Findings

Proliferative (''Erythrocytotic'') Phase

The diagnosis of PV generally is made in the initial, ''proliferative'' stage. It requires documentation of an increase in the RBC mass and exclusion of ''secondary'' causes of erythrocytosis. The diagnosis can be made from clinical and laboratory findings; morphology plays an important but largely supportive role. The most commonly employed criteria for establishing a diagnosis of PV have been those suggested by the Polycythemia Vera Study Group (PVSG), which require documentation of an increased RBC mass, normal arterial oxygen saturation, and splenomegaly. If splenomegaly is not present, two additional hematologic abnormalities, such as leukocytosis, thrombocytosis, elevated NAP scores, or elevated vitamin B12 levels, are necessary for confirmation of the diagnosis (235–237). Some believe that the PVSG criteria are too restrictive and may exclude some patients with early PV; others have argued that newer tests, such as those that can detect decreased serum EPO levels and EECs, are more specific and sensitive than the criteria proposed by the PVSG. Such concerns have led to proposals for modifications in the diagnostic criteria, such as those recently proposed by the World Health Organization (122) (Table 49.3).

Clinical Features

Polycythemia vera has a yearly incidence of 1 in 100,000 population (238), with nearly equal frequencies in the sexes

TABLE 49.3. *Proposed World Health Organization criteria for diagnosis of polycythemia vera (122)*

A1. Elevated RBC mass (>25% above mean normal predicted value) or Hgb >18.5 g/dl in men, 16.5 g/dl in women (or >99th percentile of method-specific reference range for age, sex, altitude of residence)
A2. No causes of secondary erythrocytosis, including
  1. Absence of familial erythrocytosis
  2. No elevation of EPO due to
    a. Hypoxia (arterial $pO_2 \leq 92\%$)
    b. High oxygen affinity hemoglobin
    c. Truncated EPO receptor
    d. Inappropriate EPO production by tumor
A3. Splenomegaly
A4. Clonal cytogenetic abnormality of marrow cell lines
A5. Endogenous erythroid colonies formation *in vitro*
B1. Thrombocytosis $>400 \times 10^9$/L
B2. WBC $\geq 12 \times 10^9$/L
B3. Bone marrow hyperplasia with erythroid hyperplasia and increase of megakaryocyte number and size
B4. Low serum erythropoeitin levels
Diagnosis of PV established when
  A1 + A2 + A3 or
  A1 + A2 + A4 or
  A1 + A2 + A5 or
  A1 + A2 + any two of B category

(239). The mean age at diagnosis is 60 years, and patients younger than 20 years of age rarely are reported (239–241). The major symptoms are related to hypertension or to vascular abnormalities caused by the increased RBC mass. Headache, dizziness, visual disturbances, and paresthesia are major complaints. Nearly 25% of patients are first identified after an episode of venous or arterial thrombosis, such as deep vein thrombophlebitis, myocardial ischemia, or stroke. Mesenteric and portal or splenic vein thrombosis always should prompt consideration of PV as a possible cause (242). Hemorrhage, particularly gastrointestinal bleeding, may occur and, if chronic, can mask the polycythemia. Other findings include pruritus without an accompanying rash, erythromelalgia, and gouty arthritis (235,238,239). The principal physical findings include plethora in 70% of patients, palpable splenomegaly in 70%, hepatomegaly in 40%, and hypertension in 70% (243).

Peripheral Blood

The demonstration of an elevated RBC mass, which is reflected as increases in the hematocrit and hemoglobin levels, is the key to the diagnosis of PV. The RBC mass should be measured directly whenever the hematocrit level is between 40 and 60%, because it may be normal in this hematocrit range. It almost always is elevated if the hematocrit level is above 60% (or greater than the 99th percentile of the method-specific range for altitude of residence) and rarely is elevated if the hematocrit level is less than 40% (239). RBCs usually are morphologically normal in the proliferative stage, unless hemorrhage (or phlebotomy) has produced iron deficiency, in which case microcytosis and hypochromia are seen. Nucleated RBCs and marked poikilocytosis are not features of the proliferative stage.

More than 50% of patients with PV have leukocytosis resulting from neutrophilia, with WBC counts usually between 12 and 25 $\times 10^9$ per liter, although occasionally they may exceed 50,000 $\times 10^9$ per liter (235,239). There may be a mild ''left shift,'' and 75% of patients have increased NAP scores. Mild basophilia is usual.

Platelet counts range from 400 to 800 $\times 10^9$ per liter in 50% of patients, but counts in excess of 1,000 $\times 10^9$ per liter are found in up to 10% of patients (235,239). Functional abnormalities of platelets, including decreased platelet aggregation with adenosine 5′-diphosphate and epinephrine, are a common but nonspecific finding, because patients with other CMPDs may show similar abnormalities.

Bone Marrow

The features of PV in the bone marrow are appreciated best in bone marrow biopsy specimens; marrow aspirate smears aid mainly in the assessment of cytologic detail and marrow iron stores. In the proliferative phase, the characteristic finding in bone marrow specimens is hypercellularity caused by erythroid, granulocytic, and megakaryocytic hyperplasia (103,244–246). Usually, erythroid and megakaryocytic proliferation is most prominent, and the M:E ratio often is reduced, sometimes to less than 1:1 (103,247). Erythropoiesis is normoblastic, unless there is severe iron deficiency (246). Granulopoiesis is morphologically normal, and myeloblasts are not increased in percentage. Megakaryocytes are consistently conspicuous, even in patients who have otherwise normally cellular marrow specimens. The megakaryocytes may cluster and be localized close to the marrow sinusoids (103). They are increased in size as well as in number, although they lack significant pleomorphism (Fig. 49.9A). Silver stains performed on the biopsy specimen reveal normal marrow reticulin fibers in more than two thirds of patients at the time of diagnosis, but they are increased slightly to markedly in the remainder. If found in conjunction with other features of the proliferative phase, reticulin fibrosis does not necessarily signify a worse prognosis or indicate imminent transformation to a more aggressive stage (245,246).

In some patients, bone marrow specimens lack the expected features, even if other clinical and laboratory data support the diagnosis of PV. For example, in nearly 300 cases reported by the PVSG, the cellularity of marrow biopsy specimens ranged from 37 to 100%, with a mean of 82% (246). Normal cellularity was found in 13% of the patients, and they had no other laboratory or clinical findings that distinguished them from patients with hypercellularity (246). Thus, although some morphologic findings in the marrow, such as hypercellularity, are characteristic for PV, they are not specific enough to be diagnostic without knowledge of other clinical and laboratory parameters.

A,B

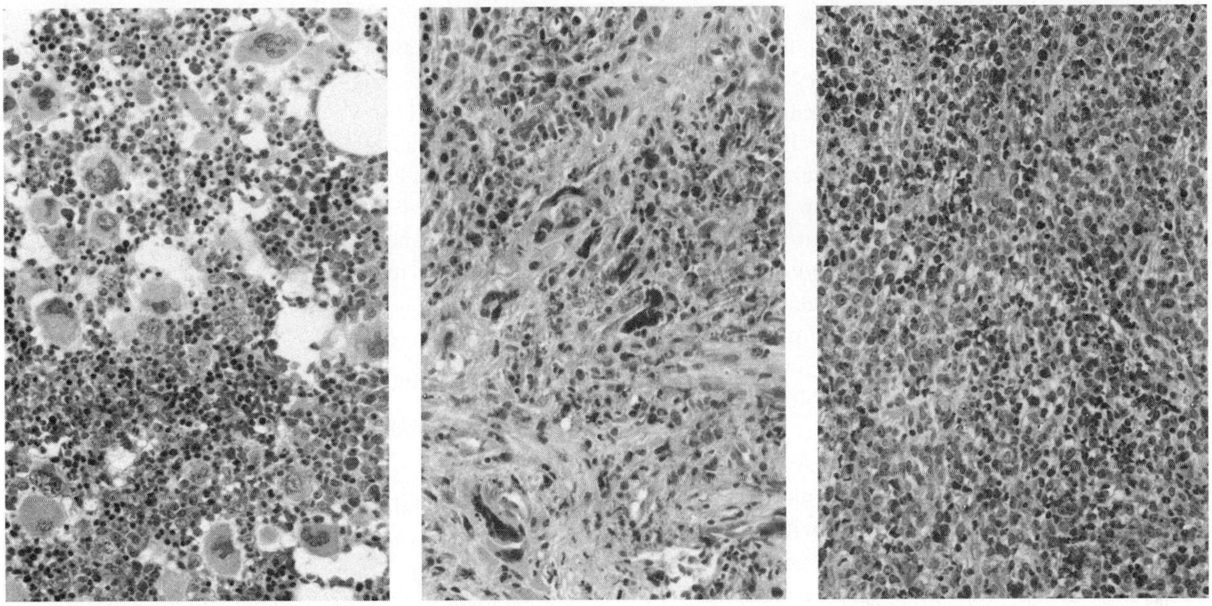

C

FIG. 49.9. Bone marrow biopsy specimens obtained over the course of illness from a patient who had polycythemia vera and was treated intermittently with phlebotomy and alkylating agents. **A:** The initial specimen shows hypercellularity with panhyperplasia. Note the prominent megakaryocytes, which are increased not only in number but also in size. The M:E is 1:1. **B:** Eight years later, the patient had a leukoerythoblastic blood smear, a markedly enlarged spleen, and a bone marrow biopsy that was less cellular, with fibrosis and changes of postpolycythemic myeloid metaplasia. **C:** The patient later developed acute myeloblastic leukemia.

Extramedullary Tissues

During the proliferative phase, splenomegaly and hepatomegaly are caused primarily by sinusoidal and cordal congestion by RBCs. Platelet pooling also may be observed in the splenic cords. Although a few islands of extramedullary hematopoiesis (EMH) may be seen in the spleen or liver, it is generally minimal during this phase (248).

Cytogenetic and Other Laboratory Findings

In contrast to CML, there are no specific cytogenetic abnormalities in PV (25,249–251). Most studies have shown abnormal karyotypes in only 10 to 20% of patients at diagnosis. The most common anomalies include del(20)(q11), +8, +9, and del(1)(p11); sometimes +8 and +9 are seen together. Chromosomal abnormalities increase in frequency during the illness and are found in nearly 80% of patients with the advanced stage of postpolycythemic myeloid metaplasia (PPMM), and in nearly 100% of patients who develop acute leukemia. In many cases, cytogenetic evolution is likely to be related to the myelosuppressive therapy used for treating the proliferative stage (240,249–251), although cytogenetic evolution also may occur in patients treated only with phlebotomy (251).

A number of other laboratory findings are helpful in confirming the diagnosis of PV. The detection of EECs in *in vitro* cultures of blood and bone marrow is characteristic of PV (228,229). The finding of EECs is not entirely specific for PV, because they are present in patients with other CMPDs, including ET and CIMF (229), but they do not occur in patients with secondary erythrocytosis. Serum EPO levels are decreased or low-normal, and the finding of elevated levels excludes the diagnosis of PV (227). A recent report that the erythroid precursors in PV have increased expression of BCL-X protein have prompted some to suggest that study of BCL-X could be used as an additional confirmatory test (233). Other abnormalities include elevated vitamin B12 and B12 binding protein levels and increased amounts of uric acid, although they are not specific for PV.

"Spent Phase" and Postpolycythemic Myeloid Metaplasia

Patients who survive the thrombotic and hemorrhagic complications of the proliferative stage may enter a phase in which the hematocrit level normalizes or anemia develops, and in which the spleen becomes markedly enlarged. Although the term *spent phase* is used widely to describe all end stages of PV, regardless of clinical or pathologic findings, some authors believe that the term should be reserved for those patients (about 5%) who develop hypersplenism with cytopenia in one or more cell lines and have persistent marrow hyperplasia without marrow fibrosis or evidence of EMH. In the cases reported, even though the RBC mass remains increased, the hematocrit falls because of increased plasma volume (252). A more common type of progression, however, is PPMM, which is characterized by marrow fibrosis and by splenomegaly that is caused by EMH. Clinical manifestations of this stage relate to anemia or other cytopenias, massive splenomegaly, and bleeding (239,246). During this period, the peripheral blood smear may show leukopenia or leukocytosis, with WBC sometimes $\geq 100 \times 10^9$ per liter (253). Immature granulocytes, nucleated RBCs, and poikilocytosis with teardrop-shaped RBCs usually are evident. Platelet counts vary but are low in at least 30% of patients because of splenic sequestration and ineffective hematopoiesis. Circulating megakaryocytes and large and abnormal, and bizarre platelets commonly are seen.

The hallmark of PPMM in the bone marrow specimen is reticulin and even collagen fibrosis (103,246). The cellularity of the bone marrow may vary, but hypocellular marrow specimens are usual, and they often display dilatation of marrow sinusoids filled with immature hematopoietic elements. Clusters of megakaryocytes, often with hyperchromatic, pleomorphic nuclei, are prominent (Fig. 49.9B). Osteosclerosis may occur. The bone marrow findings are virtually identical to those in the myelofibrotic stage of CIMF.

Splenic enlargement often is marked in PPMM, and spleens weighing more than 6,000 g have been reported (248). This enlargement is caused primarily by EMH, with granulocytic, erythroid, and megakaryocytic precursors in the red pulp sinuses. The liver and lymph nodes may demonstrate trilineage EMH (248).

Recent reports on long-term survivors of the PVSG studies reveal that the incidence of PPMM may reach 20% at 15 years and 50% at 20 years of follow-up after the initial diagnosis (218). Patients who were treated with phlebotomy, or who were phlebotomized for prolonged periods before receiving a myelosuppressive agent, are reported to have the highest incidence of PPMM. The cytogenetic abnormalities found in patients with PPMM suggest a relationship to the previous myelosuppressive therapy (249–251). Duration of survival after the onset of PPMM is reported to vary from 6 months to more than 9 years, but median durations of survival commonly reported are shorter than 5 years (218,238,246).

Myelodysplastic Syndromes and Acute Leukemia

A low incidence of AML and of MDS appears to be a part of the natural history of PV, because they occcur in about 1 to 2% of patients who received no treatment other than phlebotomy (216,218,236). Data from the PVSG, however, indicate that, in patients treated with ^{32}P or alkylating agents, the frequency of MDS or acute leukemia is much higher, approximately 10 to 15%, at 10 to 15 years of follow-up, and up to 30% at 20 years (218,236). The incidence in patients treated with hydroxyurea has been reported to approach 10% at 10 years of follow-up (216,254,255). Although AML may appear abruptly, it is preceded by a myelodysplastic phase in nearly 50% of patients (256,257). Some of the patients who have MDS die of marrow failure; in others, the condition evolves into overt acute leukemia (256,257) (Fig. 49.9C). Patients previously treated with myelosuppressive agents usually display the hallmarks of therapy-related AML or MDS, including multilineage dysplasia, and chromosomal abnormalities that include hypodiploidy, abnormalities of chromosome 5 or 7, or complex karyotypic anomolies (25,249,250,256–258). Fewer patients have cytologic and cytogenetic abnormalities characteristic of *de novo* AML, and they may represent the natural evolution of PV to acute leukemia (249,258).

Differential Diagnosis of Polycythemia Vera

Relative, Secondary, and Familial Polycythemia

The differential diagnosis of polycythemia includes relative polycythemia (''stress'' erythrocytosis), secondary polycythemia, primary familial (congenital) polycythemia, as well as PV. In relative polycythemia, a decreased plasma volume results in an elevated hematocrit, but the RBC mass is not increased. Hemoconcentration resulting from dehydration, preeclampsia, or other causes result in such a change. A common cause of polycythemia is chronic carbon monoxide toxicity caused by cigarette smoking. In such patients, carboxyhemoglobinemia causes a decrease in the plasma volume as well as tissue hypoxia, so that EPO levels may be increased. Cigarette smoking may produce features of both relative and secondary erythrocytosis (259). One should not assume that relative polycythemia is always clinically benign, because nearly 30% of patients experience thromboembolic complications (259).

In ''secondary'' polycythemia, the increased RBC mass is caused either by an appropriate increase in serum EPO secondary to tissue hypoxia (such as in cardiopulmonary insufficiency) or by an inappropriate increase in EPO secretion, such as by an EPO-producing tumor. Although the RBC mass is increased, patients with secondary polycythemia fail to meet the other criteria suggested for a diagnosis of PV. Table 49.4 outlines some of the differences between PV and secondary polycythemia.

TABLE 49.4. *Differentiation of polycythemia vera and secondary polycythemia (227,229,233,235,237)*

	Polycythemia vera	Secondary polycythemia
Red cell mass	Increased	Increased
Splenomegaly	Present	Absent
Leukocytosis	Present	Absent
Thrombocytosis	Present	Absent
Erythropoietin levels	Low, normal	Increased
Endogenous erythroid colonies	Present	Absent
Bone marrow	Panhyperplasia	Erythroid hyperplasia
Megakaryocyte size	Increased	Normal
BCLX in erythroid precursors	Increased	Normal

Primary familial (congenital) polycythemia is a rare disorder in which the RBCs of the affected patients are hypersensitive to EPO (260,261). The genetic basis for this disease may be heterogeneous. Abnormalities of the EPO receptor have been identified in some patients but not in others (260,261). In this form of polycythemia, serum EPO levels may be normal or low, and some patients even may form a few EECs (260). The restriction of the proliferation to the erythroid series and the familial history helps to distinguish such cases from PV.

Other Chronic Myeloproliferative Diseases

Occasionally, patients with CML have erythrocytosis. In such patients, the detection of the Ph chromosome or *BCR-ABL* fusion gene, a low NAP score, and the finding of small megakaryocytes in the bone marrow establish the diagnosis of CML. The cellular phases of CIMF and ET are more difficult diagnostic issues, because these may resemble PV clinically and morphologically. It is not possible to distinguish PPMM from the myelofibrotic stage of CIMF based on laboratory or morphologic features alone.

Prognosis

Without therapy, the median survival of patients with PV is only 18 months, but with currently available treatment protocols, median durations of survival longer than 10 years commonly are reported (216–218). In the earlier PVSG studies, approximately 30% of the reported deaths resulted from thromboses, 19% from acute leukemia, 15% from other neoplasms, 5% from hemorrhage, and 5% from the complications of PPMM. In follow-up studies of long-term survivors on the PVSG protocols, the death rates from acute leukemia and from PPMM were greater, however (218). Numerous investigators have attempted to find features that identify patients at risk for these complications, particularly those at risk for early death by thrombosis or hemorrhage. Neither the degree of elevation of the platelet count nor that of the hematocrit level seems to predict these events (236,253,247). A history of cytotoxic therapy increases the possibility of MDS and AML. Overall, given the age at which PV occurs, and the long median durations of survival achieved with current treatment, the average patient with PV may not experience a significantly reduced life expectancy (218). Whether newer agents such as interferon-α may improve survival rates further and eliminate the treatment-related complications remains to be established.

ESSENTIAL THROMBOCYTHEMIA

Essential thrombocythemia generally is regarded as a clonal hematopoietic disorder characterized by a sustained increase in the number of platelets in the blood and by megakaryocytic proliferation in the bone marrow (262). The major symptoms and complications are related to thromboembolic and hemorrhagic events. Discovering the reason for an elevated platelet count can be challenging, however, because thrombocytosis is frequent in the other CMPDs, and in occasional patients with MDS or AML, and also occurs as a reactive response in a number of systemic diseases, including other types of cancer. No clinical, morphologic, or laboratory marker has been identified that is specific for ET; the diagnosis is made by exclusion of the better-characterized myeloid disorders and of the possible causes of reactive thrombocytosis (262,263). Although the complications of hemorrhage or thrombosis can be catastrophic, the median durations of survival reported for patients with ET are the best among all of the CMPDs.

Etiology and Pathogenesis

The cause of ET is unknown. Rare familial cases have been reported (264), and retrovirus-like particles have been demonstrated in the platelets of some patients (224). Exposure to chemicals in hair dyes and selected occupations, such as electricians exposed to electrical fields, reportedly are more common among patients with ET than in control populations (265).

Although ET often is considered a bone marrow stem cell disorder, it resembles PV in that lineage commitment of the affected stem cell appears to be variable. Some studies using G6PD isoenzyme analyses or X-linked polymorphisms have indicated that lymphoid and myeloid cells (including megakaryocyte) are part of the clonal process; in other studies performed with similar techniques, not only were the lymphoid cells not clonal, but even granulocytic and monocytic cells were nonclonal in some patients (11,13,266,267). On the other hand, some recent reports have indicated that occasional patients who meet the usual criteria for ET have only polyclonal hematopoiesis, even in the megakaryocytic lineage (266,267). Determination of the histologic and clinical implications of these findings requires additional investigation, but they suggest that prolonged megakaryocytic stimulation or proliferation might precede clonality in some cases.

The mechanism that bestows a proliferative advantage to the megakaryocytes in ET is unknown. Recent investigations have focused on growth factors and their receptors that regulate megakaryocytic proliferation and development. Several growth factors, including EPO, stem cell factor, IL-6 , IL-11, and thrombopoietin (TPO), act synergistically to stimulate megakaryocyte growth and proliferation (268–271). TPO and its receptor, MPL, are particularly crucial to these processes. Disruption of the genes for TPO or for MPL in knockout experiments in mice result in marked diminution of the numbers of megakaryocytes and platelets (268,272). On the other hand, administration of TPO in animal models and humans leads to marked megakaryocytic hyperplasia in the marrow and an increase in the platelet count (267,273). Normally, there is an inverse relationship between TPO and the megakaryocyte and platelet mass; that is, increased numbers of megakaryocytes are associated with lower TPO levels (269–273). In ET, however, this relationship is lost. Despite the markedly increased megakaryocyte mass in ET, TPO levels are normal or elevated, implying an abnormal feedback mechanism (269,273). There is some evidence that abnormalities of MPL may be partly to blame. Normally, MPL binds TPO and removes it from the plasma, but in ET there are fewer receptors on the surface of the platelets than normally are found (274). This abnormality is apparently not limited to ET, however, because a decrease of MPL on platelets from patients with PV has been reported (275). Despite these findings, there is no current evidence of a disruption of the *TPO* or *MPL* genes in ET, nor have structural abnormalities of MPL been identified (271).

There are similarities between ET and the other CMPDs in that there is an expansion of the megakaryocyte progenitor cell pool in the blood and bone marrow specimens of patients with ET (276–278). These progenitors are capable of generating endogenous megakaryocytic colonies in *in vitro* culture systems, even if deprived of the growth factors normally required to support megakaryocyte growth and proliferation (278–280). The finding of endogenous megakaryocytic colonies is not specific for ET; however, they have been reported in patients with PV and CML. EECs also may be found in patients with ET (228,280).

Clinical and Laboratory Findings

Establishing the diagnosis of ET is largely an exercise in excluding reactive and neoplastic disorders that may be accompanied by extreme thrombocytosis. It is important to bear in mind that reactive thrombocytosis is more common than ET (281). Furthermore, among patients who have a CMPD with thrombocythemia, more have CML than ET (281). The criteria commonly employed for the diagnosis of ET are given in Table 49.5 (262).

TABLE 49.5. *Diagnostic criteria for essential thrombocythemia (262)*

1. Platelet count ≥600 × 10^9/L
2. No evidence of polycythemia vera
   a. Hct <40% or normal RBC mass
   b. Stainable iron in marrow or normal serum ferritin or normal MCV
   c. If "b" is not met, failure of iron trail to increase RBC mass into the polycythemia range
3. No evidence of CML
   a. Absent Ph chromosome
   b. Absent *BCR/ABL* fusion gene
4. No evidence of CIMF
   a. Collagen fibrosis absent
   b. Reticulin fibrosis minimal or absent
5. No evidence of MDS
   a. No del(5q), t(3;3), inv(3;3)
   b. No evidence of RARS
6. No evidence that thrombocytosis is reactive
   a. No underlying inflammatory or infectious disorder
   b. No underlying neoplasm

RARS, refractory anemia with ringed sideroblasts.

Clinical Features

Essential thrombocythemia is reported to be the least prevalent of the CMPDs, with an annual incidence of less than 1 per 100,000 population (282). It is diagnosed most commonly in the seventh decade of life but can occur at any age, including during childhood. There is nearly equal affliction of both sexes, although females predominate among younger patients (282,283).

The initial complaint often is related to thrombosis and hemorrhage, but in some series, more than one half of patients are asymptomatic when a markedly elevated platelet count is discovered fortuitously on a routine blood cell count (284). Between 20 and 50% of patients have some manifestation of vascular occlusion (283,284–289). Microvascular disturbances that lead to digital ischemia with gangrene or paresthesias, to erythromelalgia, or to transient cerebral ischemic attacks are the events reported most commonly, but thrombosis of major arteries leading to stroke or coronary infarct also occurs. Venous thrombosis involves either deep or superficial veins, and ET should be considered as a possible cause of splenic and hepatic vein thrombosis. Hemorrhage, usually at mucocutaneous sites, may occur spontaneously or be recognized first as excess bleeding after trauma or surgery (284,286–289). Most reports indicate that there is no correlation between the degree of thrombocytosis and the frequency of thrombosis in ET, but bleeding occurs more frequently if the platelet count is above 1,000 × 10^9 per liter than at lower levels (284,286). Modest splenomegaly is present in up to 50% of patients, and 15 to 20% have hepatomegaly (283,284,289).

Peripheral Blood

The most striking abnormality in the peripheral blood is marked thrombocytosis. The platelet count is at least 600 × 10^9 per liter and may reach even 5 to 10 fold higher (262). On the blood smear, platelets display anisocytosis, ranging from tiny forms to large platelets, and can have bizarre shapes, pseudopods, or agranular cytoplasm (290,291). The platelet distribution width measured on automated blood counters is significantly elevated. Several abnormalities of platelet function have been described, the most characteristic of which is loss of the primary and secondary wave of aggregation with epinephrine (290–294). This abnormality is not unique to ET, however; platelets from patients with other CMPDs may exhibit similar behavior. An abnormally elevated ratio of platelet adenosine 5′-triphosphate to adenosine 5′-diphosphate also usually is found (292,294).

The median WBC count is normal or minimally elevated (10–14 × 10^9 per liter), but counts in excess of 40 × 10^9 per liter have been reported (283,284). Rarely, a few immature granulocytes are found on the blood film. Absolute basophilia is infrequent, and its presence should prompt consideration of the other CMPDs, particularly CML. Most patients have normal NAP scores, but low and high scores may be observed (283). Anemia is sometimes present, particularly in patients who have experienced bleeding episodes, but most often the hemoglobin level is between 12 and 16 g/dL, although it has been reported to be as high as 18 g/dL (283). RBC morphology is normal, unless chronic hemorrhage has led to iron deficiency.

Bone Marrow

Bone marrow specimens in ET are usually slightly to moderately hypercellular, but hypocellular specimens are seen in approximately 5% of patients (103,283,285,295). The most consistent abnormality is marked proliferation of enlarged megakaryocytes (Fig. 49.10). In biopsy specimens, megakaryocytes often exceed 100 per square millimeter of marrow, although this number may range from less than 50 to more than 200 (291,295). The megakaryocytes may occur in small clusters throughout the specimen, but they are just as often diffusely dispersed. Megakaryocytes in ET are larger than normal, with deeply lobated, high-ploidy, dense nuclei, often with smooth nuclear outlines (103,263). Pleomorphism is not prominent. Emperipolesis often is found, with red cells, granulocytes, or their precursors present within the megakaryocytic cytoplasm. Although some authors have emphasized that there is less heterogeneity in the size of megakaryocytes in ET than in other CMPDs, immunostaining techniques for factor VIII or megakaryocyte-specific glycoproteins may uncover a population of smaller megakaryocytes (296). On bone marrow aspirate smears, clusters of large megakaryocytes and huge pools of platelets may be found. Some authors contend that granulopoiesis and erythropoiesis are unaffected in patients with ET (295), but others report erythroid or granulocytic hyperplasia in more than one half of patients (262,283). The bone marrow morphology may overlap that observed in PV and in the cellular stage of CIMF (283,285).

A significant increase in reticulin fibers in the initial bone marrow specimen speaks strongly against ET (103,262,263, 295), although a slight increase is found in 20 to 30% of patients (283,285,291). Reticulin fibrosis may increase as the disease runs its course, but even this is unusual, occuring in less than 5% of patients (103). Stainable iron is reported to be present in 40 to 70% of marrow specimens at the time of diagnosis (285,291,295).

Extramedullary Tissues

The spleen serves as a sequestration site for platelets in ET, and its removal can lead to a dramatic increase in the platelet count (297). The splenic cords may be widened because of retention of platelets, and aggregates of platelets may be seen in the sinusoids. EMH is scant, except for occasional megakaryocytes in splenic and hepatic sinuses. In patients who have experienced splenic vein thromboses, splenic atrophy is possible (297).

Cytogenetic and Other Laboratory Studies

An abnormal karyotype generally is regarded as unusual in ET (298,299). At the Third International Workshop on Chromosomes in Leukemia, only 5.3% of cases submitted as ET had an abnormal karyotype (298). Of these, one had del(13)(q22), a recurring abnormality in CMPD, but each of the remaining patients had a different anomaly. Some investigators, however, have reported cytogenetic abnormalities in as many as 25% of patients and have found that +8, with or without +9, is the most frequent abnormality in ET (287).

A,B

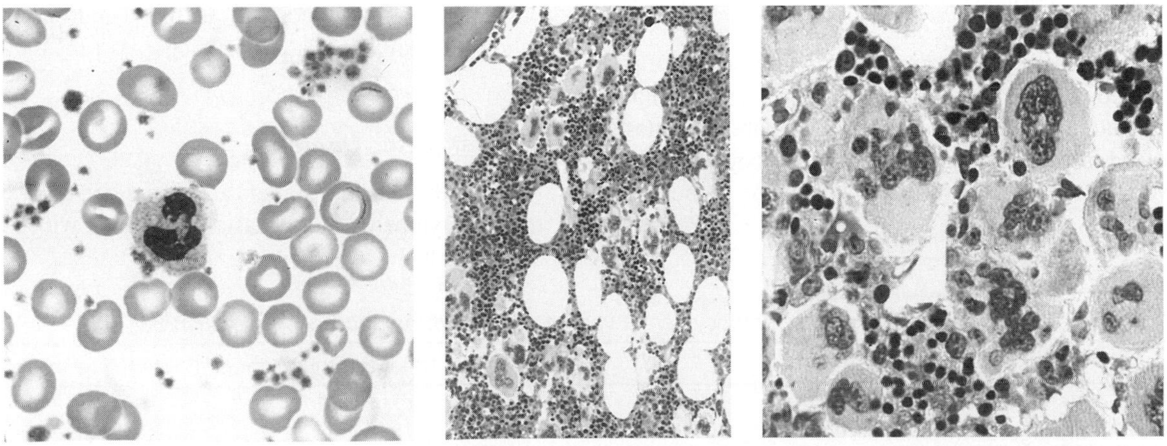

C

FIG. 49.10. These photomicrographs are taken from the blood (**A**) and bone marrow biopsy specimen (**B,C**) of a 50-year-old man with essential thrombocythemia. The platelet count was 950 $\times$ 10^9 per liter, with a normal white blood cell count and leukocyte differential, normal hemoglobin concentration, and a normal red blood cell mass study. Note the increased platelets and the platelet anisocytosis. The bone marrow biopsy specimen has increased numbers of megakaryocytes, which are enlarged with deeply lobated nuclei.

Coagulation studies are usually normal, except that bleeding times may be prolonged (287). There is a decrease in large von Willebrand factor multimers in the plasma that correlates with the degree of thrombocytosis. The decrease is most pronounced if the platelet count is at least 1,000 × 10^9 per liter, and it may play a major role in predisposing the patient to bleeding (286,300). A decrease in the amount of von Willebrand factor is not unique to ET; it occurs in other CMPDs with thrombocytosis (300).

Differential Diagnosis

In one series of more than 200 patients with platelet counts above 1,000 × 10^9 per liter, reactive thrombocytosis accounted for 82% of the cases, 4% involved a CMPD, and the remainder were of uncertain cause (281). Of those patients with a CMPD, fewer than 30% had ET. Symptoms of bleeding or vasoocclusive episodes were noted in nearly 50% of patients who had CMPDs, but only 4% of patients with reactive thrombocytosis had such events. There is therapeutic importance in distinguishing ET and the CMPDs from illnesses with reactive thrombocytosis.

Reactive Thrombocytosis

Reactive thrombocytosis can be associated with acute and chronic infection, chronic blood loss and iron deficiency anemia, chronic inflammatory disorders, solid tumors, and postsplenectomy or hyposplenic states (281). A careful history and physical examination often identifies many of these causes of reactive thrombocytosis. A history of a chronically elevated platelet count or of prior hemorrhage or thrombosis, and the finding of splenomegaly are more in keeping with a CMPD as a cause of the thrombocytosis (301). Although bone marrow biopsy findings of increased megakaryocyte number and size, clusters of megakaryocytes, and increased cellularity have statistical significance in distinguishing between ET and reactive thrombocytosis in large series of patients, individual cases may not be classified easily by morphologic features alone (285). Additional laboratory tests that may aid in establishing whether thrombocytosis is due to a CMPD or to reactive thrombocytosis are summarized in Table 49.6.

Other Chronic Myeloproliferative Diseases

Some patients who have CML initially may have thrombocytosis without significant leukocytosis. In such patients, the finding of basophilia in the peripheral blood film may provide a clue that the proper diagnosis is CML rather than ET (283). Furthermore, inspection of the bone marrow biopsy specimen permits separation of the two disorders, because the megakaryocytes in CML are smaller than normal, whereas those in ET are quite large (103) (Fig. 49.11). Still, all patients in whom the diagnosis of ET is considered should be studied for the Ph chromosome and the *BCR-ABL* fusion gene (25,262). Although the Ph chromosome has been reported to occur in ET (283,302–305), scrutiny of such reports indicates that the patients probably had CML rather than ET (262). In cases of Ph^+ CML associated with the variant fusion protein p230, thrombocytosis is prominent and may lead to confusion with ET (72,73).

The distinction between PV and ET is frequently difficult, and some authors reporting on series of patients with ET concede that patients with PV may have been included inadvertently (283–285). This difficulty arises because approximately 5 to 10% of patients with PV have platelet counts in excess of 1000 × 10^9 per liter, and a similar number of patients with ET have a hematocrit concentration above 50% (235,239,283). Determinations of the RBC mass make it possible to separate the two disorders in most instances, but in patients with PV who have chronic blood loss and a normal RBC mass, determination of serum ferritin and even a trial of iron therapy may be necessary to make the distinction.

In one study of patients with CIMF, nearly 10% initially had laboratory and clinical findings that fulfilled the criteria for ET (263). Discrimination between the cellular phase of CIMF and ET may be possible in bone marrow biopsy specimens by careful examination of the megakaryocytes, which are more pleomorphic and bizarre in CIMF than in ET. This distinction can be impossible at times, and only prolonged follow-up may allow a proper diagnosis (263).

Myelodysplastic Disorders

Myelodysplastic disorders are associated most often with thrombocytopenia, but occasional patients with MDS have

TABLE 49.6. *Essential thrombocythemia versus reactive thrombocytosis (279,281·283,292)*

Feature	Essential thrombocythemia	Reactive thrombocytosis
History of chronic thrombocytosis	+	−
History of hemorrhage or thrombosis	+	−
Splenomegaly	+	−
Endogenous erythroid colonies, endogenous megakaryocyte colonies	+	−
Megakaryocyte clusters	+	−
Platelet ATP:ADP >4 SD above normal mean	+	−
Platelet distribution width >2 SD above normal mean	+	−
Increased C-reactive protein, interleukin-6	−	+

A

B

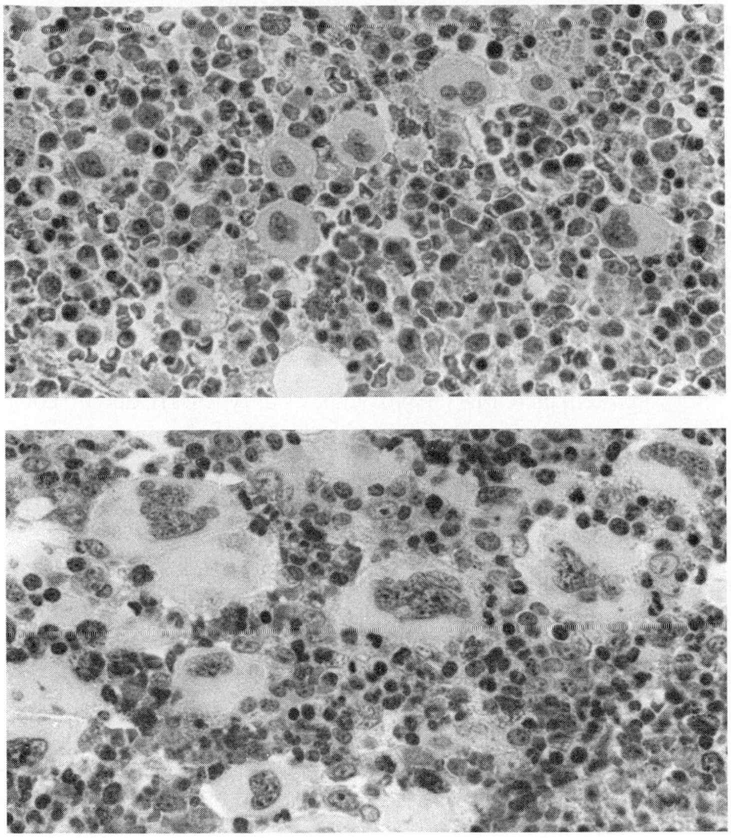

FIG. 49.11. This figure contrasts the size of the megakaryocytes in chronic myelogenous leukemia (**A**), with the megakaryocytes in essential thrombocythemia (**B**).

marked thrombocytosis, with symptoms and laboratory findings similar to those found in ET (306–309). In the setting of MDS, thrombocythemia has been reported most frequently in association with refractory anemia with ringed sideroblasts (306–308). In such patients, the megakaryocytes are increased in number and may range from small, dwarf forms to large, hyperlobated forms characteristic of those in ET. More than 15% of the erythroid precursors in such patients are ringed sideroblasts. Some patients with refractory anemia with ringed sideroblasts and thrombocythemia have been reported to have abnormalities of chromosome band 3q21 (306). Excessive thrombocythemia also may be observed in occasional patients who have the 5q− syndrome (309). In these latter patients, megakaryocytes with hypolobated nuclei predominate, and thus the megakaryocyte morphology is quite different from that of ET.

Prognosis

Essential thrombocythemia is an indolent disorder with long symptom-free intervals interrupted by occasional life-threatening thromboembolic or hemorrhagic episodes (262,283–285). Median durations of survival of 10 to 15 years commonly are reported, and because ET ususally occurs late in middle age, the life expectancy is near normal for many patients (262,284,285). Older patients often require therapy to control the complications of bleeding and thrombosis, and radioactive phosphorus, alkylating agents, hydroxyurea, interferon, and recently, anagrelide have been reported to have efficacy in ET (310,311). In young patients, however, the risk of complications from treatment with therapeutic agents that have leukemogenic potential may be more serious than the disease itself; conservative management often is recommended for younger patients (262,286,287). Management of pregnant patients with ET may be particularly challenging, but the outcome is often favorable if there is careful monitoring of the expectant mother and fetus (286,312).

Transition of ET to MDS or to acute leukemia is an uncommon event, observed in about 3 to 5% of patients (262,313). Most of the reported instances of this occur subsequent to myelosuppressive therapy (262,314). Myelomonocytic and megakaryoblastic leukemias are the most frequent types of AML reported, but all subtypes, including rare cases of acute lymphoblastic leukemia, have been described (284,313–315). A few patients with ET may develop marrow fibrosis with bone marrow failure, but this pattern of progression is rare (103,263).

CHRONIC IDIOPATHIC MYELOFIBROSIS

Chronic idiopathic myelofibrosis is an abnormal, clonal proliferation of bone marrow cells associated with deposition of bone marrow connective tissue as a secondary event. It is recognized most easily if there is splenomegaly, myelofibrosis demonstrated in a bone marrow biopsy specimen, a leukoerythroblastic peripheral blood smear, and evidence of EMH. The initial clinical, hematologic, and morphologic features are variable and, according to some investigators, may depend on the duration of the disease prior to its clinical detection (316,317). Abnormalities often regarded as hallmarks of the disease, such as myelofibrosis and leukoerythroblastosis, may not be present initially and become apparent only later in the disease course (103,263,317). Because fibrosis is a nonspecific marrow response that can be observed in a number of neoplastic and inflammatory disorders, the diagnosis of CIMF requires that other causes of stromal proliferation be excluded. Chronic idiopathic myelofibrosis is a progressive disease, and marrow failure or evolution to acute leukemia is common. In most series, the median duration of survival was only 5 to 6 years (317,263).

Etiology and Pathogenesis

The cause of CIMF is unknown. Exposure to benzene and to ionizing radiation has been documented in a few patients, and rare examples of familial myelofibrosis have been reported (318–320). For most cases, the designation *idiopathic* is appropriate.

Numerous studies have documented the clonal origin of CIMF in a multipotent myeloid stem cell and have proved that the fibroblasts are not part of the clone (12,17,20,21). The level of stem cell, however, involvement is uncertain. Some data, based on analysis of *RAS* mutations, suggest an origin in a pluripotent stem cell from which not only myeloid but also T- and B-lymphoid lineages are derived (321). It also has been reported that the lymphocyte lineage is derived clonally in some patients, but not in others (15). Whether there is variability of involvement among the myeloid lineages, similar to that observed in PV and ET, has not yet been determined (14).

Extramedullary hematopoiesis, generally regarded as a hallmark of CIMF (317), probably originates from multipotent and committed stem cells and precursor cells that escape the bone marrow in excessive numbers as a result of distortion of the blood–marrow barrier by abnormal deposition of connective tissue (322–325). Once in the circulation, these progenitors lodge in sites favorable for EMH, such as the spleen and liver (325). The progenitor cells found in the bone marrow, blood, and extramedullary organs are abnormally sensitive to, or even independent of, normal regulatory growth factors and control (229).

Myelofibrosis can be found in myeloid disorders other than CIMF, including any of the other CMPDs, MDS, and in some cases AML, but its pathogenesis is likely to be similar in each disorder. For nearly 20 years, the megakaryocyte has been thought to play a pivotal role in marrow fibrosis (22,23). This might be suspected from histologic analyses alone, because increased numbers of morphologically atypical megakaryocytes go hand-in-hand with bone marrow fibrosis. A number of biologic studies have confirmed this notion. In patients with CIMF, there is a direct correlation between an increase in serum TPO levels and the amount of marrow fibrosis that suggests an important link between regulation of megakaryocyte proliferation and connective tissue deposition (326). The most convincing evidence of the relationship between megakaryocytes and marrow fibrosis, however, is the localization of several cytokines important in fibroblastic proliferation and matrix deposition to the α-granules of megakaryocytes and platelets (323,324,327). Multiple factors, including platelet-derived growth factor, calmodulin, and platelet-derived collagenase inhibitors, play roles in collagen deposition. The abnormal production and secretion of TGF-β is particularly crucial (323,324). This protein increases the biosynthesis of type I, III, and IV collagens, fibronectin, and proteoglycans in the marrow, and it simultaneously inhibits degradation of connective tissue by blocking the expression of collagenase-like proteases. TGF-β production has been shown to be increased in the megakaryocytes in the blood and marrow of patients with CIMF (327). The mechanism by which TGF-β or other cytokines are ''leaked'' from myeloproliferative megakaryocytes is not clear, but the notion that it may be a result of an intrinsic defect in the megakaryocyte cannot be discounted. In CIMF, the megakaryocytes have increased production and secretion of TGF-β, but in ET—a disease that rarely exhibits marrow fibrosis—the megakaryocyte production of TGF-β is not abnormal, suggesting an inherent difference between the megakaryocytes in these two CMPDs (328). Of course, it is possible that accessory cells in the microenvironment could influence the transcription and excretion of TGF-β by megakaryocytes, and other cells, such as lymphocytes and macrophages, also manufacture the protein (329). It has been suggested that the increased frequency of immunologic disturbances observed in patients with CIMF may play a role in the abnormal release of cytokines from the platelets and megakaryocytes. Elevated levels of circulating immune complexes often are found in patients' sera, and these complexes could interact with the platelets to promote cytokine release (330,331).

Clinical and Laboratory Findings

It has been postulated that CIMF has a preclinical stage that can last from months to years, and that features such as splenomegaly, marrow fibrosis, and leukoerythroblastosis may appear at a relatively late stage in the natural history of the disease (263,317). Support for this notion was provided by a report that compared the clinical and hematologic findings in two groups of patients with CIMF who were diagnosed in two different decades, 1975 through 1986 and 1987 through 1997 (332). The study showed a recent trend towards finding less severe manifestations of the disease at diagnosis, probably because of earlier detection by screening procedures that are more widely available now than 20 years ago.

Clinical Findings

The annual incidence rate of CIMF is only about 0.5 per 100,000, and men are affected slightly more commonly than women (317,332–335). The peak age at diagnosis ranges from 60 to 70 years. CIMF is uncommon in children; other causes of marrow fibrosis, such as infection and other malignancies, must be excluded before the diagnosis is made in a child (336–338).

Up to 30% of patients with CIMF are asymptomatic at diagnosis. They are discovered by detection of splenomegaly during a routine physical examination, or if a routine blood count discloses some abnormality (317,332–335). The most common symptom is fatigue, but dyspnea, weight loss, night sweats, low-grade fever, and bleeding are other constitutional symptoms that may be recorded. The increased cell turnover may produce hyperuricemia, with accompanying gouty arthritis and renal stones (317). Between 70 and 90% of patients have palpable splenomegaly—often massive—but the absence of a clinically detectable spleen does not exclude the diagnosis (332–335). Abdominal discomfort, early satiety, or pain caused by splenic infarct are frequent clinical manifestations of the enlarged spleen. Hepatomegaly occurs in about 50% of patients (317,333), and in 20%, the complications of portal hypertension with esophageal and gastric varices and bleeding are present (317). EMH is very prominent in the spleen and liver and accounts for their enlargement. EMH can occur, however, in almost any organ and lead to symptoms related to the enlargement and distortion of the organ, or impairment of organ function. Fewer than 10% of patients have complaints related to the bony deposition that may occur, and almost as many have deafness caused by osteosclerosis (317,333).

Peripheral Blood

The classic blood picture of CIMF is that of leukoerythroblastosis with anisopoikilocytosis of RBCs and, most notably, teardrop-shaped RBCs. In practice, the blood findings vary considerably, and only 50 to 75% of patients have initial specimens that demonstrate the classic features (103,263).

White blood cell counts usually range from 10 to 20 $\times$ $10^{/}$ per liter but may be in excess of 60 $\times$ 10^9 per liter. Nearly 20% of patients are leukopenic, however (317,263,332). Immature granulocytes are found in more than 70% of patients, but in some, one may need to search to find even occasional myelocytes. Myeloblasts can account for up to 10% of the WBCs and are not necessarily indicative of transformation to a blast phase, although the finding of 10% or more blasts plus promyelocytes plus myelocytes is reported to predict a poor prognosis (335). Modest absolute basophilia may be observed (263,317). The NAP score may be low, normal, or increased (333).

Most patients with CIMF have at least mild anemia caused by decreased or ineffective erythropoiesis and splenic sequestration, but hemoglobin levels ranging from 2.2 to 19.0 g/dl have been recorded (263,317). Although normoblasts are present in the blood in nearly all patients, a few may not exhibit this finding, and the teardrop-shaped RBCs that accompany EMH sometimes are difficult to find (263).

Platelet counts may be decreased, normal, or elevated at diagnosis, and counts in excess of 1,000 $\times$ 10^9 per liter may occur (263,339,340). Giant or bizarrely shaped platelets that are sometimes poorly granulated, and fragments of megakaryocytes and megakaryocytic nuclei, are characteristic. Functional platelet abnormalities include defects in aggregation in response to epinephrine and adenosine 5′-diphosphate (339,340).

Bone Marrow

The variability in the peripheral blood findings in CIMF is mirrored in the spectrum of bone marrow changes observed initially. In 20 to 40% of patients, the initial bone marrow biopsy is hypercellular, with minimal if any detectable increase in reticulin or collagen fibrosis (103,263). In this prefibrotic, "cellular" phase, granulocytic and megakaryocytic hyperplasia is conspicuous (Fig. 49.12), and has led some to propose the term *granulocytic–megakaryocytic myelosis* for this disorder (103). Although erythroid precursors may be hyperplastic, they commonly are reduced in number, sometimes severely so (103,263,341). The most constant morphologic abnormalities occur in the megakaryocytic lineage. Megakaryocytes are increased in number, and clusters of 3 to 10 or more often are found around or within dilated marrow sinusoids (Fig. 49.13). The megakaryocytes tend to be more pleomorphic in CIMF than in the other CMPDs. They often are described as having "balloon-shaped" nuclei with lightly-stained nuclear chromatin, but micromegakaryocytes and megakaryocytes with hypersegmented, hyposegmented, or bare, pyknotic nuclei are also commonly noted (103,263,341). Although there may be a shift toward immaturity in the granulocytes, it is not marked, and the percentage of blasts is not increased. Eosinophils may be increased in number. Erythropoiesis is usually normoblastic, but up to 40% of patients have been reported to show a mixture of normoblastic and megaloblastic erythroid precursors (341). Proliferation of vascular structures and endothelium is usual in this stage. Lymphoid nodules comprising of small lymphocytes are found in nearly 25% of patients with CIMF, principally during the cellular phase (342).

Nearly 50 to 60% of patients initially have bone marrow specimens that demonstrate conspicuous reticulin or collagen fibrosis, or osteosclerotic change, features that characterize the "myelofibrotic" phase of CIMF. Such marrows tend to be normo- or hypocellular, and to have patches of neutrophilic granulopoiesis and erythroid precursors separated by regions of loose connective tissue or fat (Fig. 49.14). Dilatation of marrow sinusoids with intrasinusoidal hematopoieis is more obvious in this stage than in the cellular phase. Atypical megakaryocytes are often the predominant bone marrow

A,B

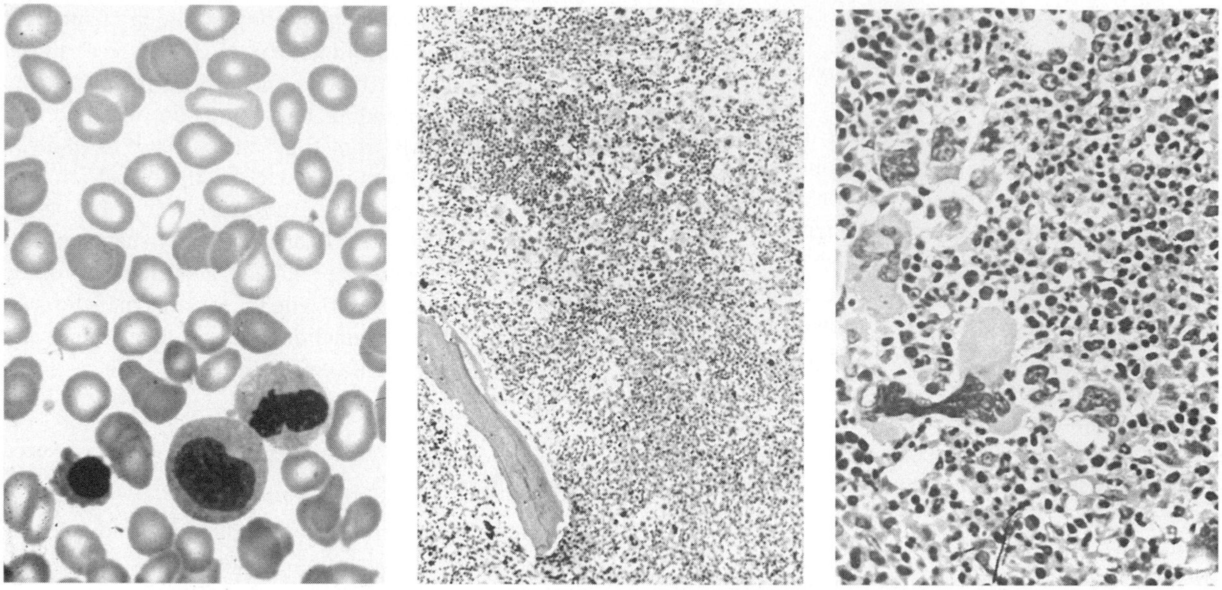

C

FIG. 49.12. These photomicrographs illustrate the blood and marrow findings from a 45-year-old man in the cellular phase of chronic idiopathic myelofibrosis with myeloid metaplasia, who presented with fatigue. He was found to have only slight splenomegaly, but his peripheral blood smear (**A**) showed some teardrop-shaped red blood cells, occasional nucleated red blood cells, and immature granulocytes. His bone marrow biopsy specimen (**B,C**) was hypercellular, with prominent granulocytosis and pleomorphic, atypical megakaryocytes.

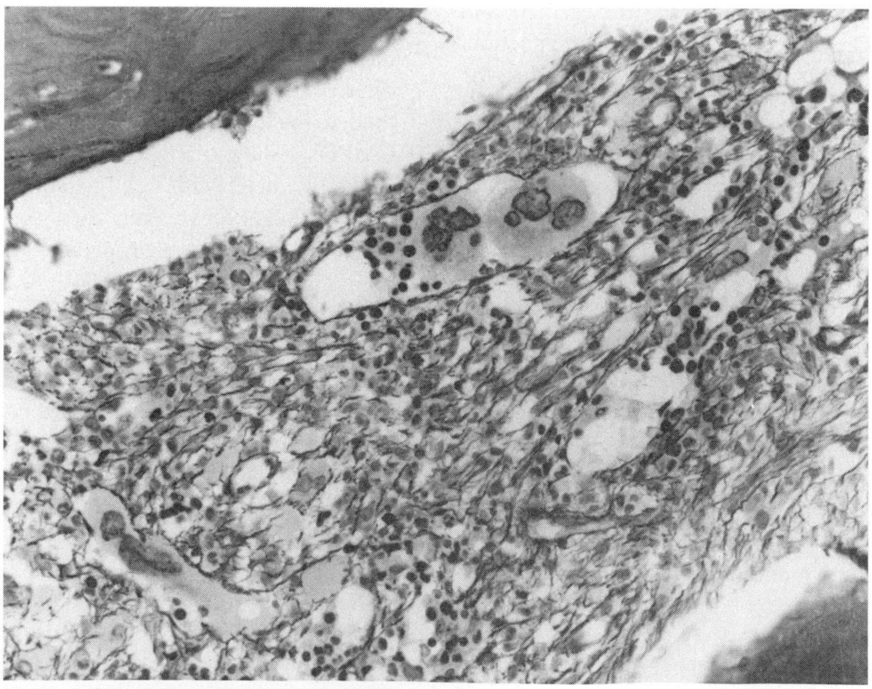

FIG. 49.13. Silver impregnation techniques often demonstrate variably increased numbers of reticulin fibers during the cellular phase of chronic idiopathic myelofibrosis with myeloid metaplasia and may accentuate sinusoidal dilatation. A characteristic feature of this condition is the finding of hematopoiesis within the marrow sinusoids. This "extramedullary hematopoiesis" in the marrow is important in the pathogenesis of hematopoiesis that occurs in extramedullary sites, such as the spleen and liver. It is most prominent in depleted, fibrotic specimens (Fig. 49.14) (Wilder's reticulin stain).

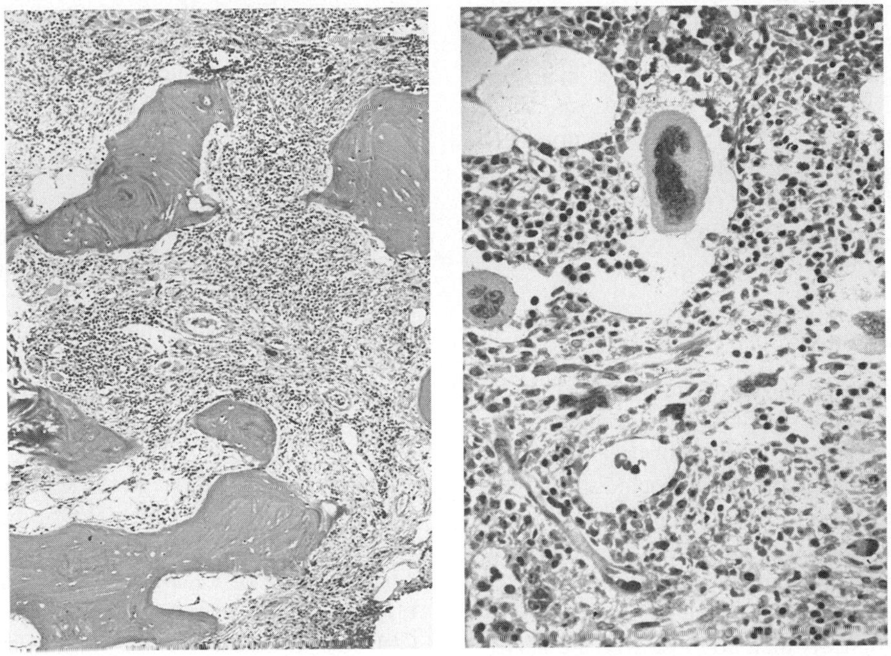

A B

FIG. 49.14. These photomicrographs are of a bone marrow specimen of a patient in the myelofibrotic stage of chronic idiopathic myelofibrosis with myeloid metaplasia. **A:** Low-power view showing that the marrow is depleted overall, with patches of hematopoiesis separated by fibrosis. Note that there is also osteosclerosis. **B:** Higher-power view in which the dilated sinusoids with "extramedullary hematopoiesis" can be appreciated readily.

element and can occur in sizable clusters or sheets or be situated mainly within the sinusoids (103,263). Some specimens are almost devoid of hematopoietic elements and consist of regions of dense reticulin or collagen fibrosis, with generous amounts of fatty marrow. Membranous or appositional new bone formation in bud-like plaques may be observed, but osteoblasts and osteoclasts are typically sparse (103,263). The osterosclerotic tissue may form broad, irregular trabeculae that occupy more than 50% of the marrow space (Fig. 49.15).

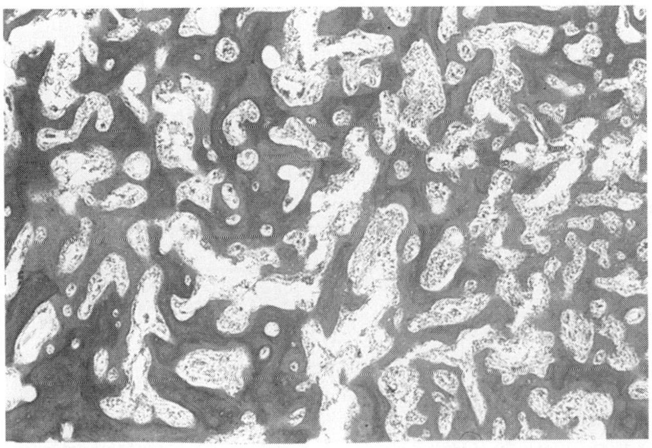

FIG. 49.15. A depleted marrow with severe osteosclerosis sometimes is seen in the bone marrow specimen of patients who have chronic idiopathic myelofibrosis with myeloid metaplasia. Such dense bony sclerosis can be detected by radiographic means.

Most authorities believe that the cellular phase of CIMF evolves to the myelofibrotic phase, but others have reported that marrow fibrosis is not uniformly distributed and does not correlate with disease progression (343). Some reports do show a correlation between bone marrow histology and the clinical and laboratory findings, in that patients with fibrotic marrow specimens tend to have larger spleens and lower hemoglobin levels and are more likely to have leukoerythroblastosis than those in the cellular phase (263,317,341, 344). In most series, however, the histology correlates poorly with the overall survival rate, so that even if extensive marrow fibrosis indicates disease of longer duration, it is not necessarily a measure of disease behavior (263,333,335).

Extramedullary Hematopoiesis

Extramedullary hematopoiesis may occur in any tissue that supports the proliferation of the progenitors that seed from the bone marrow. Such tissue includes the kidney, adrenal gland, gastrointestinal tract, lung and pleura, skin, breast, dura mater, central nervous system, and lymph nodes, although the liver and spleen are the most common sites. The spleen is diffusely enlarged, and microscopic sections reveal that the splenic trabeculae are widely separated, with diminished amounts of white pulp. The red pulp is expanded by trilineage EMH in the sinusoids. Often megakaryocytes are the most conspicuous elements. The red pulp cords may show fibrosis or contain a few developing granulocytes as well as sequestered platelets. It is the EMH that accounts for many of the peripheral blood abnormalities in CIMF, including misshapen RBCs and leukoerythroblastosis. These abnormalities diminish temporarily after splenectomy (344). Hepatic sinuses also demonstrate EMH, but fibrosis and cirrhosis of the liver also commonly occur, and they, along with the EMH, play the major role in the pathogenesis of the portal hypertension in CIMF.

Cytogenetic and Other Laboratory Findings

The reported frequency of cytogenetic abnormalities in CIMF varies from 30 to 70% (25,345–347). A consistent or specific chromosomal abnormality has not been identified, but recurring, nonrandom abnormalities include −7, +8, +9 and structural abnormalities of 1q, 20q, and 13q. Of these, del(20q) and del(13q) are the most common (345–347). The genes involved in the pathogenesis of CIMF are unknown. Patients with an abnormal karyotype at diagnosis have a worse prognosis than do those who are karyotypically normal (345–347).

Nearly one half of patients with CIMF have some disturbance of the immune system, often manifested by evidence of complement activation, circulating immune complexes, positive tests for antinuclear factors, or hemolytic autoimmune anemia (334,342). Whether these abnormalities play roles in the pathogenesis of the disease or are epiphenomena is not known. Bleeding is a common complication (317,333,335). Coagulation abnormalities include platelet dysfunction, acquired factor V deficiency, or disseminated intravascular coagulation (340,348). Liver function studies are abnormal in up to 30% of patients, and serum lactate dehydrogenase levels are almost always abnormally high (317,334). Serum levels of amino-terminal propeptides of type III collagen may correlate with disease activity, because they reflect the amount of collagen synthesized (324).

Differential Diagnosis

The diagnosis of CIMF can be difficult to establish. During the cellular phase, it can be difficult to distinguish CIMF from PV or ET. In the myelofibrotic stage, other CMPDs as well as a long list of other neoplastic and inflammatory disorders associated with marrow fibrosis must be excluded. In one survey of more than 3,000 patients with myelofibrosis, only 40% had CIMF or another CMPD. Other hematologic neoplasms, including Hodgkin's and non-Hodgkin's lymphoma, hairy cell leukemia, multiple myeloma, and acute leukemia, accounted for a similar number of patients, and nonhematopoietic tumors and inflammatory, infectious, and metabolic disorders for the remainder (349). Table 49.7 lists other myeloid disorders associated with myelofibrosis and some of their distinguishing features.

Chronic Myeloproliferative Disorders

Patients with CML may exhibit marrow reticulin or collagen fibrosis and marked megakaryocytic hyperplasia. In CML, however, the megakaryocytes are uniformly small, whereas those of CIMF are large and pleomorphic (103). Cytogenetic or molecular studies should be done in all CMPDs, and the detection of the Ph chromosome or the *BCR-ABL* fusion gene should be considered evidence for CML.

Marked thombocytosis, even in excess of $1,000 \times 10^9$ per liter, occurs in up to 20% of patients with CIMF (317,263,333). In such cases, distinguishing the cellular phase of CIMF from ET may be problematic. Differences in megakaryocyte morphology may provide a useful clue, because in ET, although the megakaryocytes are about the same size as those in CIMF, they are not as pleomorphic, and they have deeper lobulation of their nuclei and smoother nuclear contours (103,263). Furthermore, a leukoerythroblastic blood smear with teardrop RBCs and significant marrow fibrosis is not a feature of ET. Even so, in some patients only clinical and laboratory follow-up provides enough information to permit the separation of these two entities (263).

The proliferative stage of PV can be distinguished from the cellular stage of CIMF by the RBC parameters. In PV, the RBC mass is increased, and in the bone marrow the M:E ratio is usually decreased. In contrast, most patients with CIMF are anemic, including those in the cellular phase. Their

TABLE 49.7. *Myeloid disorders associated with marrow fibrosis*

	CML	CMML	CIMF	MDS,F	APMF	AML(M7)
Splenomegaly	++	++	+++	−/+	−/+	−
WBC	Increased	Variable	Variable	Decreased	Decreased	Decreased
Blasts in BM, %	CP <5–9 AP 10–19 BP ≥20	<5–19	<10	<5–19	>20	>20
Monocytes, %	≤3	≥10	<10	<10	<10	<10
Dysplasia	+ (Mega)	+ (Gran, Mega, Ery)	+/− (Mega, Ery)	++ (Gran, Mega, Ery)	++ (Gran, Ery, Mega)	++ (Gran Mega, Ery)

BM, bone marrow; CML, chronic myelogenous leukemia; MDS,F, MDS with fibrosis; CIMF, chronic idiopathic myelofibrosis; APMF, acute panmyelosis with fibrosis; CMML, chronic myelomonocytic leukemia; AML(M7), acute megakaryoblastic leukemia; CP, chronic phase; AP, accelerated phase; BP, blast phase.

marrow specimens show a higher M:E ratio than in PV, and the megakaryocytes are more pleomorphic. Serious blood loss or iron deficiency may obscure some of these features, however, and an iron trial may be required for the recognition of PV. PPMM is indistinguishable morphologically from CIMF.

Nearly 25% of patients with CMML have reticulin myelofibrosis, and occasionally there is collagen myelofibrosis (350). Such cases may be difficult to distinguish from CIMF, because the patients may have splenomegaly as well as marked megakaryocytic hyperplasia with atypia. The finding of peripheral blood and marrow monocytosis should lead one to suspect CMML, particularly if erythroid and granulocytic dysplasia is present.

Myelodysplastic Disorders and Acute Leukemia

A minority of patients with MDS, perhaps 15 to 20%, show a significant increase in reticulin fibers (350–352). Often the fibrosis is focal, and rarely is overt collagen deposition present (350). Still, because MDS with fibrosis is invariably associated with megakaryocytic abnormalities, and because megakaryocytic dysplasia, including micromegakaryocytes, may be seen in CIMF, difficulties in distinguishing between MDS with fibrosis and CIMF are not uncommon (263,334,350–353). The diagnosis of MDS with fibrosis should be reserved for patients who show multilineage (preferably trilineage) dysplasia in the blood and marrow, a significant increase in reticulin fibers as demonstrated by silver stains, and no significant hepatosplenomegaly (350–353). In contrast, although CIMF shows megakaryocytic atypia, including some small forms with hypolobated nuclei, rarely is there granulocytic dysplasia, and hepatosplenomegaly is usually present (341). A few patients have been reported who had marked hepatosplenomegaly, teardrop RBC poikilocytosis, leukoerythroblastosis, and fibrotic bone marrow specimens, as well as trilineage dyspoiesis, often severe (354). The classification of such patients is problematic because they have features of both MDS and CMPD. Whether they represent an accelerated, myelodysplastic phase of CIMF is not clear, but some investigators have suggested that such cases are a unique "transitional" group between MDS and CMPD (355).

Acute panmyelosis with myelofibrosis, also known as *malignant myelosclerosis*, *acute myelosclerosis*, *acute myelodysplasia with myelofibrosis*, and *acute myelofibrosis*, is a rare disorder that is best considered to be a specific subtype of AML (122,353,356–360). In acute panmyelosis with myelofibrosis, the peripheral blood smear is characterized by pancytopenia, usually with circulating blasts. Multilineage dysplasia is present, but, in contrast to the usual case of MDS with fibrosis, overt collagen deposition frequently is present in the biopsy specimen and often is "destructive" in nature (353). The bone marrow often appears hypocellular, but blasts of granulocytic or megakaryocytic origin usually account for 20% or more of the marrow elements, and immature erythroid precursors also sometimes are prominent. Maturation is present in these cell lines, however. Megakaryocytes vary in their maturity, but large, atypical forms as well as immature and small, dysplastic megakaryocytes are present. In contrast to the myelofibrotic stage of CIMF, organomegaly is usually absent in acute panmyelosis with myelofibrosis. A significant increase in the percentage of blasts in the marrow renders the diagnosis of CIMF untenable (353).

Any acute leukemia, including acute megakaryocytic leukemia, may be associated with marrow fibrosis. The diagnosis of acute leukemia should be made only if the percentage of blasts in the blood or marrow exceeds 20%.

Other Neoplasms

Hodgkin's and non-Hodgkin's lymphoma, multiple myeloma, hairy cell leukemia, acute and chronic lymphocytic leukemia, as well as metastatic carcinomas may be associated with marrow fibrosis, leukoerythroblastosis, and EMH (333,349). In these diseases, the markedly atypical megakaryocytes characteristic of CIMF are not present. The ready availability of a number of immunohistochemical reagents for identifying cells of myeloid, lymphoid, and epithelial origin has enhanced greatly the ability to accurately identify the origin of the cells in malignant disorders that induce myelofibrosis. Whenever there is doubt, these techniques should be applied in the identification of the neoplastic elements.

Prognosis

The duration of survival of patients with CIMF may range from months to decades. In most reports, the median survival time is approximately 5 years from the time of diagnosis (317,332,347), a statistic that has changed little over the past 30 years. Factors that influence prognosis as well as scoring systems for predicting prognosis have been reported by numerous investigators; the data are often conflicting. There is agreement, however, that features that indicate bone marrow failure indicate a poor prognosis. Severe anemia (hemoglobin concentration less than 10 g/dL) consistently is identified as a poor prognostic sign. Additional findings that have been reported to have an adverse influence on survival include thrombocytopenia (less than 100×10^9 per liter), leukocyte count greater than 20×10^9 per liter, marked granulocytic immaturity in the blood, and an abnormal karyotype (341,344–347).

In CIMF, the major causes of injury and death are related to bone marrow failure (infection and hemorrhage), thromboembolic events, portal hypertension, cardiac failure, and acute leukemia (263,317,348). The reported incidence of acute leukemia varies from 5 to 30% (263,348). Although its development may be related to prior cytotoxic therapy in some patients, acute leukemia in CIMF often occurs in patients who received no therapy; acute leukemia appears to be a part of the natural history of the disease. The acute leukemia may be derived from any of the myeloid lineages, including granulocytic, monocytic, erythroid, or megakaryoblastic; mixed-lineage phenotypes also may be observed (361,362).

MYELOPROLIFERATIVE DISEASE, UNCLASSIFIABLE

In some patients diagnosed as having a CMPD, the clinical, laboratory, or morphologic features may not be entirely characteristic of CML, PV, ET, or CIMF. Many of these are advanced cases in which the intitial underlying disease cannot be recognized reliably, and in which fibrosis and megakaryocytic hyperplasia and atypia are prominent (103). Cytogenetic or molecular genetic studies should be done in such cases, because the absence of a Ph chromosome or of the *BCR-ABL* fusion gene excludes CML as a diagnostic possibility. In other patients, a hypercellular bone marrow with panhyperplasia, prominent, large megakaryocytes, and minimal or absent fibrosis may pose diagnostic problems, if the typical clinical or peripheral blood findings of the other CMPDs are absent. In such instances, after careful correlation of the histologic findings with clinical, laboratory, and cytogenetic data, a diagnosis of myeloproliferative disorder, unclassifiable, may be appropriate, and only further evolution of the disease may clarify its nature.

MYELOPROLIFERATIVE/MYELODYSPLASTIC DISEASES

The generally accepted notion regarding CMPD and MDS is that they are fundamentally different disorders. The CMPDs are characterized, at least initially, by effective hematopoiesis, with increased numbers of one or more peripheral blood elements. In contrast, MDS has ineffective hematopoiesis, with cytopenias in the peripheral blood. Significant dysplasia is uncommon at the time of diagnosis of CMPD but is a requirement for a diagnosis of MDS. Organomegaly almost always is found in patients with CMPDs but is unusual or modest in MDS. Despite these apparent differences, some patients have hematologic disorders that have features of both MDS and CMPD. These disorders do not fit well into the usual classification schemes of either CMPD or MDS and could be considered a separate group of *myeloproliferative and myelodysplastic* disorders. The major members of this group include aCML, CMML, and JMML.

Atypical Chronic Myeloid Leukemia

The name applied to this disorder is somewhat unfortunate, because it implies that it is CML with some atypical features. Rather, aCML is a unique entity that is different in many respects from CML (83,148,152). Most importantly, the leukemic cells in aCML lack the Ph chromosome or the *BCR-ABL* fusion gene. Although the leukemia is characterized by leukocytosis comprised principally of immature and mature neutrophils, in contrast to CML there is prominent dysplasia that often involves multiple cell lineages (148,152,363). In practice, the disorder usually is distinguished readily from CML in chronic phase, but it may be more difficult to distinguish it reliably from the accelerated phase of CML, and the distinction from CMML can be even more problematic. Table 49.2 outlines some of the differences in the laboratory and morphologic findings in CML, aCML, and CMML. It is likely that the syndrome of abnormal chromatin clumping in granulocytes is a variant of aCML (364,365).

Patients with aCML tend to be elderly; in most series the median age at diagnosis was in the seventh decade of life (148,363,366). Most patients have symptoms related to anemia or sometimes to thrombocytopenia, but in others, the chief complaint may be related to splenomegaly (152, 366–368).

The median WBC count in patients with aCML often is reported to be between 30 and 50 $\times 10^9$ per liter at the time of diagnosis (83,152,367). The leukocyte count is elevated primarily by cells of the neutrophilic series. Blasts may be present but usually account for less than 5% of the WBCs. Promyelocytes, myelocytes, and metamyelocytes account for 10 to 20% of the leukocyte differential, and mature neutrophils make up most of the remaining cells. Monocytes account for only 3 to 10% of the WBCs, although they often are increased in absolute numbers (148,152,368). In some patients, monocytes are increased sufficiently in number and percentage that distinction of aCML from CMML becomes very difficult (366). Basophilia (at least 2%) is uncommon in aCML but, if present, does not necessarily exclude the diagnosis (152). The major finding that distinguishes aCML from CML is dysplasia, which is the key to the diagnosis of aCML (83,148,152,368) (Fig. 49.16). In the granulocytes, dysplasia may be observed as abnormal chromatin clumping, pseudo–Pelger-Huet nuclear abnormalities, or abnormalities in cytoplasmic granulation. NAP scores are low in most but elevated in one third of patients with aCML. Anemia is usually present. The RBCs may show changes indicative of dyserythropoiesis, such as macroovalocytosis. Platelets often are reduced in number, with median values of approximately 100 $\times 10^9$ per liter generally reported, but severe thrombocytopenia is also possible (148,152,366,369).

Bone marrow biopsy specimens in aCML are hypercellular because of granulocytic proliferation. Blasts may be increased modestly in number, but large sheets or clusters of blasts are not usually present on biopsy. Megakaryocytes may be decreased, normal, or increased in number but almost always show dysplasia (368). Erythropoiesis is variable in quantity, but in some patients erythroid precursors account for nearly 30% of the marrow elements (366). Reticulin fibers usually are not increased initially, but reticulin fibrosis has been reported, and evolution of aCML may be associated with marrow fibrosis in some patients (363,370). In the mar-

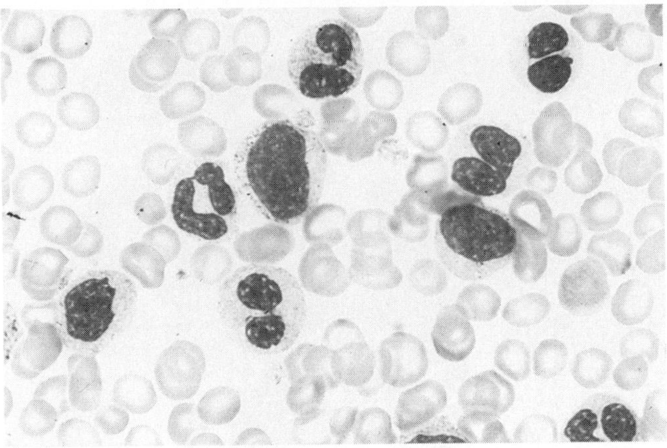

FIG. 49.16. This peripheral blood smear is from a patient with atypical chronic myelogenous leukemia. Characteristically, granulocytic dysplasia is prominent, and in this patient pseudo–Pelger-Huet neutrophils are observed readily. Immature granulocytes are seen, and sometimes monocytes are present in low percentages. Basophils usually are scarce. This patient had no Philadelphia chromosome or *BCR-ABL* fusion gene but did demonstrate trisomy 8 on karyotypic analysis.

row aspirate smears, granulocytic dysplasia is a constant finding, although it may vary in severity. Dyserythropoiesis is present in many patients, and dysmegakaryocytopoiesis, with micromegakaryocytes and abnormal nuclear segmentation, is the rule (368). Monocytes are not significantly increased in the marrow specimens (152).

By definition, aCML lacks a Ph chromosome or *BCR-ABL* fusion gene. Other cytogenetic abnormalities may be seen, but none are specific. Trisomy of chromosome 8 is probably the most commonly reported change, but trisomy 14 and isochromosome 17q are other abnormalities that may be observed (153–155,363,366,371).

Patients with aCML fare poorly. The series reported to date have included small numbers of patients, but median durations of survival were often less than 20 months (148,363,367,368). In approximately 30 to 40% of patients, aCML evolves into acute leukemia; others die of bone marrow failure.

Chronic Myelomonocytic Leukemia

Monocytosis is the defining feature of CMML. As defined by the FAB group, which placed it into the myelodysplastic group of diseases, CMML is characterized by peripheral monocytosis of 1×10^9 per liter, increased numbers of monocytic cells in the bone marrow, dysplasia of variable degrees in the erythroid, megakaryocytic, or granulocytic precursors, and fewer than 5% circulating blasts plus promonocytes and fewer than 30% blasts plus promonocytes in the marrow (372,373). Yet CMML is a very heterogeneous disease. About 50% of patients initially have leukocytosis caused by monocytosis and neutrophilia. In these patients, splenomegaly, skin infiltration, serous effusions, and minimal dyspoiesis often occur, and the disease appears more like a CMPD (152,366,374). In a nearly equal number of patients, however, the WBC count is decreased, normal, or only mildly elevated, and although absolute monocytosis is present, there may be neutropenia (152,366,374). Splenomegaly is uncommon in these latter cases, and there is often significant dyspoiesis—features that usually are found in MDS. This heterogeneity has led some authors to suggest that CMML can be divided into a myelodysplastic and a myeloproliferative type, based primarily on the WBC count (152). Despite the advantage that such a subclassification might appear to provide in addressing the heterogeneity in CMML, there is little evidence that it has any clinical relevance. Durations of survival are similar for the myeloproliferative and myelodysplastic types, and no molecular, cytogenetic, or major cellular differences between the two groups have been identified (374,375). Furthermore, some patients who initially exhibit myelodysplastic features eventually may have increasing WBC and monocyte counts, and the disease may become more myeloproliferative in nature. It is probably best to think of CMML as having a spectrum of disease manifestations, ranging from primarily dysplastic to primarily myeloproliferative.

The median leukocyte count at diagnosis for patients with CMML is usually between 15 and 30×10^9 per liter, but the WBC count may range from 2.5 to more than 200×10^9 per liter (152,148,366,367). In many patients, the absolute monocyte count is less than 5×10^9 per liter, but it may range from 1 to more than 100×10^9 per liter. Anemia is mild, with most investigators reporting median values of 10 to 11 g/dL. Severe thrombocytopenia is uncommon, and the majority of patients have platelet counts above 100×10^9 per liter (366,376). Nevertheless, marked thrombocytopenia as well as thrombocythemia is possible.

Inspection of the peripheral blood smear reveals that monocytes account for at least 10% and usually 30 to 50% of the WBCs. They may be atypical, with nuclear hyper- or hypolobulation and increased or decreased cytoplasmic granules (367). Although some degree of nuclear immaturity may be seen, blasts and promonocytes account for fewer than 5% of the peripheral WBCs. There may be neutrophilia or neutropenia, and in some series dysgranulopoiesis, including pseudo–Pelger-Huet changes, and cytoplasmic hypogranularity have been reported to be present in more than 80% of patients (366,367) (Fig. 49.17). Immature granulocytes are infrequent in the blood, usually accounting for fewer than 10 to 15% of the WBCs (368). Absolute basophilia is present in occasional patients, but in most the basophil count is normal (152,367). Macroovalocytosis is the most common abnormality noted in the RBCs. Platelet abnormalities, including large forms with granulopathies, sometimes are observed.

The bone marrow biopsy and aspirate are hypercellular and show granulocytic and monocytic proliferation. The monocytosis may be difficult to recognize in the marrow, and

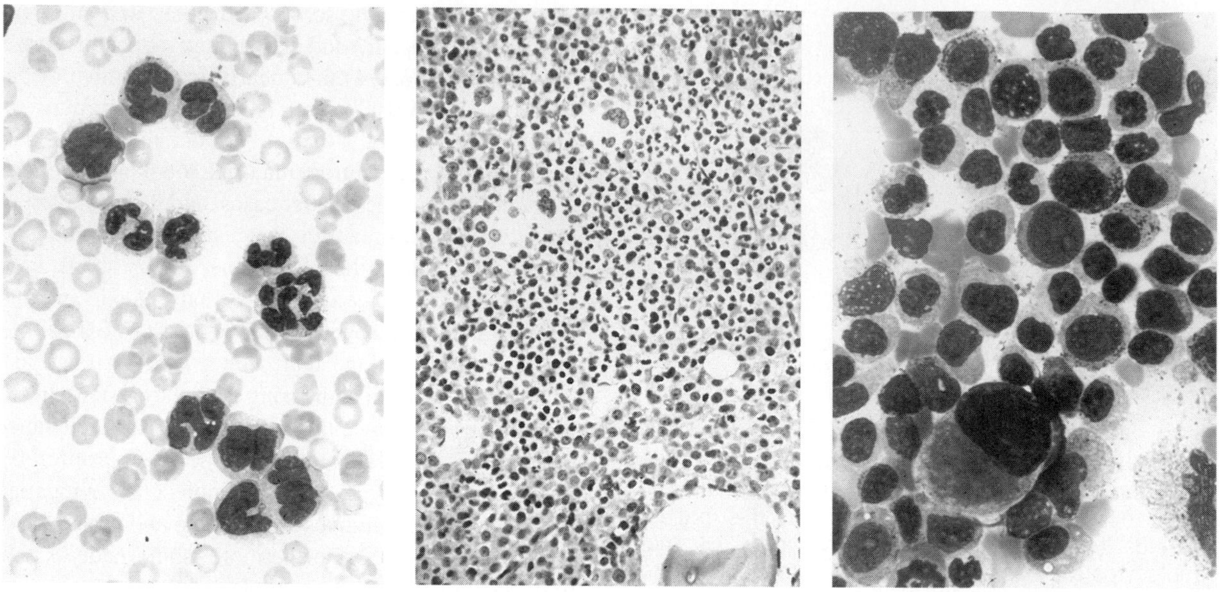

A,B C

FIG. 49.17. These photomicrographs illustrate the blood (**A**) and marrow specimens (**B,C**) of a patient with chronic myelomonocytic leukemia. Although the monocytosis is evident in the peripheral blood smear, it is often less apparent in the bone marrow biopsy specimen and marrow aspirate smears. Often, nonspecific esterase reactions are necessary to fully appreciate monocytosis in a marrow aspirate.

cytochemical studies for nonspecific esterase may be required for accurate assessment of the number of monocytes present. The number of monocytes found in the bone marrow is not stated clearly in most reported series. Some authors comment that the number of marrow monocytes rarely exceeds 20%, but studies in which esterase reactions were used for accurate enumeration of the monocytic component show a greater percentage (377). In most patients, blasts, including myeloblasts, monoblasts, and promonocytes, usually account for fewer than 5% of the marrow elements, and 20% signals transformation to acute leukemia (122). Dysgranulopoiesis, dyserythropoiesis, and dysmegakaryocytopoiesis are found in most patients (366). Nearly 30% of patients with CMML have a significant amount of reticulin fibrosis (350).

Cytogenetic studies reveal abnormal karyotypes in 20 to 30% of patients with CMML (377,378). Recurring abnormalities include trisomy 8, del(20q), monosomy 7, and del(11q), but these can be seen in other myeloproliferative or myelodysplastic disorders as well. A unique subset of patients with CMML and blood and marrow eosinophilia have a chromosomal translocation, t(5;12)(q33;p13), in their leukemic cells. This abnormality fuses the *TEL* gene on chromosome 12 with the platelet-derived growth factor receptor (*PDGFR*) gene on chromosome 5 and results in an abnormal *TEL-PDGFR* fusion transcript that may play an important role in the proliferative process, perhaps through the deregulation of RAS. Variant translocations have been reported that translocate the *PDFGR* gene to other chromosomal partners (211–213).

The differential diagnosis of CMML includes aCML and CML; the differences between these entities are summarized in Table 49.2. In some patients, it is difficult to differentiate between reactive and neoplastic monocytosis, particularly if dysplasia is minimal. Cytogenetic studies may be of help, but, if there is any doubt, it is best to wait and observe the patient rather than make a diagnosis of malignancy that is not clear-cut. Sometimes, the distinction among CMML, acute myelomonocytic leukemia, and acute monocytic leukemia with differentiation is difficult. Marked immaturity of the monocytic elements in the blood (more than 5% blasts and promonocytes) is unusual for CMML and should prompt careful examination of the marrow; the finding of 20% blasts plus promonocytes in the blood or bone marrow is sufficient for a diagnosis of acute leukemia (122).

Juvenile Myelomonocytic Leukemia

Juvenile myelomonocytic leukemia (previously referred to as *juvenile CML* or *juvenile CMML*) is a Ph^-, *BCR-ABL*-negative leukemia of childhood that is characterized by principal involvement of granulocytes and monocytes. It is a rare disorder but accounts for approximately 20 to 30% of all cases of myelodysplastic or myeloproliferative syndromes in children (149,379). The mean age at diagnosis generally is reported to be between 1.5 and 2 years, and more than 70% of the patients are children younger than 3 years of age (149,379–381). Approximately 7% of the reported cases occur in children with neurofibromatosis type 1 (149,379). JMML is considered by some to be synonymous with chronic myelomonocytic leukemia (381), but others consider it to be a unique entity.

Although the cause of JMML is unknown in most patients, some interesting and diagnostically useful information is known about the leukemic cells. In JMML, the leukemic cells are hypersensitive to the effects of GM-CSF. If placed in cell culture, circulating progenitor cells from patients with JMML form granulocyte-macrophage colonies in the absence of added growth factors (382). The formation of these colonies can be prevented by removal of monocytes and other adherent cells prior to culture of the blood or marrow mononuclear cells, as well as by antibodies to GM-CSF (382,383). It is thought that, *in vitro*, the patient's adherent cells synthesize the GM-CSF required for the spontaneous colony formation. The level of GM-CSF in the culture supernatant, however, is not elevated above that found in control studies, suggesting that the leukemic cells are hypersensitive to small quantities of the growth factor. The demonstration of spontaneous formation of granulocyte-macrophage colonies in culture, with inhibition of the growth by antibodies to GM-CSF, is a useful diagnostic test for JMML.

Of additional interest is the finding that, as in CMML in adults, in JMML nearly 30% of patients have mutations involving the *RAS* gene (384). These point mutations may lead to increased intracellular levels of RAS-GTP, which may alter the RAS signaling pathway that normally is triggered when GM-CSF binds to its receptor (385). Additional support that the RAS pathway may be involved in the pathogenesis of JMML comes from data generated by the study of patients with neurofibromatosis type 1 and JMML. In these children, loss of the normal neurofibromatosis type 1 allele is a common finding in the leukemic cells. The normal neurofibromatosis type 1 protein, neurofibromin, negatively regulates the *P21RAS* family of protooncogenes by down-regulating RAS-GTP. Inactivation of neurofibromatosis type 1 through allele loss may deregulate the RAS pathway (386).

Most patients with JMML have fever or other evidence of infection, symptoms related to bleeding, or evidence of pulmonary involvement (149,379–381). Splenomegaly is virtually always present, and hepatomegaly and lymphadenopathy are reported to occur in more than one half of patients (149,379–381). A maculopapular skin rash may be observed in up to one half of patients, although café-au-lait spots are seen in patients with neurofibromatosis type 1.

The peripheral blood is characterized by leukocytosis, anemia, and thrombocytopenia. The WBC count is greater than 10×10^9 per liter (median, $25–35 \times 10^9$ per liter) and comprises in part granulocytes, including immature myeloid precursors. The absolute monocyte count is at least 1×10^9 per liter (median, $5–7 \times 10^9$ per liter). Blasts and promonocytes usually account for fewer than 5% of the WBCs, and never for more than 20%. Nucleated red cells commonly are seen. Platelet counts at diagnosis vary, but thrombocytopenia is often severe.

Bone marrow biopsy specimens reveal cellularity that is normal or increased, with an elevated M:E ratio. Blasts and promonocytes account for fewer than 10% of the marrow elements in more than 90% of children, and never for more than 20%. Monocytes generally account for 5 to 10% of the marrow cells, but values up to 30% or more have been recorded. Megakaryocytes usually are reduced in number but rarely display atypical morphology. Dysplasia in the form of pseudo–Pelger-Huet neutrophils, hypogranularity of myeloid cytoplasm, or megaloblastic changes in the erythroid cells may be noted but is usually not prominent in JMML (149,379–381,384).

Leukemic infiltrates are common in the skin, where myelomonocytic elements infiltrate the superficial and deep dermis. In the lung, leukemic cells spread from the peribronchial lymphatics into adjacent alveolar septae. In the spleen, they infiltrate the red pulp and have a predilection for trabecular and central arteries. Lymph nodes show a leukemic pattern of infiltration in the interfollicular area (387).

An important laboratory finding is the detection of hemoglobin F levels greater than 10%, with decreased hemoglobin A2 concentration. This abnormality is found in nearly 70% of patients and may be helpful in establishing the diagnosis. In addition, most patients have polyclonal hypergammaglobulinemia (149,379–381,384).

Cytogenetic studies are normal in most children with JMML. In some series, the most commonly reported abnormal karyotype is monosomy 7. Although some authors consider the finding of monosomy 7 in a child younger than 4 years of age to indicate that the patient should be classified as having the *infantile monosomy 7 syndrome* rather than JMML, in practice these two syndromes are clinically and hematologically similar, and many authors believe that distinguishing between them is not clinically meaningful (384,388).

The diagnosis of JMML is not always easy. A number of infections, including infections with Epstein-Barr virus, cytomegalovirus, human herpesvirus-6, histoplasma, mycobacteria, and toxoplasma, may cause similar clinical and hematologic findings. Infection with EBV not only may mimic the clinical and hematologic findings but even may cause elevation of HbF (389).

The prognosis for patients with JMML generally is poor. If untreated, most patients have a rapidly fatal course; others may have more indolent disease, only to die in a fulminant relapse. Patients with JMML often respond poorly to chemotherapy, and the only currently available therapy that improves the outcome is bone marrow transplantation (379–381,387).

SUMMARY AND CONCLUSIONS

In the first edition of this text, we summarized this chapter on CMPDs by including tables that compared the features of the major entities. We also expressed our hope that such tables, in the future, would include detailed information on the molecular and genetic processes that control the abnormal cellular proliferations in each entity. We have included similar tables in this edition (Tables 49.8, 49.9), but unfortunately, despite the investigative work of hundreds of scien-

TABLE 49.8. *Clinical and cytogenetic findings in the CMD*

	CML (chronic phase) (39,79–81,159)	PV (proliferative phase) (217,235–239,243,247,251)	ET (262,283–285,257,289,298)	CIMF (263,317,332–335,346)
Clinical features				
Median age, years	46–53	53–62	50–61	60–70
Asymptomatic	20–40%	—	50%	25–30%
Hemorrhage/thrombosis	5–15%	20–25%	25–85%	20–30; pc
Splenomegaly	60–80%	60–70%	30–50%	70–90%
Cytogenetic and molecular findings	~95% Ph+, 100% *BCR/ABL*+	No Ph or *BCR/ABL*, but 10–20% have abnormal karyotype, including del(20q), +8, +9	No Ph or *BCR/ABL*, but <5% have abnormal karyotype	No Ph or BCR/ABL, but 30–70% have abnormal karyotype, including del(13q), del(20q), +8, +9
Transformation to acclerated phase	>95%	No cytotoxic therapy: 5% Cytotoxic therapy: 10%–20%	No cytotoxic therapy: <1% Cytotoxic therapy: 10%–20%	5–25%
Median survival, months	58–69	108–144	>120	45–60
Causes of death	Blast transformation	Thrombosis, hemorrhage, acute leukemia, PPMM	Thrombosis, hemorrhage,	Hemorrhage, cardiac failure, portal hypertension, acute leukemia, infection

TABLE 49.9. *Peripheral blood and bone marrow findings at diagnosis in CMPD in selected series*

	CML (chronic phase) (81,82,165)	PV (proliferative phase) (235,239,243,247)	ET (262,263,283–285)	CIMF (263,317,333,334)
Blood				
Mean WBC × 10^9/L	134–225	9.8–15.0	11–12.4	11.0–16.6
(range)	(50–500)	(2–54)	(6–41)	(1–237)
Mean Hgb	9.7–12.0	16.5–19.6	13–15	9.5–11.6
(range) (g/dL)	(5.4–14.4)	(13.5–27.0)	(10.0–18.8)	(2.2–18)
Mean platelets	399–484	419–500	897–1,300	175–580
(range) (×10^9/L)	(24–1400)	(140–3,000)	(600–4,800)	(9–3,215)
Marrow				
Cellularity	~95% marked hypercellular	~85% hypercellular ~15% normocellular	~90% normal to hypercellular ~10% hypocellular	~40% marked hypercellular 60% normo- to hypocellular
Proliferating cells	Gran +++ Meg + to +++ Ery 0 to +	Ery +++ Meg +++ Gran + to +++	Meg +++ Gran +++ Ery 0 to ++	Meg +++ Gran ++ Ery 0 to ++
Reticulin fibrosis	Slight to marked increase in 50%	Slight to marked increase in 40%	Minimal	Slightly increased in 40%, markedly increased in 60%

tists and physicians, we have not been able to add the genetic defects and the events that initiate them—this information remains unknown. The CMPDs are complex, even more so than might have been perceived initially. This complexity stems from the complex nature of the hematopoietic stem cell and progenitors, and from the factors that control their proliferation, lineage commitment, and maturation. Perhaps by the next edition we will know more.

REFERENCES

1. Dameshek W. Some speculations on the myeloproliferative syndromes. *Blood* 1951;6:372–375.

2. Whang J, Frei E III, Tijo JH, et al. The distribution of the Philadelphia chromosome in patients with chronic myelogenous leukemia. *Blood* 1963;22:664–673.
3. Rastrick JM, Fitzgerald PH, Gunz FW. Direct evidence for presence of Ph1 chromosome in erythroid cells. *Br Med J* 1968;1:96–98.
4. Golde DW, Burgaleta C, Sparkes RS, et al. The Philadelphia chromosome in human macrophages. *Blood* 1977;49:367–370.
5. Nitta M, Kato Y, Strife A, et al. Incidence of involvement of the B and T lymphocyte lineages in chronic myelogenous leukemia. *Blood* 1985;66:1053–1061.
6. Fauser AA, Kanz L, Bross KJ, et al. T cells and probably B cells arise from the malignant clone in chronic myelogenous leukemia. *J Clin Invest* 1985;75:1080–1082.
7. Al-Amin A, Lennartz K, Runde V, et al. Frequency of clonal B lymphocytes in chronic myelogenous leukemia evaluated by fluorescence in situ hybridization. *Cancer Genet Cytogenet* 1998;104:45–47.
8. Fialkow PJ, Jacobson RJ, Papayannopoulou T. Chronic myelocytic leukemia: clonal origin in a stem cell common to the granulocytic, erythrocytic, platelet and monocyte/macrophage. *Am J Med* 1977;63: 125–130.
9. Martin PJ, Najfeld V, Hansen JA, et al. Involvement of the B-lymphoid system in chronic myelogenous leukaemia. *Nature* 1980; 287:49–50.
10. Adamson JW, Fialkow PJ, Murphy S, et al. Polycythemia vera: stem-cell and probable clonal origin of the disease. *N Engl J Med* 1976; 295:913–916.
11. Fialkow PJ, Faguet GB, Jacobson RJ, et al. Evidence that essential thrombocythemia is a clonal disorder with origin in a multipotent stem cell. *Blood* 1981;58:916–918.
12. Jacobson RJ, Salo A, Fialkow PJ. Agnogenic myeloid metaplasia: a clonal proliferation of hematopoietic stem cells with secondary myelofibrosis. *Blood* 1978;51:189–194.
13. Anger B, Janssen JWG, Schrezenmeier H, et al. Clonal analysis of chronic myeloproliferative disorders using X-linked DNA polymorphisms. *Leukemia* 1990;4:258–261.
14. Gilliland DG, Blanchard KL, Levy J, et al. Clonality in myeloproliferative disorders: analysis by means of the polymerase reaction. *Proc Natl Acad Sci USA* 1991;88:6848–6852.
15. Tsukamoto N, Morita K, Maehara T, et al. Clonality in chronic myeloproliferative disorders defined by X-chromosome linked probes: demonstration of heterogeneity in lineage involvement. *Br J Haematol* 1994;86:253–258.
16. Price CM, Kanfer EJ, Colman SM, et al. Simultaneous genotypic and immunophenotypic analysis of interphase cells using dual-color fluorescence: a demonstration of lineage involvement in polycythemia vera. *Blood* 1992;80:1033–1038.
17. Buschle M, Janssen JW, Drexler H, et al. Evidence for the pluripotent stem cell origin of idiopathic myelofibrosis: clonal analysis of a case characterized by a N-ras mutation. *Leukemia* 1988;2:658–660.
18. Gay S, Gay RE, Prchal JT. Immunohistological studies of bone marrow collagen. In: Berk PD, Castro-Malaspina H, Wasserman LR, eds. *Myelofibrosis and the biology of connective tissue.* New York: Alan R. Liss, 1984:291–306.
19. Reilly JT. Pathogenesis of idiopathic myelofibrosis: present status and future directions [Annotation]. *Br J Haematol* 1994;88:1–8
20. Greenberg BR, Woo L, Veomett IC, et al. Cytogenetics of bone marrow fibroblastic cells in idiopathic chronic myelofibrosis. *Br J Haematol* 1987;66:487–490.
21. Wang JC, Lang HD, Lichter S, et al. Cytogenetic studies of bone marrow fibroblasts cultured from patients with myelofibrosis and myeloid metaplasia. *Br J Haematol* 1992;80:184–188.
22. Groopman JE. The pathogenesis of myelofibrosis in myeloproliferative disorders. *Ann Intern Med* 1980;92:857–858.
23. Castro-Malaspina H, Rabellino EM, Yen A, et al. Human megakaryocyte stimulation of proliferation of bone marrow fibroblasts. *Blood* 1981;57:781–787.
24. Martyre MC, Le Bousse-Kerdiles MC, Chevillard S, et al. Transforming growth factor-β and megakaryocytes in the pathogenesis of idiopathic myelofibrosis. *Br J Haematol* 1994;88:9–16.
25. Dewald GW, Wright PI. Chromosome abnormalities in the myeloproliferative disorders. *Semin Oncol* 1995;22:341–354.
26. Bennett JH. Two cases of disease and enlargement of the spleen in which death took place from the presence of purulent matter in the blood. *Edinburgh Med Surg J* 1845:64;413–423.
27. Virchow R. Weisses blut. *Froiep's Notizen* 1845;36:151–156.
28. Virchow R. Die Leukaemie. In: *Gesammelte abhandlugen zur wissenschaftlichen medizin.* Frankfurt: Meidinger, 1865:190–211.
29. Neumann E. Uber myelogene leukaemie. *Berl Klin Wochenschur* 1878;15:69.
30. Nowell PC, Hungerford DA. A minute chromosome in human chronic granulocytic Leukemia. *Science* 1960;132:1497–1500.
31. Caspersson T, Gahrtoin G, Lindsten J, et al. Identification of the Philadelphia chromosome as number 22 by quinacrine mustard fluorescence analysis. *Exp Cell Res* 1970;63:238–240.
32. Rowley JD. A new consistent abnormality in chronic myelogenous leukemia identified by quinicrine fluorescence and Giemsa staining. *Nature* 1973;243:290–293.
33. Bartam CR, de Klein A, Hagemeijer A, et al. Translocation of c-abl oncogene adjacent to a translocation breakpoint in chronic myelogenous leukaemia. *Nature* 1983;306: 277–280.
34. Groffen J, Stephenson JR, Heisterkamp N, et al. Philadelphia chromosomal breakpoints are clustered within a limited region bcr on chromosome 22. *Cell* 1984;36:93–99.
35. Shtivelman E, Lifshitz B, Gale RP, et al. Fused transcripts of abl and bcr genes in chronic myeloid leukaemia. *Nature* 1985;315:550–554.
36. Konopka JB, Witte ON. Detection of c-abl tyrosine kinase activity in vitro permits direct comparison of normal and altered abl gene products. *Mol Cell Biol* 1985;5:3116–3123.
37. Young JL Jr, Percy CL, Asire AJ, et al. Cancer incidence and mortality in the United States, 1973–1977. *Natl Cancer Inst Monogr* 1981;57: 1–187.
38. Call TG, Noel P, Habermann TM, et al. Incidence of leukemia in Olmstead County, Minnesota 1975 through 1989. *Mayo Clin Proc* 1994;69:315–322.
39. Cortes JE, Talpaz M, Kantarjian H. Chronic myelogenous leukemia: a review. *Am J Med* 1996;100:555–570.
40. Bergsagel DE. The chronic leukemias: a review of disease manifestations and the aims of therapy. *Can Med Assoc J* 1967;96:1615–1620.
41. Moloney WC. Natural history of chronic granulocytic leukaemia. *Clin Haematol* 1977;6:41–60.
42. Brinker H. Population-based age- and sex-specific incidence rates in the 4 main types of leukaemia. *Scand J Haematol* 1982;29:241–249.
43. Baikie AG, Garson OM, Spiers AS, et al. Cytogenetic studies in familial leukemias. *Aust Ann Med* 1969;18:7–11.
44. Jacobs EM, Luce JK, Cailleau R. Chromosome abnormalities in human cancer: report of a patient with chronic myelogenous leukemia and his non-leukemic monozygotic twin. *Cancer* 1966;19:869–876.
45. Bizzozzero OJ, Johnson KG, Ciocco A. Radiation related leukemia in Hiroshima and Nagasaki, 1946-1964: distribution, incidence and appearance time. *N Engl J Med* 1966;274:1095–2101.
46. Corso A, Lazzarino M, Morra E, et al. Chronic myelogenous leukemia and exposure to ionizing radiation: a retrospective study of 443 patients. *Ann Hematol* 1995;70:79–82.
47. Deininger MW, Bose S, Gora-Tybor J, et al. Selective induction of leukemia-associated fusion genes by high dose ionizing radiation. *Cancer Res* 1998;58:421–425.
48. Fialkow PJ, Martin PJ, Najfeld V, et al. Evidence for a multistep pathogenesis of chronic myelogenous leukemia. *Blood* 1984;63: 1318–1323.
49. Ferraris AM, Canepa L, Melani C, et al. Clonal B lymphocytes lack bcr rearrangement in Ph-positive chronic myelogenous leukemia. *Br J Haematol* 1989;73:48–50.
50. Raskin WH, Ferraris AM, Najfeld V, et al. Further evidence for the existence of a clonal Ph-negative stage in some cases of Ph-positive chronic myelocytic leukemia. *Leukemia* 1993;7:1163–1167.
51. Daley GQ, Baltimore D. Transformation of an interleukin 3-dependent hematopoietic cell line by the chronic myelogenous leukemia-specific P210bcr/abl protein. *Proc Natl Acad Sci USA* 1988;85:9312–9316.
52. Daley GQ, Van Etten RA, Baltimore D. Induction of chronic myelogenous leukemia in mice by the P210bcr/abl gene of the Philadelphia chromosome. *Science* 1990;247:824–830.
53. Gishizky ML, Johnson-White J, Witte ON. Efficient transplantation of BCR-ABL-induced chronic myelogenous leukemia-like syndrome in mice. *Proc Natl Acad Sci USA* 1993;90:3755–3759.
54. Secker-Walker LM, Summersgill BM, Swansbury GJ, et al. Philadel-

phia-positive blast crisis masquerading as acute lymphoblastic leukemia in children. *Lancet* 1976;ii:1405.
55. Torlakovic E, Litz CE, McClure JS, et al. Direct detection of the Philadelphia chromosome in CD20-positive lymphocytes in chronic myeloid leukemia by tri-color immunophenotyping/FISH. *Leukemia* 1994;8:1940–1043.
56. Knuutila S, Larramendy ML, Ruutu T, et al. Involvement of natural killer cells in chronic myeloid leukemia. *Cancer Genet Cytogenet* 1995;79:21–24.
57. Haferlach T, Winkemann M, Nickenig C, et al. Which compartments are involved in Philadelphia-chromosome positive chronic myeloid leukaemia? An answer at the single cell level by combining May-Grunwald-Giemsa staining and fluorescence in situ hybridization techniques. *Br J Haematol* 1997;97:99–106.
58. Kirk JA, Reems JA, Roecklein BA, et al. Benign marrow progenitors are enriched in the CD34 + /HLA-DRlo population but not in the CD34 + /CD38lo population in chronic myeloid leukemia: an analysis using interphase fluorescence in situ hybridization. *Blood* 1995;86:737–743.
59. Lukasova E, Kozubek S, Kozubek M, et al. Localization and distance between ABL and BCR genes in interphase nuclei of bone marrow cells of control donors and patients with chronic myeloid leukaemia. *Hum Genet* 1997;100:525–535.
60. Ferrajoli A, Fizzotti A, Liberati AM, et al. Chronic myelogenous leukemia: an update on the biological findings and therapeutic approaches. *Clin Rev Oncol Hematol* 1996;22:151–174.
61. Verfaillie CM. Biology of chronic myelogenous leukemia. *Hematol Oncol Clin North Am* 1998;12:1–29.
62. Heisterkamp N, Stam K, Groffen H, et al. Structural organization of the bcr gene and its role in the Ph1 translocations. *Nature* 1985;315:758–761.
63. Bernards A, Rubin CM, Westbrook CA, et al. The first intron in the human abl gene is at least 200 kilobases long and is a target for translocations in chronic myelogenous leukemia. *Mol Cell Biol* 1987;7:3231–3236.
64. Westbrook CA, Hooberman AL, Spino C, et al. Clinical significance of the BCR-ABL fusion gene in adult acute lymphoblastic leukemia: a Cancer and leukemia Group B study (8762). *Blood* 1992;80:2983–2990.
65. Ribeiro RC, Abromowitch M, Raimondi SC, et al. Clinical and biologic hallmarks of the Philadelphia chromosome in childhood acute lymphoblastic leukemia. *Blood* 1987;70:948–953.
66. Heisterkamp N, Jenkins R, Thibodeau S, et al. The bcr gene in Philadelphia chromosome positive acute lymphoblastic leukemia. *Blood* 1989;73:1307–1311.
67. Melo JV. The diversity of BCR-ABL fusion proteins and their relationship to leukemia phenotype. *Blood.* 1996;88:2375–2384.
68. Melo JV, Myint H, Galton DA, Goldman JM. P190BCR-ABL chronic myeloid leukemia: the missing link with chronic myelomonocytic leukemia? *Leukemia* 1994;8:1795–1796.
69. Hochhaus A, Reiter A, Skladny H, et al. A novel BCR-ABL fusion gene (e6a2) in a patient with Philadelphia chromosome-negative chronic myelogenous leukemia. *Blood* 1996;88:2236–2240.
70. Hehlmann R, Goldman JM, Cross NC. A novel BCR-ABL fusion gene (e6a2) in a patient with Philadelphia chromosome-negative chronic myelogenous leukemia. *Blood* 1996;88:2236–2240.
71. Pane F, Frigeri F, Sindona M, et al. Neutrophilic-chronic myeloid leukemia: a distinct disease with a specific molecular marker (BCR/ABL with C3/A2 junction). *Blood* 1996;88:2410–2414.
72. Yamagata T, Mitani K, Kanda Y, et al. Elevated platelet count features the variant type of BCR/ABL junction in chronic myelogenous leukaemia. *Br J Haematol* 1996;94:370–372.
73. Emilia G, Luppi M, Ferrari MG, et al. Chronic myeloid leukemia with thrombocythemic onset may be associated with different BCR/ABL variant transcripts. *Cancer Genet Cytogenet* 1998;101:75–77.
74. Anastasi J, Feng J, Dickstein JI, et al. Lineage involvement by BCR/ABL in Ph + lymphoblastic leukemias: chronic myelogenous leukemia presenting in lymphoid blast vs Ph + acute lymphoblastic leukemia. *Leukemia* 1996;10:795–802.
75. Schenk TM, Keyhani A, Bottcher S, et al. Multilineage involvement of Philadelphia chromosome positive acute lymphoblastic leukemia. *Leukemia* 1998;12:666–674.
76. Honda H, Oda H, Suzuki T, et al. Development of acute lymphoblastic leukemia and myeloproliferative disorder in transgenic mice expressing p210 bcr/abl: a novel transgenic model for human Ph-positive leukemias. *Blood* 1998;91:2067–2075.
77. Lewis ID, McDonald LA, Samuels LM, et al. Establishment of a reproducible model of chronic-phase chronic myeloid leukemia in NOD/SCID mice using blood-derived mononuclear or CD34 + cells. *Blood* 1998;91:630–640.
78. Drexler HG. Leukemic cell lines: in vitro models for the study of chronic myeloid leukemia. *Leuk Res* 1994 18:919–927.
79. Spires ASD. Clinical manifestations of chronic granulocytic leukemia. *Semin Oncol* 1995;22:380–395.
80. Kantarjian HM, Deisseroth A, Kurzrock R, et al. Chronic myelogenous leukemia: a concise update. *Blood* 1993;82:691–703.
81. Savage DG, Szydlo RM, Goldman JM. Clinical features at diagnosis in 430 patients with chronic myeloid leukemia seen at a referral center over a 16-year period. *Br J Haematol* 1997;96:111–116.
82. Spiers ASD, Bain BJ, Turner JE. The peripheral blood in chronic granulocytic leukaemia: study of 50 untreated Philadelphia-positive cases. *Scand J Haematol* 1977;18:25–38.
83. Pugh WC, Pearson MC, Vardiman JW, et al. Philadelphia chromosome-negative chronic myelogenous leukemia: a morphologic reassessment. *Br J Haematol* 1985;60:457–467.
84. Ullyot JL, Baintoin DF: Azurophil and specific granules of blood neutrophils in chronic myelogenous leukemia: an ultrastructural and cytochemical analysis. *Blood* 1974;44:469–482.
85. Okum DB, Tanaka KR. Leukocyte alkaline phosphatase. *Am J Hematol* 1978;4:293–299.
86. Brandt L. Adhesiveness to glass slide and phagocytic activity of neutrophilic leukocytes in myeloproliferative disease. *Scand J Haematol* 1965;2:126–130.
87. Banerjee TK, Senn H, Holland JF. Comparative studies on localized leukocytic mobilization in patients with chronic myelocytic leukemia. *Cancer* 1972;29:637–644.
88. Cramer E, Auclair C, Hakim J, et al. Metabolic activity of phagocytizing granulocytes in chronic granulocytic leukemia: ultrastructural observations of a degranulation defect. *Blood* 1977;50:93–106.
89. Odenberg H, Olofsson T, Olsson I. Granulocytic function in chronic granulocytic leukemia: I. Bactericidal and metabolic capabilities during phagocytosis in isolated granulocytes. *Br J Haematol* 1975;29:427–441.
90. Dowding C, Th'ng KH, Goldman JM, et al. Increased T-lymphocyte number in chronic granulocytic leukemia before treatment. *Exp Haematol* 1984;12:811–815.
91. Chang WC, Fujimiya Y, Casteel N, et al. Natural killer cell immunodeficiency in patients with chronic myelogenous leukemia: III. Defective interleukin 2 production by T-helper and natural killer cells. *Int J Cancer* 1989;43:591–597.
92. Adams T, Schultz L, Goldberg L. Platelet function abnormalities in the myeloproliferative disorders. *Scand J Haematol* 1974;13:215–224.
93. Dickstein JI, Vardiman JW. Hematopathologic findings in the myeloproliferative disorders. *Semin Oncol* 1995;22:355–373.
94. Rappaport H. Tumors of the hematopoietic system. In: *Atlas of tumor pathology.* Washington, DC: Armed Forces Institute of Pathology, 1966;263–284.
95. Lorand-Metze I, Vassalo Jsouza CA. Histological and cytological heterogeneity of bone marrow in Philadelphia-positive chronic myelogenous leukaemia at diagnosis. *Br J Haematol* 1987;67:45–49.
96. Brunning RD, McKenna RW. Tumors of the bone marrow. In: *Atlas of tumor pathology.* Washington, DC: Armed Forces Institute of Pathology, 1994:195–254.
97. Marmount AM. The autoimmune myelopathies. *Acta Haematol* 1983;69:73–77.
98. Kattlove HE, Williams JC, Gaynor E, et al. Gaucher cells in chronic myelocytic leukemia: an acquired abnormality. *Blood* 1969;33:379–390.
99. Kelsey PR, Geary CG. Sea-blue histiocytes and Gaucher cells in bone marrow of patients with chronic myeloid leukaemia. *J Clin Pathol* 1988;41:960–962.
100. Busche G, Majewski H, Schlue J, et al. Frequency of pseudo-Gaucher cells in diagnostic bone marrow biopsies from patients with Ph-positive chronic myeloid leukemia. *Virchows Arch* 1997;430:1393–1398.
101. Anastasi J, Musvee T, Roulston D, et al. Pseudo-Gaucher histiocytes identified up to 1 year after transplantation for CML are BCR/ABL-positive. *Leukemia* 1998;12:233–237.

102. Golde DW, Burgaleta C, Sparkes RS, et al. The Philadelphia chromosome in human macrophages. *Blood* 1977;49:367–370.
103. Georgii A, Vykoupil KF, Buhr T, et al. Chronic myeloproliferative disorders in bone marrow biopsies. Pathol Res Pract 1990;186;3–27.
104. Clough V, Geary CG, Hashjmi K, et al. Myelofibrosis in chronic granulocytic leukaemias. *Br J Haematol* 1979;42:515–526.
105. Dekmezian R, Kantarjian HM, Keating MJ, et al. The relevance of reticulin stain-measured fibrosis at diagnosis in chronic myelogenous leukemia. *Cancer* 1987;59:1739–1743.
106. Muehleck SD, McKenna RD, Arthur DC, et al. Transformation of chronic myelogenous leukemia: clinical, morphologic and cytogenetic features. *Am J Clin Pathol* 1984;82:1–14.
107. Rowley JD, Testa JR. Chromosome abnormalities in malignant hematologic diseases. *Adv Cancer Res* 1982;8:103–148.
108. Hagemeijer A, Bartram CR, Smit EME, et al. Is the chromosomal region 9q34 always involved in variants of the Ph1 translocation? *Cancer Genet Cytogenet* 1984;13:1–16.
109. Werner M, Ewig M, Nasarek A, et al. Value of fluorescence in situ hybridization for detecting the bcr/abl gene fusion in interphase cells of routine bone marrow specimens. *Diagn Mol Pathol* 1997;6: 282–287.
110. Morgan GJ, Wiedemann LM. Annotation: the clinical application of molecular techniques in Philadelphia-positive leukaemia. *Br J Haematol* 1992;80:1–5.
111. Westbrook CA. The role of molecular techniques in the clinical management of leukemia: lessons from the Philadelphia chromosome. *Cancer* 1992;70:1695–1700.
112. Guo JQ, Lian J, Glassman A, et al. Comparison of bcr-abl protein expression and Philadelphia chromosome analyses in chronic myelogenous leukemia. *Am J Clin Pathol* 1996;106:442–448.
113. Van Denderen J, ten Hacken P, Berendes P, et al. Antibody recognition of the tumor-specific b3-a2 junction of bcr-abl chimeric proteins in Philadelphia-chromosome-positive leukemias. *Leukemia* 1992;6: 1107–1112.
114. Sokol JE, Gomez GA, Baccarani M, et al. Prognostic significance of additional cytogenetic abnormalities at diagnosis of Philadelphia chromosome-positive chronic granulocytic leukemia. *Blood* 1988;72: 294–298.
115. Swolin B, Weinfiels A, Westin J, et al. Karyotypic evolution in Ph-positive myeloid leukemia in relation to management and disease progression. *Cancer Genet Cytogenet* 1985;18:65–79.
116. Kantarjian HM, Talpaz M, Gutterman JU. Chronic myelogenous leukemia: past, present, and future. *Hematol Pathol* 1988;2:91–120.
117. Cervantes F, Lopez-Guillermo A, Bosch F, et al. An assessment of the clinicohematological criteria for the accelerated phase of chronic myeloid leukemia. *Eur J Haematol* 1996;57:286–291.
118. Kantarjian HM, Dixon D, Keating MJ, et al. Characteristics of accelerated disease in chronic myelogenous leukemia. *Cancer* 1984;61: 1441–1446.
119. Orazi A, Neiman RS, Cualing H, et al. CD34 immunostaining of bone marrow biopsy specimens is a reliable way to classify the phases of chronic myeloid leukemia. *Am J Clin Pathol* 1994;101:426–428.
120. Bernstein R. Cytogenetics of chronic myelogenous leukemia. *Semin Hematol* 1988;25:20–34.
121. Mitelman F. The cytogenetic scenario of chronic myeloid leukemia. *Leuk Lymph* 1993;11[Suppl 1]:11–13.
122. Harris NL, Jaffe ES, Diebold J, et al. World Health Organization classification of neoplastic diseases of the hematopoietic and lymphoid tissues: Report of the clinical advisory committee meeting—Airlie House, Virginia, November 1997. *J Clin Oncol* 1999;17: 3835–3849.
123. Kantarjian HM, Keating MJ, Talpaz M, et al. Chronic myelogenous leukemia in blast crisis: analysis of 242 patients. *Am J Med* 1987;83: 445–454.
124. Griesshammer M, Heinze B, Hellmann A, et al. Chronic myelogenous leukemia in blast crisis: retrospective analysis of prognostic factors in 90 patients. *Ann Hematol* 1996;73:225–230.
125. Jacknow G, Frizzera G, Gail-Peczalska K, et al. Extramedullary presentation of the blast crisis of chronic myelogenous leukemia. *Br J Haematol* 1985;61:225–236.
126. Specchia G, Palumbo G, Pastore D, et al. Extramedullary blast crisis of chronic myeloid leukemia. *Leuk Res* 1996;20:905–908.
127. Beard MEJ, Durrant J, Catovsky D, et al. Blast crisis of chronic myeloid leukemia (CML): I. Presentation simulating acute lymphoid leukemia (ALL). *Br J Haematol* 1976;34:167–178.
128. Roman J, Andres P, Jimenez MA, et al. Lymphoid blast crisis at the onset of chronic myelogenous leukemia: molecular evidence. *Br J Haematol* 1994;87:624–626.
129. Dederian PM, Kantarjian HM, Talpaz M, et al. Chronic myelogenous leukemia in the lymphoid blastic phase: characteristics, treatment response and prognosis. *Am J Med* 1993;94:69–73.
130. Cervantes F, Villamor N, Esteve J, et al. "Lymphoid" blast crisis of chronic myeloid leukaemia is associated with distinct clinicohaematological features. *Br J Haematol* 1998;100:123–128.
131. Schmetzer HM, Gerhartz HH. Immunological classification of chronic myeloid leukemia distinguishes chronic phase, imminent blastic transformation, and acute lymphoblastic leukemia. *Exp Hematol* 1997;25: 502–508.
132. Advani SH, Malhotra H, Kadam PR, et al. T-lymphoid blast crisis in chronic myeloid leukemia. *Am J Hematol* 1991;36:86–92.
133. Parreira L, Kearney L, Rassool F, et al. Correlation between chromosomal abnormalities and blast phenotype in the blast crisis of Ph-positive CGL. *Cancer Genet Cytogenet* 1986;22:29–34.
134. Spencer A, Vulliamy T, Kaeda J, et al. Clonal instability preceding lymphoid blastic transformation of chronic myeloid leukemia. *Leukemia* 1997;11:195–201.
135. Saikia T, Advani S, Dasgupta A, et al. Characterization of blast cells during blastic phase of chronic myeloid leukaemia by immunophenotyping: experience in 60 patients. *Leuk Res* 1988;12:499–506.
136. Hernandez JM, Gonzalez-Sarmiento R, Martin C, et al. Immunophenotypic, genomic and clinical characteristics of blast crisis of chronic myelogenous leukaemia. *Br J Haematol* 1991;79:408–414.
137. Anastasi J, Feng J, Le Beau MM, et al. The relationship between secondary chromosomal abnormalities and blast transformation in chronic myelogenous leukemia. *Leukemia* 1995;9:628–633.
138. Enright H, Weisdorf D, Peterson L, et al. Inversion of chromosome 16 and dysplastic eosinophils in accelerated phase of chronic myeloid leukemia. *Leukemia* 1992;6:381–384.
139. Abuja H, Bar-Eli M, Arlin Z, et al. The spectrum of molecular alterations in the evolution of chronic myelocytic leukemia. *J Clin Invest* 1991;87:2041–2047.
140. Dann EJ, Anastasi J, Larson RA. High dose claribine therapy for chronic myelogenous leukemia in the accelerated or blast phase. *J Clin Oncol* 1998;16:1498–1504.
141. Rosenthal S, Canellos GP, Gralnick HR. Erythroblastic transformation of chronic granulocytic leukemia. *Am J Med* 1977;63:116–124.
142. Ekblom M, Borgstrom G, von Willebrand E, et al. Erythroid blast crisis in chronic myelogenous leukemia. *Blood* 1983;62:591–596.
143. Wu CD, Medeiros LJ, Miranda RN, et al. Chronic myeloid leukemia manifested during megakaryoblastic crisis. *South Med J* 1996;89: 422–427.
144. Ishikura H, Yufu Y, Yamashita S, et al. Biphenotypic blast crisis of chronic myelogenous leukemia: abnormalities of p53 and retinoblastoma genes. *Leuk Lymphoma* 1997;25:573–578.
145. Akashi K, Mizuno S, Harada M, et al. T lymphoid/myeloid bilineal crisis in chronic myelogenous leukemia. *Exp Hematol* 1993;21: 743–748.
146. Werner M, Kaloutsi V, Kausche F, et al. Evidence from molecular genetic and cytogenetic analyses that bone marrow histopathology is reliable in the diagnosis of chronic myeloproliferative disorders. *Virchows Arch Cell Pathol* 1993;63:1994–2004.
147. Costello R, Lafage M, Toiron Y, et al. Philadelphia chromosome-negative chronic myeloid leukaemia: a report of 14 new cases. *Br J Haematol* 1995;90:346–352.
148. Shepherd PCA, Ganesan TS, Galton DAG. Haematological classification of the chronic myeloid leukaemias. *Bailliers Clin Haematol* 1987; 1:887–906.
149. Arico M, Biondi A, Pui C-H. Juvenile myelomonocytic leukemia. *Blood* 1997;90:479–488.
150. Ramos FJ, Zamora F, Peres-Sicilia M, et al. Chronic granulocytic leukemia versus neutrophilic leukemoid reaction. *Am J Med* 1990;88: 83–84.
151. Frisch C, Frisch B, Beham A, et al. Comparison of bone marrow histology in early chronic granulocytic leukemia and in leukemoid reaction. *Eur J Haematol* 1990;44:154–158.
152. Bennett JM, Catovsky D, Daniel MT, et al. The chronic myeloid leukaemias: guidelines for distinguishing chronic granulocytic, atypi-

cal chronic myeloid, and chronic myelomonocytic leukaemias. Proposals by the French-American-British cooperative leukaemia group. *Br J Haematol* 1994;87:746–754.

153. Sole F, Tarabadella M, Granada I, et al. Isochromosome 17q as a sole anomaly: a distinct myelodysplastic syndrome entity? *Leuk Res* 1993; 17:717–720.
154. Becher R, Carbonell F, Bartram CR. Isochromosome 17q in Ph1-negative leukemia: a clinical, cytogenetic and molecular study. *Blood* 1990;75:1679–1683.
155. Mareni C, Sessarego M, Origone P, et al. Molecular analysis of Philadelphia-negative myeloproliferative syndromes with i(17q). *Cancer Genet Cytogenet* 1989;43:195–201.
156. You W, Weisbrot IM. Chronic neutrophilic leukemia: report of two cases and review of literature. *Am J Clin Pathol* 1979;72:233–242.
157. Secker-Walker LM, Craig JM. Prognostic implications of breakpoint and lineage heterogeneity in Philadelphia-positive acute lymphoblastic leukemia: a review. *Leukemia* 1993;7:147–151.
158. Paietta E, Racevskis J, Bennett JM, et al. Biological heterogeneity in Philadelphia chromosome-positive acute leukemia with myeloid morphology: the Eastern Cooperative Oncology Group Experience. *Leukemia* 1998;12:1881–1885.
159. Hasford J, Pfirrmann M, Hehlmann R, et al. A new prognostic score for survival of patients with chronic myeloid leukemia treated with interferon alfa. *J Natl Cancer Inst* 1998;90:850–858.
160. Sokal JE, Cox EB, Baccarani M, et al. Prognostic discrimination in "good-risk" chronic granulocytic leukemia. *Blood* 1984;63: 789–799.
161. Tefferi A, Litzow MR, Noel P, et al. Chronic granulocytic leukemia: recent information on pathogenesis, diagnosis and disease monitoring. *Mayo Clin Proc* 1997;72:445–452.
162. Hehlmann R, Heimpel H, Hasford J, et al. Randomized comparison of busulfan and hydroxyurea in chronic myelogenous leukemia: prolongation of survival by hydroxyurea. *Blood* 1993;83:398–407.
163. O'Brien S, Kantarjian H, Keating M, et al. Homoharringtonine therapy induces responses in patients with chronic myelogenous leukemia in late chronic phase. *Blood* 1995;86:3322–3326.
164. Buyssens N, Bourgeois NH. Chronic myelocytic leukemia versus idiopathic myelofibrosis: a diagnostic problem in bone marrow biopsies. *Cancer* 1977;40:1548–1561.
165. Anastasi J, Larson RA, Vardiman JW. Prominent erythroid proliferation in chronic myelogenous leukemia. *Lab Invest* 1996;74:105A.
166. Niederie N, Kloke O, Osieka R, et al. Interferon alfa-2b in the treatment of chronic myelogenous leukemia. *Semin Oncol* 1987; 1429–1435.
167. Talpaz M, Kantarjian HM, McCredie K, et al. Hematologic remission and cytogenetic improvement by recombinant human interferon alphaA, in chronic myelogenous leukemia. *N Engl J Med* 1986;314: 1065–1069.
168. Dowding C, Guo A-P, Osterholz J, et al. Interferon-alfa overrides the deficient adhesion of chronic myeloid leukemia primitive progenitor cells to bone marrow stromal cells. *Blood* 1991;78:499–505.
169. Facchetti F, Tironi A, Marocolo D, et al. Histopathological changes in bone marrow biopsies from patients with chronic myeloid leukaemia after treatment with recombinant alpha-interferon. *Histopathology* 1997;31:3–11.
170. Wilhelm M, Bueso-Ramos C, O'Brien S, et al. Effect of interferon-alpha therapy on bone marrow fibrosis in chronic myelogenous leukemia. *Leukemia* 1998;12:65–70.
171. Stock W, Westbrook CA, Peterson B, et al. Value of molecular monitoring during the treatment of chronic myeloid leukemia: a Cancer and leukemia Group B study. *J Clin Oncol* 1997;15:26–36.
172. Seong DC, Kantarjian HM, Ro JY, et al. Hypermetaphase fluorescence in situ hybridization for quantitative monitoring of Philadelphia chromosome-positive cells in patients with chronic myelogenous leukemia during treatment. *Blood* 1995;86:2343–2349.
173. Tanaka K, Arif M, Eguchi M, et al. Application of fluorescence in situ hybridization to detect residual leukemic cells with 9;22 and 15; 17 translocations. *Leukemia* 1997;11:436–440.
174. Lee SJ, Anasetti C, Horowitz MM, et al. Initial therapy for chronic myelogenous leukemia: playing the odds [Editorial]. *J Clin Oncol* 1998;16:2897–2903.
175. Rousselet M-C, Kerjean A, Guyetant S, et al. Histopathology of bone marrow after allogeneic bone marrow transplantation for chronic myeloid leukemia. *Pathol Res Pract* 1996;92:790–795.
176. Hochhaus A, Reiter A, Skladny H, et al. Molecular monitoring of residual disease in chronic myelogenous leukemia patients after therapy. *Recent Results Cancer Res* 1998; 144:36–44.
177. Radich JP, Gehly G, Gooley T, et al. Polymerase chain reaction detection of the BCR-ABL fusion transcript after allogeneic marrow transplantation for chronic myeloid leukemia: results and implications in 346 patients. *Blood* 1995;85:2632–2638.
178. Delage R, Soiffer RJ, Dear K, et al. Clinical significance of bcr-abl gene rearrangement detected by polymerase chain reaction after allogeneic bone marrow transplantation in chronic myelogenous leukemia. *Blood* 1991;78:2759–2767.
179. Lin F, van Rhee F, Goldman JM, et al. Kinetics of increasing BCR-ABL transcript numbers in chronic myeloid leukemia patients who relapse after bone marrow transplantation. *Blood* 1996;87: 4473–4478.
180. Carreras E, Sierra J, Rovira M, et al. Successful autografting in chronic myelogenous leukaemia using Philadelphia negative blood progenitor cells mobilized with rHuG-CSF alone in a patient responding to alpha-interferon. *Br J Haematol* 1997;96:421–423.
181. Smetsers TF, Linders EH, van de Locht LT, et al. An antisense Bcr-Abl phosphodiester-tailed methylphosphonate oligonucleotide reduces the growth of chronic myeloid leukaemia patient cells by a non-antisense mechanism. *Br J Haematol* 1997;96:377–381.
182. Deininger MW, Goldman JM, Lydon N, et al. The tyrosine kinase inhibitor CGP57148B selectively inhibits the growth of BCR-ABL-positive cells. *Blood* 1997;90:3691–3698.
183. Lim SH, Coleman S. Chronic myelogenous leukemia as an immunologic target. *Am J Hematol* 1997;54:61–67.
184. Podesta M, Piaggio G, Sewssarego M, et al. Spontaneous exodus of high numbers of normal early progenitors cells (Ph-negative LTC-IC) in the peripheral blood of patients with chronic myeloid leukemia at the beginning of the disease. *Br J Haematol* 1997;97:94–98.
185. Grand FH, Marley SB, Chase A, et al. BCR/ABL-negative progenitors are enriched in the adherent fraction of CD34 + cells circulating in the blood of chronic phase chronic myeloid leukemia patients. *Leukemia* 1997;11:1486–1492.
186. Tuohy EA. A case of splenomegaly with polymorphonuclear neutrophil hyperleukocytosis. *Am J Med Sci* 1920;160:18–25.
187. Zittoun R, Rea D, Ngoc LH, et al. Chronic neutrophilic leukemia: A study of four cases. *Ann Hematol* 1994;68:55–60.
188. Tursz T, Flandrin G, Brouet JC, et al. Coexistence un myelome et une leucémie granuleuse en absence de tout traitement: etude de quarte observations. *Nouv Rev Fr Hematol* 1974;14:693–704.
189. Standen GR, Jasani B, Wagstaff M, et al. Chronic neutrophilic leukemia and multiple myeloma: an association with λ light chain expression. *Cancer* 1990;66:162–166.
190. Masini L, Salvarani C, Macchioni P, et al. Chronic neutrophilic leukemia (CNL) with karyotypic abnormalities associated with plasma cell dyscrasia: a case report. *Haematologica* 1992;77:277–279.
191. Cehreli C, Undar B, Akkoc N, et al. Coexistence of chronic neutrophilic leukemia with light chain myeloma. *Acta Haematol* 1994;91: 32–34.
192. Cervantes F, Marti JM, Rozman C, et al. Chronic neutrophilic leukemia with marked myelodysplasia terminating in blast crisis. *Blut* 1988; 56:75–78.
193. Zoumbos NC, Symeonidis A, Kourakli-Symeonidis A. Chronic neutrophilic leukemia with dysplastic features: a new variant of the myelodysplastic syndromes? *Acta Haemat* 1989;82:156–160.
194. Foa P, Iurlo A, Saglio G, et al. Chronic neutrophilic leukemia associated with polycythemia vera: pathogenetic implications and therapeutic approach. *Br J Haematol* 1991;72:285–288.
195. Di Donato C, Croci G, Lazzari S, et al. Chronic neutrophilic leukemia: description of a new case with karyotypic abnormalities. *Am J Clin Pathol* 1986;85:369–371.
196. Matano S, Nakamura S, Kobayaski K, et al. Deletion of the long arm of chromosome 20 in a patient with chronic neutrophilic leukemia: cytogenetic findings in chronic neutrophilic leukemia. *Am J Hematol* 1997;54:72–75.
197. Froberg MK, Brunning RD, Dorion P, et al. Demonstration of clonality in neutrophils using FISH in a case of chronic neutrophilic leukemia. *Leukemia* 1998;12:623–626.
198. Kwong YL, Cheng G. Clonal nature of chronic neutrophilic leukemia. *Blood* 1993;82:1035–1036.
199. Yanagisawa K, Ohminami H, Sato M, et al. Neoplastic involvement

of granulocytic lineage, not granulocytic-monocytic, monocytic, or erythrocytic lineage, in a patient with chronic neutrophilic leukemia. *Am J Hematol* 1998;57:221–224.
200. Standen GR, Steers FJ, Jones L. Clonality of chronic neutrophilic leukaemia associated with myeloma: analysis using the X-linked probe M27β. *J Clin Pathol* 1993;46:297–298.
201. Hasle H, Olesen G, Kerndrup G, et al. Chronic neutrophil leukaemia in adolescence and young adulthood. *Br J Haematol* 1996;94:628–630.
202. Hardy WR, Anderson RE. The hypereosinophilic syndrome. *Ann Intern Med* 1968;68:1220–1228.
203. Chusid MJ, Dale DC, West BC, et al. The hypereosinophilic syndrome: analysis of fourteen cases with review of the literature. *Medicine* 1975;54:1–27.
204. Weller PF, Bubley GJ. The idiopathic hypereosinophilic syndrome. *Blood* 1994;83:2759–2779.
205. Bain BJ. Eosinophilic leukaemias and the idiopathic hypereosinophilic syndrome. *Br J Haematol* 1996;95:2–9.
206. Chang HW, Leong KH, Koh DR, et al. Clonality of isolated eosinophils in the hypereosinophilic syndrome. *Blood* 1999;93:1651–1657.
207. Sanderson CJ. Interleukin-5, eosinophils, and disease. *Blood* 1992; 79:3101–3109.
208. Spry CJF, Davies J, Tai PC, et al. Clinical features of fifteen patients with the hypereosinophilic syndrome. *QJM* 1983;205:1–22.
209. Flaum MA, Schooley RT, Fauci AS, et al. A clinicopathologic correlation of the idiopathic hypereosinophilic syndrome: I. Hematologic manifestations. *Blood* 1981;58:1012–1020.
210. Kueck BD, Smith RE, Parkin J, et al. Eosinophilic leukemia: a myeloproliferative disorder distinct from the hypereosinophilic syndrome. *Hematol Pathol* 1991;5:195–205.
211. Golub TR, Barker GF, Lovett M, et al. Fusion of PDGF receptor to a novel ets-like gene, tel, in chronic myelomonocytic leukemia with t(5;12) chromosomal translocation. *Cell* 1994;77:307–316.
212. Wlodarska I, Mecucci C, Maynen P, et al. TEL gene is involved in myelodysplastic syndromes with either the typical t(5;12)(q33;p13) translocation or its variant t(10;12)(q24;p13). *Blood* 1995;85: 2848–2852.
213. Baranger L, Szapiro N, Gardais J, et al. Translocation t(5;12)(q31-q33;p12-p13): a non-random translocation associated with a myeloid disorder with eosinophilia. *Br J Haematol* 1994;88:343–347.
214. Schooley RT, Flaum MA, Gralnick HR, et al. A clinicopathologic correlation of the idiopathic hypereosinophilic syndrome: II. Clinical manifestations. *Blood* 1981;58:1021–1028.
215. Lefebvre C, Bletry O, Degoulet P, et al. Facteurs pronostiques du syndrome hypereosinophilique: etude de 40 observations. *Ann Med Interne (Paris)* 1989;140:253–257.
216. Fruchtman SM, Mack K, Kaplan ME, et al. From efficacy to safety: a Polycythemia Vera Study Group report on hydroxyurea in patients with polycythemia vera. *Semin Hematol* 1997;34:17–23.
217. Najean Y, Rain JD, for the French Polycythemia Study Group. Treatment of polycythemia vera: the use of hydroxyurea and pipobroman in 292 patients under the age of 65 years. *Blood* 1997;90:3370–3377.
218. Najean Y, Rain JD. The very long-term evolution of polycythemia vera: an analysis of 318 patients initially treated by phlebotomy or 32P between 1969 and 1981. *Semin Hematol* 1997;34:6–16.
219. Brubaker JH, Wasserman LR, Goldberg JD, et al. Increased prevalence of polycythemia vera in parents of patients on Polycythemia Vera Study Group protocols. *Am J Hematol* 1984;16:367–373.
220. Miller RL, Purvis JD, Weick JK. Familial polycythemia vera. *Cleve Clin J Med* 1989;56:813–818.
221. Manoharan A, Garson OM. Familial polycythemia vera: A study in 3 sisters. *Scand J Haematol* 1976;17:10–16.
222. Caldwell GG, Kelley DB, Heath CW, et al. Polycythemia vera among participants of a nuclear weapons test. *JAMA* 1984;252:662–664.
223. Kilgore ES. Polycythemia in feather dyers. *JAMA* 1927;89:343–344.
224. Boyd MT, Maclean N, Oscier DG. Detection of retrovirus in patients with myeloproliferative disease. *Lancet* 1989;i:814–816.
225. Muta K, Drantz SB, Bondurant MC, et al. Distinct roles of erythropoietin, insulin-like growth factor I, and stem cell factor in the development of erythroid progenitor cells. *J Clin Invest* 1994;94:34–43.
226. Adamson JW. The erythropoietin hematocrit relationship in normal and polycythemic man: implications of marrow regulation. *Blood* 1968;32:597–609.
227. Remacha AF, Montserrat I, Santamaria A, et al. Serum erythropoietin in the diagnosis of polycythemia vera: a follow-up study. *Haematologica* 1997;82:406–410.
228. Prchal JF, Adamson JW, Murphy S, et al. Polycythemia vera: the in vitro response of normal and abnormal stem cell lines to erythropoietin. *J Clin Invest* 1978;61:1044–1047.
229. Weinberg RS. In vitro erythropoiesis in polycythemia and other myeloproliferative disorders. *Semin Hematol* 1997;34:64–69.
230. Correa PN, Eskinazi D, Axelrad AA. Circulating erythroid progenitors in polycythemia vera are hypersensitive to insulin-like growth factor-I in vitro: studies in an improved serum-free medium. *Blood* 1994; 83: 99–112.
231. Mirza AM, Correa PN, Axelrad AA. Increased basal and induced tyrosine phosphorylation of the insulin-like growth factor I receptor subunit in circulating mononuclear cells of patients with polycythemia vera. *Blood* 1995;86:877–882.
232. Mirza AM, Ezzat S, Axelrad AA. Insulin-like growth factor binding protein-1 is elevated in patients with polycythemia vera and stimulates erythroid burst formation in vitro. *Blood* 1997:89:1862–1869.
233. Silva M, Richard C, Benito A, et al. Expression of Bcl-x in erythroid precursors from patients with polycythemia vera. *N Engl J Med* 1998; 338:564–571.
234. Dai CH, Krantz SB, Dessypris EN, et al. Polycythemia vera II: hypersensitivity of bone-marrow erythroid, granulocyte-macrophage and megakaryocyte progenitor cells to interleukin-3 and granulocyte-macrophage colony-stimulating factor. *Blood* 1992;80:891–899.
235. Berlin NI. Diagnosis and classification of the polycythemias. *Semin Hematol* 1975;12:339–351.
236. Berk PD, Goldberg JD, Donovan PB, et al. Therapeutic recommendations in polycythemia vera based on Polycythemia Vera Study Group protocols. *Semin Hematol* 1986:23:132–143.
237. Berk PD. Epilogue: broader lessons from the study of polycythemia vera. *Semin Hematol* 1997;34:77–80.
238. Bilgrami S, Greenberg BR. Polycythemia rubra vera. *Semin Oncol* 1995;22:307–326.
239. Murphy S. Polycythemia vera. *Dis Mon* 1992(March):158–211.
240. Danish EH, Rasch CA, Harris JW. Polycythemia vera in childhood: case report and review of the literature. *Am J Hematol* 1980;9: 421–428.
241. Najean Y, Mugnier P, Dresch C, et al. Polycythaemia vera in young people: an analysis of 58 cases diagnosed before 40 years. *Br J Haematol* 1987:67:285–291.
242. Valla D, Casadevall N, Huisse MG, et al. Etiology of portal vein thrombosis in adults: a prospective evaluation of primary myeloproliferative disorders. *Gastroenterology* 1988;94:1063–1069.
243. Orlandi E, Castelli G, Brusamolino E, et al. Hemorrhagic and thrombotic complications in polycythemia vera: a clinical study. *Haematologica* 1989:74:45–49.
244. Lundin PM, Ridell B, Weinfeld A. The significance of bone marrow morphology for the diagnosis of polycythemia vera. *Scand J Haematol* 1972;9:271–282.
245. Ellis JT, Peterson P. *The bone marrow in polycythemia vera.* New York: Appleton-Century-Crofts, 1979:383–403.
246. Ellis JT, Peterson P, Geller SA, et al. Studies of the bone marrow in polycythemia vera and the evolution of myelofibrosis and second hematologic malignancies. *Semin Hematol* 1986:23:144–155.
247. Anger B, Haug U, Seidler R, et al. Polycythemia vera: a clinical study of 141 patients. *Blut* 1989:59:493–500.
248. Wolf BC, Banks PM, Mann RB, et al. Splenic hematopoiesis in polycythemia vera: a morphologic and immunohistologic study. *Am J Clin Pathol* 1988;89:69–75.
249. Rege-Cambrin G, Mecucci C, Tricot G, et al. A chromosomal profile of polycythemia vera. *Cancer Genet Cytogenet* 1987;25:233–245.
250. Swolin B, Weinfeld A, Westin J. A prospective long-term cytogenetic study in polycythemia vera in relation to treatment and clinical course. *Blood* 1988;72:386–395.
251. Diez-Martin JL, Graham DL, Petitt RM, et al. Chromosome studies in 104 patients with polycythemia vera. Mayo Clin *Proc* 1991;66: 287–299.
252. Najean Y, Arrago JP, Rain JD, et al. The ''spent'' phase of polycythaemia vera: hypersplenism in the absence of myelofibrosis. *Br J Haematol* 1984;56:163–170.
253. Ikkala E, Rapola J, Kotilainen M. Polycythaemia vera and myelofibrosis. *Scand J Haematol* 1967;4:453–464.
254. Weinfeld A, Swolin B, Westin J. Acute leukaemia after hydroxyurea

therapy in polycythaemia vera and allied disorders: prospective study of efficacy and leukaemogenicity with therapeutic implications. *Eur J Haematol* 1994;52:134–139.
255. Najean Y, Rain JD, Dresch C, et al. Risk of leukaemia, carcinoma and myelofibrosis in 32P-or chemotherapy-treated patients with polycythaemia vera: a prospective analysis of 682 cases. *Leuk Lymphoma* 1996;22:111–119.
256. Meytes D, Katz D, Ramot B. Preleukemia and leukemia in polycythemia vera. *Blood* 1976;47:237–241.
257. Najean Y, Deschamps A, Dresch C, et al. Acute leukemia and myelodysplasia in polycythemia vera: a clinical study with long-term follow-up. *Cancer* 1988;61:89–95.
258. Berger R, Bernheim A, Flandrin G, et al. Cytogenetic studies on acute nonlymphocytic leukemias following polycythemia vera. *Cancer Genet Cytogenet* 1984;11:441–451.
259. Smith JR, Landaw SA. Smoker's polycythemia. *N Engl J Med* 1978; 298:6–10.
260. Emanuel PD, Eaves CJ, Broudy VC, et al. Familial and congenital polycythemia in three unrelated families. *Blood* 1992;79:3019–3030.
261. Sokol L, Luhovy M, Guan Y, et al. Primary familial polycythemia: a frameshift mutation in the erythropoietin receptor gene and increased sensitivity of erythroid progenitors to erythropoietin. *Blood* 1995;86: 15–22.
262. Murphy S, Peterson P, Iland H, et al. Experience of the Polycythemia Vera Study Group with essential thrombocythemia: a final report on diagnostic criteria, survival, and leukemic transition by treatment. *Semin Hematol* 1997;34:29–39.
263. Thiele J, Kvasnicka HM, Werden C, et al. Idiopathic primary osteo-myelofibrosis: a clinico-pathological study on 208 patients with special emphasis on evolution of disease features, differentitation from essential thrombocythemia and variables of prognostic impact. *Leuk Lymphoma* 1996;22:303–317.
264. Eyster ME, Saletan SL, Rabellino EM, et al. Familial essential thrombocythemia. *Am J Med* 1986;80:497–501.
265. Mele A, Visani G, Pulsoni A, et al. Risk factors for esstential thrombocythemia: a case-control study. *Cancer* 1996;77:2157–2161.
266. El-Kassar N, Hetet G, Briere J, et al. Clonality analysis of hematopoiesis in essential thrombocythemia: advantages of studying T lymphocytes and platelets. *Blood* 1997;89:128–134.
267. Harrison CN, Gale RE, Machin SJ, et al. A large proportion of patients with a diagnosis of essential thrombocythemia do not have a clonal disorder and may be at a lower-risk of thrombotic complications. *Blood* 1999;93:417–424.
268. Broudy VC, Lin NL, Kaushansky K. Thrombopoietin (c-mpl ligand) acts synergistically with erythropoietin, stem cell factor and IL-11 to enhance murine megakaryocyte colony growth and increased megakaryocyte ploidy in vitro. *Blood* 1995;85:1719–1726.
269. Griesshammer M, Bangerter M, Schrezenmeier H. A possible role for thrombopoietin and its receptor c-mpl in the pathobiology of essential thrombocythemia. *Semin Thromb Hemost* 1997;23:419–423.
270. Cerutti A, Custodi P, Duranti M, et al. Thrombopoietin levels in patients with primary and reactive thrombocytosis. *Br J Haematol* 1997; 99:281–284.
271. Kiladjian JJ, Elkassar N, Hetet G, et al. Study of the thrombopoietin receptor in essential thrombocythemia. *Leukemia* 1997;11: 1821–1826.
272. Gurney AL, Carver-Moore K, de Sauvage FJ, et al. Thrombocytopenia in c-mpl-deficient mice. *Science* 1994;265:1445–1447.
273. Kutter DJ, Rosenberg RD. The reciprocal relationship of thrombopoietin (c-mpl ligand) to changes in the platelet mass during busulfan-induced thrombocytopenias in the rabbit. *Blood* 1995;85:2720–2730.
274. Li J, Xia Y, Kuter DJ. Analysis of the thrombopoietin receptor (mpl) on platelets from normal and essential thrombocythemia (ET) patients. *Blood* 1996;88[Suppl 1]:595 (abst 2168).
275. Moliterno AR, Hankins WD, Spivak JL. Impaired expression of the thrombopoietin receptor by platelets from patients with polycythemia vera. *N Engl J Med* 1998;338:572–580.
276. Komatsu N, Suda T, Sakata Y, et al. Megakaryocytopoiesis in vitro of patients with essential thrombocythaemia: effect of plasma and serum on megakaryocytic colony formation. *Br J Haematol* 1986;64: 241–252.
277. Juvonen E, Partanen S, Ruutu T. Colony formation by megakaryocytic progenitors in essential thrombocythaemia. *Br J Haematol* 1986;66: 161–164.
278. Croizat H, Amato D, McLeod DL, et al. Differences among myeloproliferative disorders in the behavior of their restricted progenitor cells in culture. *Blood* 1983;62:578–584.
279. Rolovic Z, Basara N, Gotic M, et al. The determination of spontaneous megakaryocyte colony formation is an unequivocal test for discrimination between essential thrombocythaemia and reactive thrombocytosis. *Br J Haematol* 1995;90:326–331.
280. Westwood NB, Pearson TC. Diagnostic applications of haemopoietic progenitor culture techniques in polycythaemias and thrombocythaemias. *Leuk Lymphoma* 1996;22[Suppl 1]:95–103.
281. Buss DH, Cashell AW, O'Connor ML, et al. Occurrence, etiology and clinical significance of extreme thrombocytosis: a study of 280 cases. *Am J Med* 1994;96:247–252.
282. McIntyre KJ, Hoagland HC, Silverstein MN, et al. Essential thrombocythemia in young adults. *Mayo Clin Proc* 1991;66:149–154.
283. Murphy S, Iland H, Rosenthal D, et al. Essential thrombocythemia: an interim report from the Polycythemia Vera Study Group. *Semin Hematol* 1986;23:177–182.
284. Bellucci S, Janvier M, Tobelem G, et al. Essential thrombocythemias: clinical evolutionary and biological data. *Cancer* 1986:58; 2440–2447.
285. Hehlmann R, Jahn M, Baumann B, et al. Essential thrombocythemia: clinical characteristics and course of 61 cases. *Cancer* 1988;61: 2487–2496.
286. Pearson TC. Primary thrombocythaemia: diagnosis and management. *Br J Haematol* 1991;78:145–148.
287. Colombi M, Radaelli F, Zocchi L, et al. Thrombotic and hemorrhagic complications in essential thrombocythemia: a retrospective study of 103 patients. *Cancer* 1991;67:2926–2930.
288. Mitus A, Schafer AI. Thrombocytosis and thrombocythemia. *Hematol Oncol Clin North Am* 1990;4:157–178.
289. Lengfelder E, Hochhaus A, Kronawitter U, et al. Should a platelet limit of 600×10^9/L be used as a diagnostic criterion in essential thrombocythaemia? An analysis of the natural course including early stages. *Br J Haematol* 1998;100:15–23.
290. Sehayek E, Ben-Yosef N, Modan M, et al. Platelet parameters and aggregation in essential and reactive thrombocytosis. *Am J Clin Pathol* 1988;90:431–436.
291. Buss DH, O'Connor ML, Woodruff RD, et al. Bone marrow and peripheral blood findings in patients with extreme thrombocytosis: a report of 63 cases. *Arch Pathol Lab Med* 1991;115:475–480.
292. Dudley JM, Messinezy M, Eridani S, et al. Primary thrombocythaemia: diagnostic criteria and a simple scoring system for positive diagnosis. *Br J Haematol* 1989;71:331–335.
293. Kaywin P, McDonough M, Insel PA, et al. Platelet function in essential thrombocythemia: decreased epinephrine responsiveness associated with a deficiency of platelet alpha-adrenergic receptors. *N Engl J Med* 178;299:505–509.
294. Nozaki H, Nagao T, Arimori S. Platelet volume and intraplatelet adenine nucleotides in various hematologic disorders. *Eur J Haematol* 1988;40:65–68.
295. Thiele J, Moedder B, Kremer B, et al. Chronic myeloproliferative diseases with an elevated platelet count (in excess of 1,000,000/μl): a clinicopathological study on 46 patients with special emphasis on primary (essential) thrombocythemia. *Hematol Pathol* 1987;1: 227–237.
296. Knecht H, Streuli RA. Megakaryocytopoiesis in different forms of thrombocytosis and thrombocytopenia: identification of megakaryocyte precursors by immunostaining of intracytoplasmic factor VIII-related antigen. *Acta Haematol* 1985;74:208–215.
297. Wolf BC, Neiman RS. Essential thrombocythemia. In: Disorders of the Spleen. Philadelphia: WB Saunders, 1989:173–174.
298. Third International Workshop on Chromosomes in leukemia, 1980. Report on essential thrombocythemia. *Cancer Genet Cytogenet* 1981; 4:138–142.
299. Sessarego M, Defferrari R, Dejana AM, et al. Cytogenetic analysis in essential thrombocythemia at diagnosis and at transformation: a 12-year study. *Cancer Genet Cytogenet* 1989;43:57–65.
300. Van Genderen PJJ, Budde U, Michiels JJ, et al. The reduction of large von Willebrand factor multimers in plasma in essential thrombocythaemia is related to the platelet count. *Br J Haematol* 1996;93: 962–965.
301. Tefferi A, Hoagi HC. Issues in the diagnosis and management of essential thrombocythemia. *Mayo Clin Proc* 1994;69:651–655.

302. Michiels JJ, Prins E, Hagermeijer A, et al. Philadelphia chromosome-positive thrombocythemia and megakaryoblast leukemia. *Am J Clin Pathol* 1987;88:645–652.
303. Paietta E, Rosen N, Roberts M, et al. Philadelphia chromosome positive essential thrombocythemia evolving into lymphoid blast crisis. *Cancer Genet Cytogenet* 1987;25:227–231.
304. Stoll DB, Peterson P, Esten R, et al. Clinical presentation and natural history of patients with essential thrombocythemia and the Philadelphia chromosome. *Am J Hematol* 1988;27:77–83.
305. Morris CM, Fitzgerald PH, Hollings PE, et al. Essential thrombocythaemia and the Philadelphia chromosome. *Br J Haematol* 1988;70: 13–19.
306. Carroll AJ, Poon MC, Robinson NC, et al. Sideroblastic anemia associated with thrombocytosis and a chromosome 3 abnormality. *Cancer Genet Cytogenet* 1986;22:183–187.
307. Case Reconds of the Massachusetts General Hospital: Case 17-1992. *N Engl J Med* 1992;326:1146.
308. Cazzola M, Barosi G, Gobbi G, et al. Natural history of idiopathic refractory sideroblastic anemia. *Blood* 1988;71:305–312.
309. Koike T, Uesugi Y, Toba K, et al. 5q-syndrome presenting as essential thrombocythemia: myelodysplastic syndrome or chronic myeloproliferative disorder [Letter]? *Leukemia* 1995;9:517–518.
310. Anagrelide Study Group. Anagrelide, a therapy for thrombocythemia states: experience in 577 patients. *Am J Med* 1992;92:69–76.
311. Sacchi S. The role of α-interferon in essential thrombocythaemia, polycythaemia vera and myelofibrosis with myeloid metaplasia (MMM): a concise update. *Leuk Lymphoma* 1995;19:13–20.
312. Beard J, Hillmen P, Anderson CC, et al. Primary thrombocythaemia in pregnancy. *Br J Haematol* 1991;77:371–374.
313. Shibata K, Shimamoto Y, Suga K, et al. Essential thrombocythemia terminating in acute leukemia with minimal myeloid differentiation: a brief review of recent literature. *Acta Haematol* 1994;91:84–88.
314. Sedlacek SM, Curtis JL, Weintraub J, et al. Essential thrombocythemia and leukemic transformation. *Medicine* 1986:65;353–363.
315. Murphy PT, Sivakumaran M, et al. Acute lymphoblastic transformation of essential thrombocythaemia. *Br J Haematol* 1995;89:921–922.
316. Laszlo J. Myeloproliferative disorders (MPD): myelofibrosis, myelosclerosis, extramedullary hematopoiesis, undifferentiated MPD and hemorrhagic thrombocythemia. *Semin Hematol* 1975;4:409–432.
317. Ward HP, Block MH. The natural history of agnogenic myeloid metaplasia (AMM) and a critical evaluation of its relationship with the myeloproliferataive syndrome. *Medicine* 1971;150:357–420.
318. Anderson RE, Hoshino T, Yamamoto T. Myelofibrosis with myeloid metaplasia in survivors of the atomic bomb in Hiroshima. *Ann Intern Med* 1964;1:1–17.
319. Hu H. Benzene-associated myelofibrosis. *Ann Intern Med* 1987;106: 171–172.
320. Patakfalvi A, Csete B, Horvath T. Familial myelofibrosis. *Haematologia* 1969;3:217–224.
321. Buschle M, Janssen JWG, Drexler H, et al. Evidence for pluripotent stem cell origin of idiopathic myelofibrosis and clonal analysis of a case characterised by a N-ras gene mutation. *Leukemia* 1988;2: 658–660.
322. Hibbin JA, Njoku OS, Matutes E, et al. Myeloid progenitor cells in the circulation of patients with myelofibrosis and other myeloproliferative disorders. *Br J Haematol* 1984;57:495–503.
323. Martyre MC. TGF- and megakaryocytes in the pathogenesis of myelofibrosis in myeloproliferative disorders. *Leuk Lymphoma* 1995;20: 39–44.
324. Reilly JT. Pathogenesis of idiopathic myelofibrosis: present status and future directions [Annotation]. *Br J Haematol* 1994;88:1–8.
325. Wolf BC, Neiman RS. Myelofibrosis with myeloid metaplasia: pathophysiologic implications of the correlation between bone marrow changes and progression of splenomegaly. *Blood* 1985;65:803–809.
326. Wang JC, Chen C, Lou LH, et al. Blood thrombopoietin, IL-6 and IL-11 levels in patients with agnogenic myeloid metaplasia. *Leukemia* 1997;11:1827–1832.
327. Martyre MC, Romquin N, Le Bousse-Kerdiles MC, et al. Transforming growth factor-β and megakaryocytes in the pathogenesis of idiopathic myelofibrosis. *Br J Haematol* 1994;88:9–16.
328. Zayli G, Visani C, Cateni L, et al. Reduced responsiveness of bone marrow megakaryocyte progenitors to platelet-derived transforming growth factor-β1 produced in normal amounts in patients with essential thrombocythemia. *Br J Haematol* 1993;83:14–20.
329. Rameshwar P, Chang VT, Gascon P. Implication of CD44 in adhesion-mediated overproduction of TGF- and IL-1 in monocytes from patients with bone marrow fibrosis. *Br J Haematol* 1996;93:22–29.
330. Cappio FC, Vigliani R, Novarino A, et al. Idiopathic myelofibrosis: a possible role for immune-complexes in the pathogenesis of bone marrow fibrosis. *Br J Haematol* 1981;49:17–21.
331. Rondeau E, Solal-Celigny P, Dhermy D, et al. Immune disorders in agnogenic myeloid metaplasia: relations to myelofibrosis. *Br J Haematol* 1983;53:467–475.
332. Cervantes F, Pereira A, Esteve J, et al. The changing profile of idiopathic myelofibrosis: a comparison of the presenting features of patients diagnosed in two different decades. *Eur J Haematol* 1998;60: 101–105.
333. Varki A, Lottenberg R, Griffith R, et al. The syndrome of idiopathic myelofibrosis: a clinicopathologic review with emphasis on the prognostic variables predicting survival. *Medicine* 1983;62:353–371.
334. Hasselbalch H. Idiopathic myelofibrosis: a clinical study of 80 patients. *Am J Hematol* 1990;34:291–300.
335. Visani G, Finelli C, Castelli U, et al. Myelofibrosis with myeloid metaplasia: clinical and haematological parameters predicting survival in a series of 133 patients. *Br J Haematol* 1990;75:4–9.
336. Sekhar M, Prentice HG, Popat U, et al. Idiopathic myelofibrosis in children. *Br J Haematol* 1996;93:394–397.
337. Boxer LA, Camitta BM, Berenberg W, et al. Myelofibrosis-myeloid metaplasia in childhood. *Pediatrics* 1975;55:861–865.
338. Shalev O, Goldfarb A, Ariel I, et al. Myelofibrosis in young adults. *Acta Haematol* 1983;70:396–399.
339. Geary CG. Clinical and hematological aspects of chronic myelofibrosis. In: Lewis SM, ed. *Myelofibrosis, pathophysiology and clinical management.* New York: Marcel Dekker, 1985:15–50.
340. Ellis JT, Peterson P. Myelofibrosis in the myeloproliferative disorders. In: Berk PD, Castro-Malaspina H, Wasserman LR, eds. *Myelofibrosis and the biology of connective tissue.* New York: Alan R. Liss, 1984: 19–42.
341. Ozen S, Ferhanoglu B, Senocak M, et al. Idiopathic myelofibrosis (agnogenic myeloid metaplasia): clinicopathological analysis of 32 patients. *Leuk Res* 1997;21:125–131.
342. Cervantes F, Pereira A, Marti JM, et al. Bone marrow lymphoid nodules in myeloproliferative disorders: association with the nonmyelosclerotic phases of idiopathic myelofibrosis and immunological significance. *Br J Haematol* 1988;70:279–282.
343. Wolf BC, Neiman RS. Myelofibrosis with myeloid metaplasia: pathophysiologic implications of the correlation between bone marrow changes and progression of splenomegaly. *Blood* 1985;65:803–809.
344. Kvasnicka HM, Thiele J, Werden C, et al. Prognostic factors in idiopathic (primary) osteomyelofibrosis. *Cancer* 1997:80:708–719.
345. Demory JL, Dupriez B, Fenaux P. Cytogenetic studies and their prognostic significance in agnogenic myeloid metaplasia: a report on 47 cases. *Blood* 1988;72:855–859.
346. Reilly JT, Snowden JA, Spearing RL, et al. Cytogenetic abnormalities and their prognostic significance in idiopathic myelofibrosis: a study of 106 cases. *Br J Haematol* 1997;98:96–102.
347. Dupriez B, Morel P, Demory JL, et al. Prognostic factors in agnogenic myeloid metaplasia: a report on 195 cases with a new scoring system. *Blood* 1996;88:1013–1018.
348. Tefferi A, Silverstein MN, Noel P. Agnogenic myeloid metaplasia. *Semin Oncol* 1995;22:327–333.
349. Frisch B, Bartl R. Histology of myelofibrosis and osteomyelosclerosis. In: Lewis SM, ed. *Myelofibrosis, pathophysiology and clinical management.* New York: Marcel Dekker, 1985:51–86.
350. Maschek H, Georgii A, Kaloutsi V, et al. Myelofibrosis in primary myelodysplastic syndromes: a retrospective study of 352 patients. *Eur J Haematol* 1992;48:208–214.
351. Pagliuca A, Layton DM, Manoharan A, et al. Myelofibrosis in primary myelodysplastic syndromes: a clinico-morphological study of 10 cases. *Br J Haematol* 1989;71:499–504.
352. Lambertenghi-Deliliers G, Orazi A, Luksch R, et al. Myelodysplastic syndrome with increased marrow fibrosis: a distinct clinico-pathological entity. *Br J Haematol* 1991;78:161–166.
353. Imbert M, Nguyen D, Sultan C. Myelodysplastic syndromes (MDS) and acute myeloid *Leukamias (AML) with myelofibrosis. Leuk Res* 1992;16:51–54.
354. Verhoef GEG, De Wolf-Peeters C, Ferrant A, et al. Myelodysplastic

syndromes with bone marrow fibrosis: a myelodysplastic disorder with proliferative features. *Ann Hematol* 1991;63:235–241.
355. Reilly JT, Dolan G. Proposed classification for the myelodysplasia/myelofibrosis syndromes [Letter]. *Br J Haematol* 1991;79:653.
356. Brunning RD, McKenna RW. *Atlas of tumor pathology, tumors of the bone marrow.* Washington, DC: Armed Forces Institute of Pathology, 1994:92–93.
357. Lewis SM, Szur L. Malignant myelosclerosis. *Br Med J* 1963;2: 472–477.
358. Bearman RM, Pangalis GA, Rappaport H. Acute (''malignant'') myelosclerosis. *Cancer* 1979;43:279–293.
359. Sultan C, Sigaux F, Imbert M, et al. Acute myelodysplasia with myelofibrosis: a report of eight cases. *Br J Haematol* 1981;49:11–16.
360. Bird T, Proctor SJ. Malignant myelosclerosis: Myeloproliferative disorder or leukemia? Am J Clin Pathol 1977;67:512–520.
361. Cervantes F, Tassies D, Salgado C, et al. Acute transformation in nonLeukemic chronic myeloproliferative disorders: actuarial probability and main characteristics in a series of 218 patients. *Acta Haematol* 1991;85:124–127.
362. Hernandez JM, San Miguel JF, Gonzalez M, et al. Development of acute leukaemia after idiopathic myelofibrosis. *J Clin Pathol* 1992; 45:727–730.
363. Shukrulla N, Finiewicz KJ, Roulston D, et al. Is atypical chronic myeloid leukemia a high white cell count myelodysplastic syndrome? *Mod Pathol* 1997;10:134a.
364. Felman P, Bryon P, Gentilhomme, et al. The syndrome of abnormal chromatin clumping in leucocytes: a myelodysplastic disorder with proliferative features? *Br J Haematol* 1988;70:49–54.
365. Invernizzi R, Custodi P, De Fasio P, et al. The syndrome of abnormal chromatin clumping in leucocytes: clinical and biological study of a case. *Haematology* 1990;75:532–536.
366. Michaux J, Martiat P. Chronic myelomonocytic leukaemia (CMML): a myelodysplastic or myeloproliferative syndrome? *Leuk Lymphoma* 1993;9:35–41.
367. Montefusco E, Alimena G, Lo Coco F, et al. Ph-negative and bcr-negative atypical chronic myelogenous leukemia: biological features and clinical outcome. *Ann Hematol* 1992;65:17–21.
368. Galton DAG. Haematological differences between chronic granulocytic leukemia, atypical chronic myeloid leukaemia, and chronic myelomonocytic leukaemia. *Leuk Lymph* 1992;7:343–350.
369. Oscier DG. Atypical chronic myeloid leukaemia, a distinct clinical entity related to the myelodysplastic syndrome? *Br J Haematol* 1996; 92:582–586.
370. Stewart K, Carstairs KC, Dube ID, et al. Neutrophilic myelofibrosis presenting as Philadelphia chromosome negative BCR non-rearranged chronic myeloid leukemia. *Am J Hematol* 1990;34:59–60.
371. Mertens F, Johansson B, Heim S, et al. Trisomy 14 in atypical chronic myeloid leukemia. *Leukemia* 1990;4:117–120.
372. Bennett JM, Catovsky D, Daniel MT, et al. Proposals for the classification of the myelodysplastic syndromes. *Br J Haematol* 1982;51: 189–199.
373. Storniolo AM, Moloney WC, Rosenthal DS, et al. Chronic myelomonocytic leukemia. *Leukemia* 1990;11:766–770.
374. Germing U, Gattermann N, Minning H, et al. Problems in the classification of CMML: dysplastic versus proliferative type. *Leuk Res* 1998; 22:871–878.
375. Oscier D, Chapman R. The classification of chronic myelomonocytic leukaemia. *Leuk Res* 1998;22:879–880.
376. Groupe Français de Cytogénétique Hématologique. Chronic myelomonocytic leukemia: single entity or heterogeneous disorder? A prospective multicenter study of 100 patients. *Cancer Genet Cytogenet* 1991;55:57–65.
377. Tefferi A, Hoagland HC, Therneau TM, et al. Chronic myelomonocytic leukemia: natural history and prognostic determinants. *Mayo Clin Proc* 1989;64:1246–1254.
378. Solé F, Prieto F, Badia L, et al. Cytogenetic studies in 112 cases of untreated myelodysplastic syndromes. *Cancer Genet Cytogenet* 1992; 64:12–20.
379. Luna-Fineman S, Shannon KM, Atwater SK, et al. Myelodyplastic and myeloproliferative diorders of childhood: a study of 167 patients. *Blood* 1999;93:459–466.
380. Castro-Malaspina H, Schaison G, Passe et al. Subacute and chronic myelomonocytic leukemia in children (juvenile CML): clinical and hematologic observations, and identification of prognostic factors. *Cancer* 1984;54:675–686.
381. Niemeyer CM, Arico M, Basso G, et al. Chronic myelomonocytic leukemia in childhood: a retrospective analysis of 110 cases. *Blood* 1997;89:3534–3543.
382. Emmanuel P, Bates LJ, Castleberry RP, et al. Selective hypersensitivity to granulocyte macrophage colony stimulating factor by juvenile chronic myeloid leukemia hematopoietic progenitors. *Blood* 1991;77: 925–931.
383. Emmanuel P, Bates LJ, Zy SW, et al. The role of monocyte-derived hematopoietic growth factors in the regulation of myeloproliferation in juvenile chronic myelogenous leukemia. *Exp Hematol* 1991;19: 1017–1020.
384. Haas OA, Gadner H. Pathogenesis, biology, and management of myelodysplastic syndromes in children. *Semin Hematol* 1996;33: 225–235.
385. Gallagher A, Darley R, Padua RA. RAS and the myelodysplastic syndromes. Pathol Biol 1997;45:561–568.
386. Shannon KM, O'Connell P, Martin GA, et al. Loss of the normal NF1 allele from the bone marrow of children with type 1 neurofibromatosis and malignant myeloid disorders. *N Engl J Med* 1994;330: 597–599.
387. Hess JL, Zutter MM, Castleberry RP, et al. Juvenile chronic myelogenous leukemia. *Am J Clin Pathol* 1996;105:238–248.
388. Luna-Fineman S, Shannon KM, Lange BJ. Childhood monosomy 7: epidemiology, biology, and mechanistic implications. *Blood* 1995;85: 1985–1999.
389. Pinkel D. Differentiating juvenile myelomonocytic leukemia from infectious disease. *Blood* 1998;91:365–367.

CHAPTER 50

Interpretation of Postchemotherapy and Posttransplantation Bone Marrow Specimens

M. Kathryn Foucar

Chemotherapy, with or without radiotherapy, is the treatment of choice for various hematopoietic and nonhematopoietic neoplasms. Because of the diverse actions of these treatments on cells, profound morphologic changes occur not only in neoplastic cells but also in normal proliferating bone marrow elements in response to these therapeutic agents. Practicing hematopathologists must be able to interpret therapeutic effects on both neoplastic and nonneoplastic cells in the bone marrow. The morphology of both is reviewed in this chapter, including both early and late morphologic findings. In addition to cytoablative therapy, other therapeutic agents are linked to impressive bone marrow morphologic changes. Most notable among this group are recombinant cytokines such as colony-stimulating factors and interleukins. These agents are produced endogenously and are key hematopoietic regulatory factors; pharmacologic doses of these recombinant regulatory factors cause exaggerated morphologic changes not seen under baseline physiologic conditions. This chapter also describes the morphology of bone marrow transplantation (BMT) in patients who have neoplastic and nonneoplastic disorders.

The goal of potent myeloablative therapy (with or without subsequent peripheral blood stem cell or BMT) is obviously the permanent eradication of the neoplastic clone. The bone marrow of these patients is evaluated intermittently for evidence of disease recurrence. These evaluations for minimal residual disease or early relapse are enhanced greatly by sophisticated techniques such as multicolor flow cytometric immunophenotyping, fluorescence *in situ* hybridization, and various molecular assays. Methods to detect rare neoplastic cells admixed with normal hematopoietic cells and the clinical significance of minimal residual disease are reviewed at the end of this chapter.

M. K. Foucar: Department of Pathology, University of New Mexico Health Sciences Center, Albuquerque, New Mexico 87131-5301

POSTCHEMOTHERAPEUTIC CHANGES IN BONE MARROW

Early Morphologic Changes

Depending on the tumor type, the goal of a treatment regimen may be either palliation or ablation of all neoplastic cells. The effects on the bone marrow are sequential, and, as would be expected, more profound bone marrow effects are seen in patients who receive potent myeloablative multiagent chemotherapy. To evaluate these bone marrow effects optimally, it is important to integrate findings observed on aspirate smears and biopsy sections (1–5). Although cytologic detail is superior with aspiration specimens, trephine biopsy sections are also necessary. This is because profoundly hypocellular bone marrow particles often do not aspirate readily and because chemotherapy may induce a transient increase in reticulin fibers, further compromising the quality of bone marrow aspirate smears. A good quality bone marrow biopsy specimen, therefore, may be essential for evaluating response to treatment, early regeneration, overall bone marrow cellularity, and the extent of residual blast infiltration in patients who have acute leukemia.

The morphologic features of the bone marrow after intensive chemotherapy are the result of two overlapping processes: cellular depletion and bone marrow reconstitution (1–3) (Table 50.1). Cellular death begins focally and rapidly progresses to widespread ablation, with resultant profound blood cytopenias (1,2) (Fig. 50.1). Bone marrow ablation is associated with marked edema, dilated sinuses, and multiloculated fat cells (1,3,4,6). The stroma of the bone marrow takes on an eosinophilic granular appearance secondary to fibrinoid necrosis, and mild reticulin fibrosis may develop (1,3,7) (Fig. 50.2). Macrophages are abundant and may contain pigment and other phagocytized material (Fig. 50.3; see also Color Plate 92, between pp. 1446–1447). In general, serous fat atrophy is not prominent after potent chemotherapy, although this occasionally has been reported (1,3,8).

TABLE 50.1. *Features of bone marrow after mycloablative chemotherapy (1–4)*

Cellular depletion	Bone marrow reconstitution
Earliest effect of chemotherapy is focal cell death, which rapidly progresses to widespread hypocellularity	Earliest regeneration detected 1–2 weeks after ablative therapy Granulocytic regeneration tends to be paratrabecular
Cell death associated with marked edema, dilated sinuses, multiloculated fat cells	Fat regeneration concurrent with hematopoietic recovery; islands of hematopoietic elements surround unilocular fat cells
Widespread granular appearance of stroma termed fibrinoid necrosis or fibrinoid myelitis	Variable sequence of cellular regeneration
Transient increase in stromal reticulin	Reticulin fibers decrease as regeneration occurs
Abundant pigment laden macrophages may be present	
Pronounced blood cytopenias in peripheral blood	

Hematopoietic regeneration usually begins about 1 to 2 weeks after ablative chemotherapy and tends to begin adjacent to bony trabeculae (9,10). Fat cell regeneration appears to play a key role in hematopoietic recovery, with islands of hematopoietic elements tending to surround unilocular fat cells (1,3,6). The sequence of erythroid and granulocytic recovery within the bone marrow varies, but megakaryocyte regeneration generally occurs last (6) (Fig. 50.4). In rapidly regenerating bone marrows, dyspoiesis of normal elements, especially erythroid cells, may be evident (Fig. 50.5; see also Color Plate 93, between pp. 1446–1447). As reconstitution occurs, adipose cells and reticulin fibers decrease (1,3).

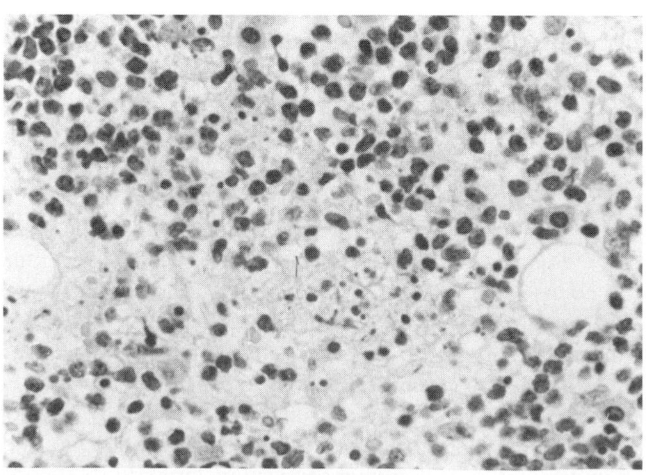

FIG. 50.1. Prominent individual cell necrosis is evident in this bone marrow biopsy specimen 1 week after initiation of induction chemotherapy for acute leukemia (hematoxylin and eosin stain, original magnification: 400× magnification).

In addition to evaluating the proportion of fat cells on bone marrow biopsy specimens, magnetic resonance imaging scans can be used to monitor the amount of fat within the bone marrow (11). After chemotherapy or radiation, a marked increase in fat cells is detected by these scans. As hematopoietic reconstitution occurs, the amount of fat decreases progressively. The advantage of a radiographic evaluation of bone marrow fat is that hematopoietic recovery within the entire bone marrow cavity can be assessed (11).

Several morphologic and hematologic features in the blood and bone marrow of acute leukemia patients whose disease is in remission have been linked with sustained complete remission and prolonged survival. Patients who demonstrate more profound bone marrow ablation, lower percentages of bone marrow blasts, and higher hematocrit values at the time of complete remission tend to experience longer duration of survival (12). Conversely, recent investigations have determined that patients with acute myeloid leukemia (AML) in whom bone marrow blasts outnumber promyelocytes or who demonstrate other atypical patterns of reconstitution experience lower remission induction rates, shortened duration of survival, and higher-risk AML subtypes (2). Likewise, persistence of circulating blasts after a week of induction chemotherapy is linked to adverse outcome (13).

A variety of factors is linked to failure of regeneration of normal hematopoietic elements. In patients with acute leukemia, failure of regeneration may reflect a persistent leukemic clone, which usually can be documented by specialized studies. Other patients may experience an idiosyncratic hypersensitivity to the therapeutic regimen. The bone marrow microenvironment must be restored in order to support and promote hematopoietic recovery. Failure to restore this microenvironment may reflect drug hypersensitivity or occult viral infection. Viruses implicated in hematopoietic suppression include parvovirus, cytomegalovirus, human herpesvirus-6, and HIV-1 (14–16). Occasional patients develop striking postmyeloablative histiocyte hyperplasia with failure of regeneration, another possible reflection of altered bone marrow microenvironment (17,18).

Effects of Chemotherapy on Regenerating Normal Bone Marrow Elements

In patients who receive potent chemotherapy for solid tumors, a wide variety of morphologic abnormalities in normal marrow elements can develop (Table 50.2, Fig. 50.5). Following radiotherapy and most types of chemotherapy, all bone marrow cell lines are suppressed, and irreversible stem cell ablation usually results from radiation of active hematopoietic sites (19). The degree of bone marrow suppression by chemotherapy is variable from patient to patient and may be related to patient age, nutritional status, and whether or not underlying bone marrow fibrosis or infiltration by tumor has occurred (20). In addition to the immediate bone marrow

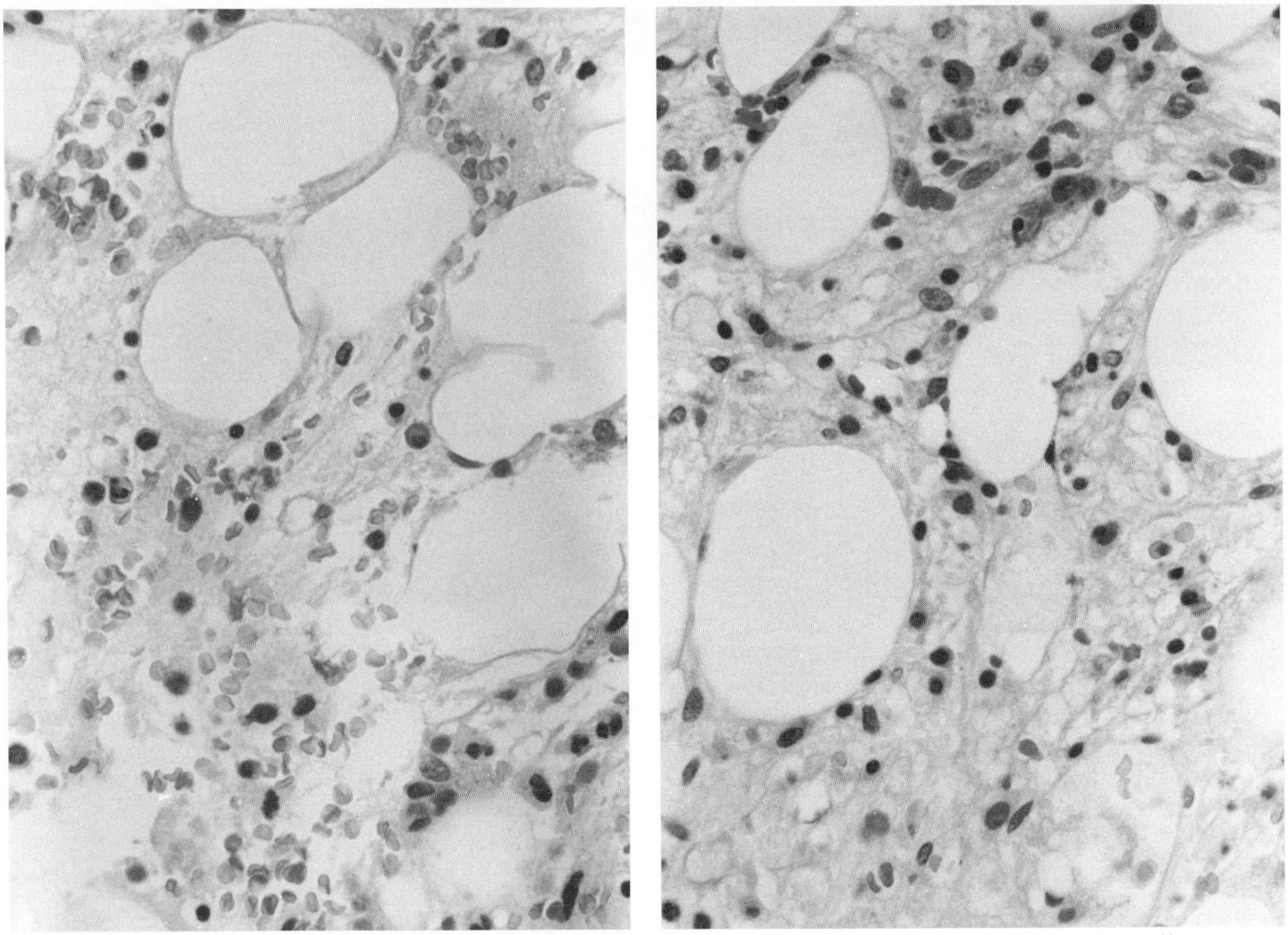

A B

FIG. 50.2. Composite photomicrograph illustrating bone marrow biopsy sections from two patients. The left portion is from day 30 of induction chemotherapy for acute lymphoblastic leukemia. The right section is from a patient who has received intensive multiagent chemotherapy for stage IV Hodgkin's disease. Note the pronounced fibrinoid necrosis of the stroma evident in both. Residual plasma cells and occasional macrophages are evident (hematoxylin and eosin stain, original magnification: 400× magnification).

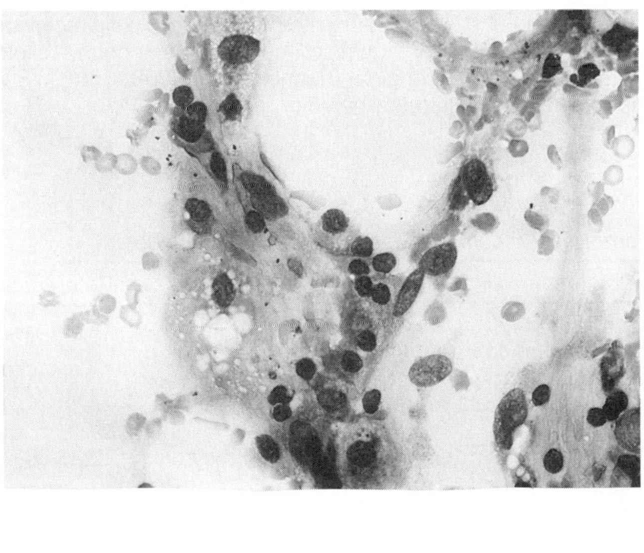

FIG. 50.3. Markedly hypocellular bone marrow particles are evident from a patient status postinduction chemotherapy for relapsed acute leukemia. Occasional macrophages contain ingested material. Endothelial cells line aspirated portions of blood vessels (Wright stain, original magnification: 1,000× magnification). See Color Plate 92, between pp. 1446–1447.

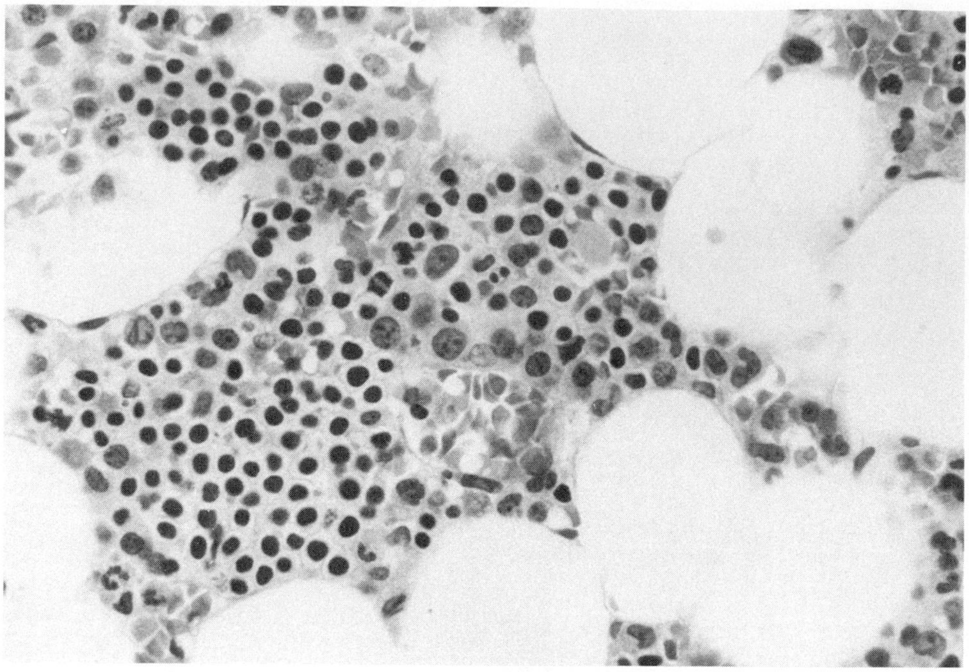

FIG. 50.4. Bone marrow clot section showing early hematopoietic regeneration with a striking predominance of erythroid elements. This patient recently had received induction chemotherapy for acute leukemia (hematoxylin and eosin stain, original magnification: 400× magnification).

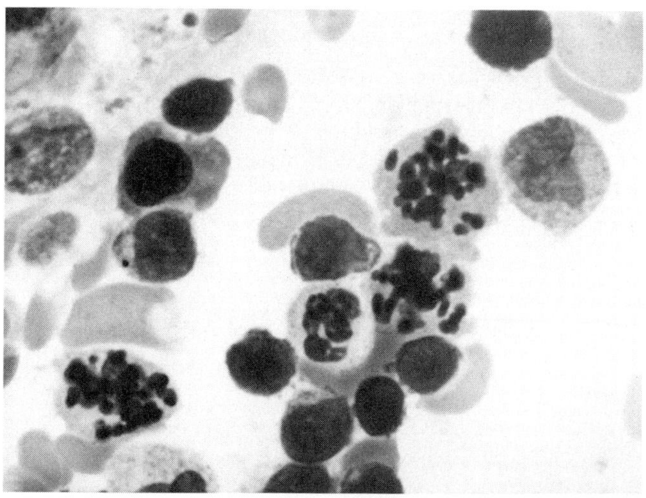

FIG. 50.5. Prominent dyserythropoiesis with apoptosis is evident on this bone marrow aspirate smear from a child receiving aggressive therapy for high risk T-cell acute lymphoblastic leukemia (Wright stain, original magnification: 1000× magnification). See Color Plate 93, between pp. 1446–1447.

TABLE 50.2. *Postchemotherapeutic morphologic abnormalities in nonneoplastic bone marrow elements*

Cell line	Comments	References
All hematopoietic cell lines	Variable degree of bone marrow suppression Radiation to marrow results in irreversible stem cell ablation Effects of chemotherapy are longstanding Prolonged defects in bone marrow microenvironment with defective production of regulatory factors	19–24
Erythroid	May exhibit marked megaloblastosis with striking karyorthexis, blood macrocytosis	20,25,26
Granulocytic	Neutropenia is dominant finding	20
Megakaryocytic	Thrombocytopenia is dominant finding	20

suppression, longstanding effects of chemotherapy have been documented in patients and in laboratory animals, suggesting that chemotherapy-induced bone marrow suppression is much more prolonged than formerly thought. In humans, persistent nuclear defects have been documented years after cessation of chemotherapy and radiotherapy (20–23). In addition, prolonged defects in the production of regulatory factors have been identified in bone marrow specimens from patients receiving potent antileukemic therapy (24).

Because many chemotherapeutic agents inhibit DNA synthesis, megaloblastic changes are common in normal hematopoietic lineages, especially in the erythroid cell line. Dyserythropoiesis can be pronounced, with nuclear–cytoplasmic dysynchrony, nuclear karyorrhexis, and multinuclearity (20,25,26) (Fig. 50.5). Mature erythrocytes may be macrocytic (20,25,26). The erythroid cell line also is more rapidly ablated by chemotherapy, and, as a consequence, the myeloid:erythroid ratio is greatly increased. One explanation for this disparity is that erythroid elements proliferate more rapidly and, therefore, are more susceptible to these chemotherapeutic agents (25). There is a greater nonmitotic granulocyte reserve in the bone marrow, which is relatively more resistant to chemotherapy. The dominant granulocytic and megakaryocytic abnormalities that follow chemotherapy for nonhematopoietic neoplasms are neutropenia and thrombocytopenia, and functional defects such as impaired regulatory factor production have been detected (24).

Uncommon Findings during Bone Marrow Recovery

Less common morphologic findings that can occur during bone marrow recovery from ablative therapy are detailed in Table 50.3. These uncommon findings are generally more significant and more problematic in patients with underlying acute leukemias who are undergoing induction chemotherapy. In these patients, a variety of morphologic findings can occur including transient blastemia, foci of blasts in an otherwise hypocellular bone marrow, persistent multilineage dyspoiesis, florid atypical megakaryocytic hyperplasia, sheets of promyelocytes, and increased benign lymphocyte precursors terms hematogones. In each of these situations, the goal of the diagnostician is to determine if this morphologic finding is linked to eminent or eventual leukemic relapse or is instead a unique feature of regenerating normal bone marrow. In occasional leukemic patients, more than 3% circulating blasts are evident transiently in the blood after the first week of induction chemotherapy is given, even though the corresponding blast count in the bone marrow is below 3% (12,13,20,27). Although remission generally is achieved in these patients, the incidence of early relapse is substantial. The identification of substantial proportions of blasts in bone marrows obtained 1 and 2 weeks following induction chemotherapy also is disconcerting. In general, high cellularity with a predominance of blasts indicates persistent leukemia (Fig. 50.6). The significance of increased blasts in a hypocellular

TABLE 50.3. *Uncommon findings during bone marrow recovery from ablative therapy*

Finding	Comments	References
Transient blastemia in leukemic patients	Occurs during the early reconstitution period; persistence of circulating blasts one week after induction chemotherapy linked to poor outcome	12,13,20,27
Foci of blasts in otherwise depleted bone marrow (leukemia patients)	Generally indicative of treatment failure, if blast percent exceeds promyelocyte percent	2
Persistent dyspoiesis (leukemia patients)	Postinduction dyspoiesis (notably granulocytic and megakaryocytic dyspoiesis) linked to eventual relapse in AML patients; may reflect therapy-induced maturation of leukemia clone. Resembles myelodysplasia	28,29
Sheets of megakaryocytes (leukemia patients)	Megakaryocytes may rarely be the dominant early regenerating element In one study, 13% of AML postinduction bone marrow specimens exhibited transient striking hyperplasia of dysplastic megakaryocytes resembling acute megakaryoblastic leukemia; not linked to adverse outcome unless myeloblasts also increased	30
Sheets of promyelocytes	Wave of early regeneration may be associated with large numbers of immature myeloid elements	31–33
Clusters of normoblasts	May be either immature or more differentiated	
Increase in hematogones	These normal B-lymphocyte precursor cells are often abundant in recovering bone marrow especially in young children Especially problematic in patients with acute lymphoblastic leukemia May be abundant after completion of several years of antileukemic therapy	34, 35
Fibrosis	May develop after therapy especially in patients with CML stable phase or blast crisis	1
Bone changes	Increased bone formation can accompany marked fibrosis	1
Persistent hypocellularity	Failure of prompt reconstitution of bone marrow may reflect idiosyncratic reaction to chemotherapy or poor nutritional status, or be a consequence of advanced age	20

AML, acute myelogenous leukemia; CML, chronic myelogenous leukemia.

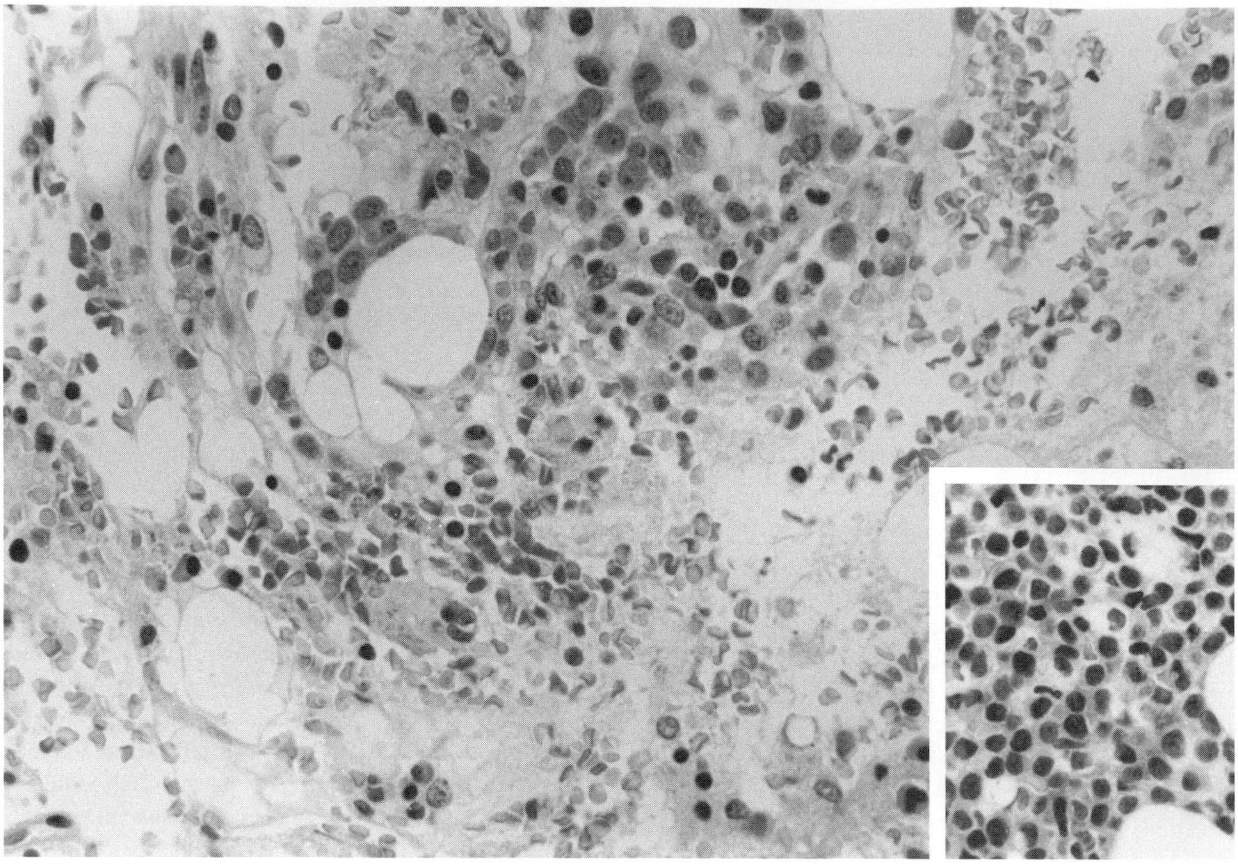

FIG. 50.6. Photomicrograph of a bone marrow biopsy speciment taken 30 days after induction chemotherapy showing residual islands of blasts, probably neoplastic cells, in an otherwise depleted bone marrow. **Inset:** Extensive bone marrow replacement by leukemia in this patient at diagnosis (hematoxylin and eosin stain, original magnification: 400× magnification).

bone marrow is more problematic. In these patients, the proportion of promyelocytes seems critical, and if promyelocytes outnumber myeloblasts, the patient is more likely to ultimately achieve a complete remission without reinduction than a patient in whom myeloblasts predominate in the hypocellular bone marrow (2).

In some patients with AML undergoing therapy, persistent and prolonged multilineage dyspoiesis is identified after the achievement of a complete remission based on the percentage of blasts within blood and bone marrow (28,29). In these patients, the blood and bone marrow pictures are identical to those in myelodysplasia, and most patients ultimately experience overt acute leukemic relapse, although there may be a relatively prolonged period with a stable blast count and persistent dyspoiesis. Another unusual finding in patients with AML undergoing induction chemotherapy is the development of profoundly dysplastic megakaryocytic hyperplasia, which was identified in approximately 13% of patients with AML in one study (30). In those specimens with megakaryocytic hyperplasia that also demonstrated increased blasts, eventual relapse was likely; the finding of isolated atypical megakaryocytic hyperplasia in the absence of increased blasts was a transient finding not linked to adverse outcome (30).

In some patients with AML who undergo induction chemotherapy, the granulocytic recovery is characterized by a wave of promyelocytes, which may cause diagnostic difficulty, especially in patients with a diagnosis of M2 or M3 AML. In general, reactive promyelocytes can be distinguished from their neoplastic counterparts by the presence of vigorous mitotic activity and a prominent paranuclear pale area or hof (31–33) (Fig. 50.7). If such a wave of promyelocytes is a reflection of early regeneration, subsequent bone marrow specimens should reveal obvious maturation of the granulocytic lineage. Similarly, a wave of regenerating normoblasts that demonstrate therapy-induced dyspoiesis occasionally can be problematic in patients with leukemia.

In patients with acute lymphoblastic leukemia undergoing chemotherapy, benign B-lymphocyte precursor cells can be difficult to distinguish from recurrent leukemia. These benign lymphocyte precursors are termed *hematogones* and can be identified in regenerating bone marrow specimens, especially from young children (34). These lymphoid cells have distinctive morphologic features, including round to notched nuclei with uniformly dense, homogeneous chromatin, inconspicuous nucleoli, and scant cytoplasm (Fig. 50.8). Hematogones may be especially numerous in the bone marrow of children who have completed several years of antileu-

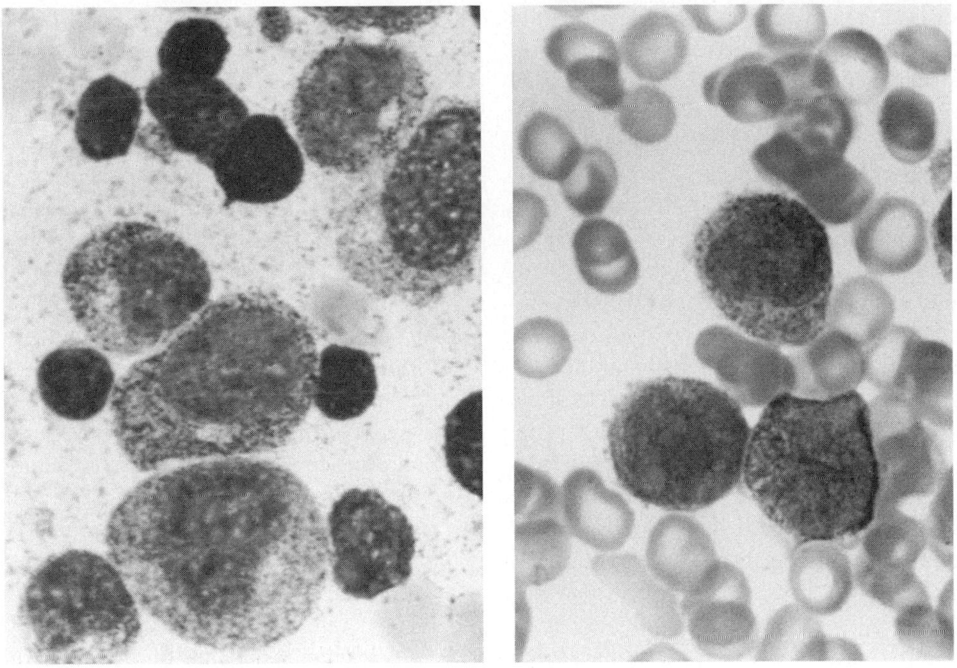

A B

FIG. 50.7. Photomicrograph comparing the morphology of regenerating promyelocytes (**left**) to leukemic promyelocytes from a patient who had acute promyelocytic leukemia (**right**). Note the prominent Golgi (hof) of the regenerating promyelocytes from a patient who had drug-induced neutropenia (Wright stain, original magnification: 1,000× magnification).

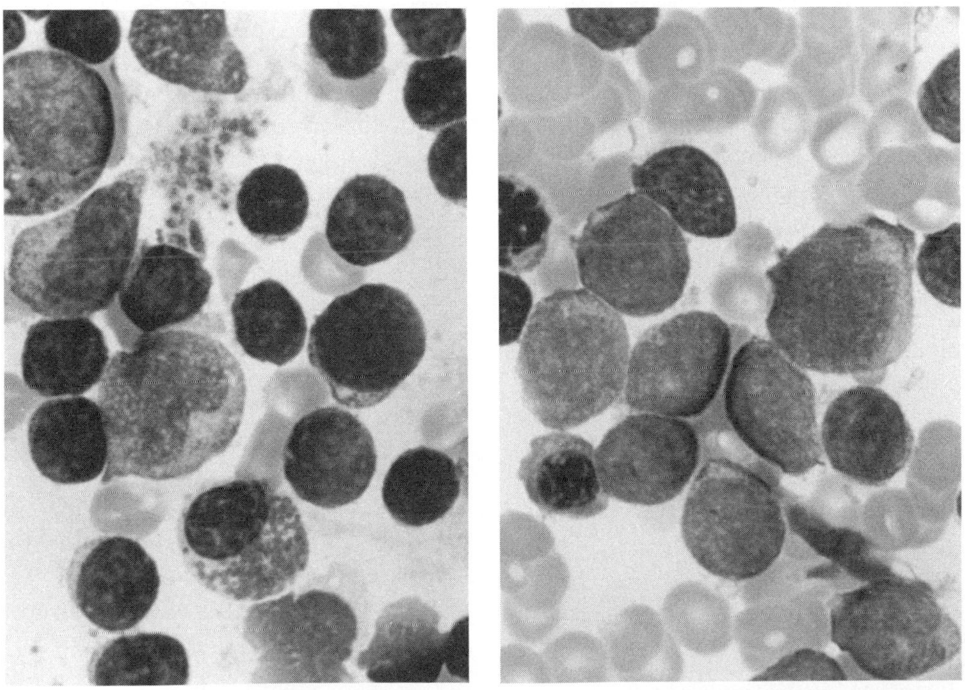

A B

FIG. 50.8. Side-by-side composite comparing the morphology of hematogones (**left**) with that of acute lymphoblastic leukemia cells (**right**). Note the highly condensed homogeneous chromatin of hematogones compared with the finely dispersed chromatin of leukemic blasts (Wright stain, original magnification: 1,000× magnification).

kemic therapy. Because these normal precursor cells exhibit an immunophenotypic profile similar to precursor B-cell acute lymphoblastic leukemia, the distinction between benign hematogones and recurrent or residual acute lymphoblastic leukemia can be challenging (34,35). The highly condensed nuclear chromatin of hematogones facilitates distinction from lymphoblasts, which generally exhibit fairly dispersed chromatin and variably prominent nucleoli. In addition, the immunophenotypic profile of hematogones demonstrates clear maturation to mature, polyclonal B lymphocytes, a finding not identified in acute lymphoblastic leukemia. Evaluation of bone marrow biopsy and clot sections by immunoperoxidase stains for CD34 and terminal deoxynucleotidyl transferase is also useful in distinguishing hematogones from residual or recurrent acute lymphoblastic leukemia (35). In patients with increased numbers of hematogones, the CD34- and terminal deoxynucleotidyl transferase–positive cells, although sometimes prominent, are dispersed individually or present in clusters of fewer than five cells; residual or recurrent acute lymphoblastic leukemia is characterized by the presence of CD34- or terminal deoxynucleotidyl transferase–positive clusters of five or more lymphoblasts. In contrast to acute lymphoblastic leukemia, there is neither cytogenetic nor molecular evidence that hematogones, even if markedly increased, are a clonal proliferation (34).

Unusual bone marrow findings may be identified in patients with nonleukemic disorders who undergo potent multiagent chemotherapy. Similar to the findings described previously in patients with acute leukemia, these nonleukemic patients can have bone marrows that contain sheets of promyelocytes, increased hematogones, clusters of normoblasts, bone marrow fibrosis, and changes in the bony trabeculae. The identification of benign lymphocyte precursors and a wave of benign regenerating promyelocytes is generally substantially less problematic in patients with underlying solid tumors rather than acute leukemia. Likewise, clusters of normoblasts are indicative of regeneration in this patient population. Bone marrow fibrosis and bone changes often are linked and are especially prevalent in patients with underlying myeloproliferative disorders. Finally, in some patients, reconstitution of the bone marrow following myeloablative therapy is delayed profoundly and may reflect an idiosyncratic reaction to the chemotherapy or underlying poor nutritional status, and this failure to regenerate normal bone marrow elements, is more likely to occur in elderly patients (20).

Unique Features of Therapy for Acute Promyelocytic Leukemia

Since the recognition in 1988 and confirmation in 1989 that all-trans retinoic acid (ATRA) could be used to induce complete remission in patients with acute promyelocytic leukemia, this agent has become used routinely in conjunction with standard chemotherapy (36,37). ATRA is postulated to overcome the block in myeloid maturation that results from the reciprocal translocation t(15;17)(q21;q21) that defines this distinctive AML subtype. The gradual ATRA-induced maturation of the leukemic clone is characterized by a spectrum of changes as the leukemic promyelocytes acquire morphologic features of more mature elements. Often it is difficult to perform differential counts on blood smears from these patients, because maturing promyelocytes may resemble unusual monocytoid cells. If necessary cytochemical stains can be utilized to distinguish these aberrant leukemic forms (strongly Sudan black B–positive, nonspecific esterase–negative) from true monocytic cells (Sudan black B–weak or negative, nonspecific esterase–positive). Using fluorescence *in situ* hybridization studies, the maturation of the leukemic clone can be documented, although eventual repopulation of the bone marrow and blood by normal hematopoietic elements does occur, usually by day 30 (38).

Prior to the recognition of the therapeutic efficacy of ATRA, standard induction chemotherapy in acute promyelocytic leukemia patients often was associated with unique features that also appear to reflect therapy-induced maturation of the leukemic clone (39,40). In some studies, the bone marrow specimens obtained during early-induction therapy in up to 40% of patients with acute promyelocytic leukemia did not demonstrate the predicted profound hypoplasia typically associated with potent myeloablative therapy (39) (Fig. 50.9). Although controversial, the relatively slow decrease in blasts and promyelocytes, in conjunction with the gradual increase in more mature granulocytic elements, suggests therapy-induced maturation, analogous to that confirmed by fluorescence *in situ* hybridization studies in patients with acute promyelocytic leukemia treated with ATRA.

Complications of ATRA therapy include hyperleukocytosis, respiratory distress, and rare reports of either extensive bone marrow necrosis or collagenous fibrosis in patients receiving ATRA, usually in conjunction with chemotherapy (41,42).

Bone Marrow Relapse and Late Effects of Chemotherapy

The majority of patients who receive myeloablative therapy for acute leukemia achieve a complete remission (43). Despite the induction of a complete remission, a substantial proportion of these patients later experience a relapse of their disease. Although relapse is generally florid, with extensive replacement of the bone marrow, early relapse occasionally can be detected by identifying rare blasts with Auer rods or small clusters of blasts in otherwise unremarkable bone marrow biopsy sections. Sophisticated immunologic or molecular markers may be needed to confirm these early relapses.

In a minority of leukemia patients experiencing relapse, there is a change in either the morphology or the immuno-

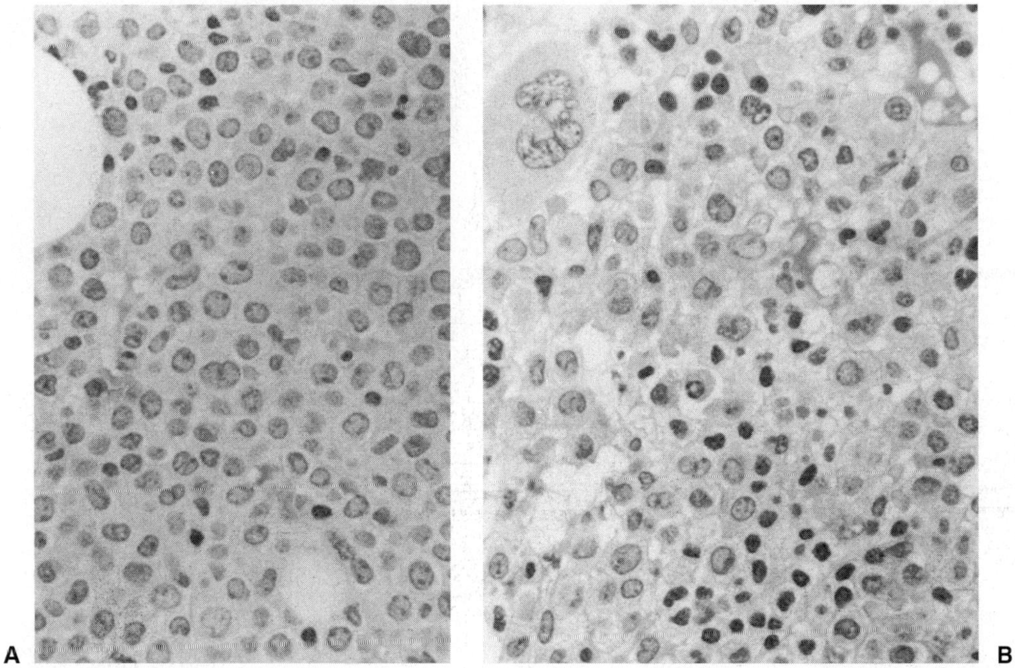

FIG. 50.9. Composite photomicrograph comparing bone marrow biopsy sections at diagnosis (**left**) and 30 days after aggressive induction chemotherapy (**right**) in a patient who had acute promyelocytic leukemia. Although minimal erythroid and megakaryocyte regeneration is evident after 30 days of chemotherapy, bone marrow hypercellularity with a predominance of promyelocytes persists (hematoxylin and eosin stain, original magnification: 400× magnification).

phenotype of the relapsed leukemic cells. One possible explanation for this phenomenon is that chemotherapy eradicated only a subpopulation of the leukemic cells, and another, more chemotherapy-resistant subpopulation of the original clone continued to proliferate.

Several late effects of ablative chemotherapy on the bone marrow have been described. A small proportion of patients who undergo potent chemotherapy for AML develop a stable blood and bone marrow picture identical to that of myelodysplasia rather than the morphologically normal appearance of a typical complete remission (28,29,44). This phenomenon of postleukemic myelodysplasia suggests that the chemotherapy has induced leukemic cell maturation rather than eradication of this cell line. This morphologic observation is substantiated by sophisticated techniques, such as X-linked DNA polymorphisms, that document ''clonal remissions'' or ''clonal hematopoiesis'' in some patients who have myeloid leukemias (45). Some patients who have AML may have a disease analogous to chronic myelogenous leukemia (CML) presenting in blast crisis, which reverts to stable-phase CML following aggressive chemotherapy; some authors postulate that the so-called clonal hematopoiesis identified in some patients in complete remission may reflect normal constitutional features (46,47).

In addition to this unique phenomenon of leukemic cell maturation, overt myelodysplasia or acute leukemia also can occur as a late event in patients who receive potent therapy for nonhematopoietic neoplasms (1,48–53). Up to 5 to 10% of patients with solid tumors who are treated successfully with multiagent chemotherapy with or without radiotherapy eventually develop clonal hematopoietic malignancies that exhibit pronounced multilineage dyspoiesis and a variable percentage of myeloblasts (see Chapters 47 and 48). The morphologic abnormalities that occur in these iatrogenic stem cell neoplasms include increased immature forms of all lineages, nuclear segmentation defects, failure of cytoplasmic maturation, and pronounced megaloblastic changes (48,54) (Fig. 50.10). Patients at greatest risk for developing this type of therapy-related myelodysplasia and leukemia are those who require multiple courses of alkylating agent therapy for their primary tumor. Recent studies document significant bone marrow abnormalities in patients who have been off therapy for as long as 5 years (21–23). Both alkylating agent therapy and radiation induce chromosome damage and instability, which may be related to the subsequent development of myelodysplasia and leukemia (50). A more recently recognized type of therapy-induced leukemia is linked to topoisomerase II inhibitor treatment (50). Compared to alkylating agent–induced leukemia, this type of leukemia is characterized by more abrupt onset and a shorter latent period from treatment to secondary leukemia. Leukemias associated with topoisomerase II inhibitor therapy typically are monocytic and lack multilineage dyspoiesis. The

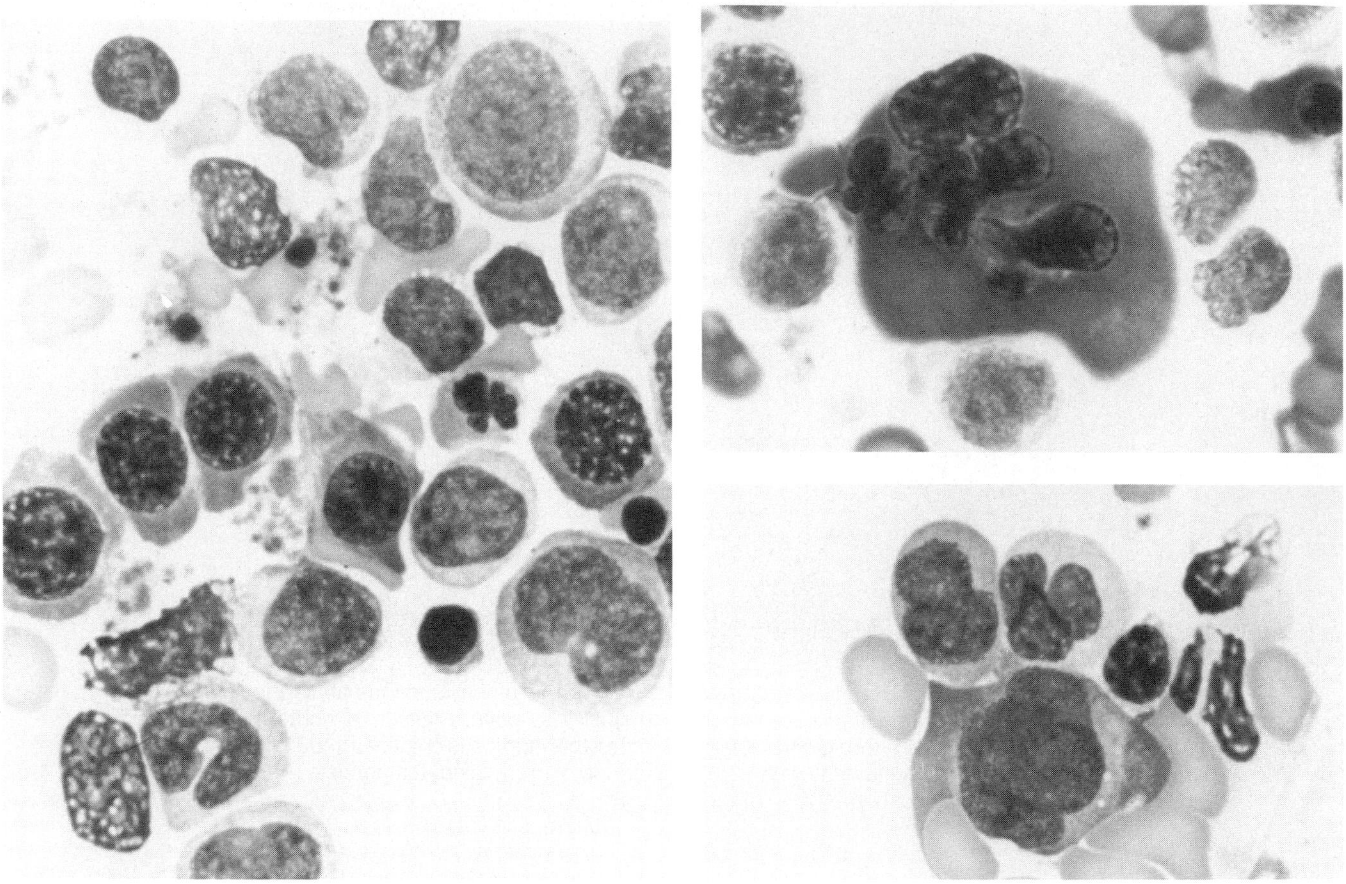

FIG. 50.10. Composite photomicrograph illustrating multilineage dyspoietic morphology characteristic of therapy-induced leukemias (Wright stain, original magnification: 1,000× magnification).

prognosis is generally poor for patients who develop either type of therapy-induced hematopoietic neoplasm (50).

BLOOD AND BONE MARROW FEATURES IN PATIENTS RECEIVING RECOMBINANT CYTOKINE THERAPY

Many hematopoietic regulatory factors such as granulocyte colony-stimulating factor, granulocyte-monocyte colony-stimulating factor, interleukin-2, interleukin-3, erythropoietin, and thrombopoietin are available in human recombinant form and can be used to either ameliorate cytopenias or stimulate immune function. Recently, evidence-based review of the literature by the American Society of Clinical Oncology has attempted to delineate the efficacy for recombinant colony-stimulating factor therapy in oncology populations. In this group, current recommendations for colony-stimulating factor therapy include patients undergoing high-dose chemotherapy with peripheral blood stem cell or autologous BMT, and patients receiving bone marrow suppressive therapy linked to a high likelihood of neutropenic fever (55–59). Colony-stimulating factor therapy is also efficacious in patients with constitutional neutropenic disorders; recombinant erythropoietin is effective in improving hemoglobin levels in patients with disease- or treatment-related anemias (60). Recombinant human thrombopoietin is being utilized in clinical trials to enhance platelet recovery after potent chemotherapy with or without progenitor cell support (61).

Several investigators have described the blood and bone marrow findings in patients receiving these various types of recombinant agents (62–70) (Table 50.4). Most emphasis has been placed on the morphologic features in blood and peripheral cell counts; bone marrow examination is not performed in most of these patients. Blood changes are most pronounced in patients receiving granulocyte and granulocyte-macrophage colony-stimulating factor therapy. Early changes include a transient increase in circulating blasts followed by eventual mature neutrophilia exhibiting striking toxic changes. Other abnormalities include nuclear-cytoplasmic asynchrony and nuclear segmentation defects of neutrophils. Changes in other lineages are less pronounced. In patients with profound bone marrow suppression, early features of colony-stimulating factor therapy consist of initial small collections of immature myeloid elements; more mature forms predominate in patients receiving several weeks of therapy (Fig. 50.11; see also Color Plate 94, between pp. 1446–1447). All stages of granulocytic maturation

TABLE 50.4. *Morphologic features of blood and bone marrow in patients receiving recombinant human growth factor therapy (62–70)*

Type of therapy	Blood	Bone marrow[a]
rh GM-CSF	Marked leukocytosis with increase in neutrophils and monocytes, with variable increase in eosinophils, lymphocytes, and sometimes basophils Prominent toxic changes in mature and immature granulocytes Left shift with circulating blasts (usually low percent) and erythroblasts Nuclear–cytoplasmic asynchrony Nuclear segmentation defects	Early changes include interstitial foci of granulocyte precursors in hypocellular bone marrow Increased cellularity with left shift in hematopoietic elements Promyelocytic hyperplasia with reactive features during early phase of therapy Rare reports of transient increase in blood and bone marrow blasts mimicking leukemia Pronounced toxic changes of immature and mature granulocytic elements Occasional binucleate promyelocytes and myelocytes More mature granulocytes predominate after several weeks of therapy Rare development of fibrosis with bony changes Histiocytic proliferation (GM-CSF plus G-CSF) (rarely described)
rh Interleukin-3	Leukocytosis with increase in all granulated cells and lymphocytes; increase in basophils variable Variable increase in platelets and reticulocytes	Increased cellularity with left shift in all hematopoietic elements Increased eosinophils Rare reports of fibrosis with bony changes
rh G-CSF	Marked leukocytosis secondary to neutrophilia Rare giant (tetraploid) neutrophils present Prominent toxic changes of neutrophils, vacuoles prominent Nuclear–cytoplasmic asynchrony Nuclear segementation abnormalities Left shift with circulating blasts Circulating myeloid cytoplasmic fragments	Early changes include interstitial foci of granulocyte precursors in hypocellular bone marrow Increased cellularity with left shift in hematopoietic elements Rare reports of transient increase in blood and bone marrow blasts mimicking leukemia Promyelocytic hyperplasia with reactive features during early phase of therapy Pronounced toxic changes of immature and mature granulocytic elements Occasional binucleate promyelocytes and myelocytes More mature granulocytes predominate after several weeks of therapy Rare development of fibrosis with bony changes Histiocytic proliferation (GM-CSF plus G-CSF) Rare development of acute bone marrow necrosis
rh Interleukin-2 (usually given in conjunction with lymphokine activated killer cell therapy)	Enhanced functional activity including increased natural killer cell activity	Numerous noncaseating epithelioid granulomas in some patients

[a] Bone marrow examination not routinely performed on most patients receiving recombinant cytokine therapy.

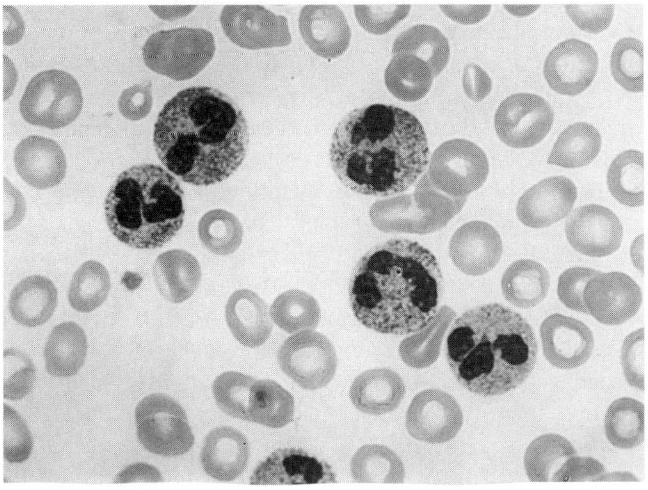

FIG. 50.11. Peripheral blood smear illustrating the prominent toxic neutrophilia that occurs in patients receiving sustained granulocyte colony-stimulating factor therapy (Wright stain, original magnification: 1,000× magnification). See Color Plate 94, between pp. 1446–1447.

exhibit marked toxic changes. Unusual findings following colony-stimulating factor therapy include diffuse histiocytic proliferation, fibrosis with associated bony changes, and a transient marked increase in blood and bone marrow blasts (68,69).

BONE MARROW TRANSPLANTATION

Indications and General Features

Clinical indications for BMT, especially autologous BMT, have increased steadily over the past several decades (Table 50.5). Although the earliest transplants were performed on patients who had severe aplastic anemia or relapsed acute leukemia, BMT currently is used successfully in patients who have various hematopoietic malignancies, constitutional hematopoietic disorders, congenital immunodeficiency states, and solid tumors refractory to conventional therapy (71–81). Although allogeneic bone marrow is used for patients with acute leukemia and constitutional disorders, autologous marrow can be used in patients who have solid tumors and in leukemia patients whose harvested peripheral blood stem cells or bone marrow specimens have been purged of the neoplastic cells (76,82,83). As efficient gene transfer techniques (with sustained expression) become a reality, greater reliance on autologous BMT is likely for the treatment of diverse constitutional disorders (71,72,77). Although results are controversial, comparisons of leukemia patient survival data generally suggest improved survival rates for patients who undergo BMT as opposed to chemotherapy alone, and relatively similar disease-free survival rates for autologous and allogeneic BMT recipients have been reported. In recent years, collection of peripheral blood stem cells has surpassed traditional autologous BMT, because of the ease of collecting these cells from the patient, cord blood, or volunteer donors (74,75,78–81). *Ex vivo* stem cell expansion techniques and the reduced (but not absent) likelihood of contamination by tumor cells make peripheral blood stem cell collection an optimal method in both autologous and allogeneic situations.

TABLE 50.5. *Indications for peripheral blood stem cell, umbilical cord blood, or bone marrow transplantation*[a] *(71–83)*

Aplastic anemia
Acute leukemias[b]
Chronic myelogenous leukemia
Myelodysplasia[b]
Myeloproliferative disorders
Non-Hodgkin's lymphoma (B and T)
Hodgkin's disease
Carcinomas
Constitutional hematopoietic disorders
Congenital immunodeficiency disorders
Chronic lymphocytic leukemia
Osteopetrosis

[a] Allogeneic blood–bone marrow transplant for all constitutional disorders, aplastic anemia, and most primary bone marrow disorders; autologous transplant generally used for solid tumors

[b] With improved bone marrow purging techniques, autologous transplantation will increase; harvesting blood stem cells may replace actual bone marrow transplantation.

The type of preparative regimen for transplantation varies, depending on the patient's disease. Chemotherapy alone is adequate for patients who have aplastic anemia. Multiagent chemotherapy plus radiation is necessary, however, to eradicate tumor cells, in addition to hematopoietic and immune cells, in patients receiving transplantation for hematopoietic malignancies and solid tumors. Complications of this rigorous preparative regimen are substantial and include mucositis, drug and radiation toxicity, interstitial pneumonitis, venoocclusive disease, and increased susceptibility to various infections (84,85). During the immediate posttransplant interval, the patient is most susceptible to bacterial and fungal infections because of profound neutropenia. From about 30 to 100 days after transplantation, the patient is most susceptible to viral infections, especially cytomegalovirus. These viral infections are toxic to the bone marrow and may contribute to rejection of the transplant. After 100 days, the most likely infectious agents include *Pneumocystis carinii*, encapsulated bacterial infections, and herpes zoster (84). In addition to infectious complications, other late complications include pulmonary disease, neurologic and endocrine defects, graft-*versus*-host disease (in allogeneic recipients), and secondary epithelial neoplasms (72,84,85). Posttransplant lymphoproliferative disorders, posttransplant myelodysplasia, and recurrent disease also can occur and are discussed in a subsequent section.

Morphology of Bone Marrow Transplantation

Similar to the recommendations for bone marrow evaluation following chemotherapy, the bone marrow biopsy, in addition to aspirate smear preparations, is essential in evaluating patients immediately after BMT. Because potent chemotherapy is part of the preparative regimen for transplantation, there are many morphologic similarities in the bone marrow between patients who receive chemotherapy for its antileukemic potential alone and those who receive it for marrow ablation preceding BMT. The addition of total body radiation to the preparative regimen in oncology patients results, however, in even more profound bone marrow ablation.

The morphologic features identified in the early period following transplantation consist of sequential features of cellular death followed by regeneration and are listed in Table 50.6 (1,84,86,87) (Fig. 50.12). The massive bone marrow damage with proteinaceous debris is similar to that seen after other ablative chemotherapy. Stromal edema, increased reticulin fibers, and small granulomas all have been noted during the early post-BMT interval (1,84,86,88). Areas of fibrosis may persist in patients who have metastatic marrow disease or various myeloproliferative disorders (86).

TABLE 50.6. *Morphologic features of early, middle, and late bone marrow transplantation periods*

Findings	Comments	References
Cell death (days 1–14)	Massive bone marrow damage with fat necrosis, proteinaceous debris, stromal edema	1,84,86–88
Early regeneration (7–14 days posttransplant)	Early nonparatrabecular monotypic colonies of erythroid and myeloid precursors; dyspoiesis of cells (erythroid >granulocytic) may be evident Erythroid and myeloid regeneration usually precede megakaryoblastic colonies	1,84,86–90
Persistence of blasts in patients transplanted during leukemic relapse	Persistence of blasts in day 7 bone marrow generally indicates residual disease	84
Complete engraftment	By day 28 all cell lines engrafted Dyserythropoietic changes may persist including ring sideroblasts Neutrotrophils may show megaloblastic changes or pseudo–Pelger-Huet nuclei Regeneration after allogeneic transplant generally faster than after autologous transplant	86,87,149, 150
Delayed engraftment or graft failure	Clinical settings Transplantation during relapse Extensive prior chemotherapy HLA partial match ABO mismatched donor T cell–depleted bone marrow Histiocytic proliferation (rare) Presumed stem cell or bone marrow microenvironment damage	17,86,87, 91
Declining cell counts (after day 28)	Possible rejection of graft, drug toxicity, viral infection, posttransplant lymphoproliferative disorder,[a] GVHD,[a] recurrent leukemia or secondary myelodysplasia[b] Morphology of rejection is nonspecific with variable features of bone marrow microenvironment damage such as fat necrosis, edema, hemorrhage, plasmacytosis, lymphocytosis, or increased histiocytes GVHD primarily affects liver, skin,and gastrointestinal tract Posttransplant lymphoproliferative disorders only occasionally involve bone marrow and are characterized by infiltration by a spectrum of lymphoid cells, plasmacellular elements, and immunoblasts; usually occurs in recipients of T cell–depleted allogeneic bone marrow Posttransplant myelodysplasia occurs in patients receiving autologous transplants and is characterized by unexplained cytopenias and highly variable trilineage dysplasias in conjunction with clonal cytogenetic abnormalities; likely the consequence of stem cell damage from prior therapy	14–16,84,86, 87,91,94, 96–112

[a] GVHD, rejection, and Epstein-Barr virus lymphoproliferative disorders do not occur in patients who undergo autologous transplants.
[b] Posttransplant myelodysplasia restricted to autologous transplant recipients.
GVHD, graft-versus-host disease.

The morphologic features of regeneration that follow BMT are somewhat different from those seen after aggressive systemic chemotherapy without transplantation. After BMT, the earliest regeneration is identified approximately 7 to 14 days after transplantation and consists predominantly of nonparatrabecular monotypic colonies of erythroid or myeloid precursors (1,84,86–90) (Figs. 50.13, 50.14). Because these colonies consist of only a single cell type, some authors have proposed that the committed progenitor cell is the first to repopulate the bone marrow after transplantation (88). Failure to develop monotypic myeloid colonies generally is associated with failure of engraftment (17,88,91). By 14 to 21 days after transplantation, the colonies are larger and consist of several lineages. Erythroid and granulocytic regenerations generally precede megakaryocytic recovery, and transient dyserythropoiesis and, to a lesser extent, dysgranulopoiesis are common (86,87) (Fig. 50.15). In general, neutrophil recovery occurs by day 21, whereas platelet recovery is expected by 25 to 30 days after BMT (84). The bone marrow cellularity in allogeneic recipients usually has recovered to approximately one half its normal level by day 21 (86,88) (Fig. 50.12). In recent studies, the relatively slower rate of hematopoietic regeneration following autologous BMT has been noted and attributed to techniques of specimen preparation or to bone marrow damage from prior therapy (87). Regeneration may be accelerated by growth

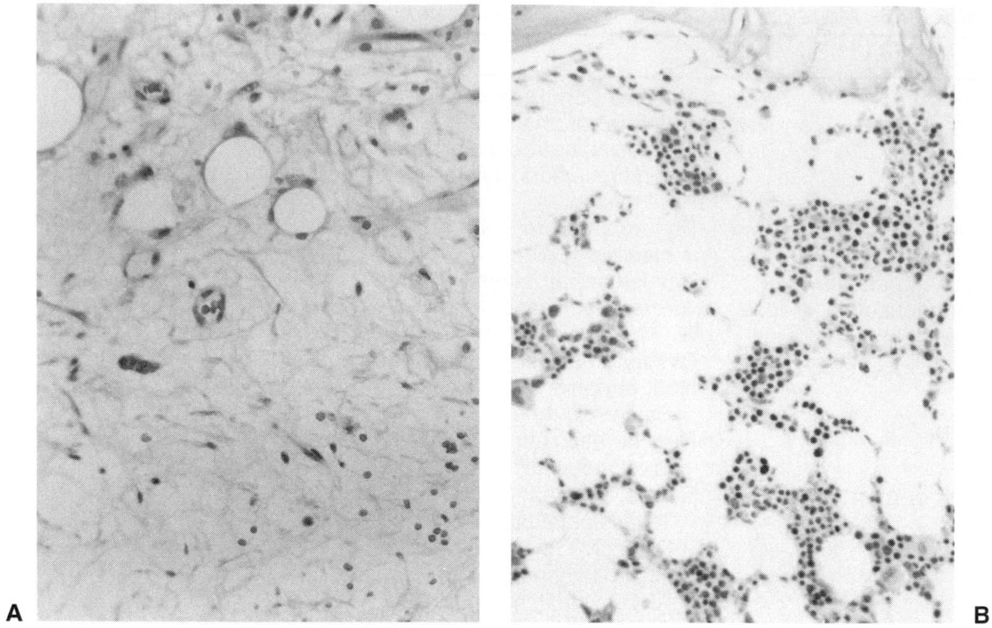

FIG. 50.12. Side-by-side comparison of a bone marrow transplant recipient showing the morphologic features 7 days (**left**) and 28 days (**right**) after transplantation. Note the pronounced stromal damage and cellular ablation shortly after transplantation, followed by hematopoietic recovery to 40% cellularity by day 28 (hematoxylin and eosin stain, original magnification: 400× magnification).

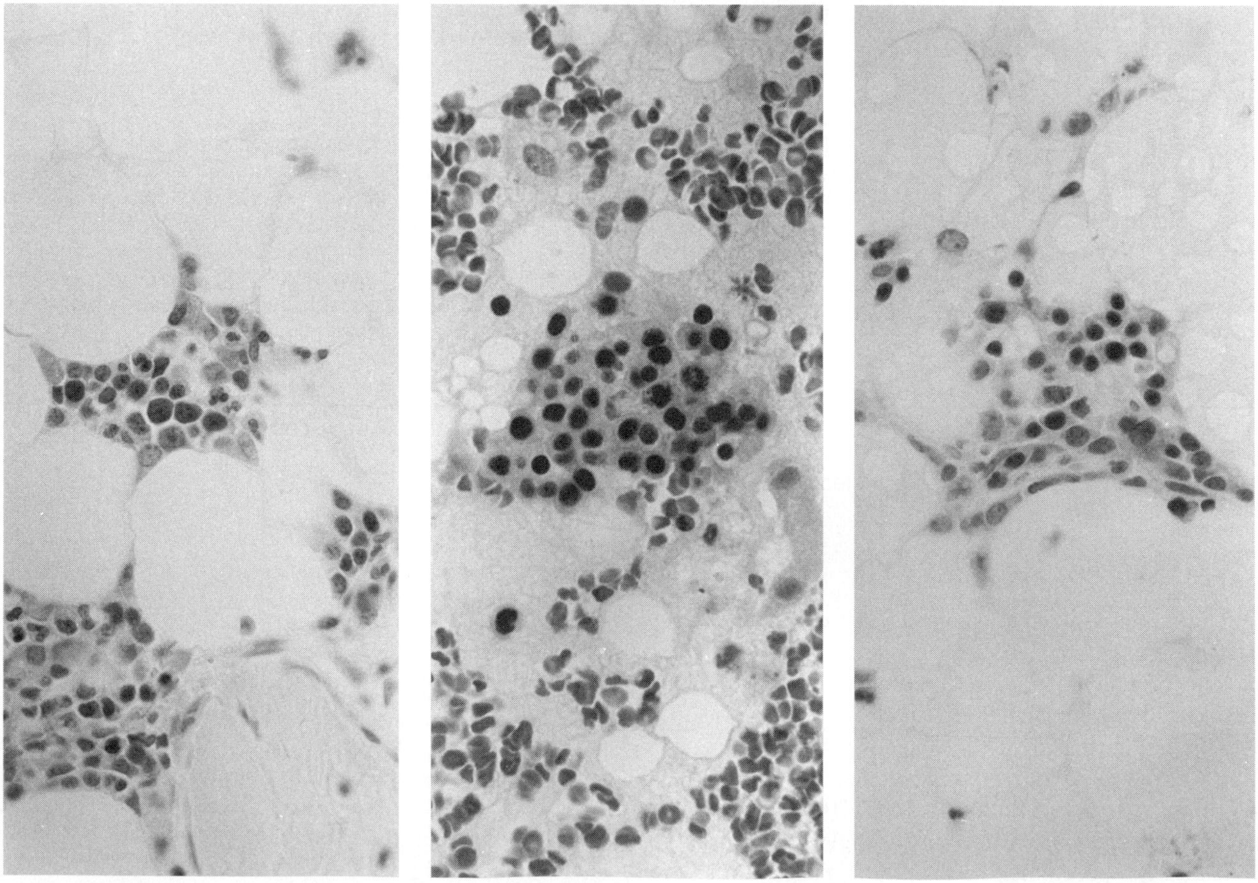

FIG. 50.13. Composite showing three areas of the bone marrow biopsy taken on day 13 after bone marrow transplantation. Although nonparatrabecular monotypic colonies predominate, a single paratrabecular colony is present. **Center:** A red cell colony. **Left, right:** Myeloid colonies (hematoxylin and eosin stain, original magnification: 400× magnification).

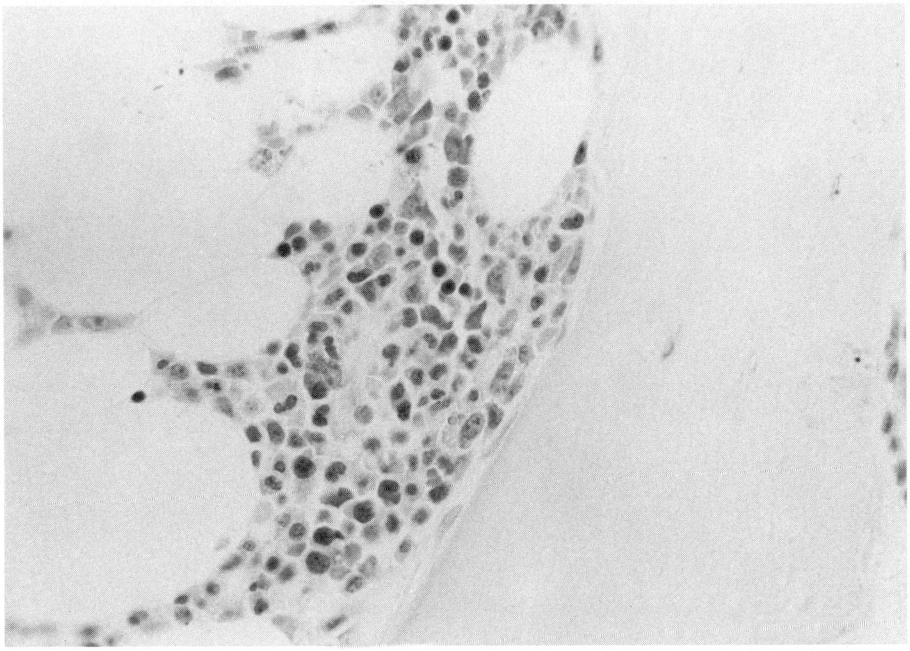

FIG. 50.14. This large paratrabecular island of regenerating hematopoietic elements shows a predominance of myeloid cells with minimal admixture of erythroid elements in a patient 13 days after bone marrow transplantation (hematoxylin and eosin stain, original magnification: 400× magnification).

factor therapy (55–57). Persistence of blasts in patients who received transplantation during leukemic relapse is an ominous sign indicating eventual florid relapse (84) (Fig. 50.16).

After successful BMT, some patients develop peripheral blood abnormalities such as monocytosis, lymphocytosis, eosinophilia, and thrombocytopenia (86,92). Although these abnormalities may be secondary to infectious complications, often no specific cause can be determined. Monitoring peripheral blood cell counts, such as absolute neutrophil count and reticulocyte count, is a reliable surrogate for bone marrow examination in assessing hematopoietic reconstitution following allogeneic, autologous, and peripheral blood stem cell transplantation (93). In a recent study, the most rapid recovery of these peripheral blood cell counts was noted in patients undergoing peripheral blood stem cell infusion (93).

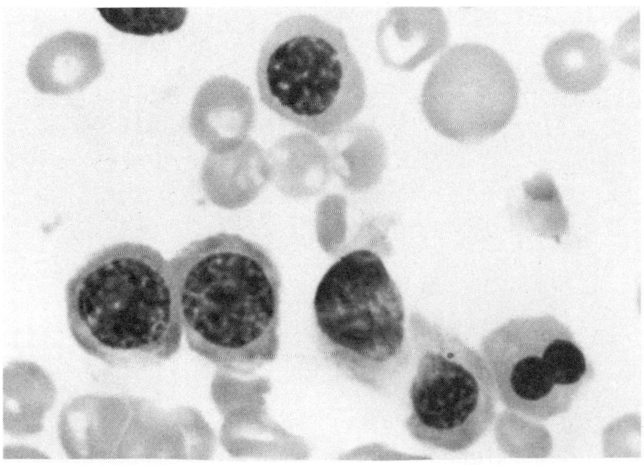

FIG. 50.15. Minimal dyserythropoiesis is evident in this aspiration smear on day 13 after bone marrow transplantation (Wright stain, original magnification: 1,000× magnification).

Some patients experience delayed engraftment that may be secondary to underlying bone marrow damage from extensive prior chemotherapy or receipt of a bone marrow that is ABO-mismatched, partially matched for human leukocyte antigens, or T cell–depleted (84,91,94) (Table 50.6). Patients receiving transplantation in relapse also are slower to engraft. Despite earlier concerns that underlying bone marrow fibrosis would interfere with hematopoietic reconstitution, recent studies document only slight delays in cell-count recovery in these patients (95). Although exceptions occur, lack of engraftment by day 28 after transplantation usually indicates that the procedure has failed (17,84) (Fig. 50.17). Although morphologic studies are limited, engraftment failure occasionally has been associated with diffuse histiocytic infiltration analogous to that seen in bone marrow specimens from patients with AIDS (17) (Fig. 50.18; see also Color Plate 95, between pp. 1446–1447). Some authors suggest that this morphologic picture may reflect widespread damage to the bone marrow microenvironment (18,91).

Causes of Bone Marrow Transplantation Failure

Once engraftment is complete, any significant decrease in the patient's peripheral blood cell counts may indicate rejection of the graft, drug toxicity, viral infections, posttransplant lymphoproliferative disorder, posttransplant mye-

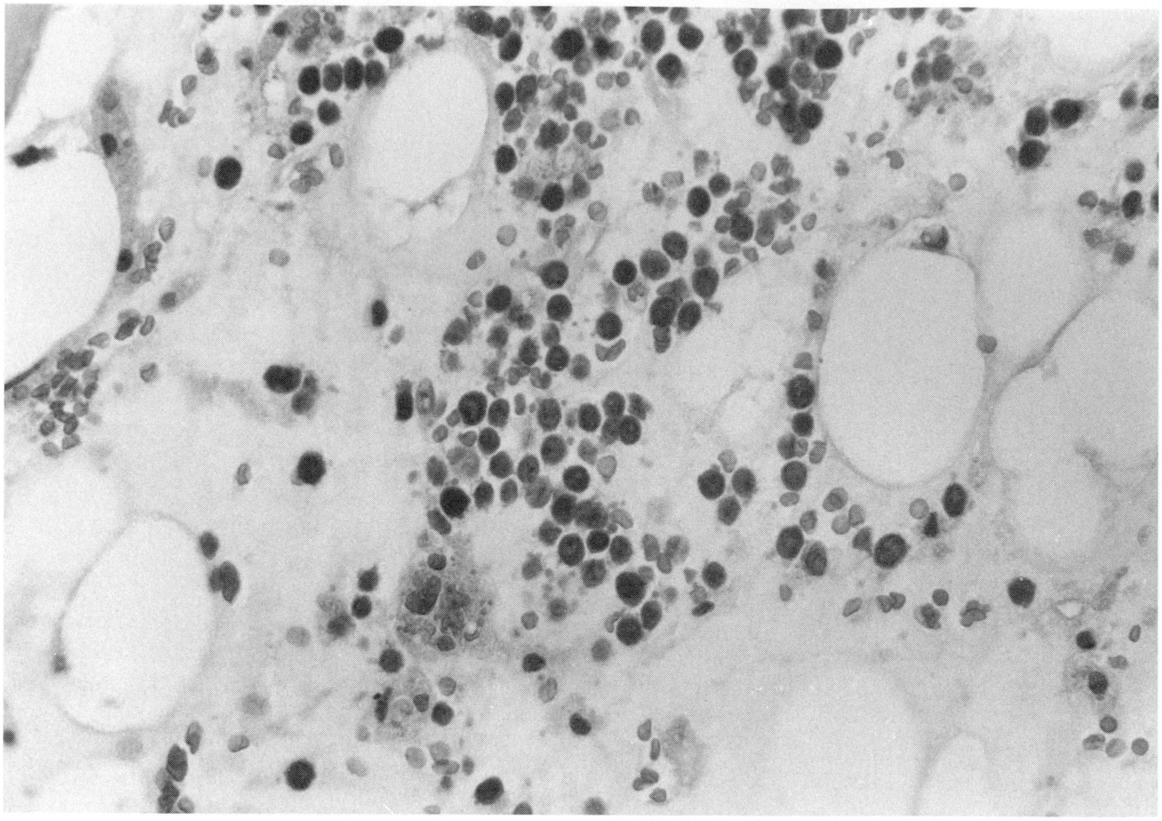

FIG. 50.16. After bone marrow transplantation for acute myelogenous leukemia, this biopsy section shows persistence of immature cells, heralding relapse (hematoxylin and eosin stain, original magnification: 400× magnification).

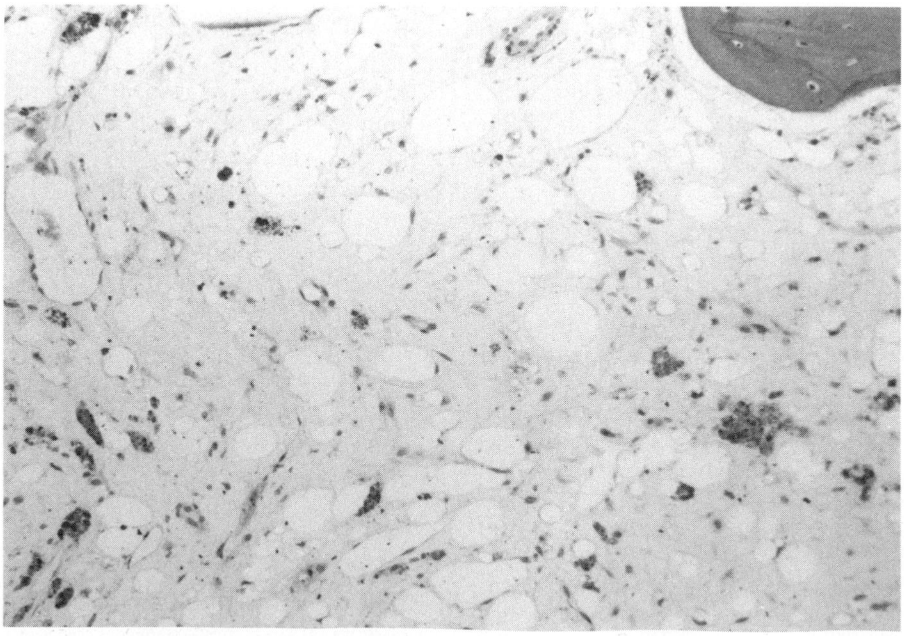

FIG. 50.17. Specimen from bone marrow biopsy performed 1 month after bone marrow transplantation, showing no evidence of hematopoietic recovery, indicative of graft failure. Note persistence of marked stromal changes, as well as abundant pigment-laden macrophages (hematoxylin and eosin stain, original magnification: 400× magnification).

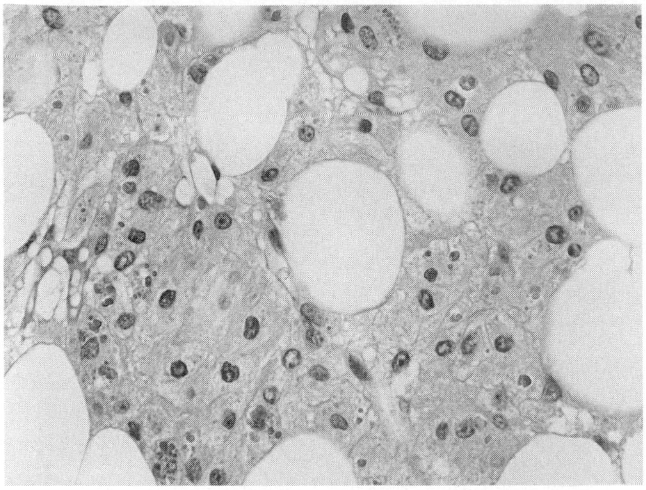

FIG. 50.18. Bone marrow biopsy speciment from a bone marrow transplant recipient shows prominent histiocytic hyperplasia; note failure of engraftment (hematoxylin and eosin stain, original magnification: 400× magnification). See Color Plate 95, between pp. 1446–1447. (Courtesy of N. Rosenthal, M.D., Department of Pathology, University of Iowa.)

lodysplasia, or recurrent disease (14–16,84,86,87,91,94, 96–112) (Table 50.6). Declining peripheral blood cell counts also may be a feature of bone marrow graft-*versus*-host disease in those patients who have congenital immunodeficiency disorders and who undergo allogeneic BMT (86). Some of these complications, such as rejection of graft, graft-*versus*-host disease, and posttransplant lymphoproliferative disorders, occur only in patients who receive allogeneic transplants; posttransplant myelodysplasia is a complication of autologous BMT (84,86,87,91,97–112).

No good morphologic predictors of bone marrow rejection are available. The pathologic features of evolving rejection include declining cellularity in conjunction with features of nonspecific bone marrow damage such as fat necrosis, edema, plasmacytosis, lymphocytosis, and increased histiocytes (84,87,91,96). Graft rejection is more frequent in patients receiving grafts either partially matched for human leukocyte antigens or depleted of T cells (91).

In addition to rejection, drug toxicity and infections can cause graft failure. After BMT, the marrow is more susceptible to infections and drug toxicities (14–16,84,86,91). Various drugs have been shown to be toxic to transplanted marrow, including methotrexate, many antibiotics, acyclovir, and cimetidine (84). In addition, viral infections, especially cytomegalovirus and human herpesvirus-6, have been linked to bone marrow stem cell suppression that eventually may lead to graft failure (14–16,84,86,91).

A well-known complication of organ transplantation is the development of morphologically and immunophenotypically heterogeneous lymphoproliferative disorders. These EBV-associated posttransplant lymphoproliferative disorders are much more prevalent in solid organ recipients but also have been described in patients undergoing allogeneic BMT, especially if T cell–depleted specimens are utilized (84,86,97–105,111,112). (Chapter 16 contains a detailed discussion.) These disorders demonstrate a morphologic spectrum from polymorphic processes including plasma cell hyperplasia to monomorphic large cell lymphoma or multiple myeloma (101–105). Immunophenotypic studies demonstrate a range from polyclonal to monoclonal B-cell proliferations; T cell–derived posttransplant lymphoproliferative disorders are very rare (105). Molecular assessment for EBV clonality and various oncogene alterations may prove useful in predicting disease course (102,104). Although generally not prominent sites of involvement, blood and bone marrow infiltration has been described in patients with posttransplant lymphoproliferative disorders and is substantially more common in pediatric patients (97,111) (Fig. 50.19). In these children (who typically have undergone solid organ transplantation), the bone marrow infiltrates range from subtle B-lymphoid aggregates to frank effacing lymphomatous lesions (97). The posttransplant lymphoproliferative disorders that occur in T cell–depleted allogeneic BMT recipients often are disseminated and biologically aggressive and show variable bone marrow and blood involvement (98,99).

A recently recognized complication of autologous transplantation (either bone marrow or peripheral blood stem cell) is the development of posttransplantation myelodysplasia or AML (105–110). This complication is presumably a consequence of prior chemoradiotherapy that these patients have received for their primary solid neoplasms, analogous to therapy-induced myelodysplasia or AML that occurs in the nontransplant setting. The cumulative incidence of myelodysplasia and AML in autologous transplant is 10 to 20% at 5 years, depending on the criteria utilized for the diagnosis. For example, if the detection of clonal cytogenetic abnormalities after transplantation (in a patient who had normal bone marrow cytogenetics beforehand) is the defining criteria for this disorder, the incidence is 20% at 5 years (108). If morphologic criteria for myelodysplasia are used, the incidence is lower. Risk factors for posttransplant myelodysplasia and AML include older age at transplant and more prolonged pretransplant chemotherapy. This complication is more frequent in patients receiving autologous peripheral blood stem cell infusions compared with those receiving bone marrow transplants (105). Morphologic features of posttransplant myelodysplasia are variable but generally include increased numbers of bone marrow blasts or single or multilineage dysplasia in the setting of unexplained cytopenias (105–107). In some patients with posttransplant clonal cytogenetic abnormalities in bone marrow, however, there are very few dysmorphic features (108). The clonal cytogenetic abnormalities are primarily numeric and identical to those described in nontransplant-related therapy-induced myelodysplasia, although the clonal abnormalities tend to be very complex and translocations may be evident (105,108).

Patients who undergo BMT for hematologic and nonhematologic neoplasms must be monitored for evidence of disease recurrence. Because BMT has been used for a long time

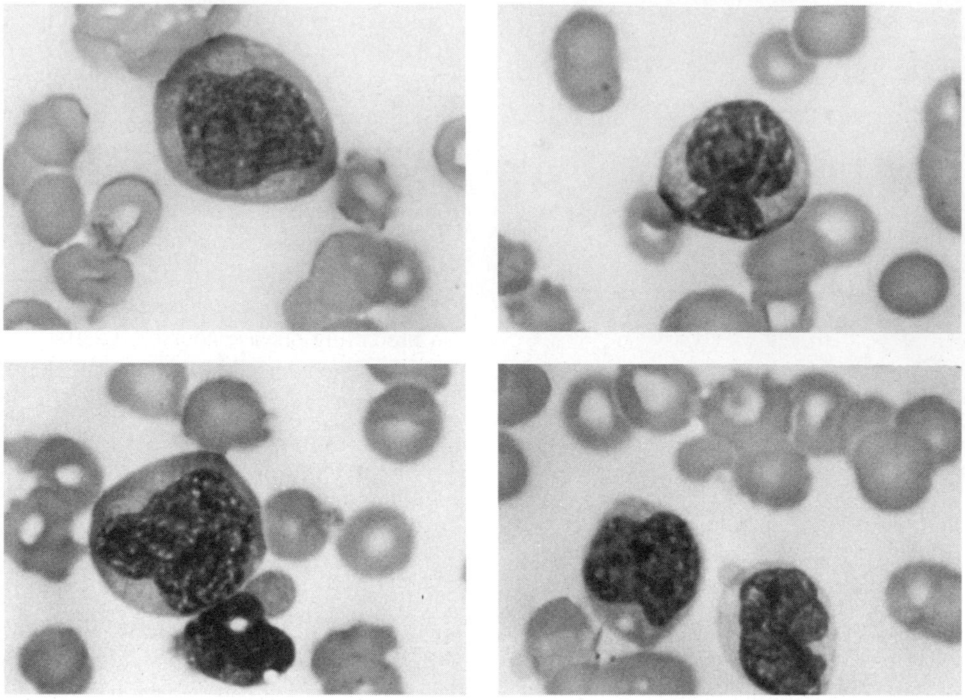

FIG. 50.19. Composite photomicrograph highlighting the types of atypical lymphoid cells present in the peripheral blood of a patient with a posttransplant lymphoproliferative disorder (Wright stain, original magnification: 1,000× magnification).

in the treatment of acute leukemia, most of the research on recurrent disease has been performed on recurrent leukemia. The incidence of leukemic recurrence is higher in patients who receive T cell–depleted bone marrow cells and in those patients who do not experience graft-*versus*-host disease (84,113). A clear-cut graft-*versus*-leukemia affect has been documented (113). Although the vast majority of recurrent leukemias are of host cell origin, well-documented cases of apparent donor cell recurrent leukemia have been described (84,105,114–116). The ability to resolve host-*versus*-donor origin of a recurrent leukemia is highly problematic, especially in the presence of recipient–donor chimerism (116). If rigorous standards to determine donor-*versus*-host origin are applied, it appears that convincing donor cell leukemia accounts for a very small number of cases (only 4 in 40,000 BMT patients assessed) (116). If leukemic relapse occurs within the first 100 days post-BMT, the prognosis is very poor, whereas later relapses of acute or chronic myeloid leukemias sometimes can be eradicated successfully by reinduction chemotherapy or immune modulation (117).

DETECTION OF MINIMAL RESIDUAL DISEASE

The detection of minimal residual disease is important in patients who receive chemotherapy alone and in those who undergo peripheral blood stem cell transplantation or BMT. For the most part, efforts at detection of minimal residual disease have focused on bone marrow specimens from patients with various leukemias and lymphomas. After ablative chemotherapy for a leukemia or lymphoma, identifying minimal residual tumor in bone marrow may be relevant to further treatment needs, predicting early relapse, determining if the patient's bone marrow can be harvested for future autologous transplantation, or determining if bone marrow purging techniques have been successful in removing neoplastic cells.

The methods that have been used to detect minimal residual disease and their relative sensitivities are detailed in Table 50.7 (35,84,118–148). These methods range from standard morphologic and cytochemical analyses to sophisticated molecular and genetic techniques. To consider the relative sensitivities to detect residual neoplastic cells admixed with normal hematopoietic elements, the differences in "tumor burden" detected by these diverse methodologies must be appreciated. For example, the detection of residual leukemia by morphologic or standard immunoperoxidase techniques reflects a substantially greater tumor burden compared with detection of disease by polymerase chain reaction (PCR) techniques. Consequently, the detection of residual leukemia by morphologic or immunoperoxidase techniques is associated much more consistently with overt relapse within a short time interval (35). Conversely, the significance of the detection of persistent leukemic cells by PCR techniques is much more variable, must be correlated with the time interval from initial diagnosis, must be assessed on sequential specimens, and in some diseases is not associated with subsequent relapse (123–125,127,129,130). The sensitivities of morphology, cytochemistry, immunophenotype,

TABLE 50.7. *Methods to detect minimal residual disease (35,84,118–148)*

Methods	Sensitivity, %	Comments
Morphology/cytochemistry	1–10	Sensitivity dependent on unique features of neoplastic clone
Immunoperoxidase	1–10	Sensitivity dependent on unique features of neoplasm Useful for detection of metastatic lesions Clusters of CD34$^+$ TdT$^+$ cells predicts imminent relapse in ALL
Multicolor flow cytometry	<1–5	Most sensitive for nonhematopoietic lesions Overlap of immunophenotypic profile between AML and normal hematopoietic precursors may be problematic
Cytogenetics	5	Dependent on proliferation and mitosis in culture Sensitivity may be enhanced by initial cell sorting by immunophenotype
Fluorescence *in situ* hybridization	≪1–5	Requires specific gene probe to investigate translocations; chromosome probes adequate for cases of ALL with hyperdiploidy; sensitivities 10^{-4} achieved with three chromosome probes in ALL Applicable to metaphase and interphase cells Careful control studies must be done to establish background levels of false positivity secondary to chromosome overlays Greater specificity if combined with other methods to assess minimal residual disease, such as RT-PCR
PCR (RT-PCR) Nested RT-PCR	≪0.01	Applicable only if probe available Can be utilized for immunoglobulin or T-cell receptor gene rearrangement studies or assessment for a specific fusion gene (translocation); junctional sequences of T-cell receptor or immunoglobulin gene rearrangements can be used as clonal markers of leukemic cells Variable clinical significance of detection of such low numbers of clonal cells; significance dependent on time of detection in disease course, type of leukemia, and persistence of detectable minimal residual disease; rare reports of fusion genes detected in normal hematopoietic elements

ALL, acute lymphoblastic leukemia; RT-PCR, reverse transcriptase-polymerase chain reaction.

and standard cytogenetics are all in the range between 1 and 10% of tumor cells admixed with normal hematopoietic elements, depending on unique features of the malignant cells. As few as one metastatic carcinoma cell in 100,000 bone marrow cells can be detected by multicolor immunophenotypic techniques (118–120). The sensitivity of immunophenotypic techniques to detect hematopoietic tumor cells is enhanced by applying multiflow cytometry, using relatively unique leukemia cell–specific antibody combinations, or using cell culture techniques to augment the neoplastic population before immunophenotypic studies (122,137). Also, the combination of a surface antigen marker with DNA content sometimes can be used to identify selectively low numbers of residual leukemia cells. Greater specificity in detecting minimal residual disease is achieved by combining two methods such as PCR and fluorescence *in situ* hybridization (135,136).

The application of a specialized cytogenetic technique like interphase *in situ* hybridization has improved greatly the sensitivity of karyotype studies in detecting rare neoplastic cells. Using fluoresceinated probes against specific chromosome regions, an excess, deletion, or translocation can be detected even in terminally differentiated cells such as neutrophils (121–123,126). If rigorous controls are utilized, as few as one tumor cell in 1,000 normal bone marrow cells can be detected by interphase cytogenetics (126,132,134). Another method to enhance the sensitivity of cytogenetics is to apply *in vitro* cell culture techniques to amplify selected types of neoplastic cells before karyotyping.

Various molecular methods have been applied to detect residual leukemia or lymphoma cells with variable sensitivities in tumor cell identification. The sensitivity of standard DNA gene rearrangement techniques ranges from 2 to 5% (84,121,122,124,125). The use of cell culture immune selection or flow-sorting techniques to amplify tumor cells before molecular analysis substantially increases sensitivity (84,122,143). Even greater sensitivity in tumor cell detection is achieved by PCR studies. If a specific probe is available to identify tumor cells, the sensitivity ranges from one neoplastic cell in 100,000 to 1 in 10×10^6 normal cells using PCR techniques (84,121, 122,128–130,144–146). Sensitivity is enhanced by utilizing clone-specific probes and a comprehensive primer set (128,144–146).

If very sensitive methods to detect minimal residual disease are applied to a bone marrow aspirate sample, the significance of very low numbers of residual tumor cells is uncertain. It is possible that host factors prevent recurrence even though minimal residual disease is present (147). Also, the proliferative potential of low numbers of residual tumor cells is not evaluated in most of the techniques currently used to detect rare tumor cells (84). In general, the detection of residual neoplastic cells in multiple sequential studies or a progressive increase in the proportion of neoplastic cells is more likely a harbinger of eventual relapse (148). Recent studies indicate a high correlation of detecting minimal residual disease by reverse transcriptase–PCR or PCR techniques and relapse in acute lymphoblastic leukemia if tumor-specific probes are utilized (138–141). The significance of minimal residual disease (detected by PCR techniques) in types of AML, however, is less clear-cut, especially because recent reports describe the finding of fusion genes such as *MLL-AF4* in normal hematopoietic elements from nonleukemic control groups (131).

SUMMARY AND CONCLUSIONS

Despite the high risks of potent chemotherapy and BMT, a substantial number of patients who undergo these aggressive treatment regimens is cured. In this chapter I detail the morphologic effects of chemotherapy and BMT, including details about morphologic changes in neoplastic and nonneoplastic bone marrow cells. Areas of particular difficulty include the distinction of reactive from neoplastic promyelocytes, the distinction of benign hematogones from acute lymphoblastic leukemia cells, and the detection of early relapse and minimal residual disease. I have emphasized the importance of detecting minimal residual disease in the bone marrow not only *after* ablative chemotherapy but also *before* BMT. Using sophisticated molecular techniques, as few as one malignant cell in 1,000,000 normal bone marrow cells can be identified. The significance of very low numbers of neoplastic cells admixed with normal hematopoietic cells is unclear and may vary by disease type, although the detection of early occult relapse may be valuable in prompting new treatment modalities in some patients prior to overt relapse.

ACKNOWLEDGMENTS

The author thanks Jerri A. Lusk for excellent manuscript preparation.

REFERENCES

1. Foucar K. Effects of therapy and transplantation, and detection of minimal residual disease. In: Foucar K, ed. *Bone marrow pathology*, 1st ed. Chicago: ASCP Press, 1995:531–552.
2. Dick FR, Burns CP, Weiner GJ, et al. Bone marrow morphology during induction phase of therapy for acute myeloid leukemia (AML). *Hematol Pathol* 1995;9:95–106.
3. Wittels B. Bone marrow biopsy changes following chemotherapy for acute leukemia. *Am J Surg Pathol* 1980;4:135–142.
4. Krech R, Thiele J. Histopathology of the bone marrow in toxic myelopathy: a study of drug induced lesions in 57 patients. *Virchows Arch A Pathol Anat Histopathol* 1985;405:225–235.
5. Browman G, Preisler H, Raza A, et al. Use of the day 6 bone marrow to alter remission induction therapy in patients with acute myeloid leukaemia: a leukemia intergroup study. *Br J Haematol* 1989;71: 493–497.
6. Islam A, Catovsky D, Galton DA. Histological study of bone marrow regeneration following chemotherapy for acute myeloid leukaemia and chronic granulocytic leukaemia in blast transformation. *Br J Haematol* 1980;45:535–540.
7. Seaman JP, Kjeldsberg CR, Linker A. Gelatinous transformation of the bone marrow. *Hum Pathol* 1978;9:685–692.
8. Feng CS. Gelatinous transformation of marrow in a case of acute myelogenous leukemia post-chemotherapy. *Am J Hematol* 1991;38: 220–222.
9. Jacobsen K, Tepper J, Osmond DG. Early B-lymphocyte precursor cells in mouse bone marrow: subosteal localization of B220 + cells during postirradiation regeneration. *Exp Hematol* 1990;18:304–310.
10. Naeim F. Topobiology in hematopoiesis. *Hematol Pathol* 1995;9: 107–119.
11. Casamassima F, Ruggiero C, Caramella D, et al. Hematopoietic bone marrow recovery after radiation therapy: MRI evaluation. *Blood* 1989; 73:1677–1681.
12. Vogler WR, Raney MR. Prognostic significance of blood and marrow findings in acute myelogenous leukemia in remission: a Southeastern Cancer Study Group report. *Cancer* 1988;61:2481–2486.
13. Gajjar A, Ribeiro R, Hancock ML, et al. Persistence of circulating blasts after 1 week of multiagent chemotherapy confers a poor prognosis in childhood acute lymphoblastic leukemia. *Blood* 1995;86: 1292–1295.
14. Bolger GB, Sullivan KM, Storb R, et al. Second marrow infusion for poor graft function after allogeneic marrow transplantation. *Bone Marrow Transplant* 1986;1:21.
15. Carrigan DR, Knox KK. Human herpesvirus 6 (HHV-6) isolation from bone marrow: HHV-6-associated bone marrow suppression in bone marrow transplant patients [see comments]. *Blood* 1994;84: 3307–3310.
16. Moses A, Nelson J, Bagby GC. The influence of human immunodeficiency virus-1 on hematopoiesis. *Blood* 1998;91:1479–1495.
17. Rosenthal NS, Farhi DC. Failure to engraft after bone marrow transplantation: bone marrow morphologic findings [see comments]. *Am J Clin Pathol* 1994;102:821–824.
18. Foucar K. Bone marrow histiocytosis and autologous graft failure: possible implications. *Am J Clin Pathol* 1994;102:713–714.
19. Dritschilo A, Sherman DS. Radiation and chemical injury in the bone marrow. Environ Health Perspect 1981;39:59–64.
20. Hoagland HC. Hematologic complications of cancer chemotherapy. *Semin Oncol* 1982;9:95–102.
21. Chang J, Geary CG, Testa NG. Long-term bone marrow damage after chemotherapy for acute myeloid leukaemia does not improve with time. *Br J Haematol* 1990;75:68–72.
22. Leitner SP, Bosl GJ, Pelus LM. Abnormal colony formation and prostaglandin E responsiveness of myeloid progenitor cells in patients cured of germ cell neoplasms after combination chemotherapy. *Cancer* 1987;60:312–317.
23. Bhavnani M, Morris Jones PH, Testa NG. Children in long-term remission after treatment for acute lymphoblastic leukaemia show persisting haemopoietic injury in clonal and long-term cultures. *Br J Haematol* 1989;71:37–41.
24. Ridgway D, Borzy MS. Defective production of granulocyte-macrophage colony-stimulating factor and interleukin-1 by mononuclear cells from children treated for acute lymphoblastic leukemia. *Leukemia* 1992;6:809–813.
25. Adelstein DJ, Hines JD. Bone marrow morphologic changes after combination chemotherapy including VP-16. *Cancer* 1985;56: 467–471.
26. Brunning RD. The effects of leukemia and lymphoma chemotherapy on hematopoietic cells. *Am J Med Technol* 1973;39:165–174.
27. Dharmasena F, Galton DA. Circulating blasts in acute myeloid leukaemia in remission. *Br J Haematol* 1986;63:211–213.
28. Foucar K, Vaughan WP, Armitage JO, et al. Postleukemic dysmyelopoiesis. *Am J Hematol* 1983;15:321–334.
29. Nagai K, Matsuo T, Atogami S, et al. Remission with morphological myelodysplasia in de novo acute myeloid leukaemia: implications for early relapse. *Br J Haematol* 1992;81:33–39.
30. Rosenthal NS, Farhi DC. Dysmegakaryopoiesis resembling acute megakaryoblastic leukemia in treated acute myeloid leukemia. *Am J Clin Pathol* 1991;95:556–560.
31. Sjogren U. Mitotic activity in acute promyelocytic leukaemia and leukaemoid reactions. *Acta Med Scand* 1976;199:181–183.
32. Levine PH, Weintraub LW. Pseudoleukemia during recovery from dapsone-induced agranulocytosis. *Ann Intern Med* 1968;68: 1060–1065.
33. Innes DJ Jr, Hess CE, Bertholf MF, et al. Promyelocyte morphology: differentiation of acute promyelocytic leukemia from benign myeloid proliferations. *Am J Clin Pathol* 1987;88:725–729.
34. Longacre TA, Foucar K, Crago S, et al. Hematogones: a multiparameter analysis of bone marrow precursor cells. *Blood* 1989;73:543–552.
35. Rimsza LM, Viswanatha DS, Winter SS, et al. The presence of CD34 + cell clusters predicts impending relapse in pediatric ALL patients on maintenance chemotherapy. *Am J Clin Pathol* 1998;110:313–320.

36. Chomienne C, Ballerini P, Balitrand N, et al. Retinoic acid therapy for promyelocytic leukaemia [Letter]. *Lancet* 1989;ii:746–747.
37. Huang ME, Ye YC, Chen SR, et al. Use of all-trans retinoic acid in the treatment of acute promyelocytic leukemia. *Blood* 1988;72: 567–572.
38. Vyas RC, Frankel SR, Agbor P, et al. Probing the pathobiology of response to all-trans retinoic acid in acute promyelocytic leukemia: premature chromosome condensation/fluorescence in situ hybridization analysis. *Blood* 1996;87:218–226.
39. Kantarjian HM, Keating MJ, McCredie KB, et al. A characteristic pattern of leukemic cell differentiation without cytoreduction during remission induction in acute promyelocytic leukemia. *J Clin Oncol* 1985;3:793–798.
40. Wallace PJ. Complete remission in acute promyelocytic leukemia despite the persistence of the 15;17 translocation. *Am J Hematol* 1989; 31:266–268.
41. Limentani SA, Pretell JO, Potter D, et al. Bone marrow necrosis in two patients with acute promyelocytic leukemia during treatment with all-trans retinoic acid. *Am J Hematol* 1994;47:50–55.
42. Hatake K, Ohtsuki T, Uwai M, et al. Tretinoin induces bone marrow collagenous fibrosis in acute promyelocytic leukaemia: new adverse, but reversible effect. *Br J Haematol* 1996;93:646–649.
43. Cheson BD, Cassileth PA, Head DR, et al. Report of the National Cancer Institute-sponsored workshop on definitions of diagnosis and response in acute myeloid leukemia. *J Clin Oncol* 1990;8:813–819.
44. Jinnai I, Nagai K, Yoshida S, et al. Incidence and characteristics of clonal hematopoiesis in remission of acute myeloid leukemia in relation to morphological dysplasia. *Leukemia* 1995;9:1756–1761.
45. Smith FO, Raskind WH, Fialkow PJ, et al. Cellular biology of acute myelogenous leukemia. *J Pediatr Hematol Oncol* 1995;17:113–122.
46. Lo Coco F, Pelicci PG, D'Adamo F, et al. Polyclonal hematopoietic reconstitution in leukemia patients at remission after suppression of specific gene rearrangements. *Blood* 1993;82:606–612.
47. Lo Coco F, Saglio G. Single or multistep origin of hemopoietic tumors: the contribution of clonality studies. *Leukemia* 1995;9: 1586–1589.
48. Foucar K, McKenna RW, Bloomfield CD, et al. Therapy-related leukemia: a panmyelosis. *Cancer* 1979;43:1285–1296.
49. Foucar K, Langdon RMd, Armitage JO, et al. Myelodysplastic syndromes: a clinical and pathologic analysis of 109 cases. *Cancer* 1985; 56:553–561.
50. Ellis M, Ravid M, Lishner M. A comparative analysis of alkylating agent and epipodophyllotoxin-related leukemias. *Leuk Lymphoma* 1993;11:9–13.
51. Park DJ, Koeffler HP. Therapy-related myelodysplastic syndromes. *Semin Hematol* 1996;33:256–273.
52. van Leeuwen FE, Klokman WJ, Hagenbeek A, et al. Second cancer risk following Hodgkin's disease: a 20-year follow-up study. *J Clin Oncol* 1994;12:312–325.
53. van Leeuwen FE, Chorus AMJ, van den Belt-Dusebout AW, et al. Leukemia risk following Hodgkin's disease: relation to cumulative dose of alkylating agents, treatment with teniposide combinations, number of episodes of chemotherapy, and bone marrow damage. *J Clin Oncol* 1994;12:1063–1073.
54. Foucar K. Acute myelogenous leukemia. In: Foucar K, ed. *Bone marrow pathology*, 1st ed. Chicago: ASCP Press, 1995:189–228.
55. American Society of Clinical Oncology. Recommendations for the use of hematopoietic colony-stimulating factors: evidence-based, clinical practice guidelines. *J Clin Oncol* 1994;12:2471–2508.
56. American Society of Clinical Oncology. Update of recommendations for the use of hematopoietic colony-stimulating factors: evidence-based clinical practice guidelines. *J Clin Oncol* 1996;14:1957–1960.
57. American Society of Clinical Oncology. 1997 update of recommendations for the use of hematopoietic colony-stimulating factors: evidence-based, clinical practice guidelines. *J Clin Oncol* 1997;15:3288.
58. Hartmann LC, Tschetter LK, Habermann TM, et al. Granulocyte colony-stimulating factor in severe chemotherapy-induced afebrile neutropenia [see comments]. *N Engl J Med* 1997;336:1776–1780.
59. Byrne JL, Haynes AP, Russell NH. Use of haemopoietic growth factors: commentary on the ASCO/ECOG guidelines: American Society of Clinical Oncology/Eastern Co-operative Oncology Group. *Blood Rev* 1997;11:16–27.
60. Vadhan-Raj S. Recombinant human erythropoietin in combination with other hematopoietic cytokines in attenuating chemotherapy-induced multilineage myelosuppression: brief communication. *Semin Hematol (Suppl)* 1996;33:16–18.
61. Vadhan-Raj S. Recombinant human thrombopoietin: clinical experience and in vivo biology [In Process Citation]. *Semin Hematol* 1998; 35:261–268.
62. Falk S, Seipelt G, Ganser A, et al. Bone marrow findings after treatment with recombinant human interleukin-3. *Am J Clin Pathol* 1991; 95:355–362.
63. Ryder JW, Lazarus HM, Farhi DC. Bone marrow and blood findings after marrow transplantation and rhGM-CSF therapy. *Am J Clin Pathol* 1992;97:631–637.
64. Campbell LJ, Maher DW, Tay DLM, et al. Marrow proliferation and the appearance of giant neutrophils in response to recombinant human granulocyte colony stimulating factor (rhG-CSF). *Br J Haematol* 1992;80:298–304.
65. Schmitz LL, McClure JS, Litz CE, et al. Morphologic and quantitative changes in blood and marrow cells following growth factor therapy. *Am J Clin Pathol* 1994;101:67–75.
66. Harris AC, Todd WM, Hackney MH, et al. Bone marrow changes associated with recombinant granulocyte-macrophage and granulocyte colony-stimulating factors: discrimination of granulocytic regeneration. *Arch Pathol Lab Med* 1994;118:624–629.
67. Kerrigan DP, Castillo A, Foucar K, et al. Peripheral blood morphologic changes after high-dose antineoplastic chemotherapy and recombinant human granulocyte colony-stimulating factor administration. *Am J Clin Pathol* 1989;92:280–285.
68. Wilson PA, Ayscue LH, Jones GR, et al. Bone marrow histiocytic proliferation in association with colony-stimulating factor therapy. *Am J Clin Pathol* 1993;99:311.
69. Meyerson HJ, Farhi DC, Rosenthal NS. Transient increase in blasts mimicking acute leukemia and progressing myelodysplasia in patients receiving growth factor. *Am J Clin Pathol* 1998;109:675–681.
70. Katayama Y, Deguchi S, Shinagawa K, et al. Bone marrow necrosis in a patient with acute myeloblastic leukemia during administration of G-CSF and rapid hematologic recovery after allotransplantation of peripheral blood stem cells. *Am J Hematol* 1998;57:238–240.
71. Beutler E. Bone marrow transplantation beyond treatment of aplasia and neoplasia. *West J Med* 1994;160:129–132.
72. Armitage JO. Bone marrow transplantation [see comments]. *N Engl J Med* 1994;330:827–838.
73. Stiff PJ, Bayer R, Kerger C, et al. High-dose chemotherapy with autologous transplantation for persistent/relapsed ovarian cancer: a multivariate analysis of survival for 100 consecutively treated patients [see comments]. *J Clin Oncol* 1997;15:1309–1317.
74. Cairo MS, Wagner JE. Placental and/or umbilical cord blood: an alternative source of hematopoietic stem cells for transplantation. *Blood* 1997;90:4665–4678.
75. Johnson FL. Placental blood transplantation and autologous banking: caveat emptor. *J Pediatr Hematol Oncol* 1997;19:183–186.
76. De Witte T, Van Biezen A, Hermans J, et al. Autologous bone marrow transplantation for patients with myelodysplastic syndrome (MDS) or acute myeloid leukemia following MDS. *Blood* 1997;90:3853–3857.
77. Parkman R. Overview: bone marrow transplantation in the 1990s. *Am J Pediatr Hematol Oncol* 1994;16:3–5.
78. To LB, Haylock DN, Simmons PJ, et al. The biology and clinical uses of blood stem cells. *Blood* 1997;89:2233–2258.
79. Piacibello W, Sanavio F, Garetto L, et al. Extensive amplification and self-renewal of human primitive hematopoietic stem cells from cord blood. *Blood* 1997;89:2644–2653.
80. Lange W, Henschler R, Mertelsmann R. Biological and clinical advances in stem cell expansion. *Leukemia* 1996;10:943–945.
81. Guillaume T, Rubinstein DB, Symann M. Immune reconstitution and immunotherapy after autologous hematopoietic stem cell transplantation [In Process Citation]. *Blood* 1998;92:1471–1490.
82. Gorin NC. Autologous stem cell transplantation in acute myelocytic leukemia [In Process Citation]. *Blood* 1998;92:1073–1090.
83. Cagnoni PJ, Shpall EJ. Mobilization and selection of CD34-positive hematopoietic progenitors. *Blood Rev* 1996;10:1–7.
84. Sale GE, Buckner CD. Pathology of bone marrow in transplant recipients. *Hematol Oncol Clin North Am* 1988;2:735–756.
85. Champlin RE, Gale RP. The early complications of bone marrow transplantation. *Semin Hematol* 1984;21:101–108.
86. Dick F, Gingrich RD. Biopsy analysis in bone marrow transplantation.

In: Kolbeck PC, McManus BM, eds. *Transplant pathology.* Chicago: ASCP, 1994:281–292.
87. Bombi JA, Palou J, Bruguera M, et al. Pathology of bone marrow transplantation. *Semin Diagn Pathol* 1992;9:220–231.
88. van den Berg H, Kluin PM, Vossen JM. Early reconstitution of haematopoiesis after allogeneic bone marrow transplantation: a prospective histopathological study of bone marrow biopsy specimens. *J Clin Pathol* 1990;43:365–369.
89. Cline MJ, Gale RP, Golde DW. Discrete clusters of hematopoietic cells in the marrow cavity of man after bone marrow transplantation. *Blood* 1977;50:709–712.
90. Naeim F, Smith GS, Gale RP. Morphologic aspects of bone marrow transplantation in patients with aplastic anemia. *Hum Pathol* 1978;9: 295–308.
91. Quinones RR. Hematopoietic engraftment and graft failure after bone marrow transplantation. *Am J Pediatr Hematol Oncol* 1993;15:3–17.
92. Anasetti C, Rybka W, Sullivan KM, et al. Graft-v-host disease is associated with autoimmune-like thrombocytopenia [see comments]. *Blood* 1989;73:1054–1058.
93. d'Onofrio G, Tichelli A, Foures C, et al. Indicators of haematopoietic recovery after bone marrow transplantation: the role of reticulocyte measurements. *Clin Lab Haematol* 1996;18[Suppl 1]:45–53.
94. Kusunoki Y, Chen W, Martin PJ. Prevention of marrow graft rejection without induction of graft-versus-host disease by a cytotoxic T-cell clone that recognizes recipient alloantigens. *Blood* 1998;91: 4038–4044.
95. Soll E, Massumoto C, Clift RA, et al. Relevance of marrow fibrosis in bone marrow transplantation: a retrospective analysis of engraftment. *Blood* 1995;86:4667–4673.
96. Sale GE, Marmont P. Marrow mast cell counts do not predict bone marrow graft rejection. *Hum Pathol* 1981;12:605–608.
97. Koeppen H, Newell K, Baunoch DA, et al. Morphologic bone marrow changes in patients with posttransplantation lymphoproliferative disorders. *Am J Surg Pathol* 1998;22:208–214.
98. Orazi A, Hromas RA, Neiman RS, et al. Posttransplantation lymphoproliferative disorders in bone marrow transplant recipients are aggressive diseases with a high incidence of adverse histologic and immunobiologic features. *Am J Clin Pathol* 1997;107:419–429.
99. Davey DD, Kamat D, Laszewski M, et al. Epstein-Barr virus-related lymphoproliferative disorders following bone marrow transplantation: an immunologic and genotypic analysis. *Mod Pathol* 1989;2:27–34.
100. Craig FE, Gulley ML, Banks PM. Posttransplantation lymphoproliferative disorders. *Am J Clin Pathol* 1993;99:265–276.
101. Knowles DM, Cesarman E, Chadburn A, et al. Correlative morphologic and molecular genetic analysis demonstrates three distinct categories of posttransplantation lymphoproliferative disorders. *Blood* 1995;85:552–565.
102. Frank D, Cesarman E, Liu YF, et al. Posttransplantation lymphoproliferative disorders frequently contain type A and not type B Epstein-Barr virus. *Blood* 1995;85:1396–1403.
103. Swerdlow SH. Classification of the posttransplant lymphoproliferative disorders: from the past to the present. *Semin Diagn Pathol* 1997; 14:2–7.
104. Chadburn A, Cesarman E, Knowles DM. Molecular pathology of posttransplantation lymphoproliferative disorders. *Semin Diagn Pathol* 1997;14:15–26.
105. Deeg HJ, Socie G. Malignancies after hematopoietic stem cell transplantation: many questions, some answers. *Blood* 1998;91: 1833–1844.
106. Stone RM, Neuberg D, Soiffer R, et al. Myelodysplastic syndrome as a late complication following autologous bone marrow transplantation for non-Hodgkin's lymphoma. *J Clin Oncol* 1994;12:2535–2542.
107. Miller JS, Arthur DC, Litz CE, et al. Myelodysplastic syndrome after autologous bone marrow transplantation: an additional late complication of curative cancer therapy [see comments]. *Blood* 1994;83: 3780–3786.
108. Wilson CS, Traweek ST, Slovak ML, et al. Myelodysplastic syndrome occurring after autologous bone marrow transplantation for lymphoma; morphologic features. *Am J Clin Pathol* 1997;108:369–377.
109. Mach-Pascual S, Legare RD, Lu D, et al. Predictive value of clonality assays in patients with non-Hodgkin's lymphoma undergoing autologous bone marrow transplant: a single institution study. *Blood* 1998; 91:4496–4503.
110. Taylor PR, Jackson GH, Lennard AL, et al. Low incidence of myelodysplastic syndrome following transplantation using autologous non-cryopreserved bone marrow. *Leukemia* 1997;11:1650–1653.
111. Lones MA, Lopez-Terrada D, Shintaku IP, et al. Posttransplant lymphoproliferative disorder in pediatric bone marrow transplant recipients: disseminated disease of donor origin demonstrated by fluorescence in situ hybridization. Arch Pathol Lab Med 1998;122:708–714.
112. Hale G, Waldmann H. Risks of developing Epstein-Barr virus-related lymphoproliferative disorders after T-cell-depleted marrow transplants: CAMPATH Users. *Blood* 1998;91:3079–3083.
113. Antin JH. Graft-versus-leukemia: no longer an epiphenomenon [Editorial]. *Blood* 1993;82:2273–2277.
114. Minden MD, Messner HA, Belch A. Origin of leukemic relapse after bone marrow transplantation detected by restriction fragment length polymorphism. *J Clin Invest* 1985;75:91–93.
115. Witherspoon RP, Schubach W, Neiman P, et al. Donor cell leukemia developing six years after marrow grafting for acute leukemia. *Blood* 1985;65:1172–1174.
116. Brown SA, Bashey A, Schey SA. Donor cell leukaemia: an unresolved problem [Letter]. *Eur J Haematol* 1995;54:198–199.
117. Boiron JM, Cony-Makhoul P, Mahon FX, et al. Treatment of hematological malignancies relapsing after allogeneic bone marrow transplantation. *Blood Rev* 1994;8:234–240.
118. Ellis G, Ferguson M, Yamanaka E, et al. Monoclonal antibodies for detection of occult carcinoma cells in bone marrow of breast cancer patients. *Cancer* 1989;63:2509–2514.
119. Porro G, Menard S, Tagliabue E, et al. Monoclonal antibody detection of carcinoma cells in bone marrow biopsy specimens from breast cancer patients. *Cancer* 1988;61:2407–2411.
120. Leslie DS, Johnston WW, Daly L, et al. Detection of breast carcinoma cells in human bone marrow using fluorescence-activated cell sorting and conventional cytology. *Am J Clin Pathol* 1990;94:8–13.
121. van Dongen JJM, Adriaansen HJ. Immunobiology of leukemia. In: Henderson ES, Lister TA, Greaves MF, eds. *Leukemia, 6th ed.* Philadelphia: WB Saunders, 1996:83–130.
122. Campana D, Pui CH. Detection of minimal residual disease in acute leukemia: methodologic advances and clinical significance [see comments]. *Blood* 1995;85:1416–1434.
123. el-Rifai W, Ruutu T, Vettenranta K, et al. Minimal residual disease after allogeneic bone marrow transplantation for chronic myeloid leukaemia: a metaphase-FISH study. *Br J Haematol* 1996;92:365–369.
124. Dibenedetto SP, Lo Nigro L, Mayer SP, et al. Detectable molecular residual disease at the beginning of maintenance therapy indicates poor outcome in children with T-cell acute lymphoblastic leukemia. *Blood* 1997;90:1226–1232.
125. Kusec R, Laczika K, Knobl P, et al. AML1/ETO fusion mRNA can be detected in remission blood samples of all patients with t(8;21) acute myeloid leukemia after chemotherapy or autologous bone marrow transplantation. *Leukemia* 1994;8:735–739.
126. Vrazas V, Ooms LM, Rudduck C, et al. Application of interphase cytogenetics to monitor bone marrow transplants. *Am J Hematol* 1995; 49:15–20.
127. Maia DM, Kell DL, Goates JJ, et al. The significance of light chain-restricted bone marrow plasma cells after peripheral blood stem cell transplantation for multiple myeloma. *Am J Clin Pathol* 1997;107: 643–652.
128. van Belzen N, Hupkes PE, Doekharan D, et al. Detection of minimal disease using rearranged immunoglobulin heavy chain genes from intermediate- and high-grade malignant B cell non-Hodgkin's lymphoma. *Leukemia* 1997;11:1742–1752.
129. Steenbergen EJ, Verhagen OJ, van Leeuwen EF, et al. Prolonged persistence of PCR-detectable minimal residual disease after diagnosis or first relapse predicts poor outcome in childhood B-precursor acute lymphoblastic leukemia. *Leukemia* 1995;9:1726–1734.
130. Zwicky CS, Maddocks AB, Andersen N, et al. Eradication of polymerase chain reaction detectable immunoglobulin gene rearrangement in non-Hodgkin's lymphoma is associated with decreased relapse after autologous bone marrow transplantation. *Blood* 1996;88:3314–3322.
131. Uckun FM, Herman-Hatten K, Crotty ML, et al. Clinical significance of MLL-AF4 fusion transcript expression in the absence of a cytogenetically detectable t(4;11)(q21;q23) chromosomal translocation [see comments]. *Blood* 1998;92:810–821.
132. Kasprzyk A, Secker-Walker LM. Increased sensitivity of minimal residual disease detection by interphase FISH in acute lymphoblastic leukemia with hyperdiploidy. *Leukemia* 1997;11:429–435.

133. el-Rifai W, Ruutu T, Elonen E, et al. Prognostic value of metaphase-fluorescence in situ hybridization in follow-up of patients with acute myeloid leukemia in remission. *Blood* 1997;89:3330–3334.
134. Dewald GW, Wyatt WA, Juneau AL, et al. Highly sensitive fluorescence in situ hybridization method to detect double BCR/ABL fusion and monitor response to therapy in chronic myeloid leukemia. *Blood* 1998;91:3357–3365.
135. Tchirkov A, Giollant M, Tavernier F, et al. Interphase cytogenetics and competitive RT-PCR for residual disease monitoring in patients with chronic myeloid leukaemia during interferon-alpha therapy. *Br J Haematol* 1998;101:552–557.
136. Vettenranta K, Huhta T, Lindlof M, et al. Combined RT-PCR and metaphase-FISH posttransplant studies in pediatric patients with chronic myeloid leukemia. *J Pediatr Hematol Oncol* 1998;20: 108–111.
137. Farahat N, Morilla A, Owusu-Ankomah K, et al. Detection of minimal residual disease in B-lineage acute lymphoblastic leukaemia by quantitative flow cytometry. *Br J Haematol* 1998;101:158–164.
138. Gruhn B, Hongeng S, Yi H, et al. Minimal residual disease after intensive induction therapy in childhood acute lymphoblastic leukemia predicts outcome. *Leukemia* 1998;12:675–681.
139. Goulden NJ, Knechtli CJ, Garland RJ, et al. Minimal residual disease analysis for the prediction of relapse in children with standard-risk acute lymphoblastic leukaemia. *Br J Haematol* 1998;100:235–244.
140. Owen RG, Goulden NJ, Oakhill A, et al. Comparison of fluorescent consensus IgH PCR and allele-specific oligonucleotide probing in the detection of minimal residual disease in childhood ALL. *Br J Haematol* 1997;97:457–459.
141. Cave H, van der Werff ten Bosch J, Suciu S, et al. Clinical significance of minimal residual disease in childhood acute lymphoblastic leukemia: European Organization for Research and Treatment of Cancer–Childhood Leukemia Cooperative Group [see comments]. *N Engl J Med* 1998;339:591–598.
142. Jacquy C, Delepaut B, Van Daele S, et al. A prospective study of minimal residual disease in childhood B-lineage acute lymphoblastic leukaemia: MRD level at the end of induction is a strong predictive factor of relapse. *Br J Haematol* 1997;98:140–146.
143. Campana D. Applications of cytometry to study acute leukemia: in vitro determination of drug sensitivity and detection of minimal residual disease. *Cytometry* 1994;18:68–74.
144. Chan DW, Liang R, Kwong YL, Chan V. Detection of T-cell receptor delta gene rearrangement in T-cell malignancies by clonal specific polymerase chain reaction and its application to detect minimal residual disease. *Am J Hematol* 1996;52:171–177.
145. Galoin S, Al Saati T, Schlaifer D, et al. Oligonucleotide clonospecific probes directed against the junctional sequence of t(14;18): a new tool for the assessment of minimal residual disease in follicular lymphomas. *Br J Haematol* 1996;94:676–684.
146. Seriu T, Hansen-Hagge TE, Erz DH, et al. Improved detection of minimal residual leukemia through modifications of polymerase chain reaction analyses based on clonospecific T cell receptor junctions. *Leukemia* 1995;9:316–320.
147. Pichert G, Roy DC, Gonin R, et al. Distinct patterns of minimal residual disease associated with graft-versus-host disease after allogeneic bone marrow transplantation for chronic myelogenous leukemia. *J Clin Oncol* 1995;13:1704–1713.
148. Orfao A, Ciudad J, Lopez-Berges MC, et al. Acute lymphoblastic leukemia (ALL): detection of minimal residual disease (MRD) at flow cytometry. *Leuk Lymphoma* 1994;13:87–90.
149. Macon WR, Tham KT, Greer JP, et al. Ringed sideroblasts: a frequent observation after bone marrow transplantation. *Mod Pathol* 1995;8: 782–785.
150. Masat T, Feliu E, Tassies D, et al. Pseudo-Pelger-Huet anomaly after bone marrow transplantation [Letter]. *Hematol Pathol* 1991;5:89–91.

CHAPTER 51

Histiocytic and Dendritic Cell Proliferations

Lawrence M. Weiss

Histiocytes (macrophages) and dendritic cells are two of the major types of nonlymphoid mononuclear cells involved in immune and nonimmune inflammatory responses. They are involved to some extent in all of the reactive and neoplastic processes of lymphoid tissue. For example, histiocytes are a major component of the reactive infiltrate of Hodgkin's disease, and a well-developed network of follicular dendritic cells is a feature of follicular lymphoma. There are some diseases of lymphoid tissue, however, in which a histiocytic or dendritic cell proliferation is the major feature. After a brief review of normal histiocytes and dendritic cells, this chapter discusses the major histiocytic and dendritic cell proliferations.

NORMAL HISTIOCYTES AND DENDRITIC CELLS

An overview of the major phenotypes of histiocytes and dendritic cells is presented in Table 51.1 (see Chapters 2 and 3). Briefly, histiocytes are derived from hematopoietic stem cells, through myeloid progenitor cells, monocyte-macrophage progenitor cells, promonocytes, and monocytes (1). They express the surface markers HLA-DR, CD45, CD11c, CD13, CD14, CD15, MAC-387, and CD4, and their cytoplasm contains CD68 and lysozyme. They may be fixed, such as the Kupffer cells of the liver or tingible body macrophages of germinal centers, or freely mobile. Morphologically, they generally have bland nuclei and a moderate to marked amount of cytoplasm (epithelioid histiocytes), depending on their functional states. Ultrastructurally, histiocytes usually have numerous vacuoles, lysosomes, and residual bodies in their cytoplasm and often show numerous folds and microvillous projections. Cytochemically, the cells show reactivity for nonspecific esterase, acid phosphatase, and lysozyme (Fig. 51.1). They have specific receptors that react with various types of immunoglobulins, complement, glycoproteins, transferrin, lipoproteins, peptides, coagulation factors, hormones, and cytokines, including tumor necrosis factor family proteins, interleukin-1, interferon-γ, and granulocyte-macrophage colony-stimulating factor (2). They internalize substances by pinocytosis or phagocytosis, in general fusing the internalized vesicles with lysosomes (3). They respond to a number of chemotactic factors, including human (particularly C5a), and foreign substances, with motility supported by an actin-based cytoskeletal apparatus. They produce a wide range of substances, most notably enzymes (including lysozyme, neutral proteases, and acid hydrolases), complement factors, coagulation factors, reactive oxygen and nitrogen species, bioactive lipids, and numerous cytokines and growth factors. They mediate resistance to intracellular microorganisms and tumors through nonimmunologic mechanisms. They gain enhanced resistance to intracellular microorgansms through a process called *activation* that is induced by lymphokines, particularly interferon-γ. They also play an important role in the recognition and clearance of apoptotic cells.

Dendritic cells are characterized by a dendritic morphology and low levels of lysosomal enzymes and do not have the capacity for significant amounts of phagocytosis. Types of dendritic cells include Langerhans cells, indeterminate cells, veiled cells, interdigitating dendritic (interdigitating reticulum) cells, follicular dendritic (dendritic reticulum) cells, and dermal dendrocytes. Dendritic cells appear to comprise at least two lineages, including myeloid and lymphoid (4). Myeloid dendritic cells are derived from CD34-positive progenitors in the bone marrow that differentiate under stimulation from granulocyte-macrophage colony-stimulating factor, tumor necrosis factor-α, and other factors into immature dendritic cells (Langerhans cells). Langerhans cells possess characteristic organelles called Birbeck granules, racket- or rod-shaped structures of about 200 to 400 nm in length and about 33 nm in width, with an osmiophilic core and a double outer sheath (Fig. 51.2). Langerhans cells express CD45, CD1, and S-100 protein and possess a high level of ATPase but have only low levels of accessory molecules

L. M. Weiss: Division of Pathology, City of Hope National Medical Center, Duarte, California 91010

TABLE 51.1. *Phenotype of histiocytes and common dendritic cells*

	Histiocytes	Langerhans' cells	Interdigitating cells	Follicular dendritic cells
Adenosine triphosphatase	1+	2+	2+	2+
α-Naphthyl acetate esterase	2+	1+	1+	1+
CD45	2+	1+	1+	0
S-100 protein	0	2+	2+	1+
Fascin	0	0	2+	2+
HLA-DR	2+	2+	2+	1+
CD1	0	2+	0	0
R4/23	0	0	0	2+

2+, strong and constant labeling; 1+, weak or inconstant labeling; 0+, no labeling.

that mediate binding and stimulation of T cells (5,6). They have abundant major histocompatibility complex II products within intracellular compartments, which represent efficient antigen-processing and antigen-presentation machines. As these cells respond to inflammation-induced cytokines or microbial substances, they become mature dendritic cells with abundant surface major histocompatibility complex II. They lose their Birbeck granules and migrate through the tissue interstitium and lymph system (as veiled cells) to the paracortical region of lymph nodes. Indeterminate cells are dendritic cells of the dermis that are morphologically and antigenically similar to Langerhans cells with the exception that Birbeck granules are not identified (7). They express CD45, CD1, and S-100 protein and may represent either direct precursors or direct successors of Langerhans cells. In the paracortical region of the lymph node, having lost CD1 expression as well, they become interdigitating cells. These cells express CD45, S-100 protein, the actin-bundling protein fascin, and many macrophage antigens but lack complement receptors. Through surface major histocompatibility complex–peptide complexes, the expression of T cell–stimulatory molecules (such as CD40 and CD86), and the secretion of an array of chemokines, interdigitating cells are responsible for the initiation of strong cellular immunity. Their ultimate fate is cell death by apoptosis, accompanied by their phagocytosis and processing by lymphoid dendritic cells.

An alternate pathway has been proposed for myeloid dendritic cells. In this hypothesis, a CD34-positive, CD45-negative marrow cell or a CD14-positive peripheral blood monocyte, under the influence of granulocyte-macrophage colony-stimulating factor, tumor necrosis factor-α, and interleukin-4, differentiates into a mature dendritic cell that may circulate in the blood or home to the peripheral interstitial spaces (a subset of which may be factor XIIIa–positive) or sites of inflammation. The dermal dendrocyte (dermal dendrophage or perivascular dermal dendrocytic cell), a dendritic cell normally present in the perivascular area of the

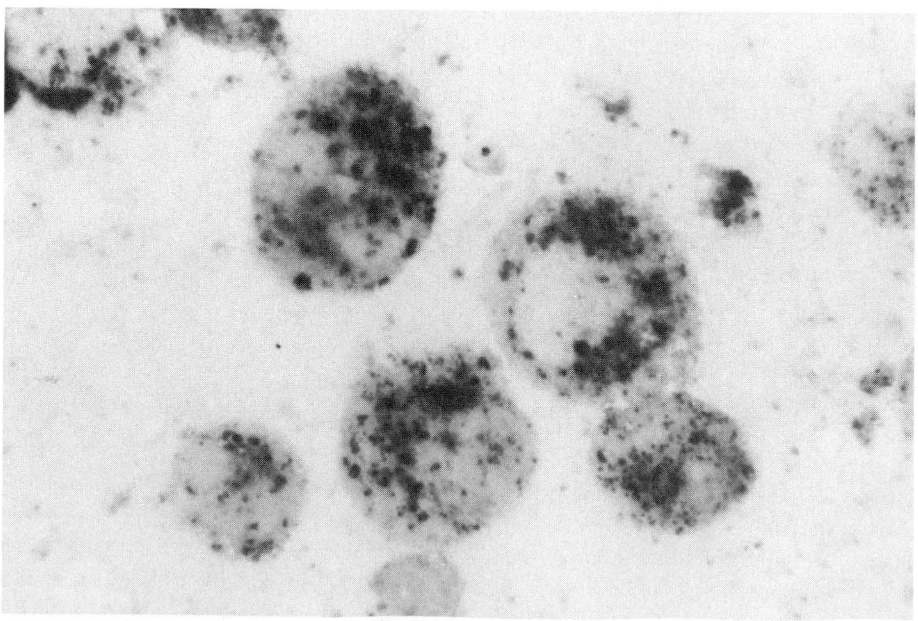

FIG. 51.1. Touch preparation showing histiocytes reactive for acid phosphatase (original magnification: 1,000× magnification). (Courtesy of Chae Koo, M.D.)

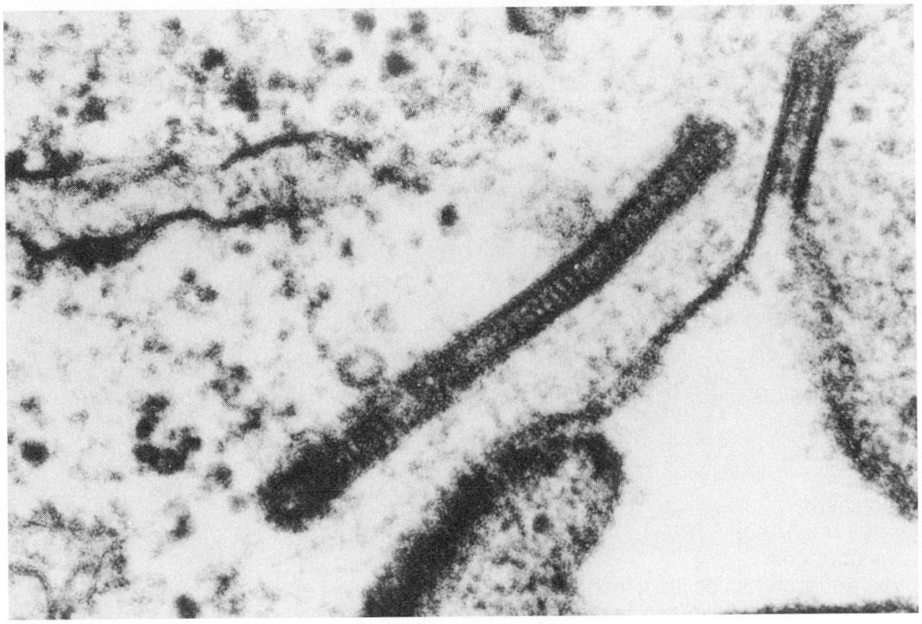

FIG. 51.2. Characteristic Birbeck granule, with a "zipper"-like appearance.

papillary dermis, may represent an example of such a cell. It has a phenotype distinct from both indeterminate cells and Langerhans cells, expressing factor XIIIa and CD68 but negative for S-100 protein and markers for follicular dendritic cells (8). It is thought that these cells have a role in humoral immunity. It is even possible that these cells are the precursors of follicular dendritic cells.

A second major lineage of dendritic cells is the lymphoid dendritic cells. These cells are derived from lymphoid-committed bone marrow stem cells that migrate to the thymic medulla and, under the influence of interleukin-3, differentiate into dendritic cells that migrate to the lymph node (9). The dendritic cells may arrive through high endothelial venules as plasmacytoid T cells. With further maturation, these lymphoid dendritic cells are thought to reside in the T-cell areas and may be indistinguishable from myeloid-derived interdigitating cells. These cells may be responsible for immune tolerance through immune regulation or deletion, through their uptake of self-peptides captured by the uptake of apoptotic myeloid dendritic cells.

Although originally thought to be of non–bone marrow origin, follicular dendritic cells now are thought to be derived from mononuclear cells expressing KIM-4 (a marker of follicular dendritic cells) that may be found in the bone marrow and peripheral blood (10). More proximally, follicular dendritic cells are thought to derive from antigen-transporting cells found in afferent lymph and the subcapsular sinuses of lymph nodes. Follicular dendritic cells form a reticulum meshwork within germinal centers, retaining immune complexes on their cell surface. They are multinucleate cells with long branching cell processes that form desmosomal attachments. They express several macrophage and B-lineage markers in addition to a cell specific antigen recognized by monoclonal antibodies R4/23, KIM-4, and BU-10 (11). They lack CD45 but express the complement receptors CD21 and CD35. They are involved intimately in memory cell formation and affinity maturation of follicle B cells.

An additional cell type, the fibroblastic reticular cell, plays a role in stromal support but has no proven role in the immune system. This cell is located in the parafollicular area and deep cortex of lymph nodes, and ultrastructural studies have demonstrated an association with the reticular network (12,13). Fibroblastic reticular cells are not derived from the bone marrow but have ultrastructural and immunohistochemical features of myofibroblasts (12–15) (see Chapter 6).

CLASSIFICATION OF HISTIOCYTIC AND DENDRITIC CELL PROLIFERATIONS

A brief classification of the histiocytic and dendritic cell proliferations discussed in this chapter is given in Table 51.2, and the classification of histiocytic and dendritic cell neoplasms given in the recently proposed World Health Organization classification is given in Table 51.3. Any proposed classification of these proliferations is by necessity arbitrary. First, one must decide what entities to include. An all-encompassing classification might include the storage disorders and inflammatory or infectious disorders such as tuberculosis or sarcoidosis; however, these entities have been omitted from this chapter. Furthermore, it is not always possible to pigeonhole an entity's biologic behavior. For example, although most cases of sinus histiocytosis with massive lymphadenopathy (SHML) are localized and show spontaneous resolution, a minority of patients have an aggressive presentation with multiple sites involved. Third, the precise cell of origin is not known for all entities. In SHML, although

TABLE 51.2. *Classification of histiocytic and dendritic cell proliferations*

Benign histiocytic proliferations
Sinus hyperplasia
Sinus histiocytosis with massive lymphadenopathy
Infection-associated hemophagocytic syndrome
Familial hemophagocytic lymphohistiocytosis
Malignant lymphoma with benign erythrophagocytosis
Hepatosplenic $\gamma\delta$ T-cell lymphoma (erythrophagocytic Tγ lymphoma)
Histiocytic necrotizing lymphadenitis
Benign dendritic cell proliferations
Dermatopathic lymphadenitis
Borderline and malignant dendritic cell proliferations
Juvenile and adult xanthogranuloma
Langerhans cell histiocytosis
Follicular dendritic cell sarcoma
Interdigitating cell sarcoma
Indeterminate cell neoplasm
Fibroblastic reticular cell neoplasm
Malignant histiocytic proliferations
Malignant histiocytosis and true histiocytic lymphoma
Malignant histiocytosis associated with mediastinal germ cell tumor
(Histiocytic medullary reticulosis)
(Regressing atypical histiocytosis)

TABLE 51.3. *Classification of histiocytic and dendritic cell neoplasms proposed in the World Health Organization classification (118)*

Dendritic cell neoplasms
Langerhans cell histiocytosis
Langerhans cell sarcoma
Interdigitating dendritic cell sarcoma or tumor
Follicular dendritic cell sarcoma or tumor
Dendritic cell sarcoma, not otherwise specified
Macrophage or histiocytic neoplasm
Histiocytic sarcoma

the light microscopic appearance is more in keeping with an origin from sinus histiocytes, the immunologic findings are conflicting, with a hybrid phenotype between histiocytes and dendritic cells seen. Finally, many entities thought previously to be histiocytic or dendritic in origin have been found on more comprehensive analysis to be better classified with the lymphoid proliferations.

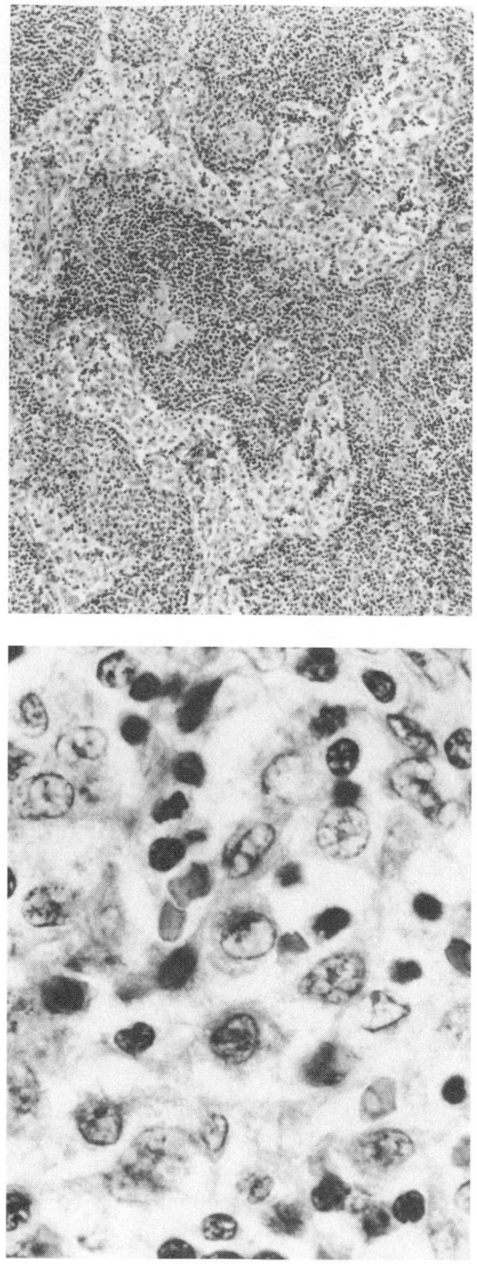

A

B

FIG. 51.3. Sinus hyperplasia. **A:** Dilated sinuses are seen (original magnification: 200× magnification). **B:** The sinuses are seen to be filled with bland histiocytic cells (original magnification: 600× magnification).

BENIGN HISTIOCYTIC PROLIFERATIONS

Sinus Hyperplasia

Sinus hyperplasia is so common that it is perhaps best regarded as a physiologic state rather than a pathologic condition. It is often prominent in lymph nodes draining the extremities as well as in the mesenteric region. It also may occur in lymph nodes draining sites of malignant neoplasms or prostheses (16). Histologically, one sees prominent lymph node sinuses distended by histiocytes with cytologically bland nuclei and abundant cytoplasm (Fig. 51.3). Rarely, the histiocytes have signet-ring features (17,18). Erythrophagocytosis may be present (17) (see Chapter 15).

Sinus Histiocytosis with Massive Lymphadenopathy

Sinus histiocytosis with massive lymphadenopathy is a rare proliferative histiocytic disorder of unknown cause only recognized since the 1960s (18–20). Although usually benign and limited to lymph nodes, the disease may involve extranodal sites. The eponym *Rosai-Dorfman disease* often has been applied to SHML, especially in the context of extranodal disease. SHML has been the subject of a recent review of over 400 cases, to which the reader is referred for a more comprehensive coverage of the subject (21).

Clinically, the patients have a median age of 20 years but a wide range of ages, from neonates presenting with congenital disease to the elderly (21). There is a male : female ratio of about 4:3, and blacks may be affected more frequently than whites. Two pairs of identical twins have developed SHML within an interval of 5 years. A minority of patients has concomitant evidence of an immune-mediated disease (22). The disease usually presents as isolated cervical lymphadenopathy, often dramatic in size (Fig. 51.4). Other lymph node groups may be involved, including axillary, inguinal, and mediastinal nodes, either alone or in conjunction with cervical disease. Fever, weight loss, malaise, joint symptoms, and night sweats may be present, but hepatosplenomegaly is not a common occurrence.

Abnormal results of laboratory studies often found in these patients include a mild normochromic and normocytic or hypochromic and microcytic anemia. A minority of patients have red cell autoantibodies, sometimes manifesting as severe hemolytic anemia. The peripheral white blood cell count is usually normal, although a reversal in the CD4 : CD8 ratio often is found. Serum protein levels are often abnormal, with a decrease in the albumin level and polyclonal elevations in IgG, IgM, or IgA levels sometimes present. The erythrocyte sedimentation rate usually is elevated. Some patients have tested positive for rheumatoid factor or produced a positive lupus erythematosus cell preparation. No consistent lymphocyte, granulocyte, or histiocyte abnormalities have been found, and lipid studies are normal.

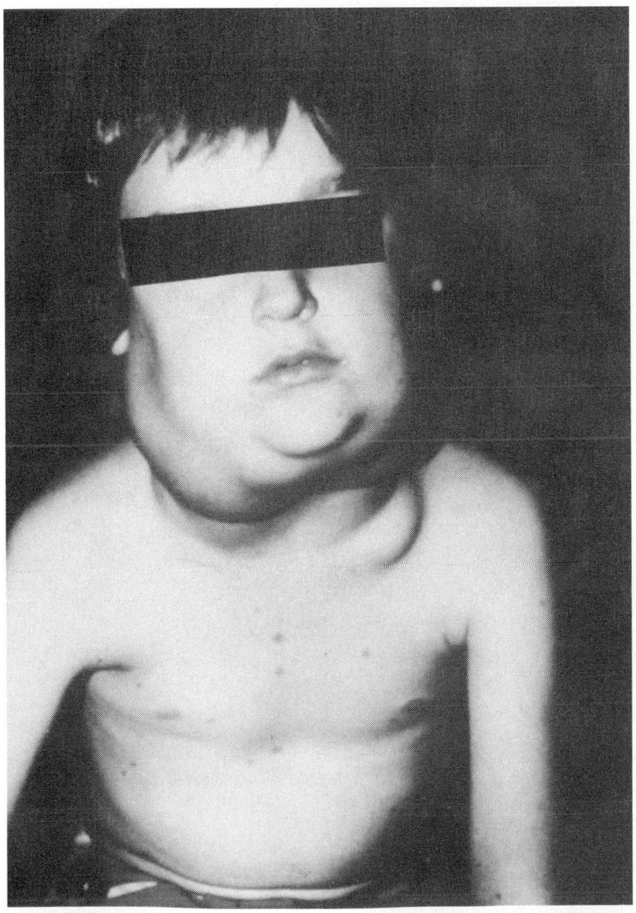

FIG. 51.4. Patient with sinus histiocytosis with massive lymphadenopathy. Massive cervical lymphadenopathy is present. Also note the cutaneous lesions. (Courtesy of Ronald Dorfman, M.D., Stanford University Medical Center.)

On gross examination, involved lymph nodes usually are enlarged. The cut surface of the node usually is described as yellow-white, with either a nodular or diffuse architecture. The histologic features are distinctive. On low-power examination, the lymph node capsule is often fibrotic, although in contrast to Hodgkin's disease, the fibrosis does not extend into the lymph node parenchyma. The most striking feature in most patients is a marked dilatation of the sinuses (Fig. 51.5). At high magnification, this expansion is found to be a result of the abundance of cells that are characteristic of this disease (Figs. 51.6, 51.7). These cells have an intermediate-sized nucleus with a vesicular chromatin pattern and one to several nucleoli. Cytologic atypia is usually lacking but is present in some patients. These cells generally have a voluminous cytoplasm, amphophilic to eosinophilic in hematoxylin and eosin stains, which often contains well-preserved lymphocytes (often termed *lymphophagocytosis* or *emperipolesis*) (Fig. 51.8). Less often, plasma cells, neutrophils, and red blood cells are found within the cell cytoplasm. Sometimes, the characteristic cells may possess a foamy cytoplasmic appearance. Plasma cells are often numerous, both within the sinuses and especially within the intervening cords (Fig. 51.9). Germinal centers are usually present, although they are not generally a prominent feature. Rarely, diffuse effacement of lymph node architecture is seen.

The histologic differential diagnosis of SHML in lymph nodes mainly involves benign sinus hyperplasia on the one hand and sinusoidal malignancies on the other. In benign sinus hyperplasia, the expansion of sinuses usually is less marked than in SHML and, more importantly, the characteristic cells of SHML with their usually prominent lymphophagocytosis are not present. Malignancies involving the sinuses, such as metastatic carcinoma and malignant melanoma, as well as sinusoidal malignant lymphoma can be distinguished from SHML by attention to the cytologic features of the proliferating cells. In SHML the degree of cytologic atypia is usually not marked. Langerhans cell histiocytosis (LCH; also known as *histiocytosis X*) also may have an appearance on low-power examination similar to SHML. Recognition of the cytologic characteristics of the proliferating Langerhans cells as well as the usual accompanying eosinophils enables distinction.

Involvement of extranodal sites occurs in approximately 40% of patients (21). This involvement usually is seen in conjunction with lymph node involvement, although SHML

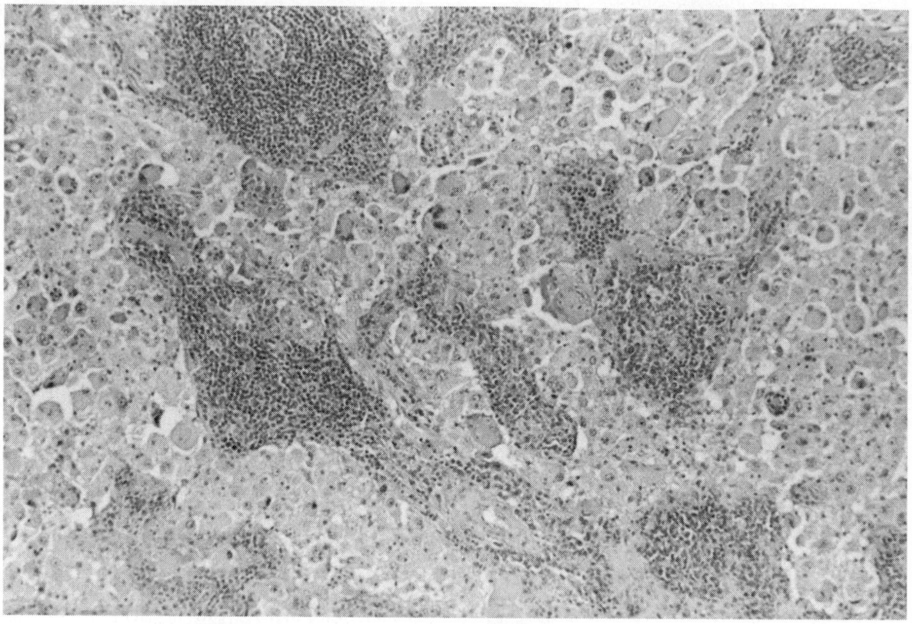

FIG. 51.5. Sinus histiocytosis with massive lymphadenopathy. A distinct sinusoidal pattern of involvement is seen (original magnification: 200× magnification).

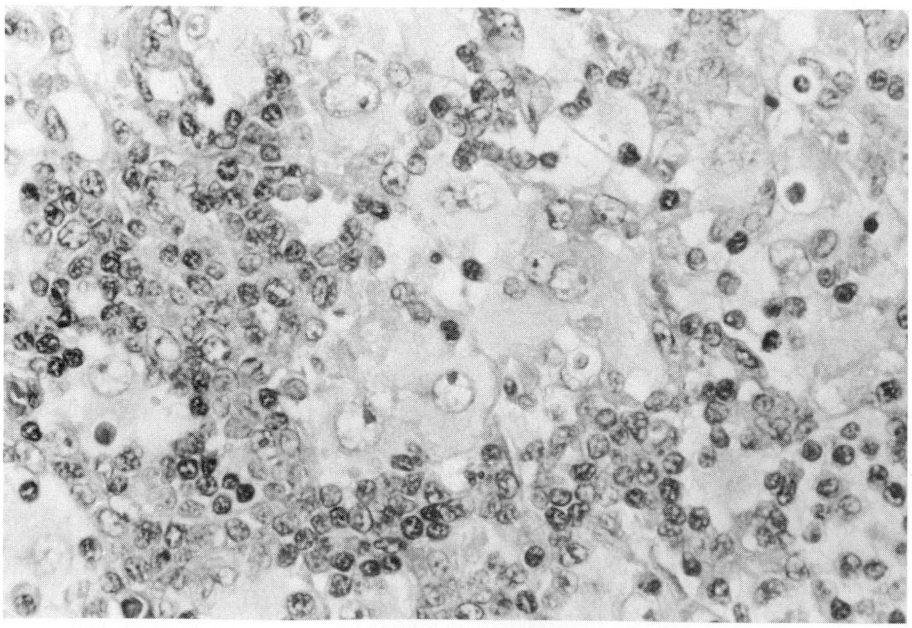

FIG. 51.6. Sinus histiocytosis with massive lymphadenopathy. The characteristic cells have abundant cytoplasm and medium-sized nuclei with one to several prominent nucleoli (original magnification: 600× magnification).

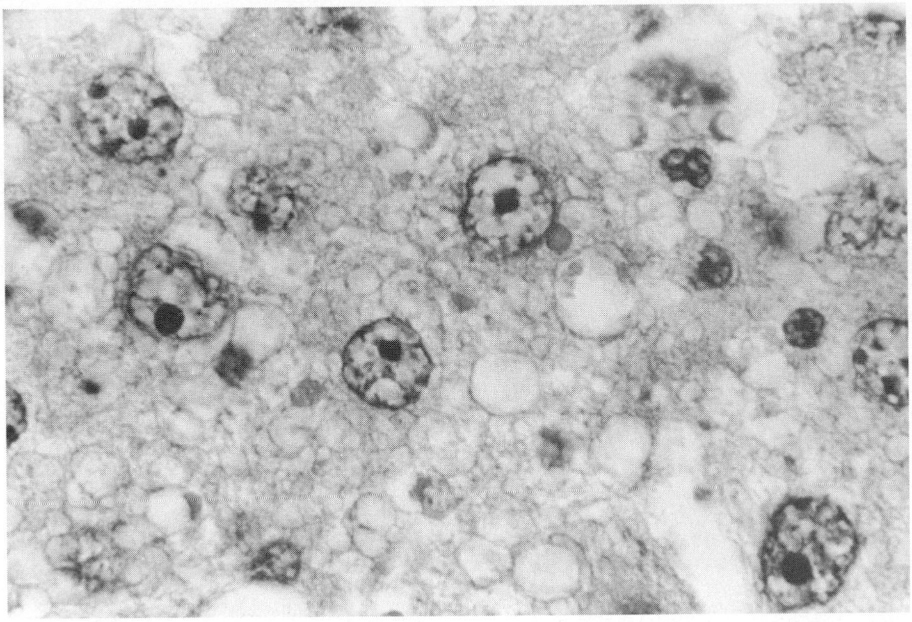

FIG. 51.7. Sinus histiocytosis with massive lymphadenopathy. The cells show the characteristic appearance. Occasional phagocytosis is seen (original magnification: 1,000× magnification).

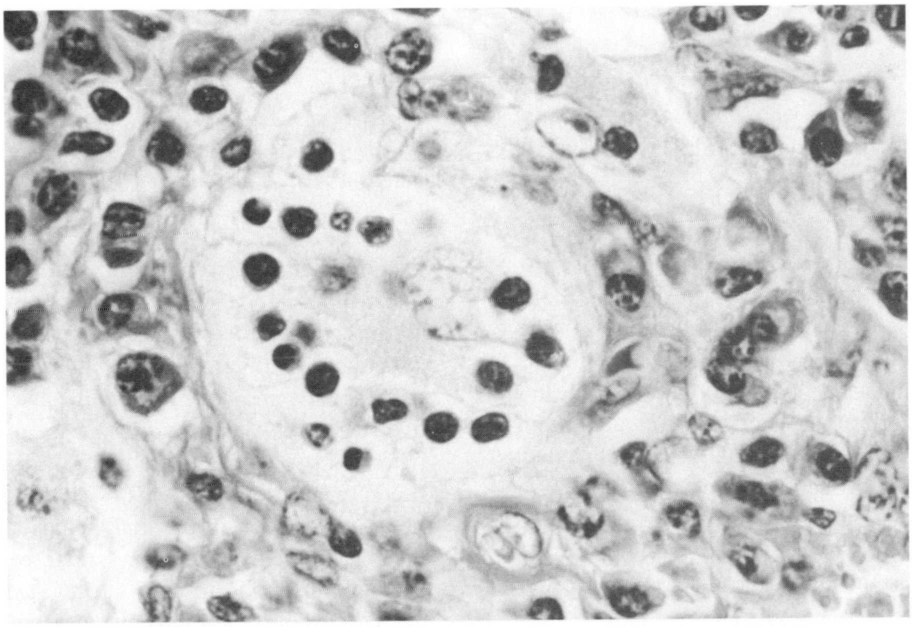

FIG. 51.8. Sinus histiocytosis with massive lymphadenopathy. This cell shows prominent lymphophagocytosis. Note the plasma cells around it (original magnification: 1,000× magnification).

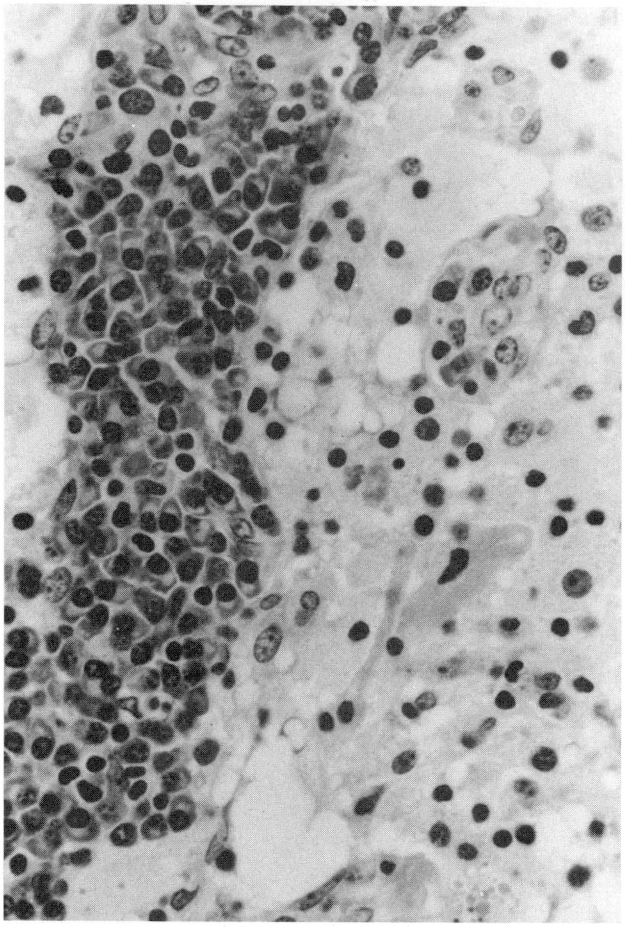

FIG. 51.9. Sinus histiocytosis with massive lymphadenopathy. The cords contain numerous plasma cells (original magnification: 600× magnification).

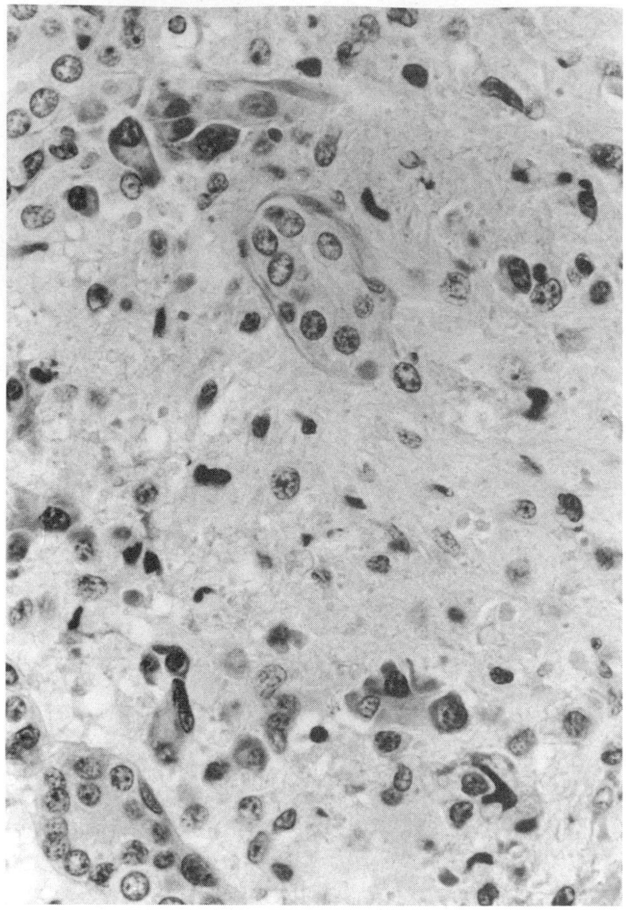

FIG. 51.10. Sinus histiocytosis with massive lymphadenopathy involving the salivary gland. Isolated ducts are seen surrounded by the proliferating histiocytes (original magnification: 600× magnification).

occasionally affects extranodal tissues alone. As seen in Table 51.4, many different sites may be involved. The histologic findings in these sites are usually strikingly similar to those seen in lymph nodes (Fig. 51.10), even to the extent of having the appearance of dilated sinuses at times. The degree of fibrosis is generally greater, however, and the number of the characteristic cells is usually smaller and their prominence less than that seen in lymph nodes.

It is likely that the majority of patients with SHML undergo spontaneous remission (21,23). Another large group of patients has persistent but stable disease not requiring

TABLE 51.4. *Extranodal organs commonly involved by sinus histiocytosis with massive lymphadenopathy, in order of frequency (21)*

Skin
Sinonasal region
Soft tissues
Orbit
Bone
Salivary gland
Central nervous system

therapy. Some patients require additional surgery beyond initial biopsy for the alleviation of obstruction or cosmetic reasons. Chemotherapy has been administered to a minority of patients. Although a combination of vinca alkaloid, alkylating agents, and corticosteroids appears to be most effective, the response rates are inferior to those seen in most other hematolymphoid neoplasms. Radiation therapy has been given to some patients, with response rates again inferior to those seen in the malignant lymphomas. A few patients have died, either from SHML or with SHML significantly contributing to their death (21–24). Patients with an aggressive course tend to have involvement of a larger number of lymph node groups and a larger number of extranodal sites. Many of these patients also have evidence of immunologic abnormalities.

The nature of the proliferating cells in SHML still has not been clarified completely. Ultrastructural studies have demonstrated the presence of lipid vacuoles and varying numbers of lysosomes in the cytoplasm as well as complex filopodia, suggesting a histiocytic character. Birbeck granules are absent. Histochemical studies have demonstrated the presence of neutral fat and diastase-resistant material that

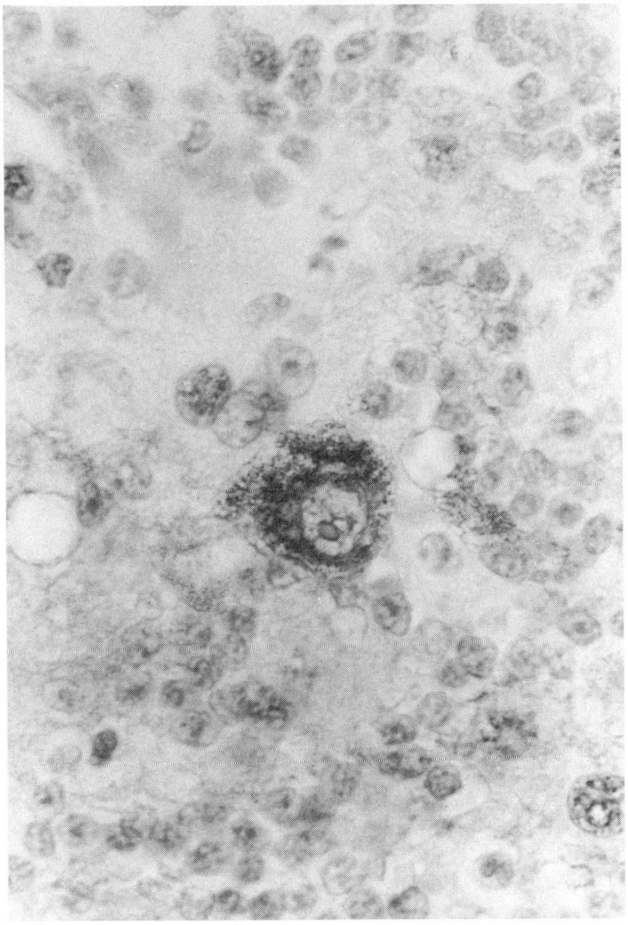

FIG. 51.11. Sinus histiocytosis with massive lymphadenopathy. This S-100 protein stain shows the atypical histiocyte in the center to be positive, characteristic for this disease (original magnification: 600× magnification).

is positive with periodic acid–Schiff staining in the cytoplasm, and reactions for acid phosphatase, α-naphthyl acetate, and α-butyrate esterase are additional evidence supporting a histiocytic differentiation (25,26).

Immunoperoxidase studies on paraffin sections have shown that the cells of SHML express S-100 protein, lysozyme, α_1-antitrypsin, α_1-antichymotrypsin, and the macrophage-specific markers HAM-56 and MAC-387 (27) (Fig. 51.11). They are also positive for the aspartic proteinases cathepsin D (expressed in macrophages) and cathepsin E (expressed in antigen-processing cells), a finding similar to the Langerhans cells of LCH (28). Expression of CD30 (the Ki-1 antigen) is seen in one half of patients (27). Frozen-section immunoperoxidase studies have demonstrated expression of numerous macrophage and macrophage-associated antigens, including several antigens not found on interdigitating dendritic cells. In addition, the cells of SHML lack expression of the CD1 antigen found on Langerhans cells and reactivity with R4/23, a monoclonal antibody specific for follicular dendritic cells. Gene rearrangement studies have shown a germline configuration for both the immunoglobulin heavy chain gene and the β gene of the T-cell receptor (26). All of the evidence to date supports a relationship between the cells of SHML and the histiocytic lineage. Because normal sinus histiocytes lack the S-100 protein, however, S-100 protein expression by the cells of SHML does not support a close relationship with these cells and may suggest some relationship to dendritic cells. Regardless of the lineage, it has been demonstrated, using X-linked polymorphic loci, that SHML is a polyclonal rather than a monoclonal proliferation and probably represents a reactive rather than a neoplastic process (29). At least two groups have reported finding evidence of human herpesvirus-6 in SHML (30,31). In one study, the late antigen p101K was found in follicular dendritic cells of germinal centers, and the late antigen gp106 exhibited an intense cytoplasmic positivity in the atypical histiocytes (31). There is no association with the Epstein-Barr virus (32).

Infection-Associated Hemophagocytic Syndrome

Infection-associated hemophagocytic syndrome (IAHS), also called *reactive hemophagocytic syndrome*, is a nonneoplastic, potentially reversible systemic proliferation of cytologically benign histiocytes. Although originally described in association with viral infections, particularly cytomegalovirus and other herpesviruses (33), it is now evident that this disease is found in association with many types of infectious agents. Gram-positive and gram-negative bacteria, mycobacteria, fungi, and Leishmaniasis organisms all have been associated with this histiocytic reaction (34,35). About one half of reported cases have occurred in Asian patients (36). It is thought that IAHS is a manifestation of an impaired immune response to an infectious process. Many but not all patients have documented immunodeficiency. It is possible that those patients without an obvious immunodeficiency who develop IAHS have a subtle deficit, possibly specific for particular types of infectious agents (35). Dysfunction of cellular cytotoxity, specifically an acquired defect in natural killer cell activity, is suspected, and lymphocyte hyperactivation also may play a role, although not more than 10% of peripheral lymphocytes express an activated phenotype (36). Interferon-γ has been shown to be a sensitive indicator of disease activity (37).

Patients who present with IAHS generally fall into one of two main categories: those without evidence of an apparent underlying disease, generally children, and those with a history of immunosuppression, including all age groups. Patients usually present with a severe systemic illness, including fever and other constitutional symptoms, and often also have hepatosplenomegaly, lymphadenopathy, a skin rash, and bilateral pulmonary infiltrates. Often, there is a prodrome of a viral-like illness several weeks before the occurrence of severe symptomatology. Laboratory evaluation usually reveals pancytopenia, liver function abnormalities, and abnormal coagulation parameters, generally characterized by prolonged partial thromboplastin and thrombin times with normal to prolonged prothrombin times. The Epstein-Barr virus is the triggering organism in the majority of patients.

The most striking findings are present in the hematolymphoid organs. Involved lymph nodes generally show an intact architecture, with numerous histiocytes present in the sinusoids and within the paracortical areas (Figs. 51.12, 51.13). The histiocytes lack cytologic atypia and often show prominent platelet phagocytosis and hematophagocytosis. Germinal centers are not generally prominent, and the lymph node often shows an overall cell-depleted appearance. The differential diagnosis generally centers on the distinction of IAHS from hematolymphoid neoplasms involving the sinuses as well as hematolymphoid neoplasms secondarily inducing benign hemophagocytosis. The former distinction generally is based on the cytologic characteristics of the proliferating cells. The histiocytes are cytologically benign in IAHS; atypicality of the proliferating cells should be evident in hematolymphoid malignancies. In some patients this distinction can be quite difficult. Repeat biopsies sometimes may allow resolution of the problem (38). Some lymphomas, particularly T-cell neoplasms, may induce an exuberant hyperplasia of benign-appearing hemophagocytizing lymphocytes (39,40). Attention to the other elements in the biopsy specimen besides the benign histiocytes is important in identifying these cases.

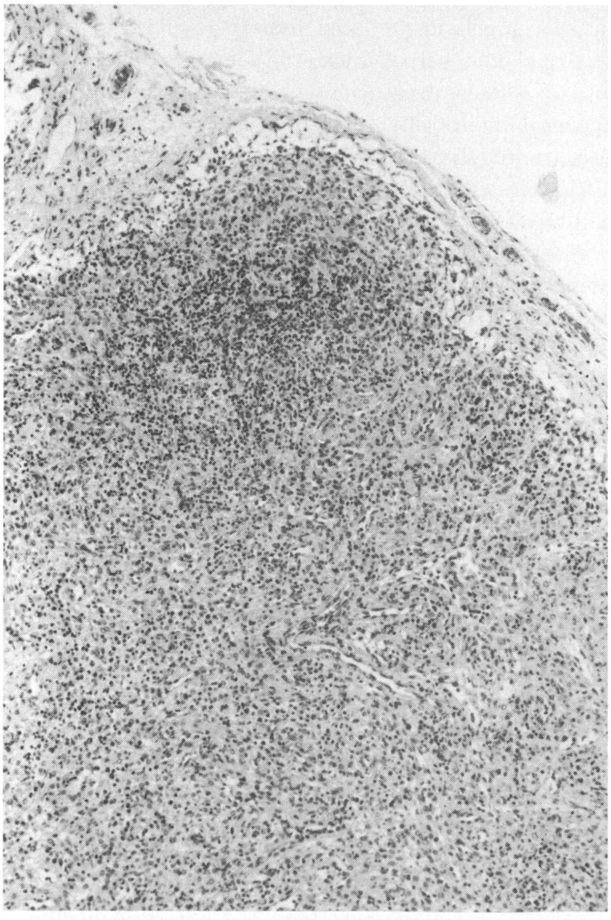

FIG. 51.12. Infection-associated hemophagocytic syndrome. At low-power magnification, a lymphocyte depleted appearance is seen (original magnification: 100× magnification).

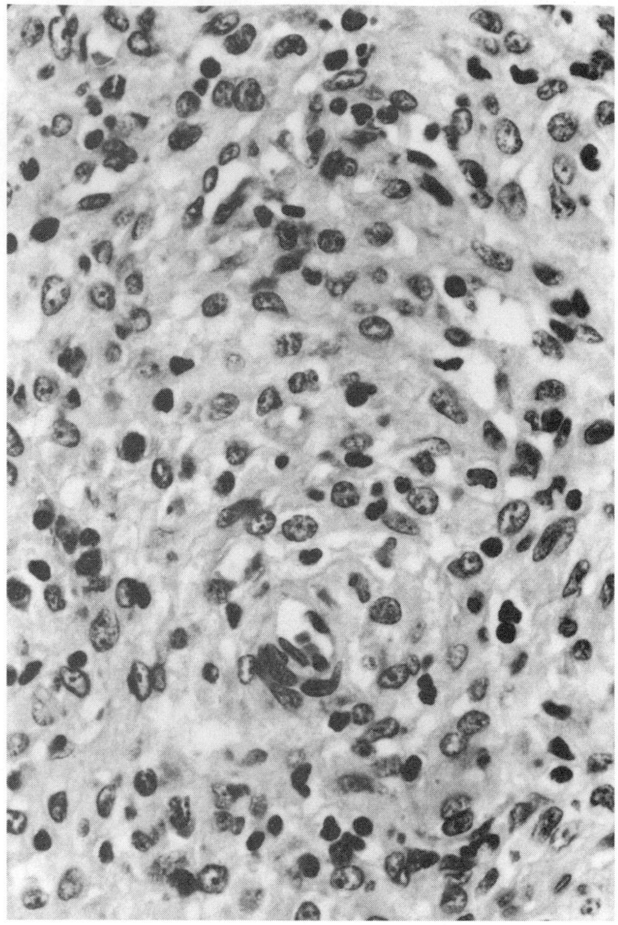

FIG. 51.13. Infection-associated hemophagocytic syndrome. At high-power magnification, numerous histiocytes are seen (original magnification: 400× magnification).

The bone marrow in IAHS usually shows hypocellularity with a decrease in the erythropoietic and granulopoietic lines, but with normal or increased numbers of megakaryocytes. Moderate to marked histiocytic hyperplasia is usually present. Again, the histiocytes are cytologically benign and often show prominent phagocytosis. Platelet and erythrophagocytosis generally predominates, but phagocytosis of other cellular debris often also is seen. A negative bone marrow examination, however, does not rule out the diagnosis (41). Histiocytic hyperplasia also may be seen in the liver and spleen. In the liver, both sinusoidal and portal areas may be involved and a lymphoid hyperplasia usually also is seen (Fig. 51.14); in the spleen, the red pulp is affected preferentially by hemophagocytosis, and lymphoid depletion is usually present. Rarely, nodular lesions may be seen. Other organs that may be involved include the thymus, lungs, and intestine.

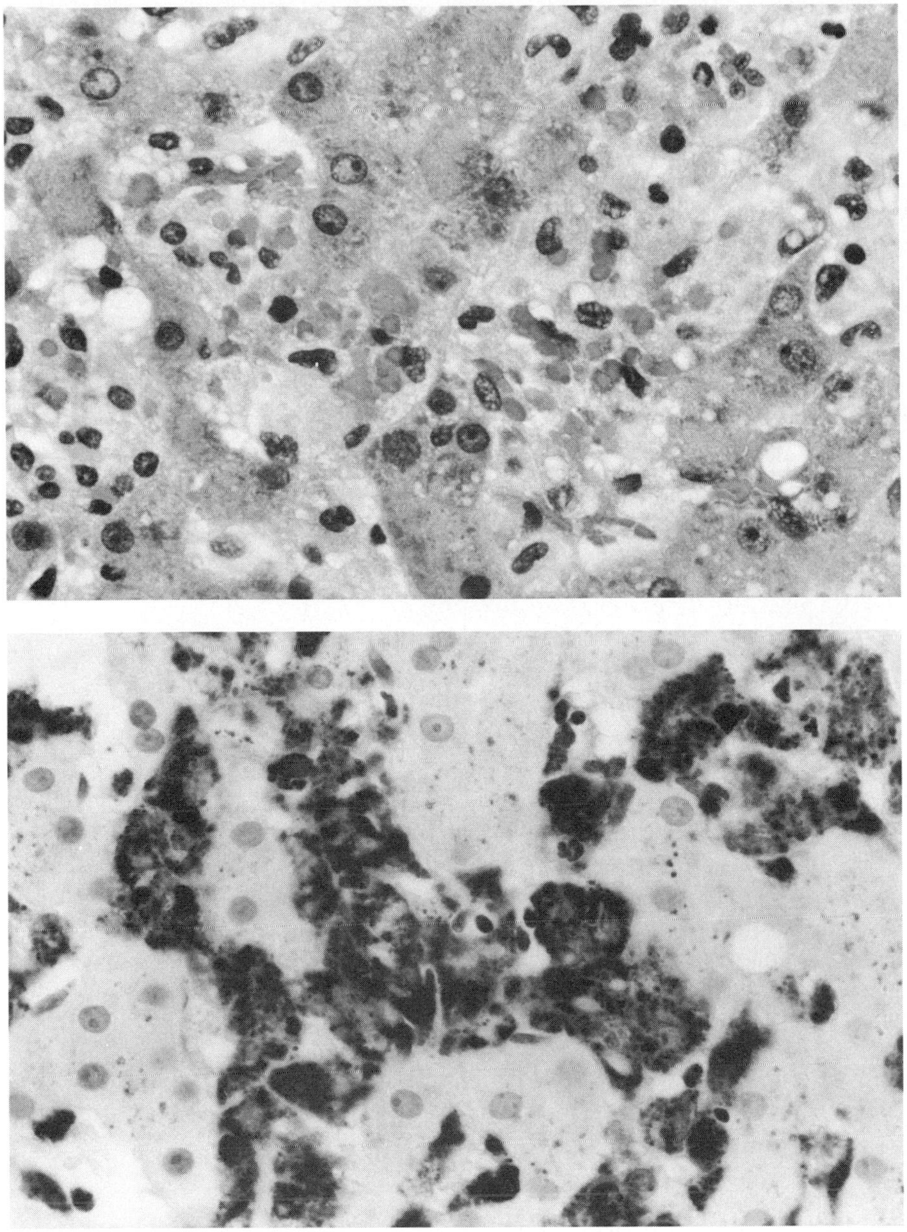

FIG. 51.14. Infection-associated hemophagocytic syndrome. **Top:** Numerous histiocytes exhibiting erythrophagocytosis are seen. **Bottom:** CD68 stain, confirming the histiocytic differentiation of the cells (original magnification: 600× magnification).

Infection-associated hemophagocytic syndrome is a benign, self-limited condition from which the patient may recover completely. About one half of these patients, however, dies with the disease, because of multisystem failure during the acute episode or infectious complications exacerbated by the underlying immunodeficiency that often exists. IAHS triggered by bacterial infections is associated with a relatively high recovery rate; the worst prognosis is found in Epstein-Barr virus infection (about a 25% survival rate).

There is no way to distinguish reliably between IAHS and familial hemophagocytic lymphohistiocytosis; many patients with familial hemophagocytic lymphohistiocytosis present with a syndrome indistinguishable from IAHS in those patients who have no known family history of the disorder (41).

Familial Hemophagocytic Lymphohistiocytosis

Familial hemophagocytic lymphohistiocytosis is an extremely rare, usually fatal disease of early childhood marked by multiorgan involvement with lymphohistiocytic infiltrates (42,43). The onset of disease, usually fever, pancytopenia, and hepatosplenomegaly, is within the first year of life in most patients (44,45), and almost always in the first 7 years (41). There is a slight male predominance. The disease occurs in all ethnic groups and is familial in about one half to three fourths of patients. In this latter group, the disease appears to be inherited as an autosomal recessive trait, and parental consanguinity is often present (41,43). The estimated overall 5-year survival rate is about 20%, but it is 66% for those patients who receive allogeneic bone marrow

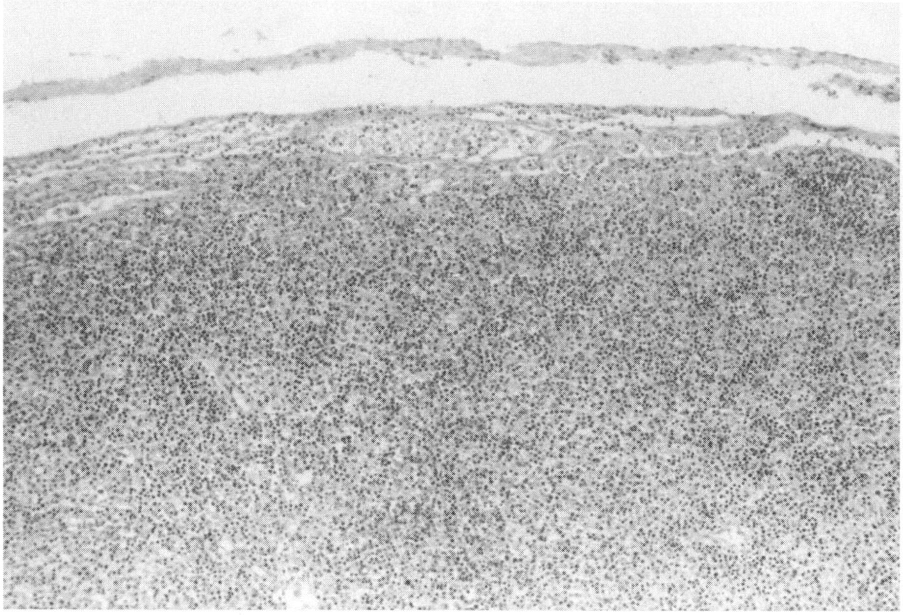

FIG. 51.15. Familial hemophagocytic lymphohistiocytosis. Similar to infection-associated hemophagocytic syndrome, a lymphocyte-depleted appearance is seen in lymph node biopsies (original magnification: 100× magnification).

transplant, in contrast to 10% for patients treated with chemotherapy alone.

The organs affected are most frequently the lymph nodes and bone marrow and less frequently the spleen, liver, and central nervous system (46). Involved lymph nodes generally show cellular depletion and distortion of the architecture by infiltrates consisting of histiocytes accompanied by lymphocytes and often also plasma cells (Fig. 51.15). The histiocytes are cytologically bland and display prominent erythrophagocytosis and often lymphophagocytosis and phagocytosis of other cellular debris as well (Fig. 51.16). Examination of the bone marrow usually reveals a hypercellular specimen with erythroid hyperplasia and myeloid hypoplasia. The most prominent finding is diffuse infiltration by cytologically bland histiocytes displaying variable degrees of erythrophagocytosis, although this may be found in fewer than

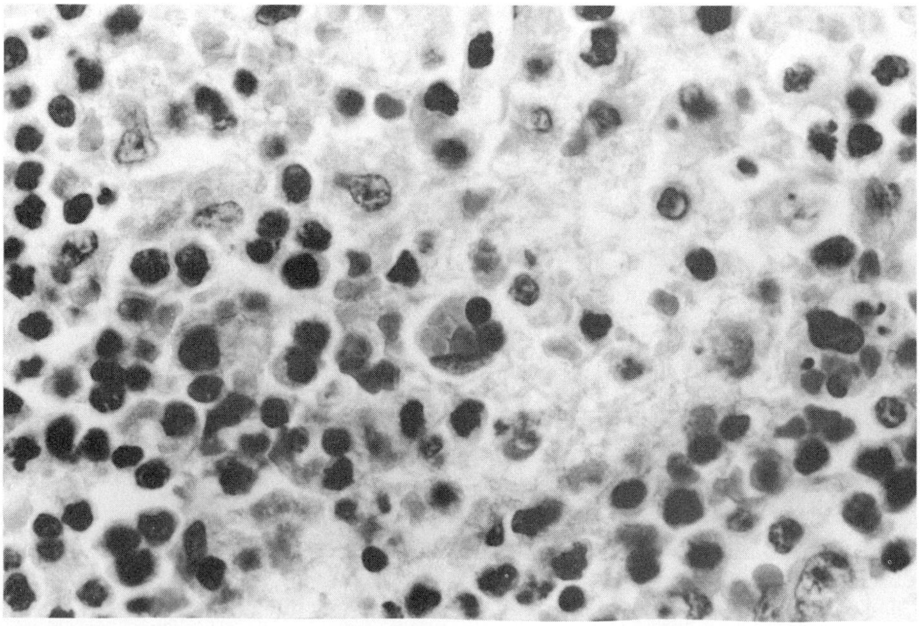

FIG. 51.16. Familial hemophagocytic lymphohistiocytosis. Numerous histiocytes, including several with erythrophagocytosis, are present (original magnification: 600× magnification).

half the patients (41,45). The spleen shows involvement of the red pulp and the liver shows sinusoidal involvement by a similar infiltrate. The central nervous system, if involved, shows diffuse infiltration of the leptomeninges and infiltration of perivascular spaces within the brain parenchyma, particularly the white matter.

Histochemically, the proliferating cells express acid phosphatase, nonspecific esterase, and lysozyme, consistent with a histiocytic derivation (45). Immunophenotypic studies have shown that the histiocytic cells express CD14 and HLA-DR, with variable expression of CD15, again consistent with tissue histiocytes (47). The cells are negative for S-100 protein and CD1 and do not show Birbeck's granules on ultrastructural examination, evidence against a dendritic cell lineage.

The exact nature of familial hemophagocytic lymphohistiocytosis has not been clarified. Some speculate that it is a primary immunodeficiency in which there is a marked predisposition to develop IAHS. Abnormalities of both cellular and humoral immunity have been demonstrated in this disorder (48,49), with impairment of natural killer activity noted in almost all patients (43). Chromosomal analysis is usually normal, but there is a decreased frequency of HLA-B7 and HLA-B8 alleles and increased frequency of HLA-B21 and HLA-DQ3.

Malignant Lymphoma with Benign Erythrophagocytosis

This disease represents a mixed process that combines features of a malignant lymphoma with a reactive disorder of histiocytes (39,40,50,51). Similar to IAHS, a widespread proliferation of benign histiocytes with prominent erythrophagocytosis is seen. Instead of being associated with a systemic infection, however, the process is associated with a malignant lymphoma, most often T-cell lymphoma, which may be segregrated physically from the proliferating histiocytes.

Malignant lymphoma with benign erythrophagocytosis has been seen in two main clinical settings. The first is in patients with known malignant lymphoma in whom a syndrome mimicking IAHS develops (39,40,50). In this group of patients, disseminated lymphoma is often present. Most lymphomas are T-cell lymphomas or natural killer cell neoplasms, including nasal T/natural killer cell lymphoma and anaplastic large cell lymphoma, but lymphomas of B-cell lineage also have been associated with this syndrome (39,51–54). The erythrophagocytotic process is physically distinct from the lymphoma and is characterized by a marked proliferation of cytologically benign histiocytes that frequently demonstrate conspicuous erythrophagocytosis as well as phagocytosis of other formed elements of the blood. This process is most evident in bone marrow, lymph node sinuses, splenic red pulp, and hepatic sinusoids. This process is usually a terminal event in a patient with advanced stage lymphoma.

In the second presentation, the hemophagocytic syndrome occurs in the absence of any preexisting disease (40). In this setting, benign hemophagocytizing histiocytes are found in intimate association with the malignant lymphoma, which often has involved the bone marrow, spleen, and liver (Fig. 51.17). Paraffin- and frozen-section immunophenotyping

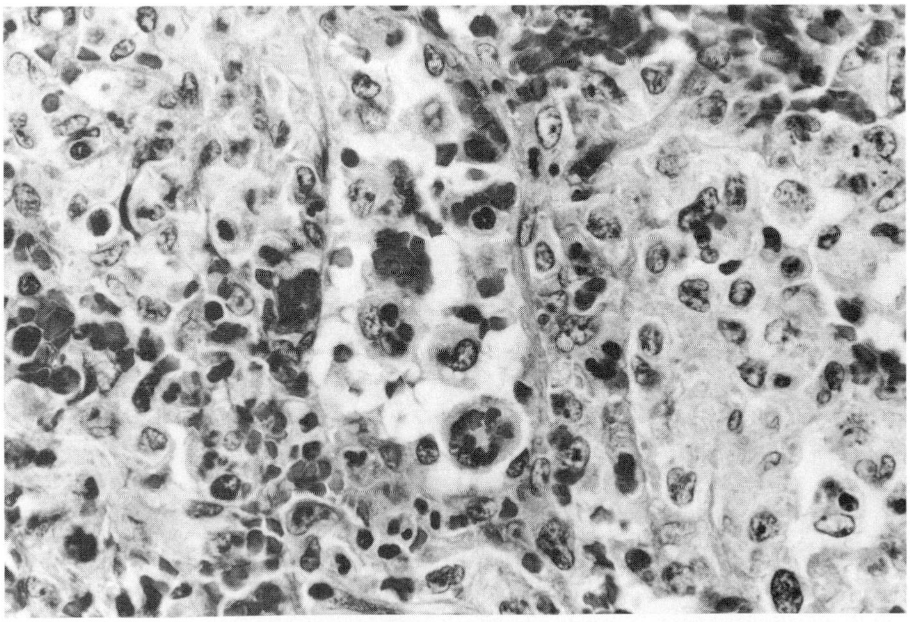

FIG. 51.17. Malignant lymphoma with benign erythrophagocytosis. The splenic cords contain numerous malignant cells; the sinuses show numerous benign histiocytes with erythrophagocytosis. Some admixture between the two populations of cells also is seen (original magnification: 400× magnification).

studies have demonstrated a T-cell lineage. Again, the prognosis is usually poor in the majority of patients.

It is suspected that the prominent phagocytosis by the benign histiocytes in this disorder is mediated by production of a lymphokine by the neoplastic cells. In support of this hypothesis, a factor that augmented the phagocytosis of IgG-coated ox red blood cells by the human monocyte–macrophage line U9437 has been identified in two patients with this disease (55). Recently, it has been shown that T-cell infection by Epstein-Barr virus selectively upregulates tumor necrosis factor-α, which, in combination with interferon-γ and probably other cytokines, can activate macrophages (56).

Hepatosplenic $\gamma\delta$ T-cell Lymphoma (Erythrophagocytic Tγ Lymphoma)

Erythrophagocytic Tγ lymphoma was described as a rare neoplasm in which the clinical and pathologic features resemble those of malignant histiocytosis (MH), but immunologic studies reveal that the malignant cells belong to a subpopulation of T-lymphocytes known as Tγ cells (57). In the two reported cases, the patients were 33- and 30-year-old men presenting with fever and hepatosplenomegaly. Histologically, there was involvement of the red pulp of the spleen and the sinusoids of the liver by large lymphoid cells, with erythrophagocytosis evident on thin sections (Fig. 51.18). The tumor cells expressed CD2 and lacked a monocytic antigen, evidence supporting a T-cell lineage. The tumor cells also were able to form rosettes with IgG-coated sheep or ox erythrocytes, consistent with Tγ cells. Similar cases have been described more recently and have been better defined with the more extended phenotyping and genotyping available. These studies have led to the conclusion that these rare cases probably represent examples of hepatosplenic $\gamma\delta$ T-cell lymphoma, a distinct clinicopathologic entity of cytotoxic $\gamma\delta$ T-cell origin (58–60). These cases may be distinguished from MH or true histiocytic tumor by the $\gamma\delta$ T-cell phenotype of the malignant cells (see Chapter 29).

Histiocytic Necrotizing Lymphadenitis

Histiocytic necrotizing lymphadenitis (HNL) (of Kikuchi and Fujimoto) is a well-defined clinicopathologic disorder with a benign clinical course that primarily affects lymph nodes. Although it first was described in Japan (61,62), numerous cases have been reported in Western countries (63–67). For a more comprehensive coverage of the topic, the reader is referred to a review by Dorfman (68) and an analysis of 108 cases by Dorfman and Berry (67).

Clinically, women are affected approximately four times as often as men (68). The median age at diagnosis is about 30 years, with a wide age range from teenagers to the elderly. The patients are generally healthy, with no obvious predisposing occupation, lifestyle, or underlying disease. Patients usually present with localized cervical or posterior cervical lymphadenopathy that may be tender to palpation. Less often, a variety of other lymph nodes are primarily affected; on occasion, two or more sites may be involved. Rarely, involvement of extranodal tissues such as skin, bone marrow, and salivary gland has been reported (69–71). In the majority of patients, lymphadenopathy is the only symptom, but occasional patients report mild fever, often associated with upper respiratory symptoms, weight loss, nausea and

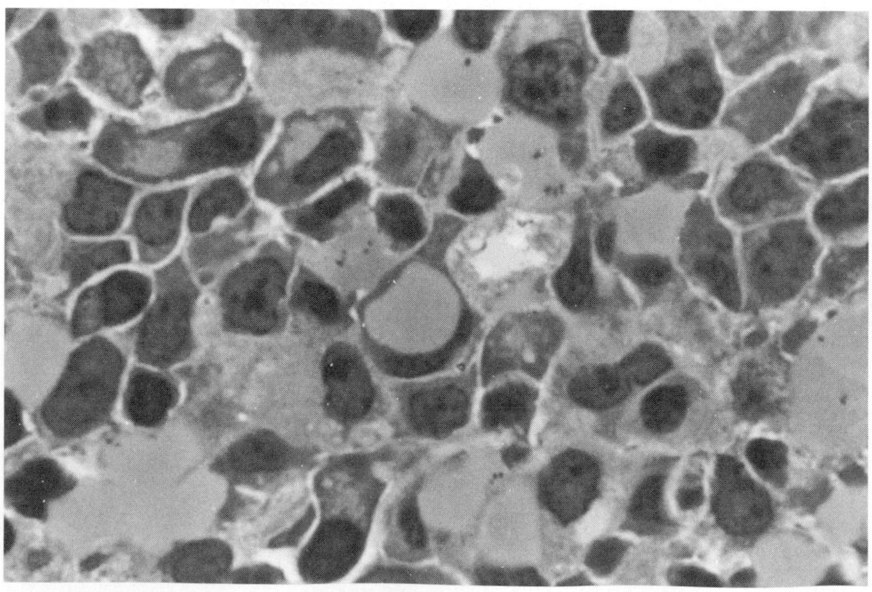

FIG. 51.18. Hepatosplenic T-cell lymphoma (erythrophagocytic Tγ lymphoma). This thin section shows prominent erythrophagocytosis (original magnification: 1,000× magnification). (Courtesy of Marshall Kadin, M.D., Beth Israel Deaconess Medical Center.)

vomiting, myalgia and arthralgia, chills, and night sweats. Rare patients report a rash with a malar distribution. The duration of symptoms prior to diagnosis is usually several months. Examination of the peripheral blood of these patients usually discloses no abnormalities, although neutropenia, a lymphocytosis, or circulating atypical lymphocytes have been reported on occasion. Serologic studies usually do not show good evidence for an infectious agent, although one group has reported three patients in whom serologic studies suggested infection with *Yersinia enterocolitica* (65).

Grossly, most lymph nodes are normal or only slightly increased in size. Areas of necrosis generally are not appreciated grossly but usually are quite striking microscopically. These foci generally are located in the paracortex and less often in the cortex (Fig. 51.19). They usually consist of irregular, circumscribed areas of deposition of an eosinophilic substance (probably representing fibrin) along with a marked degree of karyorrhexis (Fig. 51.20). Despite the widespread necrosis with karyorrhexis, there is an almost complete absence of intact neutrophils. Most of the viable cells present are macrophages, often exhibiting phagocytosis and occasionally containing foamy cytoplasm, reactive immunoblasts, and other mononuclear cells with somewhat atypical nuclear features (Fig. 51.21). The macrophages often have a distinctive appearance, with peripherally placed, crescent-shaped, twisted nuclei with abundant cytoplasm containing karyorrhectic debris (72). Plasma cells are generally few in number and eosinophils are absent. On occasion, there is very little deposition of the eosinophilic substance, but the marked karyorrhexis along with the cell population is present. Areas immediately adjacent to the foci of necrosis usually show a reactive immunoblastic proliferation. The remainder of the lymph node is usually normal and generally does not show significant reactive follicular hyperplasia. Focal distention of sinuses by monocytoid B lymphocytes has been reported (73) but is usually not a prominent finding. The lymph node capsule is sometimes thickened adjacent to the areas of necrosis. Recently, a case of HNL with cutaneous involvement has been reported (70). The histologic findings in the skin were similar to those seen in a biopsy specimen from the patient's involved cervical lymph node.

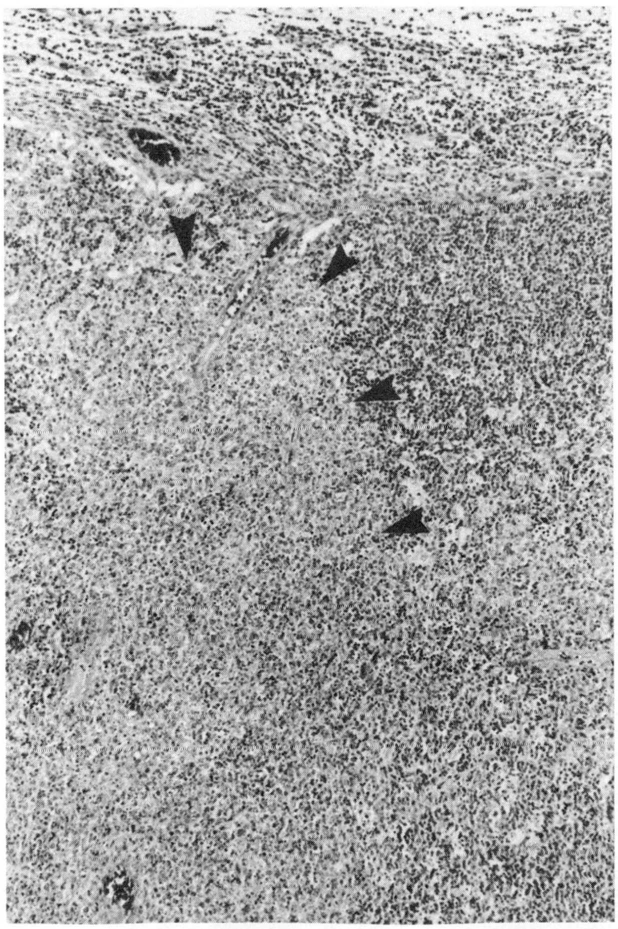

FIG. 51.19. Histiocytic necrotizing lymphadenitis. *Arrows* highlight a discrete area of necrosis in this lymph node. The adjacent area shows a mottled appearance resulting from an immunoblastic proliferation (original magnification: 100× magnification).

All of the histologic findings in HNL also may be seen in lymph nodes from patients with systemic lupus erythematosus (SLE). Features that might favor SLE would be the additional presence of basophilic necrotic material often deposited in vessel walls and sometimes forming hematoxyphilic bodies, and the presence of more than occasional plasma cells (74) (Fig. 51.22). Because the histologic findings in HNL may be indistinguishable from SLE, however, any patient given a diagnosis of HNL should be investigated clinically to rule out that possibility.

The most important entity to be distinguished from HNL is non-Hodgkin's lymphoma. The abundant karyorrhectic debris found in HNL often suggests a high-grade lymphoma at first glance. This impression may be reinforced if areas of macrophages form sheets, giving the superficial appearance of a large cell lymphoma. The characteristic clinical history often gives the first clue to a diagnosis of HNL. In addition, one should remember that the only lymphomas to have such a high degree of karyorrhexis are the high-grade lymphomas such as Burkitt's and immunoblastic lymphoma. The monotonous cellular populations found in these lymphomas, however, are not seen in HNL. Lymph node infarction, a finding that also may be associated with non-Hodgkin's lymphoma, generally shows granulation tissue at the edges of the necrotic areas (75). Sometimes, "ghosts" of cells can be seen in the necrotic areas. Hodgkin's disease and infectious agents such as *Yersinia enterocolitis* or the organism causing cat-scratch disease may be associated with stellate areas of necrosis (stellate microabscesses) but can be distinguished from HNL by the presence of neutrophils in and around the areas of necrosis in these disorders. Similarly, lymph node biopsy from patients with Kawasaki's disease also show neutrophils in association with the areas of necrosis. In addition, fibrin thrombi in small vessels are usually a prominent feature in this disorder (76).

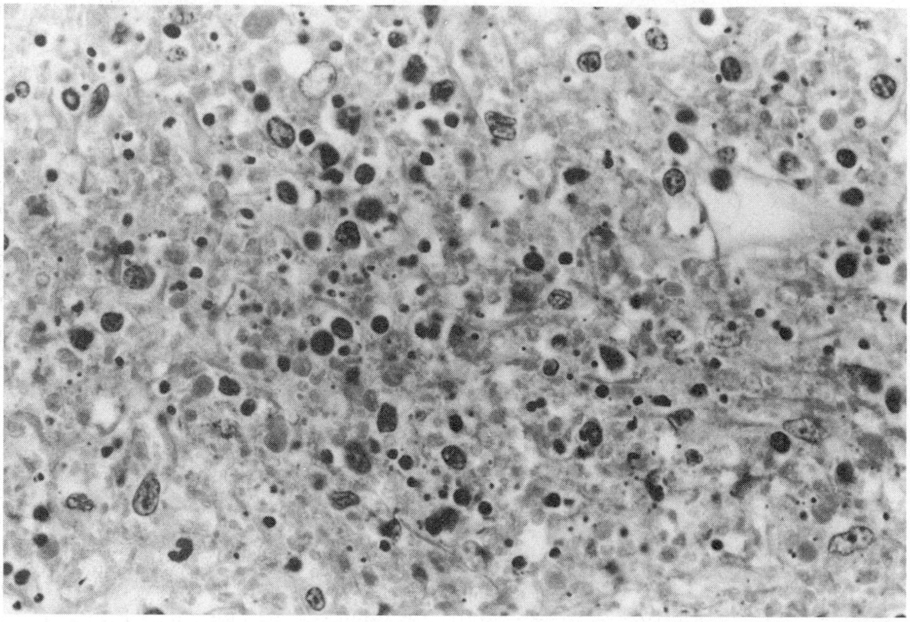

FIG. 51.20. Histiocytic necrotizing lymphadenitis. This area shows karyorrhectic debris and fibrin without viable cells (original magnification: 400× magnification).

Immunophenotyping studies have demonstrated a predominance of T cells and macrophages within involved areas of the lymph node (63,65,66). Helper or inducer T cells may predominate in early lesions; cytotoxic or suppressor T cells may be in the majority in biopsy specimens taken later after presentation (77). There is some evidence that the karyorrhectic debris may be derived from T-associated plasmacytoid cells (65).

Patients with HNL usually have a benign clinical course with spontaneous resolution of the disease in a large majority of patients (67). Rare patients have developed recurrent lymphadenopathy in which repeat biopsy has shown similar histologic features. Nonetheless, all patients probably should remain under clinical surveillance, because at least two patients have subsequently developed SLE (67).

The cause of this disease is as yet unknown. Evidence for an infectious cause has been sought, but no convincing evidence has been obtained; the studies to date have proved

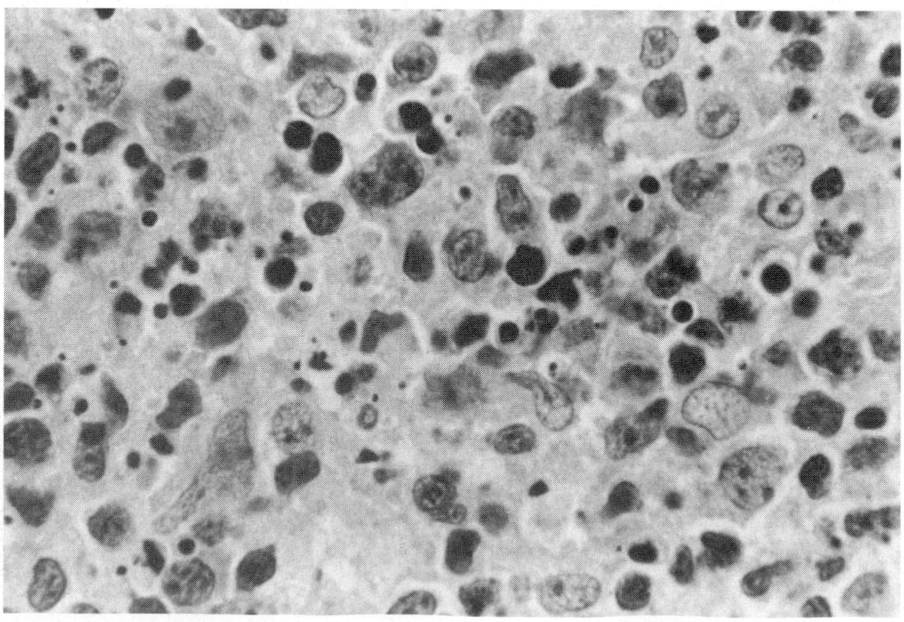

FIG. 51.21. Histiocytic necrotizing lymphadenitis. Nuclei of macrophages and immunoblasts are seen amid karyorrhectic debris. Such areas could simulate non-Hodgkin's lymphoma (original magnification: 1,000× magnification).

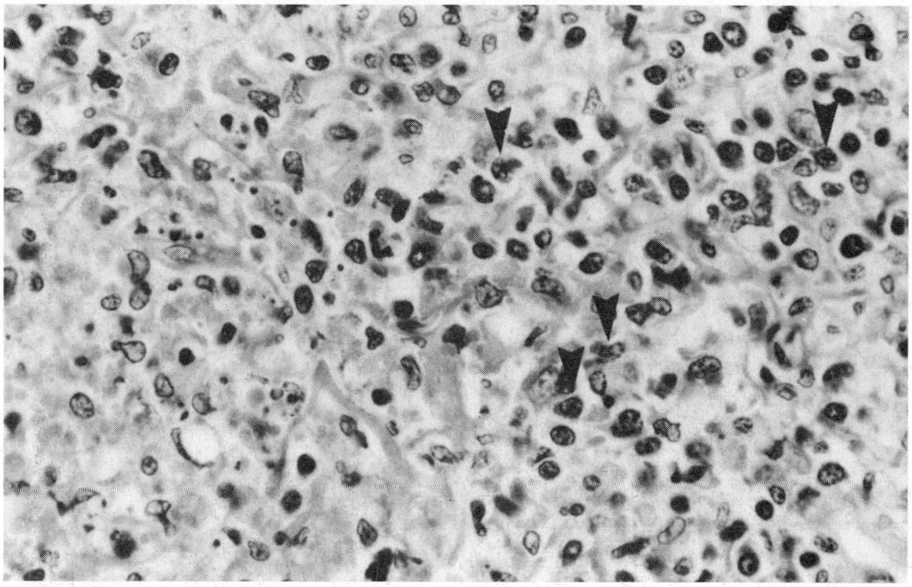

FIG. 51.22. Systemic lupus erythematosus. This field is identical to what may be seen in histiocytic necrotizing lymphadenitis, except that occasional plasma cells are evident (*arrows*) (original magnification: 400× magnification).

negative (65,78–80). Dorfman and Berry (67) have suggested that the disease may reflect a self-limited SLE-like autoimmune condition, perhaps induced by virus-infected transformed lymphocytes, but evidence to support or refute this proposal is lacking at the current time.

BENIGN DENDRITIC CELL PROLIFERATIONS: DERMATOPATHIC LYMPHADENITIS

Dermatopathic lymphadenitis refers to the lymph node reaction that occurs in lymph nodes draining areas of disruption of the skin integrity. Grossly, the lymph node is enlarged and fleshy and often has melanotic pigmentation. Histologically, the node architecture shows varying degrees of paracortical expansion, usually but not always accompanied by reactive follicular hyperplasia (Fig. 51.23). The enlarged paracortical areas contain a population of dendritic cells and histiocytes, often admixed with immunoblasts, eosinophils, and plasma cells. The numerous dendritic cells, comprising both interdigitating dendritic cells and Langerhans cells, can be highlighted with an anti-S-100 protein stain (see Chapter 15).

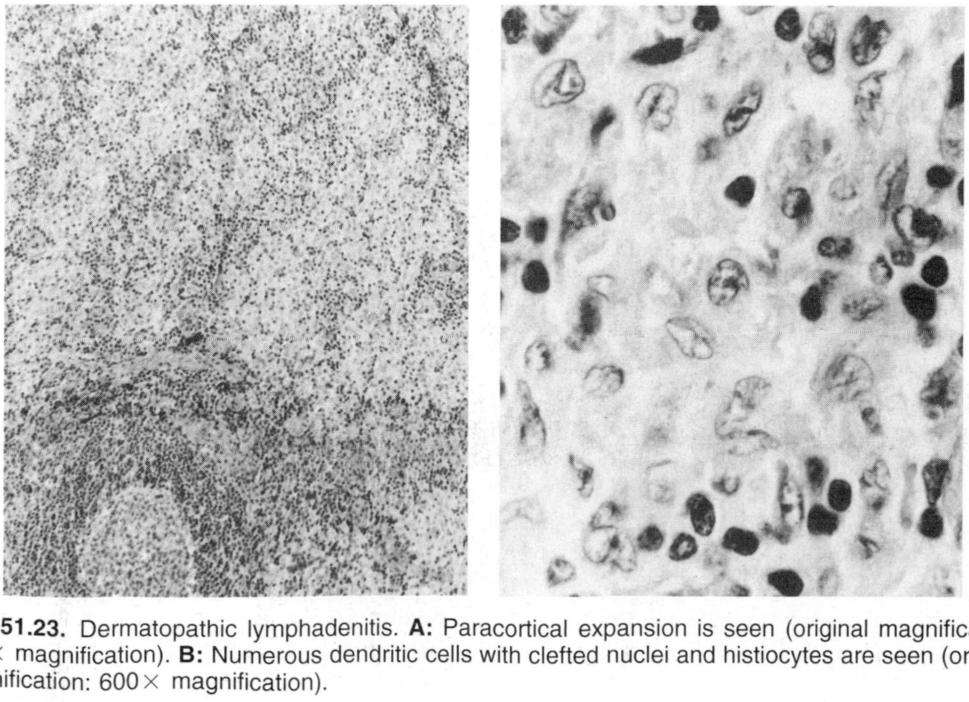

A B

FIG. 51.23. Dermatopathic lymphadenitis. **A:** Paracortical expansion is seen (original magnification: 100× magnification). **B:** Numerous dendritic cells with clefted nuclei and histiocytes are seen (original magnification: 600× magnification).

BORDERLINE AND MALIGNANT DENDRITIC CELL PROLIFERATIONS

Juvenile and Adult Xanthogranuloma

Juvenile and adult xanthogranuloma represent the most common members of a spectrum of disease that probably also includes such rare entities as xanthoma disseminatum, benign cephalic histiocytosis, progressive nodular histiocytosis, spindle cell xanthogranuloma, and generalized eruptive histiocytosis (81). The most common form, juvenile xanthogranuloma, usually presents in children with yellow to pink protuberant cutaneous nodules up to 1 cm in diameter, usually in the head and neck region. Similar lesions may occur in adults (adult xanthogranuloma). Some lesions may occur in the subcutaneous or intramuscular soft tissues or rarely in internal organs (82). The intramuscular forms have a marked predilection to occur as solitary lesions in skeletal muscles of the trunk of infants (83). Almost all lesions, including extracutaneous lesions, involute spontaneously.

Histologically, the lesions are usually well circumscribed, with an exophytic appearance if skin is involved (84). The epidermis itself is usually uninvolved, and there is usually an underlying Grenz zone. The lesions consist of variable numbers of histiocyte-like cells, spindle cells, and giant cells. The histiocyte-like cells have bland nuclei with abundant vacuolated, eosinophilic, or foamy cytoplasm (Fig. 51.24). The spindle cells are similar to the histiocyte-like cells but are spindled and form a storiform architecture. The giant cells usually are described as Touton-type (foamy periphery outside a wreathe of nuclei around central eosinophilic anucleate cytoplasm) but are just as often foreign body–type or nondescript with central eosinophilic or ground-glass cytoplasm. Early lesions tend to have more vacuolated histiocyte-like cells, intermediate lesions have more foamy cells, and late lesions tend to be more spindled. Intramuscular lesions tend to be composed of a monotonous population of histiocyte-like cells, with rare, if any, foamy macrophages or giant cells (83). Immunohistochemical studies demonstrate factor XIIIa, fascin, and CD68 positivity, particularly at the periphery of the lesion. Peanut agglutinin lectin is also present in most patients, but tests for S-100 protein are negative (see Chapter 32).

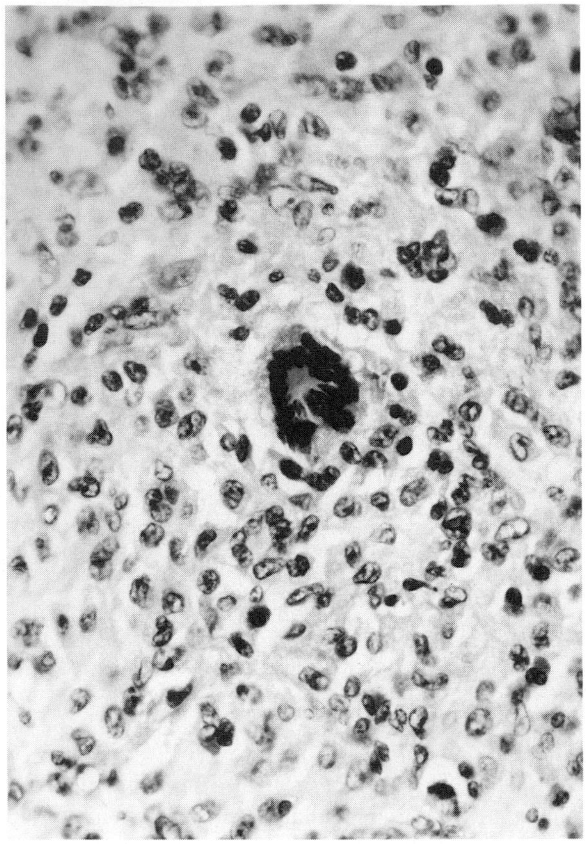

FIG. 51.24. Juvenile xanthogranuloma. A Touton-like giant cell is seen in a background of relatively bland histiocytic cells (original magnification: 400× magnification).

Langerhans Cell Histiocytosis (Histiocytosis X, Langerhans Cell Granulomatosis)

The term *Langerhans cell histiocytosis* (*LCH*) encompasses a set of closely related clinicopathologic disorders unified by a common proliferating element, the Langerhans cell (85,86). The incidence is about 5 per million, and the median age is less than 5 years (87,88). There is an association with other hematopoietic neoplasms; although much of this may be related to posttherapy leukemia, there does seem to be an unusually frequent occurrence of disseminated LCH in patients with acute nonmyelocytic leukemia (89). There may be an association among LCH and neontal infection, solvent exposure, lack of childhood vaccination, and thyroid disease (90).

Although there are many different classification systems for LCH, three overlapping clinical syndromes generally are recognized. In unifocal LCH (solitary eosinophilic granuloma), representing about two thirds of cases, a single site is involved, most commonly bone, lymph node, or lung (86). Although it most commonly occurs in children, adults also may be affected; about two thirds of affected patients are males. Bone is overwhelmingly the most common site of involvement, usually the skull, femur, pelvic bones, or ribs. The diaphyses are involved most often, with erosion of the adjacent cortical bone. It is not clear whether the unifocal involvement of the lung that sometimes occurs in adult smokers (of tobacco or marijuana) represents a form of LCH or a peculiar reactive process (91). In multifocal unisystem LCH (many cases of Hand-Schuller-Christian syndrome), several involved sites in one organ system, generally bone, are present. Patients are generally younger in age than those with unifocal involvement but still are more often males. Finally, in multifocal, multisystem histiocytosis (many cases of Letterer-Siwe syndrome), multiple sites in multiple organ systems are involved. These patients are almost always infants or young children, with a predominance of males.

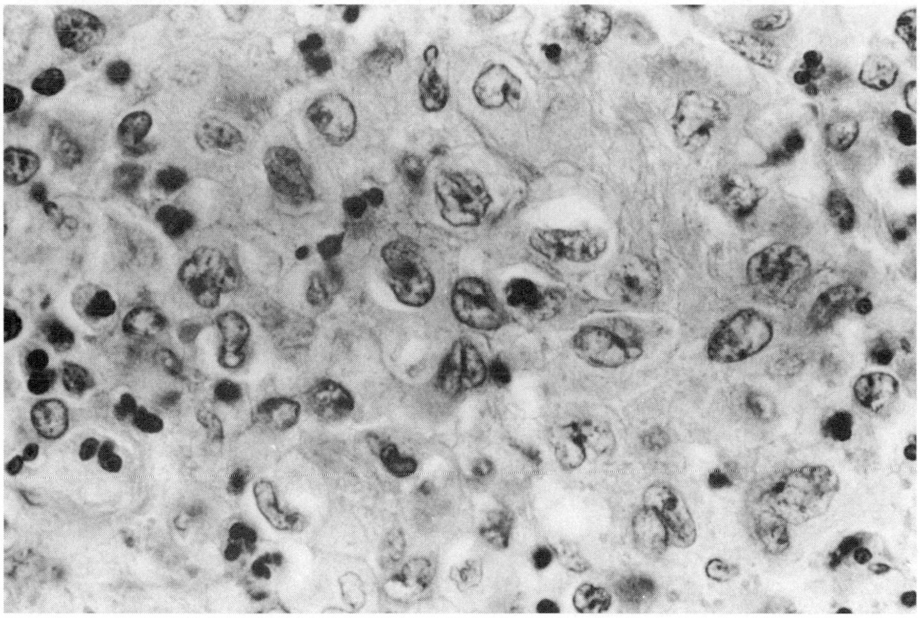

FIG. 51.25. Langerhans cell histiocytosis. The characteristic grooving and folding of the nuclei are present (original magnification: 1,000× magnification).

The histologic hallmark of all involved tissues is the presence of proliferating Langerhans cells in the appropriate cellular milieu. Morphologically, the Langerhans cells are about 10 to 12 μm in diameter and have characteristic folded, indented, or lobulated nuclei, generally with inconspicuous nucleoli (Fig. 51.25). Although some nuclear atypia may be present, the cells are cytologically benign, and mitotic figures are usually rare. A moderate amount of slightly eosinophilic cytoplasm usually is seen. The cells are almost always accompanied by a characteristic reactive infiltrate, which usually includes eosinophils, histiocytes, neutrophils, multinucleated cells (either foreign body or Langhans type), and small lymphocytes (Fig. 51.26). Necrosis may be present, often in the form of eosinophilic microabscesses (Fig. 51.27). Early lesions tend to be very cellular; late lesions tend to be more fibrotic, often with the accumulation of foamy macrophages.

Involved lymph nodes almost always show sinusoidal pat-

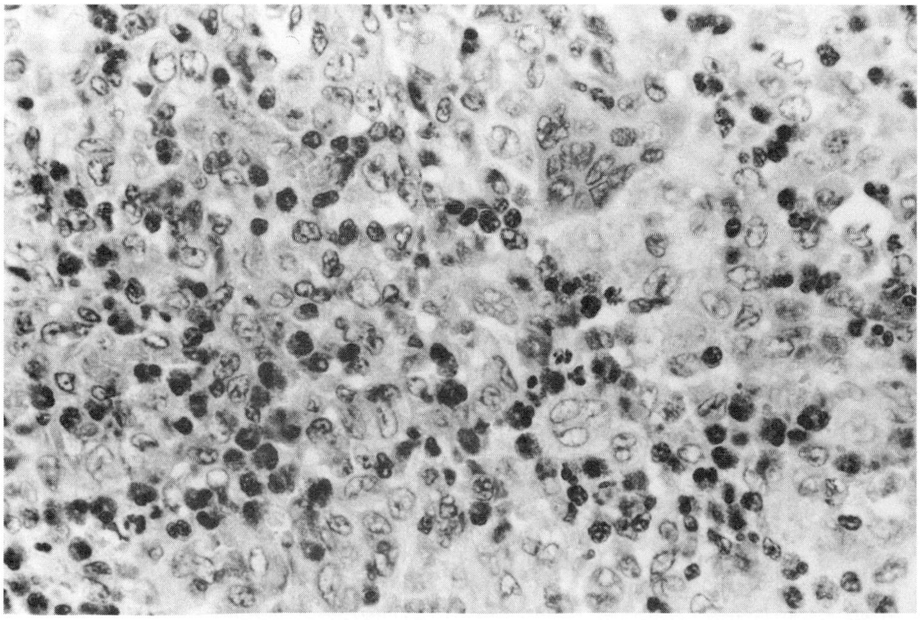

FIG. 51.26. Langerhans cell histiocytosis. A mixture of cell types, including Langerhans cells, eosinophils, macrophages, lymphocytes, and giant cells, is seen (original magnification: 400× magnification).

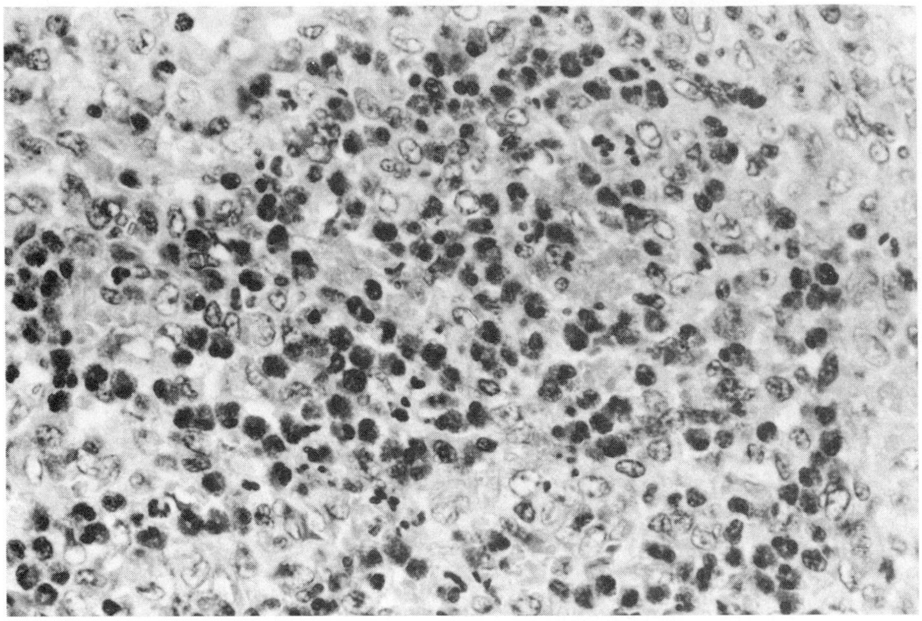

FIG. 51.27. Langerhans cell histiocytosis. An eosinophilic microabscess is present (original magnification: 400× magnification).

terns of involvement, often with marked distension of the sinuses, beginning with the subcapuslar sinuses and progressing to involvement of the medullary sinuses (92) (Fig. 51.28). The overall lymph node architecture generally is retained, but partial or even complete effacement is seen in rare advanced cases. The histologic differential diagnosis includes sinusoidal proliferations of the lymph nodes such as metastatic carcinoma, metastatic malignant melanoma, sinusoidal malignant lymphoma, SHML, and benign sinusoidal hyperplasia. The key to the diagnosis lies in the recognition of the cytologic features of the Langerhans cells. Large numbers of Langerhans cells may be seen in lymph nodes showing dermatopathic lymphadenopathy (93). In that condition, however, the Langerhans cells are seen in paracortical areas and are not prominent within the sinuses.

Rarely, a focus of LCH can be seen in lymph nodes involved by malignant lymphoma, both of non-Hodgkin's type and Hodgkin's disease (94,95). In these circumstances, the

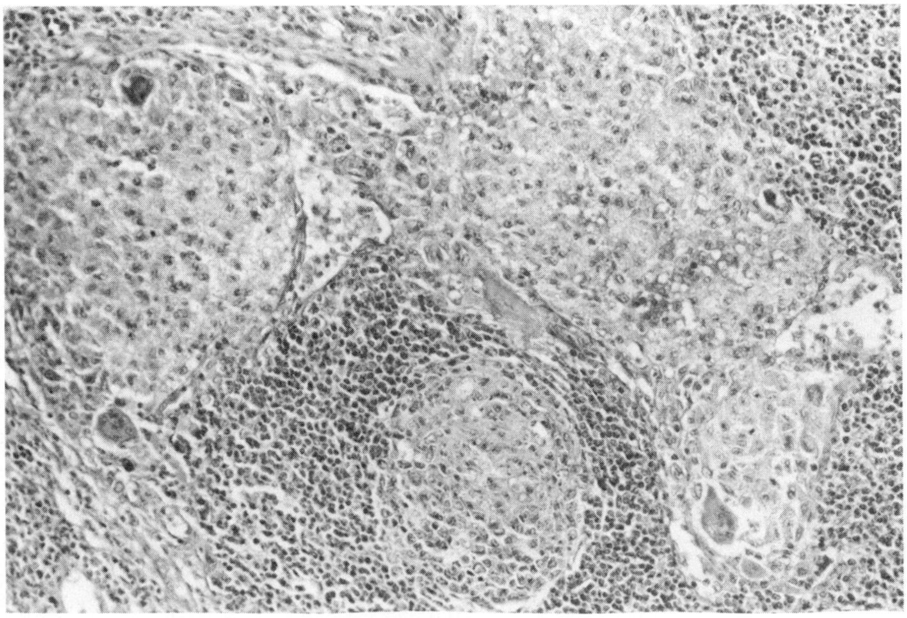

FIG. 51.28. Langerhans cell histiocytosis. A sinusoidal pattern of involvement is seen in this lymph node biopsy (original magnification: 200× magnification).

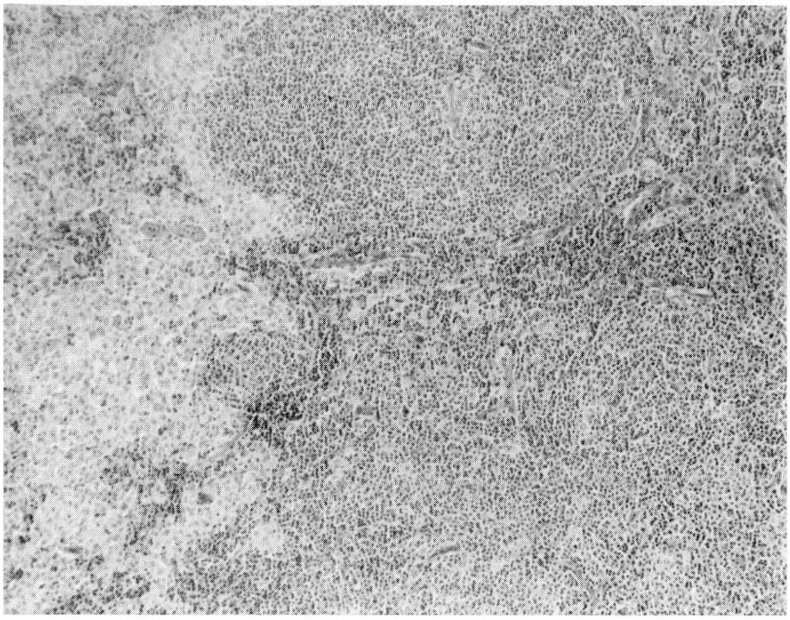

FIG. 51.29. Follicular lymphoma. A focus of Langerhans cell histiocytosis is seen at the left (original magnification: 100× magnification).

focus of disease can be quite small and not limited to the sinuses (Fig. 51.29). As in the case of pulmonary LCH occurring in smokers, it is not clear whether these instances represent a peculiar reactive phenomenon rather than true LCH.

The ultrastructural, enzyme histochemical, and immunophenotypic characteristics of the Langerhans cells in LCH are virtually identical to those of normal Langerhans cells (5,86). Ultrastructurally, the cells in LCH contain variable numbers of Birbeck granules morphologically identical to those found in normal Langerhans cells (Fig. 51.2). The nuclei are deeply cleaved or multisegmented, with finely dispersed chromatin and an inconspicuous nucleolus. The cells show expression of adenosine triphosphatase, α-naphthyl acetate esterase (with variable inhibition by sodium fluoride), α-naphthyl butyrate esterase, and acid phosphatase, and negativity for tartrate-resistant acid phosphatase, 5′-nucleotidase, peroxidase, chloroacetate esterase, and β-glucuronidase.

CD1, S-100 protein, and peanut lectin agglutinin are the markers most consistently seen in paraffin-section immunohistochemical studies, although rare patients show weak or negative staining of these markers (96). CD1 reactivity is extremely useful in terms of differential diagnosis, because only lymphoblastic malignancies share this feature. The cells also express placental alkaline phosphatase, vimentin, CDw75, and LN-3 in more than 80% of patients (97,98). Similar to the cells of SHML, the cells of LCH are positive for cathepsins D and E (28). The cells also lack CD30, LN-1, lysozyme, α_1-antitrypsin, epithelial membrane antigen, and CD15 expression in paraffin sections, although CD15 positivity may be seen after removal of sialic acid residues. A negative reaction is seen for CD45 (leukocyte common antigen) in paraffin sections, although a positive reaction generally is seen in frozen sections (5,98). In addition to expression of CD45, frozen-section immunohistochemical studies show the Langerhans cells of LCH to express cytoplasmic CD2, cytoplasmic CD3, CD4, CD14, HLA-A, HLA-B, HLA-C, and HLA-DR, and to lack expression of other markers of B- and T-cell lineages (5,97,98).

The Langerhans cells of LCH have been shown to differ from normal Langerhans cells in their expresion of cellular adhesion molecules. In contrast to normal Langerhans cells, the cells of LCH show strong expression of CD54 (ICAM-1), CD58 (LFA-3), CD11c (receptor molecule for iC3b), and CD49D (VLA-4) (99–101). The receptors for CD54 and CD58, CD2 and CD11A, also are expressed in a significant subset of cases, suggesting an autocrine effect. The cells of LCH express much more granulocyte-macrophage colony-stimulating factor, tumor necrosis factor-α, interleukin-1α and β, interferon-γ, and transforming growth factor-α and β than normal Langerhans cells (102). In addition, although normal Langerhans cells are negative for fascin, the cells of LCH are fascin positive (103,104).

Gene rearrangement studies have shown a germline configuration for the immunoglobulin heavy chain gene as well as the β, γ, and δ chains of the T-cell receptor gene (105,106). However, X-linked polymorphic DNA probes to assess clonality have demonstrated that lesions of LCH, whether unifocal, multifocal, or disseminated, represent clonal proliferations (106,107). In one study, evidence of human herpesvirus-6 was found in about one half of lesions (108); another study found no good evidence of human herpesvirus-6 or of adenovirus, cytomegalovirus, Epstein-Barr virus, herpes simplex virus, parvovirus, human T-cell viruses type I or II, or human immunodeficiency virus (109). DNA ploidy studies performed on paraffin-embedded tissue with either localized or disseminated forms of the disease have shown a diploid population in most patients (110,111).

One study utilizing a variety of techniques to study cell proliferation concluded that the cells in LCH are not actively proliferating (112).

The most important factor determining prognosis appears to be the pattern of organ involvement (113). Less than 10% of patients who present with only one involved site develop disseminated disease. Patients with multiple organs involved at presentation, particularly if the involvement leads to organ dysfunction, generally have a poor outcome (114). The number of involved organs, however, is not the only important factor. The absence of bone lesions is a poor prognostic factor, and the presence of multiple osseous lesions is associated with a favorable prognosis. Patients younger than 2 years of age generally do poorly, but age may be less important than the pattern of organ involvement in determining prognosis. Histologic grading is of much less significance in predicting prognosis than pattern of organ involvement or age. In one study, the presence of cytologic atypia or the mitotic rate could not be correlated with patient outcome (115).

There have been reports of a malignant form of LCH (116,117). This neoplasm has been termed *Langerhans cell sarcoma* in the recently proposed World Health Organization classification of hematopoietic and lymphoid neoplasms (118). In Langerhans cell sarcoma, the proliferating cells have frankly malignant cytologic features but are otherwise ultrastructurally and immunophenotypically typical for LCH. Clinically, the few reported patients have been predominantly male, have had multiorgan involvement, and have followed a rapidly progressive clinical course. It is not yet clear whether this disease represents a distinctive clinicopathologic entity, the extreme end of the morphologic and clinical spectrum of ordinary LCH, or other neoplasms that have been confused with LCH.

Follicular Dendritic Cell Sarcoma

Neoplasms of follicular dendritic cell lineage, so-called *follicular dendritic cell sarcoma,* are rare but well described, including several recent relatively large series (11,119–129). Almost all patients have been adults, with a median age of about 40 years. There is about an equal sex distribution. Most patients present with an enlarged cervical or axillary lymph node, but extranodal presentations, including oral cavity, tonsil, gastrointestinal tract, soft tissue, and breast, occur in almost half of the patients. Rare cases of neoplasms with the histologic appearance of inflammatory pseudotumors have been reported in the liver and spleen that have been shown to express one or more markers of follicular dendritic cells. It is not clear yet whether they represent true follicular dendritic cell sarcomas or a variant of inflammatory pseudotumor; these rare tumors often are associated with Epstein-Barr virus (130). Follicular dendritic cell sarcomas arising in other organs are consistently negative for Epstein-Barr virus and human herpesvirus-8 as well (131). The neoplasm arises in association with Castleman's disease in about 10% to 20% of patients; in most instances, it is associated with the hyaline vascular type, but the plasma cell type also has been reported rarely (120,132,133). The behavior of follicular dendritic cell sarcoma is more like that of a sarcoma than a hematolymphoid neoplasm, with local recurrence and occasional metastasis. Almost one half of patients have one or more recurrences; metastases have been reported in about one quarter of patients.

There is a wide range in tumor size in follicular dendritic cell sarcoma, with a mean size of about 5 cm. The largest tumors occur in the retroperitoneum and may be up to 20 cm. They are usually well circumscribed and are seen as solid tan-gray masses on cut section. Histologically, an ovoid to spindle cell–shaped morphology is seen, often in a storiform or whorled growth pattern (Fig. 51.30). Necrosis is usually absent but may occur in a geographic pattern. The individual cells are usually uniform, with occasional multinucleation. The nuclei are elongated, with vesicular or granular chromatin, distinct nucleoli, and a delicate nuclear membrane. There may be multinucleated cells or nuclear pseudoinclusions, and some patients may have moderate to marked nuclear pleomorphism. The mitotic rate is usually between 0 and 10 per 10 high-power fields but may be higher. Residual lymphoid tissue is generally present in between the spindled proliferation, either as single cells, clusters of lymphocytes often in a perivascular location, or occasional germinal centers. In occasional patients associated with hyaline-vascular Castleman's disease, the neoplasm appears to be arising in association with a dysplastic proliferation of follicular dendritic cells. Recurrences and metastases may have a greater degree of nuclear atypia, a higher mitotic rate, and a greater degree of necrosis, consistent with histologic progression.

Electron microscopy reveals numerous villous cytoplasmic extensions, often connected with each other through numerous cell junctions, which include well-formed desmosomes. Immunologically, the neoplasm shows a close resemblance to the normal follicular dendritic cell, with absent to weak CD45, variable expression of S-100 protein, consistent expression of vimentin and the C3b and C3d complement receptors (CD35 and CD21, respectively), variable expression of desmoplakin and CD68, and consistent expression of follicular dendritic cell specific markers such as R4/23. Surprisingly, epithelial membrane antigen is expressed in a majority of cases, despite the fact that normal follicular dendritic cells are negative for this marker (125). The neoplasm is consistently negative for CD1, desmin, keratin, HMB-45, and vascular markers. Gene rearrangement studies have revealed a germline configuration for the immunoglobulin heavy chain and T-cell receptor β genes.

The differential diagnosis is large and includes other dendritic cell tumors, thymoma, spindle cell carcinoma, malignant melanoma, and sarcoma. A complete immunohistochemical profile should rule out these other neoplasms and demonstrate the appropriate immunophenotype of follicular dendritic cell sarcoma.

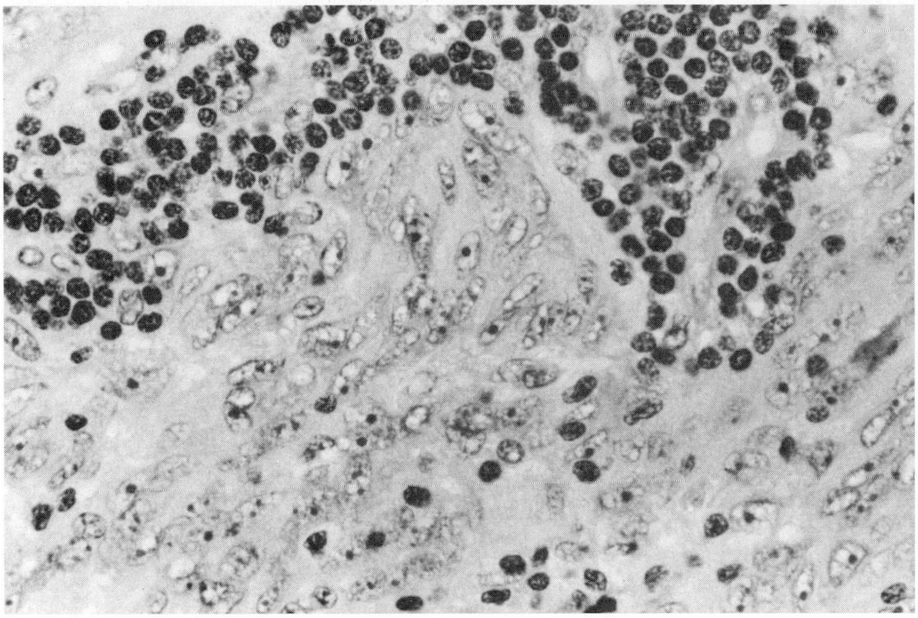

FIG. 51.30. Follicular dendritic cell sarcoma. A spindled pattern with residual lymphocytes is present (original magnification: 600× magnification).

Interdigitating Dendritic Cell Sarcoma

Rare neoplasms consistent with an interdigitating dendritic cell lineage have been reported, although the literature is somewhat confusing, because some authors have included CD1-expressing tumors within this category. In this review, these latter tumors are included within the discussion of indeterminate cell neoplasms. There have been few well-documented cases of interdigitating dendritic cell neoplasms. They have occurred in both males and females from the teens through adulthood, with a median age of about 50 years (119,121,124,134–139). The presentation has varied, from solitary lymph node enlargement to widespread disease including hepatosplenomegaly. The clinical course appears to be aggressive, with most patients dying of the disease. The median overall duration of survival is about 15 months.

These neoplasms also have been variable in their histologic appearance, ranging from spindle cell neoplasms similar in morphologic appearance to follicular dendritic cell neoplasms, to neoplasms resembling histiocytic tumors or large cell lymphomas (Fig. 51.31). There is often a paracortical localization. The fine structure of these tumors is similar to normal interdigitating cells, with elongated and complex cell processes, but no true desmosomes; Birbeck granules are not present. Immunophenotypically, the tumors typically express vimentin, CD45, S-100 protein, macrophage antigens (variable) and, by the definition used here, are negative for CD1 and follicular dendritic cell markers. Gene rearrangement studies have shown a germline configuration for the immunoglobulin heavy chain and T-cell receptor β genes.

Indeterminate Cell Neoplasm

Several examples of tumors with morphologic and immunologic characteristics of indeterminate cells have been reported (140–144). The patients have been adults, and the majority have presented with solitary or multiple cutaneous lesions, although rare patients have had presentation in lymph nodes (120). A significant subset of cases has been associated with low-grade B-cell lymphomas (145). Histologically, these lesions often have been dermal-based, occasionally with extension into the epidermis. The cells usually have abundant cytoplasm with irregularly shaped and often clefted nuclei. Lymph nodes also have been involved, either at presentation or during the course of the disease. Ultrastructurally, the cells have shown numerous dendritic processes that interdigitate with those of adjacent cells. No Birbeck granules are present. Immunophenotypically, the neoplastic cells express vimentin, CD45, CD1, S-100 protein, fascin, and macrophage antigens (146). Clinically, it is still not clear whether these lesions behave differently than LCH.

Fibroblastic Reticular Cell Neoplasm

Only three cases of fibroblastic reticular cell neoplasms have been reported (120). The two male patients and one female patient were in the second or third decades of life. In all three the neoplasm presented in lymph nodes. Follow-up available in two patients showed no evidence of recurrence or metastasis. Histologically, preferential paracortical involvement was seen in two patients, and diffuse efface-

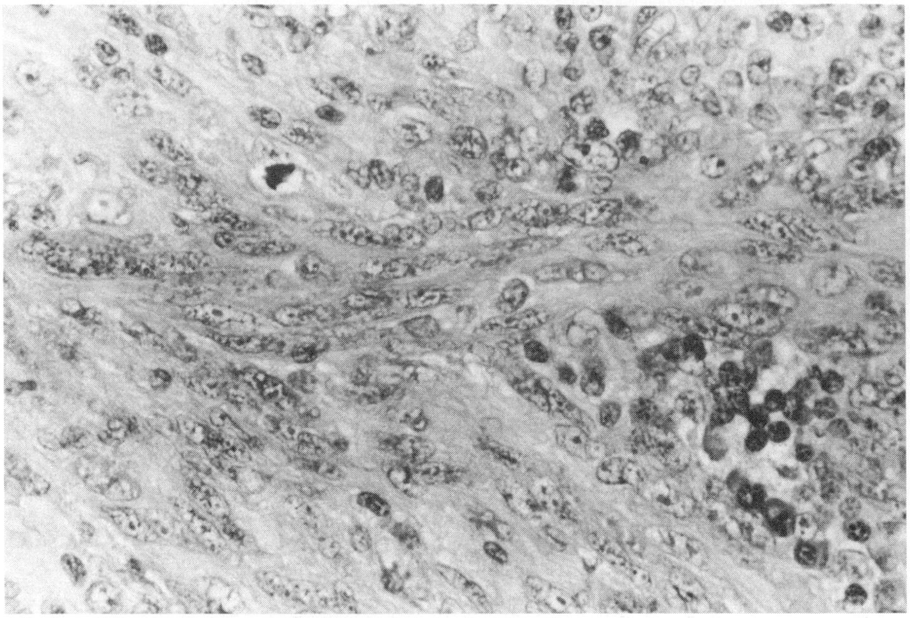

FIG. 51.31. Interdigitating dendritic cell sarcoma. A spindled pattern is seen (original magnification: 600× magnification).

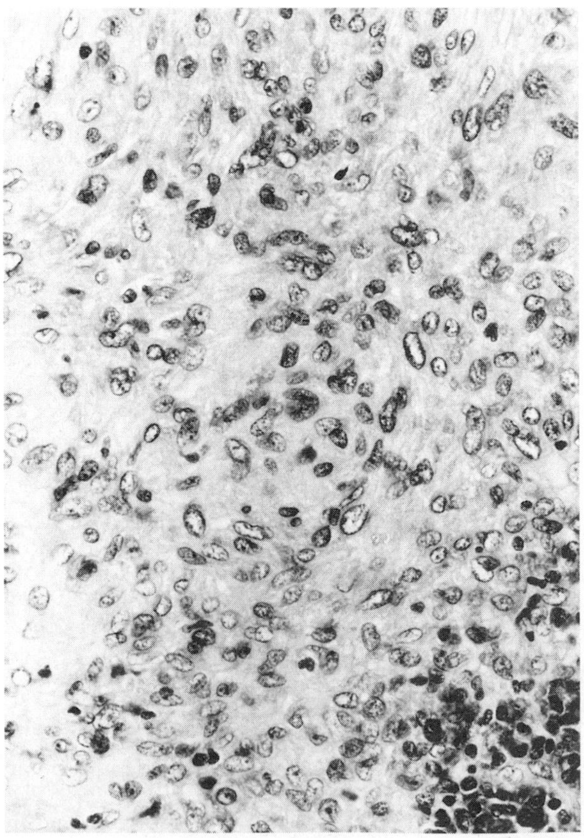

FIG. 51.32. Fibroblastic reticular cell neoplasm. This spindle cell proliferation is essentially indistinguishable from that of follicular dendritic cell sarcoma or interdigitating dendritic cell sarcoma (original magnification: 400× magnification).

ment was seen in one. At high magnification there was a spindle cell proliferation indistinguishable from other dendritic cell proliferations, although there was a finely collagenized background (Fig. 51.32). Electron microscopic studies performed in two patients showed features of myofibroblasts, with elongated tumor cells with slender cytoplasmic extensions associated with basal lamina–like material, intracytoplasmic filaments, occasional fusiform densities, and well-developed intercellular attachments. Immunohistochemical studies showed the spindle cell proliferation to have strong vimentin expression and variable smooth-muscle actin and desmin expression. There was also factor XIII staining, but the positivity was not clearly within the neoplastic population. CD45RB, S-100 protein, keratin, CD1a, CD21, CD35 and specific B- and T-cell markers were not expressed.

MALIGNANT HISTIOCYTIC PROLIFERATIONS

Malignant Histiocytosis and True Histiocytic Lymphoma

Malignant histiocytosis (MH) and true histiocytic lymphoma (THL) are neoplasms theoretically derived from true tissue macrophages. The term *MH* generally is used if a prominent sinusoidal pattern of involvement is seen; *THL* often is used for cases in which effacement of lymph node architecture is present, similar to most non-Hodgkin's lymphomas.

Most clinicopathologic studies defining MH and THL were performed prior to the availability of monoclonal antibodies, the development of modern immunohistochemistry, and the application of molecular biology to clinical material.

Therefore, in these seminal reports, the identification of these cases as histiocytic was based primarily on the assessment of the morphologic similarity of the neoplastic cells to histiocytes and their pattern of involvement (147,148). These studies suggested that MH or THL was a systemic disease of children and adults with frequent extranodal involvement, including liver, spleen, skin, bone, and gastrointestinal tract. The small intestine was thought by some to be a particularly common site for presentation (149). The overall prognosis was poor, although some good responses were seen to chemotherapeutic adriamycin containing regimens.

The results of several recent studies have cast considerable doubt on the histiocytic nature of many of the cases included in previous studies. For example, a reassessment of 15 cases reported in 1975 as MH recently was made based on paraffin-section immunophenotyping studies performed on the retrieved blocks (150). Nine cases were found to have profiles consistent with T-cell lineage, including expression of CD30 (the Ki-1 antigen); two were of B-cell lineage; three could not be classified as being of T- or B-cell lineage but expressed CD30 and lacked the macrophage marker CD68; and one case was reclassified as most consistent with the infection-associated viral hemophagocytic syndrome. Even if paraffin- and frozen-section immunophenotyping studies do not demonstrate clearly a lymphocyte lineage or even favor a histiocyte lineage, gene rearrangement studies may show evidence of T- or B-cell lineage through the demonstration of clonal T-cell receptor or immunoglobulin gene rearrangements in a majority of cases (151–154) (Fig. 51.33). Clonal rearrangements of the T-cell receptor genes appear to be found more commonly than clonal immunoglobulin gene rearrangements. Presumably, the neoplastic cells in these patients have become so poorly differentiated that they have lost expression of all their pan–T- and B-cell markers, similar to the partial loss of expression that is known to occur in T- and B-cell lymphomas, particularly in the former (155,156). Some investigators, however, favor the possibility that patients with some phenotypic evidence of histiocytic differentiation still should be regarded as having histiocyte-derived disease, regardless of the presence of clonal T-cell receptor or immunoglobulin gene rearrangements (157). Although this interpretation cannot be refuted, I urge extreme caution in the diagnosis of MH or THL, particularly because the entity has a history of confusion caused by overdiagnosis. Until more data are available in this difficult area, I recommend that the diagnosis of MH or THL be used only for patients in whom phenotyping studies show clear evidence supporting a histiocytic lineage, with the absence of specific markers of T- or B-cell lineage and with a germline configuration for the T-cell receptor and immunoglobulin genes. The demonstration of a germline configuration for these genes in the absence of strongly supportive immunophenotypic data suggestive of specific histiocytic differentiation would not constitute sufficient evidence for classifying a neoplasm as having histiocytic lineage, because a subset of peripheral T-cell lymphomas as well as other B- and T-cell neoplasms may lack detectable antigen receptor gene rearrangements (154,158,159).

Using the strict criteria delineated previously, there have been only rare reports of MH or THL (119,160–163). The neoplasm occurs most often in older adults, although it has been reported in children; there does not appear to be any sex predilection. About one half of the cases present in lymph nodes; the other half present in a variety of extranodal

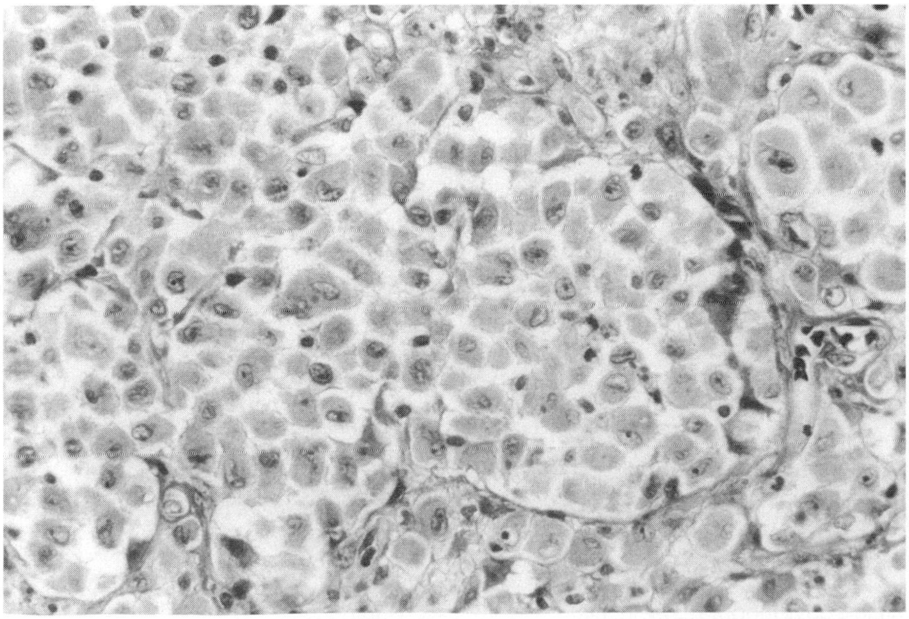

FIG. 51.33. Malignant lymphoma simulating malignant histiocytosis. This patient exhibited clonal T-cell receptor β gene rearrangements (original magnification: 400× magnification).

sites, most commonly the gastrointestinal tract and skin. Some patients have a ''systemic'' presentation. Rare cases have been associated with another hematologic malignancy, either an acute leukemia or malignant lymphoma. The clinical course is aggressive, with most reported patients dying from the disease.

Histologically, the neoplasm usually consists of a diffuse, noncohesive proliferation of round to oval neoplastic cells (Fig. 51.34). The nuclei often are placed eccentrically and have folded to pleomorphic nuclei, with prominent nucleoli. Multinucleate cells commonly are seen. The mitotic rate is generally high. Cytoplasm is usually eosinophilic and abundant but may be spindled in focal areas. Hemophagocytosis or lymphophagocytosis may be seen on occasion but is usually not prominent. Foamy cell change may be seen. Accompanying the neoplastic proliferation is a variable number of host cells, including lymphocytes, plasma cells, and eosinophils. If organs are involved, a sinusoidal or focal parenchymal pattern of infiltration may be seen. Ultrastructural studies show cytoplasmic lysosomes, but no evidence of Birbeck granules or junctions. Immunohistochemical studies, by definition, show expression of one or more markers of histiocytic differentiation, usually CD68 or lysosome. Both usually are strongly positive, often with Golgi accentuation.

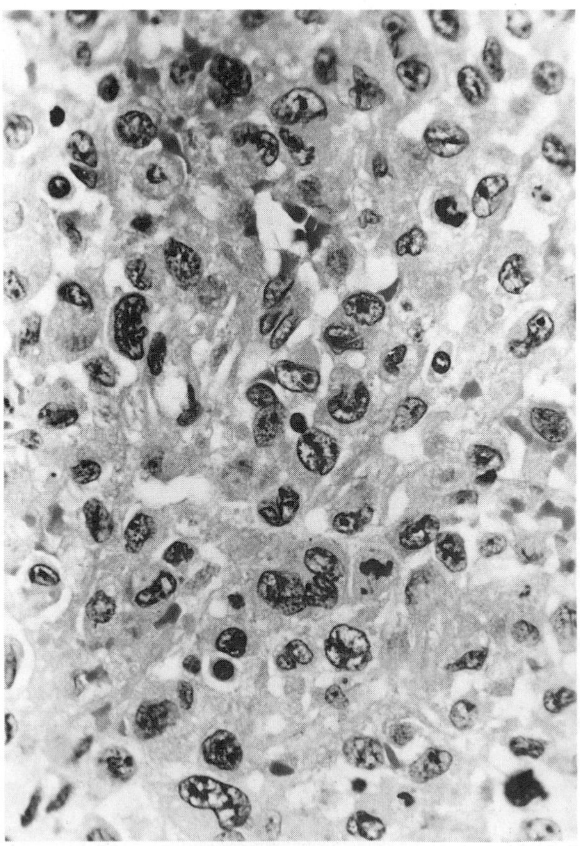

FIG. 51.34. True histiocytic lymphoma. The nuclei show irregular folds; the cytoplasm is relatively abundant (original magnification: 600× magnification).

Expression of S-100 protein is variable but usually not as strong or consistent as seen in interdigitating dendritic cell sarcoma. There usually is expression of CD45, CD45RO, and HLA-DR. By definition, there is no expression of specific B- and T-cell markers or CD30, myeloperoxidase, or follicular dendritic cell markers. Also by definition, there are no clonal rearrangements of antigen receptor genes.

In summary, MH or THL should be diagnosed with certainty only on the basis of consistent clinical, histologic, phenotypic, and molecular findings. The differential diagnosis includes malignant lymphoma of B- or T-cell types (including lymphomas associated with benign hemophagocytosis), anaplastic large cell lymphoma (Fig. 51.35), anaplastic carcinomas exhibiting hemophagocytosis, hepatosplenic $\gamma\delta$ T-cell lymphoma, acute monocytic leukemia, and a dendritic cell tumor, particularly an interdigitating dendritic cell tumor. B- and T-cell lymphomas and anaplastic large cell lymphoma can be distinguished by immunohistochemical studies for B- and T-cell antigens and CD30, respectively. IAHS and familial hemophagocytic lymphohistiocytosis lack the cytologic atypia seen in MH or THL. Tissue involvement by acute monocytic leukemia, in the absence of peripheral blood or bone marrow involvement, may be indistinguishable from MH or THL, although follow-up usually resolves these cases. Interdigitating dendritic cell tumors may show close overlap with MH or THL, particularly if patients with the latter express S-100 protein. The S-100 protein expression in interdigitating dendritic cell tumors is usually stronger and more consistent. Histologically, interdigitating dendritic cell tumors are much more likely to be spindled and ultrastructurally show complex cell processes.

Malignant Histiocytosis Associated with Mediastinal Germ Cell Tumor

There appears to be an unusually frequent association between mediastinal germ cell tumors and hematologic malignancies; this topic recently was reviewed by DeMent (164). Approximately one half of the hematologic malignancies have been characterized as MH, usually associated with a malignant teratoma, with or without yolk sac tumor differentiation. It has been suggested that the hematopoietic malignancies arise from the pluripotent germ cell, because teratocarcinoma cells are capable of differentiation along hematopoietic lines under the proper *in vitro* conditions (165). The cases reported as MH have generally not been investigated rigorously to confirm their histiocytic nature.

Histiocytic Medullary Reticulosis

Histiocytic medullary reticulosis was the term used by Scott and Robb-Smith in 1939 (166) for a clinicopathologic entity characterized by fever, weight loss, hepatosplenomegaly, and lymphadenopathy thought to be caused by widespread tissue infiltration by phagocytizing histiocytes. It has been considered by many to be synonymous with, or a var-

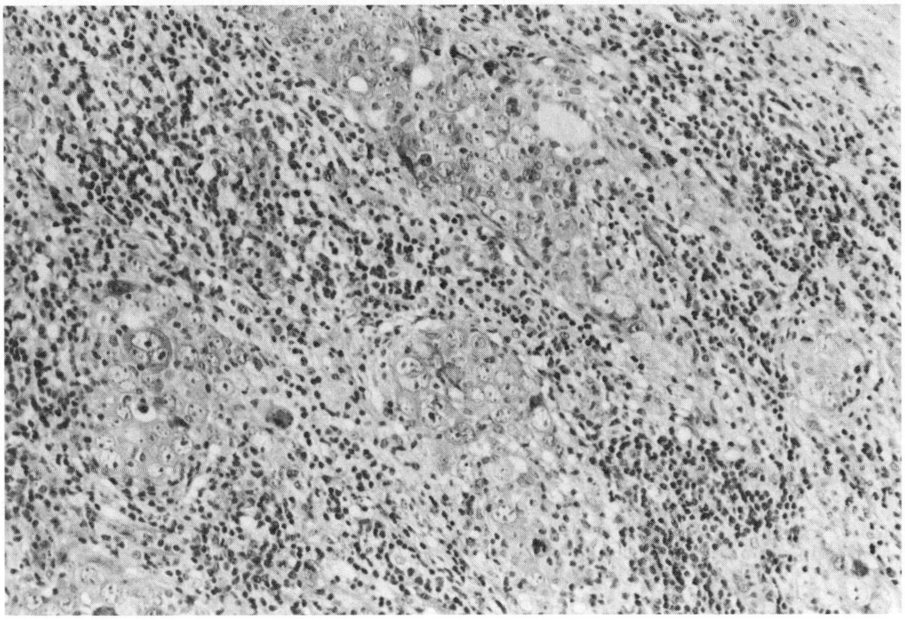

FIG. 51.35. Sinusoidal anaplastic large cell lymphoma. This lymphoma expressed markers of T-cell lineage and the CD30 (Ki-1) antigen (original magnification: 400× magnification).

iant of, MH, possibly also including some cases of IAHS. Falini and colleagues (40) restudied eight cases diagnosed by Robb-Smith during the period from 1949 to 1965. Their retrospective analysis suggested that several current entities were included within that diagnosis, including T-cell lymphoma with hemophagocytic syndrome, disseminated LCH, anaplastic large cell lymphoma, Lennert's lymphoma, Hodgkin's disease, and hyperimmune reaction. Because histiocytic medullary reticulosis appears to be superceded by MH and THL and, in current pathologic diagnosis, does not appear to represent a homogeneous disease entity, perhaps it is best not to use this designation at all.

Regressing Atypical Histiocytosis

Regressing atypical histiocytosis is a cutaneous proliferative disorder of cells histologically resembling histiocytes. Clinically, morphologically, and immunologically, regressing atypical histiocytosis shows many similarities to lymphomatoid papulosis. Each of these disorders has been shown to contain clonal rearrangements of the T-cell receptor β gene. For this reason, regressing atypical histiocytosis might be more appropriately regarded as a lymphoproliferative disorder of T lymphocytes (cutaneous CD30-positive lymphoproliferative disease), rather than a true histiocytic lesion (167). This entity is discussed further in Chapter 32.

SUMMARY AND CONCLUSIONS

The histiocytic and dendritic cell proliferative disorders are an uncommon but diverse group of diseases. The cells comprising most of these disorders show differentiation along pathways of normal differentiation, although the normal cellular counterpart for a few of them, such as SHML, has yet to be elucidated fully. Erythrophagocytic Tγ lymphoma, MH, THL, histiocytic medullary reticulosis, and atypical regressing histiocytosis have undergone intense scrutiny as we have been able to apply modern techniques of study more frequently to clinical material. This has led to redefinition of some of these disease entities, such as erythophagocytic Tγ lymphoma as hepatosplenic $\gamma\delta$ T-cell lymphoma and atypical regressing histiocytosis as CD30-positive lymphoproliferative disease; elimination of some of these disease entities, such as histiocytic medullary reticulosis, and a more precise definition of others, such as MH and THL.

REFERENCES

1. Metcalf D. The granulocyte-macrophage colony-stimulating factors. *Science* 1985;229:16–22.
2. Weinberg JB. Mononuclear phagocytes. In: Lee GR, Foerster J, Lukens J, eds. *Wintrobe's clinical hematology*. Baltimore: Williams & Wilkins, 1999:377–414.
3. Aderem A, Underhill DM. Mechanisms of phagocytosis in macrophages. *Annu Rev Immunol* 1999;17:593–623.
4. Steinman RM, Inaba K. Myeloid dendritic cells. *J Leukoc Biol* 1999; 66:205–208.
5. Beckstead JH, Wood GS, Turner RR. Histiocytosis X cells and Langerhans' cells: enzyme histochemical and immunologic similarities. *Hum Pathol* 1984;15:826–833.
6. Wood GS, Turner RR, Shiurba RA, et al. In situ immunophenotypic definition of subsets that exhibit specific morphologic and microenvironmental characteristics. *Am J Pathol* 1985;119:73–82.
7. Murphy GF, Bhan AK, Harrist TJ, et al. In situ identification of T6-positive cells in normal human dermis by immunoelectron microscopy. *Br J Dermatol* 1983;108.
8. Cerio R, Spaull J, Oliver GF. A study of Factor XIIIa and MAC

387 immunolabeling in normal and pathological skin. *Am J Dermatol* 1990;12:221–233.
9. Ardavin C. Thymic dendritic cells. *Immunol Today* 1997;18:350–161.
10. Parwaresch MR, Radzun HJ, Hansmann M-L, et al. Monoclonal antibody Ki-M4 specifically recognizes human dendritic cells (follicular dendritic cells) and their possible precursors in blood. *Blood* 1983; 62:585–590.
11. Pallesen G, Myhre-Jensen O. Immunophenotypic analysis of neoplastic cells in follicular dendritic cell sarcoma. *Leukemia* 1987;1: 549–557.
12. Gloghini A, Carbone A. The nonlymphoid microenvironment of reactive follicles and lymphomas of follicular origin as defined by immunohistology on paraffin-embedded tissues. *Hum Pathol* 1993;24: 67–76.
13. Tykocinski M, Schinnella RA, Greco MA. Fibroblastic reticulum cells in human lymph nodes: an ultrastructural study. *Arch Pathol Lab Med* 1983;107:418–422.
14. Schmitt-Graff A, Desmouliere A, Gabbiani G. Heterogeneity of myofibroblast phenotypic features: an example of fibroblastic cell plasticity. *Virchows Arch* 1994;425:3–24.
15. Pinkus GS, Warhol MJ, O'Connor EM, et al. Immunohistochemical localization of smooth muscle myosin in human spleen, lymph node, and other lymphoid tissues: unique staining patterns in splenic white pulp and sinuses, lymphoid follicles, and certain vasculature, with ultrastructural correlations. *Am J Pathol* 1986;123:440–453.
16. Albores-Saavedra J, Vuitch F, Delgado R, et al. Sinus histiocytosis of pelvic lymph nodes after hip replacement: a histiocytic proliferation induced by cobalt-chromium and titanium. *Am J Surg Pathol* 1994; 18:83–90.
17. Listinsky CM. Common reactive erythrophagocytosis in axillary lymph nodes. *Hum Pathol* 1988;89:189–192.
18. Destombes P. Adenites avec surcharge lipidique, de l'enfant ou de l'adulte jeune, observees aux antilles et au mali. Quatre observations. *Bull Soc Pathol Exot* 1965;58:1169–1175.
19. Rosai J, Dorfman RF. Sinus histiocytosis with massive lymphadenopathy: a newly recognized benign clinicopathologic entity. *Arch Pathol* 1969;87:63–70.
20. Rosai J, Dorfman RF. Sinus histiocytosis with massive lymphadenopathy: a pseudolymphomatous benign disorder. Analysis of 34 cases. *Cancer* 1972;30:1174–1188.
21. Foucar E, Rosai J, Dorfman RF. Sinus histiocytosis with massive lymphadenopathy (Rosai-Dorfman disease): review of the entity. *Semin Diagn Pathol* 1990;7:19–73.
22. Foucar E, Rosai J, Dorfman RF, et al. Immunologic abnormalities and their significance in sinus histiocytosis with massive lymphadenopathy. *Am J Clin Pathol* 1984;92:515–525.
23. Komp DM. The treatment of sinus histiocytosis with massive lymphadenopathy (Rosai-Dorfman disease). *Semin Diagn Pathol* 1990; 7:83–86.
24. Foucar E, Rosai J, Dorfman RF. Sinus histiocytosis with massive lymphadenopathy: an analysis of 14 deaths occurring in a patient registry. *Cancer* 1984;54:1834–1840.
25. Ngendahayo P, Roels H, Quatacker J, et al. Sinus hystiocytosis with massive lymphadenopathy in Rwanda: report of eight cases with immunohistochemical and ultrastructural studies. *Histopathology* 1983; 7:49–63.
26. Bonetti F, Chilosi M, Menestrina F, et al. Immunohistological analysis of Rosai-Dorfman histiocytosis: a disease of S-100 + CD1-histiocytes. *Virchows Arch* 1987;411:129–135.
27. Eisen RN, Buckley PJ, Rosai J. Immunophenotypic characterization of sinus histiocytosis with massive lymphadenopathy (Rosai-Dorfman disease). *Semin Diagn Pathol* 1990;7:74–82.
28. Paulli M, Feller AC, Boveri E, et al. Cathepsin D and E co-expression in sinus histiocytosis with massive lymphadenopathy (Rosai-Dorfman disease) and Langerhans' cell histiocytosis: further evidence of a phenotypic overlap between these histiocytic disorders. *Virchows Arch* 1994;424:601–606.
29. Paulli M, Bergamaschi G, Tonon L, et al. Evidence for a polyclonal nature of the cell infiltrate in sinus histiocytosis with massive lymphadenopathy (Rosai-Dorfman disease). *Br J Haematol* 1995;91: 415–418.
30. Levine PH, Jahan N, Murari P, et al. Detection of HHV-6 in tissues involved by sinus histiocytosis with massive lymphadenopathy (Rosai-Dorfman disease). *J Infect Dis* 1992;166:291–295.
31. Luppi M, Barozzi P, Garber R, et al. Expression of human herpesvirus-6 antigens in benign and malignant lymphoproliferative diseases. *Am J Pathol* 1998;153:815–823.
32. Tsang WYW, Yip TTC, Chan JKC. The Rosai-Dorfman disease histiocytes are not infected by Epstein-Barr virus. *Histopathology* 1994; 25:88–90.
33. Risdall RJ, McKenna RW, Nesbitt ME, et al. Virus associated hemophagocytic syndrome: a benign histiocytic proliferation distinct from malignant histiocytosis. *Cancer* 1979;44:993–1002.
34. Risdall RJ, Brunning RD, Hernandez JJ. Bacteria-associated hemophagocytic syndrome. *Cancer* 1984;54:2968–2972.
35. McKenna RW, Risdall RJ, Brunning RD. Virus associated hemophagocytic syndrome. *Hum Pathol* 1981;12:395–398.
36. Jenka G, Imashuku S, Elinder G, et al. Infection- and malignancy-associated hemophagocytic syndromes: secondary hemophagocytic lymphohistiocytosis. *Hematol Oncol Clin North Am* 1998;12: 435–444.
37. Ohga S, Matsuzaki A, Nishizaki M, et al. Inflammatory cytokines in virus-associated hemophagocytic syndrome: interferon-gamma as a sensitive indicator of disease activity. *Am J Pediatr Hematol Oncol* 1993;15:291–298.
38. Weiss LM, Azzi R, Dorfman RF, et al. Sinusoidal hematolymphoid malignancy (''malignant histiocytosis'') presenting as atypical sinusoidal proliferation: a study of nine cases. *Cancer* 1986;58:1681–1688.
39. Jaffe ES, Costa J, Fauci AS, et al. Malignant lymphoma and erythrophagocytosis simulating malignant histiocytosis. *Am J Med* 1983;75: 741–749.
40. Falini B, Pileri S, DeSolas I, et al. Peripheral T-cell lymphoma associated with hemophagocytic syndrome. *Blood* 1990;75:434–444.
41. Ost A, Nilsson-Ardnor S, J-I H. Autopsy findings in 27 children with haemophagocytic lymphohistiocytosis. *Histopathology* 1998;32: 310–316.
42. Farquhar JW, Claireaux AF. Familial hemophagocytic reticulosis. *Arch Dis Child* 1952;27:519–525.
43. Arico M, Janka G, Fischer A, et al. Hemophagocytic lymphohistiocytosis: report of 122 children from the International Registry. *Leukemia* 1998;10:197–203.
44. Stark B, Hershko C, Rosen N, et al. Familial hemophagocytic lymphohistiocytosis (FHLH) in Israel: description of 11 patients of Iranian-Iraqi origin and review of the literature. *Cancer* 1984;54:2109–2121.
45. Janka GE. Familial hemophagocytic lymphohistiocytosis: Review. *Eur J Pediatr* 1983;140:221–230.
46. Soffer D, Okon E, Rosen N, et al. Familial hemophagocytic lymphohistiocytosis in Israel: II. Pathologic findings. *Cancer* 1984;54: 2423–2431.
47. Wieczorek R, Greco A, McCarthy K, et al. Familial erythrophagocyttic lymphohistiocytosis: immunophenotypic, immunohistochemical and ultrastructural demonstration of the relation to sinus histiocytes. *Hum Pathol* 1986;17:55–63.
48. Fullerton P, Ekert H, Hosking C, et al. Hemophagocytic reticulosis: a case report with investigations of immune and white cell function. *Cancer* 1975;36:441–445.
49. Ladisch S, Holiman B, Poplack DG, et al. Immunodeficiency in familial erythrophagocytic lymphohistiocytosis. *Lancet* 1978;i:581–583.
50. Boyd AW, Ellis DW, Kannourakis G, et al. Activated killer cell lymphoma: an erythrophagocytic syndrome simulating histiocytic medullary reticulosis. *Pathology* 1988;20:265–270.
51. Wong KF, Chan JK. Reactive hemophagocytic syndrome: a clinicopathologic study of 40 patients in an Oriental population. *Am J Med* 1992;93:177–180.
52. Wong KF. Anaplastic large cell Ki-1 lymphoma involving bone marrow: marrow findings and association with reactive hemophagocytosis. *Am J Hematol* 1991;37:112–119.
53. Chubachi A, Imai H, Nishimura S, et al. Nasal T-cell lymphoma associated with hemophagocytic syndrome: immunohistochemical and genotypic studies. *Arch Pathol Lab Med* 1992;116:1209–1212.
54. Chang C-S, Wang C-H, Su I-J, et al. Hematophagic histiocytosis: a clinicopathologic analysis of 23 cases with special reference to the association with peripheral T-cell lymphoma. *J Formos Med Assoc* 1994;93:421–428.
55. Simrell CR, Margolick JB, Crabtree GR, et al. Lymphokine-induced phagocytosis in angiocentric immunoproliferative lesions (AIL) and malignant lymphoma arising in AIL. *Blood* 1985;65:1469–1476.
56. Lay JD, Tsao CJ, Chen JY, et al. Upregulation of tumor necrosis

factor-alpha gene by Epstein-Barr virus and activation of macrophages in Epstein-Barr virus-infected T cells in the pathogenesis of hemophagocytic syndrome. *J Clin Invest* 1997;100:1969–1979.
57. Kadin ME, Kamoun M, Lamberg J. Erythrophagocytic Tγ lymphoma: a clinicopathologic entity resembling malignant histiocytosis. *N Engl J Med* 1981;304:648–653.
58. Cooke CB, Krenacs L, Stetler-Stevenson M, et al. Hepatosplenic T-Cell lymphoma: a distinct clinicopathologic entity of cytotoxic $\gamma\delta$ T-Cell origin. *Blood* 1996;88:4265–4274.
59. Chang KL, Arber DA. Hepatosplenic $\gamma\delta$ T-cell lymphoma: not just alphabet soup. *Adv Anat Pathol* 1998;5:21–29.
60. Farcet JP, Gaulard P, Marolleau JP, et al. Hepatosplenic T-cell lymphoma: sinusal/sinusoidal localization af malignant cells expressing the T-cell receptor $\gamma\delta$. *Blood* 1990;75:2213–2219.
61. Kikuchi M. Lymphadenitis showing focal reticulum cell hyperplasia with nuclear debris and phagocytes: a clinico-pathological study (in Japanese). *Nippon Ketsueki Gakkai Zasshi* 1972;35:379–380.
62. Fujimoto Y, Kozima Y, Yamaguchi K. Cervical subacute necrotizing lymphadenitis: a new clinicopathologic entity. *Naika* 1972;20: 920–927.
63. Turner RR, Martin J, Dorfman RF. Necrotizing lymphadenitis: a study of 30 cases. *Am J Surg Pathol* 1983;7:115–123.
64. Pileri S, Kikuchi M, Helbron D, et al. Histiocytic necrotizing lymphadenitis without granulocytic infiltration. *Virchows Arch* 1982;395: 257–271.
65. Feller AC, Lennert K, Stein H, et al. Immunohistology and aetiology of histiocytic necrotizing lymphadenitis: report of three instructive cases. *Histopathology* 1983;7:825–829.
66. Unger PD, Rappaport KM, Strauchen JA. Necrotizing lymphadentitis (Kikuchi's disease): report of four cases of an unusual pseudolymphomatous lesion and immunologic marker studies. *Arch Pathol Lab Med* 1987;111:1031–1034.
67. Dorfman RF, Berry GJ. Kikuchi's histiocytic necrotizing lymphadenitis: an analysis of 108 cases with emphasis on differential diagnosis. *Semin Diagn Pathol* 1988;5:329–345.
68. Dorfman RF. Histiocytic necrotizing lymphadenitis of Kikuchi and Fujimoto. *Arch Pathol Lab Med* 1987;111:1026–1029.
69. Sumiyoshi Y, Kikuchi M, Ohshima K, et al. A case of histiocytic necrotizing lymphadenitis with bone marrow and skin involvement. *Virchows Arch A Pathol Anat Histopathol* 1992;420:275–279.
70. Kuo T. Cutaneous manifestation of Kikuchi's histiocytic necrotizing lymphadentitis. *Am J Surg Pathol* 1990;14:872–876.
71. Kuo TT, Jung SM, Wu WJ. Kikuchi's disease of intraparotid lymph nodes presenting as a parotid gland tumor with extranodal involvement of salivary gland. *Histopathology* 1996;28:185–187.
72. Tsang WYW, Chan JKC, Ng CS. Kikuchi's lymphadenitis: a morphologic analysis of 75 cases with special reference to unusual features. *Am J Surg Pathol* 1994;18:219–231.
73. Pileri S, Kikuchi M, Helbron D, et al. Histiocytic necrotizing lymphadenitis without granulocytic infiltration. *Virchows Arch A Pathol Anat Histopathol* 1982;395:257–271.
74. Dorfman RF, Warnke RA. Lymphadenopathy simulating the malignant lymphomas. *Hum Pathol* 1974;5:519–550.
75. Cleary KR, Osborne BM, Butler JJ. Lymph node infarction foreshadowing malignant lymphoma. *Am J Surg Pathol* 1982;6:435–442.
76. Giesker DW, Pastuszak WT, Forouhar FA, et al. Lymph node biopsy for early diagnosis in Kawasaki disease. *Am J Surg Pathol* 1982;6: 493–501.
77. Kikuchi M. Histiocytic necrotizing lymphadenitis. Clinicopathologic and immunologic study. In: Hanoaka M, Kadin ME, Mikata A, et al, eds. *Lymphoid malignancy: Immunocytology and cytogenetics*. New York: Field and Wood, 1990.
78. Sumiyoshi Y, Kikuchi M, Minematu T, et al. Analysis of herpesvirus genomes in Kikuchi's disease. *Virchows Arch* 1994;424:437–440.
79. Anagnostopoulos I, Hummel M, Korbjuhn P, et al. Epstein-Barr virus in Kikuchi-Fujimoto disease. *Lancet* 1993;341:893.
80. Hollingsworth HC, Peiper SC, Weiss LM, et al. An investigation of the viral pathogenesis of Kikuchi-Fujimoto disease (KFD): lack of evidence for Epstein-Barr virus or human herpesvirus-6 as the causative agents. *Arch Pathol Lab Med* 1994;118:134–140.
81. Favara BE, Feller AC, Paulli M, et al. A contemporary classification of histiocytic disorders. *Med Pediatr Oncol* 1997;29:157–166.
82. Freyer DR, Kennedy R, Bostrom BC, et al. Juvenile xanthogranuloma: forms of systemic disease and their clinical implications. *J Pediatr* 1996;129:227–237.
83. Nascimento AG. A clinicopathologic and immunohistochemical comparative study of cutaneous and intramuscular forms of juvenile xanthogranuloma. *Am J Surg Pathol* 1997;21:645–652.
84. Zelger B, Cerio R, Orchard G, et al. Juvenile and adult xanthogranuloma: a histological and immunohistochemical comparison. *Am J Surg Pathol* 1994;18:126–135.
85. Favara BE, McCarthy RC, Mierau GW. Histiocytosis X. *Hum Pathol* 1983;14:663–676.
86. Lieberman PH, Jones CR, Steinman RM, et al. Langerhans cell (eosinophilic) granulomatosis: a clinicopathologic study encompassing 50 years. *Am J Surg Pathol* 1996;20:519–552.
87. Carstensen H, Ornvold K. The epidemiology of Langerhans cell histiocytosis in children in Denmark. 1975–1989. *Med Pediatr Oncol* 1993;21:387–388.
88. Nicholson HS, Egeler RM, Nesbit ME. The epidemiology of Langerhans cell histiocytosis. *Hematol Oncol Clin North Am* 1998; 12:379–384.
89. Egeler RM, Neglia JP, Arico M, et al. The relation of Langerhans cell histiocytosis to acute leukemia, lymphomas, and other solid tumors: the LCH-Malignancy Study Group of the Histiocyte Society. *Hematol Oncol Clin North Am* 1998;12:369–378.
90. Bhatia S, Newbit ME, Egeler M, et al. Epidemiologic study of Langerhans cell histiocytosis in children. *J Pediatr* 1997;130: 774–784.
91. Colby TV, Lombard C. Histiocytosis X in the lung. *Hum Pathol* 1983; 14:847–856.
92. Williams JW, Dorfman RF. Lymphadenopathy as the initial manifestation of histiocytosis X. *Am J Surg Pathol* 1979;3:405–421.
93. Weiss LM, Beckstead JH, Warnke RA, et al. Leu-6-expressing cells in lymph nodes: dendritic cells phenotypically similar to interdigitating cells. *Hum Pathol* 1984;17:179–184.
94. Burns BF, Colby TV, Dorfman RF. Langerhans' cell granulomatosis (histiocytosis X) associated with malignant lymphomas. *Am J Surg Pathol* 1983;7:529–533.
95. Neuman MP, Frizzera G. The coexistence of Langerhans' cell granulomatosis and malignant lymphoma may take different forms: report of seven cases with a review of the literature. *Hum Pathol* 1986;17: 1060–1065.
96. Krenacs L, Tiszlavicz L, Krenacs T, et al. Immunohistochemical detection of CD1a antigen in formalin-fixed and paraffin-embedded tissue sections with monoclonal antibody O10. *J Pathol* 1993;171: 99–104.
97. Hage C, Willman CL, Favara BE, et al. Langerhans' cell histiocytosis (histiocytosis X): immunophenotype and growth fraction. *Hum Pathol* 1993;24:840–845.
98. Azumi N, Sheibani K, Swartz WG, et al. Antigenic phenotype of Langerhans cell histiocytosis: an immunohistochemical study demonstrating the value of LN-2, LN-3 and vimentin. *Hum Pathol* 1988; 19:1376–1382.
99. DeGraaf JH, Tamminga RYJ, Kamps WA, et al. Langerhans' cell histiocytosis: expression of leukocyte cellular adhesion molecules suggests abnormal homing and differentiation. *Am J Pathol* 1994; 144:466–472.
100. DeGraaf JH, Tamminga RYJ, Kamps WA, et al. Expression of cellular adhesion molecules in Langerhans cell histiocytosis and normal Langerhans cells. *Am J Pathol* 1995;147:1161–1171.
101. Ruco LP, Stoppacciaro A, Vitolo D, et al. Expression of adhesion molecules in Langerhans' cell histiocytosis. *Histopathology* 1993;23: 29–37.
102. DeGraaf JH, Tamminga RYJ, Dam-Meiring A, et al. The presence of cytokines in Langerhans cell histiocytosis. *J Pathol* 1996;180: 400–406.
103. Pinkus GS, Pinkus JL, Lones MA, et al. Fascin: a marker for Langerhans cell histiocytosis. *Lab Invest* 1998;78:138A (abst).
104. Pinkus GS, Pinkus JL, Langhoff E, et al. Fascin, a sensitive new marker for Reed-Sternberg cells of Hodgkin's disease: evidence for a dendritic or B cell derivation? *Am J Pathol* 1997;150:543–562.
105. Yu RC, Chu AC. Lack of T-cell receptor gene rearrangements in cells involved in Langerhans cell histiocytosis. *Cancer* 1995;75: 1162–1166.
106. Willman CL, Busque L, Griffith BB, et al. Langerhans'-cell histio-

cytosis (Histiocytosis X): a clonal proliferative disease. *N Engl J Med* 1994;331:154–160.
107. Yu RC, Chu C, Buluwela L, et al. Clonal proliferation of Langerhans cells in Langerhans cell histiocytosis. *Lancet* 1994;343:767–768.
108. Leahy MA, Krejci SM, Friedmash M, et al. Human herpsvirus 6 is present in lesions of Langerhans cell histiocytosis. *J Invest Dermatol* 1993;101:642–645.
109. McClain K, Jin H, Gresik V, et al. Langerhans cell histiocytosis: lack of a viral etiology. *Am J Hematol* 1994;47:16–20.
110. Rabkin MS, Wittwer CT, Kjeldsberg CR, et al. Flow-cytometric DNA content of histiocytosis X (Langerhans cell histiocytosis). *Am J Pathol* 1988;131:283–289.
111. Ornvold K, Carstensen H, Larsen JK, et al. Flow cytometric DNA analysis of lesions from 18 children with Langerhans cell histiocytosis (histiocytosis X). *Am J Pathol* 1990;136:1301–1307.
112. Brabencova E, Tazi A, Lorenzata M, et al. Langerhans cells in Langerhans cell granulomatosis are not actively proliferating cells. *Am J Pathol* 1998;152:1143–1149.
113. Lahey ME. Prognostic factors in histiocytosis X. *Am J Pediatr Hematol Oncol* 1981;3:57–60.
114. Greenberger JS, Crocker AC, Vawter G, et al. Results of treatment of 127 patients with systemic histiocytosis (Letterer-Siwe syndrome, Schuller-Christian syndrome and multifocal eosinophilic granuloma). *Medicine* 1981;60:311–338.
115. Risdall RJ, Dehner LP, Duray P, et al. Histiocytosis X (Langerhans' cell histiocytosis): prognostic role of histopathology. *Arch Pathol Lab Med* 1983;107:59–63.
116. Ben-Ezra J, Bailey A, Azumi N, et al. Malignant histiocytosis X: a distinct clinicopathologic entity. *Cancer* 1991;68:1050–1060.
117. Wood C, Wood GS, Deneau DG, et al. Malignant histiocytosis X: report of rapidly fatal case in an elderly man. *Cancer* 1984;54: 347–352.
118. Harris NL, Jaffe ES, Diebold J, et al. World Health Organization classification of neoplastic diseases of the hematopoietic and lymphoid tissues: report of the Clinical Advisory Committee meeting—Airlie House, Virginia, November, 1997. *J Clin Oncol* 1999; 17:3835–3849.
119. Pileri SA, Grogan TM, Banks P, et al. Tumors of histiocytes and accessory dendritic cells: a proposed classification from the International Lymphoma Study Group based on a comprehensive evaluation of 61 cases. (*submitted*).
120. Andriko JW, Kaldjian EP, Tsokos M, et al. Reticulum cell neoplasms of lymph nodes: a clinicopathologic study of 11 cases with recognition of a new subtype derived from fibroblastic reticular cells. *Am J Surg Pathol* 1998;22:1048–1058.
121. Fonseca R, Yamakawa M, Nakamura S, et al. Follicular dendritic cell sarcoma and interdigitating reticulum cell sarcoma: a review. *Am J Hematol* 1998;59:161–167.
122. Perez-Ordonez B, Rosai J. Follicular dendritic cell tumor: review of the entity. *Semin Diagn Pathol* 1998;15:144–154.
123. Monda L, Warnke R, Rosai J. A primary lymph node malignancy with features suggestive of dendritic reticulum cell differentiation. *Am J Surg Pathol* 1986;122:562–572.
124. Weiss LM, Berry GJ, Dorfman RF, et al. Spindle cell neoplasms of lymph nodes of probable reticulum cell lineage: true reticulum cell sarcoma? *Am J Surg Pathol* 1990;14:405–414.
125. Chan JKC, Fletcher CDM, Nayler S, et al. Follicular dendritic cell sarcoma: clinicopathologic analysis of 17 cases suggesting a malignant potential higher than currently recognized. *Cancer* 1997;79: 294–313.
126. Perez-Ordonez B, Erlandson RA, Rosai J. Follicular dendritic cell tumor: report of 13 additional cases of a distinctive entity. *Am J Surg Pathol* 1996;20:944–955.
127. Nguyen DT, Diamond LW, Hansmann M, et al. Follicular dendritic cell sarcoma: identification by monoclonal antibodies in paraffin sections. *Appl Immunohistochem* 1994;2:60–64.
128. Hollowood K, Stamp G, Zouvani I, et al. Extranodal follicular dendritic cell sarcoma of the gastrointestinal tract: morphologic, immunohistochemical and ultrastructural analysis of two cases. *Am J Clin Pathol* 1995;103:90–97.
129. Chan JKC, Tsang WYW, Ng CS, et al. Follicular dendritic cell tumors of the oral cavity. *Am J Surg Pathol* 1994;18:148.
130. Arber DA, Weiss LM, Chang KL. Detection of Epstein-Barr virus in inflammatory pseudotumor. *Semin Diagn Pathol* 1998;15:155–160.
131. Nayler SJ, Taylor L, Cooper K. HHV-8 is not associated with follicular dendritic cell tumours. *Mol Pathol* 1998;51:168–170.
132. Chan JKC, Tsang WYW, Ng CS. Follicular dendritic cell tumor and vascular neoplasm complicating hyaline-vascular Castleman's disease. *Am J Surg Pathol* 1994;18:517–525.
133. Perez-Ordonez B, Erlandson RA, Rosai J. Follicular dendritic cell tumor. *Am J Surg Pathol* 1996;20:944–955.
134. Luk IS, Shek TW, Tang VW, et al. Interdigitating dendritic cell tumor of the testis: a novel testicular spindle cell neoplasm. *Am J Surg Pathol* 1999;23:1141–1148.
135. Nakamura S, Koshikawa T, Kitoh K, et al. Interdigitating cell sarcoma: a morphologic and immunologic study of lymph node lesions in four cases. *Pathol Int* 1994;44:374–386.
136. Miettinen M, Fletcher CDM, Lasota J. True histiocytic lymphoma of small intestine: analysis of two S-100 protein-positive cases with features of interdigitating reticulum cell sarcoma. *Am J Surg Pathol* 1993;100:285–292.
137. Rousselet M-C, François S, Croué A, et al. A lymph node interdigitating reticulum cell sarcoma. *Arch Pathol Lab Med* 1994;118:183–188.
138. Feltkamp CA, van Heerde P, Feltkamp-Vroom TM, et al. A malignant tumor arising from interdigitating cells: light microscopical, ultrastructural, immuno- and enzyme-histochemical characteristics. *Pathol Anat* 1981;393:183–192.
139. Nakamura S, Hara K, Suchi T, et al. Interdigitating cell sarcoma: a morphologic, immunohistologic, and enzyme-histochemical study. *Cancer* 1988;61:562–568.
140. Berti E, Gianotti R, Alessi E. Unusual cutaneous histiocytosis expressing an intermediate immunophenotype between Langerhans' cells and dermal macrophages. *Arch Dermatol* 1988;124:1250–1253.
141. Kolde G, Brocker E-B. Multiple skin tumors of indeterminate cells in an adult. *J Am Acad Dermatol* 1986;15:591–597.
142. Bonetti F, Knowles DM, Chilosi M, et al. A distinctive cutaneous malignant neoplasm expressing the Langerhans cell phenotype: synchronous occurrence with B-chronic lymphocytic leukemia. *Cancer* 1985;55:2417–2425.
143. Chan WC, Zaatari G. Lymph node interdigitating cell sarcoma. *Am J Clin Pathol* 1986;85:739–744.
144. Wood GS, Hu C-H, Beckstead JH, et al. The indeterminate cell proliferative disorder: report of a case manifesting as an unusual cutaneous histiocytosis. *J Dermatol Surg Oncol* 1985;11:111–1119.
145. Vasef MA, Zaatari GS, Chan WC, et al. Dendritic cell tumors associated with low-grade B-cell malignancies: report of three cases. *Am J Clin Pathol* 1995;104:696–701.
146. Jaffe R, DeVaughn D, Langhoff E. Fascin and the differential diagnosis of childhood histiocytic lesion. *Pediatr Dev Pathol* 1998;1: 216–221.
147. Bryne GE, Rappaport H. Malignant histiocytosis. In Adazaki K, Rappaport H, Berard CW, et al, eds. *Malignant disease of the hematopoietic system.* Gann Monograph on Cancer Research, vol. 15. Tokyo: University of Tokyo Press, 1973:145–162.
148. Warnke RA, Kim H, Dorfman RF. Malignant histiocytosis (''histiocytic medullary reticulosis''): I. Clinicopathologic study of 29 cases. *Cancer* 1975;34:215–230.
149. Isaacson P, Wright DH, Jones DB. Malignant lymphoma of true histiocytic (monocyte-macrophage) origin. *Cancer* 1983;51:80.
150. Wilson MS, Weiss LM, Gatter KC, et al. Malignant histiocytosis: a reassessment of cases previously reported in 1975 based upon paraffin section immunophenotyping studies. *Cancer* 1990;66:530–536.
151. Turner RR, Wood GS, Beckstead JH, et al. Histiocytic malignancies: morphologic, immunologic, and enzymatic heterogeneity. *Am J Surg Pathol* 1984;8:482–500.
152. Weiss LM, Trela MJ, Cleary ML, et al. Frequent immunoglobulin and T-cell receptor rearrangements in ''histiocytic'' neoplasms. *Am J Pathol* 1985;121:369–373.
153. Isaacson PG, Spencer J, Connolly CE, et al. Malignant histiocytosis of the intestine: a T-cell lymphoma. *Lancet* 1985;ii:688–691.
154. Cattoretti G, Villa A, Vezzoni P, et al. Malignant histiocytosis: a phenotypic and genotypic investigation. *Am J Pathol* 1990;136: 1009–1019.
155. Weiss LM, Crabtree GS, Rouse RV, et al. Morphologic and immunologic characterization of 50 peripheral T-cell lymphomas. *Am J Pathol* 1985;118:316–324.
156. Picker LJ, Weiss LM, Medeiros LJ, et al. Immunophenotypic criteria

for the diagnosis of non-Hodgkin's lymphoma. *Am J Pathol* 1987; 128:181–201.
157. Hanson CA, Jaszcz W, Kersey JH, et al. True histiocytic lymphoma: histopathologic, immunophenotypic and genotypic analysis. *Br J Haematol* 1989;73:187–198.
158. Weiss LM, Picker LJ, Grogan TM, et al. Absence of clonal beta and gamma T-cell receptor gene rearrangements in a subset of peripheral T-cell lymphomas [published erratum appears in Am J Pathol 1988; 131:604]. *Am J Pathol* 1988;130:436–442.
159. Weiss LM, Picker LJ, Copenhaver CM, et al. Large-cell hematolymphoid neoplasms of uncertain lineage. *Hum Pathol* 1988;19:967–973.
160. Copie-Bergman C, Wotherspoon AC, Norton AJ, et al. True histiocytic lymphoma: a morphologic, immunohistochemical and molecular genetic study of 13 cases. *Am J Surg Pathol* 1998;22:1386–1392.
161. Franchino C, Reich C, Distenfeld A, et al. A clinicopathologically distinctive primary splenic histiocytic neoplasm: demonstration of its histiocytic derivation by immunophenotypic and molecular genetic analysis. *Am J Surg Pathol* 1988;12:398–404.
162. Kamel OW, Gocke CD, Kell DL, et al. True histiocytic lymphoma: a study of 12 cases based on current definition. *Leuk Lymphoma* 1995; 18:81–86.
163. Ralfkiaer E, Delsol G, O'Connor NTJ, et al. Malignant lymphomas of true histiocytic origin: a clinical, histological, immunophenotypic and genotypic study. *J Pathol* 1990;160:9–17.
164. DeMent SH. Association between mediastinal germ cell tumors and hematologic malignancies: an update. *Hum Pathol* 1990;21:699–703.
165. Cudennec CA, Johnson GR. Presence of multipotential hemopoietic cells in teratocarcinoma cultures. *J Embryol Exp Morphol* 1981;61: 51–59.
166. Scott RB, Robb-Smith AHT. Histiocytic medullary reticulosis. *Lancet* 1939;ii:194–198.
167. Weiss LM, Wood GS, Trela MJ, et al. Clonal T cell populations in lymphomatoid papulosis. Evidence for a lymphoproliferative etiology in a clinically benign disease. *N Engl J Med* 1986;315:475–479.

CHAPTER 52

Mast Cell Disease

Reza M. Parwaresch, Hans P. Horny, and Verena Schemmel

While working with aniline dyes, Paul Ehrlich discovered a new cell type in human tissue with distinct cytoplasmic granules that he interpreted as ingested nutrients, giving them the name *mast cells* (1). Salient contributions to the understanding of various biologic aspects of mast cells were made by Unna (2), who recognized the first case of cutaneous mast cell disease; Jorpes (3) and Riley (4), who discovered the abundant occurrence of heparin and histamine in mast cell granules, respectively; and Ishizaka and Ishizaka (5), who elucidated the IgE mediation of atopia. Important contributions to the identification of mast cell mediators were made by Schwartz and coworkers (6); Valent (7) provided considerable information on the immunophenotype of mast cells. The elucidation of stem cell factor (SCF) and the SCF receptor coded by the protooncogene *KIT* represents a major achievement in mast cell biology by Anderson and colleagues (8) and Rottem and associates (9). Mast cell neoplasias may involve *KIT* mutations as shown by Furitsu and coworkers (10).

Despite abundant evidence for the close relationship of mast cells to the myelomonocytic lineage, mast cells have to be distinguished clearly from their blood counterpart, the basophil granulocyte (Table 52.1). Striking similarities exist between the cell types in morphology and biochemical composition of the cytoplasmic granules (11). To avoid confusion, it is recommended that terms such as *tissue basophils* for mast cells and *blood mast cells* for basophil granulocytes be discarded.

R. M. Parwaresch: Institute of Hematopathology and Lymphnode Registry Kiel, Christian-Albrechts Universität zu Kiel, Kiel, Germany

H. P. Horny: Institute of Pathology, University of Tübingen, Tübingen, Germany

V. Schemmel: Department of Paediatric Medicine, Hochschule Hannover, Hannover, Germany

NORMAL MAST CELLS

Distribution and Morphology

In humans, mast cells are a regular constituent of connective tissue. Their frequent occurrence in pericapillary, perineural, and subepithelial spaces has been related to secretory activity during inflammatory processes. The mast cell number in various tissue types is variable, being high, for example, in loose connective tissue such as uvea and serous cavities. In the dermis, the average mast cell count amounts to 7,225 per square millimeter (SD, 2,167) in paraffin sections (12) and 12,000 to 15,100 per square millimeter in epon-embedded semithin sections (13). The average distribution density of mast cells in lung tissue, 350 per square millimeter, is considerably lower (14). Other tissue types such as spleen, kidney, liver, and adrenals may contain only a small number of or no mast cells.

Morphologically, mast cells are characterized by oval or spindle-shaped cytoplasm, sometimes with short, plump cytoplasmic protrusions. The cytoplasm is equipped richly with rounded or oval granules about 1 μm in diameter. The nucleus is oval and shows occasional indentations, although clear-cut segmentation is rare. Binucleated mast cells or mast cell mitoses are extremely rare but can be observed, especially if mast cell generation has been stimulated by destruction or massive mast cell depletion. Multinucleated or giant mast cells with irregular granule distribution and cytoplasmic vacuoles are observed in tissue areas after radiotherapy.

Rounded mast cells are found primarily in loose connective tissue, whereas the fusiform variant is localized in areas of fibrosis. In tissue sections subjected to hematoxylin and eosin, van Gieson, Goldener, or Azan staining, mast cells are hardly distinguishable. In the periodic acid–Schiff reaction, however, mast cells are stained weakly. Mast cells can be visualized selectively with acridine orange, methyl-green, and colloidal iron or by using basic dyes, such as methylene

TABLE 52.1. *Comparison of blood basophils and mast cells*

Features	Blood basophils	Mast cells
Nuclear segmentation	+	−
Water-soluble granules	+	−
Occurrence in blood	+	−
Longevity[a]	−	+
Chloroacetate esterase	−	+
Ki–M1p[b]	−	+

[a] Blood basophils are short-lived granulocytes with a half-life of 6 hours and a mean circulation time of 8.5 hours (11). Mast cells have a half-life that exceeds 3 weeks.

[b] Ki-M1p is a panmacrophage monoclonal antibody that coreacts with immature and mature mast cells.

or toluidine blue, that react with highly polymeric sulfated glycosaminoglycans, revealing a red to purple metachromasia of the granules. The metachromatic staining of mast cell granules depends on pH and ion concentration. Histochemical possibilities for demonstrating the immaturity of mast cells include application of safranin and alcian blue or recording the critical electrolyte concentration and pH of optimum staining with pure anionic dyes (15–18). Various aspects of mast cells have been studied extensively on electron microscopic images (Fig. 52.1). The most striking organelles are the specific intracytoplasmic granules densely packed throughout the cytoplasm (19,20).

Mediators, Immunophenotype, and Function

The functional activity of mast cells is expressed to a large extent in mast cell degranulation, which gives way to the extrusion of granule-matrix lipoproteins, highly sulfated glycosaminoglycans bound to basic peptides, and biogenic amines such as histamine. Under adequate stimulation, human mast cells produce and release potent cytokines and arachidonic acid metabolites. Among the complicated set of membrane proteins expressed by mast cells, those that serve as receptors for complement factor C5a and immunoglobulin E are especially important to the understanding of the role that mast cells play as amplifiers of the inflammatory response that links the noncellular initial phase of inflammation to the cellular phase and in various types of immune reactions (43–50).

Mediators synthesized and released by mast cells have been divided into three groups:

1. Those preformed and stored in granules such as histamine (4), proteoglycans: heparin and chondroitin sulfate E (3,21) and neutral proteases such as tryptase and chymase (22,23), as well as a remarkable array of acid hydrolases
2. Arachidonic acid derivatives, such as prostaglandin and the leucotriens, which are synthesized mainly after mast cell activation (6)
3. A large number of cytokines that also is produced following mast cell stimulation (24,25).

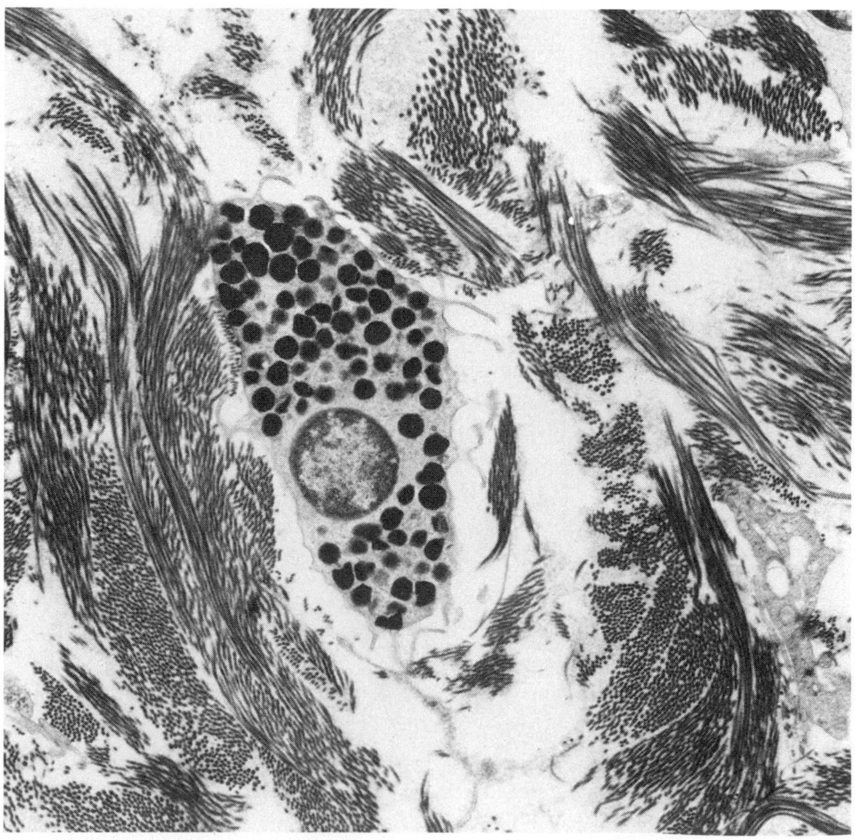

FIG. 52.1. Electronphotomicrograph of a mast cell in normal human dermis surrounded by collagen fibers. The cytoplasm contains numerous highly electron-dense granules (araldite embedding, lead citrate and uranyl acetate contrasting, original magnification: 4,500× magnification).

TABLE 52.2. *Mast cell mediators*

Preformed granule-associated mediators
- Histamine
- Heparin
- Chondroitin sulfate E
- Tryptase
- Chymase
- Cathepsin G
- Carboxypeptidase A
- Arylsulfatase A
- β-Hexosaminidase
- β-Glucuronidase
- N-Acetylglucosaminidase
- Superoxide dismutase
- Peroxidase

Arachidonic acid metabolites
- Prostaglandin D2
- Leukotriene B4, C4, D4
- Platelet-activating factor (PAF)
- 12-L-hydroxy-5,8,10-heptadecatrienoic acid (HHT)
- 5-Hydroxyeicosatetraenoic acid (HETE)

Cytokines
- IL-1, IL-3, IL-4, IL-5, IL-6, IL-8, IL-10, IL-13
- T-cell activating antigen
- Interferon-γ
- Granulocyte-macrophage colony-stimulating factor
- Tumor necrosis factor-α
- Transforming growth factor-β
- Basic fibroblast growth factor-2
- Macrophage inflammatory protein-1α and -1β
- Monocyte chemotactic factor
- Regulated on activation, normal T cell–expressed and secreted

IL, interleukin.

Table 52.2 surveys various mediators unequivocally shown in human mast cells.

In conjunction with the cells of granulopoiesis, mast cells are the only cell type that reveals a strong enzyme cytochemical activity with naphthol AS-D chloroacetate esterase (26), and elastase (27,28). Well-preserved samples processed according to the methods described by Fahimi (29) also may reveal peroxidase content, not only of the granules but also of the perinuclear envelope. Staining with alkaline phosphatase and alpha-naphthyl-acetate esterase is not positive in mast cells. Dipeptidyl-peptidase IV, aminocaproate, and acid phosphatase show a moderate reactivity in these cells, the last being resistant to tartrate inhibition. Mast cell tryptase represents a specific neutral protease that is already detectable in early stages of mast cell development. This enzyme can be employed in the detection of mast cells by its enzymatic activity or by a monoclonal antibody to the enzyme protein. A poorly defined subpopulation of mast cells may contain chymase in addition to tryptase and chloroacetate esterase. Such neutral proteases have been used to demonstrate mast cell heterogeneity in different tissue types. Tryptase- and chymase-positive mast cells occur in skin, intestinal submucosa, and synovia; tryptase-positive, chymase-negative mast cells reside in the lung and in the gastrointestinal mucosa.

Recently there has been considerable progress in the immunophenotypic characterization of human mast cells (Table 52.3). These cells reveal a negative immunohistochemical reactivity to the majority of lineage-specific monoclonal antibodies, including those reactive with T and B lymphocytes, plasma cells, fibroblasts, granulocytes, keratin, myosin, actin intermediate filaments, endothelia, and neural components, although neuron-specific enolase reveals weak activity. A small number of monoclonal antibodies reactive with monocytes and macrophages (such as those directed against CD11c, CD68, and Ki-M1p) may react positively with mast cells. Some monoclonal antibodies related to the leukocyte common antigen (CD45) with a restricted specificity to B lymphocytes and a mild coreactivity with myeloid cells also show coreactivity with human mast cells. This is the case with Ki-B3 (30). Broad-spectrum antibodies to the leukocyte common antigen react positively with human mast cells. A positive reaction also is found with antimetencephaline and antiencephaline. Although reactive with monocytes and macrophages, MAC-387, OKM-1, and antilysozyme display a negative reaction with mast cells.

Under normal conditions, tryptase and the *KIT* product CD117 are the most specific proteins of human tissue mast

TABLE 52.3. *Immunophenotypic profile of normal mast cells in comparison to basophils and monocytes*

Antigen	CD	Mast cells	Basophils	Monocytes
Tryptase	NC	+	−	−
Chymase	NC	+[a]	−	−
Histamine	NC	+	+	−
Heparin	NC	+[a]	−	−
c-kit	CD117	+	−	−
C5aR	CD88	+[a]	+	+
C3biR	CD11b	−	+	+
FceRI	NC	+	+	−
FcgRII	CDW32	−	+	+
FcgRIII	CD16	−	−	+
IL-2Ra	CD25	−	+	+/−
IL-3Ra	CD123	−	+	+
GM-CSFRa	CD116	−	+/−	+
Lactosylceramid	CDw17	−	+	+/−
Leucosialin	CD43	+	+	+
Panleucocyte	CD45	+	+	+
p24-Aggregation	CD9	+	+	+
gp 110	CD68	+	−	+
gp 67	CD33	+	+	+
Pgp-1-HR	CD44	+	+	+
LPSRr	CD14	−	−	+
3-FAL	CD15	−	+[b]	+
ICAM-1	CD54	+	+	+
b1-Integrin	CD29	+	+	+
b3-Integrin	CD61	+	−	+
MHC-class-1		+	+	+

[a] Subpopulation.
[b] Masked.
NC, not yet clustered; LPSRr, lipopolysaccharide receptor–related; 3-FAL, 3-fucosylactosamine; Pgp-1-HR, Pgp-1 homing–receptor.

cells. In Table 52.3, the immunophenotype of tissue mast cells is compared with that of blood basophils and monocytes.

Derivations

There appears to be a growing acceptance of the close relationship of mast cells to the myelomonocytic lineage. This hypothesis is supported by the following observations:

1. Mast cells contain the enzymes naphthol AS-D chloroacetate esterase, which is a highly specific feature of myelomonocytic cells (26–28,31,32).
2. Mast cell neoplasias may be associated with clonal granulocytes indicative of a stem cell aberration.
3. Malignant mastocytosis (MM) coincides in about 55% of patients with myeloid or monocytic leukemias as well as with other myeloproliferative disorders (33,34).
4. Mast cells share highly specific immunophenotypic features, such as Ki-M1p, CD11c, and CD68, with monocytes and macrophages.
5. The renewal kinetics and proliferation mode of mast cells, as far as is known, resemble those of monocyte-derived cells.
6. More than 5% of all myeloid leukemias are associated with the occurrence of atypical mast cells (35).
7. Mast cell proliferations are associated mostly with an increase of monocytes in the blood (36).

Although there is wealth of indirect evidence, few direct observations document an immediate derivation of mast cells from blood cells. Small human mast cell clones can be grown from hematopoietic precursor cells selected by the limited dilution technique. A single observation was made by Kreipe (personal communication), who was able to induce mast cell differentiation from separated blood monocytes after stimulation with media of BCG-conditioned T lymphocytes from patients with a history of active tuberculosis. McCarthy and colleagues (37) mentioned the presence of mast cells in agar cultures. Mast cell precursors may circulate in patients with chronic myeloid leukemia and systemic mastocytosis (SM) (38). This finding agrees with the observation that myeloid leukemia may be associated with atypical mast cells (35) and that MM is complicated by a myeloproliferative disorder in over 55% of patients (33,34,39).

Ample evidence indicates that tissue mast cells are of hematopoietic origin and derive from CD34-positive ($CD34^+$) stem cells as shown *in vitro* (40) and *in vivo* (41).

A probable mode of mast cell derivation is early myeloid precursors giving rise to circulating monocytes or cells indistinguishable from monocytes. Such mast cell precursors lack metachromatic granules, are weakly adherent, float at a density of 1.077 g/mL with the majority of the monocytes, migrate into tissue with adequate stimulation, and terminally differentiate into mast cells. This seems to be mediated by mast cell–generating factors produced by T lymphocytes and fibroblasts. An enhanced peripheral need is covered adequately by an increased precursor migration. Accelerated mast cell generation also is accompanied, however, by the persistent capability of precursors to undergo an average of one mitosis between their appearance in the extravascular tissue and their evolution into mast cells, analogous to monocyte-derived macrophages (42). A reasonable mode of mast cell evolution from precursor cells circulating in the blood was suggested by Rottem and colleagues, including SCF and interleukin-3, the cytokines relevant to mast cell evolution (9) (Fig. 52.2). This track of mast cell generation, however,

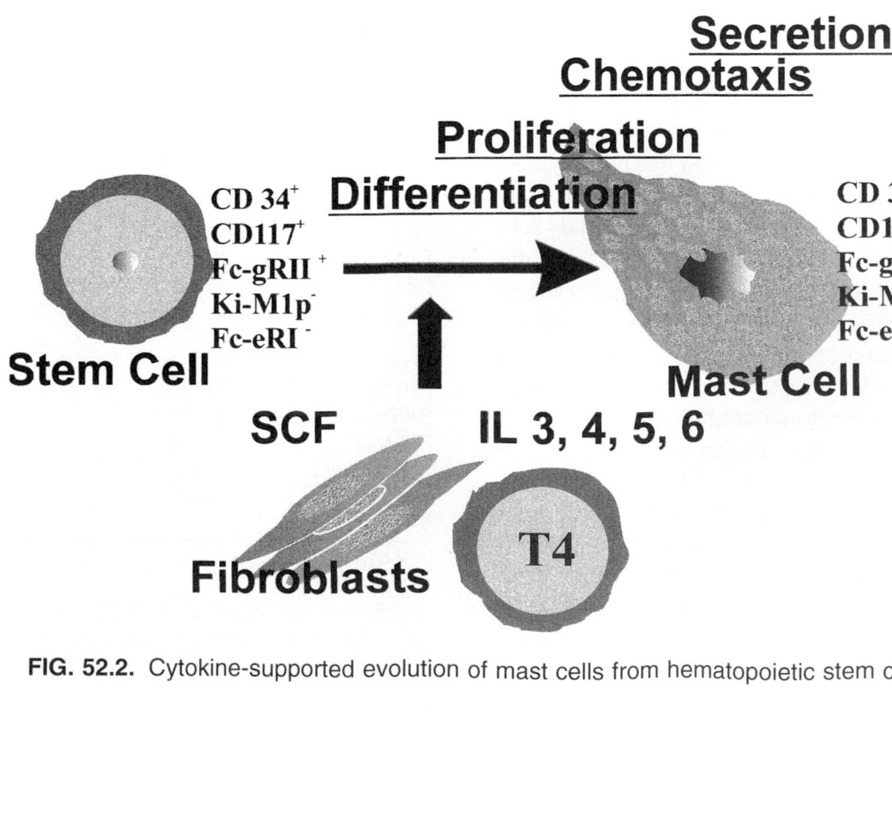

FIG. 52.2. Cytokine-supported evolution of mast cells from hematopoietic stem cell.

provides no information on the maturation stages between the stem cells and the terminally differentiated mast cells. For a prolonged survival of mast cells a concerted presence of the cytokine SCF and helper T cell 2–type cytokines such as interleukins 3 through 6 seems to be an essential requirement (51). Together with transforming growth factor-β and RANTES, SCF is the most effective chemoattractant for the mast cells promoting their adhesion to connective tissue matrix, preferably to fibronectin (52). Besides C5a and IgE, SCF is the most important factor of mast cell mediator release (53).

MAST CELL HYPERPLASIA

A focal increase in the number of mast cells occurs in a large number of inflammatory lesions, within benign or malignant tumors, and in bone marrow in connection with allergic reactions. Such alterations are referred to as *reactive mast cell hyperplasia*; others (such as mast cell increase in patients with myelodysplasia or myelomonocytic leukemias) reflect a stem cell disorder common to mast cell and myelomonocytic progenies (35).

MAST CELL NEOPLASIA

General Comments

A deregulated proliferation of mast cells in one or more tissue types has been referred to as *mastocytosis* (54), or *mast cell disease*. In patients with mastocytosis, as in proliferative disorders of other terminally differentiated forms of the monocyte-macrophage lineage, it may be difficult or even impossible to distinguish clearly between hyperplasia and neoplasia. This is partly because of the gap in our knowledge about the exact route of mast cell recruitment and the mechanisms that regulate their renewal and kinetics.

The neoplastic nature of mast cell disease has been documented using various techniques:

1. In a limited number of cases of malignant forms of mast cell disease in our files, a high level of activity for the enzyme telomerase, which is restricted to germ line, stem, and cancer cells, could be detected.
2. In nine patients (one with cutaneous mastocytoma, three with bone marrow mastocytosis, one with mast cell sarcoma, and one with systemic and three with malignant mast cell disease) clonal rearrangement for the T cell antigen receptor γ gene was found. This finding is not unusual among myeloproliferative diseases and indicates the clonal nature of the proliferation, but not its relation to the T-cell lineage.
3. In two patients with indolent systemic mast cell disease (SMCD) in our files a monoclonal methylation pattern of the X-chromosomal phosphoglycerokinase gene in granulocytes was detected, indicating an aberration on the stem cell level.
4. In a considerable number of patients, typical point mutations have been identified, which involve codon positions 560 (base 1700: GTT→GGT⇒Gly→560 Val), codon position 816 (base 2468: GAC→GTC⇒Asp→816 Val) and 820 (base 2480: GAT→GGT⇒Asp→820 Gly) on the 17th of the 21 exons of the proto-oncogene *c-KIT* on the chromosome 4q11-q21. The mutation mainly involved, the heterozygote clonal aberration Asp→816Val, has been detected in the permanent human cell line HMC1 established from a mast cell leukemia (10), in patients with malignant SMCD (55), in urticaria pigmentosa, and in benign (indolent) SMCD (56,57).

The aberration has been found in the neoplastic mast cells infiltrating skin, spleen, and bone marrow. In addition, mononuclear blood cells, monocytes, granulocytes, marrow progenitor cells, and cultured erythropoietic cells have been shown to harbor this mutation on mRNA as well as on genomic levels. Because buccal epithelia are not affected, the *KIT* aberration seems to represent an acquired somatic mutation on a ''hot spot'' region. Recent evidence has been found that the detection of an Asp→816Val mutation in mast cell disease frequently is associated with hematologic disorders and extensive systemic involvement (132).

The protooncogene *KIT* encodes a type III transmembrane tyrosine kinase, which represents the receptor for the SCF (58,59). The latter has been shown convincingly to play a key role in the processes of mast cell differentiation, proliferation, prolonged survival, chemotaxis, and mediator release. The acquired heterozygote point mutations give rise to a ligand (SCF)–independent autophosphorylation of the mutant receptor protein. The permanent activation of the SCF receptor, as the result of the mutational ''gain of function'' of the protooncogene, seems to have oncogenic bearings on the clonal evolution of the affected mast cells into a neoplastic mast cell disease.

In childhood onset of cutaneous mast cell disease, however, an inactivating *KIT* mutation substituting lysine for glutamic acid in position 839 (Glut→839Lys) with dominant loss of function seems to play a key role (133). This may explain the transient character of pediatric cutaneous mast cell disease.

In our files two patients showed karyotypic aberrations involving chromosome 8. They were a 75-year-old man with indolent SMCD, who had a translocation t(X;8), and a 42-year-old man with malignant SCMD and a trisomy of chromosome 8. Other cytogenetic aberrations have been reported in the literature (60). No relationship was found between cytogenetic abnormalities and Asp→816Val *KIT* mutation in patients with mast cell disease (134).

Neoplasias of mast cells are rare, although not as rare as commonly assumed. Lack of experience, together with the confusing range of symptoms and clinical pictures, account for the high frequency of mistaken diagnoses (more than 50%). Abnormal proliferations of mast cells most frequently involve the dermis as maculopapular disseminated skin lesions known as *urticaria pigmentosa* or small localized tu-

TABLE 52.4. *Classification of mast cell diseases*

Kiel classification[a]	Travis-Metcalfe classification[b]
1. Nonsystemic mast cell disease	1. Indolent mast cell disease
1.1. Cutaneous mast cell disease	1.A. Skin only
1.1.1. Solitary mastocytoma (mast cell nevus)	Solitary mastocytoma
1.1.2. Urticaria pigmentosa (UP)	Urticaria pigmentosa
Bullous urticaria pigmentosa	Telangiectasia macularis eruptiva persistans
Diffuse cutaneous "erythrodermic" mastocytosis	Diffuse "erythrodermic" cutaneous mastocytosis
Telangiectasia macularis eruptiva persistans	1.B. Systemic mast cell diasease (± UP)
1.2. Solitary mast cell tumor (mastocytoma)	Bone marrow
1.3. Isolated bone marrow mast cell disease	Gastrointestinal tract
1.4. Mast cell sarcoma[b]	2. Mast cell disease with an associated hematologic disorder (± UP)
2. Systemic mast cell disease	2.A. Dysmyelopoietic disorders
2.1. "Indolent" systemic mast cell disease	2.B. Myeloproliferative disorders
2.2. "Malignant" systemic mast cell disease	2.C. Acute non-lymphatic leukemia
± Myelodysplasia	2.D. Malignant lymphoma
± Myeloproliferation	2.E. Chronic neutropenia
± Mast cell leukemia	3. Mast cell leukemia
	4. Lymphadenopathic mastocytosis with eosinophilia (± UP) (aggressive mastocytosis)

[a] The classification used for our files of 196 patients.
[b] Mast cell sarcoma may be associated with a mast cell leukemia.

mors, referred to as *localized cutaneous* and *extracutaneous mastocytoma*. Solitary mast cell tumors also may occur in other regions. In rare patients, mastocytosis is restricted to the bone marrow. Mast cell proliferations may involve more than one organ, justifying the terms *systemic* or *generalized mastocytosis* (61). Other terms, such as *mast cell reticulosis* (62–65) and *systemic mast cell disease*, have been applied. SM has proved to be heterogeneous, with many overlapping features. Considerable efforts have been made to elucidate the significance of different features in predicting outcome, such as the optimal pH for metachromatic staining of mast cells in histochemical studies (39,66); the absence or presence of primary skin involvement (34); the histologic infiltration pattern in the bone marrow (67); involvement of liver, spleen, and lymph nodes; sex and age distribution (68); and the evaluation of various symptoms and associated disorders in multivariate analysis (69,70). The determination of *KIT* mRNA (135) and mutations of the *KIT* protooncogene may provide an additional approach in assessing prognosis. In our files there is a single case of SMCD occurring in a mother and daughter. A brief survey of the generally accepted entities follows (Table 52.4).

Nonsystemic Mast Cell Disease

Localized Mastocytoma (Mast Cell Nevus)

Localized mastocytoma is a firm, nodular or flat, yellow or brown tumor of the dermis. It may occur on the head or trunk or on the extremities and usually is limited to the first 3 years of life or is present at birth. In the collection of the Lymph Node Registry in Kiel we have seen one lesion about 2 cm in diameter. One lesion was localized on the major labia. One of our patients, however, was 67 years old.

The majority of patients has a solitary nodule, although multiple lesions do occur. Normally, the tumor does not exceed a few millimeters in diameter and urticates on stroking (71–73). On histologic examination, localized mastocytoma consists of dense, tumor-like accumulations of mast cells (Fig. 52.3). The infiltrates may be present throughout the whole dermis or even localized within the subcutaneous adipose tissue. The localized mastocytoma is covered by a well-preserved epidermis that may show a mild degree of acanthosis and hyperkeratosis. There is mild hyperpigmentation of the basal layer. Between the mast cell infiltrates, there are partly hyalinized streaks of collagen fibers and vessels. The latter may be surrounded closely by mast cells, although no infiltration of the vessel wall occurs. Cytologically, mast cells exhibit a broad oval or polygonal cytoplasm. Generally, spindled or fusiform mast cells do not occur in these lesions. Monomorphous small granules are faintly visible within the cytoplasm in routine hematoxylin and eosin staining. Giemsa staining is the preferred histochemical technique in detecting such lesions. Enzyme histochemistry demonstrates no major differences between localized mastocytoma and normal mast cells. On immune histochemical studies, localized mastocytoma cells show the following phenotype: The leukocyte common antigen and the antigen recognized by the panmacrophage antibody Ki-M1p, CD117, and tryptase are strongly expressed; lysozyme, CD4, MAC 378 and S-100 are regularly not expressed.

Localized mastocytoma shows a strong tendency toward spontaneous regression, disappearing within 1 or 2 years. Nevertheless, excision of the tumor is recommended because

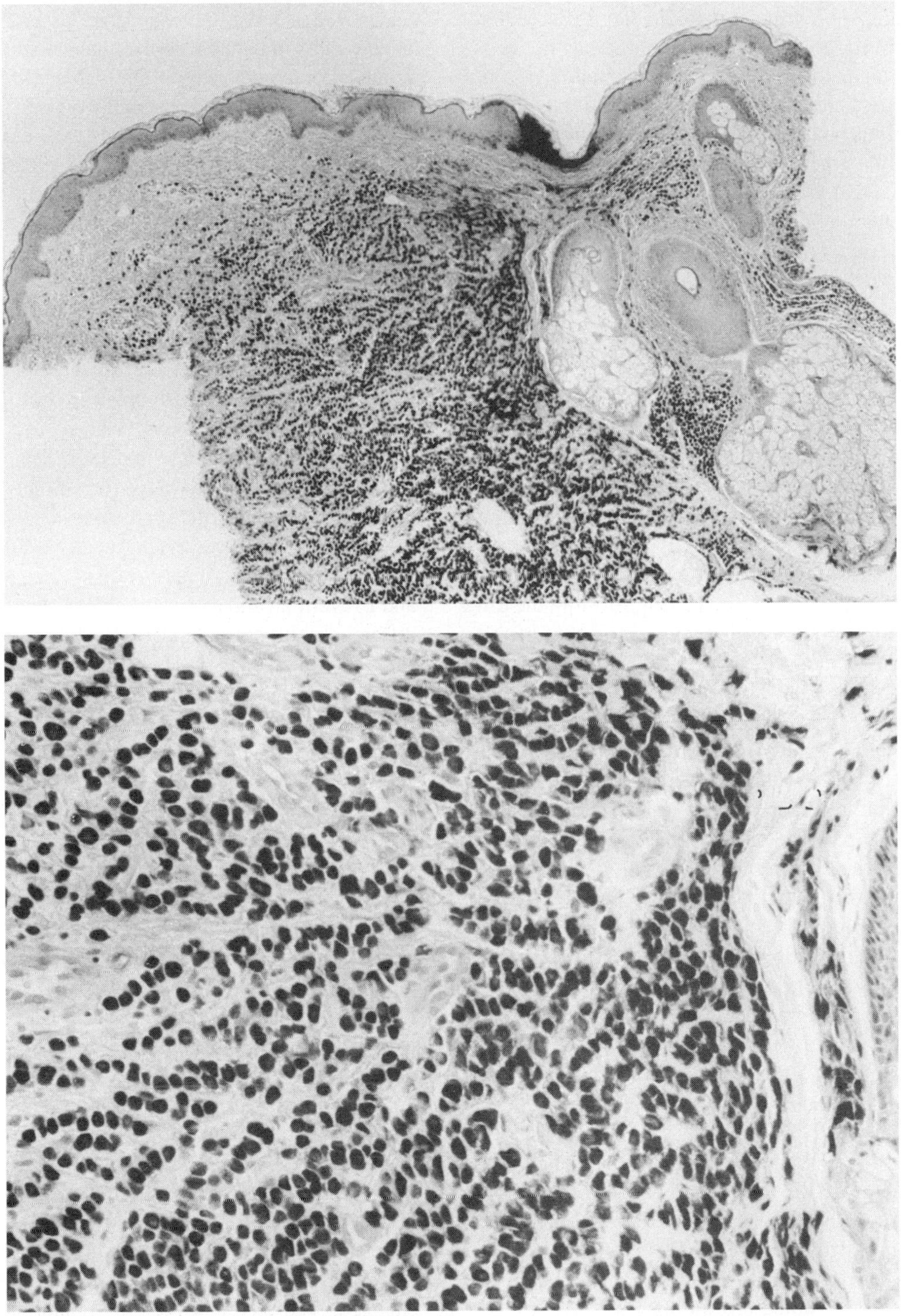

A

B

FIG. 52.3. A mastocytoma (mast cell nevus) localized to the skin of the wrist of a 1-year-old child. Note tumor-like growth pattern of monomorphous mast cells with densely packed metachromatic granules (4-μm paraffin section, Giemsa stain, original magnification: **A:** 200× magnification; **B:** 800× magnification).

it is the only means of providing a reliable diagnosis. Malignant transformation of localized mastocytoma has not been observed. No cytogenetic information is available on this benign tumor. Localized mastocytoma should be distinguished from various types of pigmented nevi, fibrous histiocytoma, the juvenile types of nevoxanthoendotheliomas, reticulohistocytoma, and vascular tumors such as pericytoma and hemangioendothelioma (73–75). Rare types of Langerhans cell granulomatosis of the dermis that present with an aggressive clinical course may be of differential diagnostic interest.

Urticaria Pigmentosa

The term *urticaria pigmentosa* was applied by Sangster (76) to an urticarial disease first described by Nettleship and Tay (77). An excellent account of the histopathologic findings of this disease was provided by Unna as early as 1887 (2).

Urticaria pigmentosa may appear as solitary or disseminated dermal lesions that may be confluent, forming the diffuse erythrodermic subtype. The various categories of this disease have been worked out by various investigators on the basis of the gross morphology of the dermal lesions and on the clinical course (78,79). Over 80% of cases begin in early childhood, and a small number are present at birth. In fewer than 20% of cases is there adult onset, in which the prevailing dermal involvement demonstrates a maculopapular character. Rare patients, mostly infants, present with pseudoxanthomatous and bullous or diffuse erythrodermic lesions. Telangiectasia macularis eruptiva perstans represents a rare form of diffuse cutaneous mastocytosis with an accentuated mast cell proliferation around the capillaries, which nearly always affects adults (80–82). In rare patients, maculopapular eruptions are accompanied by one or more mast cell nodules, called *tumorifactive cutaneous mastocytosis* (83). Familial cases are extremely rare but can occur in both monozygote twins (79, 84). Urticaria pigmentosa rarely affects blacks (69).

The diagnosis is based on clinical observations, including the appearance of macular or maculopapular reddish to brown dermal lesions that readily urticate on physical irritation. The eruptions are disseminated and exceed 100 in number at times. In addition to clinical findings, the diagnosis is best ascertained by histologic examination.

Mastocytosis is confined to the skin. The involved foci show a mild acanthosis of the epidermis and a hyperpigmentation of the basal layer, particularly in macular lesions (Fig. 52.4). The experienced pathologist readily recognizes the abnormal accumulation of mast cells in routinely processed hematoxylin and eosin staining on the basis of the typical nuclear form and the inner structure of the cytoplasm. Mast cells mainly are localized in the mid- and upper dermis, with a mild accentuation around the vessels. An infiltration of the vessel wall or other structures such as sweat or sebaceous glands, hair follicles, nerves, and smooth muscles does not occur. Some areas have a dense assembly of mast cells; others show only marginal enhancement of the mast cell number compared with normal values (85). In older lesions, fibrohyalinosis of the dermis may obscure the few mast cells present. More specific stains such as Giemsa, toluidine blue, or tryptase must be used to obtain selective demonstration of the mast cells in these patients. In patients with urticaria pigmentosa, mast cells show a normal pH range of metachromatic staining with pure basic dyes such as toluidine blue (15). Cytologically, mast cells show elongated or spindle-shaped cytoplasm with numerous monomorphous granules. The nuclei are oval or reniform, with varying degrees of indentation. Some nuclei are bilobed and contain prominent nucleoli. Mitoses are extremely rare but do occur. Binucleated mast cells may be observed in such cases. In enzyme and immune cytochemical investigations, mast cells of urticaria pigmentosa show behavior similar to that of normal mast cells and those that constitute localized mastocytoma.

The ultrastructure of the mast cells in urticaria pigmentosa has been the subject of few studies. Krueger and Nyfors (86) and Braverman and associates (87) did not find any essential difference with normal mast cells. Kobayashi and colleagues (88) underlined the lack of crystalloid inclusions in the center of the granules, in contrast to normal mast cell granules. This finding was considered to be a sign of granule immaturity. In a thorough account of the ultrastructural features of mast cells in urticaria pigmentosa, Schmidt and Leder (89) outlined the main distinctive features and described the differences between these cells and normal mast cells. These include the abundance of microvilli, hypogranulation with rather small granules, bilobed nuclei, and prominent nucleoli. Such variations from normal mast cells were considered to reflect, at least in part, functional abnormalities. From these findings, it has been inferred that urticaria pigmentosa may be a neoplastic disease. This view is confirmed by detection of the typical point mutation in codon position 816 of the protooncogene *KIT* in the affected mast cells (56,55).

Over 70% of cases of urticaria pigmentosa with an infantile onset subside with puberty, leaving only a minor irregularity of the epidermal pigmentation. The remaining cases persist, and a comparable number have an adult onset. In any case, urticaria pigmentosa should be regarded as a benign disease of chronic course. Despite the long course of the disease, the general status of the patient remains unchanged. The frequency of malignant tumors in cases of urticaria pigmentosa does not seem to be higher than in a comparable normal population. This applies also to myeloproliferations and malignant lymphomas. Considering that the number of registered or published cases exceeds 1,000, the true incidence of myeloproliferative or lymphoproliferative malignancies appears to be low. So far, only six cases of myeloproliferative disorder and three cases of malignant lymphoma have been reported in patients who suffered from typical forms of urticaria pigmentosa. Urticaria pigmentosa is a cutaneous disease in which infiltrates remain confined strictly to the dermis. A progression to other organs usually

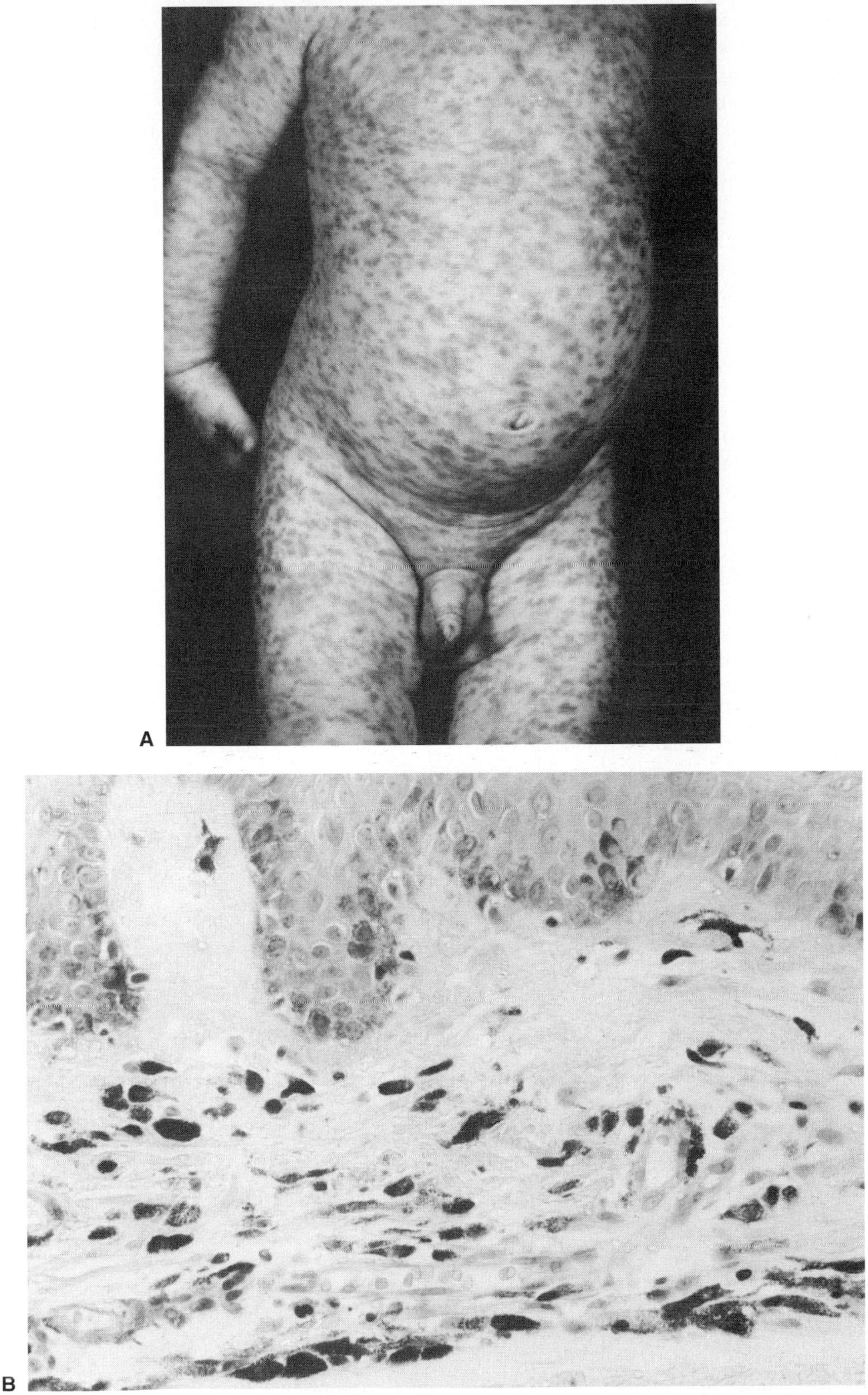

FIG. 52.4. A: Urticaria pigmentosa with abundant macular or maculopapular brown skin lesions in a 2-year-old infant. (Courtesy of Professor E. Christophers, University of Kiel, Kiel, Germany.) **B:** A skin biopsy in urticaria pigmentosa shows mast cell proliferation in papillae and perivascular areas (4-μm paraffin section, Giemsa stain, original magnification: 800$\times$ magnification).

does not occur. This applies especially to the visceral organs, including bone marrow. If a diagnosis of urticaria pigmentosa is suspected, an extensive search must be carried out to exclude involvement of other organs that would justify the diagnosis of SMCD. Transformation of urticaria pigmentosa into systemic variants or into malignant mast cell disease has not been observed reliably. Pregnancy does not influence the course of the disease. The main diseases of differential diagnostic relevance are other maculopopular allergic and nonallergic forms of dermatitis and rare cases of cutaneous Langerhans cell histiocytosis.

Mastocytosis of the Bone Marrow

In our files of patients with mast cell diseases, there exist at least six with disseminated mastocytosis restricted to the bone marrow. In the past we interpreted such cases as the initial phase of an SM, but eventually we became convinced that mastocytosis can remain confined to this tissue. The diagnostic feature is a mild involvement of the bone marrow indistinguishable from cases of benign SM (Fig. 52.5). Benign SM, however, regularly is associated with skin involvement similar to that found in urticaria pigmentosa; mastocytosis of the bone marrow lacks this feature.

Mastocytosis of the bone marrow also may affect skeletal areas such as vertebrae and pelvic bones and is associated with pain and radiologic abnormalities of the bone. In three patients from our files, moderate degrees of anemia were seen. None of the patients developed a severe hematologic disorder. We do not believe that the bone marrow–restricted mastocytosis evolves into a more generalized form.

Solitary Mast Cell Tumors

Solitary mast cell tumors are extremely rare; they have been observed in the lung in three patients (73–75). Like localized mastocytomas of the dermis, solitary mast cell tumors are round or oval soft nodules that measure from a few millimeters to 3 cm in diameter and mostly are localized beneath the pleura in the periphery of the lung. The surface of the tumor has been reported to be colored from ivory to dark red. Histologically, such lesions consist of mostly well-granulated round or oval mast cells with reniform or oval nuclei. Some of the mast cells contain only a few metachromatic granules; others lack any cytoplasmic granulation. Such cells have clear cytoplasm; may resemble hairy cells, monocytoid B lymphocytes, or immature vascular cells such as endothelia or pericytes; and probably represent immature mast cells. Mast cell tumors of the lung also have been referred to as *mast cell granuloma* or *histiocytoma* (73). On clinical observation, such lesions exhibit a benign behavior, remaining stationary for years with no sign of aggressive growth, metastasis, or recurrence after surgical treatment. In none of these cases was there any sign of spread to other organs. Urticaria pigmentosa was present. Solitary mast cell tumors also may occur in the dermis, spleen (90), and bone marrow. We are following one 30-year-old man who has disease localized to the oral mucosa (Fig. 52.6). The patient is doing well 6 years after pure surgical treatment. Whether the so-called inflammatory pseudotumors of the lung and other sites represent regressive end stages of such lesions is not clear.

Mast Cell Sarcoma

Mast cell sarcoma is a rare and clearly malignant mast cell neoplasm sporadically observed. To avoid confusion, the term should be applied to localized lesions with unequivocal signs of malignancy such as severe cytologic atypia, aggressive growth, metastasis, or leukemia. So far we have observed only two cases, one in a 63-year-old woman who presented with a solitary nodule in the upper larynx. At the time of the first diagnosis, no cutaneous lesions and no signs of other organ involvement were detectable (33,91). Cytologically, the mast cells were immature and atypical, with irregularly indented nuclei, prominent nucleoli, and a large amount of proliferation activity. The cytoplasm contained scant or no granules, as shown by light and electron microscopy. Two years after diagnosis and treatment metastatic nodules appeared in the breast and left thigh. The terminal phase of the disease assumed a leukemic course with 9,900 atypical mast cells per microliter of blood.

The second patient was an 8-year-old girl presenting with a subdural mass 3 cm in diameter seen infiltrating the cranial bones on magnetic resonance imaging and in an open biopsy specimen (Fig. 52.7). She died of local relapse 2 years after onset and 1 year after diagnosis, despite two surgical interventions including radiotherapy and systemic as well as intrathecal chemotherapy. On histopathologic examination the tumor was seen to consist of a mixture of pleomorphic mast cells with high and low amounts of metachromatic granules, tumor giant cells, macrophages, and eosinophils. Proliferation activity as assessed with the antibodies to Ki-67 (Ki-S5) or the topoisomerase II alpha (Ki-S1) amounted to 60%; assessed with anti-p100 (Ki-S2), which detects true proliferating cells traversing the cycle phases S, G_2, and M, it was 30%. The tumor had the typical point mutated *KIT* protooncogene and phenotyped to CD45, CD117, CD11c, CD68, and Ki-M1p positive. There was a positive reactivity for naphthol AS-D chloroacetate esterase and tryptase.

Systemic Mast Cell Disease

General Comments

In contrast to the restricted distribution of the nonsystemic forms of mast cell proliferations, the generalized or systemic forms may infiltrate any organ, including the central nervous system. Following the reports by Nettleship and Tay (77), Sangster (76), and Unna (2), it was Jeanselme and Touraine (61) who underlined the involvement of other organs in patients originally classified as having cutaneous mastocytosis

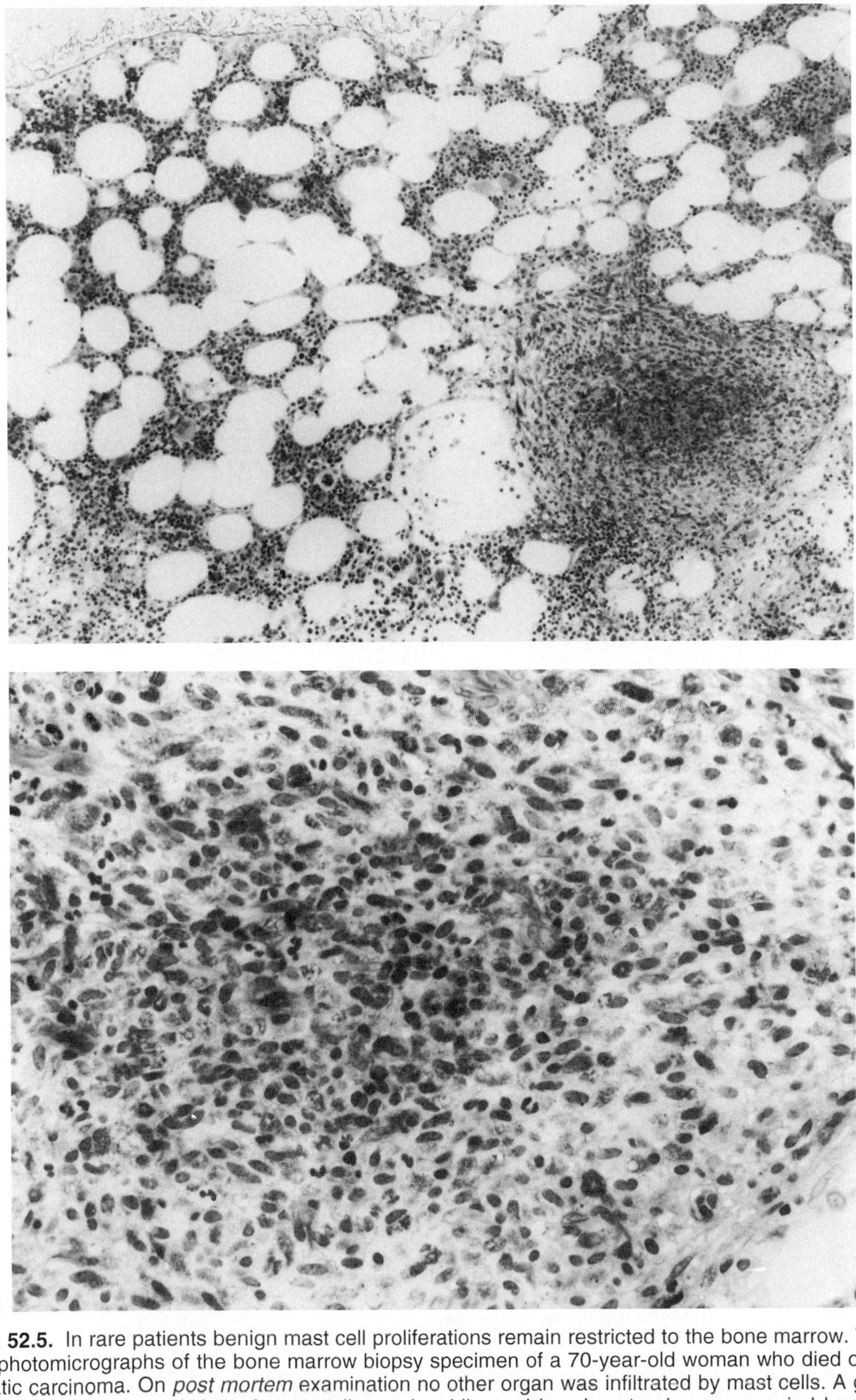

A

B

FIG. 52.5. In rare patients benign mast cell proliferations remain restricted to the bone marrow. These are photomicrographs of the bone marrow biopsy specimen of a 70-year-old woman who died of pancreatic carcinoma. On *post mortem* examination no other organ was infiltrated by mast cells. A granuloma-like infiltrate consisting of mast cells, eosinophils, and lymphocytes is accompanied by a mild fibrosis. Unaffected marrow areas display a normal distribution of hematopoiesis and fat cells (4-μm methacrylate section, Giemsa stain, original magnification: **A:** 200× magnification; **B:** 800× magnification).

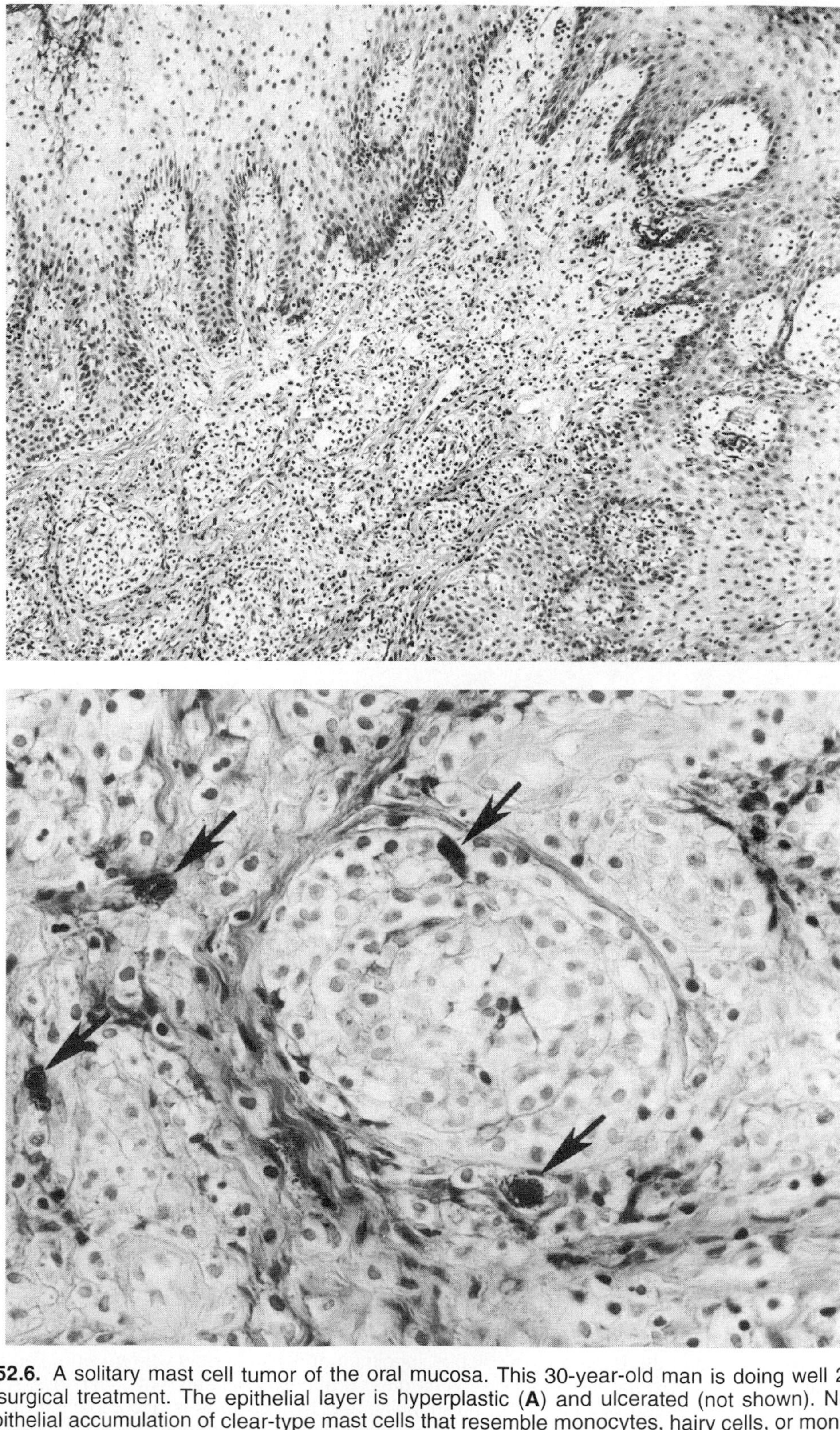

A

B

FIG. 52.6. A solitary mast cell tumor of the oral mucosa. This 30-year-old man is doing well 2 years after surgical treatment. The epithelial layer is hyperplastic (**A**) and ulcerated (not shown). Note the subepithelial accumulation of clear-type mast cells that resemble monocytes, hairy cells, or monocytoid B cells (**B**). Residual normal mast cells (*arrows*) contain large numbers of metachromatic granules (4-μm paraffin sections; **A:** Hematoxylin and eosin, original magnification: 400× magnification; **B:** Giemsa stain, original magnification: 1,600× magnification).

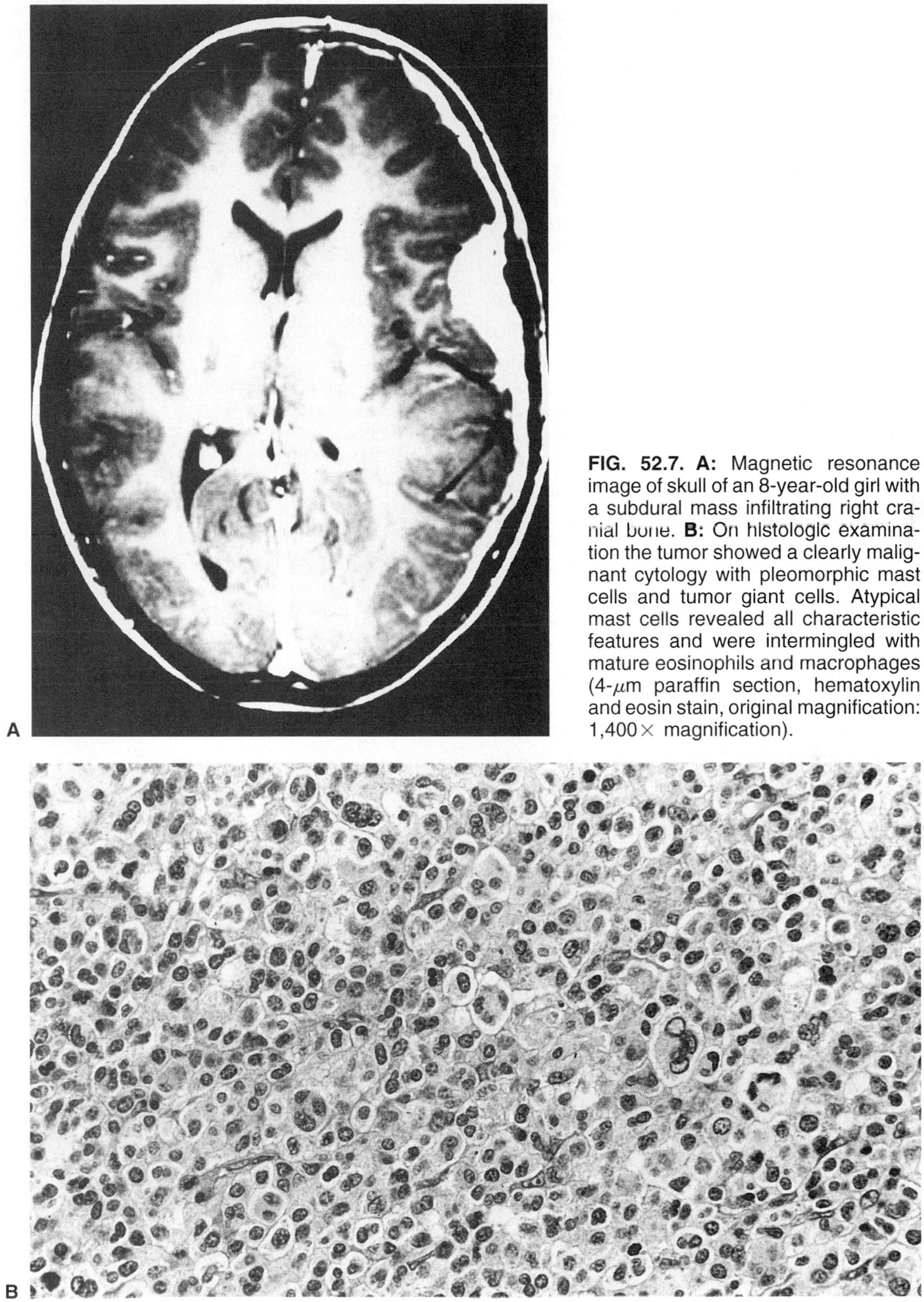

FIG. 52.7. **A:** Magnetic resonance image of skull of an 8-year-old girl with a subdural mass infiltrating right cranial bone. **B:** On histologic examination the tumor showed a clearly malignant cytology with pleomorphic mast cells and tumor giant cells. Atypical mast cells revealed all characteristic features and were intermingled with mature eosinophils and macrophages (4-μm paraffin section, hematoxylin and eosin stain, original magnification: 1,400× magnification).

(92). The term *mastocytosis* was proposed by Sezary and colleagues (54). Ellis (93) was the first to prove histologically the occurrence of mast cells in systemic involvement. Sagher and colleagues (94), Sagher and Even-Paz (79), and Stark and associates (95) described the possible concomitant bone changes in patients with SMCD.

In the files of the Lymph Node Registry in Kiel we are following a collection of 160 patients with SMCD. Reviewing the pertinent literature (34), we found that the 162 published cases showed an unpredictable and highly variable clinical course, with some patients dying within a few months after the diagnosis and others surviving over 40 years. The available data of our patients and those described in the literature were analyzed separately and jointly, considering clinical course, complications, and outcome in patients grouped according to one main feature. It became evident that patients who had primary skin involvement differed in many respects from those who lacked this feature. The behavior of our own collection was identical to that of the cases reported in the literature. Patients who had no skin involvement were, on average, 21 years older ($P < 0.0001$) and had a significantly higher incidence ($P < 0.0001$) of splenomegaly, hepatomegaly, lymphadenopathy, severe anemia, leukocytosis, and thrombocytopenia (Table 52.5). The survival probability represented the most striking difference between these two groups. For this reason we proposed to restrict the term *benign* or *indolent SM* to patients with primary skin involvement and a better prognosis, separating them from those with the other form of generalized mastocytosis, which lacks skin involvement and is distinguished by an extremely poor prognosis. This latter form was referred to as *malignant mastocytosis*. Providing a thorough report on the well-documented cases of the Mayo Clinic, Travis and coworkers (69) referred to seven patients who had skin involvement and poor outcomes (with a median duration of survival of 10 months) and to seven additional patients who lacked skin involvement but whose durations of survival ranged from 30 to 132 months (with a median duration of 66 months). It was maintained that "the absence of skin involvement is a feature of poor prognosis but skin involvement is not always a reliable predictor of outcome" (69). In their meticulous analysis, these authors suggested the use of the term *indolent*, rather than *benign*, *systemic mast cell disease*, because the term *benign* would imply an invariably good prognosis. In our studies, the categories *benign* and *malignant* were proposed only to express the growth behavior of the neoplastic cell type according to the nomenclature usual in pathology, bearing in mind that even benign tumors at critical sites could cause death. The category of *MM*, however, is generally accepted. Travis and colleagues (69) suggest the designation *aggressive systemic mast cell disease*. As stressed by these authors, the label MM implies that mast cells have undergone a malignant transformation or that, at least, their proliferation represents part of a stem cell transformation that basically accounts for the poor outcome. We believe not that patients who have malignant or aggressive mastocytosis and who develop a myelodysplasia or a myelomonocytic leukemia suffer from a second type of neoplasia, but rather that this is further evidence of a stem cell defect and is caused by a growing dedifferentiation tendency of the neoplastic lineage. Malignant mast cells may develop a true mast cell leukemia, build up a solid mast cell sarcoma, or show a diffuse or disseminated growth pattern that aggressively infiltrates various organs. With no exceptions, the patients with mast cell leukemia we examined had signs of a panmyelosis or a myeloproliferative disease. This was inferred easily from clear cytologic and enzyme cytochemical atypia encountered in neutrophils, basophils, and eosinophils, as well as in monocytes, erythropoietic cells, and megakaryocytes.

TABLE 52.5. *Frequency of various symptoms in all cases of indolent (SM) and malignant (MM) forms of systemic mast cell disease at the time of initial diagnosis*

Symptoms	SM, % (n = 97)	MM, % (n = 63)
Constitutional symptoms		
Fatigue	14	56
Fever	6	16
Weight loss	6	41
Clinical findings		
Primary skin involvement	99	—
Splenomegaly	27	78
Hepatomegaly	23	68
Lymphadenopathy	15	54
Ascites	4	14
Portal hypertension	3	8
Hematologic abnormalities		
Anemia	13	81
Thrombocytopenia	5	43
Thrombocytosis	4	2
Leukocytosis	15	43
Neutropenia	1	14
Eosinophilia	13	40
Basophilia	5	16
Monocytosis	6	25
Circulating mast cells	—	8
Mediator-related symptoms		
Flushing	16	8
Pruritus	28	11
Bronchospasm	1	5
Syncope	6	—
Nausea or vomitus	9	16
Diarrhea	15	17
Abdominal pain	11	22
Gastrointestinal bleeding	3	8
Peptic ulcer	5	11
Headache	2	2
Neuropsychic symptoms	9	9
Skeletal symptoms		
Bone pain	20	14
Arthralgia	8	2
Osteosclerosis	35	38
Osteoporosis	27	28
Osteolysis	3	16

The indolent form was separated from cases with an associated hematologic disorder (mast cell leukemia) and from cases of aggressive nonleukemic SMCD (69). This last category includes cases described as *lymphadenopathic mastocytosis with eosinophilia* (96).

In the section that follows, each category is discussed separately to underscore the differences in natural history, morphology, and outcome.

Benign, Indolent Systemic Mastocytosis (Indolent Systemic Mast Cell Disease)

Benign, indolent SM is probably the disease type first described by Ellis (93). This entity can be diagnosed only if histologic proof of a combined cutaneous and extracutaneous mast cell infiltration is provided. These patients lack features of a malignant transformation of mast cells or of their cytogenetic lineage (such as myelodysplasia and myeloproliferation) and of mast cell leukemia (34,67–69). In reviewing 162 cases from the literature and 160 from our own observations, we found that this variant of SMCD had a far better prognosis, showing no signs of malignancy of mast cells or of the closely related myelomonocytic system in all but a single patient with myelodysplasia. All cases were associated regularly with primary skin involvement indistinguishable from urticaria pigmentosa.

Travis and associates (69) have observed a few patients with benign SM who lacked primary skin involvement. Excluding the 29 patients with indolent SMCD examined by Travis and associates (69), about 130 cases have been reported in the literature to date. Including our 97 cases of benign SM, we have a collection of 227 cases that are documented well enough to be classified as benign SM.

The male-to-female ratio is about 1.3:1. The median age at onset is 38 years. In general, the diagnosis is established about 5 years after onset, as the symptoms become more evident, prompting thorough clinical investigation. The median age at the time of diagnosis is 43 years. Although pure urticaria pigmentosa is more frequent in children, benign SM (indolent SMCD) is an adult disease but may affect infants also. In our files the youngest patient was an infant 3 months of age.

The cytologic, enzymatic, immunocytochemical, and ultrastructural features of mast cells in this disease form do not differ from urticaria pigmentosa. Mast cells are nonreactive to B- and T-cell reagents such as L26, Ki-B3, Ki-B5, MB2, LN1, LN2, Leu M1, CD1a, CD3, CD4, CD5, CD8 and UCHL 1 (97). Chromosome analyses in one of our cases revealed a translocation t(X;8). Swolin and coworkers (60) observed in one patient variable chromosomal losses. In six of our patients, no *BCR* rearrangement could be detected on Southern blot analysis of the DNA extracted from blood cells. From six patients the granulocytes were analyzed for the clonal methylation pattern of the X-chromosomal gene phosphoglycerokinase; three were homozygote, one had a clear monoclonal pattern (Fig. 52.8), one patient was polyclonal, and one 40-year-old woman exhibited loss of both alleles, which never was seen before. Flowcytometric studies

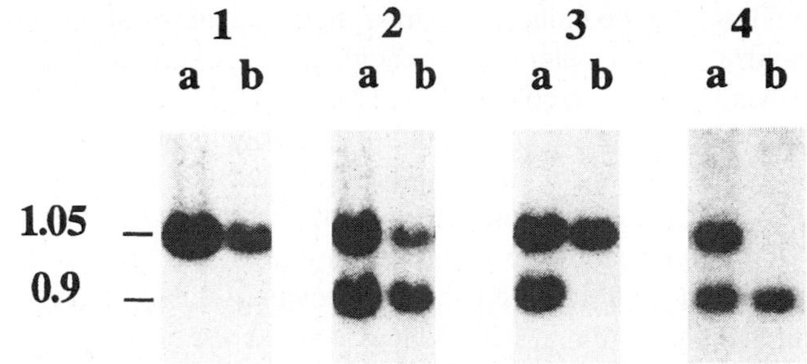

FIG. 52.8. Detection of clonal granulocytes in systemic mastocytosis documents an aberration on the level of stem cells shared by both cell types. Analysis of methylation pattern of the X-chromosomal phosphoglycerokinase gene. DNA from purified granulocytes was cut with BstXI and PstI (**A**) as well as with HpII (**B**). Healthy control subjects (numbers 1 and 2) with homozygote and heterozygote allelic bands at 1.05 and 0.9 kb, respectively. In a patient with CML (number 3), loss of heterozygosity with a remaining single allele at 0.9 kb. In a patient with systemic mastocytosis (number 4), loss of allele 1.05 kb indicates monoclonality of granulocytes.

performed by Escribano and associates (136) revealed more forward and side light scatter and higher baseline autofluorescence levels in mast cells of indolent SMCD patients compared with mast cells of healthy control subjects, signs of larger cell size and higher internal complexity. Striking findings from an immunophenotypic point of view were the constant expression of CD2 and CD25 molcules by mast cells of SMCD patients, markers that were absent from all normal controls.

Like other forms of mast cell disease, this variant has confusing clinical manifestations with a broad spectrum of different and highly variable symptoms, probably the main cause of false diagnosis (Table 52.5). Travis and colleagues (69) grouped most of the symptoms into four categories: constitutional, skin- and bone-related, and caused by mast cell mediators. Among the constitutional symptoms—fatigue, weight loss, fever, and sweats—only the first two, occurring far less frequently in cases of indolent SMCD, were found to be of value in the separation of prognostically relevant categories ($P < 0.0001$).

Mediator-Related Symptoms

A set of clinical symptoms has been related to the mediators released by these cells. For our cases these symptoms are listed in Table 52.5. Pruritus, flushing, syncope, enhanced blood level of histamine, urinary excretion of histamine and prostaglandin D2 metabolite, and episodes of diarrhea are the most frequent symptoms. Tryptase, histamine, and prostaglandin D2 and their metabolites, methylhistamine and N-methyl-imidazoleacetic acid, have been measured to assess the extent of the infiltrates (98,99). Anaphylaxis, hypotension, dyspnea, tachycardia, abdominal pain, nausea, vomitus, and headache also have been considered important signs of SMCD, in addition to cutaneous alterations. Anaphylaxis can be induced by stress, mechanical irritation, anesthesia, hymenoptera sting venom, and exposure to organic solvents, heat, or cold (100,101) and may result in death (69,102). Elevated concentration of blood histamine is a usual finding in patients with benign SM. Its degree, however, does not correlate with extent of disease (103,104). Although urinary excretion of histamine and its metabolite, N-methyl-imidazoleacetic acid, is elevated, this is not absolutely specific for SMCD. Values that exceed 50 μg per 24 hours urine volume, however, may reflect the extent of tissue infiltration. Enhanced levels of these substances have been observed in chronic myeloid leukemia, with high numbers of blood basophils or in basophil leukemias. In addition, some bacterial infections and microbially prepared food can cause an enhanced excretion of histamine and its metabolites. Other excretion products of mast cells such as prostaglandin D2 may be helpful in monitoring the course of the disease and in the differential diagnosis with other neoplasias that have mediator-induced symptoms (such as carcinoid tumors and pheochromocytoma) in which 5-hydroxyindoleacetic acid and metanephrine levels are enhanced (103,105). In our material, histamine flush occurred in 16% of the cases and lasted 20 to 30 minutes each time, with an erythema of the face, throat, and thorax, some being associated with paroxysmal tachycardia and aphasia.

Dermatologic Findings

Pruritus, urticaria, and dermatographism are common findings in these patients. All 97 patients followed up in Kiel except one 61-year-old male (Table 52.5), all 130 patients recorded in the literature, and apparently the majority of the 29 patients included in the ''indolent SMCD group''of Travis and colleagues (69) showed primary skin involvement. The initial macular and later maculopapular and, sometimes, nodular skin eruptions are mostly indistinguishable from urticaria pigmentosa, which remains confined to the skin (Fig. 52.9). Although skin involvement is present at the initial stage of disease, in four patients Travis and colleagues (69) observed skin involvement at 1 to 48 months postdiagnosis. It is essential to perform a careful dermatologic examination, because regressive foci of the skin may be overlooked easily. Histologic confirmation should be obtained. There is general agreement that primary skin involvement represents a reliable sign of favorable outcome; however, Travis and associates (69) observed seven patients who had skin involvement and did poorly, with a median duration of survival of 10 months after diagnosis. It would be interesting to analyze the immediate causes of death in these seven patients and to survey the extent and distribution pattern of the infiltrates. Travis and associates also mention seven other patients who lacked dermal involvement and who are still well, with a median duration of survival of 66 months (ranging from 32 to 132 months). We are not sure whether the marrow-restricted form can be excluded in all these patients.

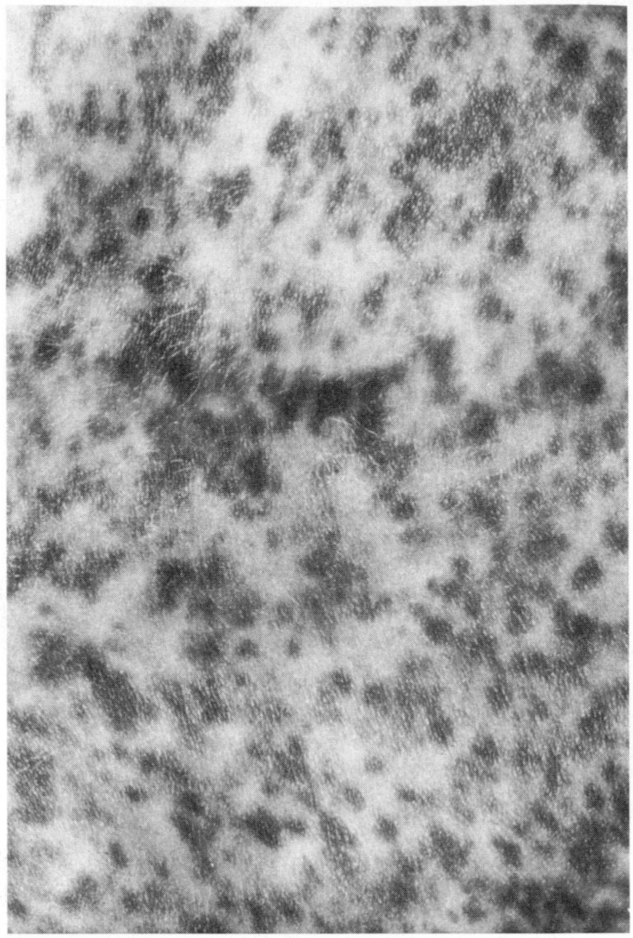

FIG. 52.9. In benign systemic mastocytosis (indolent systemic mast cell disease), brown maculopapular skin effluorescences represent the leading symptom.

These findings suggest that a minor subgroup may present with an adverse behavior in this respect.

The characteristic macular or maculopapular skin lesions sometimes are present years or even decades before the diagnosis. The skin lesions, numbering from a few to over 100, are disseminated and measure up to 5 mm in diameter. In typical areas, reddish-brown eruptions appear, localized on the trunk and extremities (Fig. 52.9). In our files two patients presented with bullous and one with diffuse erythrodermic manifestation of the skin involvement. A single 52-year-old man showed the typical picture of telangiectasia macularis eruptiva perstans. Mucous membranes usually are not affected, but exceptions do occur. On histologic examination, the epidermis is intact or partly hyperplastic. A mild degree of hyperpigmentation exists in the basal layer. Abundant mast cells are distributed preferentially in the perivascular or periadnexal areas within the dermis (Fig. 52.10). In maculopapular lesions of longer standing, there generally are more mast cells than in purely macular lesions. Sometimes lymphocytes and eosinophils may be interspersed among the mast cells. The majority of these lymphocytes represent

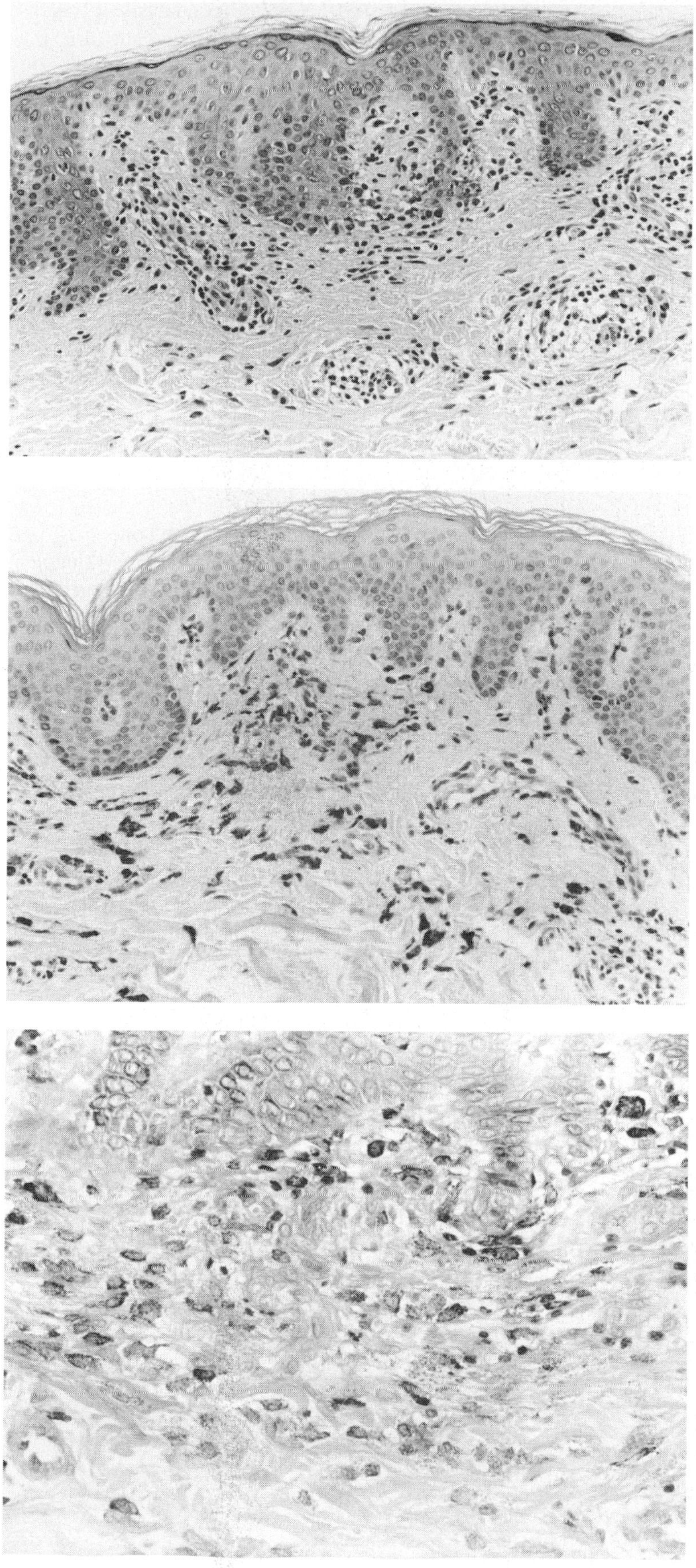

A

B

C

FIG. 52.10. Skin involvement in benign systemic mastocytosis (indolent systemic mast cell disease). Photomicrographs of a skin biopsy specimen from a 53-year-old man with a positive history of 18 years. **A:** Mast cells accumulated in papillae and around medium-sized or small venules may be missed in conventional hematoxylin and eosin–stained sections (4-μm paraffin section, original magnification: 800× magnification). **B:** In immunoalkaline phosphatase staining with the paraffin-resistant panmacrophage antibody Ki-M1p, mast cells reveal a strong reactivity (4-μm paraffin section, original magnification: 800× magnification). **C:** Metachromasia of mast cell granules is easily detectable in Giemsa staining (4-μm paraffin section, original magnification: 1,600× magnification).

CD4$^+$, CD8-negative, CD3$^+$, and CD2$^+$ T cells. In older lesions, a band-shaped subepidermal fibrohyalinosis with a limited number of single mast cells is visible. Cytologically, the majority of the mast cells appear to be round or oval, with a reniform or slightly indented nucleus. A moderate number of granules are detectable within the cytoplasm. Areas that have severe fibrosis show elongated fusiform mast cells. In addition, there are other mast cells with medium-sized and clear cytoplasm that show hardly any detectable granules, even on specific staining. Histologically, skin lesions are indistinguishable from alterations found in urticaria pigmentosa. The delineation of localized mastocytoma, however, is readily possible on a histologic basis. Localized mastocytoma is a well-defined, sharply separated tumor with a high density of mostly oval and mature mast cells heavily laden with granules (Fig. 52.3).

Hematologic Findings

The most frequent hematologic findings in our patients are leukocytosis, eosinophilia, and anemia. Anemia has been reported in the literature as the most frequent finding (34,70). The median values of hemoglobin and erythrocyte counts were normal. In individual patients, however, anemia may be severe. Completely normal hematologic findings are encountered in the majority of patients. Leukocytosis is observed in 15% of patients, eosinophilia in 13%, and monocytosis in 6%. A significant increase in the number of basophil granulocytes, which is a highly specific sign of myeloproliferation (11), occurred in none of these patients. Thrombocytopenia, bihemocytopenia, or pancytopenia occurred only in a few. A myelodysplasia leading to an acute myeloid leukemia was observed in one patient (Table 52.6). In the literature, however, 11 patients seem to have developed a myelodysplasia or a myeloproliferative disorder secondary to or coincident with this entity. These were chronic myeloproliferative disorders in six patients and acute myeloid or myelomonocytic leukemia in three. Myelodysplasia was reported in two patients. Mast cell leukemia does not occur in cases of benign SM (indolent SMCD). The proper interpretation of hematologic findings in these cases may be quite difficult. This was the case in two of our patients originally classified as having benign SM with a secondary myeloproliferative disorder. On further analysis, it was discovered that one patient originally had an urticaria pigmentosa with a mastocytosis restricted to the dermis. This patient had a concurrent monocytic leukemia with infiltration of the dermis. The intermingling of mast cells with leukemic monocytes had led to the false diagnosis. On extensive search, no mast cell infiltrates could be detected in the bone marrow or other extracutaneous sites. The second patient, classified as having benign SM (indolent SMCD) with an acute myeloid leukemia, also turned out to have a pure urticaria pigmentosa with a coincidental basophil leukemia. The atypical basophils mistakenly had been identified as tissue mast cells infiltrating bone marrow, leading to the erroneous diagnosis. In one patient a typically localized Burkitt's lymphoma was observed in the colon.

TABLE 52.6. *Associated hematologic disorders in indolent (SM) and malignant (MM) forms of systemic mast cell disease*

Hematologic disorders	SM, % (n = 97)	MM, % (n=63)
Myelodysplasia	1 [1][a]	21 [13]
Acute myelomonocytic leukemia	—	5 [3]
Chronic myeloproliferations	—	35 [22]
Mast cell leukemia	—	6 [4]
Non Hodgkin lymphoma	1 [1]	3 [2]

[a] Items in brackets indicate number of cases.

Bone Marrow Findings

Irrespective of osteologic alterations, the bone marrow is one of the major sites of involvement in benign SM (indolent SMCD). In our collection, 96% of the patients showed mast cell infiltrates in the bone marrow in addition to skin involvement (Table 52.7). In the literature, a somewhat lower frequency of mast cell infiltration in bone marrow (90%) is reported. In eight patients, no samples were available, and in four no evidence of mast cell infiltration could be obtained on the basis of cytologic or histologic evaluations. Considering this, bone marrow involvement should be regarded as an important diagnostic criterion, although, in exceptional cases, marrow involvement may be absent or, more probably, escape detection.

In smears or imprints from marrow aspirates, mast cells are found in variable numbers. In large areas, only a small number of mast cells can be seen. In others, dense clusters of strongly stained tissue mast cells are found. In many patients the diagnosis is missed because of the small number of mast cells detectable in smears. This is partly because of

TABLE 52.7. *Histologically confirmed organ involvement in indolent (SM) and malignant (MM) forms of systemic mast cell disease*

Organs involved	SM, % (n = 97)	MM, % (n = 63)
Skin	70	3[a]
Bone marrow	96	92
Liver	12	43
Spleen	6	32
Lymph node	10	52
Duodenum	2	16
Stomach	1	—
Colon	2	2
Testis	1	—
Lung	—	3
Brain	—	2
Kidney	—	2
Muscle	—	2

[a] Secondary metastatic skin infiltration.

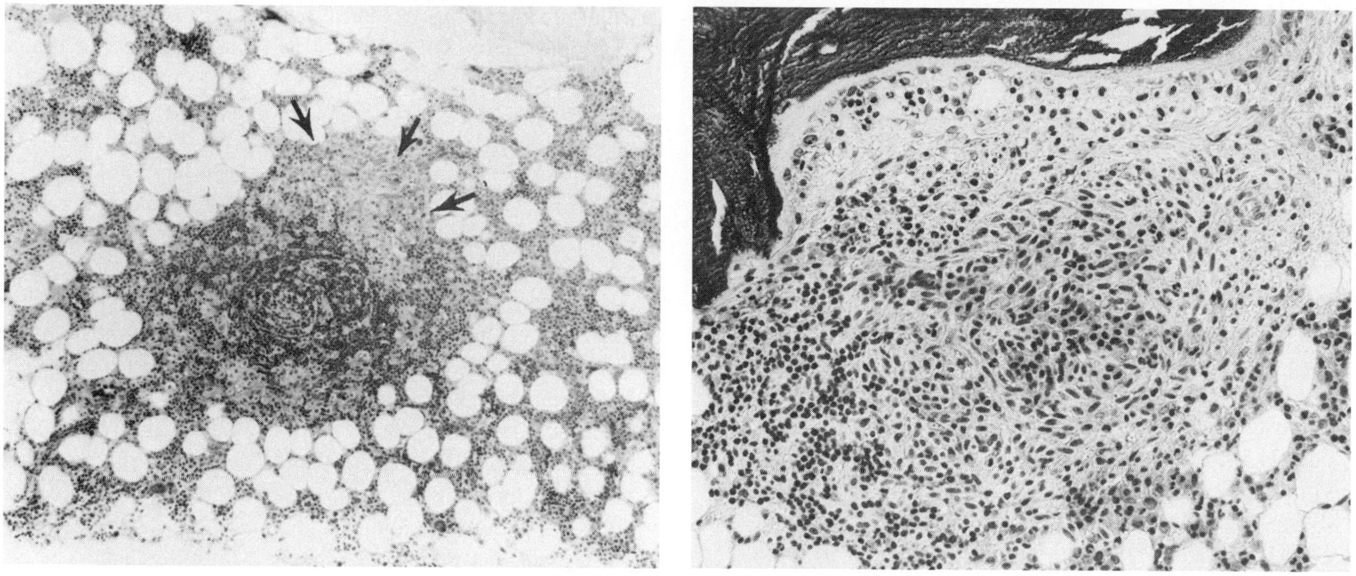

A B

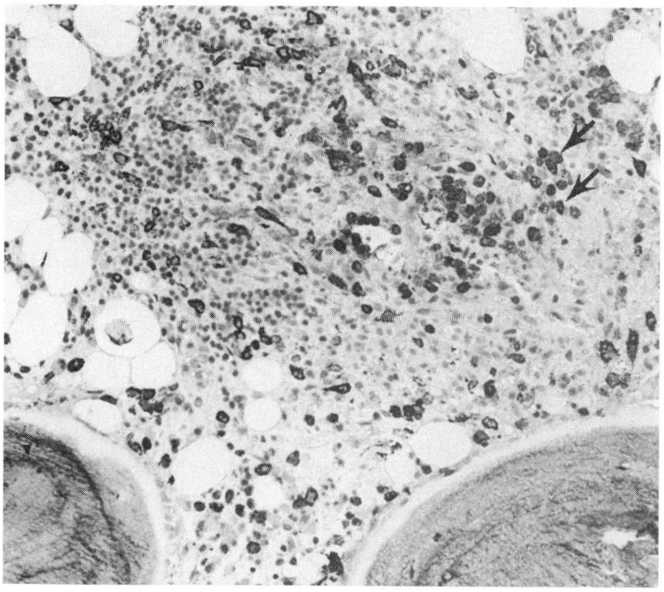

C

FIG. 52.11. In benign systemic mastocytosis (indolent systemic mast cell disease) the bone marrow is regularly infiltrated, featuring patchy, peritrabecular infiltrates that consist of fusiform or oval mast cells, focal fibrosis and osteosclerosis, accumulation of lymphocytes and eosinophils, and reactive alterations of hematopoiesis in nonaffected areas. **A:** A bone marrow biopsy specimen from a 23-year-old man that shows a mast cell infiltrate (*arrows*) and a dense accumulation of lymphocytes. Nonaffected areas display a normal distribution of fat cells and hematopoiesis (4-μm methacrylate section, Giemsa stain, original magnification: 400× magnification). **B:** Peritrabecular infiltrates in a 27-year-old man accompanied by lymphocytes, fibrosis, and osteosclerosis (4-μm methacrylate section, Giemsa stain, original magnification: 800× magnification). **C:** The same sample as in **B**. Mast cell infiltrates consist of oval mature mast cells rich in metachromatic granules (*arrows*) and of fusiform mast cells with scanty granules (4-μm methacrylate section, chloroacetate esterase reaction, original magnification: 800× magnification).

the presence of fibrosis, which prevents mast cell release. A reliable diagnosis is only possible on the basis of a marrow biopsy (Fig. 52.11). Marrow infiltrations are irregular and patchy. Some parts are densely infiltrated; others are only mildly so or lack any mast cell infiltration. The majority of mast cells are of the fusiform type and contain a variable number of granules. Some cells contain a few granules within a clear cytoplasm. Fusiform mast cells are accompanied closely by collagen fibers. Between the collagen fibers there are some spindled fusiform cells that lack granules. These cells probably represent fibroblasts or myofibroblasts. Giemsa, toluidine blue, aldehyde-fuchsin, astra blue, and chloroacetate esterase and tryptase stains are strongly positive in mast cells, with a high granule content, and are only weakly positive or even negative in clear cells. In some areas, mast cells build up granuloma-like foci intermingled with lymphocytes, a few plasma cells, and fibroblasts. Fewer than 20% of the lymphocyte accumulations represent B cells, the remainder being $CD4^+$ T lymphocytes; $CD8^+$ T lymphocytes are lacking or are few in number. Mast cell foci are partly surrounded by mature eosinophils. Histologically, benign SM (indolent SMCD) is characterized by a fairly typical pattern of marrow involvement, readily enabling a proper diagnosis according to our experience (67). This view has been debated by other investigations (69). The diagnostic criteria follow:

1. The infiltrates are disseminated and partly peritrabecular and comprise fusiform mast cells in strands or nodules.
2. Mast cell infiltrates usually are accompanied by fibrosis and sometimes by an adjacent osteosclerosis (106).
3. Abundant numbers of eosinophils and foci of lymphocytes are present near the mast cell foci.
4. Noninfiltrated marrow areas mostly show a regular dis-

tribution of blood cell precursors and fat cells, provided the involvement of marrow and spleen have not resulted in a hemocytopenia.

Skeletal Lesions

Bone lesions are not rare in patients with benign SM (indolent SMCD), although complaints of bone pain or arthralgia remain confined to about 20% of patients. Radiographic alterations, scintigraphic scans, and magnetic resonance imaging of skeletal lesions may be critical in the initial diagnosis (107). Perhaps this explains why a large number of mast cell diseases has been reported by radiologists. Skeletal changes include various degrees of osteosclerosis, especially within the infiltrated marrow areas. This accounted for over 80% of cases. Also, osteoporosis is a common finding, observed in about 30% of patients. No skeletal alterations could be found in fewer than 20% of the patients. The radiographic appearance may be osteoporotic or osteosclerotic, but detectable lytic foci are rare. In our files, 9% of the patients experienced pathologic fractures.

Gastrointestinal Symptoms

Symptoms such as abdominal pain, diarrhea, nausea and vomiting, and steatorrhea represent severe findings seen in 15% of our patients. Peptic ulcers and melena or hematemesis occur in fewer than 10% of patients. Endoscopic biopsy specimens from the gastrointestinal tract in patients with benign SM (indolent SMCD) hardly ever show clear infiltration of the gatrointestinal wall. The reactive increase of mast cells at this tissue site is never great enough, to our knowledge, to acquire differential diagnostic relevance, as claimed by some investigators (108). The mucosal abnormality may range from gastric rugal hypertrophy and flattening or loss of mucosal folds to diffuse mucosal thickening.

Liver Involvement

Symptoms such as steatorrhea, melena, ascites, and other signs of portal vein hypertension are important findings that may indicate hepatic involvement. This was the case in 23% of our own patients. Only 35% showed no liver involvement. About 66% of all patients, including those whose cases were collected from the literature, showed liver involvement (68,109). Based on autopsy data, hepatic weight ranged from 1,650 to 4,500 g, with a median value of 2,375 g. The histologic alterations found in liver biopsy specimens do not correlate well with the extent of hepatomegaly on clinical examinations. A small number of mast cells is found within the sinuses or in the immediate vicinity of the periportal fields. Mast cell infiltrates generally do not destroy the lobules. In a small number (2%) of patients, massive fibrosis or even liver cirrhosis emerges. The periportal fibrosis that frequently occurs may lead to portal hypertension and can contribute to the complex alterations found in the spleen. The cytologic findings correspond to those of other infiltrated tissue types.

Spleen Involvement

During the prediagnostic phase of the disease, splenomegaly is seen in about 27% of patients. In the postdiagnostic phase, however, the incidence increases to over 41%, which is in accord with other findings (110). The spleen is firm and shows fibrotic areas. The spleen weight in our patients ranged from 280 to 950 g, with a median value of 380 g. Including the cases from the literature, the range was 160 to 2,100 g, with a median weight of 750 g. Histologically, the lymphatic follicles are replaced partially by foci of mast cell infiltration. In part these are nodules of mast cells with abundant cytoplasm. Some cells contain only a few granules. Others lack any granules and have clear cytoplasm. The nuclei are located centrally and mostly reniform. Within and around such foci, which appear as poorly stained clear areas on low-power magnification, there are eosinophils and some lymphocytes. In other areas, mast cells acquire a fusiform, spindled shape and largely are obscured by the accompanying collagen fibers. The latter may form hyaline patches and streaks intermingled with macrophages and plasma cells as well as dense accumulations of eosinophils (106). The paucity of the cytoplasmic granules may render the recognition of mast cells difficult, and an appropriate diagnosis may be impossible. A clear disproportion seems to exist between the extent of mast cell proliferation and the degree of tissue destruction in the spleen. Splenomegaly also can cause hypersplenism with panhematocytopenia in the peripheral blood and hyperplasia of blood cell precursors in the bone marrow. Splenic fibrosis and hypersplenism might contribute even more to the complexity of the histologic alterations and hematologic findings with the appearance of blood cell precursors in the spleen and also in blood smears.

Lymph Node Involvement

Lymphadenopathy was detectable in 15% of our patients. A clear infiltration of the lymph node tissue by mast cells was histologically ascertained in only 10% of the patients. On histologic examination using low-power magnification, the typical lymph node structure is obscured slightly by the mast cell infiltrates (Fig. 52.12). Cortical and paracortical areas display more accentuated mast cell infiltrations than the medullary pulp. Mast cells partly surround vessels and sinuses, concentrically localized in various layers of the vessel wall, some underlying the endothelium. The vessel wall is largely preserved, and the lumen remains patent. In cases of mild infiltration with mostly clear mast cells, the diagnosis can be missed easily. Lymphoid B follicles mostly are surrounded or only partially infiltrated by mast cells. The capsule and the trabeculae, as well as the perinodal tissue, often remain unaltered. The majority of mast cells have a clear

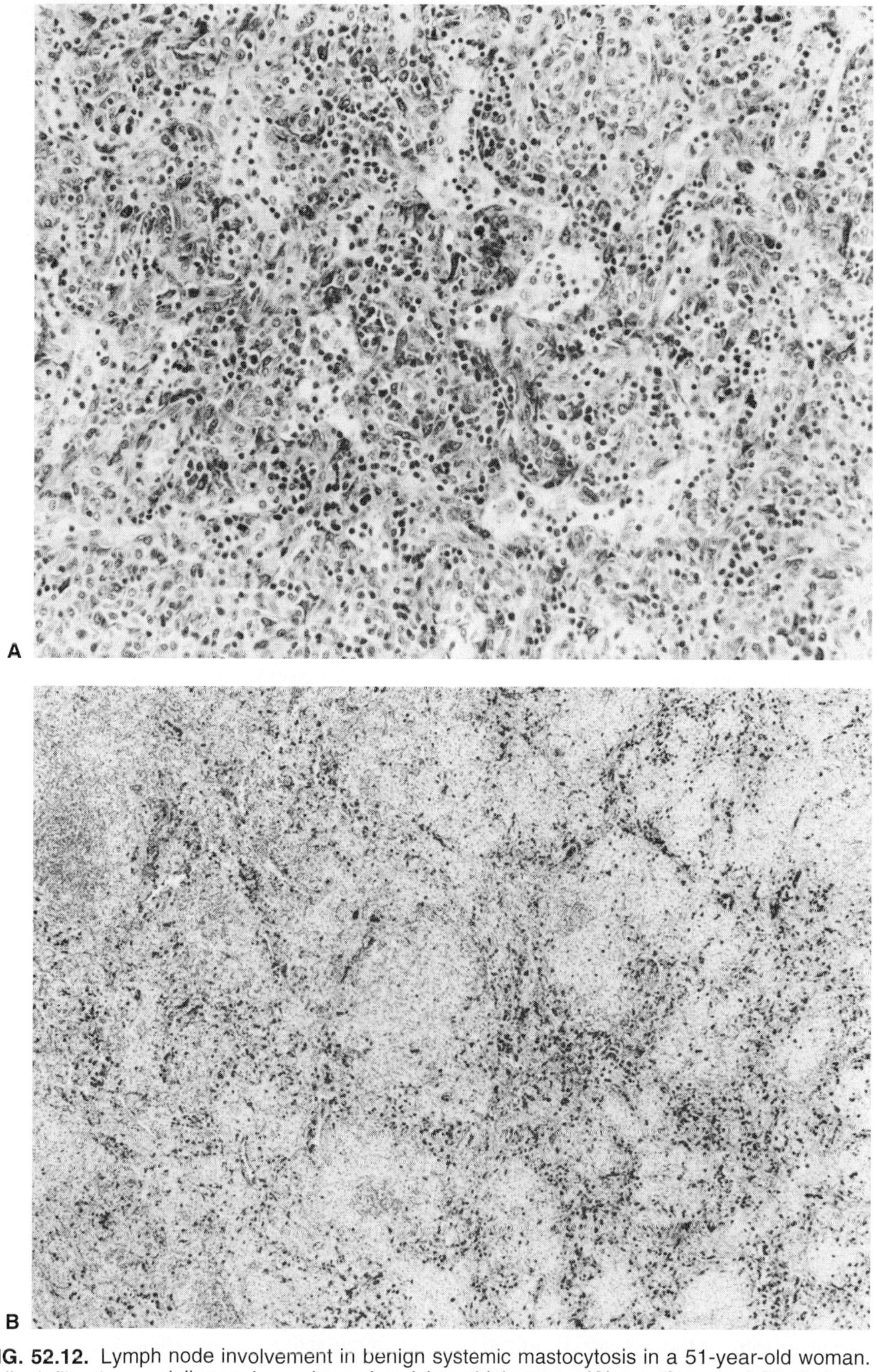

FIG. 52.12. Lymph node involvement in benign systemic mastocytosis in a 51-year-old woman. Mast cells, infiltrating medullary pulp cords, and perisinusoidal spaces (**A**) may form nodules that resemble follicular lymphoma (**B**) (4-μm paraffin sections; **A:** Giemsa stain, original magnification: 800× magnification; **B:** Immune alkaline phosphatase reaction with the antilysozyme antibody immunostaining reactive macrophages but not mast cells, original magnification: 200× magnification).

cytoplasm that contains only a few metachromatic granules. Mast cells of fusiform type are not abundant. Some infiltrates are accompanied by mature eosinophils.

Some patients have a nodular or granuloma-like infiltration pattern, as stressed by Travis and Li (110), who reported on the morphology of spleen and lymph node in a substantial number of patients. In their experience, lymph node and spleen were two of the most common organs infiltrated. Peripheral lymphadenopathy was present in 26% and central lymphadenopathy in 19% of the 58 patients examined. Mast cell infiltrates were localized in the paracortex in 88% of patients, in the perifollicular areas in 50% of patients, and within the follicles in 25% of patients. The medullary cords were infiltrated in 13% of the patients and the sinuses in 6%. Despite the meticulous description of incidence, histologic findings, and differential diagnostic implications, no reference was made to the different categories of the disease.

Cause of Death

Twenty-nine (22%) of the patients who had benign SM (indolent SMCD) died during the follow-up period. Peptic ulcers of stomach and duodenum with massive hemorrhages or perforations were found to be the immediate cause of death in five patients. Cachexia and various types of carcinomas were observed in 8 out of 97 patients. Cardiorespiratory insufficiency accounted for death in five patients. Hemorrhagic diathesis and histamine shock were additional causes in four patients. One patient died in an accident, and in the remaining patients the immediate cause of death could not be determined. In none of these patients could neoplastic mast cell infiltrates have caused death directly. For example, in none of the patients who died of perforated peptic ulcers was the stomach infiltrated by mast cells, and in no case of cardiorespiratory failure did the lungs or any other intrathoracic organ show a notable infiltration.

Malignant Mastocytosis

The term *malignant mastocytosis*, used by many authors, refers to a systemic proliferation of mast cells with unequivocal signs of malignant growth. The rapid deterioration of the patient's condition, aggressive growth features of the mast cells, high incidence of myelodysplasia, and transition into myeloproliferative disorders or mast cell leukemia document the malignant nature of this neoplasia at a stem cell level. Excluding the cases of bone marrow–restricted benign forms of mastocytosis, MM can be diagnosed based on the involvement of extracutaneous organs in the absence of urticaria pigmentosa. This demonstrates the importance of a thorough sampling of marrow, liver, lymph nodes (if enlarged), and, if possible, spleen for diagnostic survey. Among the files of the Lymph Node Registry in Kiel are 63 cases of MM defined by these criteria. Considering the high incidence of the associated hematologic disorders that comprise myelodysplasias and full-blown myeloproliferations or mast cell leukemia, this entity seems to correspond to the three subgroups:

1. SMCD with associated hematologic disorders
2. Mast cell leukemia
3. Aggressive nonleukemic forms of SMCD, as described by Travis and colleagues (69).

These types accounted for 29 of the 58 cases of SMCD examined at the Mayo clinic between 1954 and 1985. In our files covering 63 patients, the male-to-female ratio was 2.2:1, and the median age at onset of the disease was 64 years (with a range of 6–84 years). The diagnosis of MM generally is established at the onset of the disease or shortly thereafter. About 75% of the patients had a median prediagnostic phase of 11 months, whereas in only 25% the prediagnostic period exceeded 24 months, this length being significantly ($P < 0.0001$) shorter than that of benign SM or indolent SMCD.

The occurrence of MM before the age of 30 years is the exception. The youngest patient in our collection, however, was a 6-year-old girl. The age distribution curve peaked between the sixth and seventh decades. The age difference from the patients with benign SM (indolent SMCD) is statistically significant ($P < 0.0001$). Constitutional symptoms such as fatigue (56%), weight loss (41%), night sweats, and fever are common and correspond with those found in other hematopoietic malignancies. Hyperthermia was more frequent in cases of MM (16%) than in benign SM (6%).

Symptoms Related to Mast Cell Mediators

Of the symptoms attributable to the preformed or other mast cell mediators, abdominal pain, diarrhea, nausea, vomiting, and flushing were encountered in about 20% of patients. A significant difference from the patients with benign SM (indolent SMCD) is not detectable. This applies also to other symptoms of this line such as syncope, hypertension, headache, arthralgia, dizziness, hypotension, tachycardia, and respiratory distress as signs of anaphylaxis (69).

Dermatologic Findings

Because this collection did not contain any patients who had primary skin involvement, a long history of skin rash, pruritus, and wheeze was an exceptional finding in patients who had MM. In our collection, only two patients developed skin symptoms in the terminal stage of the disease because of secondary infiltration by leukemic mast cells, as described by Efrati and colleagues (63).

Hematologic Findings

Anemia as a regular finding in MM varies considerably according to the stage of disease. About 81% of our patients had a severe anemia with a median hemoglobin value of 9.8 g/dL at the time of diagnosis. Enhanced leukocyte counts over 10,000 per microliter were found in 43%, with values ranging from 10,000 to 212,000 per microliter and a median value of 20,100. Similar values have been documented in the literature (69,70). The incidence of anemia and increased leukocytes exceeds the values found in the benign forms. Granulocytopenia occurred in 14% and thrombocytopenia in 43% of the patients. Basophils were increased in 16%, eosinophils in 40%, and monocytes in 25% of patients with MM. In our series, the median values were 230, 1,840, and 2,160 per microliter, respectively. In 8%, tissue mast cells were detectable in blood smears. Six percent of the patients with MM had more than 10% mast cells in the blood and accordingly were classified as mast cell leukemia. Normal hematologic findings are extremely rare.

A considerable number of patients who have MM develop a myelodysplasia (21%), a myeloproliferation (40%), or a mast cell leukemia (6%) in the course of the disease. In our collection of 63 cases of MM, 13 patients had a myelodysplasia (Table 52.6). These were found to be consistent with refractory anemia in the French–American–British classification in four patients and with chronic myelomonocytic leukemia in eight patients. One patient was classified as refractory anemia with excess of blasts in transformation. There were 22 patients with MM with full-blown myeloproliferation, representing chronic myeloproliferative disorders, of which 13 were classified as having atypical chronic myelogenous leukemia and two as having agnogenic myeloid metaplasia with myelofibrosis (megakaryocytic myelosis). In seven patients a reliable classification of the myeloproliferation was not possible. Three patients were classified as having acute myelomonocytic leukemia. Four patients underwent a transition into mast cell leukemia (Fig. 52.13). In two patients an immunocytoma of the bone marrow was diagnosed additionally.

Mast cell diseases may be accompanied by the appearance of mast cells in circulation. Circulating mast cells, however, usually constitute a minority of leukocytes, accounting for fewer than 10% of cases. In patients with mast cell leukemia, circulating mast cells usually exceed 30% of the leukocytes. In all patients with mast cell leukemia there was a primary MM that preceded the leukemic outbreak. All patients showed concomitant atypias in granulocytes, monocytes, megakaryocytes, and erythropoieses, so that the term *panmyelosis* appeared more justified. In addition to the atypical mast cells with metachromatic granules, there were monocytoid cells with slightly lobed nuclei and weakly metachromatic cytoplasm. In contrast, Travis and coworkers (111) found that in patients with mast cell leukemia, mast cells were the only atypical cell types. In enzyme cytochemical studies, the leukemic mast cells and the monocytoid cells were seen on naphthol AS-D chloroacetate esterase, myeloperoxidase, elastase, and acid phosphatase staining. Immuno-

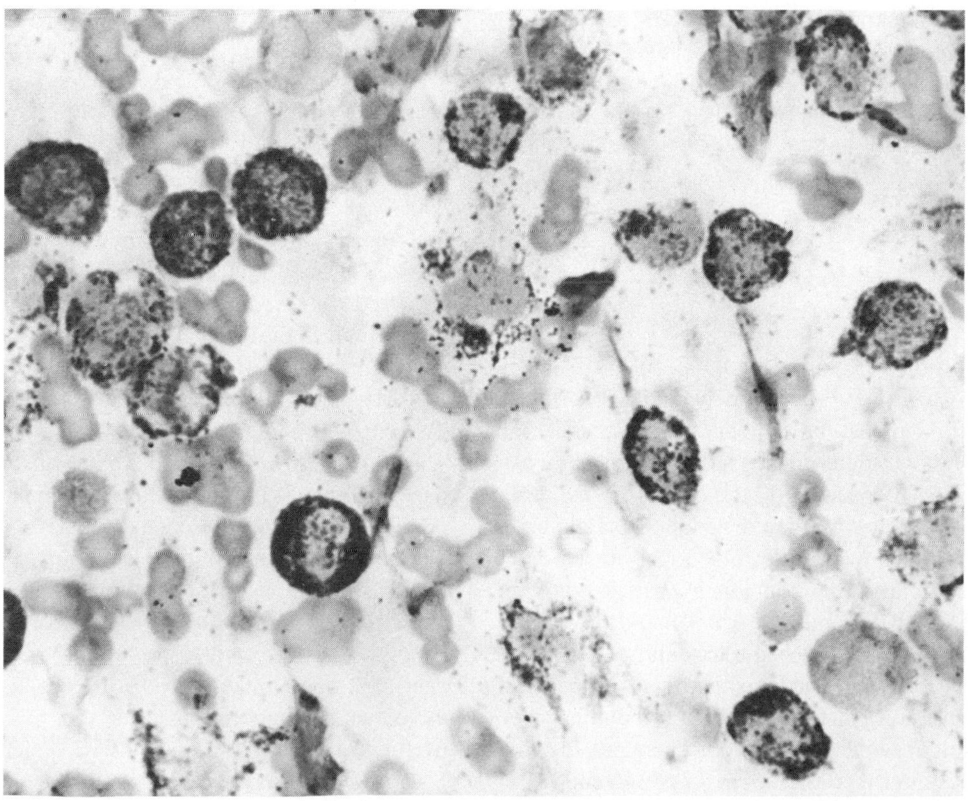

FIG. 52.13. Malignant mastocytosis may be associated with a mast cell leukemia. Atypical mast cells in blood smear of a 46-year-old man suffering from malignant mastocytosis for 5 months (Pappenheim stain, original magnification: 1,600× magnification).

cytochemically, leukemic mast cells were seen to express CD45, CD11c, CD68, Ki-M1p, tryptase, and CD117. A thorough account of this issue has been provided by Escribano and coworders (112), who found leukemic mast cells to strongly express CD11c, CD13, CD29, CD33, CD44, CD45, CD63, CD71, CD117, and to FcηRI.

The widely distributed atypias that affect all cells of myeloid lineages may suggest that the neoplastic transformation involves a genomic defect at the stem cell level. To date, however, it has not been possible to demonstrate monoclonality of blood cells or mast cells by the analysis of isoenzymes or of the restriction length polymorphism of X-chromosomal genes such as that of phosphoglycerokinase (113,114).

The association of hematopoietic malignancies with mast cell disease is a generally accepted finding (63,67,70,79,90). It is difficult to estimate the significance of such findings in relation to the subtypes of SMCD. Among the 29 patients with mastocytosis classified as belonging to the nonindolent subgroups by Travis and associates (69), 20 showed hematologic abnormalities with a broad range of variety, including myelodysplastic syndrome in nine patients, myeloproliferative disorders in five, acute nonlymphoid leukemia in two, and chronic neutropenia in one (70). A reliable comparison of our results with the data from the Mayo Clinic cases is difficult, because the delineated categories also contain hematologic alterations such as anemia and thrombocytopenia, which may be caused by other solid tumors present in at least eight patients. Such patients, classified as having SMCD with associated hematologic disorders and with skin involvement, would correspond to our patients of benign SM, despite the unfavorable outcomes. In addition, the frequency of the hematologic findings reported in the literature has not been related to the individual categories of the mast cell disease.

Bone Marrow

Hematologic abnormalities are common and mostly associated with severe alterations in the bone marrow, which was involved in 92% of our 63 patients with MM (Table 52.7). In smears and cytologic imprints, the increased number of mast cells may be masked by the excess of myeloid cells that mainly comprises poorly segmented precursors. Mast cells display reniform or atypically lobed nuclei and oval or spindled cytoplasm that contains a variable number of poorly metachromatic granules. In the majority of patients, the first appropriate diagnosis was established on histologic examination of bone marrow samples. A proper interpretation of the histologic findings in this tissue can be extremely difficult. In our collection, we encountered two different histologic patterns (67). The first type encompasses those patients with MM associated with a myelodysplasia or myeloproliferation. The characteristic histologic findings (Fig. 52.14) are as follows

1. Spindle-shaped or clear type mast cells localized in peritrabecular or intermediate marrow spaces
2. Foci of fibrosis with adjacent osteosclerosis
3. Lack of lymphoplasmacellular infiltrates
4. Marrow areas not infiltrated by mast cells that may show a depletion of fat cells because of a hyperplasia of granulopoiesis and monocytes.

In typical patients with myelodysplasia, blasts or ringed sideroblasts may be present in moderate numbers. In cases associated with a full-blown myeloproliferative disorder, the diagnosis may be made best in conjunction with blood smears.

The second type of histologic pattern seen with MM occurs in cases complicated by a mast cell leukemia. The main histologic alterations are as follow:

1. Diffuse and patchy infiltrates by pleomorphic and atypical mast cells
2. Mild focal fibrosis associated with foci of osteosclerosis
3. Lack of lymphoplasmacellular accumulations
4. Depletion of fat cells and hematopoietic precursors.

Skeletal Lesions

Skeletal alterations are common and even may give rise to spontaneous fractures (79). In our patients with MM, pathologic fractures occurred in 13%. Osteosclerosis was the most frequent alteration of the bone, occurring in 68%; it was associated with mast cell infiltrates and adjacent fibrosis on a histologic level (Fig. 52.15). A diffuse osteoporosis was observed in 50%; osteolytic foci were present in 16% of our patients and usually were associated with an acute myelomonocytic or a mast cell leukemia. Only 20% of patients with MM lacked any skeletal alterations as seen on radiologic examination. In some patients all these skeletal alterations may coincide to form a peculiar bone disorder referred to as *osteopetrosis-like osteopathia of mastocytosis*. Aberrations in the *KIT* gene locus in the mice may be associated with osteopetrosis.

Skeletal lesions have been described by several authors as occurring in up to 70% of patients with mast cell disease. The skull, vertebral column, spine, ribs, and pelvis are the most commonly involved sites. Cystic and sclerotic lesions may occur in close association (115–119). In addition to the classic imaging findings, an enhanced bone density on radiographs, an intense uptake on bone scans, and a marrow expansion on bone marrow scans generally were reported. Dual-photon absorptiometry of the skeleton has revealed very high bone mineral levels of 1.678 g/cm^2 of the lumbar vertebrae. It has been suggested that this technique may be useful in the follow-up studies of skeletal involvement in SMCD (120). It is not really possible to relate such information to the prognostically relevant categories of the disease, although a few contrary reports have been published (121,122).

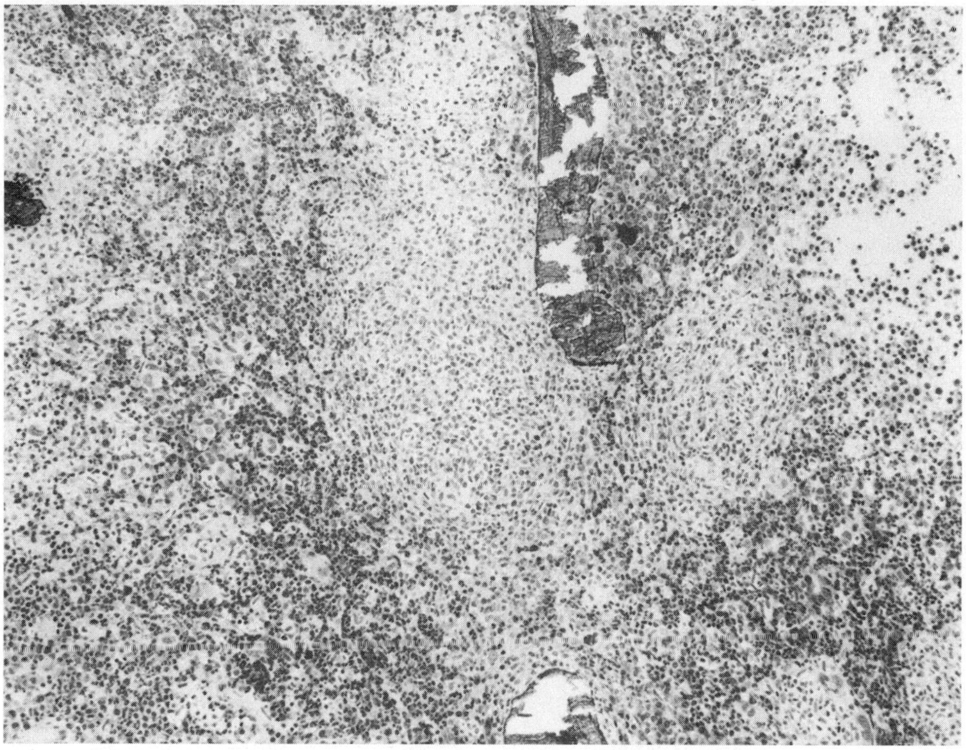

A

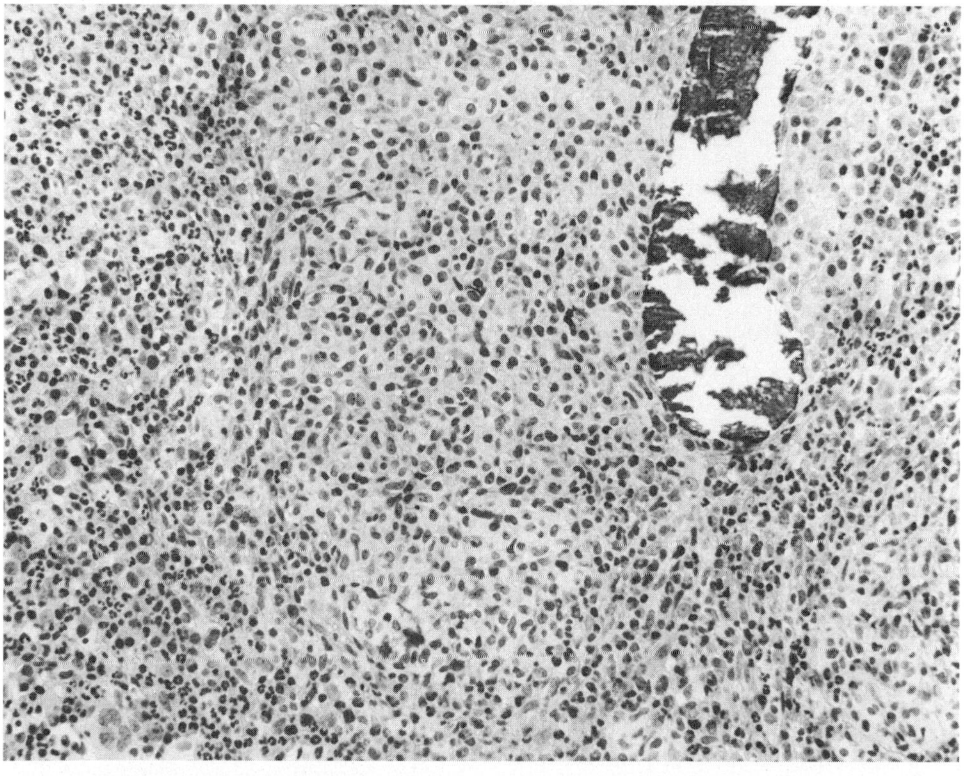

B

FIG. 52.14. Malignant mastocytosis frequently involves bone marrow characterized by peritrabecular infiltrates of atypical clear type mast cells, foci of fibrosis with adjacent osteosclerosis (not shown), lack of lymphocytic accumulations, and marrow areas not infiltrated by mast cells; patients may show signs of severe hematologic disorders such as myelodysplasia, myeloproliferation, or mast cell leukemia. Photomicrograph of bone marrow of a 52-year-old man who has malignant mastocytosis and who developed a chronic myeloid leukemia. Areas not infiltrated by mast cells display diffuse enhancement of granulocytes and some atypical megakaryocytes (4-μm methacrylate sections; **A:** Chloroacetate esterase staining, original magnification: 400× magnification; **B:** Giemsa stain, original magnification: 800× magnification).

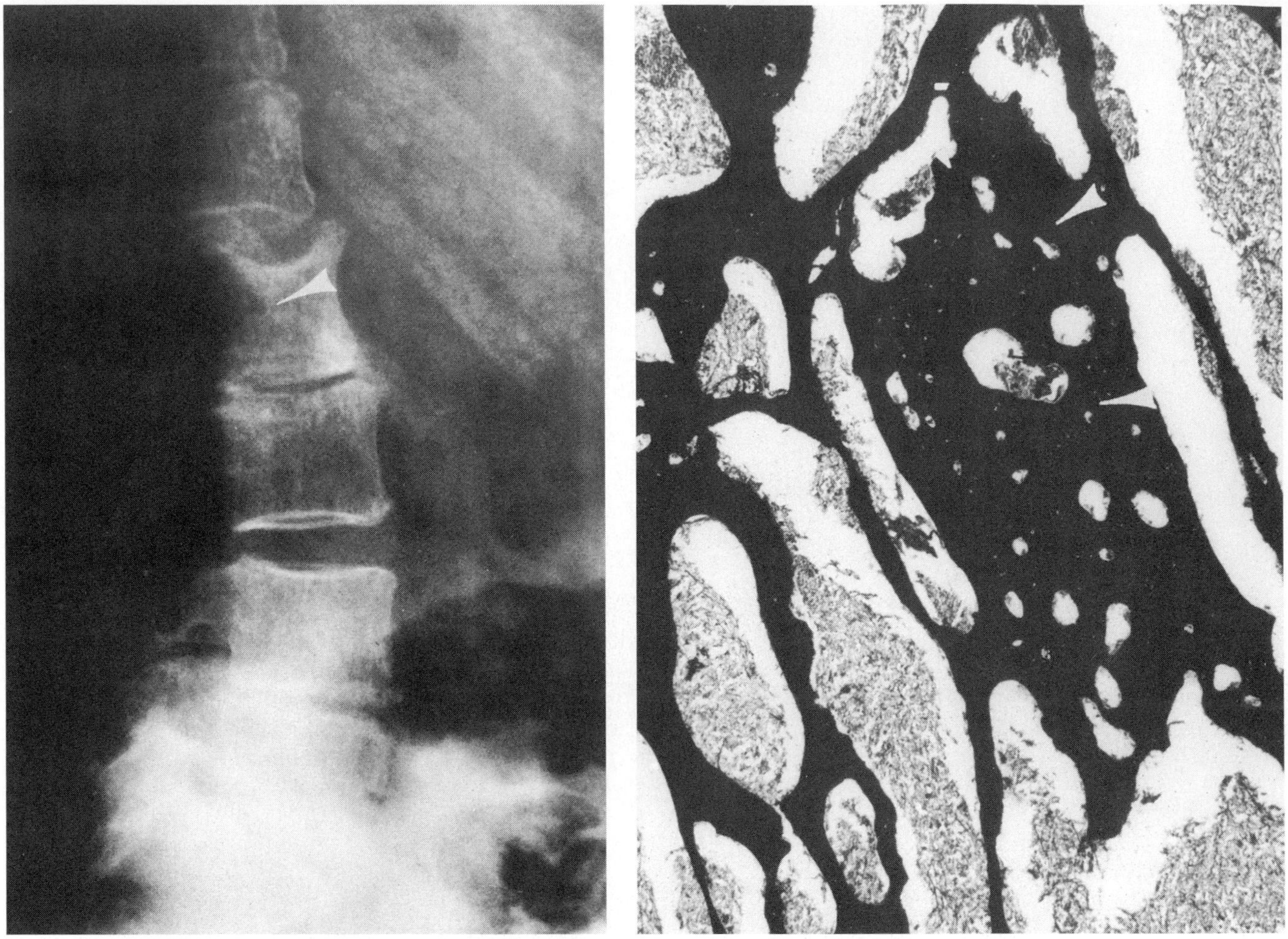

A B

FIG. 52.15. Skeletal lesions are frequent in cases of malignant mastocytosis. Radiograph (**A**) and photomicrograph (**B**) of a biopsy specimen from a spontaneously fractured vertebra of a 51-year-old woman who had malignant mastocytosis that showed a combination of osteoporosis and patchy osteosclerosis (*arrows*). In addition, irregular osteolytic foci are detectable in the body of vertebrae (*arrows*) (**B:** 4-μm methacrylate section, cossa stain, original magnification: 200$\times$ magnification).

Liver Involvement

Hepatomegaly was present in 80% of patients in whom a reliable monitoring of hepatic status was possible. In a few patients, however, the liver probably was not involved. The median weight of the liver in *post mortem* studies was 2,950 g, with a range of 1,960 to 3,860 g. On histologic examination, small foci of atypical mast cells were usually found in the sinuses and in the broadened periportal fields (Fig. 52.16). Alterations do not correlate with liver size or with liver function. In some patients, icterus indicated severe liver damage. Fibrosis was found in about 20% of patients; fully developed cirrhosis was observed in 5%. The hepatic changes hardly ever are useful in distinguishing the different categories of mast cell diseases.

Spleen Findings

Splenomegaly occurred in 91% of our patients with MM in whom reliable information on spleen size was available. Spleen weight ranged from 350 to 2,300 g, with a median of 975 g in 10 of our patients. Including the 21 spleen weights mentioned in the literature, the median amounts to 865 g. In two patients, no splenomegaly was present, although the spleen showed typical mast cell infiltrations. More recent reports stress the importance of spleen involvement in patients with mastocytosis and indicate the more frequent peritrabecular and perifollicular deposition of the mast cell infiltrates; involvement of the follicles and of the red pulp seems to be less frequent (Fig. 52.17). Some correlation ($P < 0.01$) was found between splenomegaly and a poor prognosis (110). In our files, splenomegaly occurred significantly more frequent ($P < 0.0001$) in MM than in indolent SM.

In addition to the typical infiltrates, a depletion of follicles and multiple fibrotic foci within the red pulp occurred, with or without detectable mast cell infiltrates. In patients with a coincidentally occurring myeloproliferation or a mast cell leukemia, the leukemic infiltrates also were detectable in various areas of the spleen. The microscopic alterations are

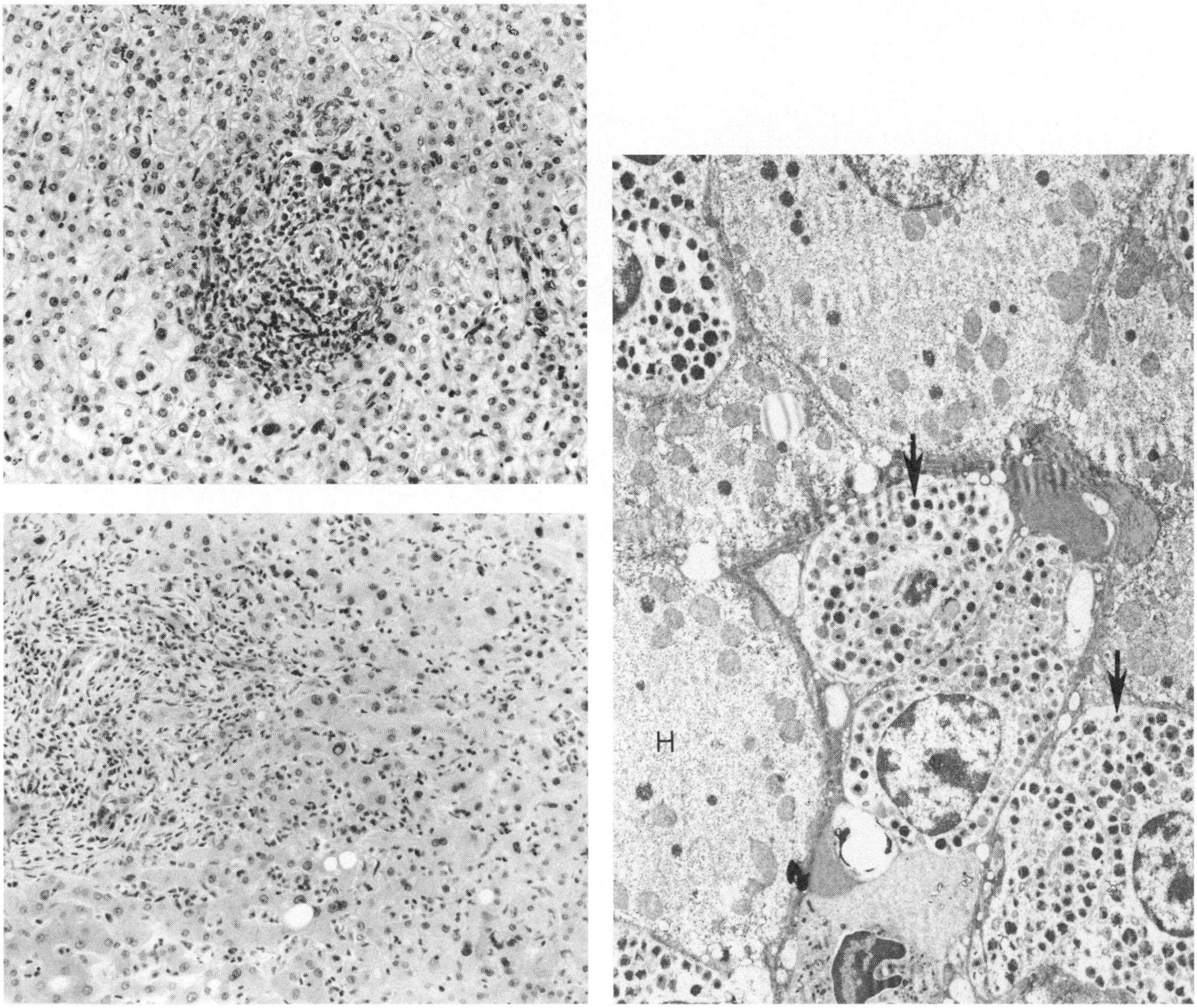

A

B

C

FIG. 52.16. A,B: A liver biopsy in a case of malignant mastocytosis. Mast cells form granuloma-like infiltrates accompanied by fibrosis and inflammatory cells. In infiltrated areas, hepatocytes are destroyed. A small number of blood cell precursors are found within the hepatic sinusoids (4-μm paraffin sections, hematoxylin and eosin stain, original magnification: 800× magnification). **C:** Atypical mast cells (*arrows*) are scattered between hepatocytes and within the hepatic sinusoids. Hepatocytes (*H*) are replaced by infiltrating mast cells (araldite embedding, lead citrate and uranyl acetate contrasting, original magnification: 6,000× magnification).

difficult to interpret and are obscured further because of the additional signs of hypersplenism, which is a regular phenomenon in these diseases. The histologic examination of the spleen does not seem to provide a reliable prediction of outcome. Splenectomy seems to exert a positive influence on the prognosis, probably because of the reduction of thrombocyte pooling in the spleen.

Lymph Nodes

Lymphadenopathy was observed in 54% of our patients with MM in whom information was available on this issue. About one third of the patients had generalized and another one third localized lymph node involvement, mostly in the retroperitoneal region. Axillary lymph nodes were not involved.

The involved lymph nodes reach an average diameter of 2 cm and rarely can grow to up to 6 cm. Generalized lymphadenopathy is about twice as frequent as in benign SM (indolent SMCD). On physical examination, lymph nodes generally are reported as firm masses, and this finding has been attributed partly to the fibrosis usually found in mast cell lesions. In 35 patients lymph node biopsy specimens could be studied histologically. Of these, 94% percent showed massive mast cell infiltrations. Mast cells built up weakly stained foci of clear cells. Such foci were distributed

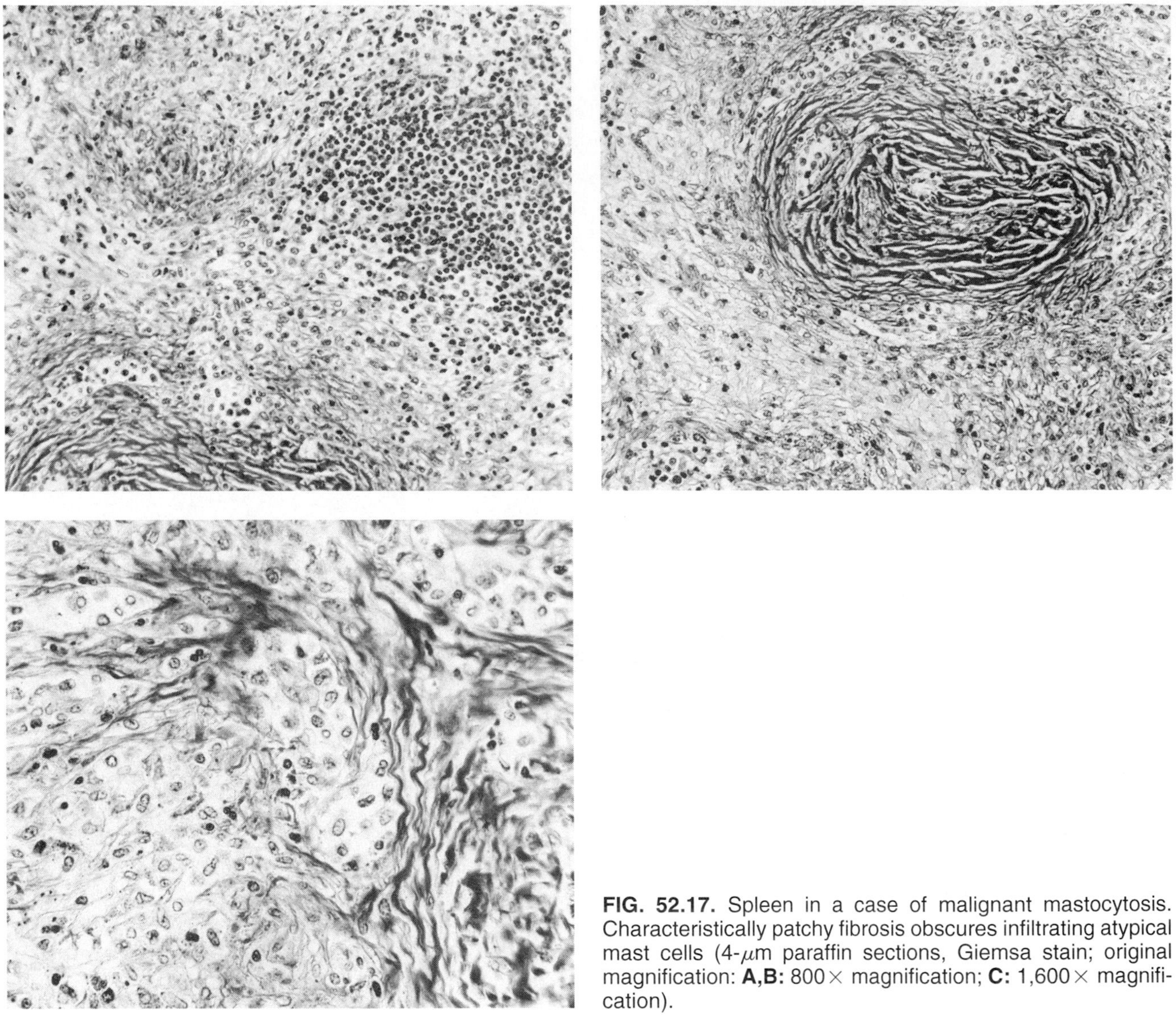

FIG. 52.17. Spleen in a case of malignant mastocytosis. Characteristically patchy fibrosis obscures infiltrating atypical mast cells (4-μm paraffin sections, Giemsa stain; original magnification: **A,B:** 800× magnification; **C:** 1,600× magnification).

irregularly, infiltrating perivascular and mostly perisinusoidal areas with no clear preference for B- or T-cell zones. Unlike benign or indolent SM, mast cell infiltrates may not be confined to the lymph node but can extend to the capsule or to the adjacent tissue areas. In many patients, mast cells are accompanied by an increase of reticulin fibers and capillary vessels. In a limited number of patients, clear-type mast cells follow the course of sinuses and form a peculiar pattern that resembles immature sinus histiocytosis or certain types of low-grade B-cell lymphomas.

In contrast to the spleen, foci of fibrosis that obscure the infiltrating mast cells do not occur in the lymph node. The diagnosis can be missed easily, however, because of the wide range of differential diagnostic possibilities and the sparse granulation of the atypical mast cells. The histopathology of lymph nodes and spleen in mast cell disease has been dealt with in a more recent work in which the broad spectrum of histologic manifestations has been analyzed in well-documented cases. These studies show that the paracortical and perifollicular areas often are involved, but medullary cords and sinuses only occasionally are infiltrated (110). According to our experience, lymph node histology rarely proves contributory in distinguishing malignant variants from more benign forms, although the occurrence of additional leukemic infiltrates that consist of myeloid or myelomonocytic blasts and of granulocytic precursors or even leukemic mast cells favors MM.

Other Organs

Mast cell infiltrates were observed sporadically in tissue sites other than those already discussed. In single patients, duodenum wall, colon, lungs, brain, kidney and muscles were infiltrated by mast cell sheets of variable size.

Cause of Death

Of the 63 patients with MM, 48 died during the follow-up period. In 75% of patients there was a combined thrombocytopenia and a significantly diminished Quick value. Fifteen had severe hemorrhagic diatheses caused by extensive marrow infiltration and depletion of megakaryocytes, leading to fatal bleeding from gastric ulcers or causing cerebal hemorrhages. Hemorrhagic diatheses developed in other patients because of extensive pooling of platelets in the spleen. Circulatory failure was the cause of death in five and hepatic failure in one patient. Three patients died of kachexia. Two died of heart infarction at an advanced stage of MM. Massive release of mast cell mediators was suspected to have caused the unexpected myocardial infarction.

In 22 patients a reliable statement on the cause of death could not be made.

Prognosis of Mast Cell Disease

The majority of mast cell neoplasias is benign lesions. This certainly applies to localized mastocytoma of the dermis and of other organs, as well as to urticaria pigmentosa and bone marrow–restricted benign mastocytosis. Many of these lesions are self-limiting, disappearing within a few years. The best example of this is urticaria pigmentosa, which subsides at puberty in over 70% of patients.

Histologic proof of mast cell infiltrates at one extracutaneous site, in addition to skin involvement, justifies the diagnosis of indolent SMCD. Cutaneous involvement in these patients is indistinguishable from that in urticaria pigmentosa. It is unclear whether pure cases of urticaria pigmentosa can evolve into SMCD or whether the systemic involvement is prone to be missed in the early stages of disease, resulting in the false diagnosis of urticaria pigmentosa. It generally is agreed that skin involvement, early onset, and lack of severe hematologic complications are signs of a favorable course, with actuarial survival rates of 98% at 1 year after diagnosis and 93% at 5 years (Fig. 52.18). This variant has been designated *benign* or *indolent SMCD.*

A sizable body of evidence indicates that an additional category of SMCD exists, distinguished by a multitude of associated hematologic findings that range from severe anemia and granulocytopenia to myelodysplasia, myelomonocytic leukemia, or mast cell leukemia in about 80% of patients. At least the majority of these cases lacks concomitant skin involvement. A poor outcome is reflected by the significantly lower 1- and 5-year survival rates of 43% and 18%, respectively, and a median duration of survival of about 11 months after the initial diagnosis. This category was referred to as MM to underline clearly the difference in clinical course and outcome.

Malignant mastocytosis seems to encompass these three categories:

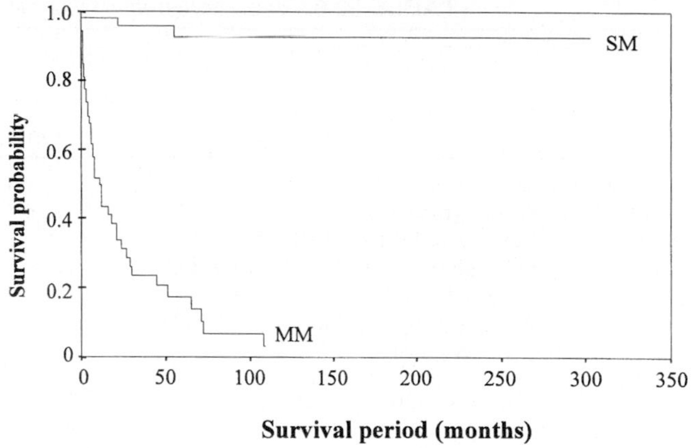

FIG. 52.18. Actuarial survival probabilities computed for 56 patients with benign (indolent) systemic mast cell disease and for 53 patients with malignant mastocytosis followed up in the Lymph Node Registry in Kiel. Mean duration of survival for patients with malignant mastocytosis was 11 months. The difference between the groups was statistically significant ($P < 0.0001$).

1. SMCD with associated hematologic disorders
2. Aggressive SMCD
3. Mast cell leukemia.

The introduction of modern therapeutic strategies has improved the median duration of survival of patients with MM from 6 months, as reported in the first edition of this book in 1992, to 11 months.

Like other neoplastic hematopoietic cells, especially monocytes or macrophages, malignancies of mast cells may appear as localized sarcoma, leading to death within 2 to 3 years from the onset and 1 to 2 years from the diagnosis.

Differential Diagnosis of Mast Cell Disease

The differential diagnostic considerations in SMCD concern, on the one hand, the separation of benign or indolent forms from the more malignant variants associated with severe hematologic diseases, aggressive mast cell growth, or mast cell leukemia. On the other hand, mast cell disease has to be distinguished from numerous other entities such as various hematologic malignancies, including lymphomas, histiocytosis, and various hyperimmune reactions. The clinical picture is prone to misinterpretation because of the broad range of symptoms (79). Those symptoms associated with histamine release have to be separated from serotonin flush, which is considerably shorter and lasts only a few minutes, with a reddish-blue erythema that appears on the head and thorax (72). The gastrointestinal symptoms include various diseases with overlapping symptoms. In most patients, the diarrhea and the celiac sprue–like episodes are interrupted by normal intervals. The skeletal changes, such as osteoporosis, osteosclerosis, and osteolysis or the combination of all three, represent nonspecific findings and can be associ-

TABLE 52.8. *Immunohistochemistry in the differential diagnosis of mast cell disease*

	Tryptase	Ki-M1p[a]	Ki-B3, Ki-B5, L-26[b]	S-100	CD30, Ber-H2[c]	CD3, β-F1, UCHL1, Ki-T1
Mast cell disease (mast cells)	+	+	+/−	−	−	−
Hairy cell leukemia (B cells)	−	+	+	−	−	−
Monocytoid B-cell lymphoma (B cells)	−	+	+	−	−	−
Langerhans cell histiocytosis (Langerhans cells)	−	+	−	+	−	−
Lymphoplasmacytoid lymphoma (B cells)	−	−	+	−	−	−
Angioimmunoblastic lymphadenopathy (T cells)	−	−	−	−	−	+
Hodgkin's disease (Hodgkin cells)	−	−	−	−	+	−

Distinctive immunoreagents appropriate for the differential diagnosis of mast cell disease and other hematopoietic neoplasias. All antibodies recognize paraffin-resistant epitopes.

[a] Ki-M1p is a monocyte–macrophage-associated monoclonal antibody that coreacts weakly with a subpopulation of B lymphocytes (130).

[b] B cell–reactive antibodies (Ki-B3 and Ki-B5) also may recognize some mast cells (30,131).

[c] Ber-H2 recognizes Hodgkin cells (123).

ated with other hematologic disorders, especially osteomyelosclerosis, multiple myeloma, and primary B-cell lymphoma of the bone marrow. Also, metastatic carcinomas or primary osteogenic disorders such as Paget's disease, osteopetrosis, and calcitonin-induced or renal osteopathia may produce similar lesions. Splenomegaly is another finding common to a large number of hematologic disorders and infectious diseases. Detection of metachromatic mast cells is the salient criterion for the diagnosis. Major problems arise in interpreting bone marrow biopsy specimens. In areas that have a disseminated or focal infiltration pattern, Hodgkin's lymphoma, histiocytosis X (Langerhans cell granulomatosis), angioimmunoblastic lymphadenopathy, and some other T-cell lymphomas represent the major differential diagnostic candidates. The recognition of Hodgkin's lymphoma in uncertain cases can be based on the immunohistochemical detection of Hodgkin's cells that use the monoclonal antibody BerH2 against the activation antigen CD30 (123). Histiocytosis X is distinguished by the typical Langerhans cells, which are positive with antibodies that recognize CD1a and S-100 protein on fresh and paraffin-embedded material. Lesions of angioimmunoblastic lymphadenopathy have a typical cellular composition that consists of T lymphocytes expressing βF_1 (124) or CD3 (125). In addition, a large number of macrophages, epithelioid cells, and histiocytes detectable with Ki-M1p or antibodies to CD11c, CD68, and lysozyme are present. Plasma cells and lymphoid blasts as well as numerous venules represent regular findings in this entity. Also critical for the diagnosis is a concomitant proliferation of follicular dendritic cells detectable with the antibodies Ki-M4p or Ki-FDC1 on frozen as well as on paraffin sections (126). In addition, there are typical alterations in the blood (127) and a generalized lymphadenopathy.

Hypercellular stages of agnogenic myeloid metaplasia with myelofibrosis (128) may resemble mast cell disease because of the enhancement of spindle shaped fibroblasts or myofibroblasts and collagen fibers. But the metachromasia and the reaction of the fusiform mast cells with Ki-M1p in addition to tryptase enable a clear separation.

Certain types of immunoreactions in the bone marrow, such as those related to the graft-versus-host reaction may produce histologic pictures similar to mast cell disease. The usual increase in lymphocytes and collagen fibers and the hemocytopenia in the blood may add to the differential diagnostic difficulties. A similar alteration, closely related to the hypersensitivity reaction, has been described by Rywlin and associates (129), who proposed the term *eosinophilic fibrohistiocytic lesion of the bone marrow*. Because of the enhanced numbers of eosinophils, mast cells, and fibroblasts, in addition to the abundance of lymphocytes, this lesion may be indistinguishable from early stages of SMCD. Among the collection of Rywlin and associates were at least one or two cases of mastocytosis. Nevertheless, the eosinophilic fibrohistiocytic lesion of the bone marrow is a rare but dis-

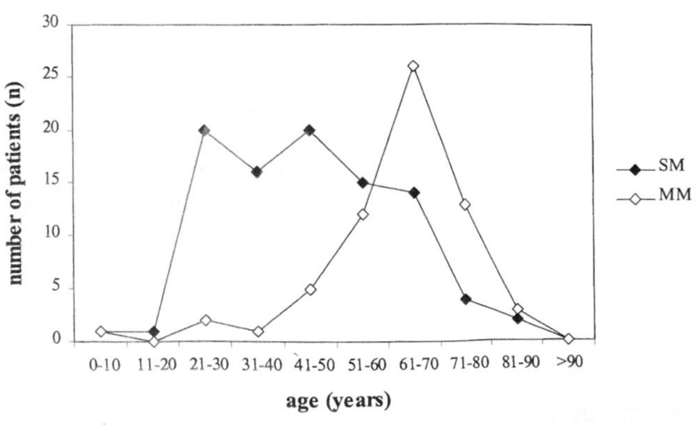

FIG. 52.19. Age distribution curves for 97 patients suffering from benign (indolent) systemic mastocytosis and for 63 patients with malignant systemic mastocytosis followed up in Lymph Node Registry in Kiel. Median ages of 43 years for benign and 64 years for malignant mastocytosis differ significantly ($P < 0.0001$).

TABLE 52.9. *Comparison of therapeutic strategies and survival time in patients with malignant systemic mast cell disease*

Therapy	1-year survival (%)	2-year survival (%)	5-year survival (%)
Interferon-α and chemotherapy (n = 4)	2/4	2/4	2/4
Interferon-α, only (n = 4)	3/4	1/4	0[a]/4
Chemotherapy, only (n = 16)	7/16 (44)	5/16 (31)	1[b]/16 (6)
Neither Interferon alpha nor chemotherapy (n = 11)	6/11 (55)	2/11 (18)	0/11 (0)

Only patients with complete clinical reports were included (n = 35).
[a] One patient still under observation.
[b] Three patients still under observation.

tinct entity mostly associated with chronic multidrug treatment or drug addiction.

Mast cell infiltrates in the liver, spleen, and lymph nodes may mimic various lymphomas, especially hairy cell leukemia, lymphoplasmacytoid lymphoma, and low-grade T-cell lymphomas. Mast cell infiltrates may resemble follicular low-grade B-cell lymphomas, especially on low-power magnification. Cytologic details easily reveal the diagnosis. In addition, the immunohistochemical application of the recently developed antibodies to paraffin-resistant antigenic epitopes can be helpful (Table 52.8).

Once the diagnosis of SMCD is established, a disease category must be decided. Important criteria are age at onset (Fig. 52.19), skin involvement, and coincidence of severe hematologic disorders.

Treatment of Mast Cell Diseases

A uniform therapeutic strategy has not been applied to patients who suffer from mast cell diseases. The majority of therapeutic regimens is aimed at relieving complaints. Patients should avoid triggers of mast cell activation such as cold, alcohol, and morphine derivatives.

Dermatologic complaints may be treated successfully with H1 blocker–type antihistamines such as diphenhydramine and chlorpheniramine. Local application of corticoids as well as photochemotherapy with psoralens and ultraviolet light A irradiation reduces dermatologic symptoms in urticaria pigmentosa and in indolent SMCD. Some H2 antagonists such as cyproheptadine, as well as cromolyn sodium, can be quite effective in relieving gastrointestinal symptoms, especially in patients with diarrhea and gastric or duodenal ulcer. Bone pain caused by mast cell foci can be treated by local irradiation.

In systemic disease, especially with hypersplenism, splenectomy reduces hemorrhagic complications considerably. In patients with severe systemic disease, oral corticoid medication generally is recommended. In patients in whom the disease has an aggressive clincal courses and in those with MM, interferon-α may lead to regression in the size of mast cell infiltrates. This was the case in four of our patients with benign SMCD and in six patients with MM. Although a standardized polychemotherapy regimen tested on an appropriately stratified collection of patients does not exist, modern strategies including hydroxyurea and the polychemotherapeutic regimens in general oncologic use may improve life quality as well as prognosis significantly. One patient who had MM that originally was mistaken for mixed cellularity Hodgkin's disease and treated accordingly, survived for over 40 years as the first patient with MM in our files treated with chemotherapy. Two male patients aged 46 and 42 years, both with MM, were treated with a combination of interferon-α, corticoids, and polychemotherapy. One patient survived 65 and the other over 146 months. A 69-year-old man who received corticoids and polychemotherapy (MCOP protocol) died 51 months after diagnosis. A comparison of groups of patients with MM treated with and without interferon-α and polychemotherapy is shown in Table 52.9.

Chemotherapy used in patients with mast cell leukemia proved ineffective (111).

Promising perspectives are expected from bone marrow transplantation. The decision for this potentially curative treatment should be made at the very early onset of the disease. In our files a 29-year-old female with MM is free of disease 4 years after successful marrow transplantation.

SUMMARY AND CONCLUSIONS

Mast cells derive from hematopoietic stem cells and are most probably of myelomonocytic lineage, populating the majority of human organs with a varying distribution density. Mast cell evolution, survival and function depend strongly on SCF and its receptor KIT (CD117). In addition, interleukins 3 through 6 seem to play important roles in mast cell biology. Using light and electron microscopic techniques, the metachromatic electrondense granules are revealed as the most distinctive features of these cells. Mast cell granules represent secondary lysosomes with a complicated biochemical composition that contains highly polymerized glycosaminoglycans, histamine, and basic peptides linked to a lipoprotein matrix. The abundance of biologically active mediators present in these cells qualifies mast cells as amplifiers of nonspecific inflammatory response, linking the noncellular and cellular phases of the inflammatory reaction. Specific receptors for complement factor C5a (CD88) and Fcη on the surface membrane of mast cells underline the importance of these cells in various immunologic reactions.

Uncontrolled mast cell proliferations are rare but distinct disorders, referred to as *mastocytoma*, *mastocytosis*, or *mast cell disease*. Neoplasias of mast cells represent clonal expansions and are associated with clonal somatic point mutations in the *KIT* gene locus. Disseminated macular skin lesions are the leading finding in urticaria pigmentosa; they are the most frequent mast cell proliferations. SMCD may affect any tissue type and can be accompanied by a wide range of hematologic and nonhematologic symptoms. Those disorders associated with skin involvement and early onset offer a far better probability of survival and are considered benign SM or indolent SMCD.

Patients who have an SM of late onset that lacks skin involvement have been shown to develop a rapidly deteriorating clinical course and a poor outcome, justifying their classification as having MM. In this type of SCMD, there is a high incidence of severe hematologic disorders that ranges from hemocytopenia (more than 80%) and myelodysplasia (21%) to full-blown myeloproliferation (40%). In 6% of patients, a mast cell leukemia results.

Recently, the prognosis of malignant mast cell disease has improved considerably, as a result of combined application of interferon-α and polychemotherapy.

Nosologically, the close relationship of mast cells to the myelomonocytic lineage assigns SMCD to the group of myeloproliferative disorders.

ACKNOWLEDGMENTS

The authors acknowledge expert photographic documentation by W. Zeiser.

REFERENCES

1. Ehrlich P. Beitraege zur kenntnis der granulierten bindegewebszellen und der eosinophilen leukozyten. *Arch Anat Physiol* 1879;3:166–169.
2. Unna PG. Beitraege zur anatomie und pathogenese der urticaria simplex und pigmentosa. *Mschr Prakt Dermat* 1887;3.H.
3. Jorpes JE. The site of formation of heparin. In: Jorpes JE, ed. *Heparin: its chemistry, physiology and application in medicine.* London: Humphrey Milford, 1939.
4. Riley JF. The relationship of the tissue mast cells to the blood vessels in the rat. *J Pathol Bacteriol* 1953;65:461–469.
5. Ishizaka K, Ishizaka T. Immune mechanisms of reversed type reaginic hypersensitivity. *J Immunol* 1969;103:588–593.
6. Schwartz LB, Austen KF. The Kaplan-Meier analysis revealed a significant difference in clinical outcome of patients with the PF pattern of FDC and the other two (GC and diffuse) pattern (p = 0.015). Structure and function of the chemical mediators of mast cells. *Prog Allergy* 1984;34:271–321.
7. Valent P. Mack-Forster Award lecture: review. Mast cell differentiation antigens. Expression in normal and malignant cells and use for diagnostic purposes. *Eur J Clin Invest* 1995;25:715–720.
8. Anderson DM, Lyman SD, Baird A, et al. Molecular cloning of mast cell growth factor, a hematopoietin that is active in both membrane bound and soluble forms [published erratum appears in *Cell* 1990; 63:1112). *Cell* 1990;63:235–243.
9. Rottem M, Okada T, Goff JP, et al. Mast cells cultured from the periphal blood of normal donors and patients with mastocytosis originate from a CD 34 + /Fc epsilon RI-cell population. *Blood* 1994;84: 2489–2496.
10. Furitsu T, Tsujimura T, Tono T, et al: Identification of mutations in the coding sequence of the proto-oncogene c-kit in a human mast cell leukemia cell line causing ligand-independent activation of c-kit product. *J Clin Invest* 1993;92:1736–1744.
11. Parwaresch MR. *The human blood basophil.* New York: Springer-Verlag, 1976.
12. Mikhail GR, Miller-Milinska A. Mast cell population in human skin. *J Invest Dermatol* 1964;43:245–249.
13. Soter NA, Mihm JR, Dvorak HF, et al. Cutaneous necrotizing venulitis: a sequential analysis of the morphologic alterations occurring after mast cell degranulation in patients in a unique syndrome. *Clin Exp Immunol* 1978;32:46–58.
14. Fox B, Bull TB, Guz A. Mast cells in human alveolar wall: an electron microscopic study. *J Clin Pathol* 1981;34:1333–1342.
15. Lennert K, Schubert JCF. Untersuchungen ueber die sauren mucopolysaccharide der gewebsmastzellen im menschlichen Knochenmark. *Frankf Ztschr Pathol* 1959;69:579–590.
16. Scott JE, Dorling J. Differential staining of acid glycosaminoglycans (mucopolysaccharides) by alcian blue in salt solutions. *Histochemie* 1965;5:221–233.
17. Parwaresch RM, Lennert K. Zur differenzierung der blutbasophilen und gewebsmastzellen nach dem reifegrad ihrer granula: eine neue modifikation der toluidinblau-pH-reihe. *Histochemie* 1969;19: 262–271.
18. Csaba G, Surjam L, Fischer J, et al. On the mechanism of mast cell formation. *Acta Biol Acad Sci Kung* 1969;20:57–74.
19. Kobayasi T, Midtgard K, Asboe-Hansen G. Ultrastructure of human mast cell granules. *J Ultrastr Res* 1968;23:153–165.
20. Ludatscher RM, Haim S, Gellei B, et al. A comparative ultrastructural study of mast cells in mastocytoma and mastocytosis. *Dermatologica* 1977;155:80–89.
21. Metcalfe DD, Kaliner M, Donlon MA. The mast cell. *Crit Rev Immunol* 1981;3:23–74.
22. Irani AA, Schechter NM, Craig SS, et al. Two types of human mast cells that have distinct neutral protease compositions. *Proc Natl Acad Sci USA* 1986;83:4464–4468.
23. Craig SS, DeBlois G, Schwartz LB. Mast cells in human keloid, small intestine, and lung by an immunoperoxidase technique using a murine monoclonal antibody against tryptase. *Am J Pathol* 1986;124: 427–435.
24. Bradding P, Feather IH, Wilson S, et al. Immunolocalization of cytokines in the nasal mucosa of normal and perinnial rhinitic subjects: the mast cell as a source of IL-4, IL-5, and IL-6 in human allergic mucosal inflammation. *J Immunol* 1993;151:3853–3865.
25. Burd PR, Thompson WC, Max EE, et al. Activated mast cells produce interleukin 13. *J Exp Med* 1995;181:1373–1380.
26. Leder L-D. Ueber die selektive fermentcytochemische Darstellung neutrophiler myeloischer Zellen und Gewebsmastzellen im Paraffinschnitt. *Klin Wochenschr* 1964;42:553.
27. Desaga JF. Der nachweis von myeloperoxidase in jungen gewebsmastzellen der ratte. *Klin Wochenschr* 1972;50:444–445.
28. Christie KN, Stoward PJ. Endogenous peroxidase in mast cells localized with a semipermeable membrane technique. *Histochem J* 1978; 10:425–433.
29. Fahimi HD. The fine structural localization of endogenous and exogenous peroxidase activity in Kupffer cells of rat liver. *J Cell Biol* 1970; 47:247–262.
30. Feller AC, Wacker HH, Moldenhauer G, et al. Monoclonal antibody Ki-B3 detects a formalin resistant antigen on normal and neoplastic B cells. *Blood* 1987;70:629–636.
31. Combs JW. Maturation of rat mast cells: an electron microscopic study. *J Cell Biol* 1966;31:563–575.
32. Desaga JF, Parwaresch RM, Mueller-Hermelink HK. Die zytochemische identifikation der mastzellvorstufen bei der ratte. *Z Zellforsch* 1971;121:292–300.
33. Lennert K, Parwaresch RM. Mast cell and mast cell neoplasia: a review. *Histopathology* 1979;3:349–365.
34. Horny HP, Parwaresch RM, Lennert K. Klinisches bild und prognose generalisierter mastozytosen. *Klin Wochenschr* 1983;61:785–793.
35. Leder L-D. Morphologie und differentialdiagnose der akuten myelogenen leukämien. *Verh Dtsch Ges Pathol* 1983;67:149–166.
36. Horny HP, Ruck M, Wehrmann M, et al. Blood findings in generalized mastocytosis: evidence of frequent simultaneous occurrence of myeloproliferative disorders [See comments]. *Br J Haematol* 1990;76: 186–193.
37. McCarthy JH, Mandel TE, Garson OM, et al. The presence of mast cells in agar cultures. *Exp Hematol* 1980;8:562–567.
38. Denburg JA, Richardson M, Telizyn S, et al. Basophil-mast cell precursors in human peripheral blood. *Blood* 1983;61:775–780.

39. Lennert K, Parwaresch RM. Zur pathologie der gewebsmastzellen. *Verh Dtsch Ges Pathol* 1978;62:546.
40. Kirshenbaum AS, Kessler SW, Goff JP, et al. Demonstration of the origin of human mast cells from CD34 + bone marrow progenitor cells. *J Immunol* 1991;146:1410–1415.
41. Foedinger M, Fritsch G, Winkler K, et al. Origin of human mast cells: development from transplanted hematopoietic stem cells after allogeneic bone marrow transplantation. *Blood* 1994;84:2954–2959.
42. Parwaresch RM, Wacker HH. Origin and kinetics of resident tissue macrophages: parabiosis studies with radio-labeled leukocytes. *Cell Tissue Kinet* 1984;17:25–39.
43. Jones TD, Mote JR. Phases of foreign protein sensitization in human beings. *N Engl J Med* 1934;210:120–123.
44. Ginsburg H. The in vitro differentiation and culture of normal mast cells from the mouse thymus. *Ann NY Acad Sci* 1963;103:20–39.
45. Dvorak HF, Dvorak AM, Simpson AM, et al. Cutaneous basophil hypersensitivity: II. A light and electron microscopic description. *J Exp Med* 1970;132:558–582.
46. Dvorak HF, Mihm MC, Dvorak AM. Morphology of delayed-type hypersensitivity reactions in man. *J Invest Dermatol* 1976;67: 391–401.
47. Kaliner MA. The mast cell: a fascinating riddle. *N Engl J Med* 1979; 301:498–499.
48. Dvorak AM, Galli SJ, Schulman ES, et al. Basophil and mast cell degranulation: ultrastructural analysis of mechanisms of mediator release. *Federal Proceedings* 1983;42:2510–2515.
49. Schwartz LB, Austen KF. Structure and function of the chemical mediators of mast cells. *Prog Allergy* 1984;34:271–321.
50. Serafin WE, Austen KF. Mediators of immediate hypersensitivity reactions. *N Engl J Med* 1987;317:30–34.
51. Yanagida M, Fukamachi H, Ohgami K, et al. Effects of T-helper 2-type cytokines, interleukin-3 (IL-3), IL-4, IL-5, and IL-6 on the survival of culrured human mast cells. *Blood* 1995;86:3705–3714.
52. Nilsson G, Butterfield JH, Nilsson K, et al. Stem cell factor is a chemotactic factor for human mast cells. *J Immunol* 1994;153: 3717–3723.
53. Columbo M, Horowitz EM, Botana LM, et al. The human recombinant c-kit receptor ligand, rhSCF, induces mediator release from human cutaneous mast cells and enhances IgE dependent mediator release from both skin mast cells and periphal blood basophils. *J Immunol* 1992;149:599–608.
54. Sezary A, Levy-Coblenz G, Chauvillon P. Dermographisme et mastocytose. *Bull Soc Franc Derm Syph* 1936;43:357–359.
55. Nagata H, Worobec AS, Oh CK, et al. Identification of a point mutation in the catalytic domain of the protooncogene c-kit in peripheral blood mononuclear cells of patients who have mastocytosis with an associated hematologic disorder. *Proc Natl Acad Sci USA* 1995;92: 10560–10564.
56. Longley BJ, Tyrrell L, Lu SZ, et al. Somatic c-kit activating mutation in urticaria pigmentosa and aggressive mastocytosis: establishment of clonality in human mast cell neoplasm. *Nat Genet* 1996;12:312–314.
57. Afonja O, Amorosi E, Takeshita K. Multilineage involvement and erythropoietin independent erythroid progenitor cells in a patient with systemic mastocytosis. *Ann Hematol* 1998;77:183–186.
58. Yarden Y, Kuang WJ, Yang-Feng, et al. Human proto-oncogene c-kit: a new cell surface receptor tyrosine kinase for an unidentfied ligand. *EMBO J* 1987;6:3341–3351.
59. Qui Fh, Ray P, Brown K, et al. Primary structure of c-kit: relationship with the CSF-1/PDGF receptor kinase family-oncogenic activation of v-kit involves deletion of extracellular domain and C terminus. *EMBO J* 1988;7:1003–1011.
60. Swolin B, Rodjer S, al-Obaidy A, et al. A follow-up study of bone marrow chromosomes and in vitro colony growth in patients with mastocytosis. *Acta Derm Venereol* 1994;74:163–167.
61. Jeanselme E, Touraine A. Urticaire pigmentaire avec hypertrophie du foie et splenomegalie, hematologie, radiotherapie. *Bull Soc Franc Derm Syph* 1919;26:98–101.
62. Asboe-Hansen G, Kaalund-Jorgensen O. Systemic mast cell disease involving skin, liver, bone-marrow, and blood associated with disseminated xanthomata. *Acta Haematol* 1956;16:273–279.
63. Efrati P, Klajman A, Spitz H. Mast cell leukemia: malignant mastocytosis with leukemia-like manifestations. *Blood* 1957;12:869–882.
64. Friedmann BI, Will JJ, Freiman DG, et al. Tissue mast cell leukemia. *Blood* 1958;13:70–78.
65. Mutter RB, Tannenbaum M, Ultman JE. Systemic mast cell disease, (Review). *Ann Intern Med* 1963;57:887–904.
66. Parwaresch MR, Lennert K. Zur differenzierung der blutbasophilen und gewebsmastzellen nach dem reifegrad ihrer granula. *Histochemie* 1969;19:262–271.
67. Horny H-P, Parwaresch RM, Lennert K. Bone marrow findings in systemic mastocytosis. *Hum Pathol* 1985;16:808–814.
68. Parwaresch RM, Horny H-P, Lennert K. Tissue mast cells in health and disease. *Pathol Res Pract* 1985;179:439–461.
69. Travis WD, Li C-Y, Bergstralh EJ, et al. Systemic mast cell disease: analysis of 58 cases and literature review. *Medicine* 1988;67:345–368.
70. Travis WD, Li C-Y, Yam LT, et al. Significance of systemic mast cell disease with associated hematologic disorders. *Cancer* 1988;62: 965–972.
71. Unna PG. *The histopathology of the skin.* New York: Macmillan, 1896.
72. Selye R. *The mast cells.* Boston: Butterworths, 1965.
73. Charrette EE, Mariano AV, Laforet EG. Solitary mast cell "tumor" of lung, its place in the spectrum of mast cell disease. *Arch Intern Med* 1966;118:358–362.
74. Sherwin RP, Kern WH, Jones JC. Solitary mast cell granuloma (histiocytoma) of the lung: a histologic, tissue culture and time-lapse cinematographic. *Cancer* 1965;18:634–641.
75. Kudo H, Morinaga S, Shimosato Y, et al. Solitary mast cell tumor of the lung. *Cancer* 1988;61:2089–2094.
76. Sangster A. An anomalous mottled rash accompanied by pruritis, factitious urticaria and pigmentation, "Urticaria pigmentosa?" *Trans Clin Soc Lond* 1878;11:161–163.
77. Nettleship E, Tay W. Rare forms of urticaria. *Br Med J* 1869;2: 323–329.
78. Klaus SN, Winkelmann RK. The clinical spectrum of urticaria pigmentosa. *Mayo Clin Proc* 1965;40:923–931.
79. Sagher F, Even-Paz Z. *Mastocytosis and the mast cell.* Basel: S Karger, 1967.
80. Robinson HM, Kile RL, Hitch JM, et al. Bullous urticaria pigmentosa. *Arch Dermatol* 1962;85:346–357.
81. Fernex M. *The mast-cell system: its relationship to atherosclerosis, fibrosis and eosinophils.* Baltimore: Williams & Wilkins, 1968.
82. Griffiths WAD, Daneshbod K. Pseudoxanthomatous mastocytosis. *Br J Dermatol* 1975;93:91–95.
83. McDermott WV, Topol BM. Systemic mastocytosis with extensive large cutaneous mastocytomas: surgical management. *J Surg Oncol* 1985;30:221–225.
84. Offidani A, Cellini A, Simonetti O, et al. Urticaria pigmentosa in monozygotic twins [Letter]. *Arch Dermatol* 1994;130:935–936.
85. Garriga MM, Friedman MM, Metcalfe DD. A survey of the number and distribution of mast cells in the skin of patients with mast cell disorders. *J Allergy Clin Immunol* 1988;82:425–432.
86. Krüger PG, Nyfors A. Phagocytosis by mast cells in urticaria pigmentosa. *Acta Derm Venerol (Stockh)* 1984;64:373–377.
87. Braverman DZ, Dollberg L, Shiner M. Clinical histological, and electron microscopic study of mast cell disease of the small bowel. *Am J Gastroenterol* 1985;80:30–37.
88. Kobayashi T, Mitgard K, Asboe-Hansen G. Ultrastructure of human mast-cell granules. *J Ultrastruct Res* 1968;23:153–165.
89. Schmidt U, Leder L-D. Ultrastrukturelle Befunde an Gewebsmastzellen bei Urticaria pigmentosa. *Z Hautkr* 1988;63:651–657.
90. Ende N, Cherniss NI. Splenic mastocytosis. *Blood* 1958;12:631–641.
91. Horny H P, Parwaresch MR, Kaiserling E, et al. Mast cell sarcoma of the larynx. *J Clin Pathol* 1986;39:596–602.
92. Touraine A, Solente G, Renault P. Urticaire pigmentaire avec reaction splenique et myelemique. *Bull Soc Franc Derm Syph* 1933;40: 1691–1694.
93. Ellis JM. Urticaria pigmentosa: a report of a case with autopsy. *Arch Pathol* 1949;48:426–435.
94. Sagher F, Cohen C, Schorr S. Concomitant bone changes in urticaria pigmentosa. *J Invest Dermatol* 1952;18:425–432.
95. Stark E, Van Buskirk FW, Daly JF. Radiologic and pathologic bone changes associated with urticaria pigmentosa. *Arch Pathol* 1956;62: 143–148.
96. Meggs WJ, Frieri M, Costello R, et al. Oligoclonal immunoglobulins in mastocytosis. *Ann Intern Med* 1985;103:894–895.
97. Kubic VL, Brunning RD. Immunohistochemical evaluation of neo-

plasms in bone marrow biopsies using monoclonal antibodies reactive in paraffin-embedded tissue. *Mod Pathol* 1989;2:618–629.
98. Granerus G, Wass U. Urinary excretion of histamine, methylhistamine (1-MeHi) and methylimidazoleacetic acid (melmAA) in mastocytosis: comparison of new HPLC methods with other present methods. *Agents Actions* 1984;14:341–345.
99. Frieri M, Alling DW, Metcalfe DD. Comparison of the therapeutic efficacy of cromolyn sodium with that of combined chlorpheniramine and cimetidine in systemic mastocytosis, results of a double-blind clinical trial. *Am J Med* 1985;78:9–14.
100. Roberts LJ, Fields JP, Oates JA. Mastocytosis without urticaria pigmentosa: a frequently unrecognized cause of recurrent syncope. *Trans Assoc Am Physicians* 1982;95:36–41.
101. Olafsson JH. Cutaneous and systemic mastocytosis in adults. A clinical, histopathological and immunological evaluation in relation to histamine metabolism. *Acta Dermatovenereologic Supplementum* 1985; 115:1–43.
102. Dodd NJ, Bond MG. Fatal anaphylaxis in systemic mastocytosis. *J Clin Pathol* 1979;32:31–34.
103. Demis DJ, Walton MD, Higdon RS. Histaminuria in urticaria pigmentosa. *Arch Dermatol* 1961;83:127–138.
104. Ridell B, Olafsson JH, Roupe G, et al. The bone marrow in urticaria pigmentosa and systemic mastocytosis. *Arch Dermatol* 1986;122: 422–427.
105. Kootte AMM, Haak A, Roberts LJ. The flush syndrome: an expression of systemic mastocytosis with increased prostaglandin D2 production. *Neth J Med* 1983;26:18–20.
106. Brunning RD, McKenna RW, Rosai J, et al. Systemic mastocytosis: extracutaneous manifestations. *Am J Surg Pathol* 1983;7:425–438.
107. Sostre S, Handler HL. Bony lesions in systemic mastocytosis. Scintigraphic evaluation. *Arch Dermatol* 1977;113:1245–1247.
108. Norris HT, Zamcheck N, Gottleib LS. The presence and distribution of mast cells in the human gastrointestinal tract at autopsy. *Gastroenterology* 1963;44:448–455.
109. Horny H-P, Kaiserling E, Campbell M, et al. Liver findings in generalized mastocytosis: a clinico-pathologic study. *Cancer* 1989;63: 532–538.
110. Travis WD, Li C-Y. Pathology of the lymph node and spleen in systemic mastocytosis. *Mod Pathol* 1988;1:4–14.
111. Travis WD, Li C-Y, Hoagland HC, et al. Mast cell leukemia: report of a case and review of the literature. *Mayo Clin Proc* 1986;61:957–966.
112. Escribano L, Orfao A, Villarrubia J, et al. Sequential immunophenotypic analysis of mast cells in a case of systemic mast cell disease evolving to a mast cell leukemia. *Cytometry* 1997;30:98–102.
113. Vogelstein B, Fearon ER, Hamilton SR, et al. Use of restriction length polymorphism to determine the clonal origin of human tumors. *Science* 1985;227:642–645.
114. Kreipe H, Radzun HJ, Bartels H, et al. Klonalitaet und stammzelldefekt in der molekularen pathologie chronischer myeloproliferativer erkrankungen. *Verh Dtsch Ges Pathol* 1990;74:1–15.
115. Poppel MH, Gruber WF, Silber R, et al. The roentgen manifestations of urticaria pigmentosa (mastocytosis). *Am J Roentgenol* 1959;82: 239–248.
116. Gagon JH, Katz F, Kadri AM, et al. Mastocytosis: unusual manifestations: clinical and radiologic changes. *JCMA* 1965;112:1329–1331.
117. Rafii M, Firooznia H, Golimbu C, et al. Pathologic fracture in systemic mastocytosis: radiographic spectrum and review of the literature. *Clin Orthop* 1983;180:260–267.
118. Ensslen RD, Jackson FI, Reid AM. Bone and gallium scans in mastocytosis: correlation with count rates, radiography, and microscopy. *J Nucl Med* 1983;24:586–588.
119. Schweitzer ME, Irwin GAI, Facr CM. Case report 561. *Skeletal Radiol* 1989;1:411–413.
120. Arrington ER, Eisenberg B, Hartshorne F, et al. Nuclear medicine imaging of systemic mastocytosis. *J Nucl Med* 1989;30:2046–2048.
121. Chen CC, Andrich MP, Mican JM, et al. A retrospective analysis of bone scan abnormalities in mastocytosis: correlation with disease category and prognosis. *J Nucl Med* 1994;35:1471–1475.
122. Delsignore JL, Dvoretsky PM, Hicks DG, et al. Mastocytosis presenting as a skeletal disorder. *Iowa Orthop J* 1996;16:126–134.
123. Schwarting R, Gerdes J, Stein H. Ber-H2: a new monoclonal antibody of the Ki-1 family for the detection of Hodgkin's disease in formaldehyde-fixed tissue sections. In: McMichael AJ, Beverley PCL, Cobbold S, et al., eds. *Leucocyte typing III.* Oxford: University Press, 1987.
124. Brenner MB, McLean J, Scheft H, et al. Characterization and expression of the human alpha/beta T-cell receptor by using a frame work monoclonal antibody. *J Immunol* 1987;138:1502–1509.
125. Mason DY, Cordell J, Brown M, et al. Detection of T cells in paraffin wax embedded tissue using antibodies against a peptide sequence from the CD3 antigen. *J Clin Pathol* 1989;42:1194–1200.
126. Tabrizchi H, Hansmann M-L, Parwaresch RM, et al. Distribution pattern of follicular dendritic cells in low grade B-cell lymphomas of the gastrointestinal tract: immunostained by Ki-FDC1p. A new paraffin-resistant monoclonal antibody. *Mod Pathol* 1990;3:470–478.
127. Zankowich R, Parwaresch RM, Lennert K. Blood findings in lymphogranulomatosis X. *Blut* 1984;48:99–107.
128. Gartner LI, Tice AA. Histamine and related compounds in urticaria pigmentosa: analysis of tissues having mast cell infiltration. *Pediatrics* 1958;21:805–806.
129. Rywlin AM, Hoffman EP, Ortega RS. Eosinophilic fibrohistiocytic lesion of bone marrow: at distinctive new morphologic finding probably related to drug hypersensitivity. *Blood* 1972;40:464–472.
130. Radzun HJ, Hansmann ML, Heidebrecht HJ, et al. Detection of a monocyte/macrophage differentiation antigen in routinely processed paraffin-embedded tissues by monoclonal antibody Ki-M1p. *Lab Invest* 1991;65:306–315.
131. Hansmann M-L, Wacker HH, Gralla J, et al. Ki-B5: a monoclonal antibody to normal and neoplastic human B cells in routine paraffin sections. *Blood* 1991;77:809–817.
132. Worobec AS, Semere T, Nagata H, et al. Clinical correlates of the presence of the Asp816Val c-kit mutation in the peripheral blood mononuclear cells of patients with mastocytosis. *Cancer* 1998;83: 2120–2129.
133. Longley BJ, Metcalfe DD, Tharp M, et al. Activating and dominant inactivating c-Kit catalytic domain mutations in distinct clinical forms of human mastocytosis. *Proc Natl Acad Sci USA* 1999;96:1609–1614.
134. Worobec AS, Akin C, Scott LM, et al. Cytogenetic abnormalities and their lack of relationship to the Asp816Val c-kit mutation in the pathogenesis of mastocytosis. *J Allergy Clin Immunol* 1998;102 (3): 523–524.
135. Nagata H, Worobec AS, Semere T, et al. Elevated expression of the proto-oncogene c-kit in patients with mastocytosis. *Leukemia* 1998; 12:175–181.
136. Escribano L, Orfao A, Diaz-Agustin B, et al. Indolent systemic mast cell disease in adults: immunophenotypic characterization of bone marrow mast cells and its diagnostic implications. *Blood* 1998;91: 2731–2736.

CHAPTER 53

Histopathologic Manifestations of Lymphoproliferative and Myeloproliferative Disorders Involving the Spleen

Richard S. Neiman and Attilio Orazi

Although the immunologic and blood filtration functions of the spleen define its importance in the hematopoietic system, it is not as well studied as the bone marrow or lymph nodes. This is related to the fact that the spleen is not as accessible as the other organs of the hematopoietic system. Biopsy can be performed easily on bone marrow and lymph nodes during the course of a given disease process. Splenectomy, however, requires a major surgical procedure and entails risks to the patient, not only during but also subsequent to it. It is not surprising that neoplastic disorders that involve the spleen are not as well characterized as those that involve the lymph nodes and bone marrow.

Because the spleen is by nature a bloody organ, attention to careful processing assumes greater importance than in many other organs. The procedure that we use to evaluate splenectomy specimens provides us with the maximum amount of information. First, a spleen should be submitted in the fresh state. Fixation in the operating room is never effective and usually results in part of the specimen being overfixed and the remainder of the organ being autolyzed. Multiple touch imprints should be made at the time that the spleen reaches the laboratory, and Romanowsky stains should be performed immediately on a minimum of two of these touch imprints. In addition, material should be obtained for flow cytometry and for immunophenotyping, and a piece should be banked for molecular genetic studies. The role of the frozen section in the diagnosis of splenic neoplasms is controversial. We believe that the procedure is of limited value. Obtaining adequate specimens is technically difficult, the cytologic detail obtained is usually inadequate to make a specific diagnosis, and there is usually little, if any, need to make a quick diagnosis in patients who will not be treated immediately after surgery.

Our preference for fixative is B5 or Zenker's, although any fixative appropriately used is satisfactory. There is a greater chance of bad fixation because of underfixation than because of the choice of fixative. Blocks should be cut a maximum of 3 mm in thickness, and the tissue blocks should never be more than 1 cm^2. Specimens should be fixed at least overnight. Penetration of fixatives in spleens is notoriously slow. The majority of disorders that involve the spleen do not require immediate diagnosis; therefore, careful attention to fixation is appropriate.

The most appropriate stain for the examination of the spleen is the periodic acid–Schiff stain. Because eosin stains red cells, hematoxylin and eosin stains frequently do not provide the best opportunity to examine the anatomy of the red pulp. The Schiff reagent does not stain red cells but does stain the ring fibers of the spleen, which can demarcate beautifully the cordal–sinusoidal relationships of the red pulp.

THE NORMAL SPLEEN

Neoplastic disorders that involve the spleen are understood best in light of the structure and function of that organ (see Chapter 6). The spleen is composed of two anatomically and functionally distinct regions. The lymphoid tissue of the spleen, called the *white pulp*, can be seen grossly as uniformly distributed white nodules. The white pulp of the spleen is associated intimately with the splenic arterial circulation. The central arteries, which arise from trabecular arter-

R. S. Neiman: Department of Pathology and Laboratory Medicine/Hematopathology, Riley Hospital for Children, Indianapolis, Indiana 46202-5200

A. Orazi: Division of Hematopathology, Columbia-Presbyterian Medical Center, Columbia University, New York, New York 10032 ies within the fibrous trabeculae, are surrounded by cylindric cuffs of lymphocytes, which are admixtures of B and T cells (1–4). Periodically, lymphoid follicles occur as outgrowths of the lymphatic sheath (5,6). The morphology of the splenic white pulp varies with the age of the patient and with the presence of antigenic stimulation. Inactive or hypoplastic white pulp, in which no germinal centers are seen, is characteristic of infancy, senescence, and the immunologically unstimulated adult spleen. In the immunologically activated state, three distinct zones are identifiable within the lymphoid follicle (7–9): The germinal center itself, composed of B lymphocytes in a meshwork of follicular dendritic cells, is surrounded by a darker rim of small lymphocytes called the *mantle zone*, which also is composed predominantly of B cells. The mantle zone is encased in the outer marginal zone, at the interface between white and red pulp. The marginal zone, which is an extension of the periarterial lymphoid sheath (PALS) and is composed of both B and T cells (4), is the site of antigen trapping and processing. The B cells, which represent the majority of the marginal zone cells, are those primarily responsible for the elaboration of opsonizing antibody (10).

The red pulp of the spleen is composed of vascular sinuses and the cords of Billroth (11–13). The structure of the splenic sinuses provides the mechanism for filtration of the peripheral blood by the spleen. The sinus-lining cells have long cytoplasmic processes that overlap. Because tight junctions are not present, there is the potential for spaces between these cells (2,14). Circulating blood cells percolate through the cords of Billroth before entering the splenic sinuses and returning to the systemic circulation. The ability of circulating blood cells to enter the venous sinuses depends on their deformability, because these cells must squeeze through the potential spaces between the sinus lining cells. Cells without the ability to deform are not able to enter the sinuses and are destroyed in the acidotic, hypoxic environment of the cords of Billroth (2,15).

The immunoarchitecture of the spleen has been studied with immunohistologic techniques, and its immunotopography has been mapped (1,4,16–20). The white pulp of the spleen is largely compartmentalized into B- and T-cell zones, although there is some intermingling, particularly in the marginal zones and the PALS (1,20,21). A few CD4-positive ($CD4^+$) helper or inducer T cells are scattered within the germinal centers and in the mantle zones. There is also some spillover of T cells into the red pulp, although the T cells in the red pulp are predominantly $CD8^+$ suppressor or cytotoxic cells (17), which rarely are found in the PALS and are virtually absent in the germinal centers. The majority of B cells is found in the germinal centers and mantle zones, although they may account for a substantial percentage of marginal zone lymphocytes (4,16,17). The distribution of immunoglobulin-containing B cells are similar to that seen in the lymph nodes. The majority of B cells in the germinal centers contain no surface or cytoplasmic immunoglobulin (16). The mantle and marginal zone B cells bear surface immunoglobulin, which is predominantly IgM and IgD. IgG expression is lacking in these areas and is limited to scattered cells in the red pulp. Only rare IgA-containing cells are found. Lymphocytes that bear surface immunoglobulin light chains also are found predominantly in the mantle and marginal zones, with a κ-to-λ ratio of 2:1 to 3:1 (4,16). The red pulp contains numerous cells of monocyte-macrophage lineage, only a few of which are found in the white pulp. Natural killer cells are scattered throughout the red pulp and within germinal centers.

Disorders of splenic lymphoid tissue usually produce a nodular pattern in the spleen, reflecting the nodular architecture of its normal lymphoid structure. In contrast, disorders that affect the red pulp of the spleen result in homogeneous enlargement of the organ because of the expansion of the red pulp and the obliteration of the white pulp. Hematologic neoplasms that affect the white pulp of the spleen are largely the same as those that affect other lymphoid organs. These disorders include Hodgkin's disease, non-Hodgkin's lymphomas, and a group of diseases associated with aberrant immunoglobulin production that may be linked loosely under the term *dysproteinemias* (Table 53.1). Neoplastic proliferations that involve the red pulp include leukemias, myeloproliferative disorders and a variety of nonhematopoi-

TABLE 53.1. *Lymphoproliferative disorders involving the spleen*

White pulp
Hodgkin's disease
Malignant lymphomas
B-cell tumors
Small lymphocytic (including immunocytoma)[a]
Mantle cell[a]
Marginal zone cell[a]
Predominantly small cleaved cell[a]
Burkitt's-like[a]
T-cell tumors
Mycosis fungoides[a]
Lymphoblastic[a]
Dysproteinemias
Systemic amyloidosis[a]
Heavy chain diseases[a]
Waldenstrom's macroglobulinemia
Red pulp
Malignant lymphomas
Peripheral T-cell[b]
Hepatosplenic T-cell lymphoma
Hepatosplenic B-cell lymphoma
Multiple myeloma
Acute lymphoblastic leukemia
Chronic lymphoid leukemia
Chronic lymphocytic leukemia
Prolymphocytic leukemia
Hairy cell leukemia
Large granular lymphocytic leukemia
Hodgkin's disease (all subtypes)
Leukemias

[a] Also may have variable degree of red pulp involvement.
[b] Also may have variable degree of white pulp involvement.

TABLE 53.2. *Myeloid proliferations involving the spleen*

Leukemias
Acute myeloid (M_0–M_7)
Chronic myeloid
Chronic myelomonocytic
Systemic mastocytosis
Myeloproliferative disorders
Essential thrombocythemia
Polycythemia vera
Chronic idiopathic myelofibrosis

etic tumors (Table 53.2). Some lymphomas may involve the splenic red pulp preferentially. These include some T-cell lymphomas formerly termed *malignant histiocytosis* and hepatosplenic T-cell lymphomas. Diseases that cause enlargement of the red pulp frequently lead to hypersplenism. Because infiltrative processes cause widening of the cords of Billroth and a proliferation of cordal macrophages, circulating blood cells have a prolonged exposure to the hostile environment of the red pulp, resulting in an increased opportunity for phagocytosis by cordal macrophages. This can lead to peripheral cytopenias. Occasionally, however, infiltrative processes result in functional asplenia, although the spleen may be normal in size or even enlarged (2). The resultant hyposplenism is associated with the presence of Howell-Jolly bodies in circulating erythrocytes, as well as target cells and acanthocytes, reflecting the lack of the red pulp filtration function (22,23). There also may be an immunologic deficit.

HODGKIN'S DISEASE

Although the spleen is the most common extranodal organ involved by Hodgkin's disease (24,25), primary Hodgkin's disease of the spleen is extremely rare (26–30). All histologic subtypes of Hodgkin's disease may involve the spleen, although nodular sclerosis and mixed cellularity are the most common (24). Involvement by lymphocyte predominance Hodgkin's disease is rare (31). Lymphocyte depletion Hodgkin's disease, an uncommon subtype difficult to distinguish from non-Hodgkin's lymphomas of large cell type, characteristically presents with subdiaphragmatic disease and usually involves the spleen (32).

Because of the lack of correlation between splenic size and involvement with Hodgkin's disease, accurate assessment of splenic involvement formerly required splenectomy (33–40). There are several risks associated with splenectomy. The procedure has been associated with an increased risk for the development of secondary acute leukemia in patients treated with chemotherapy, especially alkylating agents (41,42). A further risk is the possibility of overwhelming postsplenectomy sepsis, although preoperative pneumococcal vaccination and improved surgical techniques during the past decade have reduced the incidence of this complication greatly (43). The organisms most commonly involved in postsplenectomy infections are the encapsulated bacteria, particularly *Streptococcus pneumoniae* and *Haemophilus influenzae*, which are the organisms associated with fulminant infections in most asplenic states. To avoid complications related to splenectomy, computed tomographic scans and nuclear magnetic resonance techniques have been used to detect Hodgkin's disease in the spleen, and the frequency of staging laparotomy has decreased. In spite of arguments against its use, surgical staging still is recommended for early-stage patients, for whom the results influence the choice of treatment (44,45). In such patients, accurate assessment of splenic involvement by Hodgkin's disease requires splenectomy, because clinical and radiologic evaluation of the spleen still often is inaccurate (37,38). The documentation of splenic involvement has therapeutic and prognostic implications, although these implications appear less critical in light of the dramatic long-term remissions obtained with newer regimens of combination chemotherapy (33,34). Because involvement of the liver and bone marrow rarely are found in the absence of splenic involvement, documentation of Hodgkin's disease in the spleen suggests that other organs related to unfavorable prognosis are at risk (24).

Hodgkin's disease produces either miliary nodules or, more frequently, solitary or multiple tumor masses in the spleen (2,46) (Fig. 53.1). Splenic involvement generally is detectable grossly but may be subtle (Fig. 53.2). Foci of involvement may be only a few millimeters in size (47,48). We have seen numerous patients in whom single foci of histologically confirmed disease were no more than 2 or 3 mm in diameter. For this reason, the gross examination of the spleen must be meticulous in patients who have Hodgkin's disease, so that such small foci of involvement are not missed. The early lesions of Hodgkin's disease in the spleen are found microscopically in the PALS or the marginal zones (2,49) (Fig. 53.3). As the disease progresses, the nodules expand to efface the lymphoid follicles and also may produce involvement of the red pulp.

Sarcoidal granulomas also may be found in the spleens of patients who have Hodgkin's disease, in addition to various other disorders associated with impaired T-cell function (50–55). Several studies have suggested that these granulomas occur more frequently in spleens uninvolved by Hodgkin's disease than in those involved by Hodgkin's disease (52,53). Grossly, they may be so large as to mimic involvement by Hodgkin's disease. Microscopically, the granulomas are composed of clusters of epithelioid histiocytes that occur in the white pulp in close association with the arterial circulation (Fig. 53.4). The finding of granulomas in the spleen of a patient who has Hodgkin's disease in the absence of involvement by the tumor does not change the clinical stage or treatment regimen, although Sacks and colleagues (55) suggested that patients who have splenic sarcoidal granulomas may have a better prognosis. These granulomas are not related to prior lymphangiography, and their origin is unknown (46).

The criteria for the diagnosis of Hodgkin's disease in the spleen are the same as those as for other nonnodal sites

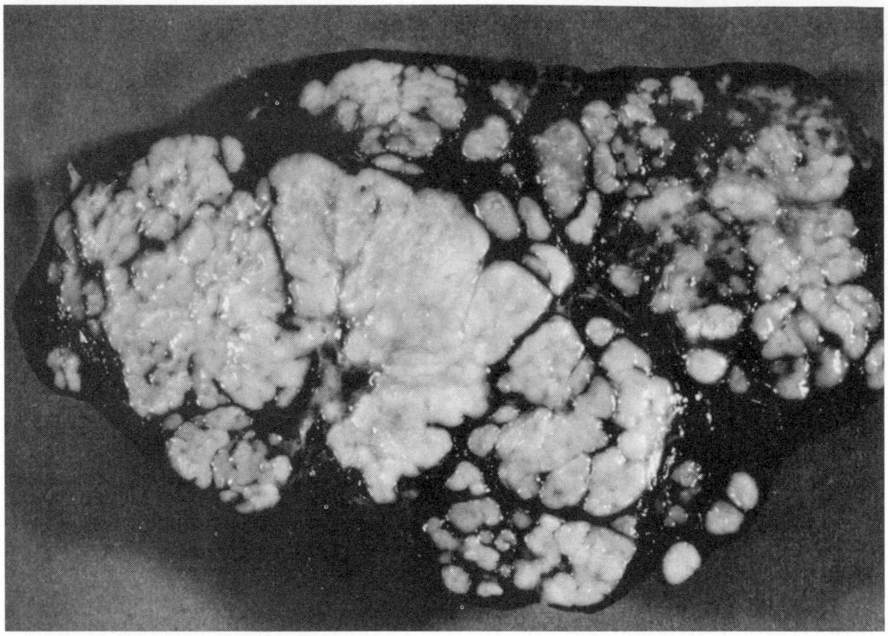

FIG. 53.1. Multiple tumor masses in a spleen involved by Hodgkin's disease. This pattern is similar to that seen in malignant lymphomas of large cell type and metastatic carcinoma.

(56,57). In a patient who has had a previous nodal diagnosis, the documentation of Hodgkin's disease in the spleen can be made if the general features of one of the histologic subtypes are found in association with one of the variants of the Reed-Sternberg cell (56,57). A classic Reed-Sternberg cell is not necessary for the diagnosis in this setting. If the patient does not have a previous nodal diagnosis, however, diagnostic Reed-Sternberg cells must be found. The subclassification of Hodgkin's disease in the spleen is sometimes difficult and is unnecessary in a patient with a previous nodal diagnosis (48). In some patients the identification of characteristic Reed-Sternberg variants such as lymphocytic and histiocytic or lacunar cells allows for the distinction of histologic subtypes in the spleen. In occasional patients, particularly those for whom the histologic preparations are suboptimal, immunohistochemical studies can be helpful in confirming the diagnosis of Hodgkin's disease by showing in cytologically atypical cells a phenotype appropriate for Reed-Sternberg cells. In classic Hodgkin's disease (nodular sclerosis, mixed cellularity), Reed-Sternberg cells usually express the myelomonocytic antigen CD15 (Leu-M1) and lymphoid activation antigen CD30 (Ki-1, Ber-H2), and do

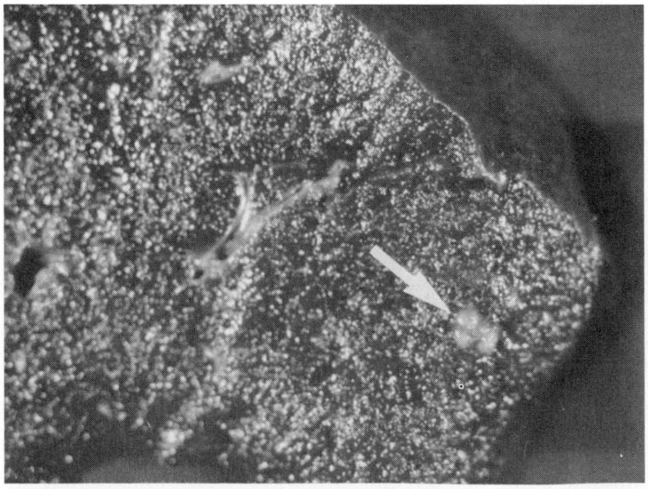

FIG. 53.2. Single focus of Hodgkin's disease (*arrow*) in an otherwise unremarkable spleen. The possibility of such subtle involvement necessitates careful gross examination of splenectomy specimens performed for the staging of Hodgkin's disease.

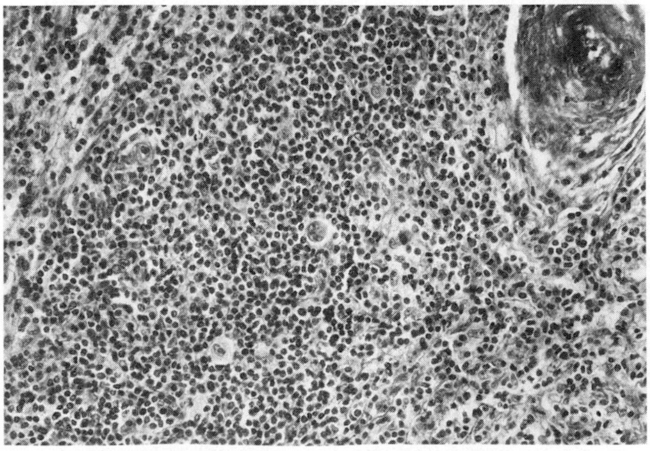

FIG. 53.3. Early involvement of the spleen in Hodgkin's disease. The focus of tumor is located in the periarterial lymphoid sheath (periodic acid–Schiff stain, original magnification: 250× magnification).

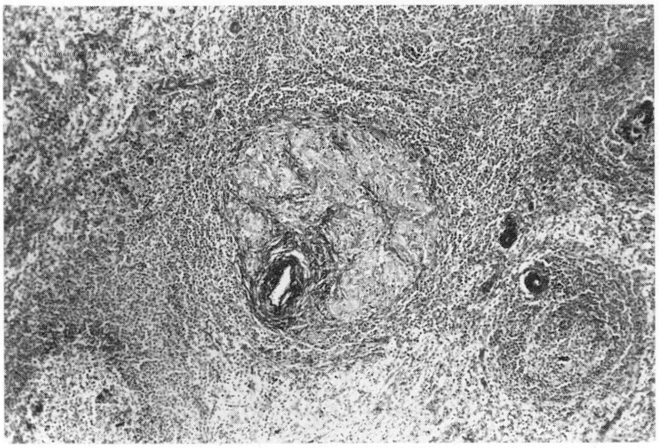

FIG. 53.4. Sarcoidal-type granuloma in the spleen of a patient with Hodgkin's disease showing the association with the arterial circulation (periodic acid–Schiff stain, original magnification: 200× magnification).

not express CD45 (leucocyte common antigen) (58–64). A second major paraffin-associated phenotype commonly is observed in nodular lymphocyte predominance Hodgkin's disease: the coexpression of a B-cell marker such as CD20 (L26) with CD45, and absence of CD15 expression (65). Reed-Sternberg cells in classic Hodgkin's disease, however, may express CD20 in a subset of patients (66–68) and may not express CD15 (68).

Although the distinction between the nodular sclerosis and mixed cellularity subtypes of Hodgkin's disease occasionally is impossible, the unique morphologic and immunologic characteristics of nodular lymphocyte predominance Hodgkin's disease allow its distinction from the classic subtypes, at least in a proportion of patients (70,71). The presence of lymphocytic and histiocytic cells that are CD45RB-negative ($CD45^-$), $CD20^-CD15^-$ in a background of a nodular proliferation of small lymphocytes and epithelioid histiocytes is uniquely characteristic of lymphocyte predominance Hodgkin's disease and is largely preserved in the rare occurrence in extranodal sites, including the spleen (70). Early involvement in lymphocyte predominance Hodgkin's disease may be difficult to recognize because of the scarcity of characteristic lymphocytic and histiocytic cells.

NON-HODGKIN'S LYMPHOMAS

Malignant lymphoma may involve the spleen in any of three clinical settings. In the first and rarest setting, termed *primary splenic lymphoma*, the tumor is confined to the spleen or splenic hilar lymph nodes, without evidence of involvement of other sites. In the second and most common setting, the organ is involved as part of generalized disease. In the third setting, patients present with prominent or predominant splenomegaly and often distinctive clinicopathologic features.

Primary Splenic Lymphoma

Primary splenic lymphoma is rare, accounting for less than 1% of all lymphomas. Because of the differences in diagnostic criteria, it is difficult to define the clinical and pathologic features of this entity. By reviewing the literature, Warnke and colleagues (72) were able to identify 47 cases of primary splenic lymphoma fulfilling the most stringent diagnostic criteria (i.e., tumor confined to the spleen and splenic hilar lymph nodes) (73–85). The patients all were adults; a slight male preponderance was noted. The most common presenting symptoms included leftsided abdominal pain and systemic symptoms such as fever, malaise, and weight loss. Two patients were HIV-positive (72,77). The gross findings and the histologic characteristics were similar to those observed in spleens secondarily involved by malignant lymphoma. The 47 cases showed the following distribution of histologic types: large cell, 30; small cell (small lymphocytic, lymphoplasmacytoid, or mantle cell type), 15; mixed cell lymphomas of follicle center cell type, 1; and small noncleaved cell, 1. A B-cell origin was found in most cases (72). A case of primary splenic $CD30^+$ anaplastic large cell lymphoma has been described in an HIV-positive patient (73). Of the 17 splenic lymphomas reported by Falk and Stutte (86) (which included patients with minimal extrasplenic involvement), three showed T-cell lineage.

The course of primary splenic lymphoma is hard to predict because of its rarity and the disparate histologic types included. The overall survival rate is approximately 50% irrespective of the histologic type, although the different therapeutic regimens (chemotherapy, radiotherapy, or both) employed and the limited number of patients treated prevent any conclusive statement in this regard (73–85).

Secondary Splenic Involvement by Lymphoma

Non-Hodgkin's lymphomas of different types involve the spleen with variable frequency. Splenic involvement is particularly frequent in low-grade lymphomas. This is probably a result of the fact that many high-grade lymphomas are localized at the time of diagnosis (87). Liver involvement by lymphoma is rare in the absence of splenic disease (19). Clinical assessment of the likelihood of splenic involvement by malignant lymphomas may be difficult. The weights of involved spleens vary widely (88). Although tumor involvement usually results in palpable splenomegaly, Goffinet and coworkers (89) found that approximately one third of nonpalpable spleens were involved by lymphoma at staging laparotomy.

B-Cell Lymphomas

The morphology of the spleen involved by malignant lymphomas of B-cell lineage has been well characterized (2,90). The B-cell lymphomas involve the spleen in one of several patterns, either with uniform expansion of all the white pulp

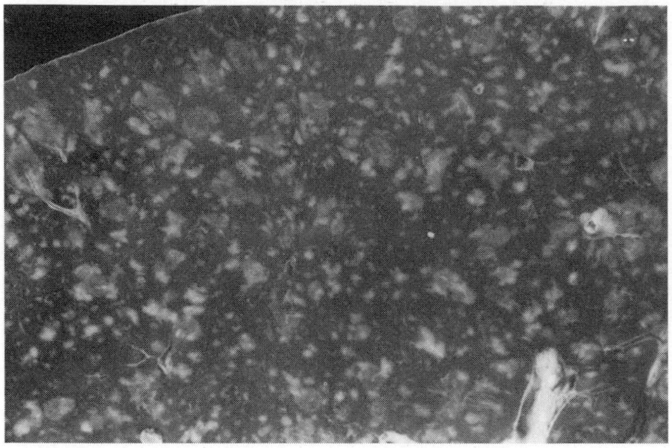

FIG. 53.5. Cut section of the spleen showing involvement by small cleaved cell lymphoma. A miliary pattern results from expansion of all the Malpighian corpuscles.

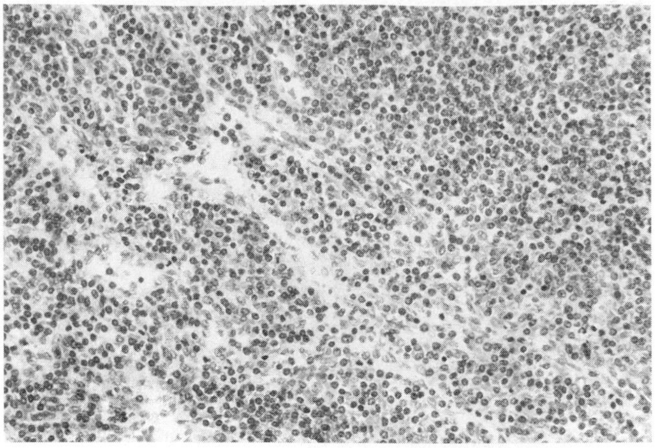

FIG. 53.7. Malignant lymphoma, small lymphocytic type. The red pulp is infiltrated to a degree that obscures the demarcation with the white pulp, which is located in the upper righthand portion of the image (hematoxylin and eosin stain, original magnification: 150× magnification).

nodules, as seen in small lymphocytic lymphoma, mantle cell lymphoma, and small cleaved cell or mixed small and large cell follicular lymphoma (Fig. 53.5); or with the formation of single or multiple tumor masses, as seen in large cell lymphoma (2,90) (Fig. 53.6). Because of the nodular architecture of the lymphoid tissue of the spleen, all types of B-cell lymphoma that involve the spleen may produce nodules. Therefore, the histologic pattern of a lymphoma, either follicular or diffuse, cannot be discerned from the pattern of splenic involvement but requires the examination of an involved lymph node (2,90). Prediction of splenic involvement on clinical grounds is difficult, because the weights of involved spleens vary widely (88). Follicular lymphomas have a higher incidence of splenic involvement at presentation than diffuse large B-cell lymphomas, probably because large cell lymphomas often are localized at the time of diagnosis (91).

The morphology of small lymphocytic lymphoma in the spleen is indistinguishable from that of B-cell chronic lymphocytic leukemia (CLL) (92) (Fig 53.7). Because the majority of patients present with stage IV disease, splenic involvement is common, and prominent splenomegaly may be the presenting feature of this disorder (93–96). Early in the course of the disease, small lymphocytic lymphoma may produce grossly visible nodules in a miliary pattern because of expansion of all the white pulp areas (2,97). As the disease progresses, red pulp involvement becomes prominent, often resulting in obliteration of the white pulp and producing a diffuse pattern of involvement. This pattern rarely is seen with other subtypes of B-cell lymphoma. Early splenic involvement by small lymphocytic lymphoma may be difficult to detect because the white pulp nodules resemble those of the immunologically unstimulated spleen (2,98). The presence of scattered prolymphocytes and infiltration of the red pulp aid, however, in the diagnosis of malignancy. In some patients, the diagnosis rests on examination of splenic hilar lymph nodes or on immunologic confirmation.

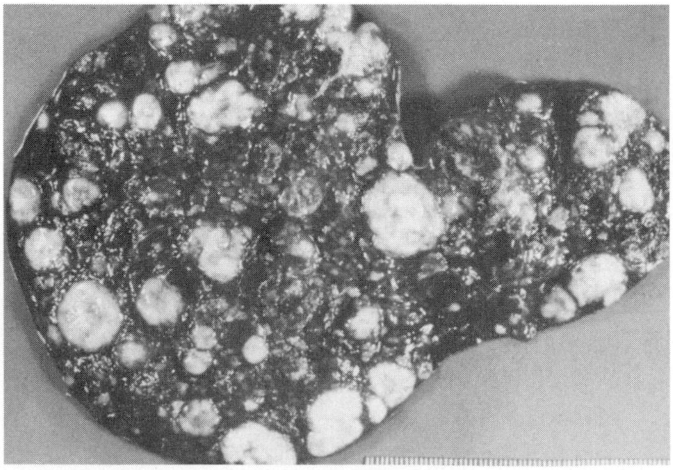

FIG. 53.6. Involvement of the spleen by malignant lymphomas of large cell type typically produce tumor masses.

Both small lymphocytic lymphoma and CLL typically show low-density expression of surface immunoglobulins. The heavy chain is most commonly μ alone in small lymphocytic lymphoma but μ plus δ in CLL. In addition, both express a variety of pan–B cell markers as well as CD5, CD43, and CD23 and do not express CD10 (99,100). Loss of CD5 expression has been reported in patients with small lymphocytic lymphoma with extranodal presentation (101) (see Chapters 21 and 40).

Some cases of small lymphocytic lymphoma show evidence of plasmacytoid differentiation, as evidenced by plasmacytoid cells and lymphocytes with intranuclear or cytoplasmic inclusions (Dutcher bodies, Russell bodies, or Mott cells) (Fig. 53.8). Tumors with these features have been termed *lymphoplasmacytic lymphoma* or *immunocytoma* (102) (Fig. 53.8). Some patients with lymphoplasmacytic

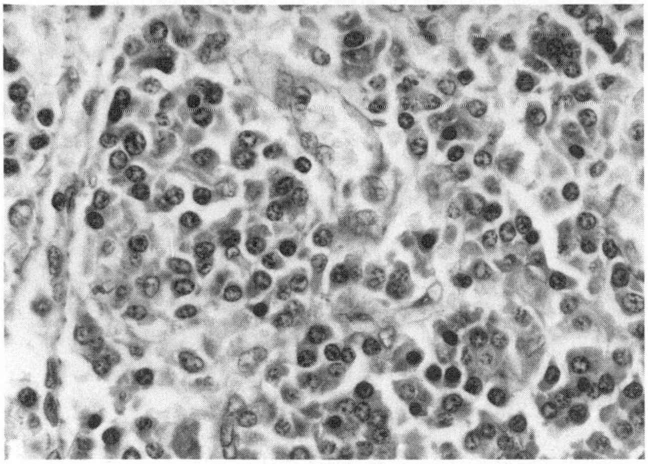

FIG. 53.8. Splenic immunocytoma. Plasma cells and plasmacytoid lymphocytes infiltrate the red pulp (hematoxylin and eosin stain, original magnification: 400× magnification).

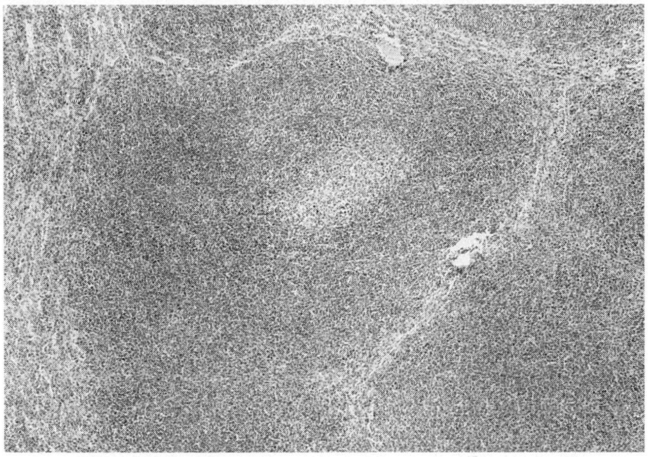

FIG. 53.9. Mantle cell lymphoma. Cells of the mantle zone proliferate in widened masses around secondary germinal centers (hematoxylin and eosin stain, original magnification: 100× magnification).

lymphoma present with prominent splenomegaly, minimal lymphadenopathy, and abnormal lymphocytes in the peripheral blood. These cases represent a proportion of those included in the clinical entity termed *splenic lymphoma with villous lymphocytes* (SLVL). Lymphoplasmacytic lymphoma typically expresses surface and cytoplasmic μ heavy chain. Most patients express CD25 and CD43 in addition to the usual B-cell markers; fewer than half coexpress CD5. Approximately 10% to 20% express CD11c or CD23 (90,100). Although patients with this disorder are usually not leukemic, they often have marrow involvement at presentation (92,97,100). These cases frequently are associated with a serum or urine paraprotein, or both, that is usually of the IgM type. The morphology of lymphoplasmacytic lymphoma is characteristic of Waldenström's macroglobulinemia (see Chapter 42).

Mantle cell lymphoma frequently involves the spleen (93,96,103). Although mantle cell lymphoma may present initially with clinically isolated splenomegaly, workup of these patients reveals that all have stage IV disease at the time of diagnosis, with bone marrow or liver involvement or both (93,96). The morphology of the disorder in the spleen is similar to that seen in involved lymph nodes (104,105). The white pulp is expanded uniformly, with tumor cells proliferating in widened mantle zones around benign, atrophic appearing germinal centers (Fig. 53.9). This pattern may mimic reactive secondary follicles. The latter are tripartite, however, with central follicles and mantle and marginal zones. The presence of small lymphocytes with irregular nuclear contours in the red pulp may aid in the diagnosis of lymphoma. In some patients, however, the diagnosis of malignancy can be made only by examination of other involved organs or by immunologic or molecular studies.

The tumor cells express bright surface immunoglobulin (IgM and usually also IgD), which is often of the λ light chain type; strongly express B-cell associated antigens and CD5, similar to CLL and small lymphocytic lymphoma; but are $CD23^-$ (99). The product of the cyclin D1 gene can be detected in the nuclei of the neoplastic cells by immunohistochemistry, and its presence is useful in distinguishing mantle cell lymphoma from other B-cell lymphomas (106,107) (see Chapter 22).

Splenic involvement is common in follicular lymphomas, particularly in the small cleaved cell type, which often is disseminated at the time of diagnosis (Fig. 53.10). Rarely, patients with follicular small cleaved cell lymphoma may present with isolated splenomegaly. Grossly, the spleen shows a miliary pattern of involvement because of expansion of the white pulp nodules, although occasionally these nodules coalesce to form larger tumor masses. Low-power microscopic examination can be deceptive because of uniform involvement of the Malpighian corpuscles (2,90,81); how-

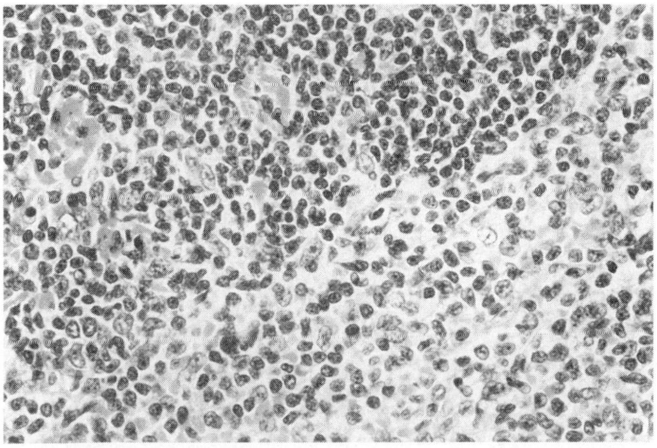

FIG. 53.10. Malignant lymphoma, small cleaved cell type. Cleaved lymphocytes occupy the center of the white pulp nodule (hematoxylin and eosin stain, original magnification: 250× magnification).

ever, high-power examination reveals a monotonous population of small cleaved lymphocytes with coarse chromatin and inconspicuous nucleoli. The diagnosis of follicular lymphoma of the mixed small and large cell type may be more difficult, because the admixture of cells may resemble reactive germinal centers superficially (108). The neoplastic follicles have a bimorphic population rather than a range of cell types as seen in reactive follicles, however, and usually lack tingible-body macrophages and mantle or marginal zones. In addition, the red pulp does not display the plasmacytosis usually seen in reactive lymphoid hyperplasia and often contains smaller nodules composed of lymphoma cells. In difficult cases, subtle red pulp involvement can be demonstrated effectively by immunostaining with CD20 or other B-cell antibodies. In other cases the diagnosis of lymphoma may depend on immunostaining with CD20 or other B-cell antibodies or on immunologic studies to demonstrate monoclonality and BCL-2 expression in neoplastic follicles (99).

Splenic involvement by monocytoid B-cell lymphoma is rare (109–111). If it occurs, it is usually in patients with advanced disease and peripheral blood involvement (112). Splenomegaly, however, may be the presenting feature (113). The involvement is predominantly in the white pulp, with a variable extension of the lymphoma cells into the red pulp. The white pulp often shows residual germinal centers and follicular mantles surrounded by pale cells with small nuclei, abundant cytoplasm, and distinct cell margins expanding the marginal zone (90,99,113). Although the lymphoma cells are cytologically similar to the cells of hairy cell leukemia (HCL), the two diseases show different patterns of splenic infiltration, that is, white versus red pulp. Immunohistochemically, monocytoid B-cell lymphoma cells express B-cell markers including Ki-B3 and CD72 (DBA.44) and are typically $CD11c^{+}CD5^{+}CD25^{-}$ and usually $CD43^{-}$. The tartrate resistant acid phosphatase reaction in monocytoid B-cell lymphoma is negative (99). Recent evidence has shown wide overlap between low-grade B-cell lymphomas of mucosa-associated lymphoid tissue and monocytoid B-cell lymphoma in terms of morphology, immunophenotype, and molecular features (114). Although splenic marginal zone lymphoma has some features that overlap with monocytoid B-cell lymphoma lymphomas, some of its specific findings justify a separate categorization (102,114) (see Chapter 23).

Large B-cell lymphomas characteristically produce solitary or multiple tumor masses in the spleen (Fig. 53.6). Prominent splenomegaly may be a presenting feature (2,72,89,96). These tumors do not show a predilection for involvement of the white pulp and may involve the red pulp as well (80). A predominant red pulp involvement with an associated reactive histiocytosis is observed in some patients (115). These cases must be distinguished from cases of malignant histiocytosis and peripheral T-cell lymphoma (72,115). A subtype of large cell lymphoma that corresponds to the morphologic variant known as *T cell–rich B-cell lymphoma* also has been reported in the spleen (116) (see Chapter 25).

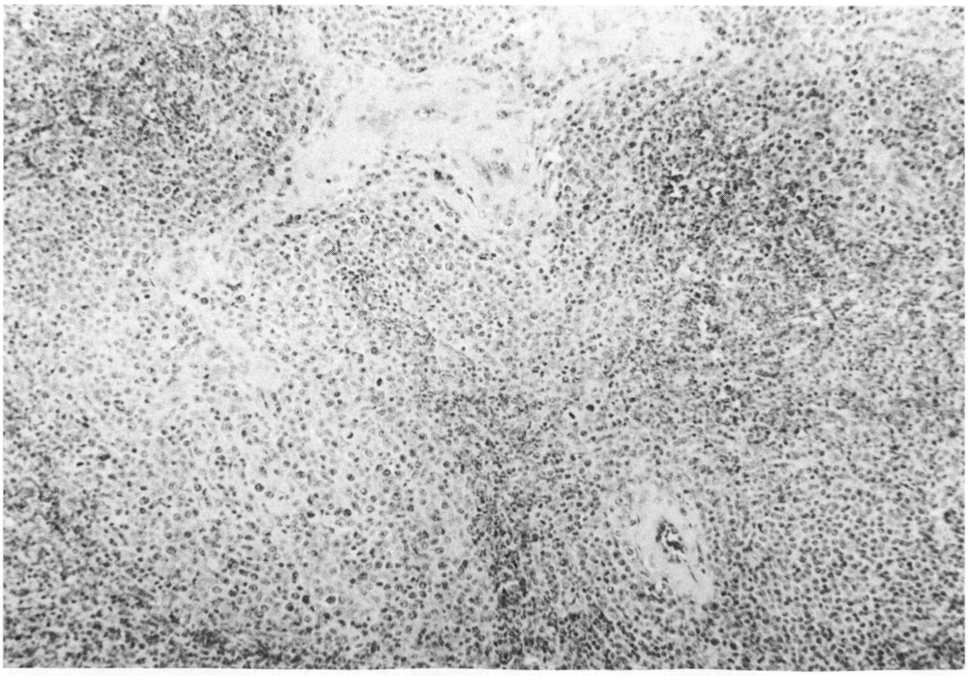

FIG. 53.11. Early involvement of the spleen in mycosis fungoides may be localized to the marginal zones and periarterial lymphoid sheaths (periodic acid–Schiff stain, original magnification: 100× magnification). (From Neiman RS, Orazi A. *Disorders of the spleen,* 2nd ed. Philadelphia: WB Saunders, 1999, with permission.)

Lymphoblastic and Burkitt's Lymphomas

Involvement of the spleen is not common in lymphoblastic lymphoma. As a result, the morphology of splenic involvement has not been well described. In early stages, the disease is localized adjacent to the white pulp, especially in the regions of the PALS (2,90). In the leukemic phase, diffuse red pulp involvement results in a homogeneous pattern with obliteration of the white pulp.

Lymphoblastic lymphoma can be confused easily with both Burkitt's lymphoma (117) and the blastoid variant of mantle cell lymphoma (118), particularly in suboptimal histologic preparations. Burkitt's lymphoma is invariably a mature B-lineage neoplasm; the majority of lymphoblastic lymphomas are of pre–T cell or pre–B cell origin. Paraffin-reactive B-cell antibodies may help identify the former (117). Terminal deoxynucleotidyl transferase, an antigen that also can be demonstrated in conventionally processed histologic material (119,120) is expressed in almost all patients with lymphoblastic lymphoma, but not in the other subtypes. CD99 (013) also may help identify lymphoblastic lymphoma in paraffin tissue sections (121) (see Chapter 26).

Involvement of the spleen, lymph nodes, or liver also is uncommon in Burkitt's lymphoma. Grogan and associates (122) reported splenic involvement in two patients, one of whom was leukemic; Banks and colleagues (123) found splenic involvement in 10 of 17 patients with sporadic Burkitt's tumor at autopsy. Most patients have both red and white pulp involvement, although occasionally more selective involvement of the white pulp, either in the Malpighian corpuscles or in the marginal zones, is seen (124). Immunohistochemistry for terminal deoxynucleotidyl transferase and CD99 can be used to separate Burkitt's lymphoma from lymphoblastic malignancies (119–121). In difficult cases, molecular demonstration of *MYC* gene rearrangement may be necessary to confirm the diagnosis (see Chapter 27).

Peripheral T-Cell Lymphomas

Because of the relatively recent characterization of the peripheral T-cell lymphomas and their rarity in Western countries (125), there have been few descriptive studies of splenic involvement in these lymphomas.

Mycosis fungoides is perhaps the best characterized disease of this type (126). Splenic involvement in this disorder usually affects the white and red pulp alike. The marginal zones are infiltrated by large atypical cells, associated with both diffuse and patchy nodular involvement in the red pulp (Fig. 53.11). Combinations of some of these patterns may occur (126,127). Not all cells have cerebriform nuclear contours, and a variable proportion of the tumor cells may appear blastic. Splenic involvement is a manifestation of disseminated disease and occurs relatively late in the course of the disorder.

The unspecified node-based peripheral T-cell lymphomas are perhaps the least well-studied group of T-cell neoplasms that occur in the spleen. Evidence suggests that the pattern of splenic involvement in these diseases is different from that in B-cell lymphomas and is more red pulp oriented (Fig. 53.12).

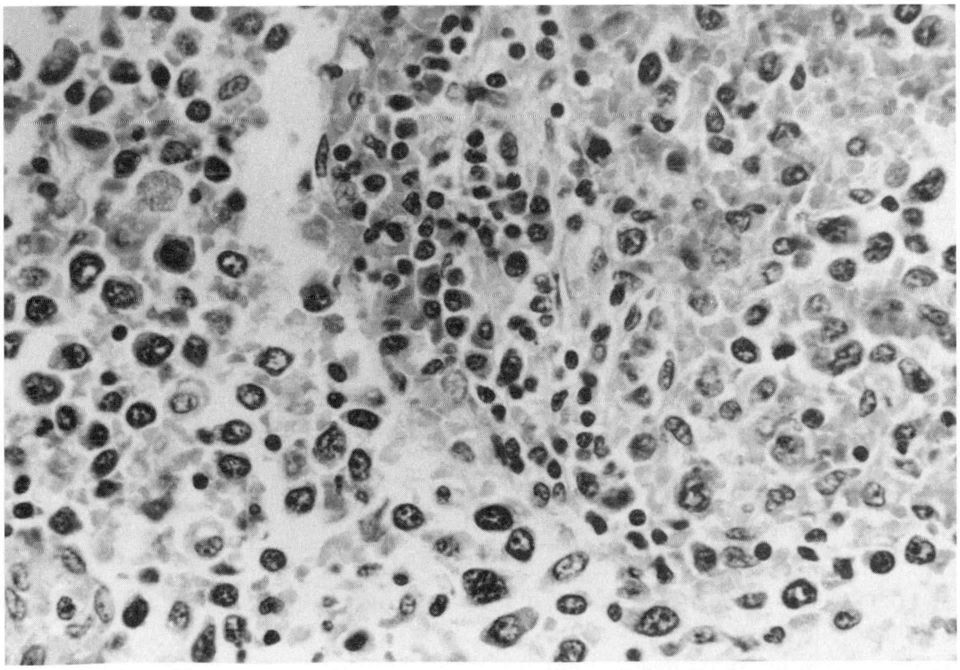

FIG. 53.12. Spleen involved with peripheral T cell lymphoma showing red pulp infiltrate of a pleomorphic population of lymphoid cells (periodic acid–Schiff stain, original magnification: 250× magnification).

In the description by Waldron and coworkers (128), three of six patients had massive splenomegaly. Brisbane and colleagues (129) described autopsy findings in one patient in whom the spleen showed coalescent masses, as well as discrete involvement of the PALS. Weinberg and Pinkus (130) described an unusual variant of T-cell lymphoma composed of large multilobulated cells with splenic involvement in 2 of 10 cases but did not describe the splenic morphology. Burke (90), however, reported several patients with immunologically confirmed T immunoblastic lymphoma in whom nodules were formed at the periphery of the white pulp, and one in whom the red pulp was the predominant site of involvement. We have seen several such cases with differing types of involvement, some expanding the PALS diffusely, some producing discrete masses, and one mimicking the pattern of involvement seen in mycosis fungoides. Lymphoepithelioid cell (Lennert's) lymphoma (131,132), a cytologic subtype of peripheral T-cell lymphoma that is characterized by a high content of epithelioid histiocytes, may produce a characteristic but not specific splenic morphology. Early involvement usually occurs in the peripheral zones of follicles and the PALS, consistent with the T-cell origin of this lymphoma. The epithelioid histiocytes tend to localize in a ring-like arrangement at the periphery of the white pulp, although they occasionally form clusters (90). Although originally thought to be characteristic of this type of lymphoma, the ring-like arrangement of epithelioid cells can be seen in other forms of lymphoma as well. The epithelioid cells may be difficult to differentiate from the sarcoidal type of granulomas sometimes seen in the spleens of patients with Hodgkin's disease (132).

MALIGNANT LYMPHOMA PRESENTING WITH PROMINENT SPLENOMEGALY

Non-Hodgkin's lymphoma presenting with prominent splenomegaly appears to be a clinical syndrome but not a specific histologic entity. Almost any histologic type of lymphoma can present initially with isolated splenomegaly. Prominent splenomegaly can be the presenting clinical feature in paients with small lymphocytic and lymphoplasmacytic lymphoma, and less commonly mantle cell lymphoma. There are, however, several types of lymphoma that present with splenomegaly and distinct clinicopathological characteristics, such as splenic marginal zone cell lymphoma, SLVL, and hepatosplenic $\gamma\delta$ T-cell lymphoma, that require separate discussion.

Splenic Marginal Zone B-Cell Lymphoma

The marginal zone of the human splenic white pulp is an anatomically and immunologically distinct B-cell region (133–136). Cells similar to splenic marginal zone lymphocytes also have been described in lymph nodes (136,137) and in Peyer's patches (138). Marginal zone cells have been postulated to be the origin of extranodal mucosa-associated lymphoid tissue–type and nodal monocytoid B-cell lymphomas (139–141). A number of patients with splenic marginal zone B-cell lymphomas (SMZCLs) have been reported (142–153). Most patients present with splenomegaly, anemia, and weight loss. The bone marrow and liver commonly are involved. Rare patients with minimal or no splenomegaly and absent bone marrow or liver involvement that have been incidentally identified through splenectomy specimens have been reported (150,153). The course of SMZCL is reported to be indolent, and splenectomy may be followed by prolonged survival (146,148).

The cut surface of the spleen in SMZCL shows miliary expansion of the white pulp. Histologically, nodular involvement of the white pulp centered on preexisting follicles is observed (Fig 53.13). Follicular centers rarely are identifiable, being often completely or partially replaced by small lymphocytes similar to mantle cells. Toward the periphery of the neoplastic nodule, the small cells give way to larger cells with irregular nuclei and pale cytoplasm (Fig 53.14). If residual follicular centers are identified, the medium-sized neoplastic cells are arranged into broad concentric bands around the germinal center (reactive or hyalinized), a pattern that superficially may resemble reactive marginal zone hyperplasia, particularly in those patients with minimal or no splenomegaly (150,153–156) (Fig. 53.15). In marginal zone hyperplasia, However, lymphoid infiltration of the follicles is not observed. In addition, red pulp involvement, which is a common feature in SMZCL, is not seen in reactive hyperplasia.

Immunohistochemically, the lymphoma cells express various B-cell markers, surface immunoglobulin, usually IgM (+ IgD), and BCL-2, but not CD5, CD10, CD23, CD11c, or CD43 (99). CD72 (DAB.44) is expressed in a minority of patients. Molecular analysis shows lack of *BCL2* or *BCL1* gene rearrangement (99).

It has been suggested that SMZCL overlaps with extranodal (mucosa-associated lymphoid tissue type) and nodal

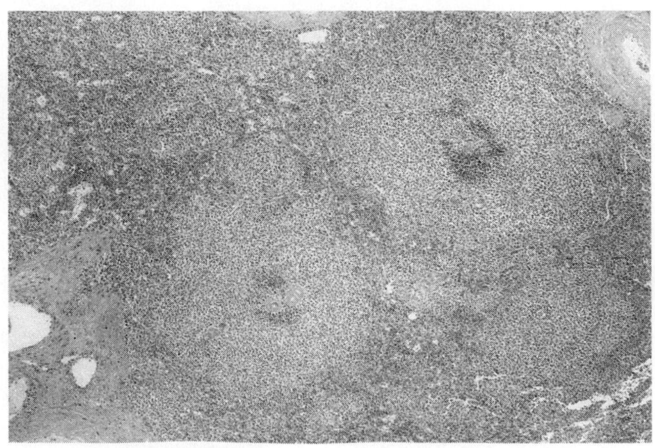

FIG. 53.13. Splenic marginal zone cell lymphoma. Marginal zones are greatly expanded and encroach upon the mantle and follicular zones of the white pulp (hematoxylin and eosin stain, original magnification: 100× magnification).

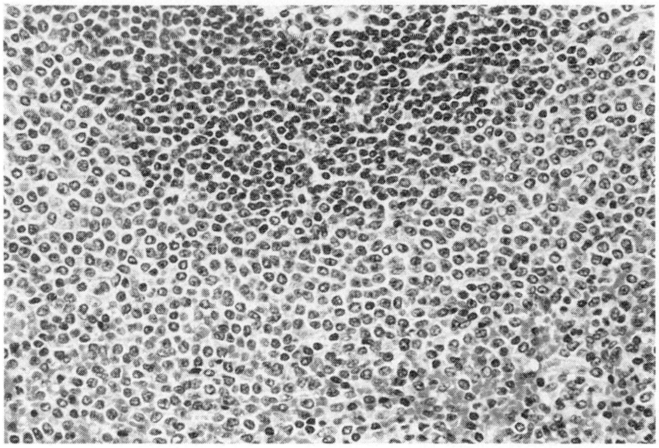

FIG. 53.14. Splenic marginal zone cell lymphoma. Marginal zone cells proliferate in the periphery of the white pulp nodule. (hematoxylin and eosin stain, original magnification: 250× magnification).

(monocytoid) marginal zone B-cell lymphoma. SMZCL, however, differs clinically from those other lymphoma types by virtue of its dissemination at presentation. In addition, the histologic and immunohistochemical findings are only partially overlapping (143,144,146,148). The low incidence of trisomy 3 in patients with SMZCL also suggests that this neoplasm may be genetically distinct from other types of marginal zone cell lymphomas (149).

Splenic Lymphoma with Circulating Villous Lymphocytes

In 1979, Neiman and colleagues (157) described 10 patients with splenic lymphomas with circulating atypical cells that mimicked hairy cell leukemia. The histologic appearance of the spleen in these patients was similar to that seen in small lymphocytic lymphoma but never demonstrated exclusive involvement of the red pulp as observed in hairy cell leukemia. Plasmacytoid differentiation was observed in 6 of 10 patients. In 1986, Spriano and associates (158) reported 8 more cases. The histologic diagnosis was lymphoplasmacytic lymphoma (immunocytoma). Similar patients were described by Melo and coworkers (159,160), who detailed the peripheral blood findings in this group of patients. They termed the disorder *splenic lymphoma with villous lymphocytes*. Histologic examination of splenic tissues in these patients was considered consistent with that observed in CLL and immunocytomas (159,160). Subsequent studies by the same group defined SLVL as a disorder that occurs predominantly in elderly men who present with splenomegaly but little or no lymphadenopathy. The disease usually runs an indolent course, splenectomy rather than chemotherapy being the most effective treatment, often resulting in long-term control even in patients with bone marrow involvement (161).

The circulating lymphoma cells in SLVL are usually larger than the lymphocytes found in CLL. The nuclei are round or ovoid, with a coarse chromatin pattern and a single small nucleolus, and sometimes are placed eccentrically. The cytoplasm is basophilic and usually abundant, although it may be scant. The most important diagnostic feature is the presence of unevenly distributed short thin villi often concentrated in one pole of the cell (159). In nearly every case there is a variable proportion of plasmacytoid cells. The cells usually lack tartrate-resistant acid phosphatase reactivity. The bone marrow is involved in 75% of patients (99). The pattern of infiltration can be focal (interstitial or nodular) or focal and diffuse. A peculiar intravascular pattern recently was described (162,163). The immunophenotypic profile of SLVL is variable, with most cases resembling lymphoplasmacytoid lymphoma (surface immunoglobulin–positive, $CD5^-CD23^-$) (99,164). Molecular analysis shows a lack of *BCL2* gene rearrangement (165); a small proportion of patients has the translocation t(11;14), with rearrangement of the *BCL1* gene and increased expression of cyclin D1 (166).

It recently was suggested by Isaacson and colleagues (142) that SLVL may represent a single clinicopathologic entity, corresponding to a leukemic variant of SMZCL. SMZCL, however, is still poorly understood and should be kept separate from other better characterized subtypes of marginal zone lymphoma (nodal, monocytoid and extranodal, mucosa-associated lymphoid tissue type). We as well as others (99,145,167,168), however, believe that SLVL represents a heterogeneous group of low-grade B-cell lymphomas. Recent evidence suggests that the leukemic cells in patients with SLVL have a remarkable morphologic and phenotypic fluctuation with time (169), resulting from their activation status.

Splenic lymphoma with villous lymphocytes has been associated with the presence of persistent polyclonal B-cell proliferation as seen in patients with chronic malarial spleno-

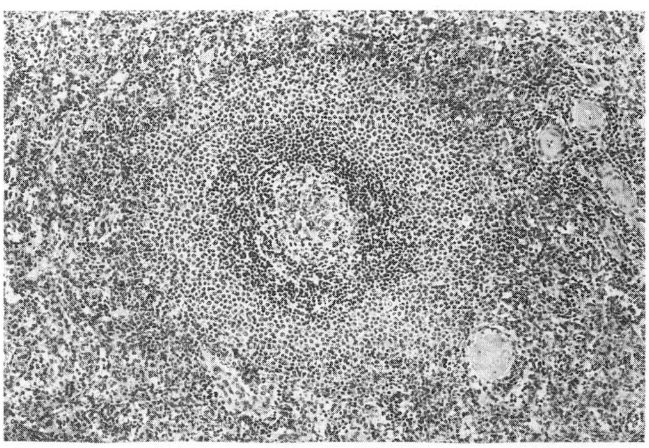

FIG. 53.15. So-called indolent marginal zone cell lymphoma. The widened marginal zone is morphologically indistinguishable from reactive marginal zone hyperplasia (hematoxylin and eosin stain, original magnification: 100× magnification).

megaly (170,171) as well as those with several autoimmune conditions (172,173).

Hepatosplenic $\gamma\delta$ T-Cell Lymphoma

Hepatosplenic $\gamma\delta$ T-cell lymphoma (HTCL) is a distinct clinical entity within the spectrum of peripheral T-cell lymphomas. It is characterized by hepatosplenomegaly, sinusoidal trophism, and a T-cell $\gamma\delta$ receptor phenotype of the malignant cells in most cases (174–178). It typically occurs in young adults, more frequently in males, and is associated with a poor prognosis. The presenting symptoms include fever, weight loss, hepatosplenomegaly, and variable cytopenias. This tumor overlaps to a certain degree with a rare type of T-cell lymphoma that also involves the spleen, termed *erythrophagocytic Tγ lymphoma* (179). In the latter disorder, the tumor cells show erythrophagocytic activity as well as CD16 (FcγRIII receptor) expression, features that also may be observed in patients with HTCL. Splenic involvement in both conditions is similar. Macroscopically, the spleen is enlarged, usually weighing 3,000 g or more, with a homogeneous cut surface and loss of white pulp markings. Histologically, the neoplastic cells infiltrate the red pulp cords and sinuses (Fig. 53.16). The lymphoid cells are medium-sized and have oval or folded nuclei, with chromatin less condensed than that of small lymphocytes, and a moderate amount of pale cytoplasm. The histologic appearance of the spleen may mimic hairy cell leukemia closely (178). In HTCL, however, blood lakes are not seen. In addition, the immunophenotypic differences are distinctive. The main histologic feature of liver as well as bone marrow involvement is an intrasinusoidal distribution of the neoplastic cells. Abdominal lymph node involvement has been observed in one patient with HTCL, in whom the lymph node showed partial infiltration by similar lymphoid cells arranged in an interfollicular and sinusoidal pattern. The neoplastic cells express various pan–T cell markers including CD3. Most patients express the $\gamma\delta$ T-cell receptor (174,175,178), although some also express the $\alpha\beta$ receptor (176). Most patients show clonal rearrangement of the γ or δ chain of the T-cell receptor gene; the T-cell receptor β chain gene may be either germline or rearranged (174,177). Recent evidence has suggested an association between HTCL and the presence of isochromosome 7a10 (178,180) (see Chapter 29).

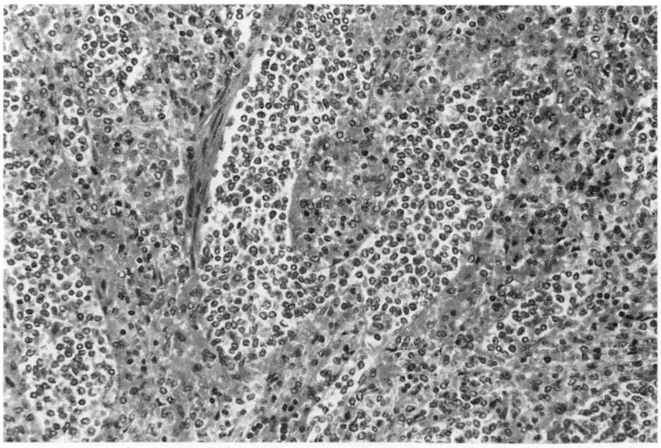

FIG. 53.16. Hepatosplenic $\gamma\delta$ T-cell lymphoma. Tumor cells infiltrate cords and sinuses. A prominent sinusoidal component is present (hematoxylin and eosin stain, original magnification: 200× magnification).

Hepatosplenic B-Cell Lymphoma

Recently, several investigators have shown that hepatitis C virus infection may be related to the pathogenesis of different types of B-cell malignancies such as Waldenström's macroglobulinemia (181), non-Hodgkin's lymphoma (182,183), and mixed cryoglobulinemia (184). Among the hepatitis-associated lymphomas, several have been described as primary hepatosplenic B-cell lymphomas (185–189). Most cases are of the large B-cell type. The direct causal relationship between the occurrence of hepatosplenic B-cell lymphomas and chronic hepatitis C virus infection is unclear; a relationship with chronic hepatitis has been suggested. A pathogenetically similar relationship between persistent infection and local development of B-cell malignancy has been demonstrated in patients with gastric mucosa-associated lymphoid tissue lymphomas (190,191).

DYSPROTEINEMIAS

The dysproteinemias are a heterogenous group of neoplastic conditions associated with monoclonal immunoglobulin production. Some of these disorders appear morphologically benign; others show histologic features of malignancy. These conditions often affect both the red and white pulp of the spleen. A common finding is evidence of immunoglobulin production, manifested by the presence of plasmacytoid lymphocytes with cytoplasmic globules positive on periodic acid–Schiff staining (Mott cells) and intranuclear and cytoplasmic immunoglobulin inclusions (Dutcher and Russell bodies, respectively).

The morphologically benign-appearing lesions are present in most cases of primary amyloidosis and γ heavy chain disease as well as some cases of μ heavy chain disease. Those that appear histologically malignant include multiple myeloma, Waldenström's macroglobulinemia, and plasma cell leukemia (see Chapter 42).

Primary Amyloidosis

Although both primary and secondary amyloidosis may involve the spleen, splenic involvement is more common in the latter. Early in the disease, amyloid is deposited in the walls of small blood vessels. A nodular deposition of amyloid in the white pulp produces the miliary, or "sago," pattern, whereas the "lardaceous" spleen results from sheets of amyloid in the sinuses of the red pulp. The white pulp in amyloidosis often contains numerous mature plasma cells and less numerous plasmacytoid lymphocytes. In a large percentage of these patients whom we have studied, the plasma cells exhibit monoclonal λ light chain restriction. Functional hyposplenism may occur with extensive amyloid deposition (192).

Heavy Chain Diseases

Splenic involvement may be a feature of both γ and μ heavy chain diseases. Patients with these disorders usually have a serum paraprotein that consists of an intact but structurally abnormal heavy chain. Gamma heavy chain (Franklin's) disease has the clinical features of a lymphoma-like disorder. In addition to involvement of Waldeyer's ring, hepatosplenomegaly and generalized lymphadenopathy are features of γ heavy chain disease (193–196). A diffuse infiltrate of lymphocytes and plasmacytoid cells results in obliteration of the white pulp (Fig. 53.17). Eosinophils and immunoblasts may be prominent. In contrast, μ heavy chain disease presents as slowly progressive CLL (197,198). The spleen is infiltrated by plasma cells that have typically vacuolated cytoplasm and Russell bodies.

Multiple Myeloma

Splenomegaly is rarely clinically significant in patients who have multiple myeloma, although the organ sometimes is involved, even in the absence of plasma cell leukemia (199). Splenomegaly in multiple myeloma also may result from amyloid deposition. In rare patients light chain deposition only and not amyloid has been described in myeloma. This can be accompanied by a foreign body type of granulomatous reaction. The myeloma cells either infiltrate the red pulp diffusely or, rarely, produce grossly visible nodules. Hepatosplenomegaly is, however, a common feature of the POEMS syndrome, in which an osteosclerotic variant of myeloma occurs in association with polyneuropathy, organomegaly, endocrinopathy, the presence of a monoclonal paraprotein, and hyperpigmentation of the skin (200–204). The pattern of involvement of the spleen in plasma cell leukemia resembles that seen in other leukemic processes. Cytopenias resulting from hypersplenism (205,206) and splenic rupture occasionally have been reported in patients with plasma cell leukemia (206,207).

Waldenström's Macroglobulinemia

Hepatosplenomegaly often is a feature of macroglobulinemia, a syndrome in which a disseminated lymphoplasmacytic lymphoma is associated with a monoclonal IgM paraprotein, anemia, and often a bleeding diathesis (208–210). The most common cellular pattern is that of a pleocytotic infiltrate of lymphocytes, plasmacytoid lymphocytes, and plasma cells that may have numerous Dutcher and Russell bodies (Fig. 53.18). Splenic involvement may be extensive in Waldenström's macroglobulinemia and may be associated with hypersplenism (211). The histologic features observed in spleen sections of patients with Waldenström's macroglobulinemia are consistent with the morphologic appearance of small lymphocytic or lymphoplasmacytic lym-

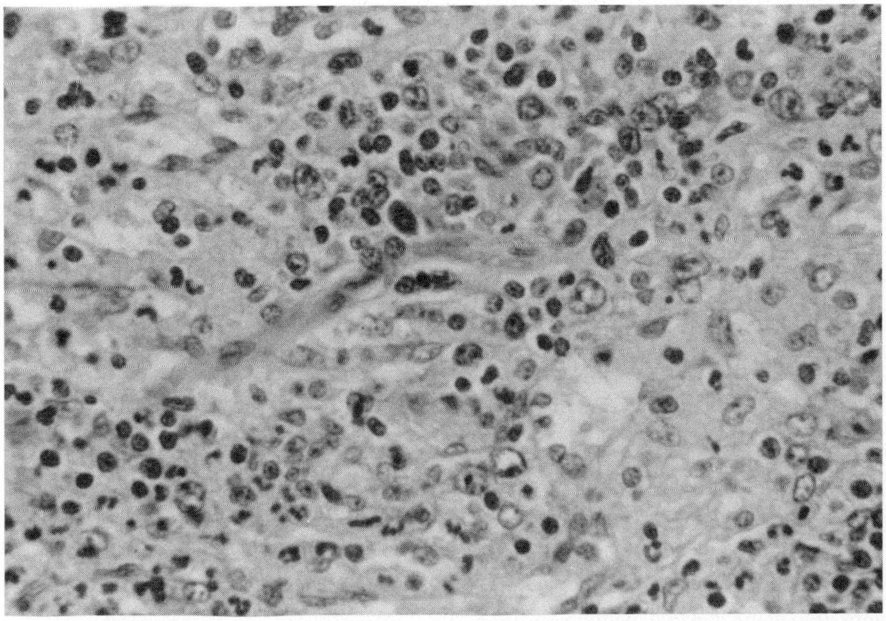

FIG. 53.17. Gamma heavy chain disease showing infiltration of the splenic red pulp by a proliferation of lymphocytes and plasmacytoid lymphocytes (periodic acid–Schiff stain, original magnification: 250× magnification).

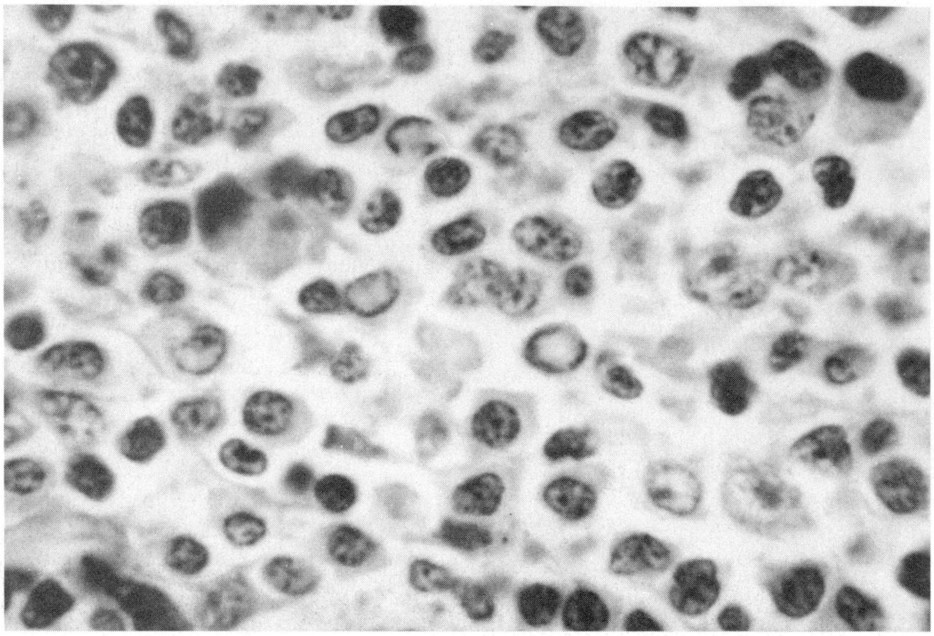

FIG. 53.18. Waldenström's macrogobulinemia. The red pulp is infiltrated by a proliferation of lymphocytes, plasmacytoid lymphocytes, and plasma cells (periodic acid–Schiff stain, original magnification: 400× magnification). (From Neiman RS, Orazi A. *Disorders of the spleen,* 2nd ed. Philadelphia: WB Saunders, 1999, with permission.)

phoma. Occasional patients have the morphologic features of CLL (212,213).

LEUKEMIAS

Red pulp disease is characteristic of splenic involvement in leukemic processes (2,214) (Fig. 53.19). The leukemic cells usually appear localized to the cords of Billroth, with secondary involvement of the sinuses. Peritrabecular and subendothelial deposits may be seen early in the course of leukemic infiltration. Although splenic disease is invariable in the leukemic disorders, the degree of splenomegaly depends on the type of leukemia and the duration of the disease. The acute leukemias usually result in mild to moderate splenic enlargement, but the chronic leukemias may produce prominent splenomegaly.

The expansion of the red pulp by leukemic infiltration often results in hypersplenism. This occurs more commonly in the chronic leukemias. Peripheral cytopenias may necessitate splenectomy, which may be effective in ameliorating the cytopenias, although removal of the spleen usually does not affect the course of the underlying disease. Splenic rupture is also a complication in patients with leukemia. This is believed to result from infiltration by tumor cells of the trabecular framework and vascular structure of the organ or from infarction within the spleen (215–217). Rupture of the spleen is far more common in the chronic leukemias (particularly myeloid leukemia) than in the acute forms.

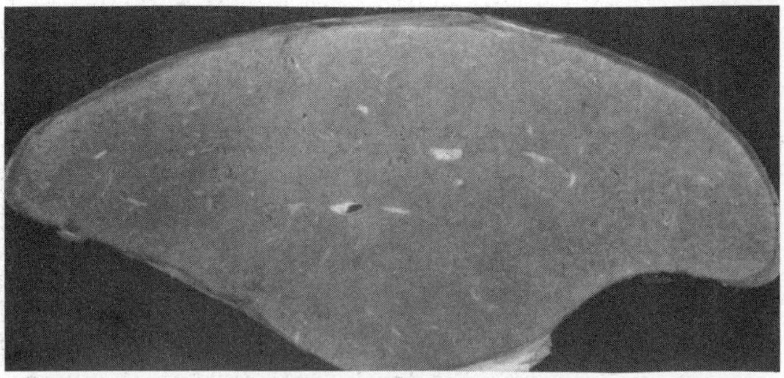

FIG. 53.19. Diffuse expansion of the red pulp with obliteration of the white pulp markings is characteristic of the splenic involvement in leukemic processes, as seen in this patient with hairy cell leukemia.

Nonlymphocytic Leukemias

The nonlymphocytic leukemias include acute and chronic forms that may be derived from the granulocytic, erythroid, monocytic, or megakaryocytic lineages (Fig. 53.20). Distinction among these forms often is difficult on examination of the spleen alone, although touch imprints and histochemical stains in tissue sections frequently are helpful. Immunohistologic studies and immunophenotypic analysis by flow cytometry may be required to characterize the leukemia. Splenic involvement in the acute myeloid leukemias may occur either as a *de novo* phenomenon or as part of the accelerated phase of a chronic myeloproliferative disorder. The existence of an underlying myeloproliferative disorder may be suggested by the presence of hematopoietic cells of

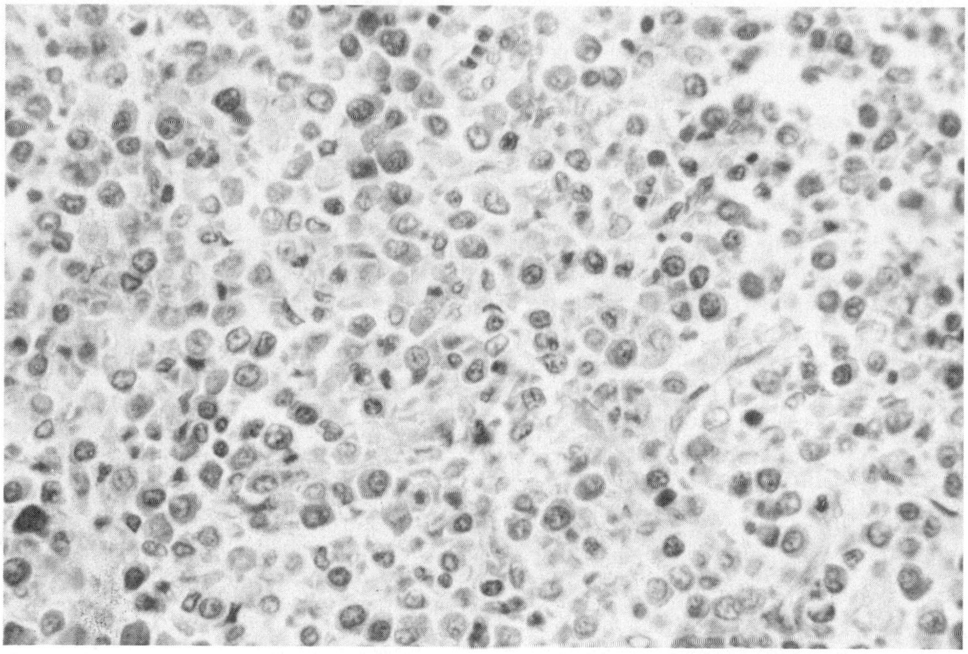

FIG. 53.20. Acute myeloblastic leukemia. The infiltrate in the red pulp obliterates the white pulp markings (periodic acid–Schiff stain, original magnification: 250× magnification).

the other cell lines, which may suggest a chronic component. All the myeloid leukemias of the French-American-British classification involve the spleen in the same topographic manner, with the exception of erythroleukemia (M6), in which the leukemic cells tend to cluster preferentially in the red pulp sinuses (2) (Fig. 53.21).

Chronic myeloid leukemia (CML) often is associated with massive splenomegaly (2). The cut surface of the spleen is deep red without visible white pulp, because CML generally obliterates the lymphoid follicles, although small remnants of white pulp may be seen. Infarcts are common because of subendothelial invasion of the splenic trabecular veins, and

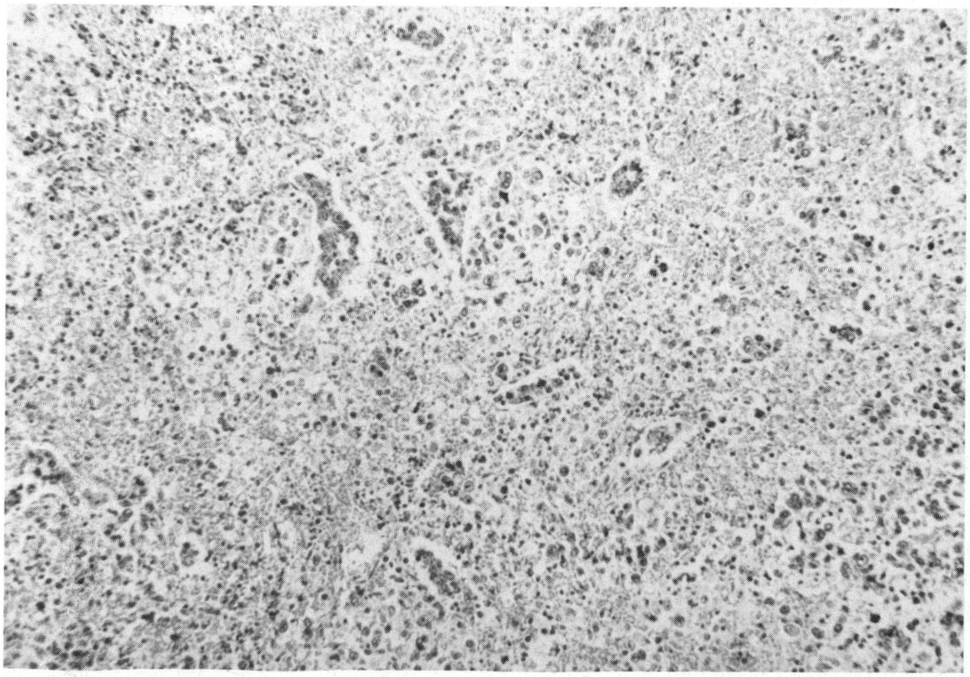

FIG. 53.21. Erythroblasts clustering in the splenic sinuses in a case of erythroleukemia (periodic acid–Schiff stain, original magnification: 100× magnification).

fibrosis of the cords may be prominent. Microscopic examination reveals a polymorphous infiltrate in the red pulp, including myeloid cells at all stages of maturation (2). Immature granulocytes can be detected in tissue sections by using immunohistologic stains for myeloperoxidase, CD15 or lysozyme; or with the enzymatic chloroacetate esterase reaction (Leder stain). In our experience, myeloperoxidase is the most sensitive and specific immunohistologic myeloid marker (218). Results with this marker frequently are positive although cytochemical myeloperoxidase is negative.

The majority of CML cases terminate with the development of an accelerated phase that resembles a *de novo* acute leukemia (219,220). Approximately one third of the cases of blast crisis arise in a clone in an extramedullary site, the most common of which is the spleen (221–225). Several studies have indicated that the myeloid cells in the spleen may develop additional cytogenetic abnormalities before those present in other sites (226–228). These studies also have suggested that a clone may proliferate in the spleen more rapidly than in other sites (229,230). Splenic blast crisis in CML may result in a dramatic increase in the size of the organ (231). Gross examination usually reveals a homogeneous cut surface. In some patients, however, blast transformation may be a localized phenomenon, with nodules on the cut surface that represent collections of blasts (2). Most often these are myeloblasts, although in approximately 25% of patients the blast cells in the accelerated phase are lymphoblasts (232) or, in rare patients, megakaryoblasts or erythroblasts (232). Occasionally, nodules may be seen on the cut surface of a spleen from a patient with CML that represent localized collections of ceroid-containing histiocytes (233).

Splenectomy once was advocated in CML because it was believed that removal of the organ might delay blast transformation (234,235). This has not been confirmed. Splenectomy is performed occasionally in CML to alleviate the symptoms of massive splenomegaly and hypersplenism. It is also performed routinely in patients who undergo bone marrow transplantation.

Chronic monocytic leukemia may be accompanied by prominent splenomegaly with hypersplenism, which may be a presenting manifestation of this disorder. Bearman and colleagues (236) described five patients whose spleens were infiltrated by apparently mature monocytes that demonstrated phagocytosis.

Lymphoid Leukemias

Splenomegaly is seldom prominent in acute lymphoblastic leukemia. Although enlargement of the spleen often occurs during the course of the disease, it rarely approaches clinical significance. Microscopic examination reveals a sparse infiltrate in the red pulp. Splenomegaly, however, may be an early feature of CLL, although the degree of splenomegaly is rarely as prominent as that seen in CML (237). Patients with CLL have been reported in whom the presenting feature is prominent splenomegaly with an insignificant peripheral blood lymphocytosis (238). Hypersplenism may result from splenic enlargement in CLL (240). Prominent splenomegaly, particularly if associated with cytopenias, has been reported to be a poor prognostic sign (240,241). Splenectomy usually is reserved for patients who have advanced disease and severe hypersplenism (242,243). Splenectomy may accelerate the disease in certain patients (244).

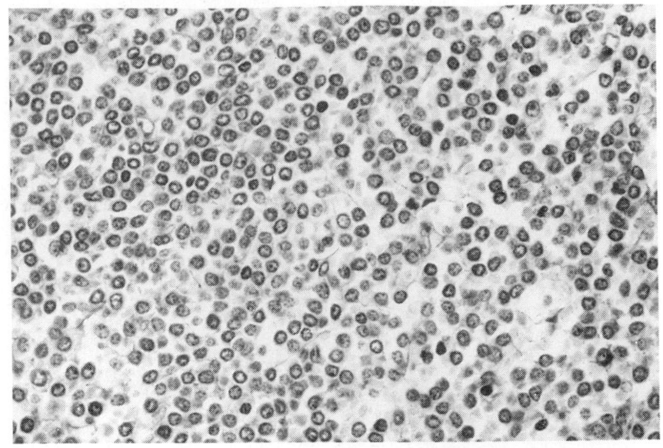

FIG. 53.22. Chronic lymphocytic leukemia. Splenic involvement includes both the white and red pulp. In this patient with advanced disease, the red pulp is diffusely infiltrated by tumor cells and the white pulp is indistinct (periodic acid–Schiff stain, original magnification: 250× magnification).

Most CLLs are of B cell lineage. The morphologic features in the spleen are histologically identical to those seen in malignant lymphoma, small lymphocytic type (92). CLL and its variants are the only forms of leukemia in which the splenic white pulp is involved (2,90) (Fig. 53.22). Early in the course of the disease, the replacement of the lymphoid follicles by small lymphocytes may be difficult to distinguish from the immunologically unstimulated adult spleen. In these early cases, the diagnosis of malignancy may rest on the demonstration of clonality by immunophenotyping or on gene rearrangement studies, although the presence of prolymphocytes and infiltration of the red pulp can be subtle clues to the diagnosis.

A small number of CLLs are of T-cell origin. These disorders appear to represent an exception to the rule that lymphoid disorders involve the white pulp, for in both $CD4^+$ and $CD8^+$ subtypes, involvement is predominantly in the red pulp.

The term *lymphoproliferative disease of granular lymphocytes*, or *large granular lymphocytosis* (LGL), defines a spectrum of proliferations of large granular lymphocytes of T- or natural killer cell phenotype that were formerly termed *T-cell* or *T8 lymphocytosis with neutropenia* (245–247).

Large granular lymphocytosis is a common occurrence, present in over 30% of blood samples analyzed in a recent study (248). It occurs most frequently in patients with aplastic anemia, rheumatoid arthritis, or other autoimmune disorders (249–251). Some patients with LGL have only a moderate lymphocytosis with neutropenia and minimal splenomegaly. Others have progressive disease with marked blood and bone marrow lymphocytosis and prominent splenomegaly (252,253). The presence of clonal cytogenetic abnormalities as well as clonal T-cell receptor gene rearrangements in some cases of LGL indicates that many of these proliferations are neoplastic (253,254). Because distinct criteria to differentiate these conditions have not been determined with certainty, it has been proposed that the diagnostic criteria for LGL leukemia be the presence of more than 2 $\times 10^3$ large granular lymphocytes per microliter occurring for at least a 6-month period (252). Clonal (neoplastic) proliferations occur in patients who do not meet these criteria (255).

Large granular lymphocytic leukemia is divided into two subtypes based on the immunophenotype of the cells and clinical presentation (247,253,256). T-cell lymphocytic leukemia is $CD3^+CD8^+CD16^+CD57^+$ but does not express CD56. It occurs in adults and affects males and females equally. It is relatively indolent and is characterized by recurrent bacterial infections associated with the neutropenia characteristic of the disorder. There is usually only a modest absolute lymphocytosis, but the neutropenia may be severe. Splenic involvement occurs in approximately one half of these patients. The majority of these patients require no specific chemotherapy (253), although an aggressive variant has been reported (253,257).

The other subtype of LGL leukemia, referred to as *$CD3^-$* or *natural killer cell* LGL leukemia, is $CD3^+CD4^+CD8^+CD57^-$, but the cells express CD16 and CD56. The median age in natural killer cell LGL leukemia is younger than that in T-cell LGL leukemia; they occur with equal frequencies in both sexes. Cytopenias and infections are less common in natural killer cell LGL leukemia, but hepatitis, splenomegaly, and B symptoms are quite common, and the peripheral blood large granular lymphocyte count is frequently quite high. The course is more rapid than that in T-cell LGL, and patients usually die with progressive disease within 1 year.

Splenic involvement in both types of LGL is similar (258). It is confined to the red pulp, in which LGL cells infiltrate both cords and sinuses (Fig. 53.23). The histopathologic features of LGL mimic hairy cell leukemia, but the blood lakes characteristic of hairy cell leukemia are not present in LGL. Immunophenotypic findings are distinctively different between the two disorders.

Prolymphocytic leukemia, a variant of CLL, is characterized by a lymphocytosis in which more than 55% of the lymphocytes are prolymphocytes (259). Splenomegaly is prominent even at the time of diagnosis, with hypersplenism, peripheral cytopenias, and the absence of significant lymphadenopathy-associated features (259–261). The white blood cell count is elevated markedly, with a predominance of prolymphocytes that have large vesicular nuclei and single

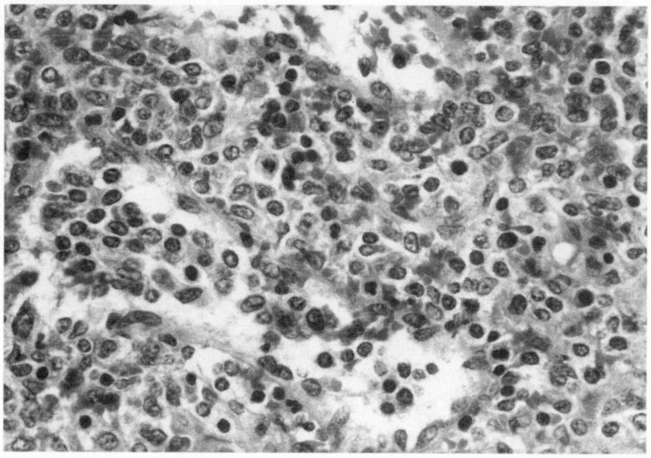

FIG. 53.23. Large granular lymphocytic leukemia showing infiltration of the splenic red pulp (periodic acid–Schiff stain, original magnification: 250× magnification).

prominent nucleoli. The majority of these cases are of B-cell origin, but about 25% have the T-cell immunophenotype (261,262). The pattern of infiltration in the spleen is similar to that seen in B-cell CLL in that, in addition to red pulp involvement, the splenic white pulp may be involved (259,263) (Fig. 53.24). Bearman (263) and coworkers reported a nodular pattern of involvement in B-cell prolymphocytic leukemia.

Prominent splenomegaly is also characteristic of hairy cell leukemia, which usually is associated with cytopenias and insignificant lymphadenopathy (264–266). The gross appearance of the spleen is homogeneous and dark red because of prominent pooling of blood (Fig. 53.19). The white pulp is inconspicuous. Tumor cells infiltrate both the cords of Billroth and the red pulp sinuses (Fig. 53.25), and subendothelial invasion of the trabecular veins may be prominent (264,267,268). The infiltrate in hairy cell leukemia may resemble myeloid leukemias or may mimic closely those in LGL leukemia and hepatosplenic $\gamma\delta$ T-cell lymphoma. Characteristic tartrate-resistant acid phosphatase positivity, however, can be demonstrated on touch imprints of the spleen (269,270) and in tissue sections by immunohistochemistry (270,271). In addition, hairy cells characteristically express CD11c and CD25. Microscopic examination usually demonstrates pseudosinuses or blood lakes (272) (Fig. 53.26). These structures occur in the red pulp, range in size from microscopic to grossly visible, and resemble a hemangioma. These pseudosinuses lack endothelial linings and appear to be lined with hairy cells (see Chapter 41).

Several investigators have described a variant of hairy cell leukemia in which prominent splenomegaly is a feature. This disorder is characterized by a high white blood cell count (273,274). The tumor cells of hairy cell leukemia variant demonstrate tartrate-resistant acid phosphatase positivity but have a higher nuclear-to-cytoplasmic ratio than typical hairy cells, more condensed chromatin, and often a prominent nucleolus (see Chapter 41).

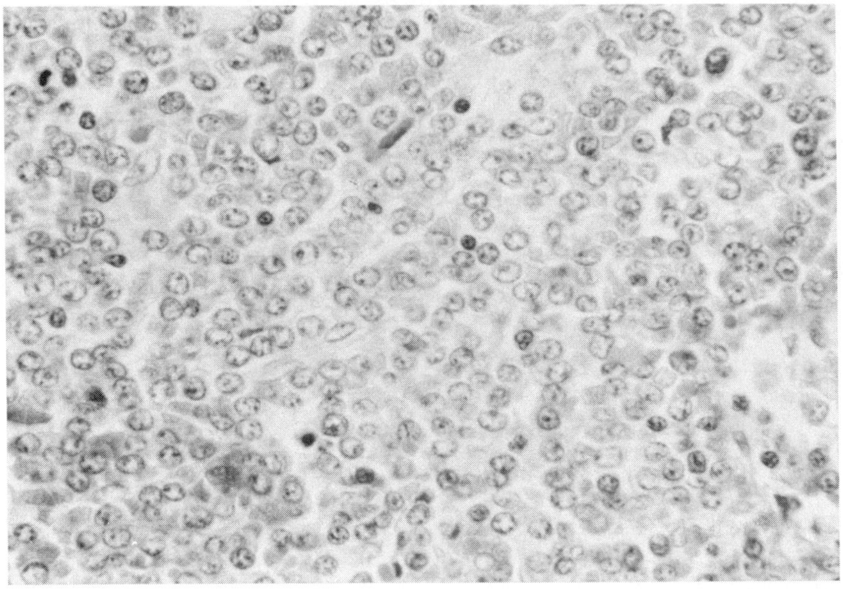

FIG. 53.24. Prolymphocytic leukemia. Tumor cells in the red pulp show characteristic prominent nucleoli. In some patients, involvement may be localized to the white pulp (periodic acid–Schiff stain, original magnification: 250× magnification).

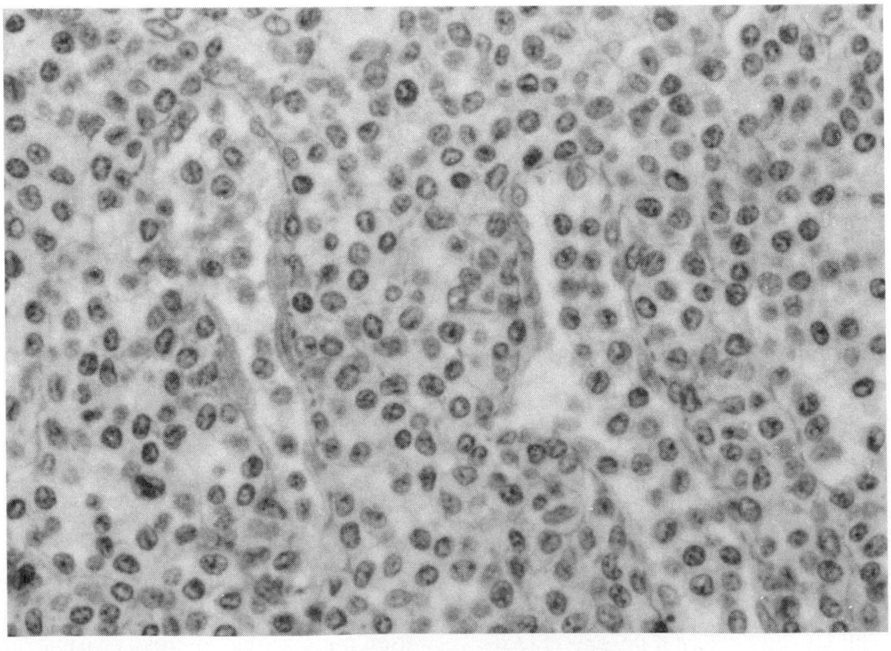

FIG. 53.25. The red pulp of the spleen in hairy cell leukemia is diffusely infiltrated by cells with round to oval nucleoli, rare mitotic figures, and copious cytoplasm (periodic acid–Schiff stain, original magnification: 250× magnification).

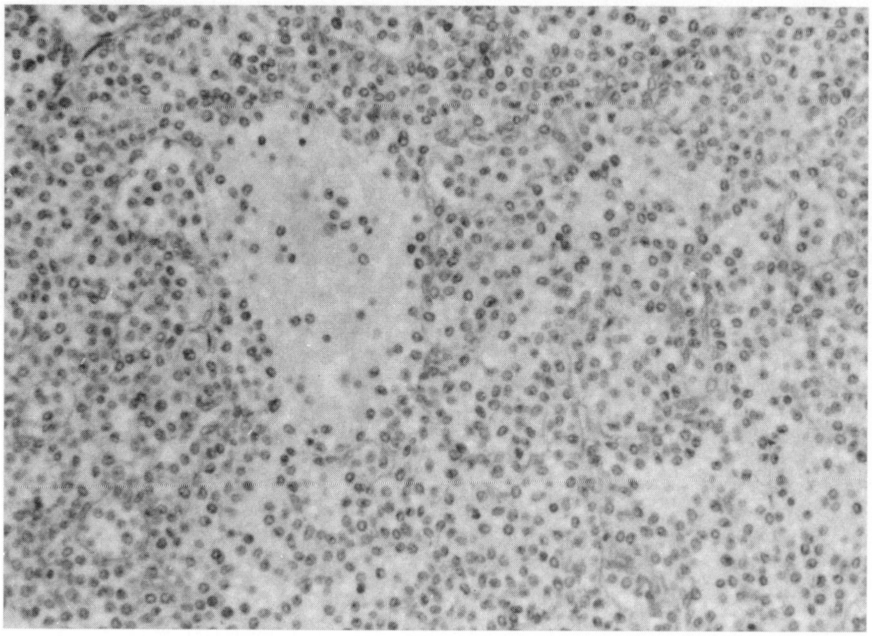

FIG. 53.26. Splenic pseudosinuses in a case of hairy cell leukemia. These structures lack ring fibers and are lined by tumor cells (periodic acid–Schiff stain, original magnification: 100× magnification).

The spleen usually is involved in patients with systemic mastocytosis, even in the absence of mast cell leukemia, although the degree of splenomegaly usually is mild to moderate. Splenic involvement occasionally results in hypersplenism. Hepatosplenomegaly at the time of diagnosis has been reported in approximately 50% of patients (275–277). The pattern of involvement of the spleen in mast cell disease is variable (275–279). Early involvement may show striking localization to the marginal zone of the white pulp associated with thickening of the trabeculae and fibroblastic reaction (Fig. 53.27), resulting in a concentric rimming of the lymphoid follicles. Mast cells that typically appear cuboidal, with pale nuclei and grayish cytoplasm are present. Spindle-shaped forms also may be seen (Fig. 53.28). Other investigators have reported a diffuse infiltration of the red pulp, and nodular perivascular or perifollicular infiltrates have been described (279). Mast cell granules can be demonstrated with the Leder stain and are metachromatic with toluidine blue. They also can be seen with tissue Giemsa stains. Systemic mast cell disease may be associated with other hematologic disorders, most notably acute leukemia and myeloproliferative disorders (280,281) (see Chapter 52).

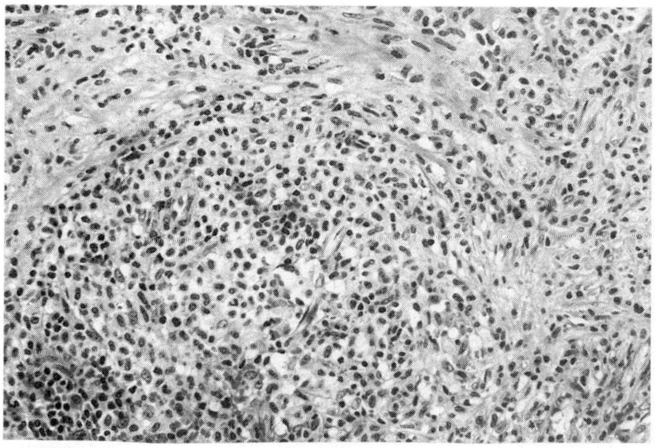

FIG. 53.27. Splenic mastocytosis. There is fibrosis of the white pulp with expansion of cellular infiltrate in to the periphery of the red pulp (hematoxylin and eosin stain, original magnification: 100× magnification).

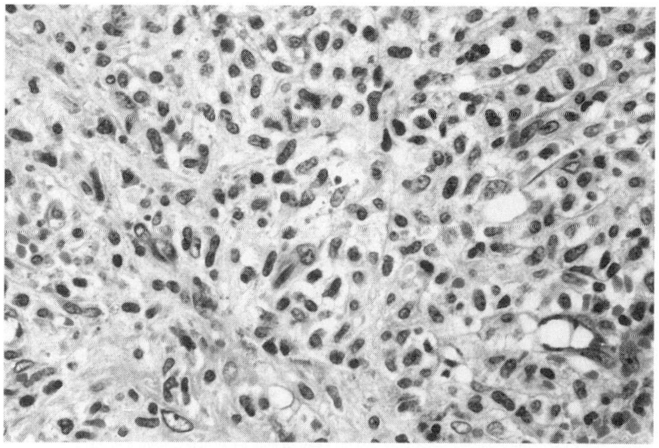

FIG. 53.28. Splenic mastocytosis. The proliferating mast cells show a biphasic morphology, some cells being oval with abundant cytoplasm, and others spindle-shaped (hematoxylin and eosin stain, original magnification: 250× magnification).

MYELOPROLIFERATIVE DISORDERS

The chronic myeloproliferative disorders are a group of interrelated clonal disorders of the hematopoietic stem cell (282–284). These disorders include polycythemia vera, chronic idiopathic myelofibrosis (CIMF), essential thrombocythemia, and CML (see Chapter 49). Variable degrees of splenomegaly occur in all of these disorders. Although each has characteristic morphologic findings in the spleen, a specific diagnosis of one of the myeloproliferative disorders cannot be made on morphologic examination of the spleen in the absence of relevant clinical and laboratory data as well as the examination of bone marrow and a peripheral blood smear (285,286).

This section includes a discussion of the morphology of the spleen in polycythemia vera, CIMF, and essential thrombocythemia.

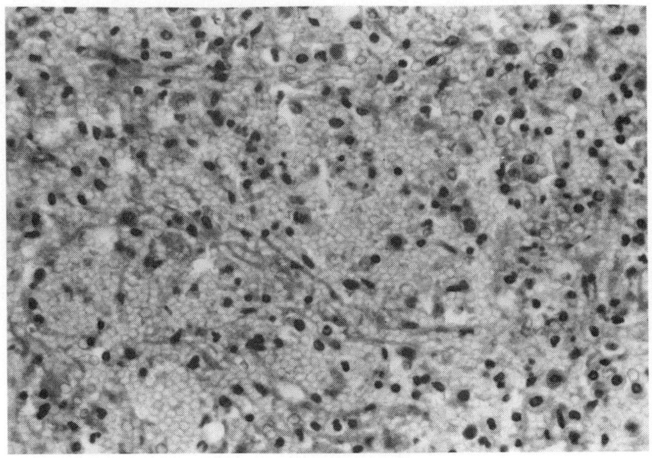

FIG. 53.29. The spleen in the erythrocytotic phase of polycythemia vera shows intense congestion of the cords and sinuses without extramedullary hematopoiesis (periodic acid–Schiff stain, original magnification: 200× magnification).

Polycythemia Vera

Splenomegaly occurs in the majority of patients who have polycythemia vera and is one of the major criteria for diagnosis (287–289). In the uncomplicated, or erythrocytotic, phase of this disorder, an elevated red blood cell mass occurs in the absence of hypoxic stimulation and usually is accompanied by leukocytosis and thrombocytosis. In approximately 15% of patients, however, polycythemia vera evolves to the spent phase, also called *postpolycythemic myeloid metaplasia*, in which the development of reticulin fibrosis in the bone marrow is accompanied by leukoerythroblastosis and increasing splenomegaly (290,291).

The degree of splenomegaly in the erythrocytotic phase of polycythemia vera usually is mild or moderate, with the size of the spleen correlating with the duration of the disease (291–294). Although it previously was believed that splenic enlargement in polycythemia vera resulted from myeloid metaplasia, we have demonstrated that extramedullary hematopoiesis is not a feature of this disease before the development of reticulin fibrosis in the bone marrow (293). Because splenectomy is contraindicated in the erythrocytotic phase of polycythemia vera because of postoperative thrombocythemia, spleens are rarely available for study in this phase. We have found, however, that spleens obtained in the erythrocytotic phase show intense congestion of the cords of Billroth and the sinuses of the red pulp, accompanied by a proliferation of cordal macrophages without myeloid metaplasia (Fig. 53.29). In contrast, spleens obtained from patients whose disease has evolved to postpolycythemic myeloid metaplasia show the presence of hematopoietic precursors indistinguishable from the morphology of the spleen in *de novo* CIMF (295). The development of myeloid metaplasia in polycythemia vera correlates with the evolution of the disease to postpolycythemic myeloid metaplasia and with the development of leukoerythroblastosis and reticulin fibrosis in the bone marrow.

Chronic Idiopathic Myelofibrosis

The degree of splenomegaly in CIMF, also termed *agnogenic myeloid metaplasia* or *myelofibrosis with myeloid metaplasia*, is the most striking among the myeloproliferative disorders. In CIMF, reticulin fibrosis in the bone marrow is accompanied by splenomegaly and leukoerythroblastosis (285,286,292,293,296). Splenomegaly may be the presenting feature of this disorder and may cause symptoms related to massive enlargement of the organ. The degree of splenomegaly usually increases during the course of the disease. Although the rate of splenic enlargement varies widely, the degree of splenomegaly has been shown to correlate with the duration of disease (292,293,296). Increasing splenomegaly may be arrested transiently by splenic irradiation or chemotherapy.

Splenomegaly in CIMF results from the presence of trilinear extramedullary hematopoiesis in the red pulp and secondary proliferation of cordal macrophages (285–287,293). The gross appearance therefore is indistinguishable from the other red pulp diseases. The spleen is greatly enlarged and deep purple to red, with indistinct white pulp markings. Infarcts are common (Fig. 53.30). Microscopic examination reveals all three hematopoietic cell lines in the red pulp sinuses and in the cords of Billroth, in which they may be accompanied by a variable degree of fibrosis. The hematopoietic precursors usually are distributed uniformly throughout the red pulp (Fig. 53.31). In some patients, however, focal proliferations may result in grossly recognizable nodules, usually composed predominantly of one cell type. Although the hematopoiesis present is always trilinear, one cell line may predominate in a given patient. Erythroid precursors occur in easily recognizable clusters, frequently in the sinuses. Megakaryocytes show the same dysplastic features as those in the bone marrow. Although granulocytic precur-

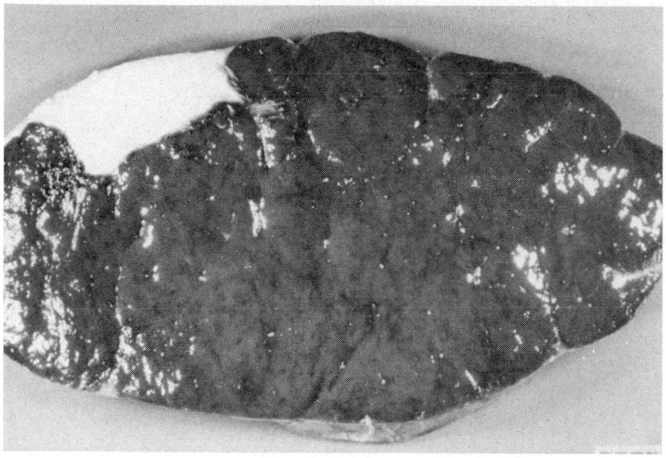

FIG. 53.30. Massive splenomegaly is characteristic of long-term chronic idiopathic myelofibrosis.

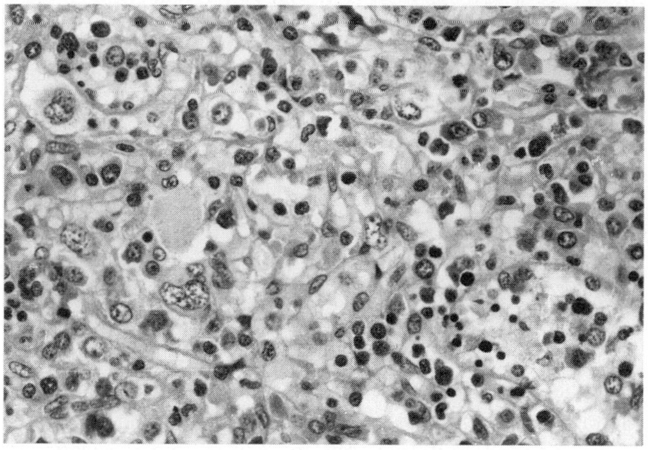

FIG. 53.31. The spleen in chronic idiopathic myelofibrosis shows extramedullary hematopoiesis (periodic acid–Schiff stain, original magnification: 250× magnification).

sors may be difficult to distinguish from cordal macrophages, they can be recognized in touch imprints or in tissue sections by using the immunoperoxidase technique with antibodies to myeloperoxidase or lysozyme. The presence of extramedullary hematopoiesis is accompanied by a proliferation of the cordal macrophages, and phagocytosis of hematopoietic precursors often is seen (292). The trilinear nature of the hematopoiesis seen in CIMF aids in the distinction of this disorder from CML, in which the bone marrow morphology may mimic that of CIMF.

In addition to CML, the differential diagnosis of myeloid metaplasia in the spleen includes various disorders that may cause secondary bone marrow fibrosis with leukoerythroblastosis and the resultant filtration of circulating hematopoietic precursors from the peripheral blood by the spleen. Metastatic carcinoma and infectious disorders that involve the bone marrow are well-known causes of bone marrow fibrosis that may mimic CIMF (297).

Essential Thrombocythemia

Essential, or primary, thrombocythemia is characterized by a marked megakaryocytic hyperplasia in the bone marrow associated with a thrombocytosis, usually in excess of one million platelets per cubic millimeter (285,286,298–300). Clinical manifestations include hemorrhagic or, less commonly, thrombotic phenomena (298). The degree of splenomegaly in essential thrombocythemia usually is less marked than that seen in the other chronic myeloproliferative disor-

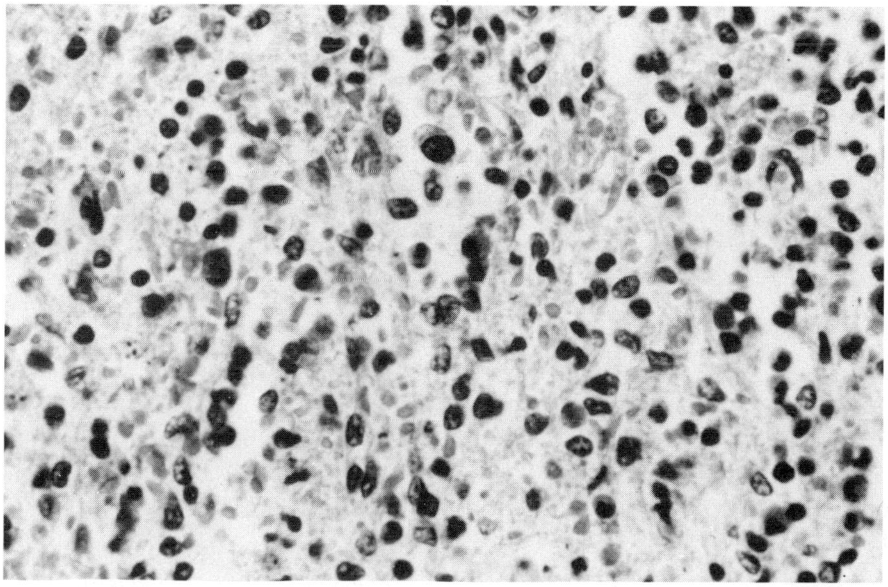

FIG. 53.32. The spleen in essential thrombocythemia shows widening of the cords of Billroth because of masses of platelets (periodic acid–Schiff stain, original magnification: 100× magnification).

ders. Because of the spleen's ability to sequester large numbers of platelets, the organ provides a protective effect in this disorder. Splenectomy therefore is contraindicated, because removal of the spleen may result in a marked increase in the peripheral platelet count, with resultant thrombotic complications. Because of the scarcity of splenectomy specimens, there is no large study of the pathology of the spleen in essential thrombocythemia. In the few patients we have studied, the most notable finding is the widening of the cords of Billroth, which may appear hypocellular at low power because of the presence of large masses of platelets, which also may be seen in the sinuses (Fig. 53.32). Touch preparations of the spleen are useful for demonstrating the sequestration and phagocytosis of platelets. In our experience, no significant extramedullary hematopoiesis is seen. Occasionally, however, the bone marrow shows significant reticulin deposition, and hematopoietic precursors may be seen in the spleen.

Although mild to moderate splenomegaly is characteristic of most cases of essential thrombocythemia, hypersplenism is not a common clinical manifestation. In advanced cases, the spleen may become atrophic and nonfunctional, with atrophy probably resulting from infarction caused by the pooling of platelets (301). The presence of fibrosis and Gamma-Gandi bodies may mimic the morphology of the spleen in advanced sickle cell disease. Functional asplenia may be heralded by the appearance of Howell-Jolly bodies in the peripheral blood.

OTHER TUMORS

Follicular dendritic cell sarcoma, or follicular dendritic cell tumor, is a rare neoplasm derived from the follicular dendritic cell of the germinal center that has been observed to occur rarely in the spleen (302–304). The cells are typically $CD21^+CD35^+HLA\text{-}DR^+CD11a^+CD18^+CD1a^-$. These tumors resemble soft tissue sarcomas, with oval or spindle cells usually growing in bundles and whorls. Nuclei are bland in appearance and have a low mitotic rate. The clinical behavior of these tumors appears to be more aggressive than the relatively bland cytology would suggest (305).

Interdigitating dendritic cell sarcoma is a rare tumor that is thought to arise from lymph node interdigitating dendritic cells (304). The disease usually involves lymph nodes, but splenic involvement may occur. In a variable portion of patients the disease is disseminated, with involvement of spleen, bone marrow, skin, liver, kidney, and lung (306). The histologic features are similar to those described for follicular dendritic cell sarcoma. In paraffin sections, the cells express S-100 protein and CD68 and lack CD1a, B-cell, T-cell, and specific follicular dendritic cell antigen expression (see Chapter 51).

BENIGN LESIONS THAT SIMULATE HEMATOPOIETIC MALIGNANCIES

Immune Reactions

Various benign conditions that affect the splenic white or red pulp can simulate hematopoietic malignancies (Table 53.3). Most notably, some of the patterns of reaction of the splenic lymphoid tissue can be difficult to distinguish histologically from malignant lymphoma. Reactive follicular hyperplasia, seen in the evolving activated immune response, usually is recognized easily as benign (2). The marginal zones, however, may become widely expanded in more chronic cases, and their fusion may result in grossly visible nodules, a phenomenon that has been referred to as *splenic marginal zone hyperplasia* (2,153–156). It may be impossible, on morphologic grounds alone, to distinguish these cases from cases of so-called indolent marginal zone cell lymphoma (150,153). The so-called early activated immune reaction, or reactive nonfollicular lymphoid hyperplasia, which is characteristic of infectious mononucleosis as well as herpes simplex and other viral infections, can simulate Hodgkin's disease and non-Hodgkin's lymphoma (2,307–309) (Fig. 53.33). The white pulp in these conditions lacks germinal centers and, on low-power examination, resembles the immunologically unstimulated spleen (2,7,49,

TABLE 53.3. *Benign lesions of the spleen that simulate hematopoietic malignancies*

Early activated immune reaction
Disorders of the monocyte–macrophage system
Storage diseases
Hemophagocytic syndromes
Infection-associated
Familial
Langerhans cell histiocytosis
Angioimmunoblastic lymphadenopathy
Systemic Castleman's disease
Nonhematopoietic lesions
Cysts
Hamartomas
Inflammatory pseudotumors

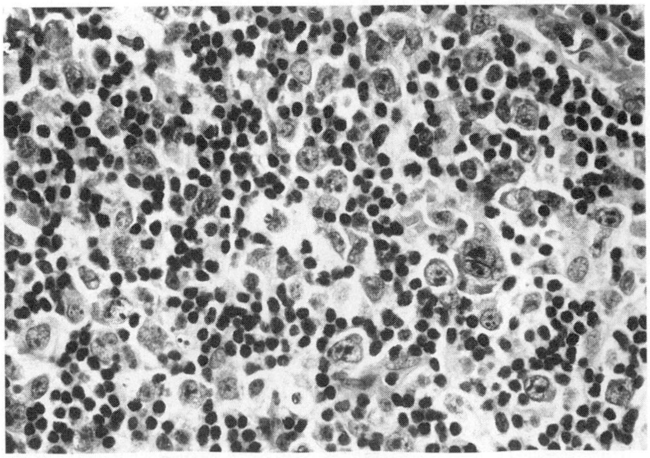

FIG. 53.33. The early activated immune reaction in the spleen of a patient with infectious mononucleosis. The white pulp is expanded by transformed lymphocytes and immunoblasts (periodic acid–Schiff stain, original magnification: 400× magnification).

90). Higher-power examination, however, reveals morphologic evidence of antigenic stimulation characterized by the presence of lymphocytes in varying stages of transformation, including small and large lymphocytes and immunoblasts. Transformed lymphocytes and immunoblasts also proliferate around the penicilliary arterioles and may infiltrate the subendothelial zones of the trabecular veins and the connective tissue framework, resulting in splenic rupture in extreme cases (310). The finding of tingible body macrophages and a pleocytotic cell population that involves all white pulp nodules points to the correct diagnosis of a reactive condition. Steroid-treated immune thrombocytopenic purpura and autoimmune hemolytic anemia also may show this pattern of immunologic activation (311,312).

Proliferations of the Monocyte-Macrophage System

The hemophagocytic syndromes are a group of disorders characterized by the proliferation of cordal macrophages associated with prominent phagocytosis of hematopoietic elements (313). Some cases are familial, affecting infants and children younger than 2 years of age (314–317). They have no immediately apparent cause and are usually acute in their clinical course (318). Because of the acute clinical course with death in many cases, the lack of obvious cause, the systemic distribution, and the striking proliferation of cells in all lymphoreticular organs, these patients usually were considered to have malignancies, and there condition often was called *malignant histiocytosis* (319). The distinction of these disorders from true malignant histiocytosis was complicated by the fact that no reliable criteria for identifying clonality in histiocytes were available. Risdall and colleagues (320) were the first to define the disorder in detail. They described a distinct clinical syndrome characterized by a proliferation of benign histiocytes demonstrating prominent hemophagocytosis, and a fulminant clinical course characterized by fever and varying cytopenias in a clinical context of underlying immunosuppression in most cases. They termed the disorder *viral-associated hemophagocytic syndrome*. A later publication from the same group reported a bacterial association with this syndrome (321), and numerous subsequent studies have revealed that it may be associated with a wide variety of organisms as well as with a variety of tumors (322).

Spleens in the hemophagocytic syndromes are usually only moderately enlarged, although significant enlargement to more than 1 kg does occur. The red pulp displays a proliferation of macrophages and prominent hemophagocytosis, most characteristically of erythrocytes but also of granulocytes, lymphocytes, and platelets (Fig. 53.34). Fibrosis, focal infarctions, and gradual obliteration of the white pulp may occur. The phagocytic histiocytes may be accompanied by more primitive cells of similar lineage, but these cells do not display cytologic evidence of malignancy. Hemophagocytic syndromes associated with malignancies of the hematopoietic system differ morphologically and contain a component of malignant cells. This is particularly true in patients with hemophagocytic syndromes associated with T-cell lymphoma. In patients in whom the neoplastic T cells diffusely infiltrate the splenic red pulp, the resemblance to malignant histiocytosis may be considerable. The diagnosis of T-cell lymphoma in these patients can be confirmed by molecular studies.

Langerhans cell histiocytosis has multiple clinical presentations, ranging from an isolated lytic lesion of bone to a fulminating, disseminated disorder mimicking leukemia. This latter disorder is most common in children and is the form of the disease in which splenic involvement occurs (323). Children with Letterer-Siwe disease usually present with fever and skin lesions (324). Hepatosplenomegaly is common, and splenomegaly is a poor prognostic factor (325–327). Cytopenias result from hypersplenism and from infiltration of the bone marrow. The spleen may be massive and often shows areas of hemorrhage, necrosis, and infarction. Involvement occurs in the red pulp and may be in the form of a diffuse infiltrate of ill-defined tumor aggregates resembling loosely formed granulomas (Fig. 53.35). The characteristic cell of this disorder is large with abundant pale

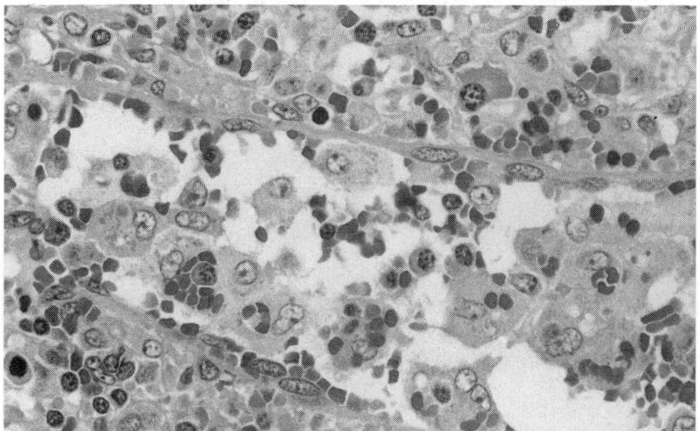

FIG. 53.34. Hemophagocytosis is readily apparent in the red pulp of this spleen from a patient with the infection-associated hemophagocytic syndrome (hematoxylin and eosin stain, original magnification: 400× magnification).

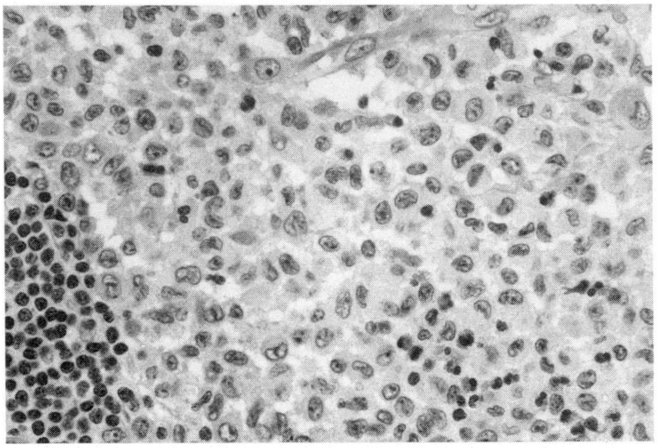

FIG. 53.35. Langerhans cell histiocytosis. The proliferating Langerhans cells fill the red pulp and encroach on the white pulp (in the lower lefthand portion of the image) (hematoxylin and eosin stain, original magnification: 250× magnification.)

and sometimes vacuolated cytoplasm (328). Nuclei frequently are deeply indented or grooved, with regular chromatin and one or two small nucleoli. Electron microscopy usually reveals characteristic structures, termed *Birbeck* or *Langerhans granules*, within the cytoplasm of the cells (329,330). Cells in Langerhans cell histiocytosis typically express S-100 and CD1a and express HLA-DR, CD74, vimentin, CD68, and peanut agglutinin (331–335) in most patients. Recently, molecular studies using X-linked DNA probes capable of detecting inactivation patterns in tissues from female patients have demonstrated that Langerhans cell histiocytosis is a proliferation of CD1a^{+} clonal histiocytes (336,337).

Rare patients with so-called malignant Langerhans cell histiocytosis have been reported (338,339). These patients have a male predominance, an older age, disseminated involvement with frequent splenic distribution, and cytologically malignant-appearing cells. Not all occurrences of cytologic atypia are associated with a malignant clinical course (see Chapter 51).

The existence of a clinically malignant disseminated proliferation of histiocytes first was noted by Scott and Robb-Smith (340). It is now recognized that this disorder is heterogeneous, composed of a variety of neoplastic and nonneoplastic proliferations (341,342). The morphology of the spleen in "malignant histiocytosis" resembles that in an acute leukemia, with diffuse infiltration of the red pulp sometimes obliterating the white pulp. The infiltrate is pleomorphic with the proliferating cells showing a variable degree of differentiation and cytologic atypia (337).

Recent studies have indicated that many diseases once considered malignant histiocytosis are in fact malignant lymphomas (343–345), including such subtypes as anaplastic large cell lymphoma (346), erythrophagocytic Tγlymphoma (347), and Epstein-Barr virus–related (348,349) and non–Epstein-Barr virus–related T-cell lymphomas (350). The proliferation of histiocytes presumably is related to the elaboration by tumor cells of cytokines such as tumor necrosis factor-α or macrophage colony-stimulating factor that induce macrophage proliferation. The hemophagocytic syndromes also probably have been diagnosed mistakenly as malignant histiocytosis in many patients (351–353).

"Malignant Histiocytosis" associated with Mediastinal Germ Cell Tumor

An unusual association occurs between mediastinal nonseminomatous germ cell tumors and hematologic malignancies (354). Approximately one half of the hematologic malignancies have been characterized as malignant histiocytosis (355–357). These proliferations of histiocytes may occur either diffusely or in the form of ill-defined nodules of CD68^{+} cells within the red pulp of the spleen. They are thought to represent an unusual form of metastasis from hematologic elements originating within the germ cell tumor through aberrant hematologic differentiation of malignant germ cells (356). The histiocytes may be reactive however, because it has not been shown by cytogenetic or other means that they are clonal.

Angioimmunoblastic Lymphadenopathy

In addition to generalized lymphadenopathy, fever, weight loss, and a pruritic rash, hepatosplenomegaly often is a presenting feature in patients who have angioimmunoblastic lymphadenopathy (358–360). This is a poorly characterized disorder that originally was believed to be a hyperimmune B-cell proliferation. More recent studies have suggested, however, that most cases of angioimmunoblastic lymphadenopathy represent malignant lymphomas, usually of peripheral T-cell type (angioimmunoblastic T-cell lymphoma) (361–366). The majority of descriptions of the morphology of the spleen in this disorder have come from autopsy series, although splenectomy occasionally is performed in patients with severe hemolytic anemia (367). The descriptions of spleens obtained as surgical specimens vary widely. Some have shown histologic changes predominantly in the marginal zones, with a cellular infiltrate similar to that seen in lymph nodes, although focal aggregates of transformed lymphoid cells also were seen in the red pulp (359,367). There may be an increased reticulin content in the marginal zones with a prominent perifollicular fibrosis (Fig 53.36). Other investigators have described nonspecific reactive follicular hyperplasia (367). Some cases have shown more extensive red pulp involvement. The arborizing vascular network typically seen in lymph nodes has not been reported in the spleen. The majority of reports of spleens in autopsy series have reflected end-stage disease and changes that may be related to chemotherapy, including lymphoid depletion and fibrosis in the spleen as well as in the lymph nodes (360) (see Chapter 16).

The original descriptions of malignant lymphomas that

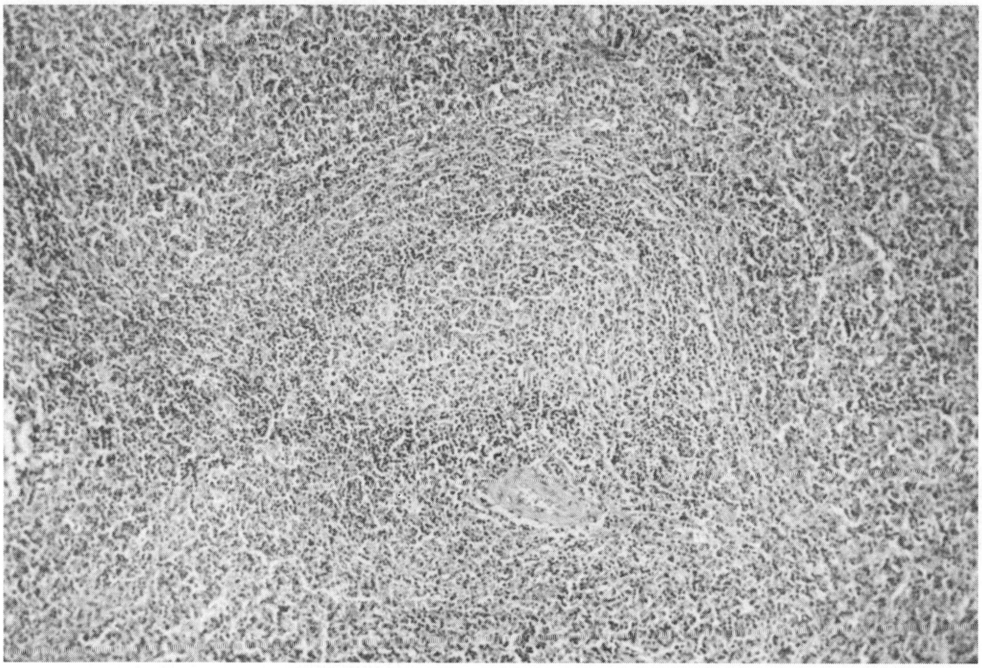

FIG. 53.36. The morphology of the spleen in angioimmunoblastic lymphadenopathy is variable. In this patient, note the fine perifollicular fibrosis resulting in an indistinct demarcation between the red and white pulp (periodic acid–Schiff stain, original magnification: 100× magnification).

arise in patients who have angioimmunoblastic lymphadenopathy included a predominance of immunoblastic plasmacytoid subtypes. Nathwani and colleagues (368) described the morphology of the spleen in 25 patients with angioimmunoblastic lymphadenopathy and lymphoma. These spleens showed a miliary pattern of involvement, with nodules involving both white and red pulp. This pattern of involvement rarely is seen in large cell lymphomas, which usually produce tumor masses. More recent reports have described immunologically or molecularly confirmed T-cell lymphomas (362–366), and the entity is generally accepted as a subtype of peripheral T-cell lymphoma (366).

Castleman's Disease

Patients with multicentric Castleman's disease involving the spleen have been reported (369,370). The original descriptions of Castleman's disease included two subtypes. The more common is the hyaline-vascular type, characterized by atrophic lymphoid follicles surrounded by small lymphocytes in a concentric configuration and containing hyalinized blood vessels. The multicentric plasma cell variant form of Castleman's disease is a rare systemic B-cell lymphoproliferative disorder commonly associated with systemic symptoms, including hypergammaglobulinemia and splenomegaly (370–372). This variant recently has been associated with the presence of Kaposi's sarcoma–associated herpes virus (KSHV) (373) and the overexpression derived from it of interleukin-6 (374), a cytokine considered of pathogenetic significance in Castleman's disease (375,376). In some patients, the clinical and morphologic features of the two subtypes overlap.

The majority of cases reported in the spleen are of the plasma cell type (370,371), although Gaba and colleagues (377) reported a case in which the morphology was more typical of the hyaline-vascular variant. Weisenburger (371) described the morphology of seven patients with Castleman's disease that involved the spleen, five of whom had features typical of the plasma cell variant, although there were admixed atrophic follicles with hyaline-vascular germinal centers. One patient had expansion of the marginal zones with plasma cells, similar to the morphology in three of the four cases reported by Frizzera and colleagues (372). Grossly visible masses composed of hyperplastic nodules of white pulp surrounded by dense fibrous tissue were seen in the two patients in Weisenburger's study in whom the morphology was that of the hyaline-vascular subtype (see Chapter 16).

Nonhematopoietic Lesions

Several benign lesions involving the spleen can mimic malignant lymphoma by virtue of the production of mass lesions that may be associated with hypersplenism, although their benign nature usually is readily apparent microscopically. Splenic cysts are most commonly single and unilocular. The majority of these are so-called false cysts that lack

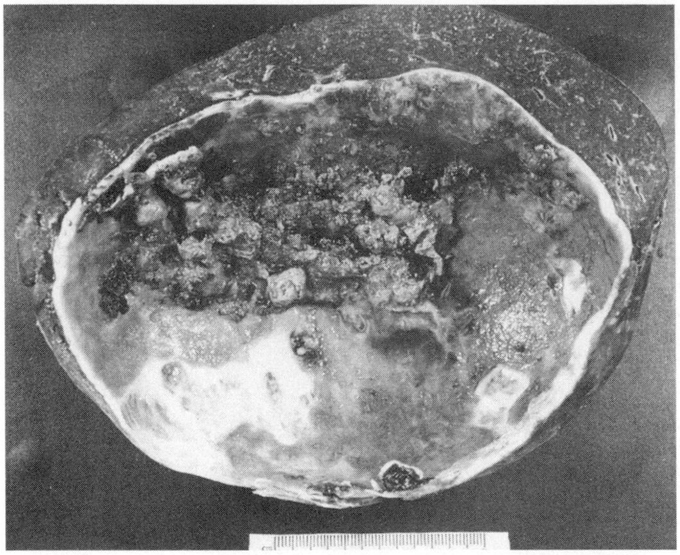

FIG. 53.37. Splenic pseudocyst. These cysts lack an epithelial lining on microscopic examination. (Courtesy of Otelo Solis, MD.)

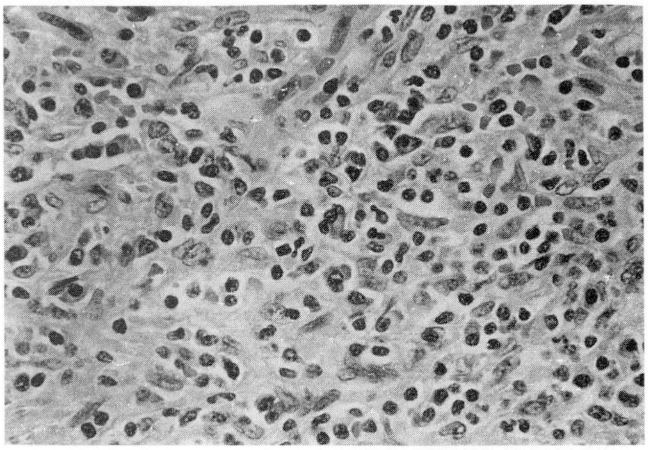

FIG. 53.39. Inflammatory pseudotumors are characterized by a proliferation of spindle cells, macrophages, lymphocytes, and often numerous plasma cells (periodic acid–Schiff stain, original magnification: 250× magnification).

epithelial linings (378) (Fig. 53.37). Approximately 20% of splenic cysts have an epithelial lining, which usually is of stratified squamous type (379–383). These are termed *true* or *epidermoid* cysts. Rarely, true cysts result in hypersplenism.

Similarly, splenic hamartomas occasionally result in hypersplenism (384), although they are more commonly incidental findings at autopsy or in spleens removed for unrelated causes (385). Splenic hamartomas are well-circumscribed nodules that resemble normal red pulp histologically, with slit-like vascular spaces lined by plump endothelial cells (Fig. 53.38). Splenic trabeculae and white pulp rarely are seen in hamartomas, although scattered lymphocytes often are found.

Inflammatory pseudotumor is a rare lesion of the spleen that can mimic malignant lymphoma both clinically and histologically (386,387). Inflammatory pseudotumors present as mass lesions that usually are poorly circumscribed and that infiltrate surrounding structures. Microscopically, they are composed of a variable admixture of spindle-shaped mesenchymal cells, including numerous myofibroblasts and a pleocytotic inflammatory infiltrate that may include foamy histiocytes and numerous plasma cells and lymphocytes (Fig 53.39). Occasional multinucleated giant cells are seen. In spite of their infiltrative nature, inflammatory pseudotumors are cured by surgical removal.

Metastatic tumors are uncommon in the spleen, perhaps because of the absence of splenic afferent lymphatics. Most cause tumor masses, but some may infiltrate the organ diffusely (Fig. 53.40).

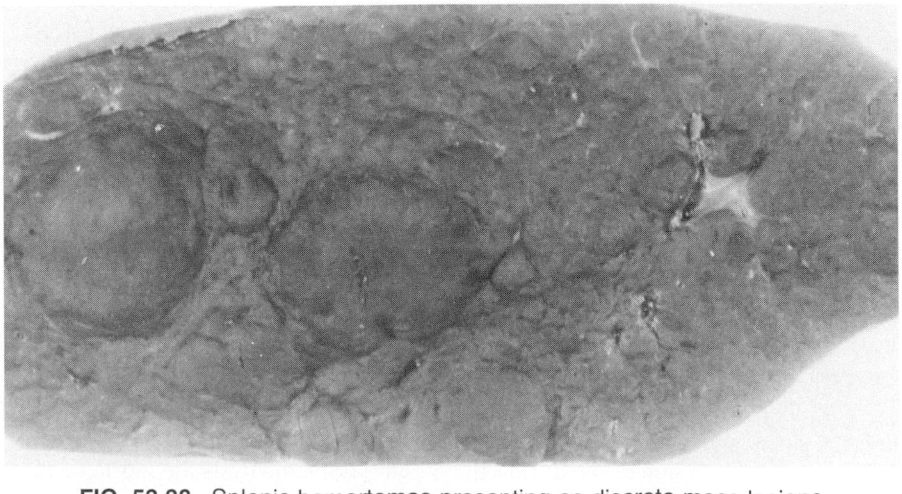

FIG. 53.38. Splenic hamartomas presenting as discrete mass lesions.

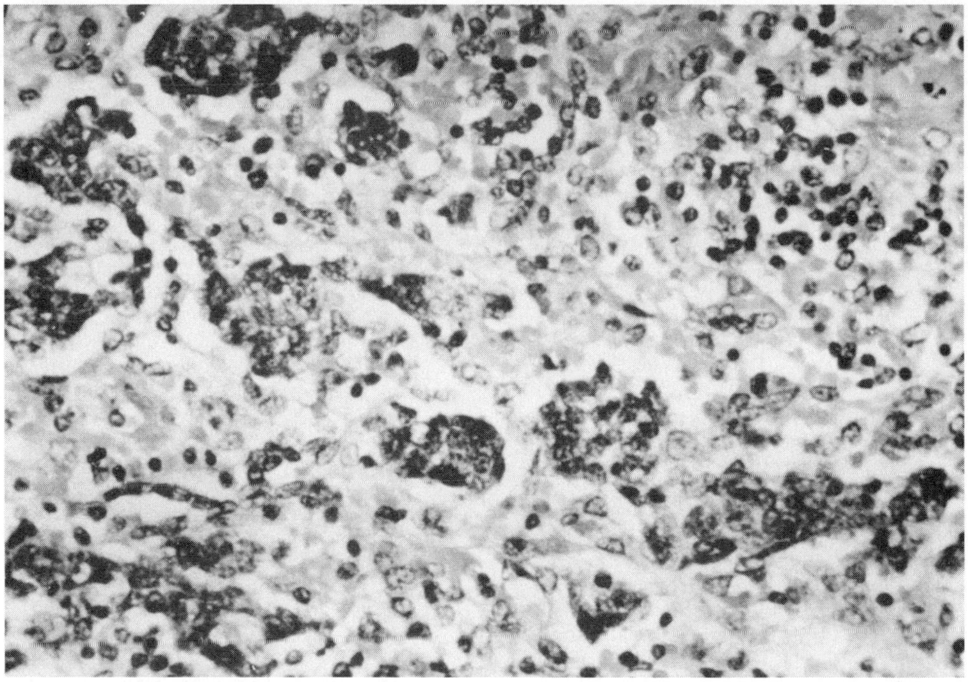

FIG. 53.40. Metastatic small cell carcinoma of the lung showing infiltration of the red pulp sinuses (periodic acid–Schiff stain, original magnification: 250× magnification).

SUMMARY AND CONCLUSIONS

Neoplastic disorders of the spleen are predominantly of hematopoietic origin. They rarely occur as isolated phenomena but are, in most patients, part of a systemic pattern of disease. They include various malignant lymphomas, lymphoid and myeloid leukemias, and myeloproliferative disorders. Lymphoid neoplasms almost invariably involve the white pulp but may involve the red pulp if leukemic or in certain T-cell malignancies. Leukemic and myeloproliferative disorders involve the red pulp. Most nonhematopoietic tumors of the spleen are benign and are composed of tissue elements that make up the vascular tissue of that organ (i.e., angiomas). Malignant nonhematopoietic tumors are uncommon and usually are vascular. Metastatic neoplasms in the spleen are uncommon.

REFERENCES

1. van Krieken JH, te Velde J. Normal histology of the human spleen. *Am J Surg Pathol* 1988;12:777–785.
2. Neiman RS, Orazi A. *Disorders of the spleen,* 2nd ed. Philadelphia: WB Saunders, 1998.
3. Grogan TM, Jolley CS, Rangel CS. Immunoarchitecture of the human spleen. *Lymphology* 1983;16:72–82.
4. Grogan TM, Rangel CS, Richter LC, et al. Further delineation of the immunoarchitecture of the human spleen. *Lymphology* 1984;17: 61–68.
5. Bishop MB, Lansing LS. The spleen: A correlative overview of normal and pathologic anatomy. *Hum Pathol* 1980;13:334–342.
6. Raviola E. Spleen. In: Fawcett DW, ed. *A textbook of histology,* 12th ed. New York: Chapman and Hall, 1994:460.
7. Lukes RJ. The pathology of the white pulp of the spleen. In: Lennert K, Harms D, eds. *Die milz.* Berlin: Springer-Verlag, 1970:130–138.
8. Millikin PD. Anatomy of germinal centers in human lymphoid tissue. *Arch Pathol* 1966;82:499–503.
9. Millikin PD. The nodular white pulp of the human spleen. *Arch Pathol* 1969;87:247–258.
10. Nossal GJV, Abbot A, Mitchell J, et al. Antigens in immunity: XV. Ultrastructural features of antigen capture in primary and secondary lymphoid follicles. *J Exp Med* 1968;127:277–290.
11. Hirasaw Y, Tokuhiro H. Electron microscopic studies on the normal human spleen: especially on the red pulp and the reticulo-endothelial cells. *Blood* 1970;35:201–212.
12. Rappaport H. The pathologic anatomy of the splenic red pulp. In: Lennert K, Harms D, eds. *Die milz.* Berlin: Springer-Verlag, 1970: 25–41.
13. Wennberg E, Weiss L. The structure of the spleen and hemolysis. *Annu Rev Med* 1969;20:29–40.
14. Weiss L. A scanning electron microscopic study of the spleen. *Blood* 1974;43:665–691.
15. Crosby WH. Splenic remodeling of red cell surfaces. *Blood* 1977;50: 643–645.
16. Hsu SM, Cossman J, Jaffe ES. Lymphocyte subsets in normal human lymphoid tissue. *Am J Clin Pathol* 1883;80:21–30.
17. Timens W, Poppema S. Lymphocyte compartments in human spleen. An immunohistologic study in normal spleens and non-involved spleens in Hodgkin's disease. *Am J Pathol* 1985;120:443–453.
18. Van Ewijk W, Nieuwenhuis P. Compartments, domains and migration pathways of lymphoid cells in the splenic pulp. *Experentia* 1985;41: 199–208.
19. Gutman GA, Weissman IL. Lymphoid tissue architecture: experimental analysis of the origin and distribution of T cells and B cells. *Immunology* 1972;23:465–479.
20. Stein H, Bonk A, Tolksdorf G, et al. Immunohistologic analysis of the organization of normal lymphoid tissue in non-Hodgkin's lymphomas. *J Histochem Cytochem* 1980;26:746–760.
21. Tonder P, Morse PA, Humphrey LJ. Similarities of Fc receptors in human malignant tissue and normal lymphoid tissue. *J Immunol* 1974; 113:1162–1169.
22. Lipson RL, Bayrd ED, Watkins CH. The postsplenectomy blood picture. *Am J Clin Pathol* 1959;32:526–532.
23. Singer K, Miller EB, Dameshek W. Hematologic changes following splenectomy in man with particular reference to target cells, hemolytic index and lysolecithin. *Am J Med Sci* 1941;202:171–187.

24. Kadin ME, Glatstein E, Dorfman RF. Clinicopathologic studies of 117 untreated patients subjected to laparotomy for the staging of Hodgkin's disease. *Cancer* 1971;27:1277–1294.
25. Mauch PM, Kalish LA, Kadin M, et al. Patterns of presentation of Hodgkin's disease. *Cancer* 1993;71:2062–2071.
26. Martinazzi M, Palatini M. A casual finding of primary splenic Hodgkin's disease in a case of traumatic rupture of the spleen. *Tumor* 1978; 64:639–643.
27. Kreamer BB, Osborne BM, Butler JJ. Primary splenic presentation of malignant lymphoma and related disorders. *Cancer* 1984;53: 1606–1613.
28. Re G, Lambertina F, Bucchi ML, et al. Primary splenic Hodgkin's disease: case report. *Pathologica* 1986;78:335–340.
29. Zellers RA, Thibodeau SN, Banks PM. Primary splenic Lymphocyte depletion Hodgkin's disease. *Am J Clin Pathol* 1990;94:453–457.
30. Brissette M, Dhru RD. Hodgkin's disease presenting as spontaneous splenic rupture. *Arch Pathol Lab Med* 1992;116:1077–1078.
31. Trudel M, Krikorian J, Neiman RS. Lymphocyte predominance Hodgkin's disease: clinical and morphologic heterogeneity. *Cancer* 1987; 59:99–106.
32. Neiman RS, Rosen PJ, Lukes RJ. Lymphocyte depletion Hodgkin's disease: a clinicopathologic entity. *N Engl J Med* 1973;288:751–755.
33. Hoppe RT, Cox RS, Rosenberg SA, et al. Prognostic factors in stage III Hodgkin's disease. *Cancer Treat Rep* 1982;66:743–749.
34. Hoppe RT, Rosenberg SA, Kaplan HS, et al. Prognostic factors in pathological state IIIA Hodgkin's disease. *Cancer* 1980;46: 1240–1246.
35. Askergren J, Bjorkholm M, Holm G, et al. On the size and tumor involvement of the spleen in Hodgkin's disease. *Acta Med Scand* 1981;209: 217– 220.
36. Colby TV, Hoppe RT, Warnke RA. Hodgkin's disease at autopsy: 1972–1977. *Cancer* 1981;47:1852–1862.
37. Glatstein E, Guernsey JM, Rosenberg SA, et al. The value of laparotomy and splenectomy in the staging of Hodgkin's disease. *Cancer* 1969;24:709–718.
38. Glatstein E, Trueblood HW, Enright LP, et al. Surgical staging of abdominal involvement in unselected patients with Hodgkin's disease. *Radiology* 1970;97:425–432.
39. Larson RA, Ultmann JE. The strategic role of laparotomy in staging Hodgkin's disease. *Cancer Treat Rep* 1982;66:767–773.
40. Sweet DL Jr, Kinnealey A, Ultmann JE. Hodgkin's disease. Problems of staging. *Cancer* 1978;42:957–970.
41. Rosenberg SA. Exploratory laparotomy and splenectomy for Hodgkin's disease: a commentary. *J Clin Oncol* 1988;6:574–575.
42. Dietrich PY, Henry-Amar M, Cosset JM, et al. Second primary cancers in patients continuously disease-free from Hodgkin's disease: a protective role for the spleen? *Blood* 1994;84:1209–1215.
43. Jockovich M, Mendenhall NP, Sombeck MD, et al. Long-term complications of laparotomy in Hodgkin's disease [Review]. *Ann Surg* 1994; 219:615–621.
44. Mauch P, Somers R. Controversies in the use of diagnostic staging laparotomy and splenectomy in the management of Hodgkin's disease. *Ann Oncol* 1992;4[Suppl 3]:41–43.
45. Marble KR, Deckers PJ, Kern KA. Changing role of splenectomy for hematologic disease. *J Surg Oncol* 1993;52:169–171.
46. Neiman RS. Current problems in the histopathologic diagnosis and classification of Hodgkin's disease. *Pathol Annu* 1978;2:289–328.
47. Desser PK, Moran EM, Ultmann JE. Staging of Hodgkin's disease and lymphoma. *Med Clin North Am* 1973;57:479–498.
48. Farrer-Brown G, Bennett MH, Harrison CV, et al. The diagnosis of Hodgkin's disease in surgically excised spleens. *J Clin Pathol* 1972; 25:294–300.
49. Neiman RS, Orazi A. *Disorders of the spleen,* 2nd ed. Philadelphia: WB Saunders, 1999.
50. Brincker H. Sarcoid reactions and sarcoidosis in Hodgkin's disease and other malignant lymphomata. *Br J Cancer* 1972;26:120–128.
51. Collins RD, Neiman RS. Granulomatous diseases of the spleen. In: Ioachim HL, ed. *Pathology of granulomas.* New York: Raven Press, 1983;189–207.
52. Kadin ME, Donaldson SS, Dorfman RF. Isolated granulomas in Hodgkin's disease. *N Engl J Med* 1970;283:859–861.
53. Neiman RS. Incidence and importance of splenic sarcoidal-like granulomas. *Arch Pathol Lab Med* 1977;101:518–521.
54. O'Connell MJ, Schimpff SC, Kirschner RH, et al. Epithelioid granulomas in Hodgkin's disease: a favorable prognostic sign. *JAMA* 1975; 233:886–890.
55. Sacks EL, Donaldson SS, Gordon J, et al. Epithelioid granulomas associated with Hodgkin's disease: clinical correlations in 55 previously untreated patients. *Cancer* 1978;41:562–567.
56. Lukes RJ. Criteria for involvement of lymph nodes, bone marrow, spleen and liver in Hodgkin's disease. *Cancer Res* 1971;31: 1755–1767.
57. Rappaport H, Berard CW, Butler JJ, et al. Report of the committee on histopathological criteria contributing to staging of Hodgkin's disease. *Cancer Res* 1971;31:1864–1865.
58. Hsu SM, Yang K, Jaffe ES. Phenotypic expression of Hodgkin's and Reed-Sternberg cells in Hodgkin's disease. *Am J Pathol* 1985;118: 209–217.
59. Dorfman RF, Gatter KC, Pulford KAF, et al. An evaluation of the utility of anti-granulocyte and anti-leukocyte monoclonal antibodies in the diagnosis of Hodgkin's disease. *Am J Pathol* 1986;123: 508–513.
60. Stein H, Uchanska-Ziegler B, Gerdes J, et al. Hodgkin and Sternberg-Reed cells contain antigens specific to late cells of granulopoiesis. *Int J Cancer* 1982;29:283–290.
61. Falini B, Stein H, Pileri S, et al. Expression of lymphoid-associated antigens on Hodgkin's and Reed-Sternberg cells of Hodgkin's disease: an immunocytochemical study on lymph node cytospins using monoclonal antibodies. *Histopathology* 1987;11:1229–1242.
62. Chittal SM, Caveriviere P, Schwarting R, et al. Monoclonal antibodies in the diagnosis of Hodgkin's disease. *Am J Surg Pathol* 1988;12: 9–21.
63. Stauchen JA. Leucocyte common antigen in the differential diagnosis of Hodgkin's disease. *Hematol Oncol* 1989;7:149–151.
64. Strickler JG, Michie SA, Warnke RA, et al. The "syncytial variant" of nodular sclerosing Hodgkin's disease. *Am J Surg Pathol* 1986;10: 470–477.
65. Nicholas DS, Harris S, Wright DH. Lymphocyte predominance Hodgkin's disease: an immunohistochemical study. *Histopathology* 1990; 16:157–165.
66. Schmid C, Pan L, Diss T, et al. Expression of B cell antigens by Hodgkin's and Reed-Sternberg cells in Hodgkin's disease. *Am J Pathol* 1991;139:701–707.
67. Zukerberg LR, Collins AB, Ferry JA, et al. Coexpression of CD15 and CD20 by Reed-Sternberg cells in Hodgkin's disease. *Am J Pathol* 1991;139:475–483.
68. Orazi A, Jiang B, Lee C-H, et al. Correlation between presence of clonal rearrangements of immunoglobulin heavy chain genes and B cell antigen expression in Hodgkin's disease. *Am J Clin Pathol* 1995; 104:413–418.
69. Arber DA, Weiss LM. CD15: a review. *Appl Immunohistochem* 1993; 1:17–25.
70. Siebert JD, Stuckey JH, Kurtin PJ, et al. Extranodal lymphocyte predominance Hodgkin's disease: clinical and pathologic features. *Am J Clin Pathol* 1995;103:485–491.
71. Chang KL, Kamel OW, Arber DA, et al. Pathologic features of nodular lymphocyte predominance Hodgkin's disease in extranodal sites. *Am J Surg Pathol* 1995;19:1313–1324.
72. Warnke RA, Weiss LM, Chan JKC, et al. Primary splenic lymphoma. In: *Atlas of tumor pathology: tumors of the lymph nodes and spleen.* Series 3, Fascicle 14. Washington: Armed Forces Institute of Pathology, 1995:411.
73. Bellamy CO, Krajewski AS. Primary splenic large cell anaplastic lymphoma associated with HIV infection. *Histopathology* 1994;24: 481–483.
74. Brox A, Bishinsky JI, Berry G. Primary non-Hodgkin lymphoma of the spleen. *Am J Hematol* 1991;38:95–100.
75. Brox A, Shustik C. Non-Hodgkin's lymphoma of the spleen. *Leuk Lymphoma* 1993;11:165–171.
76. Das Gupta T, Coombes B, Brasfeld RD. Primary malignant neoplasms of the spleen. *Surg Gynecol Obstet* 1965;120:947–959.
77. Falk S, Karhoff M, Takeshita M, et al. Primary pleomorphic T cell lymphoma of the spleen. *Histopathology* 1990;16:191–2.
78. Fausel R, Sun NC, Klein S. Splenic rupture in HIV-infected patient with primary splenic lymphoma. *Cancer* 1990;66:2414–2416.
79. Hara K, Ito M, Shimizu K, et al. Three cases of primary splenic lymphoma: case report and review of the Japanese literature. *Acta Pathol Jpn* 1985:35:419–435.

80. Harris NL, Aisenberg AC, Meyer JE, et al. Diffuse large cell (histiocytic) lymphoma of the spleen: clinical and pathologic characteristics of ten cases. *Cancer* 1984;53:2460–2467.
81. Ishihara T, Takahashi M, Uchino F, et al. A filiform large cell lymphoma of the spleen: a case report with immunohistochemical and electron microscopic study. *Ultrastruct Pathol* 1990:14:193–199.
82. Kobrich U, Falk S, Karhoff M, et al. Primary large cell lymphoma of the splenic sinuses: a variant of angiotropic B cell lymphoma (neoplastic angioendotheliomatosis)? *Hum Pathol* 1992;23:1184–1187.
83. Montanaro A, Patten R. Primary splenic malignant lymphoma, histiocytic type, with sclerosis. *Cancer* 1976;38:1625–1628.
84. Spier CM, Kjeldsberg CR, Eyre HJ, et al. Malignant lymphoma with primary presentation in the spleen: a study of 20 patients. *Arch Pathol Lab Med* 1985;109:1076–1080.
85. Weide R, Gorg C, Pfluger KH, et al. Concomitant primary low grade non-Hodgkin's lymphoma of the spleen and breast carcinoma. *Leuk Lymphoma* 1992;7:337–339.
86. Falk S, Stutte JJ. Primary malignant lymphomas of the spleen, a morphologic and immunohistochemical analysis of 17 cases. *Cancer* 1990;66:2612–2613.
87. Kim H, Dorfman RF. Morphological studies of 84 untreated patients subjected to laparotomy for the staging of non-Hodgkin's lymphomas. *Cancer* 1974;33:657–676.
88. Lotz MJ, Chabner B, DeVita VT, et al. Pathological staging of 100 consecutive untreated patients with non-Hodgkin's lymphomas. *Cancer* 1976;37:266–270.
89. Goffinet DR, Warnke R, Dunnick NR, et al. Clinical and surgical (laparotomy) evaluation of patients with non-Hodgkin's lymphomas. *Cancer Treat Rep* 1977;61:981–992.
90. Burke JS. Diagnosis of lymphoma and lymphoid proliferations in the spleen. In: Jaffe ES, ed. *Surgical pathology of the lymph nodes and related organs,* 2nd ed. Philadelphia: WB Saunders, 1995:448.
91. Mann RB. Follicular lymphoma and lymphocytic lymphoma of intermediate differentiation. In: Jaffe ES, ed. *Surgical pathology of the lymph nodes and related organs.* Philadelphia: WB Saunders, 1985: 165–202.
92. Pangalis GA, Nathwani BN, Rappaport H. Malignant lymphoma, well differentiated lymphocytic: its relationship with chronic lymphocytic leukemia and macroglobulinemia of Waldenström. *Cancer* 1977;39: 999–1010.
93. Narang S, Wolf BC, Neiman RS. Malignant lymphoma presenting with prominent splenomegaly: a clinicopathologic study with special reference to intermediate cell lymphoma. *Cancer* 1985;55: 1948–1957.
94. Ahmann DL, Kiely JM, Harrison EG Jr, et al. Malignant lymphoma of the spleen: a review of 49 cases in which the diagnosis was made at splenectomy. *Cancer* 1966;19:461–469.
95. Long JC, Aisenberg AC. Malignant lymphoma diagnosed at splenectomy and idiopathic splenomegaly. *Cancer* 1974;33:1053–1061.
96. Arber DA, Rappaport H, Weiss LM. Non-Hodgkin's lymphoproliferative disorders involving the spleen. *Mod Pathol* 1997;10:18–32.
97. Evans HL, Butler JJ, Youness EL. Malignant lymphoma, small lymphocytic type: a clinicopathologic study of 84 cases with suggested criteria for intermediate lymphocytic lymphoma. *Cancer* 1978; 41:1440–1455.
98. Palutke M, Tabaczka P, Mirchandani I, et al. Lymphocytic lymphoma simulating hairy cell leukemia: a consideration of reliable and unreliable diagnostic features. *Cancer* 1981;48:2047–2055.
99. Malignant lymphoma, small lymphocytic and diffuse small cleaved cell (centrocytic). In: Warnke RA, Weiss LM, Chan JKC, et al, eds. *Atlas of tumor pathology: tumors of the lymph nodes and spleen.* Series 3, Fascicle 14. Washington: Armed Forces Institute of Pathology, 1995:119.
100. Dick FR. Small lymphocytic malignancies and related immunoproliferative disorders. In: Jaffe ES, ed. *Surgical pathology of the lymph nodes and related organs,* 2nd ed. Philadelphia: WB Saunders, 1995: 205.
101. Sundeen JT, Longo DL, Jaffe ES. CD5 expression in B cell small lymphocytic malignancies: correlations with clinical presentation and sites of disease. *Am J Surg Pathol* 1992:16:130–137.
102. Harris NL, Jaffe ES, Stein H, et al. A revised European-American classification of lymphoid neoplasms: a proposal from the International Lymphoma Study Group. *Blood* 1994;84:1361–1392.
103. Pittaluga S, Verhoef G, Criel A, et al. "Small" B cell non-Hodgkin's lymphomas with splenomegaly at presentation are either mantle cell lymphoma or marginal zone cell lymphoma. *Am J Surg Pathol* 1996; 20:211–223.
104. Weisenburger DD, Linder J, Daley DT, et al. Intermediate lymphocytic lymphoma: an immunohistologic study with comparison to other lymphocytic lymphomas. *Hum Pathol* 1987;18:781–790.
105. Weisenburger DD, Kim H, Rappaport H. Mantle zone lymphoma: a follicular variant of intermediate lymphocytic lymphoma. *Cancer* 1982;49:1429–1438.
106. Yang WI, Zukerberg LR, Motokura T, et al. Cyclin D1 (BCL-1, PRAD1) protein expression in low-grade B cell lymphomas and reactive hyperplasia. *Am J Pathol* 1994;145:86–96.
107. Zukerberg LR, Yang WI, Arnold A. Cyclin D1 expression in non-Hodgkin's lymphomas: detection by immunohistochemistry. *Am J Clin Pathol* 1995;103:756–760.
108. Lukes RJ, Parker JW, Taylor CR, et al. Immunologic approach to non-Hodgkin's lymphomas and related leukemias: analysis of the results of multiparameter studies of 425 cases. *Semin Hematol* 1978;15: 322–325.
109. Sheibani K, Burke JS, Swartz WG, et al. Monocytoid B cell lymphoma: clinicopathologic study of 21 cases of a unique type of low-grade lymphoma. *Cancer* 1988;62:1531–1538.
110. Agnarsson BA, Kadin ME. An unusual B cell lymphoma simulating hairy cell leukemia. *Am J Clin Pathol* 1987;88:752–759.
111. Ngan B-Y, Warnke RA, Wilson M, et al. Monocytoid B cell lymphoma: a study of 36 cases. *Hum Pathol* 1991;22:409–421.
112. Traweek ST, Sheibani K. Monocytoid B cell lymphoma: the biologic and clinical implications of peripheral blood involvement. *Am J Clin Pathol* 1992;97:591–598.
113. Vasef M, Katzin WE. Monocytoid B cell lymphoma with a distinctive clinical presentation. *Hum Pathol* 1993;24:558–561.
114. Mollejo M, Menarguez J, Cristobal E, et al. Monocytoid B cells: a comparative clinical pathological study of their distribution in different types of low-grade lymphomas. *Am J Surg Pathol* 1994;18: 1131–1139.
115. Stroup RM, Burke JS, Sheibani K, et al. Splenic involvement by aggressive malignant lymphomas of B cell and T cell types: a morphologic and immunophenotypic study. *Cancer* 1992;69:413–420.
116. Betman HF, Vardiman JW, Lau J. T cell rich B cell lymphoma of the spleen. Letter to the editor. *Am J Surg Pathol* 1994;18:323–324.
117. Brownell MD, Sheibani K, Battifora H, et al. Distinction between undifferentiated (small noncleaved) and lymphoblastic lymphoma: an immunohistologic study on paraffin-embedded, fixed tissue sections. *Am J Surg Pathol* 1987;11:779–787.
118. Lardelli P, Bookman MA, Sundeen J, et al. Lymphocytic lymphoma of intermediate differentiation: morphologic and immunophenotypic spectrum and clinical correlations. *Am J Surg Pathol* 1990;14: 752–763.
119. Orazi A, Cattoretti G, John K, et al. Terminal deoxynucleotidyl transferase staining of malignant lymphomas in paraffin sections. *Mod Pathol* 1994:7:582–763.
120. Orazi A, Cotton J, Cattoretti G, et al. Terminal deoxynucleotidyl transferase staining in acute leukemia and normal bone marrow in routinely processed paraffin sections. *Am J Clin Pathol* 1994;102:640–645.
121. Robertson PB, Neiman RS, Worapongpaiboon S, et al. 013 (CD99) positivity in hematologic proliferations correlates with TdT positivity. *Mod Pathol* 1997;10:277–282.
122. Grogan TM, Warnke RA, Kaplan HS. A comparative study of Burkitt's and non-Burkitt's "undifferentiated" malignant lymphoma: immunologic, cytochemical, ultrastructural, histopathologic, clinical and cell culture features. *Cancer* 1982;49:1817–1828.
123. Banks PM, Arseneau JC, Gralnick HR, et al. American Burkitt's lymphoma: a clinicopathologic study of 30 cases. II. Pathologic correlations. *Am J Med* 1975;58:322–329.
124. Mann RB, Jaffe ES, Braylan RC, et al. Non-endemic Burkitt's lymphoma: a B cell tumor related to germinal centers. *N Engl J Med* 1976;295:685–691.
125. Jaffe ES. Post-thymic lymphoid neoplasia. In: Jaffe ES, ed. *Surgical pathology of the lymph nodes and related organs,* 2nd ed. Philadelphia: WB Saunders, 1985:344.
126. Rappaport H, Thomas LB. Mycosis fungoides: the pathology of extracutaneous involvement. *Cancer* 1974;34:1198–1129.
127. Variakojis D, Rosas-Uribe A, Rappaport H. Mycosis fungoides:

pathologic findings in staging laparotomies. *Cancer* 1974;33: 1589–1600.
128. Waldron JA, Leech JH, Glick AD, et al. Malignant lymphoma of peripheral T-lymphocyte origin: immunologic, pathologic, and clinical features in six patients. *Cancer* 1977;40:1604–1617.
129. Brisbane JU, Berman LD, Neiman RS. Peripheral T cell lymphoma: a clinicopathologic study of nine cases. *Am J Clin Pathol* 1983;79: 285–293.
130. Weinberg DS, Pinkus GS. Non-Hodgkin's lymphoma of large multilobated cell type: a clinicopathologic study of ten cases. *Am J Clin Pathol* 1981;76:190–196.
131. Lennert K, Mestdagh J. Lymphogranulomatoses mit konstant hohem epithelioid zell gehalt. *Virchows Arch* 1968;344:1–20.
132. Burke JS, Butler JJ. Malignant lymphoma with a high content of epithelioid histiocytes (Lennert's lymphoma). *Am J Clin Pathol* 1976; 66:1–3.
133. Gray D, Kumararatne DS, Lortan J, et al. Relation of intra-splenic migration of marginal zone B cells to antigen localization on follicular dendritic cells. *Immunology* 1984;52:659–663.
134. Hsu SM. Phenotypic expression of B lymphocytes: III. Marginal zone B cells in the spleen are characterized by the expression of Tac and Alkaline Phosphatase. *J Immunol* 1985;135:123–130.
135. MacLennan ICM, Liu YJ, Oldfield S, et al. The evolution of B cell clones. *Curr Top Microbiol Immunol* 1990;159:37–63.
136. van Krieken JHJM, von Schilling C, Kluin M, et al. Splenic marginal zone lymphocytes and related cells in the lymph node: a morphologic and immunohistochemical study. *Hum Pathol* 1989;20:320–325.
137. Van den Oord JJ, De Wolf-Peeters C, Desmet VJ. The marginal zone in the human reactive lymph node. *Am J Clin Pathol* 1986;86: 475–479.
138. Spencer J, Finn T, Pulford KAF, et al. The human gut contains a novel population of B lymphocytes which resemble marginal zone cells. *Clin Exp Immunol* 1985;62:607–612.
139. Myhre MJ, Isaacson PG. Primary B cell gastric lymphoma: a reassessment of its histogenesis. *J Pathol* 1987;152:1–11.
140. Smith-Ravin J, Spencer J, Beverley PCL, et al. Characterization of two monoclonal antibodies (UCL4D12 and UCL3D3) that discriminate between human mantle zone and marginal zone B cells. *Clin Exp Immunol* 1990;82:181–187.
141. Spencer J, Diss TC, Isaacson PG. A study of the properties of a low-grade mucosal B cell lymphoma using a monoclonal antibody specific for the tumor immunoglobulin. *J Pathol* 1990;160:231–238.
142. Isaacson PG, Matutes E, Burke M, et al. The histopathology of splenic lymphoma with villous lymphocytes. *Blood* 1994;84:3828–3834.
143. Schmid C, Kirkham N, Diss T, et al. Splenic marginal zone cell lymphoma. *Am J Surg Pathol* 1992;16:455.
144. Pawade J, Wilkins BS, Wright DH. Low-grade B cell lymphomas of the splenic marginal zone: a clinicopathological and immunohistochemical study of 14 cases. *Histopathology* 1995;27:129–137.
145. Swerdlow SH, Zukerberg LR, Yang W-I, et al. The morphologic spectrum of non-Hodgkin's lymphomas with BCL-1/Cyclin D1 gene rearrangements. *Am J Surg Pathol* 1996;20:627–640.
146. Mollejo M, Menarguez J, Lloret E, et al. Splenic marginal zone lymphoma: a distinctive type of low-grade B cell lymphoma. A clinicopathological study of 13 cases. *Am J Surg Pathol* 1995;19:1146–1157.
147. Palutke M, Eisenberg L, Narang S, et al. B lymphocytic lymphoma (large cell) of possible splenic marginal zone origin presenting with prominent splenomegaly and unusual cordal red pulp distribution. *Cancer* 1988;62:593–600.
148. Cousar JB, McKee LC, Greco FA, et al. Report of an unusual B cell lymphoma, probably arising from the perifollicular cells (marginal zone) of the spleen. *Lab Invest* 1980;42;109A(abst).
149. Sendelbach KM, Pugh WC, Rodriguez J, et al. Splenic marginal zone lymphoma (MGZL): clinical and pathologic characteristics of 11 cases. *Mod Pathol* 1994;7:120A(abst).
150. Rosso R, Neiman RS, Paulli M, et al. Splenic marginal zone cell lymphoma: report of an indolent variant without massive splenomegaly presumably representing an early phase of the disease. *Hum Pathol* 1995;26:39–46.
151. Dierlamm J, Pittaluga S, Wlodarska I, et al. Marginal zone B cell lymphomas of different sites share similar cytogenetic and morphologic features. *Blood* 1996;87:299–307.
152. Mollejo M, Lloret E, Menarguez J, et al. Lymph node involvement by splenic marginal zone lymphoma: morphological and immunohistochemical features. *Am J Surg Pathol* 1997;21:772–780.
153. Dunphy CH, Bee C, McDonald JW, et al. Incidental early detection of a splenic marginal zone lymphoma by polymerase chain reaction analysis of paraffin-embedded tissue. *Arch Pathol Lab Med* 1998; 122:84–86.
154. Harris S, Wilkins BS, Jones DB. Splenic marginal zone expansion in B cell lymphomas of gastrointestinal mucosa-associated lymphoid tissue (MALT) is reactive and does not represent homing of neoplastic lymphocytes. *J Pathol* 1996;179:49–53.
155. Farhi DC, Ashfaq R. Splenic pathology after traumatic injury. *Am J Clin Pathol* 1996;105:474–478.
156. Kroft SH, Singleton TP, Dahiya M, et al. Ruptured spleens with expanded marginal zones do not reveal occult B cell clones. *Mod Pathol* 1997;10:1214–1220.
157. Neiman RS, Sullivan AL, Jaffe R. Malignant lymphoma simulating leukemic reticuloendotheliosis. *Cancer* 1979;43:329–342.
158. Spriano P, Barosi G, Invernizzi R, et al. Splenomegalic immunocytoma with circulating hairy cells: review of eight cases and revision of the literature. *Haematologica* 1986;71:25–33.
159. Melo JV, Hegde U, Parreira A, et al. Splenic B cell lymphoma with circulating villous lymphocytes: differential diagnosis of B cell leukaemias with large spleens. *J Clin Pathol* 1987;40:642– 651.
160. Melo JV, Robinson DS, Gregory C, et al. Splenic B cell lymphoma with "villous" lymphocytes in the peripheral blood: a disorder distinct from hairy cell leukemia. *Leukemia* 1987;1:294–298.
161. Mulligan SP, Catovsky D. Splenic lymphoma with villous lymphocytes. *Leuk Lymphoma* 1992;6:97–103.
162. Franco V, Florena AM, Campesi G. Intrasinusoidal bone marrow infiltration: a possible hallmark of splenic lymphoma. *Histopathology* 1996;29:571–575.
163. Labouyrie E, Marit G, Vial J, et al. Intrasinusoidal bone marrow involvement by splenic lymphoma with villous lymphocytes: a helpful immunohistologic feature. *Mod Pathol* 1997;10:1015–1020.
164. Matutes E, Morilla R, Owusu-Ankomah K, et al. The immunophenotype of splenic lymphoma with villous lymphocytes and its relevance to the differential diagnosis with other B cell disorders. *Blood* 1994; 83:1558–1562.
165. Dyer MJ, Zani VJ, Lu WZ, et al. BCL-2 translocations in leukemias of mature B cells. *Blood* 1994;83:3682–3688.
166. Jadayel D, Matutes E, Dyer MJ, et al. Splenic lymphoma with villous lymphocytes: analysis of BCL-1 rearrangements and expression of the cyclin D1 gene. *Blood* 1994;83:3664–3671.
167. Sun T, Susin M, Brody J, et al. Splenic lymphoma with circulating villous lymphocytes: report of seven cases and review of the literature. *Am J Hematol* 1994;45:39–50.
168. Sun T, Dittmar K, Koduru P, et al. Relationship between hairy cell leukemia variant and splenic lymphoma with villous lymphocytes: Presentation of a new concept. *Am J Hematol* 1996;51:282–288.
169. Dargent JL, Delville JP, Kornreich A, et al. Morphologic and phenotypic changes of the leukemic cells in a case of marginal zone B cell lymphoma. *Ann Hematol* 1997;74:149–153.
170. Bates I, Bedu-Addo G, Rutherford TR, et al. Circulating villous lymphocytes: a link between hyperreactive malarial splenomegaly and splenic lymphoma. *Trans R Soc Trop Med Hyg* 1997;91:171–174.
171. Bates I, Bedu-Ado G. Chronic malaria and splenic lymphoma: clues to understanding lymphoma evolution. *Leukemia* 1997;11:2162–2167.
172. de Figueiredo M, Lima M, Macedo G, et al. Association of splenic lymphoma with villous lymphocytes and primary biliary cirrhosis in a man [Letter]. *Sangre* 1996:41:71.
173. Murakami H, Irisawa H, Saitoh T, et al. Immunological abnormalities in splenic marginal zone cell lymphoma. *Am J Hematol* 1997;56: 173–178.
174. Farcet JP, Gaulard P, Marolleau JP, et al. Hepatosplenic T cell lymphoma: sinusal/sinusoidal localization of malignant cells expressing the T cell receptor $\gamma\delta$. *Blood* 1990;75;2213–2219.
175. Cooke CB, Greiner T, Raffeld M, et al. Gamma delta T cell lymphoma, a distinct clinicopathologic entity. *Mod Pathol* 1994;7:106A(abst).
176. Krishnan J, Goodman Z, Frizzera G. Primary hepatic sinusoidal presentation of malignant T cell lymphoma. *Mod Pathol* 1992;5: 81A(abst).
177. Sun T, Brody J, Susin M, et al. Extranodal T cell lymphoma mimicking malignant histiocytosis. *Am J Hematol* 1990;35:269–274.
178. Wong KF, Chan JK, Matutes E, et al. Hepatosplenic gamma delta T

cell lymphoma: a distinctive aggressive lymphoma type. *Am J Surg Pathol* 1995;6:718–726.
179. Kadin ME, Kamoun M, Lamberg J. Erythrophagocytic T-gamma lymphoma: a clinicopathologic entity resembling malignant histiocytosis. *N Engl J Med* 1981;304:648–653.
180. Francois A, Lesesve J-F, Stamatoullas A, et al. Hepatosplenic gamma/delta T cell lymphoma: a report of two cases in immunocompromised patients, associated with isochromosome 7q. *Am J Surg Pathol* 1997; 21:781–790.
181. Santini GF, Crovatto M, Modolo ML, et al. Waldenström macroglobulinemia: a role of HCV infection? *Blood* 1993;82:2932.
182. Ferri C, Caracciolo F, Zignego AL, et al. Hepatitis C virus infection in patients with non-Hodgkin's lymphoma. *Br J Haematol* 1994;88: 392–386.
183. Pozzato G, Mazzaro C, Crovatto M, et al. Low-grade malignant lymphoma, hepatitis C virus infection, and mixed cryoglobulinemia. *Blood* 1994;84:3047–3053.
184. Mussini C, Ghini M, Mascia MT, et al. Monoclonal gammopathies and hepatitis C virus infection. *Blood* 1995;85:1144–1145.
185. Murakami Y, Hotei H, Tsumura H, et al. A case of primary splenic malignant lymphoma and a review of 98 cases reported in Japan. *J Jpn Soc Clin Surg* 1988;49:716–723.
186. Naschitz JE, Zuckerman E, Elias N, et al. Primary hepatosplenic lymphoma of the B cell variety in a patient with hepatitis C liver cirrhosis. *Am J Gastroenterol* 1994;89:1915–1916.
187. De Vita S, Sansonno D, Dolcetti R, et al. Hepatitis C virus within a malignant lymphoma lesion in the course of type II mixed cryoglobulinemia. *Blood* 1995;86:1887–1992.
188. Izumi T, Sasaki R, Miura Y, et al. Primary hepatosplenic lymphoma: association with hepatitis C virus infection. *Blood* 1996;87: 5380–5381.
189. Izumi T, Sasaki R, Tsunoda S, et al. B cell malignancy and hepatitis C virus infection. *Leukemia* 1997;11:516–518.
190. Wotherspoon AC, Ortiz-Hidalgo C, Falzon MR, et al. Helicobacter pylori-associated gastritis and primary B cell gastric lymphoma. *Lancet* 1991;338:1175–1176.
191. Hussel T, Isaacson PG, Crabtree JE, et al. The response of cells from low-grade B cell gastric lymphomas of mucosa-associated lymphoid tissue to *Helicobacter pylori*. *Lancet* 1993;342:571–574.
192. Boyko WJ, Pratt R, Wass H. Functional hyposplenism, a diagnostic clue in amyloidosis: report of six cases. *Am J Clin Pathol* 1982;77: 745–748.
193. Frangione B, Franklin EC. Heavy chain diseases: clinical features and molecular significance of the disordered immunoglobulin structure. *Semin Hematol* 1973;10:53–64.
194. Kyle RA, Greipp PR, Banks PM. The diverse picture of gamma heavy-chain diseases: report of seven cases and review of the literature. *Mayo Clin Proc* 1981;56:439–451.
195. Kyle RA, Greipp PR. Heavy chain diseases, section III: myeloma and related disorders. In: Wiernik PH, Canellos GP, Kyle RA, et al, eds. *Neoplastic diseases of the blood,* 2nd ed. New York: Churchill Livingston, 1991:153.
196. Seligmann M, Mihaesco E, Preud'homme JL, et al. Heavy chain disease: current findings and concepts. *Immunol Rev* 1979;48;145–167.
197. Franklin EC. Mu chain disease. *Arch Intern Med* 1975;153;71–72.
198. Jonsson V, Videbaek A, Axelsen NH, et al. Mu chain disease in a case of chronic lymphocytic leukemia and malignant histyocytoma: I. Clinical aspects. *Scand J Haematol* 1976;16:209–217.
199. Azar HA. Plasma cell myelomatosis and other monoclonal gammapathies. *Pathol Annu* 1972;7;1–17.
200. Schey S. Osteosclerotic myeloma and "POEMS" syndrome. *Blood Rev* 1996;10:75–80.
201. Bardwick PA, Zvaifler NG, Gill GN, et al. Plasma cell dyscrasia with polyneuropathy, organomegaly, endocrinopathy, M protein and skin changes: the POEMS syndrome. *Medicine* 1980;59:311–322.
202. Kobayashi H, Ii K, Sono T, et al. Plasma-cell dyscrasia with polyneuropathy and endocrine disorders associated with dysfunction of salivary glands. *Am J Surg Pathol* 1985;9:759–768.
203. Takatsuki K, Sanada I. Plasma cell dyscrasia with polyneuropathy and endocrine disorders (clinical aspects). *Pathol Clin Med* 1983;12: 1663–1668.
204. Takatsuki K, Yodoi J, Uchiyama T, et al. Plasma cell dyscrasia with polyneuropathy and endocrine disorders: review of 36 cases. *Neurol Med* 1977:483–493.
205. Polliack A, Rachmilewitz D, Zlotnick A. Plasma cell leukemia. *Arch Intern Med* 1974;134:131–134.
206. Stephens PJT, Hudson P. Spontaneous rupture of the spleen in plasma cell leukemia. *Can Med Assoc J* 1969;100:31–34.
207. Ustun C, Sungur C, Akbas O, et al. Spontaneous splenic rupture as the initial presentation of plasma cell leukemia: a case report. *Am J Hematol* 1998;57:266–267.
208. Cohen RJ, Bohannon RA, Wallerstein RO. Waldenström's macroglobulinemia: a study of ten cases. *Am J Med* 1966;41:274–284.
209. MacKenzie MR, Fudenberg HH. Macroglobulinemia: an analysis of forty patients. *Blood* 1972;39:874–889.
210. Waldenström J. Incipient myelomatosis or "essential" hyperglobulinemia with fibrinogenopenia a new syndrome? *Acta Med Scand* 1944; 117:216–244.
211. Cohen RJ, Bohannon RA, Wallerstein RO. Waldenström's macroglobulinemia: a study of ten cases. *Am J Med* 1966;41:274–284.
212. Berman HH. Waldenström's macroglobulinemia with lytic osseous lesions and plasma-cell morphology. *Am J Clin Pathol* 1975;63: 397–402.
213. Rywlin AM, Civantos F, Ortega RS, et al. Bone marrow histology in monoclonal macroglobulinemia. *Am J Clin Pathol* 1975;63:769–778.
214. Burke JS. Surgical pathology of the spleen: an approach to the differential diagnosis of splenic lymphomas and leukemias. Part II. Diseases of the red pulp. *Am J Surg Pathol* 1981;5:681–694.
215. Flood MJ, Carpenter RA. Spontaneous rupture of the spleen in acute myeloid leukemia. *Br Med J* 1961;1:35–36.
216. Greenfield MM, Lund II. Spontaneous rupture of the spleen in chronic myeloid leukemia. *Ohio Med J* 1944;40:950–951.
217. Sarin LR, Sarin JC. Spontaneous rupture of the spleen in chronic myeloid leukemia. *J Indian Med Assoc* 1957;29:286–289.
218. Pinkus GS, Pinkus JL. Myeloperoxidase: a specific marker for myeloid cells in parraffin sections. *Mod Pathol* 1991; 4:733.
219. Rosenthal S, Canellos GP, DeVita VT, et al. Characteristics of blast crisis in chronic granulocytic leukemia. *Blood* 1977;49:705–714.
220. Shaw MT, Bottomley RH, Grozea PN, et al. Heterogeneity of morphological, cytochemical, and cytogenetic features in the blastic phase of chronic granulocytic leukemia. *Cancer* 1975;35:199–207.
221. Baccarani M, Zaccaria A, Santucci AM, et al. A simultaneous study of bone marrow, spleen, and liver in chronic myeloid leukemia: evidence for differences in cell composition and karyotypes. *Ser Haematol* 1975;8:81–112.
222. Brandt L. Comparative study of bone marrow and extramedullary haematopoietic tissue in chronic myeloid leukaemia. *Ser Haematol* 1975;8:75–80.
223. Brandt L, Schnell CR. Granulopoiesis in bone marrow and spleen in chronic myeloid leukaemia. *Scand J Haematol* 1969;6:65–68.
224. Mitelman F. Comparative cytogenetic studies of bone marrow and extramedullary tissues in chronic myeloid leukemia. *Ser Haematol* 1975;8:113–117.
225. Stoll C, Oberling F, Flori E. Chromosome analysis of spleen and/or lymph node of patients with chronic myeloid leukemia. *Blood* 1978; 52:828–838.
226. Mitelman F, Brandt L, Nilsson PG. Cytogenetic evidence for splenic origin of blastic transformation in chronic myeloid leukemia. *Scand J Haematol* 1974;13:87–92.
227. Zaccaria A, Baccarani M, Barbieri E, et al. Differences in marrow and spleen karyotype in early chronic myeloid leukemia. *Eur J Cancer* 1975;11:123–126.
228. Griesshammer M, Heinze B, Bangerter M, et al. Karyotype abnormalities and their clinical significance in blast crisis of chronic myeloid leukemia. *J Mol Med* 1997;75:836–838.
229. Brandt L. Differences in the proliferative activity of myelocytes from bone marrow, spleen, and peripheral blood in chronic myeloid leukemia. *Scand J Haematol* 1969;6:105–112.
230. Brandt L. Difference in uptake of tritiated thymidine by myelocytes from bone marrow and spleen in chronic myeloid leukaemia. *Scand J Haematol* 1973;11:23–26.
231. Bouvet M, Babiera GV, Termuhlen PM, et al. Splenectomy in the accelerated or blastic phase of chronic myelogenous leukemia: a single-institution, 25-year experience. *Surgery* 1997;122:20–25.
232. Boggs DR. Hematopoietic stem cell theory in relation to possible lymphoblastic conversion of chronic myeloid leukemia. *Blood* 1974; 44:449–453.

233. Hogan SF, Osborne BM, Butler JJ. Unexpected splenic nodules in leukemic patients. *Hum Pathol* 1989;20:62–68.
234. Idhe DC, Canellos GP, Schwartz JA, et al. Splenectomy in the chronic phase of chronic granulocytic leukemia. *Ann Intern Med* 1976;84: 17–21.
235. Spiers ASD, Baikie AG, Galton DAG, et al. Chronic granulocytic leukemia: effect of elective splenectomy and the course of the disease. *Br Med J* 1975;1:175–179.
236. Bearman RM, Kjeldsberg CR, Pangalis GA, et al. Chronic monocytic leukemia in adults. *Cancer* 1981; 48:2239–2255.
237. Hansen MM. Chronic lymphocytic leukemia: clinical studies based on 189 cases followed for a long time. *Scand J Haematol* 1973[Suppl 18]:3–152.
238. Videbaek A, Christensen BE, Jonsson V. *The spleen in health and disease.* Chicago: Year Book Medical Publishers, 1982:79.
239. Christensen BE. Effects of an enlarged splenic erythrocyte pool in chronic lymphocytic leukemia: mechanism of erythrocyte sequestration in the spleen and liver. *Scand J Haematol* 1971;8:92–103.
240. Binet JL, Leporrier M, Dighiero G, et al. A clinical staging system for chronic lymphocytic leukemia: prognostic significance. *Cancer* 1977;40:855–864.
241. Rai KR, Sawitsky A, Cronkite EP, et al. Clinical staging of chronic lymphocytic leukemia. *Blood* 1975;46:219–234.
242. Adler S, Stutzman L, Sokal JE, et al. Splenectomy for hematologic depression in lymphocytic lymphoma. *Cancer* 1975;35:521–528.
243. Seymour JF, Cusack JD, Lerner SA, et al. Case/control study of the role of splenectomy in chronic lymphocytic leukemia. *J Clin Oncol* 1997;15:52–60.
244. Neal TF Jr, Tefferi A, Witzig TE, et al. Splenectomy advances chronic lymphocytic leukemia: a single institution experience with 50 patients. *Am J Med* 1992;93:435–440.
245. Aisenberg AE, Wilkes BM, Harris NL, et al. Chronic T cell lymphocytosis with neutropenia: report of a case study with monoclonal antibody. *Blood* 1981;58:812–822.
246. Brisbane JU, Berman LD, Osband ME, et al. T8 chronic lymphocytic leukemia: a distinctive disorder related to T8 lymphocytosis. *Am J Clin Pathol* 1983;80:391–396.
247. Pandolfi F, Loughran TP Jr, Starkebaum G, et al. Clinical course and prognosis of the lymphoproliferative disease of granular lymphocytes: a multicenter study. *Cancer* 1990;65:341–348.
248. Scott CS, Richards SJ, Sivakumaran M, et al. Transient and persistent expansions of large granular lymphocytes (LGL) and NK-associated (Nka) cells: the Yorkshire Leukaemia Group Study. *Br J Haematol* 1993;83:505–515.
249. Okuno SH, Tefferi A, Hannson CA, et al. Spectrum of diseases associated with increased proportions or absolute numbers of peripheral blood natural killer cells. *Br J Haematol* 1996;93:810–812.
250. Maciejewski JP, Hibbs JR, Anderson S, et al. Bone marrow and peripheral blood lymphocyte phenotype in patients with bone marrow failure. *Exp Hematol* 1994;22:1102–1110.
251. Loughran TP Jr, Kadin ME, Starkebaum G, et al. Leukemia of large granular lymphocytes: association with clonal chromosomal abnormalities and auto-immune neutropenia, thrombocytopenia and hemolytic anemia. *Ann Intern Med* 1985;102:169–175.
252. Semenzato G, Pandolfi F, Chisesi T, et al. The lymphoproliferative disease of granular lymphocytes: a heterogeneous disorder ranging from indolent to aggressive conditions. *Cancer* 1987;60:2971–2978.
253. Dhodapkar MV, Li CY, Lust JA, et al. Clinical spectrum of clonal proliferations of T-large granular lymphocytes: a T cell clonopathy of undetermined significance? *Blood* 1994;84:1620–1627.
254. Loughran P Jr. Clonal diseases of large granular lymphocytes. *Blood* 1993;82:1–14.
255. Semenzato G, Zambello R, Starkebaum G, et al. The lymphoproliferative disease of granular lymphocytes: updated criteria for diagnosis. *Blood* 1997;89:256–260.
256. Chan WC, Link S, Mawle A, et al. Heterogeneity of large granular lymphocyte proliferations: delineation of two major subsets. *Blood* 1986;68:1142–1153.
257. Gentile TC, Uner AH, Hutchinson RE, et al. CD3 positive, CD56 positive aggressive variant of large granular lymphocyte leukemia. *Blood* 1994;84:2315–2321.
258. Agnarsson BA, Loughran TP Jr, Starkebaum G, et al. The pathology of large granular lymphocyte leukemia. *Hum Pathol* 1989;20:643–651.
259. Galton DA, Goldman JM, Wiltshaw E, et al. Prolymphocytic leukemia. *Br J Haematol* 1974;27:7–23.
260. Stone RM. Prolymphocytic leukemia. *Hematol Oncol Clin North Am* 1990;4:457–471.
261. Matutes E, Brito-Babapulle V, Swansbury J, et al. Clinical and laboratory features of 78 cases of T-prolymphocytic leukemia. *Blood* 1991; 78:3269–3274.
262. Catovsky D, Galetto J, Okos A, et al. Prolymphocytic leukemia of B and T cell type. *Lancet* 1973;ii:232–234.
263. Bearman RM, Pangalis GA, Rappaport H. Prolymphocytic leukemia: clinical, histopathologic, and cytochemical observations. *Cancer* 1978;42:2360–2372.
264. Burke JS, Byrne GE Jr, Rappaport H. Hairy cell leukemia (leukemic reticuloendotheliosis): I. A clinical pathologic study of 21 patients. *Cancer* 1974;33:1399–1416.
265. Catovsky D, Pettit JE, Galton DAG, et al. Leukaemic reticuloendotheliosis (hairy cell leukemia): a distinct clinicopathologic entity. *Br J Haematol* 1974;26:9–27.
266. Brunning RD, McKenna RW. Tumors of the bone marrow. In: *Atlas of tumor pathology.* Series 3, Fascicle 9. Washington: Armed Forces Institute of Pathology, 1994: 276.
267. Burke JS, MacKay B, Rappaport H. Hairy cell leukemia (leukemic reticuloendotheliosis): II. Ultrastructure of the spleen. *Cancer* 1976; 37:2267–2274.
268. Pilon VA, Davey FR, Gordon GB, et al Splenic alterations in hairy cell leukemia: II. An electron microscopic study. *Cancer* 1982;49: 1617–1623.
269. Mover S, Li CY, Yam LT. Semiquantitative evaluation of tartrate resistant acid phosphatase activity in human blood cells. *J Lab Clin Med* 1972;80:711–717.
270. Janckila AJ, Cradwell EM, Yam LT, et al. Hairy cell identification by immunohistochemistry of tartrate-resistant acid phosphatase. *Blood* 1995; 85:2839–2844.
271. Hoyer JD, Li C-Y, Yam LT, et al. Immunohistochemical demonstration of acid phosphatase isoenzyme 5 (tartrate-resistant) in paraffin sections of hairy cell leukemia and other hematologic disorders. *Am J Clin Pathol* 1997;108:308–315.
272. Nanba K, Soban EJ, Bowling MC, et al. Splenic pseudosinuses and hepatic angiomatous lesions: distinctive features of hairy cell leukemia. *Am J Clin Pathol* 1977;67:415–426.
273. Catovsky D, O'Brien M, Melo JV, et al. Hairy cell leukemia (HCL) variant: an intermediate disease between HCL and B prolymphocytic leukemia. *Semin Oncol* 1984;11;362–369.
274. Cawley JC, Burns GF, Hayhoe FGJ. A chronic lymphoproliferative disorder with distinctive features: a distinct variant of hairy cell leukaemia. *Leukemia* 1980;4:537–559.
275. Travis WD, Li CY, Bergstrallh J, et al. Systemic mast cell disease: analysis of 58 cases and literature review. *Medicine (Baltimore)* 1988; 67:345–368.
276. Horny H-P, Ruck MT, Kaiserling E. Spleen findings in generalized mastocytosis. *Cancer* 1992;70:459–468.
277. Brunning RD, McKenna RW, Rosai J, et al. Systemic mastocytosis extracutaneous manifestations. *Am J Surg Pathol* 1983;7:425–438.
278. Travis WD, Li-CY. Pathology of the lymph node and spleen in systemic mast cells disease. *Mod Pathol* 1988;1:4–14.
279. Diebold J, Riviere O, Gosselin B, et al. Different patterns of spleen involvement in systemic and malignant mastocytosis: a histological and immunohistochemical study of three cases. *Virchows Arch* 1991; 419:273–280.
280. Travis W, Li C-Y, Yam LT, et al. Significance of systemic mast cell disease with associated hematologic disorders. *Cancer* 1988;62: 965–972.
281. Horny HP, Ruck M, Wehrmann M, et al. Blood findings in generalized mastocytosis: evidence of frequent simultaneous occurrence of myeloproliferative disorders. *Br J Haematol* 1990;76:186–193.
282. Adamson JW, Fialkow PJ, Murphy S, et al. Polycythemia vera: Stem-cell and probable clonal origin of the disease. *N Eng J Med* 1976; 295:913–916.
283. Fialkow PJ, Faguet GB, Jacobson RJ, et al. Evidence that essential thrombocythemia is a clonal disorder with origin in a multipotent stem cell. *Blood* 1981;58:916–919.
284. Jacobson RJ, Salo A, Fialkow PJ. Agnogenic myeloid metaplasia: a clonal proliferation of hematopoietic stem cells with secondary myelofibrosis. *Blood* 1978;51:189–194.

285. Dickstein JI, Vardiman JW. Hematopathologic findings in the myeloproliferative disorders. *Semin Oncol* 1995;22:355–373.
286. Dickstein JI, Vardiman JW. Issues in the pathology and diagnosis of the chronic myeloproliferative disorders and the myelodysplastic syndromes. *Am J Clin Pathol* 1993;99:513–525.
287. Neiman RS, Orazi A. *Disorders of the spleen,* 2nd ed. Major problems in pathology, vol 38. Philadelphia: WB Saunders, 1999:220.
288. Peterson P, Wasserman LR. The natural history of polycythemia vera. In: Wasserman LR, Berk PD, Berlin NI, eds. *Polycythemia and the myeloproliferative disorders.* Philadelphia: WB Saunders, 1995:14.
289. Berlin NI. Classification of the polycythemias and initial clinical features in polycythemia vera. In: Wasserman LR, Berk PD, Berlin NI, eds. *Polycythemia and the myeloproliferative disorders.* Philadelphia: WB Saunders, 1995:22.
290. Ellis JT, Peterson P, Geller SA, et al. Studies of the bone marrow in polycythemia vera and the evolution of myelofibrosis and second hematologic malignancies. *Semin Hematol* 1986;23:144–155.
291. Peterson P, Ellis JT. The bone marrow in polycythemia vera. In: Wasserman LR, Berk PD, Berlin NI, eds. *Polycythemia and the myeloproliferative disorders.* Philadelphia: WB Saunders, 1995:31.
292. Ward HP, Block MH. The natural history of agnogenic myeloid metaplasia (AMM) and a critical evaluation of its relationship with the myeloproliferative syndrome. *Medicine* 1971;50:357–420.
293. Wolf BC, Neiman RS. Myelofibrous with myeloid metaplasia: pathophysiologic implications of the correlation between bone marrow changes and progression of splenomegaly. *Blood* 1985;65:803–809.
294. Westin J, Lanner L-O, Larsson A, et al. Spleen size in polycythemia: a clinical and scintigraphic study. *Acta Med Scand* 1972;191:263–271.
295. Wolf BC, Banks PM, Mann RB, et al. Splenic hematopoiesis in polycythemia vera: a morphologic and immunohistologic study. *Am J Clin Pathol* 1988;89:69–75.
296. Thiele J, Kvasnicka H-M, Werden C, et al. Idiopathic Primary Osteomyelofibrosis: a clinico-pathological study on 208 patients with special emphasis on evolution of disease features, differentiation from essential thrombocythemia and variables of prognostic impact. *Leuk Lymphoma* 1996;22:303–317.
297. O'Keane JC, Wolf BC, Neiman RS. The pathogenesis of splenic extramedullary hematopoiesis in metastatic carcinoma. *Cancer* 1989;63: 1539–1533.
298. McIntyre KJ, Hoagland HC, Silverstein MN, et al. Essential thrombocythemia in young adults. *Mayo Clin Proc* 1991;66:149–153.
299. van Genderen PJ, Michiels JJ. Primary thrombocythemia: diagnosis, clinical manifestations and management. *Ann Hematol* 1993;67: 57–62.
300. Tefferi A, Silverstein MN, Hoagland HC. Primary thrombocythemia. *Semin Oncol* 1995;22:334–340.
301. Marsh GW, Lewis SM, Szur L. The use of 15Cr-labelled heat-damaged red cells to study splenic function: II. Splenic atrophy in thrombocythaemia. *Br J Haematol* 1966;12:167–171.
302. Gastineau DA, Banks PM, Knowles DM. Primary splenic neoplasm. *Am J Surg Pathol* 1989:13:989.
303. Perez-Ordonez B, Erlandson RA, Rosai J. Follicular dendritic cell tumor: report of 13 additional cases of a distinctive entity. *Am J Surg Pathol* 1996;20:944–955.
304. Warnke RA, Weiss LM, Chan JKC, et al. Tumors of lymph nodes and spleen. In: *Atlas of tumor pathology.* Series 3, Fascicle 14. Washington: Armed Forces Institute of Pathology, 1966:360.
305. Chan JKC, Fletcher CDM, Nayler SJ, et al. Follicular dendritic cell sarcoma: clinicopathologic analysis of 17 cases suggesting a malignant potential higher than currently recognized. *Cancer* 1997;79: 294–313.
306. Chan WC, Zaatari G. Lymph node interdigitating reticulum cell sarcoma. *Am J Clin Pathol* 1986;85:739–744.
307. Tindle BH, Parker JW, Lukes RJ. ''Reed-Sternberg cells'' in infectious mononucleosis. *Am J Clin Pathol* 1972;58:607–617.
308. McMahon NJ, Gordon HW, Rosen RB. Reed-Sternberg cells in infectious mononucleosis. *Am J Dis Child* 1970;120:148–50.
309. Lukes RJ, Tindle BH, Parker JW. Reed-Sternberg like cells in infectious mononucleosis. *Lancet* 1969;ii:1003–1004.
310. Smith EB, Custer RP. Rupture of the spleen in infectious mononucleosis: a clinicopathologic report of seven cases. *Blood* 1946;1:317–333.
311. Slavin RE, Santos GW. The graft versus host reaction in man after bone marrow transplantation: pathology, pathogenesis, clinical features and implications. *Clin Immunol Immunopathol* 1973;1:472–498.
312. Hassan NMR, Neiman RS. The pathology of the spleen in steroid-treated immune thrombocytopenic purpura. *Am J Clin Pathol* 1985; 84:433–438.
313. Reiner AP, Spivak JL. Hematophagic histiocytosis: a report of 23 new patients and a review of the literature. *Medicine* 1988;67:369–388.
314. Farquhar JW, Claireauu AE. Familial hemophagocytic reticulosis. *Arch Dis Child* 1952;27:519–522.
315. Janka G. Familial hemophagocytic lymphohistiocytosis. *Eur J Pediatr* 1983;140:221–230.
316. Henter J-I, Elinder G, Ost A, and the FHL Study Group of the Histiocyte Society. Diagnostic guidelines for hemophagocytic lymphohistiocytosis. *Semin Oncol* 1991;18:29–33.
317. The Writing Group of the Histiocyte Society. Histiocytosis syndromes in children. *Lancet* 1987;i:208–209.
318. Henter J-I, Elinder G, Soder O, et al. Incidence and clinical features of familial hemophagocytic lymphohistiocytosis. *Acta Paediatr Scand* 1991;80:428–435.
319. Manoharan A, Painter D. Histiocytic medullary reticulosis. *Lancet* 1992; 2:881.
320. Risdall RJ, McKenna RW, Nesbit ME, et al. Virus-associated hemophagocytic syndrome: a benign histiocytic proliferation distinct from malignant histiocytosis. *Cancer* 1979;44:993–1002.
321. Risdall RJ, Brunning RD, Hernandez JI, et al. Bacteria-associated hemophagocytic syndrome. *Cancer* 1984;53:2968–2972.
322. Neiman RS, Orazi A. *Disorders of the spleen: disorders of the monocyte-macrophage system,* 2nd ed. Philadelphia: WB Saunders, 1999: ch 11.
323. Callihan TR. Langerhans cell histiocytosis (histiocytosis X). In: Jaffe ES, ed. *Surgical pathology of the lymph nodes and related organs.* Philadelphia: WB Saunders, 1995:534.
324. A multicentre retrospective survey of Langerhans cell histiocytosis: 348 cases observed between 1983 and 1993. The French Langerhans Cell Histiocytosis Study Group. *Arch Dis Childhood* 1996;75:17–24.
325. Komp DM. Langerhans cell histiocytosis. *N Engl J Med* 1987;316: 747–748.
326. Komp DM, Herson J, Starling KA, et al. A staging system for histiocytosis X: a Southwest Oncology Group Study. *Cancer* 1981;47: 798–800.
327. Lahey ME. Prognostic factors in histiocytosis X. *Am J Pediatr Hematol Oncol* 1981;3:57–60.
328. Jaffe R. Pathology of histiocytosis X. *Perspect Pediatr Pathol* 1987; 9:4–47.
329. Basset F, Escaig J, LeCrom M. A cytoplasmic membranous complex in histiocytosis X. *Cancer* 1972;29:1380–1386.
330. Mierau GW, Favara BE, Brenman JM. Electron microscopy in histiocytosis X. *Ultrastruct Pathol* 1982;3:137–142.
331. Chu T, Jaffe R. The normal Langerhans cell and the LCH cell. *Br J Cancer Suppl* 1994;70:S4–10.
332. Azumi N, Sheibani K, Swartz WG, et al. Antigenic phenotype of Langerhans cell histiocytosis: an immunohistochemical study demonstrating the value of LN-2, LN-3, and vimentin. *Hum Pathol* 1988; 19:1376–1382.
333. Ornvold K, Ralfkiaer E, Carstensen H. Immunohistochemical study of the abnormal cells in Langerhans cell histiocytosis (histiocytosis X). *Virchows Arch* 1990;416:403–410.
334. Hage C, Willman CL, Favara BE, et al. Langerhans cell histiocytosis (histiocytosis X): immunophenotype and growth fraction. *Hum Pathol* 1993;24:840–845.
335. Ruco LP, Pulford KAF, Mason DY, et al. Expression of macrophage-associated antigens in tissues involved by Langerhans cell histiocytosis (histiocytosis X). *Am J Clin Pathol* 1989;92:273–279.
336. Willman CL. Detection of clonal histiocytes in Langerhans cell histiocytosis: biology and clinical significance. *Br J Cancer Suppl* 1994; 23:S29–33.
337. Willman CL, Busque L, Griffith BB, et al. Langerhans cell histiocytosis (histiocytosis X): a clonal proliferative disease. *N Engl J Med* 1994;331:153–160.
338. Wood C, Wood GS, Deneau DG, et al. Malignant histiocytosis X. Report of a rapidly fatal case in an elderly man. *Cancer* 1984;53: 347–352.
339. Ben-Ezra J, Bailey A, Azumi N, et al. Malignant histiocytosis X: a distinct clinicopathologic entity. *Cancer* 1991;68:1050–1060.
340. Scott RB, Robb-Smith AH. Histiocytic medullary reticulosis. *Lancet* 1939;ii:194–199.

341. Robb-Smith AH. Before our time: half a century of histiocytic medullary reticulosis. A T cell teaser? *Histopathology* 1990;17:279–283.
342. Warnke RA, Weiss LM, Chan JKC, et al. Tumors of lymph nodes and spleen. In: *Atlas of tumor pathology.* Series 3, Fascicle 14. Washington: Armed Forces Institute of Pathology, 1995:371.
343. Wilson MS, Weiss LM, Gatter KC, et al. Malignant histiocytosis: a reassessment of cases previously reported in 1975 based on paraffin section immunophenotyping studies. *Cancer* 1990;66:530–536.
344. Weiss LM, Trela MJ, Cleary ML, et al. Frequent immunoglobulin and T cell receptor gene rearrangements in "histiocytic" neoplasms. *Am J Pathol* 1985;121:369–373.
345. Cattoretti G, Villa A, Vezzoni P, et al. Malignant histiocytosis: a phenotypic and genotypic investigation. *Am J Pathol* 1990;136: 1009–1019.
346. Chan JK, Ng CS, Hui PK, et al. Anaplastic large cell lymphoma: delineation of two morphological types. *Histopathology* 1989;15: 11–34.
347. Kaneko Y, Frizzera G, Edamura S, et al. A novel translocation t(2:5)(p23;q35) in childhood phagocytic large T cell lymphoma mimicking malignant histiocytosis. *Blood* 1989;73:806–813.
348. Su IJ, Hsu YH, Lin MT, et al. Epstein-Barr virus-containing T cell lymphoma presents with hemophagocytic syndrome mimicking malignant histiocytosis. *Cancer* 1993;72:2019–2027.
349. Su IJ, Wang CH, Cheng AL, et al. Hemophagocytic syndrome in Epstein-Barr virus-associated T-lymphoproliferative disorders: disease spectrum, pathogenesis, and management. *Leuk Lymphoma* 1995; 19:401–406.
350. Isaacson PG, O'Connor NT, Spencer J, et al. Malignant histiocytosis of the intestine: a T cell lymphoma. *Lancet* 1985;ii:688–691.
351. Chan JK, Ng CS, Law CK, et al. Reactive hemophagocytic syndrome, a study of seven fatal cases. *Pathology* 1987;19:43–50.
352. Wong KF, Chan JK. Hemophagocytic disorders: a review. *Hematol Rev* 1991;5:5.
353. Wong KF, Chan JK. Reactive hemophagocytic syndrome: a clinicopathologic study of 40 patients in an Oriental population. *Am J Med* 1992;93:177–180.
354. Nichols CR, Roth BJ, Heerema N, et al. Hematologic neoplasia associated with primary mediastinal germ-cell tumors. *N Engl J Med* 1990; 322:1425–1429.
355. DeMent SH. Association between mediastinal germ cells tumors and hematologic malignancies: an update. *Hum Pathol* 1990;21:699–703.
356. Orazi A, Neiman RS, Ulbright TM, et al. Hematopoietic precursor cells within the yolk sac tumor component are the source of secondary hematopoietic malignancies in patients with mediastinal germ cell tumors. *Cancer* 1993;71:3873–3881.
357. Landanyj M, Indrojit R. Mediastinal germ cell tumors and histiocytosis. *Hum Pathol* 1988;19:586–590.
358. Frizzera G, Moran EM, Rappaport H. Angioimmunoblastic lymphadenopathy with dysproteinemia. *Lancet* 1974;i:1070–1073.
359. Frizzera G, Moran EM, Rappaport H. Angioimmunoblastic lymphadenopathy. Diagnosis and clinical course. *Am J Med* 1975;59:803–818.
360. Lukes RJ, Tindle BH. Immunoblastic lymphadenopathy: a hyperimmune entity resembling Hodgkin's disease. *N Engl J Med* 1975;292: 1–8.
361. Lukes RJ, Tindle BH. Immunoblastic lymphadenopathy: a prelymphomatous state of immunoblastic sarcoma. *Cancer Res* 1978;64: 241–246.
362. Weiss LM, Strickler JG, Dorfman RF, et al. Clonal T cell populations in angioimmunoblastic lymphadenopathy-like lymphoma. *Am J Pathol* 1986;122:392–397.
363. Namikawa R, Suchi T, Ueda R, et al. Phenotyping of proliferating lymphocytes in angioimmunoblastic lymphadenopathy and related lesions by the double immunoenzymatic staining technique. *Am J Pathol* 1987;127:279–287.
364. Feller AC, Griesser H, Schilling CV, et al. Clonal gene rearrangement patterns correlate with immunophenotype and clinical parameters in patients with angioimmunoblastic lymphadenopathy. *Am J Pathol* 1988;133:539–556.
365. O'Connor NT, Crick JA, Wainscoat JS, et al. Evidence for monoclonal T lymphocyte proliferation in angioimmunoblastic lymphadenopathy. *J Clin Pathol* 1986;39:1229–1232.
366. Nathwani BN, Jaffe ES. Angioimmunoblastic lymphadenopathy (AILD) and AILD-like T cell Lymphomas. In: Jaffe ES, ed. *Surgical pathology of the lymph nodes and related organs,* 2nd ed. Major problems in pathology, vol 16. Philadelphia: WB Saunders, Philadelphia, 1995:390.
367. Neiman RS, Dervan P, Haudenschild C, et al. Angioimmunoblastic lymphadenopathy: an ultrastructural and immunologic study with review of the literature. *Cancer* 1978;41:507–518.
368. Nathwani BN, Rappaport H, Moran EM, et al. Malignant lymphoma arising in angioimmunoblastic lymphadenopathy. *Cancer* 1978;41: 578–606.
369. Keller AR, Hochholzer L, Castleman B. Hyaline vascular and plasma-cell types of giant lymph node hyperplasia of the mediastinum and other locations. *Cancer* 1972;29:670–683.
370. Schnitzer B. Reactive lymphoid hyperplasias. In: Jaffe ES, ed. *Surgical pathology of lymph nodes and related organs,* 2nd ed. Philadelphia: WB Saunders, 1995:98–132.
371. Weisenburger DD. Multicentric angiofollicular lymph node hyperplasia: Pathology of the spleen. *Am J Surg Pathol* 1988;12:176–181.
372. Frizzera G, Massarelli G, Banks PM, et al. A systemic lymphoproliferative disorder with morphologic features of Castleman's disease. *Am J Surg Pathol* 1983;7:211–231.
373. Cesarman E, Knowles DM. Kaposi's sarcoma-associated herpesvirus: a lymphotropic human herpesvirus associated with Kaposi's sarcoma, primary effusion lymphoma, and multicentric Castleman's disease. *Semin Diagn Pathol* 1997;14:53–66.
374. Parravicini C, Corbellino M, Paulli M, et al. Expression of a virus-derived cytokine, KSHV vIL-6, in HIV-seronegative Castleman's disease. *Am J Pathol* 1997;151:1517–1522.
375. Yoshizaki K, Matsuda T, Nishimoto N, et al. Pathogenic significance of interleukin-6 (IL-6/BSF2) in Castleman's disease. *Blood* 1989;74: 1360–1367.
376. Brandt SJ, Bodine DM, Dunbar CE, et al. Dysregulated interleukin 6 expression produces a syndrome resembling Castleman's disease in mice. *J Clin Invest* 1990;86:592–599.
377. Gaba AR, Stein RS, Sweet DL, et al. Multicentric giant lymph node hyperplasia. *Am J Clin Pathol* 1978;69:86–90.
378. Garvin DF, King FM. Cysts and nonlymphomatous tumors of the spleen. *Pathol Annu* 1981;16:61–80.
379. Blank E, Campbell JR. Epidermoid cysts of the spleen. *Pediatrics* 1973;51:75–84.
380. Burrig K-F. Epithelial (true) splenic cysts: pathogenesis of the mesothelial and so-called epidermoid cyst of the spleen. *Am J Surg Pathol* 1988;12:275–281.
381. Robbins FG, Yellin AE, Lingua RW, et al. Splenic epidermoid cysts. *Ann Surg* 1968;187:231–235.
382. Talerman A, Hart S. Epithelial cysts of the spleen. *Br J Surg* 1972; 57:201–204.
383. Tsakraklides V, Hadley TW. Epidermoid cysts of the spleen: a report of five cases. *Arch Pathol* 1973;96:251–253.
384. Ross CF, Schiller KFR. Hamartoma of the spleen associated with thrombocytopenia. *J Pathol* 1971;105:62–64.
385. Silverman ML, LiVolsi VA. Splenic hamartoma. *Am J Clin Pathol* 1978;70:224–229.
386. Cotelingham JD, Jaffe ES. Inflammatory pseudotumor of the spleen. *Am J Surg Pathol* 1984;81:375–380.
387. Sheahan K, Wolf BC, Neiman RS. Inflammatory pseudotumor of the spleen: a clinicopathologic study of three cases. *Hum Pathol* 1988; 19:1024–1029.

Subject Index

Note: Page numbers followed by f indicate figures; those followed by t indicate tables.

C

D

F

I

M

N

O

U

V